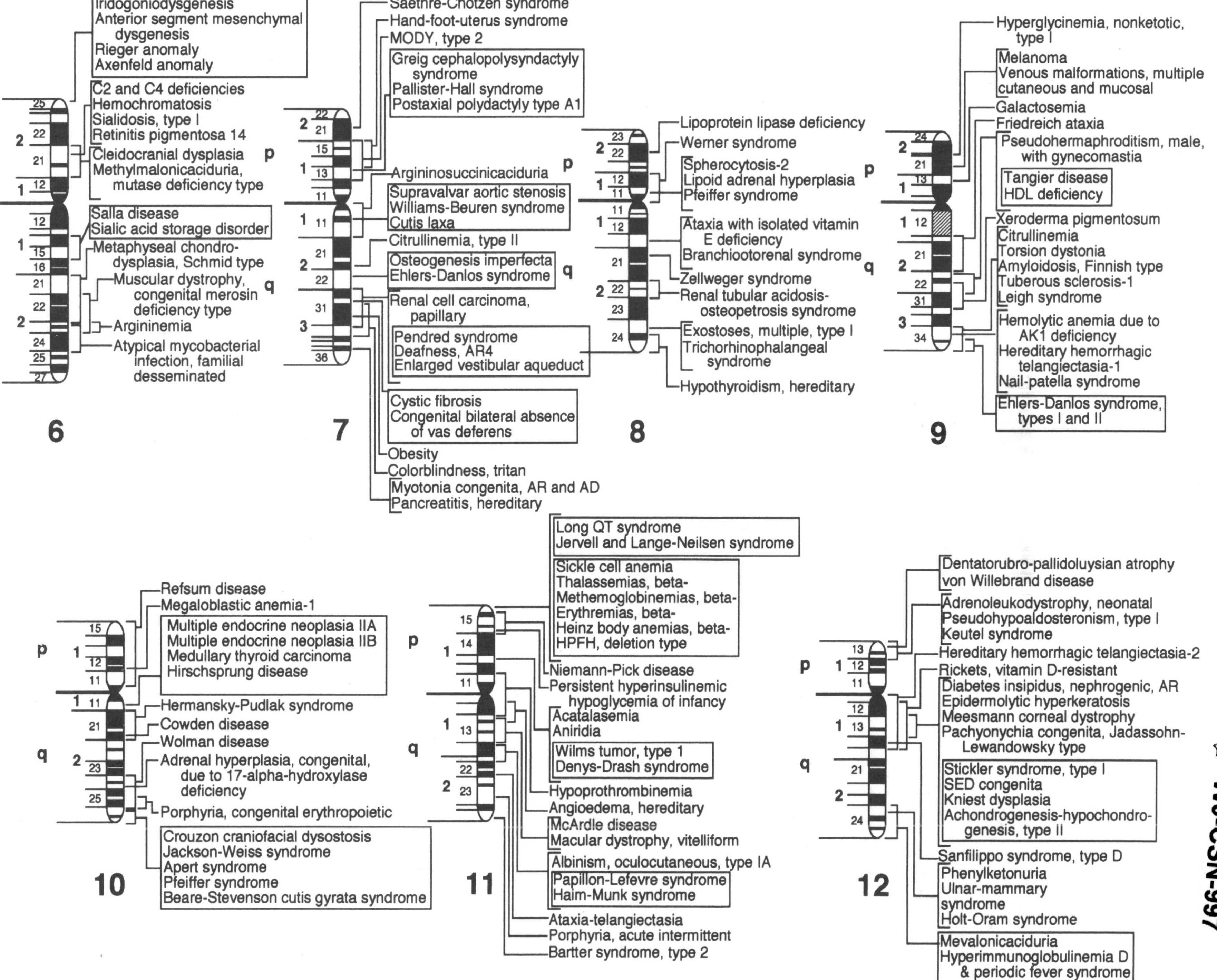

6
Iridogoniodysgenesis
Anterior segment mesenchymal dysgenesis
Rieger anomaly
Axenfeld anomaly
C2 and C4 deficiencies
Hemochromatosis
Sialidosis, type I
Retinitis pigmentosa 14
Cleidocranial dysplasia
Methylmalonicaciduria, mutase deficiency type
Salla disease
Sialic acid storage disorder
Metaphyseal chondrodysplasia, Schmid type
Muscular dystrophy, congenital merosin deficiency type
Argininemia
Atypical mycobacterial infection, familial desseminated
7
Saethre-Chotzen syndrome
Hand-foot-uterus syndrome
MODY, type 2
Greig cephalopolysyndactyly syndrome
Pallister-Hall syndrome
Postaxial polydactyly type A1
Argininosuccinicaciduria
Supravalvar aortic stenosis
Williams-Beuren syndrome
Cutis laxa
Citrullinemia, type II
Osteogenesis imperfecta
Ehlers-Danlos syndrome
Renal cell carcinoma, papillary
Pendred syndrome
Deafness, AR4
Enlarged vestibular aqueduct
Cystic fibrosis
Congenital bilateral absence of vas deferens
Obesity
Colorblindness, tritan
Myotonia congenita, AR and AD
Pancreatitis, hereditary
8
Lipoprotein lipase deficiency
Werner syndrome
Spherocytosis-2
Lipoid adrenal hyperplasia
Pfeiffer syndrome
Ataxia with isolated vitamin E deficiency
Branchiootorenal syndrome
Zellweger syndrome
Renal tubular acidosis-osteopetrosis syndrome
Exostoses, multiple, type I
Trichorhinophalangeal syndrome
Hypothyroidism, hereditary
9
Hyperglycinemia, nonketotic, type I
Melanoma
Venous malformations, multiple cutaneous and mucosal
Galactosemia
Friedreich ataxia
Pseudohermaphroditism, male, with gynecomastia
Tangier disease
HDL deficiency
Xeroderma pigmentosum
Citrullinemia
Torsion dystonia
Amyloidosis, Finnish type
Tuberous sclerosis-1
Leigh syndrome
Hemolytic anemia due to AK1 deficiency
Hereditary hemorrhagic telangiectasia-1
Nail-patella syndrome
Ehlers-Danlos syndrome, types I and II
10
Refsum disease
Megaloblastic anemia-1
Multiple endocrine neoplasia IIA
Multiple endocrine neoplasia IIB
Medullary thyroid carcinoma
Hirschsprung disease
Hermansky-Pudlak syndrome
Cowden disease
Wolman disease
Adrenal hyperplasia, congenital, due to 17-alpha-hydroxylase deficiency
Porphyria, congenital erythropoietic
Crouzon craniofacial dysostosis
Jackson-Weiss syndrome
Apert syndrome
Pfeiffer syndrome
Beare-Stevenson cutis gyrata syndrome
11
Long QT syndrome
Jervell and Lange-Neilsen syndrome
Sickle cell anemia
Thalassemias, beta-
Methemoglobinemias, beta-
Erythremias, beta-
Heinz body anemias, beta-
HPFH, deletion type
Niemann-Pick disease
Persistent hyperinsulinemic hypoglycemia of infancy
Acatalasemia
Aniridia
Wilms tumor, type 1
Denys-Drash syndrome
Hypoprothrombinemia
Angioedema, hereditary
McArdle disease
Macular dystrophy, vitelliform
Albinism, oculocutaneous, type IA
Papillon-Lefevre syndrome
Haim-Munk syndrome
Ataxia-telangiectasia
Porphyria, acute intermittent
Bartter syndrome, type 2
12
Dentatorubro-pallidoluysian atrophy
von Willebrand disease
Adrenoleukodystrophy, neonatal
Pseudohypoaldosteronism, type I
Keutel syndrome
Hereditary hemorrhagic telangiectasia-2
Rickets, vitamin D-resistant
Diabetes insipidus, nephrogenic, AR
Epidermolytic hyperkeratosis
Meesmann corneal dystrophy
Pachyonychia congenita, Jadassohn-Lewandowsky type
Stickler syndrome, type I
SED congenita
Kniest dysplasia
Achondrogenesis-hypochondrogenesis, type II
Sanfilippo syndrome, type D
Phenylketonuria
Ulnar-mammary syndrome
Holt-Oram syndrome
Mevalonicaciduria
Hyperimmunoglobulinemia D & periodic fever syndrome

The Metabolic & Molecular Bases of Inherited Disease

eighth edition

EDITORS

Charles R. Scriver, M.D.C.M.
Alva Professor of Human Genetics, Professor of Pediatrics, Faculty of Medicine, Professor of Biology, Faculty of Science, McGill University; Director (retired), deBelle Laboratory of Biochemical Genetics and Biochemical Genetics Clinical Unit, McGill University–Montreal Children's Hospital Research Institute, McGill University Health Centre, Montreal, Quebec, Canada

Arthur L. Beaudet, M.D.
Henry and Emma Meyer Professor and Chair, Department of Molecular and Human Genetics, Professor, Departments of Pediatrics and Molecular and Cellular Biology, Baylor College of Medicine, Houston, Texas

William S. Sly, M.D.
Alice A. Doisy Professor of Biochemistry and Molecular Biology, Chair, Edward A. Doisy Department of Biochemistry and Molecular Biology, Professor of Pediatrics, St. Louis University School of Medicine, St. Louis, Missouri

David Valle, M.D.
Professor of Pediatrics and Molecular Biology, Howard Hughes Medical Institute, McKusick-Nathans Institute of Genetic Medicine. The Johns Hopkins University School of Medicine, Baltimore, Maryland

ASSOCIATE EDITORS

Barton Childs, M.D.
Emeritus Professor of Pediatrics, The Johns Hopkins University School of Medicine, Baltimore, Maryland

Kenneth W. Kinzler, Ph.D.
Professor of Oncology, The Johns Hopkins University School of Medicine, Baltimore, Maryland

Bert Vogelstein, M.D.
Investigator, Howard Hughes Medical Institute, Clayton Professor of Oncology and Pathology, The Johns Hopkins University School of Medicine, Baltimore, Maryland

The Metabolic & Molecular Bases of Inherited Disease

eighth edition

VOLUME I

EDITORS

Charles R. Scriver, M.D.C.M.
Arthur L. Beaudet, M.D.
William S. Sly, M.D.
David Valle, M.D.

ASSOCIATE EDITORS

Barton Childs, M.D.
Kenneth W. Kinzler, Ph.D.
Bert Vogelstein, M.D.

McGRAW-HILL
Medical Publishing Division

New York St. Louis San Francisco Auckland Bogotá Caracas Lisbon London Madrid Mexico City Milan Montreal New Delhi San Juan Singapore Sydney Tokyo Toronto

McGraw-Hill 
A Division of The **McGraw-Hill** *Companies*

The Metabolic and Molecular Bases of Inherited Disease, 8th Edition

1234567890 KGPKGP 09876543210

ISBNs
0-07-913035-6
0-07-136319-X (vol. 1)
0-07-136320-3 (vol. 2)
0-07-136321-1 (vol. 3)
0-07-136322-X (vol. 4)
This book was set in Times Roman by Progressive Information Technologies, Inc.
The editors were Martin J. Wonsiewicz, Susan R. Noujaim, and Peter J. Boyle;
the production supervisor was Richard Ruzycka; the text designer was José R. Fonfrias;
the cover designer was Elizabeth Schmitz; Barbara Littlewood prepared the index.
Quebecor Printing/Kingsport was printer and binder.
This book is printed on acid-free paper.

Library of Congress Cataloging-in-Publication Data

The metabolic and molecular bases of inherited disease / editors,
Charles R. Scriver . . . [et al.].–8th ed.
p.; cm.
Includes bibliographical references and index.
ISBN 0-07-913035-6 (set)
1. Metabolism, Inborn errors of 2. Medical genetics. 3. Pathology, Molecular. I. Scriver, Charles R.
[DNLM: 1. Hereditary Diseases. 2. Metabolic Diseases. 3. Metabolism, Inborn Errors.
WD 200 M5865 2001]
RC627.8 . M47 2001
616′.042–dc21

00-060957

INTERNATIONAL EDITION
ISBNs 0-07-116336-0
0-07-118833-9 (vol. 1)
0-07-118834-7 (vol. 2)
0-07-118835-5 (vol. 3)
0-07-118836-3 (vol. 4)

Notice

CONTENTS

VOLUME I

PART 1
INTRODUCTION

PART 2
PERSPECTIVES

PART 5
CHROMOSOMES

PART 6
DIAGNOSTIC APPROACHES

PART 7
CARBOHYDRATES

VOLUME II

PART 8
AMINO ACIDS

PART 9
ORGANIC ACIDS

PART 10
DISORDERS OF MITOCHONDRIAL FUNCTION

PART 11
PURINES AND PYRIMIDINES

PART 12
LIPIDS

VOLUME III

PART 16
LYSOSOMAL DISORDERS

PART 17
VITAMINS

PART 18
HORMONES

PART 19
BLOOD

PART 20
IMMUNE AND DEFENSE SYSTEMS

PART 21
MEMBRANE TRANSPORT DISORDERS

VOLUME IV

PART 22
CONNECTIVE TISSUE

PART 23
CARDIOVASCULAR SYSTEM

PART 24
KIDNEY

PART 25
MUSCLE

PART 26
LUNG

PART 27
SKIN

PART 28
NEUROGENETICS

PART 29
EYE

PART 30
MULTISYSTEM INBORN ERRORS OF DEVELOPMENT

CONTRIBUTORS

Lauri A. Aaltonen, M.D. [34]*
Senior Fellow, Academy of Finland, Dept. of Medical Genetics, Haartman Institute, Finland
Lauri.aaltonen@helsinki.fi

Frank Accurso, M.D. [201]
Dept. of Pediatrics, University of Colorado School of Medicine; Director, The Mike McMorris Cystic Fibrosis Center, The Children's Hospital, Denver, Colorado
accurso.frank@tchden.org

Milton B. Adesnik, Ph.D. [16]
Professor of Cell Biology, Dept. of Cell Biology, New York University School of Medicine, New York, New York
Adesnm01@popmail.med.nyu.edu

Björn A. Afzelius, M.D. [187]
Professor Emeritus, Wenner-Gren Institute, Stockholm University, Arrhenius Laboratories, Stockholm, Sweden
Bjorn.Afzelius@zub.su.se

Naji Al-Dosari, M.D. [57]
Duke University, Durham, North Carolina
naji@acpub.duke

Rando L. Allikmets, Ph.D. [243]
Dept. of Ophthalmology, Columbia University, New York, New York
rla22@columbia.edu

Robert J. Alpern, M.D. [195]
Dean, Southwestern Medical School, Ruth W. and Milton P. Levy, Sr., Chair in Molecular Nephrology, Atticus James Gill Chair in Medical Science, Div. of Nephrology, UT Southwestern Medical Center at Dallas, Dallas, Texas
Robert.alpern@email.swmed.edu

Wallace L.M. Alward, M.D. [242]
Dept. of Opthalmology and Visual Sciences, University of Iowa College of Medicine, Iowa City, Iowa
wallace-alward@uiowa.edu

Joanna S. Amberger, M.D. [1]
McKusick-Nathans Institute of Genetic Medicine, Johns Hopkins University School of Medicine, Baltimore, Maryland
joanna@peas.welch.jhu.edu

Donald C. Anderson, M.D. [188]
Professor, Dept. of Pediatrics, Baylor College of Medicine, Vice President and Chief Scientific Officer, Pharmacia & Upjohn, Kalamazoo, Michigan
donald.c.anderson@pnu.com

Karl E. Anderson, M.D. [124]
Professor of Preventive Medicine and Community Health, Internal Medicine, and Pharmacology and Toxicology, Dept. of Preventive Medicine and Community Health, University of Texas Medical Branch, Galveston, Texas
karl.anderson@utmb.edu

Mary E. Anderson, Ph.D. [96]
Assistant Professor, Dept. of Microbiology and Molecular Cell Sciences, University of Memphis, Memphis, Tennessee
Mary@mmcs.memphis.edu

*The numbers in brackets following each contributor's name refer to chapters written or co-written by that contributor.

Generoso Andria, M.D. [152]
Professor of Pediatrics, Department of Pediatrics, Federico II University, Naples, Italy

Stylianos E. Antonarakis, M.D., D.Sc. [13, 172]
Professor and Director of Medical Genetics, Div. of Medical Genetics, University of Geneva Medical School, Geneva, Switzerland
stylianos.antonarakis@medicine.unige.ch

Irwin M. Arias, M.D. [125]
Professor and Chairman, Dept. of Physiology, Tufts University, Boston, Massachusetts
irwin.arias@tufts.edu

Gerd Assmann, M.D., F.R.C.P [118, 122, 142]
Professor of Medicine, Director, Institute for Clinical Chemistry and Lab Medicine, Director, Institute for Arteriosclerosis Research, Westfälische Wilhelms-University, Münster, Germany
assmann@uni-muenster.de

Arleen D. Auerbach, Ph.D. [31]
Associate Professor, Laboratory of Human Genetics and Hematology, The Rockefeller University, New York, New York
auerbac@rockvax.rockefeller.edu

Perti Aula, M.D. [141, 200]
Professor of Medical Genetics, Medical Genetics Dept., University of Helsinko, Haartman Institute, Haartmaninkatu, Finland
Perti.aula@helsinki.fi

Salvatore Auricchio, M.D. [75]
Professor, Dept. di Pediatria, Università Federico II Napoli, Italy

Andrea Ballabio, M.D. [149, 166, 225]
Professor of Medical Genetics, Second University of Naples, Director, Telethon Institute of Genetics and Medicine (TIGEM), Naples, Italy
ballabio@tigem.it

Peter G. Barth [130]
Professor of Pediatric Neurology, University of Amsterdam Academic Medical Centre, Emma Children's Hospital and Clinical Chemistry, Amsterdam, The Netherlands
p.g.barth@amc.uva.nl

Stephen B. Baylin, M.D. [58]
Professor of Oncology and Medicine, Associate Director for Research, The Johns Hopkins Oncology Center, Baltimore, Maryland
sbaylin@jhmi.edu

Philip A. Beachy, M.D. [205]
Professor of Molecular Biology and Genetics, Howard Hughes Medical Institute, The Johns Hopkins University School of Medicine, Baltimore, Maryland
pbeachy@jhmi.edu

Arthur L. Beaudet, M.D. [1, 229]
Henry and Emma Meyer Professor and Chair, Dept. of Molecular and Human Genetics, Professor, Depts. of Pediatrics and Molecular and Cellular Biology, Baylor College of Medicine, Houston, Texas
abeaudet@bcm.tmc.edu

Michael A. Becker, M.D. [106]
Professor of Medicine
Dept. of Medicine University of Chicago School of Medicine, Chicago, Illinois
mbecker@medicine.bsd.uchicago.edu

David M.O. Becroft, M.D. [113]
Dept. of Obstetrics and Gynecology, University of Auckland School of Medicine, Auckland, New Zealand
David.Genevieve.Becroft@extra.co.nz

Lenore K. Beitel, Ph.D. [161]
Research Scientist, Lady Davis Institute for Medical Research, Sir M.B. Davis–Jewish General Hospital, Montreal, Quebec, Canada
mdtm001@musica.mcgill.ca

John W. Belmont, M.D., Ph.D. [185]
Dept. of Molecular and Human Genetics, Baylor College of Medicine, Houston, Texas
jbelmont@bcm.tmc.edu

Merrill D. Benson, M.D. [209]
Professor of Medicine, Pathology and Medical Genetics, Dept. of Medical and Molecular Genetics, Indiana University School of Medicine, Indianapolis, Indiana
mdbenson@iupui.edu

Wolfgang Berger, M.D. [239]
Max-Planck-Institute for Molecular Genetics, Berlin, Germany
berger@molgen@mpg.de

Michel Bergeron, M.D. [196]
Professor of Physiology, Dept. of Physiology, Université de Montréal, Montreal, Quebec, Canada
Bergermi@ere.umontreal.ca

Sten Erik Bergstrom, M.D. [187]
Dept. of Pediatrics, Huddinge University Hospital, Stockholm, Sweden

Ernest Beutler, M.D. [127, 146, 182]
Chairman, Dept. of Molecular and Experimental Medicine, Scripps Clinic and Research Foundation, La Jolla, California
beutler@scripps.edu

Daniel G. Bichet, M.D. [163]
Professor of Medicine, University of Montreal,
Director, Clinical Research Unit, Hopital du Sacre-Coeur de Montreal, Montreal, Quebec, Canada
D-Binette@crhsc.umontreal.ca

Sandra H. Bigner, M.D. [57]
Professor of Pathology, Dept. of Pathology, Duke University Medical Center, Durham, North Carolina
Bigne002@mc.duke.edu

David F. Bishop, Ph.D. [124]
Professor of Human Genetics, Dept. of Human Genetics, Mount Sinai School of Medicine, New York, New York
David.bishop@mssm.edu

Ingemar Björkhem, M.D., Ph.D. [123]
Professor and Head Physician, Dept. of Medical Laboratory Sciences and Technology, Division of Clinical Chemistry, Karolinska Institutet, Huddinge University Hospital, Huddinge, Sweden
Ingemar.Bjorkhem@chemlab.hs.sll.se

E. Joan Blanchette-Mackie, M.D. [145]
Chief, Sect. of Lipid Cell Biology, Laboratory of Cell Biochemistry and Biology, National Institute of Diabetes and Digestive and Kidney Diseases, Bethesda, Maryland
eb78u@nih.gov

Nenad Blau, M.D., Ph.D. [78]
Associate Professor, Div. of Clinical Chemistry and Biochemistry, Dept. of Pediatrics, University Children's Hospital, Zurich, Switzerland
blau@access.unizh.ch

Kirsten Muri Boberg, M.D., Ph.D. [123]
Dept. of Clinical Chemistry, Rikshospitalet, Oslo, Norway
kirsten.boberg@online.no

Sir Walter F. Bodmer, M.D., Ph.D., F.R.C.Path, F.R.S. [11]
Imperial Cancer Research Fund Laboratories, University of Oxford, Institute of Molecular Medicine, John Radcliffe Hospital, Oxford, United Kingdom
walter.bodmer@hertford.ox.ac.uk

C. Richard Boland, M.D. [32]
Professor of Medicine; Chief, Gastroenterology, University of California, San Diego, La Jolla, California
CRBOLAND@UCSD.EDU

Dirk Bootsma, M.D. [28]
Dept. of Cell Biology and Genetics, Erasmus University, Rotterdam, The Netherlands
Bootsma@gen.fgg.eur.nl

Thomas H. Bothwell, M.D., D.Sc. [127]
Emeritus Professor of Medicine, Honorary Professorial Research Fellow, Faculty of Medicine, University of Witwatersrand, Medical School, Johannesburg, South Africa
014jozo@chiron.wits.ac.za

G. Steven Bova, M.D. [56]
Assistant Professor, Depts. of Pathology, Urology and Oncology, Johns Hopkins Hospital, Pelican Laboratory, Baltimore, Maryland
gbov@jhmi.edu

Bernard Brais, M.D., MPhil, Ph.D. [216]
Direction de L'IREP, Centre de recherche du CHUM, Hopital Notre-Dame, Montreal, Quebec, Canada

David S. Bredt, M.D., Ph.D. [168]
Associate Professor of Physiology, Dept. of Physiology, University of California, San Francisco
bredt@phy.ucsf.edu

Jan L. Breslow, M.D. [121]
Frederick Henry Leonhardt Professor, Director, Laboratory of Biochemical Genetics and Metabolism, The Rockefeller University, New York, New York
breslow@rockvax.rockefeller.edu

Martijn H. Breuning, M.D. [248]
Dept. of Clinical Genetics, Centre for Human and Clinical Genetics, Leiden University Medical Centre, Leiden, The Netherlands M.H.Breuning@kgc.azl.nl

H. Bryan Brewer, Jr., M.D. [118, 122]
Chief, Molecular Disease Branch, National Heart, Lung, and Blood Institute, Bethesda, Maryland
bryan@mdb.nhlbi.nih.gov

Garrett M. Brodeur, M.D. [21, 60]
Div. of Oncology, Children's Hospital of Philadelphia, Philadelphia, Pennsylvania
brodeur@email.chop.edu

Dieter Brömme, Ph.D. [137]
Associate Professor of Human Genetics, Mount Sinai School of Medicine, New York, New York
brommd01@doc.mssm.edu

Michael D. Brown [105]
Assistant Professor, The Center for Molecular Medicine, Emory University School of Medicine, Atlanta, Georgia
mdbrown@gen.emory.edu

Michael S. Brown, M.D. [120]
Regental Professor, Johnson Center for Molecular Genetics, University of Texas Southwestern Medical Center, Dallas, Texas
mike.brown@utsouthwestern.edu

George J. Broze, Jr., M.D. [175]
Professor of Medicine, Cell Biology and Physiology, Washington University School of Medicine, Barnes-Jewish Hospital at Washington University, St. Louis, Missouri
gbroze@im.wustl.edu

John D. Brunzell, M.D. [117]
Professor of Medicine, Program Director, General Clinical Research Center, Dept. of Medicine, University of Washington School of Medicine, Seattle, Washington
brunzell@u.washington.edu

Saul W. Brusilow, M.D. [85]
Professor of Pediatrics Emeritus, The Johns Hopkins Hospital, Baltimore, Maryland
sbru@jhmi.edu

Manuel Buchwald, O.C., Ph.D., F.R.S.C. [31]
Professor, Molecular and Medical Genetics, University of Toronto, Chief of Research and Director, Research Institute, Hospital for Sick Children, Toronto, Ontario, Canada
Manuel.Buchwald@sickkids.on.ca

Peter H. Byers, M.D. [205]
Professor, Dept. of Pathology and Medicine, Dept. of Pathology, University of Washington, Seattle, Washington
pbyers@u.washington.edu

Daniel P Cahill, M.D., Ph.D. [22]
Dept. of Oncology, The Johns Hopkins University School of Medicine, Baltimore, Maryland

Paul Cairns, M.D. [54]
Fox Chase Cancer Center, Philadelphia, Pennsylvania 19111

Giovanna Camerino, Ph.D. [62]
Professor Biologia Generale E Genetica Medica, Universitá Di Pavia, Pavia, Italy
camerino@unipv.it

Hubert Carchon, Ph.D. [74]
Assistant Professor, University of Leuven, Centre for Metabolic Disease, Leuven, Belgium
hubert.carchon@med.kuleuven.ac.be

Eugene D. Carstea, M.D. [145]
Director, Saccomanno Research Institute, St. Mary's Hospital and Medical Center, Grand Junction, Colorado
gcarstea@stmarygj.com

Webster K. Cavenee, M.D. [36]
Director, Ludwig Institute for Cancer Research, University of California, San Diego, La Jolla, California

Aravinda Chakravarti, Ph.D. [251]
Henry J. Knott Professor and Director, McKusick-Nathans Institute of Genetic Medicine, Johns Hopkins University School of Medicine, Baltimore, Maryland
aravinda@jhmi.edu

Arlene B. Chapman, M.D. [215]
Associate Professor of Medicine, Director, Hypertension and Renal Disease Research Center, Emory University School of Medicine, Atlanta, Georgia
arlene_chapman@emory.org

Robert W. Charlton, M.D. [127]
Emeritus Professor, University of Witwatersrand Medical School, Johannesburg, South Africa
014jozo@chiron.wits.ac.za

Christiane Charpentier, Ph.D. [66]
Biologist, INSERM-Paris France, Metabolic/Diabetes Unit-Dept. of Pediatrics, Hopital Necker Enfants Malades, Paris, France
Elisabeth.saudubray@nck.ap_hop_paris.fr

Yuan-Tsong Chen, M.D., Ph.D. [71]
Professor of Pediatrics and Genetics, Chief, Div. of Medical Genetics, Duke University Medical Center, Durham, North Carolina
chen0010@mc.duke.edu

Russell W. Chesney, M.D. [194]
Le Bonheur Professor and Chair, Dept. of Pediatrics, Le Bonheur Children's Medical Center, University of Tennessee, Memphis, Tennessee
rchesney@utmem.edu

Barton Childs, M.D. [2, 3, 4]
Emeritus Professor of Pediatrics, The Johns Hopkins University School of Medicine, Baltimore, Maryland

Kathleen R. Cho, M.D. [53]
Associate Professor, Depts. of Pathology and Internal Medicine, University of Michigan Medical School, Ann Arbor, Michigan
kathcho@umich.edu

Streamson C. Chua, Jr. [157]
Dept. of Medicine, Columbia University College of Physicians and Surgeons, New York, New York

David T. Chuang, Ph.D. [87]
Associate Professor, Dept. of Biochemistry, University of Texas Southwestern Medical Center, Dallas, Texas
david.chuang@utsouthwestern.edu

Dominic W. Chung, Ph.D. [171]
Dept. of Biochemistry School of Medicine, University of Washington, Seattle, Washington
chung@u.washington.edu

Carmen Cifuentes-Diaz, Ph.D. [231]
Laboratoire de Neurogénétique Molécularie, INSERM, GENOPOLE, Evry, France
c.diaz@genopole.inserm.fr

James E. Cleaver, M.D. [28]
Dept. of Dermatology, University of California at San Francisco Cancer Center, San Francisco, California
jcleaver@cc.ucsf.edu

J.B. Clegg [181]
Institute of Molecular Medicine, John Radcliffe Hospital, Oxford, United Kingdom

Bruce E. Clurman, M.D. [23]
Assistant Professor, Fred Hutchinson Cancer Research Center, Seattle, Washington
bclurman@fhcrc.org

Anne-Marie Codori, Ph.D. [49]
Dept. of Psychiatry and Behavioral Sciences, The Johns Hopkins University School of Medicine, Baltimore, Maryland

Joy D. Cogan, M.D. [162]
Research Assistant Professor of Pediatric Genetics, Div. of Genetics, Vanderbilt University School of Medicine, Nashville, Tennessee
joy.cogan@mcmail.vanderbilt.edu

Francis S. Collins, M.D., Ph.D. [39]
National Human Genome Research Institute, Bethesda, Maryland
Fc23@nih.gov

Mary Ellen Conley, M.D. [184]
St. Jude Children's Research Hospital, University of Tennessee School of Medicine, Memphis, Tennessee
maryellen.conley@stjude.org

David N. Cooper, Ph.D. [13]
Professor of Human Molecular Genetics, Institute of Medical Genetics, University of Wales College of Medicine, Cardiff, Wales, United Kingdom
cooperdn@cardiff.ac.uk

Valerie Cormier-Daire, M.D., Ph.D. [99]
Dept. of Medical Genetics, Hopital Necker Enfants Malades, Paris, France
cormier@necker.fr

Richard G.H. Cotton, Ph.D., D.Sc. [1, 78]
Professor, Mutation Research Centre, Director, Mutation Research Centre, St. Vincent's Hospital, Fitzroy, Victoria, Australia
cotton@ariel.ucs.unimelb.edu.au

Fergus J. Couch, M.D. [47]
Assistant Professor, Dept. of Laboratory Medicine and Pathology, Mayo Foundation and Clinic, Rochester, Minnesota
Couch.Fergus@mayo.edu

Diane Wilson Cox, M.D., Ph.D. [219]
Professor and Chair, Dept. of Medical Genetics, Genetics Sect. Head, Child Health, Capital Health Authority, Dept. of Medical Genetics, University of Alberta, Edmonton, Alberta, Canada
diane.cox@ualberta.ca

Rody P. Cox, M.D., Ph.D. [86]
Professor of Internal Medicine, Dept. of Internal Medicine, University of Texas, Southwestern Medical Center, Attending Physician, Parkland Memorial Hospital and St. Paul University Hospital, Dallas, Texas
rcox@mednet.swmed.edu

William J. Craigen, M.D., Ph.D. [14]
Dept. of Molecular and Human Genetics, Baylor College of Medicine, Houston, Texas
wcraigen@bcm.tmc.edu

Donnell J. Creel, Ph.D. [220]
Research Professor, Moran Eye Center, University of Utah School of Medicine, Salt Lake City, Utah
Donnell.creel@hsc.utah.edu

Frans P.M. Cremers, Ph.D. [236]
Associate Professor, Dept. of Human Genetics University Medical Center Nymegen, Nymegen, The Netherlands
F.Cremers@Antrg.azn.nl

Valeria Cizewski Culotta, Ph.D. [126]
Associate Professor, Dept. of Environmental Health Sciences, Johns Hopkins University, School of Hygiene and Public Health, Baltimore, Maryland
vculotta@JHSPH.edu

Garry R. Cutting, M.D. [201]
Professor of Pediatrics and Medicine, McKusick-Nathan Institute of Genetic Medicine, The Johns Hopkins University, Baltimore, Maryland
gcutting@jhmi.edu

Christopher J. Danpure, Ph.D. [133]
Professor of Molecular Cell Biology, MRC Laboratory for Molecular Cell Biology, University College London, London, United Kingdom
c.danpure@ucl.ac.uk

Earl W. Davie, Ph.D. [169]
Dept. of Biochemistry School of Medicine, University of Washington, Seattle, Washington

Alessandra d'Azzo, Ph.D. [152]
Professor, Member, Dept. of Genetics, St. Jude Children's Research Hospital, Memphis, Tennessee
sandra.dazzo@stjude.org

Samir S. Deeb, Ph.D. [117, 238]
Research Professor of Medicine and Genetics, Dept. of Genetics, University of Washington School of Medicine, Seattle, Washington
deeb@genetics.washington.edu

Robert J. Desnick, Ph.D., M.D. [124, 137, 139, 144, 150]
Professor and Chairman, Human Genetics, Professor of Pediatrics; Attending Physician, Dept. of Human Genetics, Mount Sinai School of Medicine, New York, New York
rjdesnick@mcvax.mssm.edu

Harry C. Dietz, M.D. [206]
Associate Investigator, Howard Hughes Medical Institute, Professor, Dept. of Pediatrics, Medicine and Molecular Biology and Genetics, McKusick-Nathan Institute of Genetic Medicine, Johns Hopkins University School of Medicine, Baltimore, Maryland
hdietz@jhmi.edu

Mary C. Dinauer, M.D., Ph.D. [189]
Novz Letzter Professor of Pediatrics and Medical and Molecular Genetics, Riley Hospital for Children, Indiana University School of Medicine, Director, Herman B. Wells Center for Pediatric Research, Indianapolis, Indiana
mdinauer@iupui.edu

Jiahuan Ding, M.D., Ph.D. [101]
Director, Molecular Diagnostics, Senior Scientist, Associate Professor, Baylor University, Waco, Texas, Institute of Metabolic Disease, Baylor University Medical Center, Dallas, Texas
j.ding@baylordallas.edu

Michael J. Dixon, M.D. [246]
Professor of Dental Genetics, School of Biological Sciences, Dept. of Dental Medicine and Surgery, University of Manchester, Manchester, United Kingdom
mdixon@fs1.scg.man.ac.uk

Patricia A. Donohoue, M.D. [159]
Associate Professor, Dept. of Pediatrics, Div. of Endocrinology, University of Iowa Hospitals, Dept. of Pediatrics, The Children's Hospital of Iowa, Iowa City, Iowa
patricia-donohoue@uiowa.edu

Thaddeus P. Dryja, M.D. [235]
Professor of Ophthalmology, Harvard Medical School, Dept. of Ophthalmology, Massachusetts Eye and Ear Infirmary, Boston, Massachusetts
dryja@helix.mgh.harvard.edu

Louis Dubeau, M.D., Ph.D. [51]
Professor, Dept. of Pathology, USC/Norris Comprehensive Cancer Center, Keck School of Medicine of USC, Los Angeles, California
ldubeau@hsc.usc.edu

Thomas D. DuBose, Jr., M.D. [195]
Peter T. Bohan Professor and Chair, Dept. of Internal Medicine, Professor of Molecular and Integrative Physiology, University of Kansas School of Medicine, Kansas City, Kansas
tdubose@kumc.edu

Jacques E. Dumont, M.D., Ph.D. [158]
Professor of Biochemistry, Head, Institut de Recherche interdisciplinaire, Faculté de Medecine, Université Libre de Bruxelles, Brussels, Belgium
jedumont@ulb.ac.be

Marinus Duran, M.D. [128]
Academic Medical Center, Laboratory Genetic Metabolic Diseases, University of Amsterdam, Amsterdam, The Netherlands
m.duram@amc.uva.nl

Michael J. Econs, M.D. [197]
Associate Professor of Medicine and Medical and Molecular Genetics, Indiana University School of Medicine, Indianapolis, Indiana
mecons@iupui.edu

Lora Hedrick Ellenson, M.D. [52]
Associate Professor and Director, Div. of Gynecologic Pathology, Weill Medical College of Cornell University, New York, New York
lhellens@med.cornell.edu

Nathan A. Ellis, M.D. [59]
Associate Member, Dept. of Human Genetics, Memorial Sloan-Kettering Cancer Center, New York, New York
n-ellis@ski.mskcc.org

Lynne W. Elmore, Ph.D. [59]
Research Associate, Dept. of Pathology, School of Medicine, Virginia Commonwealth University, Richmond, Virginia
LWElmore@hsc.vcu.edu

Charis Eng, M.D., Ph.D. [45]
Assoc. Professor of Medicine and Human Cancer Genetics, The Ohio State University; Hon. Fellow, CRC, Human Cancer Genetics Research Group, Univ. of Cambridge, United Kingdom; Director, Clinical Cancer Genetics Program, Ohio State University, Columbus, Ohio
Eng-1@medctr.osu.edu

Christine M. Eng, M.D. [150]
Associate Professor, Dept. of Molecular and Human Genetics, Baylor College of Medicine, Houston, Texas
ceng@bcm.tmc.edu

Charles J. Epstein, M.D. [63]
Professor of Pediatrics, Co-Director, Program of Human Genetics, Chief, Div. of Medical Genetics, Dept. of Pediatrics, University of California at San Francisco, California
cepst@itsa.ucsf.edu

Charles T. Esmon, Ph.D. [170]
Head, Cardiovascular Biology Research Program, Oklahoma Medical Research Foundation, Investigator, Howard Hughes Medical Institute, Oklahoma Medical Research Foundation, Oklahoma City, Oklahoma
charles-esmon@omrf.ouhsc.edu

Lindsay A. Farrer, Ph.D. [234]
Genetics Program, Boston University School of Medicine, Boston, Massachusetts
farrer@neugen.bu.edu

Eric R. Fearon, M.D. [26]
Div. of Molecular Medicine and Genetics, University of Michigan Medical Center, Ann Arbor, Michigan
fearon@umich.edu

Andrew P. Feinberg, M.D., M.P.H. [18]
King Fahd Professor of Medicine, Oncology and Molecular Biology and Genetics, Johns Hopkins Medical School, Baltimore, Maryland
afeinberg@jhu.edu

Anthony H. Fensom, Ph.D. [143]
Prince Philip Laboratory, Guy's Hospital, London, United Kingdom

Wayne A. Fenton, Ph.D. [94, 155]
Dept. of Genetics, Yale University School of Medicine, New Haven, Connecticut
wayne.fenton@yale.edu

Malcolm A. Ferguson-Smith, F.R.S. [62]
Professor, Dept. of Clinical Veterinary Medicine, University of Cambridge, Centre for Veterinary Science, Cambridge, United Kingdom

Clair A. Francomano, M.D. [210]
National Center for Human Genome Research, National Institutes of Health, Bethesda, Maryland
clairf@nhgri.nih.giv

Deborah L. French, Ph.D. [177]
Assistant Professor of Medicine and Immunobiology, Div. of Hematology, Mount Sinai School of Medicine, New York, New York
dfrench@mssm.edu

Frank E. Frerman, Ph.D. [95, 103]
Professor of Pediatrics, Dept. of Pediatrics, University of Colorado Health Science Center, Denver, Colorado
Frank.frerman@uchsc.edu

Carol Freund, Ph.D. [240]
Dept. of Clinical Bioethics, National Institutes of Health, Bethesda, Maryland
cfreund@nih.gov

Theodore Friedmann, M.D. [107]
Dept. of Pediatric/Molecular Genetics, University of California, San Diego, Center for Molecular Genetics, La Jolla, California
tfriedmann@ucsd.edu

Tony Frugier, MSc [231]
Laboratoire de Neurogénétique Moléculaire, INSERM, GENOPOLE, Evry, France
t.frugier@genopole.inserm.fr

Elaine Fuchs, Ph.D. [221]
Amgen Professor of Basic Sciences, HHMI, Dept. of Molecular Genetics and Cell Biology, University of Chicago, Chicago, Illinois
lain@midway.uchicago.edu

Lars Fugger, M.D., Ph.D. [12]
Professor, Dept. of Clinical Immunology, Aarhus University Hospital, Aarhus, Denmark
fugger@inet.uni2.dk

T. Mary Fujiwara, MSc [163]
Assistant Professor, Depts. of Human Genetics and Medicine, McGill University, Div. of Medical Genetics, Montreal General Hospital, Montreal, Quebec, Canada
fujiwara@bagel.epi.mcgill.ca

Toshiyuki Fukao, M.D., Ph.D. [102]
Department of Pediatrics, Gifu University School of Medecine, Gifu, Japan
toshi-gif@umin.ac.jp

William A. Gahl, M.D., Ph.D. [199, 200]
Head, Sect. on Human Biochemical Genetics, Heritable Disorders Branch, National Institute of Child Health and Human Development, Bethesda, Maryland
bgahl@helix.nih.gov

David Gailani, M.D. [175]
Assistant Professor of Pathology and Medicine, Director, Clinical Coagulation Laboratory, Vanderbilt Hospital, Hematology/Oncology Div., Vanderbilt University, Nashville, Tennessee
dave.gailani@mcmail.vanderbilt.edu

Hans Galjaard, M.D., Ph.D. [152]
Professor of Clinical Genetics, Dept. of Clinical Genetics, Erasmus University Medical Faculty, Rotterdam, The Netherlands
galjaard@algm.azr.nl

Carlos A. Garcia, M.D. [227]
Professor, Dept. of Psychiatry and Neurology, Tulane University Health Sciences Center, New Orleans, Louisiana
cgarcia2@tulane.edu

Paolo Gasparini, M.D. [191]
Medical Genetics Service, IRCCS-Ospedale CSS, San Giovanni Rotondo, Foggia, Italy
genetcss@fg.nettuno.it

Richard A. Gatti, M.D. [29]
Professor, Dept. of Pathology, School of Medicine, University of California, Los Angeles, Los Angeles, California
rgatti@mednet.ucla.edu

Bruce D. Gelb, M.D. [137]
Associate Professor of Pediatrics and Human Genetics, Mount Sinai School of Medicine, New York, New York
gelbb01@doc.mssm.edu

James L. German, III, M.D. [30]
Professor, Dept. of Pediatrics, Weill Medical College of Cornell University, New York, New York
jlg2003@mail.med.cornell.edu

Gregory G. Germino, M.D. [215]
Associate Professor of Medicine, Div. of Nephrology, Johns Hopkins University School of Medicine, Baltimore, Maryland
ggermino@welch.jhu.edu

Ali Gharavi, M.D. [211]
Assistant Professor of Medicine, Mount Sinai School of Medicine, New York, New York; Visiting Assistant Professor, Dept. of Genetics, Yale University School of Medicine, New Haven, Connecticut
ali.gharavi@yale.edu

K. Michael Gibson, Ph.D. [91]
Director, Biochemical Genetics Laboratory, Associate Professor, Dept. of Molecular and Medical Genetics, Biochemical Genetics Lab, Oregon University Health Sciences, Portland, Oregon
gibsonm@ohsu.edu

Volkmar Gieselmann, M.D. [148]
Professor and Director, Biochemisches Institut, Christian-Albrechts-Universitat Zu Kiel, Kiel, Germany
office@biochem.uni-kiel.de

Rachel H. Giles, Ph.D. [248]
Dept. of Immunology, University Medical Center Utrecht, Utrecht, The Netherlands
R.Giles@lab.azu.nl

David Ginsburg, M.D. [178]
Warner-Lambert/Parke-Davis Professor of Medicine and Human Genetics, Investigator, Howard Hughes Medical Institute, The University of Michigan Medical Center, Ann Arbor, Michigan
ginsburg@umich.edu

Jonathan David Gitlin, M.D. [126]
Helene B. Roberson Professor of Pediatrics, Professor of Pathology and Immunology, Director, Division of Pediatric Immunology and Rheumatology, Washington University School of Medicine, St. Louis Children's Hospital, St. Louis, Missouri
gitlin@kidsal.wustl.edu

Richard Gitzelmann, M.D. [70]
Professor Emeritus, Div. of Metabolic and Molecular Pediatrics, University Children's Hospital, University of Zurich, Zurich, Switzerland

M. Goedert, M.D., Ph.D. [234]
MRC Laboratory of Molecular Biology, Cambridge, England, United Kingdom
mg@mrc-lmb.cam.ac.uk

Joseph L. Goldstein, M.D. [120]
Paul J. Thomas, Professor of Genetics and Chair, Dept. of Molecular Genetics, University of Texas Southwestern Medical Center, Dallas, Texas
joseph.goldstein@utsouthwestern.edu

Peter N. Goodfellow, B.Sc., D.Phil. [62]
Senior Vice President, Discovery Biopharmaceutical Research and Development, SmithKline Beecham, Harlow, Essex, United Kingdom
peter_n_goodfellow@sbphrd.com

Stephen I. Goodman, M.D. [95, 103]
Chief, Sect. of Genetics, Metabolism, and Birth Defects, Professor of Pediatrics, Dept. of Pediatrics, School of Medicine, University of Colorado Health Science Center, Denver, Colorado
stephen.goodman@uchsc.edu

Paul Goodyer, M.D. [191]
Professor of Pediatrics, McGill University, Montreal Children's Hospital, Nephrology Dept., Montreal, Quebec, Canada
paul.goodyer@muhc.mcgill.ca

Jerome L. Gorski, M.D. [247]
Professor of Pediatrics and Human Genetics, Director, Div. of Pediatric Genetics, Div. of Clinical Genetics, Dept. of Pediatrics, University of Michigan, Ann Arbor, Michigan
jlgorski@umich.edu

André Gougoux, M.D. [196]
Professor of Medicine, CHUM (Pavillon Notre Dame), Université de Montréal, Montreal, Quebec, Canada

Stephen J. Gould, Ph.D. [129]
Associate Professor, Dept. of Biological Chemistry, The Johns Hopkins University School of Medicine, Baltimore, Maryland
sgould@jhmi.edu

Gregory A. Grabowski, M.D. [146]
Director, Div. and Program in Human Genetics, Children's Hospital Research Foundation, Cincinnati, Ohio
grabg0@chmcc.org

Denis M. Grant, Ph.D. [9]
Genetics and Genomic Biology Programme, Research Institute, Hospital for Sick Children, Toronto, Ontario, Canada
grant@sickkids.on.ca

Roy A. Gravel, Ph.D. [94, 153]
Professor, Cell Biology and Anatomy, University of Calgary, Calgary, Alberta, Canada
rgravel@ucalgary.ca

Eric D. Green, M.D., Ph.D [10]
Chief, Genome Technology Branch, Director, NIH, Intramural Sequencing Center, National Human Genome Research Institute, Bethesda, Maryland
egreen@nhgri.nih.gov

Daniel L. Greenberg, M.D. [169]
Dept. of Medicine, University of Washington Medical Center, Division of Hematology, Seattle, Washington
robin@u.washington.edu

James E. Griffin, M.D. [160]
Professor of Internal Medicine, Diana and Richard C. Strauss Professor in Biomedical Research, University of Texas Southwestern Medical Center, Dallas, Texas
jgrif2@mednet.swmed.edu

Markus Grompe, M.D. [79]
Dept. of Molecular/Medical Genetics and Dept. of Pediatrics, Oregon Health Sciences University, Portland, Oregon
grompem@ohsu.edu

James Gusella, M.D. [40]
Molecular Neurogenetics Unit, Massachusetts General Hospital, Charlestown, Massachusetts

David H. Gutmann, M.D., Ph.D. [39]
Associate Professor, Director, Neurofibromatosis Program, St. Louis Children's Hospital, Dept. of Neurology, Washington University, St. Louis, Missouri
gutmannd@neuro.wustl.edu

Daniel A. Haber, M.D., Ph.D. [38]
Associate Professor of Medicine, Harvard Medical School, Director, Center for Cancer Risk Analysis, Massachusetts General Hospital Cancer Center, Lab of Molecular Genetics, Charlestown, Massachusetts
haber@helix.mgh.harvard.edu

Theodora Hadjistilianou, M.D. [36]
Associate Professor, Dept. of Ophthalmology, University of Siena School of Medicine, Siena, Tuscany, Italy

Judith G. Hall, M.D. [15]
Dept. of Pediatrics, British Columbia Children's Hospital, Vancouver, British Columbia, Canada
judyhall@interchange.ubc.ca

Ada Hamosh, M.D., M.P.H. [1, 90]
Associate Professor of Pediatric, McKusick-Nathans Institute of Genetic Medicine, The Johns Hopkins University School of Medicine, Johns Hopkins Hospital, Baltimore, Maryland
ahamosh@jhmi.edu

Folker Hanefeld, M.D. [84]
Professor of Pediatrics and Child Neurology, Georg-August-Universitat, Zentrum Kinderheilkunde, Abt. Padiatrie, Schwerpunkt Neuropadiatrie, Germany

Isabel Hanson, M.D. [240]
Molecular Medicine Center, Western General Hospital, Edinburgh, United Kingdom
isabel.hanson@ed.ac.uk

Jean-Pierre Hardelin [254]
Unite de Genetique des Deficits Sensoriels, Institut Pasteur, Paris, France

Peter S. Harper, M.D. [217]
Professor and Consultant in Medical Genetics, University of Wales College of Medicine, Heath Park Institute of Medical Genetics, Cardiff, United Kingdom
harperps@cardiff.ac.uk

Curtis C. Harris, M.D. [59]
Chief, Laboratory of Human Carcinogenesis, National Cancer Institute, Bethesda, Maryland
Curtis_Harris@NIH.GOV

Klaus Harzer, M.D. [134]
Professor, Neurochemical Laboratory, University of Tübingen, Institut für Hirnforschung, Tübingen, Germany
hirnforschung@uni-tuebingen.de

Richard J. Havel, M.D. [114, 115]
Professor Emeritus, Cardiovascular Research Institute, University of California School of Medicine, San Francisco, California
dargank@curi.ucsf.edu

J. Ross Hawkins, Ph.D. [62]
Principal Scientist of Development Incyte Genomics, Ltd. Cambridge, United Kingdom
Ross.Hawkins@incyte.com

Michael R. Hayden, M.D., ChB, Ph.D., FRCP(C), FRSC [223]
Professor of Medical Genetics, Centre for Molecular Medicine and Therapeutics, University of British Columbia, Vancouver, British Columbia, Canada
mrh@cmmt.ubc.ca

Vincent J. Hearing, M.D. [220]
Laboratory of Cell Biology, National Institutes of Health, Bethesda, Maryland

Jacqueline T. Hecht, Ph.D. [210]
Dept. of Pediatrics, University of Texas Medical School, Houston, Texas
jhecht@ped1.med.uth.tmc.edu

Peter Hechtman, Ph.D. [82]
Associate Professor of Biology, Human Genetics, and Pediatrics, McGill University, Dept. of Biochemical Genetics, Montreal Children's Hospital, Montreal, Quebec, Canada
Peter@uww.debelle.mcgill.ca

James F. Hejtmancik, M.D., Ph.D. [241]
National Eye Institute, National Institutes of Health, Bethesda, Maryland
f3h@helix.nih.gov

Raoul C. M. Hennekam, Ph.D., M.D. [248, 249]
Pediatrician and Clinical Geneticist, Dept. of Pediatrics and Institute for Human Genetics, Academic Medical Center, University of Amsterdam, Amsterdam, The Netherlands
r.c.hennekam@amc.uva.nl

Meenhard Herlyn, Ph.D. [44]
Professor, The Wistar Institute, Philadelphia, Pennsylvania
herlynm@wistar.upenn.edu

Michael S. Hershfield, M.D. [109]
Dept. of Medicine and Biochemistry, Duke University Medical Center, Durham, North Carolina
msh@biochem.duke.edu

Hugo S.A. Heymans [130]
Professor of Pediatrics, Director and Chairman. Emma Children's Hospital and Clinical Chemistry, University of Amsterdam Academic Medical Centre, Amsterdam, The Netherlands
h.s.heymans@amc.uva.nl

Howard H. Hiatt, M.D. [73]
Professor of Medicine, Harvard Medical School, Senior Physician, Div. of General Medicine, Dept. of Medicine, Brigham and Women's Hospital, Boston, Massachusetts
hhiatt@partners.org

D.R. Higgs [181]
Institute of Molecular Medicine, John Radcliffe Hospital, Oxford, United Kingdom
drhiggs@molbiol.ox.ac.uk

Katherine A. High, M.D. [173]
William H. Bennett Professor of Pediatrics, UPENN School of Medicine, Director of Research, Hematology Div., Director, Hematology and Coagulation Laboratories, Children's Hospital of Philadelphia, Philadelphia, Pennsylvania
high@email.chop.edu

Adrian V. S. Hill, D.Phil., D.M. [7]
Professor of Human Genetics, Wellcome Trust Centre for Human Genetics, Headington, Oxford, United Kingdom
adrian.hill@imm.ox.ac.uk

Akira Hirono, M.D., Ph.D. [182]
Research Associate, Okinaka Memorial Institute for Medical Research, Tokyo, Japan
Ncc01353@nifty.nc.jp

Rochelle Hirschhorn, M.D. [135]
Professor of Medicine and Cell Biology, Chief, Div. of Medical Genetics, Dept. of Medicine, New York University School of Medicine, New York, New York
hirscr01@mcrcr0.med.nyu.edu

Helen H. Hobbs, M.D. [120]
Professor, Depts. of Internal Medicine and Molecular Genetics, The University of Texas Southwestern Medical Center at Dallas, Dallas, Texas
helen.hobbs@utsouthwestern.edu

Jan H.J. Hoeijmakers, M.D. [28]
Dept. of Cell Biology and Genetics, Erasmus University, Rotterdam, The Netherlands
hoeijmakers@gen.fgg.eur.nl

Sandra L. Hofmann, M.D., Ph.D. [154]
Associate Professor of Internal Medicine, Hamon Center for Therapeutic Oncology Research, University of Texas Southwestern Medical Center, Dallas, Texas
hofmann@simmons.swmed.edu

Jeffrey M. Hoeg, M.D. [118]
Chief, Section on Molecular Biology, Molecular Disease Branch, National Institutes of Health, Bethesda, Maryland
Deceased 7/21/98.

Michael D. Hogarty, M.D. [21]
Div. of Oncology, The Children's Hospital of Philadelphia, Philadelphia, Pennsylvania
hogartym@email.chop.edu

Edward J. Hollox, Ph.D. [76]
Institute of Genetics, University of Nottingham, Queens Medical Centre Nottingham, United Kingdom
Ed.Hollox@Nottingham.ac.uk

Edward W. Holmes, M.D. [110]
Vice Chancellor and Dean, School of Medicine, University of California, San Diego, California

John B. Holton, Ph.D. [72]
Emeritus Consultant Clinical Scientist, Clinical Biochemistry, Southmean Hospital, Bristol, United Kingdom

John J. Hopwood, Ph.D. [149]
Professor & Head, Lysosomal Diseases Research Unit, Dept. of Chemical Pathology, Women's and Children's Hospital, North Adelaide, South Australia
john.hopwood@adelaide.edu.au

Ourania Horaitis, B.Sc. [1]
Co-ordinator, HUGO Mutation Database Initiative, Mutation Research Centre, St. Vincent's Hospital, Fitzroy, Melbourne, Victoria, Australia
horaitis@ariel.ucs.unimelb.edu.au

D. Jonathan Horsford, B.Sc. [240]
Program in Developmental Biology, Hospital for Sick Children, Toronto, Ontario, Canada
djhors@sickkids.on.ca

Arthur L. Horwich, M.D. [85]
Professor of Genetics and Pediatrics, Investigator, HHMI, Yale School of Medicine/HHMI, New Haven, Connecticut
horwich@csb.yale.edu

James R. Howe, M.D. [35]
Assistant Professor, Dept. of Surgery, University of Iowa College of Medicine, Iowa City, Iowa
James_howe@uiowa.edu

Ralph H. Hruban, M.D. [50]
Professor of Pathology and Oncology, The Johns Hopkins University, School of Medicine, Dept. of Oncology and Pathology, Baltimore, Maryland
rhruban@jhmi.edu

Chien-an A. Hu, Ph.D. [81]
Research Associate, McKusick-Nathans Institute of Genetic Medicine, Johns Hopkins University School of Medicine, Baltimore, Maryland
cahu@welch.jhu.edu

Lynn D. Hudson, Ph.D. [228]
Acting Chief, Lab of Developmental Neurogenetics, National Institute of Neurologic Disorders and Stroke, National Institutes of Health, Bethesda, Maryland
hudsonl@ninds.nih.gov

Donald E. Hultquist [180]
Associate Chair, Dept. of Biological Chemistry, University of Michigan Medical School, Ann Arbor, Michigan
hultquis@umich.edu

Keith Hyland, Ph.D. [78]
Associate Professor, Baylor University, Associate Professor, University of Texas Southwestern Medical Center, Senior Research Scientist, Baylor University Medical Center, Institute of Metabolic Diseases, Dallas, Texas
k.hyland@baylordallas.edu

Akitada Ichinose, M.D., Ph.D. [171]
Professor and Chairman, Dept. of Molecular Pathological Biochemistry, Yamagata University School of Medicine, Yamagata, Japan
aichinos@med.id.yamagata-u.ac.jp

Yiannis A. Ioannou, Ph.D. [150]
Associate Professor, Dept. of Human Genetics, Mount Sinai School of Medicine, New York, New York
yiannis.ioannou@mssm.edu

William B. Isaacs, Ph.D. [56]
Professor of Urology and of Oncology, Dept. of Urology, The Johns Hopkins University School of Medicine, Baltimore, Maryland
wisaacs@mail.jhmi.edu

Dirk Isbrandt, M.D. [84]
Research Scientist, Universitat Hamburg, Zentrum fur Molekulare Neurobiologie Hamburg, Institut fur Neurale Signalverarbeitung, Hamburg, Germany
isbrandt@uni-hamburg.de

Jaak Jaeken, M.D., Ph.D. [74, 112, 148]
Professor of Pediatrics, University of Leuven; Director, Center for Metabolic Disease, University Hospital Gasthuisberg, Leuven, Belgium
Jaak.jacken@uz.kuleuven.ac.be

Ernst R. Jaffe, M.D. [180]
Distinguished University Professor of Medicine Emeritus, Albert Einstein College of Medicine, Bronx, New York
(Deceased)

Cornelis Jakobs, Ph.D. [91, 132]
Associate Professor, Head Metabolic Unit, Dept. of Clinical Chemistry, Vrije Universiteit Medical Centre, Amsterdam, The Netherlands
C.Jakobs@AZVU.nl

Anu Jalanko, Ph.D. [141]
Senior Scientist, Dept. of Human Molecular Genetics, National Public Health Institute, Helsinki, Finland
Anu.jalanko@ktl.fi

Joanna C. Jen, M.D. [204]
Assistant Professor, Dept. of Neurology, UCLA School of Medicine, Los Angeles, California
jjen@ucla.edu

Gerardo Jimenez-Sanchez, M.D., Ph.D. [3,4]
McKusick-Nathans Institute of Genetic Medicine, Johns Hopkins University School of Medicine, Baltimore, Maryland
gjimenez@jhmi.edu

H.A. Jinnah, M.D., Ph.D. [107]
Assistant Professor, Dept. of Neurology, Johns Hopkins Hospital, Baltimore, Maryland
hjinnah@welch.jhu.edu

Hans Joenje, Ph.D. [31]
Senior Scientist, Dept. Clinical and Human Genetics, Free University Medical Center, Amsterdam, The Netherlands
H.Joenje.HumGen@med.vu.nl

Jean L. Johnson, M.D. [128]
Assistant Research Professor, Dept. of Biochemistry, Duke University Medical Center, Durham, North Carolina
jean_johnson@biochem.duke.edu

Keith J. Johnson, Ph.D. [217]
Professor of Genetics, Head, Div. of Molecular Genetics, Institute of Biomedical and Life Sciences, University of Glasgow, Glasgow, United Kingdom
K.Johnson@bio.gla.ac.uk

Michael V. Johnston, M.D. [90]
Professor of Neurology and Pediatrics, The Johns Hopkins University School of Medicine, Kennedy Krieger Institute, Baltimore, Maryland
johnston@kennedykrieger.org

Michael M. Kaback, M.D. [153]
Professor, Depts. of Pediatrics and Reproductive Medicine, University of California, San Diego, Children's Hospital and Health Center, San Diego, California
mkaback@ucsd.edu

Steven E. Kahn, M.B., Ch.B. [67]
Associate Professor of Medicine, University of Washington, Staff Physician, VA Puget Sound Health Care System, Seattle, Washington
skahn@u.washington.edu

Muriel I. Kaiser-Kupfer, M.D. [241]
Chief, Ophthalmic Genetics, National Eye Institute, Bethesda, Maryland
kaiserm@box-k.nih.gov

Anne Kallioniemi, M.D. [20]
Cancer Genetics Branch, National Human Genome Research Institute, Bethesda, Maryland

Werner Kalow, M.D. [9]
Professor Emeritus, Dept. of Pharmacology, University of Toronto, Toronto, Ontario, Canada
w.kalow@utoronto.ca

Naoyuki Kamatani, M.D. [108]
Professor and Director, Institute of Rheumatology, Tokyo Women's Medical University, Tokyo, Japan
kamatani@ior.twmu.ac.jp

Alexander Kamb, Ph.D. [44]
Chief Scientific Officer, Arcaris, Inc., Salt Lake City, Utah
kamb@arcaris.com

John P. Kane, M.D., Ph.D. [114, 115]
University of California, San Francisco, California
Kane@itsa.ucsf.edu

Hitoshi Kanno, M.D., Ph.D. [182]
Assistant Professor, Dept. of Biochemistry, Nihon University School of Medicine, Tokyo, Japan
hikanno@med.nihon-u.ac.jp

Josseline Kaplan [237]
Unite de Recherches sur les Handicaps, Genetiques de L'Enfant, INSERM, Hôpital des Enfants Malades, Paris, Cedex, France

George Karpati, M.D., FRCP(C), FRS(C) [216]
Director, Neuromuscular Research, Dept. Neurology/ Neurosurgery, Montreal Neurological Institute, McGill University, Montreal, Quebec, Canada
mcgk@musica.mcgill.ca

Seymour Kaufman, Ph.D. [77]
Emeritus Chief, Laboratory of Neurochemistry, National Institute of Mental Health, National Institutes of Health, Bethesda, Maryland
kaufman@codon.nih.gov

Haig H. Kazazian, Jr., M.D. [172]
Chairman, Dept. of Genetics, University of Pennsylvania School of Medicine, Philadelphia, Pennsylvania
kazazian@mail.med.upenn.edu

Mark T. Keating, M.D. [203]
Professor of Medicine and Human Genetics, Eccles Institute of Human Genetics, University of Utah/Howard Hughes Medical Institute, Eccles Institute of Human Genetics, Salt Lake City, Utah
mark@howard.genetics.utah.edu

Richard I. Kelley, M.D., Ph.D. [249]
Associate Professor of Pediatrics, Johns Hopkins University, Director of Metabolism, Kennedy Krieger Institute, Baltimore, Maryland
kelle_ri@jhuvms.hcf.jhu.edu

Scott E. Kern, M.D. [50]
Associate Professor of Oncology, Johns Hopkins University School of Medicine, Baltimore, Maryland
sk@jhmi.edu

Keith Kerstann, M.A. [105]
The Center for Molecular Medicine, Emory University School of Medicine, Atlanta, Georgia
kkersta@gen.emory.edu

Richard A. King, M.D. [220]
Professor, University of Minnesota, Minneapolis, Minnesota
kingx002@tc.umn.edu

Kenneth W. Kinzler, Ph.D. [17, 27, 48]
Professor of Oncology, The Johns Hopkins University School of Medicine, Baltimore, Maryland
kinzlke@jhmi.edu

D. Richard Klausner, M.D. [41]
Director, National Cancer Institute, Bethesda, Maryland
Klausner@helix.nih.gov

Michael Koenig, M.D. [232]
Professor of Medical Genetics, University of Louis Pasteur, Strasbourg; Adjunct Director of the Genetics Diagnosis Laboratory, Institute de Genetique et de Biologie Moleculaire et Cellulaire, CNRS-INSERM-ULP, Illkirch, Strasbourg, France
mkoenig@igbmc.u-strasbg.fr

Thomas Kolter, Ph.D. [134]
Kekule-Institut für Organische Chemie und Biochemie, der Reinnischen Friedrich-Wilhelms Universität Bonn, Bonn, Germany
kolter@snchemie1.chemie.uni-bonn.de

Stuart Kornfeld, M.D. [138]
Professor of Medicine, Div. of Hematology-Oncology, Dept. of Medicine, Washington University School of Medicine, St. Louis, Missouri
skornfel@im.wustl.edu

Kenneth H. Kraemer, M.D. [28]
Research Scientist, Basic Research Laboratory, National Cancer Institute, Bethesda, Maryland
kraemerk@nih.gov

Jan P. Kraus, Ph.D. [88]
Professor of Pediatrics and Cellular/Structural Biology, Dept. of Pediatrics, University of Colorado School of Medicine, Denver, Colorado
jan.kraus@uchsc.edu

Michael Krawczak, M.D. [13]
Professor, Institute of Medical Genetics, University of Wales College of Medicine, Cardiff, Wales, United Kingdom
krawczak@cardiff.ac.uk

Berry Kremer, M.D., Ph.D. [223]
Professor, Dept. of Neurology, University Medical Center Nijmegen, The Netherlands
h.kremer@czzoneu.azn.nl

Anjli Kukreja, Ph.D. [69]
Research Associate, Weill College of Medicine, Cornell University, New York
anjlik@hotmail.com

Bert N. La Du, Jr., M.D., Ph.D. [92]
Emeritus Professor of Pharmacology, Dept. of Pharmacology, University of Michigan Medical School, Ann Arbor, Michigan
bladu@umich.edu

Marie Lambert, M.D. [79]
Service de genetique medicale, Centre de recherche, Ste-Justine Hospital, Montreal, Quebec, Canada
lamberma@medclin.umontreal.ca

Risto Lappatto, M.D., Ph.D. [111]
Consultant Pediatrician, University of Helsinki, Helsinki, Finland
Risto.Lapatto@helsinki.fi

Agne Larsson, M.D., Ph.D. [96]
Professor of Pediatrics, Chairman, Dept. of Pediatrics, Children's Hospital, Karolinska Institutet, Huddinge University Hospital, Stockholm Sweden
agne.larsson@klinvet.ki.se

David H. Ledbetter, Ph.D. [65]
Professor and Chair, Dept. of Human Genetics, The University of Chicago, Chicago, Illinois
dhl@genetics.uchicago.edu

Rudolph L. Leibel, M.D. [157]
Chief, Division of Molecular Genetics, Co-Director, Naomi Berrie Diabetes Center, Professor of Pediatrics and Medicine, Columbia University College of Physicians & Surgeons, New York, New York
RL232@columbia.edu

Eran Leitersdorf, M.D. [123]
Professor of Medicine, Dorothy and Maurice Bucksbaum Chair in Molecular Genetics, Head, Center for Research, Prevention, and Treatment of Atherosclerosis, Dept. of Medicine, Hadassah University Hospital, Jerusalem, Israel
eran1@hadassah.org.il

Christoph Lengauer, M.D. [22]
The Johns Hopkins Oncology Center, Baltimore, Maryland
lengauer@jhmi.edu

Thierry Levade, Ph.D. [143]
Laboratoire de Biochemie, Maladies Metaboliques, CJF INSERM, Institut Louis Bugnard, Toulouse, France

Jacqueline Levilliers [254]
Unite de Genetique des Deficits Sensoriels, Institut Pasteur, Paris, France

Harvey L. Levy, M.D. [80, 88, 193]
Associate Professor of Pediatrics, Harvard Medical School, Senior Associate in Medicine and Genetics, Children's Hospital, Boston, Massachusetts
levy_h@al.tch.harvard.edu

Richard Alan Lewis, M.D. [243]
Professor, Dept. of Ophthalmology, Medicine, Pediatrics and Molecular Human Genetics, Baylor College of Medicine, Houston, Texas
rlewis@bcm.tmc.edu

Roland Libau, M.D. [12]
Postdoctoral Fellow, Dept. of Microbiology and Immunology, Stanford University School of Medicine, Stanford, California

Uri A. Liberman, M.D., Ph.D. [165]
Professor of Physiology and Medicine, Head, Dept. of Endocrinology and Metabolism, Rabin Medical Center, Beilinson Campus, Sackler School of Medicine, Tel-Aviv University, Petach-Tikvah, Israel
uliberman@clalit.org.il

Richard P. Lifton, M.D. [211]
Associate Investigator, Howard Hughes Medical Institute, Chair, Dept. of Genetics, Professor of Genetics, Internal Medicine & Molecular Biophysics, Yale University School of Medicine, New Haven, Connecticut
richard.lifton@yale.edu

W. Marston Linehan, M.D. [41]
Chief, Urologic Oncology Branch, National Cancer Institute, Bethesda, Maryland
Wml@nih.gov

Thomas Linke, M.D. [143]
Institute fur Organisch Chemie, Bonn, Germany

A. Thomas Look, M.D. [19]
Dept. of Experimental Oncology, St. Jude Children's Research Hospital, Memphis, Tennessee
Thomas.look@stjude.org

Marie T. Lott, M.A. [105]
Research Specialist, Supervisor, Center for Molecular Medicine, Emory University School of Medicine, Atlanta, Georgia
mtlott@gen.emory.edu

James R. Lupski, M.D., Ph.D. [65, 227, 243]
Cullen Professor of Molecular and Human Genetics and Professor of Medicine, Dept. of Molecular and Human Genetics, Baylor College of Medicine, Houston, Texas
jlupski@bcm.tmc.edu

Andreas Lux, Ph.D. [212]
Research Associate, Dept. of Genetics, Duke University Medical Center, Durham, North Carolina

Samuel E. Lux, IV, M.D. [183]
Robert A. Stranahan Professor of Pediatrics, Harvard Medical School Chief, Div. of Hematology/Oncology, Children's Hospital, Boston, Massachusetts
lux@genetics.med.harvard.edu

Lucio Luzatto, M.D., Ph.D. [179]
Scientific Director, Instituo Nazionale per la Ricerca sul Cancro, Genova, Italy
luzzatto@hp380.ist.unige.it

Stanislas Lyonnet, M.D., Ph.D. [251]
Professor of Genetics, University of Paris, Dept. de Genetique et Unite, INSERM, Hospital Necker-Enfants Malades, Paris, France
lyonnet@necker.fr

Mack Mabry, M.D. [58]
Div. of Radiology, The Johns Hopkins Hospital, Baltimore, Maryland

Mia MacCollin, M.D. [40]
Assistant Professor of Neurology, Massachusetts General Hospital, Charlestown, Massachusetts
maccollin@helix.mgh.harvard.edu

Noel Keith Maclaren, M.D. [69]
Professor of Pediatrics, Director, Juvenile Diabetes, Weill College of Medicine, Cornell University, New York
NKMaclaren@aol.com

Edward R. B. McCabe, M.D., Ph.D [97, 167]
Professor and Executive Chair, Dept. of Pediatrics UCLA School of Medicine; Physician-in-Chief, Mattel Children's Hospital at UCLA, Los Angeles, California
emccabe@pediatrics.medsch.ucla.edu

Hugh O. McDevitt, M.D. [12]
Professor of Microbiology and Immunology, Stanford University School of Medicine, Stanford, California
hughmcd@stanford.edu

Roderick R. McInnes, M.D., Ph.D. [80, 240]
University of Toronto Tanenbaum Chair in Molecular Medicine, Professor of Pediatrics and Molecular Genetics, University of Toronto, Head, Program in Developmental Biology, Research Institute, Hospital for Sick Children, Toronto, Ontario, Canada
mcinnes@sickkids.on.ca

Victor A. McKusick, M.D. [1]
Professor , McKusick-Nathans Institute of Genetic Medicine, Johns Hopkins University School of Medicine, Baltimore, Maryland
McKusick@peas.welch.jhu.edu

Roger E. McLendon, M.D. [57]
Associate Professor; Director of Anatomic Pathology Services; Chief, Sect. of Neuropathology, Duke University Medical Center, Durham, North Carolina
roger.mclendon@duke.edu

Michael J. McPhaul, M.D. [160]
Professor, Dept. of Internal Medicine, Div. of Endocrinology and Metabolism, University of Texas Southwestern Medical Center, Dallas, Texas
mcphaul@pop3.utsw.swmed.edu

Robert W. Mahley, M.D., Ph.D. [119]
Director, Gladstone Institute of Cardiovascular Disease, Professor of Pathology and Medicine, University of California, San Francisco
rmahley@gladstone.ucsf.edu

David Malkin, M.D. [37]
Associate Professor of Pediatrics, University of Toronto, Program in Cancer and Blood Research, Research Institute, Hospital for Sick Children, Toronto, Ontario, Canada
David.malkin@sickkids.on.ca

Ned Mantei, Ph.D. [75]
Professor, Swiss Federal Institute of Technology, Institute for Cell Biology, Zurich, Switzerland
mantei@cell.biol.ethz.ch

Douglas A. Marchuk, Ph.D. [212]
Assistant Professor, Dept. of Genetics, Duke University Medical Center, Durham, North Carolina
march004@mc.duke.edu

Sandrine Marlin [254]
Unite de Genetique des Deficits Sensoriels, Institut Pasteur, Paris, France

Karen L. Marsh, Ph.D. [246]
University of Manchester, School of Biological Sciences, Manchester, United Kingdom

George M. Martin, M.D. [8]
Professor of Pathology, Adjunct Professor of Genetics, Director, Alzheimer's Disease Research Center, Attending Pathologist, Medical Center, University of Washington School of Medicine, Seattle, Washington
gmmartin@u.washington.edu

Martín G. Martín, M.D. [190]
Dept. of Pediatrics, Gastroenterology, UCLA School of Medicine, Los Angeles, California
mmartin@mednet.ucla.edu

Paula Martin, Ph.D. [214]
Dept. of Biochemistry, University of Oulu, Finland
paula.martin@oula.fi

Stephen J. Marx, M.D. [43, 165]
Chief, Genetics and Endocrinology Sect., National Institutes of Health, Bethesda, Maryland
stephenm@intra.niddk.nih.gov

Gert Matthijs, Ph.D. [74]
Assistant Professor, Center for Human Genetics, University Hospital of Leuven, Centre for Human Genetics, Leuven, Belgium
gert.matthijs@med.kuleuven.ac.be

Atul Mehta, M.D. [179]
Consultant Hematologist, Dept. of Hematology, Royal Free Hospital, London, United Kingdom
atul.mehta@rfh.nthames.nhs.uk

Judith Melki, M.D., Ph.D. [231]
Neurogénétique Moléculaire, INSERM, GENOPOLE, Evry, France
j.melki@genopole.inserm.fr

Paul S. Meltzer, M.D., Ph.D. [20]
Sect. of Molecular Cytogenetics, Lab of Cancer Genetics, National Institutes of Health, Bethesda, Maryland

Claude J. Migeon, M.D. [159]
Professor of Pediatrics, Div. of Pediatric Endocrinology, The Johns Hopkins University School of Medicine, Baltimore, Maryland
cmigeon@welchlink.welch.jhu.edu

Tetsuro Miki, Ph.D. [33]
Geriatric Research Education and Clinical Center, University of Washington, Seattle, Washington

Beverly S. Mitchell [109]
Wellcome Professor of Cancer Research, University of North Carolina, Lineberger Comprehensive Cancer Center, Chapel Hill, North Carolina

Grant A. Mitchell, M.D. [79, 102]
Div. of Medical Genetics, Hopital Ste-Justine, Montreal, Quebec, Canada
mitchell@justine.umontreal.ca

Shiro Miwa, M.D. [182]
Director, Okinaka Memorial Institute for Medical Research, Tokyo, Japan

Maria Judit Molnar, M.D., Ph.D. [216]
Dept. of Neurology, Medical University of Debrecen, National Institute of Psychiatry and Neurology, Budapest, Hungary
molnarm@jaguar.dote.hu

Jill A. Morris, Ph.D. [145]
Senior Research Biologist, Dept. of Pharmacology, Merck Research Laboratories, West Point, Pennsylvania
jill_morris@merck.com

Ann B. Moser, BA [131]
Kennedy Krieger Institute, Baltimore, Maryland
mosera@kennedykrieger.org

Hugo W. Moser, M.D. [131, 143]
Professor of Neurology and Pediatrics, Johns Hopkins University, Director of Neurogenetics, Kennedy Krieger Institute, Baltimore, Maryland
moser@kennedykrieger.org

Björn Mossberg, M.D., Ph.D. [187]
Chief Physician, Dept. of Respiratory Medicine and Allerology, Huddinge University Hospital Stockholm, Sweden
bjorn.mossberg@lungall.hs.sll.se

Arno G. Motulsky, M.D., D.Sc. [127, 238]
Professor Emeritus Active of Medicine and Genetics, Attending Physician, University of Washington Hospital, Div. of Medical Genetics, Dept. of Medicine, University of Washington, Seattle, Washington
agmot@u.washington.edu

S. Harvey Mudd, M.D. [88]
Guest Scientist, Laboratory of Molecular Biology, National Institute of Mental Health, National Institutes of Health, Bethesda, Maryland
sbm@codon.nih.gov

Maximilian Muenke, M.D. [245, 250]
Chief, Medical Genetics Branch, National Human Genome Research Institute, National Institutes of Health, Bethesda, Maryland
muenke@nih.gov

Joseph Muenzer, M.D., Ph.D. [136]
Associate Professor of Pediatrics, Dept. of Pediatrics, University of North Carolina at Chapel Hill, North Carolina
muenzer@css.unc.edu

Arnold Munnich, M.D., Ph.D. [99, 237]
Professor, Dept. of Pediatrics, INSERM, Hopital des Enfants Malades, Hopital Necker, Paris, France
munnich@necker.fr

Jun Nakura, M.D., Ph.D. [33]
Department of Geriatric Medicine, School of Medicine, Ehime University, Ehime, Japan
nakura@ m.ehime-u.ac.jp

Eiji Nanba, M.D. [151]
Associate Professor, Gene Research Center, Tottori University, Yonago, Japan
enanba@grape.med.tottori-u.ac.jp

William M. Nauseef, M.D. [189]
Professor, Inflammation Program and Dept. of Medicine, University of Iowa, Iowa City, Iowa
william-nauseef@uiowa.ed

Barry D. Nelkin, Ph.D. [58]
Associate Professor of Oncology, Johns Hopkins University School of Medicine, Baltimore, Maryland
bnelkin@jhmi.edu

Edward B. Neufeld, Ph.D. [145]
National Heart, Lung, and Blood Institute, Bethesda, Maryland
neufelde@mail.nih.gov

Elizabeth F. Neufeld, Ph.D. [136]
Professor and Chair Biological Chemistry, Dept. of Biological Chemistry, UCLA School of Medicine, Los Angeles, California
eneufeld@mednet.ucla.edu

Peter E. Newburger, M.D. [189]
Professor of Pediatrics and Molecular, Genetics/Microbiology; Director, Pediatric Hematology/Oncology, University of Massachusetts Medical School, Worcester, Massachusetts
peter.newburger@ummed.edu

Peter J. Newman, Ph.D. [177]
Senior Investigator, Vice President and Assoc. Director for Research, The Blood Center, Milwaukee, Wisconsin
pjnewman@bcsew.edu

Irene F. Newsham, Ph.D. [36]
Dept. of Anatomy and Pathology, Medical College of Virginia, Richmond, Virginia
inewsham@hsc.vcu.edu

Jeffrey L. Noebels, M.D., Ph.D. [230]
Professor of Neurology, Neuroscience, and Molecular and Human Genetics, Dept. of Neurology, Baylor College of Medicine, Houston, Texas
jnoebels@bcm.tmc.edu

Josette Noël, M.D. [196]
Assistant Professor, Dept. of Physiology, Université de Montréal, Montreal, Quebec, Canada
josette.noel@umontreal.ca

Lawrence M. Nogee, M.D. [218]
Associate Professor, Dept. of Pediatrics, Div. of Neonatology, Johns Hopkins University School of Medicine, Baltimore, Maryland
lnogee@welch.jhu.edu

Virginia Nunes, Ph.D. [191]
Medical and Molecular Genetics Center, L'Hospitalet de Llobregat, Barcelona, Catalunya, Spain
vnunes@iro.es

Robert L. Nussbaum, M.D. [252]
Chief, Genetic Diseases Research Branch, National Human Genome Research Institute, Bethesda, Maryland
rlnuss@nhgri.nih.gov

William S. Oetting, M.D. [220]
Assistant Professor, University of Minnesota, Minneapolis, Minnesota
bill@lenti.med.umn.edu

Harry T. Orr, M.D. [226]
University of Minnesota, Institute of Human Genetics, Minneapolis, Minnesota
harry@lenti.med.umn.edu

Akihiro Oshima, M.D. [151]
Visiting Investigator, Dept. of Veterinary Science, National Institute of Infectious Diseases, Tokyo, Japan
oshima@nih.go.jp

Manuel Palacín, M.D. [191]
Professor, Biochemistry and Molecular Biology, Faculty of Biology, Dept. of Biochemistry and Physiology, University of Barcelona, Barcelona, Spain
mnpalacin@porthos.bio.ub.es

Cristina Panozzo, Ph.D. [231]
Laboratoire de Neurogénétique Moléculaire, INSERM, GENOPOLE, Evry, France
c.panozzo@genopole.inserm.fr

Lucie Parent, M.D. [196]
Associate Professor, Dept. of Physiology, Université de Montréal, Montreal, Quebec, Canada
lucie.parent@umontreal.ca

Peter Parham, Ph.D. [12]
Professor of Structural Biology and of Microbiology and Immunology, Stanford University, Stanford, California
Peropa@leland.stanford.edu

Morag Park, M.D. [25]
Molecular Oncology Group, Royal Victoria Hospital, Montreal, Quebec, Canada
morag@lan1.molonc.mcgill.ca

Keith L. Parker, M.D., Ph.D. [159]
Professor of Internal Medicine and Pharmacology, Dept. of Internal Medicine, UT Southwestern Medical Center, Dallas, Texas
kparke@mednet.swmed.edu

Ramon Parsons, M.D., Ph.D. [45]
Assistant Professor, Columbia Institute of Cancer Genetics, Columbia University, New York, New York
rep15@columbia.edu

Marc C. Patterson, M.D. [145]
Consultant, Div. of Child and Adolescent Neurology, Mayo Clinic, Rochester, Minnesota
mpatterson@mayo.edu

Leena Peltonen, M.D., Ph.D. [141, 154]
Professor and Chair of Human Genetics, Dept. of Human Genetics, UCLA School of Medicine, Los Angeles, California
lpeltonen@mednet.ucla.edu

Peter G. Pentchev, Ph.D. [145]
Chief, Sect. of Cellular and Molecular Pathophysiology, Developmental and Metabolic Neurology Branch, National Institutes of Neurological Disorders and Stroke, Bethesda, Maryland
peter.pentchev@xtra.co.nz

Isabelle Perrault, M.D. [237]
Unite de Recherches sur les Handicaps, Genetiques de L'Enfant, INSERM, Hôpital des Enfants Malades, Paris, France

Gloria M. Petersen, Ph.D. [49]
Professor of Clinical Epidemiology, Consultant, Mayo Foundation, Mayo Clinic, Rochester, New York
peterg@mayo.edu

Christine Petit [254]
Unite de Genetique des Deficits Sensoriels, Institut Pasteur, Paris, France
cpetit@pasteur.fr

Fred Petrij, M.D. [248]
Clinical Genetics Registrar, Dept. of Clinical Genetics, Erasmus University, Rotterdam, The Netherlands
petrij@kgen.azr.nl

James M. Phang, M.D. [81]
Chief, Metabolism and Cancer Susceptibility Sect., Basic Research Laboratory, Div. of Basic Sciences, National Cancer Institute, Frederick, Maryland
phang@mail.ncifcrf.gov

John A. Phillips, III, M.D. [162]
Professor of Pediatrics and Biochemistry, Div. of Medical Genetics, Vanderbilt University School of Medicine, Nashville, Tennessee
john.phillips@mcmail.vanderbilt.edu

Joram Piatigorsky, Ph.D. [241]
Chief, Laboratory of Molecular and Developmental Biology, National Eye Institute, Bethesda, Maryland
joramp@intra.nei.nih.gov

Leonard Pinsky, M.D. [161]
Professor, Depts. of Medicine, Human Genetics, Biology and Pediatrics, McGill University, Lady Davis Institute for Medical Research, Sir M.B. Davis–Jewish General Hospital, Montreal, Quebec, Canada
rrosenzw@ldi.jgh.mcgill.ca

Eleanor S. Pollak, M.D. [173]
Assistant Professor of Pathology and Laboratory Medicine, Hospital of the University of Pennsylvania, Associate Director, Clinical Coagulation Laboratory, The Children's Hospital of Philadelphia, Philadelphia, Pennsylvania
pollak@mail.med.upenn.edu

Bruce A.J. Ponder, Ph.D., F.R.C.P. [42]
CRC Professor of Oncology, University of Cambridge, Cambridge Institute for Medical Research, Cambridge, United Kingdom
bajp@mole.bio.cam.ac.uk

Mortimer Poncz, M.D. [177]
Professor of Pediatrics, University of Pennsylvania Medical Center, Philadelphia, Pennsylvania

Daniel Porte, Jr., M.D. [67]
Professor of Medicine, University of California San Diego; Staff Physician, VA San Diego Health Care System, San Diego, California
dporte@ucsd.edu
poncz@email.chop.edu

Steven M. Powell, M.D. [55]
Assistant Professor of Medicine, Div. of Gastroenterology, University of Virginia Health Systems, Charlottesville, Virginia
SMP8N@virginia.edu

James M. Powers, M.D. [131]
Dept. of Pathology, University of Rochester Medical Center, Rochester, New York

Richard L. Proia, Ph.D. [153]
Chief, Genetics of Development and Disease Branch, National Institute of Diabetes and Digestive and Kidney Diseases, National Institutes of Health, Bethesda, Maryland
proia@nih.gov

Kathleen P. Pratt, Ph.D. [171]
Instructor, Department of Biochemistry, University of Washington, Seattle
kpratt@u.washington.edu

Stanley B. Prusiner, M.D. [224]
Director, Institute for Neurodegenerative Diseases, Professor of Neurology and Biochemistry, Dept. of Neurology, University of California, San Francisco, California

Louis J. Ptáček, M.D. [204]
Associate Professor, Associate Investigator, Dept. of Neurology Human Genetics, Howard Hughes Medical Institute, University of Utah, Salt Lake City, Utah
ptacek@genetics.utah.edu

Jennifer M. Puck, M.D. [185]
Head Chief, Immunologic Genetics Sect., National Human Genome Research Institute, Genetics and Molecular Biology Branch, Bethesda, Maryland
jpuck@nhgri.nih.gov

Leena Pulkkinen, Ph.D. [222]
Jefferson Institute of Molecular Medicine, Dept. of Dermatology and Cutaneous Biology, Jefferson Medical College, Thomas Jefferson University, Philadelphia, Pennsylvania
leena.pulkkinen@mail.tju.edu

Reed E. Pyeritz, M.D., Ph.D. [206]
Professor of Human Genetics, MCP Hahnemann School of Medicine, Philadelphia, Pennsylvania
pyeritz@yahoo.com

Kari O. Raivio, M.D. [111]
Professor of Perinatal Medicine, School of Medicine, University of Helsinki, Helsinki, Finland
kari.raivio@helsinki.fi

Stanley C. Rall, Jr., Ph.D. [119]
Investigator, Gladstone Institute of Cardiovascular Disease, San Francisco, California

Bonnie W. Ramsey, M.D. [201]
Dept. of Pediatrics, University of Washington School of Medicine, Children's Hospital Regional Medical Center, Seattle, Washington
bramsey@u.washington.edu

Ahmed Rasheed [57]
Research Assistant Professor, Duke University Medical Center, Durham, North Carolina
a.rasheed@duke.edu

Gerald V. Raymond, M.D. [129]
Assistant Professor, Neurology, Kennedy Krieger Institute, Johns Hopkins University School of Medicine, Baltimore, Maryland
raymond@kennedykrieger.org

Andrew P. Read, MA, Ph.D., FRC Path, FmedSci [244]
Professor of Human Genetics, Dept. of Medical Genetics, St. Mary's Hospital, University of Manchester, Manchester, United Kingdom
andrew.read@man.ac.uk

Jonathan J. Rees, MBBS, FRCP [46]
Professor and Chairman, Dept. of Dermatology, The University of Edinburgh, Edinburgh, Scotland, United Kingdom
Jonathan.rees@ed.ac.uk

Samuel Refetoff, M.D. [158]
Professor of Medicine and Pediatrics, Director, Endocrinology Laboratory, Depts. of Medicine and Pediatrics and the J.P. Kennedy Jr. Mental Retardation Research Center, The University of Chicago, Chicago, Illinois
refetoff@medicine.bsd.uchicago.edu

Arnold J.J. Reuser, Ph.D. [135]
Associate Professor of Cell Biology, Erasmus University Rotterdam, Dept. of Clinical Genetics, Rotterdam, The Netherlands
reuser@ikg.fgg.eur.nl

William B. Rizzo, M.D. [98]
Professor of Pediatrics, Human Genetics, Biochemistry, and Molecular Biophysics, Dept. of Pediatrics, Medical College of Virginia, Virginia Commonwealth University, Richmond, Virginia
wrizzo@hsc.vcu.edu

James M. Roberts, M.D. [23]
Div. of Basic Sciences, Fred Hutchinson Cancer Research Center, Seattle, Washington 98104

Brian H. Robinson, Ph.D. [100]
Professor, Depts. of Biochemistry and Pediatrics, Program Head, Metabolism, Senior Scientist, Genetics and Genomic Biology, Hospital for Sick Children, Toronto, Ontario, Canada
bhr@sickkids.on.ca

Charles R. Roe, M.D. [101]
Institute of Metabolic Disease, Baylor University Medical Center, Dallas, Texas
cr.roe@baylordallas.edu

Hans-Hilger Ropers, M.D., Ph.D. [236, 239]
Professor, Dept. of Human Genetics, Max-Planck-Institute fuer Molekulare Genetik, Berlin, Germany
Ropers@molgen.mpg.de

Michael Rosenbaum, M.D. [157]
Associate Professor of Clinical Pediatrics and Clinical Medicine, Div. of Molecular Genetics, Russ Berrie Research Center, Columbia University College of Physicians and Surgeons, New York, New York
mr475@columbia.edu

David S. Rosenblatt, M.D. [94, 155]
Professor of Human Genetics, Medicine, Pediatrics, and Biology, Director, Div. of Medical Genetics, McGill University Health Centre, Royal Victoria Hospital, Montreal, Quebec, Canada
mc74@musica.mcgill.ca

Agnes Rötig, Ph.D. [99]
Dept. of Genetics, INSERM, Hopital Necker, Paris, France
roetig@necker.fr

Jayanta Roy Chowdhury, M.D., M.R.C.P. [125]
Professor of Medicine and Molecular Genetics, Dept. of Medicine and Molecular Genetics, Albert Einstein College of Medicine at Yeshiva University, Bronx, New York
chowdhur@aecom.yu.edu

Namita Roy Chowdhury, Ph.D. [125]
Professor of Medicine and Molecular Genetics, Albert Einstein College of Medicine, Bronx, New York

Jean-Michel Rozet, M.D. [237]
Unite de Recherches sur les Handicaps, Genetiques de L'Enfant, INSERM, Hôpital des Enfants Malades, Paris, France

Edward M. Rubin, M.D., Ph.D. [121]
Head, Genome Sciences Dept., Lawrence, Berkeley Laboratory, University of California at Berkeley, Berkeley, California
emrubin@lbl.gov

Charles M. Rudin, M.D. [24]
Assistant Professor of Medicine, University of Chicago Medical Center, Chicago, Illinois
crudin@medicine.bsd.uchicago.edu

Elena I. Rugarli, M.D. [225]
Researcher, Telethon Institute of Genetics and Medicine (TIGEM), Milan, Italy
rugarli@tigem.it

David W. Russell, Ph.D. [160]
Eugene McDermott Distinguished Professor of Molecular Genetics, University of Texas Southwestern Medical Center Dallas, Texas
russell@utsw.swmed.edu

Pierre Rustin, Ph.D. [99]
Dept. of Genetics, INSERM, Hopital Des Enfants-Malades, Paris, France
rustin@necker.fr

David D. Sabatini, M.D., Ph.D. [16]
Frederick L. Ehrman Professor and Chairman, Dept. of Cell Biology, New York University School of Medicine, New York, New York
Sabatd01@popmail.med.nyu.edu

Richard L. Sabina, Ph.D. [110]
Associate Professor of Biochemistry, Dept. of Biochemistry, Medical College of Wisconsin, Milwaukee, Wisconsin
sabinar@mcw.edu

J. Evan Sadler, M.D., Ph.D. [174]
Professor, Depts. Of Medicine, Biochemistry and Molecular Biophysics; Investigator, Howard Hughes Medical Institute, Washington University School of Medicine, St. Louis, Missouri
esadler@im.wustl.edu

Amrik S. Sahota, Ph.D., F.A.C.M.G. [108]
Dept. of Genetics, Nelson Biological Laboratories, Rutgers University, Piscataway, New Jersey
sahota@nel-exchange.vutgers.edu

Mika Saksela, M.D. [111]
Research Associate, Children's Hospital, University of Helsinki, Helsinki, Finland
Mika.Saksela@Helsinki.fi

Julian R. Sampson, M.D. [233]
Professor of Medical Genetics Institute of Medical Genetics, University of Wales, College of Medicine, Cardiff, United Kingdom
wmgjrs@cardiff.ac.uk

Konrad Sandhoff, Ph.D. [134, 143, 153]
Director and Professor of Biochemistry, Kekule-Institut fur Organische Chemie und Biochemie, Universitat Bonn, Bonn, Germany
sandhoff@uni-bonn.de

Michael C. Sanguinetti, Ph.D. [203]
University of Utah, Eccles Institute of Human Genetics, Salt Lake City, Utah
mike.sanguinetti@hci.utah.edu

Silvia Santamarina-Fojo, M.D, Ph.D. [118]
Chief, Section on Cell Biology, Molecular Disease Branch, National Institutes of Health, Bethesda, Maryland
silvia@mdb.nhlbi.nih.gov

Carmen Sapienza, Ph.D. [15]
Professor of Pathology and Laboratory Medicine, Associate Director, Fels Institute for Cancer Research, Temple University School of Medicine, Philadelphia, Pennsylvania
sapienza@unix.temple.edu

Shigeru Sassa, M.D., Ph.D. [124]
Emeritus Head, Laboratory of Biochemical Hematology, The Rockefeller University, New York, New York
sassa@rockvax.rockefeller.edu

Jean-Marie Saudubray, M.D. [66]
Director of the Metabolic/Diabetes Unit, Professor, Dept. of Pediatrics, Hopital Necker Enfants Malades, Paris, France
Elisabeth.saudubray@nck.ap_hop_paris.fr

Alan J. Schafer, Ph.D. [253]
Vice President Genetics, Incyte Genomics, Cambridge, United Kingdom
alan.schafer@incyte.com

Gerard Schellenberg, Ph.D. [33]
Veterans Affairs Medical Center, Seattle, Washington
zachdad@u.washington.edu

Detlev Schindler, M.D. [139]
Director, Cell Culture, Biochemistry and Flowcytometry Div.; Associate Professor of Human Genetics, Dept. of Human Genetics, University of Wuerzburg, Wuerzburg, Germany
schindler@biozentrum.uni-wuerzburg.de

Jerry A. Schneider, M.D. [199]
Professor of Pediatrics; Benard L. Maas Chair in Inherited Metabolic Disease, Dean for Academic Affairs, Office of the Dean, School of Medicine, University of California, San Diego School of Medicine, La Jolla, California
jschneider@ucsd.edu

Edward H. Schuchman, Ph.D. [144]
Professor of Human Genetics, Dept. of Human Genetics, Mount Sinai School of Medicine, Member, Institute for Gene Therapy and Molecular Medicine, New York, New York
schuchman@msvax.mssm.edu

C. Ronald Scott, M.D. [89]
Professor, Dept. of Pediatrics, University of Washington School of Medicine, Seattle, Washington
crscott@u.washington.edu

Charles R. Scriver, M.D.C.M. [1, 5, 77]
Alva Professor of Human Genetics, Professor of Pediatrics, Faculty of Medicine, Professor of Biology, Faculty of Science, McGill University; McGill University-Montreal Children's Hospital Research Institute, McGill University Health Centre, Montreal, Quebec, Canada
mc77@musica.mcgill.ca

Udo Seedorf, M.D. [142]
Institut fur Klinische Chemie and Laboratoriumsmedizin, Zentrallaboratorium Westfalische Wilhelms-Universitat, Munster, Germany
seedorfu@uni-muenster.de

Christine E. Seidman, M.D. [213]
Investigator, Howard Hughes Medical Institute
Professor Medicine and Genetics, Director, Cardiovascular Genetics Center, Dept. of Medicine, Brigham and Women's Hospital, Harvard Medical School, Boston, Massachusetts
cseidman@rascal.med.harvard.edu

Jonathan G. Seidman, Ph.D. [213]
Henrietta B. and Frederick H. Bugher Professor of Cardiovascular Genetics, Investigator, Howard Hughes Medical Institute, Harvard Medical School, Boston, Massachusetts

Giorgio Semenza, M.D. [75]
Professor, Dept. of Biochemistry, Swiss Institute of Technology, Laboratorium fur Biochemie, Zurich, Switzerland; Professor, Dept. of Chemistry and Medical Biochemistry, University of Milan, Milan, Italy
giorgio.semenza@unimi.it
semenza@bc.biol.ethz.ch

Gul N. Shah, Ph.D. [208]
Assistant Research Professor, Edward A. Doisy Dept. of Biochemistry and Molecular Biology, Saint Louis University School of Medicine, St. Louis, Missouri
shahgn@slu.edu

Lisa G. Shaffer, Ph.D. [65]
Associate Professor, Dept. of Molecular and Human Genetics, Baylor College of Medicine, Houston, Texas
lshaffer@bcm.tmc.edu

Larry J. Shapiro, M.D. [166]
W.H. and Marie Wattis Distinguished Professor, Chairman, Dept. of Pediatrics, University of California Medical Center, San Francisco, California
Lshapiro@peds.ucsf.edu

Val C. Sheffield, M.D., Ph.D. [242]
Professor of Pediatrics, Associate Investigator, Howard Hughes Medical Institute, Dept. of Pediatrics, Div. of Medical Genetics, University of Iowa Hospital and Clinic, Iowa City, Iowa
Val-sheffield@uiowa.edu

Stephanie L. Sherman, Ph.D. [64]
Dept. of Genetics Emory University School of Medicine, Atlanta, Georgia
ssherman@genetics.emory.edu

Vivian E. Shih, M.D. [87]
Professor of Neurology, Harvard Medical School, Director, Amino Acid Disorder Laboratory/Metabolic Disorders Unit, Massachusetts General Hospital, Charlestown, Massachusetts
vshih@partners.org

John M. Shoffner, M.D. [104]
Director, Molecular Medicine, Molecular Medicine Laboratory, Children's Healthcare of Atlanta, Atlanta, Georgia
john.shoffner@choa.org

David Sidransky, M.D. [54]
Dept. of Otolaryngology-HNS, The Johns Hopkins University School of Medicine, Baltimore, Maryland
dsidrans@jhmi.edu

Olli Simell, M.D. [83, 192]
Professor of Pediatrics, Dept. of Pediatrics, University of Turku, Turku, Finland
Olli.simell@utu.fi

H. Anne Simmonds, Ph.D. [108]
Purine Research Unit, Guy's Hospital, London Bridge, London, United Kingdom
anne.simmonds@kcl.ac.uk

Ola H. Skjeldal, M.D., Ph.D. [132]
Div. of Pediatrics, Ullevaal University Hospital, Oslo, Norway
ola.skjeldal@klinmed.uio.no

William S. Sly, M.D. [1, 138, 208]
Alice A. Doisy Professor of Biochemistry and Molecular Biology, Chair, Edward A. Doisy Dept. of Biochemistry and Molecular Biology, Professor of Pediatrics, St. Louis University School of Medicine, St. Louis, Missouri
slyws@slu.edu

C. Wayne Smith, M.D. [188]
Head, Sect. of Leukocyte Biology; Professor, Depts. of Pediatrics, Microbiology and Immunology, Sect. of Leukocyte Biology, Children's Nutrition Research Center, Baylor College of Medicine Houston, Texas
cwsmith@bcm.tmc.edu

Kirby D. Smith, Ph.D. [131]
Professor of Pediatrics, Kennedy Krieger Institute, McKusick-Nathans Institute of Genetic Medicine, The Johns Hopkins University School of Medicine, Baltimore, Maryland
smithk@mail.jhmi.edu

Oded Sperling, Ph.D. [198]
Professor and Chairman of Clinical Biochemistry, Dept. of Clinical Biochemistry, Rabin Medical Center, Petah-Tikva, Israel
odeds@post.tau.ac.il

Allen M. Spiegel, M.D. [164]
Director, National Institute of Diabetes and Digestive and Kidney Diseases, Bethesda, Maryland
allens@amb.niddk.nih.gov

Peter H. St. George-Hyslop, M.D. [234]
Professor, Dept. of Medicine, Center for Research in Neurodegenerative Diseases, University of Toronto, Toronto, Ontario, Canada
p.hyslop@utoronto.ca

Beat Steinmann, M.D. [70]
Professor, Div. of Metabolism and Molecular Pediatrics, University Children's Hospital, Zurich, Switzerland
beat.steinmann@kispi.unizh.ch

Sylvia Stöckler-Ipsiroglu, M.D. [84]
Dept. of Pediatrics, University Hospital Vienna, Laboratory for Inherited Metabolic Diseases, Wahringergurtel, Vienna, Austria

Edwin M. Stone, M.D., Ph.D. [242]
Dept. of Ophthalmology and Visual Sciences, University of Iowa College of Medicine, Iowa City, Iowa
edwin-stone@viowa.edu

Pietro Strisciuglio, M.D. [152]
Associate Professor of Pediatrics, Dept. of Pediatrics, "Magna Graecia", Catanzaro, Italy
strisciuglio_unicz@libero.it

Sharon F. Suchy, Ph.D. [252]
Staff Scientist, Genetic Disease Research Branch, National Human Genome Research Instit, Bethesda, Maryland
suchy@nhgri.nih.gov

Kathleen E. Sullivan, M.D., Ph.D. [186]
Assistant Professor of Pediatrics, Children's Hospital of Philadelphia, Philadelphia, Pennsylvania

Andrea Superti-Furga, M.D. [202]
Div. of Metabolism and Molecular Pediatrics, University of Zurich, Universitaets-Kinderklinik, Zurich, Switzerland
asuperti@access.unizh.ch

Kinuko Suzuki, M.D. [145, 147, 153]
Professor of Pathology and Lab Medicine, Dept. of Pathology and Lab Medicine, School of Medicine, University of North Carolina at Chapel Hill
kis@med.unc.edu

Kunihiko Suzuki, M.D. [147, 153]
Director Emeritus, Neuroscience Center, Professor of Neurology and Psychiatry, School of Medicine,
University of North Carolina at Chapel Hill, North Corolina
Kuni.Suzuki@attglobal.net

Yoshiyuki Suzuki, M.D. [147, 151]
Professor and Director, Nasu Institute for Developmental Disabilities, Clinical Research Center, International University of Health and Welfare, Otawara, Japan
suzukiy@iuhw.ac.jp

Dallas M. Swallow, Ph.D. [76]
Professor of Human Genetics, The Galton Laboratory, Dept. of Biology, University College London, London, United Kingdom
dswallow@hgmp.mrc.ac.uk

Lawrence Sweetman, Ph.D. [93]
Professor, Institute of Biomedical Studies, Baylor University; Director, Mass Spectrometry Lab, Institute of Metabolic Disease, Baylor University Medical Center, Dallas, Texas
l.sweetman@baylordallas.edu

Alan Richard Tall, M.D. [121]
Tilden Weger Bieler Professor of Medicine, Dept. of Medicine, Div. of Molecular Medicine, Columbia University College of Physicians and Surgeons, New York, New York
art1@columbia.edu

Robert M. Tanguay, Ph.D. [79]
Laboratoire de genetique cellulaire et developpementale, Pavillon Charles-Eugene Marchand, Université Laval, Ste-Foy, Quebec, Canada
robert.tanguay@rsvs.ulaval.ca

Robin G. Taylor, Ph.D. [80]
Dept. of Genetics, The Hospital for Sick Children Research Institute, Toronto, Canada
rgtaylor@alumni.haas.org

Simeon I. Taylor, M.D., Ph.D. [68]
Lilly Research Fellow, Lilly Research Laboratories, Indianapolis, Indiana

Harriet S. Tenenhouse, Ph.D. [197]
Professor of Pediatrics and Human Genetics, Auxiliary Professor of Biology, Div. of Medical Genetics,
McGill University, Montreal Children's Hospital Research Institute, Montreal, Quebec, Canada
mdht@www.debelle.mcgill.ca

Jess G. Thoene, M.D. [199]
Karen Gore Professor; Director, Hayward Genetics Center, Human Genetics Program, Tulane University School of Medicine, New Orleans, Louisiana
jthoene@mailhost.tcs.tulane.edu

George H. Thomas, Ph.D. [140]
Professor of Pediatrics, Pathology and Medicine, The Johns Hopkins University School of Medicine, Director of Kennedy Krieger Institute Genetics Laboratory Baltimore, Maryland
thomasg@kennedykrieger.org

Craig B. Thompson, M.D. [24]
Abramson Family Cancer Research Institute, University of Pennsylvania, Philadelphia, Pennsylvania
drt@mail.med.upenn.edu

Beat Thöny, Ph.D. [78]
Associate Professor, Division of Clinical Chemistry & Biochemistry, Div. of Chemistry and Biochemistry, University of Zurich, Zurich, Switzerland
bthony@kispi.unizh.ch

Roland Tisch, Ph.D. [12]
Postdoctoral Fellow, Dept. of Microbiology and Immunology, Stanford University School of Medicine, Stanford, California

Jay A. Tischfield, Ph.D. [108]
MacMillan Professor and Chair, Dept. of Genetics, Rutgers University, Professor of Pediatrics and Psychiatry, Robert Wood Johnson Medical School, Piscataway, New Jersey

John A. Todd, M.D. [6]
Professor, Dept. of Medical Genetics, Cambridge University; Institute for Medical Research, Addenbrooke's Hospital, Cambridge, United Kingdom
john.todd@cimr.cam.ac.uk

Douglas M. Tollefsen, M.D., Ph.D. [176]
Professor of Medicine, Hematology Div., Washington University Medical School, St. Louis, Missouri
tollefsen@im.wustl.edu

Eileen P. Treacy, M.D. [5]
Associate Professor of Human Genetics and Pediatrics; Director, Biochemical Genetics Unit, Div. of Medical Genetics, Dept. of Biochemical Genetics, Montreal Children's Hospital, Montreal, Quebec, Canada
mcet@musica.mcgill.ca

Jeffrey M. Trent, M.D., Ph.D. [20]
Chief, Lab of Cancer Genetics, National Human Genome Research Institute, Bethesda, Maryland
jtrent@nih.gov

Mark A. Trifiro, Ph.D. [161]
Associate Professor, Dept. of Medicine, McGill University; Associate Physician, Dept. of Medicine, Lady Davis Institute for Medical Research, Sir Mortimer B. Davis Jewish General Hospital, Montreal, Canada, Quebec
mdtm@musica.mcgill.ca

Karl Tryggvason, M.D. [214]
Div. Matrix Biology, Dept. of Medical Biochemistry and Biophysics, Karolinska Institut, Stockholm, Sweden
karl.tryggvason@mbb.ki.se

William T. Tse, M.D., Ph.D. [183]
Children's Hospital/Dana-Farber Cancer Institute, Div. of Hematology/Oncology, Boston, Massachusetts
William_tse@dfci.harvard.edu

Edward G.D. Tuddenham, M.D. [172]
Professor, MRC/CSC, Hammersmith Hospital, London, United Kingdom
etuddenh@rpms.ac.uk

Eric Turk, Ph.D. [190]
Dept. of Physiology, UCLA School of Medicine, Los Angeles, California
eturk@mednet.ucla.edu

Linda A. Tyfield, M.D. [72]
Consultant Clinical Scientist, Hon. Sr. Research Fellow, Dept. of Child Health, University of Bristol, Molecular Genetics Unit, The Lewis Laboratories, Southmead Hospital, Bristol, United Kingdom
linda.tyfield@bristol.ac.uk

Jouni Uitto, M.D., Ph.D. [222]
Jefferson Institute of Molecular Medicine, Dept. of Dermatology and Cutaneous Biology, Jefferson Medical College, Philadelphia, Pennsylvania
jouni.uitto@mail.tju.edu

Gerd M. Utermann, M.D. [116]
Professor and Chair, Institute for Medical Biology and Human Genetics, Leopold-Franzens University of Innsbruck, Innsbruck, Austria
Gerd.Utermann@uibk.ac.at

David Valle, M.D. [1, 3, 4, 5, 81, 83, 129]
Professor of Pediatrics Genetics and Molecular Biology, Investigator Howard Hughes Medical Institute, McKusick-Nathans Institute of Genetic Medicine, The Johns Hopkins University, Baltimore, Maryland
dvalle@jhmi.edu

Georges Van den Berghe, M.D. [70, 112]
Professor, Dept. of Biochemistry and Cellular Biology, University of Louvain Medical School, Director of Research, Laboratory of Physiological Chemistry, Christian de Duve Institute of Cellular Pathology, Brussels, Belgium
vandenberghe@bchm.ucl.ac.be

Peter van Endert, M.D. [12]
Postdoctoral Fellow, Dept. of Microbiology and Immunology, Stanford University School of Medicine, Stanford, California

Albert H. van Gennip, M.D. [113]
Laboratory Genetic Metabole Diseases, Academic Medical Center, University of Amsterdam, Amsterdam, The Netherlands

Veronica van Heyningen, D.Phil., F.R.S.E. [240]
Head of Cell and Molecular Genetics Sect., MRC Human Genetics Unit, Western General Hospital, Edinburgh, Scotland, United Kingdom
v.vanheyningen@hgu.mrc.ac.uk

Marie T. Vanier, M.D., Ph.D. [145]
Directeur de Recherche INSERM, Lyon-Sud Medical School, Oullins, France
vanier@univ-lyonl.fr

André B.P. Van Kuilenburg, M.D. [113]
Laboratory Genetic Metabole Diseases, Academic Medical Center, University of Amsterdam, Amsterdam, The Netherlands

Emile Van Schaftingen, M.D., Ph.D. [74]
Professor of Biochemistry, Laboratory of Physiological Chemistry, ICP, Universite Catholique de Louvain, Brussels, Belgium
vanschaftingen@bchm.ucl.ac.be

Gilbert Vassart, M.D., Ph.D. [158]
Head, Dept. of Medical Genetics, Institut de Recherche Interdisciplinaire, Universite Libre de Bruxelles, Brussels, Belgium
gvassart@ulb.ac.be

Bert Vogelstein, M.D. [17, 27, 48]
Investigator, Howard Hughes Medical Institute, Clayton Professor of Oncology and Pathology, The Johns Hopkins University School of Medicine, Baltimore, Maryland
vogelbe@welch.jhu.edu

Arnold von Eckardstein, M.D. [122]
Institut für Klinische Chemie und Laboratoriumsmedizin, Zentrallaboratorium, Westfälische Wilhelms-Universität Münster, Münster, Germany
vonecka@uni-muenster.de

Kurt von Figura, Ph.D. [84, 148]
Director and Professor, Institute of Biochemistry II Zentrum Biochemie und Molekulare Zellbiologie Georg-August-Universitat Gottingen, Gottingen, Germany
kfigura@gwdg.de

Tom Vulliamy, Ph.D. [179]
Clinical Scientist, Honorary Lecturer, Dept. of Hematology, Imperial College of School of Medicine, Hammersmith Hospital, London, United Kingdom
t.vulliamy@ic.ac.uk

Douglas C. Wallace, Ph.D. [105]
Robert W. Woodruff, Professor of Molecular Genetics, Professor and Director, Center for Molecular Medicine, Emory University School of Medicine, Atlanta, Georgia
dwallace@gen.emory.edu

John H. Walter, M.D. [72]
Consultant Pediatrician, Willink Biochemical Genetics Unit, Royal Manchester Children's Hospital, Pendlebury, Manchester, United Kingdom
john@jhwalter.demon.co.uk

Ronald J.A. Wanders, Ph.D. [130, 132]
Professor of Clinical Enzymology and Inherited Diseases, University of Amsterdam Academic Medical Centre, Emma Children's Hospital and Clinical Chemistry, Amsterdam, The Netherlands
wanders@amc.uva.nl

Stephen T. Warren, Ph.D. [64]
Rollins Research Center, Emory University School of Medicine, Atlanta, Georgia
swarren@bimcore.emory.edu

Paul A. Watkins, M.D., Ph.D. [131]
Associate Professor, Neurology, Dept. of Neurogenetics, Kennedy Krieger Institute, Johns Hopkins University, Baltimore, Maryland
watkins@kennedykrieger.org

Sir David J. Weatherall, M.D., FRS [181]
Regius Professor of Medicine, Institute of Molecular Medicine, John Radcliffe Hospital, Headington, Oxford, United Kingdom
janet.watt@imm.ox.ac.uk

Barbara L. Weber, M.D. [47]
Professor of Medicine and Genetics; Director, Breast Cancer Program; Assoc. Director, Cancer, Control and Population Science, University of Pennsylvania Cancer Center, Philadelphia, Pennsylvania
weberb@mail.med.upenn.edu

Dianne R. Webster, Ph.D [113]
National Testing Center, Lab Plus Auckland Hospital, Auckland, New Zealand

Lee S. Weinstein, M.D. [164]
Investigator, Metabolic Disease Branch, National Institute of Diabetes and Digestive Kidney Diseases, Bethesda, Maryland

Michael J. Welsh, M.D. [201]
Investigator, Howard Hughes Medical Institute, Dept. of Internal Medicine, University of Iowa College of Medicine, Iowa City, Iowa
mjwelsh@blue.weeg.uiowa.edu

David A. Wenger, Ph.D. [147]
Professor of Neurology and Biochemistry and Molecular Pharmacology, Jefferson Medical College, Philadelphia, Pennsylvania
David.wenger@mail.tju.edu

Jeffrey A. Whitsett, M.D. [218]
Div. of Pulmonary Biology, Children's Hospital Medical Center, Cincinnati, Ohio
jeff.whitsett@chmcc.org

Michael P. Whyte, M.D. [207]
Professor of Medicine, Pediatrics, and Genetics, Div. of Bone and Mineral Diseases, Washington University School of Medicine, Barnes-Jewish Hospital, Medical Scientific Director, Center for Metabolic Bone Disease and Molecular Research, Shriners Hospital for Children, St. Louis, Missouri
mwhyte@shrinenet.org

Andrew O.M. Wilkie, M.D., F.R.C.P. [245]
Senior Research Fellow in Clinical Science, Wellcome Trust, Institute of Molecular Medicine, John Radcliffe Hospital, Headington, Oxford, United Kingdom
awilkie@worf.molbiol.ox.ac.uk

Douglas Wilkin, Ph.D. [210]
Medical Genetics Branch, National Human Genome Research Institute, Bethesda, Maryland

Huntington F. Willard, Ph.D. [61]
Henry Wilson Payne Professor and Chairman of Genetics, Director, Center for Human Genetics, Case Western Reserve University School of Medicine, Cleveland, Ohio
hfw@po.cwru.edu

Julian C. Williams, M.D., Ph.D. [93]
Associate Professor of Pediatrics, USC School of Medicine, Head, Div. Of Med. Genetics, Children's Hospital LA, Med. Dir., Dept. of Pathology and Laboratory Medicine Genetics Laboratories, Los Angeles, California
jwilliams@chlais.usc.edu

Jean D. Wilson, M.D. [160]
Charles Cameron Sprague Distinguished Chair in Biomedical Science, Clinical Professor of Internal Medicine, Dept. of Internal Medicine, University of Texas Southwestern Medical Center, Dallas, Texas
jwils1@mednet.swmed.edu

Jerry A. Winkelstein, M.D. [186]
Dept. of Pediatrics, Johns Hopkins University School of Medicine, Baltimore, Maryland
jwinkels@welchlink.welch.jhu.edu

Barry Wolf, M.D., Ph.D. [156]
Associate Chair for Research, Head, Div. of Pediatric Research, Professor, Div. of Human Genetics, University of Connecticut School of Medicine, Director of Pediatric Research, Connecticut Children's Medical Center, Hartford, Connecticut
bwolf@hsc.vcu.edu

Allan W. Wolkoff, M.D. [125]
Professor, Albert Einstein College of Medicine, Liver Research Center Bronx, New York
wolkoff@aecom.yu.edu

W.G. Wood [181]
Institute of Molecular Medicine, John Radcliffe Hospital, Oxford, United Kingdom

Ronald G. Worton, C.M., Ph.D., F.R.S.C. [216]
CEO and Scientific Director, Ottawa General Hospital Research Institute, University of Ottawa, Ottawa, Ontario, Canada
rworton@ogh.on.ca

Ernest M. Wright, D.Sc. [190]
Professor and Chair, Dept. of Physiology, UCLA School of Medicine, Los Angeles, California
ewright@mednet.ucla.edu

Charles John Yeo, M.D. [50]
Professor and Attending Surgeon, Dept. of Surgery and Oncology, The Johns Hopkins Hospital, Baltimore, Maryland
cyeo@jhmi.edu

Chang-En Yu, M.D., Ph.D. [33]
Veterans Affairs Puget Sound Health Care System, Seattle Div. and the Dept. of Medicine, University of Washington, Seattle, Washington
changeyu@u.washington.edu

Berton Zbar, M.D. [41]
Chief, Laboratory of Immunology, National Cancer Institute-Frederick Cancer, Research Facility, Frederick, Maryland
zbar@mail.ncifcrf.gov

Huda Y. Zoghbi, M.D. [226, 255]
Professor, Dept. of Pediatrics and Molecular and Human Genetics; Investigator Howard Hughes Medical Institute, Baylor College of Medicine, Houston, Texas
hzoghbi@bcm.tmc.edu

PREFACE TO THE EIGHTH EDITION

Following "the new synthesis" of Mendelism and Darwinism, Theodosins Dobzhansky stated that biology makes sense only in the light of evolution.[1] A corollary to that opinion would say that medicine without biology does not make sense. This book, now in its eighth edition, presents evidence that biology, as we come to know it in the era of genomics, is helping to make better sense of medicine.

In its first edition,[2] this book, then known as *The Metabolic Basis of Inherited Disease* (MBID), focused almost exclusively on the Mendelian diseases falling into the category known as "inborn errors of metabolism." For the next five editions, MBID served as a medical companion to human biochemical genetics which had its own seminal text.[3] Then, to acknowledge the increasing relevance of molecular biology and molecular genetics, for the seventh edition we changed its title to: *The Metabolic and Molecular Bases of Inherited Disease* (*MMBID*). There were further changes in the seventh edition: complex genetic traits were increasingly recognized, cancer being a notable new section of the book, and even more so in the CD-ROM update of the print edition. Chromosomal disorders had appeared in the sixth edition and they increased their presence in the seventh, along with a chapter dedicated to imprinting.

The eighth edition of MMBID, now appearing in the first year of the twenty-first century, contains new chapters on the history of the inborn errors of metabolism (Chapter 3), their impact on health (Chapter 4) and their response to treatment (Chapter 5). This edition further reveals how genetics is contributing to the understanding of complex traits and birth defects as well as the Mendelian diseases with nominal pathways of metabolism or development. It is not surprising then that MMBID-8 should have chapters on aging and hypertension or on Hirschsprung disease, for example. In brief, this book is becoming a "textbook of medicine," as predicted by one reviewer of an earlier edition.[4]

Five questions formulated as such by Victor McKusick among others have been of abiding interest in medicine since at least the time of Osler: (1) What is the problem? (2) How did it happen? (3) What is the cause? (4) What can be done? (5) Will it happen again? The questions address the corresponding issues of diagnosis, pathogenesis, ultimate and proximal cause, treatment and prevention, and inherited risks of recurrence. As for cause, the theme of special interest shared by every entity discussed in this book is *mutation*: mutation that modifies phenotype, contributes to pathogenesis of the disease and, in various ways, identifies a key component in a "pathway" or "network" responsible for homeostasis and functional integrity.

MMBID-8 is being published as genome projects, both human and nonhuman, yield information and knowledge about the organization and nucleotide sequences of genomes. The allied field of research, now called genomics, has been called "a journey to the center of biology."[5] Comparative genomics reveals that homeostasis of energy metabolism and many aspects of intermediary metabolism are encoded in genes with a very long evolutionary history (see Chapter 4). Moreover, a number of the human disorders can be analyzed functionally in yeast in a manner some will call "biochemical genomics"[6] and there is a corresponding database cross-referencing human and yeast phenotypes.[7] Accordingly, Dobzhansky's angle of vision is increasingly validated.

At the same time, the genomes of *C. elegans* and *Drosophila* are telling us that development of multicellular organisms is controlled by the major portion of the corresponding genomes and each organism has particular programs for particular body plans. New sections and chapters in MMBID-8 are devoted to various disorders of development in *H. sapiens*.

It follows that biology is indeed a shared language for medicine.[8] However, shared language does not preclude particular language to deal with variant phenotypes (the diseases), their clinical consequences, and the specialization in clinical expertise required to address them. In recognition of this, the book contains material in the particular languages of counseling, testing and screening, and treatment; indeed, in a language increasingly accessed on Web sites by patients who want to know. The particular language extends beyond phenotype, counseling, and so on; it reaches the patient. Every patient who has one of the so-called "single-gene" diseases described in this book has an "orphan" disease; furthermore, because of biological individuality, each patient has his or her own private (orphan) form of unhealth. In other words, this book is an ultimate guidebook for *individualized medicine*.

MMBID-8 will contribute to an instauration of the clinician-investigator, a colleague who has been much marginalized by successes in the basic science and molecular and cellular biology and the corresponding contributions to medical science. The original editions of MBID were written largely by clinician-investigators; or by basic scientists who still retained a familiarity with patients or did research that was patient-oriented and disease-oriented.[9] However, in the more recent editions of MMBID, the chapters themselves and the majority of the references cited in them were more often than not authored by persons doing basic research, sometimes rather remote from the patient's primary problem. But, as the "genome project" moves from its structural to a functional phase and into biochemical- and pharmacogenomics, the editors of MMBID recognize a need for the return of the clinician-investigator. The latter must share equal status with the basic scientist so that science can be translated quickly into benefits for patients. That is why some chapters in MMBID-8 (e.g., 66 and 99) are devoted to clinical algorithms.

The prefaces to MBID-6 and MMBID-7 described how the editors chose material for Chapters and Parts of these editions. In the seventh edition, we said: "If there is an identifiable molecular explanation for the disease — and it affects a dynamic phenotype, metabolic or otherwise — then it is a candidate for inclusion .... The expansion of topics here is selective and obviously not inclusive of all possibilities." Although MMBID-8 has not changed its title, it has changed in many other ways. It has three new associate editors (Barton Childs, Kenneth Kinzler, and Bert Vogelstein), new chapters have appeared (the total is now 255) and the number of authors now exceeds 500. That the printed and bound book exceeds 7000 pages is not really a surprise, but it is an abiding reason to have portable and online versions of the book.

A survey undertaken by some of the editors, by some of our readers and owners of the seventh edition showed that 70% used the book at least once per week. Half those persons believed the book should grow beyond its original domain; that content of MMBID-7 was appropriate; and over 90% of the readers welcomed the prospect of a Web version.

The editors intend to keep MMBID-8 "user friendly;" and also to keep it up to date. We hope a portable version of MMBID-8 will be available for those who wish to have something they can carry home; there will be a Web version. In this latter format, MMBID will become a "continuous book," able to update all material and to incorporate new topics as they become pertinent to our stated mission. Accordingly, as more and more scientific print literature goes "on line" in one format or another, MMBID will do likewise;

the web version will allow MMBID to reincarnate itself through a long and healthy life.

So much seems to change between editions of MMBID; for example, a new team — Susan Noujaim, Peter Boyle, Marty Wonsiewicz, and others at McGraw-Hill — have translated formidable stacks of typescript into a book agreeable to the publisher. On the other hand, stability can still be found in the life of this book; the editors are still working with the same colleagues: Lynne Prevost and Huguette Rizziero (CRS), Grace Watson (AB), Elizabeth Torno (WS), Sandy Muscelli (DV); while Kathy Helwig helped the new editors (BC, KK, and BV). The process of reading manuscripts and proofs was yet again lightened by the tolerant support of our families and by colleagues at the places of business.

REFERENCES

1. Dobzhansky TH: "Nothing in biology makes sense except in the light of evolution." *Am Biol Teach* **35**:125, 1973.
2. Stanbury JB, Wyngaarden JB, Fredrickson DS (eds.): *The Metabolic Basis of Inherited Disease*. McGraw-Hill Book Co., New York. 1960.
3. Harris H: The principles of human biochemical genetics. *Frontiers of Biology* (Neuberger A, Tatum EL (eds.), Vol. 19. North Holland Pub. Co., London, 1970. North-Holland Research Monographs.
4. Childs B: Book Review. *The Metabolic Basis of Inherited Disease*. 6th ed. 2 volumes. Scriver CR, Beaudet AL, Sly WS, Valle D (eds.). *Am J Hum Genet* **46**:848, 1990.
5. Lander ES, Weinberg RA: Genomics: Journey to the center of biology. *Science* **287**:1777, 2000.
6. Carlson M: The awesome power of yeast biochemical genomics. *Trends Genet* **16**:49, 2000.
7. Bassett DE Jr., Boguski MS, Spencer F, Reeves R, Kim SH, Weaver T, Hieter P: Genome cross-referencing and XREFdb: Implications for the identification and analysis of genes mutated in human disease. *Nat Genet* **15**:339, 1997.
8. Scriver CR: American Pediatric Society Presidential Address 1995. Disease, war and biology: Language for medicine — and pediatrics. *Pediatric Res* **38**:819, 1995.
9. Goldstein JL, Brown MS: The clinical investigator: Bewitched, bothered, and bewildered — but still beloved. Editorial. *J Clin Invest* **99**:2803, 1997.

PREFACE TO THE SEVENTH EDITION

The sixth edition of *The Metabolic Basis of Inherited Disease* experienced "transition, transformation, and challenge." Transition continues in the seventh edition with the arrival of many new authors. Challenge remains, like the mountain whose peak is never in view while the climb proceeds. And there is transformation again, not least with the title: *The Metabolic and* Molecular *Bases of Inherited Disease*. The new word is significant.

A reviewer of the sixth edition reminds us of the original plan for the book: to present "the pertinent clinical, biochemical, and genetic information concerning those metabolic anomalies grouped under Garrod's engaging term 'inborn errors of metabolism.' "[1] The term *molecular* is a belated but natural homecoming for Garrod. During his lifetime, Garrod's views grew to encompass inherited susceptibility to any disease originating in our chemical individuality. These ideas emerged fully developed, for their time, in Garrod's second book. *The Inborn Factors in Disease*. That we have been slow to perceive the reach of his thinking is a theme of his recent biographer.[2] To accept it and put it to use requires the means to test its validity. Molecular analysis of the genetic variation causing or predisposing to disease provides the opportunity. The inborn errors of metabolism are simply our most obvious illustrations of the genetic variation that affects health and the molecular underpinnings of that variation. A corresponding analysis of multifactorial diseases is the obvious next step in the understanding of disease.[3] Need we say that MMBID-7 is nothing less than a textbook of molecular medicine, encompassing the diseases about which we know most? We predict that the "classic" textbooks of medicine in the future will look more and more like MMBID.

Change in the title of MBID did something else: it solved a problem the editors created for themselves in MBID-6, again commented on by the above-mentioned reviewer.[1] When we included topics not overtly "metabolic" in the sixth edition, for example, Down and fragile X syndromes, primary ciliary dyskinesia, collagen disorders and the muscular dystrophies, we moved well beyond the canonical theme of inborn errors of *metabolism*. The nonmetabolic topics are further expanded in this edition because they conform to a *logic of disease*, as it is called by Barton Childs in Chapter 2. The manifestations of any "genetic" disease are explained by a process (pathogenesis) that originates in part or in full form an intrinsic cause (mutation); and, since genotype is one of the determinants of the phenotype (disease), it follows that diagnosis, treatment, and counseling should be motivated form the genetic point of view because the disease involves both the patient and his or her family.

If there is an identifiable molecular explanation for the disease — and it affects a dynamic phenotype, metabolic or otherwise — then it is a candidate for inclusion in the seventh edition. The expansion of topics here is selective and obviously not inclusive of all possibilities. If this were the case, the table of contents would resemble the McKusick catalog, *Mendelian Inheritance in Man*! Nevertheless, yet a further 32 chapters are new to this edition of MBID while 31 others were introduced in the sixth edition; new ideas appear again and again in virtually all "old" chapters. Will it be three volumes — or more — for the eighth edition? (A CD-ROM format is under serious consideration for the next edition.) The Summary Table, immediately preceding Chapter 1, surveys the information in MMBID-7.

In the first section of the book, the following major new themes appear:

- A logic of disease based on genetic and evolutionary concepts that challenges conventional medical thinking (Chapter 2).
- Mutational mechanisms, including dynamic mutations (elastic or unstable DNA) (Chapter 3) and the methods to detect them (Chapter 1).
- Pharmacogenetics (Chapter 4) as a classical illustration of multifactorial disease (with ultimate and proximate causes) and of the "idiosyncratic reaction to drugs" — to recall Garrod's felicitous phrase.
- Diagnostic algorithms for the patient with an inborn error of metabolism (Chapter 5).
- Mapping of genes (genomics) (Chapter 6), along with an increased awareness that mutant gene expression may involve more than conventional Mendelian inheritance: for example, imprinting and mosaicism (Chapter 7).
- How cellular organelles, protein targeting and posttranslational modification, and the HLA complex affect expression of "genetic" disease (the subjects of Chapters 8 and 9, respectively).
- Cancer appears as a major theme for the first time in this edition (Chapters 10 to 15). Cancers are products of genetic damage. Modified events in pathways release cells from the normal controls of replication and growth. The cascades of events controlled by proto-oncogenes are counterparts of Garrod's pathways of metabolism. Because cancers can involve constitutional mutations, somatic mutations, or both, they further expand the conceptual boundaries of the book.
- Processes of inactivation harbored on the X chromosome (Chapter 16) and knowledge about the testis-determining factor and primary sex reversal (Chapter 17) are topics new to the section on chromosomes, itself an innovation of the sixth edition.

An awesome expansion of information continues in old and new chapters. The new chapters include, for example, insulin gene defects (Chapter 22); a completely new look at nonketotic hyperglycinemia (Chapter 37); diseases of the mitochondrial genome (Chapter 46); the apolipoprotein (a) molecule and its association with heart disease (Chapter 58); oxalosis as a peroxisomal disorder (Chapter 75); lysosomal enzyme activator proteins (Chapter 76); Pompe disease as a disease of lysosome function (Chapter 77) rather than a disease of carbohydrate metabolism; Lowe syndrome, separated from the Fanconi syndrome, following positional cloning of the gene (Chapter 123); Marfan syndrome, a disease of fibrillin dysfunction (Chapter 135); the muscular dystrophies (Chapters 140 and 141), and hypertrophic cardiomyopathy (Chapter 142). All is not new; in recognition of tradition, the spelling of *alcaptonuria* has reverted to *alkaptonuria* (Chapter 39).

A new section on disease of the eye (Chapters 143 to 146) includes retinitis pigmentosis, choroideremia, and disorders of color vision and crystallins. Discussions of epidermolysis bullosa (Chapter 149). Huntington disease (Chapter 152), and prion-related diseases (Chapter 153) reflect emerging molecular information on diseases of skin and brain. Chapter 154, the last in the book, catches recent developments involving half a dozen diseases.

The authors of chapters about particular diseases were asked to remember the needs of physicians and families, and they provide up-to-date information on diagnosis, treatment, and counseling. (These aspects are dealt with an even greater depth in a book that functions as our companion — the excellent *Inborn Metabolic*

Diseases: Diagnosis and Treatment, edited by J. Fernandes, J-M. Saudubray, and K. Tada.)

Some 200 authors wrote for MBID-6; 302 have written for MMBID-7; they have achieved the continuing transformation of this text. While so much seems to change overnight in molecular biology and genetics, stability can be found in the life of this book. Gail Gavert, Mariapaz Ramos-Englis, J. Dereck Jeffers, Peter McCurdy, and their colleagues have translated formidable stacks of typescript into a book agreeable to the publisher. The editors are still working with the same colleagues: Lynne Prevost and Huguette Rizziero (CRS), Grace Watson (AB), Elizabeth Torno (WS), and Sandy Muscelli (DV), Loy Denis was again our editorial coordinator until the last stages of this edition; her successor is Catherine Watson. The process of reading manuscripts and proofs was lightened by the tolerant support of our families and by colleagues at the place of business.

As this edition went to press, Harry Harris died. A giant in our field, his imprint is apparent everywhere in the book.

REFERENCES

1. Childs B: Book Review: *The Metabolic Basis of Inherited Disease*, 6th ed. *Am J Hum Genet* **66**:848, 1990.
2. Bearn AG: *Archibald Garrod and the Individuality of Man*. New York, Oxford University Press, 1993, 227 pp.
3. King RA, Rutter JI, Motulsky AG: *The Genetic Basis of Common Diseases*. New York, Oxford University Press, 1993, 978 pp.

PREFACE TO THE SIXTH EDITION

This edition of *The Metabolic Basis of Inherited Disease* marks a transition, a changing of the guard, as it were, among the editors. The sixth edition also reflects a transformation in the field of endeavor it encompasses; and there is a challenge too — for future editions. Transitions can be difficult and transformations sometimes produce unhappy results; neither need be the case here. Challenges can invigorate.

THE TRANSITION

Stanbury-Wyngaarden-'n-Fredrickson, collectively, were one famous "author" known to everyone in the field. This extraordinary editorial organism piloted the novel and timely book they had introduced and then edited through four successful editions. By a remarkable fision — or was it fusion? — the fifth edition was placed under the care of Stanbury-Wyngaarden-'n-Fredrickson, Goldstein 'n Brown. Now that giant has stepped aside, handing the challenge to a new team. The new editors have discovered how great the former ones were — if they hadn't known it before. Very large shoes had to be filled!

THE TRANSFORMATION

The sixth edition has many new features, notably the evidence of molecular genetics in one chapter after another. If *The Metabolic Basis of Inherited Disease* has had an abiding rationale, it was that the cause of all diseases listed in it was Mendelian and the diseases (so-called inborn errors of metabolism) were exceptions to be treasured for their illumination of human biology and for the insight they gave into pathogenesis of disease. But always there was a feeling that one did not understand cause as well as one should because not much was known about the genes. That situation is changing. There are new data about loci and structures of numerous normal genes and about the mutations affecting the phenotype encoded by them.

With 31 new chapters, the book is approximately one-third larger than it was. Accordingly, this edition appears for the first time in a two-volume format. It is a change undertaken with reluctance, but size of type, weight of paper, and the like had been adapted to the limit in the previous edition to accommodate the mass of information presented there. We elected to revise and print all chapters instead of using a précis of some, as in the last edition. Authors were encouraged to focus on up-to-date material and to use previous editions as archives of older material. But the wealth of new information neutralized contraction of the old. Hence the option taken here; to divide the book into two volumes, between separate covers.

New topics in the sixth edition include the following: There is a formal discussion of gene mapping and the medical use of genome markers (Chapter 6). Down syndrome (Chapter 7) and fragile X syndrome (Chapter 8) illustrate how any genetic disorder can eventually accommodate to our views of molecular genetics. They are the thin edge of the wedge toward understanding a great deal about human genetic disease and the editors introduce these chapters with some trepidation, realizing they could well be the very thin edge of a very big wedge — one of our challenges for future editions. One new chapter (122) covers the lactose deficiency polymorphism. This disorder does not fit the paradigm of a rare inborn error because it is so common; on the other hand, it does represent a Mendelian disadaptive phenotype for some individuals. There is a whole new section on peroxisomal diseases (Chapters 57–60) and Chapter 3 covers organelle biogenesis. Contiguous gene syndromes appear in this edition for the first time. The retinoblastoma story (Chapter 9) began as a contiguous gene syndrome; the new chapter encompasses this and analogous phenomena. Chapter 5 on oncogenes is new. The genes for retinoblastoma, chronic granulomatosus disease, and Duchenne muscular dystrophy are now known through techniques of "reverse" or "indirect" genetics. They are harbingers of what is to come in other diseases and they are topics developed at some length in this edition. Two appendices to Chapter 1, experiments in this edition, list: (1) the Mendelian disorders that can be diagnosed at the DNA level through oligonucleotide probes or by tightly linked markers that associate with alleles encoding mutant gene products; useful probes and their sources are catalogued in this appendix; (2) the mapped loci and their chromosomal assignments in the most current version of Victor McKusick's famous catalog available as we went to press. Perhaps a future edition will also catalog what we know about the mutant alleles at the loci encoding disease. Meanwhile the summary table grows in Chapter 1. It was introduced for the first time in the fifth edition and it is continued here for two reasons: first to show, in a simple manner, the growth of subject material between the last and present editions; second, to show how the white spaces in the fifth edition table are being filled in.

THE CHALLENGE

The future holds the potential for a separate chapter delineating the biochemical basis of each variant listed in McKusick's *Mendelian Inheritance in Man*. If this is the case, there will be many hundred chapters in subsequent editions of MBID. In addition, most monogenic disorders are not monogenic but modified through other loci by definable biochemical mechanisms; and most diseases are caused by polygenic and multifactorial mechanisms which also have a biochemical basis. Cytogenetic disorders have a biochemical basis as well, and in some instances the phenotypes may be determined by one or a few loci. These all represent effects of the constitutional genotypes on the phenotype, but there is also the role of somatic mutation in the pathogenesis of malignancies whether inherited or sporadic. With the explosion of information virtually assured, the challenge of how to focus and mold future editions is a daunting one.

This book has not grown unattended. In addition to the herculean efforts of some 200 authors and their assistants, others assured a safe passage during the development of the book, notably Dereck Jeffers and Gail Gavert at McGraw-Hill; Loy Denis, who served as coordinator for the editors and authors; and our own assistants: Lynne Prevost and Huguette Rizziéro (CRS), Grace Watson (AB), Elizabeth Torno (WS), and Sandy Muscelli (DV). But especially we thank our extraordinary predecessors for their nurture and care of a book many of us have come to admire and need. If this edition meets with the approval of its former editors, we will have partially done the job we acquired; the readers will ultimately decide whether it was done satisfactorily.

Last, an acknowledgment to our families; they know more about this book than they bargained for . . .!

Charles R. Scriver
Arthur L. Beaudet
William S. Sly
David Valle

The Metabolic & Molecular Bases of Inherited Disease

eighth edition

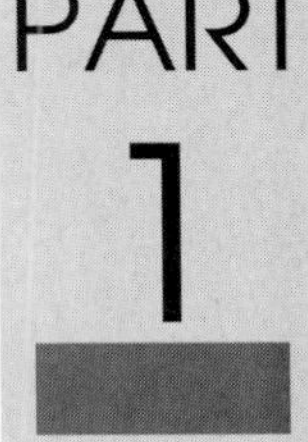

INTRODUCTION

Coding region

Intervening sequence

3′

DNA strand

5′

RNA transcript

Poly A

Cap

m RNA

Spliced mRNA

Polypeptide chain

H_2N

COOH

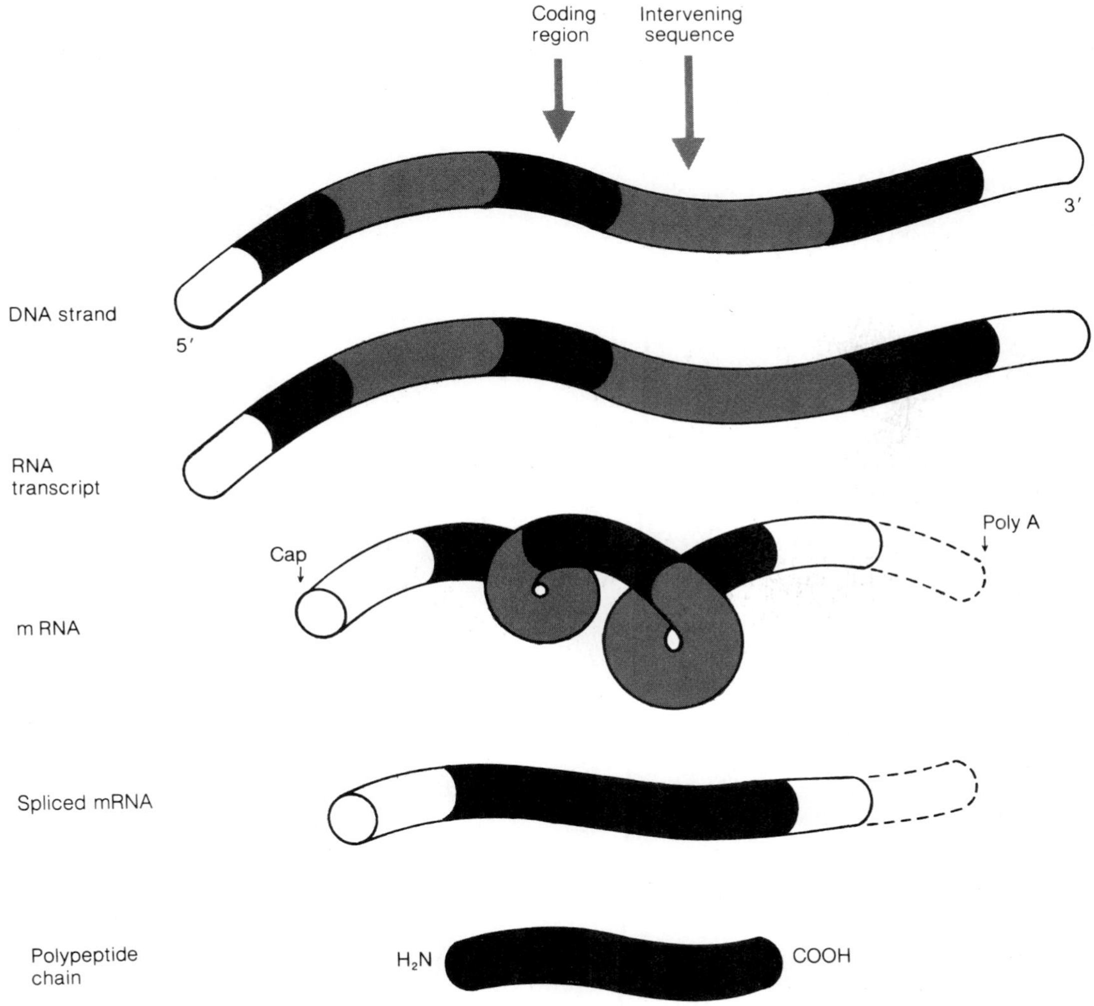

Gene splicing

CHAPTER

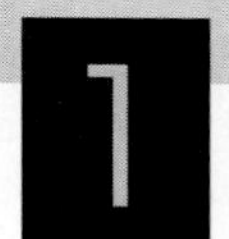

Genetics, Biochemistry, and Molecular Bases of Variant Human Phenotypes

Arthur L. Beaudet ▪ Charles R. Scriver
William S. Sly ▪ David Valle

Nature is nowhere accustomed more openly to display her secret mysteries than in cases where she shows traces of her workings apart from the beaten path; nor is there any better way to advance the proper practice of medicine than to give our minds to discovery of the usual law of Nature by careful investigation of cases of rarer forms of disease. For it has been found, in almost all things, that what they contain of useful or applicable is hardly perceived unless we are deprived of them, or they become deranged in some way. (Taken from Garrod[1] quoting a letter written by William Harvey in 1657 to emphasize the value of studying human variants.)

The medical model of disease holds that *manifestations* are the result of a *process* that has a *cause*. The manifestations of disease are assembled in *diagnosis* and they constitute a *taxonomy*. The process which underlies them is the pathogenesis of disease. The cause of disease comprises either an event that overwhelms homeostatic mechanisms (an extrinsic cause) or one that undermines them (an intrinsic cause). Most diseases involve a combination of both (a multifactorial cause).

This text has three unifying themes. The first, and central, theme is that the causes of the diseases described are mutations (intrinsic). Because these mutations are often expressed as *disadaptive phenotypes* (i.e., clinical manifestations) in the universal environment, they may cause diseases that are simply inherited and classified as *Mendelian* or *single-gene disorders*. Some chapters describe more complex causes with non-Mendelian inheritance, as in the cases of Down syndrome (Chap. 63, a chromosomal disease) and diabetes mellitus (Chaps. 6 and 67 to 69, a multifactorial disease). The discussion of LDL-receptor deficiency (Chap. 120) and other lipoprotein disorders illustrates how a disease of heterogeneous etiology (coronary artery disease) is being broken down into its component causes, some cases being caused primarily by a defect in a single gene, and some cases being of multifactorial etiology. The text is now greatly expanded to encompass cancer, in which somatic mutation and environmental exposures play a more prominent role along with germ line mutations. Any of these three factors — germ line mutation, somatic mutation, or environmental factors — may predominate in a single individual or type of cancer. Germ line mutation is the major contributor in retinoblastoma (Chap. 36) and polyposis of the colon or hereditary nonpolyposis colon cancer (Chaps. 32 and 48). Somatic mutations and environment are usually entwined, but stochastic somatic mutation independent of environment may be more prominent, as perhaps is true for many cases of breast cancer (Chap. 47) or pancreatic cancer (Chap. 50), while environmental factors causing somatic mutations may be more obvious, as in the case of smoking and lung cancer or asbestosis and mesothelioma (Chap. 58). Each recent edition of this text, when compared with the previous edition, reveals an enormous increase in our knowledge about genetic cause at the molecular level. This knowledge is applied increasingly through the use of recombinant DNA methods in clinical diagnosis and counseling. Although the study of single-gene disorders has been the traditional focus of this book, the understanding of the molecular and biochemical basis of common, multifactorial disorders is increasing rapidly and will have a growing impact on the practice of medicine.

This text's second unifying theme deals with pathogenesis in great detail. Knowledge of the pathophysiology of a disease explains its manifestations, is necessary for rational treatment, and may even suggest that treatment is not feasible.[2,3] It can be taken for granted that at least partial knowledge of pathogenesis is important for the treatment of most inborn errors of metabolism. The successive editions of this book document the expansion of knowledge about cause and about pathogenesis of inherited diseases. In due course, this book, or one like it, should become a fundamental textbook for the theory and practice of medicine, because most diseases in developed societies have genetic determinants. Every individual is a deviant in terms of biochemical individuality,[4] meaning that every person has an inherited predisposition to disease (diathesis) in a particular circumstance. This is not a new idea; Garrod expounded it thoroughly and clearly in his second book.[5] The difference between then and now is simply that molecular methods have made it possible to see in our DNA, our inherited predispositions. We can either avoid the occurrence of serious disease genotypes through genetic counseling procedures or ameliorate symptoms through treatment.

Therapy of inherited diseases constitutes the third unifying theme of this text as outlined in Chap. 5 and in chapters throughout the book for specific diseases. In the metabolic context, we think first of dietary therapy as in phenylketonuria, but therapy for genetic disease is now very broad, encompassing organ transplantation, enzyme replacement, pharmacologic intervention, avoidance of genotype-specific risk factors, surgical correction or amelioration, and a multitude of other strategies. Attempts to provide treatment through somatic gene therapy have barely begun, but there is hope that this approach could provide dramatic new therapeutic avenues as discussed in recent reviews[6–8] and texts,[9–11] despite the unfortunate, gene therapy-related death of a patient with an inborn error of metabolism in late 1999.[12]

The power of current cellular, molecular, and metabolic techniques is that they provide a vast amount of new information. There is the astounding prospect of identifying the biochemical

A list of standard abbreviations is located immediately preceding the index in each volume.

defects for most or all of the thousands of disease phenotypes catalogued by McKusick in *Mendelian Inheritance in Man*[13] and its electronic version, OMIM (www.ncbi.nlm.nih.gov/Omim/). A detailed map of the human genome is now a reality (see Chap. 10), and about half of human genes were reported to be identified by late 1998.[14] Efforts are underway to develop a full set of human full-length cDNA clones and sequences.[15]

GENOMIC MEDICINE

Genomic medicine can be defined as the use of genotypic analysis (DNA testing) to enhance the quality of medical care, including presymptomatic identification of susceptibility to disease, preventive intervention, selection of pharmacotherapy, and individual design of medical care based on genotype. The progress of the human genome project and research in molecular medicine have made genomic medicine an important strategy. Genotype can be deduced by analysis of protein (e.g., hemoglobin or α_1-antitrypsin), RNA, or DNA, but analysis of DNA is the usual method. It can be argued that there are no new principles or concepts involved in genomic medicine, but that it will change the way medicine is practiced, particularly in regard to intervention for common diseases. Testing for predisposition to disease does have the potential for harm because it opens the possibility of various forms of discrimination; however, it also has the potential of extraordinary benefits. Primary care physicians and genetic specialists are in pivotal positions to provide the benefits and minimize the harm. Genotypic analysis is standard practice for diseases in which a single gene plays a prominent role, but the role of genetic testing in complex disease traits—where multiple genes and nongenetic factors are implicated—is less established. Nevertheless, genomic medicine has the potential to reduce the burden of these disorders. Genotypic information has two broad applications: first, to modify the medical care provided to the individual; and second, to make possible reproductive counseling to couples who wish to have children. It is important to distinguish those genotypic results that provide potential for benefit and/or intervention (e.g., hemochromatosis) as compared to those situations where no clear intervention is available (e.g., Alzheimer or Huntington disease). Most disorders, however, fall in an intermediate category (e.g., hereditary nonpolyposis colon cancer) where opportunity for treatment or prevention is significant but by no means simple or 100 percent effective.

The concept that it is good medical practice to screen the population to identify individuals with risks and to intervene to prevent disease processes in such persons is well established. For example, blood pressure and cholesterol are measured for screening purposes to identify individuals who are asymptomatic but who have a predisposition to cardiovascular disease, and attempts are made to intervene in such individuals through pharmacology and changes in lifestyle. Although treatment is not always effective, there is frequent benefit to individuals and to society. Likewise, in perinatal medicine, population-based screening is used to identify individuals with particular genotypes who can benefit from prompt intervention, as exemplified by phenylketonuria. The rationales for routine mammography, screening for blood in the stool, measurement of prostate-specific antigen, and glaucoma screening are based on similar principles that early diagnosis can lead to beneficial intervention. Although some of these procedures test for disease rather than for predisposition to disease, all such strategies are based on the concept that early recognition and intervention can provide a medical benefit. The boundary between predisposition to disease and presymptomatic disease is not a clear one. Is hypertension a disease or a predisposition to a symptomatic event such as a stroke? Is a mutation in the breast and ovarian cancer gene *BRCA1* a predisposition to breast cancer or an early phase of the disease process? As with any medical strategy, intervention based on genotypic information is valid only if the benefit to the individual outweighs the potential harm of genotypic analysis (see "Discrimination, Ethical Concerns, and Excessive Costs" below). An example in which opportunities for genomic medicine have been largely unused is population-based screening to identify individuals with predisposition to emphysema because of α_1-antitrypsin deficiency (Chap. 219); such individuals can be identified by analysis of protein or DNA and should be counseled regarding the certainty of injury from smoking. The application and follow-up of widespread screening of this type may require major reorganization of medical care and its financing, but the potential benefits are enormous. We must strive to identify many adult diseases where population-based screening and intervention are as effective as is newborn screening for PKU. Hemochromatosis (Chap. 127) may provide such an opportunity, although arguments have been made for[16,17] and against[18] immediate implementation of screening.

Recombinant DNA methods, the polymerase chain reaction (PCR), the human genome project, new technologies for analyzing DNA, and research in molecular medicine make it feasible to obtain large amounts of genotypic information at very low cost using current and developing technologies. The DNA information is useful in providing medical care for an individual only to the extent that we can use it to implement a therapeutic or preventive intervention. As DNA information becomes routine, it should be incorporated into medical practice and into the medical record in the same way that blood pressure, cholesterol level, and hemoglobin electrophoresis are currently utilized. Proposals that DNA information be held in a separate medical record and treated differently than other medical information are inappropriate, impractical, and would have a negative impact on medical care. Such suggestions reflect an exaggerated view of the predictive power of most DNA information. Indeed, many relatively public pieces of information, such as obesity, alcohol intake, smoking, past medical conditions, and parental health history, are likely to have greater predictive implications than most DNA analyses.

A Continuum of Genetic Disease and Susceptibility

Genetic disease, apart from chromosomal disorders, is often thought of as falling into two groups: single-gene disorders or complex disease traits, the latter also known as multifactorial diseases. However, there is, in reality, a complex continuum involving (a) the number of loci, (b) the relative contribution of each allele, (c) nongenetic factors, and (d) very different contributions in individuals with a similar or virtually identical phenotype. This continuity is also discussed in Chap. 2 (see "Continuity of Monogenic, Multifactorial Modes of Inheritance"). Figure 1-1 is an attempt to symbolize the circumstances for a single-gene disorder, which is in fact a misnomer, because other loci almost always act as modifiers of the phenotype; a major gene disorder, implying that one locus has a predominant effect, but other loci also have more obvious effects; and a complex disease trait, meaning that multiple loci contribute to the phenotype with no one locus playing a predominant role. The phenotype resulting from all of these germ line genotypes may be modified to varying degrees by nongenetic factors such as diet and smoking, by stochastic factors such as random X inactivation or immunoglobulin gene rearrangements, and by somatic mutation. Particular phenotypes may fall into one or another group, but, importantly, different individuals with the same phenotype may fall into varying categories.

Genomic Medicine for Single-Gene Disorders

Genotypic analysis is available for the diagnosis, counseling, and management of many so-called Mendelian or single-gene disorders, in which one gene plays a predominant role in determining disease. The relevant genes have been cloned, and mutations have been identified for most common genetic disorders, including neurofibromatosis, Marfan syndrome, familial hypercholesterolemia, osteogenesis imperfecta, myotonic dystrophy, achondroplasia, familial polyposis of the colon, Huntington disease, adult polycystic kidney disease, cystic fibrosis, and globin

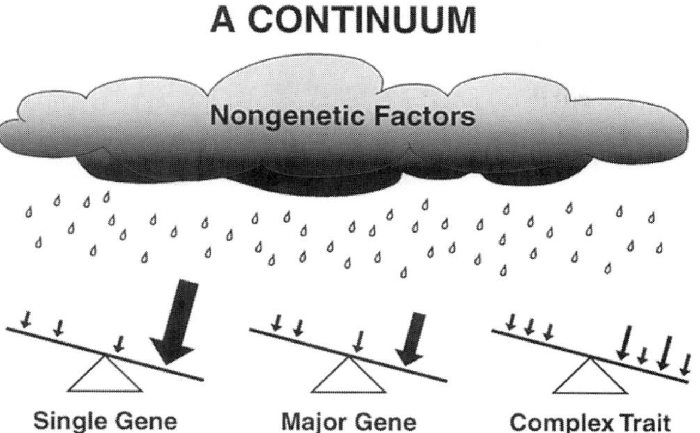

Fig. 1-1 A continuum of genetic complexity. As described in the text, this continuum can be considered among disorders ranging from single gene, to major gene, to complex trait, and can also be considered in the context of individual subjects within a single phenotype such as Hirschsprung disease, hypertension, or coronary atherosclerosis. The arrows in the lower portion of the figure depict the relative effects of the germline alleles at different loci (in proportion to size of the arrow) in causing the phenotype or disease susceptibility. The raindrops depict the contributions of factors other than germline genotype such as environmental differences (diet, smoking, drug exposure), stochastic factors (random X inactivation or immunoglobulin rearrangements), and somatic mutation.

disorders. All are discussed in detail in various chapters of this text. At the time of the preparation of this edition, familial Mediterranean fever,[19,20] Tangier disease,[21–23] and Rett syndrome[24] were relatively recent additions to the cohort of disorders whose mutant genes are known. For these "single-gene disorders," genotypic analysis can confirm the diagnosis, determine the status of relatives at risk, sometimes predict severity, provide the option of presymptomatic diagnosis, and provide the basis for genetic counseling. An excellent example of the benefits of genotypic analysis is multiple endocrine neoplasia type 2 (Chap. 42) where mutation analysis can eliminate the need for burdensome, expensive, and imprecise endocrine screening for large numbers of family members not carrying the mutation and makes possible improved preventive and therapeutic strategies for individuals found to have the mutant gene. Similar benefits attributable to precise diagnosis are now available for many genetic disorders. Single-gene mutations also can influence pharmacogenetic susceptibilities where administration of a drug may result in catastrophic side effects among a subgroup of patients with a susceptible genotype. Examples include glucose-6-phosphate dehydrogenase deficiency (Chap. 179), suxamethonium sensitivity, malignant hyperthermia, 5-fluorouracil sensitivity, 6-mercaptopurine sensitivity, and others (see Chap. 9).

Genomic Medicine for Complex Disease Traits

In complex disease traits, multiple genes and nongenetic factors interact to contribute to the presence or absence of a disease phenotype. Complexity can arise under two distinct circumstances. The first circumstance is when multiple loci, sometimes quantitative trait loci (QTL), and nongenetic factors contribute to the crossing of a threshold, giving rise to a phenotype or disease susceptibility in a single individual. Multifactorial diseases and quantitative trait loci are discussed at length in Chap. 6, which focuses on type I or insulin-dependent diabetes mellitus, one of the best-documented examples of complexity with multiple loci contributing to the phenotype in a single individual. In this form of diabetes, familial clustering is thought to involve as many as 10 genes, including the HLA region and the insulin gene (see also Chap. 69). No one gene appears to contribute the major effect for type I diabetes. In the second circumstance, complexity may be present because mutations at different loci can give rise to single-gene disorders with the same or similar phenotypes, but a single gene has the major effect in any one individual. The first category is complexity due to the interactive effects of quantitative trait loci and the second category is complexity due to locus heterogeneity. There are more numerous well-documented examples of locus heterogeneity, where a single gene has a predominant effect in any one individual or family. Examples of locus heterogeneity include maturity onset diabetes of youth (MODY), where the causative gene may be the glucokinase gene or any of three hepatocyte nuclear-transcription factors mapped to other chromosomes (Chap. 67); hereditary breast cancer, which can be due to mutations in the *BRCA1* gene on chromosome 17 or the *BRCA2* gene on chromosome 13 (Chaps. 47 and 51); and colon cancer, which can be caused by mutations in the gene for hereditary polyposis of the colon on chromosome 5, or to mutations in other genes that cause hereditary nonpolyposis colon cancer (Chaps. 32 and 48). Coronary artery disease (and perhaps most other common adult disorders) may involve both quantitative trait loci and single-gene cases with locus heterogeneity resulting in a continuum of complexity that is very difficult to unravel. Some individuals may have early onset coronary artery disease primarily due to mutations at a single locus, as for familial hypercholesterolemia or apolipoprotein E abnormalities, while disease in most individuals is thought to be due to interactions of nongenetic factors (e.g., smoking and diet) with variations in multiple genes including apolipoprotein (a); apolipoprotein B; other apolipoproteins; lipoprotein receptors; lipoprotein lipase; the intracellular cholesterol transporter mutated in Tangier disease and familial HDL deficiency; low angiotensin converting enzyme; genes affecting homocysteine levels; genes affecting the clotting system; leukocyte and endothelial cell adhesion genes; and many others (see multiple chapters in Part 12). Even when a single gene has a predominant effect as in heterozygous familial hypercholesterolemia, other genes have secondary or modifier effects. That there may be both major and minor effects in an individual disorder blurs the boundary between the concepts of complex disease traits and genetic heterogeneity. Figure 1-1 attempts to depict the interactions between various loci in the germ line genotype and other factors (nongenetic and somatic mutation) as they might occur for phenotypes determined predominantly by a single gene, a major gene, or multiple loci.

Hypertension is a complex trait in which the relative contribution of multiple loci in a single individual versus locus heterogeneity is less clear. Hypertension with a major or single gene effect is well documented as a exemplified by the β or γ subunit of the renal amiloride-sensitive sodium channel, the enzyme 11β-hydroxy steroid dehydrogenase, dysregulated fusion genes (aldosterone synthase/11β-hydroxylase) leading to aldosterone synthesis under the control of ACTH, the renal thiazide-sensitive Na-Cl cotransporter, or many other loci (Chap. 211). These disorders demonstrate dominant effects in some cases and recessive in others, considerable variation in findings even within a single family, and the need for different therapeutic intervention based on the specific defect. The extensive discoveries in the genetic basis of hypertension are shrinking the concept of "essential hypertension" and illustrate the potential for the practice of genomic medicine.

The extent to which the strategies of genomic medicine may be applied to complex disease traits, as they can for single gene disorders such as phenylketonuria or hemochromatosis, will depend on our ability to unravel complex etiology and understand its differences in patients of apparently similar phenotype. The challenge is certainly a daunting one.

Discrimination, Ethical Concerns, and Excessive Costs

There are widespread fears that discrimination in employment, health care, and insurance underwriting will be based on the results of genetic testing. Such concerns are analogous to those related to other medical information including hypertension, hypercholesterolemia, family history of a specific genetic disorder such as Huntington disease, or strong family history of breast cancer or coronary artery disease. It is imperative that individuals not be discriminated against based on genotype, and it is a challenge for society and for the medical profession to procure the benefits of genomic medicine and to prevent discrimination. Societal, governmental, and legal steps should be taken as needed to prohibit such discrimination (particularly based on genotype or predisposition) in the case of employment and health care. Many societies guarantee universal access to health care, and it is likely that genetic testing will increase the impetus in the United States for universal access to health care at standardized costs. The issues involved in discrimination are complex, are not unique to genetics, and will continue to be debated. Anonymous genetic testing has been suggested as one option if individuals wish to obtain predictive information and minimize the risk of breech of confidentiality (e.g., anonymous testing for Huntington disease or cancer susceptibility). Anonymous testing creates difficulties in assuring that individuals with burdensome results will be provided with proper interpretation, supportive counseling, and medical care, but there are some parallels to the experience with anonymous HIV testing. In future generations, children increasingly will be born to parents who already know their genotype as relevant to specific risks, and the focus may eventually be on parental genotypic information rather than population based screening.

There is increasing concern that excessive royalties tied to patents on gene discoveries and testing methods will limit the practice of genomic medicine, particularly at a population-based level.[25,26] Unfortunately, these costs could delay the benefits of genomic medicine by a generation if not controlled.

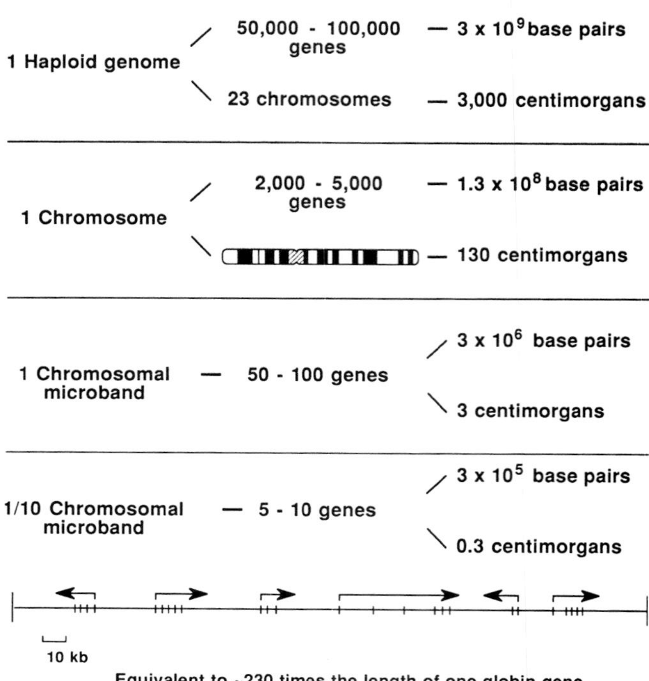

Fig. 1-2 Perspectives on the amount of DNA, number of genes, and genetic distance in the human genome. The arrows in the lowest panel indicate hypothetical transcripts, with vertical lines indicating exons within genes.

MOLECULAR BASIS OF GENE EXPRESSION

The human genome is estimated to contain 50,000 to 100,000 genes, with one recent estimate of 140,000 (www.Incyte.com),[27] each of which is composed of a linear polymer of DNA. The genes are assembled into lengthy linear strands that, together with the proteins of chromatin, form the *chromosomes*. All normal nucleated human cells other than sperm or ova contain 46 chromosomes, arrayed in 23 pairs, 1 of each pair derived from each of the individual's parents. The discovery that genes are not contiguous sequences of DNA but, instead, consist of coding sequences (exons) interrupted by intervening sequences (introns), led to a more complex view of gene expression.

Some approximations regarding the magnitude and organization of the human genome are presented in Fig. 1-2. The estimated 50,000 to 140,000 genes are encoded within the 3 billion base pairs (bp) of DNA that comprise a haploid genome. DNA length is ordinarily quantitated in kilobase (kb) units of 1000 bp or megabase (Mb) units of 1 million bp. Linkage studies indicate that the human genome is comprised of approximately 3000 centimorgans in recombination distance. A centimorgan (1/100 of a Morgan) is a measure of genetic distance that reflects the probability of a crossover between two loci during meiosis. One centimorgan approximates a 1 percent chance of a crossover during meiosis. Thus, an average chromosome contains 2000 to 7000 genes within 130 million base pairs of DNA and is equivalent to about 130 centimorgans of genetic material. A typical microband on a chromosome (stained at the 800-band level of resolution) should contain 3 to 5 million base pairs and 60 to 140 genes. This formulation oversimplifies many issues. Estimates of the total number of genes are imprecise, and although the average recombination distance is approximately 1 centimorgan per million base pairs of DNA, there is wide variation in this rate over shorter distances, and differences in recombination distance with sex. Genes range in size from small (1.5 kb for a globin gene) to large (approximately 2000 kb for the Duchenne muscular dystrophy locus). *Cis*-acting regulatory elements (i.e., on the contiguous DNA strand) may be a considerable distance from the coding region, for example, 50 kb 5′ and 20 kb 3′ to the β-globin gene, thus extending the functional domains of genes and complicating the definition of boundaries. The human genome also contains numerous highly reiterated sequences of unknown function.

If one were to print *one copy* of *one strand* of the haploid human genome, it would fill a text 250 times the size of one of the three volumes of the seventh edition of this text. The analogy of the human genome to a large text can be carried further. The text can be envisioned as being bound into 23 separate volumes of various sizes, each the equivalent of one chromosome. Individuals would inherit one paternal set of 23 volumes and one maternal set of 23 volumes. The mutation that causes sickle cell anemia would be the equivalent of changing a single letter on one page of one volume from each of the sets, while deletion of the α-globin gene cluster in α-thalassemia would be equivalent to the loss of one or two pages of text in each set. This text can also be envisioned as having been copied over and over again for thousands of generations with multiple errors or alterations (mutations) being introduced and passed to the progeny copies (see discussion and reference for single nucleotide polymorphisms or SNPs under "Genetic Diversity in Humans" below). Finally, to carry this analogy to the concept of crossing-over and linkage, each volume of each set can exchange parts with its corresponding partner at 1 to 6 sites per volume, so that a unique 23-volume text comprised of mixed portions of the 2 available sets is passed to the next generation. This results in the unique genotype that is the basis of our genetic individuality.

The Molecular Flow of Information

Much is known about how living organisms store, transmit, and utilize genetic information. Two excellent textbooks[28,29] provide a more systematic and comprehensive treatment of cellular and molecular biology; two texts, *Discovering Molecular Genetics* by Miller[30] and *Genes VII* by Lewin,[31] provide a detailed view of molecular genetics.

The genetic information carried on chromosomes is transmitted to daughter cells under two different sets of circumstances. *Mitosis* occurs each time a somatic cell (i.e., a nongerm cell) divides and functions to transmit two identical copies of each gene to each daughter cell, thus maintaining a uniform genetic composition in all cells of a single organism. The other set of circumstances, *meiosis*, prevails when genetic information is to be transmitted from one individual to an offspring. In meiosis, the 46 chromosomes of an immature germ cell arrange themselves in 23 pairs at the center of the nucleus, each pair being composed of one chromosome derived from the mother and its homologous chromosome derived from the father. During the meiotic process, the two partner chromosomes separate, only one of each pair going into each gamete. Thus, meiosis reduces the number of chromosomes from 46 to 23, with each gamete receiving 1 chromosome from each of the 23 pairs. The assortment of each pair of chromosomes is random, so that each gamete receives a different combination of maternal and paternal chromosomes. Fusion at fertilization of ovum and sperm cell, each of which has 23 chromosomes, produces an individual with 46 chromosomes.

The independent assortment of chromosomes into gametes during meiosis produces an enormous diversity among the possible genotypes of the progeny. For each 23 pairs of chromosomes, there are 2^{23} different combinations of chromosomes that could occur in a gamete, and the likelihood that one set of parents will produce two offspring with the identical complement of chromosomes is 1 in 2^{23} or 1 in 8.4 million (except in the case of monozygotic twins). Adding even further to the enormous genetic diversity in humans is the phenomenon of *genetic recombination* resulting in meiotic crossing over (see "The Genetic Map and the Principle of Genetic Linkage" below).

The Structure of DNA

Most organisms store their genetic information in *deoxyribonucleic acid* (DNA). DNA is a linear polymer of four different monomeric units, collectively called *deoxyribonucleotides*, or simply *nucleotides*, that are linked together in a chain by phosphodiester bonds. A typical DNA molecule consists of two interwoven polynucleotide chains, each containing many thousand to several million base pairs. Each nucleotide in one chain is specifically linked by hydrogen bonds to a nucleotide in the other chain. Only two nucleotide pairings are found in DNA: deoxyadenosine monophosphate with thymidine monophosphate (A-T pairs) and deoxyguanosine monophosphate with deoxycytidine monophosphate (G-C pairs). Thus, the sequence of nucleotides of one chain fixes the sequence of the other, and the two chains are therefore said to be *complementary* to each other.

The sequence of the four nucleotides along a polynucleotide chain varies among the DNAs of unrelated organisms and, indeed, is the molecular basis of their genetic diversity. Because most genetic characteristics are stably transmitted from parent to progeny, the sequence of nucleotides in DNA must be faithfully copied or replicated as the organism reproduces itself. This occurs by unwinding of the two chains and polymerization of two daughter chains along the separated parental strands. The nucleotide sequence and the genetic information are conserved during this process because each nucleotide in the daughter chains is paired specifically with its complement in the parental or template chains before polymerization occurs.

The actual replication process is mechanically complex but conceptually simple. The two strands of DNA separate, and each is copied by a series of enzymes that inserts a complementary base opposite each base on the original strand of DNA. Thus, two identical double helices are generated from one. Extensive reviews of the biochemical mechanisms of DNA replication are available.[32]

The Genetic Code

The sequence of bases in a gene ultimately dictates the sequence of amino acids in a specific protein (Fig. 1-3). This colinearity

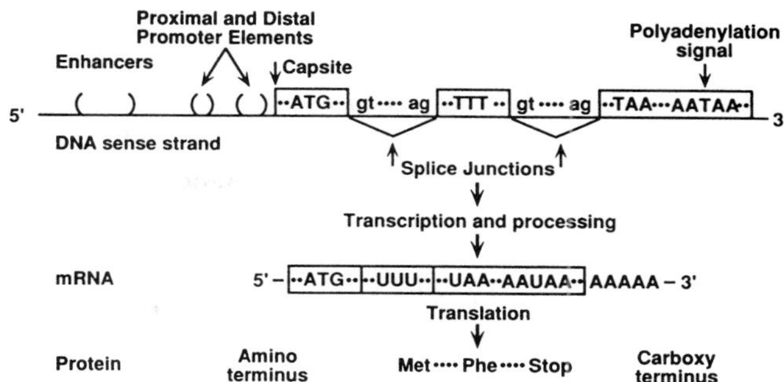

Fig. 1-3 Prototypical eukaryotic gene. In schematic form, a cellular gene is depicted in which exons or coding regions (boxes) are separated by intervening sequences (introns). Introns begin with the dinucleotide GT and end with AG. A short motif of AATAA (or modified versions) direct endonucleolytic cleavage and polyadenylation of nascent RNAs. Promoter elements, shown as empty parentheses, lie upstream from the start of the gene and are often multiple in nature. Common promoter elements include motifs such as TATA and CCAAT (TATA and CAT boxes) and GGCGGG (the Spl nuclear factor binding site). Additional sequences, known as enhancers, augment transcription and can lie either before, within, or downstream from the gene. After transcription, the RNA is processed to yield mature mRNA, which is translated to yield protein.

between the DNA molecule and the protein sequence is achieved by means of the *genetic code*. The four types of bases in DNA are arranged in groups of three, each triplet forming a code word, or *codon*, that ultimately signifies a single amino acid. Triplet codons exist for each of the 20 amino acids that occur in proteins (Fig. 1-4); there are slight differences in the genetic code in mitochondria (see Chaps. 104 and 105). Because 64 different triplets can be generated from the 4 bases and only 20 amino acids exist, the genetic code is said to be *degenerate*. That is, most amino acids are specified by more than one codon, each of which is completely specific. Thus, the double-stranded sequence adenine-adenine-adenine (or AAA) in the antisense (complementary to messenger RNA, mRNA) strand, and thymine-thymine-thymine (or TTT) in the sense (same sequence as mRNA) strand of DNA code for uridine-uridine-uridine (or UUU) in mRNA, which is translated to phenylalanine in protein.

$$\text{DNA} \rightarrow \text{RNA} \rightarrow \text{Protein}$$

To translate its genetic information into a protein, a segment of DNA is first transcribed into mRNA. The mRNA contains a sequence of purine and pyrimidine bases that is complementary to the bases of the antisense strand of the DNA. By this mechanism, each adenine of DNA becomes a uridine of RNA, each cytosine of DNA becomes a guanine of RNA, each thymine of DNA becomes an adenine of RNA, and each guanine of DNA becomes a cytosine of RNA. Thus, each DNA triplet codon is translated into a corresponding RNA triplet codon.

The messenger RNA for each gene is processed extensively within the cell nucleus including splicing to remove intronic sequences. It then crosses the nuclear membrane and enters the cytoplasm, where it serves as a template for the synthesis of a specific protein. To translate the messenger RNA code into a protein, the messenger RNA binds to a complex structure called a ribosome, which is composed of a different type of RNA (ribosomal RNA or rRNA) and a large number of proteins. To be inserted in its proper place in the protein sequence, each of the 20 amino acids is attached in the cytoplasm to an additional type of RNA (transfer RNA or tRNA). Each transfer RNA contains an anticodon loop, which includes a sequence of three bases that is complementary to a specific codon in the corresponding mRNA. For example, phenylalanine is attached to a tRNA whose anticodon loop contains the sequence AAA, which is complementary to the mRNA codon UUU, which codes for phenylalanine.

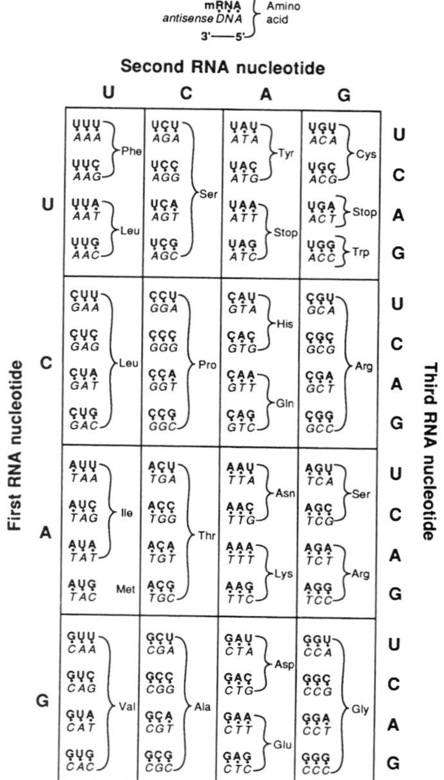

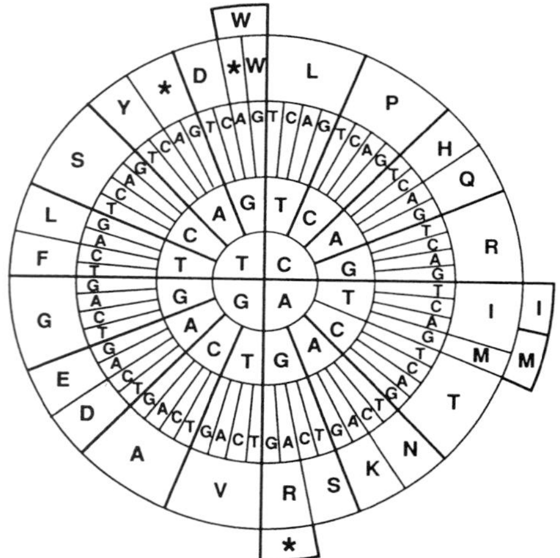

Fig. 1-4 The eukaryotic nuclear genetic code. *A*, The RNA codons appear in boldface type; the complementary DNA codons are in italics. A = adenine; C = cytosine; G = guanine; T = thymine; U = uridine (replaces thymine in RNA). In RNA, adenine is complementary to thymine of DNA; uridine is complementary to adenine of DNA; cytosine is complementary to guanine and vice versa. "Stop" = peptide chain termination. The three-letter and single-letter abbreviations for the amino acids are as follows: Ala (A) = alanine; Arg (R) = arginine; Asn (N) = asparagine; Asp (D) = aspartic acid; Cys (C) = cysteine; Gln (Q) = glutamine; Glu (E) = glutamic acid; Gly (G) = glycine; His (H) = histidine; Ile (I) = isoleucine; Leu (L) = leucine; Lys (K) = lysine; Met (M) = methionine; Phe (F) = phenylalanine; Pro (P) = proline; Ser (S) = serine; Thr (T) = threonine; Trp (W) = tryptophan; Tyr (Y) = tyrosine; Val (V) = valine. *B*, The outermost complete circle represents the amino acid in single letter code or a stop codon (*); the DNA sense strand for the triplet codon for each amino acid is given on the radial, starting with the first base of the codon in the center. Differences in the mitochondrial genetic code are shown in the outermost boxes.

Under the influence of cytoplasmic factors (initiation factors, elongation factors, and termination factors), peptide bonds are formed between the various amino acids that are aligned along the mRNA. Eventually, a terminator codon is reached, and the completed polypeptide is released from the ribosome. Because the primary sequence of bases in the coding regions of the DNA determines the sequence of amino acids in the protein, the gene and its protein are said to be *collinear*. This means that any alteration of the sequence of bases in the gene causes an alteration of the protein at a specific point in its sequence.

Control of Gene Expression

The control of gene expression at a transcriptional level is complex. The *cis*-acting regulatory DNA sequences are part of the same duplex DNA molecule as the coding sequence and *trans*-acting factors (usually proteins) are encoded by other genes. The *trans*-acting factors interact with the *cis* sequences to control the process of transcription. Many *cis*-acting transcriptional control elements are short distances upstream from the initiation site for transcription, but some occur at great distances upstream and downstream from the initiation site for transcription, for example, 5 to 50 kb. Extensive reviews of transcriptional gene regulation and transcription factors are available.[33–36] Regulation of gene expression also occurs at a posttranscriptional level, including regulation of export of mRNA from nucleus to cytoplasm, alternative splicing of transcripts, polyadenylation of transcripts, translation of mRNA, and stabilization of mRNA.

MUTATION AS THE ORIGIN OF NORMAL VARIATION AND GENETIC DISEASE

Mutation was traditionally defined as a stable, heritable change in DNA, a definition that does not depend on the functional significance of the change. This definition implies a change in primary nucleotide sequence, with other changes, such as those involving methylation, usually being referred to as epigenetic events. Mutations in somatic cells may be relevant to cancer or aging and otherwise may be of less phenotypic significance. Mutations in germ cells have their impact on offspring of an individual. The concept that mutations are stable changes remains generally true, but the discovery of expanding triplet repeat mutations emphasizes that some mutations can be unstable either in somatic or in germ cells. Some mutations are genetically lethal and cannot be passed from one generation to the next, while others are less deleterious and are tolerated in the descendants. From the viewpoint of evolution, mutations provide sufficient genetic diversity to permit species to adapt to environmental changes through the mechanism of natural selection.

Mutations are quite diverse (Table 1-1) and can involve gross alterations (millions of base pairs) in the structure of a chromosome; these include duplications, deletions, and translocations of a portion of one chromosome to another (see Chap. 13). Mutations can even involve the entire genome (3 billion base pairs) as in triploidy, where there is a third copy of the whole chromosome constitution. On the other hand, mutations can be minute, involving deletion, insertion, or replacement of a single base. Single base or very small mutations are called *point mutations*. If deletions or insertions of one or two bases occur in a coding region, they give rise to *frameshift mutations* because they alter the reading frame of the triplet genetic code in the mRNA so that every codon distal to the mutation in the same gene is read in the wrong frame. Frameshift mutations alter the protein sequence and usually result in premature termination of the peptide chain because of the occurrence of a termination codon in the altered reading frame. Small deletions or insertions can also affect transcription, splicing, or RNA processing depending on their location.

When one base is replaced by another in the coding region, the resulting point mutation may be of three types: (a) a *synonymous* or *silent mutation* (comprising about 23 percent of random base

Table 1-1 Common Mechanisms of Mutation

Type	Usual Effect	Examples	Chapter
Large Mutation			
Deletions	Null*	Duchenne dystrophy	216
		Contiguous gene	65
Insertions	Null	Hemophilia A/LINE repeat	172
Duplications	Null, gene disrupted	Duchenne dystrophy	216
	Dosage, gene intact	Charcot-Marie-Tooth	227
Inversions	Null	Hemophilia A	172
Expanding triplet	Null	Fragile X	64
	?Gain of function	Huntington	223
Point Mutation			
Silent (in or out of coding)	None	Cystic fibrosis	201
Missense or in-frame deletion	Null, hypomorphic, altered function, benign	Globin	181
Nonsense	Null	Cystic fibrosis	201
Frameshift	Null	Cystic fibrosis	201
Splicing (ag/gt)†	Null	Globin	181
Splicing (outside ag/gt)†	Hypomorphic	Globin	181
Regulatory (TATA, other)	Hypomorphic	Globin	181
Regulatory (poly A site)	Hypomorphic	Globin	181

*"Null" indicates no functional gene product.
†"ag/gt" indicates mutations in the almost absolutely canonical first two and last two base pairs of each intron, while "outside ag/gt" indicates splicing mutations in less canonical sequences of introns or exons.

substitutions in coding regions) in which the base replacement does not lead to a change in the amino acid, but only to the substitution of a different codon for the same amino acid (e.g., a replacement of a single base pair in the DNA so that a RNA codon for phenylalanine is transcribed into RNA as UUC, not as UUU, which still codes for phenylalanine); (b) a *missense mutation* (about 73 percent of base substitutions in coding regions) in which the base replacement changes the codon for one amino acid to another (e.g., the replacement of a base pair in DNA in the codon for phenylalanine such that it is transcribed into RNA as UUA, not as UUU, which would change the codon to leucine); and (c) a *nonsense mutation* (about 4 percent of base substitutions in coding regions) in which the base replacement changes the codon to one of the termination codons (e.g., the replacement of a base pair in the codon for tyrosine such that it is transcribed into RNA as the stop codon UAA, not as UAU). Occasionally, a base substitution in the coding region alters RNA splicing either by creating a cryptic splice site or by interfering with function of a normal splice site. For missense mutations, the single-letter amino acid code is often used to indicate substitutions, such that R560T indicates replacement of arginine (R) at position 560 in the protein by threonine (T). Additional guidelines for mutation nomenclature are available.[37,38]

Larger deletions may affect a portion of a gene, an entire gene, or a set of contiguous genes. Contiguous gene syndromes are discussed in Chap. 65. Such deletion mutations may interrupt or remove the coding region of a gene, causing the absence of its protein product. Alternatively, a deletion can bridge between the coding regions of two genes and produce a fusion resulting in the production of a hybrid protein containing the initial sequence of one protein followed by the terminal sequence of another protein. This latter type of mutation may occur particularly by unequal crossing over between tandemly repeated homologous genes such as the globin genes. The range of mutations seen at the human β-globin locus provides a good perspective on the heterogeneity of possible mutations. More than 200 missense mutations cause amino acid substitutions in the β-globin locus, and various $\delta\beta$ and $\beta\delta$ fusions can occur. Numerous transcriptional, splicing, and RNA processing mutations cause β-thalassemia as depicted in Fig. 1-5.[39] The reciprocal products of deletions caused by unequal crossover are duplications, and such duplications are the most common form of mutation causing type IA Charcot-Marie-Tooth disease; the mutations are related to the presence of low-copy repeat sequences at the borders of duplication. The reciprocal deletion of the Charcot-Marie Tooth duplication causes the phenotype of hereditary neuropathy with liability to pressure palsies (see Chap. 227). Insertions in genomic DNA also occur by retrotransposition as exemplified by the appearance of a repeat sequence in the factor VIII gene as a cause of hemophilia A. Inversion affecting the factor VIII gene related to the presence of a repeat sequence is a common cause of severe hemophilia A.

Expanding triplet repeat mutations are known to cause fragile X mental retardation, myotonic dystrophy, spinobulbar muscular atrophy, Huntington disease, multiple types of spinocerebellar ataxia, and other disorders. These triplet repeat sequences can occur in the 5′ untranslated, coding, intronic, or 3′ untranslated regions. Longer repeat sequences are generally associated with a more severe and/or earlier onset phenotype, and repeat sequences slightly longer than normal may function as premutations in asymptomatic individuals. The premutant and mutant expanded triplet repeats are unstable and may become more unstable when transmitted from females, as in the case of fragile X syndrome and myotonic dystrophy, or when transmitted from males, as in Huntington disease and spinocerebellar ataxia type 1. For many of the neurodegenerative disorders (Huntington disease, spinobulbar muscular atrophy, spinocerebellar ataxia type 1, and others), the expanded triplet repeat encodes a polyglutamine tract in the protein, but the mechanism by which this repeat causes neurodegeneration is not known. Expanding triplet repeat mutations are one mechanism underlying the phenomenon of anticipation, in which the phenotype of a disease may worsen over successive generations within a family.

The type and frequency of human mutations are complex topics (see Chap. 13). Mutations that cause chromosomal aneuploidy

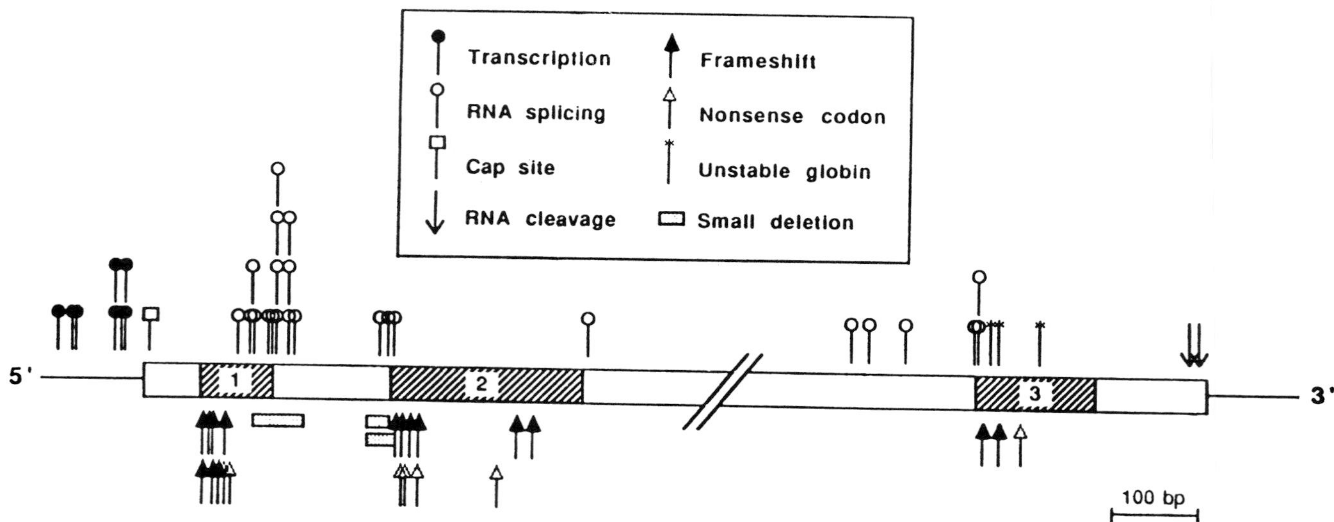

Fig. 1-5 Point mutations in β-thalassemia. The β-globin gene is shown with numbered hatched areas representing the coding regions of exons. Boxed open areas between the exons are introns, and boxed open areas at the 5′ and 3′ ends of the gene are untranslated regions that appear in the messenger RNA. The various types of mutations are depicted by different symbols. (*From Kazazian and Boehm.*[39] *Used by permission.*)

occur at increasing frequency with advancing age of the mother. Some classes of mutations occur with increased frequency with advancing age of the father. Some loci, such as those for Duchenne muscular dystrophy and achondroplasia, are subject to high rates of new mutation. In Duchenne dystrophy, this may be related in part to the unusually large size of the gene. The structure of a gene, its position within the genome, and the constraints on the gene product may contribute to the frequency of new mutations. The occurrence of 5-methylcytosine at the sites of CpG base pairs provides sites of increased mutational frequency due to spontaneous deamination of 5-methylcytosine to yield a thymine base. This propensity leads to increased frequency of polymorphisms at CpG sites in the genome and accounts for certain mutational hot spots; in achondroplasia one specific C to T base change is remarkably frequent (see Chap. 210), but similar alterations also occurs for hemophilia A and B, and many, if not most, other disorders. The availability of recombinant DNA techniques makes possible the definition of the exact nature of mutations, determination of whether they arose from a maternal or paternal gamete, and analysis of whether the mutation is of recent or ancient origin. Mutations that are widespread in the population but that are descended from a single event, can be recognized by the occurrence of specific haplotypes of DNA polymorphisms surrounding the mutations, as is well-studied for thalassemia, phenylketonuria, and cystic fibrosis. A haplotype is a group of genetic markers linked together on a single chromosome, such as a group of close DNA polymorphisms or a group of human leukocyte antigen (HLA) alleles.

When mutations occur in germ cells, the altered expression of the mutant gene does not affect the phenotype of the individual in whom the mutation occurs, but is manifest in subsequent generations. Usually such *new mutations* are sporadic events in human populations, but a mutation that occurs in somatic cells at an early developmental stage may affect the individual harboring the mutation, and may or may not be passed to subsequent generations. The individual harboring such a somatic cell mutation is said to be a *mosaic* because two populations of cells are present: normal cells and cells harboring the mutant gene. Mutations occurring in an early germ line cell can give rise to gonadal mosaicism so that numerous mutant gametes may be descended from a single event. Gonadal mosaicism is documented in osteogenesis imperfecta and in Duchenne muscular dystrophy, and presumably occurs at some frequency for the majority of single-gene disorders. The reason for the more frequent occurrence of gonadal mosaicism for osteogenesis imperfecta (Chap. 205) compared to its rarity for disorders such as achondroplasia (Chap. 210) is unknown, but mutations arising at meiosis (e.g., unequal crossing over) or later in life should not show gonadal mosaicism. Mutations directly associated with advanced paternal age (e.g., achondroplasia) are *unlikely* to involve gonadal mosaicism.

In the clinical context, human mutations fall into two general categories. Some mutations are relatively ancient, and the same mutation is found in thousands or millions of individuals, as in the case of sickle cell anemia, the Z allele for α_1-antitrypsin deficiency, and the common mutation for cystic fibrosis. These ancient mutations either tend to be recessive, or dominant with little effect on reproductive fitness, so that the mutant allele persists in the population in heterozygous recessive form or is a sufficiently benign dominant allele to permit reproduction. The presence of the same mutant allele in large numbers of individuals has implications for strategies in DNA diagnosis and screening (see "Analysis of Mutations" below). If genetic predisposition to common adult disorders were associated with ancient mutations (e.g., hemochromatosis, Chap. 127), population screening with molecular methods would be feasible. Other human mutations are either recent or new to the first case diagnosed in a family. This circumstance is most common for autosomal dominant mutations with reduced reproductive fitness and for X-linked mutations that impair or prevent reproduction in males. These mutations tend to be heterogeneous with a different mutation in each family studied with only rare recurrence of identical mutations. This scenario is typical for disorders such as Duchenne muscular dystrophy, neurofibromatosis, retinoblastoma, and many other disorders that have an effect on reproductive fitness. New mutations are discussed further below (see "Dominant New Mutations" and "X-Linked New Mutations").

GENETIC DIVERSITY IN HUMANS: GARROD'S CHEMICAL INDIVIDUALITY AND THE CONCEPT OF POLYMORPHISM

At the start of the twentieth century, Garrod[40] recognized that the aberrant metabolism seen in a condition such as alkaptonuria might imply far more extensive chemical individuality. Garrod's concept of chemical individuality has found its explanation with the realization that the gene for a given protein frequently exists in different forms in different normal individuals and with the recognition that even more extensive variation exists in the DNA sequence of genomes among individuals. The widespread nature of genetic diversity was first apparent when it became possible to study enzymes by electrophoresis of cell extracts and thereby to detect structurally variant forms of enzymes without the necessity of purification. With the use of this technique, it was demonstrated that many proteins exist in two or more forms in the population. These multiple forms are due to the existence in the population of multiple variations of a gene (called *alleles*) at the same genetic locus coding for the same protein. For most loci, each individual possesses two alleles, one derived from each parent. If the two alleles are identical, the individual is said to be *homozygous*; if they differ, the individual is *heterozygous*. The various alleles have been derived from a single precursor allele by mutations during the evolution of the species; in general, they differ from each other only in the substitution of one base for another (missense mutations). In most cases, the proteins produced by both alleles at a given locus are equally functional; that is, the amino acid difference is "neutral" or nearly so from the standpoint of natural selection.

At the level of protein sequence, many genetic loci (such as that for the β chain of hemoglobin) have a standard sequence/allele that accounts for the majority of alleles in the population, whereas the other alleles are rare. At other genetic loci, no single allele occurs with sufficient frequency to be designated as standard or normal. Variation in the α chain of haptoglobin and in apolipoprotein (a) represent examples of such extreme genetic polymorphism. A polymorphic locus (or nucleotide site) is one at which the most common allele has a frequency < 0.99. Note that this definition is concerned only with the frequency of variants at a locus and not with the functional consequences of the variant, and thus polymorphisms may be benign or disease causing. It is a common error in genetic jargon to equate polymorphism with a benign effect.

The recognition of polymorphism has been extended by the discovery of extraordinary variation at the DNA sequence level. One in 100 to 1 in 200 base pairs in the human genome is polymorphic; this is consistent with heterozygosity at 1 in 250 to 1 in 500 base pairs. It is possible to detect single-base DNA polymorphisms that represent synonymous differences or amino acid polymorphisms in coding regions, and DNA polymorphisms occur with even greater frequency outside of coding regions in parts of the genome that have little or no effect on gene expression. DNA polymorphisms include, in addition to single-base differences, insertions, deletions, and variation in numbers of tandemly repeated sequences. The latter are termed variable number tandem repeats (VNTR) if the repeats are long, or short tandem repeats (STR) if the repeats are very short, for example, tetra-, tri-, di-, or mononucleotide repeats. The gene for lipoprotein lipase (Chap. 117) was studied extensively by sequencing a 9.7 kb region.[41,42] Sequencing of this region from 71 individuals, or 142 chromosomes, identified 88 variable sites, or 1/500 bp. This included 79 single nucleotide polymorphisms (SNPs), of which 4 changed amino acids in the coding sequence. Nine insertion/deletion variants were identified. Extensive data such as this are potentially extremely valuable, but there is a great challenge to decipher the biologic and medical significance, or lack thereof, for each variation.

With the recognition of the extent of DNA polymorphism (millions of nucleotide differences between two random haploid genomes), it is clear that the DNA of each individual contains millions of differences compared to the DNA of another individual except in the case of identical twins. These DNA differences can be divided into four broad categories: (a) those with no phenotypic effect (e.g., DNA polymorphisms used for identity testing); (b) those causing phenotypic differences without affecting disease susceptibility (e.g., differences in height, hair color, etc.); (c) those making minor or modest contributions to disease processes (e.g., as for complex diseases involving quantitative trait loci); and (d) those having a major role in causing a disease phenotype (e.g., as for single gene disorders). There is great interest in trying to use SNPs to unravel the genetic contribution to complex traits.[43] These polymorphisms might themselves contribute to disease susceptibility or be in linkage disequilibrium with disease-related variations.

METHODS FOR ANALYSIS OF HUMAN DNA

Molecular analyses of clinical relevance rely on multiple features and strategies, including: (a) the ability to clone genes and DNA fragments using recombinant methods; (b) determination of the sequence of DNA fragments; (c) the specificity of nucleic acid hybridization; (d) the specificity of recognition sites of restriction endonucleases; (e) the power of DNA amplification using the polymerase chain reaction; and (f) the ability to transcribe and translate DNA in vitro for analysis of the protein product. Various combinations of these approaches are used for diagnostic procedures, and some methods use mRNA rather than DNA as the starting material.

MOLECULAR CLONING AND SEQUENCING

The size, complexity, and variability of the human genome constitute barriers to the analysis of individual traits and genes. The feasibility for such analysis was greatly enhanced by the development of recombinant DNA technology, which allows for isolation of small DNA fragments and production of unlimited amounts of the cloned material. Hundreds of human genes have been cloned, including the genes for cystic fibrosis, Marfan syndrome, polyposis of the colon, neurofibromatosis, myotonic dystrophy, fragile X mental retardation, Huntington disease, breast cancer (BRCA1), hereditary nonpolyposis colon cancer, and many other disorders. Once cloned, the various genes and gene products can be utilized for studies of gene structure and function in normal and disease states with diagnostic, therapeutic, counseling, and research implications.

The cloning of DNA involves isolation of DNA fragments and their insertion into the nucleic acid from another biologic source (vector) for manipulation and propagation. These vectors can accommodate DNA fragments of tens to hundreds of kb in size. Various methods for DNA cloning are described in greater detail elsewhere.[44–48]

Most genes are divided into coding exons and intervening introns in the genomic DNA. The mRNA from a gene is spliced to link the coding segments, and mRNA can be copied in vitro to synthesize cDNA (DNA complementary to mRNA) for analysis and cloning. Genomic DNA and cDNA clones have been isolated for hundreds of human genes, and for thousands of gene fragments and *anonymous* sequences. The anonymous genomic DNA regions represent unique sites in the genome and often are associated with polymorphic markers that map to that site. Complete cDNA clones, or even fragments thereof, can be deduced to encode protein sequences that may be homologous to known proteins. Radioactive, biotinylated, or otherwise modified copies of DNA can be prepared from any cloned or amplifiable fragment, and can serve as a specific molecular *probe*. Radioactive probes can be detected by autoradiography, whereas biotinylated probes can be detected using avidin and secondary nonradioactive detection methods. Some of the fruits of molecular cloning are the availability of probes for analytical procedures, the availability of DNA sequence data both to deduce protein sequence and to allow for DNA amplification (see "Polymerase Chain Reaction" below), and the ability to analyze for disease mutations.

Nucleic Acid Hybridization

Many of the steps in recombinant DNA analysis take advantage of the complementary nature of nucleic acid interaction that is so essential for the synthesis of DNA and RNA. Linear pieces of

*Hae*III	5′ – G – G ❘ C – C – 3′ 3′ – C – C ↓ G – G – 5′	*Hind*III	5′ – A ❘ A – G – C – T – T – 3′ 3′ – T – T – C – G – A ↓ A – 5′	*Mst*II	5′ – C – C ❘ T – N – A – G – G – 3′ 3′ – G – G – A – N – T ↓ C – C – 5′

Fig. 1-6 DNA sequence specificity and nuclease activity for three restriction endonucleases. *Hae*III leaves a blunt end while the other enzymes leave single-stranded ends.

double-stranded (native) DNA can be treated with heat or alkali to dissociate the two strands to yield single-stranded (denatured) DNA. The denatured DNA can be incubated under conditions that allow for nucleic acid hybridization; that is, the recognition of two complementary strands and reformation of double-stranded molecules by base pairing. Nucleic acid hybridization is so sensitive that a single-stranded DNA molecule can be hybridized specifically to a complementary strand of RNA or DNA and detected if present at about 1 part in 10,000. It is possible to identify and distinguish fully homologous sequences and partially homologous sequences. The specificity of nucleic acid hybridization, often in combination with fractionation or amplification procedures, allows detection of a single gene among tens of thousands, or of nucleic acid from an infectious organism, which may be present at a frequency of less than one copy per human cell. The majority of hybridization probes have been prepared in radioactive form, but the use of nonradioactive detection methods is increasing.

A particularly useful variation of nucleic acid hybridization involves the use of allele-specific oligonucleotides (ASO). The ASO probe is a synthetic, single-stranded oligonucleotide that is usually 15 to 20 bases in length. Two probes are synthesized usually differing at the mutation site by a single base, one perfectly matching the normal sequence and one perfectly matching the mutant sequence, with the variable nucleotide in the midportion of the oligonucleotide. Hybridization conditions are adjusted so that the oligonucleotide detects a perfectly matched sequence but fails to hybridize if there is a single base mismatch. Allele-specific oligonucleotides are widely used to analyze amplified DNA.

Restriction Endonucleases

The discovery in microorganisms of restriction endonucleases, commonly known as restriction enzymes, facilitated recombinant DNA manipulations. Each enzyme recognizes a specific short sequence in double-stranded DNA, typically 4 to 8 base pairs, and cleaves the DNA at this site. Hundreds of enzymes are known, each recognizing a unique DNA sequence (Fig. 1-6). For example, one enzyme (*Hae*III) that recognizes sequences only 4 base pairs in length cleaves the sequence 5′-GGCC-3′. The sequence specificity of restriction enzymes is a powerful tool in dissection of large genomes. When human DNA is digested with a particular restriction enzyme, hundreds of thousands of DNA fragments are reproducibly generated, varying from a few base pairs to several thousand base pairs in length depending on the enzyme used. Restriction enzymes that recognize a sequence only 4 base pairs long cleave the DNA into smaller fragments than enzymes that recognize longer sequences because shorter recognition sites occur more often. With the use of multiple restriction enzymes, it is possible to define a detailed map of restriction endonuclease cleavage sites for a particular segment of DNA. Such a map can span a region of several hundred to tens of thousands of base pairs of DNA. Enzymes that cut the DNA infrequently can be used to prepare DNA maps over megabase distances. As described below, variations in the sequences of cleavage sites may reveal polymorphisms or mutations in the human genome.

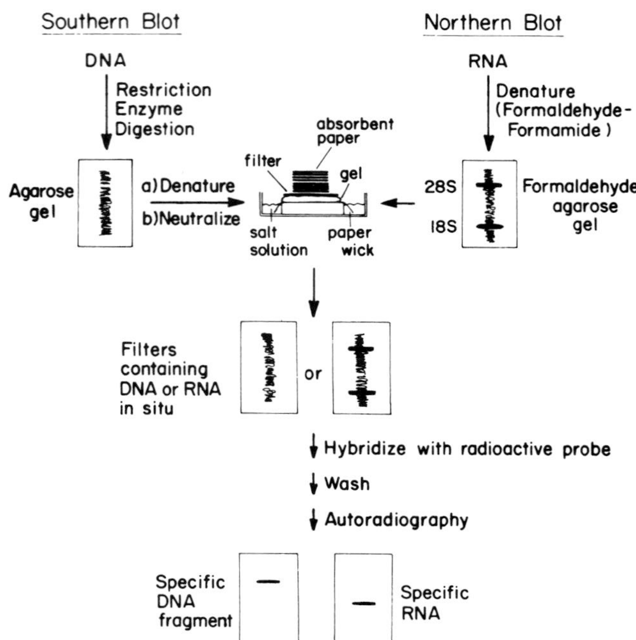

Fig. 1-7 Procedures for Southern and northern blot analysis.

Southern Blotting

Many analyses of the human genome utilize the blotting procedure developed by E. M. Southern, which involves hybridizing DNA in solution to DNA fixed on a membrane support. For clinical analysis, *Southern blotting* (Fig. 1-7) begins with the isolation of genomic DNA from sources such as peripheral leukocytes or fetal cells. The sensitivity of Southern blotting is achieved by splitting the DNA into small segments, fractionating the fragments by electrophoresis on agarose gels, and applying a sensitive detection method to identify specific fragments (nucleic acid hybridization). Overall, this method can detect unique genomic DNA fragments that typically represent about 1 part in 1 million in the genome. The clinical power of Southern blotting resides in the capacity to analyze a specific small portion of the primary structure of human genomic DNA from an individual. The procedure is useful for detecting gross rearrangements in DNA and some point mutations, but most point mutations are not detected by routine Southern blotting.

An analogous procedure starting with RNA for analysis has been termed *northern* (in contrast to Southern) *blotting*. In this procedure, the presence or absence and approximate size of a particular mRNA can be determined. The term *immunoblotting* or *western blotting* describes a procedure designed to analyze protein antigens. Proteins are separated by electrophoresis and transferred to a solid membrane through a blotting procedure. The membrane is analyzed by incubation with antibodies followed by a second step for enzymatic or radioactive detection of bound antibody. Thus, Southern blotting, northern blotting, and immunoblotting or western blotting each combines a fractionation and a detection method to provide a sensitive technique for the analysis of DNA, RNA, and protein, respectively.

Polymerase Chain Reaction (PCR)

The technique of PCR for DNA amplification has had a revolutionary impact on molecular diagnosis. The technique is based on knowing the nucleic acid sequence for a region which, for a diagnostic application, is to be analyzed repeatedly from different individuals. Oligonucleotide primers are prepared that are complementary to opposite strands of the DNA and are separated by up to a few hundred base pairs (Fig. 1-8). The oligonucleotide primers are incubated with the target DNA to be

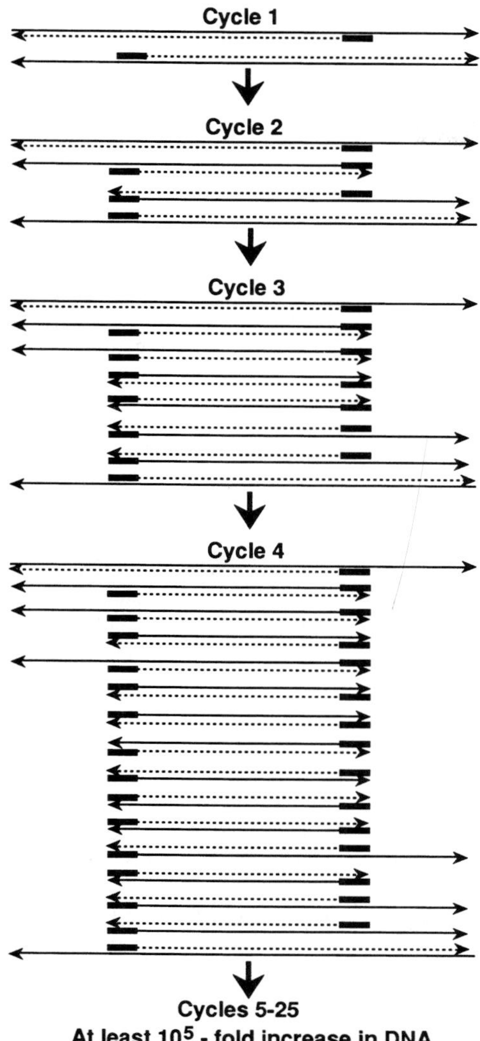

Fig. 1-8 Polymerase chain reaction for amplification of DNA. The target DNA is shown as a solid line in cycle 1. Newly synthesized DNA is indicated by dotted lines in each cycle. Primer oligonucleotides are indicated by solid rectangles. Each DNA strand is marked with an arrow indicating 5′ to 3′ orientation.

amplified and with a DNA polymerase that synthesizes a complementary strand in a 5′-to-3′ direction. Considerable specificity is provided by the requirement that primers must lead to convergent synthesis for amplification to be effective. The reaction is subjected to a series of temperature variations, including a denaturing temperature where double-stranded DNA is dissociated to single-stranded DNA, an annealing temperature where oligonucleotide primers hybridize to target DNA, and a polymerization temperature for the synthetic step. The reaction is usually carried out using a thermostable polymerase so that the polymerase remains active during the temperature cycles (usually ranging from 50°C to 95°C). After a number of such cycles, typically 20 to 30 or more, hundreds of thousands of copies of the original target sequence are synthesized as depicted in Fig. 1-8. The bulk of the product is a double-stranded DNA fragment of specific length. The technique is so sensitive that it can be used to amplify and analyze DNA from a single human sperm that contains one duplex target DNA molecule. PCR is easily performed with minimal preparation of crude and even degraded samples allowing analysis from whole blood, dried blood filters, mouthwash, old tissue sections, and other sources. PCR can be performed starting with genomic DNA as the template; alternatively, RNA can be reverse transcribed to yield cDNA for use as a template, a procedure known as reverse transcription-PCR (RT-PCR). Molecular diagnosis with PCR can include: (a) determining the presence or the absence of an amplified product; (b) digesting the amplified product with a restriction enzyme; (c) hybridizing the PCR product with allele-specific oligonucleotides; (d) direct sequencing of the PCR product; (e) analyzing the ratio of RNA from two alleles using RT-PCR; and (f) analysis for expression in vitro to search for truncation mutations. Variations and modifications include synthesis of single-stranded DNA by altering the ratio of the oligonucleotide primers, preparation of recombinant DNA constructs, mutagenesis of cloned DNA, detection of rare nucleotide sequences, and detection of nucleotide sequences of infectious agents. The PCR method offers extremely rapid analysis (single day), ease of automation, relative economy, and extraordinary specificity.

Protein Truncation Tests

The protein truncation test (PTT) can be used to detect any mutation that results in premature termination of the peptide during protein synthesis; these are primarily nonsense, frameshift, and some splicing mutations (Fig. 1-9). In protein truncation testing, the amplified genomic DNA encoding an exon or amplified cDNA is transcribed and translated in vitro, and the protein products are analyzed using gel electrophoresis to detect truncated proteins. Protein truncation testing has been used mostly to detect heterozygous mutations in autosomal dominant disorders, but the method is generally applicable and is particularly suited for detection of loss of function mutations.

Analysis of Mutations

The challenge of detecting unknown mutations is different than diagnostic testing for the presence of known mutations. Large mutations are more easily detected, using Southern blotting or PCR to detect expansions of triplet repeats, deletions, insertions, and other rearrangements. RT-PCR is useful to detect absence or major reduction in mRNA from a mutant allele; common polymorphisms are used to identify heterozygosity within an exon of genomic DNA followed by analysis of the ratio of mRNA from the two alleles. Using this strategy detects any mutation that profoundly reduces the level of mRNA. More discriminating methods are required for detection of point mutations. Well-characterized methods for detection of unknown mutations include ribonuclease cleavage, denaturing gradient-gel electrophoresis (DGGE), carbodiimide modification, chemical cleavage of mismatches, single-strand conformation polymorphism (SSCP) analysis, heteroduplex analysis, and sequencing of DNA, as reviewed elsewhere.[49] These methods involve chemical or enzymatic recognition of mismatches in nucleic acid duplexes, electrophoretic separation of single- or double-stranded DNA, or sequencing. DNA sequencing can be performed directly on PCR products or on individual clones or pools of clones. The sensitivity for detection of mutations varies from 80 to virtually 100 percent, and analysis can be performed on genomic DNA or mRNA (cDNA) depending on specific circumstances. A newer method of denaturing, high-performance liquid chromatography (DHPLC),[50] is reported to consistently detect 100 percent of nucleotide changes[51,52] and is supplanting many other methods. Fig. 1-10 is an example of using DHPLC to detect a single nucleotide substitution causing Angelman syndrome.[53] This method combines the advantages of a denaturing gradient with the fractionation of HPLC. Protein truncation tests detect a subset of mutations, primarily nonsense and frameshift mutations. In the case of ancient mutations that are widely distributed in the population, diagnostic methods focus on the presence or absence of particular mutations. These methods include allele-specific oligonucleotide (ASO) hybridization, allele-specific amplification, ligase amplification or assay, primer extension sequencing, and restriction enzyme analysis (including artificial introduction of restriction sites). These methods all

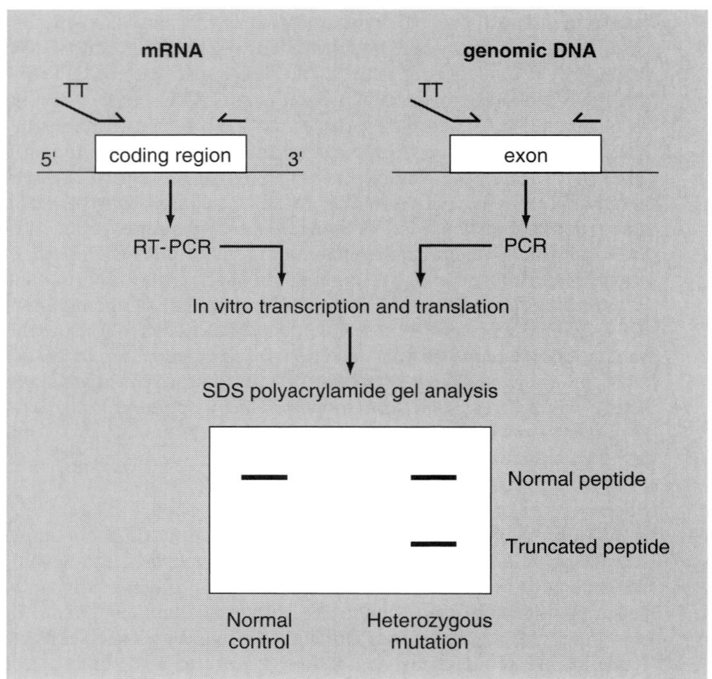

Fig. 1-9 Protein truncation testing. PCR is performed starting with genomic DNA or RT-PCR is performed using mRNA. Sequences for transcription and translation (TT) are introduced at the 5′-end of the coding segments. Mutations leading to truncation of a protein are detected by gel analysis.

depend on a hybridization or enzymatic reaction to distinguish nucleic acid sequences differing by as little as a single base.

DNA Chips

The term DNA chip refers to methods based on the preparation of large arrays of oligonucleotides on miniaturized solid supports for analysis of DNA sequence (Fig. 1-11). In one strategy, a very large number of oligonucleotides (e.g., all possible 65,536 octamer nucleotides or each sequential decanucleotide to analyze the known sequence of a gene; see Southern[54] for details) can be arrayed on a small surface using adaptations of photolithographic methods. The use of DNA chips offers the promise of enormously expanded opportunity for comparison of sequence of disease genes among individuals and of automated and cost-effective mutation analysis. Although DNA chips have not yet achieved the status of routine diagnostic practical application, these devices may become a key component of medical diagnosis in the future.

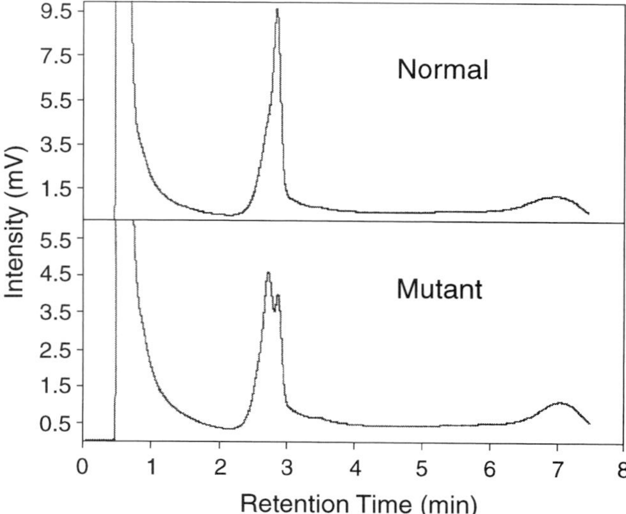

Fig. 1-10 Denaturing high performance liquid chromatography (DHPLC). Exon 9 of the E6-AP ubiquitin-protein ligase gene was amplified as described elsewhere,[53] and DHPLC detects an abnormal pattern of a 2997 T→A mutation causing Angelman syndrome. The analysis was performed using the WAVE equipment of Transgenomic, Inc., Omaha, NE. (*Figure courtesy of Dr. Dani Bercovich.*)

ANALYZING THE HUMAN GENOME

The topographic map of our genomic DNA can be divided into regions corresponding to the chromosomal bands visually identified by standard cytogenetic analysis of the 24 chromosomes (22 autosomes and X and Y). As of September 1999, over 5700 loci were assigned to specific positions on the human genetic map according to *Online Mendelian Inheritance in Man* (electronic address: www3.ncbi.nlm.nih.gov/omin/). Two kinds of maps describing the relative order and distance of genetic markers and their position within a defined region have been developed: the genetic and the physical maps. The genetic map is an indirect statistical analysis based on genetic recombination, whereas the physical map hinges on direct measurement of the length of DNA.

The Genetic Map and the Principle of Genetic Linkage

Genetic linkage is essential for preparation of the map of the human genome and is used routinely for molecular diagnosis. Genetic distance, which is expressed in centimorgans (cM), is a measure of the likelihood of crossover between two loci. Two loci are 1 cM apart if there is a 1 percent probability of a crossover between them at meiosis. There are on average 30 to 35 crossovers during meiosis in males and perhaps twice as many during meiosis in females.

The feasibility of human linkage analysis was revolutionized by the demonstration of genetic variation in the size of fragments generated by digestion of normal human DNA with restriction endonucleases. These restriction fragment length polymorphisms (RFLPs) are the consequence of the DNA sequence polymorphisms and are inherited according to Mendelian principles (Fig. 1-12). Restriction enzyme digestion and Southern blotting make it possible to use these polymorphisms as genetic markers for sites within the genome. If one of the base pairs in the recognition sequence for a restriction enzyme differs between individual

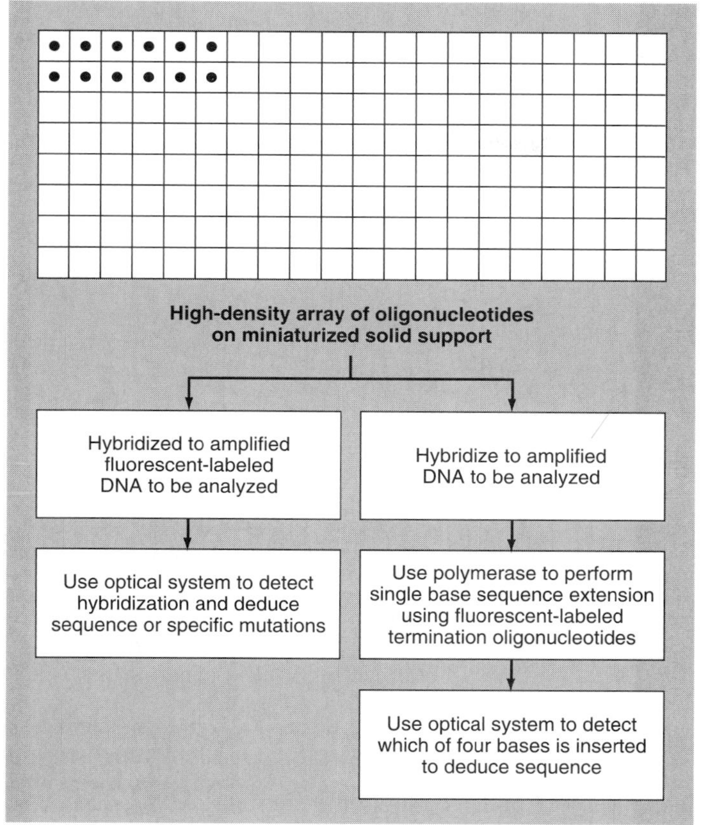

Fig. 1-11 Use of DNA chips for molecular analysis. Large numbers of unique oligonucleotides are arrayed on a solid support and analyzed as indicated. See Southern[54] for detailed discussion.

copies of the genome, or if there is a length variation in the DNA, there will be variation in the size of DNA fragments generated by the restriction enzyme digestion.

A particularly informative subset of RFLPs is the result of VNTR. These are sites of length variation in which a DNA sequence is variably and tandemly repeated on different chromosomes, so that many different sizes of DNA fragments can be regarded as different alleles at a VNTR site. The repeat unit in VNTRs can be tens or hundreds of bases in length with variation arising through unequal crossing-over. In the case of the gene for the apolipoprotein (a), a VNTR repeat unit includes two exons and gives rise to polymorphism in both the length of the gene and the protein. STRs are repeats of tetra-, tri-, di-, and mononucleotides in the genome in which variation has arisen through "slippage" of the DNA polymerase at replication to increase or decrease the number of repeat units on a chromosome. STRs are highly polymorphic, easily analyzed, and widely distributed in the genome (Fig. 1-13). An essential feature of linkage analysis, whether for construction of the human gene map or for clinical diagnosis, is that DNA markers have different alleles at the marker locus of interest, so that the two chromosomes of the individual can be distinguished.

Genetic linkage can be assessed between any pair (or more) of markers, one of which may represent a mutation that causes a disease phenotype. For autosomal genes, each new individual inherits one copy of each chromosome from each parent. Panel A of Fig. 1-14 depicts one pair of chromosomes ready to enter meiosis with one normal copy of a gene (open rectangle) and one defective copy of the same gene (hatched rectangle). Four DNA markers, typically dinucleotide repeat polymorphisms, with A/B, F/G, K/L, and R/S alleles are depicted at 0, 1, 10, and >50 cM from the disease gene. After meiosis and three crossover events, gametes are formed containing one chromosome with various segments of the original chromosomes. Alleles A and F are at

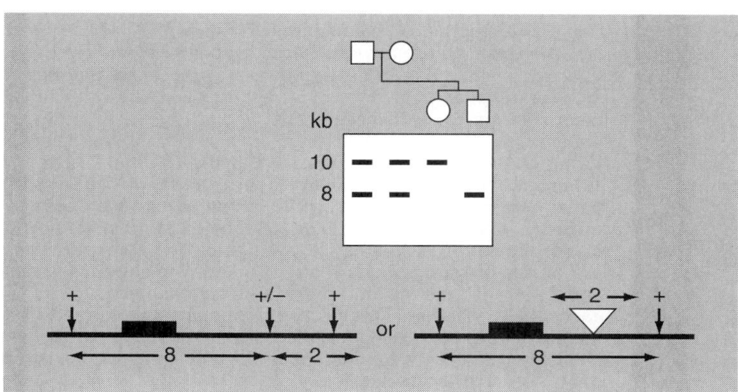

Fig. 1-12 Example of restriction fragment length polymorphism (RFLP) in human DNA using Southern blotting. The solid blocks indicate segments of DNA used as probe. Parents are heterozygous and children are homozygous for the RFLP. Symbols above the arrows indicate cutting (+) or noncutting (−) by the restriction endonuclease. The "2" above the open triangle depicts a 2-kb insertion/deletion polymorphism. Numbers indicate DNA length in kilobases.

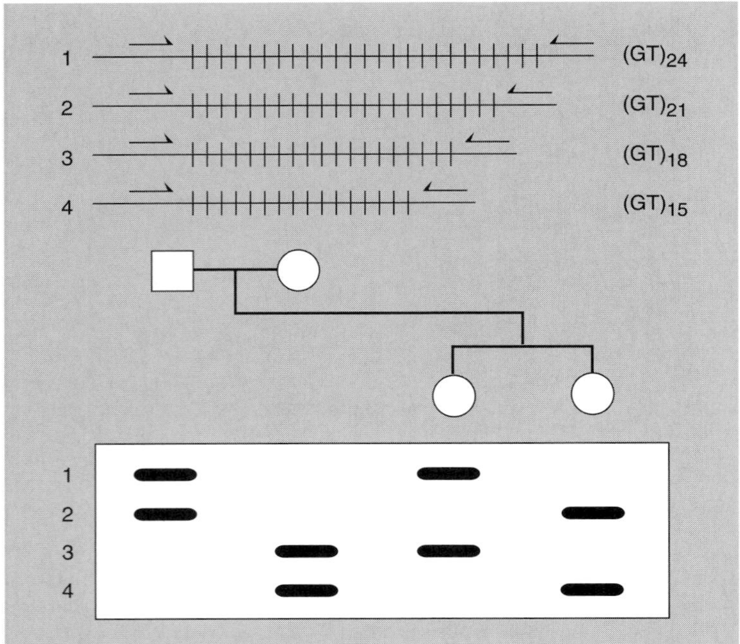

Fig. 1-13 Depiction of a short tandem repeat (STR) polymorphism for a dinucleotide $(GT)_n$ repeat. Each repeat is separated by a vertical line. Sites for two primers for PCR are indicated by arrows. Four alleles of 24, 21, 18, and 15 GT repeats are indicated. Inheritance of the alleles in a family as detected by PCR is shown below.

DNA markers within (A) or close to (F) the gene of interest and remain on the chromosome with the normal copy of the gene. DNA markers further away have a greater probability of undergoing crossover, and the L allele of one DNA marker is now on the chromosome with the normal copy of the gene, although it was previously on the chromosome with the defective copy of the gene. The greater the distance between markers and genes, the greater the probability of crossovers. Alleles for a gene and markers on different chromosomes are inherited in a completely independent fashion.

Panel B of Fig. 1-14 depicts the analysis of DNA markers in a family with an autosomal dominant disorder such as Huntington disease. Data are shown for the K/L DNA marker that is 10 cM from the disease gene, and for a Y/Z DNA marker on a different

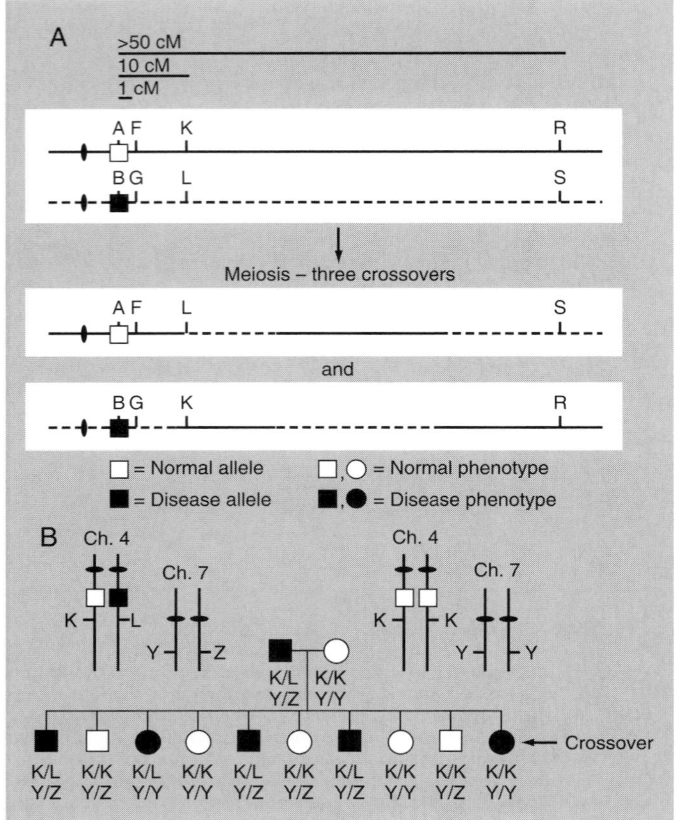

Fig. 1-14 Depiction of meiotic crossing over and linkage analysis. The upper panel shows two copies of one chromosome (one in solid line and one in dashed line) from an individual before (above) and after (below) meiotic crossing over. The individual is heterozygous for a disease locus with a normal allele (open square) and a disease allele (filled square) and is heterozygous for four DNA markers with alleles A/B, F/G, K/L, and R/S at 0, 1, 10, and >50 cM from the disease locus, respectively. The lower panel depicts analysis in a family for an autosomal dominant disorder. The DNA marker with K/L alleles at 10 cM from the disease locus on chromosome 4 and another DNA marker with Y/Z alleles on chromosome 7 are depicted. The chromosomes 4 and 7 for each parent are shown and the genotypes given for each family member. The disease phenotype is inherited from the father with the L allele for the DNA marker except for the last child who represents a crossover of the type shown in the upper panel. See text for discussion.

chromosome. A researcher trying to map a disease gene is likely to study many DNA markers, like the Y/Z marker, that show no correlation between which allele of the critical gene is inherited and whether the disease phenotype is inherited. Eventually a marker is discovered, such as K/L, that is close to the disease gene. Analysis of additional families can provide conclusive statistical evidence that a polymorphic DNA marker is near a disease gene and makes possible immediate application of the marker for diagnosis within a family such as that shown in Fig. 1-14 (see "Diagnosis by Linkage Analysis" below) and opens the way for positional cloning of the disease gene (see "Cloning and Identifying Human Disease Genes" below). The frequency of crossovers as shown for the last offspring in Fig. 1-14 is a measure of the genetic distance between the DNA marker and the disease gene. Once a linked DNA marker is found, closer DNA markers can be identified rapidly.

The Physical Map

The physical map is based on direct DNA analysis and is not influenced by regional differences in recombination frequency. A physical map facilitates both the isolation of abundant DNA markers and the identification and cloning of the genes in a region.

Major strategies for physical mapping of the human genome include *in situ* hybridization, deletion mapping, long range restriction mapping, and isolation of yeast artificial chromosome (YAC) or other large insert clones. With *in situ* hybridization, the direct hybridization of a DNA marker to a chromosome allows the assignment of the marker to a specific chromosomal band. With the advent of fluorescent *in situ* hybridization (FISH), it is now possible to use different colored probes for simultaneous mapping of more than one DNA marker. Hybridization to interphase nuclei allows determination of the order of markers within a particular chromosomal region. This technique is also very effective for the identification of chromosomal abnormalities (see Chap. 65).

Deletion mapping is based on the presence or absence of a particular region or locus in the DNA from patients with chromosomal abnormalities or from human/rodent somatic cell hybrids that contain defined segments of the human chromosomes. Deletion mapping was particularly useful for mapping of the X chromosome because deletions of the X chromosome frequently result in a disease phenotype in males and because the nullisomic regions can be defined without having to separate the abnormal chromosome in somatic cell hybrids. Deletion mapping is also useful in establishing relative orders of sets of markers in the genome, although it does not provide precise information as to the distance involved.

Long-range restriction mapping provides information about physical distance. In this technique, high-molecular-weight DNA is cut into large fragments (from 100 kb up to 4 Mb), using restriction enzymes that cut very rarely in the genome, and these fragment are separated by pulsed-field gel electrophoresis (PFGE) and hybridized to several DNA markers using Southern blotting procedures. If, for example, two DNA probes hybridize to the same 200-kb restriction fragment, it can be concluded that the maximum distance between the two loci is 200 kb.

Another strategy in physical mapping uses yeast artificial chromosome (YAC) clones, which carry large fragments of genomic DNA (from 50 kb to 1 or 2 Mb in length). These YAC vectors contain yeast telomeres and centromeres, and the clones are actually propagated as separate chromosomes in a yeast host.

The Human Genome Project

A "first draft" of the sequence of the human genome is expected to be completed before this book appears, and this will revolutionize our level of knowledge regarding human genes and disease. The human genome project, described in greater detail in Chap. 10, is an international effort, started in the mid-1980s, aimed at the complete characterization of human genomic DNA. Specific goals include: (a) development of detailed physical and genetic maps; (b) cloning of the entire genome in overlapping large insert vectors; (c) identification and characterization of all genes; (d) sequencing of all the haploid human genome; and (e) biologic interpretation of the information encrypted in the nucleotide sequence. This project will almost certainly enhance knowledge both in basic biology and in medicine. In the latter field, an important goal is the identification of genes involved in genetic predisposition to cancer and to complex diseases such as hypertension and atherosclerosis.

As of September 1999, a detailed map of the human genome was available with the analysis of many thousand highly informative, short tandem repeat polymorphisms. Sequencing has been performed for thousands of fragments of cDNA (expressed sequence tags, ESTs), and this sequence information makes it possible to perform computerized searches of DNA and to deduce protein sequences. Numerous electronic databases are available to access the information accumulating from the human genome project. The pace of the human genome project quickened in 1999 with the formation of a commercial venture that challenged both the strategy and the rate of human genomic sequencing[55] such that a "draft sequence" of the human genome is expected to be available about the time of publication of this text, with more refined versions following quickly. The complete genomic sequence for a human chromosome was reported for chromosome 22 in late 1999.[56]

Cloning and Identifying Human Disease Genes

There are four general strategies for cloning human disease genes: (a) starting with knowledge and availability of the protein; (b) using the ability to select for function of the gene; (c) determining the precise genetic location (positional cloning); and (d) some combination of biologic information regarding the phenotype and the genetic map location of the disease compared to the genetic map location of relevant genes (a positional candidate gene approach). Increasingly, a combination of minimal linkage data for chromosomal localization of the disease phenotype and extensive searching of databases to identify candidate genes (cloning *in silico*) leads to rapid identification of disease genes. This approach promises to become predominant with the availability of the sequence of the entire genome. Many of the early gene cloning successes relied on purification of a protein, determination of partial amino acid sequence, preparation of antibodies, and development of enzymatic or other assays. Using this information, cDNA clones were isolated using approaches such as mRNA purification, hybridization screening with oligonucleotides based on available amino acid sequence, PCR amplification based on similar oligonucleotides, immunologic screening of expression cDNA libraries, and other related approaches. Currently, expressed DNA sequences can often be found in databases if minimal amino acid sequence is available. In some instances, genes have been cloned based on a functional property without knowing the protein or the genetic map location. For example, various genes involved in DNA repair disorders have been isolated using selection in tissue culture to identify clones that correct the cellular phenotype of defective DNA repair.

Positional cloning is the isolation of a disease gene based on its location in the genome with no knowledge of its function. This strategy depends on the analysis of DNA samples from affected families to find a DNA marker that is located close to the disease locus as discussed above and illustrated in the lower panel of Fig. 1-14. Having localized the disease gene in a general way, it is possible to isolate the DNA of the relevant region in overlapping clones, identify genes in the region, and eventually prove which is the disease gene, often by identifying small mutations within one of the genes (Fig. 1-15). This strategy is facilitated if chromosomal translocations are available to assist in mapping and identifying the disease gene. This approach yielded landmark successes as in the identification of the genes for Duchenne muscular dystrophy, cystic fibrosis, retinoblastoma, polyposis of the colon, neurofibromatosis, Huntington disease, and breast cancer (BRCA1 and BRCA2).

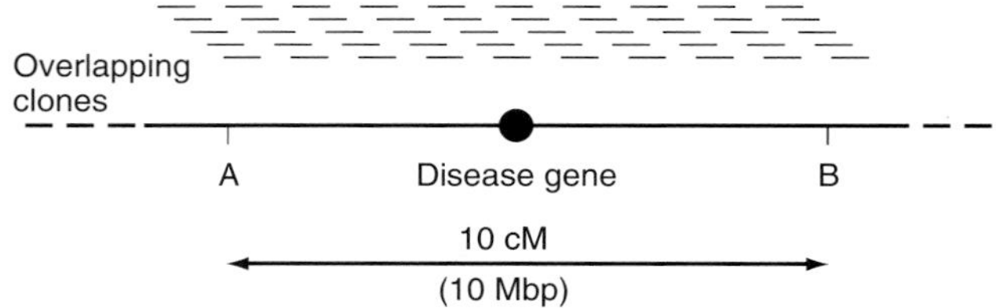

Fig. 1-15 A positional cloning strategy. DNA markers at sites A and B are found to flank a disease gene. Overlapping DNA clones are isolated for the region, and the disease gene is identified within the region.

As more genes are described, the positional candidate gene approach has become very productive for identifying disease genes. A pure candidate gene strategy occasionally involves guessing the disease gene from among known proteins based on the disease phenotype, but more often, the candidate gene approach requires an approximate genetic mapping, but much less specific than would be adequate for a strictly positional cloning effort. Based on the limited mapping information, on knowledge about relevant genes mapping to the same region, and perhaps taking into account information from other species such as the mouse, one can formulate and test the hypothesis that a particular gene is mutated in a specific disease by amplification and/or cloning of the gene in question from affected patients to search for mutations. Such an approach led to the identification of mutations in the cardiac myosin heavy chain genes that cause familial hypertrophic cardiomyopathy, in the fibrillin gene in Marfan syndrome, in the *RET* proto-oncogene in multiple endocrine neoplasia type 2, and in various mismatch DNA repair genes in hereditary nonpolyposis colon cancer. Use of information from the mouse led to the recognition that the *PAX3* gene is mutated in Waardenburg syndrome. The identification of mutations in a gene encoding a thiamine transporter as causing the syndrome of thiamine-responsive anemia with diabetes and deafness is an excellent example of the *in silico* strategy.[57] One variation on the candidate gene approach involves the production of mice with targeted mutations and identifying candidate genes based on phenotypes in the mice that resemble a human phenotype. The map locations for many of disorders are shown in Appendix I of this chapter, and many mouse homologies are tabulated in Chap. 14.

Transgenic and Mutant Mice

Gene structure and function are usually similar in mouse and human, and studies in the mouse can often be of value in understanding human disease. Chapter 14 has an extensive discussion and tabulation of mouse models. After microinjection of cloned DNA sequences into the male pronucleus of fertilized mouse eggs, the injected DNA becomes integrated into the mouse chromosomal DNA in a fraction of the injected cells, including the germ cells, so that a series of descendant animals will express the transgene. Each site of integration of foreign DNA behaves as a single Mendelian trait, and heterozygous and homozygous animals can be bred. This strategy can be used to produce mouse models of human disease in the case of dominant negative or gain-of-function alleles, as has been done for osteogenesis imperfecta and spinocerebellar ataxia type 1.

Transgenic animals are particularly useful for the evaluation of *cis*-acting regulatory DNA sequences that control tissue-specific and temporal aspects of gene expression. Putative regulatory sequences are linked to a reporter gene that encodes an easily detectable product. Using this strategy, it has been shown that short DNA sequences provide exquisite tissue specificity for genes such as insulin and elastase, and that more complex and distant regulatory sequences control the expression of globin genes. The transgenic method has also been utilized to introduce viral or cellular oncogenes in animals to induce tumors, opening up approaches for the study of tumor biology. For example, a tissue-specific regulatory sequence linked to the SV40 T antigen produces tumors in specific cell types. Another transgenic mouse strategy involves linking of regulatory sequences to a toxin that will selectively kill cells that express the sequence. As an example, linking of insulin regulatory sequences to diphtheria toxin can generate mice with selective absence of pancreatic β cells. In yet another application, larger transgenic animals can be used for production of pharmaceuticals to be harvested from milk or blood. Cloning of large animals to produce recombinant proteins is a newer variation on this theme.[58]

It is also possible to induce mutations in mice, and treatment of male animals with ethylnitrosourea is quite effective in inducing small mutations. Because integration of transgenic DNA is relatively random, such insertions can occasionally interrupt normal mouse genes. Retroviruses can also be used to infect mouse embryonic cells to produce relatively random insertional mutagenesis. Mutant phenotypes can then be ascertained in the resulting heterozygous or homozygous mice, including identification of defects that are benign in heterozygotes but are embryonic lethals in the homozygous state. Because the retrovirus inserts at the site of the affected gene, it is possible to identify many new mutations and to clone the relevant genes. A gene-trapping strategy using retroviral vectors has been effective in identifying new genes.[59]

Homologous recombination with mouse embryonic stem (ES) cells provides additional opportunities. ES cells are totipotent cells that can be manipulated in culture and then reintroduced into mouse embryos. Using homologous recombination in ES cells, it is possible to target a specific gene for subtle mutation or inactivation ("knockout"). Altered ES cells are injected into recipient blastocysts and give rise to chimeric animals composed partially of mutant cells derived from the ES cell culture. The genetically altered cells are often represented in the sperm of the resulting chimeric animals, and mutant mice can be obtained and bred to study the gene in heterozygotes and homozygotes. The technique has allowed the production of mouse models of retinoblastoma, p53 oncogene deficiency (Li-Fraumeni familial cancer syndrome), cystic fibrosis, Lesch Nyhan syndrome, Gaucher disease, apolipoprotein E deficiency, and others (see Chap. 14 for a more detailed list). In some instances, there are phenotypic differences for the same mutation in mouse and human, providing an opportunity for important biologic insights; in others, the phenotype in mice and humans is very similar, so that the animals are valuable for studies of pathogenesis and for therapeutic trials. Mutant mice of these types will be useful for unraveling the genetic factors in complex disease processes such as atherosclerosis and for analysis of neurologic functions. The ability to obtain mouse mutants for virtually any cloned gene provides an opportunity for analyzing the function of the increasing number of cloned genes whose biologic roles are not delineated. This strategy can be used to introduce point mutations[60,61] and duplications,[62] as well as null alleles. There is an increasing focus on producing conditional mutations in the mouse that would be cell type-specific or inducible by ligands after birth.[63–65]

CATEGORIES OF GENETIC DISORDERS

Genetic diseases generally fall into one of three categories: (a) *Chromosomal disorders* involve the lack, excess, or abnormal arrangement of one or more chromosomes, producing large amounts of excessive or deficient genetic material and affecting many genes. (b) *Mendelian or monogenic disorders* are determined primarily by a single mutant gene. These disorders display simple (Mendelian) inheritance patterns that can be classified into autosomal dominant, autosomal recessive, or X-linked types. (c) *Complex disease traits* are caused by an interaction of multiple genes and multiple exogenous or environmental factors. Although many of these complex traits, such as diabetes mellitus, gout, and

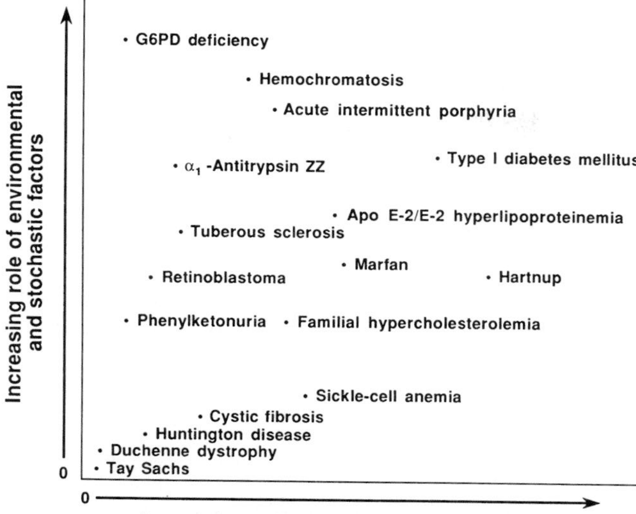

Fig. 1-16 Depiction of estimated roles of modifier genes and nongenetic factors in influencing the phenotypes for "monogenic" disorders. Extensive variation is due to allelic heterogeneity, and the intent is to indicate crude estimates of the contributions that might occur in addition to allelic variation.

cleft lip and palate, exhibit familial clustering, the inheritance pattern is complex, and the risk to relatives is less than in the single gene disorders. Each of these categories of genetic disease presents different problems with respect to pathogenesis, prevention, diagnosis, genetic counseling, and treatment. Furthermore, this classification is in fact an oversimplification. For example, small chromosomal deletions can cause contiguous gene syndromes (Chap. 65) with the simultaneous presence of multiple Mendelian or monogenic disorders as exemplified by males with cytogenetically visible deletions in the short arm of the X chromosome in association with Duchenne muscular dystrophy, chronic granulomatous disease, retinitis pigmentosa, and the McLeod phenotype.[66] Deletions of the retinoblastoma locus on chromosome 13 may be visible or submicroscopic and may extend to nearby loci such as esterase D (Chap. 36). Thus, these defects bridge the gap between chromosomal and monogenic disorders. The phenotype cased by chromosomal disorders obviously is due to the altered expression of single genes within the abnormal region. Chromosomal translocations may interrupt single genes as exemplified by some women with Duchenne muscular dystrophy due to X/autosomal translocations.

The phenotypes of many monogenic disorders are modified by the genes at other loci and by environmental factors (Fig. 1-16). Indeed, a single locus *entirely* determines the disease phenotype in relatively few monogenic disorders. Examples of effects of nongenetic factors that influence monogenic disorders include drug exposure for glucose-6-phosphate dehydrogenase deficiency and acute intermittent porphyria, iron intake and blood loss for hemochromatosis, smoking for α_1-antitrypsin deficiency, and diet for lipoprotein lipase deficiency. Similarly, genes at other loci can modify the phenotype as exemplified by the effect of the genotype at the α-globin cluster on sickle cell anemia (Chap. 181). The border between monogenic disorders and complex traits is not a sharp one, because other genes frequently modify the phenotype of monogenic disorders and major genes often play a role in complex traits (e.g., HLA genotype and type I diabetes mellitus), as discussed under "A Continuum of Genetic Disease and Susceptibility" above. Whereas monogenic disorders provide an excellent starting point for the study of human genetic disease, an even greater challenge is to understand the more common complex disease traits.

Frequency of Genetic Disease

In studies in Montreal, Baltimore, and Newcastle, 6 to 8 percent of diseases among hospitalized children were attributable to single-gene defects, and 0.4 to 2.5 percent were due to chromosomal abnormalities; another 22 to 31 percent were considered to be gene influenced.[67,68] The overall frequency of monogenic disorders is about 1 percent, and about 5.3 percent of individuals below age 25 will have a disease with an important genetic component (single gene, chromosomal, or complex trait).[68] If complex traits of late onset are included, about 60 percent of individuals have genetically influenced diseases at some time.[69,70] One study[70] evaluated survival of adoptees relative to the survival of their biologic and adoptive parents. The results indicated that premature death in adults has a strong genetic component for death from all causes, from natural causes, from infections, and from cardiovascular causes. Premature death of a biologic parent (less than age 50) resulted in a relative risk of death in the adoptees of 1.71 (95 percent confidence interval, 1.14 to 2.57). Genetic factors contribute in a significant way to an even larger fraction of diseases in a population when common infections disorders are controlled.

Chromosomal Disorders

The *karyotype* of an individual (i.e., the number and structure of the chromosomes) can be ascertained from readily accessible somatic cells, such as peripheral blood lymphocytes or skin fibroblasts, by growing them in tissue culture until active proliferation occurs, and then preparing single metaphase cells for examination by microscopy. By the 1970s, it became possible to identify each individual chromosome by special staining methods using fluorescent dyes or Giemsa staining after treatment with proteolytic enzymes (trypsin). These techniques produce characteristic *banding patterns* for each chromosome (Fig. 1-17). The number of chromosomes in normal individuals is 46, of which 44 are the 22 pairs of *autosomes* and the other 2 are the *sex chromosomes*. Females have two X chromosomes (XX), and males have one X chromosome and one Y chromosome (XY). Each of the 22 pairs of autosomes and the 2 sex chromosomes can be distinguished on the basis of size, location of the centromere (which divides the chromosome into arms of equal or unequal length), and the unique banding pattern (Fig. 1-17). More details regarding cytogenetic concepts[71] and methodology[72–74] are

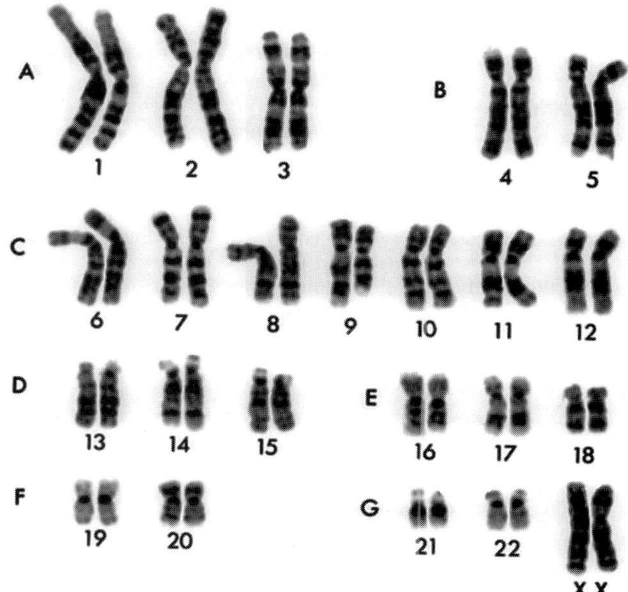

Fig. 1-17 A trypsin G-banded normal human female karyotype. (*Courtesy of David H. Ledbetter.*)

available elsewhere, and selected chromosomal disorders are discussed in Chaps. 61 to 65.

Most chromosomal disorders found in humans can be classified into one of four groups: (a) excess or loss of one or more intact chromosomes (*aneuploidy*); (b) breakage and loss of a piece of a chromosome (*deletion*); (c) breakage of two chromosomes, with transfer and fusion of parts of the broken fragments onto each other (*translocation*); and (d) abnormal splitting of the centromere during mitosis so that one arm is lost and the other is duplicated to form one symmetric chromosome with two genetically identical arms (*isochromosome formation*). In addition, chromosomal *mosaicism* may occur such that a single individual may possess two or more cell lines, or *clones*, each differing in its chromosomal constitution. For example, many patients with the Turner syndrome have been shown to possess some cells with a 45,X constitution and other cells with a normal 46,XX. Their karyotype is symbolized 45,X/46,XX.

The major *autosomal* trisomies responsible for specific clinical syndromes include: trisomy 21 (Down syndrome, Chap. 63), characterized by mental retardation, a characteristic facies, marked hypotonia, and many other abnormalities; trisomy 13, characterized by ocular defects, brain malformation, cleft lip and palate, polydactyly, and an average life span of less than 6 months; and trisomy 18, characterized by micrognathia, severe failure to thrive, multiple malformations, and an average life span similar to trisomy 13.

The common aneuploidies involving sex chromosomes (Chap. 61) include 47,XXY and 47,XYY in phenotypic males; aneuploidies in phenotypic females include 47,XXX and 45,X with or without associated mosaicism. The XXY karyotype is found in patients with the Klinefelter syndrome, who are phenotypic males with testicular dysgenesis, infertility, gynecomastia, tall stature, and behavioral changes. Most individuals with a 47,XYY karyotype are normal fertile males; however, some may be unusually tall and show tendencies to criminality or other behavior abnormalities. Most individuals with the 47,XXX karyotype are clinically normal females, except that somewhat more than half of patients have mild or moderate mental retardation, and fertility is reduced. The 45,X karyotype is found in about one-half of patients with the Turner syndrome, who are phenotypic females with ovarian dysgenesis, failure of secondary sexual development, short stature, cardiovascular malformations, renal anomalies, and webbed neck. Patients with the Turner syndrome who do not have a 45,X karyotype may have either mosaicism (45,X/46,XX or 45,X/46,XY) or a structural abnormality such as an isochromosome of the long arm of the X chromosome.

Little is known about the factors that cause chromosomal disorders in humans. The most important finding is the association between increasing maternal age and nondisjunction syndromes such as Down syndrome (trisomy 21) and the other autosomal trisomies. As discussed in Chap. 63, there is evidence that the majority of nondisjunction events causing trisomy involve errors in maternal meiosis I. There is also evidence that nondisjunction is correlated with a reduced frequency of recombination for the involved chromosomes.

Chromosomal aberrations are common. The detected frequency of chromosomal aberrations in karyotypes of unselected newborn infants is about 1 in 200 (0.5 percent); Table 1-2[71,75] lists the most frequently encountered chromosomal abnormalities occurring among liveborn infants. Among recognized first-trimester spontaneous abortions, the frequency of chromosomal defects is 50 to 60 percent. Given a 20 percent rate of spontaneous abortion in recognized conceptions, at least 10 percent of all conceptions are affected by chromosomal aberrations. The vast majority of affected fetuses do not survive the apparently intense in utero selection and are lost early in gestation. Despite this, a high frequency of chromosomal aberrations has, however, been observed in patients with several clinical abnormalities, including (a) multiple congenital malformations (2 to 20 percent); (b) infertility and sterility (1 to 10 percent); (c) mental retardation (1 to 3 percent); and (d) certain forms of malignancy, such as chronic myelogenous leukemia, in which the long arm of chromosome 22 is translocated to one of the larger chromosomes, most often to the long arm of chromosome 9, producing the so-called *Philadelphia* chromosome.

Table 1-2 Frequency of Chromosomal Disorders Among Liveborn Infants

Disorders	Frequency
Autosomal abnormalities	
Trisomy 21 (Down syndrome)	1 in 600
Trisomy 18	1 in 5,000
Trisomy 13	1 in 15,000
Sex chromosome abnormalities	
Klinefelter syndrome (47,XXY)	1 in 700 males
XYY syndrome (47,XYY)	1 in 800 males
Triple X syndrome (47,XXX)	1 in 1000 females
Turner syndrome (45,X or 45X/46XX) or 45X/46,XY or isochromosome Xq)	1 in 1500 females

SOURCE: Modified from Vogel and Motulsky[71] and Galjaard.[75]

Chromosomal aberrations occur with extremely high frequency in various malignancies. In these instances, the constitutional karyotype is usually normal, but the tumor cells show abnormal findings as mentioned above for the Philadelphia chromosome. Numerous chromosomal translocations are now known to be found with some specificity for a variety of tumors (Chaps. 19 and 20).[76] In some instances, a constitutional genetic abnormality may represent a first step in a two-step process leading to malignancy. The second step in this process occurs in a single somatic cell and may often be a gross chromosomal aberration that contributes to the development of a tumor. This is best documented for retinoblastoma (Chap. 36), but also occurs in Wilms tumor (Chap. 38), polyposis of the colon (Chaps. 32 and 48), von Hippel-Lindau disease (Chap. 41), and other disorders. The locus involved in hereditary tumors is often also involved in sporadic tumors as documented for colon tumors, retinoblastoma, renal cell carcinoma, and other tumors.

Chromosomal disorders often occur as new mutations. Both parents are usually normal, and the risk of recurrence in sibs is low, although slightly increased for common trisomies. However, when the aberration involves an unbalanced translocation, one parent is a balanced translocation carrier in about a third of the cases. In this instance, the recurrence risk for subsequent children may be as high as 20 percent, and additional members of the extended family may also be balanced translocation carriers at high risk for having an offspring with an unbalanced chromosomal complement.

One important disorder involving a fragile site on the X chromosome is often considered with chromosomal abnormalities, although it represents an expanding triplet repeat mutation at a specific locus (Chap. 64). Fragile sites are regions of chromosomes that are subject to narrowing or breakage when cells are cultured under conditions that slow or inhibit DNA replication. The fragile X mental retardation syndrome is a common important form of mental retardation associated with the occurrence of a fragile site at Xq28. The disorder shows unusual features of inheritance, now explainable at a molecular level based on the unstable mutations, with a high frequency of clinical expression in hemizygous males and a lower frequency of clinical expression in heterozygous females.

The indications for complete chromosomal analysis have expanded with the growth of information and with the improved resolution of the analysis. Chromosome analysis is clinically indicated in these situations: (a) in children with two or more major malformations including prenatal or postnatal growth failure as a major malformation; (b) in children with mental retardation of unknown cause with or without malformations; (c) in all children with features of recognized chromosomal syndromes including trisomies, deletions, and duplications; (d) in couples with a poor reproductive history (infertility, increased numbers of spontaneous abortions, or stillbirths); (e) in antecedents and offspring of individuals with chromosomal translocations; (f) in individuals with sexual malformations or abnormalities of sexual development; and (g) in patients with various malignancies (analysis of tumor cells). The quality of chromosome analysis is important, and subtle abnormalities are easily missed.

Molecular analysis using Southern blotting and/or PCR is more definitive when the specific diagnostic concern relates to fragile X mental retardation. Small deletions occur in conditions such as hereditary retinoblastoma, Prader-Willi syndrome, Angelman syndrome, Miller-Dieker syndrome, Di George/velocardiofacial syndrome, and other conditions, such that use of fluorescence *in situ* hybridization (FISH) with molecular probes from critical regions is more definitive than high-resolution cytogenetic analysis if a clinical diagnosis known to be associated with deletion of a specific region. The role of the FISH methodology in general cytogenetics and in cancer cytogenetics has grown rapidly and allows for many novel diagnostic approaches. Analysis of malignancies also requires the use of special techniques to obtain adequate analysis on tumor cells of various types (see Chaps. 19 and 20). Cytogenetic changes in tumors may assist in establishing diagnostic categories, in devising treatment protocols, and in long-term follow-up. The role of chromosome analysis in prenatal diagnosis has grown such that the number of analyses performed on prenatal samples now exceeds the number of analyses performed on postnatal samples in most Western countries. While prenatal cytogenetic analysis may be performed because of the previous occurrence of cytogenetic abnormalities or because of known familial translocations, the majority of studies are performed for advanced maternal age or abnormal values for various analytes in the so-called triple screen (maternal serum levels of α-fetoprotein, human chorionic gonadotropin, and unconjugated estriol) alone or in combination with ultrasound measurement of fetal nuchal translucency or humerus length.[77–79] There is a progressive trend towards increased utilization of cytogenetic analysis for prenatal diagnosis, which can now be carried out using amniocentesis or chorionic villus sampling as discussed below.

A number of newer techniques are being reported for microscopic analysis. Each individual chromosome can be "painted" to characterize complex rearrangements, and this can be done simultaneously, so that each chromosome is a different color.[80,81] FISH using probes for all of the telomeres promises to improve the detection of submicroscopic chromosome rearrangements in children with idiopathic mental retardation.[82–84] The technique of rolling-circle amplification can be used to detect point mutations in cytologic preparations.[85]

For a more complete discussion of the etiology and clinical features of chromosome abnormalities affecting humans, the reader is referred to the *Clinical Atlas of Human Chromosomes*[86] and the *Catalogue of Unbalanced Chromosome Aberrations in Man*.[87] A registry of *Chromosomal Variation in Man* is available online (www.wiley.com/products/subject/life/borgaonkar/). More general texts on birth defects, including cytogenetic abnormalities, are also useful.[88–90]

Monogenic Disorders

Although few phenotypes are entirely determined by a single locus, the concept of monogenic disorders is still valuable. Such disorders ordinarily exhibit one of three patterns of inheritance: (a) autosomal dominant; (b) autosomal recessive; or (c) X-linked. The overall population frequency of monogenic disorders is about 10 per 1000 live births, comprising approximately 7 in 1000 dominant, approximately 2.5 in 1000 recessive, and approximately 0.4 in 1000 X-linked conditions (excluding color blindness). Table 1-3 lists some of the more common Mendelian disorders.[75,91,92]

Table 1-3 Frequency of Some Common Monogenic Disorders

Disorder	Estimated Frequency*	Chapter
Autosomal dominant		
Familial hypercholesterolemia	1 in 500 heterozygote	120
Hereditary nonpolyposis colon cancer	1 in 200–1000	32, 48
Polyposis of the colon	1 in 15,000	48
BRCA1 and BRCA2 breast cancer	1 in 1000; 1 in 100 in Ashkenazim	47
Marfan syndrome	1 in 20,000	206
Hereditary spherocytosis	1 in 5000	183
Adult polycystic kidney disease	1 in 1250	215
Huntington chorea	1 in 2500	223
Acute intermittent prophyria	1 in 15,000	124
Osteogenesis imperfecta	1 in 20,000	205
Von Willebrand disease	1 in 8000	174
Myotonic dystropy	1 in 10,000	217
Familial hypertrophic cardiomyopathy	1 in 5000	213
Neurofibromatosis I	1 in 3000	39
Tuberous sclerosis	1 in 15,000	233
Achondroplasia	1 in 50,000	210
Autosomal recessive		
Deafness	1 in 500–1000	254
Albinism	1 in 10,000	220
Wilson disease	1 in 50,000	126
Hemochromatosis	1 in 500 (Europeans)	127
Sickle cell anemia	1 in 655 (U.S. blacks)	181
β Thalassemia	Very high in malaria regions	181
Cystic fibrosis	1 in 2500 (Europeans)	201
Hereditary emphysema (α_1-antitrypsin ZZ)	1 in 3500	219
Friedreich ataxia	1 in 75,000	232
Phenylketonuria	1 in 12,000 (average)	77
Spinal muscular atrophy	1 in 10,000	231
Gaucher disease type 1	1 in 600 in Ashkenazim	146
X-linked		
Hemophilia A	1 in 10,000 males	172
Glucose 6-phosphate dehydrogenase deficiency	Variable up to 1 in 10 males	179
Duchenne/Becker muscular dystrophy	1 in 3000 males	216
Fabry disease	1 in 40,000	150
Testicular feminization	1 in 64,000	160
Chronic granulomatous disease	1 in 750,000	189
Hypophosphatemic rickets	1 in 20,000	197
Fragile X syndrome	1 in 1250 males	64
Color blindness	1 in 12 males	238

*The frequency of some disorders varies widely between ethnic groups (e.g., sickle cell anemia, cystic fibrosis, Tay-Sachs disease, α_1-antitrypsin deficiency, and phenylketonuria) but is less variant for others, perhaps particularly when new mutations are frequent (e.g., achondroplasia, Duchenne muscular dystrophy, and hemophilia A).

Source: Data modified from Galjaard,[75] Carter,[91] Motulsky,[92] and various chapters in this book.

If a particular disease shows one of the three Mendelian patterns of inheritance, its pathogenesis, no matter how complex, must be due to an abnormality at a single site in the genome, usually involving a single protein. For example, in sickle cell anemia, the entire clinical syndrome, including such seemingly unrelated disturbances as anemia, pain crises, nephropathy, and

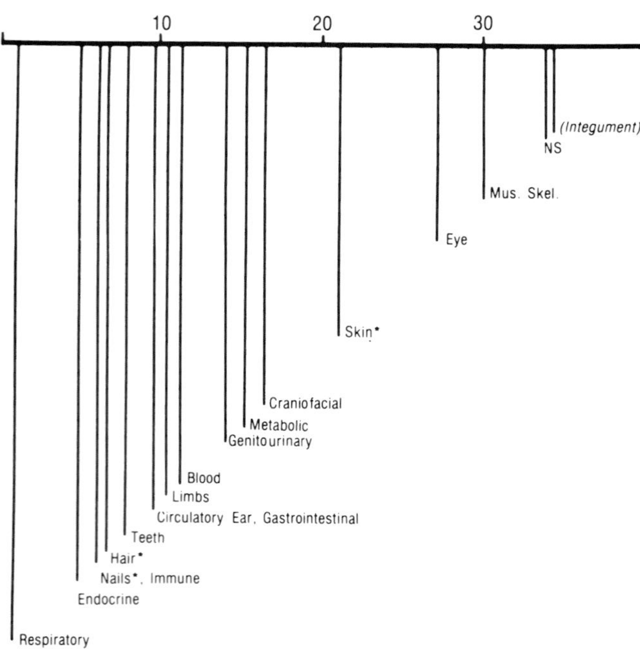

Fig. 1-18 Rank order (abscissa is percentage of phenotypes involving system) for the involvement of a particular anatomic/functional system by Mendelian disease in humans (see Costa et al.[93] for likelihood that more than one system is involved). Skin, hair, and nails are shown both individually and as a group-designated integument. Mus Skel = musculoskeletal; NS = nervous system. (*From Costa et al.*[93] *Used by permission.*)

predisposition to pneumococcal infections, is the physiological consequence of having a single base change at a specific site in the gene that codes for the β-chain of hemoglobin, producing a substitution of a valine for a glutamic acid in the sixth amino acid position in the protein sequence. The mutant gene and protein for many common Mendelian disorders are known even when the full pathogenesis of a disorder is not known.

The basic biochemical lesions in monogenic disorders involve defects in a wide variety of proteins, including enzymes, receptors, transport proteins, peptide hormones, immunoglobulins, collagens, transcription factors, and coagulation factors. Defects in genes that do not encode proteins (e.g., defects in genes for transfer RNA in the mitochondrial genome) are rare.

The impact of Mendelian disease on human health has been reviewed in detail.[93] It was found that 25 percent of disadaptive Mendelian phenotypes were apparent at birth and over 90 percent by the end of puberty. Slightly more than half of phenotypes involved more than one anatomic or functional system. Life span was reduced in 57 percent of disorders, more often in autosomal recessive and X-linked diseases. Reproductive capacity was reduced in 69 percent of phenotypes. Most phenotypes compatible with prolonged survival were associated with handicaps that limited the access to schooling and work. The distribution of phenotypes by systems affected is presented in Fig. 1-18; the distribution pattern indicates a high frequency of central nervous system involvement.

Significance of Dominance or Recessiveness. Unless otherwise specified, the terms dominant and recessive refer to the clinical phenotype associated with a particular allele. This distinction is useful for clinical diagnosis, for linkage analysis, and for genetic counseling, but there are a number of complexities inherent in the use of the terms dominant and recessive. The circumstance is relatively simple if the heterozygous individual is indistinguishable from one or the other homozygote. In this case, the dominant trait (disease) or allele (mutation) is the one that prevails in the heterozygote. In true recessive disorders, the phenotype in heterozygotes is indistinguishable from normal, and in true dominant disorders, heterozygous individuals have a disease phenotype that is indistinguishable from homozygous affected individuals. Although many recessive medical disorders appear on the surface to qualify as true recessives, heterozygotes for many of these conditions exhibit subtle differences in phenotype and these may be enhanced by environmental factors. Such subtle phenotypic consequences may be advantageous or disadvantageous. Even when clinically "normal," individuals who are heterozygous for recessive loss of function alleles often have demonstrable metabolic differences and always have demonstrable differences at the protein level. These complexities are exemplified by sickle cell anemia, which is clinically a recessive disorder in that heterozygotes are usually normal healthy individuals. Nevertheless, heterozygotes exhibit a selective advantage for resistance to malaria and have subtle physiological abnormalities in renal concentrating ability and at high altitude in cardiopulmonary function (Chap. 181). Subtle phenotypic effects in heterozygotes for recessive disorders may be more common than is generally recognized and may contribute to phenotypes usually considered to be complex disease traits. For example, heterozygotes for ataxia telangiectasia and other DNA repair disorders may be at increased risk of malignancy (Chaps. 27 to 29), heterozygosity for homocystinuria is probably a risk factor in vascular disease (Chap. 88), and heterozygosity for α_1-antitrypsin deficiency may predispose to pulmonary disease (Chap. 219). Heterozygosity for known recessive disorders may make a major contribution to biochemical and medical individuality.

The situation is different for dominant phenotypes. Very few conditions qualify as true dominants, but such may be the case for Huntington disease (Chap. 223). Homozygotes for most dominant disorders are ascertained rarely, and when recognized the disease is usually more severe than in heterozygotes, indicating that most such disorders are actually semidominant (incompletely or partially dominant) traits (e.g., familial hypercholesterolemia and achondroplasia). The term codominant has relatively little clinical applicability and describes a situation such as the A and B blood group alleles in which the presence of one antigenic determinant does not affect the presence or absence of the other.

Additional complexities arise from the fact that the phenotypic consequences of heterozygosity may be inconsistent and cause uncertainty as to whether the disorder is dominant or recessive. Heterozygotes may display symptoms in only a very fraction of cases, or heterozygotes may have subtle and mild symptoms that do not qualify as a disease diagnosis. Homozygotes for these traits typically have clear-cut disease manifestation. From a clinical and counseling vantage point, most medical disorders fall into the dominant or recessive category despite this classification being an arbitrary division of a continuum rather than a true biologic demarcation.

Although there is a tendency for a given disease locus to be considered as typically involving dominant or recessive mutations, the classification of a mutation or trait as dominant or recessive must be made on an allele by allele basis and not on a locus by locus basis, as in the case of osteogenesis imperfecta, where different mutations in the same gene can have dominant or recessive effects. When two different mutant alleles are present at the same locus, patients are referred to as compound heterozygotes or genetic compounds. This is distinct from a double heterozygote individual who is heterozygous at two different loci. Most compound heterozygous genotypes involve different recessive alleles at a locus, but phenotypic homozygotes for dominant traits (such as familial hypercholesterolemia) may be compound heterozygotes at a molecular level as well. Alternatively, compound heterozygotes may have one recessive allele and one dominant allele such that heterozygotes for the recessive allele are phenotypically normal, heterozygotes for the dominant allele have a disease process, and the compound heterozygote individuals have a disease process that is distinct (usually more severe) from the disease in heterozygotes for the dominant allele. Such instances are likely for osteogenesis imperfecta (Chap. 205).

Mutant alleles may cause a total or partial loss of function (referred to as null or hypomorphic alleles, respectively), may exhibit altered function, or may gain a novel function. In general, most loss of function alleles tend to be recessive, as in the case of the majority of enzyme deficiencies in humans and most null mutations produced in mice. However, some null alleles have phenotypic effects and cause human disease if a half-normal level of the encoded protein is insufficient for normal physiology. Whether a mutation generates a dominant or recessive disorder is determined by two factors: (a) the effect of the mutation on the function of the gene product, and (b) the tolerance of the biologic system to perturbation of that particular gene product. In this reductionist era, it is important to realize that gene products work in systems and that the phenotype — be it normal development and physiological homeostasis or maldevelopment and dyshomeostasis — is, at a first approximation, the result of the normal or abnormal functioning of the system (e.g., the blood glucose homeostatic system or the connective tissue extracellular matrix system). Tolerant systems tend to result in recessive phenotypes; less-tolerant systems tend to result in dominant phenotypes. Loci that encode enzymes usually result in recessive phenotypes because of the catalytic nature of enzymes and because enzymes are usually present in amounts considerably in excess of that required to maintain a relatively normal phenotype. Kacser and Burns[94] described the sensitivity coefficient as the fractional change in flux in a pathway over the fractional change in enzyme activity. Quantitative analysis demonstrates that a large change in enzyme activity results in a negligible change in flux for most pathways, explaining why most enzyme mutants are recessive. This approach is particularly applicable to metabolic pathways and emphasizes *control analysis*, which is a quantitative assessment of flux in a metabolizing system.[95] The concept can be extended to noncatalytic processes by recognizing that the impact of a mutant allele depends on its relative contribution to the overall functioning of the system, be it a pathway, a network, or a structure. Examples where a heterozygous loss-of-function mutation causes a disease phenotype include several forms of porphyria (Chap. 124), familial hypercholesterolemia (Chap. 120), and type I osteogenesis imperfecta (Chap. 205). In the case of recessive disorders the presence of protein with residual function, hypomorphic mutations can result in mild forms of disorders, as exemplified by many disorders of amino acid metabolism and lysosomal storage diseases.

The term *dominant negative* is applied to mutant alleles in which a mutant protein interferes in one way or another with the function of normal protein being produced from the normal allele in a heterozygote. Dominant negative alleles occur when proteins are involved in subunit structures or when proteins interact with other proteins or nucleic acids. Numerous examples of complex mechanisms that can underlie dominant negative alleles are described elsewhere.[96] In general, the term *dominant negative* is appropriate when a mutant allele causes a more severe phenotype than that caused by a null allele. This results from an adverse effect of the product of the abnormal allele on the function of the product from the normal allele. Again, excellent examples are found in the case of collagen and osteogenesis imperfecta, where many missense mutations interfere with fiber assembly and cause lethal osteogenesis imperfecta type II in heterozygotes, while null alleles cause a much milder form of the disease (Chap. 205). Most dominant negative mutations might be considered as altered function alleles or as a particular subset of gain-of-function alleles. In other instances, gain-of-function alleles might acquire totally new properties that have little or nothing to do with the normal function of the protein. Amyloidosis (Chap. 209) may represent a reasonably good example of such an instance, where the abnormal folding properties of the mutant protein lead to a harmful, extracellular deposition of material that appears to be unrelated to the normal function of the protein. The expanded polyglutamine tracts in the mutant alleles for Huntington disease, spinocerebellar ataxia, and spinobulbar muscular atrophy may represent clear gain-of-function alleles, but the pathogenesis is not yet understood.

Exceptions to the Rules: Unstable Mutations, Uniparental Disomy, Imprinted Genes, and Transmission Ratio Distortion. The traditional formulation of single-gene disorders involved assumptions that are generally correct, including the stability of mutations, the inheritance of one allele from each parent for an autosomal locus, the equal expression of both alleles at an autosomal locus, and the random transmission of either allele to an offspring. Genetic counseling, linkage analysis, and interpretation of genetic data are based on these assumptions. However, evidence for relatively rare examples of exceptions to these rules now abound.

As mentioned above, the clearest examples of unstable mutations involve the expanding triplet repeats that cause fragile X syndrome, myotonic dystrophy, Huntington disease, spinobulbar muscular atrophy, multiple spinocerebellar ataxias, and other disorders. Previously, the significance of anticipation (defined as the worsening of a disease phenotype over generations within a family) was uncertain, and molecular documentation was lacking for the concept of premutation. Expanding triplet mutations have demonstrated that premutations can exist as modest expansions of triplet repeats (perhaps including minor sequence differences from stable alleles). These premutations do not themselves cause clear phenotypic effects but are prone to further expansion and causation of disease. The phenomenon of anticipation is due to increasing size of repeats, which causes earlier onset of disease or a more severe phenotype.

Recognition that individuals can inherit two copies of part or all of a chromosome from one parent and no copy from the other parent is also a rare departure from Mendelian inheritance. This phenomenon of *uniparental disomy* is relatively rare but contributes to the occurrence of Prader-Willi and Angelman syndromes (Chap. 65). The significance of uniparental disomy is in large part due to the existence imprinting, whereby the maternal copy of a gene and the paternal copy of a gene are differentially expressed (Chap. 15). The copy of the genes for insulin-like growth factor 2 (*IFG2*) and small nuclear ribonucleopolypeptide N (*SNRPN*) that are inherited from the father are expressed, while the copies inherited from the mother are silenced in mouse and human; in contrast, the maternal copy of the H19 gene is expressed, and the paternal copy is silenced in mouse and human. The gene(s) causing Prader-Willi syndrome appear to be expressed from the paternal copy, while that causing Angelman syndrome is expressed from the maternal copy. In the case of Angelman syndrome, the imprinting is tissue-specific involving the brain, and based on combined human and mouse data, probably particularly Purkinje cells and hippocampal neurons.[97] Patterns of inheritance for diseases involving mutations in imprinted genes deviate from usual Mendelian patterns (see "Disorders of Imprinted Genes" below). Uniparental disomy and loss of imprinting can occur in somatic cells and result in mosaicism with relevance to Beckwith-Wiedemann syndrome in particular and to cancer more generally (Chap. 18).

Further deviations from simple Mendelian rules probably exist. Transmission ratio distortion (or meiotic drive) describes the circumstance where there is preferential transmission of an allele to the offspring from a heterozygous parent. This phenomenon is well documented for various alleles at the *T* locus in the mouse and may occur in humans. Despite some evidence for transmission ratio distortion for a number of human loci, an indisputable example is lacking.[98–101] Imprinted gene expression is only one aspect of epigenetic phenomena that are well described in plants, *Drosophila*, and other organisms, as is discussed in a series of

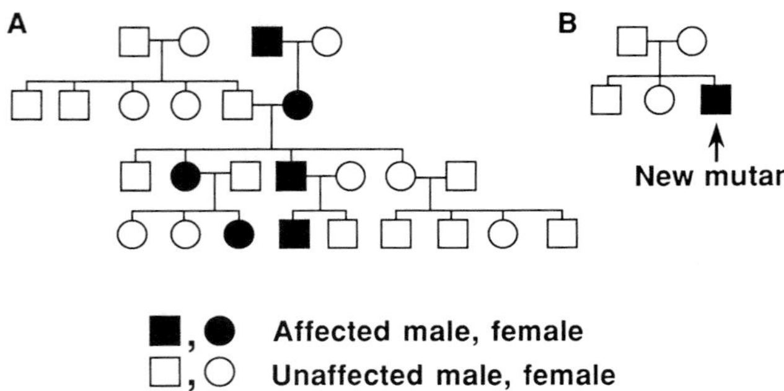

Fig. 1-19 Pedigree pattern for an autosomal dominant trait. Note the vertical pattern of inheritance; compare new mutation and inherited pedigrees.

Table 1-4 Approximate Percentage of Patients Affected by New Mutations in Some Autosomal Dominant Disorders

Disorder	Percentage
Achondroplasia	80
Tuberous sclerosis	80
Neurofibromatosis	40
Marfan syndrome	30
Polyposis of the colon	30
Myotonic dystrophy	Anticipation*
Huntington chorea	Anticipation*
Adult polycystic kidney disease	1
Familial hypercholesterolemia	Very low
BRCA1 breast cancer	Very low

*Anticipation is intended to indicate a multistep process from normal allele to premutation to mutation. A very high percentage of cases are inherited.

reviews.[102] It is likely that many epigenetic phenomena remain to be discovered in human genetics.

Autosomal Dominant Disorders. Dominant diseases are manifest in the heterozygous state; that is, when only one abnormal gene (*mutant allele*) is present and the corresponding allele on the homologous chromosome is normal. By definition, the gene responsible for an autosomal dominant disorder must be located on one of the 22 autosomes; hence, both males and females can be affected. Because alleles segregate independently at meiosis, there is a 1 in 2 chance that the offspring of an affected heterozygote will inherit the mutant allele.

Figure 1-19 shows typical pedigrees involving an autosomal dominant trait: (a) Each affected individual has an affected parent, unless the condition arose by a new mutation in the sperm or ovum that formed the individual, or unless the mutant allele is present but without phenotypic effect in the affected parent, as discussed under "Penetrance and Expressivity" below; (b) an affected individual has a 50 percent probability of passing the trait to each offspring; (c) normal children of an affected individual have only normal offspring; (d) males and females are affected in equal proportions except in sex-limited disorders; (e) each sex is equally likely to transmit the condition to male and female offspring, including male-to-male transmission; and (f) vertical transmission of the condition through successive generation occurs, especially when the trait does not impair reproductive capacity. Autosomal dominant disorders can be inherited in a sex-limited or sex-modified pattern, as exemplified by breast/ovarian cancer in women caused by the *BRCA1* and *BRCA2* loci (Chap. 47) and by familial male precocious puberty caused by constitutively activating mutations of the luteinizing hormone receptor gene (MIM 176410).

Dominant New Mutations. For autosomal dominant diseases, a certain proportion of cases are due to new mutations rather than to inherited mutations. Because a rough estimate of the frequency of mutation is 5×10^{-6} mutations per gene per generation and because there are two copies of each autosomal gene, one would expect that about 1 in 100,000 newborn persons possess a new mutation at any given genetic locus. Many of these mutations either do not impair the function of the gene product or involve a recessive effect, so that the mutation is clinically silent. Others, however, give rise to dominant traits. The parent in whose germ cells the mutation arose is clinically normal, and the sibs of the affected individual are usually normal, because the mutation affects one or only a few germ cells. Given the nature of germ cell proliferation, mutations are most likely to occur at one of the later cell divisions, but multiple mutant gametes may be descended from a single mutational event in some cases (gonadal mosaicism). Given these factors, and because humans have few offspring, the probability of a recurrence of the disorder among the sibs of an individual with a new mutation generally is quite low. The presence of the identical mutation in sibs when neither parent has the mutation in somatic cells, can occur through gonadal mosaicism and will cause a higher recurrence risk in sibs, as has been well documented for osteogenesis imperfecta (Chap. 205) and Duchenne muscular dystrophy (Chap. 216). In some cases, it is possible to assess the proportion of gonadal mosaicism by molecular analysis of sperm. Individuals affected with new dominant mutations are able to transmit the disease, and each offspring is at 50 percent risk for the condition.

The proportion of dominant disorders due to new mutations is inversely proportional to the effect on biologic fitness (Table 1-4). *Biologic fitness* refers to the ability of an individual to produce children who survive to adult life and reproduce. In the extreme case, if a dominant mutation causes infertility, then all observed cases, of necessity, represent new mutations, and there would be no evidence of familial transmission. Thanatophoric dysplasia (Chap. 210) represents such a disorder. In moderately severe disorders, as in tuberous sclerosis, biologic fitness is approximately 20 percent of normal, and approximately 80 percent of cases are due to new mutations. In disorders such as familial hypercholesterolemia, hereditary breast and ovarian cancer (BRCA1 or BRCA2), or hereditary nonpolyposis colon cancer, in which there is relatively little reduction in biologic fitness, almost all affected persons have a pedigree showing classic vertical transmission. The incidence of a dominant disorder is dependent both on the biologic fitness and on the mutation frequency for the locus, which is widely variable. Although the proportion of cases due to new mutation is directly related to biologic fitness, genetic counseling and reproductive planning now can alter this proportion. For example, if a large proportion of patients with neurofibromatosis or Marfan syndrome were to avoid affected offspring through prenatal or preimplantation diagnosis, the proportion of cases due to new mutation would be sharply increased.

Many new mutations occur in the germ cells of fathers who are of advanced age. For example, in the Marfan syndrome (Chap. 206), the average age of fathers of sporadic or "new mutation" cases (37 years) is in excess of the age of fathers who transmit the disease as an inherited mutation (30 years). The paternal age effect is also prominent in achondroplasia (Chap. 210). There is evidence that the mutations associated with advanced paternal age are frequently point mutations, often C to T transitions at CpG dinucleotides. Differences in mutation rates for male and female gametes are discussed below under "X-linked New Mutations and Heterozygote Detection."

Before one concludes that a dominant disorder in a patient with unaffected parents is the result of a new mutation, it is important to consider two other possibilities: (a) the gene may be carried by one parent, in whom the mutant allele is not penetrant, and (b) nonpaternity may have occurred (i.e., the father is someone other than the putative father), as occurs in 3 to 5 percent of randomly studied children in many cultures.

Penetrance and Expressivity. These terms are frequently the subject of confusion and slight variations in usage. In the medical context, penetrance is the proportion of individuals with a given genotype that present with *any* phenotypic features of the disorder (i.e., it is an all or none phenomenon). Although in one sense penetrance may vary with age, as in the case of Huntington disease, variation in age of onset is most often considered as an aspect of variable expression. In some cases, penetrance depends on environmental exposure, e.g., medications or fava beans in glucose-6-phosphate dehydrogenase deficiency. In the autosomal dominant context, it is instructive to consider the concept of penetrance from a counseling perspective and in terms of molecular diagnosis. Penetrance is the question at issue when the apparently unaffected offspring of an individual with a dominant disorder wishes to know if they carry the mutant gene and if they are at risk of having affected offspring. The mutant gene is not penetrant if an individual carrying the mutant gene shows no phenotypic effects. In molecular terms, the presence or absence of the mutant gene can be determined with appropriate diagnostic tests, and a person without the mutant gene can be distinguished from one carrying the nonpenetrant mutant gene. Clinically, penetrance often depends on the quality of clinical methodologies; for example, magnetic resonance imaging might demonstrate findings not previously recognizable. In the medical context, the gene is usually considered penetrant if diagnostic abnormalities can be demonstrated even if the individual is asymptomatic. In the biologic context, the gene can be considered penetrant if it affects the structure or function of the individual.

Expressivity or variability in clinical expression describes the range of phenotypic effects in individuals carrying a given mutation. This variability can include the type and severity of symptoms and the age of onset of symptoms. Variability in clinical expression is illustrated dramatically the multiple endocrine neoplasia, type I. Patients in the same family with the same abnormal gene may have hyperplasia or neoplasia of one or all of a wide variety of endocrine tissues, including the pancreas, parathyroid glands, pituitary gland, or adipose tissue. The resulting manifestations are extremely diverse; different members of the same family may develop peptic ulcers, hypoglycemia, kidney stones, or pituitary tumors. In the case of other dominant disorders characterized by tumor formation, random second mutations in tumor-suppressor genes may explain some of the clinical variability.

Variation in age of onset is seen in disorders such as Huntington disease and adult polycystic kidney disease. These disorders often do not become symptomatic until adulthood, even though the mutant gene is present throughout life. Whether variation in age of onset is considered as a form of variation in expression is somewhat arbitrary. In one sense, it cannot be said that the mutant gene was nonpenetrant in an individual until the person has had a complete evaluation and has died from other causes. Lack of penetrance can be considered as the absolute mildest end of the spectrum of expression so that no phenotypic effects are observed. In the counseling context, variation in expression, as distinct from penetrance, is the point in question when an individual with a dominant disorder wishes to know whether an offspring who carries the mutation would have mild or severe symptoms. In molecular terms, analysis of the single gene locus will not answer this question (i.e., predict variation in expression within a family), but it can determine whether the mutant gene is present and not penetrant.

At least three factors underlie lack of penetrance and variability in expression: (a) the effects of genes at the same or other loci; (b) exogenous or environmental factors; and (c) stochastic factors. Effects within the same gene locus can be seen with mutations in α-spectrin where a polymorphism involving a high-expressing or low-expressing promoter affects the phenotype (Chap. 183). The low-expression allele moderates the phenotype of hereditary elliptocytosis when in *cis* with the mutation, but worsens the phenotype when in *trans* in a heterozygote for the mutation. In the case of cystic fibrosis, the phenotypic severity of the R117H mutation varies through a *cis* effect on the level of functional mRNA due to a splice junction polymorphism that influences skipping of an exon (Chap. 201). The genotype at the α-globin locus that affects the sickle cell anemia phenotype and various loci that affect the monogenic hyperlipidemias are examples of effects by genes at other loci. The phenotypes in the monogenic hyperlipidemias, the porphyrias, and hemochromatosis can be affected by diet, drug exposure, alcohol use, smoking, and exercise. The effects of stochastic factors, perhaps particularly somatic mutations, are exemplified by variability in the severity and distribution of lesions among identical twins with retinoblastoma, neurofibromatosis, or tuberous sclerosis. Differences in random X chromosome inactivation among identical twin female heterozygotes for an X-linked disorder, and somatic rearrangements and mutations associated with expression of immunoglobulins and T cell receptors are other examples of stochastic events that can affect phenotypes. Although the issues of penetrance and expressivity are often defined in the context of autosomal dominant disorders, these principles are relevant to chromosomal disorders, autosomal recessive and X-linked disorders, and complex disease traits as well.

Biochemical Basis of Dominant Alleles. The biochemical and/or molecular defects causing dominant disorders such as familial hypercholesterolemia, amyloidosis, hereditary spherocytosis, osteogenesis imperfecta, hereditary retinoblastoma, neurofibromatosis, Marfan syndrome, and Huntington disease have been determined. A number of mechanisms can account for an abnormal phenotype in the presence of one mutant gene. One mechanism is haploinsufficiency, meaning that a half-normal amount of gene product is insufficient to maintain a normal phenotype (i.e., the process is sensitive to reduced dosage). This is true, for example, when gene products regulate complex metabolic pathways, such as membrane receptors and rate-limiting enzymes in biosynthetic pathways under feedback control (e.g., familial hypercholesterolemia and dominant porphyrias in Chaps. 120 and 124, respectively). In other cases, a dosage effect due to gene duplication can cause a dominant phenotype as in the case of the common mutation in type IA Charcot-Marie-Tooth disease where triploid dosage for the *PMP22* gene causes the condition (Chap. 227). This means that homeostasis is disrupted by the expression of 150 percent of the normal level of gene product. Another mechanism involves abnormalities of structural proteins where a complex network of direct protein interactions is involved (e.g., collagens in osteogenesis imperfecta and erythrocyte cytoskeleton proteins in spherocytosis and elliptocytosis). Dominant negative mutations are instances where the molecules of mutant gene product interfere with the function of the normal gene products. Many mutations involving structural proteins have a dominant negative component, and some missense mutations may be more deleterious than null mutations, as in the case of osteogenesis imperfecta. Dominant phenotypic effects can also occur when the remaining normal copy of a gene is mutated at a single-cell level so that both copies of the locus are inactivated (e.g., hereditary retinoblastoma). These defects may be considered dominant at the pedigree level and recessive at the single-cell level. Conceptually, it is useful to distinguish dominant mutations that generate products with new or neomorphic biologic properties and that cause a harmful effect (e.g., amyloidosis) from those due to deficiency of normal gene product (e.g., familial hypercholesterolemia and porphyrias). In the former group, restoration of a normal level of gene product does not negate the effect of the mutant gene.

Disorders of Imprinted Genes. If an autosomal locus is imprinted such that it is expressed from one allele and silenced/repressed

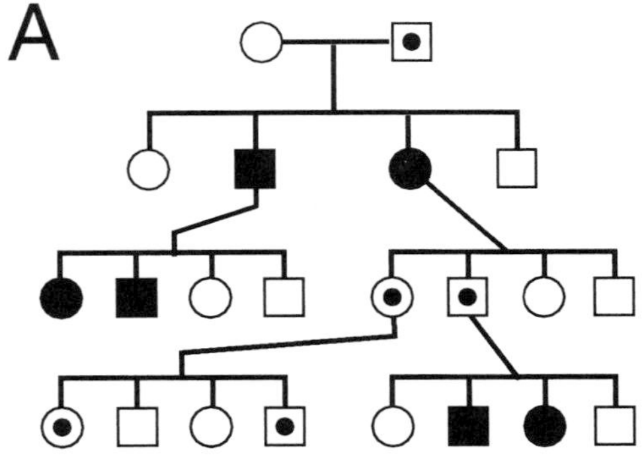

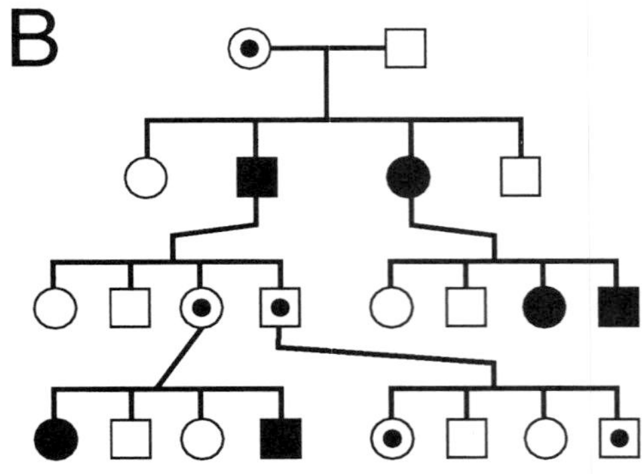

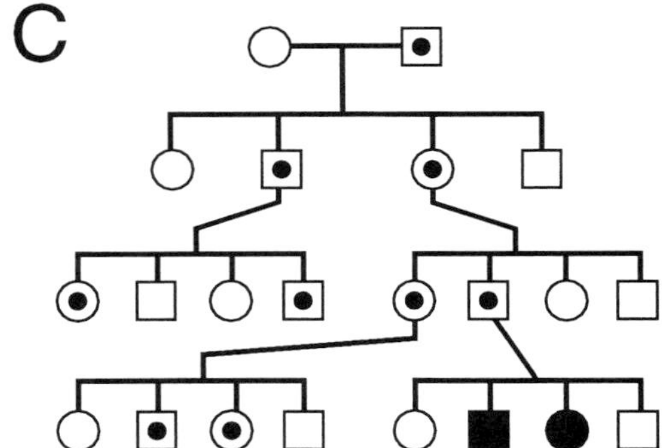

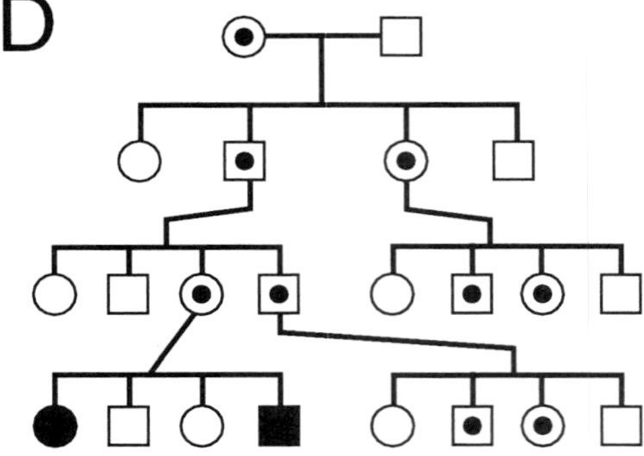

Fig. 1-20. Pedigree patterns that might be observed with an abnormal phenotype involving an imprinted gene. Open symbols are individuals without a mutation; open symbols with a dot in the center are individuals who have the mutation but with a normal phenotype; and solid symbols are individuals with the mutation and an abnormal phenotype. *Panel A* could represent a loss-of-function mutation for a paternally expressed gene leading to dwarfism; alternatively, it could depict a mutation causing constitutive expression (derepression) of a paternally silenced gene leading to gigantism. *Panel B* could depict a loss-of-function mutation for a maternally expressed gene leading to lighter pigmentation; alternatively, it could depict a mutation causing constitutive expression (derepression) of a maternally silenced gene leading to darker pigmentation. *Panel C* could depict a mutation such that the chromosome begins in the pedigree functionally normal and is able to switch from paternal to maternal expression pattern but is unable to switch from maternal to paternal expression pattern leading either to a loss of function of a paternally expressed gene causing dwarfism or to constitutive expression (derepression) of a paternally silenced gene leading to gigantism. *Panel D* could depict a mutation such that the chromosome begins in the pedigree functionally normal and is able to switch from maternal to paternal expression pattern but is unable to switch from paternal to maternal expression pattern leading either to loss of function for a maternally expressed gene causing lighter pigmentation or to constitutive expression (derepression) of a maternally silenced gene leading to darker pigmentation.

from the other, there is no question of a dominant or recessive effect at the level of the protein product, because the gene is functionally hemizygous. However, heterozygous mutations may cause a phenotype (i.e., appear dominant) or not (i.e., appear recessive) depending on the parent of origin of the mutation for an individual subject. This can result in many complex patterns of inheritance over multiple generations considering that mutations may involve gain or loss of function mutations in structural genes, loss of silencing or loss of expression for an allele, or defects in the switching or maintenance of imprinting (Fig. 1-20 and legend). With defects in switching, the chromosome may be unable to switch from paternal to maternal epigenotype, or vice versa, such that the mutant allele may act as a premutation that will only cause a phenotype after being switched into an epigenotype in which it becomes fixed. The familial pattern can result in quite distantly related individuals having the same disease genotype and phenotype. There are good examples of large pedigrees with inherited phenotypes involving imprinted genes. Hereditary paragangliomas is a disorder in which the phenotype is expressed only when the mutant allele is inherited from the father.[103] In contrast, Angelman syndrome is expressed only when the mutant allele is inherited from the mother[97] (Chaps. 19 and 65).

Autosomal Recessive Disorders. Autosomal recessive conditions are clinically apparent only in the homozygous or compound heterozygous state; that is, when both alleles at a particular genetic locus are mutant. It is useful to distinguish phenotypic "homozygotes" (perhaps better referred to as affected individuals) in whom both copies of the gene are defective in contrast to molecular homozygotes where DNA analysis reveals identical mutations in both copies of the gene. By definition, the gene responsible for an autosomal recessive disorder must be located on one of the 22 autosomes so that both males and females can be affected.

Figure 1-21 shows two pedigrees for families with an autosomal recessive trait. Monoplex families (pedigree A) are the most common, but families with multiple affected individuals occur. These features are characteristic: (a) the parents are clinically normal; (b) only sibs are affected, and vertical transmission usually does not occur; (c) males and females are affected in equal proportions except for sex-limited effects; and (d) consanguinity can be a contributing factor.

The variety of recessive alleles and the requirement for two abnormal copies for clinical expression create special conditions for autosomal recessive inheritance: (a) the more infrequent the mutant gene in the population, the stronger the likelihood that affected individuals are the product of consanguineous matings (see "Consanguinity" below); (b) if both parents are carriers for the same autosomal recessive gene, the probability for disease in offspring is 0.25, for a heterozygote (carrier) the probability is

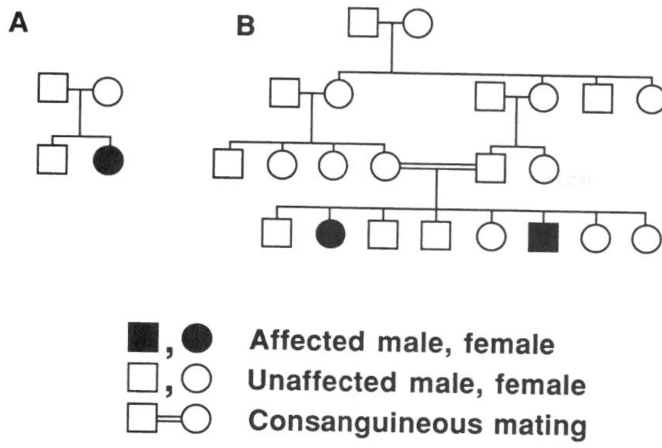

Fig. 1-21 **Pedigree pattern for an autosomal recessive trait. Note the horizontal pattern of inheritance and consanguinity in the multiplex pedigree (*B*) in comparison to the more common monoplex pedigree (*A*).**

0.50, and for a normal (noncarrier) the probability is 0.25; (c) if an affected individual mates with a heterozygote, there is a 50 percent probability of disease for each child, and a pedigree simulating dominant inheritance may result; and (d) if two individuals with the same recessive disease mate, all the children will be affected.

The clinical features of autosomal recessive disorders tend to be more uniform than those of dominant diseases, and recessive disorders are more commonly diagnosed in children. Many autosomal recessive disorders present or cause major morbidity in adulthood including hemochromatosis (Chap. 127), α_1-antitrypsin deficiency (Chap. 219), some forms of hyperlipidemia (Chaps. 114 to 122), and late onset lysosomal storage diseases (Chaps. 134 to 154).

Because the probability is that only one in four individuals in a sibship will be affected, most cases of autosomal recessive disease may occur as isolated individuals, particularly when small families are common. Consider, for example, 16 families in which both parents are heterozygous for the same recessive disorder, such as cystic fibrosis. If each family has 2 children, the probability is that 9 of the 16 families will have no affected children, 6 will have 1 affected and 1 normal child, and only 1 of the 16 families will have 2 affected children. Because of the modern tendency toward smaller families, physicians usually see isolated cases of a recessive disease without an affected sib to alert them to the possibility of a genetic disorder. Fortunately, because of the relatively uniform manifestations of recessive disorders and because many conditions can be diagnosed directly by biochemical or molecular tests, the diagnosis of a genetic disease can frequently be made even when no other members of a family are clinically affected. Autosomal recessive disorders can be inherited in a sex-limited manner as exemplified by steroid 5α-reductase 2 deficiency (Chap. 160), where only 46,XY males are phenotypically abnormal.

Biochemical Basis of Recessive Alleles. The biochemical defects underlying many autosomal recessive disorders have been identified. Most alleles are complete or partial loss-of-function mutations, often involving enzymatic proteins. In these conditions, recessive inheritance occurs because a mutation that impairs the catalytic activity of an enzyme usually does not impair the health of a heterozygote. Regulatory mechanisms function to avert clinical consequences of this 50 percent deficiency, and so heterozygotes for enzyme defects usually are clinically normal, as discussed above. On the other hand, when an individual inherits abnormal alleles at both copies of the locus specifying an enzyme, a disease results.

Many of the enzyme deficiencies in recessive diseases involve enzymes in catabolic pathways, frequently enzymes that degrade organic molecules in the diet, such as galactose (galactosemia, Chap. 72), phenylalanine (phenylketonuria, Chap. 77), and phytanic acid (Refsum syndrome, Chap. 132). When deficiency affects an acid hydrolase (lysosomal storage disorders), the substrate, usually a complex lipid or polysaccharide, accumulates within swollen lysosomes (Chaps. 134 to 154). Examples of such lysosomal diseases include the mucopolysaccharidoses, such as Hurler syndrome (α-iduronidase deficiency), and the sphingolipidoses, such as Gaucher disease (glucocerebrosidase deficiency).

Population Genetics of Recessive Alleles. Many recessive alleles or milder dominant alleles occur at higher frequency in particular geographic areas or ethnic groups (Table 1-5). In general, recessive diseases are rare because the reduced biologic fitness of homozygotes serves to remove the mutant gene from the population. A few lethal recessive disorders, such as cystic fibrosis, thalassemia, and sickle cell anemia are common. To explain this paradox, it has been postulated that the biologic fitness of heterozygotes is greater than that of noncarriers for these genes. In such a case, the frequency of the gene in the population depends on the balance between the increased fitness of the relatively numerous heterozygotes and the reduced fitness of the less common homozygotes. A small selective advantage of the heterozygote, in terms of reproductive advantage, results in a high gene frequency, and hence a high birth frequency of homozygotes, even when the disease is lethal (see Chap. 12 in Vogel and Motulsky).[71] Thus, about 1 in 25 Caucasians is heterozygous (a carrier) for the genetically lethal disease cystic

Table 1-5 **Examples of Simply Inherited Disorders That Occur with Increased Frequency in Specific Ethnic Groups**

Ethnic group	Simply inherited disorder
African blacks	Hemoglobinopathies, especially Hb S, Hb C, persistent Hb F, α and β thalassemia, glucose 6-phosphate dehydrogenase deficiency
Armenians	Familial Mediterranean fever
Ashkenazic Jews	Abetalipoproteinemia
	Bloom syndrome
	Dystonia musculorum deformans (recessive form)
	Tay-Sachs disease
	Breast ovarian cancer BRCA1 (specific mutation)
Chinese	α Thalassemia
	Glucose 6-phosphate dehydrogenase deficiency
	Adult lactase deficiency
Eskimos (Inuit)	Pseudocholinesterase deficiency
	Adrenogenital syndrome
Finns	Congenital nephrosis
	Aspartylglucosaminuria
French Canadians	Tyrosinemia
	Familial hypercholesterolemia
Japanese	Acatalasemia
Lebanese	Familial hypercholesterolemia
Mediterranean peoples (Italians, Greeks, Sephardic Jews)	β Thalassemia
	Glucose 6-phosphate dehydrogenase deficiency
	Familial Mediterranean fever
	Glycogen storage disease, type III
Europeans	Cystic fibrosis
Scandinavians	α_1-Antitrypsin deficiency
	LCAT (lecithin:cholesterol acyltransferase) deficiency
South African whites	Porphyria variegata
	Familial hypercholesterolemia

fibrosis, and the disease occurs in about 1 in 2500 Caucasian births. To maintain such a high gene frequency, heterozygotes for cystic fibrosis may have a selective advantage over noncarriers, and this advantage may involve protection against death from childhood diarrhea. Alternatively, there could be a slight transmission ratio distortion (meiotic drive), that is, gametes carrying the mutant gene could have a slightly greater probability of achieving fertilization compared to gametes with the normal gene, or disorders might achieve a high frequency without a selective advantage, that is, by chance. Haplotype data indicate that chromosomes carrying the common ΔF508 allele for cystic fibrosis are descended from a single mutational event, but this does not resolve why the mutant gene is so frequent. In sickle cell anemia, another recessive disorder with high frequency among certain populations, heterozygotes have increased resistance to falciparum malaria (Chap. 181).

Consanguinity. By definition, a recessive disease requires the inheritance of a mutant allele at the same genetic locus from each parent. When the genes are rare, the likelihood of unrelated parents being carriers for the same defect is small. If the parents have a common ancestor who carried a recessive gene, the likelihood that two of the descendants inherited the same allele is enhanced. The less frequent the recessive gene, the stronger the likelihood that an affected individual is the product of a consanguineous mating. On the other hand, when recessive genes are common in the population, the likelihood of two unrelated parents being carriers is great enough to minimize the role of consanguinity. For common traits, such as sickle cell anemia, phenylketonuria, cystic fibrosis, and Tay-Sachs disease, consanguinity is uncommon in the parents.

Recessive New Mutations. New mutations for recessive disorders can rarely be identified because such mutations usually generate asymptomatic heterozygotes. Only generations later will the descendants of individuals with that mutation mate with another heterozygote at the same locus. The selective pressure to eliminate deleterious recessive traits from the population is low because these traits are easily passed on in heterozygous form. Most recessive diseases appear to be due to mutations that occurred many generations earlier, as indicated from haplotype analysis of mutations causing phenylketonuria, β-thalassemia, sickle cell anemia, Tay-Sachs disease, cystic fibrosis, and other disorders.

X-Linked Disorders. The genes responsible for X-linked disorders are located on the X chromosome, and the clinical risks are different for the two sexes. Because a female has two X chromosomes, she may be either heterozygous or homozygous for a mutant gene, and the mutant allele may demonstrate either recessive or dominant expression. Expression in females is often variable and influenced by random X chromosome inactivation. Males, on the other hand, have only one X chromosome, so they are more likely to display the full phenotype, regardless of whether the mutation produces a recessive or dominant allele in the female. Thus, the terms *X-linked dominant* and *X-linked recessive* refer only to the expression of the gene in women.

The distinction of dominant and recessive X-linked disorders is complicated by the effect of X chromosome inactivation. In both ornithine transcarbamoylase deficiency (Chap. 85), often described as an X-linked dominant, and Fabry disease (Chap. 150), often described as an X-linked recessive, phenotypic abnormalities are relatively frequent in heterozygotes. Because there is no clear convention, it may be best to consider such disorders as simply X-linked without a dominant or recessive designation. The recessive or dominant descriptors are more useful for X-linked disorders in which heterozygotes are consistently asymptomatic (e.g., X-linked recessive Hunter mucopolysaccharidosis, Chap. 136) or consistently symptomatic in a manner similar to hemizygous males (e.g., X-linked dominant hypophosphatemic rickets, Chap. 197).

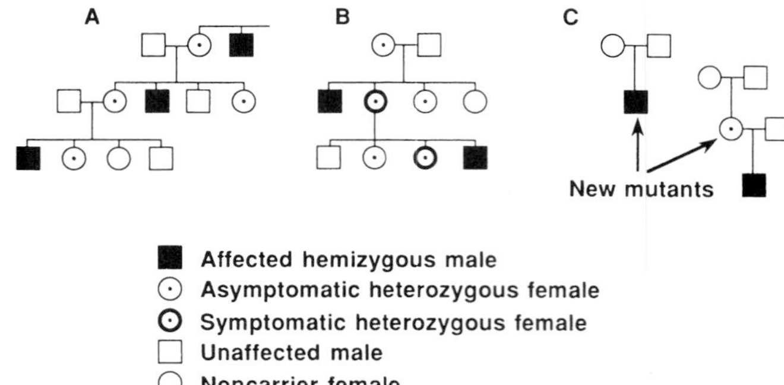

Fig. 1-22 Pedigree pattern for an X-linked trait. *A*, Note the oblique pattern of inheritance. *B*, Note the occurrence of symptomatic and asymptomatic heterozygous females in the same pedigree. Heterozygotes are consistently asymptomatic in some disorders (recessive) and are variably symptomatic in other disorders (see text). *C*, New mutations can give rise to either affected males or heterozygous females.

An important feature of all X-linked inheritance is the absence of male-to-male (i.e., father-to-son) transmission of the trait. This follows because a male contributes his Y chromosome to his son and does not contribute an X chromosome. On the other hand, because a male contributes his sole X chromosome to each daughter, all daughters of a male with an X-linked disorder will inherit the mutant allele.

X-Linked Pedigrees. The pedigrees in Fig. 1-22 illustrate some of the characteristic features of X-linked inheritance. (a) In contrast to the vertical distribution in dominant traits (parents and children affected) and the horizontal distribution in autosomal recessive traits (sibs affected), the pedigree pattern in X-linked recessive traits tends to be oblique; that is, the trait occurs in the maternal uncles of affected males and in male cousins who are descended from the mother's sisters who are carriers (Fig. 1-22A). (b) Male offspring of carrier females have a 50 percent chance of being affected. (c) All female offspring of affected males are carriers, and affected males do not transmit the disease to their sons. (d) Unaffected males do not transmit the trait to any offspring. (e) Affected homozygous females occur only when an affected male mates with a carrier female.

Examples of X-linked recessive disorders in humans include the Lesch-Nyhan syndrome, glucose-6-phosphate dehydrogenase deficiency, testicular feminization, and Hunter mucopolysaccharidosis. Color blindness is a frequent X-linked recessive trait (occurring in about 8 percent of white males), so that the occurrence of homozygous color-blind females is no rarity. A pedigree for an X-linked disorder with variable symptomatology in females is depicted in Fig. 1-22B, and X-linked disease because of new mutation is shown by the pedigree in Fig. 1-22C (see "X-linked New Mutations and Heterozygote Detection" below).

X-linked dominant inheritance is illustrated by the pedigree in Fig. 1-23: (a) females are affected about twice as often as males; (b) an affected female has a 50 percent probability of transmitting the disorder to her sons or daughters; (c) an affected male transmits the disorder to all of his daughters and to none of his sons; and (d) the phenotype may be more variable and less severe in heterozygous affected females than in hemizygous affected males. One common trait, the Xg (a+) blood group, is inherited as an X-linked dominant trait, as are a few diseases, such as hypophosphatemic rickets (Chap. 197).

Some rare conditions may be inherited as X-linked dominant traits in which there is lethality in the hemizygous male (Fig. 1-24): (a) the disorder occurs only in females who are heterozygous for the mutant gene; (b) an affected mother has a 50 percent probability of transmitting the trait to her daughters; (c) an increased frequency of spontaneous abortions occurs in affected women, the abortions representing affected male fetuses. An

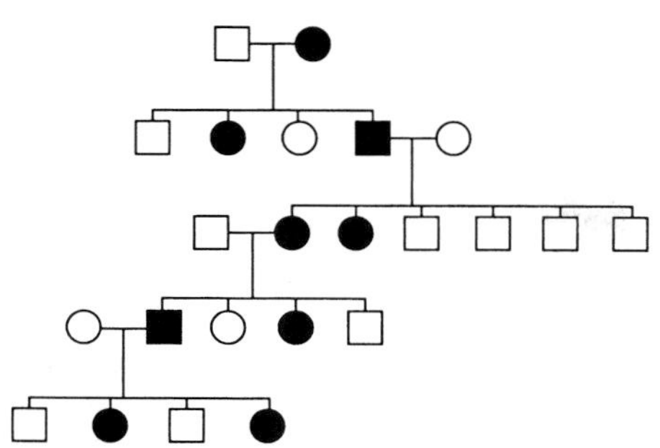

■ Affected hemizygous male
● Affected heterozygous female
□, ○ Unaffected male, female

Fig. 1-23 Pedigree pattern of an X-linked dominant trait.

example of a condition that is transmitted by this mode of inheritance is incontinentia pigmenti. Some X-linked disorders are lethal in utero in males and impair reproduction in females so that a condition occurs primarily or exclusively as a sporadic disorder in females due to new mutation. The syndromes of microphthalmia with linear skin defects (MIM 309801), Aicardi (MIM 304050), and Goltz (MIM 305600) may represent such examples. Rett syndrome may also represent such an example, and the recent identification of the mutant gene will now allow determination of whether hemizygous males die before birth or have a previously unrecognized more severe phenotype.[24]

Genes in the pseudoautosomal region of the X chromosome have a homologous copy on the Y chromosome, and the pattern of inheritance of these genes is indistinguishable from autosomal circumstances, as the term implies.

X Inactivation and Impact on X-linked Disorders. Phenotypic expression of X-linked traits in females is greatly influenced by the phenomenon of random X chromosome inactivation. Early in embryonic development, one of the two X chromosomes in each somatic cell of a female is randomly inactivated so that for each cell there is an equal probability that the paternal or maternal X chromosome will be inactivated (Chap. 61). The inactivation is stable so that all progeny of the initial cell inherit the same active and inactive X chromosomes. Thus, each female is a mosaic; on the average, half of the cells express the X chromosome of the father, and half express the X chromosome of the mother. If a mutation in a gene is carried on one of the X chromosomes, about one-half of the cells in each tissue will be normal and the other half will manifest the mutant phenotype. Chance or preferential survival of one clone of cells may alter these proportions in any given individual. Depending on the proportions of mutant and normal X chromosomes that are active in each tissue, a genetically heterozygous female may be clinically normal or have mild or severe manifestations of disease.

In each female cell, the nonfunctional X chromosome can be identified as a condensed clump of chromatin—the Barr body. The inactive X chromosome is late replicating, and its DNA is more highly methylated. Methylation of DNA is thought to play a role in maintenance of X inactivation. The XIST gene [for X (inactive) specific transcripts] is transcribed exclusively from inactive X chromosomes and is required for X inactivation; the molecular mechanism of X inactivation is becoming better understood (Chap. 61).[104]

Random X inactivation is the most important determinant of expression in females for many X-linked disorders. Many individuals are asymptomatic, some have mild symptoms, and others have severe manifestations. The frequency of detectable phenotypic alterations depends on how carefully heterozygotes are examined and, in some instances, on the age at examination. Ornithine transcarbamoylase deficiency exhibits variable phenotypic expression in heterozygotes. Many heterozygotes are asymptomatic; some have minimal protein intolerance; and others experience intermittent hyperammonemic coma, occasionally with fatal outcome. Hemizygous affected males are more consistently and more seriously symptomatic than are heterozygous females. Other examples in which clinical expression may occur in females include Duchenne muscular dystrophy, hemophilia A, and Fabry disease. In some cases, the biochemical defect behaves in a cell autonomous fashion resulting in a mosaic tissue pattern as in choroideremia and certain forms of X-linked ocular albinism. If the defect involves a product that is secreted by cells, the phenotypic effect is an average for the relevant somatic tissues, as for factor VIII levels in hemophilia A. As discussed under "X-Linked Disorders" above, it is preferable to describe these conditions as X-linked without applying the dominant or recessive descriptor because the literature is inconsistent.

X-Linked New Mutations and Heterozygote Detection. Identification of new mutations in X-linked genes is an important counseling issue in families ascertained because of an isolated affected male (monoplex families). In these families, the mother may be a noncarrier and may have contributed an egg with a new mutation. The father cannot contribute the new mutation, because he contributes a Y chromosome. Alternatively, the mother may be a carrier who received a gamete with a preexisting mutation from a carrier mother or father (if the disorder is not male-lethal), or who received a gamete with a new mutation from either her father or her mother. In the case of male-lethal disorders, a larger fraction of mothers of isolated male cases are carriers. As formulated by Haldane,[105,106] assuming that affected males do not reproduce, approximately two-thirds of mothers of isolated male cases are expected to be carriers, if the mutation rates for male and female gametes are identical (see pp. 407 to 410 in Vogel and Motulsky).[71] This proportion increases, if the mutation rate for male gametes exceeds that for female gametes, a fact that is often misunderstood or ignored. Mutation rates for male and female gametes are similar for Duchenne dystrophy (a disorder predominantly due to large deletions), and the mutation rates for male gametes are higher than for female gametes for hemophilia A and B (disorders largely due to point mutations). Thus, more mothers of isolated hemophilia cases are carriers than are mothers of isolated Duchenne dystrophy cases.

Heterozygous females can sometimes be detected using biochemical methods, as in the Lesch-Nyhan syndrome, Fabry disease, Hunter syndrome, hemophilia A, hemophilia B, ornithine transcarbamoylase deficiency, and Duchenne muscular dystrophy. These biochemical methods are rarely completely accurate because random X inactivation may lead to a relatively normal biochemical result. Accuracy may be increased by sampling relatively clonal cells such as hair roots or cloned skin fibroblasts. Molecular methods can circumvent the problems of biochemical analysis of the gene product when the mutation can be detected directly.

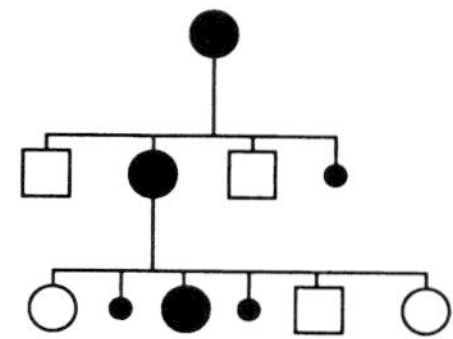

●,○ Affected and unaffected female
□ Unaffected male
Spontaneous abortion

Fig. 1-24 Pedigree pattern of an X-linked dominant trait lethal in the hemizygous male.

Y-Linked Disorders. Only a few genes are known on the Y chromosome, the gene encoding the sex-region determining Y (SRY) factor (also called the testis-determining factor, TDF) being the most salient. Translocations between X and Y chromosomes can result in XY females where the Y chromosome is missing the SRY gene. The reciprocal situation exists in which XX males possess an X chromosome that carries a copy of the SRY gene. Point mutations that impair the function of the SRY factor can also result in XY females. For Y-linked genes, fathers pass the trait to all sons and to no daughters. The male phenotype is the most obvious Y-linked trait. The number of Y-linked disorders is likely to remain limited because of the small number of genes on the Y chromosome, but as many as 18 percent of men with severe oligospermia/azoospermia have microdeletions of the long arm of the Y chromosome that involve the azoospermia factor (AZF).[107]

Mitochondrial Inheritance. There are many genetic disorders affecting mitochondrial function (Chaps. 104 and 105). Mitochondria contain a 16.6 kb circular DNA genome that encodes the ribosomal RNAs and tRNAs for the distinct mitochondrial protein synthesis. This genome also encodes some of the proteins essential for oxidated phosphorylation, but many of the mitochondrial proteins are encoded in the nuclear genome, synthesized in the cytoplasm, and transported into mitochondria. Genetic disorders affecting mitochondria can be divided into two classes: mutations in the nuclear genome and mutations in the mitochondrial genome. For mutations in the nuclear genome, the inheritance is as for other nuclear genes, but mutations in the mitochondrial genome display a distinct pattern of inheritance.

There is wide variation in the number of mitochondria per cell and in the number of mitochondrial DNA genomes per mitochondrion (typically 2 to 10), so that each cell contains thousands of copies of mitochondrial DNA. Mitochondrial DNA is maternally inherited with 200,000 to 300,000 copies per egg and insignificant contributions from sperm. This means that all individuals inherit their mitochondrial genome from their mothers. If a pathologic mutation is present in the mitochondrial genome, this typically affects some proportion of the mitochondrial genomes per cell, and this heterogeneity of mitochondrial DNA within a single cell and within an individual is referred to as heteroplasmy. If a woman carries a mutation in the mitochondrial genome, she will potentially transmit this mutation to all of her children, while the man with such a mutation will not transmit the trait to any of his children. This can give rise to a typical pattern of inheritance with vertical transmission and the disease trait being passed to most or all of the offspring of affected women. The proportion of mutant to wild-type mitochondria may vary among individuals in a pedigree leading to phenotypic heterogeneity. Disorders of the mitochondrial genome include chronic progressive external ophthalmoplegia, Kearns-Sayre syndrome, myopathy, Leber hereditary optic neuropathy, myoclonic epilepsy, and other disorders (see Chaps. 104 and 105).

GENETIC HETEROGENEITY

Genetic heterogeneity can result from different mutations at a single locus (*allelic heterogeneity*) or from mutations at different genetic loci (*nonallelic or locus heterogeneity*). For example, Charcot-Marie-Tooth neurogenic atrophy, congenital sensorineural deafness, and retinitis pigmentosa all have autosomal dominant, autosomal recessive, and X-linked forms. Nonallelic heterogeneity is responsible in many cases, but allelic mutation also can account for dominant and recessive variation at a single locus. A similar bleeding disorder can be caused by mutations at either of two loci on the X chromosome, one causing deficiency of factor VIII (classic hemophilia, hemophilia A) and the other a deficiency of factor IX (Christmas disease, hemophilia B). Hereditary methemoglobinemia, once regarded as a homogeneous clinical entity, is the result of many different mutations involving at least four distinct loci: one coding for the α-chain of hemoglobin, a second encodes the β-chain of hemoglobin, and two involving deficiency of cytochrome b5 or its reductase (Chap. 180). Most, if not all, hereditary diseases are genetically heterogeneous.

The extent of allelic heterogeneity is particularly impressive. Indeed, a large number of mutations have been characterized as causing hemoglobinopathies and thalassemias, cystic fibrosis, familial hypercholesterolemia, phenylketonuria, and breast cancer via the BRCA1 locus. A great deal of clinical heterogeneity is due to different mutations at a single locus. With detailed molecular characterization, many patients with autosomal recessive disorders are compound heterozygotes at a molecular level. Compound heterozygotes have different mutations in the mutant alleles, as exemplified by SC hemoglobinopathy or cystic fibrosis due to a ΔF508/G542X genotype. Exceptions to this generalization occur when a patient is the product of a consanguineous mating or when particular mutant alleles are present in high frequency in the population, for example, sickle cell anemia with SS genotype or cystic fibrosis with a ΔF508/ΔF508 genotype.

Variation in manifestations due to allelic heterogeneity is particularly important. For example, Hurler mucopolysaccharidosis and Scheie mucopolysaccharidosis were thought to be different genetic conditions based on the severe, lethal phenotype in Hurler disease and the milder phenotype of bone and joint disease in Scheie disease. In fact, these conditions are both due to deficiency of L-iduronidase. Similarly, the severe Duchenne muscular dystrophy and milder Becker muscular dystrophy are allelic disorders, each of which can be caused by gene deletions, most often out-of-frame for Duchenne and in-frame for Becker. The classical and attenuated forms of adenomatous polyposis coli have about 15 years difference in the age of onset so that the attenuated disorder has minimal impact on reproduction, and unrecognized alleles of this type may be a major contributor to the risk of colon cancer. Additional examples of different clinical manifestations due to allelic heterogeneity are found throughout genetics. In many instances, a classical phenotype occurs when no functional gene product is produced, and there is frequently a continuum of milder expression arising from mutations that partially impair the function of the gene product. Compound heterozygotes contribute to the complexity of the clinical continuum. At the mild end of the continuum, mutant alleles encode a product that leads to a nearly normal clinical phenotype or to a phenotype that is normal under most environmental circumstances. This continuum includes detectable biochemical variation that is ordinarily not associated with clinical effect. Obviously, the amount of functional gene product required to prevent clinical symptoms depends on other genetic and environmental factors. As an example, an individual with "benign" methylmalonic acidemia is at risk during major catabolic disorders so that the benign designation is merely conditional. This type of genetic heterogeneity forms a part of the border between monogenic disorders and multifactorial diseases.

COMPLEX DISEASE TRAITS

The common chronic diseases of adults (such as essential hypertension, gout, coronary heart disease, diabetes mellitus, peptic ulcer disease, and schizophrenia), and the common birth defects (such as cleft lip and palate, spina bifida, and congenital heart disease) have long been known to "run in families," indicating a genetic contribution to etiology. These disorders are *complex disease traits* or *multifactorial genetic diseases* as discussed, with emphasis on the distinction between complexity involving quantitative trait loci and complexity involving locus heterogeneity (see "Genomic Medicine for Complex Traits" above). The principles of diseases caused by quantitative trait loci are discussed in detail in Chap 6. It is important to recognize the extraordinary heterogeneity of etiology for disorders such as cleft lip and palate; some cases are due to single-gene defects, some to chromosome abnormalities, some to specific in utero drug exposures, and the majority, presumably, to poorly understood, complex interactions of multiple genes and environmental factors.

In complex disease traits, *constitutional (polygenic) components* consist of multiple genes at independent loci whose effects interact in a cumulative fashion. An individual who inherits a particular combination of these genes has a relative risk that may combine with an *environmental component* to cross a "threshold" of biologic significance so that the individual is affected with a disease. For another individual in the same family to express the same syndrome, a similar combination of genes would present similar risks. Because sibs share half of their genes, the probability of a sib inheriting the same combination of genes is $(2)^n$, where n is the number of genes required to express the trait (assuming that none of the genes is linked).

The number of genes responsible for polygenic traits is unknown, and risk estimates are based on empiric risk figures (i.e., a direct tally of the proportion of affected relatives in previously reported families). In contrast to the monogenic disorders, in which 25 or 50 percent of the first-degree relatives of an affected proband are at genetic risk, complex disease traits usually affect no more than 5 to 10 percent of first-degree relatives. Moreover, the recurrence risk for these conditions varies from family to family and is influenced by two factors: the greater number of affected relatives and the more severe their disease, the higher the risk to other relatives. For example, the risk of cleft lip in the sibs of a child with unilateral cleft lip is about 2.5 percent, but if the lesion in the index case is bilateral, the risk in the sibs rises to 6 percent.

Multifactorial etiology is thought to be important for many diseases that develop after adolescence, and diseases with later age of onset may have decreased heritability on average. This is discussed in greater detail in Chap. 2 (see "Continuity of Monogenic, Multifactorial Modes of Inheritance" and Table 2-5).

The hypothesis of a polygenic component in the inheritance of multifactorial diseases is supported by the findings that a large fraction of all gene loci harbor polymorphic alleles. This variation in normal genes provides a substrate for variations in response to environmental factors. At present, the genetic loci most strikingly associated with predisposition to specific diseases are those that constitute the major histocompatibility or HLA (human leukocyte antigen) gene complex located on the short arm of chromosome 6 and consisting of multiple closely linked but distinct loci (A, B, DR, DQ, and DP; see Chap. 12). The products of these genes are proteins on the surface of cells involved in cellular immune recognition. Each HLA locus in the population consists of multiple alleles, each of which produces an immunologically distinct protein. For example, an individual may inherit any 2 of more than 36 alleles at the HLA-B locus. The inheritance of certain alleles predisposes to the development of certain diseases when the individual is exposed to an environmental challenge.

Complex disease traits are heterogeneous in etiology in the sense that the relative contribution of genetic ("risk genes") and environmental factors vary from patient to patient. As discussed above, among common phenotypes that are largely multifactorial, some cases may be due to monogenic or chromosomal abnormalities. For example, although coronary heart disease is usually of complex etiology, about 5 percent of subjects with premature myocardial infarctions are heterozygotes for familial hypercholesterolemia, a single-gene disorder that produces atherosclerosis in the absence of an extraordinary environmental factor (see Chap. 120). However, even in a single-gene disorder such as familial hypercholesterolemia, other loci (e.g., the genes for apolipoprotein B, apolipoprotein (a), lipoprotein lipase, and apolipoprotein E) and nongenetic factors (diet and smoking) can influence the phenotype. The complexity of the etiology for coronary artery disease is detailed in multiple chapters in Part 12 of this text. Multiple genetic and nongenetic factors affect the risk. An appreciation of this etiologic heterogeneity and careful investigation of each patient are prerequisites for counseling families at risk for these disorders.

Methods for unraveling the molecular basis of multifactorial etiology include the analysis of candidate genes using association studies, sib-pair analysis, and other complex strategies. The advantages of focusing on molecular variations that are important in gene function have been emphasized. The complexity of these approaches is daunting, but major loci have been identified for a number of multifactorial diseases, including hypertension (see "Complex Disease Traits" under "Genomic Medicine" above and Chap. 211) and insulin-dependent diabetes mellitus (see Chaps. 6 and 69) in which several loci in addition to HLA are involved.

PHARMACOGENETICS AND INTERACTION BETWEEN GENETIC TRAITS AND ENVIRONMENTAL FACTORS

The term *pharmacogenomics* has been popularized to describe a somewhat diverse set of concepts including 1) pharmacogenetics (to be discussed immediately below), 2) the potential to resurrect drugs abandoned because of adverse effects by distinguishing individuals with genotypes causing susceptibility to side effects, 3) identification of responder subgroups based on genotype, 4) development of disease-specific therapies (e.g., hematin in porphyria), and 5) using data from the Human Genome Project to identify novel gene products as drug targets.

As discussed in Chap. 9, many single-gene mutations can cause abnormal responses to environmental factors as illustrated by pharmacogenetic disorders that produce major, often life-threatening, idiosyncratic responses to drugs (Table 1-6). There is significant genetic variation in response to drugs such as isoniazid, some beta-adrenergic blockers, and tricyclic antidepressants. Other important interactions between genotype and drugs include glucose-6-phosphate dehydrogenase deficiency (Chap. 179), acute intermittent porphyria (Chap. 124), hemochromatosis (iron supplements; Chap. 127), and muscle diseases with susceptibility to malignant hyperthermia (Chap. 9).

Misinterpretation of adverse drug reactions can cause serious harm to patients, and unusual or idiosyncratic reactions should be considered as genetically determined until proven otherwise. Fortunately, the pharmacogenetic disorders are a group of diseases for which therapy is straightforward: avoidance of the noxious drug by the patient and relatives at risk.

In addition to drugs, environmental factors may aggravate specific genetic traits. Cigarette smoke is particularly deleterious to persons homozygous (and possibly heterozygous) for α_1-antitrypsin deficiency, who are predisposed to the development of emphysema. Patients with xeroderma pigmentosum are sensitive to the ultraviolet exposure of sunlight. Avoidance of milk at an early age prevents the life-threatening complications of galactosemia, and diet is an important variable for most forms of hyperlipidemia. Unfortunately, a modern society is subjected to an endless array of novel environmental exposures. The current widespread utilization of aspartame is an example of a special risk for subjects with phenylketonuria.

TAKING THE FAMILY HISTORY

Recording a *family history* should be a routine part of primary care (Fig. 1-25) and should be performed in greater detail in patients with a likely genetic disorder. The first step is to obtain certain information on the *proband* or *index case*, and on each of the *first-degree relatives* (i.e., the parents, siblings, and offspring of the proband). This information includes the given name, surname, maiden name, birth date or current age, age at death, cause of death, and name or description of any disease or defect. Similar information should be recorded on reproductive partners where appropriate. More distant relatives should be included for autosomal dominant disorders, X-linked disorders, and chromosomal translocations. For reproductive counseling, the reproductive plans for a couple should be recorded including use of contraception or previous sterilization procedure. It is important to ask specifically about spontaneous abortions, stillbirths, and childhood deaths, because these are frequently omitted and may

Table 1-6 Examples of Inherited Disorders Involving an Abnormal Response to Drugs

Disorder	Molecular abnormality	Mode of inheritance	Frequency	Clinical effect	Drugs producing abnormal response
Slow inactivation of isoniazid	Isoniazid acetylase in liver	Autosomal recessive	50% of U.S. population	Polyneuritis	Isoniazid, sulfamethazine, sulfamaprine, phenalzine, dapsone, hydralazine
Suxamethonium sensitivity	Pseudocholinesterase in plasma	Autosomal recessive	Several mutant alleles; most common affects 1 in 2500	Apnea	Suxamethonium, succinylcholine
Malignant hyperthermia	Ryanodine receptor	Autosomal dominant	1 in 20,000 anesthetized	Severe, hyperpyrexia, muscle rigidity, death	Such anesthetics as halothane, succinylcholine, methoxyflurane, ether, cyclopropane
Debrisoquine sensitivity	Cytochrome P450, CYP2D6	Autosomal recessive	5–10%; range 0–18% in ethnic groups	Toxicity of drug; e.g., postural hypotension	Antiarrhythmics, beta blockers, neuroleptics, tricyclic antidepressants
Glucose 6-phosphate dehydrogenase deficiency	Glucose 6-phosphate dehydrogenase in erythrocytes	X-linked	~500 million affected persons in world; common in persons of African, Mediterranean, Asiatic origin; multiple mutant alleles	Hemolysis	Analgesics, sulfonamides, antimalarials, nitrofurantoin, other drugs

provide information of great relevance. Pedigrees should be drawn in a manner that distinguishes siblings and half siblings.

Direct inquiry regarding possible consanguinity should be a routine part of recording the family history and is of particular relevance to the occurrence of autosomal recessive disorders. Reproductive couples can be asked whether they may be related in any way, and this information should be supplemented by inquiries regarding surnames, ethnic status, and geographic origin of families. Cousin marriages are common in many societies and in isolated areas. Incest is an extreme form of consanguinity and may occur in the context of sexual abuse of children and teenagers. The risk of autosomal recessive disorders, including mental retardation, is high for incestuous matings.[71,108]

Interpreting the family history is aided by understanding the variation in expression in specific genetic disorders. Assuming that the family history is focused on the presence of a specific disorder within the family, meticulous questioning regarding possible manifestations in relatives is important. In addition to recording the general health status of all first-degree relatives, inquiry should be made about other genetically determined conditions in the family. This is often best done by asking whether any relatives have experienced genetic diseases, rare conditions, mental retardation, birth defects, childhood deaths, or occurrence of common adult disorders at a young age. The philosophy of the physician should be to identify any genetic issues of potential importance for all family members and to urge evaluation, education, counseling, and intervention as appropriate.

Ethnic and geographic origin of family members can be an important part of the family history, because monogenic and complex disease traits occur at different frequencies in different

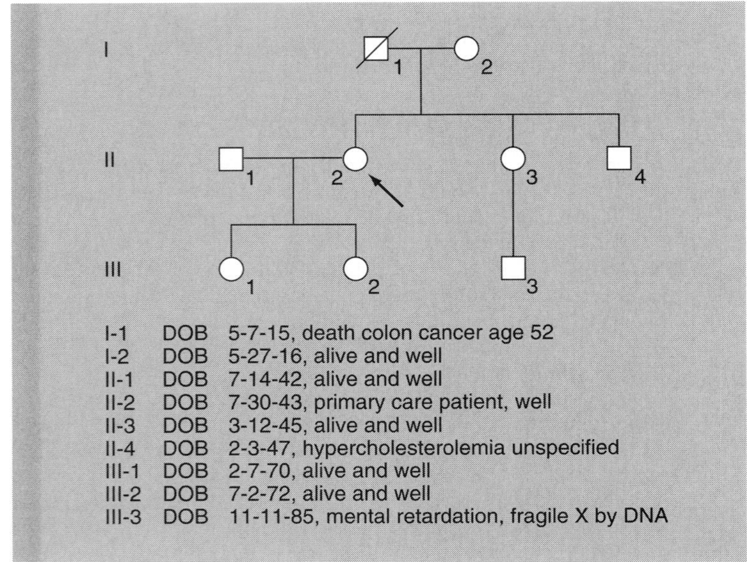

Fig. 1-25 Suggested style for routine recording of family history. Individual II-2 is intended to represent a healthy individual (the patient) in a primary care setting.

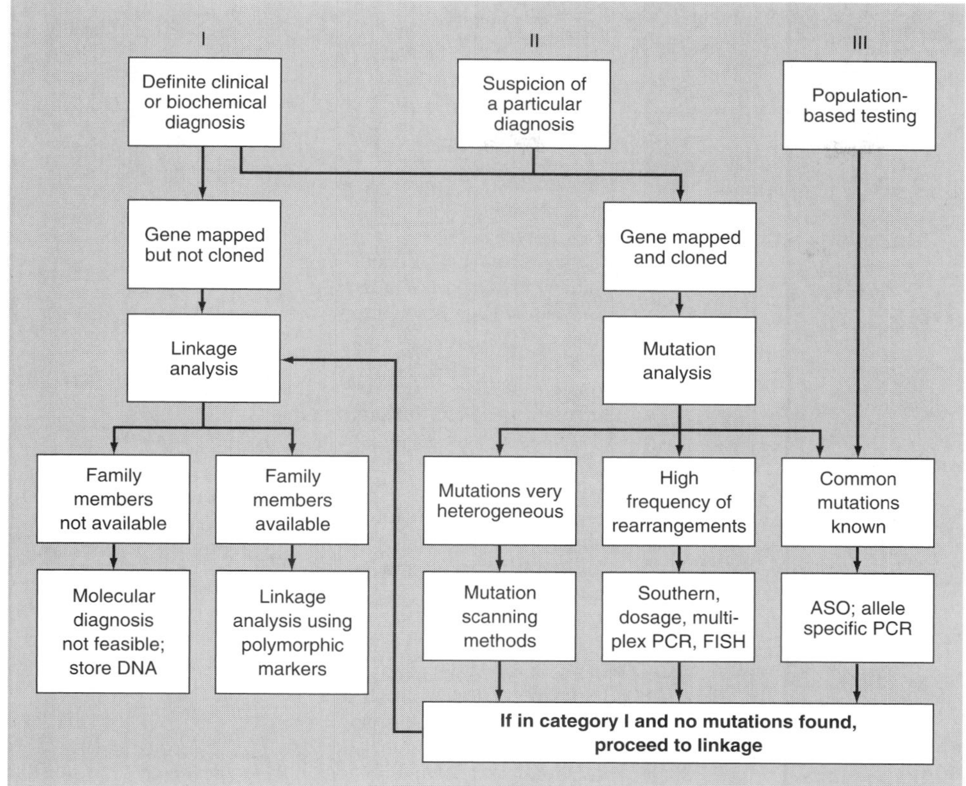

Fig. 1-26 A scheme for utilization of DNA analysis for genetic diagnosis.

populations (Table 1-5). Screening for diabetes mellitus, hypertension, and hyperlipidemia is particularly important in high-risk populations (e.g., the high incidence of diabetes mellitus in some native North American populations), and different options for reproductive screening are offered to different ethnic groups (e.g., Tay-Sachs testing for Ashkenazic Jews, thalassemia testing for Mediterranean populations, sickle cell testing for populations of African descent, and perhaps cystic fibrosis testing for populations of European descent).

MOLECULAR STRATEGIES FOR ANALYSIS OF MENDELIAN DISORDERS

As for any form of clinical diagnosis, a detailed history (including family history) and clinical examination is the appropriate starting point. In some cases, the phenotype of the patient may be characteristic of a specific genetic disease, and the diagnostic information may be supplemented by the family history or by specific biochemical tests. A general scheme for utilization of molecular methods for diagnosis is depicted in Fig. 1-26. Although such techniques are powerful and provide precise information, the studies are often performed by research laboratories, academic laboratories, and commercial laboratories with variable levels of experience and attention to quality assurance. One report found that 35 percent of 136 laboratories incorrectly typed one or more alleles from 12 alleles included in a trial.[109] It is essential that clinicians are familiar with the quality of work in diagnostic laboratories and interpret data cautiously in the full context of the medical circumstance.

Definite Clinical and/or Biochemical Genetic Diagnosis

In many cases, a clinical genetic diagnosis is established before undertaking DNA analysis to confirm the clinical diagnosis and provide molecular definition. The goals in such cases may include genotype/phenotype correlation; that is, predicting the severity of the disease based on the mutations. For example, some mutations cause nonneuronopathic Gaucher disease, and others cause neuronopathic disease (see Chap. 146). Predicting the phenotype, future risks, and complications from the genotype is complex. Extensive studies are necessary, and great caution must be exercised to avoid overinterpretation or misinterpretation of molecular data. In principle, important therapeutic decisions can be based on genotypic data (e.g., α_1-antitrypsin deficiency or familial hypercholesterolemia), but exact predictions for individuals may be hazardous, due to variation in expression, even when detailed molecular knowledge is available (i.e., triplet repeat length in Huntington disease). Extensive studies are in progress for Marfan syndrome and breast cancer due to BRCA1 mutations, but the power and the limitations of genotype/phenotype correlations have not been defined for many disorders. Genotype/phenotype correlation and confirmation of diagnosis rely on mutation analysis and generally cannot be based on linkage analysis. Additional applications of molecular diagnosis include heterozygote detection, presymptomatic diagnosis, prenatal diagnosis, and preimplantation diagnosis. Family studies should be performed using mutation analysis if possible, reserving linkage analysis as a secondary option.

Clarification of a Possible Genetics Diagnosis

In some cases, there may be a suspicion of a particular genetic disease, but the findings may be inconclusive, because it is too early in the clinical course or the findings are atypical in some way. This frequently occurs when it is possible to detect some mutations causing a disease, but when it is impractical to rule out the possibility of an undetected mutation. In the case of dominant disorders or X-linked diseases in males, a diagnosis may be established by demonstration of deletion, frameshift, nonsense mutation, expanded triplet repeat, or unspecified truncation mutation. Failure to find a mutation does not rule out the diagnosis but makes it less likely if analysis is known to detect most disease mutations. Molecular analysis is particularly useful in the

Table 1-7 Examples of the Role of Molecular Analysis for Diagnosis of Genetic Disease

Disease	Detection Mutation*	Linkage Analysis	Comments
Sickle cell anemia	++++		PCR with ASO
Other globin disorders	++++	+	PCR with ASO
Hemophilia A & B	+++	+	Mutation scanning & sequencing
Phenylketonuria	++	++	PCR with ASO
α_1-Antitrypsin ZZ	++++		PCR with ASO
Familial hypercholesterolemia	++++		Mutation scanning & sequencing
Lesch-Nyhan syndrome	++++		Mutation scanning & sequencing
Tay-Sachs disease	+++	+	PCR with ASO in Ashkenazim
Duchenne muscular dystrophy	+++	++	Multiplex PCR, Southern
Retinoblastoma	+++	+	Mutation scanning & sequencing
Huntington disease	++++		Southern & PCR for expanding triplet
Myotonic dystrophy	++++		Southern & PCR for expanding triplet
Adult polycystic kidney disease	++	++	Mutation scanning & sequencing
Fragile X syndrome	++++		Southern & PCR for expanding triplet
Cystic fibrosis	+++	+	PCR with ASO
Neurofibromatosis 1	++	++	Mutation scanning & sequencing, PTT
BRCA1 breast cancer	+++	+	Mutation scanning & sequencing
Polyposis of colon	+++	+	Mutation scanning & sequencing, PTT
Marfan syndrome	++	++	Mutation scanning & sequencing
Gaucher disease	++++	+	PCR with ASO in Ashkenazim
Glycogen storage disease 1a	+++	+	PCR with ASO
Familial hypertrophic cardiomyopathy	++++	+	Southern & mutation scanning
Spinal muscular atrophy	+++	+	Southern and PCR for deletions
Charcot-Marie-Tooth disease IA	++++	+	PFGE or FISH for duplication
Prader-Willi	++++		FISH for deletion & methylation testing
Angelman	+++		FISH for deletions, methylation, mutation scanning & sequencing
DiGeorge/velocardiofacial syndrome	++++		FISH for deletion
Rett syndrome	++++		Mutation scanning & sequencing

*Symbols of + to ++++ indicate relative importance of an approach as of 2000; the status for disorders could change rapidly. PCR = polymerase chain reactions; ASO = allele-specific oligonucleotide or other method to detect point mutations; PFGE = pulsed-field gel electrophoresis; STR = short tandem repeat; FISH = fluorescence in situ hybridization; PTT = protein truncation test; mutation scanning often done by DHPLC.

differential diagnosis of triplet repeat disorders, because virtually all clinically important expansions can be identified. Likewise, protein truncation testing can be helpful in evaluating possible cases of neurofibromatosis or hereditary breast cancer, but will not detect all mutations. For autosomal recessive disorders, the situation may be complex (e.g., a phenotype of bronchiectasis possibly related to cystic fibrosis). Identification of pathologic mutations in both copies of the gene establishes a diagnosis, whereas identification of a pathologic mutation in one allele only increases the probability but does not prove that the suspect phenotype is related to mutation at this locus. Failure to identify any pathologic mutations lessens the likelihood that the disease is related to mutation at this locus but does not eliminate that possibility because mutations can occur outside the coding sequence or otherwise be undetected by the method utilized.

Population-Based DNA Testing

Utilization of DNA testing as a population-based screening method is similar to nonmolecular methods of population screening such as newborn screening; cholesterol measurements; mammography; prostate specific antigen testing; carrier screening for Tay-Sachs, sickle cell, or thalassemia; and screening for maternal serum α-fetoprotein and related analytes. As with established screening methods, DNA testing could be applied for (a) presymptomatic detection of disease susceptibility with plans for intervention, (b) carrier screening to offer reproductive counseling, or (c) prenatal testing. Many forms of genotypic analysis based on protein methods (e.g., sickle cell, α_1-antitrypsin and Tay-Sachs testing) might be performed more specifically or economically in the future using DNA methods. Whether screening by DNA analysis for carriers of cystic fibrosis mutations should be offered routinely is being debated; such testing is likely to increase and offspring or relatives of known carriers are likely to seek testing preferentially. With DNA variation of known or likely disease significance in the loci for hemochromatosis, apolipoprotein E, apolipoprotein Lp (a), angiotensinogen, angiotensin-converting enzyme, α_1-antitrypsin, and many other genes, population-based DNA screening might become a powerful preventive approach by providing possible pharmacologic, lifestyle, and other (e.g., phlebotomy in hemochromatosis) interventions for individuals with high-risk genotypes. There is debate as to the appropriateness of population-based screening for disorders in which the definition of risk and potential for intervention are not fully known, as exemplified by BRCA1 mutations. Testing for disorders where specificity is low and/or there is no potential for intervention is generally discouraged (e.g., apolipoprotein E genotype and Alzheimer risk).

Examples of Mutation Detection

As indicated in the section designated "Gene Mapped and Cloned" in Fig. 1-26, different methods of analysis are employed for molecular diagnosis depending on the most common type of mutation for a particular disorder, whether the mutations are large rearrangements or point mutations, and whether the mutations are of predictable type from ancient origins or are more heterogeneous and more recent in origin. Examples of common genetic disorders are listed in Table 1-7 with the type of analysis that is most applicable.

Examples of large molecular defects that can be detected by Southern blotting include α-thalassemia, some forms of

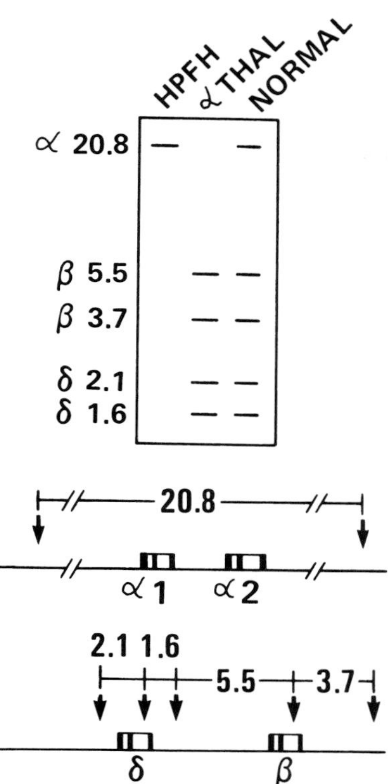

Fig. 1-27 Depiction of Southern blot analysis of human globin genes. *Above*, DNA was isolated from a normal individual and from patients with homozygous hereditary persistence of fetal hemoglobin (HPFH) or homozygous α-thalassemia (α THAL). DNA was digested with the enzyme *Eco*RI. A mixed DNA probe was prepared by reverse transcription of reticulocyte globin mRNA. *Below*, arrows indicate *Eco*RI cut sites in the α- and β-globin regions, and numbers indicate DNA fragment size in kilobases. (*Adapted from Kan and Dozy.*[110] *Used by permission.*)

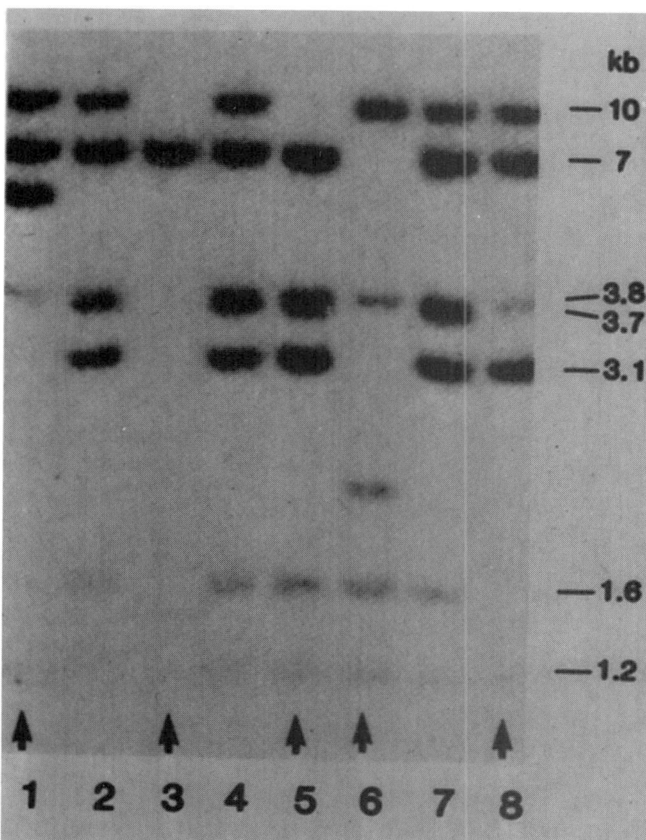

Fig. 1-28 Detection of deletions in the DNA isolated from Duchenne muscular dystrophy patients using a dystrophin cDNA probe. Southern blot analysis detects deletions (absence of fragments) in five of eight patients (arrows). A junction fragment is clearly demonstrated in patients 1 and 6. (*From Koenig et al.*[111] *Used by permission.*)

β-thalassemia, and hereditary persistence of fetal hemoglobin (Fig. 1-27).[110] For Duchenne/Becker muscular dystrophy, 60 to 70 percent of cases involve large deletions that are easily detected by Southern blotting (Fig. 1-28).[111] If one considers Fig. 1-28 in the context of carrier detection for family members, a case such as lane 1 with a novel, junctional DNA fragment is optimal because the presence of this fragment is absolutely diagnostic for carrier status for females in this family. For cases such as lane 3, heterozygote detection depends on dosage analysis with one copy of the deleted fragments in carrier females, and two copies of the nondeleted fragments. Dosage analysis is more difficult and requires meticulous quantitation and attention to internal controls. For families of the type depicted in lane 2, where Southern blotting is normal and does not detect a presumed point mutation in the gene, this analysis is not useful for carrier detection. Deletions such as those seen in Duchenne/Becker dystrophy can also be detected using PCR to test for the presence or absence of various sites in the gene (Fig. 1-29). Deleted segments are identified by the absence of particular PCR products in a multiplex reaction testing for the presence of various sites along the length of the gene.

Expanding triplet repeat mutations are the cause of myotonic dystrophy, fragile X mental retardation, Huntington disease, X-linked spinobulbar muscular atrophy, and other neurodegenerative disorders. With fragile X mental retardation and myotonic dystrophy, severity of the disease increases as premutation progresses to mutation and mild mutation progresses to severe mutation, the phenomenon of anticipation. Depending on the size of the expanded triplet repeat, these mutations can be detected by Southern blotting and/or PCR analysis. Fig. 1-30 is an example of an expanded triplet repeat mutation with more severe disease in later generations. Although the size of a triplet repeat expansion has potential information for genotype/phenotype correlations, experience and caution are needed to make phenotypic predictions.

For many disorders, typically including any autosomal recessive disorders and autosomal dominant and X-linked disorders with minimal effect on reproduction, mutations of ancient origin may be present in many people in the population. Even when these are common traits, there may still be extensive molecular heterogeneity as for β-thalassemia (Fig. 1-5). Likewise, in cystic fibrosis, the common ΔF508 mutation accounts for

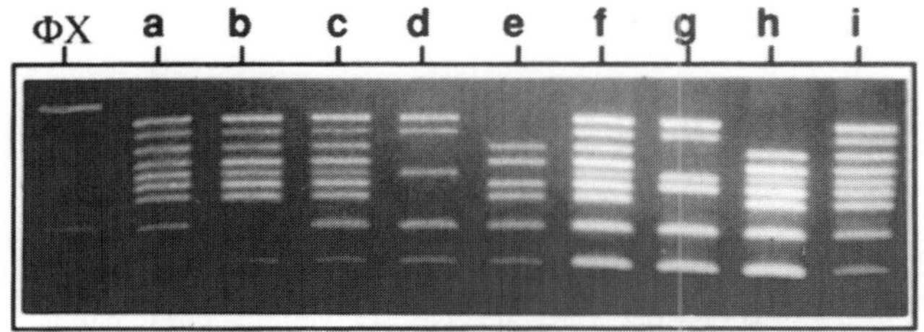

Fig. 1-29 Multiplex amplification of DNA using PCR to detect deletions in the dystrophin gene. Nine amplifications detecting fragments of nine different exons are performed in a single tube and analyzed on an agarose gel. Deletions can be seen as missing fragments for the Duchenne dystrophy patients shown in lanes b, d, e, g, and h, while no deletion is detected in lanes a, c, f, and i. ϕX indicates DNA markers. (*Used by permission. Multicenter Study Group: JAMA 267:2609, 1992.*)

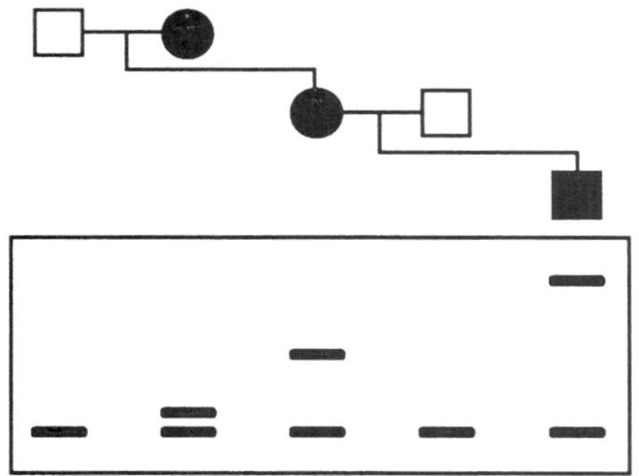

Fig. 1-30 Representation of Southern blot analysis revealing an expanding triplet repeat mutation in a myotonic dystrophy family. A grandmother and mother with the adult form of the disease and a child with the infantile form of the disease are shown. The normal-size genomic DNA fragment (lowest band) is present in homozygous form in the unaffected individuals and in heterozygous form in the affected family members. The larger mutant fragment is present in all affected individuals, with its size increasing from grandmother to mother to child. (*From Beaudet AL, Ballabio A: Harrison's Principles of Internal Medicine 13th ed. New York, McGraw-Hill, 1994, p 349. Used by permission.*)

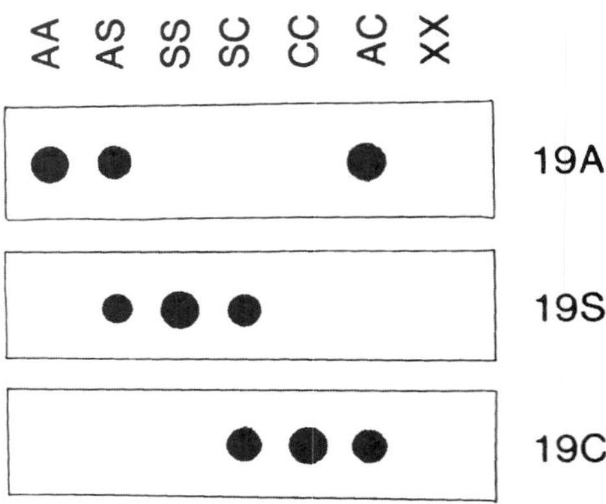

Fig. 1-31 Genotype analysis of PCR-amplified genomic DNA using allele-specific oligonucleotide (ASO) probes. DNA was extracted from the blood of individuals of β-globin genotypes AA, AS, SS, SC, CC, and AC, and homozygous deletion (XX). The DNA was applied to replicate filters for hybridization with ASO as follows: β^A probe (19A), β^S probe (19S), or β^C probe (19C). (*From Mullis K et al. Specific enzymatic amplification of DNA in vitro: The polymerase chain reaction. Cold Spring Harbor Symp Quant Biol 51:263, 1986. Used by permission.*)

approximately 70 percent of mutations in most populations, but hundreds of different mutations have been identified among the remaining 30 percent of mutant chromosomes. Common mutations of this type are usually best tested using some allele-specific method such as hybridization with allele specific oligonucleotides. Typically, such analysis for a single disease may require testing for only a few alleles as in α_1-antitrypsin deficiency or for 10 to 30 or more mutations in the case of β-thalassemia or cystic fibrosis (Figs. 1-31 and 1-32).

Mutation analysis is difficult because most patients carry heterogeneous point mutations including autosomal dominant disorders that impair reproductive fitness and X-linked disorders that limit reproduction in males. The factors influencing the proportion of cases of autosomal dominant disorders due to new mutation are discussed above. In these cases of heterogeneous mutations, some method for analyzing the entire gene is needed. Sequencing all of the exons of a gene is feasible if the coding region of the gene is small, and this approach is being used increasingly even for genes such as BRCA1 and BRCA2 with many exons. However, full-length sequencing is expensive, and identification of mutations depends on a variety of procedures designed to detect small mutations in DNA as discussed above (see "Analysis of Mutations"). The protein truncation test is useful for detecting certain classes of mutations and is quite useful for polyposis of the colon (Fig. 1-33) and breast cancer due to BRCA1 mutations. In many cases, searching for mutations is an activity for

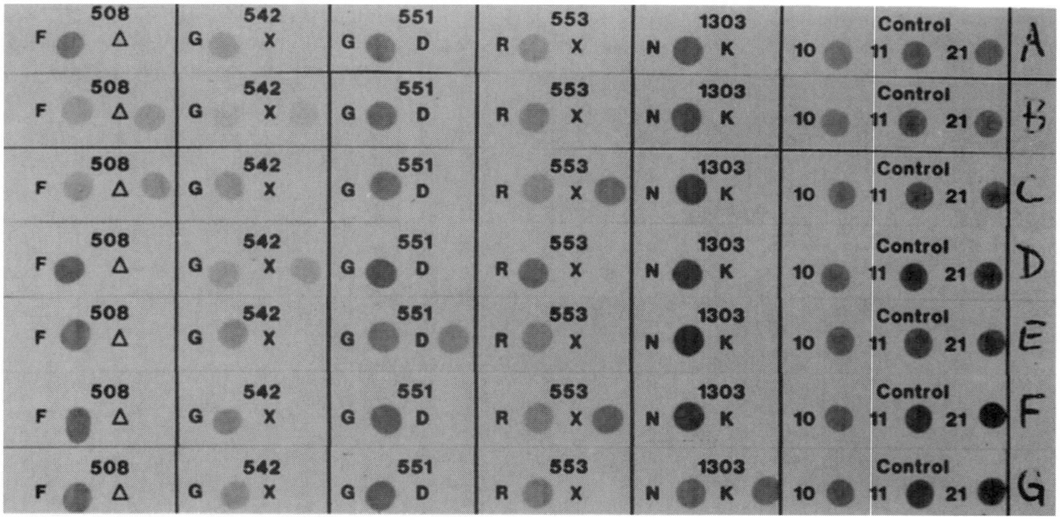

Fig. 1-32 Reverse-dot ASO analysis for various point mutations causing cystic fibrosis. For each mutation, the PCR product is hybridized to an ASO dot on the left for normal allele and on the right for the mutant allele. The positions for each ASO are indicated as follows: F and Δ for the ΔF508 mutation; G and X for the G542X mutation; G and D for the G551D mutation; R and X for the R553X mutation; N and K for the N1303K mutation; and 10 or 11 or 21 under control for the ASO to detect the amplification of exons of those numbers. Mutations are designated by single letter amino acid code (X = nonsense), with the normal amino acid followed by the position number followed by the substituted amino acid. Thus, G551D is substitution of aspartic acid (D) for glycine (G) at position 551. ΔF508 is deletion of phenylalanine at position 508. Letters at the right margin identify individuals of the following genotypes: A = no mutation; B = ΔF508/G542X compound heterozygote; C = ΔF508/R553X compound heterozygote; D = G542X heterozygote; E = G551D heterozygote; F = R553X heterozygote; and G = N1303K heterozygote. (*Provided by H. Erlich, Roche Molecular Systems.*)

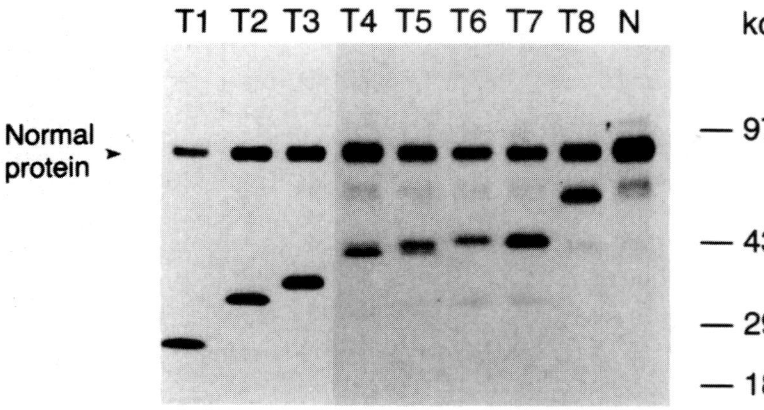

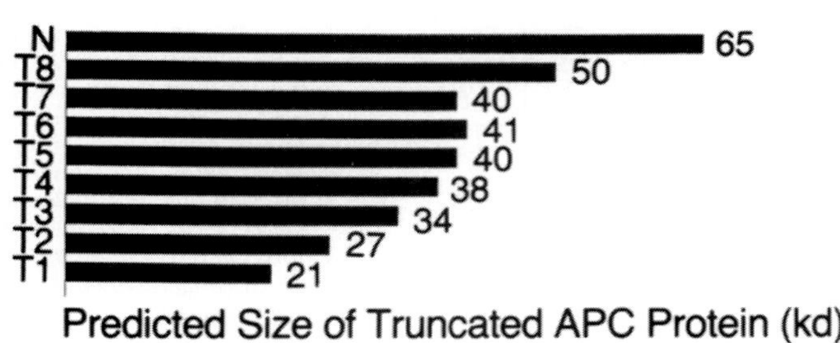

Fig. 1-33 Protein assay for the detection of known truncating mutations causing familial polyposis. Representative samples of sporadic colorectal tumors (T1 through T8), known to have truncating mutations from sequence analysis, demonstrate the expected truncated APC (adenomatous polyposis coli) proteins. A substantial amount of normal, full-length APC protein is noted in the remaining normal alleles. A sample of normal tissue (N) is also shown. The numbers to the right of the horizontal bars indicate the predicted size of the truncated APC protein (*From Powell SM et al. Molecular diagnosis of familial adenomatous polyposis. N Engl J Med 329:1982, 1993.*)

research laboratories and beyond the capacity of routine clinical service.

Diagnosis by Linkage Analysis

When a gene is cloned but it is not practical to identify the mutation or mutations in a given family, it is sometimes possible to perform molecular diagnosis using linkage analysis. In other cases, mutation analysis is impossible because the disease gene is not cloned, but informative DNA markers may be available. In such cases, linkage diagnosis can be performed with a negligible possibility of crossovers (see Fig. 1-13). For linkage analysis, some genetic marker near the disease locus must be *informative*, namely key individuals in the pedigree must have two different alleles at the marker locus. Linkage analysis is appropriate when an individual carries one mutant gene and one normal gene, and when the goal is to determine which has been transmitted to the next generation. Many such analyses are informative because highly polymorphic short tandem repeat polymorphisms are frequently present within and near genes causing diseases.

A second requirement for linkage analysis is that of *phase* information between the marker locus and the disease locus for genetic analysis. If an individual is heterozygous for a marker that is tightly linked to a mutation, it must be determined which allele for the marker is on the chromosome with the disease allele and which is on the homologous chromosome with the normal allele. When the genetic marker is informative and the phase is known, genetic diagnosis can include heterozygote detection, presymptomatic diagnosis, detection of lack of penetrance, and prenatal diagnosis. When the DNA probe or marker is within the mutant gene, crossing-over between the genetic marker and the disease causing mutation usually is negligible. Duchenne muscular dystrophy is an exception because the responsible gene is extremely large, and crossing-over occurs at a detectable frequency within the gene.

Fig. 1-34 shows examples of molecular diagnosis by linkage, when there is negligible recombination between the loci. Genetic marker data are presented as letters that might represent simple marker alleles or haplotypes of markers. A *haplotype* is a cluster of tightly linked specific alleles on a chromosome. Phase can usually be determined from a single index case for autosomal recessive disorders (Fig. 1-34A). Fetuses of AC genotype are predicted to be affected in Fig. 1-34A while fetuses of AA or BC genotype are predicted to be carriers and those of AB genotype to be noncarriers. In Fig. 1-34B, carrier detection is sought for the aunt and uncle of the affected. The data on the maternal side require analysis of the grandparents and predict the aunt is a noncarrier. Although the paternal grandparents are deceased, it is still possible to conclude that the uncle is a noncarrier because he does not inherit the C haplotype that is linked to disease allele on the paternal side. For autosomal dominant disorders, linkage phase usually cannot be determined from a single affected individual (Fig. 1-34C). Exceptions occur in retinoblastoma, when analysis of tumor DNA may distinguish the allele on the abnormal chromosome (often retained in the tumor) from the allele on the normal chromosome (often lost in the tumor). Linkage phase for autosomal dominant disorders can be determined from two appropriate individuals and it is not essential that both be affected if penetrance is complete. Fetuses of AA and AC genotype are predicted to be affected in Fig. 1-34D and fetuses of AB and BC genotype are predicted to be unaffected. In Fig. 1-34E, fetuses of AB or BC genotype are predicted to be affected, and fetuses of AA or AC genotype are predicted to be unaffected. For X-linked disorders, phase information can be obtained from a single affected male individual (Fig. 1-34F). In general, although linkage information can predict the genotype of offspring of individuals of known genotype, it cannot be used consistently to determine the genotype of antecedents of individuals of known genotypes because of the possibility of new mutation from one generation to the next. This is exemplified by an X-linked disorder, where linkage information will not clarify whether or not the mother of an isolated affected male is a heterozygote (Fig. 1-34G). This limitation is an important difference between direct detection of a mutation and linkage analysis; but occasionally, linkage analysis can suggest the genotype of an antecedent. Note in Fig. 1-34G that

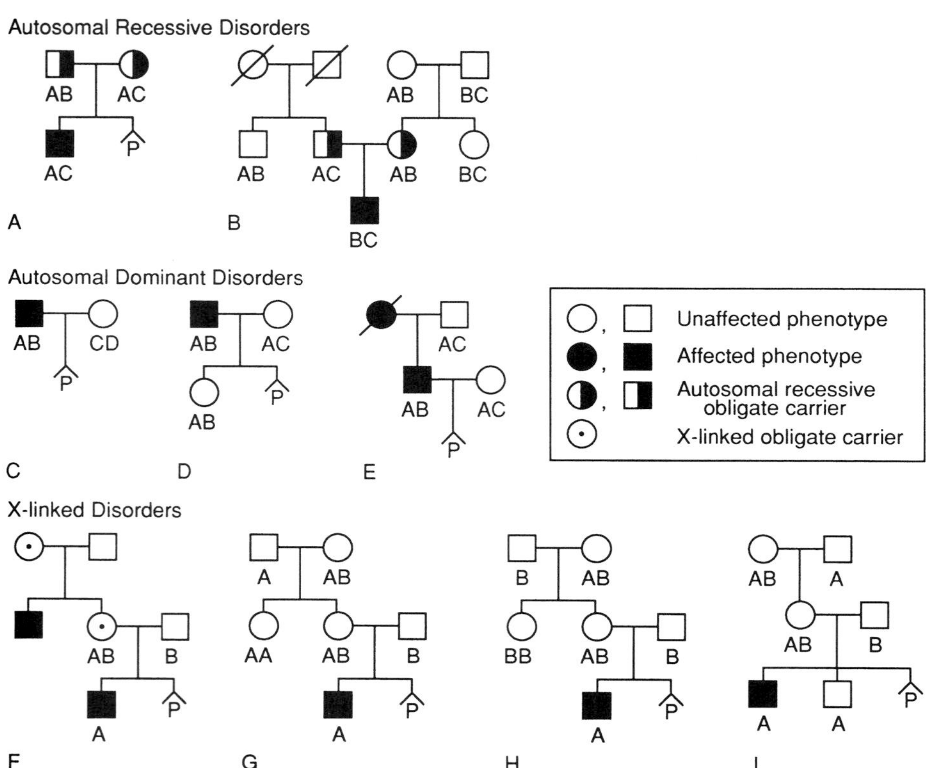

Fig. 1-34 Examples of molecular diagnosis by genetic linkage with negligible recombination between the DNA probe and the disease locus. Letters below pedigree symbols indicate alleles for a DNA marker. Families A and B depict autosomal recessive disorders; C through E depict autosomal dominant disorders; and F through I depict X-linked disorders. Complete penetrance is assumed. See text for discussion. (*From Beaudet AL, Ballabio A: in Harrison's Principles of Internal Medicine 13th ed. New York, McGraw-Hill, 1994, p 349. Used by permission*).

the mutation arose on the chromosome from the unaffected maternal grandfather; it can be predicted that the maternal grandmother and the maternal aunt of the index case do not carry the mutation and that either the mother or the index case is the recipient of the new mutation. The situation is similar in Fig. 1-34H, except that the mutation is on the chromosome from the maternal grandmother and the new mutation could go back further in the family. Still by linkage analysis, the maternal aunt is not a carrier of the mutation. The genotype of an antecedent also can be inferred when a woman has two sons with the same DNA marker, one son being affected and one son being unaffected with the X-linked disorder (Fig. 1-34I). In this instance, the mother is not a heterozygote for the X-linked disorder, although the possibility of gonadal mosaicism (i.e., some proportion of the maternal germ cells have the new mutation) is not eliminated.

Linkage analysis also can be performed with DNA markers that show detectable recombination with a disease locus, but this introduces probabilities of misdiagnosis due to recombination. Problems with recombination in linkage diagnosis become less common as innumerable highly informative markers are identified.

DIAGNOSIS AND PREVENTION OF GENETIC DISEASES

The present trend for couples to have smaller families, the increased availability of genetic testing, and increased public awareness require that health care providers give attention and priority to genetic services. Primary-care physicians are called upon to play a more active role in informing patients of genetic and reproductive risks and options. In many clinical situations, the primary physician can give genetic advice after the relatively simple principles of medical genetics and genetic counseling have been mastered. In other situations, the complexities may make referral to a genetic specialist a necessity, but a good genetic history is essential even for identification of families for appropriate referral. For a more in-depth discussion of these principles, the reader is referred to Vogel and Motulsky's *Human Genetics: Problems and Approaches*[71] and Harper's *Practical Genetic Counselling*.[112] Genetic counseling may be provided because of the occurrence of an affected individual (index case) in a family. Other types of programs are population based and may include newborn screening, heterozygote screening, prenatal screening, and screening for disease in later life.

Genetic Counseling with an Index Case

Proper counseling for genetic diseases requires the advance identification of matings that are capable of producing genotypes associated with medical disorders. These may involve matings in which one of the two individuals is carrying a dominant or X-linked mutation or a balanced translocation, or matings in which both individuals carry a deleterious recessive allele at the same locus. Such individuals have usually been identified through the birth of an affected child or near relative, in which case retrospective genetic counseling can be provided.

When advising family members about the risk of transmitting a disorder that has already affected someone in the family, the counselor's first step is to be certain of the *correct diagnosis*, in particular to make certain that the problem in question is truly of genetic origin. This is especially important in disorders that may have either a genetic or nongenetic etiology, such as deafness or mental retardation. Second, if the disease has a hereditary element, the possibility of genetic heterogeneity must be considered.

Estimation of the *recurrence risk* of a disease requires knowledge of the genetic mechanisms controlling the relevant disorder. When more than one genetic mechanism exists, or when environmental factors can cause clinically indistinguishable traits, the *relative probabilities* of the different mechanisms operating in the particular family are computed. For conditions determined by simple Mendelian inheritance, there is no difficulty in predicting the probability of an offspring's being affected, provided the genotypes of the parents can be deduced. Identification of the parental genotype is easiest if a biochemical or molecular test is available to detect the mutant gene.

For autosomal dominant disorders, identification of the parental genotype is often more difficult because of the occurrence of *lack of penetrance* and *variation in expression*. In counseling a family in which one relative is affected with a dominant disorder, it is important that appropriate clinical examination of all first-degree relatives and appropriately selected distant relatives be carried out. If relatives appear unaffected, there is the possibility that the gene is present but not penetrant or the possibility of delayed age of onset or mild expression. When no relatives are affected, the possibility of a new dominant mutation must be entertained. It is increasingly feasible to determine genotypes using biochemical and molecular methods for many but not all disorders.

When advising families about multifactorial genetic diseases, such as diabetes mellitus, in which the inheritance pattern is not simple, the physician must resort to empiric risk estimates that have been derived from retrospectively assembled data.[71] Even within a multifactorial disorder such as diabetes mellitus, the genotype at the HLA cluster can be used to greatly modify the risk for insulin dependent diabetes, and the primary mutation can be identified in other cases as for families with defects in glucokinase (see Chap. 67).

Once the parental genotypes are deduced, the genetic prognosis is usually presented in terms of probability that a given couple will produce an affected offspring. The physician providing genetic counseling must make certain that the couple understands not only the meaning of such absolute risk figures but also the severity of the disease and the variability in clinical expression. In other words, in dealing with a disorder such as α_1-antitrypsin deficiency, it is important for the parents to realize that they have a 25 percent risk of producing a child with this disorder and that a certain proportion of children with the disorder have severe disease with both liver and pulmonary manifestations, a certain proportion have mild disease with only pulmonary manifestations, and so forth. They should also have an understanding of the potential impact of the disease on their family. This is evidence that perception of the burden of a disorder is an important factor in the decision-making process for couples with increased genetic risks.[113,114]

Heterozygote Detection

Heterozygote testing is one form of genetic screening. The efficiency of a genetic screening test is related to its sensitivity (detection rate), and its false positive rate (equivalent to 1 minus specificity).[115,116] Sensitivity is defined as the ability of the test to identify those with the mutant genotype. Such persons yield either a positive test (with frequency a) or a normal (false negative) test (with frequency c).

$$\text{Sensitivity} = \frac{a}{a + c}$$

Specificity is defined as the ability to exclude those with the normal genotype (with frequency d) from a false-positive classification (with frequency b).

$$\text{Specificity} = \frac{d}{b + d}$$

The false positive rate is 1 minus specificity. Binary discrimination yields perfect specificity and sensitivity (value = 1 for each). In practice, discrimination of most biochemical tests is statistical (i.e., dependent on the distribution of metrical parameters), hence specificity and sensitivity are less than perfect. There is thus no overlap of values between classes (e.g., heterozygotes and normals) for a binary test, but there are overlapping values for a statistical test. Molecular tests tend to be binary in testing for the presence or absence of a known mutation, often within a family, but tend to be statistical in regard to whether any mutation might be present in a gene or not, because methods to test for all possible mutations often are not available. For example, molecular carrier testing for the sib of a cystic fibrosis patient homozygous for the ΔF508 mutation is binary while carrier testing for cystic fibrosis in the general population has a sensitivity of about 0.9 but a specificity of 1.0 if 20 to 30 specific mutations are tested.

Detection of heterozygotes is an important part of counseling families where a known genetic disorder has occurred. This arises most frequently in the case of X-linked disorders or autosomal recessive traits, but analogous questions arise in the case of autosomal dominant disorders where an enzyme assay is available, and the phenotype is not always obvious clinically (e.g., acute intermittent porphyria). The ideal method for heterozygote detection is the direct demonstration of the mutant gene or gene product (i.e., binary discrimination with a specificity and sensitivity both with a value of 1). This is possible for some disorders using protein electrophoresis as for hemoglobin or α_1-antitrypsin. This is also possible when the disease mutation can be directly detected by molecular techniques. As discussed above, heterozygote detection is also possible using linkage analysis in which case the accuracy will depend upon the possibility of recombination between the linked marker and the disease mutation.

Another method for heterozygote detection involves the detection of half-normal levels of the mutant gene product. In such a statistical discrimination, the values for specificity and sensitivity are both less than 1. This approach usually involves enzyme assay on blood or tissue samples. The ability to separate heterozygotes from normals is extremely dependent upon the coefficient of variation for the determination in question. A high degree of variation may be due to unavoidable biologic variation in the human population. In many instances, the variation can be reduced by appropriate strategies. For example analysis of mixed leukocytes may give a wide variation because of heterogeneity in differential white blood cell count, while analysis of a specific leukocyte population such as granulocytes or lymphocytes may reduce the variation. For many enzyme deficiencies causing inborn errors of metabolism, the data sets for determining the normal and heterozygote ranges are suboptimal, in part due to lack of adequate numbers of obligate heterozygote samples and in part due to infrequent demand for the procedures. In the case of Tay-Sachs disease, the ability to distinguish heterozygotes by enzyme assay is unusually good. This is due in part to the excellent data sets available, but perhaps also in part to the intrinsic circumstances where the deficiency of α subunits both reduces hexosaminidase A activity and increases hexosaminidase B activity through the formation of β_2 dimers. Despite this, combined enzyme testing and DNA testing are more sensitive and specific than either is alone.[117] Heterozygote detection tests are frequently interpreted as positive or negative, and this is appropriate for a relatively absolute or binary test such as hemoglobin electrophoresis. When significant doubt is present, it is preferable to use the results to modify the probability that an individual is a carrier based on the range of values observed in heterozygotes and normal individuals.[118] Again, the data are frequently inadequate to pursue this optimal approach, but it should be recognized that many enzyme determinations for heterozygote detection do not provide absolute diagnoses. These same issues apply when diagnosing affected individuals with autosomal dominant enzyme disorders as for acute intermittent porphyria. As more molecular tests become available, heterozygote detection is moving increasingly from a statistical to a binary discrimination.

In the case of X-linked disorders, heterozygote detection at the level of the gene product is complicated by the Lyon mechanism for random X inactivation as discussed above. Strategies for circumventing the problems of X inactivation include analysis of clonal cell populations which can include individual hair roots, randomly isolated cultured cell clones, and cell clones isolated by selection methods. In the case of the Lesch-Nyhan syndrome, toxic purine antimetabolites such as thioguanine or azaguanine can be used to select for, and thereby demonstrate the presence of, deficient cells in a mixed population from a heterozygote female.

Heterozygote detection can also be based on various metabolic studies. In general, these tests (again statistical discriminations), which are more removed from the defective gene, are less reliable. For example, in heterozygotes for cystinuria, the excretion of dibasic amino acids in the urine is elevated, but not as much as in the patient with the homozygous disease (Chap. 191). Appropriate measurements of the ratio of blood phenylalanine to tyrosine before the noon meal provide a useful heterozygote test for phenylketonuria (Chap. 77). In the case of ornithine transcarbamoylase deficiency, urinary excretion of orotic acid and orotidine is significantly increased in heterozygotes after a protein-loading test or after administration of allopurinol (Chap. 85). These metabolic heterozygote tests can be quite accurate, although molecular data offer a binary discrimination when informative.

Antenatal Diagnosis of Genetic Disease

During the 1960s, transabdominal amniocentesis came into widespread use for the purpose of diagnosis of certain genetic diseases at a stage early enough to permit parents the option of terminating the pregnancy. This procedure gives high-risk couples the opportunity to have unaffected children and avoid the birth of an affected child if they are willing to terminate the pregnancy if an abnormal fetus is detected. Since the 1960s, there has been a progressive expansion of prenatal diagnostic techniques with improved resolution by prenatal ultrasound, measurement of amniotic fluid α-fetoprotein and other analytes, fetal blood sampling, and the development of transcervical and transabdominal chorionic villus sampling.

Amniocentesis consists of the transabdominal aspiration of amniotic fluid from the uterus. The procedure involves minimal risk. Maternal mortality has not been observed, and morbidity has been minor. Fetal loss (due to death or spontaneous abortion) is minimally different from that in controls matched for maternal age, gravidity, parity, race, religion, socioeconomic group, gestational age, and other features.[71,119–123] If a diagnostic amniocentesis is performed at the fifteenth or sixteenth week of gestation, the delay required for culture of an adequate number of cells for biochemical or cytogenetic study brings one only to the eighteenth to twentieth week, when pregnancy may still be terminated safely.

Direct examination of the amniotic fluid itself may be diagnostic. For example, an elevated level of α-fetoprotein is a relatively good indicator of the presence of spina bifida or some other related neural tube abnormality.[123] More frequently, prenatal diagnosis requires culture of the fetal cells in vitro. By this means, the karyotype of the fetus can be determined to ascertain fetal sex and to detect various chromosomal aberrations such as Down syndrome. Fluorescence *in situ* hybridization can be used for rapid analysis of interphase cells from amniotic fluid with a high degree of accuracy,[124] and this approach is likely to be used increasingly given decreased cost, more rapid results, and reports of high accuracy in large-scale evaluations.[125]

Transcervical or transabdominal chorionic villus sampling (CVS) can be used to obtain tissue of fetal origin, and multiple collaborative assessments have been performed.[126–130] CVS can be performed at 9 to 12 weeks gestation (only 5 to 8 weeks after the first missed menstrual period). Chorionic villi can be analyzed directly using cytogenetic, biochemical, or molecular techniques. In addition, cells can be cultured from chorionic villi and again subjected to any of these forms of analysis. The major advantage of CVS is the earlier sampling time and the availability of larger amounts of tissue which allow for direct analysis, so that a woman undergoing CVS at 9 weeks gestation might have final diagnostic information at 10 weeks gestation in comparison to up to 20 weeks gestation for amniocentesis. The earlier results are substantially more attractive to many high-risk families. Virtually all cytogenetic disorders can be detected using either amniocentesis or CVS. A large collaborative analysis of 11,473 procedures emphasizes the reliability of CVS but also the complexity of variables such as direct analysis of cells versus analysis of cultured cells, transcervical versus transabdominal sampling, maternal cell contamination, and mosaic results.[127] Many biochemical genetic disorders can be detected by suitable assays of specific enzyme activities in cultured fetal cells or in chorionic villi. In general, most of the disorders detectable by enzyme assay in cultured amniotic fluid cells are also detectable using CVS, but the relative expression of genes in these tissues differs slightly, and the reliability of each cell type for each enzymatic assay must be documented carefully.[131,132] The safety of CVS is related primarily to a low risk of inducing miscarriage and to the risk of causing a fetal malformation. The procedure is quite safe, with a statistically nonsignificant risk of miscarriage in most studies.[127,129,130] Concerns about fetal limb defects resulting from CVS have been raised,[133,134] but the risks are uncertain,[135] and the procedure is widely utilized because of the early results and overall reliability and relative safety. The feasibility, safety, and reliability of early amniocentesis at 7 to 14 weeks gestation has been evaluated as an alternative procedure to CVS, but careful comparison studies suggest that CVS and mid-trimester amniocentesis remain preferable to early amniocentesis.[136,137]

DNA can be obtained from any of the cell sources, and molecular diagnosis has assumed an expanding role using direct detection of mutations and linkage analysis as discussed above under "Molecular Strategies for Analysis of Mendelian Disorders." Increasingly, the disease gene itself is used as the diagnostic molecular probe or as the target for amplification. Molecular diagnosis does not require that the gene product be expressed in the fetal cells. For some disorders such as Tay-Sachs disease, Lesch-Nyhan syndrome, and sickle cell anemia, prenatal diagnosis is extremely reliable. In some instances, diagnosis traditionally was accomplished by enzyme assay, but molecular diagnosis is now the primary method. In some instances, molecular diagnosis may be available for only a proportion of families, because of inability to detect all possible mutations directly (currently exemplified by Duchenne muscular dystrophy and a small fraction of families with hemophilia A). When the disease mutation cannot be found, linkage analysis is an option in some cases. Fetal blood sampling is useful for prenatal diagnosis of hemophilia if molecular analysis is uninformative. In many cases prenatal diagnosis for specific disorders has been markedly improved by molecular methods as exemplified by fragile X syndrome, although even now it is not possible to predict the presence or extent of mental retardation completely, particularly in heterozygous females. It is virtually certain that the number of disorders that can be diagnosed will continue to increase rapidly and that the accuracy of diagnosis will improve in instances where it is still troublesome. Specific details for prenatal diagnosis can be found in chapters throughout this book and in standard texts.[138–140]

Population-Based Genetic Screening

Genetic screening represents the search in a population for persons possessing certain genotypes that are known to be associated with or to predispose to disease in the individuals or their descendants.[115,141] Screening is also employed for research purposes in order to ascertain distributions of traits, for example, polymorphisms, not known to be associated with disease. In this section, we are concerned only with the identification of deleterious genes in individual members of populations.

Population-based genetic screening is considered under the headings of newborn screening (usually for disease), heterozygote screening, prenatal screening, and screening for disease later in life. Newborn screening involves the identification of genetic disease in an infant to allow the institution of a prophylactic or therapeutic program to prevent injury to the child. Heterozygote screening and prenatal screening are designed to identify couples at high risk of transmitting a serious genetic disease in order to provide the couple with the option to forestall the birth of affected children. In heterozygote screening programs, reproductive options for carrier couples (autosomal recessive disorders) or for carrier females (X-linked disorders) are numerous and include avoidance of pregnancy, adoption, artificial insemination by noncarrier donor, selective abortion after prenatal diagnosis, and acceptance of the birth of affected infants. In instances such as Tay-Sachs disease and β-thalassemia where carrier testing has led to a substantial reduction in the number of affected births, prenatal diagnosis and selective termination of pregnancy has been the most widely used option. Screening for disease is designed to detect individuals in the population under circumstances where some prophylactic or therapeutic program may avert or reduce the burden of the disease. This strategy is similar to newborn screening, but is applied later in life.

Detailed discussions of genetic screening are available in a report published by the United States National Academy of Sciences in 1975,[141] and in the report of an international workshop held in 1982.[115] The recommendations from the workshop were:

1. The specific rationale for genetic screening should be defined, namely whether the goal is medical intervention, family planning, or research.
2. Population screening for medical intervention should not be performed outside an integrated program capable of information dispersal, screening, retrieval of persons with positive tests, diagnosis, counseling, medical management, and outcome evaluation.
3. The screening procedure should maximize specificity (by counting false positive tests), sensitivity (by counting false negative tests), and predictive efficiency (ratio of true positive to false positive tests) of the test. Proficiency testing should be implemented to monitor performance. (See explanation of specificity and sensitivity above under "Heterozygote Detection" above).
4. The contribution of ethnic and geographic factors to variation of phenotype (and mutation type and frequency) should be considered when designing and implementing programs.
5. Participation should be informed and in keeping with the relevant mores of the society; participants should acquire accurate information relevant to their needs.
6. Information about the rationale and goal of the program and the meaning of test results should be available to participants, physicians, and all other personnel affected by the program.
7. Outcome and impact of the program, whether for service or research in medical, economic, social, and legal contexts, should be evaluated. Policy should be sufficiently flexible so that practice can be modified in keeping with developments and findings.

A more recent report from the Institute of Medicine of the US National Academy of Sciences[142] focuses on the use of molecular methods and on the risks and benefits that might derive from more widespread genetic analysis. The report distinguishes genetic testing (analysis of symptomatic individuals or those with a positive family history) from genetic screening (population-based approaches).

Newborn Screening. The goal of newborn screening is almost always to make a specific diagnosis for the purpose of providing medical intervention to avoid or ameliorate symptoms. Newborn screening first evolved to identify phenylketonuria in infants in time to institute a low-phenylalanine diet and thus prevent the devastating effects of the untreated disease.[143] Newborn screening for phenylketonuria is discussed in detail in Chap. 77. Subsequently newborn screening has been implemented for many other disorders including amino acidopathies, galactosemia, congenital hypothyroidism, sickle cell anemia, cystic fibrosis, α_1-antitrypsin deficiency, and Duchenne muscular dystrophy. Almost all disorders detected by newborn screening represent Mendelian conditions except congenital hypothyroidism, which has a heterogeneous etiology, and HIV status, which is infectious. For some disorders, the evidence for efficacy of early medical intervention is overwhelming, as for phenylketonuria, for congenital hypothyroidism, and for survival in galactosemia. In other instances, the benefits of medical intervention are less dramatic but probably significant. Examples include sickle cell anemia, cystic fibrosis, and α_1-antitrypsin deficiency. In the case of Duchenne muscular dystrophy, no significant medical intervention is available. Newborn screening is more widely accepted and practiced for the disorders where intervention is most beneficial. The frequency of disorders based on newborn screening (Table 1-8)[115] is often found to be higher than was previously appreciated, and mild or variant forms of disorders frequently are discovered. There are potential genetic counseling benefits for early detection of disorders such as Duchenne muscular dystrophy.

Table 1-8 Frequency of Some Inborn Errors of Metabolism Based on Experience from Newborn Screening

Disorder	Average frequency in liveborn infants*
Cystic fibrosis	1 in 2500
Congenital hypothyroidism	1 in 6000
Cystinuria	1 in 7000
α_1-Antitrypsin deficiency	1 in 8000
Phenylketonuria	1 in 12,000
Histidinemia	1 in 17,000
Iminoglycinuria	1 in 20,000
Hartnup disorder	1 in 26,000
Hyperprolinemia	1 in 40,000
Galactosemia	1 in 57,000
Biotinidase deficiency	1 in 60,000
Adenosine deaminase deficiency	$<$1 in 100,000
Maple syrup urine disease	1 in 200,000
Homocystinuria	1 in 200,000

*These frequencies often vary widely among ethnic groups (e.g., about 1 in 5000 in Dublin compared with 1 in 200,000 in Japan for phenylketonuria; see Ref. 115 for details.)

SOURCE: Data modified from Galjaard[75] and various chapters in this book.

Heterozygote Screening. The general recommendations for genetic screening in populations cited above apply to heterozygote screening as well. The usual goal for heterozygote screening in this context is to provide options for family planning. The specificity and sensitivity of the heterozygote test are important variables. Qualitative or binary tests, such as hemoglobin electrophoresis for sickle cell anemia, provide relatively absolute diagnosis, while quantitative or statistical tests may provide lower specificity and sensitivity as discussed under "Heterozygote Detection," above.

Tay-Sachs Disease. The carrier frequency of this lethal disorder is about 1 in 30 in the American Jewish population of northeastern European ancestry, approximately tenfold higher than in the population at large. Detection of Tay-Sachs heterozygotes is accomplished by quantitative analysis of hexosaminidase A in serum, plasma, or leukocytes using a ratio to hexosaminidase B or by analysis for specific mutations (Chap. 153). Tay-Sachs disease is an ideal disorder for screening for reproductive counseling for these reasons: (a) it is limited mainly to a defined population; (b) there are simple, reliable, automated, and relatively inexpensive tests for identifying the carrier state; and (c) there are reproductive alternatives for couples, both of whom are carriers, because the disorder can be diagnosed antenatally at a time when induced abortion can be safely performed. Thus, such couples can plan to have unaffected children while avoiding having children with the disease. Heterozygote screening has led to a marked reduction of the frequency of Tay-Sachs disease in the Jewish and French Canadian populations as detailed in Chap. 153. A combination of enzymatic and molecular analysis now makes carrier detection very efficient. The advent of reliable screening procedures for heterozygote detection and antenatal diagnosis is particularly valuable in Tay-Sachs disease, in which 80 percent of cases are the first affected in the family, but amniocentesis also enables the prevention of the birth of a second affected child in a family in which one Tay-Sachs case has appeared, and in which both parents are therefore known heterozygotes.

Hemoglobinopathies. Heterozygote screening programs for β-thalassemia have been well received in various parts of the Mediterranean and North America. Major reductions in the frequency of β-thalassemia have occurred.[144,145] Heterozygote screening programs for β-thalassemia and α-thalassemia may be appropriate in various parts of Asia as other health care needs are met with further economic development.

Many heterozygotes for sickle cell anemia are being diagnosed as a relatively incidental component of newborn screening programs designed to detect homozygotes. In addition, heterozygote screening programs are being offered in many cities in the United States and elsewhere.[146] The most usual procedure for heterozygote detection is hemoglobin electrophoresis, which will also screen for other hemoglobinopathies, although molecular methods can be used as well. Molecular techniques have made prenatal diagnosis for sickle cell anemia completely reliable. The three favorable features of screening for Tay-Sachs disease listed above apply here also. There is a major difference, however, in regard to the severity and burden of sickle cell anemia in comparison to Tay-Sachs disease. There is considerable variation in expression for sickle cell disease, and some individuals experience mild disease, which is compatible with a long and productive life. In addition, there are major cultural, educational, and socioeconomic differences between the Jewish and African populations. Due to some combination of these reasons, perhaps primarily due to the milder expression, heterozygote screening and prenatal diagnosis have not been used in combination to reduce the frequency of sickle cell anemia to anywhere near the extent that this approach has been applied for Tay-Sachs disease. While heterozygote screening for sickle cell anemia may be successful at an educational level or for individual couples, it has not reduced substantially the burden of disease in the population up to the present time. This may provide important lessons for milder disorders such as α_1-antitrypsin deficiency and cystic fibrosis where individuals in the population may be more attracted to therapeutic strategies and may show little interest in avoidance approaches which make extensive use of selective abortion.

Cystic Fibrosis and Other Disorders. The cloning of the cystic fibrosis gene initiated an immediate debate regarding whether carrier testing should be offered in the general population. Testing for 10 to 20 mutations detects 60 to 95 percent of carriers with approximately 95 percent detection in Ashkenazic Jews, 90 percent detection in northern Europeans and North Americans, and lesser sensitivity in various southern European populations. Reproductive decisions regarding risks for cystic fibrosis are complex, because the disorder has a wide range of expression, intelligence is normal, and supportive treatment has tended to improve. The pitfalls and merits of population based screening have been debated extensively, but an NIH Consensus Conference recommends offering carrier testing to couples planning a pregnancy.[147] It will be of interest to follow the level of utilization of carrier testing for cystic fibrosis by various communities over the coming years.

With the identification of the molecular defect in fragile X syndrome, the question has also been raised as to whether population-based screening to identify heterozygote females could be considered.[148] Preliminary data regarding the prevalence of fragile X premutations in the population are being gathered.[149] Population-based carrier testing for Duchenne muscular dystrophy might also become an option if laboratory methods provided sufficient sensitivity and specificity at some time in the future.

Prenatal Screening. Major forms of population-based prenatal screening in use today include cytogenetic prenatal diagnosis for advanced maternal age, maternal serum analysis for α-fetoprotein and other analytes, and routine prenatal ultrasound. These methods represent a growing approach to monitor the health of the fetus by various means before delivery, usually in conjunction with the option of elective abortion of abnormal fetuses to avoid disease. Utilization of cytogenetic prenatal diagnosis for women of advanced maternal age has grown steadily since it became generally available in the 1960s. The procedure is widely used, but utilization is quite variable depending on urban compared to rural location, educational level, and religious preference.[150] Maternal serum α-fetoprotein screening was instituted with the goal of prenatal detection of anencephaly and meningomyelocele.[151,152] Subsequently, it was recognized that low levels of maternal serum α-fetoprotein and changes in levels of other analytes may be associated with increased risk of Down syndrome. This has led to strategies that calculate the risk of Down syndrome based on maternal age in combination with maternal serum levels of α-fetoprotein, unconjugated estriol, and chorionic gonadotropin to determine who should be offered cytogenetic prenatal diagnosis.[153] Using this strategy, it was possible to detect approximately 60 percent of Down syndrome pregnancies through maternal serum screening. Fetal ultrasound studies during the second trimester have become widespread and are routine in some settings. Careful ultrasound evaluation can detect a very broad range of fetal anatomic abnormalities.[154–156] Although heterozygote screening would optimally be implemented prior to conception, such testing is frequently delayed until the time of pregnancy. Strategies for prenatal screening are likely to continue to expand.

Screening for Disease in Later Life. Screening for genotypes that are associated with increased risk of disease in the individual or in their offspring or relatives is assuming many different forms. Newborn screening programs are detecting individuals who will have major disease risks later in life (e.g., sickle cell anemia and cystic fibrosis). Screening institutionalized populations for genetic disorders can lead to genetic counseling for relatives. For example, detection of fragile X syndrome, chromosomal translocations, or Lesch-Nyhan syndrome can lead to anticipatory genetic counseling for numerous relatives.

However, the primary focus of screening for disease later in life would be to detect adults or children for whom medical intervention would be beneficial. Widespread use of laboratory screening in adult populations is leading to the identification of numerous individuals with disorders such as hyperlipidemia. Identification of disorders such as heterozygous familial hypercholesterolemia has both major therapeutic implications for the individual detected and has implications for disease risk in their offspring. The impetus to screen for diseases increases as therapeutic options improve. Genetic screening of individuals in the workplace is beginning to occur and may become more frequent. It is appropriate to consider whether individuals with heterozygous or homozygous α_1-antitrypsin deficiency should work in environments with pulmonary risks (e.g., coal mines). Genetic screening of populations carries many potential risks and benefits for the future as reviewed in the recent Institute of Medicine report.[142] Optimistically one might envision the day when widespread population screening would be well understood and well accepted and would identify individuals with high-risk genotypes who would then benefit from specific preventative interventions.

TREATMENT OF GENETIC DISEASE

The treatment of genetic disease takes many forms and is discussed at length in Chap. 5.

ACKNOWLEDGMENTS

This chapter represents the evolution of the cumulative contributions to chapters that have appeared in *Harrison's Principles of Internal Medicine* and in the *Metabolic and Molecular Bases of Inherited Disease*. Past contributors have included John B. Stanbury, James B. Wyngaarden, Donald S. Fredrickson, Joseph L. Goldstein, Michael S. Brown, Stuart Orkin, and Andrea Ballabio. The authors gratefully acknowledge the contributions of these predecessors and colleagues.

REFERENCES

1. Garrod A: The lessons of rare maladies. *Lancet* **1**:1055, 1928.
2. Hayes A, Costa T, Scriver CR, Childs B: The effect of Mendelian disease on human health. II: Response to treatment. *Am J Med Genet* **21**:243, 1985.
3. Treacy E, Childs B, Scriver CR: Response to treatment in hereditary metabolic disease: 1993 survey and 10-year comparison. *Am J Hum Genet* **56**:359, 1995.
4. Williams RJ: *Biochemical Individuality*. New York, Wiley, 1956.
5. Garrod AE: *Inborn Factors in Disease*. London, Oxford University Press, 1931.
6. Wivel NA, Wilson JM: Methods of gene delivery. *Hematol Oncol Clin North Am* **12**:483, 1998.
7. Emery DW, Stamatoyannopoulos G: Stem cell gene therapy for the beta-chain hemoglobinopathies. *Ann N Y Acad Sci* **872**:94, 1999.
8. Chowdhury JR. Foreward: prospects of liver cell transplantation and liver-directed gene therapy. *Semin Liver Dis* **19**:1, 1999.
9. Jain KK, Kewal K: *Textbook of Gene Therapy*. Seattle, WA, Hogrefe and Huber, 1998.
10. Blankenstein T: *Gene Therapy: Principles and Applications*. Boston, Birkhauser, 1999.
11. Lemoine NR, Cooper DN: *Gene Therapy*. Herndon, Bios Scientific, 1996.
12. Marshall E: Gene therapy death prompts review of adenovirus vector. *Science* **286**:2244, 1999.
13. McKusick VA: *Mendelian Inheritance in Man*, 12th ed. Baltimore, MD, The Johns Hopkins University Press, 1998.
14. Deloukas P, Schuler GD, Gyapay G, Beasley EM, Soderlund C, Rodriguez-Tome P, Hui L, Matise TC, McKusick KB, Beckmann JS, Bentolila S, Bihoreau M, Birren BB, Browne J, Butler A, Castle AB, Chiannilkulchai N, Clee C, Day PJR, Dehejia A, Dibling T, Drouot N, Duprat S, Fizames C, Fox S: A physical map of 30,000 human genes. *Science* **282**:744, 1998.
15. Strausberg RL, Feingold EA, Klausner RD, Collins FS: The mammalian gene collection. *Science* **286**:455, 1999.
16. Beaudet AL: 1998 ASHG Presidential Address. Making genomic medicine a reality. *Am J Hum Genet* **64**:1, 1999.
17. Witte DL, Crosby WH, Edwards CQ, Fairbanks VF, Mitros FA: Practice guideline development task force of the College of American Pathologists. Hereditary hemochromatosis. *Clin Chim Acta* **245**:139, 1996.
18. Burke W, Thomson E, Khoury MJ, McDonnell SM, Press N, Adams PC, Barton JC, Beutler E, Brittenham G, Buchanan A, Clayton EW, Cogswell ME, Meslin EM, Motulsky AG, Powell LW, Sigal E, Wilfond BS, Collins FS: Hereditary hemochromatosis: Gene discovery and its implications for population-based screening. *JAMA* **280**:172, 1998.
19. The French FMF Consortium. A candidate gene for familial Mediterranean fever. *Nat Genet* **17**:25, 1997.
20. The International FMF Consortium. Ancient missense mutations in a new member of the RoRet gene family are likely to cause familial Mediterranean fever. *Cell* **90**:797, 1997.
21. Brooks-Wilson AR, Marcil M, Clee SM, Zhang LH, Roomp K, van Dam M, Yu L, Brewer C, Collins JA, Molhuizen HO, Loubser O, Ouelette BF, Fichter K, Ashbourne-Excoffon KJ, Sensen CW, Scherer S, Mott S, Denis M, Martindale D, Frohlich J, Morgan K, Koop B, Pimstone S, Kastelein JJ, Hayden MR: Mutations in ABC1 in Tangier disease and familial high-density lipoprotein deficiency. *Nat Genet* **22**:336, 1999.
22. Bodzioch M, Orso E, Klucken J, Langmann T, Bottcher A, Diederich W, Drobnik W, Barlage S, Buchler C, Porsch-Ozcurumez M, Kaminski WE, Hahmann HW, Oette K, Rothe G, Aslanidis C, Lackner KJ, Schmitz G: The gene encoding ATP-binding cassette transporter 1 is mutated in Tangier disease. *Nat Genet* **22**:347, 1999.
23. Rust S, Rosier M, Funke H, Real J, Amoura Z, Piette JC, Deleuze JF, Brewer HB, Duverger N, Denefle P, Assmann G: Tangier disease is caused by mutations in the gene encoding ATP-binding cassette transporter 1. *Nat Genet* **22**:352, 1999.
24. Amir RE, Van den Veyver IB, Wan M, Tran CQ, Francke U, Zoghbi HY: Rett syndrome is caused by mutations in X-linked *MECP2*, encoding methyl-CpG-binding protein 2. *Nat Genet* **23**:185, 1999.
25. Merz JF: Disease gene patents: Overcoming unethical constraints on clinical laboratory medicine. *Clin Chem* **45**:324, 1999.
26. Paxton A: Gene patents push labs to their limits. *CAP Today* **13**:30, 1999.
27. Zweiger G: Knowledge discovery in gene-expression-microarray data: Mining the information output of the genome. *Trends Biotechnol* **17**:429, 1999.
28. Alberts B, Bray D, Lewis J, Raff M, Roberts K, Watson JD: *Molecular Biology of the Cell* 3rd ed. New York, Garland, 1994.
29. Lodish H, Baltimore D, Berk AJ, Zepursky SL: 3rd ed. *Molecular Cell Biology*, New York, Scientific American Books, 1995.
30. Miller JH: *Discovering Molecular Genetics: A Case Study Course with Problems & Scenarios*. Plainview, NY, Cold Spring Harbor Laboratory Press, 1996.
31. Lewin B: *Genes VII*. New York, Oxford University Press, 1997.
32. DePamphilis ML: *DNA Replication in Eukaryotic Cells*. Plainview, NY, Cold Spring Harbor Laboratory Press, 1996.
33. Sauer F, Tjian R: Mechanisms of transcriptional activation: Differences and similarities between yeast, *Drosophila*, and man. *Curr Opin Genet Dev* **7**:176, 1997.
34. Ranish JA, Hahn S: Transcription: Basal factors and activation. *Curr Opin Genet Dev* **6**:151, 1996.
35. Berk AJ: Activation of RNA polymerase II transcription. *Curr Opin Cell Biol* **11**:330, 1999.
36. Struhl K: Fundamentally different logic of gene regulation in eukaryotes and prokaryotes. *Cell* **98**:1, 1999.
37. Antonarakis SE: Recommendations for a nomenclature system for human gene mutations. Nomenclature Working Group. *Hum Mutat* **11**:1, 1998.
38. Ad Hoc Committee on Mutation Nomenclature. Update of nomenclature for human gene mutations. *Hum Mutat* **8**:197, 1996.
39. Kazazian HH Jr, Boehm CD: Molecular basis and prenatal diagnosis of β-thalassemia. *Blood* **72**:1107, 1988.
40. Garrod AE: The incidence of alkaptonuria: A study in chemical individuality. *Lancet* **2**:1616, 1902.
41. Clark AG, Weiss KM, Nickerson DA, Taylor SL, Buchanan A, Stengard J, Salomaa V, Vartiainen E, Perola M, Boerwinkle E, Sing CF: Haplotype structure and population genetic inferences from nucleotide-sequence variation in human lipoprotein lipase. *Am J Hum Genet* **63**:595, 1998.
42. Nickerson DA, Taylor SL, Weiss KM, Clark AG, Hutchinson RG, Stengard J, Salomaa V, Vartiainen E, Boerwinkle E, Sing CF: DNA sequence diversity in a 9.7-kb region of the human lipoprotein lipase gene. *Nat Genet* **19**:233, 1998.
43. Collins A, Lonjou C, Morton NE: Genetic epidemiology of single-nucleotide polymorphisms. *Proc Natl Acad Sci U S A* **96**:15173, 1999.
44. Sambrook J, Fritsch EF, Maniatis T: *Molecular Cloning. A Laboratory Manual*. Cold Spring Harbor, NY, Cold Spring Harbor Laboratory, 1989.
45. Birren B, Green ED, Klapholz S, Myers RM, Roskams J: Vol 1. *Analyzing DNA: A Laboratory Manual*. Plainview, NY, Cold Spring Harbor Laboratory Press, 1997.
46. Birren B, Green ED, Myers RM, Roskams J: Vol. 2. *Detecting Genes: A Laboratory Manual*. Plainview, NY, Cold Spring Harbor Laboratory Press, 1998.
47. Birren B, Green ED, Myers RM, Riethman H, Roskams J: Vol. 3. *Cloning Systems: A Laboratory Manual*. Plainview, NY, Cold Spring Harbor Laboratory Press, 1999.
48. Birren B, Green ED, Klapholz S, Myers RM, Riethman H, Roskams J: Vol. 4. *Mapping Genomes: A Laboratory Manual*. Plainview, NY, Cold spring Harbor Laboratory Press, 1999.
49. Cotton RG. Mutation detection and mutation databases. *Clin Chem Lab Med* **36**:519, 1998.
50. Underhill PA, Jin L, Lin AA, Mehdi SQ, Jenkins T, Vollrath D, Davis RW, Cavalli-Sforza LL, Oefner PJ: Detection of numerous Y chromosome biallelic polymorphisms by denaturing high-performance liquid chromatography. *Genome Res* **7**:996, 1997.
51. Liu WO, Oefner PJ, Qian C, Odom RS, Francke U: Denaturing HPLC-identified novel FBN1 mutations, polymorphisms, and sequence

variants in Marfan syndrome and related connective tissue disorders. *Genet Test* **1**:237, 1997.

52. Arnold N, Gross E, Schwarz-Boeger U, Pfisterer J, Jonat W, Kiechle M: A highly sensitive, fast, and economical technique for mutation analysis in hereditary breast and ovarian cancers. *Hum Mutat* **14**:333, 1999.
53. Fang P, Lev-Lehman E, Tsai T-F, Matsuura T, Benton CS, Sutcliffe JS, Christian SL, Kubota T, Halley DJ, Meijers-Heijboer H, Langlois S, Graham JM, Beuten J, Willems P, Ledbetter DH, Beaudet AL: The spectrum of mutations in *UBE3A* causing Angelman syndrome. *Hum Mol Genet* **8**:129, 1999.
54. Southern EM: DNA chips: Analysing sequence by hybridization to oligonucleotides on a large scale. *Trends Genet* **12**:110, 1996.
55. Pennisi E: Academic sequencers challenge Celera in a sprint to the finish. *Science* **283**:1822, 1999.
56. Dunham I, Shimizu N, Roe BA, Chissoe S, Hunt AR, Collins JE, Bruskiewich R, Beare DM, Clamp M, Smink LJ, Ainscough R, Almeida JP, Babbage A, Bagguley C, Bailey J, Barlow K, Bates KN, Beasley O, Bird CP, Blekey S, Bridgeman AM, Buck D, Burgess J, Burrill WD, O'Brien KP: The DNA sequence of human chromosome 22. *Nature* **402**:489, 1999.
57. Fleming JC, Tartaglini E, Steinkamp MP, Schorderet DF, Cohen N, Neufeld EJ: The gene mutated in thiamine-responsive anaemia with diabetes and deafness (TRMA) encodes a functional thiamine transporter. *Nat Genet* **22**:305, 1999.
58. Wilmut I: Cloning for medicine. *Sci Am* **279**:58, 1998.
59. Zambrowicz BP, Friedrich GA, Buxton EC, Lilleberg SL, Person C, Sands AT: Disruption and sequence identification of 2,000 genes in mouse embryonic stem cells. *Nature* **392**:608, 1998.
60. Hasty P, Ramirez-Solis R, Krumlauf R, Bradley A: Introduction of a subtle mutation into the *Hox*-2.6 locus in embryonic stem cells. *Nature* **350**:243, 1991.
61. Lewis J, Yang B, Detloff P, Smithies O: Gene modification via "plug and socket" gene targeting. *J Clin Invest* **97**:3, 1996.
62. Smithies O, Kim HS: Targeting gene duplication and disruption for analyzing quantitative genetic traits in mice. *Proc Natl Acad Sci U S A* **91**:3612, 1994.
63. Lobe CG, Nagy A: Conditional genome alteration in mice. *Bioessays* **20**:200, 1998.
64. Rajewsky K, Gu H, Kuhn R, Betz UA, Muller W, Roes J, Schwenk F: Conditional gene targeting. *J Clin Invest* **98**:600, 1996.
65. Sauer B: Inducible gene targeting in mice using the Cre/lox system. *Methods* **14**:381, 1998.
66. Francke U, Ochs HD, de Martinville B: Minor XP-21 chromosome deletion in a male associated with expression of Duchenne muscular dystrophy, chronic granulomatous disease, retinitis pigmentosa, and McLeod syndrome. *Am J Hum Genet* **37**:250, 1985.
67. Scriver CR, Neal JL, Saginur R, Clow A: The frequency of genetic disease and congenital malformation among patients in a pediatric hospital. *Can Med Assoc J* **108**:1111, 1973.
68. Baird PA, Anderson TW, Newcombe HB, Lowry RB: Genetic disorders in children and young adults: A population study. *Am J Hum Genet* **42**:677, 1988.
69. UNSCEAR : *Genetic and Somatic Effects of Ionizing Radiation*. New York, United Nations, 1986.
70. Sorensen TIA, Nielsen GG, Andersen PK, Teasdale TW: Genetic and environmental influences on premature death in adult adoptees. *N Engl J Med* **318**:727, 1988.
71. Vogel F, Motulsky AG: *Human Genetics: Problems and Approaches*, 3rd ed. New York, Springer-Verlag, 1997.
72. Rooney DE, Czepulkowski BH: *Human Cytogenetics: A Practical Approach. Vol. 1. Constitutional Analysis*. New York, Oxford University Press, 1994.
73. Rooney DE, Czepulkowski BH: *Human Cytogenetics: A Practical Approach*. Vol. 2, 2nd ed. New York, Oxford University Press, 1994.
74. Verma RS, Babu A: *Human Chromosomes: Principals and Techniques*. New York, McGraw-Hill, 1995.
75. Galjaard H: *Genetic Metabolic Diseases: Early Diagnosis and Prenatal Analysis*. Amsterdam, Elsevier, 1980.
76. Heim S, Mitelman F: *Cancer Cytogenetics*. 2nd ed. New York, Wiley-Liss, 1995.
77. Maymon R, Dreasen E, Rozinsky S, Bukovsky I, Weinraub Z, Herman A: Comparison of nuchal translucency measurement and second-trimester triple serum screening in twin versus singleton pregnancies. *Prenat Diagn* **19**:727, 1999.
78. Bahado-Singh RO, Oz AU, Kovanci E, Deren O, Copel J, Baumgarten A, Mahoney J: New Down syndrome screening algorithm: ultrasonographic biometry and multiple serum markers combined with maternal age. *Am J Obstet Gynecol* **179**:1627, 1998.
79. Wald NJ, Kennard A, Hackshaw A, McGuire A: Antenatal screening for Down's syndrome. *J Med Screen* **4**:181, 1997.
80. Speicher MR, Ward DC: The coloring of cytogenetics. *Nat Med* **2**:1046, 1996.
81. Schermelleh L, Thalhammer S, Heckl W, Posl H, Cremer T, Schutze K, Cremer M: Laser microdissection and laser pressure catapulting for the generation of chromosome-specific paint probes. *BioTechniques* **27**:362, 1999.
82. Flint J, Wilkie AO, Buckle BJ, Winter RM, Holland AJ, McDermid HE: The detection of subtelomeric chromosomal rearrangements in idiopathic mental retardation. *Nat Genet* **9**:132, 1995.
83. Ghaffari SR, Boyd E, Tolmie JL, Crow YJ, Trainer AH, Connor JM: A new strategy for cryptic telomeric translocation screening in patients with idiopathic mental retardation. *J Med Genet* **35**:225, 1998.
84. Slavotinek A, Rosenberg M, Knight S, Gaunt L, Fergusson W, Killoran C, Clayton-Smith J, Kingston H, Campbell RH, Flint J, Donnai D, Biesecker L: Screening for submicroscopic chromosome rearrangements in children with idiopathic mental retardation using microsatellite markers for the chromosome telomeres. *J Med Genet* **36**:405, 1999.
85. Lizardi PM, Huang X, Zhu Z, Bray-Ward P, Thomas DC, Ward DC: Mutation detection and single-molecule counting using isothermal rolling-circle amplification. *Nat Genet* **19**:225, 1998.
86. de Grouchy J, Turleau C: *Clinical Atlas of Human Chromosomes*. New York, Wiley, 1984.
87. Schinzel A: *Catalogue of Unbalanced Chromosome Aberrations in Man*. New York, Walter de Gruyter, 1983.
88. Jones KL: *Smith's Recognizable Patterns of Human Malformations. 5th ed.*Philadelphia, WB Saunders, 1997.
89. Buyse ML: *Birth Defects Encyclopedia*. Dover, U.K., Blackwell Scientific, 1990.
90. Stevenson RE, Hall JG, Goodman RM: *Human Malformations and Related Anomalies*. New York, Oxford University Press, 1993.
91. Carter CO: Monogenic disorders. *J Med Genet* **14**:316, 1977.
92. Motulsky AG: Frequency of sickling disorders in U.S. Blacks. *N Engl J Med* **288**:31, 1973.
93. Costa T, Scriver CR, Childs B: The effect of Mendelian disease on human health: A measurement. *Am J Med Genet* **21**:231, 1985.
94. Kacser H, Burns JA: The molecular basis of dominance. *Genetics* **97**:639, 1981.
95. Kacser H, Porteous JW: Control of metabolism: What do we have to measure? *Trends Biochem Sci* **12**:5, 1987.
96. Herskowitz I: Functional inactivation of genes by dominant negative mutations. *Nature* **329**:219, 1987.
97. Jiang Y-H, Lev-Lehman E, Bressler J, Tsai T-F, Beaudet AL: Genetics of Angelman syndrome. *Am J Hum Genet* **65**:1, 1999.
98. Contu L, Arras M, Mulargia M, La Nasa G, Carcassi C, Leone AL, Leda A, Goddi F: Study of HLA segregation in 479 thalassemic families. *Tissue Antigens* **39**:58, 1992.
99. Munier FL, Arabien L, Flodman P, Spence MA, Pescia G, Rutz HP, Murphree AL: Putative non-Mendelian transmission of retinoblastoma in males: A phenotypic segregation analysis of 150 pedigrees. *Hum Genet* **94**:484, 1994.
100. Naumova AK, Leppert M, Barker DF, Morgan K, Sapienza C: Parental origin-dependent, male offspring-specific transmission-ratio distortion at loci on the human X chromosome. *Am J Hum Genet* **62**:1493, 1998.
101. MacMillan JC, Voisey J, Healey SC, Martin NG: Mendelian segregation of normal CAG trinucleotide repeat alleles at three autosomal loci. *J Med Genet* **36**:258, 1999.
102. Henikoff S, Matzke MA: Exploring and explaining epigenetic effects. *Trends Genet* **13**:293, 1997.
103. Heutink P, van Schothorst EM, van der Mey AG, Bardoel A, Breedveld G, Pertijs J, Sandkuyl LA, van Ommen GJ, Cornelisse CJ, Oostra BA: Further localization of the gene for hereditary paragangliomas and evidence for linkage in unrelated families. *Eur J Hum Genet* **2**:148, 1994.
104. Brockdorff N: The role of Xist in X-inactivation. *Curr Opin Genet Dev* **8**:328, 1998.
105. Haldane JBS: The mutation rate of the gene for haemophilia, and its segregation ratios in males and females. *Ann Eugen* **13**:262, 1947.
106. Haldane JBS: The spread of harmful autosomal recessive genes in human populations. *Ann Eugen* **9**:232, 1939.
107. Ferlin A, Moro E, Garolla A, Foresta C: Human male infertility and Y chromosome deletions: Role of the AZF-candidate genes DAZ, RBM and DFFRY. *Hum Reprod* **14**:1710, 1999.

108. Jancar J, Johnston SJ: Incest and mental handicap. *J Ment Defic Res* **34**:483, 1990.
109. Dequeker E, Cassiman JJ: Evaluation of CFTR gene mutation testing methods in 136 diagnostic laboratories: Report of a large European external quality assessment. *Eur J Hum Genet* **6**:165, 1998.
110. Kan YW, Dozy AM: Polymorphism of DNA sequence adjacent to human β-globin structural gene: Relationship to sickle mutation. *Proc Natl Acad Sci U S A* **75**:5631, 1978.
111. Koenig M, Hoffman EP, Bertelson CJ: Complete cloning of the Duchenne muscular dystrophy (DMD) cDNA and preliminary genomic organization of the DMD gene in normal and affected individuals. *Cell* **50**:509, 1987.
112. Harper PS: *Practical Genetic Counseling*. Boston, Butterworth-Heinemann, 1998.
113. Leonard CO, Chase GA, Childs B: Genetic counseling: A consumers' view. *N Engl J Med* **287**:433, 1972.
114. Chase GA, Faden RR, Holtzman NA, Chwalow AJ, Leonard CO, Lopes C, Quaid K: Assessment of risk by pregnant women: Implications for genetic counseling and education. *Soc Biol* **33**:57, 1986.
115. Scriver CR and Committee: Population screening: Report of a workshop, in Marios M, Bennett HS, Klingberg MS, Brent RL, Lander J, Saxen L (eds): *Prevention of Physical and Mental Congenital Defects: Part B: Epidemiology. Early Detection and Therapy, and Environmental Factors*. New York, Alan R. Liss, 1985.
116. Black ER, Panzer RJ, Mayewski RJ, Griner PF: Characteristics of diagnostic tests and principles for their use in quantitative decision making, in Panzer RJ, Black ER, Griner PF (eds): *Diagnostic Strategies for Common Medical Problems*. Philadelphia, American College of Physicians, 1991.
117. Fernandes MJG, Kaplan F, Clow CL, Hechtman P, Scriver CR: Specificity and sensitivity of hexosaminidase assays and DNA analysis for the detection of Tay-Sachs disease gene carriers among Ashkenazic Jews. *Genet Epidemiol* **9**:169, 1992.
118. Kaback MM, Rimoin DL, O'Brien JS: *Tay-Sachs Disease: Screening and Prevention*. New York, Alan R. Liss, 1977.
119. NICHD National Registry for Amniocentesis Study Group. Midtrimester amniocentesis for prenatal diagnosis. *JAMA* **236**:1471, 1976.
120. Tabor A, Madsen M, Obel EB, Philip J, Bang J, Naergaard-Pedersen B: Randomised controlled trial of genetic amniocentesis in 4606 low risk women. *Lancet* **1**:1287, 1986.
121. Milunsky A: *Genetic Disorders and the Fetus: Diagnosis, Prevention, and Treatment*. 3rd ed.Baltimore, MD, Johns Hopkins University Press, 1992.
122. Simpson JL, Elias S: *Essentials of Prenatal Diagnosis*. New York, Churchill Livingston, 1993.
123. Brock DJH, Rodeck CH, Ferguson-Smith AC, Weatherall DJ: *Prenatal Diagnosis and Screening*. New York, Churchill Livingstone, 1992.
124. Ward BE, Gersen SL, Carelli MP, McGuire NM, Dackowski WR, Weinstein M, Sandlin C, Warren R, Klinger KW: Rapid prenatal diagnosis of chromosomal aneuploidies by fluorescence in situ hybridization. Clinical experience with 4,500 specimens. *Am J Hum Genet* **53**:526, 1993.
125. Eiben B, Trawicki W, Hammans W, Goebel R, Pruggmayer M, Epplen JR: Rapid prenatal diagnosis of aneuploidies in uncultured amniocytes by fluorescence *in situ* hybridization. Evaluation of $>3{,}000$ cases. *Fetal Diagn Ther* **14**:193, 1999.
126. MCR Working Party on the Evaluation of Chorion Villus Sampling. Medical research council European trial of chorion villus sampling. *Lancet* **337**:1491, 1991.
127. Ledbetter DH, Zachary JM, Simpson JL, Golbus MS, Pergament E, Jackson L, Mahoney MJ, Desnick RJ, Schulman J, Copeland KL, Verlinsky Y, Yang-Feng T, Schonberg SA, Babu A, Tharapel A, Dorfmann A, Lubs HA, Rhoads GG, Fowler SE, De La Cruz F: Cytogenetic results from the U.S. collaborative study on CVS. *Prenat Diagn* **12**:347, 1992.
128. Wapner RJ, Simpson JL, Golbus MS, Zachary JM, Ledbetter DH, Desnick RJ, Fowler SE, Jackson LG, Lubs H, Mahony RJ, Pergament E, Rhoads GG, Schulman JD, Zachary J: Chorionic mosaicism: Association with fetal loss but not with adverse perinatal outcome. *Prenat Diagn* **12**:373, 1992.
129. Golbus MS, Simpson JL, Fowler SE, De La Cruz F, Desnick RJ, Wapner R, Ledbetter DH, Lubs H, Mahoney MJ: Risk factors associated with transcervical CVS losses. *Prenat Diagn* **12**:373, 1992.
130. Lippman A, Tomkins DJ, Shime J, Hamerton JL: Canadian multicentre randomized clinical trial of chorion villus sampling and amniocentesis. *Prenat Diagn* **12**:385, 1992.
131. Poenaru L: First trimester prenatal diagnosis of metabolic diseases. A survey in countries from the European community. *Prenat Diagn* **7**:333, 1987.
132. Desnick RJ, Schuette JL, Golbus MS, Jackson L, Lubs HA, Ledbetter DH, Mahoney MJ, Pergament E, Simpson JL, Zachary JM, Fowler SE, Rhoads GG, De La Cruz F: First-trimester biochemical and molecular diagnoses using chorionic villi: High accuracy in the U.S. collaborative study. *Prenat Diagn* **12**:357, 1992.
133. Firth HV, Boyd PA, Chamberlain P, MacKenzie IZ, Lindenbaum RH, Huson SM: Severe limb abnormalities after chorion villus sampling at 56–66 days' gestation. *Lancet* **337**:762, 1991.
134. Burton BK, Schulz CJ, Burd LI: Limb anomalies associated with chorionic villus sampling. *Obstet Gynecol* **79**:726, 1992.
135. Mahoney MJ: Limb abnormalities and chorionic villus sampling. *Lancet* **337**:1422, 1991.
136. Johnson JM, Wilson RD, Singer J, Winsor E, Harman C, Armson BA, Benzie R, Dansereau J, Ho MF, Mohide P, Natale R, Okun N: Technical factors in early amniocentesis predict adverse outcome. Results of the Canadian early (EA) versus mid-trimester (MA) amniocentesis trial. *Prenat Diagn* **19**:732, 1999.
137. Nagel HT, Vandenbussche FP, Keirse MJ, Oepkes D, Oosterwijk JC, Beverstock G, Kanhai HH: Amniocentesis before 14 completed weeks as an alternative to transabdominal chorionic villus sampling: a controlled trial with infant follow-up. *Prenat Diagn* **18**:465, 1998.
138. Reece EA, Hobbins JC: *Medicine of the Fetus and Mother. 2nd ed.*Philadelphia, Lippincott-Raven, 1999.
139. Creasy RK, Resnik R: *Maternal-Fetal Medicine. 4th ed.*Philadelphia, WB Saunders, 1999.
140. Milunsky A: *Genetic Disorders and the Fetus: Diagnosis, Prevention, and Treatment. 4th ed.*Baltimore, MD, Johns Hopkins University Press, 1998.
141. National Research Council (U.S). Committe for the Study of Inborn Errors of Metabolism: *Genetic Screening: Programs, Principles and Research*. Washington, D.C., National Academy of Sciences, 1975.
142. Anderson LB, Fullerton JE, Holtzman NA, Motulsky AG: *Assessing Genetic Risks: Implementation for Health and Social Policy*. Washington, D.C., National Academy Press, 1994.
143. MacCready RA, Hussey MG: Newborn phenylketonuria detection program in Massachusetts. *Am J Public Health* **54**:2075, 1999.
144. Cao A, Rosatelli C, Pirastu M, Galanello R: Thalassemias in Sardinia: Molecular pathology, phenotype-genotype correlation, and prevention. *Am J Pediatr Hematol Oncol* **13**:179, 1964.
145. Scriver CR, Bardanis M, Cartier L, Clow CL, Lancaster GA, Ostrowsky JT: β-thalassemia disease prevention: Genetic medicine applied. *Am J Hum Genet* **36**:1024, 1984.
146. Rucknagel DL: A decade of screening in the hemoglobinopathies: Is a national program to prevent sickle cell anemia possible? *Am J Pediatr Hematol Oncol* **5**:373, 1983.
147. Genetic testing for cystic fibrosis. National Institutes of Health Consensus Development Conference Statement on genetic testing for cystic fibrosis. *Arch Intern Med* **26**:159, 1999.
148. Palomaki GE, Haddow JE: Is it time for population-based prenatal screening for fragile-X? *Lancet* **341**:373, 1993.
149. Rousseau F, Rehel R, Rouillard P, DeGrandpre P, Morgan K, Khandjian EW: Mutational prevalence of fragile X premutations in 10,624 females from the general population by Southern blotting. *Am J Hum Genet* **53(Suppl)**:3, 1993.
150. Sokal DC, Byrd JR, Chen ATL, Goldberg MF, Oakley GP: Prenatal chromosomal diagnosis: Racial and geographic variation for older women in Georgia. *JAMA* **244**:1355, 1980.
151. Brock DJH: Biochemical and cytological methods in the diagnosis of neural tube defects. *Prog Med Genet* **2**:1, 1977.
152. U.K. Collaborative Study on α-Fetoprotein in Relation to Neural Tube Defects. Maternal serum α-fetoprotein measurement in antenatal screening for anencephaly and spina bifida in early pregnancy. *Lancet* **1**:1323, 1977.
153. Haddow JE, Palomaki GE, Knight GJ, Williams J, Pulkkinen A, Canick JA, Saller DN Jr, Bowers GB: Prenatal screening for Down syndrome with use of maternal serum markers. *N Engl J Med* **327**:636, 1992.
154. Chervenak FA, Isaacson GC, Campbell S: *Ultrasound in Obstetrics and Gynecology*. Boston, Little, Brown, 1993.
155. Bowerman RA: *Atlas of Normal Fetal Ultrasonographic Anatomy*. Boston, Mosby Year Book, 1992.
156. Meizner I, Bar-Ziv J: *In Utero Diagnosis of Skeletal Disorders. An Atlas of Prenatal Sonographic and Postnatal Radiologic Correlation*. Boca Raton, FL, CRC Press, 1993.

APPENDIX 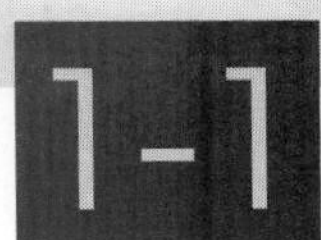

Morbid Anatomy of the Human Genome

Joanna S. Amberger ■ Ada Hamosh ■ Victor A. McKusick

The Morbid Anatomy of the Human Genome is a list of mapped loci for which there is a known clinical association. It is derived from the Synopsis of the Human Gene Map which was published in the 7th edition of MMBID and which is available with Online Mendelian Inheritance in Man (OMIM), a continuously updated catalog of genetic disorders and genes (http://www.ncbi.nlm.nih.gov/omim). The gene map and morbid map are periodically published as part of Mendelian Inheritance in Man (Johns Hopkins University Press, 12th edition, 1998).

The morbid map provides a view of the genome with a focus on disease. By indicating where each mapped disease is located along each chromosome, it provides a ready reference associating cloned genes with diseases, an overview of the range of diseases associated with mutations in a particular gene or gene family, insight into gene function based on the disease etiology and vice versa, and a ready list of phenotypes relevant to cytogenetic rearrangements and contiguous gene syndromes.

Table A1-1 Overview of the Morbid Map

Total number of loci with clinical association	1734
Total number of mapped phenotypes	2253
Number of phenotypes mapped by the wildtype gene	191
Number of phenotypes mapped by linkage or chromosome analysis	699
Number of phenotypes with molecular basis defined	1363

The fields of the Morbid Map are as follows:

A. Location. Chromosomal location.
B. Symbol. Gene or locus symbol(s).
C. Status. The certainty of mapping is represented by 3 symbols:
   C = confirmed
   P = provisional
   L = limbo or tentative
D. Locus Name. Title of gene or locus.
E. MIM#. This is a unique identification number of the entry in Mendelian Inheritance in Man that describes the gene or locus, including any information known about gene function or disease pathogenesis.
F. Disorder. This field lists the disorders associated with the particular locus, including those disorders or conditions that may be caused by mutations in the gene. MIM numbers after diseases indicate that the description of the disorder is contained in a MIM entry separate from that of the gene or locus. The numbers after the name of the disorder signify: (1) the phenotype was placed on the map by association with a mapped gene; (2) the phenotype itself was mapped usually by family linkage studies; (3) the molecular basis of the disorder has been identified. Brackets, [ ], signify "nondisease"; braces, { }, indicate susceptibilities.

Additional information, including methods of mapping and homologous mouse loci, are available online from the Synopsis of the Human Gene Map (http://www.ncbi.nlm.nih.gov/omim).

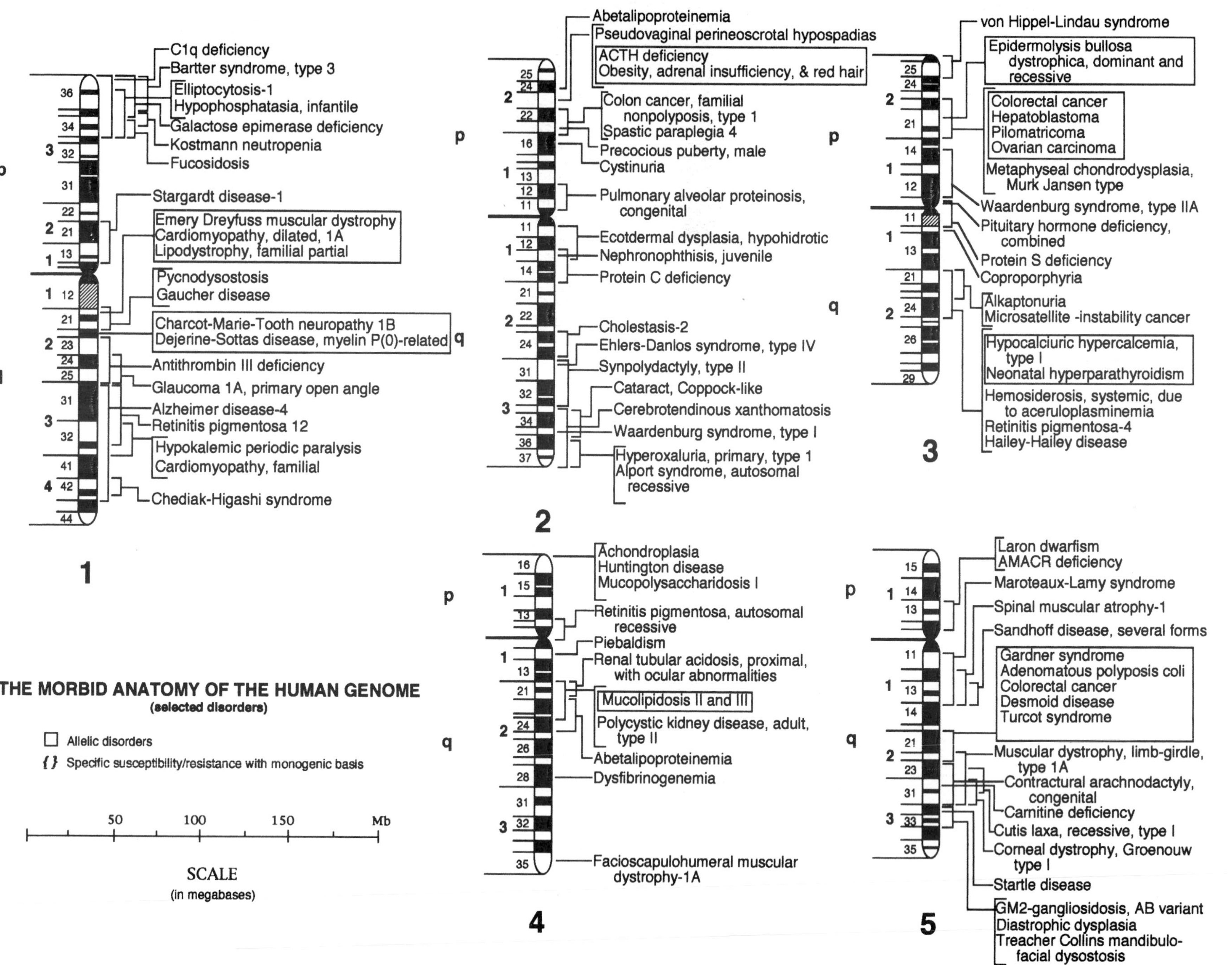

Fig. A1-1 The morbid anatomy of the human genome as of 2000. See the chromosome tables that follow for details by individual chromosomes, disease and adjacent normal loci, location by banding pattern, and gene symbol MIM number.

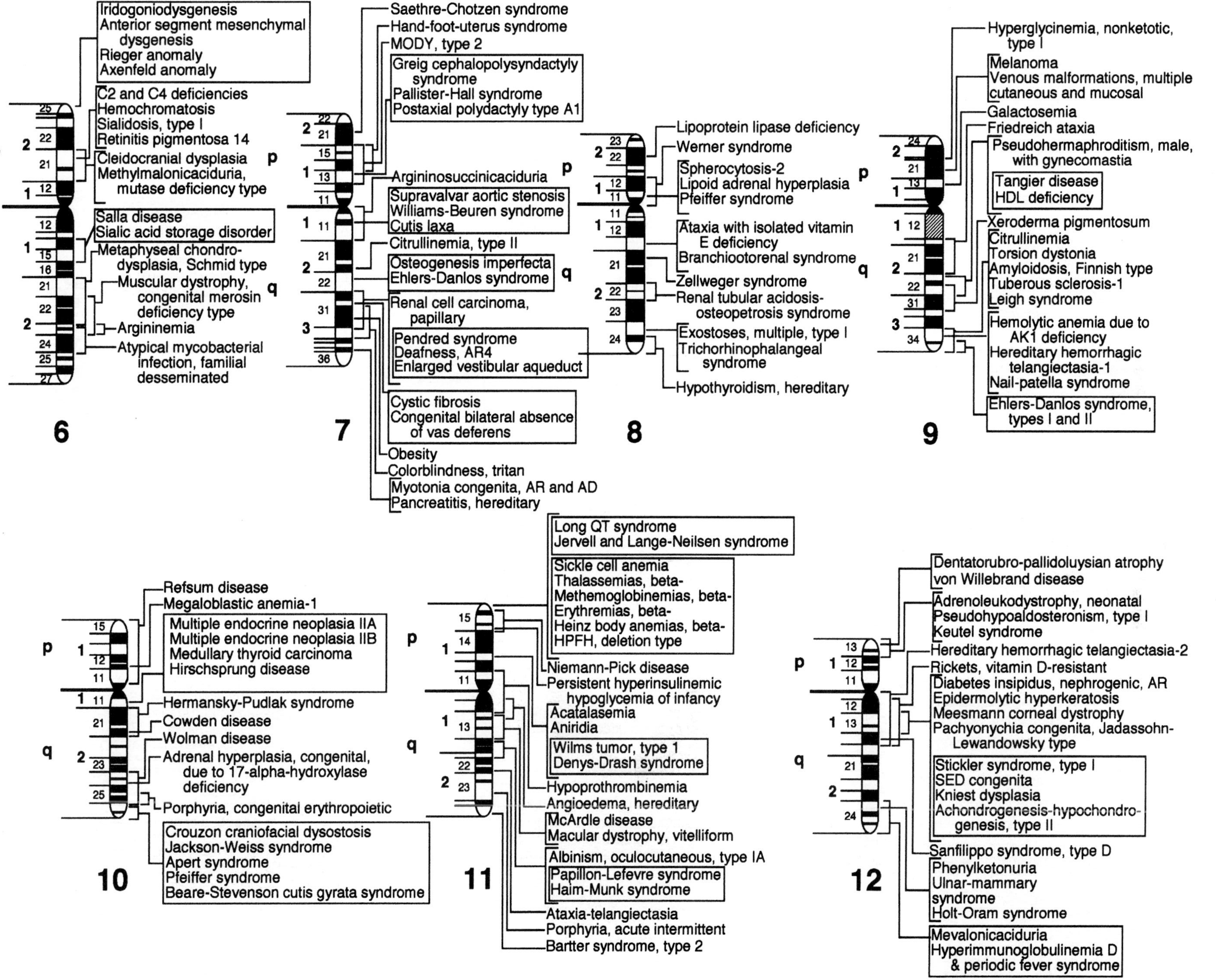

Fig. A1-1 (Continued)

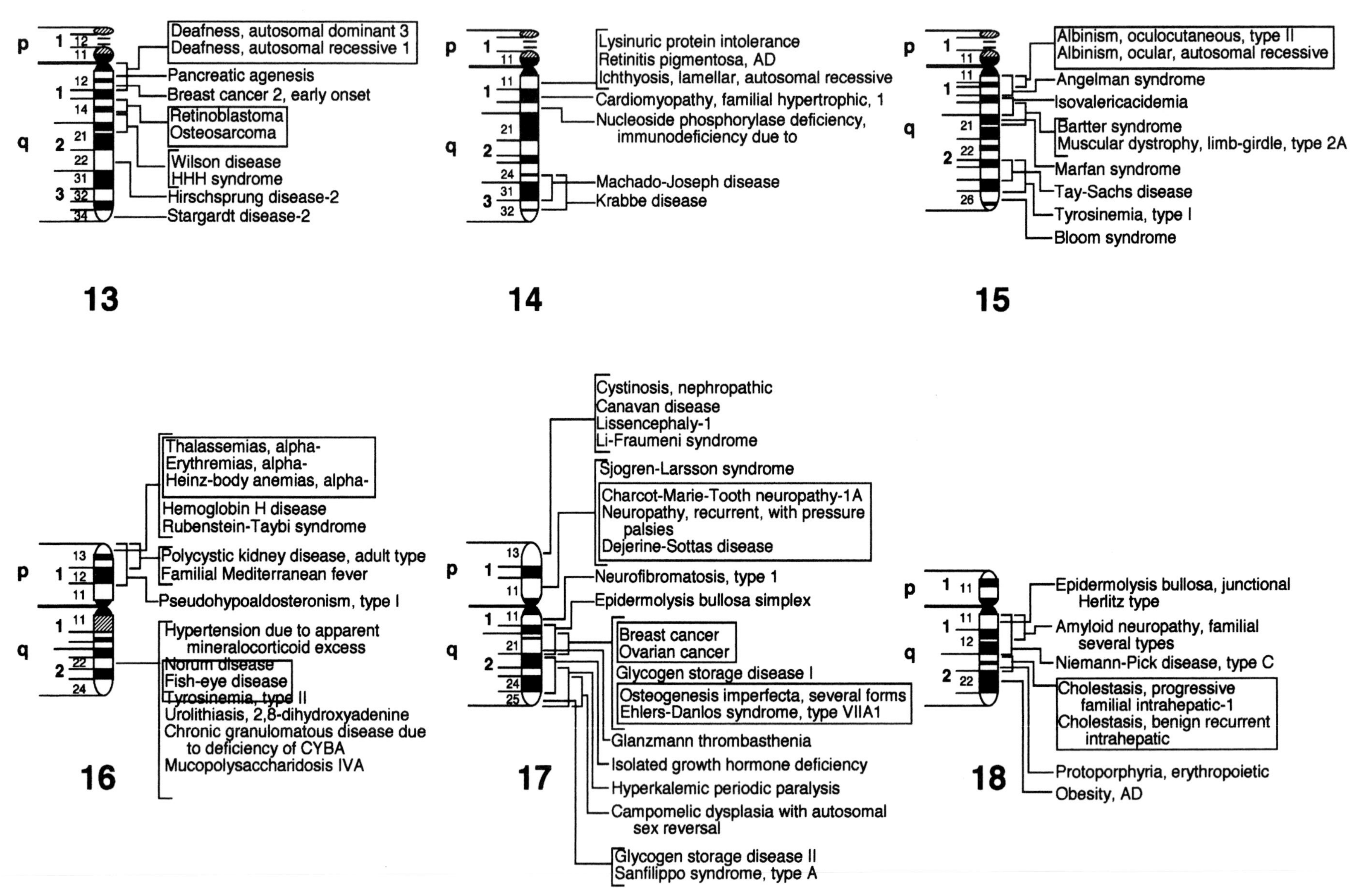

Fig. A1-1 (Continued)

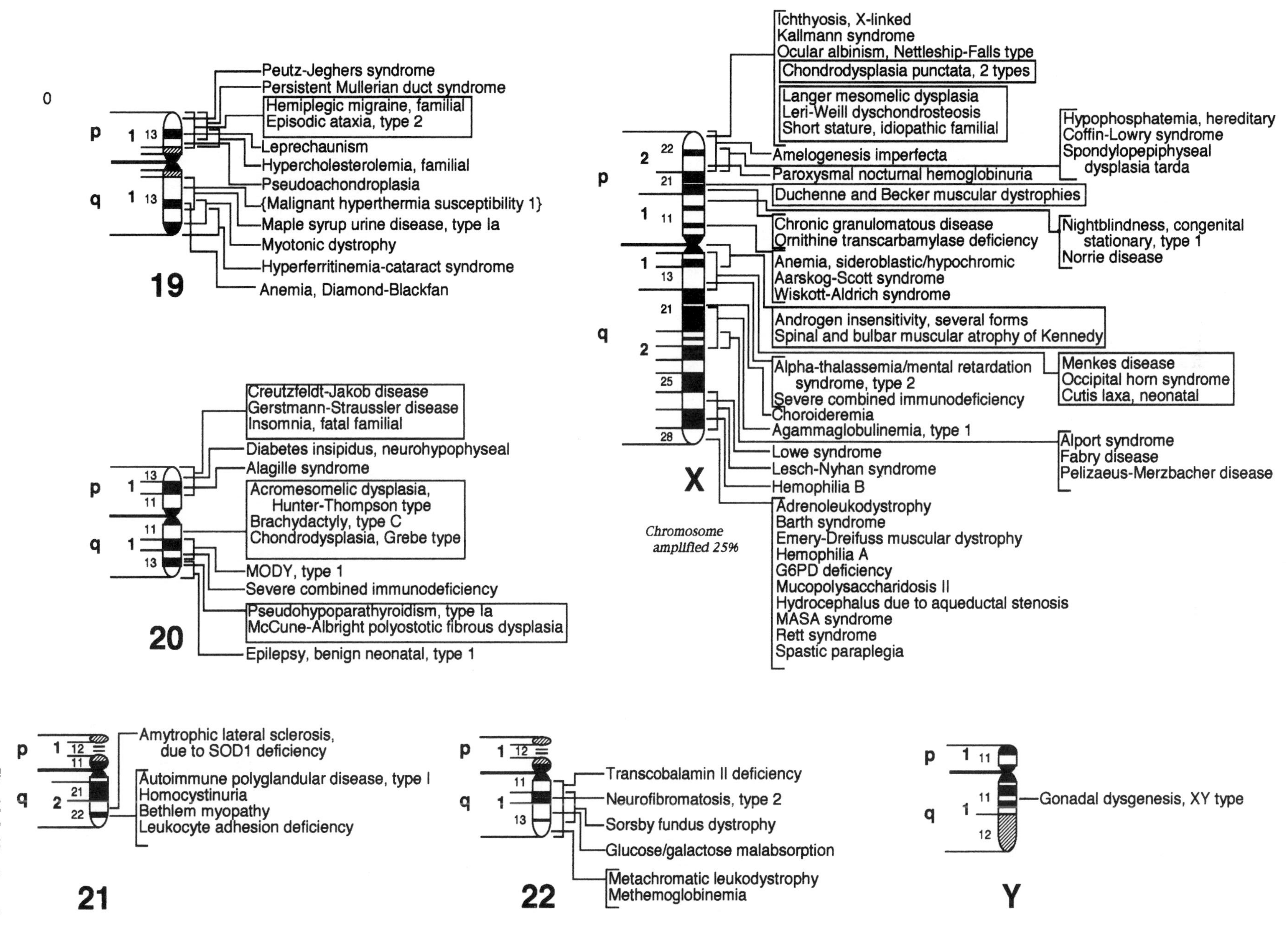

Fig. A1-1 (Continued)

Table A1-2 The Morbid Map

Location	Symbol	Status	Locus Name	MIM#	Disorder
1pter-p36.13	CCV	P	Cataract, congenital, Volkmann type	115665	Cataract, congenital, Volkmann type (2)
1pter-p36.13	ENO1, PPH	C	Enolase-1, alpha	172430	Enolase deficiency (1)
1pter-p36.1	CTPP, CPP, CTPA	P	Cataract, posterior polar	116600	Cataract, posterior polar (2)
1pter-p33	HMGCL	P	3-hydroxy-3-methylglutaryl-Coenzyme A lyase	246450	HMG-CoA lyase deficiency (3)
1p36.3	MTHFR	P	Methylenetetrahydrofolate reductase	236250	Homocystinuria due to MTHFR deficiency (3)
1p36.3-p36.2	NB, NBS	C	Neuroblastoma (neuroblastoma suppressor)	256700	Neuroblastoma (2)
1p36.3-p36.2	PLOD	P	Procollagen-lysine, 2-oxoglutarate 5-dioxygenase (lysine hydroxylase)	153454	Ehlers-Danlos syndrome, type VI, 225400 (3)
1p36.3-p34.1	C1QA	C	Complement component-1, q subcomponent, alpha polypeptide	120550	C1q deficiency, type A (3)
1p36.3-p34.1	C1QB	C	Complement component-1, q subcomponent, beta polypeptide	120570	C1q deficiency, type B (3)
1p36.3-p34.1	C1QG	P	Complement component-1, q subcomponent, gamma polypeptide	120575	C1q deficiency, type C (3)
1p36.2-p36.12	PAX7	C	Paired box homeotic gene-7	167410	Rhabdomyosarcoma, alveolar, 268220 (3)
1p36.2-p36.1	GLC3B	P	Glaucoma 3, primary infantile, B	600975	Glaucoma 3, primary infantile, B (2)
1p36.2-p34	EPB41, EL1	C	Erythrocyte surface protein band 4.1	130500	Elliptocytosis-1 (3)
1p36.1	ECE1	C	Endothelin converting enzyme 1	600423	Hirschsprung disease, cardiac defects, and autonomic dysfunction (3)
1p36.1-p35	SDHB, SDH1, SDHIP	C	Succinate dehydrogenase complex, subunit B, iron sulfur (Ip)	185470	?Myopathy due to succinate dehydrogenase deficiency (1)
1p36.1-p34	SJS, SJA	P	Schwartz-Jampel syndrome	255800	Schwartz-Jampel syndrome (2)
1p36.1-p34	ALPL, HOPS	C	Alkaline phosphatase, liver/bone/kidney	171760	Hypophosphatasia, infantile, 241500 (3); Hypophosphatasia, childhood, 241510 (3); ?Hypophosphatasia, adult, 146300 (1)
1p36	ALDH4, P5CDH	P	Aldehyde dehydrogenase-4 (delta-1-pyrroline 5-carboxylate dehydrogenase)	239510	Hyperprolinemia, type II (3)
1p36	BRCD2	P	Breast cancer, ductal	211420	Breast cancer, ductal (2)
1p36	CLCNKB	C	Chloride channel, kidney, B	602023	Bartter syndrome, type 3 (3)
1p36	CMM, MLM, DNS	P	Cutaneous malignant melanoma/ dysplastic nevus	155600	Malignant melanoma, cutaneous (2)
1p36	PCBC, CAPB	P	Prostate cancer-brain cancer susceptibility	603688	{Prostate cancer-brain cancer susceptibility} (2)
1p36	TP73	P	p53-related protein	601990	?Neuroblastoma (1)
1p36-p35	CMT2A	P	Charcot-Marie-Tooth neuropathy-2A (hereditary motor sensory neuropathy II)	118210	Charcot-Marie-Tooth neuropathy-2A (2)
1p36-p35	GALE	C	UDP galactose-4-epimerase	230350	Galactose epimerase deficiency (3)
1p36-p35	RSMD1, MDRS1	P	Muscular dystrophy, congenital, with early spine rigidity	602771	Muscular dystrophy, congenital, with early spine rigidity (2)
1p36-p34.1	SCCD	P	Schnyder crystalline corneal dystrophy	121800	Corneal dystrophy, crystalline, Schnyder (2)
1p35.1	GJB3, CX31, DFNA2	P	Gap junction protein, beta-3	603324	Erythrokeratodermia variabilis, 133200 (3); Deafness, autosomal dominant 2, 600101 (3); Deafness, autosomal recessive (3)
1p35	PLA2G2A, PLA2B, PLA2L, MOM1	C	Phospholipase A2, group IIA, platelets, synovial fluid	172411	{?Colorectal cancer, resistance to} (1)

Table A1-2 (Continued)

Location	Symbol	Status	Locus Name	MIM#	Disorder
1p35-p34.3	CSF3R, GCSFR	C	Colony-stimulating factor-3 receptor (granulocyte)	138971	Kostmann neutropenia, 202700 (3)
1p35-p34.3	LCK	C	Lymphocyte-specific protein tyrosine kinase	153390	SCID due to LCK deficiency (1)
1p35-p31.3	SLC2A1, GLUT1	C	Solute carrier family 2 (facilitated glucose transporter), member 1	138140	Glucose transport defect, blood-brain barrier (3)
1p34.1-p32	FH3	P	Hypercholesterolemia, familial, 3	603776	Hypercholesterolemia, familial, 3 (2)
1p34.1-p32	PTOS1	P	Ptosis, congenital 1, autosomal dominant	178300	Ptosis, hereditary congenital, 1 (2)
1p34	DFNA2	C	Deafness, autosomal dominant 2	600101	Deafness, autosomal dominant 2 (2)
1p34	ELAVL4, HUD, PNEM	C	Embryonic lethal, abnormal vision, Drosophila, homolog of, like-4 (Hu antigen D)	168360	Neuropathy, paraneoplastic sensory (1)
1p34	FUCA1	C	Fucosidase, alpha-L- 1, tissue	230000	Fucosidosis (3)
1p34	KCNQ4, DFNA2	P	Potassium voltage-gated channel, KQT-like subfamily, member 4	603537	Deafness, autosomal dominant 2, 600101 (3)
1p34	MPL, TPOR, MPLV	P	Myeloproliferative leukemia virus, homolog of	159530	Thrombocytopenia, congenital amegakaryocytic, 604498 (3)
1p34	UROD	C	Uroporphyrinogen decarboxylase	176100	Porphyria cutanea tarda (3); Porphyria, hepatoerythropoietic (3)
1p34-p32	MEB	P	Muscle-eye-brain disease	253280	Muscle-eye-brain disease (2)
1p33-p32.2	COL9A2, EDM2	C	Collagen IX, alpha-2 polypeptide	120260	Epiphyseal dysplasia, multiple, type 2, 600204 (3); Intervertebral disc disease, 603932 (3)
1p32	C8A	C	Complement component-8, alpha polypeptide	120950	C8 deficiency, type I (2)
1p32	C8B	C	Complement component-8, beta polypeptide	120960	C8 deficiency, type II (3)
1p32	CPT2	C	Carnitine palmitoyltransferase II	600650	Myopathy due to CPT II deficiency, 255110 (3); CPT deficiency, hepatic, type II, 600649 (3)
1p32	PPT, CLN1	C	Palmitoyl-protein thioesterase	600722	Ceroid lipofuscinosis, neuronal-1, infantile, 256730 (3); Ceroid lipofuscinosis, neuronal, variant juvenile type, with granular osmiophilic deposits (3)
1p32	PTCH2	P	Patched, drosophila, homolog of, 2	603673	Medulloblastoma, 155255 (3); Basal cell carcinoma, 109400 (3)
1p32	RAD54L, HR54, HRAD54	P	RAD54, S. cerevisiae, homolog-like	603615	Lymphoma, non-Hodgkin (3); Breast cancer, invasive intraductal (3); Colon adenocarcinoma (3)
1p32	TAL1, TCL5, SCL	C	T-cell acute lymphocytic leukemia-1	187040	Leukemia-1, T-cell acute lymphocytic (3)
1p32-q12	M1S1	P	Membrane component, chromosome 1, surface marker 1 (40kD glycoprotein, identified by monoclonal antibody GA733)	137290	Corneal dystrophy, gelatinous drop-like, 204870 (3)
1p31	ACADM, MCAD	P	Acyl-Coenzyme A dehydrogenase, C-4 to C-12 straight chain	201450	Acyl-CoA dehydrogenase, medium chain, deficiency of (3)
1p31	AIR	P	Acute insulin response	601676	Acute insulin response (2)
1p31	BSND	P	Bartter syndrome, infantile, with sensorineural deafness	602522	Bartter syndrome, infantile, with sensorineural deafness (2)
1p31	DBT, BCATE2	C	Dihydrolipoamide branched chain transacylase (E2 component of branched chain ketoacid dehydrogenase complex)	248610	Maple syrup urine disease, type II (3)
1p31	RPE65, RP20	C	Retinal pigment epithelium-specific protein, 65kD	180069	Leber congenital amaurosis-2, 204100 (3); Retinal dystrophy, autosomal recessive, childhood-onset (3); Retinitis pigmentosa-20 (3)

(Continued on next page)

Table A1-2 (Continued)

Location	Symbol	Status	Locus Name	MIM#	Disorder
1p31-p21	AVSD, AVCD	P	Atrioventricular canal defect 1	600309	Atrioventricular canal defect-1 (2)
1p22	BCL10	P	B-cell leukemia/lymphoma 10	603517	Lymphoma, MALT (3); Lymphoma, follicular (3); Mesothelioma (3); Germ cell tumor (3); Sezary syndrome (3); Colon cancer (3)
1p22	DPYD, DPD	C	Dihydropyrimidine dehydrogenase	274270	Thymine-uraciluria (3); {Fluorouracil toxicity, sensitivity to} (3)
1p22	UOX	P	Urate oxidase	191540	[Urate oxidase deficiency] (1)
1p22-p21	ABCD3, PXMP1, PMP70	P	ATP-binding cassette, subfamily D, member 3 (peroxisomal membrane protein 1, 70 kD)	170995	Zellweger syndrome-2 (3)
1p22-p21	VMGLOM	P	Venous malformations with glomus cells (glomus tumors, multiple)	138000	Glomus tumors, multiple (2)
1p21	AGL, GDE	C	Amylo-1,6-glucosidase, 4-alpha-glucanotransferase (glycogen debranching enzyme)	232400	Glycogen storage disease IIIa (3); Glycogen storage disease IIIb (3)
1p21	COL11A1	C	Collagen XI, alpha-1 polypeptide	120280	Stickler syndrome, type III, 108300 (3); Marshall syndrome, 154780 (3)
1p21	OPTA2	P	Osteopetrosis, autosomal dominant, type II	166600	Osteopetrosis, AD, type II (2)
1p21-p13	ABCA4, ABCR, STGD1, FFM, RP19	C	ATP-binding transporter, retina-specific	601691	Stargardt disease-1, 248200 (3); Retinitis pigmentosa-19, 601718 (3); Cone-rod dystrophy 3 (3); Macular dystrophy, age-related, 2, 153800 (3); Fundus flavimaculatus, 248200 (2)
1p21-p13	AMPD1	P	Adenosine monophosphate deaminase-1, muscle	102770	Myoadenylate deaminase deficiency (3)
1p21-p13.3	WS2B	P	Waardenburg syndrome, type 2B	600193	Waardenburg syndrome, type 2B (2)
1p13.2	NRAS	C	Neuroblastoma RAS viral (v-ras) oncogene homolog	164790	Colorectal cancer (3)
1p13.1	HSD3B2	C	Hydroxy-delta-5-steroid dehydrogenase, 3 beta- and steroid delta-isomerase, type 2 (adrenal, gonadal)	201810	3-beta-hydroxysteroid dehydrogenase, type II, deficiency (3)
1p13	TSHB	C	Thyroid-stimulating hormone, beta polypeptide	188540	Hypothyroidism, nongoitrous (3)
1p13-p12	HMGCS2	P	3-hydroxy-3-methylglutaryl-Coenzyme A synthase 2	600234	HMG-CoA synthase-2 deficiency (1)
1p13-q23	RP18	P	Retinitis pigmentosa-18	601414	Retinitis pigmentosa-18 (2)
1p	CSE, DYT9	P	Choreoathetosis/spasticity, episodic (paroxysmal choreoathetosis/spasticity)	601042	Choreoathetosis/spasticity, episodic (2)
1p	PCHC	P	Pheochromocytoma	171300	Pheochromocytoma (2)
1cen-q21	PSORS4	P	Psoriasis susceptibility 4	603935	{Psoriasis, susceptibility to} (2)
1q	HFE2	P	Hemochromatosis, type 2	602390	Hemochromatosis, type 2 (2)
1q11-q21	LGMD1B	P	Limb-girdle muscular dystrophy-1B, autosomal dominant	159001	Muscular dystrophy, limb-girdle, type 1B (2)
1q21	AF1Q	P	ALL1-fused gene from chromosome 1q	604684	Leukemia, acute myelomonocytic (3)
1q21	CTSK	P	Cathepsin K	601105	Pycnodysostosis, 265800 (3)
1q21	FLG	C	Filaggrin	135940	?Ichthyosis vulgaris, 146700 (1)
1q21	GBA	C	Glucosidase, acid beta	230800	Gaucher disease (3); Gaucher disease with cardiovascular calcification (3)
1q21	LOR	C	Loricrin	152445	Vohwinkel syndrome with ichthyosis, 604117 (3); Erythrokeratoderma, progressive symmetric, 602036 (3)
1q21	MCKD1	P	Medullary cystic kidney disease 1, autosomal dominant	174000	Medullary cystic kidney disease 1 (2)
1q21	PKLR, PK1	C	Pyruvate kinase, liver and RBC type	266200	Anemia, hemolytic, due to PK deficiency (3)

Table A1-2 (Continued)

Location	Symbol	Status	Locus Name	MIM#	Disorder
1q21	PRCC, RCCP1	C	Papillary renal cell carcinoma, translocation-associated	179755	Renal cell carcinoma, papillary, 1 (2)
1q21	SPTA1	C	Spectrin, alpha, erythrocytic-1	182860	Elliptocytosis-2 (3); Pyropoikilocytosis (3); Spherocytosis, recessive (3)
1q21-q22	FY, GPD	C	Duffy blood group	110700	{Vivax malaria, susceptibility to} (1)
1q21-q22	NTRK1, TRKA	C	Neurotrophic tyrosine kinase, receptor, type 1	191315	Insensitivity to pain, congenital, with anhidrosis, 256800 (3)
1q21-q23	APCS, SAP	C	Amyloid P component, serum	104770	{?Amyloidosis, secondary, susceptibility to} (1)
1q21-q23	APOA2	C	Apolipoprotein A-II	107670	Apolipoprotein A-II deficiency (3)
1q21-q23	DFNA7	P	Deafness, autosomal dominant 7	601412	Deafness, autosomal dominant 7 (2)
1q21-q23	FCGR2A, IGFR2, CD32	C	Fc fragment of IgG, low affinity IIa, receptor for (CD32)	146790	{Lupus nephritis, susceptibility to} (3)
1q21-q23	HYPLIP1	P	Hyperlipidemia, familial combined, 1	602491	Hyperlipidemia, familial combined, 1 (2)
1q21-q23	MHP2	P	Migraine, familial hemiplegic, 2	602481	Migraine, familial hemiplegic, 2 (2)
1q21-q32	HRPT2	C	Hyperparathyroidism 2, with jaw tumor	145001	Hyperparathyroidism-jaw tumor syndrome (2); Hyperparathyroidism, familial primary, 145000 (2)
1q21.1	GJA8, CX50, CAE1	C	Gap junction membrane channel protein alpha-8 (connexin 50)	600897	Cataract, zonular pulverulent-1, 116200 (3)
1q21.1-q21.3	RFX5	C	Regulatory factor X, 5 (influences HLA class II expression)	601863	MHC class II deficiency, complementation group C, 209920 (3)
1q21.2	LMNA, LMN1, EMD2, FPLD, CMD1A	C	Lamin A/C	150330	Emery-Dreifuss muscular dystrophy, autosomal dominant, 181350 (3); Cardiomyopathy, dilated, 1A, 115200 (3); Lipodystrophy, familial partial, 151660 (3)
1q21.2-q21.3	FCGR1A, IGFR1, CD64	C	Fc fragment of IgG, high affinity Ia, receptor for (CD64)	146760	[IgG receptor I, phagocytic, familial deficiency of] (1)
1q22	FCGR2B, CD32	P	Fc fragment of IgG, low affinity IIb, receptor for	604590	Lymphoma, progression of (3)
1q22	MPZ, CMT1B	C	Myelin protein zero	159440	Charcot-Marie-Tooth neuropathy-1B, 118200 (3); Dejerine-Sottas disease, myelin P(0)-related, 145900 (3); Hypomyelination, congenital (3)
1q22	PPOX	P	Protoporphyrinogen oxidase	600923	Porphyria variegata, 176200 (3)
1q22-q23	CD3Z, TCRZ	C	CD3Z antigen, zeta polypeptide (TiT3 complex)	186780	CD3, zeta chain, deficiency (1)
1q22-q23	TPM3, NEM1	C	Tropomyosin 3	191030	Nemaline myopathy 1, autosomal dominant, 161800 (3)
1q23	F5	C	Coagulation factor V (proaccelerin, labile factor)	227400	Hemorrhagic diathesis due to factor V deficiency (1); {Thromboembolism susceptibility due to factor V Leiden} (3)
1q23	FCGR3A, CD16, IGFR3	C	Fc fragment of IgG, low affinity III, receptor for (CD16)	146740	{Lupus erythematosus, systemic, susceptibility}, 152700 (1); Neutropenia, alloimmune neonatal (3); {Viral infections, recurrent} (3)
1q23	PBX1	C	Pre-B cell leukemia transcription factor-1	176310	Leukemia, acute pre-B-cell (2)
1q23	TNFSF6, APT1LG1, FASL	C	Tumor necrosis factor ligand superfamily, member 6	134638	{Systemic lupus erythematosus, susceptibility}, 152700 (3)
1q23-q25	AT3	C	Antithrombin III	107300	Antithrombin III deficiency (3)
1q23-q25	FMO3	P	Flavin-containing monooxygenase 3	136132	[Fish-odor syndrome], 602079 (3)
1q23-q25	SELE, ELAM1	C	Selectin E (endothelial leukocyte adhesion molecule-1)	131210	{Atherosclerosis, susceptibility to} (2)

(Continued on next page)

Table A1-2 (Continued)

Location	Symbol	Status	Locus Name	MIM#	Disorder
1q23-q25	SELP, GRMP	C	Selectin P (granulocyte membrane protein, 140kD; antigen CD62)	173610	Platelet alpha/delta storage pool deficiency (1)
1q23.3	SLC19A2, THTR1	C	Solute carrier family 19 (folate transporter), member 2	603941	Thiamine-responsive megaloblastic anemia syndrome, 249270 (3)
1q24-q25	PRCA1, HPC1	C	Prostate cancer, hereditary, 1	601518	Prostate cancer, hereditary, 1, 176807 (2)
1q24.3-q25.2	MYOC, TIGR, GLC1A, JOAG, GPOA	C	Myocilin (trabecular meshwork-induced glucocorticoid response protein)	601652	Glaucoma 1A, primary open angle, juvenile-onset, 137750 (3); Glaucoma 1A, primary open angle, recessive (3)
1q25	NCF2	C	Neutrophil cytosolic factor-2, 65kD	233710	Chronic granulomatous disease due to deficiency of NCF-2 (3)
1q25-q31	ARMD1	P	Macular degeneration, age-related, 1	603075	Macular degeneration, age-related, 1 (2)
1q25-q31	CACP, MSF, SZP	P	Megakaryocyte stimulating factor	604283	Camptodactyly-arthropathy-coxa vara-pericarditis syndrome, 208250 (3)
1q25-q31	LAMC2, LAMNB2, LAMB2T	C	Laminin, gamma-2 (nicein, 100kD; kalinin, 105kD; BM600, 100kD)	150292	Epidermolysis bullosa, Herlitz junctional type, 226700 (3)
1q25-q31	PDCN, NPHS2, SRN1	P	Podocin	604766	Nephrotic syndrome, steroid-resistant, 600995 (3)
1q25-q31	SRN1	P	Nephrotic syndrome, idiopathic, steroid-resistant	600995	Nephrotic syndrome, idiopathic, steroid-resistant (2)
1q31-q32	CHIT	C	Chitotriosidase	600031	[Chitotriosidase deficiency] (3)
1q31-q32.1	CRB1, RP12	P	Crumbs, drosophila, homolog of, 1	604210	Retinitis pigmentosa-12, autosomal recessive, 600105 (3)
1q31-q32.1	F13B	C	Coagulation factor XIII, B polypeptide	134580	Factor XIIIB deficiency (3)
1q31-q42	PHA2A, PHA2	P	Pseudohypoaldosteronism type II	145260	Pseudohypoaldosteronism, type II (2)
1q31-q42	PSEN2, AD4, STM2	P	Presenilin 2	600759	Alzheimer disease-4 (3)
1q32	CACNA1S, CACNL1A3, CCHL1A3	C	Calcium channel, voltage-dependent, L type, alpha 1S subunit	114208	Hypokalemic periodic paralysis, 170400 (3); {Malignant hyperthermia susceptibility 5}, 601887 (3)
1q32	CMD1D, CMPD2	P	Cardiomyopathy, dilated-1D, autosomal dominant	601494	Cardiomyopathy, familial, dilated-2 (2)
1q32	CR1, C3BR	C	Complement component (3b/4b) receptor-1	120620	CR1 deficiency (1); {?SLE susceptibility} (1)
1q32	GFND	P	Glomerulopathy with fibronectin deposits	601894	Glomerulopathy, fibronectin (2)
1q32	HF1, CFH, HUS	C	H factor-1 (complement factor H)	134370	Factor H deficiency (1); Membroproliferative glomerulonephritis (1); Hemolytic-uremic syndrome, 235400 (3); Nephropathy, chronic hypocomplementemic (3)
1q32	LAMB3	P	Laminin, beta-3 (nicein, 125kD; kalinin, 140kD; BM600, 125kD)	150310	Epidermolysis bullosa, Herlitz junctional type, 226700 (3); Epidermolysis bullosa, generalized atrophic benign, 226650 (3)
1q32	MCP, CD46	C	Membrane cofactor protein (CD46, trophoblast-lymphocyte cross-reactive antigen)	120920	{Measles, susceptibility to} (1)
1q32	REN	C	Renin	179820	[Hyperproreninemia] (3)
1q32	TNNT2, CMH2	C	Troponin-T2, cardiac	191045	Cardiomyopathy, familial hypertrophic, 2, 115195 (3)
1q32	VWS, LPS, PIT	C	van der Woude syndrome (lip pit syndrome)	119300	van der Woude syndrome (2)
1q32-q44	PKP1	P	Plakophilin-1	601975	Ectodermal dysplasia/skin fragility syndrome, 604536 (3)
1q41	RMD1	C	Rippling muscle disease 1	600332	Rippling muscle disease-1 (2)
1q41	USH2A	C	Usher syndrome-2A, autosomal recessive, mild	276901	Usher syndrome, type 2 (3)

Table A1-2 (Continued)

Location	Symbol	Status	Locus Name	MIM#	Disorder
1q41-q42	SLEB1, SLE1	P	Systemic lupus erythematosus, susceptibility to, 1	601744	{Systemic lupus erythematosus, susceptibility to, 1} (2)
1q42	ADPRT, PPOL	C	ADP-ribosyltransferase NAD(+)	173870	?Fanconi anemia (1); ?Xeroderma pigmentosum (1)
1q42	MDC1B	P	Muscular dystrophy, congenital, 1B	604801	Muscular dystrophy, congenital, 1B (2)
1q42-q43	AGT	C	Angiotensinogen	106150	{Hypertension, essential, susceptibility to} (3); {Preeclampsia, susceptibility to} (3)
1q42-q43	ARVD2	P	Arrhythmogenic right ventricular dysplasia-2 (arrhythmogenic right ventricular cardiomyopathy)	600996	Arrhythmogenic right ventricular dysplasia-2 (2)
1q42-q43	HRD	P	Hypoparathyroidism-retardation-dysmorphism syndrome (Sanjad-Sakati syndrome)	241410	Hypoparathyroidism-retardation-dysmorphism syndrome (2)
1q42-q43	KCS, KCS1	P	Kenny-Caffey syndrome-1	244460	Kenny-Caffey syndrome-1 (2)
1q42.1	ACTA1, ASMA, NEM2, NEM1	C	Actin, alpha-1, skeletal muscle	102610	Myopathy, nemaline, 161800, 256030 (3); Myopathy, actin (3)
1q42.1	EPHX1	C	Epoxide hydroxylase 1, microsomal xenobiotic	132810	?Fetal hydantoin syndrome (1); Diphenylhydantoin toxicity (1)
1q42.1	FH	C	Fumarate hydratase	136850	Fumarase deficiency (3)
1q42.1	TGFB4, EBAF, LEFTY1	C	Transforming growth factor, beta-4 (endometrial bleeding-associated factor; LEFTY A)	601877	Left-right axis malformation (3)
1q42.1-q42.2	CHS1, LYST	C	Lysosomal trafficking regulator	214500	Chediak-Higashi syndrome (3)
1q42.2-q43	PCAP, PRCA2, HPC2	P	Prostate cancer, hereditary, 2	602759	Prostate cancer, hereditary, 2, 176807 (2)
1q43	MTR	C	5-methyltetrahydrofolate-homocysteine methyltransferase 1	156570	Methylcobalamin deficiency, cbl G type (3)
1q44	MWS	P	Muckle-Wells syndrome	191900	Muckle-Wells syndrome (2)
Chr.1	GNPAT, DHAPAT	P	Glyceronephosphate O-acyltransferase	602744	Chondrodysplasia punctata, rhizomelic, type 2, 222765 (3)
Chr.1	PEX10, NALD	P	Peroxisome biogenesis factor 10	602859	Zellweger syndrome, 214100 (3); Adrenoleukodystrophy, neonatal, 202370 (3)
2p25.3	D2S448, MG50, D2S448E	P	Melanoma associated gene	600134	?Melanoma (1)
2p25	TPO, TPX	C	Thyroid peroxidase	274500	Thyroid iodine peroxidase deficiency (1); Goiter, congenital (3); Hypothyroidism, congenital (3)
2p25-p22	ETM2	C	Tremor, familial essential, 2	602134	Tremor, familial essential, 2 (2)
2p24	APOB	C	Apolipoprotein B (including Ag(x) antigen)	107730	Hypobetalipoproteinemia (3); Abetalipoproteinemia (3); Hyperbetalipoproteinemia, 144400 (3); Apolipoprotein B-100, ligand-defective, 144010 (3)
2p24-p23	ODED, MODED	P	Oculodigitoesophagoduodenal syndrome	164280	Oculodigitoesophagoduodenal syndrome (2)
2p23.3	POMC	C	Proopiomelanocortin (adrenocorticotropin/beta-lipotropin)	176830	ACTH deficiency (1); Obesity, adrenal insufficiency, and red hair (3)
2p23.3-p23.2	KHK	P	Ketohexokinase (fructokinase)	229800	[Fructosuria] (1)
2p23	HADHA, MTPA	C	Hydroxyacyl-Coenzyme A dehydrogenase/3-ketoacyl-Coenzyme A thiolase/enoyl-Coenzyme A hydratase (trifunctional protein), alpha subunit	600890	LCHAD deficiency (3); Trifunctional protein deficiency, type 1 (3); HELLP syndrome, maternal, of pregnancy (3); Fatty liver, acute, of pregnancy (3)
2p23	HADHB	C	Hydroxyacyl-Coenzyme A dehydrogenase/3-ketoacyl-Coenzyme A thiolase /enoyl-Coenzyme A hydratase (trifunctional protein), beta subunit	143450	Trifunctional protein deficiency, type II (3)

(Continued on next page)

Table A1-2 (Continued)

Location	Symbol	Status	Locus Name	MIM#	Disorder
2p23	SRD5A2	C	Steroid-5-alpha-reductase, alpha polypeptide-2 (3-oxo-5 alpha-steroid delta 4-dehydrogenase alpha-2)	264600	Pseudovaginal perineoscrotal hypospadias (3)
2p23-p22	OTOF, DFNB9, NSRD9	C	Otoferlin	603681	Deafness, autosomal recessive 9, 601071 (3)
2p23-p22	XDH	C	Xanthine dehydrogenase (xanthine oxidase)	278300	Xanthinuria, type I (3)
2p22-p21	CYP1B1, GLC3A	C	Cytochrome P450, subfamily I, dioxin-inducible, polypeptide 1	601771	Glaucoma 3A, primary infantile, 231300 (3)
2p22-p21	MSH2, COCA1, FCC1	C	mutS, E. coli, homolog of, 2	120435	Colorectal cancer, hereditary, nonpolyposis, type 1 (3); Ovarian cancer (3); Muir-Torre syndrome, 158320 (3)
2p22-p21	SPG4, SPAST	C	Spastin	604277	Spastic paraplegia-4, 182601 (3)
2p21	GF1, HGF	P	Gingival fibromatosis, hereditary, 1	135300	Fibromatosis, gingival (2)
2p21	LHCGR	P	Luteinizing hormone/ choriogonadotropin receptor	152790	Precocious puberty, male, 176410 (3); Pseudohermaphroditism, male, with Leydig cell hypoplasia (3); Hypogonadotropic hypogonadism (3); Micropenis (3); Leydig cell adenoma, with precocious puberty (3)
2p21	SIX3, HPE2	C	Sine oculis homeo box, drosophila, homolog of, 3	603714	Holoprosencephaly-2, 157170 (3)
2p21	STSL	P	Sitosterolemia	210250	Sitosterolemia (2)
2p21-p16	FSHR, ODG1	C	Follicle stimulating hormone receptor	136435	Ovarian dysgenesis, hypergonadotropic, with normal karyotype, 233300 (3)
2p16.3	SLC3A1, ATR1, D2H, NBAT	C	Solute carrier family 3 (cystine, dibasic and neutral amino acid transporters), member 1	104614	Cystinuria, 220100 (3)
2p16	CNC, CNC1	C	Carney complex 1	160980	Carney myxoma-endocrine complex (2)
2p16	EFEMP1, FBNL, DHRD	C	EGF-containing fibulin-like extracellular matrix protein 1 (fibrillin-like)	601548	Doyne honeycomb degeneration of retina, 126600 (3)
2p16	MSH6, GTBP, HNPCC5	P	MutS, E. coli, homolog of, 6	600678	{Cancer susceptibility} (3); Endometrial carcinoma (3)
2p16-p15	DYX3	P	Dyslexia, specific, 3	604254	Dyslexia, specific, 3 (2)
2p15	PEX13, ZWS, NALD	P	Peroxisome biogenesis factor 13 (peroxin 13)	601789	Zellweger syndrome, 214100 (3); Adrenoleukodystrophy, neonatal, 202370 (3)
2p13.3-p13.1	DYSF, LGMD2B	C	Dysferlin	603009	Muscular dystrophy, limb-girdle, type 2B, 253601 (3); Miyoshi myopathy, 254130 (3); Myopathy, distal, with anterior tibial onset (3)
2p13	ALMS1, ALSS	C	Alstrom syndrome	203800	Alstrom syndrome (2)
2p13	OFC2	P	Orofacial cleft-2	602966	Orofacial cleft-2 (2)
2p13	PEE1	P	Preeclampsia/eclampsia	189800	Preeclampsia (2)
2p13	PARK3	P	Parkinson disease, type 3	602404	Parkinson disease, type 3 (2)
2p13	WDM	P	Welander distal myopathy	604454	Welander distal myopathy (2)
2p12	GGCX	P	Gamma-glutamyl carboxylase	137167	Vitamin K-dependent coagulation defect, 277450 (3)
2p12	IGKC	C	Immunoglobulin kappa constant region	147200	[Kappa light chain deficiency] (3)
2p12-p11.2	SFTPB, SFTB3	C	Pulmonary surfactant-associated protein B, 18 kD	178640	Pulmonary alveolar proteinosis, congenital, 265120 (3)
2cen-q13	ATP6B1, VPP3	C	ATPase, H+ transporting, lysosomal, beta polypeptide, 58 kD (vacuolar proton pump, subunit 3)	192132	Renal tubular acidosis with deafness, 267300 (3)
2cen-q13	GLC1B	P	Glaucoma 1, open angle, B (adult-onset)	137760	Glaucoma 1B, primary open angle, adult onset (2)

Table A1-2 (Continued)

Location	Symbol	Status	Locus Name	MIM#	Disorder
2q	NIDDM1	P	Non-insulin-dependent diabetes mellitus (common, type 2)	601283	{Diabetes mellitus, non-insulin dependent, 1} (2)
2q11	CNGA3, CNG3, ACHM2	P	Cyclic nucleotide-gated channel, alpha-3	600053	Achromatopsia-2, 216900 (3)
2q11	TMD	P	Tibial muscular dystrophy	600334	Tibial muscular dystrophy (2)
2q11-q13	DL, ED3, EDA3	C	Downless, mouse, homolog of	604095	Ectodermal dysplasia, hypohidrotic, autosomal dominant, 129490 (3); Ectodermal dysplasia, hypohidrotic, autosomal recessive, 224900 (3)
2q12	ZAP70, SRK, STD	C	Zeta-chain associated protein kinase, 70 kD (syk-related tyrosine kinase)	176947	Selective T-cell defect (3)
2q12-q13	OADIP, DIPOA	L	Osteoarthritis of distal interphalangeal joints	140600	?Osteoarthritis of distal interphalan geal joints (2)
2q12-q14	PAX8	C	Paired box homeotic gene-8	167415	Hypothyroidism, congenital, due to thyroid dysgenesis or hypoplasia (3)
2q13	NPHP1, NPH1	C	Nephronophthisis-1 gene	256100	Nephronophthisis, juvenile (3)
2q13-q14	PROC	C	Protein C (inactivator of coagulation factors Va and VIIIa)	176860	Thrombophilia due to protein C deficiency (3); Purpura fulminans, neonatal (1)
2q14	BUB1	C	Budding uninhibited by benzimidazoles 1, S. cerevisiae, homolog of (mitotic checkpoint gene BUB1)	602452	Colorectal cancer with chromosomal instability (3)
2q14-q21	LCO	P	Liver cancer oncogene	165320	?Hepatocellular carcinoma (1)
2q14-q22	CMD1H	P	Cardiomyopathy, dilated, 1H	604288	Cardiomyopathy, dilated, 1H (2)
2q21	ERCC3, XPB	C	Excision-repair cross-complementing rodent repair deficiency, complementation group 3	133510	Xeroderma pigmentosum, group B (3); Trichothiodystrophy (3)
2q21-q31	SCP	P	Spastic cerebral palsy, symmetric, autosomal recessive	603513	Spastic cerebral palsy, symmetric (2)
2q22	NEB	C	Nebulin	161650	Nemaline myopathy 2, autosomal recessive, 256030 (3)
2q23-q24	3-Feb	P	Convulsions, familial febrile, 3	604403	Convulsions, familial febrile, 3 (2)
2q23-q24.3	DFNA16	P	Deafness, autosomal dominant 16	603964	Deafness, autosomal dominant 16 (2)
2q24	ABCB11, BSEP, SPGP, PFIC2	C	ATP-binding cassette, subfamily B, member 11 (bile salt export pump)	603201	Progressive intrahepatic cholestasis-2, 601847 (3)
2q24	SCN1A, GEFSP2	C	Sodium channel, voltage-gated, type I, alpha polypeptide	182389	Epilepsy, generalized, with febrile seizures plus, type 2, 604233 (3)
2q24-q31	MPRM	P	Myopathy, proximal, with early respiratory muscle involvement (Edstrom myopathy)	603689	Myopathy, proximal, with early respiratory muscle involvement (2)
2q24-q32	CHRNA1	C	Cholinergic receptor, nicotinic, alpha polypeptide-1, muscle	100690	Myasthenic syndrome, slow-channel congenital, 601462 (3)
2q24-q32	MMDK, MDK	P	Mesomelic dysplasia, Kantaputra type	156232	Mesomelic dysplasia, Kantaputra type (2)
2q24.1	GPD2	C	Glycerol-3-phosphate dehydrogenase 2 (mitochondrial)	138430	{Diabetes mellitus, type II} (3)
2q24.3	TTN	C	Titin	188840	Cardiomyopathy, familial hypertrophic, 9 (3)
2q31	AGPS, ADHAPS	P	Alkylglycerone-phosphate synthase	603051	Rhizomelic chondrodysplasia punctata, type 3, 600121 (3)
2q31	BBS5	P	Bardet-Biedl syndrome 5	603650	Bardet-Biedl syndrome 5 (2)
2q31	CMD1G	P	Cardiomyopathy, dilated, 1G	604145	Cardiomyopathy, dilated, 1G (2)
2q31	COL3A1	C	Collagen III, alpha-1 polypeptide	120180	Ehlers-Danlos syndrome, type IV, 130050 (3); Ehlers-Danlos syndrome, type III, 130020 (3); Aneurysm, familial arterial (3)
2q31	COL5A2	C	Collagen V, alpha-2 polypeptide	120190	Ehlers-Danlos syndrome, type I, 130000 (3)
2q31	DURS2	P	Duane retraction syndrome 2	604356	Duane retraction syndrome 2 (2)
2q31	GAD1	C	Glutamate decarboxylase-1, brain, 67 kD	266100	?Pyridoxine dependency with seizures (1)

(Continued on next page)

Table A1-2 (Continued)

Location	Symbol	Status	Locus Name	MIM#	Disorder
2q31	IDDM7	P	Insulin-dependent diabetes mellitus-7	600321	{Diabetes mellitus, insulin-dependent, 7} (2)
2q31-q32	HOXD13, HOX4I, SPD	C	Homeo box-D13	142989	Synpolydactyly, type II, 186000 (3)
2q31-q32	PPH1	C	Primary pulmonary hypertension 1	178600	Pulmonary hypertension, familial primary (2)
2q31-q33	PMS1, PMSL1	P	Postmeiotic segregation increased, S. cerevisiae, like 1	600258	Colorectal cancer, hereditary nonpolyposis, type 3 (3)
2q32	CP1, CP	P	Cleft palate, isolated	119540	Cleft palate, isolated (2)
2q32	NEUROD1, NIDDM	C	Neurogenic differentiation 1	601724	Diabetes mellitus, type II, 125853 (3)
2q32	WSS	P	Wrinkly skin syndrome	278250	Wrinkly skin syndrome (2)
2q32.1-q32.3	ARVD4	P	Arrhythmogenic right ventricular dysplasia-4	602087	Arrhythmogenic right ventricular dysplasia-4 (2)
2q33	ALS2	C	Amyotrophic lateral sclerosis-2, juvenile recessive	205100	Amyotrophic lateral sclerosis, juvenile recessive (2)
2q33	IDDM12	P	Insulin-dependent diabetes mellitus-12	601388	{Diabetes mellitus, insulin-dependent, 12} (2)
2q33-q34	CHRNG, ACHRG	C	Cholinergic receptor, nicotinic, gamma polypeptide	100730	Myasthenia gravis, neonatal transient (2)
2q33-q34	NDUFS1	P	NADH dehydrogenase (ubiquinone), Fe-S protein-1, 75 kD	157655	Lactic acidosis due to defect in iron-sulfur cluster of complex I (1)
2q33-q35	CRYGC, CRYG3, CZP1, CAE1	C	Crystallin, gamma C	123680	Cataract, Coppock-like, 604307 (3)
2q33-q35	CRYGD, CRYG4	C	Crystallin, gamma D	123690	Cataracts, punctate, progressive juvenile-onset (3); Cataract, crystalline aculeiform, 115700 (3)
2q33-q35	ICR2B, LI2	P	Ichthyosis congenita IIB	601277	Ichthyosis, lamellar, type 2 (2)
2q33-q35	PCC, CCP	P	Cataract, polymorphic congenital, autosomal dominant nonnuclear	601286	Cataract, polymorphic congenital (2)
2q33-q35	PNKD, FPD1, PDC, DYT8	P	Paroxysmal nonkinesiogenic dyskinesia	118800	Choreoathetosis, familial paroxysmal (2)
2q33-q37	FLNMS	P	Finnish lethal neonatal metabolic syndrome	603358	Finnish lethal neonatal metabolic syndrome (2)
2q33-qter	CYP27A1, CYP27, CTX	P	Cytochrome P450, subfamily XXVIIA, polypeptide 1 (sterol 27-hydroxylase)	213700	Cerebrotendinous xanthomatosis (3)
2q34	FN1	C	Fibronectin-1	135600	?Ehlers-Danlos syndrome, type X, 225310 (1)
2q34	IDDM13	P	Insulin-dependent diabetes mellitus-13	601318	{Diabetes mellitus, insulin-dependent, 13} (2)
2q34	TCL4	P	T-cell leukemia/lymphoma-4	186860	Leukemia/lymphoma, T-cell (2)
2q34-q35	ACADL, LCAD	P	Acyl-Coenzyme A dehydrogenase, long chain	201460	Acyl-CoA dehydrogenase, long chain, deficiency of (3)
2q34-q36	BJS, PTD	P	Bjornstad syndrome (pili torti and deafness)	262000	Bjornstad syndrome (2)
2q35	CPS1	C	Carbamoyl-phosphate synthetase 1, mitochondrial	237300	Carbamoylphosphate synthetase I deficiency (3)
2q35	DES, CMD1I	C	Desmin	125660	Myopathy, desmin-related, cardioskeletal, 601419 (3); Cardiomyopathy, dilated, 1I, 604765 (3)
2q35	PAX3, WS1, HUP2, CDHS	C	Paired box homeotic gene-3	193500	Waardenburg syndrome, type I (3); Waardenburg syndrome, type III, 148820 (3); Rhabdomyosarcoma, alveolar, 268220 (3); Craniofacial-deafness-hand syndrome, 122880 (3)
2q35	NRAMP1, NRAMP	C	Natural resistance-associated macrophage protein	600266	?Resistance/susceptibility to TB, etc. (1)
2q35-q36	BDA1	P	Brachydactyly, type A1	112500	Brachydactyly, type A1 (2)
2q36	IRS1	P	Insulin receptor substrate-1	147545	{Diabetes mellitus, noninsulin-dependent} (3)
2q36-q37	AGXT, SPAT	C	Alanine-glyoxylate aminotransferase, liver-specific peroxisomal	604285	Hyperoxaluria, primary, type 1, 259900 (3)

Table A1-2 (Continued)

Location	Symbol	Status	Locus Name	MIM#	Disorder
2q36-q37	COL4A3	C	Collagen IV, alpha-3 polypeptide (Goodpasture antigen)	120070	Alport syndrome, autosomal recessive, 203780 (3)
2q36-q37	COL4A4	C	Collagen IV, alpha-4 polypeptide	120131	Alport syndrome, autosomal recessive, 203780 (3); Hematuria, familial benign (3)
2q36-q37	GCG	C	Glucagon	138030	[?Hyperproglucagonemia] (1)
2q37	BDE	L	Brachydactyly type E	113300	?Brachydactyly type E (2)
2q37	BDMR	P	Brachydactyly-mental retardation syndrome	600430	Brachydactyly-mental retardation syndrome (2)
2q37	COL6A3	C	Collagen VI, alpha-3 polypeptide	120250	Bethlem myopathy, 158810 (3)
2q37.1	SAG	C	S-antigen; retina and pineal gland (arrestin)	181031	Oguchi disease-1, 258100 (3)
Chr.2	ITGA6	P	Integrin, alpha-6	147556	Epidermolysis bullosa, junctional, with pyloric stenosis, 226730 (3)
Chr.2	LSFC	P	Leigh syndrome, French-Canadian type	220111	Leigh syndrome, French-Canadian type (2)
Chr.2	UGT1, UGT1A1, GNT1	P	UDP glycosyltransferase 1	191740	Crigler-Najjar syndrome, type I, 218800 (3); [Gilbert syndrome], 143500 (3)
3p26-p25	VHL	C	von Hippel-Lindau syndrome	193300	von Hippel-Lindau syndrome (3); Renal cell carcinoma (3)
3p26-p24.2	MYMY	P	Moyamoya disease	252350	Moyamoya disease (2)
3p26-p22	FANCD, FACD, FAD	P	Fanconi anemia, complementation group D	227646	Fanconi anemia, type D (2)
3p25	CAV3, LGMD1C	C	Caveolin-3	601253	Muscular dystrophy, limb-girdle, type IC (3)
3p25	BTD	P	Biotinidase	253260	Biotinidase deficiency (3)
3p25	PPARG, PPARG1, PPARG2	C	Peroxisome proliferator activated receptor, gamma	601487	Obesity, severe, 601665 (3); [Obesity, protection against] (3); Diabetes mellitus, insulin-resistant, with acanthosis nigricans and hypertension, 604367 (3)
3p25	XPC, XPCC	C	Xeroderma pigmentosum, complementation group C	278720	Xeroderma pigmentosum, group C (3)
3p25-p24.2	MFS2	P	Marfan-like connective tissue disorder	154705	Marfan-like connective tissue disorder (2)
3p25-p22	CMD1E, CDCD2, CMPD2	P	Cardiomyopathy, dilated, 1E, autosomal dominant	601154	Cardiomyopathy, dilated, 1E (2)
3p24.3	THRB, ERBA2, THR1	C	Thyroid hormone receptor, beta (avian erythroblastic leukemia viral (v-erb-a) oncogene homolog-2)	190160	Thyroid hormone resistance, 274300, 188570 (3)
3p24.2	COLQ, EAD	C	Collagenic tail of endplate acetylcholinesterase	603033	Endplate acetylcholinesterase deficiency, 603034 (3)
3p23	ARVD5, ARVC5	P	Arrhythmogenic right ventricular dysplasia-5	604400	Arrhythmogenic right ventricular dysplasia-5 (2)
3p23-p22	ACAA1	P	Acetyl-Coenzyme A acyltransferase 1 (peroxisomal 3-oxoacyl-Coenzyme A thiolase)	604054	Pseudo-Zellweger syndrome, 261510 (1)
3p23-p21	SCLC1	C	Small-cell cancer of lung	182280	Small-cell cancer of lung (2)
3p22	TGFBR2, HNPCC6	P	Transforming growth factor, beta receptor II, 70–80 kD	190182	Colon cancer (3); Colorectal cancer, familial nonpolyposis, type 6 (3)
3p22-p21.3	CTNNB1	C	Catenin (cadherin-associated protein), beta 1, 88 kD	116806	Colorectal cancer (3); Hepatoblastoma (3); Pilomatricoma (3); Ovarian carcinoma, endometrioid type (3)
3p22-p21.1	PTHR1, PTHR	C	Parathyroid hormone receptor-1	168468	Metaphyseal chondrodysplasia, Murk Jansen type, 156400 (3)
3p21.33	GLB1	C	Galactosidase, beta-1	230500	GM1-gangliosidosis (3); Mucopolysaccharidosis IVB (3)
3p21.31	CACT, CAC	P	Carnitine-acylcarnitine translocase	212138	Carnitine-acylcarnitine translocase deficiency (3)
3p21.3	GPX1	C	Glutathione peroxidase-1	138320	Hemolytic anemia due to glutathione peroxidase deficiency (1)

(Continued on next page)

Table A1-2 (Continued)

Location	Symbol	Status	Locus Name	MIM#	Disorder
3p21.3	MLH1, COCA2	P	mutL, E. coli, homolog of, 1	120436	Colorectal cancer, hereditary nonpolyposis, type 2 (3); Turcot syndrome with glioblastoma, 276300 (3); Muir-Torre family cancer syndrome, 158320 (3); Leukemia (3)
3p21.3-p21.2	HYAL1	C	Hyaluronoglucosaminidase 1	601492	Mucopolysaccharidosis type IX (3)
3p21.2-p21.1	AMT	P	Aminomethyltransferase (glycine cleavage system protein T)	238310	Hyperglycinemia, nonketotic, 2 (1)
3p21.2-p21.1	HESX1, RPX	P	Homeo box gene expressed in ES cells	601802	Septooptic dysplasia, 182230 (3)
3p21.2-p14.1	PEO2	P	Progressive external ophthalmoplegia, type 2	601226	Progressive external ophthalmoplegia, type 2 (2)
3p21.1	ARP	P	Arginine-rich protein	601916	Pancreatic cancer (2)
3p21.1-p14.1	LRS1, LAR1	P	Larsen syndrome 1, autosomal dominant	150250	Larsen syndrome, autosomal dominant (2)
3p21.1-p12	SCA7, OPCA3	C	Spinocerebellar ataxia 7 (olivopontocerebellar atrophy with retinal degeneration)	164500	Spinocerebellar ataxia-7 (3)
3p21	CMKBR2, CCR2	C	Chemokine (C-C) receptor 2	601267	{HIV infection, susceptibility/ resistence to} (3)
3p21	CMKBR5, CCCKR5	P	Chemokine (C-C) receptor 5	601373	{HIV infection, susceptibility/ resistance to} (3)
3p21	GNAI2, GNAI2B, GIP	C	Guanine nucleotide-binding protein (G protein), alpha-inhibiting activity polypeptide-2	139360	Pituitary ACTH-secreting adenoma (3); Ventricular tachycardia, idiopathic, 192605 (3)
3p21	IECN2, NCIE2	P	Ichthyosiform erythroderma, congenital, nonbullous, 2	604780	Ichthyosiforme erythroderma, congenital, nonbullous, 2 (2)
3p21	GNAT1	C	Guanine nucleotide-binding protein (G protein), alpha-transducing (transducin) activity polypeptide-1	139330	Night blindness, congenital stationary (3)
3p21	SCN5A, LQT3, IVF, HB2	C	Sodium channel, voltage-gated, type V, alpha polypeptide	600163	Long QT syndrome-3, 603830 (3); Brugada syndrome, 601144 (3); Heart block, progressive, 2, 604559 (3); Heart block, nonprogressive, 604559 (3)
3p21-p14	DFNB6	P	Deafness, autosomal recessive 6	600971	Deafness, autosomal recessive 6 (2)
3p14.3	TKT	P	Transketolase	277730	{Wernicke-Korsakoff syndrome, susceptibility to} (1)
3p14.1-p12.3	MITF, WS2A	C	Microphthalmia-associated transcription factor	156845	Waardenburg syndrome, type IIA, 193510 (3); Waardenburg syndrome/ocular albinism, digenic, 103470 (3); Tietz syndrome, 103500 (3)
3p13-p12	BBS3	P	Bardet-Biedl syndrome 3	600151	Bardet-Biedl syndrome 3 (2)
3p12	GBE1	P	Glycogen branching enzyme	232500	Glycogen storage disease IV (3)
3p11.1-q11.2	DMT1	P	Dementia, familial, nonspecific	600795	Dementia, familial, nonspecific (2)
3p11.1-q11.2	PROS1	C	Protein S, alpha	176880	Protein S deficiency (3)
3p11	POU1F1, PIT1	C	POU domain, class 1, transcription factor 1 (Pit1, growth hormone factor 1)	173110	Pituitary hormone deficiency, combined (3)
3p	MYL3	P	Myosin, light polypeptide-3, alkali; ventricular, skeletal, slow	160790	Cardiomopathy, hypertrophic, mid-ventricular chamber type (3)
3p	TRH	P	Thyrotropin-releasing hormone	275120	Thyrotropin-releasing hormone deficiency (1)
3q	DFNB15	P	Deafness, autosomal recessive 15	601869	Deafness, autosomal recessive 15 (2)
3q	DM2	P	Myotonic dystrophy 2	602668	Myotonic dystrophy 2 (2)
3q	PCLN1	P	Paracellin 1	603959	Hypomagnesemia, primary, 248250 (3)
3q12	CPO	P	Coproporphyrinogen oxidase	121300	Coproporphyria (3); Harderoporphyrinuria (3)

Table A1-2 (Continued)

Location	Symbol	Status	Locus Name	MIM#	Disorder
3q13	ETM1, FET1	P	Tremor, familial essential, 1	190300	Tremor, familial essential, 1 (2)
3q13	FIH	L	Hypoparathyroidism	146200	Hypoparathyroidism, familial (2)
3q13	UMPS, OPRT	C	Uridine monophosphate synthetase (orotate phosphoribosyl transferase and orotidine-5\(fm-decarboxylase)	258900	Oroticaciduria (3)
3q13-q22	CMT2B	P	Charcot-Marie-Tooth neuropathy 2B	600882	Charcot-Marie-Tooth neuropathy-2B (2)
3q13.1	HMSNO, HMSNP	P	Neuropathy, hereditary motor and sensory, Okinawa type	604484	Neuropathy, hereditary motor and sensory, Okinawa type (2)
3q13.1	MHS4	P	Malignant hyperthermia susceptibility 4	600467	{Malignant hyperthermia susceptibility 4} (2)
3q13.3	DRD3	P	Dopamine receptor D3	126451	{?Schizophrenia, susceptibility to} (2)
3q13.3-q21	CASR, HHC1, PCAR1	C	Calcium-sensing receptor	601199	Hypocalciuric hypercalcemia, type I, 145980 (3); Neonatal hyperparathyroidism, 239200 (3); Hypocalcemia, autosomal dominant, 601198 (3)
3q21	PSORS5	P	Psoriasis susceptibility 5	604316	{Psoriasis susceptibility} (2)
3q21	TF	C	Transferrin	190000	Atransferrinemia (1)
3q21-q22	MBS2	P	Moebius syndrome 2	601471	Moebius syndrome-2 (2)
3q21-q22	PCCB	C	Propionyl Coenzyme A carboxylase, beta polypeptide	232050	Propionicacidemia, type II or pccB type (3)
3q21-q23	HGD, AKU	C	Homogentisate 1,2-dioxygenase (homogentisate oxidase)	203500	Alkaptonuria (3)
3q21-q23	LTF	C	Lactotransferrin	150210	?Lactoferrin-deficient neutrophils, 245480 (1)
3q21-q24	ATP2C1, BCPM, HHD	C	ATPase, Ca(2+)-sequestering	604384	Hailey-Hailey disease, 169600 (3)
3q21-q24	GLC1C	P	Glaucoma 1, open angle, C	601682	Glaucoma 1C, primary open angle (2)
3q21-q24	RHO, RP4	C	Rhodopsin	180380	Retinitis pigmentosa-4, autosomal dominant (3); Retinitis pigmentosa, autosomal recessive (3); Night blindness, congenital stationary, rhodopsin-related (3)
3q21-q25	AGTR1, AGTR1A, AT2R1	C	Angiotensin receptor 1	106165	Hypertension, essential, 145500 (3)
3q21-q25	USH3	C	Usher syndrome-3	276902	Usher syndrome, type 3 (2)
3q22	NPHP3, NPH3	P	Nephronophthisis, adolescent	604387	Nephronophthisis, adolescent (2)
3q22-q23	BPES, BPES1	C	Blepharophimosis, epicanthus inversus, and ptosis 1	110100	Blepharophimosis, epicanthus inversus, and ptosis, type 1 (2)
3q23-q24	CP	C	Ceruloplasmin	117700	[Hypoceruloplasminemia, hereditary] (1); Hemosiderosis, systemic, due to aceruloplasminemia (3)
3q25-q26	SI	P	Sucrase-isomaltase	222900	Sucrose intolerance (3)
3q25.1	MLF1	P	Myeloid leukemia factor-1	601402	Leukemia, myeloid, acute (1)
3q25.2-q27	CCM3	P	Cerebral cavernous malformations-3	603285	Cerebral cavernous malformations-3 (2)
3q26	EVI1	C	Ectropic viral integration site-1 (oncogene EVI1)	165215	3q21q26 syndrome (1)
3q26	MDS1	P	Myelodysplasia syndrome-1	600049	Myelodysplasia syndrome-1 (3)
3q26	PI12	P	Protease inhibitor 12	602445	Encephalopathy, familial, with neuroserpin inclusion bodies, 604218 (3)
3q26.1-q26.2	BCHE, CHE1	C	Butyrylcholinesterase	177400	Apnea, postanesthetic (3)
3q26.1-q26.3	SLC2A2, GLUT2	C	Solute carrier family 2 (facilitated glucose transporter), member 2	138160	{Diabetes mellitus, noninsulin-dependent} (3); Fanconi-Bickel syndrome, 227810 (3)
3q26.3	CDL1	L	Cornelia de Lange syndrome 1	122470	?Cornelia de Lange syndrome (2)
3q26.3	PIK3CA	P	Phosphatidylinositol 3-kinase, catalytic, alpha polypeptide	171834	Ovarian cancer (1)
3q26.3-q27	THPO, MGDF, MPLLG, TPO	C	Thrombopoietin (megakaryocyte growth and development factor)	600044	Thrombocythemia, essential, 187950 (3)

(Continued on next page)

Table A1-2 (Continued)

Location	Symbol	Status	Locus Name	MIM#	Disorder
3q27	BCL6	P	B-cell CLL/lymphoma-6	109565	Lymphoma, B-cell (2); Lymphoma, diffuse large cell (3)
3q27	EHHADH, PBFE	C	Enoyl-Coenzyme A, hydratase/3-hydroxyacyl Coenzyme A dehydrogenase	261515	Peroxisomal bifunctional enzyme deficiency (1)
3q27	HRG	C	Histidine-rich glycoprotein	142640	Thrombophilia due to HRG deficiency (3); ?Thrombophilia due to elevated HRG (1)
3q27	KNG	C	Kininogen	228960	[Kininogen deficiency] (3)
3q27	LMS	P	Limb-mammary syndrome	603543	Limb-mammary syndrome (2)
3q27	LVWM, CACH	C	Leukoencephalopathy with vanishing white matter	603896	Leukoencephalopathy with vanishing white matter (2)
3q27	TP63, KET, EEC3	P	Tumor protein p63	603273	Ectrodactyly, ectodermal dysplasia, and cleft lip/palate syndrome 3, 604292 (3)
3q28	LPP	P	Lipoma-preferred-partner gene	600700	Lipoma (1)
3q28-q29	OPA1	C	Optic atrophy 1, autosomal dominant	165500	Optic atrophy 1 (2)
Chr.3	GP9	P	Glycoprotein IX, platelet	173515	Bernard-Soulier syndrome, type C (3)
4p16.3	CRBM	C	Cherubism	118400	Cherubism (2)
4p16.3	DFNA6	P	Deafness, autosomal dominant 6	600965	Deafness, autosomal dominant 6 (2)
4p16.3	FGFR3, ACH	C	Fibroblast growth factor receptor-3	134934	Achondroplasia, 100800 (3); Hypochondroplasia, 146000 (3); Thanatophoric dysplasia, types I and II, 187600 (3); Crouzon syndrome with acanthosis nigricans (3); Muencke syndrome, 602849 (3); Bladder cancer, 109800 3); Cervical cancer, 603956 (3)
4p16.3	HD, IT15	C	Huntingtin	143100	Huntington disease (3)
4p16.3	IDUA, IDA	P	Iduronidase, alpha-L-	252800	Mucopolysaccharidosis Ih (3); Mucopolysaccharidosis Is (3); Mucopolysaccharidosis Ih/s (3)
4p16.3	PDE6B, PDEB, CSNB3	C	Phosphodiesterase-6B, cGMP-specific, rod, beta	180072	Night blindness, congenital stationary, type 3, 163500 (3); Retinitis pigmentosa, autosomal recessive (3)
4p16.3	WHCR	C	Wolf-Hirschhorn syndrome chromosome region	194190	Wolf-Hirschhorn syndrome (2)
4p16.2-p12	PROML1, AC133	P	Prominin, mouse, homolog-like 1	604365	Retinal degeneration, autosomal recessive, prominin-related (3)
4p16.1	MSX1, HOX7	C	msh, Drosophila, homeo box homolog of, 1 (formerly homeo box 7)	142983	Hypodontia, autosomal dominant, 106600 (3); Hypodontia with orofacial cleft, 106600 (3)
4p16.1	WFS1, WFRS, WFS	C	Wolframin	222300	Wolfram syndrome (3)
4p16	CRSA, CRS3	P	Craniosynostosis, Adelaide type	600593	Craniosynostosis, Adelaide type (2)
4p16	EVC	P	Ellis-van Creveld syndrome gene	225500	Ellis-van Creveld syndrome (3); Weyers acrodental dysostosis, 193530 (3)
4p15.31	QDPR, DHPR	C	Quinoid dihydropteridine reductase	261630	Phenylketonuria due to dihydropteridine reductase deficiency (3)
4p15.3	HLN2	P	Huntington-like neurodegenerative disorder 2	604802	Huntington-like neurodegenerative disorder 2 (2)
4p14	UCHL1	P	Ubiquitin C-terminal esterase L1	191342	Parkinson disease, familial, 168600 (3)
4p13-q12	TAPVR1	P	Total anomalous pulmonary venous return	106700	Total anomalous pulmonary venous return (2)
4p12-cen	CNGA1, CNCG1	C	Cyclic nucleotide gated channel, alpha 1	123825	Retinitis pigmentosa, autosomal recessive (3)
4p	MHW1	P	Mental health wellness 1	603663	{Mental health wellness-1} (2)
4p	STGD4	P	Stargardt disease 4	603786	Stargardt disease 4 (2)

Table A1-2 (Continued)

Location	Symbol	Status	Locus Name	MIM#	Disorder
4q	DTDP2	P	Dentin dysplasia, Shields type II	125420	Dentin dysplasia, type II (2)
4q	MHW2	P	Mental health wellness 2	603664	{Mental health wellness-2} (2)
4q	PSORS3	P	Psoriasis susceptibility 3	601454	{Psoriasis susceptibility 3} (3)
4q11-q13	AFP, HPAFP	C	Alpha-fetoprotein	104150	[AFP deficiency, congenital] (1); [Hereditary persistence of alpha-fetoprotein] (3)
4q11-q13	ALB	C	Albumin	103600	Analbuminemia (3); [Dysalbuminemic hyperthyroxinemia] (3); [Dysalbuminemic hyperzincemia], 194470 (3)
4q11-q13	JPD	P	Periodontitis, juvenile	170650	Periodontitis, juvenile (2)
4q11-q21	AIH2	P	Amelogenesis imperfecta-2, hypocalcification, autosomal dominant	104500	Amelogenesis imperfecta-2, hypoplastic local type (2)
4q11-q12	BTL	P	Brx-like gene translocated in leukemia	604332	{Leukemia, acute myeloid} (3)
4q12	SGCB, LGMD2E	C	Sarcoglycan, beta (43 kD dystrophin-associated glycoprotein)	600900	Muscular dystrophy, limb-girdle, type 2E, 604286 (3)
4q12	KIT, PBT	C	Hardy-Zuckerman 4 feline sarcoma (v-kit) oncogene	164920	Piebaldism (3); Mast cell leukemia (3); Mastocytosis with associated hematologic disorder (3)
4q13-q21	DGI1	C	Dentinogenesis imperfecta-1	125490	Dentinogenesis imperfecta-1 (2)
4q21	HIES	P	Hyper-IgE syndrome	147060	Hyper-IgE syndrome (2)
4q21	SLC4A4, NBC1, KNBC, SLC4A5	P	Solute carrier family 4, sodium bicarbonate cotransporter, member 4	603345	Renal tubular acidosis, proximal, with ocular abnormalities, 604278 (3)
4q21	SNCA, NACP, PARK1	C	Synuclein, alpha (non A4 component of amyloid precursor)	163890	Parkinson disease, type 1, 601508 (3)
4q21-q23	GNPTA	P	UDP-N-acetylglucosamine-lysosomal-enzyme N-acetylglucosamine phosphotransferase	252500	Mucolipidosis II (1); Mucolipidosis III (1)
4q21-q23	PKD2, PKD4	C	Polycystin-2	173910	Polycystic kidney disease, adult, type II (3)
4q21-q25	RAP1GDS1	P	RAP1, GTP-GDP dissociation stimulator 1	179502	Lymphocytic leukemia, acute T-cell (3)
4q21.2	GNRHR	C	Gonadotropin-releasing hormone receptor	138850	Hypogonadotropic hypogonadism (3)
4q22	ADH2	C	Alcohol dehydrogenase (class I), beta polypeptide	103720	{Alcoholism, susceptibility to} (1)
4q22-q24	MTP	P	Microsomal triglyceride transfer protein, 88 kD	157147	Abetalipoproteinemia, 200100 (3)
4q22-q25	MANBA, MANB1	C	Mannosidase, beta A, lysosomal	248510	Mannosidosis, beta- (3)
4q23	TYS, HRZ	P	Sclerotylosis	181600	Huriez syndrome (2)
4q25	IF	C	I factor (complement component I)	217030	C3b inactivator deficiency (3)
4q25-q26	PITX2, IDG2, RIEG1, RGS, IGDS2	C	Paired-like homeodomain transcription factor-2	601542	Rieger syndrome, 180500 (3); Iridogoniodysgenesis syndrome-2, 137600 (3)
4q25-q27	LQT4	P	Long QT syndrome-4	600919	Long QT syndrome-4 with sinus bradycardia (2)
4q26-q27	IL2	C	Interleukin-2	147680	Severe combined immunodeficiency due to IL2 deficiency (1)
4q27-q31	FOP	P	Fibrodysplasia ossificans progressiva	135100	Fibrodysplasia ossificans progressiva (2)
4q28	FGA	C	Fibrinogen, alpha polypeptide	134820	Dysfibrinogenemia, alpha type, causing bleeding diathesis (3); Dysfibrinogenemia, alpha type, causing recurrent thrombosis (3); Amyloidosis, hereditary renal, 105200 (3); Afibrinogenemia (3)
4q28	FGB	C	Fibrinogen, beta polypeptide	134830	Dysfibrinogenemia, beta type (3)

(Continued on next page)

Table A1-2 (Continued)

Location	Symbol	Status	Locus Name	MIM#	Disorder
4q28	FGG	C	Fibrinogen, gamma polypeptide	134850	Dysfibrinogenemia, gamma type (3); Hypofibrinogenemia, gamma type (3)
4q28-q31	ASMD	P	Anterior segment mesenchymal dysgenesis	107250	Anterior segment mesenchymal dysgenesis (2)
4q28-q31	HCL2, RHC	P	Hair color 2, red	266300	[Hair color, red] (2)
4q31.1	NR3C2, MLR, MCR	C	Nuclear receptor subfamily 3, group C, member 2 (mineralocorticoid receptor; aldosterone receptor)	600983	Pseudohypoaldosteronism type I, autosomal dominant, 177735 (3)
4q32-q33	AGA	C	Aspartylglucosaminidase	208400	Aspartylglucosaminuria (3)
4q32-qter	ETFDH	P	Electron transfer flavoprotein: ubiquinone oxidoreductase	231675	Glutaricaciduria, type IIC (3)
4q32.1	HVBS6	P	Hepatitis B virus integration site-6	142380	Hepatocellular carcinoma (3)
4q33-qter	HCA	P	Hypercalciuria, absorptive	143870	Hypercalciuria, absorptive (2)
4q34-q35	PEO3	P	Progressive external ophthalmoplegia, type 3	601227	Progressive external ophthalmoplegia, type 3 (2)
4q35	BHD, BFHD	P	Beukes familial hip dysplasia	142669	Hip dysplasia, Beukes type (2)
4q35	F11	C	Coagulation factor XI (plasma thromboplastin antecedent)	264900	Factor XI deficiency (3)
4q35	FSHMD1A, FSHD1A	C	Facioscapulohumeral muscular dystrophy-1A	158900	Facioscapulohumeral muscular dystrophy-1A (2)
4q35	KLKB1, KLK3	P	Kallikrein B plasma 1 (Fletcher factor)	229000	Fletcher factor deficiency (1)
Chr.4	LAG5	P	Leukocyte antigen group 5	151450	Neutropenia, neonatal alloimmune (1)
5p15.3	SLC6A3, DAT1	C	Solute carrier family 6 (neurotransmitter transporter, dopamine), member 3	126455	{Attention-deficit hyperactivity disorder, susceptibility to}, 143465 (2)
5p15.3-p15.2	MTRR	P	Methionine synthase reductase	602568	Homocystinuria-megaloblastic anemia, cbl E type, 236270 (3)
5p15.2	CTNND2, NPRAP	P	Catenin, delta-2	604275	Mental retardation in cri-du-chat syndrome, 123450 (2)
5p15.2-p14.1	CMDJ	P	Craniometaphyseal dysplasia, Jackson type	123000	Craniometaphyseal dysplasia (2)
5p15	CCAL2, CPPDD	C	Chondrocalcinosis 2 (calcium pyrophosphate dihydrate deposition disease)	118600	Chondrocalcinosis, familial articular (2)
5p15	PTC	P	Phenylthiocarbamide taste	171200	[Phenylthiocarbamide tasting] (2)
5p15	SDHA, SDH2, SDHF	C	Succinate dehydrogenase complex, subunit A, flavoprotein	600857	Leigh syndrome (3)
5p14	FST, FS	P	Follistatin	136470	Polycystic ovary syndrome, 184700 (2)
5p14-p12	NPR3, ANPRC	P	Natriuretic peptide receptor C	108962	?Hypertension, salt-resistant (1)
5p13.2-q11.1	AMACR	P	Alpha-methylacyl-CoA racemase	604489	Alpha-methylacyl-CoA racemase deficiency (3)
5p13.1-p12	GDNF	C	Glial cell line derived neurotrophic factor	600837	Hirschsprung disease, 142623 (3)
5p13	C6	C	Complement component-6	217050	C6 deficiency (1); Combined C6/C7 deficiency (1)
5p13	C7	C	Complement component-7	217070	C7 deficiency (1)
5p13	C9	C	Complement component-9	120940	C9 deficiency (3)
5p13	IL7R	P	Interleukin-7 receptor	146661	Severe combined immunodeficiency, T-cell negative, B-cell/natural killer cell-positive type, 600802 (3)
5p13	SCOT, OXCT	P	Succinyl CoA:3-oxoacid CoA transferase	245050	Ketoacidosis due to SCOT deficiency (3)
5p13-p12	GHR	C	Growth hormone receptor	600946	Laron dwarfism, 262500 (3); Short stature, idiopathic (3); Short stature, autosomal dominant, with normal serum growth hormone binding protein (3)

Table A1-2 (Continued)

Location	Symbol	Status	Locus Name	MIM#	Disorder
5p	MHS6	P	Malignant hyperthermia susceptibility 6	601888	{Malignant hyperthermia susceptibility 6} (2)
5q	MPD2, CMT2C, HMSN2C	P	Myopathy, distal, with vocal cord and pharyngeal weakness	158580	Myopathy, distal 2 (2)
5q	PROP1	P	Prophet of Pit1, paired-like homeodomain transcription factor	601538	Pituitary hormone deficiency, combined (3)
5q11	MOCS2, MPTS	P	Molybdenum cofactor synthesis-2	603708	Molybdenum cofactor deficiency, type B, 252150 (3)
5q11-q12	MSH3	P	mutS, E. coli, homolog of, 3	600887	Endometrial carcinoma (3)
5q11-q13	ARSB	C	Arylsulfatase B	253200	Maroteaux-Lamy syndrome, several forms (3)
5q11.1	NDUFS4, AQDQ	P	NADH dehydrogenase (ubiquinone) Fe-S protein 4, 18 kD (NADH-coenzyme Q reductase)	602694	Complex I deficiency (3)
5q11.2	KFS	L	Klippel-Feil syndrome	214300	?Klippel-Feil syndrome (2)
5q11.2-q13.2	DHFR	C	Dihydrofolate reductase	126060	?Anemia, megaloblastic, due to DHFR deficiency (1)
5q11.2-q13.3	SCZD1	L	Schizophrenia susceptibility locus, chromosome 5-related	181510	{?Schizophrenia}, 181500 (2)
5q12.2-q13.3	SMN1	C	Survival of motor neuron 1, telomeric	600354	Spinal muscular atrophy-1, 253300 (3); Spinal muscular atrophy-2, 253550 (3); Spinal muscular atrophy-3, 253400 (3)
5q13	HEXB	C	Hexosaminidase B, beta polypeptide	268800	Sandhoff disease, infantile, juvenile, and adult forms (3); Spinal muscular atrophy, juvenile (3)
5q13-q14	WGN1, ERVR	P	Wagner syndrome (erosive vitreoretinopathy)	143200	Wagner syndrome (2); Erosive vitreoretinopathy (2)
5q13.3	RASA1, GAP	C	RAS p21 protein activator 1 (GTPase activating protein)	139150	Basal cell carcinoma (3)
5q14-q15	FEB4	P	Convulsions, familial febrile, 4	604352	Convulsions, familial febrile, 4 (2)
5q15-q21	PCSK1, NEC1, PC1, PC3	P	Proprotein convertase subtilisin/kexin type 1	162150	Obestiy with impaired prohormone processing, 600955 (3)
5q2	HSD17B4	P	Hydroxysteroid (17-beta) dehydrogenase 4	601860	D-bifunctional protein deficiency (3)
5q21	MCC	C	Mutated in colorectal cancers	159350	Colorectal cancer (3)
5q21-q22	APC, GS, FPC	C	Adenomatous polyposis coli	175100	Gardner syndrome (3); Adenomatous polyposis coli (3); Colorectal cancer (3); Desmoid disease, hereditary, 135290 (3); Turcot syndrome, 276300 (3); Adenomatous polyposis coli, attenuated (3); Gastric cancer, 137215 (3); Adenoma, periampullary (3)
5q23	DTR, DTS, HBEGF, HEGFL	C	Diphtheria toxin receptor (heparin-binding EGF-like growth factor)	126150	{Diphtheria, susceptibility to} (1)
5q23-q31	FBN2, CCA	P	Fibrillin-2	121050	Contractural arachnodactyly, congenital (3)
5q23-q31	ITGA2, CD49B, BR	P	Integrin, alpha-2 (CD49B; alpha-2 subunit of VLA-2 receptor; platelet antigen Br)	192974	Neonatal alloimmune thrombocytopenia (2); ? Glycoprotein Ia deficiency (2)
5q23-q31	UBE2B, RAD6B	P	Ubiquitin-conjugating enzyme E2B (RAD6 homolog)	179095	?Male infertility (1)
5q23.3-q31.2	LOX	C	Lysyl oxidase	153455	Cutis laxa, recessive, type I, 219100 (1)
5q31	ACS2	P	Long-chain acyl-CoA synthetase 2	604443	Myelodysplastic syndrome (3); Myelogenous leukemia, acute (3)
5q31	DIAPH1, DFNA1, LFHL1	C	Diaphanous, Drosophila, homolog of, 1	602121	Deafness, autosomal dominant nonsyndromic sensorineural, 1, 124900 (3)

(Continued on next page)

Table A1-2 (Continued)

Location	Symbol	Status	Locus Name	MIM#	Disorder
5q31	LGMD1A, LGMD1	C	Limb-girdle muscular dystrophy-1A, autosomal dominant	159000	Muscular dystrophy, limb-girdle, type 1A (2)
5q31	NR3C1, GCR, GRL	C	Nuclear receptor subfamily 3, group C, member 1 (glucocorticoid receptor)	138040	Cortisol resistance (3)
5q31	POU4F3, BRN3C	C	POU domain, class 4, transcription factor-3	602460	Deafness, autosomal dominant 15, 602459 (3)
5q31	TGFBI, CSD2, CDGG1, CSD, BIGH3	C	Transforming growth factor, beta-induced, 68 kD	601692	Corneal dystrophy, Groenouw type I, 121900 (3); Corneal dystrophy, lattice type I, 122200 (3); Corneal dystrophy, Reis-Bucklers type, 121900 (3); Corneal dystrophy, Avellino type (3); Corneal dystrophy, lattice type IIIA (3)
5q31-q33	BHR1	P	Bronchial hyper-responsiveness-1 (bronchial asthma)	600807	Bronchial asthma (2)
5q31-q33	EOS	P	Eosinophilia, familial	131400	Eosinophilia, familial (2)
5q31-q33	HCI, HEMC	P	Hemangioma, capillary infantile	602089	Hemangioma, capillary infantile (2)
5q31-q33	PFBI	P	Plasmodium falciparum blood infection levels	248310	{Plasmodium falciparum parasitemia, intensity of} (2)
5q31-q33	PPP2R2B	P	Protein phosphatase 2, regulatory subunit B, beta	604325	Spinocerebellar ataxia 12, 604326 (3)
5q31-q33	SM1	C	Schistosoma mansoni infection, susceptibility/resistance to	181460	{Schistosoma mansoni infection, susceptibility/resistance to} (2)
5q31.1	IGES	P	Immunoglobulin E concentration, serum	147061	?{Allergy and asthma susceptibility} (2)
5q31.1	IRF1, MAR	C	Interferon regulatory factor-1	147575	Macrocytic anemia refractory, of 5q- syndrome, 153550 (3); Myelodysplastic syndrome, preleukemic (3); Myelogenous leukemia, acute (3) ; Gastric cancer, 137215 (3); Nonsmall cell lung cancer (3)
5q31.1-q33.1	IL12B, NKSF2	C	Interleukin-12B (natural killer cell stimulatory factor-2, cytotoxic lymphocyte maturation factor-2, p40)	161561	BCG and salmonella infection, disseminated, 209950 (1)
5q31.2-q34	PDE6A, PDEA	C	Phosphodiesterase-6A, cGMP-specific, rod, alpha	180071	Retinitis pigmentosa, autosomal recessive (3)
5q31.3-q33.1	GM2A	C	GM2 ganglioside activator protein	272750	GM2-gangliosidosis, AB variant (3)
5q32	CMTND	C	Charcot-Marie-Tooth neuropathy, demyelinating	601596	Charcot-Marie-Tooth neuropathy, demyelinating (2)
5q32	GLRA1, STHE	C	Glycine receptor, alpha-1 polypeptide	138491	Startle disease/hyperekplexia, autosomal dominant, 149400 (3); Startle disease, autosomal recessive (3); Hyperekplexia and spastic paraparesis (3)
5q32	NETS, NS	P	Netherton syndrome	256500	Netherton syndrome (2)
5q32-q33.1	SLC26A2, DTD, DTDST, D5S1708	C	Solute carrier family 26 (sulfate transporter), member 2 (diastrophic dysplasia sulfate transporter)	222600	Diastrophic dysplasia (3); Atelosteogenesis II, 256050 (3); Achondrogenesis Ib, 600972 (3); Epiphyseal dysplasia, multiple, 226900 (3)
5q32-q33.1	TCOF1, MFD1	C	Treacher Collins-Franceschetti syndrome-1 (TREACLE)	154500	Treacher Collins mandibulofacial dysostosis (3)
5q32-q34	ADRB2	C	Adrenergic, beta-2-, receptor, surface	109690	{Asthma, nocturnal, susceptibility to} (3); {Obesity, susceptibility to} (3)
5q33	SGCD, SGD, LGMD2F	C	Sarcoglycan, delta (35 kD dystrophin-associated glycoprotein)	601411	Muscular dystrophy, limb-girdle, type 2F, 601287 (3)
5q33-qter	F12, HAF	C	Coagulation factor XII (Hageman factor)	234000	Factor XII deficiency (3)

Table A1-2 (Continued)

Location	Symbol	Status	Locus Name	MIM#	Disorder
5q33.1	SLC22A5, OCTN2, CDSP, SCD	C	Solute carrier, family 22 (organic cation transporter), member 5	603377	Carnitine deficiency, systemic primary, 212140 (3)
5q33.2-q33.3	CSF1R, FMS	C	Colony-stimulating factor-1 receptor; oncogene FMS (McDonough feline sarcoma)	164770	Myeloid malignancy, predisposition to (3)
5q34	CSX	C	Cardiac-specific homeo box	600584	Atrial septal defect with atrioventricular conduction defects, 108900 (3)
5q34-q35	MSX2, CRS2, HOX8	C	msh, Drosophila, homeo box homolog of, 2	123101	Craniosynostosis, type 2, 604757 (3); Parietal foramina 1, 168500 (3)
5q35	AMCN, AMCN1	P	Arthrogryposis multiplex congenital, neurogenic	208100	Arthrogryposis multiplex congenita, neurogenic (2)
5q35	LTC4S	P	Leukotriene C4 synthase	246530	Leukotriene C4 synthase deficiency (1)
5q35	NPM1	P	Nucleophosmin 1 (nucleolar phosphoprotein B23, numatrin)	164040	Leukemia, acute promyelocytic, NPM/RARA type (3)
5q35.1-q35.3	B4GALT7, XGALT1, XGPT1	P	Xylosylprotein 4-beta-galactosyltransferase, polypeptide 7	604327	Ehlers-Danlos syndrome, progeroid form, 130070 (3)
5q35.3	FLT4, VEGFR3, PCL	C	fms-related tyrosine kinase-4 (vascular endothelial growth factor receptor 3)	136352	Lymphedema, hereditary I, 153100 (3)
Chr.5	ADTB3A, AP3B1	P	Adaptin, beta-3A	603401	Hermansky-Pudlak syndrome due to defect in beta-3A-adaptin (3)
Chr.5	CKN1	P	Cockayne syndrome 1, classical	216400	Cockayne syndrome-1 (3)
6p25	FKHL7	C	Forkhead, drosophila, homolog-like 7	601090	Iridogoniodysgenesis, 601631 (3); Anterior segment mesenchymal dysgenesis (3); Rieger anomaly (3); Axenfeld anomaly (3)
6p25	IRF4, MUM1	P	Interferon regulatory factor-4 (multiple myeloma oncogene-1)	602028	Multiple myeloma (3)
6p25-p24	F13A1, F13A	C	Coagulation factor XIII, A polypeptide	134570	Factor XIIIA deficiency (3)
6p24.3	OFC1, CL	C	Orofacial cleft-1 (cleft lip with or without cleft palate; isolated cleft palate)	119530	Orofacial cleft-1 (2)
6p24	DSP, KPPS2, PPKS2	P	Desmoplakin	125647	Keratosis palmoplantaris striata II (3)
6p23	ATX1, SCA1	C	Ataxin-1	601556	Spinocerebellar ataxia-1, 164400 (3)
6p23	DEK, D6S231E	P	DEK oncogene	125264	Leukemia, acute nonlymphocytic (2)
6p23	SCZD3	P	Schizophrenia susceptibility locus, chromosome 6-related	600511	{Schizophrenia}, 181500 (2)
6p22.3	TPMT	P	Thiopurine S-methyltransferase	187680	6-mercaptopurine sensitivity (3)
6p22	SSADH	P	Succinic semialdehyde dehydrogenase	271980	Succinic semialdehyde dehydrogenase deficiency (3)
6p22-p21	BCKDHB, E1B	C	Branched chain keto acid dehydrogenase E1, beta polypeptide	248611	Maple syrup urine disease, type Ib (3)
6p22-p21	FANCE, FACE	P	Fanconi anemia, complementation group E	600901	Fanconi anemia, complementation group E (2)
6p21.3	ABCB3, TAP2, RING11, PSF2	C	ATP-binding cassette, subfamily B, member 3	170261	Bare lymphocyte syndrome, type I, due to TAP2 deficiency (1)
6p21.3	AS, ANS	P	Ankylosing spondylitis	106300	Ankylosing spondylitis (2)
6p21.3	ASD1, ASD2	P	Atrial septal defect, secundum type	108800	Atrial septal defect, secundum type (2)
6p21.3	C2	C	Complement component-2	217000	C2 deficiency (3)
6p21.3	C4A, C4S	C	Complement component-4A	120810	C4 deficiency (3)
6p21.3	C4B, C4F	C	Complement component-4B	120820	C4 deficiency (3)

(Continued on next page)

Table A1-2 (Continued)

Location	Symbol	Status	Locus Name	MIM#	Disorder
6p21.3	COL11A2	C	Collagen XI, alpha-2 polypeptide	120290	Stickler syndrome, type II, 184840 (3); OSMED syndrome, 215150 (3); Weissenbacher-Zweymuller syndrome, 277610 (3); Deafness, nonsyndromic sensorineural 13, 601868 (3)
6p21.3	CYP21A2, CYP21, CA21H	C	Cytochrome P450, subfamily XXIA, polypeptide 2 (steroid 21-hydroxylase)	201910	Adrenal hyperplasia, congenital, due to 21-hydroxylase deficiency (3)
6p21.3	DYX2, DYLX2, DLX2	P	Dyslexia 2	600202	Dyslexia, specific, 2 (2)
6p21.3	GLYS1	P	Renal glucosuria-1	233100	[Renal glucosuria] (2)
6p21.3	HFE	C	Hemochromatosis	235200	Hemochromatosis (3); Porphyria variegata, 176200 (3)
6p21.3	HLA-DPB1	C	Major histocompatibility complex, class II, DP beta-1	142858	{Beryllium disease, chronic, susceptibility to} (3)
6p21.3	HLA-DR1B	C	Major histocompatibility complex, class II, DR beta-1	142857	{Pemphigoid, susceptibility to} (2)
6p21.3	IDDM1	L	Insulin-dependent diabetes mellitus-1	222100	{?Diabetes mellitus, insulin-dependent-1} (2)
6p21.3	IGAD1	P	Immunoglobulin A deficiency	137100	Immunoglobulin A deficiency (2)
6p21.3	MOCS1, MOCOD	C	Molybdenum cofactor synthesis-1	603707	Molybdenum cofactor deficiency, type A, 252150 (3)
6p21.3	NEU1, NEU	C	Neuraminidase 1 (lysosomal sialidase)	256550	Sialidosis, type I (3); Sialidosis, type II (3)
6p21.3	PBLT	P	Panbronchiolitis, diffuse	604809	Panbronchiolitis, diffuse (2)
6p21.3	PDB	L	Paget disease of bone	167250	?Paget disease of bone (2)
6p21.3	PSORS1	C	Psoriasis susceptibility 1	177900	{Psoriasis susceptibility-1} (2)
6p21.3	RWS	L	Ragweed sensitivity	179450	?Ragweed sensitivity (2)
6p21.3	TNF, TNFA	P	Tumor necrosis factor (cachectin)	191160	{Malaria, cerebral, susceptibility to} (3)
6p21.3	TNXA, HXBL, TNX	C	Tenascin XA	600261	Ehlers-Danlos-like syndrome (3)
6p21.3	TULP1, RP14	C	Tubby-like protein-1	602280	Retinitis pigmentosa-14, 600132 (3)
6p21.3-p21.2	LAP	L	Laryngeal adductor paralysis	150270	?Laryngeal adductor paralysis (2)
6p21.2-p12	PLA2G7, PAFAH	C	Phospholipase A2, group VII (platelet-activating factor acetylhydrolase)	601690	Platelet-activating factor acetylhydrolase deficiency (3)
6p21.1	GUCA1A, GCAP	P	Guanylate cyclase activator 1A, retina	600364	Cone dystrophy-3, 602093 (3)
6p21.1	PEX6, PXAAA1, PAF2	C	Peroxisomal biogenesis factor 6 (peroxisomal AAA-type ATPase 1)	601498	Peroxisomal biogenesis disorder, complementation group 4 (3)
6p21.1-p12	PKHD1, ARPKD	C	Polycystic kidney and hepatic disease-1, autosomal recessive	263200	Polycystic kidney disease, autosomal recessive (2)
6p21.1-p11	RHAG, RH50A	C	Rhesus blood group-associated glycoprotein	180297	Anemia, hemolytic, Rh-null, suppressor type, 268150 (3); Rh(mod) syndrome (3)
6p21.1-cen	RDS, RP7	C	Retinal degeneration, slow (peripherin)	179605	Retinitis pigmentosa-7, peripherin-related (3); Retinitis punctata albescens (3); Macular dystrophy (3); Retinitis pigmentosa, digenic (3); Butterfly dystrophy, retinal (3); Macular dystrophy, vitelliform (3); Retinitis pigmentosa with bull's-eye maculopathy (3); Foveomacular dystrophy, adult-onset, with choroidal neovascularization (3); Pattern dystrophy of retina (3)
6p21	HMGIY	P	High-mobility group (nonhistone chromosomal) protein isoforms I and Y	600701	?Lipoma (1)
6p21	MUT, MCM	C	Methylmalonyl Coenzyme A mutase	251000	Methylmalonicaciduria, mutase deficiency type (3)

Table A1-2 (Continued)

Location	Symbol	Status	Locus Name	MIM#	Disorder
6p21	RUNX2, CBFA1, PEBP2A1, AML3	C	Runt-related transcription factor 2	600211	Cleidocranial dysplasia, 119600 (3); Dental anomalies, isolated (3)
6p21-p12	CHAR	P	Char syndrome (patent ductus arteriosus with facial dysmorphism and abnormal fifth digits)	169100	Char syndrome (2)
6p12	GLCLC	C	Glutamate-cysteine ligase (gamma-glutamylcysteine synthetase), catalytic (72.8 kD)	230450	Hemolytic anemia due to gamma-glutamylcysteine synthetase deficiency (1)
6p12	NYS2, NYSA	P	Nystagmus-2, autosomal dominant	164100	Nystagmus-2, autosomal dominant (2)
6p	GSE, CD	P	Gluten-sensitive enteropathy (celiac disease)	212750	Celiac disease (2)
6p	PUJO	C	Pelviureteric junction obstruction	143400	Pelviureteric junction obstruction (2)
6cen-q14	CORD7	P	Cone-rod dystrophy 7	603649	Cone-rod dystrophy-7 (2)
6cen-q14	STGD3	P	Stargardt disease 3, autosomal dominant	600110	Stargardt disease-3 (2)
6p	IBD3	P	Inflammatory bowel disease 3	604519	Inflammatory bowel disease 3 (2)
6q	MPSH	P	Mixed polyposis syndrome, hereditary	601228	Mixed polyposis syndrome, hereditary (2)
6q11-q16	LCA5	P	Leber congenital amaurosis, type V	604537	Leber congenital amaurosis 5 (2)
6q13-q15	OA3, OAR	L	Ocular albinism, autosomal recessive	203310	?Ocular albinism, autosomal recessive (2)
6q13-q26	SCZD5	P	Schizophrenia susceptibility locus, chromosome 6q-related	603175	{Schizophrenia}, 181500 (2)
6q14-q15	SLC17A5, SIASD, SLD	C	Solute carrier family 17 (sodium phosphate), member 5	604322	Salla disease, 604369 (3); Sialic acid storage disorder, infantile, 269920 (3)
6q14-q16.2	PBCRA, CRAPB	P	Progressive bifocal chorioretinal atrophy	600790	Chorioretinal atrophy, progressive bifocal (2)
6q14-q16.2	MCDR1	P	Macular dystrophy, retinal, 1, North Carolina type	136550	Macular dystrophy, North Carolina type (2)
6q14-q21	RP25	P	Retinitis pigmentosa-25	602772	Retinitis pigmentosa-25 (2)
6q16.3-q21	SIM1	C	Single-minded, drosophila, homolog of, 1	603128	Obesity, severe (3)
6q21	IDDM15	P	Insulin-dependent diabetes mellitus-15	601666	{Diabetes mellitus, insulin-dependent, 15} (2)
6q21-q22.3	COL10A1	C	Collagen X, alpha-1 polypeptide	120110	Metaphyseal chondrodysplasia, Schmid type (3); Spondylometaphyseal dysplasia, Japanese type (3)
6q22-q23	LAMA2, LAMM	C	Laminin, alpha-2 (merosin)	156225	Muscular dystrophy, congenital merosin-deficient (3)
6q22-q23	PDNP1, NPPS, M6S1, PCA1, OPLL	P	Phosphodiesterase I/nucleotide pyrophosphatase 1 (homologous to mouse Ly-41 antigen)	173335	Ossification of posterior longitudinal ligament of spine, 602475 (3)
6q22-q23	WISP3, PPAC, PPD	C	Wnt-1 inducible signaling pathway protein 3	603400	Arthropathy, progressive pseudorheumatoid, of childhood, 208230 (3)
6q22-q24	ODDD, SDTY3, ODOD	P	Oculodentodigital dysplasia (syndactyly type III)	164200	Oculodentodigital dysplasia (2); Syndactyly, type III, 186100 (2)
6q22-q24	PEX7, RCDP1	P	Peroxisomal biogenesis factor-7	601757	Rhizomelic chondrodysplasia punctata, type 1, 215100 (3)
6q22.3-q23.1	HPFH	P	Hereditary persistence of fetal hemoglobin, heterocellular	142470	[Hereditary persistence of fetal hemoglobin, heterocellular] (2)
6q22.2-q23.3	DFNA10	P	Deafness, autosomal nonsyndromic sensorineural, 10	601316	Deafness, autosomal dominant 10 (2)
6q23	ARG1	P	Arginase, liver	207800	Argininemia (3)
6q23	CMD1F, CDCD3	P	Cardiomyopathy, dilated-1F, autosomal dominant	602067	Cardiomyopathy, dilated, 1F (2)
6q23-q24	IFNGR1	C	Immune interferon, receptor for	107470	Mycobacterial infection, atypical, familial disseminated, 209950 (3); BCG infection, generalized familial (3); {Tuberculosis, susceptibility to} (3)

(Continued on next page)

Table A1-2 (Continued)

Location	Symbol	Status	Locus Name	MIM#	Disorder
6q24	EPM2A, MELF, EPM2	C	Laforin	254780	Epilepsy, myoclonic, Lafora type (3)
6q24	TNDM, DMTN	C	Diabetes mellitus, transient neonatal	601410	{Diabetes mellitus, transient neonatal} (2)
6q24-q27	IDDM5	P	Insulin-dependent diabetes mellitus-5	600320	{Diabetes mellitus, insulin-dependent, 5} (2)
6q25-q26	RCD1	L	Retinal cone dystrophy-1	180020	?Retinal cone dystrophy-1 (2)
6q25-q27	IDDM8	P	Insulin-dependent diabetes mellitus-8	600883	{Diabetes mellitus, insulin-dependent, 8} (2)
6q25.1	ESR1, ESR	C	Estrogen receptor 1	133430	Breast cancer (1); Estrogen resistance (3)
6q25.2-q27	PRKN, PARK2, PDJ	C	Parkin	602544	Parkinson disease, juvenile, type 2, 600116 (3)
6q25.3-q26	ACAT2	P	Acetyl-Coenzyme A acetyltransferase 2 (acetoacetyl Coenzyme A thiolase)	100678	?ACAT2 deficiency (1)
6q26	IGF2R, MPRI	C	Insulin-like growth factor-2 receptor (mannose-6-phosphate receptor, cation-independent)	147280	Hepatocellular carcinoma (3)
6q26	PLG	C	Plasminogen	173350	Plasminogen Tochigi disease (3); Thrombophilia, dysplasminogenemic (1); Plasminogen deficiency, types I and II (1); Conjunctivitis, ligneous, 217090 (3)
6q26-q27	ST8, OVCS	P	Suppression of tumorigenicity-8, ovarian	167000	Ovarian cancer, serous (2)
6q27	LPA	C	Apolipoprotein Lp(a)	152200	{Coronary artery disease, susceptibility to} (1)
6q27	TBP	C	TATA box binding protein	600075	Complex neurologic disorder, 117200 (3)
Chr.6	GCNT2	P	Glucosaminyl (N-acetyl) transferase 2, I-branching enzyme	600429	[Ii blood group, 110800] (1)
Chr.6	PBCA	P	Pancreatic beta cell, agenesis of	600089	?Diabetes mellitus, insulin-dependent, neonatal (2)
Chr.6	POLH, XPV	P	Polymerase, DNA, eta	603968	Xeroderma pigmentosum, variant type, 278750 (3)
7p22	PMS2, PMSL2	P	Postmeiotic segregation increased, S. cerevisiae, 2, homolog of	600259	Turcot syndrome with glioblastoma, 276300 (3); Colorectal cancer, hereditary nonpolyposis, type 4 (3)
7p21.3-p21.2	CRS, CSO	C	Craniosynostosis, type I	123100	Craniosynostosis, type 1 (2)
7p21	IL6, IFNB2, BSF2	C	Interleukin-6 (interferon, beta-2)	147620	Osteopenia/osteoporosis, 166710 (2)
7p21	TWIST, ACS3, SCS	C	TWIST, drosophila, homolog of	601622	Saethre-Chotzen syndrome, 101400 (3)
7p21-p15	MDDC	P	Macular dystrophy, dominant cystoid	153880	Macular dystrophy, dominant cystoid (2)
7p21-p13	BPES2	P	Blepharophimosis, epicanthus inversus, and ptosis 2	601649	Blepharophimosis, epicanthus inversus, and ptosis, type 2 (2)
7p15.1-p13	RP9	P	Retinitis pigmentosa-9	180104	Retinitis pigmentosa-9 (2)
7p15	DFNA5	C	Deafness, autosomal dominant 5	600994	Deafness, autosomal dominant 5 (3)
7p15-p14	GHRHR	C	Growth hormone releasing hormone receptor	139191	Growth hormone deficient dwarfism (3)
7p15-p14.2	HOXA13, HOX1J	C	Homeo box-A13	142959	Hand-foot-uterus syndrome, 140000 (3)
7p15-p13	CCM2	P	Cerebral cavernous malformations-2	603284	Cerebral cavernous malformations-2 (2)
7p15-p13	GCK	C	Glucokinase (hexokinase-4)	138079	MODY, type 2, 125851 (3); Hyperinsulinism, familial, 602485 (3)
7p15-p11.2	WTSL, WT5	C	Wilms tumor suppressor locus	601583	{Wilms tumor susceptibility-5} (2)
7p14	AQP1, CHIP28, CO	C	Aquaporin-1 (channel-forming integral protein, 28 kD)	107776	Colton blood group, 110450 (3); [Aquaporin-1 deficiency] (3)

Table A1-2 (Continued)

Location	Symbol	Status	Locus Name	MIM#	Disorder
7p14	CMT2D	C	Charcot-Marie-Tooth neuropathy, neuronal type, D	601472	Charcot-Marie-Tooth neuropathy-2D (2)
7p14-p13	OGDH	C	Oxoglutarate dehydrogenase (lipoamide)	203740	Alpha-ketoglutarate dehydrogenase deficiency (1)
7p13	GLI3, PAPA, PAPB	C	GLI-Kruppel family member GLI3 (oncogene GLI3)	165240	Greig cephalopolysyndactyly syndrome, 175700 (3); Pallister-Hall syndrome, 146510 (3); Polydactyly, preaxial, type IV, 174700 (3); Polydactyly, postaxial, types A1 and B, 174200 (3)
7p13-p12.3	PGAM2, PGAMM	C	Phosphoglycerate mutase, muscle form	261670	Myopathy due to phosphoglycerate mutase deficiency (3)
7p12-p11.2	GRB10	C	Growth factor receptor-bound protein-10	601523	?Russell-Silver syndrome, 180860 (1)
7p	GHS	L	Goldenhar syndrome	141400	?Goldenhar syndrome (2)
7p	SMAD1	P	Spinal muscular atrophy, distal, with upper limb predominance	600794	Spinal muscular atrophy, distal, with upper limb predominance (2)
7cen-q11.2	ASL	C	Argininosuccinate lyase	207900	Argininosuccinicaciduria (3)
7q	AUT	P	Autism, susceptibility to	209850	{Autism, susceptibility to} (2)
7q	LGMD1D	P	Limb-girdle muscular dystrophy-1D, autosomal dominant	603511	Muscular dystrophy, limb-girdle, type 1D (2)
7q11.2	CD36	P	CD36 antigen (collagen type I)	173510	[Macrothrombocytopenia] (1); Platelet glycoprotein IV deficiency (3)
7q11.2	ELN	C	Elastin	130160	Supravalvar aortic stenosis, 185500 (3); Williams-Beuren syndrome, 194050 (3); Cutis laxa, 123700 (3)
7q11.2-q21	CCM1, CAM, KRIT1	C	KREV interaction trapped 1	604214	Cerebral cavernous malformations-1, 116860 (3)
7q11.2-q21.3	EEC1	L	Ectrodactyly, ectodermal dysplasia, cleft lip/palate, 1	129900	?EEC syndrome-1 (2)
7q11.23	NCF1	P	Neutrophil cytosolic factor-1, 47 kD	233700	Chronic granulomatous disease due to deficiency of NCF-1 (3)
7q11.23	PTPN12, PTPG1	P	Protein tyrosine phosphatase, non-receptor type 12	600079	Colon cancer (3)
7q21	EPO	C	Erythropoietin	133170	?Erythremia (1)
7q21-q22	MHS3	P	Malignant hyperthermia susceptibility 3	154276	{Malignant hyperthermia susceptibility 3} (2)
7q21-q22	PEX1, ZWS1	C	Peroxisome biogenesis factor-1	602136	Zellweger syndrome-1, 214100 (3); Adrenoleukodystrophy, neonatal, 202370 (3); Refsum disease, infantile, 266510 (3)
7q21.1	ABCB4, PGY3, MDR3	P	ATP-binding cassette, subfamily B, member 4 (P-glycoprotein-3/ multiple drug resistance-3)	171060	Cholestasis, progressive familial intrahepatic, type III, 602347 (3); Cholestasis, familial intrahepatic, of pregnancy, 147480 (3)
7q21.1	ABCB1, PGY1, MDR1	C	ATP-binding cassette, subfamily B, member 1 (P-glycoprotein-1/ multiple drug resistance-1)	171050	Colchicine resistance (3)
7q21.11	GUSB	C	Glucuronidase, beta-	253220	Mucopolysaccharidosis VII (3)
7q21.2-q21.3	SHFM1, SHFD1, SHSF1	C	Split hand/foot malformation (ectrodactyly) type 1	183600	Split hand/foot malformation, type 1 (2)
7q21.3	CALCR, CRT	C	Calcitonin receptor	114131	{Osteoporosis, postmenopausal, susceptibility}, 166710 (3)
7q21.3	PON1, PON, ESA	C	Paraoxonase-1	168820	{Coronary artery disease, susceptibility to} (3)
7q21.3	PON2	C	Paraoxonase-2	602447	{Coronary artery disease, susceptibility to} (3)
7q21.3	SLC25A13, CTLN2	P	Solute carrier family 25 (mitochondrial carrier, citrin), member 13	603859	Citrullinemia, adult-onset type II, 603471 (3)
7q21.3-q22	PAI1, PLANH1	C	Plasminogen activator inhibitor, type I	173360	Thrombophilia due to excessive plasminogen activator inhibitor (1); Hemorrhagic diathesis due to PAI1 deficiency (1)

(Continued on next page)

Table A1-2 (Continued)

Location	Symbol	Status	Locus Name	MIM#	Disorder
7q22	MUC3	P	Mucin 3, intestinal	158371	{Ulcerative colitis, susceptibility to}, 191390 (1)
7q22-q31.1	DRA, CLD	C	Down-regulated in adenoma	126650	?Colon cancer (1); Chloride diarrhea, congenital, Finnish type, 214700 (3)
7q22.1	COL1A2	C	Collagen I, alpha-2 polypeptide	120160	Osteogenesis imperfecta, 3 clinical forms, 166200, 166210, 259420 (3); Ehlers-Danlos syndrome, type VIIA2, 130060 (3); Osteoporosis, idiopathic, 166710 (3); Marfan syndrome, atypical (3)
7q3	CMH6	P	Cardiomyopathy, hypertrophic 6	600858	Cardiomyopathy, familial hypertrophic with Wolff-Parkinson-White syndrome (2)
7q31	DFNB14	P	Deafness, autosomal recessive 14	603678	Deafness, autosomal recessive 14 (2)
7q31	DFNB17	P	Deafness, autosomal recessive 17	603010	Deafness, autosomal recessive 17 (2)
7q31	MET	C	Oncogene MET	164860	Renal cell carcinoma, papillary, familial and sporadic (3); Hepatocellular carcinoma, childhood type, 114550 (3)
7q31	PDS, DFNB4	C	Pendrin	274600	Pendred syndrome (3); Deafness, autosomal recessive 4, 600791 (3); Enlarged vestibular aqueduct, 603545 (3)
7q31	SPCH1	P	Speech-language disorder-1	602081	Speech-language disorder-1 (2)
7q31-q32	DLD, LAD, PHE3	C	Dihydrolipoamide dehydrogenase (E3 component of pyruvate dehydrogenase complex, 2-oxo-glutarate complex)	246900	Lipoamide dehydrogenase deficiency (3)
7q31-q32	SMOH, SMO	P	Smoothened, drosophila, homolog of	601500	Basal cell carcinoma, sporadic (3)
7q31-q34	BPGM	P	2,3-bisphosphoglycerate mutase	222800	Hemolytic anemia due to bisphosphoglycerate mutase deficiency (1)
7q31-q35	RP10	C	Retinitis pigmentosa-10, autosomal dominant	180105	Retinitis pigmentosa-10 (2)
7q31.1-q31.3	LAMB1	C	Laminin, beta-1	150240	?Cutis laxa, marfanoid neonatal type (1)
7q31.2	ABCC7, CFTR, CF, MRP7	C	ATP-binding cassette, subfamily C, member 7 (cystic fibrosis transmembrane conductance regulator)	602421	Cystic fibrosis, 219700 (3); Congenital bilateral absence of vas deferens, 277180 (3); Sweat chloride elevation without CF (3)
7q31.3	LEP, OB	C	Leptin (murine obesity homolog)	164160	Obesity, severe, due to leptin deficiency (3); Obesity, morbid, with hypogonadism (3)
7q31.3-q32	BCP, CBT	C	Blue cone pigment	190900	Colorblindness, tritan (3)
7q33-q34	RTA1C, RTADR, RDRTA2	P	Renal tubular acidosis, distal, autosomal recessive	602722	Renal tubular acidosis, distal, autosomal recessive (2)
7q34	TBXAS1	C	Thromboxane A synthase 1, platelet	274180	Thromboxane synthase deficiency (2)
7q34-q36	DFNB13	P	Deafness, autosomal recessive 13	603098	Deafness, autosomal recessive 13 (2)
7q35	CLCN1	P	Chloride channel-1, skeletal muscle	118425	Myotonia congenita, recessive, 255700 (3); Myotonia congenita, dominant, 160800 (3); Myotonia levior, recessive (3)
7q35	PRSS1, TRY1	C	Protease, serine, 1 (trypsin 1)	276000	Trypsinogen deficiency (1); Pancreatitis, hereditary, 167800 (3)
7q35-q36	GLC1F	P	Glaucoma 1, open angle, F	603383	Glaucoma 1F (2)

Table A1-2 (Continued)

Location	Symbol	Status	Locus Name	MIM#	Disorder
7q35-q36	GPDS1, PDS1	P	Glaucoma-related pigment dispersion syndrome-1	600510	Pigment dispersion syndrome (2)
7q35-q36	KCNH2, LQT2, HERG	C	Potassium channel, voltage-gated, subfamily H, member 2 (human ether-a-go-go-related gene)	152427	Long QT syndrome-2 (3)
7q36	HLXB9, HOXHB9, SCRA1	C	Homeo box-HB9	142994	Currarino syndrome, 176450 (3)
7q36	HPFH2	L	Hereditary persistence of fetal hemoglobin, heterocellular, Indian type	142335	?Hereditary persistence of fetal hemoglobin, heterocellular, Indian type (2)
7q36	NOS3	C	Nitric oxide synthase 3, endothelial cell	163729	{Preeclampsia, susceptibility to, 189800} (2); {Coronary spasm, susceptibility to} (3)
7q36	SCRA1	P	Sacral agenesis, autosomal dominant (Currarino triad)	176450	Sacral agenesis-1 (2)
7q36	SHH, HPE3, HLP3	C	Sonic hedgehog, Drosophila, homolog of	600725	Holoprosencephaly-3, 142945 (3)
7q36	TPTPS, TPT	C	Triphalangeal thumb-polysyndactyly syndrome	190605	Triphalangeal thumb-polysyndactyly syndrome (2)
8pter-p22	CLN8, EPMR	P	CLN8 gene	600143	Epilepsy, progressive, with mental retardation (2)
8pter-p22	MCPH1	P	Microcephaly, primary autosomal recessive 1	251200	Microcephaly, autosomal recessive 1 (2)
8p23-p22	KWE	P	Keratolytic winter erythema	148370	Keratolytic winter erythema (2)
8p22	LPL, LIPD	C	Lipoprotein lipase	238600	Hyperlipoproteinemia I (1); Lipoprotein lipase deficiency (3); Chylomicronemia syndrome, familial (3); Combined hyperlipemia, familial (3)
8p22	N33	P	Putative prostate cancer tumor suppressor	601385	?Prostate cancer (1)
8p22-p21.3	ASAH, AC	P	N-acylsphingosine amidohydrolase (acid ceramidase)	228000	Farber lipogranulomatosis (3)
8p22-p21.3	PDGFRL, PDGRL, PRLTS	P	Platelet-derived growth factor receptor-like	604584	Hepatocellular cancer, 114550 (3); Colorectal cancer, 114500 (3)
8p22-p21	HMU	P	Hypotrichosis, Marie Unna type	146550	Hypotrichosis, Marie Unna type (2)
8p21.2	HR, AU	C	Hairless, mouse, homolog of	602302	Alopecia universalis, 203655 (3); Atrichia with papular lesions, 209500 (3)
8p21.1	GSR	C	Glutathione reductase	138300	Hemolytic anemia due to glutathione reductase deficiency (1)
8p21.1	GULOP, GULO	P	Gulonolactone (L-) oxidase pseudogene	240400	Scurvy (3)
8p21	SCZD6	P	Schizophrenia susceptibility locus, chromosome 8p-related	603013	{Schizophrenia}, 181500 (2)
8p21-p11.2	GNRH1, LNRH	P	Gonadotropin-releasing hormone-1 (leutinizing-releasing hormone)	152760	?Hypogonadotropic hypogonadism due to GNRH deficiency, 227200 (1)
8p21-q22	DYT6	P	Dystonia-6 (torsion dystonia, adult onset, of mixed type)	602629	Dystonia-6, torsion (2)
8p12	PLAT, TPA	C	Plasminogen activator, tissue type	173370	Plasminogen activator deficiency (1)
8p12-p11.2	RECQL3, WRN	C	RecQ protein-like 3	604611	Werner syndrome, 277700 (3)
8p12-q13	SPG5A	P	Spastic paraplegia-5A, autosomal recessive	270800	Spastic paraplegia-5A (2)
8p11.2	ANK1, SPH2	C	Ankyrin-1, erythrocytic	182900	Spherocytosis-2 (3)
8p11.2	STAR	P	Steroidogenic acute regulatory protein	600617	Lipoid adrenal hyperplasia, 201710 (3)
8p11.2-p11.1	FGFR1, FLT2	C	Fibroblast growth factor receptor-1 (fms-related tyrosine kinase-2)	136350	Pfeiffer syndrome, 101600 (3)
8q	CCAL1	P	Chondrocalcinosis 1	600668	Chondrocalcinosis with early-onset osteoarthritis (2)

(Continued on next page)

Table A1-2 (Continued)

Location	Symbol	Status	Locus Name	MIM#	Disorder
8q11	PRKDC, HYRC1, DNPK1	C	Protein kinase, DNA-activated, catalytic polypeptide (hyperradiosensitivity of murine SCID mutation, complementing-1)	600899	?Severe combined immunodeficiency, type I, 202500 (1)
8q11-q13	RP1, ORP1	C	Oxygen-regulated photoreceptor protein-1 (retinitis pigmentosa-1)	603937	Retinitis pigmentosa-1, 180100 (3)
8q12	SGPA, PSA	P	Salivary gland pleomorphic adenoma	181030	Salivary gland pleomorphic adenoma (2)
8q13	CRH	C	Corticotropin releasing hormone	122560	ACTH deficiency, 201400 (2)
8q13	DURS1, DUS	P	Duane retraction syndrome 1	126800	Duane syndrome (2)
8q13-q21	FEB1	P	Convulsions, familial febrile, 1	602476	Convulsions, familial febrile, 1 (2)
8q13-q21.1	CMT4A	C	Charcot-Marie-Tooth neuropathy-4A, autosomal recessive	214400	Charcot-Marie-Tooth neuropathy-4A (2)
8q13.1-q13.3	TTPA, TTP1, AVED	C	Tocopherol, alpha, transfer protein	600415	Ataxia with isolated vitamin E deficiency, 277460 (3)
8q13.3	EYA1, BOR	C	Eyes absent, Drosophila, homolog of, 1	601653	Branchiootorenal syndrome, 113650 (3); Branchiootic syndrome (3); Anterior segment anomalies and cataract (3); Branchiootorenal syndrome with cataract, 113650 (3)
8q21	CYP11B1, P450C11	C	Cytochrome P450, subfamily XIB, polypeptide 1 (11-beta-hydroxylase; corticosteroid methyl-oxidase II (CMO II))	202010	Adrenal hyperplasia, congenital, due to 11-beta-hydroxylase deficiency (3); Aldosteronism, glucocorticoid-remediable (3)
8q21	CYP11B2	C	Cytochrome P450, subfamily XIB, polypeptide 2	124080	CMO II deficiency (3)
8q21	NBS1, NBS	C	Nibrin	602667	Nijmegen breakage syndrome, 251260 (3)
8q21-q22	ACHM3	C	Achromatopsia-3	262300	Achromatopsia-3 (2)
8q21.1	PXMP3, PAF1, PMP35, PEX2	C	Peroxisomal membrane protein-3, 35 kD	170993	Zellweger syndrome-3 (3); Refsum disease, infantile form, 266510 (3)
8q21.3	CYP7B1	P	Oxysterol 7-alpha-hydroxylase	603711	Giant cell hepatitis, neonatal, 231100 (3)
8q21.3	DECR1	P	2,4-dienoyl CoA reductase	222745	?DECR deficiency (2)
8q21.3-q22	RAD54B	P	RAD54, S. cerevisiae, homolog of, B	604289	Lymphoma, non-Hodgkin (3); Colon adenocarcinoma (3)
8q22	CA2	C	Carbonic anhydrase II	259730	Renal tubular acidosis-osteopetrosis syndrome (3)
8q22	DPYS, DHP	P	Dihydropyrimidinase	222748	Dihydropyrimidinuria (3)
8q22-q23	COH1	P	Cohen syndrome 1	216550	Cohen syndrome (2)
8q22.2	SGM1, KFSL	P	Segmentation syndrome 1 (Klippel-Feil syndrome with laryngeal malformation)	148900	Klippel-Feil syndrome with laryngeal malformation (2)
8q23	GLC1D	P	Glaucoma 1, open angle, D	602429	Glaucoma 1D, primary open angle (2)
8q23-q24	SPG8	P	Spastic paraplegia-8	603563	Spastic paraplegia-8 (2)
8q23.3-q24.11	MEBA, BAFME	P	Myoclonic epilepsy, benign adult familial	601068	Epilepsy, myoclonic, benign adult familial (2)
8q24	EBS1	C	Epidermolysis bullosa simplex-1, Ogna type	131950	Epidermolysis bullosa, Ogna type (2)
8q24	ECA1	P	Epilepsy, childhood absence, 1	600131	Epilepsy, childhood absence, 1 (2)
8q24	EGI	P	Epilespy, generalized, idiopathic	600669	Epilepsy, generalized, idiopathic (2)
8q24	HMSNL, NMSL	P	Hereditary motor and sensory neuropathy, Lom type	601455	Hereditary motor and sensory neuropathy, Lom type (2)
8q24	KCNQ3, EBN2, BFNC2	C	Potassium voltage-gated channel, KQT-like subfamily, member-3	602232	Epilepsy, benign neonatal, type 2, 121201 (3)
8q24	PLEC1, PLTN	C	Plectin 1, intermediate filament binding protein, 500 kD	601282	Muscular dystrophy with epidermolysis bullosa simplex, 226670 (3)
8q24	VMD1	C	Macular dystrophy, atypical vitelliform	153840	Macular dystrophy, atypical vitelliform (2)

Table A1-2 (Continued)

Location	Symbol	Status	Locus Name	MIM#	Disorder
8q24.1	THM	L	Tibial hemimelia	275220	?Tibial hemimelia (2)
8q24.1	TRC8, RCA1, HRCA1	P	Translocation-related gene on chromosome 8	603046	Renal cell carcinoma, 144700 (3)
8q24.11-q24.13	EXT1	C	Exostoses, multiple, 1	133700	Exostoses, multiple, type 1 (3); Chondrosarcoma, 215300 (3)
8q24.11-q24.13	LGCR, LGS, TRPS2	C	Langer-Giedion syndrome chromosome region	150230	Langer-Giedion syndrome (2)
8q24.12	TRPS1	C	Trichorhinophalangeal syndrome type I zinc finger protein	604386	Trichorhinophalangeal syndrome, type I, 190350 (3)
8q24.12-q24.13	MYC	C	Avian myelocytomatosis viral (v-myc) oncogene homolog	190080	Burkitt lymphoma, 113970 (3)
8q24.2-q24.3	TG	C	Thyroglobulin	188450	Hypothyroidism, hereditary congenital (3); Goiter, adolescent multinodular (1); Goiter, nonendemic, simple (3)
8q24.3	RECQL4, RTS, RECQ4	P	RecQ protein-like 4 (DNA helicase, RecQ-like, type 4)	603780	Rothmund-Thomson syndrome, 268400 (3)
8qter	MDM	P	Meleda disease (mal de Meleda)	248300	Meleda disease (2)
9p24.3	DMRT1, DMT1	P	Double sex and mab-3-related transcription factor-1	602424	XY sex reversal (1)
9p24	SLC1A1, EAAC1	P	Solute carrier family 1, member 1 (high-affinity glutamate transporter; excitatory amino acid carrier 1)	133550	?Dicarboxylicaminoaciduria, 222730 (1)
9p24	OVC	P	Oncogene OVC (ovarian adenocarcinoma oncogene)	164759	Ovarian carcinoma (2)
9p24	SRA2, TDFA	C	Sex-reversal, autosomal, 2 (testis-determining factor, autosomal)	154230	XY sex reversal (2)
9p23	TYRP1, CAS2, GP75	C	Tyrosinase-related protein 1	115501	Albinism, brown, 203290 (1); Albinism, rufous, 278400 (3)
9p22	GLDC, HYGN1, GCSP	C	Glycine dehydrogenase (decarboxylating; glycine decarboxylase, glycine cleavage system protein P)	238300	Hyperglycinemia, nonketotic, 1 (3)
9p22	IFNA1, IFNA@	C	Interferon, alpha-1	147660	Interferon, alpha, deficiency (1)
3p25	ST11, PETS1	P	Suppression of tumorigenicity 11, pancreas	602011	?Pancreatic endocrine tumors (1)
9p22-p21	DMSFH, BDMF	P	Diaphyseal medullary stenosis with malignant fibrous histiocytoma	112250	Diaphyseal medullary stenosis with malignant fibrous histiocytoma (2)
9p22-p21	LALL	P	Lymphomatous acute lymphoblastic leukemia	247640	Leukemia, acute lymphoblastic (2)
9p21	CDKN2A, MTS1, P16, MLM, CMM2	C	Cyclin-dependent kinase inhibitor 2A (p16, inhibits CDK4)	600160	Melanoma, 155601 (3)
9p21	MFT, TEM	P	Trichoepithelioma, multiple familial	601606	Trichoepithelioma, multiple familial (2)
9p21	TEK, TIE2, VMCM	C	TEK tyrosine kinase, endothelial	600221	Venous malformations, multiple cutaneous and mucosal, 600195 (3)
9p21-p13	DNAI1	P	Dynein, axonemal, intermediate chain 1	604366	Immotile cilia syndrome-1, 242650 (3)
9p21-q21	AMCD1, DA1	P	Arthrogryposis multiplex congenita, distal, type 1	108120	Arthrogryposis multiplex congenita, distal, type 1 (2)
9p13	CHH	P	Cartilage-hair hypoplasia	250250	Cartilage-hair hypoplasia (2)
9p13	GALT	C	Galactose-1-phosphate uridyltransferase	230400	Galactosemia (3)
9p13	XRCC9, FANCG	C	X-ray repair, complementing defective, in Chinese hamster, 9	602956	Fanconi anemia, complementation group G (3)
9p13-p12	AMDM	P	Acromesomelic dysplasia, Maroteaux type	602875	Acromesomelic dysplasia, Maroteaux type (2)
9p12-p11	GNE, GLCNE	P	UDP-N-acetylglucosamine 2-epimerase/N-acetylmannosamine kinase	603824	Sialuria, 269921 (3)

(Continued on next page)

Table A1-2 (Continued)

Location	Symbol	Status	Locus Name	MIM#	Disorder
9p11	MROS	L	Melkersson-Rosenthal syndrome	155900	?Melkersson-Rosenthal syndrome (2)
9p1-q1	IBM2	P	Inclusion body myopathy, autosomal recessive	600737	Inclusion body myopathy, autosomal recessive (2)
9cen	GRHPR, GLXR	P	Glyoxylate reductase/ hydroxypyruvate reductase	604296	Hyperoxaluria, primary, type II, 260000 (3)
9q12-q22.2	HOMG, HSH, HMGX	P	Hypomagnesemia with secondary hypocalcemia	602014	Hypomagnesemia with secondary hypocalcemia (2)
9q13	CMD1B, CMPD1, FDC	C	Cardiomyopathy, dilated-1B, autosomal dominant	600884	Cardiomyopathy, familial dilated 1B (2)
9q13	FRDA, FARR	C	Frataxin	229300	Friedreich ataxia (3); Friedreich ataxia with retained reflexes (2)
19q13	SPG12	P	Spastic paraplegia 12, autosomal dominant	604805	Spastic paraplegia-12 (2)
9q13-q21	DFNB7	P	Deafness, autosomal recessive 7	600974	Deafness, autosomal recessive 7 (2)
9q13-q21	GSM1, GSP	P	Geniospasm 1	190100	Geniospasm (2)
9q21	CHAC	P	Choreoacanthocytosis	200150	Choreoacanthocytosis (2)
9q21	GNAQ	P	Guanine nucleotide-binding protein (G protein), q	600998	Bleeding diathesis due to GNAQ deficiency (1)
9q21.3-q22	HPLH1	P	Hemophagocytic lymphohistiocytosis, familial, 1	603552	Hemophagocytic lymphohistiocytosis, familial, 1 (2)
9q22	CSMF	C	Chondrosarcoma, extraskeletal myxoid, fused to EWS in	600542	Chondrosarcoma, extraskeletal myxoid (1)
9q22	FKHL15, TITF2, TTF2	C	Forkhead, drosophila, homolog-like 15 (thyroid transcription factor-2)	602617	Bamforth-Lazarus syndrome, 241850 (3)
9q22	HSD17B3, EDH17B3	P	Hydroxysteroid (17-beta) dehydrogenase 3	264300	Pseudohermaphroditism, male, with gynecomastia (3)
9q22	ROR2, BDB1, BDB, NTRKR2	C	Receptor tyrosine kinase-like orphan receptor 2	602337	Brachydactyly, type B1, 113000 (3)
9q22-q31	ABCA1, ABC1, HDLDT1, TGD	C	ATP-binding cassette 1	600046	Tangier disease, 205400 (3); HDL deficiency, familial, 604091 (3)
9q22-q31	NPHP2, NPH2	P	Nephronophthisis-2 (infantile)	602088	Nephronophthisis, infantile (2)
9q22.1-q22.3	HSN1, HSAN1	P	Hereditary sensory neuropathy, type 1	162400	Neuropathy, hereditary sensory and autonomic, type 1 (2)
9q22.2-q22.3	FBP1	C	Fructose-bisphosphatase 1	229700	Fructose-bisphosphatase deficiency (1)
9q22.3	ALDOB	C	Aldolase B, fructose-bisphosphatase	229600	Fructose intolerance (3)
9q22.3	FANCC, FACC	C	Fanconi anemia, complementation group C	227645	Fanconi anemia, type C (3)
9q22.3	PTCH, NBCCS, BCNS	C	Patched, Drosophila, homolog of	601309	Basal cell nevus syndrome, 109400 (3); Basal cell carcinoma, sporadic (3)
9q22.3	XPA	C	Xeroderma pigmentosum, complementation group A	278700	Xeroderma pigmentosum, group A (3)
9q31	FCMD	C	Fukuyama congenital muscular dystrophy	253800	Muscular dystrophy, Fukuyama congenital (3); ?Walker-Warburg syndrome, 236670 (2)
9q31	MSSE, ESS1	P	Epithelioma, self-healing, squamous 1, Ferguson-Smith type	132800	Epithelioma, self-healing, squamous 1, Ferguson-Smith type (2); ? Basal cell carcinoma (2)
9q31	NBCCS, BCNS	C	Nevoid basal cell carcinoma syndrome	109400	Basal cell nevus syndrome (2)
9q31	TAL2	P	T-cell acute lymphocytic leukemia-2	186855	Leukemia-2, T-cell acute lymphoblastic (3)
9q31-q33	DYS	C	Dysautonomia (Riley-Day syndrome, hereditary sensory autonomic neuropathy type III)	223900	Dysautonomia, familial (2)
9q31-q34.1	LGMD2H	P	Limb-girdle muscular dystrophy 2H	254110	Muscular dystrophy, limb-girdle, type 2H (2)
9q32	AFD1, AFDN	L	Acrofacial dysostosis-1, Nager type	154400	?Acrofacial dysostosis, Nager type (2)

Table A1-2 (Continued)

Location	Symbol	Status	Locus Name	MIM#	Disorder
9q33	FTZF1, FTZ1, SF1	P	Fushi tarazu factor, Drosophila, homolog of, 1	184757	Sex reversal, XY, with adrenal failure (3)
9q33-q34	SARDH, SARD, SAR	L	Sarcosine dehydrogenase	604455	[Sarcosinemia], 268900 (2)
9q34	ALAD	C	Aminolevulinate, delta-, dehydratase	125270	Porphyria, acute hepatic (3); {Lead poisoning, susceptibility to} (3)
9q34	ALS4	P	Amyotrophic lateral sclerosis-4, juvenile dominant	602433	Amyotrophic lateral sclerosis-4, juvenile dominant (2)
9q34	ASS	C	Argininosuccinate synthetase	603470	Citrullinemia, 215700 (3)
9q34	DBH	C	Dopamine-beta-hydroxylase	223360	Dopamine-beta-hydroxylase deficiency (1)
9q34	DYT1	C	Dystonia-1, torsion, autosomal dominant	128100	Dystonia-1, torsion (3)
9q34	GSN	P	Gelsolin	137350	Amyloidosis, Finnish type, 105120 (3)
9q34	LCCS	P	Lethal congenital contracture syndrome	253310	Lethal congenital contracture syndrome (2)
9q34	MCPH3	P	Microcephaly, primary autosomal recessive, 3	604804	Microcephaly, primary autosomal recessive, 3 (2)
9q34	SURF1	C	Surfeit-1	185620	Leigh syndrome, due to COX deficiency, 256000 (3)
9q34	TSC1	C	Tuberous sclerosis-1	191100	Tuberous sclerosis-1 (3)
9q34.1	ABL1	C	Abelson murine leukemia viral (v-abl) oncogene homolog 1	189980	Leukemia, chronic myeloid (3)
9q34.1	AK1	C	Adenylate kinase-1	103000	Hemolytic anemia due to adenylate kinase deficiency (3)
9q34.1	C5	C	Complement component-5	120900	C5 deficiency (1)
9q34.1	CRAT, CAT1	P	Carnitine acetyltransferase	600184	?Carnitine acetyltransferase deficiency (1)
9q34.1	D9S46E, CAN, CAIN, NUP214	P	CAIN gene	114350	Leukemia, acute myeloid (2)
9q34.1	ENG, END, HHT1, ORW	C	Endoglin	131195	Hereditary hemorrhagic telangiectasia-1, 187300 (3)
9q34.1	EPB72	C	Erythrocyte membrane protein band 7.2 (stomatin)	133090	?Stomatocytosis I, 185000 (1)
9q34.1	LMX1B, NPS1	C	LIM homeo box transcription factor 1, beta	602575	Nail-patella syndrome, 161200 (3); Nail-patella syndrome with open-angle glaucoma, 137750 (3)
9q34.2-q34.3	COL5A1	C	Collagen V, alpha-1 polypeptide	120215	Ehlers-Danlos syndrome, type II, 130010 (3); Ehlers-Danlos syndrome, type I, 130000 (3)
9q34.3	JBTS1	P	Joubert syndrome-1	213300	Joubert syndrome-1 (2)
9q34.3	NOTCH1, TAN1	C	Notch, Drosophila, homolog of, 1, translocation-associated	190198	Leukemia, T-cell acute lymphoblastic (2)
10pter-p11.2	PHYH, PAHX	P	Phytanoyl-CoA hydroxylase	602026	Refsum disease, 266500 (3)
10pter-p11.2	RDPA	P	Refsum disease, adult, with increased pipecolicacidemia	600964	Refsum disease, adult, with increased pipecolicacidemia (2)
10pter-q11	ST12, PAC1	P	Suppression of tumorigenicity 12, prostate	601188	Prostate adenocarcinoma (2)
10p15.1-p14	HDR	P	Hypoparathyroidism, sensorineural deafness, renal dysplasia	146255	HDR syndrome (2)
10p15-p14	IL2RA, IL2R	C	Interleukin-2 receptor	147730	Interleukin-2 receptor, alpha chain, deficiency of (3)
10p14-p13	DGCR2, DGS2	C	DiGeorge syndrome chromosome region-2	601362	DiGeorge syndrome/velocardiofacial syndrome complex-2 (2)
10p14-p12	ARVD6	P	Arrhythmogenic right ventricular dysplasia-6	604401	Arrhythmogenic right ventricular dysplasia-6 (2)
10p12-p11.2	THC2	P	Thrombocytopenia 2	188000	Thrombocytopenia-2 (2)
10p12.1	CUBN, IFCR, MGA1	C	Cubilin (intrinsic factor-cobalamin receptor)	602997	Megaloblastic anemia-1, 261100 (3)
10p11-q11	IDDM10	P	Insulin-dependent diabetes mellitus-10	601942	{Diabetes mellitus, insulin-dependent, 10} (2)
10p	OB10	P	Obesity, susceptibility to, on chromosome 10	603188	{Obesity, susceptibility to}, 601665 (2)

(Continued on next page)

Table A1-2 (Continued)

Location	Symbol	Status	Locus Name	MIM#	Disorder
10p	SCIDA	P	Severe combined immunodeficiency disease, Athabascan type	602450	Severe combined immunodeficiency disease, Athabascan type (2)
10q	USH1D	P	Usher syndrome-1D, autosomal recessive, severe	601067	Usher syndrome, type 1D (2)
10q11	ERCC6, CKN2	P	Excision repair cross complementing rodent repair deficiency, complementation group 6	133540	Cockayne syndrome-2, type B (3)
10q11.1	SDF1	P	Stromal cell-derived factor 1	600835	{AIDS, resistance to} (3)
10q11.2	RET, MEN2A	C	RET transforming sequence; oncogene RET	164761	Multiple endocrine neoplasia IIA, 171400 (3); Medullary thyroid carcinoma, 155240 (3); Multiple endocrine neoplasia IIB, 162300 (3); Hirschsprung disease, 142623 (3)
10q11.2-q21	MBL2, MBL, MBP1	C	Mannose-binding lectin 2, soluble (opsonic defect)	154545	{Chronic infections, due to opsonin defect} (3)
10q21	D10S170, H4, TST1, PTC, TPC	C	RET-activating gene H4	601985	Thyroid papillary carcinoma, 188550 (1)
10q21-q22	DFNB12	P	Deafness, autosomal recessive 12	601386	Deafness, autosomal recessive 12 (2)
10q21-q23	CMD1C, CMPD3	P	Cardiomyopathy, dilated-1C, autosomal dominant	601493	Cardiomyopathy, dilated 1C (2)
10q21.1-q22.1	EGR2, KROX20	P	KROX-20, Drosophila, homolog of (early growth response-2)	129010	Neuropathy, congenital hypomyelinating, 1 (3)
10q22	HK1	C	Hexokinase-1	142600	Hemolytic anemia due to hexokinase deficiency (3)
10q22	MAT1A, MATA1, SAMS1	P	Methionine adenosyltransferase I, alpha	250850	Hypermethioninemia, persistent, autosomal dominant, due to methionine adenosyltransferase I/III deficiency (3)
10q22	PCBD, DCOH	C	Pterin-4a-carbinolamine dehydratase (dimerization cofactor of hepatic nuclear factor 1-alpha)	126090	Hyperphenylalaninemia due to pterin-4a-carbinolamine dehydratase deficiency, 264070 (3)
10q22	PRF1, HPLH2	P	Perforin	170280	Hemophagocytic lymphohistiocytosis, familial, 2, 603553 (3)
10q22.1	PSAP, SAP1	C	Prosaposin (sphingolipid activator protein-1)	176801	Metachromatic leukodystrophy due to deficiency of SAP-1 (3); Gaucher disease, variant form (3)
10q23	RGR	C	Retinal G protein coupled receptor	600342	Retinitis pigmentosa, autosomal recessive (3); Retinitis pigmentosa, autosomal dominant (3)
10q23-q24	ATPSK2	P	ATP sulfurylase/APS kinase 2	603005	SEMD, Pakistani type (3)
10q23-q24	UFS	P	Urofacial syndrome (Ochoa syndrome)	236730	Urofacial syndrome (2)
10q23.1-q23.3	HPS	C	Hermansky-Pudlak syndrome gene	203300	Hermansky-Pudlak syndrome (3)
10q23.2	BLNK, SLP65	P	B-cell linker protein (SH2 domain-containing leukocyte protein, 65 kD)	604515	Hypoglobulinemia and absent B cells (3)
10q23.3	GLUD1	C	Glutamate dehydrogenase-1	138130	Hyperinsulinism-hyperammonemia syndrome (3)
10q23.3	PTEN, MMAC1	C	Phosphatase and tensin homolog (mutated in multiple advanced cancers 1)	601728	Cowden disease, 158350 (3); Lhermitte-Duclos syndrome (3); Bannayan-Zonana syndrome, 153480 (3); Endometrial carcinoma (3); Polyposis, juvenile intestinal, 174900 (3); Prostate cancer (3); Bannayan-Riley-Ruvalcaba syndrome (3)
10q23.3-q24.1	EPT	C	Epilepsy, partial	600512	Epilepsy, partial (2)

Table A1-2 (Continued)

Location	Symbol	Status	Locus Name	MIM#	Disorder
10q23.3-q24.1	SPG9	P	Spastic paraplegia-9 (spastic paraparesis with amyotrophy, cataracts and gastroesophageal reflux)	601162	Spastic paraplegia-9 (2)
10q23.3-q24.3	PEO1, PEO	P	Progressive external ophthalmoplegia, type 1	157640	PEO with mitochondrial DNA deletions, type 1 (2)
10q24	ABCC2, CMOAT	P	ATP-binding cassette, subfamily C, member 2 (canalicular multispecific organic anion transporter)	601107	Dubin-Johnson syndrome, 237500 (3)
10q24	CDB2, CDTB	P	Corneal dystrophy, Thiel-Behnke type	602082	Corneal dystrophy, Thiel-Behnke type (2)
10q24	CYP2C9	P	Cytochrome P450, subfamily IIC (mephenytoin 4-hydroxylase), polypeptide 9	601130	Tolbutamide poor metabolizer (3); Warfarin sensitivity, 122700 (3)
10q24	HOX11, TCL3	C	Homeo box-11 (T-cell leukemia-3 associated breakpoint, homologous to Drosophila Notch)	186770	Leukemia, T-cell acute lymphocytic (2)
10q24	IOSCA, SCA8	P	Infantile-onset spinocerebellar ataxia	271245	Spinocerebellar ataxia, infantile-onset, with sensory neuropathy (2)
10q24	RBP4	C	Retinol-binding protein-4, interstitial	180250	Retinol binding protein, deficiency of (3)
10q24	SHFM3, DAC	C	Split hand/foot malformation, type 3 (dactylin)	600095	Split hand/foot malformation, type 3 (2)
10q24-q25	LIPA	C	Lipase A, lysosomal acid, cholesterol esterase	278000	Wolman disease (3); Cholesteryl ester storage disease (3)
10q24.1	TNFRSF6, APT1, FAS, CD95	C	Tumor necrosis factor receptor superfamily, member 6	134637	{Autoimmune lymphoproliferative syndrome} (3)
10q24.1-q24.3	CYP2C, CYP2C19	C	Cytochrome P450, subfamily IIC (mephenytoin 4\(fm-hydroxylase)	124020	Mephenytoin poor metabolizer (3)
10q24.3	COL17A1, BPAG2	C	Collagen XVII, alpha-1 polypeptide	113811	Epidermolysis bullosa, generalized atrophic benign, 226650 (3)
10q24.3	CYP17, P450C17	C	Cytochrome P450, subfamily XVII (steroid 17-alpha-hydroxylase)	202110	Adrenal hyperplasia, congenital, due to 17-alpha-hydroxylase deficiency (3)
10q24.3	PYCS, GSAS	C	Pyrroline-5-carboxlate synthetase	138250	?P5CS deficiency (1)
10q24.3-q25.1	PAX2	C	Paired box homeotic gene-2	167409	Optic nerve coloboma with renal disease, 120330 (3)
10q25	IDDM17	P	Insulin-dependent diabetes mellitus-17	603266	{Diabetes mellitus, insulin-dependent, 17} (2)
10q25	MXI1	C	MAX-interacting protein 1	600020	Prostate cancer, 176807 (3); Neurofibrosarcoma (3)
10q25	PITX3	P	Paired-like homeodomain transcription factor-3	602669	Anterior segment mesenchymal dysgenesis and cataract, 107250 (3); Cataract, congenital (3)
10q25.2-q26.3	UROS	P	Uroporphyrinogen III synthase	263700	Porphyria, congenital erythropoietic (3)
10q25.3-q26.1	DMBT1	P	Deleted in malignant brain tumors 1	601969	Glioblastoma multiforme, 137800 (3); Medulloblastoma, 155255 (3)
10q26	DEC	C	Deleted in endometrial carcinoma	602084	Endometrial carcinoma (2)
10q26	FGFR2, BEK, CFD1, JWS	C	Fibroblast growth factor receptor-2 (bacteria-expressed kinase)	176943	Crouzon syndrome, 123500 (3); Jackson-Weiss syndrome, 123150 (3); Beare-Stevenson cutis gyrata syndrome, 123790 (3); Pfeiffer syndrome, 101600 (3); Apert syndrome, 101200 (3); Saethre-Chotzen syndrome (3); Antley-Bixler syndrome (3); Craniosynostosis, nonspecific (3)
10q26	OAT	C	Ornithine aminotransferase	258870	Gyrate atrophy of choroid and retina with ornithinemia, B6 responsive or unresponsive (3)
10q26.1	EMX2	P	Empty spiracles, Drosophila, homolog of, 2	600035	Schizencephaly (3)

(Continued on next page)

Table A1-2 (Continued)

Location	Symbol	Status	Locus Name	MIM#	Disorder
10q26.1	PNLIP	P	Pancreatic lipase	246600	Pancreatic lipase deficiency (1)
Chr.10	GLC1E	P	Glaucoma 1, open angle, E	602432	Glaucoma 1E, primary open angle, adult-onset (2)
Chr.10	NODAL	P	Nodal, mouse, homolog of	601265	Situs ambiguus (3)
Chr.10	USH1F	P	Usher syndrome-1F, autosomal recessive, severe	602083	Usher syndrome, type IF (2)
11pter-p15.4	BWS, WBS	C	Beckwith-Wiedemann syndrome	130650	Beckwith-Wiedemann syndrome (2)
11pter-p13	AMPD3	P	Adenosine monophosphate deaminase-3, isoform E	102772	[AMP deaminase deficiency, erythrocytic] (3)
11p15.5	AMCD2B, DA2B, FSSV	P	Arthrogryposis multiplex congenita, distal, type 2B (Freeman-Sheldon syndrome variant)	601680	Arthrogryposis multiplex congenita, distal, type 2B (2)
11p15.5	CDKN1C, KIP2	C	Cyclin-dependent kinase inhibitor 1C (p57, Kip2)	600856	Beckwith-Wiedemann syndrome, 130650 (3)
11p15.5	CLN2	C	Ceroid-lipofuscinosis, neuronal 2, late infantile (Jansky-Bielschowsky disease)	204500	Ceroid-lipofuscinosis, neuronal 2, classic late infantile (2)
11p15.5	DRD4	C	Dopamine receptor D4	126452	Autonomic nervous system dysfunction (3); [Novelty seeking personality], 601696 (1)
11p15.5	IDDM2	C	Insulin-dependent diabetes mellitus-2	125852	{Diabetes mellitus, insulin-dependent, 2} (2)
11p15.5	KCNQ1, KCNA9, LQT1, KVLQT1	C	Potassium voltage-gated channel, KQT-like subfamily, member 1	192500	Long QT syndrome-1 (3); Jervell and Lange-Nielsen syndrome, 220400 (3)
11p15.5	HBB	C	Hemoglobin beta	141900	Sickle cell anemia (3); Thalassemias, beta- (3); Methemoglobinemias, beta- (3); Erythremias, beta- (3); Heinz body anemias, beta- (3); HPFH, deletion type (3)
11p15.5	HBD	C	Hemoglobin delta	142000	Thalassemia, delta- (3); Thalassemia due to Hb Lepore (3)
11p15.5	HBG1	C	Hemoglobin, gamma A	142200	HPFH, nondeletion type A (3)
11p15.5	HBG2	C	Hemoglobin, gamma G	142250	HPFH, nondeletion type G (3)
11p15.5	HRAS	C	Harvey rat sarcoma viral (v-Ha-ras) oncogene homolog	190020	Bladder cancer, 109800 (3)
11p15.5	INS	C	Insulin	176730	Diabetes mellitus, rare form (1); MODY, one form (3); Hyperproinsulinemia, familial (3)
11p15.5	MTACR1, WT2	C	Multiple tumor associated chromosome region-1	194071	Wilms tumor, type 2 (2); Adrenocortical carcinoma, hereditary, 202300 (2)
11p15.5	SLC22A1L, BWSCR1A, IMPT1	P	Solute carrier family 22, member 1-like (Beckwith-Wiedemann region 1A; organic-cation transporter-like 2)	602631	Breast cancer, 114480 (3); Rhabdomyosarcoma, 268210 (3); Lung cancer, 211980 (3)
11p15.5	TH, TYH	C	Tyrosine hydroxylase	191290	Segawa syndrome, recessive (3)
11p15.4	LDHA, LDH1	C	Lactate dehydrogenase A	150000	Exertional myoglobinuria due to deficiency of LDH-A (3)
11p15.4-p15.1	SMPD1, NPD	P	Sphingomyelin phosphodiesterase-1, acid lysosomal	257200	Niemann-Pick disease, type A (3); Niemann-Pick disease, type B (3)
11p15.3-p15.1	PTH	C	Parathyroid hormone	168450	Hypoparathyroidism, autosomal dominant(3); Hypoparathyroidism, autosomal recessive (3)
11p15.2-p15.1	CALCA, CALC1	C	Calcitonin/calcitonin-related polypeptide, alpha	114130	Osteoporosis (3)
11p15.2-p15.1	TSG101	P	Tumor susceptibility gene 101	601387	Breast cancer (3)
11p15.1	ABCC8, SUR, PHHI, SUR1	C	ATP-binding cassette, subfamily C, member 8 (sulfonylurea receptor)	600509	Persistent hyperinsulinemic hypoglycemia of infancy, 256450 (3)

Table A1-2 (Continued)

Location	Symbol	Status	Locus Name	MIM#	Disorder
11p15.1	KCNJ11, BIR, PHHI	P	Potassium inwardly-rectifying channel, subfamily J, member 11	600937	Persistent hyperinsulinemic hypoglycemia of infancy, 256450 (3)
11p15.1	USH1C	C	Usher syndrome-1C, autosomal recessive, severe	276904	Usher syndrome, type 1C (2)
11p15.1-p14	DFNB18	P	Deafness, autosomal recessive 18	602092	Deafness, autosomal recessive 18 (2)
11p15	AA	P	Atrophia areata	108985	Atrophia areata (2)
11p15	FANCF	P	Fanconi anemia, complementation group F	603467	Fanconi anemia, complementation group F (3)
11p15	LMO1, RBTN1, RHOM1	C	LIM domain only 1 (rhombotin 1)	186921	Leukemia, T-cell acute lymphoblastic (2)
11p15	NUP98	C	Nucleoporin, 98 kD	601021	Leukemia, lymphycytic, acute T-cell (1)
11p14-p13	HVBS1	C	Hepatitis B virus integration site-1	114550	Hepatocellular carcinoma (1)
11p13	CAT	C	Catalase	115500	Acatalasemia (3)
11p13	CD59, MIC11	C	CD59 antigen (p18-20)	107271	CD59 deficiency (3)
11p13	FSHB	C	Follicle-stimulating hormone, beta polypeptide	136530	?Male infertility, familial (1)
11p13	LMO2, RBTNL1, RHOM2, TTG2	P	LIM domain only 2 (rhombotin-like 1)	180385	Leukemia, acute T-cell (2)
11p13	PAX6, AN2	C	Paired box homeotic gene-6	106210	Aniridia (3); Peters anomaly, 603807 (3); Cataract, congenital, with late-onset corneal dystrophy (3); Foveal hypoplasia, isolated, 136520 (3); Ectopia pupillae, 129750 (3); Keratitis, 148190 (3); Eye anomalies, multiplex (3)
11p13	PDX1	C	Pyruvate dehydrogenase complex, lipoyl-containing component X	245349	Lacticacidemia due to PDX1 deficiency (3)
11p13	RAG1	C	Recombination activating gene-1	179615	Severe combined immunodeficiency, B cell-negative, 601457 (3); Reticulosis, familial histiocytic, 267700 (3); Omenn syndrome, 603554 (3)
11p13	RAG2	C	Recombination activating gene-2	179616	Severe combined immunodeficiency, B cell-negative, 601457 (3); Omenn syndrome, 603554 (3)
11p13	TCL2	P	T-cell leukemia/lymphoma-2	151390	Leukemia, acute T-cell (2)
11p13	WT1	C	Wilms tumor-1	194070	Wilms tumor, type 1 (3); Denys-Drash syndrome (3); Frasier syndrome, 136680 (3)
11p12-p11.2	MAPK8IP1, IB1	P	Mitogen-activated protein kinase 8-interacting protein 1	604641	Diabetes mellitus, noninsulin-dependent, 125853 (3)
11p12-p11.12	PFM, FPP	P	Foramina parietalia permagna (Catlin marks)	168500	Parietal foramina (2)
11p12-p11	ACP2	C	Acid phosphatase 2, lysosomal	171650	?Lysosomal acid phosphatase deficiency (1)
11p12-p11	DDB2	P	Damage-specific DNA binding protein 2, 48 kD	600811	Xeroderma pigmentosum, group E, DDB-negative subtype, 278740 (3)
11p12-p11	EXT2	C	Exostoses, multiple, 2	133701	Exostoses, multiple, type 2 (3)
11p11.2	MYBPC3, CMH4	C	Myosin-binding protein C, cardiac	600958	Cardiomyopathy, familial hypertrophic, 4, 115197 (3)
11p11.2	KAI1, ST6, CD82, SAR2	P	Kangai 1 (suppression of tumorigenicity 6, prostate)	600623	Prostate cancer, 176807 (2)
11p11-q11	SCA5	P	Spinocerebellar ataxia 5	600224	Spinocerebellar ataxia-5 (2)
11p11-q12	F2	C	Coagulation factor II (thrombin)	176930	Hypoprothrombinemia (3); Dysprothrombinemia (3)
11p	HYPLIP2	P	Hyperlipidemia, combined, 2	604499	Hyperlipidemia, combined, 2 (2)
11p	NNO1	P	Nanophthalmos 1	600165	Nanophthalmos-1 (2)
11q11-q13.1	C1NH	C	Complement component-1 inhibitor	106100	Angioedema, hereditary (3)

(Continued on next page)

Table A1-2 (Continued)

Location	Symbol	Status	Locus Name	MIM#	Disorder
11q12-q13	DDB1	P	Damage-specific DNA binding protein 1, 127 kD	600045	Xeroderma pigmentosum, group E, subtype 2 (1)
11q12-q13	DHCR7, SLOS	P	Delta-7-dehydrocholesterol reductase	602858	Smith-Lemli-Opitz syndrome, type I, 270400 (3); Smith-Lemli-Opitz syndrome, type II, 268670 (3)
11q12-q13	HBM	P	High bone mass	601884	[High bone mass] (2)
11q12-q13	IGER, APY	C	IgE responsiveness, atopic	147050	Atopy (2)
11q12-q13	OPTB1	P	Osteopetrosis, autosomal recessive	259700	Osteopetrosis, recessive (2)
11q12-q13	OPPG	P	Osteoporosis-pseudoglioma syndrome	259770	Osteoporosis-pseudoglioma syndrome (2)
11q13	BBS1	C	Bardet-Biedl syndrome 1	209901	Bardet-Biedl syndrome 1 (2)
11q13	CCND1, PRAD1	C	Cyclin D1	168461	Parathyroid adenomatosis 1 (2); Centrocytic lymphoma (2); Multiple myeloma, 254500 (2)
11q13	CPT1A	C	Carnitine palmitoyltransferase I, liver	600528	CPT deficiency, hepatic, type I, 255120 (3)
11q13	GIF	C	Gastric intrinsic factor	261000	Anemia, pernicious, congenital, due to deficiency of intrinsic factor (1)
11q13	IDDM4	C	Insulin-dependent diabetes mellitus-4	600319	{Diabetes mellitus, insulin-dependent, 4} (2)
11q13	MEN1	C	Menin	131100	Multiple endocrine neoplasia I (3); Hyperparathyroidism, AD, 145000 (3); Prolactinoma, hyperparathyroidism, carcinoid syndrome (2); Carcinoid tumor of lung (3); Parathyroid adenoma, sporadic (3); Lipoma, sporadic (3); Angiofibroma, sporadic (3); Adrenal adenoma, sporadic (3)
11q13	MKS2	P	Meckel syndrome, type 2	603194	Meckel syndrome, type 2 (2)
11q13	MS4A1, FCER1B	C	Membrane-spanning 4-domains, subfamily A, member 1 (Fc fragment of IgE, high affinity I, receptor for, beta polypeptide)	147138	{Asthma, atopic, susceptibility to} (3)
11q13	NDUFS8	C	NADH dehydrogenase (ubiquinone) Fe-S protein 8, 23 kD (NADH-coenzyme Q reductase)	602141	Leigh syndrome, 256000 (3)
11q13	NDUFV1, UQOR1	P	NADH dehydrogenase (ubiquinone) flavoprotein 1, 51 kD	161015	Leigh syndrome, 256000 (3); Alexander disease, 203450 (3)
11q13	NUMA1	C	Nuclear mitotic apparatus protein-1	164009	Leukemia, acute promyelocytic, NUMA/RARA type (3)
11q13	PYGM	C	Phosphorylase, glycogen, muscle	232600	McArdle disease (3)
11q13	ROM1, ROSP1	P	Rod outer segment membrane protein-1	180721	Retinitis pigmentosa, digenic (3)
11q13	RT6	P	RT6 antigen, rat, homolog of	180840	?{Susceptibility to IDDM} (1)
11q13	SMTPHN	P	Somatotrophinoma	102200	Somatotrophinoma (2)
11q13	ST3	C	Suppression of tumorigenicity-3 (tumor-suppressor gene, HELA cell type)	191181	Cervical carcinoma (2)
11q13	VMD2	C	Vitelliform macular dystrophy (Best disease)	153700	Macular dystrophy, vitelliform type (3)
11q13	VRNI	P	Vitreoretinopathy, neovascular inflammatory	193235	Vitreoretinopathy, neovascular inflammatory (2)
11q13-q21	SMARD1	P	Spinal muscular atrophy with respiratory distress 1	604320	Spinal muscular atrophy with respiratory distress 1 (2)
11q13-q23	EVR1, FEVR	C	Exudative vitreoretinopathy-1, autosomal dominant (Criswick-Schepens syndrome)	133780	Vitreoretinopathy, exudative, familial (2)
11q13.1	PGL2	P	Paraganglioma or familial glomus tumors 2	601650	Paraganglioma, familial nonchromaffin, 2 (2)
11q13.2	FEOM2, CFEOM2	P	Fibrosis of extraocular muscles, congenital, 2, autosomal recessive	602078	Fibrosis of extraocular muscles, congenital, 2 (2)

Table A1-2 (Continued)

Location	Symbol	Status	Locus Name	MIM#	Disorder
11q13.3	BCL1	C	B-cell CLL/lymphoma-1	151400	Leukemia/lymphoma, B-cell, 1 (2)
11q13.3-q13.5	FOLR1	C	Folate receptor-1, adult	136430	{?Congenital anomalies, susceptibility to} (2)
11q13.4-q13.5	PC	C	Pyruvate carboxylase	266150	Pyruvate carboxylase deficiency (3)
11q13.5	MYO7A, USH1B, DFNB2, DFNA11	C	Myosin VIIA	276903	Usher syndrome, type 1B (3); Deafness, autosomal recessive 2, neurosensory, 600060 (3); Deafness, autosomal dominant 11, neurosensory, 601317 (3)
11q14	CLTH	P	Clathrin assembly lymphoid-myeloid leukemia gene	603025	Leukemia, myeloid/lymphoid or mixed lineage (2)
11q14	PALS, PLS	C	Papillon-Lefevre syndrome	245000	Papillon-Lefevre syndrome (2)
11q14-q21	SCZD2	L	Schizophrenia susceptibility locus, chromosome 11-related	603342	{?Schizophrenia}, 181500 (2)
11q14-q21	TYR	C	Tyrosinase	203100	Albinism, oculocutaneous, type IA (3); Waardenburg syndrome/ ocular albinism, digenic, 103470 (3)
11q14.1-q14.3	CTSC, CPPI, PALS, PLS	C	Cathepsin C	602365	Papillon-Lefevre syndrome, 245000 (3)
11q21-q22	FSGS2	P	Focal segmental glomerulosclerosis 2	603965	Glomerulosclerosis, focal segmental, 2 (2)
11q21	MRE11A, MRE11, ATLD	P	Meiotic recombination 11, S. cerevisiae, homolog A of	600814	Ataxia-telangiectasia-like disorder, 604391 (3)
11q22.1	CMT4B	C	Charcot-Marie-Tooth neuropathy 4B	601382	Charcot-Marie-Tooth neuropathy-4B (2)
11q22-q24	PPP2R1B	P	Protein phosphatase 2, structural/regulatory subunit A, beta	603113	Lung cancer, 211980 (3)
11q22-q24	TECTA, DFNA8, DFNA12, DFNB21	P	Tectorin, alpha	602574	Deafness, autosomal dominant 8, 601543 (3); Deafness, autosomal dominant 12, 601842 (3); Deafness, autosomal recessive 21, 603629 (3)
11q22-qter	ANC	L	Anal canal carcinoma	105580	?Anal canal carcinoma (2)
11q22.3	ATM, ATA, AT1	C	Ataxia-telangiectasia mutated (includes complementation groups A, C, D, and E)	208900	Ataxia-telangiectasia (3); T-cell prolymphocytic leukemia, sporadic (3); B-cell non-Hodgkin lymphoma, sporadic (3)
11q22.3-q23.1	ACAT1	C	Acetyl-Coenzyme A acetyltransfer ase-1 (acetoacetyl Coenzyme A thiolase)	203750	3-ketothiolase deficiency (3)
11q22.3-q23.1	CRYAB, CRYA2	C	Crystallin, alpha B	123590	Myopathy, desmin-related, cardioskeletal, 601419 (3)
11q22.3-q23.3	PTS	P	6-pyruvoyltetrahydropterin synthase	261640	Phenylketonuria due to PTS deficiency (3)
11q23	APOA1	C	Apolipoprotein A-I	107680	ApoA-I and apoC-III deficiency, combined (3); Hypertriglyceridemi, one form (3); Hypoalphalipo-proteinemia (3); Corneal clouding, autosomal recessive (3); Amyloidosis, 3 or more types (3)
11q23	APOC3	C	Apolipoprotein C-III	107720	Hypertriglyceridemia (3)
11q23	BRCA3	P	Breast cancer, 11;22 translocation associated	600048	Breast cancer-3 (2)
11q23	CD3E	P	CD3E antigen, epsilon polypeptide (TiT3 complex)	186830	Immunodeficiency, T-cell receptor/ CD3 complex (3)
11q23	CD3G	C	CD3G antigen, gamma polypeptide (TiT3 complex)	186740	Immunodeficiency due to defect in CD3-gamma (3)
11q23	DRD2	C	Dopamine receptor D2	126450	Dystonia, myoclonic, 159900 (3)
11q23	ECB2	P	Erythrocytosis, autosomal recessive benign	263400	Erythrocytosis, autosomal recessive benign (2)
11q23	ED4	P	Ectodermal dysplasia, type 4 (ectodermal dysplasia, Margarita type)	225060	Ectodermal dysplasia, type 4 (2)

(Continued on next page)

Table A1-2 (Continued)

Location	Symbol	Status	Locus Name	MIM#	Disorder
11q23	G6PT1	C	Glucose-6-phosphate transporter-1	602671	Glycogen storage disease Ib, 232220 (3); Glycogen storage disease Ic, 232240 (3)
11q23	HOMG2	P	Hypomagnesemia, renal	154020	Hypomagnesemia, renal (2)
11q23	JBS	C	Jacobsen syndrome	147791	Jacobsen syndrome (2)
11q23	MLL, HRX, HTRX1	C	Myeloid/lymphoid or mixed-lineage leukemia (trithorax, Drosophila, homolog)	159555	Leukemia, myeloid/lymphoid or mixed-lineage (2)
11q23	SDHD, PGL1	P	Succinate dehydrogenase complex, subunit D, integral membrane protein	602690	Paragangliomas, familial nonchromaffin, 1, 168000 (3)
11q23	TCPT	L	Thrombocytopenia, Paris-Trousseau type (deletion 11q23 syndrome)	188025	?Thrombocytopenia, Paris-Trousseau type (2)
11q23	TSG11	P	Tumor suppressor gene on chromosome 11	603040	{Nonsmall cell lung cancer} (2)
11q23-q25	HLS	P	Hydrolethalus syndrome	236680	Hydrolethalus syndrome (2)
11q23.1	PLZF	P	Promyelocytic leukemia zinc finger	176797	Leukemia, acute promyelocytic, PL2F/RARA type (3)
11q23.1	PORC	P	Porphyria, acute, Chester type	176010	Porphyria, Chester type (2)
11q23.3	HMBS, PBGD, UPS	C	Hydroxymethylbilane synthase	176000	Porphyria, acute intermittent (3)
11q23.3	LARG	P	Rho guanine nucleotide exchange factor, leukemia-associated	604763	Leukemia, acute myeloid (3)
11q24	KCNJ1, ROMK1	C	Potassium inwardly-rectifying channel, subfamily J, member 1	600359	Bartter syndrome, type 2 (3)
11q25	HJCD	P	Histiocytosis with joint contractures and sensorineural deafness	602782	Faisalabad histiocytosis (2)
11q25-qter	DFNB20	P	Deafness, autosomal recessive 20	604060	Deafness, autosomal recessive 20 (2)
12pter-p12	CD4	C	CD4 antigen (p55)	186940	[CD4(+) lymphocyte deficiency] (2); {Lupus erythematosus, susceptibility to} (2)
12p13.31	DRPLA	C	Atrophin 1	125370	Dentatorubro-pallidoluysian atrophy (3)
12p13.3	ADHR, HPDR2	P	Hypophosphatemia vitamin D-resistant rickets-2, autosomal dominant	193100	Hypophosphatemic rickets, autosomal dominant (2)
12p13.3	PXR1, PEX5, PTS1R	C	Peroxisome receptor 1	600414	Adrenoleukodystrophy, neonatal, 202370 (3)
12p13.3	VWF, F8VWF	C	Coagulation factor VIII VWF (von Willebrand factor)	193400	von Willebrand disease (3)
12p13.3-p12.3	A2M	C	Alpha-2-macroglobulin	103950	Emphysema due to alpha-2-macroglobulin deficiency (1); {Alzheimer disease, susceptibility to} (3)
12p13.3-p11.2	ACLS	L	Acrocallosal syndrome	200990	?Acrocallosal syndrome (2)
12p13.2	TNFRSF1A, TNFR1, TNFAR	C	Tumor necrosis factor receptor superfamily, member 1A	191190	Periodic fever, familial, 142680 (3)
12p13.2-q24.1	IBD2	C	Inflammatory bowel disease-2	601458	Inflammatory bowel disease-2 (2)
12p13.1-p12.3	MGP	C	Matrix Gla protein	154870	Keutel syndrome, 245150 (3)
12p13	C1R	C	Complement component-1, r subcomponent	216950	C1r/C1s deficiency, combined (1)
12p13	C1S	C	Complement component-1, s subcomponent	120580	C1r/C1s deficiency, combined (1); C1s deficiency, isolated (3)
12p13	ETV6, TEL	C	ETS variant gene-6 (TEL oncogene)	600618	Leukemia, acute lymphoblastic (1)
12p13	FPF	C	Familial periodic fever (Hibernian fever)	142680	Periodic fever, familial (2)
12p13	GNB3	C	Guanine nucleotide-binding protein, beta polypeptide-3	139130	{Hypertension, essential, susceptibility to}, 145500 (3)
12p13	KCNA1, AEMK, EA1	C	Potassium voltage-gated channel, shaker-related subfamily, member 1	176260	Episodic ataxia/myokymia syndrome, 160120 (3)

Table A1-2 (Continued)

Location	Symbol	Status	Locus Name	MIM#	Disorder
12p13	MPE	L	Malignant proliferation, eosinophil	131440	?Eosinophilic myeloproliferative disorder (2)
12p13	SCNN1A	C	Sodium channel, nonvoltage-gated 1, alpha	600228	Pseudohypoaldosteronism, type I, 264350 (3)
12p13	TPI1	C	Triosephosphate isomerase-1	190450	Hemolytic anemia due to triosephosphate isomerase deficiency (3)
12p12.2	GYS2	C	Glycogen synthase-2, liver	138571	Glycogen storage disease, type 0, 240600 (3)
12p12.2-p12.1	LDHB	C	Lactate dehydrogenase B	150100	Lactate dehydrogenase-B deficiency (3)
12p12.2-p11.2	HTNB	C	Hypertension with brachydactyly	112410	Hypertension with brachydactyly (2)
12p12.1	KRAS2, RASK2	C	Kirsten rat sarcoma-2 viral (v-Ki-ras2) oncogene homolog	190070	Colorectal adenoma (1); Colorectal cancer (1)
12p12.1-p11.2	PTHLH	P	Parathyroid hormone-like hormone	168470	?Humoral hypercalcemia of malignancy (1)
12p12	BCAT1, BCT1	C	Branched chain aminotransferase-1, cytosolic	113520	?Hyperleucinemia-isoleucinemia or hypervalinemia (1)
12p11.23-q13.12	AD5	P	Alzheimer disease, familial, type 5	602096	Alzheimer disease-5 (2)
12p11.2-q12	FEOM1, CFEOM1, FEOM1	P	Fibrosis of extraocular muscles, congenital, 1, autosomal dominant	135700	Fibrosis of extraocular muscles, congenital, 1 (2)
12q11-q13	KRT2A, KRT2E	P	Keratin-2A	600194	Ichthyosis bullosa of Siemens, 146800 (3)
12q11-q13	PPKB	P	Palmoplantar keratoderma, Bothnia type	600231	Palmoplantar keratoderma, Bothnia type (2)
12q11-q14	ACVRL1, ACVRLK1, ALK1, HHT2	C	Activin A receptor, type II-like kinase 1	601284	Hereditary hemorrhagic telangiectasia-2, 600376 (3)
12q12-q14	VDR	P	Vitamin D (1,25-dihydroxyvitamin D3) receptor	601769	Rickets, vitamin D-resistant, 277440 (3); ?Osteoporosis, involutional (1)
12q13	AAA	P	Achalasia-addisonianism-alacrimia syndrome (Allgrove syndrome)	231550	Achalasia-addisonianism-alacrimia syndrome (2)
12q13	AMHR2, AMHR	P	Anti-Mullerian hormone receptor, type II	600956	Persistent Mullerian duct syndrome, type II, 261550 (3)
12q13	AQP2	C	Aquaporin-2 (collecting duct)	107777	Diabetes insipidus, nephrogenic, autosomal recessive, 222000 (3); Diabetes insipidus, nephrogenic, autosomal dominant, 125800 (3)
12q13	KRTHB1, HB1	P	Keratin, hair, basic, 1	602153	Monilethrix, 158000 (3)
12q13	KRTHB6, HB6	C	Keratin, hair, basic, 6	601928	Monilethrix, 158000 (3)
12q13	ITGA7	P	Integrin, alpha-7	600536	Myopathy, congenital (3)
12q13	KRT1	C	Keratin-1	139350	Epidermolytic hyperkeratosis, 113800 (3); Keratoderma, palmoplantar, nonepidermolytic (3); Cyclic ichthyosis with epidermolytic hyperkeratosis (3)
12q13	KRT3	C	Keratin-3	148043	Meesmann corneal dystrophy, 122100 (3)
12q13	KRT4, CYK4	C	Keratin-4	123940	White sponge nevus, 193900 (3)
12q13	KRT5	P	Keratin-5	148040	Epidermolysis bullosa simplex, Koebner, Dowling-Meara, and Weber-Cockayne types, 131900, 131760, 131800 (3)
12q13	KRT6A	P	Keratin-6A	148041	Pachyonychia congenita, Jadassohn-Lewandowsky type, 167200 (3)
12q13	KRT18	C	Keratin-18	148070	{?Liver disease, susceptibility to, from hepatotoxins or viruses} (1)
12q13-q14	RDH5	P	Retinol dehydrogenase-5	601617	Fundus albipunctatus, 136880 (3)
12q13-q15	GAS41	P	Glioma-amplified sequence-41	602116	Glioma (1)
12q13-q21	ENUR2	P	Enuresis, nocturnal, 2	600808	Enuresis, nocturnal, 2 (2)

(Continued on next page)

Table A1-2 (Continued)

Location	Symbol	Status	Locus Name	MIM#	Disorder
12q13.1-q13.2	DDIT3, GADD153, CHOP10	C	DNA-damage-inducible transcript-3	126337	Myxoid liposarcoma (3)
12q13.11-q13.2	COL2A1	C	Collagen II, alpha-1 polypeptide	120140	Stickler syndrome, type I, 108300 (3); SED congenita (3); Kniest dysplasia (3); Achondrogenesis, type II, 200610 (3); Osteoarthrosis, precocious (3); Wagner syndrome, type II (3); SMED Strudwick type, 184250 (3); Spondyloepiphyseal dysplasia, congenita, 183900 (3); Osteoarthritis with mild chondrodysplasia (3); Hypochondrogenesis (3); Kniest dysplasia, 156550 (3); Spondylometaphyseal dysplasia, 184252 (3); Wagner syndrome, 143200 (3); Epiphyseal dysplasia, multiple, with myopia and conductive deafness, 132450 (3); Spondyloperipheral dysplasia, 271700 (3)
12q13.3	PFKM	P	Phosphofructokinase, muscle type	232800	Glycogen storage disease VII (3)
12q13.3-q15	SPPM, SPMD	P	Scapuloperoneal syndrome, myopathic type	181430	Scapuloperoneal syndrome, myopathic type (2)
12q14	CDK4, CMM3	C	Cyclin-dependent kinase 4	123829	Melanoma (3)
12q14	CYP27B1, PDDR, VDD1	C	Cytochrome P450, subfamily XXVIIB, polypeptide 1	264700	Pseudovitamin D deficiency rickets 1 (3)
12q14	GNS, G6S	P	N-acetylglucosamine-6-sulfatase	252940	Sanfilippo syndrome, type D (1)
12q14	IFNG	C	Interferon, gamma	147570	Interferon, immune, deficiency (1)
12q15	HMGIC, BABL, LIPO	C	High-mobility group protein HMGI-C	600698	Lipoma (3); Salivary adenoma (3); Uterine leiomyoma (3); ?Lipomatosis, mutiple, 151900 (2)
12q21	CNA2	C	Cornea plana 2, autosomal recessive	217300	Cornea plana congenita, recessive (2)
12q21-q23	MYP3	P	Myopia, high grade, autosomal dominant 2	603221	Myopia-3 (2)
12q22	MGCT	C	Male germ cell tumor	273300	Male germ cell tumor (2)
12q22-q23	HAL, HSTD	C	Histidine ammonia-lyase (histidase)	235800	[Histidinemia] (1)
12q22-q24.1	IGF1	C	Insulin-like growth factor-1, or somatomedin C	147440	Growth retardation with deafness and mental retardation (3)
12q22-qter	ACADS, SCAD	C	Acyl-Coenzyme A dehydrogenase, C-2 to C-3 short chain	201470	Acyl-CoA dehydrogenase, short-chain, deficiency of (3)
12q23-q24	SMAL	P	Spinal muscular atrophy, congenital nonprogressive, of lower limbs	600175	Spinal muscular atrophy, congenital nonprogressive, of lower limbs (2)
12q23-q24.1	ATP2A2, ATP2B, DAR	C	ATPase, Ca++ dependent, slow-twitch, cardiac muscle-2	108740	Darier disease, 124200 (3)
12q23-q24.3	MYL2	P	Myosin, light polypeptide-2, regulatory, cardiac, slow	160781	Cardiomyopathy, hypertrophic, mid-left ventricular chamber type (3)
12q24	ATX2, SCA2	C	Ataxin-2	601517	Spinocerebellar ataxia-2, 183090 (3)
12q24	BDC	P	Brachydactyly, type C	113100	Brachydactyly, type C (2)
12q24	MVK, MVLK	C	Mevalonate kinase	251170	Mevalonicaciduria (3); Hyperimmunoglobulinemia D and periodic fever syndrome, 260920 (3)
12q24	NS1, CFC	C	Noonan syndrome 1	163950	Noonan syndrome-1 (2); Cardiofaciocutaneous syndrome, 115150 (2)

Table A1-2 (Continued)

Location	Symbol	Status	Locus Name	MIM#	Disorder
12q24	SMA4, HMN2	P	Spinal muscular atrophy-4	158590	Spinal muscular atrophy-4 (2)
12q24-qter	HPD	C	4-hydroxyphenylpyruvate dioxygenase	276710	Tyrosinemia, type III (1)
12q24.1	PAH, PKU1	C	Phenylalanine hydroxylase	261600	Phenylketonuria (3); [Hyperphenylalaninemia, mild] (3)
12q24.1	BCL7A, BCL7	P	B-cell CLL/lymphoma-7A	601406	B-cell non-Hodgkin lymphoma, high-grade (3)
12q24.1	TBX3	C	T-box 3	601621	Ulnar-mammary syndrome, 181450 (3)
12q24.1	TBX5	C	T-box 5	601620	Holt-Oram syndrome, 142900 (3)
12q24.1-q24.31	SPSMA	P	Scapuloperoneal spinal muscular atrophy, New England type	181405	Scapuloperoneal spinal muscular atrophy, New England type (2)
12q24.2	ALDH2	C	Aldehyde dehydrogenase-2, mitochondrial	100650	Alcohol intolerance, acute (3); {?Fetal alcohol syndrome} (1)
12q24.2	TCF1, HNF1A, MODY3	C	Interferon production regulator factor (HNF1), albumin proximal factor	142410	MODY, type 3, 600496 (3); {Diabetes mellitus, noninsulin-dependent, 2}, 601407 (2) {Diabetes mellitus, insulin-dependent} (3)
Chr.12	LYZ	P	Lysozyme	153450	Amyloidosis, renal, 105200 (3)
13q11-q12	GJB2, CX26, DFNB1	C	Gap junction protein, beta-2, 26 kD (connexin 26)	121011	Deafness, autosomal recessive 1, 220290 (3); Deafness, autosomal dominant 3, 601544 (3); Vohwinkel syndrome, 124500 (3)
13q11-q12	GJA3, CX46, CZP3, CAE3	C	Gap junction protein, alpha-3, 46 kD (connexin 46)	121015	Cataract, zonular pulverulent-3, 601885 (3)
13q11-q12	ZNF198, SCLL, RAMP, FIM	C	Zinc finger protein-198	602221	Stem-cell leukemia/lymphoma syndrome (3)
13q11-q12.1	ED2, HED, EDH	C	Ectodermal dysplasia 2, hidrotic	129500	Ectodermal dysplasia 2, hidrotic (2)
13q12	GJB6, CX30, DFNA3	C	Gap junction protein, beta-6 (connexin-30)	604418	Deafness, autosomal dominant non syndromic sensorineural 3, 601544 (3)
13q12	SACS, ARSACS	P	Sacsin	604490	Spastic ataxia, Charlevoix-Saguenay type, 270550 (3)
13q12	SGCG, LGMD2C, DMDA1, SCG3	C	Sarcoglycan, gamma (35 kD dystrophin-associated glycoprotein)	253700	Muscular dystrophy, limb-girdle, type 2C (3)
13q12.1	IPF1	P	Insulin promoter factor 1, homeodomain transcription factor	600733	Pancreatic agenesis, 260370 (3); MODY, type IV (3)
13q12.2-q13	MBS	L	Moebius syndrome	157900	?Moebius syndrome (2)
13q12.3	BRCA2	C	Breast cancer-2, early onset	600185	Breast cancer 2, early onset (3); Pancreatic cancer (3)
13q13-q14.3	ENUR1	P	Enuresis, nocturnal, 1	600631	Enuresis, nocturnal, 1 (2)
13q14	D13S25, DBM	P	Disrupted in B-cell neoplasia	109543	Leukemia, chronic lymphocytic, B-cell (2)
13q14	ITM2B, BRI, ABRI, FBD	P	Integral membrane protein 2B (BRI gene)	603904	Dementia, familial British, 176500 (3)
13q14	RFXAP	P	Regulatory factor X-associated protein	601861	MHC class II deficiency, group B, 209920 (3)
13q14	RIEG2, RGS2	C	Rieger syndrome, type 2	601499	Rieger syndrome, type 2 (2)
13q14	SLC25A15, ORNT1, HHH	C	Solute carrier family 25 (mitochondrial carrier), member 15 (ornithine transporter 1)	603861	Hyperornithinemia-hyperammonemia-homocitrullinemia syndrome, 238970 (3)
13q14.1	FKHR	P	Forkhead, Drosophila, homolog of, 1	136533	Rhabdomyosarcoma, alveolar, 268220 (3)
13q14.1-q14.2	RB1	C	Retinoblastoma-1	180200	Retinoblastoma (3); Osteosarcoma, 259500 (2); Bladder cancer, 109800 (3); Pinealoma with bilateral retinoblastoma (2)
13q14.12-q14.2	DICE1	P	Deleted in cancer 1	604331	{Nonsmall cell lung cancer} (2)
13q14.3-q21.1	ATP7B, WND	C	ATPase, Cu++ transporting, beta polypeptide	277900	Wilson disease (3)

(Continued on next page)

Table A1-2 (Continued)

Location	Symbol	Status	Locus Name	MIM#	Disorder
13q21	SCA8	P	Spinocerebellar ataxia 8	603680	Spinocerebellar ataxia 8 (3)
13q21-q32	PAPA2	P	Postaxial polydactyly, type A2	602085	Postaxial polydactyly, type A2 (2)
13q21.1-q32	CLN5	C	Ceroid-lipofuscinosis, neuronal-5	256731	Ceroid-lipofuscinosis, neuronal-5, variant late infantile (3)
13q22	EDNRB, HSCR2	C	Endothelin receptor type B	131244	Hirschsprung disease-2, 600155 (3)
13q31-q32	MCOR	P	Microcoria, congenital	156600	Microcoria, congenital (2)
13q32	PCCA	C	Propionyl Coenzyme A carboxylase, alpha polypeptide	232000	Propionicacidemia, type I or pccA type (3)
13q32	SCZD7	P	Schizophrenia susceptibility locus, chromosome 13q-related	603176	{Schizophrenia}, 181500 (2)
13q32	ZIC2, HPE5	P	ZIC family member 2	603073	Holoprosencephaly-5 (3)
13q33	ERCC5, XPG	C	Excision-repair, complementing defective, in Chinese hamster, number 5	133530	Xeroderma pigmentosum, group G, 278780 (3)
13q33	SLC10A2, NTCP2	C	Solute carrier family 10 (sodium/ bile acid cotransporter family), member 2	601295	Bile acid malabsorption, primary (3)
13q34	F7	C	Coagulation factor VII	227500	Factor VII deficiency (3)
13q34	F10	C	Coagulation factor X	227600	Factor X deficiency (3)
13q34	RHOK, RK, GRK1	P	Rhodopsin kinase	180381	Oguchi disease-2, 258100 (3)
13q34	STGD2	P	Stargardt disease 2, autosomal dominant	153900	Stargardt disease-2 (2)
Chr.13	BRCD1	P	Breast cancer, ductal, suppressor-1	211410	Breast cancer, ductal (2)
14q	BCH	P	Chorea, hereditary benign	118700	Chorea, hereditary benign (2)
14q	MNG1	P	Multinodular goiter-1	138800	Multinodular thyroid goiter-1 (2)
14q	MPD1	P	Myopathy, distal 1	160500	Myopathy, distal (2)
14q11-q12	DAD1	P	Defender against cell death 1	600243	Temperature-sensitive apoptosis (1)
14q11.1-q11.2	NRL, D14S46E	C	Neural retina leucine zipper	162080	Retinitis pigmentosa, autosomal dominant (3)
14q11.2	SLC7A7, LPI	C	Solute carrier family 7 (cationic amino acid transporter, y+ system), member 7	603593	Lysinuric protein intolerance, 222700 (3)
14q11.2	TCRA	C	T-cell antigen receptor, alpha polypeptide	186880	Leukemia/lymphoma, T-cell (3)
14q11.2	TGM1, ICR2, LI	C	Transglutaminase-1 (K polypeptide epidermal type I, protein-glutamine gamma-glutamyltransferase)	190195	Ichthyosis, lamellar, autosomal recessive, 242300 (3); Ichthyosiform erythroderma, congenital, 242100 (3)
14q11.2-q13	PABP2, PAB2	C	Poly(A)-binding protein-2	602279	Oculopharyngeal muscular dystorphy, 164300 (3); Oculopharyngeal muscular dystrophy, autosomal recessive, 257950 (3)
14q11.2-q24.3	SPG3A	C	Spastic paraplegia-3A	182600	Spastic paraplegia-3A (2)
14q12	DFNB5	P	Deafness, autosomal recessive 5	600792	Deafness, autosomal recessive 5 (2)
14q12	MYH7, CMH1	C	Myosin, heavy polypeptide-7, cardiac muscle, beta	160760	Cardiomyopathy, familial hypertrophic, 1, 192600 (3); ?Central core disease, one form (3)
14q12-q13	COCH, DFNA9	C	Cochlin	603196	Deafness, autosomal dominant 9, 601369 (3); Meniere disease, 156000 (3)
14q12-q13	PAX9	P	Paired box homeotic gene-9	167416	Oligodontia, 604625 (3)
14q12-q22	ARVD3	P	Arrhythmogenic right ventricular dysplasia-3	602086	Arrhythmogenic right ventricular dysplasia-3 (2)
14q13	TITF1, NKX2A, TTF1	P	Thyroid transcription factor 1 (NK-2, Drosophila, homolog of, A)	600635	Goiter, familial, due to TTF-1 defect (1)
14q13	TMIP	L	Tetramelic mirror-image polydactyly	135750	?Tetramelic mirror-image polydactyly (2)
14q13.1	NP	C	Nucleoside phosphorylase	164050	Nucleoside phosphorylase deficiency, immunodeficiency due to (3)
14q21	MGAT2, CDGS2	P	Mannosyl (alpha-1,6-)-glycoprotein beta-1,2-N-acetylglucosaminyl-transferase	602616	Carbohydrate-deficient glycoprotein syndrome, type II, 212066 (3)
14q21-q22	PYGL	P	Phosphorylase, glycogen, liver	232700	Glycogen storage disease VI (3)

Table A1-2 (Continued)

Location	Symbol	Status	Locus Name	MIM#	Disorder
14q22-q23.2	SPTB	C	Spectrin, beta, erythrocytic	182870	Elliptocytosis-3 (3); Spherocytosis-1 (3); Anemia, neonatal hemolytic, fatal and near-fatal (3)
14q22.1-q22.2	GCH1, DYT5	P	GTP cyclohydrolase 1	600225	Phenylketonuria, atypical, due to GCH1 deficiency, 233910 (1); Dystonia, DOPA-responsive, 128230 (3)
14q23-q24	ARVD1	C	Arrhythmogenic right ventricular dysplasia-1	107970	Arrhythmogenic right ventricular dysplasia-1 (2)
14q24	LCA3	P	Leber congenital amaurosis, type III	604232	Leber congenital amaurosis, type III (2)
14q24	LTBP2, LTBP3	P	Latent transforming growth factor beta binding protein-2	602091	Marfan syndrome, atypical (3)
14q24-qter	CTAA1	L	Cataract, anterior polar, 1	115650	?Cataract, anterior polar-1 (2)
14q24.3	GSTZ1, MAAI	P	Glutathione S-transferase, zeta-1 (maleylacetoacetate isomerase)	603758	Tyrosinemia, type Ib (1)
14q24.3	PSEN1, AD3	C	Presenilin 1	104311	Alzheimer disease-3 (3)
14q24.3-q31	IDDM11	P	Insulin-dependent diabetes mellitus-11	601208	{Diabetes mellitus, insulin-dependent, 11} (2)
14q24.3-q31	MJD, SCA3	C	Machado-Joseph disease (spinocerebellar ataxia 3, olivopontocerebellar ataxia 3, autosomal dominant); ataxin-3	109150	Machado-Joseph disease (3)
14q31	GALC	C	Galactosylceraminidase	245200	Krabbe disease (3)
14q31	TSHR	C	Thyroid-stimulating hormone receptor	603372	Hypothyroidism, congenital, due to TSH resistance, 275200 (3); Thyroid adenoma, hyperfunctioning (3); Graves disease, 275000 (1); Hyperthroidism, congenital (3)
14q32	CKBE	P	Creatine kinase, ectopic expression	123270	[Creatine kinase, brain type, ectopic expression of] (2)
14q32	MCOP	P	Microphthalmia, autosomal recessive	251600	Microphthalmia, autosomal recessive (2)
14q32	USH1A, USH1	C	Usher syndrome-1A, autosomal recessive, severe	276900	Usher syndrome, type 1A (2)
14q32.1	AACT	C	Alpha-1-antichymotrypsin	107280	Alpha-1-antichymotrypsin deficiency (3); Cerebrovascular disease, occlusive (3)
14q32.1	CBG	C	Corticosteroid-binding globulin	122500	[Transcortin deficiency] (1)
14q32.1	PCI, PLANH3	C	Protein C inhibitor (plasminogen activator inhibitor-3)	601841	Protein C inhibitor deficiency (2)
14q32.1	PI, AAT	C	Protease inhibitor (alpha-1-antitrypsin)	107400	Emphysema-cirrhosis (3); Hemorrhagic diathesis due to 'antithrombin' Pittsburgh (3); Emphysema (3)
14q32.1	TCL1A, TCL1	C	T-cell lymphoma/leukemia 1A	186960	Leukemia/lymphoma, T-cell (2)
14q32.33	IGHG2	C	Constant region of heavy chain of IgG2	147110	IgG2 deficiency, selective (3)
14q32.33	IGHM, MU	C	Constant region of heavy chain of IgM	147020	Agammaglobulinemia, 601495 (3)
14q32.33	IGHR	L	Immunoglobulin heavy chain regulator	144120	?Hyperimmunoglobulin G1 syndrome (2)
Chr.14	ACHM1, RMCH1	P	Achromatopsia-1	603096	Achromatopsia-1 (2)
Chr.14	MPS3C	L	Mucopolysaccharidosis, type IIIC	252930	?Sanfilippo syndrome, type C (2)
15q	HYT2	P	Hypertension, essential, susceptibility to, 2	604329	Hypertension, essential, susceptibility to, 2 (2)
15q11	PWCR, PWS	C	Prader-Willi syndrome chromosome region	176270	Prader-Willi syndrome (2)
15q11-q13	AHO2	L	Albright hereditary osteodystrophy-2	103581	?Albright hereditary osteodystrophy-2 (2)
15q11-q13	BCL8	P	B-cell CLL/lymphoma-8	601889	Lymphoma, diffuse large cell (3)
15q11-q13	NDN	C	Necdin	602117	Prader-Willi syndrome, 176270 (3)
15q11-q13	UBE3A, ANCR	C	Ubiquitin protein ligase E3A	601623	Angelman syndrome (3)
15q11-q15	EYCL3	P	Eye color 3, brown	227220	[Eye color, brown] (2)

(Continued on next page)

Table A1-2 (Continued)

Location	Symbol	Status	Locus Name	MIM#	Disorder
15q11-q15	HCL3	P	Hair color 3, brown	601800	[Hair color, brown] (2)
15q11.1	SPG6	P	Spastic paraplegia-6	600363	Spastic paraplegia-6 (2)
15q11.2-q12	OCA2, P, PED, D15S12	C	Oculocutaneous albinism II (pink-eye dilution, murine, homolog of)	203200	Albinism, oculocutaneous, type II (3); Albinism, ocular, autosomal recessive (3)
15q12	SNRPN	P	Small nuclear ribonucleoprotein polypeptide N	182279	Prader-Willi syndrome, 176270 (3)
15q13-q15	ACCPN	P	Agenesis of corpus callosum and peripheral neuropathy (Andermann syndrome)	218000	Andermann syndrome (2)
15q13-q15	SPG11	P	Spastic paraplegia 11, autosomal recessive	604360	Spastic paraplegia-11 (2)
15q14	ACTC	C	Actin, alpha, cardiac muscle	102540	Cardiomyopathy, dilated, 115200 (3); Cardiomyopathy, familial hypertrophic, 192600 (3)
15q14	CHRNA7	C	Cholinergic receptor, nicotinic, alpha polypeptide-7	118511	Schizophrenia, neurophysiologic defect in (2)
15q14	EJM1, JME	P	Epilepsy, juvenile myoclonic 1	254770	Epilepsy, juvenile myoclonic (2)
15q14-q15	IVD	P	Isovaleryl Coenzyme A dehydrogenase	243500	Isovalericacidemia (3)
15q14-q21.3	SCA11	P	Spinocerebellar ataxia 11	604432	Spinocerebellar ataxia-11 (2)
15q15	EPB42	C	Erythrocyte surface protein band 4.2	177070	Spherocytosis, hereditary, Japanese type (3)
15q15-q21	MCPH4	P	Microcephaly, primary autosomal recessive 4	604321	Microcephaly, primary autosomal recessive 4 (2)
15q15-q21.1	SLC12A1, NKCC2	C	Solute carrier family 12 (sodium/potassium/chloride transporters), member 1	600839	Bartter syndrome, 241200 (3)
15q15.1-q15.3	CDAN1, CDA1	P	Congenital dyserythropoietic anemia, type I	224120	Dyserythropoietic anemia, contenital, type I (2)
15q15.1-q21.1	ALS5	P	Amytrophic lateral sclerosis-5, juvenile recessive	602099	Amytrophic lateral sclerosis-5, juvenile recessive (2)
15q15.1-q21.1	CAPN3, CANP3	C	Calpain, large polypeptide L3	114240	Muscular dystrophy, limb-girdle, type 2A, 253600 (3)
15q15.3	SORD, SORD1	C	Sorbitol dehydrogenase	182500	?Cataract, congenital (2)
15q21	CDAN3, CDA3	P	Congenital dyserythropoietic anemia, type III	105600	Dyserythropoietic anemia, congenital, type III (2)
15q21	DYX1	P	Dyslexia-1	127700	Dyslexia-1 (2)
15q21	MYO5A, MYH12	C	Myosin, heavy polypeptide kinase	160777	Griscelli disease, 214450 (3)
15q21-q22	B2M	C	Beta-2-microglobulin	109700	Hemodialysis-related amyloidosis (1)
15q21-q22	DFNB16	C	Deafness, autosomal recessive 16	603720	Deafness, autosomal recessive 16 (2)
15q21-q23	CLN6	C	Ceroid-lipofuscinosis, neuronal 6, late infantile, variant	601780	Ceroid-lipofuscinosis, neuronal-6, variant late infantile (2)
15q21-q23	LIPC	C	Lipase, hepatic	151670	Hepatic lipase deficiency (3)
15q21.1	CYP19, ARO	C	Cytochrome P450, subfamily XIX (aromatization of androgens)	107910	Gynecomastia, familial, due to increased aromatase activity (1); Virilization, maternal and fetal, from placental aromatase deficiency (3)
15q21.1	FBN1, MFS1	C	Fibrillin-1	134797	Marfan syndrome, 154700 (3); Shprintzen-Goldberg syndrome, 182212 (3); Ectopia lentis, familial (3)
15q22	PML, MYL	C	Promyelocytic leukemia, inducer of	102578	Leukemia, acute promyelocytic, PML/RARA type (3)
15q22-qter	MPI, PMI1	C	Mannosephosphate isomerase (phosphomannose isomerase 1)	154550	Carbohydrate-deficient glycoprotein syndrome, type Ib, 602579 (3)
15q22.1	TPM1, CMH3	C	Tropomyosin 1, alpha	191010	Cardiomyopathy, familial hypertrophic, 3, 115196 (3)
15q22.3-q23	BBS4	C	Bardet-Biedl syndrome 4	600374	Bardet-Biedl syndrome 4 (2)
15q23	NR2E3, PNR, ESCS	P	Nuclear receptor subfamily 2, group E, member 3	604485	Enhanced S-cone syndrome, 268100 (3)

Table A1-2 (Continued)

Location	Symbol	Status	Locus Name	MIM#	Disorder
15q23-q24	CYP11A, P450SCC	C	Cytochrome P450, subfamily XIA (cholesterol side chain cleavage enzyme)	118485	?Polycystic ovary syndrome, 184700 (2)
15q23-q24	HEXA, TSD	C	Hexosaminidase A, alpha polypeptide	272800	Tay-Sachs disease (3); GM2-gangliosidosis, several forms (3); [Hex A pseudodeficiency] (3)
15q23-q25	ETFA, GA2	P	Electron transfer flavoprotein, alpha polypeptide	231680	Glutaricaciduria, type IIA (1)
15q23-q25	FAH	C	Fumarylacetoacetase	276700	Tyrosinemia, type I (3)
15q24	CHRNA3	C	Cholinergic receptor, neuronal nicotinic, alpha polypeptide-3	118503	?Megacystis-microcolon-intestinal hypoperistalsis syndrome, 249210 (1)
15q24	ENFL2	P	Epilepsy, nocturnal frontal lobe, type 2	603204	Epilepsy, nocturnal frontal lobe, type 2 (2)
15q24	MRST	P	Mental retardation, severe, with spasticity and tapetoretinal degeneration	602685	Mental retardation, severe, with spasticity and tapetoretinal degeneration (2)
15q25-q26	FHCB1, ARH1	P	Hypercholesterolemia, familial, autosomal recessive	603813	Hypercholesterolemia, familial, autosomal recessive (2)
15q26	IDDM3	C	Insulin-dependent diabetes mellitus-3	600318	{Diabetes mellitus, insulin-dependent, 3} (2)
15q26	RLBP1	P	Retinaldehyde-binding protein-1, cellular	180090	Retinitis pigmentosa, autosomal recessive (3)
15q26.1	RECQL2, BLM, BS	C	RecQ protein-like 2	604610	Bloom syndrome, 210900 (3)
15q26.1-qter	OTS	P	Otosclerosis	166800	Otosclerosis (2)
16pter-p13.3	HBA1	C	Hemoglobin alpha-1	141800	Thalassemias, alpha- (3); Methemoglobinemias, alpha- (3); Erythremias, alpha- (3); Heinz body anemias, alpha- (3)
16pter-p13.3	HBA2	C	Hemoglobin alpha-2	141850	Thalassemia, alpha- (3); Erythrocytosis (3); Heinz body anemia (3); Hemoglobin H disease (3); Hypochromic microcytic anemia (3)
16pter-p13.3	HBHR, ATR1	C	Alpha-thalassemia/mental retardation syndrome, type 1	141750	Alpha-thalassemia/mental retardation syndrome, type 1 (1)
16p13.3	ABAT, GABAT	P	4-aminobutyrate aminotransferase	137150	GABA-transaminase deficiency (3)
16p13.3	AXIN1, AXIN	P	Axis inhibitor 1	603816	Hepatocellular carcinoma, 114550 (3)
16p13.3	CATM	P	Cataract, congenital, with microphthalmia	156850	Cataract, congenital, with microphthalmia (2)
16p13.3	CREBBP, CBP, RSTS	C	CREB binding protein	600140	Rubenstein-Taybi syndrome, 180849 (3)
16p13.3	PKDTS	P	Polycystic kidney disease, infantile severe, with tuberous sclerosis	600273	Polycystic kidney disease, infantile severe, with tuberous sclerosis (3)
16p13.3	TSC2	C	Tuberous sclerosis-2 (tuberin)	191092	Tuberous sclerosis-2 (3)
16p13.3-p13.2	PMM2, CDG1	C	Phosphomannomutase 2	601785	Carbohydrate-deficient glycoprotein syndrome, type I, 212065 (3)
16p13.3-p13.13	ERCC4, XPF	C	Excision-repair, complementing defective, in Chinese hamster, number 4	133520	Xeroderma pigmentosum, group F, 278760 (3)
16p13.3-p13.12	PKD1	C	Polycystin-1	601313	Polycystic kidney disease, adult type I, 173900 (3)
16p13.11	SAH	P	SA (rat hypertension-associated) homolog	145505	{?Hypertension, essential} (1)
16p13.1	PXE, PXE1	C	Pseudoxanthoma elasticum	264800	Pseudoxanthoma elasticum (2)
16p13	HAGH, GLO2	C	Hydroxyacyl glutathione hydrolase; glyoxalase II	138760	[Glyoxalase II deficiency] (1)
16p13	MEFV, MEF, FMF	C	Pyrin (marenostrin)	249100	Familial Mediterranean fever (3)
16p13	MHC2TA, C2TA	P	MHC class II transactivator	600005	MHC class II deficiency, complementation group A, 209920 (3)

(Continued on next page)

Table A1-2 (Continued)

Location	Symbol	Status	Locus Name	MIM#	Disorder
16p13-p12	SCNN1B	C	Sodium channel, nonvoltage-gated 1, beta	600760	Liddle syndrome, 177200 (3); Pseudohypoaldosteronism, type I, 264350 (3)
16p13-p12	SCNN1G, PHA1	C	Sodium channel, nonvoltage-gated 1, gamma	600761	Liddle syndrome, 177200 (3); Pseudohypoaldosteronism, type I, 264350 (3)
16p12.3-p12.1	RP22	P	Retinitis pigmentosa-22	602594	Retinitis pigmentosa-22 (2)
16p12.1	CLN3, BTS	C	Ceroid-lipofuscinosis, neuronal-3, juvenile (Batten disease)	204200	Ceroid-lipofuscinosis, neuronal-3, juvenile (3)
16p12.1-p11.2	IL4R, IL4RA	P	Interleukin-4 receptor	147781	{Atopy, susceptibility to} (3)
16p12.1-p11.2	MVP, PMV	P	Mitral valve prolapse, familial	157700	Mitral valve prolapse, familial (2)
16p12.1-p11.2	PHKG2	P	Phosphorylase kinase, gamma 2 (testis/liver)	172471	Glycogenosis, hepatic, autosomal (3)
16p12	ATP2A1, SERCA1	C	ATPase, Ca++ transporting, fast-twitch, 1	108730	Brody myopathy, 601003 (3)
16p12	MCKD2, ADMCKD2	P	Medullary cystic kidney disease 2, autosomal dominant	603860	Medullary cystic kidney disease 2 (2)
16p12-q12	ICCA	C	Infantile convulsions and paroxysmal choreoathetosis	602066	Convulsions, infantile and paroxysmal choreoathetosis (2)
16p12-q13	IBD1	P	Inflammatory bowel disease-1 (Crohn disease)	266600	Inflammatory bowel disease-1 (2)
16p12-q21	ACUG, BLAU	P	Arthrocutaneouveal granulomatosis (Blau syndrome)	186580	Arthrocutaneouveal granulomatosis (2)
16p11.2	SLC5A2, SGLT2	P	Solute carrier family 5 (sodium/glucose cotransporter), member 2	182381	?Renal glucosuria, 233100 (1)
16p11.2-q12.1	PKC, DYT10	P	Paroxysmal kinesigenic choreoathetosis	128200	Paroxysmal kinesigenic choreoathetosis (2)
16q	WT3	P	Wilms tumor-3	194090	Wilms tumor, type 3 (2)
16q12-q13	CYLD1, CDMT, EAC	P	Cylindromatosis 1, turban tumor syndrome	132700	Cylindromatosis (2)
16q12-q13	PHKB	C	Phosphorylase kinase, beta polypeptide	172490	Phosphorylase kinase deficiency of liver and muscle, autosomal recessive, 261750 (3)
16q12.1	HYD2	P	Hypodontia, autosomal recessive	602639	Hypodontia, autosomal recessive (2)
16q12.1	SALL1, HSAL1, TBS	P	Sal-like 1	602218	Townes-Brocks syndrome, 107480 (3)
16q12.2	SLC6A2, NAT1, NET1	C	Solute carrier family 6 (neurotransmitter transporter, noradrenalin), member 2, cocaine- and antidepressant-sensitive	163970	Orthostatic intolerance, 604715 (3)
16q13	SLC12A3, NCCT, TSC	C	Solute carrier family 12 (sodium/potassium/chloride transporters), member 3	600968	Gitelman syndrome, 263800 (3)
16q13-q22.1	CES1, SES1	P	Carboxylesterase 1 (monocyte/macrophage serine esterase 1)	114835	?Monocyte carboxyesterase deficiency (1)
16q21	BBS2	C	Bardet-Biedl syndrome 2	209900	Bardet-Biedl syndrome 2 (2)
16q21	CETP	P	Cholesteryl ester transfer protein, plasma	118470	[CETP deficiency] (3)
16q22	AMLCR2	P	Acute myeloid leukemia chromosome region 2	602439	Leukemia, acute myelogenous (2)
16q22	CBFB	C	Core-binding factor, beta subunit	121360	Myeloid leukemia, acute, M4Eo subtype (2)
16q22	HSD11B2, HSD11K	C	Hydroxysteroid (11-beta) dehydrogenase 2	218030	Apparent mineralocorticoid excess, hypertension due to (3); Hypertension, mild low-renin (3)
16q22	MCDC1	P	Macular dystrophy, corneal, 1	217800	Macular corneal dystrophy (2)
16q22-q24	ALDOA	C	Aldolase A, fructose-bisphosphatase	103850	Aldolase A deficiency (3)
16q22.1	CDH1, UVO	C	Cadherin-1 (E-cadherin; uvomorulin)	192090	Endometrial carcinoma (3); Ovarian carcinoma (3); Breast cancer, lobular (3); Gastric cancer, familial, 137215 (3)
16q22.1	CTM	C	Cataract, Marner type	116800	Cataract, Marner type (2)

Table A1-2 (Continued)

Location	Symbol	Status	Locus Name	MIM#	Disorder
16q22.1	DIA4, NMOR1	C	Diaphorase-4	125860	{Benzene toxicity, susceptibility to} (3); {Leukemia, post-chemotherapy, susceptibility to} (3)
16q22.1	HP	C	Haptoglobin	140100	[Anhaptoglobinemia] (3); [Hypohaptogloginemia] (3)
16q22.1	LCAT	C	Lecithin-cholesterol acyltransferase	245900	Norum disease (3); Fish-eye disease (3)
16q22.1	SCA4	P	Spinocerebellar ataxia 4	600223	Spinocerebellar ataxia-4 (2)
16q22.1-q22.3	TAT	C	Tyrosine aminotransferase, cytosolic	276600	Tyrosinemia, type II (3)
16q23-q24	DHS	P	Dehydrated hereditary stomatocytosis	194380	Dehydrated hereditary stomatocytosis (2); Pseudohyperkalemia, familial, 177720 (2)
16q24	CYBA	C	Cytochrome b-245, alpha polypeptide	233690	Chronic granulomatous disease, autosomal, due to deficiency of CYBA (3)
16q24	MLYCD, MCD	P	Malonyl-CoA decarboxylase	248360	Malonyl-CoA decarboxylase deficiency (3)
16q24.1	GAN, GAN1	C	Giant axonal neuropathy-1	256850	Giant axonal neuropathy-1 (2)
16q24.2-q24.3	FEOM3	P	Fibrosis of extraocular muscles, congenital, 3	604361	Fibrosis of extraocular muscles, congenital, 3 (2)
16q24.3	APRT	C	Adenine phosphoribosyltransferase	102600	Urolithiasis, 2,8-dihydroxyadenine (3)
16q24.3	FANCA, FACA, FA1, FA, FAA	C	Fanconi anemia, complementation group A	227650	Fanconi anemia, type A (3)
16q24.3	GALNS, MPS4A	C	Galactosamine (N-acetyl)-6-sulfate sulfatase	253000	Mucopolysaccharidosis IVA (3)
16q24.3	LD	P	Lymphedema with distichiasis	153400	Lymphedema with distichiasis (2)
16q24.3	MC1R	C	Melanocortin-1 receptor (alpha melanocyte-stimulating hormone receptor)	155555	{UV-induced skin damage, vulnerability to} (3); [Red hair/fair skin] (3)
16q24.3	PGN, SPG7	P	Paraplegin	602783	Spastic paraplegia-7 (3)
Chr.16	CTH	P	Cystathionase	219500	[Cystathioninuria] (1)
17pter-p13	ASPA	P	Aspartoacylase (aminoacylase-2)	271900	Canavan disease (3)
17pter-p12	GP1BA	P	Glycoprotein Ib, platelet, alpha polypeptide	231200	Bernard-Soulier syndrome (3)
17pter-p12	PLI	P	Alpha-2-plasmin inhibitor	262850	Plasmin inhibitor deficiency (3)
17p13.3	BCPR	P	Breast cancer-related regulator of TP53	113721	Breast cancer (1)
17p13.3	MDCR, MDS	C	Miller-Dieker syndrome chromosome region	247200	Miller-Dieker lissencephaly syndrome (2)
17p13.3	PAFAH1B1, LIS1	C	Platelet-activating factor acetylhydrolase, isoform 1B, alpha subunit	601545	Lissencephaly-1 (3); Subcortical laminar heterotopia (3)
17p13.3	RP13	C	Retinitis pigmentosa-13	600059	Retinitis pigmentosa-13 (2)
17p13.1	AIPL1, LCA4	C	Arylhydrocarbon-interacting receptor protein-like 1	604392	Leber congenital amaurosis, 604393 (3)
17p13.1	GUCY2D, GUC2D, LCA1, CORD6	C	Guanylate cyclase 2D, membrane, retina-specific	600179	Leber congenital amaurosis, type I, 204000 (3); Cone-rod dystrophy 6, 601777(3)
17p13.1	TP53	C	Tumor protein p53	191170	Colorectal cancer, 114500 (3); Li-Fraumeni syndrome (3)
17p13	CTAA2	P	Cataract, anterior polar, 2	601202	Cataract, anterior polar-2 (2)
17p13	CTNS	C	Cystinosis	219800	Cystinosis, nephropathic (3)
17p13	MGI, FIMG	P	Myasthenia gravis, familial infantile	254210	Myasthenia gravis, familial infantile (2)
17p13	SLC2A4, GLUT4	P	Solute carrier family 2 (facilitated glucose transporter), member 4	138190	{Diabetes mellitus, noninsulin-dependent} (3)
17p13-p12	CORD5	C	Cone rod dystrophy 5	600977	Cone dystrophy, progressive (2)
17p12	BRKS, TLH1	P	Telopeptide lysyl hydroxylase, bone-specific	259450	Bruck syndrome (2)
17p12-p11	CHRNB1, ACHRB	C	Cholinergic receptor, nicotinic, beta polypeptide-1, muscle	100710	Myasthenic syndrome, slow-channel congenital, 601462 (3)

(Continued on next page)

Table A1-2 (Continued)

Location	Symbol	Status	Locus Name	MIM#	Disorder
17p11.2	ALDH10, SLS, FALDH	C	Aldehyde dehydrogenase-10 (fatty aldehyde dehydrogenase)	270200	Sjogren-Larsson syndrome (3)
17p11.2	MYO15, DFNB3	C	Myosin XV	602666	Deafness, autosomal recessive 3, 600316 (3)
17p11.2	PMP22, CMT1A	C	Peripheral myelin protein-22	601097	Charcot-Marie-Tooth neuropathy-1A, 118220 (3); Dejerine-Sottas disease, 145900 (3); Neuropathy, recurrent, with pressure palsies, 162500 (3); Charcot-Marie-Tooth disease with deafness, 118300 (3)
17p11.2	SMCR	C	Smith-Magenis syndrome chromosome region	182290	Smith-Magenis syndrome (2)
17p11.2-p11.1	ACADVL, VLCAD	C	Acyl-Coenzyme A dehydrogenase, very long chain	201475	VLCAD deficiency (3)
17p	CACD	P	Choroidal dystrophy, central areolar	215500	Choroidal dystrophy, central areolar (2)
17p	RCD2	P	Retinal cone dystrophy-2	601251	Retinal cone dsytrophy 2 (2)
17cen-q21.3	TCF2, HNF2	C	Transcription factor-2, hepatic; LF-B3; variant hepatic nuclear factor	189907	MODY, type V (3); MODY5 with non-diabetic renal disease and Mullerian aplasia (3)
17q	HYT1	P	Hypertension, essential, susceptibility to, 1	603918	{Hypertension, essential, susceptibility to, 1}, 145500 (2)
17q	PSORS2, PSS1	P	Psoriasis susceptibility 2	602723	{Psoriasis susceptibility-2} (2)
17q11-q12	WHN	P	Winged helix nude	600838	T-cell immunodeficiency, congenital alopecia, and nail dystrophy (3)
17q11-qter	ITGB4	P	Integrin, beta-4	147557	Epidermolysis bullosa, junctional, with pyloric atresia, 226730 (3)
17q11.1-q11.2	TAF2N, RBP56	P	TATA box-binding protein-associated factor 2N (RNA-binding protein 56)	601574	Chondrosarcoma, extraskeletal myxoid (1)
17q11.1-q12	CRYBA1, CRYB1	C	Crystallin, beta A1	123610	Cataract, congenital zonular, with sutural opacities, 600881 (3)
17q11.1-q12	SLC6A4, HTT	C	Solute carrier family 6 (neurotransmitter transporter, serotonin), member 4	182138	Anxiety-related personality traits (3)
17q11.2	BLMH, BMH	P	Bleomycin hydrolase	602403	{Alzheimer disease, susceptibility to} (3)
17q11.2	NF1, VRNF, WSS	C	Neurofibromin (neurofibromatosis, type I)	162200	Neurofibromatosis, type 1 (3); Watson syndrome, 193520 (3); Leukemia, juvenile myelomonocytic (3)
17q11.2	VBCH	P	Van Buchem disease	239100	Van Buchem disease (2)
17q11.2-q12	SCYA5, D17S136E, TCP228	P	Small inducible cytokine A5 (RANTES)	187011	{HIV-1 disease, delayed progression of} (2)
17q11.2-q24	MHS2	P	Malignant hyperthermia susceptibility 2	154275	{Malignant hyperthermia susceptibility 2} (2)
17q12	KRT12	C	Keratin-12	601687	Meesmann corneal dystrophy, 122100 (3)
17q12	RARA	C	Retinoic acid receptor, alpha polypeptide	180240	Leukemia, acute promyelocytic (1)
17q12	TCAP, LGMD2G	C	Telethonin	604488	Muscular dystrophy, limb-girdle, type 2G, 601954 (3)
17q12-q21	KRT9, EPPK	C	Keratin-9	144200	Epidermolytic palmoplantar keratoderma (3)
17q12-q21	KRT14	P	Keratin-14	148066	Epidermolysis bullosa simplex, Koebner, Dowling-Meara, and Weber-Cockayne types, 131900, 131760, 131800 (3); Epidermolysis bullosa simplex, recessive, 601001 (3)
17q12-q21	KRT16	C	Keratin-16	148067	Pachyonychia congenita, Jadassohn-Lewandowsky type, 167200 (3); Nonepidermolytic palmoplantar keratoderma, 600962 (3)

Table A1-2 (Continued)

Location	Symbol	Status	Locus Name	MIM#	Disorder
17q12-q21	KRT17, PCHC1	C	Keratin-17	148069	Pachyonychia congenita, Jackson-Lawler type, 167210 (3); Steatocystoma multiplex, 184500 (3)
17q12-q21	SOST	P	Sclerosteosis	269500	Sclerosteosis (2)
17q12-q21	WT4	C	Wilms tumor-4	601363	Wilms tumor, type 4 (2)
17q12-q21.33	SGCA, ADL, DAG2, LGMD2D	C	Sarcoglycan, alpha (50 kD dystrophin-associated glycoprotein; adhalin)	600119	Muscular dystrophy, Duchenne-like, type 2 (3); Adhalinopathy, primary (1)
17q21	ACACA, ACAC, ACC1	C	Acetyl-Coenzyme A carboxylase, alpha	200350	Acetyl-CoA carboxylase deficiency (1)
17q21	BRCA1	C	Breast cancer-1, early onset	113705	Breast cancer-1 (3); Ovarian cancer (3)
17q21	G6PC, G6PT	C	Glucose-6-phosphatase, catalytic	232200	Glycogen storage disease I (3)
17q21	NAGLU	P	N-acetylglucosaminidase, alpha-	252920	Sanfilippo syndrome, type B (3)
17q21	PHB	C	Prohibitin	176705	Breast cancer, sporadic (3)
17q21	PPND	P	Parkinsonism-dementia with pallidopontonigral degeneration	168610	Parkinsonism-dementia with pallidopontonigral degeneration (2)
17q21-q22	GPSC	P	Gliosis, familial progressive subcortical	221820	Gliosis, familial progressive subcortical (2)
17q21-q22	KRT10	C	Keratin-10	148080	Epidermolytic hyperkeratosis, 113800 (3)
17q21-q22	KRT13	P	Keratin-13	148065	White sponge nevus, 193900 (3)
17q21-q22	PHA2B	P	Pseudohypoaldosteronism type II	601844	Pseudohypoaldosteronism type II (2)
17q21-q22	PNMT, PENT	C	Phenylethanolamine N-methyltransferase	171190	?Hypertension, essential, 145500 (1)
17q21-q22	PTLAH, FPAH	P	Patella aplasia or hypoplasia	168860	Patella aplasia or hypoplasia (2)
17q21-q22	SLC4A1, AE1, EPB3	C	Solute carrier family 4, anion exchanger, member 1 (erythrocyte membrane protein band 3, Diego blood group)	109270	[Acanthocytosis, one form] (1); [Elliptocytosis, Malaysian-Melanesian type] (3); Spherocytosis, hereditary (3); Hemolytic anemia due to band 3 defect (3); Renal tubular acidosis, distal, 179800 (3)
17q21.31-q22	COL1A1	C	Collagen I, alpha-1 polypeptide	120150	Osteogenesis imperfecta, 4 clinical forms, 166200, 166210, 259420, 166220 (3); Ehlers-Danlos syndrome, type VIIA1, 130060 (3); Osteoporosis, idiopathic, 166710 (3); {Dissection of cervical arteries, susceptibility to} (3)
17q21.1	MAPT, MTBT1, DDPAC, MSTD	C	Microtubule-associated protein tau	157140	Dementia, frontotemporal, with parkinsonism, 601630 (3)
17q21.3	NME1, NM23	C	Non-metastatic cells 1, protein (NM23A) expressed in	156490	Neuroblastoma (3)
17q21.3-q22	DLX3, TDO	C	Distal-less homeo box-3	600525	Trichodontoosseous syndrome, 190320 (3)
17q21.32	ITGA2B, GP2B, CD41B	C	Integrin, alpha-2b (platelet glycoprotein IIb of IIb/IIIa complex, antigen CD41B)	273800	Glanzmann thrombasthenia, type A (3); Thrombocytopenia, neonatal alloimmune (1)
17q21.32	ITGB3, GP3A	C	Integrin, beta-3 (platelet glycoprotein IIIa; antigen CD61)	173470	Glanzmann thrombasthenia, type B (3)
17q22	NOG, SYM1, SYNS1	C	Noggin, mouse, homolog of	602991	Symphalangism, proximal, 185800 (3); Synostoses syndrome, multiple, 1, 186500 (3)
17q22	RP17	C	Retinitis pigmentosa-17	600852	Retinitis pigmentosa-17 (2)
17q22-q23	MKS1, MKS	C	Meckel syndrome, type 1	249000	Meckel syndrome, type 1 (2)
17q22-q23	MUL	C	Mulibrey nanism	253250	Mulibrey nanism (2)
17q22-q23.2	PRKCA, PKCA	C	Protein kinase C, alpha polypeptide	176960	Pituitary tumor, invasive (3)
17q22-q24	CSH1, CSA, PL	C	Chorionic somatomammotropin hormone-1	150200	[Placental lactogen deficiency] (1)

(Continued on next page)

Table A1-2 (Continued)

Location	Symbol	Status	Locus Name	MIM#	Disorder
17q22-q24	GH1, GHN	C	Growth hormone-1	139250	Isolated growth hormone deficiency, Illig type with absent GH and Kowarski type with bioinactive GH (3)
17q23	DCP1, ACE1	C	Dipeptidyl carboxypeptidase-1 (angiotensin I converting enzyme)	106180	{Myocardial infarction, susceptibility to} (3); {Alzheimer disease, susceptibility to}, 104300 (3)
17q23-qter	APOH	C	Apolipoprotein H (beta-2-glycoprotein I)	138700	[Apolipoprotein H deficiency] (3)
17q23.1	MPO	C	Myeloperoxidase	254600	Myeloperoxidase deficiency (3)
17q23.1-q25.3	SCN4A, HYPP, NAC1A	C	Sodium channel, voltage-gated, type IV, alpha polypeptide	603967	Hyperkalemic periodic paralysis, 170500 (3); Paramyotonia congenita, 168300 (3); Myotonia congenita, atypical, acetazolamide-responsive (3); Cramps, familial, potassium-aggravated (3)
17q24	CCA1	P	Cataract, congenital, cerulean type	115660	Cataract, cerulean, type 1 (2)
17q24	GALK1	C	Galactokinase-1	604313	Galactokinase deficiency with cataracts, 230200 (3)
17q24	SSTR2	C	Somatostatin receptor-2	182452	Lung cancer, small cell (3)
17q24	TOC, TEC	C	Tylosis with esophageal cancer	148500	Tylosis with esophageal cancer (2)
17q24.3-q25.1	SOX9, CMD1, SRA1	C	SRY (sex-determining region Y)-box 9	114290	Campomelic dysplasia with autosomal sex reversal (3)
17q25	ACOX1, ACOX	C	Acyl-Coenzyme A oxidase 1	264470	Adrenoleukodystrophy, pseudoneonatal (2)
17q25	DFNA20	P	Deafness, autosomal dominant 20	604717	Deafness, autosomal dominant 20 (2)
17q25	GCGR	P	Glucagon receptor	138033	Diabetes mellitus, type II (3)
17q25	MSF, MSF1	P	MLL septin-like fusion gene	604061	Leukemia, acute myeloid, therapy-related (1)
17q25	NAPB	C	Neuralgic amyotrophy with predilection for brachial plexus	162100	Neuralgic amyotrophy with predilection for brachial plexus (2)
17q25.2-q25.3	GAA	C	Glucosidase, acid alpha-	232300	Glycogen storage disease II (3)
17q25.3	SGSH, MPS3A, SFMD	P	N-sulfoglucosamine sulfohydrolase (sulfamidase)	252900	Sanfilippo syndrome, type A (3)
Chr.17	CHRNE	P	Cholinergic receptor, nicotinic, epsilon polypeptide	100725	Myasthenic syndrome, slow-channel congenital, 601462 (3)
18p11.32	MCL	L	Multiple hereditary cutaneous leiomyoma	150800	?Leiomyoma, multiple hereditary cutaneous (2)
18p11.31	MYP2	P	Myopia, high grade, autosomal dominant 1	160700	Myopia-2 (2)
18p11.31-p11.2	NDUFV2	C	NADH dehydrogenase (ubiquinone) flavoprotein 2, 24 kD	600532	{Parkinson disease, susceptibility to}, 168600 (3)
18p11.3	TGIF, HPE4	P	TG-interacting factor	602630	Holoprosencephaly-4, 142946 (3)
18p11.2	MC2R	C	Melanocortin-2 receptor (ACTH receptor)	202200	Glucocorticoid deficiency, due to ACTH unresponsiveness (1)
18p	DYT7	P	Dystonia-7 (torsion dystonia, adult-onset, focal)	602124	Dystonia-7, torsion (2)
18p	MAFD1, BPAD, MD1	L	Major affective disorder 1	125480	Bipolar affective disorder (2)
18p	SCZD8	P	Schizophrenia susceptibility locus, chromosome 18-related	603206	{Schizophrenia}, 181500 (2)
18q	OHDS	P	Orthostatic hypotensive disorder of Streeten	143850	Orthostatic hypotensive disorder of Streeten (2)
18q11-q12	LCFS2	L	Lynch cancer family syndrome II	114400	?Lynch cancer family syndrome II (2)
18q11-q12	NPC1, NPC	C	Niemann-Pick disease, type C	257220	Niemann-Pick disease, type C1 (3); Niemann-Pick disease, type D, 257250 (3)
18q11.2	LAMA3	P	Laminin, alpha-3 (nicein, 150 kD; kalinin, 165 kD; BM600, 150 kD; epilegrin)	600805	Epidermolysis bullosa, junctional, Herlitz type (3)

Table A1-2 (Continued)

Location	Symbol	Status	Locus Name	MIM#	Disorder
18q11.2	SSXT, SYT	C	Synovial sarcoma, translocated to X chromosome	600192	Sarcoma, synovial (1)
18q11.2-q12.1	TTR, PALB	C	Transthyretin (prealbumin)	176300	Amyloid neuropathy, familial, several allelic types (3); [Dystransthyretinemic hyperthyroxinemia](3); Amyloidosis, senile systemic (3); Carpal tunnel syndrome, familial (3)
18q12.1-q12.2	DSG1	C	Desmoglein-1	125670	Keratosis palmoplantaris striata I, 148700 (3)
18q21	FIC1, BRIC, PFIC1	P	Familial intrahepatic cholestasis-1	602397	Cholestasis, progressive familial intrahepatic-1, 211600 (3); Cholestasis, benign recurrent intrahepatic, 243300 (3)
18q21	IDDM6	P	Insulin-dependent diabetes mellitus-6	601941	{Diabetes mellitus, insulin-dependent, 6} (2)
18q21-q22	LOH18CR1, OSTS	P	Loss of heterozygosity, 18, chromosomal region 1 (osteosarcoma tumor suppressor)	603045	Osteosarcoma, 259500 (2)
18q21.1	MADH4, DPC4, SMAD4, JIP	P	Mothers against decapentaplegic, Drosophila, homolog of, 4	600993	Pancreatic cancer (3); Polyposis, juvenile intestinal, 174900 (3)
18q21.1-q21.3	CORD1, CRD1	P	Cone rod dystrophy 1, autosomal dominant	600624	Cone-rod retinal dystrophy-1 (2)
18q21.3	BCL2	C	B-cell CLL/lymphoma-2	151430	Leukemia/lymphoma, B-cell, 2 (2)
18q21.3	CNSN	P	Carnosinemia (carnosinase)	212200	Carnosinemia (2)
18q21.3	DCC	C	Deleted in colorectal carcinoma	120470	Colorectal cancer (3)
18q21.3	FECH, FCE	C	Ferrochelatase	177000	Protoporphyria, erythropoietic (3); Protoporphyria, erythropoietic, recessive, with liver failure (3)
18q21.3	FVT1	P	Follicular lymphoma, variant translocation 1	136440	Lymphoma/leukemia, B-cell, variant (1)
18q21.3-q22	LMAN1, ERGIC53, F5F8D, MCFD1	C	Lectin, mannose-binding, 1	601567	Combined factor V and VIII deficiency, 227300 (3)
18q22	MC4R	C	Melanocortin-4 receptor	155541	Obesity, autosomal dominant (3)
18q22.1	TNFRSF11A, RANK, ODFR, OFE	C	Tumor necrosis factor receptor superfamily, member 11A	603499	Osteolysis, familial expansile, 174810 (3); Paget disease of bone, 602080 (3)
18q23	CYB5	C	Cytochrome b5	250790	Methemoglobinemia due to cytochrome b5 deficiency (3)
18q23-qter	CCFDN	P	Congenital cataract, facial dysmorphism, and neuropathy syndrome	604168	Congenital cataract, facial dysmorphism, and neuropathy syndrome (2)
19p13.3	ATCAY, CLAC	P	Ataxia, cerebellar, Cayman type	601238	Cerebellar ataxia, Cayman type (2)
19p13.3	ELA2	C	Elastase-2, neutrophil	130130	Cyclic hematopoiesis, 162800 (3)
19p13.3	FEB2	P	Convulsions, familial febrile, 2	602477	Convulsions, familial febrile, 2 (2)
19p13.3	FUT6	P	Fucosyltransferase 6 (alpha (1,3) fucosyltransferase)	136836	Fucosyltransferase-6 deficiency (3)
19p13.3	GAMT	P	Guanidinoacetate methyltransferase	601240	GAMT deficiency (3)
19p13.3	HHC2, FHH2	P	Hypocalciuric hypercalcemia-2	145981	Hypocalciuric hypercalcemia, type II (2)
19p13.3	MDRV	P	Muscular dystrophy with rimmed vacuoles	601846	Muscular dystrophy with rimmed vacuoles (2)
19p13.3	NRTN, NTN	P	Neurturin	602018	Hirschsprung disease, 142623 (3)
19p13.3	STK11, PJS, LKB1	C	Serine/threonine protein kinase-11	602216	Peutz-Jeghers syndrome, 175200 (3)
19p13.3	TBXA2R	C	Thromboxane A2 receptor	188070	Bleeding disorder due to defective thromboxane A2 receptor (3)
19p13.3	TCF3, E2A	C	Transcription factor-3 (E2A immunoglobulin enhancer-binding factors E12/E47)	147141	Leukemia, acute lymphoblastic (1)
19p13.3-p13.2	AMH, MIF	P	Anti-Mullerian hormone	600957	Persistent Mullerian duct syndrome, type I, 261550 (3)
19p13.3-p13.2	ATHS, ALP	P	Atherosclerosis susceptibility (lipoprotein associated)	108725	{Atherosclerosis, susceptibility to} (2)

(Continued on next page)

Table A1-2 (Continued)

Location	Symbol	Status	Locus Name	MIM#	Disorder
19p13.3-p13.2	C3	C	Complement component-3	120700	C3 deficiency (3)
19p13.3-p13.2	EPOR	C	Erythropoietin receptor	133171	[Erythrocytosis, familial], 133100 (3)
19p13.3-p13.2	ICAM1	C	Intercellular adhesion molecule-1	147840	{Malaria, cerebral, susceptibility to} (3)
19p13.3-p13.2	ML4	P	Mucolipidosis IV	252650	Mucolipidosis IV (2)
19p13.2	GCDH	P	Glutaryl-Coenzyme A dehydrogenase	231670	Glutaricaciduria, type I (3)
19p13.2	INSR	C	Insulin receptor	147670	Leprechaunism, 246200 (3); Rabson-Mendenhall syndrome, 262190 (3); Diabetes mellitus, insulin-resistant, with acanthosis nigricans (3)
19p13.2	TCO	P	Thyroid carcinoma, nonmedullary, with cell oxyphilia	603386	Thyroid carcinoma, nonmedullary, with cell oxyphilia (2)
19p13.2-p13.1	INLNE	P	Ichthyosis, nonlamellar and nonerythrodermic, congenital, autosomal recessive	604781	Ichthyosis, nonlamellar and nonerythrodermic, congenital (2)
19p13.2-p13.1	LDLR, FHC, FH	C	Low density lipoprotein receptor	143890	Hypercholesterolemia, familial (3)
19p13.2-p13.1	LYL1	C	Lymphoblastic leukemia derived sequence-1	151440	Leukemia, T-cell acute lymphoblastoid (2)
19p13.2-p13.1	NOTCH3, CADASIL, CASIL	C	Notch, Drosophila, homolog of, 3	600276	Cerebral arteriopathy with subcortical infarcts and leukoencephalopathy, 125310 (3)
19p13.2-p12	SLC5A5, NIS	P	Solute carrier family 5 (sodium iodide symporter), member-5	601843	Hypothyroidism, congenital, 274400 (3)
19p13.2-q13.3	LPSA, D19S381E	P	Oncogene liposarcoma (DNA segment, single copy, expressed, probes MC15, MC6)	164953	Liposarcoma (1)
19p13.1	COMP, EDM1, MED, PSACH	P	Cartilage oligomeric matrix protein	600310	Pseudoachondroplasia, 177170 (3); Epiphyseal dysplasia, multiple 1, 132400 (3)
19p13.1	IL12RB1	P	Interleukin-12 receptor, beta-1	601604	{Mycobacterial and salmonella infections, susceptibility to} (3)
19p13.1	JAK3, JAKL	P	Janus kinase 3 (Janus kinase, leukocyte)	600173	SCID, autosomal recessive, T-negative/B-positive type (3)
19p13	CACNA1A, CACNL1A4, SCA6	C	Calcium channel, voltage-dependent, P/Q type, alpha 1A subunit	601011	Hemiplegic migraine, familial, 141500 (3); Episodic ataxia, type 2, 108500 (3); Spinocerebellar ataxia-6, 183086 (3); Cerebellar ataxia, pure (3)
19p13	NDUFS7, PSST	P	NADH dehydrogenase (ubiquinone) Fe-S protein 7, 20 kD (NADH-coenzyme Q reductase)	601825	Leigh syndrome, 256000 (3)
19p13	SH3GL1, EEN	P	SH3 domain GRB2-like 1 (Extra 11-19 leukemia fusion gene)	601768	Leukemia, acute myeloid (1)
19p12	RFXANK	P	Regulatory factor X, ankyrin repeat-containing	603200	MHC class II deficiency, complementation group B, 209920 (3)
19p12-q12	LI3	P	Ichthyosis congenita III	604777	Ichthyosis, lamellar, type 3 (2)
19p	EXT3	P	Exostoses, multiple, 3	600209	Exostoses, multiple, type 3 (2)
19cen-q12	MAN2B1, MANB	C	Mannosidase, alpha, class 2B, member 1	248500	Mannosidosis, alpha-, types I and II (3)
19cen-q13.11	PEPD	C	Peptidase D (prolidase)	170100	Prolidase deficiency (3)
19cen-q13.2	AD2	C	Alzheimer disease-2, late-onset	104310	Alzheimer disease-2, late onset (2)
19q	BFIC	P	Benign familial infantile convulsions	601764	Benign familial infantile convulsions (2)
19q13	ACTN4, FSGS1, FSGS	C	Actinin, alpha-4	604638	Glomerulosclerosis, focal segmental, 1, 603278 (3)
19q13	BCAT2, BCT2	C	Branched chain aminotransferase-2, mitochondrial	113530	?Hypervalinemia or hyperleucine-isoleucinemia (1)
19q13	BCL3	C	B-cell CLL/lymphoma-3	109560	Leukemia/lymphoma, B-cell, 3 (2)
19q13	DFNA4	P	Deafness, autosomal dominant 4	600652	Deafness, autosomal dominant 4 (2)

Table A1-2 (Continued)

Location	Symbol	Status	Locus Name	MIM#	Disorder
19q13	DLL3, SCDO1	C	Delta, drosophila, homolog of	277300	Spondylocostal dysostosis, autosomal recessive, 1, 277300 (3)
19q13	HHC3, FBH3	P	Hypercalcemia, familial benign, 3 (hypercalcemia, familial benign, Oklahoma type)	600740	Hypercalciuric hypercalcemia, type III (2)
19q13	OFC3	P	Orofacial cleft-3	600757	Orofacial cleft-3 (2)
19q13.1	SLC7A9, CSNU3	C	Solute carrier family 7 (cationic amino acid transporter, y+ system), member 9	604144	Cystinuria, type III (3); Cystinuria, type II (3)
19q13.1	GPI	C	Glucose phosphate isomerase; neuroleukin	172400	Hemolytic anemia due to glucosephosphate isomerase deficiency (3); Hydrops fetalis, one form (1)
19q13.1	NPHN, NPHS1	P	Nephrin	602716	Nephrosis-1, congenital, Finnish type, 256300 (3)
19q13.1	PLOSL	C	Polycystic lipomembranous osteodysplasia with sclerosing leukencephalopathy	221770	Polycystic lipomembranous osteodysplasia with sclerosing leukencephalopathy (2)
19q13.1	RYR1, MHS, CCO	C	Ryanodine receptor-1, skeletal	180901	{Malignant hyperthermia susceptibility 1}, 145600 (3); Central core disease, 117000 (3)
19q13.1	SCN1B	C	Sodium channel, voltage-gated, type I, beta polypeptide	600235	Generalized epilepsy with febrile seizures plus (3)
19q13.1-q13.2	AKT2	P	Murine thymoma viral (v-akt) homolog-2	164731	Ovarian carcinoma, 167000 (2)
19q13.1-q13.2	BCKDHA, MSUD1	C	Branched chain keto acid dehydrogenase E1, alpha polypeptide	248600	Maple syrup urine disease, type Ia (3)
19q13.1-q13.2	MCPH2	P	Microcephaly, primary autosomal recessive 2	604317	Microcephaly, autosomal recessive 2 (2)
19q13.1-q13.3	DPD1, CED	P	Diaphyseal dysplasia 1, progressive (Camurati-Engelmann disease)	131300	Camurati-Engelmann disease (2)
19q13.2	APOE	C	Apolipoprotein E	107741	Hyperlipoproteinemia, type III (3); {Myocardial infarction susceptibility} (3)
19q13.2	APOC2	C	Apolipoprotein C-II	207750	Hyperlipoproteinemia, type Ib (3)
19q13.2	CYP2A6, CYP2A3	C	Cytochrome P450, subfamily IIA, phenobarbital-inducible, polypeptide 6	122720	Coumarin resistance, 122700 (3); {Nicotine addiction, protection from} (3)
19q13.2	RPS19, DBA	C	Ribosomal protein S19	603474	Anemia, Diamond-Blackfan, 105650 (3)
19q13.2-q13.3	DMPK, DM, DMK	C	Dystrophia myotonica-protein kinase	160900	Myotonic dystrophy (3)
19q13.2-q13.3	ERCC2, EM9	C	Excision repair cross complementing rodent repair deficiency, complementation group-2	126340	Xeroderma pigmentosum, group D, 278730 (3); Trichothiodystrophy, 601675 (3)
19q13.2-q13.3	HB1, PFHB1	C	Heart block, progressive familial, type I	113900	Heart block, progressive familial, type I (2)
19q13.2-q13.3	LIG1	C	Ligase I, DNA, ATP-dependent	126391	DNA ligase I deficiency (3)
19q13.2-q13.3	OPA3, MGA3	P	Optic atrophy 3 (Iraqi-Jewish 'optic atrophy plus')	258501	3-methylglutaconicaciduria, type III (2)
19q13.2-q13.3	PVR, PVS	C	Polio virus receptor	173850	{Polio, susceptibility to} (2)
19q13.2-q13.4	CFM1	P	Cystic fibrosis modifier-1	603855	Meconium ileus in cystic fibrosis, susceptibility to (2)
19q13.3	CRX, CORD2, CRD	C	Cone-rod homeo box-containing gene	602225	Cone-rod retinal dystrophy-2, 120970 (3); Leber congenital amaurosis due to defect in CRX, 204000 (3); Retinitis pigmentosa, late-onset dominant (3)
19q13.3	ETFB	C	Electron transfer flavoprotein, beta polypeptide	130410	Glutaricaciduria, type IIB (3)
19q13.3	GYS1, GYS	C	Glycogen synthase	138570	{Diabetes mellitus, noninsulin-dependent} (2)

(Continued on next page)

Table A1-2 (Continued)

Location	Symbol	Status	Locus Name	MIM#	Disorder
19q13.3-q13.4	BAX	C	BCL2-associated X protein	600040	Colorectal cancer (3); T-cell acute lymphoblastic leukemia (3)
19q13.3-q13.4	FTL	C	Ferritin, light chain	134790	Hyperferritinemia-cataract syndrome, 600886 (3)
19q13.3-q13.4	HYDM	P	Hydatidiform mole	231090	Hydatidiform mole (2)
19q13.32	LHB	C	Luteinizing hormone, beta polypeptide	152780	Hypogonadism, hypergonadotropic (3); ?Male pseudohermaphroditism due to defective LH (1)
19q13.4	RP11	C	Retinitis pigmentosa-11, autosomal dominant	600138	Retinitis pigmentosa-11 (2)
19q13.4	TNNI3	C	Troponin-I, cardiac	191044	Cardiomyopathy, familial hypertrophic (3)
Chr.19	EEC2	P	Ectrodactyly, ectodermal dysplasia, cleft lip/palate-2	602077	Ectrodactyly, ectodermal dysplasia, cleft lip/palate-2 (2)
20pter-p12	PRNP, PRIP	C	Prion protein (p27-30)	176640	Creutzfeldt-Jakob disease, 123400 (3); Gerstmann-Straussler disease, 137440 (3); Insomnia, fatal familial (3)
20p13	AVP, AVRP, VP	C	Arginine vasopressin (neurophysin II, antidiuretic hormone)	192340	Diabetes insipidus, neurohypophyseal, 125700 (3)
20p13	CHED2	C	Congenital hereditary endothelial dystrophy of cornea	121700	Congenital hereditary endothelial dystrophy of cornea (2)
20p13-p12.3	NBIA1	P	Neurodegeneration with brain iron accumulation 1 (Hallervorden-Spatz syndrome)	234200	Neurodegeneration with brain iron accumulation (2)
20p12	BMP2, BMP2A	C	Bone morphogenetic protein-2	112261	?Fibrodysplasia ossificans progressiva (1)
20p12	MKKS, HMCS, KMS, MKS	P	Hydrometrocolpos (McKusick-Kaufman syndrome)	236700	McKusick-Kaufman syndrome (2)
20p12	JAG1, AGS, AHD	C	Jagged 1	601920	Alagille syndrome, 118450 (3)
20p11.2	CST3	C	Cystatin C	604312	Cerebral amyloid angiopathy, 105150 (3)
20p11.2	THBD, THRM	C	Thrombomodulin	188040	Thrombophilia due to thrombomodulin defect (3); {Myocardial infarction, susceptibility to} (3)
20p11.2-q11.2	PPCD, PPD	P	Posterior polymorphous corneal dystrophy	122000	Corneal dystrophy, posterior polymorphous (2)
20p	HLN1	P	Huntington-like neurodegenerative disorder 1	603218	Huntington-like disorder 1 (2)
20p	ITPA	C	Inosine triphosphatase-A	147520	[Inosine triphosphatase deficiency] (1)
20q11.2	CDAN2, HEMPAS	P	Congenital dyserythropoietic anemia II	224100	Congenital dyserythropoietic anemia II (2)
20q11.2	DNMT3B, ICF	C	DNA methyltransferase 3B	602900	Immunodeficiency-centromeric instability-facial anomalies syndrome, 242860 (3)
20q11.2	GDF5, CDMP1	P	Growth/differentiation factor-5 (cartilage-derived morphogenetic protein-1)	601146	Acromesomelic dysplasia, Hunter-Thompson type, 201250 (3); Brachydactyly, type C, 113100 (3); Chondrodysplasia, Grebe type, 200700 (3)
20q11.2	GHRH, GHRF	C	Growth hormone releasing hormone (somatocrinin)	139190	?Isolated growth hormone deficiency due to defect in GHRF (1); Gigantism due to GHRF hypersecretion (1)
20q11.2	GSS, GSHS	P	Glutathione synthetase	601002	Hemolytic anemia due to glutathione synthetase deficiency, 231900 (3); 5-oxoprolinuria, 266130 (3)
20q12-q13	SRC, ASV, SRC1	C	Protooncogene SRC, Rous sarcoma	190090	Colon cancer, advanced (3)

Table A1-2 (Continued)

Location	Symbol	Status	Locus Name	MIM#	Disorder
20q12-q13.1	HNF4A, TCF14, MODY1	C	Hepatocyte nuclear factor 4, alpha (transcription factor-14)	600281	MODY, type 1, 125850 (3); {Diabetes mellitus, noninsulin-dependent}, 125853 (3)
20q12-q13.1	NIDDM3	P	Noninsulin-dependent diabetes mellitus 3	603694	Diabetes mellitus, noninsulin-dependent, 3 (2)
20q13.1	PPGB, GSL, NGBE, GLB2, CTSA	C	Protective protein for beta-galactosidase (cathepsin A)	256540	Galactosialidosis (3)
20q13.11	ADA	C	Adenosine deaminase	102700	Severe combined immunodeficiency due to ADA deficiency (3); Hemolytic anemia due to ADA excess (1)
20q13.11	GRD2	C	Graves disease, susceptibility to, 2	603388	{Graves disease, susceptibility to, 2} (2)
20q13.11-q13.2	OQTL	C	Obesity quantitative trait locus (Obesity susceptibility locus on chromosome 20)	602025	{Obesity/hyperinsulinism, susceptibility to} (2)
20q13.2	GNAS1, GNAS, GPSA	C	Guanine nucleotide-binding protein (G protein), alpha-stimulating activity polypeptide-1	139320	Pseudohypoparathyroidism, type Ia, 103580 (3); McCune-Albright polyostotic fibrous dysplasia, 174800 (3); Somatotrophinoma (3); Pituitary ACTH secreting adenoma (3)
20q13.2-q13.3	CHRNA4, ENFL1	C	Cholinergic receptor, nicotinic, alpha polypeptide-4	118504	Epilepsy, nocturnal frontal lobe, 600513 (3)
20q13.2-q13.3	EDN3	C	Endothelin-3	131242	Shah-Waardenburg syndrome, 277580 (3)
20q13.3	COL9A3, EDM3	C	Collagen IX, alpha-3 polypeptide	120270	Epiphyseal dysplasia, multiple, 3, 600969 (3); Epiphyseal dysplasia, multiple, with myopathy (3)
20q13.3	KCNQ2, EBN1	C	Potassium voltage-gated channel, KQT-like subfamily, member 2	602235	Epilepsy, benign, neonatal, type 1, 121200 (3)
20q13.3	PHP1B	P	Pseudohypoparathyroidism, type IB	603233	Pseudohypoparathyroidism, type IB (2)
20q13.31	PCK1	C	Phosphoenolpyruvate carboxykinase-1 (soluble)	261680	?Hypoglycemia due to PCK1 deficiency (1)
21q11.2	TAM, MST	P	Myeloproliferative syndrome, transient (transient abnormal myelopoiesis)	159595	Leukemia, transient, of Down syndrome (2)
21q21	APP, AAA, CVAP, AD1	C	Amyloid beta (A4) precursor protein	104760	Amyloidosis, cerebroarterial, Dutch type (3); Alzheimer disease-1, APP-related (3); Schizophrenia, chronic (3)
21q21	PRSS7, ENTK	P	Protease, serine, 7 (enterokinase)	226200	Enterokinase deficiency (1)
21q21	USH1E	P	Usher syndrome-1E, autosomal recessive, severe	602097	Usher syndrome, type 1E (2)
21q22.1	HLCS, HCS	C	Holocarbyoxylase synthetase	253270	Multiple carboxylase deficiency, biotin-responsive (3)
21q22.1	KCNE2, MIRP1	P	Potassium voltage-gated channel, Isk-related family, member 2	603796	Long QT syndrome-6 (3)
21q22.1	SOD1, ALS1	C	Superoxide dismutase-1, soluble	147450	Amytrophic lateral sclerosis, due to SOD1 deficiency, 105400 (3)
21q22.1-q22.2	IFNGR2, IFNGT1, IFGR2	C	Interferon gamma receptor-2 (interferon gamma transducer 1)	147569	Mycobacterial infection, atypical, familial disseminated, 209950 (3)
21q22.1-q22.2	KCNE1, JLNS, LQT5	C	Potassium voltage-gated channel, Isk-related subfamily, member 1	176261	Jervell and Lange-Nielsen syndrome, 220400 (3); Long QT syndrome-5 (3)
21q22.3	AIRE, APECED	C	Autoimmune regulator	240300	Autoimmune polyglandular disease, type I (3)
21q22.3	CBS	C	Cystathionine beta-synthase	236200	Homocystinuria, B6-responsive and nonresponsive types (3)
21q22.3	COL6A1	C	Collagen VI, alpha-1 polypeptide	120220	Bethlem myopathy, 158810 (3)
21q22.3	COL6A2	C	Collagen VI, alpha-2 polypeptide	120240	Bethlem myopathy, 158810 (3)
21q22.3	CRYAA, CRYA1	C	Crystallin, alpha A	123580	Cataract, congenital, autosomal dominant (3)

(Continued on next page)

Table A1-2 (Continued)

Location	Symbol	Status	Locus Name	MIM#	Disorder
21q22.3	CSTB, STFB, EPM1	P	Cystatin B (stefin B)	601145	Epilepsy, progressive myoclonic 1, 254800 (3)
21q22.3	DFNB8	P	Deafness, autosomal recessive 8	601072	Deafness, autosomal recessive 8 (2)
21q22.3	DCR, DSCR	C	Down syndrome chromosome region	190685	Down syndrome (1)
21q22.3	HPE1	P	Holoprosencephaly-1, alobar	236100	Holoprosencephaly-1 (2)
21q22.3	ITGB2, CD18, LCAMB, LAD	C	Integrin, beta-2 (antigen CD18 (p95), lymphocyte function-associated antigen-1; macrophage antigen, beta polypeptide)	600065	Leukocyte adhesion deficiency, 116920 (3)
21q22.3	KNO, KS	P	Knobloch syndrome	267750	Knobloch syndrome (2)
21q22.3	PFKL	C	Phosphofructokinase, liver type	171860	Hemolytic anemia due to phosphofructokinase deficiency (1)
21q22.3	RUNX1, CBFA2, AML1	C	Runt-related transcription factor 1 (aml1 oncogene)	151385	Leukemia, acute myeloid (1); Platelet disorder, familial, with associated myeloid malignancy, 601399 (3)
22q11	CECR, CES	C	Cat eye syndrome	115470	Cat eye syndrome (2)
22q11	CTHM	L	Conotruncal cardiac anomalies	217095	?Conotruncal cardiac anomalies (2)
22q11	DGCR, DGS, VCF	C	DiGeorge syndrome chromosome region (velocardiofacial syndrome)	188400	DiGeorge syndrome (2); Velocardiofacial syndrome, 192430 (2)
22q11	HCF2, HC2	C	Heparin cofactor II	142360	Thrombophilia due to heparin cofactor II deficiency (3)
22q11	NAGA	C	Acetylgalactosaminidase, alpha-N- (alpha-galactosidase B)	104170	Schindler disease (3); Kanzaki disease (3); NAGA deficiency, mild (3)
22q11	SMARCB1, SNF5, INI1, RDT	C	SWI/SNF related, matrix associated, actin dependent regulator of chromatin, subfamily b, member 1	601607	Rhabdoid tumors (3); Rhabdoid predisposition syndrome, familial (3)
22q11-q12	FPEVF	P	Epilepsy, partial, with variable foci	604364	Epilepsy, partial, with variable foci (2)
22q11-q13	SCZD4	P	Schizophrenia susceptibility locus, chromosome 22-related	600850	{Schizophrenia}, 181500 (2)
22q11.1-q11.2	GGT1, GTG	C	Gamma-glutamyltransferase-1	231950	Glutathioninuria (1)
22q11.1	GGT2	P	Gamma-glutamyltransferase-2	137181	[Gamma-glutamyltransferase, familial high serum] (2)
22q11.2	GP1BB	C	Glycoprotein Ib, platelet, beta polypeptide	138720	Bernard-Soulier syndrome, type B, 231200 (2); Giant platelet disorder, isolated (3)
22q11.2	OGS2, BBBG2, GBBB2	C	Opitz G syndrome, type II	145410	Opitz G syndrome, type II (2)
22q11.2	PRODH	C	Proline dehydrogenase (proline oxidase)	239500	Hyperprolinemia, type I (1)
22q11.2-q12.2	CRYBB2, CRYB2	C	Crystallin, beta-B2	123620	Cataract, cerulean, type 2, 601547 (3)
22q11.2-qter	TCN2, TC2	C	Transcobalamin II	275350	Transcobalamin II deficiency (3)
22q11.21	BCR, CML, PHL	C	Breakpoint cluster region	151410	Leukemia, chronic myeloid (3)
22q12	EWSR1, EWS	C	Ewing sarcoma breakpoint region-1	133450	Ewing sarcoma (3); Neuroepithelioma (2)
22q12	HMOX1	C	Heme oxygenase, decycling, 1	141250	Heme oxygenase-1 deficiency (3)
22q12.1	CHK2, RAD53	P	Checkpoint kinase 2	604373	Li-Fraumeni syndrome, 151623 (3)
22q12.1-q13.2	FTNS	P	Fechtner syndrome	153640	Fechtner syndrome (2)
22q12.1-q13.2	TIMP3, SFD	C	Tissue inhibitor of metalloproteinase-3	188826	Sorsby fundus dystrophy, 136900 (3)
22q12.2	NEFH	C	Neurofilament, heavy polypeptide	162230	{Amyotrophic lateral sclerosis, susceptibility to}, 105400 (3)
22q12.2	NF2	C	Neurofibromatosis-2 (bilateral acoustic neuroma); merlin	101000	Neurofibromatosis, type 2 (3); Meningioma, NF2-related, sporadic (3) Schwannoma, sporadic (3); Neurolemmomatosis (3); Malignant mesothelioma, sporadic (3)

Table A1-2 (Continued)

Location	Symbol	Status	Locus Name	MIM#	Disorder
22q12.2-q13.1	CSF2RB	P	Colony-stimulating factor-2 receptor, beta, low-affinity	138981	Pulmonary alveolar proteinosis, 265120 (3)
22q12.2-q13.3	DFNA17	P	Deafness, autosomal dominant 17	603622	Deafness, autosomal dominant 17 (2)
22q12.3-q13.1	LARGE	P	Acetylglucosaminyltransferase-like protein	603590	?Meningioma (2)
22q12.3-q13.1	PDGFB, SIS	C	Platelet-derived growth factor, beta polypeptide (oncogene SIS)	190040	Meningioma, SIS-related (3); Dermatofibrosarcoma protuberans (3); Giant-cell fibroblastoma (3)
22q12.3-q13.2	MHA	P	May-Hegglin anomaly	155100	May-Hegglin anomaly (2)
22q12.3-qter	MGCR, MN1	P	Meningioma chromosome region	156100	Meningioma (2)
22q13	EP300	P	E1A-binding protein, 300 kD	602700	Colorectal cancer, 114500 (3)
22q13	SCA10	P	Spinocerebellar ataxia 10	603516	Spinocerebellar ataxia-10 (2)
22q13	SCO2	P	SCO2, S. cerevisiae, homolog of	604272	Cardioencephalomyopathy, fatal infantile, due to cytochrome c oxidase deficiency, 604377 (3)
22q13	SOX10, WS4	C	SRY (sex-determining region Y)-box-10	602229	Waardenburg-Shah syndrome, 277580 (3); Yemenite deaf-blind hypopigmentation syndrome, 601706 (3)
22q13-qter	ACR	P	Acrosin	102480	?Male infertility due to acrosin deficiency (2)
22q13.1	ADSL	C	Adenylosuccinate lyase	103050	Adenylosuccinase deficiency (1); Autism, succinylpurinemic (3)
22q13.1	CYP2D@, CYP2D, P450C2D	C	Cytochrome P450, subfamily IID	124030	{?Parkinsonism, susceptibility to} (1); Debrisoquine sensitivity (3)
22q13.1	SLC5A1, SGLT1	C	Solute carrier family 5 (sodium/glucose transporter), member 1	182380	Glucose/galactose malabsorption (3)
22q13.31-qter	ARSA	C	Arylsulfatase A	250100	Metachromatic leukodystrophy (3)
22q13.31-qter	DIA1	C	Diaphorase (NADH); cytochrome b-5 reductase	250800	Methemoglobinemia, type I (3); Methemoglobinemia, type II (3)
22q13.32-qter	ECGF1	C	Endothelial cell growth factor-1, platelet-derived	131222	Myoneurogastrointestinal encephalomyopathy syndrome, 603041 (3)
Xpter-p22.32	SHOX, GCFX, SS, PHOG	C	Growth control factor, X-linked (pseudoautosomal homeo box-containing osteogenic gene)	312865	Short stature, idiopathic familial (3); Leri-Weill dyschondrosteosis, 127300 (3); Langer mesomelic dysplasia, 249700 (3)
Xpter-p22.32	HDPA	P	Hodgkin disease, susceptibility, pseudoautosomal	300221	{Hodgkin disease susceptibility, pseudoautosomal} (2)
Xp22.32	CSF2RA	C	Colony-stimulating factor-2 receptor, alpha, low-affinity, granulocyte-macrophage	306250	Leukemia, acute myeloid, M2 type (1)
Xp22.32	STS, ARSC1, ARSC, SSDD	C	Steroid sulfatase, microsomal (arylsulfatase C, isozyme S)	308100	Ichthyosis, X-linked (3); Placental steroid sulfatase deficiency (3)
Xp22.31	MLS, MIDAS	P	Microphthalmia with linear skin defects	309801	Microphthalmia with linear skin defects (2); Microphthalmia, dermal aplasia, and sclerocornea (2)
Xp22.3	ARSE, CDPX1, CDPXR	C	Arylsulfatase E	300180	Chondrodysplasia punctata, X-linked recessive, 302950 (3); Chondrodysplasia punctata, brachytelephalangic, 302940 (3)
Xp22.3	EMWX	P	Episodic muscle weakness, X-linked	300211	Episodic muscle weakness, X-linked (2)
Xp22.3	KAL1, KMS, ADMLX	C	Kallmann syndrome-1 sequence (anosmin-1)	308700	Kallmann syndrome (3)
Xp22.3	MRX49	C	Mental retardation, X-linked-49	300114	Mental retardation, X-linked-49 (2)
Xp22.3	OA1	C	Ocular albinism-1, Nettleship-Falls type	300500	Ocular albinism, Nettleship-Falls type (3)
Xp22.3	OASD	P	Ocular albinism and sensorineural deafness	300650	Ocular albinism with sensorineural deafness (2)
Xp22.3-p22.2	OFD1	C	Oral-facial-digital syndrome 1	311200	Oral-facial-digital syndrome 1 (2)

(Continued on next page)

Table A1-2 (Continued)

Location	Symbol	Status	Locus Name	MIM#	Disorder
Xp22.3-p22.1	AMELX, AMG, AIH1, AMGX	C	Amelogenin	301200	Amelogenesis imperfecta (3)
Xp22.3-p21.3	MRX29	P	Mental retardation, X-linked-29	300077	Mental retardation, X-linked 29 (2)
Xp22.3-p21.1	NHS	C	Nance-Horan cataract-dental syndrome	302350	Nance-Horan syndrome (2)
Xp22.3-p21.1	POLA	C	Polymerase (DNA directed), alpha	312040	?N syndrome, 310465 (1)
Xp22.2	CMTX2	P	Charcot-Marie-Tooth disease, X-linked-2, recessive	302801	Charcot-Marie-Tooth neuropathy, X-linked-2, recessive (2)
Xp22.2	FCP1, FCPX, FCP	P	F-cell production 1	305435	Heterocellular hereditary persistence of fetal hemoglobin, Swiss type (2)
Xp22.2-p22.13	KFSD	C	Keratosis follicularis spinulosa decalvans	308800	Keratosis follicularis spinulosa decalvans (2)
Xp22.2-p22.1	PDHA1, PHE1A	C	Pyruvate dehydrogenase, E1-alpha polypeptide-1	312170	Pyruvate dehydrogenase deficiency (3)
Xp22.2-p22.1	PHEX, HYP, HPDR1	C	Phosphate regulating gene with homologies to endopeptidases on the X chromosome	307800	Hypophosphatemia, hereditary (3)
Xp22.2-p22.1	PHKA2, PHK	C	Phosphorylase kinase deficiency, liver (glycogen storage disease type VIII)	306000	Glycogenosis, X-linked hepatic, type I (3); Glycogenosis, X-linked hepatic, type II (3)
Xp22.2-p22.1	PRTS, MRXS1	P	Partington syndrome (mental retardation, X-linked, syndromic-1, with dystonic movements, ataxia, and seizures)	309510	Mental retardation, X-linked, syndromic-1, with dystonic movements, ataxia, and seizures (2)
Xp22.2-p22.1	RPS6KA3, RSK2, MRX19	C	Ribosomal protein S6 kinase, 90 kD, polypeptide 3	300075	Coffin-Lowry syndrome, 303600 (3); Mental retardation, X-linked nonspecific, type 19 (3)
Xp22.2-p22.1	RS1, XLRS1	C	Retinoschisis	312700	Retinoschisis (3)
Xp22.2-p22.1	SEDL, SEDT	C	Sedlin	300202	Spondyloepiphyseal dysplasia tarda, 313400 (3)
Xp22.13-p22.11	RP15	P	Retinitis pigmentosa-15	300029	Retinitis pigmentosa-15 (2)
Xp22.13-p21.1	MEHMO	P	MEHMO syndrome (Mental retardation, epileptic seizures, hypogonadism and hypogenitalism, microcephaly, and obesity)	300148	MEHMO syndrome (2)
Xp22.11-p21.2	GDXY, TDFX, SRVX	P	Gonadal dysgenesis, XY female type	306100	Gonadal dysgenesis, XY female type (2)
Xp22.1	PIGA	P	Phosphatidylinositol glycan, class A	311770	Paroxysmal nocturnal hemoglobinuria (3)
Xp22.1-p21.3	IL1RAPL, MRX1, MRX21	C	Il-1 receptor accessory protein-like	300206	Mental retardation, X-linked 1, non-dysmorphic, 309530 (3)
Xp22.1-p21.3	ISSX	C	Infantile spasm syndrome, X-linked	308350	Infantile spasm syndrome, X-linked (2)
Xp22	AGMX2, XLA2, IMD6	P	Agammaglobulinemia, X-linked 2 (with growth hormone deficiency)	300310	Agammaglobulinemia, type 2, X-linked (2)
Xp22	AIC	C	Aicardi syndrome	304050	Aicardi syndrome (2)
Xp22	CFNS, CFND	C	Craniofrontonasal syndrome	304110	Craniofrontonasal dysplasia (2)
Xp22	DFN6	P	Deafness, X-linked 6, sensorineural	300066	Deafness, X-linked 6, sensorineural (2)
Xp22	MID1, OGS1, BBBG1, GBBB1, OSX	C	Midline-1	300000	Opitz G syndrome, type I (3)
Xp22	SGBS2	P	Simpson-Golabi-Behmel syndrome, type 2	300209	Simpson-Golabi-Behmel syndrome, type 2 (2)
Xp22-p21	PDR	P	Pigment disorder, reticulate	301220	Partington syndrome II (2)
Xp22-q12	MRX58	P	Mental retardation, X-linked nonspecific, 58	300210	Mental retardation, X-linked nonspecific, 58 (2)
Xp21.3-p21.2	DAX1, AHC, AHX, NROB1	C	DSS-AHC critical region on the X chromosome, gene 1	300200	Adrenal hypoplasia, congenital, with hypogonadotropic hypogonadism (3); Dosage-sensitive sex reversal, 300018 (3)
Xp21.3-p21.2	GK	C	Glycerol kinase deficiency	307030	Glycerol kinase deficiency (3)

Table A1-2 (Continued)

Location	Symbol	Status	Locus Name	MIM#	Disorder
Xp21.3-p21.2	RP6	L	Retinitis pigmentosa-6, X-linked recessive	312612	?Retinitis pigmentosa-6 (2)
Xp21.2	DFN4	C	Deafness 4, congenital sensorineural	300030	Deafness, X-linked 4, congenital sensorineural (2)
Xp21.2	DMD, BMD	C	Dystrophin (muscular dystrophy, Duchenne and Becker types)	310200	Duchenne muscular dystrophy (3); Becker muscular dystrophy (3); Cardiomyopathy, dilated, X-linked (3)
Xp21.2-p21.1	XK	C	Kell blood group precursor	314850	McLeod phenotype (3)
Xp21.1	CYBB, CGD	C	Cytochrome b-245, beta polypeptide	306400	Chronic granulomatous disease, X-linked (3)
Xp21.1	OTC	C	Ornithine transcarbamylase	311250	Ornithine transcarbamylase deficiency (3)
Xp21.1	RPGR, RP3, CRD	P	Retinitis pigmentosa GTPase regulator	312610	Retinitis pigmentosa-3 (3)
Xp21.1-q22	WTS, MRXS6	P	Wilson-Turner syndrome (mental retardation, X-linked, syndromic-6, with gynecomastia and obesity)	309585	Mental retardation, X-linked, syndromic-6, with gynecomastia and obesity (2)
Xp21	GTD	L	Gonadotropin deficiency	306190	?Gonadotropin deficiency (2); ?Cryptorchidism (2)
Xp21	SRS, MRSR	P	Snyder-Robinson X-linked mental retardation syndrome	309583	Mental retardation, Snyder-Robinson type (2)
Xp21-q13	MRX9	P	Mental retardation, X-linked-9	309549	Mental retardation, X-linked 9 (2)
Xp11.4	COD1, PCDX	C	Cone dystrophy-1, X-linked	304020	Cone dystrophy, progressive X-linked, 1 (2)
Xp11.4	NDP, ND	C	Norrin	310600	Norrie disease (3); Exudative vitreoretinopathy, X-linked, 305390 (3); Coats disease, 300216 (3)
Xp11.4-p11.23	AIED, OA2	C	Aland island eye disease (ocular albinism, Forsius-Eriksson type)	300600	Ocular albinism, Forsius-Eriksson type (2)
Xp11.4-p11.23	PFC, PFD	C	Properdin P factor, complement	312060	Properdin deficiency, X-linked (3)
Xp11.4-p11.21	OPA2	P	Optic atrophy, X-linked	311050	Optic atrophy, X-linked (2)
Xp11.4-p11.2	RENS1, MRXS8	P	Renpenning syndrome-1	309500	Renpenning syndrome-1 (2)
Xp11.4	CSNB1	C	Congenital stationary night blindness-1 (CSNB, complete)	310500	Night blindness, congenital stationary, type 1 (2)
Xp11.3	RP2	C	Retinitis pigmentosa-2, X-linked recessive	312600	Retinitis pigmentosa-2 (2)
Xp11.3-p11.21	MRX50	P	Mental retardation, X-linked nonspecific, type 50	300115	Mental retardation, X-linked nonspecific, type 50 (2)
Xp11.3-q11.2	AMCX1	P	Arthrogryposis multiplex congenita, X-linked (spinal muscular atrophy, infantile, X-linked)	301830	Arthrogryposis, X-linked (spinal muscular atrophy, infantile, X-linked) (2)
Xp11.3-q13.3	MRX14	P	Mental retardation, X-linked-14	300062	Mental retardation, X-linked 14 (2)
Xp11.3-q22	MRXS7	P	Mental retardation, X-linked, syndromic 7	300218	Mental retardation, X-linked, syndromic 7 (2)
Xp11.23	CACNA1F, CSNB2	P	Calcium channel, voltage-dependent, alpha-1F subunit	300110	Night blindness, congenital stationary, X-linked, type 2, 300071 (3)
Xp11.23	GATA1, GF1, ERYF1, NFE1	C	GATA-binding protein-1 (globin transcription factor-1)	305371	Dyserythropoietic anemia with thrombocytopenia (3)
Xp11.23	MAOA	C	Monoamine oxidase A	309850	Brunner syndrome (3)
Xp11.23-p11.22	EBP, CDPX2, CPXD, CPX	P	Emopamil-binding protein	300205	Chondrodysplasia punctata, X-linked dominant, 302960 (3)
Xp11.23-p11.22	WAS, IMD2, THC	C	Wiskott-Aldrich syndrome	301000	Wiskott-Aldrich syndrome (3); Thrombocytopenia, X-linked, 313900 (3)
Xp11.23-q21.1	AIID	P	Autoimmunity-immunodeficiency syndrome, X-linked	304930	Autoimmunity-immunodeficiency syndrome, X-linked (2)

(Continued on next page)

Table A1-2 (Continued)

Location	Symbol	Status	Locus Name	MIM#	Disorder
Xp11.22	CLCN5, CLCK2, NPHL2, DENTS	C	Chloride channel-5	300008	Dent disease, 300009 (3); Nephrolithiasis, type I, 310468 (3); Hypophosphatemia, type III (3); Proteinuria, low molecular weight, with hypercalciuric nephrocalcinosis (3)
Xp11.21	ALAS2, ASB, ANH1	C	Aminolevulinate, delta-, synthase-2	301300	Anemia, sideroblastic/ hypochromic (3)
Xp11.21	FGD1, FGDY, AAS	C	Faciogenital dysplasia (Aarskog-Scott syndrome)	305400	Aarskog-Scott syndrome (3)
Xp11.2	CAMR, MRXS10	P	Chorioathetosis with mental retardation and abnormal behavior	300220	Chorioathetosis with mental retardation and abnormal behavior (2)
Xp11.2	RCCP2	C	Renal cell carcinoma, papillary	312390	Renal cell carcinoma, papillary, 2 (2)
Xp11.2	SSX1, SSRC	C	Synovial sarcoma, X breakpoint 1	312820	Sarcoma, synovial (3)
Xp11.2	SSX2	P	Sarcoma, synovial, X breakpoint 2	300192	Sarcoma, synovial (1)
Xp11	IDDMX	P	Diabetes mellitus, insulin-dependent, X-linked, susceptibility to	300136	{Diabetes mellitus, insulin-dependent, X-linked} (2) (2)
Xp11	MRXA	L	Mental retardation, X-linked nonspecific, with aphasia	309545	?Mental retardation, X-linked nonspecific, with aphasia (2)
Xp11-q21	MRX20	P	Mental retardation, X-linked-20	300047	Mental retardation, X-linked 20 (2)
Xp11-q21	PRS, MRXS2	P	Prieto syndrome (mental retardation, X-linked, syndromic-2, with dysmorphism and cerebral atrophy)	309610	Mental retardation, X-linked, syndromic-2, with dysmorphism and cerebral atrophy (2)
Xp11-q21.3	SHS, MRXS3	P	Sutherland-Haan syndrome (mental retardation, X-linked, syndromic-3, with spastic diplegia)	309470	Mental retardation, X-linked, syndromic-3, with spastic diplegia (2)
Xp	CCT	L	Cataracts, congenital total	302200	?Cataract, congenital total (2)
Xp	SMAX2	P	Spinal muscular atrophy, X-linked lethal infantile	300021	Spinal muscular atrophy, X-linked lethal infantile (2)
Xq	CGF1	P	Cognitive function-1, social	300082	[Social cognition] (2)
Xq	MFTS	P	Migraine, familial typical, susceptibility to	300125	{Migraine, familial typical, susceptibility to, 1} (2)
Xq11	TM4SF2, MXS1, A15	C	Transmembrane 4 superfamily, member 2	300096	Mental retardation, X-linked nonspecific (3)
Xq11-q12	AR, DHTR, TFM, SBMA, KD	C	Androgen receptor (dihydrotestosterone receptor)	313700	Androgen insensitivity, several forms, 300068 (3); Spinal and bulbar muscular atrophy of Kennedy, 313200 (3); Prostate cancer (3); Perineal hypospadias (3); Breast cancer, male, with Reifenstein syndrome (3)
Xq12	OPHN1	P	Oligophrenin-1	300127	Mental retardation, X-linked, 60 (3)
Xq12-q13	ATP7A, MNK, MK, OHS	C	ATPase, Cu^{++} transporting, alpha polypeptide	300011	Menkes disease, 309400 (3); Occipital horn syndrome, 304150 (3); Cutis laxa, neonatal (3)
Xq12-q13.1	ED1, EDA, HED	C	Ectodermal dysplasia-1, anhidrotic	305100	Ectodermal dysplasia-1, anhidrotic (3)
Xq12-q21.31	FGS1	C	FG syndrome 1	305450	FG syndrome (2)
Xq13	ATRX, XH2, XNP, MRXS3	C	ATR-X gene (helicase 2; X-linked nuclear protein)	300032	Alpha-thalassemia/mental retardation syndrome, 301040 (3); Juberg-Marsidi syndrome, 309590 (3); Sutherland-Haan syndrome, 309470 (3); Smith-Fineman-Myers syndrome, 309580 (3)
Xq13	IL2RG, SCIDX1, SCIDX, IMD4	C	Interleukin-2 receptor, gamma	308380	Severe combined immunodeficiency, X-linked, 300400 (3); Combined immunodeficiency, X-linked, moderate, 312863 (3)

Table A1-2 (Continued)

Location	Symbol	Status	Locus Name	MIM#	Disorder
Xq13	PGK1, PGKA	C	Phosphoglycerate kinase-1	311800	Hemolytic anemia due to PGK deficiency (3); Myoglobinuria/ hemolysis due to PGK deficiency (3)
Xq13	PHKA1	C	Phosphorylase kinase, muscle, alpha polypeptide	311870	Muscle glycogenosis (3)
Xq13-q21	WWS	P	Wieacker-Wolff syndrome	314580	Wieacker-Wolff syndrome (2)
Xq13-q22	MCS, MRXS4	P	Miles-Carpenter syndrome (mental retardation, X-linked, syndromic-4, with congenital contractures and low fingertip arches)	309605	Mental retardation, X-linked, syndromic-4, with congenital contractures and low fingertip arches (2)
Xq13.1	DYT3	C	Torsion dystonia-parkinsonism, Filipino type	314250	Dystonia-3, torsion, with parkinsonism, Filipino type (2)
Xq13.1	GJB1, CX32, CMTX1	C	Gap junction protein, beta-1, 32 kD (connexin 32)	304040	Charcot-Marie-Tooth neuropathy, X-linked-1, dominant, 302800 (3)
Xq13.1-q13.3	ABCB7, ABC7, ASAT	P	ATP-binding cassette-7	300135	Anemia, sideroblastic, with ataxia, 301310 (3)
Xq13.2	XIC, XCE, XIST	C	X chromosome controlling element (X-inactivation center)	314670	X-inactivation, familial skewed (3)
Xq21	AHDS	P	Allan-Herndon-Dudley mental retardation syndrome	309600	Allan-Herndon syndrome (2)
Xq21	POF1, POF	P	Premature ovarian failure-1	311360	Ovarian failure, premature (2)
Xq21.1	POU3F4, DFN3	P	POU domain, class 3, transcription factor 4	300039	Deafness, X-linked 3, conductive, with stapes fixation, 304400 (3)
Xq21.2-q24	ARTS	P	Arts syndrome	301835	Arts syndrome (2)
Xq21.2	CHM, TCD	C	Choroideremia	303100	Choroideremia (3)
Xq21.3	CPX	C	Cleft palate and/or ankyloglossia	303400	Cleft palate, X-linked (2)
Xq21.3-q22	BTK, AGMX1, IMD1, XLA, AT	C	Bruton agammaglobulinemia tyrosine kinase	300300	Agammaglobulinemia, type 1, X-linked (3); ?XLA and isolated growth hormone deficiency, 307200 (3)
Xq21.3-q22	MGC1, MGCN	P	Megalocornea-1, X-linked	309300	Megalocornea, X-linked (2)
Xq21.3-q24	PAK3	C	p21-activated kinase-3	300142	Mental retardation, X-linked 30 (3)
Xq22	DFN2	P	Deafness, X-linked 2, perceptive, congenital	304500	Deafness, X-linked 2, perceptive congenital (2)
Xq22	DIAPH2, DIA	C	Diaphanous, Drosophila, homolog of, 2	300108	Premature ovarian failure, 311360 (3)
Xq22	EFMR	P	Epilepsy, female restricted, with mental retardation (Juberg-Hellman syndrome)	300088	Epilepsy, female restricted, with mental retardation (2)
Xq22	GLA	C	Galactosidase, alpha	301500	Fabry disease (3)
Xq22	PLP, PMD	C	Proteolipid protein	312080	Pelizaeus-Merzbacher disease (3); Spastic paraplegia-2, 312920 (3)
Xq22	TIMM8A, DFN1, DDP, MTS, DDP1	C	Translocase of inner mitochondrial membrane 8, yeast, homolog of, A	304700	Deafness, X-linked 1, progressive (3); Mohr-Tranebjaerg syndrome (3); Jensen syndrome, 311150 (3)
Xq22-q24	PRPS1	C	Phosphoribosyl pyrophosphate synthetase-1	311850	Phosphoribosyl pyrophosphate synthetase-related gout (3)
Xq22-q28	AIH3	L	Amelogenesis imperfecta-3, hypomaturation or hypoplastic type	301201	?Amelogenesis imperfecta-3, hypoplastic type (2)
Xq22.2	TBG	C	Thyroxine-binding globulin	314200	[Euthyroidal hyper- and hypothyroxinemia] (1)
Xq22.3	AMMECR1	P	Alport syndrome, mental retardation, midface hypoplasia, and elliptocytosis chromosomal region gene 1	300195	Alport syndrome, mental retardation, midface hypoplasia, and elliptocytosis, 300194 (2)
Xq22.3	COL4A5, ATS, ASLN	C	Collagen IV, alpha-5 polypeptide	303630	Alport syndrome, 301050 (3)
Xq22.3	COL4A6	C	Collagen IV, alpha-6 polypeptide	303631	Leiomyomatosis, diffuse, with Alport syndrome, 308940 (3)
Xq22.3-q23	DCX, DBCN, LISX	C	Doublecortin	300121	Lissencephaly, X-linked, 300067 (3); Subcortical laminal heteropia, X-linked, 300067 (3)

(Continued on next page)

Table A1-2 (Continued)

Location	Symbol	Status	Locus Name	MIM#	Disorder
Xq23-q24	MRX23	P	Mental retardation, X-linked-23	300046	Mental retardation, X-linked 23, nonspecific (2)
Xq24-q26.1	NAMSD, CMT2D, NADMR	P	Neuropathy, axonal motor-sensory, with deafness and mental retardation (Cowchock syndrome)	310490	Cowchock syndrome (2)
Xq24-q27	BZX	P	Bazex syndrome	301845	Bazex syndrome (2)
Xq24-q27.1	HTC2, HCG, CGH	P	Hypertrichosis, congenital generalized	307150	Hypertrichosis, congenital generalized (2)
Xq24-q27.1	MRGH	C	Mental retardation with isolated growth hormone deficiency	300123	Mental retardation with isolated growth hormone deficiency (2)
Xq25	SH2D1A, LYP, IMD5, XLP, XLPD	C	SH2 domain protein 1A	308240	Lymphoproliferative syndrome, X-linked (3)
Xq25-q26	PHP, GHDX, PHPX	P	Panhypopituitarism, X-linked	312000	Panhypopituitarism, X-linked (2)
Xq25-q26.1	THAS, TAS	P	Thoracoabdominal syndrome	313850	Thoracoabdominal syndrome (2)
Xq25-q27	PGS, MRXS5	P	Pettigrew syndrome (mental retardation, X-linked, with Dandy-Walker malformation, basal ganglia disease, and seizures)	304340	Mental retardation, X-linked, syndromic-5, with Dandy-Walker malformation, basal ganglia disease, and seizures (2)
Xq26	GPC3, SDYS, SGB	C	Glypican 3	300037	Simpson-Golabi-Behmel syndrome, type 1, 312870 (3)
Xq26	GUST	P	Gustavson mental retardation syndrome (with microcephaly, optic atrophy, deafness)	309555	Gustavson syndrome (2)
Xq26	SHFM2, SHFD2	P	Split hand/foot malformation, type (ectrodactyly) 2	313350	Split hand/foot malformation, type 2 (2)
Xq26	TNFSF5, CD40LG, HIGM1, IGM	C	Tumor necrosis factor ligand superfamily, member 5	308230	Immunodeficiency, X-linked, with hyper-IgM (3)
Xq26-q27	HPT, HPTX, HYPX	P	Hypoparathyroidism	307700	Hypoparathyroidism, X-linked (2)
Xq26-q27	NYS1	I	Nystagmus 1, congenital	310700	Nystagmus 1, congenital (2)
Xq26-q27	RP24	P	Retinitis pigmentosa-24	300155	Retinitis pigmentosa-24 (2)
Xq26-q27	SMRXS	P	Shashi X-linked mental retardation syndrome	300238	Mental retardation, X-linked, Shashi type (2)
Xq26-q27.2	HPRT1, HPRT	C	Hypoxanthine phosphoribosyltransferase 1	308000	Lesch-Nyhan syndrome (3); HPRT-related gout (3)
Xq26-qter	INDX	P	Immunoneurologic syndrome X-linked, of Wood, Black, and Norbury	300076	Wood neuroimmunologic syndrome (2)
Xq26.1	OCRL, LOCR, OCRL1	C	Oculocerebrorenal syndrome of Lowe	309000	Lowe syndrome (3)
Xq26.2	ZIC3, HTX1, HTX	C	Zic family member-3	306955	Heterotaxy, X-linked visceral (3)
Xq26.3	BFLS	C	Borjeson-Forssman-Lehmann syndrome	301900	Borjeson-Forssman-Lehmann syndrome (2)
Xq26.3-q27.1	ADFN, ALDS	P	Albinism-deafness syndrome	300700	Albinism-deafness syndrome (2)
Xq27	COD2	P	Cone dystrophy-2, X-linked	300085	Cone dystrophy, progressive X-linked, 2 (2)
Xq27	TGCT1	P	Testicular germ cell tumor 1	300228	Testicular germ cell tumor (2)
Xq27-q28	ANOP1	L	Anophthalmos-1 (with mental retardation but without anomalies)	301590	?Anophthalmos-1 (2)
Xq27-q28	HPCX	P	Prostate cancer, hereditary, X-linked	300147	{Prostate cancer susceptibility, X-linked} (2)
Xq27.1-q27.2	F9, HEMB	C	Coagulation factor IX (plasma thromboplastic component)	306900	Hemophilia B (3); Warfarin sensitivity (3)
Xq27.3	FMR1, FRAXA	C	Fragile X mental retardation-1	309550	Fragile X syndrome (3)
Xq28	ABCD1, ALD, AMN	C	ATP-binding cassette, subfamily D, member 1	300100	Adrenoleukodystrophy (3); Adrenomyeloneuropathy (3)
Xq28	AVPR2, DIR, DI1, ADHR	C	Arginine vasopressin receptor-2	304800	Diabetes insipidus, nephrogenic (3)
Xq28	CBBM, BCM	C	Blue-monochromatic colorblindness (blue cone monochromacy)	303700	Colorblindness, blue monochromatic (3)

Table A1-2 (Continued)

Location	Symbol	Status	Locus Name	MIM#	Disorder
Xq28	CVD1, XMVD	P	Cardiac valvular dysplasia-1 (myxomatous valvular dystrophy, X-linked)	314400	Cardiac valvular dysplasia-1 (2)
Xq28	DKC1, DKC	C	Dyskerin	300126	Dyskeratosis congenita-1, 305000 (3); Hoyeraal-Hreidarsson, 300240 (3)
Xq28	EMD, EDMD	C	Emery-Dreifuss muscular dystrophy	310300	Emery-Dreifuss muscular dystrophy (3)
Xq28	F8C, HEMA	C	Coagulation factor VIIIc, procoagulant component	306700	Hemophilia A (3)
Xq28	FLNA, FLN1, ABPX, NHBP	C	Filamin A, alpha (actin-binding protein-280)	300017	Heterotopia, periventricular, 300049 (3)
Xq28	FMR2, FRAXE, MRX2	P	Fragile site, X-linked, E	309548	Mental retardation, X-linked, FRAXE type (3)
Xq28	FRAXF	P	Fragile site, folic acid type, rare, fra(X)(q28)	300031	Mental retardation, X-linked, FRAXF type (3)
Xq28	G6PD, G6PD1	C	Glucose-6-phosphate dehydrogenase	305900	G6PD deficiency (3); Favism (3); Hemolytic anemia due to G6PD deficiency (3)
Xq28	GDI1, RABGD1A, MRX41, MRX48	P	GDP dissociation inhibitor 1	300104	Mental retardation, X-linked nonspecific, 309541 (3)
Xq28	HMS1, GAY1	L	Homosexuality, male	306995	[?Homosexuality, male] (2)
Xq28	GCP, CBD	C	Green cone pigment	303800	Colorblindness, deutan (3)
Xq28	IDS, MPS2, SIDS	C	Iduronate 2-sulfatase (Hunter syndrome)	309900	Mucopolysaccharidosis II (3)
Xq28	IP2	C	Incontinentia pigmenti-2, familial, male-lethal type	308310	Incontinentia pigmenti, familial (2)
Xq28	IPOX, CIIPX	P	Intestinal pseudoobstruction, neuronal, primary idiopathic	300048	Intestinal pseudoobstruction, neuronal, X-linked (2)
Xq28	L1CAM, CAML1, HSAS1	C	L1 cell adhesion molecule	308840	Hydrocephalus due to aqueductal stenosis, 307000 (3); MASA syndrome, 303350 (3); Spastic paraplegia, 312900 (3)
Xq28	MAFD2, MDX	L	Major affective disorder-2	309200	?Manic-depressive illness, X-linked (2)
Xq28	MECP2, RTT	C	Methyl-CpG-binding protein-2	300005	Rett syndrome, 312750 (3)
Xq28	MRSD, CHRS	P	Mental retardation-skeletal dysplasia	309620	Mental retardation-skeletal dysplasia (2)
Xq28	MTM1, MTMX	C	Myotubularin	310400	Myotubular myopathy, X-linked (3)
Xq28	MYP1, BED	P	Myopia, X-linked (Bornholm eye disease)	310460	Myopia-1 (2); Bornholm eye disease (2)
Xq28	OPD1	P	Otopalatodigital syndrome, type I	311300	Otopalatodigital syndrome, type I (2)
Xq28	PPMX	P	Mental retardation with psychosis, pyramidal signs, and macroorchidism	300055	Mental retardation with psychosis, pyramidal signs, and macroorchidism (2)
Xq28	RCP, CBP	C	Red cone pigment	303900	Colorblindness, protan (3)
Xq28	TAZ, EFE2, BTHS, CMD3A	C	Tafazzin	302060	Endocardial fibroelastosis-2 (2); Barth syndrome (3); Cardiomyopathy, X-linked dilated, 300069 (3); Noncompaction of left ventricular myocardium, isolated, 300183 (3)
Xq28	TKCR, TKC	C	Torticollis, keloids, cryptorchidism and renal dysplasia	314300	Goeminne TKCR syndrome (2)
Xq28	TKTL1, TKT2, TKR	P	Transketolase-like 1	300044	{?Wernicke-Korsakoff syndrome, susceptibility to} (1)
Xq28	WSN, BGMR	P	Waisman syndrome (basal ganglion disorder with mental retardation)	311510	Waisman parkinsonism-mental retardation syndrome (2)
Chr.X	CLA2, OPCA	P	Cerebellar ataxia-2	302500	Cerebellar ataxia-2 (2)
Yp11.3	SRY, TDF	C	Sex-determining region Y (testis determining factor)	480000	Gonadal dysgenesis, XY type (3)
Yq11	AZF1, SP3	C	Azoospermia factor 1	415000	?Sertoli-cell-only syndrome (1)
Yq11	DAZ	P	Deleted in azoospermia	400003	?Sertoli-cell-only syndrome (1)
Yq11.2	USP9Y, DFFRY	P	Ubiquitin-specific protease-9, Y chromosome (Drosophila fat facets related, Y-linked)	400005	Azoospermia (3)

APPENDIX 1-2

Mutation Databases: Overview and Catalogues

Rania Horaitis ■ Charles R. Scriver ■ Richard G.H. Cotton

Genetics is the study of inheritance, genomics is the study of genomes,[1] and mutations, or nucleotide changes, occur at the interface between the two. Mutations are the source of genetic variation and diversity, and by their effect some are pathogenic while others are neutral. By definition, the majority of mutations documented in this eighth edition of *The Metabolic and Molecular Bases of Inherited Disease* are pathogenic.

As the genome projects enter the final stages of their structural phases, they will yield integrated chromosomal, genetic, and physical maps for the host organisms. In the poststructural era, genomics will continue as "functional genomics"; a new term describing the old domains of, for example, embryology, physiology, biochemistry, and pathology. Meanwhile, structural genomics will benefit from cross-referencing of genes in different species[2] and, in this regard, "expression genomics"[3] is relevant because it will include systematic analysis and documentation of gene expression in organisms while revealing patterns of host gene expression, in natural and mutant states, and in organs, tissues, and cell types during development and at maturity of the organism. All of this presupposes knowledge of individual genes and the corresponding knowledge bases. Genomes, mutations, and the Internet have come together.[4]

If a typical human locus contains 100 different alleles—a reasonable estimate based on current information—then the human genome containing an estimated 35,000–120,000 genes or, for the sake of argument, 80,000 genes[5] will harbor at least 8 million different alleles. Informatics is necessary to capture, record, and distribute information of this magnitude about variation in the human or any other genome. The HUGO Mutation Database Initiative[6] (http://ariel.ucs.unimelb.edu.au:80/~cotton/mdi.htm) is a significant initiative to catalogue, store, and deploy data about genetic variation, primarily human in nature. Mutation databases will thus be essential resources for the era of functional genomics.

ALLELES

The tools for mutation detection,[7–9] which include scanning and diagnostic methods, are enhancing the rate of discovery which, in the human genome, already exceeds the ability of the print literature to keep pace. Mutational databases thus serve both as tools for biologic taxonomy and as respositories for essential genetic data. Accordingly, "*in silico* genetics" is the latest step in the journey of modern human genetics whose milestones, as Victor McKusick has noted, include cytogenetics, somatic cell genetics, molecular genetics, and transgenic manipulation.

The term *mutation* is understood in many ways. Here we use it to mean allelic variant, explained by a variation in DNA nucleotide sequence. The allele might be disease causing, or pathogenic, and modify phenotype (see "Proof of Causation" below); or it might be neutral without apparent effect on gene expression and phenotype. The frequency of pathogenic alleles tends to be low in human populations ($q < 0.01$), while neutral alleles, or those that confer a selective advantage, tend to occur at higher frequency, and are designated polymorphic when q exceeds 0.01. Because a polymorphic allele might either modify parent gene expression under certain circumstances, or simply be a silent component of genomic variation, we see reason to record all allelic variation in the human genome.

In broad terms, three types of polymorphic alleles are recognized at the DNA level: (a) biallelic variation in length of a DNA segment revealed by restriction enzyme digestion (an RFLP); (b) multiallelic variation in length (so-called minisatellite VNTRs and microsatellite STRs); and (c) single nucleotide variation (SNP) detected either by sequencing or scanning methods. These alleles are detected by the appropriate use of unique sequence probes, restriction enzymes, the polymerase chain reaction and direct nucleotide sequencing or scanning (by chips). Mutation databases can record the position of these polymorphic alleles and the corresponding haplotypes. The importance of SNPs in the final stages of the genome projects is already recognized by dedicated databases.

A TAXONOMY FOR ALLELES

Taxonomy takes place at three different levels, each essential:

The Chromosome: The chromosomal constitution of an individual is named according to an international convention.[10] It describes the diploid number, sex chromosome constitution, and variation in number and structure of chromosomes. Individual loci on chromosomes are identified in association with banded regions on a particular arm of a particular chromosome.

The Gene (locus): Recommendations exist for naming homologous genes in different organisms[11] and for naming human genes.[12]

The Allele: Guidelines exist for naming alleles[13] (http://journals.wiley.com/humanmutation/nomenclature.html) and *their use is recommended by the HUGO Mutation Database Initiative. A controlled vocabulary to describe an allele and its components is also recommended (see www2.ebi.ac.uk/mutations/recommendations/mutclass.txt).*

Nomenclature for alleles operates at two levels. The systematic name is centered on the change in the nucleotide sequence. The trivial name recognizes change in the gene product. A Web-based tool exists to validate naming of alleles (www2.ebi.ac.uk/cgi-bin/mutations/check.cgi).

In the example (see Table A2-1) the complete classification of the disease-causing allele begins at the level of species and ends with the McKusick number for the disease. The HUGO Mutation Database Initiative[6] encourages authors to use the appropriate nomenclature; journals increasingly require authors to do so. Further ideas about nomenclature, particularly for complex mutations, continue to evolve, for example:

www.dmd.nl/mutnomen.html;
www2.ebi.ac.uk/mutations/recommendations/naming.html;
www.ncbi.nlm.nih.gov/collab/FT/index.html

Authors are also encouraged to consult Antonarakis for advice (stylianos.antonarakis@medicine.unige.ch).

Table A2-1 Taxonomy of an Allele: An Illustration*

The Entity	The Name
Species	*Homo sapiens*
Chromosome	12
Locus	12q24.1
Gene (Symbol)	Phenylalanine hydroxylase (*PAH*)
Reference Nucleotide Sequence	cDNA, GenBank U49897
Allele Name	c.1222C → T (systematic) R408W (trivial)
Product (enzyme)	L-Phenylalanine-4-monooxygenase (EC 1.14.16.1)
Disease	PKU and non-PKU HPA
OMIM	261600
Online database	www.mcgill.ca/pahdb

*Adapted from Scriver and Nowacki[4] and illustrated by a prevalent mutation in the human gene for phenylalanine hydroxylase (symbol *PAH*) causing the disease phenylketonuria (PKU); see Chap. 77.

PROOF OF CAUSATION

What is the evidence that an allele modifies phenotype, either constitutionally or under particular conditions, and how does one provide reliable annotation?[14] The question is relevant in a context such as the book in which this essay appears.

Missense alleles are the principal, but not the only, challenge. Artifacts include errors introduced by PCR; every allele newly discovered should be confirmed on a second PCR product. A variant allele may indeed be confirmed, but it may not be the allele directly responsible for the variant phenotype; the whole functional gene sequence should be analyzed accordingly, and the extent of DNA sequence analyzed stated. Ambiguity can be resolved if necessary by *in vitro* expression analysis.[15]

Criteria for pathogenicity include information on the mutation type; an allele that produces "functional hemizygosity"[16] is likely to modify phenotype when combined with an homologous allele in an autosomal recessive trait. Segregation analysis should reveal a consistent association with the variant phenotype. A missense mutation affecting a conserved amino acid is likely to have functional significance. Frequency of the variant allele in a panel of alleles from 100 normal chromosomes is useful information; a polymorphic allele ($q > 0.01$) is less likely to have a constitutional effect on phenotype, although it may be a modifier of gene expression or part of a complex trait.

Information about mutability of the gene in question is also useful. There is a Web-based program for that purpose (www.hgu.mrc.ac.uk/softdata/mutability/muthelp/htm). A software program (MUTPRED) to analyze predicted mutability is also available from its authors.[17]

MUTATION DATABASES

Types

Two types of mutation databases exist: (a) omnifarious, general, and inclusive (genomic) and (b) particular (locus-specific). The genomic database will eventually contain complete records of all known alleles in the genome of the organism; examples exist for *Drosophila melanogaster* (http://Flybase.bio.indiana.edu/); for the mouse genome (www.informatics.jax.org/); and for the human genome (www.uwcm.ac.uk/uwcm/mg/htmd0.html). The alternative, while waiting for completion of the relevant genomic database, is to proceed locus by locus with specialized databases while attempting to achieve seamless integration between the two types of databases (genomic and locus-specific).[18] At the current stage of the Mutation Database Initiative, one hopes to: (a) maximize the locus-specific database approach for particular usefulness and interoperability; (b) expand the inclusive genomic mutation database initiative in all possible ways; and (c) develop disease-centered databases for complex traits that involve multiple loci and the corresponding interactions and associations. In each case, decisions are required about core data types, to be shared by the different databases.

Content

Annotated mutation databases are likely to contain widely different sets of information. However only four types of information are needed to enable sharing among different database types: (a) *a unique identifier* for the allele; (b) *source* of the information (published article, investigator, etc.); (c) *context* of the allele (species, gene, reference sequence); and (d) the *allele* itself (name, type, nucleotide change, etc.).

Design

There is no single or correct way to design a database. In the accompanying Catalogue of Mutation Databases and in the Molecular Biology Database List,[19] the reader will discover an array of databases with a variety of designs. Design is a challenge for the inexpert and one that is usually met by colleagues skilled in informatics and computer science. Elsewhere the issues of design and deployment of databases have been discussed in the form of Guidelines.[20] Protocols for entering alleles into a database have been developed.[21] Curators who do not wish to design a unique database have the option of acquiring Universal Mutation Database Software (at www.umd.necker.fr/ or at MuStar at www.hgu.mrc.ac.uk/softdata/mutability/).

Links

Locus-specific mutation databases should provide a minimum set of cross-references (active links and pointers) for the user to access additional information. Important links include: MedLine/Pubmed, OMIM, GenBank/EMBL/DDBJ, SwissProt/TrEMBL, GeneCard, and the like; the Molecular Biology Database List[19] is a useful catalog of these resources.

MUTATION DATABASES: A CATALOGUE

Table A2-2 is compiled here from the HUGO Mutation Database Initiative whose ongoing catalogue can be assessed at: http://ariel.ucs.unimelb.edu.au:80/~cotton/mdi.htm. Some genes, for example p53, have several independent locus-specific databases and conversely some databases represent numerous genes. The majority of databases are locus-specific but general databases which collect variation in hundreds of genes are also listed. Databases focussed on regional and ethnic variation are also listed and databases for complex traits are beginning to appear. Clinical databases, as well as databases in other species, are mentioned where known and relevant to this work. The reader is also referred to the Molecular Biology Database List.[19]

Table A2-2 Locus-Specific Databases Listed According to Gene Designation

Gene Designation/ OMIM No.	Database name	Internet address	Curator(s)
ABCD1 300100	Mutation Database for X-Linked Adrenoleukodystrophy	www.x-ald.nl	Hugo W. Moser, Dept. of Neurogenetics, Kennedy Krieger Inst. Baltimore, USA, & Stephen Kemp & Ronald RJA Wanders, Lab. of Genetic Metabolic Diseases Academic Medical Ctr, Amsterdam, The Netherlands
ABCR 601691	Keio Mutation Database for Eye Disease Genes (KMEYEDB)	mutview.dmb.med.keio.ac.jp	S. Minoshima, S. Mitsuyama, S. Ohno, T. Kawamura, & N. Shimizu, Keio Univ. School of Med., Tokyo, Japan
ABO 110300 ACHE 100740	Blood Group Antigen Mutation Database	www.bioc.aecom.yu.edu/ bgmut/index.htm	Olga O. Blumenfeld, Dept. of Biochemistry & Santoch Patnaik, Dept. of Cell Biology, Albert Einstein College of Medicine, New York, NY, U.S.A.
ADL 600119	Alpha-Sarcoglycan	www.dmd.nl/asg_home.html	Johan T. den Dunnen & Bert E. Bakker, Leiden Univ. Med. Centre, Leiden, The Netherlands
ALB 103600	Albumin Mutation Database	www.albumin.org	Eugene W. Holowachuk, The Mary Imogene Bassett Hospital Research Institute, Cooperstown, NY, U.S.A.
ALDH1 100640	Human Polymorphisms of ALDH Genes	www.uchsc.edu/sp/sp/alcdbase/ hpol-aldh.html	Vasilis Vasiliou & Agi Pappa Univ. Colorado Health Sci. Center, Denver, CO, U.S.A.
ALDH2 100650			
ALDH3 100660			
ALDH4 NO OMIM No.			
ALDH9 NO OMIM No.			
ALDOB 229600	Hereditary Fructose Intolerance/Aldolase	www.bu.edu/aldolase/	Dean R. Tolan, Boston Univ., Boston, MA, U.S.A.
APC 175100 No. 1	Adenomatous Polyposis Coli	perso.curie.fr/Thierry.Soussi/ APC.html	Thierry Soussi, INSERM, Hopital Necker Enfants Malades, Paris, France
APC 175100 No. 2	Adenomatous Polyposis Coli at GeneDis	www.tau.ac.il/~racheli/genedis/ apc/apc.html	Cyril Iegum, Avi Orr-Urtreger Rachel Kreisberg-Zakarin, Tel Aviv Univ., Tel Aviv, Israel
AQP1 107776	Blood Group Antigen Mutation Database	www.bioc.aecom.yu.edu/ bgmut/index.htm	Olga O. Blumenfeld, Dept. of Biochemistry & Santoch Patnaik, Dept. of Cell Biology, Albert Einstein College of Medicine, New York, NY, U.S.A.
AQP2 222000 125800 107777	Neurogenic Diabetes Insipidus	www.medcor.mcgill.ca/ ~nephros/	Mary Fujiwara & Daniel G. Bichet, McGill Univ. & Univ. de Montreal, Montreal, Canada
AR 313700	Androgen Receptor	www.mcgill.ca/androgendb/	Bruce Gottlieb & L. Pinsky, Lady Davis Inst. Med, Res, Montreal, Canada
ARSB 253200	Mucopolysaccharidosis Mutation Database	www.peds.umn.edu/gene	Chester B. Whitley, Univ. of Minnesota, U.S.A.
AT3 107300	Antithrombin IIII Mutation Database	www.med.ic.ac.uk/dd/ddhc/	David A. Lane, Imperial College School of Medicine, London, UK

(Continued on next page)

Table A2-2 (Continued)

Gene Designation/ OMIM No.	Database name	Internet address	Curator (s)
ATP7B 277900 No. 1	Wilson Disease Mutation Database	www.medgen.med.ualberta.ca/database.html	Susan Kenney & Diane Cox, Dept. Med. Gen., Univ. Alberta, Canada
ATP7B 277900 No. 2	Colon Cancer database at GeneDis	www.tau.ac.il/~racheli/genedis/apc/apc.html	Batsheva Bonne-Tamir, Rachel Kreisberg-Zakarin, Tel Aviv Univ. Tel Aviv, Israel
ATM 208900 No. 1	Ataxia-Telangiectasia	www.vmmc.org/vmrc/atm.htm	Patrick Concannon, Virginia Mason Research Center, Seattle, Washington & Richard A. Gatti, Dept. of Pathology UCLA, U.S.A.
ATM 208900 No. 2	ATM Mutation Database	www.mec.jhv.edu/ataxia/mutate.htm	Ataxia-Telangiectasia Children's Project, Boca Raton, FL, U.S.A.
AVP 125700 192340	Neurogenic Diabetes Insipidus	www.medcor.mcgill.ca/~nephros/	Mary Fujiwara & Daniel G. Bichet, McGill Univ. & Univ. de Montreal, Montreal, Canada
AVPR2 304800			
BCHE 177400	ESTHER - ESTerases & α/β Hydrolase Enzymes & Relatives	Meleze.ensam.inra.fr/cholinesterase/	Xavier Cousin, Institut National de la Recherche Agronomique, Montpellier, France
BRCA1 113705	Breast Cancer	www.nhgri.nih.gov/Intramural_research/Lab_transfer/Bic/Member/index.html	Laurence Brody & Breast Cancer Information Core, NCHGR/NIH Bethesda, MD, U.S.A.
BRCA2 600185			
BTK 300300	Bruton Agammaglobulinemia (BTKbase)	helsiniki.fi/science/signal/btkbase.html	Mauno Vihinen, Univ. of Tampere, Helsinki, Finland
CANP3 114240	Limb-Girdle Muscular Dystrophy, Type 2A	www.dmd.nl/canp3_home.html	Johan T. den Dunnen & Bert E. Bakker, Leiden Univ. Med. Centre, Leiden, The Netherlands
CASR 601199	Calcium Sensing Receptor Locus Mutation Database	data.mch.mcgill.ca/casrdb/	Geoff Hendy, L. D'Souza-Li & Xing Zeng, McGill Univ., Montreal, Canada
CAV3 601253	Limb-Girdle Muscular Dystrophy, Type 1c	www.dmd.nl/cav3_home.html	Johan T. den Dunnen & Bert E. Bakker, Leiden Univ. Med. Centre, Leiden, The Netherlands
CBS 236200	Cystathione beta-Synthase Database	www.uchsc.edu/sm/cbs	Jan P. Kraus, Univ. of Colorado, Denver, CO, U.S.A.
CD3E 186830	CD3Ebase: Mutation Registry for Autosomal Recessive CD3ϵ Immunodeficiency	www.uta.fi/imt/bioinfo/CD3Ebase/	Mauno Vihinen & José R. Regueiro, Univ. of Tampere, Helsinki, Finland
CD3G 186740	CD3Gbase: Mutation Registry for Autosomal Recessive CD3 γ Immunodeficiency	www.uta.fi/imt/bioinfo/CD3Gbase/	Mauno Vihinen & José R. Regueiro, Univ. of Tampere, Helsinki, Finland
CD40L No OMIM No.	CD40Lbase: Mutation Registry for X-Linked Hyper-IgM Syndrome	www.uta.fi/imt/bioinfo/CD40Lbase/	Luigi D. Notrangelo, Manuel C. Peitsch & Mauno Vihinen, Univ. of Tampere, Helsinki, Finland

Table A2-2 (Continued)

Gene Designation/ OMIM No.	Database name	Internet address	Curator (s)
CD40LG 308230	Immunodeficiency with Increased IgM-The European CD40 Defect Database	www.expasy.ch/www/ cd40lbase.htm	European Society for Immunodeficiencies
CDKN2A 600160	Cyclin dependent kinase Inhibitor A	pcdnr83.uio.no/	Eivind Hovig, The Norwegian Radium Hospital, Oslo, Norway
CFTR 219700	Cystic Fibrosis Database	www.genet.sickkids.on.ca/cftr/	Lap Chee Tsui, The Hospital for Sick Children, Toronto, Canada
CHM 303100	Keio Mutation Database for Eye Disease Genes (KMEYEDB)	mutview.dmb.med.keio.ac.jp	S. Minoshima, S. Mitsuyama, S. Ohno, T. Kawamura, & N. Shimizu, Keio Univ. School of Med., Tokyo, Japan
CHS1 214500	Albinism Database	www.cbc.umn.edu/tad	William S. Oetting, Int. Albinism Center, Univ. of Minnesota, U.S.A.
CLN1 – CLN2 204500 CLN3 – CLN4 204300 CLN5 256731 CLN6 CLN7 CLN8	Neuronal Ceroid Lipofuscinosis NCL Mutations	www.ucl.ac.uk/ncl	Sara E. Mole, Dept. Paediatrics, Univ. College, London Medical School, The Rayne Institute, London, UK
CNCG1 123825	Keio Mutation Database for Eye Disease Genes (KMEYEDB)	mutview.dmb.med.keio.ac.jp	S. Minoshima, S. Mitsuyama, S. Ohno, T. Kawamura, & N. Shimizu, Keio Univ. School of Med., Tokyo, Japan
COCH 601369	Hereditary Hearing Loss Homepage	dnalab-www.uia.ac.be/ dnalab/hhh	Guy van Camp, Univ. of Antwerp, Antwerp, Belgium, & Richard JH Smith, Univ. of Iowa Hospitals & Clinics, Iowa, U.S.A.
COL1A1 120150 COL1A2 120160 COL3A1 120180	Collagen Type I & III	www.le.ac.uk/genetics/ collagen/	Raymond Dalgleish & Collaborative Group, Leicester, UK
COLQ 603033	ESTHER - ESTerases & α/β Hydrolase Enzymes & Relatives	Meleze.ensam.inra.fr/ cholinesterase/	Xavier Cousin, Institut National de la Recherche Agronomique, Montpellier, France
CXB2 121011	Hereditary Hearing Loss at GeneDis	www.tau.ac.il/~racheli/genedis/ deafness/deafness.html	Karen Avraham, Noa Davis, Rachel Kreisberg-Zakarin, Tel Aviv Univ, Israel
CYBA 233690	Autosomal Recessive Chronic Granulomatous Disease (CGD) Deficiency of p22phox CYBAbase	www.uta.fi/imt/bioinfo/ CYBAbase/	Dirk Roos, Mauno Vihinen, Univ. of Helsinki, Helsinki, Finland
CYBB 306400	X-linked Granulomatous Disease	www.helsinki.fi/science/signal/ databases/x-cgdbase.html	Univ. of Helsinki, Helsinki, Finland
CYP1B1 601771	Keio Mutation Database for Eye Disease Genes (KMEYEDB)	mutview.dmb.med.keio.ac.jp	S. Minoshima, S. Mitsuyama, S. Ohno, T. Kawamura, & N. Shimizu, Keio Univ. School of Med., Tokyo, Japan

(Continued on next page)

Table A2-2 (Continued)

Gene Designation/ OMIM No.	Database name	Internet address	Curator (s)
CYP 610637 123960 124070	Human Cytochrome P450 (CYP)	www.imm.ki.se/CYPalleles/	Magnus Ingelman-Sundberg, Ann K. Daly, Daniel E. Nebert
DIAPH1 602121	Hereditary Hearing Loss Homepage	dnalab-www.uia.ac.be/ dnalab/hhh	Guy van Camp, Univ. of Antwerp, Antwerp, Belgium, & Richard JH Smith, Univ. of Iowa Hospitals & Clinics, Iowa, U.S.A.
DMD 310200	Duchenne & Becker Muscular Dystrophy	www.dmd.nl/database.html	Johan T. den Dunnen & Bert E. Bakker, Leiden Univ. Med. Centre, Leiden, The Netherlands
DYSF 603009	Limb-Girdle muscular dystrophy Type 2B	www.dmd.nl/dysf_home.html	Johan T. den Dunnen & Bert E. Bakker, Leiden Univ. Med. Centre, Leiden, The Netherlands
EGR2 129010	Mutation Database of Inherited Peripheral Neuropathies	molgen-www.uia.ac.be/ CMTMutations/	Eva Nelis, Univ. of Antwerp, Antwerp, Belgium
EMD 310300	Emery-Dreifuss Muscular Dystrophy	www.path.cam.ac.uk/emd	Manfred Wehnert & John Yates, Cambridge, UK
ENG 131195	Endoglin Hereditary Haemorrhagic Telangiectasia, HHT	genetics.ms.duke.edu/hht/	Doulas Marchuk, Dept. of Genetics, Duke Univ. Medical Center, Durham, NC, U.S.A.
F7 227500	Factor VII Mutation Database	europium.mrc.rpms.ac.uk/	Haemostasis Res. Group, MRC Clinical Sci. Center, London, UK
F8 306700	The Haemophilia A Mutation, Structure, Test and Resource Site (HAMSTeRS)	europium.mrc.rpms.ac.uk/	Haemostasis Res. Group, MRC Clinical Sci. Center, London, UK
F9 306900	Haemophilia B Mutation Database	www.umds.ac.uk/molgen/ haemBdatabase.html	PM Green, F. Gianelli & Consortium
FANCA 227650 FANCC 227645	Fanconi Anaemia	www.rockefeller.edu/fanconi/ mutate/	Arleen Auerbach, Christopher Matthew & Consortium
FBN1 134797	Marfan Database-Fibrillin-1 Gene Mutations	www.umd.necker.fr/ Sire%20Marfan/ Marfan_Home_Page.html	G. Collod-Beroud, C. Boileau, & C. Beroud, INSERM, Hopital Necker Enfants Malades, Paris, France
FY 110700	Blood Group Antigen Mutation Database	www.bioc.aecom.yu.edu/ bgmut/index.htm	Olga O. Blumenfeld, Dept. of Biochemistry & Santoch Patnaik, Dept. of Cell Biology, Albert Einstein College of Medicine, New York, NY, U.S.A.
G6PD 305900	Glucose-6-Phosphate-Dehydrogenase	rialto.com./favism/mutat.htm	E. Beutler, Scripps Res. Inst., La Jolla, Ca, U.S.A., T. Vuillamy RPMS, London UK, & L. Luzzato, Dept. Hum. Gen. NY, NY U.S.A.
GAA 232300	Glycogen Storage Disease Type II, Pompe Disease	www.eur.nl/FGG/CH1/pompe/	AJJ Reuser, Erasmus Univ, Rotterdam, The Netherlands
GALB 104170	Mutations in the α-N-Acetylgalactosaminidase Gene Causing Schindler disease	www.mssm.edu/crc/mutations/ schindler.html	Kenneth H. Astrin & Robert J. Desnick, Dept. of Human Genetics, Mt. Sinai School of Medicine, New York, NY, U.S.A.
GALC 245200	Krabbe Disease, at GeneDis	–	Karen Avraham, Noa Davis, Rachel Kreisberg-Zakarin, Tel Aviv Univ., Iel Aviv, Israel

Table A2-2 (Continued)

Gene Designation/ OMIM No.	Database name	Internet address	Curator (s)
GALNS 253000	Mucopolysaccharidosis Mutation Database	www.peds.umn.edu/gene	Chester B. Whitley, Univ. of Minnesota, U.S.A.
GALT 230400	Galactosaemia	www.ich.bris.ac.uk/galtdb/	Linda Tyfield & David Carmichael, Inst. Child Health, Univ. Bristol, Bristol, UK
GBA 230800	Tel-Aviv Univ. Human Genetic Disease Database (Gaucher Disease)	www.tau.ac.il/~racheli/ genedis/gaucher/gaucher.html	Metsada Pasmanik-chor, Mia Horowitz & Rachel Kreigsberg-Zakarin, Wise Faculty of Life Sciences, Tel Aviv Univ., lel Aviv, Israel, & Ernest Beutler, Scripps Res. Inst., La Jolla, CA, U.S.A.
GCH1 600225	GTP Cyclohydrolase I Deficiency -BIOMED/BIODEF DATABASE	www.unizh.ch/%7eblau/ biomdb1.html	N. Blau, Univ. Children's Hospital, Zurich, Switzerland, JL Dhont, Faculté libre de Médicine, Lille, France, & I. Dianzani, Univ., of Torino, Torino, Italy
GJB1 304040	Mutation Database of Inherited Peripheral Neuropathies	molgen-www.uia.ac.be/ CMTMutations/	Eva Nelis, Univ. of Antwerp, Antwerp, Belgium
GJB2 121011	Hereditary Hearing Loss Homepage	dnalab-www.uia.ac.be/ dnalab/hhh	Guy van Camp, Univ. of Antwerp, Antwerp, Belgium, & Richard JH Smith, Univ. of Iowa Hospitals & Clinics, Iowa, U.S.A.
GNAS1 139320	GNAS1 Mutations in Albright Hereditary Osteodystrophy	mammary.nih.gov/aho/	Lee S. Weinstein, Metabolic Diseases Branch, Bethesda, MD, U.S.A.
GPA 111300 GPB 111740	Blood Group Antigen Mutation Database	www.bioc.aecom.yu.edu/ bgmut/index.htm	Olga O. Blumenfeld, Dept. of Biochemistry & Santoch Patnaik, Dept. of Cell Biology, Albert Einstein College of Medicine, New York, NY, U.S.A.
GRL 138040	Glucocorticoid Receptor Resource Database	nrr.georgetown.edu/GRR/ mutation/mutation.html	S. Stoney Simons & Mark Danielson, Georgetown Univ., Georgetown, MD, U.S.A.
GSN 137350	Keio Mutation Database for Eye Disease Genes (KMEYEDB)	mutview.dmb.med.keio.ac.jp	S. Minoshima, S. Mitsuyama, S. Ohno, T. Kawamura, & N. Shimizu, Keio Univ. School of Med., Tokyo, Japan
GUSB 253220	Mucopolysaccharidosis Mutation Database	www.peds.umn.edu/gene	Chester B. Whitley, Univ. of Minnesota, U.S.A.
HBA1 141800 HBA2 141850 HBB 141900 HBD 142000 HBG1 142200 HBG2 142250	A Syllabus of Human Haemoglobin Variants & A Syllabus of Thalassemia Mutations	globin.cse.psu.edu/ & http://globin.cse.psu.edu/ globin/html/huisman/thals/	Ross Hardison Pennsylvania State Univ. U.S.A., Titus HJ Huisman, Marianne FH Carver, United Kingdom & Georgi D. Efemrov, Macedonian Academy of Sciences and Arts Skopje, Former Yugoslav Republic of Macedonia, & Erol Baysal, Dubai Thalassemia and Genetic Center, Dubai, United Arab Emirates
HEXA 272800 No. 1	Hexosaminidase A, Tay-Sachs Disease	data.mch.mcgill.ca/hexadb/	F. Kaplan, P. Nowacki & K. Hechtman, McGill Univ., Montreal, Canada
HEXA 272800 No. 2	Tay-Sachs at GeneDis	–	Ruth Navon, Rachel Kresberg-Zakarin, Tel Aviv Univ., Tel Aviv, Israel
HPRT1 308000	Hypoxanthine Guanine Phosphoribosyltransferase 1, Lesch-Nyhan Syndrome	sunsite.unc.edu/dnam/ mainpage.html	Neil Cariello, Univ. North Carolina, U.S.A.

(Continued on next page)

Table A2-2 (Continued)

Gene Designation/ OMIM No.	Database name	Internet address	Curator (s)
HPS 203300	Albinism Database	www.cbc.umn.edu/tad	William S. Oetting, Int. Albinism Center, Univ. of Minnesota, U.S.A.
HSP60 118190 HSPE1 600141	Mutations in GroEL & GroES	bioc09.uthscsa.edu/~seale/ Chap/mut.html	Jeff Seale
IDS 309900 IDUA 252800	Mucopolysaccharidosis Mutation Database	www.peds.umn.edu/gene	Chester B. Whitley, Univ. of Minnesota, U.S.A.
IGHV 147070 IGHD 147170 IGHJ 147010 IGKV 146980 IGKJ 146970 IGLV 147240 IGLJ 147230	IMGT, The International ImMunoGeneTics database	imgt.cnusc.fr:8104	Marie-Paule Lefranc, CNRS, Université Montpellier II, Montpellier, France
IL2RG 308380	X-Linked Severe Combined Immunodeficiency, SCID	www.nhgri.nih.gov/DIR/ LGT/SCID/	Jeniffer Puck, Joie Davies, Roxanne Fisher & Amy Pepper, NHGRI/NIH, Bethesda, Md, U.S.A.
JAK3 600173	JAK3base: Mutation Registry for Autosomal Recessive Severe Combined Immunodeficiency	www.uta.fi/imt/bioinfo/ JAK3base/	Luigi D. Notrangelo, & Mauno Vihinen, Univ. of Tampere, Helsinki, Finland
JK(SLC14A1) 111000	Blood Group Antigen Mutation Database	www.bioc.aecom.yu.edu/ bgmut/index.htm	Olga O. Blumenfeld, Dept. of Biochemistry & Santoch Patnaik, Dept. of Cell Biology, Albert Einstein College of Medicine, New York, NY, U.S.A.
KCNE1 176261 KCNH2 152427 KCNQ1 192500	Long QT Syndrome Database	www.ssi.dk/en/forskning/ lqtsdb.htm	Michael Christiansen, Lars A. Larsen, & Paal Skytt Andersen, Molecular Cardiology Grp, Statens Serum Institut, Copenhagen, Denmark
KEL 110900	Blood Group Antigen Mutation Database	www.bioc.aecom.yu.edu/ bgmut/index.htm	Olga O. Blumenfeld, Dept. of Biochemistry & Santoch Patnaik, Dept. of Cell Biology, Albert Einstein College of Medicine, New York, NY, U.S.A.
–	KinMutBase: Mutation Registry for Disease-Causing Mutations in Tyrosine Kinase domains	www.uta.fi/imt/bioinfo/ KinMutBase/	Mauno Vihinen & Kaj Stenberg, Univ. of Tampere, Helsinki, Finland
L1CAM 308840	L1 Cell Adhesion Molecule	dndlab-www.uia.ac.be/ dnalab/l1/	PJ Willems, Univ. of Antwerp, Antwerp, Belgium
LDLR 143890 No. 1	Hypercholesterolemia, familial	www.ucl.ac.uk/fh/	S. Humphries
LDLR 143890 No. 2	Low-density Lipoprotein Receptor Mutation Database	www.umd.necker.fr:2004/	M. Varret, C. Boileau & C. Beroud, INSERM, Hopital Necker Enfants Malades, Paris, France

Table A2-2 (Continued)

Gene Designation/ OMIM No.	Database name	Internet address	Curator (s)
LQTS 192500	Long QT Syndrome Database	www.ssi.dk/en/forskning/lqtsdb.htm	Michael Christiansen, Lars A. Larsen, & Paal Skytt Andersen, Molecular Cardiology Grp, Statens Serum Institut, Copenhagen, Denmark
LU 111200 LW 111250	Blood Group Antigen Mutation Database	www.bioc.aecom.yu.edu/bgmut/index.htm	Olga O. Blumenfeld, Dept. of Biochemistry & Santoch Patnaik, Dept. of Cell Biology, Albert Einstein College of Medicine, New York, NY, U.S.A.
MEFV 249100	Familial Mediterranean Fever at GeneDis	www.tau.ac.il/~racheli/genedis/fmf/fmf.html	Nurit Magal, Mordechai Shohat, & Rachel Kreisberg-Zakarin, Tel Aviv Univ., Tel Aviv Israel
MLH1 120436 MSH2 120435 MSH6	Hereditary Non-Polyposis Colorectal Cancer, HNPCC	www.nfdht.nl/database/mdbchoice.htm	Collaborative Group, The Netherlands
MPZ 159440	Mutation Database of Inherited Peripheral Neuropathies	molgen-www.uia.ac.be/CMTMutations/	Eva Nelis, Univ. of Antwerp, Antwerp, Belgium
MYBPC3 600958 MYH7 160760 MYL2 160781	FHC Mutation Database	www.angis.org.au/Databases/Heart/heartbreak.html	David C. Fung, Bing Yu, & Ronald J. Trent, Dept. Molecular & Clinical Genetics, Royal Prince Alfred Hospital, Sydney, Australia
MYO7A 276903 MYO15 600316 602266	Hereditary Hearing Loss Homepage	dnalab-www.uia.ac.be/dnalab/hhh	Guy van Camp, Univ. of Antwerp, Antwerp, Belgium, & Richard JH Smith, Univ. of Iowa Hospitals & Clinics, Iowa, U.S.A.
MYOC 601652	Keio Mutation Database for Eye Disease Genes (KMEYEDB)	mutview.dmb.med.keio.ac.jp	S. Minoshima, S. Mitsuyama, S. Ohno, T. Kawamura, & N. Shimizu, Keio Univ. School of Med., Tokyo, Japan
NAGA 104170	Mutations in the α-N-Acetylgalactosaminidase Gene Causing Schindler Disease	www.mssm.edu/crc/mutations/schindler.html	Kenneth H. Astrin & Robert J. Desnick, Dept. of Human Genetics, Mt. Sinai School of Med. New York, NY, U.S.A.
NAGLU 252920	Mucopolysaccharidosis Mutation Database	www.peds.umn.edu/gene	Chester B. Whitley, Univ. of Minnesota, U.S.A.
NBS1 602667	Nijmegen Breakage Syndrome Mutation Database	www.vmresearch.org/nbs.htm	Pat Concannon, Virginia Mason Research Center, Seattle, WA, U.S.A.
NF1 162200	Neurofibromatosis Type I	www.nf.org/nf1gene/nf1gene.home.html	BR Korf & NF1 Genetic Analysis Consortium, Harvard, MA, U.S.A.
NF2 101000	Neurofibromatosis Type II	neuro-trials1.mgh.harvard.edu/nf2/index.htm	Massachusetts General Hospital, Boston, MA, U.S.A.
OA1 300500 OCA1 203100 OCA2 203200 OCA3 203290	Albinism Database	www.cbc.umn.edu/tad	William S. Oetting, Int. Albinism Center, Univ. of Minnesota, U.S.A.
OTC 311250	Ornithine Transcarbamylase	www.peds.umn.edu/otc/	Mendel Tuchman, Univ. of Minnesota, U.S.A.

(Continued on next page)

Table A2-2 (Continued)

Gene Designation/ OMIM No.	Database name	Internet address	Curator (s)
PAH 261600	Phenylalanine Hydroxylase Locus Database	www.mcgill.ca/pahdb/	Charles Scriver, Piotr Nowacki, Saeed Teebi, Xing Zeng, Lynne Prevost, & PAH Mutation Analysis Consortium, McGill Univ., Montreal, Canada
PAX2 167409	PAX2 Mutation Database	www.hgu.mrc.ac.uk/Softdata/ PAX2/	Les McNoe, Cancer Genetics Lab., Univ. of Otago, Dunedin, New Zealand
PAX6 106210	PAX6 Mutation Database, Aniridia Type II	www.hgu.mrc.ac.uk/Softdata/ PAX6/	Isabel Hanson, MRC, HGM, Edinburgh, Scotland
PCBD 126090 PCD 176430	Pterin-4a-Carbionolamine Dehydratase Deficiency Premature Centromere Division	www.unizh.ch/%7eblau/biomdb1. html	N. Blau, Univ. Children's Hospital, Zurich, Switzerland, JL Dhont, Faculté Libre de Médicine, Lille, France, & I. Dianzani, Univ. Torino, Torino, Italy
PDE6A 180071 PDE6B 180072	Keio Mutation Database for Eye Disease Genes (KMEYEDB)	mutview.dmb.med.keio.ac.jp	S. Minoshima, S. Mitsuyama, S. Ohno, T. Kawamura, & N. Shimizu, Keio Univ. School of Med., Tokyo, Japan
PDS 600791 274600	Hereditary Hearing Loss Homepage	dnalab-www.uia.ac.be/ dnalab/hhh	Guy van Camp, Univ. of Antwerp, Antwerp, Belgium, & Richard JH Smith, Univ. of Iowa Hospitals & Clinics, Iowa, U.S.A.
PHEX 307800	PHEX Locus Database	data.mch.mcgill.ca/phexdb	Y. Sabbagh, AO Jones, & HS Tenenhouse, McGill Univ., Montreal, Canada
PKD1 601313 PKD2 173910	Polycystic Kidney Research Foundation	www.pkdcure.org/res/index. html	?
PLP 312080	Proteolipid Protein Mutation Database	www.med.wayne.edu/Neurology/ plp.html	James Garbern, Dept. Neurology, Wayne State Univ., Detroit, MI, U.S.A.
POU3F4 300039 POU4F3 602460 602459	Hereditary Hearing Loss Homepage	dnalab-www.uia.ac.be/ dnalab/hhh	Guy van Camp, Univ. of Antwerp, Antwerp, Belgium, & Richard JH Smith, Univ. of Iowa Hospitals & Clinics, Iowa, U.S.A.
PMI 154550 PMM2 601785	Carbohydrate Deficient Glycoprotein Syndrome Types Ia & Ib Mutation database	www.med.kuleuven/cme/ cdg.htm	Gert Matthijs, Center for Human Genetics, Leuven, Belgium
PMP22 601097	Mutation Database of Inherited Peripheral Neuropathies	molgen-www.uia.ac.be/ CMTMutations/	Eva Nelis, Univ. of Antwerp, Antwerp, Belgium
PMS1 PMS2	Hereditary Non-Polyposis Colorectal Cancer, HNPCC	www.nfdht.nl/database/ mdbchoice.htm	Collaborative Group, The Netherlands
PSAP 176801	Tel-Aviv Univ. Human Genetic Disease Database (Gaucher Disease)	www.tau.ac.il/~racheli/genedis/ gaucher/gaucher.html	Metsada Pasmanik-Chor, Mia Horowitz & Rachel Kreigsberg-Zakarin, Wise Faculty of Life Sciences, Tel-Aviv Univ., lel Aviv, Israel, & Ernest Beutler, Scripps Res. Inst., La Jolla, CA, U.S.A.
PRNP 176640	Prion Protein/CJD Database	www.mad-cow.org/~tom/ prion_point_mutations.html	Sperling Biomedical Foundation, O, U.S.A.

Table A2-2 (Continued)

Gene Designation/ OMIM No.	Database name	Internet address	Curator (s)
PTCH1 601309	PTCH Mutation Database	www.cybergene.se/PTCH/	Rune Toftgard, Karolinska Institutet, Sweden, Georgia Chenevix-Trench, QIMR, Brisbane, Australia, & Mike Dean, National Cancer Institute, Bethesda, MD, U.S.A.
PTS 261640 QDPR 261630	6-Pyruvoyl-Tetrahydropterin Synthase Deficiency Quinoid dihydropteridine Rreductase Deficiency	www.unizh.ch/%7eblau/ biomdb1.html	N. Blau, Univ. Children's Hospital, Zurich, Switzerland, JL Dhont, Faculté Libre de Médicine, Lille, France, & I. Dianzani, Univ. of Torino, Torino, Italy
RAG1 179615	RAG1base: Mutation Registry for Autosomal Recessive RAG1 Immunodeficiency	www.uta.fi/imt/bioinfo/RAG1base/ index.html	Mauno Vihinen & Anna Villa, Univ. of Tampere, Helsinki, Finland
RAG2 179616	RAG2base: Mutation Registry for Autosomal Recessive RAG2 Immunodeficiency	www.uta.fi/imt/bioinfo/RAG2base/ index.html	Mauno Vihinen & Anna Villa, Univ. of Tampere, Helsinki, Finland
RB1 180200 No. 1	Retnoblastoma, RB1 Mutation Database	www.d-lohmann.de/Rb/ mutations.htm	Dietmar Lohmann, Institut fuer Humangenetik, Essen, Germany
RB1 180200 No. 2	Keio Mutation Database for Eye Disease Genes (KMEYEDB)	mutview.dmb.med.keio.ac.jp	S. Minoshima, S. Mitsuyama, S. Ohno, T. Kawamura, of N. Shimizu, Keio Univ. School of Med., Tokyo, Japan
RDS 179605 No. 1	Retinal Degeneration Slow	mol.ophth.uiowa.edu/ MOL_WWW/RDStab.html	Univ. of Iowa
RDS 179605 No. 2	Keio Mutation Database for Eye Disease Genes (KMEYEDB)	mutview.dmb.med.keio.ac.jp	S. Minoshima, S. Mitsuyama, S. Ohno, T. Kawamura, & N. Shimizu, Keio Univ. School of Med., Tokyo, Japan
RHAG 180297 RHCE 111700 RHD 111680	Blood Group Antigen Mutation Database	www.bioc.aecom.yu.edu/ bgmut/index.htm	Olga O. Blumenfeld, Dept. of Biochemistry & Santoch Patnaik, Dept. of Cell Biology, Albert Einstein College of Medicine, New York, NY, U.S.A.
RHO 180380 No. 1	Rhodopsin	mol.ophth.uiowa.edu/ MOL_WWW/Rhotab.html	Univ. of Iowa
RHO 180380 No. 2 RHOK 180381	Keio Mutation Database for Eye Disease Genes (KMEYEDB)	mutview.dmb.med.keio.ac.jp	S. Minoshima, S. Mitsuyama, S. Ohno, T. Kawamura, & N. Shimizu, Keio Univ. School of Med., Tokyo, Japan
RS1 312700 No. 1	x-Linked Juvenile Retinoschisis	www.dmd.nl/rs/rs.html	Thirsa Kraayenbrink & Johan T. den Dunnen, Leiden Univ. Medical Center, Leiden, The Netherlands
RS1 312700 No. 2 RP3 312610	Keio Mutation Database for Eye Disease Genes (KMEYEDB)	mutview.dmb.med.keio.ac.jp	S. Minoshima, S. Mitsuyama, S. Ohno, T. Kawamura, & N. Shimizu, Keio Univ. School of Med., Tokyo, Japan
SCN5A 600163	Long QT Syndrome Database	www.ssi.dk/en/forskning/ lqtsdb.htm	Michael Christiansen, Lars A. Larsen, & Paal Skytt Andersen, Molecular Cardiology Grp, Statens Serum Institut, Copenhagen, Denmark

(Continued on next page)

Table A2-2 (Continued)

Gene Designation/ OMIM No.	Database name	Internet address	Curator (s)
SGCC – SGCA 600119 SGCB 600900 SGCD 601411	Limb-Girdle Muscular Dystrophy, Type 2C, 2D, 2E, 2F	www.dmd.nl/sgcc_home.html www.dmd.nl/sgca_home.html www.dmd.nl/sgcb_home.html www.dmd.nl/sgcd_home.html	Johan T. den Dunnen, Leiden Univ. Medical Center, Leiden, The Netherlands
SLC14A1 111000	Blood Group Antigen Mutation Database	www.bioc.aecom.yu.edu/ bgmut/index.htm	Olga O. Blumenfeld, Dept. of Biochemistry & Santoch Patnaik, Dept. of Cell Biology, Albert Einstein College of Medicine, New York, NY, U.S.A.
TECTA 602574	Hereditary Hearing Loss Homepage	dnalab-www.uia.ac.be/ dnalab/hhh	Guy van Camp, Univ. of Antwerp, Antwerp, Belgium, & Richard JH Smith, Univ. of Iowa Hospitals & Clinics, Iowa, U.S.A.
TNNT2 191045 TNN13 191044 TPM1 191010	FHC Mutation Database	www.angis.org.au/Databases/ Heart/heartbreak.html	David C. Fung, Bing Yu & Ronald J. Trent, Dept. of Molecular & Clinical Genetics, Royal Prince Alfred Hospital, Sydney, Australia
TP53 191170 No. 1	P53 Somatic Mutations in Tumours & Cell Lines	www.iarc.fr/p53/ Homepage.htm	T. Hernandez, P. Hainaut, R. Montesano, T. Soussi, B. Shomer, M. Hollstein, M. Greenblatt, E. Hovig & C.C. Harris, IARC, Lyon, France
TP53 191170 No. 2	P53 Mutation in Human Cancer	perso.curie.fr/Thierry.Soussi/ p53_mutation.html	Thierry Soussi, C. Beroud, INSERM, Hopital Necker Enfants Malades, Paris, France
TP53 191170 No. 3	Human HPRT & p53 Mutations	sunsite.unc.edu/dnam/ mainpage.html	Neil Cariello, Univ. North Carolina, U.S.A.
TP53 191170 No. 4	P53 Tumour Protein	www.mayo.edu/research/papers /P53%20Mutations	Mayo Clinic, U.S.A.
TP53 191170 No. 5	Database of Germline p53 Mutations	www.lf2.cuni.cz/projects/ germline_mut_p53.htm	Z. Sedlacek, A. Poustka, & P. Goetz, Charles Univ., Prague, Czech Republic
TP53 191170 No. 6	P53 Mutation Database, Analysis & Search	p53.genome.ad.jp/	Human Genome Center, Tokyo, Japan
TRAV TRBD TRGV TRGJ TRGC TRDV TRDD TRDJ NO OMIM ENTIRE	IMGT, The International ImMunoGeneTics Database	imgt.cnusc.fr:8104	Marie-Paule Lefranc, CNRS, Université Montpellier, Montpellier, France
TSC1 19100	Tuberous Sclerosis Mutation Listings	zk.bwh.harvard.edu/ts/	Mary-Pat Reeve, WEHI, Melbourne, Australia

Table A2-2 (Continued)

Gene Designation/ OMIM No.	Database name	Internet address	Curator (s)
TSC2 191092	The Cardiff-Rotterdam Tuberous Sclerosis Mutation Database	www.uwcm.ac.uk/uwcm/mg/tsc_db/	S. Verhoef, Inst. of Medical Genetics, Cardiff, Edinburgh, Scotland
TSHR 603372	TSH Receptor Mutation Database	www.uni-leipzig.de/innere/TSH	Ralf Paschke, 3rd Med. Dept. Univ. of Leipzig, Leipzig, Germany
VHL 193300	Von Hippel-Lindau Disease Gene	www.umd.necker.fr:20051	C. Beroud, INSERM, Hopital Necker Enfants Malades, Paris, France
VMD2 155370	Vitelliform Macular Dystrophy Mutation Database	www.uni-wuerzberg.de/humangenetics/vmd2.html	Bernhard HF Weber, Inst. of Human Genetics, Wuerzburg, Germany
VWF 193400	Von Willebrand Factor Database	mmg2.im.med.umich.edu/vWF/	D. Ginsburg & JE Sadler, Univ. of Michigan, U.S.A.
WRN 277700	Database of WS associated WRN mutations	www.pathology.washington.edu/werner/ws_wrn.html	Mike Moser, Univ. of Washington, Seattle, U.S.A.
WT1 194070	Wilm's Tumour Database	www.umd.necker.fr:2003/	C. Jeanpierre & C. Beroud, INSERM, Hopital Necker Enfants Malades, Paris, France
X-CGD 306400	X-CGDbase: Mutation Registry for X-Linked Chronic Granulomatous Disease	www.helsinki.fi/science/signal/databases/x-cgdbase.html	Dirk Roos & Mauno Vihinen, Univ. of Tampere, Helsinki, Finland
XK 314850	Blood Group Antigen Mutation Database	www.bioc.aecom.yu.edu/bgmut/index.htm	Olga O. Blumenfeld, Dept. of Biochemistry & Santoch Patnaik, Dept. of Cell Biology, Albert Einstein College of Medicine, New York, NY, U.S.A.
XLRS 312700	X-Linked Juvenile Retinoschisis	www.dmd.nl/rs.html	Johan T. den Dunnen, Leiden Univ. Medical Center, Leiden, The Netherlands
ZAP70 176947	ZAP70base: Mutation Registry for Autosomal Recessive ZAP70 Immunodeficiency	www.uta.fi/imt/bioinfo/ZAP70base/index.html	Mauno Vihinen, Univ. of Tampere, Helsinki, Finland

This list, which is continually updated, may be found online at: http://ariel.ucs.unimelb.edu.au:80/~cotton/glsdb.htm

REFERENCES

1. Goodfellow P: A celebration and a farewell. *Nat Genet* **16**:209, 1997.
2. Bassett DEJ, Boguski MS, Spencer F et al: Genome cross-referencing and XREFdb: Implications for the identification and analysis of genes mutated in human disease. *Nat Genet* **15**:339, 1997.
3. Strachan T, Abitbol M, Davidson D et al: A new dimension for the human genome project: Towards comprehensive expression maps [Commentary]. *Nat Genet* **16**:126, 1997.
4. Scriver CR, Nowacki PM: Genomics, mutations and the Internet: The naming and use of parts. *J Inherit Metab Dis* **22**:519, 1999.
5. Aparico SAJR: How to count . . . human genes. *Nat Genet* **25**:129, 2000.
6. Cotton RGH, McKusick VA, Scriver CR: The HUGO mutation database initiative. *Science* **279**:10, 1998.
7. Cotton RGH: Current methods of mutation detection. *Mutat Res* **285**:125, 1993.
8. Grompe M: The rapid detection of unknown mutations in nucleic acids. *Nat Genet* **5**:111, 1993.
9. Cotton RGH: *Mutation Detection*. New York, Oxford University Press, 1997.
10. Mitelman F: *ISCN-1995: An International System for Human Cytogenetic Nomenclature*. Basel, S. Karger, 1995.
11. Blake JA, Davisson MT, Eppig JT et al: A report on the International Nomenclature Workshop held May 1997 at the Jackson Laboratory, Bar Harbour, Maine, U.S.A. *Genomics* **45**:464, 1997.
12. White A, McAlpine PJ, Antonarakis S et al: Guidelines for human gene nomenclature (1997). *Genomics* **45**:468, 1997.
13. Antonarakis SE, The Nomenclature Working Group: Recommendations for a nomenclature system for human gene mutations. *Hum Mutat* **11**:1, 1998.
14. Cotton RGH, Scriver CR: Proof of "disease-causing" mutation. *Hum Mutat* **12**:1, 1998.
15. Waters PJ, Parniak MA, Nowacki P et al: In vitro expression analysis of mutations in phenylalanine hydroxylase: Linking genotype to phenotype and structure to function. *Hum Mutat* **11**:14, 1998.
16. Guldberg P, Mikkelsen I, Henriksen KF et al: In vivo assessment of mutations in the phenylalanine hydroxylase gene by phenylalanine loading: Characterization of seven common mutations *Eur J Pediatr* **154**:551, 1995.
17. Cooper DN, Krawczak M: *Human Gene Mutation*. Oxford, U.K., Bios Scientific Publishers, 1993.
18. Gelbart WM: Databases in genome research. *Science* **282**:659, 1998.
19. Burks C: Molecular biology database list. *Nucleic Acids Res* **27**:1, 1999.
20. Scriver CR, Nowacki PM, Lehvaslaiho H et al: Guidelines and recommendations for content, structure and deployment of mutation databases. *Hum Mutat* **13**:344, 1999.
21. Horaitis R, Cotton RGM: Human mutation databases. Unit 7.11. *Current Protocols in Human Genetics*, 1999.

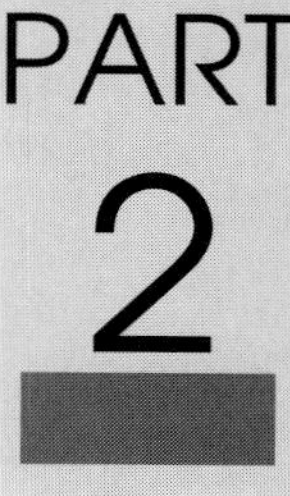

PERSPECTIVES

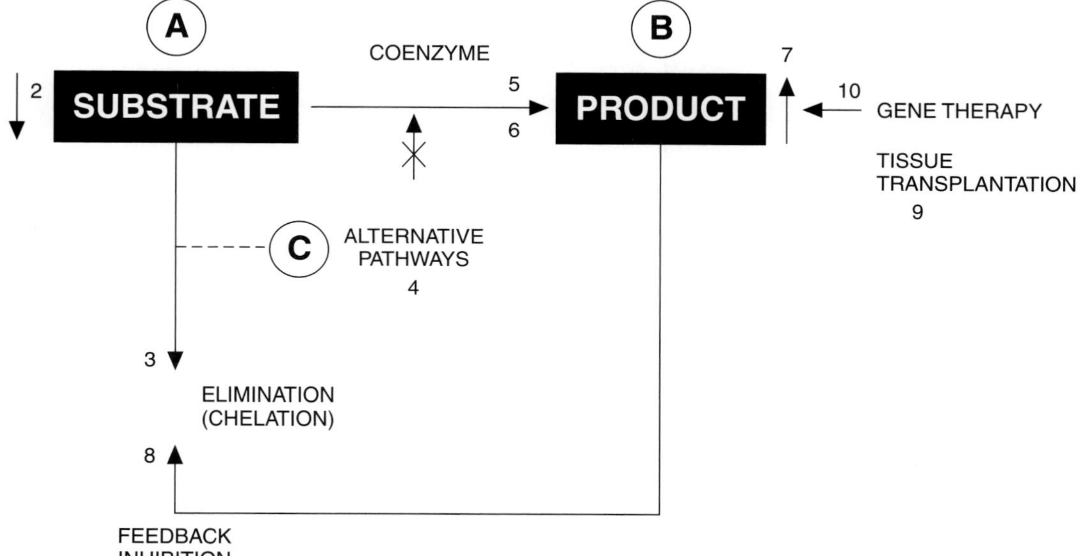

CHAPTER 2

A Logic of Disease

Barton Childs

INBORN ERRORS AND CHEMICAL INDIVIDUALITY

It might be claimed that what used to be spoken of as a diathesis is nothing else but chemical individuality. But to our chemical individualities are due our chemical *merits* as well as our chemical shortcomings; and it is more nearly true to say that the factors which confer upon us our predispositions to and immunities from the various mishaps which are spoken of as diseases, are inherent in our very chemical structure: and even in the molecular groupings which confer upon us our individualities, and which went to the making of the chromosomes from which we sprang.—A. E. Garrod[5]

The Inborn Error as a Central Theme in Medicine

The Metabolic and Molecular Bases of Inherited Disease is now in its eighth edition. It is an account of the origins and characteristics of diverse diseases, and being a human enterprise, the book has an ontogeny. The chief attribute of this development is the shift from biochemical explanations of pathogenesis to molecular descriptions of abnormality of structure and function, and with it has come a recognition that disease cannot be described simply as a consequence of a chance encounter with an inimical environment. Rather, it is individual variation in homeostatic range and flexibility that differentiates the disease-prone individual. So the ontogeny of MMBID is the history of the integration of genetics and medicine.

The first edition appeared in 1960, with the inborn error as its central theme. The editors advanced their intention to present "the pertinent clinical, biochemical and genetic information concerning those metabolic anomalies which have been grouped under Garrod's engaging term 'the inborn errors of metabolism.'"[1] They also recognized that the existing list of inborn errors was not exhaustive. This sensitivity to undiscovered disease was extended in later editions to a much enlarged definition of the inborn error, which at the start was limited to enzyme deficiencies. For example, the second edition included defects of serum proteins and of hemostasis, and in the fourth the immune system made its appearance. By the sixth edition 374 disorders were listed, and the definition of the inborn error had been extended to cancer and developmental defects due to chromosomal anomalies.[2] So in the face of such a proliferation, logic leads us to the conclusion that the inborn error is a central idea in medicine.

In this vein the editors of the sixth edition gave notice that the book ought to embrace any disease as soon as some glimmering of its biochemical-genetic attributes were perceived. Obviously, this definition of the inborn error embraces disorders called multifactorial, which constitute the chief bane of humankind, and it imposes no barrier to the inclusion of, say, prostatic hypertrophy and varicose veins, which in the general consensus are hardly perceived as due to inborn errors. Surely we are witnessing a change in medical thought no less profound than that in which morbid anatomy gave way to biochemical interpretations of pathogenesis. It is a change in the canon.

The idea of the inborn error crystallized in Garrod's mind while he studied patients with alkaptonuria.[3,4] In such patients, he said, the inborn error lay in their inability to degrade the benzene ring of homogentisic acid because the enzyme assigned to that step in the pathway was wanting. This idea led Garrod to infer that alkaptonuria was only one of what must be a nearly limitless list of variations that account for a chemical individuality that must identify each human being no less definitively than the more obvious physical properties by which each of us is known. Over the next several years he added several more inborn variants, which he suggested were merely a visible but trifling fragment of a great many more, which he confessed he was unable to find.[5] Few of these variants were diseases defined by disability or threat to life. Indeed, had Garrod perceived these inborn errors as diseases, the extension to chemical individuality might have had less appeal. That is, had he had to define inborn errors as we have done, in the context of overwhelming, often lethal, diseases, it is palpably less likely that he would have seen such catastrophes as simply one end of an uninterrupted distribution of the variation that characterizes the species.

Garrod perceived immediately the evolutionary implications of his ideas. He pointed to the diversity of protein structure that differentiates one species from others and then proposed that such variation did not stop at species borders but continued on into chemical individuality, so that it was not interspecies but intraspecies diversity, it was chemical individuality, that formed the substrate for natural selection and evolution.[4,5] Much later he summarized the thoughts of a lifetime in a second book—*Inborn Factors in Disease*.[6] In this book he relegated the rare inborn errors to a lesser role, as opposed to more frequent disorders, for which he used the term *diathesis*, a word that had been discredited, he said, because the idea was lacking in substance. But redefined as susceptibility based on chemical individuality, the concept is infused with meaning. Such individuality must be a vital ingredient in the cause of any disease, since "in every case of every malady there are two sets of factors at work in the formation of the morbid picture, namely, internal or constitutional factors inherent in the sufferer and usually inherited from his forebears, and external ones which fire the train." He thought that these internal inherited factors were generally latent and "are apt to be revealed sooner or later by the effects produced by external influences which are innocuous to the average man." Indeed, "For some individuals, those trifling traumata which go to make up the wear and tear of daily life are apparently the provoking cause of grave disorders." Many of these thoughts were drawn together in the last paragraph of *Inborn Factors*, which appears at the beginning of this chapter.

We cannot know what Garrod meant by "molecular groupings which confer. . . . " Certainly he didn't mean the DNA. In fact he never attained any particular interest in genetics.[4] Nor could he have meant amino acid sequence in proteins, since the recognition that such sequences confer specificity came only in the 1940s.[7] But it is clear that he saw that people differ in susceptibility to disease as a result of hereditary chemical variation, itself both a product of evolution and a substrate for natural selection. Obviously Garrod could not have imagined how today we can give genetic and molecular body to the concept of diathesis, and should a historian quarrel with a too-modern interpretation of an idea that is really an adumbration of a concept of disease that is just now taking shape, such a critic might at least agree that Garrod has given us a powerful metaphor to use to compare with that which informs our thoughts and practices today.

So the enlarging conception of the inborn error as it is taking shape in MMBID is something Garrod anticipated and would have been delighted to have observed. And it is the basis for the reorientation of our thinking about disease. Unlike Garrod, we do know about the DNA that specifies the proteins that constitute the homeostatic systems that characterize our species, and we know a little about the variation therein that confers biochemical uniqueness on each human being. And, in principle, we know how to use that knowledge to explain the origins of disease. Such an expanded definition of the inborn error tells us that all diseases arise out of some condition of incongruence between a chemical constitution and the factors of the environment that "fire the train." So we shall be practicing a medicine of genotypes rather than a medicine of phenotypes, a proposition to which the chapters of this book already attest.

Garrod and Osler: A Contrast

Archibald Garrod succeeded William Osler as Regius Professor of Medicine at Oxford.[4] There is a prophetic symbolism in this succession. Osler—or the Oslerian ideal; it is not easy to separate the man from the myth—dominated medicine in his time as few have done before or since.[8] And in large degree the ideal persists to this day. What is the Oslerian ideal? Disease is accepted as simply a fact of life, and it is the doctor's duty to deal with it. Osler's book, *The Principles and Practice of Medicine*, begins on page 1 with the diagnosis and treatment of typhoid fever.[9] There is no preliminary discussion of the nature of disease, of who is likely to be sick, who escapes, or why anyone should ever be sick at all. Indeed, it would have been thought eccentric to have started the book in any such way. As for medical education, "the student begins with the patient, continues with the patient, and ends his studies with the patient, using books and lectures as tools, as means to an end."[10] Osler put his considerable weight behind the idea of bedside teaching, of student participation in hospital care. Indeed, he said, "It is a safe rule to have no teaching without a patient for a text, and the best teaching is taught by the patient himself."[11] Such experiences with hospitalized patients, often heightened by the drama of life-threatening illness, formed the embryonic doctor's conception of disease as a puzzle to be solved. The solution must be always in the patient's interest—Osler was forceful in promoting humane care—but the illness was no less an interesting puzzle for all that.

To solve the conundrum the clinician was expected to use all five senses, a profound knowledge of pathology, and a broad experience of disease to arrive at a diagnosis that accurately reflects the pathologic process that accounts for the signs and symptoms. That is, in Osler's time, diagnosis was based on morbid anatomy, and then, as now, knowledge of pathogenesis was needed to formulate any more than symptomatic treatment. The skill of Oslerian clinicians was often of a high degree, and the histrionic talent displayed in matching wits with the pathologist in the drama of the Clinical Pathological Conference (CPC) enhanced for the student an absorbing educational experience.

We adhere to the Oslerian ideal today, and if morbid anatomy, the CPC, and finely honed senses have given way to biochemical and molecular diagnosis, aided by visual techniques that peer into the most remote recesses of the body, we still adapt our treatments to what we can learn about pathogenesis. And although we often fall short, we are still exhorted to pay at least as much attention to the needs, the fears, and the comfort of the patient as to the products of technological devices. In the Oslerian vein we ask the questions: What disease does the patient have? and How do I treat it? The emphasis is on the disease and how its effects are to be reversed. The patient, who is perceived as representative of the class of people with the disease at hand, might be anybody. Like Garrod, Osler perceived disease as "chemicophysical," but unlike the situation in Garrod's time, the idea of biologic individuality among patients was not prominent, indeed was perhaps never advanced. The function of a medical school, Osler said, was "to instruct men about disease, what it is, what are its manifestations, how it may be prevented and how it may be cured."[12] The emphasis here is wholly on disease; the patient is a battleground whereon a medical Saint George tilts with the dragon of disease.

The same questions phrased in the Garrodian context might be: What disease does this particular human being have? In what way does this patient differ from other people among whom he lives? and What can I do to restore this person's unique orientation to the environment? So, although both physicians wore striped trousers and a black coat when seeing patients in consultation, their ideas were literally poles apart. The difference between them is this: Osler, the activist, saw in a patient a broken machine and was at pains to tell the world how to fix it. Garrod, a contemplative man, saw the patient not as a broken machine but as a less well adapted product of evolution and the disease as a consequence of an encounter of a unique individual with an environment for which he was uniquely unfit. Osler's knowledge of evolution is not in question; rather his silence on the subject suggests that he gave it minor emphasis, whereas Garrod perceived evolution as a starting point in education.

Osler taught us how to practice medicine, Garrod how to think about it. Osler conjured with facts, Garrod with ideas. Oslerian thinking is organized around treatment and management. It is a practical approach in which the student is perceived as an apprentice who is learning what he needs to know to practice medicine. It is pretty much what we do in residency training. Garrodian thinking, in contrast, is about concepts: what diseases are and why they exist. So in the ontogeny of MMBID we are witnessing a transition from an Oslerian medicine to ideas that represent a natural elaboration of Garrod's thoughts about inborn errors, chemical individuality, and inborn susceptibility as a natural outcome of human evolution. No one would deny that Osler was the hero of the medicine of the 20th century. It is likely that Garrod will be the chief icon of the 21st.

THE TRANSITION FROM OSLERIAN TO GARRODIAN MEDICINE

Some of the contrasts in the thinking of the two Regius professors have been outlined. This section will be devoted to how these alternatives affect medical thought today.

Some may say that we have already attained the Garrodian state of mind, that the rich lore of human biology and genetics is sufficient to inform a logic of disease. There is no doubt that we are on our way to that goal, most notably perhaps through our grasp of the disorders included in this book, but in more complex diseases, too; the discovery of chemical individuality in atherosclerosis, high blood pressure, and cancer shows how our gaze is shifting from populations to the individual. But examination of medical textbooks, for example, suggests that we still have a long way to go; and while it is true that genetics, the branch of biology that embraces the idea of individuality, has become a medical watchword, there is every reason to believe that human genetics has been adapted to existing medical thinking, rather than having been allowed to change it.

In what follows, the basis for present medical thinking will be compared with an alternative. No doubt stark contrasts do not exist; reality is likely to reside somewhere in between.

But a contrast is most informative when polarities are brought out. Nor are the alternatives exclusionary. The best of all worlds is attained in the doctor who cleaves to the Oslerian ideal in practice and the Garrodian in thinking.

Prevalent Medical Thought

Human society is based on ideas; ideas inform and shape all our actions. They are often deeply embedded and interlaced with our identity and self-esteem. They lie there unarticulated and unexamined, and when threatened by a contrary idea, however rational, they are likely to be fiercely defended. Medical practices are based on such firmly rooted ideas, and they are seldom examined with the possibility of conscious change in mind. But discoveries in human biology, especially in genetics, compel just such an examination.

The Body as a Machine. The prevailing metaphor of medicine is that of the body as a machine which the doctor is called on to fix when it breaks; the latter's role is that of an engineer who uses technology in the service of practical utility.[13,14] And because it is expected that the engineer will indeed fix the disabled machine, the governing criterion of this view of medicine is cure. Of course, reality requires that amelioration be accepted, if only until the discovery of the details of the breakage that point to the actual cure. And there is faith in the capacity of science to find a cure. This optimism has been expressed by Lewis Thomas, our most lyrical expositor of high technology, who has said, "I cannot imagine any category of human disease that we are precluded by nature from thinking our way around."[15] "Disease," he says, "comes as a result of biological mistakes," and "the mechanisms of disease are quite open to intelligent intervention and reversal whenever we learn more about how they operate." Indeed, medicine has been defined by Seldin in just such a context.[16] The goals of medicine, he said, are "the relief of pain, the prevention of disability and the postponement of death by the application of the theoretical knowledge incorporated in medical science." The basic sciences, he said, furnish a theoretical framework for clinical medicine, a framework that consists of physiological homeostasis with its powers of communication and sensitive regulatory devices. So medicine uses biology to provide insights that lead to the discovery and explanation of pathogenesis, the better to invent an appropriate treatment. And, of course, herein lie the triumphs of medicine; cell and molecular biology show where and how disease has distorted homeostasis. This is where Lewis Thomas' "thinking around" is going on, where the virtuosi of the laboratory score their glittering successes. Indeed, it seems almost as if biology and medicine are one. Clinical investigators are doing basic science, and basic scientists contribute notably to the solution of clinical problems, and the rate at which information accumulates is such as to ensure that no one can encompass more than some limited fragment of the whole. For example, Osler carried his book *Principles and Practice of Medicine* through eight editions by himself. Now in its 22nd edition, the book has five editors and 159 contributors.[17] And this pattern is the rule now, whatever the subject of the book; MMBID is no exception. So when observed from some Olympian height, there is an inescapable sense that here, at last, in all this concerted effort, the promise of continuous and open-ended progress is being fulfilled, and if there is an end to it, it will be only after all the questions have been answered. If we know the sequence of base pairs in the entire human genome shall we not be well on our way to the millennium?[18]

Signs of Unease. This engineering mentality has dominated medical thought for 200 years or more, and through its influence on the classification of disease it has shaped medical institutions. For example, specialization has followed the classification of diseases by organ systems, etiology, age, and sex, with consequent influence on the organization of departments and divisions in medical schools and hospitals and with obvious reflection on medical teaching and training as well as on how medical care is provided. Nor is the rising cost of medical care exempted; efforts to diagnose disease and effect a cure have become increasingly dependent on expensive technology. It is a system that is generally agreed to have worked to public advantage, but given the rapidity of recent change, it can surprise no one that there are signs of strain. These signs are expressed in misgivings about medical education, the doctor-patient relationship, the fragmentation of the medical enterprise, and an apparent inability to accommodate prevention easily. Numerous committees of thoughtful physicians, educators, ethicists, and others have considered these strains and have reported their concerns.[19–30] One of these perceives "a continuing and accelerating erosion in the education of physicians," and cites a need for a "general professional education for physicians."[22]

The questions that emerged from the deliberations of these bodies were of two kinds. First, how is it possible to encompass the mountain of facts generated by molecular biology, the better to use them to medical ends? These facts, in all their baroque detail, are said to be too great a burden for any mind to bear, so some sort of framework of theory or logic must be found to bring out relationships, determine relative importance, and form hierarchies of knowledge. And it is evident that the massive accumulation of information about cause and pathogenesis of so many disorders has engendered centrifugal forces that have fragmented the medical enterprise into many self-contained subdisciplines, without at the same time providing a countervailing logic to hold them all together. Some might say that the seeds of this logic are near at hand. They are the DNA and the variation encoded within it. But although investigators in such unrelated disciplines as urology and ophthalmology are cloning genes and doing linkage studies, there is still little evidence that this is more than the application of technology to parochial problems.

Second, the committees ask, by what means can we bring the benefits of science to bear on disease without omitting the identity and human qualities of patients? Evidently, the technology has come between the patient and the doctor, distorting how each sees the other.[19]

Many suggestions for change have been advanced. These include fewer lectures, less emphasis on facts and more on independent thought, better integration of basic and clinical teaching, and more attention to the humanities and ethics. But such suggestions, while useful, may not be coming to grips with all that is wrong. It is as if the germ of change is not in the metaphor of the machine, which is not fertile and does not generate ideas or principles. It is not that the metaphor is not based on principles; the rules of biological homeostasis are certainly implied. Rather, there is nothing in the metaphor that allows us to infer where the machine came from, how it reproduces itself, how all the machines are related one to another, or how they all fit into the economy of the rest of the biological and social world. And we need such information if we are to understand why breakages occur, how or why they take the forms they do, why they affect one individual rather than another, and whether and how either breakage or individual fits into any grand biological scheme. And it may be that answers to these seemingly peripheral questions of where and how will reveal biological constraints that limit what can be done or that move the disposition from treatment to prevention. So it may be that what is needed is a new outlook in which the reasons why disease occurs at all, and the forms it takes, can be seen to be a consequence of how human beings have evolved.

An Alternative

Evolution is the touchstone of biological thought; nothing in biology makes sense apart from evolution. The criterion of cure leads to an ever narrower focus on the job at hand, but evolutionary thinking broadens the enquiry to include relationships of individuals to the past, to one another, and to the environment, even to the future. Apropos of medicine it raises questions of why anyone gets sick at all, what forms illnesses can take, and which particular human beings are likely to come down with which disease.

Congruence-Incongruence. Since evolution proceeds by descent with modification, the fates of individual human beings depend on their adaptation to the environments they meet. Through selection a species perfects its adaptation, so it is the molecular mechanisms by which this adaptive success is attained that occupy the minds of biological scientists: how molecules, cells, organs, and systems are integrated to attain the harmony required to fulfill a reproductive destiny in an indifferent environment. So biology, including genetics, which is its foundation, is the study of congruence, and it is in the framework of selection and evolution that the rules for the organization and behavior of living organisms are elaborated. The attainment of congruence for the species requires a stock of variation from which to choose. Some of it, in some individuals, leads not to harmony but to dissonance, which may lead to disease.[31] So disease is a consequence of incongruence with some aspect of the environment, internal or external, that is expressed in difficulty carrying out daily life or as a threat to life or reproduction or that may lead to residual handicap. It is an expression in microcosm of processes that in macrocosm account for evolution.

Representing disease as a consequence of incongruence gives it a biological as well as a social definition, and if it is biological and deriving from an evolutionary context, the rules that provide a logic of life must also provide a logic of disease, a set of principles that at the same time accommodate all diseases and the qualities that distinguish them. The basis for this logic is, on the one hand, our humanness, which will determine which diseases are possible and which not, and on the other hand, our individuality, which must determine who experiences them and in what degree. The concept of disease as an outcome of incongruence is the antithesis of that of the broken machine. If congruence represents a favorable ecological relationship that disease disrupts, then the doctor, who must be no less ardent in interventions to repair the dislocation, must see as his or her primary concern that of conservation. Accordingly, this concept is far more tolerant of prevention than is the concept of the doctor as engineer. Indeed, the role of conservator flows naturally from the principle of a favorable ecological balance. When the primary job of the doctor is perceived as treating disease, then prevention must accept a secondary position. But when the necessity to fix something broken is perceived to be due to failure of that which is believed to be the primary aim of medicine, then adaptation and prevention rise to preeminence.

Other Contrasts. Other contrasts between these concepts involve how individuality is defined, the relative importance accorded causes, and how these alternative positions influence traditional concepts of disease.

Individuality. Each of us expresses two kinds of individuality. First, we are each indivisible units of classes: sex, nationality, political party, occupation, and the like. The distinction here is that of the class, not of the persons of which the class is composed. At the same time, each of us is in a class of our own, in which we express a unique endowment and unique experiences by virtue of which we impart variety to the classes to which we belong. This means that each class is characterized by a range of expressions of class, and empirical observation reveals that although consensus is common, outliers are infrequent and may even be considered as classes themselves. So the first kind of individuality is distinguished by types or categories and the second by the ranges of qualities expressed by individuals in populations, and these differences inform our thinking. We think first in types and categories; we classify, and then deal with the members of each class individually—or we should. But the instinct for simplicity and order induces a powerful urge to classify and then, overlooking individuality, to characterize populations in terms of abstract mean values, to the neglect of dispersions constituted of real individuals. The contrasts between these two ways of thinking have been emphasized by Ernst Mayr.[32] Typological thinking he sees as inimical to biology, since it overlooks the variation that is the wherewithal of evolution. Population thinking, as he calls its antithesis, accommodates to individuality and its origins.

The concept of the body as a machine implies typological thinking; machines, even when hand-made, are built undeviatingly to a blueprint, so all are identical, or nearly so. But the Garrodian concept implies population thinking that embraces individual particularity; each unique human open system accommodates uniquely to a unique pattern of environments and experiences. Garrod put it, "each is an individual and not merely a member of the human race."[6] The medicine of today tilts toward the typological. Indeed, it is ironic that a profession so devoted to the care of individuals should care so little about individuality.

Causes. Ernst Mayr distinguishes two principal currents of biological thought by the kinds of questions they raise.[32] One of these, of which medicine is representative, is functional biology, which is concerned primarily with the structure and function of elements from molecules to organisms. So the questions a functional biologist asks are generally preceded by "how": How do organs work? How do cells communicate? How do molecules interact? The focus in functional studies is on the type; variability is not of interest. For example, biochemists and molecular biologists are interested in species-specific mechanisms, while medical investigators concentrate on the details of pathogenesis; both probe deeply, but narrowly. Natural history, the second current, is the realm of the evolutionary biologist, who asks questions preceded by "why": Why is a species the way it is, particularly in its adaptations and in its variation?[32,33] These two currents of thought coincide at the level of the genetic program. Functional biologists' questions have to do with everything that happens consequent on the decoding of the DNA. They are interested in immediate causes. Evolutionary biologists are interested in the history of the DNA, in mutation, gene duplication, chromosome organization, sex determination, segregation, selection, and the dynamics of the gene pool; they are concerned with remote causes—remote because they represent the mechanisms whereby, through selection of variable individuals, the species evolves. But genetic causes are not all. Obviously, an open system is in and of the environment and experiences it throughout life. So immediate and remote causes must also reside in a no less evolving social and cultural environment—immediate in experiences of the moment, remote in the cultural tradition and social organization that make experiences possible. So if we wish to explain disease, both kinds of causes are germane—the remote to account for (1) the origins of the agents of disease, (2) what forms diseases can take, and (3) how vulnerability is attained; the immediate to account for the characteristics of the illness itself.

Evidently it is the remote causes that set the rules of disease, but they may be of little interest to the doctor attending a patient in the intensive care unit. What matters there is the present state of pathogenesis and what can be done about it. In contrast, to the preventive mentality the presence of the patient in the hospital may be due to a failure to pay attention to the patient's genetic and cultural particularities, a failure to distinguish individuality and to use the information in the patient's best interest.

Traditional Definitions of Disease. How do we define the idea of disease in a way that includes these concepts of individuality and cause? This is far from a new question, alternative answers having been argued from antiquity. Each such answer has been appropriate to the concepts of its time, but throughout, two polar positions have been advanced.[34–41] In one, called "ontological" or "essentialist," each disease is accorded specific entity. Each is visited more or less randomly on previously healthy persons, has a specific, usually external cause, and is expressed in more or less constant form; each case is exemplary of a universal prototype. Infections fit this design very well, and hereditary diseases, despite their internal causes, fulfill the definition too. The latter are called "genetic" diseases in contrast to the former, which are called "environmental," and both are in consonance with the questions posed by the thoroughgoing Oslerian: What disease does this patient have? and How is it to be treated? The distinction among patients is subsidiary to the choice of treatment, which is directed to the disease, not the patient.

The second concept, called variously "nominal," "historical," or "physiological," describes disease not as entity but as quantitative deviation; the extreme version says there are no diseases, only sick people. Here the origins of disease have to do with peculiar qualities of each individual and are rooted in the general nature of humankind. A modern expression of this "historical" view might be that the causes of illness are not of themselves harmful but that they are expressed selectively in people with limited adaptive powers; sometimes, the limitation runs to everyone. It follows that the expressions of illness are dictated by the special qualities and experiences of each afflicted person but that similarities are observed because genes and experiences are shared, sometimes by everyone, sometimes by only a few related persons. The Garrodian questions pertinent to this view of disease are, How and why is this particular human being ill? and What treatment is appropriate for so peculiar a constitution? or What differentiates this patient from the population from which he or she is drawn?

The first of these definitions, and its questions, are clearly typological and appropriate to engineering thinking; individuality is that of the class, and emphasis is on immediate causes. But the second definition and its question are exemplary of population thinking. The individuality is that of the particular person with unique genes and experiences, and the immediate precipitating causes are perceived as deriving from the convergence of biological and cultural currents channeled into families by inheritance of both genes and mores.

The strength of the essentialist view lies in its perception of unity and homogeneity of entities. Since the differences between patients are merely variations on a single theme, one treatment should be suitable for all. But in its strength lies its weakness: there is the risk of overlooking heterogeneity of causes, which may dictate treatments appropriate for each. The strength of the historical view lies in the attention it draws to the particularities of each person. For example, it accommodates very well the complexity and heterogeneity of both cause and pathogenesis currently being uncovered by the use of the methods of molecular biology. Furthermore, since disease is defined as quantitative variation rather than separate entity, the physiological view accommodates easily the shifting, indefinable point at which health becomes disease or disease becomes health as well as the broad margin at which there is disagreement as to whether such disabling conditions as, say, alcoholism or panic attacks are to be called diseases at all; the individual is emphasized, not the entity. The essentialist tradition requires us to say that a person has a disease or does not, or else resort is made to the designation of "subclinical" or social deviation, which does nothing to help the "either-or" quality of the definition. The weakness of the nominalist position lies in an overemphasis on the individual. After all, if we did not classify, we should be nowhere at all, and if we did not try to group cases for treatment, we would be in worse financial straits than we are.

Conclusion

In summary, these two ways of looking at disease reveal some salient contrasts. The Oslerian view is essentialist; is approached typologically; emphasizes likeness between cases, means as opposed to dispersions, and proximate causes (especially abnormalities in the molecular composition of homeostatic systems); and conceives the body as a machine to be fixed by the doctor when it breaks.

The Garrodian view sees disease as a consequence of some incongruence between a patient's individuality and his or her environment, is approached in a populational turn of mind, emphasizes individual variation in the biological constitution of the patient, and while not neglecting proximate causes, seeks their origin in remote causes deriving from biological and cultural history, which is to say that disease in individuals is a byproduct of the processes necessary to preserve the species. And the role of the physician is to use his or her grasp of individuality to find ways to skirt the proximate causes and to make prevention the primary aim of medicine.

The prevailing concept today lies somewhere between these extremes. The pressures exerted by our understanding of the molecular basis and extent of human genetic diversity in both health and disease are pushing us toward the second of these polar positions. This view is more firmly based in biology than that of the body as a machine, so it should be possible to employ biological rules to compose a logic of incongruence that may do for disease what the rules of congruence do for normal biological development, structure, and function. And since congruence is an evolutionary concept, so must be incongruence.

A LOGIC OF DISEASE

Definition

What exactly is meant by a "logic of disease"? Webster's defines the word *logic* variously: (1) "a statement of the formal principles of a branch of knowledge," and (2) "interrelationships or connections or sequences of facts and events seen by rational analysis as inevitable, necessary or predictable." The questions here are, Are there principles of disease that flow by means of predictable connections and sequences from the facts of evolution and natural selection? Are there regularities in the nature, frequency, and characteristics of diseases that can be shown to be consequences of the human genetic and cultural condition? and Have the whole range of diseases some common properties that stem from the human substrate they all share? If such a logic can be demonstrated it should prove useful, perhaps principally to the medical teacher in offering the students both a framework for the facts and a philosophy, defining that word as embodying principles and causes of reality.[38] For the practitioner it should be useful in demystifying imponderables that must be confronted even in "straightforward" cases. The idea of such a logic of disease is well within the Garrodian canon and altogether foreign to that of Osler. Indeed, it might be said with reason that *Inborn Factors*[6] is an argument for just such a logic.

A critic might protest that human physiology and the pathogenesis of disease are far too complex to allow the elaboration of such a logic. There is too much randomness. Living organisms are not simple linear systems; their moment-to-moment behavior depends on their own state. So predictions can be only probabilistic at best. But even in chaotic systems like the weather, where conditions may change hourly, long-range predictions of climate are usually fulfilled. It is the rules of "climate" rather than "weather" that constitute the logic of disease. A critic might also say that any such logic must defy composition. The facts are too many and too diverse, the diseases too varied, the homeostasis too complex to be embraced in a set of principles. If such principles are truly comprehensive, they must be banal, and if not, then no logic will be apparent. But the authors of *Molecular Biology of the Cell*, a book of 1200 pages that comprehends much of what is known about the structure and function of cells, say in their preface, "There is a paradox in the growth of scientific knowledge. As information accumulates in ever more intimidating quantities, disconnected facts and impenetrable mysteries give way to rational explanations and simplicity emerges from chaos."[42] If simplicity emerges from chaos in the biology of normal cells, why not from the biology of cells caught up in the processes of disease?

Such a logic can evolve only when the thinking of biologists and that of physicians are so interlaced as to have attained the identity of a new discipline. This evolution is occurring rapidly as contrasts between the aims of cell and molecular biology and those of medicine are resolved. Some of these contrasts and convergences are reviewed below.

Biology and Medicine: Some Contrasts

In the practice of medicine the physician is confronted by outcomes of individual incongruence. Medical thought is not primarily concerned with such general biological aims as how the species has become attuned to the environment but with how patients have come to represent discordant notes in nature's harmony. So the physician tries to describe the behavioral, physiological, biochemical, and molecular attributes of individuals dissonant with life. That is not to say that physicians are altogether indifferent to the evolutionary forces that have led to adaptation and congruence or that biologists are indifferent to incongruence. Rather, the rules for a logic of disease must originate in an emphasis unlike that of either molecular biology or medicine. It is an emphasis perhaps more congenial to the population biologist or geneticist, whose views accommodate both the characterization of species and genetic individuality. If so, it will be useful to begin by contrasting the aims of biology with those of medicine and to show how they are coming to coincide.

Individuality. Biological thinking perceives individuals as vehicles for the transmission of genes and a means for generation of the variability required to maintain the species. In this view individuals represent the variegated materials from which an indifferent nature creates the fabric of species. In sharp contrast, medical thought perceives each human being as an individual person with an option to pursue life, liberty, and happiness, and it is the business of medicine to correct individual encumbrances to those pursuits. Molecular genetics is modifying this view of the individual to include uniqueness: a Garrodian chemical individuality that is expressed in disease no less than in other aspects of life.

Classification. In studying the elements of congruence, the questions biologists ask are given largely typological answers: this is how replication is achieved in *Escherichia coli*, homeotic genes control body segmentation, and so on. Further, although physiology is a strongly quantitative discipline, biochemistry is less so, and molecular biology is almost altogether qualitative. So for molecular biology, the classes are the species, and for the quantitative disciplines, individuality is disguised in means and deviations. Typological thinking in these disciplines is natural; variation is noise and biologists are interested in elaborating general rules of development and homeostasis. But a logic of disease requires population thinking; individuals are ill because their particular qualities are at odds with their particular experiences. The differences in goals between biology and medicine are also reflected in the language employed. In traditional medical thinking much attention is given to proximate causes. This preoccupation is revealed in our classification of diseases as "genetic" or "environmental." Although these typological classes are losing their sharp definition as the genetic contribution to "nongenetic" disorders is affirmed, we still call monogenic phenotypes "genetic," and we often refer to "genes for" even such ill-defined conditions as hypertension or schizophrenia. Molecular biologists are less likely to think of their phenotypes as genetic or nongenetic. Their interest in proximate causes derives from a need, not to circumscribe and classify, but to show how gene-specific molecules integrate in structure and function.[42] But when both are working at the level of the DNA and its products, even when pursuing quite different ends, differences in language and concept disappear. One result of this confluence of purpose is a growing interest among molecular biologists in "medical" problems as they are expressed in molecular aberration. This infusion was observed in the sixth edition of MMBID, in which, in the "General Themes" section, authors with nonmedical degrees were nearly equal in number to those with MDs, while among the rest, people with nonmedical degrees made up only 25 percent of the authors.

Families. A central feature of biology is the union of two gametes to engender a zygote. Population biology is much taken up with mating systems and families, reproductive fitness, ethnicity, and migration, all marginal to traditional medical thought. Physicians focus on people one at a time and deal only exceptionally (e.g., pediatrics or obstetrics) with couples or families; examples are couples plagued by infertility or whole families exposed to malign infections. But consanguinity, ethnicity, and history of illness among relatives are now staples of the encounter of patient and doctor. They represent the recognition of remote causes with their significance in preventive thinking. Whole families are also the basis for linkage studies that lead to the detection and description of genes of medical moment.

Time. A salient difference between biological and medical thought lies in the significance of time. To the biologist everything is "time-bound."[43] The organism "is not a particular expression of an ideal organism, but one thread in an infinite web of all living forms, all interrelated and all interdependent."[43] Biologists perceive ontogeny as a prelude to phylogeny; the development of each individual represents a test of the robustness and viability of the species. But in traditional medical thinking, species and the history of the DNA are of marginal interest or are irrelevant. The physician's attention is held by the here and now, by what must be done now. In biology, "To every thing there is a season, and a time to every purpose under the heaven, a time to be born and a time to die . . . " (Eccles. 3:1, 2). Not so in medicine, in which if imminent birth will be harmful, the time to be born must be changed, and a primary aim is to defer death as long as possible. To these ends medicine is practiced cross sectionally, the lifetime is stratified; obstetrics, pediatrics, adolescent medicine, internal medicine, and geriatrics all represent compartments wherein the nature of the work is determined by the age at onset of the disease. Such a narrow focus is likely to minimize the physician's appreciation of the unity of a lifetime that proceeds from zygote to dissolution, as well as to obscure the historical quality of development in which the attributes of today carry the stamp of the past.

But here too our thinking is beginning to change, and in two ways. The first is in the recognition of the predictive powers of genetics, which provide the wherewithal for reproductive decisions for individuals and families found to harbor undesirable mutants, as well as for probabilities for recurrence of many diseases associated with specific genes known to contribute to diseases of complex origin. These perceptions of the influence of genetic variation on disease are affecting the compartmentalization of medicine. Divisions and departments of genetics cross age boundaries to reveal patients as people with a past that begins in the lives of their ancestors and with a future that will be colored by genes inherited from those predecessors. Here the biologist's idea of time is imposed on the pragmatism of medicine.

The second way our thinking is changing is in our recognition that predispositions to diseases of late onset reside not only in the genes but in experiences of early life, beginning with conception and including intrauterine life.[44] Once the natural history of disease included only its history from some overt onset to its end. Now the natural history may be traced to conditions of hereditary susceptibility with early onset of subtle expressions that show a steady progression from genetic potential to pathogenesis. It is as if people grow into their diseases. Atherosclerosis and hypertension are examples.

Definition of Evolution

What is it specifically about evolution that suggests a logic of disease? After defining evolution, the argument will be presented in a series of propositions, each based on some aspect of the definition and each capable of expansion to include subsections and examples.

How is evolution defined? It is the process biological organisms undergo to attain the morphological and physiological characteristics that identify the species. It proceeds by descent with such modification as may be necessary to achieve adaptive flexibility in unstable environments. The modifications are a result of a process of sorting through stocks of genetic variation to find that which facilitates the broad range of congruence required for development and reproduction, and for the continuity of life both between and within species. The success or failure of such variants in fulfilling this mission is likely to be reflected in their frequencies in subsequent generations. Words in this definition most pertinent to the logic of disease are (1) species identity, (2) adaptive flexibility and development, (3) descent with modification, and (4) congruence and continuity. These key words and phrases can be elaborated into propositions that embody the concepts of the logic.

Elements of the Logic

Species Identity. Evolution is the record of biological history. Life has proceeded from the simple to the complex by integrating simple systems into more complicated aggregates, leading, at each new level of integration, to new constraints as well as new qualities.[45,46] The constraints are imposed because the new level of integration represents only one of several or many that might have occurred but did not, and new qualities emerge because old systems have been aggregated to interact in new and not necessarily predictable ways.[45,46] The basic biochemical elements of these systems took form very early in evolution, and diversification was made possible by new variation on old themes, including the differential use of existing biochemical mechanisms, the elaboration of new genes and gene families, and the development of more complex and refined controlling elements. Thus, phylogeny represents an uninterrupted continuum in which both change and stability are reflected in the sequences of units in the molecules of both DNA and protein, and despite the morphological and reproductive discontinuity that is observed in species, the molecular continuity remains. So, although species identity is sharply defined, shared properties that transcend species identity are retained, with implications for the logic of disease. This chemical continuity both between and within species was noted by Garrod.[5]

Lessons from Phylogeny: The Constraints of Evolution. Toward the end of Pope's "An Essay on Man," appears the line, "Whatever is, is right." We need not subscribe to the 18th-century ideology that informed the "Essay" to see the line as a metaphor for the relationship between a species and its environment. If a quality exists, it has stood the test of selection and is likely to serve, or to have served, some useful function.[47] It need not be the best possible adaptation; evolution is a process of tinkering. But whatever is selected is likely at some time and condition to represent some advantage. The search for such useful functions is the essence of what evolutionary biologists call "The adaptationist program."[47]

Adaptation is defined in relation to some environment or particular experiences, and however flexible the homeostatic defenses, adaptation to one environment or experience is likely to represent a constraint for another. Some such constraints may lead to incongruences: Some are species-specific; others, because of shared molecular identity, may cross species. There is preventive significance in such observations. That is, where particular experiences lead to disease in one species, they may do so in others. Similarly, environments and experiences that are foreign to one species are likely to be alien to individuals of related species. Two examples are given below. In one, a popular human experience shared by no other species has proven to be harmful to many individuals. In a second, a species-specific adaptation has proved to exert an unexpected constraint.

1. The Use of Tobacco. Nowhere among plants and animals do we find any who seek or tolerate an atmosphere of smoke; no species other than *Homo sapiens* purposefully dilutes inspired oxygen with carbon monoxide. A biologically alert society might have made these observations and taken warning; for example, today no substance capable of the degree of damage plainly caused by tobacco could possibly be widely advertised and legitimately sold — except tobacco. So, if it had been observed that inhalation of smoke is natural to no organism, the possibility of harm to human beings might have been carefully examined. But, as it happened, the hazard of smoking became apparent in Britain only when it was observed to be strongly associated with an otherwise unaccountable rise in the incidence of bronchogenic cancer, and in the United States only when a surgeon observed the frequency ofheavy smokers among his patients with lung cancer.[48–50] The observations were entirely empirical; no one had tested the hypothesis that smoking might be damaging. Evidence of the relationship of smoking and chronic obstructive pulmonary disease and heart attack came later, after suspicion about the bad effects of smoking had been aroused.

Today we know that smoking is associated with cancer of several organs other than the lung — with chronic pulmonary disorders, atherosclerosis and heart attack, reproductive hazards, and indeed with abnormality of nearly every organ system. It is an imposing list, and in an appraisal of data gathered from 31 "developed" countries, Peto et al. concluded that about 30 percent of deaths of individuals between 35 and 69 years of age in these countries during the 1990s are attributable to smoking.[51] So it is now a principal contributor to early mortality. Medical educators might do well to teach the virtues of nature's examples.

2. Breast-Feeding. No one would deny that human milk is the "natural" food for newly born human babies; again, evolution has seen to that.[52] To begin with, breast-feeding leads to temporary amenorrhea in the mother and a natural spacing of pregnancies of around 2 years.[53] Failure of this natural contraception and more frequent childbearing may promote disease and mortality for all infants embraced within the narrowed interval.[53,54] But for many reasons, some necessary, some trivial, infants may be fed nonhuman milk.

Although we act as if birth represents a discrete discontinuity from intrauterine life, it is in fact a far less abrupt change than it seems; it is more like doing the same business under new conditions. At birth the infant assumes responsibility for its own physiology and development but must still conform to the trajectory set *in utero* and supported by the maternal environment. Some of the infant's physiological equipment needs time to adapt to the new environment, and it is human milk that has been designed by nature to supply the antibodies, nutrients, and other substances that the infant lacks. Cow's milk is the most popular substitute, but is it appropriate? Perhaps not, at least not for all infants. For example, the rate of development of the brain of the human newborn infant is well behind that of a newborn calf, so we may question whether cow's milk, which is adapted to the needs of calves, is attuned to the dynamics of early postnatal human development. That it is not is suggested by the discovery that average attainments on tests of cognitive development of premature infants fed cow's milk were significantly less than their breast-fed coevals.[55] Further, a comparison of learning-disabled children with controls showed that significantly fewer of the former were breast-fed,[56] and scores in language attainment tests of 15-year-old children were significantly higher among those who had been breast-fed.[57] Table 2-1 is a sample of a growing literature on the protective effects of human as opposed to cow's milk. The

Table 2-1 Diseases Prevented or Ameliorated by Human Milk

Disorder	References
Type I diabetes mellitus	168–170
Allergies	61, 62
Necrotizing enterocolitis	63
Urinary tract infection	64
Infectious diarrhea	59, 60, 65
α_1-Antitrypsin and infantile liver disease	66, 67
Otitis media	68
Childhood lymphoma	69
Sudden infant death syndrome	70

reasons for these effects are not always clear. Protection against diabetes is attained by avoiding cow's milk proteins,[58] but the evolutionary origin of protection against diarrhea is demonstrated by the discovery in human milk of a glycolipid receptor analogue that binds to Shiga toxin, thereby preventing its adherence to its target receptors.[59] Another example of protection against microorganisms is a human milk mucin that specifically binds rotaviruses,[60] and still another is an enhancement of response to *Haemophilus influenzae* vaccine in breast-fed babies.[71] So human milk is best for human babies. No data exist to attest to the dangers of human milk when fed to calves, but we have every reason to suppose they exist. Oddly enough, the evolutionary significance of human milk has been remarked on for years, but until recently medical thinking managed to ignore it, so we have been given all sorts of milk substitutes, some facsimiles, some representing "improvements." But human milk is a cardinal example of Pope's principle, or possibly of that of a later, less elegant poet who said, "If it ain't broke, don't fix it."

Adaptive Flexibility: Homeostasis and Development. Human beings are open systems in and of the world around them, so the species has evolved physiological mechanisms to ensure protective responses to environmental fluctuation. The qualities of the molecules that compose these systems reflect relationships of individuals to family, populations, species, and phylogeny. These same molecules are also engaged in the processes of development and change as individuals move through life. So homeostasis has several faces.

Homeostasis. It is amusing to think of Claude Bernard, W. B. Cannon, and L. J. Henderson whiling away an afternoon at the bar of some celestial Harvard Club examining the sixth edition of MMBID. Who can doubt their pleasure in observing that although the word *homeostasis* does not appear in the index, the ideas are so deeply woven into the thinking of the authors of all the articles that each disease is perceived as a genetic flaw in some homeostatic system. All this they would approve with enthusiasm, even while envying today's biological scientist the ideas, the information, and the technology available to pursue aims they could only imagine. Bernard, who perceived a *milieu interieure* that defended the integrity of the cells, and Henderson, who saw the blood as an agent of integration that governed the fluxes of gases, water, and ions into and out of Bernard's milieu, would be delighted with mechanisms of transport that include gates and channels through which the flow of ions and metabolites is controlled by the contortions of proteins responding to signals that start and stop the flow. And Cannon would rejoice in the complexity of the endocrine system, the peptide hormones that penetrate to the nuclei of cells to influence genes to transcribe RNA. And they might above all applaud the modern description of the integration of components to form and protect the whole organism, since it was the whole organism that was the object of their interest.[72–76] Henderson in particular emphasized that stability lay in complexity; the greater the number of components and the more intricate their interrelationships, the greater the stability of the whole.[74,75]

But they might regret the lack of attention to the relationships of social homeostasis to disease.[72,75,76] They would say that since physiological homeostasis is the means whereby an open system maintains its integrity in its environment, some knowledge of how that environment is organized is essential to a full understanding of the internal milieu. After all, it is the outside that tests the inside. All three were much taken by the idea that societies were organized around mechanisms of self-regulation.[72,74–76] They recognized the necessity for integration of the elements of society in a government that controls communication, regulation, and protection; individuals, families, and communities can survive only by organizing and integrating systems to preserve the common weal.

At some point they might be joined by C. H. Waddington, who would add that physiological homeostasis would be at risk were it not for the genes whose strategy it is to guide and preserve homeostasis through a lifetime and to connect each person with an ordered past and a possible future.[77] Waddington was interested in working out a synthesis of genetics, evolutionary biology, and embryology.[78] Lacking knowledge of the molecules involved, he envisioned this interaction in the form of "epigenetic landscapes," in which he attempted to give dynamic visual form to the differentiation, under genetic guidance, of homogeneous cells into diverse cell types.[77] Today, insights into determination, differentiation, and morphogenesis have been given molecular and biochemical body, and the synthesis Waddington visualized in the abstract is a reality.[79,80] So there is a homeostasis of the genes that constrains the physiological homeostasis of the individuals who compose the species. Accordingly, Waddington would say, no biological story can ever be complete unless it is told in three time frames at once — that of the moment, that of the lifetime, and that of evolution.[77]

In introducing the genes into the discussion Waddington would be adding a dimension not emphasized by the others. The study of the mechanisms of physiological homeostasis is the study of proximate causes, but by connecting the momentary time frame with that of the past, Waddington introduces remote causes that regulate whether and how the proximate causes can work. It is through evolution, genetic variation, selection, and adaptation that physiological homeostatic systems have attained the perfection we observe. And it is in these same processes that the remote causes of disease are to be found.

Of the three time frames, Waddington was primarily interested in that of the lifetime.[77] Here the strategy of the genes embraces yet another homeostasis, that of ontogeny, wherein the genes help both to promote and to constrain development through early life and on into aging, wherein the integration of physiological homeostasis is loosened. This relationship of development to physiological homeostasis was observed by Cannon, who remarked that people "grow into" their regulatory processes.[76] And, he might have added, in aging they grow out of them. So, since physiology changes throughout development, moment-to-moment homeostasis could be said to represent a cross-sectional account of developmental homeostasis. That is, as development proceeds, the matrix wherein the interactions of the genes and experiences take place changes. Early in development, newly activated genes begin their mission, adjusting later to new conditions. Thus, moment-to-moment phenotypes are outcomes of hierarchies of causes derived from three systems of organization — the genes, the environment, and development — each with its own imperatives. And inevitably, each such phenotype exerts a reciprocal influence on the forces that shaped it; there is a dialectical process. This idea has been expounded by Lewontin, who has pointed out how organisms not only adapt to their surroundings but do much to shape them.[81]

1. The Present: The Phenotype. The word *phenotype* is being used here as a stand-in for moment-to-moment homeostasis and its effects. It may be taken to include all the enzyme pathways and cascades, receiving and signaling systems, transporting mechanisms, and other means whereby metabolic business is done. It embraces also the means whereby such systems are integrated in the whole organism to protect the interior from adverse experiences. The molecular details of moment-to-moment homeostasis is the principal subject of the authors of the sections of this book. Less attention has been given to the relationships of physiological homeostasis to the elements of the other time frames.

2. The Past: Genetic and Cultural Homeostasis. **Genetic homeostasis** — The purpose of life, as opposed to that of individual lives, is reproduction. To this end each species has a gene pool whose stability is maintained by reproduction, through which both losses and replenishment are attained. The instruments of this stability are the individuals of the species, who as recipients of aliquots of the pool act as filters, transmitting whatever genes and combinations of genes are workable and discarding those that are not by reproductive failure. So there is a genetic homeostasis, which in serving the purpose of reproducing the species serves that of individual lives too, but with the proviso that the preservation of the gene pool comes first. That is, the necessity for replenishment and variation brings in new mutants and new combinations of genes, many inviable, some conditionally tolerable, and perhaps a few even useful. All of these must be submitted to the test of life, so the necessity to replenish and preserve the stability of the gene pool is an overriding remote cause of diseases whose proximate causes are the mutants themselves.

The means whereby the stability of the gene pool is both conserved and promoted is the province of evolutionary biologists. Genetics is first of all a predictive discipline, so it can be no surprise that theories of natural selection and evolution were advanced even before there were data to test them. These data were supplied by Lewontin for *Drosophila* and Harris for *H. sapiens* when, after examining the mobility of soluble enzymes in electrophoresis, they found that nearly a third of the loci specifying soluble enzymes of both species were polymorphic and that there was a great deal of rare variation as well.[82,83] These studies of enzyme polymorphism have been extended to many hundreds of species with similar results,[84] so we know, at least in regard to soluble enzymes, how variable the species are, and it is well attested that the average human being is heterozygous for 7–10 percent of such loci.[82,83] And now we know that the polymorphism of the DNA is far greater still.

It is not yet clear to what degree all this variation, particularly that of proteins, has been attained by selection and how much by chance. But theory suggests it is mainly by chance, and theory is made plausible by the observation that allelic differences in enzyme mobility are not usually reflected in significant differences in activity.[83] But the question remains whether there is selective advantage in some heterozygotes.[84,85] That is, substantial heterozygosity would reduce species variability, enhancing conformity to the average and reducing the number of anomalous outliers. This is an old question that has engendered much controversy, and it is still unsettled, although studies of many species have demonstrated the reduced variability and enhanced developmental stability anticipated in the hypothesis.[84–86] The alternative, that heterozygosity contributes to a "genetic load," or debt to be paid in illness or death, while clearly not applicable to much of the common polymorphism, retains some validity in regard to heterozygosity for a few mutants associated with recessive disease.[87,88] That is, although Kacser and Burns have demonstrated that heterozygotes for most recessive mutants show no deficiency in the flux through a pathway, there are a few such heterozygotes that express modified forms of the diseases observed in homozygotes or unexpected susceptibility to other disorders.[88–91]

Cultural homeostasis—If remote causes of disease are engendered by the requirement of species for genetic variation, the organization of the environment must be no less a source of such causes. Both the gene pool and the cultural traits that characterize societies evolve. Cultural traits are the ideas, beliefs, and values by which we live, and they motivate society, so there are analogies between cultural traits and genes on the one hand and between social organization and biological integration on the other.[92–95] Culture is to society what genes are to physiology. This analogy between the evolution of biological qualities and that of cultural traits has been given serious attention by several workers in the past decade.[92–95] Some of their thinking is summarized below.

Cultural traits may be perceived as units of transmission and as being capable of mutation. They may be transmitted vertically like the genes, but also horizontally, as between sibs or coevals, and obliquely, as between aunt and nephew. Other departures from the Mendelian-like pattern involve the transmission of ideas or behaviors from one central figure to many pupils or fans as well as from many to one, as in the pressure on individuals to accept the conventional wisdom. The cultural units may also vary in frequency as genes do and are subject to selection, proliferating to prevalence or diminishing to extinction. And their frequencies may be changed by migration—adoption of foreign styles, say—or by chance. But unlike biological qualities, which change at glacial rates, cultural change may be very rapid, a difference in tempo likely to create incongruence and risks for disease.

There is much interaction between the behaviors determined by culture and the homeostatic qualities promoted by the genes; the former may constitute risk factors for disease. And there is a complex relationship in the evolution, or coevolution, of both. Apposite examples are given by Durham.[95] One is the persistence of lactase in the intestinal mucosa of some populations. This persistence varies directly with latitude and inversely with skin pigmentation and ultraviolet radiation exposure. The hypothesis is that in areas of low ultraviolet radiation precursors may not be converted to active vitamin D and there is the threat of rickets, which, untreated, may reduce reproductive fitness. But rickets can be averted by lactose, which promotes the intestinal absorption of Ca^{2+}; hence the persistence of lactase. But where the intensity of ultraviolet radiation is high, rickets is not a threat, so lactase is unneeded. So cultural and biological traits have evolved together.

Durham's second example is that of the well-known advantage of hemoglobin S in malarial areas. In some parts of Africa the frequency of the hemoglobin S gene is influenced by diet. The highest frequency of the gene is found where yams are cultivated for food. Yams require sunlight, which means cleared forests and warm sunlit pools wherein the mosquitos thrive. Populations that live in forests and eat other food have fewer mosquitoes, less malaria, and less hemoglobin S.

So there are intimate relationships between gene frequencies and the way people live. Gene-determined molecules work in cellular environments, themselves influenced by cultural traits that determine social environments. Sometimes these are at cross purposes and therefore of interest in medicine. The tobacco industry and human health are again an example. The tobacco enterprise has its own internal homeostasis that includes farmers, manufacturers, wholesalers, retailers, advertisers, marketers, and lobbyists. And it is a part of a larger homeostatic system consisting of community, state, and international trade. The livelihoods of all the workers named above, as well as taxes and the economy, all depend on smokers who imperil their health by smoking and do so in the face of growing social disapprobation. So in this case, physiological homeostasis, subject to injury by smoke, is opposed by a social homeostasis, and we are observing how difficult it is, when there is a clash of values, to change the prevalent custom, even when it is manifestly harmful. Social homeostatic systems are as stubborn and defensive as the physiological version.

Medical educators often stress the need for an infusion of "humanities" into the medical curriculum. The inheritance and evolution of cultural traits, their influence on social homeostasis, and how these interact with their biological counterparts would seem an appropriate answer to their concern.

3. The Lifetime: Developmental Homeostasis. Nature imposes three tests on us all: (1) We must survive long enough to (2) attain fertility, which should lead to (3) successful reproduction. To fail any is to fail nature's intent, but only the first compromises individual life irretrievably. Obviously, nature's expectations can be fulfilled only by a fully developed person acting independently, so human development may be seen as a path to independence. Although it is useful to think of development in stages, it is in fact seamlessly continuous. Birth and puberty, however apparently discrete, are merely transitional phases that lead to fertility and reproduction. Aging is more insidious, more indistinct, and miscellaneous in its choice of organ systems. There is some question whether aging is a part of development at all, but if not, it is inalienably coupled with it.

The human path to independence lasts longer than that of even our nearest phylogenetic relatives. It is characterized by neoteny, an evolutionary program wherein juvenility is much prolonged and, in comparison with related organisms, retained in adult features.[96] For example, not only is the time of growth and maturation of human beings longer than that of, say, the chimpanzee, but as adults we have features that resemble those of their young. This prolonged growth and maturation has promoted bipedal posture as well as enlargement and increased complexity and plasticity of the brain; the latter persists into adult life, even into old age. The advantages are obvious. Extended exposure of a gradually maturing nervous system to experiences of a variable environment, together with the mental resiliency to continue to learn at all ages, is a recipe for the adaptive agility that has enabled human beings to live in all latitudes and climates and so to exploit the earth's resources to construct civilizations and to be aesthetically creative. These achievements are a consequence of the nature of learning. Learning is not a static process of piling block on block. Rather it is integrative; what we learn today has been determined by what we learned yesterday, and tomorrow's learning will be influenced by today's. So the store of learning accumulates and takes the learners into diverse fields of information and behavior. Learning is a metaphor for development, which is also a historical process.[97] The effects of experience are accumulative and, within constraints set by diverse genotypes, lead to variable developmental paths — "canalization," Waddington called it. So development is a formative process in which we move through life from the general to the specific, the unspecialized to the particular, the simple to the complex, defining and refining our distinctions and risking, in old age, becoming caricatures of ourselves.

Early life — It is the special triumph of molecular biology to have replaced the phenomenology of embryology with molecular explanations of mechanisms.[98] Induction, fields, and gradients have given way to descriptions of the molecules engaged in fertilization and cell division and in cell determination and differentiation.[98,99] Molecular mechanisms of intercellular communication, migration, adhesion, association, morphogenesis, and selective cell death have been discovered, and lineages of cells have been traced to their final roles in the coordinated assembly of specialized cells in the tissues and organs of the embryo.[99] All these processes are under rather strict genic control, and while chance enters in, for example, in the choice of which cells migrate in which direction and which die off (called "developmental noise" by Waddington), there is little leeway for mistakes that would result in distortions. So embryogenesis is more nearly programmed than later fetal and postnatal development, in which the opportunities for variation due to experiences are progressively greater. And postnatal development shows it. For example, attainment of postnatal milestones is increasingly variable with age; nearly all babies sit unaided at or around 6 months, but walking and talking vary by several months, and even broader limits are observed around the onset of menses and puberty. Social development is more variable still. Very young infants respond only to stimuli imposed on them; later, babies learn to evoke responses and still later to create for themselves an environment in which to react.[100] So by slowing the process of our development into whatever each of us is to become, neoteny provides opportunities for shaping that outcome, some of it by choice and some by the imposition of outside influences, adding thereby to individuality and to the diversity of the species. Neoteny allows us to escape the tyranny of our genes, or at least to modulate their rule.

Maternal effects on gestational life — There is another source of individuality in development. Although fetal life is shielded from the outside by the uterus and maternal circulation, intrauterine life is marked by maternal effects, some of which leave a lifelong stamp. Table 2-2 lists some of these.

(1) Since all of the cytoplasm of the fertilized ovum is maternal, the events of the first cell divisions are governed not by the embryo but by the mother. (2) The transfer of maternal mitochondria may have an impact on developmental direction and disease. (3) Maternal-fetal incompatibilities make the embryo a potentially incompatible graft. Results of blood group antigen incompatibility are well known, and while polymorphism of the MHC antigens makes inconsonance the rule, paradoxically, maternal-paternal compatibility for these proteins reduces fertility.[101] (4) Imprinting of parental genes is reflected in inheritance of disease according to the sex of one or the other parent, the imprinting having created a species of haploidy.[102,103] If imprinting is a consequence of the necessity to defend the integrity of membranes and embryo, then such a biological necessity is a remote cause of disorders whose proximate causes are traceable to the haploid effect. (5) Variations in the intrauterine environment may have profound effects on development; maternal age and birth rank are examples with effects that may not be apparent until postnatal life. For example, onset of both insulin-dependent diabetes mellitus (IDDM) and schizophrenia is influenced by the age of the mother at the birth of the patient. Further, maternal disease may reduce fertility or have adverse fetal consequences. Phenylketonuria (PKU) and IDDM are examples. (6) Disorders due to external influences are too well known to review here. Their often profound effects prejudice the lives of their victims, and the differences in effects depending on the timing of the insult is further evidence of the historical nature of development. (7) Neotenous delay means that the newborn human infant, as compared with those of other primate species, is still a fetus, so the continuation of an intimate maternal-infant tie is paramount. The virtues of human milk in this regard have been reviewed above.

Table 2-2 Maternal Effects on Development of Embryo, Fetus, and Newborn

	In Utero	Postnatal
Maternal genes	Mitochondria Imprinting Maternal–fetal incompatibility	
Maternal environment	Cytoplasm of zygote Nutrition Maternal age Birth rank Disease Teratogens Drugs	Breast milk Cultural environment

These aspects of fetal and early infant life have been recounted one at a time, but in fact every embryo and fetus is subject to some version of each of these variables and to many others besides, including its own genes. And the course such an individual takes must depend both on the qualities of all these influences and on how they interact with one another at which times in ontogeny. What happens in embryogenesis is the coalescence of parts into a unique individual. Each embryonic phase represents another choice, a further canalization, another irretrievable ordination to be supplanted by yet another, each reducing the range of choices for the next. The fertilized ovum represents the earliest and most versatile array of matrixes for homeostatic development and change. As embryogenesis and postnatal growth continue, each matrix is influenced by the last, and each influences the next so that no characteristic can escape the mark of individual history. So a salient feature of ontogeny is the continuous creation of new matrixes for the interaction of genes and experiences, an internal environment that is strongly influential in the shaping of phenotypes, that they cannot be analyzed apart from it.

Later life — The path to independence peters out somewhere in early adult life; the first two tests have been passed and the third is or is not an option. All systems are at peak performance and seemingly ready to go on forever. But, insidiously and variously, aging begins in the third decade, hardly recognized by the individual and for most purposes compensated by homeostasis, whose only sign of aging is a modest delay in return to baseline after perturbation.[104] Early expressions are followed by increasing homeostatic disorder; some see aging as a kind of entropy. The uniqueness of individual aging is composed of individual patterns of affected homeostatic systems, indeed of individual cells,[104] so if it is dust from which we arise and dust to which we return, each aliquot thereof will have traveled a different route. Evidences of this uniqueness are derived from both cross-sectional and longitudinal studies.[105] The former reveal increasing variances with age for physiological measurements, while the latter make clear that patterns and rates of aging in different organ systems vary independently both within and among individuals. That is, few individuals follow the patterns of change predicted by averages of many subjects, and the age of an individual is a poor predictor of performance in tests of physical function. Evidently, cleaving to the central tendency is a criterion for passing the three tests; afterward we are at liberty to pursue an individual path compounded of not entirely wholesome gene effects and possibly destructive experiences.

Why do we age and what causes it? More than 300 theories of aging have been reported.[106] If anything is favored, it is that selection bears most heavily on life before reproduction ends and, as it were, loses interest after that.[107,108] Williams has suggested that genes that are at a selective advantage in youth are less useful, even damaging, in later life.[107] Kirkwood has explained this seeming paradox by proposing that nature wisely invests energy resources in youth and reproduction rather than in the very expensive enzymatic and metabolic equipment required to continue indefinitely to repair the random and cumulative ravages of life's experiences.[108] And it is this damage, whether due to oxidants, free radicals, radiation, or other causes, that leads to such metabolic aberrations as reduced protein synthesis and degradation, changes in posttranslational modification, and failure of DNA repair.[109] So is aging itself a form of disease, or does it provide a favorable substrate for the agents of disease? This is a moot question and may always be.[110,111] Homeostatic abnormality, due either to mutations in the germ line or to aging, creates a substrate for disease, which becomes overt, perhaps as a consequence of other mutants or of cumulative damage or, more likely, of both. For example, do the dominant diseases of later years emerge because of aging? The mutants date to conception but may express themselves only when some homeostatic inhibition is weakened by aging.[112] This relationship of disease to aging was foreseen by Garrod, who proposed that susceptibility might become overt disease in individuals who encounter "the innumerable minimal insults that constitute the wear and tear of living."

A Conclusion. A logic of disease must be based on relationships between physiological, genetic, and developmental homeostasis and on prevalent cultures. Susceptibility, made up of accumulating effects of genes and experiences, becomes a disease whose form depends on the specificity of the genes and experiences as well as on the individuality of ontogeny. These elements, which can be seen to comprehend Waddington's three time frames—the present, the lifetime, and the biological past—can be listed as in Table 2-3, in an arrangement that allows the physician to analyze each case according to the individual array of constituents, which is to say, to the individuality of the case, which itself should help in the choice of treatment. Is it not also plausible that so individual an analysis of a patient's disease must lead the doctor to observe the specificity of the patient as a person?

Descent with Modification. If evolution proceeds by descent with modification, the basis for the latter is the mutable gene. Genetic novelty arises in point mutations and the meiotic reconstitution of chromosomes. Variations in chromosomal conformation and number occur also and may be important in speciation.

Table 2-3 Elements Contributing to the Individuality of Phenotypes

Genes	Developmental Matrix	Environment (Experiences)
Major gene	Age	Geography
Modifiers	Sex	Time
	Parental effects	Climate
	Ethnic group	Education
	Cognition	Occupation
	Behavioral attributes	Diet
		Habits
		Socioeconomic status
		Disease

If the inborn error is a central theme in medicine, the gene must be at the heart of the logic that gives the inborn error such a position. What is a gene? Although the word has not changed since Johanssen's coinage, the ideas it embodies have evolved, always in consonance with the techniques available to pursue the question. So this section on descent with modification must begin with some definitions.

Definitions of the Gene. It is significant that the ideas of the gene originated in an evolutionary context. For example, Mendel did not set out to invent genetics; he was attempting to give mathematical rigor to experiments on hybrids that were expected to elucidate speciation, and the Ancestrian-Mendelist controversy of the first decade of this century turned on whether the genetic contribution to evolution was continuous or discontinuous.[113,114] Genetic explanations of natural selection and evolution were the subject of the lucubrations of Fisher, Wright, and Haldane in the 1920s and 1930s, and Delbruck, the physicist, was drawn to study the replication of genes in bacteriophages because therein might lie the answer to the "riddle of life."[115] Indeed, it is generally accepted that nothing in biology makes sense apart from evolution. So the salience of mutable genes and chromosomes in the origins of disease locks the logic of disease into evolution. Accordingly, this section will be devoted to how this need for variation leads to inborn errors that, broadly defined, originate the pathogenesis of disease.

Initial definitions of the gene were statistical and abstract. It is not easy today to grasp the thinking of Bateson, whose heritable "unit character" was actually a phenotype, not a gene, or the ideas of Johanssen, who distinguished genotype from phenotype but could not accept that the gene represented more than a statistical concept. But the drosophilists and maize geneticists, whose experiments led to an operational definition of the gene, located heritable units in chromosomes and demonstrated linkage, recombination, allelism, and mutation, which, in turn, led them to propose that specific entities would be found in the chromosomes that would add a functional definition to the statistical and operational versions.[116] Such a concept was clarified by Beadle and Tatum's elaboration of Garrod's inborn error to include a unitary relationship of specificity between genes and enzymes. And finally, the acceptance of DNA as the genetic material, together with the recognition of the information latent in its structure, led to a structural definition, with the collinearity of nucleotide sequence in DNA with amino acid sequence in protein at its core.[117] Later discoveries of new features of the DNA—exons, introns, flanking sequences, promoters, enhancers, repeating sequences, and the like—led to an enlarged definition of the gene to include everything that is transcribed into RNA, which, in omitting that which goes untranscribed, omits a good deal of "genetic material."[118]

The Uses of These Definitions. In analyzing the genetic contribution to a disease phenotype we follow the historical path of the definition of the gene. We begin with a comparison of the recurrence rate of the disorder in families with the incidence in the general population. This is often followed by tests of twin concordance, path analysis, and calculation of heritability. These statistical processes ignore the physical reality of genes. Segregation analysis and tests of phenotypic heterogeneity or even of linkage with another defined phenotype provide operational definition—evidence that a physical gene exists. Next, the association of a biochemical attribute that segregates with the phenotype provides a functional dimension directing attention to some abnormal protein, which in turn channels the search for chromosomal location and a structural dissection of its originator gene. So the diagnostic process, defined in this instance as characterization of the phenotype by specific cause, has imitated the historical in its progression from a statistical definition by way of operational and functional descriptions to a structural reality. Diagnosis is an ontogenetic process that recapitulates the phylogeny of gene definition.

In the process of descent of the definition of the gene from an abstract heritability to DNA, a concept of gene action evolved in which information was shown to flow in the opposite direction, that is, from base-pair sequences to physiological levels of ever-increasing complexity, ending with some property of biologic, social, and evolutionary significance. Most of the inborn errors listed in MMBID have been characterized by following the path of phenotype to DNA, but today it is possible to omit the steps between the phenotype and the DNA and, beginning with the latter, to proceed to the discovery of an affected protein and so to elucidate pathogenesis. Examples are muscular dystrophy, chronic granulomatous disease, and cystic fibrosis. These successes suggest that as the fruits of the human genome initiative become available the latter pathway may come to prevail. But even then, history will not be denied. Phenotypic descriptions will always be necessary, and statistical and operational evidences of genetic influences will always be useful in detecting linkage with some marker of known genetic provenance. So this example of cultural evolution resembles its biologic counterpart in patching together something useful from that which history offers as well as that which is new. If there is a revolution in genetics it is in the methods; the ideas have evolved.

Mutation: Whatever Is, Is Variable. If the gene is the central focus of evolution, it is because of its capacity for variation. The mutability of the DNA, its versatility in response to the agencies of mutation, and the studied imprecision of the instruments of its repair provide the wherewithal for nature the tinkerer to try out what she will.[46] Perhaps most of the trials turn out to be errors that remain in the untranslated DNA or are lost by chance, but those that remain in translatable DNA are constrained by the consequences of previous tinkering, which, having turned out to work in particular conditions, is likely to be intolerant of further novelty. But some changes, representing neither better nor worse in the homeostasis of the moment, do attain such population frequencies as to constitute a reserve of variation against unforeseen need.

Mutation is both random and extravagant in its variety. These properties are reviewed in Chap. 3; it is enough to observe here that since nothing we know exempts any part of the DNA, or any part of any chromosome, no gene product is immune to genetic variation. So the question for medicine is how random mutation is reflected in overt or potential disease. Many of the answers to this question are given in Chap. 1. Here I wish to emphasize some implications of the observation that all DNA is susceptible to mutation.

The first such implication is the vulnerability of all elements in all homeostatic systems. A second is that the specificity of expression of disease and the severity thereof must depend on both the nature of the mutation involved and how critical it is to optimal homeostasis—for example, whether it is highly conserved or rate-limiting, and so on. These implications are under test. Figure 2-1

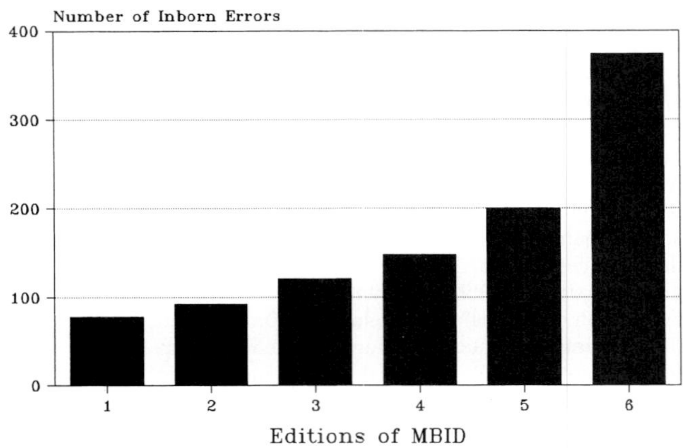

Fig. 2-1 Inborn errors being described at a rapid rate.

shows the rate at which single-gene inborn errors have been accumulated in the editions of MMBID. The curve will surely continue to rise, and at some point it will be useful to ask questions about which genes are proving to be most prone to cause what kinds of disease. In the meantime an implication for the medical educator is the necessity to bring about a change in mentality; the expectation of type causes variation to be squeezed and kneaded into existing classes, whereas the flexibility to see variation rather than type leads to the description of new disorders. A visceral grasp of the extent and variety of mutation promotes the latter frame of mind.

Heterogeneity. A further implication of the randomness of mutation is the heritability of genetic heterogeneity. The subject is given appropriate prominence in Chap. 1; it is enough to say here that unilocal heterogeneity will certainly be found in all monogenic diseases, while multilocal heterogeneity is equally inevitable whenever more than one gene is required for expression of disease.

We are accustomed to thinking of heterogeneity as distinguishing families. At the clinical level heterogeneity is suspected when there is within-family likeness and between-family difference for any of many manifestations of a disorder. But when a disease is a consequence of the effects of two or more genes, heterogeneity becomes more and more difficult, at the clinical level, to sort out, partly because there is likely to be allelic variety for each locus and partly because the heterogeneity may be as much within families as between.

Nor is that all. There is heterogeneity in experiences of the environment as well. Smoking is again an example. There are smokers, former smokers, and nonsmokers, and the smokers and former smokers vary according to intensity of exposure to smoke—for example, the number and type (filter, nonfilter) of cigarettes smoked per day, how completely they are smoked, whether or not the smoke is inhaled, and the duration of the smoking experience, sometimes expressed as pack-years. And of course other experiences, with their own variations in kind, duration, and intensity, act as modifiers of the heterogeneity of the experience of smoking—to say nothing of providing variables in which genetic heterogeneity may be expressed.

Summary. In this section we have been dealing with the means to attain a balance between a teeming variety in the DNA and the necessity for homeostatic stability. Most of the alternatives proffered by the DNA cannot contribute to such an end, so the remote causes of individual disease reside in the freedom of the DNA to experiment in the interest of a resilient homeostasis for the species.

Sexual Reproduction and Its Consequences. Only at the level of gene-protein specificity is bimodality commonly observed in human biology. Most human phenotypes are readily accommodated in continuous distributions; evidently nature prefers continuity, which is to say, variability. But sex is a nearly complete dichotomy, and paradoxically, the complete differentiation of the sexes is an important reason for the continuity and variability of other phenotypes and as such must be included among remote causes of disease.

The Diploid State. Diploidy enables eukaryotes to tolerate a greater range of mutational variation than is allowed to prokaryotes, and so to submit a broader compass of options to selective test. The consequences of diploidy expressed in dominant, recessive, and sex-linked phenotypes are discussed in detail in Chap. 1. The emphasis here is on the origins of human disease as a consequence of the possession of a double chromosome set.

Physiological Differences. A diploid zygote is compounded from sexually differentiated gametes. This differentiation has three kinds of implications for disease: (1) Sex chromosome differences are compensated by inactivation of one X chromosome in females. But even though such inactivation equates the number of active genes in each cell, populations of cells may reflect both allelic differences and variable inactivation, giving females sources of variation denied males. (2) Physiological differentiation leads to increasing divergence of the sexes in body conformation and structure, as well as in the function of homeostatic systems susceptible to hormonal influence, some of which work in ways not directly related to reproduction or sexually differentiated behavior. (3) Behavioral development is codified in sexual characteristics that differentiate the outcomes of the kinds, intensities, and durations of experiences to which the sexes are exposed.

So genetic, physiological, and social influences create aspects of the developmental matrix that condition and modify not only normal homeostasis but how, where, and when it breaks down under the influence of mutant genes and experiences. That is why in characterizing the clinical and physiological qualities of diseases at all ages, sex is always included as an important variable.

The Frequency of Disease. What accounts for the frequency of a disease? Why are some rare while others retain frequencies of 1–10 percent of a population, occasionally even more, despite their harmful effects?

The answer is in no way surprising if asked in an evolutionary context. Given a species that is well accommodated to environments commonly encountered, rare diseases must be a consequence of (1) breaches of adaptation, due to genetic mistakes that invariably make their victims unfit, or (2) chance encounters with "foreign" environments infrequently met. The common diseases, for their part, are due mainly to encounters with environments that have been systematically changed from those to which the species had become reconciled or changed in response to social and cultural imperatives that are at odds with biological adaptation and that lead to both deficiency and intolerance. Some of these changes are poverty, increased population densities that have changed the population dynamics of microorganisms, and dietary habits for which human beings are not genetically prepared.[31] These social changes represent provocations that single out the genetically vulnerable, who may be fairly frequent for two reasons — because the genes that contribute to their vulnerability are not intrinsically as noxious as the rare genes and because such genes may have, under other conditions, contributed something useful.[119,120] Of course, assortative mating and inbreeding play some part, but perhaps less and less as the world becomes increasingly panmictic.

Why do people not have several diseases at once? The answer is some do, but where genetic differences are influential the frequencies are multiples of those of the genes involved. So there should be a frequency distribution in the population in which unlucky outliers on one side have several or many genetic susceptibilities, some or several of which are overtly expressed, while their more fortunate brethren at the other end have none at all. The former die prematurely, the latter live to a healthy old age. Since it is the nature of such distributions to decline from the mean, outliers are infrequent. The modal position is currently unknown. Do we all have some genes that put us at risk for something? Perhaps, but maybe only under conditions that require other genes, too, or complicated concatenations of genes and experiences acting only at particular phases of the lifetime. It is a promise of the human genome initiative to provide lists of such genes. But whether or not such lists are either desired or desirable remains to be seen.[121]

So, if disease is to be perceived as a consequence of incongruence between homeostasis and experiences of the environment, the forces that account for the qualities and frequencies of both the specific genes and the experiences that have interacted to produce a disease represent remote causes that have set the stage for proximate causes that lead to pathogenesis. The conditions that engender those forces have been recounted in the section on "Homeostasis" above. The point to be made here is that the frequency of most diseases is not randomly attained. Its variability is commensurate with the selective values of genes, values that are determined by the congruence of their effects with experiences of the environment, a congruence that may be nil from conception or, of more consequence in medicine, be overwhelmed by the consequences of choices offered in a society all of whose diverse motivations are not necessarily compatible with human biology.

CONGRUENCE AND INCONGRUENCE; UNITY AND CONTINUITY IN EXPRESSION OF DISEASE

Textbooks of medicine are all alike; they dispense their information in tight compartments. Nowhere are we given evidence of unity and continuity in disease. Textbooks of biology, in contrast, begin at the beginning to elaborate principles that unify the whole subject. Logic suggests that what is possible in biology can be done in medicine; if biological congruence exemplifies unity and continuity, so must incongruence.

In this section we examine salient features shared by all disease for evidence of unity and continuity. Do these features show relationships with one another? Are there ways they can be arranged in some sort of order? These characteristics are set out in Table 2-4. Measures of all these qualities are distributed continuously both between and within diseases. For example, each disorder is characterized by an age at onset and a degree of burden, so that they can be arranged in order from the earliest onset to the latest and from the most perilous to the least. These features also vary within diseases, sometimes widely and often together. And so it is with the other qualities included in the table.

A Gradient of Selective Effect

How are these qualities related? Can we compose a coherent account of why we have disease at all and of its great variability? We begin with (1) the constraints set by evolution that make the species incongruent with some aspects of the environment. Add

Table 2-4 Characteristics of Disease

Mode of inheritance	Number of diseases
Age at onset	Burden
Frequency	Sex differences
Latency	Influence of migration
Affected relatives	Secular change
Diagnostic specificity	Effects of SES

(2) the variability of kind and frequency of mutants in the population and (3) the kinds, frequencies, intensities, and possible durations of exposures to experiences of the environment that can interact within (4) the variable contexts of individual developmental qualities and directions, and there emerges a recipe for a gradient of selective effect that wanes over the lifetime of a cohort of individuals and that accommodates all the qualities listed in Table 2-4. The device of the cohort contributes coherence to the argument, because changes in its composition and behavior may be traced from the simultaneous conception of all to the death of its last member. Further, it allows unambiguous comparisons to be made both between individuals and across the lifetime of each. The bases for the selective gradient are the variation in detrimental effects of both genes and experiences from something lethal to none at all and the relationship of these effects to individual ontogenies.

But why should there be a gradient of selective effect? There are several reasons. First, the controlled imperfection of mutational and recombinational events at meiosis is species business and it is transacted in perfect indifference to the life or happiness of individual inheritors. And much of such novelty makes its heirs the object of "purifying" selection. So we human beings lead two lives. In one we are inheritors, generators, and transmitters of the variation that maintains the species. In the other we each use our unique endowment to make a life of individual expression. It is a remarkable device and one that works well in the interest of the species and of most individuals too, but sometimes these purposes conflict and incongruence arises. Second, since the mutations range in damage to the DNA from losses of whole chromosomes to harmless base substitutions, their potential for impact on the developing organism must vary from lethal to none. Third, the evolutionary significance of mutated genes may make a difference. For example, mutations in genes specifying housekeeping enzymes, histones, or chaperoning proteins may exert more physiological impact than those, say, that differentiate the alleles of the blood group substances. Fourth, since some genes are active only in some cell types, and that only at some times in ontogeny, the effects of disruptive mutants, although concentrated early in life, must be distributed throughout development and aging. And fifth, since it is the business of homeostasis to modulate less than optimal influences, incongruence may be buffered and overt consequences deferred until some change in development or in experience, or both, proves too taxing.

The logic is as follows. The most destructive mutants, measured by burden and reproductive impairment, must be the first to be selected against, the next most destructive next, and so on. In primitive populations, such selection would be expressed in mortality, but in the developed world, onset of disease is a surrogate. So the contribution of genetic variation to disease declines continuously throughout the life of the cohort, even while exposure to experiences capable of promoting disease increases, and their effects accumulate. This means that the cohort is at its most variable genetically at conception and at its least at its end, while variation due to experiences is least at conception and increases and accumulates throughout. These reciprocal trends are shown schematically in Fig. 2-2A, which appears adjacent to a distribution by age of mortality rates (Fig. 2-2B). The latter is a continuous U-shaped distribution that resembles that made by the intersecting lines of Fig. 2-2A. Everyone knows that the diseases contributing to mortality in the two arms of the distribution of mortality rates are quite different. Figure 2-2A suggests a reason why they differ, and Table 2-5 lists the characteristics that differentiate them. As it happens, the antimode of the distribution of mortality coincides pretty well with puberty, so the list distinguishes prepubertal and postpubertal disease.

Continuity of Monogenic, Multifactorial Modes of Inheritance. The list in Table 2-5 represents confirmation of expectations raised by the selective gradient. The most obvious implication of the genetic gradient is the strong association of monogenic disease with early onset and of multifactorial causes with later onset. But, in fact, there is no discontinuity: (1) There are multifactorial disorders of childhood and monogenic diseases with onset in late adult life. (2) Monogenic conditions are subject to modification by other genes. (3) Some monogenic inborn errors are made overt only in specific circumstances. So, in a very real sense, all phenotypes are multifactorial, and the multiple genes that contribute to multifactorial phenotypes are constrained by nature to behave qualitatively in the same way as those that contribute to Mendelizing phenotypes; at some level of gene action they too produce segregating effects. So what do we find at the interface? One example is PKU (Chap. 77). What causes this disease—the mutant that specifies an ineffective enzyme or the phenylalanine, which is toxic in doses tolerable to the unaffected? Obviously both are required, and in a quantitative balance. A second example is G-6-PD deficiency (Chap. 179) in African-Americans, in whom the cause of the (usually) mild hemolysis in deficient individuals is the interaction of the mutant and one of several drugs. Favism also depends on G-6-PD deficiency, but for hemolysis some other genetic factor is needed too. So if PKU and G-6-PD deficiency are prototypical multifactorial disorders, favism is a prototype of multigenic, multifactorial disorders.

But it is not only the genes that distinguish these prototypical examples; so do the provocative experiences. PKU is precipitated by intolerance to phenylalanine and only phenylalanine; nothing else will do. So the environmental component in this disorder is unitary and of general prevalence, in consonance with most other inborn errors in which the "environmental" component consists of the intracellular homeostasis with which the mutant effect is incongruent. In contrast, the agents of hemolysis in African-Americans with G-6-PD deficiency are neither unitary nor prevalent; they are mainly drugs with no counterpart in nature, and they are numerous. So these two interface disorders are embraced in a continuum in which incompatible environments or provocative experiences vary from intrinsic and unitary to unnatural and numerous. PKU looks back in the continuum to, say, Tay-Sachs disease, while G-6-PD deficiency in African-Americans looks ahead to conditions with causes that are likely to be more variable, less pervasive, and cumulative.

Typological thinkers may reject the idea that monogenic phenotypes could be multifactorial, perhaps on the grounds that the former mendelize while the latter do not. But even the typologist must accept that PKU and G-6-PD deficiency represent a prelude to complex interactions to be observed in other diseases and that they are unambiguous evidence of a seamless continuity between the Mendelian and multifactorial modes of inheritance. And if this is true, then phenotypes of the latter mode may be seen as special cases of the former and our approach to analysis is guided accordingly. That is, we know that the genes will behave the same in both cases; they will specify or regulate protein products, act epistatically, vary in influence with gene dosage, and cause dominant or recessive effects, and our aim is, no less in one case than in the other, to discover the genes and to characterize them as to both their primary effects and their contributions to the complex physiological aberrations represented in pathogenesis.

Monogenic Disorders. What of the other characteristics in Table 2-5? How are they accommodated in the selective gradient? That monogenic disorders should tend to be numerous, be infrequent, have an early onset, carry heavy burdens, and be relatively impervious to the effects of socioeconomic status, migration, and secular change is to be expected. They should also show sex differences when the mutant is sex-linked, and diagnostic specificity should be high, given how discretely the homeostasis is distorted by the mutants. But all of these qualities are variable. For example, Garrod's inborn errors, while rare, were low on the scale of burden; no one has yet found a disease manifestation in people with pentosuria. And single-gene diseases of late onset are well known.

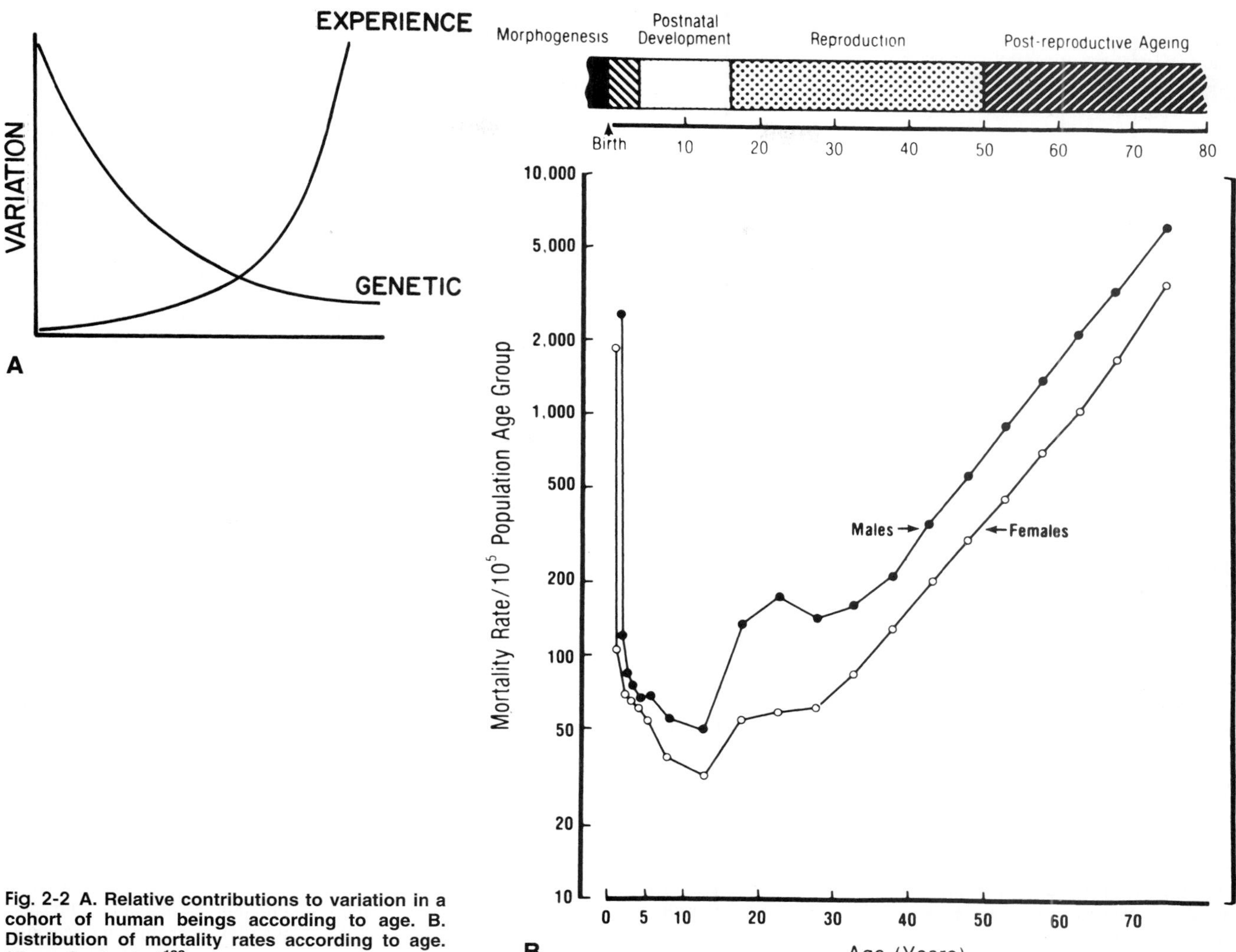

Fig. 2-2 A. Relative contributions to variation in a cohort of human beings according to age. B. Distribution of mortality rates according to age. (*From Costa et al.*[122])

A Test of the Gradient: Monogenic Disorders. An empirical test of these expectations was made by Costa, who studied a sample of entries in the fifth edition of *Mendelian Inheritance in Man.*[122] The study showed that 90 percent of monogenic entries had onset before puberty and only 1 percent after 40 years of age (Fig. 2-3). Onsets of the recessives were aggregated in the early years, while most disorders of late onset were dominants. Burden, as measured by threat to life, diminished fertility, and residual handicap, followed the pattern of age at onset of the recessives and dominants, with expression of X-linked disorders in between.

Table 2-5 **Differences between Prepubertal and Postpubertal Diseases**

	Prepubertal	Postpubertal
Mode of inheritance	Monogenic	Multifactorial
Age at onset	Early	Late
Frequency	Rare	Frequent
Latency	Short	Long
Affected relatives	Numerous	Few
Diagnostic specificity	High	Low
Number of diseases	Very many	Fewer
Burden	Great	Less
Sex differences	Occasional	Frequent
Influences of migration	No	Yes
Secular change	No	Yes
Effects of SES	Some	More
Success in treatment	Some	More

Figure 2-3 shows an uninterrupted decline in number of disorders by age at onset, but a distribution of burden as measured by reduced longevity according to age at onset (Fig. 2-4) shows two distinct peaks that coincide with significant developmental milestones: one with birth and the assumption of responsibility for one's own metabolism, and the second with postpubertal adjustment to the necessity to make one's own way in a life of stresses and exposure. Yet another distribution, that of dominant disorders according to age at onset, showed three peaks—one corresponding with fetal life, one with childhood, and a third with late adult life. Presumably, the dis-integration of homeostasis associated with aging has provided a favorable substrate for the emergence of effects of genes causing these late-onset monogenic conditions; Huntington's disease is an example.[112] Although the study was not designed to show it, it follows that genetic heterogeneity would introduce variation in each attribute; inborn errors characterized by onset at birth would have milder forms with later onset, perhaps even as late as adult life. For example, ornithine transcarbamylase deficiency, a sex-linked inborn error characterized by an explosive onset in newborn males, has been known to declare itself, with fatal consequences, after 40 years of age.[123]

To return to Fig. 2-4, why are there fewer lethal conditions with onset in fetal life than in the newborn period? A plausible reason is

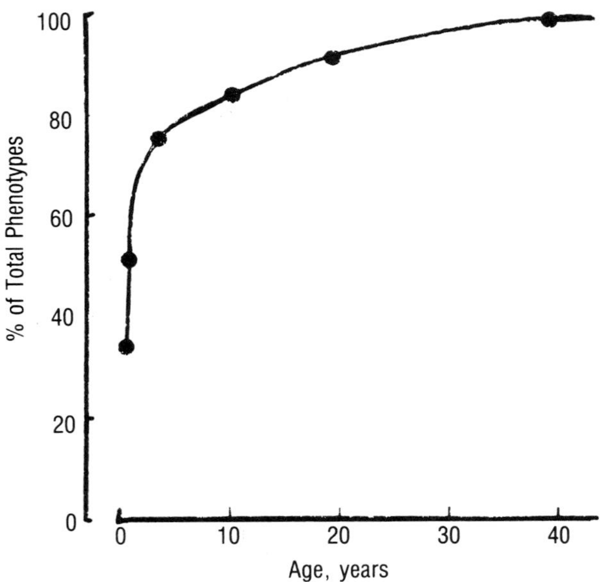

Fig. 2-3 Most Mendelian phenotypes are expressed early in life. (*Adapted from data in Costa et al.*[122])

that the latter represent only the backwash of a heavy intrauterine mortality. Indirect evidence suggests that as many as 70–80 percent of conceptuses never make it to term, while more direct evidence indicates that as many as 40 percent of implanted embryos are lost; most of the latter cases are due to chromosomal aneuploidy.[124–126] So, had it been possible to add the data representing mortality *in utero* to Fig. 2-4, there would be three modes, corresponding to morphogenesis and intrauterine development, the perinatal period, and young to midadult life, all times when new pressures are applied to homeostatic vulnerability. Evidently there is a new spate of monogenic variation presented for selection early in each developmental stage, with a greater contribution of variation in experience in its latter phase. For example, stillbirths and late abortions are usually associated with abnormality of the maternal environment; mortality in childhood is often due to accidents and mayhem, and that of old age is commonly associated with infections, malnutrition, and the entropy of time.

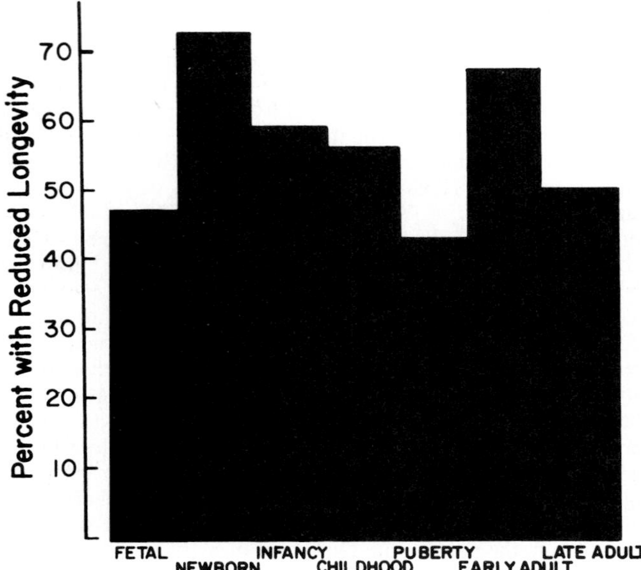

Fig. 2-4 Effect of Mendelian disease on longevity in relation to age at onset. (*Adapted from data in Costa et al.*[122])

Treatment of Monogenic Disorders. Success in treatment of monogenic diseases reflects the extent of homeostatic damage. A study of 65 inborn errors with a known defect of an enzyme or other protein revealed that treatment was ineffective in about half, somewhat ameliorative in 40 percent, and restorative to something like normal in the rest (12 percent).[127] A moment's reflection reveals why these inborn errors are so intractable. Evolution leads to increasing integration, complexity, and stability, but only at the expense of increasing constraint. So we cannot expect an easy conquest of imperfections in that which required millions of years to construct. Gene therapy will help, but the virtues of prevention are nowhere more evident.

Multifactorial Disorders. Evidence tends to support the gradient idea in the case of monogenic disorders. What should we expect of multifactorial disease? Although each of the multigenes expresses no qualitative differences from those implicated in monogenic disorders, each cannot of itself produce a disease phenotype. The latter is a consequence, as it were, of a chorus of modifiers, each contributing something different in both quality and intensity to the whole. So these genes must be positioned farther down the selective gradient, and in consequence the diseases would be expected to have a later onset, affect fewer relatives, and impose a lesser burden as measured by threat to life and fertility; to be fewer in number; to respond to variations in socioeconomic status, migration, and secular change; to show more variation according to sex; and to be more responsive to management.

All this is expressive of a greater individuality in disease expressed along a continuum of diagnostic specificity. For example, although there is a modest variability in clinical expression of Tay-Sachs disease, and no dearth of allelic variability, each patient is, within pretty narrow limits, representative of all. In contrast, when a patient is said to have atherosclerosis, no very particular clinical expression is conjured up by the name, and such are the degree of both multilocal and allelic genetic heterogeneity and the variation in kind, intensity, and duration of experiences that we can say that a patient given such a diagnosis is representative only of self.

A Test of the Gradient: Multifactorial Disorders. A test of the gradient hypothesis in relation to several multifactorial conditions was reported.[128] Several expectations were tested. In this trial no effort was made to arrange the diseases themselves in any order. The question was of the existence of a selective gradient within diseases.

The assumption was that since such disorders are likely to be heterogeneous as to kinds and number of both mutants and experiences, the selective declivity should express itself in several ways: (1) Age-specific age at onset should reach a peak and then decline. By some age or other most of those possessing the requisite genes are likely to have the disease. (2) Cases of early onset are more likely to have affected first-degree relatives, to be associated with "major" genes, and to express the disease with greater severity. That is, the most disadaptive mutants, and aggregations thereof, should be salient in cases with early onset, while those with late onset should be characterized by accumulation of experiences. As a result, the frequency of affected relatives should fall continuously. A further consequence is a decline in concordance of monozygotic twin pairs with increasing age at onset for the first twin. (3) Family history and age at onset should vary with migration, secular change, and socioeconomic status. When the homeostasis of a population is taxed by experiences of some new cultural environment, the salience of the genetic contribution to the disorder in the population is likely to be reduced. But when the pressure on homeostasis is relieved, the apparent contribution of the genes in the remaining cases must rise. (4) In diseases that show a sex difference in incidence, the cases of the less frequently affected sex should have an early onset and more affected relatives.[129] The idea is that a more powerful genetic impulse is required to affect a member of the less frequently involved sex. (5) Late-onset cases should be milder, more readily prevented, and more responsive to treatment. An overtaxed homeostasis is bound to be easier to manage than one that was faulty from the start.

To provide a test of the hypothesis, nine diseases were chosen only because each had been a frequent object of epidemiological and genetic study — duodenal ulcer, non-insulin-dependent diabetes mellitus (NIDDM), Crohn's disease, gout, Parkinson's disease, celiac disease, systemic lupus erythematosus, rheumatoid arthritis (RA), and Alzheimer's disease. All but Parkinson's disease, Alzheimer's disease, and RA reached a peak for age-specific age at onset and then declined, but for each of these three, at least one study showed such a peak. In all but duodenal ulcer, the cases of earlier onset were more severe, and in all, including duodenal ulcer, early onset was more often accompanied by positive family history. The presence of some associated polymorphic genes was noted in duodenal ulcer (ABO blood groups), celiac disease, lupus erythematosus, and RA (HLA alleles). The effect of sex was well illustrated in gout, in which women with onset at ages 30–50, although greatly outnumbered by men, had more attacks of gout per year, higher serum uric acid levels, and more affected relatives.[130] The salience of experience in cases of late onset was illustrated in gout, in which hyperuricemia and arthritis were associated, in older males and females alike, with the use of diuretics in the treatment of hypertension, and in the effects of obesity and parity in type II diabetes.[131] Lean patients with this disease are more likely to have affected relatives than obese patients, and parity follows the same pattern; nulliparous diabetic women are more likely to have affected relatives, a quality that declines with parity.[131,132] As for the effects of migration, secular change, and socioeconomic status, although it is clear that cultural changes have greatly increased the incidence of type II diabetes and gout in certain populations, we have no comparative data as to family history or age at onset before the change and so can draw no conclusion. But the position apropos of socioeconomic status was well illustrated in a study by Marmo et al., who contrasted mortality rates due to heart attack across four grades of civil servants in London.[133] Although risk factors and mortality were inversely related to socioeconomic status, family history varied directly.

Success in treatment follows the expected pattern; there is an inverse relationship between intensity of selection against gene effects and success. For example, dietary change alone often suffices in treating late-onset patients with type II diabetes, patients with iatrogenic gout — usually late onset — are relieved by a change in medication, and the generally mild rheumatoid arthritis of late onset is more susceptible to suppressive therapy.

The study outlined above suffers the handicap of looking for answers to questions that were never asked; the data are often nowhere to be found. In addition, the diseases included may not be representative and in any case are a small sample of the universe. But there is no dearth of additional evidence. For example, there is an uninterrupted decline in number of affected relatives with rising age at onset of major depression, and early onset of schizophrenia is also associated with familial aggregation.[134,135] Salient genes contributing to early-onset NIDDM have been discovered, as have at least two genes associated with early-onset hypertension.[136–138] And early-onset forms of cancer of the breast, prostate, and large bowel have been described.[139–141]

Both investigations reviewed above were intended to test the idea of an unbroken continuity in the expression of disease. And both were efforts to explore the unity in medicine, to discover threads of thought about disease that can be woven into a comprehensive fabric. Each was an exercise in Garrodian thinking that began with the assumption that a student of medicine should examine that which holds medicine together before disappearing into one of its byways.

Heritability

There is a further dimension useful in defining the unity and continuity of disease — that of heritability. Heritability is an expression of the quantitative contribution of genetic variation to a trait. It is based on correlations of measurements of a property between various kinds of pairs of individuals — monozygotic twins, dizygotic twins, parent-child, sib-sib, and so on — and it is representative of no single individual but of a particular population at a particular time. Now, since populations are always in a dynamic state as to their components, including the number, ages, and sexes of its constituent individuals; the composition of its gene pool; the availability, frequency, and intensity of exposure to experiences; and the variations in the interactions between these genes and experiences, the heritability of traits must vary between and, over time, within populations. So the concept is useful in this context of unity and continuity because it tells us something about the shifting contributions of genes and experiences in influencing the salience of the characteristics of our cohort as it pursues its destiny through time. First, we have seen that there is a decline with age in the heritability of disease experienced by the cohort, punctuated by upward shifts at particular times in ontogeny. Second, cultural changes, whether secular or associated with migration or socioeconomic status, raise or lower it. It is lowered when some new and provocative experiences raise a latent genetic susceptibility to phenotypic expression, and it is raised when just such experiences are removed — that is, as the provocation is eased, the least genetically vulnerable are the first to drop out of the data, leaving in the end only the most genetically blighted. How do we demonstrate changes in heritability? Quantitative expressions of phenotypes vary around means in gaussian distributions whose shapes are strongly influenced by selection that eliminates on both sides those who possess the most disadaptive genes or have suffered the most disadaptive experiences. But it is never clear just where in the distribution selective incongruity begins or ends. That is, there must be a provisional zone of uncertain but decreasing vulnerability as the curve climbs toward the mean. If so, shifts in heritability are likely to be expressed in changes in the shapes of distributions. That is, as pressures on homeostasis are intensified, the limits of vulnerability will move up the curve toward the mean, while when pressures are relieved, vulnerability moves down toward the limiting cases among the outliers.

Heritability of Birth Weight. One example of the effect of easing of provocative experiences is the reduction of infant mortality as a result of affluence in the developed nations.[142] These provocations are deficiencies of education, diet, housing, and medical care. Both birth weight and perinatal mortality are influenced by these deficiencies. Terrenato, Ulizzi, and others have compared perinatal mortality according to birth weight of babies born in Italy in 1960 and in 1980.[142,143] Mortality was much reduced during these 20 years, and the distribution of birth weights among the dead babies showed two revealing differences: The variance was significantly reduced, and what had been a well-defined antimode of least mortality (or optimal birth weight) had flattened out. The reduced variance means that some among the outliers on both sides have been saved, and the flattening out of the antimode means reduced selection at the middle of the distribution as well. Ulizzi's most recent paper, which extends the study a further 5 years, shows that the rate of change in heritability has slowed as infant mortality approaches a minimum.[144]

The only changes in this period are the remedy of some of the deficiencies, particularly in diet and medical care, which means that mortality in the 1980s was more strongly influenced by the genes. Indeed, it may be that in the developed nations today, most disease and mortality among babies born at term, with average weight who become ill in the first day or two of life is "genetic." Most such babies have classic inborn errors of metabolism.[145]

Deficiency and Intolerance. Until recently most rickets in the United States was associated with lack of dietary vitamin D, but in a remarkable reversal of form, monogenic types of rickets, all but unnoticed when deficiency rickets was prevalent, are now prominently represented; there has been a rise in heritability.[146] This is a consequence of increased affluence, which, in supplying vitamin D and reducing the incidence of vitamin D deficiency rickets, makes salient the various kinds and degrees of innate insensitivity to vitamin D. In contrast to the decline in rickets, affluence is accompanied by an increase of atherosclerosis associated with an excess of dietary fat, smoking, and indolence, and the withdrawal of these provocations may have a good deal to do with the decline in coronary thrombosis during the past decade or so.[146,147] One explanation of this decline might be that as the provocations are withdrawn, the variation in the population contributing to heart attack is more and more genetic, so while heritability rises with both the disappearance of vitamin D deficiency rickets and reduction in the extrinsic causes of atherosclerosis, there is a paradoxical effect—the heritability of rickets is raised when something is supplied, while that of atherosclerosis is raised when something is withdrawn.[146,147] It is the difference between deficiency and intolerance, and it is an illuminating example of nature's central tendency and of stabilizing selection.[148] There is a further paradox: The genetic forms of deficiency diseases are most prominent under conditions of plenty, while those of intolerance are most easily distinguishable under conditions of want.

Other Examples. Reye's syndrome and infantile cortical hyperostosis are conditions of uncertain origin and are usually nonfamilial. For reasons that remain obscure, the incidence of both has declined, with the result that hereditary forms have emerged.[149,150] For example, cases of inborn errors of the urea cycle have become prominent among residual cases of Reye's syndrome.[149]

Iron deficiency anemia, once so frequent among the undernourished, is now a relatively less common cause of microcytosis, which at least in certain places is more likely to be found among heterozygotes for thalassemia or as a result of other, even less frequent genetic causes.[151] And pellagra, now a rare disease in the United States, is occasionally seen in people who are homozygous for Hartnup's disorder and whose plasma amino acid levels, presumably under polygenic control, are on the low side of a gaussian distribution of such levels.[146] Such people are those for whom a modest deprivation is enough to precipitate the signs of vitamin deficiency. Also in this vein of nutritional deficiencies is cretinism, associated most frequently with a lack of dietary iodine. It is a deficiency now nearly universally supplied in the developed nations, so the genetic causes of the disorder now predominate.[146]

Summary

The principle of a selective gradient suggests that continuity is the rule. Discontinuities in distributions are a result of homeostatic competence rather than a lack of graded mutant effect. For example, Kacser and Burns have shown how the reduced enzyme activity in heterozygotes for recessive diseases is compensated so that the flux through a pathway is unimpaired even when the activity imparted by the mutant is nil.[89] Consequently, in distributions of enzyme activity that include normals and mutant heterozygotes and homozygotes, the homozygous mutants are usually completely separated. But not all heterozygotes are so compensated; for example, some heterozygotes for homocystinuria show mutant effect.[90] And it may be that sufficient pressure would find a few vulnerable heterozygotes in many more recessive disorders.

The discontinuities of form observed in congenital anomalies may also seem to be an exception, but they are believed to represent a threshold effect, not a discontinuity in the developmental process. It is simply that what seems a trivial departure in some aspect of development is grossly exaggerated and distorted by growth and subsequent development.

Continuity: Infections and Cancer

Textbooks of medicine list infections as "environmental" diseases, and epidemiologists claim cancer as their own. But, in fact, both are comfortably embraced within the concepts of continuity, the selective gradient, heritability, the inborn error, and Garrod's chemical individuality.

Infections. Infections are usually perceived, perhaps principally in medical textbooks, as the archetype of environmental diseases. And so they are, in one sense. But when observed from another point of view they are seen to resemble other diseases, since they derive from incongruence between the human genotype and the environment, represented in this case by the microbial genotype and modified by the matrix of the development and special experiences of the human being involved; susceptibility to infection is influenced by age, nutrition, socioeconomic status, and so on.

Archibald Garrod leaves us in no doubt about his recognition of infections as products of the individuality of both human and microbial species. In *Inborn Factors* he put it: "In our fight against the infective diseases we are not confronted with blind forces, acting at random, but with the disciplined offensive of highly trained foes. Whilst on the one hand the weapons of attack have been improved by evolution, there has been a corresponding evolution of protective mechanisms of great ingenuity, and of no small efficiency, for the defense of the individual attacked."[6] So human susceptibility and immunity are a consequence of the human genes that define individuals and account for variability in populations, and of those of the microorganisms that have "their own careers to work out. . . ."[6] And when successful, those careers have a powerful impact on the numerical density and distribution of animals, including human beings. So an infection must be seen as "a struggle of conflicting interests," and outcomes have to do with individual incongruities between these systems that evolve together, albeit at different rates. Anthropocentrism causes us to see microorganisms as implacable enemies, and although we inherit an efficient means to oppose them, no small effort is devoted to enhancing our defensive weaponry by invention. But a deeper understanding of the position of man and microbe may be attained by entertaining, if only for a moment, an alternative view, in which microorganisms are perceived as victims and the human immune system and antibiotics as offensive weapons, so that the human species is the bane and ruthless scourge of microorganisms who are only struggling to work out "their own careers."

The genes of both agonists in the contest specify proteins, and as genes, they must vary. Accordingly, there must be variation in both the capacity of microorganisms to express virulence and that of human partner to resist or to succumb.[152] So virulence and pathogenicity are relative properties; if we say an organism is virulent, we must ask for whom, and if an individual is said to be susceptible, we should specify to what. As it happens, the organisms we commonly call "pathogenic" are likely to have adapted not to individual differences in human defenses but to the prevailing versions thereof, so some organisms may be virulent for nearly all human beings; but even so, virulence is a property that is fully understood only with the above provisos.

It is often supposed that coevolution must end in an amicable coexistence in which human beings tolerate microorganisms, even assisting in their spread, without disease.[153,154] The latter might even pay rent in the form, say, of vitamins useful in human metabolism, and many organisms have attained this nirvana. But some have worked out no scheme to uncouple virulence from dissemination and so are doomed to infect so as to be transmitted.[153,154] So coevolution can attain any of many degrees of accommodation for species, and we may assume an additional range of variation for individuals within the species. All of this means that our relationships with microbial life remain fluid; the latter can mutate to forms for which our defenses are not prepared, even while we enjoy the advantage of an intelligence capable sometimes of inventing the means to thwart their designs. But invention is not always immediately successful — the acquired immunodeficiency syndrome (AIDS) is an example — and the power of viruses, particularly, to mutate is great. So as long as parasitic organisms continue to pursue their careers, the human species is under an unrelenting threat.[155–157]

No doubt individual variation and selection have led through phylogeny to our high degree of resistance; for example, the adaptive immune response appears to have evolved after such primitive effector mechanisms as the alternative complement pathway and natural killer cells were already in place.[158] But individual variation has contributed to susceptibility as well. Although Garrod acknowledged differences in resistance and susceptibility, he knew of no specific disorders of immune defense. How could he? The very high prevalence of infection and mortality would have made them inapparent; heritability was low. Now, MMBID has six chapters covering disorders of defense. But however many separate entities have been described, given the number of molecules embraced within the immune system, its complexity, and the extensive genetic polymorphism of its components, what we know today is likely to be dwarfed by what we will know tomorrow.

What have been discovered so far are the most profound deficiencies, easily perceived as inborn errors and as typologically distinguishable from "normal." But here too the continuity of the distribution of vulnerability is demonstrated. The results of some investigations even raise the question of how immunodeficiency is to be defined.[159] For some people, infection with *Haemophilus influenzae* is familial; they have a quantitative variation, not a deficiency, in their immune response.[159] There is also evidence of multigenic control of the magnitude of the response to vaccines.[159] This is a relative immune deficiency; it is evidence of continuity in vulnerability. Further testimony for such continuity is given in an investigation into the causes of death of people who had been separated from their biological parents very early in life.[160] When a biological parent died of infection at or before age 70, the relative risk of dying of the same cause for their children was five times higher than average. That is, the correlation in cause of death was between the biologically related but separated persons, not the adopted child and adoptive parent. There was no conventional immunodeficiency here, only enhanced susceptibility.

In a more recent paper it was reported that the probability that patients hospitalized for pneumococcal pneumonia would be readmitted for the same disease was more than five times the probability of other patients being readmitted for their particular illnesses.[161] Evidently, there are people especially susceptible to the pneumococcus. And why not? Each of us must have a unique set of molecules pertaining to responses to all sorts of infection, and what we know of mutation tells us that where there are devastating inborn errors there are usually also lesser grades of deviation. That the potential for such differences is likely to lurk in our gene pool was demonstrated by Biozzi et al., who after 15 generations of selection succeeded in breeding strains of mice that were either high or low responders to a specific antigen.[162]

What about genetic variations in microorganisms? Inborn errors in *Neurospora* and *E. coli* played salient roles in defining what genes are and do.[163,164] Such organisms are not likely to go far in the business of infection, but a mutation leading to an advantage might make itself known; for example, a variant was discovered in a strain of *Neisseria meningococcus* that produced localized epidemics of meningitis in England, Wales, and elsewhere.[165] This strain was found to differ from others in a single base substitution in a gene that specifies the outer membrane protein of the meningococcus. Evidently, this point mutation gave this strain a sufficient advantage to account for most of the cases of meningitis in the affected areas.

Cancer. The genes associated with cancer are described in a familiar context. Oncogenes, which are mutant forms of protooncogenes, produce dominant effects, chief of which is to promote cell proliferation.[166–168] Mutants of repressor genes have recessive, or sometimes intermediate dominant, effects; they release the brakes on proliferation.[166–168] Not surprisingly, then, it is mutants of the repressors that are most directly associated with such early-onset, hereditary cancers as retinoblastoma, Wilms' tumor, and neuroblastoma as recessive deficiency disorders with mutant or absent proteins. These may be classified as inborn errors of metabolism,[166–169] but with a twist — only one of the repressor mutants is in the germ line. No doubt there are true germ-line recessives, but they should be lethal. More than one locus may be involved, notably in Wilms' tumor, but the number of both loci and steps to malignancy are presumed to be at a minimum in the hereditary, early-onset recessive disorders.

Both oncogenes and repressors are involved in cancers of later onset, which include among their number some of the best-understood examples of multifactorial diseases. These later-onset cancers are associated principally with somatic oncogenes.[166–168] Several such mutants coexist in malignant tissues, often in association with repressor mutants too.[170] In the case of colon cancer, mutations of several such genes occur one after another, producing precancerous adenomas along the way.[170,171] The mutations need not occur in a particular order, but all are required if malignancy is to be attained.[170,171]

There is much variation in age at onset and clinical expression in the cancers of late onset. Cases with early onset are more likely to be familial; cancer of the breast and prostate are examples, and the early-onset cases are more rapidly progressive and, in the case of breast cancer, bilateral.[139,140] Later-onset disease is less severe, and although it is often nonfamilial, aggregation in families is sometimes found.

Somatic mutations are presumed to be a consequence of mutagenic experiences. Only a few such mutagens are known, but the steady increase in age-specific incidence of so many cancers suggests long and continuous exposure to carcinogenic stimuli.[172] That is, while the early-onset cancers are associated with a germ-line mutation, nonfamilial, late-onset disorders and cases of late onset of diseases in which early-onset cases are familial are no less due to environmental causes for all their being "genetic" in their pathogenesis. So in these ways — association of earliest disorders with germ-line mutants, less and less (germ-line) genetic contribution to disease with age, and ever-decreasing familial representation and burden with age — cancer conforms to the pattern of other multifactorial diseases. But there is a notable exception. As a consequence of the ever-increasing variety, intensity, and duration of experiences and the accumulating wear and tear of living, aging, and surviving exemplified, for example, in smoking, alcohol drinking, dietary excess, exposure to radiation, and so on, there is an ever-increasing number of somatic mutations, representing late in life a sort of mirror image of the extravagant genetic variety of intrauterine life. Fortunately for all of us, the expression of such mutational diversity is limited to the systems of control of cell growth.

There is no mention of cancer in Garrod's *Inborn Factors in Disease.* No doubt in his time it was a disease of less moment than today, hardly remarkable in a population with an average life expectancy of around 50 years. But perhaps it is surprising that Garrod omitted cancer from his book, because given that so many people did not live long enough to experience the disease, the familial cancers should have stood out. Now they do not, which is to say that with a rising life expectancy, the heritability of cancer has declined.

APPLICATIONS OF THE LOGIC

The application of a logic of disease is likely to be in the shaping of a mentality, in how we think about medical problems. So, by way of conclusion, some examples will be given that conform to the three time frames — the moment, the lifetime, and biological history — and that show how in thinking about disease we do so in the context of all three at once.

Analysis of Cases

Diagnosis follows the assembly of historical information, signs, symptoms, and laboratory data so as to name a disease that experience tells us responds to a particular treatment. When a disease is not well understood, many cases are investigated to discover its causes, to characterize its properties, and to describe risk factors in the form of experiences and qualities that characterize susceptibility. In these too-often-typological exercises, the qualities described are those of the disease, and it is assumed that any individual patient will resemble, although variably, the average or common character.

How does the logic outlined above help in this practical pursuit? The aim is to discern not only what disease a patient has but to characterize his or her particular version of it. The analysis begins with a single patient, whose disease is represented as a consequence of homeostatic incongruence, itself a result of interactions of unique genetic variation with no less unique experiences — interactions that have been transacted in a unique developmental matrix. So at least three sets of factors must go into the analysis (see Table 2-3). The next step is to characterize the patient according to his or her particular constellation of the qualities listed in the table. Type I diabetes will serve as an example.

The Present: Type I Diabetes Mellitus. Type I diabetes is a transitional disorder, having in cases of early onset the infrequency, severity, and biochemical detail of the classic inborn errors of infancy and childhood and in cases of later onset that are milder and more treatable resembling the multifactorial disorders of adult life. So we should expect a continuity of characteristics along the axis of age at onset, which stands in here for the gradient of selective effect. The cases with earliest and latest onset should be the easiest to differentiate and perhaps the easiest to make predictions about, but specificity and sensitivity will deteriorate as we approach the middle of this distribution, so there is practical use in individual assessments.

In Table 2-6 the elements of cause are arranged in three columns. How do these genes, and presumably others, interact with these and other elements of experience in the context of these and other developmental influences? All but one of the genes listed belong to the immune system: DR4 is an immunological specificity, which is a surrogate for a DQ allele thought to be directly involved in pathogenesis.[173] The non-HLA genes are perhaps modifiers; at least the GM alleles are presumed to contribute only through their association with MHC alleles.[174] In any case, no one believes this list to be exhaustive. Reports incriminate a fragment in the insulin gene region[175] and at least five loci in a mouse analogue (NOD).[176] On the right of Table 2-6 are factors of the environment. Infection may be the first incident in a chain of events leading to autoimmune destruction of islet cells, but it is not clear why the incidence of the disease, which varies geographically, appears to be rising generally as well as locally.[177,178] Several reports suggest a protective effect of human milk, and antibodies to cow's milk albumin are often found in the blood of newly diagnosed diabetics who have been fed cow's milk.[179–181] Among the developmental factors are age at onset, maternal age at the birth of the diabetic, and segregation distortion when the father of a diabetic is affected.[182] Such fathers transmit a surplus of their DR4 alleles to their offspring. The origin of this effect is unclear, but it is said not to be due to imprinting.[183] Associations of some of these factors are reflected in clinical expression. For example, when the onset is before puberty, there are a concentration of genes (DR4/DR3, bf, gm, etc.), higher titers of antiinsulin antibodies, recurrence rates of up to 10 percent, and a higher monozygotic twin concordance.[184–187] Late onset, especially after 40 years, is just the opposite — milder expression, much less representation of DR3, and infrequent affected sibs.[185,188] In a study of 190 patients with type I diabetes with onset later than 20 years of age, 16 percent were reported to lack either DR3 or DR4, to be less severely affected, to have low levels of antibody, and to have few affected relatives. The authors offered etiologic heterogeneity by way of explanation and cited these patients as evidence of the need for individual analysis of cases.[189] Winter onset is also associated with severe disease and more DR3/DR4 genotypes, but it is unclear whether the winter-onset cases are also of early onset.[190] If not, when the disease has onset in the winter in the very young, is it worse than when onset in very young patients is in the summer? Other associations are still unexplored; for example, we do not know the particulars of the diabetes of patients born to elderly mothers, only that there are more of them.[191] Also, if breast-feeding reduces the incidence of diabetes, what characterizes patients who get the disease despite such feeding? And if the incidence is rising, are the patients observed in the years with higher frequency in some way different? Is the heritability changing?

Table 2-6 Factors Involved in Type I Diabetes

Genes	Development	Environment
HLA-DR3, DR4, DR2	Age	Infection
GM types	Maternal age	Season
Complement alleles	Sex of affected parent	Geography
Other genes		Year
		Human milk feeding

In its focus on the particular set of variables possessed by each of many individuals, such an analysis goes beyond epidemiology, which characterizes populations. Each different combination of such variables must be expressed in a unique version of the disease. Subtle differences may have little impact on the treatment, which may be equally appropriate for some, or many, of the versions, but is it not likely that the characteristics we admire in superior clinicians derive from their intuitive perception of just such subtleties? And clearly, their careful adjustment of treatment to the apparent need of each patient represents a response to individuality, an expression of what we all applaud as the "art" of medicine. Curiously, this attention to detail was exemplified by Osler, but what we know of Garrod suggests he was not much interested in clinical medicine.[4]

The Lifetime. Individuality evolves over the lifetime; that of the conceptus is almost wholly genetic, that of the embryo is chiefly genetic, and that of the centenarian, while constrained by early development, is strongly influenced by a lifetime of experiences. So we are never so like our parents, or like each other, as at conception and never so much our own selves as in old age. But outcomes of the experiences of each life are always constrained by the way the genes internalized them and wove them into the fabric of individuality, a fabric that derives its distinctive character from subtle modifications of a trajectory established early in life. Some of that fabric is likely to represent incongruence, made overt from the start in the unlucky few but with consequences that for most may be averted by chance or prevented by choice. So the proclivity for disease evolves over the lifetime no less than that for health.

The Impact of Early Life. There is a growing literature on the impact of early life on later diseases. Atherosclerosis, some cancers, pulmonary disease, and essential hypertension are all traceable to events of early life.[192–198] And many behavioral qualities originate in early life.[199,200] Here, the genes must act merely to put limits on the variation of such qualities; studies of temperament in newborn twin pairs show negligible heritability.[201,202]

An Example. A particularly instructive example of lifetime impact is in variations in homeostasis of bone that lead to fractures in old people. The state of bone at any moment is a result of a balance between bone formation and destruction that is influenced by stresses, nutrition, and hormones, including vitamin D and parathyroid and sex hormones. All of the cellular mechanisms — including the absorption and excretion of calcium; the synthesis, secretion, and degradation of hormones; and the processes of bone formation and destruction — are mediated by protein products of genes susceptible to mutation, so it can be no surprise that the heritability of bone mass is high.[203,204] The implication of this heritability is that osteoporosis and fracture may turn out to be familial.

But most of the genetic variation is expressed in the attainment of peak bone mass, while most of the variation in the loss of bone is associated with experiences.[203] Peak bone mass is reached in early adult life, and twin studies show the heritability to be high.[203–205] In males, bone mass is influenced by testosterone, so men with delayed puberty or hypogonadism attain a lesser peak.[206–208] Bone mass in both sexes is then maintained until an indeterminate time when, with great individual variability, it begins a very slow descent, hastened in women by the loss of estrogen at the menopause. Much of the individual variation has to do with poor nutrition, lack of exercise, alcohol, smoking, and other influences, aided by variations in the way people age.[204,209–211] A twin study in which mono- and dizygotic twin pairs were compared both before and after a 15-year interval reported a low heritability, attesting to the predominant contribution of these nongenetic variables.[212]

Fractures, pain, and disability are usually reserved for old age, but it is the people whose peak bone mass was low to begin with who are most vulnerable to the effects of estrogen lack, alcohol, smoking, or lack of exercise. So the genetic variation expressed early in life provides a range of probabilities, varying from nil to near certainty, for events to occur 50 years later, events that can be hastened, deferred, or prevented by experiences — some random, some a consequence of habits — and behaviors within the choice of the individual.

The moral of the story is plain. An elderly grandmother who has shrunk a few inches or had a fracture is a signal to her daughters and granddaughters to look to their own bones and to think of exercise as a useful preventive measure and perhaps to consider estrogen after the menopause to preserve a bone mass that might have little margin for loss. Similarly, a grandson whose puberty was delayed might see salvation in exercise and add this to a dozen other reasons for not smoking. The limitation of medical practice that is engaged only when a patient is already sick is nowhere so starkly evident as in these impacts of early life on later disease. First, disease is likely to be a family matter — even when only one person is affected, others may be liable. Second, as molecular pathogenesis is exposed, and as we learn how particular experiences interact with the products of specific genotypes over the lifetime, medical education and practice can hardly fail to accept the primacy of prevention.

Biological and Social History. Waddington's historical dimension was biological, but since biology makes no sense apart from a context composed of the cultural, social, and physical environments, the history we confront here is that of living open systems, discrete but confluent with an environment that is, in part, of their own making. Biological history is slow, measured in hundreds of millions of years. Social and cultural history are more likely to be reckoned in generations and seem now to be measured in decades or less.

The asynchrony of these two histories has significant human consequences. Human ingenuity has added social adaptation to that of biological evolution, enabling us to broaden our experiences of the planet, even giving ourselves social definition as people with names, identities, attainments, and many other characteristics — definitions that transcend but do not defy biology. At least when we do the latter, as in our "conquest" of space, it is at no small cost.

In the developed nations, cultural and social history has brought adjustments in housing, nutrition, education, and medicine that have reduced sickness and mortality and doubled the average life expectancy, with significant and unanticipated changes in our demography; for example, no one foresaw that today the oldest old — 85 years and over — would be the fastest-growing segment of the population.[213] At the same time, this evolutionary asynchrony gives origin to much of our disease.[31,147] Examples are unintended ecological disruptions that lead to incongruence and disease — fouling of the atmosphere, a damaged ozone layer, desertification of arable land, pollution of the seas, and misuse of drugs. And iatrogenic disease is by no means unknown; drugs said to be sovereign for a particular disease prove to be intolerable for some individuals. But nowhere is the clash more evident than in the disorders associated with the habits and modes of living enjoyed in the developed nations.[31,119,147] The excesses of the present overtax the tolerance of a homeostasis designed for the past.

A CONTEXT FOR MEDICAL TEACHING AND PRACTICE

So here, it seems, is a context for medical education and an alternative to the metaphor of the body as a machine. It is a context of three levels, in which the first is embraced within the second and both within the third like a set of Chinese boxes, and there is an uninterrupted continuity of thought as one moves from one level to the next. In the innermost box is diagnosis and treatment of a particular patient whose genetic and developmental individuality is incongruent with experience. But the individuality of the patient cannot be clearly perceived apart from the second box. Indeed, individuality is defined only in the comparison of one to others. So individuality is first tested in the family, which ought to be the primary focus of the physician — primary because it is in the family setting that individuality takes shape and where the most significant developmental events occur, including the inheritance of genes, the most explosive growth and maturation, the beginning of acculturation, and the origin of the developmental trajectories that differentiate individuals. Sibs share parental genes, parental culture, and household experiences. These are all sources of within-family likeness in vulnerability, and since different families are likely to vary in constellations of both genes and experiences, a better sense of the future for any individual is likely to derive from observations of a whole family than from those of any single person. The third box includes the elements of which incongruence is made — the wherewithal the species uses to get on with its business of living and reproduction (mutation, recombination, genetic polymorphism) and the composition of the gene pool, as well as the cultural and social attributes that characterize and differentiate ethnic groups and larger communities. These are remote causes that tell us why human beings must suffer disease at all and how incongruities arise.

The continuities in going from one box to the next are obvious. The first starts from the present — the patient in box 1 — and goes, by way of the lifetime of development within the influence of the family (box 2), to biological and cultural history (box 3). Second, in passing from the first box to the third, kinship is diluted; relatives share peculiarities of both genes and experiences, and so, in progressively lesser degree, do members of ethnic groups and larger communities. But the diversity within such groups is greater than that between them; in the end our humanness transcends our ethnic or other differentiation. So at the basis of ideas about disease that include genetic variation there is always a powerful constraint. Remote causes inherent in evolution lead to disease but also constrain its forms.

In a third continuity, there is a progression of forms of management. Treatment in the form of medication or surgery is focused sharply on individual patients (box 1). Prevention is most easily perceived and executed in families of individuals who share genes and habits (box 2), and preventive medicine and public health are most comfortably embraced in box 3, among the remote causes.

A fourth continuity is critical for medical teaching, in which a tension exists between education and practical training. Education is defined here as disposing principles and ideas — their relationships, how they evolved, and how they inform practical training. Training is defined as teaching how to care for patients and includes diagnosis and management, which is rote learning unless taught in the context of ideas. Practice (box 1) taught unclothed in the ideas of boxes 2 and 3 risks limiting the doctor-patient encounter to technology. Perhaps it is a lack of reconciliation between education and practice that has so stirred the critics of medical education, whose view is that failure to observe the patient's social integration — and biologic too, they might have added — leads to omission of ethical and humanistic dimensions essential for good management. Confirmation of the critics' contention is given by Kunitz, who observed that the physicians most attentive to patients' values and sensibilities were family practitioners and pediatricians, that is, those whose mission includes the family (box 2) as a primary concern.[214] So unity of ideas and practice is most naturally attained in the context of the family, wherein development and the experiences of the lifetime are also most readily comprehended.

Such continuities flow naturally from the different ideas expressed in the three boxes, and I believe some such medicine of ideas was in Garrod's mind when he sat down to write *Inborn Factors in Disease*.[6] The idea of the inborn error, limited at its inception to alkaptonuria, soon took in three more variants, and today there are hundreds. While it is unlikely that anyone could, or would want to, recite from memory the whole list of their names, all medical students should be comfortable with the concept and perceive how central it is in our thinking today. Logic took Garrod's thinking from the inborn error to chemical individuality, which, transcending individuals, can be seen to characterize species too. From there it was only a short step to the perception that chemical individuality is the wherewithal for selection, which defines our evolutionary advantages as well as the disadvantages that may constitute disease. What Garrod lacked to test his ideas was the rich detail of today's cell and molecular biology. This the writers of the articles of MMBID have at hand, and they are showing how seemingly trivial changes in chemical individuality can be translated into devastating disease. In doing so, they recount new mechanisms and generalizations that Garrod could not even have imagined, but rather than leading to significant departures from original principles, these novelties give them new meaning, lending coherence and logic to explanations of disease. And such coherence and logic cannot fail to be helpful in the recasting of the medical curriculum now at hand.

REFERENCES

1. Stanbury JB, Wyngaarden JB, Fredrickson DS (eds): *The Metabolic Basis of Inherited Disease*. New York, McGraw-Hill, 1960.
2. Scriver CR, Beaudet AL, Sly WS, Valle D (eds): *The Metabolic Basis of Inherited Disease* 6th ed. New York, McGraw-Hill, 1989.
3. Garrod AE: The incidence of alkaptonuria: A study in chemical individuality. *Lancet* **2**:1616, 1902.
4. Bearn AB: *Archibald Garrod and the Individuality of Man*. Oxford, Oxford University Press, 1993.
5. Garrod AG: *Inborn Errors of Metabolism*. Oxford, Oxford University Press, 1909.
6. Scriver CR, Childs B: *Garrod's Inborn Factors in Disease*. Oxford, Oxford University Press, 1989.
7. Fruton, JS: *Molecules and Life*. New York, Wiley, 1972.
8. Cushing H: *The Life of Sir William Osler*. Oxford, Oxford University Press, 1926, vols 1 and 2.
9. Osler W: *The Principles and Practice of Medicine*. New York, Appleton, 1892.
10. Osler W: The natural method of teaching the subject of medicine. *JAMA* **36**:1673, 1901.
11. Osler W: On the need of a radical reform in our methods of teaching medical students. *Med News* **82**:49, 1904.
12. Osler W: Teaching and thinking. An address given at McGill Medical School, Oct. 1894, in McGovern JP, Roland CG (eds): *The Collected Essays of Sir William Osler*. Birmingham, Classics of Medicine Library, 1985, vol 2, p 111.
13. Powles J: On the limitations of modern medicine. *Sci Med Man* **1**:1, 1973.
14. McKeown T: *The Role of Medicine*. London, Nuffield Trust, 1976.
15. Thomas L: The future impact of science and technology on medicine. *Bioscience* **24**:99, 1974.
16. Seldin DW: The boundaries of medicine. *Trans Assoc Am Physicians* **94**:75, 1981.
17. Harvey AM, Johns RJ, McKusick VA, Owens AH Jr, Ross RS: *The Principles and Practice of Medicine* 22d ed. New York, Appleton-Century-Crofts, 1988.
18. Hood L: Biology and medicine in the 21st century, in Keveles D, Hood L (eds): *The Code of Codes*. Cambridge, MA, Harvard University Press, 1992, p 136.
19. Reiser SJ: *Medicine and the Reign of Technology*. New York, Cambridge University Press, 1978.
20. Freymann JG: The origins of disease orientation in American medical education. *Prev Med* **10**:663, 1981.
21. Council on Medical Education: AMA House of Delegates. Future directions for medical education. *JAMA* **248**:3225, 1982.
22. Muller S, Cooper JAD: Physicians for the twenty-first century. *J Med Educ* **59(suppl)**:1, 1984.
23. Ebert RH: Medical education at the peak of the era of experimental medicine. *Daedalus* **115**:55, 1986.
24. Rothstein WG: *American Medical Schools and the Practice of Medicine*. New York, Oxford University Press, 1987.
25. White KL: *The Task of Medicine*. Menlo Park, CA, Kaiser Family Foundation, 1988.
26. Schroeder SA, Zones JS, Showstack JA: Academic medicine as a public trust. *JAMA* **262**:803, 1989.
27. Tosteson DC: New pathways in medical education. *N Engl J Med* **322**:234, 1990.
28. White KL, Connelly JE: The medical school's mission and the population's health. *Ann Intern Med* **115**:968, 1991.
29. Cantor JC, Cohen AB, Barker DC, Shuster AL, Reynolds RC: Medical educators' views on medical education reform. *JAMA* **265**:1002, 1991.
30. Marston RQ, Jones RM: *Commission on medical education: The sciences of medical practice: Medical education in transition*. Princeton, NJ, Robert Wood Johnson Foundation, 1992.
31. Eaton SB, Shostak M, Konner M: *The Paleolithic Prescription*. New York, Harper & Row, 1988.
32. Mayr E: *The Growth of Biological Thought*. Cambridge, MA, Harvard University Press, 1982, p 45.
33. Mayr E: Cause and effect in biology. *Science* **134**:1501, 1961.
34. Cohen H: The evolution of the concept of disease. *Proc R Soc Med* **48**:159, 1955.
35. Temkin O: The scientific approach to disease: Specific entity and individual sickness, in Crombie AC (ed): *Scientific Change*. New York, Basic Books, 1963.
36. Copeland DA: Concepts of disease and diagnosis. *Perspect Biol Med* **20**:528, 1977.
37. Campbell EJM, Scadding JG, Roberts RS: The concept of disease. *Br Med J* **2**:757, 1979.
38. Greaves D: What is medicine? Towards a philosophical approach. *J Med Ethics* **5**:29, 1979.
39. King LS: *Medical Thinking*. Princeton, NJ, Princeton University Press, 1982.
40. Nordenfelt L: Health and disease: Two philosophical perspectives. *J Epidemiol Community Health* **41**:281, 1986.
41. Cassell EJ: Ideas in conflict: The rise and fall (and rise and fall) of new views of disease. *Daedalus* **115**:19, 1986.
42. Alberts B, Bray D, Lewis J, Raff M, Roberts K, Watson JD: *Molecular Biology of the Cell*. New York, Garland, 1989, p VII.
43. Delbruck M: A physicist looks at biology, in Cairns J, Stent GS, Watson JD (eds): *Phage and the Origins of Molecular Biology*. Cold

Spring Harbor, NY, Cold Spring Harbor Laboratory of Quantitative Biology, 1966, p 9.

44. Bock GR, Whelan J: *The Childhood Environment and Adult Disease*. Ciba Foundation Symposium 156. New York, Wiley, 1991.
45. Jacob F: *The Logic of Life*. New York, Pantheon, 1973.
46. Jacob F: Evolution and tinkering. *Science* **196**:1161, 1977.
47. Williams GC, Neese RM: The dawn of Darwinian medicine. *Q Rev Biol* **66**:1, 1991.
48. Ochsner A, DeBakey M: Carcinoma of the lung. *Arch Surg* **42**:209, 1941.
49. Doll R, Hill AB: Smoking and carcinoma of the lung. *Br Med J* **2**:739, 1950.
50. Anon.: Conversation with Sir Richard Doll. *Br J Addict* **86**:365, 1991.
51. Peto R, Lopez AD, Boreham J, Thun M, Heath C Jr: Mortality from tobacco in developed countries. *Lancet* **339**:1268, 1992.
52. Dugdale AE: Evolution and infant feeding. *Lancet* **1**:670, 1986.
53. Palloni A, Tienda M: The effects of breast feeding and pace of childbearing on mortality at early ages. *Demography* **23**:31, 1986.
54. Thapa S, Short RV, Potts M: Breast feeding, birth spacing and their effects on child survival. *Nature* **335**:679, 1988.
55. Lucas A, Morely R, Cole TJ, Lister G, Leeson-Payne C: Breast milk and subsequent intelligence quotient in children born pre-term. *Lancet* **1**:261, 1992.
56. Menkes JH: Early feeding history of children with learning disorders. *Dev Med Child Neurol* **19**:169, 1977.
57. Rodgers B: Feeding in infancy and later ability and attainment: A longitudinal study. *Dev Med Child Neurol* **20**:421, 1978.
58. Karjalainen J, Martin JM, Knip M, Ilonen J, Robinson B, Savilahti E, Akerblow HK, Dosh H-M: A bovine albumin peptide as a possible trigger of insulin-dependent diabetes mellitus. *N Engl J Med* **327**:302, 1992.
59. Newberg DS, Ashkenazc S, Clearly TG: Human milk contains the Shiga toxin and Shiga-like toxin receptor glycolipid Gb3. *J Infect Dis* **166**:832, 1992.
60. Yolken RH, Peterson JA, Vonderfecht SL, Fouts ET, Midthun K, Newburg DS: Human milk mucin inhibits rotavirus replication and prevents experimental gastroenteritis. *J Clin Invest* **90**:1984, 1992.
61. Pabst HF, Spady DW: Effect of breast feeding on antibody response to conjugate vaccine. *Lancet* **2**:269, 1990.
62. Atherton DJ: Breast feeding and atopic eczema. *Br Med J* **287**:775, 1983.
63. Bjorksten B: Does breast feeding prevent the development of allergy? *Immunol Today* **4**:215, 1983.
64. Lucas A, Cole TJ: Breast milk and neonatal necrotizing enterocolitis. *Lancet* **2**:1519, 1990.
65. Pisacane A, Graziano L, Mazzarella G, Scarpellino B, Zona G: Breast feeding and urinary tract infection. *J Pediatr* **120**:87, 1992.
66. Howie PW, Forsyth JS, Ogston SA, Clark A, Florey CduV: Protective effect of breast feeding against infection. *Br Med J* **300**:11, 1990.
67. Udall JN, Dixon M, Newman AP, Wright JA, James B, Block KJ: Liver disease in alpha 1-antitrypsin deficiency. *JAMA* **253**:2679, 1985.
68. Sveger T: Breast feeding, alpha-1-antitrypsin deficiency and liver disease. *JAMA* **254**:3036, 1985.
69. Teele DW, Klein JO, Rosner B: Epidemiology of otitis media during the first seven years of life in children in Greater Boston. *J Infect Dis* **160**:83, 1989.
70. Davis MK, Savitz DA, Graubard BI: Infant feeding and childhood cancer. *Lancet* **2**:365, 1988.
71. Dwyer T, Ponsonby AL: Sudden infant death syndrome — insights from epidemiological research. *J Epidemiol Community Health* **46**:98, 1992.
72. Bernard C: *Lectures on the Phenomena of Life*. Hoff HE, Guillemin R, Guillemin L (eds): Springfield IL, Charles C Thomas, 1974, vol 1.
73. Holmes FL, Bernard C: The Milieu Interieux and regulatory physiology. *Hist Phil Life Sci* **8**:3, 1986.
74. Cannon WB: Lawrence Joseph Henderson. *Natl Acad Sci Biogr Memoirs* **23**:31, 1943.
75. Parascandola J: Organismic and holistic concepts in the thought of L. J. Henderson. *J Hist Biol* **4**:63, 1971.
76. Cannon WB: *The Wisdom of the Body*. Cambridge, MA, Harvard University Press, 1939.
77. Waddington CH: *The Strategy of the Genes*. London, Allen & Unwin, 1957.
78. Gilbert SF: Epigenetic landscaping: Waddington's use of cell fate bifurcation diagrams. *Biol Phil* **6**:135, 1991.
79. Davidson EH: Understanding embryonic development: A contemporary view. *Am Zool* **27**:581, 1987.
80. Gurdon J: The generation of diversity and pattern in animal development. *Cell* **68**:185, 1992.
81. Lewontin RC: Gene, organism and environment, in Bendall DS (ed): *Evolution: From Molecules to Man*. New York, Cambridge University Press, 1983.
82. Lewontin RC: Population genetics. *Annu Rev Genet* **19**:81, 1985.
83. Harris H: *The Principles of Human Biochemical Genetics* 3d ed. New York, Elsevier, 1980, p 316.
84. Mitton JB, Grant MC: Associations among protein heterozygosity, growth rate, and developmental homeostasis. *Annu Rev Ecol Syst* **15**:479, 1984.
85. Lerner IM: *Genetic Homeostasis*. Edinburgh, Oliver & Boyd, 1954.
86. Livshits G, Kobyliansky E: Lerner's concept on developmental homeostasis and the problem of heterozygosity level in natural population. *Heredity* (Edinburgh) **55**:341, 1985.
87. Muller HJ: Our load of mutations. *Am J Hum Genet* **2**:111, 1950.
88. Vogel F: Clinical consequences of heterozygosity for autosomal-recessive diseases. *Clin Genet* **25**:381, 1984.
89. Kacser H, Burns JA: The molecular basis of dominance. *Genetics* **97**:639, 1981.
90. Boers GHJ, Smals AGJ, Trijbels FJM, Fowler B, Bakkeren JAJM, Schoonderwaldt HC, Kleijer WJ, Kloppenberg PWC: Heterozygosity for homocystinuria in premature peripheral and cerebral occlusive arterial disease. *N Engl J Med* **313**:709, 1985.
91. Swift M, Cohen J, Pinkham R: A maximum likelihood method for estimating the disease predisposition of heterozygotes. *Am J Hum Genet* **26**:304, 1974.
92. Cavalli-Sforza LL, Feldman MW: *Cultural Transmission and Evolution*. Princeton, NJ, Princeton University Press, 1981.
93. Cavalli-Sforza LL: Cultural evolution. *Am Zool* **26**:845, 1986.
94. Boyd R, Richerson PJ: *Culture and the Evolutionary Process*. Chicago, University of Chicago Press, 1985.
95. Durham WH: *Coevolution: Genes, Culture and Human Diversity*. Stanford, CA, Stanford University Press, 1991.
96. Gould SJ: *Ontogeny and Phylogeny*. Cambridge, MA, Harvard University Press, 1977, p 352.
97. Stent GS: Strength and weakness of the genetic approach to the development of the nervous system, in Cowan WM (ed): *Studies in Developmental Neurobiology*. New York, Oxford University Press, 1981.
98. Davidson EH: Understanding embryonic development: A contemporary view. *Am Zool* **27**:581, 1987.
99. Gurdon JB: Embryonic induction, molecular prospects. *Development* **99**:285, 1987.
100. Scarr S, McCartney K: How people make their own environments: A theory of genotype — environment effects. *Child Dev* **54**:424, 1983.
101. Hill JA: Immunological mechanisms of pregnancy maintenance and failure: A critique of theories and therapy. *Am J Reprod Immunol* **22**:33, 1990.
102. Reik W: Genomic imprinting and genetic disorders in man. *Trends Genet* **5**:331, 1989.
103. Hall JG: Genomic imprinting: Review and relevance to human disease. *Am J Hum Genet* **46**:857, 1990.
104. Shock N: Systems integration, in Finch CE, Schneider EI (eds): *Handbook of the Biology of Aging* 1st ed. New York, Van Nostrand Reinhold, 1977, p 639.
105. Shock NW: Longitudinal studies of aging in humans, in Finch CE, Schneider EI (eds): *Handbook of the Biology of Aging* 2d ed. New York, Van Nostrand Reinhold, 1985, p 721.
106. Medvedev ZA: An attempt at a rational classification of theories of aging. *Biol Rev Camb Philos Soc* **65**:375, 1990.
107. Williams GC: Pleiotropy, natural selection, and the evolution of senescence. *Evolution* **11**:398, 1957.
108. Kirkwood TBL: The nature and causes of aging, in *Research and the Aging Population*. Ciba Foundation Symposium 134. Chichester, Wiley, 1988, p 193.
109. Olson CB: A review of how and why we age: A defense of multifactorial aging. *Mech Ageing Dev* **41**:1, 1987.
110. Brody JA, Schneider EL: Diseases and disorders of aging: An hypothesis. *J Chron Dis* **39**:871, 1986.
111. Evans JG: Aging and disease, in *Research and the Aging Population*. Ciba Foundation Symposium 134. Chichester, Wiley, 1988, p 38.
112. Farrer LA, Conneally PM: Predictability of phenotype in Huntington's disease. *Arch Neurol* **44**:109, 1987.
113. Monaghan FV, Corcos AF: The real objective of Mendel's paper. *Biol Phil* **5**:267, 1990.

114. Froggatt P, Nevin NC: The "law of ancestral heredity" and the Mendelian-ancestrian controversy in England, 1889–1906. *J Med Genet* **8**:1, 1971.
115. Delbruck M: A physicist's renewed look at biology: Twenty years later. *Science* **168**:1312, 1970.
116. Muller HJ: The gene. *Proc R Soc Lond [Biol]* **134**:1, 1947.
117. Yanofsky C: Gene structure and protein structure. *Harvey Lect* **61**:145, 1965.
118. Watson JD, Hopkins NH, Roberts JW, Steitz JA, Weiner AM (eds): *Molecular Biology of the Gene*. Menlo Park, CA, Benjamin/Cummings, 1987, p 233.
119. Neel JV: Diabetes mellitus: A thrifty genotype rendered detrimented by "progress." *Am J Hum Genet* **14**:353, 1962.
120. Dowse G, Zimmet P: The thrifty genotype in non-insulin dependent diabetes. *Br Med J* **306**:532, 1993.
121. Holtzman NA: *Proceed with Caution*. Baltimore, Johns Hopkins Press, 1989.
122. Costa T, Scriver CR, Childs B: The effect of Mendelian disease on health: A measurement. *Am J Med Genet* **21**:231, 1985.
123. Finkelstein JE, Hauser ER, Leonard CO, Brusilow SW: Late onset ornithine transcarbamylase deficiency in male patients. *J Pediatr* **117**:897, 1990.
124. Roberts CJ, Lowe CR: Where have all the conceptions gone? *Lancet* **1**:498, 1975.
125. Edmonds DK, Lindsay KS, Miller JF, Williamson E, Wood PJ: Early embryonic mortality in women. *Fertil Steril* **38**:447, 1982.
126. Simpson JL: Incidence and timing of pregnancy losses. *Am J Med Genet* **35**:165, 1990.
127. Hayes A, Costa T, Scriver CR, Childs B: The effect of Mendelian disease on human health. II. Response to treatment. *Am J Med Genet* **21**:243, 1985.
128. Childs B, Scriver CR: Age at onset and causes of disease. *Perspect Biol Med* **29**:437, 1986.
129. Carter CO: Genetics of common disorders. *Br Med Bull* **25**:52, 1969.
130. Yu T-F: Diversity of clinical features in gouty arthritis. *Semin Arthritis Rheum* **13**:360, 1984.
131. Kobberling J: Studies on the genetic heterogeneity of diabetes mellitus. *Diabetologia* **7**:46, 1971.
132. Fitzgerald MG, Malins JM, O'Sullivan DJ, Wally M: The effect of sex and parity on the incidence of diabetes mellitus. *Q J Med* **30**:57, 1961.
133. Marmot MG, Shipley MJ, Rose G: Inequalities in death-specific explanations of a general pattern. *Lancet* **1**:1003, 1984.
134. Weissman M, Wikramaratne P, Merikangas KR: Onset of major depression in early adulthood. *Arch Gen Psychiatry* **41**:1136, 1984.
135. Pulver AE, Liang KY: Estimating effects of proband characteristics on familial risk. II. The association between age at onset and familial risk in the Maryland schizophrenia sample. *Genet Epidemiol* **8**:339, 1991.
136. Velho G, Groguel P, Clement K, Pueyo ME, Rabotoambinina B, Zouali H, Passa P, Cohen D, Robert J-J: Primary pancreatic beta-cell secretory defect caused by mutations in glucokinase gene in kindreds of maturity onset diabetes of the young. *Lancet* **340**:444, 1992.
137. Jeunemaitre X, Soubrier F, Kotelertser YV, Lifton RP, Williams CS, Charru A, Hunt SC, Hopkins PN, Williams RR, Lalouel JM, Corvol P: Molecular basis of human hypertension: Role of angiotensinogen. *Cell* **71**:169, 1992.
138. Lifton RP, Dluhy RG, Powers M, Rich GM, Gutkin M, Fallo F, Gill JR Jr, Feld L, Ganguly A, Laidlaw JC, Murnaghan DJ, Kaufman C, Stockigt JR, Vlick S, Lalouel JM: Hereditary hypertension caused by chimeric gene duplications and ectopic expression of aldosterone synthase. *Nature Genet* **2**:66, 1992.
139. Hall JM, Friedman L, Guenther C, Lee MK, Weber JL, Black DM, King MC: Closing in on a breast cancer gene on chromosome 17q. *Am J Human Genet* **50**:1235, 1992.
140. Carter BS, Beaty TH, Steinberg GD, Childs B, Walsh PC: Mendelian inheritance of familial prostate cancer. *Proc Natl Acad Sci USA* **89**:3367, 1992.
141. Houlston RS, Collins A, Slack J, Morton NE: Dominant genes for colorectal cancer are not rare. *Ann Hum Genet* **56**:99, 1992.
142. Terrenato L, Gravina MF, San Martini A, Ulizzi L: Natural selection associated with birth weight. III. Changes over the last twenty years. *Ann Human Genet* **45**:267, 1981.
143. Ulizzi L, Terrenato L: Natural selection associated with birth weight. V. The secular relaxation of the stabilizing component. *Ann Hum Genet* **51**:205, 1987.
144. Ulizzi L, Terrenato L: Natural selection associated with birth weight. VI. Towards the end of the stabilizing component. *Ann Hum Genet* **56**:113, 1992.
145. Brusilow SW, Valle DL, Arn P: Symptomatic inborn errors of metabolism. *Curr Ther Neonat Perinat Med* **2**:164, 1990.
146. Scriver CR: Changing heritability of nutritional disease: Another explanation for clustering, in Simopoulos AP, Childs B (eds): *Genetic Variation and Nutrition*. Basel, Karger, 1990, p 60.
147. Leaf A: Preventive medicine for our ailing health care system. *JAMA* **269**:616, 1993.
148. Cavalli-Sforza LL, Bodmer WF: *The Genetics of Human Populations*. San Francisco, Freeman, 1971, p 602.
149. Rowe PC, Valle D, Brusilow SW: Inborn errors of metabolism in children referred with Reye's syndrome. *JAMA* **260**:3167, 1988.
150. Maclachlan AK, Gerrard JW, Houston CS, Ives EJ: Familial infantile cortical hyperostosis in a large Canadian family. *Can Med Assoc J* **130**:1173, 1984.
151. Bannerman RM: Of mice and men and microcytes. *J Pediatr* **98**:760, 1981.
152. Childs B, Moxon ER, Winkelstein JA: Genetics and infectious disease, in King RA, Rotter JI, Motulsky AG (eds): *Genetic Basis of Common Disease*. New York, Oxford University Press, 1992, p 71.
153. Anderson RM, May RM: Population biology of infectious diseases: Part I. *Nature* **280**:361, 1979.
154. Anderson RM, May RM: Population biology of infectious diseases: Part 2. *Nature* **280**:455, 1979.
155. Kilbourne ED: New viral diseases. *JAMA* **264**:68, 1990.
156. Littlefield J: Short analytical review. Possible supplemental mechanisms in the pathogenesis of AIDS. *Clin Immunol Immunopathol* **65**:35, 1992.
157. Lederberg J: Medical science, infectious disease, and the unity of mankind. *JAMA* **260**:684, 1988.
158. Janeway C Jr: The immune system evolved to discriminate infectious nonself from noninfectious self. *Immunol Today* **13**:11, 1992.
159. Winkelstein JA, Childs B: Genetically determined variation in the immune system: Implications for host defense. *Pediatr Infect Dis J* **8**:S31, 1989.
160. Sorenson TIA, Nielsen GG, Anderson PK, Teasdale TW: Genetic and environmental influences on premature death in adult adoptees. *N Engl J Med* **318**:727, 1988.
161. Hedlund JU, Ortquist AB, Kalin M, Scalia-Tomba G, Gieseke J: Risk of pneumonia in patients previously treated in hospital for pneumonia. *Lancet* **340**:396, 1992.
162. Biozzi G, Mouton D, Stiffel C, Bouthillier Y: Major role of macrophages in quantitative genetic regulation of immuno responsiveness and anti-infectious immunity. *Adv Immunol* **36**:189, 1984.
163. Beadle GW: Genes and chemical reactions in Neurospora. *Science* **129**:1715, 1959.
164. Tatum EL: Indole and serine in the biosynthesis and breakdown of tryptophan. *Proc Natl Acad Sci* **30**:30, 1944.
165. McGuinness BJ, Clarke IN, Lambden PR, Barlow AK, Poolman JT, Jones DM, Heckels JE: Point mutation in meningococcal por A gene associated with increased endemic disease. *Lancet* **337**:514, 1991.
166. Knudson AG Jr: Hereditary cancer, oncogenes and antioncogenes. *Cancer Res* **45**:1437, 1985.
167. Weinberg RA: Oncogenes, antioncogenes, and the molecular basis of multistep carcinogenesis. *Cancer Res* **49**:3713, 1989.
168. Bishop JM: Molecular themes in oncogenesis. *Cell* **64**:235, 1991.
169. Ponder BAJ: Inherited predisposition to cancer. *Trends Genet* **6**:213, 1990.
170. Fearon ER, Vogelstein B: A genetic model for colorectal tumorigenesis. *Cell* **61**:759, 1990.
171. Vogelstein B, Kinzler KW: p53 and dysfunction. *Cell* **70**:523, 1992.
172. Peto R, Roe FJC, Lee PN, Levy L, Clack J: Cancer and aging in mice and men. *Br J Cancer* **32**:411, 1975.
173. Nepom G: A unified hypothesis for the complex genetics of HLA associations with IDDM. *Diabetes* **39**:1153, 1990.
174. Field LL, Dizier M-H, Anderson CE, Spence MA, Rotter JI: HLA dependent GM effects in insulin-dependent diabetes: Evidence from pairs of affected siblings. *Am J Hum Genet* **39**:640, 1986.
175. Bain SC, Prins JB, Hearne CM, Rodrigues NR, Rowe BR, Pritchard LE, Ritchie RJ, Hall JRS, Undlien DE, Ronningen KS, Dunger DB, Barnett AH, Todd JA: Insulin gene region-encoded susceptibility to type I diabetes is not restricted to HLA-DR4-positive individuals. *Nature Genet* **2**:212, 1992.
176. Todd JA, Aitman TJ, Cornall RJ, Ghosh S, Hall JRS, Hearne CM, Knight AM, Love JM, McAleer MA, Prins J-B, Rodriguez N, Lathrop M, Pressey A, DeLarato NH, Peterson LB, Wicker LS: Genetic analysis of autoimmune Type I diabetes mellitus in mice. *Nature* **351**:542, 1991.

177. Diabetes Epidemiology Research Group: Secular trends in incidence of childhood IDDM in 10 countries. *Diabetes* **39**:858, 1990.
178. Rewers M, LaPorte RE, Walczak M, Dmochowski K, Bogaczynska E: Apparent epidemic of insulin-dependent diabetes mellitus in mid western Poland. *Diabetes* **36**:106, 1987.
179. Borch-Johnsen K, Jones G, Mandrup-Poulsen T, Christy M, Zachau B, Kastrup K, Nerup J: Relation between breast-feeding and incidence rates of insulin-dependent diabetes mellitus. *Lancet* **2**:1083, 1984.
180. Mayer EJ, Hamman RF, Gay EC, Lezotte DC, Savitz DA, Klingensmith GJ: Reduced risk of IDDM among breast fed children. *Diabetes* **37**:1625, 1988.
181. Glathaar C, Whittall DE, Welborn TA: Diabetes in Western Australian children. *Med J Aust* **148**:117, 1988.
182. Vadheim CM, Rotter JI, Maclaren NK, Riley WS, Anderson CE: Preferential transmission of diabetic alleles within the HLA gene complex. *N Engl J Med* **315**:1314, 1986.
183. McCarthy BJ, Dorman JS, Aston CE: Investigating genomic imprinting and susceptibility to insulin-dependent diabetes-mellitus. *Genet Epidemiol* **8**:117, 1991.
184. Rubinstein P, Walker M, Ginsberg-Fellner F: Excess of DR3/4 in type I diabetes: What does it portend? *Diabetes* **35**:985, 1986.
185. Karjalainen J, Salmela P, Ilonen J, Surcel H-M, Knip M: A comparison of childhood and adult type I diabetes mellitus. *N Engl J Med* **320**:881, 1989.
186. Chern MM, Anderson VE, Barbosa J: Empirical risk for insulin-dependent diabetes in sibs. *Diabetes* **31**:1115, 1982.
187. Johnston C, Pyke DA, Cudworth AG, Wolf E: HLA-DR typing in identical twins with insulin-dependent diabetes. *Br Med J* **286**:253, 1983.
188. Pittman WB, Acton R, Barger BO, Bell R, Go CP, Murphy CC, Roseman IM: HLA B and DR associations in type I diabetes mellitus with onset after age 40. *Diabetes* **31**:122, 1984.
189. Zucman-Caillet S, Garchon H-J, Timsit J, Assan R, Boitard C, Djlalli-Saiah I, Bougneres P, Bach J-F: Age dependent HLA genetic heterogeneity of type I insulin-dependent diabetes mellitus. *J Clin Invest* **90**:2242, 1992.
190. Ludvigsson J, Afoke AO: Seasonality of type I diabetes mellitus. *Diabetologia* **32**:84, 1989.
191. Wagener DK, LaPorte RE, Orchard TJ, Cavender D, Kuller LH, Drash AL: The Pittsburgh diabetes study: An increased prevalence with older maternal age. *Diabetologia* **25**:82, 1983.
192. Barker DJP: The intrauterine environment and adult cardiovascular disease, in Bock GR, Whelen GR (eds): *The Childhood Environment and Adult Disease*. Ciba Foundation Symposium 156. Chichester, Wiley, 1991, p 3.
193. Berensen GS, Srinivasan SR, Hunter SM, Niklas TA, Freedman DS, Shear CL, Webber LS: Risk factors in early life as predictors of adult heart disease: The Bogalusa heart study. *Am J Med Sci* **298**:141, 1989.
194. Wang XL, Wilcken DEL, Dudman NPD: Early expression of the apolipoprotein (a) gene: Relationship between infants and their parents' serum apolipoprotein (a) levels. *Pediatrics* **89**:401, 1992.
195. Ekborn R, Trichopoulos D, Adami H-O, Hsieh C-C, Lan S-J: Evidence of prenatal influences on breast cancer risk. *Lancet* **340**:1015, 1992.
196. Martyn CN: Childhood infection and adult disease, in Bock GR, Whelen GR (eds): *The Childhood Environment and Adult Disease*. Ciba Foundation Symposium 156. Chichester, Wiley, 1991, p 93.
197. Lever AF, Harrap SB: Essential hypertension: A disorder of growth with origins in childhood. *J Hypertens* **10**:101, 1992.
198. Labarthe DR, Eissa M, Varas C: Childhood precursors of high blood pressure and elevated cholesterol. *Annu Rev Public Health* **12**:519, 1991.
199. Rutter M: Childhood experiences and adult psychosocial functioning, in Bock GR, Whelen GR (eds): *The Childhood Environment and Adult Disease*. Ciba Foundation Symposium 156. Chichester, Wiley, 1991, p 189.
200. Greenough WT, Black JE, Wallace CS: Experience and brain development. *Child Dev* **58**:539, 1987.
201. Riese ML: Neonatal temperament in monozygotic and dizygotic twin pairs. *Child Dev* **61**:1230, 1990.
202. Riese ML: Genetic influences on neonatal temperament. *Acta Genet Med Gemellol* (Roma) **39**:207, 1990.
203. Pocock NA, Eisman JA, Hopper JL, Yeates MG, Sambrook PN, Eberl S: Genetic determinants of bone mass in adults. *J Clin Invest* **80**:706, 1987.
204. Chesnut CH III: Theoretical overview: Bone development, peak bone mass, bone loss, and fracture risk. *Am J Med* **91(suppl 5B)**:2S, 1991.
205. Seeman E, Hopper JL, Bach LA, Cooper ME, Parkinson E, McKay J, Jerums G: Reduced bone mass in daughters of women with osteoporosis. *N Engl J Med* **320**:554, 1989.
206. Jackson JA, Kleerskoper M: Osteoporosis in men: Diagnosis, pathophysiology, and prevention. *Medicine* (Baltimore) **69**:137, 1990.
207. Finkelstein J, Neer R, Biller BMK, Crawford JD, Klibanski A: Osteopenia in men with a history of delayed puberty. *N Engl J Med* **326**:600, 1992.
208. Slemenda CW, Christian JC, Reed T, Reister TK, Williams CJ, Johnston CC: Long-term bone loss in men: Effects of genetic and environmental factors. *Ann Intern Med* **117**:286, 1992.
209. Eisman JA, Sambrook PN, Kelly PJ, Pocock NA: Exercise and its interaction with genetic influences in the determination of bone mineral density. *Am J Med* **91(suppl 5B)**:5S, 1991.
210. Felson DT, Sloutskia D, Anderson JJ, Anthony JM, Kiel DP: Thiazide diuretics and the risk of hip fracture. *JAMA* **265**:370, 1991.
211. Sowers MR, Clark MK, Jannausch ML, Wallace RB: A prospective study of bone mineral content and fracture in communities with differential fluoride exposure. *Am J Epidemiol* **133**:649, 1991.
212. Christian JC, Yu P-L, Slemenda CW, Johnston CC Jr: Heritability of bone mass: A longitudinal study in aging male twins. *Am J Hum Genet* **44**:429, 1989.
213. Binstock RH: The oldest old: A fresh perspective or compassionate ageism revisited. *Milbank Mem Fund Q* **63**:420, 1985.
214. Kunitz SJ: The historical roots and ideological functions of disease concepts in three primary care specialties. *Bull Hist Med* **57**:412, 1983.

CHAPTER 3

The Inborn Error and Biochemical Individuality

Barton Childs ▪ David Valle ▪ Gerardo Jimenez-Sanchez

INTRODUCTION

In the seventh edition of MMBID there is a table of 50 pages listing 469 entries perceived by the editors as inborn errors of metabolism, descendants of what Archibald Garrod described in 1909. The table consists of eight columns that itemize the qualities of each inborn error. One of these, headed "Mutant gene product," lists the names of the variant proteins that lie at the root of the pathogenesis of each disease. These proteins comprehend principally enzymes, but there are also receptors, transporting and structural proteins, hormones, clotting factors, immunoproteins, hemoglobins, and the like. Other columns lodge the variant in its homeostatic system and allude to its phenotype, while still others reveal the chromosomal locus occupied by the gene of its origin.

So the data comprise gene, gene locus, gene product, homeostatic system, and the results of dysfunction. Naturally the data are not complete. Of the total, the crucial variant protein is missing for 71, and for even more, chromosomal localization and other properties are missing. Why are those incomplete entries included? Because the disease phenotypes segregate and biochemical and other attributes predict that gene and gene product will soon be manifest. Such is the power of segregation!

Of course, the list was out of date when the seventh edition emerged in 1994, and the list in the present edition, despite the addition of many more entries, will also be out of date; the rate of increase is exponential. Even so, we may be confident that although the new list embraces new kinds of protein variants and new homeostatic systems, it does not deviate in principle from the old. But the significance for medicine of this expanding list of proteins and homeostatic devices lies not in their number or rate of increase but in the hypothesis that no homeostatic element is invulnerable, so that, as defined by the editors of MMBID, the list of inborn errors must expand until all variants of all protein components of all homeostatic systems have been included.

There is a further hypothesis, more embracing, more profound. It is that the protein variants of homeostasis, each a unit step in a physiological mechanism, are the points of origin of all disease. Descriptions of pathogenesis focus on cellular dysfunction as it originates in the protein elements of the cells wherein they are integrated into physiological systems. Proteins take their specificity from their genes, so pathogenesis, explained in terms of variation in unit steps of homeostasis, is a reflection of genotype, which is to say, all diseases originate in relationships of incongruence between genetically specified protein unit steps of homeostasis and experiences of the environment, whether within the cells or without.

This hypothesis has been tested repeatedly in that fraction of disease we call the inborn error of metabolism. But this comprises only a fraction of all disease; most is comprehended in diseases called *multifactorial, multigenic*, or *complex*. What of them? Inasmuch as their pathogenesis conforms to that observed in the inborn errors, complex diseases might be perceived as special cases of the inborn error but differentiated by a pathogenesis originating in two, several, or many unit steps of one, two, or many homeostatic devices. That is the hypothesis that informs the investigations of those who seek the origins of atherosclerosis, hypertension, cancer, and infections too.

The confidence with which these investigators can proceed is based on the unassailable validity of the monogenic inborn error. But there are manifest differences between our concepts of the inborn error and complex disease. Many of these have been described in Chaps. 1 and 2. So what do we call the complex diseases? Type II inborn errors? After all, the genes of both mendelize. The previous chapters have also shown that close scrutiny of the monogenic inborn errors reveals variation in their expression that can be ascribed to genes other than the principal one, genes often called *modifiers*. So there is a continuity that joins the monogenic with the multigenic into a seamless fabric conveniently embraced in Garrod's second, and more profound, idea, that of chemical individuality. But the concepts of both the inborn error and chemical individuality are limited by their having originated in the intellectual contexts of other times, and concepts change even when words do not. L. C. Dunn made a point of this in relation to genetic concepts in his book *A Short History of Genetics*, published in 1965.[1] In the reductionist atmosphere of today, the focus is on the variant unit step of homeostasis and its reflection into pathogenesis, which means that what the phrase *inborn error of metabolism* means today is likely to differ in many ways from what it meant to its originator, or to others who have used it since. Perhaps we need new words more suitable for today's reality, or if the words continue to suit, we need new definitions. But if we are to change old concepts, we must know whence they came and through what steps they passed to attain their present significance. We should know their history. Accordingly, this chapter is organized as follows: We begin with some implications of the unit step of homeostasis as the central focus in defining disease and pathogenesis, then take up the history of the concepts of the inborn error and of chemical, or today we would say biochemical, individuality in the contexts of developments in genetics on the one hand and in medicine on the other. And finally, we will show how the convergence of the inborn error and chemical individuality on the unit step of homeostasis form the basis for the alternative to the metaphor of the body as a machine outlined in Chap. 2.

THE UNIT STEP OF HOMEOSTASIS

"Unit step of homeostasis," words less felicitous and infinitely less elegant than "inborn error of metabolism," suit the broader mission of a locution that must at once express: a) a unitary relationship of a protein or peptide to its gene, b) the role of the protein as a unitary, singular element in a homeostatic device that has stood the test of selection, and c) all degrees of qualitative and quantitative variation of both structure and function of the protein in its homeostatic role. That is, the phrase is applicable whether as the basis of a monogenic disease, a contributor to a multigenic disease, or a part of a system functioning adaptively. In modern usage, "inborn error of metabolism" also implies a one-to-one relationship of a gene to a protein engaged in homeostatic business, but the word *error* is defined by Webster's as a deviation, a mistake, a lapse, all words suitable for dysfunction. In the end, variation of the unit step of homeostasis is more compatible with Garrod's concept of chemical individuality than with that of the inborn error. Like the unit step, biochemical individuality is inclusive of all variation regardless of adaptive quality. A fuller explication of the concept of the unit step follows.

The Qualities of the Unit Step of Homeostasis

As a unit of history. We tend to think of proteins only in relation to their functions, but they are a link to both the immediate and the phylogenetic past, memories of other lives, even other species, and as such they are a focus of history. Just as social and cultural history focus on pivotal events, so phylogenetic history focuses on milestones of homeostatic history; and just as the history of a culture has its remote past, its intermediate past, and its immediate phases, so does that of the protein elements of human homeostasis. The proteins that give us life today descend not only from our parents and other human antecedents but, in varying degrees of conservation, from those of other species.

As an effector of genetic "intention." In ordinary parlance genes are said to be "for" something, a usage that is perhaps defensible when the pathway from gene to phenotype is clear. Then it is useful as a way of thinking about the connection between mendelism, including segregation and the dynamics of the gene pool, and the protein products that form the structural elements of homeostasis. It is a way of connecting remote with proximate causes and may be helpful in the clinician's duty to explain and the patient's need to understand. But at the molecular and physiological level it is inaccurate, because the only "intention" of the gene is to transmit its information to the transcript that sees to the translation of that information into protein product. The career of that product, however, is determined not by its gene nor even by itself, but by how well it fits into its homeostatic device and how well that device assembles and integrates with others, all acting in concert to promote the adaptation of an open system in an indifferent environment. Unit steps act as both choreographers and dancers; they are mediators and effectors of regulation and development. Assemblies of protein elements are sometimes called protein machines, and they may include 50 or more such elements.[2] The DNA, after specifying its products, then responds to signals from those products, while the latter lose their identity in their service to the larger aims of the machines and still larger integrated systems. The unit step is like a private soldier serving faithfully and anonymously. But no army, no matter how glittering the reputation of its commander, ever prevailed in battle except through the will and determination of its private soldiers. It is sometimes said that one of the fruits of the genome project will be a representation of our humanity, and so it will, in a flat, two-dimensional way. But such a list of genes cannot represent the three-dimensional human being, nor can it predict or represent its efflorescence in the dimension of time. These qualities are informed by the actions and interactions, independent of the DNA, of the unit steps of homeostasis.

The unit step as interface. The importance of the unit step is exemplified in its role as interface between diverse elements.

a) The previous section established the primacy of the gene product as effector of the gene's intention, but in a way not predicted by information residing in the gene. So the unit step acts at the interface between the gene and its phenotype.

b) The description of the unit step is the end of the quest of the molecular biologist, whose path goes from the gene upward to its protein and its fate in cellular business, there to meet the outcome of the aims of the clinician, who proceeds downward toward the protein by way of signs and symptoms and their associated physiological and biochemical qualities. It is to be noted that the science of the clinician is physiological, which is to say integrative, while that of the molecular biologist is reductive. The junctional node is the unit step. This interface is also conceptually critical for the physician, who observes on the one hand a molecular analysis of the disease of an individual patient, whose identity may be reduced to that of his or her abnormal molecules, and on the other hand the integrated person, expressed in the whole of the homeostatic apparatus. It is the job of the physician to reconcile these philosophically opposed analyses in the interest of the patient.

c) The unit steps are the junction, or point of union, of the thinking characterized by the concept of the body as a machine with the alternative outlined in Chap. 2, in which disease is perceived as an unavoidable by-product of the necessity to a species of variability. Variant unit steps are the site of proximate causes that represent the origins of pathogenesis, but proximate causes necessarily reflect the remote causes that individualize them. The unit steps are, therefore, the focus of investigators, who would elucidate homeostatic dysfunction in such detail as to expose points of vulnerability in pathogenesis and study the dynamics of the gene pool, as well as the social and cultural milieus that are incongruent with the variant protein.

Individuality. Human beings are open systems, exchanging matter and energy with the environment in the interest of growth and maintenance. The individuality of such open systems resides in the variation of the proteins that constitute its unit steps, themselves a reflection of the genes that specified them. This uniqueness is expressed in differences in how homeostatic systems meet the demands made upon them by the experiences they encounter in a career marked initially by development, later by aging. Now, since the whole organism is constituted by the integration of many homeostatic systems, mutational variation in one is likely to be reflected in others, each of which will respond according to its own genetic and developmental variation. So in the matter of description of a disease, it is safe to say that each individual suffers his or her own version of it.

In its role of element in integrated systems that lead to emergent qualities unpredicted by its gene, the variant unit step acts as determiner of both individuality and the range of qualities accepted as normal. The genes cannot do this, since they do not control the outcomes of the actions of their products in the complexity of the cell. So usages like "normal" or "mutant" gene, while acceptable for ordinary discourse, neither plumb the depths nor encompass the extent of the influences of their products.

As units of natural selection. It is the qualities of the elements of homeostasis and their integration that determine whether or not genes survive and spread in populations. Although it is individuals that are the units of selection, the proteins dictate the qualities of their phenotypes by virtue of their effectiveness in carrying out their allotted function, as well as by how well they integrate with other steps in their system, and in turn, how well their system integrates with still others. This effectiveness must vary according to a) allelic differences within the loci that specify each single step and b) variations in how the associated elements in the system work together. So a molecule that works well within the requirements and constraints exerted by the variations of others must be the most effective, and its retention in species will be favored in selection by virtue of its contribution to the success of the whole. Conversely, the failure of a variant unit step to fulfill expectation may make its dysfunctional phenotype the object of a different kind of selection, that of elimination, in what is sometimes called "purifying" selection.

As antidote to the mythical powers of the gene. The symbolism of the gene has led to such locutions as "gene-environment interaction," when in fact interactions with conditions of the environment occur only at the site of, and through the specificities of, the unit steps. Recognition of the pivotal place of homeostatic proteins must strike a heavy blow to the idea of genetic determinism, since it is not the gene that determines phenotype but its product, at work with others in the integrated organism. The use of expressions like "genes for" intelligence, hypertension, or atherosclerosis is meaningless apart from knowledge of the proteins the genes specify and their roles in some homeostatic device. Loci discovered by linkage analysis are not "genes for" until their proteins are known. Then they are discovered to be "for" receptors, transcription factors, enzymes, or other protein molecules, variations of which contribute to the disease in question.

The point is that "gene-environmental interaction" is a drosophiline usage that originated in times when the action of genes was unclear. It may be that those who know the reality of the interaction use the phrase as a shorthand notation, but when the complexity of the physiology involved is unknown, its use can lead to such absurdities as genes for success in business or even for happiness.[3]

As preserver of coherence. Not the least of the qualities of the unit step is its usefulness as a point of departure for keeping up with medical advances. New knowledge about disease must build upon the basis of variation of the unit step and its reflection into homeostasis. Knowing that, we are immediately au courant even though the disease be ophthalmologic, urologic, or psychiatric. The concept of the unit step is an instrument of coherence.

THE HISTORY OF THE GENE PRODUCT IN DISEASE

A Justification for a Historical Approach

The perception of the primacy of the gene product in cellular life was not a consequence of one or two explosive epiphanies. It represents a coalescence of the thinking and actions of investigators who would say that they were asking questions in botany, or microbiology, or evolutionary biology, or physics, or biochemistry, or medicine. So the idea has a variegated history to which many disciplines have contributed, and while each has imposed some characteristics of its own, those of each have been modified by those of others. Perhaps the history of the central position of the protein gene product in medicine is best represented as an ontogeny, a developmental process. Ontogeny is a dynamic, cumulative process; today's qualities are a consequence of what happened yesterday, and tomorrow's must depend upon those of today. So if development is represented as a linear structure of ever-changing qualities, cross-sectional samples should reveal a series of developmental matrices composed of outcomes of the forces, both genetic and of experience, bearing on the ontogeny of that moment. Developmental history then, is a description of such cross-sectional samples, an account of both the progress attained at each stage and an interpretation of its meanings in regard to the whole.

An important characteristic of such development is the retention of aspects of prior stages, even as they are modified to become the new; aspects of early development are always to be observed in later ontogeny. A second quality is flexibility, the capacity to change direction, although always within the trajectory set at the start. That is, although there may be what seem revolutionary changes, when viewed from a later perspective they are recognized to have been more evolutionary than radical.[4] So there is every reason to take this ontogenetic path, beginning with the idea of the inborn error as it took form in Archibald Garrod's mind and tracing it to today's version of the variable gene product as it is expressed not only in the diseases described in MMBID but also in the form of risk factors or merely harmless variation. And in so doing we will observe that this development was guided on the one hand by advances in genetics, especially in the progressive refinement of the definition of the gene, and on the other by changes in medicine, in which the pursuit of conventional aims in both research and patient care became more and more technological.

The Ontogeny of the Inborn Error and Chemical Individuality

Introduction. When, in his Nobel Prize paper, George Beadle proclaimed Archibald Garrod to be the originator of the one gene-one enzyme hypothesis, he was imposing his 1940s view on the history of 40 years before.[5] In fact, Garrod did not propose exactly that; he never came to grips with genetics, even in his book *Inborn Factors in Disease*, published in 1931.[6] So Beadle simply interpreted a medical observation of 40 years before as a biologist of his own time might do. In this chapter we begin with Garrod the physician, who made some astute clinical observations using his understanding of the biochemistry of the time to do so.

Garrod's Definition. In his elegant and perceptive biography of Garrod, Alexander Bearn has assembled all of Garrod's writings and has given us a penetrating analysis of his character and his work.[7] Inevitably, we have drawn heavily upon Bearn's book in our analysis of the ontogeny of the inborn error.

Although Garrod knew nothing of genes, he contributed to genetics. He was the first to give a mendelian interpretation to a human trait and, with Bateson's help, the first to show the effects of "consanguinity."[8] So medicine, biochemistry, and genetics all were involved in the first description of the inborn error, and all, plus molecular biology, must be reckoned with in its history. No doubt adherents of each discipline will perceive the inborn error in their own context, but since our aim is to examine how the concept has fared in medicine, we will be looking at how these other sciences have contributed to the *medical* meaning of the concept.

We begin with Garrod's formulation of the concept of the inborn error of metabolism. Bearn tells how Garrod advanced the idea of the inborn error in papers about alkaptonuria published between 1898 and 1902, both before and after the rediscovery of Mendel.[8] Garrod did not then use the words "inborn error,"preferring "metabolic alternative," which in the 1902 paper was defined as a rare, hereditary, recessive biochemical variation, lifelong and harmless although inferior to type, all a consequence of a block in an enzymatic pathway due to the loss of an enzyme. That is, such variations were not defined as diseases.

Evidence was adduced for each point, first in relation to alkaptonuria and then in relation to three other such metabolic alternatives. And then, toward the end of the 1902 paper, where today the investigator expounds the significance of the reported work in light of the position of the field at the moment, there appears the following: "If it be, indeed the case that in alkaptonuria and the other conditions mentioned we are dealing with individualities of metabolism and not with the results of morbid processes, the thought naturally presents itself that these are merely extreme examples of variations of chemical behavior which are probably everywhere present in minor degree and that just as no two individuals of a species are absolutely identical in bodily structure neither are their chemical processes carried out on exactly the same lines."[8] And this inter-individual variation he called chemical individuality, supporting the idea, Bearn tells us, by reference to a paper by C. H. Huppert of Prague, who alluded to the well-known inter-species variations in proteins.[7] Huppert said nothing, however, of intra-species variation. That was Garrod's idea, and it originated in the observations on alkaptonuria and the other more or less harmless metabolic aberrations.

One point to emphasize here is that Garrod saw that the idea of chemical individuality transcends that of the inborn error. This priority is clearly stated in the title of the 1902 paper, which reads, "The incidence of alkaptonuria: A study in chemical individuality." This emphasis is repeated in his first book, "Inborn Errors of Metabolism," published in 1909, in which, in Chap. 1, the significance of the inborn errors as components of chemical individuality is again stressed; and finally, in his 1931 book, called *Inborn Factors in Disease*, the inborn errors, whose definition had been modified to include disease in the 2nd edition of *Inborn Errors*, published in 1923, are relegated to a single chapter representing about one sixth of a book dedicated to the proposition that human disease is an outcome of hereditary vulnerabilities, mostly brought to overt expression by special experiences.[6]

It is noteworthy that Garrod did not call these hereditary vulnerabilities "inborn errors." That term he reserved for qualities that fulfilled the definition given above. That is, in this book, at a time when the idea of diathesis was waning fast, he revived it, clothing it in chemical individuality, which to him is clearly the paramount idea. There is an irony here. Had Garrod's four examples been drawn from today's list of mainly lethal or crippling inborn errors, it is unlikely that he would have perceived their continuity with chemical individuality. These ideas of Garrod's sound very modern, but historians warn us against giving the words of the past a modern meaning.[1] That is why we have to observe how these ideas fared in the contexts of genetics, biochemistry, molecular biology, and medicine and how the inborn error, conceived in medicine, moved into genetics and then back to medicine in the form of biochemical descriptions of metabolic diseases and differences in hemoglobins, at first without reference to the idea of the inborn error. Chemical individuality, in the meantime, faded into the background, only to re-emerge, first in variations in blood group substances, then in the genetic idea of protein polymorphism, and finally in medicine in the guise of risk factors and genetic vulnerability associated with diseases of complex origin. Accordingly, we turn now to contemporaneous events in medicine and genetics that formed the milieu within which the inborn error concept developed during the years 1900–1950.

Developments in Medicine and Genetics

Developments in Medicine 1900–1950. What was happening in medicine from the time of the description of the inborn error and chemical individuality until the 1950s? Although readers of the 8th edition of MMBID will find the medicine of the first half of the 20th century quaint and uncomplicated, their awareness of the knowledge and technology of today may give them some insight into the failure of earlier physicians to grasp the significance of Garrod's observations. To them it had no meaning; there was no context into which to fit it. Even Garrod himself was unsure where his ideas might go. He saw no obvious way to expand them. To gather more inborn errors and to fill in the repertory of chemical individuality was his aim, but there was no way to do it. So what happened in medicine that led, in time, to the recognition and acceptance of the inborn error (Table 3.1)?

All living entities have the same growth curve: a long slow climb toward an exponential phase, to be followed by a flattening as the growth is completed.[9] It is arguable that although the exponential phase is more spectacular, the early slow climb includes the most significant novelties, the wherewithal without which the later explosion could not have taken place. Applying this description to medical change, the exponential phase of its development began in earnest in the 1950s. Before that, medicine was engaged in a process of redefinition that set the pattern for the second half of the 20th century. We all know the cardinal features of the second half: the explosion in technology, not only in the biochemical and molecular perception of pathogenesis but also in radiologic, sonographic, and endoscopic appreciation of disease. These methods led to a reductionist analysis that increased the necessity for a specialism that materially changed medical practice and education.

What characterized that developmental period? It was a time of reconstitution. Medicine came out of the 19th century with an essentialist concept of disease and a mono-etiologic mentality based on infection and morbid anatomy. But in the first 50 years of the 20th, in conjunction with biochemistry, molecular biology, physiology, and microbiology, medicine refined its scientific basis, perceiving itself as a university subject with the intellectual stature accorded other sciences and the humanities.[10–12] This took the shape of the full-time system, which itself promoted clinical investigation, raising research to equality with teaching and patient care.

The model of infections, disease by assault; essentialist in character, was extended to disease as deficiency, so in the first 30 or 40 years of the century, disorders due to lack of vitamins or other essential factors yielded to biochemical attack with solutions that reduced their incidence. At the same time, a conceptual trend toward a nominalist (adaptive failure) interpretation of disease was propelled by emphasis on the internal causes of disease, causes that had to be understood and described as disturbing integrated functions. During this time W. B. Cannon and L. J. Henderson were developing their ideas of homeostasis, and endocrinology was an important part of it.[13,14] Accordingly, the pathology of disease was increasingly perceived as a consequence of disrupted physiology, a failure of regulation. Sinding has used Albright's study of resistant rickets to illustrate this transition from external to internal.[15] Although the disorder is familial, Albright did not see it as an inborn error or genetic disease. But he did see it in the nominalist light of individuality, and as Sinding points out, "After 1937, this history progressed by successively separating new individual entities, affecting smaller and smaller groups of individuals in each case." A geneticist would say that the goal of genetic heterogeneity was being pursued, but that is an anachronism. What was going on was the creation of a foundation for a rapprochement between medicine and genetics as equals. Without the concepts of homeostasis and regulation, human biochemical genetics would not have gone very far.[16]

So American investigators, often trained in Germany, began to see pathogenesis as a result of abnormalities of biochemical and physiological processes that ended in morbid anatomy. In 1931, Cohn spoke of medicine as ". . . the study of diseases as biological systems."[12] This emphasis on metabolism led to a refocus of attention from the organs to the cell, which became medicine's "unifying principle."[12] Whatever the disease, cells were its seat. Many diseases were organ specific, but it was the disability of its cells that impaired the organ's function. And once inside the cell, disease was perceived as molecular disorder.

We are fortunate to have a summary of the position of American medical research in 1955. In that year an extensive study of medical schools, universities, and independent institutes was published by the American Foundation.[17] Representatives of many such institutions were interviewed, and a record was compiled of the nature and scope of the research then underway.

What did the investigators find? First, the principles that governed the duty of medical schools to support research were that a) *all* disease would be shown to originate in disordered metabolism at the cellular level; b) the names of diseases, often based on affected organ systems, did not reflect what was going on in the cells — not only those of the apparently affected organ, but of others too; c) the discovery of proximate causes would explain the pathogenesis and lead to an appropriate treatment.

Second, there was at the time no strong tie between the basic sciences and medicine, even though the departments of the former were usually lodged in medical schools. That is, ideas engendered by basic scientists were applied to human beings by physician investigators, whose aims were quite different from those who originated them. In addition, since finding the mechanisms of pathogenesis for all cases was the goal, the idea of individuality never came up. It simply wasn't on the agenda.

Third, although the study was not oblivious to genetics, there was very little recognition at the medical institutions surveyed in the study of genetic ideas that might prove to have any practical use, nor any vision of genetics' future impact. In an introduction to the report, entitled "Biological basis of medicine," after a perfunctory notice of the DNA as being involved in "heredity within the cell," there appears the following: "Obviously the relation to human medicine of such findings may be apparently remote, may be direct, or may consist of analogies in plant and animal life." No resounding conviction there! There were also in

Table 3-1 Chronology of ideas and events in genetics, medicine and the history of the inborn error.

DECADES	GENETICS		INBORN ERRORS		MEDICINE	
	CONCEPTUAL	EVENTS	CONCEPTUAL	EVENTS	CONCEPTUAL	EVENTS
1902–1910	Abstract gene	Rediscovery of mendelism	Inborn error inherited recessive enzyme deficiences with visible & permanent phenotype Chemical individuality	Alkaptonuria, cystinuria, albinism, pentosuria Cuenot—coat colors	Body as machine Essentialist disease Monoetiologic mentality Morbid anatomy Flexner report	Infections Few treatments ABO blood groups Congenital anomalies
1910–1930	Operational gene	Chromosome theory Recombination Linkage Allellsm		Anthocyanins S. Wright—coat colors	Biochemistry Disease at cellular level	Vitamins Nutritional deficiencies Hormones
1930–1950	Functional gene One gene-one peptide	Physiological (biochemical) genetics Population genetics Textbooks	Unit biochemical process One gene-one peptide		Enter genetics in *Drosophilia* guise Nominalist disease Clinical investigation Concept of homeostasis	Antibiotics Rh blood groups Biochemical physiological study of homeostatic abnormality Endocrinology Electrolyte physiology Immunology
1950–1970	Structural gene Colinearity Genetic individuality	Biochemical genetics Polymorphism Variety of mutants (including chromosomal)	Phenotype derives from variant protein Relation to environment Inborn error includes non-enzyme proteins	Hemoglobin variants >100 inborn errors described	Recognition of medical genetics and "genetic disease"	Medical genetics in textbooks & curricula: 15% of schools have depts, 75% divisions Reduced infections, increased chronic disease Changes in fertility
1970–Present	Molecular gene defined as exons, introns and non-transcribed control elements	Fine structure of genes and chromosomes Linkage analysis Fine structure of proteins Microdeletion syndromes Genomics	Inborn error as variant unit step of homeostasis Variant represented as vulnerability which in appropriate conditions becomes disease Variant unit steps as risk Continuity of mono- and multigenetic disease Genetic individuality	Structure of variant genes & mutants known Candidate protein and linkage analysis >400 IEMs known Analysis of diseases of complex origin New forms of treatment Nominalist disease	"Genetic disease" Genes in multifactorial disease Synthesis of machine mentality with genetic thinking Population genetics Molecular pathogenesis Prevention looms Ethical issues	95% American schools teach genetics Board of Medical Genetics College of Medical Genetics 20% of schools have Departments of Genetics Risk factors Screening, antenatal diagnosis Recognition of role of genes in complex, chronic disease

the introduction accounts of visits to Beadle and Pauling without mention of how their discoveries or the ideas they embraced could be incorporated into medical thinking. It must be said that the study took several years to carry out, and so the investigators may have visited Pauling before his work on hemoglobin, which appeared in 1949, but Beadle published his one gene-one enzyme hypothesis in 1941. A visit was also made to Avery, and the visitor recounts only how the DNA had proved to be the transforming factor for pneumococci. So genetics was not uppermost in the minds of the representatives of the Foundation, and by extension in those of physicians in general.

This indifference to genetics in medical research is further attested in the citation of only 24 references (3%) related to genetics among a total of 715. Of those 24, only 5, or less than 1%, had anything to do with genetics in medicine. These 715 references included reports of the most recent work in biochemistry, physiology, and virology and must be taken as the latest in the work and thinking of investigators in and around medicine.

But perhaps this study, however comprehensive, did not represent the reality of the presence of genetics in medicine. That it did so is attested by the observation that citations to articles on human heredity in the *Index Medicus* did not exceed those to papers on hernias until 1962, after which the numbers of the former soared into the many hundreds.[18] Even so, genetics was not completely neglected in American medicine. A survey in 1955 revealed that seven medical schools gave courses in genetics, and there were at least two departments of that name.[19] And Great Britain, although not as advanced in the biochemical analysis of pathogenesis, was ahead of the U.S. in the application of mendelian ideas to human disease.[20]

Why should medicine have been so impervious to genetic ideas? Many reasons have been given. One is that human genetics was identified by physicians with the follies of eugenics of the 1920s and 1930s.[21] Another, perhaps promoted by geneticists to whom the central feature of research was the controlled mating, was that human material was unsuited for genetic study.[22] Yet another was that physician interest in heredity, which had been based on the discredited idea of diathesis, actually declined, even while *Drosophila* genetics prospered. And the rare familial case of arcane disease hardly commanded much interest.[23]

Perhaps it was not yet time; there was no context into which to receive anything beyond the occasional pedigree, no receptors for new ideas such as genetic and molecular individuality, which by 1955 were beginning to be perceived, however dimly. If so, it should surprise no one, inasmuch as the focus of pathogenesis had so recently passed from organs and morbid anatomy to cells and the deranged metabolism therein. What was needed was the techniques of biochemical analysis for a further descent to perceive diseases as deviations in molecular homeostasis, a result of variation in the protein elements of the homeostatic apparatus, at which time it would be noticed that the variant proteins were the product of variant genes. That this was happening was demonstrated in the American Foundation study in reviews of the current position of research in several diseases. In atherosclerosis, lipoproteins were under study; in hypertension, renin; and in rheumatic syndromes, "protein metabolism in connective tissue."[17] But developments in a science are more often evolutionary than revolutionary, and we should applaud the flights of thought and ingenuity that led to the discoveries in medicine of the first half of the 20th century rather than impatiently wonder how they could have overlooked the importance of the inborn error.

Developments in Genetics: The Definition of the Gene. If medicine failed to take up genetics during the first half of the 20th century, it may have been because genetics was not ready for medicine; it could offer little beyond pedigrees of rare disorders. There was not much to fit into conventional diagnosis and treatment, nor anything conceptual either, at first. Genetics was a new science and had to develop its own explanatory principles[24] (Table 3.1).

Mendel's contribution was the formulation of the laws of segregation and independent assortment. That was all that was known when Garrod advanced the idea of the inborn error and its parent concept of chemical individuality, so, since the gene hadn't been defined yet — indeed was not even fully distinguished from its phenotype — Garrod could not have been proposing any gene-enzyme relationship. So the gene remained a statistical entity until around 1920, by which time it had been given an operational definition as an element in a chromosome that could mutate, recombine, segregate, and control a phenotype.[25] This was the position until the Beadle and Tatum hypothesis gave the gene a biochemical-functional definition; that is, the function of the operationally defined gene was to specify an enzyme.[26]

For some time, the genes themselves had been assumed to be proteins. In 1917, Troland proposed that the protein genes had both auto- and heterocatalytic properties, fulfilling thereby the functions of replication and control of the life of the cell.[27]

So the one gene-one enzyme idea was not utterly outside the canon. It is also easy to see why Beadle and Tatum should have found Garrod and the inborn error so compatible with the one gene–one enzyme concept. Their method consisted of *creating* inborn errors in *Neurospora*, which they then detected by curing them with the metabolite that was lacking due to the failure of the defective gene. The first such deficiency was of pyridoxine, later shown to be an inborn error of all humanity and treatable equally in both species by growing the organisms on a complete medium.

The next step was a structural definition of the gene. This required acceptance of the DNA as the genetic material and the identification of a code that governed the sequence of amino acids in proteins. Taking advantage of an inborn error in tryptophane synthetase in *E. coli*, Yanofsky showed a colinear relationship between mutations at a specific locus and the amino acid sequence at a corresponding site in a protein gene product.[28] A final molecular definition of the gene as all of the transcribable, plus some non-transcribable, DNA required to specify a peptide brings us up the moment.[29] It is in the context of this ontogeny of the definition of the gene that the conflicting accounts of the inborn error can be reconciled. Each step in the progression of the meaning of the word *gene* leads to a new conceptual level, at which the words *inborn error* and *chemical individuality* must be re-evaluated for meanings unfathomable in the context of previous definitions. This sequence also suggests why there was no rapprochement with medicine until after the functional definition and until the development of methods to study biochemical attributes in human body fluids.

Today's reader will have no difficulty imagining how dependent these advances in gene definition were on contemporaneous developments, both conceptual and technological, in biochemistry and molecular biology. But of course, each of the latter were dependent upon the advances in genetics that they themselves had produced. Indeed, so intertwined did genetics and molecular biology become that the former was often defined in terms of the latter, overlooking genetics' historical populational and analytical roles.

Now, having reviewed the developments in medicine and genetics that made it possible, we turn to the events of the evolution of the concepts of inborn error and biochemical individuality.

The Inborn Error and Biochemical Individuality. The "neglect" of Garrod's observations or their "prematurity" has been a matter for conjecture. Although more inborn errors might have been added to the list; Garrod himself added hematoporphyria and steatorrhea; the ideas could not become a part of any useful generalization until there was some genetic context into which to fit them. So the path from the inborn error and chemical individuality to the unit step of homeostasis could proceed only by way of that of the definition of the gene up to the functional version, after which Garrod's concepts could be fitted into the thinking of both the genetics and the medicine of the time.

Table 3-2 Chronology of the gene-enzyme-phenotype relationship.

			Inborn Error		
Contributor	Date	Definition of Gene	Gene	Enzyme	Chemical Phenotype
Garrod	1902	Statistical	−	+	+
Cuenot	1903	Statistical	±	±	±
Onslow	1909–1915	Operational	+	−	+
Wright	1917	Operational	+	±	+
Beadle-Tatum	1941	Functional	+	+	+

Initially genes were called "factors" and weren't differentiated from their phenotypes, which may be why the question of their function arose immediately. Bateson's explanation was that of presence-absence.[24] A recessive trait was a consequence of a loss of a dominant factor, a proposition Garrod's absent enzyme did nothing to dispel. Table 3-2 lists contributors to the gene-enzyme-phenotype idea. Although his hypothesis lacked reference to genes, Garrod appears in the table because the relationship of enzyme deficiency to a biochemical phenotype was clear.

The first reference to a gene-enzyme-phenotype relationship was that of Cuenot in 1902.[30] He suggested that genetic differences in coat color in mice could be a consequence of enzymatic differentiation of chromogens. So, however ambiguous his idea was, Cuenot deserves mention for an early adumbration of gene function involving enzymes and color phenotypes. But he did not develop his hypothesis and soon lost interest in mendelism, so in Table 3-2, the lack of experimental support is signaled by ±. It could hardly be otherwise given the lack of grasp of both genes and enzymes of the time.

The first unequivocal demonstration of a one-to-one affinity between an operationally defined gene and a biochemical phenotype is that of Onslow, Scott-Moncrieff, and others in work carried out during the second decade of the 20th century and again in the 1930s.[31] Curiously, despite intimate knowledge of the biochemistry of the pigments and their behavior as genetic segregants, the issue of enzyme variants never came up. Therefore, in the diagram there is a — under the enzyme heading.

The next step in the progression was Wright's work on coat colors in guinea pigs in 1917.[32] Although the gene-enzyme-biochemical phenotype is for the first time unambiguously stated, the work was handicapped by the undeveloped state of knowledge of enzymes. But the concept was more complete than that of Garrod, as well as of both Cuenot and Onslow, and very little less so than that of Beadle and Tatum.

Finally, the demonstration by Beadle and Tatum of a straightforward relationship among a gene, an enzyme, and a biochemical phenotype was influential in making the idea of the inborn error accessible to medicine.[33] First, it provided a functional definition for the gene: The control exerted by a gene over a biochemical phenotype was mediated by a protein that bore a one-to-one affinity to its gene. It was still unclear what genes were, but there was now insight into what they did. Second, that definition made clear how both inborn error and biochemical individuality were to be perceived. That is, the principle of a linear relationship among a gene, its product, and a biochemical phenotype is still observed today, whether the approach is from the phenotype to the gene or from the gene to the phenotype. Always in between is the protein product, the unit step of homeostasis.

The Beadle-Tatum work appeared in the 1940s, a period described by Dunn as beginning "a new period of rapid increase of knowledge."[1] We have already shown how during the decades from 1945 to 1965 the definition of the gene passed from operational to structural and was well on its way to its final molecular description. We cite these developments again here to emphasize their contemporaneity with the rise in medicine of clinical investigation and the proliferation of ideas and techniques in both biochemistry and molecular biology. Now in the late 1940s and early 1950s, knowledge and technology in genetics, biochemistry, molecular biology, and medicine were such as to begin to promote new perceptions of both inborn error and chemical individuality not only in molecular detail but also as concepts that could recast the idea of the body as a machine in a broad biological context to include remote causes, individuality, and appeal to natural selection and evolution.

At this point, acknowledging that the conceptual development of the inborn error and biochemical individuality pursued different paths, we intend to recount their evolution separately.

The Inborn Error. While both the genetic and medical milieu were moving toward conditions favorable for rapprochement, what was happening to the idea of the inborn error? Most of its maturation was due to Garrod himself. He maintained his interest, publishing the first edition of *Inborn Errors of Metabolism* in 1909 and a second edition in 1923 even while giving numerous prestige-laden lectures on the same subject.[7] But then in 1931 he took a second, and for medicine a more portentous, leap into the future in his book *Inborn Factors in Disease*, a work dedicated to the principle that disease is a consequence of chemical individuality, which he defined as molecular.[6]

Was there much else? There were reports of fructosuria and glycosuria, ideal candidates for the list, but no mention of inborn errors or Garrod.[34–37] A long article by Van Crevald on glycogen storage disease (of which MMBID lists 12 varieties) makes no mention of inborn error or Garrod.[38] But Medes published her celebrated case of tyrosinosis, and Marble reported some new cases of pentosuria both in 1932 and within Garrod's framework.[39,40] And while in 1935 Fölling overlooked Garrod in describing what today we know as phenylketonuria (PKU),[41] Jervis reported 50 cases of Fölling's disease 2 years later, citing Garrod and calling it an inborn error.[42] Bearn reports that Garrod wrote to Fölling for a reprint. In his reply Fölling professed to be proud that "... the author of *Inborn Errors in Metabolism* ..." should wish to read of his work, so he knew of inborn errors, although perhaps after the fact.[7] Penrose also cited Garrod in a paper on PKU published in 1935.[43] He had ignored Garrod in a review of human genetics published in 1934, but Bearn tells us that Garrod wrote Penrose a letter about his misattribution of the consanguinity effect and that thereafter Penrose was a Garrod enthusiast.[7,43,44] J. B. S. Haldane, who had a longstanding interest in human genetics and biochemistry, knew of Garrod and the inborn error and wrote of them in a paper in 1937 and in his book *New Paths in Genetics* published in 1941.[45,46] Gowland Hopkins in the U.K. and Bodansky in the U.S. were biochemists who also cited Garrod, but none of this was likely to have much impact on medical thinking. Mendelian genetics was taught in British medical schools from at least the 1930s, and such volumes as we have examined omit Garrod and inborn errors.[47,48] Osler mentioned the inborn errors in several editions of his textbook of medicine, but only as rare and insignificant disorders. In the 1940s Gibson wrote several papers on methemoglobinemia, a clearly defined inborn error, without reference to Garrod;[49,50,51] nor was there any allusion to inborn errors in Pauling's paper in 1949 on the specificity of hemoglobin S.[52] Pauling called sickle cell disease a "molecular" disease and predicted that there were others. At first glance there appears little to choose between these two phrases, *inborn error* and *molecular disease*, each of which approaches the molecular deficiency from a different vantage. Garrod's way is the one that became the classic phenotype-to-molecule view traditional in medicine, consonant with his medical origins, while Pauling takes the road from the gene to the molecule, perhaps most comfortable for a physicist. Pauling tried for a while to popularize the molecular disease idea but soon lost interest. Today Pauling's concept is tautologous, since all disease engages protein molecules. The inborn error, however, retains a place, embracing monogenic disorders in which an association among gene, protein, and phenotype is clearly demonstrated.

There was another important difference between the inborn error as defined by Beadle and Tatum and by Pauling. The former perceived a direct relationship between gene and enzyme, while Pauling saw a more roundabout association. In his 1949 paper he said, "... we can identify the gene responsible for the sickling process with one of an alternative pair of alleles, capable through some *series of reactions* of introducing the modification into the hemoglobin molecule that distinguishes sickle cell anemia hemoglobin from the normal protein [italics ours]."[52]

In 1947 the American Society of Human Genetics was founded for the express purpose of fostering an understanding of genetics among physicians and a better appreciation of the problems of medicine among geneticists.[53] The first issue of the Society's journal appeared in 1949, and the first paper, written by J. V. Neel, was about carrier states in human beings.[54] Neel cited Garrod, but only in relation to gout, and the words *inborn error* did not appear. A similar review, also by Neel, had appeared in 1947 in the journal *Medicine*, then among the most prominent journals in medicine, suggesting an awakening of interest in genetics.[55] An article in the *British Medical Bulletin*, also published in 1947, provided a glimpse of the future; metabolic disorders were described as inborn errors in the model of Garrod, whose views were liberally cited.[56] And in 1949 a symposium of the Biochemical Society in London was devoted exclusively to biochemical genetics. Two of the seven articles in the report of the symposium were about inborn errors.[57,58] In one, Penrose pointed to the limitation of the term *inborn error*, which is inappropriate for normal traits like red hair.[57] As an alternative he suggested *inborn specificity*. Penrose also alluded to "a second extension of Garrod's views, namely, the general aim of genetics to express, as far as possible, all genetic differences in chemical terms," and he suggested that myopathies and red cell disorders would soon be perceived as inborn errors. He ended his remarks in the following way: "Garrod's pioneer work has provided human genetics with two most valuable principles. First, to measure genetical differences whenever possible, by chemical test. Secondly, to assume that, if we knew enough, every gene would be found to have a specific chemical effect in the body." So by 1950, for those whose minds were receptive, human biochemical genetics had been established, and generally in the Garrodian model, and Penrose, at least, saw the extension to biochemical individuality.

But what do we make of the publication in 1952 of a paper on glycogen storage disease as a consequence of a deficiency of glucose-6-phosphatase and in 1956 of another on galactosemia associated with deficiency of galactose-1-phosphate uridyl transferase, both without reference to Garrod or the words *inborn error*.[59,60] These investigators, both biochemists, may be said to have re-invented the inborn error out of the logic of their observations of genetic deficiencies of enzyme function. But neither offered any such generalization.

Perhaps by then it no longer mattered. Human biochemical genetics was established and would soon be called by that name. In 1953, Harris published a monograph called *An Introduction to Human Biochemical Genetics* with numerous references to inborn errors;[61] in 1959, the Ciba Foundation sponsored a symposium, *Biochemistry of Human Genetics*,[62] and in the same year, Harris' book, called *Human Biochemical Genetics*, appeared,[63] to be followed in 1965 by a reprinting of Garrod's *Inborn Errors of Metabolism* with commentary by Harris[64] and beginning in 1970 by three editions of a book called *The Principles of Human Biochemical Genetics*, also by Harris.[65] And in 1960 the first edition of *The Metabolic Basis of Inherited Disease* emerged, with its editors' statement in the preface of their intention to assemble all known inborn errors as defined by Garrod.[66] As we know, they were not constrained by their own definition, because even in the first edition they included hemoglobin variants and each edition since has revised the definition further. And today's editors have announced their intention to make the final leap to include multigenic disorders as well. Are the latter inborn errors, assuming the 1990s definition of them as variations in gene products that are incongruent with the steady state? Can the concept include variations in gene products that are incongruent under one condition and not another? The answer to both questions is yes. But suppose that the incongruent state depends upon variants of more than one — several or even many — loci and that disease appears only under conditions of living of specific kind, intensity, and duration? It seems that "inborn error" does not fit here, because the variants are incongruent only in particular combinations and under certain conditions. The holders of such variant genes in some combinations are not threatened; each variant, on its own, may be congruent with the steady state. Here we may wish to fall back on "biochemical individuality," words that do not distinguish normal from abnormal.

Biochemical Individuality. What happened to chemical individuality in the years after 1902? Garrod continued to think about it, and it is the central theme of *Inborn Factors*. The epigraph for Chap. 2, taken from *Inborn Factors*, summarizes his vision of chemical individuality. "Our chemical shortcomings," he says, "are a property of our chemical individuality, and it is to the latter that we owe our diatheses, our propensities to disease." But how did he visualize diathesis? As an assembly of chemical properties, including those of proteins and other molecules, all perceived through a veil of ignorance that has since been lifted to allow us to see such liabilities to disease in the form of variant protein gene products that exert variable effects on the metabolic properties of the organism.

The Blood Groups. There was another discovery, of the same vintage as Garrod's 1902 paper, that generated an immunologic definition of chemical individuality. In 1901, Landsteiner reported the ABO blood group system.[67] That its immunologic differences in erythrocytes were heritable was established in 1910, and the three-allele system we know today was reported in 1924.[67] Later still, Morgan and Watkins showed A and B substances to be mucoproteins, widely distributed beyond the red cells, and enzymatic products of H substance, which when unmodified is immunologically blood group O.[68,69] The original work on blood groups was done in ignorance of Garrod, but he cited them in *Inborn Factors*, saying, "... it can hardly be doubted that they testify to chemical or physico-chemical differences within the boundaries of the species."[6] Other blood groups were discovered, the MN group also by Landsteiner. By 1950 there were eight, and more have been discovered since.[70] Some blood groups — Diego and Gerbich are examples — are found only in some populations, and the principal ones vary in frequency all over the world from one population to another.[70] So inter-person individuality is reflected in that between populations.

Interest in the blood groups was spurred by transfusion reactions and by maternal-fetal immunization of which that due to RH incompatibility is the chief, but ABO and Kell are also dangerous antigens. These incompatibilities can generate serious, even lethal, disease. Should they be called inborn errors? Remember that the diseases depend in one case upon mismatched transfusions and in the other upon maternal immunization by an incompatible fetus. There is no inborn error here. The variants themselves are selectively favored; they are simply incompatible, and in each case the disease could be avoided by careful matching to prevent transfusion reactions or by compatible mating to prevent erythroblastosis. As it happens, for the latter we have taken the more reasonable expedient of preventing the immunization. So inborn error does seem inapt, but are these not diseases of biochemical individuality? It is the proteins that generate the immune responses, the gene products that are fulfilling roles in some cellular homeostatic device. So there are causes of disease that do not fulfill the definition of the inborn error. But such disorders, although not qualifying as inborn errors, are not less mediated by variant protein unit steps of homeostasis. So perhaps we should change the relationship between the monogenic inborn error and the multigenic disease suggested in the Introduction to read that the inborn error and multigenic disease are both special cases of diseases of biochemical individuality.

Although the blood grouping industry came into being mainly because of threats to human health, it has also had a vital role in teaching human genetics, in anthropology, and in the study of the genetics of populations. A common device in teaching is to show that, given certain frequencies of the alleles of the blood groups, the probability of the identity of any two non-twins is, if not nil, exceedingly small. This is impressive, but the blood groups are a specialized set of proteins. What of other proteins, what of all? Perhaps this question was asked by many, but an approach to its answer was undertaken in two laboratories.

Polymorphism. In the mid-1960s, after two decades of observing human genetic variation, Harris began to ask himself just how extensive that variation is. This question he attacked with starch-gel electrophoresis of cellular extracts, staining the gels for soluble enzymes.[71] The answer by this method was more than one allele in a frequency of more than 1% at about 30% of the loci, which means that 7–10% of individuals are heterozygous for alleles at those loci. Such loci are said to be polymorphic and the sets of alleles to be polymorphisms.* And of course there were infrequent variants too.

At exactly the same time, the same question was asked of *Drosophila* by Richard Lewontin, this time to settle a contention in genetics in which one side claimed that there was very little variability in any species, the other that there was a great deal. The results of the *Drosophila* study, as well as those of many other species, resembled the human work almost exactly; one third of the loci were polymorphic, 7–10% of the individuals heterozygous.[72] This degree of variation in all species raised the question of its origin in the evolutionary alternatives of selection or drift, a question of epic proportions in biology. But of greater interest to us in medicine is the discovery of an unsuspected degree of *common* human biochemical diversity expressed in structural variation of protein gene products, only a few of which are directly associated with inborn errors. This was the first overt evidence of *continuity* between inborn errors and this presumably normal variation now called biochemical individuality. But is it normal?

Measurements of the activity of polymorphic enzymes were only occasionally found by Harris, Lewontin, and others to be outside the normal range, but before long, polymorphic alleles began to appear in association with diseases in frequencies well above prevalence rates. Perhaps the association of the highly polymorphic HLA alleles with autoimmune disease was the first. Soon, polymorphic alleles at other loci would be called "susceptibility genes," "genetic vulnerabilities," or "risk factors."

*This is a special usage of the word *polymorphism*, first employed by E. B. Ford and defined as a frequency for the least common allele of at least 1%, a level unattainable by mutation alone.

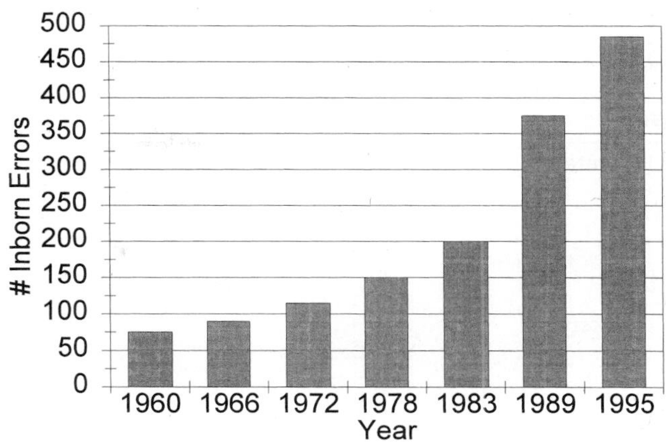

Fig. 3-1 Exponential rise in inborn errors listed in the seven editions of MMBID.

The Ontogeny of MMBID. We have seen how diseases due to immunologic incompatibility threaten the conceptual comprehensiveness of the inborn error, but the immunologic disorders could be said to be merely exceptions to the rule. Genetic polymorphism, however, suggests that the immunologic exception is a part of a continuity that is best expressed as biochemical individuality. The ontogeny of MMBID reveals the evolution of this continuity as nothing else can.

Originating in 1960 for reasons already stated, the book has grown steadily by including new inborn errors accumulated between editions. This growth is shown in Fig. 3-1. Each chapter of the book gives an account of a different disorder or set of allied conditions, outlining the biochemistry and molecular biology of pathogenesis and their correlation with clinical expression and treatment. At the start, the genetic details were likely to be limited to pedigree analysis: Was the disorder dominant, recessive, or sex-linked? But genetics has been so insistently pervasive that in recent editions pathogenesis and clinical details have become inseparable from the qualities of the relevant gene products. This change is shown in Table 3-3, which shows a crude estimate of the amount of text devoted to genetics as opposed to biochemistry, molecular biology, or clinical detail in two samples consisting of the same chapters appearing in the first and sixth editions. Nowhere is the incursion of genetics into medicine more plainly demonstrated.

In the first edition, the definition of the inborn error was essentially that of Garrod, modified by Beadle and Tatum, but soon, in addition to the hemoglobin variants, other non-enzyme molecules were added. And then, in consonance with a final molecular definition of the gene in which alleles are defined by nucleotide sequences rather than amino acid content of proteins, cancer and chromosome abnormalities were included: One chapter of the sixth edition was called "Molecular Cytogenics: The interface of cytogenics and monogenetic disease." So this book, which started out in a strongly medical vein with a half-patronizing nod to genetics, has grown more genetic with each edition, and now the editors proclaim that if there is an identifiable

Table 3-3 A rough estimate of the amount of space given to genetics as opposed to biochemical or clinical detail in the same sample of articles in the 1st and 6th edition of MBID.

	Space Devoted to Genetics	
Edition	**Average**	**Range**
First	$<10\%$	5–15%
Sixth	30%	7–70%

Table 3-4 Factors involved in analysis of origin of heart attack in individuals.

Genes	Developement and Homeostasis	Environment
Lipoproteins	Sex	Smoking
APO A	Age	Diet
APO B	Ethnic	Exercise
APO E	Circadian rhythm	Alcohol
Lp(a)	Intrauterine nutrition	Vitamins
LDL	Other diseases	Fatty acids
LDL receptor	Hypertension	Aspirin
	Diabetes	SES
	Obesity	
Clotting Factors		
Fibrinogen		
Protein C		
Factor VII		
von Willebrand		
Platelets		
Plasminogen		
Growth Factors		
Endothelins		
Other Factors		
Cystathionine synthase		
ACE		
Prostaglandins		

ACE, angiotension converting enzyme; SES, socioeconomic status.

molecular explanation for any disease, it will be included in MMBID. What is meant by "molecular explanation" is the presence of a protein gene product as proximate cause. And the editors have made plain their recognition that the more they move away from canonical definitions of the inborn error, the more they are moving into chemical individuality. And this has led, in turn, to "a corresponding analysis of multifactorial diseases as the next step in the understanding of disease."[73]

The investigation of the gene-specified protein molecules that lead, under appropriate conditions, to complex diseases is an inquiry into biochemical and molecular individuality, and it is going on apace. Numerous variant gene products have been shown to contribute, for example, to atherosclerosis—proteins from several different and seemingly unrelated homeostatic systems, including cholesterol transport, the clotting cascade, the renin-angiotensin system, variant endothelins, and platelet and tissue growth factors (Table 3-4). Most of the loci involved are polymorphic, so only certain of the alleles they specify are involved in pathogenesis and represent a risk factor. The table, which is certainly incomplete, reveals a list of genes, a list of experiences, and a list of factors that constitute a homeostatic matrix within which gene products interact with influences of the environment. Such interactions occur in health as in disease; the table simply lists the elements involved.

In a disease, it is the physician's business to sort out the variant proteins that, in their adverse impact on their own homeostatic devices, exert a deleterious influence on others. Each such consequence must react upon still others, interfering with integrated mechanisms, challenging adaptive powers, perhaps reaching some new steady state or going on to overt disease. In heart attacks, there is an interaction between elements that have led to atherosclerosis and those of the clotting mechanism. It has been demonstrated that certain variants of both systems turn up more often than others in people who have heart attacks. The obvious response is to use the information preventively, but first, observations have to be made of which factors play the most salient roles in which victims of heart attack, as well as the frequency of each. Such information may tell us which combinations of gene products interacting with which combinations of experiences of the environment in which conditions of the homeostatic matrix are most likely to be represented among patients with coronary occlusion. But given the number and frequencies of even the most prominent factors involved, it is evident that nearly everyone will attain his or her heart attack by means of an independent path. So it looks as if, while inborn errors are a consequence of rare variant gene products that carry all before them to produce monogenic disease, disorders of complex origin are outcomes of the collaboration of numerous common variant gene products drawn from the store of biochemical individuality. But is there really a difference? The answer is that while in one sense there is, in another and more profound sense there is none.

The difference is genetic, the identity is physiological. The difference lies in the distinction given segregating monogenic diseases (inborn errors) as opposed to non-segregating multigenic (multifactorial or complex) disorders, and it is undeniable that, with exceptions, there *are* differences in phenotype, including segregation, age at onset, threat to longevity and reproduction, and so on. Those are the differences, and they represent a residuum of an analysis like that done for *Drosophila* appropriate for the operational definition of the gene. The identity, on the other hand, is apparent in the observation that both are products of physiological dysfunction due to variant gene products that act as unit steps in one or more homeostatic systems. The clinical differences are associated with a *gradient* of selective effect in which the most disadaptive variants produce the most devastating consequences, most often in utero (see Chap. 2). Indeed, it is probable that most human disease with the greatest loss of human life occurs there; estimates vary, but it may be that 60–80% of all conceptuses never reach term.[74] Among the inborn errors that appear after birth, 90% have expressed themselves by puberty (Chap. 2). And so the gradient declines, with fewer monogenic and more multigenic disorders, to the end of life. It is a continuum, but there is overlap; there are multigenic diseases in childhood and monogenic disorders in adulthood, even in old age, but there is no interruption. There cannot be, since close examination of post-natal diseases reveals that although there are variant proteins that are so destructive as to harrow up homeostasis on their own, in fact all are modified by the qualities of the proteins that constitute the other unit steps in the whole of the integrated homeostasis, as well as by the individuality of experiences in development and in daily life. In fact, all phenotypes are in varying degrees complex; all must be described in the context of phylogeny, of maturation, and of daily life. So disease of any kind is defined as a consequence of *incongruence* between variable homeostatic devices and the conditions to which they must try to adapt.

Now, if we can accept this principle of the origin of all disease in variant unit steps of homeostasis, what unifying generalizations flow from it? Heart attacks, PKU, and cancer of the large bowel are rooted in variant unit steps of homeostasis of systems that, when diseased, are attended by physicians in three different disciplines and departments, so one virtue of a unitary principle of disease is that of coherence in the midst of reductive abundance, a centripetal force to counter centrifugal scatter. A second outcome is a new classification of disease arising from a common principle, the variant step of homeostasis, rather than as at present from etiology, organ system, or age at onset. This unity is exemplified in MMBID, in which most of the diseases are classified according to molecular variation. Third, it may enable us to establish in medical education a mentality inclusive of variability and individuality to counter that of the body as a machine, in which it is too easy to perceive all machines as the same. Fourth, it is even conceivable that the principle of individuality might contribute to a return to the now quaint notion, all but forgotten, that the patient is actually a unique person, the only one of his or her kind that ever was or will be. And fifth, the risk factor, the inherited vulnerability, will surely become the core of sensitive understanding of the advantages, as well as the complexities, of prevention, perhaps in time raising prevention to primacy in medicine.

CONCLUSION

What, then, of the inborn error of metabolism? The more we have learned about the genes and their actions, the more restricting the concept of the inborn error seems, even when, as in MMBID, it includes a broad array of defects of gene products other than enzymes. If the word *error* has any meaning, then the locution cannot embrace genetically specified variants that confer resistance, say to infections, nor is it satisfactory in relation to the multigenic disorders, in which the disease is contingent upon some specific combination of gene products acting in developmental matrices characterized by experiences of particular kinds, intensities, and durations. It might be said that the complex disease is a consequence of a concatenation of contingent inborn errors, but that stretches the definition of "error" beyond tolerance, since the effect of at least some of the contributory "errors" are likely to fall within a range that we must all agree is "normal." Of course, we could give up the idea of blockage of pathways or even of contingent errors and assign the deviance to the gene itself, ignoring its functional significance. This works only when the gene specifies a product that inevitably leads to an inborn error all by itself. But even there it is the product, not the gene, that is engaged in the pathology. In addition, genes, in specifying their products, give no indication of their contingencies. For example, an examination of the hundreds of variants at the *G6PD* locus gives no indication of which will provoke hemolytic anemia permanent and severe, which hemolysis in the presence of fava beans, and which no disorder at all. So the gene is no help. Where then in this continuum does the inborn error begin, where end? The answer is that no matter at what level it is defined, the inborn error is a special case of biochemical individuality whose mediator is the protein gene product, the unit step of homeostasis. So if we wish to generalize, we are thrust back upon the concept of biochemical individuality, itself a property of variation of the genes, their products, and the impact of those products on the integrated homeostasis of the open system, which is to say that in thinking about the variable molecular aspects of the biochemistry and physiology of pathogenesis of disease, we must begin with what is known about occupants of the loci involved and the range of competences and incompetences of the products thereof. The words "inborn error of metabolism" should remain useful in relation to monogenic diseases; they have, in that regard, an honorable place in our lexicon; but they are of little use in constructing the nature and range of pathogenesis and symptomatology of complex diseases.

This leaves the variable protein gene product at the conceptual center of disease. Its virtues were detailed at the beginning of this chapter. It remains to ask how it relates to the alternative to the metaphor of the body as a machine, discussed in Chap. 2. In this alternative view, the machine is perceived to be a product of evolution and natural selection. Disease is represented as a consequence of incongruence between a variable homeostasis and conditions of the environment. Variation is required for the survival of species, which must maintain adaptability in changing environments. In the formation of gametes, mutation is unconstrained, but after fertilization, selection begins—selection of phenotypes expressed in individuals. In the case of human individuals, or, as we call ourselves, people, selection makes favorable choices of the congruent and unfavorable choices of the incongruent. And, as we have seen, both congruence and incongruence are mediated by the gene-specified protein unit steps of homeostasis.

Representing disease as an outcome of homeostatic incongruence with experiences of the environment gives it a social dimension, an aspect sometimes overlooked in concentrating on molecular analysis. But it is by way of this social connection that the doctor gains access to patients to whom the molecular details, however essential to a grasp of pathogenesis, are of less moment than their feelings or illness and their concern with the prognosis. It seems that analysis has outstripped synthesis here and that medicine needs a new set of ideas and principles with which to accommodate both the molecular analysis of disease and its impact on the integrated patient who harbors it. Perhaps the place to start is medical education, and it will be immediately apparent that the foundation upon which to build an edifice of such concepts is the unit step of homeostasis in its junctional position, looking down to the gene and further analytical detail and up to a synthesis of pathogenesis and symptomatology in the patient as a whole person. And in this, the unit step attains a further distinction: that of giving molecular body to Garrod's penetrating vision into biochemical individuality.

REFERENCES

1. Dunn LC: *A Short History of Genetics*. New York, McGraw-Hill, 1965.
2. Alberts B: The cell as a collection of protein machines. *Cell* **92**:291, 1998.
3. Nelkin D, Lindee MS: *The DNA Mystique. The Gene as a Cultural Icon*. New York, Freeman, 1995.
4. Toulmin S: *Human Understanding*. Princeton, NJ, Princeton University Press, 1977.
5. Beadle GW: Genes and chemical reactions in *Neurospora*. *Science* **129**:1715, 1959.
6. Scriver CR, Childs B: *Garrod's Inborn Factors in Disease*. Oxford, Oxford University Press, 1989.
7. Bearn AG: *Archibald Garrod and the Individuality of Man*. Oxford, Oxford University Press, 1993.
8. Garrod AE: The incidence of alkaptonuria: A study in chemical individuality. *Lancet* **2**: 1616, 1902.
9. DeSolla Price: *Little Science, Big Science*. New York, Columbia University Press, 1963, p. 1.
10. Lush B: *Concepts of Medicine*. Oxford, Pergamon Press, 1961.
11. Beecher HK: *Disease and the Advancement of Science*. Cambridge, Harvard University Press, 1960.
12. Cohn AE: *Medicine, Science and Art*. Chicago, University of Chicago Press, 1931, p. 138.
13. Cannon WB: *The Wisdom of the Body*. Cambridge, Harvard University Press, 1939.
14. Parascandola J: Organismic and holistic concepts in the thought of L. J. Henderson. *J Hist Biol* **4**:631971.
15. Sinding C: The history of resistant rickets: A model for understanding the growth of biomedical knowledge. *J Hist Biol* **22**:461, 1989.
16. Bearn AG: The contribution of clinical medicine to biochemical genetics, in Beecher HK (ed): *Disease and the Advancement of Basic Science*. Cambridge, Harvard University Press, 1960.
17. American Foundation: *Medical Research: A Midcentury Survey*. Boston, Little Brown, 1955.
18. Childs B: Garrod, Galton and clinical medicine. *Yale J Biol Med* **46**:297, 1973.
19. Herndon CN: Genetics in medical education. *J Med Ed* **30**:407, 1955.
20. Penrose LS: The influence of the English tradition in human genetics, in Crow JF, Neel JV (eds): *Proceedings of the 3rd International Congress on Human Genetics*. Baltimore, Johns Hopkins University Press, 1967.
21. Dunn LC: The study of genetics in man—retrospect and prospect. *Birth Defects Original Article Series* **1**:5, 1965.
22. Wagner RP, Mitchell HK: *Genetics and Metabolism*. New York, Wiley, 1955, p. 400.
23. Rushton AR: *Genetics and Medicine in the United States 1800–1922*. Baltimore, Johns Hopkins University Press, 1994.
24. Glass B: A century of biochemical genetics. *Proc Am Phil Soc* **109**:227, 1965.
25. Sturtevant AH: *A History of Genetics*. New York, Harper & Row, 1965, p 39.
26. Tatum EL: A case history in biological research. **129**:1711, 1959.
27. Troland LT: Biological enigmas and the theory of enzyme action. *Am Nat* **51**:321, 1917.
28. Yanofsky C: Gene structure and protein structure. *Harvey Lectures* **51**:145, 1965–1966.
29. Berg P, Singer M: *Dealing with Genes. The Language of Heredity*. Mill Valley, University Science Books, 1992, p 134.
30. Wagner RP: On the origins of the gene-enzyme hypothesis. *J Hered* **80**:503, 1989.
31. Scott-Mancrieff R: The classical period in chemical genetics. *Notes & Records, Roy Soc London* **36–37**:125, 1981–1983.

32. Wright S: Color inheritance in mammals. *Jour Hered* **8**:224, 1917.
33. Beadle GW, Tatum EL: Genetic control of biochemical reactions in *Neurospora*. *Proc Natl Acad Sci USA* **27**:499, 1941.
34. Lasker M: Essential fructosuria. *Hum Biol* **13**:51, 1941.
35. Heeres PA, Vos H: Fructosuria. *Arch Intern Med* **44**:47, 1929.
36. Silver S, Reiner M: Essential fructosuria. *Arch Intern Med* **54**:412, 1934.
37. Parkes-Weber F: A glycosuric family without hyperglycaemia. *Lancet* **2**:71, 1931.
38. Van Crevald: Glycogen disease. *Medicine* **18**, 1, 1939.
39. Medes G: A new error of tyrosine metabolism: Tyrosinosis. The intermediary metabolism of tyrosine and phenylalanine. *Biochem J* **26**:916, 1932.
40. Marble A: Chronic essential pentosuria. *Am J Med Sci* **183**:827, 1932.
41. Fölling A: Uber Ausscherdung von Phenylbrenztraubensaur in den Harn auf Stoffwechselanomalie in Verbindung mit Imbezieritat *J Physiol Chem* **277**: 169, 1934.
42. Jervis GA: Phenylpyruvic oligophrenia. *Arch Neurol Psychol* **38**:944, 1937.
43. Penrose LS: Inheritance of phenylpyruvic amentia (phenylketonuria). *Lancet* **2**:192, 1935.
44. Penrose LS: Phenylketonuria: A problem in eugenics. *Lancet* **1**:949, 1946.
45. Haldane JBS: The biochemistry of the individual, in Needham J, Green DE (eds): *Perspectives in Biology*. Cambridge, Cambridge University Press, 1937.
46. Haldane JBS: *New Pathways in Genetics*. London, George Allen and Unwin, 1953, p. 47.
47. Crew FAE: *Genetics in Relation to Clinical Medicine*. Edinburgh, Oliver and Boyd, 1947.
48. Ford EB: *Genetics for Medical Students*. London, Methuen, 1942.
49. Barcroft H, Gibson QH, Harrison DC, McMurray J: Familial idiopathic methemoglobinemia and its treatment with ascorbic acid. *Clin Sci* **5**:145, 1945.
50. Gibson QH, Harrison DC: Familial idiopathic methaemoglobinemia. *Lancet* **2**:941, 1947.
51. Gibson QH: The reduction of methemoglobin in red cells and studies on the cause of idiopathic methemoglobinemia. *Biochem J* **42**:13, 1940.
52. Pauling L, Itano HA, Singer SJ, Wells IC: Sickle cell anemia, a molecular disease. *Science* **110**:543, 1949.
53. Muller H: Progress and prospects in human genetics. *Am J Hum Genet* **1**:1, 1949.
54. Neel JV: The detection of genetic carriers of human disease. *Am J Hum Genet* **1**:19, 1949.
55. Neel JV: The clinical detection of the genetic carriers of inherited disease. *Medicine* **26**:115, 1947.
56. Tracey MV: Human biochemical genetics. *Br Med Bull* **5**:325, 1947–1948.
57. Penrose LS: Garrod's conception of inborn error and its development. *Biochem Soc Symposia* **4**:10, 1950.
58. Rimington C: The interpretation of biochemical detail revealed by inborn errors. *Biochem Soc Symposia* **5**:16, 1950.
59. Cori GT, Cori CF: Glucose-6-phosphatase of the liver in glycogen storage disease. *J Biol Chem* **199**:661, 1952.
60. Isselbacher KJ, Anderson EP, Kurahashi K, Kalckar HM: Congenital galactosemia, a single enzymatic block in galactose metabolism. *Science* **123**:635, 1956.
61. Harris H: *An Introduction to Human Biochemical Genetics*. Cambridge, Cambridge University Press, 1953.
62. Wolstenholme GEW, O'Connor G (eds): *Biochemistry of Human Genetics. Ciba Foundation Symposium*. London, Churchill, 1959.
63. Harris H: *Human Biochemical Genetics*. Cambridge, Cambridge University Press, 1959.
64. Harris H: *Garrod's Inborn Errors of Metabolism*. Oxford University Press, 1965.
65. Harris H: *The Principles of Human Biochemical Genetics*. New York, Elsevier, 1970, 1974, 1980.
66. *The Metabolic Basis of Inherited Disease*. Stanbury JB, Wyngaarden JB, Fredrickson DS (eds): New York, McGraw-Hill, 1960.
67. Race RR, Sanger R: *Blood Groups in Man*. Oxford, Blackwell, 1950.
68. Morgan WTJ: Some immunochemical aspects of the products of the human blood group genes, in Wolstenholme, GEW, O'Connon CM (eds): *Ciba Symposium, Biochemistry of Human Genetics*. London, Churchill, 1959 pp 194–216.
69. Yamamoto F, Clausen H, White T, Marken J, Hakamori S: Molecular genetic basis of the histo-blood group ABO system. *Nature* **345**:229, 1990.
70. Mourant AE: *Blood Relations. Blood Groups and Anthropology*. Oxford, Oxford University Press, 1985.
71. Harris H: Enzyme polymorphisms in man. *Proc Roy Soc* **164**:298, 1966.
72. Lewontin RC, Hubby JL: A molecular approach to the study of genic heterozygosity in natural populations. *Genetics* **54**:595, 1966.
73. Scriver CR, Beaudet AL, Sly W, Valle D (eds): *The Metabolic and Molecular Bases of Inherited Disease* 7th ed. New York, McGraw-Hill, 1995, p XXXV.
74. Kane JP, Havel RJ: Disorders of the biogenesis and secretion of lipoproteins containing the B apolipoproteins, in Scriver CR, Beaudet AL, Sly WS, Valle D (eds): *The Metabolic and Molecular Bases of Inherited Disease* 7th ed. New York, McGraw-Hill, 1995, p 1853.
75. Uterman G: Lipoprotein (a), in Scriver CR, Beaudet AL, Sly WS, Valle D (eds): *The Metabolic and Molecular Bases of Inherited Disease* 7th ed. New York, McGraw-Hill, 1995, p 1887.
76. Goldstein JL, Hobbs HH, Brown MS: Familial hypercholesterolemia, in Scriver CR, Beaudet AL, Sly WS, Valle D (eds): *The Metabolic and Molecular Bases of Inherited Disease* 7th ed. New York, McGraw-Hill, 1995, p 1981.
77. Breslow J: Familial disorders of high-density lipoprotein metabolism, in Scriver CR, Beaudet AL, Sly WS, Valle D (eds): *The Metabolic and Molecular Bases of Inherited Disease* 7th ed. New York, McGraw-Hill, 1995, p 2031.
78. Gunby P: Lipoprotein patterns, plaque, homocysteine, and hormones among ongoing cardiology studies. *JAMA* 1996, 276, 1122.
79. Ross R: Atherosclerosis: A defense mechanism gone awry. *Am J Path* **143**:987, 1993.
80. Newman PJ: Platelet alloantigens: cardiovascular as well as immunological risk factors? *Lancet* **349**:370, 1997.
81. McCaffrey TA, Basheng D, Consigli S, Szabo P, Bray PJ, Hartner L, Weksler B, Sanborn TA, Bergman G, Bush HL Jr: Genomic instability in the type 2TGF-B1 receptor gene in atherosclerotic and restenotic vascular cells. *J Clin Invest* **100**:2182, 1997.
82. Iacoriello L, DiCastelnuevo A, DeKnigff P, D'Orazio A, Amore C, Arboretti R, Kluft C, Donati MB: Polymorphisms in the coagulation factor VII gene and the risk of myocardial infarction. *N Engl J Med* **338**:79, 1998.
83. Keating MT, Sanguinetti MC: Molecular genetic insights into cardiovascular disease. *Science* **272**:681, 1996.
84. Cambien F, Poirier O, Lecerf L, et al: Deletion polymorphism in the gene for angiotensin-converting enzyme is a potent risk-factor for myocardial infarction. *Nature* **359**:641-, 1992.
85. Welch GN, Loscalgo J: Homocysteine and atherosclerosis. *N Engl J Med* **338**:1042, 1998.
86. Fowkes FGR, Connor JM, Smith FB, Wood J, Donnan PT, Lowe GDO: Fibrinogen genotype and risk of peripheral atherosclerosis. *Lancet* **339**:693, 1992.
87. Jacobs PA: Chromosome abnormalities: Origin and etiology in abortions and live births, in Vogel F, Sperling K (eds): *Human Genetics: Proc. 7thInt. Cong.* Springer-Verlag, 1987, p 233.

CHAPTER 4

The Effect of Mendelian Disease on Human Health

Gerardo Jimenez-Sanchez ▪ Barton Childs ▪ David Valle

In Chap. 3, we emphasized the prominence in disease of the protein gene products that serve as unit steps of homeostasis. Variant proteins are salient proximate causes of disease, impairing the function of the homeostatic devices they serve. It is characteristic of an integrated whole that no single element stands out, but when the harmony is disrupted by the failure of one of its parts, the specificity of the variant unit step is likely to be reflected by the nature of the failed function. However, other qualities may be distinguishing, too: age at onset of symptoms, burden as measured by threat of life, impaired reproduction or permanent disability, or frequency in populations.

Physicians characterize and classify diseases according to the most prominent expressions, principally of organ systems. Hospitals and specialties have been organized accordingly. But molecular biology and medicine have shifted our attention to molecular causes and their role in pathogenesis, so that some diseases, particularly monogenic disorders, are both characterized and classified according to the homeostatic system or molecules involved in proximate cause, as for example lysosomal storage diseases (see Part 16 of this text) or disorders of oxidative phosphorylation (see Part 10). Some are named for the variant molecule, as is G6PD deficiency (see Chap. 179). These designations do not contravene the old classification, which is likely to persist. Rather they represent subclasses, revealing of cause in their names.

Table 4-1 documents the exponential rate of increase in our recognition of classical inborn errors over the history of this book. Chapters in the current edition also tell of the discovery of variant gene products engaged in the pathogenesis of disorders of more complex etiology. Moreover, the once distant rumble of the promise of the Human Genome Project has given way to a roar with a crescendo to come in 2 to 3 years, or sooner. With the sequence in hand, attention will turn to describing the protein products of the sequenced genes, their function, and their homeostatic position. Proteomics[1,2] will uncover increasing levels of complexity resulting from amplification of the encoded information by alternative splicing, transcriptional regulation, a myriad of posttranslational modifications, and by the intricate roles the proteins play in what Goldstein calls the "dialectic" between molecules and integrating physiology.[3] Anomalies of this discourse due to mutant gene products will occur and the aberrant physiology will be characterized in the context of the diseases of heart, lung, kidney, and so on. The benefits to medicine of such an analysis cannot be overstated, but there are other benefits to be gained, too.

The premise of our study was that from an examination of a large sample, perhaps thousands, of variant gene products, each identified because they are associated with one or more specific diseases, we may expect to learn the fundamental explanatory principles of disease. For the most part in medicine, our attention is constrained to individual diseases; for example, one looks in vain for descriptions of the general properties of disease in medical textbooks. But it is only through characterization of such properties that we can bring coherence to the diverse ideas and aims that distinguish today's medicine. Such coherence should be imposed at the earliest time in medical education, the better to accommodate at the same time to the diversity of careers open to the students and the biologic individuality of the patients they meet in those careers.

A study of disease that includes disorders caused by mutants at thousands of loci is some way off, but it is not too early to begin to think of the questions that could be asked of it nor even to undertake prototypical versions of the study. Some of those questions are: (a) How do diseases differ according to the qualities of the variant proteins that are their proximate causes? (b) Are all types of gene products represented equally in disease, or even represented at all? And if they are, are they represented in the same proportion in disease as in health? (c) Is there a disease for every locus, and if not, do those that escape have anything in common? (d) What is the relationship to disease of evolutionarily conserved sequences in genes and their protein products? Are mutations in conserved sequences more, or less, likely to disrupt homeostasis and so to appear as proximate causes of disease? (e) Developmental constraints reduce the probability of further evolution of conserved processes. But Kirschner and Gerhart have pointed to processes of "deconstraint" that allow for accumulation of genetic variation even in complex systems.[4] These mechanisms enhance evolability, but what is their consequence for disease? On the one hand, the deconstraining processes reduce the phenotypic consequences of mutation; on the other hand, they allow accumulation of the genetic variation that ultimately may contribute to disorders of complex etiology. (f) Are the genes frequently associated with diseases of complex origin also associated with monogenic disorders? Intuitively one might say yes, and indeed, there are examples. Genes recognized in homozygotes with rare recessive inborn errors of homocysteine metabolism are, in the heterozygous state, risk factors for complex vascular thrombolic disorders (Chap. 88).[5,6] Similarly, mutant alleles of the *ABCR* gene that cause a rare early onset macular degeneration in the homozygous state appear to contribute to common age-related macular degeneration in the heterozygous state (Chap. 243).[7,8] But is this common or is there something about the evolution of physiological mechanisms, or about the pathology involved, that constrains the genetic effects in one direction or the other? (g) Elucidation of the genetic contribution to aging has only just begun. Oxidative damage to DNA, lipids and proteins and disturbances in protein glycosylation may be contributing factors (see Chap. 8).[9,10] Are all proteins equally susceptible to these modifications and are certain "normal" variants more or less likely to be affected? (h) The ultimate list of our genes will include some active only in fetal life and occupied in the processes of development. If human fecundity is of the order of only 25 percent, then most human disease occurs *in utero*—out of sight and out of mind—but no less a vital contribution to our understanding of the whole range of human disease. But what are the genetic contributions to this *in utero* carnage? A good deal, perhaps most, of fetal disease is associated with chromosomal abnormality.[11] In addition, there must be a good many classical

Table 4-1 Evolution of MMBID from Its First to Seventh Editions

	Edition						
	1st	2nd	3rd	4th	5th	6th	7th
Year	1960	1966	1972	1978	1983	1989	1995
No. of inborn errors listed	78	92	121	148	200	374	469
No. of contributors	46	72	93	113	137	221	300
No. of pages	1477	1434	1778	1862	2048	3006	4603
Weight (g)	2150	3200	2400	3002	3060	7100	12,000

inborn errors and developmental disorders of complex origin, about which we know nothing, that produce fetal disease. The recent recognition of developmental defects caused by inborn errors in the sterol synthetic pathway and the hedgehog signaling pathway are consistent with this assertion.[12–14]

Answers to these and other questions must await a more complete elaboration of our genome and its complement of proteins, but it would be well to start the effort now, to provide a baseline for future studies made possible by compilation of diseases stimulated by completion of the Human Genome Project. In fact, a start was made 15 years ago when Costa and her colleagues characterized a sample of monogenic disorders taken from the fifth edition of *Mendelian Inheritance in Man*.[15] We reasoned that the seventh edition of *The Metabolic and Molecular Bases of Inherited Disease* (MMBID7) would be a better source for a similar study, in as much as it includes descriptions of the clinical details and of the molecular aspects, and, most importantly, of the deviant proteins and their effect on development and homeostasis.

ANALYSIS OF MMBID7

We analyzed the disorders included in MMBID7 (1995) with the aim of characterizing the genes and proteins so identified and of describing the burden of this group of diseases on human health. We also asked whether the genes in MMBID7, identified by their association with a human phenotype, are a representative sample of the entire human gene repertoire. Our results reflect the evolution and expansion of this field and put it in perspective with medicine as a whole. They also highlight areas where our understanding of disease is limited and where future studies will be of value.

We first examined the growth and contents of MMBID as a reflection of the expansion of the study of inborn errors of metabolism. Since its first edition in 1960, MMBID has enlarged considerably as new diseases have been identified and as the editors expanded their view of the types of disorders includible under the heading of inborn errors. This is reflected in a threefold increase in pages and chapters and a fivefold increase in disorders, contributors, weight, and thickness! The original editors (John B. Stanbury, James B. Wyngaarden, and Donald Frederickson with later assistance from Michael S. Brown and Joseph L. Goldstein) served through the fifth edition; the sixth and seventh editions were compiled by the current editorial team, which has continued to widen the scope of the book, reasoning that virtually all monogenic disorders result from a specific change in a protein that perturbs its function in specific homeostatic or developmental systems. The criteria set by the editors for inclusion in MMBID7 included a clinical phenotype plus a biochemical and/or molecular phenotype. On this basis, 460 genes were included in MMBID7. Coincident with this evolution of editorial perspective, there has been an increase in the number of biomedical professionals interested in the study of the biochemical and molecular basis of human disease. Together, these factors have led to a gradual transition of MMBID from a book devoted to small numbers of rare inherited metabolic diseases to one that has a view of medicine that embraces all diseases in terms of their biochemical and molecular bases. This evolution in our thinking about inborn errors was anticipated by A.E. Garrod who saw rare inborn errors as "merely extreme examples of variations of chemical behavior which are probably everywhere present."[16]

Burden of Inborn Errors of Metabolism in Human Health

In a study performed nearly 20 years ago, Costa and colleagues assessed the impact of monogenic disorders in human health.[15] They studied 351 confirmed monogenic disorders, selected in an unbiased way from the fifth edition (1978) of *Mendelian Inheritance in Man*.[17] Using information from the literature, they characterized this set of disorders in terms of inheritance, age at onset, organ systems involved and impact on life span, reproductive capability, and permanent disability. Their results showed that most of the disorders they surveyed became apparent early in life, most involved multiple organ systems, and more than half reduced life span and reproductive capacity, and limited life opportunities.

For this review, we evaluated all the disorders described in MMBID7 by criteria developed from those used by Costa and colleagues.[15] In contrast to their study, we were able to include more extensive molecular information and we made no attempt to review additional literature; all information was extracted from MMBID7. Of the 460 monogenic disorders in MMBID7, we excluded those with so little information that they could not be scored (n = 30). The definition of the categories and the scoring system for each disease is presented in Table 4-2. Because information pertinent to each of the categories was not included for every disease, the denominator may vary from one category to another.

Inheritance Patterns and Frequency

Information on mode of inheritance was available for 413 of the 430 disorders (Fig. 4-1A). Most (~60 percent) were inherited as autosomal recessive traits while approximately 20 percent were inherited as autosomal dominants, with X-linked recessives and mitochondrial traits still lower. The threefold excess of recessives over dominants is the converse of large surveys of all Mendelian phenotypes (e.g., see the twelfth edition of MIM, v. 1, p. xviii).[18] This difference likely derives from a traditional emphasis of MMBID on enzyme deficiencies, nearly all of which are inherited as recessive traits. For example, of the 44 chapters dealing with specific disorders in the first edition, 25 (57 percent) described enzyme deficiencies. Despite an expanding view of inborn errors, this tradition continues in MMBID7 where 76 (55 percent) of 138 chapters devoted to specific disorders involve enzyme deficiencies.

Population frequency information was supplied for about two-thirds of the disorders in our study (n = 284). The lack of reliable frequency data for such a large number of disorders (n = 156 or 36 percent) is an indication of the difficulty in obtaining this information, particularly for rare diseases. Population-based screening is performed for only a few disorders (e.g., in the state of Maryland, only six inherited disorders are included in the Newborn Screening Program). The recent development of tandem

Table 4-2 List of Categories Scored in Entries from MMBID7

1. Mode of inheritance. Unknown, autosomal recessive, autosomal dominant, X-linked, mitochondrial, multifactorial or complex

2. Frequency. Unknown, common (< 10,000), rare (10–100,000), very rare (> 100,000)

3. Ethnic aggregation. Yes/No

4. Age at onset. Not reported; *in utero*; birth to 1 yr; [to puberty,] early adulthood (puberty to 50 yr); late adulthood (> 50 yr); no recognized clinical manifestations. We used the age at onset for the typical phenotype to classify each disorder.

5. Systems and organs involved in phenotype. See text.

6. Reduction of life expectancy. None; mild; moderate; severe; not reported.

7. Chromosome mapped. Yes/No

8. Gene cloned. Yes/No

9. Mutations described. Not described; point mutations; gross rearrangements; expansion alleles.

10. Molecular mechanism of inheritance pattern. Unknown; haploinsufficiency; gain of function; dominant negative; recessive loss of function; other.

11. Function of deficient gene product. Unknown; enzyme; transcription factor; receptor; hormone; channel protein; transmembrane; transporters; extracellular transporter; modulator of protein function; extracellular matrix; intracelllular structural protein.

mass spectrometry as a screening tool offers the promise of providing prospective frequency data on scores of disorders, but these results are not yet available.[19–21] Thus, in the absence of direct measures, disease frequency is usually estimated by extrapolation from the number of recognized cases. This underestimates frequency, in part, because patients who are more mildly affected or whose phenotype otherwise varies from the "classical" are less likely to be recognized. Thus, there is consistent underestimation of disease frequency and a distorted view of phenotypic severity, skewed to the severe, easily recognized end of the spectrum. With these limitations, the range of frequencies for the diseases in MMBID7 was wide; the most common disorders had frequencies on the order of 0.0001 in a particular target population (e.g., cystic fibrosis in northern Europeans; type I Gaucher disease in Ashkenazi Jews), while more than 80 percent of the disorders were rare or very rare with frequencies < 0.0001 (Fig. 4-1B).

We designated ethnic aggregation when the incidence of the disorder was higher in populations of substantial size (≥5 million) with a common biologic background. Only 14 percent of the disorders had a clear ethnic predomination in well-characterized ethnic groups such as Ashkenazi Jews and Finns. Nearly all (> 80 percent) of these were inherited as autosomal recessive traits.

Clinical Phenotypes

Age at onset of clinical manifestations of a disease has medical and biological significance. Physicians categorize diseases by age at onset and organ system involvement. Indeed, these features determine what sort of doctor a patient is likely to see. The biological significance of age at onset for genetic disease is that it reflects the timing of the development of incongruence between the genetic program of an individual and the developmental, homeostatic, and environmental demands placed on that individual. For some disorders, compensatory mechanisms may postpone the onset of overt clinical manifestations for years or even decades (e.g., certain lysosomal storage diseases) while for others, the adaptive mechanisms are overwhelmed in short order (e.g., acute metabolic diseases of the newborn). A related biologic variable is the extent to which a particular mutation disrupts the protein's function as a unit step in homeostasis. Thus, some patients with completely inactivating mutations at the ornithine transcarbamylase locus present within 24 to 48 h after birth, while others with some residual function do not come to medical attention until childhood or even young adult life.[22]

We enumerated age at onset for the diseases identified in MMBID7 scoring the age when clinical manifestations appear in the standard presentation dividing life into five stages: *in utero*; birth to the first birthday; 1 year to puberty; early adulthood (puberty to 50 years); and late adulthood (> 50 years). Of the 389 phenotypes we were able to analyze for this characteristic, the vast majority (85 percent) showed clinical manifestations in the prereproductive age (Fig. 4-2). Age at onset for the remainder was mainly during early adulthood. This result is similar to that of Costa *et al.*[15] who found that 25 percent of the disadaptative Mendelian phenotypes in their study were apparent at birth and over 90 percent by the end of puberty. Parsing the age at onset distribution according to mode of inheritance (Fig. 4-3) has little consequence for autosomal recessive and X-linked disorders, but autosomal dominant phenotypes have a bimodal age distribution with the modes occurring during the first year of life and early adulthood.

Thus, for most of the disorders in MMBID, the consequences for development and homeostasis are severe and disadaptive early in extrauterine life. This explains the more rapid invasion of genetics into pediatrics as compared to internal medicine,[23] and predicts difficulty with treatment. The bimodal distribution of the autosomal dominants is of special interest (Fig. 4-2C). Some in the late onset group may reflect new age-related demands on homeostatic systems revealing previously asymptomatic functional deficits (e.g., Chap. 124). Other disorders in this group may

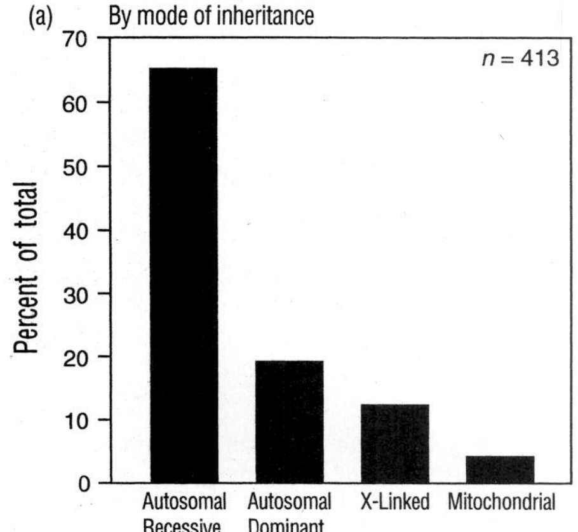

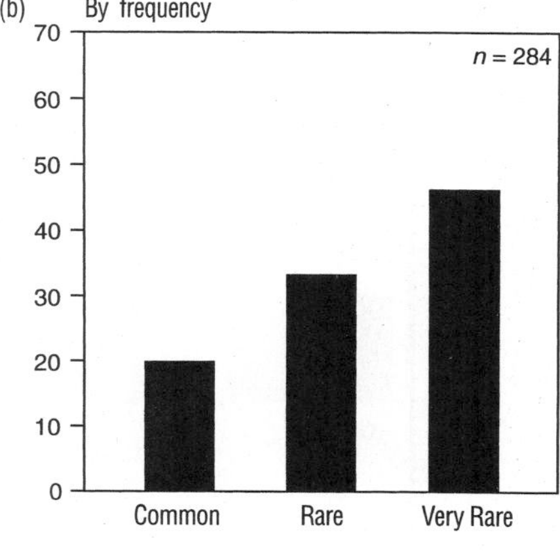

Fig. 4-1 Distribution of MMBID7 disorders by (*A*) mode of inheritance and (*B*) frequency. See Table 4-2 for definition of categories.

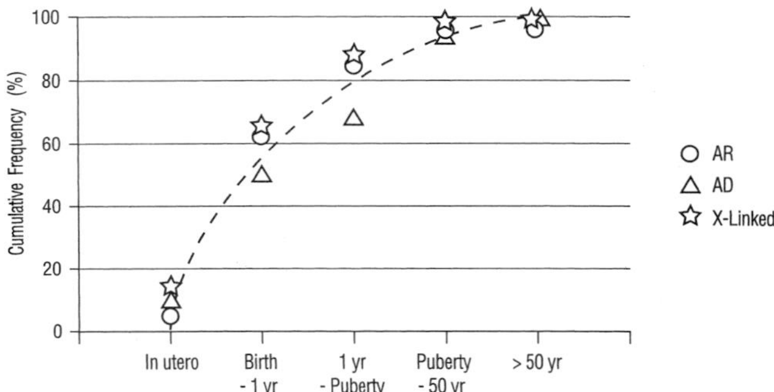

Fig. 4-2 The relationship between age at onset of clinical symptoms and cumulative frequency of the disorder grouped by mode of inheritance.

be caused by partial alterations in protein function and homeostatic abilities that gradually produce cell damage leading to cell death and eventually to system failure (e.g., Chaps. 223 and 234).

Figure 4-4 shows a relationship between age at onset and frequency of disease. The figure reveals that when diseases are frequent, ages at onset vary widely, even while those of infancy and childhood predominate. But as frequency declines, the range of onsets narrows. If we compare Figs. 4-4A and 4-4C, we see that for the very rare disorders onsets *in utero* are reduced by half, those in infancy almost double, and those over 50 disappear altogether. It is perhaps what one expects. The more damaging the gene effect, the earlier the onset and the more subject to negative selection. On the other hand a gene effect associated with disease of late onset is more likely to be conditional, dependent upon collaboration with others and with experiences of the environment and so less subject to selection. A geneticist would say that the heritability of disease varies directly with severity and indirectly with age at onset.

Organs and Systems Affected

One difference among genes is their pattern of expression. For some, expression is exquisitely limited to one cell type (e.g., rhodopsin in photoreceptors; phenylalanine hydroxylase in hepatocytes), while others are broadly expressed, apparently required by nearly all cell types (so-called housekeeping genes). How does this difference in expression relate to involvement in disease? Or does it? One clue might come from an examination of the number and type of organs and systems affected in each genetic disease, with the caveat that pattern of gene expression is but one of several variables that determines pathophysiology and hence organ and system involvement.

We scored organ and system involvement for each disease according to abnormalities detected by clinical history, physical exam, and routine laboratory investigation (Table 4-2). For practical reasons, we limited the number of organs and systems scored to three, selecting those that cause the most severe problems for the patient and added an additional category for those disorders with ≥ 4 organs or systems involved. We divided the organs and systems into 20 categories: blood included plasma proteins and all blood cells; reticuloendothelial included spleen, lymph nodes, Kupffer cells, and macrophages; nervous system was scored for both central and peripheral neuropathies; genitourinary refers to kidneys and the genitourinary tract; digestive included alimentary tract but not liver and exocrine pancreas; circulatory

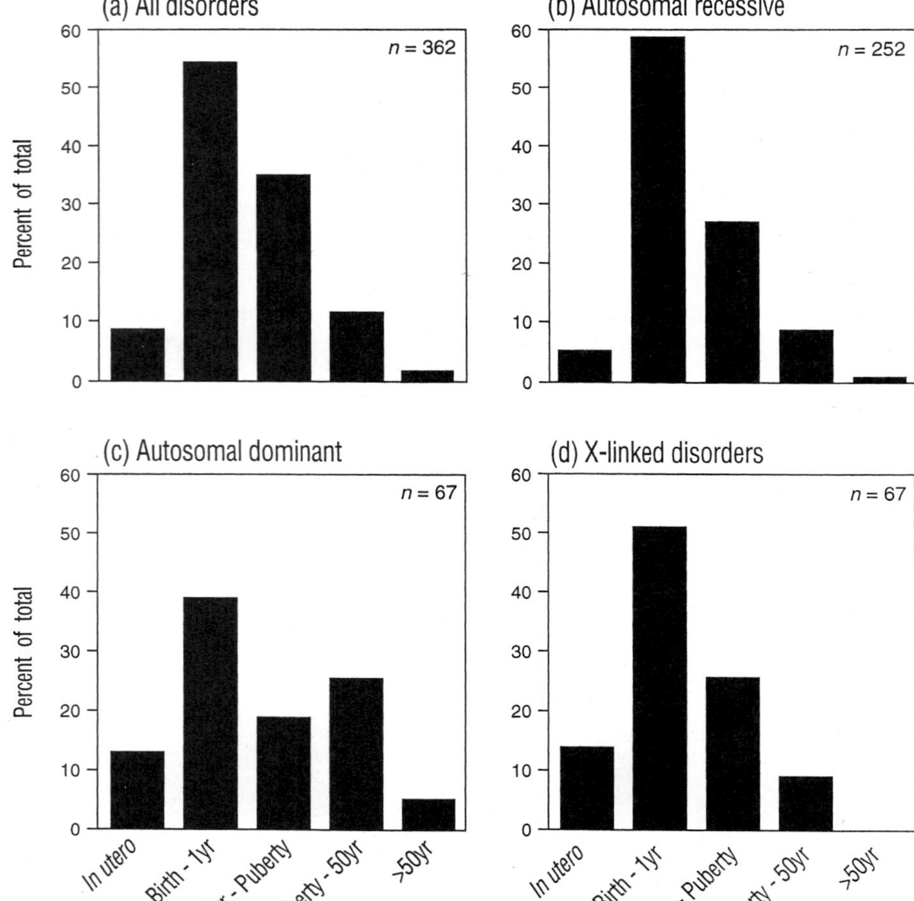

Fig. 4-3 Age at onset of clinical symptoms: *A*, all disorders; *B*, autosomal recessive; *C*, autosomal dominant; *D*, X-linked.

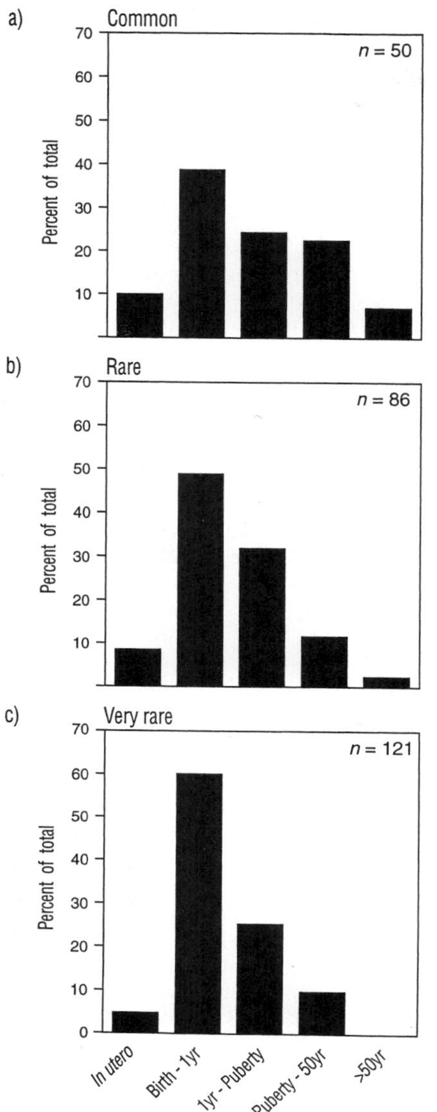

Fig. 4-4 Age at onset for (*A*) common, (*B*) rare, and (*C*) very rare disorders.

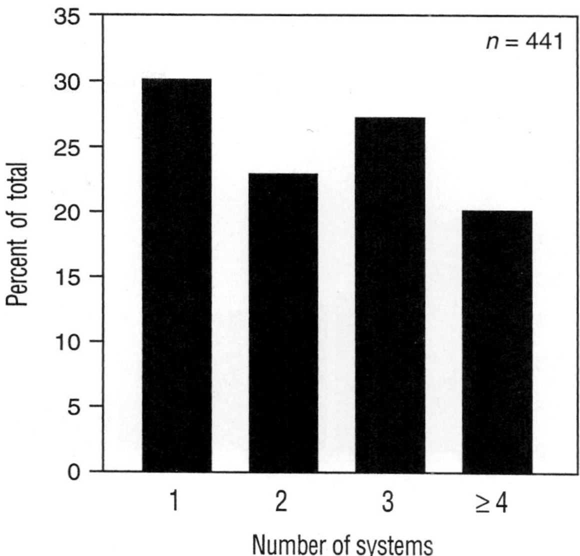

Fig. 4-5 Distribution of MMBID7 phenotypes by number of organs and systems affected.

included the heart and blood vessels; muscular was limited to striated muscle; integument included skin, nails, hair, and mammary glands; and limbs included developmental defects. In the category designated metabolic, we included disturbances in the total body water concentration of small molecules such as amino acids, sugars, and organic acids. The remaining categories are self-explanatory.

Our results showed that 70 percent of the phenotypes were multisystemic (Fig. 4-5). Metabolic was the most frequent (47 percent) followed closely by the nervous system (43 percent). None of the organs and systems we analyzed was immune from genetic disease (Fig. 4-6). Thus, pleiotropism is the rule for nearly all (>70 percent) the phenotypes in MMBID7. It is hardly surprising that most diseases affect more than one tissue. The multiplicity of affected cells and organs is simply a reflection of how tightly integrated the body is. Indeed, it is a tribute to the versatility of homeostasis that more are not involved.

Reduction of Life Expectancy

We scored the impact of the disorders in MMBID7 on life span by considering the typical life expectancy of the untreated patient with the most frequent form of the disease. Adequate information was available for 332 (77 percent) of the 430 disorders. We defined four categories: no reduction; mild, for those in which patients usually reach middle age; moderate, for those diseases where death occurs between age 10 and 30; and severe, for those where mortality occurs before age 10.

We found that about two-thirds of the disorders had an effect on lifespan (Fig. 4-7). Of these, about 75 percent were moderate to severe reductions with death before age 30. These results are consistent with the expectation that the disorders in which the gene effect is the most obtrusive and independent of modification have the earliest onset and the most disrupted phenotype.

Molecular Characterization

The interval of medical history corresponding to the birth, development, and maturation of MMBID spans the molecular revolution. The first edition appeared in 1960, just 16 years after the description by Avery, McCloud, and McCarty of DNA as the hereditary material,[24] and just 7 years after the elucidation of the antiparallel double-stranded structure of DNA by Watson and Crick (1953).[25] MMBID7, by contrast, appeared 35 years later in 1995, 5 years after the start of the Human Genome Project and 5 years before we expect to have a draft of the entire human sequence.[26]

Not surprisingly, the first edition of MMBID had virtually no molecular information; aside from X-linked traits, no genes were mapped to chromosomes and there was no information about causative mutations. By contrast, MMBID7, as emphasized by the insertion of "Molecular" into its title, has substantial molecular information. Of the 430 disorders in our study, nearly 70 percent were mapped, and for more than half, the responsible gene was cloned and disease-producing mutations identified. Of these, 94 percent were point mutations (nucleotide substitutions, insertion or deletions of less than 20 bp); 4 percent were gross rearrangements often affecting more than one gene, and 2 percent consisted of those diseases caused by expansion of short repeat sequences. This distribution of causative mutations is similar to other large collections of mutations (e.g., see the Cardiff Human Gene Mutation Database http://www.uwcm.ac.uk/uwcm/mg/hgmd0.html), so at the molecular level mutations associated with monogenic disease are indistinguishable from mutations in general.

Thus, our knowledge of the proximate cause of disease is increasing dramatically. The molecular information in MMBID8 is

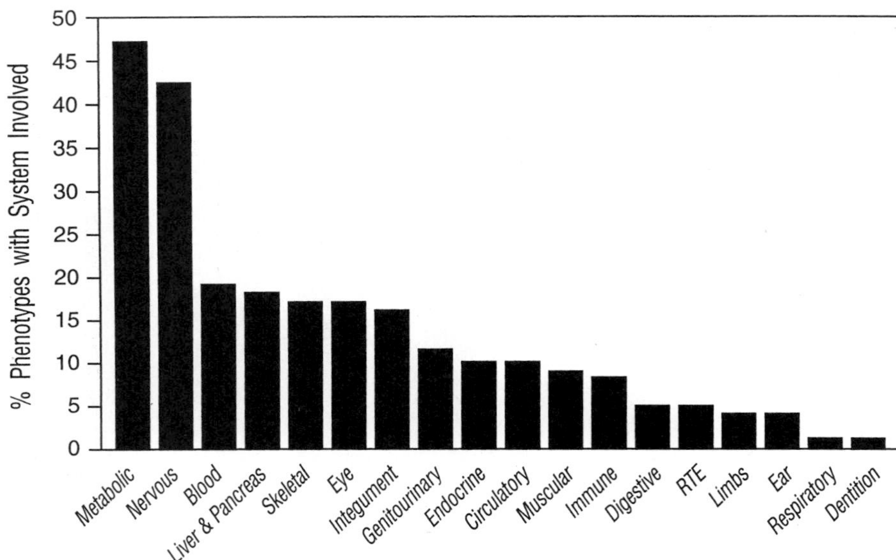

Fig. 4-6 Involvement of organs and systems in MMBID7 phenotypes.

greater still and in future editions, we can reasonably expect a nearly complete enumeration of the genes and mutations responsible for monogenic disorders. Identification of the genes and alleles contributing to complex traits will come along at a slower pace. The paradox is that our ability to treat genetic disease is improving at a much slower rate (see Chap. 5). Proximate cause is but one piece of the puzzle, useful for diagnosis and as a starting point for understanding pathogenesis but of limited value for developing treatment.

The Protein Product

Proteins do the work of the genes; understanding their function will provide more insight into disease, especially pathophysiology. Of the 430 disorders we analyzed, the nature of the protein product was identified for 348 (81 percent). We classified these according to function: enzymes, transporters, transcription factors, and so forth. Not surprisingly (and in part for the historical biases mentioned earlier), almost half were enzymes involved in intermediary metabolism. The distribution of the remaining categories is broad; that is, proteins performing virtually any function can be involved in disease (Fig. 4-8).

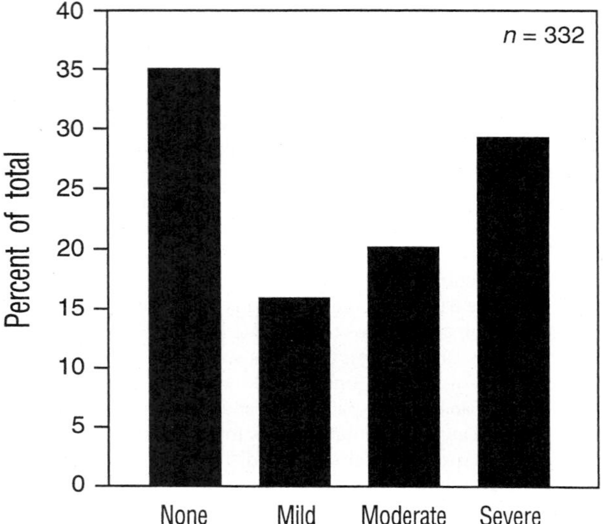

Fig. 4-7 Consequences of the MMBID7 disorders on life expectancy. See Table 4-2 for definition of categories.

How does this set of proteins, identified by their association with disease phenotypes, compare to the complete repertoire of human proteins? Are some gene products more often involved in disease or is the distribution simply a mirror of the protein products of our complete genome? Answers to these questions must wait for completion of the sequence and annotation of the human genome.

In an effort to foretell the answers to these questions, however, we took advantage of the recent completion of the yeast and worm whole-genome sequence.[27,28] Chervitz and colleagues compared the full complement of the predicted protein sequences encoded by these genomes and identified a set of about 3000 orthologous proteins that carry out core biologic processes in each organism (Fig. 4-8A).[29] These comprise about 40 percent of the yeast proteins and 20 percent of the worm proteins. The remainder appear to be involved in specialized function related to the special biologic requirements of each organism: one a multicellular creature that utilizes coordinated patterns of gene expression to produce specialized cell types; the other a single cell that turns batteries of genes on and off to adapt to environmental variables. We reasoned that a similar core would hold for all organisms and asked how the human proteins identified by association with disease in MMBID compared to the core biologic set identified by the yeast-worm comparison (Fig. 4-8A). Again, the MMBID7 set has a greater percentage of enzymes, we think in part for historical and technical biases rather than for entirely biologic reasons (Fig. 4-8B). If we arbitrarily set the percentage encoding enzymes as equal in both (Fig. 4-8C), then the adjusted distribution of the remainder is more similar except for the extracellular proteins (not represented in the yeast/worm set) and the larger fraction of unclassified proteins in the MMBID7 set (perhaps reflecting more complexity and less understanding of the human organism). This general similarity of the kinds of proteins identified in the MMBID7 set and the yeast/worm set suggests that, at least for the core set of proteins, all functional categories are equally likely to be involved in disease. It will be of great interest to follow the course of this trend as the numbers increase. Similarly, it will be interesting to compare the disease involvement of the conserved core set with the specialized nonorthologous proteins characteristic of each type of organism.

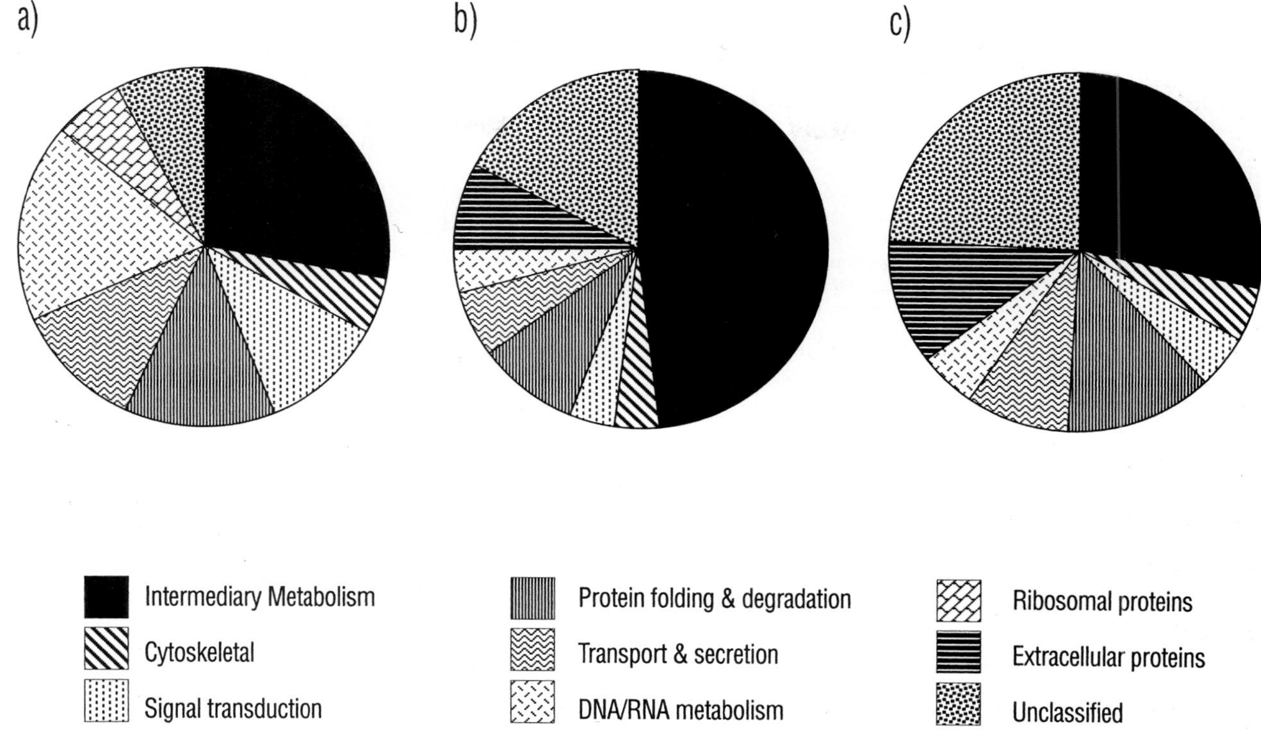

Fig. 4-8 Functional classification of proteins identified as: *A*, the conserved set of orthologous proteins that carry out core biologic processes in *S. cerevisiae* and *C. elegans* (see reference 29); *B*, the primary defects in the disorders in MMBID7; *C*, the MMBID7 set adjusted so that the fraction that are enzymes in intermediary metabolism is set equal to the same category in the yeast/worm set.

CONCLUSION

In addition to the analyses described above, there were many others that we would have liked to do, but in which differences could not reach significance because of the scarcity of cases in the various categories. For example, one might wish to characterize the diseases associated with the different variant proteins, transporters, transcription factors, cytoskeletal proteins, and so on; or to compare them one against the other, for all of the characteristics: age at onset, frequency, severity, mode of inheritance, and so on. But the numbers prohibited any such treatment. Still, the purpose of our work was to emphasize the value of such a study and the kinds of questions it will answer.

Obviously new questions will arise as earlier ones are answered, the proteins engaged in the diseases of complex origin will enter the analyses, and we will work our way slowly toward a molecular grasp, not only of disease as opposed to diseases, but of the relationship of human disease to human evolution. The product of the Genome Project will supply the wherewithal. One challenge for the leaders of the Genome Project will be to organize and annotate the product in ways that will enable and facilitate these studies.

REFERENCES

1. Burley SK, Almo SC, Bonanno JB, Capel M, Chance MR, Gaasterland T, Lin D, Sali A, Studier FW, Swaminathan S: Structural genomics: Beyond the human genome project. *Nat Genet* **23**:151, 1999.
2. Abbott A: A post-genomic challenge: Learning to read patterns of protein synthesis. *Nature* **402**:715, 1999.
3. Goldstein DS: On the dialectic between molecular biology and integrative physiology: Toward a new medical science. *Persp Biol Med* **40**:505, 1997.
4. Kirschner M, Gerhart J: Evolvability. *Proc Natl Acad Sci U S A* **95**:8420, 1998.
5. Hankey GJ, Eikelboom JW: Homocysteine and vascular disease. *Lancet* **354**:407, 1999.
6. American Society of Human Genetics/American College of Medical Genetics Test and Technology Transfer Committee Working Group: ASHG/ACMG statement: Measurement and use of total plasma homocysteine. *Am J Hum Genet* **63**:1541, 1998.
7. Allikmets R, Singh N, Sun H, Shroyer NF, Hutchinson A, Chidambaram A, Gerrard B, Baird L, Stauffer D, Peiffer A, Rattner A, Smallwood P, Li Y, Anderson KL, Lewis RA, Nathans J, Leppert M, Dean M, Lupski JR: A photoreceptor cell-specific ATP-binding transporter gene (ABCR) is mutated in recessive Stargardt macular dystrophy. *Nat Genet* **15**:236, 1997.
8. Lewis RA, Shroyer NF, Singh N, Allikmets R, Hutchinson A, Li Y, Lupski JR, Leppert M, Dean M: Genotype/phenotype analysis of a photoreceptor-specific ABC transporter gene, *ABCR*, in Stargardt disease. *Am J Hum Genet* **64**:422, 1999.
9. Martin GM, Austad SN, Johnson TE: Genetic analysis of ageing: Role of oxidative damage and environmental stresses. *Nat Genet* **13**:25, 1996.
10. Kuro-o M, Matsumura Y, Aizawa H, Kawaguchi H, Suga T, Utsugi T, Ohyama Y, Kurabayashi M, Kaname T, Kume E, Iwasaki H, Shiraki-Iida T, Nishikawa S, Nagai R, Nabeshima YL: Mutation of the mouse klotho gene leads to a syndrome resembling ageing. *Nature* **390**:45, 1997.
11. Jacobs PA, Hassold TJ: Chromosome abnormalities: Origin and etiology in abortions and live births, in Vogel F, Sperling K (eds): *7th International Congress of Genetics*. Berlin, 1986, p 233.
12. Braverman N, Lin P, Moebius FF, Obie C, Moser A, Glossmann H, Wilcox WR, Rimoin DL, Smith M, Kratz L, Kelley RI, Valle D: Mutations in the gene encoding 3β-hydroxysteroid-Δ^8,Δ^7-isomerase cause X-linked dominant Conradi-Hünermann syndrome. *Nat Genet* **22**:291, 1999.
13. Fitzky BU, Witsch-Baumgartner M, Erdel M, Lee JN, Paik YK, Glossmann H, Utermann G, Moebius FF: Mutations in the Delta7-sterol reductase gene in patients with the Smith-Lemli-Opitz syndrome. *Proc Natl Acad Sci U S A* **95**:8181, 1998.
14. Liu XY, Dangel AW, Kelley RI, Zhao W, Denny P, Botcherby M, Cattanach B, Peters J, Hunsicker PR, Mallon A-M, Strivens MA, Bate R, Miller W, Rhodes M, Brown SDM, Herman GE: The gene mutated in bare patches and striated mice encodes a novel 3β-hydroxysteroid dehydrogenase. *Nat Genet* **22**:182, 1999.
15. Costa T, Scriver CR, Childs B: The effect of Mendelian disease on human health: A measurement. *Am J Hum Genet* **21**:231, 1985.

16. Garrod AE: The incidence of alkaptonuria, a study in chemical individuality. *Lancet* **ii**:1616, 1902.
17. McKusick VA: *Mendelian Inheritance in Man*, 5th ed. Baltimore: Johns Hopkins Press, 1978.
18. McKusick VA: *Mendelian Inheritance in Man*, 12th ed. Baltimore: Johns Hopkins Press, 1998.
19. Levy HL: Newborn screening by tandem mass spectrometry: A new era. *Clin Chem* **44**:2401, 1998.
20. Naylor EW, Chace DH: Automated tandem mass spectrometry for mass newborn screening for disorders in fatty acid, organic acid and amino acid metabolism. *J Child Neurol* **14**:S4, 1999.
21. Chace DH, DiPerna JC, Naylor EW: Laboratory integration and utilization of tandem mass spectrometry in neonatal screening: A model for clinical mass spectrometry in the next millennium. *Acta Paediatr Suppl* **88**:45, 1999.
22. Tuchman M, Morizono H, Rajagopal BS, Plante RJ, Allewell NM: The biochemical and molecular spectrum of ornithine transcarbamylase deficiency. *J Inherit Metab Dis* **21**:40, 1998.
23. Childs B, Huether CA, Murphy EA: Human genetics teaching in U.S. medical schools. *Am J Hum Genet* **33**:1, 1981.
24. Avery OT, MacLeod CM, McCarty M: Studies on the chemical nature of the substance inducing transformation of pneumococcal types. *J Exp Med* **79**:137, 1944.
25. Watson JD, Crick FHC: Molecular structure of nucleic acids. *Nature* **171**:737, 1953.
26. Collins FS, Patrinos A, Jordan E, Chakravarti A, Gesteland R, Walters L: New goals for the U.S. Human Genome Project: 1998–2003. *Science* **282**:682, 1998.
27. *C. elegans* Sequencing Consortium: Genome sequence of the nematode *C. elegans*: A platform for investigating biology. *Science* **282**:2012, 1998.
28. Goffeau A, Barrell BG, Bussey H, Davis RW, Dujon B, Feldmann H, Galibert F, Hoheisel JD, Jacq C, Johnston M, Louis EJ, Mewes HW, Murakami Y, Philippsen P, Tettelin H, Oliver SG: Life with 6000 genes. *Science* **274**:546, 1996.
29. Chervitz SA, Aravind L, Sherlock G, Ball CA, Koonin EV, Dwight SS, Harris MA, Dolinski K, Mohr S, Smith T, Weng S, Cherry JM, Botstein D: Comparison of the complete protein sets of worm and yeast: Orthology and divergence. *Science* **282**:2022, 1998.

CHAPTER 5

Treatment of Genetic Disease

Eileen P. Treacy ▪ David Valle ▪ Charles R. Scriver

1. **Genetic diseases have ultimate causes that undermine normal phenotypes associated with homeostatic functions and structures.**
2. **The goal of treatment, as we know it, is to restore homeostasis, currently and usually by modalities that modify proximate events. These *euphenic* strategies attempt to modify phenotype; they do not alter genotype.**
3. **The modalities include restriction of (toxic) substrates, replacement of (deficient) products, activation or stabilization of mutant enzymes with pharmacologic doses of coenzymes or other agents, replacement of normal protein (by several approaches, including tissue transplantation); surgical repair; and combinations of these approaches.**
4. **The effectiveness of these modalities has been measured in a series of studies over the past two decades. The response to treatment was only partial at best in the majority of genetic diseases but is steadily improving as new knowledge of pathogenesis is combined with new strategies and tactics for treatment. The prospects for combinatorial drug design to fit therapy to phenotype are encouraging.**
5. **There are no unequivocal examples yet of persistent success with somatic gene therapy for a human genetic disease.**

INTRODUCTION

Science, in its simplest definition, is an assault on ignorance.[1] Society expects the assault to produce results in the form of concepts, verifiable data, and technologies. In the case of genetics, and particularly in medical genetics, a chief expectation is that new knowledge will lead to new and better treatments of genetic diseases.

Homo sapiens is the only species on earth that intentionally modifies experience, thereby modifying natural selection on itself. *Homo sapiens* as such is *Homo modificans*, and increasingly we manipulate experience to maintain health. Treatment of genetic disease involves modified selection and directed adaptation; it is focused on individuals and, in many ways, is a cultural as well as a scientific activity.

Is There a Problem?

The goal of treatment for genetic diseases is to restore the normal metrical trait value in the target area of the treatment effect,[2] that is, to restore normal *homeostasis*, the term introduced by Walter B. Cannon in the 1930s to describe the central tendency of a complex trait value.[3] In the previous century, the French physiologist Claude Bernard had recognized that maintenance of the steady state in the *milieu interieur* is a universal feature of living systems. Accordingly, the ultimate goal of treatment in genetic disease is to restore normal homeostasis *in the appropriate space*. All too often, the treatment, as we have known it up to now, fails to reach that objective and that is the core of the problem. Two examples illustrate it.

Type I diabetes mellitus (Chap. 69) used to kill affected children before insulin was discovered in 1921. It was widely believed at that time that the discovery of insulin would soon solve the problem of type I diabetes, but it has not done that (even though the development of insulin led to a Nobel Prize). At the end of the 20th century, the long-term complications of the disease, such as retinopathy, renal failure, and neuropathy and the effects of maternal diabetes on the fetus, continue to be serious complications with insulin treatment.

The Diabetes Control and Complications Trial Research Group (DCCT) has studied and compared outcomes in patients treated with the older conventional methods and with the newly recommended intensive treatment protocol.[4] The latter requires much more aggressive control of blood glucose level, either with an external continuous infusion insulin pump or by means of multiple daily intramuscular injections of insulin. The DCCT study shows that intensive treatment achieves better control of capillary blood glucose, less glycosylation of hemoglobin (as a marker of long-term control), and significantly fewer complications involving eyes, kidneys, and peripheral nerves. The study introduces an additional message: better treatment of diabetes and compliance with the intensive protocol is difficult and demanding.

Our second example is taken from phenylketonuria (PKU), an inborn error of metabolism, one of a set of diseases called *Mendelian* (under the control of a single major locus) and considered to be less complex in their mechanisms of pathogenesis than is the case in type I diabetes mellitus. Modifying strategies for the treatment of Mendelian inborn errors of metabolism are the major focus of our chapter, because they constitute the group of genetic diseases with the greatest experience of treatment, which involves altering extrinsic environment, restoring intrinsic homeostasis by whatever means and, in some cases, by replacing the mutant gene product with the normal counterpart. PKU illustrates these general principles (Chap. 77).

In its broadest terms, treatment of PKU is a genuine success story, and it is one of the flagships in the armada being assembled for the campaign on treatment of genetic disease in general. Early dietary treatment of PKU prevents severe mental retardation. A generation of experience, however, reveals that cognitive development in treated patients is half a standard deviation below normal; and premature termination of treatment, in adolescence, for example, can have unfavorable consequences in some patients. Accordingly, new guidelines for earlier, more aggressive, and potentially lifelong treatment of PKU have been recommended, guidelines that are not compatible with the wishes of many patients who seek a better lifestyle, even if they could have access to improved low phenylalanine dietary treatment products. Besides their poor organoleptic properties, the current treatment diet products may lack essential nutrients such as the fatty acid docosahexaenoic acid, which is necessary for normal brain development. One of the alternatives for PKU therapy might be to restore phenylalanine homeostasis, not by a better diet, but by enzyme therapy with phenylalanine ammonia lyase to degrade excess phenylalanine. The enzyme that converts phenylalanine to *trans*-cinnamic acid could be given by mouth in a protected formulation. Pilot studies show that oral delivery of a recombinant phenylalanine ammonia lyase in a mouse model of PKU effectively lowers blood phenylalanine.[5]

The Message in the Problem

The treatments of type I diabetes mellitus and PKU illustrate an important message: whereas the *principles* for treatment of genetic disease are quite clear and reasonably well understood, the *practices* to restore homeostasis are often difficult and less well achieved. There is a reason: biologic homeostasis in *Homo sapiens* is the result of fine-tuning by evolutionary processes. Accordingly, one cannot expect a treatment invented today to be instantly successful if it is supposed to replace or repair a design achieved by millions of years of evolution. On the other hand, detailed knowledge of pathogenesis behind the genetic disease, as described in chapter after chapter of this work, both in this and previous editions, will always help. Here are three examples.

- Dramatically improved treatment of familial hypercholesterolemia with statins and bile acid-binding resins[6] came about through research revealing the pathogenesis of hypercholesterolemia in low-density lipoprotein (LDL) receptor deficiency (Chap. 120).
- The treatment of hereditary tyrosinemia type I by diets low in phenylalanine and tyrosine content was ultimately a failure until pathogenesis of this disease was more clearly understood. Artificial inhibition of the tyrosine pathway with a synthetic chemical (NTBC)[7] to block synthesis of a toxic tyrosine metabolite has changed the natural history of this disease (Chap. 79).
- The treatment of osteogenesis imperfecta (Chap. 205), particularly for the allelic variants that affect the structure of collagen rather than its synthesis, was unsatisfying until the use of bisphosphonate pamidronate decreased bone turnover, increased bone density, and reduced frequency of fractures.[8]

As we develop our overview on treatment of genetic disease in this chapter, there are two encompassing ideas to keep in mind. First, the phenomenon of allelic heterogeneity implies that each patient has his or her own disease in a subcategory of the generic form; accordingly, if there were a drug therapy for cystic fibrosis, for example, there might be a need for a specific form of it to modify the pathogenic effects of different mutant genotypes at the CFTR locus.[9] The second idea follows from the first. If allelic variation produces different phenotypes, then combinatorial drug design[10] is a development to fit the treatment to the phenotype. The idea could be posed as a question: If evolution learned to make combinatorial molecules called antibodies, can *Homo sapiens* learn to make combinatorial drugs to treat genetic diseases? That is a fascinating challenge, not yet met by any of the treatments we describe later in this chapter.

A Context for Interest in Treatment of Genetic Disease

The human genome is a by-product of evolutionary tinkering,[11] and the nucleotide sequences of its expressed loci have been selected for their contributions to the processes of phenotypic homeostasis in both developmental and mature functions of the organism. Pathogenic mutations (Chap. 13) disrupt homeostasis, and *Homo sapiens sapiens* has been increasingly inclined not to accept their unfavorable effects. *Homo modificans* has turned its attention to the maintenance of health and the prevention and treatment of disease.

One result of this concern for health and disease has been an improvement in child, maternal, and public health in many human societies, particularly in the 20th century.[12] This change has been accompanied by a corresponding rise in the heritability of human disease, such that awareness of the relative importance of genetic components in human disease now coincides with the appearance of the Human Genome Project and all its implications. At the risk of "medicalizing" human genetic variation, and of "geneticizing" health and disease,[13] it is no surprise that treatment of genetic disease is seen as just another step in the journey that has up to now focused on epidemic and endemic causes of disease — causes that *overwhelm* homeostasis. *Homo modificans* chooses to address, with equivalent interest, those causes that *undermine* homeostasis.[14]

There is good reason to take this step. By age 25 years, 5 percent of the population, in developed societies, will experience the disadaptive effects of genetic variation and, during a lifetime, almost two thirds of the population will experience disease in which a genetic component is a contributing factor.[15] Whereas to call a disease *genetic* was at one time a prescription for despair, now it is seen as a challenge that perhaps can be met.

The Third International Congress of Human Genetics, held in Chicago in 1966, discussed many genetic problems of the day on its scientific program. Among them was "Treatment in Medical Genetics,"[16] for which there was an emerging sense of optimism at the time. As already mentioned, dietary treatment of PKU, which had begun in the decade before, was showing evidence that it could prevent the mental retardation associated with this Mendelian disease, and Rh blood group incompatibility, an important cause of neonatal jaundice and kernicterus, was also yielding to preventive measures. Environmental engineering (so-called euphenic therapy) was seen as a reasonably effective way to neutralize the effects of many different mutant human alleles. There were many other examples to encourage optimism, and a simple algorithm for treatment based on toxic substrate restriction, deficient product replacement, coenzyme supplementation (to activate dormant mutant enzymes) or protein (or enzyme) replacement, in the particular context of treating inborn errors of metabolism, seemed to offer great promise.[16] Pharmacogenetics (Chap. 9), a new branch of medical genetics, fitted nicely into the paradigm; even *genetic engineering* was not out of bounds. Many review articles soon documented efficacious treatment of various genetic diseases. However, treatment has not always kept pace with advances in understanding the molecular basis of the diseases, and the gap between the science of medicine and its applications (in diagnosis and treatment) has not been closed as completely as desired.

A Challenge Beyond the Mendelian Diseases

Multifactorial common diseases are the major proportion of *genetic diseases* in society. The more salient their genetic component, the earlier is their age at onset and the more likely to affect family members. Such disease also constitutes an important proportion of *disability* in our aging population. The relevance of rethinking how therapy might change our current outlook on disease in this population is introduced as follows:[17]

1. New biotechnologies can reduce the age-adjusted chronic disability prevalence rate.
2. Improved understanding of human biology may make conventional care and treatment less necessary; new approaches changes the status of the medical paradigm from palliative to halfway technology and then to high technology with improved health.
3. The revolution in pharmaceutical research and development (miniaturization robotic and combinatorial chemistry) will reduce drug development costs and improve drug design (see the foregoing).

The authors then develop their argument to predict the economic benefits of improved prediction, diagnosis, prevention, and treatment of human disability notably in the real world of living longer. Accordingly, all that can be learned about treatment of patients with genetic diseases, such as the hereditary disorders described in this book, will benefit a much larger population of individuals with similar needs.

TREATMENT: MEASUREMENTS OF SUCCESS

The McKusick Catalogs of Mendelian Inheritance in Man (MIM) in printed and on-line formats (OMIM),[18] are genomic databases of variant human phenotypes; the latter are mainly, but not necessarily, pathogenic with consequences for health that are usually perceived to be unfavorable.[19] The catalogs record conditions and traits inherited conventionally as autosomal dominants or recessives, or by linkage to the X chromosome; or unconventionally — as alleles on the mitochondrial chromosome, as expanded trinucleotide repeats in expressed nuclear genes or with an imprinting effect (Chap. 15). As of October 27, 1998, for example, OMIM had recorded 9861 allelic variants in 845 genes, the corresponding gene locus had been mapped in well over 600 of these entities, and at least one mutant pathogenic allele had been characterized in 494 of these disorders, although several dozen genes harbor more than 25 known mutant alleles, and some loci contain hundreds of disease-causing mutations.

Does treatment of genetic disease really work—when it is available? The medical arena of medical genetics tends to be more anecdotal than its scientific arena, and measurements of treatment efficacy in general tend to be rare. An attempt was made in the early 1980s to rectify this dearth of information—first, by measuring the phenotypic consequences of Mendelian inheritance[20] and then by measuring the effect of treatment on Mendelian disease.[21] When it was found that treatment of such disease as a whole was not as successful as had been hoped,[21] the measurements of efficacy were narrowed to focus on the class of Mendelian disease recognized as *inborn errors of metabolism*, where there is a great deal of knowledge about cause, pathogenesis, and manifestations of the disease.[21] Measurements in this subset were then pursued systematically through the 1980s[21] and 1990s[22] to monitor progress. Whereas some have found a clear message in these analyses (treatment is not so good), there is evidence over time of a different and more optimistic message: treatments are getting better. Most treatments are still halfway technologies, but the combination of improved compliance and better technology is making a difference.

The Effect of Mendelian Disease on Human Health

To perform the first study,[20] carried out in 1983, the authors used the 5th (printed) edition of the McKusick Catalogs. Phenotypes were selected from the catalogs. Only entries with a confirmed mode of inheritance were used, and every third entry in this category was then taken; a number of the selected disorders were then discarded because they were either neutral polymorphisms or there was insufficient information. By this approach, 351 Mendelian *disease* phenotypes were available for analysis. The MIM entry was then used to find articles in the literature: 1200 articles were thus selected and read to describe the impact of Mendelian disease on human individuals. All disorders, by definition, were disadaptive and caused some form of impairment, disability, or handicap, according to the definitions of the World Health Organization.[19] Phenotypic effects were scored to measure their impact on two biologic parameters (life span and reproductive capability), two developmental parameters (cognitive and somatic), and three social parameters (the ability to attend school, to obtain regular employment, and to endure cosmetic blemish).

From their review of the literature up to 1983, the authors found the following.[20] One-quarter of the disadaptive Mendelian phenotypes were apparent at birth, and over 90 percent had become manifest by the end of puberty. Age at onset was trimodal in distribution for the whole set, essentially unimodal for autosomal recessive and X-linked diseases, and clearly trimodal for autosomal dominant conditions, with modes appearing in the life intervals of morphogenesis, infancy, and early adult life. Over half of the phenotypes involved more than one anatomic or functional system; some diseases affected more than five organ or functional systems. Life span of patients was reduced in over half the diseases, particularly in those where onset was in pre-adult life. Reproductive capability was impaired in over two-thirds of phenotypes. The vast majority of diseases compatible with life beyond infancy caused psychosocial handicap and limited access to schooling and work.

These findings also bear on the treatment of the genetic disease. Since the distribution of age at onset is not random and one of its frequency modes occurs during intrauterine life of the fetus, and because important phases of ontogeny representing morphogenesis are occurring during this time, treatment would have to offset the prenatal effects of the mutant allele. A second mode for age at onset occurs in infancy when the patient is assuming self-directed metabolism and development; here again, the efficacy of treatment must take into account both the vulnerability of the organism and the dynamic nature of growth and development in all parameters at this stage of life. A third frequency mode, identified in early adulthood, implies that onset of a genetic disease at this time of life could have major consequences for the economic and social dimensions of life. Although the emphasis in this project was on *Mendelian* disease, a relationship was noticed between salience of the gene and its contribution to homeostasis. Thus, it could be argued that there is a continuous distribution of genes contributing to disease (Chap. 2) and a similar relationship would exist between age at onset and the characteristics of *multifactorial* diseases.[23] Forms of the latter when associated with readily discernible *major* gene effects would be likely to have an earlier age at onset and a stronger family history than those forms of the disease in which this is not the case. This hypothesis has supporting evidence,[23] and again it is relevant to any thoughts about the treatment of so-called genetic diseases.

Efficacy of Treatment: The 1985 Report

After measuring the effects of Mendelian diseases on human health, it was appropriate to measure the response to treatment.[21] A scoring system was developed that would allow the effect of treatment to be measured by comparing pretreatment and posttreatment scores: the system quantified the seven parameters of phenotype (biologic, developmental, and social) (Table 5-1). A score was first calculated for the untreated disease and then for the

Table 5-1 Impact of Mendelian Disease on Phenotype Parameter: Descriptors for Scoring System*

Component and Manifestations	0	1	2	3
Effect on biological selection				
Longevity	None	Premature postreproductive death	Death during reproductive interval	Death before reproductive age
Reproductive capability	None	Impaired	—	Inability to reproduce or death before reproductive age
Effect on development				
Somatic growth	None	Impaired	—	Height/weight < 3rd centile
Intellectual development	None	Mild (IQ 70–80)	Moderate (IQ 50–70)	Severe (IQ < 50)
Effect on social adaption				
Learing handicap	None	Remedial schooling	Special program	Uneducable
Work handicap	None	Mild restriction	Sheltered workshop	No capability
Cosmetic impairment	None	Mild	Moderate	Major

*The scoring system is used to measure effect of the genetic disease before and after treatment.[21]

Table 5-2 Summary of Treatment Effects on Inborn Errors of Metabolism: The 1993 Study/1995 Report [21]

Component (Manifestation)	Disease Impact (% of Diseases)		
	Prevented	Modified	Unchanged
Longevity	21	9	70
Reproductive capability	15	15	70
Development			
Growth	15	12	73
Intelligence	11	9	80
Social			
Schooling	16	8	76
Work	13	12	75
Cosmetic	15	17	68

SOURCE: From Treacy et al.[22]

treated disease, based on published reports of the *best* results of treatment. The study, based on the reading of 1500 additional reports, was carried out in two parts: the first, on the set of Mendelian diseases as a whole,[20] and the second, on a subset of 65 inborn errors of metabolism contained in the whole set.[21]

The response to treatment on *Mendelian disease* as a whole was slight. Treatment extended life span to normal in only 15 percent of the diseases (when longevity was seen to be reduced in the untreated state); reproductive capability was improved in only 11 percent and social adaptation in only 6 percent. At the time of the study (1983), the mutant gene and its product had been identified in only 15 percent of the 351 conditions. Since the mutant polypeptide is known, or surmised with reasonable accuracy, in most inborn errors of metabolism, it was recognized that these diseases could be studied separately, with the expectation (a hypothesis) that treatment would be more beneficial in this set because knowledge about pathogenesis, on average, was greater than for Mendelian diseases in general.

Even in the inborn errors of metabolism, though, the effect of treatment overall was disappointing, and no parameter in the set as a whole yielded completely to treatment (Table 5-2). When the scores were pooled for all parameters, however, they revealed some successes; a complete response to treatment (relaxation of selection) occurred in 12 percent of the 65 diseases in the sample. On the other hand, there was only a partial response in 40 percent and none whatsoever in 48 percent of the diseases.[21]

If the goal of treatment is to restore chemical and physiological homeostasis, and if it can be done by substrate restriction, product replacement, coenzyme supplementation, or protein replacement, one has to ask why so few diseases were successfully treated. The answer lies in the ability to restore homeostasis. Treatment was likely to be successful when the modality of treatment could penetrate to the locus of its essential effect and homeostasis can be restored in that space, organelle, or organ (see the diseases listed in Table 5-3). Treatment was ineffective when the deviant phenotype was expressed prenatally or at a site of cellular homeostasis that could not be reached; for example, Tay-Sachs disease would not yield to enzyme replacement therapy unless the enzyme could penetrate a neuronal lysosome in the developing fetus. Thus, outcome of current modes of treatment will probably be poor for phenotypes affecting highly adapted metabolic systems such as glycolysis or energy metabolism and for diseases affecting development. The poorer long-term outcomes of treatment for patients with severe disorders of lactate metabolism, the urea cycle and ganglioside turnover, for example (Chaps. 100, 85, and 153, respectively) — corroborate this simplified interpretation.

Table 5-3 Examples of Genetic Disease Where Treatment Completely Removes Its Effects*

Catalog No. (MIM-12)	
223000	Disaccharide Intolerance II (congenital lactose intolerance)
226200	Enterokinase deficiency
229600	Fructose intolerance (aldolase deficiency)
231900	Glutathionine synthetase deficiency (erythrocyte)
232800	Glycogen storage disease VII (phosphofructokinase deficiency)
237450	Hyperbilirubinemia (rotor type)
251100/251110	Methylmalonic aciduria, vitamin B_{12} responsive
276000	Trypsinogen deficiency

*Treatment modality can penetrate space where disease is expressed; homeostasis is thus achievable.

SOURCE: From Hayes.[21] Used by permission.

Efficacy of Treatment: The 1995 Report

By using and repeating the same measurements, a follow-up analysis was performed in 1993–1994[22] on the 65 diseases previously studied. Although a number of disorders had been reclassified in the 10th edition of MIM, these entities could still be studied; all articles pertaining to these entities (listed in *Medline* and OMIM) were used to measure efficacy as described in the earlier study[21] (Table 5-4).

The new analysis[22] showed that manifestations and effects of the disease on all metrical parameters had been diminished by treatment more effectively in the decade that followed the original study[21] than in the years before it (Fig. 5-1; Table 5-4). Treatments in the decade leading up to the 1995 report had almost uniformly improved scores in each parameter yet did not result in more "cures" of hereditary metabolic diseases (Fig. 5-2): only 12 percent of the diseases again fell into this category, meaning it had not enlarged; however, the number achieving a partial benefit had increased to 57 percent and those showing no benefit had decreased to 31 percent (Fig. 5-2). The modest average improvement in treatment responses for many of these entities could be attributed to better protocols, supervision, and compliance rather than better modalities of and products for treatment.

Disappointments in the efficacy of treatment persisted notably, for example, in the treatment of galactosemia (Chap. 72) and disorders of the urea cycle (Chap. 85). In the latter conditions, treatment had indeed substantially reduced *mortality* associated with the diseases but also had left a substantial residue of chronic *morbidity*. Thus, the knowledge at hand and its use were still insufficient for effective euphenic treatment for many inborn errors of metabolism.

Tissue transplantation was a major new modality accounting for improved outcomes in the 1993 analysis.[22] It benefited a number of disorders but also introduced its own potential morbidity. Moreover, in a number of diseases, components of the mutant phenotype persisted after transplantation, for example, acitrullinemia in carbamoyl phosphate synthetase deficiency[24] and

Table 5-4 Effect of Treatment on Mendelian Disease (65 Inborn Errors of Metabolism): A 10-Year Comparison

Category (Response)	1983 Study* (%)	1993 Study (%)
A (Full benefit)	12	12
B (Partial benefit)		
Change in score > 10	14	14
Change in score < 0	26	43
C (No benefit)	48	31
Total	100	100

*SOURCE: From Hayes et al.[21] and Treacy et al.[22] Used by premission.

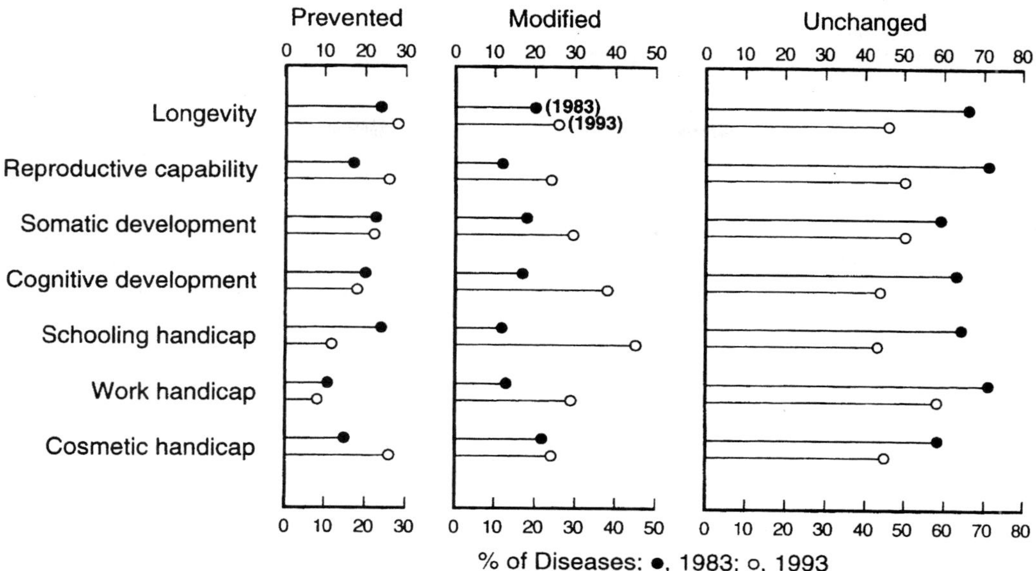

Fig. 5-1 The effect of treatment on 65 inborn errors of metabolism measured with seven parameters (see Table 5-1) and the experience in 1995[22] (*open circles*) compared with that reported in 1985[21] (*solid circles*). The diseases in which the responses were measured are grouped under three categories: effects of disease are completely prevented, are modified, or are unchanged. Improvement in treatment responses during the decade is revealed. (*From Treacy et al.*[22] *Used by permission.*)

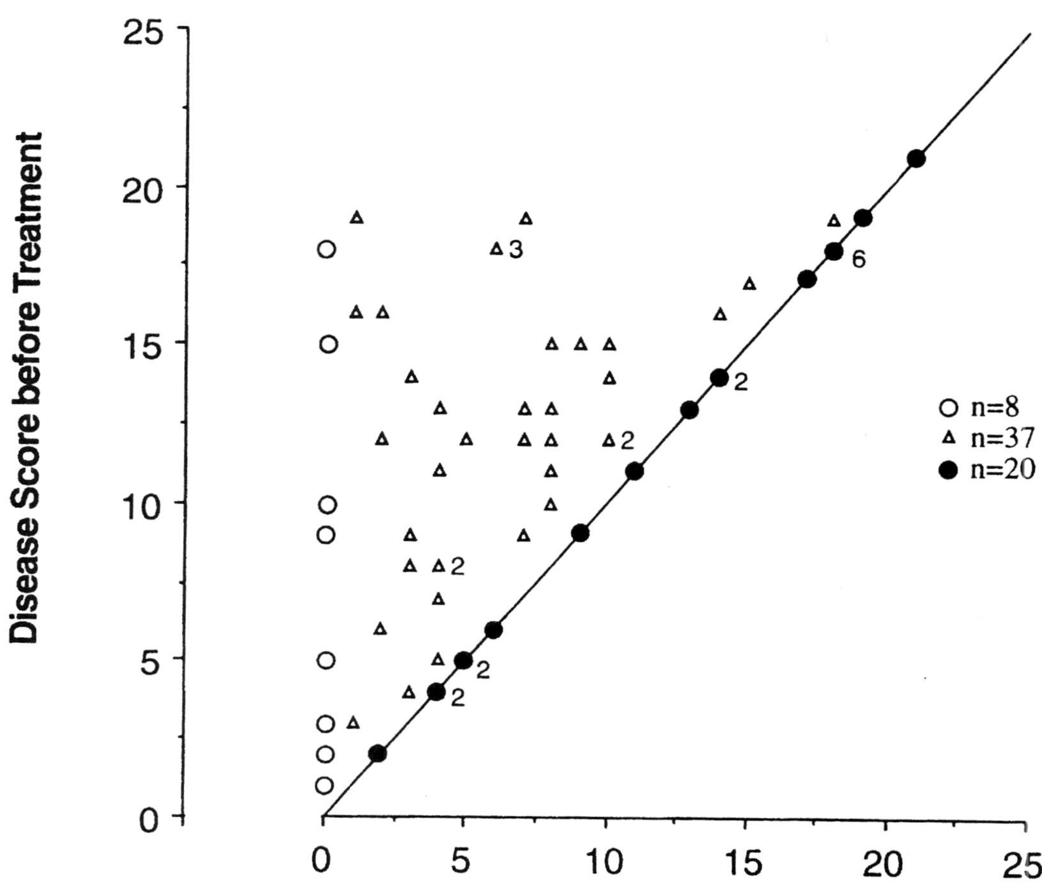

Fig. 5-2 Disease scores in 65 inborn errors of metabolism, before (*ordinate*) and after treatment (*abscissa*).[22] Eight diseases (12 percent of the sample) completely responded to treatment (*open circles*), 57 percent of the diseases only partially responded to therapy (*open triangles*), and 31 percent of the total did not respond (*solid circles*). Nonetheless, the overall response had improved in the decade since the earlier study by Hayes et al[21] on the same diseases set. (*From Treacy et al.*[22] *Used by permission.*)

hypoargininemia in argininosuccinic acid lyase deficiency.[25] In some diseases, the disease progressed in the nontransplanted organs of the host, as in the case of oxalosis type 1 and infantile nephropathic cystinosis. Bone marrow transplantation did not benefit the central nervous system in four diseases where it improved the phenotype in other organs. On the other hand, there has been significant progress with *protein replacement therapy* (by transplantation and cell implantation) as we show in the third part of this chapter.

A Third Analysis: Findings in MMBID-7

The 7th edition of the *Metabolic and Molecular Bases of Inherited Disease* (MMBID-7), published in 1995, documents 475 distinct disorders in 154 chapters, with recent additions in the CD-ROM edition published in 1997. From a total of 517 well-defined entities, we again derived new scores by using the previous criteria. (Diseases due to allelic mutations were counted as one entity, and benign entries were excluded, as were disorders where treatment options were not discussed.) Outcome scores were based on information provided solely in the text of MMBID-7 and its CD-ROM update. The altered DNA diagnosis was known in at least 70 percent of conditions (Fig. 5-3), 12 percent of the entries (now 46 different disorders) responded completely to therapy (e.g., biotinidase deficiency), 200 disorders (54 percent of the total and now the major class) showed a partial benefit (e.g., the urea cycle disorders), and 126 diseases (34 percent) had no significant response to treatment (e.g., disorders of peroxisomal biogenesis, carbohydrate-deficient glycoprotein syndrome, and the majority of lysosomal disorders). Figure 5-4 illustrates the different modalities of treatment used for these entities and the range of modalities now in use either individually or in various combinations. Progress in treatment is the result of what is being done and how carefully it is done.

How the DNA mutation alters protein function and whether there is any redundancy in that function will have much bearing on future treatments, as will our understanding of protein and cellular chemistry and how that will influence drug design.[9,26–28] Meanwhile, generic approaches to treatment, as they have been used up to now, will remain the mainstays in management of *genetic disease* and, for that reason, we provide an overview of these approaches.

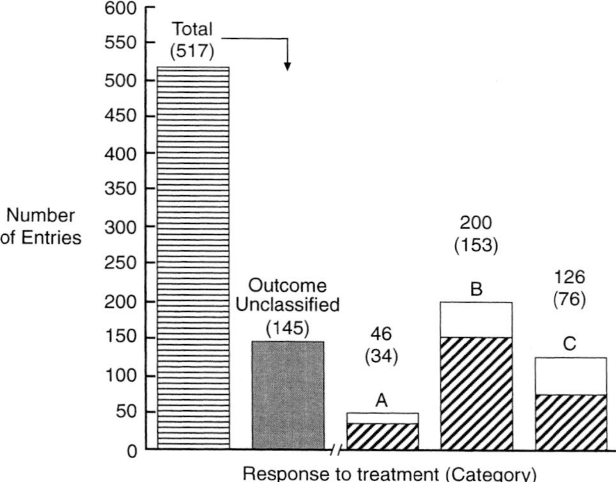

Fig. 5-3 The effect of treatment of disease entities as listed in MMBID-7 and CD-ROM additions. Of 517 total entities, it was not possible to designate a treatment outcome in 145 disorders, because of insufficient information in the text. Of the resulting 372 disorders, 46 (12 percent) demonstrated complete response to treatment (*category A*), 200 (54 percent) showed partial benefit, and 126 (39 percent) showed no response to treatment. The altered DNA structure was known in more than 70 percent of the total number of entities (seen as the *hatched boxes*, and the number for each subgroup is given in parentheses).

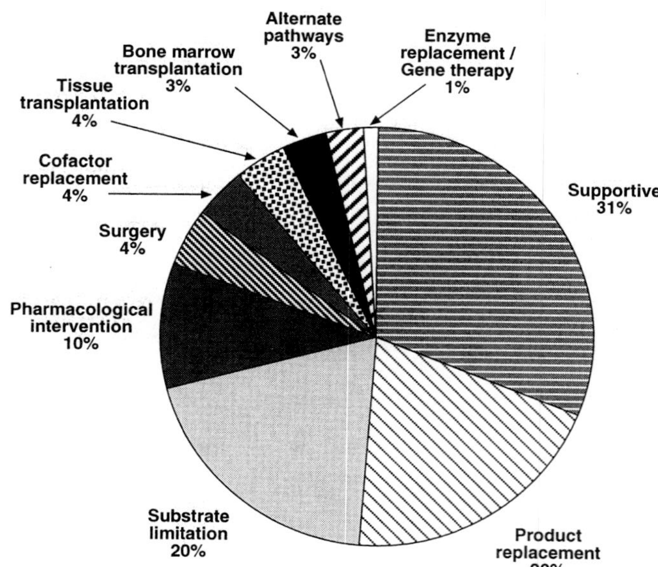

Fig. 5-4 Illustrated are the different modalities of treatment utilized for the 372 disorders as listed in Fig 5-3. Each disorder may have been amenable to one or more therapies. The percentages indicate the relative overall contribution of each form of therapy.

GENERAL PRINCIPLES FOR TREATMENT OF GENETIC DISEASE*

Genetic disease results from inherited abnormalities in the workings of complex systems that program the components of normal development and physiological homeostasis. Environmental factors contribute variably to the disease phenotype by stressing defective systems. Treatment of genetic disorders requires accurate diagnosis, early intervention, and intimate knowledge of the pathogenesis of the disorder. Expanding knowledge regarding the molecular basis of genetic diseases, and continued advances in analytic and diagnostic technologies (e.g., fast-atom-bombardment mass spectrometry, the use of stable isotopes as tracers, nuclear magnetic resonance spectrometry, and mutation analysis), have greatly enhanced our ability to interpret and diagnose genetic disease.

Our understanding of pathogenesis also increases, but at a slower pace, principally because of the difficulties in studying the intact organism. Murine (and other animal) models of human genetic disorders, produced by homologous recombination and other methods, are providing better opportunities to study whole-organism disease phenotypes[29,30] (see the section "Animal Models"). For example, the mucopolysaccharide type VII mouse has served as a very useful model to develop therapeutic approaches to lysosomal storage disorders.[31–36]

Therapy of genetic disease can be viewed in a biologic model, starting from the clinical phenotype and working back to the level of the defective gene. If our objectives are to *cure* the disease by ablating its cause, at this date, there are no cures of genetic diseases to report. The alternatives are to *control* (or *prevent*) its effects as well as we can; there are generic modalities to do that. Sometimes the best we can do is to provide supportive *care* (for patient and family).

Treatment at the Level of the Clinical Phenotype

Therapy at the level of clinical phenotype includes a variety of conventional medical practices and depends on a thorough understanding of the natural history of the disorder. Instruction and education of the patients, and use of various pharmacologic

*Adapted from Chapter 1 of this book's 7th edition.

interventions and surgical procedures, are all examples of symptomatic treatment. The basic genetic defect is not corrected, but a patient's problems are often ameliorated. Examples include education of patients about pharmacogenetic susceptibilities, instruction to limit exposure to ultraviolet radiation for patients with the various forms of albinism and xeroderma pigmentosa, administration of β-adrenergic blocking agents to patients with Marfan syndrome in attempts to prevent or delay dilation of the aortic root, and use of anticonvulsants for a variety of patients with neurodegenerative genetic disorders. A host of surgical interventions can provide benefits for patients with malformations, chondrodystrophies, and disorders with increased risk of malignancy in a particular organ.

Treatment at the Metabolite Level

Therapy at this level often involves nutritional or pharmacologic approaches and is closely dependent on an understanding of pathogenesis. Deficient function of a mutant enzyme may cause a disease phenotype (Fig. 5-5) because (1) the substrate accumulates to toxic levels (precursor toxicity), (2) an alternative metabolite is produced in excessive amounts (alternative pathway overflow), (3) there is reduced formation of the reaction product or some downstream metabolite (product deficiency), or (4) some combination of these possibilities coexists. Although this paradigm is most easily visualized for the effect of a mutant enzyme on fluxes through a metabolic pathway, it holds for all gene products that participate in dynamic molecular or biochemical interactions. The following are modalities of treatment as they relate to the pathophysiological process.

Substrate Restriction. Dietary alterations designed to restrict intake of a particular substrate may be effective if the pathophysiology involves accumulation of a toxic precursor when its major source can be controlled. Diets restricted in phenylalanine or in the branched-chain amino acids are effective in preventing the mental retardation associated with PKU and maple syrup urine disease, respectively, if the diets are started soon after birth and monitored in such a way that amounts of these substances just sufficient for normal growth are supplied (Chaps. 77 and 87). In addition to substrate restriction, it is often necessary to replace the deficient end product. Tyrosine supplementation to avoid tyrosine deficiency is a consideration in the treatment of PKU.[37] For reviews of dietary management of disorders of intermediary metabolism, see references 38–40. Patients on restricted diets, as in the treatment of maple syrup urine disease and hyperphenylalaninemia, have been noted to have decreased serum levels of trace elements such as zinc and selenium; also vitamin B_{12} deficiency has been observed.[38,41] It is also now recognized

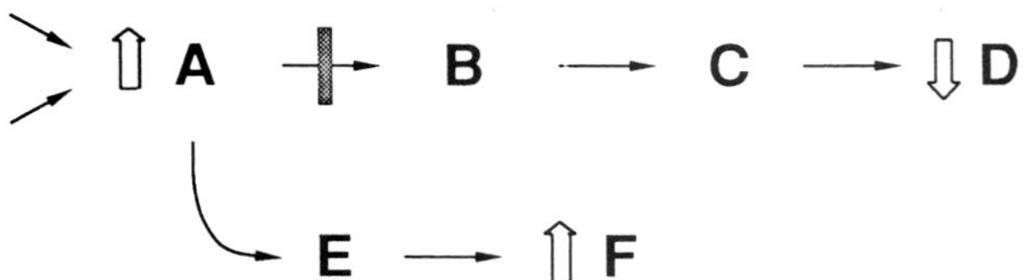

Fig. 5-5 Potential consequences of pathophysiological significance when there is a genetic defect in a metabolic pathway. A series of intermediates are formed from substrate A during its conversion to the pathway product, D. The enzymes catalyzing these reactions are indicated by *arrows*. A genetically inherited dysfunction of the enzyme converting metabolite A to B (indicated by the *hatched rectangle*) can lead to conversion of A to by products E and F via an alternative pathway. The enzyme deficiency may have pathophysiological consequences related to one of four possibilities: (1) accumulation of metabolite A (precursor toxicity), (2) overflow to products E or F (alternative, potentially toxic metabolites), (3) reduced formation of metabolite D (product deficiency), or (4) some combination of these three possibilities. (*Adapted from Chapter 1, 7th edition, of this work.*)

that long-chain polyunsaturated fatty acids such as arachidonic acid and docosahexaenoic acids (both present in breast milk) are involved in myelination and their supplementation, particularly in fat-restricted semisynthetic dietary formulas,[42,43] is a new consideration in the treatment of PKU, for example (Chap. 77).

Episodes of net protein catabolism (e.g., associated with intercurrent infections or trauma) complicate the therapy of organic acidurias by releasing large amounts of offending substrates and precursors from endogenous sources. Hospitalization for intravenous parenteral or nasogastric feeding or even dialysis may be required.

Propionic and methymalonic acidemia (Chap. 99) are two examples of inborn errors of metabolism involving disordered catabolism of the branched-chain amino acids: isoleucine, valine, and also methionine and threonine. Whereby mortality rates for these disorders was previously deemed high, affected individuals are now more effectively managed with a diet restricted in propionic acid precursors along with management of intercurrent illnesses. A favorable outcome is achieved if compliance is closely adhered to early in the course of the illness and with the assistance of nasogastric feeding and other adjunctive therapies.[44–48]

Early treatment of galactosemia (transferase-deficient form) reduces the infantile mortality rate of this disease, and lifetime restriction of dietary galactose corrects growth failure, prevents cataracts, and reduces, but does not completely prevent, harm to cognitive development (Chap. 72). Despite these overall improvements, early-treated galactosemic females also exhibit ovarian failure as a long-term complication of their disease.

Use of Alternative Pathways to Remove Toxic Metabolites. For disorders in which the pathophysiology involves accumulation of a toxic precursor or alternative pathway overflow, conversion of the offending metabolite can sometimes be promoted to a readily eliminated and less harmful substance. The effectiveness of this approach may be limited by the capacity of the converting system, and it is often combined with some dietary restriction of the offending substrate. Administration of benzoate, phenylbutyrate, or phenylacetate to patients with inborn errors of ureagenesis illustrates this approach (Chap. 87). Benzoate and phenylacetate (phenylbutyrate is converted to phenylacetate) undergo conjugation reactions with glycine and glutamine, respectively, forming hippurate and phenylacetylglutamine; the conjugates are readily excreted in urine, and they contain more waste nitrogen than their precursors, thereby providing a way to eliminate excess nitrogen. When used in conjunction with restrictions of dietary protein, this therapy reduces the accumulation of the toxic precursor (ammonium ion) characteristic of the urea-cycle disorders. Similar approaches include the use of glycine to conjugate with isovaleryl coenzyme A (CoA) in isovaleric acidemia (Chap. 93), carnitine to conjugate with accumulated CoA esters in various defects of fatty acid (Chap. 101) and organic acid metabolism, cysteamine to help eliminate cystine in cystinosis (Chap. 199), penicillamine to remove stored copper in Wilson disease (Chap. 126), and phlebotomy to remove iron in hemochromatosis (Chap. 127).

Metabolic Inhibitors. In certain disorders, such as those in which an alternative pathway overflows and produces a toxic level of a particular metabolite, toxicity can be reduced by inhibiting a prior step in the pathway. This may lead to accumulation of upstream substrates, which may be better tolerated if this approach is to be successful. Allopurinol is used to inhibit xanthine oxidase in gout and other situations characterized by excessive purine degradation and uric acid accumulation (Chaps. 106 and 107). Inhibition of xanthine oxidase lowers the level of uric acid and reduces the likelihood of nephropathy and gouty arthritis. Accumulation of xanthine is the biochemical consequence of xanthine oxidase inhibition, but this consequence is tolerated because xanthine is more soluble. Heterozygotes for mutations at the locus for the LDL receptor experience significant reductions in plasma cholesterol when treated with statin-type inhibitors of 3-hydroxy-3-methylglutaryl-CoA reductase, the enzyme catalyzing early- and rate-limiting steps in the synthesis of cholesterol (Chap. 120).

An outstanding example of effective therapy with an enzyme inhibitor is seen in the use of 2-(2-nitro-4-trifluoromethylbenzoyl)-1,3-cyclohexanedione (NTBC), an inhibitor of 4-hydroxyphenylpyruvate dioxygenase; its use in the treatment of type I hereditary tyrosinemia is dramatically changing the prognosis for affected patients (Chap. 79).

Replacement of Deficient Product. For those disorders in which the pathophysiology involves a product deficit, nutritional or pharmacologic approaches to replenish the metabolite may be effective. For example, deficient hepatic glucose production in patients with glycogen storage disease, type Ia, is treated by frequent feeding with glucose or glucose polymers (Chap. 71). Cornstarch, a slowly digested glucose polymer, acts as a timed-release source of glucose and is helpful in these patients. Similarly, administration of uridine to patients with impaired pyrimidine synthesis owing to hereditary orotic aciduria provides a source for the deficient product and corrects the macrocytic anemia caused by pyrimidine deficiency (Chap. 115); furthermore, product replacement here depresses pyrimidine biosynthesis by reducing orotic acid production and decreases orotic acid nephrolithiasis.

Two newly recognized metabolic disorders illustrate response to replacement therapy. The first is a deficiency in the synthesis of creatinine involving the enzyme guanidinoacetate methyltransferase (GAMT); supplementation with arginine and creatinine monohydrate increases brain creatinine and guanidinoacetate.[49] In the second disorder, 3-phosphoglycerate dehydrogenase deficiency, synthesis of serine (a nonessential amino acid) from 3-phosphoglycerate is affected, involving many other metabolic pathways[50]; oral treatment with serine supplements relieves symptoms of the disease.

Several inborn errors in hormone biosynthesis respond well to pharmacologic replacement of the deficient hormone. Examples include thyroid hormone replacement for patients with cretinism (Chap. 158) and corticosteroid administration in patients with the adrenogenital syndrome (Chap. 159). Biotin treatment of biotinidase-deficient patients is another example of product replacement therapy (Chap. 156): biotinidase deficiency disrupts recovery of biotin from biotinylated proteins, resulting in biotin loss and eventually biotin deficiency and impairment of the biotin-dependent carboxylases. Early diagnosis and treatment prevents all manifestation of this genetic disease.

Therapy at the Level of the Dysfunctional Protein

Therapy at this level involves either activation of a mutant enzyme or replenishment with its normal counterpoint.

Enzyme Activation with Vitamin Cofactors. Enhancement of the activity of a dysfunctional enzyme may be possible when the protein uses a vitamin cofactor that can be tolerated by a patient in pharmacologic amounts.

The enzymatically inactive enzyme protein (apoenzyme), when associated with its cofactor, is the active holoenzyme. The coenzyme is a small molecule; the polypeptide apoenzyme is a macromolecule with a tertiary or quarternary structure. The specific spatial relationship of coenzyme and apoenzyme enhances the catalytic action of the polypeptide toward its substrate.

Vitamin-responsive inborn errors of metabolism can result from a variety of mechanisms (Fig. 5-6). Coenzyme-dependent apoproteins are more likely to respond to pharmacologic doses of coenzyme when the aberrant state is the result of a "leaky" mutant phenotype involving synthesis of the coenzyme from the precursor vitamin or the result of (missense) mutations that either decrease the affinity of the apoenzyme for its cofactor or destabilize the protein in a way that can be partially overcome by substantially increasing the cofactor concentration in the environment of the

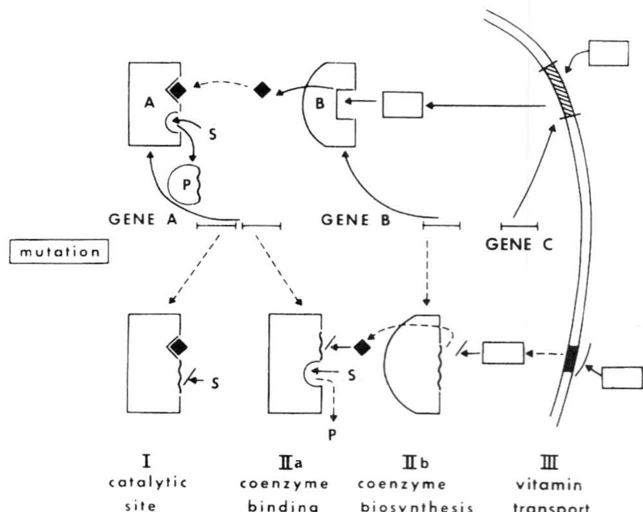

Fig. 5-6 Possible mechanisms to account for inherited dependence on pharmacologic doses of vitamin supplements. Gene A encodes apoenzyme A, which converts a metabolic substrate to a product. Gene B encodes an apoenzyme that converts a vitamin precursor to its coenzyme structure. Gene C encodes a membrane transport system responsible for uptake into the cell of the vitamin or coenzyme molecule. *Model I:* If mutation (e.g., missense) affects the function of the apoenzyme A, depressed residual function might be augmented by saturating the mutant apoenzyme with coenzyme to reduce its turnover. *Model IIa:* Mutation at locus A specifically perturbs the normal binding of coenzyme by apoenzyme. *Model IIb:* Mutation in gene B impairs biosynthesis of coenzyme from vitamin precursor; the kinetics of a leaky mutant are offset by increasing the cellular concentration of vitamin precursor. *Model III:* Mutation in gene C impairs uptake of coenzyme (or vitamin) by the cell. (*Adapted from Scriver.*[163] *Used by permission.*)

apoprotein. For example, about one-third of the cases of homocystinuria caused by a deficiency of cystathionine β-synthase recover a functionally significant amount of enzyme activity when treated with large doses of vitamin B_6 (50 to 500 mg pyridoxine/day) (Chap. 88). The actual increment in enzyme activity may be small but is sufficient to improve or even normalize metabolic flux in the *trans*-sulfuration pathway; activation of residual enzyme both reduces precursor (homocysteine) accumulation and increases product (cystathionine and cysteine supply). Other examples of this type of therapy include the use of thiamine in some cases of maple syrup urine disease (Chap. 87) and thiamine, biotin, or riboflavin for certain forms of lactic acidosis (Chap. 100). Thus, vitamin-responsive disorders may reflect either replacement of a deficient product (biotinidase deficiency) or enhancement of apoprotein function (cystathionine β-synthase deficiency).

To illustrate, at least 10 different inherited defects are known to impair the pathways of cobalamin (Cbl) transport and metabolism in humans: three affect its absorption and transport; the others affect utilization and coenzyme production (Chap. 165). In abnormalities of adenosine (Ado)-Cbl synthesis, most but not all respond to pharmacologic supplementation with cyanocobalamin or hydroxycobalamin.

Mutations creating defective binding of cofactor affect ornithine amino acid transferase (Chap. 83), holocarboxylase synthetase (Chap. 156), pyruvate dehydrogenase (Chap. 100), and branched-chain keto acid dehydrogenase enzymes (Chap. 87). At least four frequent mutations in the holocarboxylase synthetase gene affect the putative biotin-binding domain (Chap. 156). In one of the thiamine-responsive variants of maple syrup urine disease (Chap. 87), where the E1 α-subunit of the dehydrogenase contains the thiamine pyrophosphate (TPP)-binding site, the F215C mutation in the E2 subunit impairs interactions between E1 and

E2 subunits and alters efficient binding of thiamine coenzyme (thiamine pyrophosphate) on the E1 α-subunit.[51]

Vitamin Therapy for Complex Traits. The study of individuals with recessive vitamin-responsive inborn errors of metabolism has relevance for understanding the pathophysiology of complex traits. Rare severe mutations in the methylene tetrahydrofolate reductase gene result in an inborn error of metabolism with hypomethioninemia and hyperhomocystinemia (Chap. 158). On the other hand, a prevalent nucleotide polymorphism in the gene (c.677C → T) is associated with thermolability of the enzyme and, when combined with subnormal folate levels, is now seen to be associated with hyperhomocystinemia and an increased relative risk for coronary artery and peripheral vascular disease (Chap. 158).

Normal vascular homeostasis depends on endothelial elaboration of paracrine factors that prevent both platelet adhesion to the endothelial surface and inappropriate vasospasm. One important factor responsible for this is endothelium-derived nitric oxide (EDNO); the documentation of this effect merited a 1998 Nobel Prize in Medicine and Physiology.[52] Antioxidants improve EDNO-mediated arterial relaxation.[53–55] Reduced arterial tissue glutathione is found in experimental atherosclerosis.[56] EDNO activity may be improved by administration of the vitamin ascorbic acid, a potent free-radical scavenger in plasma, also known to reciprocally interchange with and spare glutathione.[55,57–59] An inverse relationship exists between dietary intake of flavonoids and mortality from coronary artery disease, and the use of vitamin C and the risk of coronary artery disease.[60–62] Cellular redox state may thus be an important regulator of EDNO action,[63] a potential target for therapy in patients with coronary artery disease that may become the chief cause of morbidity and mortality worldwide early in the next century.[64]

Protein Replacement Therapies.† Replacement of the mutant protein by the normal counterpart continues to be a major area of interest, but currently accounts for less than 1 percent of available therapies. To have some hope of success, the normal protein must be able to reach its appropriate physiological compartment. This is readily achieved when the target space is extracellular such as the gastrointestinal tract or plasma.

Delivery of exogenous enzyme to lysosomes is possible owing to organelle fusion.[65] The encouraging results in treatment of nonneuronopathic Gaucher disease with macrophage-targeted glucocerebrosidase illustrate how targeting a particular enzyme to a desired location (the lysosomes of macrophages), by taking advantage of a specific receptor (the mannose *N*-acetylglucosamine-specific receptor present on activated macrophages and reticular endothelial cells), can alter the disease phenotype (Chap. 146).

Other considerations for protein replacement therapies include the availability, stability, and immunogenicity of the protein administered. In a few instances, recombinant DNA technology is used to supply sufficient amounts of pure protein (e.g., human growth hormone): factor VIII for the treatment of hemophilia A (Chap. 172), α_1-antitrypsin for the treatment of its deficiency (Chap. 219), and phenylalanine ammonia lyase to degrade excess phenylalanine in PKU (Chap. 77) are produced by recombinant technology. This approach ensures adequate supplies of unique proteins and avoids the risk of transmitting contaminating pathogens to the recipients.

Cell-mediated protein replacement had been attempted earlier. Enzyme replacement for lysosomal diseases by infusions of plasma with leukocytes in patients with mucopolysaccharidoses types I and II was not sufficiently effective,[66] the use of transplanted fibroblasts was also unsuccessful[67] and amniotic transplantation treatment proved to be unpromising.[68]

†We thank Lisa Sniderman for assistance with retrieval of information for this and the following section.

An innovative approach to the problems of stability and avoidance of immune recognition exists in the treatment of severe combined immunodeficiency caused by adenosine deaminase deficiency (Chap. 109). Bovine adenosine deaminase covalently crosslinked to polyethylene glycol (PEG) is administered by intramuscular injection; the bulky hydrophilic PEG molecules coat the surface of the enzyme, preventing immune recognition while substrates and products can still diffuse through the PEG layer. Intramuscular injections weekly are sufficient to maintain high blood adenosine deaminase levels and achieve gradual improvement in immune function over several months.

Lysosomal storage material was diminished by direct replacement of the deficient lysosomal enzyme[69–71] in Hunter syndrome (MPS II), Hurler syndrome (MPS I), and Pompe disease fibroblasts. In addition, substantial headway has been reported in the treatment of animal models of mucopolysaccharidoses and other lysosomal disorders, such as Fabry disease[72] (leading in this case to a current phase I trial),[73] MPS VI,[74] MPS VII,[31] and in Niemann-Pick disease type B with amniotic cell implantation.[75] Intravenous recombinant α-L-iduronidase has been shown to reduce lysosomal storage in a canine model of MPS I.[74] Mutant MPS VII mice have received recombinant enzyme, with documented improvements in performance and reduction in hearing loss. Intravenous injections of recombinant β-glucuronidase, initiated at birth, significantly improved the histopathologic findings in brain and ear,[76] with relatively high levels of enzyme activity detected in many tissues, including the central nervous system, after 6 weeks of injections initiated at birth. Success in replacing recombinant α-L-iduronidase in mucopolysaccharidosis I with improvement of the somatic manifestations has also been reported.[77]

Pompe disease is a fatal disease of striated muscle caused by a deficiency of acidic α-glucosidase (GAA), a glycogen-degrading lysosomal enzyme (Chap. 135). Acid maltase-deficient Japanese quails served as a useful animal model for studies of enzyme replacement.[78] Exogenous recombinant human enzyme (rhGAA) dramatically improved the clinical symptoms and corrected glycogen accumulation in the heart. This study is the first to demonstrate that an exogenous enzyme can be targeted to muscle and produce muscle improvement; rhGAA is apparently taken up by muscle cells via mannose 6-phosphate-mediated endocytosis.

Organ Transplantation

Organ transplantation (or implantation of cells or stem cells) lies on the borderline between therapy by directed replacement of protein and by gene therapy. On the one hand, a transplanted organ or cell can supply the desired protein; on the other, it also brings new genetic information, although this is not integrated into the recipient's genome. Allogenic organ transplantation has been used with increasing success in the past decade and is probably the single most important modality to improve treatment of genetic disease in the past decade and a half.[22]

Transplantation of kidney, bone marrow, or liver has been used in a variety of genetic diseases. The development of more effective and specific immunosuppressants (particularly cyclosporine and FK506), and inadequacies of the more conventional therapies, both contribute to the increased interest in transplantation therapy. One-year graft and patient survival rates are at least 85 to 90 percent after liver transplantation in pediatric patients when the newer immunosuppressant regimens are used.[79–82] Innovative strategies, such as the use of transgenic animals as organ sources, are being proposed to resolve and overcome the immunologic barriers.[83] Small-scale trials are in progress involving the transplantation of fetal porcine central nervous tissue for the treatment of Parkinson disease, and islets of Langerhans for the treatment of diabetes.[84,85]

Residual long-term concerns of transplantation include higher risks of malignancies (especially lymphomas) associated with prolonged immunosuppression and the risk of kidney damage caused by cyclosporine. Shortage of donor organs is a practical limitation. Xenogeneic organ transplants are being considered, particularly as *bridge transplants* while awaiting donor organs.

Liver transplantations have been performed for patients with maple syrup urine disease, propionic acidemia, methylmalonic acidemia, and tyrosinemia.[86–88] The results indicate that liver transplantation can "cure" or at least greatly ameliorate hepatic and extrahepatic metabolic disorders.

In some instances, transplantation is done only to supply the recipient with a tissue that can provide a missing protein; in others, the transplant also replaces a damaged organ or protects the function of organs. Examples of the former include bone marrow transplants for lysosomal storage diseases, β thalassemia, and X-linked adrenoleukodystrophy, and liver transplantation for type I glycogen storage disease, familial hypercholesterolemia, and ornithine transcarbamoylase deficiency; examples of the latter include liver transplants in α_1-antitrypsin deficiency and hepatorenal tyrosinemia and kidney transplants in cystinosis. The distinction between protein and tissue replacement is relevant: when the intent is simply to provide a source of the required protein, partial liver transplants or even hepatocyte infusion into the portal vein or peritoneal cavity may be possible.

When the purpose of transplantation is to provide a source of the protein, the latter must be able to reach the tissue or organelle of pathophysiological significance. This is of special concern with bone marrow transplantation for lysosomal storage diseases. Here the transplanted marrow will presumably provide cells capable of repopulating the recipient's reticuloendothelial system; lysosomal enzymes released from the donor cells will then enter host cells by systems that deliver the enzyme to the proper subcellular compartment (i.e., lysosomes). Evidence from marrow transplants in patients with mucopolysaccharidosis indicates that both of these desired results will occur. What is not clear, however, is whether the transplant-derived cells or the enzymes they contain can cross the blood-brain barrier and repair the cerebral component of the disease phenotype. Since central nervous system involvement is a prominent feature of most lysosomal storage diseases, any failure to reach this tissue would severely limit the applicability of bone marrow transplantation, particularly in view of the attendant morbidity and mortality rates. Current experience with early bone marrow transplantation for Hurler syndrome shows the potential for success;[89,90] so also with early hematopoietic stem-cell transplantation in globoid cell leukodystrophy (galactocerebrosidase deficiency) with correction of somatic and cerebral phenotypes.[91]

Bone Marrow Transplantation: A Particular Illustration

Allogenic bone marrow transplantation has been used to treat blood dyscrasias, hematologic malignancies, and immunodeficiency states.[92] Transplantation of hematopoietic stem cells alters the course of some, but not all, lysosomal and peroxisomal disorders.

Bone marrow transplantation involves the replacement of enzymatically deficient cells with enzymatically normal cells that may be beneficial if the mononuclear phagocytic cell system is affected, as in Gaucher disease, or by transfer of an enzyme from normal cells to the enzyme-deficient cells by cell-cell contact. A major limitation occurs in the treatment of disorders affecting the central nervous system when donor enzyme is unable to penetrate the blood-brain barrier to enter brain tissue.

Trials of bone marrow transplantation have been used for a number of lysosomal disorders without significant effect (Tay-Sachs disease, Sandhoff disease, GM_1 gangliosidosis, and Farber disease),[93] although infiltration of donor-derived cells and circulating enzyme into brain tissue can still contribute to metabolic correction.[93,94]

Early onset of hematopoietic stem-cell transplantation, using bone marrow or umbilical cord blood, has been the only effective long-term treatment for Hurler syndrome.[89,95] Prior attempts at treatment produced minimal effects on skeletal abnormalities,[96–98] and long-term evaluations of psychomotor function yielded differing outcomes from deterioration to stabilization to improvement.[95,96,99,100] Peters and colleagues recently reported encouraging results,[89,101] with substrate reduction in liver, tonsils, conjunctiva, lung and, most importantly, in central nervous system consistent with maintenance of normal intelligence in a number of patients who underwent transplantation. The procedure, however, seldom results in improvement of skeletal or neurologic symptoms that are already established at the time of transplantation. Fleming and colleagues described their 5-year median follow-up experience using partially mismatched donors for allogenic bone marrow transplantation; the overall success in infants is 64 percent, with a graft failure rate of 36 percent. Success depends on matching donor enzyme levels.[102] The ultimate neuropsychological function is significantly lower when the donor is a carrier or the recipient engraftment of normal cells is incomplete.[95]

Bone marrow transplantation was not effective for the treatment of the skeletal abnormalities in Morquio disease (MPS IV);[103] it improved cardiopulmonary function, but not neurologic function or auditory capacity, in MPS VI (Maroteaux-Lamy).[103] Bone marrow transplantation has not been shown to affect outcome substantially for early-onset metachromatic leukodystrophy.[104–106] Adult-onset disease has been successfully engrafted at an early onset with correction not only of the enzyme deficiency but also stabilization and even reversal of some symptoms demonstrated by longitudinal neurologic, neuropsychological, neurophysiological, and neuroradiologic studies.[104,105] Treatment is most effective when it begins early in the course of the disease; response is related to genotype and familial history of the disease.[102,104,107]

Cell therapy, another approach that has emerged as a treatment for many diseases, involves placement of characterized mature cells or embryonic stem cells in a target organ in sufficient number to restore the function of damaged tissue or organs.[108] Differentiated cells may be replaced by regenerated cells from residual cycling stem cells. This includes hepatocytes and skeletal muscle and endothelial cells. The hematopoietic cell lineage is the prototypical example of the replacement of differentiated functioning cells. The donor cell may be genetically engineered to synthesize and to secrete a missing entity. The strategy used is as for *ex vivo* gene therapy. Accessible cells, such as fibroblasts or myoblasts for autografts, avoid the immunologic problems as demonstrated in animal models such as β-glucuronidase deficiency and mucopolysaccharidosis type VII.[109,110] Examples of cell therapy have been the use of pancreatic cells, delivery of factor IX to muscle or skin, and transplantation to the brain or spinal cord of cells engineered to secrete neurotropic factors. The primary sources of hematopoietic stem cells for clinical transplantation include bone marrow. More recently, umbilical cord blood has been used as an alternative source of hematopoietic support.[111]

Somatic Gene Therapy

Our views about the role of somatic gene therapy and the mechanisms for its implementation have evolved in recent years.[112–116] The range of disorders that might be considered amenable to this type of therapy has expanded from single-gene disorders to include cancer, AIDS, other infectious diseases, and atherosclerosis; in addition, recombinant protein therapies (e.g., with insulin, erythropoietin, or clotting factor) could be converted to *in vivo* production via somatic gene therapy. During the past 10 years, more than 300 clinical protocols and over 3000 patients have experienced somatic gene therapy (see references for gene therapy trial in progress at Wiley: http://www.wiley.co.uk/genetherapy; NIH database: http://www.nih.gov/od/ordc/protocol/htm); the experience with the genetic diseases discussed here is far less.

There are three approaches to somatic cell gene therapy:[113,117] (1) *ex vivo*, where cells are removed from the body and incubated with a vector, and the gene-engineered cells are then returned to the body; (2) *in situ*, where the vector is placed directly into the affected tissues; and (3) *in vivo*, where a vector would be injected directly into the bloodstream. Figure 5-6 describes the *in vivo* and *in vitro* strategies.

The repertoire of delivery systems, which began with retroviral vectors, has expanded to include vectors based on adenovirus, adeno-associated virus, herpes virus, vaccinia, and other agents, and nonviral systems such as liposomes, DNA-protein conjugates, and DNA-protein-defective virus conjugates. Emphasis has shifted from *ex vivo* modification of cells to *in vivo* delivery, although the pursuit continues in the attempt to achieve *ex vivo* manipulation of bone marrow cells, tumor cells, and cultured fibroblasts and epithelium.

Retroviral vectors efficiently integrate at random sites in the genome of dividing cells, permanently altering the recipient. Typically one or a few integrated copies of the recombinant vectors are found in each transduced cell. Currently, about 60 percent of approved clinical protocols for somatic gene therapy use retroviral vectors (see http://www.wiley.co.uk/genetherapy). Despite this, retroviral vectors have several disadvantages: first, they require dividing cells as a target; second, they are difficult to produce at titers high enough for most *in vivo* approaches; and, third, depending on its location, retroviral integration may adversely alter the expression of a gene in the area (e.g., a proto-oncogene) and produce a transformed cellular phenotype. Adenovirus vectors, in contrast, offer a high titer and a better ability to infect large numbers of cells *in vivo*, but there is concern about toxic effects on infected cells, and the therapeutic effect is transient, with expression for only days or weeks. Recent results with newer adenoviral vectors, in which nearly all adenoviral sequences have been removed, show promise for reduced toxicity and much longer expression (several months).[118,119] Vectors based on adeno-associated virus have the potential to provide high titer, safety, and long-term expression. Recent reports using adeno-associated viral vectors introduced into liver and skeletal muscle have shown long-term high-level expression.[120] It is believed that the recombinant virus persists as an episome in these cells, reducing the risk of malignant transformation. Vaccinia vectors and nonviral systems provide only transient expression, since they do not provide for DNA integration. Transient expression may be perfectly acceptable for some applications, such as eliciting an altered immune response to malignant cells or treatment of an acute disease process. There is need for new delivery systems or vectors that can be delivered efficiently *in vivo* (preferably by intravenous injection), can be targeted to specific cell types, can alter resting or dividing cells, and will persist indefinitely, whether by integration into the chromosome or by an extrachromosomal (episomal) mechanism.

Recent studies with lentiviral vectors are also promising in these regards.[121,122] DNA vectors may also be delivered directly without the aid of viruses by using pharmaceutical methods to target DNA vectors to specific cells and the nucleus. The approaches include the use of purified DNA via intramuscular injection (naked DNA, particles coated with DNA, cationic lipids, or other ligands) to target DNA to cell types and enhance their activity.

Gene Therapy Strategies

For somatic gene therapy, at least three strategies for regulation of expression of the therapeutic DNA can be distinguished. (1) A cDNA under the control of a foreign promotor can be utilized so that the product is synthesized at high levels but without normal regulation. (2) Alternatively, genomic DNA including the sequences necessary for proper regulation of the level and tissue specificity of expression of the therapeutic gene can be used. (3) Lastly, artificial *minigenes* that link genomic regulatory regions with cDNA encoding the entire open reading frame provide constructs that are of manageable size yet confirm proper regulation can be used. All of these strategies would typically involve random insertion of DNA sequences into the genome of the recipient, although expression of extrachromosomal sequences is also a possibility. An alternative strategy would be to use site-specific recombination so that the region of a gene containing the mutation would be replaced by the normal DNA sequence. This approach is in theory the best and, although challenging, is more feasible now that homologous recombination has been achieved in cultured cells. The choice of strategy will vary depending on the expression requirements of the disorder to be treated. In the case of enzyme or other protein deficiencies, where a modest increment in function may result in much improved homeostasis, any of the three nonhomologous approaches might suffice. By contrast, for hemoglobin disorders, the relative accessibility of bone marrow stem cells and the advantages of maintaining all the normal regulatory mechanisms make homologous recombination an extremely attractive goal. Various *in vivo* strategies for gene therapy are being explored. Several single-gene disorders are now candidates for gene therapy (see http://www.wiley.co.uk/genetherapy and reference 113) and a number of phase I clinical trials are in process (see NIH: http://www.nih.gov/od/ordc/protocol/hcm).

Life-threatening, recessive diseases involving marrow-derived cells (e.g., adenosine deaminase deficiency, chronic granulomatous disease, and leukocyte adhesion deficiency) are considered the preferred targets for somatic gene therapy, as are disorders in which extracellular products such as hormones, clotting factors, or other serum proteins might be produced by transfected cells. Dominant, neurologic disorders, such as Huntington disease, appear to be the least approachable at present. If proper regulation of globin genes could be achieved, sickle cell anemia and thalassemia would constitute important opportunities because of the accessibility of bone marrow for in vitro treatment, the frequency of the diseases, and their serious nature.

The following disorders illustrate progress:

- In *maple syrup urine disease*, retroviral gene transfer of a normal E1α cDNA was achieved in cultured lymphoblasts from a Mennonite patient homozygous for Y393N mutation.[123] The E1α construct completely restored decarboxylation activity in the transduced lymphoblasts and this activity persisted for up to 14 weeks (the duration of the study).
- In the *lethal X-linked disorder*, ornithine transcarboxylase deficiency adenovirus-mediated gene transfer was attempted.[124] A significant difference between treated and untreated mice in response to an NH_4Cl challenge in metabolic and behavioral parameters was observed. Protection lasted for at least 14 days. Phase I clinical trials are being considered for adults.
- Transfer of stable, functional acid β-glucosidase into cultured fibroblasts and transformed lymphoblasts, using a retroviral vector, has been accomplished for Gaucher disease (Chap. 146). Phase I gene therapy trials are currently under way for this disease.
- Gene therapy trials are currently under way in animal models, and with *in vitro* systems, for many lysosomal disorders, including globoid cell leukodystrophy, metachromatic leukodystrophy, and Niemann-Pick type A.[125–129] Retroviral transfer and high levels of expression of the human α-subunit gene have been achieved in murine Hex A-deficient (Tay-Sachs) fibroblasts.[130] The transduced cells showed restoration of the enzymatic activity following heterodimer formation between the human α chain and the murine β chain. The α chain was secreted in the culture medium and taken up by Hex A-deficient cells via mannose 6-phosphate receptor binding, allowing for the restoration of intracellular Hex A activity in nontransduced cells.

Gene Therapy for Cancer, AIDS, Atherosclerosis, and Pharmacotherapy. Several protocols for gene-based treatment of cancer have been initiated. Strategies include alteration of cancer cells or other host cells to produce cytokines or other molecules to alter the host response to the malignant cells;

expression of antigens (e.g., allogeneic HLA proteins) on cancer cells to induce a host immune response; insertion of tumor suppressor gene sequences or other sequences to slow cell growth; introduction of genes into tumor cells to allow selective killing by chemotherapy (e.g., selective killing by ganciclovir of tumor cells transfected with thymidine kinase); and introduction of drug resistance genes into normal cells (e.g., marrow) to facilitate more aggressive chemotherapy. The *immunomodulatory* approaches show significant promise and are the basis of numerous research protocols.

Strategies for gene therapy of marrow stem cells to introduce resistance to HIV, or otherwise blunt expression of its effects, have been proposed. There is evidence in transgenic mice that overexpression of apolipoprotein A-I can protect against atherosclerosis,[131] and various strategies are being proposed for preventing and reversing atherosclerosis, whether of single-gene or multifactorial origin. As previously mentioned, recombinant proteins could be produced *in vivo* rather than *ex vivo* with repeated injection. Transient and rapid expression of therapeutic proteins after injection of a viral or nonviral vector could greatly expand current therapeutic avenues.

Gene therapy protocols have been applied to prevalent genetic disorders such as cystic fibrosis and Duchenne muscular dystrophy. Recently, the delivery of angiogenic factors into ischemic heart of muscle tissue has provided an indication of potential applicability to previously untreatable problems.[132,133]

ANIMAL MODELS

Much of the remarkable progress in genetic research over the last two decades has resulted from reductive strategies focusing on specific genes or proteins. Ultimately, however, we must understand how individual genes and their protein products function in intact organisms, interacting with other genes and gene products in the complex networks that achieve normal development and physiological homeostasis. As regards treatment, we want to understand how defects in one or a few genes disrupt normal development and/or physiological homeostasis to produce genetic disease; that is, we want to understand pathogenesis and use this knowledge to devise rational and effective treatments for our patients. These goals require integrative rather than reductive strategies and depend heavily on the use of animal models of genetic disease.

Until about a decade ago, identification of animals with genetic disorders depended on the recognition by astute observers of deviant phenotypes arising spontaneously, as the result of random mutagenesis methods, or as products of selective breeding strategies aimed at producing animals with phenotypes such as obesity or hypertension. Although inefficient, these methods led to the identification of useful models for a host of human genetic disorders in a variety of animal species. In particular, breeders of the laboratory mouse, *Mus musculus*, have identified scores of spontaneously arising mutants, many of which have been established as models of human genetic diseases.[134,135]

More recently, advances in technologies for the manipulation of mouse gametes and pluripotent embryonic stem cells have opened the way for the rational, preplanned development of specific models, greatly reducing dependence on serendipity.[136,137] Methods include transgenic approaches in which the introduced DNA inserts randomly in the host genome, and homologous recombination in which the introduced DNA inserts precisely into its normal genomic location. Depending on the structure of the introduced DNA (the targeting construct), this can result in disruption of the endogenous wild-type gene (a *knockout*) or replacement of the wild-type target gene by a specific mutant allele (a *knockin*). The extensive collection and characteristics of spontaneous and induced mutants now available has led to the mouse becoming the leading model for studying biologic processes in mammals.[136]

Relevant databases are the Harwell MRC and Jackson Laboratory databases (http://www.jax.org/; http:/www.gsf.de/isg/groups/enu/enu_cpt.html; http://www.mgc.har.mrc.ac.uk/mutabase/).

In addition to their value in disease gene identification and in sorting out the variables involved in complex traits, mouse models have played a major role in the recent progress in treating genetic disease. They provide the opportunity to investigate whole animal pathophysiology and to perform experimental trials under highly controlled conditions.

How a particular molecular or biochemical defect produces a particular clinical phenotype often requires an integrative approach only possible with *in vivo* systems. Low disease frequency, genetic heterogeneity, variation in clinical severity, and difficulty in obtaining samples of affected tissue at all stages of a disease are some of the problems that make these studies difficult to perform in human patients, and mouse models provide an excellent alternative. For example, although we have considerable knowledge regarding the clinical features, biochemical abnormalities, and molecular defects in PKU, we still are unsure of the mechanism(s) by which elevation in blood phenylalanine produces the principal phenotypic feature: severe mental retardation. The recently described ethylnitrosourea-induced mouse models[138] of PKU enable one to study neurotransmitter metabolism and myelin formation, for example, and they provide insight into the pathogenesis of the mental retardation in human PKU.

An observation from certain gene knockout experiments is particularly relevant to understanding pathogenesis: null mutations in some genes cause markedly different phenotypic consequences in humans and mice.[134,137] For example, mice with a complete knockout of the hypoxanthine phosphoribosyltransferase (HPRT) gene exhibit little, if any, of the mental defects and self-injurious behavior characteristic of human patients with the same genetic defect (Lesch-Nyhan syndrome), and the dystrophin-deficient *mdx* mouse does not have the obvious, progressive muscle weakness characteristic of the cognate human disorder: Duchenne muscular dystrophy. These examples of discordance in clinical phenotypes are every bit as interesting and useful as models with well-matched phenotypes. Metabolic and genetic redundancy, short absolute life span, and environmental differences are all possible explanations for this lack of concordance.[139] It should be obvious that elucidation of the basis for these species-dependent differences in response to a particular genetic defect will reveal important information about pathogenesis and may suggest therapeutic strategies.

Animal models also provide opportunities to study novel treatments of genetic diseases. For example, the recent explosion in activity in gene therapy research is linked closely to availability of animal models. Gene therapy successes have been reported in animal models for hypercholesterolemia,[140,141] cystic fibrosis,[142] ornithine transcarbamoylase deficiency,[124] and MPS VII.[33,36] In careful and well-controlled studies, these investigators have examined the efficacy of enzyme infusions, bone marrow transplantation, and germ-line and somatic gene therapies of various durations and in animals of various ages. Studies of this type are necessary steps along the way from laboratory bench to treatment trials in human patients.

TREATMENT IN TRANSITION

Phenotypes of genetic disease have a taxonomy, as documented in the McKusick Catalogs. Phenotypic taxonomy is accounted for by two forms of genotypic variation: allelic heterogeneity, and locus heterogeneity. From this, it follows that treatment must be adapted to the patient with the disease — that is, to the person's particular genotype — while recognizing that the treatment will be designed to modify the disease process that the patient has. This is not a new idea. Successful treatment of bacterial pneumonia depends on identification of the organism responsible for the particular illness and determination of the antibiotic sensitivity of the particular strain of the organism infecting the patient, considerations that lead to informed selection of the appropriate antibiotic for the treatment.

In addition to selecting the particular modality of therapy, and the specific agent in the generic modality, there is the additional problem of compliance with the treatment. Patients require counseling and support.[143] In the treatment of genetic disease, *care* is as important as *control* until such time as there are *cures*. As the majority of genes for the conditions without a response to treatment described in the previous studies[22] are now mapped, prenatal diagnosis may be provided by molecular testing. Prenatal diagnosis and early detection will also provide opportunities for treatment, as has been shown for multiple carboxylase deficiency,[144] methylmalonic acidemia (B_{12} responsive),[145,146] methylcobalamin deficiency,[147] and congenital adrenal hyperplasia.[148]

Meantime, new developments bring encouragement as illustrated by the following examples:

- The design and use of specific drugs to match the specific options associated with allelic variation are nicely illustrated in the case of cystic fibrosis.[9] Different drugs can be considered to match the particular effect of the mutation on the biosynthesis and function of the CFTR gene product if one cannot modify the function of the mutant protein itself. There may be drugs to compensate, by amplifying activities of redundant physiological functions such as other ion channels. In this or any other disease where a missense mutation alters folding of the protein, thus affecting its function, synthetic chaperones such as glycerol[149] might restore some degree of function.
- Wherever there are redundant genes or functions, there is the possibility to amplify their activities to substitute for loss of the primary function. For example, 5-azocytidine, hydroxyurea, sodium butyrate, and sodium 4-phenylbutyrate amplify fetal hemoglobin production and can play a role in the treatment of hemoglobinopathies.[150–152] 4-Phenylbutyrate has been used in cultured cells to stimulate synthesis of a protein with a function that overlaps with that of the deficient protein in X-linked adrenoleukodystrophy.[153] Studies of Tay-Sachs disease by using knockout models[154,155] suggest that amplification of sialidase activity could prevent GM_2-ganglioside accumulation. In these examples, the approach is either experimental, even hypothetical, or still very limited in its application to human patients. The examples are illustrations to show how more detailed knowledge of the variant and normal cellular biology and biochemistry might lead to new therapies.
- In a number of genetic diseases, particularly slowly progressive neurodegenerative disorders, the phenotype appears to be mediated by aberrant apoptosis, a process dependent on activation of cellular caspases. Specific inhibitors of caspase function prevent apoptosis-associated liver failure in an animal model of hereditary tyrosinemia type I.[156] Caspase inhibitors may thus prove to be adjunctive therapy for certain genetic diseases.
- Certain syndromes of mysterious origin are newly recognized to be specific disorders of metabolic and developmental pathways, and thus accessible to therapy in ways we had not considered previously. For example, the carbohydrate-deficient glycoprotein syndrome, in at least one of its forms, responds to mannose supplementation.[157] A patient with Niemann-Pick type C, perhaps with a particular form of that disease, has responded to statin therapy with altered progression of the neurologic features of that disease.[158] The Smith-Lemli-Opitz syndrome is explained by deficient function of microsomal 7-dehydrocholesterol δ-reductase; aggressive cholesterol supplementation improves the clinical and metabolic phenotype in this disease.[159,160]
- The value of an improved understanding of the pathophysiological mechanisms of disease is also exemplified by recent studies of hypertrophic cardiomyopathy. Olson and his colleagues[161,162] have shown that a variety of pathologic stimuli (e.g., hypertension, myocardial infarction, and genetic defects in the contractile proteins) ultimately produce hypertrophic cardiomyopathy by a common pathway involving the calcium-dependent phosphatase, calcineurin, which in turn activates certain transcription factors. Previous work done for other reasons had shown that calcineurin is inhibited by cyclosporine and FK506, drugs currently in use for prevention of organ rejection following transplantation. In convincing studies done in a variety of animal models, these investigators have shown that cyclosporine or FK506 can completely prevent the development of certain forms of hypertrophic cardiomyopathy. These results have led to ongoing clinical trials in humans and show how increased understanding of pathophysiology may identify previously unsuspected and highly approachable targets for pharmacologic intervention.

Further illustrations of successful *transitions in therapy* can be found in both old and new chapters in the current edition of this work.

CONCLUSION

The term *Homo modificans* is used in this chapter to describe a feature of *Homo sapiens sapiens*; it recognizes that human beings purposefully modify their experience. In the 20th century, one result has been an increase in the heritability of our diseases. Accordingly, the relative importance of genetic causes in human disease is relatively greater than it was in the past. As our ability to recognize and identify those diseases and their causes increases, our ability to treat them successfully should also increase.

General principles for the treatment of genetic disease were established a generation ago. Those principles identify modalities that, in practice, modify the effect of a mutant gene in the affected individual. Although the principles of treatment are reasonably well understood, consistent and successful application of those principles in practice for many of these disorders remains elusive.

The goal of treatment for genetic diseases, in every case, is to restore homeostasis through time and in the particular compartment relevant to the pathogenic process. Experience proves that it has been difficult with the existing modalities of treatment to reestablish normal homeostasis in most genetic diseases. Failure to do so is usually explained by the inability of the modality to penetrate the compartment where dishomeostasis begins or to introduce the process of treatment early enough to prevent deviant development and function. Measurements of the outcome of treatment undertaken over the past 15 years in three separate studies show significant progress but, where there is disappointment, it is usually because treatment does not restore homeostasis adequately.

The basic modalities of treatment, up to now, have operated at four general levels: (1) At the clinical level are opportunities for surgical corrections and repairs. (2) At the metabolic level, it may be possible to prevent substrate accumulation and toxicity or to repair product depletion and the effects of the corresponding deficiency. (3) At the protein level, it may be possible to activate or stabilize a mutant protein with pharmacologic doses of coenzyme or replace lost function with normal protein. (4) At the cellular level, organ, tissue, or cellular transplantation/implantation may repopulate the body with integrated and regulated gene product activity. The major progress accounting for improved treatment of human genetic diseases over the past decade is explained by transplantation in its various forms.

At present, there are no unambiguous examples of successful somatic gene therapy.

As we proceed from structural genomics to functional genomics, the focus will shift from DNA to proteins. How a mutation affects the structure and function of a protein is already a major area of inquiry. It follows that therapies to neutralize the effect of mutation on the protein itself will be of increasing interest. Some of this knowledge will be converted through combinatorial drug design techniques into agents that fit and modify the variant protein phenotype (either structural or functional). Early work in this direction looks promising with applications to patient care.[26–28]

Complex traits account for the majority of patients with genetic disease. As their pathogenic mechanisms are broken down into their components, the principles and practices developed for single-gene diseases will find new applications in the vastly larger community of patients with complex trait diseases. Again, there is reason for optimism as shown by progress with treatment of coronary artery disease over the past generation. There are thoughtful scientists who dare to pose this question with some optimism: "Heart attacks: Gone by the end of the 20th century?"[6] Perhaps, then it is reasonable to expect an affirmative answer to this question: "Can we greatly improve the treatment of genetic diseases within the next quarter-century?"

REFERENCES

1. Ridley M: A survey of science: The edge of ignorance. *Economist* **16**:1, 1991.
2. Scriver CR: Treatment of inborn errors of metabolism: The nature:nurture argument specified, in Crawfurd MD, Gibbs DA, Watts RWE (eds): *Advances in the Treatment of Inborn Errors of Metabolism*. New York, John Wiley and Sons, 1982, p 289.
3. Cannon WB: *The Wisdom of the Body*. New York, WW Norton, 1932.
4. Diabetes Control and Complications Trial Research Group: The effect of intensive treatment of diabetes on the development and progression of long-term complications in insulin-dependent diabetes mellitus. *N Engl J Med* **329**:977, 1993.
5. Sarkissian CN, Shao Z, Blain F, et al: A different approach to treatment of phenylketonuria: Phenylalanine degradation with recombinant phenylalanine ammonia lyase. *Proc Natl Acad Sci USA* **96**:2339, 1999.
6. Brown MS, Goldstein JL: Heart attacks: Gone with the century? *Science* **272**:629, 1996.
7. Lindstedt S, Holme E, Lock EA, et al: Treatment of hereditary tyrosinemia type 1 by inhibition of 4-hydrophenylpyruvate dioxygenase. *Lancet* **340**:813, 1992.
8. Glorieux FH, Bishop NJ, Plotkin H, et al: Cyclic administration of pamidronate in children with severe osteogenesis imperfecta. *N Engl J Med* **329**:947, 1998.
9. Delaney SJ, Wainwright BJ: New pharmaceutical approaches to the treatment of cystic fibrosis. *Nat Med* **92**:392, 1996.
10. Plunkett MJ, Ellman JA: Combinatorial chemistry and new drugs. *Sci Am* **276**:68, 1997.
11. Jacob F: Evolution and tinkering. *Science* **196**:1161, 1977.
12. Scriver CR: American Pediatric Society Presidential Address 1995: Disease, war and biology: Languages for medicine — and pediatrics. *Pediatr Res* **38**:819, 1995.
13. Harper PS, Clarke AJ: Genetics, society and clinical practice. *Nat Med* **4**:857, 1998.
14. Scriver CR: The Canadian Rutherford Lecture: An evolutionary view of disease in man. *Proc R Soc Lond [Biol]* **220**:273, 1984.
15. Baird PA, Anderson TW, Newcombe HB, et al: Genetics disorders in children and young adults: A population study. *Am J Hum Genet* **42**:677, 1988.
16. Scriver CR: Treatment in medical genetics, in Crow JF, Neel JV (eds): *Proceedings of the Third International Congress Human Genetics*. Baltimore, Johns Hopkins University Press, 1967, p 45.
17. Pardes H, Manton KG, Lander ES, et al: Effects of medical research on healthcare and the economy. *Science* **283**:36, 1999.
18. OMIM (Online Mendelian Inheritance in Man): http://www.ncbi.nlm.nih.gov/omim, 1998.
19. World Health Organization (WHO): *International Classification of Impairments, Disabilities, and Handicaps*. Geneva, WHO, 1980.
20. Costa T, Scriver CR, Childs B: The effect of Mendelian disease on human health: A measurement. *Am J Med Genet* **21**:231, 1985.
21. Hayes A, Costa T, Scriver CR, et al: The effect of Mendelian disease on human health: II. Response to treatment. *Am J Med Genet* **21**:243, 1985.
22. Treacy E, Childs B, Scriver CR: Response to treatment in hereditary metabolic disease: 1993 survey and 10-year comparison. *Am J Hum Genet* **56**:359, 1995.
23. Childs B, Scriver CR: Age at onset and cause of disease. *Perspect Biol Med* **29**:437, 1986.
24. Tuchman M: Persistent Acitrullinemia after liver transplantation for carbamylphosphate synthetase deficiency. *N Engl J Med* **320**:1498, 1989.
25. Rabier D, Narcy C, Bardet J, et al: Arginine remains an essential amino acid after liver transplantation in urea cycle enzyme deficiencies. *J Inherited Metab Dis* **14**:277, 1991.
26. Charlton BG: Natural kinds, natural history and the clinician-researcher. *Q J Med* **90**:707, 1997.
27. Goldstein JL, Brown MS: The clinical investigator — bewitched, bothered, and bewildered — but still beloved. *J Clin Invest* **99**:2803, 1997.
28. Flowers CR, Melman KL: Clinical investigators as critical determinants in pharmaceutical innovation. *Nat Med* **3**:136, 1997.
29. Paigen K: A miracle enough: The power of mice. *Nat Med* **1**:215, 1995.
30. Searle AG, Edwards JH, Hall JG: Mouse homologues of human hereditary disease. *J Med Genet* **31**:1, 1994.
31. Sands MS, Vogler C, Kyle JW, et al: Enzyme replacement for murine mucopolysaccharidosis type VII leads to improvements in behaviour and auditory function. *J Clin Invest* **93**:2324, 1994.
32. Snyder EY, Taylor RM, Wolfe JH: Neuronal progenitor cell engraftment corrects lysosomal storage throughout the MPS VII mouse brain. *Nature* **374**:367, 1995.
33. Wolfe JH, Sands MS, Barker JE, et al: Reversal of pathology in murine mucopolysaccharidosis type VII by somatic gene transfer. *Nature* **360**:753, 1992.
34. Li T, Davidson BL: Phenotypic correction in retinal pigment epithelium in murine mucopolysaccharidosis VII by adenovirus-mediated gene transfer. *Proc Natl Acad Sci USA* **92**:7700, 1995.
35. Taylor RM, Wolfe JM: Decreased lysosomal storage in the adult MPS VII mouse brain in the vicinity of grafts of retroviral vector-corrected fibroblasts secreting high levels of β-glucuronidase. *Nat Med* **3**:771, 1997.
36. Vogler C, Sands MS, Levy B, et al: Enzyme replacement with recombinant β-glucuronidase in murine mucopolysaccharidosis type VII: Impact of therapy during the first six weeks of life on subsequent lysosomal storage, growth and survival. *Pediatr Res* **39**:1050, 1996.
37. Koch R: Tyrosine supplementation for phenylketonuria treatment. *Am J Clin Nutr* **64**:974, 1996.
38. Acosta PB: Nutrition studies in treated infants and children with phenylketonuria: Vitamins, minerals, trace elements. *Eur J Pediatr* **155**:S136, 1996.
39. Francis DEM: *Diets for Sick Children*. 4th ed. Oxford, Blackwell Scientific, 1998.
40. Prasad C, Dalton L, Levy H: Role of diet therapy in management of hereditary metabolic diseases. *Nutr Res* **18**:391, 1998.
41. Hanley WB, Feigenbaum ASJ, Clarke JTR, et al: Vitamin B_{12} deficiency in adolescents and young adults with phenylketonuria. *Eur J Pediatr* **155**:S145, 1996.
42. Farquharson J, Cockburn F, Patrick WA, et al: Infant cerebral cortex phospholipid fatty-acid composition and diet. *Lancet* **340**:810, 1992.
43. Galli C, Agostini C, Mosconi C, et al: Reduced plasma C-20 and C-22 fatty acids in children with phenylketonuria during dietary intervention. *J Pediatr* **119**:562, 1991.
44. Leonard JV: The management and outcome of propionic and methylmalonic acidaemia. *J Inherit Metab Dis* **18**:430, 1995.
45. Van der Meer SB, Poggi F, Spada M, et al: Clinical outcome and long-term management of 17 patients with propionic acidemia. *Eur J Pediatr* **155**:205, 1996.
46. Van der Meer SB, Poggi F, Spada M, et al: Clinical outcome of long-term management of patients with vitamin B_{12}-unresponsive methylmalonic acidemia. *J Pediatr* **125**:903, 1994.
47. Dixon MA, Leonard JV: Intercurrent illness in inborn errors of intermediary metabolism. *Arch Dis Child* **67**:1387, 1992.
48. Treacy E, Arbour L, Chessex P, et al: Glutathione deficiency as a complication of methylmalonic acidemia: Response to high doses of ascorbate. *J Pediatr* **129**:445, 1996.
49. Stockler S, Isbrandt D, Hanefeld F, et al: Guanidinoacetate methyltransferase deficiency: The first inborn error of creatine metabolism in man. *Am J Hum Genet* **58**:914, 1996.
50. Jaeken J, Detheux M, Van Maldergem L, et al: 3-Phosphoglycerate dehydrogenase deficiency: An inborn error of serine biosynthesis. *Arch Dis Child* **74**:542, 1996.
51. Fischer CW, Lau KS, Fischer CR, et al: A 17-bp insertion and a $Phe^{215} \rightarrow Cys$ missense mutation in the dihydrolipoyl transacetylase (E2) mRNA from a thiamine-response maple syrup urine disease patient WG-34. *Biochem Biophys Res Commun* **174**:804, 1991.

52. Furchgott RF, Ignarro LJ, Murad F: Physiology or medicine: A versatile gas. *Sci Am* January 18, 1999.
53. Keaney JF Jr, Gaziano JM Jr, Xu A, et al: Dietary antioxidants preserve endothelium-dependent vessel relaxation in cholesterol-fed rabbits. *Proc Natl Acad Sci USA* **90**:11880, 1993.
54. Simon BC, Haudenschild CC, Cohen RA: Preservation of endothelium-dependent relation in atherosclerotic rabbit aorta by probucol. *J Cardiovasc Pharmacol* **21**:893, 1993.
55. Vita JA, Frei B, Holbrook M, et al: L-2-oxothiazolidine-4-carboxylic acid reverses endothelial dysfunction in patients with coronary artery disease. *J Clin Invest* **6**:1408, 1998.
56. Ma XL, Lopez BL, Liu GL, et al: Hypercholesterolemia impairs a detoxification mechanism against peroxynitrate and renders the vascular tissue more susceptible to oxidative injury. *Circ Res* **80**:894, 1997.
57. Martensson JJ, Han EW, Gokce N, et al: Glutathione delays the onset of scurvy in ascorbate-deficient guinea pigs. *Proc Natl Acad Sci USA* **90**:317, 1993.
58. Levine GN, Frei B, Koulouris SN, et al: Ascorbic acid reverses endothelial vasomotor dysfunction in patients with coronary artery disease. *Circulation* **96**:1107, 1996.
59. Ting HH, Timimi FK, Haley EA, et al: Vitamin C improves endothelium-dependent vasodilation in forearm resistance vessels of humans with hypercholesterolemia. *Circulation* **95**:2617, 1997.
60. Hertoz MG, Kromhout D, Aravanis C, et al: Flavonoid intake and long-term risk of coronary heart disease and cancer in the seven countries study. *Arch Intern Med* **155**:381, 1995.
61. Knekt P, Jarvinen R, Reutenen A, et al: Flavonoid intake and coronary mortality in Finland: A cohort study. *BMJ* **312**:478, 1996.
62. Todd S, Woodward M, Bolton-Smith C: An investigation of the relationship between antioxidant vitamin intake and coronary heart disease in men and women using logistic regression analysis. *J Clin Epidemiol* **48**:307, 1995.
63. Kinsella JE, Frankel EN, German JB, et al: Possible mechanisms for the protective role of antioxidants in wine and plant foods. *Food Technol* **47**:85, 1993.
64. Reddy KS, Yusuf S: Emerging epidemic of cardiovascular disease in developing countries. *Circulation* **97**:596, 1998.
65. Rattazzi MC, Dobrenis K: Enzyme replacement: Overview and prospects, in Desnick RJ (ed): *Treatment of Genetic Diseases*. London, Churchill Livingstone, 1991, p 131.
66. Di Ferrante N, Nichols BL, Donnelly PV: Induced degradation of glycosaminoglycans in Hurler's and Hunter's syndromes by plasma infusion. *Proc Natl Acad Sci USA* **68**:303, 1971.
67. Gibbs DA, Spellacy E, Tompkins R et al: A clinical trial of fibroblast transplantation for the treatment of mucopolysaccharidoses. *J Inherit Metab Dis* **6**:67, 1983.
68. Yeager AM, Singer HS, Buck JR, et al: A therapeutic trial of amniotic epithelial cell implantation in patients with lysosomal storage diseases. *Am J Med Genet* **22**:347, 1985.
69. Bielicki J, Hopwood JJ, Wilson PJ, et al: Recombinant human iduronate 2-sulphatase: Correction of mucopolysaccharidosis type II fibroblasts and characterization of the purified enzyme. *Biochem J* **289**:241, 1993.
70. Unger EG, Durrant J, Anson DS, et al: Recombinant α-L-iduronidase: Characterization of the purified enzyme and correction of mucopolysaccharidosis type 1 fibroblasts. *Biochem J* **304**:43, 1994.
71. Fuller M, Van der Ploeg A, Reuser JJ, et al: Isolation and characterization of a recombinant, precursor form of lysosomal acid α-glucosidase. *Eur J Biochem* **234**:903, 1995.
72. Ioannou YA, Zeidner KM, Friedman B, et al: Fabry disease: Enzyme replacement therapy in α-galactosidase A-deficient mice. *Am J Hum Genet* **59**:15(A71), 1996.
73. Kakkis ED, McEntee MF, Schmidtchen A, et al: Long term and high-dose trials of enzyme replacement in the canine model of mucopolysaccharidosis type I. *Biochem Mol Med* **58**:156, 1996.
74. Crawley AC, Niedzielski KH, Isaac EL, et al: Enzyme replacement therapy from birth in a feline model of mucopolysaccharidosis type VI. *J Clin Invest* **99**:651, 1997.
75. Bembi B, Comelli M, Scaggiante B, et al: Treatment of sphingomyelinase deficiency by repeated implantations of amniotic epithelial cells. *Am J Med Genet* **44**:527, 1992.
76. O'Connor LH, Erway LC, Vogler CA, et al: Enzyme replacement therapy for murine mucopolysaccharidosis type VII leads to improvements in behaviour and auditory function. *J Clin Invest* **10**:1394, 1998.
77. Kakkis E, Muenzer J, Tiller G, et al: Recombinant α-L-iduronidase replacement therapy in mucopolysaccharidosis: I. Results of a human clinical trial [abstr]. *Am J Hum Genet* **63**:58(A128), 1998.
78. Kikuchi T, Yang HW, Pennybacker M, et al: Clinical and metabolic correction of Pompe disease by enzyme therapy in acid maltase-deficient quail. *J Clin Invest* **101**:827, 1998.
79. Lee H, Vacanti JP: Liver transplantation and its long-term management in children. *Pediatr Clin North Am* **43**:99, 1996.
80. Tzakis AG, Fung JJ, Todo S, et al: Use of FK506 in pediatric patients. *Transplant Proc* **23**:924, 1991.
81. Salt A, Noble-Jamieson G, Barnes ND, et al: Liver transplantation in 100 children: Cambridge and King's College Hospital Series. *BMJ* **304**:416, 1992.
82. Kalayoglu M, Stratta RJ, Sollinger HW, et al: Liver transplantation in infants and children. *J Pediatr Surg* **24**:70, 1989.
83. Platt JL: New directions for organ transplantation. *Nature* **392**:11, 1998.
84. Deacon T, Schumacher J, Dinsmore J, et al: Histological evidence of fetal pig neural cell survival after transplantation into a patient with Parkinson's disease. *Nat Med* **3**:350, 1997.
85. Groth CG: Transplantation of porcine fetal pancreas to diabetic patients. *Lancet* **345**:735, 1995.
86. Jan D, Laurent J, Lacaille F, et al: Liver transplantation in children with inherited metabolic disorders. *Transplant Proc* **27**:1706, 1995.
87. Rabier D, Narcy C, Revillon HP, et al: Normalization of plasma branched-chain amino acids (BCAAs) after liver transplantation in maple syrup urine disease (MSUD) [abst]. Proceedings of 29th Meeting of Society for the Study of Inborn Errors of Metabolism, London, Sept 10–13, 1991. **129**, 1991.
88. Schlenzig JS, Poggi-Travert F, Laurent J, et al: Liver transplantation in two cases of propionic acidaemia. *J Inherit Metab Dis* **18**:448, 1995.
89. Peters C, Balthazor M, Shapiro E, et al: Outcome of unrelated donor bone marrow transplantation in 40 children with Hurler syndrome. *Blood* **87**:4894, 1996.
90. Peters C, Shapiro EG, Krivit W: Hurler syndrome: Past, present, and future. *J Pediatr* **133**:7, 1998.
91. Krivit W, Shapiro EG, Peters C, et al: Hematopoietic stem-cell transplantation in globoid-cell leukodystrophy. *N Engl J Med* **338**:1119, 1998.
92. Hong R: Bone marrow transplantation. *Adv Pediatr* **40**:101, 1993.
93. Hoogerbrugge PM, Vossen JMJJ: Bone marrow transplantation in the treatment of lysosomal storage diseases, in Fernandez JM, Saudubray J-M, Tada K (eds): *Inborn Metabolic Diseases, Diagnosis and Treatment*. Berlin Heidelberg, Springer, 1996.
94. Krivit W, Sung JH, Shapiro EG, et al: Microglia: The effector cell for reconstitution of the central nervous system following bone marrow transplantation for lysosomal and peroxisomal diseases. *Cell Transplant* **4**:385, 1995.
95. Peters C, Shapiro EG, Krivit W: Neuropsychological development in children with Hurler syndrome following hematopoietic stem cell transplantation. *Pediatr Transplant* **2**:1, 1998.
96. Hopwood JJ, Vellodi A, Scott HS, et al: Long-term clinical progress in bone marrow transplanted mucopolysaccharidosis type I patients with a defined genotype. *J Inherit Metab Dis* **16**:1024, 1993.
97. Vellodi A: Bone marrow transplantation for mucopolysaccharidoses, in Ringden O, Hobbs JR, Stelsand GG (eds): *Correction of Genetic Diseases by Transplantation*. London, Cogent, 1997.
98. Downie C, Hancock MR, Hobbs JR: Longterm outcome after BMT for Hurler's syndrome, in Hobbs JR, Riches PG (eds): *Correction of Genetic Diseases by Transplantation*. London, Cogent, 1991, p 1.
99. Krivit W, Lockman LA, Watkins PA, et al: The future for treatment of bone marrow transplantation for adrenoleukodystrophy, metachromatic leukodystrophy, globoid cell leukodystrophy and Hurler syndrome. *J Inherit Metab Dis* **18**:398, 1995.
100. Marshall E: Gene therapy's growing pains. *Science* **269**:1050, 1995.
101. Peters C, Shapiro E, Anderson J, et al: Hurler syndrome: II. Outcome of HLA-genotypically identical sibling and HLA-haploidentical related donor bone marrow transplantation in fifty-four children. The Storage Disease Collaborative Study Group. *Blood* **91**:2601, 1998.
102. Fleming DR, Henslee-Downey PJ, Ciocci G, et al: The use of partially HLA-mismatched donors for allogenic transplantation in patients with mucopolysaccharidosis-1. *Pediatr Transplant* 2, 1998.
103. Krivit W, Shapiro E: Bone marrow transplantation for storage diseases, in Desnick RJ (ed): *Treatment of Genetic Diseases*. New York, Livingstone, 1991, p 203.
104. Navarro C, Fernandez Fernandez JM, Dominguez C, et al: Late juvenile metachromatic leukodystrophy treated with bone marrow transplantation: A 4-year follow-up study. *Neurology* **46**:254, 1996.
105. Guffon N, Souillet G, Maire I, et al: Juvenile metachromatic leukodystrophy: Neurological outcome two years after bone marrow transplantation. *J Inher Metab Dis* **18**:159, 1995.

106. Dhuna A, Toro C, Torres F, et al: Longitudinal neurophysiologic studies in a patient with metachromatic leukodystrophy following bone marrow transplantation. *Arch Neurol* **49**: 1088, 1992.
107. Malm G, Ringden O, Winiarski J, et al: Clinical outcome in four children with metachromatic leukodystrophy treated by bone marrow transplantation. *Bone Marrow Transplant* **17**: 1003, 1996.
108. Gage FH: Cell therapy. *Nature* **392**: 18, 1998.
109. Naffakh N, Pinset C, Montarras D, et al: Longterm secretion of therapeutic proteins from genetically modified skeletal muscles. *Hum Gene Ther* **7**: 11, 1996.
110. Taylor RM, Wolfe JH: Decreased lysosomal storage in the adult MPS VII mouse brain in the vicinity of grafts of retroviral-corrected fibroblasts secreting high levels of β-glucuronidase. *Nat Genet* **3**: 771, 1997.
111. Broxmeyer HE, Kurtzberg J, Gluckman E, et al: Umbilical cord blood hematopoietic stem and replicating cells in human clinical transplantation. *Blood Cells* **17**: 313, 1991.
112. Kay MA, Liu D, Hoogerbrugge PM: Gene therapy. *Proc Natl Acad Sci USA* **94**: 12744, 1997.
113. Anderson WF: Human gene therapy. *Nature* **392**: 25, 1998.
114. Friedmann T: Overcoming the obstacles to gene therapy. *Sci Am* **276**: 96, 1997.
115. Blau H, Khavari P: Gene therapy: Progress, problems, prospects. *Nat Med* **3**: 612, 1997.
116. Touchette N: News: Gene therapy: Not ready for prime time. *Nat Med* **1**: 7, 1996.
117. Ledley FD: Somatic gene therapy, in Fernandes J, Saudubray J-M, Van den Berghe G (eds): *Inborn Metabolic Diseases. Diagnosis and Treatment.* New York, Springer-Verlag, 1996, p 429.
118. Morral N, Parks RJ, Zhou H, et al: High doses of a helper-dependent adenoviral vector yield supraphysiological levels of alpha-antitrypsin with negligible toxicity. *Hum Gene Ther* **9**: 2709, 1998.
119. Schiedner G, Morral N, Parks RJ, et al: Genomic DNA transfer with a high capacity adenovirus vector results in improved in vivo gene expression and decreased toxicity. *Nat Genet* **18**: 180, 1998.
120. Snyder RO, Miao CH, Patijn GA, et al: Persistent and therapeutic concentrations of human factor IX in mice after hepatic gene transfer of recombinant AAV vectors. *Nat Genet* **16**: 270, 1997.
121. Kafri T, Blomer U, Peterson DA, et al: Sustained expression of genes delivered directly into liver and muscle by lentiviral vectors. *Nat Genet* **17**: 314, 1997.
122. Miyoshi H, Smith KA, Mosier DE, et al: Transduction of human CD34+ cells that mediate long-term engraftment of NOD/SCID mice by HIV vectors. *Science* **283**: 682, 1999.
123. Koyata H, Cox RP, Chuang DT: Stable correction of maple syrup urine disease in cells from a Mennonite patient by retroviral-mediated gene transfer. *Biochem J* **295**: 635, 1998.
124. Xuehai YE, Robinson MD, Pabin C, et al: Adenovirus-mediated in vivo gene transfer rapidly protects ornithine transcarbamoylase deficient mice from an ammonium challenge. *Pediatr Res* **41**: 527, 1997.
125. Rafi MA, Fugaro J, Amini S, et al: Retroviral vector-mediated transfer of the galactocerebrosidase (GALC) cDNA leads to overexpression and transfer of GALC activity to neighbouring cells. *Biochem Mol Med* **58**: 142, 1996.
126. Gama Sosa MA, De Gasperi R, Undevia S, et al: Correction of the galactocerebrosidase deficiency in globoid cell leukodystrophy-cultured cells by SL3-3 retroviral-mediated gene transfer. *Biochem Biophys Res Commun* **218**: 766, 1996.
127. Ohashi T, Eto Y, Learish R, et al: Correction of enzyme deficiency in metachromatic leukodystrophy fibroblasts by retroviral-mediated transfer of the human arylsulphatase A gene. *J Inherit Metab Dis* **16**: 881, 1993.
128. Ohashi T, Watabe K, Sato Y, et al: Successful transduction of oligodendrocytes and restoration of arylsulfatase A deficiency in metachromatic leukodystrophy fibroblasts using an adenovirus vector. *Gene Ther* **2**: 443, 1995.
129. Yeyati PL, Agmon V, Fillat C: Fluorescence-based selection of retrovirally transduced cells in the absence of a marker gene: Direct selection of transduced type B Niemann-Pick disease cells and evidence for bystander correction. *Hum Gene Ther* **6**: 975, 1995.
130. Guidotti J-E, Akli S, Castelnau-Ptakhine L, et al: Retrovirus-mediated enzymatic correction of Tay-Sachs defect in transduced and non-transduced cells. *Hum Mol Genet* **7**: 831, 1998.
131. Rubin EM, Krauss RM, Sprangler EA, et al: Inhibition of early atherogenesis in transgenic mice by human apolipoprotein A1. *Nature* **353**: 265, 1991.
132. Tsurumi Y, Kearney M, Chen D, et al: Treatment of acute limb ischemia by intramuscular injection of vascular endothelial growth factor gene. *Circulation* **96**: 382, 1997.
133. Magovern C, Mack CA, Zhang J, et al: Regional angiogenesis induced in nonischemic tissue by an adenoviral vector expressing vascular endothelial growth factor. *Hum Gene Ther* **8**: 215, 1997.
134. Darling SM, Abbott CM: Mouse models of human single gene disorders: I. Non-transgenic mice. *Bioessays* **14**: 359, 1992.
135. Lyon M, Searle AG. *Genetic Variants and Strains of the Laboratory Mouse*, 2d ed. New York, Oxford University Press, 1989.
136. Battey J, Jordon E, Cox D, et al: An action plan for mouse genomics. *Nat Genet* **21**: 73, 1999.
137. Smithies O: Animal models of human genetic diseases. *Trends Genet* **9**: 112, 1993.
138. Shedlovsky A, McDonald JD, Symula D, et al: Mouse models of human phenylketonuria. *Genetics* **134**: 1205, 1993.
139. Erickson RP: Why isn't a mouse more like a man? *Trends Genet* **5**: 1, 1989.
140. Chowdhury JR, Grossman M, Gupta S, et al: Long-term improvement of hypercholesterolemia after ex vivo gene therapy in LDLR-deficient rabbits. *Science* **254**: 1802, 1991.
141. Ishibashi S, Brown MS, Goldstein JL, et al: Hypercholesterolemia in low density lipoprotein receptor knockout mice and its reversal by adenovirus-mediated gene delivery. *J Clin Invest* **92**: 883, 1993.
142. Hyde SC, Gill DR, Higgins CF, et al: Correction of the ion transport defect in cystic fibrosis transgenic mice by gene therapy. *Nature* **362**: 250, 1993.
143. Harris JC: Psychosocial care of the child and family, in Fernandes M, Saudubray J, Van den Berghe G (eds): *Inborn Metabolic Diseases: Diagnosis and Treatment*. Berlin, Springer-Verlag, 1996, p 57.
144. Roth KS, Yang W, Allan L, et al: Prenatal administration of biotin in biotin responsive multiple carboxylase deficiency. *Pediatr Res* **16**: 126, 1992.
145. Ampola MG, Mahoney MJ, Nakamura E, et al: Prenatal therapy of a patient with vitamin B_{12}-responsive methylmalonic acidemia. *N Engl J Med* **293**: 313, 1975.
146. Zab R, Leupold D, Fernandez MA, et al: Evaluation of prenatal treatment in newborns with cobalamin-responsive methylmalonic acidaemia. *J Inherit Metab Dis* **18**: 100, 1995.
147. Rosenblatt DS, Cooper BA, Schmutz SM, et al: Prenatal vitamin B_{12} therapy of a fetus with methylcobalamin deficiency (cobalamin E disease). *Lancet* **1**: 1127, 1985.
148. Pang S, Clark A: Newborn screening, prenatal diagnosis and prenatal treatment of congenital adrenal hyperplasia due to 21-hydroxylase deficiency. *Trends Endocrinol Metab* **1**: 300, 1990.
149. Sato S, Ward CL, Krouse ME, et al: Glycerol reverses the misfolding phenotype of the most common cystic fibrosis mutation. *J Biol Chem* **271**: 635, 1996.
150. Charache S, Dover G, Smith K, et al: Treatment of sickle cell anemia with S-azacytidine results in increased fetal hemoglobin production and is associated with nonrandom hypomethylation of DNA around the gamma-delta-beta-globin gene complex. *Proc Natl Acad Sci USA* **80**: 4842, 1983.
151. Dover GJ, Humphries RK, Moore JG, et al: Hydroxyurea induction of hemoglobin F product in sickle cell disease: Relationship between cytotoxicity and F cell production. *Blood* **67**: 735, 1986.
152. Dover GJ, Brusilow S, Charache S: Induction of fetal hemoglobin production in subjects with sickle cell anemia by oral sodium phenylbutyrate. *Blood* **84**: 339, 1994.
153. Kemp S, Wei H, Lu J, et al: Gene redundancy and pharmacological gene therapy: Implications for X-linked adrenoleukodystrophy. *Nat Med* **4**: 1261, 1998.
154. Phaneuf D, Wakamatsu N, Huang JQ, et al: Dramatically different phenotypes in mouse models of human Tay-Sachs and Sandhoff diseases. *Hum Mol Genet* **5**: 1, 1996.
155. Sango K, Yamanaka A, Hoffmann A, et al: Mouse models of Tay-Sachs and Sandhoff diseases differ in neurologic phenotype and ganglioside metabolism. *Nat Genet* **11**: 170, 1995.
156. Kubo S, Sun M, Miyahara M, et al: Hepatocyte injury in tyrosinemia type 1 is induced by fumarylacetoacetate and is inhibited by caspase inhibitors. *Proc Natl Acad Sci USA* **95**: 9552, 1998.
157. Niehues R, Hasilik M, Alton G, et al: Carbohydrate-deficient glycoprotein syndrome type 1b: Phosphomannose isomerase deficiency and mannose therapy. *J Clin Invest* **101**: 1414, 1998.
158. Sylvain M, Arnold DL, Scriver CR, et al: Magnetic resonance spectroscopy in Niemann-Pick disease type C: Correlation with

diagnosis and clinical response to cholestyramine and lovastatin. *Pediatr Nephrol* **10**:228, 1994.

159. Linck L, Lin D, Connor WE, et al: Cholesterol supplementation with egg yolk decreases plasma 7-dehydrocholesterol in Smith-Lemli-Opitz syndrome [abstr]. *Am J Hum Genet* **63**:A270 (1555), 1998.
160. Irons M, Elias ER, Tint GS, et al: Abnormal cholesterol metabolism in the Smith-Lemli-Opitz syndrome: Report of the clinical and biochemical findings in 4 patients and treatment in one patient. *Am J Med Genet* **50**:347, 1994.
161. Molkentin JD, Lu JR, Antos CL, et al: A calcineurin-dependent transcriptional pathway for cardiac hypertrophy. *Cell* **93**:215, 1998.
162. Sussman MA, Lim HW, Gude N, et al: Prevention of cardiac hypertrophy in mice by calcineurin inhibition. *Science* **281**:1690, 1998.
163. Scriver CR: Vitamin responsive inborn errors of metabolism (progress in endocrinology and metabolism). *Metabolism* **22**:1329, 1973.

CHAPTER 6

Multifactorial Diseases: Ancient Gene Polymorphism at Quantitative Trait Loci and a Legacy of Survival During Our Evolution

John A. Todd

Multifactorial diseases are common quantitative traits underpinned by the interaction of common alleles of several genetic polymorphisms, each a quantitative trait locus (QTL), and by environmental factors. Affected individuals have inherited a threshold of liability, the penetrance of which is usually much less than 100 percent. The number and interactions of disease protective and predisposing alleles that are inherited from both parents determine the threshold, and the penetrance is affected by developmental, stochastic, and environmental factors. With the emergence of dense, easily typed genetic maps, the search for genes with etiologically associated alleles with measurable effects is in full swing. But because most QTLs have small effects, the approach of meiotic mapping used successfully in rare, fully penetrant, single-gene diseases is not practical. Rapid progress in identifying the molecular basis of common disease requires a catalogue of all of the common polymorphisms in or near all genes, a goal currently within the budgetary and technical grasp of the genome project, combined with large, well-characterized collections of patients, relatives, and genetically-matched controls. The difficulties encountered in the genetic and functional analysis of human common disease continue to highlight the necessity of mapping and identifying QTLs in rodent models of these diseases. Progress and strategies in the identification of etiologic variants in common disease is illustrated using type 1 diabetes as an example.

TERMS OF REFERENCE

Penrose introduced the term "multifactorial" to describe traits or diseases that did not exhibit a clear Mendelian mode of inheritance owing to their reduced penetrance.[1] Possession of the disease-associated genotype bestows only a risk of developing the disorder. It is presumed that these traits are the result of the combined action of several or many genetic variants or alleles. Alleles of QTL are common in the general population and mostly ancient in origin, and account for a large proportion of the normal variation within the population. Certain combinations of QTLs, however, constitute the predisposition to multifactorial diseases such as diabetes, asthma, autoimmunity, obesity, and cardiovascular disease, which are "threshold characters."[2] Individual QTL alleles or polymorphisms have modest or subtle effects compared to the mutant alleles that cause rare Mendelian diseases. Mutant alleles usually have major consequences on gene functions.

FAMILIAL CLUSTERING

Cystic fibrosis is a clear example of a fully genetically determined disease. If an individual inherits two copies of a defective *CFTR* gene, then the disease will develop in that individual. In a family in which both parents are carriers, the risk of cystic fibrosis in the sibling of an affected sibling is 0.5 (the probability of inheriting the mutant allele from the father) $\times$ 0.5 (the probability of inheritance from the mother), or 0.25. Depending on the population, the frequency of cystic fibrosis carriers can be 0.04 percent, so the relative risk K or λs for the sibling is 25/0.04, or 625. The sibling, therefore, has a 625 times greater risk of developing cystic fibrosis than a randomly selected member of the population. This high value of 625 is due to the nearly complete penetrance of CFTR mutations. If the penetrance of a mutation is reduced substantially, it cannot produce a disease unless certain alleles at other loci are present (or absent in the case of resistance alleles). Accordingly, λs drops precipitously by an order of magnitude or more. λs for type 1 diabetes is about 15: a 0.4 percent population prevalence in a sibling risk of 6 percent. In general, the more common the disease, the smaller the λs value.[2–5]

An allele of a multifactorial disease locus will have low penetrance because the functional variant has only a modest influence on protein structure or expression. Mutations with major functional consequences and high penetrance are simply not compatible with the common occurrence of multifactorial disease and their low λs values. This is why rare diseases occur in pedigrees in which many affected members can be identified and traced back several generations. In contrast, such large pedigrees are rarely found in multifactorial disease in which at least 90 percent of patients usually have no family history of the disease at all.

A list of standard abbreviations is located immediately preceding the index in each volume. Additional abbreviations used in this chapter include: AEC = angiotensin-converting enzyme; IGF2 = insulin-like growth factor 2; IDDM = insulin-dependent diabetes mellitus; INS = insulin gene; LD = linkage disequilibrium; SLE = systemic lupus erythematosus; SNP = single nucleotide polymorphism; TDT = transmission/disequilibrium test; Th = T helper lymphocyte; QTL = quantitative trait locus; and VNTR = variable number of tandem repeats.

GENE MAPPING AND IDENTIFICATION

Owing to the near complete penetrance of single-gene disorders and, consequently, that healthy people never have the disease-causing mutation, tremendous progress in their mapping and identification has been made. Meiotic mapping using living family members can be used to locate the disease locus by identifying contemporary recombination break points. In contrast, the incomplete penetrance of multifactorial disease polymorphisms seriously compromises their mapping and identification because unaffected members of families and controls will have the candidate disease-associated allele. This means that a recombination in a family may not be relevant to the refinement of the location of the disease locus because the sibling with the recombinant chromosome may have developed the disease without any contribution from the allele at the disease locus. Because of this, huge numbers of families, the number being proportional to the effect of the locus, are required to narrow a disease locus-containing interval to less than 1 cM, a distance amenable to detailed sequence analysis of genes within the interval. This is not practical. Instead, methods that depend on detection of linkage disequilibrium or allelic association between alleles of markers or candidate genes and disease alleles have to be employed.

THE FUNCTIONAL CANDIDATE GENE APPROACH

The functional candidate gene approach using the case-control study design continues to dominate research on the genetics of type 1 diabetes[6,7] and other common diseases. The case-control design is simple: allele and genotype frequencies at a candidate gene polymorphism are evaluated in cases and matched controls to test the hypothesis that a particular polymorphism in a gene, which could have a function relevant to disease development, is associated with occurrence of the disease. Differences in the frequencies between the two groups indicate an association, the strength of which is measured as an odds ratio with a χ^2 test of statistical significance. This approach has identified the only two known loci in type 1 diabetes: the *insulin-dependent diabetes mellitus 1 locus* (*IDDM1*) in the major histocompatibility complex (MHC) human leukocyte antigen (HLA) region on chromosome 6p21 and the *IDDM2* locus at the insulin gene (*INS*) on chromosome 11p15.

IDDM1 AND IDDM2

IDDM1 is most closely associated with functional polymorphisms, encoding the peptide-binding sites of the HLA class molecules DQ and DR (these molecules allow T lymphocytes to distinguish self and foreign proteins in form of peptides).[8–10] Scanning of the whole human genome for linkage of type 1 diabetes using easily typed PCR-analyzed maps of highly polymorphic simple tandem repeat microsatellite markers has shown that in European or European-derived populations *IDDM1* is the major locus.[11,12] Susceptibility and resistance have been mapped to the HLA class II loci (*HLA-DQB1, -DQA1, -DRB1* and probably *-DPB1/DPA1*), which regulate T lymphocyte activity in normal immune responses (during infection) and in abnormal immune responses (during autoimmune attack or uncontrolled inflammatory activity). *IDDM1* could account for about 40 percent of the familial clustering of the disease by itself.[4,11] This estimate assumes that type 1 diabetes is a "polygenic" threshold character with several, if not many, constituent QTLs interacting according to a epistatic multiplicative model on a linear scale or additively on a log scale. More than 95 percent of European type 1 diabetic cases possess either of two most common predisposing haplotypes marked by alleles HLA-DRB1*04 and -DRB1*03 compared to 55 percent of the general population. These frequencies give an attributable risk (or δ value—the proportion of disease that might be prevented if the risk factor could be removed) of about 90 percent.

Scanning of the mouse genome in experimental crosses of the spontaneously type 1 diabetic strain NOD laid the foundation for later efforts in humans.[13] Studies in mice showed that although the mouse MHC was the major locus, it alone was not sufficient to cause diabetes and that it required the joint action of other loci spread throughout the rest of the genome.[14,15] A polygenic threshold model or a multiplicative model fitted the mouse backcross data well.[16]

The *IDDM2* locus is most closely associated with the variable number of tandem repeats (VNTR) polymorphism 596 bp upstream of the methionine codon of *INS*. Both the *INS* VNTR and the HLA class II loci now have extensive biological data supporting their candidacy as etiologic determinants of type 1 diabetes.[8,18–20] As the first QTLs identified for any common disease, their mapping and identification provides guidelines for the identification of the other QTLs involved in the development of type 1 diabetes and of other multifactorial diseases.

LINKAGE DISEQUILIBRIUM

In the MHC, the first association was detected at the class I locus *HLA-B*,[21–23] but it became clear that this was not a primary association.[24] Instead, the association was caused by linkage disequilibrium (LD) between alleles of *HLA-B* and alleles of the etiologic locus, which mapped much closer to the HLA class II loci, 1.45 Mb telomeric of *HLA-B*.[6] LD is said to occur when two alleles at neighboring loci occur together on the same chromosome or haplotype more often than would be expected by chance (which is the product of their individual allele frequencies in the population, when the alleles are at equilibrium).

Sequencing of alleles of the class II loci from controls and patients indicated that certain amino acid polymorphisms within their active sites correlate with resistance and susceptibility to disease.[25] These correlations, taking into account allelic variation at the three polymorphic class II genes *HLA-DQB1, -DQA1*, and *-DRB1,* account for most features of the association of the HLA region with type 1 diabetes in different ethnic groups.[8–10] A lesson from these studies is that even if a statistically significant association is obtained between a candidate polymorphism and disease, it need not necessarily reflect an etiologic role for that locus; instead it could be indicative of the primary action of another locus in LD with it. Hence, it is important to test the other polymorphisms that flank the candidate polymorphism for association, and if the flanking polymorphisms are associated, then this can be explained by LD with the candidate variant. It is expected that other common polymorphisms flanking the etiologic QTL will show association because the likely selective pressure will have dragged them along on the functional activity of the QTL (called hitchhiking) and by random genetic drift. Because genetics can only give a probabilistic evaluation of a candidacy, analyses of the difference in function of the two (or more) alleles of the candidate polymorphisms, as shown at *IDDM1* and at *IDDM2,* is essential. Nevertheless, genetics, even in humans, and certainly in mice using congenic strains, can exclude certain polymorphisms as candidates for the disease-associated QTL.

"CROSS-MATCH" ANALYSIS OF CANDIDATE POLYMORPHISMS

Almost all of the functional variation of class II molecules that affects CD4+ T lymphocyte recognition is encoded by exon 2 of these homologous genes. There are now hundreds of recognized alleles of these and of the HLA class I molecules (which allow CD8+ lymphocytes to distinguish self and foreign proteins). This enormous diversity has obviously been generated and maintained by the survival advantages of having an immune system capable of responding effectively to a wide range of infectious diseases. In type 1 diabetes, particular exon 2-encoded amino acid polymorphisms were correlated with both disease susceptibility and resistance to disease by comparing the occurrence of exon 2-encoded amino acid variants associated with disease to those not associated (or protective) with disease. This "cross-matching" revealed that a particular amino acid polymorphism at position 57 of the HLA-DQβ chain correlated well,[25] but not completely,[26] with the known associations of HLA class II alleles and haplotypes:[17] alleles of *HLA-DQB1* that are negatively associated with type 1 diabetes or had no association (neutral) tend to have an aspartic acid codon at position 57 compared to predisposing alleles that tend to have a noncharged amino acid, such as alanine or valine. This position, in the peptide-binding site, is a "hot spot" for selection because there are class II alleles that differ only at this position.[27] Remarkably, this correlation was conserved in inbred mice where the NOD strain is the only diabetic strain known, and was the only one that did not have aspartic acid at position 57.[17] Subsequently, it has been shown that there are tenfold differences in peptide-binding capacity between allotypes with different amino acids at position 57.[19] Asp57-positive class II molecules bind peptides with different amino acid composition than molecules with a noncharged amino acid at position 57[28] and the Asp57 forms a salt bridge across one end of the peptide-binding site with Arg79 in the α chain of this α,β heterodimeric receptor.

Provided all the polymorphisms of the candidate gene are known and the associations of each polymorphism and haplotype are known, this cross-match approach will yield a subset of loci that are candidates for the etiologic polymorphism. Polymorphisms with alleles that do not begin to explain the observed associations of haplotypes can be excluded with some degree of confidence. This strategy will fail if the region containing the etiologic variant has not been included in the analysis. It will be complicated if there is more than one common etiologic variant in the gene or region, as is the case for *IDDM1*. All three of the class II loci *HLA-DQB1, -DQA1*, and *-DRB1* are etiologic, each a QTL influencing the specificity and magnitude of the T-lymphocyte response to infectious disease and, in the case of autoimmune disease, to self proteins.[8–10,29] A primary role for the polymorphism in the *HLA-DRB1* locus was deduced by identification of *DQB1* and *DQA1* haplotypes that had the same DQ alleles but different *DRB1* alleles and that had different associations with disease.[9,30–34] Also, the analysis of patients and controls matched for DQ alleles provided further evidence for heterogeneity outside the DQ region, mapping to the *HLA-DRB1* locus.[34] Polymorphism of the third class II molecule HLA-DP may also be involved.[35] The analysis is very complicated by having genes (generated by duplication during evolution) of very similar function within 700 kb of each other. The story does not end here because the class II region explains most but not all of the HLA haplotype associations. Other QTLs within the MHC, and possibly closely flanking it, remain to be identified.[26,36,37] This is not surprising because the MHC contains over 100 genes, many of which have a function in antigen recognition, T cell activity, and in the immune response.[38] Nevertheless, in the case of the HLA class II genes, LD and haplotype analyses have led to a model for the etiology of the *IDDM1* QTL that is consistent with the genetic and biologic data.

ANCESTRAL HAPLOTYPE MAPPING

A recombination event has never been observed in living families between the *HLA-DQB1* and *-DRB1* loci. These loci are 100 to 200 kb apart but are in very strong LD. We can, however, observe ancient recombination events between them by characterizing recombinant haplotypes of the class II genes in which the alleles have been recombined form new haplotypes (Fig. 6-1). By evaluating the association of different, but closely related, haplotypes made up of identical-by-descent allelic segments of DNA, it is possible to construct a correlation or cross-match between ancestral segments and disease association (Fig. 6-1).

The most informative examples of this approach for the HLA class II region were reported in a comparison of European and African chromosomes. Two type 1 diabetes-predisposing HLA class II haplotypes are common in Africa but very rare in Europe. Comparison of the allelic content of the African haplotypes with their related European recombinant haplotypes by DNA sequencing of exon 2 DNA (to confirm identity-by-descent) and by restriction fragment length polymorphism mapping, pinpointed

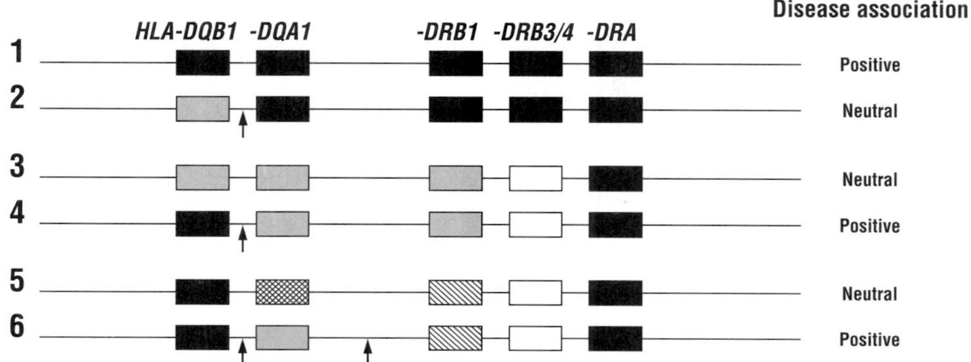

Fig. 6-1 The *HLA-DRB1, -DQA1, -DRB1, -DRB3/4*, and *-DRA* loci are encoded by a 350 kb region of the MHC.[38] There is strong LD between these loci, and characteristic haplotypes can be identified and their association with type 1 diabetes evaluated.[39,40] Each box type (hatched or solid) is a different allele of the particular locus. Pairwise comparison of haplotypes 1 and 2, and 3 and 4 indicate that these haplotypes arose by a recombination event as indicated by the arrows between the *HLA-DQB1* and *-DQA1* loci during the history of the human population. Because they differ in their disease association, it can be estimated that the substitution of the *DQB1* allele contributed to the change of disease association of these otherwise highly related haplotypes. Haplotype 6 required more than one recombination event to give rise to its close relative, haplotype 5; in this comparison, allelic variation at the *DQA1* locus appears to be important. Taken together, these data and other studies support a model in which allelic variation at these loci explains a good part of the association of type 1 diabetes with HLA. The approach, which has been termed "haplotype cross-matching" can be applied to genes, as is the case here, or single nucleotide polymorphisms in a chromosome region showing LD with the disease in order to locate polymorphisms that could be active in disease etiology, and to exclude polymorphisms that cannot explain the association of the region.

both the *HLA-DQB1* and *-DQA1* loci as plausible sites of susceptibility determinants.[39,40] The presence or absence of different allelic versions of exon 2 of the *HLA-DQB1* and *-DQA1* loci could account for the different disease associations of the haplotypes. Further similar analyses in Sardinian[32,33] and Norwegian[29] case-controls confirmed earlier studies[30,41] that the predisposing effects of the major susceptibility DQ-defined haplotypes could be (dominantly) overridden by certain alleles of the *HLA-DRB1* locus, resulting in a protective or neutral haplotype overall. Ancestral haplotype mapping of the HLA region in common disease has been studied by Dawkins and colleagues,[42,43] and the same basic principle underlies phylogeny haplotype mapping by cladograms or trees of haplotypes.[44,45]

The requirements for this approach include very large case-control or family studies, preferably from several distinct ethnic groups, such as Europeans, Africans, and Asians. The most informative haplotypes might be relatively rare, in the order of 1 to 5 percent, and it is important to be confident that the true association of the haplotype has been identified. The second requirement is that all the polymorphisms in the region are known or can be guessed with near certainty by knowing the patterns of LD between markers that are very close to each other. Much cheaper technologies for finding polymorphisms and scoring them in large sample sizes are required. With a very dense map of single nucleotide polymorphisms (SNPs), in the order of 1 per 5 to 10 kb, it is possible to construct an ancestral map of any region with confidence that the regions being claimed as identical-by-descent are indeed just that and not identical-by-state. A dense enough map avoids the ambiguities and possible bias introduced by guessing haplotypes when the information is incomplete. Logically, and this is the implication from the published data for *IDDM1* and at *IDDM2*,[8,46,47] a map of all polymorphisms, including and flanking the etiologic locus, allows precise mapping of the disease-associated QTL by measuring the association of each polymorphism in a pointwise fashion. The predisposing allele of the QTL will be the most associated allele in the region with decreasing associations extending outwards on both sides. LD decays with increasing physical and genetic distance between loci (at a rate of $(1 - r)^n$, where r = recombination fraction and n = number of generations). A less dense map, say of unevenly spaced microsatellite markers only, could be misleading as to the location of the QTL because the association of a marker locus with disease that is not the disease locus itself is dependent on the distribution of marker alleles on disease-predisposing chromosomes and nonpredisposing chromosomes.[48] If, for example, a rare allele of a microsatellite marker occurred almost exclusively on the predominant susceptibility haplotype, then this allele would be strongly associated with disease, but the marker could be some distance from the QTL. This problem of marker informativity accounts for the irregular shape of single-point LD curves in which the low points are markers that have alleles equally distributed on predisposing and nonpredisposing haplotypes (e.g., mapping of the hemochromatosis gene telomeric of the *HLA-A* locus[49]). But if the map is dense, dense enough to include the actual QTL, then a small patch of markers closest to the QTL should show a consistent and high association, and be consistent with the pattern of ancestral recombination breakpoints mapped in the region.

Key information comes from identification of the points along present-day haplotypes where in the past a recombination event has occurred between two chromosomes and a recombinant chromosome has survived in the population by drift, or by selection, or both. It may be that in present-day populations, both the parental chromosomes can be detected but more likely one or other will have been lost by drift. In fact, the vast majority of mutations or recombinant haplotypes have been lost by random genetic drift. HLA may be a very extreme case in that a high degree of functional polymorphism was essential for survival and hence many polymorphisms and haplotypes have survived over 150,000 years of human evolution and population growth. Haplotypes 1 and 2 in Fig. 6-1 are highly likely to have arisen from each other by a recombination event between the *HLA-DQB1* and *-DQA1* loci (marked with an arrow), thereby mapping the susceptibility determinant to the left (centromeric) of this ancestral breakpoint. Pairwise comparison of haplotypes 3 and 4, and of 5 and 6, give consistent results, mapping susceptibility to both the *HLA-DQB1* and *-DQA1* loci. It is also possible that gene conversion has contributed the observed haplotypic diversity, making it essential to have analyzed the DNA flanking the candidate gene or region with an equally dense set of polymorphisms. It is a matter of luck how informative haplotype similarities and differences with ancestral breakpoints will be in any particular chromosome region. This type of mapping will be increasingly informative the more patients and controls or families from distinct populations can be studied and compared, because haplotype and allele frequencies vary considerably between populations (by chance via drift or because different environmental factors have imposed different selection pressures). Admixed populations, such as Mexican Americans, which have a mixture of European and native-American haplotypes, have advantages in association and haplotype mapping if the disease is more prevalent in one of the populations, as is the case for type 1 diabetes in Europeans compared to native Americans.[50]

Such a systematic analysis of the MHC, which could be focused on genes and their flanking DNA, would be of enormous benefit to the identification of the etiologic polymorphisms responsible for the association of at least 50 MHC-different diseases, including dyslexia, multiple sclerosis, psoriasis, and rheumatoid arthritis. Ancestral haplotype or identity-by-descent content mapping should be carried out for QTLs identified for other common diseases; e.g., the angiotensin converting enzyme (*ACE*) locus in cardiovascular disease, and the *APOE* locus in Alzheimer disease, in order to map the etiologic locus for the ACE gene, and to confirm that the amino acid or promoter polymorphisms of the APOE molecule are, in fact, the etiologic sites. Ancestral haplotype mapping has already begun at the *ACE* locus.[45]

Once a chromosome segment has been associated with disease-candidate polymorphisms, it can be analyzed in more detail as carried out for exon 2 of HLA class II genes and for the 20 kb of DNA containing the *INS* and *insulin-like growth factor 2* (*IGF2*) genes at *IDDM2*,[7,46,47,51] again using the cross-matching approach. Assuming there is one etiologic locus in the region, all haplotypes containing the predisposing allele should be positively associated with disease; conversely, all haplotypes with the nonassociated allele should not be associated with disease. Functional studies of the remaining short list of candidates can then be undertaken to reinforce genetic data. It should be evident early in the association analysis whether there are two or more etiologic variants in a candidate gene at detectable frequencies, as haplotypes cluster into two main families (because it is unlikely that two functional alleles arose on the same haplotype). Taking into account the history of human populations over the last 100,000 years and the effects of random genetic drift (see "How Far Does LD Extend?"), it seems unlikely that two functional alleles at two different sites affecting the activity or expression of the same gene would survive to become frequent in modern populations (unless there was strong selection pressure on polymorphism of the gene as found in HLA class II and class I genes).

IDDM2

Many of the same approaches have been applied to the tyrosine hydroxylase-*INS-IGF2* region of chromosome 11p15. Here the problem was that despite many positive case-control studies there was no apparent evidence of linkage (although this depends on the populations studied: *INS* shows reasonable evidence of linkage in affected sib-pairs from the UK[11,52] but not from the USA[53] or France[54]). Moreover, controls can be drawn inadvertently from a group with a different genetic background than the patients, giving rise to false positive results. Thomson was the first to use family-based association studies to demonstrate that the *INS* VNTR type 1 diabetes association was a true one.[55] Ewens and Spielman formalized this approach in the transmission disequilibrium test (TDT) in a further confirmation that VNTR was genuinely associated with type 1 diabetes.[56] The TDT evaluates the departure of transmission of alleles (from heterozygous parents) from the expected random transmission of 50 percent. It is robust to admixture in populations, and avoids the pitfalls of mismatching the controls and the cases. The TDT and modified versions of it, including analysis of sibs (when parents are not available)[57–59] is now widely used to confirm case-control results and to search for new associations in functional candidate genes[60] or in linked regions.[61] TDT can also be used to evaluate the association of haplotypes and ancestral segments.[48] In the case of the TDT, the strength of the association is measured as the percentage transmission of an allele from heterozygous parents to affected offspring. In this test, it is very important to also measure transmission to the unaffected offspring to control for segregation distortion.[56] In type 1 diabetes, considerable support for the existence of the *IDDM4* locus on chromosome 11q13 was obtained from the analysis of transmission of a protective haplotype to both affected and unaffected siblings.[62]

The common polymorphisms for 20 kb around *INS* were determined and typed in case-control sets[63] and in families,[7,46] revealing that the VNTR polymorphism at −596 bp (5′ of the *INS* ATG codon) is the most associated polymorphism in the region, with the −23 bp SNP a close second, owing to its near complete LD with the VNTR. In the most associated region of 4.1 kb all polymorphisms were typed to determine the association of haplotypes of the core region. By cross-match analysis, as described above, the VNTR emerged as the most plausible candidate. The flanking diallelic SNPs were ruled as unlikely candidates for *IDDM2* because some of them had disease-associated alleles that also occurred on protective haplotypes. Furthermore, three categories of haplotype were identified—susceptible/neutral, protective, and very protective—indicative of a multiallelic etiological polymorphism and not consistent with the model of IDDM2 as a single SNP.

A criticism of these studies was that the region analyzed, including the 20 kb region and its core 4.1 kb, was too small.[64] The effect of the *IDDM2* locus on the familial clustering of type 1 diabetes in the UK population is much less (about 10 percent) than that of *IDDM1*. Therefore, the *IDDM2* locus, with its relatively modest effect, is an important test case for the mapping of QTLs in common disease. A much more extensive region should be examined on either side of the *INS* VNTR to ensure that the VNTR is indeed the most associated polymorphism and that its allelic variants dictate the associations of haplotypes and ancestral identical-by-descent segments. This should include all genes in the region and perhaps 200 kb of DNA on either side of the VNTR in the first instance. This is made more feasible because the genomic clones containing this region are being sequenced (as part of the Human Genome Project effort; http://gestec.swmed.edu/chromoso.htm). Also, the homologous mouse DNA is being sequenced,[65] facilitating identification of conserved regulatory regions and genes by cross-comparison of the sequences from the two species. Nevertheless, the resequencing (or rescanning using methods to detect polymorphisms rather than direct DNA sequencing) is an expensive and still labor-intensive task. Advances in technology and in automation are required.

Ongoing functional studies of the *INS* VNTR have shown that the VNTR regulates the expression of both *INS* and of *IGF2* in various tissues.[7,66] Most interestingly, because it provides a plausible biologic mechanism for the protective effects of the VNTR class III alleles (those that have more than 200 repeats), the VNTR has been shown to influence *INS* expression in the thymus.[18,67] The thymus is the organ that ensures self-tolerance by deleting potentially harmful autoreactive T cells through an interaction of the T-cell antigen receptor, self proteins in the thymus, and HLA class II and I molecules. *INS* VNTR class III alleles are associated with increased thymic expression of *INS*, which could lead to an increase in T cell deletion of clones capable of recognizing insulin or its precursor, preproinsulin. The *INS* VNTR is, therefore, likely to be the *IDDM2* QTL modulating tolerance to preproinsulin and its peptides. This model is consistent with extensive experiments in rodents.[17]

AN EVOLUTIONARY PERSPECTIVE

Both *IDDM1* and *IDDM2* are common and ancient polymorphisms: the *INS* class I/I, I/III and III/III genotype frequencies in European populations are 47 percent, 43 percent, and 9.4 percent, respectively. The two allele classes are globally distributed, although in Asians, for example, class III alleles are very rare. In Central African Pygmies, the class III allele is by far the more common (Livak K, Todd JA 1995). The *INS* VNTR polymorphism is found in higher primates but not in rodents or in lower primates.[46] Key associated alleles of the *HLA-DRB1* and *-DQB1* loci, such as the predisposing alleles DRB1*0401, DRB1*03, and DQB1*0302, and the protective alleles DQB1*0301 and DQB1*0602, are at frequencies of 10 to 20 percent. Fifty-five percent of the population is either DRB1*04- or DRB*03-positive as compared to 95 percent of type 1 diabetic cases. Owing to drift, and perhaps to differential selection forces in different geographical regions, some *HLA-DRB1* alleles, such as the DRB1*0405 allele, is common in some European populations (e.g., 8 percent in Sardinia[32]) but significantly rarer in northern European populations such as Norway.[29] The DRB1*0405 allele is highly predisposing for type 1 diabetes so its fluctuation in frequency is an important factor.

At HLA how did so many alleles occur and be maintained during millions of years of evolution and survive the emergence of a small population from Africa about 100,000 years ago? For HLA, part of the answer is that amino acid polymorphism in the T-cell recognition site of the class II and class I molecules has been selected to ensure survival from infectious disease at the population level.[68] HLA class II and class I polymorphism contributes to the normal QTL variation of immune responses characteristic of a randomly breeding population. Probably many genes, non-MHC and MHC, contribute to this normal variation, and these are the polymorphisms that underpin susceptibility and resistance to inflammatory or autoimmune diseases.[17] Susceptibility to these diseases is the cost of having individuals in the population with particularly vigorous or prolonged immune responses.[17] Type 1 diabetes and other diseases, such as multiple sclerosis and rheumatoid arthritis, which run in the same families as those with type 1 diabetes, are believed to be caused by defective activity of T cells that secrete cytokines such as interferon-γ and interleukin-2 (IL-2).[69] This type of lymphocyte, the T helper 1 subset (Th1), is also responsible for the cell-mediated inflammatory response to infection.[70] The other arm of the T helper cell response, Th2, is characterized by IL-4 and is associated with antibody production (or humoral immunity) during infection. The cytokines of the Th1 and Th2 subsets are counter-regulatory, promoting and inhibiting growth and differentiation of the other cell type.[70] Type 1 diabetes is inhibited by Th2-associated cytokines.[69] It is expected that different types of infectious disease would have resulted in selection of alleles of genes in the pathways of both Th subsets to potentiate the ability to survive a variety of infections. This is perhaps one explanation why protective haplotypes for type 1 diabetes are such a common feature, most recently illustrated at the *IDDM4* locus on chromosome 11q13.[62] Haplotypes protective for type 1 diabetes may have alleles that provide resistance to certain infectious diseases by increasing Th2 subset activity, whereas diabetes-susceptible haplotypes may tend to have alleles that increase Th1 activity, which is beneficial in fighting disease requiring a Th1-mediated immune response. It is interesting to note that the *IDDM4* region contains the high affinity IgE Fc receptor locus, which has been linked to, and associated with, atopy (high IgE production).[71,72] Atopy and asthma are associated with Th2 responses; their prevalence today could be an evolutionary consequence of Th2-dependent resistance to infectious diseases. Hence, alleles predisposing to atopy could be protective for type 1 diabetes. Clinically, it is suspected that type 1 diabetes may occur less in individuals affected with atopy and vice versa.

For the *INS* VNTR, evidence of a potential mechanism of selection for its common polymorphism was only recently published.[73] The *INS* VNTR III/III genotype has been associated with increased weight, head circumference, and length at birth. Low birth-weight is a major risk factor for infant mortality. Even in the 1920s in the UK, the infant mortality rate was over 100 infants/1000 compared to 6 infants/1000 now. Possession of the *INS* VNTR III/III genotype results in about a 200 g difference in birth-weight,[73] predicting a 30 percent reduction in morality in the lowest birth-weight group of 2.95 kg or less (6.5 lb; Dunger D, unpublished). Hence the *INS* VNTR could be a "surviving small baby" genotype,[74] which could have had a large effect in the past when the chances of survival were really low. Why then is the frequency of the class III not 100 percent? It is possible that this locus has other functions that are not yet understood (for example, the class I allele may affect early postnatal growth; Todd JA, 1998). It is also possible that the *INS* VNTR class I allele is subject to segregation distortion. There is evidence (unpublished) that the class I allele is transmitted more than 50 percent of the time from parents to normal offspring (Eaves I, Todd JA, 1998). *IGF2,* the transcription of which may also be controlled by allelic variation of the VNTR,[66] is expressed (and imprinted) in the preimplantation embryo.[75] Polymorphisms in genes like these, with known functions in growth and development, are strong candidates for loci that affect fertility (gamete and zygote viability, pre- and postimplantation success).

HOW FAR DOES LD EXTEND?

This question is important because it influences the map density required to detect association in the first place; for example, when scanning a linkage peak with a denser set of markers. This, in turn, affects directly the power of any association study. Unfortunately, without actually measuring the LD in the genome, it is almost impossible to predict its pattern owing to the variable parameters that affect LD: mutation rate of polymorphisms; the rate of population growth; founder events that have occurred during human history and selection; and other effects, such as nonrandom mating. In general, LD has been found to extend out to about 2 cM,[76] but much larger distances have been reported.[77,78] Power calculations have been made for TDT studies of association but this assumed that the marker was the etiologic variant.[79,80]

Selection of functional alleles of closely linked loci can have a large effect on LD. In the HLA region, multiple genes of related function are closely linked within 3.5 Mb of DNA. Functionally active polymorphisms in two or more of these genes could act together to promote even greater chances of survival during infection. This is likely to be the case, and is a plausible explanation for the high levels of LD observed in the MHC. Strong LD is seen between certain class II and class I alleles, even though the loci are at least 1.45 Mb apart (that is 1.45 percent recombination every generation). Early workers were able to find the association between the *HLA-B* locus and type 1 diabetes because of the significant LD between the HLA-B8 and -B15 alleles and the HLA-DRB1*03 and HLA-DRB1*04 alleles, respectively. How often this occurs outside the MHC is unknown, but there are many examples of genes of related function being clustered (e.g., several immune response genes on chromosome 5q31), partly through gene duplication, and the occurrence of closely linked polymorphisms could give rise to extended regions of LD. Obviously, for extended LD there must be more than one selected polymorphism in the region. These questions can be answered only by empirical observation. Currently, the LD profile of the human genome according to different populations is "uncharted territory."

One model for the origin of modern humans is that a small group of *Homo sapiens* came out of Africa about 100,000 years ago.[81] Before this the polymorphic diversity of the stable and ancient population in Africa would have been large (as it is in primates) and equilibrium would have been reached between many loci, according to the recombination distance between them and the total number of generations (which may have been many thousands). But when *H. sapiens* emerged from Africa, and the number of individuals is thought to have been small, LD would have been re-established. A huge amount of polymorphism and haplotypes would have been lost (unless they were under strong selection pressure). There is direct experimental evidence for this model from the analysis of LD between two polymorphisms in the *CD4* gene. Much less LD was observed in African populations.[81] This kind of "bottleneck" would also have occurred during the colonization of Europe 50,000 years ago, as humans encountered different climates and infectious organisms. Again, LD would have been reset. Only 700 years ago, more than 50 percent of people in parts of Europe were killed by plague, which may have contributed to increased LD between markers. The immune response gene alleles that helped the survivors of plague are not known, but their frequencies presumably increased during this time. Perhaps the immune response resistance alleles for plague are susceptibility alleles for type 1 diabetes. Presumably selection is acting today in Africa where millions of individuals are dying from HIV. It is known that polymorphisms in immune-response genes, such as the chemokine receptors and in the HLA region, influence susceptibility and resistance to the progression of AIDS and, presumably, to early infection by HIV. In populations that are endemic for AIDS, allele and haplotype frequencies at resistance/susceptibility loci must be changing. In an extreme example, Finland was founded by only about 2000 individuals about 2000 years ago (the story is more complicated than this[82]), thereby creating higher levels of LD than present in other European populations for common polymorphisms.

Uncertainty about the power of LD mapping in common diseases would be partially alleviated if there were an extensive catalogue of the potentially functional polymorphisms in all genes. Nevertheless, it is known that microsatellite markers can be used to detect association at *IDDM2/INS* and at *IDDM1* in non-founder European and European-derived populations[7,54] (Herr M, Koeterman B, Todd JA, unpublished; 1999). It seems highly likely, based on results from *IDDM1* and *IDDM2,* that other QTLs can be mapped using the same approaches in the same populations, using a number of distinct populations with a range of LD, for example, from Finland to Africa.

WHOLE GENOME SCANNING

The evidence so far from linkage scanning studies using affected sib-pairs to detect increased marker allele sharing suggests that several regions could potentially contain type 1 diabetes loci.[52,53,83] The problem is that even for the true locus *IDDM2* some sib-pair sets show very little or no evidence of linkage,[53] proving that for loci with modest effects, linkage is not a sensitive approach. In contrast, TDT detects *IDDM2* easily even in the same sib-pair families that did not show conventional linkage.[7,56] The message here is that efforts should be focused on using TDT or LD-based methods to extend and confirm linkage results rather than performing more linkage studies. If we had a large catalogue of gene-associated SNPs, it might be beneficial to abandon linkage studies, if no major loci are evident from the scan (major meaning something as strong as HLA in type 1 diabetes). As more and more (potentially) functional SNPs are discovered, TDT analysis of these will be the approach where the linkage-based positional data is just one piece of information in the case for investigating a region further.

Testing extensive regions or large numbers of genes with SNPs for association carries with it the burden of multiple testing. *P* values for association of 10^{-8} should be attained because eventually very large numbers of markers will be typed. A *P* value at this level is quite easily achieved at the *INS* VNTR.[7] One strategy is to seek replication of primary results in additional independent data sets in which a hypothesis is generated based on the transmission of a specific allele and tested specifically in the other data sets.

Improved technology will be important for these studies. The Human Genome Project is planning to harvest large numbers of SNPs. We need technology to use these in our own laboratories or to outsource their genotyping. Better methods for multiplexing PCR reactions will reduce costs and conserve diminishing DNA resources. PCR-independent methods should be developed for SNP scoring. In the meantime, LD analyses of the named putative IDDM loci and of other chromosome regions implicated by linkage should be carried out, as well as systematic analysis of all candidate genes, as SNPs become available.

THE UTILITY OF MICE IN MAPPING QTLs

As in humans, the chromosome regions containing type 1 diabetes QTLs in mice cannot be accurately mapped by linkage analysis.[13] Linkage peaks are broad[13] and could contain multiple QTLs, which is the case for at least two of the mapped loci, *insulin-dependent diabetes 3* (*Idd3*), now four separate linked loci on chromosome 3)[15,84,85] and *Idd5* (chromosome 1).[86,87] But in mice, congenic strains can be constructed by standard breeding methods in which the chromosome segment of interest is selected by using markers that distinguish the chromosomes of the parental strains.[15] Congenic stocks can be developed to determine the effect of any particular chromosome segment on disease, providing firm boundaries for the QTL location. Congenic strains have been used in the MHC to prove that there is another gene or genes outside the class II region that influences type 1 diabetes.[88] They have been used to show that the separate loci of *Idd3* can interact synergistically.[84] In a mouse model of systemic lupus erythematosus (SLE), the SLE-resistant parental strain was converted to a sensitive strain by breeding in three chromosome segments of DNA containing three of the mapped *SLE* loci. This demonstrated that three of the several mapped *SLE* loci are sufficient to cause disease.[89] Congenic strains can be used to exclude functional candidate genes and narrow the interval containing the QTL.[15,90] Using this approach, *Idd3* has been localized to a 0.15 cM 750 kb interval containing the interleukin-2 structural gene, a strong candidate gene for *Idd3*.[15] But even with an interval as small as 750 kb, it is still a formidable task to identify the gene with certainty, especially if only a fraction of the genes are known in the interval. Nevertheless, a major advantage of congenic strains is that they can be used to study the biologic effects of the QTL without knowing the identity of the QTL. Identification of mouse QTLs will be greatly facilitated by determination of the sequence of the mouse genome, which will allow identification of all genes and their allelic variants, as well as comparison of the murine and human sequences to detect conserved regulatory regions.

CONCLUSION

The molecular identification of QTLs is just beginning. It will allow the inheritance and mechanisms of common disease to be explained specifically and will offer new insights to their prevention. As Haldane wrote in his defence of "beanbag genetics," the collection of the data "will be expensive,"[91] but, in my view, worth every penny.

ACKNOWLEDGMENTS

I thank my colleagues, including F. Cucca, D. Dunger, J. Edwards, D. Clayton, G. te Meerman, W. Bodmer, and Martin Farrall, for discussion, and the Wellcome Trust, the Medical Research Council, the British Diabetic Association, and the Juvenile Diabetes Foundation for support.

REFERENCES

1. Penrose LS: A further note on the sib-pair method. *Ann Eugen* **13**:120, 1947.
2. Cavalli-Sforza LL, Bodmer WF: *The Genetics of Human Populations*. San Francisco, W.H. Freeman, 1971.
3. Newcombe HB: in Fishbein M (ed): Paper and Discussions of the Second International Conference on Congenital Malformations. New York, International Medical Congress, 1964.
4. Risch N: Assessing the role of HLA-linked and unlinked determinants of disease. *Am J Hum Genet* **40**:1, 1987.
5. Todd JA: Genetic analysis of type 1 diabetes using whole genome approaches. *Proc Natl Acad Sci USA* **92**:8560, 1995.
6. Todd JA, Bell JI, McDevitt HO: A molecular basis for genetic susceptibility to insulin-dependent diabetes mellitus. *Trends Genet* **4**:129, 1988.
7. Bennett ST, Lucassen AM, Gough SCL, Powell EE, Undlien DE, Pritchard LE, Merriman ME, et al: Susceptibility to human type 1 diabetes at *IDDM2* is determined by tandem repeat variation at the insulin gene minisatellite locus. *Nat Genet* **9**:284, 1995.
8. Cucca F, Todd JA: HLA susceptibility to type 1 diabetes: Methods and mechanisms, in Browning MJ, McMichael AJ (eds): *HLA/MHC: Genes, Molecules and Function*. Oxford, βIOS Scientific Publishers, 1996, p 383.
9. She J-X: Susceptibility to type 1 diabetes: HLA-DQ and DR revisited. *Immunol Today* **17**:323, 1996.
10. Thorsby E, Undlien D: The HLA associated predisposition to type 1 diabetes and other autoimmune diseases. *J Pediatr Endocrinol Metab* **9**:75, 1996.
11. Davies JL, Kawaguchi Y, Bennett ST, Copeman JB, Cordell HJ, Pritchard LE, Reed PW, et al: A genome-wide search for human type 1 diabetes susceptibility genes. *Nature* **371**:130, 1994.
12. Hashimoto L, Habita C, Beressi J, Delepine M, Besse C, Cambon-Thomsen A, Deschamps I, et al: Genetic mapping of a susceptibility locus for insulin-dependent diabetes mellitus on chromosome 11q. *Nature* **371**:161, 1994.
13. Todd JA, Aitman TJ, Cornall RJ, Ghosh S, Hall JRS, Hearne CM, Knight AM, et al: Genetic analysis of autoimmune type 1 diabetes mellitus in mice. *Nature* **351**:542, 1991.
14. Wicker LS, Todd JA, Peterson LB: Genetic control of autoimmune diabetes in the NOD mouse. *Ann Rev Immunol* **13**:179, 1995.
15. Lyons PA, Wicker LS: Localising quantitative trait loci in the NOD mouse model of type 1 diabetes, in Theofilopoulos A (ed): *Genetics of Autoimmunity. Current Directions in Autoimmunity*. Basel, Karger, 1999; p 208.
16. Risch N, Ghosh S, Todd JA: Statistical evaluation of multiple locus linkage data in experimental species and relevance to human studies: Application to murine and human IDDM. *Am J Hum Genet* **53**:702, 1993.
17. Todd JA: From genomics to aetiology in a multifactorial disease, type 1 diabetes. *Bioessays* **21**:164, 1999.
18. Vafiadis P, Bennett ST, Todd JA, Nadeau J, Grabs R, Goodyer CG, Wickramasinghe S, et al: Insulin expression in human thymus is modulated by INS VNTR alleles at the *IDDM2* locus. *Nat Genet* **15**:289, 1997.
19. Nepom BS, Nepom GT, Coleman M, Kwok WW: Critical contribution of β chain residue 57 in peptide binding ability of both HLA-DR and -DQ molecules. *Proc Natl Acad Sci USA* **93**:7202, 1996.
20. Schmidt D, Verdaguer J, Averill N, Santamaria P: A mechanism for the major histocompatibility complex-linked resistance to autoimmunity. *J Exp Med* **186**:1059, 1997.
21. Nerup J, Platz P, Andersson OO, Christy M, Lyngsoe J, Poulson JE, Ryder LP, et al: HL-A antigens and diabetes mellitus. *Lancet* **II**:864, 1974.
22. Cudworth A, Woodrow J: HL-A system and diabetes mellitus. *Diabetes* **24**:345, 1974.
23. Singal DP, Blajchman MA: Histocompatability antigens, lymphocytotoxic antibodies and tissue antibodies in patients with diabetes mellitus. *Diabetes* **22**:429, 1973.
24. Cudworth AG, Gorsuch AN, Wolf E, and Festenstein H: A new look at HLA genetics with particular reference to type-1 diabetes. *Lancet* **II**:389, 1979.

25. Todd JA, Bell JI, McDevitt HO: HLA-DQ β gene contributes to susceptibility and resistance to insulin-dependent diabetes mellitus. *Nature* **329**:599, 1987.
26. Valdes AM, McWeeney S, Thomson G: HLA class II DR-DQ amino acids and insulin-dependent diabetes mellitus: Application of the haplotype method. *Am J Hum Genet* **60**:717, 1997.
27. Apple RJ, Erlich HA: HLA class II genes: Structure and diversity, in Browning M, McMichael AJ (eds): *HLA and MHC: Genes, Molecules and Function*. Oxford, βIOS Scientific Publisher, 1996, p 97.
28. Reizis B, Eisenstein M, Mor F, Cohen IR: The peptide-binding strategy of the MHC class II I-A molecules. *Immunol Today* **19**:212, 1998.
29. Undlien DE, Friede T, Rammensee H-G, Joner G, Dahl-Jorgensen K, Sovik O, Akselsen HE, et al: HLA-encoded genetic predisposition in IDDM: DR4 subtypes may be associated with different degrees of protection. *Diabetes* **46**:143, 1997.
30. Sheehy MJ, Scharf SJ, Rowe JR, Neme de Gimenez MH, Meske LM, Erlich HA, Nepom BS: A diabetes-susceptible HLA haplotype is best defined by a combination of HLA-DR and -DQ alleles. *J Clin Invest* **83**:830, 1989.
31. Todd JA, Fukui Y, Kitagawa T, Sasazuki T: The A3 allele of the HLA-DQA1 locus is associated with susceptibility to type 1 diabetes in Japanese. *Proc Natl Acad Sci* **87**:1094, 1990.
32. Cucca F, Lampis R, Frau F, Macis M, Angius E, Masile P, Chessa M, et al: The distribution of DR4 haplotypes in Sardinia suggests a primary association of type 1 diabetes with DRB1 and DQB1 loci. *Hum Immunol* **43**:301, 1995.
33. Cucca F, Muntoni F, Lampris R, Frau F, Argiolas L, Silvetti M, Angius E, et al: Combinations of specific DRB1, DQA1, DQB1 haplotypes are associated with insulin-dependent diabetes mellitus in Sardinia. *Hum Immunol* **37**:85, 1993.
34. Undlien DE, Friede T, Rammensee H-G, Joner G, Dahl-Jorgensen K, Sovik O, Akselsen HE, Knitsen I, Ronningen KS, Thorsby E: HLA-encoded genetic predisposition in IDDM: DR4 subtypes may be associated with different degrees of protection. *Diabetes* **46**:143, 1997.
35. Noble JA, Valdes AM, Cook M, Klitz W, Thomson G, Erlich HA: The role of HLA class II genes in insulin-dependent diabetes mellitus: Molecular analysis of 180 Caucasian, multiplex families. *Am J Hum Genet* **59**:1134, 1996.
36. Robinson WP, Barbosa J, Rich SS, Thomson G: Homozygous parent affected sib pair method for detecting disease predisposing variants: Application to insulin-dependent diabetes mellitus. *Genet Epidemiol* **10**:273, 1993.
37. Langholz B, Tuomilehto-Wolf E, Thomas D, Pitkaniemi J, Tuomilehto J, Group DS: Variation in HLA-associated risks of childhood insulin-dependent diabetes in the Finnish population. *Genet Epidemiol* **12**:441, 1995.
38. Browning MJ, McMichael AJ: *HLA and MHC: Genes, Molecules and Function*. Oxford, βIOS Scientific Publishers, 1996.
39. Todd JA, Mijovic C, Fletcher J, Jenkins D, Bradwell AR, Barnett AH: Identification of susceptibility loci for insulin-dependent diabetes mellitus by trans-racial gene mapping. *Nature* **338**:587, 1989.
40. Todd JA: The role of MHC class II genes in susceptibility to insulin-dependent diabetes mellitus. *Curr Top Microbiol Immunol* **164**:17, 1990.
41. Sheehy M: HLA and insulin-dependent diabetes. *Diabetes* **41**:123, 1992.
42. Degli-Esposti MA, Andreas A, Christiansen FT, Schalke B, Albert E, Dawkins RL: An approach to the localisation of the susceptibility genes for generalised myasthenia gravis by mapping recombinant ancestral haplotypes. *Immunogenetics* **35**:355, 1992.
43. Degli-Esposti MA, Abraham LJ, McCann V, Spies T, Christiansen FT, Dawkins RL: Ancestral haplotypes reveal the role of the central MHC in the immunogenetics of IDDM. *Immunogenetics* **36**:345, 1992.
44. Templeton AR: A cladistic analysis of phenotypic associations with haplotypes inferred from restriction endonuclease mapping of DNA sequencing. V. Analysis of case/control sampling designs: Alzheimer's disease and the apoprotein E locus. *Genetics* **140**:403, 1995.
45. Keavney B, McKenzie CA, Connell JMC, Julier C, Ratcliffe PJ, Sobel E, Lathrop GM, Farral MC et al: Measured haplotype analysis of the angiotensin-1 converting enzyme (ACE) gene. *Hum Mol Genet* **7**:1745, 1998.
46. Bennett ST, Todd JA: Human type 1 diabetes and the insulin gene: Principles of mapping polygenes. *Ann Rev Genet* **30**:343, 1996.
47. Julier C, Lucassen A, Villedieu P, Delepine M, Levy-Marchal C, Danzé PM, Bianchi F, et al: Multiple DNA variant association analysis: Application to the insulin gene region in type 1 diabetes. *Am J Hum Genet* **55**:1247, 1994.
48. Merriman T, Eaves IA, Twells RCJ, Merriman ME, Danoy PAC, Muxworthy CE, Hunter KMD, et al: Transmission of haplotypes of microsatellite markers rather than single marker alleles in the mapping of a putative type 1 diabetes susceptibility gene (*IDDM6*). *Hum Mol Genet* **7**:517, 1998.
49. Feder JN, Gnirke A, Thomas W, Tsuchihashi Z, Ruddy DA, Basava A, Dormishian F, et al: A novel MHC class I-like gene is mutated in patients with hereditary haemochromatosis. *Nat Genet* **13**:399, 1996.
50. Cruickshanks KJ, Jobim LF, Lawler-Heavner J, Neville TG, Gay EC, Chase HP, Klingensmith G, et al: Ethnic differences in human leukocyte antigen markers of susceptibility to IDDM. *Diabetes Care* **17**:132, 1994.
51. Owerbach D, Gabbay K: Localisation of a Type 1 diabetes susceptibility locus to the variable tandem repeat region flanking in the insulin gene. *Diabetes*. **42**:1708, 1993.
52. Mein CA, Esposito L, Dunn MG, Johnson GCL, Timms AE, Goy JV, Smith AN, et al: A search for type 1 diabetes susceptibility genes in families from the United Kingdom. *Nat Genet* **19**:297, 1998.
53. Concannon P, Gogolin-Ewens KJ, Hinds DA, Wapelhorst B, Morrison VA, Stirling B, Mitra M, et al: A second-generation screen of the human genome for susceptibility to insulin-dependent diabetes mellitus. *Nat Genet* **19**:292, 1998.
54. Julier C, Hyer RN, Davies J, Merlin F, Soularu P, Briant L, Cathelineau G, et al: Insulin-IGF2 region on chromosome 11p encodes a gene implicated in HLA-DR4-dependent diabetes susceptibility. *Nature* **354**:155, 1991.
55. Thomson G, Robinson W, Kuhner M, Joe S, Klitz W: HLA and insulin gene associations with IDDM. *Genet Epidemiol* **6**:155, 1989.
56. Spielman R, McGinnis R, Ewens W: Transmission test for linkage disequilibrium: The insulin gene region and insulin-dependent diabetes mellitus (IDDM). *Am J Hum Genet* **52**:506, 1993.
57. Curtis D: Use of siblings as controls in case-control association studies. *Ann Hum Genet* **61**:319, 1997.
58. Boehnke M, Langefeld CD: Genetic association mapping based on discordant sib pairs: The discordant-alleles test. *Am J Hum Genet* **62**:950, 1998.
59. Spielman RS, Ewens WJ: A sibship test for linkage in the presence of association: The sib transmission/disequilibrium test. *Am J Hum Genet* **62**:450, 1998.
60. Garchon H-J, Djabiri F, Viard J-P, Gajdos P, Bach J-F: Involvement of human muscle acetylcholine receptor α-subunit gene (CHRNA) in susceptibility to myasthenia gravis. *Proc Natl Acad Sci USA* **91**:4668, 1994.
61. Copeman JB, Cucca F, Hearne CM, Cornall RJ, Reed PW, Rønningen KS, Undlien DE, et al: Linkage disequilibrium mapping of a type 1 diabetes susceptibility gene (*IDDM7*) to human chromosome 2q31-q33. *Nat Genet* **9**:80, 1995.
62. Nakagawa Y, Kawaguchi Y, Twells RCJ, Muxworthy C, Hunter KMD, Wilson A, Merriman ME, et al: Fine mapping of the diabetes-susceptibility locus, *IDDM4,* on chromosome 11q13. *Am J Hum Genet* **63**:547, 1998.
63. Lucassen A, Julier C, Beressi J-P, Boitard C, Froguel P, Lathrop G, Bell J: Susceptibility to insulin-dependent diabetes mellitus maps to a 4.1 kb segment of DNA spanning the insulin gene and associated VNTR. *Nat Genet* **4**:305, 1993.
64. Doria A, Lee J, Warram JH, Krolewski AS: Diabetes susceptibility at *IDDM2* cannot be positively mapped to the VNTR locus of the insulin gene. *Diabetologia* **39**:594, 1996.
65. Paulsen M, Davies KR, Bowden LM, Villar AJ, Franck O, Fuermann M, Dean WL, et al: Syntenic organisation of the mouse distal chromosome 7 imprinting cluster and the Beckwith-Wiedemann syndrome region in chromosome 11p15.5. *Hum Mol Genet* **7**:1149, 1998.
66. Paquette J, Giannoukakis N, Polychronakos C, Vafiadis P, Deal C: The INS 5′ variable number of tandem repeats is associated with IGF2 expression in humans. *J Biol Chem* **273**:14158, 1998.
67. Pugliese A, Zeller M, Fernandez A, Zalcberg LJ, Bartlett RJ, Ricordi C, Pietropaolo M, et al: The insulin gene is transcribed in the human thymus and transcriptional levels correlate with allelic variation at the INS VNTR-*IDDM2* susceptibility locus for type 1 diabetes. *Nat Genet* **15**:293, 1997.
68. Kaufman J: Evolution of the major histocompatibility complex and MHC-like molecules, in Browning MJ, McMichael AJ (eds): *HLA and MHC: Genes, Molecules and Function*. Oxford, βIOS Scientific Publishers, 1996, p. 1–21
69. Tisch R, McDevitt H: Insulin-dependent diabetes mellitus. *Cell* **85**:291, 1996.
70. Janeway JCA, Travers P: Immunobiology: The Immune System in Health and Disease. Garland, New York, 1997.

71. Hill MR, Cookson WOCM: A new variant of the β subunit of the high affinity receptor for immunoglobulin E (FcεRI-β E237G): associations with measures of atopy and bronchial hyper-responsiveness. *Hum Mol Genet* **5**:959, 1996.
72. Barnes KC, Marsh DG: The genetics and complexity of allergy and asthma. *Immunol Today* **19**:325, 1998.
73. Dunger DB, Ong KKL, Huxtable SJ, Sherriff A, Woods KA, Ahmed ML, Golding J, et al: Association of the *INS* VNTR with size at birth. *Nat Genet* **19**:98, 1998.
74. McCance DR, Pettitt DJ, Hanson RL, Jacobsson LT, Knowler WC, Bennett PH: Birth-weight and non-insulin-dependent diabetes: Thrifty genotype, thrifty phenotype or surviving small baby genotype? *BMJ* **308**:942, 1994.
75. Lighten AD, Hardy K, Winston RML, Moore GE: IGF2 is parentally imprinted in human preimplantation embryos. *Nat Genet* **15**:122, 1997.
76. Jorde LB: Linkage disequilibrium mapping as a gene-mapping tool. *Am J Hum Genet* **56**:11, 1995.
77. Peterson AC, Di Rienzo A, Lehesjoki A-E, de la Chapelle A, Slatkin M, Freimer NB: The distribution of linkage disequilibrium over anonymous genome regions. *Hum Mol Genet* **4**:887, 1995.
78. Crouau-Roy B, Sevice S, Slatkin M, Fremer N: A fine-scale comparison of the human and chimpanzee genomes: Linkage, linkage disequilibrium and sequence analysis. *Hum Mol Genet* **5**:1131, 1996.
79. Risch N, Merikangas K: The future of genetic studies of complex human diseases. *Science* **273**:1516, 1996.
80. Muller-Myhsok B, Abel L: Genetic analysis of complex diseases. *Science* **275**:1328, 1997.
81. Tishkoff SA, Dietzsch E, Speed W, Pakstis AJ, Kidd JR, Cheung K, Bonne-Tamir B, et al: Global patterns of linkage disequilibrium at the CD4 locus and modern human origins. *Science* **271**:1380, 1996.
82. Kittles RA, Perola M, Peltonen L, Bergen AW, Aragon RA, Virkkunen M, Linnoila M, et al: Dual origins of Finns revealed by Y chromosome haplotype variation. *Am J Hum Genet* **62**:1171, 1998.
83. Cucca F, Goy JV, Kawaguchi Y, Esposito L, Merriman ME, Wilson AJ, Cordell HJ, et al: A male-female bias in type 1 diabetes and linkage to chromosome Xp in MHC HLA-DR3-positive patients. *Nat Genet* **19**:301, 1998.
84. Wicker LS, Todd JA, Prins J-B, Podolin PL, Renjilian RJ, Peterson LB: Resistance alleles at two non-major histocompatibility complex-linked insulin-dependent diabetes loci on chromosome 3, *Idd3* and *Idd10,* protect nonobese diabetic mice from diabetes. *J Exp Med* **180**:1705, 1994.
85. Podolin PL, Armitage N, Lord CJ, Levy ER, Peterson LB, Todd JA, Wicker LS, et al: Localization of two insulin-dependent diabetes (*Idd*) genes to the *Idd10* region on mouse chromosome 3. *Mamm Genome* **9**:283, 1998.
86. Cornall RJ, Prins J-B, Todd JA, Pressey A, DeLarato NH, Wicker LS, Peterson LB: Type 1 diabetes in mice is linked to the interleukin-1 receptor and *Lsh/Ity/Bcg* genes on chromosome 1. *Nature* **353**:262, 1991.
87. Garchon H-J, Luan J-J, Eloy L, Bedossa P, Bach J-F: Genetic analysis of immune dysfunction in non-obese diabetic (NOD) mice: Mapping of a susceptibility locus close to the *Bcl-2* gene correlates with increased resistance of NOD T cells to apoptosis induction. *Eur J Immunol* **24**:380, 1994.
88. Ikegami H, Makino S, Yamato E, Kawaguchi Y, Ueda H, Sakamoto T, Takekawa K, et al: Identification of a new susceptibility locus for insulin-dependent diabetes mellitus by ancestral haplotype congenic mapping. *J Clin Invest* **96**:1936, 1995.
89. Wakeland EK, Morel L, Mohan C, Yui M: Genetic dissection of lupus nephritis in murine models of SLE. *J Clin Immunol* **17**:272, 1997.
90. Podolin PL, Denny P, Lord CJ, Hill NJ, Todd JA, Peterson LB, Wicker LS, et al: Congenic mapping of the insulin-dependent diabetes (*Idd*) gene, *Idd10,* localizes two genes mediating the *Idd10* effect, and eliminates the candidate gene *Fcgr1*. *J Immunol* **159**:1835, 1997.
91. Haldane JBS: A defense of beanbag genetics. *Perspect Biol Med* **7**:343, 1964.

CHAPTER 7

Genes and Susceptibility to Infectious Diseases

Adrian V. S. Hill

It has been recognized since ancient times that people vary in their susceptibility to infectious diseases and before the relevant microbe was identified some such diseases were regarded as familial.[1] Earlier in this century, twin studies began to provide some estimates of the magnitude of the host genetic component to variable susceptibility. It is now clear that genetic variation in the host has a substantial influence on the course of disease caused by many infectious microorganisms. Such interactions have been particularly well studied in human infectious diseases where both the pathogen and the host genome are well characterized.

Over the last 10 years, the methodologies available for analyzing human genetic variation have advanced rapidly, leading to the identification of a large number of genes associated with altered susceptibility to infectious pathogens. However, it is likely that those characterized so far represent only a small fraction of a very large number of genes that influence susceptibility to one or other infection. Indeed susceptibility to most infectious diseases in humans is likely to be highly polygenic, and this has both attractions and disadvantages for those attempting to identify relevant genes. A large number of genes increases the probability of success with a candidate-gene approach but makes it more difficult to map genes by linkage analysis of multicase families. Another complicating factor in attempts to identify infectious disease susceptibility genes is genetic variation in the infectious pathogen. Nonetheless, a surprising amount of progress has been made in identifying susceptibility and resistance genes, and this is providing new insights into disease pathogenesis and resistance mechanisms. Conversely, it appears increasingly likely that a substantial proportion of the functional variation in the human genome has evolved to facilitate defense against infectious pathogens, leading to the observed polygenic variation in susceptibility between individuals and populations. In this chapter, after an outline of research approaches, specific susceptibility and resistance genes are reviewed before data relevant to particular infectious diseases are summarized.

MEASURING GENETIC EFFECTS ON INFECTIOUS DISEASE

Many different types of studies have been undertaken to search for genetic effects on susceptibility to infectious diseases. Most of these have focused on particular candidate genes, and more recently some genome-wide studies have been undertaken, However, different approaches are required to estimate the magnitude of the genetic component to variable susceptibility.

Family Clustering

For some infections, such as leprosy, family clustering is well recognized,[2] but with infectious diseases it is particularly difficult to assess the relative importance of shared environment and shared genes. In a highland New Guinea population where the community rather than the family is the basic social unit, it was demonstrated that closeness of kin to a case of leprosy was still the main determinant of risk.[3] However, such opportunities are rare. More generally, some correction for exposure needs to be applied as has been done, for example, by measurement of water contact in epidemiologic studies of schistosomiasis risk.[4] A parameter widely used in analysis of complex diseases is λ_s, the increased risk of disease in a sibling of a case compared with the general population risk.[5] It is a useful measure of the possible extent of the genetic component to an infectious disease, even though it is influenced by both environmental and genetic factors. Although few field studies have attempted to measure this directly, λ_s may often be of the order of 1.5 to 5.0 for common infectious diseases.

Population Comparisons

Apparent interpopulation and racial differences in susceptibility have also been noted. Because of their lack of the Duffy blood group chemokine receptor on erythrocytes, most sub-Saharan Africans are completely resistant to *Plasmodium vivax* malaria.[6] Within the same country in West Africa, differences between ethnic groups have been found in both susceptibility and immune responsiveness to malaria.[7] A study of tuberculosis in nursing homes in Arkansas found blacks to be more susceptible to *Mycobacterium tuberculosis* infection than were whites after correcting for socioeconomic variables.[8] In a primary school outbreak in Missouri, however, black children were found to be more susceptible to pulmonary radiographically defined disease but not to infection.[9] Examples of marked susceptibility of populations newly exposed to an infectious pathogen have been reported with suggestions that these may have been genetically determined. High mortality rates were observed following the introduction of several viral infections to small Pacific island populations and, more recently, isolated Amerindian populations in South America have been well studied.[10] Among the Qu'Appelle Indians of Saskatchewan, annual mortality rates of almost 1 percent were observed after the introduction of tuberculosis to the settlement in the 1880s. After some decades of exposure to tuberculosis, rates of disease dropped 50-fold,[11] and selection for resistance genes may in part have been responsible. The high frequency of lysosomal lipid storage diseases in Ashkenazi Jews has led to the suggestion that carriers of these disorders may have been selected for resistance to tuberculosis,[12] but no direct evidence of the tuberculosis susceptibility of individuals with these genotypes is available. Human leukocyte antigen (HLA) data on the descendants of survivors of epidemics of typhoid and yellow fever in Surinam have been used to argue that these infectious diseases have selected particular protective alleles.[13] Although interesting and often strongly suggestive, uncontrolled population comparisons rarely provide compelling evidence that the apparent susceptibility differences observed are due to human genetic variation. Comparisons of individuals directly in terms of their susceptibility to infectious pathogens have also suggested some substantial genetic effects. In the 1920s and 1930s, malaria therapy was fairly widely used for the treatment of syphilis, and marked differences in susceptibility to both *Plasmodium vivax* and *Plasmodium falciparum* were observed in these malaria nonimmune individuals.[14] The

Table 7-1 Twin Studies of Infectious Diseases Showing Significantly Higher Concordances in Monozygotic (MZ) than Dizygotic (DZ) Twin Pairs

		Concordance		
Disease	Population	MZ	DZ	Reference
Tuberculosis	Germany	65	25	127
	U.S.A.	62	18	128
	U.K.	32	14	9
Leprosy	India	52	22	11
Helicobacter pylori	Sweden	81	63	13
Poliomyelitis	U.S.A.	36	6	10
Hepatitis B	Taiwan	35	4	12

accidental vaccination of a large number of children with *M. tuberculosis* rather than bacillus Calmette-Guérin (BCG) in Lubeck, Germany, also provided direct evidence of interindividual differences in susceptibility to the same dose and strain of this pathogen.

Twin and Adoptee Studies

In addition to these observational data, two types of studies have provided more direct quantification of the importance of host genetics in susceptibility to infectious diseases: adoptee and twin studies. In an important study of over 900 Scandinavian adoptees, early death of a biologic parent from an infectious disease was associated with an almost sixfold increase in risk of an infectious cause of death in the adoptee, consistent with a substantial role for host genetics.[15] In contrast, early death of an adoptive parent had little effect on the risk of an infectious death of the adoptee. In this study, the effect of host genetics on the mortality rate from infectious causes was slightly higher than that from cardiovascular disease and much higher than from cancer. Probably the most important data on the overall role of genetic factors in susceptibility to infectious disease have come from twin studies. Several such studies have found higher concordance rates among monozygotic than dizygotic twin pairs who share, respectively, 100 percent and, on average, 50 percent of their genes (Table 7-1). The disease most frequently studied has been tuberculosis, with several large studies carried out over 40 years ago[16–18] all showing significantly higher concordances in monozygotic twin pairs. Similar results have been reported for poliomyelitis[19] and leprosy,[20] but the latter study has been criticized because an overrepresentation of monozygotic twins reflected some ascertainment bias. A study of Taiwanese twins found a higher concordance rate for persistent carriage of hepatitis B virus (HBV) but not for HBV infection in monozygotic twins.[21] A recent Swedish study of *Helicobacter pylori* infection studied both twins reared apart and reared together.[22] A high heritability was found in the monozygotic twins reared apart, and sharing of the rearing environment was shown to add a separate smaller component to the familial clustering. A twin study of malaria in West Africa found evidence of a genetic influence on fever induced by malaria but not on risk of parasite infection.[23] Studies of common viral infections of childhood have mainly shown very high concordance rates in both types of twins.[24] In general, it has been easier to demonstrate a significant role for host genetic factors in infections where only a proportion of those infected develop disease and in chronic rather than acute infectious diseases. As with studies of candidate genes, a stronger effect of host genetic variation in twin studies may be found by studying severe clinical cases rather than susceptibility to infection per se.

APPROACHES TO GENE IDENTIFICATION

Many different approaches may be taken to identifying genes determining susceptibility to complex disease, and these are discussed in detail in Chapter 5. Several different and usually complementary approaches have been taken to identifying genes involved in susceptibility to infectious diseases. By far, the most widely used has been the assessment of candidate genes in case-control studies. In this approach, the frequencies of variants of a gene with a suspected role in variable susceptibility are compared in individuals with and without the disease. In general, large sample sizes are required, particularly to assess rare alleles or multiallelic genes. Control populations need to be selected carefully to avoid false-positive or false-negative associations due to population stratification. Parental controls may be used to avoid this potential problem.[25] The number of candidate genes available for study is large and rapidly increasing, and attractive candidate genes have been suggested by a variety of approaches. A particular geographical distribution of certain hemoglobin variants suggested that they might play a role in malaria resistance.[26] A few genes have been identified as affecting susceptibility to infection in different strains of mice, leading to assessment of their human homologues.[27,28] A larger number of candidate genes have recently been suggested by studies of the susceptibility of various gene knockout mice to infectious pathogens. Finally, genes known to play roles in immune or innate resistance to infection, such as HLA, tumor necrosis factor, and mannose-binding lectin variants, have been assessed based on their known function.

A different and more recent approach in the study of infectious diseases is to search for genetic linkage to, rather than association with, a disease in family studies. Identification of a genetic marker linked to susceptibility indicates that there is a susceptibility gene somewhere in that region.[5] In molecular terms, however, regions mapped in this way are large, of the order of many megabases, and much further work is required to actually identify the causative gene. The advantage of this approach is that unknown genes may be mapped and identified without prior information on their function. The statistical power of this approach is generally lower than that of case-control studies, in part because it is usually far easier to recruit individual cases than multicase families, but it does enable a comprehensive screen of the whole genome to be undertaken for major susceptibility genes. A similar approach in mice has led to the mapping of numerous susceptibility genes,[29] and a few of these, such as the natural resistance-associated macrophage protein 1 (*Nramp1*) gene have then been identified[28] The human homologue in this case, *NRAMP1*, was found to affect susceptibility to pulmonary tuberculosis,[30] but the human homologue of other murine susceptibility genes, such as the *Mx* influenza resistance gene,[27] have not been shown to be functionally polymorphic in humans. It remains unclear how generally useful the mapping of mouse susceptibility genes will be as a route to identifying relevant human genes.

A family linkage approach has also been taken to map and identify genes causing rare monogenic susceptibility phenotypes. For example, mutations in the genes for the γ-interferon receptor chain 1 and the interleukin 12 (IL-12) receptor β1 chain have been shown to underlie susceptibility to weakly pathogenic mycobacteria in rare cases and families.[31–34] Mutations in other genes producing more generalized immunodeficiency are described in other chapters, but these are almost all found at nonpolymorphic frequencies, i.e., at an allele frequency of less than 1 percent.

SUSCEPTIBILITY AND RESISTANCE GENES

Blood Groups

ABO blood groups were among the first genetic markers to have been investigated in a large number of infectious diseases. Probably the most consistent association has been that of blood group O with increased severity of cholera symptoms (Table 7-2).[35,36] Blood group O was associated with peptic ulceration in early studies, and peptic ulceration is now known to be associated with *H. pylori* infection. A possible mechanism for this association

Table 7-2 Some Susceptibility and Resistance Genes Implicated in Bacterial Diseases

Gene	Variant	Disease	Effect
HLA-DR	HLA-DR2	Tuberculosis	Susceptibility
NRAMP1	5′ and 3′ Variants	Tuberculosis	Susceptibility
VDR	3′ Variant	Tuberculosis	Resistance
HLA-DR	HLA-DR2	Leprosy	Susceptibility
TNF	Promoter −308	Lepromatous leprosy	Susceptibility
ABO	Blood group O	Cholera	Susceptibility
FUT2	Nonsecretors	Urinary tract infection	Susceptibility
MBL	Coding variants	*Pneumococcus*	Susceptibility
γ-Interferon receptor	Various mutations	Disseminated *bacillus Calmette-Guérin*	Susceptibility
IL-12 receptor	Various mutations	Intracellular bacteria	Susceptibility

IL-12, interleukin 12; MBL; manose-binding lectin; NRAMP1, natural resistance-associated macrophage protein 1; TNF, tumor necrosis factor; VDR, vitamin-D receptor.

was suggested by the finding that fucosylation of the Le^b receptor for *H. pylori* in the gastric mucosa, found only in individuals with A or B blood groups, impaired binding of this bacterium.[37] However *H. pylori* infection is not clearly influenced by ABO blood group type,[38] and the blood group O association with peptic ulceration may therefore be independent of this infection. The ability to secrete blood group substances into saliva as well as at other mucosal surfaces is inherited as a monogenic trait. Most individuals are secretors, but about 20 percent of most populations are nonsecretors due to mutation in the fucosyltransferase-2 (*FUT2*) gene.[39] In relatively small studies, nonsecretion has been suggested to be associated with susceptibility to some bacterial and fungal infections and with resistance to certain common viral infections.[40,41] The most convincing association is between nonsecretor status and susceptibility to recurrent urinary tract infection,[42] and a possible mechanism for this has been proposed.[43]

The most striking blood group association is that relating the Duffy blood group and susceptibility to *P. vivax* malaria (Table 7-3). This malaria parasite uses the Duffy blood group antigen as the receptor to invade erythrocytes.[6] The Duffy blood group antigen has more recently been found to be a promiscuous chemokine receptor.[44] Most sub-Saharan Africans and most American blacks are Duffy blood group negative due to homozygosity for a mutation in the promoter of this gene. They are thus completely resistant to *P. vivax* infections. This is one of the few examples of a variant that is completely protective against an infectious pathogen. Interestingly, Duffy-negative individuals express the Duffy antigen on some other tissues, because the promoter mutation, which is in the recognition site for an erythroid-specific enhancer, is tissue specific.[45] It is perhaps surprising that the one mutation that is completely protective against malaria is specific for the much less virulent parasite *P. vivax* and apparently does not affect susceptibility to *P. falciparum*. The latter species would be expected to have been a more powerful selective agent. In historical terms, however, it is unclear whether preexisting Duffy-negative genotypes prevented *P. vivax* ever entering Africa or whether an earlier, more virulent form of this parasitic infection might have selected the variant in Africa.

Hemoglobin Gene Variants

The hemoglobinopathies have provided the classic examples of human infectious disease resistance genotypes. Noting the distribution of thalassemia in the Mediterranean, Haldane proposed that certain hemoglobin gene variants might have reached high frequencies in malarious regions by providing resistance to this disease.[26] The protective efficacy of sickle hemoglobin in heterozygotes against *P. falciparum* malaria was discovered a few years later[46] and was soon confirmed.[47] The greatest protection is afforded against death and severe life-threatening malaria,[48] with somewhat less protection against uncomplicated disease and least protection against becoming infected. This pattern of greater protection against disease than infection appears to be found for many infectious disease resistance genes. *In vitro* studies have found both decreased parasite invasion of hemoglobin AS erythrocytes and impaired parasite growth in these cells at low oxygen tensions.[49–51]

Table 7-3 Susceptibility and Resistance Genes Implicated in Malaria and Leishmaniasis. (Pf, *Plasmodium falciparum*; and Pv, *Plasmodium vivax*)

Gene	Variant	Disease	Effect
Duffy chemokine receptor	Promoter variant	Malaria (Pv)	Resistance
α-Globin	Thalassemias	Malaria (Pf)	Resistance
β-Globin	Sickle, thalassemias	Malaria (Pf)	Resistance
Erythrocyte band 3	27-bp Deletion	Malaria (Pf, Pv)	Resistance
G-6-PD	Deficiency variants	Malaria (Pf)	Resistance
HLA-B	HLA-B53	Malaria (Pf)	Resistance
HLA-DR	HLA-DRB1*1302	Malaria (Pf)	Resistance
ICAM-1	Kilifi variant	Malaria (Pf)	Susceptibility
TNF	Promoter −308	Malaria (Pf)	Susceptibility
	Promoter −308	Leishmaniasis	Susceptibility

G-6-PD, glucose-6-phosphate dehydrogenase; ICAM-1, intercellular adhesion molecule 1; TNF, tumor necrosis factor.

The α and β thalassemias are extremely common disorders of hemoglobin synthesis that lead to imbalanced globin-chain production. The mild forms of thalassemia are among the most prevalent single-gene disorders. Both the α and β thalassemias have been shown to afford some protection against *P. falciparum* malaria in keeping with their geographical distribution,[52,53] but the mechanism of protection associated with the thalassemias remains unknown. There is no marked impairment of parasite growth *in vitro*,[54,55] and other mechanisms that have been suggested include decreased rosetting of parasitized cells[56] and increased expression of a major parasite antigen on the erythrocyte surface, leading to more effective parasite clearance.[57] In a prospective study on a Melanesian island, the rate of malaria caused by both *P. falciparum* and *P. vivax* was found to be higher among young children homozygous for α^+ thalassemia than among nonthalassemic controls, suggesting that the protective mechanism may be quite complex.[58] In a hospital-based study in New Guinea, however, homozygous children appeared to be protected against clinical malaria.[59] The geographical distribution of hemoglobins C and E suggests that they may also protect against malaria, but this has not been demonstrated.[60] However, hemoglobin E behaves as a mild form of β thalassemia,[61] suggesting that it is probably weakly protective. Thus, although the relationship of the hemoglobinopathies to malaria resistance has been extensively investigated, some key questions, particularly in relation to the molecular mechanisms of protection, remain to be resolved.

Glucose-6-Phospate Dehydrogenase Deficiency

Erythrocyte glucose-6-phosphate dehydrogenase (G-6-PD) deficiency is found at high frequencies in many tropical and subtropical populations (Chap. 179). This is an X-linked disorder that is associated with red cell destruction under certain conditions.[62] A variety of drugs, some infections, and ingestion of fava beans can trigger acute hemolysis, and male G-6-PD-deficient infants may have neonatal jaundice. Over 100 different mutations of G-6-PD have been described by using molecular analysis, and a small group of uncommon variants is associated with chronic hemolytic anemia in the absence of any environmental agents. The majority of G-6-PD variants are associated with lesser degrees of enzyme deficiency and are found at higher frequency. As for the hemoglobinopathies, the geographical distribution of G-6-PD deficiency in the "malaria belt" suggested its selective advantage.[11] In several locations, populations with malarial exposure in previous generations had significantly higher frequency of G-6-PD deficiency when compared with genetically similar populations who had not been exposed to malarial selection. As with the hemoglobinopathies, a variety of molecular mutations are associated with this enzyme deficiency: in Africans, G-6-PD A^-; in the Mediterranean basin, G-6-PD-Med; and, in Asia and Melanesia, several different G-6-PD variants.[63] In some studies, malaria parasite densities and counts were found to be lower in enzyme-deficient males and, sometimes, females. However, studies of severe malaria in both East and West Africa have shown that both hemizygous males and heterozygous females are significantly protected.[64] This is in keeping with the results of in vitro studies of erythrocytic cultures of *P. falciparum*, which showed impaired growth in G-6-PD-deficient red cells.[65]

Human Leukocyte Antigens

The pivotal position of HLAs in the initiation and regulation of immune responses together with their well-documented polymorphism has led to numerous studies of their influence on infectious disease susceptibility. The first evidence of HLA effects came from studies of the mycobacterial diseases leprosy and tuberculosis.[66] The HLA class II antigen HLA-DR2 was found to be both associated with and genetically linked to susceptibility to tuberculoid leprosy in India.[67,68] Although initially it appeared that HLA might predominantly influence leprosy type, most studies now indicate that HLA-DR2 in Asian populations predisposes individuals to the development of leprosy per se.[69,70] In several Asian populations, but not in other continents, the same HLA-DR2 has been associated with susceptibility to tuberculosis.[71–73] The mechanism of these susceptibility associations remains unclear, but it has been speculated that HLA-DR2 may influence the type of immune response developed, leading to stronger humoral but weaker protective cellular responses to mycobacterial antigens.

Studies of malaria susceptibility in African children identified protective associations between particular HLA types and this disease. In a large Gambian study, the HLA class I antigen HLA-B53 (now denoted B*5301) was associated with resistance to severe malaria.[48] This HLA type is particularly common in Africans, possibly as a result of natural selection by malaria. Cytotoxic T lymphocytes restricted by this HLA class I molecule recognize a peptide epitope from the liver stage of the malaria parasite's life cycle and may mediate this protective association.[74] In the same study, an HLA class II molecule, HLA-DRB1*1302, a subtype of HLA-DR13 in the older nomenclature, was also associated with resistance to a form of severe malaria, presumably indicating a protective action of CD4+ T cells restricted by this HLA-DR molecule.[48]

In a subsequent study, this same HLA type, HLA-DRB1*1302, was associated with resistance to persistent HBV infection in West Africans (Table 7-4).[75] In European populations, HLA-DR11 has been associated with resistance to persistent hepatitis C virus (HCV) infection.[76] Strong evidence of HLA associations with disease manifestations has also been presented for human papilloma virus infection.[77,78] Numerous studies of HLA and HIV infection have been undertaken. Although there appears to be relatively little consistency between most published associations, in some populations there probably are real associations between HLA type and the rate of disease progression to AIDS (see below). An overall effect of polymorphism in the major histocompatibility complex (MHC) was most convincingly demonstrated in a study of pairs of HIV-infected hemophiliac brothers. Pairs sharing two HLA haplotypes had a more similar rate of CD4 T-cell decline than those sharing only one or zero haplotypes.[79]

The accumulating evidence that particular HLA types are associated with altered susceptibility to infectious disease supports the view that the remarkable diversity of HLA types has been generated and maintained through natural selection by infectious

Table 7-4 Susceptibility and Resistance Genes Implicated in Some Viral Diseases

Gene	Variant	Disease	Effect
HLA-DR	HLA-DRB1*1302	HBV persistence	Resistance
HLA-DR	HLA-DRB1*11	HCV persistence	Resistance
CCR5	32-bp Deletion	HIV infection/progression	Resistance
CCR2	Codon 64	HIV progression	Resistance
SDF-1	3′-Untranslated region	HIV progression	Resistance
PRPN	Codon 129	Creutzfeldt-Jakob disease	Susceptibility

SDF-1, stromal-derived factor 1.

pathogens. The relatively modest magnitude of the reported associations, compared with some HLA associations with autoimmune disease, is in keeping with this possibility. Small selective effects can over time markedly change allele frequencies. The observation that cellular immune responses are restricted by HLA molecules suggested an attractive mechanism whereby heterozygosity for HLA type might be evolutionarily advantageous.[80] Heterozygotes should be able to recognize more peptide epitopes in a foreign pathogen than homozygotes, generating a more protective immune response. However, a protective effect of heterozygosity has been observed only in relation to HLA class II antigens and clearance of HBV infection.[81] Another feature of HLA associations with infectious disease is that they often vary geographically. In some cases, this may result from geographical strain variation in the infectious pathogen, and an HLA association with the strain of parasite causing infection has been reported in malaria.[82] More detailed analysis of the mechanisms of identified associations should explain further this population diversity and provide insights to immune mechanisms of protection and pathogenesis.

Cytokine Genes

Increasing understanding of the pleiotropic effects of various cytokines in immune defense has led analysis of cytokine genes in several infectious diseases. Studies of the tumor necrosis factor (TNF) gene, located in the class III region of the MHC, have been most rewarding. Several point mutations are found in the promoter of this gene which may affect the level of TNF production. A variant at position − 308 has been associated with susceptibility to cerebral malaria in Africa,[83] mucocutaneous leishmaniasis in South America,[84] and lepromatous leprosy in India.[85] Interestingly, serum levels of TNF have been found to be elevated in all of these conditions, and the genetic associations suggest that the elevated TNF levels may play a pathogenic role. These genetic associations were identified before there was in vitro evidence that this promoter variant is associated with increased levels of TNF gene expression.[86] Associations have also been described with susceptibility to trachoma[87] and to persistent HBV infection. Other promoter variants may also be associated with altered susceptibility to infectious diseases.[88] Studies of children with meningococcal disease found that those from families with low TNF and high IL-10 production in response to endotoxin stimulation in vitro had much higher mortality rates,[89] implying a protective role for a proinflammatory cytokine profile.

Searches for infectious disease associations with variants of other cytokine genes have thus far been less fruitful, but a susceptibility gene for worm burden in schistosomiasis has been mapped to a region of the long arm of chromosome 5 that encodes a large number of cytokine genes, and it has been suggested that one of these may be causative.[90] Also, rare defects in the genes for the IL-12 $\beta 1$ receptor chain and the interferon-γ receptor 1 have been associated with marked susceptibility to some avirulent mycobacteria and to *Salmonella* infection.[31,32]

Chemokine Receptors

The relatively recent discovery that certain chemokine receptors act as coreceptors for invasion of macrophages and lymphocytes by human immunodeficiency viruses has led to numerous studies of the role of polymorphism in these genes in variable susceptibility to both HIV infection and disease progression to AIDS. A 32-bp deletion in the CCR5 chemokine receptor is found at allele frequencies of up to 0.10 in European and derived populations.[91] This variant is rare or absent in other parts of the world.[92] CCR5 is the coreceptor for the macrophage-tropic strains of HIV-1 involved in viral transmission. Heterozygotes for the 32-bp deletion progress more slowly to AIDS but are not at reduced risk of HIV infection.[93] In contrast, homozygotes for this variant have very substantial resistance to HIV infection, and only a few infected homozygotes have been identified. Another rarer variant of this gene has been associated with resistance to infection.[94] An amino acid change in the linked CCR2 gene is also associated with slower disease progression to AIDS,[95] but this might be secondary to linkage disequilibrium with variants of the CCR5 gene. Lymphotropic HIV viruses which appear later in the course of infection use the CXCR4 rather than the CCR5 receptor. The natural ligand for the CXCR4 receptor is stromal-derived factor 1 (SDF-1), and variation in the 3′-untranslated region of this gene has also been associated with altered rates of disease progression to AIDS.[96]

The high prevalence of the CCR5 32-bp deletion in northern Europeans is intriguing. Analysis of flanking molecular markers has shown that this deletion is found on a rare background haplotype and suggests an origin in the last few thousand years.[97,98] This argues strongly that the variant allele has been subject to positive selection, but HIV appeared too recently to have been the selective agent. It has been speculated that various other infectious pathogens, including the plague bacillus, may have been involved.

Mannose-Binding Lectin

Mannose-binding lectin (MBL) is a serum protein that plays a role in innate immunity. It is a collagenous lectin with at least two important roles in host defense.[99] It binds to sugars, particularly *N*-acetylglucosamine and mannose, on the surface of microorganisms and facilitates their opsonization by macrophages. It also activates complement by means of two MBL-associated serine proteases. Perhaps surprisingly, inactivating mutations of this gene are quite prevalent in various populations. Three single amino acid changes are found at codons 52, 54 and 57, each of which leads to a substantial reduction in MBL concentration in heterozygotes. Homozygotes or compound heterozygotes for these variants have absent or extremely low MBL levels in serum. Variation in the promoter of the gene has less marked but detectable functional effects.[100] It was originally proposed that mannose-binding lectin (MBL) might play a key role in immune defense in late infancy after maternal antibodies had waned and before acquired immunity had been well developed. However, this remains to be established. Case reports and small-scale studies suggested that MBL deficiency might predispose individuals to a variety of infectious diseases,[101] but initial studies of individual diseases, meningococcal disease, malaria, tuberculosis, and persistent HBV infection failed to show clear associations.[102,103] A recent study of pneumococcal invasive disease, however, revealed a threefold higher frequency of individuals homozygous for codon changes in mannose-binding ligand (Roy et al. submitted 2000). Heterozygotes for these deficiency alleles were not at increased risk of disease. A study of London children with a variety of infections also found increased frequencies of MBL deficiency alleles,[104] but an increase in both heterozygotes and homozygotes for MBL deficiency alleles was reported in the infected children as well as an unexplained high prevalence of compound heterozygotes.

NRAMP1

The relevance of natural resistance-associated macrophage protein 1 (*NRAMP1*) to tuberculosis susceptibility was discovered by an unusual route. In studies of mouse strains, susceptibility to species of *Salmonella*, *Leishmania,* and some mycobacteria was found to be influenced by a single major gene that was mapped and identified by positional cloning.[28] The human homologue of this murine gene *Nramp1* is termed *NRAMP1*. Several sequence changes in *NRAMP1* have been associated with susceptibility to severe pulmonary tuberculosis in West Africa, and these variants may also affect the leprosy manifestations.[30] It is more likely that this gene affects susceptibility to clinical tuberculosis than to infection by *M. tuberculosis*, but this has not been demonstrated. The function of the *NRAMP1* gene product remains to be clarified, but it is present only in macrophages and found on the membrane of the phagolysosome in which *M. tuberculosis* grows.[105] *NRAMP1* is homologous to the recently described *NRAMP2* gene that encodes a divalent ion transporter,[106] and the former may influence intraphagosomal iron concentrations and thus mycobacterial growth.

Other Susceptibility Genes

Twin studies have indicated that most of the genetic component of variation in cellular and humoral immune responses to some common infectious pathogens appears to map to genes outside of the MHC.[107] These genes are likely to be numerous and may affect susceptibility to several infectious diseases but are unidentified. One candidate for this type of role is the vitamin-D receptor (VDR). The active form of vitamin D (D_3) has immunoregulatory functions as well as an important role in calcium metabolism.[108] The VDR is expressed in macrophages and activated lymphocytes, and vitamin D_3 leads to increased macrophage activation and a shift in the cytokine secretion profile of lymphocytes to a more TH2-like pattern. Variation in the vitamin D receptor has been associated with resistance to tuberculosis and persistent HBV infection[108a] and appears to influence the type of leprosy developed, possibly by an influence of the polarization of CD4 T-cell responses. As with the VDR association with osteoporosis, gene-environment interactions are likely to be important so that some population differences in the magnitude of such genetic associations are to be expected.

Creutzfeldt-Jakob disease (CJD) is caused by infection with prions, proteinaceous particles that appear to lack all nucleic acid. Rare familial forms of the disease have been related to variation in the host human prion protein (PRNP) gene.[109,110] In both French and U.S. patients iatrogenically infected with the CJD agent, a marked effect of a very common variation in PRNP genotype on susceptibility to disease was observed.[111,112] Homozygotes for either of the amino acids, methionine or valine, commonly found at position 129 were markedly more susceptible to disease than were heterozygotes. In U.K. patients with new-variant CJD, presumably related to infection with the bovine prion that causes bovine spongiform encephalopathy in cattle, only methionine homozygotes have been found among cases.[111]

Cystic fibrosis is the commonest life-threatening autosomal recessive disorder in populations of European origin. Causative mutations in the cystic fibrosis transmembrane conductance regulator (CFTR) are found at frequencies of up to 0.04 in these populations. It is likely, but probably not necessary,[113] that some selective advantage has contributed to the high frequencies of mutations in this gene.[114] Studies in a mouse model of cystic fibrosis led to the suggestion that cholera may have been the selective agent,[115] but more recent studies have provided stronger support for selection by typhoid rather than by cholera.[116,117] The CFTR molecule was found to be the receptor used by *Salmonella typhi* to enter intestinal epithelial cells.[116] As yet, there are no data on CFTR variation and susceptibility to typhoid in humans.

DISEASES

Malaria

More genes have been implicated in differential susceptibility to malaria than to any other disease of humans or other animals (Table 7-2). This in part reflects the early success in identifying the relevance of the sickle hemoglobin polymorphism and the geographical distribution of some malaria resistance alleles.[46] Early evidence of differential susceptibility to malaria in nonimmunes came from studies of the use of malaria therapy in the management of syphilis.[14] Marked differences in susceptibility to the same dose and strain of malaria parasite were observed between individuals. Numerous studies of sickle hemoglobin and G-6-PD deficiency have provided clear-cut evidence of their protective relevance against *P. falciparum* malaria,[47,64] but it is uncertain whether hemoglobin C, which is common in parts of West Africa, and hemoglobin E, widely distributed in Southeast Asia, are protective. A few studies have demonstrated protection associated with heterozygosity for β thalassemia and various α thalassemia genotypes, but the nature of protective effects and mechanisms of protection remain to be established.[52,53,58]

There have been relatively few useful interpopulation comparisons of malaria susceptibility. However, a study of different ethnic groups in Mali, West Africa, has found significant differences in immune responses to *P. falciparum* and in malaria susceptibility between these that appears to be genetic in origin.[7] The differences could not be explained by the known malaria resistance alleles.

HLA class I and II alleles have both been found to influence malaria susceptibility in Africa in large case-control studies,[48,118] but it is likely that the particular alleles showing associations will differ between populations, and there is some evidence that this is so. Such interpopulation heterogeneity can result from many causes, but a prominent one in malaria is likely to be the marked polymorphism of immunodominant malaria antigens. Indeed, HLA has also been found to influence the strain of malaria parasite associated with clinical malaria, and the complex interaction between HLA and parasite strain may lead to further variability in HLA associations.[82] It seems likely that the predominant immune protective mechanisms against malaria may vary geographically with transmission patterns.

Malaria parasites vary in their capacity to form rosettes with uninfected erythrocytes and to sequester in capillary beds, and both of these phenotypes have been implicated in increased malaria severity.[119,120] Recently, evidence has been provided that a polymorphic host receptor involved in parasite sequestration, intercellular adhesion molecule 1 (ICAM-1), may influence susceptibility to cerebral malaria.[121] Homozygotes for an African-specific variant, ICAM-Kilifi, were surprisingly found more frequently among cases of cerebral malaria in Kenya. In a more recent West African study, no effect of ICAM-Kilifi on malaria susceptibility was detected.[121a] Furthermore, the polymorphic complement receptor, CD35, has been found to play a role in rosetting of parasitized erythrocytes.[122] Thus, such host receptors that interact with the surface of the parasitized erythrocyte may add to the list of malaria resistance genes.

Although most genes that influence susceptibility to infectious disease have relatively small effects, a few malaria resistance genes are exceptions. The strength of the protective effect of heterozygosity for hemoglobin S is one, with about a 90 percent reduction in risk of severe malaria.[48] The protection from *P. vivax* afforded by the Duffy-negative blood group is complete, as this parasite is unable to invade Duffy-negative erythrocytes.[123] Finally, Melanesian carriers of a 27-bp deletion in the erythrocyte band 3 gene appear to be very strongly protected from *P. falciparum*,[124] maintaining the deletion at frequencies of up to 0.35 even though homozygous fetuses do not survive gestation.[125]

The large number of genes implicated in malaria resistance have all been identified through case-control studies or in vitro analyses. Apart from one study showing genetic linkage of malaria to the MHC,[126] linkage approaches have not been employed. A thorough genome-wide search, however, would likely reveal many new resistance genes. Malaria provides perhaps the best example of population variation in susceptibility and resistance genes. In West Africa, for example, sickle hemoglobin, the A^- allele of G-6-PD, HLA-B53, and an HLA-DR13 allele are associated with protection, but all of these alleles are either rare or absent in Southeast Asia and Melanesia. In the latter region, hemoglobin E, ovalocytosis, other G-6-PD alleles, and both α and β thalassemias are more prevalent.

Mycobacterial Diseases

Genetic susceptibility studies of mycobacterial diseases have been relatively common for several reasons. Familial clustering of leprosy and tuberculosis has been well recognized, and leprosy was regarded by some as a genetic disorder before *Mycobacterium leprae* was identified.[2] An accident in Lubeck, Germany, in which children were immunized with *M. tuberculosis* rather than BCG provided early evidence for variable susceptibility to tuberculosis. This was substantiated by several large twin studies that found higher concordance rates among monozygotic than dizygotic twin pairs (Table 7-1).[18] A large twin study of leprosy in India also reported higher concordance rates for leprosy in monozygotic twins but was inconclusive on the question of genetic susceptibility to leprosy type.[20] Observations on the introduction of tuberculosis to some populations previously free of the infection and disease suggested that the decline in frequency of the disease over time might in part reflect some selection for resistance genes.[11] In contrast to malaria, there is evidence that blacks may be more susceptible to infection with *M. tuberculosis* than are Caucasians. The clearest data were obtained in a comparison of rates of skin test conversion among socioeconomically matched nursing-home residents in the United States.[8] Studies of large pedigrees with multiple cases of leprosy or tuberculosis by complex segregation analysis techniques have suggested that just one or two major genes might account for much of the genetic component of susceptibility to these diseases,[127] but this suggestion remains to be evaluated in genome-wide studies. Recently, analysis of the *M. tuberculosis* genome has revealed remarkable sequence conservation between isolates with a lack of single nucleotide changes, suggesting that host polymorphism might be relatively important.[128] Finally, the chronicity of these diseases and the existence of control programs in many countries have facilitated the recruitment of families as well as unrelated cases.

Early studies of HLA variation established the relevance of HLA variation in susceptibility to both tuberculosis and leprosy.[66,68] HLA-DR2 was associated with susceptibility to tuberculoid leprosy in India, and more recent data support an association of this HLA type with susceptibility to both tuberculoid and lepromatous forms of leprosy as well as to tuberculosis in several Asian populations.[69–72] Outside of Asia, no clear HLA association has been identified and HLA-DR2 appears not to be associated with susceptibility. Variation in the promoter of the TNF gene has been associated with susceptibility to lepromatous but not tuberculoid leprosy in Bengal, India.[85] In the same population, allelic variation in the VDR has also been associated with leprosy type.[128a]

The natural resistance-associated macrophage protein-1 gene (*NRAMP1*) was suggested as a candidate gene for human mycobacterial disease by identification of its homologue as a susceptibility gene for some intracellular pathogens in mice.[28] Variation in both the 3′-untranslated region and the promoter region of the human *NRAMP1* gene has been associated with susceptibility to pulmonary tuberculosis in West Africans.[30] However, the magnitude of the effect observed in human tuberculosis is relatively modest compared with that suggested by studies of susceptibility to BCG in mice. Genes with larger effects may be identified by genome-wide linkage studies of multicase families, and these have suggested that an X-linked gene may influence susceptibility to tuberculosis.[128b]

Rare genetic disorders have frequently been informative indicators of disease mechanisms, and this also applies to mycobacterial disease. Children homozygous for mutations in the interferon-γ receptor gene have been found to be remarkably susceptible to weakly pathogenic mycobacteria, including the BCG vaccine, and have a poor prognosis.[31,32] Whether these children have increased susceptibility to tuberculosis and leprosy is unknown. Rare knockout mutations in an IL-12 receptor gene produces a similar phenotype of marked susceptibility to atypical mycobacterial disease,[33,34] directly implicating this cytokine and pathway in resistance to these bacteria.

HIV and AIDS

Studies of cohorts exposed to HIV infection have identified a small proportion of individuals who, despite repeated exposure to infection from infected sexual partners, remain HIV seronegative.[129] Some such resistant sex workers have immunologic evidence of exposure to the virus. There is also clear evidence that individuals vary in the rate of disease progression to AIDS once infected, and several genes have now been found to influence this rate.

A large number of studies of HLA type and rate of disease progression have been reported. Although there are marked differences between studies, some alleles have now been associated with susceptibility or resistance in more than one population. HLA-B35 and the HLA-A1-B8-DR3 haplotype have been associated with more rapid disease progression in several studies.[130,131] Similarly, HLA-B27 and HLA-B57 may be associated with a lower rate of progression.[132] Particular combinations of HLA class I and II alleles and variants of the transporter associated with antigen processing (TAP) genes have also been implicated.[133] Evidence of linkage of the MHC to rate of CD4 T-cell decline provides support for the relevance of polymorphism in this region.[79] However, part of the difficulty in assessing individual studies is the small size of most samples studied, usually with fewer than 200 individuals in each group. Further heterogeneity between studies may be attributed to genetic variation in HIV, because variation in viral epitopes for HLA molecules is well described both between and within individuals.

The discovery of the role of chemokine receptors as coreceptors with CD4 for viral entry into macrophages and lymphocytes has given rise to numerous studies of genetic variants of these receptors and their ligands. The CCR5 associations with risk of infection and rates of disease progression are now well established,[93] and variants in the *CCR2* and *SDF-1* gene have also been associated with altered disease progression (see above).[95,96] However, it seems likely that several other relevant genes have yet to be discovered, as the known variants of CCR5 can account for only a minority of Caucasians and none of the African individuals found to be resistant to HIV infection. Indeed, almost all available information on genetic susceptibility comes from studies of susceptibility to clade B virus in North Americans or Europeans, and little is known about genes determining susceptibility in high-prevalence African and Asian populations where other clade types are found.

Persistent Hepatitis

HBV was discovered during population genetic studies, and it was noted that carriage of hepatitis B surface antigen tended to run in families.[134,135] Some population and family studies suggested the presence of a major autosomal recessive gene. The ability or inability to clear HBV is one of the most striking immunogenetic dichotomies in medicine, with 10 to 20 percent of infected individuals becoming chronic carriers. One relatively small twin study in Taiwan provided evidence that susceptibility to HBV chronic carriage, but not HBV infection, is genetically determined.[21]

Several studies of HLA class I and II genes in HBV infection initially appeared to show little consistency. A two-stage study of Quatari patients found HLA-DR2 associated with viral clearance and HLA-DR7 with viral persistence.[136] A larger study of persistently infected Gambians found a protective association with the HLA-DRB1*1302 allele as well as a protective effect of heterozygosity in the class II region.[75,137] The same HLA-DR13 allele may be associated with protection in Europeans.[138] HLA class II antigens have also been associated with the outcome of HCV infection. In contrast to HBV infection, most individuals fail to clear HCV, and HLA-DRB1*1101 and the linked HLA-DQB1*0301 allele have been associated with higher rates of clearance in Europeans.[76]

In single studies, some non-HLA genes, TNF,[88] MBL,[139] and the VDR[108a] have also been associated with susceptibility to HBV persistence, and haptoglobin genotype may influence clearance of HCV infection.[140] The high prevalence of persistent HBV infection in some populations may make it possible to identify major non-MHC genes by using family linkage studies. The major complication of these persistent viral infections is chronic liver disease and a high incidence of hepatocellular carcinoma. Other genes may be relevant to these outcomes. In particular, the liver detoxification enzymes, epoxide hydrolase and glutathione S-transferase M1, metabolize aflatoxin, a cofactor with persistent HBV infection for risk of hepatocellular carcinoma. A synergistic interaction between these environmental risk factors and genetic variants of the detoxification enzymes has been described.[141]

Other Infectious Diseases

The genetic linkage approach has been successfully applied to the study of the host genetics of susceptibility to helminths. A study of a relatively small number of extended Brazilian families with *Schistosoma mansoni* infection found evidence of linkage of worm burden to a region of the long arm of chromosome 5.[90] The analysis allowed for the effects of some environmental variables, such as contact with infected water. No other region of the genome showed significant linkage in this model-based analysis. This chromosome 5 region may also be relevant in Senegalese families[142] and encodes numerous cytokine genes, including IL-4, IL-9, and IL-13. Interestingly, this cytokine gene cluster has also shown evidence of linkage to atopy and asthma—linkage consistent with the speculation that a gene selected for resistance to helminthic infections might predispose individuals to asthma or atopy. A promoter variant of the TNF gene has been associated with mucocutaneous leishmaniasis,[84] a disease where high levels of TNF production may be of pathogenic importance. It is unclear, however, whether this TNF-promoter association is independent of polymorphism in flanking HLA genes.

Although some mouse studies suggested that mutations of the CFTR might affect susceptibility to cholera,[115,117] recent work has identified the CFTR as the human intestinal receptor for *Salmonella typhi*, raising the possibility that heterozygotes for this disease may be resistant to typhoid.[116] Studies in humans will be required to evaluate this interesting possibility, but it may be difficult to find a region with sufficiently high prevalence of typhoid and cystic fibrosis carriers to perform a definitive case-control study. Studies of the prion diseases, new-variant CJD attributed to infection with the bovine spongiform encephalopathy agent,[143] sporadic CJD,[144] and iatrogenic CJD[111] have all shown strong associations with variation in the human prion protein (PRNP) gene.

Genetic variation in the FcγRII immunoglobulin receptor, CD32, affects the ability of neutrophils to clear Ig G_2-opsonized bacteria. Small studies of recurrent bacterial respiratory infection and systemic meningococcal infection[145,146] have suggested that alleles encoding histidine at amino acid position 132, which are associated with greater opsonic activity, may be less frequent in the disease group. However, larger studies are required. In a family study of meningococcal disease, children with first-degree relatives who had low TNF and high IL-10 production in ex vivo assays were more likely to die, suggesting a role for genes regulating production of these cytokines.[89] Little is known of the genetic basis of variable susceptibility to various fungal infections, but polymorphism in the mannose-binding ligand gene and the blood group secretor gene may be relevant.[147,148]

EVOLUTION OF POLYGENIC RESISTANCE

The information summarized in this chapter suggests that susceptibility to most infectious diseases in outbred human populations will prove to be highly polygenic. Such polygenic susceptibility has also been found in extensive analyses of the genetic basis of susceptibility to autoimmune diseases in both humans and mice,[149] but in many of these diseases major gene effects are detectable. However, it has also been suggested that there may be a few major single genes for some human infectious diseases. In this context, a major gene is one that accounts for a substantial proportion of the overall degree of genetic variation in susceptibility, not simply a susceptibility allele with a major effect. Thus, a major gene must have a relatively high frequency of variants in the population. The major-single-gene hypothesis is based on complex segregation analysis of large and sometimes highly selected pedigrees.[127] Some limitations of this approach have been highlighted,[150] and there is, as yet, no example of a major identified gene in common human infectious diseases.

The finding that multiple genes affect susceptibility to many infectious diseases probably reflects the major role that infectious pathogens have played in shaping variation in the human genome through natural selection. Indeed, it appears that genes playing a role in host defense against infectious pathogens evolve at a higher rate than any other class of genes.[151] Natural selection for resistance to infectious pathogens may also explain why the observed effects of most individual genes are relatively modest in magnitude and therefore relatively difficult to detect in small studies. Alleles that markedly increased or decreased susceptibility to major infectious disease would be quickly eliminated or selected to very high frequency or to fixation, thereby eliminating polymorphism.

Given the pressure for fixation of selectively advantageous variants, one of the major questions in evolutionary biology is related to the mechanisms maintaining substantial genetic diversity in populations. Polymorphisms that influence susceptibility to pathogens that produce high mortality rates might be expected to be lost particularly quickly. Some aspects of this evolutionary issue are particularly well addressed in human populations where the host genome and the infectious pathogens have been characterized in most detail. Heterozygote advantage is an attractive mechanism by which two alleles may be maintained in a population and is classically exemplified by the sickle hemoglobin polymorphism and resistance to malaria. Heterozygote advantage may occasionally also apply to HLA variation.[137] However, this appears to be a relatively unusual means of maintaining genetic diversity, and other mechanisms may be more generally important. These include frequency-dependent selection, whereby new or low-frequency alleles are advantageous because pathogens have not had time to adapt to them, or fluctuating selection, which may result from epidemics of different pathogens and may in some cases preserve genetic polymorphism in the host. Another relevant factor is likely to be variation in the genome of infectious pathogens. As more variants of immunologic and other functional importance are identified in pathogen genomes, increasing attention is being paid to specific interactions between variants of the host and the parasite. Interactions between polymorphic T epitopes in pathogens and variable HLA molecules in the host have been well studied in vitro. More recently, genetic studies have been undertaken in populations. Particular HLA types have been associated with disease caused by specific serotypes of human papilloma virus,[77] and HLA type may also influence the strain of *P. falciparum* causing malaria.[82]

A variety of mechanisms are used by pathogens, particularly viruses, to interfere with the antigen processing and presentation mechanisms of the host cellular immune response. One mechanism that shows specificity for genetic variants of the pathogen is altered peptide ligand antagonism of the T-cell receptor.[152] This mechanism appears to underlie complex interactions between parasite strains in malaria that may in turn affect the protective efficacy of particular HLA types.[82] There may be exquisite specificity in some of these host-parasite interactions, leading to coevolution of genetic variation in the host and pathogen. Thus, the emerging picture is that individual susceptibility to a particular infectious disease will be the result of a variety of genetic factors in both host and pathogen, tempered by environmental variables. It is likely that many polygenes will interact nonindependently or epistatically, so that their effects will depend on variation in other genes. Very large population studies will be needed to document such epistatic effects. One implication of this evolutionary perspective is that the genes affecting susceptibility to an infectious disease may show significant interpopulation heterogeneity due to geographical variation in the pathogen genome, in the environment, and in the frequencies of interacting genes in the host. This prediction is consistent with available data on malaria susceptibility and has a practical implication for the conduct of host genetic studies. With significant heterogeneity in susceptibility genes expected, it may be difficult to combine data from different study populations to provide confirmatory results. Thus, very large studies in a single population will often be more useful than a series of smaller studies in different geographical regions. This constraint applies particularly to studies of host genes, such as HLA, that interact directly or indirectly with polymorphic pathogen sequences. Wherever possible, pathogen genetic diversity should be studied in parallel with host genetics to determine whether there is strain specificity in disease associations.

CLINICAL UTILITY

There are several potential advantages to applying the power of modern molecular genetics to understand susceptibility to infectious disease more fully. One application is in risk prediction. This might influence behavior, travel patterns, or the use of prophylactic antimicrobials and immunizations. It is likely that in the future it will be possible to offer a genetic profiling test to estimate individual susceptibility to particular pathogens. It has already been proposed that widespread screening for mannose-binding ligand deficiency alleles might be valuable, but more extensive studies of the susceptibility profile of homozygotes and heterozygotes are required. It is unlikely that most of the genetic component to any common infectious disease can be accounted for by the polymorphisms and associations identified to date. For example, the recently identified *NRAMP1* association can account for less than 2 percent of the overall host genetic component to tuberculosis susceptibility found in twin studies. But, as genes with larger effects or more genes with effects of similar magnitude are identified, screening for susceptibility to some diseases will become more useful. It seems likely that in the future some of the same genetic variants will be typed in evaluating susceptibility to autoimmune and infectious disease.

Association of functional polymorphisms in genes encoding cytokines or their receptors with disease susceptibility may lead to attempts to modulate the activity of these mediators in patients. The upregulatory variant of the polymorphism at position -308 of the TNF promoter[86] was associated with susceptibility to severe malaria,[83] and agents that may reduce the activity of this cytokine are under assessment.[153,154] Another application is in the understanding of specific immune defenses used in host resistance to infection. For example, the HLA-B53 association with resistance to malaria[48] supported a protective role for CD8 T cells in this disease. This led to the identification of epitope in malaria antigens for inclusion in subunit CD8 T-cell-inducing vaccines by using an approach known as reverse immunogenetics.[74,155] However, the utility of the genetic association with HLA-B53 was principally to provide evidence that HLA class I-restricted T cells are of protective relevance in human malaria. The enhanced susceptibility to nonvirulent mycobacteria in children with mutations in the γ-interferon receptor has highlighted the importance of this pathway in controlling these mycobacteria, but the observation that these children appear to have no alteration in their susceptibility to other common pathogens, particularly many common viruses, has been equally interesting. The comparison of disease susceptibility in individuals with and without mannose-binding ligand deficiency has illustrated how this molecule plays a key role in resistance to some, but not to other, infectious agents.

An increasingly important application will be the identification of molecules and pathways that are targets for pharmacologic intervention. This is the main applied goal of current attempts to identify new major susceptibility genes through genome-wide analyses. An illustration of the rapid application of a finding in host genetics comes from the HIV field. The demonstration of the very substantial resistance to HIV infection of homozygotes for a deletion in the CCR5 gene has underpinned recent attempts to develop pharmacologic blockers of this viral coreceptor. The *NRAMP1* gene product may also turn out to be amenable to specific pharmacologic interventions. New techniques of genome-wide analysis offer the prospect of many new target molecules discovered through linkage analysis and positional cloning, but how many of these can be usefully employed remains to be seen. Of the many malaria resistance genes known (Table 7-3) only a few have led to new approaches to disease intervention. Yet the potentially very large number of infectious disease resistance genes and the increasing power of methods of identifying these suggest that several useful new molecular targets should be identifiable in the near future.

REFERENCES

1. Harboe M: Gerhard Henrik Armauer Hansen—still of current interest. *Tidsskr Nor Laegeforen* **112**:3795, 1992.
2. Fine PE: Immunogenetics of susceptibility to leprosy, tuberculosis, and leishmaniasis: An epidemiological perspective. *Int J Lepr Other Mycobact Dis* **49**:437, 1981.
3. Shields ED, Russell DA, Pericak-Vance MA: Genetic epidemiology of the susceptibility to leprosy. *J Clin Invest* **79**:1139, 1987.
4. Abel L, Demenais F, Prata A, et al: Evidence for the segregation of a major gene in human susceptibility/resistance to infection by *Schistosoma mansoni*. *Am J Hum Genet* **48**:959, 1991.
5. Weeks DE, Lathrop GM: Polygenic disease: Methods for mapping complex disease traits. *Trends Genet* **11**:513, 1995.
6. Miller LH, Mason SJ, Clyde DF, et al: The resistance factor to *Plasmodium vivax* in blacks: The Duffy-blood-group genotype, FyFy. *N Engl J Med* **295**:302, 1976.
7. Modiano D, Petrarca V, Sirima BS, et al: Different response to *Plasmodium falciparum* malaria in West African sympatric ethnic groups. *Proc Natl Acad Sci USA* **93**:13,206, 1996.
8. Stead WW, Senner JW, Reddick WT, et al: Racial differences in susceptibility to infection by *Mycobacterium tuberculosis*. *N Engl J Med* **322**:422, 1990.
9. Hoge CW, Fisher L, Donnell HD Jr, et al: Risk factors for transmission of *Mycobacterium tuberculosis* in a primary school outbreak: Lack of racial difference in susceptibility to infection. *Am J Epidemiol* **139**:520, 1994.
10. Black FL: Why did they die? *Science* **258**:1739, 1992.
11. Motulsky AG: Metabolic polymorphisms and the role of infectious diseases in human evolution. *Hum Biol* **32**:28, 1960.
12. Motulsky AG: Jewish diseases and origins. *Nat Genet* **9**:99, 1995.
13. De Vries RR, Meera Khan P, Bernini LF, et al: Genetic control of survival in epidemics. *J Immunogenet* **6**:271, 1979.
14. James SP, Nicol WD, Shute PG: A study of induced malignant tertian malaria. *Proc R Soc Med* **25**:1153, 1932.
15. Sorensen TI, Nielsen GG, Andersen PK, et al: Genetic and environmental influences on premature death in adult adoptees. *N Engl J Med* **318**:727, 1988.
16. Diehl K, Von Verscheur O: *Der Erbeinfluss bei den Tuberkulose*. Jena, Gustav Fischer, 1936.
17. Kallmann FJ, Reisner D: Twin studies on the significance of genetic factors in tuberculosis. *Am Rev Tuberculosis* **47**:549, 1942.
18. Comstock GW: Tuberculosis in twins: A re-analysis of the Prophit survey. *Am Rev Respir Dis* **117**:621, 1978.
19. Herndon CN, Jennings RG: A twin-family study of susceptibility to poliomyelitis. *Am J Hum Genet* **3**:17, 1951.
20. Chakravarti MR, Vogel F: *A Twin Study on Leprosy*, vol 1. Stuttgart, Thieme, 1973.
21. Lin TM, Chen CJ, Wu MM, et al: Hepatitis B virus markers in Chinese twins. *Anticancer Res* **9**:737, 1989.
22. Malaty HM, Engstrand L, Pedersen NL, et al: *Helicobacter pylori* infection: Genetic and environmental influences—A study of twins. *Ann Intern Med* **120**:982, 1994.
23. Jepson AP, Banya WA, Sisay-Joof F, et al: Genetic regulation of fever in *Plasmodium falciparum* malaria in Gambian twin children. *J Infect Dis* **172**:316, 1995.
24. Vogel F, Motulsky AG: *Human Genetics: Problems and Approaches*, 3d ed. New York, Springer, 1996.
25. Flanders WD, Khoury MJ: Analysis of case-parental control studies: Method for the study of associations between disease and genetic markers. *Am J Epidemiol* **144**:696, 1996.
26. Haldane JBS: Disease and evolution. *Ric Sci* **19**(Suppl):68, 1949.
27. Staeheli P, Grob R, Meier E, et al: Influenza virus-susceptible mice carry *Mx* genes with a large deletion or a nonsense mutation. *Mol Cell Biol* **8**:4518, 1988.

28. Vidal SM, Malo D, Vogan K, et al: Natural resistance to infection with intracellular parasites: Isolation of a candidate for Bcg. *Cell* **73**:469, 1993.
29. McLeod R, Buschman E, Arbuckle LD, et al: Immunogenetics in the analysis of resistance to intracellular pathogens. *Curr Opin Immunol* **7**:539, 1995.
30. Bellamy R, Ruwende C, Corrah T, et al: Variations in the *NRAMP1* gene and susceptibility to tuberculosis in West Africans. *N Engl J Med* **338**:640, 1998.
31. Newport MJ, Huxley CM, Huston S, et al: A mutation in the interferon-gamma-receptor gene and susceptibility to mycobacterial infection. *N Engl J Med* **335**:1941, 1996.
32. Jouanguy E, Altare F, Lamhamedi S, et al: Interferon-gamma-receptor deficiency in an infant with fatal bacille Calmette-Guerin infection. *N Engl J Med* **335**:1956, 1996.
33. Jong R, Altare F, Haagen IA, et al: Severe mycobacterial and salmonella infections in interleukin-12 receptor-deficient patients. *Science* **280**:1435, 1998.
34. Altare F, Durandy A, Lammas D, et al: Impairment of mycobacterial immunity in human interleukin-12 receptor deficiency. *Science* **280**:1432, 1998.
35. Levine MM, Nalin DR, Rennels MB, et al: Genetic susceptibility to cholera. *Ann Hum Biol* **6**:369, 1979.
36. Glass RI, Holmgren J, Haley CE, et al: Predisposition for cholera of individuals with O blood group. Possible evolutionary significance. *Am J Epidemiol* **121**:791, 1985.
37. Boren T, Falk P, Roth KA, et al: Attachment of *Helicobacter pylori* to human gastric epithelium mediated by blood group antigens. *Science* **262**:1892, 1993.
38. Umlauft F, Keeffe EB, Offner F, et al: *Helicobacter pylori* infection and blood group antigens: Lack of clinical association. *Am J Gastroenterol* **91**:2135, 1996.
39. Kelly RJ, Rouquier S, Giorgi D, et al: Sequence and expression of a candidate for the human secretor blood group alpha(1,2)fucosyltransferase gene (FUT2): Homozygosity for an enzyme-inactivating nonsense mutation commonly correlates with the non-secretor phenotype. *J Biol Chem* **270**:4640, 1995.
40. Blackwell CC, Jonsdottir K, Hanson M, et al: Non-secretion of ABO antigens Predisposing to infection by *Neisseria meningitidis* and *Streptococcus pneumoniae*. *Lancet* **2**:284, 1986.
41. Raza MW, Blackwell CC, Molyneaux P, et al: Association between secretor status and respiratory viral illness. *BMJ* **303**:815, 1991.
42. Sheinfeld J, Schaeffer AJ, Cordon-Cardo C, et al: Association of the Lewis blood-group phenotype with recurrent urinary tract infections in women. *N Engl J Med* **320**:773, 1989.
43. Stapleton A, Nudelman E, Clausen H, et al: Binding of uropathogenic *Escherichia coli* R45 to glycolipids extracted from vaginal epithelial cells is dependent on histo-blood group secretor status. *J Clin Invest* **90**:965, 1992.
44. Horuk R, Chitnis CE, Darbonne WC, et al: A receptor for the malarial parasite *Plasmodium vivax*: The erythrocyte chemokine receptor. *Science* **261**:1182, 1993.
45. Tournamille C, Colin Y, Cartron JP, et al: Disruption of a GATA motif in the Duffy gene promoter abolishes erythroid gene expression in Duffy-negative individuals. *Nat Genet* **10**:224, 1995.
46. Allison AC: Protection afforded by sickle-cell trait against subtertian malarial infection. *BMJ* **1**:290, 1954.
47. Allison AC: Polymorphism and natural selection in human populations. *Cold Spring Harbor Symp Quant Biol* **29**:137, 1964.
48. Hill AV, Allsopp CE, Kwiatkowski D, et al: Common west African HLA antigens are associated with protection from severe malaria. *Nature* **352**:595, 1991.
49. Pasvol G, Weatherall DJ, Wilson RJ: Cellular mechanism for the protective effect of haemoglobin S against *P. falciparum* malaria. *Nature* **274**:701, 1978.
50. Friedman MJ: Erythrocytic mechanism of sickle cell resistance to malaria. *Proc Natl Acad Sci USA* **75**:1994, 1978.
51. Friedman MJ: Oxidant damage mediates variant red cell resistance to malaria. *Nature* **280**:245, 1979.
52. Flint J, Hill AVS, Bowden DK et al: High frequencies of α thalassemia are the result of natural selection by malaria. *Nature* **321**:744, 1986.
53. Willcox M, Bjorkman A, Brohult J, et al: A case-control study in northern Liberia of *Plasmodium falciparum* malaria in haemoglobin S and beta-thalassaemia traits. *Ann Trop Med Parasitol* **77**:239, 1983.
54. Luzzi GA, Torii M, Aikawa M, et al: Unrestricted growth of *Plasmodium falciparum* in microcytic erythrocytes in iron deficiency and thalassaemia. *Br J Haematol* **74**:519, 1990.
55. Senok AC, Li K, Nelson EA, et al: Invasion and growth of *Plasmodium falciparum* is inhibited in fractionated thalassaemic erythrocytes. *Trans R Soc Trop Med Hyg* **91**:138, 1997.
56. Udomsangpetch R, Sueblinvong T, Pattanapanyasat K, et al: Alteration in cytoadherence and rosetting of *Plasmodium falciparum*-infected thalassemic red blood cells. *Blood* **82**:3752, 1993.
57. Luzzi GA, Merry AH, Newbold CI, et al: Surface antigen expression on *Plasmodium falciparum*-infected erythrocytes is modified in alpha- and beta-thalassemia. *J Exp Med* **173**:785, 1991.
58. Williams TN, Maitland K, Bennett S, et al: High incidence of malaria in alpha-thalassaemic children. *Nature* **383**:522, 1996.
59. Allen SJ, O'Donnell A, Alexander ND, et al: alpha$^+$-Thalassemia protects children against disease caused by other infections as well as malaria. *Proc Natl Acad Sci USA* **94**:14,736, 1997.
60. Guinet F, Diallo DA, Minta D, et al: A comparison of the incidence of severe malaria in Malian children with normal and C-trait hemoglobin profiles. *Acta Trop* **68**:175, 1997.
61. Orkin SH, Kazazian HH Jr, Antonarakis SE, et al: Abnormal RNA processing due to the exon mutation of beta E-globin gene. *Nature* **300**:768, 1982.
62. Motulsky AG, Stamatoyannopoulos G: Clinical implications of glucose-6-phosphate dehydrogenase deficiency. *Ann Intern Med* **65**:1329, 1966.
63. Vulliamy T, Beutler E, Luzzatto L: Variants of glucose-6-phosphate dehydrogenase are due to missense mutations spread throughout the coding region of the gene. *Hum Mutat* **2**:159, 1993.
64. Ruwende C, Khoo SC, Snow RW, et al: Natural selection of hemi- and heterozygotes for G6PD deficiency in Africa by resistance to severe malaria. *Nature* **376**:246, 1995.
65. Roth EF Jr, Raventos-Suarez C, Rinaldi A, et al: Glucose-6-phosphate dehydrogenase deficiency inhibits in vitro growth of *Plasmodium falciparum*. *Proc Natl Acad Sci USA* **80**:298, 1983.
66. De Vries RR, Fat RF, Nijenhuis LE, et al: HLA-linked genetic control of host response to *Mycobacterium leprae*. *Lancet* **2**:1328, 1976.
67. De Vries RR, Mehra NK, Vaidya MC, et al: HLA-linked control of susceptibility to tuberculoid leprosy and association with HLA-DR types. *Tissue Antigens* **16**:294, 1980.
68. Singh SP, Mehra NK, Dingley HB, et al: Human leukocyte antigen (HLA)-linked control of susceptibility to pulmonary tuberculosis and association with HLA-DR types. *J Infect Dis* **148**:676, 1983.
69. Todd JR, West BC, McDonald JC: Human leukocyte antigen and leprosy: Study in northern Louisiana and review. *Rev Infect Dis* **12**:63, 1990.
70. Rani R, Fernandez Vina MA, Zaheer SA, et al: Study of HLA class II alleles by PCR oligotyping in leprosy patients from north India. *Tissue Antigens* **42**:133, 1993.
71. Brahmajothi V, Pitchappan RM, Kakkanaiah VN, et al: Association of pulmonary tuberculosis and HLA in south India. *Tubercle* **72**:123, 1991.
72. Bothamley GH, Beck JS, Schreuder GM, et al: Association of tuberculosis and *M. tuberculosis*-specific antibody levels with HLA. *J Infect Dis* **159**:549, 1989.
73. Khomenko AG, Litvinov VI, Chukanova VP, et al: Tuberculosis in patients with various HLA phenotypes. *Tubercle* **71**:187, 1990.
74. Hill AV, Elvin J, Willis AC, et al: Molecular analysis of the association of HLA-B53 and resistance to severe malaria. *Nature* **360**:434, 1992.
75. Thursz MR, Kwiatkowski D, Allsopp CE, et al: Association between an MHC class II allele and clearance of hepatitis B virus in the Gambia. *N Engl J Med* **332**:1065, 1995.
76. Zavaglia C, Bortolon C, Ferrioli G, et al: HLA typing in chronic type B, D and C hepatitis. *J Hepatol* **24**:658, 1996.
77. Apple RJ, Erlich HA, Klitz W, et al: HLA DR-DQ associations with cervical carcinoma show papillomavirus-type specificity. *Nat Genet* **6**:157, 1994.
78. Wank R, Thomssen C: High risk of squamous cell carcinoma of the cervix for women with HLA-DQw3. *Nature* **352**:723, 1991.
79. Kroner BL, Goedert JJ, Blattner WA, et al: Concordance of human leukocyte antigen haplotype-sharing, CD4 decline and AIDS in hemophilic siblings: Multicenter Hemophilia Cohort and Hemophilia Growth and Development Studies. *AIDS* **9**:275, 1995.
80. Doherty PC, Zinkernagel RM: A biological role for the major histocompatibility antigens. *Lancet* **1**:1406, 1975.

81. Thursz MR, Kwiatkowski D, Torok ME, et al: Association of hepatitis B surface antigen carriage with severe malaria in Gambian children. *Nat Med* **1**:374, 1995.
82. Gilbert SC, Plebanski M, Gupta S, et al: Association of malaria parasite population structure, HLA, and immunological antagonism. *Science* **279**:1173, 1998.
83. McGuire W, Hill AV, Allsopp CE, et al: Variation in the TNF-alpha promoter region associated with susceptibility to cerebral malaria. *Nature* **371**:508, 1994.
84. Cabrera M, Shaw M-A, Sharples C, et al: Polymorphism in tumor necrosis factor genes associated with mucocutaneous leishmaniasis. *J Exp Med* **182**:1259, 1995.
85. Roy S, McGuire W, Mascie-Taylor CG, et al: Tumor necrosis factor promoter polymorphism and susceptibility to lepromatous leprosy. *J Infect Dis* **176**:530, 1997.
86. Wilson AG, Symons JA, McDowell TL, et al: Effects of a polymorphism in the human tumor necrosis factor alpha promoter on transcriptional activation. *Proc Natl Acad Sci USA* **94**:3195, 1997.
87. Conway DJ, Holland MJ, Bailey RL, et al: Scarring trachoma is associated with polymorphism in the tumor necrosis factor alpha (TNF-alpha) gene promoter and with elevated TNF-alpha levels in tear fluid. *Infect Immun* **65**:1003, 1997.
88. Hohler T, Kruger A, Gerken G, et al: A tumor necrosis factor-alpha (TNF-alpha) promoter polymorphism is associated with chronic hepatitis B infection. *Clin Exp Immunol* **111**:579, 1998.
89. Westendorp RG, Langermans JA, Huizinga TW, et al: Genetic influence on cytokine production and fatal meningococcal disease. *Lancet* **349**:170, 1997.
90. Marquet S, Abel L, Hillaire D, et al: Genetic localization of a locus controlling the intensity of infection by *Schistosoma mansoni* on chromosome 5q31-q33. *Nat Genet* **14**:181, 1996.
91. Liu R, Paxton WA, Choe S, et al: Homozygous defect in HIV-1 coreceptor accounts for resistance of some multiply-exposed individuals to HIV-1 infection. *Cell* **86**:367, 1996.
92. Martinson JJ, Chapman NH, Rees DC, et al: Global distribution of the CCR5 gene 32-basepair deletion. *Nat Genet* **16**:100, 1997.
93. Dean M, Carrington M, Winkler C, et al: Genetic restriction of HIV-1 infection and progression to AIDS by a deletion allele of the CKR5 structural gene: Hemophilia Growth and Development Study, Multicenter AIDS Cohort Study, Multicenter Hemophilia Cohort Study, San Francisco City Cohort, ALIVE Study. *Science* **273**:1856, 1996.
94. Quillent C, Oberlin E, Braun J, et al: HIV-1-resistance phenotype conferred by combination of two separate inherited mutations of CCR5 gene. *Lancet* **351**:14, 1998.
95. Smith MW, Dean M, Carrington M, et al: Contrasting genetic influence of CCR2 and CCR5 variants on HIV-1 infection and disease progression: Hemophilia Growth and Development Study (HGDS), Multicenter AIDS Cohort Study (MACS), Multicenter Hemophilia Cohort Study (MHCS), San Francisco City Cohort (SFCC), ALIVE Study. *Science* **277**:959, 1997.
96. Winkler C, Modi W, Smith MW, et al: Genetic restriction of AIDS pathogenesis by an SDF-1 chemokine gene variant: ALIVE Study, Hemophilia Growth and Development Study (HGDS), Multicenter AIDS Cohort Study (MACS), Multicenter Hemophilia Cohort Study (MHCS), San Francisco City Cohort (SFCC). *Science* **279**:389, 1998.
97. Libert F, Cochaux P, Beckman G, et al: The deltaccr5 mutation conferring protection against HIV-1 in Caucasian populations has a single and recent origin in Northeastern Europe. *Hum Mol Genet* **7**:399, 1998.
98. Stephens JC, Reich DE, Goldstein DB, et al: Dating the origin of the CCR5-delta32 AIDS-resistance allele by the coalescence of haplotypes. *Am J Hum Genet* **62**:1507, 1998.
99. Turner MW: Mannose-binding lectin: The pluripotent molecule of the innate immune system. *Immunol Today* **17**:532, 1996.
100. Madsen HO, Garred P, Thiel S, et al: Interplay between promoter and structural gene variants control basal serum level of mannan-binding protein. *J Immunol* **155**:3013, 1995.
101. Summerfield JA, Ryder S, Sumiya M, et al: Mannose binding protein gene mutations associated with unusual and severe infections in adults. *Lancet* **345**:886, 1995.
102. Garred P, Michaelsen TE, Bjune G, et al: A low serum concentration of mannan-binding protein is not associated with serogroup B or C meningococcal disease. *Scand J Immunol* **37**:468, 1993.
103. Bellamy R, Ruwende C, McAdam KP, et al: Mannose binding protein deficiency is not associated with malaria, hepatitis B carriage nor tuberculosis in Africans. *Q J Med* **91**:13, 1998.
104. Summerfield JA, Sumiya M, Levin M, et al: Association of mutations in mannose binding protein gene with childhood infection in consecutive hospital series. *BMJ* **314**:1229, 1997.
105. Gruenheid S, Pinner E, Desjardins M, et al: Natural resistance to infection with intracellular pathogens: The *Nramp1* protein is recruited to the membrane of the phagosome. *J Exp Med* **185**:717, 1997.
106. Gunshin H, Mackenzie B, Berger UV, et al: Cloning and characterization of a mammalian proton-coupled metal-ion transporter. *Nature* **388**:482, 1997.
107. Jepson A, Banya W, Sisay-Joof F, et al: Quantification of the relative contribution of major histocompatibility complex (MHC) and non-MHC genes to human immune responses to foreign antigens. *Infect Immun* **65**:872, 1997.
108. Tsoukas CD, Provvedini DM, Manolagas SC: 1,25-Dihydroxyvitamin D_3: A novel immunoregulatory hormone. *Science* **224**:1438, 1984.
108a. Bellamy R, Ruwende C, Corrah T, McAdam KP, Thursz M, Whittle HC, Hill AVS: Tuberculosis and chronic hepatitis B virus infection in Africans and variation in the vitamin D receptor gene. *J Infect Dis* **179**:721, 1999.
109. Goldfarb LG, Brown P, Haltia M, et al: Creutzfeldt-Jakob disease cosegregates with the codon 178Asn PRNP mutation in families of European origin. *Ann Neurol* **31**:274, 1992.
110. Chen SG, Parchi P, Brown P, et al: Allelic origin of the abnormal prion protein isoform in familial prion diseases. *Nat Med* **3**:1009, 1997.
111. Deslys J-P, Jaeglyy A, d'Aignaux JH, et al: Genotype at codon 129 and susceptibility to Creutzfeldt-Jacob disease. *Lancet* **351**:1251, 1998.
112. Brown P, Cervenakova L, Goldfarb LG, et al: Iatrogenic Creutzfeldt-Jakob disease: An example of the interplay between ancient genes and modern medicine. *Neurology* **44**:291, 1994.
113. Thompson EA, Neel JV: Allelic disequilibrium and allele frequency distribution as a function of social and demographic history. *Am J Hum Genet* **60**:197, 1997.
114. Bertranpetit J, Calafell F: Genetic and geographical variability in cystic fibrosis: Evolutionary considerations. *Ciba Found Symp* **197**:97, 1996.
115. Gabriel SE, Brigman KN, Koller BH, et al: Cystic fibrosis heterozygote resistance to cholera toxin in the cystic fibrosis mouse model. *Science* **266**:107, 1994.
116. Pier GB, Grout M, Zaidi T, et al: *Salmonella typhi* uses CFTR to enter intestinal epithelial cells. *Nature* **393**:79, 1998.
117. Cuthbert AW, Halstead J, Ratcliff R, et al: The genetic advantage hypothesis in cystic fibrosis heterozygotes: A murine study. *J Physiol (Lond)* **482**(Pt 2):449, 1995.
118. Hill AV, Yates SN, Allsopp CE, et al: Human leukocyte antigens and natural selection by malaria. *Philos Trans R Soc Lond [Biol]* **346**:379, 1994.
119. Carlson J, Helmby H, Hill AV, et al: Human cerebral malaria: Association with erythrocyte rosetting and lack of anti-rosetting antibodies. *Lancet* **336**:1457, 1990.
120. Marsh K, Snow RW: Host-parasite interaction and morbidity in malaria endemic areas. *Philos Trans R Soc Lond [Biol]* **352**:1385, 1997.
121. Fernandez-Reyes D, Craig AG, Kyes SA, et al: A high frequency African coding polymorphism in the N-terminal domain of ICAM-1 predisposing to cerebral malaria in Kenya. *Hum Mol Genet* **6**:1357, 1997.
121a. Bellamy R, Kwiatkowski D, Hill AVS: Absence of an association between ICAM-1, complement receptor 1 and interleukin 1 receptor antagonist gene polymorphisms and severe malaria in a West African population. *Trans R Soc Trop Med Hyg* **92**:312, 1998.
122. Rowe JA, Moulds JM, Newbold CI, et al: *P. falciparum* rosetting mediated by a parasite-variant erythrocyte membrane protein and complement-receptor 1. *Nature* **388**:292, 1997.
123. Miller LH, Mason SJ, Dvorak JA, et al: Erythrocyte receptors for (*Plasmodium knowlesi*) malaria: Duffy blood group determinants. *Science* **189**:561, 1975.
124. Genton B, al-Yaman F, Mgone CS, et al: Ovalocytosis and cerebral malaria [Letter]. *Nature* **378**:564, 1995.
125. Mgone CS, Koki G, Paniu MM, et al: Occurrence of the erythrocyte band 3 (AE1) gene deletion in relation to malaria endemicity in Papua New Guinea. *Trans R Soc Trop Med Hyg* **90**:228, 1996.
126. Jepson A, Sisay-Joof F, Banya W, et al: Genetic linkage of mild malaria to the major histocompatibility complex in Gambian children: Study of affected sibling pairs. *BMJ* **315**:96, 1997.

127. Abel L, Demenais F: Detection of major genes for susceptibility to leprosy and its subtypes in a Caribbean island: Desirade island. *Am J Hum Genet* **42**:256, 1988.
128. Sreevatsan S, Pan X, Stockbauer KE, et al: Restricted structural gene polymorphism in the *Mycobacterium tuberculosis* complex indicates evolutionarily recent global dissemination. *Proc Natl Acad Sci USA* **94**:9869, 1997.
128a. Roy AS, Frodsham A, Saha B, Hazra SK, Mascie-Taylor CGN, Hill AVS: Association of vitamin D receptor genotype with leprosy type. *J Infect Dis* **179**:187, 1999.
128b. Bellamy R, Beyers N, McAdam KP, et al: Genetic susceptibility to tuberculosis in Africans: a genome-wide scan. *Proc Natl Acad Sci USA* **97**:8005, 2000.
129. Fowke KR, Nagelkerke NJ, Kimani J, et al: Resistance to HIV-1 infection among persistently seronegative prostitutes in Nairobi, Kenya. *Lancet* **348**:1347, 1996.
130. Scorza Smeraldi R, Fabio G, Lazzarin A, et al: HLA-associated susceptibility to acquired immunodeficiency syndrome in Italian patients with human-immunodeficiency-virus infection. *Lancet* **2**:1187, 1986.
131. Kaslow RA, Duquesnoy R, Van Raden M, et al: A1, Cw7, B8, DR3 HLA antigen combination associated with rapid decline of T-helper lymphocytes in HIV-1 infection: A report from the Multicenter AIDS Cohort Study. *Lancet* **335**:927, 1990.
132. McNeil AJ, Yap PL, Gore SM, et al: Association of HLA types A1-B8-DR3 and B27 with rapid and slow progression of HIV disease. *Q J Med* **89**:177, 1996.
133. Kaslow RA, Carrington M, Apple R, et al: Influence of combinations of major histocompatibility genes on the course of HIV-1 infection. *Nat Med* **2**:405, 1996.
134. Blumberg BS: The nature of Australia antigen: Infectious and genetic characteristics. *Prog Liver Dis* **4**:367, 1972.
135. Blumberg BS, Melartin L, Guint RA, et al: Family studies of a human serum isoantigen system (Australia antigen). *Am J Hum Genet* **18**:594, 1966.
136. Almarri A, Batchelor JR: HLA and hepatitis B infection. *Lancet* **344**:1194, 1994.
137. Thursz MR, Thomas HC, Greenwood BM, et al: Heterozygote advantage for HLA class-II type in hepatitis B virus infection. *Nat Genet* **17**:11, 1997.
138. Hohler T, Gerken G, Notghi A, et al: HLA-DRB1*1301 and *1302 protect against chronic hepatitis B. *J Hepatol* **26**:503, 1997.
139. Thomas HC, Foster GR, Sumiya M, et al: Mutation of gene of mannose-binding protein associated with chronic hepatitis B viral infection. *Lancet* **348**:1417, 1996.
140. Louagie HK, Brouwer JT, Delanghe JR, et al: Haptoglobin polymorphism and chronic hepatitis C. *J Hepatol* **25**:10, 1996.
141. McGlynn KA, Rosvold EA, Lustbader ED, et al: Susceptibility to hepatocellular carcinoma is associated with genetic variation in the enzymatic detoxification of aflatoxin B_1. *Proc Natl Acad Sci USA* **92**:2384, 1995.
142. Muller-Myhsok B, Stelma FF, Guisse-Sow F, et al: Further evidence suggesting the presence of a locus, on human chromosome 5q31-q33, influencing the intensity of infection with *Schistosoma mansoni*. *Am J Hum Genet* **61**:452, 1997.
143. Zeidler M, Stewart G, Cousens SN, et al: Codon 129 genotype and new variant CJD. *Lancet* **350**:668, 1997.
144. Palmer MS, Dryden AJ, Hughes JT, et al: Homozygous prion protein genotype predisposes to sporadic Creutzfeldt-Jakob disease. *Nature* **352**:340, 1991.
145. Bredius RG, Derkx BH, Fijen CA, et al: Fc gamma receptor IIa (CD32) polymorphism in fulminant meningococcal septic shock in children. *J Infect Dis* **170**:848, 1994.
146. Sanders LA, van de Winkel JG, Rijkers GT, et al: Fc gamma receptor IIa (CD32) heterogeneity in patients with recurrent bacterial respiratory tract infections. *J Infect Dis* **170**:854, 1994.
147. Thom SM, Blackwell CC, MacCallum CJ, et al: Non-secretion of blood group antigens and susceptibility to infection by *Candida* species. *FEMS Microbiol Immunol* **1**:401, 1989.
148. Tabona P, Mellor A, Summerfield JA: Mannose binding protein is involved in first-line host defence: Evidence from transgenic mice. *Immunology* **85**:153, 1995.
149. Vyse TJ, Todd JA: Genetic analysis of autoimmune disease. *Cell* **85**:311, 1996.
150. McGuffin P, Huckle P: Simulation of Mendelism revisited: The recessive gene for attending medical school. *Am J Hum Genet* **46**:994, 1990.
151. Murphy PM: Molecular mimicry and the generation of host defense protein diversity. *Cell* **72**:823, 1993.
152. Sette A, Alexander J, Ruppert J, et al: Antigen analogs/MHC complexes as specific T cell receptor antagonists. *Annu Rev Immunol* **12**:413, 1994.
153. Kwiatkowski D, Molyneux ME, Stephens S, et al: Anti-TNF therapy inhibits fever in cerebral malaria. *Q J Med* **86**:91, 1993.
154. Van Hensbroek MB, Palmer A, Onyiorah E, et al: The effect of a monoclonal antibody to tumor necrosis factor on survival from childhood cerebral malaria. *J Infect Dis* **174**:1091, 1996.
155. Davenport M, Hill AVS: Reverse immunogenetics: From HLA-disease associations to vaccine candidates. *Mol Med Today* **2**:38, 1996.

CHAPTER 8

Genetics and Aging

George M. Martin

1. The current unprecedented rate of growth of the population over age 85 years underscores the importance of investigating genetic factors modulating age-related disabilities and diseases. An equally important and neglected task, however, is to discover genetic factors leading to unusual degrees of maintenance of structure and function in late life (*successful* or *elite* aging).
2. There are six stages in the life cycle of humans: developing, maturing, reproducing, *sageing* (characterized by extensive use of physiological and behavioral compensations), senescing (characterized by increasing degrees of homeostatic failures), and dying. Gene action at all of these stages is relevant to the biology of aging.
3. Senescence can occur in the absence of overt specific disease entities but cannot easily be dissociated from disease states. Senescent changes in tissues may be direct precursors of common late-onset diseases via mechanisms that remain to be fully elucidated. One example is somatic mutation, a precursor of the many neoplasms that emerge in late life. Late-onset diseases may therefore be viewed as senescent phenotypes.
4. Senescent phenotypes are nonadaptive traits that occur because of the decline in the force of natural selection with respect to the age of gene effects. Senescence is not "programmed" in the sense that determinative, sequential gene action programs development.
5. Two broad classes of gene action are postulated to differentially modulate senescent phenotypes and life span. The first involves constitutional mutations with neutral effects on reproductive fitness but with deleterious effects late in the life course, thus escaping the force of natural selection. These modulations can be regarded as *private* in that their frequencies in various populations are largely functions of genetic drift. The second involves genes with antagonistic pleiotropic actions. These involve allelic variants selected to enhance reproductive fitness but with deleterious effects late in the life course. Because such alleles are likely to spread widely within many populations, they can be considered to lead to *public* modulations of senescence. Polymorphisms, rather than rare mutations, are more likely to be responsible for differential public modulations within populations.
6. It is probably the case that variants at thousands of genetic loci have the potential to modulate the pathobiology of senescence. These can be divided into two classes: variants that lead to *segmental progeroid syndromes*, which impact upon multiple senescent phenotypes, and variants that lead to *unimodal progeroid syndromes*, which impact upon a single tissue or phenotype. The prototypic example of a segmental progeroid syndrome is the Werner syndrome ("Progeria of The Adult"). It is caused by null mutations at a member of the RecQ class of DNA helicases and leads to accelerated replicative senescence and a mutator phenotype. Although it is best viewed as a private modulation of aging, polymorphic forms of the gene might prove to be of more general significance. Examples of unimodal progeroid syndromes include familial forms of dementias of the Alzheimer type. These are also rare private modulations, but these may inform us as to general pathogenetic mechanisms. The apolipoprotein E locus, however, serves as an example of a public polymorphic modulation of that disorder.
7. A highly polygenic basis for senescence does not necessarily mean that there are very large numbers of distinct mechanisms of senescence. A single generic mechanism—oxidative damage to macromolecules—can be influenced by variations at numerous genetic loci. The possibility of a single dominating pathway to senescence is supported by the results of caloric restriction experiments in rodents. These have yet to be replicated in nonhuman primates, however.
8. Single gene mutations in *Caenorhabditis elegans* and in *Drosophila melanogaster* have been shown to result in substantial increments in life span. The former, however, may simply be the result of lowered metabolic rates and the latter the result of complementation for a particular genetic abnormality of genetically inbred laboratory strains. Other experiments with hybrid nematodes and genetically heterogeneous flies provide evidence of a polygenic basis for life span.
9. Great opportunities for new directions of research on genetic aspects of the pathobiology of aging include quantitative trait analysis of longevity in experimental animals, investigations of mouse models of human senescent disorders, including searches for suppressor and enhancer genes, genetic aspects of comparative gerontology, and a variety of investigations in humans, including sib-pair analyses of unusually well-preserved structure and function in specific physiological domains (*elite* aging).

THE DEMOGRAPHIC IMPERATIVE

Physicians are faced with the care of an exponentially growing population of people over the age of 85 years[1] (Fig. 8-1), who account for an increasing proportion of medical care. For example, in 1992, 88.2 percent of individuals over the age of 65 had sought consultation from a physician within the previous year (Fig. 8-2). To what extent do inborn genetic susceptibilities contribute to the large range of morbidities exhibited by our geriatric patients? Medical geneticists are usually preoccupied with gene action in the early stages of the life history. The unprecedented growth of the elderly population, particularly of the "old old" (the subset over age 85), is changing the patterns of medical practice in virtually all specialties. It should be the same for medical geneticists. Moreover, primary care physicians and geriatricians will require a deeper understanding of biologic aspects of aging, including relevant concepts of evolutionary biology and genetics. This chapter summarizes these principles for our readership and point outs the need for more research on the mechanisms of biologic aging; these surely serve as substrates for virtually all of the common disorders of late life. A major theme for such future

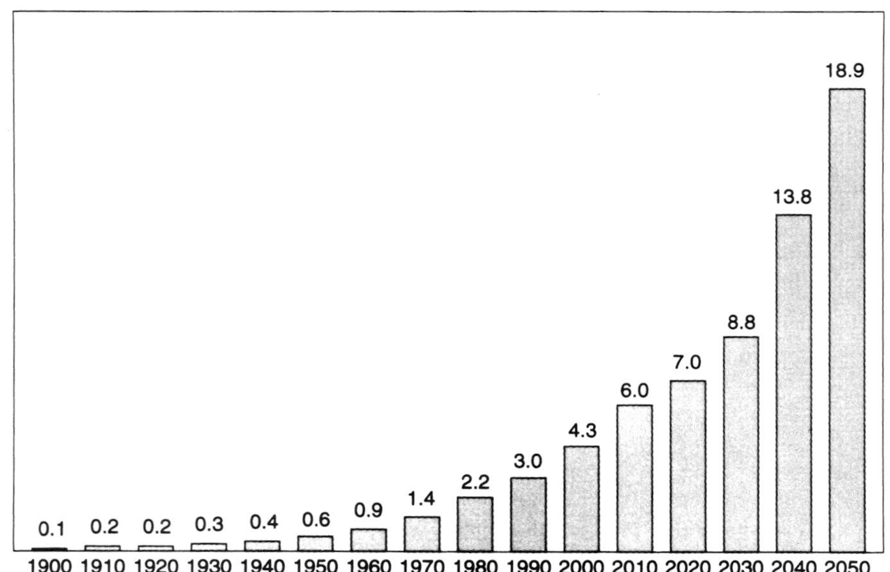

Fig. 8-1 Past and projected future numbers of individuals in U.S. population ages 85 years and over (in millions). (*From Hobbs and Damon.*[1] *Used by permission.*)

research will be the search for alleles that confer unusual protection against specific components of aging and of age-related disorders. Until very recently, this area of inquiry has been almost entirely neglected by physician scientists.

THE SIX STAGES OF THE LIFE CYCLE OF *HOMO SAPIENS*

There is considerable confusion concerning definitions of aging. Botanists use that term to refer to all changes in structure and function within an organism, from conception to death.[2] They have a more restricted use of the term *senescence*, using it to refer to the deleterious alterations that precede tissue or organismal death. Mammalian gerontologists, however, generally use *aging* and *senescence* interchangeably to refer to the changes in structure and function that gradually and insidiously unfold after the attainment of the fully mature adult phenotype, including sexual maturity. Thus, for mouse experiments, the "young" animals are 6 months old. Observations with "young" human subjects typically utilize subjects in their third decade. This is not to say that gene action in development is not of great significance to the biology of aging. Clearly, how one "builds" an organism makes a great deal of difference in how long it lasts and how well it functions. Conceptually, however, there is a major difference between gene action in development and gene action in senescence. The former clearly involves adaptive, determinative, sequential gene action, although with some stochastic elements. (For example, the random inactivation, early in development, of one of the two X chromosomes could lead to skewed distributions; in the case of female identical twins, this could manifest as significant differences in gene expression.) By contrast, senescence is nonadaptive and not "programmed" in the sense that development is programmed. These conclusions derive from evolutionary biologic concepts discussed below.

Not all changes in structure and function that unfold during the last half of the usual life span of humans are deleterious. Some (both behavioral and biologic) may be compensations for functional declines. The biologic mechanisms that are employed for such compensations are likely to be those that evolved as adaptations to periodic exogenous and endogenous stresses in young organisms. We might refer to them as being in "part-time" use in the young organism. There are reasons to believe that these adaptations are invoked more often when an organism is past the prime of reproductive activity, but not yet overtly senescent. These compensations may be invoked on a "full-time" basis. Let me cite two possible examples. Research by Ed Lakatta and his colleagues,[3] using subjects in the Baltimore Longitudinal Study of Aging, has shown that subjects selected because of a lack of evidence of ischemic heart disease are capable of maintaining normal cardiac output. They manage to achieve this happy status by the full-time use of the Starling phenomenon, which leads to an increased diastolic filling and stroke volume. A second example comes from observations of human brains stained by the Golgi method. Paul Coleman and his colleagues have provided statistical evidence for enhanced focal neuritic sprouting of pyramidal neurons, presumably as compensations for loss of synapses previously provided by atrophic or deleted neighboring neurons.[4,5] For human subjects, this stage would be roughly between ages 50 and 75. These various compensations ultimately fail, however, leading to a stage that might be more properly referred to as senescence. The loss of the ability to maintain homeostasis, coupled with the increased vulnerability to major geriatric disorders such as cancer, stroke, diabetes, infections, and heart failure, inevitably leads to organismal death. These concepts are summarized in Fig. 8-3.[6]

Senescence may occur in the absence of overt disease but is difficult to dissociate from late-life diseases, which are highly prevalent. An interesting line of evidence that demonstrates subtle

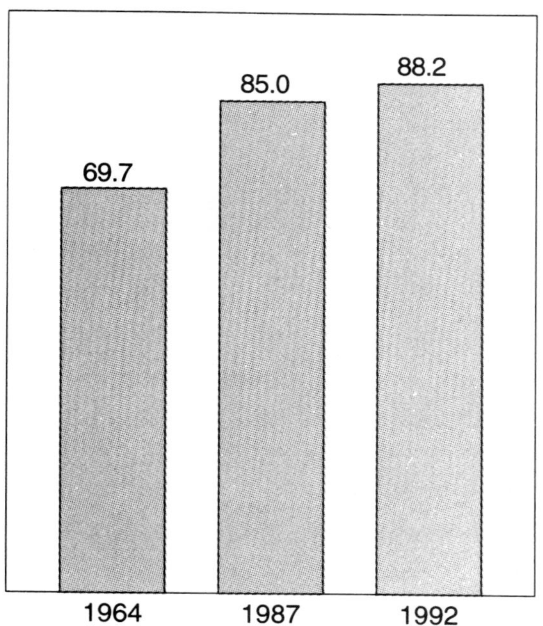

Fig. 8-2 Percent of elderly U.S. residents visiting a physician in the years prior to 1964, 1987, and 1992. (*From Hobbs and Damon.*[1] *Used by permission.*)

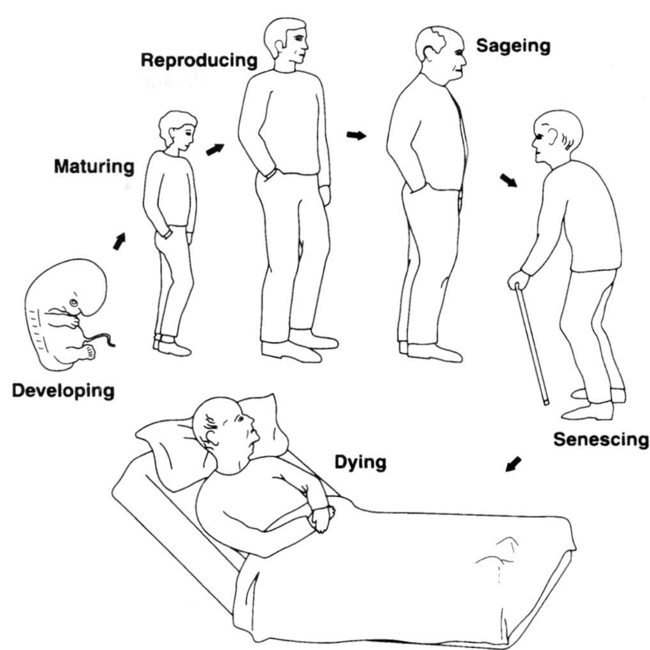

Fig. 8-3 The six stages in the life history of *Homo sapiens*. (*From Martin.*[6] *Used by permission.*)

and progressive declines in function is presented in Fig. 8-4, which charts the record times for marathon races as a function of age.[7] This "bioassay" serves nicely as a probe for essentially all body systems. We can assume that cohorts of exceptionally healthy individuals free of clinically significant disease have achieved these records, at least until the most advanced ages. How might these declines in function, which must have some structural basis, "set the stage" for the emergence of late-life disease? This raises the question of *how* we age, which is briefly discussed at the end of this chapter. We do not know the answers to this question, but there are likely to be many. We can cite two plausible examples, however. The first deals with the pathogenesis of neoplasms. Except for a subset of childhood neoplasms, the prevalence of malignancies, particularly of carcinomas, appears to be coupled to the biology of aging in that rates of increase appear to scale to life span for a number of mammalian species. Particularly compelling data come from comparisons of age-specific rates of malignancies in beagles compared with populations of human subjects.[8] Somatic mutations in tumor suppressor genes and oncogenes are now exceedingly well-documented components of the pathogenesis of cancer. Somatic mutations are also known to accumulate in the tissues of aging mammals.[9–11] Although we need a great deal more information on quantitative and qualitative aspects of these age-related mutations, it is a reasonable assumption that they do indeed set the stage for the emergence of late-life cancers. The

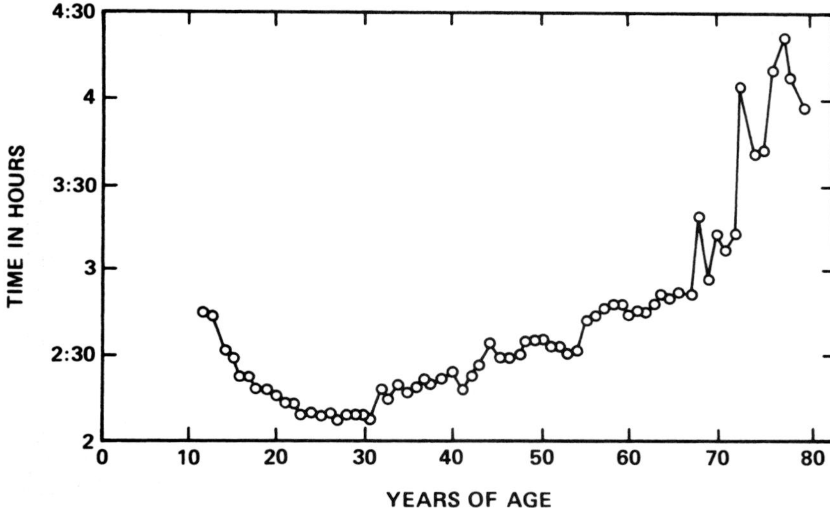

Fig. 8-4 Records for marathon runners as a function of age. (*From Fries and Crapo.*[7] *Used by permission.*)

pathogenesis of "senile" ocular cataracts may serve as a second example. Proteins with little turnover are subject to a variety of posttranslational alterations. These steadily accumulate with age and are considered to be among the basic mechanisms of aging. Lens crystallins are in this class.[12] A common such posttranslational alteration involves the glycation and glycoxidation of proteins.[13] Thus, there may be a line of continuum of aging processes and late-life disease.

THE EVOLUTIONARY BIOLOGIC BASIS FOR *WHY* WE AGE

Evolutionary biologists are confident that they have a satisfactory explanation for *why* we age, although they can tell us little about *how* we age (i.e., the proximal mechanisms of aging). Readers wishing a more thorough analysis of this most crucial aspect of the science of gerontology are referred to the excellent popular expositions by Steven N. Austad,[14,15] the more mathematically oriented monographs by Brian Charlesworth,[16] Michael R. Rose,[17] and the writings by T. B. Kirkwood and his colleagues.[18–22] The essence of the evolutionary theory of aging is that we age because of the decline in the force of natural selection with respect to the age of gene effects. The theory applies to age-structured populations with repeated rounds of reproduction. This would apply to all placental mammals and to numerous other species, including fruit flies and nematodes. For such populations in the wild, one finds very few old adults. This is because such phenomena as predation, infectious disease, accidents, malnutrition, and droughts deplete individuals as functions of time even in the absence of any natural aging processes. These ecologic considerations (operating over thousands of years) were in fact the prime determinants of the very different life history strategies found among extant species. For species that have evolved under conditions of high hazard, there was strong selective pressure for alleles that conferred rapid growth, development, and sexual maturation and large numbers of progeny over short periods. This was coupled with relatively short life spans, for reasons that are discussed below. As environmental hazards decrease, there is the opportunity to evolve different life history strategies, including those that are associated with longer life spans. These ideas have been confirmed by field studies of sibling species of Virginia opossums.[23] One species evolved under the hazardous conditions of the mainland while its sibling species evolved in an insular environment free of predators The island species exhibited a decrease in its actuarial rate of aging[23] (Fig. 8-5).

Now let us consider the degree to which alleles that reach expressions at different ages within age-structured populations are passed on to the subsequent generation. Let us start with the lucky

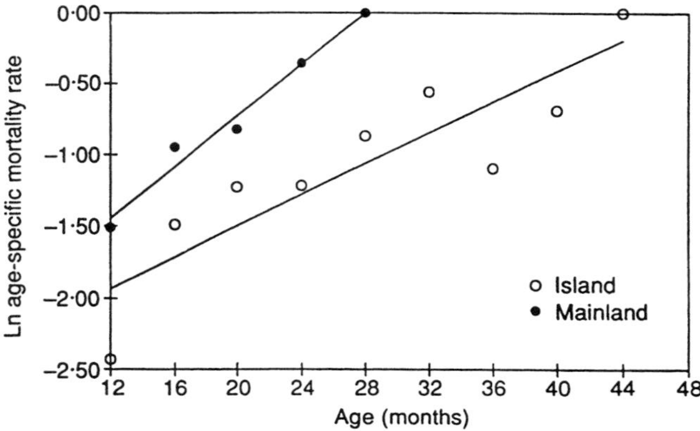

Fig. 8-5 The rate of aging of two sibling species of Virginia opossums. The species that evolved under the protected insular environment has a slower rate of aging. (*From Austad.*[23] *Used by permission.*)

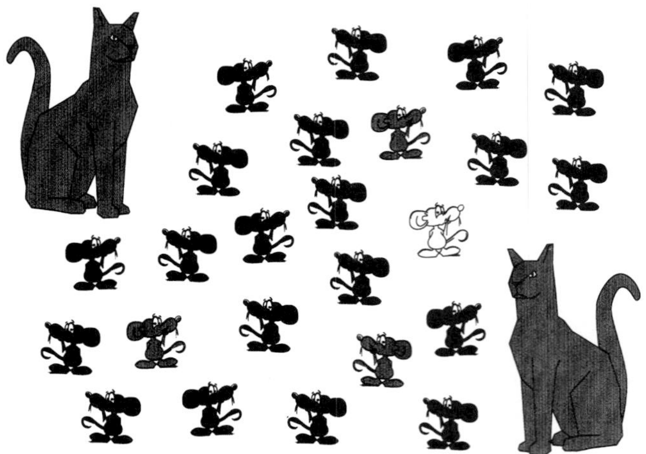

Fig. 8-6 A diagrammatic illustration of a fundamental principle of the evolutionary biologic theory of aging. We illustrate a population of rodents and its natural predator, felines. Even in the absence of any biologic aging, the predominant members of the population will be young (*black*). With time, very few middle-aged rodents (*gray*) will have survived predation and other environmental hazards and only very rare old rodents (*white*) will have survived. Neither beneficial nor deleterious alleles that reach phenotypic expression *only* in the middle-aged or old members of the population will have any significant impact upon the genetic structure of future populations and thus will have escaped the force of natural selection.

few that manage to survive numerous environmental hazards for exceptionally long periods. It should become obvious that any allele that reaches phenotypic expression only in those few surviving older members will have a substantially smaller representation in the following generation, as compared with the alleles contributed by the much more numerous younger members of the population. This concept is caricaturized in Fig. 8-6. A more quantitative analysis for the case of humans is presented in Fig. 8-7.[24] A striking conclusion of that analysis is that there is virtually no contribution to the next generation of alleles that do

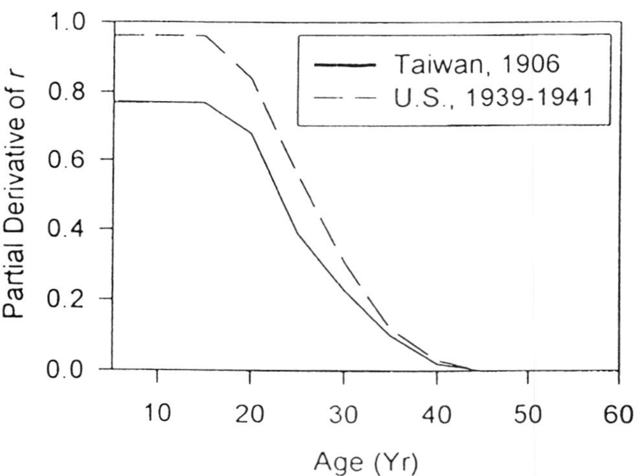

Fig. 8-7 A quantitative expression of the principle illustrated in Fig. 8-6 for the case of two human populations. On the *y*-axis is plotted a partial derivative of the Malthusian parameter, *r*. Age brackets are plotted on the *x*-axis. The *curve* represents the decline in the force of natural selection with age. For both populations (exhibiting different mortality rates), the force of natural selection approaches zero by about age 45. For details of the derivation, which is based on earlier work of William Hamilton and Brian Charlesworth, see Martin et al.[24] and citations therein.

not reach phenotypic expression until after the age of around 45 years. This finding has important implications for new directions of genetic research on aging discussed at the end of this chapter.

Two classes of gene action are thought to underlie senescence. The first class invokes constitutional mutations that have neutral effects during the early phases of the life history but that eventually achieve deleterious types of gene action late in the life span, when they escape the force of natural selection. This concept was best articulated by Peter B. Medawar,[25–27] who cites J. B. S. Haldane as having given the first exposition of the idea, using the Huntington disease mutation as an example. Medawar also pointed out that even if such mutations did impact upon reproductive fitness, there would be strong selection pressure to postpone the phenotypic effects via the evolution of suppressor alleles at other loci. Eventually, however, such suppression would become ineffectual because of the waning of the force of natural selection at older ages. My colleagues and I have referred to this type of gene action as leading to *private* modulations of aging, as the individual mutations, though collectively numerous, would be individually rare, the prevalence being determined as functions of genetic drift.[24]

The second class of gene action thought to be responsible for senescence invokes alleles selected because of beneficial effects early in the life course but with deleterious effects in late life. This phenomenon has been referred to as *antagonistic pleiotropy*.[17] The idea was first clearly articulated by George C. Williams.[28] Such genes can be considered to lead to *public* modulations of aging as, once selected, these alleles should spread throughout the population.[24] Moreover, one can imagine that at least a subset of such alleles will have appeared independently during evolution within many species. Because rare mutations at such loci are more likely to be deleterious than beneficial, I suggest that polymorphisms, rather than mutations, are what lead to *public* modulations of aging for that particular class of genes. Here again we have a principle that could serve as a guide to future research on the genetics of aging, particularly in our species, which is so rich in polymorphisms and which offers such diverse opportunities for the study of gene action as functions of environment and genetic background.

IMPLICATIONS OF THE EVOLUTIONARY BIOLOGIC THEORY OF AGING

There are a number of very important implications of the evolutionary biologic theory of aging. First of all, the theory predicts that life span is plastic. There is no fixed species-specific maximum life span (although one can certainly specify some range for a given genotype in a given environment). There is strong experimental confirmation of this prediction for the case of *D. melanogaster*, using both indirect[29–32] and direct[33] selection for increased life span. Second, given the conclusion that aging is not subject to determinative, sequential gene action (there are no "switches" that evolved for the purpose of inducing aging), the theory anticipates strong stochastic elements in the playing out of senescence. Third, the theory predicts that many genes should be involved in the determination of life span and the age-related disorders that limit life span. Although still an active area of research, the aforementioned fruit fly experiments clearly involve polygenes.[34,35] The same is true of life span determination in *C. elegans*.[36] (See below, however, for a discussion of single gene mutations in *C. elegans* and *D. melanogaster* that lead to enhanced life span.) Fourth, there is the expectation that a variety of mechanisms are likely to be involved in the genesis of senescent phenotypes and life span, as the constitutional mutations and antagonistic pleiotropic gene actions could be quite varied. Fifth, these mechanisms may well vary among different species. Although, as just indicated, there could well be commonalities, consider the striking differences in mating behaviors among various species. Antagonistic pleiotropic alleles impacting upon such behavior are likely to involve very different biochemical pathways. Thus, while the probable existence of a subset of public mechanisms of aging provides a strong rationale for research on aging in a wide range of organisms, in the last analysis, we will have to investigate specific processes in our own species. Sixth, the theory predicts substantial intraspecific variation in patterns of aging. Documentation of this prediction for the case of *Homo sapiens* is given in the following section.

There have been several challenges to the evolutionary biologic theory of aging. The first derives from the fact that single gene mutations can result in substantial increments in the life spans of animals. While a highly polygenic basis of life span is predicted by the evolutionary theory of aging, several single gene mutations leading to enhanced life spans have been found in *C. elegans*. These mutations involve loci concerned with a signal transduction pathway that functions in the implementation of an alternative life strategy, the dauer stage.[37–39] A second set of "clock" mutants appear to impact upon a different pathway.[40,41] Wild-type nematodes, when faced with nutritional deprivation, cease reproductive activities and exhibit extended periods of survival as dauers. There is evidence, however, that all of the mutants in each of these pathways exhibit decreased metabolic rates.[42] Thus, their increased life spans could be analogous to the enhanced life spans resulting from maintaining such poikilothermic animals at lower temperatures. I therefore do not regard these mutants as serious challenges to evolutionary theory. Moreover, the mutants would not likely survive competition with wild-type organisms under nonlaboratory conditions. Nevertheless, long-lived mutants with low metabolic rates are of interest in that they are consistent with an important role for oxidative damage in the genesis of aging.

Simple genetic manipulations have also been claimed to increase the life spans of *D. melanogaster*. The first such report, involving introduction of additional genetic information for the synthesis of a component of the protein synthesis apparatus (elongation factor 1α)[43] could not be confirmed.[44] Two other reports have indicated that relatively simple genetic manipulations can significantly increase the life spans of fruit flies. One used overexpression of both superoxide dismutase 1 and catalase[45] and another of superoxide dismutase 1 alone (expressed in motor neurons).[46] All of these experiments were performed on laboratory stocks. As such, a genetic manipulation that enhanced life span might function by complementing a particular and special deficiency of that strain. Inbred laboratory strains of flies are typically developed from a small number of breeding founders and selected for reproductive fitness in an artificial laboratory environment. It would thus not be surprising to discover that such strains might exhibit private modulations of aging. Nevertheless, it is certainly of interest that the experiments by Orr and Sohal[45] and Parkes et al.[46] provide support for the oxidative damage theory of aging. The same is true of *C. elegans* mutants.[47,48]

Caloric restriction experiments in rodents (most of them performed on genetically defined inbred lines) result in substantial increments in life span, with concomitant delays in the expression of the major causes of death of these animals (for mice, mostly B-cell lymphomas and renal disease).[49,51] The finding that a single environmental manipulation (moderate caloric restriction) can enhance life span argues for a single major mechanism underlying mammalian aging. By contrast, as we have already noted, an implication of the evolutionary theory is that there exist multiple mechanisms of aging. Although there are important ongoing experiments with rhesus and squirrel monkeys,[52] it remains to be determined whether caloric restriction increases the life spans of long-lived organisms. The life history strategies of higher primates and other long-lived organisms are quite different that those of short-lived species such as rodents, which is a reason for caution in extrapolating the results of experiments in mice to humans. Some skeptics also argue that the control animals in caloric restriction experiments are overfed. By such a view, the restricted animals may represent a state more appropriate for their ancestral genes under wild-type conditions. On the other hand, caloric restriction may have evolved as a particularly useful mechanism for many species in order to temporarily shunt energetic resources from reproduction to survival.[53]

The best current evidence in rodents is that caloric restriction, except for a transient reduction in metabolic rate, does not have its effect via a reduction in the oxygen consumption per gram of lean body mass.[54] It is conceivable, however, that caloric restriction leads to a more efficient utilization of the electron transport system of mitochondria, resulting in a lower rate of production of univalent modes of oxygen reduction. Upregulation of mechanisms to protect against oxidative damage may also accompany caloric reduction.[51] This line of experimentation thus supports the *free radical* or *oxidative stress* theory of aging.[51,55]

VARIANTS AT NUMEROUS GENETIC LOCI HAVE THE POTENTIAL TO MODULATE THE PATHOBIOLOGY OF AGING IN *HOMO SAPIENS*

As indicated in the introductory paragraph, physicians have rarely investigated the Mendelian basis of unusually well-preserved structure and function. This should have a high priority for future research in aging. Meanwhile, we can take advantage of a large body of literature concerning mutations and allelic variations that lead to premature and severe expressions of senescent phenotypes. Many of these are severe loss or gain of function mutations that impact upon reproductive fitness and, therefore, would not fit the evolutionary definition of the types of alleles that impact upon senescence. For each such highly deleterious allele, however, there may be a number of "leaky alleles" or polymorphic variants whose phenotypic effects do indeed escape the force of natural selection. Moreover, alleles that confer unusual *resistance* to senescent phenotypes may exist in some individuals. Given this rationale, the author examined McKusick's *Mendelian Inheritance in Man* for loci that impacted upon a limited number of senescent phenotypes and concluded that almost 7 percent of entries had the potential to modulate the pathobiology of aging.[56] Assuming a total of 100,000 genes, it became apparent that variants at many thousands of loci could potentially explain, in part, clinical observations indicating considerable variations in patterns of senescence among the geriatric population. A more recent unpublished preliminary study, based on a search of a computerized version of that catalogue, addressed certain deficiencies of the 1978 study, which considered only a limited numbers of phenotypes and which included several nonphenotypic criteria (relevance to certain postulated mechanisms of aging). This more recent study suggests that an even larger proportion of the human genome could play a role in the modulation of senescent phenotypes. Nevertheless, there remains the possibility that a subset of such loci could be of major importance, either because of an impact upon multiple senescent phenotypes or because of a potential to elucidate the pathogenesis of a single, but exceptionally common, senescent phenotype. The first category leads to what have been termed *segmental progeroid syndromes*.[56] The second category leads to what have been termed *unimodal progeroid syndromes*.[57] The prototypic example of a segmental progeroid syndrome is the Werner syndrome (WS).[58] It is also known as "Progeria of the Adult" in order to distinguish it from the Hutchinson-Gilford syndrome ("Progeria of Childhood" or "Progeria," a clinically and genetically distinct entity).[59]

WS is a rare autosomal recessive disorder discussed in detail in Chap. 33. For the reader of this chapter, however, it will be helpful to briefly review the phenotype in order to give some specific examples of important *senescent phenotypes*. WS patients appear normal until about the time of puberty, when they fail to undergo the usual adolescent growth spurt. They subsequently develop premature graying and thinning of scalp hair, atrophy of the skin, regional atrophy of subcutaneous fat, bilateral ocular cataracts, several varieties of arteriosclerosis (atherosclerosis, arteriolosclerosis, medial calcinosis), severe calcifications of heart valves, type-2 diabetes mellitus, osteoporosis, benign and malignant neoplasms, and gonadal atrophy. Caucasian WS subjects typically die of a myocardial infarction, at a median age of 47 years.[58] Cancer appears to be a more common case of death among Japanese patients.[60] It is important to point out that there are a number of clinical and cell biologic discordances with what is seen in "usual" aging, however.[56] To cite just one example of a clinical discordance, the ratio of epithelial-mesenchymal neoplasms in WS is approximately 1:1, whereas the ratio in usual aging is about 10:1.[61] Moreover, WS patients are extraordinarily susceptible to certain rare neoplasms. For example, acral lentiginous melanoma is about 1000 times more common than in controls in a Japanese series.[61] There are cell biologic discordances as well. For example, while WS somatic cells exhibit a striking acceleration of replicative senescence,[62] transcription of the *cFOS* gene in senescent WS cells is quite responsive to mitogenic stimulation, unlike senescent cells from control subjects.[63] WS subjects have null mutations at a member (*WRN*) of the *RecQ* family of DNA helicases.[64–66] The WRN protein may therefore play a role in such basic DNA transactions as replication, recombination, repair, transcription, and chromosomal segregation. WS somatic cells are genetically unstable.[67] These findings provide a reasonable explanation for the enhanced susceptibility to neoplasia. Perhaps more surprising, however, is this new evidence for a role of aberrant DNA metabolism and somatic mutation in the many other WS phenotypes. For example, posttranslational alterations in lens proteins have long been regarded as the cause of ocular cataracts.[12] Research with WS, however, provides support for an alternative pathogenetic pathway, perhaps operative in a minor proportion of the population, involving aberrations in DNA transactions of lens epithelial cells. The research on WS has also revived interest in the somatic mutational hypothesis of the origin of atheromas.[68]

The discordances between the features of aging in WS and in "usual" aging suggest that the null mutations found in WS patients are best interpreted as leading to a private modulation of aging.[67] In keeping with our introductory remarks, however, we should now ask whether there is any evidence that "leaky" mutations or polymorphisms at *WRN* can result in more modest modulations of senescent phenotypes, either deleterious or beneficial. Certain of these, particularly polymorphisms, might lead to more public modulations of aging. There are only hints that this may be the case. There is a single case-control association study that provides evidence that a polymorphic form of *WRN* may protect Japanese patients from myocardial infarction.[69] There is also evidence that heterozygous carriers are hypersensitive to a genotoxic, carcinogenic agent, 4-nitroquinoline-1-oxide.[70] This finding is consistent with a clinical study indicating a high prevalence of malignancies in first-degree relatives of WS patients.[71]

The three autosomal dominant mutations leading to early onset familial Alzheimer disease are good examples of unimodal progeroid syndromes.[72–74] There is as yet no compelling evidence that these mutations have any significant systemic peripheral effects. These mutations are individually and collectively exceedingly rare and are best regarded as leading to private modulations of the senescent phenotype. However, the associated neuropathology usually cannot be differentiated from what is observed in the vastly more prevalent late-onset, "sporadic" forms of Alzheimer disease. Thus, like so many inborn errors of metabolism, these rare "experiments of nature" may reveal a pathogenetic pathway or relevance to a senescent phenotype that may impact upon as many as 47 percent of individuals who live past the age of 85 years.[75] A variety of lines of evidence support this contention and indicate that the pathway involves the metabolism of the β-amyloid precursor protein.[76] There is one well-accepted polymorphic locus, *APOE*, that modulates the common late-onset form.[77] It can be regarded as leading to a public modulation of a senescent phenotype. Gene action at the *APOE* locus may be an example of antagonistic pleiotropy.[78] If this is the case, the allele that is associated with increased susceptibility to Alzheimer disease (the epsilon 4 allele) may have provided enhanced reproductive fitness to ancestral carriers in some environments. It is a challenge for the future to discover the molecular basis and the environmental milieu for a putative beneficial effect early in life but a deleterious effect late in life. One highly speculative candidate area for research would be resistance to an infectious agent (e.g., *Mycobacterium tuberculosis*) on the basis of an altered lipid metabolism.

A BRIEF OVERVIEW OF GENETIC AND CELL BIOLOGIC ASPECTS OF *HOW* WE AGE

Given the present paucity of definitive information as to *how* we age, this section is of necessity brief. The study of genetic variants in a wide variety of organisms, however, has provided a surprising degree of evidence for a major role for oxidative damage as an underlying mechanism of aging. Interested readers should consult a recent review for details of this evidence.[24] Mutations and polymorphisms at a very large number of genetic loci can modulate the rates at which such oxidative damage can accumulate. These genes fall into seven classes (Table 8-1). The macromolecular targets of oxidative damage include lipids, proteins, and DNA, both mitochondrial and nuclear. Somatic mutations in mitochondrial DNA may be of particular importance to the aging of postreplicative cells such as skeletal muscle and neurons.[79] Replicating populations of normal diploid cells have finite replicative potentials. The bulk of the evidence indicates that the replicative potential of mammalian cells declines as functions of donor age. This is particularly evident when sensitive methods are used, such as primary cloning or clone size distribution assays.[80,81] Transfection experiments have provided strong evidence that the epigenetic silencing of telomerase is the primary cause of this limited replicative life span.[82] Depletion of telomere repeat units is thought to lead more directly to the exit from the cell cycle, but the precise mechanism is not clear. Telomerase is active in the germ line, consistent with its indefinite replicative potential. The enzyme is also active in most cancers.[83] Although intuitively attractive, there is as yet little evidence linking a limited replicative life span as causal in senescent phenotypes. An interesting line of investigation links focal replicative senescence to the emergence of atherosclerosis.[84]

Replicatively senescent cells overexpress a variety of gene products. For the case of skin fibroblasts, these include gene products capable of altering the structure and function of connective tissue (via collagenases and elastases) and of regional epithelial cells (via cytokines).[85] Campisi has pointed out that only a few such cells would be capable of initiating a significant "field effect" in the contiguous tissues. Using a histochemical marker of replicatively senescent cells, she and her colleagues have indeed found evidence for such cells in vivo.[86]

Table 8-1 Classification of Genetic Loci of Potential Relevance to the Oxidative Damage Theory of Aging

Class I	Structural and regulatory genes modulating genesis of free radicals
Class II	Structural and regulatory genes for scavenger enzymes
Class III	Genes regulating flux of nonenzymatic free radical scavengers
Class IV	Genes regulating target copy number
Class V	Genes specifying target structure
Class VI	Structural and regulatory genes for repair of target macromolecules
Class VII	Genes specifying the orderly replacement of effete cells

SOURCE: From Martin et al.[24] Used by permission.

SOME FUTURE DIRECTIONS FOR RESEARCH ON GENETIC ASPECTS OF AGING

Given the enormous progress in mapping and genotyping, we are now in a position to do quantitative trait locus analysis of life span and of various senescent phenotypes in experimental organisms. There are great opportunities for such research in *D. melanogaster*. There are also possibilities of useful results in *Mus domesticus* (although the usual laboratory strains represent only a small sample of the genetic variance of *M. musculus*). Methods for the creation of mouse models of dysfunction and disease should increasingly address issues relevant to the geriatric population. For recessive alleles, these should include studies of heterozygous carriers, as phenotypes may not emerge until late in the life course. They should also include efforts to map and positionally clone suppressors and enhancers of senescent phenotypes of major importance to man.

Comparative gerontology is also a neglected area from a genetic point of view. A promising avenue of research, for example, will be the delineation of avian loci responsible for their unusual resistance to oxidative stress.[87]

There is currently great interest in genetic association studies with centenarians.[88,89] It has been shown, for example, that the *APOE* epsilon 2 allele is enriched in such populations.[90] It is likely, however, that a very large number of such associations will be uncovered and that the subsets of such associations will vary among different populations. Perhaps a more useful approach will be to carry out sib-pair analyses for extreme discordances and concordances of the rates of change of highly specific physiological traits known to be impacted by aging. As can be inferred from the results of Fig. 8-7, such research could utilize middle-aged subjects. This will have the advantage of potential access to parental and filial generations, in order to obtain information on phase relationships of markers. It would also have the advantage of avoiding the complications of comorbidity for various diseases that commonly emerge much later in the life span. Such research would give us the potential of defining alleles and haplotypes that are contributing to unusually successful aging (*elite* aging).

REFERENCES

1. Hobbs FB, Damon BL: *65+ in the United States*. Washington, DC, US Department of Commerce, 1996, pp 2–8.
2. Leopold AC: The biological significance of death in plants, in Behnke JA, Finch CE, Moment GB (eds): *Biology of Aging*. New York, Plenum, 1978, pp 101–114.
3. Lakatta EG: Heart and circulation, in Finch CE, Schneider EL (eds): *Handbook of the Biology of Aging*. New York, Van Nostrand Reinhold, 1985, pp 377–413.
4. Flood DG, Buell SJ, Defiore CH, Horwitz GJ, Coleman PD: Age-related dendritic growth in dentate gyrus of human brain is followed by regression in the oldest old. *Brain Res* **345**:366, 1985.
5. Coleman PD, Rogers KE, Flood DG: Neuronal plasticity in normal aging and deficient plasticity in Alzheimer's disease: A proposed intercellular and signal cascade. *Prog Brain Res* **86**:75, 1990.
6. Martin GM: Genetics and the pathobiology of ageing. *Philos Trans R Soc Lond [Biol]* **352**:1773, 1997.
7. Fries JF, Crapo LM: *Vitality and Aging: Implications of the Rectangular Curve*. San Francisco, WH Freeman, 1981, p 115.
8. Albert RE, Benjamin SA, Shukla R: Life span and cancer mortality in the beagle dog and humans. *Mech Ageing Dev* **74**:149, 1994.
9. Trainor KJ, Wigmore DJ, Chrysostomou A, Dempsey JL, Seshadri R, Morley AA: Mutation frequency in human lymphocytes increases with age. *Mech Ageing Dev* **27**:83, 1984.
10. Martin GM, Smith AC, Ketterer DJ, Ogburn CE, Disteche CM: Increased chromosomal aberrations in first metaphases of cells isolated from the kidneys of aged mice. *Isr J Med Sci* **21**:296, 1985.
11. Martin GM, Ogburn CE, Colgin LM, Gown AM, Edland SD, Monnat RJ Jr: Somatic mutations are frequent and increase with age in human kidney epithelial cells. *Hum Mol Genet* **5**:215, 1996.
12. Taylor A, Davies KJ: Protein oxidation and loss of protease activity may lead to cataract formation in the aged lens. *Free Radic Biol Med* **3**:371, 1987.

13. Sell DR, Lane MA, Johnson WA, Masoro EJ, Mock OB, Reiser KM, Fogarty JF, et al: Longevity and the genetic determination of collagen glycoxidation kinetics in mammalian senescence. *Proc Natl Acad Sci USA* **93:**485, 1996.
14. Austad S: On the nature of aging. *Nat Hist* **2:**25, 1992.
15. Austad SN: *Why we age: What Science Is Discovering About the Body's Journey Through Life*. New York, John Wiley and Sons, 1997.
16. Charlesworth B: *Evolution in age-structured populations,* 2d ed. New York, Cambridge University Press, 1994.
17. Rose MR: *Evolutionary biology of aging*. New York, Oxford University Press, 1991.
18. Kirkwood TB, Holliday R: The evolution of ageing and longevity. *Proc R Soc Lond [Biol]* **205:**531, 1979.
19. Kirkwood TB: The nature and causes of ageing. *Ciba Found Symp* **134:**193, 1988.
20. Kirkwood TB, Rose MR: Evolution of senescence: Late survival sacrificed for reproduction. *Philos Trans R Soc Lond [Biol]* **332:**15, 1991.
21. Lithgow GJ, Kirkwood TB: Mechanisms and evolution of aging. *Science* **273:**80, 1996.
22. Kirkwood TB: The origins of human ageing. *Philos Trans R Soc Lond [Biol]* **352:**1765, 1997.
23. Austad SN: Retarded senescence in an insular population of Virginia possums (*Didelphis virginiana*). *J Zool Lond* **229:**695, 1993.
24. Martin GM, Austad SN, Johnson TE: Genetic analysis of ageing: Role of oxidative damage and environmental stresses. *Nat Genet* **13:**25, 1996.
25. Medawar PB: Old age and natural death. *Mod Q* **1:**30, 1946.
26. Medawar PB: *An unsolved problem of biology*. London, HK Lewis, 1952.
27. Medawar PB: An unsolved problem of biology, in *The Uniqueness of the Individual*. London, Methuen, 1957.
28. Williams GC: Pleiotrophy, natural selection, and the evolution of senescence. *Evolution* **11:**398, 1957.
29. Rose MR, Charlesworth B: Genetics of life history in *Drosophila melanogaster*: II. Exploratory selection experiments. *Genetics* **97:**187, 1981.
30. Rose MR: Laboratory evolution of postponed senescence in *Drosophila melanogaster. Evolution* **38:**1004, 1984.
31. Lukinbill LS, Clare MJ: Selection for life span in *Drosophila melanogaster. Heredity* **55:**9, 1985.
32. Lukinbill LS, Clare MJ: Successful selection for increased longevity in *Drosophila*: Analysis of the survival data and presentation of a hypothesis on the genetic regulation of longevity. *Exp Gerontol* **22:**221, 1987.
33. Zwaan B, Bulsma R, Hoekstra RF: Direct selection on life in *Drosophila melanogaster. Evolution* **49:**649, 1995.
34. Hutchinson EW, Rose MR: Quantitative genetic analysis of postponed aging in *Drosophila melanogaster*, in Harrison DL (ed): *Genetic Effects of Aging II*. New Jersey, Telford, 1990, pp 65–85.
35. Fleming JE, Spicer GS, Garrison RC, Rose MR: Two-dimensional protein electrophoretic analysis of postponed aging in *Drosophila*. *Genetica* **91:**183, 1993.
36. Johnson TE, Wood WB: Genetic analysis of *Caenorhabditis elegans*. *Proc Natl Acad Sci USA* **79:**6603, 1982.
37. Kenyon C, Chang J, Gensch E, Rudner A, Tabtiang R: A *C. elegans* mutant that lives twice as long as wild type. *Nature* **366:**461, 1993.
38. Larsen PL, Albert PS, Riddle DL: Genes that regulate both development and longevity in *Caenorhabditis elegans*. *Genetics* **139:**1567, 1995.
39. Dorman JB, Albinder B, Shroyer T, Kenyon C: The age-1 and daf-2 genes function in a common pathway to control the lifespan of *Caenorhabditis elegans*. *Genetics* **141:**1399, 1995.
40. Lakowski B, Hekimi S: Determination of life-span in *Caenorhabditis elegans* by four clock genes. *Science* **272:**1010, 1996.
41. Lin K, Dorman JB, Rodan A, Kenyon C: Daf-16: An HNF-3/forkhead family member that can function to double the life-span of *Caenorhabditis elegans*. *Science* **278:**1319, 1997.
42. Van Voorhies WA, Ward S: Genetic and environmental conditions that increase longevity in *caenorhabditis elegans* decrease metabolic rate. *Proc Natl Acad Sci USA* **96:**11399, 1999.
43. Shepherd JC, Walldorf U, Hug P, Gehring WJ: Fruit flies with additional expression of the elongation factor EF-1 alpha live longer. *Proc Natl Acad Sci USA* **86:**7520, 1989.
44. Stearns SC, Kaiser M: The effects of enhanced expression of elongation factor EF-1 alpha on lifespan in *Drosophila melanogaster*: IV. A summary of three experiments: *Genetica* **91:**167, 1993.
45. Orr WC, Sohal RS: Extension of life-span by overexpression of superoxide dismutase and catalase in *Drosophila melanogaster. Science* **263:**1128, 1994.
46. Parkes TL, Elia AJ, Dickinson D, Hilliker AJ, Phillips JP, Boulianne GL: Extension of *Drosophila* lifespan by overexpression of human SOD1 in motorneurons. *Nat Genet* **19:**171, 1998.
47. Larsen PL: Aging and resistance to oxidative damage in *Caenorhabditis elegans. Proc Natl Acad Sci USA* **90:**8905, 1993.
48. Murakami S, Johnson TE: A genetic pathway conferring life extension and resistance to UV stress in *Caenorhabditis elegans. Genetics* **143:**1207, 1996.
49. Masoro EJ: Dietary restriction and aging. *J Am Geriatr Soc* **41:**994, 1993.
50. Masoro EJ: Possible mechanisms underlying the antiaging actions of caloric restriction. *Toxicol Pathol* **24:**738, 1996.
51. Sohal RS, Weindruch R: Oxidative stress, caloric restriction, and aging. *Science* **273:**59, 1996.
52. Lane MA, Ingram DK, Roth GS: Beyond the rodent model: Calorie restriction in rhesus monkeys. *Age* **20:**45, 1997.
53. Masoro EJ, Austad SN: The evolution of the antiaging action of dietary restriction: A hypothesis. *J Gerontol [A Biol Sci Med Sci]* **51:**B387, 1996.
54. McCarter R, Masoro EJ, Yu BP: Does food restriction retard aging by reducing the metabolic rate? *Am J Physiol* **248:**E488, 1985.
55. Harman D: Aging: A theory based on free radical and radiation chemistry. *J Gerontol* **11:**298, 1956.
56. Martin GM: Genetic syndromes in man with potential relevance to the pathobiology of aging. *Birth Defects* **14:**5, 1978.
57. Martin GM: Syndromes of accelerated aging. *Natl Cancer Inst Monogr* **60:**241, 1982.
58. Epstein CJ, Martin GM, Schultz AL, Motulsky AG: Werner's syndrome: A review of its symptomatology, natural history, pathologic features, genetics and relationship to the natural aging process. *Medicine (Baltimore)* **45:**177, 1966.
59. Brown WT, Kieras FJ, Houck GE Jr, Dutkowski R, Jenkins EC: A comparison of adult and childhood progerias: Werner syndrome and Hutchinson-Gilford progeria syndrome. *Adv Exp Med Biol* **190:**229, 1985.
60. Goto M: Hierarchical deterioration of body systems in Werner's syndrome: Implications for normal aging. *Mech Ageing Dev* **98:**239, 1997.
61. Goto M, Miller RW, Ishikawa Y, Sugano H: Excess of rare cancers in Werner syndrome (adult progeria). *Cancer Epidemiol Biomarkers Prev* **5:**239, 1996.
62. Martin GM, Sprague CA, Epstein CJ: Replicative life-span of cultivated human cells: Effects of donor's age, tissue, and genotype. *Lab Invest* **23:**86, 1970.
63. Oshima J, Campisi J, Tannock TC, Martin GM: Regulation of c-fos expression in senescing Werner syndrome fibroblasts differs from that observed in senescing fibroblasts from normal donors. *J Cell Physiol* **162:**277, 1995.
64. Yu CE, Oshima J, Fu YH, Wijsman EM, Hisama F, Alisch R, Matthews S, et al: Positional cloning of the Werner's syndrome gene. *Science* **272:**258, 1996.
65. Oshima J, Yu CE, Piussan C, Klein G, Jabkowski J, Balci S, Miki T, et al: Homozygous and compound heterozygous mutations at the Werner syndrome locus. *Hum Mol Genet* **5:**1909, 1996.
66. Yu CE, Oshima J, Wijsman EM, Nakura J, Miki T, Piussan C, Matthews S, et al: Mutations in the consensus helicase domains of the Werner syndrome gene. *Am J Hum Genet* **60:**330, 1997.
67. Martin GM: The Werner mutation: Does it lead to a 'public' or 'private' mechanism of aging. *Mol Med* **3:**356, 1997.
68. Benditt EP, Benditt JM: Evidence for a monoclonal origin of human atherosclerotic plaques. *Proc Natl Acad Sci USA* **70:**1753, 1973.
69. Ye L, Miki T, Nakura J, Oshima J, Kamino K, Rakugi H, Ikegami H, et al: Association of a polymorphic variant of the Werner helicase gene with myocardial infarction in a Japanese population. *Am J Med Genet* **68:**494, 1997.
70. Ogburn CE, Oshima J, Poot M, Chen R, Hunt KE, Gollahon KA, Rabinovitch PS, et al: An apoptosis-inducing genotoxin differentiates heterozygotic carriers for Werner helicase mutations from wild-type and homozygous mutants. *Hum Genet* **101:**121, 1997.
71. Goto M, Tanimoto K, Horiuchi Y, Sasazuki T: Family analysis of Werner's syndrome: A survey of 42 Japanese families with a review of the literature. *Clin Genet* **19:**8, 1981.
72. Goate A, Chartier-Harlin MC, Mullan M, Brown J, Crawford F, Fidani L, Giuffra L, et al: Segregation of a missense mutation in the amyloid precursor protein gene with familial Alzheimer's disease. *Nature* **349:**704, 1991.

73. Sherrington R, Rogaev EI, Liang Y, Rogaeva EA, Levesque G, Ikeda M, Chi H, et al: Cloning of a gene bearing missense mutations in early-onset familial Alzheimer's disease. *Nature* **375:**754, 1995.
74. Levy-Lahad E, Wasco W, Poorkaj P, Romano DM, Oshima J, Pettingell WH, Yu CE, et al: Candidate gene for the chromosome 1 familial Alzheimer's disease locus. *Science* **269:**973, 1995.
75. Evans DA, Funkenstein HH, Albert MS, Scherr PA, Cook NR, Chown MJ, Hebert LE, et al: Prevalence of Alzheimer's disease in a community population of older persons; higher than previously reported. *JAMA* **262:**2551, 1989.
76. Hardy J: The Alzheimer family of diseases: Many etiologies, one pathogenesis. *Proc Natl Acad Sci USA* **94:**2095, 1997.
77. Higgins GA, Large CH, Rupniak HT, Barnes JC: Apolipoprotein E and Alzheimer's disease: A review of recent studies. *Pharmacol Biochem Behav* **56:**675, 1997.
78. Charlesworth B: Evolution of senescence: Alzheimer's disease and evolution. *Curr Biol* **6:**20, 1996.
79. Wallace DC: Mitochondrial DNA in aging and disease. *Sci Am* **277:**40, 1997.
80. Martin GM, Ogburn CE, Wight TN: Comparative rates of decline in the primary cloning efficiencies of smooth muscle cells from the aging thoracic aorta of two murine species of contrasting maximum life span potentials. *Am J Pathol* **110:**236, 1983.
81. Pendergrass WR, Li Y, Jiang D, Fei RG, Wolf NS: Caloric restriction: Conservation of cellular replicative capacity in vitro accompanies life-span extension in mice. *Exp Cell Res* **217:**309, 1995.
82. Bodnar AG, Ouellette M, Frolkis M, Holt SE, Chiu CP, Morin GB, Harley CB, et al: Extension of life-span by introduction of telomerase into normal human cells. *Science* **279:**349, 1998.
83. Shay JW, Werbin H, Wright WE: Telomerase assays in the diagnosis and prognosis of cancer. *Ciba Found Symp* **211:**148, 1997.
84. Chang E, Harley CB: Telomere length and replicative aging in human vascular tissues. *Proc Natl Acad Sci USA* **92:**11190, 1995.
85. Campisi J: Aging and cancer: The double-edged sword of replicative senescence. *J Am Geriatr Soc* **45:**482, 1997.
86. Dimri GP, Lee X, Basile G, Acosta M, Scott G, Roskelley C, Medrano EE, et al: A biomarker that identifies senescent human cells in culture and in aging skin in vivo. *Proc Natl Acad Sci USA* **92:**9363, 1995.
87. Ogburn CE, Austad SN, Holmes DJ, Kiklevich JV, Gollahon K, Rabinovitch PS, Martin GM: Cultured renal epithelial cells from birds and mice: Enhanced resistance of avian cells to oxidative stress and DNA damage. *J Gerontol [Biol Sci Med Sci]*, 1998 (in press).
88. Akisaka M, Suzuki M, Inoko H: Molecular genetic studies on DNA polymorphism of the HLA class II genes associated with human longevity. *Tissue Antigens* **50:**489, 1997.
89. Perls TT, Bubrick E, Wager CG, Vijg J, Kruglyak L: Siblings of centenarians live longer. *Lancet* **351:**1560, 1998.
90. Schachter F, Faure-Delanef L, Gu'enot F, Rouger H, Froguel P, Lesueur-Ginot L, Cohen D: Genetic associations with human longevity at the APOE and ACE loci. *Nat Genet* **6:**29, 1994.

CHAPTER 9

Pharmacogenetics

Werner Kalow ■ Denis M. Grant

1. Pharmacogenetics has been defined as the science that deals with pharmacologic responses and their modification by hereditary influences. Much clinical work has been done under this broad label. Variation of drug-metabolizing enzymes, responsible for a large section of pharmacogenetics, represents person-to-person differences within the chemical defense systems. These differences and the variations that affect susceptibility to infectious diseases (e.g., tuberculosis and malaria) may have comparable biologic effects: They will aid the survival of populations exposed to toxins or to infectious agents, respectively.
2. The history and scope of pharmacogenetics have been outlined briefly. Various chapters in this book might have been classified by their contents as part of pharmacogenetics [e.g., glucose-6-phosphate dehydrogenase (G-6-PD) deficiency] but they are treated as independent entities and presented on their own merits. This chapter on pharmacogenetics presents three selected case studies that are of unquestioned clinical importance and, at the same time, illustrate a wide range of problems.
3. Malignant hyperthermia (MH) is the most feared complication of general anesthesia, observed in about 1:15,000 children and 1:100,000 adults; it occurs on the basis of genetic predisposition affecting skeletal muscle. It is not a uniform disease, but its common parameter is pathologic elevation of ionized calcium in the sarcoplasm. This calcium triggers muscle rigidity, elevation of body temperature, acidosis, tachycardia, and other secondary events. Clinically, an MH attack is most frequently triggered by halothane and succinylcholine; for diagnostic purposes, contractures of muscle biopsy specimens on exposure to caffeine and/or halothane are utilized. An equivalent abnormality in pigs is caused by a Cys for Arg^{615} substitution in the ryanodine receptor, the calcium release channel of the sarcoplasmic reticulum. Predisposition to MH in humans is often but not always caused by the same mutation.
4. In the 1950s, a variant (*atypical*) form of butyrylcholinesterase (BChE) was found to be responsible for the prolongation of action of the muscle relaxant succinylcholine. Any physiological function of BChE is still not known, but it is known to be a homotetramer produced by a single gene on chromosome 3 at q26.1-26.2. Mutations with an allele frequency of 0.017 in Caucasians may affect its capacities for substrate binding, its turnover numbers, or both combined in linkage disequilibrium; some *silent* variants are inactive, and some represent frameshift mutations with absence of enzyme protein. Originally, the clinical interest in BChE deficiency centered on the prolonged action of the normally short-acting succinylcholine when given during anesthesia. Of recent interest is the metabolism of cocaine by BChE; infusions of purified BChE promise to relieve cocaine toxicity, particularly when the drug has been applied in multiple doses or in forms designed for rapid absorption. Recent areas of study are questions of a role of BChE in Alzheimer disease, or of BChE variants as contributors to the Gulf War syndromes because of abnormalities of pyridostigmine action.
5. A genetic polymorphism now known to affect the oxidative biotransformation of debrisoquine, sparteine, and over 60 other therapeutic agents was first described in the mid-1970s. This genetic defect affects the function of a specific isozyme of cytochrome P_{450}, namely, CYP2D6, and it has been intensively investigated with respect to both its clinical and toxicologic implications and its underlying biochemical and molecular mechanisms. The *CYP2D* gene cluster, located on chromosome 22q13.1, is highly polymorphic in the human population. It may contain from two to four genes, only one of which (*CYP2D6*) produces functional enzyme in individuals of the *extensive metabolizer* (EM) phenotype. *Poor metabolizers* (PMs) of debrisoquine possess two of the almost 60 known mutant *CYP2D6* alleles. Of these, the four most common mutants account for about 90 percent of defective alleles in Caucasian populations and lead to impairment in expression of functional CYP2D6 protein by mechanisms ranging from deletion of the entire gene to single nucleotide substitutions that lead to premature translation termination. The clinical importance of genetically variable CYP2D6 function for the response to a given drug or other foreign chemical will depend on the quantitative significance of CYP2D6 in governing the compound's fate, its therapeutic window, the extent of its use in clinical practice, and the availability of therapeutic alternatives.

This chapter starts with definitions and an outline of the history and state of pharmacogenetics in biology and medicine, followed by a brief discussion and characterization of its scope. This introduction is followed by three case studies, which were chosen for their diversity and because of their established clinical significance. These are (1) malignant hyperthermia, discovered as a fatal response to general anesthesia, which arises from faulty intracellular calcium metabolism in skeletal muscle; (2) variation of butyrylcholinesterase, with consequences for the use of succinylcholine and apparently for cocaine; and (3) debrisoquine

A list of standard abbreviations is located immediately preceding the index in each volume. Additional abbreviations used in this chapter include: ALDH = aldehyde dehydrogenase; BChE = butyrylcholinesterase, also known as plasma cholinesterase; CICR = calcium-induced calcium release; CSC = caffeine-specific concentration, i.e., the caffeine concentration causing a contracture of specified magnitude in a specimen of muscle biopsy (used for MH diagnosis); CSC-H = like CSC, but in the presence of halothane; CYP2D6 = cytochrome P_{450}2D6, also referred to as debrisoquine 4-hydroxylase or sparteine monooxygenase, a polymorphic cytochrome P_{450}; EM = extensive metabolizer, i.e., normal CYP2D6 activity; MH = malignant hyperthermia; MHE, malignant hyperthermia equivocal; MHN = malignant hyperthermia normal, i.e., no predisposition to MH; MHS = malignant hyperthermia susceptible; MR = metabolic ratio, the ratio of the amount of a drug over that of its metabolite excreted in the same sample of urine; NAT = *N*-acetyltransferase; PM = poor metabolizer, i.e., CYP2D6 activity low or absent; PSEP = pale, soft, exudative pork; PSS = porcine stress syndrome; SR = sarcoplasmic reticulum; TPMT = thiopurine methyltransferase; TT = transverse tubule.

4-hydroxylase, a highly variable human enzyme, the deficiency of which accounts for failures of metabolism of numerous drugs. Other examples of pharmacogenetic variation [e.g., glucose-6-phosphate dehydrogenase (G-6-PD) deficiency] are treated as independent topics in various chapters of this book.

HISTORY

Three discoveries in the 1950s gave rise to the hybrid discipline that we now call *pharmacogenetics*:[1] the discoveries of primaquine sensitivity (G-6-PD deficiency), of the slow metabolism of isoniazid (acetylation polymorphism), and of atypical plasma cholinesterase giving rise to prolonged effects of succinylcholine. In 1957, Motulsky[2] wrote an article outlining what might be called the basic concepts of pharmacogenetics. In 1959, Vogel[3] was the first to use the word *pharmacogenetics* in print. Kalow[4] summarized the field in a book in 1962. In the mid-1960s, Vesell and Page[5] showed in family studies that genetic control of drug metabolism is a common occurrence. Independent discoveries in Bonn[6] and in London[7] of the debrisoquine/sparteine polymorphism helped the field of pharmacogenetics to its current status, a status symbolized by the foundation in 1991 of the journal *Pharmacogenetics*.[8] The future of pharmacogenetics may be symbolized by an increasing use of the word *pharmacogenomics*; whereas pharmacogenetics told us that genetic factors can modify drug action, pharmacogenomics indicates the aim to find the right drug for the right person who suffers from a common disease with numerous genetic roots.

DEFINITIONS

An original definition by a pharmacologist[4] reads, "Pharmacogenetics deals with pharmacologic responses and their modification by hereditary influences." Broadly defined, a pharmacologic response could be any functional alteration in any living organism produced by any exogenous chemical; such a response could be intentional, and classified as medical or therapeutic, or it could be unintentional and often toxic. With this definition, pharmacogenetics is characterized neither by the nature of biologically active chemicals nor by the biochemistry of a response but by the fact that a response may lack uniformity, and that this lack of uniformity has a genetic basis. With this liberal definition, pharmacogenetics can be looked at as a circumscribed element of the nature-nurture interface. However, more restricted definitions are frequently used.

In the first place, the term *pharmaco-* often conjures up a picture of drugs and medicines. Hence, when the concepts of pharmacogenetics are applied to biologically active nondrugs, the term *ecogenetics* is sometimes used.[9] Second, practical usage of the word pharmacogenetics has narrowed its most frequent application to humans rather than other creatures (see, however, reference 10), and here most often in reference to deficient or abnormal responses to drug therapy.[8] In choosing the contents of this chapter, we had to restrict ourselves even more by dwelling only on cases that some physicians will have to know in order to avoid damaging or killing patients with certain drugs.

SCOPE

Pharmacogenetic variability deserves comparison with inborn differences in susceptibilities to infectious disease.[11] A piece of knowledge that is still startling to many physicians is that susceptibility to tuberculosis is much dependent on a dominant gene that controls the function of macrophages;[12,13] it is found in mice, cattle, and humans. The same gene may affect susceptibility to infections with *Salmonella* and with *Leishmania*[14] and may participate in the resistance to leprosy.[15] Some particularly well-established examples of genetic control of susceptibility to infection have come from studies of malaria. Thus, G-6-PD deficiency (Chap. 179) is frequent in tropical countries because it conveys resistance to *Plasmodium falciparum* malaria.[16] Also, part of the high variability of the histocompatibility genes (Chap. 12) is associated with defense against malaria,[17] preventing human deaths caused by a malaria epidemic. Studies in mice suggest that cystic fibrosis protects against cholera[18] and, more recently, that it protects against salmonella-caused typhus.[19] A nucleotide deletion in the chemokine receptor 5 gene makes 1 percent of Caucasians immune against AIDS by protecting against HIV infection.[20,21] Most plagues have left survivors because susceptibility to infectious disease is probably always affected by genetic factors.[22]

Similarly, our defenses against chemical intruders must be variable from person to person and from race to race if the preservation of humanity in the face of a chemical catastrophe is to be ensured. Because of such variation, flies and mosquitoes have survived the onslaught of DDT and other chemicals. For our chemical defense systems, drugs are just like any other chemical intruder. A driving force for variability may be an ever-present animal-plant "warfare."[23] Pharmacogenetic variability of the human drug-metabolizing systems (Table 9-1) is ubiquitous and deeply ingrained in humanity.

There are other examples of human variability in the face of the environment: genetic variants in the perception of bitter taste[24] and various odors[25] are often considered to be part of pharmacogenetics. The variations in cone pigments[26] indicate that there are true person-to-person differences in visual perception.

In contrast to the rich metabolizing variations of any organism that interfaces with the environment, pharmacogenetic variation of

Table 9-1 Drug-Metabolizing Enzymes Known to be Genetically Variable

Esterases	**Oxidases**
Butyrylcholinesterase	Alcohol dehydrogenase
Paraoxonase/arylesterase	Aldehyde dehydrogenase
Transferases	Monoamine oxidase B
N-Acetyltransferases	Catalase
Sulfotransferases	Superoxide dismutase
Thiol methyltransferase	Trimethylamine *N*-oxidase
Thiopurine methyltransferase	Dihydropyrimidine dehydrogenase
Catechol-*O*-methyltransferase	**Cytochromes P_{450}**
Glutathione-*S*-transferases	CYP1A1
UDP-glucuronosyltransferases	CYP2A6
Glucosyltransferase	CYP2C8
Histamine methyltransferase	CYP2C9
Reductases	CYP2C19
NAD(P)H:quinone oxidoreductase	CYP2D6
Glucose-6-phosphate dehydrogenase	CYP2E1
	CYP3A5

receptors of hormones and neurotransmitters is relatively rare. The rarity might have technical reasons because the methods for determining genetic receptor variation (e.g., by studying receptor genes in white blood cells) are relatively new. More likely, the comparative rarity might have biologic reasons, because receptor variants might tend to produce disease rather than merely pharmacogenetic individuality.[27] Structural variation of a receptor may readily lead to functional failure because the receptor has to fit, on the one hand, to the messenger molecule and, on the other, to a G protein or some other second messenger. Thus, mutations interfering with the efficiency of an internal information system may be rare because they are not compatible with health [e.g., insulin receptor (Chap. 68)]. On the other hand, the dopamine D4 receptor contains a hypervariable segment that shows large person-to-person and interethnic differences without obvious consequences.[28] Receptor structures are sufficiently similar between species[29,30] so that animals can be used for pharmaceutical drug development.

A number of case studies in pharmacogenetics have become medical projects in their own right. Many chapters in this book contain examples of those that could be (or sometimes have been) considered part of pharmacogenetics. Examples are pentosuria (Chap. 73), lactase polymorphism (Chap. 76), sulfuration disorders (Chap. 88), glutathione synthetase deficiency (Chap. 96), porphyria (Chap. 124), sulfatase deficiency (Chap. 149), G-6-PD (Chap. 179), cytochrome-b_5 reductase (Chap. 180), and hemoglobinopathies (Chap. 181). For some additional examples of pharmacogenetics, compilations in books and reviews may be consulted (e.g., references 31–36). Many or most of the well-defined pharmacogenetic variants represent Mendelian (monogenic) traits. Hence, the rate of occurrence of such a variant in a population can be defined in terms of an allele frequency. These frequencies tend to differ between racially or ethnically defined populations,[37] accounting for some of the geographic and anthropologic differences in drug safety.[38]

Multifactorial variation is mathematically characterized, not by measurements of a frequency, but by the mean and standard deviation of some measured quantity. Multifactorial variation accounts for innumerable differences between individuals as well as between populations. In a comparison between populations, the items of toxicologic interest are often the edges of comparable distribution curves rather than their means (i.e., a comparison between the outliers in response to a drug).[37,39]

CHOICE OF EXAMPLES

In the context of this chapter on pharmacogenetics, it is impossible to cover all potential topics. Instead, three examples of clinical importance have been selected for special review. They are not new discoveries, yet they are still the subject of intensive investigations at both the clinical and genetic levels. They represent a variety of problems and thereby illustrate the scope of the field. We hope that the relatively thorough coverage of these three important topics will be more useful to most readers than would be a superficial review of many observations.

Topics that we omit with particular regret are those dealing with three of the drug-metabolizing enzymes (see Table 9-1):[39] namely, *N*-acetyltransferase (NAT), thiopurine methyltransferase (TPMT), and aldehyde dehydrogenase (ALDH). In studies of NAT (reviewed in references 40 and 41), two separate enzymes, NAT1 and NAT2, and their genes have been identified. The classic polymorphic enzyme is NAT2, although allelic variation in NAT1 has also now been demonstrated. DNA-based genotyping and probe-drug phenotyping of both NAT1[42–45] and NAT2[46–51] have become frequently pursued projects in cancer research.[52–57] Patients deficient in TPMT may die as a result of treatment of neoplastic or autoimmune diseases with thiopurines.[58] ALDH deficiency in Oriental populations is a deterrent against alcoholism.[59] These and other data indicate that pharmacogenetics of drug metabolism is a field in lively development.[39]

Not long ago, there was a lack of analytic capabilities to detect drug metabolites in body fluids. It was understandable that physicians handed out medicines as if all people were alike. At this time, we are still struggling to learn when — or to what extent or under what circumstances — we can afford to neglect human diversity in drug treatment. The study of pharmacogenetics represents this learning process.

MALIGNANT HYPERTHERMIA

History, Status, and Incidence

The pharmacogenetic entity *malignant hyperthermia* (MH; sometimes called *malignant hyperpyrexia*) is surely as old as is general anesthesia with ether or chloroform. However, if a pathologic event is rare enough to be seen not even once in a lifetime by most physicians, it is not easily recognized as a particular disease entity. Harrison and Isaacs[60] traced MH in a human family through four generations back to 1915. The merit of having recognized MH as an entity with a genetic basis belongs to Denborough and Lovell,[61] whose patient in 1960 survived an MH attack, and who took seriously the patient's tale of events in his family. In the meantime, MH has become the topic of 10 books and at least 15 review articles.[62–67]

In spite of its rarity, MH has excited considerable medical interest for the following reasons: The fulminant, classic MH attack is a dramatic medical event, with the key features of muscle rigidity, high fever, tachycardia, and acidosis. With a mortality rate of 70 to 80 percent at the outset, it has been the most serious and the most feared complication of general anesthesia. The mortality rate has dropped to 10 percent or less because of early diagnosis of an incipient attack, good management of MH crises, and the discovery of the curative effects of dantrolene.[68–72] The ability to recognize the genetically dominant predisposition to MH [MH susceptibility (MHS)] by in vitro tests[73,74] offered the opportunity to avoid MH attacks, besides initiating fundamental investigations of skeletal muscle with emphasis on the functional roles of ionized calcium. Last but not least, the discovery of MH in swine[75] and the economic impact of this discovery [pale, soft, exudative pork (PSEB)] stimulated research with benefits for treatment of human MH.

Incidence estimates of MH episodes during anesthesia depend on many factors but have been on the order of 1:15,000 in children's hospitals[63] to 1:100,000 or less in most locations.[76] The majority of cases represent dominant inheritance (see the section on "Human Malignant Hyperthermia").

The fact that MHS represents an affliction of skeletal muscle seems to be mirrored by the fact that acute MH episodes predominate in the prime of life, when muscle strength is greatest. Ellis[77] states, "Undoubtedly a proportion of our probands fall into the 'elitist athlete' category, and many others have obvious and well developed musculature." Males from the teens to the early thirties are the ones most often affected, although MH attacks have occurred in all age groups. The proportion of males with MH attacks outnumbers females 2.5:1.[77] There is no formal explanation, but there are hormonal influences during muscle development,[78] and there are gender differences in that excised fibers of muscles from females respond less to caffeine and to the caffeine-halothane combination than do specimens from males.[79] Furthermore, the responsiveness to caffeine contractures is distinctly heritable from father to son but not from mother to daughter.[79]

Biochemical Aspects of the Malignant Hyperthermia Defect

At the outset of this discussion, it needs to be understood that MH in humans is a syndrome, not a uniform disease,[80] so one can expect a variety of pathophysiological factors to play a role at some time or other, or in some patient or other.[67,81–87] By contrast, a primary defect has been identified that seems to determine every case of porcine MH in all breeds of pigs investigated.[88,89] This observation has sharpened the search for the causes of human MHS. An excellent overview of the many biochemical questions raised by MH has been provided recently by Loke and MacLennan.[90]

Ionized Calcium. Before discussing the defect(s) of MH, a brief look at muscle physiology[91–94] and pharmacology[95–97] is helpful. It has long been known that intracellular calcium metabolism regulates muscle contraction, which consists of bonding between the proteins actin and myosin. Troponin, which along with actin and tropomyosin is a component of the thin filament, is the calcium-binding site, and the amount of Ca^{2+} available for binding regulates the interaction between the actin and myosin filaments. Besides regulating muscle contraction, ionized calcium also activates the glycolytic pathway by binding to phosphorylase kinase and thereby favors the replenishment of adenosine triphosphate (ATP). The muscle machinery composed of myosin-troponin-tropomyosin-actin is not altered or disturbed in MH; a given calcium concentration causes the same contraction of "skinned fibers" from malignant hyperthermia normal (MHN) and MHS subjects.[98] An MH attack is caused by an excess of ionized calcium in the sarcoplasm. The only question is what causes the calcium accumulation?

The structure within the muscle cell that regulates the concentration of ionized calcium in the sarcoplasm is the sarcoplasmic reticulum (SR).[82,96] The SR is an organelle in skeletal muscle equivalent to the endoplasmic reticulum in other cells. The SR consists of longitudinal segments and of bulging terminal structures called *cisternae*. What counts is the function of these cisternae: they contain the release channels[99,100] that discharge calcium from the stores within the SR into the sarcoplasm.[101] A Ca^{2+}-ATPase pumps calcium back into the longitudinal section of the SR.[96,102] The calcium concentration in the sarcoplasm is primarily determined by the balance between release of calcium from the SR and reuptake into the SR. Thus, in skeletal muscle, the regulator of the sarcoplasmic calcium concentration that determines normal muscle function is not the sarcolemma itself, nor is it the calcium storage system of the mitochondria. This does not exclude the possibility that disturbances of sarcolemmal or mitochondrial functions could contribute to MHS.[103]

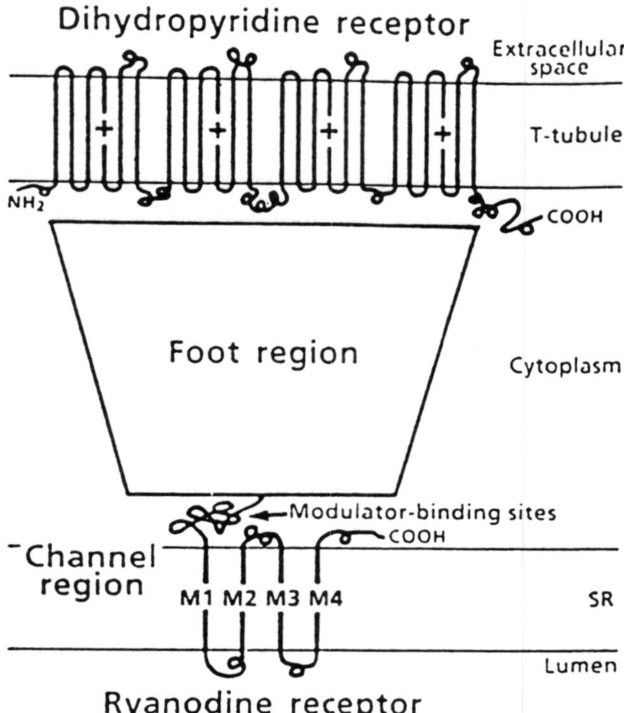

Fig. 9-1 Ryanodine receptor. Structural features of the skeletal muscle ryanodine receptor; proposed transmembrane topology and molecular architecture of the ryanodine receptor in the triad junction of skeletal muscle. The C-terminal channel region, including the putative transmembrane segments M1 to M4 and the putative modulator binding sites, and the large cytoplasmic region corresponding to the foot structure of the ryanodine receptor are shown schematically. The putative transmembrane segments of the T-tubular dihydropyridine receptor (segments S1 to S6 in each of the four repeated homology units) are also shown, and the putative voltage sensor segment S4 in each repeat is indicated by a *plus sign*. (*From Takeshima et al.*[108] *Used by permission of the author and Nature 339:439–445; © 1989 Macmillan Magazines Ltd.*)

Excitation-Contraction Coupling. Since it is the nervous system that determines muscular activity, the question arises as to how the function of the SR is regulated by nerve impulses or, in other words, how does the excitation-contraction coupling proceed?[104] If a nerve impulse arrives at a neuromuscular end plate, it causes release of acetylcholine and a consequent opening of local sodium and potassium channels, and this in turn causes a depolarization at the end plate, which then spreads from its local origins over the whole muscle membrane. This membrane extends at regular intervals toward the interior of the muscle fiber and ends in the sarcolemma at the opposite side of the fiber; these extensions of the membrane are referred to as *transverse tubules* (T tubules or TTs). The TT membrane contains dihydropyridine receptors that serve as voltage sensors and calcium channels.[105,106] The TT meets with structures called *feet*, which extend from the cisternae of the SR to serve as calcium release channels and which constitute the *ryanodine receptor*,[100,107] so called because it is the binding site of the toxic alkaloid ryanodine. The meeting between the TT and the SR via the foot is the location of excitation-contraction coupling (Fig. 9-1).[108]

When the membrane depolarization arrives at the end of the TT, it may liberate a small pulse of ionized calcium from within it. It may be that these calcium ions are the messengers that stimulate the ryanodine receptor to release calcium into the sarcoplasma for muscle contraction. This is *calcium-induced calcium release* (CICR), and caffeine has been shown to enhance CICR.[82,109–111] It is easy to imagine that CICR represents the essence of excitation-contraction coupling. Thus, it was disturbing news that dantrolene, the drug that specifically counteracts an MH attack, has been stated to inhibit caffeine-induced calcium release but not CICR.[112] However, newer investigations indicate that, depending on concentration, dantroline can activate or inhibit the ryanodine receptor.[72]

The Ryanodine Receptor. As already mentioned, the ryanodine receptor is a calcium release channel that was identified by using the labeled toxic alkaloid ryanodine as a ligand. The ryanodine receptor is a tetramer of an already exceptionally large protein (molecular weight, 565 kDa).[113] It extends from the SR cisternae to close proximity with the dihydropyridine receptor in the T tubule (see Fig. 9-1). Its function as the calcium release channel of the SR can be modulated pharmacologically.[66,95,110,112] It must have an important bridging function in excitation-contraction coupling, although the function is not yet precisely definable. The ryanodine receptor[114] is the target of caffeine[112,115–118] and of halothane[119] when stimulating the CICR[102,110,120] (Table 9-1). The selective binding to it of 4-chloro-*m*-cresol is a more recent finding.[121] In the presence of caffeine, a given amount of inducing calcium causes more calcium release than in the absence of caffeine; in other words, caffeine reduces the threshold of CICR.

Salviati et al[119] concluded that halothane activates the calcium efflux from the SR by interacting with calmodulin, a specific calcium-binding protein. If so, caffeine should be postulated to act differently. If caffeine and halothane had the same mode of action, their joint application would yield a summation of effects. Since combination of the two drugs shows potentiation (i.e., a multiplicative synergism),[122] their points of attack must be different; there must be more than one way to modulate calcium release. Perhaps caffeine binds to the ryanodine receptor protein, whereas halothane affects the lipid membrane of both the sarcolemma and the SR.[123]

The ryanodine receptor is changed in MH muscle:[96] the enhancing effect of caffeine and/or halothane is greater than in normal muscle, presumably by an increased duration of the opening of the calcium release channel in MHS muscle.

All observations taken together indicate that the increased responsiveness of the ryanodine receptor is the quintessence of MHS in most cases.[84,124,125] A given depolarization produced by succinylcholine, any given impulse in the presence of halothane, or the combination of stimuli, produces excessive calcium release by the SR and, thereby, muscle rigidity, heat production, acidosis, and ATP loss, so that eventually the integrity of the muscle membrane cannot be maintained.

These observations indicate that the current investigations of MH are still intense and not always without controversy. The studies promise benefits not only by improving the treatment of MH patients, but by raising the understanding of normal muscle function.

Genetics of Malignant Hyperthermia in Swine and in Humans

Genetic investigations of MHS in humans[77,126,127] are handicapped if based solely on clinical observations. MH attacks are rare, and multiple cases within one family are rarer still. The diversity of the signs and symptoms of an MH episode may make the clinical diagnosis enigmatic, particularly in the case of aborted or semiaborted attacks. An additional difficulty is that many patients have uneventful anesthesias with triggering agents before they suffer an MH episode;[128] this means that besides genetic susceptibility and a triggering drug, there must be a particular trigger (PSEP) before an attack occurs. As a consequence, most genetic studies of MH rely on either a combination of clinical assessments and the results of diagnostic muscle biopsies or on the latter alone.

Porcine Malignant Hyperthermia. At present, the genetics of MH in pigs is well defined and thus will be presented first. Historically,[129] the concern was the porcine stress syndrome (PSS). This syndrome refers to the sudden death of pigs with hyperthermia and rigidity in stressful situations (e.g., during transport, fighting, or mating); their meat is devalued (PSEP). MHS pigs show all features of PSS, that is, an acute attack of hyperthermia and rigidity may be caused by stress as well as by drugs (e.g., halothane or succinylcholine). Thus, MHS means PSS susceptibility with all its economic implications; it also seems that PSS always means MH.

There have been massive genetic studies of MH in several breeds of swine.[130–134] Suffice it to state that studies that relied on a 3-min exposure of young pigs to halothane to distinguish between MHS and MHN individuals gave clear-cut evidence for a recessive inheritance, at least in terms of the contracture response.[135] However, halothane exposure for longer periods combined with an injection of succinylcholine may also cause MH in heterozygotes. Thus, the classification of MHS inheritance in pigs as either dominant or recessive can be a matter of testing conditions.

MacLennan and coworkers[88,89,136] have produced new and straightforward data of satisfying simplicity. These investigators concentrated on the ryanodine receptor. Their investigations of the ryanodine receptor gene RYR1 showed 18 nucleotide differences between MHS and MHN pigs, but only one of these nucleotide substitutions resulted in a difference of amino acids: it was defined as the C.1843T $C \rightarrow T$ mutation, giving rise to the substitution R615C in the amino acid sequence (the human counterpart is R614C).

DNA-based tests developed to study this mutant revealed it in all affected individuals from five different breeds, while haplotyping suggested that the abnormal gene had arisen in a founder animal.[88] In a large-scale comparison using 376 British-Landrace pigs from the Animal Breeding Research Organisation in Edinburgh,[130,137] the MHS (n/n) animals as defined by halothane responsiveness and flanking marker haplotyping were homozygotes for this mutation, whereas the heterozygotes were classified as N/n (Lod score 101.75 for linkage at $\text{Theta}_{max} = 0.0$). The test was in complete agreement with clinical observation and is used widely in agriculture.

There has been selection for the porcine MH mutation because it is associated with leanness and heavy muscling. This may result because the abnormal Ca^{2+} release channel leads to continued toning of the muscle and to subsequent muscle hypertrophy. The location of the ryanodine receptor gene on chromosome 6q11-q21 in pigs,[134] however, indicates its close proximity plus a possible linkage to genes controlling lipid metabolism and muscle growth (*APOE, LIPE,* and *TGFB-1*). The linkage may account for the increased frequency in leanness and heavy muscling in MHS pigs.[89]

The recognition of the mutant ryanodine receptor as the principal cause of MH in swine will give pig breeders the opportunity to eliminate the gene from their stock. On the other hand, some breeders might wish deliberately to leave the gene in heterozygous form in their herds. If increased activity of the calcium release channel in heterozygotes increases muscle bulk, it would produce features desired by the pig breeders. The less desirable PSEP resulting from the PSS occurs at the highest rate in affected homozygotes.

Human Malignant Hyperthermia. In 1960, Denborough and Lovell[61] had a patient who gave a family history of death associated with anesthesia. Further inquiries[138] indicated that there were in this family several anesthesia-related fatalities, which seemed to occur on the basis of a dominantly inherited predisposition. In review articles written many years later and with many more data at hand,[128,139,140] it was estimated that approximately 50 percent of MH cases occurred on the basis of a dominantly inherited trait. There was evidence of an MH attack having occurred on the basis of recessive inheritance[140] in perhaps 20 percent of cases.[139] About 30 percent of the cases collected by Britt were solitary cases.[62] In most of these, it was probably because affected relatives were not available for testing. The familial and the solitary cases did not differ statistically in their response to diagnostic tests with caffeine or caffeine plus halothane.[79]

Human MHS is usually a dominant trait,[141] whereas the defect in pigs is always recessive. The reason could be that the combination of halothane and succinylcholine is a most effective stimulant, and that use of this drug combination is common in humans during anesthesia. From that point, there is no necessity to look for different causes of human and porcine MHS.

Only 1 of 35 human families with the MHS trait had exactly the same mutation in the ryanodine receptor as did the MHS pigs.[142] This receptor is an exceptionally large protein molecule, and a variety of mutations exist.[90,143,144] Linkage between MHS and the ryanodine receptor gene *RYR1* (Fig. 9-2) has been shown in approximately half of MHS families.[90,136,142,145] Thus, human MHS is often caused by a mutation of the ryanodine receptor, but it usually would be a different mutation from that in pigs.

There are some families in whom MHS is not associated with ryanodine receptor variation.[67,85] While the ryanodine receptor gene (*RYR1*) is on chromosome 19, there are some indications that variant genes on chromosome 3,[87] chromosome 7,[146] or chromosome 17[147] may have responsibility for MH. Variation of a sodium channel gene might be a culprit.[148,149] There are suggestions of defective cation transport in the sarcolemma,[103] but Everts et al[150] found a normal content of the Na^+/K^+-ATPase in the sarcolemma of MH muscle. There are observations of a mutation[151] and of an

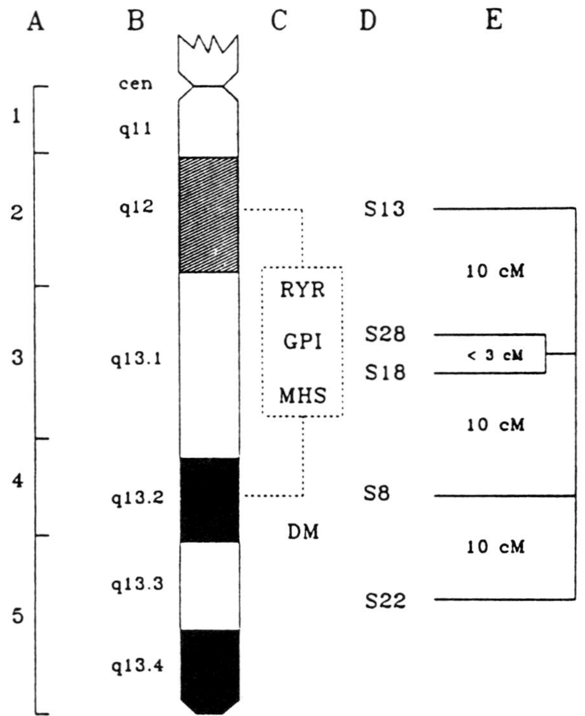

Fig. 9-2 Long arm of chromosome 19. *A*, physical distances; *B*, cytogenetic bands; *C*, area of the genes for the ryanodine receptor (RYR), glucose phosphate isomerase (GPI), and susceptibility for malignant hyperthermia (MHS); *D*, available DNA markers; and *E*, genetic distances. (*From Lehmann-Horn et al.*[65] *Used by permission.*)

altered binding of the TT dihydropyridine receptor[152] and of a role of a G protein in the SR.[153] There is possibly a membrane defect with perhaps general consequences.[154,155] Seewald et al[156] found altered phospholipid and fatty-acid composition in muscle membranes of MHS pigs. Free fatty acids are released from skeletal muscle homogenates by the activity of an endogenous lipase, and this release is elevated in preparations from MHS pigs and humans.[154] It may be that the elevation of free fatty acids sensitizes the release of calcium from the SR.[157] Levitt et al[158] suggested an abnormal function of the hormone-sensitive lipase as the cause of altered lipid metabolism in MH. The gene for this lipase is located near the ryanodine receptor gene. The proximity between MH and lipid-controlling genes is present in humans as in pigs.[65]

In some of the clinically severe MH attacks, biopsy tests of the probands' father and mother revealed that one parent's test results showed the expected gross abnormalities in response to caffeine and halothane, while the other parent's response suggested a minor deviation from normal,[122,140] i.e., there was no response to either caffeine or halothane indicative of MHS, but an unusually strong potentiation of the caffeine effect by halothane when both drugs were given at the same time (the *K variant*, named for Kalow[140]). This observation raises the question of whether the genetically dominant MHS may result in a particularly severe MH reaction if there is a supporting genetic background. If so, it could mean that more than one gene may contribute to the trait of MHS.

The frequency of the gene or gene combination accounting for the proportion of MHS subjects in a population must be far higher than the frequency of MH attacks. The frequency of surgical procedures in populations grouped by age and gender may vary with time and location, anesthesia does not always involve the use of MH-triggering agents, and a large proportion of MH attacks occur only during a second or third anesthesia even when triggering agents are used. If the frequency of MH attacks is on the order of 1:100,000 anesthesias,[76] the population frequency of MHS is probably closer to 1:1000 or 1:10,000.

Functional Diagnosis of Malignant Hyperthermia Susceptibility

Initial biochemical efforts in the 1960s to recognize susceptibility to MH had been unsuccessful. Only after various frustrating histologic and biochemical investigations was a pharmacologic diagnosis attempted as a last resort (Fig. 9-3).[73] That is, small specimens of skeletal muscle were collected from survivors of an MH attack and their contracture response to caffeine,[73] and later to halothane,[74] was measured. These in vitro measurements are still the most widely used MH tests in spite of their invasiveness, cost, and inconvenience.[159] They offer fair reliability as a diagnostic tool[160,161] and, in that respect, cannot yet be replaced.

The Caffeine-Halothane Contracture Tests. In the course of the widespread use and adaptation of the caffeine-halothane contracture tests,[77,122,162] the technical aspects of testing have been improved[163,164] and data interpretation has been standardized to some extent:[165,166] there is now a North American MH

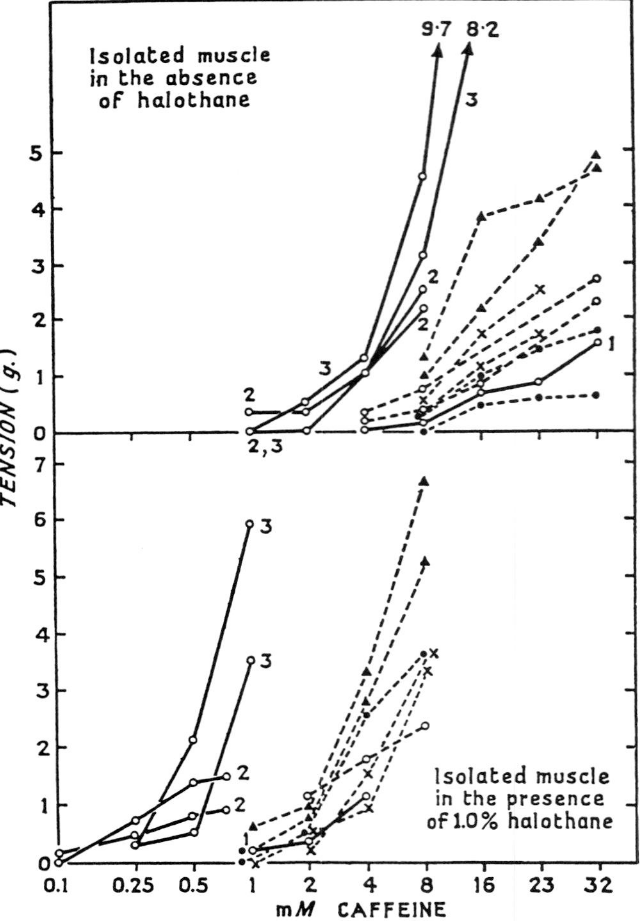

Fig. 9-3 Caffeine contracture of isolated muscle from volunteers disposed to malignant hyperthermia and from controls. The *abscissa* (log scale) indicates the concentration of caffeine in the tissue bath, whereas the *ordinate* gives the maximal increase of isometric contracture produced by caffeine. The *bottom plot* shows the measurements obtained when 1% halothane was added to the oxygen-carbon dioxide mixture bubbling through the bath. *Broken line*, control muscle; *solid line*, patient's muscle; *1*, patient without rigidity; *2* and *3*, patients with rigidity; *o*, quadriceps; *x*, soleus; *solid triangle*, gastrocnemius. (*From Kalow et al.*[73] *Used by permission.*)

protocol[167–170] and a somewhat different European protocol[171–174] for caffeine-halothane contracture tests.

Essentials of the North American protocol may be summarized as follows. The subjects tested are patients with a clinical history of unequivocal or suspected MH and relatives of such patients. Under regional anesthesia, muscle is removed from the vastus lateralis or other large mixed-type I/II muscle belly. The muscle specimen must be large enough that several strips about 1- to 5-mm thick and 10- to 20-mm long, each weighing between 100 and 300 mg, can be produced. With minimum delay, each muscle strip is placed for testing into a small glass chamber with Krebs Ringer solution, which is continuously aerated with a gas consisting of 95% oxygen and 5% CO_2. Halothane vapor can be introduced into this gas in measured concentrations. The bath fluid is maintained at 37°C and at a pH of 7.4. Isometric muscle contraction is measured with the help of a transducer. Incremental doses of caffeine are added to the muscle bath in both absence and presence of 1% halothane; the caffeine additions are to produce concentrations of 0.5, 1.0, 2.0, and 4.0 mM (8 mM if needed), and finally 32 mM to assess the maximum contracture. The protocol also calls for exposure of a muscle strip to a fixed dose of 3% halothane in the gas mixture.

Three types of data evaluation are used. First, the measured tensions are plotted on a semilogarithmic graph, and the dose of caffeine required to raise the tension by 1 g is derived by interpolation. This dose is termed the *caffeine specific concentration*, abbreviated CSC in the absence and CSC-H in the presence of halothane. CSC values above 4.0 mM and CSC-H above 1.0 mM are considered normal in most laboratories (see, however, reference 167). The difficulty of the test interpretation is that the frequency distributions do not show clear-cut divisions between MHS and MHN subjects (see Fig. 9-4 with CSC data from almost 1200 subjects[79]). Second, the tension increase after addition of 2 mM caffeine is reported in grams and also as percentage increase, whereby the response to 32 mM is taken as 100 percent. Third, the presence or absence of a contracture response to 3% halothane is registered and measured when present. Any response to 3% halothane is regarded as the most specific indicator of MHS, but it is also the least sensitive test, giving many false-negative diagnoses. By contrast, CSC-H test results are the least specific but most sensitive indicators. An indication of MHS by any of the tests leads to the classification of the subject as MHS,[62,77] since a wrong positive classification is considered safer for the patient than a wrong negative one. For the record, however, MHS subjects have been subdivided by test results into those with H-MH, C-MH, K-MH, and combinations thereof, where H indicates a positive response to halothane, C to caffeine (CSC, < 4 mM), and K to the caffeine-halothane combination (CSC-H, < 1 mM); for instance, HCK-MH would indicate a positive response to all three tests.[62,168]

The European Protocol has been outlined by Ording and colleagues.[174–176] Incremental doses of caffeine are used similarly as for the North American CSC measurements. CSC-H tests are not performed. Instead, incremental doses of halothane are used (0.5, 1.0, and 2.0% vol/vol in the oxygenating gas, specified to produce concentrations of 0.11, 0.22, and 0.44 mM in the tissue bath). Using these same concentrations of halothane, an additional *dynamic halothane test* is performed in many centers, in which the muscle fibers are subjected to cycles of mechanical stretching and relaxing in association with halothane exposure. The response to halothane is thereby increased, but this does not necessarily enhance its power of discrimination.[176]

The philosophy and practice of data interpretation are different from those in North America.[177] Threshold concentrations are determined for both caffeine and halothane; they are defined as the concentrations eliciting a sustained increase in tension of 0.2 g. The concentrations denoting abnormal reactions are taken to be 0.44 mM (2.0% vol/vol) halothane or less, and 2 mM caffeine or less. Four test results are possible: If both halothane and caffeine are below threshold, it indicates MHS. Both values above threshold are registered as MHN, i.e., absence of the MH trait. Discrepancies between the caffeine and halothane thresholds are

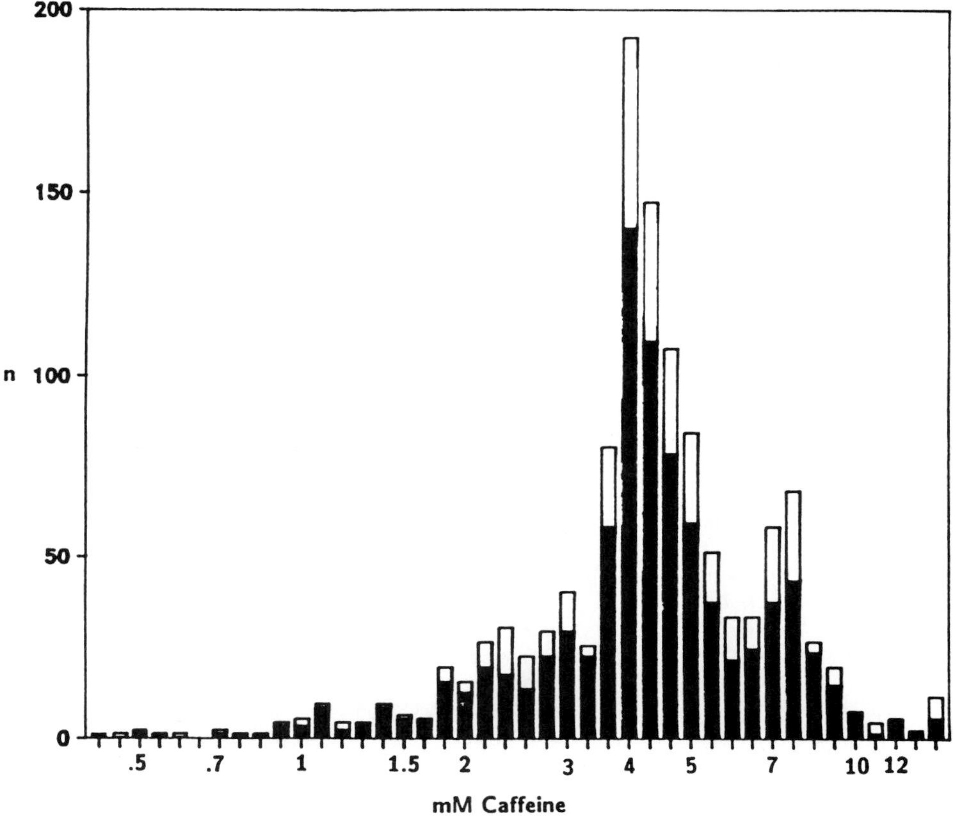

Fig. 9-4 Frequency distribution of muscle responsiveness to caffeine. The measured parameter is the caffeine specific concentration (CSC) in millimoles (mM), that is, the caffeine concentration producing a contracture of standardized magnitude in biopsy specimens of human skeletal muscle. The study comprised 1192 subjects. The *bar graph* represents the distribution of the logarithmically converted data (ln CSC). The *x*-axis indicates the caffeine concentration (mM) on a logarithmically distorted scale. The *shaded* part of each column indicates 855 subjects for whom pedigree data are available. (*From Kalow et al.*[79] *Used by permission.*)

registered as MH equivocal (MHE); MHE occurs in two varieties: MHEc with only the caffeine effect abnormal and MHEh with only the halothane effect abnormal. By using the designation MHE, a diagnosis regarding MHS is avoided. For the sake of caution, however, the subjects are treated clinically like MHS patients.[161]

The caffeine-halothane contracture tests are usually not performed on small children in order to avoid the scarring from muscle biopsy.[178]

It is appropriate that both caffeine and halothane are used in the diagnostic contracture tests; it is not a surprise that the test results are usually but not always alike or equivalent. Test results of 967 patients screened in Europe[176] showed 560 MHN, 278 MHS, 113 MHEh, and 22 MHEc. The occurrence of such a large proportion of MHE subjects fits with the pharmacologic evidence[79,122] that caffeine and halothane have different points of attack. The predisposition to MH in humans is neither clinically, biochemically, nor genetically uniform.

Because of the nonuniformity of predisposition to MH, it is not surprising that the *in vitro* tests with caffeine or halothane give sometimes deviating results.[179] Several investigations explored genotype/phenotype relations or the sensitivity and specificity of the *in vitro* tests.[167,170,174,180,181] The evidence indicates that exclusion of MHS is achieved with near certainty, while the presence of MHS is diagnosed with acceptable reliability.

Other in Vitro Tests. Many attempts have been made to replace the described contracture tests by other *in vitro* methods. The skinned-fiber test uses single muscle fibers that can be obtained by needle biopsy and that can be stored.[62] The fibers are mechanically or chemically skinned, i.e., the sarcolemma and mitochondria are removed and the excitation-contraction coupling site is eliminated. Unfortunately, the tests are too technically demanding for widespread use.

Britt[62,182] and Ording[175] cite various other *in vitro* procedures that have been recommended at some time or other, such as the ATP depletion test, the calcium uptake test by muscle, and tests measuring halothane-induced calcium accumulation in lymphocytes.[183,184] Hofmann[185] summarized all tests involving blood cells. Particular effort by various investigators went into studying blood platelets that resemble muscle cells in that they contain contractile elements, calcium storage vesicles, and a calcium-dependent ATPase. To date, all in vitro tests (except the contracture tests) have had sufficient drawbacks that they have not gained general acceptance.

The apparent variety of the biochemical lesions responsible for human MH makes it unlikely that DNA-based tests will be able to eliminate functional tests in the near future. However, as new discoveries of MHS-causing DNA alterations will be forthcoming, genotyping may replace phenotyping within families after identification of the mutation in a propositus.[67]

Many attempts have been made to find histologic alterations in MHS muscle that would characterize it sufficiently to serve as a diagnostic criterion. This goal has not been achieved. Harnden-Mayor et al[186] found a muscle fiber hypertrophy affecting all fiber types, which might be specific but is difficult to quantify. Nonspecific alterations have been repeatedly observed.[64,187]

***In Vivo* Tests.** The observation of creatine kinase (CK) elevation in MH families goes back to studies by Isaacs and Barlow.[188] Many attempts by various authors were made to find ways and means to utilize this observation (see references 189–192), although the unreliability of the test in some families had been recognized and reported.[193] In general, use of the CK test is justified only when the danger of false-negative assessments is fully appreciated.

One proposed test using nuclear magnetic resonance (NMR) deserves attention.[194–196] The metabolic reserves of finger muscles are noninvasively assessed by measuring exercise-induced changes in pH and inorganic phosphate. The test has a sound scientific basis. A proposed noninvasive test using ultrasound[197] has been criticized.[198,199]

Britt[200] has compiled lists of clinical manifestations that appeared to be statistically associated with MHS; these included squint, tendency for muscle cramps, and bone and joint diseases. Smith and Ellis[201] confirmed that the trait of MHS tends to be associated with minor pathologies. It remains to be seen to what extent such associations can be utilized for diagnostic purposes in conjunction with physical examinations.

Clinical Aspects of Malignant Hyperthermia

MH may occur in its classic form as an acute crisis or in more or less abortive forms. All events are initiated by a persisting elevation of ionized calcium in the sarcoplasm, accounting for the rigidity and the sustained glycolytic and anaerobic metabolism and the consequences thereof. Table 9-2 lists the biochemical events that underlie an MH attack.

The Acute Crisis. The classic cardinal manifestations are tachycardia, muscle rigidity, and a rapidly rising body temperature.[200–205] These symptoms may develop suddenly to produce the clinical picture of a fulminant MH episode. If succinylcholine is used, the muscle rigidity tends to start with masseter spasm but may develop any degree of severity, in extreme cases to opisthotonus, so that the arched body is supported by the heels and the head. The temperature may rise at a rate of more than 2°C/h. Tachycardia and cardiac arrhythmias are perhaps the most consistent early signs of MH, but they are initially often ascribed to other causes and thus at first are not recognized as part of an MH attack.

Metabolic changes noticeable at the very early stages of the crisis are a marked increase in carbon dioxide production and a consequent tachypnea.[82,206,207] As the oxygen demand of the hypermetabolic tissues exceeds oxygen availability, an anaerobic metabolic pattern develops, with increased lactate production and metabolic acidosis. In other words, there is a mixed respiratory and metabolic acidosis. If the patient is breathing spontaneously, end-tidal carbon dioxide increases despite the rise in ventilation. Pulmonary edema may occur as the episode progresses, and cardiac failure becomes apparent.

Typical for the early phase of the crisis is a release of potassium into the blood, which contributes to the production of cardiac arrhythmias.

Table 9-2 Biochemical Events during a Malignant Hyperthermia Attack

1. Prolonged opening of the calcium release channels of the sarcoplasmic reticulum (SR) floods the sarcoplasm with Ca^{2+}.
2. The Ca^{2+} has four effects:
   a. The Ca-ATPase pumps calcium back into the SR at maximal rate, thereby consuming ATP and producing ADP.
   b. Myosin ATPase causes actin-myosin interaction, which produces muscle contraction with ATP consumption and production of heat.
   c. Phosphorylase kinase activation produces anaerobic glycogen metabolism to form lactic acid, producing ATP from ADP.
   d. Stimulation of aerobic metabolism in mitochondria together with influx of lactic acid produces ATP, CO_2, and heat.
3. Immediate consequences are rigidity, heat production, and acidosis.
4. The ATP turnover, though very high, may become insufficient to maintain energy sufficiency of the cell. The cell membrane becomes leaky for electrolytes and certain proteins.

With the crisis tends to come a release of muscle proteins into the blood, such as CK, and myoglobin; such release is a sign that the sarcolemma, the muscle membrane, is damaged. The myoglobin release may be massive enough to damage kidney function. The CK measurement may reach extreme levels, but usually only after the crisis. A frequent late event is a coagulopathy, which may be either due to a preexisting platelet defect or to diffuse intravascular coagulation with factor depletion triggered by the crisis.

A fatal outcome of the crisis is likely due to brain death, coagulopathy, or renal failure. Initially, about 80 percent of MH attacks ended fatally. This number is now reduced to less than 10 percent. This reflects appropriate management of the MH crises and dantrolene treatment (see below). However, this improved survival also reflects the increased medical awareness of MH, and therefore improved diagnosis of abortive cases of MH.

Survivors of a crisis usually suffer from severe muscle pains, sometimes for months. Neurologic defects may take any form, including any form of brain damage, particularly in patients with the most fulminant reactions.

Unusual, Abortive, and Borderline Cases. Susceptibility to MH seems to go along with a change of the human masseter muscle, which is put into spasm by succinylcholine in MHS subjects, particularly when halothane is used as an anesthetic. Thus, when succinylcholine is used, masseter spasm is a fairly regular sign of a beginning MH crisis, particularly in children.[208] Moreover, roughly half the cases (75 of 141) of clinically observed masseter spasm without any other or with only mild symptoms (temperature $< 38.6°C$ and pH > 7.3) turned out to be MH susceptible by the caffeine-halothane tests.[209] Mild symptoms of that magnitude by themselves were rarely indicative of MHS.

The timing of MH in relation to the triggering anesthesia can be peculiar. Although some signs of MH are evident within minutes, onset of an MH crisis may occur only hours after the beginning of anesthesia, particularly when only inhalational agents, and no succinylcholine, were used. Recrudescent MH, which is a flare-up of an attack, has occurred up to 30 h after an apparently successful treatment.

An obviously separate disease is nonrigid MH, which was responsible for several anesthesia-related deaths in a Wisconsin family.[210,211] The disease is clearly much more rare than "ordinary" MH; its biochemistry must be different, since muscle biopsy indicates relative resistance to caffeine, and not increased sensitivity as usual. The major difference in the symptomatology of the crisis was the absence of muscle rigidity.

MH and central core disease are clearly related items.[90] According to Mortier et al,[212] some patients with Noonan syndrome and with apparently nonspecific myopathies are highly susceptible; none of the various muscular dystrophies regularly predispose individuals to MH, but some dystrophic patients nevertheless register as MHS. Poels et al[213] have added cases with unexplained recurrent rhabdomyolysis to the list of MHS subjects. Brownell[214] has provided a list of diseases with suspected MH association and the reasons for the suspicions. The failure of a suspected MH case to respond to the therapeutic use of dantrolene has been used to exclude the diagnosis of MHS.[215]

Considerable effort has gone into studies of whether the malignant neuroleptic syndrome (MNS)[216] is related to MH.[217] MNS is a rare complication of treatment with neuroleptics and is characterized by hyperthermia, rigor, and stupor and an epidemiology similar to MH in that most patients were young males; lethality was in the order of 20 percent. Only 11 of 23 MNS patients did register as susceptible to MH by caffeine-halothane tests.[218] Some Japanese authors[219,220] considered MNS and MH to have only superficial similarities. However, dantrolene, the lifesaving drug in MH attacks, has also helped MNS victims.[218] One must conclude that MH and MNS pull the same metabolic trigger in muscle, even if the primary defect of MNS lies in the central nervous system.

Heat stroke[217] (the inability to deal with excessive ambient temperature) may lead to body temperatures above 40°C, which in turn may cause agitation, rigor, and coma. Children and old or sick people are those most often affected. This contrasts with exercise-induced heat stroke, which most often tends to affect apparently healthy young men (e.g., athletes running or soldiers marching), when heat loss cannot compensate for the heat produced by muscular exercise. This may lead to hyperthermia, tachycardia, metabolic acidosis, and secondarily to rhabdomyolysis and myoglobinuria, which in turn may cause renal failure[217] (and see above). There are case reports of MH attacks having been initiated not by drugs but by excessive exercise in subjects who were later tested with caffeine and halothane and found to be MHS.[221] Thus, some cases of heat stroke may represent MHS, analogous to PSS, representing a non-drug-induced MH attack.

Prevention and Treatment of Malignant Hyperthermia

Since early recognition of an MH crisis is vital for successful treatment, each patient undergoing anesthesia must be subject to routine monitoring of heart rate, blood pressure, cardiac rhythm, tidal volume, airway pressure, respiratory rate, end-tidal CO_2, pulse oximetry, airway oxygen, and body temperature.[222]

The elements of treatment of an MH crisis are items of general agreement:[62,222–225] (1) stop the anesthetic, (2) administer 100% oxygen, (3) start dantrolene (initially, 2.5 mg/kg intravenously), (4) cool the patient, (5) counteract abnormalities (acidosis, hyperkalemia, failing renal output, cardiac arrhythmias), and (6) continue dantrolene postoperatively.

Caution and flexibility in the application of the various treatments are needed, because the extent and severity of an MH crisis may vary considerably from case to case.[226,227] For details regarding the application of any of the recommended treatments, consult the specialized literature.

Prevention of MH means the choice of anesthetic procedures that will not produce an MH attack in MHS subjects. The MH-triggering drugs[228] include all halogenated volatile anesthetics; halothane is a more potent trigger than are enflurane or isoflurane. The triggering effect of succinylcholine has been described above; it is probably due to its depolarizing action, and it is the only depolarizing relaxant in common use. These drugs are sufficiently valuable for most patients that they cannot be simply discarded for the sake of the rare cases of MH.

Nitrous oxide, barbiturates, benzodiazepines, opiates, or opioids like fentanyl, sulfanilamide, or alfentanil, and droperidol do not trigger MH.[228] Jantzen and Kleemann[227] have specialized in providing anesthesia to MHS patients. They also register nondepolarizing muscle relaxants and all local anesthetics as nontriggers, although they are aware of some contradictory reports.

The provision of surgical anesthesia to MHS subjects calls for many considerations[229] besides the simple choice of nontriggering agents — for example, whether or not to give dantrolene prophylactically, how deeply to anesthetize, or choices affecting the use of incidental drugs.

VARIATION OF BUTYRYLCHOLINESTERASE

Nomenclature and History

The cholinesterase in plasma (EC 3.1.1.8: acylcholine acylhydrolase) was originally called pseudocholinesterase[230] and is often referred to as plasma cholinesterase or more recently and formally as *butyrylcholinesterase* (BChE), in distinction from acetylcholinesterase and because it hydrolyzes butyrylcholine more readily than it does acetylcholine. The abbreviation for the protein is BChE, for the gene *BCHE*.[231]

The discovery in the 1950s of genetic variants of plasma cholinesterase was one of the events that initiated the development of pharmacogenetics.[1] Preceding were the discoveries of the

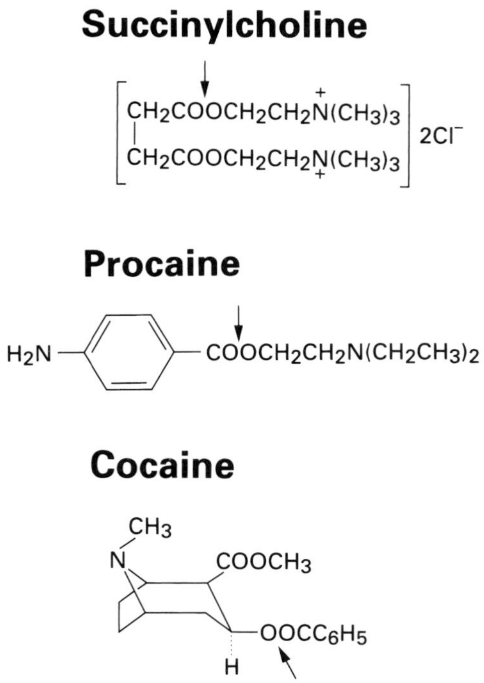

Succinylcholine

$$\left[\begin{array}{l} CH_2COOCH_2CH_2\overset{+}{N}(CH_3)_3 \\ | \\ CH_2COOCH_2CH_2\underset{+}{N}(CH_3)_3 \end{array}\right] 2Cl^-$$

Procaine

$H_2N-C_6H_4-COOCH_2CH_2N(CH_2CH_3)_2$

Cocaine

CH_3, N, $COOCH_3$, $OOCC_6H_5$, H

Fig. 9-5 Structures of some prominent substrates of butyrylcholinesterase (BChE). The *arrows* indicate the ester bonds hydrolyzed by BChE. The succinylmonocholine formed as the initial product by BChE is virtually inactive; it is subject to slow hydrolysis by BChE.

muscle-relaxant properties of succinylcholine (also referred to as suxamethonium)[232] and of its brief duration of action due to rapid hydrolysis by plasma cholinesterase.[232,233] Studies of procaine toxicity revealed that procaine was hydrolyzed by cholinesterase.[234,235] These studies led to the development of a then radically new method for measuring cholinesterase activity.[236] It was this method and its extensions that enabled the identification of cholinesterase variants in homozygotes and heterozygotes.[237–239] This knowledge provided the means to avoid fatalities and permitted the safe use of succinylcholine in spite of esterase deficiencies.

Over time, the subsequent investigations amalgamated aspects of molecular biology, enzymology, drug metabolism, pharmacokinetics, anesthesia, and population genetics, rendering the BChE variations and their consequences a particularly clear example of pharmacogenetics. The variants are still important for the fate of succinylcholine, and for cocaine among other ester-type drugs (Fig. 9-5). The book by Whittaker[240] contains much biochemical and clinical information that cannot be covered here. The review by Lockridge[241] provides broad and balanced information with special emphasis on enzymology and genetics of BChE and some related enzymes.

Occurrence and Nature of Butyrylcholinesterase

In humans as in several other mammalian species, BChE is an enzyme that occurs in plasma and in most tissues, including liver and brain.[242–244] Its active center contains a catalytic site with a serine molecule and an anionic site,[241] making it particularly suitable for cationic substrates. The physiological function of BChE is unknown.

BChE is a tetramer consisting of four identical monomeric subunits with one active center per subunit. Each subunit has 574 amino acids and has a molecular weight of 85,544, including nine carbohydrate chains.[245] The serine molecule of the active center is in position 198.[243,246] The sequence around the active site serine is Phe-Gly-Glu-Ser-Ala-Gly-Ala, and this was present in all mammalian species tested, as was aspartate 70 as a component of the anionic site.[247] BChE is determined by one copy of a single gene containing four exons.[248] It is located on chromosome 3 at q26.1-26.2.[249,250] The linkage group includes the genes for transferrin, BChE, ceruloplasmin, and α-2HS glycoprotein.[241]

Table 9-3 Some Causes of Decreased Plasma Cholinesterase Activity

Type	Condition
Inherited	Rare cholinesterase variants
Physiological	Pregnancy Puerperium Newborns and infants
Acquired	Liver diseases (acute hepatitis) Collagen diseases Acute infection Carcinoma Chronic debilitating diseases Malnutrition Burn injury Kidney dialysis Myxedema
Iatrogenic	Monoamine oxidase inhibitors Ecothiopate iodide Neostigmine Organophosphate insecticides Plasmapheresis Cyclophosphamide

SOURCE: Adapted from Whittaker.[240] Used by permission.

A second gene[251] that explains the occurrence of the so-called C5+ variant[252] is not a cholinesterase gene[241] but that of another protein that occurs in some people and is capable of binding BChE. The C5+ variant appears to be clinically unimportant and will not be dealt with in this review. Different genes control the formation of BChE and of acetylcholinesterase.[253–255]

Independent of the genetic control of its structure, the cholinesterase concentration in plasma is subject to variation[256–258] (Table 9-3). Females of reproductive age have somewhat lower levels of cholinesterase activity than do males; pregnancy may reduce the level by as much as one-third or even one-half. There are nutritional effects: values tend to be high in obese subjects and drop substantially with poor nutrition. In cases of malnutrition, shrinkage of the blood volume may reduce the amount of enzyme in the blood much more drastically than the lowering of enzyme concentration would suggest.[235]

Listings of pathologic or toxicologic causes of reduced BChE activity can be found in several reviews[240,241,259] and are summarized in Table 9-3. The enzyme is produced in the liver, and the level is therefore subject to disturbances of liver function. Indeed, cholinesterase synthesis seems to be a good indicator of the capacity for protein synthesis, which may be disturbed also in malignancies. In patients with severe burn injuries, BChE activity is always low. Furthermore, the enzyme may be inhibited, for example by bambuterol (see below), by organophosphates used as insecticides,[260] or by eyedrops used in glaucoma therapy.[261]

Pharmacogenetics of Butyrylcholinesterase Variants

Diagnostic and clinical aspects of the cholinesterase variants have been studied for many years in specialized research units established in England by Whittaker and Berry[262] and in Denmark by Viby-Mogensen and Hanel.[263] La Du et al[231] in Michigan, Lockridge[241] in Nebraska, and Soreq and Gnatt[253] in Israel have used the techniques of molecular biology to identify the structural changes that characterize the different genetic variants of cholinesterase. Table 9-4 is based on compilations of Lock-

Table 9-4 Nomenclature for Homozygous Forms of Human Butyrylcholinesterase (BChE) Variants*

Common Name	Phenotypic Description	DNA and AA Alterations	Formal Name for Genotype	Frequency of Homozygotes†	References
Usual	Normal	None	BCHE	96:100	240, 241
Atypical‡	Dibucaine resistant	209 (GAT to CGT) 70 Asp-Gly	BCH*70G	1:3500	239, 331, 332, 333
Silent 1§	No activity	351 (GGG to GGAG) 117 Gly-Frameshift	BCHE*FS117	1:100,000	334, 335
Silent 8*	Trace activity	1411 (TGG-CGG) 471 Trp-Arg	BCHE*471R		
Fluoride 1	Fluoride resistant	728 (ACG to ATG) 243 Thr-Met	BCHE*243M	1:150,000	284, 336
Fluoride 2	Fluoride resistant	1169 (CGT to GTT) 390 Gly-Val	BCHE*390V		337
K variant‡	66% Activity	1615 (GCA to ACA) 539 Ala-Thr	BCHE*539T	1:100	271, 337, 272
J variant‡	33% Activity	1490 (GAA to GTA) 497 Glu-Val	BCHE*497V	1:150,000	338, 273, 339

*Compiled with information from La Du et al,[231] Lockridge,[241] and Bartels et al.[273] Additional very rare variants are not listed. BChE is determined by one copy of a single gene containing four exons.[247] It is located on chromosome 3 at q26.1-26.2.

†Approximate frequencies in Caucasian populations.

‡The change that characterizes the K variant was also present in all investigated J variants and in 90 percent of atypical variants (*linkage disequilibrium*).

§Primo-Parmo et al.[264] have defined most of the 17 known silent alleles. The frequency quotation refers to the series and not only to Silent 1.

ridge,[241] supplemented with two data as examples of the 17 mutations leading to "silent cholinesterase."[264] The table omits a number of very rare variants that have been seen in only a few isolated families. Two of these variants are enzymes with somewhat greater than normal catalytic activity: the Cynthiana[265–267] and the Johannesburg[268] variants. Reduced activity is seen in the Newfoundland variant[269] and the H variant.[270] These unlisted rare variants and the listed J variant (Table 9-4) are not discussed further in this chapter.

Clinical Classification. It should be sufficient in this section to refer to the allelic forms of cholinesterase, which are known by common names as the usual cholinesterase, the K variant, and the silent, atypical, and fluoride-resistant variants; these may be designated by the letters U, K, S, A, and F, respectively. In this abbreviation system, the atypical variant may be subdivided to be designated either as A if there is one amino acid change ($Asp^{70}Gly$) or as AK if there are two amino acid changes ($Asp^{70}Gly$ as in A and $Ala^{539}Thr$ as in K). The gene is autosomal so that there are six homozygotes (UU, KK, SS, AA, AK/AK, and FF) and 15 heterozygotes and compound heterozygotes (UK, US, UA, U/AK, UF, KS, KA, K/AK, KF, SA, S/AK, SF, A/AK, AF, and F/AK). Because of rarity (Table 9-4), not all of these 21 genotypes have been actually encountered, but enough is known to allow their classification for clinical purposes.

The UU genotype has only the normal ("usual") form of cholinesterase with all its characteristic catalytic capabilities. The U variant is the standard of comparison. The genotypes UU, UK, KK, and UF represent phenotypes that are functionally not distinguishable from each other because there is considerable interindividual variability of enzyme activity within any population with the same genotype.

The K variant was discovered as an allozyme that binds substrates with the same affinity as does the usual BChE but has about 30 percent lower activity.[271,272] The amino acid alteration ($Ala^{439}Thr$) characterizing the K variant is also present in most A and J variants and similarly reduces activity without changing affinities.[273] The K variant is by far the most frequent mutation of BChE. Its allele frequency in Caucasians is approximately 9 percent[274] and, in Japanese, 17.5 percent.[275]

The S variants have virtually no cholinesterase activity. There are two biochemically and immunologically distinguishable classes of S variants:[276,277] those with inactive (or trace activity) enzyme protein, and those characterized by an absence of the protein. Primo-Parma et al[264] have listed most of the mutations associated with S variants.

The maximal reaction velocities (or the turnover numbers) are alike for the pure A and U variants but are reduced by about 30 percent for the AK variant. About 90 percent of the atypical cholinesterase genes are AK and only about 10 percent are pure A variants. Atypical phenotypes are the genotypes AA, A/AK, AK/AK, AS, and AK/S.

The atypical variants A and AK have a reduced affinity for all tertiary and quaternary amines because the mutation $Asp^{70}Gly$ weakens the anionic binding site.[278] In AK, there is in addition the V_{max}-reducing $Ala^{539}Thr$ mutation. If the apparent affinity (K_m) of any monocationic substrate is known for the usual enzyme, the affinity for the atypical variant can be calculated.[279,280] For many substances with intermediate affinities, the atypical K_m or K_i exceeds the usual one by an order of magnitude. Succinylcholine as a bisquaternary agent does not follow this rule, since the K_m differs by two orders of magnitude. By contrast, *O*-nitrophenylbutyrate has the same affinity for both variants.[280] Organophosphate inhibitors that do not bind to the anionic site inhibit the usual and atypical variants to the same extent;[279] however, the atypical variants A and AK are not reactivated by 2-aldoxime methiodide (PAM).[281]

The enzyme kinetics of the two F variants are the least understood of the variants investigated. Both variants are rare, but F-2 is the more frequent one. *In vitro* comparisons between U and F variants have always been difficult, since comparative properties depend on the buffer used.[282] Kinetic studies with recombinant F-2 conclusively demonstrated nonlinear enzyme kinetics. Inhibition studies suggested a sixfold reduction of the usual affinity of the F-2 variant for succinylcholine, but only when succinylcholine was present at low concentrations.[283] This observation explains the clinical experiences of prolonged succinylcholine action in the presence of fluoride-resistant BChE.

In heterozygotes, the characteristics of BChE activity are generally close to that of the sum of the contributing variants. Slight deviations can occur because most BChE tetramers will consist of a mixture of two variants whose actions may not be entirely independent of each other. Dominant negative phenotypes do not seem to exist. Moderately prolonged effects of succinylcholine may be expected from the heterozygotes AF, AK/F, SF, and perhaps KF and AK/K. The activity reduction in UA, UK, and

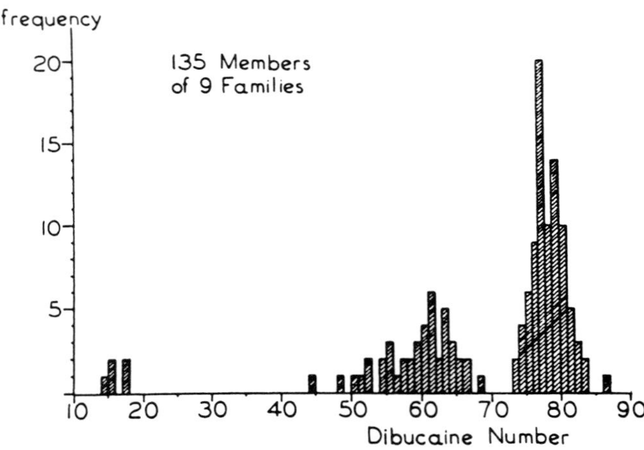

Fig. 9-6 Frequency distribution of dibucaine numbers in families ascertained through persons with low or intermediate dibucaine numbers. (*From Kalow and Staron.*[239] *Used by permission.*)

U/AK is usually not clinically important but may be so under some circumstances (see below in discussions of succinylcholine and cocaine).

Screening Tests and Allele Frequencies. In principle, the variants with altered affinity, i.e., the atypical and fluoride-resistant cholinesterase types, can be recognized by measuring the Michaelis constants (K_m) for suitable substrates. In practice, this has proven difficult when attempting to sort out the heterozygotes. However, it turned out that all the affinity differences could be easily recognized by using enzyme inhibitors.[238] Inhibitors useful for that purpose were the amide-type local anesthetic dibucaine[238] (Fig. 9-6) and the salt sodium fluoride.[284] When these were used for cholinesterase phenotyping under standardized conditions, the percentage inhibition was referred to as *dibucaine number* or *fluoride number*. These index numbers, plus the more recently introduced *RO2-0683 number* are still being used for phenotypic classification of the BChE variants.[273] RO2-0683 is the dimethylcarbamate of (2-hydroxy-5-phenylbenzyl)trimethylammonium bromide and a selective inhibitor of BChE of exceptional potency.[279]

Dibucaine numbers have been tested in more than 100,000 people. Since they enable the detection of heterozygotes (see Fig. 9-6), they have formed the basis for estimates of gene frequency in many populations.[240] One may briefly summarize[38] some of the extensive investigations by stating that the gene frequency for the atypical variant is greatest in Caucasians (0.0170), much less in Africans (0.0046), and very rare in Orientals (0.0002). By contrast, the fluoride-resistant variants have the highest frequency in Africa (0.0135). There are population pockets with high frequency of any of the classic variants. As stated previously, the K variant has double the frequency in Japan than in Europe.

Substrates of Butyrylcholinesterase

Substrates selected to be of either diagnostic or potentially clinical interest are listed in Table 9-5.

Succinylcholine. The medical value of succinylcholine is its ability to eliminate any undesirable contraction of skeletal muscle for a short time, thereby allowing physicians to perform brief, vital manipulations of patients.[223] Its main use is at the beginning of anesthesia for major surgery, when it greatly facilitates cannulation of the patient's airway. Another use is during electroconvulsive therapy for drug-resistant mental disease, when succinylcholine prevents muscle stimulation by the electric current. No drug other than succinylcholine combines as rapid an onset with a normally short duration of action.

Succinylcholine is a powerful muscle relaxant; to ensure its rapid onset of action, it is normally given as a bolus injection intravenously. Thereby, the onset of action is on the order of a circulation time, that is, about 45 s. From the moment the drug enters the bloodstream to the time of its exit from the blood toward its target — the neuromuscular end plate — the drug is exposed to attack by the BChE in plasma. With usual cholinesterase type and average activity, most of the injected drug molecules are destroyed before they can reach the end plate. Termination of action appears to be a physicochemical process, probably simply a dispersal of the drug molecules by diffusion away from the end-plate region so that the succinylcholine concentration becomes low enough for the end-plate to resume function.

Table 9-5 K_m Values and Turnover Numbers for Substrates of Usual and Atypical Butyrylcholinesterase

	K_m (mM)			
	Usual	**Atypical**	**Turnover Number**	**Reference**
Positively charged				
Acetylcholine	1.4	9.0	33,200	340
Butyrylcholine	0.91	1.7	80,000	340
Benzoylcholine	0.004	0.022	15,000	340
Succinyldithiocholine	0.035	1.08	600	341
Succinylcholine	0.1	40	300	342
Procaine	0.0066	0.10	255	343
Tetracaine	0.00014	0.008	74	343
Meprylcaine	—	—	2750	344
Cocaine	0.044	0.4*	0.4	292
Heroin	0.11	0.45	500	345
Aspirin $CaCl_2$	4.2	16	7200	343
Methylprednisolone acetate	1.0	—	25	315
Mivacurium	—	—	—	316

*Estimated value.

NOTE: Most of the contents of this table consist of information condensed from Lockridge.[241]

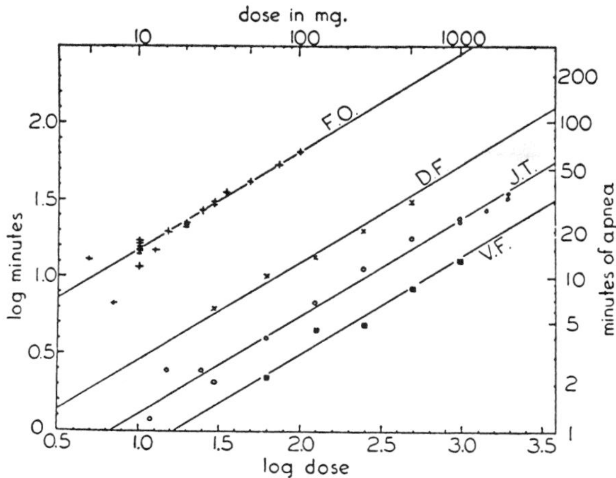

Fig. 9-7 Relation between dose of succinylcholine chloride and duration of apnea in four representative patients. Subject F.O. represents atypical BChE, D.F. represents genotype UF, and J.T. and V.F. represent lowest and highest BChE activity, respectively, of healthy subjects with the UU genotype. (*From Kalow and Gunn.*[285] *Used by permission.*)

If cholinesterase activity is low or absent, the proportion of drug molecules reaching the end plate increases, and the dispersal of the excess takes time: the greater the excess of succinylcholine molecules in the end-plate region, the longer the time. This mode of action is indicated by plotting on logarithmic scales the dose of succinylcholine versus duration of effect:[285] esterase activity determines the intercept but not the slope of individual curves (Fig. 9-7). In Fig. 9-7, the duration of succinylcholine action was registered as time of apnea, that is, the duration of paralysis of the respiratory muscles. The modern method of assessing the paralyzing action (*phase-I* or *phase-II block*) uses electrical stimuli as for example the *train of four* stimulus of the ulnar nerve while the local muscle response is being recorded.[286]

Comparing phenotypes of usual and atypical variants, the K_m of the latter for succinylcholine is larger by about two orders of magnitude.[4,241,279] At the point of injection, the succinylcholine concentration reaches or approaches its K_m value with the usual form of cholinesterase, so hydrolysis can proceed rapidly, but its concentration is too low to combine with the atypical variant, so it cannot be hydrolyzed. The genotypes AA, AK/AK, A/AK, SS, S/AK, and AS are virtually unable to hydrolyze succinylcholine; their combined frequency is approximately 1 in 3000 in the Caucasian population (Table 9-4). The difference between the biochemical mechanisms that cause these functional failures is clinically immaterial.

Kalow and Gunn[285] and Viby-Mogensen[287,288] tried to determine the extent to which quantitative alterations of enzyme activity (Table 9-3) affect the fate of succinylcholine. An approximate answer can be given by a rule of thumb: the duration of action of succinylcholine is inversely proportional to the remaining enzyme activity. For instance,[285] an intravenous dose of 100 mg of succinylcholine injected over a 30-s period into a subject with average cholinesterase activity caused apnea for about 3 min. In a subject with only half the average enzyme activity, the duration of apnea would average about 6 min—double the normal time but a clinically insignificant prolongation of the paralysis. By this rule, it takes a reduction to 5 percent of normal enzyme activity for succinylcholine to cause paralysis for about 1 h. A reduction in the usual cholinesterase activity to such low levels is possible through enzyme inhibition but not through physiological or pathologic modifiers of enzyme concentration. In other words, for the fate of succinylcholine, the occurrence of genetic determinants of cholinesterase activity is more important than are most functional alterations of enzyme activity.

For the sake of clinical perspective, one has to keep in mind that the homozygous presence of atypical BChE always leads to prolonged effects of succinylcholine, but that only about two-thirds of cases with a prolonged effect can be explained by a definable BChE failure.[289] A variety of factors associated with anesthesia (e.g., anesthetic dose) may affect the behavior of succinylcholine,[285] thereby simulating the impact of a BChE variant. However, unexplained gross prolongations occur more frequently in UA than in UU genotypes.[288]

The first-pass metabolism of a drug is usually thought of as an event that takes place in the liver, but the prolongation of the effects of succinylcholine in the presence of esterase variants represents a failure of the normal first-pass metabolism of this drug in plasma. It needs to be emphasized that this prolongation of drug action is a function of its administration by intravenous injection.

What should anesthetists do to prevent or overcome trouble with succinylcholine when BChE activity fails? The safest action is simply to make sure that the paralyzed patient gets proper artificial ventilation until the paralysis disappears. Only if a phase-II block can be diagnosed through electrophysiological testing may treatment with neostigmine be initiated.[223] In the 1950s, fatalities from succinylcholine in the presence of atypical BChE were due to desperate but misguided attempts by frightened physicians to resuscitate patients, whereas increased knowledge saved lives.

Procaine and Congeners. Procaine may be considered a prototype of a series of local anesthetics that are substrates of plasma cholinesterase (see Fig. 9-5). It has a K_m of 7 mM with the usual cholinesterase and of 100 mM with the atypical variant. Its normal rate of hydrolysis is similar to that of succinylcholine, but the rate will be slowed in the presence of any of the BChE variants that hydrolyze succinylcholine with a reduced V_{max}. Thus, there are distinct differences between the variants' capacities to hydrolyze procaine.

It is not surprising to see a description of a metabolically caused prolongation of an epidural block with 2-chloroprocaine,[290] a drug normally hydrolyzed very rapidly. However, there are few convincing cases of toxicity of procaine, chloroprocaine, or related drugs due to cholinesterase variants.[291] Usually, the duration of action of local anesthetics like procaine is not determined by metabolic degradation but by blood flow; to prolong the local action of procaine, one does not add a cholinesterase inhibitor to the injectable procaine solution, but a vasoconstrictor.

Cocaine. Cocaine is hydrolyzed by human plasma cholinesterase to form methylecgonine.[292,293] The apparent affinity of the naturally occurring (−)-cocaine with the usual enzyme averaged $K_m = 44$ mM;[292] when measured via inhibition, the K_i was 7.6 to 9 mM.[294] The hydrolysis rate is very slow in comparison with that of many other substrates: its turnover number of 0.4196 indicates a hydrolysis rate of approximately 1/750 that of succinylcholine. The cocaine kinetics with atypical cholinesterase could not be directly determined but, on general principles,[279] the K_m and K_i values may be assumed to be about tenfold larger with the atypical than with the usual enzyme type. Because of the comparatively slow rate of cocaine hydrolysis by cholinesterase even under normal conditions, this metabolism has been overlooked or disregarded for a long time. Is this justified?

Methylecgonine, the pharmacologically inactive product of BChE activity, accounts for 30 to 50 percent of administered cocaine.[295–297] Cocaine can also be hydrolyzed to methylecgonine by an unidentified esterase in human liver; however, the K_m is somewhat above 1000 mM,[292] so the participation of this liver enzyme is presumably negligible under most circumstances. Between 2 and 6 percent of cocaine is demethylated to the active norcocaine, which is then also hydrolyzed by cholinesterase. Less than 10 percent of cocaine is excreted unchanged in the urine; the rest is nonenzymatically hydrolyzed to benzoylecgonine.[292]

An association between cocaine toxicity and reduced activity of BChE has often been suspected. Some cocaine addicts have prolonged their high by deliberately inhibiting their BChE with organophosphate insecticides.[298] Hoffman et al[299] showed particularly low BChE activity in subjects who had survived life-threatening cocaine toxicity. Thus, even though the cholinesterase-catalyzed metabolism of cocaine is slow compared with that of other BChE substrates, this metabolism appears to be a major determinant of the fate of cocaine in humans.[300]

It therefore has been suggested to use intravenous injection of purified BChE to counteract cocaine toxicity, regardless of the presence or absence of any genetic variant of the enzyme.[301–303] So far, the efficacy and safety of this procedure have been demonstrated only in animals. However, looking into the future, Grunwald et al[304] have described an improved method to purify and concentrate human BChE to be used as a potential bioscavenger drug.

Cocaine is readily absorbed from all surfaces. It is widely used by otolaryngologists and plastic surgeons for topical anesthesia and control of bleeding during nasal surgery.[305,306] The standard concentrations of cocaine for this purpose are between 1 and 4 percent, but dosages above 400 mg are not rare. Nevertheless, 40 percent of the iatrogenic fatalities occurred after a "safe" dose of less than 200 mg of intranasal cocaine; in other words, these were non-dose-dependent toxicities.[305] Cholinesterase activity was not tested.

TAC, a combination of tetracaine 0.5%, adrenaline 0.05%, and cocaine 11.8%, has become a favorite for application to wounds in order to prevent the pain from laceration repair in children.[307] Since both tetracaine and cocaine are substrates of BChE, it needs to be investigated to what extent the two drugs are mutually inhibiting their metabolism and how their fate is affected by BChE deficiency. Fatalities from the use of TAC have been recorded.[307]

Toxicity has been frequently reported in young healthy cocaine users[308,309] who used average street doses. The reported size of dose in recreational use is notoriously unreliable. Even when a single dose is not particularly high, however, frequent repetition of cocaine administration is typical for addicts;[310] if slow metabolism is immaterial when only a single dose is used, slow metabolism plus repeated administration can set the stage for drug cumulation with toxic consequences.

Myocardial infarction after cocaine use[311] is a function of cocaine-induced vasoconstriction.[312] Such vasoconstriction may not be dose dependent in terms of milligrams of cocaine consumed but may be dependent on the plasma concentration of cocaine achieved; this could vary with the speed with which cocaine enters the bloodstream (e.g., as "crack," snorting, or intravenous injection) and with the speed of its metabolism. If cocaine reaches the bloodstream very quickly, analogies with intravenously injected succinylcholine become apparent; in other words, the importance of cholinesterase variation for the fate of cocaine may well vary with the mode of its administration.

As already explained, a 50 percent decrease in BChE activity tends to be clinically unimportant for the fate of succinylcholine. The situation could be different with respect to cocaine: any decrease of BChE activity that prolongs the normal 1-h half-life of cocaine would automatically favor accumulation of cocaine in blood and tissues, particularly if there is repeated cocaine intake, and particularly by methods that favor its rapid absorption. Thus, all genetic[241] and all environmentally produced alterations of the activity of BChE (e.g., liver damage[313]) are potentially able to affect the fate of cocaine.

Other Substrates. Some other prominent drug substrates of cholinesterase are heroin and aspirin.[241] There is no information on altered action of heroin in the presence of esterase variants, although the drug is metabolized at a reduced rate by atypical BChE. The explanation might lie in the fact that there is also metabolism by an erythrocyte enzyme that in whole blood accounts for 50 to 70 percent of heroin hydrolysis.[241]

Low esterase activity has been associated with aspirin sensitivity[314] but without proving that the low activity was that of BChE and not of any other contributing esterase. Further studies seem to be warranted.

Only about 25 percent of the deacetylation (activation) of methylprednisolone acetate is due to cholinesterase.[315] No pharmacogenetic information seems to be available with regard to mivacurium,[316] although they are both metabolized by cholinesterase. Bambuterol[317] is a prodrug that has been developed as a specialized substrate of cholinesterase with a nanomolar K_i[318] to achieve a slow release of the active bronchodilator terbutaline. Bambuterol is not only a substrate but a potent inhibitor of BChE.[317,319,320]

Butyrylcholinesterase and Alzheimer Disease

β-Amyloid may exist in the brain for many years before leading to neuritic degeneration and dementia. Guillozet et al[321] described a role of BChE in the conversion of β-amyloid to plaques in brains with Alzheimer disease. Gomez-Ramos and Moran[322] described the deposition of this enzyme in senile plaques. Lehmann et al[274] described a synergy between the genes for the K variant of BChE and for apolipoprotein E-4, particularly in late-onset Alzheimer cases, but this association could not be confirmed by two other groups of investigators.[323,324] The cholinesterase inhibitor tacrine is used to treat Alzheimer cases on the theory that its inhibition of acetylcholinesterase leads to a beneficial increase in the transmitter substance acetylcholine.[325] In any case, BChE is present in human amygdala and hippocampus, and its distribution differs from that of acetylcholinesterase.[326] Since tacrine also inhibits BChE, one may wonder whether it is inhibition of acetyl- or of butyrylcholinesterase that is responsible for the benefit of those patients with Alzheimer disease who respond to it.[327]

Gulf War Syndrome

Some veterans of the Gulf War, the international war of 1991 against Iraq, complained afterward of often ill-defined conditions designated by investigators as "impaired cognition" or "confusion-ataxia." An agent widely used to protect troops against chemical warfare with cholinesterase inhibitors was pyridostigmine, an antidote to the toxic esterase-inhibiting organophosphates sarin or tabun. As mentioned earlier in this chapter, atypical BChE is inhibited like the normal form by the organophosphates but is not reactivated like normal by the antidotes.[328] It is therefore of interest to learn that an Israeli soldier homozygous for atypical BChE suffered severe symptoms following pyridostigmine exposure.[329] An American statistical account lends support to the idea of adverse effects from pyridostigmine bromide,[330] but there has been no phenotyping or genotyping in search of BChE variants. A contradicting hypothesis states that the Gulf War syndrome may be a consequence of acute stress, which can cause changes affecting acetylcholine function.

POLYMORPHISM OF DEBRISOQUINE HYDROXYLASE (CYTOCHROME P_{450}2D6)

Several features distinguish the pharmacogenetic defect affecting the function of cytochrome P_{450}2D6 (CYP2D6) from the previous two examples: (1) It represents a considerably more recent discovery of a pharmacogenetic entity. (2) It involves a defect in drug oxidation by one of the expressed products of the cytochrome-P_{450} gene superfamily, which is regarded as quantitatively one of the most important enzyme systems in mediating drug biotransformation reactions in general. (3) It affects the function of an enzyme localized predominantly (although not exclusively) to the liver, the organ generally considered to be one of the most important anatomic sites of xenobiotic biotransformation. (4) It is a polymorphism rather than a rare defect and thus affects a significant proportion of the individuals in most populations. (5) The importance of the CYP2D6 polymorphism in clinical practice, drug development, and toxicology is currently an area of intense investigation and considerable controversy. Recent reviews have summarized our current state of knowledge with regard to the clinical, toxicologic, and mechanistic aspects of this intensively studied subject area.[345–349]

Discovery

In retrospect, it is not surprising that it was not until the mid-1970s that the first clear-cut instance of genetically determined variation in drug oxidation by a member of the microsomal cytochrome-P_{450} monooxygenase enzyme system was observed. The cytochrome-P_{450} gene superfamily[350] is now known to encode the expression of a remarkably large number of related membrane-bound hemoproteins that have evolved to possess a broad substrate specificity enabling them to biotransform, at least to some degree, chemicals with widely divergent structures. This combination of P_{450} enzyme multiplicity and substrate promiscuity tends to ensure that not only are most substrates unlikely to escape some form of oxidative biotransformation (not to mention unrelated reactions that also have the ultimate goal of increasing hydrophilicity), but that most substrates will also be acted on by several competing or cooperating enzymes either at the same time or sequentially to produce multiple products. Thus, the metabolic fate of a typical xenobiotic substrate tends to be governed by the action of multiple gene products, making the detection of defects in single enzymes less likely.

Nonetheless, notable exceptions to the foregoing generalizations concerning substrates for oxidative biotransformation led two groups in the mid-1970s to the separate discoveries of a genetic polymorphism that was ultimately shown to affect a specific isozyme of cytochrome P_{450}, which is now designated CYP2D6. During studies by British investigators into the pharmacokinetics of the sympatholytic antihypertensive agent debrisoquine, a marked and prolonged postural hypotensive episode experienced by one of the primary investigators prompted a series of detailed investigations into the metabolic fate of this agent.[7] It soon became apparent that the side effects were dose related, and resulted from an inability of the patient to eliminate debrisoquine efficiently via conversion to its inactive 4-hydroxylated metabolite.[351,352] Family studies[353] and further population screens verified the genetic nature of this defect and established its polymorphic nature—approximately 5 to 10 percent of the individuals in healthy Caucasian populations are distinguishable as phenotypically *poor metabolizers* (PMs) based on the molar ratio of unchanged debrisoquine to 4-hydroxydebrisoquine detected in pooled urine samples collected following drug administration (Fig. 9-8A).

At the same time, independent investigations into variations in response to the antiarrhythmic and oxytocic alkaloid sparteine produced the observation that a similar proportion of a healthy German population sample was unable to convert sparteine enzymatically to its 2- and 5-dehydrosparteine metabolites[6] (Fig. 9-8B). Subsequent correlation studies demonstrated that the defective biotransformations of debrisoquine and sparteine were under identical genetic control[354–356] (Fig. 9-8C) and further substantiated the observation that the PM phenotype appeared to display an autosomal recessive inheritance pattern.

Occurrence and Prevalence of Defective Debrisoquine Oxidation Tests for Determining Metabolizer Phenotype. As already noted, numerous in vivo studies using probe drugs that are affected by the genetic defect (see below) have established the polymorphic nature of defective debrisoquine oxidation in several human populations. The two tests that were originally applied for this purpose involved the administration of either debrisoquine or sparteine, collection of urine for a defined interval following drug intake, and calculation of the ratio of unchanged drug to its oxidized metabolite(s) measured in urine by gas chromatography or high-performance liquid chromatography. This urinary *metabolic ratio* (MR), when plotted in the form of a frequency histogram or a probit transformation, yielded a distinctly bimodal distribution from which antimodes separating the *extensive metabolizer* (EM) and PM phenotypes could be defined (see Fig. 9-8). However, considering that the debrisoquine and sparteine polymorphisms were first discovered by the observation

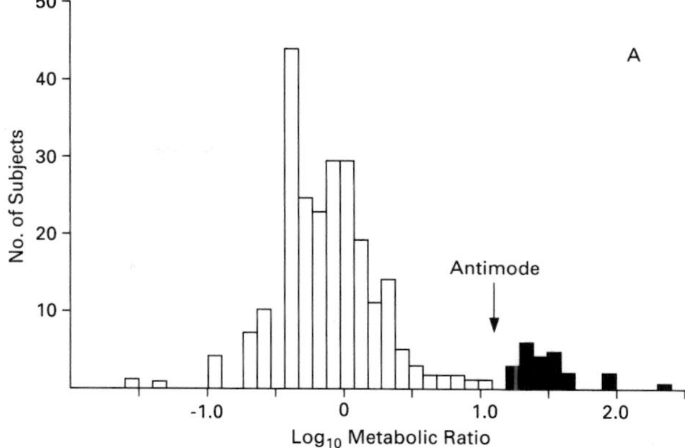

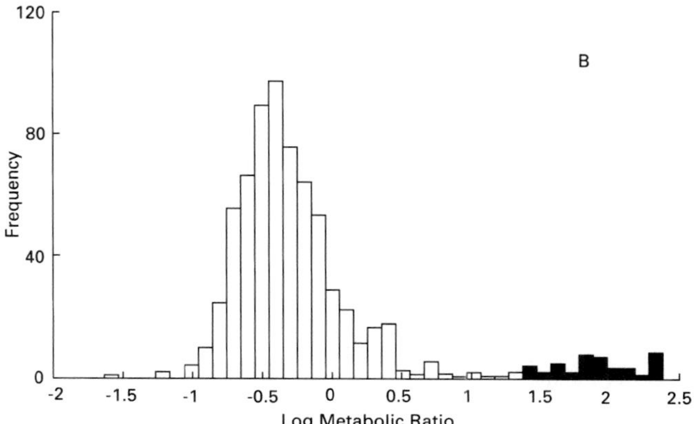

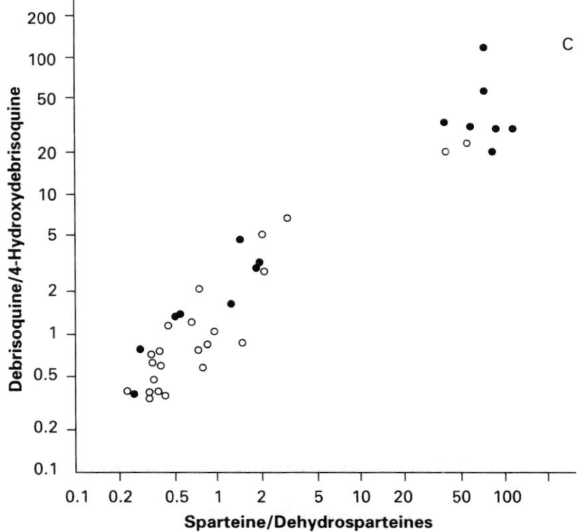

Fig. 9-8 ***A*: Population frequency histogram of urinary debrisoquine/4-hydroxydebrisoquine ratios after debrisoquine administration to 258 individuals in a healthy British population. (*From Evans et al.*[353] *Used by permission.*) *B*: Population frequency histogram of sparteine/dehydrosparteine ratios after sparteine administration to 735 individuals in a healthy German population. (*From Eichelbaum et al.*[478] *Used by permission.*) *C*: Cosegregation of debrisoquine and sparteine metabolic ratios in a Canadian population. (*From Inaba et al.*[356] *Used by permission.*)**

of adverse drug effects in individuals now known to be of the PM phenotype, such tests for screening healthy populations carried a finite risk of imparting such adverse reactions. Phenotyping with dextromethorphan[357] has largely supplanted tests using debrisoquine or sparteine as in vivo probes, since it is a relatively innocuous antitussive agent commonly used in over-the-counter cough remedies. More recently, advances in the elucidation of the molecular genetic mechanisms underlying the polymorphism have led to the promotion of molecular tests for mutant alleles at the CYP2D6 gene locus as alternatives to the use of probe drugs. The advantages and limitations of each of these approaches are discussed in the sections "Genotyping Tests for Mutant Alleles" and "Genotyping Versus Phenotyping Tests."

Interethnic Differences in Poor Metabolizer Phenotype Frequencies. There is considerable variation in the incidence of the PM phenotype between populations of different ethnic origins.[348,358] Populations of European origin, from which the bulk of the available data have been obtained, display PM phenotype frequencies ranging from 3 to 10 percent, with an overall mean of about 7.5 percent. However, it should be appreciated that the accuracy of reported frequency estimates in single population samples is often limited by small sample sizes and heterogeneity in the ethnic origin of recruited population samples. Nonetheless, it appears clear that certain non-Caucasian groups possess PM phenotype frequencies that are markedly different from those observed in Caucasians: The Cuna Amerindians of Panama, for example, represent one group in which the PM phenotype has not been detected,[359] whereas almost 20 percent of San Bushmen are PMs.[360] On the other hand, studies in Nigerians[361] have provided evidence for nonconcordance in the metabolism of probe drugs that are equally effective markers of the PM phenotype in Caucasian populations. It has also been observed in phenotyping studies that Chinese populations possess metabolic ratios that are generally shifted toward lower apparent CYP2D6 activities than those observed in Caucasians.[358] In combination with genotype analysis studies, it is now evident that such observations may result from the existence of particular variant alleles that are more prevalent among certain ethnic groups (see the section "Characterization of Mutant Alleles of Cytochrome P_{450}2D6"). It is therefore important to exercise caution in the extrapolation of conclusions from pharmacogenetic studies in one race to others that may exhibit both quantitatively and qualitatively distinct metabolic capabilities.

Table 9-6 Drugs Whose Metabolism is Affected by the Debrisoquine Oxidation (CYP2D6) Defect

Antiarrhythmics	**Other drugs**
Aprindine	Carvedilol
Encainide	Cinnarizine
Flecainide	Codeine
Mexiletine	Debrisoquine
N-Propylajmaline	Dexfenfluramine
Procainamide	Dextromethorphan
Propafenone	Dihydrocodeine
Sparteine	Dolasetron
β-Adrenergic receptor blockers	Flunarizine
Alprenolol	Guanoxon
Bufuralol	Hydrocodone
Bunitrolol	Indoramin
Metoprolol	MDMA (ecstasy)
Propranolol	Mequitazine
Timolol	Methoxyamphetamine
Neuroleptics	Methoxyphenamine
Haloperidol	MPTP
Perphenazine	Nicergoline
Risperidone	Perhexiline
Sertindole	Orphenadrine
Thioridazine	Phenformin
Zuclopenthixol	Promethazine
Antidepressants	Tamoxifen
Amiflamine	Tolterodine
Amitriptyline	Tropisetron
Brofaromine	Tramadol
Citalopram	
Clomipramine	
Desipramine	
Fluoxetine	
Ifoxetine	
Imipramine	
Maprotiline	
Mianserin	
Nortriptyline	
Paroxetine	
Selegiline	
Tomoxetine	

Substrates for CYP2D6

In the years since the discovery that debrisoquine and sparteine oxidations are affected by the same genetic defect, evidence for impairment in the biotransformations of more than 60 other therapeutic agents in individuals of the PM phenotype has been presented[362,363] (Table 9-6 and Fig. 9-9). In many cases associations with the debrisoquine oxidation defect have been established, after observing unusual patterns of variability in the disposition or efficacy of a therapeutic agent, through the use of a *typed panel* approach. Thus, the pharmacokinetics or metabolic fate of a suspected polymorphic substrate are tested in a selected group of subjects of known EM and PM phenotypes, and significant correlations are then taken as strong evidence for cosegregation with the defect. In other instances, *in vitro* studies using isozyme-selective substrates, inhibitors, and recombinant expression systems have been used to provide evidence for CYP2D6 involvement. It is important to emphasize that although the biotransformation of a considerable number of xenobiotics is affected by the CYP2D6 polymorphism, biochemical and molecular studies have shown that this is by no means a generalized impairment of drug oxidation; indeed, the metabolic fates of the large majority of foreign chemicals are completely unaffected by the polymorphism. It is also worth noting that deficient metabolism of some drugs (e.g., propranolol) by CYP2D6 is of no pharmacokinetic or clinical importance because of compensatory elimination pathways mediated by independently expressed biotransformation enzymes.

Structure-Activity Predictions. Because of the potential clinical consequences associated with the debrisoquine hydroxylase defect (see the section "Clinical Consequences of Defective Cytochrome P_{450}2D6"), it may be of value in new drug development to predict whether a given chemical is likely to be a substrate for polymorphic oxidation by CYP2D6. Although the structures of affected compounds (see Fig. 9-9) do not at first glance exhibit similarities that would enable such predictions, closer examination reveals several common elements.[364–366] First, all substrates contain one or more basic nitrogen atom, and it appears that CYP2D6 accepts only basic compounds as substrates. Second, independently derived models had earlier proposed that the basic nitrogen atom and the site of oxygen addition are separated by a planar hydrophobic region and that the distance between the two is either 5 or 7 Å. More recent active site predictions have been derived for CYP2D6 that accommodate substrates fitting both the 5-Å and 7-Å models by postulating an interaction of the basic nitrogen with either one of the two oxygen atoms on the carboxylic acid side chain of Asp[301] on the protein. This interaction serves to align the oxidation site on the substrate molecule in close proximity with the catalytic heme moiety. As well, favorable van der Waals and electrostatic interactions between the protein

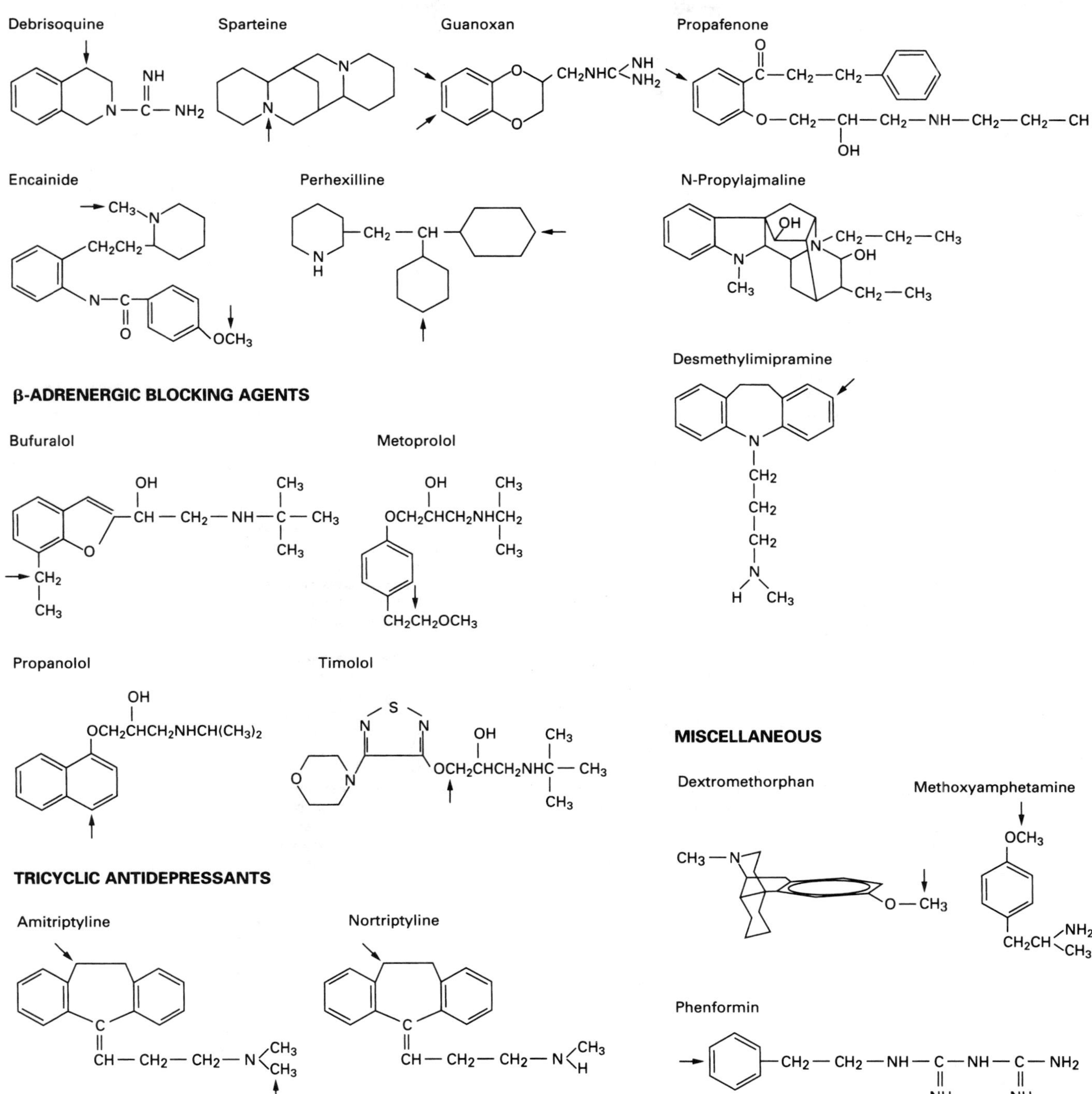

Fig. 9-9 Structures of some chemicals whose biotransformation is affected by the CYP2D6 polymorphism. (*From Meyer et al.*[363] *Used by permission.*)

and oxidation site appear to occur when substrate molecules can assume a planar conformation in this region. This model has been used thus far to predict CYP2D6 involvement in the biotransformations of several previously untested chemicals with a reasonable degree of accuracy. Further studies using a combination of site-directed mutagenesis and computer modeling have identified additional structural and functional features of the CYP2D6-active site region.[367–370] Refinement of such active site models may prove helpful in rational drug design, although it should be mentioned that evidence for polymorphic biotransformation by CYP2D6 is not in and of itself grounds for avoiding development of drugs, especially those with great therapeutic potential. Rather, such knowledge could serve equally well as a starting point for guiding the appropriate design of phase-I and phase-II clinical trials.[362]

Molecular Mechanism of the Cytochrome-P_{450}2D6 Defect Biochemical Studies. *In vitro* studies of the biotransformations of debrisoquine,[371] sparteine,[372] and bufuralol[373] by human liver microsomes had established early on that the genetic defect was related to functional alterations in the catalytic activity of a specific isozyme of P_{450}. It remained to be determined which of the multiple P_{450} species was affected and whether such alterations were the result of quantitative or qualitative differences in the enzyme protein in human liver. Kinetic analyses of microsomal debrisoquine and bufuralol oxidations indicated the presence of at least two contributing catalytic activities, one of which (a high-affinity, stereoselective enzyme) was deficient in livers from individuals with the PM phenotype.[374,375] Ultimately, the use of highly sensitive and specific assays allowed for the purification of sufficient quantities of the affected P_{450} isozyme, now designated as CYP2D6, to allow partial protein sequence information to be obtained.[376] At the same time, it was observed that a polyclonal antiserum directed against a rat orthologue of human CYP2D6 specifically cross-reacted with the human enzyme, enabling it to be used both for immunoquantitation of CYP2D6 in human liver microsomes[377] and for expression cloning of a full-length human CYP2D6 cDNA.[376] The immunoquantitation studies in human liver microsomes showed that the PM phenotype is in most instances characterized at the protein level by a specific absence of CYP2D6 enzyme rather than a functional difference in an expressed enzyme.[378] More recently, however, variant alleles at the CYP2D gene locus have been isolated (see the section "Characterization of Mutant Alleles of Cytochrome P_{450}2D6") that encode the synthesis of forms of CYP2D6 that may produce the PM phenotype as a result of single amino acid changes that impair the function rather than the expression of CYP2D6 by a variety of possible mechanisms.[348]

Cloning of *CYP2D* Genes. As previously mentioned, a polyclonal antiserum directed against a rat orthologue of *CYP2D6* was used to isolate a full-length human *CYP2D6* cDNA clone. Somatic cell hybrid analysis using the cDNA probe established the location of the gene encoding *CYP2D6* to human chromosome 22q13.1,[376,379] in agreement with the results of linkage studies in families of PM individuals.[380] The cDNA probe was also used in Southern blot hybridizations of human genomic DNA, most notably those generated by digestion with the endonuclease *Xba*I, to detect restriction fragment length polymorphisms (RFLPs) that were associated with the PM phenotype.[381] However, such analyses are not highly predictive of phenotype, since one-half of the mutant alleles in PMs display an *Xba*I RFLP pattern identical to that seen in EMs.

Subsequent genomic cloning and sequencing studies using DNA isolated from EM and PM individuals have yielded a wealth of information concerning the structure, organization, and interindividual variation in what is now known to be a cluster of *CYP2D* genes residing on a contiguous region of chromosome 22.[382,383] The *CYP2D* gene cluster on a given allelic DNA fragment (excluding those in ultrarapid metabolizers; see below) may contain between two and four genes, each possessing nine exons and eight introns. However, since three of the possible genes (*CYP2D7P*, *CYP2D7P′*, and *CYP2D8P*) are considered to be nonexpressed pseudogenes,[384] mutations affecting the functional *CYP2D6* gene ultimately determine the expression of the debrisoquine metabolizer phenotype.

Characterization of Mutant Alleles of Cytochrome P_{450}2D6. To date, a total of at least 64 different allelic variants have been detected at the *CYP2D* gene cluster in human populations,[385] of which 26 have so far been characterized in any detail with respect to their functional consequences (Table 9-7).[348,386] Of this large number of variant alleles, most are rare, and almost half have been observed only once in

Table 9-7 Variant Alleles at the CYP2D6 Gene Locus

Allel	Trivial Name	Effect on Gene	Effect on Protein	Activity	Freq*
Functional alleles					
*1A	Wild type			Normal	34
*1B		1 Point mutation	None	Normal	
*2A	2D6-L	2 Point mutations	2 Amino acid changes	Normal	28
*2B		3 Point mutations	3 Amino acid changes	Normal	5
*2×N		Gene duplication	Increased production	Increased	
Defective alleles†					
*3	2D6-A	1 Base deletion	Truncation	None	1
*4A	2D6-B				
*4B	2D6-B′	Splice site mutation	Truncation	None	20
*4C	K-29-1				
*4D					
*5	2D6-D	Gene deleted	No protein	None	5
*6A	2D6-T	1 Base deletion	Truncation	None	1.5
*6B					
*7	2D6-E	1 Point mutation	1 Amino acid change	None	<1
*8	2D6-G	1 Point mutation	Truncation	None	<1
*9	2D6-C	3 Base deletion	1 Amino acid deletion	Decreased	2
*10A	2D6-J				
*10B	2D6-Ch1	1 Point mutation	1 Amino acid change	Decreased	3
*10C	2D6-Ch2				
*11	2D6-F	Splice the mutation	Truncation	None	<1
*12		1 Point mutation	1 Amino acid change	None	<1
*13		2D6/2D7 hybrid gene	Truncation	None	<1
*14		1 Point mutation	1 Amino acid change	None	<1
*15		1 Base insertion	Truncation	None	<1
*16	2D6-D2	2D6/2D7 hybrid gene	Truncation	None	<1
*17	2D6-Z	2 Point mutations	2 Amino acid change	Decreased	<1

*Allele frequencies are from Meyer and Zarger,[348] and are estimated for Caucasian populations only.
†For defective alleles, only the gene and protein alterations directly related to functional consequences are listed.
SOURCE: Adapted from Meyer and Zarger[348] and Daly et al.[386]

population-screening studies. The four most frequently occurring mutant alleles are *CYP2D6*4* (formerly the 2D6-B variant), *CYP2D6*5* (formerly 2D6-D), *CYP2D6*6* (formerly 2D6-T), and *CYP2D6*3* (formerly 2D6-A), which together account for about 90 percent of all mutant alleles in Caucasian PMs. The *CYP2D6*4* allele produces the PM phenotype due to a single point mutation in a consensus splice site in intron 3, which shifts splicing by one base, produces an mRNA with a premature stop codon, and leads to a complete absence of functional CYP2D6 protein expression.[387,388] In contrast, *CYP2D6*5* also results in a complete abolition of protein expression, but this is due to deletion of a large fragment of genomic DNA, including the entire CYP2D6 coding region.[389] The *CYP2D6*6* and *CYP2D6*3* variants produce the same lack of functional protein due to single base deletions within exon sequences that lead to premature translation termination.

Other more rare variant alleles with distinctive functional consequences have also been observed. For example, *CYP2D6*7* possesses a single amino acid change, His^{324}Pro, which results in a catalytically inactive enzyme probably due to its inability to incorporate heme properly.[390] *CYP2D6*18* contains a nine-base insertion that produces a protein with reduced affinity for bufuralol.[391] *CYP2D6*9* (formerly 2D6-C) has a three-base deletion that leads to loss of Lys^{281} (see reference 392) and association with an "intermediate" metabolic ratio,[393] even though the activity of the recombinant expressed product of this allele is functionally normal. Another variant that associates with a partially impaired level of enzyme function is *CYP2D6*10* (formerly 2D6-Ch1/2 or 2D6-J), which has a Pro^{34}Ser mutation that abolishes activity in recombinant expression systems[388] but correlates with an EM phenotype *in vivo*. This variant is much more frequent in Oriental than in Caucasian populations, and is thought to be partly responsible for the general shift in metabolic ratios in Orientals toward lower CYP2D6 activity. The *CYP2D6*17* variant contains three amino acid substitutions. Two of these are required to produce impaired enzyme function for the oxidation of bufuralol, whereas only one is sufficient to impair codeine metabolism.[394]

In contrast, recent reports have indicated that there exist individuals with metabolic ratios indicating *ultrarapid* metabolism by CYP2D6, which is caused by the selective amplification of the functional *CYP2D6*2* allele to two, three, or as many as 13 copies,[395,396] resulting in elevated protein expression. The frequency of the twofold-amplified allelic variant also varies widely among different populations, ranging from 0.8 percent in Danes[397] to 13 percent in Ethiopians.[398]

Genotyping Tests for Mutant Alleles. Assuming that a knowledge of debrisoquine oxidation status is of value in the design of rational drug therapies and for molecular epidemiologic studies of chemical toxicity (see the section "Clinical Consequences of Defective Cytochrome P_{450}2D6"), the development of molecular tests to detect the presence of specific mutant alleles at the CYP2D6 gene locus, and thereby to predict phenotype, has been advocated.[399,400] As already mentioned, RFLP analysis alone is not particularly informative in predicting PM phenotype. This has led to the development of a variety of rapid and specific polymerase chain reaction-based allele-specific amplification[401–403] and/or single-strand conformation polymorphism tests,[404,405] often in combination with RFLP analysis,[381] to detect the presence of the most common variant alleles. Current testing procedures correctly identify 98 to 99 percent of all mutant alleles of CYP2D6, allowing for the accurate prediction of about 95 percent of PM phenotypes.[385]

Genotyping Versus Phenotyping Tests. The advent of molecular testing to predict the PM phenotype has led to considerable discussion as to the relative merits and drawbacks of this approach as compared with the traditional use of probe drugs as *in vivo* markers for pharmacogenetic variation. Proponents of molecular tests cite the potential for adverse drug reactions or for noncompliance from administration of probe drugs to healthy subjects or patients, time-consuming and complex sample collection protocols, and the confounding effects of disease or concurrent drug administration on metabolic ratios as sufficiently important weaknesses of the *in vivo* approach to lead to exclusion of subjects from such procedures. On the other hand, proponents of probe-drug phenotyping could argue, at least in the case of CYP2D6 polymorphism, that allelic multiplicity has made the accurate prediction of phenotype from genotyping information exceedingly complex and cumbersome, with the need for multiple simultaneous tests to determine the presence of any of the great number of variant alleles known to exist at the *CYP2D6* gene cluster. Moreover, the introduction of safer *in vivo* probes, such as dextromethorphan, alleviates most of the problems with potential toxicity and therefore with obtaining patient consent. On the whole, however, phenotyping and genotyping methods are certainly complementary for basic mechanistic studies, and each also has its specific applications. For example, a precise knowledge of genotype may not be either necessary or sufficient in clinical situations, where the goal is simply optimization of drug dosage, if other current patient variables have the potential to affect the functional expression of that genotype significantly. On the other hand, the validity of epidemiologic studies to evaluate associations of metabolizer phenotype with disease states would seriously suffer from misclassification of subjects due to the effects of nongenetic variables on *in vivo* metabolic ratios.

Clinical and Toxicologic Consequences of Defective CYP2D6

One of the main features that distinguishes pharmacogenetic defects of drug biotransformation from most other inborn errors of metabolism is that they are completely silent in the absence of drug challenge, and it is likely to be this weak selective pressure that allows many such defects to reach high frequencies in populations. Because of this and because certain of the agents affected by the CYP2D6 defect have a wide therapeutic window, the clinical importance of defects such as the CYP2D6 polymorphism has from time to time been questioned. However, the very fact that the CYP2D6 polymorphism was discovered as a result of observations of drug-induced toxicity in clinical studies would argue against this contention. The suggestion that polymorphisms are not clinically important may be more a function of the physician's unawareness of the possibility that complications arising during treatment of disease might be related to the drug therapy employed. Although it has been argued that even in PM individuals the incidence of toxicity may be low for many drugs, the high frequency of the pharmacogenetic defect itself, when compared with most other inborn errors, makes the occurrence of adverse reactions significant in the population as a whole. Moreover, the list of drugs whose disposition is affected by the CYP2D6 defect (Table 9-6) has grown considerably since the relevance of the polymorphism for drug therapy was first called into question in the mid-1980s, and it continues to grow.

Earlier[362,406] and more recent[346,347,349] reviews have summarized many of the recognized instances in which the CYP2D6 polymorphism is of clinical significance. In addition, they have provided a set of criteria under which this significance can be assessed for any given therapeutic agent. Generally speaking, genetically impaired metabolism of a drug may be clinically important under the following circumstances: (1) Either the defective metabolic pathway is quantitatively significant in determining the overall fate of the active agent in the body, or it produces a minor but highly active or toxic metabolite. (2) The drug displays a narrow enough therapeutic range that alterations in its disposition can lead to drug accumulation to levels above those considered safe. (3) The drug's therapeutic and toxic effects cannot be easily assessed and titrated by clinical monitoring. (4) The drug is widely used in clinical practice. (5) Therapeutic alternatives are limited or absent.

There also exist several possible manifestations of defective drug oxidation by CYP2D6. These include decreased first-pass metabolism leading to increased bioavailability and increased peak therapeutic response or toxicity; decreased drug elimination leading to prolonged drug half-life, accumulation with repeated dosing, and increased response or toxicity; decreased formation of active metabolites leading to therapeutic failure; and alterations in the formation or elimination of toxic chemicals leading to epidemiologic associations with apparently "spontaneous" disorders. Examples of each of these situations are discussed below.

Dose-Related Toxicity. As already noted, the CYP2D6 polymorphism was initially discovered as a result of investigations into the reason for marked variations in therapeutic responses to debrisoquine and sparteine. In the case of debrisoquine, individuals with the PM phenotype exhibited peak plasma concentrations and AUC (area under the curve) values about fourfold greater than those seen in EM subjects, reflecting a marked decrease in first-pass metabolism of debrisoquine in the former group.[351,352] Thus, at doses that produced no adverse effects in EM subjects, severe postural hypotension could be observed in PM subjects. Sparteine, on the other hand, probably never gained widespread use as an antiarrhythmic agent because most EM subjects were unable to reach sufficient steady-state plasma concentrations to achieve a therapeutic response.[362] In addition, it has been suggested that the 6 to 7 percent incidence of severe side effects from use of this drug for the induction of labor[407] likely represented predominantly patients of the PM phenotype. However, since neither debrisoquine nor sparteine is widely used at present, they merit mostly historical and diagnostic importance in the context of the CYP2D6 polymorphism and its clinical relevance.

On the other hand, as can be seen from Table 9-6, antiarrhythmic agents, β-adrenergic receptor antagonists, neuroleptics, and antidepressants represent major therapeutic classes with currently used drugs whose disposition is significantly affected by the CYP2D6 polymorphism. Of these groups, perhaps the greatest controversy surrounds the contention that defective metabolism of β-receptor blockers by CYP2D6 is of clinical importance,[408–410] since these agents are known to have a rather wide therapeutic window in the treatment of hypertension and a correspondingly low incidence of serious side effects. A large part of the disagreement, however, appears to center on discrepant definitions of *clinically significant* variation. Certainly, life-threatening complications of β-blocker therapy are exceedingly rare, but it has been estimated that 15 to 20 percent of patients who undertake therapy with these agents are forced to discontinue their use due to adverse reactions that are not particularly dangerous. Evidence against a significant clinical effect of metabolizer phenotype has been reported for metoprolol,[411] although more recent reports of disconcordance between the oxidation of metoprolol and that of debrisoquine or sparteine in certain populations[361,412] imply that this may be due to the variable presence of compensatory pathways. On the other hand, excessive β-blockade has been observed following the application of timolol eyedrops in PM subjects or in individuals taking the CYP2D6 inhibitor quinidine (see below).[413,414]

In contrast, there is general agreement that pharmacogenetic variation in CYP2D6 affecting the elimination of certain of the currently used antiarrhythmic agents listed in Table 9-6 is of definite clinical relevance because of a higher incidence of dose-related toxicity in PM individuals.[415] Flecainide and propafenone, for example, require careful monitoring because low plasma levels are ineffective in suppressing potentially life-threatening rhythm disturbances, and high levels may produce proarrhythmias leading to ventricular tachycardia or fibrillation.[362] Although impaired flecainide metabolism in PM individuals is partly compensated for by renal elimination, in PM patients with renal failure one would expect drug accumulation and toxic side effects. The marked first-pass metabolism of propafenone is impaired in PM patients, leading to higher steady-state plasma drug concentrations and a greater incidence of central nervous system side effects that are likely due to partial β-receptor blockade.[416] On the other hand, although side effects from *N*-propylajmaline are also greater in PM individuals and therapeutic failure more common in EM subjects, this agent is not widely available for use in clinical practice, so the general importance of the effect is reduced.

The clinical implications of variable oxidation of antidepressants, most notably those of the tricyclic class, have been discussed extensively.[417–419] Because of the rather narrow therapeutic window and long lag phase before clinical improvement is observed during tricyclic antidepressant therapy, it is estimated that, without careful plasma-level monitoring and dosage adjustments, 20 to 30 percent of patients are at risk due to either dose-related toxicity or subtherapeutic failure. A crucial factor lies in the ambiguous nature of the clinical improvement that clinicians expect to observe during therapy with such agents. Symptoms of overdose (e.g., sedation and tremors) that could be expected with higher frequency in PM individuals administered standard doses of agents such as nortriptyline and desipramine may easily be misinterpreted as symptoms of the original depression and lead to inappropriate increases in dosage. Thus, a lack of dose individualization based on metabolizer phenotype could result both in underdosing of rapid, or particularly of ultrarapid, metabolizer patients[420] and overdosing of PM patients (often leading to cessation of therapy in the latter group because of drug intolerance), with a similar ultimate clinical course of recurring depression in both groups. Many of the newer generation of antidepressant agents, the selective serotonin reuptake inhibitors (SSRIs) such as paroxetine and fluoxetine, are also either metabolized by CYP2D6 or are potent and selective inhibitors of the enzyme.[421,422] This has important implications for managing the therapy of depression with combinations of these drugs and tricyclic antidepressants.

The metabolism of certain neuroleptics such as haloperidol[423] and perphenazine[424] is also significantly impaired *in vivo* in persons with the PM phenotype. Although it has been suggested that this impairment results in an increased incidence of adverse effects, such as extrapyramidal symptoms,[425,426] the fact that these agents are often prescribed in conjunction with tricyclic antidepressants may also lead to drug-drug interactions as a result of mutual competitive inhibition (see section "Inhibition of Cytochrome P_{450}2D6 by Alternate Substrates and Other Chemicals"), as has been observed both *in vivo*[427] and *in vitro*.[428]

Lack of Efficacy. As implied in several of the examples in the previous section, individuals of either the homozygous or the ultrarapid EM phenotype have the potential to eliminate any of the compounds listed in Table 9-6 more rapidly than those with intermediate or PM phenotypes, resulting in decreased intensity or duration of the intended effect and therapeutic failure. On the other hand, codeine and encainide represent examples of drugs that require metabolic activation by CYP2D6 before certain of their therapeutic effects can be fully realized. Thus, for these drugs it is the PM subjects who may experience therapeutic failure. CYP2D6-mediated *O*-demethylation of codeine to morphine[429] represents a minor pathway in codeine biotransformation but appears to account for most of its analgesic properties; codeine is therefore an ineffective analgesic in the 5 to 10 percent of the population who have the PM phenotype.[430,431] Encainide is metabolized by CYP2D6 to a metabolite that has a tenfold higher therapeutic potency, and in PM patients this pathway is impaired.[432] In these subjects, much higher levels of the parent drug are therefore required to achieve a therapeutic response than in EM patients, in whom the active metabolite produces most of the effect of the drug treatment;[433] this difference in pharmacokinetic profile between the metabolizer phenotypes must be recognized and correctly interpreted during therapeutic drug monitoring.

Inhibition of Cytochrome P_{450}2D6 by Alternate Substrates and Other Chemicals. A useful method for predicting the involvement of CYP2D6 in the biotransformation of chemicals is to test for their ability to inhibit competitively the *in vitro* metabolism of known CYP2D6 substrates such as sparteine, debrisoquine, dextromethorphan, or bufuralol.[428,434,435] From the results of such studies, the involvement of CYP2D6 can definitively be excluded if no inhibition is observed, but involvement must still be directly proven if inhibition is seen, since certain compounds (e.g., quinidine[436]) are potent inhibitors without being substrates for CYP2D6. Such competitive interactions, when extrapolated to the clinical situation, obviously suggest the potential for drug interactions during polytherapy and for misclassification of subjects during phenotyping procedures when alternative substrates for the enzyme are coadministered for therapeutic purposes.

For example, as previously noted, it has long been known that dopamine-receptor-blocking neuroleptics such as haloperidol can inhibit the metabolism of tricyclic antidepressants *in vivo*,[437] an effect of some relevance, since the two classes of drugs are often used together. This inhibition has been shown to interfere significantly with standard phenotyping tests,[438] potentially converting EM subjects into phenocopies of PM subjects. It has been determined that CYP2D6 is involved in the oxidation of reduced haloperidol (a metabolite produced by ketoreduction) back to the parent drug,[439] and also that CYP2D6 is expressed in brain[440–442] and may be competitively inhibited by dopamine uptake blockers such as (−)cocaine, *d*-amphetamine, and methylphenidate. This localization to the central nervous system has led to the speculation that neuronal CYP2D6 may play a role not only in drug biotransformation in proximity to sites of action but also possibly in the catabolism and processing of neurotransmitters or other endogenous compounds.[443] Thus, it has been suggested that genetically based variations in CYP2D6 could play a dual role in affecting the response to certain centrally acting CYP2D6 substrates, including drugs of abuse such as codeine and hydrocodone, by both local and systemic availability mechanisms.[444,445]

Associations with Parkinson Disease. Following an initial report[446] suggesting an association between impaired debrisoquine oxidation and both increased incidence and earlier age of onset of Parkinson disease, a large body of conflicting epidemiologic data has been generated in an attempt to confirm these findings.[447,448] A mechanistic model to explain such an association postulates that environmental toxins may play an important role in producing the nigrostriatal neuronal damage that is a common feature of this disorder, and that genetically based variations in the metabolic activation or detoxification of such toxins would be significant risk modulators. Indeed, experimental studies have indicated that 1-methyl-4-phenyl-1,2,3,6-tetrahydropyridine (MPTP), a neurotoxin known to induce nigrostriatal cell death and a parkinsonian syndrome in animals, is both a substrate and a competitive inhibitor of human CYP2D6.[442,449] However, epidemiologic studies have failed to find a consistent association between CYP2D6 phenotypes or genotypes and Parkinson disease, with roughly equal numbers of studies showing either a positive association[447,450–454] or no association.[448,455–460] Thus, it would appear that the effect of CYP2D6 on risk for the occurrence of Parkinson disease is modest at best. More recently, genetic studies have suggested that the *CYP2D* gene locus may be in linkage disequilibrium with an as yet unidentified Parkinson disease susceptibility locus,[461] which may explain the lack of concordance among the studies to date.

Associations with Lung Cancer. In theory, genetically based variations in xenobiotic biotransformation may be risk factors for cancer at two levels. First, differences in the metabolic activation of procarcinogens to electrophilic DNA-binding species could affect mutation frequencies and thus alter processes of tumor initiation or progression. Second, genetically based variations in the disposition of cancer chemotherapeutic agents could influence the effectiveness of therapeutic interventions for existing tumors. The latter possibility has not been directly demonstrated for the CYP2D6 polymorphism, although several drugs used in chemotherapy have been shown to be competitive inhibitors of CYP2D6.[462]

On the other hand, evidence that CYP2D6 may play a role in the metabolic activation of procarcinogens was first obtained from the report of an association between the EM phenotype and increased risk for lung cancer.[463] Subsequent to this publication, several groups published conflicting results concerning the validity of the association (see earlier reviews on the subject by Nebert,[464] Caporaso et al,[465] Idle,[466] and Shields and Harris[467]). Possible problems with study design and methodology aside,[468] perhaps the greatest factor contributing to the uncertainty of this association is that, unlike the situation with defective *N*-acetylation of known arylamine carcinogens and bladder cancer, it has not been possible to definitively identify a potential causative agent that is a substrate for CYP2D6. It has been suggested that the tobacco smoke-derived carcinogen 4-(methylnitrosamino)-1-(3-pyridyl)-1-butanone (NNK) is metabolized by CYP2D6,[469] although not at rates as high as those displayed by other P_{450} isoforms. Indeed, molecular modeling and inhibition studies[470] have suggested that NNK is not likely to be a particularly good substrate for CYP2D6. Moreover, recent studies have failed to find evidence for the expression of CYP2D6 in human lung, where one would expect to observe localized bioactivation of procarcinogens.[471] The most recent reports using improved study designs indicate that the association between CYP2D6 activity and lung cancer risk is weak to nonexistent,[405,472–475] although it should be remembered that procarcinogen metabolic activation processes may require a complex interplay of several risk modulatory factors of modest impact[476] that in combination produce significantly elevated risk.[477] Also, cancer risk in such instances is driven largely by carcinogen exposure, a parameter that is often difficult to quantify accurately in human epidemiologic studies.

CONCLUDING COMMENTARY

There were several common elements in the three case studies presented here. First, we were dealing with healthy subjects whose differences became apparent only on standardized exposure to chemicals—in these cases, drugs. Second, each of these pharmacogenetic conditions has stimulated investigations that otherwise would not have been undertaken; several of these studies have substantially contributed to the understanding of normal human genetics, biochemistry, and physiology. Third, discovery and identification of each of these three conditions has saved some lives and may prevent future fatalities or morbidities. Although we have focused on specific topics, we hope to have shown essential elements of pharmacogenetics.

REFERENCES

1. Kalow W: Pharmacogenetics: Past and future. *Life Sci* **47**:1385, 1990.
2. Motulsky AG: Drug reactions, enzymes, and biochemical genetics. *JAMA* **165**:835, 1957.
3. Vogel F: Moderne Probleme der Humangenetik. *Ergeb Inn Med Kinderheilkd* **12**:65, 1959.
4. Kalow W: *Pharmacogenetics: Heredity and the Response to Drugs*. Philadelphia, London, WB Saunders, 1962.
5. Vesell ES, Page JG: Genetic control of drug levels in man: Antipyrine. *Science* **161**:72, 1968.
6. Dengler VHJ, Eichelbaum M: Polymorphismen und Defekte des Arzneimittelstoffwechsels als ursache toxischer Reaktionen. *Arzneimittelforschung* **27**:1836, 1977.
7. Mahgoub A, Dring LG, Idle JR, Lancaster R, Smith RL: Polymorphic hydroxylation of debrisoquine in man. *Lancet* **2**:584, 1977.
8. Motulsky AG: Pharmacogenetics and ecogenetics in 1991. *Pharmacogenetics* **1**:2, 1991.
9. Grandjean P, Kello D, Rohrborn G, Tarkowski S: *Ecogenetics: Genetic Predisposition to the Toxic Effects of Chemicals* Geneva, World Health Organization/Chapman and Hall, 1991.

10. Crabbe JC, Belknap JK: Genetic approaches to drug dependence. *Trends Pharmacol Sci* **13**:212, 1992.
11. Kalow W: Pharmacogenetics in biological perspective. *Pharmacol Rev* **49**:369, 1997.
12. Skamene E: Population and molecular genetics of susceptibility to tuberculosis, in Sorg C (ed): *Natural Resistance to Infection*. Stuttgart, Gustav Fischer, 1990, p 1.
13. Skamene E: The Bcg gene story. *Immunobiology* **191**:451, 1994.
14. Skamene E, Schurr E, Gros P: Infection genomics: Nrampl as a major determinant of natural resistance to intracellular infections. *Annu Rev Med* **49**:275, 1998.
15. Lagrange PH, Abel L: The genetic susceptibility to leprosy in humans. *Acta Leprol (Geneve)* **10**:11, 1996.
16. Luzzatto L: Glucose-6-phosphate dehydrogenase and other genetic factors interacting with drugs, in Kalow W, Goedde HW, Agarwal D (eds): *Ethnic Differences in Reactions to Drugs and Xenobiotics*. New York, Alan R Liss, 1986, p 385.
17. Hill AVS, Allsopp CEM, Kwiatkowski D, Anstey NM, Twumasi P, Rowe PA, Bennett S, et al: Common West African HLA antigens are associated with protection from severe malaria. *Nature* **352**:595, 1991.
18. Gabriel SE, Brigman KN, Koller BH, Boucher RC, Strutts MJ: Cystic fibrosis heterozygote resistance to cholera toxin in the cystic fibrosis mouse model. *Science* **266**:107, 1994.
19. Pier GB, Grout M, Zaidi T, Meluleni G, Mueschenborn SS, Banting G, Ratcliff R, et al: *Salmonella typhi* uses CFTR to enter intestinal epithelial cells. *Nature* **393**:79, 1998.
20. Huang Y, Paxton WA, Wolinsky SM, Neumann AU, Zhang L, He T, Kang S, et al: The role of a mutant CCR5 allele in HIV-1 transmission and disease progression. *Nat Med* **2**:1240, 1996.
21. Dean M, Carrington M, Winkler C, Huttley GA, Smith MW, Allikmets R, Goedert JJ, et al: Genetic restriction of HIV-1 infection and progression to AIDS by a deletion allele of the CKR5 structural gene. *Science* **273**:1856, 1996.
22. Skamene E, Kongshavn PAL, Landy M: *Genetic Control of Natural Resistance to Infection and Malignancy*. New York, Academic, 1980.
23. Gonzalez FJ, Nebert DW: Evolution of the P450 gene superfamily: Animal-plant 'warfare', molecular drive and human genetic differences in drug oxidation. *Trends Genet* **6**:182, 1990.
24. Whissell-Buechy D: Genetic basis of the phenylthiocarbamide polymorphism. *Chem Sens* **15**:27, 1990.
25. Lison M, Blondheim SH, Melmed RN: A polymorphism of the ability to smell urinary metabolites of asparagus. *BMJ* **281**:20, 1980.
26. Merbs SL, Nathans J: Absorption spectra of human cone pigments. *Nature* **356**:433, 1992.
27. Dreyer M, Rudiger HW: Genetic defects of human receptor function. *Trends Pharmacol Sci* **9**:98, 1988.
28. Lichter JB, Barr CL, Kennedy JL, Van Tol HH, Kidd KK, Livak KJ: A hypervariable segment in the human dopamine receptor D4 (DRD4) gene. *Hum Mol Genet* **2**:767, 1993.
29. Bonner TI, Young AC, Brann MR, Buckley MJ: Cloning and expression of the human and rat m5 muscarinic acetylcholine receptor genes. *Neuron* **1**:403, 1988.
30. Zhou Q-Y, Grandy DK, Thambi L, Kushner JA, Van Tol HHM, Cone R, Pribnow D, et al: Cloning and expression of human and rat D1 dopamine receptors. *Nature* **347**:76, 1990.
31. Goedde HW, Lentner C: Pharmacogenetics and ecogenetics. *Geigy Sci Tables* **4**:289, 1986.
32. Weber WW: *The Acetylator Genes and Drug Response*. New York, Oxford University Press, 1987.
33. Nebert DW, Weber WW: Pharmacogenetics, in Pratt WB, Taylor P (eds): *Principles of Drug Action: The Basis of Pharmacology*. New York, Churchill Livingstone, 1990, p 469.
34. Price Evans DA: *Genetic Aspects of Drug Therapy*. Cambridge, Cambridge University Press, 1992.
35. Gibaldi M: Pharmacogenetics: Parts I and II. *Ann Pharmacother* **26**:121,255, 1992.
36. Weber WW: *Pharmacogenetics*. Oxford: Oxford University Press, 1997.
37. Kalow W, Bertilsson L: Interethnic factors affecting drug response. *Adv Drug Res* **25**:1, 1994.
38. Kalow W: Interethnic variation of drug metabolism. *Trends Pharmacol Sci* **12**:102, 1991.
39. Kalow W (ed): *International Encyclopedia of Pharmacological Therapy*, Sect. 137: *Pharmacogenetics of Drug Metabolism*. New York, Pergamon, 1992.
40. Grant DM, Hughes NC, Janezic SA, Goodfellow GH, Chen HJ, Gaedigk A, Yu VL, Grewal R: Human acetyltransferase polymorphisms. *Mutat Res* **376**:61, 1997.
41. Grant DM, Spielberg SP: Genetic regulation of drug metabolism, in Polin RA, Fox WW (eds): *Fetal and Neonatal Physiology*, 2d ed. Philadelphia, WB Saunders, 1998, p 161.
42. Vatsis KP, Weber WW: Structural heterogeneity of Caucasian *N*-acetyltransferase at the NAT1 gene locus. *Arch Biochem Biophys* **301**:71, 1993.
43. Weber WW, Vatsis KP: Individual variability in *p*-aminobenzoic acid *N*-acetylation by human *N*-acetyltransferase (NAT1) of peripheral blood. *Pharmacogenetics* **3**:209, 1993.
44. Deitz AC, Doll MA, Hein DW: A restriction fragment length polymorphism assay that differentiates human *N*-acetyltransferase-1 (NAT1) alleles. *Anal Biochem* **253**:219, 1997.
45. Hughes NC, Janezic SA, McQueen KL, Jewett MA, Castranio T, Bell DA, Grant DM: Identification and characterization of variant alleles of human acetyltransferase NAT1 with defective function using *p*-aminosalicylate as an in-vivo and in-vitro probe. *Pharmacogenetics* **8**:55, 1998.
46. Tang BK, Kadar D, Qian L, Iriah J, Yip J, Kalow W: Caffeine as a metabolic probe: Validation of its use for acetylator phenotyping. *Clin Pharmacol Ther* **49**:648, 1991.
47. Fuhr U, Rost KL, Engelhardt R, Sachs M, Liermann D, Belloc C, Beaune P, et al: Evaluation of caffeine as a test drug for CYP1A2, NAT2 and CYP2E1 phenotyping in man by in vivo versus in vitro correlations. *Pharmacogenetics* **6**:159, 1996.
48. Doll MA, Fretland AJ, Deitz AC, Hein DW: Determination of human NAT2 acetylator genotype by restriction fragment-length polymorphism and allele-specific amplification. *Anal Biochem* **231**:413, 1995.
49. Delomenie C, Sica L, Grant DM, Krishnamoorthy R, Dupret JM: Genotyping of the polymorphic *N*-acetyltransferase (NAT2*) gene locus in two native African populations. *Pharmacogenetics* **6**:177, 1996.
50. Agundez JA, Olivera M, Martinez C, Ladero JM, Benitez J: Identification and prevalence study of 17 allelic variants of the human NAT2 gene in a white population. *Pharmacogenetics* **6**:423, 1996.
51. Smith CA, Wadelius M, Gough AC, Harrison DJ, Wolf CR, Rane A: A simplified assay for the arylamine *N*-acetyltransferase 2 polymorphism validated by phenotyping with isoniazid. *J Med Genet* **34**:758, 1997.
52. Bell DA, Stephens EA, Castranio T, Umbach DM, Watson M, Deakin M, Elder J, et al: Polyadenylation polymorphism in the acetyltransferase 1 gene (NAT1) increases risk of colorectal cancer. *Cancer Res* **55**:3537, 1995.
53. Probst-Hensch NM, Haile RW, Li DS, Sakamoto GT, Louie AD, Lin BK, et al: Lack of association between the polyadenylation polymorphism in the NAT1 (acetyltransferase 1) gene and colorectal adenomas. *Carcinogenesis* **17**:2125, 1996.
54. Okkels H, Sigsgaard T, Wolf H, Autrup H: Arylamine *N*-acetyltransferase 1 (NAT1) and 2 (NAT2) polymorphisms in susceptibility to bladder cancer: The influence of smoking. *Cancer Epidemiol Biomarkers Prev* **6**:225, 1997.
55. Risch A, Wallace DM, Bathers S, Sim E: Slow *N*-acetylation genotype is a susceptibility factor in occupational and smoking related bladder cancer. *Hum Mol Genet* **4**:231, 1995.
56. Cascorbi I, Brockmoller J, Mrozikiewicz PM, Bauer S, Loddenkemper R, Roots I: Homozygous rapid arylamine *N*-acetyltransferase (NAT2) genotype as a susceptibility factor for lung cancer. *Cancer Res* **56**:3961, 1996.
57. Hunter DJ, Hankinson SE, Hough H, Gertig DM, Garcia-Closas M, Spiegelman D, Manson JE, et al: A prospective study of NAT2 acetylation genotype, cigarette smoking, and risk of breast cancer. *Carcinogenesis* **18**:2127, 1997.
58. Lennard L, Lilleyman JS, Van Loon J, Weinshilboum RM: Genetic variation in response to 6-mercaptopurine for childhood acute lymphoblastic leukaemia. *Lancet* **336**:225, 1990.
59. Goedd HW, Agarwal DP: Aldehyde dehydrogenase polymorphism: Molecular basis and phenotypic relationship to alcohol sensitivity. *Alcohol Alcohol Suppl* **1**:47, 1987.
60. Harrison GG, Isaacs H: Malignant hyperthermia: An historical vignette. *Anaesthesiology* **47**:54, 1992.
61. Denborough MA, Lovell RRH: Anaesthetic deaths in a family. *Lancet* **2**:45, 1960.
62. Britt BA: *Malignant Hyperthermia*. Boston, Martinus Nijhoff, 1987.
63. Britt BA: Malignant hyperthermia: A review, in Schoenbaum E, Lomax P (eds): *Thermoregulation: Pathology, Pharmacology and Therapy*. New York, Pergamon, 1991, p 179.
64. Heiman-Patterson TD: Malignant hyperthermia. *Semin Neurol* **11**:220, 1991.

65. Lehmann-Horn F, Klein W, Spittelmeister W: Neurologisch relevante Aspekte der malignen Hyperthermie. *Aktuel Neurol* **18**:117, 1991.
66. Joffe M, Savage N, Silove M: The biochemistry of malignant hyperthermia: Recent concepts. *Int J Biochem* **24**:387, 1992.
67. MacLennan DH, Phillips MS: Malignant hyperthermia. *Science* **256**:789, 1992.
68. Harrison GG: Control of the malignant hyperpyrexia syndrome in MHS swine by dantrolene sodium. *Br J Anaesth* **47**:62, 1975.
69. Weber G: Dantrolen: Wirkungen, Nebenwirkungen, Interaktionen. *Beitr Anaesthesiol Intensivmed* **27**:166, 1989.
70. Roed A: Separate sites for the dantrolene-induced inhibition of contracture of the rat diaphragm preparation due to depolarization or to caffeine. *Eur J Pharmacol* **209**:33, 1991.
71. Fruen BR, Mickelson JR, Louis CF: Dantrolene inhibition of sarcoplasmic reticulum Ca^{2+} release by direct and specific action at skeletal muscle ryanodine receptors. *J Biol Chem* **272**:26,965, 1997.
72. Nelson TE, Lin M, Zapata-Sudo G, Sudo RT: Dantrolene sodium can increase or attenuate activity of skeletal muscle ryanodine receptor calcium release channel: Clinical implications. *Anesthesiology* **84**:1368, 1996.
73. Kalow W, Britt BA, Terreau ME, Haist C: Metabolic error of muscle metabolism after recovery from malignant hyperthermia. *Lancet* **2**:895, 1970.
74. Ellis FR, Harriman DGF, Keaney NP, Kyei-Mensah K, Tyrrell JH: Halothane-induced muscle contracture as a cause of hyperpyrexia. *Br J Anaesth* **43**:721, 1971.
75. Hall LW, Woolf N, Bradley JW, Jolly DW: Unusual reaction to suxamethonium chloride. *BMJ* **2**:1305, 1966.
76. Morio M, Kikuchi H, Yuge O, Kawachi S: Incidence of malignant hyperthermia, in Bergmann H, Steinbereithner K (eds): *Seventh European Congress of Anaesthesiology*. Vienna, Wilhelm Maudrich, 1987, p 82.
77. Ellis FR: Natural history and genetics of MH. *Beitr Anaesthesiol Intensivmed* **27**:41, 1989.
78. Rubinstein NA, Lyons GE, Kelly AM: Hormonal control of myosin heavy chain genes during development of skeletal muscles. *Ciba Found Symp* **138**:35, 1988.
79. Kalow W, Sharer S, Britt B: Pharmacogenetics of caffeine and caffeine-halothane contractures in biopsies of human skeletal muscle. *Pharmacogenetics* **1**:126, 1991.
80. Lehmann-Horn F, Knorr-Held S: Muscle diseases relevant to the anesthetist. *Acta Anaesthesiol Belg* **41**:113, 1990.
81. Gronert GA, Mott J, Lee J: Aetiology of malignant hyperthermia. *Br J Anaesth* **60**:253, 1988.
82. Heffron JJA, Brickley KD: Pathobiochemistry of malignant hyperthermia. *Beitr Anaesthesiol Intensivmed* **27**:24, 1989.
83. Gericke GS, Isaacs H: An association between certain congenital abnormalities and the malignant hyperthermia trait. *S Afr Med Assoc* **77**:570, 1990.
84. Valdivia HH, Hogan K, Coronado R: Altered binding site for Ca^{2+} in the ryanodine receptor of human malignant hyperthermia. *Am J Physiol* **261**:C237, 1991.
85. Levitt RC, Nouri N, Jedlicka AE, McKusick VA, Marks AR, Shutack JG, Fletcher JE, et al: Evidence for genetic heterogeneity in malignant hyperthermia susceptibility. *Genomics* **11**:543, 1991.
86. Robinson R, Curran JL, Hall WJ, Halsall PJ, Hopkins PM, Markham AF, Stewart AD, et al: Genetic heterogeneity and HOMOG analysis in British malignant hyperthermia families. *J Med Genet* **35**:196, 1998.
87. Sudbrak R, Procaccio V, Klausnitzer M, Curran JL, Monsieurs K, van Broeckhoven C, Ellis R, et al: Mapping of a further malignant hyperthermia susceptibility locus to chromosome 3q13.1. *Am J Hum Genet* **56**:684, 1995.
88. Fujii J, Otsu K, Zorzato F, De Leon S, Khanna VK, Weiler JE, O'Brien PJ, MacLennan DH: Identification of a mutation in porcine ryanodine receptor associated with malignant hyperthermia. *Science* **253**:448, 1991.
89. Otsu K, Khanna V, Archibald AL, MacLennan DH: Consegregation of porcine malignant hyperthermia and a probable causal mutation in the skeletal muscle ryanodine receptor gene in backcross families. *Genomics* **11**:744, 1991.
90. Loke J, MacLennan DH: Malignant hyperthermia and central core disease: Disorders of Ca^{2+} release channels. *Am J Med* **104**:470, 1998.
91. Entman ML, Van Winkle WB: *Sarcoplasmic Reticulum in Muscle Physiology.* Boca Raton, FL, CRC, 1986.
92. Sugi H, Pollack GH: *Molecular Mechanism of Muscle Contraction.* New York, Plenum, 1986.
93. Volpe P: The unraveling of the junctional sarcoplasmic reticulum. *J Bioenerg Biomembr* **21**:215, 1989.
94. Ikemoto N, Ronjat M, Meszaros LG: Kinetic analysis of excitation-contraction coupling. *J Bioenerg Biomembr* **21**:247, 1989.
95. Palade P: Drug-induced Ca^{2+} release from isolated sarcoplasmic reticulum. *J Biol Chem* **262**:6135, 1987.
96. Nelson TE: Skeletal muscle targets for the action of anesthetic agents, in Blanck TJJ, Wheeler DM (eds): *Mechanisms of Anesthetic Action in Skeletal, Cardiac, and Smooth Muscle*. New York, Plenum, 1991, p 3.
97. Pessah IN, Lynch C III, Gronert GA: Complex pharmacology of malignant hyperthermia. *Anesthesiology* **84**:1275, 1996.
98. Donaldson SK: Mechanisms of excitation-contraction coupling in skinned muscle fibers. *Med Sci Sports Exerc* **21**:411, 1989.
99. Smith JS, Imagawa T, Ma J, Fill M, Campbell KP, Coronado R: Purified ryanodine receptor from rabbit skeletal muscle is the calcium-release channel of sarcoplasmic reticulum. *Gen Physiol* **92**:1, 1988.
100. McGrew SG, Wolleben C, Siegl P, Inui M, Fleischer S: Positive cooperativity of ryanodine binding to the calcium release channel of sarcoplasmic reticulum from heart and skeletal muscle. *Biochemistry* **28**:1686, 1989.
101. Lai FA, Meissner G: The muscle ryanodine receptor and its intrinsic Ca^{2+} channel activity. *J Bioenerg Biomembr* **21**:227, 1989.
102. Nelson TE: SR function in malignant hyperthermia. *Cell Calcium* **9**:257, 1988.
103. Heffron JJA: Biochemistry of the malignant hyperthermia syndrome, in Hofmann JG, Schmidt A (eds): *Malignant Hyperthermia: An Update*. Berlin, Volk und Gesundheit, 1989, p 212.
104. Ebashi S: Excitation-contraction coupling and the mechanism of muscle contraction. *Annu Rev Physiol* **53**:1, 1991.
105. Tanabe T, Takeshima H, Mikami A, Flockerzi V, Takahashi H, Kangawa K, Kojima M, et al: Primary structure of the receptor for calcium channel blockers from skeletal muscle. *Nature* **328**:313, 1987.
106. Tsien RW, Ellinor PT, Horne WA: Molecular diversity of voltage-dependent Ca^{2+} channels. *Trends Pharmacol Sci* **12**:349, 1992.
107. Agnew WS: Cloning of the SR foot. *Nature* **339**:422, 1989.
108. Takeshima H, Nishimura S, Matsumoto T, Ishida H, Kangawa K, Minamino N, Matsuo H, et al: Primary structure and expression from complementary DNA of skeletal muscle ryanodine receptor. *Nature* **339**:439, 1989.
109. Endo M, Yagi S, Ishizuka T, Horiuti K, Koga Y, Amaha K: Changes in the Ca-induced Ca release mechanism in the sarcoplasmic reticulum of the muscle from a patient with malignant hyperthemia. *Biomed Res* **4**:83, 1983.
110. Ohnishi ST, Taylor S, Gronert GA: Calcium-induced Ca^{2+} release from sarcoplasmic reticulum of pigs susceptible to malignant hyperthermia. *FEBS Lett* **161**:103, 1983.
111. Endo M: Calcium release from sarcoplasmic reticulum. *Curr Top Membr Transp* **25**:181, 1985.
112. Palade P, Dettbarn C, Brunder D, Stein P, Hals G: Pharmacology of calcium release from sarcoplasmic reticulum. *J Bioenerg Biomembr* **21**:295, 1989.
113. Coronado R, Morrissette J, Sukhareva M, Vaughan DM: Structure and function of ryanodine receptors. *Am J Physiol* **266**:C1485, 1994.
114. Ma J, Fill M, Knudson CM, Campbell KP, Coronado R: Ryanodine receptor of skeletal muscle is a gap junction-type channel. *Science* **242**:99, 1988.
115. Sekiguchi T, Shimizu H: Caffeine-induced calcium release from sarcoplasmic reticulum of a skeletal muscle. *J Pharmacobiodyn* **10**:55, 1987.
116. O'Brien PJ: Microassay for malignant hyperthermia susceptibility: Hypersensitive ligand-gating of the Ca channel in muscle sarcoplasmic reticulum causes increased amounts and rates of Ca-release. *Mol Cell Biochem* **93**:53, 1990.
117. McPherson PS, Kim Y-K, Valdivia H, Knudson CM, Takekura H, Franzini-Armstrong C, Coronado R, Campbell KP: The brain ryanodine receptor: A caffeine-sensitive calcium release channel. *Neuron* **7**:17, 1991.
118. Petersen OH: Actions of caffeine. *News Physiol Sci* **6**:98, 1991.
119. Salviati G, Ceoldo S, Fachechi-Cassano G, Betto R: Ca release from skeletal muscle SR: Effects of volatile anesthetics, in Blanck TJJ, Wheeler DM (eds): *Mechanisms of Anesthetic Action in Skeletal, Cardiac, and Smooth Muscle*. New York, Plenum, 1991, p 31.
120. O'Brien PJ: Porcine malignant hyperthermia susceptibility: Hypersensitive calcium-release mechanism of skeletal muscle sarcoplasmic reticulum. *Can J Vet Res* **50**:318, 1986.
121. Herrmann-Frank A, Richter M, Lehmann-Horn F: 4-Chloro-*m*-cresol: A specific tool to distinguish between malignant hyperthermia-susceptible and normal muscle. *Biochem Pharmacol* **52**:149, 1996.

122. Kalow W, Britt BA, Richter A: The caffeine test of isolated human muscle in relation to malignant hyperthermia. *Can Anaesth Soc J* **24**:678, 1977.
123. Thomas MA, Rock E, Viret J: Membrane properties of the sarcolemma and sarcoplasmic reticulum of pigs susceptible to malignant hyperthermia: Action of halothane. *Clin Chim Acta* **200**:201, 1991.
124. Davies K: Malignant hyperthermia be due to a defect in a large Ca^{2+} release channel protein. *Trends Genet* **6**:171, 1990.
125. Fill M, Coronado R, Mickelson JR, Vilven J, Ma J, Jacobson BA, Louis CF: Abnormal ryanodine receptor channels in malignant hyperthermia. *Biophys J* **57**:471, 1990.
126. King JO, Denborough MA, Zapf PW: Inheritance of inherited malignant hyperpyrexia. *Lancet* **1**:365, 1972.
127. Kelstrup J, Reske-Nielsen E, Haase J, Jorni J: Malignant hyperthermia in a family: A clinical and serological investigation of 139 members. *Acta Anaesthesiol Scand* **18**:58, 1974.
128. Kalow W, Britt BA, Chan F: Epidemiology and inheritance of malignant hyperthermia. *Int Anesthesiol Clin* **17**:119, 1979.
129. Gordon RA, Britt BA, Kalow W: *International Symposium on Malignant Hyperthermia.* Springfield, IL, Charles C Thomas, 1973.
130. Simpson SP, Webb AJ, Wilmut I: Performance of British Landrace pigs selected for high and low incidence of halothane sensitivity: 1. Reproduction. *Anim Prod* **43**:485, 1986.
131. Archibald AL, Imlah P: The halothane sensitivity locus and its linkage relationships. *Anim Blood Groups Biochem Genet* **16**:253, 1985.
132. Brenig B, Jurs S, Brem G: The porcine PHIcDNA linked to the halothane gene detects a HindIII and XbaI RFLP in normal and malignant hyperthermia susceptible pigs. *Nucleic Acids Res* **18**:388, 1990.
133. Gahne B, Juneja RK: Prediction of the halothane (Hal) genotypes of pigs by deducing Hal, Phi, Po2, Pgd haplotypes of parents and offspring: Results from a large-scale practice in Swedish breeds. *Anim Blood Groups Biochem Genet* **61**:265, 1985.
134. Harbitz I, Chowdhary B, Thomsen P, Davies W, Kaufman U, Kran S, Gustavsson I, et al: Assignement of the porcine calcium release channel gene, a candidate for the malignant hyperthermia locus, to the 6p11-q21 segment of chromosome 6. *Genomics* **8**:243, 1990.
135. Gallant EM, Mickelson JR, Roggow BD, Donaldson SK, Louis CF, Rempel WE: Halothane-sensitivity gene and muscle contractile properties in malignant hyperthermia. *Am J Physiol* **257**:C781, 1989.
136. MacLennan DH, Duff C, Zorzato F, Fujii J, Phillips M, Korneluk RG, Frodis W, et al: Ryanodine receptor gene is a candidate for predisposition to malignant hyperthermia. *Nature* **343**:559, 1990.
137. Webb AJ, Simpson SP: Performance of British Landrace pigs selected for high and low incidence of halothane sensitivity: 2. Growth and carcass traits. *Anim Prod* **43**:493, 1986.
138. Denborough MA, Forster JFA, Lovell RRH, Maplestone PA, Villiers JD: Anaesthetic deaths in a family. *Br J Anaesth* **34**:395, 1962.
139. McPherson E, Taylor CA: The genetics of malignant hyperthermia: Evidence for heterogeneity. *Am J Med Genet* **11**:273, 1982.
140. Kalow W: Inheritance of malignant hyperthermia: A review of published data, in Britt BA (ed): *Malignant Hyperthermia.* Boston, Martinus Nijhoff, 1987, p l55.
141. Fagerlund TH, Islander G, Ranklev Twetman E, Berg K: Malignant hyperthermia susceptibility, an autosomal dominant disorder? *Clin Genet* **51**:365, 1997.
142. Gillard EF, Otsu K, Fujii J, Khanna VK, De Leon S, Derdemezi J, Britt BA, et al: A substitution of cysteine for arginine 614 in the ryanodine receptor is potentially causative of human malignant hyperthermia. *Genomics* **11**:751, 1991.
143. Quane KA, Ording H, Keating KE, Manning BM, Heine R, Bendixen D, Berg K, et al: Detection of a novel mutation at amino acid position 614 in the ryanodine receptor in malignant hyperthermia. *Br J Anaesth* **79**:332, 1997.
144. Manning BM, Quane KA, Ording H, Urwyler A, Tegazzin V, Lehane M, O'Halloran J, et al: Identification of novel mutations in the ryanodine-receptor gene (RYR1) in malignant hyperthermia: Genotype-phenotype correlation. *Am J Hum Genet* **62**:599, 1998.
145. McCarthy TV, Healy JMS, Heffron JJA, Lehane M, Deufel T, Lehmann-Horn F, Farrall M, Johnson K: Localization of the malignant hyperthermia susceptibility locus to human chromosome 19q12-13.2. *Nature* **343**:562, 1990.
146. Iles DE, Lehmann-Horn F, Scherer SW, Tsui LC, Olde Weghuis D, Suijkerbuijk RF, Heytens L, et al: Localization of the gene encoding the alpha 2/delta-subunits of the L-type voltage-dependent calcium channel to chromosome 7q and analysis of the segregation of flanking markers in malignant hyperthermia susceptible families. *Hum Mol Genet* **3**:969, 1994.
147. Levitt RC, Olckers A, Meyers S, Fletcher JE, Rosenberg H, Isaacs H, Meyers DA: Evidence for the localization of a malignant hyperthermia susceptibility locus (MHS2) to human chromosome 17q. *Genomics* **14**:562, 1992.
148. Olckers A, Meyers DA, Meyers S, Taylor EW, Fletcher JE, Rosenberg H, Isaacs H, Levitt RC: Adult muscle sodium channel alpha-subunit is a gene candidate for malignant hyperthermia susceptibility. *Genomics* **14**:829, 1992.
149. Fletcher JE, Wieland SJ, Karan SM, Beech J, Rosenberg H: Sodium channel in human malignant hyperthermia. *Anesthesiology* **86**:1023, 1997.
150. Everts ME, Ording H, Hansen O, Nielsen PA: Ca^{2+}-ATPase and Na^{+}-K^{+}-ATPase content in skeletal muscle from malignant hyperthermia patients. *Muscle Nerve* **14**:162, 1992.
151. Monnier N, Procaccio V, Stieglitz P, Lunardi J: Malignant-hyperthermia susceptibility is associated with a mutation of the alpha 1-subunit of the human dihydropyridine-sensitive L-type voltage-dependent calcium-channel receptor in skeletal muscle. *Am J Hum Genet* **60**:1316, 1997.
152. Ervasti JM, Claessens MT, Mickelson JR, Louis CF: Altered transverse tubule dihydropyridine receptor binding in malignant hyperthermia. *J Biol Chem* **264**:2711, 1989.
153. Hasegawa T, Kumagai S: A G-protein of sarcoplasmic reticulum of skeletal muscle is activated by caffeine or inositol trisphosphate. *FEBS Lett* **244**:283, 1989.
154. Wieland SJ, Fletcher JE, Gong Q, Rosenberg H: Effects of lipid-soluble agents on sodium channel function in normal and MH-susceptible skeletal muscle cultures, in Blanck TJJ, Wheeler DM (eds): *Mechanisms of Anesthetic Action in Skeletal, Cardiac and Smooth Muscle.* New York, Plenum, 1991, p 9.
155. Shah A, Sahgal V, Subramani V: Membrane abnormality in malignant hyperthermia. *Acta Neuropathol (Berl)* **78**:86, 1989.
156. Seewald MJ, Eichinger HM, Iaizzo PA: Malignant hyperthermia: An altered phospholipid and fatty acid composition in muscle membranes. *Acta Anaesthesiol Scand* **35**:380, 1991.
157. Fletcher JE, Rosenberg H, Beech J: Interactions of fatty acids with the calcium release channel in malignant hyperthermia, in Blanck TJJ, Wheeler DM (eds): *Mechanisms of Anesthetic Action in Skeletal, Cardiac and Smooth Muscle.* New York, Plenum, 1991, p 57.
158. Levitt RC, McKusick VA, Fletcher JE, Rosenberb H: Gene candidate. *Nature* **345**:297, 1990.
159. Ording H, Hedengran AM, Skovgaard LT: Evaluation of 119 anaesthetics received after investigation for susceptibility to malignant hyperthermia. *Acta Anaesthesiol Scand* **35**:711, 1991.
160. Nelson TE: Diagnosing malignant hyperthermia. *Plast Reconstr Surg* **84**:699, 1989.
161. Ellis FR, Halsall PJ, Christian AS: Clinical presentation of suspected malignant hyperthermia during anaesthesia in 402 probands. *Anaesthesia* **45**:838, 1990.
162. Kalow W, Britt BA, Peters P: Rapid simplified techniques for measuring caffeine contraction for patients with malignant hyperthermia, in Aldrete JA, Britt BA (eds): *Second International Symposium on Malignant Hyperthermia.* New York, Grune and Stratton, 1978, p 339.
163. Iaizzo PA, Wedel DJ, Gallagher WJ: In vitro contracture testing for determination of susceptibility to malignant hyperthermia: A methodologic update. *Mayo Clin Proc* **66**:998, 1991.
164. Urwyler A, Funk B, Censier K, Drewe J: Effect of halothane equilibration kinetics on in vitro muscle contractures for malignant hyperthermia screening. *Acta Anaesthesiol Scand* **36**:115, 1992.
165. Melton AT, Martucci RW, Kien ND, Gronert GA: Malignant hyperthermia in humans: Standardization of contracture testing protocol. *Anesth Analg* **69**:437, 1989.
166. Rosenberg H: Standards for halothane/caffeine contracture test. *Anesth Analg* **69**:429, 1989.
167. Larach MG, Landis JR, Bunn JS, Diaz M: Prediction of malignant hyperthermia susceptibility in low-risk subjects. *Anesthesiology* **76**:16, 1992.
168. Britt BA: The North American caffeine halothane contracture test, in Nalda Felipe MA, Gottmann S, Khambatta HJ (eds): *Malignant Hyperthermia: Current Concepts, International Course, Spain, Sept. 15–17, 1988.* Bad Homburg, Germany, Normed, 1989, p 53.
169. Larach MG: Standardization of the caffeine halothane muscle contracture test. *Anesth Analg* **69**:511, 1989.
170. Allen GC, Larach MG, Kunselman AR: The sensitivity and specificity of the caffeine-halothane contracture test: A report from the North American Malignant Hyperthermia Registry of MHAUS. *Anesthesiology* **88**:579, 1998.

171. European MH Group: Laboratory diagnosis of malignant hyperpyrexia susceptibility (MHS). *Br J Anaesth* **57**:1038, 1985.
172. Ording H: In-vitro contracture tests: State of the art. *Beitr Anaesthesiol Intensivmed* **27**:67, 1989.
173. Ording H: Disposition for malignant hyperthermia: Diagnostic procedures, in Mortier W, Breucking E (eds): *Malignant Hyperthermia Neuromuscular Diseases and Anaesthesia*. New York, Georg Thieme, 1990, p 35.
174. Ording H, Brancadoro V, Cozzolino S, Ellis FR, Glauber V, Gonano EF, Halsall PJ, et al: In vitro contracture test for diagnosis of malignant hyperthermia following the protocol of the European MH group: Results of testing patients surviving fulminant MH and unrelated low-risk subjects. The European Malignant Hyperthermia Group. *Acta Anaesthesiol Scand* **41**:955, 1997.
175. Ording H: The European MH Group: Protocol for in vitro diagnosis of susceptibility to MH and preliminary results, in Britt BA (ed): *Malignant Hyperthermia*. Boston, Martinus Nijhoff, 1987, p 269.
176. Ording H: In-vitro diagnosis of malignant hyperthermia, in Bergmann H, Steinbereithner K (eds): *Seventh European Congress of Anaesthesiology*. Vienna, Wilhelm Maudrich, 1987, p 62.
177. Fletcher JE, Conti PA, Rosenberg H: Comparison of North American and European malignant hyperthermia group halothane contracture testing protocols in swine. *Acta Anaesthesiol Scand* **35**:483, 1991.
178. Krivosic-Horber R, Adnet P, Krivosic I, Reyford H, Gouyet L: The in-vitro determination of susceptibility to malignant hyperthermia in children, in Mortier W, Breucking E (eds): *Malignant Hyperthermia Neuromuscular Diseases and Anaesthesia*. New York, Georg Thieme, 1990, p 41.
179. Urwyler A, Censier K, Kaufmann MA, Drewe J: Genetic effects on the variability of the halothane and caffeine muscle contracture tests. *Anesthesiology* **80**:1287, 1994.
180. MacKenzie AE, Allen G, Lahey D, Crossan ML, Nolan K, Mettler G, Worton RG, et al: A comparison of the caffeine halothane muscle contracture test with the molecular genetic diagnosis of malignant hyperthermia. *Anesthesiology* **75**:4, 1991.
181. Loke JC, MacLennan DH: Bayesian modeling of muscle biopsy contracture testing for malignant hyperthermia susceptibility. *Anesthesiology* **88**:589, 1998.
182. Britt BA: Elective diagnosis of malignant hyperthermia: Review, in Hofmann JG, Schmidt A (eds): *Malignant Hyperthermia: An Update*. Berlin, Volk und Gesundheit, 1989, p 42.
183. Klip A, Elliott ME, Frodis W, Britt BA, Pegg W, Scott E: Anaesthetic-induced increase in ionised calcium in blood mononuclear cells from malignant hyperthermia patients. *Lancet* **1**:463, 1987.
184. O'Brien PJ, Kalow BI, Brown BD, Lumsden JH, Jacobs RM: Porcine malignant hyperthermia susceptibility: Halothane-induced increase in cytoplasmic free calcium in lymphocytes. *Am J Vet Res* **50**:131, 1989.
185. Hofmann JG: Blood cells in diagnosing MH susceptibility: The platelet model, in Hofmann JG, Schmidt A (eds): *Malignant Hyperthermia: An Update*. Berlin, Volk und Gesundheit, 1989, p 121.
186. Harnden-Mayor P, Franks AJ, Halsall PJ, Howell DM, Ellis FR: Histomorphologic changes in malignant hyperpyrexia. *Beitr Anaesthesiol Intensivmed* **27**:45, 1989.
187. Stadhouders AM, Viering WAL, Sengers RCA: Histochemical aspects of malignant hyperthermia. *Beitr Anaesthesiol Intensivmed* **27**:50, 1989.
188. Isaacs H, Barlow MB: Malignant hyperpyrexia during anaesthesia: Possible association with subclinical myopathy. *BMJ* **1**:275, 1970.
189. Ellis FR, Clarke IMC, Modgill M, Currie S: Evaluation of creatinine phosphokinase in screening patients for malignant hyperpyrexia. *BMJ* **3**:511, 1975.
190. Amaranath L, Lavin TJ, Trusso RA, Boutros AR: Evaluation of creatinine phosphokinase screening as a predictor of malignant hyperthermia. *Br J Anaesth* **55**:531, 1983.
191. Lehmann-Horn F: Creatine kinase elevation in serum: Consequence for diagnosis and anaesthesia, in Mortier W, Breucking E (eds): *Malignant Hyperthermia Neuromuscular Diseases and Anaesthesia*. New York, Georg Thieme, 1990, p 1.
192. Kojima Y, Oku S, Takahashi K, Mukaida K: Susceptibility to malignant hyperthermia manifested as delayed return of increased serum creatine kinase activity and episodic rhabdomyolysis after exercise. *Anesthesiology* **87**:1565, 1997.
193. Britt BA, Endrenyi L, Peters PL, Kwong FH, Kadijevic L: Screening of malignant hyperthermia susceptible families by creatine phosphokinase measurement and other clinical investigations. *Can Anaesth Soc J* **23**:263, 1977.
194. Kozak-Reiss G, Gascard JP: Comparison of contracture test and ^{31}P-NMR spectrometry, in Hofmann JG, Schmidt A (eds): *Malignant Hyperthermia: An Update*. Berlin, Volk und Gesundheit, 1989, p 104.
195. Allsop P, Jorfeldt L, Rutberg H, Hall GM: Muscle pH recovery after high intensity cycle exercise in malignant hyperthermia susceptible subjects. *Biochem Soc Trans* **19**:131S, 1991.
196. Olgin J, Rosenberg H, Allen G, Seestedt R, Chance B: A blinded comparison of noninvasive, in vivo phosphorus nuclear magnetic resonance spectroscopy and the in vitro halothane/caffeine contracture test in the evaluation of malignant hyperthermia susceptibility. *Anesth Analg* **72**:36, 1991.
197. Von Rohden L, Steinbicker V, Krebs P, Wiemann D, Koditz H: The value of ultrasound for the diganosis of malignant hyperthermia. *J Ultrasound Med* **9**:291, 1990.
198. Ortlepp VK, Seidel U, Hofmann JG: Maligne Hyperthermie: In-vivo-Diagnostik mit Ultraschall. *Z Klin Med* **44**:1153, 1989.
199. Hassler F, Wysocki J, Kandler U, Beckmann K: Maligne hyperthermie: In-vivo-diagnostik mittels myosonographie. *Z Klin Med* **46**:1175, 1991.
200. Britt BA: Malignant hyperthermia: A review. *Handb Exp Pharmacol* **60**:547, 1982.
201. Smith RJ, Ellis FR: Non-invasive screening for MH. *Beitr Anaesthesiol Intensivmed* **27**:85, 1989.
202. Gronert GA: Malignant hyperthermia. *Anesthesiology* **53**:395, 1980.
203. Ellis FR, Heffron JJA: Clinical and biochemical aspects of malignant hyperpyrexia. *Recent Adv Anaesth Analg* **15**:173, 1985.
204. Fletcher R: Clinical patterns of MH. *Beitr Anaesthesiol Intensivmed* **27**:87, 1989.
205. Jantzen J-P, Kleemann JP, Dick W: Klinische differentialdiagnose der malignen hyperthermie (MH). *Beitr Anaesthesiol Intensivmed* **27**:121, 1989.
206. Hall GM: Biochemical aspects of malignant hyperthermia, in Bergmann H, Steinbereithnar K (eds): *Seventh European Congress of Anaesthesiology Proceedings, III*. Vienna, Wilhelm Maudrich, 1987, p 58.
207. Heffron JJA: Malignant hyperthermia: Biochemical aspects of the acute episode. *Br J Anaesth* **60**:274, 1988.
208. Meakin G, Walker RWM, Dearlove OR: Myotonic and neuromuscular blocking effects of increased doses of suxamethonium in infants and children. *Br J Anaesth* **65**:816, 1990.
209. Christian AS, Ellis FR, Halsall PJ: Masseteric muscle spasm and malignant hyperthermia, in Hofmann JG, Schmidt A (eds): *Malignant Hyperthermia: An Update*. Berlin, Volk und Gesundheit, 1989, p 112.
210. Britt BA, Locher WG, Kalow W: Hereditary aspects of malignant hyperthermia. *Can Anaesth Soc J* **16**:89, 1969.
211. Allen PD, Ryan JF, Sreter FA, Malbuchi K: Rigid vs. nonrigid MH: Studies of Ca^{2+} uptake and actomyosin ATPase. *Anesthesiology* **53**:S251, 1986.
212. Mortier W, Breucking E, Pothmann R: Malignant hyperthermia and neuromuscular diseases. *Beitr Anaesthesiol Intensivmed* **27**:92, 1989.
213. Poels PJE, Joosten EMG, Sengers RCA, Stadhouders AM, Veerkamp JH, Benders AAGM: In vitro contraction test for malignant hyperthermia in patients with unexplained recurrent rhabdomyolysis. *J Neurol Sci* **105**:67, 1991.
214. Brownell AKW: Malignant hyperthermia: Relationship to other diseases. *Br J Anaesth* **60**:303, 1988.
215. Ong RO, Rosenberg H: Malignant hyperthermia-like syndrome associated with metrizamide myelography. *Anesth Analg* **68**:795, 1989.
216. Delay J, Deniker P: Drug-induced extrapyramidal syndromes. *Handb Clin Neurol* **16**:248 1968.
217. Spiess-Kiefer C: MH-verwandte Krankheitsbilder. *Beitr Anaesthesiol Intensivmed* **27**:97, 1989.
218. Krivosic-Horber R, Adnet PJ: MH and neuroleptic malignant syndrome. *Beitr Anaesthesiol Intensivmed* **27**:108, 1989.
219. Matsui K, Fujioka Y, Takahashi M, Fujii K, Morio M: Differences in calcium related functions in skeletal muscle between MH and neuroleptic malignant syndrome, in Hofmann JG, Schmidt A (eds): *Malignant Hyperthermia: An Update*. Berlin, Volk und Gesundheit, 1989, p 160.
220. Miyatake R, Iwahashi K, Matsushita M, Nakamura K, Suwaiki H: No association between the neuroleptic malignant syndrome and mutations in the RYR1 gene associated malignant hyperthermia. *J Neurol Sci* **143**:161, 1996.
221. Hackl W, Winkler M, Mauritz W, Sporn P, Steinbereithner K: Muscle biopsy for diagnosis of malignant hyperthermia susceptibility in two patients with severe exercise-induced myolysis. *Br J Anaesth* **66**:138, 1991.

222. Jones DE, Ryan JF: Treatment of acute hyperthermia crises, in Britt BA (ed): *Malignant Hyperthermia*. Boston, Martinus Nijhoff, 1987, p 393.
223. Bevan DR, Bevan JC, Donati F: *Muscle Relaxants in Clinical Anesthesia*. Chicago, Year Book Medical, 1988.
224. Mauritz W, Hackl W, Steinbereithner K: Therapie der malignen Hyperthermie (MH). *Beitr Anaesthesiol Intensivmed* **27**:173, 1989.
225. Krivosic-Horber R: Treatment of the acute episode. *Acta Anaesthesiol Belg* **41**:83, 1990.
226. Ranklev E, Fletcher R: Treatment of malignant hyperthermia, in Mortier W, Breucking E (eds): *Malignant Hyperthermia Neuromuscular Diseases and Anaesthesia*. New York, Georg Thieme, 1990, p 83.
227. Jantzen J-PAH, Kleemann PP: Anaesthesia in malignant hyperthermia susceptible patients, in Mortier W, Bruecking E (eds): *Malignant hyperthermia, Neuromuscular Diseases and Anaesthesia*. New York, Georg Thieme, 1990, p 72.
228. Mauritz W: Drugs relevant to malignant hyperthermia. *Beitr Anaesthesiol Intensivmed* **21**:71, 1987.
229. Steinbereithner K, Sporn P, Hackl W, Mauritz W: Narkoseführung bei bekannter MH-Anlage. *Beitr Anaesthesiol Intensivmed* **27**:156, 1989.
230. Mendel B, Rudney H: Studies on cholinesterase: I. Cholinesterase and pseudocholinesterase. *Biochem J* **37**:59, 1943.
231. La Du BN, Bartels CF, Nogueira CP, Arpagaus M, Lockridge O: Proposed nomenclature for human butyrylcholinesterase genetic variants identified by DNA sequencing. *Cell Mol Neurobiol* **11**:79, 1991.
232. Bovet D, Bovet-Nitti F, Guarino S, Longo VG, Marotta M: Proprieta farmacodinamiche di alcuni deravati della succinilcolina dotatie di azione curarica. *R C 1st Sup Sanita* 12:106, 1949 (quoted in *Biol Abstr* **24**:3276, 1949).
233. Bourne JC, Collier HO, Somers GF: Succinylcholine (succinoylcholine): Muscle relaxant of short action. *Lancet* **1**:1225, 1952.
234. Kalow W: Hydrolysis of local anesthetics by human serum cholinesterase. *J Pharmacol Exp Ther* **104**:122, 1952.
235. Kalow W: Entwicklungen der Pharmakogenetik: Ein Ruckblick zum 75 — Geburtstag von Hans Herken. *Klin Wochenschr* **66**:229, 1988.
236. Kalow W, Lindsay HA: A comparison of optical and manometric methods for the assay of human serum cholinesterase. *Can J Biochem Physiol* **35**:568, 1955.
237. Kalow W: Familial incidence of low pseudocholinesterase level. *Lancet* **2**:576, 1956.
238. Kalow W, Genest K: A method for the detection of atypical forms of human serum cholinesterase: Determination of dibucaine numbers. *Can J Biochem Physiol* **35**:339, 1957.
239. Kalow W, Staron N: On distribution and inheritance of atypical forms of human serum cholinesterase, as indicated by dibucaine numbers. *Can J Biochem Physiol* **35**:1305, 1957.
240. Whittaker M: Cholinesterase. *Monogr Hum Genet* 11, 1986.
241. Lockridge O: Genetic variants of human serum butyrylcholinesterase influence the metabolism of the muscle relaxant succinylcholine, in Kalow W (ed): *International Encyclopedia of Pharmacological Therapy*, Sect. 137: *Pharmacogenetics of Drug Metabolism*. New York, Pergamon, 1992, p 15.
242. Brimijoin S, Hammond P: Butyrylcholinesterase in human brain and acetylcholinesterase in human plasma: Trace enzymes measured by two-site immunoassay. *J Neurochem* **51**:1227, 1988.
243. Prody CA, Zevin-Sonkin D, Gnatt A, Goldberg O, Soreq H: Isolation and characterization of full-length cDNA clones coding for cholinesterase from fetal human tissues. *Proc Natl Acad Sci USA* **84**:3555, 1987.
244. McTiernan C, Adkins S, Chatonnet A, Vaughan TA, Bartels CF, Kott M, Rosenberry TL, et al: Brain cDNA clone for human cholinesterase. *Proc Natl Acad Sci USA* **84**:6682, 1987.
245. Lockridge O, Bartels CF, Vaughan TA, Wong CK, Norton SE, Johnson LL: Complete amino acid sequence of human serum cholinesterase. *J Biol Chem* **262**:549, 1987.
246. Lockridge O, La Du BN: Amino acid sequence of the active site of human serum cholinesterase from usual, atypical, and characteristic-silent genotypes. *Biochem Genet* **24**:485, 1986.
247. Arpagaus M, Chatonnet A, Masson P, Newton M, Vaughan TA, Bartels CF, Nogueira CP, et al: Use of the polymerase chain reaction for homology probing of butyrylcholinesterase from several vertebrates. *J Biol Chem* **266**:6966, 1991.
248. Arpagaus M, Kott M, Vatsis KP, Bartels CF, La Du BN, Lockridge O: Structure of the gene for human butyrylcholinesterase: Evidence for a single copy. *Biochemistry* **29**:124, 1990.
249. Allderdice PW, Gardner HAR, Galutira D, Lockridge O, La Du BN, McAlphine PJ: The cloned butyrylcholinesterase (BCHE) gene maps to a single chromosome site, 3q26. *Genomics* **11**:452, 1991.
250. Gaughan G, Park H, Priddle J, Craig I, Craig S: Refinement of the localization of human butyrylcholinesterase to chromosome 3q26.l-q26.2 using a PRC-derived probe. *Genomics* **11**:455, 1991.
251. Soreq H, Zamir R, Zevin-Sonkin D, Zakut H: Human cholinesterase genes localized by hybridization to chromosomes 3 and 16. *Hum Genet* **77**:325, 1987.
252. Robson EB, Harris H: Further data on the incidence and genetics of the serum cholinesterase phenotype C5+. *Am J Hum Genet* **29**:403, 1966.
253. Soreq H, Gnatt A: Molecular biological search for human genes encoding cholinesterases. *Mol Neurobiol* **1**:47, 1987.
254. Chatonnet A, Lockridge O: Comparison of butyrylcholinesterase and acetylcholinesterase. *Biochem J* **260**:625, 1989.
255. Gnatt A, Ginzberg D, Lieman-Hurwitz J, Zamir R, Zakut H, Soreq H: Human acetylcholinesterase and butyrylcholinesterase are encoded by two distinct genes. *Cell Mol Neurobiol* **11**:91, 1991.
256. Brown SS, Kalow W, Pilz W, Whittaker M, Woronick CL: The plasma cholinesterases: A new perspective. *Adv Clin Chem* **22**:1, 1981.
257. Brock A: Immunoreactive plasma cholinesterase (EC 3.1.1.8) substance concentration, compared with cholinesterase activity concentration and albumin: Inter- and intra-individual variations in a healthy population group. *J Clin Chem Clin Biochem* **28**:851, 1990.
258. Brock A, Brock V: Plasma cholinesterase activity in a healthy population group with no occupational exposure to known cholinesterase inhibitors: Relative influence of some factors related to normal inter- and intra-individual variations. *Scand J Clin Lab Invest* **50**:401, 1990.
259. Viby-Mogensen J: Abnormal plasma cholinesterase activity: Implications for the anaesthetist, in Zorab JSM (ed): *Lectures in Anaesthesiology*. London, Blackwell Scientific/Oxford University Press, 1985, p 63.
260. Guillermo FP, Pretel CMM, Royo FT, Marcias MJP, Ossorio RA, Gomez JAA, Vidal CJ: Prolonged suxamethonium-induced neuromuscular blockade associated with organophosphate poisoning. *Br J Anaesth* **61**:233, 1988.
261. De Roetth A, Wong A, Dettbarn WD, Rosenberg P, Wilensky JG: Cholinesterase activity of glaucoma patients treated with phospholine iodide. *Am J Ophthalmol* **62**:634, 1966.
262. Whittaker M, Berry M: The pseudocholinesterase variants: A family segregating for two homozygotes with the fluoride resistant gene. *Hum Hered* **22**:243, 1972.
263. Viby-Mogensen J, Hanel HK: Prolonged apnoea after suxamethonium: An analysis of the first 225 cases reported to the Danish Cholinesterase Research Unit. *Acta Anaesthesiol Scand* **22**:371, 1978.
264. Primo-Parmo SL, Bartels CF, Wiersema B, van der Spek AF, Innis JW, La Du BN: Characterization of 12 silent alleles of the human butyrylcholinesterase (BCHE) gene. *Am J Hum Genet* **58**:52, 1996.
265. Neitlich HW: Increased plasma cholinesterase activity and succinylcholine resistance: A genetic variant. *J Clin Invest* **45**:380, 1966.
266. Yoshida A, Motulsky AG: A pseudocholinesterase variant (E Cynthiana) associated with elevated plasma enzyme activity. *Am J Hum Genet* **21**:486, 1969.
267. Delbruck A, Henkel E: A rare genetically determined variant of pseudocholinesterase in two German families with high plasma enzyme activity. *Eur J Biochem* **99**:65, 1979.
268. Krause A, Lane AB, Jenkins T: A new high activity plasma cholinesterase variant. *J Med Genet* **25**:677, 1988.
269. Simpson NE, Elliott CR: Cholinesterase Newfoundland: A new succinylcholine-sensitive variant of cholinesterase at locus 1. *Am J Hum Genet* **33**:366, 1981.
270. Whittaker M, Britten JJ: E_1^h, a new allele at cholinesterase locus 1. *Hum Hered* **37**:54, 1987.
271. Rubinstein HM, Dietz AA, Lubrano T: E_1^k, another quantitative variant at cholinesterase locus l. *J Med Genet* **15**:27, 1978.
272. Whittaker M, Britten J: Recognition of two new phenotypes segregating the E_1^k allele for plasma cholinesterase. *Hum Hered* **38**:233, 1988.
273. Bartels CF, James K, La Du BN: DNA mutations associated with the human butyrylcholinesterase J-variant. *Am J Hum Genet* **50**:1104, 1992.
274. Lehmann DJ, Johnston C, Smith AD: Synergy between the genes for butyrylcholinesterase K variant and apolipoprotein E4 in late-onset confirmed Alzheimer's disease. *Hum Mol Genet* **6**:1933, 1997.
275. Maekawa M, Sudo K, Dey DC, Ishikawa J, Izumi M, Kotani K, Kanno T: Genetic mutations of butyrylcholine esterase identified from phenotypic abnormalities in Japan. *Clin Chem* **43**:924, 1997.

276. Altland K, Goedde HW: Heterogeneity in the silent gene phenotype of pseudocholinesterase of human serum. *Biochem Genet* **4**:321, 1970.
277. Rubinstein HM, Dietz AA, Hodges LK, Lubrano T, Czebotar V: Silent cholinesterase gene: Variations in the properties of serum enzyme in apparent homozgotes. *J Clin Invest* **49**:479, 1970.
278. Masson P, Legrand P, Bartels CF, Froment MT, Schopfer LM, Lockridge O: Role of aspartate 70 and tryptophan 82 in binding of succinyldithiocholine to human butyrylcholinesterase. *Biochemistry* **36**:2266, 1997.
279. Kalow W, Davies RO: The activity of various esterase inhibitors towards atypical human serum cholinesterase. *Biochem Pharmacol* **1**:183, 1958.
280. Masson P, Froment MT, Bartels CF, Lockridge O: Asp70 in the peripheral anionic site of human butyrylcholinesterase. *Eur J Biochem* **235**:36, 1996.
281. Neville LF, Gnatt A, Loewenstine Y, Soreq H: Aspartate-70 to glycine substitution confers resistance to naturally occurring and synthetic anionic-site ligands on in-ovo produced human butyrylcholinesterase. *J Neurosci Res* **27**:452, 1990.
282. Garry PJ, Owen GM, Lubin AH: Identification of serum cholinesterase fluoride variants by differential inhibition in tris and phosphate buffers. *Clin Chem* **18**:105, 1972.
283. Masson P, Adkins S, Govet P, Lockridge O: Recombinant human benzoylcholinesterase G 390V, the fluoride-2 variant expressed in CHO cells is a low affinity variant. *J Biol Chem* **268**:14329, 1993.
284. Harris H, Whittaker M: Differential inhibition of human serum cholinesterase with fluoride: Recognition of two new phenotypes. *Nature* **191**:496, 1961.
285. Kalow W, Gunn DR: The relation between dose of succinylcholine and duration of apnea in man. *J Pharmacol Exp Ther* **120**:203, 1957.
286. Vickers MD, Morgan M, Spencer PSJ: *Drugs in Anaesthetic Practice,* 7th ed. Butterworth Heinemann, 1991.
287. Viby-Mogensen J: Correlation of succinylcholine duration of action with plasma cholinesterase activity in subjects with the genotypically normal enzyme. *Anesthesiology* **53**:517, 1980.
288. Viby-Mogensen J: Succinylcholine neuromuscular blockade in subjects heterozygous for abnormal plasma cholinesterase. *Anesthesiology* **55**:231, 1981.
289. Whittaker M: Pharmacogenetic studies of suxamethonium sensitivity, in Quartino AR, Cominetti M, DeBellis P (eds): *Pharmacogenetics and Anaesthetics.* Genoa, Silver, 1988, p 59.
290. Kuhnert BR, Philipson EH, Pimental R, Kuhnert PM: A prolonged chloroprocaine epidural block in a postpartum patient with abnormal pseudocholinesterase. *Anesthesiology* **56**:477, 1982.
291. Raj PP, Rosenblatt R, Miller J, Katz RL, Carden E: Dynamics of local-anesthetic compounds in regional anesthesia. *Anesth Analg* **56**:110, 1977.
292. Stewart DJ, Inaba T, Tang BK, Kalow W: Hydrolysis of cocaine in human plasma by cholinesterase. *Life Sci* **20**:1557, 1977.
293. Stewart DJ, Inaba T, Lucassen M, Kalow W: Cocaine metabolism: Cocaine and norcocaine hydrolysis by liver and serum esterases. *Clin Pharmacol Ther* **25**:464, 1979.
294. Gatley SJ: Activities of the enantiomers of cocaine and some related compounds as substrates and inhibitors of plasma butyrylcholinesterase. *Biochem Pharmacol* **41**:1249, 1991.
295. Inaba T, Stewart DJ, Kalow W: Metabolism of cocaine in man. *Clin Pharmacol Ther* **23**:547, 1978.
296. Ambre J, Ruo TI, Nelson J, Belknap S: Urinary excretion of cocaine, benzoylecgonine, and ecgonine methyl ester in humans. *J Anal Toxicol* **12**:301, 1988.
297. Inaba T: Cocaine: Pharmacokinetics and biotransformation in man. *Can J Physiol Pharmacol* **67**:1154, 1989.
298. Aaron CK, Hirschman Z, Smilkstein MJ: Street pharmacology: A dangerous new way to prolong the high [abstr]. *Vet Hum Toxicol* **31**:375, 1989.
299. Hoffman RS, Henry GC, Howland MA, Weisman RS, Weil L, Goldfrank LR: Association between life-threatening cocaine toxicity and plasma cholinesterase activity. *Ann Emerg Med* **21**:247, 1992.
300. Kalow W: Genetic mechanisms of idiosyncratic drug reactions, in Naranjo CA, Jones JK (eds): *Idiosyncratic Adverse Drug Reactions.* New York, Elsevier Science, 1990, p 159.
301. Mattes CE, Lynch TJ, Singh A, Bradley RM, Kellaris PA, Brady RO, Dretchen KL: Therapeutic use of butyrylcholinesterase for cocaine intoxication. *Toxicol Appl Pharmacol* **145**:372, 1997.
302. Gorelick DA: Enhancing cocaine metabolism with butyrylcholinesterase as a treatment strategy. *Drug Alcohol Depend* **48**:159, 1997.
303. Lynch TJ, Mattes CE, Singh A, Bradley RM, Brady RO, Dretchen KL: Cocaine detoxification by human plasma butyrylcholinesterase. *Toxicol Appl Pharmacol* **145**:363, 1997.
304. Grunwald J, Marcus D, Papier Y, Raveh L, Pittel Z, Ashani Y: Large-scale purification and long-term stability of human butyrylcholinesterase: A potential bioscavenger drug. *J Biochem Biophys Methods* **34**:123, 1997.
305. Johns ME, Henderson RL: Cocaine use by the otolaryngologist: A survey. *Trans Am Acad Ophthamol Otol* **84**:969, 1976.
306. Jones R: The pharmacology of cocaine. *NIDA Res Monog Ser* **50**:34, 1984.
307. Tipton GA, DeWitt GW, Eisenstein SJ: Topical TAC (tetracaine, adrenaline, cocaine) solution for local anesthesia in children: Prescribing inconsistency and acute toxicity. *South Med J* **82**:1344, 1989.
308. Cregler LL, Mark H: Medical complications of cocaine abuse. *N Engl J Med* **315**:1495, 1989.
309. Loper KA: Clinical toxicology of cocaine. *Med Toxicol Adverse Drug Exp* **4**:174, 1989.
310. Washton AM, Gold MS: *Cocaine: A Clinician's Handbook.* Chichester, NY, John Wiley and Sons, 1987.
311. Lange F, Cigarroa R, Yancy C, Willard J, Popma J, Sills M, McBride W, et al: Cocaine-induced coronary-artery vasoconstriction. *N Engl J Med* **321**:1557, 1986.
312. Isner JM, Chokshi SK: Cocaine and vasospasm. *N Engl J Med* **321**:1604, 1989.
313. Cregler LL: Protracted elimination of cocaine metabolites. *Am J Med* **86**:632, 1989.
314. Williams FM, Asad SI, Lessol MH, Rawlins MD: Plasma esterase activity in patients with aspirin-sensitive asthma or urticaria. *Eur J Clin Pharmacol* **33**:387, 1987.
315. Myers C, Lockridge O, La Du BN: Hydrolysis of methylprednisolone acetate by human serum cholinesterase. *Drug Metab Dispos* **10**:279, 1982.
316. Savarese JJ, Hassan HH, Basta SJ, Embree PB, Scott RPF, Sunder N, Weakly JN, et al: The clinical neuromuscular pharmacology of mivacurium chloride (BW 1090U): A short-acting nondepolarizing ester neuromuscular blocking drug. *Anesthesiology* **68**:723, 1988.
317. Tunek A, Svensson LA: Bambuterol, a carbamate ester prodrug of terbutaline, as inhibitor of cholinesterases in human blood. *Drug Metab Dispos* **16**:759, 1988.
318. Fisher DM, Caldwell JE, Sharma M, Wiren JE: The influence of bambuterol (carbamated terbutaline) on the duration of action of succinylcholine-induced paralysis in humans. *Anesthesiology* **69**:757, 1988.
319. Bang U, Viby-Mogensen J, Wiren JE: The effect of bambuterol on plasma cholinesterase activity and suxamethonium-induced neuromuscular blockade in subjects heterozygous for abnormal plasma cholinesterase. *Acta Anaesthesiol Scand* **34**:600, 1990.
320. Bang U, Viby-Mogensen J, Wiren JE, Skovgaard LT: The effect of bambuterol (carbamylated terbutaline) on plasma cholinesterase activity and suxamethonium-induced neuromuscular blockade in genotypically normal patients. *Acta Anaesthesiol Scand* **34**:596, 1990.
321. Guillozet AL, Smiley JF, Mash DC, Mesulam MM: Butyrylcholinesterase in the life cycle of amyloid plaques. *Ann Neurol* **42**:909, 1997.
322. Gomez-Ramos P, Moran MA: Ultrastructural localization of butyrylcholinesterase in senile plaques in the brains of aged and Alzheimer disease patients. *Mol Chem Neuropathol* **30**:161, 1997.
323. Singleton AB, Smith G, Gibson AM, Woodward R, Perry RH, Ince PG, Edwardson JA, Morris CM: No association between the K variant of the butyrylcholinesterase gene and pathologically confirmed Alzheimer's disease. *Hum Mol Genet* **5**:937, 1998.
324. Brindle N, Song Y, Rogaeva E, Premkumar S, Levesque G, Yu G, Ikeda M, et al: Analysis of the butyrylcholinesterase gene and nearby chromosome 3 markers in Alzheimer disease. *Hum Mol Genet* **7**:933, 1998.
325. Lawrence AD, Sahakian BJ: The cognitive psychopharmacology of Alzheimer's disease: Focus on cholinergic systems. *Neurochem Res* **23**:787, 1998.
326. Darvesh S, Grantham DL, Hopkins DA: Distribution of butyrylcholinesterase in the human amygdala and hippocampal formation. *J Comp Neurol* **393**:374, 1998.
327. Farlow MR, Lahiri DK, Poirier J, Davignon J, Schneider L, Hui SL: Treatment outcome of tacrine therapy depends on apolipoprotein genotype and gender of the subjects with Alzheimer's disease. *Neurology* **50**:669, 1998.

328. Bolioli B, Costello ME, Jerusalinsky D, Rubinstein M, Medina J, Dajas F: Neurochemical and behavioral correlates of unlateral striatal acetylcholinesterase inhibition by fasciculin in rats. *Brain Res* **504**:1, 1989.
329. Loewenstein-Lichtenstein Y, Schwarz M, Glick D, Norgaard-Pedersen B, Zakut H, Soreq H: Genetic predispostion to adverse consequences of anti-cholinesterases in 'atypical' BCHE carriers. *Nat Med* **10**:1082, 1995.
330. Haley RW, Kurt TL: Self-reported exposure to neurotoxic chemical combinations in the Gulf War: A cross-sectional epidemiologic study. *JAMA* **277**:231, 1997.
331. McGuire MC, Nogueira CP, Bartels CF, Lightstone H, Hajra A, Van der Spek AFL, Lockridge O, La Du BN: Identification of the structural mutation responsible for the dibucaine-resistant (atypical) variant form of human serum cholinesterase. *Proc Natl Acad Sci USA* **86**:953, 1989.
332. Kalow W, Gunn DR: Some statistical data on atypical cholinesterase of human serum. *Ann Hum Genet* **23**:239, 1959.
333. Liddell J, Lehmann H, Silk E: A silent pseudocholinesterase gene. *Nature* **193**:561, 1962.
334. Nogueiria CP, McGuire MC, Graeser C, Bartels CF, Arpagaus M, Van der Spek AFL, Lightstone H, et al: Identification of a frameshift mutation responsible for the silent phenotype of human serum cholinesterase, Gly 117 (GGT-GGAG). *Am J Hum Genet* **46**:934, 1990.
335. Bartels CF, Nogueira CP, McGuire MC, Adkins S, Rubinstein HM, Lubrano T, Van der Spek AFL, et al: Identification of two different mutations associated with human butyrylcholinesterase fluoride resistance in serum, in *Proceedings of the Third Internation Meeting on Cholinesterases, La Grande Motte, France, May 12–16, 1990*. Washington, DC, American Chemical Society, 1990.
336. Bartels CF, Jensen FS, Lockridge O, Van der Spek AFL, Rubinst ein HM, Lubrano T, La Du BN: DNA mutation associated with the human butyrylcholinesterase K-variant and its linkage to the atypical variant mutation and other polymorphic sites. *Am J Hum Genet* **50**:1086, 1992.
337. Garry P, Dietz AA, Lubrano T, Ford PC, James K, Rubinstein HM: New allele at cholinesterase locus 1. *J Med Genet* **13**:38, 1976.
338. Evans RT, Wardell J: On the identification and frequency of the J and K cholinesterase phenotypes in a Caucasian population. *J Med Genet* **21**:99, 1984.
339. Davies RO, Marton AV, Kalow W: The action of normal and atypical cholinesterase of human serum upon a series of esters of choline. *Can J Biochem Physiol* **38**:545, 1960.
340. Hersch LB, Raj PP, Ohlweiler D: Kinetics of succinyldithiocholine hydrolysis by serum cholinesterase: Comparison to dibucaine and succinylcholine numbers. *J Pharmacol Exp Ther* **189**:544, 1974.
341. Goedde HW, Held KR, Altland K: Hydrolysis of succinyldicholine and succinylmonocholine in human serum. *Mol Pharmacol* **4**:274, 1968.
342. Valentino RJ, Lockridge O, Eckerson HW, La Du BN: Prediction of drug sensitivity in individuals with atypical serum cholinesterase based on in vitro biochemical studies. *Biochem Pharmacol* **30**:1643, 1981.
343. Foldes FF, Davidson GM, Duncalf D, Kuwabara S: The intravenous toxicity of local anesthetic agents in man. *Clin Pharmacol Ther* **6**:328, 1965.
344. Lockridge O, Mottershaw-Jackson N, Eckerson HW, La Du BN: Hydrolysis of diacetylmorphine (heroin) by human serum cholinesterase. *J Pharmacol Exp Ther* **215**:1, 1980.
345. Cholerton S, Daly AK, Idle JR: The role of individual human cytochromes P450 in drug metabolism and clinical response. *Trends Pharmacol Sci* **13**:434, 1992.
346. Lennard MS: Genetically determined adverse drug reactions involving metabolism. *Drug Saf* **9**:60, 1993.
347. Kroemer HK, Eichelbaum M: "It's the genes, stupid": Molecular bases and clinical consequences of genetic cytochrome P450 2D6 polymorphism. *Life Sci* **56**:2285, 1995.
348. Meyer UA, Zanger UM: Molecular mechanisms of genetic polymorphisms of drug metabolism. *Annu Rev Pharmacol Toxicol* **37**:269, 1997.
349. Grant DM, Spielberg SP: Genetic regulation of drug metabolism, in Polin RA, Fox WW (eds): *Fetal and Neonatal Physiology, 2d ed.* Philadelphia, WB Saunders, 1998, p 161.
350. Nelson DR, Kamataki T, Waxman DJ, Guengerich FP, Estabrook RW, Feyereisen R, Gonzalez FJ, et al: The P450 superfamily: Update on new sequences, gene mapping, accession numbers, early trivial names of enzymes, and nomenclature. *DNA Cell Biol* **12**:1, 1993.
351. Silas JH, Lennard MS, Tucker GT, Smith AJ, Malcolm SL, Marten TR: Why hypertensive patients vary in their response to oral debrisoquine. *BMJ* **1**:422, 1977.
352. Idle JR, Maghoub A, Lancaster R, Smith RL: Hypotensive response to debrisoquine and hydroxylation phenotype. *Life Sci* **22**:979, 1978.
353. Evans DAP, Maghoub A, Sloan TP, Idle JR, Smith RL: A family and population study of the genetic polymorphism of debrisoquine oxidation in a white British population. *J Med Genet* **17**:102, 1980.
354. Bertilsson L, Dengler HJ, Eichelbaum M, Schulz H-U: Pharmacogenetic covariation of defective N-oxidation of sparteine and 4-hydroxylation of debrisoquine. *Eur J Clin Pharmacol* **17**:153, 1980.
355. Eichelbaum M, Bertilsson L, Sawe B, Zekorn C: Polymorphic oxidation of sparteine and debrisoquine: Related pharmacogenetic entities. *Clin Pharmacol Ther* **31**:184, 1982.
356. Inaba T, Vinks A, Otton SV, Kalow W: Comparative pharmacogenetics of sparteine and debrisoquine. *Clin Pharmacol Ther* **33**:394, 1983.
357. Küpfer A, Schmid B, Preisig R, Pfaff G: Dextromethorphan as a safe probe for debrisoquine hydroxylation polymorphism. *Lancet* **1**:517, 1984.
358. Bertilsson L: Geographical/interracial differences in polymorphic drug oxidation: Current state of knowledge of cytochromes P450 (CYP) 2D6 and 2C19. *Clin Pharmacokinet* **29**:192, 1995.
359. Arias TD, Jorge LF, Lee D, Barranres R, Inaba T: The oxidative metabolism of sparteine in the Cuna Amerindians of Panama: Absence of evidence for deficient metabolizers. *Clin Pharmacol Ther* **43**:456, 1988.
360. Sommers DK, Moncrieff J, Avenant J: Polymorphism of the 4-hydroxylation of debrisoquine in the San Bushmen of Southern Africa. *Hum Toxicol* **7**:273, 1988.
361. Lennard MS, Iyun AO, Jackson PR, Tucker GT, Woods HF: Evidence for a dissociation in the control of sparteine, debrisoquine and metoprolol metabolism in Nigerians. *Pharmacogenetics* **2**:89, 1992.
362. Eichelbaum M, Gross AS: The genetic polymorphism of debrisoquine/sparteine metabolism: Clinical aspects, in Kalow W (ed): *Pharmacogenetics of Drug Metabolism, ed.* New York, Pergamon, 1992, p 625.
363. Meyer UA, Skoda RC, Zanger UM, Heim M, Broly F: Genetic polymorphisms of drug metabolism: Molecular mechanisms, in Kalow W (ed): *Pharmacogenetics of Drug Metabolism*, ed. New York, Pergamon, 1992, p 609.
364. Wolff T, Distlerath LM, Worthington MT, Groopman JD, Hammons GJ, Kadlubar FF, Prough RA, et al: Substrate specificity of human liver cytochrome P-450 debrisoquine 4-hydroxylase probed using immunochemical inhibition and chemical modelling. *Cancer Res* **45**:2116, 1985.
365. Koymans L, Vermuelen NPE, van Acker SABE, te Koppele JM, Heykants JJP, Lavrijsen K, Meuldermans W, et al: A predictive model for substrates of cytochrome P450-debrisoquine (2D6). *Chem Res Toxicol* **5**:211, 1992.
366. De Groot MJ, Bijloo GJ, Martens BJ, van Acker FA, Vermeulen NP: A refined substrate model for human cytochrome P450 2D6. *Chem Res Toxicol* **10**:41, 1997.
367. Mackman R, Tschirret-Guth RA, Smith G, Hayhurst GP, Ellis SW, Lennard MS, Tucker GT, et al: Active-site topologies of human CYP2D6 and its aspartate-301 → glutamate, asparagine, and glycine mutants. *Arch Biochem Biophys* **331**:134, 1996.
368. Modi S, Paine MJ, Sutcliffe MJ, Lian LY, Primrose WU, Wolf CR, Roberts GC: A model for human cytochrome P450 2D6 based on homology modeling and NMR studies of substrate binding. *Biochemistry* **35**:4540, 1996.
369. Lewis DF, Eddershaw PJ, Goldfarb PS, Tarbit MH: Molecular modelling of cytochrome P450 2D6 (CYP2D6) based on an alignment with CYP102: Structural studies on specific CYP2D6 substrate metabolism. *Xenobiotica* **27**:319, 1997.
370. Smith G, Modi S, Pillai I, Lian LY, Sutcliffe MJ, Pritchard MP, Friedberg T, et al: Determinants of the substrate specificity of human cytochrome P-450 CYP2D6: Design and construction of a mutant with testosterone hydroxylase activity. *Biochem J* **331**:783, 1998.
371. Davies DS, Khan GC, Murray S, Brodie MG, Boobis AR: Evidence for an enzymatic defect in the 4-hydroxylation of debrisoquine by human liver. *Br J Clin Pharmacol* **11**:89, 1981.
372. Inaba T, Nakano M, Otton SV, Mahon WA, Kalow W: A human cytochrome P-450 characterized by inhibition studies as the sparteine-debrisoquine monooxygenase. *Can J Physiol Pharmacol* **62**:860, 1984.
373. Gut J, Gasser R, Dayer P, Kronbach T, Catin T, Meyer UA: Debrisoquine-type polymorphism of drug oxidation: Purification from human liver of a cytochrome P450 isozyme with high activity for bufuralol hydroxylation. *FEBS Lett* **173**:287, 1984.
374. Dayer P, Gasser R, Gut J, Kronbach T, Robertz G-M, Eichelbaum M, Meyer UA: Characterization of a common genetic defect of cytochrome P-450 function (debrisoquine-sparteine type polymorph-

ism): Increased Michaelis constant (Km) and loss of stereoselectivity of bufuralol 1′-hydroxylation in poor metabolizers. *Biochem Biophys Res Commun* **125**:374, 1984.
375. Boobis A, Murray S, Hampden C, Davies D: Genetic polymorphism in drug oxidation: In vitro studies of human debrisoquine 4-hydroxylase and bufuralol 1′-hydroxylase activities. *Biochem Pharmacol* **34**:66, 1985.
376. Gonzalez FJ, Vilbois F, Hardwick JP, McBride OW, Nebert DW, Gelboin HV, Meyer UA: Human debrisoquine 4-hydroxylase (P450IID1): cDNA and deduced amino acid sequence and assignment of the *CYP2D* locus to chromosome 22. *Genomics* **2**:174, 1988.
377. Zanger UM, Vilbois F, Hardwick JP, Meyer UA: Absence of hepatic cytochrome P450bufI causes genetically deficient debrisoquine oxidation in man. *Biochemistry* **27**:5447, 1988.
378. Gonzalez FJ, Skoda RC, Kimura S, Umeno M, Zanger UM, Nebert DW, Gelboin HV, et al: Characterization of the common genetic defect in humans deficient in debrisoquine metabolism. *Nature* **331**:442, 1988.
379. Gough AC, Smith CA, Howell SM, Wolf CR, Bryant SP, Spurr NK: Localization of the CYP2D gene locus to human chromosome 22q13.1 by polymerase chain reaction, in situ hybridization, and linkage analysis. *Genomics* **15**:430, 1993.
380. Eichelbaum M, Baur MP, Osikowska-Evers BO, Tieves G, Zekorn C, Rittner C: Chromosomal assignment of human cytochrome P450 (debrisoquine/sparteine type) to chromosome 22. *Br J Clin Pharmacol* **23**:455, 1987.
381. Skoda RC, Gonzalez FJ, Demierre A, Meyer UA: Two mutant alleles of the human cytochrome P-450db1 gene (*P4502D1*) associated with genetically deficient metabolism of debrisoquine and other drugs. *Proc Natl Acad Sci USA* **85**:5240, 1988.
382. Broly F, Gaedigk A, Heim M, Eichelbaum M, Morike K, Meyer UA: Debrisoquine/sparteine hydroxylation genotype and phenotype: Analysis of common mutations and alleles of *CYP2D6* in a European population. *DNA Cell Biol* **10**:545, 1991.
383. Heim MH, Meyer UA: Evolution of a highly polymorphic human cytochrome P450 gene cluster: CYP2D6. *Genomics* **14**:49, 1992.
384. Kimura S, Umeno M, Skoda RC, Gelboin HV, Meyer UA, Gonzalez FJ: The human debrisoquine 4-hydroxylase (CYP2D) locus: Sequence and identification of the polymorphic CYP2D6 gene, a related gene, and a pseudogene. *Am J Hum Genet* **45**:889, 1989.
385. Marez D, Legrand M, Sabbagh N, Guidice JM, Spire C, Lafitte JJ, Meyer UA, et al: Polymorphism of the cytochrome P450 CYP2D6 gene in a European population: Characterization of 48 mutations and 53 alleles, their frequencies and evolution. *Pharmacogenetics* **7**:193, 1997.
386. Daly AK, Brockmoller J, Broly F, Eichelbaum M, Evans WE, Gonzalez FJ, Huang JD, et al: Nomenclature for human CYP2D6 alleles. *Pharmacogenetics* **6**:193, 1996.
387. Hanioka N, Kimura S, Meyer UA, Gonzalez FJ: The human CYP2D locus associated with a common genetic defect in drug oxidation: A G_{1934} to A base change in intron 3 of a mutant CYP2D6 allele results in an aberrant splice recognition site. *Am J Hum Genet* **47**:994, 1990.
388. Kagimoto M, Heim M, Kagimoto K, Zeugin T, Meyer U: Multiple mutations of the human cytochrome P4502D6 gene (*CYP2D6*) in poor metabolizers of debrisoquine: Study of the functional significance of individual mutations by expression of chimeric genes. *J Biol Chem* **265**:17209, 1990.
389. Gaedigk A, Blum M, Gaedigk R, Eichelbaum M, Meyer UA: Deletion of the entire cytochrome P450 CYP2D6 gene as a cause of impaired drug metabolism in poor metabolizers of the debrisoquine/sparteine polymorphism. *Am J Hum Genet* **48**:943, 1991.
390. Evert B, Eichelbaum M, Haubruck H, Zanger UM: Functional properties of CYP2D6 1 (wild-type) and CYP2D6 7 (His324Pro) expressed by recombinant baculovirus in insect cells. *Naunyn Schmiedebergs Arch Pharmacol* **355**:309, 1997.
391. Yokoi T, Kosaka Y, Chida M, Chiba K, Nakamura H, Ishizaki T, Kinoshita M, et al: A new CYP2D6 allele with a nine base insertion in exon 9 in a Japanese population associated with poor metabolizer phenotype. *Pharmacogenetics* **6**:395, 1996.
392. Tyndale R, Aoyama T, Broly F, Matsunaga T, Inaba T, Kalow W, Gelboin HV, et al: Identification of a new variant CYP2D6 allele lacking the codon encoding Lys-281: Possible association with the poor metabolizer phenotype. *Pharmacogenetics* **1**:26, 1991.
393. Broly F, Meyer UA: Debrisoquine oxidation polymorphism: Phenotypic consequences of a 3-base-pair deletion in exon 5 of the CYP2D6 gene. *Pharmacogenetics* **3**:123, 1993.
394. Oscarson M, Hidestrand M, Johansson I, Ingelman-Sundberg M: A combination of mutations in the CYP2D6*17 (CYP2D6Z) allele causes alterations in enzyme function. *Mol Pharmacol* **52**:1034, 1997.
395. Johansson I, Lundqvist E, Bertilsson L, Dahl ML, Sjoqvist F, Ingelman-Sundberg M: Inherited amplification of an active gene in the cytochrome P450 CYP2D locus as a cause of ultrarapid metabolism of debrisoquine. *Proc Natl Acad Sci USA* **90**:11825, 1993.
396. Dahl ML, Johansson I, Bertilsson L, Ingelman-Sundberg M, Sjoqvist F: Ultrarapid hydroxylation of debrisoquine in a Swedish population: Analysis of the molecular genetic basis. *J Pharmacol Exp Ther* **274**:516, 1995.
397. Bathum L, Johansson I, Ingelman-Sundberg M, Horder M, Brosen K: Ultrarapid metabolism of sparteine: Frequency of alleles with duplicated CYP2D6 genes in a Danish population as determined by restriction fragment length polymorphism and long polymerase chain reaction. *Pharmacogenetics* **8**:119, 1998.
398. Akullu E, Persson I, Bertilsson L, Johansson I, Rodrigues F, Ingelman-Sundberg M: Frequent distribution of ultrarapid metabolizers of debrisoquine in an Ethiopian population carrying duplicated and multiduplicated functional CYP2D6 alleles. *J Pharmacol Exp Ther* **278**:441, 1996.
399. Meyer UA: Molecular genetics and the future of pharmacogenetics, in Kalow W (ed): *Pharmacogenetics of Drug Metabolism,* New York, Pergamon, 1992, p 879.
400. Gonzalez FJ, Idle JR: Pharmacogenetic phenotyping and genotyping: Present status and future potential. *Clin Pharmacokinet* **26**:59, 1994.
401. Heim M, Meyer UA: Genetic polymorphism of debrisoquine oxidation: Analysis of mutant alleles of CYP2D6 by restriction fragment analysis and by allele specific amplification. *Methods Enzymol* **206**:173, 1991.
402. Stuven T, Griese EU, Kroemer HK, Eichelbaum M, Zanger UM: Rapid detection of CYP2D6 null alleles by long distance- and multiplex-polymerase chain reaction. *Pharmacogenetics* **6**:417, 1996.
403. Sachse C, Brockmoller J, Bauer S, Roots I: Cytochrome P450 2D6 variants in a Caucasian population: Allele frequencies and phenotypic consequences. *Am J Hum Genet* **60**:284, 1997.
404. Broly F, Marez D, Sabbagh N, Legrand M, Millecamps S, Lo Guidice JM, Boone P, et al: An efficient strategy for detection of known and new mutations of the CYP2D6 gene using single strand conformation polymorphism analysis. *Pharmacogenetics* **5**:373, 1995.
405. Legrand-Andreoletti M, Stucker I, Marez D, Galais P, Cosme J, Sabbagh N, Spire C, et al: Cytochrome P450 CYP2D6 gene polymorphism and lung cancer susceptibility in Caucasians. *Pharmacogenetics* **8**:7, 1998.
406. Brosen K, Gram LF: Clinical significance of the sparteine/debrisoquine oxidation polymorphism. *Eur J Clin Pharmacol* **36**:537, 1989.
407. Newton BW, Benson RC, McCarriston CC: Sparteine sulphate: A potent capricious oxytocic. *Am J Obstet Gynecol* **94**:234, 1966.
408. Jack D, Wilkins M: Protecting the poor metabolizer—from what? *Br J Clin Pharmacol* **17**:488, 1984.
409. Smith RL: Polymorphic metabolism of the β-adrenoceptor blocking drugs and its clinical relevance. *Eur J Clin Pharmacol* **28**(Suppl):77, 1985.
410. Lennard MS: The polymorphic oxidation of beta-adrenoceptor antagonists. *Pharmacol Ther* **41**:461, 1989.
411. Clark D, Morgan A, Waal-Manning H: Adverse effects from metoprolol are not generally associated with oxidation status. *Br J Clin Pharmacol* **18**:965, 1984.
412. Al-Hadidi HF, Irshaid YM, Rawashdeh NM: Metoprolol alpha-hydroxylation is a poor probe for debrizoquine oxidation (CYP2D6) polymorphism in Jordanians. *Eur J Clin Pharmacol* **47**:311, 1994.
413. Edeki TI, He H, Wood AJ: Pharmacogenetic explanation for excessive beta-blockade following timolol eye drops: Potential for oral-ophthalmic drug interaction. *JAMA* **274**:1611, 1995.
414. Higginbotham EJ: Topical beta-adrenergic antagonists and quinidine: A risky interaction. *Arch Ophthalmol* **114**:745, 1996.
415. Buchert E, Woosley RL: Clinical implications of variable antiarrhythmic drug metabolism. *Pharmacogenetics* **2**:2, 1992.
416. Siddoway L, Thompson K, McAllister B, Wang T, Wilkinson G, Roden D, Woosley R: Polymorphism of propafenone metabolism and disposition in man: Clinical and pharmacokinetic consequences. *Circulation* **4**:785, 1987.
417. Brosen K: Drug-metabolizing enzymes and therapeutic drug monitoring in psychiatry. *Ther Drug Monit* **18**:393, 1996.
418. Meyer UA, Amrein R, Balant LP, Bertilsson L, Eichelbaum M, Guentert TW, Henauer S, et al: Antidepressants and drug-metabolizing enzymes: Expert group report. *Acta Psychiatr Scand* **93**:71, 1996.

419. Bertilsson L, Dahl ML, Tybring G: Pharmacogenetics of antidepressants: Clinical aspects. *Acta Psychiatr Scand Suppl* **391**:14, 1997.
420. Kraus RP, Diaz P, McEachran A: Managing rapid metabolizers of antidepressants. *Depress Anxiety* **4**:320, 1996.
421. DeVane CL: Pharmacogenetics and drug metabolism of newer antidepressant agents. *J Clin Psychiatry* **55**(Suppl):38, 1994.
422. Nemeroff CB, DeVane CL, Pollock BG: Newer antidepressants and the cytochrome P450 system. *Am J Psychiatry* **153**:311, 1996.
423. Llerena A, Dahl ML, Ekqvist B, Bertilsson L: Haloperidol disposition is dependent on the debrisoquine hydroxylation phenotype: Increased plasma levels of the reduced metabolite in poor metabolizers. *Ther Drug Monit* **14**:261, 1992.
424. Jerling M, Dahl ML, Aberg-Wistedt A, Liljenberg B, Landell NE, Bertilsson L, Sjoqvist F: The CYP2D6 genotype predicts the oral clearance of the neuroleptic agents perphenazine and zuclopenthixol. *Clin Pharmacol Ther* **59**:423, 1996.
425. Arthur H, Dahl ML, Siwers B, Sjoqvist F: Polymorphic drug metabolism in schizophrenic patients with tardive dyskinesia. *J Clin Psychopharmacol* **15**:211, 1995.
426. Andreassen OA, MacEwan T, Gulbrandsen AK, McCreadie RG, Steen VM: Non-functional CYP2D6 alleles and risk for neuroleptic-induced movement disorders in schizophrenic patients. *Psychopharmacology (Berlin)* **131**:174, 1997.
427. Llerena A, Herraiz AG, Cobaleda J, Johansson I, Dahl ML: Debrisoquin and mephenytoin hydroxylation phenotypes and CYP2D6 genotype in patients treated with neuroleptic and antidepressant agents. *Clin Pharmacol Ther* **54**:606, 1993.
428. Otton S, Inaba T, Kalow W: Inhibition of sparteine oxidation in human liver by tricyclic antidepressants and other drugs. *Life Sci* **32**:795, 1983.
429. Dayer P, Desmeules J, Leemann T, Striberni R: Bioactivation of the narcotic drug codeine in human liver is mediated by the polymorphic monooxygenase catalyzing debrisoquine 4-hydroxylation. *Biochem Biophys Res Commun* **152**:1988.
430. Sindrup SH, Brosen K: The pharmacogenetics of codeine hypoalgesia. *Pharmacogenetics* **5**:335, 1995.
431. Poulsen L, Brosen K, Arendt-Nielsen L, Gram LF, Elbaek K, Sindrup SH: Codeine and morphine in extensive and poor metabolizers of sparteine: Pharmacokinetics, analgesic effect and side effects. *Eur J Clin Pharmacol* **51**:289, 1996.
432. Wang T, Roden D, Wolfenden H, Woosley R, Wood A, Wilkinson G: Influence of genetic polymorphism on the metabolism and disposition of encainide in man. *J Pharmacol Exp Ther* **228**:605, 1984.
433. Woosley R, Roden D, Dai G, Wang T, Altenbern D, Oates J, Wilkinson G: Co-inheritance of the polymorphic metabolism of encainide and debrisoquine. *Clin Pharmacol Ther* **39**:282, 1986.
434. Otton S, Inaba T, Kalow W: Competitive inhibition of sparteine oxidation in human liver by β-adrenoceptor antagonists and other cardiovascular drugs. *Life Sci* **34**:73, 1984.
435. Fonne-Pfister R, Meyer UA: Xenobiotic and endobiotic inhibitors of cytochrome P450db1 function, the target of the debrisoquine/sparteine type polymorphism. *Biochem Pharmacol* **37**:3829, 1988.
436. Ono S, Hatanaka T, Hotta H, Satoh T, Gonzalez FJ, Tsutsui M: Specificity of substrate and inhibitor probes for cytochrome P450s: Evaluation of in vitro metabolism using cDNA-expressed human P450s and human liver microsomes. *Xenobiotica* **26**:681, 1996.
437. Gram L, Overo K: Drug interaction: Inhibitory effect of neuroleptics on metabolism of tricyclic antidepressants in man. *BMJ* **163**:463, 1972.
438. Syvülahti E, Lindberg R, Kallio J, de Vocht M: Inhibitory effects of neuroleptics on debrisoquine oxidation in man. *Br J Clin Pharmacol* **22**:89, 1986.
439. Tyndale R, Kalow W, Inaba T: Oxidation of reduced haloperidol to haloperidol: Involvement of human P4502D6 (sparteine/debrisoquine monooxygenase). *Br J Clin Pharmacol* **31**:655, 1991.
440. Niznik H, Tyndale R, Sallee F, Gonzalez F, Hardwick J, Inaba T, Kalow W: The dopamine transporter and cytochrome P450IID1 (debrisoquine 4-hydroxylase) in brain: Resolution and identification of two distinct [^{3}H]GBR-12935 binding proteins. *Arch Biochem Biophys* **276**:424, 1990.
441. Tyndale R, Sunahara R, Inaba T, Kalow W, Gonzalez F, Niznik H: Neuronal cytochrome P450IID1 (debrisoquine/sparteine type): Potent inhibition of activity by (−)-cocaine and nucleotide sequence identity to human hepatic P450 gene *CYP2D6*. *Mol Pharmacol* **40**:63, 1991.
442. Gilham DE, Cairns W, Paine MJ, Modi S, Poulsom R, Roberts GC, Wolf CR: Metabolism of MPTP by cytochrome P4502D6 and the demonstration of 2D6 mRNA in human foetal and adult brain by in situ hybridization. *Xenobiotica* **27**:111, 1997.
443. Martinez C, Agundez JA, Gervasini G, Martin R, Benitez J: Tryptamine: A possible endogenous substrate for CYP2D6. *Pharmacogenetics* **7**:85, 1997.
444. Sellers EM, Otton SV, Tyndale RF: The potential role of the cytochrome P-450 2D6 pharmacogenetic polymorphism in drug abuse. *NIDA Res Monogr* **173**:6, 1997.
445. Tyndale RF, Droll KP, Sellers EM: Genetically deficient CYP2D6 metabolism provides protection against oral opiate dependence. *Pharmacogenetics* **7**:375, 1997.
446. Barbeau A, Cloutier T, Roy M, Plasse L, Paris S, Poirier J: Ecogenetics of Parkinson's disease: 4-Hydroxylation of debrisoquine. *Lancet* **2**:1213, 1985.
447. McCann SJ, Pond SM, James KM, Le Couteur DG: The association between polymorphisms in the cytochrome P-450 2D6 gene and Parkinson's disease: A case-control study and meta-analysis. *J Neurol Sci* **153**:50, 1997.
448. Riedl AG, Watts PM, Jenner P, Marsden CD: P450 enzymes and Parkinson's disease: The story so far. *Mov Disord* **13**:212, 1998.
449. Fonne-Pfister R, Bargetzi MJ, Meyer UA: MPTP, the neurotoxin inducing Parkinson's disease is a potent competitive inhibitor of human and rat cytochrome P450 isozymes (P450bufl, P450db1) catalysing debrisoquine 4-hydroxylation. *Biochem Biophys Res Commun* **148**:1144, 1987.
450. Armstrong M, Daly AK, Cholerton S, Bateman DN, Idle JR: Mutant debrisoquine hydroxylation genes in Parkinson's disease. *Lancet* **339**:1017, 1992.
451. Smith CA, Gough AC, Leigh PN, Summers BA, Harding AE, Maraganore DM, Sturman SG, et al: Debrisoquine hydroxylase gene polymorphism and susceptibility to Parkinson's disease. *Lancet* **339**:1375, 1992.
452. Rempfer R, Crook R, Houlden H, Duff K, Hutton M, Roberts GW, Raghavan R, et al: Parkinson's disease, but not Alzheimer's disease, Lewy body variant associated with mutant alleles at cytochrome P450 gene. *Lancet* **344**:815, 1994.
453. Agundez JA, Jimenez-Jimenez FJ, Luengo A, Bernal ML, Molina JA, Ayuso L, Vazquez A, et al: Association between the oxidative polymorphism and early onset of Parkinson's disease. *Clin Pharmacol Ther* **57**:291, 1995.
454. Lucotte G, Turpin JC, Gerard N, Panserat S, Krishnamoorthy R: Mutation frequencies of the cytochrome CYP2D6 gene in Parkinson disease patients and in families. *Am J Med Genet* **67**:361, 1996.
455. Steiger MJ, Lledo P, Quinn NP, Marsden CD, Turner P, Jenner PG: Debrisoquine hydroxylation in Parkinson's disease. *Acta Neurol Scand* **86**:159, 1992.
456. Bordet R, Broly F, Destee A, Libersa C, Lafitte JJ: Lack of relation between genetic polymorphism of cytochrome P-450IID6 and sporadic idiopathic Parkinson's disease. *Clin Neuropharmacol* **19**:213, 1996.
457. Diederich N, Hilger C, Goetz CG, Keipes M, Hentges F, Vieregge P, Metz H: Genetic variability of the CYP 2D6 gene is not a risk factor for sporadic Parkinson's disease. *Ann Neurol* **40**:463, 1996.
458. Gasser T, Muller-Myhsok B, Supala A, Zimmer E, Wieditz G, Wszolek ZK, Vieregge P, et al: The CYP2D6B allele is not overrepresented in a population of German patients with idiopathic Parkinson's disease. *J Neurol Neurosurg Psychiatry* **61**:518, 1996.
459. Sandy MS, Armstrong M, Tanner CM, Daly AK, Di Monte DA, Langston JW, Idle JR: CYP2D6 allelic frequencies in young-onset Parkinson's disease. *Neurology* **47**:225, 1996.
460. Tsuneoka Y, Matsuo Y, Ichikawa Y, Watanabe Y: Genetic analysis of the CYP2D6 gene in patients with Parkinson's disease. *Metabolism* **47**:94, 1998.
461. Wilhelmsen K, Mirel D, Marder K, Bernstein M, Naini A, Leal SM, Cote LJ, et al: Is there a genetic susceptibility locus for Parkinson's disease on chromosome 22q13? *Ann Neurol* **41**:813, 1997.
462. Le Guellec C, Lacarelle B, Catalin J, Durand A: Inhibitory effects of anticancer drugs on dextromethorphan-*O*-demethylase activity in human liver microsomes. *Cancer Chemother Pharmacol* **32**:491, 1993.
463. Ayesh R, Idle JR, Ritchie JC, Crothers MJ, Hetzel MR: Metabolic oxidation phenotypes as markers for susceptibility to lung cancer. *Nature* **312**:169, 1984.
464. Nebert DW: Role of genetics and drug metabolism in human cancer risk. *Mutat Res* **247**:267, 1991.
465. Caporaso N, Landi MT, Vineis P: Relevance of metabolic polymorphisms to human carcinogenesis: Evaluation of epidemiologic evidence. *Pharmacogenetics* **1**:4, 1991.
466. Idle JR: Is environmental carcinogenesis modulated by host polymorphism? *Mutat Res* **247**:259, 1991.

467. Shields PG, Harris CC: Molecular epidemiology and the genetics of environmental cancer. *JAMA* **266**:681, 1991.
468. N, DeBaun MR, Rothman N: Lung cancer and CYP2D6 (the debrisoquine polymorphism): Sources of heterogeneity in the proposed association. *Pharmacogenetics* **5**:S129, 1995.
469. Crespi C, Penman B, Gelboin H, Gonzalez F: A tobacco smoke-derived nitrosamine, 4-(methylnitrosamino)-1-(3-pyridyl)-1-butanone, is activated by multiple human cytochrome P450s including the polymorphic human cytochrome P4502D6. *Carcinogenesis* **12**:1197, 1991.
470. Islam S, Wolf C, Lennard M, Sternberg M: A three-dimensional molecular template for substrates of human cytochrome P450 involved in debrisoquine 4-hydroxylation. *Carcinogenesis* **12**:2211, 1991.
471. Kivisto KT, Griese EU, Stuven T, Fritz P, Friedel G, Kroemer HK, Zanger UM: Analysis of CYP2D6 expression in human lung: Implications for the association between CYP2D6 activity and susceptibility to lung cancer. *Pharmacogenetics* **7**:295, 1997.
472. Shaw GL, Falk RT, Deslauriers J, Frame JN, Nesbitt JC, Pass HI, Issaq HJ, et al: Debrisoquine metabolism and lung cancer risk. *Cancer Epidemiol Biomarkers Prev* **4**:41, 1995.
473. Christensen PM, Gotzsche PC, Brosen K: The sparteine/debrisoquine (CYP2D6) oxidation polymorphism and the risk of lung cancer: A meta-analysis. *Eur J Clin Pharmacol* **51**:389, 1997.
474. London SJ, Daly AK, Leathart JB, Navidi WC, Carpenter CC, Idle JR: Genetic polymorphism of CYP2D6 and lung cancer risk in African-Americans and Caucasians in Los Angeles County. *Carcinogenesis* **18**:1203, 1997.
475. Shaw GL, Falk RT, Frame JN, Weiffenbach B, Nesbitt JC, Pass HI, Caporaso NE, et al: Genetic polymorphism of CYP2D6 and lung cancer risk. *Cancer Epidemiol Biomarkers Prev* **7**:215, 1998.
476. Caporaso N, Goldstein A: Cancer genes: Single and susceptibility—Exposing the difference. *Pharmacogenetics* **5**:59, 1995.
477. El-Zein R, Zwischenberger JB, Wood TG, Abdel-Rahman SZ, Brekelbaum C, Au WW: Combined genetic polymorphism and risk for development of lung cancer. *Mutat Res* **381**:189, 1997.
478. Eichelbaum M, Reetz K-P, Schmidt EK, Zekorn C: The genetic polymorphism of sparteine metabolism. *Xenobiotica* **16**:465, 1986.

PART 3

GENERAL THEMES

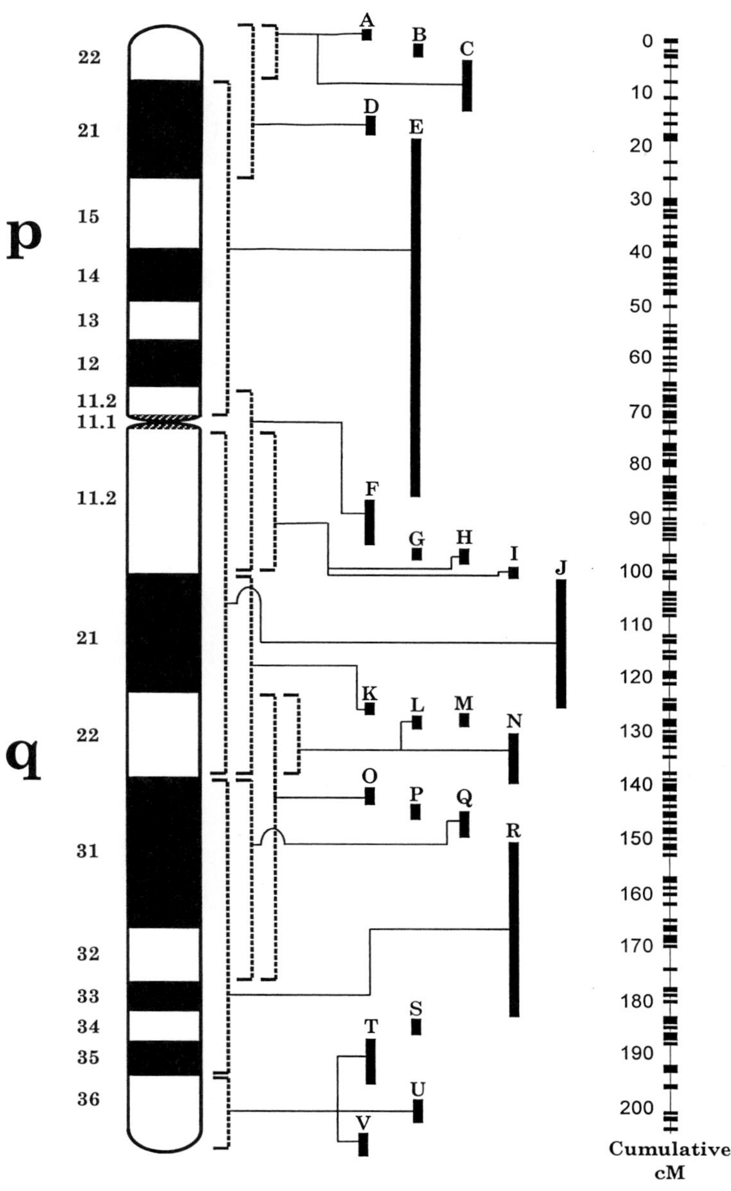

CHAPTER 10

The Human Genome Project and Its Impact on the Study of Human Disease

Eric D. Green

1. **For many human diseases, the fundamental defect resides in a simple alteration in the genome — the master *blueprint* of DNA that orchestrates the basic operation of a cell and an organism. Genetic studies often provide the ability to define at a molecular level the nature of such DNA alterations (i.e., mutations). Knowledge of the normal and abnormal forms of genes is invaluable for understanding the basis of many human genetic diseases.**
2. **The haploid human genome consists of ~3 billion base pairs (bp) of DNA that are distributed among 24 distinct chromosomes (22 autosomes and 2 sex chromosomes). Within this vast array of nucleotides are encoded an estimated 50,000 to 100,000 genes and the necessary elements that control the regulation of their expression.**
3. **Analyzing a genome involves the construction of various types of maps that reflect different features of the DNA, with the major classes being cytogenetic maps, genetic maps, and physical maps. The highest-resolution physical map is the DNA sequence map, which reflects the precise order of nucleotides along a chromosome. Important technological advances have produced a number of powerful methods that greatly facilitate the ability to analyze genomes.**
4. **The Human Genome Project (HGP) is a large, coordinated effort to elucidate the genetic architecture of the human genome and, in parallel, that of several model organisms. The initial phase of this endeavor has mostly involved constructing relatively low-resolution genomic maps and refining the approaches for large-scale DNA sequencing. The next phase of the HGP will focus more on establishing the complete nucleotide sequence of the human and other genomes as well as beginning to decipher the encoded information systematically.**
5. **The products of the HGP are providing a detailed working knowledge about the organization of human DNA and that of several model organisms as well as an infrastructure (in the form of biologic, informational, and technological tools) that is already ushering in a spectacular new era of biomedical inquiry. From a clinical viewpoint, this infrastructure is facilitating the identification and characterization of genes that directly and indirectly lead to human disease, which in turn should ultimately improve the ability to diagnose and treat affected individuals.**

A list of standard abbreviations is located immediately preceding the index in each volume. Additional abbreviations used in this chapter include: BAC = bacterial artificial chromosome; bp = base pair; EST = expressed-sequence tag; HGP = Human Genome Project; kb = kilobase pair; LINE = long interspersed nucleotide element; Mb = megabase pair; PAC = P1-derived artificial chromosome; SINE = short interspersed nucleotide element; SNP = single-nucleotide polymorphism; STS = sequence-tagged site; Web = World Wide Web.

GENETICS AS A PARADIGM FOR STUDYING HUMAN BIOLOGY AND DISEASE

Diseases are associated with alterations of normal biologic processes and can be caused by infectious agents, environmental influences, genetic anomalies, or combinations of these factors. Human disease is classically studied by comparing affected tissues with their unaffected counterparts. Such studies often reveal biochemical and physiological differences, and this information can, in some cases, be used to formulate appropriate therapies. Though this approach has led to the development of a successful treatment for many diseases, it frequently fails to identify the fundamental etiology of the disorder itself. Indeed, the differences encountered in affected tissues are often due to secondary effects rather than consequences of the primary defect. However, in cases where DNA sequence alterations (i.e., mutations) are responsible for the disease, it is possible to identify the fundamental defect by a completely different route, one that uses genetics. Studying diseases by a genetic approach takes advantage of the fact that all humans have an almost identical *DNA blueprint*. Alterations at one or a few positions in the DNA sequence itself are often necessary and sufficient to cause the symptoms of a genetic disease. The identification of such causative mutations provides an opportunity to study and understand the basic biologic defect responsible for that disease.

In humans, genetic studies often start by identifying traits, usually diseases, that appear to cluster in families. Of course, not all diseases that appear multiple times in the same family are genetic in origin, and possible contributions from nongenetic factors must also be considered. In the case of genetic disorders, the challenge is to identify what is often a single-base-pair alteration among the ~3 billion base pairs in the haploid human genome. Causative mutations for only a few of the thousands of human genetic diseases have been identified by the use of hints from biochemical or physiological differences between affected and unaffected individuals. Because this approach is difficult to apply to most genetic diseases, an alternative strategy, called *positional cloning*, has been developed that enables a disease gene to be identified without relying on knowledge or suppositions about the encoded protein.[1–8] Rather, in this strategy, the disease gene is identified on the basis of its location in the genome (see the section "Background on Positional Cloning").

A positional cloning strategy has been used to isolate the causative genes for numerous genetic diseases (see http://genome.nhgri.nih.gov/clone), including relatively common ones such as cystic fibrosis,[9,10] Huntington disease,[11] and hereditary hemochromatosis.[12] To date, however, the strategy has been mostly applied to those diseases caused by defects in a single gene. Many common disorders (e.g., cardiovascular, autoimmune, and psychiatric) have a genetic etiology, but their inheritance is genetically complex, such that mutations in more than one gene are likely required to produce the phenotype.[13–17] In these cases, the responsible genes are difficult to identify by traditional positional cloning for two reasons. First, the strategy must be successfully implemented for the identification of multiple genes. Second, these diseases are complicated by the frequent absence of a strict correlation between genotype and phenotype; instead, an interplay between genetic and environmental factors is typically encountered. Nonetheless, there is increasing optimism that new technologies can be applied in conjunction with increasingly powerful statistical tools to elucidate the genetic bases of complex diseases[13–17] (see Chap. 6).

All the steps involved in the isolation of human disease genes are labor intensive and require the marshaling of extensive resources and specialized skills. A central rationale for the Human Genome Project — an intense, international effort to clone, map, and sequence all of the DNA in the human genome — is to simplify the task of identifying human disease genes. This chapter provides an overview of how the information and reagents being generated by the HGP and related efforts are being used to advance our understanding of genetic disease and human biology. Because it is important to be aware of some basic concepts and the language of geneticists and genomicists, the chapter begins with some background on DNA structure and function, the general "anatomy" of the human genome, and information about genes and other relevant sequences. A major emphasis of the chapter is to describe the experimental approaches that are being used to generate maps, to determine DNA sequence, and to identify genes. Also discussed is the strategic plan for the HGP and how this carefully crafted endeavor is affecting the study of genetic diseases and other biologic problems. An overview of the important role of studying the genomes of model organisms is also provided. Finally, the potential impact of the HGP on the diagnosis and treatment of genetic disease is outlined, and the important ethical, legal, and social issues that are coming to the forefront as a consequence of the HGP are highlighted.

STRUCTURE AND ORGANIZATION OF THE HUMAN GENOME

DNA Basics

DNA is a macromolecule composed of a linear array of deoxyribonucleotides, each of which consists of three components: a nitrogenous base, a sugar (deoxyribose), and phosphate. Each base is linked to adjacent bases on the same strand by the sugar and phosphate groups. The bases in DNA are either purines [adenine (A) and guanine (G)] or pyrimidines [cytosine (C) and thymine (T)], and together these nucleotides constitute the "four-letter alphabet" of DNA that is universal among organisms. In the Watson-Crick helical structure of double-stranded DNA, first reported in 1953,[18] pairing occurs between a purine base on one strand and a pyrimidine base on the opposite strand (i.e., G pairs with C, and A pairs with T), thereby making each strand complementary to the other. It is the order of these bases that encodes the genetic information contained within DNA. Physical lengths of DNA are frequently discussed as individual base pairs, thousands of base pairs (kilobase pairs, or kb), or millions of base pairs (megabase pairs, or Mb). An excellent source of background information on DNA biochemistry and recombinant DNA technology is *Recombinant DNA* by Watson et al.[19]

General Structure of the Human Genome

The human genome contains an estimated 3000 Mb of DNA[20] (Fig. 10-1) divided among 22 autosomes and 2 sex chromosomes (X and Y), which range in size from ~50 to ~260 Mb,[20,21] as well as the DNA present in mitochondria. Human somatic cells are typically diploid (containing 22 pairs of autosomes and 1 pair of sex chromosomes), whereas germ cells (i.e., sperm and egg) are haploid (containing a single copy of each autosome and one sex chromosome). The physical length of the DNA contained in each human cell is remarkably large, theoretically stretching out for about 1 m if fully "unpacked" from the associated proteins. The amount of encoded information within the human genome is even more daunting. In fact, a listing of the nucleotide sequence of the ~3000 Mb in single-letter symbols (G, A, T, C) would fill 13 sets of the *Encyclopaedia Britannica*,[22] 750 megabytes of computer disk space, or roughly 1 CD-ROM.[23]

Subchromosomal Organization of Human DNA

Structural Components of Chromosomes. Human chromosomes are highly organized structures. At the ends of each chromosome are telomeres, which contain sequences thought to stabilize the chromosome, prevent fusion with other DNA, and permit DNA replication without loss of chromosomal material.[24,25] The DNA within a telomere consists of highly reiterated, simple sequence repeats, with the predominant motif in human telomeres being 5′TTAGGG3′.[26] Various human telomeres have been isolated in cloned form,[27–33] allowing more precise dissection of their molecular features and corresponding function. Each chromosome also contains a single centromere, defined functionally by the attachment site of the spindle apparatus during mitosis.[24,34] Human centromeres contain large blocks of repetitive DNA, called *alphoid DNA*,[35–37] which, together with other sequences, span for several megabases. As with telomeres, the cloning and characterization of human centromeric DNA should provide greater insight about the role of specific repetitive sequences in chromosome structure and function.

Interspersed Repetitive DNA Sequences. In contrast to the large and extended blocks of repetitive DNA present in human telomeres and centromeres, most of the remaining regions of human chromosomes contain repetitive sequences that are interspersed among unique segments of DNA.[38,39] The two major classes of interspersed repetitive DNA in the human genome are the short interspersed nucleotide element (SINE) and the long interspersed nucleotide element (LINE). The major SINE is the *Alu* sequence, an ~300-bp segment that is estimated to be present, on average, every 3 to 10 kb (occurring upward of 10^6 times in the human genome). The major LINE is the L1 sequence, a segment that spans up to 6.4 kb in length. Often, only a portion of an L1 sequence is present at a particular site, with an estimated 10^4 to 10^5 L1 copies (complete or partial) present in the human genome. Together, *Alu* and L1 sequences are thought to account for 10 to 25 percent of human DNA. In general, copies of the same repeat (*Alu* or L1) present at different sites in the genome are very similar (but typically not identical) in sequence. However, prototypic consensus sequences have been established for the most common human repetitive elements,[40] thereby allowing their identification within stretches of human DNA sequence.

Coding Versus Noncoding DNA. Within the human genome are an estimated 50,000 to 100,000 genes, which can be as small as 100 bp (e.g., the $tRNA^{Tyr}$ gene) to over 2.3 Mb long (e.g., the dystrophin gene). However, most human genes are thought to span between 1 and 200 kb of genomic DNA. The amino-acid-encoding portions of genes (i.e., coding DNA) represent a small component of the human genome. In fact, some estimates predict that less than 10 percent of human DNA reflects coding sequences and their regulatory elements[41,42]; however, a more meaningful assessment of this number awaits more detailed analysis. The remaining noncoding DNA in the human genome consists of repetitive DNA and other sequences whose importance is not completely understood and undoubtedly not fully appreciated.

A. TOTAL SIZE

Human Genome

3,000,000,000 bp

Human Chromosome (average)

130,000,000 bp

Fruit Fly Genome

160,000,000 bp

Nematode Genome

100,000,000 bp

Yeast Genome

15,000,000 bp

E. coli Genome

5,000,000 bp

B. CLONING CAPACITY

YAC

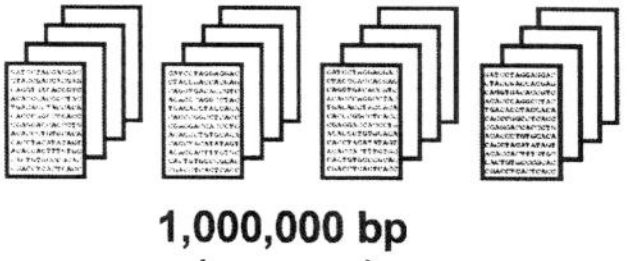

1,000,000 bp (or more)

BAC

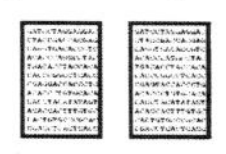

100,000 bp

Cosmid

45,000 bp

Bacteriophage

25,000 bp

Fig. 10-1 Relative sizes of genomes, chromosomes, and cloned DNA segments. A: The estimated total sizes of various DNA sources, along with corresponding schematic representations by using books that contain the written DNA sequence. Each book represents ~50,000,000 bp of DNA sequence. B: The total cloning capacities of a yeast artificial chromosome (YAC), a bacterial artificial chromosome (BAC), a cosmid, and a bacteriophage clone, along with corresponding schematic representations by using pages of books that contain the written DNA sequence. Each page represents ~50,000 bp of DNA sequence, which is roughly 16 times the number of characters on a typical page of this book. (*Adapted from Green and Waterston.*[474] *Used by permission.*)

Gene Structure. Human genes (also called *transcription units*) are complex structures containing several major components. *Exons* are the segments of DNA in a gene that include the sequences encoding amino acids. Between adjacent exons of a gene are intervening sequences known as *introns*, which in some cases extend for hundreds of kilobase pairs. Following generation of the corresponding messenger RNA (mRNA) from a gene by transcription, the introns are removed from the mRNA in a series of steps known as *splicing*. The processed mRNA is then used to direct the sequential and precise addition of amino acids to yield a specific polypeptide chain by a process known as *translation*. Because different mRNAs can be produced from the same gene by alternate splicing of the primary transcript, there is a larger number of gene products than there are genes — adding to the complex and combinatorial nature of the genome. Interestingly, some introns have been found to contain whole, smaller genes transcribed from the opposite DNA strand.[43,44] Also associated with genes are adjacent regulatory sequences (including promoters, enhancers, inhibitory sequences, and others) that interact with cellular proteins and other components to determine when, where, and to what level transcription (i.e., gene expression) occurs.

CpG Islands. The dinucleotide CpG (i.e., 5′CG3′) is relatively underrepresented in the human genome, for example, in contrast to the dinucleotide GpC. Among the various enzymes that cleave DNA at precise sequences (called *restriction enzymes*) is a class that cuts relatively infrequently within the human genome (called *rare cutters*), most of which contain a CpG dinucleotide within their recognition sequence. Many such rare-cutting restriction enzymes will not cleave the DNA if the nucleotides within the recognition sequence have been modified by the addition of a methyl group (i.e., if they are methylated). Interestingly, at the 5′ end of many human genes are DNA segments that contain an overabundance of unmethylated CpG dinucleotides.[45] These genomic regions are called *CpG islands* (or *HTF islands* for "*Hpa*II tiny fragments," since numerous small DNA fragments are produced from such segments by digestion with the restriction enzyme *Hpa*II). Thus, methylation-sensitive, rare-cutting restriction enzymes can be used to identify undermethylated CpG islands that essentially mark the 5′ ends of many (but not all) genes.[45–47]

Distribution of Genes, CpG Islands, and Repetitive DNA. The distribution of genes, CpG islands, and interspersed repetitive sequences is not uniform across the human genome. Rather, several interesting patterns are evident that provide some insight about chromosomal organization.[46,48–51] Chromosome preparations can be stained with various agents and examined microscopically, for example, revealing the presence of lighter- and darker-staining regions (or bands) after Giemsa staining (see the section "Cytogenetic Maps"). There is evidence that Giemsa-negative (light) bands tend to contain a greater proportion of housekeeping and tissue-specific genes, CpG islands, DNA sequence with a higher GC content, and SINEs. In contrast, Giemsa-positive (dark) bands tend to contain fewer genes and CpG islands, consist of DNA sequence with a lower GC content, and have more LINEs. Another level of chromosomal organization is the presence of DNA blocks that span over 300 kb in length with relatively homogeneous GC compositions (called *isochores*). Interestingly, the composition of genes among different isochores is not uniform, with the highest gene content being associated with the GC-richest isochores.[52–55] Furthermore, there is evidence that many of the gene-richest isochores are located near the ends of human chromosomes (in the subtelomeric regions).[53,56]

CRITICAL TECHNOLOGIES FOR GENOME ANALYSIS

Central to the HGP has been the development of a number of technologies that are critical for analyzing genomes. A basic understanding of these methods and approaches is necessary to comprehend the experimental bases of most genome mapping and sequencing efforts. Virtually all the techniques described here represent standard tools in the armamentarium of investigators performing genome research as well as those searching for and characterizing human disease genes. An excellent source of information on the technologies and experimental methods intrinsic to the study of genomes is the four-volume series *Genome Analysis: A Laboratory Manual*.[57]

Basic Recombinant DNA Techniques

The isolation and characterization of DNA involve the utilization of a fundamental set of techniques that have been refined over the past two decades.[58,59] Most often, the source DNA (e.g., human DNA) is purified and fragmented to yield more manageable-sized pieces. The tools most often used for the latter step are restriction enzymes, each of which cuts double-stranded DNA at a defined sequence of nucleotides. The size of the recognition sequence varies among restriction enzymes (typically from 4 to 8 nucleotides), with those requiring a fewer number of nucleotides cutting more often than those requiring a greater number (the latter being the rare cutters described in the section "CpG Islands"). Often, it is necessary to reproduce one or more of the resulting DNA fragments, thereby obtaining sufficient quantities for detailed studies. One way this can be done is by *cloning*, whereby foreign DNA is inserted into a rapidly growing organism that is essentially "tricked" into synthesizing the incorporated DNA along with its own. Another way DNA can be reproduced is by the polymerase chain reaction (PCR).

Polymerase Chain Reaction

Few (if any) experimental techniques have had as dramatic an impact on biomedical research as PCR.[60–62] In the simplest view, PCR involves the in vitro enzymatic synthesis of large amounts of a specific DNA segment. The target DNA is defined by two short (typically 18 to 25 bases each), single-stranded oligonucleotides (primers) that anneal to complementary sequences on opposite strands of the template DNA and initiate (i.e., prime) synthesis back toward one another. The synthesized DNA thus consists of the two oligonucleotides and the sequence between them. Following DNA synthesis, the sample is heated (to greater than 90°C), causing the double-stranded DNA molecules to denature and become single stranded. Upon cooling, unused oligonucleotides (which are present in excess) anneal to available target DNA molecules, and DNA synthesis is once again allowed to proceed.

The standard cycle (DNA synthesis, denaturation, and primer annealing) is repeated 25 to 40 times, with the products of each cycle serving as templates during subsequent cycles. This results in the exponential accumulation (or amplification) of the target DNA sequence defined by the two flanking primers, with the production of as many as a million copies of the target DNA molecule. The size of the DNA segment that can be amplified is typically between 60 and 4000 bp, although segments as large as 10 to 30 kb can be amplified under special conditions. It is important to stress that the critical aspect of PCR is the specificity of the oligonucleotide primers. The ability to amplify a particular DNA sequence often depends on designing an appropriate pair of primers that will uniquely and faithfully anneal to the target DNA under the proper conditions, even when present in a complex mixture such as total genomic DNA.

Like other areas of molecular biology, several important advances have catalyzed the explosive growth of PCR in genome research.[63] These include (1) the generation of improved thermostable DNA polymerases[64] and PCR-enhancing reagents, (2) the design of more sophisticated instrumentation that improves the efficiency with which PCR assays can be subjected to thermal cycling, and (3) the development of more robust and automated methods for chemically synthesizing large numbers of oligonucleotide primers,[65,66] which in turn has dramatically reduced the cost of synthesizing PCR primers. Together, these and other advances have catapulted PCR to become one of the most widely used experimental methods in research today, including its use for a wide array of tasks inherent to the study of genomes.[63] As a result, the HGP has benefited tremendously from the use of PCR; ironically, PCR was not yet invented[60,62] when the initial proposals and earliest plans for the HGP were first discussed.[67–69] In retrospect, the thought of embarking on the HGP without PCR is terrifying.

DNA Cloning Systems

Standard Bacterial Cloning Systems. Traditional DNA cloning systems are based in prokaryotic cells, typically the bacterium *Escherichia coli*. For example, plasmids are extrachromosomal DNA molecules that can be engineered to contain relatively small pieces (most often less than 10 kb) of exogenous DNA.[58] A modified form of plasmids, called *cosmids*, can accommodate cloned DNA segments upward of 40 to 45 kb[58,70] (Fig. 10-1). Bacteriophages are viruses that infect bacteria, and certain types, such as phage lambda, can be modified to carry up to 25 kb of foreign DNA in cloned form[58] (Fig. 10-1). Because of their capacity for intermediate amounts of cloned DNA, cosmid (and, to some extent, bacteriophage) clones have played important roles in some aspects of genome mapping. For example, strategies for using cosmids to isolate and map large segments of human DNA have been developed;[71–74] however, these efforts have rarely resulted in contiguous cloned coverage extending much beyond 300 to 500 kb. Nonetheless, cosmid and bacteriophage clones

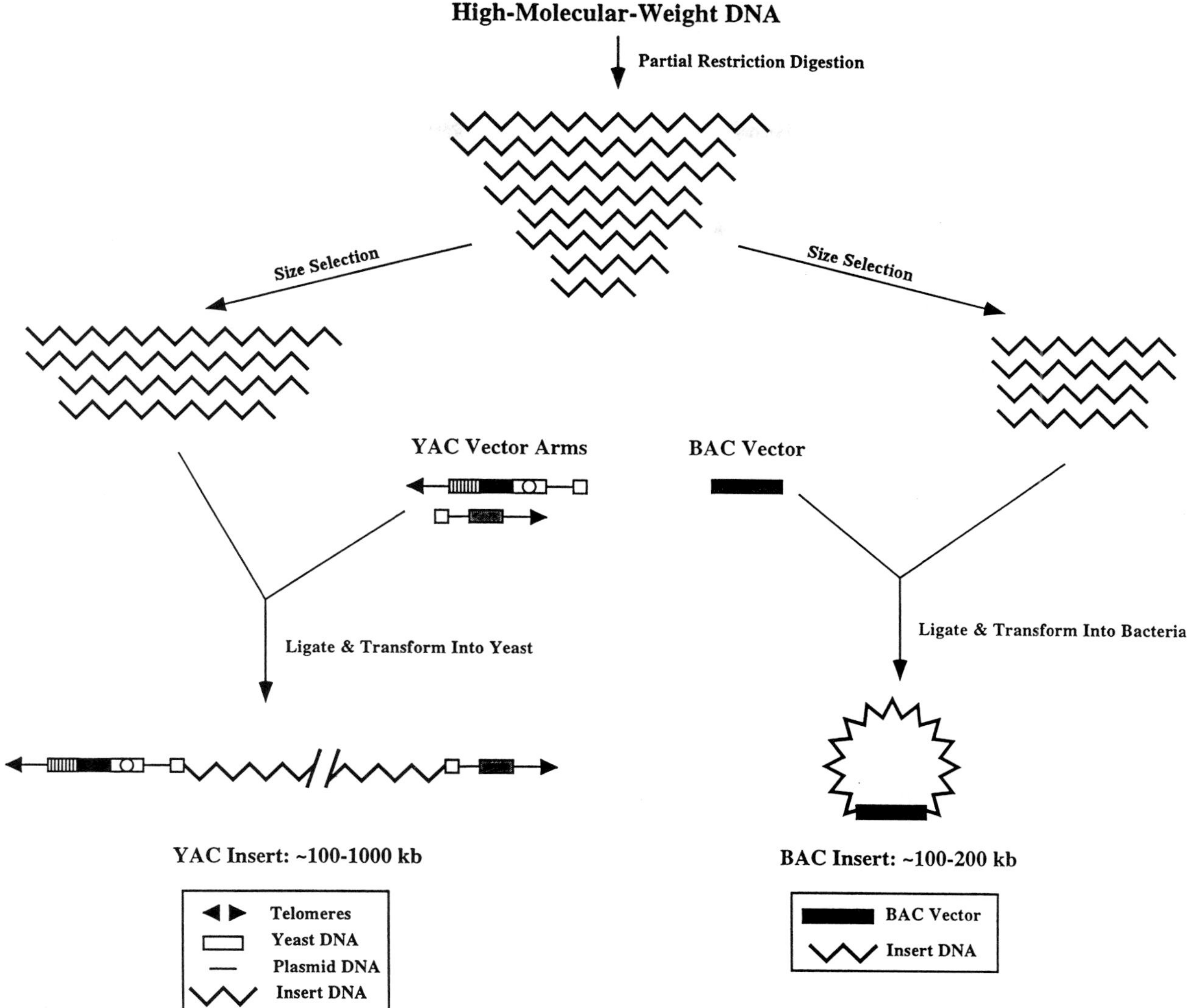

Fig. 10-2 YAC and BAC cloning systems. The general steps involved in the construction of yeast artificial chromosome (YAC, *left*) and bacterial artificial chromosome (BAC, *right*) clones are summarized. Specifically, high-molecular-weight source DNA (e.g., human DNA) is carefully prepared, partially digested with a restriction enzyme, and size selected to yield large DNA fragments (e.g., typically about 200 to 1000 kb for YACs and about 100 to 300 kb for BACs). Appropriate vector sequences are then ligated to the size-selected, insert DNA. For YACs, this consists of two vector arms that together contain all the structural elements necessary for the propagation of a chromosome in yeast (see Green et al.[76] for details). For BACs, this consists of a single vector fragment that contains a suitable antibiotic-resistance gene (see Birren et al.[114] for details). The ligated DNA is then transformed into appropriately prepared yeast or bacterial cells, respectively. The systems are set up such that the only cells that grow are those containing the appropriate yeast-selectable markers (in the case of YACs) or antibiotic-resistance gene (in the case of BACs). Note that the resulting YACs and BACs are linear and circular DNA molecules, respectively.

serve a valuable supplementary role in the study of human DNA and the isolation of genes of interest.

Yeast Artificial Chromosomes. The yeast artificial chromosome (YAC) cloning system was developed in 1987[75] and provides the ability to isolate DNA segments that are significantly larger than those cloned in traditional bacterial-based systems.[76] In this case, the host is the yeast *Saccharomyces cerevisiae* (a eukaryotic cell), and the cloned DNA is contained within a linear artificial chromosome rather than an extrachromosomal DNA molecule (Fig. 10-2). The cloned DNA contained in YACs can range in size from less than 100 kb to over 1000 kb, which is roughly 10 to 20 times larger than the capacity of more traditional bacterial cloning systems, such as cosmids (Fig. 10-1). A number of comprehensive YAC libraries have been constructed from human DNA[77–84] and that of numerous other organisms (for review, see Green et al.[76]), and efficient PCR-based strategies for YAC library screening have been developed.[85]

By providing the means to isolate large segments of cloned DNA, YACs have greatly simplified the process of constructing long-range physical maps of DNA. This capability has now been demonstrated by mapping numerous medically relevant regions of the human genome (e.g., those containing the cystic fibrosis gene,[86,87] the dystrophin gene,[88,89] the HLA class I segment,[90] and the Huntington disease gene,[91,92] just to name a few) as well as whole human chromosomes[93–107] (see the section "Highlights of the Human Genome Project"). Another novel feature of YAC cloning is the ability to use the yeast host for reconstructing large human genes by the sequential recombination of smaller, overlapping YACs,[76] as has been performed to generate single YACs containing the entire ~200-kb cystic fibrosis gene,[86] the ~230-kb *BCL2* proto-oncogene,[108] and the ~2.3-Mb dystrophin gene.[109]

YAC cloning is not, however, without its associated problems. One disadvantage is the difficulty in purifying large amounts of YAC DNA away from the endogenous yeast DNA. Thus, it often becomes necessary to isolate smaller-insert, bacterial-based clones corresponding to the YAC insert prior to performing manipulations such as DNA sequencing, gene identification, and other routine experimental procedures.[76] A more troubling problem associated with YACs is the frequent presence of two unrelated segments of DNA within a single cloned insert. Such *chimeric* YACs constitute half (or more) of the clones in most libraries made from human genomic DNA.[110] Though chimeric clones do not prevent the utilization of YACs for mapping large genomic regions, they can hinder the efficiency and accuracy with which the maps are constructed. A major mechanism by which chimeric YACs form involves recombination between homologous regions (e.g., repetitive DNA) present in unrelated DNA segments.[110] Such yeast-based recombination events likely lead to another problem observed with YACs—the deletion of internal segments within the cloned insert. In the case of chimeric YACs, two different approaches have been successfully used to decrease the problem: the construction of YACs from individual human chromosomes residing within human-rodent hybrid cell lines[76] (see the section "Somatic Hybrid Cell Lines") and the use of recombination-defective yeast strains as hosts.[76] The latter approach has also proved effective at reducing the occurrence of internal deletions in YAC inserts.

Large-Insert Bacterial Cloning Systems. Since the advent of YAC cloning, several new large-insert bacterial cloning systems have been developed. Among these are the bacteriophage P1 system, with a cloning capacity of roughly 75 to 100 kb,[111,112] as well as the bacterial artificial chromosome (BAC)[113,114] and closely related P1-derived artificial chromosome (PAC)[115] systems, with the latter two providing cloning capacities upward of 200 to 300 kb.

In particular, BAC cloning has rapidly emerged as a critical tool for genome analysis (Figs. 10-1 and 10-2). Numerous BAC libraries, with clones averaging 100 to 200 kb in size, have been constructed[116,117] (also see http://bacpac.med.buffalo.edu). These can be screened by PCR- and hybridization-based methods[114,118]; the latter has proved particularly robust and involves the use of membranes containing immobilized clone DNA arrayed at very high densities by robotic workstations.[72,119–123] Furthermore, BAC inserts appear to be quite stable during propagation.[113] As a result, BACs are being used for constructing high-resolution maps of human chromosomes[124–126] and numerous other genomes. Such BAC-based physical maps will undoubtedly supplant the first-generation YAC-based maps as well as provide the necessary templates for systematic sequencing of the human and other genomes (see the section "Genomic Sequencing").

Pulsed-Field Gel Electrophoresis

An important adjunct technology that played a critical role in the development of YACs, BACs, and other large-insert cloning systems is a technique that enables the separation of high-molecular-weight DNA molecules. Conventional approaches for gel electrophoresis (typically in agarose gels) can resolve DNA molecules that are upward of 50 kb in size; however, such methods are incapable of separating significantly larger DNA fragments. To overcome this limitation, techniques have been developed whereby the direction of the electric field applied to the DNA within an agarose gel is periodically alternated.[127–129] This method, called *pulsed-field gel electrophoresis*, can be used to separate DNA fragments up to 10 Mb in size. Numerous refinements and modifications of the basic approaches for pulsed-field gel electrophoresis have been made, making it a routine and straightforward method.[130–132] As a result, pulsed-field gel electrophoresis has been used to study the genomes of model organisms such as yeast,[133,134] to establish long-range restriction maps of human DNA using rare-cutting restriction enzymes,[135–139] to characterize the DNA in large-insert clones such as YACs[75,76,140,141] and BACs,[114] and to detect certain types of mutations causing human genetic diseases.[142]

Fluorescence *in Situ* Hybridization

A common step in the characterization of a cloned DNA segment is the identification of the approximate site in the genome from which it originated (i.e., its location on a particular chromosome). The most direct route for obtaining such information involves hybridizing the DNA segment to preparations of intact chromosomes from metaphase cells using protocols that enable the structural features of the condensed chromosomes to be preserved. If the DNA probe is labeled appropriately, the position(s) of hybridization can be identified by microscopic examination of the chromosomes, thereby allowing assignment of the DNA segment to a particular subchromosomal region. Previously, radioactive labels were employed, which required lengthy exposure of the chromosomes to film and resulted in poor precision of the chromosomal assignments. Major advances in this technology have occurred in recent years, including the development of protocols for using fluorescent tags to label the DNA probes and fluorescence microscopy to establish the positions of hybridization,[143] a technique referred to as *fluorescence* in situ *hybridization* (FISH) (Fig. 10-3).

Continued improvements in the protocols used for performing FISH analysis have greatly enhanced the technology. In general, the basic approaches are now quite efficient and reliable.[144–148] Furthermore, the ability to resolve closely spaced DNA segments has also improved. For example, standard FISH analysis with metaphase-chromosome preparations can be used to discriminate between regions separated by roughly 5 to 10 Mb.[148–150] However,

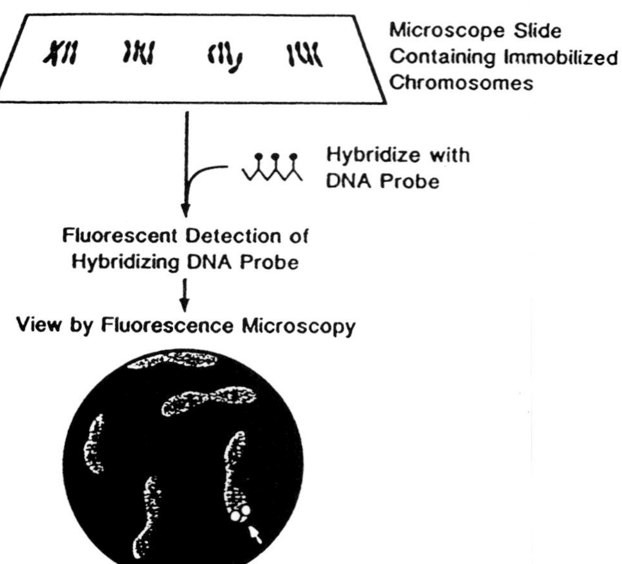

Fig. 10-3 Establishing the chromosomal position of a DNA segment by fluorescence *in situ* hybridization (FISH). Intact chromosomes from cells at metaphase are carefully immobilized on a microscope slide. An appropriate DNA probe (e.g., genomic clone) is labeled with a detectable moiety, such as biotin (depicted as *dark circles*), and hybridized to the immobilized chromosomes. The position(s) of the hybridizing DNA probe is then detected by using an appropriate fluorescence-based system (e.g., fluorescently labeled avidin, which binds to biotin). When examined by fluorescence microscopy, the hybridizing probe (indicated by the *white arrow*) typically appears as two bright yellow spots (one on each chromatid) against an orange background of the chromosome. The approximate chromosomal position of the hybridizing probe can be assessed by parallel examination of the same metaphase chromosomes following appropriate staining.[145–148] *(Adapted from Hozier and Davis.[144] Used by permission.)*

the use of fluorescent tags of different colors in conjunction with specialized methods for preparing the immobilized chromosomes now allows more closely spaced DNA segments to be resolved.[145–148,151–153] Since FISH analysis can establish the position of a cloned DNA segment relative to the source chromosome, this technique has played an important role in genome mapping by spatially organizing clones being used for constructing long-range maps of human chromosomes[154,155] (see the section "Cytogenetic Maps"). Variant methods have been developed for making FISH an even more powerful technology, including techniques that allow each human chromosome to be visualized in a different color.[156–158] Such methods offer great promise for more accurate, robust, and potentially automated karyotypic analysis of human chromosomes.

Somatic Hybrid Cell Lines

Various somatic cell lines have been constructed that contain the entire genome of the host species (e.g., rodent) along with some amount of foreign DNA from another species (e.g., human). In particularly useful cases, the foreign DNA consists of a single, intact chromosome. For example, such a monochromosomal human-rodent hybrid cell line has been derived for each human chromosome (see http://locus.umdnj.edu/nigms). In some cases, sets of hybrid cell lines, each containing a defined portion (but not all) of a particular human chromosome, are also available. Human-rodent hybrid cell lines thus provide access to more limited parts of the human genome. Of course, the human DNA is not "pure"; rather it is mixed within a background of the entire rodent genome (which is roughly the same size as the human genome). The stability of human DNA within human-rodent hybrid cell lines varies widely, especially since there is typically no selective pressure for the rodent cells to retain all the human DNA. As a result, investigators must be cautious when using such cell lines, which typically should include the routine assessment of the presence and intactness of the human chromosome (or fragment) in the cell line (e.g., by cytogenetic analysis). Human-rodent hybrid cell lines have been used extensively to generate genomic clones (e.g., cosmids, YACs, and BACs) from more limited regions of the human genome (e.g., see the section "Yeast Artificial Chromosomes") and as starting material for the development of DNA markers (see the section "Generation of Sequence-Tagged Sites").

One specialized use of somatic hybrid cell line technology is for constructing radiation hybrid cell lines. Specifically, this involves the recovery of radiation-generated chromosome fragments (e.g., from human chromosomes) within a heterologous cell line (e.g., rodent). The resulting cell lines can be used to construct landmark-based physical maps of large genomic regions[159,160] (see the section "Radiation Hybrid Mapping").

DNA Sequencing

A handful of techniques has been developed for determining the precise sequence of nucleotides within a stretch of DNA. Some of these methods have been successfully used to generate large amounts of DNA sequence data, whereas others remain in more developmental stages.[161] The approach described by Sanger and coworkers in 1977,[162] termed *dideoxy chain-termination sequencing*, is the most widely used sequencing method. This technique involves the in vitro synthesis of DNA molecules in the presence of artificial (dideoxy) nucleotides, which prevent chain extension when incorporated into a growing DNA strand. The resulting population of DNA molecules, which terminate at different nucleotide positions, is then analyzed by gel electrophoresis. The relative migration of the various DNA fragments is used to deduce the sequence of the starting DNA template. DNA fragments can be detected by the incorporation of radioactive or fluorescent tags[163,164] into the DNA (Fig. 10-4). Following radioactive sequencing, the gels are exposed to x-ray film to enable detection of the DNA fragments. In contrast, fluorescence-based sequencing involves semiautomated, real-time detection of

A.

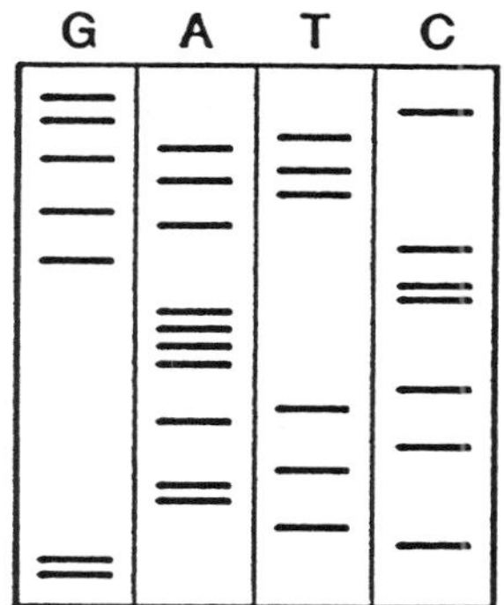

B. GGCTAATCATCAAAACCGCAGTATGATGCG

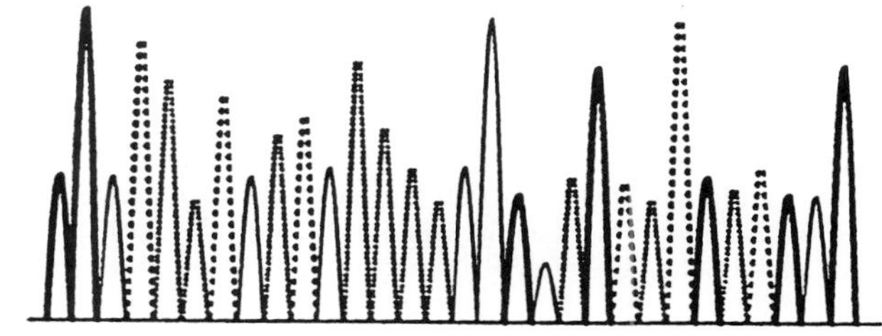

C. GGCTAATCAT
CAAAACCGCA
GTATGATGCG

Fig. 10-4 DNA sequencing by the dideoxy-chain-termination method. The dideoxy-chain-termination sequencing method yields a population of DNA segments of different lengths, each terminated by a particular type of dideoxy nucleotide (i.e., G, A, T, or C) that marks the position of that base in the starting template.[162] The resulting products are then separated by gel electrophoresis. A: The detection of radioactively labeled DNA fragments by autoradiography. In this case, each lane contains the DNA segments generated with a single type of dideoxy nucleotide, with the presence of a band at a particular *rung* position of the sequencing *ladder* reflecting the base at that position in the starting DNA template (the corresponding sequence is shown in C). B: The automated detection of fluorescently labeled DNA fragments. In this case, a laser is used to detect the migration of the fluorescently labeled, dideoxy-terminated DNA fragments as they are electrophoresed through the gel.[163,166] Each type of peak (indicated by *thick, dotted, dashed,* and *thin lines*) reflects the base (G, A, T, and C, respectively) at that position in the starting DNA template (the corresponding sequence is shown in C).

DNA fragments during electrophoresis by laser-based instrumentation.[163,165]

Numerous advances in fluorescence-based sequencing have been made in recent years that make this approach for large-scale DNA sequencing remarkably efficient and robust.[166] These have included the generation of fluorescent-dye-labeled primer[167–169] and fluorescent-dye-labeled terminator[170,171] molecules with improved spectral characteristics and sequencing enzymes that yield longer reads of higher accuracy.[166] Newer sequencing instruments, such as those that employ capillaries rather than slab gels for separating the DNA fragments, are now available, as are better sequencing enzymes and associated reagents.

DNA Chips

A rapidly evolving area of genome research involves the development and utilization of miniaturized DNA microarrays (called *DNA chips*) for performing DNA analysis.[172–177]

Essentially, various standard molecular genetics methods (e.g., PCR, DNA-DNA hybridization, and fluorescence-based image acquisition) are implemented on a microscale, allowing large numbers of analyses to be performed in a massively parallel fashion. Several distinct, although interrelated, DNA chip technologies have emerged and will undoubtedly evolve into powerful new tools for performing genome analysis.

One major type of DNA chip contains a high-density array of short, single-stranded oligonucleotides (~20 nucleotides long).[178–180] These are typically immobilized during their synthesis by a process known as photolithography.[178,179] Very high densities of oligonucleotides can be created (e.g., 100,000 to 400,000 oligonucleotides within a 1.28-cm^2 area). Target DNA, typically PCR amplified and labeled with a fluorescent tag, is hybridized to the immobilized oligonucleotides. The resulting hybridization pattern is then captured with the aid of a microscope and analyzed with suitable software, allowing the precise sequence of the target DNA to be deduced. Thus, in a simple sense, oligonucleotide-based DNA chips should be regarded as *resequencing* chips. This technology has been developed most extensively by the company Affymetrix. Numerous applications are readily apparent for such an efficient chip-based, resequencing method, with successful implementation already demonstrated for analyzing important sequences within pathogens such as HIV-1[181] and *Mycobacterium*,[182] mapping genomic clones,[183] resequencing human mitochondrial DNA,[184] performing mutation screens for human disease genes,[185] comparing sequences of closely related organisms,[186] simultaneously studying the expression of large numbers of genes,[187,188] and performing large-scale analysis of polymorphisms,[189] such as single-nucleotide polymorphisms (SNPs)[190] (see the section "Genetic Markers").

The other major type of DNA chip contains a high-density array of short, double-stranded DNA fragments.[191–196] Typically, these are first derived by PCR amplification and then immobilized onto glass or nylon surfaces by high-speed robotic workstations. A common implementation scheme for this involves the arraying of cDNA fragments on glass microscope slides at densities of greater than 1000 per 1 cm^2. For gene expression studies, hybridization is typically performed with fluorescently labeled mRNA probes and often includes the use of a two-color fluorescence detection strategy that enables the simultaneous examination of parallel mRNA samples derived from different sources. Once again, the resulting hybridization patterns are captured microscopically, with the resulting data analyzed using appropriate software and assimilated in suitable database systems.[197] Thus, this technology can be used to study the expression of literally thousands of genes in different cells or tissues, all within a single experiment. cDNA microarrays have been used to examine gene expression patterns in cells grown under distinct metabolic conditions[193,195,196] and in human cancer.[194] The true power of such expression profiling technology comes in the ability to monitor very large numbers of genes in parallel, thereby gaining insight about the global and integrated networks regulating gene expression.

Variant types of DNA chips include those that contain highly sophisticated, microfabricated systems for performing standard DNA analyses (e.g., PCR, gel electrophoresis, DNA sequencing, and genotyping) on a microscale.[198–205] Here, various technologies have been engineered to enable the handling and analysis of very small DNA samples in a rapid and automated fashion. The development and refinement of such microsystems have tremendous potential to yield important genome analysis tools for use in both research and diagnostic applications.

Computational Genomics

Among the key genomic technologies are those involving the computational analysis of mapping and sequencing data. The rapidly growing field of computational genomics (or bioinformatics), which encompasses everything from computer-based tools that are required for generating genomic data to those that are essential for using it, now represents a well-respected discipline of biomedical research.[206–210] Most major areas of computational genomics are (in some fashion) heavily dependent on the World Wide Web (Web). It is quite fitting, therefore, that the HGP and a major growth spurt of the Web are occurring at the same time; certainly, the former would be greatly weakened by the absence of the latter.

The generation of genomic maps and sequences relies extensively on the use of ever-improving computational tools.[206–210] These include a wide array of data management and analysis programs that have proved instrumental for performing large-scale genome analysis, particularly for the construction of genomic maps and the generation of genomic sequence data.[211–215] In addition, the availability of Web-based mechanisms for data dissemination allows less refined, evolving data to be made available long before they are at a stage suitable for final publication. The latter has been tremendously important to numerous investigators, who have used such preliminary data to accelerate their ongoing studies.

The use of massive amounts of accumulating genome mapping and sequencing data is also critically reliant on the availability of powerful and user-friendly computational tools.[206–210] Among these are systems for data storage and retrieval, such as the public databases that house nucleotide and protein sequences.[207,216–223] These databases and associated tools provide a critical service to the biomedical research community by storing, analyzing, cross-referencing, and disseminating all publicly available mapping and sequencing data, including those being produced by the HGP. In addition, there are ever-improving programs for performing sequence comparisons[224–228] and for predicting the presence of genes[229–235] and promoters[236] within genomic sequence. Also available are various Web sites that provide suites of programs for facilitating routine sequence analysis[237] (e.g., see http://gc.bcm.tmc.edu:8088/search-launcher/launcher.html). In fact, numerous sites on the Web are available for accessing and analyzing genomic data; especially good sites include the National Center for Biotechnology Information (http://www.ncbi.nlm.nih.gov), which operates the premiere genomic database (GenBank), and the National Human Genome Research Institute (http://www.nhgri.nih.gov/Data), which provides a listing of Web sites particularly relevant to genome analysis and the HGP.

Already, biomedical researchers spend sizable amounts of their time in front of computer screens retrieving, analyzing, and manipulating genome mapping and sequencing data. This trend will undoubtedly intensify over time, as increasing amounts of genomic information about numerous organisms are generated at an unprecedented rate.

GENOME MAPPING AND SEQUENCING: EXPERIMENTAL STRATEGIES

Genomic maps are linear representations of DNA that reflect the organization of landmarks based on some coordinate system. The construction of such maps is critical for attaining a global understanding of genome structure and function. There are three major classes of genomic maps: cytogenetic maps, genetic maps, and physical maps (Fig. 10-5). In each case, the coordinates on which the maps are based reflect the experimental method(s) used to establish the order and intervening distances between landmarks. Importantly, the various mapping methods are associated with characteristic resolution ranges (Fig. 10-6) that dictate the utility of the resulting maps. The development of highly integrated cytogenetic, genetic, and physical maps represents a central activity of the HGP.

Cytogenetic Maps

A cytogenetic map represents the appearance of a chromosome when properly stained and examined microscopically. Particularly important is the resulting appearance of differentially staining regions (called *bands*) that render each chromosome uniquely identifiable (Figs. 10-5 and 10-6). In the case of human

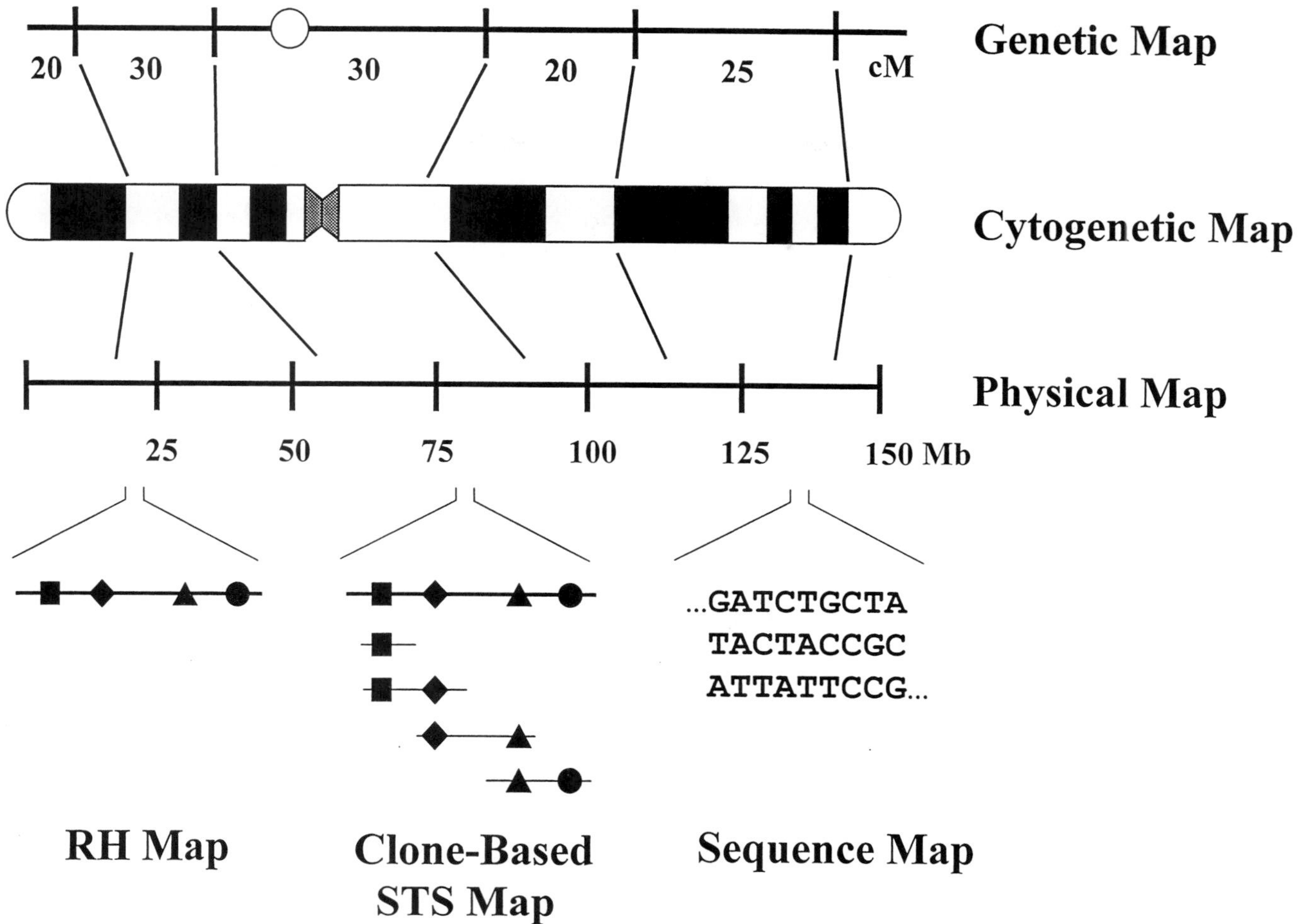

Fig. 10-5 Schematic representations of the genetic, cytogenetic, and physical maps of a human chromosome. For the genetic map, the positions of several hypothetical genetic markers are indicated, along with the distances in centimorgans (cM) between them. The *circle* indicates the position of the centromere. For the cytogenetic map, the classic Giemsa-banding pattern of a chromosome is shown. For the physical map, the approximate physical locations of the above genetic markers are indicated, along with the relative distances between them in megabase pairs (Mb). The three types of physical maps [radiation hybrid (RH), clone-based sequence-tagged site (STS), and sequence] depicted along the *bottom* are discussed in the text. (*Adapted from Green and Waterston.*[474] *Used by permission.*)

chromosomes, individual bands can be specifically discerned and are associated with well-defined names.[238] The most conventional cytogenetic maps depict the 23 chromosomes of the haploid human genome as containing a total of 350 to 500 bands at metaphase (and the amount of DNA split roughly equally between light and dark bands), with each band containing an average of about 5 to 10 Mb of DNA. More sophisticated, higher-resolution methods can be used to detect and represent over 1000 bands in the cytogenetic map of the human genome.[144]

Cytogenetic maps have played a classic role in the diagnosis and study of human genetic diseases. A karyotype, for example, is a visual representation of an individual's cytogenetic map, which may reveal chromosomal deletions, rearrangements, translocations, or other abnormalities. In some cases, the close association between such a cytogenetic abnormality and a particular genetic disorder has served as the starting point for the isolation of the defective gene (e.g., chronic granulomatous disease,[239] Duchenne muscular dystrophy,[240] and fragile X syndrome[241]).

On the surface, cytogenetic maps would appear to have a limited role in genome mapping, in that they are relatively low-resolution (e.g., about 5 to 10 Mb) representations of chromosomes (Figs. 10-5 and 10-6) and they are observational in nature, providing neither cloned DNA for additional studies nor significant assistance in obtaining it. However, cytogenetic mapping serves an important adjunct role in the construction of detailed genomic maps. By dividing the human genome into distinguishable units of 5 to 10 Mb each, cytogenetic maps provide a framework for the construction of other types of maps. For example, cloned DNA segments can be efficiently assigned to specific chromosomal bands by FISH analysis (see the section "Fluorescence *in Situ* Hybridization"), thereby providing the ability to coalign (or integrate) other types of maps (e.g., physical and genetic) with the established cytogenetic maps.[154,155] Similarly, FISH analysis can be used to monitor the quality of evolving physical maps. For example, while mapping a particular chromosomal region, newly obtained clones can be analyzed by FISH, with any evidence of hybridization to some other genomic region alerting the investigator to a potential problem. In addition, the orientation of evolving maps with respect to the centromere and telomeres can often be established by FISH analysis using representative clones from each end of the map.[242] Thus, while the basic cytogenetic map of the human genome is essentially established, efforts continue to localize DNA clones and landmarks to precise chromosomal positions by FISH analysis, so as to ensure that the resulting genomic maps are highly accurate and integrated with one another.

Genetic Maps

Genetic maps (also known as *linkage maps* or *meiotic maps*) depict the relative locations of genetic (as opposed to physical) markers

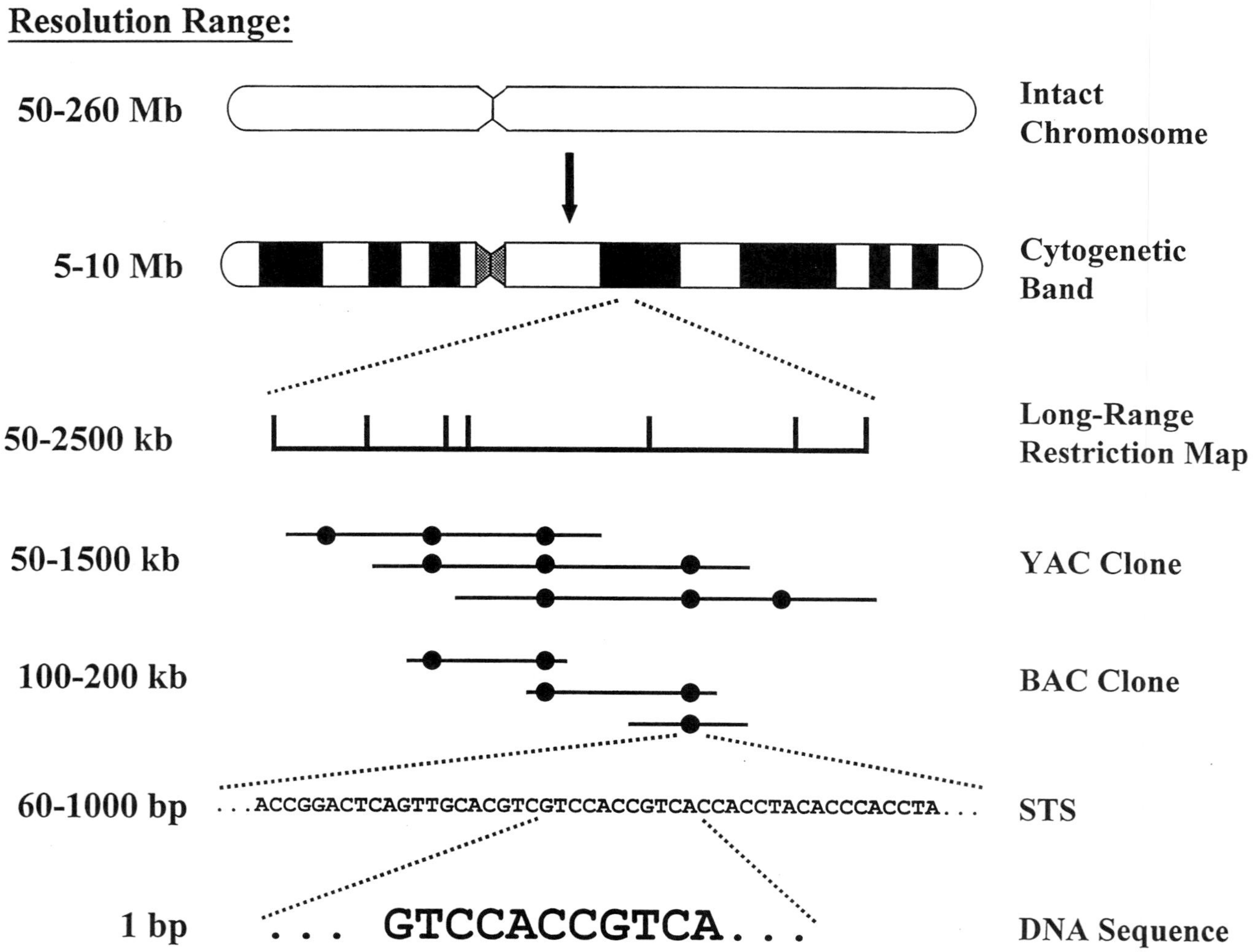

Fig. 10-6 Characteristic resolution ranges in human genome mapping. Individual human chromosomes range in size from about 50 to 260 Mb. When properly stained and examined microscopically, the characteristic cytogenetic banding pattern gives a unique appearance to each chromosome, with each band containing about 5 to 10 Mb of DNA. Physical mapping techniques, such as long-range restriction mapping by pulsed-field gel electrophoresis, yeast artificial chromosome (YAC) cloning, and bacterial artificial chromosome (BAC) cloning are associated with successively decreasing resolution ranges, as indicated. Individual DNA landmarks typically represent much smaller DNA segments [e.g., about 60 to 1000 bp for a sequence-tagged site (STS)]. The highest level of resolution is the single base pair of DNA sequence. (*Adapted from Rossiter and Caskey.*[475] *Used by permission.*)

across a stretch of DNA. These maps have a more abstract meaning than do physical or cytogenetic maps, since the order and spacing of markers is related to the complex events involved in the transmission of DNA from one generation to the next.

Theory of Genetic Mapping. Most human cells contain two sets of homologous chromosomes, one inherited paternally and one inherited maternally. Thus, for a particular DNA segment (or marker), there can exist two alleles — one on each of the two homologous chromosomes. During the formation of germ cells, the diploid set of chromosomes is divided during a process known as *meiosis*, which results in the generation of gametes with only one of each of the pairs of homologous chromosomes (a total of 23 chromosomes). Markers on nonhomologous chromosomes assort randomly during meiosis. Markers on homologous chromosomes tend to be inherited together (i.e., they are *linked*). Often, a recombination event occurs between two homologous chromosomes (i.e., there is an exchange of chromosomal material between the homologues inherited from the mother and the father), resulting in two new hybrid chromosomes, each containing portions of the starting homologous chromosomes (Fig. 10-7). Following such a recombination event, some previously linked markers may no longer cosegregate.

Genetic mapping is simply the process of measuring the probability that two closely spaced markers on a chromosome will remain together during meiosis. This is accomplished by analyzing multiple members of known families and measuring the frequency of recombination between markers. The greater the frequency of recombination observed between two markers, the larger is the genetic distance separating them, and vice versa (Fig. 10-7). The resulting genetic map depicts the genetic distance between different markers and, therefore, their relative order (Figs. 10-5 and 10-7). The unit of measure in human genetic maps is the centimorgan (cM), with 1 cM corresponding to a probability of 1 percent that a recombination event will occur in a single meiosis (i.e., 1 recombination event, on average, every 100 meioses). The human genome consists of 3300 cM in genetic distance. The correlation between genetic distance and physical distance varies throughout the genome, since some regions are more susceptible to meiotic recombination than others. As a very rough guide, 1 cM in genetic disease, on average, corresponds to ~1 Mb in physical distance.

Genetic Markers. Genetic markers serve the function of discriminating between homologous chromosomes, thereby allowing recombination events to be detected. To be useful, a genetic

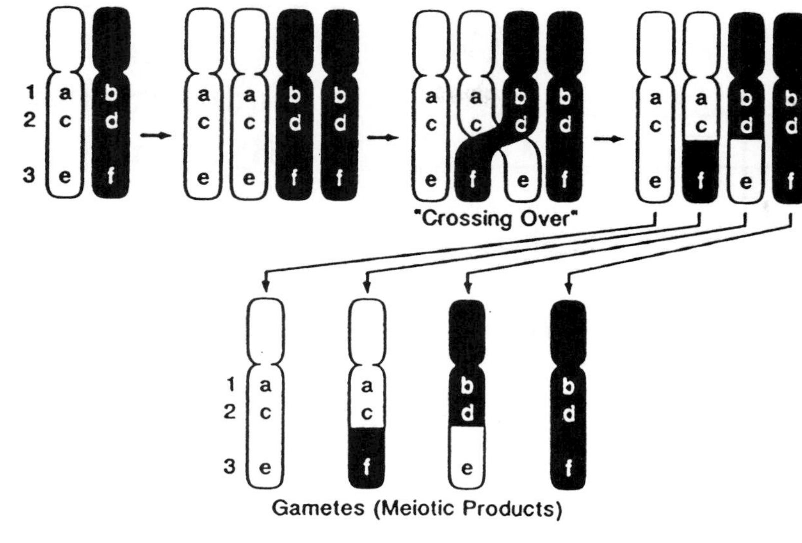

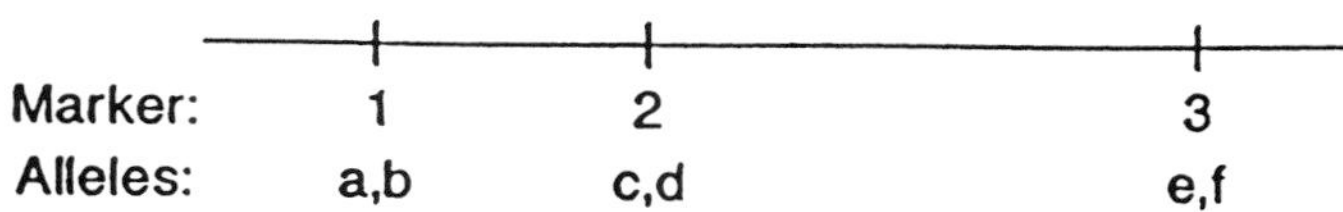

Fig. 10-7 Fundamental basis of genetic mapping. A: During meiosis, each chromosome lines up with its homologous partner and is replicated. Paired chromosomes can break and rejoin with each other at one or more points in common (called *crossing over* or *meiotic recombination*), leading to the exchange of DNA. Such a recombination event can thus result in the reassortment of alleles that were previously on the same chromosome. Three hypothetical markers (1, 2, and 3) on the chromosome are indicated, each with two alleles (a/b, c/d, and e/f, respectively). A crossover event is depicted as occurring between markers 2 and 3, yielding two recombinant chromosomes (a,c,f and b,d,e) among the four meiotic products. B: The depicted genetic map is based on the measured meiotic recombination events, such as that shown in A. The distance between markers reflects the frequency with which they are inherited together (i.e., the closer two markers are to one another, the less likely is it that a recombination event will occur between them, and vice versa). (*Adapted from Rossiter and Caskey.*[475] *Used by permission.*)

marker must display variance among different copies of the same chromosome (i.e., it must be polymorphic), thereby allowing it to be followed during passage from one generation to the next. The informativeness of a genetic marker reflects the actual likelihood that it will be different on two homologous chromosomes (i.e., the likelihood that each chromosome will contain a distinct allele). A number of different types of genetic markers have been used for constructing genetic maps. One type of genetic marker is an inherited disease itself (e.g., Huntington disease, neurofibromatosis, cystic fibrosis, and sickle cell anemia). Other biologic features can also serve as genetic markers (e.g., blood cell surface antigens, serum proteins, and tissue markers). However, most markers used for genetic mapping are DNA sequence differences that are neutral with respect to the phenotypic status of the organism.

There are several major classes of DNA-sequence-based genetic markers. Restriction fragment length polymorphisms (RFLPs) reflect sequence variations that result in DNA fragments of different sizes following restriction digestion, Southern blotting,[243] and hybridization with an appropriate probe[244–247] (Fig. 10-8). Since most RFLPs reflect two or very few distinct variants, these markers are typically not very informative, which limits their usefulness. Another class of genetic markers consists of tandemly repeated DNA segments. Included among these markers are those containing a variable number of tandem repeats[248] (VNTRs) or *minisatellites*, with each repeat unit containing 11 to 60 bp (Fig. 10-8). The latter polymorphisms are most often detected by agarose gel electrophoresis, Southern blotting,[243] and hybridization with an appropriate probe. Since a greater number of alleles are typically encountered (reflecting different numbers of repeated units), these markers are generally more informative than RFLPs.

In the case of human genetic maps, RFLPs and VNTRs have been largely supplanted by a newer type of genetic marker, termed the *short tandem repeat*[249–251] (STR) or *microsatellite*. These polymorphisms are based on differences in the lengths of DNA tracts composed of tandemly repeated di-, tri-, or tetranucleotides (typically repeated a total of about 5 to 30 times) (Fig. 10-8). STRs are particularly useful for genetic mapping because they tend to be more informative than other types of genetic markers. For detecting an STR, PCR primers that flank the tandem repeat are used to amplify the entire segment, and the size of the variable fragment is measured by gel electrophoresis[252] (Figs. 10-8 and 10-9). The most commonly encountered STR in the human genome consists of the dinucleotide CA (or GT on the opposite strand). STRs are now widely used for constructing genetic maps due to their frequent occurrence in the human genome (e.g., estimated every 30 to 60 kb for CA repeats), informativeness, and efficient detection by PCR-based analyses.

The final class of genetic marker is the single-nucleotide polymorphism (SNP). With these markers, a single base is variant at a particular site, typically being one of two possible nucleotides (i.e., biallelic; Fig. 10-8). SNPs can be readily detected by PCR amplification of the surrounding DNA, followed by analysis of the resulting PCR product by one of many possible methods, ranging from direct DNA sequencing to various non-gel-based approaches.[190,252–254] In the human genome, SNPs occur relatively frequently, roughly every 500 to 1000 bp of genomic DNA (slightly less often in coding sequences), and appear to be distributed in a relatively uniform fashion. However, because each SNP is typically associated with only two alleles, these genetic markers are not as informative as STRs. Thus, to generate the same amount of data required for performing genetic mapping studies, a larger number of SNPs are required compared to STRs.[253,255] However, the ability to use automated, non-gel-based detection methods,[252–254] such as DNA chips[190] (see the section "DNA Chips"), will almost certainly make SNPs the genetic markers of choice for performing large-scale human genetic mapping studies in the future.[255–258] Indeed, high-throughput, SNP-based genetic mapping methods are envisioned as being critical for unraveling the underlying bases of genetically complex diseases.[13–17]

Construction of Genetic Maps. The process of constructing genetic maps of human DNA is relatively complicated and tedious[259] because many of the desirable features found with other experimental organisms (e.g., large numbers of offspring, controlled matings, and relatively rapid generation times) are not

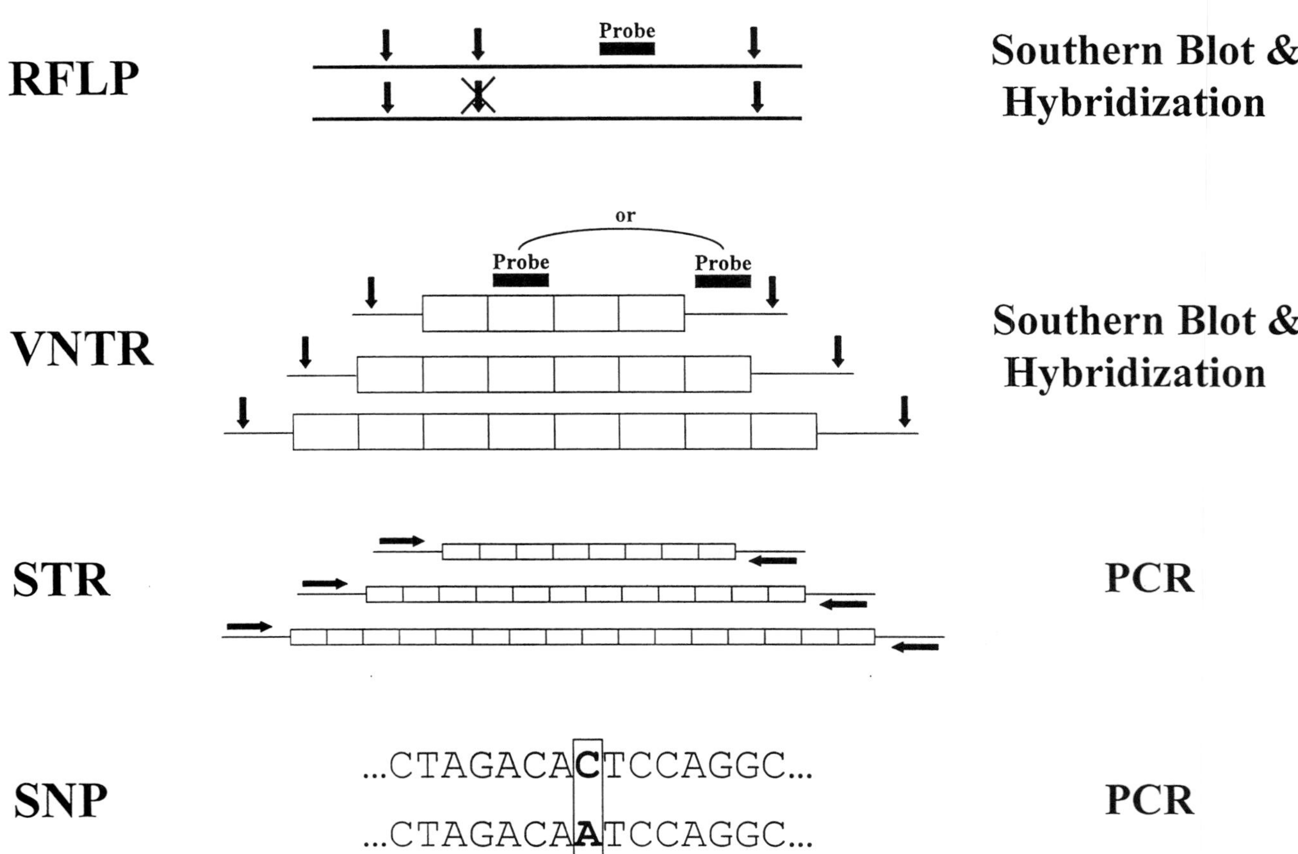

Fig. 10-8 Genetic markers and their detection. Four major types of genetic markers used for genetic mapping are depicted, along with the experimental method used for their detection. Restriction fragment length polymorphisms (RFLPs) are typically associated with the variable presence of a restriction site(s) (indicated by *vertical arrows*) in a stretch of DNA and are detected by restriction digestion, Southern blotting, and hybridization with a suitable probe. Variable numbers of tandem repeats (VNTR markers) reflect variable sizes of DNA tracts harboring a repeated DNA segment, again typically detected by digestion with a restriction enzyme, Southern blotting, and hybridization with a probe. Short tandem repeat (STR) markers consist of smaller simple-sequence (e.g., di-, tri-, or tetranucleotide) repeats, which can be detected by polymerase chain reaction (PCR) with primers (depicted as *horizontal arrows*) that flank the repeated region (see Fig. 10-9). Single nucleotide polymorphisms (SNPs) reflect differences of a single nucleotide at a defined position (shown here as a C vs A) and are typically detected by PCR amplification of the DNA segment harboring the polymorphism, followed by an analytical step that enables discrimination between the different sequences. (*Adapted from Rossiter and Caskey.*[475] *Used by permission.*)

available. Nonetheless, by using multigeneration families containing large sibships along with living parents and grandparents, sufficient data can be generated to build high-quality genetic maps. A French research group [CEPH (Centre d'Etude du Polymorphisme Humain)] was established to facilitate the distribution of cells and DNA from carefully collected and documented families.[260] Thus, different investigators around the world can use the same families for constructing genetic maps, thereby enabling different data sets to be more readily compared and integrated.

Provided the availability of genetic markers and DNA from large families, the process of constructing genetic maps is now well established. Each DNA sample is analyzed with an appropriate set of genetic markers by using a suitable detection method(s) (see Fig. 10-8), and the resulting data are carefully collected and recorded. Sophisticated computational tools have been developed for assessing the inheritance patterns of the markers and for deducing the resulting genetic maps.[261] A first-generation genetic map of the human genome was reported in 1987 and consisted of markers (predominantly RFLP based) that were spaced, on average, every 10 cM.[262] As part of the HGP, second-generation, higher-resolution genetic maps consisting of STR-type markers have now been constructed for the human genome[263–268] (see the section "Highlights of the Human Genome Project").

Uses of Genetic Maps. Genetic maps facilitate the search for genes associated with human disease. In conventional positional cloning strategies, the disease gene itself can serve as one genetic marker whose linkage to other genetic markers is assessed by the analysis of affected families. In the ideal cases, more closely linked genetic markers are identified that allow the genomic region containing the disease gene to be limited to an interval that can be readily studied by physical mapping methods (see the section "Background on Positional Cloning"). Such an approach is particularly well suited for single-gene disorders. In the future, human genetics studies will increasingly focus on the analysis of more genetically complex diseases. This will be accompanied by a shift away from the use of individual families and toward the use of large-scale association studies, whereby common genetic variants will be correlated with specific traits by analyzing large numbers of individuals (as opposed to families).[14,256] Such efforts

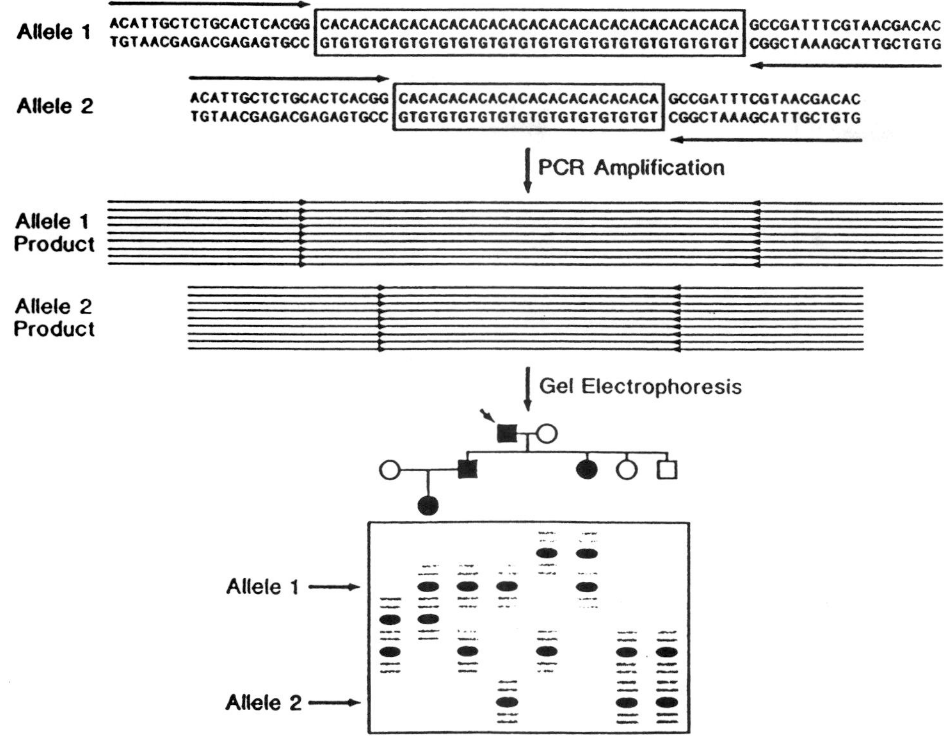

Fig. 10-9 A short tandem repeat (STR) genetic marker reflecting a variable number of CA repeats. Regions of the human genome that contain stretches of reiterated CA dinucleotides are often polymorphic with respect to the number of repeat units.[249–251] One hypothetical segment is depicted, along with polymerase chain reaction (PCR) primers (indicated by *horizontal arrows*) that can be used to amplify the CA-repeat unit. The two alleles (1 and 2) present in one of the family members (indicated with an *arrow*) are shown. PCR amplification of the STR marker in that individual yields two products of different sizes, which can be resolved on a high-resolution polyacrylamide gel. The results of analyzing the entire family for this genetic marker reveal the presence of multiple alleles, which is characteristic of STRs. A common finding with PCR amplification of CA repeats is the presence of shadow (or stutter) bands (depicted as *light lines*) smaller and/or larger than the expected product. (*Adapted from Germino and Somlo.[600] Used by permission.*)

will depend on the availability of large sets of SNP markers, an associated catalog of known human sequence variants (see http://www.ncbi.nlm.nih.gov/SNP), and more robust technologies for large-scale SNP detection[255–258] (see the section "DNA Chips").

Genetic maps are also important for at least two other applications. First, they are valuable as a framework for assembling physical maps. While genetic and physical maps provide different information about the corresponding DNA, they are colinear with respect to the order of markers. Thus, genetic mapping can complement physical mapping by providing information about the order of physical landmarks based on their genetic positions. For example, this can be accomplished by simply localizing mapped genetic markers on a physical map[154] (see the section "Generation of Sequence-Tagged Sites"). Second, genetic maps are valuable for studying subtle aspects of inheritance. For example, there is no uniform relationship between genetic distance (i.e., recombination frequency) and physical distance; in the case of human DNA, the rough correlation of 1 cM to 1 Mb represents an estimated average, with considerable variation occurring throughout the genome. Interestingly, the relative recombination frequencies per physical length of DNA are higher near the ends of chromosomes (telomeres) and lower near the centromeric regions. The availability of higher-resolution genetic maps in conjunction with more complete physical maps is allowing the molecular bases for these observations to be studied more rigorously.[106,107]

Physical Maps

Physical maps depict the relative locations of physical landmarks across a stretch of DNA, much like a travel map indicates the locations of cities along a highway. Physical maps are constructed either with the total genomic DNA of an organism or with smaller pieces derived from that genome. The conventional approach for the latter involves fragmenting and then cloning the DNA, so as to purify and analyze individual DNA fragments. By fragmenting the DNA, however, the order of the DNA segments is lost, leaving the challenge of correctly putting the pieces back together to create an accurate map. Hence, the analogy is often made to a jigsaw puzzle; however, there are some important differences. Instead of just one copy of every DNA fragment, many copies are present within the collection of clones. In addition, the same DNA segment may be present on a number of different-sized, overlapping clones. In assembling such a clone-based physical map, individual clones are analyzed for the presence of landmarks and then compared with other clones. When two clones are found to have one or more landmarks in common, they can be conceptually overlaid (or overlapped), and because such clones are typically not identical (only overlapping), a slightly larger segment is reconstructed. A collection of ordered, overlapping clones is called a *contig*, since the clones together contain a contiguous segment of DNA. Thus, a clone-based physical map (i.e., a contig map) reflects both a collection of overlapping clones and an ordered set of DNA landmarks.

Restriction Sites as Landmarks. Various types of landmarks can be used to construct physical maps of DNA. A simple one is the restriction site, which reflects the site of cleavage by a specific restriction enzyme(s). Since a large number of restriction enzymes are available, each recognizing and cutting DNA at a defined sequence, detailed restriction maps can be theoretically constructed by using several different enzymes. Long-range, low-resolution restriction maps of uncloned genomic DNA can be constructed by using rare-cutting restriction enzymes and pulsed-field gel electrophoresis;[135–137,139] however, the resulting maps are usually not very detailed and provide no direct access to the DNA itself. More typical is the detection of restriction sites within cloned DNA. Here, individual clones are analyzed, and the physical distances between restriction sites established. This information provides a restriction-site-based *fingerprint* for each clone, which in turn can be compared with other clones to deduce overlap relationships. Such an approach was particularly effective for constructing physical maps of several model organism genomes[269–271] and is now being adapted for use in constructing high-resolution physical maps en route to systematic sequencing of the human and other genomes[124–126,272] (see the section "Genomic Sequencing").

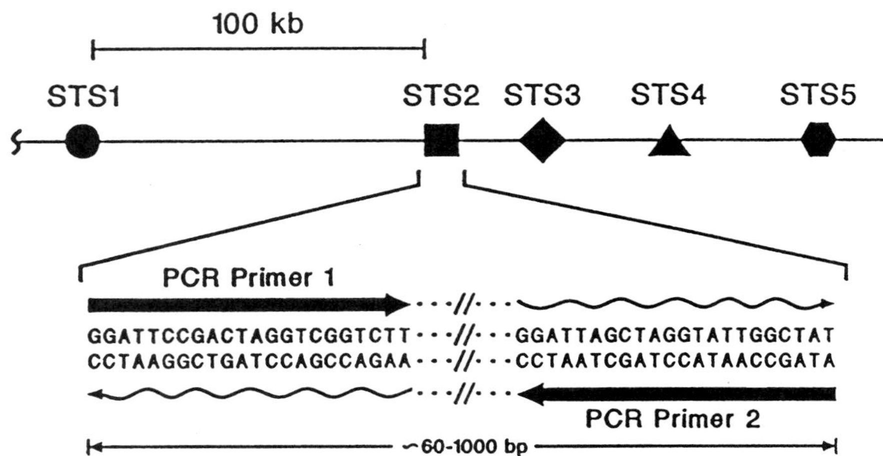

Fig. 10-10 Sequence-tagged sites (STSs) and STS maps. An STS is a unique DNA sequence in the size range of about 60 to 1000 bp that can specifically be detected by a polymerase chain reaction (PCR) assay employing two oligonucleotide primers (indicated by *horizontal arrows*). physical map of a human chromosome can be represented by the relative positions of STSs (depicted as *unique symbols*), each of which is associated with a specific PCR assay. (*Adapted from Green and Olson*[86] *and Green and Green.*[274] *Used by permission.*)

Sequence-Tagged Sites as Landmarks. Early in the HGP and shortly after the advent of PCR, a new type of DNA landmark was envisioned: the *sequence-tagged site* (STS).[273] STSs are short stretches (e.g., about 60 to 1000 bp) of unique DNA sequence that can be specifically detected by a PCR assay (Fig. 10-10); in essence, STSs are the physical landmarks, and PCR is the experimental method used to detect them. STS maps simply represent the relative positions of STSs across a stretch of DNA[86,274] (Figs. 10-5 and 10-10). STSs provide several key advantages over other landmarks (e.g., restriction sites and hybridization probes) that make them well suited for use in physical mapping. First, the use of PCR as the front-line analytical tool for detecting DNA landmarks is highly desirable because of its high sensitivity, specificity, and potential for automation. Second, all the relevant information about an STS (e.g., the sequence of the two oligonucleotide primers, reaction components, and temperature-cycling parameters) can be stored and accessed electronically (such as in the dbSTS database; see http://www.ncbi.nlm.nih.gov/dbSTS), thereby making that STS experimentally accessible to any laboratory. As a result, the DNA segment corresponding to a particular STS can be generated simply by synthesizing the appropriate oligonucleotide primers and performing PCR under the described conditions.[275] This facilitates the assimilation and comparison of STS maps constructed in different laboratories and/or by different methods. Similarly, the availability of a PCR assay specific for each STS provides the means to isolate readily a clone containing the corresponding genomic region; this offers a desirable element of flexibility with respect to the ability to utilize different cloning systems or new, improved clone libraries. Finally, since STSs are, by definition, sequence-based, physical maps assembled with STSs as the landmarks can be readily integrated with evolving sequence maps by simple computer analysis. Because of these features, STSs rapidly ascended to become the dominant landmark for constructing physical maps of mammalian chromosomes. STSs are most commonly mapped using large-insert clones, such as YACs (see the section "Yeast Artificial Chromosome-Based Sequence-Tagged Site-Content Mapping"), or radiation hybrid cell lines (see the section "Radiation Hybrid Mapping").

Generation of Sequence-Tagged Sites. To construct detailed physical maps of large genomic regions (such as human chromosomes), many thousands of STSs must be developed. The generation of an STS involves determining a small amount of DNA sequence (about 100 to 400 bp), developing a PCR assay that will specifically amplify the corresponding DNA segment (including the design[276] and synthesis of the two oligonucleotide primers), and demonstrating that the site is functionally unique within the genome.[275,277,278] A key step in this process is the generation of DNA sequence, which can be obtained either from a totally random piece of genomic DNA or from a more targeted DNA segment, with the latter being technically more demanding.

Several methods have been established for generating DNA sequence from targeted genomic regions, such as individual human chromosomes. Many of these approaches involve the use of human-rodent hybrid cell lines containing a single human chromosome or portion thereof (see the section "Somatic Hybrid Cell Lines"). Several strategies can be used to isolate the human DNA away from the rodent DNA background. For example, lambda or cosmid clones derived from such hybrid cell lines can be screened for the presence of human-specific repetitive sequences. Since most segments of human DNA present in lambda (15 to 25 kb) or cosmid (35 to 45 kb) clones should harbor at least one repetitive sequence (e.g., *Alu*), clones containing human DNA can be identified by hybridization with radioactively labeled human-DNA probes.[275,277] Alternatively, segments of human DNA within the hybrid cell lines can be amplified by using a variant type of PCR, called *Alu*-PCR[279–281] (Fig. 10-11). In this method, total DNA from the hybrid cell line is used as template in PCR assays employing oligonucleotide primers specific to consensus *Alu* sequences.[40] The PCR products generated are enriched for DNA segments residing between adjacent *Alu* repeats.[279–281] *Alu*-PCR can thus be used to amplify the human but not the rodent DNA from a hybrid cell line, with the resulting DNA segments then utilized for developing STSs.[277,282] A second approach for isolating targeted genomic regions uses the technique of flow sorting,[283–285] which separates individual chromosomes based on quantitation of the laser-induced fluorescence following staining. Typically, flow sorting yields very small quantities of DNA, which must then be subcloned prior to analysis.[283–285] Though flow-sorted DNA has been successfully used for developing STSs from individual human chromosomes,[275,277,286,287] the presence of irrelevant DNA segments has in some cases hindered the utility of this approach.[275,277] Other strategies for targeted STS generation include the use of 3′ untranslated regions of cDNAs[288] and sequences derived from the ends of large-insert clones, such as YACs.[289,290]

Efficient strategies for developing STSs have been established[98,274,275,277,278,286,287] and utilized for many large-scale physical mapping projects. In the case of the human genome, large collections of STSs have been generated in both genome-wide[98,291–293] and targeted fashions (see http://www.ncbi.nlm. nih.gov/dbSTS). It is also important to note that the large collections of developed PCR-based human genetic markers[263–268,294] (specifically STRs; see the section "Genetic Markers") are also STSs; that is, each is a unique sequence associated with a PCR assay. These markers can thus serve as

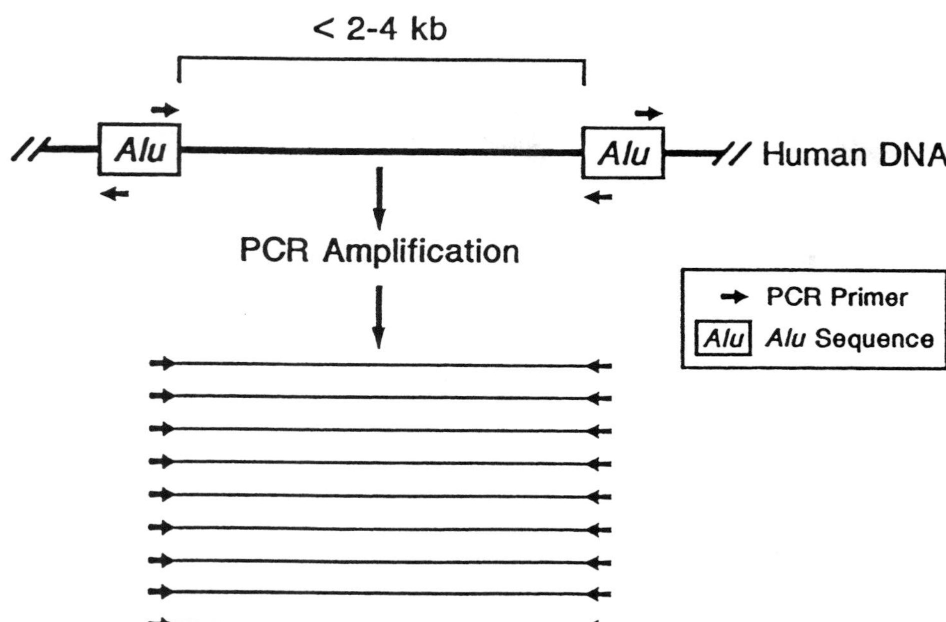

Fig. 10-11 Amplification of DNA by *Alu*-polymerase chain reaction (*Alu*-PCR). Interspersed repetitive sequences in human DNA, such as *Alu* repeats, are often closely spaced to one another (due to their high frequency in the genome). These repeated sequences represent potential annealing sites for PCR primers (depicted as *horizontal arrows*), in particular those that are complementary to known consensus *Alu* sequences and point outward from the repeat units. When two *Alu* repeats are in close enough proximity to one another (e.g., less than 2 to 4 kb apart), the region between them can be amplified by *Alu*-PCR.[279–281] The resulting PCR product consists of the outermost portions of the *Alu* repeat together with the intervening DNA segment. Typically, *Alu*-PCR is performed on samples of human DNA that contain numerous *Alu* repeats, resulting in the amplification of a heterogeneous collection of different PCR products.

landmarks on both the genetic map and the physical map, with their presence on both serving to integrate the two maps together.

Yeast Artificial Chromosome-Based Sequence-Tagged Site-Content Mapping. The major approach employed for constructing the first-generation clone-based physical maps of the human genome has involved the use of STSs as the landmarks and YACs as the source of the cloned DNA.[86,274] Because of their large insert size, YACs simplify the process of assembling contigs covering large genomic regions (much as jigsaw puzzles made of larger pieces are easier to assemble than those made of smaller pieces). In this strategy, YAC clones are isolated from appropriate libraries (typically by using an STS-specific PCR assay[85]) and analyzed for the presence of additional STSs (Fig. 10-12). An *STS content* is thus established for each YAC. Two clones are assumed to overlap if they have one or more STSs in common. By establishing the overlaps among a group of YACs, contig maps can be deduced that reflect both the relationships among the clones as well as the relative order of the STSs (Fig. 10-12). This general strategy, called *STS-content mapping*,[86,274] has been used to construct large YAC contigs corresponding to a number of regions of the human genome, including segments encompassing important disease genes[86–89,91,92] (e.g., see Fig. 10-13) and whole human chromosomes.[93–95,98, 100,101,103–107] A global view of the

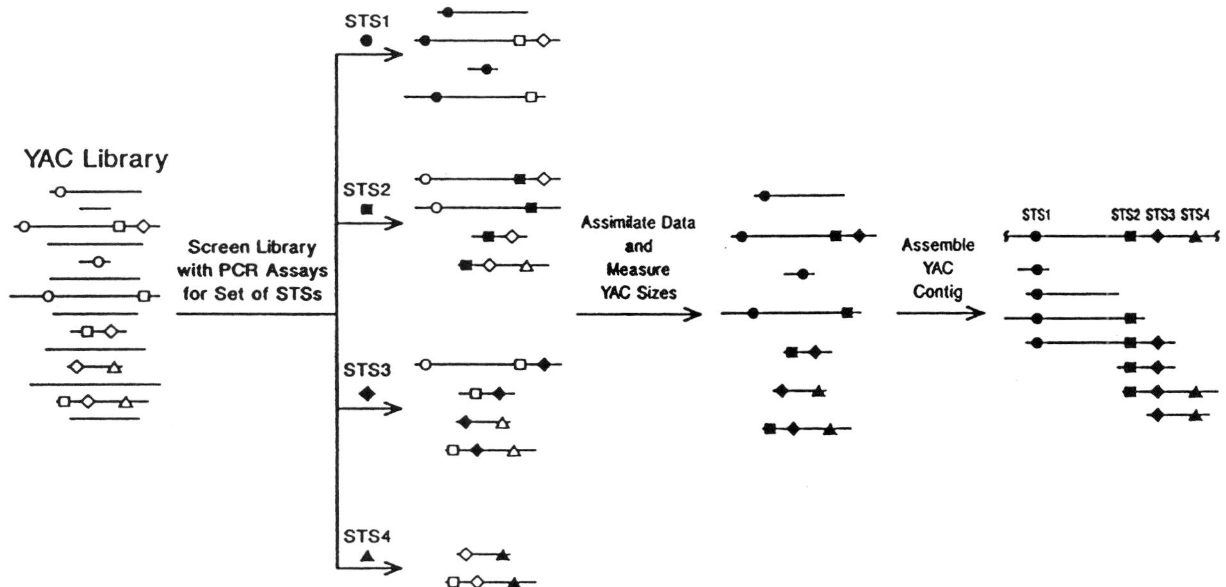

Fig. 10-12 General strategy for constructing yeast artificial chromosome (YAC)-based sequence-tagged site (STS)-content maps. A YAC library, consisting of clones of various sizes and unknown compositions of STSs (depicted as *open symbols*), is screened for a set of STSs using a polymerase chain reaction (PCR)-based screening method.[85] For each group of isolated clones, only the STS whose corresponding PCR assay was used to perform the library screen is known to be present in the positive YACs (depicted as *solid symbols*). However, data about which YACs contain which STSs can then be assimilated and the size of each YAC measured by pulsed-field gel electrophoresis. The resulting information can be used to assemble a YAC contig, reflecting both the overlap relationships among the clones and the relative order of the STSs. (*Adapted from Green and Olson*[86] *and Green and Green.*[274] *Used by permission.*)

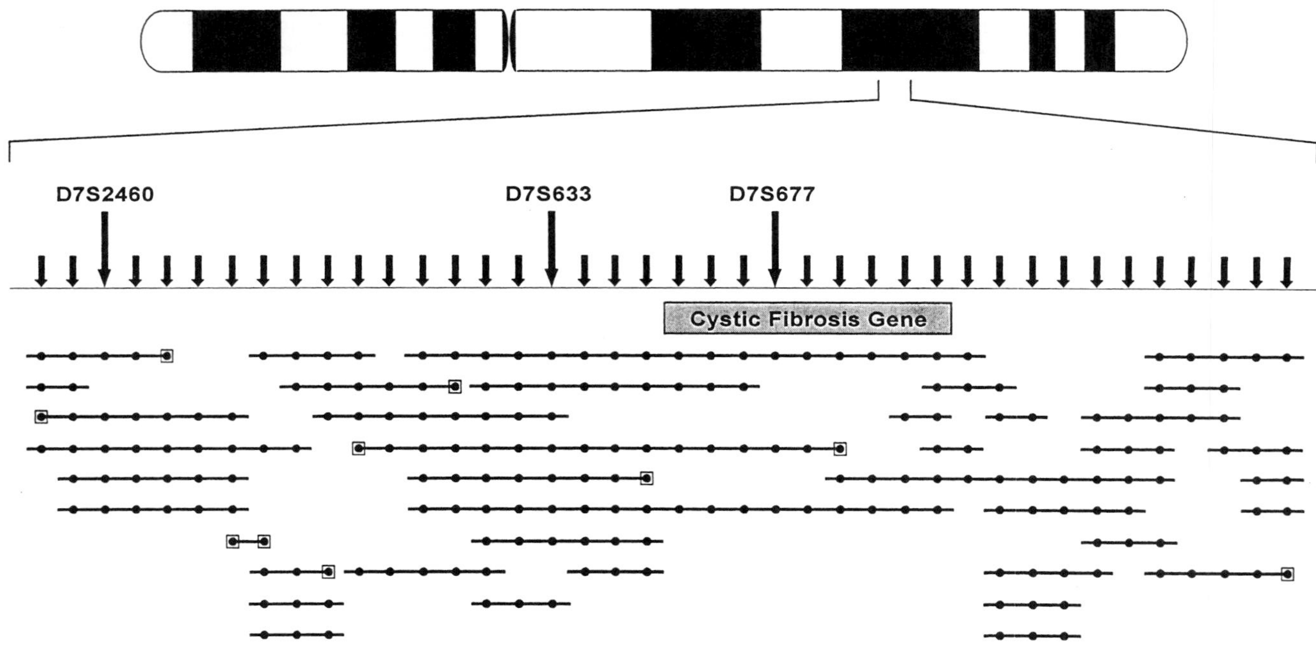

Fig. 10-13 A yeast artificial chromosome (YAC)-based sequence-tagged site (STS)-content map of the human genomic region containing the cystic fibrosis gene. A YAC contig map of the region of human chromosome 7 containing the cystic fibrosis gene is depicted. The *vertical arrows* along the *top* indicate the relative positions of the STSs, while the *horizontal bars* represent YACs. For simplicity, the STSs are spaced equidistantly and only a representative subset of mapped YACs is shown. The presence of an STS in a YAC is indicated by a *solid circle* at the appropriate position on the corresponding horizontal bar. When an STS corresponds to the insert end of a YAC, an *open square* is placed around that circle at the end of the YAC from which it was derived. The indicated overlap relationships among YACs were established by the presence of one or more common STSs. The contig spans across ~2.0 Mb of DNA, with the approximate position of the ~200-kb cystic fibrosis gene indicated. The relative position of this physical map on the chromosome 7 cytogenetic map was established by performing fluorescence *in situ* hybridization (FISH) analysis with several YACs from the contig.[154] Similarly, the localization of several genetic markers (D7S2460, D7S633, and D7S677) on the YAC contig allows integration of the genetic and physical maps at these positions.[154] Additional details about this physical map have been reported[86,107] (also see http://genome.nhgri.nih.gov/CHR7).

YAC-based STS-content map constructed for human chromosome 7 is provided in Fig. 10-14.

Radiation Hybrid Mapping. Other, non-clone-based approaches are available for establishing the relative order of landmarks (such as STSs) across a stretch of DNA. One technique, called *radiation hybrid mapping*,[159,160,295,296] exploits the ability to recover chromosome fragments in rodent cells. In one application of this method, human chromosomes in cultured cells are fragmented by irradiation, and individual pieces are recovered by fusion of the irradiated cells with a rodent cell line. Each of the resulting cell lines typically contains numerous, disjointed fragments of the starting chromosome(s). A set of such radiation hybrid cell lines (typically ~90), each containing a different assortment of human chromosomal fragments, is then isolated and analyzed for the presence or absence of DNA landmarks. An efficient approach for the latter involves the use of PCR for detecting STSs within the cell lines.[160] The relative spacing between two STSs can be deduced based on analyzing the data about their coexistence within the collection of cell lines. The fundamental principle is that the frequency of radiation-induced chromosomal breaks between STSs is proportional to the distance between them; thus, closely spaced STSs tend to coexist in a larger fraction of cell lines compared with those that are far apart on a chromosome or that are on separate chromosomes. Statistical analyses are used to order the STSs and to estimate the relative distances between them,[159,295,297–299] resulting in the assembly of a radiation hybrid map.

Radiation hybrid mapping represents an important adjunct approach for physical mapping. For example, this method facilitated the assembly of a YAC-based physical map of the human genome.[98] In these studies, the resulting STS-based radiation hybrid map was used to confirm the STS order deduced by YAC-based STS-content mapping, to order individual YAC contigs, and to orient YAC contigs relative to the centromere and telomeres. Thus, the combined use of independent methods for ordering STSs helped in the construction of an overall more consistent map. Radiation hybrid mapping has also been used extensively to map genes in the human genome[292,293] (see http://www.ncbi.nlm.nih.gov/genemap98 and the section "cDNA Sequencing"). Furthermore, STS-based radiation hybrid maps of increasing resolution are actively being constructed for the human[291,300] (also see http://shgc-www.stanford.edu) and mouse[301] genomes. Finally, radiation hybrid mapping provides an approach for the comparative mapping of genomes from different animal species.[302]

Sequence Maps. The highest-resolution physical map is the DNA sequence map (Figs. 10-5 and 10-6), which depicts the precise order of nucleotides across a stretch of DNA. There are two major types of data generated for constructing sequence maps: that derived from cDNA (copies of mRNA molecules; i.e., expressed sequences) and that from genomic DNA. Each type of sequence has its relative value and limitations, with both types frequently generated for analyzing genomes.

cDNA Sequencing. Sequence data generated from cDNA provide an enriched source of information about the small part of the genome that is expressed and encodes protein. Refinements in the methods for large-scale DNA sequencing[166] coupled with improved protocols for generating *normalized* cDNA libraries (where individual transcripts are more equally represented[303–307]) have resulted in the efficient generation of large numbers of sequences from randomly selected cDNA clones. Such sequences are called *expressed-sequence tags* (ESTs), since they correspond to partial tags of expressed sequences.[308] Literally hundreds of

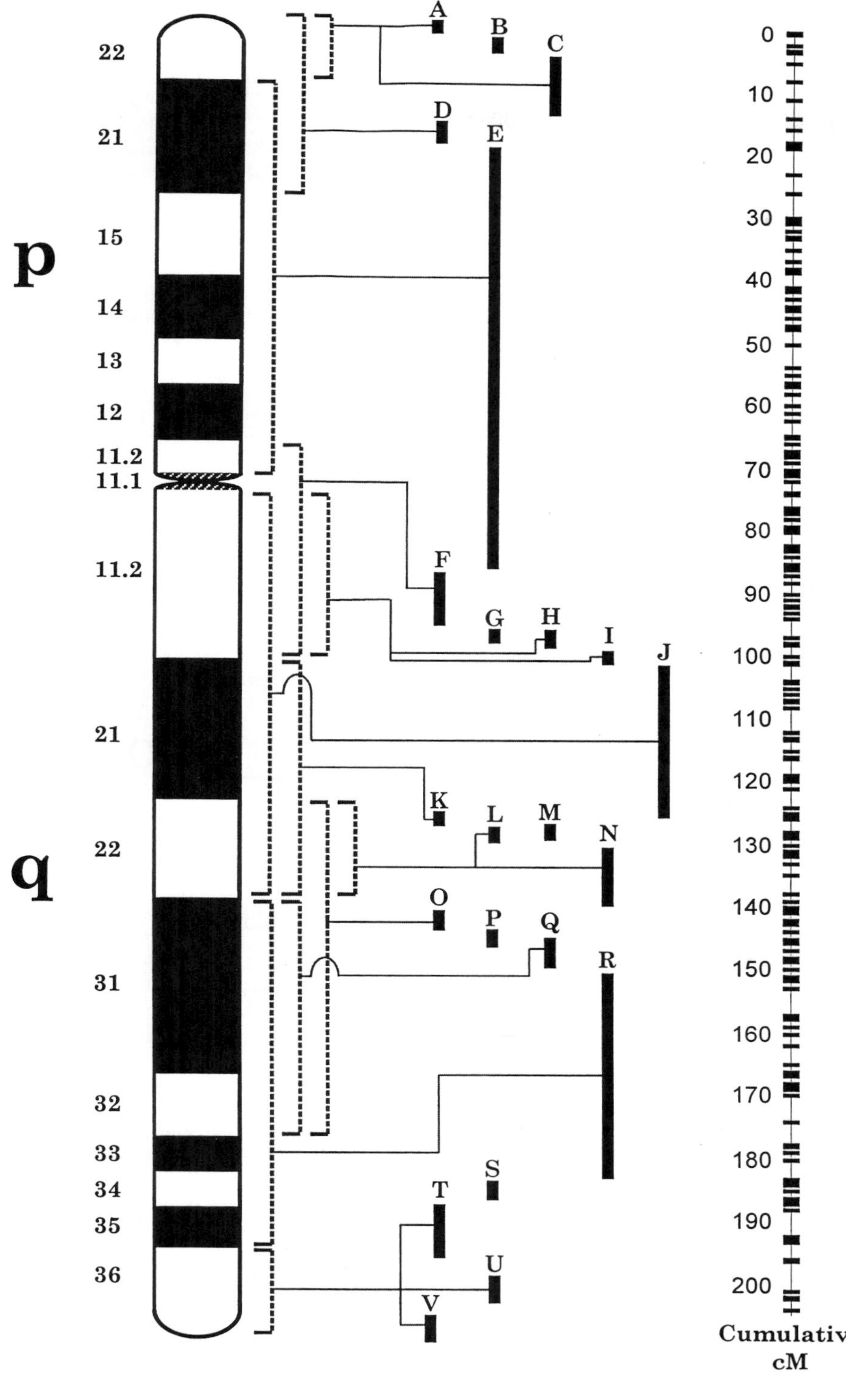

Fig. 10-14 Physical map of a human chromosome. A global overview of a first-generation physical map of a human chromosome constructed by the Human Genome Project is depicted. Specifically, a yeast artificial chromosome (YAC)-based sequence-tagged site (STS)-content map of human chromosome 7 is aligned relative to the cytogenetic map (*left*) and genetic map (*right*).[107] Each of the *vertical bars* in the middle (labeled A to V) corresponds to an individual YAC contig (see Fig. 10-13 for a more detailed view of a very small portion of contig O). Some of the contigs are quite large (e.g., contig E spans ~50 Mb or ~30 percent of the chromosome). Note that the positions of virtually all of the YAC contigs on the cytogenetic and genetic maps have been established. For additional details, see Bouffard et al.[107] and http://genome.nhgri.nih.gov/CHR7.

thousands of human ESTs have been generated[309,310] and are available in the public databases[311–314] (e.g., dbEST, see http://www.ncbi.nlm.nih.gov/dbEST). Together, these ESTs likely represent a major part of the human gene catalog. Furthermore, just under 4,000,000 ESTs (from numerous organisms) were present in dbEST as of April 2000.

ESTs can be used as a vehicle for mapping the corresponding genes in the genome. Most often, an STS is generated from the EST sequence[98,288,292,293,300,315,316] and mapped by YAC-based STS-content mapping[98] and/or radiation hybrid mapping.[98,292,293,300] The latter strategy has been applied in a large-scale fashion to construct a gene map (also called a *transcript map*) of the human genome[292,293] (see http://www.ncbi.nlm.nih.gov/genemap98).

The generation and mapping of large numbers of human ESTs enhance the ability to perform various types of studies, such as acquiring an initial exposure to the gene repertoire of the human genome,[317,318] facilitating the isolation of human disease genes by positional cloning (see the section "Isolation of Disease Genes by Positional Cloning"), and studying the differential expression of genes in various organisms, tissues, and disease states.[319,320] ESTs are not, however, without their limitations. First, since most ESTs reflect single-pass sequence reads, the corresponding sequence is generally of lower accuracy and less contiguity compared with high-quality genomic sequence (see the section "Genomic Sequencing"). Second, the data associated with an EST provide little to no information about the structure or regulation of the corresponding gene. Similarly, there is typically no insight about complex situations such as the production of multiple mRNAs from the same gene or the production of the same mRNA from multiple genes. Finally, ESTs are limited to those mRNA molecules that are present during the construction of a cDNA library, with rare transcripts or those not expressed in the tissue at the time of harvesting being difficult to identify. Thus, though large-scale EST generation provides an important source of biologically relevant DNA sequence, it should be regarded as a supplement (rather than a substitute) to complete genomic sequencing.

A variant form of EST analysis, called *serial analysis of gene expression* (SAGE),[321,322] involves the construction of libraries with clones containing concatemerized short sequence tags (e.g., 9 to 10 bp) derived from cDNA. Large numbers of sequence reads are then generated from individual clones, and the frequency of different short tags is assessed. The resulting data thus allow a quantitative cataloging and comparison of expressed genes from a defined biologic source (e.g., tissue, organism, or developmental stage). This methodology, which in essence is a sequence-based approach for monitoring gene expression levels, offers great promise for numerous applications.

Genomic Sequencing. The ability to establish the complete sequence of large genomes has advanced tremendously in recent years as a result of the experience gained in sequencing the genomes of model organisms, such as the yeast *S. cerevisiae*[323–329] (e.g., see http://genome-www.stanford.edu/Saccharomyces), the bacterium *E. coli*,[330] and the nematode *Caenorhabditis elegans*[331–335] (see http://www.sanger.ac.uk, http://genome.wustl.edu/gsc, and the section "Studying the Genomes of Model Organisms"). These accomplishments have been associated with a steady accumulation of incremental improvements in the approaches used for performing large-scale sequencing by fluorescence-based methods, rather than any individual revolutionary advance. As a result, the HGP is now firmly focused on the important task of sequencing the human genome[336–342] (see the section "Sequencing the Human Genome"), with plans to then sequence the mouse genome and inevitably many others thereafter.

The general strategy that is currently being used for systematic sequencing of large genomes (e.g., the human genome) can be broadly divided into several major steps.[342] First, suitable clones must be selected for sequencing. For a variety of reasons, YACs are not the clones of choice for use in genomic sequencing, despite their central role in the construction of long-range physical maps. Rather, BACs (and similarly PACs; note that only BACs are further mentioned below) are associated with a number of features that make them well suited as sequencing templates (see the section "Large-Insert Bacterial Cloning Systems"). Most often, available STSs (previously ordered by using YACs or radiation hybrid cell lines) are used to isolate BACs, which in turn are analyzed to establish overlap relationships among the clones and to assemble BAC contigs (Fig. 10-15). The latter typically involves some type of restriction-enzyme-based fingerprint analysis.[124–126,272] From

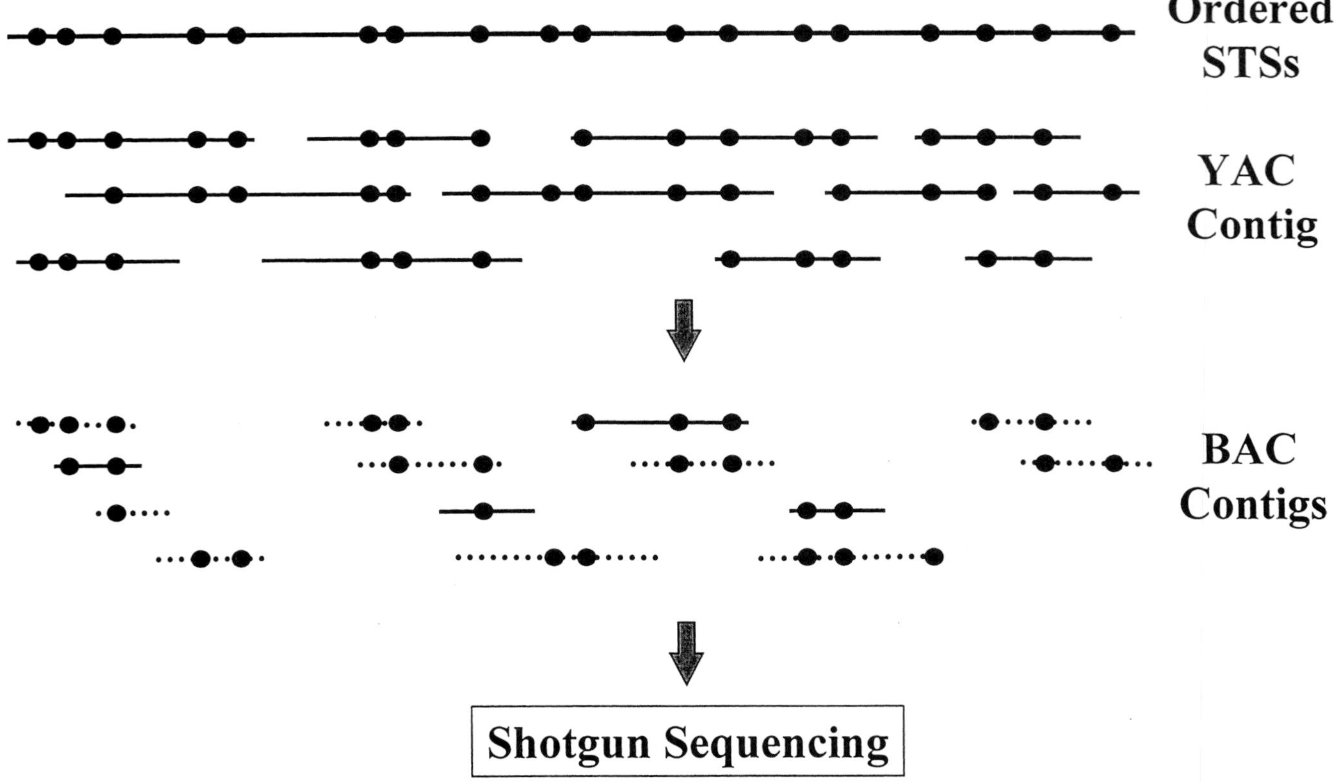

Fig. 10-15 Construction of clone-based physical maps suitable for sequencing the human genome. The first-generation physical maps of human chromosomes constructed in the Human Genome Project are predominantly yeast artificial chromosome (YAC)-based sequence-tagged site (STS)-content maps, which provide both collections of overlapping YAC clones and ordered sets of STSs. For various technical reasons, YACs are not ideal templates for DNA sequencing. Instead, the mapped STSs can be used to isolate smaller-insert bacterial artificial chromosome (BAC) (or P1-derived artificial chromosome [PAC]) clones, which in turn can be analyzed[124,125,272] and assembled into contigs. Typically, the resulting nascent BAC contigs are smaller than the corresponding YAC contig. However, the gaps between BAC contigs can be filled by various methods (e.g., by developing new STSs from appropriate BAC ends and then isolating additional overlapping clones). From the resulting BAC contigs, minimally overlapping BACs (shown as *dotted lines*) can be selected and individually subjected to shotgun sequencing (see the text and Fig. 10-16).

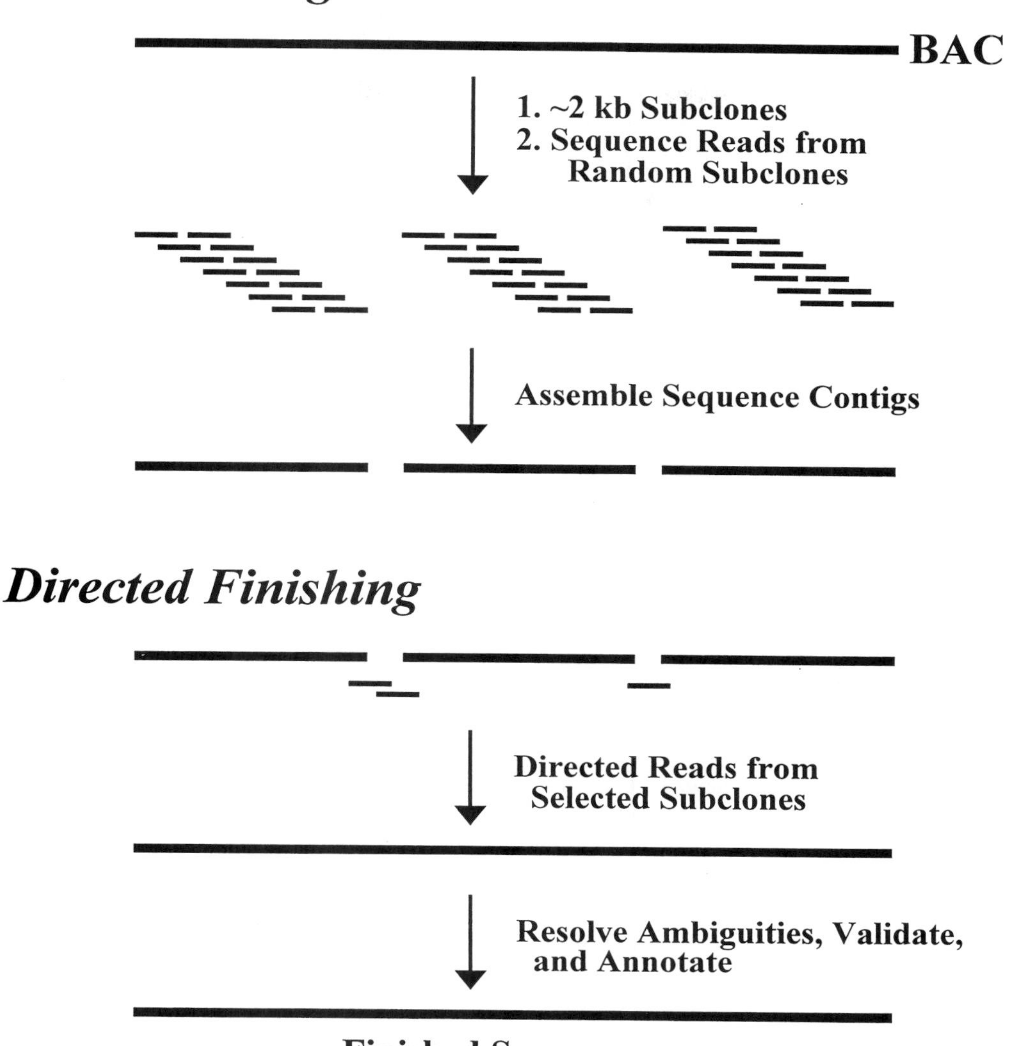

Fig. 10-16 Shotgun DNA sequencing. The dominant genomic sequencing strategy being used in the Human Genome Project is shotgun sequencing, which consists of two major phases. In the first, *random shotgun phase*, a genomic clone [e.g., a bacterial artificial chromosome (BAC)] is subcloned into ~2-kb fragments. Sequence reads are then obtained from one or both ends of a large number of randomly selected subclones. Sufficient sequence data are generated such that each nucleotide of the starting clone is read, on average, about 5 to 10 times. These redundant sequence data are then analyzed with various computational tools, enabling the assembly of sequence contigs. Typically, only a handful of gaps between sequence contigs remain at this stage. In the second, *directed finishing phase*, additional data are generated to complete the sequence, most often by obtaining directed reads from strategically selected subclones that provide sequence into or across the remaining gaps. This typically allows the merger of the remaining sequence contigs to yield a final, contiguous (i.e., finished) sequence, which is then analyzed to resolve ambiguities, validated by various tests, and annotated with respect to the location of known genes, expressed-sequence tags (ESTs), repetitive sequences, and other sequence features of interest.

the resulting BAC contig maps, minimally overlapping sets of clones that together span a genomic region of interest are selected for sequencing. Such high-resolution, bacterial-clone-based maps, which are usually highly redundant with respect to clone coverage and provide the ability to select clones that share very small overlapping regions, are commonly referred to as *sequence-ready maps* (Fig. 10-16).

In the second step of this process, selected clones are individually subjected to complete, high-accuracy sequencing. The most commonly used strategy for this step is called *shotgun sequencing*[343] (Fig. 10-16) (although a small number of groups are using a variant approach that employs transposons[344]). Shotgun sequencing begins with the construction of a subclone library, consisting of subclones that each contain a small (e.g., about 1 to 3 kb), random piece of the starting template (e.g., BAC). Sequence reads are then obtained from one or both ends of a large number of subclones. Sufficient sequence data are generated such that each base position of the starting template is read, on average, 5 to 10 times (sometimes referred to as 5× to 10× coverage). Computational tools are then used to analyze the resulting sequences, so as to identify those that overlap to form sequence contigs (each consisting of an assembled consensus sequence). This process has been greatly facilitated by powerful new software that assesses the quality of the data associated with each nucleotide of sequence and provides a user-friendly set of tools for reviewing and editing the resulting sequence assemblies.[211–213] With this software, an increasing amount of the data production and monitoring process can be more automated, thereby increasing the overall efficiency of the shotgun sequencing strategy. The initial shotgun sequencing data typically result in the assembly of a small number of sequence contigs, the order and orientation of which may or may not be known. The next phase involves generating sequence data in a highly directed fashion, so as to fill in the remaining gaps and merge the sequence contigs together. This *finishing* process (as it is often called) uses a number of specialized computational and experimental tools, requires highly trained technical personnel, and often involves generating sequence reads from particularly difficult sequences (e.g., repeated structures).[343]

The last step of genomic sequencing involves a final review of the entire assembled sequence, which includes both checking for any ambiguities or problem areas and analyzing the sequence for features of interest, such as the presence of genes, ESTs, repetitive elements, and other matching sequences. This latter activity is referred to as *sequence annotation*. Finally, the complete sequence and its associated annotations are submitted to a public database, such as GenBank.

STUDYING THE GENOMES OF MODEL ORGANISMS

Mapping and sequencing the human genome will, in principle, reveal all the information needed for the biologic development of a human being. However, the ability to interpret most of this information will be heavily dependent on parallel studies of nonhuman organisms used extensively in research laboratories as model systems. Experimentation in humans is rightly limited by ethical considerations, not to mention many practical factors. In contrast, model organisms such as bacteria, yeasts, worms, flies, and mice can be easily manipulated, especially genetically. Importantly, the knowledge gained from mapping and sequencing the genomes of these other organisms is directly relevant to understanding the human genome and many aspects of human biology, both in normal and abnormal states[319,345] (see the section "Comparative Study of the Biology of Humans and Other Organisms").

Model organisms have another important feature: most have much smaller genomes than that of humans. This feature makes comprehensive genome analysis more straightforward. As illustrated in Fig. 10-1, the genomes of *E. coli*, yeast, nematode, and fruit fly are roughly 1/600, 1/200, 1/30, and 1/20 the size of the human genome, respectively. With smaller genomes, newly developed approaches can be tested more readily. Indeed the experiences gained by mapping the yeast[269,346] and nematode[270] genomes have heavily influenced the strategies adopted for analyzing the human and mouse genomes. The smaller genomes of *E. coli*, yeast, nematode, and fruit fly are densely packed with genes, so the relative amount of information derived from systematic DNA sequencing is high. Importantly, these smaller genomes actually contain many of the same genes that are found in the human genome[319,345] (see the section "Comparative Study of the Biology of Humans and Other Organisms"), making their study of particular interest. For the early phases of the HGP, a limited set of model organisms was designated for priority study, and each of these is detailed below.

From the earliest days of molecular biology, studies with the simple prokaryote *E. coli* have revealed many of the fundamental processes of life. A physical map of the single, circular chromosome in the form of overlapping bacteriophage clones was completed in 1987,[271] and systematic efforts have now produced the complete sequence for the ~5 Mb of DNA in the *E. coli* genome.[330] This DNA sequence is proving valuable for identifying many of the essential functions needed to maintain independent life as well as for comparing with other bacterial genome sequences (see the section "Highlights of the Human Genome Project").

Eukaryotic organisms, with their DNA compartmentalized in nuclei, are evolutionarily very distant from *E. coli.* The yeast *S. cerevisiae*, with a genome size of ~15 Mb, is the simplest model organism with a nucleus. Comparison between it and *E. coli* is revealing the additional basic functions that distinguish eukaryotes from prokaryotes. The 16 chromosomes of *S. cerevisiae* can be separated by pulsed-field gel electrophoresis,[133] a set of overlapping bacteriophage clones representing most of the genome have been assembled,[269] and both long-range[134] and high-resolution[346] restriction maps have been constructed for each chromosome. In turn, the latter physical map proved extremely valuable to many yeast researchers, including those involved in the sequencing of the entire yeast genome. In 1996, the sequence of the yeast genome was completed[323–329] (e.g., see http://genome-www.stanford.edu/Saccharomyces). Yeast geneticists are now devising myriad approaches for exploiting a complete genomic sequence for studying complex genetic problems and for probing subtle aspects of yeast biology.[347–349]

Next in terms of complexity are the nematode *C. elegans* and the fruit fly *Drosophila melanogaster,* with genomes of ~100 Mb (in 6 chromosomes) and ~160 Mb (in 4 chromosomes), respectively. As multicellular animals, these organisms share with mammals specialized cell types such as nerve, muscle, intestine, and gonad. With the combination of molecular and mutational capabilities in the context of detailed biologic information, these two organisms have become powerful systems for studying the role of numerous genes in development and behavior. For *C. elegans*, a detailed physical map and corresponding clone set for virtually the entire genome have been assembled with cosmids[270] and YACs.[350,351] These clones provided the necessary templates for systematic genomic sequencing[331–335] (see http://www.sanger.ac.uk and http://genome.wustl.edu/gsc), which by the end of 1998 yielded the first complete genomic sequence of a multicellular organism. This sequence is profoundly enhancing studies with *C. elegans* in numerous ways.[352,353] For *D. melanogaster*, a well-established cytogenetic map has been available since the 1930s—in the form of the famous polytene chromosomes of the salivary gland. These structures represent a thousand or more aligned copies of each chromosome in an extended conformation, so that segments as close as 20 kb can be resolved, thereby providing a framework for organizing other mapping information.[354,355] Physical mapping of the *Drosophila* genome is well under way[356,357] and is being enhanced by efforts to perform systematic gene disruptions using *P* transposable elements.[358] The sequencing of the *Drosophila* genome[354,355] is now largely complete (see http://flybase.harvard. edu:7081).

Among the model organisms, the mouse (as a mammal) is the most closely related to humans in terms of developmental program and biologic complexity. This animal provides the closely related features of mammalian development and physiology, but in a system that is powerful in terms of its potential for genetic manipulation. The availability of fully inbred strains and a generation time of a few months make classic genetic studies feasible.[359–361] Furthermore, the ability to manipulate the mouse germ line, including the capacity to add or delete specific genes en route to the creation of transgenic mice,[362–367] is providing the means for establishing the function of many genes present in mice and humans[361,368,369] (see Chap. 14). Also important is the close evolutionary homology in the arrangement of gene segments along the chromosomes.[360,361,370–376] These features have prompted a systematic effort to construct genetic and physical maps of the mouse genome[359,377–381] (e.g., see http://www-genome.wi.mit.edu), which is roughly the same size as the human genome, as well as to develop increasingly robust computational tools for accessing and analyzing mouse genomic information.[382,383] The long-term goal is to establish the complete sequence of the mouse genome which, by comparison with the human genome sequence, will enable more precise identification of genes and their regulatory elements.[359,360,384–387] In fact, many believe that the rigorous interpretation of the human genome sequence will be possible only by comparison with the mouse genome sequence (and perhaps the genomic sequences of other more distantly related organisms). Such comparisons should reveal important evolutionarily conserved sequences, such as those that encode key structural features of proteins and those that control the regulation of gene expression. Already, significant insight has been gained from pilot-scale comparative analyses of human and mouse cDNA[388,389] and genomic[390–393] sequences.

While the organisms just detailed are included under the official umbrella of the currently planned HGP, the successes in genome mapping and sequencing have catalyzed genome analysis initiatives for a number of other organisms, including the fission yeast (*Schizosaccharomyces pombe*),[394,395] the laboratory rat (*Rattus novegicus*),[396–398] the zebrafish (*Danio rerio*),[399–403] the pufferfish (*Fugu rubripes*),[404–409] various plant species[410] (in particular, *Arabidopsis thaliana*[411–414]), and numerous bacteria and other microbes (see the section "Highlights of the Human Genome Project"). Such studies aim to exploit the unique and specialized aspects of the particular organisms for various research applications, to provide a broader collection of organisms from different points in evolution for comparative analyses, and to strengthen the ability to perform genetic-based studies in a larger set of organisms.

THE HUMAN GENOME PROJECT

History of the Human Genome Project

The official beginning of the HGP in the United States was heralded on October 1, 1990. However, the intellectual and administrative processes responsible for the initiation of the project had already been operating for a number of years before this.[415,416] Detailed historical accounts of the HGP have been compiled.[415–424] In brief, the origins of the HGP are thought by most to date back to a meeting in Alta, Utah, in 1984, where the discussion focused on the analysis of DNA for the purpose of detecting mutations among atomic bomb survivors.[67] Shortly after this meeting, the concept of a comprehensive program of genome study was entertained by two groups. First, a 1985 conference in Santa Cruz, California, was convened to examine the feasibility of sequencing the human genome.[68] Second, Charles DeLisi initiated discussions within the Department of Energy about the merits of genome-wide sequencing.[425] Because of its interest in the health effects of radiation and other types of environmental hazards, the Department of Energy viewed establishing the sequence of the human genome as critically important for programs aimed at monitoring DNA sequence changes. Furthermore, DeLisi contended that the Department of Energy, with its expertise in a diversity of complementary fields (e.g., analytical chemistry, applied physics, engineering, and computer science) and experience at directing large-scale projects, would be a strong participant for such an endeavor.[425] Additional support for the HGP came independently from Renato Dulbecco, who argued in 1986 that sequencing the human genome and identifying all the encoded genes would be an efficient way to expedite cancer research.[69] Importantly, he stressed that it would be more desirable to elucidate all this information at once, rather than obtaining it piecemeal over an extended period.

Two highly influential reports published in 1988 guided the development of the structure and scope of the early phases of the HGP in the United States — one by the National Research Council Committee on Mapping and Sequencing the Human Genome[426] and the other by a committee operating under the auspices of the United States Congress Office of Technology Assessment.[427] Together, these reports called for a systematic effort of genome mapping and sequencing, provided recommendations about the scope and goals of the effort, outlined the roles for both the National Institutes of Health (NIH) and the Department of Energy in administering the project in the United States, and recommended funding levels for the endeavor. Of note, the general program outlined by these reports has remained fundamentally unchanged, despite numerous advances in the technologies available for genome analysis. Amidst all these discussions was a significant amount of intense debate within the scientific community as to the merits of the HGP,[42,428–438] although virtually all the negative aspects of this have since waned. The Department of Energy's Office of Health and Environmental Research initiated its formal program in 1987. The Office for Human Genome Research at the NIH was created in 1988; later that year, this office became the National Center for Human Genome Research [NCHGR; note that in 1997, NCHGR became an NIH Institute, the National Human Genome Research Institute (NHGRI)]. Appropriations for both the Department of Energy and NIH programs were initiated in 1988 (although the Department of Energy's program started the previous year using funds diverted from other sources). The first set of formal goals for the project in the United States was established in 1990,[439] at which time the project officially began.

While the historic roots of the HGP are largely based in the United States, the project is international in structure and spirit. In addition to the NIH and Department of Energy orchestrating the HGP in the United States, analogous agencies are coordinating efforts under way in other countries, particularly England, France, Germany, Italy, Canada, Australia, Japan, and China. In this regard, the project is truly international in terms of collaboration and coordination.

As an aside, the inclusion of "human" in the name Human Genome Project is, of course, a misnomer, since it does not accurately reflect the breadth of the overall initiative. Rather, from the beginning, parallel mapping and sequencing of nonhuman model organisms have been central components of the HGP (see the sections "Studying the Genomes of Model Organisms" and "Comparative Study of the Biology of Humans and Other Organisms").

Scientific Plan of the Human Genome Project

In the United States, the currently planned HGP has a 15-year timetable. Since its inception, the project has been associated with carefully crafted milestone-oriented goals that reflect current and realistic near-term capabilities, including an initial set established in 1990[420–422,439] and two successive sets of 5-year goals starting in 1993[440] and 1998.[441] The key elements of these goals have focused on establishing infrastructure, developing requisite technologies, and generating the necessary inventories of data. At the same time, the goals have attempted to be visionary, flexible, and integrated with the ongoing planning process but openly acknowledged as transient in nature, due to the continual advances in the technologies for genome analysis.[442] Finally, the formulation of these goals has been accompanied by critical discussions of the evolving plans for the project by some of the key participants.[256,336,342,442]

A summary of the 1998–2003 goals for the U.S. HGP[441] is provided in Table 10-1. A number of important points about these goals should be emphasized. First, completing the human genome sequence by 2003 represents the highest-priority goal (see the section "Sequencing the Human Genome"). In fact, the initiation of this effort occurred 2 years earlier than originally anticipated. Second, associated with sequencing the human genome are plans to improve further DNA sequencing technology, so as to make the sequencing of other genomes as well as the resequencing of human DNA as efficient and cost-effective as possible. Third, plans to catalog common human sequence variants are included within the HGP for the first time. Studies of human sequence variation represent a critical and rapidly evolving growth area in human genetics.[256] New initiatives will include the construction of a third-generation, SNP-based genetic map of the human genome (with the first two generation genetic maps being composed of RFLPs/VNTRs and STRs, respectively; see the section "Construction of Genetic Maps" and http://www.ncbi.nlm.nih.gov/SNP). Fourth, also emphasized within the HGP goals are a series of activities falling under the general category of *functional genomics*,[443] an area of genome research that broadly deals with the development and implementation of technologies for exploiting complete

Table 10-1 Summary of the 1998–2003 Goals for the U.S. Human Genome Project

Human genome sequence
Complete the human genome sequence by the end of 2003 while emphasizing the establishment of a *working draft* version for at least 90% of the genome by 2000, the development of a sustainable capacity for large-scale sequencing, the generation of large contiguous stretches of high-quality sequence, and the provision of ready access to the data.

Sequencing technology
Continue incremental improvements in current sequencing methods so as to increase the throughput and reduce the cost of sequencing, with emphasis on automation, miniaturization, and process integration. In parallel, support interdisciplinary research for developing novel sequencing technologies and the means for implementing such technologies into established sequence-producing operations.

Human sequence variation
Develop the technology for rapid, large-scale identification and scoring of single-nucleotide polymorphisms (SNPs), with the aims of identifying and cataloging the common variants in the coding regions of the majority of human genes and creating a human SNP map of at least 100,000 markers. In addition, establish the intellectual foundations and requisite public resources of DNA samples and cell lines for studying human variation.

Technology for functional genomics
Generate complete sets of full-length cDNA clones for humans and model organisms, develop the technology for defining the spatial and temporal patterns of gene expression, design new strategies for the global study of noncoding sequences, design new approaches for systematic mutagenesis of genes, and advance the understanding of protein function on a genome-wide basis.

Comparative genomics
Complete the sequence of the *Caenorhabditis elegans* genome by 1998 and the *Drosophila* genome by 2002. For mouse genome analysis, develop more detailed physical and genetic maps, construct additional cDNA resources, and, by 2005, complete the genomic sequence. Identify and initiate studies on other model organisms that will markedly contribute to the understanding of the human genome.

Ethical, legal, and social implications
Examine the issues surrounding the completion of the human genome sequence and the study of human genetic variation, study the issues raised by the integration of genetic technologies and information into health care, public health activities, and non-clinical settings, and explore how the new genetic information will influence various societal issues related to genetics.

Bioinformatics and computational biology
Develop better tools for data generation and capture, improve the content and utility of databases, create mechanisms for sharing and disseminating exportable software, and construct appropriate tools and databases for dealing with comprehensive studies of gene expression and function as well as with sequence homology and variation.

Training and personnel
Facilitate the training of new scientific specialists with expertise in genomics research (including the recruitment of nonbiologic scientists from fields such as computer science, engineering, mathematics, physics, and chemistry) and aid in the establishment of academic career paths for genome scientists. Increase the number of scholars who are knowledgeable both in genetics and in ethics, law, and social sciences.

SOURCE: From Collins et al.[441] Used by permission.

genomic sequence. For example, this includes techniques for examining gene expression on a genome-wide scale (e.g., see the section "DNA Chips"). At the forefront of many areas of functional genomics are yeast, *C. elegans*, and *D. melanogaster* geneticists, who are fortunate to have complete genomic sequences for their organisms of study. Included among the numerous initiatives in functional genomics are efforts to generate improved (e.g., full-length) cDNA libraries and derive complete cDNA sequences for comprehensive sets of human and other organisms' genes. Fifth, the HGP will continue to emphasize comparative genome analysis of model organisms, for the first time including explicit plans for obtaining the complete mouse genomic sequence. Finally, the HGP goals include efforts to support a range of associated activities, including those aiming to foster the development of improved computational genomics tools, those addressing the important ethical, legal, and social issues relating to genome mapping and sequencing (see the section "Ethical, Legal, and Social Implications of the Human Genome Project"), and those supporting the training of individuals in genome research. Of note, the latter will intentionally include the recruitment of investigators with expertise outside biology (e.g., engineering, chemistry, and physics) into the field.[444]

Highlights of the Human Genome Project

To date, the HGP has achieved virtually all its well-formulated goals. Various reviews have charted this progress.[23,424,445–447] While numerous individual accomplishments can be cited, several major areas of highlights should be emphasized. These are best appreciated when considered within the context of the planned timetable for the HGP with respect to the construction of genetic, physical, and sequence maps of the human genome (Fig. 10-17).

With respect to genetic map construction, a high-resolution human genetic map consisting of PCR-based, STR-type markers has been assembled[263–267] (e.g., see http://www.genethon.fr/genethon_en.html), with the total number of markers generated to date far exceeding the number proposed for the HGP. Specifically, the original goal for the HGP was the development of ~1500 microsatellite-based genetic markers (thus providing a genetic marker, on average, every 2 to 5 cM); to date, over 20,000 such markers have been generated.

With respect to physical map construction, the initial goals of the HGP included establishing complete clone coverage of the human genome and mapping an STS, on average, every ~100 kb across all human chromosomes. Targeted efforts to construct YAC-based physical maps (mostly by STS-content mapping) have been completed for a handful of individual human chromosomes.[93–95,99–107] In addition to these studies there have been analogous genome-wide mapping efforts[95,96,98] (e.g., see http://www-genome.wi.mit.edu and http://www.cephb.fr/bio/ceph-genethon-map.html). Attainment of better than 100-kb average STS spacing has been reported for two human chromosomes, X[106] and 7.[107] Supplementing the YAC-based physical map of the human genome is an evolving STS-based radiation hybrid map[291,300] (also see http://shgc-www.stanford.edu).

In parallel to human genome mapping have been efforts to construct genetic and physical maps of the mouse genome. In particular, markedly improved STR-based genetic maps of the mouse genome have been assembled.[377–380] Similarly, a first-generation YAC-based physical map of the mouse genome has been constructed (e.g., see http://www-genome.wi.mit.edu).

With respect to DNA sequencing, the initial emphasis of the HGP was to improve the efficiency of existing methods, to develop new technologies, and to begin systematic sequencing of model organisms. These efforts produced the complete DNA sequences of the *S. cerevisiae*[323–329] (e.g., see http://genome-www.stanford.edu/Saccharomyces), *E. coli*,[330] *C. elegans*[331–335] (see http://www.sanger.ac.uk and http://genome.wustl.edu/gsc), and *D. melanogaster* genomes.

The refinement of strategies for performing large-scale DNA sequencing within the HGP has led to another major set of

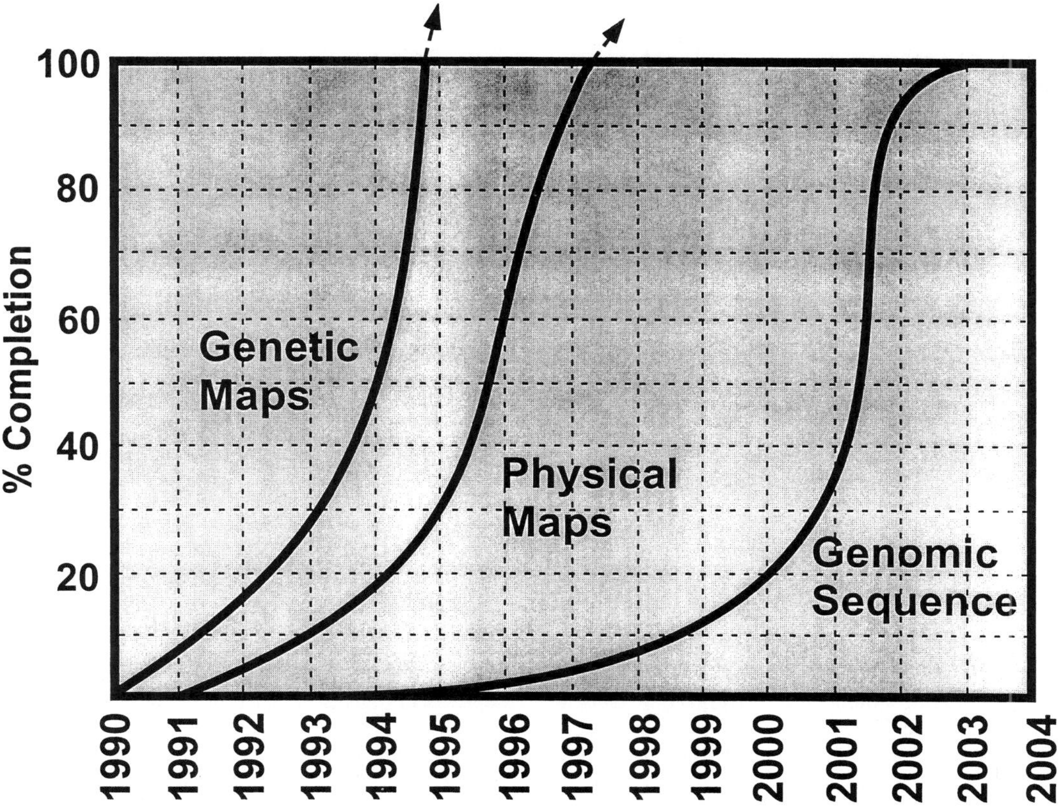

Fig. 10-17 Timetable for human genome analysis in the Human Genome Project (HGP). The approximate schedule for completing the human genetic, physical, and sequence maps in the HGP is depicted.

accomplishments: the complete genomic sequencing of numerous microorganisms.[448–456] In fact, elucidating the sequence of a whole microbial genome is now considered a relatively straightforward endeavor. Among the sequenced microbes are bacteria of major medical importance, such as *E. coli*,[330] *Haemophilus influenzae*,[457] *Mycobacterium tuberculosis*,[458] *Helicobacter pylori*,[459] *Borrelia burgdorferi*,[460] *Mycoplasma genitalium*,[461] *Treponema pallidum*,[462] *Chlamydia trachomatis*,[463] and many others. Similar efforts to sequence the genomes of medically important parasitic pathogens, such as *Trypanosoma brucei* and *Plasmodium falciparum*, are also being performed. An updated listing of sequenced microbial and parasitic genomes is available on the Web (http://www.tigr.org/tdb). In addition to providing insight about the genetic bases of microbial physiology, evolution, and virulence, studying the complete genomic sequence of important infectious pathogens should facilitate the development of more robust diagnostic tests, the design of improved antimicrobial agents, and the identification of candidate vaccine targets.[449,451,453]

In the case of sequencing human DNA, the early emphasis was on the generation of ESTs (see the section "cDNA Sequencing"). Large collections of human ESTs have been established[309,310] (see http://www.ncbi.nlm.nih.gov/dbEST), which in turn have been used to construct a radiation-hybrid-mapping-based transcript map of the human genome[292,293] (see http://www.ncbi.nlm.nih.gov/genemap98) that may already contain upward of half the human genes. Perhaps the most striking highlight of the HGP related to DNA sequencing, however, is the realization that the human genome will be sequenced shortly after we enter the next century[336,338,342] (see the section "Sequencing the Human Genome").

A final highlight of the HGP worth noting is the continual and consistent emphasis on generating high-quality mapping and sequencing data. For example, criteria for monitoring progress and completeness of physical maps have been established.[464,465] Similarly, the maintenance of rigorous accuracy standards for DNA sequencing, in particular for the generated human genome sequence, is viewed as a high priority.[466]

Sequencing the Human Genome

The early phases of the HGP have brought major advances in the approaches for performing large-scale DNA sequencing. Numerous factors have contributed to this, including subtle improvements in instrumentation, optimized experimental methods, and refined operation of large production groups (see the section "Genomic Sequencing"). These developments, in conjunction with the successful construction of physical maps of human chromosomes, resulted in the earlier-than-anticipated launching of efforts to sequence the human genome,[336–342] with the aim of completing the first-generation sequence by 2003 (Fig. 10-17). The year 2003 is particularly significant, since it will mark the 50th anniversary of the discovery of the double-helix structure of DNA by James Watson and Francis Crick.[18]

Within the HGP, sequencing of the human genome is being performed using a clone-by-clone approach, whereby individual mapped clones (BACs or PACs) are sequenced, most often by a shotgun sequencing strategy[342,343] (see Figs. 10-15 and 10-16). However, other options have been proposed. For example, some have advocated applying a shotgun sequencing strategy to the entire human genome en masse (a *whole genome shotgun*).[467] Although strong arguments against such a strategy have been made,[468] at least one private company is pursuing this general plan using a recently developed sequencing instrument.[469]

Several additional points about the ongoing efforts to sequence the human genome deserve mention. First, this activity is being carefully coordinated at an international level,[470] so as to complete the sequence as rapidly as possible, avoid unnecessary duplication, and share technical advances and expertise. Second, all sequence data being generated by the publicly funded HGP are made available regularly (typically nightly) via the Web. Note that this includes both the final, finished sequence of individual clones as well as the evolving, preliminary sequence data of clones whose analysis is still in progress (see Fig. 10-16). Such a policy of immediate data release has been widely supported by the participating groups,[471,472] although this has not been without some debate about its desirability.[473] Third, en route to completing the human genome sequence, a major effort is being made to generate as much preliminary sequence data as rapidly as possible, with the aim of producing a *working draft* version of the sequence for at least 90 percent of the human genome by the end of 2001.[441] Fourth, care has been taken to protect the individuals whose DNA is being sequenced by the HGP; specifically, several new BAC libraries designated for use in sequencing the human genome have been constructed from the DNA of anonymous individuals. In this regard, it is worth noting that the first-generation sequence of the human genome will consist of a patchwork of sequences from multiple individuals. Finally, the HGP aims to generate a highly accurate sequence of the human genome, with an error rate of 10^{-4} (or less) accepted as the standard for finished sequence.[466] Available data indicate that such an accuracy level is being achieved.

IMPACT OF THE HUMAN GENOME PROJECT ON THE STUDY OF HUMAN DISEASE

The HGP promises to provide a number of interrelated benefits to biology and clinical medicine. These include an improved ability to isolate, characterize, and manipulate the genes involved in normal physiology and human disease. Numerous reviews have detailed how the HGP will impact various areas of clinical medicine.[474–486]

Impact of the Human Genome Project on the Positional Cloning of Human Disease Genes

Background on Positional Cloning. Thousands of genes are known to cause disease when present in a mutated form (see http://www.ncbi.nlm.nih.gov/omim). Of course, the number of genes that influence human diseases more indirectly is undoubtedly much higher. A major effort of modern molecular genetics is to identify the genes that are in some way associated with human disease.

Human disease genes have been identified and isolated largely by one of two basic strategies: functional cloning and positional cloning[1–3] (Fig. 10-18). With functional cloning, the disease gene is isolated as a result of preexisting knowledge of the fundamental physiological defect, which provides sufficient insight about the function of the protein encoded by the defective gene. Often, the cloning of the gene is preceded by the purification of its protein product or by the acquisition of sufficient information about the protein's function. Thus, in functional cloning, mapping the gene follows its isolation (Fig. 10-18). Classic examples of disease genes identified by a functional cloning strategy include β-thalassemia,[487] phenylketonuria,[488] and glucose-6-phosphate dehydrogenase (G-6-PD) deficiency.[489]

For most of the myriad genetic disorders (including the probable thousands not yet uncovered), there is little to no advanced insight about the function of the defective gene. In the great majority of cases, biochemical studies fail to provide any meaningful clues. For studying these more typical genetic diseases, the strategy of positional cloning has been refined in recent years[1–8] and successfully employed for isolating numerous disease genes (see http://genome.nhgri.nih.gov/clone). With positional cloning, isolation of the gene follows the establishment of its position within the genome by genetic and/or physical mapping techniques. In most cases, these efforts proceed with limited knowledge of the gene's function or the nature of the underlying pathologic process. Thus, in this strategy, mapping precedes cloning (moving in the opposite direction as functional cloning), and gene function is defined only after the gene has been isolated and characterized (Fig. 10-18). This process was originally called *reverse genetics*,[490–493] but this somewhat incorrect terminology has now been abandoned.[1]

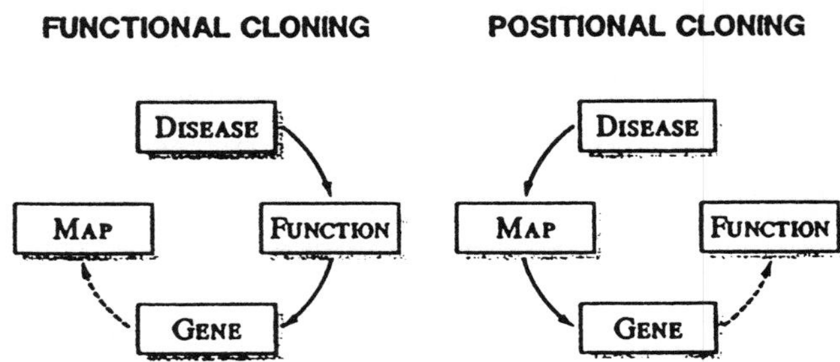

Fig. 10-18 Functional versus positional cloning of disease genes. In functional cloning, the study of gene function precedes gene identification. In positional cloning, gene mapping precedes gene identification. The last step in each case (gene mapping and defining gene function, respectively) is not critical for the isolation of the disease gene itself. (*Adapted from Collins.*[1] *Used by permission.*)

Isolation of Disease Genes by Positional Cloning. The identification and isolation of disease genes by a positional cloning strategy can be conceptually divided into the series of steps depicted in Fig. 10-19, each of which is discussed below.

The starting point for positional cloning is the collection of families with multiple affected individuals, preferably in several generations. Of critical importance is the establishment of the correct phenotype for as many family members as possible and the isolation of DNA from these individuals. Discrepancies between an individual's phenotype and genotype can be due to (1) an incorrect diagnosis (i.e., phenotype assignment), (2) genetic heterogeneity (defects in more than one gene being associated with the phenotype), (3) incomplete penetrance (some individuals inheriting the defective gene do not express the phenotype or at least not at the time of evaluation), or (4) a mix-up of the DNA sample(s). Thus, significant effort must be invested during the

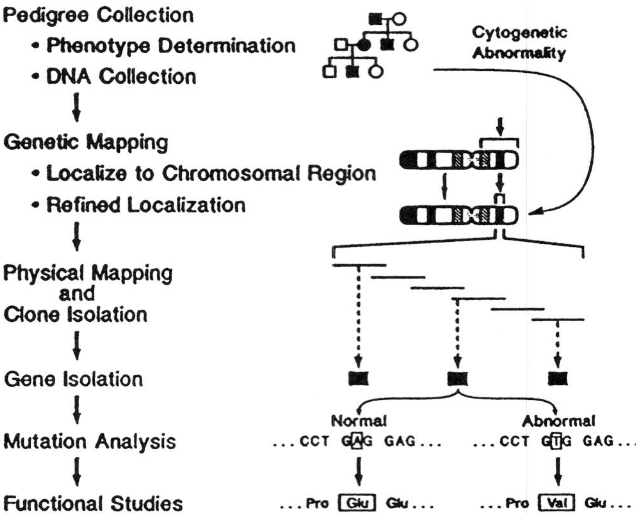

Fig. 10-19 Positional cloning of human disease genes. The major steps involved in the isolation of human disease genes by a positional cloning strategy are depicted (additional details are provided in the text). In the hypothetical example shown, a single base change (A → T) results in an amino acid change (Glu → Val) in the encoded protein, which in turn causes the disease. Remarkably, such a single-base-pair change in the 3-billion-bp human genome can be lethal.

collection of family resources to minimize errors, especially those caused by preventable mistakes.

In the next stage of positional cloning, the general region of the genome containing the defective gene is identified. In the ideal case, the disease is closely associated with a cytogenetic abnormality, which immediately defines the critical region harboring the gene (since such a cytogenetic alteration is likely to have interrupted the gene or its regulatory element). Examples of diseases associated with cytogenetic abnormalities include genetic disorders (e.g., Duchenne muscular dystrophy,[240] neurofibromatosis,[44,494] fragile X syndrome,[241] and Lowe syndrome[495]) and various types of cancer[496] (see http://www.ncbi.nlm.nih.gov/CCAP/mitelsum.cgi).

The great majority of genetic diseases are not, however, associated with cytogenetic abnormalities. For these disorders, genetic mapping is used as the front-line tool for identifying the general genomic region containing the gene. At first, DNA samples from multiple family members are analyzed for a set of genetic markers spread across the genome, searching for one (or a few) that shows linkage (coinheritance) with the disease. If successful, this typically assigns the defective gene to a rough chromosomal location, usually spanning tens of millions of base pairs. More refined localization is then accomplished using additional genetic markers that map nearby. The extent to which the region can be delimited by genetic mapping depends on a number of factors, such as the quality of the family resources (e.g., family size and availability of DNA) as well as the number, distribution, and informativeness of the genetic markers in the region. A critical component of this type of genetic mapping is the use of sophisticated computational tools for calculating the various parameters to determine whether sufficient data have been collected to allow confident establishment of linkage using the available pedigrees.[261]

In the best cases, genetic mapping allows the critical region to be limited to ~1 cM; however, the corresponding physical size of such a region can vary widely due to regional and sex-specific differences in recombination rates. Typically, ~1 cM in genetic distance corresponds to roughly 1 to 3 Mb, and such a DNA interval can then usually be analyzed by physical mapping methods. Most often, the closest mapping genetic markers are used as the starting points for clone isolation (e.g., YACs and BACs). If necessary, new markers can be derived from the ends of isolated clones and then used to identify new, overlapping clones. The iterative isolation of adjacent, overlapping clones by such a strategy is called *chromosome walking*. Additional markers can also be derived from the targeted region by other strategies (see the section "Generation of STSs") and used for clone isolation. In the ideal cases, the entire genomic interval between the flanking genetic markers is isolated in cloned form. The resulting clones can be used for developing additional genetic markers (to reduce further the critical region by genetic mapping) and, importantly, for gene isolation.

A particularly challenging step in a positional cloning approach is the identification of encoded genes within the critical region.[7,8,497–501] A number of different strategies have been developed for detecting genes in large genomic clones (e.g., YACs, BACs, PACs, P1s, and cosmids) (Table 10-2). In general, each of these methods is relatively labor intensive, suffers from a number of inherent limitations, and is rarely used alone during the search for a disease gene.

One major class of techniques for identifying coding regions within genomic clones employs DNA-DNA hybridization-based methods (Table 10-2). For example, small DNA fragments derived from a starting genomic clone can be used to probe DNA from a variety of different animal species (immobilized on a membrane referred to as a *zoo blot*). Detection of cross-hybridizing (i.e., presumed homologous) DNA suggests the presence of sequences that may have been evolutionarily conserved and therefore are likely to be essential for biologic function. The same probes can also be hybridized to mRNA derived from various human tissues

Table 10-2 Strategies for Identifying Genes in Large Genomic Regions

DNA-DNA hybridization based

Using small DNA fragments
- Analysis of DNA from other organisms (*zoo blots*)
- Analysis of RNA from individual tissues by northern blotting
- Identification of CpG islands

Using large genomic clones (e.g., yeast artificial chromosomes, bacterial artificial chromosomes, P1-derived artificial chromosomes, P1s, and cosmids)
- Hybridization-based screening of cDNA libraries
- *Direct selection* of cDNAs with immobilized DNA

Function based
- Exon trapping/amplification
- PolyA signal trapping
- Gene transfer and transcript identification

DNA sequence based
- Comparison to sequence databases (expressed-sequence tags and known genes)
- Detection of open reading frames
- Prediction of coding sequences
- Comparison to sequences from other organisms

SOURCE: Adapted from Collins.[1] Used by permission.

(immobilized on a membrane referred to as a *northern blot*[502]) to detect the presence of expressed sequences. A wide survey of tissues is advisable, especially since the expression pattern of the gene is generally unknown at this stage. Finally, the probes can be used in conjunction with rare-cutting restriction enzymes to search for the presence of CpG islands, which often (but not always) mark the 5′ ends of genes.[45–47,503]

Alternatively, genomic clones can be used either to probe directly cDNA libraries[503] (made from the mRNA of particular tissues) or to capture cDNA sequences by a method known as *direct cDNA selection*.[504–509] In the latter technique, DNA from the genomic clone is used as an affinity matrix to capture complementary sequences present in mRNA mixtures or cDNA libraries. There are a number of important issues regarding the source of mRNA or cDNA libraries for gene isolation. First, a particular gene will be identified only if it is expressed in the tissue from which the mRNA or cDNA library was derived. Second, not all mRNA molecules are expressed at equal levels in a particular tissue. In fact, some genes are expressed at exceedingly low levels, and these can be particularly difficult to isolate. One route for overcoming this general problem is to use *normalized* libraries that contain a more equal representation of different cDNA sequences, regardless of the initial levels of the corresponding mRNA molecules.[303–307]

A second class of strategies for gene isolation exploits particular aspects of gene structure or function (Table 10-2). In one approach, the presence of sequences necessary for proper removal of introns (called *splice junctions*) allows the isolation of the adjacent exon by a technique called *exon amplification* or *exon trapping*.[510–515] Similar approaches for trapping the most 3′-terminal exon in a gene (by using the associated polyA tract as the signal) have also been developed.[515,516] Alternatively, some genes can be isolated by transferring the cloned genomic DNA into an appropriate mammalian cell and selecting for the function of the gene. Of course, the latter approach requires some prior information about the likely function of the gene itself.

A final class of gene identification strategies involves the analysis of DNA sequence derived from the critical region (Table 10-2). Approaches for examining both partial (incomplete) or finished (complete) sequence data are available. For example, one strategy for gene identification involves generating random sequences from a clone(s) of interest such that each nucleotide is read, on average, one to two times (similar to the first phase of a shotgun sequencing project; see Fig. 10-16 and the section "Genomic Sequencing"). All resulting sequence data, which mostly consist of unassembled individual sequence reads, are then compared with available databases (e.g., dbEST; see http://www.ncbi.nlm.nih.gov/dbEST and the section "cDNA Sequencing") by using various computational tools.[225,226,517] Resulting sequence matches are suggestive of genes and require more careful analysis and follow-up studies. This general strategy, called *sample sequencing*, has proved effective for the identification of important human disease genes.[518,519] Completed genomic sequence is, of course, even more amenable to computational analyses for identifying genes, with increasingly sophisticated tools becoming available for predicting the presence of genes[229–235] and performing complex sequence comparisons[224–228] (see the section "Computational Genomics").

All genes identified within a critical region become candidate genes for that disease. Proof that a particular gene is the correct one requires demonstration that the disease is associated with mutations in that gene. Thus, the next stage of analysis involves the difficult task of searching for mutations within candidate genes[520,521] and demonstrating that such mutations show the proper inheritance (e.g., recessive or dominant) relative to the disease. These genetic alterations can range from single-base-pair changes to more gross aberrations (e.g., large deletions[522] or expanded tracts of trinucleotide repeats[523–525]). While mutations can occur anywhere within a gene (including its regulatory elements and introns), the majority of mutations reported to date have been within coding regions.

Often, the initial screening for mutations in affected individuals involves analyzing the gene for gross rearrangements by conventional and pulsed-field gel electrophoresis. Most often, this fails to demonstrate a mutation, and the effort then shifts to searching for more subtle DNA alterations involving one or a few nucleotides.[520,521] A number of techniques have been developed for this purpose, including denaturing gradient gel electrophoresis (DGGE),[526–528] RNase[529,530] or chemical[531] cleavage of mismatches, single-strand conformation polymorphism (SSCP) analysis,[532] and direct DNA sequencing. Ultimately, DNA sequencing must be used to establish the precise nature of any mutation. With improved methods now available, direct DNA sequencing is increasingly being used for mutation detection rather than these other methods.

An issue that must be continually addressed during the mutation-detection stage of a positional cloning project is the discrimination between innocent sequence polymorphisms (which may simply be linked to the nearby disease gene) and actual mutations (which cause the disease). Insight about the potential effect of a given mutation (e.g., changing an amino acid at a predicted key site in the protein) can often provide strong supportive evidence for its role in the disease. However, the ultimate proof that a candidate gene is the correct one often requires evidence that the normal form of the gene can correct the abnormal phenotype and/or that the mutant form of the gene can cause the abnormal phenotype.

Impact of the Human Genome Project on Positional Cloning. The HGP is dramatically simplifying the process of positional cloning by improving virtually every one of its steps. First, the availability of higher-resolution genetic maps, better sets of informative STR-type markers, and more efficient methods for genotype analysis is allowing human disease genes to be assigned to more precise genetic locations. Similarly, the construction of comprehensive physical maps of each chromosome, including the assembly of associated clone sets and the localization of genes and ESTs, is dramatically reducing the time it takes to isolate and characterize critical regions for genes of interest. Finally, advances in DNA sequencing are making sequence-based gene discovery and mutation detection more routine and robust.

With the increased mapping of genes and ESTs throughout the human genome, a variant form of positional cloning, termed *positional candidate cloning*,[2] has come to the forefront. In this strategy, a genetically defined critical region for a disease gene is identified and then evaluated for the presence of already mapped, viable candidate genes. Should such an available candidate gene turn out to be the disease gene of interest, then the steps involving the cloning of the region and the isolation of genes can be skipped entirely. Thus, in this approach, information about both the physical position and the likely candidacy of a gene is used to implicate it as the cause of a genetic disease. As a result of the increased number of mapped and characterized genes, it is now more common to identify a human disease gene by a positional candidate approach than by a pure positional cloning approach.

Overall, there is a strong correlation between the amount of mapping and sequencing data generated by the HGP and the rate at which human disease genes have been identified by a positional cloning or positional candidate approach (e.g., compare Fig. 10-17 and http://genome.nhgri.nih.gov/clone). In many cases the contribution by the HGP to the identification of the gene has been subtle, whereas in other cases it has been critical.[533–538]

Important future studies in human genetics will involve unraveling the genetic bases of diseases that are particularly complicated to study, such as those that are rare (and have limited family resources available), are caused by defects in more than one gene (polygenic diseases), or are a consequence of combined genetic and nongenetic factors (multifactorial)[13–17] (see Chap. 6). Perhaps the greatest ultimate impact of the HGP will be to improve the capacity for defining the genetic alterations associated with such medically important, genetically complex diseases. For example, studying polygenic disorders is inherently difficult in humans, in part because of the small pedigree sizes and lack of controlled matings. More detailed genomic maps [including a dense SNP map (see http://www.ncbi.nlm.nih.gov/SNP) and, eventually, a whole-genome sequence map] should help to overcome such limitations, enabling more precise correlation between sequence variation and heritable phenotypes.[13–17] In addition, newer technology may eventually allow specific steps in a standard positional cloning strategy to be bypassed. One such technique is genome-mismatch scanning,[539,540] which is a sophisticated method that allows the regions that are identical between different genomes (such as those concordant for a particular trait) to be isolated.[539,541,542] This technique, which can be combined with DNA chip detection schemes to identify corresponding clones containing the DNA of interest,[543] may allow the genetic-mapping stage of positional cloning (i.e., marker-by-marker genotyping) to be skipped. Thus, such a method may enable the rapid isolation of those genomic regions containing genes for genetically complex diseases. Together, the improved genomic infrastructure provided by the HGP coupled with more sophisticated technologies should greatly help to define the polygenic factors underlying human disease susceptibilities and predispositions.

Comparative Study of the Biology of Humans and Other Organisms

From the onset, a major component of the HGP has been to map and sequence the genomes of model organisms whose biologic properties have been examined for decades by geneticists, biochemists, and physiologists (see the section "Studying the Genomes of Model Organisms"). In fact, analyzing the genomes of model organisms has played a critical role in developing the strategies, technologies, and infrastructure needed for studying human DNA. However, the actual mapping and sequencing of the human genome will almost certainly be more straightforward than the difficult and challenging task of determining the functions of genes and the bases of human genetic disease. In this regard, the knowledge gained from research on model organisms will provide a framework for utilizing the reagents and information produced from human genome studies. The strong emphasis on studying model organisms within the HGP is based on the fundamental feature of biology that all organisms are related through a common evolutionary tree and share the same general type of DNA blueprint, with a tremendous degree of conservation of gene structure and function existing across a diverse array of organisms.

The accomplishments of the HGP have catalyzed several major efforts aiming to make connections between gene structure and function in model organisms and that in humans. For example, the availability of the complete yeast sequence[323–329] (e.g., see http://genome-www.stanford.edu/Saccharomyces) is allowing the systematic cross-referencing of yeast genes with those in the human genome,[544–546] with particular emphasis on identifying, cataloging, and studying those genes associated with human disease.[547–551] A similar effort is under way for comparing fruit fly (*Drosophila*) and human genes.[552]

As a result of these and various other studies, there are now numerous examples where the study of a gene in bacteria, yeast, worms, fruit flies, and/or mice has provided important insight about the function of a particular human gene.[319,345] Remarkably, it is often the case that the human gene can functionally substitute for its counterpart, even in the distantly related yeast *S. cerevisiae*. A very small but illustrative sampling of cases where sequence homology and/or cross-species functional studies have proved valuable includes the following:

1. The yeast *STE6* gene, which encodes a protein required for secreting a peptide pheromone factor involved in yeast mating,[553] is highly homologous to the human *MDR1* (multidrug resistance) gene, which encodes a protein that renders tumor cells resistant to a number of chemotherapeutic agents.[554] This strong sequence similarity motivated researchers to transfer the mouse homologue of the *MDR1* gene into a mutant yeast strain defective in the *STE6* gene; remarkably, the mouse gene was able to correct the mutant phenotype in the yeast.[555]

2. The gene mutated in neurofibromatosis type 1, a common autosomal dominant disease associated with a constellation of symptoms (including characteristic neurofibromas), was cloned[44,494] and found to be highly homologous to the mammalian RAS GTPase-activating gene[556,557] and two yeast genes called *IRA1* and *IRA2*.[557,558] Gene transfer experiments demonstrated that a segment of the mammalian neurofibromatosis type 1 gene can complement (i.e., correct) the function of defective *IRA* genes in yeast.[557]

3. The human *ERCC-3* gene encodes a presumed DNA helicase involved in repairing specific types of DNA damage, and defects in this gene are responsible for two rare genetic diseases: xeroderma pigmentosum and Cockayne syndrome.[559] A *Drosophila* gene called *haywire* appears to be the fruit fly equivalent of *ERCC-3*, and mutations in *haywire* result in some of the same effects as those seen in xeroderma pigmentosum.[560] However, not all *haywire* alleles are associated with the identical phenotype. This information may help to explain the variability in symptoms seen in different xeroderma pigmentosum and Cockayne patients.

4. The yeast *SGS1* gene, which encodes another DNA helicase, is closely related to the human Werner syndrome gene.[561] Mutations in these genes result in a premature-aging phenotype in yeast and humans, respectively, revealing a conserved mechanism of cellular aging.

5. There are now numerous examples where the close evolutionary relationship between mice and humans has been exploited to understand the function of particular human genes. In fact, such studies provide a key rationale for the comparative mapping[374–376] and sequencing[384–386] of the human and mouse genomes.[359,360,387] Increasingly, gene-characterization studies in either human or mouse quickly broaden to include examining the gene in the other species. This scenario has been particularly valuable for the study of human disease genes[361] (see Chap. 14). Myriad examples can be cited where important biologic insight was gained by combined human and mouse genetic analysis; however, a strikingly dramatic example is the study of mouse obesity mutants.[562] Here, the complicated task of unraveling the genetic bases of human obesity[563] was aided by the identification of the mouse *ob* gene,[564] which encodes the protein leptin. This discovery has revealed a new physiological pathway for weight control and catalyzed numerous new experimental initiatives aimed at examining the role of leptin in human obesity, identifying the other critical components in the leptin pathway, and developing possible pharmacologic agents for therapeutic weight control.[565]

In short, it is now clear that comparative genome analysis is a powerful approach for characterizing gene structure and function. In this regard, knowledge of the complete sequence of the human genome and that of an increasing number of other organisms should be regarded as the ultimate framework for deciphering the functional information encoded in DNA.

Advances in Molecular Diagnostics Resulting from the Human Genome Project

Molecular diagnostics can be broadly defined as the testing of DNA (or RNA) within a clinical context, and this medical discipline is rapidly growing in scope and importance.[566–571] The applications of molecular diagnostics span a wide range of human disorders, including tests for hereditary, neoplastic, and infectious diseases.

The HGP will accelerate the growth of molecular diagnostics in two respects. First, by facilitating the identification of disease genes (see the section "Impact of the Human Genome Project on Positional Cloning"), an increasing number of clinically relevant, human mutations will be uncovered. With this growing insight about the genetic bases of disease will come increased opportunities to make diagnostic and prognostic assessments based on examination of an individual's DNA. Second, many of the same methods and instruments being developed to construct genetic, physical, and sequence maps of the human genome are finding immediate utility for testing DNA in a clinical setting.[566–571] A prelude of this phenomenon is already evident with PCR, which is already being used extensively for clinical testing. A typical molecular diagnostic laboratory in the future will likely perform hundreds, if not thousands, of PCR assays per day, with any refinements made by the HGP for high-throughput PCR testing being of immediate utility. However, it is likely that such a laboratory will not have benches filled with PCR machines, gels, and power supplies; rather, there will inevitably be numerous advances with respect to automation and miniaturization, such as the implementation of various types of DNA chips (see the section "DNA Chips"). Thus, the insight gained about the genetic bases of human disease in conjunction with the continued developments in experimental genetic technologies should dramatically enhance the ability to perform diagnostic DNA testing.

Prospects for Therapeutic Benefits from the Human Genome Project

The HGP promises to transform the ability to understand human genetic diseases by providing a unique interplay between genetics and clinical medicine. For all the aforementioned reasons discussed, physicians and scientists should gain new insights about the genetic components that contribute to disease and acquire better means for establishing whether a patient has inherited a genetic defect. However, the full impact of the HGP should extend beyond these areas and, in the long run, enhance the ability to treat patients with genetic abnormalities.

A number of interrelated aspects of the HGP offer the potential for having a positive impact on patient care. First, for some genetic disorders, presymptomatic knowledge of an inherited defect can provide meaningful opportunities for the use of preventive measures (e.g., lifestyle alterations, increased surveillance to aid early diagnosis, and targeted intervention) that may serve to minimize morbidity (see Chap. 5). As the HGP progresses, an increasing number of genes for diseases in this category are being discovered. Second, the improved capacity to define the precise molecular defects causing genetic diseases should aid efforts to elucidate the underlying pathophysiology. Such knowledge should facilitate the design of more rational treatments for genetic diseases, which could include the development of better pharmacologic agents, the exogenous synthesis and delivery of a missing gene product, or the introduction of the normal form of a gene into an affected patient (i.e., gene therapy;[572–574] see Chap. 5). Of note, the latter might eventually include the use of *mammalian artificial chromosome* (MAC) vectors[575–579] for gene therapy; some of these vectors are being adapted from cloning systems used for genome mapping (e.g., YACs).

One notable and rapidly evolving area of therapeutics that directly relates to the HGP involves unraveling the genetic basis of drug responsiveness. Specifically, this discipline (called *pharmacogenomics* or *pharmacogenetics*) focuses on elucidating the genetic determinants that affect drug action, with the long-term goal of establishing diagnostic tests and customized therapeutic regimens that will allow drugs to be prescribed more safely and more effectively[580,581] (see Chap. 9). This involves correlating drug responsiveness with genetic variation, which often will be subtle and complex.[582,583] However, the products of the HGP should make this task more approachable. Successes in pharmacogenomics may help to remove the empirical nature associated with many aspects of drug therapy and provide more rational approaches for predicting how individuals will respond to particular therapeutic modalities.

ETHICAL, LEGAL, AND SOCIAL IMPLICATIONS OF THE HUMAN GENOME PROJECT

With the fruits of the HGP, including both the mapping and sequencing data and the improved technologies for studying DNA, has come the identification of numerous substantive ethical and policy issues. For example, one of the early anticipated benefits of the HGP—the ability to identify and isolate genes that play important roles in human disease—has indeed become a reality. In most cases, however, cloning a human disease gene is only the first step in the long process toward developing a rational therapy. Since the latter almost always lags behind the generation of new diagnostic tests, the identification of disease genes typically provides the ability to identify individuals at risk for disorders that are associated with limited therapeutic options. Furthermore, with increasing emphasis being placed on the study of human variation and the development of improved technologies for identifying such variation (see Table 10-1), the potential availability of genetic information about individuals will undoubtedly increase. How such information will or should be used by patients, physicians, and society raises a number of issues that require immediate, thoughtful consideration.

To address these concerns, the architects of the U.S. HGP established the Ethical, Legal, and Social Implications (ELSI) Program as an integral component of the HGP.[584] This program provides a novel approach to the study of ethical, legal, and social issues by carefully integrating its agenda with that of the ongoing genome mapping and sequencing efforts[446,585] (see http://www.nhgri.nih.gov/ELSI). By design, the ELSI Program has brought together individuals with diverse areas of expertise (e.g., medical geneticists, ethicists, historians, theologians, legal scholars, policy analysts, and sociologists). The program's mission includes both research studies and education projects for addressing ELSI issues as well as policy analysis and development efforts for translating the empirical research findings into pragmatic policy and programmatic recommendations. The NIH committed initially 3 percent and later 5 percent of its total HGP budget to the ELSI Program. The U.S. Department of Energy also established an ELSI Program (see http://www.ornl.gov/TechResources/Human_Genome/resource/elsi.html).

The central mission of the ELSI Program has been to identify and address the key ethical, legal, and social issues relating to the HGP (and other associated genomic and genetic research activities) and to facilitate the establishment and institution of appropriate safeguards[446,585] (see http://www.nhgri.nih.gov/ELSI). The program has focused on four high-priority areas of study: (1) privacy and fair use of genetic information, (2) safe and effective integration of new genetic technologies into clinical practice, (3) issues surrounding genetics research, and (4) public and professional education.

The increased availability of genetic data raises numerous issues about who should have access to this potentially powerful information. Several surveys have shown that this is a real concern to people.[586–588] In the past, genetic information has indeed been used to discriminate against individuals (e.g., sickle-cell anemia carriers). Of particular concern is the fear of losing or being denied health insurance because of a genetic predisposition to a disease. Ironically, the substantive issues surrounding health insurance discrimination threaten both the potential usage of new genetic technologies to improve human health and the ability to conduct the very research needed to understand, treat, and prevent genetic disease. In 1995, the National Action Plan on Breast Cancer (NAPBC) in conjunction with the ELSI Program developed detailed policy recommendations to prohibit genetic discrimination in health insurance.[589] As a result of these recommendations, the Health Insurance Portability and Accountability Act of 1996 [104 Public Law 104-191, 701, 110 STAT, 1936 (1996)], which includes prohibitions on the use of genetic information in the group health insurance market, became the first U.S. federal law enacted to protect against the misuse of genetic information. Efforts are ongoing to pass additional federal legislation that would broaden this protection to those with individual health insurance coverage and would in a more general way prohibit health insurers from asking for or using genetic information. In the United States, 30 states have now enacted laws to prevent the use of genetic information by health insurers[590] [Barbara Fuller (NHGRI), personal communication]. Finally, initial policy recommendations to address concerns about the use of genetic information in the workplace have been formulated[591] (see also http://www.nhgri.nih.gov/HGP/Reports/genetics_workplace.html).

Genetic testing is increasingly becoming an integral component of health care. As a result, the ELSI Program has examined the key issues surrounding the introduction of new genetic tests into clinical practice. An initial set of studies explored the testing and counseling for cystic fibrosis mutations, with the aim of examining alternative approaches for genetic education, testing, and counseling.[592] Based on these studies, a 1997 NIH Consensus Conference recommended optimal practices for performing cystic fibrosis genetic testing (see http://odp.od.nih.gov/consensus/statements/cdc/106/106_stmt.html). Similarly, in anticipation of the discovery of cancer-predisposing genes, the ELSI Program sponsored studies to examine the psychosocial and clinical impact of genetic testing in families with heritable forms of breast, ovarian, and colon cancer. These studies have resulted in the development of valuable experience-based guidance for implementing genetic tests for cancer susceptibility.[593–596] Similar investigations relating to genetic testing for Alzheimer disease[597] and hemochromatosis[598] have also been performed. In 1994, the NIH and the Department of Energy created the Task Force on Genetic Testing to evaluate genetic testing in the United States and to make recommendations for ensuring that such tests are safe and effective. The resulting report contains recommendations for federal agencies, testing laboratories, and health professionals[599] (see http://www.nhgri.nih.gov/ELSI/TFGT_final).

As genetic testing increases, the use and interpretation of those tests will become the responsibility of a wider array of health professionals beyond those considered to be "genetics specialists," including primary care physicians, nurses, physician assistants, nurse practitioners, psychologists, and social workers. In addition, public policy makers and the general public will increasingly be called upon to consider critical issues relating to genetic testing. In anticipation of these situations, the ELSI Program has initiated various educational efforts that aim to train health care professionals in interpreting new DNA-based diagnostic tests, to increase public genetic literacy through both the schools and the media, to encourage public discussion about genetic issues, and to provide genetic education for appropriate public policy makers. One such initiative is the establishment of the National Coalition for Health Professional Education in Genetics (NCHPEG), a coordinated effort to promote health professional education about advances in human genetics. While health professionals are the primary target audience for NCHPEG, the program plans to include efforts that aim to provide appropriate materials and guidance for educating policy makers and, through health care providers, patients, families, and the general public.

Adequate consideration of the ethical, legal, and social issues concerning human genome research and the HGP is critical for the successful introduction of genetic information into the mainstream of medical practice and society. The ELSI Program has established a solid foundation for addressing these issues and will undoubtedly continue to provide critical leadership in this area.

CONCLUSION

The HGP is one of the most important projects—if not *the* most important project—ever undertaken in biomedical research. It is fundamentally an endeavor aiming to develop tools for the study of biology and medicine. These tools reflect both an information resource in the form of genetic, physical, and sequence maps of the human genome and of several model organisms, as well as an ever-increasing number of experimental technologies that are becoming standard techniques in the armamentarium of biomedical researchers. In this regard, an exciting new genomic revolution has started, and it is permanently changing the way research is performed. The new and powerful foundation of genetic information is empowering investigators to tackle complex problems relating to disease, development, and evolution that were previously unapproachable. The direct impact of the HGP on clinical medicine is already being realized, with both a dramatic acceleration in the identification of human disease genes and the continual development of new approaches for analyzing patient DNA. Ultimately, though, the true legacy of the HGP will be to provide future generations of scientists and clinicians an unprecedented resource—the human *genetic blueprint*—that will enable them to define better the genetic bases of disease and to use that information for designing more effective therapies.

ACKNOWLEDGMENTS

I thank Francis Collins, David Schlessinger, Kathy Hudson, Maynard Olson, Andy Baxevanis, Mark Boguski, Gerry Bouffard, and Gabriela Adelt Green for helpful suggestions, Rick Myers and David Cox for contributions to the earlier version of this chapter, Renee Gamborg and Rob Lazott for administrative assistance, and Maggie Green for her dedicated and loyal support.

REFERENCES

1. Collins FS: Positional cloning: Let's not call it reverse anymore. *Nat Genet* **1**:3, 1992.
2. Ballabio A: The rise and fall of positional cloning? *Nat Genet* **3**:277, 1993.
3. Collins FS: Positional cloning moves from perditional to traditional. *Nat Genet* **9**:347, 1995.
4. Nelson DL: Positional cloning reaches maturity. *Curr Opin Genet Dev* **5**:298, 1995.
5. Foote S: Genetic analysis of disease susceptibility (disease susceptibility). *Aust NZ J Med* **25**:757, 1995.
6. Wolff RK: Positional cloning: A review and perspective. *Drug Dev Res* **41**:129, 1997.
7. Boehm T: Positional cloning and gene identification. *Methods* **14**:152, 1998.
8. Ballabio A, Brown S, Fischer E: Strategies for gene discovery in mammalian systems, in Birren B, Green ED, Klapholz S, Myers RM, Roskams J (eds): *Genome Analysis: A Laboratory Manual,* vol 2: *Detecting Genes.* Cold Spring Harbor, NY, Cold Spring Harbor Laboratory, 1998, p 1.
9. Rommens JM, Iannuzzi MC, Kerem B, Drumm ML, Melmer G, Dean M, Rozmahel R, et al.: Identification of the cystic fibrosis gene: Chromosome walking and jumping. *Science* **245**:1059, 1989.
10. Riordan JR, Rommens JM, Kerem B, Alon N, Rozmahel R, Grzelczak Z, Zielenski J, et al.: Identification of the cystic fibrosis gene: Cloning and characterization of complementary DNA. *Science* **245**:1066, 1989.
11. Huntington's Disease Collaborative Research Group: A novel gene containing a trinucleotide repeat that is expanded and unstable on Huntington's disease chromosomes. *Cell* **72**:971, 1993.
12. Feder JN, Gnirke A, Thomas W, Tsuchihashi Z, Ruddy DA, Basava A, Dormishian F, et al.: A novel MHC class I-like gene is mutated in patients with hereditary haemochromatosis. *Nat Genet* **13**:399, 1996.
13. Bell JI: Polygenic disease. *Curr Opin Genet Dev* **3**:466, 1993.
14. Lander ES, Schork NJ: Genetic dissection of complex traits. *Science* **265**:2037, 1994.
15. Kruglyak L, Lander ES: High-resolution genetic mapping of complex traits. *Am J Hum Genet* **56**:1212, 1995.
16. Lander E, Kruglyak L: Genetic dissection of complex traits: Guidelines for interpreting and reporting linkage results. *Nat Genet* **11**:241, 1995.
17. Zhang H, Zhao H, Merikangas K: Strategies to identify genes for complex diseases. *Ann Med* **29**:493, 1997.
18. Watson JD, Crick FHC: Molecular structure of nucleic acids: A structure for deoxyribose nucleic acid. *Nature* **171**:737, 1953.
19. Watson JD, Gilman M, Witkowski J, Zoller M: *Recombinant DNA.* New York, WH Freeman, 1992.
20. Morton NE: Parameters of the human genome. *Proc Natl Acad Sci USA* **88**:7474, 1991.
21. Trask B, van den Engh G, Mayall B, Gray JW: Chromosome heteromorphism quantified by high-resolution bivariate flow karyotyping. *Am J Hum Genet* **45**:739, 1989.
22. McKusick VA: Mapping and sequencing the human genome. *N Engl J Med* **320**:910, 1989.
23. Olson MV: The Human Genome Project. *Proc Natl Acad Sci USA* **90**:4338, 1993.
24. Tyler-Smith C, Willard HF: Mammalian chromosome structure. *Curr Opin Genet Dev* **3**:390, 1993.
25. Biessmann H, Mason JM: Telomeric repeat sequences. *Chromosoma* **103**:154, 1994.
26. Moyzis RK, Buckingham JM, Cram LS, Dani M, Deaven LL, Jones MD, Meyne J, et al.: A highly conserved repetitive DNA sequence, $(TTAGGG)_n$, present at the telomeres of human chromosomes. *Proc Natl Acad Sci USA* **85**:6622, 1988.
27. Riethman HC, Moyzis RK, Meyne J, Burke DT, Olson MV: Cloning human telomeric DNA fragments into *Saccharomyces cerevisiae* using a yeast-artificial chromosome vector. *Proc Natl Acad Sci USA* **86**:6240, 1989.
28. Brown WRA: Molecular cloning of human telomeres in yeast. *Nature* **338**:774, 1989.
29. Cross SH, Allshire RC, McKay SJ, McGill NI, Cooke HJ: Cloning of human telomeres by complementation in yeast. *Nature* **338**:771, 1989.
30. Cheng J-F, Smith CL, Cantor CR: Isolation and characterization of a human telomere. *Nucleic Acids Res* **17**:6109, 1989.
31. Dobson MJ, Brown WRA: Cloning human telomeres in yeast artificial chromosomes, in Anand R (ed): *Techniques for the Analysis of Complex Genomes*. London, Academic, 1992, p 81.
32. National Institutes of Health and Institute of Molecular Medicine Collaboration: A complete set of human telomeric probes and their clinical application. *Nat Genet* **14**:86, 1996.
33. Riethman H: Closing in on telomeric closure. *Genome Res* **7**:853, 1997.
34. Murphy TD, Karpen GH: Centromeres take flight: Alpha satellite and the quest for the human centromere. *Cell* **93**:317, 1998.
35. Devilee P, Slagboom P, Cornelisse CJ, Pearson PL: Sequence heterogeneity within the human alphoid repetitive DNA family. *Nucleic Acids Res* **14**:2059, 1986.
36. Waye JS, Willard HF: Nucleotide sequence heterogeneity of alpha satellite repetitive DNA: A survey of alphoid sequences from different human chromosomes. *Nucleic Acids Res* **15**:7549, 1987.
37. Choo KH, Vissel B, Nagy A, Earle E, Kalitsis P: A survey of the genomic distribution of alpha satellite DNA on all the human chromosomes, and derivation of a new consensus sequence. *Nucleic Acids Res* **19**:1179, 1991.

38. Jurka J, Pethiyagoda C: Simple repetitive DNA sequences from primates: Compilation and analysis. *J Mol Evol* **40**:120, 1995.
39. Jurka J: Repeats in genomic DNA: Mining and meaning. *Curr Opin Struct Biol* **8**:333, 1998.
40. Jurka J, Walichiewicz J, Milosavljevic A: Prototypic sequences for human repetitive DNA. *J Mol Evol* **35**:286, 1992.
41. Ohno S: An argument for the genetic simplicity of man and other mammals. *J Hum Evol* **1**:651, 1972.
42. Gall JG: Human genome sequencing. *Science* **233**:1367, 1986.
43. Levinson B, Kenwrick S, Lakich D, Hammonds G Jr, Gitschier J: A transcribed gene in an intron of the human factor VIII gene. *Genomics* **7**:1, 1990.
44. Wallace MR, Marchuk DA, Andersen LB, Letcher R, Odeh HM, Saulino AM, Fountain JW, et al.: Type 1 neurofibromatosis gene: Identification of a large transcript disrupted in three NF1 patients. *Science* **249**:181, 1990.
45. Bird AP: CpG-rich islands and the function of DNA methylation. *Nature* **321**:209, 1986.
46. Cross SH, Bird AP: CpG islands and genes. *Curr Opin Genet Dev* **5**:309, 1995.
47. John RM, Cross SH: Gene detection by the identification of CpG islands, in Birren B, Green ED, Klapholz S, Myers RM, Roskams J (eds): *Genome Analysis: A Laboratory Manual,* vol 2: *Detecting Genes*. Cold Spring Harbor, NY, Cold Spring Harbor Laboratory, 1998, p 217.
48. Korenberg JR, Rykowski MC: Human genome organization: *Alu*, Lines, and the molecular structure of metaphase chromosome bands. *Cell* **53**:391, 1988.
49. Bickmore WA, Sumner AT: Mammalian chromosome banding: An expression of genome organization. *Trends Genet* **5**:143, 1989.
50. Craig JM, Bickmore WA: The distribution of CpG islands in mammalian chromosomes. *Nat Genet* **7**:376, 1994.
51. Gardiner K: Human genome organization. *Curr Opin Genet Dev* **5**:315, 1995.
52. Bernardi G: The vertebrate genome: Isochores and evolution. *Mol Biol Evol* **10**:186, 1993.
53. Bernardi G: The human genome: Organization and evolutionary history. *Annu Rev Genet* **29**:445, 1995.
54. Saccone S, Caccio S, Kusuda J, Andreozzi L, Bernardi G: Identification of the gene-richest bands in human chromosomes. *Gene* **174**:85, 1996.
55. Zoubak S, Clay O, Bernardi G: The gene distribution of the human genome. *Gene* **174**:95, 1996.
56. Saccone S, De Sario A, Della Valle G, Bernardi G: The highest gene concentrations in the human genome are in telomeric bands of metaphase chromosomes. *Proc Natl Acad Sci USA* **89**:4913, 1992.
57. Green ED, Birren B, Klapholz S, Myers RM, Hieter P (eds): *Genome Analysis: A Laboratory Manual*, vols 1–4. Cold Spring Harbor, NY, Cold Spring Harbor Laboratory, 1997.
58. Sambrook J, Fritsch EF, Maniatis T: *Molecular Cloning: A Laboratory Manual*, 2d ed. Cold Spring Harbor, NY, Cold Spring Harbor Laboratory, 1989.
59. Wolff R, Gemmill R: Purifying and analyzing genomic DNA, in Birren B, Green ED, Klapholz S, Myers RM, Roskams J (eds): *Genome Analysis: A Laboratory Manual,* vol 1: *Analyzing DNA*. Cold Spring Harbor, NY, Cold Spring Harbor Laboratory, 1997, p 1.
60. Mullis K, Faloona F, Scharf S, Saiki R, Horn G, Erlich H: Specific enzymatic amplification of DNA in vitro: The polymerase chain reaction. *Cold Spring Harb Symp Quant Biol* **51**:263, 1986.
61. Mullis KB, Faloona FA: Specific synthesis of DNA in vitro via a polymerase-catalyzed chain reaction. *Methods Enzymol* **155**:335, 1987.
62. Saiki RK, Scharf S, Faloona F, Mullis KB, Horn GT, Erlich HA, Arnheim N: Enzymatic amplification of β-globin genomic sequences and restriction site analysis for diagnosis of sickle cell anemia. *Science* **230**:1350, 1985.
63. Fanning S, Gibbs RA: PCR in genome analysis, in Birren B, Green ED, Klapholz S, Myers RM, Roskams J (eds): *Genome Analysis: A Laboratory Manual,* vol 1: *Analyzing DNA*. Cold Spring Harbor, NY, Cold Spring Harbor Laboratory, 1997, p 249.
64. Saiki RK, Gelfand DH, Stoffel S, Scharf SJ, Higuchi R, Horn GT, Mullis KB, et al.: Primer-directed enzymatic amplification of DNA with a thermostable DNA polymerase. *Science* **239**:487, 1988.
65. Lashkari DA, Hunicke-Smith SP, Norgren RM, Davis RW, Brennan T: An automated multiplex oligonucleotide synthesizer: Development of high-throughput, low-cost DNA synthesis. *Proc Natl Acad Sci USA* **92**:7912, 1995.
66. Rayner S, Brignac S, Bumeister R, Belosludtsev Y, Ward T, Grant O, O'Brien K, et al.: MerMade: An oligodeoxyribonucleotide synthesizer for high throughput oligonucleotide production in dual 96-well plates. *Genome Res* **8**:741, 1998.
67. Cook-Deegan RM: The Alta Summit, December 1984. *Genomics* **5**:661, 1989.
68. Sinsheimer RL: The Santa Cruz Workshop—May 1985. *Genomics* **5**:954, 1989.
69. Dulbecco R: A turning point in cancer research: Sequencing the human genome. *Science* **231**:1055, 1986.
70. Evans GA: Cosmids, in Birren B, Green ED, Klapholz S, Myers RM, Riethman H, Roskams J (eds): *Genome Analysis: A Laboratory Manual,* vol 3: *Cloning Systems*. Cold Spring Harbor, NY, Cold Spring Harbor Laboratory, 1998, p 87.
71. Evans GA, Lewis KA: Physical mapping of complex genomes by cosmid multiplex analysis. *Proc Natl Acad Sci USA* **86**:5030, 1989.
72. Nizetic D, Zehetner G, Monaco AP, Gellen L, Young BD, Lehrach H: Construction, arraying, and high-density screening of large insert libraries of human chromosomes X and 21: Their potential use as reference libraries. *Proc Natl Acad Sci USA* **88**:3233, 1991.
73. Stallings RL, Torney DC, Hildebrand CE, Longmire JL, Deaven LL, Jett JH, Doggett NA, et al.: Physical mapping of human chromosomes by repetitive sequence fingerprinting. *Proc Natl Acad Sci USA* **87**:6218, 1990.
74. Ivens AC, King TF, Little PFR: Cosmid clones and generation of detailed DNA maps of large chromosomal regions, in Adolph KW (ed): *Methods in Molecular Genetics,* part A: *Gene and Chromosome Analysis*. San Diego, Academic, 1993, p 173.
75. Burke DT, Carle GF, Olson MV: Cloning of large segments of exogenous DNA into yeast by means of artificial chromosome vectors. *Science* **236**:806, 1987.
76. Green ED, Hieter P, Spencer FA: Yeast artificial chromosomes, in Birren B, Green ED, Klapholz S, Myers RM, Riethman H, Roskams J (eds): *Genome Analysis: A Laboratory Manual,* vol 3: *Cloning Systems*. Cold Spring Harbor, NY, Cold Spring Harbor Laboratory, 1998, p 297.
77. Burke DT, Olson MV: Preparation of clone libraries in yeast artificial-chromosome vectors. *Methods Enzymol* **194**:251, 1991.
78. Brownstein BH, Silverman GA, Little RD, Burke DT, Korsmeyer SJ, Schlessinger D, Olson MV: Isolation of single-copy human genes from a library of yeast artificial chromosome clones. *Science* **244**:1348, 1989.
79. Imai T, Olson MV: Second-generation approach to the construction of yeast artificial-chromosome libraries. *Genomics* **8**:297, 1990.
80. Albertsen HM, Abderrahim H, Cann HM, Dausset J, Le Paslier D, Cohen D: Construction and characterization of a yeast artificial chromosome library containing seven haploid genome equivalents. *Proc Natl Acad Sci USA* **87**:4256, 1990.
81. Dausset J, Ougen P, Abderrahim H, Billault A, Sambucy J-L, Cohen D, Le Paslier D: The CEPH YAC library. *Behring Inst Mitt* **91**:13, 1992.
82. Anand R, Riley JH, Butler R, Smith JC, Markham AF: A 3.5 genome equivalent multi access YAC library: Construction, characterisation, screening and storage. *Nucleic Acids Res* **18**:1951, 1990.
83. Anand R, Villasante A, Tyler-Smith C: Construction of yeast artificial chromosome libraries with large inserts using fractionation by pulsed-field gel electrophoresis. *Nucleic Acids Res* **17**:3425, 1989.
84. Larin Z, Monaco AP, Lehrach H: Yeast artificial chromosome libraries containing large inserts from mouse and human DNA. *Proc Natl Acad Sci USA* **88**:4123, 1991.
85. Green ED, Olson MV: Systematic screening of yeast artificial-chromosome libraries by use of the polymerase chain reaction. *Proc Natl Acad Sci USA* **87**:1213, 1990.
86. Green ED, Olson MV: Chromosomal region of the cystic fibrosis gene in yeast artificial chromosomes: A model for human genome mapping. *Science* **250**:94, 1990.
87. Anand R, Ogilvie DJ, Butler R, Riley JH, Finniear RS, Powell SJ, Smith JC, et al.: A yeast artificial chromosome contig encompassing the cystic fibrosis locus. *Genomics* **9**:124, 1991.
88. Coffey AJ, Roberts RG, Green ED, Cole CG, Butler R, Anand R, Giannelli F, et al.: Construction of a 2.6-Mb contig in yeast artificial chromosomes spanning the human dystrophin gene using an STS-based approach. *Genomics* **12**:474, 1992.
89. Monaco AP, Walker AP, Millwood I, Larin Z, Lehrach H: A yeast artificial chromosome contig containing the complete Duchenne muscular dystrophy gene. *Genomics* **12**:465, 1992.
90. Geraghty DE, Pei J, Lipsky B, Hansen JA, Taillon-Miller P, Bronson SK, Chaplin DD: Cloning and physical mapping of the *HLA* class I

region spanning the *HLA-E*-to-*HLA-F* interval by using yeast artificial chromosomes. *Proc Natl Acad Sci USA* **89**:2669, 1992.

91. Zuo J, Robbins C, Taillon-Miller P, Cox DR, Myers RM: Cloning of the Huntington disease region in yeast artificial chromosomes. *Hum Mol Genet* **1**:149, 1992.
92. Bates GP, Valdes J, Hummerich H, Baxendale S, Le Paslier DL, Monaco AP, Tagle D, et al.: Characterization of a yeast artificial chromosome contig spanning the Huntington's disease gene candidate region. *Nat Genet* **1**:180, 1992.
93. Foote S, Vollrath D, Hilton A, Page DC: The human Y chromosome: Overlapping DNA clones spanning the euchromatic region. *Science* **258**:60, 1992.
94. Vollrath D, Foote S, Hilton A, Brown LG, Beer-Romero P, Bogan JS, Page DC: The human Y chromosome: A 43-interval map based on naturally occurring deletions. *Science* **258**:52, 1992.
95. Chumakov IM, Rigault P, Guillou S, Ougen P, Billaut A, Guasconi G, Gervy P, et al.: Continuum of overlapping clones spanning the entire human chromosome 21q. *Nature* **359**:380, 1992.
96. Cohen D, Chumakov I, Weissenbach J: A first-generation physical map of the human genome. *Nature* **366**:698, 1993.
97. Chumakov IM, Rigault P, Le Gall I, Bellanne-Chantelot C, Billault A, Guillou S, Soularue P, et al.: A YAC contig map of the human genome. *Nature* **377**:175, 1995.
98. Hudson TJ, Stein LD, Gerety SS, Ma J, Castle AB, Silva J, Slonim DK, et al.: An STS-based map of the human genome. *Science* **270**:1945, 1995.
99. Gemmill RM, Chumakov I, Scott P, Waggoner B, Rigault P, Cypser J, Chen Q, et al.: A second-generation YAC contig map of human chromosome 3. *Nature* **377**:299, 1995.
100. Krauter K, Montgomery K, Yoon S-J, LeBlanc-Straceski J, Renault B, Marondel I, Herdman V, et al.: A second-generation YAC contig map of human chromosome 12. *Nature* **377**:321, 1995.
101. Collins JE, Cole CG, Smink LJ, Garrett CL, Leversha MA, Soderlund CA, Maslen GL, et al.: A high-density YAC contig map of human chromosome 22. *Nature* **377**:367, 1995.
102. Korenberg JR, Chen X-N, Mitchell S, Fannin S, Gerwehr S, Cohen D, Chumakov I: A high-fidelity physical map of human chromosome 21q in yeast artificial chromosomes. *Genome Res* **5**:427, 1995.
103. Bell CJ, Budarf ML, Nieuwenhuijsen BW, Barnoski BL, Buetow KH, Campbell K, Colbert AME, et al.: Integration of physical, breakpoint and genetic maps of chromosome 22: Localization of 587 yeast artificial chromosomes with 238 mapped markers. *Hum Mol Genet* **4**:59, 1995.
104. Quackenbush J, Davies C, Bailis JM, Khristich JV, Diggle K, Marchuck Y, Tobin J, et al.: An STS content map of human chromosome 11: Localization of 910 YAC clones and 109 islands. *Genomics* **29**:512, 1995.
105. Qin S, Nowak NJ, Zhang J, Sait SNJ, Mayers PG, Higgins MJ, Cheng Y-J, et al.: A high-resolution physical map of human chromosome 11. *Proc Natl Acad Sci USA* **93**:3149, 1996.
106. Nagaraja R, MacMillan S, Kere J, Jones C, Griffin S, Schmatz M, Terrell J, et al.: X chromosome map at 75-kb STS resolution, revealing extremes of recombination and GC content. *Genome Res* **7**:210, 1997.
107. Bouffard GG, Idol JR, Braden VV, Iyer LM, Cunningham AF, Weintraub LA, Touchman JW, et al.: A physical map of human chromosome 7: An integrated YAC contig map with average STS spacing of 79 kb. *Genome Res* **7**:673, 1997.
108. Silverman GA, Green ED, Young RL, Jockel JI, Domer PH, Korsmeyer SJ: Meiotic recombination between yeast artificial chromosomes yields a single clone containing the entire *BCL2* protooncogene. *Proc Natl Acad Sci USA* **87**:9913, 1990.
109. Den Dunnen JT, Grootscholten PM, Dauwerse JG, Walker AP, Monaco AP, Butler R, Anand R, et al.: Reconstruction of the 2.4 Mb human DMD-gene by homologous YAC recombination. *Hum Mol Genet* **1**:19, 1992.
110. Green ED, Riethman HC, Dutchik JE, Olson MV: Detection and characterization of chimeric yeast artificial-chromosome clones. *Genomics* **11**:658, 1991.
111. Sternberg N: Bacteriophage P1 cloning system for the isolation, amplification, and recovery of DNA fragments as large as 100 kilobase pairs. *Proc Natl Acad Sci USA* **87**:103, 1990.
112. Sternberg N: Cloning into bacteriophage P1 vectors, in Birren B, Green ED, Klapholz S, Myers RM, Riethman H, Roskams J (eds): *Genome Analysis: A Laboratory Manual,* vol 3: *Cloning Systems*. Cold Spring Harbor, NY, Cold Spring Harbor Laboratory, 1998, p 203.
113. Shizuya H, Birren B, Kim U-J, Mancino V, Slepak T, Tachiiri Y, Simon M: Cloning and stable maintenance of 300-kilobase-pair fragments of human DNA in *Escherichia coli* using an F-factor-based vector. *Proc Natl Acad Sci USA* **89**:8794, 1992.
114. Birren B, Mancino V, Shizuya H: Bacterial artificial chromosomes, in Birren B, Green ED, Klapholz S, Myers RM, Riethman H, Roskams J (eds): *Genome Analysis: A Laboratory Manual,* vol 3: *Cloning Systems*. Cold Spring Harbor, NY, Cold Spring Harbor Laboratory, 1998, p 241.
115. Ioannou PA, Amemiya CT, Garnes J, Kroisel PM, Shizuya H, Chen C, Batzer MA, et al.: A new bacteriophage P1-derived vector for the propagation of large human DNA fragments. *Nat Genet* **6**:84, 1994.
116. Kim U-J, Birren BW, Slepak T, Mancino V, Boysen C, Kang H-L, Simon MI, et al.: Construction and characterization of a human bacterial artificial chromosome library. *Genomics* **34**:213, 1996.
117. Asakawa S, Abe I, Kudoh Y, Kishi N, Wang Y, Kubota R, Kudoh J, et al.: Human BAC library: Construction and rapid screening. *Gene* **191**:69, 1997.
118. Dunham I, Dewar K, Kim U-J, Ross M: Bacterial cloning systems, in Birren B, Green ED, Klapholz S, Myers RM, Riethman H, Roskams J (eds): *Genome Analysis: A Laboratory Manual,* vol 3: *Cloning Systems*. Cold Spring Harbor, NY, Cold Spring Harbor Laboratory, 1998, p 1.
119. Bentley DR, Todd C, Collins J, Holland J, Dunham I, Hassock S, Bankier A, et al.: The development and application of automated gridding for efficient screening of yeast and bacterial ordered libraries. *Genomics* **12**:534, 1992.
120. Ross MT, Hoheisel JD, Monaco AP, Larin Z, Zehetner G, Lehrach H: High-density gridded YAC filters: Their potential as genome mapping tools, in Anand R (ed): *Techniques for the Analysis of Complex Genomes*. London, Academic, 1992, p 137.
121. Cox RD, Meier-Ewert S, Ross M, Larin Z, Monaco AP, Lehrach H: Genome mapping and cloning of mutations using yeast artificial chromosomes. *Methods Enzymol* **225**:637, 1993.
122. Olsen AS, Combs J, Garcia E, Elliott J, Amemiya C, de Jong P, Threadgill G: Automated production of high density cosmid and YAC colony filters using a robotic workstation. *BioTechniques* **14**:116, 1993.
123. Copeland A, Lennon G: Rapid arrayed filter production using the 'ORCA' robot. *Nature* **369**:421, 1994.
124. Marra MA, Kucaba TA, Dietrich NL, Green ED, Brownstein B, Wilson RK, McDonald KM, et al.: High throughput fingerprint analysis of large-insert clones. *Genome Res* **7**:1072, 1997.
125. Gregory SG, Howell GR, Bentley DR: Genome mapping by fluorescent fingerprinting. *Genome Res* **7**:1162, 1997.
126. McPherson JD: Sequence ready—or not? *Genome Res* **7**:1111, 1997.
127. Schwartz DC, Cantor CR: Separation of yeast chromosome-sized DNAs by pulsed field gradient gel electrophoresis. *Cell* **37**:67, 1984.
128. Carle GF, Frank M, Olson MV: Electrophoretic separations of large DNA molecules by periodic inversion of the electric field. *Science* **232**:65, 1986.
129. Chu G, Vollrath D, Davis RW: Separation of large DNA molecules by contour-clamped homogenous electric fields. *Science* **234**:1582, 1986.
130. Birren B, Lai E: *Pulsed Field Gel Electrophoresis: A Practical Guide*. San Diego, Academic, 1993.
131. Wrestler JC, Lipes BD, Birren BW, Lai E: Pulsed-field gel electrophoresis. *Methods Enzymol* **270**:255, 1996.
132. Riethman H, Birren B, Gnirke A: Preparation, manipulation, and mapping of HMW DNA, in Birren B, Green ED, Klapholz S, Myers RM, Roskams J (eds): *Genome Analysis: A Laboratory Manual,* vol 1: *Analyzing DNA*. Cold Spring Harbor, NY, Cold Spring Harbor Laboratory, 1997, p 83.
133. Carle GF, Olson MV: An electrophoretic karyotype for yeast. *Proc Natl Acad Sci USA* **82**:3756, 1985.
134. Link AJ, Olson MV: Physical map of the *Saccharomyces cerevisiae* genome at 110-kilobase resolution. *Genetics* **127**:681, 1991.
135. Smith DR: Genomic long-range restriction mapping. *Methods* **1**:195, 1990.
136. Poustka A: Physical mapping by PFGE. *Methods* **1**:204, 1990.
137. Evans GA: Physical mapping of the human genome by pulsed field gel analysis. *Curr Opin Genet Dev* **1**:75, 1991.
138. Burmeister M: Strategies for mapping large regions of mammalian genomes, in Burmeister M, Ulanovsky L (eds): *Methods in Molecular Biology,* vol 12: *Pulsed-Field Gel Electrophoresis*. Totowa, NJ, Humana, 1992, p 259.
139. Bickmore W: Analysis of genomic DNAs by pulsed-field gel electrophoresis, in Anand R (ed): *Techniques for the Analysis of Complex Genomes*. London, Academic, 1992, p 19.
140. Chandrasekharappa SC, Marchuk DA, Collins FS: Analysis of yeast artificial chromosome clones, in Burmeister M, Ulanovsky L (eds):

Methods in Molecular Biology, vol 12: *Pulsed-Field Gel Electrophoresis.* Totowa, NJ, Humana, 1992, p 235.

141. Bentley DR: The analysis of YAC clones, in Anand R (ed): *Techniques for the Analysis of Complex Genomes.* London, Academic, 1992, p 113.
142. Den Dunnen JT, van Ommen G-JB: Application of pulsed-field gel electrophoresis to genetic diagnosis, in Mathew C (ed): *Methods in Molecular Biology,* vol 9: *Protocols in Human Molecular Genetics.* Clifton, NJ, Humana, 1991, p 313.
143. Pinkel D, Straume T, Gray JW: Cytogenetic analysis using quantitative, high-sensitivity, fluorescence hybridization. *Proc Natl Acad Sci USA* **83**:2934, 1986.
144. Hozier JC, Davis LM: Cytogenetic approaches to genome mapping. *Anal Biochem* **200**:205, 1992.
145. Buckle VJ, Kearney L: New methods in cytogenetics. *Curr Opin Genet Dev* **4**:374, 1994.
146. Van Ommen G-JB, Breuning MH, Raap AK: FISH in genome research and molecular diagnostics. *Curr Opin Genet Dev* **5**:304, 1995.
147. Heng HH, Spyropoulos B, Moens PB: FISH technology in chromosome and genome research. *BioEssays* **19**:75, 1997.
148. Trask B: Fluorescence in situ hybridization, in Birren B, Green ED, Hieter P, Klapholz S, Myers RM, Riethman H, Roskams J (eds): *Genome Analysis: A Laboratory Manual,* vol 4: *Mapping Genomes.* Cold Spring Harbor, NY, Cold Spring Harbor Laboratory, 1999, p 303.
149. Cherif D, Julier C, Delattre O, Derre J, Lathrop GM, Berger R: Simultaneous localization of cosmids and chromosome R-banding by fluorescence microscopy: Application to regional mapping of human chromosome 11. *Proc Natl Acad Sci USA* **87**:6639, 1990.
150. Lichter P, Chang Tang C-J, Call K, Hermanson G, Evans GA, Housman D, Ward DC: High-resolution mapping of human chromosome 11 by in situ hybridization with cosmid clones. *Science* **247**:64, 1990.
151. Palotie A, Heiskanen M, Laan M, Horelli-Kuitunen N: High-resolution fluorescence in situ hybridization: A new approach in genome mapping. *Duodecim* **28**:101, 1996.
152. Heiskanen M, Peltonen L, Palotif A: Visual mapping by high resolution FISH. *Trends Genet* **12**:379, 1996.
153. Michalet X, Ekong R, Fougerousse F, Rousseaux S, Schurra C, Hornigold N, van Slegtenhorst M, et al.: Dynamic molecular combing: Stretching the whole human genome for high-resolution studies. *Science* **277**:1518, 1997.
154. Green ED, Idol JR, Mohr-Tidwell RM, Braden VV, Peluso DC, Fulton RS, Massa HF, et al.: Integration of physical, genetic and cytogenetic maps of human chromosome 7: Isolation and analysis of yeast artificial chromosome clones for 117 mapped genetic markers. *Hum Mol Genet* **3**:489, 1994.
155. Bray-Ward P, Menninger J, Lieman J, Desai T, Mokady N, Banks A, Ward DC: Integration of the cytogenetic, genetic, and physical maps of the human genome by FISH mapping of CEPH YAC clones. *Genomics* **32**:1, 1996.
156. Schrock E, du Manoir S, Veldman T, Schoell B, Wienberg J, Ferguson-Smith MA, Ning Y, et al.: Multicolor spectral karyotyping of human chromosomes. *Science* **273**:494, 1996.
157. Speicher MR, Gwyn Ballard S, Ward DC: Karyotyping human chromosomes by combinatorial multi-fluor FISH. *Nat Genet* **12**:368, 1996.
158. Ried T, Schrock E, Ning Y, Wienberg J: Chromosome painting: A useful art. *Hum Mol Genet* **7**:1619, 1998.
159. Cox DR, Burmeister M, Price ER, Kim S, Myers RM: Radiation hybrid mapping: A somatic cell genetic method for constructing high-resolution maps of mammalian chromosomes. *Science* **250**:245, 1990.
160. Matise TC, Wasmuth JJ, Myers RM, McPherson JD: Somatic cell genetics and radiation hybrid mapping, in Birren B, Green ED, Hieter P, Klapholz S, Myers RM, Riethman H, Roskams J (eds): *Genome Analysis: A Laboratory Manual,* vol 4: *Mapping Genomes.* Cold Spring Harbor, NY, Cold Spring Harbor Laboratory, 1999, p 259.
161. Adams MD, Fields C, Venter JC (eds): *Automated DNA Sequencing and Analysis.* San Diego, Academic, 1994.
162. Sanger F, Nicklen S, Coulson AR: DNA sequencing with chain-terminating inhibitors. *Proc Natl Acad Sci USA* **74**:5463, 1977.
163. Smith LM, Sanders JZ, Kaiser RJ, Hughes P, Dodd C, Connell CR, Heiner C, et al.: Fluorescence detection in automated DNA sequence analysis. *Nature* **321**:674, 1986.
164. Prober JM, Trainor GL, Dam RJ, Hobbs FW, Robertson CW, Zagursky RJ, Cocuzza AJ, et al.: A system for rapid DNA sequencing with fluorescent chain-terminating dideoxynucleotides. *Science* **238**:336, 1987.
165. Hunkapiller T, Kaiser RJ, Koop BF, Hood L: Large-scale and automated DNA sequence determination. *Science* **254**:59, 1991.
166. Wilson RK, Mardis ER: Fluorescence-based DNA sequencing, in Birren B, Green ED, Klapholz S, Myers RM, Roskams J (eds): *Genome Analysis: A Laboratory Manual,* vol 1: *Analyzing DNA.* Cold Spring Harbor, NY, Cold Spring Harbor Laboratory, 1997, p 301.
167. Ju J, Ruan C, Fuller CW, Glazer AN, Mathies RA: Fluorescence energy transfer dye-labeled primers for DNA sequencing and analysis. *Proc Natl Acad Sci USA* **92**:4347, 1995.
168. Ju J, Glazer AN, Mathies RA: Energy transfer primers: A new fluorescence labeling paradigm for DNA sequencing and analysis. *Nat Med* **2**:246, 1996.
169. Glazer AN, Mathies RA: Energy-transfer fluorescent reagents for DNA analyses. *Curr Opin Biotechnol* **8**:94, 1997.
170. Rosenblum BB, Lee LG, Spurgeon SL, Khan SH, Menchen SM, Heiner CR, Chen SM: New dye-labeled terminators for improved DNA sequencing patterns. *Nucleic Acids Res* **25**:4500, 1997.
171. Heiner CR, Hunkapiller KL, Chen S-M, Glass JI, Chen EY: Sequencing multimegabase-template DNA with BigDye terminator chemistry. *Genome Res* **8**:557, 1998.
172. Johnston M: Gene chips: Array of hope for understanding gene regulation. *Curr Biol* **8**:R171, 1998.
173. Ramsay G: DNA chips: State-of-the art. *Nat Biotechnol* **16**:40, 1998.
174. Marshall A, Hodgson J: DNA chips: An array of possibilities. *Nat Biotechnol* **16**:27, 1998.
175. Castellino AM: When the chips are down. *Genome Res* **7**:943, 1997.
176. Strachan T, Abitbol M, Davidson D, Beckmann JS: A new dimension for the Human Genome Project: Towards comprehensive expression maps. *Nat Genet* **16**:126, 1997.
177. Lillie J: Probing the genome for new drugs and targets with DNA arrays. *Drug Dev Res* **41**:160, 1997.
178. Fodor SPA, Read JL, Pirrung MC, Stryer L, Lu AT, Solas D: Light-directed, spatially addressable parallel chemical synthesis. *Science* **251**:767, 1991.
179. Fodor SPA: Massively parallel genomics. *Science* **277**:393, 1997.
180. Southern EM: DNA chips: Analysing sequence by hybridization to oligonucleotides on a large scale. *Trends Genet* **12**:110, 1996.
181. Kozal MJ, Shah N, Shen N, Yang R, Fucini R, Merigan TC, Richman DD, et al.: Extensive polymorphisms observed in HIV-1 clade B protease gene using high-density oligonucleotide arrays. *Nat Med* **2**:753, 1996.
182. Gingeras TR, Ghandour G, Wang E, Berno A, Small PM, Drobniewski F, Alland D, et al.: Simultaneous genotyping and species identification using hybridization pattern recognition analysis of generic *Mycobacterium* DNA arrays. *Genome Res* **8**:435, 1998.
183. Sapolsky RJ, Lipshutz RJ: Mapping genomic library clones using oligonucleotide arrays. *Genomics* **33**:445, 1996.
184. Chee M, Yang R, Hubbell E, Berno A, Huang XC, Stern D, Winkler J, et al.: Accessing genetic information with high-density DNA arrays. *Science* **274**:610, 1996.
185. Hacia JG, Brody LC, Chee MS, Fodor SPA, Collins FS: Detection of heterozygous mutations in *BRCA1* using high density oligonucleotide arrays and two-colour fluorescence analysis. *Nat Genet* **14**:441, 1996.
186. Hacia JG, Makalowski W, Edgemon K, Erdos MR, Robbins CM, Fodor SPA, Brody LC, et al.: Evolutionary sequence comparisons using high-density oligonucleotide arrays. *Nat Genet* **18**:155, 1998.
187. Lockhart DJ, Dong H, Byrne MC, Follettie MT, Gallo MV, Chee MS, Mittmann M, et al.: Expression monitoring by hybridization to high-density oligonucleotide arrays. *Nat Biotechnol* **14**:1675, 1996.
188. Wodicka L, Dong H, Mittmann M, Ho MH, Lockhart DJ: Genome-wide expression monitoring in *Saccharomyces cerevisiae.* *Nat Biotechnol* **15**:1359, 1997.
189. Winzeler EA, Richards DR, Conway AR, Goldstein AL, Kalman S, McCullough MJ, McCusker JH, et al.: Direct allelic variation scanning the yeast genome. *Science* **281**:1194, 1998.
190. Wang DG, Fan J-B, Siao C-J, Berno A, Young P, Sapolsky R, Ghandour G, et al.: Large-scale identification, mapping, and genotyping of single-nucleotide polymorphisms in the human genome. *Science* **280**:1077, 1998.
191. Schena M, Shalon D, Davis RW, Brown PO: Quantitative monitoring of gene expression patterns with a complementary DNA microarray. *Science* **270**:467, 1995.
192. Schena M: Genome analysis with gene expression microarrays. *BioEssays* **18**:427, 1996.
193. Schena M, Shalon D, Heller R, Chai A, Brown PO, Davis RW: Parallel human genome analysis: Microarray-based expression monitoring of 1000 genes. *Proc Natl Acad Sci USA* **93**:10,614, 1996.

194. DeRisi J, Penland L, Brown PO, Bittner ML, Meltzer PS, Ray M, Chen Y, et al.: Use of a cDNA microarray to analyse gene expression patterns in human cancer. *Nat Genet* **14**:457, 1996.
195. DeRisi JL, Iyer VR, Brown PO: Exploring the metabolic and genetic control of gene expression on a genomic scale. *Science* **278**:680, 1997.
196. Lashkari DA, DeRisi JL, McCusker JH, Namath AF, Gentile C, Hwang SY, Brown PO, et al.: Yeast microarrays for genome wide parallel genetic and gene expression analysis. *Proc Natl Acad Sci USA* **94**:13,057, 1997.
197. Ermolaeva O, Rastogi M, Pruitt KD, Schuler GD, Bittner ML, Chen Y, Simon R, et al.: Data management and analysis for gene expression arrays. *Nat Genet* **20**:19, 1998.
198. Woolley AT, Mathies RA: Ultra-high-speed DNA fragment separations using microfabricated capillary array electrophoresis chips. *Proc Natl Acad Sci USA* **91**:11,348, 1994.
199. Woolley AT, Hadley D, Landre P, de Mello AJ, Mathies RA, Northrup MA: Functional integration of PCR amplification and capillary electrophoresis in a microfabricated DNA analysis device. *Anal Chem* **68**:4081, 1996.
200. Woolley AT, Sensabaugh GF, Mathies RA: High-speed DNA genotyping using microfabricated capillary array electrophoresis chips. *Anal Chem* **69**:2181, 1997.
201. Burns MA, Mastrangelo CH, Sammarco TS, Man FP, Webster JR, Johnson BN, Foerster B, et al.: Microfabricated structures for integrated DNA analysis. *Proc Natl Acad Sci USA* **93**:5556, 1996.
202. Burke DT, Burns MA, Mastrangelo C: Microfabrication technologies for integrated nucleic acid analysis. *Genome Res* **7**:189, 1997.
203. Simpson PC, Roach D, Woolley AT, Thorsen T, Johnston R, Sensabaugh GF, Mathies RA: High-throughput genetic analysis using microfabricated 96-sample capillary array electrophoresis microplates. *Proc Natl Acad Sci USA* **95**:2256, 1998.
204. Kopp MU, de Mello AJ, Manz A: Chemical amplification: Continuous-flow PCR on a chip. *Science* **280**:1046, 1998.
205. Burns MA, Johnson BN, Brahmasandra SN, Handique K, Webster JR, Krishnan M, Sammarco TS, et al.: An integrated nanoliter DNA analysis device. *Science* **282**:484, 1998.
206. Doolittle RF (ed): *Methods in Enzymology*, vol 266: *Computer Methods for Macromolecular Sequence Analysis*. San Diego, Academic, 1996.
207. Fischer C, Schweigert S, Spreckelsen C, Vogel F: Programs, databases, and expert systems for human geneticists: A survey. *Hum Genet* **97**:129, 1996.
208. Baxevanis AD, Boguski MS, Ouellette BFF: Computational analysis of DNA and protein sequences, in Birren B, Green ED, Klapholz S, Myers RM, Roskams J (eds): *Genome Analysis: A Laboratory Manual*, vol 1: *Analyzing DNA*. Cold Spring Harbor, NY, Cold Spring Harbor Laboratory, 1997, p 533.
209. Baxevanis AD, Ouellette BFF (eds): *Bioinformatics: A Practical Guide to the Analysis of Genes and Proteins*. New York, Wiley, 1998.
210. Bishop M (ed): *Guide to Human Genome Computing*. London, Academic, 1998.
211. Ewing B, Hillier L, Wendl MC, Green P: Base-calling of automated sequencer traces using *Phred*: I. Accuracy assessment. *Genome Res* **8**:175, 1998.
212. Ewing B, Green P: Base-calling of automated sequencer traces using *Phred*: II. Error probabilities. *Genome Res* **8**:186, 1998.
213. Gordon D, Abajian C, Green P: *Consed*: A graphical tool for sequence finishing. *Genome Res* **8**:195, 1998.
214. Bonfield JK, Smith KF, Staden R: The new DNA sequence assembly program. *Nucleic Acids Res* **23**:4992, 1995.
215. Dear S, Durbin R, Hillier L, Marth G, Thierry-Mieg J, Mott R: Sequence assembly with CAFTOOLS. *Genome Res* **8**:260, 1998.
216. Benson DA, Boguski MS, Lipman DJ, Ostell J, Ouellette BFF: GenBank. *Nucleic Acids Res* **26**:1, 1998.
217. Stoesser G, Moseley MA, Sleep J, McGowran M, Garcia-Pastor M, Sterk P: The EMBL nucleotide sequence database. *Nucleic Acids Res* **26**:8, 1998.
218. Tateno Y, Fukami-Kobayashi K, Miyazaki S, Sugawara H, Gojobori T: DNA data bank of Japan at work on genome sequence data. *Nucleic Acids Res* **26**:16, 1998.
219. Ouellette BFF, Boguski MS: Database divisions and homology search files: A guide for the perplexed. *Genome Res* **7**:952, 1997.
220. Barker WC, Garavelli JS, Haft DH, Hunt LT, Marzec CR, Orcutt BC, Srinivasarao GY, et al.: The PIR-international protein sequence database. *Nucleic Acids Res* **26**:27, 1998.
221. Bairoch A, Apweiler R: The SWISS-PROT protein sequence data bank and its supplement TrEMBL in 1998. *Nucleic Acids Res* **26**:38, 1998.
222. Borsani G, Ballabio A, Banfi S: A practical guide to orient yourself in the labyrinth of genome databases. *Hum Mol Genet* **7**:1641, 1998.
223. Gelbart WM: Databases in genomic research. *Science* **282**:659, 1998.
224. Pearson WR, Lipman DJ: Improved tools for biological sequence comparison. *Proc Natl Acad Sci USA* **85**:2444, 1988.
225. Altschul SF, Gish W, Miller W, Myers EW, Lipman DJ: Basic local alignment search tool. *J Mol Biol* **215**:403, 1990.
226. Altschul SF, Boguski MS, Gish W, Wootton JC: Issues in searching molecular sequence databases. *Nat Genet* **6**:119, 1994.
227. Altschul SF, Madden TL, Schaffer AA, Zhang J, Zhang Z, Miller W, Lipman DJ: Gapped BLAST and PSI-BLAST: A new generation of protein database search programs. *Nucleic Acids Res* **25**:3389, 1997.
228. Zhang J, Madden TL: PowerBLAST: A new network BLAST application for interactive or automated sequence analysis and annotation. *Genome Res* **7**:649, 1997.
229. Uberbacher EC, Mural RJ: Locating protein-coding regions in human DNA sequences by a multiple sensor-neural network approach. *Proc Natl Acad Sci USA* **88**:11,261, 1991.
230. Hutchinson GB, Hayden MR: The prediction of exons through an analysis of spliceable open reading frames. *Nucleic Acids Res* **20**:3453, 1992.
231. Xu Y, Mural R, Shah M, Uberbacher E: Recognizing exons in genomic sequence using GRAIL II. *Genet Eng* **16**:241, 1994.
232. Solovyev VV, Salamov AA, Lawrence CB: Predicting internal exons by oligonucleotide composition and discriminant analysis of spliceable open reading frames. *Nucleic Acids Res* **22**:5156, 1994.
233. Burge C, Karlin S: Prediction of complete gene structures in human genomic DNA. *J Mol Biol* **268**:78, 1997.
234. Claverie J-M: Computational methods for the identification of genes in vertebrate genomic sequences. *Hum Mol Genet* **6**:1735, 1997.
235. Burge CB, Karlin S: Finding the genes in genomic DNA. *Curr Opin Struct Biol* **8**:346, 1998.
236. Fickett JW, Hatzigeorgiou AG: Eukaryotic promoter recognition. *Genome Res* **7**:861, 1997.
237. Smith RF, Wiese BA, Wojzynski MK, Davison DB, Worley KC: BCM search launcher: An integrated interface to molecular biology data base search and analysis services available on the World Wide Web. *Genome Res* **6**:454, 1996.
238. Harnden DG, Klinger HP (eds): *ISCN: An International System for Human Cytogenetic Nomenclature. Birth Defects: Original Article Series*, vol 21(1). New York, Karger, 1985.
239. Royer-Pokora B, Kunkel LM, Monaco AP, Goff SC, Newburger PE, Baehner RL, Cole FS, et al.: Cloning the gene for an inherited human disorder — chronic granulomatous disease — on the basis of its chromosomal location. *Nature* **322**:32, 1986.
240. Monaco AP, Neve RL, Colletti-Feener C, Bertelson CJ, Kurnit DM, Kunkel LM: Isolation of candidate cDNAs for portions of the Duchenne muscular dystrophy gene. *Nature* **323**:646, 1986.
241. Verkerk AJMH, Pieretti M, Sutcliffe JS, Fu Y-H, Kuhl DPA, Pizzuti A, Reiner O, et al.: Identification of a gene (FMR-1) containing a CGG repeat coincident with a breakpoint cluster region exhibiting length variation in fragile X syndrome. *Cell* **65**:905, 1991.
242. Trask BJ, Massa H, Kenwrick S, Gitschier J: Mapping of human chromosome Xq28 by two-color fluorescence in situ hybridization of DNA sequences to interphase cell nuclei. *Am J Hum Genet* **48**:1, 1991.
243. Southern EM: Detection of specific sequences among DNA fragments separated by gel electrophoresis. *J Mol Biol* **98**:503, 1975.
244. Botstein D, White RL, Skolnick M, Davis RW: Construction of a genetic linkage map in man using restriction fragment length polymorphisms. *Am J Hum Genet* **32**:314, 1980.
245. White R, Leppert M, Bishop DT, Barker D, Berkowitz J, Brown C, Callahan P, et al.: Construction of linkage maps with DNA markers for human chromosomes. *Nature* **313**:101, 1985.
246. Donis-Keller H, Barker DF, Knowlton RG, Schumm JW, Braman JC, Green P: Highly polymorphic RFLP probes as diagnostic tools. *Cold Spring Harb Symp Quant Biol* **51**:317, 1986.
247. Lander ES, Botstein D: Mapping complex genetic traits in humans: New method using a complete RFLP linkage map. *Cold Spring Harb Symp Quant Biol* **51**:49, 1986.
248. Nakamura Y, Leppert M, O'Connell P, Wolff R, Holm T, Culver M, Martin C, et al.: Variable number of tandem repeat (VNTR) markers for human gene mapping. *Science* **235**:1616, 1987.
249. Weber JL, May PE: Abundant class of human DNA polymorphisms which can be typed using the polymerase chain reaction. *Am J Hum Genet* **44**:388, 1989.

250. Litt M, Luty JA: A hypervariable microsatellite revealed by in vitro amplification of a dinucleotide repeat within the cardiac muscle actin gene. *Am J Hum Genet* **44**:397, 1989.
251. Weber JL: Human DNA polymorphisms based on length variations in simple-sequence tandem repeats, in Davies KE, Tilghman SM (eds): *Genome Analysis,* vol 1: *Genetic and Physical Mapping*. Cold Spring Harbor, NY, Cold Spring Harbor Laboratory, 1990, p 159.
252. Dietrich WF, Weber JL, Nickerson DA, Kwok P-Y: Identification and analysis of DNA polymorphisms, in Birren B, Green ED, Hieter P, Klapholz S, Myers RM, Riethman H, Roskams J (eds): *Genome Analysis: A Laboratory Manual,* vol 4: *Mapping Genomes*. Cold Spring Harbor, NY, Cold Spring Harbor Laboratory, 1999, p 135.
253. Nickerson DA, Whitehurst C, Boysen C, Charmley P, Kaiser R, Hood L: Identification of clusters of biallelic polymorphic sequence-tagged sites (pSTSs) that generate highly informative and automatable markers for genetic linkage mapping. *Genomics* **12**:377, 1992.
254. Landegren U, Nilsson M, Kwok P-Y: Reading bits of genetic information: Methods for single-nucleotide polymorphism analysis. *Genome Res* **8**:769, 1998.
255. Kruglyak L: The use of a genetic map of biallelic markers in linkage studies. *Nat Genet* **17**:21, 1997.
256. Collins FS, Guyer MS, Chakravarti A: Variations on a theme: Cataloging human DNA sequence variation. *Science* **278**:1580, 1997.
257. Schafer AJ, Hawkins JR: DNA variation and the future of human genetics. *Nat Biotechnol* **16**:33, 1998.
258. Weiss KM: In search of human variation. *Genome Res* **8**:691, 1998.
259. Chakravarti A, Lynn A: Meiotic mapping in humans, in Birren B, Green ED, Hieter P, Klapholz S, Myers RM, Riethman H, Roskams J (eds): *Genome Analysis: A Laboratory Manual,* vol 4: *Mapping Genomes*. Cold Spring Harbor, NY, Cold Spring Harbor Laboratory, 1999, p 1.
260. Dausset J, Cann H, Cohen D, Lathrop M, Lalouel J-M, White R: Centre d'Etude du Polymorphisme Humain (CEPH): Collaborative genetic mapping of the human genome. *Genomics* **6**:575, 1990.
261. Terwilliger JD, Ott J: *Handbook of Human Genetic Linkage*. Baltimore, Johns Hopkins University Press, 1994.
262. Donis-Keller H, Green P, Helms C, Cartinhour S, Weiffenbach B, Stephens K, Keith TP, et al.: A genetic linkage map of the human genome. *Cell* **51**:319, 1987.
263. Weissenbach J, Gyapay G, Dib C, Vignal A, Morissette J, Millasseau P, Vaysseix G, et al.: A second-generation linkage map of the human genome. *Nature* **359**:794, 1992.
264. Gyapay G, Morissette J, Vignal A, Dib C, Fizames C, Millasseau P, Marc S, et al.: The 1993–94 Genethon human genetic linkage map. *Nat Genet* **7**:246, 1994.
265. Dib C, Faure S, Fizames C, Samson D, Drouot N, Vignal A, Millasseau P, et al.: A comprehensive genetic map of the human genome based on 5,264 microsatellites. *Nature* **380**:152, 1996.
266. Murray JC, Buetow KH, Weber JL, Ludwigsen S, Scherpbier-Heddema T, Manion F, Quillen J, et al.: A comprehensive human linkage map with centimorgan density. *Science* **265**:2049, 1994.
267. Buetow KH, Weber JL, Ludwigsen S, Scherpbier-Heddema T, Duyk GM, Sheffield VC, Wang Z, et al.: Integrated human genome-wide maps constructed using the CEPH reference panel. *Nat Genet* **6**:391, 1994.
268. Utah Marker Development Group: A collection of ordered tetranucleotide-repeat markers from the human genome. *Am J Hum Genet* **57**:619, 1995.
269. Olson MV, Dutchik JE, Graham MY, Brodeur GM, Helms C, Frank M, MacCollin M, et al.: Random-clone strategy for genomic restriction mapping in yeast. *Proc Natl Acad Sci USA* **83**:7826, 1986.
270. Coulson A, Sulston J, Brenner S, Karn J: Toward a physical map of the genome of the nematode *Caenorhabditis elegans*. *Proc Natl Acad Sci USA* **83**:7821, 1986.
271. Kohara Y, Akiyama K, Isono K: The physical map of the whole *E. coli* chromosome: Application of a new strategy for rapid analysis and sorting of a large genomic library. *Cell* **50**:495, 1987.
272. Wong GK-S, Yu J, Thayer EC, Olson MV: Multiple-complete-digest restriction fragment mapping: Generating sequence-ready maps for large-scale DNA sequencing. *Proc Natl Acad Sci USA* **94**:5225, 1997.
273. Olson M, Hood L, Cantor C, Botstein D: A common language for physical mapping of the human genome. *Science* **245**:1434, 1989.
274. Green ED, Green P: Sequence-tagged site (STS) content mapping of human chromosomes: Theoretical considerations and early experiences. *PCR Methods Appl* **1**:77, 1991.
275. Green ED, Mohr RM, Idol JR, Jones M, Buckingham JM, Deaven LL, Moyzis RK, et al.: Systematic generation of sequence-tagged sites for physical mapping of human chromosomes: Application to the mapping of human chromosome 7 using yeast artificial chromosomes. *Genomics* **11**:548, 1991.
276. Hillier L, Green P: OSP: A computer program for choosing PCR and DNA sequencing primers. *PCR Methods Appl* **1**:124, 1991.
277. Green ED: Physical mapping of human chromosomes: Generation of chromosome-specific sequence-tagged sites, in Adolph KW (ed): *Methods in Molecular Genetics,* vol 1: *Gene and Chromosome Analysis* (part A). San Diego, Academic, 1993, p 192.
278. Vollrath D: DNA markers for physical mapping, in Birren B, Green ED, Hieter P, Klapholz S, Myers RM, Riethman H, Roskams J (eds): *Genome Analysis: A Laboratory Manual,* vol 4: *Mapping genomes*. Cold Spring Harbor, NY, Cold Spring Harbor Laboratory, 1999, p 187.
279. Nelson DL, Ledbetter SA, Corbo L, Victoria MF, Ramirez-Solis R, Webster TD, Ledbetter DH, et al.: *Alu* polymerase chain reaction: A method for rapid isolation of human-specific sequences from complex DNA sources. *Proc Natl Acad Sci USA* **86**:6686, 1989.
280. Nelson DL: Interspersed repetitive sequence polymerase chain reaction (IRS PCR) for generation of human DNA fragments from complex sources. *Methods* **2**:60, 1991.
281. Kass DH, Batzer MA: Inter-*Alu* polymerase chain reaction: Advancements and applications. *Anal Biochem* **228**:185, 1995.
282. Cole CG, Goodfellow PN, Bobrow M, Bentley DR: Generation of novel sequence tagged sites (STSs) from discrete chromosomal regions using *Alu*-PCR. *Genomics* **10**:816, 1991.
283. Deaven LL, Van Dilla MA, Bartholdi MF, Carrano AV, Cram LS, Fuscoe JC, Gray JW, et al.: Construction of human chromosome-specific DNA libraries from flow-sorted chromosomes. *Cold Spring Harb Symp Quant Biol* **51**:159, 1986.
284. Collins C, Kuo WL, Segraves R, Fuscoe J, Pinkel D, Gray JW: Construction and characterization of plasmid libraries enriched in sequences from single human chromosomes. *Genomics* **11**:997, 1991.
285. Shimizu N, Minoshima S: Gene mapping and fine-structure analysis of the human genome using flow-sorted chromosomes, in Adolph KW (ed): *Advanced Techniques in Chromosome Research*. New York, Marcel Dekker, 1991, p 135.
286. Goold RD, di Sibio GL, Xu H, Lang DB, Dadgar J, Magrane GG, Dugaiczyk A, et al.: The development of sequence-tagged sites for human chromosome 4. *Hum Mol Genet* **2**:1271, 1993.
287. Smith MW, Clark SP, Hutchinson JS, Wei YH, Churukian AC, Daniels LB, Diggle KL, et al.: A sequence-tagged site map of human chromosome 11. *Genomics* **17**:699, 1993.
288. Wilcox AS, Khan AS, Hopkins JA, Sikela JM: Use of 3′ untranslated sequences of human cDNAs for rapid chromosome assignment and conversion to STSs: Implications for an expression map of the genome. *Nucleic Acids Res* **19**:1837, 1991.
289. Kere J, Nagaraja R, Mumm S, Ciccodicola A, d'Urso M, Schlessinger D: Mapping human chromosomes by walking with sequence-tagged sites from end fragments of yeast artificial chromosome inserts. *Genomics* **14**:241, 1992.
290. Bouffard GG, Iyer LM, Idol JR, Braden VV, Cunningham AF, Weintraub LA, Mohr-Tidwell RM, et al.: A collection of 1814 human chromosome 7-specific STSs. *Genome Res* **7**:59, 1997.
291. Stewart EA, McKusick KB, Aggarwal A, Bajorek E, Brady S, Chu A, Fang N, et al.: An STS-based radiation hybrid map of the human genome. *Genome Res* **7**:422, 1997.
292. Schuler GD, Boguski MS, Stewart EA, Stein LD, Gyapay G, Rice K, White RE, et al.: A gene map of the human genome. *Science* **274**:540, 1996.
293. Deloukas P, Schuler GD, Gyapay G, Beasley EM, Soderlund C, Rodriguez-Tome P, Hui L, et al.: A physical map of 30,000 human genes. *Science* **282**:744, 1998.
294. Sheffield VC, Weber JL, Buetow KH, Murray JC, Even DA, Wiles K, Gastier JM, et al.: A collection of tri- and tetranucleotide repeat markers used to generate high quality, high resolution human genome-wide linkage maps. *Hum Mol Genet* **4**:1837, 1995.
295. Walter MA, Spillett DJ, Thomas P, Weissenbach J, Goodfellow PN: A method for constructing radiation hybrid maps of whole genomes. *Nat Genet* **7**:22, 1994.
296. McCarthy LC: Whole genome radiation hybrid mapping. *Trends Genet* **12**:491, 1996.
297. Lunetta KL, Boehnke M: Multipoint radiation hybrid mapping: Comparison of methods, sample size requirements, and optimal study characteristics. *Genomics* **21**:92, 1994.
298. Lange K, Boehnke M, Cox DR, Lunetta KL: Statistical methods for polyploid radiation hybrid mapping. *Genome Res* **5**:136, 1995.

299. Lunetta KL, Boehnke M, Lange K, Cox DR: Experimental design and error detection for polyploid radiation hybrid mapping. *Genome Res* **5**:151, 1995.
300. Gyapay G, Schmitt K, Fizames C, Jones H, Vega-Czarny N, Spillett D, Muselet D, et al.: A radiation hybrid map of the human genome. *Hum Mol Genet* **5**:339, 1996.
301. McCarthy LC, Terrett J, Davis ME, Knights CJ, Smith AL, Critcher R, Schmitt K, et al.: A first-generation whole genome-radiation hybrid map spanning the mouse genome. *Genome Res* **7**:1153, 1997.
302. Yang Y-P, Womack JE: Parallel radiation hybrid mapping: A powerful tool for high-resolution genomic comparison. *Genome Res* **8**:731, 1998.
303. Travis GH, Sutcliffe JG: Phenol emulsion-enhanced DNA-driven subtractive cDNA cloning: Isolation of low-abundance monkey cortex-specific mRNAs. *Proc Natl Acad Sci USA* **85**:1696, 1988.
304. Patanjali SR, Parimoo S, Weissman SM: Construction of a uniform-abundance (normalized) cDNA library. *Proc Natl Acad Sci USA* **88**:1943, 1991.
305. Soares MB, Bonaldo MF, Jelene P, Su L, Lawton L, Efstratiadis A: Construction and characterization of a normalized cDNA library. *Proc Natl Acad Sci USA* **91**:9228, 1994.
306. Bonaldo MF, Lennon G, Soares MB: Normalization and subtraction: Two approaches to facilitate gene discovery. *Genome Res* **6**:791, 1996.
307. Soares MB, Bonaldo MF: Constructing and screening normalized cDNA libraries, in Birren B, Green ED, Klapholz S, Myers RM, Roskams J (eds): *Genome Analysis: A Laboratory Manual,* vol 2: *Detecting Genes*. Cold Spring Harbor, NY, Cold Spring Harbor Laboratory, 1998, p 49.
308. Adams MD, Kelley JM, Gocayne JD, Dubnick M, Polymeropoulos MH, Xiao H, Merril CR, et al.: Complementary DNA sequencing: Expressed sequence tags and Human Genome Project. *Science* **252**:1651, 1991.
309. Hillier L, Lennon G, Becker M, Bonaldo M, Chiapelli B, Chissoe S, Dietrich N, et al.: Generation and analysis of 280,000 human expressed sequence tags. *Genome Res* **6**:807, 1996.
310. Adams MD, Kerlavage AR, Fleischmann RD, Fuldner RA, Bult CJ, Lee NH, Kirkness EF, et al.: Initial assessment of human gene diversity and expression patterns based upon 83 million nucleotides of cDNA sequence. *Nature* **377**:3, 1995.
311. Boguski MS, Lowe TM, Tolstoshev CM: dbEST: Database for "expressed sequence tags." *Nat Genet* **4**:332, 1993.
312. Boguski MS, Schuler GD: ESTablishing a human transcript map. *Nat Genet* **10**:369, 1995.
313. Boguski MS: The turning point in genome research. *Trends Biochem Sci* **20**:295, 1995.
314. Schuler GD: Pieces of the puzzle: Expressed sequence tags and the catalog of human genes. *J Mol Med* **75**:694, 1997.
315. Khan AS, Wilcox AS, Polymeropoulos MH, Hopkins JA, Stevens TJ, Robinson M, Orpana AK, et al.: Single pass sequencing and physical and genetic mapping of human brain cDNAs. *Nat Genet* **2**:180, 1992.
316. Berry R, Stevens TJ, Walter NAR, Wilcox AS, Rubano T, Hopkins JA, Weber J, et al.: Gene-based sequence-tagged-sites (STSs) as the basis for a human gene map. *Nat Genet* **10**:415, 1995.
317. Gerhold D, Caskey CT: It's the genes! EST access to human genome content. *BioEssays* **18**:973, 1996.
318. Okubo K, Matsubara K: Complementary DNA sequence (EST) collections and the expression information of the human genome. *FEBS Lett* **403**:225, 1997.
319. Tilghman SM: Lessons learned, promises kept: A biologist's eye view of the genome project. *Genome Res* **6**:773, 1996.
320. Marra MA, Hillier L, Waterston RH: Expressed sequence tags: ESTablishing bridges between genomes. *Trends Genet* **14**:4, 1998.
321. Velculescu VE, Zhang L, Vogelstein B, Kinzler KW: Serial analysis of gene expression. *Science* **270**:484, 1995.
322. Adams MD: Serial analysis of gene expression: ESTs get smaller. *BioEssays* **18**:261, 1996.
323. The Yeast Genome Directory. *Nature* **387S**:1, 1997.
324. Goffeau A, Barrell BG, Bussey H, Davis RW, Dujon B, Feldmann H, Galibert F, et al.: Life with 6000 genes. *Science* **274**:546, 1996.
325. Hieter P, Bassett DE Jr, Valle D: The yeast genome: A common currency. *Nat Genet* **13**:253, 1996.
326. Johnston M: Genome sequencing: The complete code for a eukaryotic cell. *Curr Biol* **6**:500, 1996.
327. Dujon B: The yeast genome project: What did we learn? *Trends Genet* **12**:263, 1996.
328. Walsh S, Barrell B: The *Saccharomyces cerevisiae* genome on the World Wide Web. *Trends Genet* **12**:276, 1996.
329. Thomas K: Yeasties and beasties: 7 years of genome sequencing. *FEBS Lett* **396**:1, 1996.
330. Blattner FR, Plunkett G III, Bloch CA, Perna NT, Burland V, Riley M, Collado-Vides J, et al.: The complete genome sequence of *Escherichia coli* K-12. *Science* **277**:1453, 1997.
331. Sulston J, Du Z, Thomas K, Wilson R, Hillier L, Staden R, Halloran N, et al.: The *C. elegans* genome sequencing project: A beginning. *Nature* **356**:37, 1992.
332. Wilson R, Ainscough R, Anderson K, Baynes C, Berks M, Bonfield J, Burton J, et al.: 2.2 Mb of contiguous nucleotide sequence from chromosome III of *C. elegans*. *Nature* **368**:32, 1994.
333. Hodgkin J, Plasterk RHA, Waterston RH: The nematode *Caenorhabditis elegans* and its genome. *Science* **270**:410, 1995.
334. Waterston R, Sulston J: The genome of *Caenorhabditis elegans*. *Proc Natl Acad Sci USA* **92**:10,836, 1995.
335. Berks M and the *C. elegans* Genome Mapping and Sequencing Consortium: Around the genomes: The *C. elegans* genome sequencing project. *Genome Res* **5**:99, 1995.
336. Olson MV: A time to sequence. *Science* **270**:394, 1995.
337. Gibbs RA: Pressing ahead with human genome sequencing. *Nat Genet* **11**:121, 1995.
338. Boguski M, Chakravarti A, Gibbs R, Green E, Myers RM: The end of the beginning: The race to begin human genome sequencing. *Genome Res* **6**:771, 1996.
339. Gibbs RA: Hares and tortoises in the race to sequence the human genome: Expectations and realities. *Trends Genet* **13**:381, 1997.
340. Rowen L, Mahairas G, Hood L: Sequencing the human genome. *Science* **278**:605, 1997.
341. Beck S, Sterk P: Genome-scale DNA sequencing: Where are we? *Curr Opin Biotechnol* **9**:116, 1998.
342. Waterston R, Sulston JE: The Human Genome Project: Reaching the finish line. *Science* **282**:53, 1998.
343. Wilson RK, Mardis ER: Shotgun sequencing, in Birren B, Green ED, Klapholz S, Myers RM, Roskams J (eds): *Genome Analysis: A Laboratory Manual,* vol 1: *Analyzing DNA*. Cold Spring Harbor, NY, Cold Spring Harbor Laboratory, 1997, p 397.
344. Kimmel BE, Palazzolo MJ, Martin CH, Boeke JD, Devine SE: Transposon-mediated DNA sequencing, in Birren B, Green ED, Klapholz S, Myers RM, Roskams J (eds): *Genome Analysis: A Laboratory Manual,* vol 1: *Analyzing DNA*. Cold Spring Harbor, NY, Cold Spring Harbor Laboratory, 1997, p 455.
345. Miklos GLG, Rubin GM: The role of the genome project in determining gene function: Insights from model organisms. *Cell* **86**:521, 1996.
346. Riles L, Dutchik JE, Baktha A, McCauley BK, Thayer EC, Leckie MP, Braden VV, et al.: Physical maps of the six smallest chromosomes of *Saccharomyces cerevisiae* at a resolution of 2.6 kilobase pairs. *Genetics* **134**:81, 1993.
347. Bassett DE Jr, Basrai MA, Connelly C, Hyland KM, Kitagawa K, Mayer ML, Morrow DM, et al.: Exploiting the complete yeast genome sequence. *Curr Opin Genet Dev* **6**:763, 1996.
348. Botstein D, Chervitz SA, Cherry JM: Yeast as a model organism. *Science* **277**:1259, 1997.
349. Hudson JR Jr, Dawson EP, Rushing KL, Jackson CH, Lockshon D, Conover D, Lanciault C, et al.: The complete set of predicted genes from *Saccharomyces cerevisiae* in a readily usable form. *Genome Res* **7**:1169, 1997.
350. Coulson A, Waterston R, Kiff J, Sulston J, Kohara Y: Genome linking with yeast artificial chromosomes. *Nature* **335**:184, 1988.
351. Coulson A, Kozono Y, Lutterbach B, Shownkeen R, Sulston J, Waterston R: YACs and the *C. elegans* genome. *BioEssays* **13**:413, 1991.
352. Hodgkin J, Herman RK: Changing styles in *C. elegans* genetics. *Trends Genet* **14**:352, 1998.
353. Walhout M, Endoh H, Thierry-Mieg N, Wong W, Vidal M: A model of elegance. *Am J Hum Genet* **63**:955, 1998.
354. Rubin GM: Around the genomes: The *Drosophila* genome project. *Genome Res* **6**:71, 1996.
355. Rubin GM: The *Drosophila* genome project: A progress report. *Trends Genet* **14**:340, 1998.
356. Hartl DL: Genome map of *Drosophila melanogaster* based on yeast artificial chromosomes, in Davies KE, Tilghman SM (eds): *Genome Analysis,* vol 4: *Strategies for Physical Mapping*. Cold Spring Harbor, NY, Cold Spring Harbor Laboratory, 1992, p 39.
357. Kimmerly W, Stultz K, Lewis S, Lewis K, Lustre V, Romero R, Benke J, et al.: A P1-based physical map of the *Drosophila* euchromatic genome. *Genome Res* **6**:414, 1996.

358. Spradling AC, Stern DM, Kiss I, Roote J, Laverty T, Rubin GM: Gene disruptions using *P* transposable elements: An integral component of the *Drosophila* genome project. *Proc Natl Acad Sci USA* **92**: 10,824, 1995.
359. Dietrich WF, Copeland NG, Gilbert DJ, Miller JC, Jenkins NA, Lander ES: Mapping the mouse genome: Current status and future prospects. *Proc Natl Acad Sci USA* **92**: 10,849, 1995.
360. Meisler MH: The role of the laboratory mouse in the Human Genome Project. *Am J Hum Genet* **59**: 764, 1996.
361. Fisher EM: The contribution of the mouse to advances in human genetics. *Adv Genet* **35**: 155, 1997.
362. Jaenisch R: Transgenic animals. *Science* **240**: 1468, 1988.
363. Capecchi MR: Altering the genome by homologous recombination. *Science* **244**: 1288, 1989.
364. Robbins J: Gene targeting. The precise manipulation of the mammalian genome. *Circ Res* **73**: 3, 1993.
365. Wynshaw-Boris A: Model mice and human disease. *Nat Genet* **13**: 259, 1996.
366. Thomas KR, Capecchi MR: Site-directed mutagenesis by gene targeting in mouse embryo-derived stem cells. *Cell* **51**: 503, 1987.
367. Brown SDM, Nolan PM: Mouse mutagenesis: Systematic studies of mammalian gene function. *Hum Mol Genet* **7**: 1627, 1998.
368. Rubin EM, Barsh GS: Biological insights through genomics: Mouse to man. *J Clin Invest* **97**: 275, 1996.
369. Rubin EM, Smith DJ: Optimizing the mouse to sift sequence for function. *Trends Genet* **13**: 423, 1997.
370. Nadeau JH: Maps of linkage and synteny homologies between mouse and man. *Trends Genet* **5**: 82, 1989.
371. O'Brien SJ: Mammalian genome mapping: Lessons and prospects. *Curr Opin Genet Dev* **1**: 105, 1990.
372. Cox RD, Lehrach H: Genome mapping: PCR based meiotic and somatic cell hybrid analysis. *BioEssays* **13**: 193, 1991.
373. O'Brien SJ, Womack JE, Lyons LA, Moore KJ, Jenkins NA, Copeland NG: Anchored reference loci for comparative genome mapping in mammals. *Nat Genet* **3**: 103, 1993.
374. Eppig JT, Nadeau JH: Comparative maps: The mammalian jigsaw puzzle. *Curr Opin Genet Dev* **5**: 709, 1995.
375. DeBry RW, Seldin MF: Human/mouse homology relationships. *Genomics* **33**: 337, 1996.
376. Carver EA, Stubbs L: Zooming in on the human-mouse comparative map: Genome conservation re-examined on a high-resolution scale. *Genome Res* **7**: 1123, 1997.
377. Dietrich W, Katz H, Lincoln SE, Shin H-S, Friedman J, Dracopoli NC, Lander ES: A genetic map of the mouse suitable for typing intraspecific crosses. *Genetics* **131**: 423, 1992.
378. Dietrich WF, Miller JC, Steen RG, Merchant M, Damron D, Nahf R, Gross A, et al.: A genetic map of the mouse with 4,006 simple sequence length polymorphisms. *Nat Genet* **7**: 220, 1994.
379. Dietrich WF, Miller J, Steen R, Merchant MA, Damron-Boles D, Husain Z, Dredge R, et al.: A comprehensive genetic map of the mouse genome. *Nature* **380**: 149, 1996.
380. Rhodes M, Straw R, Fernando S, Evans A, Lacey T, Dearlove A, Greystrong J, et al.: A high-resolution microsatellite map of the mouse genome. *Genome Res* **8**: 531, 1998.
381. Herman GE: Physical mapping of the mouse genome. *Methods* **14**: 135, 1998.
382. Eppig JT, Blake JA, Davisson MT, Richardson JE: Informatics for mouse genetics and genome mapping. *Methods* **14**: 179, 1998.
383. Seldin MF: Genome surfing: Using Internet-based informatic tools toward functional genetic studies in mouse and humans. *Methods* **13**: 445, 1997.
384. Hood L, Koop B, Goverman J, Hunkapiller T: Model genomes: The benefits of analysing homologous human and mouse sequences. *Trends Biotechnol* **10**: 19, 1992.
385. Koop BF: Human and rodent DNA sequence comparisons: A mosaic model of genomic evolution. *Trends Genet* **11**: 367, 1995.
386. Mallon A-M, Strivens M: DNA sequence analysis and comparative sequencing. *Methods* **14**: 160, 1998.
387. Eisen JA: Phylogenomics: Improving functional predictions for uncharacterized genes by evolutionary analysis. *Genome Res* **8**: 163, 1998.
388. Makalowski W, Zhang J, Boguski MS: Comparative analysis of 1196 orthologous mouse and human full-length mRNA and protein sequences. *Genome Res* **6**: 846, 1996.
389. Makalowski W, Boguski MS: Evolutionary parameters of the transcribed mammalian genome: An analysis of 2,820 orthologous rodent and human sequences. *Proc Natl Acad Sci USA* **95**: 9407, 1998.
390. Koop BF, Hood L: Striking sequence similarity over almost 100 kilobases of human and mouse T-cell receptor DNA. *Nat Genet* **7**: 48, 1994.
391. Galili N, Baldwin HS, Lund J, Reeves R, Gong W, Wang Z, Roe BA, et al.: A region of mouse chromosome 16 is syntenic to the DiGeorge, velocardiofacial syndrome minimal critical region. *Genome Res* **7**: 17, 1997.
392. Oeltjen JC, Malley TM, Muzny DM, Miller W, Gibbs RA, Belmont JW: Large-scale comparative sequence analysis of the human and murine Bruton's tyrosine kinase loci reveals conserved regulatory domains. *Genome Res* **7**: 315, 1997.
393. Ansari-Lari MA, Oeltjen JC, Schwartz S, Zhang Z, Muzny DM, Lu J, Gorrell JH, et al.: Comparative sequence analysis of a gene-rich cluster on human chromosome 12p13 and its syntenic region in mouse chromosome 6. *Genome Res* **8**: 29, 1998.
394. Mizukami T, Chang WI, Garkavtsev I, Kaplan N, Lombardi D, Matsumoto T, Niwa O, et al.: A 13 kb resolution cosmid map of the 14 Mb fission yeast genome by nonrandom sequence-tagged site mapping. *Cell* **73**: 121, 1993.
395. Hoheisel JD, Maier E, Mott R, McCarthy L, Grigoriev AV, Schalkwyk LC, Nizetic D, et al.: High resolution cosmid and P1 maps spanning the 14 Mb genome of the fission yeast *S. pombe*. *Cell* **73**: 109, 1993.
396. Jacob HJ, Brown DM, Bunker RK, Daly MJ, Dzau VJ, Goodman A, Koike G, et al.: A genetic linkage map of the laboratory rat, *Rattus norvegicus*. *Nat Genet* **9**: 63, 1995.
397. James MR, Lindpaintner K: Why map the rat? *Trends Genet* **13**: 171, 1997.
398. Brown DM, Matise TC, Koike G, Simon JS, Winer ES, Zangen S, McLaughlin MG, et al.: An integrated genetic linkage map of the laboratory rat. *Mamm Genome* **9**: 521, 1998.
399. Felsenfeld AL: Defining the boundaries of zebrafish developmental genetics. *Nat Genet* **14**: 258, 1996.
400. Postlethwait JH, Talbot WS: Zebrafish genomics: From mutants to genes. *Trends Genet* **13**: 183, 1997.
401. Knapik EW, Goodman A, Ekker M, Chevrette M, Delgado J, Neuhauss S, Shimoda N, et al.: A microsatellite genetic linkage map for zebrafish (*Danio rerio*). *Nat Genet* **18**: 338, 1998.
402. Postlethwait JH, Yan Y-L, Gates MA, Horne S, Amores A, Brownlie A, Donovan A, et al.: Vertebrate genome evolution and the zebrafish gene map. *Nat Genet* **18**: 345, 1998.
403. Beier DR: Zebrafish: Genomics on the fast track. *Genome Res* **8**: 9, 1998.
404. Brenner S, Elgar G, Sandford R, Macrae A, Venkatesh B, Aparicio S: Characterization of the pufferfish (*Fugu*) genome as a compact model vertebrate genome. *Nature* **366**: 265, 1993.
405. Mileham P, Brown SDM: The pufferfish genome: Small is beautiful? *BioEssays* **16**: 153, 1994.
406. Koop BF, Nadeau JH: Pufferfish and a new paradigm for comparative genome analysis. *Proc Natl Acad Sci USA* **93**: 1363, 1996.
407. Elgar G: Quality not quantity: The pufferfish genome. *Hum Mol Genet* **5**: 1437, 1996.
408. Elgar G, Sandford R, Aparicio S, Macrae A, Venkatesh B, Brenner S: Small is beautiful: Comparative genomics with the pufferfish (*Fugu rubripes*). *Trends Genet* **12**: 145, 1996.
409. Angrist M: Less is more: Compact genomes pay dividends. *Genome Res* **8**: 683, 1998.
410. Dean C, Schmidt R: Plant genomes: A current molecular description. *Annu Rev Plant Physiol Plant Mol Biol* **46**: 395, 1995.
411. Goodman HM, Ecker JR, Dean C: The genome of *Arabidopsis thaliana*. *Proc Natl Acad Sci USA* **92**: 10,831, 1995.
412. Settles AM, Byrne M: Opportunities and challenges grow from *Arabidopsis* genome sequencing. *Genome Res* **8**: 83, 1998.
413. Schmidt R: Physical mapping of the *Arabidopsis thaliana* genome. *Plant Physiol Biochem* **36**: 1, 1998.
414. Bevan M, Bancroft I, Bent E, Love K, Goodman H, Dean C, Bergkamp R, et al.: Analysis of 1.9 Mb of contiguous sequence from chromosome 4 of *Arabidopsis thaliana*. *Nature* **391**: 485, 1998.
415. Watson JD, Jordon E: The human genome program at the National Institutes of Health. *Genomics* **5**: 654, 1989.
416. Watson JD: The Human Genome Project: Past, present, and future. *Science* **248**: 44, 1990.
417. Cantor CR: Orchestrating the Human Genome Project. *Science* **248**: 49, 1990.
418. Cook-Deegan RM: The genesis of the Human Genome Project, in Friedmann T (ed): *Molecular Genetic Medicine,* vol 1. San Diego, Academic, 1991, p 1.

419. Watson JD, Cook-Deegan RM: Origins of the Human Genome Project. *FASEB J* **5**:8, 1991.
420. Jordan E: Organization and long-range plan. *Anal Chem* **63**:420A, 1991.
421. Jordan E: Invited editorial: The Human Genome Project: Where did it come from, where is it going? *Am J Hum Genet* **51**:1, 1992.
422. Engel LW: The Human Genome Project: History, goals, and progress to date. *Arch Pathol Lab Med* **117**:459, 1993.
423. Haq MM: Medical genetics and the Human Genome Project: A historical review. *Tex Med* **89**:68, 1993.
424. McKusick VA: Genomics: Structural and functional studies of genomes. *Genomics* **45**:244, 1997.
425. DeLisi C: The Human Genome Project. *Am Sci* **76**:488, 1988.
426. National Research Council (Committee on Mapping and Sequencing the Human Genome): *Mapping and Sequencing the Human Genome*. Washington, DC, National Academy, 1988.
427. Office of Technology Assessment (OTA): *Mapping Our Genes: Genome Projects—How Big? How Fast?* Washington, DC, OTA; 61-OTA-BA-373, 1988.
428. Watson JD: The human genome initiative: A statement of need. *Hosp Pract* **26**:69, 1991.
429. Gilbert W: Towards a paradigm shift in biology. *Nature* **349**:99, 1991.
430. Berg P: All our collective ingenuity will be needed. *FASEB J* **5**:75, 1991.
431. Yager TD, Nickerson DA, Hood LE: The Human Genome Project: Creating an infrastructure for biology and medicine. *Trends Biochem Sci* **16**:454, 1991.
432. Martin RG: We gnomes find the project an atlas but no treasure. *New Biol* **2**:385, 1990.
433. Rechsteiner MC: The Human Genome Project: Misguided science policy. *Trends Biochem Sci* **16**:455, 1991.
434. Davis BD, Colleagues: The human genome and other initiatives. *Science* **249**:342, 1990.
435. Tauber AI, Sarkar S: The Human Genome Project: Has blind reductionism gone too far? *Perspect Biol Med* **35**:221, 1992.
436. Rosenberg LE: The Human Genome Project. *Bull NY Acad Med* **68**:113, 1992.
437. Richardson WC: Summary, conference on the Human Genome Project: An agenda for science & society. *Bull NY Acad Med* **68**:162, 1992.
438. Koshland DE: Sequences and consequences of the human genome. *Science* **246**:189, 1989.
439. U.S. Department of Health and Human Services, U.S. Department of Energy (DOE): *Understanding Our Genetic Inheritance: The U.S. Human Genome Project—The First Five Years, FY 1991–1995*. Springfield, IL, National Technical Information Service, DOE; DOE/ER-0452P, 1990.
440. Collins F, Galas D: A new five-year plan for the U.S. Human Genome Project. *Science* **262**:43, 1993.
441. Collins FS, Patrinos A, Jordan E, Chakravarti A, Gesteland R, Walters L, and Members of the DOE and NIH Planning Groups: New goals for the U.S. Human Genome Project: 1998–2003. *Science* **282**:682, 1998.
442. Lander ES: The new genomics: Global views of biology. *Science* **274**:536, 1996.
443. Hieter P, Boguski M: Functional genomics: It's all how you read it. *Science* **278**:601, 1997.
444. Olson MV: A tale of two cities. *Anal Chem* **63**:416A, 1991.
445. Collins FS: Ahead of schedule and under budget: The Genome Project passes its fifth birthday. *Proc Natl Acad Sci USA* **92**:10,821, 1995.
446. Guyer MS, Collins FS: How is the Human Genome Project doing, and what have we learned so far? *Proc Natl Acad Sci USA* **92**:10,841, 1995.
447. Uddhav K, Ketan S: Advances in the Human Genome Project. *Mol Biol Rep* **25**:27, 1998.
448. Koonin EV, Mushegian AR, Rudd KE: Sequencing and analysis of bacterial genomes. *Curr Biol* **6**:404, 1996.
449. Smith DR: Microbial pathogen genomes: New strategies for identifying therapeutics and vaccine targets. *Trends Biotechnol* **14**:290, 1996.
450. Koonin EV: Big time for small genomes. *Genome Res* **7**:418, 1997.
451. Fraser CM, Fleischmann RD: Strategies for whole microbial genome sequencing and analysis. *Electrophoresis* **18**:1207, 1997.
452. Koonin EV, Galperin MY: Prokaryotic genomes: The emerging paradigm of genome-based microbiology. *Curr Opin Genet Dev* **7**:757, 1997.
453. Jenks PJ: Sequencing microbial genomes: What will it do for microbiology? *J Med Microbiol* **47**:375, 1998.
454. Doolittle RF: Microbial genomes opened up. *Nature* **392**:339, 1998.
455. Koonin EV, Tatusov RL, Galperin MY: Beyond complete genomes: From sequence to structure and function. *Curr Opin Struct Biol* **8**:355, 1998.
456. Saier MH Jr: Genome sequencing and informatics: New tools for biochemical discoveries. *Plant Physiol* **117**:1129, 1998.
457. Fleischmann RD, Adams MD, White O, Clayton RA, Kirkness EF, Kerlavage AR, Bult CJ, et al.: Whole-genome random sequencing and assembly of *Haemophilus influenzae* Rd. *Science* **269**:496, 1995.
458. Cole ST, Brosch R, Parkhill J, Garnier T, Churcher C, Harris D, Gordon SV, et al.: Deciphering the biology of *Mycobacterium tuberculosis* from the complete genome sequence. *Nature* **393**:537, 1998.
459. Tomb J-F, White O, Kerlavage AR, Clayton RA, Sutton GG, Fleischmann RD, Ketchum KA, et al.: The complete genome sequence of the gastric pathogen *Helicobacter pylori*. *Nature* **388**:539, 1997.
460. Fraser CM, Casjens S, Huang WM, Sutton GG, Clayton R, Lathigra R, White O, et al.: Genomic sequence of a Lyme disease spirochaete, *Borrelia burgdorferi*. *Nature* **390**:580, 1997.
461. Fraser CM, Gocayne JD, White O, Adams MD, Clayton RA, Fleischmann RD, Bult CJ, et al.: The minimal gene complement of *Mycoplasma genitalium*. *Science* **270**:397, 1995.
462. Fraser CM, Norris SJ, Weinstock GM, White O, Sutton GG, Dodson R, Gwinn M, et al.: Complete genome sequence of *Treponema pallidum*, the syphilis spirochete. *Science* **281**:375, 1998.
463. Stephens RS, Kalman S, Lammel C, Fan J, Marathe R, Aravind L, Mitchell W, et al.: Genome sequence of an obligate intracellular pathogen of humans: *Chlamydia trachomatis*. *Science* **282**:754, 1998.
464. Olson MV, Green P: Criterion for the completeness of large-scale physical maps of DNA. *Cold Spring Harb Symp Quant Biol* **58**:349, 1993.
465. Cox DR, Green ED, Lander ES, Cohen D, Myers RM: Assessing mapping progress in the Human Genome Project. *Science* **265**:2031, 1994.
466. Olson M, Green P: A "quality-first" credo for the Human Genome Project. *Genome Res* **8**:414, 1998.
467. Weber JL, Myers EW: Human whole-genome shotgun sequencing. *Genome Res* **7**:401, 1997.
468. Green P: Against a whole-genome shotgun. *Genome Res* **7**:410, 1997.
469. Venter JC, Adams MD, Sutton GG, Kerlavage AR, Smith HO, Hunkapiller M: Shotgun sequencing of the human genome. *Science* **280**:1540, 1998.
470. Bentley DR, Pruitt KD, Deloukas P, Schuler GD, Ostell J: Coordination of human genome sequencing via a consensus framework map. *Trends Genet* **14**:381, 1998.
471. Statement on the rapid release of genomic DNA sequence. *Genome Res* **8**:413, 1998.
472. Bentley DR: Genomic sequence information should be released immediately and freely in the public domain. *Science* **274**:533, 1996.
473. Adams MD, Venter JC: Should non-peer-reviewed raw DNA sequence data release be forced on the scientific community? *Science* **274**:534, 1996.
474. Green ED, Waterston RH: The Human Genome Project: Prospects and implications for clinical medicine. *JAMA* **266**:1966, 1991.
475. Rossiter BJF, Caskey CT: The Human Genome Project and clinical medicine. *Oncology* **6**:61, 1992.
476. Caskey CT: DNA-based medicine: Prevention and therapy, in Kevles DJ, Hood L (eds): *The Code of Codes: Scientific and Social Issues in the Human Genome Project*. Cambridge, Harvard University Press, 1992, p 112.
477. Hood L: Biology and medicine in the twenty-first century, in Kevles DL, Hood L (eds): *The Code of Codes: Scientific and Social Issues in the Human Genome Project*. Cambridge, Harvard University Press, 1992, p 136.
478. Whittaker LA: The implications of the Human Genome Project for family practice. *J Fam Pract* **35**:294, 1992.
479. Guyer MS, Collins FS: The Human Genome Project and the future of medicine. *Am J Dis Child* **147**:1145, 1993.
480. Sawicki MP, Samara G, Hurwitz M, Passaro E Jr: Human genome project. *Am J Surg* **165**:258, 1993.
481. Charo RA: Effect of the human genome initiative on women's rights and reproductive decisions. *Fetal Diagn Ther* **8**:148, 1993.
482. Sachs BP, Korf B: The Human Genome Project: Implications for the practicing obstetrician. *Obstet Gynecol* **81**:458, 1993.
483. Burn J: Relevance of the Human Genome Project to inherited metabolic disease. *J Inherited Metab Dis* **17**:421, 1994.
484. Cui K-H: Genome project and human reproduction. *Mol Hum Reprod* **10**:1275, 1995.

485. Williams JK, Lessick M: Genome research: Implications for children. *Pediatr Nurs* **22**:40, 1996.
486. Ellsworth DL, Hallman DM, Boerwinkle E: Impact of the Human Genome Project on epidemiologic research. *Epidemiol Rev* **19**:3, 1997.
487. Orkin SH, Nathan DG: The molecular genetics of thalassemia. *Adv Hum Genet* **11**:233, 1981.
488. Kwok SCM, Ledley FD, DiLella AG, Robson KJH, Woo SLC: Nucleotide sequence of a full-length complementary DNA clone and amino acid sequence of human phenylalanine hydroxylase. *Biochemistry* **24**:556, 1985.
489. Persico MG, Viglietto G, Martini G, Toniolo D, Paonessa G, Moscatelli C, Dono R, et al.: Isolation of human glucose-6-phosphate dehydrogenase (G6PD) cDNA clones: Primary structure of the protein and unusual 5′ non-coding region. *Nucleic Acids Res* **14**:2511, 1986.
490. Orkin SH: Reverse genetics and human disease. *Cell* **47**:845, 1986.
491. Ruddle FH: The William Allan Memorial Award address: Reverse genetics and beyond. *Am J Hum Genet* **36**:944, 1984.
492. Orkin SH: "Forward" and "reverse" genetics of inherited human disorders: The thalassemia syndromes and chronic granulomatous disease. *Harvey Lect* **83**:57, 1989.
493. Friedmann T: Opinion: The Human Genome Project: Some implications of extensive "reverse genetic" medicine. *Am J Hum Genet* **46**:407, 1990.
494. Cawthon RM, Weiss R, Xu G, Viskochil D, Culver M, Stevens J, Robertson M, et al.: A major segment of the neurofibromatosis type 1 gene: cDNA sequence, genomic structure, and point mutations. *Cell* **62**:193, 1990.
495. Attree O, Olivos IM, Okabe I, Bailey LC, Nelson DL, Lewis RA, McInnes RR, et al.: The Lowe's oculocerebrorenal syndrome gene encodes a protein highly homologous to inositol polyphosphate-5-phosphatase. *Nature* **358**:239, 1992.
496. Mitelman F, Mertens F, Johansson B: A breakpoint map of recurrent chromosomal rearrangements in human neoplasia. *Nat Genet* **15S**:417, 1997.
497. Parrish JE, Nelson DL: Methods for finding genes: A major rate-limiting step in positional cloning. *Genet Anal Tech Appl* **10**:29, 1993.
498. Chen E, d'Urso M, Schlessinger D: Functional mapping of the human genome by cDNA localization versus sequencing. *BioEssays* **16**:693, 1994.
499. Brennan MB, Hochgeschwender U: So many needles, so much hay. *Hum Mol Genet* **4**:153, 1995.
500. Gardiner K, Mural RJ: Getting the message: Identifying transcribed sequences. *Trends Genet* **11**:77, 1995.
501. Monaco AP: Isolation of genes from cloned DNA. *Curr Opin Genet Dev* **4**:360, 1994.
502. Thomas PS: Hybridization of denatured RNA and small DNA fragments transferred to nitrocellulose. *Proc Natl Acad Sci USA* **77**:5201, 1980.
503. Elvin P, Butler R, Hedge PJ: Transcribed sequences within YACs: HTF island cloning and cDNA library screening, in Anand R (ed): *Techniques for the Analysis of Complex Genomes*. London, Academic, 1992, p 155.
504. Lovett M, Kere J, Hinton LM: Direct selection: A method for the isolation of cDNAs encoded by large genomic regions. *Proc Natl Acad Sci USA* **88**:9628, 1991.
505. Parimoo S, Patanjali SR, Shukla H, Chaplin DD, Weissman SM: cDNA selection: Efficient PCR approach for the selection of cDNAs encoded in large chromosomal DNA fragments. *Proc Natl Acad Sci USA* **88**:9623, 1991.
506. Tagle DA, Swaroop M, Lovett M, Collins FS: Magnetic bead capture of expressed sequences encoded within large genomic segments. *Nature* **361**:751, 1993.
507. Lovett M: Fishing for complements: Finding genes by direct selection. *Trends Genet* **10**:352, 1994.
508. Parimoo S, Patanjali SR, Kolluri R, Xu H, Wei H, Weissman SM: cDNA selection and other approaches in positional cloning. *Anal Biochem* **228**:1, 1995.
509. Peterson AS: Direct cDNA selection, in Birren B, Green ED, Klapholz S, Myers RM, Roskams J (eds): *Genome Analysis: A Laboratory Manual,* vol 2: *Detecting Genes*. Cold Spring Harbor, NY, Cold Spring Harbor Laboratory, 1998, p 159.
510. Duyk GM, Kim S, Myers RM, Cox DR: Exon trapping: A genetic screen to identify candidate transcribed sequences in cloned mammalian genomic DNA. *Proc Natl Acad Sci USA* **87**:8995, 1990.
511. Buckler AJ, Chang DD, Graw SL, Brook JD, Haber DA, Sharp PA, Housman DE: Exon amplification: A strategy to isolate mammalian genes based on RNA splicing. *Proc Natl Acad Sci USA* **88**:4005, 1991.
512. Hamaguchi M, Sakamoto H, Tsuruta H, Sasaki H, Muto T, Sugimura T, Terada M: Establishment of a highly sensitive and specific exon-trapping system. *Proc Natl Acad Sci USA* **89**:9779, 1992.
513. Andreadis A, Nisson PE, Kosik KS, Watkins PC: The exon trapping assay partly discriminates against alternatively spliced exons. *Nucleic Acids Res* **21**:2217, 1993.
514. Church DM, Stotler CJ, Rutter JL, Murrell JR, Trofatter JA, Buckler AJ: Isolation of genes from complex sources of mammalian genomic DNA using exon amplification. *Nat Genet* **6**:98, 1994.
515. Krizman DB: Exon trapping, in Birren B, Green ED, Klapholz S, Myers RM, Roskams J (eds): *Genome Analysis: A Laboratory Manual,* vol 2: *Detecting Genes*. Cold Spring Harbor, NY, Cold Spring Harbor Laboratory, 1998, p 191.
516. Krizman DB, Berget SM: Efficient selection of 3′-terminal exons from vertebrate DNA. *Nucleic Acids Res* **21**:5198, 1993.
517. Claverie J-M: A streamlined random sequencing strategy for finding coding exons. *Genomics* **23**:575, 1994.
518. Chandrasekharappa SC, Guru SC, Manickam P, Olufemi S-E, Collins FS, Emmert-Buck MR, Debelenko LV, et al.: Positional cloning of the gene for multiple endocrine neoplasia-type 1. *Science* **276**:404, 1997.
519. International FMF Consortium: Ancient missense mutations in a new member of the RoRet gene family are likely to cause familial Mediterranean fever. *Cell* **90**:797, 1997.
520. Cotton RG: Slowly but surely towards better scanning for mutations. *Trends Genet* **13**:43, 1997.
521. Myers RM, Hedrick Ellenson L, Hayashi K: Detection of DNA variation, in Birren B, Green ED, Klapholz S, Myers RM, Roskams J (eds): *Genome Analysis: A Laboratory Manual,* vol 2: *Detecting Genes*. Cold Spring Harbor, NY, Cold Spring Harbor Laboratory, 1998, p 287.
522. Lupski JR: Genomic disorders: Structural features of the genome can lead to DNA rearrangements and human disease traits. *Trends Genet* **14**:417, 1998.
523. Caskey CT, Pizzuti A, Fu Y-H, Fenwick RG Jr, Nelson DL: Triplet repeat mutations in human disease. *Science* **256**:784, 1992.
524. Richards RI, Sutherland GR: Heritable unstable DNA sequences. *Nat Genet* **1**:7, 1992.
525. Nelson DL, Warren ST: Trinucleotide repeat instability: When and where? *Nat Genet* **4**:107, 1993.
526. Fischer SG, Lerman LS: DNA fragments differing by single base-pair substitutions are separated in denaturing gradient gels: Correspondence with melting theory. *Proc Natl Acad Sci USA* **80**:1579, 1983.
527. Myers RM, Lumelsky N, Lerman LS, Maniatis T: Detection of single base substitutions in total genomic DNA. *Nature* **313**:495, 1985.
528. Myers RM, Maniatis T, Lerman LS: Detection and localization of single base changes by denaturing gradient gel electrophoresis. *Methods Enzymol* **155**:501, 1987.
529. Winter E, Yamamoto F, Almoguera C, Perucho M: A method to detect and characterize point mutations in transcribed genes: Amplification and overexpression of the mutant c-Ki-*ras* allele in human tumor cells. *Proc Natl Acad Sci USA* **82**:7575, 1985.
530. Myers RM, Larin Z, Maniatis T: Detection of single base substitutions by ribonuclease cleavage at mismatches in RNA:DNA duplexes. *Science* **230**:1242, 1985.
531. Cotton RGH, Rodrigues NR, Campbell RD: Reactivity of cytosine and thymine in single-base-pair mismatches with hydroxylamine and osmium tetroxide and its application to the study of mutations. *Proc Natl Acad Sci USA* **85**:4397, 1988.
532. Orita M, Iwahana H, Kanazawa H, Hayashi K, Sekiya T: Detection of polymorphisms of human DNA by gel electrophoresis as single-strand conformation polymorphisms. *Proc Natl Acad Sci USA* **86**:2766, 1989.
533. Wooster R, Bignell G, Lancaster J, Swift S, Seal S, Mangion J, Collins N, et al.: Identification of the breast cancer susceptibility gene *BRCA2*. *Nature* **378**:789, 1995.
534. Polymeropoulos MH, Lavedan C, Leroy E, Ide SE, Dehejia A, Dutra A, Pike B, et al.: Mutation in the alpha-synuclein gene identified in families with Parkinson's disease. *Science* **276**:2045, 1997.
535. Everett LA, Glaser B, Beck JC, Idol JR, Buchs A, Heyman M, Adawi F, et al.: Pendred syndrome is caused by mutations in a putative sulphate transporter gene (*PDS*). *Nat Genet* **17**:411, 1997.
536. Yamagata K, Furuta H, Oda N, Kaisaki PJ, Menzel S, Cox NJ, Fajans SS, et al.: Mutations in the hepatocyte nuclear factor-4alpha gene in maturity-onset diabetes of the young. *Nature* **384**:458, 1996.
537. Coffey AJ, Brooksbank RA, Brandau O, Oohashi T, Howell GR, Bye JM, Cahn AP, et al.: Host response to EBV infection in X-linked lymphoproliferative disease results from mutations in an SH2-domain encoding gene. *Nat Genet* **20**:129, 1998.

538. Van Laer L, Huizing EH, Verstreken M, van Zuijlen D, Wauters JG, Bossuyt PJ, van de Heyning P, et al.: Nonsyndromic hearing impairment is associated with a mutation in *DFNA5*. *Nat Genet* **20**: 194, 1998.
539. Nelson SF, McCusker JH, Sander MA, Kee Y, Modrich P, Brown PO: Genomic mismatch scanning: A new approach to genetic linkage mapping. *Nat Genet* **4**: 11, 1993.
540. Brown PO: Genome scanning methods. *Curr Opin Genet Dev* **4**: 366, 1994.
541. Cheung VG, Nelson SF: Genomic mismatch scanning identifies human genomic DNA shared identical by descent. *Genomics* **47**: 1, 1998.
542. McAllister L, Penland L, Brown PO: Enrichment for loci identical-by-descent between pairs of mouse or human genomes by genomic mismatch scanning. *Genomics* **47**: 7, 1998.
543. Cheung VG, Gregg JP, Gogolin-Ewens KJ, Bandong J, Stanley CA, Baker L, Higgins MJ, et al.: Linkage-disequilibrium mapping without genotyping. *Nat Genet* **18**: 225, 1998.
544. Tugendreich S, Boguski MS, Seldin MS, Hieter P: Linking yeast genetics to mammalian genomes: Identification and mapping of the human homolog of CDC27 via the expressed sequence tag (EST) data base. *Proc Natl Acad Sci USA* **90**: 10,031, 1993.
545. Tugendreich S, Bassett DE Jr, McKusick VA, Boguski MS, Hieter P: Genes conserved in yeast and humans. *Hum Mol Genet* **3**: 1509, 1994.
546. Bassett DE Jr, Boguski MS, Spencer F, Reeves R, Goebl M, Hieter P: Comparative genomics, genome cross-referencing and XREFdb. *Trends Genet* **11**: 372, 1995.
547. Bassett DE Jr, Boguski MS, Hieter P: Yeast genes and human disease. *Nature* **379**: 589, 1996.
548. Mushegian AR, Bassett DE Jr, Boguski MS, Bork P, Koonin EV: Positionally cloned human disease genes: Patterns of evolutionary conservation and functional motifs. *Proc Natl Acad Sci USA* **94**: 5831, 1997.
549. Bassett DE Jr, Boguski MS, Spencer F, Reeves R, Kim S, Weaver T, Hieter P: Genome cross-referencing and XREFdb: Implications for the identification and analysis of genes mutated in human disease. *Nat Genet* **15**: 339, 1997.
550. Foury F: Human genetic diseases: A cross-talk between man and yeast. *Gene* **195**: 1, 1997.
551. Andrade MA, Sander C, Valencia A: Updated catalogue of homologues to human disease-related proteins in the yeast genome. *FEBS Lett* **426**: 7, 1998.
552. Banfi S, Borsani G, Rossi E, Bernard L, Guffanti A, Rubboli F, Marchitiello A, et al.: Identification and mapping of human cDNAs homologous to *Drosophila* mutant genes through EST database searching. *Nat Genet* **13**: 167, 1996.
553. Kuchler K, Sterne RE, Thorner J: *Saccharomyces cerevisiae STE6* gene product: A novel pathway for protein export in eukaryotic cells. *EMBO J* **8**: 3973, 1989.
554. McGrath JP, Varshavsky A: The yeast *STE6* gene encodes a homologue of the mammalian multidrug resistance P-glycoprotein. *Nature* **340**: 400, 1989.
555. Raymond M, Gros P, Whiteway M, Thomas DY: Functional complementation of yeast *ste6* by a mammalian multidrug resistance *mdr* gene. *Science* **256**: 232, 1992.
556. Bollag G, McCormick F: Differential regulation of rasGAP and neurofibromatosis gene product activities. *Nature* **351**: 576, 1991.
557. Ballester R, Marchuk D, Boguski M, Saulino A, Letcher R, Wigler M, Collins F: The *NF1* locus encodes a protein functionally related to mammalian GAP and yeast *IRA* proteins. *Cell* **63**: 851, 1990.
558. Han J-W, McCormick F, Macara IG: Regulation of Ras-GAP and the neurofibromatosis-1 gene product by eicosanoids. *Science* **252**: 576, 1991.
559. Weeda G, van Ham RCA, Vermeulen W, Bootsma D, van der Eb AJ, Hoeijmakers JHJ: A presumed DNA helicase encoded by *ERCC-3* is involved in the human repair disorders xeroderma pigmentosum and Cockayne's syndrome. *Cell* **62**: 777, 1990.
560. Mounkes LC, Jones RS, Liang B-C, Gelbart W, Fuller MT: A *Drosophila* model for xeroderma pigmentosum and Cockayne's syndrome: *haywire* encodes the fly homolog of *ERCC3*, a human excision repair gene. *Cell* **71**: 925, 1992.
561. Sinclair DA, Mills K, Guarente L: Accelerated aging and nucleolar fragmentation in yeast *sgs1* mutants. *Science* **277**: 1313, 1997.
562. Fisler JS, Warden CH: Mapping of mouse obesity genes: A generic approach to a complex trait. *J Nutr* **127**: 1909S, 1997.
563. Comuzzie AG, Allison DB: The search for human obesity genes. *Science* **280**: 1374, 1998.
564. Zhang Y, Proenca R, Maffei M, Barone M, Leopold L, Friedman JM: Positional cloning of the mouse *obese* gene and its human homologue. *Nature* **372**: 425, 1994.
565. Friedman JM, Halaas JL: Leptin and the regulation of body weight in mammals. *Nature* **395**: 763, 1998.
566. Korf B: Molecular diagnosis: 1. *N Engl J Med* **332**: 1218, 1995.
567. Korf B: Molecular diagnosis: 2. *N Engl J Med* **332**: 1499, 1995.
568. Shikata H, Utsumi N, Kuivaniemi H, Tromp G: DNA-based diagnostics in the study of heritable and acquired disorders. *J Lab Clin Med* **125**: 421, 1995.
569. Korf BR: Advances in molecular diagnosis. *Curr Opin Obstet Gynecol* **8**: 130, 1996.
570. Kiechle FL: Diagnostic molecular pathology in the twenty-first century. *Clin Lab Med* **16**: 213, 1996.
571. Wagener C: Molecular diagnostics. *J Mol Med* **75**: 728, 1997.
572. Miller AD: Human gene therapy comes of age. *Nature* **357**: 455, 1992.
573. Mulligan RC: The basic science of gene therapy. *Science* **260**: 926, 1993.
574. Anderson WF: Human gene therapy. *Nature* **392**: 25, 1998.
575. Ascenzioni F, Donini P, Lipps HJ: Mammalian artificial chromosomes: Vectors for somatic gene therapy. *Cancer Lett* **118**: 135, 1997.
576. Huxley C: Mammalian artificial chromosomes and chromosome transgenics. *Trends Genet* **13**: 345, 1997.
577. Willard HF: Human artificial chromosomes coming into focus. *Nat Biotechnol* **16**: 415, 1998.
578. Vos J-MH: Mammalian artificial chromosomes as tools for gene therapy. *Curr Opin Genet Dev* **8**: 351, 1998.
579. Grimes B, Cooke H: Engineering mammalian chromosomes. *Hum Mol Genet* **7**: 1635, 1998.
580. Housman D, Ledley FD: Why pharmacogenomics? Why now? *Nat Biotechnol* **16**: 492, 1998.
581. Marshall A: Getting the right drug into the right patient. *Nat Biotechnol* **15**: 1249, 1997.
582. Martinez FD, Graves PE, Baldini M, Solomon S, Erickson R: Association between genetic polymorphisms of the beta2-adrenoceptor and response to albuterol in children with and without a history of wheezing. *J Clin Invest* **100**: 3184, 1997.
583. Kleyn PW, Vesell ES: Genetic variation as a guide to drug development. *Science* **281**: 1820, 1998.
584. Cook-Deegan R: *The Gene Wars: Science, Politics, and the Human Genome*. New York, WW Norton, 1994.
585. Meslin EM, Thomson EJ, Boyer JT: The ethical, legal, and social implications research program at the National Human Genome Research Institute. *Kennedy Inst Ethics J* **7**: 291, 1997.
586. Billings PR, Kohn MA, de Cuevas M, Beckwith J, Alper JS, Natowicz MR: Discrimination as a consequence of genetic testing. *Am J Hum Genet* **50**: 476, 1992.
587. Alper JS, Geller LN, Barash CI, Billings PR, Laden V, Natowicz MR: Genetic discrimination and screening for hemochromatosis. *J Public Health Policy* **15**: 345, 1994.
588. Lapham EV, Kozma C, Weiss JO: Genetic discrimination: Perspectives of consumers. *Science* **274**: 621, 1996.
589. Hudson KL, Rothenberg KH, Andrews LB, Kahn MJ, Collins FS: Genetic discrimination and health insurance: An urgent need for reform. *Science* **270**: 391, 1995.
590. Rothenberg K: Genetic information and health insurance: State legislative approaches. *J Law Med Ethics* **23**: 312, 1995.
591. Rothenberg K, Fuller B, Rothstein M, Duster T, Ellis Kahn MJ, Cunningham R, Fine B, et al.: Genetic information and the workplace: Legislative approaches and policy changes. *Science* **275**: 1755, 1997.
592. Wilfond BS, Nolan K: National policy development for the clinical application of genetic diagnostic technologies: Lessons from cystic fibrosis. *JAMA* **270**: 2948, 1993.
593. Wilfond B, Rothenberg K, Thomson E, Lerman C: Cancer genetic susceptibility testing: Ethical and policy implications for future research and clinical practice. *J Law Med Ethics* **25**: 243, 1997.
594. Burke W, Petersen G, Lynch P, Botkin J, Daly M, Garber J, Kahn MJ, et al.: Recommendations for follow-up care of individuals with an inherited predisposition to cancer: I. Hereditary nonpolyposis colon cancer. Cancer Genetics Studies Consortium. *JAMA* **277**: 915, 1997.
595. Burke W, Daly M, Garber J, Botkin J, Kahn MJ, Lynch P, McTiernan A, et al.: Recommendations for follow-up care of individuals with an inherited predisposition to cancer: II. BRCA1 and BRCA2. Cancer Genetic Studies Consortium. *JAMA* **277**: 997, 1997.

596. Geller G, Botkin JR, Green MJ, Press N, Biesecker BB, Wilfond B, Grana G, et al.: Genetic testing for susceptibility to adult-onset cancer: The process and content of informed consent. *JAMA* **277**:1467, 1997.
597. Post SG, Whitehouse PJ, Binstock RH, Bird TD, Eckert SK, Farrer LA, Fleck LM, et al.: The clinical introduction of genetic testing for Alzheimer disease: An ethical perspective. *JAMA* **277**:832, 1997.
598. Burke W, Thomson E, Khoury MJ, McDonnell SM, Press N, Adams PC, Barton JC, et al.: Hereditary hemochromatosis: Gene discovery and its implications for population-based screening. *JAMA* **280**:172, 1998.
599. Holtzman NA, Murphy PD, Watson MS, Barr PA: Predictive genetic testing: From basic research to clinical practice. *Science* **278**:602, 1997.
600. Germino GG, Somlo S: A positional cloning approach to inherited renal disease. *Semin Nephrol* **12**:541, 1992.

CHAPTER 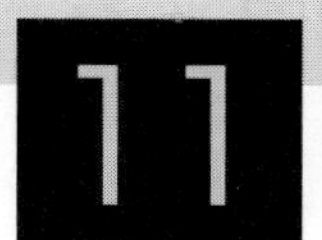

Population Genetics

Walter F. Bodmer

The extent of genetic variability in human populations is enormous. It is reflected outwardly in the unique characteristics of all individuals, other than identical twins who, of course, share a common inheritance. This variability includes differential disease susceptibility for both common and rare diseases, including those with clear-cut recessive or dominant patterns of inheritance, the main concerns of this work.

The first clear-cut Mendelian genetic examples of this human variability were the red cell blood groups, starting with Landsteiner's discovery of the ABO types in 1900, the year of the rediscovery of Mendel's work. The first common disease-related genetic variant was probably the rhesus-negative condition associated with hemolytic disease of the newborn, now a preventable disease. With the development of techniques for identifying protein variability, using starch gel and other types of electrophoresis, it became clear that many proteins including, of course, enzymes, had common genetic variants. The most extreme level of genetic variability is still associated with the major histocompatibility or HLA system, with its many loci and many hundreds of alleles—some of which show striking associations with autoimmune diseases such as ankylosing spondylitis, rheumatoid arthritis, and juvenile onset insulin-dependent diabetes mellitus (IDDM).

In parallel with the discovery of these common genetic variants, generally called polymorphisms as long as an allele has a frequency of more than 1 percent, came the description of rare clear-cut Mendelian inherited diseases, starting with Archibald Garrod's description of alkaptonuria as an "inborn error of metabolism." Some categories of inherited disease, notably the hemoglobinopathies—starting with the sickle cell trait and anemia, the first disease to be clearly defined at a molecular level—are clearly polymorphic, but only in certain populations, notably in this case those in and originating from West Africa. Gradually, some of the rare inherited diseases were defined in terms of enzyme deficiencies or other protein abnormalities, such as the hemoglobinopathies or collagen abnormalities.

It was recognized many years ago, notably by R.A. Fisher and J.B.S. Haldane in the late 1920s and early 1930s, that linkage analysis using common polymorphisms would be a very powerful tool for the analysis of inherited diseases. The limitation of this method, which Fisher and Haldane then could not easily see being overcome, was the very limited availability of usable genetic polymorphisms, largely at the time restricted to half a dozen or so red cell blood group systems. That limitation has been completely removed by the recombinant DNA revolution.

Soon after the development of the first approaches to DNA cloning and the use of restriction enzymes, together with the development of DNA sequencing techniques by Sanger, and by Maxam and Gilbert, it became clear that there was extensive variability that could be detected in all species at the DNA level, initially using restriction fragment length polymorphisms (RFLPs). As pointed out by Solomon and Bodmer in 1979[1] and Botstein and colleagues in 1980,[2] this immediately made available an essentially unlimited range of polymorphisms at the DNA level that could be used for tracing diseases within families, and so establishing the position of a mutated gene along the chromosome, thereby forming the basis for positional cloning. This revolutionized the identification of the genetic basis of disease. Now the approach comes purely from the genetics without the need for a prior understanding of the functional basis and, often, leads to wild guesses as to the protein involved. One need only remember the number of times different proteins were suggested to be the basis for cystic fibrosis until the gene itself was cloned and all previous guesses as to function were shown to have been false. Now, polymorphisms are detected using PCR technology. High levels of polymorphism, useful for genetic analysis, are found at positions of "CA" repeats. More stable variation is, however, now being extensively identified at the level of single or simple nucleotide polymorphisms (SNPs) mostly using ARMS or allele-specific PCR. This depends on the fact that polymerase extension in a PCR is much less efficient if there is a base pair mismatch at the 3′ end of the oligonucleotide primer. The availability of an essentially unlimited extent of polymorphism at the DNA level has revitalized human population genetics and shown the importance of many of the classical ideas of quantitative population genetics developed by the three great pioneers of the subject, R.A. Fisher, J.B.S. Haldane, and Sewall Wright. This chapter provides a basis for understanding the origin and maintenance of genetic variability in human populations, especially as it relates to disease.

THE HARDY-WEINBERG LAW AND ITS EXTENSIONS

Given the existence of a polymorphism, such as the ABO blood groups, or more simply the MN blood groups considered as a two-allele system, what are the implications of Mendelian genetics for the distributions of the genotypes in the population? How might these change from generation to generation? The geneticist R.C. Punnett posed these fundamental questions in Cambridge in the early years of this century to the mathematician G.H. Hardy. He solved the simple algebraic problem to give the formula that we know as the Hardy-Weinberg Law because the German physician Weinberg also independently solved it. It is ironic that G.H. Hardy will be better known to millions around the world for this trivial piece of mathematics than for all his other mathematical contributions.

The Hardy-Weinberg Law in its simplest form shows that, in a population in which individuals mate at random with respect to their genotype, and in the absence of selection, and ignoring random variation, the frequencies of genotypes, for example, *MM*, *MN*, and *NN* in the population are p^2, 2pq, and q^2 respectively, where p and q are the frequencies of the genes *M* and *N* respectively. Simply counting genes in the population gives the result that

$$p = (\text{frequency of MM}) + \tfrac{1}{2}\,(\text{the frequency of MN})$$

while

$$q = 1 - p = (\text{frequency of } NN) + \tfrac{1}{2}\,(\text{the frequency of } MN)$$

This distribution is achieved in one generation and then remains the same for all future generations (see Table 11-1).

The result is equivalent to combining at random a pool of *M* and *N* genes, where the frequency of *M* in the pool is p and of *N*, q. Thus, the result of the Hardy-Weinberg Law is that random mating is equivalent to random union of gametes, namely of the *M* and *N*

Table 11-1 Hardy-Weinberg Equilibrium for a One Locus 2 Allele Polymorphism *M, N*

Genotypes	*MM*	*MN*	*NN*	
initial frequencies	u	v	w	u + v + w = 1
After one or more generations of random mating	p^2	2pq	q^2	

where $p = u + \frac{1}{2}v$ = gene frequency of *M*
$q = \frac{1}{2}v + w = 1 - p$ = gene frequency of *N*

Random union of gametes gives the same result

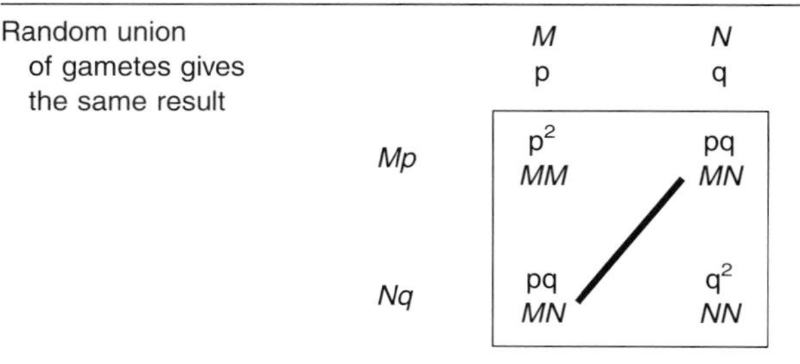

genes. This can be shown to be completely general with respect to almost any complexity of genotypes. For example, if the *A*, *B*, and *O* genes occur in a population with frequencies p, q, and r, which can be calculated from the frequencies of the genotypes just as before

$$p = (\text{frequency of } AA) + \tfrac{1}{2}\,(\text{frequency of } AO) + \tfrac{1}{2}\,(\text{the frequency of } AB) \text{ etc}$$

then the frequencies of genotypes *AA, AO, AB,* and so on are p^2, 2pr, 2pq, and so on.

Although the conditions for satisfying the Hardy-Weinberg seem quite restrictive, in practice the law is quite robust with respect to variations in the conditions. Thus, for example, the effects of inbreeding or population subdivision, which generally tend to reduce the frequency of heterozygotes compared to that expected under the Hardy-Weinberg Law, are usually too small to give a significant deviation. Indeed, testing for genotypes to fit the Hardy-Weinberg Law is extremely important in practice, as deviations are nearly always due to technical problems in establishing genotypes rather than deviations from the Hardy-Weinberg assumptions.

The Hardy-Weinberg Law has another very important implication, namely that genetic variability, once it is established in a population, tends to remain and is not dissipated. This is effectively a result of Mendelian segregation. Maintenance of variability in a population is an essential requirement for Darwin's theory of evolution by natural selection. Yet in his day, the prevailing theories of inheritance included, for example, the blending theory under which variability was quickly lost from generation to generation. Darwin realized that this was inconsistent with his theory, as did some others of his contemporaries, but they did not come up with the right answer—this came from Mendelian inheritance only rediscovered in 1900. It was R.A. Fisher, one of the founders of population genetics based on Mendelian inheritance, who first clearly pointed out that not only was Mendelian inheritance consistent with Darwin's theory of evolution by natural selection, but that the theory essentially required a discrete model of inheritance as described by Mendel. It is an irony of history that Darwin was so convinced of the correctness of evolution by natural selection that he persisted with his view even in the face of a demonstrably inadequate theory of inheritance. (For a more detailed background to the basic quantitative ideas of population genetics see, for example, Cavalli-Sforza and Bodmer,[3] or at a more elementary level Bodmer and Cavalli-Sforza,[4] or a recent text on population genetics such as Hartl and Clark.[5])

THE BALANCE BETWEEN MUTATIONS AND SELECTION

The ultimate source of all genetic variation is mutation, namely an alteration in the DNA sequence that may be induced chemically or by external radiation such as x-rays or ultraviolet light, or that may occur spontaneously, often as a result of mistakes made during DNA replication. When the mutation occurs, for example, in the middle of an intervening sequence, or in a flanking region between genes, or in a third base-pair coding position that does not give rise to a changed amino acid (a synonymous substitution), it almost certainly has no functional consequence and so is selectively "neutral." It may also be that some amino acid changes or changes in 5′ or 3′ untranslated regions of an expressed gene similarly have no functional consequence and so are effectively neutral. The fate of a neutral mutation is strictly determined by chance, sometimes referred to as "random genetic drift," a phenomenon that is discussed in more detail later. Occasional mutations are functionally advantageous, and so give rise to a positive selective advantage that may be expressed, for example, as improved viability or improved fertility. Such mutations are the basis for the adaptive process underlying Darwin's theory of evolution by natural selection. If the selective advantage persists, then generally such mutations will increase in frequency in a population until they replace the version of the gene from which they were derived, and this is the basic process of gene substitution during evolution by natural selection.

The vast majority of new mutations in expressed genes, especially those that change an amino acid in a coding region, are likely to disrupt the function of a gene at least to some extent, and therefore lead to a selective disadvantage. This disadvantage will generally lead, usually quite rapidly, to the disappearance of the mutant gene from the population. However, new mutations continuously arise each generation, and so a balance is achieved between mutation giving rise to new deleterious variants of a gene and selection removing them from the population. This is the source of nearly all of the rare inherited human diseases, including the "inborn errors of metabolism" first described by Garrod. Because mutation rates are generally quite small and their selective disadvantages appreciable, the frequencies of genes maintained by the balance between mutation and selection are generally very low, and hence the corresponding diseases are comparatively rare.

Well-known examples of dominantly inherited diseases maintained by mutation selection balance include the colorectal cancer susceptibility, familial adenomatous polyposis (FAP). This occurs with a frequency of approximately 1 in 8000 in those populations where there is essentially complete registration for the trait, and probably with a similar frequency in all human populations. Individuals with severe disruptive mutations in most of the first half of the corresponding gene, *APC*, develop hundreds to thousands of small adenomatous polyps in their large intestine, usually starting in the early teens. One or more of these inevitably develops into a colorectal cancer usually by the mid-twenties to thirties, and if untreated leads to an early death often, therefore, during or before the normal reproductive period. Now, if families with FAP are monitored and a colectomy is performed sufficiently early to prevent the development of colorectal cancers, FAP individuals can have an almost normal life expectancy and good quality of life. However, under "primitive" conditions, including even those of more than 30 to 50 years ago, FAP was clearly a severe selective disadvantage. Thus, the low frequency of FAP in the population reflects this balance between its selective disadvantage and yet the continuing production of new mutations. (For a review of FAP see reference 6.)

The simple approximate formula relating mutation rates, selective disadvantages and gene frequencies was first derived by Danforth and then J.B.S. Haldane, one of the great founders of mathematical population genetics, in the early 1920s. For a dominant disadvantageous condition determined by a gene *A* such that all heterozygotes *Aa* have the condition, and as a result have a fitness 1 − s compared to 1 for normal *aa* individuals, and ignoring random fluctuation, it can be shown that the balance between the overall mutation rate μ to the dominant disadvantageous gene *A* and the selective disadvantage, is related to the gene frequency p of *A* at equilibrium, by the formula

$$p = \mu/s \qquad (11\text{-}1)$$

The frequency of the mutant heterozygotes *Aa*, is, from the Hardy-Weinberg Law, $2pq = 2p(1 - p)$, which is approximately just 2p when p is small and terms in p^2 can be ignored. Thus the frequency of the affected individuals is approximately 2 μ/s. If, for example, there are good estimates of the frequency of affecteds in a population and of their selective disadvantage s, then the mutation rate can be estimated from the rearranged formula

$$\mu = \tfrac{1}{2} \times (\text{the frequency of affected individuals}) \times s \qquad (11\text{-}2)$$

For example, for FAP, assuming its population incidence is approximately 1 in 10,000 and the selective disadvantage about 30 percent or 0.3 then the mutation rate is estimated as

$$\mu = \tfrac{1}{2} \times (1/10{,}000) \times 0.3 = 1.5 \times 10^{-5}$$

which is a relatively high mutation rate but reflects the combined frequency of all mutations in the gene that could give rise to FAP. Even for an overall mutation rate as high as 10^{-5} and a selective disadvantage as small as 1 percent, the estimated frequency of affected individuals is still only 2 per 1,000. Thus, the balance between mutation and a dominant trait with a selective disadvantage will always give rise to gene frequencies that are substantially less than 1 percent, the conventionally accepted level for the definition of a polymorphism, and usually, at most, a hundredth of this, namely about 1 in 10,000.

If there is reliable information on the proportion of affected individuals *Aa* who are new mutants because both their parents are normal *aa*, then the selective disadvantages can be estimated simply from the proportion of these "sporadic" cases, namely those that do not have mutant parents and so are new mutations. This only applies, of course, to a fully penetrant trait.

The situation for a recessive trait is substantially different. Suppose the abnormality was recessive *aa* with a frequency, following the Hardy-Weinberg Law, of p^2. If the dominant homozygote normal genotype *AA* and the heterozygote for the mutant *Aa* generally have identical fitnesses of 1, while the fitness of the mutant homozygotes *aa* is 1 − s, then now the balance between loss of genes to a population by selection and gain by mutation is achieved when the trait frequency q^2, where q is the frequency of the gene a, is equated to μ/s, namely

$$\text{trait frequency} = q^2 = \mu/s \qquad (11\text{-}3)$$

The gene frequency at equilibrium will therefore be given by

$$q = \sqrt{(\mu/s)} \qquad (11\text{-}4)$$

which will always be substantially greater than the corresponding equilibrium frequency for a dominant gene. This is because most of the mutant genes are present in the heterozygote, and yet the only elimination is of the affected homozygotes, which is a much less efficient selective process. Thus, for example, assuming a mutation rate of 10^{-6} and a recessive lethal, for which s = 1, the frequency of the affected homozygotes would be 1 in 1,000,000 and the gene frequency of the recessive mutant therefore 1 in 1,000. For a dominant lethal with the same mutation rate the gene frequency would itself be 1 in 1,000,000.

How then, with reasonable mutation rates, which certainly are not expected to be higher on average than 10^{-5} or 10^{-6} per generation per gene overall, can a recessive lethal such as cystic fibrosis (which surely would have been sufficiently severe before recent improvements in medical treatment to preclude individuals having any offspring) ever reach the high frequency of between 1 in 2,000 and 1 in 3,000, corresponding to a gene frequency of around 2 percent, which it does in Northern Europe? It must be emphasized that this high frequency refers only to one particular mutant allele, ΔF508, amongst the very large number of possible *CFTR* mutants which can, in principle, give rise to cystic fibrosis. One answer is that the balance between mutation and selection for a true recessive is very sensitive to any departure from the assumption of recessiveness, since the effects of selection on the heterozygote *Aa* are so much greater than on the homozygote *aa*. This is only helpful if one assumes that there may, ironically, be some advantage to the heterozygote at a very low level that somehow compensates for the disadvantage of the homozygote and allows a relatively higher gene frequency to be attained. The basis for this explanation will become clearer after the forthcoming discussion of the classical mechanisms by which a polymorphism can be maintained at a high frequency purely by balancing selection. A totally different explanation, however, becomes possible if we take into account the extent to which chance, namely random drift, can occasionally give rise to an increased frequency of a mutant gene that is neutral with respect to selection, or very nearly so. That is the situation for the cystic fibrosis ΔF508 mutation, and so perhaps it is pure chance that this particular mutation has increased to the extent it has in northern Europe but not elsewhere. The counterargument will be, that this is highly unlikely, in general, because the probability of any particular mutant increasing in frequency to such an extent by chance is necessarily small. But then we must also take into account the inevitable ascertainment bias involved in identifying and analyzing such mutant traits. The chance of a disease being studied is, effectively, proportional to its frequency in the population. Therefore, inevitably, the more common abnormal traits will come to our notice first and foremost. There could be hundreds or thousands of genes that give rise to inborn errors comparable to cystic fibrosis, but it is cystic fibrosis and perhaps one or two other conditions, like PKU, which have achieved this relatively high frequency and so been brought starkly to our attention in European populations. Had the original studies on genetic abnormalities been done, for example, in China, then neither of these traits would have rated any particular attention.

One consequence of this interpretation is that, when the frequency of a rare inherited disease varies substantially by a factor of 10, or even of 100, in frequency between populations, as is the case, for example, for cystic fibrosis and PKU, then these high frequencies will be associated with particular alleles that, by chance, have drifted up in frequency substantially, compared to all other alleles present in the population with similar effects. This is only likely to apply to recessive traits because of the effective neutrality of heterozygotes for the mutant gene. (However we shall later discuss an apparent exception to this notion for dominant genes with less than full penetrance and relatively mild selective disadvantages). Dominant traits, on the other hand, maintained by the balance between mutation and selection and with a relatively severe disadvantage are unlikely to vary substantially in their incidence from one population to another. This is because, in that case, drift effects will be too weak to counteract the selective disadvantage of the new mutant present in a heterozygote, and so the overall mutation rate of the gene and its average selective disadvantage in heterozygotes will, according to the formula given above, determine the population frequency. As neither the overall mutation rate nor the overall selective disadvantage is likely to vary substantially from one population to another, this means that the incidence also is unlikely to vary. This is clearly the case, for example, for the dominantly inherited or FAP syndrome.

The effect of chance, or stochastic variation on gene frequencies in populations of finite size was first classically analyzed by R.A. Fisher and Sewall Wright, and involves for its full understanding a complex mathematical development. The basic idea behind genetic drift can however be explained simply.

Suppose we start with a population of 10 genes, 5 of which are *A*, and 5 of which are *a*. We then choose 10 new genes by choosing

A and *a* on each occasion with equal frequencies, for example, by tossing a coin. By chance this new population of genes may, for example, contain only three *A*s and seven *a*s. We now form a new population of 10 genes choosing *A* with a probability each time of 3 of 10 and *a* with a probability of 7 of 10. One could imagine doing this with a biased coin or using a computer to choose a random number between 0 and 1 and assigning *A*, if it is <0.3, and *a*, if it is bigger than 0.7. If this process is repeated many times, reflecting many generations of random mating amongst the 10 genes (or 5 individuals), eventually a situation will arise where all 10 genes are either *A* or *a* and then, in the absence of mutation, no further change can take place. In that case, gene *A* is said to be fixed. For a pair of neutral alleles in a finite population however large, the eventual outcome is bound to be that one or the other is fixed and the proportion of times they are fixed is simply proportional to their initial frequency. So, for example, starting always with 10 genes, 5 of which are *A* and 5, *a*, over many such experiments of going to fixation, half the time the result will be that *A* is fixed and half that *a* is fixed. However, supposing we had started with 3 *A* genes and 7 *a*, then the result would have been that 30 percent of the time *A* is fixed and 70 percent *a*. Taking this to its limit, a single new mutation in a population of N individuals has a gene frequency of 1/2N, and this then will be the probability that it eventually gets fixed. Clearly this probability becomes very small when N, the population size, becomes large, but it is always there. That is why random fluctuations can give rise to increases in the frequency of a gene simply by chance, although the probability that this happens for any particular gene is always small. The mean time taken for the gene to be fixed, if it is, can be shown to be about 4N generations, where N is the population size, and so may be very large for large populations. The distribution of the frequencies of different mutants due to drift is heavily skewed. In other words, only a very small proportion of new mutants will reach polymorphic frequencies, while the vast majority of the mutants hover around very low frequencies with a high probability of being lost.

A particular form of chance effect is associated with populations that have gone through a "bottle-neck," namely a severe reduction in size followed by a comparatively rapid expansion. In that case, there will be a "founder" effect in that those mutations that happen to be present in the reduced population at the time of the bottle-neck will be there at a relatively high frequency, which, on the whole, will be retained when the population expands rapidly. Thus, populations that have gone through a bottle-neck may contain a relatively larger number of alleles that have apparently drifted up in frequency than would be expected in a large homogeneous population. This accounts, presumably, for the relatively large number of comparatively frequent mutant alleles, for example, for Tay-Sachs disease and for one or two alleles of the breast cancer *BRCA1* gene in Ashkenazi Jewish populations. A somewhat similar phenomenon is seen in Finnish populations.

The first serious attempt to estimate human mutation rates was made by J.B.S. Haldane in the 1930s using the mutation-selection balance formula (Eq. 11-1) for deleterious dominant genes, (as modified for x-linked recessives) and estimates of the incidence of the abnormality and its selective advantage, as already discussed. Apart from the obvious problems of getting good estimates of the trait incidence and its selective disadvantage, the difficulty of this approach, understandably not realized at the time, is that a mutation rate when applied to a whole gene consisting of maybe 5000 to 10,000 base pairs is not itself a meaningful concept. This is because at the DNA level, different positions within the gene may have different mutation rates. In addition, mutations may vary considerably in their expression, and so selective effect, depending on the particular disruptive effect of any particular mutation. Haldane initially used hemophilia as his example and it is now clear that different mutations disrupting the function of factor VIII can have varying phenotypic consequences on clotting efficiency, leading not only to variability in the disease manifestation, but also clearly in the selective disadvantage associated with any particular mutation. Thus, the mutation rate is really the aggregate rate with which all mutations that give rise to a collective phenotype called hemophilia occur. This aggregate rate is, in general, an inextricable mixture of varying mutation rates at different positions of the gene and different selective disadvantages associated with different categories of mutations. The only general comment that perhaps can be made is that the larger the gene the higher the expected overall mutation rate. This may explain the prominence of genetic diseases such as the X-linked Duchenne muscular dystrophy and the inherited colorectal cancer susceptibility, FAP, both associated with relatively big expressed genes.

There is one condition under which this confounding between mutation rates at the DNA level and different selective effects can be resolved, namely if a phenotype is made up of a set of mutations all of which have the same, or more or less the same, effect and so can be assumed for practical purposes to have the same selective disadvantage. It can then be shown by an extension of the classical mutation-selection balance theory (personal observation), that the relative frequency with which different categories of mutation are observed is proportional to their mutation rates. In that case, given an accurate overall estimate of the incidence of the phenotype in the population, and of its selective disadvantage, for example, estimated from the proportion of sporadic cases, then absolute estimates of the mutation rate at the DNA level are obtainable.

The dominantly inherited cancer susceptibilities associated with tumor suppressor genes and Knudson's classical hypothesis on the relationship between germ line and somatic mutations may satisfy these conditions. Thus, clearcut florid polyposis arises almost entirely through truncation mutations in the *APC* gene that disrupt the function of the protein specifically between approximately amino acids 200 and 1600 out of the total 2843 amino acids that make up the protein. Several hundred germline mutations have been sequenced, nearly all of which are truncating due to either nonsense or frameshift mutations. These can be categorized into types with respect to probable mutation rates, for example; single base pair transversions, which have been seen only once; mutations at CpG positions (which often have C methylated), in particular from CGA to TGA, which replace an arginine by a stop codon; and one or two individually extremely common mutations, notably at amino acids position 1061 and 1309. For each defined category of mutations, it is possible to count the number of potential sites in that category at which truncating or frameshift mutations could occur. Using reliable estimates of the population incidence of FAP from Scandinavian registries (about 1 in 8000) and an estimate of the selective disadvantage of FAP of about 30 percent gives rise to an estimate of the germline mutation rate at the DNA level for single base pair transversion mutations of about 3 to 5×10^{-9} per base pair per generation.

Methylated CpG positions give a mutation rate estimate that is about 40 times as high as this, while the estimate of the mutation rate at the 5 base pair duplication around amino acid position 1309, which accounts for some 10 to 15 percent of all germline mutations, is a thousand-fold higher. This range of mutation rates illustrates the complexity of estimating the rate at the DNA level and emphasizes the distinctive value of the FAP/*APC* data for this purpose.[6,7]

These are perhaps the first valid direct mutation-rate estimates for human populations at the DNA level. This approach still involves some averaging assumptions because it is known, for example, that the 1309 mutation has a more severe effect than many others. A significant part of the observed phenotypic heterogeneity in FAP is due to the differential effects of mutations in different positions within the gene, which can, to some extent, begin to be explained by the protein's multifunctional role. When mutations with different phenotypic effects occur with different frequencies, then this can also explain patterns of heterogeneity with respect to a trait caused by mutations in a given gene. Beyond this, heterogeneity may arise as a result of differential environmental effects, the effects of genetic modifiers (which, however, unless they are closely linked to the primary locus, should not segregate with FAP in families), and, often most troublesome, heterogeneity due to mutations in different loci giving an essentially similar phenotype. This was initially the situation reported for xeroderma pigmentosum.

There is another aspect of the heterogeneous effects of different mutations within a given gene that is well illustrated by FAP. As already mentioned, only mutations within the region amino acids 200 to 1600 give rise to classical polyposis. Mutations near the beginning of the gene and occasional mutations beyond amino acid 1600 have been shown to give rise to a much milder phenotype, which has been called AAPC for attenuated adenomatous polyposis coli. This is exemplified by a much smaller number of polyps and a later age of onset of the disease. Recently, paralleling these observations, missense variants in the central portion of the gene have been described that have a clearly lower penetrance and may give rise to a somewhat milder phenotype. One of these (I1307K) has been found so far only in Ashkenazi Jews with colorectal cancer, or people with adenomas, at a threefold or more higher incidence than the control frequency of 5 to 10 percent in Ashkenazi Jews with no overt colorectal cancers or adenomas.[8,9] The second variant (E1317Q) has been found in patients with multiple adenomas and also with early onset of colorectal cancer with a frequency of a few percent, but has not so far been seen at all in relevant control populations.[9] The selective disadvantage (presumably mainly with respect to fertility) of these missense variants will be minimal at worst, and possibly nonexistent. Thus, these mutations can drift up in frequency by chance in just the same way that recessive mutations, such as the cystic fibrosis, ΔF508, mutation can. This explains their relatively high frequency in some populations and not others, and can account for mild sporadic early onset cases without a family history. This is because, with a relatively low penetrance, perhaps $\frac{1}{3}$ to $\frac{1}{2}$, pairs of sibs will only be affected with a probability of 1 in 16 to, roughly, 1 in 36 and therefore will mostly not show up as families, but usually only as sporadic cases.

Thus there are two quite contrasting explanations for genetically based early onset sporadic cancers. The first is that these are new mutations, but in that case the effects must be severe enough to account for the proportion of new mutations as the selective disadvantage. The other extreme arises, as in the case of the 1307 and 1317 mutants, when the effect is of sufficiently low penetrance and severity, that disease in first-degree relatives has not been detected. The relatively moderate effects of these missense variants can also account for the fact that they are not seen at the somatic level, namely as mutations in sporadic cancers. Mutations that occur in the germline are, of course, present in every cell in the body. Thus, they have a higher probability of contributing to the development of a tumor even if their selective advantage at the cellular level is relatively weak. The mutations that occur sporadically, however, generally occur in just one cell and therefore are much more likely to contribute to the somatic evolution of a cancer if they have a higher selective advantage. The overall probability of success must be proportional to the number of cells that have the mutation times its selective advantage, hence the difference between the mild germline mutations, still acting at the cellular level, and the more severe sporadic mutations, which in *APC* occur predominantly in a small central portion of the gene.

This notion may explain other situations such as for the *BRCA1* and *BRCA2* mutations in breast cancer, where germline mutations are found conferring a pronounced increase in the risk of breast cancer in genes that apparently should be behaving like tumor suppressor genes, but for which mutations are not found in sporadic cancers.

The overall frequency of these "subpolymorphic" missense variants, such as I1307K and E1307Q for *APC*, may be substantially higher than the combined frequency of the more severe truncating mutations. Thus, even though these missense variants may have a lower penetrance, their overall contribution to colorectal cancer susceptibility may at least equal, if not exceed, the overall contribution of the severe mutants maintained by mutation selection balance in the population. These missense variants thus appear to represent a new intermediate category of susceptibility between rare mutations kept at bay by their selective disadvantage, and common polymorphisms associated with comparatively common chronic diseases such as in the case of the HLA and disease associations.

The type of subpolymorphic tumor predisposing variation represented by these missense variants in the *APC* gene might be found quite generally in a wide range of disease-causing genes. Thus, in any situation where severe nonfunctional mutations in a gene cause an obvious Mendelian disease susceptibility, there could be such polymorphic or subpolymorphic variants with a much lesser, but nevertheless significant effect. These may be likely to occur particularly when the relevant protein product functions as a dimer or in a complex with other proteins, so that missense mutations can have significant dominant negative or gain of function effects (see Bodmer[6] for further background to these ideas).

POLYMORPHISM DUE TO BALANCING SELECTION

Chance fluctuations in gene frequencies, in the absence of natural selection can, as shown, lead to substantial and so clearly polymorphic gene frequencies. The extent to which this applies to any particular genetic variant is dependent on features of a population's properties, such as its size, the extent of subdivision, patterns of migration between subpopulations, and inbreeding effects. All these phenomena are a part of a population's "structure," which affects all genes equally. Furthermore, chance fluctuations always lead, eventually, to fixation of one or other allele and so cannot, in the long-term, explain how polymorphism can be attained and sustained.

The classic mechanism for the stable maintenance of a polymorphism in a population was first proposed and analyzed by R.A. Fisher in 1922. He showed that in a random mating population and ignoring chance fluctuations, if the heterozygote for two alleles at a single locus has a selective advantage over both the homozygotes, then a stable balanced polymorphism is always reached and maintained. The equilibrium gene frequencies are dependent on the relative extent to which the heterozygote is fitter than each of the two homozygotes. The prime example of such a polymorphism is still that for the human sickle cell hemoglobin variant allele *S* and its normal counterpart *A*. Under the relatively primitive conditions prevailing in West Africa when the sickle cell trait evolved, the anemic *SS* homozygotes almost certainly had a near-zero fitness, mostly dying early in life if not *in utero*, and certainly not achieving reproductive age. Following, however, J.B.S. Haldane's original suggestion, the *AS* heterozygotes have an advantage over the normal *AA* homozygotes with respect to their resistance to malaria. This situation fits precisely Fisher's analysis of balanced polymorphism achieved by heterozygote advantage. The straightforward algebra for the equilibrium situation is shown in Table 11-2. The sickle cell allele *S* is predicted to achieve an equilibrium frequency $s/(s + t)$ where t is the selective disadvantage of the anemic homozygote and s the selective disadvantage of the normal homozygote *AA* relative to the heterozygote *AS* due to differential resistance to malaria. When, for example, the anemia is lethal, $t = 1$ to give *SS* a fitness of 0, a frequency of 20 percent

Table 11-2 Equilibrium Gene Frequencies Under Heterozygote Advantage

If genotypes	*AA*	*AS*	*SS*
have fitnesses	$1 - s$	1	$1 - t$
then at equilibrium, alleles	*A*		*S*
will have frequencies	$t/(s + t)$		$s/(s + t)$

For heterozygote advantage, both *s* and *t* must be positive

Table 11-3 Summary of Sequence Changes in *CDH1* in Korean Gastric and Colon Cancer Patients and Controls

Codon	Nucleotide change	Consequence	Frequency* patients (n = 131)	Korean controls (n = 88)
Intron 4	gaaag → gaaac		4	ND
340	**A**CG → **G**CG	Thr → Ala	2	0
599	**C**TA → **G**TA	Leu → Val	4	1
Intron 12	a**t**tgc → a**c**tgc		5	ND
692	GC**C** → GC**T**	Ala → Ala	43	ND
751	AA**C** → AA**T**	Asn → Asn	10	ND
782	GT**G** → GT**A**	Val → Val	1	0

ND = not determined
Neither alleles T340A nor L599V were found in tumor specimens of 40 non-Korean sporadic colorectal cancer patients or in the germ line of 80 non-Korean controls. These alleles may be associated with an increased cancer risk.[11]
*Based on diploid chromosome number.

for the carriers could be explained by s = 0.25, giving the sickle cell heterozygote a 25 percent advantage over the normal homozygote. This gives an equilibrium gene frequency of 0.25/ 1 + 0.25 for allele *S*, namely 0.2 and so, from the Hardy-Weinberg Law, a frequency of *AS* heterozygotes of 2 × 0.2 × 0.8 or 32 percent. A smaller selective advantage for the heterozygote *AS* over *AA*, of, for example, only 10 percent gives an equilibrium frequency for *S* of 9.1 percent and a sickle cell trait heterozygote frequency of 16.6 percent. Either of these results can provide a plausible explanation for the maintenance of the sickle cell polymorphism at its extraordinarily high frequency in West Africa when malaria was rampant, notwithstanding the severe anemia of the *SS* homozygote.

There are many generalizations of this simple model for the selective maintenance of a balanced polymorphism all of which, however, imply some form of balancing selection where on average heterozygotes are fitter than homozygotes. These include, for example, fluctuations in selective advantage with time where sometimes one allele may be at an advantage and at other times another, as possibly for differential resistance and susceptibility to different pathogens. In that case, so long as generally over time, the heterozygote is fitter than either homozygote, a balanced polymorphism will be attained. A particular example of this is that either allele is always at an advantage when rare and, effectively, the selective advantage varies inversely with the frequency of the allele. Selection acting in opposite directions in the two sexes can also lead to a balanced polymorphism.

The proper definition of fitness takes into account the probability of an individual surviving to different ages, together with the probability with which offspring are produced at different ages. These two distributions when combined together define an intrinsic rate of increase as used by demographers and called by R.A. Fisher, who first introduced these ideas into genetics, the "Malthusian parameter."[10] Most of the mathematical models of population genetics are formulated in terms of an affect on viability, but it can be shown under quite broad assumptions that if the viability and the fertility parameters can be multiplied together, then equivalent results are obtained. Occasionally, however, there may be differential genetic effects on fertility and viability, and this can be another form of balance leading to a stable polymorphism.

The observed polymorphisms in a population can be there for a variety of reasons. Some may just be neutral alleles that have drifted up in frequency and so remain there for long periods, others may be polymorphisms maintained actively by selection, and yet others may be transient polymorphisms in the sense that a gene has been caught in the midst of an evolutionary process involving one allele replacing another. There has been a major argument over many years between the "selectionists," who maintained that nearly all polymorphism was due to selection; and the "neutralists," notably Motto Kimura following Sewall Wright, who argued that most polymorphisms were due to drift and simply there by chance. These arguments took place at a time long before DNA technology had developed and when most of the polymorphisms were for blood groups or enzymes, and by their nature had involved amino acid substitutions. For these, the selectionist argument, as we shall see, was probably correct. However, as soon as the new DNA technologies revealed an extraordinary level of polymorphism at the DNA sequence level, it became clear that most of this variation is indeed likely to be neutral. This is consistent with the fact that most DNA level polymorphisms are in introns or flanking regions, or give rise to synonymous substitutions, all of which are expected generally to be "neutral" in their selective effects. This pattern is strikingly revealed by the searches for germline mutations in candidate genes to explain patterns of disease inheritance in families. A typical example of data obtained in searching for cancer susceptibility mutations in the E-cadherin (*CDH1*) gene is shown in Table 11-3. The notable feature of this data, as found for many other genes, is that those variations that occur as polymorphisms with appreciable frequency are nearly all in introns or give rise to synonymous changes, for example, in a third base pair position in a codon without changing the amino acid. Since the techniques used to search for DNA variation are not biased towards any particular type of change, this suggests strongly that those mutations that change amino acids mostly give rise to a sufficient selective disadvantage to prevent their chance increase by genetic drift. For a population of size N the selective disadvantage needs only to be greater than 1/2N, which is generally quite small, to counter the effects of drift. It is only the occasional mutation causing an amino acid substitution with minimal effects that will increase to the sort of subpolymorphic frequencies discussed in relation to the *APC* variants, and which may then be associated with a functional effect reflected in an increased disease susceptibility, as for the *CDH1* alleles T340A and L599V shown in Table 11-3.

THE HLA SYSTEM AS A MODEL FOR THE STUDY OF POPULATION VARIABILITY, NATURAL SELECTION AND LINKAGE DISEQUILIBRIUM

The HLA system of genetically determined antigens, present on human white blood cells and most nucleated cells in the body, was discovered in the search for polymorphic antigens to match for transplantation, by analogy with the human red cell blood groups. The system was discovered by virtue of the fact that it was polymorphic, initially using antibodies from multiparous women produced against their fetus during pregnancy. The HLA system is now almost completely characterized at the DNA level, and polymorphism is detected using DNA typing procedures. The extent of HLA polymorphism was apparent even from the earliest

Table 11-4

Locus	Number of alleles	
	1995	1997
HLA-A	60	83
HLA-B	125	186
HLA-C	36	42
HLA-E	4	5
HLA-G	5	7
HLA-DRA	2	2
HLA-DRB1	132	184
HLA-DRB3	5	11
HLA-DRB4	4	9
HLA-DRB5	6	12
HLA-DQA1	16	18
HLA-DQB1	25	31
HLA-DOB	1	1
HLA-DMA	4	4
HLA-DMB	4	5
HLA-DNA	1	1
HLA-DPA1	8	10
HLA-DPB1	63	77
TAP1	5	5
TAP2	4	4
TOTAL	**510**	**698**

A, B, C, E, and *G* are the Class I loci, the remaining loci starting with *D* from *DRA* to *DPB1* are the Class II loci and *TAP1* and *TAP2* are the associated transporter loci. Based on the 1997 data, the total number possible of genotypes that could be formed is 1.4537×10^{42}.

studies and is now seen to be quite remarkable, as shown in Table 11-4, which lists the HLA Class I and Class II loci (together with one or two others) and the number of alleles found at each in 1995 and 1997 (see, for example, reference 12). These are all defined at the DNA sequence level, and the number is still increasing at the same rate.

One of the most striking features of the data is the enormous variability between the loci in the number of alleles found in human populations. As discussed earlier, population structure effects such as population size, patterns of migration and admixture, and levels of inbreeding affect all genes equally. The Class I and Class II loci each have very similar structures and sizes, so that it is inconceivable that this variation could be explained by differential rates of mutation. Cavalli-Sforza first pointed out more than 30 years ago, that if there is differential variability either within a gene or between genes in any population feature such as the number of alleles or their frequency distribution, then this cannot be due to population structure, which does not discriminate between genes or alleles. Thus, excluding mutation rate differences, the marked variability between the *HLA* genes in the number of alleles found can only be explained by natural selection, which presumably is discriminating between the functional effects of variants at the different gene loci.

There is another feature of the *HLA* sequence data that supports this conclusion. This is the fact that the polymorphisms found, especially in the most highly polymorphic loci, all involve amino acid substitutions and are mostly localized to the key functional part of the HLA molecule, namely its cleft, which binds peptides to be presented in immune interactions to the T-cell receptor. This is another extraordinary level of differential variability within the gene that unequivocally can only be explained through the action of natural selection. In the case of the *HLA* system, this is most probably a result of differential immune responses associated with differential resistance to infectious pathogens. This principle of differential variability is an extremely powerful approach to identifying which polymorphic variants may be selected for and which are probably neutral. Differential variation between populations, and gene frequency gradients related, for example, to latitude may often, therefore, be evidence for the action of natural selection.

The evidence suggests that HLA alleles may often have two or more regions of variation in relation to other alleles, and these can be considered as epitopes. These epitopes must be quite old in evolutionary terms, since the same epitopes can, for example, be found in quite distantly related mammalian species. New alleles can be formed from old by recombination. If different epitope combinations are present in a population at low frequencies, then when the selective situation requires it, a new combination may quickly increase in frequency to cope with a new selective challenge. This form of fluctuating selection gives rise to average heterozygote advantage over time. It is therefore a mechanism that can maintain high levels of polymorphism over long periods, without the specific requirement that particular heterozygotes are at any given time always at an advantage over the homozygotes.

LINKAGE DISEQUILIBRIUM—POPULATION ASSOCIATION BETWEEN ALLELES AT DIFFERENT LOCI

As soon as the first two loci, *A* and *B*, of the *HLA* system were properly defined it became clear that there was extensive association between pairs of alleles at different loci. This is due to the phenomenon now called linkage disequilibrium and first analyzed by Jennings in 1917.[13] The basic underlying ideas are illustrated in Table 11-5 in terms of the behavior of two linked loci each with two alleles (*A, a*: *B, b*) separated by a recombination fraction r. There are four gametes or haplotypes, *AB, Ab, aB*, and *ab*. (The now-familiar term "haplotype," which is a confluence of the terms haploid and genotype, was coined by Ceppellini in 1967 specifically to describe combinations of alleles at linked loci in the *HLA* system and also in relation to immunoglobulin gene variation.) In the absence of any association between the two loci, the haplotype frequencies x_1, and so on, would simply equal the product of the frequencies of the constituent alleles, namely $x_1 = PQ$, and so on. In this case there is statistical independence between the loci; and if, for example, A and B referred to detectable antigens or phenotypes at the two loci then, given random mating, it is easy to show that there would be no association between the two phenotypes A and B in the population. In general, however, the haplotype frequencies will depart from this random combination by a quantity $D = x_1x_4 - x_2x_3$, which is a measure of the association between the alleles at the two loci, and is called the "linkage disequilibrium" parameter. D is a measure of the association between alleles on a haplotype. That is why it is also sometimes called the "gametic association." The haplotype frequencies can be expressed quite generally in terms of the gene frequencies, and D as a measure of departure from

Table 11-5 Linkage Disequilibrium Between Alleles *A, a* and *B, b* at Two Linked loci

	AB	***Ab***	***aB***	***ab***
Gametes or haplotypes frequencies	x_1	x_2	x_3	x_4
or	$PQ + D$	$Pq - D$	$pQ - D$	$pq + D$
where	$P = x_1 + x_2 = 1 - p$			
	$Q = x_1 + x_3 = 1 - q$			
	define the gene frequencies of *A, a, B, b*			
and	$D = x_1\,x_4 - x_2\,x_3$ is the measure of linkage disequilibrium.			

In the absence of selection D decreases by (1−r) each generation, where r is the recombination fraction between the (A, *a*) and (*B, b*) loci.

independence, as shown in Table 11-5. As long as D is not zero, the gametic association imposes a phenotypic association between A and B in the population. The larger is D, the stronger the linkage disequilibrium and the stronger the association between traits A and B in the population. Jennings's classic result was to show that, in a random mating population with no other forces acting on the genes, the value of D decreases by a factor of 1 − r in each generation. For example, if r is 0.003, corresponding on average to 300,000 base pairs, then D declines by a factor of between 5 and 10 in about 1000 generations, or for humans 25,000 years. This is comparable to the time when it is presumed that, for example, modern humans, *Homo sapiens*, first came to Europe. In practice, therefore, for human populations, in the absence of selection or other disturbing factors, including population admixture, linkage disequilibrium is only likely to be substantial if the recombination fraction between the loci is less than about 0.5 percent. In the case of the *HLA* system, for example, there are some pairs of alleles at the *HLA-A* and *B* loci which show significant linkage disequilibrium with r about 0.01, but this tends to vary substantially from one population group to another. For example, *A1* and *B8* are strongly associated in northern European populations, less so in southern European populations and not at all in India, even though *A1* and *B8* occur there with comparable frequencies. On the other hand, alleles at the *HLA-B* and *C* loci nearly all show strong pairwise linkage disequilibrium and to a similar extent in most populations throughout the world. This contrast between the two pairs of loci is explained by the fact that the genetic (and physical) distance between *HLA-B* and *C* is only about one-quarter of that between *HLA-A* and *B*.

A striking feature of the *HLA* system is that many studies have shown population associations between particular *HLA* types and certain diseases, notably autoimmune diseases including, for example, ankylosing spondylitis, rheumatoid arthritis, and juvenile onset insulin-dependent diabetes mellitus (IDDM). One of the most striking associations remains that between *HLA-B27* and ankylosing spondylitis, where well over 90 percent of ankylosing spondylitis patients have *B27*, whose population frequency, for example, in Europeans is only slightly more than 5 percent. Nevertheless, the incidence of ankylosing spondylitis in the population is sufficiently low that only a few percent of people who have *B27* will, in fact, get the disease. This is a classical example of multifactorial disease susceptibility, identified nevertheless with a particular genetic factor. The low penetrance of the *B27* effect must be due to the effects of other genes and, of course, of the environment, on the probability of getting ankylosing spondylitis. In other cases, such as the association of DR4 with rheumatoid arthritis the increased relative risk associated with the presence of the antigen, while still very significant, is of the order of 3 to 4, as compared to nearly 100 for the association between *B27* and ankylosing spondylitis. In that case, therefore, one must question if the DR4 effect is direct or is associated, through linkage disequilibrium, with variation at another locus nearby. It was the interpretation of the manifest HLA and disease associations that led Bodmer (see, e.g., reference 14) to suggest that these could, in at least some cases, be due to linkage disequilibrium between an allele at a closely linked locus in the *HLA* system and the particular marker allele being studied. This was always a possibility, because of the number of functionally relevant genes that happen to be close to each other within the *HLA* system. As it became clear that the genetic map could be saturated with DNA polymorphisms, it was soon realized that the HLA model could be quite generally applied to the search for population associations between DNA markers and a disease even when the genetic effect had a relatively low penetrance, as in the case of the association between *B27* and ankylosing spondylitis. Population associations that, as discussed, are only likely to be significant at recombination fractions of less than half a percent, will therefore bring one closer to a locus of interest than could ever reasonably be achieved with linkage studies in human families. The experimental approach is a simple case-control study, comparing the frequency of DNA markers in diseased individuals with that in control populations.

The key question of interpretation is the extent to which such an association would necessarily be due to linkage disequilibrium with an allele at a nearby locus. Factors influencing linkage disequilibrium include recent population admixture, inbreeding, random drift effects, and variation due simply to the inevitably limited sizes of population samples. All these factors, however, even including population admixture, can be shown to have only relatively minor effects on linkage disequilibrium compared to the major effect of very close linkage in the absence of any other factors. Nevertheless, the most critical issue is the proper choice of control populations. A spread of carefully chosen populations throughout a geographic area is really needed to give some indication of the scope for variation in control populations being able to explain an observed association. This, I believe, is a much more robust approach to marker and disease association studies than the recent, widely promoted transmission disequilibrium test, which aims to combine recombination and linkage disequilibrium testing through the use of parent and offspring combinations, and so effectively requires a new set of controls for each disease study. It is through population association studies, for example, that the *APO-E* polymorphism has been associated with Alzheimer disease.

THE ANALYSIS OF MULTIFACTORIAL INHERITANCE

Many individual attributes, though they do not follow any simple Mendelian pattern of inheritance, nevertheless are clearly influenced by genetic factors. Some like ankylosing spondylitis or congenital malformations such as anencephaly and spina bifida are discrete characteristics, and others such as height or weight or blood pressure are quantitative measures. The association between *HLA-B27* and ankylosing spondylitis illustrates the way a well-defined single genetic difference can have a substantial influence on the incidence of a disease whose inheritance is nevertheless very far from following simple Mendelian laws. The same can be true for a quantitative character. For example, the association between *HLA-DQ* alleles and IDDM will be reflected in an influence of HLA types on the distribution of blood sugar levels. Such patterns of inherited susceptibility are generally referred to as multifactorial, implying that an attribute may be influenced by more than one genetic difference, perhaps several, as well as by environmental factors. The term polygenic is sometimes also used simply to indicate that several genes may be involved in the determination of a multifactorial trait. The term polygene was introduced more than 50 years ago by Mather to describe a category of genes that he postulated to affect quantitative traits, and that was distinct from other types of genes. That is now an untenable hypothesis, which is why the term multifactorial inheritance is to be preferred, not having any such historically biased overtones and including necessarily the all-important reference to environmental effects.

One of the first challenges of the study of quantitative inheritance is to establish what fraction of the variance of a quantitative trait can be attributed to genetic factors, a quantity referred to, in general, as its "heritability." There is an extensive literature on approaches to calculating heritability, particularly in relation to plant and animal breeding, but also in human populations using data on the correlation between relatives such as brothers and sisters, including twins, and parents and offspring, for a quantitative trait to predict its heritability. (See, for example, Chapter 9 of Cavalli-Sforza and Bodmer,[3] and Lynch and Walsh.[15]) Clearly, if a significant fraction, even 5 or 10 percent, of the distribution of a quantitative trait such as height, weight, or blood pressure in the normal human population can be attributable to genetic factors, then this implies that there are relatively common polymorphic genes which have differential effects on the quantitative trait. In some cases, the quantitative effect of a given simple genetic difference may be readily detectable. Thus, given two alleles A, a at a single locus, there may be significant differences in the average value of the trait between the genotypes AA, Aa, and aa. In that case, the nature of the genetic difference may give some clue to the functional basis for at least a part of the multifactorial inheritance of the quantitative trait. An example might be the influence of different alleles for the *ACE* enzyme, and the resulting genotypes, on blood pressure.

A quantitative trait can be turned into a discrete characteristic by the use of a threshold. For example, diabetic individuals could be simply defined as those whose blood sugar concentration lies above a certain threshold, and similarly hemochromatosis could be defined as having a blood iron concentration above a certain threshold. There is then a relationship between the inherited susceptibility to having the trait defined by the threshold, and the heritability, namely the proportion of the variance of the underlying quantitative trait that can be attributed to genetic factors. A major difficulty with the study of multifactorial inheritance, in addition to the complexity of the mixture of several genetic factors and the environment being involved, is the problem of heterogeneity. Even such apparently clear-cut inherited recessive traits as xeroderma pigmentosum turned out to be heterogeneous, in the sense that the apparent same clinical entity could be due to recessive mutations in several different genes. This makes straightforward genetic linkage analysis in families difficult especially when, as now in many populations, family sizes are small and so the number of affecteds in any pedigree is also small. It may, therefore, be hard to accumulate enough examples of any one category of a disease to show different patterns of genetic linkage with different genetically identified forms of the disease. This problem is clearly made more difficult for multifactorial traits, whose inheritance patterns can require quite sophisticated statistical procedures for their analysis, whether they are considered as quantitative characters, threshold characters derived from a quantitative distribution, or discrete traits. The difficulties that have been faced in trying to identify genetic factors for schizophrenia are most probably an example of such problems of heterogeneity.

At the end of their chapter on quantitative inheritance, Cavalli-Sforza and Bodmer[3] said that, "The ultimate goal of genetic understanding, however, is always the identification of major distinct genes affecting a character and so in fact the elimination of the need to apply statistical concepts of quantitative genetics as we have developed them here." This statement, I believe, is still valid, if not more so, nearly 30 years later. The difference now is that the extensive polymorphisms that can be identified at the DNA level, and extensions of the ideas of positional cloning, make it possible to devise strategies for identifying the individual genes contributing to a multifactorial character, provided the effect is sufficiently large.

The basic approach to positional cloning is first to locate, by some form of linkage analysis, the position on the chromosome that carries the gene whose one or more alleles have a statistically significant measurable effect on the trait being studied. The ultimate identification of the genetic difference itself then depends, as in all positional cloning, on testing the hypothesis that a given genetic difference at the DNA level is itself having the effect on the trait. This may often require a functional analysis of the relevant gene product and the effects of mutations on its function. Where, as in the case of the *HLA* system, several plausible candidate genes are found closely linked together in the region identified by the linkage analysis, the problem of identifying which is the correct one may be particularly difficult.

Two main, mutually supportive approaches are now commonly used in the attempt to identify specific gene effects on multifactorial traits. The first, most simply described as a sib-pair analysis, depends on the analysis of genetic markers in families with more than one affected individual, while the second depends on population associations between the trait and genetic markers, as exemplified in the HLA and disease associations already discussed.

The use of sib pairs for the analysis of linkage was first suggested by Penrose in 1935. His idea was that a simple pairwise association amongst the sibs, between the presence or absence of a given genetic marker and the presence or absence of a given inherited trait could give estimates of the recombination fraction. The extension of this idea to the analysis of linkage of a genetic marker with a multifactorial trait, but using only data on those who are "affected" was first applied to the search for linkage between *HLA* and spina bifida, leukemia, and IDDM. Only in the latter case were the results significant, confirming the already established association between HLA types and IDDM. The basic idea for the search is simply to ask whether the distribution of HLA types amongst affected sibs is distorted relative to Mendelian expectations. By studying only those who are affected, it is possible to avoid the problem of distinguishing unaffected individuals without the relevant gene from individuals who carry the relevant gene but do not express the disease.

Consider as an example data on HLA and Hodgkin disease, which was the first disease studied in the search for HLA association. Associations with Hodgkin disease were found with *HLA-B* locus determined antigens, but at a relative risk of only 1.3 to 1.6. Because of the extent of *HLA* polymorphism, it is nearly always possible to establish whether a given pair of sibs have received the identical *HLA* haplotype combinations from their two parents, or if they share one haplotype, or share none. (If the cross is represented as AB $\times$ CD, then sibs who are, for example, both AC share two haplotypes, sibs who are AC and AD share one, and sibs who are AC and BD share none.) Following Mendel's laws, the expected proportions of sib pairs in these three categories are one-quarter sharing both haplotypes, one-half sharing one haplotype and one-quarter sharing no haplotype. If the observed distribution of sib pairs is significantly different from Mendelian expectation then this is prima facie evidence of a linked gene with an influence on the trait. Observations of 18 sib pairs with Hodgkin disease, summarized by Dausset, Colombani, and Hors in 1982, showed that 11 were *HLA* identical, 5 shared one *HLA* haplotype, and 2 shared no haplotype, giving a χ^2 of 12.6 for two degrees of freedom for departure from Mendelian expectation, which is highly significant. The data thus clearly confirmed the involvement of an *HLA*-linked gene having an affect on susceptibility to Hodgkin disease and, because of the excess of *HLA* identical sib pairs, suggested a predominantly recessive effect. The data can be interpreted in terms of a rare gene with a frequency of approximately 1 in 1000, in which homozygotes nearly always get Hodgkin disease, whereas on average only 1 in 20 of the heterozygotes get the disease and all those without the relevant allele are unaffected.[7] The example shows how there can be a gene-determining susceptibility to a disease in such a way that there is effectively no detectable familial clustering because of the low penetrance of the heterozygote effect. This fits in with observations that suggest that at most a few percent of Hodgkin disease cases occur in families with two or more affecteds. Nevertheless, even a small number of families with sib pairs can yield a significant linkage provided the approach of using marker associations only with the affected sib pairs is followed.

The challenge now is to move in more decisively to the gene actually causing the susceptibility. In the case of Hodgkin disease, therefore, the question was asked, "Are there other markers than those of the *HLA-B* locus that might show a stronger association with Hodgkin disease and so either be the determinants of the inherited susceptibility themselves or be genetically closer to them?" Following this rationale, the association between Hodgkin disease and alleles at the *HLA-DP* locus was studied, since *DP* is at the other end of the *HLA* region and generally not in strong linkage disequilibrium with *HLA-B*. A combined international study found significant evidence of increased associations with *HLA-DP* alleles but still not enough to be convincing at a functional level.[16] Further studies would be needed to decide whether there was a direct, but small, functional effect of *HLA-DP*, for example, on immune response in relation to Epstein-Barr virus; or whether there was heterogeneity in Hodgkin disease such that only a subset was strongly *HLA* associated (unlikely because this would have significantly diluted the sib pair linkage effect), and finally, whether there is another nearby locus whose variation explains the apparent genetic susceptibility to Hodgkin disease.

The HLA and disease association studies suggest a general rationale for positional cloning of genes with a significant effect on a multifactorial trait. (See Bodmer,[17,18] and Tomlinson and Bodmer[14] for a historical account and overview of these issues.) The first step in this strategy is the careful definition of the trait, such as by objective clinical criteria defining presence or absence of a disease, or using a quantitative measure with a threshold above, or below which the trait is defined to exist. (An approach to the investigation of linkage between a quantitative trait and a marker locus using sib pairs was proposed by Haseman and Elston in 1972[19] using variance analysis, which, however, makes the definition of specific candidate loci somewhat more difficult.) After the definition of the trait, the next step is to search for linkage using the affected sib-pair approach and marker loci. These may either be spread throughout the genome, or focused on suspected areas associated with candidate genes or with the effects of chromosome deletions and translocations. Once the approximate position of a gene affecting the trait in question has been found, then closer linkage can be sought by looking for associations with a set of polymorphic markers that saturates the genetic region where linkage has been detected. This is much more efficient than seeking closer linkage using family data where the resolution is unlikely to be even as low as a 1 percent recombination fraction. The rate of decline of linkage disequilibrium, namely $(1 - r)^n$ where n is the number of generations, amplifies the effect of a small recombination fraction in population association data and, in principle, may allow resolution down to a distance of the order of 50 kb. At that level, direct testing of candidate genes for polymorphisms with plausible functional effects becomes feasible. It is this strategy for finding disease susceptibility genes that has fueled the recent surge of interest in the use of single nucleotide polymorphisms, or SNPs. Their value is that their mutation rate is likely to be very low and so they provide much more stable markers for population association studies than the more conventional highly polymorphic CA repeats.

The most important resource for such studies, apart from the availability of sufficient closely linked DNA polymorphic markers, is a good collection of control populations. The distribution of markers across widely separated population groups itself provides important information as to their age. Furthermore, the use of different control populations relevant to the disease group can indicate the potential variation in relative risk that could be attributed to heterogeneity in a control population. Theoretical calculations and empirical data on the linkage disequilibrium between markers within genes obtained from a variety of sources, suggest that very strong associations will nearly always be found between markers separated by even 50 to 100 kb. A fully saturated human genetic map at this level would contain 30,000 markers, though somewhat more may be needed to get adequate levels of polymorphism. On the other hand, the intervals over which linkage disequilibrium can readily be detected may be somewhat larger.

These various approaches to the analysis of multifactorial traits can, of course, be applied to normal, as well as to pathologic, differences. For example, we still do not know the proper genetics of skin-color differences, and yet these are the major genetic determinants of skin cancer, at least in populations of European origin. The similarity of facial features of identical twins strongly suggests that the face is almost entirely genetically determined. Furthermore, recognition of the face has special regions of the brain and has probably evolved under strong evolutionary pressure to identify membership of a family or larger grouping. The genetics of the face certainly should be analyzable using the combination of approaches we have been discussing. Craniofacial abnormalities may provide a clue as to which are the candidate genes whose polymorphism contributes to the genetic determination of the face. Special abilities, such as for music or mathematics, surely have strong genetic components as may be the case also for a variety of other behavioral attributes. Amongst these may be mild disorders such as dyslexia and mild early deafness, which can be compensated for by appropriate education.

THE RECENT EVOLUTION OF *HOMO SAPIENS*

The present structure of human populations has been determined by patterns of migration and admixture over the last 150,000 to 200,000 years, patterns subject to selective pressures connected especially with sources of food, predators, variation in the natural environment, including especially climate and its effects, and infections. These factors will all have shaped the distribution of polymorphic genes in different populations, and so have a major influence on the overall genetics of disease susceptibility. Bottlenecks and founder effects have led to the distinctive distribution of rare inherited abnormalities in populations such as the Ashkenazi Jews and the Finns. The need for vitamin D in conditions of relatively low sunlight has no doubt influenced the evolution of fair skin in northern caucasoids and, perhaps independently, in Orientals. Patterns of disease resistance, some perhaps relatively recent, for example, connected with the plagues associated with urbanization, have no doubt shaped the distribution of HLA variants. Another well-known example is that of the world-wide distribution of the hemoglobinopathies and other red cell defects, such as glucose-6-phosphate dehydrogenase deficiency, that have been determined by the incidence of malaria. The analysis of gene frequency similarities and differences in different human populations can tell us a great deal about their origins. One of the main architects of this approach to understanding our own recent evolution has been Cavalli-Sforza, and his magisterial book written with his colleagues Menozzi and Piazza is a description of some of the major conclusions that can be drawn from such analyses.[20]

The genetic or biologic definition of a population is by the pattern of gene frequencies it gives rise to, and this definition inevitably becomes more precise the more variable genes are studied. Genetic distances between populations can be measured in terms of the average differences between their gene frequency distributions, and these can be used to calculate relationships between populations that resemble phylogenetic evolutionary trees. Patterns of migration can be identified by coordinated gradients of gene frequencies, and population admixture can sometimes be estimated directly by equating the gene frequencies of the mixed population to those of linear combinations of the frequencies of two or more other populations from which it is presumed to be derived.

One of the most striking results to come out of the genetic analysis of human populations is the conclusion that modern *Homo sapiens* came out of Africa some 150,000 to 200,000 years ago, a conclusion consistent with the paleontological data. The evolution of language and intellectual ability may have fueled this dispersal and given modern humans the capacity to survive under more rigorous conditions than, for example, their close homo counterparts, *Homo neanderthalis*. The initial outward migration must have been largely to the Middle East, the Caucasus, and perhaps west Asia, with the major migrations into Europe and the rest of Asia and elsewhere, starting only some 50,000 years ago. These early migrations must have been strongly influenced by the changing climate associated with the end of the last Ice Age. As also shown by Cavalli-Sforza and colleagues, the development of agriculture in the Fertile Crescent led to a further major radical migration associated with population expansion. This started some 10,000 years ago and, for example, reached the northern limits of Europe in Britain and elsewhere some 5000 to 6000 years ago.

The biologic definition of a population must be clearly distinguished from its cultural definition. Thus, while much of the culture of Britain was surely shaped by the Roman occupation, the Romans, wherever the invaders came from, most probably left rather few of their genes. It is however the biologic and genetic definition of populations that influences the study of genetic susceptibility to disease, especially using the approach of studying population associations between multifactorial traits and genetic markers. These studies depend on linkage disequilibrium as observed. In addition to the important effect of time already discussed, selection itself can lead to strong transient linkage disequilibrium.[21] Thus, if an allele is strongly selected for, closely linked alleles will be pulled into the population due to linkage disequilibrium,[22] a phenomenon that has been called "hitchhiking."[23] When selection is strong, and the rate of increase of the allele therefore comparatively rapid, linkage disequilibrium can be maintained transiently over relatively large distances. This is because, during the increase in frequency of the selected allele, there is not enough time for recombination to disrupt the association between a selected allele and other alleles on the haplotype with which the selected allele is initially associated. Thus, comparatively recent selective events associated, for example, with epidemics, food shortages, or climatic changes may have led to changes in the pattern of linkage disequilibrium even between markers that are old and so are widely distributed in different human populations.

Whenever an association between a marker and a disease has been found, and especially when it has been interpreted at the functional level, it is worth considering the evolutionary antecedents in terms of our knowledge of modern human evolution. Thus, for example, the associations between HLA and autoimmune chronic diseases such as ankylosing spondylitis and rheumatoid arthritis are almost certainly the residue of previous selection for HLA types in relation to resistance against infectious pathogens. There may be other associations, for example, connected with nutritional effects on heart disease that could be due to human genetic adaptation being originally under sparse and perhaps mainly vegetarian food conditions. It was the human geneticist James Neel who on this basis suggested that the genetic susceptibility to diabetes could be characterized as a "thrifty" genotype. Will there be similar explanations for variation in analytical ability, or even in behavioral attributes, balancing the needs in human society for leaders and followers?

REFERENCES

1. Solomon E, Bodmer WF: Evolution of sickle variant gene. *Lancet* **1**:923, 1979.
2. Botstein D, White RL, Skolnick M, Davis RW: *Am J Hum Genet* **32**:314, 1980.
3. Cavalli-Sforza LL, Bodmer WF: *The Genetics of Human Populations*. San Francisco, WH Freeman, 1971 (reprinted with corrections New York, Dover Publications, 1999).
4. Bodmer WF, Cavalli-Sforza LL: *Genetics, Evolution and Man*. San Francisco, WH Freeman, 1976.
5. Hartl DL, Clark AG: *Principles of Population Genetics*, 3rd ed. Sunderland, MA, Sinauer Associates, 1997.
6. Bodmer WF: Familial adenomatous polyposis (FAP) and its gene, APC. *Cytogenet Cell Genet* **86**:99, 1999.
7. Bodmer WF: Cancer genetics. *Brit Med Bull* **50**:517, 1994.
8. Laken SJ, Petersen GM, Gruber SB, Oddoux C, Ostrer H, Giardello FM, Hamilton S, et al.: Familial colorectal cancer in Ashkenazim due to a hypermutable tract in APC. *Nat Genet* **17**:79, 1997.
9. Frayling IM, Beck N, Ilyas M, Dove-Edwin I, Goodman P, Pack K, Bell JA, et al.: The APC variants I1307K and E1317Q are associated with colorectal tumors, but not always with a family history. *Proc Natl Acad Sci U S A* **95**:10722, 1998.
10. Fisher RA: *The Genetical Theory of Natural Selection*. London, Oxford University Press, 1930.
11. Kim HC, Wheeler JMD, Kim JC, et al.: The E-cadherin gene (CDH1) variants T340A and L599V in gastric and colorectal cancer patients in Korea. *Gut* **47**:262, 2000.
12. Bodmer WF: HLA polymorphism: Origin and maintenance, in Terasaki PI, Gjertson DW (eds): *HLA 1997*. UCLA Tissue Typing Lab, Los Angeles, 1997, p 1.
13. Jennings HS: The numerical results of diverse systems of breeding with respect to two pairs of characters, linked or independent, with special relation to the effects of linkage. *Genetics* **2**:97, 1917.
14. Tomlinson IPM, Bodmer WF: The HLA System and the analysis of multifactorial genetic disease. *Trends Genet* **11**:493, 1995.
15. Lynch M, Walsh B: *Genetics and Analysis of Quantitative Traits*. Sunderland, MA, Sinauer Associates, 1998.
16. Bodmer JG, Tonks S, Oza AM, Mikata A, Takenouchi J, Lister TA: Hodgkin's disease study, in Tsuji K, Aizawa M, Sasazuki T (eds): *HLA 1991*. Oxford, Oxford University Press, 1992, p 701.
17. Bodmer WF: DNA polymorphisms and genetic markers in population and family studies of genetic predisposition, in Omenn GS (ed): *Banbury Report 16: Genetic Variability in Responses to Chemical Exposure*. New York, Cold Spring Harbor Laboratory, 1984, p 287.
18. Bodmer WF: Human genetics—The molecular challenge. *Cold Spring Harb Symp Quant Biol* **51**:1, 1986.
19. Haseman JK, Elston RC: The investigation of linkage between a quantitative trait and a marker locus. *Behav Genet* **2**:3, 1972.
20. Cavalli-Sforza LL, Menozzi P, Piazza A: *The History and Geography of Human Genes*. Princeton, NJ, Princeton University Press, 1994.
21. Thomson G, Bodmer WF, Bodmer J: The HL-A system as a model for studying the interaction between selection, migration and linkage, in *Proceedings of the International Conference on Population Genetics and Ecology 1975*. New York, Academic Press, 1976, p 465.
22. Bodmer WF, Parsons PA: Linkage and recombination in evolution. *Adv Genet* **11**:1, 1962.
23. Maynard-Smith J, Haigh J: The hitch-hiking effect of a favourable gene. *Genet Res* **23**:23, 1974.

CHAPTER 12

The Role of Human Major Histocompatibility Complex (HLA) Genes in Disease

Lars Fugger ▪ Roland Tisch
Roland Libau ▪ Peter van Endert ▪ Hugh O. McDevitt

The human major histocompatibility complex (MHC), also designated the human leukocyte antigen (HLA) system, was initially characterized using maternal antisera that identified paternal transplantation antigens expressed in the offspring. HLA typing was originally developed to facilitate organ and tissue transplantation, particularly renal transplantation. The discovery that the ability of mice to make an immune response to synthetic polypeptides was linked to the murine MHC, designated H-2,[1] and the earlier demonstration that susceptibility to Gross-virus-induced leukemogenesis was also linked to H-2,[2] stimulated a search for direct or indirect effects of MHC genes on susceptibility to many different diseases.

This search was highly productive, and within a few years it was shown that susceptibility to a wide variety of diseases was preferentially increased in individuals of particular HLA genotypes. Associations between HLA and disease were initially reported for systemic lupus erythematosus (SLE),[3] ankylosing spondylitis,[4] multiple sclerosis (MS),[5] and insulin-dependent diabetes mellitus (IDDM).[6] In the ensuing 20 years, susceptibility to more and more diseases was shown to be determined in part by HLA genotype; linkage of HLA type with disease was demonstrated in family studies; and a bewildering array of new genes was described and characterized in the MHC. There are now more than 30 diseases associated with HLA genotype, and more than 35 to 50 expressed genes that map in the HLA region. This makes the task of determining with certainty which genes in the HLA region predispose to which diseases extremely complex. This task is further complicated by the fact that very little genetic recombination occurs over long stretches of the MHC, which in humans extends over 4000 kbs (4 Mbp). The lack of recombination results in the phenomenon of linkage disequilibrium, in which particular combinations of alleles of the various loci in the MHC remain linked together in the population as a haploid set or haplotype, and show very little recombination either in family or population studies. Thus, relatively weak associations between IDDM and HLA class I alleles, for example, HLA-B8 (i.e., HLA-B*0801), were later shown to be due to a much stronger association of this disease with the HLA class II allele HLA-DR3 (i.e., HLA-DRB1*0301), which is in linkage disequilibrium with HLA-B8 (HLA-B*0801). Because HLA-DR3 (HLA-DRB1*0301) is itself in linkage disequilibrium with other genes in the class II region of the MHC, this assignment is also necessarily tentative and must be confirmed by detailed mechanistic studies of disease pathogenesis. Understanding associations between HLA and disease is further complicated because most of the associated diseases are of unknown etiology, are complex, and have a poorly understood pathogenesis. Fortunately, during the past 10 years there has been considerable progress in determining the structure, allelic variation, and functional role of most of the currently known genes in the MHC. This functional understanding, combined with the ability to manipulate the genes and gene products in vitro and the opportunity to apply molecular biology to studies of the pathogenesis of disease, has led to a preliminary understanding of the detailed molecular mechanisms underlying the association between the HLA system and disease. Before describing the current state of our knowledge of these mechanisms, it is useful to consider some general characteristics which apply to most, though not all, HLA-associated diseases.

PRINCIPAL CHARACTERISTICS OF HLA-ASSOCIATED DISEASES

HLA-associated diseases share (with some exceptions) a number of important characteristics that must be kept in mind when considering this type of genetic control of disease susceptibility.[7] An awareness of these characteristics facilitates an understanding of the complex patterns of inheritance of this group of diseases.

Most HLA-Associated Diseases Are Autoimmune in Nature. While this statement is true for the vast majority of HLA-associated diseases, there are notable exceptions, including Hodgkin disease, cervical squamous cell carcinoma, and narcolepsy. In the former two cases, it is conceivable that the association with the HLA system is due to genes affecting the immune response to the tumor. Discovery of an association with the HLA system has led to the discovery of the autoimmune nature of the disease in a number of instances, most notably that of IDDM. Whether the same will be true for the recently described, very strong association between HLA-DR2 (i.e., HLA-DRB1*1501) and narcolepsy remains to be seen.

A list of standard abbreviations is located immediately preceding the text in each volume. Additional abbreviations used in this chapter include: AAD = autoimmune Addison disease; AD = Addison disease; AS = ankylosing spondylitis; CD = celiac disease; CVI = common variable immunodeficiency; EAE = experimental autoimmune encephalomyelitis; EOPA JCA = early-onset polyarticular juvenile chronic arthritis; GAD = glutamic acid decarboxylase; GD = Graves disease; HSP = heat shock protein; IFN = interferon; IDDM = insulin-dependent diabetes mellitus; JCA = juvenile chronic arthritis; LPS = lipopolysaccharide; LMP = low-molecular-mass polypeptide; MBP = myelin basic protein; MS = multiple sclerosis (PCP = primarily chronic progressive form; RR = relapsing/remitting form); NOD = nonobese diabetic; PBC = primary biliary cirrhosis; PGA = polyglandular autoimmune syndrome; PV = pemphigus vulgaris; RA = rheumatoid arthritis; RD = Reiter disease; RR = relative risk; SLE = systemic lupus erythematosus; SS = Sjögren syndrome; TAP = transporters associated with antigen processing; TCR = T-cell receptor; TNF = tumor necrosis factor.

Environmental Factors Play a Critical Role in Development of Disease. The most dramatic example of the role of an environmental factor is the now well described association between enteric infection with several gram-negative organisms (*Shigella, Salmonella,* and *Yersinia*) and the subsequent development of Reiter syndrome or reactive arthritis. Almost all individuals who develop Reiter disease or reactive arthritis following gram-negative enteric infection are HLA-B27-positive. Further evidence for the role of environmental factors comes from the observation in monozygotic twin pairs that concordance for IDDM, SLE, rheumatoid arthritis (RA), and a number of other HLA-associated autoimmune diseases is never 100 percent, but varies from 20 to 70 percent. Thus, even in an individual with a proven susceptible genotype, variation in environmental factors (of unknown nature) may prevent development of the autoimmune disease.

Disease Susceptibility Is Determined by Multiple Genes. Comparison of concordance rates for IDDM, RA, and other HLA-associated diseases shows that the concordance rate is always several times lower in HLA-identical sibs than in monozygotic twin pairs. Concordance in monozygotic twins for IDDM is about 50 percent, whereas it is no more than 10 percent in HLA-identical sibs. This difference is almost certainly due to the effect of other genes that determine susceptibility but are not linked to the MHC. Even more convincing evidence of this relation is seen in the spontaneous murine model of IDDM in the nonobese diabetic (NOD) mouse. In this strain, susceptibility is determined by at least six genes, one mapping in the MHC on chromosome 17, and the others mapping on chromosomes 1, 3, 9, and 11. At least two and possibly three of these additional IDDM susceptibility genes appear to be either recessive or dominant with very low penetrance, which is also true of the MHC-mediated susceptibility in this disease. Therefore, for disease to develop in the NOD strain with any frequency, the mice must be homozygous at three to five loci. From this it is apparent, first, that the MHC susceptibility gene(s) is a necessary but not sufficient requirement for development of disease and, second, that possession of an MHC susceptibility gene will lead to development of disease in only a very small percentage of all individuals carrying that particular MHC allele. This polygenic inheritance is the major reason why HLA-associated autoimmune diseases appear to occur sporadically in the population, with no clear-cut pattern of inheritance and a relatively low familial incidence. Thus, in IDDM, although there are many multiple-case families, 85 percent of all cases of IDDM occur in families with no previous family history of this disease. Indeed, prior to the discovery of the association of these diseases with HLA, most of them were thought to have no genetic component whatsoever.

Table 12-1 HLA-Associated Diseases

Disease	HLA	Relative Risk
HLA class I associated diseases		
Ankylosing spondylitis	B27	90
Reiter disease	B27	35
Psoriatic spondylitis	B27	12
Idiopathic hemochromatosis	A3	8
Psoriasis vulgaris	Cw6	13
Behçet disease	B51	16
HLA class II associated diseases		
Rheumatoid arthritis		
Caucasian-Americans	DR4	6
Israeli Jews	DR1	4
Pauciarticular juvenile	DRB1*0801	5
rheumatoid arthritis	DPB1*0201	5
SLE	DRB1*1501	3
	DRB1*0301	3
Sjögren disease	DQB1*0201	12
IDDM	DR3	5
	DR4	6
	DR3/4	15
	DR2	0.2
Addison disease	DR3	6
Graves disease	DR3	3
Hashimoto disease	DQw7	5
Celiac disease	DRB1*0301	11
Primary biliary cirrhosis	DR3	3
Pemphigus vulgaris	DR4	25
Epidermolysis bullosa acquisita	DR5	?
Hodgkin disease	DPw2	0.1
Cervical squamous cell carcinoma	DQw3	7
Multiple sclerosis	DRB1*1501	6
	DQB1*0602/ DQB1*0602	6
Optic neuritis	DRB1*1501	4
Narcolepsy	DRB1*1501	29
Myasthenia gravis	DR3	7
Goodpasture syndrome	DR2	13
Alopecia areata	DQw7	6

More than One MHC-Linked Gene May Play a Role in Disease. Because of the large number of genes in the MHC and the fact that many of them affect immune function directly or indirectly, there is every reason to expect that in some diseases two or more different MHC-linked genes will play a role. There is evidence for this situation in SLE, where HLA-DR2 (HLA-DRB1*1501) and HLA-DR3 (HLA-DRB1*0301) have been shown to predispose the carrier to disease, and, at the same time, there is clear evidence that heterozygous or homozygous null alleles for C2 and C4 play a major role in increasing the susceptibility to SLE. A number of other genes in the MHC, in addition to the class I and class II MHC alleles, are currently under study with respect to their role in disease susceptibility.

The Initiating Event and the Target Autoantigen Are Unknown for Most Autoimmune Diseases. This statement is true for almost all the HLA-associated diseases listed in Table 12-1, except Graves disease and myasthenia gravis. While progress has been made in identifying candidate autoantigens in IDDM and MS, and some progress has been made in RA, at present the primary targets of the autoimmune response in these diseases have not been definitely established. Without knowing the critical target antigens, it is difficult to analyze the role of HLA class I and class II molecules in presenting peptides from these self antigens to the T-cell immune system. Without this information, assignments of disease susceptibility to specific HLA loci and alleles, and hypotheses concerning disease pathogenesis, must remain provisional. Once target self antigens have been identified, available techniques can be used to analyze the role of HLA class I and class II molecules and other HLA linked genes in disease pathogenesis. It is likely that this goal will be achieved for the most frequent autoimmune diseases (IDDM, RA, and MS) in the near future.

GENETICS AND STRUCTURE OF HLA PROTEINS

In all vertebrate organisms, HLA antigens are highly polymorphic cell surface proteins that present peptides to T lymphocytes and thereby affect specific T-cell immune responses. HLA class I and class II antigens form structurally related membrane-anchored heterodimers, each consisting of two membrane-proximal domains with homology to the immunoglobulin (Ig) superfamily and two

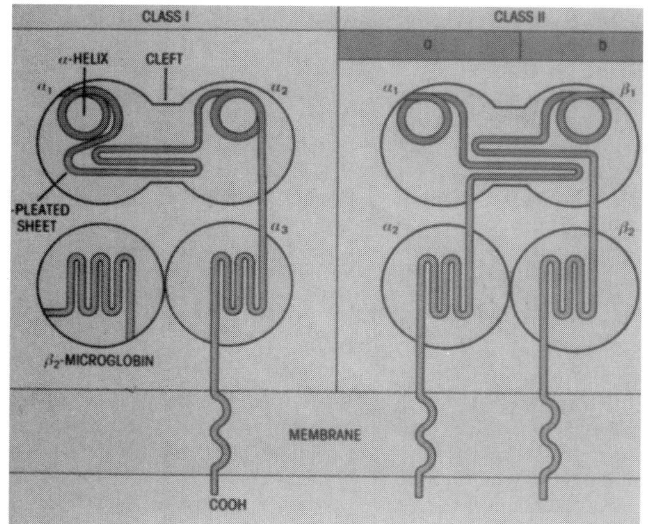

Fig. 12-1 Schematic illustration of the domain structure of class I and class II major histocompatibility molecules. (*Reprinted from Roitt's Essential Immunology, 7th ed., with permission of Blackwell Scientific Publications Limited.*)

membrane-distal domains with a peptide-binding site. HLA class I antigens consist of a polymorphic heavy chain associated with an invariant light chain, which is called β_2 microglobulin, whereas HLA class II proteins are formed by a pair of polymorphic proteins, the α or heavy chain and the β or light chain (Fig. 12-1).

The genes encoding HLA antigens reside within a 4.2-Mb region on the short arm of human chromosome 6, where at least 23 class II genes and 15 class I genes can be found (Fig. 12-2). Although most of these loci are either nonfunctional or of unknown function, the major expressed HLA genes are among the most polymorphic loci in the genome, with the polymorphism concentrated in the peptide-binding site. X-ray crystallography of this antigen-binding site, together with recent information on the nature of peptides bound in it, have produced a detailed molecular picture of antigen presentation by HLA molecules, thus providing the basis for understanding the fundamental molecular events in immune recognition.

HLA CLASS I PROTEINS

Structure

All class I antigens have a characteristic protein structure and gene organization.[8,9] The 44-kDa heavy chain, the product of the class I gene in the MHC complex, consists of three extracellular domains, the α_1, α_2, and α_3 domains (Fig. 12-1); the membrane-proximal α_3 domain is connected by a short (four-amino-acid) hydrophilic peptide to the hydrophobic transmembrane region (25 to 28 amino acids), which is followed by a C-terminal cytoplasmic tail (30 amino acids). The N-terminal α_1 (90 amino acids) and α_2 (92 amino acids) domains are exposed on the surface of the molecule, display most of the polymorphic class I variability, and together form the cleft-like peptide-binding site (for details of the HLA class I crystal structure, see "Structure of Crystallized HLA Class I Molecules" below and reference 10). Invariably, an N-linked glycosylation site is found at residue 86, together with a disulfide bridge between residues 101 and 164. Another disulfide bridge is

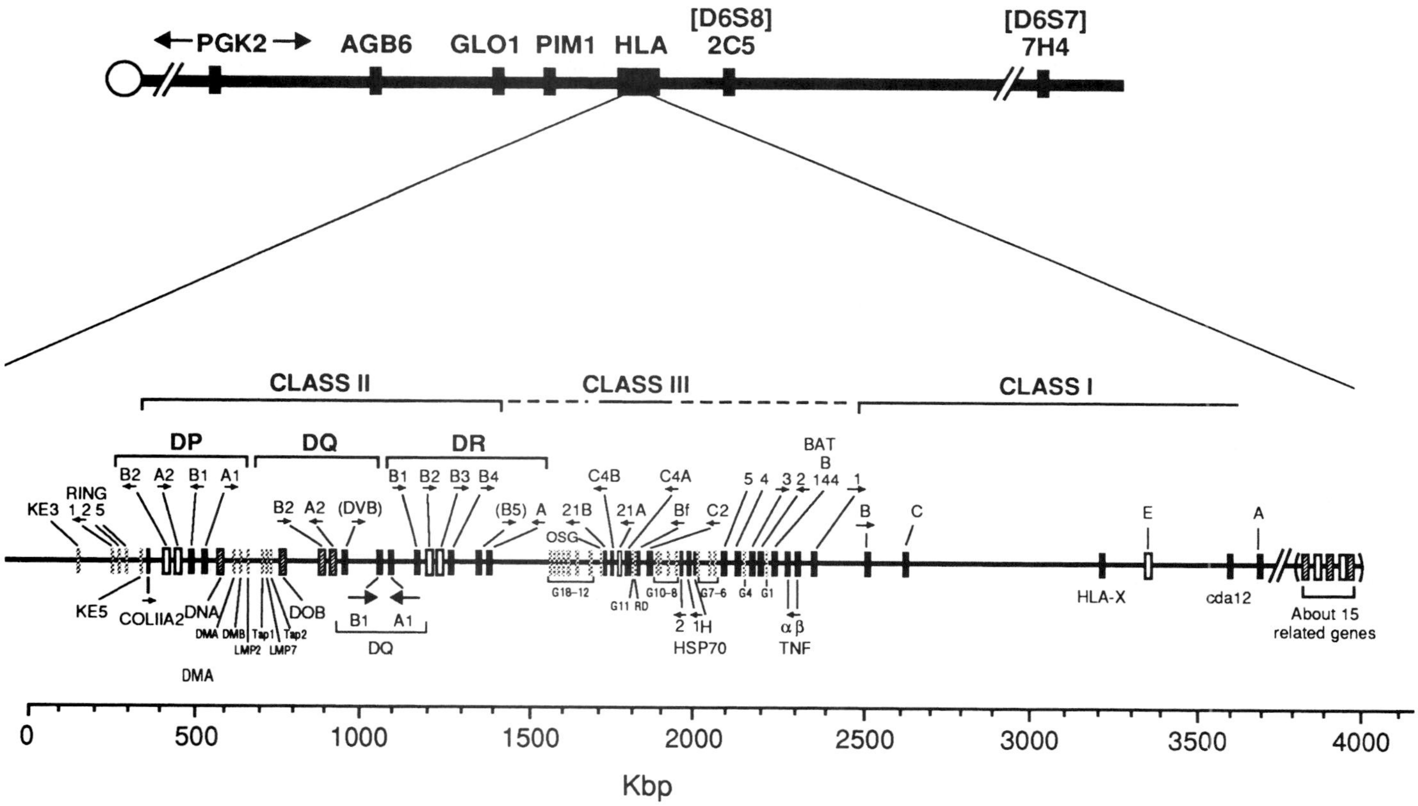

PGK2 AGB6 GLO1 PIM1 HLA [D6S8] 2C5 [D6S7] 7H4

CLASS II CLASS III CLASS I

DP DQ DR

0 500 1000 1500 2000 2500 3000 3500 4000

Kbp

Fig. 12-2 Map of the human major histocompatibility complex on the short arm of chromosome 6. Genes are shown as boxes: filled boxes = expressed genes; open boxes = pseudogenes; cross-hatched boxes = genes which are potentially expressible. Recently discovered genes are shown in gray. Many of the new genes were discovered at the same time by several laboratories and have therefore been variously named. The relationship and the product encoded by these genes have only been established to a limited extent.

located in the less polymorphic α_3 domain (92 amino acids), which is also the major binding site for the accessory molecule CD8; this protein is found on the surface of cytotoxic T cells and contributes to the specific interaction of the T cell receptor (TCR) on these cells with HLA class I molecules.

Located under the complex of the α_1 and α_2 domains, the α_3 domain is noncovalently linked to β_2 microglobulin, a virtually nonpolymorphic 12-kDa protein encoded on human chromosome 15. Structurally, both the α_3 domain and β_2 microglobulin belong to the Ig superfamily, a group of proteins which in general are involved in cellular interactions and which exhibit homology at the levels of DNA and protein.[11] Besides Igs and the membrane-proximal domains of HLA class I and class II proteins, other lymphocyte cell-surface proteins, such as the TCR, CD1, CD2, CD4, and CD8 molecules belong to this family. Members of the Ig superfamily typically have a sandwich-like structure that consists of two sheets of β-pleated strands that are linked by a disulfide bond. Hydrophobic and hydrophilic residues alternate in the three or four β strands of each sheet, with hydrophobic side chains pointing into the space between the sheets.

The conserved domain composition of HLA class I antigens is paralleled by an invariant gene organization.[12] Of the seven exons, the first encodes a 20-amino-acid leader peptide that directs nascent class I proteins into the endoplasmic reticulum and is then removed. Exons 2, 3, and 4 encode the α_1, α_2, and α_3 domains, respectively. The fifth exon encodes the connecting peptide, the transmembrane region, and the first 7 residues of the cytoplasmic tail, the rest of which is encoded by exons 6 and 7.

Gene Organization and Loci in the HLA Class I Region

The HLA class I region comprises the telomeric 2 to 2.2 Mb of the HLA gene complex (Fig. 12-2).[13] Among the 15 detected class I genes,[14] only three — the HLA-A, HLA-B, and HLA-C loci — constitute the core of the so-called classic HLA class I genes. These genes are highly polymorphic, are expressed on virtually all nucleated cells, and are known, at least in the case of HLA-A and -B, to restrict T cell responses to intracellular antigens. Whereas numerous examples of the presentation of antigenic fragments to T cells by HLA-A and -B molecules have been described,[15] no such evidence has yet been provided for HLA-C proteins. In addition, the fact that the degree of polymorphism in HLA-C genes, particularly in their antigen-binding site, is significantly lower than in HLA-A and -B genes has raised the speculation that this locus may be on its way toward the "junkyard of evolution."[8]

The other class I loci show little or no polymorphism.[16] Some of these loci — the "nonclassic" class I genes (HLA-E, -G, and -F) — are transcribed, and their gene products, which are associated with β_2 microglobulin, can be detected. However, the function of these proteins is not known. There are only a few cases in which a function is known for a nonclassic gene. For example, the murine Qa-1 protein presents some synthetic peptide copolymers to $\gamma\delta$ T cells, a class of T cells which is known to recognize antigens in a largely non-HLA-allele restricted manner.[17] Furthermore, recent evidence suggests that some nonclassic MHC class I proteins may have become specialized to present peptides that are derived from certain intracellularly replicating bacteria (e.g., *Listeria monocytogenes*) and have the unusual feature of an N-formylated N-terminus.[18] The apparently non-polymorphic HLA-G gene seems to be expressed exclusively in early-gestation human cytotrophoblasts, which are devoid of classic HLA class I proteins.[19] The HLA-G molecule may be involved in placental-maternal interactions.

Other class I genes include four pseudogenes, which are not transcribed owing to deleterious mutations, as well as some gene fragments of not fully characterized loci (HLA-X, cda 12). The HLA-H gene is transcribed but its protein is most likely nonfunctional because of structural abnormalities in the α_2 domain as well as a frameshift mutation in the α_3 domain.[16] Although all these genes may not have functional importance, their investigation has yielded some insight into probable evolutionary mechanisms associated with HLA genes (see "Evolution in HLA Genes," below).

Because of the large size of the HLA class I region, the distances and orientation of the loci in it have not been fully established. In particular, some uncertainty remains regarding the exact distances between the HLA-C and HLA-A genes. Linkage maps of entire chromosomal regions, such as the HLA complex, have been generated by cloning and mapping of large overlapping genomic fragments in cosmid libraries or, more recently, yeast artificial chromosomes.[20,21]

Polymorphism in HLA Class I Genes

A key feature of classic HLA class I genes is their extraordinary degree of polymorphism. This feature is considered to make it possible for such a wide range of antigenic peptides to be recognized and dealt with by the immune system of the species, although not always by the immune system of a particular individual or small group (see "Malaria," below). The wealth of recently obtained nucleotide sequence data, together with the analysis of HLA class I protein crystal structure, has revealed the molecular basis for the polymorphic recognition system provided by HLA proteins.

At present, 125 alleles of the HLA-A, -B, and -C genes have been officially acknowledged by the WHO Nomenclature Committee for Factors of the HLA System. Given the increasing number of studies of HLA sequences from individuals with a greater diversity of ethnic backgrounds, this number certainly will increase in the future. With 61 alleles, the HLA-B locus is more polymorphic than the HLA-A locus (41 alleles) and considerably more polymorphic than the HLA-C locus (18 alleles).[14] A special feature of the polymorphism in the HLA-A gene is the predominance of a single allele and its closely related variant, HLA-A2, which is found in 50 percent of Caucasian individuals.

An HLA sequence is assigned to the HLA-A, -B, or -C loci on the basis of conserved residues: Of the 330 residues in an HLA class I heavy chain, 62 are conserved among alleles of an individual locus but vary between the different loci. Most of these conserved residues[51] are found in the α_3 domain and in the transmembrane and cytoplasmic portions of the class I protein; in contrast, the polymorphic positions that distinguish alleles of the same locus are in the α_1 and α_2 domains.[22]

Most of the allelic polymorphism in HLA class I genes is clustered in the membrane-distal α_1 and α_2 domains (Fig. 12-3), which constitute the peptide-binding site and contact the polymorphic antigen receptor of T cells.[22,23] Individual class I alleles differ by 13 to 30 substitutions in these domains from a consensus sequence for all α_1 and α_2 domains of classic HLA class I proteins. Fifty percent of the 182 residues in these domains are polymorphic. In most of these polymorphic positions, only two or three amino acids can be found when all known alleles are compared. In 20 positions, however, a particularly high number of substitutions can be observed. Nearly all (19) of these positions are located in or close to the antigen binding site and presumably are involved in contact with a bound peptide or the TCR. Polymorphism in HLA class I (and class II) genes thus is highly focused in the functional center of the proteins, where differences in the size, charge, polarity, and hydrophobicity of amino acid side chains are likely to influence the interaction with the two ligands for HLA molecules — antigenic peptides and antigen-specific TCRs.

Evolution in HLA Genes

The availability of HLA complex maps and HLA nucleotide sequences for a number of species has made possible some interesting insights into the evolution of complexity and polymorphism in the HLA genes.[8,24] HLA class I and class II genes are thought to have evolved from a single common ancestor gene, which consisted of an Ig-like membrane-proximal domain and a peptide-binding, membrane-distal domain. The multiplicity

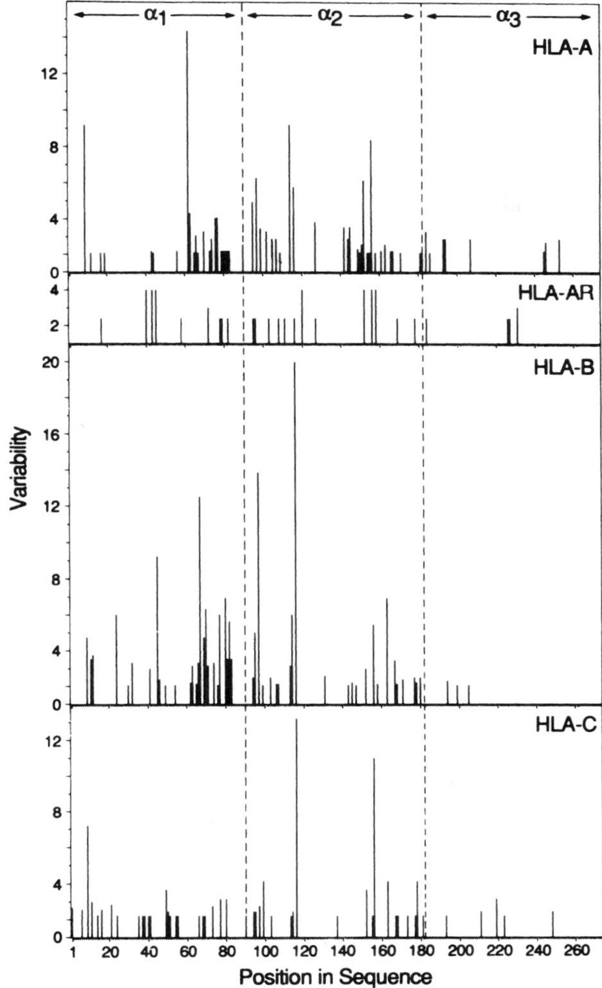

Fig. 12-3 Variability plot of the predicted products of the HLA-A, HLA-AR, HLA-B, and HLA-C alleles. Variability is the quotient of the number of amino acids found at a position in the sequence divided by the most common. The HLA-AR alleles are HLA-A related pseudogenes. (*Reproduced from Lawlor et al. Evolution of class-I MHC genes and proteins: From natural selection to thymic selection. Ann Rev Immunol 8:23, 1990, with permission.*)

of gene loci in the class I and class II regions is likely the result of gene duplications. While such duplications lead to an increase in the number of functional loci, the reverse process can also be observed in HLA genes: inactivation of certain loci, such as the HLA-H gene, resulting in a reduction in the number of functional HLA genes. Polymorphism in HLA genes has generally been interpreted as an evolutionary advantage, since a larger spectrum of antigen-binding sites should enable the species to recognize a wider array of pathogens, such as viruses, bacteria, and parasites. Although the theory of "pathogen-driven diversification" is an attractive hypothesis, epidemiologic evidence supporting it is scarce (see "Malaria," below).

A comparison of allelic nucleotide sequences yields additional evidence for an evolutionary advantage from polymorphism in HLA proteins. The rate of silent nucleotide substitutions, in other words, substitutions that do not change the amino acid encoded by a nucleotide triplet, is considered to reflect the overall mutation rate in a gene. The number of such substitutions found in positions contributing to the antigen-recognition site and in other parts of the extracellular class I molecule is roughly equivalent, arguing that the rate of mutations is equal in these regions. However, when the ratio of productive substitutions (ones that code for a different amino acid) to silent substitutions is compared, a striking difference between these regions becomes apparent: this ratio is about 3 in the antigen-recognition site, but 0.5 in other regions of the molecule.[25] Thus, evolutionary pressure has conserved most regions of HLA class I molecules but has selected for productive substitutions in the antigen-recognition site.

Polymorphism in HLA genes appears to have occurred relatively early in evolution. For example, not only the evolution of the HLA-A and -B loci but also the allelic diversification into certain HLA-A and -B alleles seems to have taken place in a common ancestor of humans and chimpanzees. Conservation of allelic elements dates back even farther than primates. In a comparison of murine and human class II molecules, the amino acid and nucleotide sequences of the hypervariable regions appear to be derived from a common pool of allelic elements that existed in a common ancestor of the two species.[26] Thus, the most variable regions of HLA proteins may have been generated relatively early in evolution, and more recent evolutionary modification may have entailed mainly exchange and shuffling of the previously generated elements.

Several mechanisms are considered to have contributed to polymorphism in HLA proteins. Point mutations, originally thought to be the major cause of allelic diversification, appear to be only one of these mechanisms. Others include homologous recombination, whereby gene segments are exchanged between alleles of the same locus or different loci, and gene conversion, which entails copying gene segments from one allele or locus to another.[27] Gene segments transferred by conversion can be as short as 44 nucleotides. An example of a reciprocal recombination is the HLA-Aw69 allele; it carries the α_1 domain of A68, while the α_2 and α_3 domains originate from the A2 allele.[28]

Structure of Crystallized HLA Class I Molecules

Our understanding of the function of HLA class I molecules has been greatly advanced by the availability of detailed crystallographic data on the protein structure. Two HLA-A proteins, HLA-A2.1[10] and HLA-Aw68,[29] were solubilized by papain cleavage at a site 13 residues from the transmembrane region, and the crystallized material was subjected to x-ray analysis (Fig. 12-4). Additional high-resolution structural data have been obtained on the HLA-B27 protein; in this case, the analysis focused on the antigen-binding site and the peptide material contained in it.[30] Very recently, high-resolution analyses have also been performed on a murine class I molecule that had been crystallized together with a single peptide species,[31] as opposed to the peptide mixture found in the binding sites of natural molecules.

Analysis of the Ig-like α_3 domain and the associated β_2 microglobulin molecule of HLA-A2 did not reveal major surprising features;[10] both showed the sandwich structure typical of members of the Ig superfamily of proteins, with two antiparallel β-pleated sheets connected by disulfide bonds. The α_1 and α_2 domains form a symmetrical structure in a manner that has been termed "intramolecular dimerization." Each domain consists of an N-terminal β sheet followed by a long α-helical region (Figs. 12-4 and 12-5). The β sheets and α helices of the two domains contact each other in a dyad symmetrical fashion, such that the two β sheets form a single extended sheet, which is topped by two parallel α helices. Between the two α helices runs a deep groove about 25 Å long and 10 Å wide, which is the predicted antigen-binding site of HLA class I molecules. It is filled with a large, continuous region of electron-dense material, which represents the mixture of peptides bound in the groove.

When the polymorphic residues in the α_1 and α_2 domains are localized in the HLA-A2 crystal, the significance of the polymorphism in class I proteins for the interaction with the TCR and the bound peptide becomes immediately apparent.[23] Of the 17 positions in which more than six different amino acids have been found in HLA alleles, only two are outside the binding site. Five are located in the β sheet that forms the bottom of the binding site; their side chains point upward and thus are predicted to

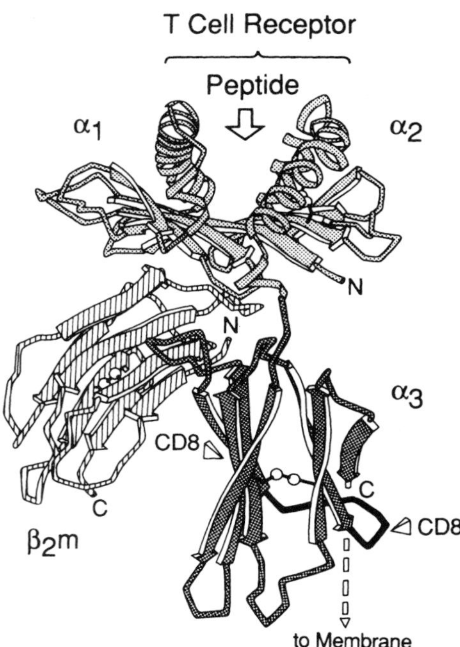

Fig. 12-4 Structure of an HLA class I molecule (HLA-A2) based on x-ray crystallographic analysis. β Strands are shown as thick arrows pointing in the amino-to-carboxy direction, and α helices are shown as helical ribbons. The loop of the α_3 domain implicated in CD8 binding is shown in black and indicated with arrowheads. The peptide-binding groove and the hypothesized area of interaction with the T cell receptor are indicated. β_2m = β_2 microglobulin. *(Reproduced from Lawlor et al. Evolution of class-I MHC genes and proteins: From natural selection to thymic selection. Ann Rev Immunol 8:23, 1990, with permission.)*

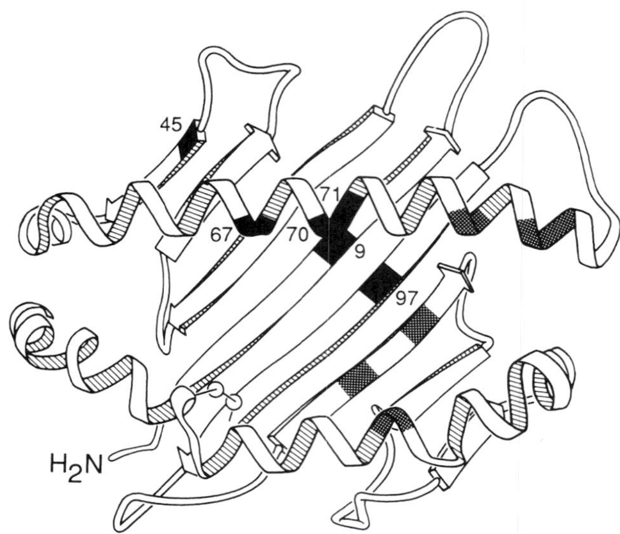

Fig. 12-5 Location of conserved (black) and polymorphic residues of the HLA-B27 alleles. The pattern of substitutions at positions 9, 45, 67, 70, 71, and 97 distinguishes the HLA-B27 alleles from other HLA-A, -B, and -C molecules and may be of importance for HLA-27 related diseases. *(Reproduced from Benjamin & Parham. Guilt by association: HLA-B27 and ankylosing spondylitis [see comments]. Immunol Today 11:137, 1990, with permission.)*

interact with peptides in the groove. Another six are found in the sides of the α helices that face the groove and thus can contact the peptide as well as the TCR. Three polymorphic residues point upward from the α helices and presumably bind only to the TCR.

The analysis of HLA-Aw68 crystals showed that the structure of A2 and Aw68 is extremely similar.[29] A striking difference, however, was found in the antigen-binding groove. Allelic substitutions in positions flanking the antigen-binding site of Aw68 result in the formation of a negatively charged pocket deep within the binding site. Similarly, a high-resolution analysis of the antigen-binding site of HLA-B27 revealed six pocket-like structures, again partly formed by polymorphic residues. Peptide material was detectable in the B27 antigen-binding site; peptides seemed to be bound in an extended conformation, and the three-dimensional shape of the "peptide cloud" closely matched the shape of the surrounding binding site.[30] Further refinement of the crystallographic analysis of HLA-B27,[32] together with the study of a murine class I molecule crystallized with one of two defined peptides, revealed the network of atomic interactions that contribute to the peptide/MHC binding.[31,33] Thus, peptides seem to be tightly fitted into the binding site only in some deep pockets at its ends, which accommodate the N- and C-terminal residue of the peptide, and at the "anchor residue," a characteristic residue required at a certain peptide position for binding to a specific class I allele (see "Peptides Bound in the Antigen-Binding Site," below). All other peptide residues contribute little to the high-affinity binding of peptide to MHC, which explains high variability at these positions. The ends of the peptide are held in the pockets by hydrogen bonds between the main-chain atoms of the peptide and side chain atoms of the MHC residues that form the pocket; the latter are highly conserved. Again, the involvement of the peptide main chain (instead of its side chains) in the most important bonds provides a mechanism by which the number of potential binders is greatly increased. Taken together, these data demonstrate that polymorphism in the HLA class I binding site is reflected morphologically as variation in the geometry and chemistry of pocket-like structures that restrict the range of peptides that can be accommodated in the groove. The molecular construction of the peptide-binding site combines allele-specific high-affinity binding of some peptide residues with great variability permitted for the others; on the functional level, these features translate into a peptide-binding molecule the various alleles of which are each able to firmly bind a defined but large set of peptides.

Peptides Bound in the Antigen-Binding Site

In order to be assembled with β_2 microglobulin and transported to and expressed on the cell surface, an HLA class I molecule requires the presence of peptides that bind to that specific HLA allele.[34,35] The peptides are provided by a process termed antigen processing, blockage of which results in low or absent expression of class I molecules. Thus, in a natural class I molecule, the antigen-binding site seems always to be occupied by a peptide. Direct sequencing of peptide material eluted from purified HLA class I molecules by acid treatment has provided information about the characteristics of peptides generated by natural antigen processing. Surprisingly, it was found that these natural peptides are significantly shorter than most of the peptides that had previously been used in in vitro experiments on antigen presentation by HLA class I molecules. From two human and three murine HLA class I molecules, only peptides with a length between 8 and 10 residues were recovered, with a predominance of 9-mers.[36–38] This finding is supported by the observation that 9-mers are 100- to 1000-fold more efficient than 12- to 16-mers with an identical core sequence when the binding of peptides to, and the assembly of, an HLA class I molecule are measured in vitro.[39]

Comparisons of the sequences in the eluted peptide pool and of the sequences of fractionated peptide peaks with the sequences of peptides known to bind the class I alleles under investigation have revealed that the chemical and geometrical properties of individual class I alleles (see "Structure of Crystallized HLA Class I Molecules," above) result in allele-specific peptide motifs that restrict the range of potential peptide ligands. All the peptides investigated contain at least two "anchor positions" in which only a single amino acid or a few amino acids with closely related side chains have been detected.[36,38] Invariably, one of these anchors was the C-terminal position, in which only a few hydrophobic amino acids have been found in peptide material from all class I proteins. In both human class I molecules analyzed so far (HLA-A2 and HLA-B27), peptide position 2 seems to be the dominant anchor residue; in B27 only an arginine, and in A2 only leucine, isoleucine, or methionine are allowed at this position. Greater but not unlimited variation has been found in the other positions; in HLA-B27, variation seems to be more limited at the positions where the side chain points into the antigen-binding site. Despite the restricted variation of amino acids in all peptide positions, the total number of different peptide sequences that could bind in the HLA-B27 groove according to the peptide motif was calculated to be 13 million. Although this figure demonstrates the wide array of peptides that can be presented by class I molecules, it is less than 1/3000 of the 500 billion possible different sequences of a nine-amino-acid peptide. As expected from the investigations on antigen processing, the peptides bound in the B27 binding site were derived from abundant cytosolic or nuclear proteins, such as members of the 90-kDa heat-shock protein family, histones, and ribosomal proteins.[40]

HLA CLASS II PROTEINS

Structure of Class II Molecules

HLA class II molecules are structurally highly related to class I molecules; this relatedness includes the domain organization and probably also the antigen-binding site.[41] Like class I molecules, they have been shown to bind antigenic peptides and to present them to T cells that display specific antigen receptors.[42] Nevertheless, the restricted expression and distinct pathway of antigen processing associated with class II molecules gives them a very different role in immune recognition from that of class I molecules. Class II molecules are predominantly involved in the interaction between specific cell types that regulate immune responses. Among these are B cells, activated T cells, dendritic cells, and cells of the myelomonocytoid lineage (macrophages). Most cell types (including most T cells) are usually class II negative, but the expression of class II proteins can be induced by the lymphokines interferon γ (IFN-γ) and tumor necrosis factor α (TNFα) on many cells of nonlymphoid lineages, including fibroblasts and many tumor cells.

Class II proteins are heterodimers composed of two membrane-anchored proteins that are encoded in the class II region of the MHC complex (Fig. 12-1). One α or heavy chain (30 to 32 kDa) associates with one β or light chain (27 to 29 kDa) to form a class II molecule. Both α and β chains have four protein domains, which are encoded by separate exons. Two extracellular domains (α_1/β_1 and α_2/β_2) are linked to a third domain that comprises a short hydrophilic peptide (13 amino acids) and the hydrophobic transmembrane region. This domain is followed by the C-terminal cytoplasmic domain, a short tail of 3 to 20 amino acids.

As in class I molecules, the N-terminal α_1 and β_1 domains of the two chains contain the antigen-binding site, and it is this region which has a high degree of polymorphism. The α_1 domain consists of 85 to 88 amino acids and has a conserved glycosylation site at position 78 (two *N*-linked glycosylation sites in DRα). The β_1 domain, composed of 95 amino acids, contains a disulfide loop that connects residues 15 and 79, and an *N*-linked glycan at position 19. The membrane-proximal α_2 and β_2 domains correspond to β_2 microglobulin and α_3 of class I molecules and exhibit sequence and structural homology with the Ig superfamily. Both domains have a length of 95 amino acids and have the characteristic disulfide loop, which spans 56 amino acids (residues 107 to 163 in α_2 and 117 to 173 in β_2).

Three isotypes, called DR, DQ, and DP, are distinguished among the class II proteins. For each of these isotypes, one α chain and one or several β chains are encoded in close proximity to each other in the class II region of the HLA complex. Generally, α and β chains of the same isotype combine to form a class II molecule; transfection experiments, however, have shown that α and β chains of mixed isotypes, e.g., DRα chains with DQβ chains, can form "hybrid" molecules, thus increasing the number of heterodimeric antigen-binding sites on class II molecules. The formation of such interisotypic pairs seems to occur between specific alleles only.[43] It has been proposed that such hybrid class II molecules may be important in certain MHC-associated autoimmune diseases.[44]

In DR molecules, only the β chain is polymorphic, whereas in DQ and DP molecules, both chains contribute polymorphic residues to the antigen-binding site. Since most individuals are heterozygous, DQ and DP heterodimers can be formed by a combination of different α and β chains on the same (*cis*-) or different (*trans*-complementation) chromosomes, resulting in a possible total of four DQ and four DP proteins for a heterozygous individual.

Unlike the situation with HLA class I molecules, crystallographic data on the structure of class II proteins are not yet available. However, taking advantage of the significant structural homologies between class I and class II proteins, a model for the class II antigen-binding site has been constructed.[45] This model makes it possible to localize polymorphic residues and, in turn, to predict which residues are likely to interact with the TCR and/or the bound peptide. The model depicts the antigen-binding site of class II molecules as an internal cavity that is lined by two α helices and closed at the bottom by a sheet of eight β-pleated strands; the α_1 and β_1 chains each contribute one α helix as a side wall and a β sheet as part of the bottom layer of the binding site. The most polymorphic residues in the α_1 and β_1 domains, which are clustered in three "hypervariable regions" (HVR), are expected to be located in the β sheet (HVR1 and HVR2) as well as in the α helix (HVR3), where they point into or up from the binding site. As in class I molecules, the polymorphism in class II molecules is predicted to affect both peptide binding and TCR recognition/binding.

Biosynthesis and Peptide Loading

In parallel to the distinct functions of class I and class II molecules, the assembly and intracellular transport of these molecules follow different rules.[46] Class I proteins are loaded in the endoplasmic reticulum (ER) with peptides derived from intracellular proteins; in the absence of these peptides, assembly of β_2 microglobulin and the class I heavy chain does not occur, and class I proteins are unstable and rapidly degraded.[35] Properly assembled class I proteins are glycosylated in the Golgi stack before they appear on the cell surface. Most class II proteins, however, seem neither to be loaded with peptides in the ER nor to be dependent (at least initially) on peptides for correct assembly. Soon after the nascent class II α and β chains are inserted into the membrane of the endoplasmic reticulum, a complex of the class II chains and a third protein, the invariant chain (Ii), is assembled.[47] Ii is a nonpolymorphic protein that has several intracellular forms ranging in molecular mass from 25 to 41 kDa, and that is not encoded in the HLA complex. Complexing of the newly synthesized class II chains with the Ii seems to serve several purposes. First, the Ii chain appears to contain several peptide sequences that act as routing signals for the class II/Ii complex.[48] Ii chains that occur alone or associated with monomeric class II chains are shuttled to a cellular compartment where they are degraded. In a correctly proceeding assembly, however, differently modified forms of Ii first aggregate as an Ii trimer in the ER. This trimer is then sequentially complexed with HLA class IIα/β dimers, resulting in a final complex of nine protein chains. These nonamers are routed first to the Golgi stack and then to a peripheral cellular compartment that is related to early endosome

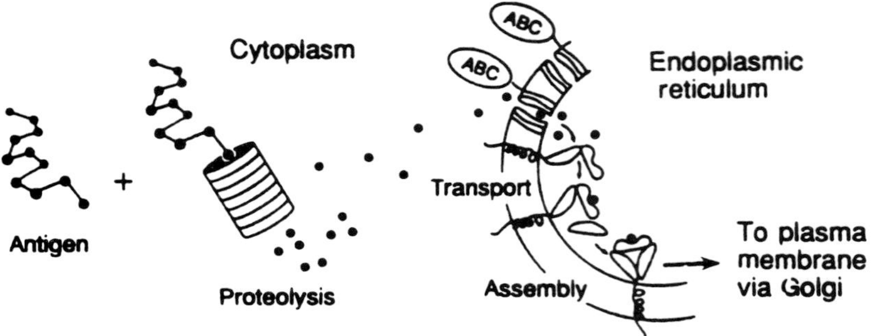

Fig. 12-6 Degradation of a cytoplasmic antigen into peptides, their transport from cytoplasm to the endoplasmic reticulum, and their assembly with class I MHC molecules. (*Reproduced from Parham. Transporters of delight. Nature 348:674, 1990, with permission © 1990 Macmillan Magazines Ltd.*)

or lysosome vesicles.[49] In the latter compartment, class II molecules encounter peptide fragments of endocytosed proteins, which are presumably broken down in these acidic vesicles in order to bind to class II.

Before the class II proteins can bind exogenously derived peptides, however, Ii has to be removed. In vitro studies have shown that antigenic peptides cannot bind to class II molecules unless Ii has been removed.[50] Solubilized Ii can in turn bind to class II proteins and can compete for binding with peptides.[51] Removal of Ii from the trimeric complex and subsequent degradation of Ii is known to occur in the endosomal peripheral vesicles; consequently, class II proteins on the cell surface are not associated with Ii. Thus, Ii not only directs class II proteins to peripheral endocytotic compartments, it also seems to prevent peptides from binding to class II molecules before the latter enter these compartments. Nevertheless, class II proteins have been shown to present some peptides derived from intracellular virus proteins. At present, it is not clear whether these peptides are generated in or transported into the endosomes or whether they bind in the ER to a minor fraction of class II molecules that are not blocked by Ii.

Although most class II molecules seem to bind first to Ii and then to peptides derived from exogenous proteins, neither of the latter is required for surface expression of class II. Cells that do not synthesize Ii can display normal amounts of class II proteins on the surface.[47] In contrast to HLA class I molecules, for some HLA class II alleles, empty molecules (i.e., molecules with an empty peptide-binding site) can be expressed on the surface of cells that are incapable of supplying peptides for class II loading.[52] Thus, assembly of stable class II heterodimers is possible in the absence of peptide.

Peptide binding to class II proteins, however, seems to affect the steric conformation and the lifetime of class II molecules. Class II molecules can assume a "compact" or a "floppy" conformation, as determined by their mobility in nondenaturing polyacrylamide gels.[53] In the absence of peptide, class II proteins assume the floppy conformation, but upon binding of peptide, they adopt the compact form. Binding of peptide and transition to the compact form stabilizes the class II proteins, reducing their tendency to denature and aggregate in vitro. Although most floppy class II molecules are degraded before reaching the cell surface, empty molecules in the floppy conformation can be found on the cell surface. These observations suggest that the stability and lifetime of class II molecules depend on the availability of peptide ligands.[54] This differs from class I molecules, in which peptides are critical for assembly and surface expression.

Initial data providing insight into the nature of the peptides that are found bound to class II molecules suggest that they tend to be longer and less restricted than the peptides that bind to class I molecules. Elution from two murine class II molecules analogous to the human DR and DQ proteins yielded peptides 13 to 17 amino acids long that seemed to be variably truncated at the C-terminus.[55] No obvious peptide motif was detectable. These results suggest that the antigen-binding site of class II molecules (unlike that of class I molecules) is open on one end, and that the C-terminus of a bound peptide protrudes from this open end and therefore is susceptible to successive trimming. Interestingly, the sequences of the bound peptides revealed that class II molecules may present predominantly peptides derived from endogenous cellular proteins, thereby resembling class I molecules. More recent data on peptides eluted from the human DR1 molecule confirmed that endogenous proteins contribute most (19 out of 20 sequenced) of the peptides found in class II molecules.[56] It has been suggested that many of these proteins are membrane proteins that encounter MHC class II during recycling. Peptides eluted from DR1 molecules were truncated at both ends; moreover, a peptide sequence motif, although less precise than that of class I molecules, was identified.

Gene Organization and Loci in the HLA Class II Region

Besides class II genes, the 900-kb class II region contains several other genes, most of which have recently been discovered as a result of systematic screenings of this genomic region for new genes (Fig. 12-2). Further genes will probably be discovered in all regions of the HLA complex. Some of the novel genes in the class II region (in particular those located centromeric to the DP genes) have functions that are not known or are not related to the immune system; these genes will not be dealt with here. Four novel genes, the TAP1, TAP2, LMP2, and LMP7 genes, have either been shown to be or are likely to be involved in the processing of antigens that are presented by class I proteins. The TAP1 and TAP2 genes code for membrane transporter proteins with an ATP-binding cassette; these proteins pair to form a heterodimer,[57] are required for proper HLA class I molecule assembly, and are thought to transport peptides into the ER.[58] The LMP2[59] and LMP7[60] genes encode subunits of a large protease that may be involved in proteolytic cleavage of antigenic proteins in the cytosol (Fig. 12-6).

Three sets of loci comprising pairs of α and β genes in the class II region are known to be expressed as class II heterodimers, which can present peptides to class II-restricted T cells. These are the DR, DQ(A1/B1), and DP(A1/B1) loci. (Numbers are used in the last place in these designations when more than one homologous gene is known at the given locus; for example, the five DRB genes are called DRB1 to DRB5.[14]) The DR subregion contains a gene for a nonpolymorphic α chain plus nine β chain genes, of which five are nonfunctional pseudogenes. These DRβ chain genes are never found all together on the same chromosome; instead, the number and the types of DRB genes in an individual HLA class II region depend on the DR "haplotype." This term is used to designate the whole set of HLA genes on one chromosome; because of the strong linkage disequilibrium between DR, DQ, and often also HLA-B genes, a specific DR allele in an individual of a given ethnic origin will often indicate a whole set of DR/DQ/B alleles; the term "DR haplotype" is used to mean this typical set of class II (and sometimes class I) alleles. Different DR haplotypes carry different numbers of DRB genes.[61] For example, the DRB2 pseudogene is found in most haplotypes, but the DRB genes 3, 4, and 5 are found only in certain haplotypes (see Fig. 12-2). The DRB1 gene is the most polymorphic locus in the class II region, whereas the additional expressed DRB loci exhibit limited polymorphism (DRB3, DRB5) or none at all (DRB4).

In the DQ (formerly DC or DS) subregion, two α chain and three β chain loci are known. Only the DQA1 and DQB1 loci are transcribed and expressed as functional heterodimers; the nonpolymorphic DQA2 and DQB2 (formerly DXA2 and DXB2) genes are not transcribed, although no obvious defect has been found in their structure.[62] The DQB3 (also called DV) gene is a pseudogene with deleterious mutations. The DP (formerly SB) subregion contains two pairs of A and B genes; the A1 and B1 genes are expressed, while the A2 and B2 genes are pseudogenes.[63]

Several additional class II genes are transcribed and are probably expressed as proteins, but their function is not yet known. The DOB and DNA genes both lack an identified partner to form a heterodimer. The nonpolymorphic DNA gene (formerly called DZ or DOA) is transcribed at low levels; because it has a nonconsensus polyadenylation signal, most of the resulting mRNA is inefficiently polyadenylated.[64] The DO gene is the only class II gene for which transcription is not induced by IFN-γ. Another unusual feature is its hydrophobic β_1 domain, which may indicate that the DOβ chain does not contribute to the formation of a typical class II antigen binding site.[65] The murine counterpart of DO, Ob, has been shown to be expressed as a heterodimer with a novel α chain in a very restricted range of cell types (B cells, medullary T cells).[66]

The DMA and DMB genes are the most recently discovered members of the HLA class II family; both are inducible by IFN-γ and are nearly as closely related to HLA class I genes as to class II genes.[67] Several disulfide bridges are predicted to span the antigen-binding site of dimers of DMα and DMβ, possibly restricting the range of peptide ligands. To date, no DM proteins have been described.

Polymorphism in HLA Class II Genes

With the exception of DRA and DRB4, all expressed class II genes are polymorphic. Both the distribution of polymorphic positions in class II genes and the evolutionary mechanisms thought to have generated class II polymorphism are similar to those for HLA class I genes. Thus, the N-terminal α_1 and β_1 domains (analogous to α_1 and α_2 in class I proteins) contain most of the polymorphic residues, many of them clustered in three "hypervariable regions" located close to the predicted peptide binding site.[68] Again, the mutation rate in the two extracellular domains (e.g., β_1 and β_2) is equal, but conservative nucleotide substitutions are dominant only in the membrane-proximal domain. Substitutions of single nucleotides or dinucleotides are common; gene conversion events can be traced, and evidence for reciprocal translocations and trans-species evolution can be found (see "Polymorphism in HLA Class I Genes," above, and Gyllensten et al.[69]).

A great number of allelic sequences of class II genes have been obtained and assigned to official HLA class II alleles, as acknowledged by the WHO committee for factors of the HLA system.[14] As of 1991, 60 alleles were acknowledged for the DRB1 gene. The DRB3 (corresponding to the serologic specificity DRw52) and DRB5 genes each have four alleles, while the DRB4 gene (specificity DRw53) is nonpolymorphic. The DQA1 gene has 14 alleles, and the DQB1 gene 19 alleles. In the DP loci, 8 alleles are defined in the A1 gene, and in the B1 gene 38 alleles are known.

MHC CLASS III GENES

The HLA class III region is located between the class I and class II regions and spans approximately 1 Mb of DNA. The class III region contains a heterogeneous collection of genes encoding components of the complement system, the 21-hydroxylase genes,[70] three HSP70 genes,[71] two TNF genes,[72] and a cluster of so-called BAT and G genes,[73–75] which are partly overlapping, and as yet have unknown function (Fig. 12-2).

Complement Genes

Three of the components of the complement system, C2, C4, and factor B (Bf), are encoded by genes within the HLA class III region (Fig. 12-2). The C4 component has two isotypes, which are encoded by the C4A and C4B loci respectively. These loci are separated by 10 kb and are located approximately 350 kb telomeric to the DRA locus. The C2 and Bf genes are separated by less than 1 kb and are located approximately 30 kb telomeric to the C4A locus.[76]

Electrophoretic and genetic analyses have revealed that C2, factor B, C4A, and C4B are polymorphic. Because of marked linkage disequilibrium, specific combinations of C2, Bf, and C4 alleles are inherited as single genetic units, referred to as complotypes.

C2 and C4 are both members of the classical pathway of complement activation. The activation of this pathway starts with the binding of the C1 component to the Fc region of IgG- or IgM-class immunoglobulins involved in immune complexes. Activated C1 then cleaves C4 at position 77 of the α chain, releasing in the fluid phase a small fragment called C4a. The larger fragment, C4b, has an exposed internal thioester bond that is reactive towards hydroxyl or amino groups on nearby cell surfaces or soluble macromolecules. Once covalently bound, C4b expresses binding sites for C2. Bound C2 is then cleaved by nearby activated C1s with the release of a C2 fragment of MW 30,000. The larger fragment remains associated with C4b to form the classical-pathway C3 convertase. This larger fragment has an active proteolytic site and will cleave C3 to continue the complement cascade by activation of the terminal components (C5 to C9) that form the cytotoxic membrane attack complex.

The cleavage of C3 allows a small fraction of C3b to bind to surrounding surfaces. The bound C3b can initiate the alternative pathway of complement activation by allowing the binding of factor B. Factor B is then cleaved by factor D with release of a Ba fragment. Bb remains bound to C3b to form the alternative-pathway C3 convertase, which cleaves additional native C3 to yield C3b, generating an amplification loop that is strictly controlled.

The major functions of the complement system are: (a) to promote the opsonization and phagocytosis of complement-coated microorganisms and the clearance of immune complexes by complement-receptor-expressing cells; (b) to initiate and maintain the inflammatory process through the release of anaphylatoxins; and (c) to cause direct lysis of microorganisms by the terminal components of the cascade.

C2 is a plasma serine protease of 734 amino acid residues (MW 95,000) that is secreted by hepatocytes, fibroblasts, and monocytes. The genomic organization of the 18-kb C2 gene is not known, but it shares a high degree of sequence homology with the factor B gene. Both the C2 and the factor B genes encode contiguous internal repeats at the N-terminal end of the molecule and a C-terminal serine protease domain. The two proteins have 40 percent sequence homology. This similarity in structure and function and the close linkage of their genes suggest that C2 and factor B arose by gene duplication. Polymorphism of C2 has been detected both by isoelectric focusing[77] and by Southern blot analysis of genomic DNA,[78] although the precise number of C2 alleles is not yet known. Among the variants of C2, the common one, C2C, has a frequency of 0.96.[77] These allelic variants also include a null allele, C2Q0, the frequency of which in Caucasians is 0.01.[79] The C2 null allele is usually present in a particular HLA extended haplotype, namely HLA-A25, B18, C2Q0, BfS, C4A4, C4B2, DR2, suggesting that most C2Q0 alleles result from the same mutation. In fact, two distinct molecular mechanisms have been shown to result in C2 deficiency.[79a] The first and most common of these is present in patients with the HLA-A25, B18, C2Q0, BfS, C4A4, C4B2, DR2 extended haplotype. It is due to a specific defect in C2 protein translation that results from a 28-bp deletion of the C2 gene. In the rarer form, the deficiency is related to a selective block in C2 secretion and is accompanied by accumulation of C2 protein in the cells.

An inherited C2 deficiency, that is, homozygosity for the C2Q0 allele, is the most frequent complement deficiency in humans, with more than 100 cases reported.[79,80] Almost half of C2-deficient individuals are asymptomatic. The pathologic conditions associated with C2 deficiency include lupus erythematosus, Henoch-Schonlein purpura, polymyositis, and recurrent pyogenic infections.[80,81] Factor B is a plasma protein of 739 amino acids (MW 93,000). Its 6-kb gene is split into 18 exons and has extensive sequence homology with the C2 gene. Several allelic variants of factor B have been described.[82] The F and S alleles, defined by differences in charges, are the most frequent.[83] Their respective frequency is 0.71 and 0.27. Sixteen other rare alleles (gene frequencies <0.01) are known. Exceptional cases of heterozygous deficiency in factor B have been reported, but no cases of homozygous deficiency are known.[84]

The two isotypes of the C4 protein (C4A and C4B) are each synthesized by hepatocytes, fibroblasts, and monocytes as a single-chain protein that is cleaved by a posttranslational event into a three-chain structure. The three disulfide-linked chains, α, β, and γ, have respective MW of 93,000, 78,000, and 33,000. The two C4 genes, C4A and C4B, code for the two C4 isotypes. The number of C4 loci on chromosome 6 can, in fact, vary due to gene deletion or duplication. Thus, instead of having two C4 loci on one haplotype, the presence of one or three C4 loci is not uncommon.[85,86] The size of the C4B gene is also variable: The C4A gene is always 22.5 kb long, but the C4B gene can be either 22.5 kb (C4B long) or 16 kb (C4B short) owing to the presence or absence of an intron near the 5′ end of the gene.[87] The C4A and C4B genes are highly homologous, having 99 percent homology at the nucleotide level. Most of the differences are clustered in the C4d region. The structural differences between the two C4 isotypes lead to functional consequences as activated C4A preferentially binds to free amino groups of proteins, whereas activated C4B preferentially forms ester bonds with carbohydrates.[88] Conversion by site-specific mutagenesis of the His residue at position 1106 of C4B to an Asp (as in C4A) converts the binding properties of C4B to those of C4A.[89] C4A is more effective than C4B in promoting the inhibiting immune complex precipitation and promoting the binding of immune complexes to the complement receptor on erythrocytes. Moreover, injection of human C4A, but not C4B, can reverse the impaired humoral response of C4-deficient guinea pigs.[90] The binding of the C4d fragment of C4A and C4B to erythrocytes is responsible for the HLA-linked Rodgers and Chido blood group antigens, respectively.[91]

The C4 protein is particularly polymorphic, with more than 13 C4A and 22 C4B alleles described.[92] C4 null alleles are frequent in the normal population, with the C4AQ0 allele present at a frequency of 0.07 to 0.19 and the C4BQ0 allele at a frequency of 0.07 to 0.25.[93] It has been calculated that only about 60 percent of the normal population have four functional C4 genes; the remainder have one, two, or three expressed C4 genes. The C4 serum level very roughly reflects the number of functional genes. Most null alleles result from a large deletion of the C4 gene, usually encompassing the flanking 21-hydroxylase gene, as revealed by Southern blot analysis of genomic DNA.[86] Null alleles can also be generated by point mutations, by small deletions or insertions, or (as is frequently the case for C4BQ0) by gene conversion, leading to the presence on one haplotype of two copies of the C4A gene and no C4B gene.[94] These null alleles are found in specific extended HLA haplotypes, such as the HLA-A1, Cw7, B8, C2C, BfS, C4AQ0, C4B1, DR3 and HLA-A30, Cw5, B18, C2C, BfF1, C4A3, C4BQ0, DR3 haplotypes. Complete serum C4 deficiency, which requires homozygosity for null alleles at both C4 loci, is a rare primary immunodeficiency; there are only 17 recorded cases.[93,95] Deficiency of C4 is associated with different HLA haplotypes, suggesting that different genetic events have led to null alleles in these patients. This was indeed proven in an RFLP study of patients with complete C4 deficiency.[96] Almost all patients with complete C4 deficiency have systemic or discoid lupus erythematosus or other types of immune complex disease. Some also have severe bacterial infections.

Tumor Necrosis Factor (TNFα) and Lymphotoxin (TNFβ)

The human TNFα and TNFβ genes are located in tandem approximately 200 kb centromeric of the HLA-B locus (Fig. 12-2).[97] The major sources of TNFα are monocytes and activated macrophages, though other cells, such as cytotoxic T lymphocytes and keratinocytes, also express the gene. These cells produce TNFα when challenged with lipopolysaccharide (LPS) or other cytokines. Two forms of TNFα seem to exist: a 17-kDa secretory component, and a 26-kDa integral transmembrane form,[98] which is a precursor of the 17-kDa component. TNFβ is a 25-kDa protein that is produced primarily by CD8+ as well as CD4+ T lymphocytes in response to MHC-restricted antigen presentation, T cell mitogens, and other cytokines. The mechanism by which TNFα and TNFβ mediate their action is largely unknown, but binding to specific cell-surface receptors is an initial event. Two TNF receptors exist, with molecular weights of 55 and 75 kDa, respectively. Both receptors bind TNFα and TNFβ,[99] and they are coexpressed in several cell lines from different tissues.[100] Both receptors appear to occur in a soluble form, which is found in the plasma of both normal subjects and patients with inflammatory diseases. At least two roles for the soluble TNF receptors have been suggested: (a) a slow-release reservoir that maintains a steady, low concentration of free TNF, and (b) absorption and inactivation of TNF that spills out of localized inflammatory sites.[101]

There is evidence that TNFα is involved in the control of diverse cellular immune reactions including: (a) activation of T lymphocytes, which in turn produce other cytokines, such as interleukin-2 (IL-2) and lymphotoxin (the induced T cells also express additional TNF receptors, HLA-DR, and high-affinity IL-2 receptors); (b) regulation of human B-cell proliferation and antibody production;[102] and (c) an autocrine-type stimulation of TNFα production by macrophages. Recently it has been shown that TNFα plays a role in lymphocyte development and differentiation. De Kossodo et al. have reported that administration of anti-TNFα to newborn mice results in lymphoid and thymic atrophy,[103] while Giroir et al. have shown that the only site of constitutive TNFα expression is in the newborn thymus.[104]

Both TNFα and TNFβ up-regulate expression of adhesion molecules (ELAM-1 and ICAM-1) on vascular endothelial cells, thereby enhancing the migration of neutrophils into damaged tissue and their subsequent killing of bacteria. Furthermore, in neutrophils, TNFα enhances phagocytic activity, the production of superoxide anion and the release of lysozyme and hydrogen peroxide, and degranulation.[105,106] TNFβ has been shown to be one of the mediators of cytolytic T-cell killing of antigen-expressing cells, although the mechanism by which this occurs is unclear.[105] Other effects of TNFα include induction of necrosis in vascularized tumors and defense against viral diseases and parasitic diseases such as malaria and schistosomiasis.[107–109] A number of pathophysiological systemic effects have been shown to be induced by TNFα. These effects include: (a) cachexia, which is typically seen in cancer patients and patients who are chronically ill and which results from the inhibition by TNFα of the lipogenic enzyme lipoprotein lipase;[108,109] (b) fever, which results from the induction by TNFα of prostaglandin E2 in the thermoregulatory center in the hypothalamus;[110] and (c) septic shock that is induced by the LPS of gram-negative organisms and involves hypotension and disseminated intravascular coagulation. For example, patients with severe meningococcal infections who have relatively high blood levels of TNFα are more prone to shock than patients with no detectable levels of TNFα.[111]

The potential involvement of TNF in genetic predisposition to certain autoimmune diseases is discussed in "TNFα and Autoimmunity," below.

Other MHC Class III Genes

Other MHC class III genes that may have a role in autoimmunity are the three loci encoding heat shock proteins (HSPs) of the HSP70 family that have been mapped to the HLA class III region. These genes are located approximately 30 kb telomeric to the C2 gene.[112] The exact function of these HSP70 is unknown. However, the HSP70 are generally believed to play a key role in the folding, unfolding, and intracellular trafficking of proteins. The HSP70 gene products have been implicated in the class II antigen processing pathway through a set of experiments in which presentation of antigen to a T-helper cell clone was blocked by an antibody that reacted with a presumed HSP70-like molecule.[112]

In addition to the TNF and HSP70 genes, several novel genes in the class III region have recently been reported, including nine BAT (HLA-B associated transcripts) genes (Fig. 12-2),[73] all of which are unique single-copy genes located between C2 in the complement gene cluster and HLA-B. The BAT1 through BAT5 genes are contained in a 160-kb segment that also includes the TNF loci, with the BAT1 gene being telomeric and the BAT2 to BAT5 genes centromeric. The BAT6 through BAT9 genes are contained in a 120-kb segment that includes the HSP70 loci; the BAT6 gene is telomeric and the BAT7 to BAT9 genes centromeric.[73,74] At present, the function of the products encoded by the BAT genes is unknown. However, these genes are transcribed in a variety of cell lines, indicating ubiquitous expression.[73,74] On the basis of DNA sequencing, two of the BAT genes, BAT2 and BAT3, have been predicted to encode large, proline-rich proteins of approximately 228 kDa and 120 kDa, respectively, neither of which appear to be members of any known family of proteins.[113] BAT3 bears some resemblance to the family of stress-response genes. However, there is no functional evidence that BAT3 is regulated by heat shock in the way that HSP70 or ubiquitin is. Whether this limited homology to the stress-response genes has any other functional correlate, such as chaperoning, is unknown.[113] The BAT2 protein sequence includes four Arg-Gly-Asp motifs. This motif functions in cell adhesion by mediating the interaction of the integrin receptor superfamily with their ligands.

RFLP studies of the BAT1 and BAT2 genes have revealed only limited polymorphism.

HLA AND DISEASE ASSOCIATIONS

A large number of diseases of unknown etiology and pathogenesis exhibit an association with specific HLA alleles.[114,115] In particular, susceptibility to most autoimmune disorders appears to be strongly influenced by genes encoded in the HLA system (Table 12-1). That is, the frequency of certain class I or II alleles is significantly higher or lower among patients with a given autoimmune disease than in a control population. A disease association can be expressed as a relative risk (RR): the increased (or decreased) chance of contracting the disease for individuals bearing the HLA allele relative to those lacking it. Thus, RR is merely another term for relative incidence. By definition, if a represents the frequency of patients carrying a particular HLA allele, b the frequency of patients lacking this allele, c the frequency of control subjects carrying this allele, and d the frequency of control subjects lacking this allele, then the RR is ad/bc.

The associations suggest that a genetic susceptibility or resistance to these diseases maps at least in part to the HLA complex. Nevertheless, most individuals with disease-associated class I and class II alleles do not develop autoimmune disorders, indicating that the mode of inheritance is complicated and that additional factors play a role in the disease process.[114]

The nomenclature for factors of the HLA system has recently been revised and has become much more specific.[14] We attempt to use this new nomenclature in the following sections. However, because many disease association studies were performed with antisera that had a broad specificity corresponding to several specificities in the new nomenclature, in some cases it is not possible to use the new nomenclature. Therefore, both the old (e.g., HLA-B8, HLA-DR3) and the new (HLA-B*0801, HLA-DRB1*0301) nomenclatures are used.

HLA-B27-Related Disorders

A common feature of patients with ankylosing spondylitis (AS), reactive arthritis, and psoriatic arthritis is that many of them are HLA-B27-positive. Here we shall focus on AS and briefly comment on Reiter disease (RD) as representative of the reactive arthritides. Psoriatic arthritis is dealt with in the "Psoriasis" section.

The classic clinical manifestations of RD consist of acute arthritis, conjunctivitis, and nonspecific urethritis. RD commonly affects young men and is often preceded by an infection in the gastrointestinal or genitourinary tract. The arthritis is commonly a monoarthritis, usually of the knee, developing 2 to 6 weeks after the infection. The organisms that have been clearly implicated in RD include *Shigella, Salmonella*, and *Yersinia* with respect to the gastrointestinal infection and (less clearly) *Chlamydia* and *Mycoplasma* in the venereal infection. While there is little evidence from family studies that a genetic element exists in the development of RD, population studies have consistently shown that 60 to 90 percent of RD patients are HLA-B27-positive, as compared to 8 percent of the normal population. Furthermore, the frequency of RD in a population generally reflects the frequency of HLA-B27, strongly implicating HLA-B27 as an allele conferring susceptibility for RD.[116] The precise role of HLA-B27 in the pathogenesis of RD is unknown, although the studies on AS described below may apply to RD as well. AS is an inflammatory arthritis that predominantly affects the spine of young men. The etiology and mechanism of the disease is unknown. AS is associated with HLA-B27, and it seems likely that HLA-B27 itself confers susceptibility to the HLA-B27-associated spondylarthropathies. The disease association with HLA-B27 is very strong (approximately 95 percent of affected Caucasians carry the HLA-B27 allele) and is seen in all races. There is also a definite correlation between the prevalence of the disease and that of HLA-B27. Finally, there is no strong linkage disequilibrium between HLA-B27 and other HLA genes.[117]

The frequency of HLA-B27 among Caucasian patients with AS is 95 percent as compared to only 8 percent of the normal population. The prevalence of AS in HLA-B27-positive individuals is less than 2 percent, although it is 10 times higher in HLA-B27-positive family members of HLA-B27-positive AS patients. Thus, most HLA-B27-positive individuals do not get AS, indicating that additional genetic and/or environmental factors are involved.[117] Recently, it was shown that another class I molecule, HLA-Bw60, may confer increased risk to AS in individuals whose other HLA-B allele is B27. However, this association could be due to other HLA-B alleles conferring negative risk, whereas HLA-Bw60 may be neutral.[116]

At least six subtypes of HLA-B27 exist (HLA-B*2701 to -2706). All subtypes have been linked with AS, and they all share a combination of six amino acid residues at positions 9, 45, 67, 70, 71, and 97 that distinguishes the HLA-B27 molecules from other class I molecules.[117] These residues are situated in the antigen-binding pocket, indicating that HLA-B27 molecules may have an antigen-presenting function for a particular peptide(s) which is different from that of other class I molecules (Fig. 12-6). On this basis, it has been suggested that peptides derived from joint-specific proteins and bound by HLA-B27 molecules may both stimulate and be the target for autoreactive T cells.[117]

Recent crystallographic studies show that the peptide backbone of HLA-B27 is essentially the same as that of HLA-A2 and HLA-Aw68.[30] Furthermore, the peptide bound in the antigen-binding groove appears to be an extended chain of nine amino acids.[30]

	67			70				74
Susceptible DRB1*0401	Leu	Leu	Glu	Gln	Lys	Arg	Ala	Ala
Susceptible DRB1*0404	-	-	-	-	Arg	-	-	-
Susceptible DRB1*0101	-	-	-	-	Arg	-	-	-
Not susceptible DRB1*0402	Ile	-	-	Asp	Glu	-	-	-
Not susceptible DRB1*0407	-	-	-	-	Arg	-	-	Glu

Fig. 12-7 The amino acid sequence at residues 67 to 74 in RA-associated and nonassociated haplotypes. For details see text.

Pockets in the antigen-binding cleft bind the N- and C-terminal ends and four side chains of the peptide. Sequencing of endogenous peptides isolated from HLA-B27 molecules has shown that these self peptides derive from abundant cytosolic proteins (ribosomal and heat shock proteins) or nuclear proteins (histones and helicases).[38] This approach may pave the way for the identification of potential "arthritogenic" peptide(s) by sequencing the peptides bound to the HLA-B27 molecules expressed in joint tissues. However, if the arthritogenic peptides are cryptic and only represent a small part of the pool of peptides presented by HLA-B27, they may not be easily identified using this approach.

Recently, a case was reported in which the antigen-presenting function of HLA-B27 molecules appears to be modulated by additional genetic factors.[118] Peripheral blood cells from a healthy donor were unable to present three peptides known to be presented by HLA-B27 to cytotoxic T lymphocytes, even though normal amounts of HLA-B27 were expressed on the cell surface. This phenotype was not the result of a mutation in the HLA-B27 molecule itself, and cells from all HLA-B27 members of this individual's family showed the same behavior. Interestingly, two family members have AS and a third has had an episode of anterior uveitis, an AS-related syndrome. The nonpresenting phenotype found in this family, for which the molecular basis is as yet unknown, may therefore be associated with an increased risk of developing AS.

Molecular mimicry between HLA-B27 and microbes that trigger HLA-B27-associated disorders has been considered as a potential mechanism of disease induction. A number of antigens with potential cross-reactivity have been identified and are expressed by *Yersinia, Salmonella, Shigella*, and *Klebsiella*. These proteins all share with HLA-B27 a short linear or nonlinear sequence identity of four to six amino acids. The area of identity for all these microbial proteins is found in the proposed antigenic peptide-binding site of the HLA-B27 molecule between amino acids 70 and 78 in the variable region of the α_1 helix.[119] Although this finding is striking, its significance is unclear. Furthermore, the molecular mimicry model it suggests is difficult to reconcile with the tissue specificity of AS in view of the fact that HLA-B27, like other class I molecules, is expressed on essentially all nucleated cells.

The pathogenic consequences of expression of HLA-B27 have been assessed in transgenic rats. Two of six lines of HLA-B27 transgenic animals spontaneously develop multiple inflammatory disease manifestations including arthritis, axial enthesitis, gut inflammation, male genital inflammation, psoriasiform skin and nail lesions, and myocarditis.[120] These manifestations resemble rather closely the symptoms of human spondylarthropathies, although the mechanism of disease in the rats remains unclear.

Rheumatoid Arthritis

RA is a chronic systemic inflammatory disease that affects primarily the synovial tissue in joints. The etiology of RA is unknown but is likely to be multifactorial. Family and twin studies have shown that RA clusters in families and that the concordance rate is 30 percent for monozygotic twins and 9 percent for dizygotic twins, suggesting a polygenic inheritance of susceptibility to the disease. Epstein-Barr virus, *Mycobacterium tuberculosis*, and recently human T-cell leukemia virus type I (HTLV-I) have been implicated as exogenous factors in the pathogenesis of RA, although the evidence is only circumstantial.[7]

In several ethnic groups, susceptibility to RA is associated with the serologically defined HLA-DR4 or HLA-DR1 groups. In general, 70 to 75 percent of Caucasian RA patients are HLA-DR4-positive, compared to a normal background frequency of 25 to 30 percent. Most HLA-DR4-negative RA patients in this group, as well as in other ethnic and racial groups, are HLA-DR1-positive.[114] The serologically defined HLA-DR4 group is divided into at least 5 subtypes—DRB1*0401, DRB1*0404, and DRB1*0405, which confer susceptibility to RA, and DRB1*0402 and DRB1*0403, which do not. DRB1*0401 and DRB1*0404 are the predominant alleles found in Caucasian RA patients, while DRB1*0405 predisposes to RA in Japanese. In other racial groups, such as Israeli Jews, DRB1*01 accounts for susceptibility to RA.[121] The disease-associated alleles DRB1*0401, DRB1*0404, DRB1*0405, and DRB1*01 share sequences in the third hypervariable region of the DRB1 gene (Fig. 12-7). This region of the β chain, located between amino acid residues 67 and 74, differs by only a single conservative change (position 71, arginine to lysine) between DRB1*0404, DRB1*0405, and DRB1*01 on the one hand and DRB1*0401 on the other. The DRB1*0402 allele has two nonconservative substitutions in this region (position 70, glutamine to aspartic acid, and position 71, arginine to glutamic acid). Similarly, the DRB1*0403 allele has a nonconservative substitution of glutamic acid for alanine at position 74. These findings have led to the hypothesis that the third HVR of the DRB1*0401, DRB1*0404, DRB1*0405, and DRB1*01 genes is at least in part responsible for the genetic susceptibility to RA. Further support for this hypothesis comes from a recent study showing that a rare allele, DRB1*1401, belonging to the HLA-DR6 family, and sharing the same third HVR as DRB1*0404, DRB1*0405, and DRB1*01, is found in high frequency in Yakima Indians with RA.[7]

A hypothetical model of the antigen-binding site of class II molecules[45] indicates that residues 67 to 74 of the β chain are located in the proposed binding site (Fig. 12-8). Thus, the expression of a common RA-associated sequence may allow one or more putative self-antigen(s) to be presented to helper T cells, initiating an immune response that leads to disease.

Examination of the antigen specificity of DRB1*0401-restricted T-cell clones isolated from rheumatoid arthritis synovial fluid has demonstrated that these clones are reactive with a component of synovial fluid. This result suggests that an HLA-DR-restricted antigen may be present in the rheumatoid arthritis synovial compartment. The precise nature of this antigen remains to be identified.[122] In other, similar studies, including animal studies of RA, the mycobacterial GroEL stress protein has been implicated as a potential target autoantigen.[123,124] Interestingly, determinants on *Mycobacterium tuberculosis* cross-react with a proteoglycan determinant.[125]

Because class II molecules are expressed ectopically on synovial cells in RA, it has been argued that synovial cells may act as antigen-processing and presenting cells and may thus induce a local immune response that ultimately leads to RA. However, it is not known whether this aberrant class II expression is a primary event that initiates the RA process, or is merely a result of the increased level of cytokines in a compartment with an ongoing immune response. It is known that various cytokines such as IFN-γ and TNF have the ability to induce class II expression on the surface of certain cells that are normally class II negative.[7] In this regard it is interesting that TNFα and, to a lesser degree, TNFβ

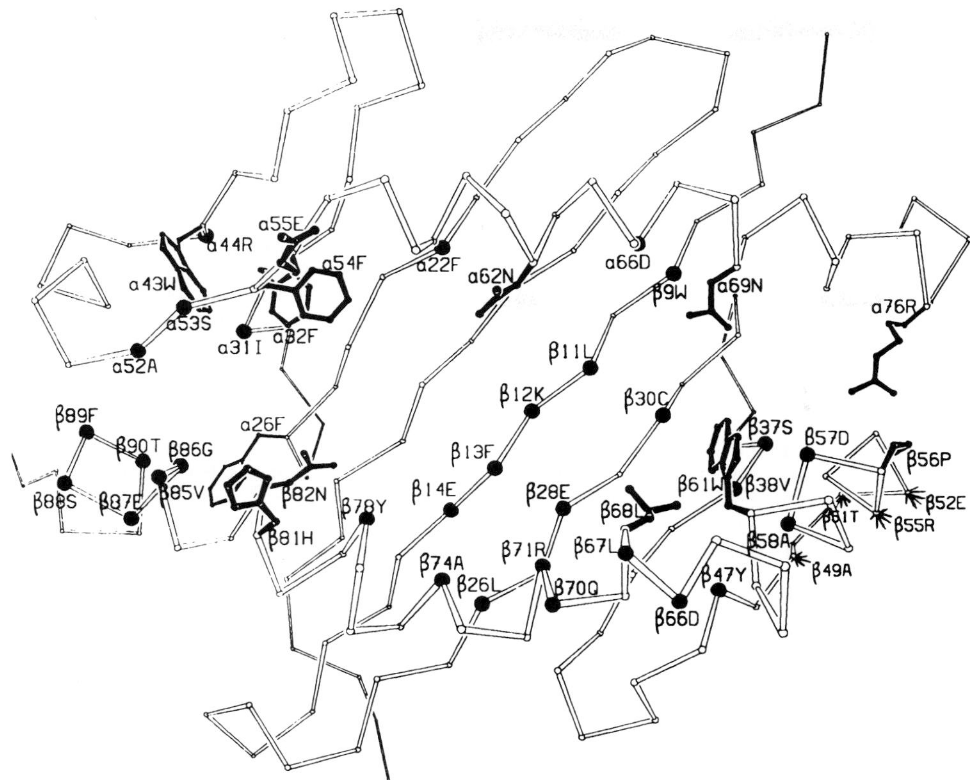

Fig. 12-8 The MHC class II α1 and β1 domains as viewed from above, showing all polymorphic positions (dark circles) and those conserved positions facing the antigen-binding groove (all atoms of chain shown). Amino-acid residues, in one letter code, and positions are given for DRA/DRB1*0101. Positively charged amino acids Gln70 and Arg71 of the DRB1 chain are associated with susceptibility to RA. Resistance to IDDM is associated with Asp57 of the DQB1 chain that may form a salt bridge with a conserved Arg79 of the DQA chain. Susceptibility to IDDM is associated with Val, Ser, or Ala at position 57 of the DQB1 chain that cannot form a salt bridge with Arg79 of the DQA chain. (*Reprinted with permission from Brown et al. Nature 364:33, 1993. © 1993 Macmillan Magazines Ltd.*)

have been shown in vitro to stimulate the resorption and inhibit the synthesis of cartilage proteoglycan and bone, respectively.[126,127] Further, TNFα (along with IL-1 and IL-6) can be detected in rheumatoid arthritis synovial fluid, particularly from patients with seropositive or active disease,[128] suggesting that TNF probably plays a role in inflammatory joint diseases.

Juvenile Chronic Arthritis

Juvenile chronic arthritis (JCA) is defined as an inflammatory arthritis that commences before the age of 16 years. Three principal forms of JCA, for which the etiology is unknown, are associated with certain HLA antigens and are immunogenetically distinct: (a) the juvenile rheumatoid arthritis form, which represents RA occurring in childhood and is thus associated with HLA-DR4; (b) the polyarticular form, which is most common in young girls and has in one study been associated with HLA-DPw3; and (c) the pauciarticular form. There are two types of pauciarticular JCA.[129] The first type, early-onset pauciarticular JCA (EOPA-JCA), is the most common form of JCA; it affects mainly young girls, who often produce anti-nuclear antibody and develop chronic iridocyclitis. This disease is associated with HLA-DR5, DR6, DR8 (DRB1*0801), and DPB1*0201. The second type of pauciarticular JCA affects older boys, is HLA-B27-associated, and represents a juvenile form of AS.[129] Here we shall focus on the EOPA form, as it is the most common and is the best studied in terms of HLA associations. In the EOPA form, the DRB1*0801 allele is more strongly associated with the disease than the DR5 and DR6 alleles. While DRB1*0801 has been confirmed in several studies to confer susceptibility to disease, there are conflicting data concerning the influence of the DR5 and DR6 alleles in the pathogenesis of JCA.[130] Whether this discrepancy reflects the different ethnic backgrounds of the patients, different diagnostic criteria, or different etiologic agents is unclear. Interestingly, all three alleles share a unique sequence in the first hypervariable region of the DRB1 gene (nucleotides 25 to 37), which represents a site in the presumed antigen-binding pocket of the class II molecule. This observation led to the suggestion that the shared-epitope hypothesis may also play a role in this disease. However, the non-disease-associated HLA-DR3 allele also shares the same sequence, a finding which, on the one hand, may argue against the importance of the shared-epitope hypothesis in JCA, but, on the other, may simply indicate that the expression of this epitope is necessary but not sufficient for developing disease.[129] The combined presence of (a) two of the three implicated HLA-DR alleles and/or (b) DPB1*0201 and DR5 and/or DRB1*0801 is associated with a further increased risk of developing JCA compared to individuals carrying only one of the risk factors. This association indicates that there is an additive effect between HLA-DR alleles as well as a possible interaction between the DP and DR gene products (e.g., in the form of a hybrid molecule).[131] Furthermore, one recent study showed that HLA-DR5 confers an increased risk of developing iridocyclitis while HLA-DR1 protects against this symptom.[132]

It is important to note that the DPB1*0201 association is independent of linkage disequilibrium with any other class II allele.[133,134] Moreover, DPB1*0201 differs from the non-JCA-associated HLA-DPB1*0402 allele by only one amino acid at position 69 in the first domain of the HLA-DP β chain. The DPB1*0201 chain has a positively charged lysine at position 69, while the DPB1*0402 chain has a negatively charged glutamic acid. These two molecules are, however, recognized as being biologically different by T lymphocytes. Thus, the DPB1*0201 molecule may have biological properties concerning peptide binding and presentation that are different from those of the DPB1*0402 molecule, and these properties may confer disease susceptibility to JCA.

The contribution of other immunologically relevant genes, such as TNF and TCR genes, has also been considered, but there is no evidence yet that these genes confer susceptibility to JCA.[135,136]

Systemic Lupus Erythematosus

Systemic lupus erythematosus (SLE) is a systemic autoimmune disorder that affects mostly young women and is characterized by a large spectrum of clinical manifestations and autoantibodies.

Most of the genes that have been associated to date with predisposition to SLE map in the HLA region; they include HLA class II genes, C2 and C4 genes, and the TNFα gene. In population studies, SLE is associated in Caucasians with the haplotypes HLA-DRB1*1501, DQA1*0102, DQB1*0602 and/or HLA-B8, DRB1*0301, DQA1*0501, DQB1*0201, whereas in Japanese the association appears to correlate with the HLA-DR2, DQw1 haplotype.[137] In most other ethnic groups, no HLA class II association has been found. A negative association with the HLA-DRB1*04, DQB1*0301 or 0302 haplotypes has been found in patients with lupus nephritis.[138] In family studies, however, sib pairs concordant for SLE do not share HLA haplotypes more frequently than expected, suggesting that HLA-linked genes play little role in the susceptibility to familial SLE. Recently, a stronger association has been described between HLA class II alleles and the presence of certain autoantibodies rather than SLE itself.[137] This phenomenon is referred to as class II restriction of autoantibody production. For example, anti-Ro/SSA antibodies are associated with serologically defined DR2 and DR3 alleles, and the presence of both anti-Ro/SSA and anti-La/SSB antibodies is associated with DR3.[139] This association was later found to be stronger with DQ alleles; anti-Ro/SSA and anti-La/SSB antibodies correlate with the presence of DQA1 alleles that code for a glutamic acid at position 34 (i.e., DQA1*0102, DQA1*0201, DQA1*0401, DQA1*0501) and DQB1 alleles that code for a leucine at position 26 (i.e., DQB1*0201, 0302, 0602, 0603, 0604, and 0605).[140] Production of anti-U1RNP antibodies is associated with DQB1 alleles (DQB1*0301, 0302, 0303, 0601, and 0604) that code for shared residues in the third hypervariable region of the DQβ chain, and production of anti-dsDNA antibody is associated withDQB1 alleles bearing a methionine at position 14 and a leucine at position 26 (DQB1*0201, 0302, and 0602).[137] Moreover, patients with anti-phospholipid antibody frequently carry the DQB1*0301 allele or other DQB1 alleles (DQB1*0302, 0602, 0603) that share with the DQB1*0301 allele a sequence motif in the third hypervariable region of the DQβ chain.[141] Because the presence of these autoantibodies correlates with specific clinical manifestations, it has been proposed that SLE is a heterogeneous disease that is made of numerous overlapping clinically, serologically, and genetically defined entities.

Although patients with deficiencies in proteins of the classical pathway of complement represent a minority of all SLE patients, C2 and C4 null alleles are the strongest susceptibility genes for the development of SLE. The prevalence of SLE or SLE-like syndrome is 70 percent in C4-deficient subjects and 35 percent in C2-deficient individuals.[142,143] Some clinical and serologic peculiarities characterize SLE in C2- or C4-deficient patients. They include an early age of onset and a high frequency of skin lesions such as atypical discoid lupus and photosensitivity.[142] Deposition of complement and Igs at the dermoepidermal junction is often lacking in these cases. Furthermore, C2- or C4-deficient patients tend to exhibit a low incidence of renal involvement; a low titer of anti-nuclear antibody and the presence of anti-DNA antibody are seen in only 25 percent of cases, whereas rheumatoid factor anti-SSA (Ro) antibodies seem to occur frequently, as does an association with severe pyogenic bacterial infections.

The strong association of SLE with complete C2 and C4 deficiency has led several groups to investigate whether a partial deficiency (i.e., one C2 null allele or one to three C4 null alleles) is also a risk factor. A significant increase in the prevalence of the C4 null allele, mainly at the C4A locus, has been found in SLE patients. The reported prevalence of homozygous C4A deficiency in SLE patients is 10 to 15 percent, and the prevalence of heterozygosity for the C4AQ0 allele is 25 to 60 percent.[144,145] However, given that, in Caucasians, the C4AQ0 allele is in linkage disequilibrium with the HLA-DR3 allele, these data do not make it possible to define the relative contribution of the two loci. Recent studies have shown that C4AQ0 confers susceptibility to SLE independently of HLA-DR3. SLE patients selected for the absence of the HLA-DR3 allele still show an increased frequency of C4 null alleles.[146] Furthermore, the prevalence of C4 null alleles is increased in non-Caucasian SLE patients despite the fact that SLE is not associated with HLA-DR3 in these populations.[145,147]

Several lines of argument strongly suggest that C2 and C4 null alleles themselves predispose to SLE and that this effect is not due to linkage disequilibrium with other immunologically relevant genes in the HLA complex. First, C2 and C4 deficiencies are extremely rare in the normal population, which eliminates the possibility that an ascertainment bias is the cause of the association between complement deficiency and SLE. Second, an increased prevalence of SLE is seen not only in subjects having C2 or C4 deficiency but also in subjects with an inherited deficiency of other complement proteins such as C1q, C1r/s, and C3, which are encoded by genes located on different chromosomes. Third, as already discussed, C4AQ0 and not HLA-DR alleles seem to be associated with SLE. There is a preliminary report of successful treatment of complement-deficient SLE patients with the deficient complement protein; this finding may provide additional support for a direct link between complement deficiency and SLE.[148]

The exact mechanism by which complement deficiency promotes SLE is not yet known. However, complement has an important role in the processing of immune complexes in the circulation and in tissues. Therefore, it is likely that complement deficiency directly favors the emergence of SLE by allowing immune complexes to deposit in tissues and to initiate inflammation, resulting in the secondary release of self-antigens that, in turn, stimulate the production of autoantibodies. An immune system that is defective because of a complement deficiency may also favor infections, a well-known triggering factor for the development of autoimmunity.

Sjögren Syndrome

Sjögren syndrome (SS) is a chronic autoimmune exocrinopathy of unknown etiology which primarily affects middle-aged women, leading to keratoconjunctivitis sicca and/or xerostomia. SS is often associated with RA, SLE, or other connective tissue disorders such as progressive systemic sclerosis and polymyositis, at which point it is referred to as secondary SS (sSS). The diagnosis of primary SS (pSS) is used when keratoconjunctivitis sicca and/or xerostomia occur(s) without other inflammatory connective tissue disorders. Since the HLA association of sSS is similar to that of the accompanying disease, we shall focus primarily on pSS.

Primary SS is associated with several HLA antigens in Caucasian populations — HLA-B*0801, DRB1*0301, DQB1*0201, and DQA1*0501 — while HLA-DRw53 is associated with this disease in Japanese. It is likely that most Caucasoid primary SS patients carry HLA-B*0801, DRB1*0301, DQA1*0501, and DQB1*0201 on one haplotype. Even though it has yet to be determined which, if any, of these antigens are primarily associated with disease, one study found the strongest association to be with HLA-DQB1*0201. The possibility of additive effects resulting from the presence of two or more of the associated antigens has been tested, but no evidence was found that suggested that a synergistic interplay occurs.[149]

One of the immunologic abnormalities of SS is the production of a variety of autoantibodies. In pSS and sSS, the ability to produce autoantibodies to the small ribonucleoproteins Ro and La is associated with the same HLA antigens as those associated with disease. However, these autoantibodies tend to be more strongly associated with HLA than are their parent diseases. Anti-Ro and anti-La antibodies were initially reported to be most closely associated with HLA-B*0801 and DRB1*0301, although recent studies suggest that a stronger association exists with HLA-DQ. The mechanism for this association has yet to be elucidated.[150]

Insulin-Dependent Diabetes Mellitus

Insulin-dependent diabetes mellitus (IDDM) is the result of autoimmune-mediated destruction of insulin-secreting pancreatic

β cells and is characterized by lymphocytic infiltrates of the islets of Langerhans (insulitis), autoantibodies to β cell components, an association with other immune disorders, and a strong association with the HLA system. Studies in NOD mice, an animal model for IDDM, have given evidence that IDDM is a T-cell-dependent and T-cell-mediated disease in which both CD4 + and CD8 + T cells are necessary for disease induction.[151] It is likely that autoantigen-specific and class II-restricted CD4 + T-cells (a) help B cells to produce autoantibodies to β cell components and (b) help class-I-restricted CD8+ T cells to destroy β cells. Six potential autoantigens in IDDM have recently been identified by characterizing the autoantibodies that develop in diabetic humans and the NOD mouse. (a) Glutamic acid decarboxylase (GAD) is an enzyme that is responsible for the production of γ-aminobutyric acid (GABA), an inhibitory neurotransmitter in the central nervous system. GAD exists in two isoforms, GAD1 (65 kDa) and GAD2 (67 kDa), which have been shown to be pancreatic β cell proteins.[152] What role GAD-aided GABA synthesis may have in pancreatic β cells is unclear, although pancreatic α cells do appear to have GABA receptors on their surface. (b) Peripherin is a 59-kDa cytoskeleton protein that is expressed by pancreatic β cells and neurons associated with the peripheral nervous system.[153] (c) Carboxypeptidase H (52 kDa) is expressed in the insulin secretory granules of pancreatic β cell and is believed to be involved in the maturation of insulin.[154] (d) Heat-shock protein 60 (HSP60) and (e) HSP69 are two potential pancreatic β cell autoantigens that are recognized by antibodies in the sera of IDDM patients and that also appear to cross-react with bovine serum albumin in milk.[155] As mentioned above, much of the evidence that implicates these antigens as targets of the diabetogenic process in humans has been based on studies showing that IDDM patients have antibodies in their sera that are reactive with these proteins. However, recent studies indicate that T cells responding to GAD2 can also be detected in IDDM patients.[156] Numerous family and population studies have demonstrated an association between the HLA system and IDDM. However, the differences in concordance rates for HLA-identical sibs (10 percent) and monozygotic twins (30 to 70 percent, depending on HLA type) suggest that additional genes as well as environmental factors contribute to disease susceptibility.[157] In population studies, IDDM was originally reported to be associated with HLA-B15 and HLA-B8. Further studies, however, showed that the class I associations were due to linkage disequilibrium between these antigens and the more strongly associated class II antigens HLA-DR3 and HLA-DR4. An interesting observation was that HLA-DR3/4 heterozygotes had a higher risk of IDDM than either DR3/3 or DR4/4 homozygotes. Moreover, it was found that IDDM is negatively associated with HLA-DR2. Family studies have confirmed the results of the population studies and have further demonstrated the linkage of IDDM to HLA by showing segregation of HLA haplotypes with disease and preferential sharing of certain haplotypes among affected sibs.[157]

Studies performed within the last 5 years have given increasing evidence that certain HLA-DQ antigens play a stronger role than the HLA-DR antigens in conferring susceptibility and/or resistance to IDDM. Thus, of the six commonly defined DR4 haplotypes, only three (DRB1*0401, DRB1*0402, and DRB1*0404) are positively associated with IDDM. All three haplotypes have in common the DQB1*0302 allele, which is not found on DR4 haplotypes not associated with IDDM and which accounts for the association of HLA-DR4 with disease. About 90 percent of DR4-positive diabetics (and 70 percent of Caucasian IDDM patients) carry the DQB1*0302 allele, as compared to approximately 65 percent of DR4-positive control subjects (and about 30 percent of all Caucasians). These findings suggest that the DQB1*0302 allele is a major susceptibility element in IDDM.[158]

Amino acid sequence comparisons of several haplotypes either associated or not associated with IDDM have revealed a striking correlation between IDDM susceptibility and substitutions at position 57 of the HLA-DQβ chain. In Caucasoids, HLA-DQβ chains having aspartic acid at position 57 are associated with dominant resistance to diabetes, whereas HLA-DQβ chains with other amino acids at position 57 are associated with susceptibility (Fig. 12-8).[159] This association also extends to NOD mice, in which the presumed murine DQ homologue, I-ANOD, has a unique β chain with serine at position at 57, whereas the corresponding molecule in all other inbred strains has aspartic acid at position 57.[160] Recent studies in Blacks and Japanese have provided evidence that the DQA1*03 allele is also involved in susceptibility to IDDM, and it is the combination of specific DQA and DQB alleles that correlates best with susceptibility.[161] It should be noted that the HLA-DR7 and DR9 alleles, which are associated with IDDM in Blacks, both have an alanine at position 57 of the DRβ chain. These studies suggest a molecular association between HLA-DQ and IDDM, but do not account for the high disease risk of HLA-DR3/4 heterozygotes or the unusually high disease resistance associated with the HLA-DRB1*1501 haplotype. In the former case, it was originally suggested that the molecular basis for the HLA-DR3/4 synergism is the formation of an HLA-DQ hybrid class II molecule encoded in *trans*. Such hybrid molecules, consisting of a DQα chain from the DR3 haplotype and a DQβ molecule from the DR4 haplotype, have since been detected in diabetics, although a direct causal relationship has yet to be shown.[158] In the latter case, it is presumed that other amino acid residues coded for by the HLA-DQB1*0602 allele on the DR2 haplotype, as well as aspartic acid at position 57 of the DQβ chain, mediate resistance.

A second susceptibility region for IDDM not linked to the HLA region has been mapped to chromosome 11 at the insulin gene/insulin-like growth factor II gene cluster.[162] Fine mapping has shown that the insulin gene is most likely responsible for the IDDM susceptibility mediated by this gene cluster. The precise mechanism(s) that cause the insulin gene susceptibility has yet to be determined.

Recently, several new candidate IDDM susceptibility genes not linked to the insulin gene or the HLA region have been identified and mapped in the NOD mouse. Idd-3 and Idd-4, which influence the onset of IDDM in the NOD mouse, have been mapped to chromosomes 3 and 11.[163] The human homologue of Idd-3 may reside on human chromosome 1 or 4, and the homologue of Idd-4 on chromosome 17. The identity of these genes remains to be determined. Idd-5 has been mapped to a region of mouse chromosome 1 that is highly homologous to human chromosome 2q.[164] This region contains at least two candidate susceptibility genes: (a) the interleukin-1 (IL-1) receptor gene, which is a candidate IDDM susceptibility gene because IL-1 is important for T cell activation and has been implicated directly in the pathogenesis of IDDM; and (b) the Lsh/Ity/Bcg locus, which controls susceptibility to a number of infectious diseases and affects the functioning of macrophages, which are essential for the development of IDDM in the NOD mouse.

Primary Biliary Cirrhosis

Primary biliary cirrhosis (PBC) is a chronic liver disorder primarily affecting middle-aged women that is characterized by nonsuppurative destructive cholangitis.

The etiology of PBC is unknown, but an immunoinflammatory pathogenesis is likely, given that PBC is associated with a number of immunologic abnormalities, such as the production of autoantibodies that recognize various targets (e.g., mitochondria), skin test anergy, and other autoimmune disorders.

Despite several studies investigating a potential association between PBC and HLA class II antigens, no consensus has been reached. In Caucasian PBC patients, increased frequencies of HLA-DR3 and HLA-DRw8 have been reported, although other groups have not been able to confirm these results. No association with HLA-DQ or DP alleles seems to exist.[165]

A possible association between PBC and proteins encoded in the HLA class III region has also been studied. One group reported an increased frequency of an RFLP-defined TNFβ allele in PBC patients, although another study found no such association.[166]

Finally, an increased frequency of the complement variant C4B2 has also been reported. However, the significance of this finding is uncertain.[167] These differences in HLA associations may reflect genetically different forms of PBC or different diagnostic criteria.

Three enzymes of the 2-oxo-acid dehydrogenase family have recently been identified as the targets of autoantibodies to mitochondria in PBC patients. The major reactive autoantigen is the E2 subunit of pyruvate dehydrogenase.[168] Other potential mitochondrial autoantigens have been reported but are less well characterized. The identification of these autoantigens should allow further studies on the immunopathology of PBC and prove helpful in developing animal models for PBC.

Celiac Disease

Celiac disease (CD) is an enteropathy caused by the ingestion of wheat gluten in genetically susceptible individuals. The mechanism by which gluten induces damage to the intestinal mucosa is poorly understood. However, CD is considered to be an autoimmune disorder because (a) CD patients have cell-mediated and humoral immune reactions to gluten, suggesting that an immunologic reaction to gluten or its derivatives causes damage to the intestinal mucosa; (b) autoimmune disorders have also been shown to be associated with CD; and (c) CD is strongly associated with certain HLA antigens.

Eighty percent of CD patients bear the HLA-DRB1*0301, DQA1*0501, DQB1*0201 haplotype (the former DR3, DQw2 haplotype), compared to 30 percent of healthy control subjects. The remaining CD patients are predominantly DRB1*11, DQA1*0501, DQB1*0301/DRB1*07, DQA1*0201, DQB1*0201 heterozygotes (the former DR5, DQw7/DR7, DQw2 haplotypes).[169] DNA sequencing studies have shown that the DQα chain encoded by the DRB1*11, DQA1*0501, DQB1*0301 haplotype is identical to the DQα chain encoded by the HLA-DRB1*0301, DQA1*0501, DQB1*0201 haplotype, and that the DQβ chain encoded by the DRB1*07, DQA1*0201, DQB1*0201 haplotype is virtually identical to the DQβ chain encoded by the HLA-DRB1*0301, DQA1*0501, DQB1*0201 haplotype.[170] The associations suggest that the primary disease molecule in CD is a DQ heterodimer (DQA1*0501/DQB1*0201), encoded either in *cis* by the HLA-DRB1*0301, DQA1*0501, DQB1*0201 haplotype or in *trans* by DRB1*11, DQA1*0501, DQB1*0301/DRB1*07, DQA1*0201, DQB1*0201 heterozygotes (Fig. 12-9). Interestingly, the DQα chain encoded by the DRB1*08, DQB1*04 haplotype is similar to the DQα chain encoded by the HLA-DRB1*0301, DQA1*0501, DQB1*0201 haplotype, differing only at amino acid residues 69 and 75. However, there is no over-representation of DRB1*08, DQB1*04/DRB1*07, DQA1*0201, DQB1*0201 heterozygotes among CD patients, suggesting that residues 69 and 75 of the DQα chain, which are located in the presumed antigen-binding pocket, are important in the presentation of peptides involved in the pathogenesis of CD, for example, peptides of gluten.

A minority of CD patients who are neither HLA-DRB1*0301 nor DRB1*07-positive are DR4-positive. In one study, the DQA and DQB alleles from a DR4-positive CD patient were sequenced and found to differ from those found on the HLA-DRB1*0301, DRB1*11, and DRB1*07 haplotypes.[169] This result may reflect the presence of two genetically distinct forms of CD.

An association between CD and certain HLA-DP alleles has also been reported[171] but has not been confirmed,[172] and may be due to linkage disequilibrium between certain HLA-DP alleles and HLA-DR haplotypes.

Autoimmune Adrenalitis

Primary hypoadrenalism, or Addison disease (AD), is caused by destruction of the adrenal glands leading to deficient synthesis of steroid hormones. The destruction may be caused, for example, by infarction, metastasis, tuberculosis, or autoimmunity. Tuberculosis was formerly the most common cause of AD, but now autoimmune destruction is the major cause, at least in areas where the incidence of tuberculosis is low. The etiology of autoimmune AD (AAD) is unknown, and the pathogenesis is only poorly understood. Immunologically relevant characteristics of AAD include an association with the HLA system, lymphocytic infiltrates of the adrenal cortex, and abnormal T-cell-mediated and humoral reactivity against the adrenal cortex.[173] Recently, 17α-hydroxylase, which is one of the key enzymes in the biosynthesis of steroids, has been identified as an autoantigen associated with AD.[174] AAD may appear either alone or in association with a variety of other autoimmune endocrinopathies, such as IDDM, hyperthyroidism, hypothyroidism, primary hypoparathyroidism, and chronic mucocutaneous candidiasis. The latter form of AAD has been further subdivided into two groups on the basis of the associated autoimmune disorder: (a) a more common form, polyglandular autoimmune syndrome II (PGA II), in which patients also have autoimmune thyroid diseases and/or IDDM; and (b) a rarer form, PGA I, which is associated with primary hypoparathyroidism and chronic mucocutaneous candidiasis.[173] For all three groups, it has been consistently reported that HLA-DR3 is more common in patients than in control subjects. Furthermore, there is some preliminary evidence that HLA-DR4 as well as HLA-DR3 is associated with PGA I.[175] This finding may indicate immunogenetic heterogeneity within AAD.

Analysis of HLA-DQB1 alleles in HLA-DR4 patients with and without IDDM has shown that HLA-DQB1*0302 is associated with AAD and IDDM, whereas HLA-DQB1*0301 is associated with AAD without IDDM.[176] It therefore appears that substitutions at position 57 of the HLA-DQβ chain are also associated with either resistance or susceptibility to IDDM in AAD.

Autoimmune Thyroid Disease

The two major forms of autoimmune thyroid disease are Graves disease (GD) and chronic autoimmune thyroiditis. Even though GD is characterized by thyroid hormone hypersecretion and

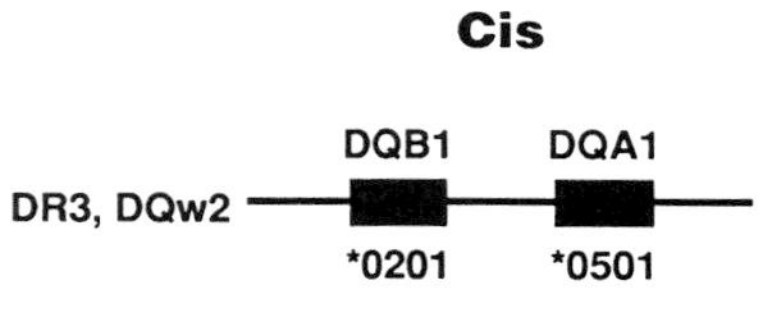

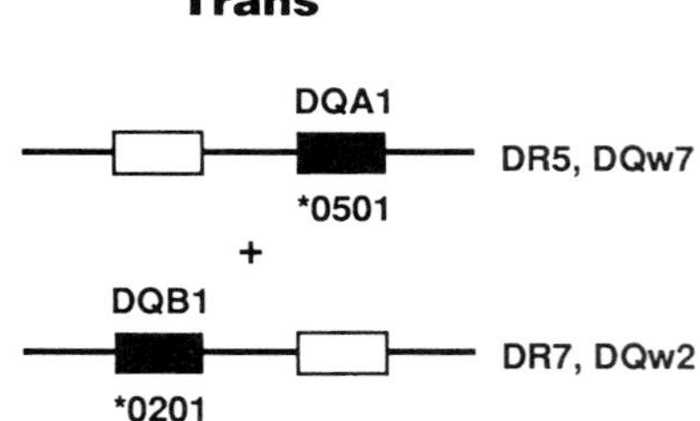

Fig. 12-9 DQ heterodimer model in celiac disease. Most CD patients bear the HLA-DRB1*0301, DQA1*0501, DQB1*0201 haplotype (the former DR3, DQw2 haplotype). The remaining CD patients are predominantly DRB1*11, DQA1*0501, DQB1*0301/DRB1*07, DQA1*0201, DQB1*0201 heterozygotes (the former DR5, DQw7/DR7, DQw2 haplotypes). The DQα chain encoded by the DRB1*11, DQA1*0501, DQB1*0301 (=DR5, DQw7) haplotype is identical to the DQα chain encoded by the HLA-DRB1*0301, DQA1*0501, DQB1*0201 (=DR3, DQw2) haplotype and the DQβ chain encoded by the DRB1*07, DQA1*0201, DQB1*0201 (=DR7, DQw2) haplotype is virtually identical to the DQβ chain encoded by the HLA-DRB1*0301, DQA1*0501, DQB1*0201 (=DR3, DQw2) haplotype.

cellular hyperplasia, while chronic autoimmune thyroiditis is often characterized by thyroid-cell destruction, the two diseases have similarities in their pathogenesis. Common features of both diseases include autoantibodies to thyroid-cell proteins, thyroid-infiltrating T lymphocytes, and an association with certain HLA antigens, the identity of which depends on the ethnic population involved.

In GD, hyperthyroidism is caused by thyroid-stimulating autoantibodies that bind to and stimulate the thyroid-stimulating receptor on thyroid follicular cells. In contrast, hypothyroidism in chronic autoimmune thyroiditis may be the result of autoantibodies to the thyroid-stimulating receptor, which have no intrinsic stimulating effect but appear to inhibit the action of TSH. Other major thyroid autoantigens against which antibodies have been found include thyroglobulin and thyroid peroxidase. While the function of antithyroglobulin antibodies is uncertain in both diseases, antithyroid peroxidase antibodies may at least in part cause the hypothyroidism in chronic autoimmune thyroiditis by inhibiting thyroid peroxidase and mediating cytotoxicity by natural killer cells.[177]

In both GD and chronic autoimmune thyroiditis, accumulations of T lymphocytes of both the CD4 and CD8 subtypes have been found in the thyroid gland, indicating that T cells are involved in the pathogenesis of these diseases. There is evidence that TCR Vα genes in T cells isolated from autoimmune thyroid glands have less variability than peripheral blood TCR Vα genes from the same patient. Even though the predominantly expressed Vα genes differ from patient to patient, this finding may indicate that administration of specific TCR antibodies may be useful in the treatment of GD and chronic autoimmune thyroiditis in the future.[178]

GD and chronic autoimmune thyroiditis are associated with certain HLA alleles. However, different studies have yielded different associations, making it difficult to reach a consensus.

Population studies in Caucasian GD patients have shown an association with HLA-DR3, whereas in China and Japan the HLA association seems rather to be with two HLA-B antigens, HLA-Bw46 and HLA-B35, respectively. The reason for these different associations is poorly understood, but may involve differences in the pathogenesis of GD in different ethnic groups.

Family studies have shown that GD runs in families and that HLA haplotypes are shared by affected sib pairs. Furthermore, the lower concordance rates for GD in HLA-identical sibs (7 percent) than in monozygotic twins (25 to 50 percent) imply that one or more other unlinked genes contribute to disease susceptibility. Moreover, the high rate of discordance between monozygotic twins suggests that environmental factors also influence susceptibility.

In contrast to GD, chronic autoimmune thyroiditis has been found to be associated with the serologically defined HLA-DR4 and DR5 specificities.[177,179] A recent study, however, found that the association is rather with the DQw7 specificity, and that this marker also accounts for the HLA-DR associations as a consequence of linkage disequilibrium.[180]

Psoriasis

Psoriasis is a skin disease of unknown etiology that is characterized by increased proliferation of keratinocytes and rapid epidermal turnover leading to the characteristic thickened scaly plaques. The pathogenesis of psoriasis is suspected to be autoimmune in nature for the following reasons: (a) Immunosuppressive drugs such as cyclosporin A, methotrexate, and corticosteroids have an antipsoriatic effect; (b) lymphocytes infiltrate the skin prior to clinical changes; and (c) psoriasis has an association with the class I antigens HLA-B13, HLA-B17, and Cw6, the association with Cw6 being the strongest.[181] The concordance rate for psoriasis in monozygotic twins is 40 to 65 percent, suggesting that as yet unidentified environmental factors also play a role in the pathogenesis of psoriasis.

Approximately 7 percent of patients with psoriasis develop an inflammatory, seronegative arthritis. Several subgroups of psoriatic arthritis are recognized, including a psoriatic spondylitis, which, like AS, is associated with HLA-B27, and an arthritis that resembles RA and that also exhibits an association with HLA-DRB1*04.

The HLA association of psoriasis is interesting because psoriasis, AS, and Reiter disease are the only known class I-associated autoimmune disorders. Furthermore, psoriasis is the only disease associated with the HLA-C locus. The class I association indicates that CD8+ cells have a critical role in the development of psoriasis. This assumption is further substantiated by the fact that in the aggressive AIDS-related psoriasis, the lymphocyte infiltrate in the dermis is deficient in CD4+ T cells and consists predominantly of CD8+ T cells. Various cytokines have also been implicated in the pathogenesis of psoriasis. For instance, epidermal keratinocytes found in a psoriatic lesion have receptors for the cytokines IL-1 and IL-6, both of which can stimulate keratinocytes to increase proliferation.[182]

Pemphigus Vulgaris

Pemphigus vulgaris (PV) is a disorder of the mucosa and the skin that is characterized by intraepidermal blister formation. The blister formation is caused by autoantibodies that bind to keratinocyte surface antigens and thereby interfere with normal cell-to-cell adhesion, resulting in a separation of epidermal cells in the basal layers of the epidermis. The target autoantigen for the autoantibodies has recently been identified as a new member of the cadherin family of calcium-dependent cell adhesion molecules, which is mostly related to desmoglein I.[183] On this basis it seems reasonable to assume that the autoantibodies do disrupt cell-to-cell adhesion in the epidermis and that this is one pathophysiologic mechanism in PV. However, it has also been suggested that the autoantibodies induce keratinocytes to produce proteolytic enzymes, which may target intercellular substances.[183]

PV, which is relatively common among Jews, particularly Ashkenazi Jews, is strongly associated with the serotypes HLA-DR4 and HLA-DRw6. The DR4 association can be accounted for by the DRB1*0402 allele, which, as mentioned above in the "Rheumatoid Arthritis" section, belongs to the DR4 family but differs from the other DR4 alleles by three amino acids at positions 67, 70, and 71 in the third hypervariable domain of the DRβ chain. The DRw6 association, on the other hand, is most strongly associated with a rare DQB1 allele, which, interestingly, has aspartic acid at position 57 in the third hypervariable domain (see "Insulin-Dependent Diabetes Mellitus," above).[184] Thus, at least two different HLA alleles from two different isotypes confer susceptibility to PV. Further studies are needed to assess the role of these alleles in generating an autoimmune response to the epithelial cadherin.

Narcolepsy

Narcolepsy is a syndrome of excessive sleepiness and abnormalities in rapid-eye-movement sleep that is often associated with cataplexy. Serologic and DNA typing have shown that narcolepsy is strongly associated with the HLA-DR2, Dw2 (i.e., DRB1*1501, DQA1*0102, DQB1*0602) haplotype.[185,186] This association can be demonstrated by a number of observations. First, the association of narcolepsy with the DRB1*1501, DQA1*0102, DQB1*0602 haplotype has been found worldwide (Japan, USA, France, Great Britain, Germany, Sweden, and Israel). No other HLA haplotype(s) are associated with the disease. Second, this association is very strong. The DRB1*1501, DQA1*0102, DQB1*0602 haplotype is found in 90 to 100 of narcolepsy patients but has a frequency of only 12 to 34 percent in control populations.[187] This haplotype confers a relative risk for narcolepsy of 29 in Caucasians and 409 in Japanese.[188,189] However, the DRB1*1501, DQA1*0102, DQB1*0602 haplotype is neither necessary nor sufficient for development of narcolepsy. Indeed, patients negative for DRB1*1501, DQA1*0102, DQB1*0602, as well as monozygotic twins discordant for the disease, have been described.[188] The presence of the DQB1*0602 allele in a number of DR2-negative patients suggests that the location of the narcolepsy-susceptibility gene is closer to the DQ locus than to the DR locus, and may be DQ itself. The finding that the association with the DQB1*0602 allele is much stronger in African Americans than the association with the DR2 allele is consistent with such a possibility.[190,191] The DRB1*1501 and DQB1*0602 molecules of narcoleptic patients do not appear to differ structurally from the corresponding molecules in normal subjects, as determined by isoelectrofocusing and gene sequencing.[192]

The etiology and pathophysiology of narcolepsy are still unclear, as is the role of a gene in the HLA complex in the development of the disease.[187] As biological and autopsy studies provide no evidence for the involvement of an inflammatory or autoimmune process, it has been suggested that a gene that produces a product essential for sleep control is located in the HLA complex in close linkage with the DR and DQ loci. However, the recently found genetic linkage of autosomal recessive canine narcolepsy with the Ig switch region gives strength to the hypothesis of an immunologic basis for narcolepsy.[193] Evidence for such an inflammatory lesion might only be present prior to or at the time of onset of the disease, with subsequent resolution or scarring, as is seen in type 1 diabetes.

Multiple Sclerosis

Multiple sclerosis (MS) is a chronic inflammatory demyelinating disease of the central nervous system. Its etiology and pathophysiology are still unclear. The prevailing hypothesis is that MS is a T-cell-mediated autoimmune disorder in which myelin-specific components target the response. Alternatively, an immune response directed against an oligodendrocyte-infecting virus may lead to demyelination. The two major clinical forms of MS are the relapsing/remitting form, in which the course of disease is characterized by bouts and remissions, and the primarily chronic progressive form, in which the disease progresses continuously from its onset. Several genetic factors, including Ig, TCR, and myelin basic protein (MBP) genes, have been implicated in the predisposition to MS, but the best characterized susceptibility-associated genes have been mapped to the HLA complex.

The suggestion that the HLA complex contributes to genetic MS susceptibility was derived from the initial observations in the early 1970s showing an association of MS with the HLA-A3 and B7 alleles. Since then, a closer association has been established in northern Europeans and North Americans between MS and the HLA-DRB1*1501, DQA1*0102, DQB1*0602 haplotype, which is in linkage disequilibrium with HLA-A3 and B7 alleles.[115] In other ethnic groups, different HLA-DR alleles are associated with MS. In Japanese and Mexicans, MS is associated with HLA-DRw6[194,195] and in Jordanian Arabs and Sardinians with HLA-DR4.[196,197] More recently, it has been proposed that the relapsing/remitting and primarily chronic progressive forms of MS are distinct disease entities not only clinically but also immunogenetically.[198] Indeed, the primarily chronic relapsing form has been found to have a positive association with the HLA-DRB1*04, DQB1*0302 haplotype in addition to its well-established association with the HLA-DRB1*1501, DQA1*0102, DQB1*0602 haplotype. In contrast, relapsing/remitting MS appears to have no association with the DRB1*04, DQB1*0302 haplotype. A second haplotype, HLA-DRB1*0301, DQB1*0201, has been found to be associated with relapsing/remitting MS, although these results require confirmation.

A significant association with HLA-DPw4, independent of the HLA-DRB1*1501 association, has also been found in two studies of Scandinavian MS patients. However, this association has not been confirmed in numerous subsequent studies,[199] and therefore it has been suggested that the MS-susceptibility gene(s) lie(s) telomeric to the HLA-DP loci. The telomeric end of the susceptibility region is not precisely known but does not seem to extend to the complement genes.[200]

Which locus or loci within this region encode(s) the MS-susceptibility gene has been a topic of intensive study. Partial sequence analysis of the DRB1, DQA1, and DQB1 genes from MS patients and control subjects has shown that there are no HLA class II sequences unique to MS patients.[201] Several RFLP studies have indicated a stronger association with the DQ loci than with the DRB1 locus. This is analogous to the situation in mice, where the I-A molecule (the murine equivalent of DQ) confers susceptibility to experimental autoimmune encephalomyelitis, an induced autoimmune disease that is considered to be a model for MS. In other studies, however, the association with DQB1*0602 was thought to be secondary to the association with the HLA-DRB1*1501 allele.[199] Since MS is associated with different HLA haplotypes in different ethnic groups, the hypothesis was proposed that the DRβ, DQα, or DQβ chains encoded by these MS-associated haplotypes share polymorphic sequences. However, the HLA-DRB1*1501, DRB1*04, and DRw6 alleles do not share polymorphic sequences in the N-terminal domain of the DRB1 gene. As a result, DQA1 and DQB1 alleles found in linkage disequilibrium with these three DR alleles were analyzed. Extensive sharing of hypervariable residues was found among DQB1 alleles.[202] Moreover, almost all patients studied had DQA1 alleles encoding glutamine at position 34.[203] This finding strongly suggested that the MS-associated genes in the HLA class II region are the DQA1 and DQB1 genes themselves. However, subsequent studies have shown that the association with shared sequences on the DQβ chain and glutamine at position 34 of the DQα chain was probably secondary to the association of MS with the HLA-DRB1*1501, DQA1*0102, DQB1*0602 haplotype.[199] Since the data suggesting that HLA class II genes confer susceptibility to MS are somewhat ambiguous, other genes that map in the HLA complex and encode proteins involved in the immune response have been proposed as candidates. There is evidence that TNFα may have functional role in the disease process.[204,205] However, no TNFα gene polymorphism has to date been associated with MS.[206] Additional genes, including TAP1, TAP2, LMP2, and LMP7, have most recently been analyzed in DR2-positive MS patients and control subjects, but, again, no significant differences were detected between the two groups.[207]

Malaria

Plasmodium falciparum is hyperendemic in West Africa and is responsible for the death of 1 percent of children under 5 years of age. Even though this mortality is high, it represents only a small fraction of the malaria-infected population. Thus, other factors, exogenous and genetic, are likely to affect the outcome of a malarial infection. Of the genetic factors that influence the infection, the hemoglobin variant HbS is the best known.

A recent study investigated the influence of HLA class I and II variation on susceptibility to *P. falciparum* in West Africa.[208] It was shown that the class I antigen HLA-Bw53 and the class II haplotype DRB1*1303, DQB1*0501 are independently associated with protection from severe malaria. Interestingly, the HLA-Bw53 antigen and the DRB1*1303, DQB1*0501 haplotype are common in malarial regions of West Africa but rare in other racial groups.[208] This geographic variation strongly supports the hypothesis that these alleles have a protective role, and also indicates that MHC polymorphism can be driven by infectious diseases.

The class I and II protective mechanisms are presumably different. The class I association suggests that cytotoxic T lymphocytes play a role in providing immunity (which is probably directed against the liver-stage malaria parasite, as erythrocytes do not express class I antigens), whereas the class II association may be interpreted as representing an antibody response mediated by T helper cells and resulting in a more rapid clearance of the blood-stage parasite.

The degree of protection conferred on an individual by the HLA alleles in question is less than that conferred by HbS. However, the higher frequency of the HLA alleles indicates that they have an overall larger protective effect.

TNF production in response to *P. falciparum* infection also appears to influence the outcome of malarial infection, which is interesting because of the association between TNF production and certain HLA alleles. TNF production is considered to be a normal and helpful host response to *P. falciparum* infection, but excessive production may predispose to cerebral malaria and a fatal outcome.[107] The beneficial effects of TNF in response to the malarial infection include activation of macrophages and neutrophils and the induction of fever, which may suppress parasite growth. The harmful effects of TNF when released in large amounts are not well understood but may be due to metabolic changes such as hypoglycemia and lactic acidosis, and inflammatory changes.[107]

Malignant Diseases

Studies have shown that associations exist between the major histocompatibility complex and malignant diseases associated with certain viruses.[209] These associations more than likely exist because certain viral antigens are presented to T cells by specific HLA molecules. Recent evidence suggests that Hodgkin disease and nasopharyngeal carcinoma, both of which have been associated with Epstein-Barr virus, are also associated with the HLA system. Hodgkin disease was originally reported to be associated with HLA-Bw35, and more recent studies suggest that HLA-DPw2 confers a weak resistance to Hodgkin disease.[210]

Nasopharyngeal carcinoma is 100 times more frequent in China than in Europe. Family studies in China have given strong evidence that nasopharyngeal carcinoma is associated with specific HLA haplotypes, even though the actual HLA gene(s) conferring the increased risk have not yet been identified.[211a] Furthermore, squamous cell carcinoma of the cervix and its precursor state, cervical dysplasia, are believed to be of viral origin, and human papilloma virus of the subtypes 16, 18, and 33 are thought to be causally involved in its pathogenesis. An association of squamous cell carcinoma and its precursor state with serologically defined HLA-DQw3 was recently reported.[211] This DQ specificity encompasses three different alleles, DQB1*0301, DQB1*0302, and DQB1*0303, which are distinguishable by sequence-specific oligonucleotide probes (SSOP). Additional studies using SSOP have shown that the DQB1*0301 and DQB1*0303 alleles account for the disease susceptibility. The DQB1*0302 allele is almost absent in the disease group, whereas it is present in 36 percent of healthy control subjects, suggesting that this allele may confer resistance to disease. DQB1*0303 differs from DQB1*0302 by only one codon, which codes for aspartic acid at position 57 in DQβ and is present on DQB1*0301 as well as DQB1*0303. This finding again confirms the functional importance of this residue, presumably in permitting certain specific immune responses (e.g., IDDM, PV, IgA deficiency, and cervical carcinoma). Another interesting question yet to be resolved is whether the HLA associations differ among patients infected with different subtypes of human papilloma virus.

The importance of studying the association between the HLA system and malignant diseases is further underscored by a recent study in which skin warts and invasive carcinomas were induced in rabbits by rabbit papillomavirus.[212] The authors demonstrated that regression and malignant conversion of rabbit viral papillomas were linked with MHC class II genes. However, because the MHC system in rabbits is poorly known, it was difficult to assign the linkage to individual MHC alleles.

Taken together, these studies suggest that HLA-encoded products influence the immune response against at least some, probably virally induced, tumors.

Selective IgA Deficiency and Common Variable Immunodeficiency

Selective IgA deficiency and common variable immunodeficiency (CVI) are the two most common primary immunodeficiencies in Caucasians. Several arguments suggest that these two entities are related. First, both are defined by low Ig serum levels—low IgA levels in the case of selective IgA deficiency (although an associated deficiency in one or several IgG subclasses is not rare), and low levels of IgA, IgG, and sometimes IgM in the case of CVI. Second, the two diseases share clinical manifestations, including recurrent respiratory infections, gastrointestinal malabsorption, and autoimmune disorders. Third, both diseases can occur in the same family.[213] Finally, they share HLA-associated genetic susceptibility.[214,215]

Selective IgA deficiency has been shown to be associated with MHC alleles and haplotypes. The association of selective IgA deficiency with HLA-DR3 and with HLA-B8 (which is in linkage disequilibrium with HLA-DR3) has been shown in different regions of the world.[216–220] Evidence for linkage of IgA deficiency with the HLA-A1, B8 haplotype has been suggested from some family studies[221] but not by all.[217]

The association of selective IgA deficiency with the HLA-A1, B8, DR3 haplotype has raised much interest, as this haplotype is associated with numerous autoimmune diseases. Although no large-scale study has compared the frequency of the HLA-A1, B8, DR3 haplotype in IgA-deficient subjects with or without autoimmunity, IgA-deficient patients with autoimmune diseases often carry this haplotype. Autoimmune disorders and selective IgA deficiency may therefore be associated by virtue of a common association with an HLA allele or haplotype, rather than by an effect of an IgA deficiency.[222]

Several other HLA alleles, most of which fall into two extended haplotypes, are also positively associated with selective IgA deficiency.[220,223] These haplotypes, as well as the A1, Cw7, B8, C4AQ0, C4B1, BfS, DR3 haplotype, have unusual MHC class III regions due to deletion or duplication of the C4A and C4B genes (encoding the complement component C4) and the steroid 21-hydroxylase gene. This situation has led one group to postulate that gene(s) regulating serum IgA concentration may be present in the central MHC region close to the C4 genes, and that defective expression of these genes caused by genomic rearrangement results in an imbalance of Ig production.[223] Other studies have confirmed the high frequency of C4A null alleles and C4A and 21-hydroxylase gene deletions in selective IgA deficiency and in CVI.[214,223a] A causal relationship between C4A deletion and selective IgA deficiency is unlikely, and the precise location of the susceptibility locus for selective IgA deficiency in the MHC has still to be established.[215] The recent discovery of numerous new genes in this region may permit the identification of this gene.

It has been shown recently that selective IgA deficiency is associated with non-Asp residues at position 57 of the β chain of the HLA-DQ molecule,[224] a feature also described in IDDM.[159] This finding was thought to explain the association between selective IgA deficiency and IDDM and led to the suggestion that the shared alleles at the HLA-DQB1 locus may themselves also confer susceptibility to selective IgA deficiency. However, it should be noted that HLA-DQB1 alleles conferring susceptibility to the two diseases, despite sharing a non-Asp at position 57, do not completely overlap. For example, IDDM is strongly associated with DQB1*0302 (DQw8) but selective IgA deficiency is not. Moreover, IDDM has yet to be shown conclusively to be associated with selective IgA deficiency.[225]

TNFα and Autoimmunity

On the basis of studies in humans and mice, it has been suggested that genetic polymorphism in the TNF gene may play a role in the associations between MHC antigens and certain autoimmune diseases. Functional studies support this hypothesis, although the exact role of TNF in autoimmunity is poorly understood. For example, in MS lesions, TNFα and TNFβ have been demonstrated by immunochemistry in astrocytes and T cells, respectively.[226] Furthermore, in vitro, recombinant human TNFα kills oligodendrocytes (the myelin-producing cells of the central nervous system),[227,228] and in vivo it mediates changes in myelin sheaths that are compatible with early steps in demyelination.[228] Moreover, astrocytes from EAE-susceptible rats produce more TNFα

than astrocytes from EAE-resistant rats in response to stimulation with IFN-γ and IL-1β.[229] In addition, transfer of EAE by T cells can be prevented by treating the recipients with a polyclonal antibody to TNFα and TNFβ.[230] Taken together, these studies indicate that TNFα and TNFβ may have a role in immune-mediated demyelination in MS, and that inhibition of TNFα and TNFβ could prevent MS/EAE.

In NZB × NZW F_1 mice, low production of TNFα may be involved in the pathogenesis of autoimmune "lupus" nephritis.[231] This notion is substantiated by the fact that RFLP patterns within the TNFα gene appear to correlate with reduced levels of TNFα production. TNFα therapy in NZB × NZW F_1 mice is also able to markedly slow progression of this autoimmune disease. These studies have been confirmed by other laboratories.[232] However, recent studies have identified this RFLP in several outbred, non-autoimmune-prone mice.[233] One report found that TNFα has a deleterious rather than a beneficial effect in murine lupus.[234] The role of TNFα in murine lupus is therefore unclear. TNFα may have opposite effects depending on timing, dose, and route of injection.

Of the HLA-alleles associated with human SLE, namely, HLA-DR2 and HLA-DR3, HLA-DR2-positive patients exhibit an increased risk of developing lupus nephritis.[138] This is interesting in light of the fact that mononuclear cells from HLA-DR2-positive individuals secrete significantly less TNFα after an LPS stimulus than do cells from HLA-DR2-negative donors.[235] There is suggestive evidence that low TNFα production may actually be involved in the genetic predisposition to lupus nephritis in humans, but accepting this interpretation is premature because many SLE patients are on steroid therapy, which reduces the levels of TNFα mRNA and protein.[236] Thus, a precise role for TNFα in the development of murine and human lupus nephritis remains to be established.

The role of TNFα in the development of IDDM in the NOD mouse has also been studied. Originally, it was shown by Bendtzen et al.[237] that IL-1 is toxic to pancreatic β cells in vitro, and that TNFα enhances this cytotoxicity.[238] In vivo studies have, however, shown that recombinant TNFα has a protective effect against development of diabetes in the NOD mouse.[239,240] Whether these data are contradictory or simply reflect a difference between in vitro and in vivo studies is unknown.

Thus, there is evidence that TNF is involved in the pathogenesis of certain autoimmune diseases. However, a more precise role for TNF in these diseases needs to be defined.

MECHANISMS OF AUTOIMMUNITY AND THE ROLE OF HLA-ENCODED ANTIGENS

A breakdown in self-tolerance leading to an autoimmune state involves both genetic and environmental elements. Normally, tolerance to self is achieved through complex mechanisms that down-regulate the activity of the anti-self T and B lymphocytes that develop in an individual. These mechanisms include clonal anergy and clonal deletion (negative selection) of populations of anti-self B, T helper, and T cytotoxic cells. In view of their role in facilitating the cellular interactions necessary for establishing tolerance to self, the class I and class II molecules encoded by the HLA complex are excellent candidates to function in the pathogenesis of autoimmune disease. In addition to these and other genetic elements, environmental factors such as pathogens or toxins are thought to trigger many of the disease processes. This triggering event may give the immune system access to a normally sequestered self antigen(s), and, if the appropriate genetic elements are in place (e.g., disease-susceptible HLA class I or II alleles), an autoimmune attack may be initiated and sustained.[241]

The Nature of HLA Peptide Binding and the Autoimmune Process

The HLA class I and II molecules function by binding antigenic peptides and presenting them to CD8+ and CD4+ T cells, respectively. It is therefore very likely that certain HLA alleles confer susceptibility to autoimmune diseases at the molecular level by binding specific antigenic peptides that other alleles do not bind. Indeed, an example of this is seen in EAE. This disease can be induced in mice by immunization with MBP plus adjuvants. Studies of antigenic epitopes within MBP in mice have shown that the N-terminal peptide (Ac1-11) binds to the murine class II molecule I-A^u (homologous to DQ in humans) and that this peptide alone is sufficient to induce EAE upon immunization in I-A^u mice. The MBP-derived peptide 89-101 binds I-A^s and is able to cause disease in mice of this haplotype. However, I-A^u does not bind 89-101, and this peptide is unable to cause disease in animals that carry the I-A^u haplotype.[242] IDDM and RA provide two additional examples of diseases for which differences in peptide binding may explain the HLA associations (Fig. 12-8). Sequence analysis of susceptible and protective alleles in IDDM suggests that the aspartic acid at position 57 of the DQβ chain may have a critical function in resistance to IDDM. By modeling the structure of these DQ class II molecules, it can be deduced that this aspartic acid residue likely forms a salt bridge with a conserved arginine on the α chain. Breaking this salt bridge could alter the ability of the groove to bind various peptides. For example, a peptide that interacts with the conserved arginine via a negative charge on the peptide would be bound with higher affinity by molecules that lack Asp 57. If this peptide were the trigger for IDDM, then this mechanism would help explain the association of non-Asp 57 alleles with IDDM.[159]

Susceptibility to RA appears to be associated with a region of amino acid residues from positions 67 to 74 in the DRβ chain. Whereas the DRB1*0401 and DRB1*0404 molecules have positively charged residues at positions 70 and 71 (Fig. 12-8), DRB1*0402 has acidic residues there. This finding suggests that a positively charged region in these molecules may be necessary for developing RA.[7]

The discovery of the HLA-encoded molecules LMP (low-molecular-mass polypeptide) and TAP (transporters associated with antigen processing) molecules, which are believed to be involved in the generation and transport, respectively, of peptides, provides a new avenue for assessing HLA associations with disease. It is possible that these molecules dictate the nature and accessibility of peptides that are destined to be bound by class I antigens. If so, self peptides may be generated that, in the presence of the appropriate HLA class I or molecule(s), may elicit an autoimmune response. Support for this notion comes from the observation that in the rat, two different alleles of the TAP heterodimer complex appear to be responsible for the efficient binding of antigenically distinct peptides to the same class I molecule alleles.[243] Moreover, a recent study examining HLA-B27-positive EBV B cell lines from a family with a history of AS and related diseases showed that these B cells were unable to present a known peptide epitope to cytotoxic T lymphocytes. The HLA-B27 molecule was shown to contain no mutations, suggesting that the defect may reside at the level of peptide synthesis and/or transport.[118] The question of whether the LMP and TAP molecules indeed have a direct association with disease still requires elucidation. Similar systems dedicated to the synthesis and transport of peptides destined for class II presentation undoubtedly exist.

Inability to Tolerize to Self Antigens

A number of mechanisms operate to ensure that a response to self is not normally elicited. One of these is the induction of tolerance in the T cell compartment. T cells can be made tolerant by three general mechanisms: clonal deletion, clonal anergy, and antigen-specific immune suppression.[244] Each of these mechanisms is dependent on the nature of the HLA molecules with which these T cells come into contact and, therefore, may provide a molecular mechanism for the association between HLA genes and disease.

A number of models of immunologic tolerance have demonstrated that clones of autoreactive T cells are deleted during their development in the thymus. For example, the relatively high frequency in mice of T cells that bear specific TCRβ chains reactive to "superantigens" derived from self has facilitated the detection of their deletion as they mature in a host that contains the necessary self superantigen. Similar results have been obtained in transgenic mice in which most of the T cells express an identical receptor specific for a self protein that is expressed in the thymus. A critical aspect of all of these studies is that tolerance is only established following an interaction between the test antigen and an MHC molecule.

Clonal deletion is not the sole mechanism by which T cells become tolerized to self antigens. Anergy has been well documented in both the B and T cell compartments.[245] Anergy in T cells has been postulated to be due to the ligation of a TCR with its cognate MHC-antigen complex but without an additional stimulus provided by the antigen-presenting cell (APC). Through the use of either environmental superantigens or transgenic mice, a number of groups have found that tolerance to antigens expressed in the periphery and not in the thymus is achieved by the induction of a state of functional unresponsiveness within the autoreactive T cell population and not by the deletion of those cells.

An additional means by which the immune system is believed to establish a state of tolerance to self is through active suppression of autoreactive T cells found in the periphery. The molecular mechanisms of suppression are at best ill defined. One hypothesis suggests an interaction with the MHC via secreted TCR molecules. Peripheral tolerance in the T cell compartment may also be gained through "immunologic ignorance" to self. An example of this is believed to occur in EAE, where MBP-reactive T cells are present in the periphery but do not cause disease unless they are stimulated by exogenous MBP plus adjuvants. These T cells normally do not encounter MBP because of the blood-brain barrier and, therefore, normally maintain a resting state.

The genetic nature of an HLA-disease association can provide clues into the role(s) that tolerance induction (or lack thereof) may have in the autoimmune process. For most autoimmune diseases, the presence of one susceptibility allele tends to confer the same risk as the presence of two, suggesting that the susceptibility allele acts like a Mendelian dominant trait. The ability to act as a restriction element for a given peptide is also inherited as a simple dominant trait, and this fact provides the simplest (but not the only) interpretation of such HLA-disease associations. The susceptibility allele serves as a restriction element for the autoantigenic peptide. In some diseases, however, two susceptibility alleles are required for the development of disease. This situation implies that the protective alleles are functioning as dominant traits and that susceptibility functions as a recessive one. Where this situation is observed, it is possible that susceptibility is the result of a failure of a particular allele to induce tolerance to the autoantigen. Therefore, a single protective allele that is able to successfully induce tolerance is dominant over a susceptibility allele that fails to do so.[7] There are instances where there is a requirement for two susceptibility alleles that are different. This situation suggests that epistatic interactions between the different loci on the two haplotypes are necessary. Such an occurrence could be explained by having a heterodimer composed of an α chain carried by one haplotype and a β chain carried by the other. This mixed heterodimer is then likely to be the actual molecule directly involved in disease susceptibility. Three diseases have been associated with hybrid molecules — P-JRA, CD, and IDDM. In IDDM, both HLA-DR3 and HLA-DR4 confer a relative risk (RR) of 5. However, heterozygotes for HLA-DR3 and HLA-DR4 have a significantly greater risk of developing IDDM (RR = 14). There is evidence that this heterozygote effect is due to a hybrid HLA-DQ molecule formed between the DQβ chain from the HLA-DR4 haplotype and the DQα chain from the HLA-DR3 haplotype.[158]

Mechanisms by Which the Immune System Targets Self Antigens

To date, three general mechanisms have been put forth by which a self antigen can elicit an anti-self response. In the first case, tissue damage brought on by bacterial or viral infections causes sequestered antigens from immunologically "privileged" sites to become accessible to surrounding cells that express HLA class II molecules. Indeed, a number of viruses have been implicated in MS, and an increased incidence of IDDM has been reported in DR3-positive patients with a history of congenital rubella infection.[241]

A second mechanism involves ectopic expression of class II molecules by cell types normally considered not to be immunocompetent, thereby allowing the immune system access to normally sequestered antigens.[246] The acquisition of class II expression by a cell is thought to be the result of the inductive effects of various cytokines, especially IFN-γ. In the presence of autoreactive T cells, presentation of a self antigen may lead to an autoimmune response. Various examples have been described in which class II molecules are expressed on target tissues that are normally class II-negative. Aberrant class II expression has been detected on synovial cells in RA, on pancreatic β cells in IDDM, and on thyrocytes in glands from patients with Graves disease and Hashimoto thyroiditis. It is unclear, however, whether ectopic expression of class II is an initiating event for these diseases or simply reflects a secondary event. Class II expression, for instance, can be induced on normal thyrocytes and β cells by IFN-γ and/or TNFα, cytokines that are produced and secreted by T cells and/or monocytes that are present in autoimmune inflammatory sites.

In an attempt to determine whether ectopic class II expression is a primary or secondary event in IDDM, transgenic mice expressing MHC class II molecules in pancreatic β cells have been produced.[247] A clinical diabetic state developed, although these mice exhibited no signs of immune-mediated diabetes, suggesting that ectopic class II expression alone is not sufficient to induce autoimmunity in this animal model.

A self antigen is thought to be targeted by the immune system by a third mechanism based on the observation that some bacterial and viral proteins share regions of amino acid sequence with mammalian proteins. The molecular mimicry hypothesis of autoimmunity proposes that an antigenic determinant, when shared between a pathogen and host, can result in the targeting of the host "self" determinant by an immune response initially directed against the pathogen.[248]

Despite the fact that a number of examples have been described in which molecular mimicry is thought to be the inductive event in the disease process, a direct causal relationship has yet to be established. For example, the two isoforms of GAD, recently identified as β islet cell autoantigens in IDDM, have a striking sequence similarity to a coat protein expressed by coxsackievirus, a virus that has been associated with IDDM in humans. Whether this similarity is merely a coincidence or indeed has a functional significance in the disease process requires further elucidation.

The mechanism(s) that enable molecular mimicry to break tolerance to self molecules is not well understood. One possibility is that molecular mimicry ensues when the pathogen and host determinants are sufficiently similar to induce a cross-reactive response yet different enough to override B and T cell immunologic tolerance. Whether a particular peptide meets these criteria would be determined to a large extent by the class I or II molecules to which it is bound. For example, a class I/II allele associated with disease susceptibility may bind an antigenic peptide that results in an epitope that is highly cross-reactive with a self molecule. In contrast, a neutral or protective allele may either not bind the self-mimicking peptide or may bind the peptide in such a manner that the resulting conformation may minimize the peptide's potential for cross-reactivity.

Yet another scenario by which molecular mimicry may break tolerance could involve a pathogen that carries a protein that contains an amino acid sequence similar to a "cryptic" self peptide. Normally, a self protein is processed into several peptides, some of which are incapable of efficiently competing for binding to the appropriate HLA molecule. Consequently, these cryptic peptides are unable to induce tolerance or elicit an autoimmune response.[249] Following infection with a pathogen, however, T cells may become sufficiently sensitized by a cross-reacting peptide to detect the cryptic self peptide and initiate an anti-self response.[249] The extent of homology between a self and cross-reacting peptide may consist of as few as six amino acid residues. For example, EAE can be induced by immunization with an MBP peptide only six residues in length (Gautam and McDevitt, unpublished results).

An often-cited example of molecular mimicry that may have a role in autoimmunity is the strong association found between AS and HLA-B27. It has been demonstrated that the nitrogenase enzyme of *K. pneumoniae*, a bacterium found in the bowels of most individuals including AS patients, contains a sequence of six amino acid residues identical to that found in the HLA-B27 molecule. Although this finding is striking, it is difficult to reconcile with the fact that AS is mainly limited to the synovial joints of the spine, whereas HLA-B27 molecules, like other class I molecules, are expressed on most somatic cell types.[117]

Another possibility is that an "arthritogenic peptide" that is found only in the joint tissues binds preferentially to the HLA-B27 molecule. Under normal conditions, this peptide may be a cryptic peptide. However, infection with bacteria could sensitize the appropriate T cells and result in an anti-self response to the arthritogenic peptide. Clearly, further investigation is required to identify the mechanism(s) involved.

The three mechanisms that lead to targeting of self antigens by the immune system — tissue damage, ectopic class II expression, and molecular mimicry — need not be mutually exclusive. It is likely that each mode may operate to a varying degree depending on the situation.

Failure to tolerize may also result from an inability of the immune system to effectively purge autoreactive B and T cells during clonal deletion. Clonal deletion is believed to involve physiological cell death or apoptosis. It is conceivable that blocking of the signals that trigger apoptosis or overriding of those signals upon transduction could, in turn, reduce the efficiency of the clonal deletion event. MRL mice, which are prone to SLE, provide such an example. The lpr mutation that is characteristic of these mice and which is manifested by a lymphoproliferative disorder maps to a defect in the gene of Fas, a transmembrane antigen that can normally trigger programmed cell death when it binds to antibody.[250] Studies using in vitro established cell lines and transgenic model systems have shown that apoptosis can also be abrogated by elevated levels of expression of the bcl-2 proto-oncogene protein.[251,252]

AUTOANTIGENS

Direct knowledge of the autoantigen(s) that targets an autoimmune response is essential to gaining insight into the disease process, as well as for establishing possible therapeutic modalities. For most autoimmune disorders, very little is known about the self antigen(s) that HLA susceptibility alleles present to T cells. However, as shown in Table 12-2, several candidate autoantigens have recently been reported. Many of these have been identified because they are targets for the humoral response in their respective diseases. The thyroid-stimulating hormone (TSH) receptor and acetylcholine receptor have direct roles in the pathogenesis of Graves disease and myasthenia gravis, respectively. However, their roles in the initiation of the disease process and their interactions with regulatory T cells are unclear. GAD and peripherin, which are candidate autoantigens in IDDM,[152,153] were both identified by characterizing the autoantibodies which develop in diabetic humans (GAD only) and the NOD mouse (both). These results are particularly interesting in light of recent findings in stiff-man syndrome,[253] in which antibodies to GAD can also be detected. About one-third of anti-GAD-positive patients also develop IDDM. Both of these antigens have yet to be studied for their role in MHC binding or T cell immunity.

Table 12-2 Candidate Autoantigens in Autoimmune Disease

Disease	Antigens
Autoimmune adrenalitis	17α-Hydroxylase
Chronic autoimmune thyroiditis	Thyroid peroxidase
Graves disease	TSH receptor
IDDM	GAD, peripherin, carboxypeptidase H, HSP60, HSP69
Myasthenia gravis	Acetylcholine receptor
Multiple sclerosis	MBP
Pemphigus vulgaris	Cadhedrin family member
Primary biliary cirrhosis	2-oxo-acid dehydrogenases
Rheumatoid arthritis	HSP65

Of the antigens shown in Table 12-2, only two have been studied in relation to T cells and MHC molecules. The role of MBP in EAE was mentioned before, and, whereas T cells specific for MBP are present in the cerebral spinal fluid of MS patients, similar T cells are also found in the peripheral blood of healthy individuals.[242] The 65-kDa heat-shock protein (HSP65) of *Mycobacterium tuberculosis* has been implicated in more than one autoimmune disease.[112,125] T cells with specificity for HSP65 have been isolated from the synovial tissues of patients with RA, and HSP65 specific T cells can cause diabetes in certain strains of mice. Finally, HSP65 has been used in adjuvants to induce arthritis in experimental animals. Analysis of the epitopes in this protein may show that the autoantigen is from a region that is conserved between a mycobacterial and a human (or rodent) HSP, and that infection with mycobacteria species or other microbes is an initiating event in these diseases. Alternatively, both disease processes may lead to the release of normally sequestered murine or human HSP, resulting in a response to it that cross-reacts with the mycobacterial protein.

It is likely that there are several antigens that are able to initiate an autoimmune process, while others may act only to perpetuate and/or focus the destruction. However, the associations with particular class II allelic hypervariable regions may imply that a single antigen, and a single immunodominant peptide, initiates the process in most patients.

Initial data providing insight into the nature of the peptides that are found bound to class II molecules suggest that they tend to be longer and less restricted than the peptides that bind to class I molecules. Elution from two murine class II molecules analogous to the human DR and DQ proteins.

ADDENDUM: A CURRENT VIEW OF THE HLA COMPLEX AND ITS RELATIONSHIP TO DISEASE

Peter Parham and Hugh O. McDevitt

Introduction. Since publication in 1995 of the seventh edition of *The Metabolic and Molecular Bases of Inherited Disease*, knowledge of the HLA complex and its role in the pathogenesis of autoimmune and metabolic diseases has greatly increased. The advances are described briefly here, with pertinent references and short commentaries, to help readers find their way in what continues to be a rapidly moving field.

Polymorphism in HLA Class I and Class II Genes. In humans, the major histocompatibility complex (MHC) is situated on the short arm of chromosome 6 at 6p21.3. It is also called the HLA complex because it was first defined as the site for genes encoding highly polymorphic *H*uman *L*eukocyte *A*ntigens, now known to be a consequence of allelic differences at HLA class I and II genes. These genes encode similarly structured molecules that bind antigenic peptides and present them to cytotoxic CD8 T cells and helper CD4 T cells, respectively. There are three class I isoforms — HLA-A, -B, and -C — and three class II isoforms — HLA-DP, -DQ, and -DR. Class I molecules comprise an

Table 12-3 Numbers of Alleles Defined for HLA Class I and II Genes

HLA class I alleles	
HLA-A	151
HLA-B	301
HLA-C	83
HLA-E	5
HLA-F	1
HLA-G	14
HLA-class II alleles	
HLA-DRA*	2
HLA-DRB1*	228
HLA-DRB3	23
HLA-DRB4	9
HLA-DRB5	14
HLA-DRB6	3
HLA-DRB7	2
HLA-DQA1	20
HLA-DQB1	43
HLA-DPA1	18
HLA-DPB1	87
HLA-DMA	4
HLA-DMB	6
HLA-DOA	8
HLA-DOB	3

*Genes encoding α chains are designated A and genes encoding β chains B.
Courtesy of Steven GE Marsh, October 1999.

HLA-encoded polymorphic heavy chain and β_2-microglobulin (invariant and encoded by a gene on chromosome 15). By contrast class II molecules comprise HLA-encoded α and β chains, of which the β chain is polymorphic in all three isoforms, whereas the α chain is invariant in HLA-DR and polymorphic in HLA-DQ.

Because of the practical benefits obtained from matching transplant recipients and donors for HLA type, alleles of the polymorphic HLA genes continue to be intensively studied, increasingly at the level of nucleotide sequence. The numbers of alleles currently defined for each locus are shown in Table 12-3 and more detailed descriptions for each allele are to be found in the HLA FactsBook.[254] "New" alleles continue to be discovered on a monthly basis. These data are collected in a specialized database that is accessible via the World Wide Web (www.ebi.ac.uk/imgt/hla/) and regularly updated.[255]

The polymorphic HLA class I and II gene products present peptides to α/β T cells and provide adaptive immunity against infections. The extraordinary polymorphism of these genes is believed to reflect the accumulated response of human populations to the mechanisms by which pathogens can change to evade an immune response. The pressure from pathogens selects for novel variants of HLA-A, -B, -C, -DR, -DQ, and -DP genes that, as a result of point mutation or recombination, have antigen-presenting function to which pathogens have yet to adapt.[256]

The Complete Sequence of an HLA Complex. The genetic markers provided by the highly polymorphic HLA class I and II genes enabled susceptibility to many diseases to be associated with the complex, which, in turn, led to the discovery of additional genes within the HLA complex. The central importance of the HLA complex in the immune response and disease susceptibility naturally led this bit of the human genome to be one of the first targets for physical mapping and complete nucleotide sequencing. A contiguous sequence for 3600 kilobases was recently reported[257] that includes all the genes that were previously defined as HLA genes. In addition, the study revealed many new genes as well as much information relating to the organization of genes within the complex. Of the 224 genes that were identified, 128 are expressed genes and 96 are pseudogenes. In comparison to those other parts of the human genome that have been sequenced, the HLA complex is densely packed with genes. To a considerable degree, these genes are related to inflammation, immunity, and defense: ≈40 percent of the expressed genes. The gene associated with susceptibility to hemochromatosis was recently shown to be a class I gene, positioned 4000 kilobases on the telomeric side of where the HLA complex was previously thought to end. This discovery thus doubled the size of the human MHC. The sequence for the full 8000 kilobases is expected to be completed shortly. Rhodes and Trowsdale[258] provide a review of the organization of genes in the HLA complex, while Parham[259] also includes articles on the MHCs of other vertebrate species. The latest information on all aspects of HLA genomics can be obtained from the Sanger Center in Cambridge, UK (www.sanger.ac.uk).

New Crystal Structures of HLA Class II Proteins. The crystal structures of a large number of human and murine MHC class I and class II molecules have been published over the past 5 years. For class I MHC molecules, these crystal structures include both the classical, polymorphic class I molecules, and some of the nonclassical class I molecules, including H2-M3, CD1d, and several nonantigen-presenting molecules that possess the MHC class I-like fold. The latter include the neonatal rat Fc receptor (FcRn) and HFE, which is the candidate gene for hereditary hemochromatosis.[260]

The structures of a large number of murine and human class II molecules have also been published during the past 5 years, including the structure of the class II-related molecule H2-DM α/β. The latter molecule functions in the MIIC endosomal compartment to catalyze the removal of the invariant chain CLIP peptide from the MHC class II peptide-binding groove, thus opening the groove for binding of other peptides in this compartment. Nelson and Fremont[261] present a review of these structures, details of the interaction of bound peptides with these structures, and the various roles of the invariant chain and DM.

The crystal structure of a T cell receptor complexed with a peptide bound to an MHC molecule has now been presented for several T cell receptors interacting with MHC class I molecules, and one such complex for a T cell receptor interacting with an MHC class II molecule was recently published.[262] (This article includes references to all of the TCR/MHC/peptide cocrystals published to date.)

Most recently, the crystal structure of murine I-A^{g7} has been solved. This molecule mediates susceptibility to type I diabetes in the nonobese diabetic (NOD) mouse, and shares with HLA DQ2 and DQ8 the characteristic of lacking aspartic acid in position 57 in the beta chain, a sequence polymorphism with a major effect on susceptibility to type I diabetes in both the NOD mouse and in man.[263] Further study of the binding of peptides from islet cell proteins by I-A^{g7}, DQ8, and DQ2, combined with functional studies of the effect of these polymorphisms on the immune response to these islet cell proteins, offers the possibility of gaining new insights into the mechanism by which this sequence polymorphism increases susceptibility to type I diabetes in susceptible individuals.

New Functions of MHC Gene Products

Class I Related. Since 1994 it has become generally appreciated that HLA class I molecules not only determine the response of cytolytic CD8 T cells, but also that of natural killer (NK) cells, lymphocytes of innate immunity that provide defense from the beginning of infection. NK cells have many properties in common with cytolytic T cells and, like them, are implicated in defense against viruses. NK cells express two distinct types of receptors for HLA class I: one type that has structural similarities with C-type lectins (for example, mannose-binding protein) and is encoded by genes within the Natural Killer Complex (NKC) on chromosome 12; another type that is assembled from immunoglobulin-like domains and encoded by genes in the Leukocyte Receptor Complex (LRC) on chromosome 19. The latter receptors are known as Killer cell Immunoglobulin-like Receptors (KIR). Both the NKC and the LRC have properties in common with the MHC, including a specialization in defense genes, an unusual amount of polymorphism, and species-specific differences.[264]

The lectin-like receptors of NK cells are heterodimers of CD94 with either NKG2A or NKG2C. These receptors have specificity for HLA-E, a relatively nonpolymorphic class I molecule (Table 12-3). HLA-E has a hydrophobic peptide binding site, with an almost exclusive preference for binding peptides derived from the leader sequences of HLA-A, -B, and -C heavy chains. Although leader peptides from all HLA-A, -B, and -C heavy chains bind to HLA-E, only those with methionine at position -21 engage the CD94:NKG2 receptors. By contrast, KIR interact directly with polymorphic determinants of HLA-A, -B, and -C molecules and four different specificities have been defined. A characteristic of both NK-cell receptor families is the existence of inhibitory and activating receptors for HLA class I molecules. For example, CD94:NKG2A is inhibitory and CD94:NKG2C is activating. The former ensures NK-cell tolerance of healthy cells while the latter is believed to respond to specific features of infected cells. However, the principle by which NK cells recognize cells as being infected is not clear. Functions for two other relatively non-polymorphic class I genes, HLA-F and HLA-G (Table 12-3), remain obscure, but analogy with HLA-E suggests they may be candidate ligands for other types of NK-cell receptors (Table 12-3).

Within the HLA complex is a family of genes related in structure to class I genes. They have been called MIC for MHC class I-like Chain. MICA and MICB are expressed and polymorphic while MICC, D, and E are pseudogene fragments. Distinguishing MICA and MICB from class I heavy chains is their lack of association with β_2-microglobulin. MICA is expressed on intestinal epithelium and binds NKG2D, another type of lectin-like receptor of NK cells.

The gene associated with hemochromatosis, HFE, encodes a class I heavy chain that associates with β_2-microglobulin and is expressed in intestinal epithelium. Through interactions with the transferrin receptor, this molecule regulates the uptake of iron from the gut. The cause of hemochromatosis is an overloading of the body with iron and many patients with the disease have inherited two nonfunctional alleles of HFE. Although the HFE gene is separated from the HLA-A gene by more than 4000 kilobases, the disease was first associated with HLA-A3. Such association was only possible because the recombination rate in the region between the HFE and HLA-A is approximately one-fifth of that seen elsewhere in the human genome.[258]

Class II Related. Genes in the HLA complex encode five different types of class II molecule. In addition to the highly polymorphic HLA-DP, -DQ, and -DR genes, there are the less polymorphic HLA-DM and DO genes (Table 12-3). The latter molecules are not involved directly in presenting peptide antigens to CD4 T cells, but act inside the cell to facilitate the binding of peptides by HLA-DP, -DQ, and -DR. After synthesis and translocation to the endoplasmic reticulum, the α and β chains of HLA-DP, -DQ, and -DR bind a third polypeptide called the invariant chain. This interaction serves first to prevent peptide binding in the endoplasmic reticulum, and second to target the class II molecules to endocytic vesicles where the invariant chain is degraded, leaving a part of it (the so-called CLIP fragment) in the peptide-binding groove. In these vesicles, called MIIC for MHC class II Compartment, HLA-DO and -DM molecules associate with HLA-DP, -DQ, and -DR and catalyze the release of the CLIP fragment and its replacement with high-affinity peptides derived from lysosomal and endosomal degradation of antigenic material taken in from the environment. The HLA-DO molecule is selectively found in B cells and is believed to facilitate the loading of HLA class II molecules with peptides derived from antigens bound to and internalized as antigen-antibody complex with cell-surface immunoglobulin. This control mechanism would favor maintenance of cognate interactions between B and T cells specific for the same antigenic moiety.[265]

Table 12-4 Sequence Polymorphisms in DR4 Subtypes in Relation to Type I Diabetes

DRB1 sequence:	37	57	67	70	71	74	86	IDDM Susceptibility
DRB1*0405	Y	S	L	Q	R	A	G	Highly susceptible
DRB1*0401	Y	D	L	Q	K	A	G	Susceptible
DRB1*0404	Y	D	L	Q	R	A	V	Permissive/neutral
DRB1*0403	Y	D	L	Q	R	E	V	Protective
DRB1*0406	S	D	L	Q	R	E	V	Protective

Further Progress in Defining the Relations of HLA Complex Gene Polymorphisms to Disease

Susceptibility to Type I Diabetes Mellitus. Extensive population studies in many different ethnic groups around the world have revealed increasing complexity in the role of MHC class II genes in susceptibility and resistance to the development of type I diabetes. Earlier studies documented the primary role of HLA-DQ polymorphisms in susceptibility and resistance to type I diabetes, with DQ8 and DQ2 being the strongest susceptibility factors.[266] Some of these studies had shown that HLA-DR alleles also played an important modifying role in influencing susceptibility and resistance to type I diabetes.[267] More recently, it has become apparent that some HL-DR4 subtypes can play a dominant role, particularly in resistance to type I diabetes. This is shown in Table 12-4.

DRB1*0403 is a particularly striking example of this dominant protective effect of a DR molecule in HLA DQ-mediated susceptibility to type I diabetes.[268] The 0403 subtype differs from the highly susceptible 0405 subtype only at positions 57, 74, and 86 in the beta chain. 0403 expresses aspartic acid at position 57, glutamic acid at position 54, and valine in place of glycine at position 86. The remaining sequence of these two DR4 subtype beta chains is identical, as are the alpha chains for each molecule. The presence of DRB1*0403, even in individuals expressing DQ8 and DQ2 (the most highly susceptible DQ allelic combination), is strongly protective, and almost no individuals with this genotype develop type I diabetes.[269] Identification of the peptides from critical islet cell proteins, which are presented by the 0405 and 0403 gene products, and the functional effect of this peptide presentation, will have to be analyzed to understand how the 0403 sequence polymorphism mediates such strong protection. (While it is beyond the scope of this brief commentary, it should be noted that polymorphisms in MHC class I molecules and in HLA-DP class II molecules can also play a minor modifying role in determining susceptibility to type I diabetes.)

Polymorphism in Other Genes in the HLA Complex in Relation to Disease. Recent studies have shown association between polymorphisms in the TNF promoter and flanking regions in susceptibility to cerebral malaria.[270]

New Findings in the HLA-DR2-Related Disease, Narcolepsy. Extensive studies of narcoleptic patient populations have documented an extremely strong association with the HLA-DR2 haplotype. Ninety-five to 100 percent of these patients carry the HLA-DR2 haplotype, and detailed analysis of this patient population in different ethnic groups indicates that the HLA-DQB1*0602 allele is the responsible MHC class II polymorphism mediating susceptibility to this disease.[271] Recently, analysis of Doberman pinschers with an inherited, recessive form of narcolepsy has shown a defect in the gene encoding a neurotransmitter—orexin or hypocretin.[271] Studies of patients with narcolepsy have shown that these individuals have very low or undetectable levels of orexin in their spinal fluid, and much lower levels than found in normal controls.[272] These results indicate that the defect in this disease is a lack of ability to produce orexin. The mechanism responsible for this deficiency is unclear, but the characteristics of the narcoleptic patient population suggest that the disease may be autoimmune in nature. As is true for many autoimmune diseases, narcolepsy first becomes apparent at or near puberty and shows a strong MHC class II association (see above) and a concordance rate of approximately 30 percent in monozygotic twins. These latter statistics are similar to those for many MHC class II-associated autoimmune diseases, including type I diabetes.

Future Directions. The "complete sequence and gene map of a human major histocompatibility complex" reported by the MHC Sequencing Consortium is a pastiche in which different parts of the sequence derive from libraries made from DNA of individuals having different HLA types. Thus the sequence does not correspond to a natural haplotype and it is therefore called a virtual HLA haplotype. What it provides is a working plan for future analysis of real haplotypes and, in particular, those that are associated with diseases. The next stage is to compare different haplotypes, work that is already in hand because the DNA libraries used to get the first sequence were made from heterozygous individuals. It is to be hoped that at least one real HLA haplotype will be completely sequenced. The best candidate for such an effort is the A1-B8-DR3 haplotype, which is associated with many different autoimmune diseases. Another profitable type of analysis should focus on sequence comparison of those parts of the HLA complex which have differences in gene content between haplotypes, for example the segment between the DRA and DRB1 genes which contains a variable number of additional DRB genes (Table 12-1).

To good approximation, the virtual HLA sequence defines the set of genes that can cause a disease to be associated with HLA. Comparison of haplotypes has already shown that the HLA region is well covered with nucleotide substitutions and they will provide a much-expanded set of genetic markers with which to map disease associations within the HLA region and identify candidate genes. Soon we should know which of the diseases are truly associated with functional polymorphisms of the antigen presenting class I and class II molecules, and which are the more conventional genetic diseases associated with rare defective alleles of nonpolymorphic genes. A further division to be made will be between diseases involving immune system genes and those involving other types of genes. These distinctions may not always be so clear, as is well illustrated by hemochromatosis, which is a conventional genetic disease that involves a class I molecule with functions in both defense and metabolism.

Using the expanded array of genetic markers — single nucleotide polymorphisms and microsatellites as well as class I and II polymorphisms — it will be possible from family studies and population analysis to define the rates of recombination throughout the HLA region and to determine how that varies from one haplotype to another. The potential for this approach is that it will help distinguish whether linkage disequilibriums are due to natural selection for advantageous combinations of alleles or are the consequence of haplotypic differences that physically prevent recombination.

With the progression of genomic analysis on all of the human chromosomes, it became possible to identify regions on chromosomes 1, 9, and 19 that share similarities in organization to the MHC. Thus, members of certain gene families, for example Notch and RING 3, were found in the different regions and in similar order. The existence of such paralogous regions to the MHC is consistent with a model in which early vertebrate evolution involved two duplications of the entire genome. Class II genes are found only in the MHC, indicating that they evolved *in* the MHC after the two duplications of the genome. In contrast, MHC class I genes are found in some of the paralogous regions, and elsewhere, suggesting that they existed prior to one or both of the duplications and are older than class II genes. This correlation is also consistent with the wide range of functions that class I molecules perform, whereas class II molecules appear strictly concerned with the processing and presentation of antigenic peptides to CD4 T cells.[273]

The Thirteenth International Histocompatibility Workshop will focus on single nucleotide polymorphisms (SNPs) in MHC chains and their possible role in disease, in addition to the currently identified allelic associations with disease susceptibility.

We hope that the next decade will also see rapid progress in methods for cheap, efficient, DNA-sequence-based population-wide genotyping at or near birth. The development of such techniques would permit the identification of individuals with susceptibility to diseases such as type I diabetes, rheumatoid arthritis, and many others. This is particularly important for diseases like type I diabetes, in which the first clinical evidence of disease appears when the autoimmune process leading to destruction of the insulin-producing islet beta cells is already complete.

These studies, in combination with ongoing studies of the target autoantigens in many of these diseases, offer the prospect for a much more detailed understanding of the pathogenesis of these diseases and the development of new methods for both preventing and treating these diseases.

REFERENCES

1. McDevitt HO, Tyan ML: Genetic control of the antibody response in inbred mice. Transfer of response by spleen cells and linkage to the major histocompatibility (H-2) locus. *J Exp Med* **128**:1, 1968.
2. Lilly F, Boyse EA, Old LJ: Genetic basis of susceptibility to viral leukaemogenesis. *Lancet* **2**:1207, 1964.
3. Grumet FC, Coukell A, Bodmer JG, Bodmer WF, McDevitt HO: Histocompatibility (HL-A) antigens associated with systemic lupus erythematosus. A possible genetic predisposition to disease. *N Engl J Med* **285**:193, 1971.
4. Schlosstein L, Terasaki PL, Bluestone R, Pearson CM: High association of an HL-A antigen, W27, with ankylosing spondylitis. *N Engl J Med* **228**:704, 1973.
5. Jersild C, Svejgaard A, Fog T: HL-A antigens and multiple sclerosis. *Lancet* **1**:1240, 1972.
6. Nerup J, Platz, Andersen OO, Christy M, Lyngso J, Poulsen JE, Svejgaard A: HL-A antigens and diabetes mellitus. *Lancet* **2**:864, 1974.
7. Todd JA, Acha-Orbea H, Bell JI, Chao N, Fronek Z, Jacob CO, McDermott M, Sinha AA, Timmerman L, McDevitt HO: A molecular basis for MHC class II-associated autoimmunity. *Science* **240**:1003, 1988.
8. Lawlor DA, Zemmour J, Ennis PD, Parham P: Evolution of class-I MHC genes and proteins: From natural selection to thymic selection. *Annu Rev Immunol* **8**:23, 1990.
9. Bjorkman PJ, Parham P: Structure, function, and diversity of class I major histocompatibility complex molecules. *Annu Rev Biochem* **59**:253, 1990.
10. Bjorkman PJ, Saper MA, Samraoui B, Bennett WS, Strominger JL, Wiley DC: Structure of the human histocompatibility antigen, HLA-A2. *Nature* **329**:506, 1987.
11. Williams AF: A year in the life of the immunoglobulin superfamily. *Immunol Today* **8**:298, 1987.
12. Malissen M, Malissen B, Jordan BR: Exon/intron organization and complete nucleotide sequence of an HLA gene. *Proc Natl Acad Sci U S A* **79**:893, 1982.
13. Ragoussis J, Bloemer K, Pohla H, Messer G, Weiss EH, Ziegler A: A physical map including a new class I gene (cda12) of the human major histocompatibility complex (A2/B13 haplotype) derived from a monosomy 6 mutant cell line. *Genomics* **4**:301, 1989.
14. Bodmer JG, Marsh SGE, Albert ED, Bodmer WF, Dupont B, Erlich HA, Mach B, Mayr WR, Parham P, Sasazuki T, Schreuder GMT, Strominger JL, Svejgaard A, Terasaki PI: Nomenclature for factors of the HLA system, 1991. *Tissue Antigens* **39**:161, 1992.
15. Gotch F, Rothbard JB, Howland K, Townsend A, McMichael A: Cytotoxic T lymphocytes recognize a fragment of influenza virus matrix protein in association with HLA-A2. *Nature* **326**:881, 1987.
16. Zemmour J, Koller BH, Ennis PD, Geraghty DE, Lawlor DA, Orr HT, Parham P: HLA-AR, an inactivated antigen-presenting locus related to HLA-A. Implications for the evolution of the MHC. *J Immunol* **144**:3619, 1990.

17. Vidovic D, Roglic M, McKune K, Guerder S, MacKay C, Dembic Z: Qa-1 restricted recognition of foreign antigen by a gamma delta T-cell hybridoma. *Nature* **340**:646, 1989.
18. Pamer EG, Wang CR, Flaherty L, Fischer Lindahl K, Bevan MJ: H-2M3 presents a Listeria monocytogenes peptide to cytotoxic T lymphocytes. *Cell* **70**:215, 1992.
19. Kovats S, Main EK, Librach D, Stubblebine M, Fisher SJ, DeMars R: A class I antigen, HLA-G, expressed in human trophoblasts. *Science* **248**:220, 1990.
20. Bronson SK, Pei J, Taillon-Miller P, Chorney M, Geraghty DE, Chaplin DD: Isolation and characterization of yeast artificial chromosome clones linking the HLA-B and HLA-C loci. *Proc Natl Acad Sci U S A* **88**:1676, 1991.
21. Shukla H, Gillespie GA, Srivastava R, Collins F, Chorney MJ: A class I jumping clone places the HLA-G gene approximately 100 kilobases from HLA-H within the HLA-A subregion of the human MHC. *Genomics* **10**:905, 1991.
22. Parham P, Lomen CE, Lawlor DA, Ways JP, Holmes N, Coppin HL, Salter RD, Wan AM, Ennis PD: Nature of polymorphism in HLA-A, -B, and -C molecules. *Proc Natl Acad Sci U S A* **85**:4005, 1988.
23. Bjorkman PJ, Saper MA, Samraoui B, Bennett WS, Strominger JL, Wiley DC: The foreign antigen binding site and T cell recognition regions of class I histocompatibility antigens. *Nature* **329**:512, 1987.
24. Erlich HA, Gyllensten UB: Shared epitopes among HLA-class II alleles: Gene conversion, common ancestry and balancing selection. *Immunol Today* **12**:411, 1991.
25. Hughes AL, Nei M: Pattern of nucleotide substitution at major histocompatibility complex class I loci reveals overdominant selection. *Nature* **335**:167, 1988.
26. Lundberg AS, McDevitt HO: Evolution of major histocompatibility complex class II allelic diversity: Direct descent in mice and humans. *Proc Natl Acad Sci U S A* **89**:6545, 1992.
27. Holmes N, Ennis P, Wan AM, Denney DW, Parham P: Multiple genetic mechanisms have contributed to the generation of the HLA-A2/A28 family of class I MHC molecules. *J Immunol* **139**:936, 1987.
28. Holmes N, Parham P: Exon shuffling in vivo can generate novel HLA class I molecules. *EMBO J* **4**:2849, 1985.
29. Garrett TPJ, Saper MA, Bjorkman PJ, Strominger JL, Wiley DC: Specificity pockets for the side chains of peptide antigens in HLA-Aw68. *Nature* **342**:692, 1989.
30. Madden DR, Gorga JC, Strominger JL, Wiley DC: The structure of HLA-B27 reveals nonamer self-peptides bound in an extended conformation. *Nature* **353**:321, 1991.
31. Fremont DH, Matsumura M, Stura EA, Peterson PA, Wilson IA: Crystal structure of two viral peptides in complex with murine MHC class I H-2Kb. *Science* **257**:919, 1992.
32. Madden DR, Gorga JC, Strominger JL, Wiley DC: The three-dimensional structure of HLA-B27 at 2.1 Å resolution suggests a general mechanism for tight peptide binding to MHC. *Cell* **70**:1035, 1992.
33. Matsumura M, Fremont DH, Peterson PA, Wilson IA: Emerging principles for the recognition of peptide antigens by MHC class I molecules. *Science* **257**:927, 1992.
34. Townsend A, Elliott T, Cerundolo V, Foster L, Barber B, Tse A: Assembly of MHC class I molecules analyzed in vitro. *Cell* **62**:285, 1990.
35. Silver ML, Parker KC, Wiley DC: Reconstitution by MHC-restricted peptides of HLA-A2 heavy chain with beta2-microglobulin, in vitro. *Nature* **350**:619, 1991.
36. Falk K, Rotzschke O, Stefanovic S, Jung G, Rammensee HG: Allele-specific motifs revealed by sequencing of self-peptides from MHC molecules. *Nature* **351**:290, 1991.
37. van Bleek GM, Nathenson SG: Isolation of an endogenously processed immunodominant viral peptide from the class I H-2Kb molecule. *Nature* **348**:213, 1990.
38. Jardetzky TS, Lane WS, Robinson RA, Madden DR, Wiley DC: Identification of self peptides bound to purified HLA-B27. *Nature* **353**:326, 1991.
39. Schumacher TNM, DeBruijn MLH, Vernie LN, Kast WM, Neefjes JJ, Ploegh HL: Peptide selection by MHC class I molecules. *Nature* **350**:703, 1991.
40. Frankel WN, Rudy C, Coffin JM, Huber BT: Linkage of Mls genes to endogenous mammary tumour viruses of inbred mice. *Nature* **349**:526, 1991.
41. Kaufman JF, Auffray C, Korman AJ, Shackelford DA, Strominger JL: The class II molecules of the human and murine major histocompatibility complex. *Cell* **36**:1, 1984.
42. Buus S, Sette A, Colon SM, Jenis DM, Grey HM: Isolation and characterization of antigen-Ia complexes involved in T cell recognition. *Cell* **47**:1071, 1986.
43. Germain RN, Quill H: Unexpected expression of a unique mixed-isotype class II MHC molecule by transfected L-cells. *Nature* **320**:72, 1986.
44. Nepom BS, Schwarz D, Palmer JP, Nepom GT: Transcomplementation of HLA genes in IDDM. HLA-DQ alpha- and beta-chains produce hybrid molecules in DR3/4 heterozygotes. *Diabetes* **36**:114, 1987.
45. Brown JH, Jardetzky T, Saper MA, Samraoui B, Bennett WS, Bjorkman PJ, Wiley DC: A hypothetical model of the foreign antigen binding site of class II histocompatibility molecules. *Nature* **332**:845, 1988.
46. Brodsky FM, Guagliardi LE: The cell biology of antigen processing. *Annu Rev Immunol* **9**:707, 1991.
47. Miller J, Germain RN: Efficient cell surface expression of class II MHC molecules in the absence of associate invariant chain. *J Exp Med* **164**:1478, 1986.
48. Lotteau V, Teyton L, Peleraux A, Nilsson T, Karlsson L, Schmid SL, Quaranta V, Peterson PA: Intracellular transport of class II MHC molecules directed by invariant chain. *Nature* **348**:600, 1990.
49. Hartley SB, Crosbie J, Brink R, Kantor AB, Basten A, Goodnow CC: Elimination from peripheral lymphoid tissues of self-reactive B lymphocytes recognizing membrane-bound antigens. *Nature* **353**:765, 1991.
50. Roche PA, Cresswell P: Invariant chain association with HLA-DR molecules inhibits immunogenic peptide binding. *Nature* **345**:615, 1990.
51. Teyton L, O'Sullivan D, Dickson PW, Lotteau V, Sette A, Fink P, Peterson PA: Invariant chain distinguishes between the exogenous and endogenous antigen presentation pathways. *Nature* **348**:39, 1990.
52. Stern LJ, Wiley DC: The human class II MHC protein HLA-DR1 assembles as empty alpha/beta heterodimers in the absence of antigenic peptide. *Cell* **68**:465, 1992.
53. Sadegh-Nasseri S, Germain RN: A role for peptide in determining MHC class II structure. *Nature* **353**:167, 1991.
54. Germain RN, Hendrix LR: MHC class II structure, occupancy and surface expression determined by post-endoplasmic reticulum antigen binding. *Nature* **353**:134, 1991.
55. Rudensky A, Preston-Hurlburt P, Hong S-C, Barlow A, Janeway CA: Sequence analysis of peptides bound to MHC class II molecules. *Nature* **353**:622, 1991.
56. Chicz RM, Urban RG, Lane WS, Gorga JC, Stern LJ, Vignali DAA, Strominger JL: Predominant naturally processed peptides bound to HLA-DR1 are derived from MHC-related molecules and are heterogeneous in size. *Nature* **358**:764, 1992.
57. Kelly A, Powis SH, Kerr L-A, Mockridge I, Elliott T, Bastin J, Uchanska-Ziegler B, Ziegler A, Trowsdale J, Townsend A: Assembly and function of the two ABC transporter proteins encoded in the human major histocompatibility complex. *Nature* **355**:641, 1992.
58. Spies T, DeMars R: Restored expression of major histocompatibility class I molecules by gene transfer of a putative peptide transporter. *Nature* **351**:323, 1991.
59. Kelly A, Powis SH, Glynne R, Radley E, Beck S, Trowsdale J: Second proteasome-related gene in the human MHC class II region. *Nature* **353**:667, 1991.
60. Glynne R, Powis SH, Beck S, Kelly A, Kerr L-A, Trowsdale J: A proteasome-related gene between the two ABC transporter loci in the class II region of the human MHC. *Nature* **353**:357, 1991.
61. Andersson G, Larhammar D, Widmark E, Servenius B, Peterson PA, Rask L: Class II genes of the human major histocompatibility complex. Organization and evolutionary relationship of the DRbeta genes. *J Biol Chem* **262**:8748, 1987.
62. Jonsson A-K, Hyldig-Nielsen JJ, Servenius B, Larhammar D, Andersson G, Jorgensen F, Peterson PA, Rask L: Class II genes of the human major histocompatibility complex. Comparisons of the DQ and DX alpha and beta genes. *J Biol Chem* **262**:8767, 1987.
63. Gustafsson K, Widmark E, Jonsson A-K, Servenius B, Sachs DH, Larhammar D, Rask L, Peterson PA: Class II genes of the human major histocompatibility complex. Evolution of the DP region as deduced from nucleotide sequences of the four genes. *J Biol Chem* **262**:8778, 1987.
64. Trowsdale J, Kelly A: The human HLA class II alpha chain gene DZalpha is distinct from genes in the DP, DQ and DR subregions. *EMBO J* **4**:2231, 1985.

65. Tonnelle C, DeMars R, Long EO: DO β: A new β chain gene in HLA-D with a distinct regulation of expression. *EMBO J* **4**:2839, 1985.
66. Karlsson L, Surh CD, Sprent J, Peterson PA: A novel class II MHC molecule with unusual tissue distribution. *Nature* **351**:485, 1991.
67. Kelly AP, Monaco JJ, Cho S, Trowsdale J: A new human HLA class II-related locus, DM. *Nature* **353**:571, 1991.
68. Bell JI, Denney D, Foster L, Belt T, Todd JA, McDevitt HO: Allelic variation in the DR subregion of the human major histocompatibility complex. *Proc Natl Acad Sci U S A* **84**:6234, 1987.
69. Gyllensten UB, Sundvall M, Erlich HA: Allelic diversity is generated by intraexon sequence exchange at the DRB1 locus of primates. *Proc Natl Acad Sci U S A* **88**:3686, 1991.
70. White PC, Grossberger D, Onufer BJ, Chaplin DD, New MI, Dupont B, Strominger JL: Two genes encoding 21-hydroxylase are located near the genes encoding the fourth component of complement in man. *Proc Natl Acad Sci U S A* **82**:1089, 1985.
71. Sargent CA, Dunham I, Trowsdale J, Campbell RD: Human major histocompatibility complex contains genes for the major heat-shock protein HSP70. *Proc Natl Acad Sci U S A* **86**:1968, 1989.
72. Spies T, Morton CC, Nedospasov SA, Fiers W, Pious D, Strominger JL: Genes for the tumor necrosis factors α and β are linked to the human major histocompatibility complex. *Proc Natl Acad Sci U S A* **85**:8699, 1986.
73. Spies T, Blanck G, Bresnahan M, Sands J, Strominger JL: A new cluster of genes within the human major histocompatibility complex. *Science* **243**:214, 1989.
74. Spies T, Bresnahan M, Strominger JL: Human major histocompatibility complex contains a minimum of 19 genes between the complement cluster and HLA-B. *Proc Natl Acad Sci U S A* **83**:8955, 1990.
75. Sargent CA, Dunham I, Campbell RD: Identification of multiple HTF-island associated genes in the human major histocompatibility complex class III region. *EMBO J* **8**:2305, 1989.
76. Campbell DR: The molecular genetics of components of the complement system. *Bailliere's Clin Rheumatol* **2**:547, 1988.
77. Alper CA: Inherited structural polymorphism in human C2, evidence for genetic linkage between C2 and Bf. *J Exp Med* **144**:1111, 1976.
78. Bentley DR, Campbell RD, Cross SJ: DNA polymorphism of the c2 locus. *Immunogenetics* **22**:377, 1985.
79. Colten HR, Rosen FS: Complement deficiencies. *Annu Rev Immunol* **10**:809, 1992.
79a. Johnson CA, Densen P, Wetsel RA, Cole FS, Goeken NE, Colten HR: Molecular heterogeneity of C2 deficiency. *N Engl J Med* **326**:871, 1992.
80. Ruddy S: Complement deficiencies. The second component. *Progr Allergy* **39**:250, 1986.
81. Ross SC, Densen P: Complement deficiency states and infection: Epidemiology, pathogenesis and consequences of neisserial and other infections in an immune deficiency. *Medicine* **63**:243, 1984.
82. Alper CA, Boenisch T, Watson L: Genetic polymorphism in human glycine-rich beta-glycoprotein. *J Exp Med* **135**:68, 1972.
83. Mauff G, Hauptmann G, Hitzeroth HW, Gauchel F, Scherz R: The nomenclature of properdin factor B allotypes. *Z Immun-Forsch* **154**:115, 1978.
84. Mauff G, Federmann G, Hauptmann G: A haemolytically inactive gene product of factor B. *Immunobiology* **158**:96, 1980.
85. Raum D, Awdeh Z, Anderson J, Strong L, Granados J, Pevan L, Giblett E, Yunis EJ, Alper CA: Human C4 haplotypes with duplicated C4A or C4B. *Am J Hum Genet* **36**:72, 1984.
86. Schneider PM, Caroll MC, Alper CA, Rittner C, Whitehead AS, Yunis EJ, Colten HR: Polymorphism of human complement C4 and steroid 21-hydroxylase genes. *J Clin Invest* **78**:650, 1986.
87. Yu CY, Belt KT, Giles CM, Campbell RD, Porter RR: Structural basis of the polymorphism of human complement component C4A and C4B, gene size, reactivity and antigenicity. *EMBO J* **5**:2873, 1986.
88. Law SKA, Dodds AW, Porter RR: A comparison of the properties of the two classes, C4A and C4B, of the human complement component C4. *EMBO J* **3**:1819, 1984.
89. Caroll MC, Fathallah DM, Bergamaschini L, Alicot EM, Isenman DE: Substitution of a single amino acid converts the functional activity of complement C4B to C4A. *Proc Natl Acad Sci U S A* **87**:6868, 1990.
90. Finco O, Li S, Cuccia M, Rosen FS, Caroll MC: Structural differences between the two human complement C4 isotypes affect the humoral immune response. *J Exp Med* **175**:537, 1992.
91. Yu CY, Campbell RD, Porter RR: A structural model for the location of the Rodgers and the Chido antigenic determinants and their correlation with the human complement component C4A/C4B isotypes. *Immunogenetics* **27**:399, 1988.
92. Caroll MC, Belt KT, Palsdottir A, Yu CY: Molecular genetics of the fourth component of human complement and steroid 21-hydroxylase. *Immunol Rev* **87**:39, 1985.
93. Hauptman G, Tappeiner G: Inherited deficiency of the fourth component of human complement. *Immunodef Rev* **1**:3, 1988.
94. Braun L, Schneider PM, Giles CM, Bertrams J, Rittner C: Null alleles of human complement C4. *J Exp Med* **171**:129, 1990.
95. Morgan BP, Walport MJ: Complement deficiency and disease. *Immunol Today* **12**:301, 1991.
96. Hauptman G, Uring-Lambert B, Vegnaduzzi-Lamouche N, Massart-Lemone F: RFLP studies of 3 complete C4-deficient patients. *Complement* **4**:166, 1987.
97. Ragoussis J, Bloeme K, Weiss EH, Ziegler A: Localization of the genes for tumor necrosis factor and lymphotoxin between the HLA class I and III region by field inversion gel electrophoresis. *Immunogenetics* **27**:66, 1988.
98. Kriegler M, Perez C, DeFay K, Albert I, Lu SD: A novel form of TNF/cachectin is a cell surface cytotoxic transmembrane protein: Ramifications for the complex physiology of TNF. *Cell* **53**:45, 1988.
99. Creasey AA, Yamamoto R, Vitt CR: A high molecular weight component of the tumour necrosis factor is associated with cytotoxicity. *Proc Natl Acad Sci U S A* **84**:3293, 1987.
100. Thoma B, Grell M, Pfizenmaier K, Scheurich P: Identification of a 60 kD tumor necrosis factor receptor as the major signal transducing component in the TNF responses. *J Exp Med* **172**:1019, 1990.
101. Chouaib S, Branellec D, Buurman WA: More insights into the complex physiology of TNF. *Immunol Today* **12**:141, 1991.
102. Kehrl JH, Miller A, Fauci AS: Effect of tumour necrosis factor alpha on mitogen-activated human B cells. *J Exp Med* **166**:786, 1987.
103. De Kossodo S, Grau GE, Daneva T, Pointaire P, Fossati L, Ody C, Zapf J, Piguet P-F, Gaillard RC, Vassalli P: Tumor necrosis factor α is involved in mouse growth and lymphoid tissue development. *J Exp Med* **179**:1259, 1992.
104. Giroir B, Brown T, Beutler B: Constitutive synthesis of tumor necrosis factor in the thymus. *Proc Natl Acad Sci U S A* **89**:4864, 1992.
105. Paul NL, Ruddle NH: Lymphotoxin. *Annu Rev Immunol* **6**:407, 1988.
106. Ruddle NH, Homer R: The role of lymphotoxin in inflammation. *Prog Allergy* **40**:162, 1988.
107. Old LJ: Tumor necrosis factor. *Sci Am* **258**:41, 1988.
108. Beutler B, Cerami A: Cachectin and tumour necrosis factor as two sides of the same biological coin. *Nature* **329**:584, 1986.
109. Cerami A, Beutler B: The role of cachectin/TNF in endotoxic shock and cachexia. *Immunol Today* **9**:28, 1988.
110. Bendtzen K: Interleukin 1, interleukin 6 and tumor necrosis factor in infection, inflammation and immunity. *Immunol Lett* **19**:183, 1988.
111. Waage A, Halstensen A, Espevik T: Association between tumour necrosis factor in serum and fatal outcome in patients with meningococcal disease. *Lancet* **1**:355, 1987.
112. Young RA: Stress proteins and immunology. *Annu Rev Immunol* **8**:401, 1990.
113. Banerji J, Strominger JL, Spies T: A gene pair from the human major histocompatibility complex encodes large proline-rich proteins with multiple repeated motifs and a single ubiquitin-like domain. *Proc Natl Acad Sci U S A* **83**:2374, 1990.
114. Svejgaard A, Platz P, Ryder LP: HLA and disease—A survey. *Immunol Rev* **70**:193, 1983.
115. Tiwari JL, Terasaki PI: *HLA and Disease Association*. New York, Springer-Verlag, 1985.
116. Lipsky P, Taurog JD: The second international Simmons center conference on HLA-B27-related disorders. *Arthritis Rheum* **34**:1476, 1991.
117. Benjamin R, Parham P: Guilt by association, HLA-B27 and ankylosing spondylitis. *Immunol Today* **11**:137, 1990.
118. Pazmany L, Rowland-Jones S, Huet S, Hill A, Sutton J, Murray R, Brooks J, McMichael A: Genetic modulation of antigen presentation by HLA-B27 molecules. *J Exp Med* **175**:361, 1992.
119. Lahesmaa R, Skurnik M, Vaara M, Leirisalo-Repo M, Nissila M, Granfors K, Toivanen P: Molecular mimicry between HLA-B27 and *Yersinia, Salmonella, Shigella* and *Klebsiella*, within the same region of HLA α1-helix. *Clin Exp Immunol* **86**:399, 1991.
120. Hammer RE, Maika SD, Richardson JA, Tang J-P, Taurog JD: Spontaneous inflammatory disease in transgenic rats expressing HLA-B27 and human β2m: An animal model of HLA-B27-associated human disorders. *Cell* **63**:1099, 1990.

121. Nepom GT, Byers P, Seyfried S, Healey LA, Wilske D, Stage D, Nepom BS: HLA genes associated with rheumatoid arthritis. Identification of susceptibility alleles using specific oligonucleotide probes. *Arthritis Rheum* **32**:15, 1989.
122. Devereux D, O'Hehir R, McGuire J, van Schooten WCA, Lamb JR: HLA-DR4Dw4-restricted T cell recognition of self antigen(s) in the rheumatoid synovial compartment. *Int Immunol* **3**:635, 1991.
123. Res PCM, Schaar CG, Breedveld FC, van Eden W, van Embden JDA, Cohen IR, de Vries RRP: Synovial fluid T cell reactivity against 65 kD heat shock protein of mycobacteria in early chronic arthritis. *Lancet* **2**:478, 1988.
124. Lamb JR, Bal V, Mendez-Samperio P, Mehlert A, So A, Rothbard JB, Jindal S, Young RA, Young DS: Stress proteins may provide a link between the immune response to infection and autoimmunity. *Int Immunol* **1**:191, 1988.
125. Strober S, Holoshitz J: Mechanisms of immune injury in rheumatoid arthritis: Evidence for the involvement of T cells and heat shock protein. *Immunol Rev* **118**:233, 1990.
126. Saklatvala J: Tumor necrosis factor-alpha stimulates resorption and inhibits synthesis of proteoglycan in cartilage. *Nature* **332**:547, 1986.
127. Bertolini DR, Nedwin G, Bringman T, Smith D, Mundy GR: Stimulation of bone resorption and inhibition of bone formation in vitro by human tumor necrosis factor. *Nature* **319**:516, 1986.
128. Saxne T, Palladino MA Jr, Heinegaard D, Talal N, Wollheim FA: Detection of tumor necrosis factor alpha but not tumor necrosis factor beta in rheumatoid arthritis synovial fluid and serum. *Arthritis Rheum* **31**:1041, 1988.
129. Fernandez-Vina MA, Fink CW, Stastny P: HLA antigens in juvenile arthritis. *Arthritis Rheum* **33**:1787, 1990.
130. Morling N, Friis J, Fugger L, Georgsen J, Heilmann C, Karup-Pedersen F, Ødum N, Svejgaard A: DNA polymorphism of HLA class II genes in pauciarticular juvenile rheumatoid arthritis. *Tissue Antigens* **38**:16, 1991.
131. Ødum N, Morling N, Friis J, Heilmann C, Hyldig-Nielsen JJ, Jakobsen BK, Pedersen FK, Platz P, Ryder LP, Svejgaard A: Increased frequency of HLA-DPw2 in pauciarticular onset juvenile chronic arthritis. *Tissue Antigens* **28**:245, 1986.
132. Giannini EH, Malagon CN, Van Kerckhove C, Taylor J, Lovell DJ, Levinson JE, Passo MH, Ginsberg J, Burke MJ, Glass DN: Longitudinal analysis of HLA associated risks for iridocyclitis in juvenile rheumatoid arthritis. *J Rheumatol* **18**:1394, 1991.
133. Begovich AB, Bugawan TL, Nepom BS, Klitz W, Nepom GT, Erlich HA: A specific HLA-DPB allele is associated with pauciarticular juvenile rheumatoid arthritis but not adult rheumatoid arthritis. *Proc Natl Acad Sci U S A* **86**:9489, 1989.
134. Fugger L, Ryder LP, Morling N, Ødum N, Friis J, Karup-Pedersen F, Friis J, Sandberg-Wollheim M, Svejgaard A: DNA typing for HLA-DPB1*02 and -DPB1*04 in multiple sclerosis and juvenile rheumatoid arthritis. *Immunogenetics* **32**:150, 1990.
135. Fugger L, Morling N, Ryder LP, Georgsen J, Jakobsen BK, Svejgaard A, Andersen V, Oxholm P, Karup-Pedersen F, Friis J, Halberg P: NcoI Restriction fragment length polymorphism (RFLP) of the tumor necrosis factor (TNFα) region in four autoimmune diseases. *Tissue Antigens* **34**:17, 1989.
136. Nepom BS, Malhotra U, Schwarz DA, Nettles JW, Schaller JG, Concannon P: HLA and T cell receptor polymorphisms in pauciarticular-onset juvenile rheumatoid arthritis. *Arthritis Rheum* **34**:1260, 1991.
137. Arnett FC: Genetic aspects of human lupus. *Clin Immunol Immunopathol* **63**:4, 1992.
138. Fronek Z, Timmerman LA, Alper CA, Hahn BH, Kalunian K, Peterlin BM, McDevitt HO: Major histocompatibility complex association with systemic lupus erythematosus. *Am J Med* **85**:42, 1988.
139. Hamilton RG, Harley JB, Bias WB, Roebber M, Reichlin M, Hochberg MC, Arnett FC: Ro (SS-A) autoantibody responses in systemic lupus erythematosus. *Arthritis Rheum* **31**:496, 1988.
140. Reveille JD, Macleod MJ, Whittington K, Arnett FC: Specific amino acid residues in the second hypervariable region of HLA-DQA1 and DQB1 chain genes promote the Ro (SS-A)/La (SS-B) autoantibody responses. *J Immunol* **146**:3871, 1991.
141. Arnett FC, Olsen ML, Anderson KL, Reveille JD: Molecular analysis of major histocompatibility complex alleles associated with the lupus anticoagulant. *J Clin Invest* **87**:1490, 1991.
142. Agnello V: Lupus diseases associated with hereditary and acquired deficiencies of complement. *Springer Semin Immunopathol* **9**:161, 1986.
143. Borradori L, Gueissaz F, Frenk E, Rohner R, Scherz R, Lantin J-P, Spatth PJ: Lupus érythemateux systémique associe à un déficit homozygote en C2. *Schweiz Med Wochenschr* **121**:418, 1991.
144. Schur PH, Marcus-Bagley D, Awdeh Z, Yunis EJ, Alper CA: The effect of ethnicity on major histocompatibility complex complement allotypes and extended haplotypes in patients with systemic lupus erythematosus. *Arthritis Rheum* **33**:985, 1990.
145. Christiansen FT, Zhang WJ, Griffiths M, Mallal SA, Dawkins RL: Major histocompatibility complex (MHC), complement deficiency, ancestral haplotypes and systemic lupus erythematosus: C4 deficiency explains some but not all the influence of the MHC. *J Rheumatol* **18**:1350, 1991.
146. Batchelor JR, Fielder AHL, Walport MJ, David J, Lord DK, Davey N, Dodi IA, Malasit P, Wanachiwanawin W, Berstein R, Mackworth-Young C, Isenberg D: Family study of the major histocompatibility complex in HLA DR3 negative patients with systemic lupus erythematosus. *Clin Exp Immunol* **70**:364, 1987.
147. Olsen ML, Goldstein R, Arnett FC, Duvic M, Pollack M, Reveille JD: C4A gene deletion and HLA associations in black Americans with systemic lupus erythematosus. *Immunogenetics* **30**:27, 1989.
148. Steinsson K, Erlendsson K, Valdimarsson H: Successful plasma infusion treatment of a patient with C2 deficiency and systemic lupus erythematosus: Clinical experience over forty-five months. *Arthritis Rheum* **32**:906, 1989.
149. Morling N, Andersen V, Fugger L, Georgsen J, Halberg P, Oxholm P, Ødum N, Svejgaard A: Immunogenetics of rheumatoid arthritis and primary Sjögren's syndrome: DNA polymorphism of HLA class II genes. *Dis Markers* **9**:289, 1991.
150. Arnett FC: Immunogenetics of the connective tissue diseases, in Talal N (ed): *Molecular Autoimmunity*. Orlando, FL: Academic Press, 1991, p 31.
151. Miller BJ, Appel MC, O'Neil JJ, Wicker LS: Both the Lyt-2 + and L3T4 + T cell subsets are required for the transfer of diabetes in nonobese diabetic mice. *J Immunol* **140**:52, 1988.
152. Baekkeskov S, Aanstoot H-J, Christgau S, Reetz A, Solimena M, Cascalho M, Folli F, Richter-Olesen H, DeCamilli P: Identification of the 64K autoantigen in insulin dependent diabetes as the GABA-synthesizing enzyme glutamic acid decarboxylase. *Nature* **347**:151, 1990.
153. Boitard C, Villa MC, Becourt C, Gia HP, Huc C, Sempe P, Portier MM, Bach J-F: Peripherin: An islet antigen that is cross-reactive with nonobese diabetic mouse class II gene products. *Proc Natl Acad Sci U S A* **89**:172, 1992.
154. Castano H, Russo E, Zhou L, Lipes MA, Eisenbarth GS: Identification and cloning of a granule autoantigen, carboxypetidase H, associated with type I diabetes. *J Clin Endocrinol Metab* **73**:1197, 1991.
155. Karjalainen J, Martin JM, Knip M, Ilonen J, Robinson BH, Savilahti E, Akerblom HK, Dosch HM: A bovine albumin peptide as a possible trigger of insulin dependent diabetes mellitus. *N Engl J Med* **327**:302, 1992.
156. Honeyman MC, Cram DS, Harrison LC: Glutamic acid decarboxylase 67 reactive T cells: A marker for insulin-dependent diabetes. *J Exp Med* **177**:535, 1993.
157. Svejgaard A, Ryder LP: HLA and insulin-dependent diabetes: An overview. *Genet Epidemiol* **6**:1, 1989.
158. Todd JA: Genetic control of autoimmunity in type 1 diabetes. *Immunol Today* **11**:137, 1990.
159. Todd JA, Bell JI, McDevitt HO: HLA-DQβ gene contributes to susceptibility and resistance to insulin-dependent diabetes mellitus. *Nature* **329**:599, 1987.
160. Acha-Orbea H, McDevitt HO: The first external domain of the non-obese diabetic mouse class II Ab chain is unique. *Proc Natl Acad Sci U S A* **84**:2435, 1987.
161. Todd JA, Mijovic C, Fletcher J, Jenkins D, Bradwell AR Barnett AH: Identification of susceptibility loci for insulin-dependent diabetes mellitus by trans-racial gene mapping. *Nature* **338**:587, 1989.
162. Julier C, Hyer RN, Davies J, Merlin, F, Soularu P, Briant L, Cathelineau G, Deschamps I, Rotter JI, Froguel P, Boitard C, Bell JI, Lathrop GM: Insulin-IGF2 region on chromosome 11p encodes a gene implicated in HLA-DR4-dependent diabetes susceptibility. *Nature* **354**:155, 1991.
163. Todd JA, Aitman TJ, Cornall RJ, Ghosh S, Hall JR, Hearne CM, Knight AM, Love JM, McAleer MA, Prins JB: Genetic analysis of autoimmune type 1 diabetes mellitus in mice. *Nature* **351**:542, 1991.
164. Cornall RJ, Prins JB, Todd JA, Pressey A, DeLarato NH, Wicker LS, Peterson LB: Type 1 diabetes in mice is linked to the interleukin-1

receptor and Lsh/Ity/Bcg genes on chromosome 1. *Nature* **353**:262, 1991.

165. Morling N, Dalhoff K, Fugger L, Georgsen J, Jakobsen BK, Ranek L, Ødum N, Svejgaard A: DNA polymorphism of HLA class II genes in primary biliary cirrhosis. *Immunogenetics* **35**:112, 1992.
166. Fugger L, Morling N, Ryder LP, Platz P, Georgsen J, Jakobsen BK, Svejgaard A, Dalhoff K, Ranek L: *Nco*I restriction fragment length polymorphism (RFLP) of the tumor necrosis factor (TNFα) region in primary biliary cirrhosis and in healthy Danes. *Scand J Immunol* **30**:185, 1989.
167. Briggs DC, Donaldson PT, Hayes P, Welsh KI, Williams R, Neuberger JM: A major histocompatibility class II allotype (C4B2) associated with primary biliary cirrhosis (PBC). *Tissue Antigens* **29**:141, 1987.
168. Gershwin ME, Mackay IR: Primary biliary cirrhosis: Paradigm or paradox for autoimmunity. *Gastroenterology* **100**:822, 1991.
169. Nepom GT, Erlich HA: HLA and disease. *Annu Rev Immunol* **9**:493, 1991.
170. Sollid LM, Markussen G, Ek J, Gjerde H, Vartdal F, Thorsby E: Evidence for a primary association of coeliac disease to a particular HLA-DQ A/B heterodimer. *J Exp Med* **169**:345, 1989.
171. Bugawan TL, Angelini G, Larrick J, Auricchio S, Ferrara GB, Erlich HA: A combination of a particular HLA-DPB allele and an HLA-DQ heterodimer confers susceptibility to coeliac disease. *Nature* **339**:470, 1989.
172. Rosenberg WMC, Wordsworth BP, Jewell DP, Bell JI: A locus telomeric to HLA-DPB encodes susceptibility to coeliac disease. *Immunogenetics* **30**:307, 1989.
173. Latinne D, Vandeput Y, De Bruyere M, Bottazzo GF, Sokal G, Crabbe J: Addison's disease: Immunological aspects. *Tissue Antigens* **30**:23, 1987.
174. Krohn K, Uibo R, Aavik E, Peterson P, Savilahti K: Identification by molecular cloning of an autoantigen associated with Addison's disease as steroid 17α-hydroxylase. *Lancet* **339**:770, 1992.
175. Weetman AP, Zhang L, Tandon N, Edwards OM: HLA associations with autoimmune Addison's disease. *Tissue Antigens* **38**:31, 1992.
176. Boehm BO, Manfras B, Seidl S, Holzenberger G, Kuhnl P, Rosak C, Schoffling K, Trucco M: The HLA-DQβ non-Asp-57 allele: A predictor of future insulin dependent diabetes mellitus in patients with autoimmune Addison's disease. *Tissue Antigens* **37**:130, 1991.
177. Utiger RD: The pathogenesis of autoimmune thyroid disease. *N Engl J Med* **325**:278, 1991.
178. Davies TF, Martin A, Concepcion ES, Graves P, Cohen L, Ben-Nun A: Evidence of limited variability of antigen receptors on intrathyroidal T cells in autoimmune thyroid disease. *N Engl J Med* **325**:138, 1991.
179. Farid NR: Understanding the genetics of autoimmune thyroid disease — Still an elusive goal [Editorial]. *J Clin Endocrinol Metab* **74**:495A, 1992.
180. Badenhoop K, Schwarz G, Walfish PG, Drummond V, Usadel KH, Bottazzo GF: Susceptibility to thyroid autoimmune disease: Molecular analysis of HLA-D region genes identifies new markers for goitrous Hashimoto's thyroiditis. *J Clin Endocrinol Metab* **71**:1131, 1990.
181. Gottlieb AB, Krueger JG: HLA region genes and immune activation in the pathogenesis of psoriasis. *Arch Dermatol* **126**:1083, 1990.
182. Baadsgaard O, Fisher G, Voorhees JJ, Cooper KD: The role of the immune system in the pathogenesis of psoriasis. *J Invest Dermatol* **95**:32S, 1990.
183. Amagai M, Klaus-Kovtun V, Stanley J: Autoantibodies against a novel epithelial cadherin in pemphigus vulgaris, a disease of cell adhesion. *Cell* **67**:869, 1991.
184. Sinha AA, Brautbar C, Szafer F, Friedmann A, Tzfoni E, Todd JA, Steinman L, McDevitt HO: A newly characterized HLA-DQB allele associated with pemphigus vulgaris. *Science* **239**:1026, 1988.
185. Juji T, Satake M, Honda Y, Doi Y: HLA antigens in Japanese patients with narcolepsy. *Tissue Antigens* **24**:316, 1984.
186. Billard M, Seignalet J: Extraordinary association between HLA-DR2 and narcolepsy. *Lancet* **1**:226, 1985.
187. Aldrich MS: Narcolepsy. *N Engl J Med* **323**:389, 1990.
188. Guilleminault C, Mignot E, Grumet FC: Familial patterns of narcolepsy. *Lancet* **2**:1376, 1989.
189. Kuwata S, Tokunaga K, Jin F, Juji T, Sasaki T, Honda Y: Letter to the editor. *N Engl J Med* **324**:271, 1991.
190. Neely S, Rosenberg R, Spire J-P, Antel J, Arnason BGW: HLA antigens in narcolepsy. *Neurology* **37**:1858, 1987.
191. Matsuki K, Grumet FC, Lin X, Gelb M, Guilleminault C, Dement WC, Mignot E: DQ (rather than DR) gene marks susceptibility to narcolepsy. *Lancet* **2**:1052, 1992.
192. Lock CB, So AKL, Welsh KI, Parkes JD, Trowsdale J: MHC class II sequences of an HLA-DR2 narcoleptic. *Immunogenetics* **27**:449, 1988.
193. Mignot E, Wang C, Rattazzi C, Gaiser C, Lovett M, Guilleminault C, Dement WC, Grumet FC: Genetic linkage of autosomal recessive canine narcolepsy with a μ immunoglobulin heavy-chain switch-like segment. *Proc Natl Acad Sci U S A* **88**:3475, 1991.
194. Naito S, Kuroiwa Y, Itoyama T: HLA and Japanese multiple sclerosis. *Tissue Antigens* **12**:19, 1978.
195. Gorodezky C, Najera R, Rangel BE, Castro LE, Flores J, Velazquez G, Granados J, Sotelo J: Immunogenetic profile of multiple sclerosis in Mexicans. *Hum Immunol* **16**:364, 1986.
196. Kurdi A, Ayesh I, Abdaller A, Ayesh I, Abdaller A, Maayta U, McDonald WI, Compston DAS, Batchelor JR: Different B-lymphocyte alloantigens associated with multiple sclerosis in Arabs and north Europeans. *Lancet* **1**:1123, 1977.
197. Marrosu MG, Muntoni F, Murru MR, Spinicci G, Pischedda MP, Goddi F, Cossu P, Pirastu M: Sardinian multiple sclerosis is associated with HLA-DR4. *Neurology* **38**:1749, 1988.
198. Olerup O, Hillert J, Fredrikson S, Olsson T, Kam-Hansen S, Moller E, Carlsson B, Wallin J: Primarily chronic progressive and relapsing/remitting multiple sclerosis: Two immunogenetically distinct disease entities. *Proc Natl Acad Sci U S A* **86**:7113, 1989.
199. Olerup O, Hillert J: HLA class II-associated genetic susceptibility in multiple sclerosis: A critical evaluation. *Tissue Antigens* **38**:1, 1991.
200. Hauser SL, Fleischnick E, Weiner HL, Marcus D, Awdeh Z, Yunis EJ, Alper CA: Extended major histocompatibility complex haplotypes in patients with multiple sclerosis. *Neurology* **39**:275, 1989.
201. Cowan EP, Pierce ML, McFarland HF, McFarlin DE: HLA-DR and -DQ allelic sequences in multiple sclerosis patients are identical to those found in the general population. *Hum Immunol* **32**:203, 1991.
202. Vartdal F, Sollid LM, Vandvik B, Markussen G, Thorsby E: Patients with multiple sclerosis carry DQB1 genes which encode shared polymorphic amino acid sequences. *Hum Immunol* **25**:103, 1989.
203. Spurkland A, Ronningen KS, Vandvik B, Thorsby E, Vartdal F: HLA-DQA1 and HLA-DQB1 genes may jointly determine susceptibility to develop multiple sclerosis. *Hum Immunol* **30**:69, 1991.
204. Hofman FM, Hinton DR, Johnson K, Merrill JE: Tumor necrosis factor identified in multiple sclerosis brain. *J Exp Med* **170**:607, 1989.
205. Sharief MK, Hentges R: Association between tumor necrosis factor-α and disease progression in patients with multiple sclerosis. *N Engl J Med* **325**:467, 1991.
206. Fugger L, Morling N, Sandberg-Wollheim M, Ryder LP, Svejgaard A: Tumor necrosis factor alpha gene polymorphism in multiple sclerosis and optic neuritis. *J Neuroimmunol* **27**:85, 1990.
207. Liblau R, van Endert PM, Sandberg-Wollheim M, Patel SD, Lopez MT, Land S, Fugger L, McDevitt HO: Antigen processing gene polymorphisms in HLA-DR2 multiple sclerosis. *Neurology* **43**:1192, 1993.
208. Hill AV, Allsopp CE, Kwiatkowski D, Anstey NM, Twumasi P, Rowe PA, Bennett S, Brewster D, McMichael AJ, Greenwood BM: Common West African HLA antigens are associated with protection from severe malaria. *Nature* **352**:595, 1991.
209. Klitz W: Viruses, cancer and the MHC. *Nature* **356**:17, 1992.
210. Bodmer JG, Tonks S, Oza AM, Lister TA, Bodmer WF: HLA-DP based resistance to Hodgkin's disease. *Lancet* **2**:1455, 1989.
211. Lu S-J, Day NE, Degos L, Lepage V, Wang P-C, Chan S-H, Simons M, McKnight B, Easton D, Zeng Y, de-The G: Linkage of a nasopharyngeal carcinoma susceptibility locus to the HLA region. *Nature* **346**:470, 1990.

211a. Wank R, Thomssen C: High risk of squamous cell carcinoma of the cervix for women with HLA-DQw3. *Nature* **352**:723, 1991.

212. Han R, Breitburd F, Marche PN, Orth G: Linkage of regression and malignant conversion of rabbit viral papillomas to MHC class II genes. *Nature* **356**:66, 1992.
213. Cunningham-Rundles C: Clinical and immunologic analysis of 103 patients with common variable immunodeficiency. *J Clin Immunol* **9**:12, 1989.
214. Schaffer FM, Palermos J, Zhu ZB, Barger BO, Cooper MD, Volanakis JE: Individuals with IgA deficiency and common variable

immunodeficiency share polymorphisms of major histocompatibility complex class III genes. *Proc Natl Acad Sci U S A* **86**:8015, 1989.

215. Olerup O, Smith CIE, Hammarstrom L: Is selective IgA deficiency associated with central HLA genes or alleles of the DR-DQ region? *Immunol Today* **12**:134, 1991.
216. Ambrus M, Hernadi E, Bajtai G: Prevalence of HLA-A1 and HLA-B8 antigens in selective IgA deficiency. *Clin Immunol Immunopathol* **7**:311, 1977.
217. Oen K, Petty RE, Schroeder ML: Immunoglobulin A deficiency: Genetic studies. *Tissue Antigens* **19**:174, 1982.
218. Hammarstrom L, Smith CIE: HLA-A, B, C and DR antigens in immunoglobulin A deficiency. *Tissue Antigens* **21**:75, 1983.
219. Heikkila M, Koistinen J, Lohman M, Koskimies S: Increased frequency of HLA-A1 and -B8 in association with total lack, but not with deficiency of serum IgA. *Tissue Antigens* **23**:280, 1984.
220. Wilton AN, Cobain TJ, Dawkins RL: Family studies of IgA deficiency. *Immunogenetics* **21**:333, 1985.
221. Lakhanpal S, O'Duffy JD, Homburger HA, Moore SB: Evidence for linkage of IgA deficiency with the major histocompatibility complex. *Mayo Clinic Proc* **63**:461, 1988.
222. Liblau R, Bach JF: Selective IgA deficiency and autoimmune diseases. *Int Arch Allergy Immunol* **99**:16, 1992.
223. French MAH, Dawkins RL: Central MHC genes, IgA deficiency and autoimmune disease. *Immunol Today* **11**:271, 1990.
223a. Cunningham-Rundles C, Fotino M, Rosina O, Peter JB: Selective IgA deficiency, IgG subclass deficiency, and the major histocompatibility complex. *Clin Immunol Immunopathol* **61**:S61, 1991.
224. Olerup O, Smith CIE, Hammarstrom L: Different amino acids at position 57 of the HLA-DQb chain associated with susceptibility and resistance to IgA deficiency. *Nature* **347**:289, 1990.
225. Liblau R, Caillat-Zucman S, Fischer A-M, Back J-F, Boitard C: The prevalence of selective IgA deficiency in type 1 diabetes mellitus. *APMIS* **100**:709, 1992.
226. Selmaj K, Raine CS, Cannella B, Brosnan CF: Identification of lymphotoxin and tumor necrosis factor in multiple sclerosis lesions. *J Clin Invest* **87**:949, 1990.
227. Robbins DS, Shirazi Y, Drysdale B-E, Lieberman A, Shin HS, Shin ML: Production of cytotoxic factor for oligodendrocytes by stimulated astrocytes. *J Immunol* **139**:2593, 1987.
228. Selmaj K, Raine CS: Tumor necrosis factor mediates myelin and oligodendrocyte damage in vitro. *Ann Neurol* **23**:339, 1988.
229. Chung IY, Norris JG, Benveniste EN: Differential tumor necrosis factor alpha expression by astrocytes from experimental allergic encephalomyelitis-susceptible and -resistant rat strains. *J Exp Med* **173**:801, 1991.
230. Ruddle NH, Bergman CM, McGrath KM, Lingenheld EG, Grunnet ML, Padula SJ, Clark RB: An antibody to lymphotoxin and tumor necrosis factor prevents transfer of experimental allergic encephalomyelitis. *J Exp Med* **172**:1193, 1990.
231. Jacob CO, McDevitt HO: Tumor necrosis factor-alpha in murine autoimmune "lupus" nephritis. *Nature* **331**:356, 1988.
232. Gordon C, Ranges GE, Greenspan JS, Wofsy D: Chronic therapy with recombinant tumor necrosis factor-α in autoimmune NZB/NZW F1 mice. *Clin Immunol Immunopathol* **52**:421, 1989.
233. Richter G, Qin ZH, Diamantstein T, Blankenstein T: Analysis of restriction fragment length polymorphism in lymphokine genes in normal and autoimmune mice. *J Exp Med* **170**:1439, 1989.
234. Brennan DC, Yui MA, Wuthrich RP, Kelley VE: Tumor necrosis factor and IL-1 in New Zealand Black/White mice. Enhanced gene expression and acceleration of renal injury. *J Immunol* **143**:3470, 1989.
235. Bendtzen K, Morling N, Fomsgaard A, Svenson M, Jakobsen B, Ødum N, Svejgaard A: Association between HLA-DR2 and production of tumor necrosis factor alpha and interleukin 1 by mononuclear cells activated by lipopolysaccharide. *Scand J Immunol* **28**:599, 1988.
236. Jacob CO, Fronek Z, Lewis GD, Koo M, McDevitt HO: Heritable major histocompatibility complex class-II associated differences in production of tumor necrosis factor alpha: Relevance to genetic predisposition to systemic lupus erythematosus. *Proc Natl Acad Sci U S A* **87**:1233, 1990.
237. Bendtzen K, Mandrup-Poulsen T, Nerup J, Nielsen JH, Dinarello CA, Svenson M: Cytotoxicity of human pI7 interleukin-1 for pancreatic islets of Langerhans. *Science* **232**:1545, 1986.
238. Mandrup-Poulsen T, Bendtzen K, Dinarello CA, Nerup J: Human TNF potentiates IL-1 mediated pancreatic β-cell cytotoxicity. *J Immunol* **139**:4077, 1987.
239. Jacob CO, Aiso S, Michie SA, McDevitt HO, Acha-Orbea H: Prevention of diabetes in non-obese diabetic mice by tumor necrosis factor. Similarities between TNF alpha and IL-1. *Proc Natl Acad Sci U S A* **87**:968, 1990.
240. Satoh J, Seino H, Abo T, Tanaka S, Shintani S, Ohta S, Tamura K, Sawai T, Nobunaga T, Otchi T, Kumagai K, Toyato T: Recombinant human tumor necrosis factor alpha suppresses autoimmune diabetes in NOD mice. *J Clin Invest* **84**:1345, 1989.
241. Sinha AA, Lopez MT, McDevitt HO: Autoimmune diseases: The failure of self-tolerance. *Science* **248**:1380, 1990.
242. Smilek DE, Lock CB, McDevitt HO: Antigen recognition and peptide mediated immunotherapy in autoimmune diseases. *Immunol Rev* **118**:37, 1990.
243. Livingstone AM, Powis SJ, Diamond AG, Butcher GW, Howard JC: A *trans*-acting major histocompatibility complex linked gene whose alleles determine gain and loss changes in the antigenic structure of a classical class I molecule. *J Exp Med* **170**:777, 1989.
244. Blackman M, Kappler J, Marrack P: The role of the T cell receptor in positive and negative selection of developing T cells. *Science* **248**:1335, 1990.
245. Schwartz RH: A cell culture model for T lymphocyte clonal anergy. *Science* **248**:1349, 1990.
246. Deuss U, Ciampolillo A, Marini V, Mirakian R, Bottazzo GFB: MHC molecule expression in nonlymphoid tissue: Implication for autoimmunity, in Farid NR (ed): *The Immunogenetics of Autoimmune Disease*. Ann Arbor, MI, CRC Press, 1991, p 135.
247. Burkly LC, Lo D, Flavell RA: Tolerance in transgenic mice expressing major histocompatibility molecules extrathymically on pancreatic cells. *Science* **248**:1364, 1990.
248. Oldstone MBA: Molecular mimicry as a mechanism for the cause and as a probe uncovering etiological agent(s) of autoimmune disease. *Curr Topics Microbiol Immunol* **145**:127, 1989.
249. Gammon G, Sercarz E: How some T cells escape tolerance induction. *Nature* **342**:183, 1989.
250. Watanabe-Fukunaga R, Brannan CI, Copeland NG, Jenkins NA, Nagata S: Lymphoproliferative disorder in mice explained by defects in Fas antigen that mediate apoptosis. *Nature* **356**:314, 1992.
251. Vaux DL: Toward an understanding of the molecular mechanisms of physiological cell death. *Proc Natl Acad Sci U S A* **90**:786, 1993.
252. Hartley SB, Cooke ME, Fulcher DA, Harris AW, Cory S, Bastan A, Goodnow CC: Elimination of self-reactive B lymphocytes proceeds in two stages: Arrested development and cell death. *Cell* **72**:325, 1993.
253. Solimena M, Folli F, Aparisi R, Pozza G, De Camilli P: Autoantibodies to GABA-ergic neurons and pancreatic beta cells in stiff-man syndrome. *N Engl J Med* **322**:1555, 1990.
254. Marsh SGE, Parham P, Barber LD: *The HLA FactsBook*. San Diego, Academic Press, 2000, p 1.
255. Robinson J, Malik A, Parham P, Bodmer JG, Marsh SGE: IMGT/HLA Database-a sequence database for the human major histocompatibility complex. *Tissue Antigens* **55**: 280, 2000.
256. Parham P, Ohta T: Population biology of antigen presentation by MHC class I molecules. *Science* **272**:67, 1996.
257. The MHC Sequencing Consortium: Complete sequence and gene map of a human major histocompatibility complex. *Nature* **401**:921, 1999.
258. Rhodes DA, Trowsdale J: Genetics and molecular genetics of the MHC. *Rev Immunogenet* **1**:21, 1999.
259. Parham P (ed.): Genomic organisation of the MHC: Structure, origin and function. *Immunol Rev* **167**:1, 1999.
260. Natarajan K, Li H, Mariuzza RA, Margulies DH: MHC class I molecules, structure and function. *Rev Immunogenet* **1**:32, 1999.
261. Nelson CA, Fremont DH: Structural principles of MHC class II antigen presentation. *Rev Immunogenet* **1**:47, 1999.
262. Reinherz EL, Tan K, Tang L, Kern P, Liu J-h, Xiong Y, Hussey RE, et al.: The crystal structure of a T cell receptor in complex with peptide and MHC class II. *Science* **286**:1913, 1999.
263. Corper AL, Stratmann T, Apostolopoulos V, Scott CA, Garcia KC, Kang A, Wilson IA, et al.: A structural framework for deciphering the link between I-Ag7 and murine autoimmune diabetes. *Science* **288**: 505, 2000.
264. Lanier LL: NK cell receptors. *Annu Rev Immunol* **16**:359, 1998.
265. Watts C, Powis S: Pathways of antigen processing and presentation. *Rev Immunogenet* **1**:60, 1999.
266. Parham P (ed): Pathways of antigen processing and presentation. *Immunol Rev* **172**:1, 2000.

267. Thorsby E, Ronningen KS: Particular HLA-DQ molecules play a dominant role in determining susceptibility or resistance to Type I (insulin-dependent) diabetes mellitus. *Diabetologia* **36**:371, 1993.

268. Nepom GT, Nepom BS, Antonelli P, Mickelson E, Silver J, Goyert SM, Hansen JA: The HLA-DR4 family of haplotypes consists of a series of distinct DR and DS molecules. *J Exp Med* **159**:394, 1984.

269. Van der Auwera B, Van Waeyenberge C, Schuit F, Heimberg H, Vandewalle C, Gorus F, Flament J: DRB1*0403 protects against IDDM in Caucasians with the high-risk heterozygous DQA1*0301-DQB1*0302/DQA1*0501-DQB1*0201 genotype. Belgian Diabetes Registry. *Diabetes* **44**:527, 1995.

270. Knight JC, Kwiatkowski D: Inherited variability of tumor necrosis factor production and susceptibility to infectious disease. *Proc Assoc Am Physicians* **111**:290, 1999.

271. Lin L, Faraco J, Li R, Kadotani H, Rogers W, Lin X, Qiu X, et al.: The sleep disorder canine narcolepsy is caused by a mutation in the hypocretin (orexin) receptor 2 gene. *Cell* **98**:365, 1999.

272. Nishino S, Ripley B, Overeem S, Lammers GJ, Mignot E: Hypocretin (orexin) deficiency in human narcolepsy. *Lancet* **355**:39, 2000.

273. Kasahara M (ed): *Major Histocompatibility Complex: Evolution, Structure and Function*. Tokyo, Springer, 2000, p 1.

CHAPTER 13

The Nature and Mechanisms of Human Gene Mutation

Stylianos E. Antonarakis ▪ Michael Krawczak ▪ David N. Cooper

1. **There are a variety of different types of mutations in the human genome and many diverse mechanisms for their generation.**
2. **Single-base-pair substitutions account for the majority of gene defects. Among them, the hypermutability of CpG dinucleotides represents the most important and frequent cause of mutation in humans.**
3. **Point mutations may affect transcription and translation, as well as mRNA splicing and processing. Mutations in regulatory elements are of particular significance, since they often reveal the existence of DNA domains that are bound by regulatory proteins. Similarly, mutations that affect mRNA splicing can contribute to our understanding of the splicing mechanism.**
4. **We describe mechanisms of gene deletion and the DNA sequences that may predispose to such lesions, as well as potential mechanisms underlying insertions, duplications, or inversions, with representative examples.**
5. **Retrotransposition is a rare but biologically fascinating phenomenon that can lead to abnormal phenotypes if the double-stranded DNA is inserted in functionally important regions of a gene. Long interspersed repeat elements (LINEs) and *Alu* repetitive elements and pseudogenes have been shown to function as retrotransposons, and their *de novo* insertion in the genome can produce disease.**
6. **The expansion of trinucleotide repeats represents a relatively novel category of mutations in humans. There is a growing list of disorders that result from an abnormal copy number of trinucleotides within the 5′ or 3′ untranslated regions, coding sequences, and introns of genes. The pathophysiologic effects of the expansion of the trinucleotide repeat are unknown. Additionally, at least one disorder is caused by expansion of a 12mer repeat (progressive myoclonus epilepsy).**
7. **The study of mutations in human genes is of paramount importance in understanding the pathophysiology of hereditary disorders, in providing improved diagnostic tests, and in designing appropriate therapeutic approaches.**

The study of naturally occurring gene mutations is important for a number of reasons, not the least being that the process of mutational change is fundamental to an understanding of the origins of genetic variation and the mechanisms of evolution. Knowledge of the nature, relative frequency, and DNA sequence context of different gene lesions improves our understanding of the underlying mutational mechanisms and provides valuable insights into the intricacies of DNA replication and repair. It also contributes to the elucidation of the function of proteins and the importance of their structural motifs. Finally, the understanding of the ground rules for assessing and predicting the relative frequencies and locations of specific types of gene lesions may contribute to improvements in the design and efficacy of mutation search strategies. Over the past 20 years, the application of novel DNA technologies has enabled remarkable progress in the analysis and diagnosis of human inherited disease by the characterization of the underlying gene lesions. Many different types of mutation (single-base-pair substitutions, deletions, insertions, duplications, inversions, and repeat expansions) have been detected and characterized in a large number of different human genes. The incidence/prevalence of human genetic diseases is variable; therefore, it is not surprising that the nature, frequency, and location of pathologic gene lesions in the human genome are highly specific. This specificity is largely sequence dependent; thus, some DNA sequences are not only more mutable than others, but they also mutate in characteristic ways. In this chapter, the various types of human gene mutations and their underlying mechanisms are discussed in the order presented in Table 13-1.

NOMENCLATURE OF HUMAN GENE MUTATIONS

Recommendations for the nomenclature of human gene mutations have been published[1] by the Nomenclature Working Group sponsored by the Human Genome Organization (HUGO). These recommendations were the result of a consensus reached after a series of meetings and revisions of the final document, and approved during the 1997 meeting of the American Society of Human Genetics in Baltimore.

It is obvious that the most unambiguous nomenclature system is that based on genomic DNA. Even in that case, however, length polymorphisms can create a problem in the numbering of nucleotides and therefore a standard reference sequence ought to be established, preferably by experts for each gene. Unfortunately, the entire genomic sequence is known for only a minority of human genes. For the vast majority, only the cDNA sequence is available. The existence of more than one transcription start site, alternative splicing, and the utilization of alternative exons and variable number of repeats complicate the nucleotide numbering. Thus, here too, a reference sequence needs to be established. The nomenclature, at least in the present state of the human genome project, needs to be accurate and unambiguous, but flexible. The nucleotide change must always be included in the original report; however, other terms may be used (for example, specifying the amino acid change). The recommendations of the working group are as follows:

- For genomic DNA and cDNA, the A of the ATG of the initiator Met codon is denoted nucleotide +1. There is no

A list of standard abbreviations is located immediately preceding the index in each volume. Additional abbreviations used in this chapter include: ARE = androgen-response element; C1I = complement component-1 inhibitor; CV = consensus value; CVA = activated cryptic splice site; CVN = consensus value for normal, wild-type splice site; DHFR = dihydrofolate reductase; DMD = Duchenne muscular dystrophy; EBP = enhancer-binding protein; GBA = glucocerebrosidase; GH, growth hormone; HGMD, Human Gene Mutation Database; hnRNP = heterogeneous nuclear ribonucleoprotein; HPFH = hereditary persistence of fetal hemoglobin; HUGO = Human Genome Organization; LCR = locus control region; LINEs = long interspersed repeat elements; OAT = ornithine- -aminotransferase; ORF = open reading frame; ss = splice site; STS = steroid sulfatase; TPI1, triosephosphate isomerase I.

Table 13-1 Different Categories of Human Mutations Discussed in This Chapter

Single-base-pair substitutions
Types of nucleotide substitutions and hypermutable nucleotides
mRNA splice-junction mutations
mRNA processing (other than splicing) and translation mutations
Regulatory mutations
Deletions
Insertions
Duplications
Inversions
Expansion of unstable repeat sequences

nucleotide zero (0). The nucleotide 5′ to +1 is numbered −1. If there is more than one potential ATG, a reference consensus may be used. The numbering of nucleotides in the reference sequence in the databases should not be changed and remains associated with the same (original) accession number.

- The use of lowercase g (for genomic) or c (for cDNA) in front of the nucleotide number is recommended. To avoid confusion, a dot should separate these from the nucleotide number (g. or c. for genomic or cDNA, respectively). The accession number in primary sequence databases (GenBank, EMBL, and DDJB) should also be included in the original publication/database submission of mutations.
- Nucleotide changes start with the nucleotide number, and the change follows this number. 1997G > T denotes that at nucleotide 1997 of the reference sequence, G, is replaced by T.
- Deletions are designated by del after the nucleotide number: 1997delT denotes the deletion of T at nucleotide (nt) 1997, and 1997–1999del denotes the deletion of 3 nts. Alternatively, this mutation can be denoted as 1997–1999delTTC. For deletions in short tandem repeats, the most 3′ position is arbitrarily assigned; e.g., a TG deletion in the sequence AATGTGTGCC is designated 1997–1998delTG or 1997–1998del (where 1997 is the first T before C).
- Insertions are designated by ins after the nucleotide interval number. 1997–1998insT denotes that T was inserted in the interval between nts 1997 and 1998. For insertions in short repeats, the most 3′ nt interval is arbitrarily assigned; e.g., a TG insertion in the sequence AATGTGTGCC is designated 1997–1998insTG (where 1997 is the last G of the short TG repeat).
- Variability of short sequence repeats is designated as $1997(GT)_{6-22}$. In this case, 1997 is the first nucleotide of the dinucleotide GT, which is repeated 6 to 22 times in the population.
- A unique identifier for each mutation should be obtained. The Online Mendelian Inheritance in Man (OMIM) (http://www.ncbi.nlm.nih.gov/Omim/) unique identifier can be used, or database curators may assign such unique identifiers. Other existing databases such as the Human Gene Mutation Database (HGMD; http://www.uwcm.ac.uk/uwcm/mg/hgmd0.html), for example, could also be used as a reference source for cataloged mutations.
- When the full genomic sequence is not known, intron mutations can be designated by the intron intervening sequence (IVS) number, positive numbers starting from the G of the donor site invariant GT, negative numbers starting from the G of the acceptor site invariant AG. IVS4+1G > T denotes the G-to-T substitution at nt +1 of intron 4. IVS4−2A > C denotes the A-to-C substitution at nt −2 of intron 4. Alternatively, the cDNA nucleotide numbering may be used to designate the location of the mutation in the adjacent intron. For example, c.1997+1G > T denotes the G-to-T substitution at nt +1 after nucleotide 1997 of the cDNA. Similarly, c.1997−2A > C denotes the A-to-C substitution at nt −2 upstream of nucleotide 1997 of the cDNA. When the full-length genomic sequence is known, the mutation can be designated by the nt number of the reference sequence.
- Two mutations in the same allele can be listed within brackets as follows: [1997G > T;2001A > C]. This will also enable (1) the designation of mutations that are only deleterious when they occur in the same allele with additional nucleotide substitutions, and (2) the designation of haplotypes of different alleles.
- For amino-acid-based systems, the codon for the initiator *methionine* is codon 1.
- The single-letter amino acid code is recommended, but the three-letter code is also acceptable.
- For the amino-acid-based nomenclature, the format is Y97S (*tyrosine* at codon 97 substituted by *serine*). The *wild-type* amino acid is given before and the mutant amino acid after the codon number. Therefore, there is no confusion as to the significance of G, C, T, and A.
- Stop codons are designated by X, e.g., R97X (*arginine* codon 96 substituted by a termination codon).
- Deletions of amino acids are designated as: T97del denotes that the codon 97 for *threonine* is deleted.
- Insertions of amino acids are designated as: T97–98ins denotes that a codon for *threonine* is inserted at the interval between codons 97 and 98 of the reference amino acid sequence.
- The first report of a mutation in the literature should contain both a nucleotide-based and amino-acid-based name, when appropriate.

No recommendations have yet been made for complex mutations. Detailed description of such mutations and nomenclature proposals can usually be found in the original report or by the unique identifier. A second phase of recommendations will deal with such issues in the future. A discussion paper with further recommendations has recently been published.[2] In addition, the consequences of a mutation (frameshift, particular splicing abnormality, exon skipping, etc.) are not addressed in this nomenclature. However, investigators who maintain mutation databases are encouraged to include a field of mutation consequences or mechanisms (if known) in their databases.

The foregoing recommendations did not always represent a full consensus of the scientific community or the investigators involved in the discussions. Among the numerous other proposals/criticisms, it is worth mentioning the following:

- The "^" sign may be used to determine the interval of an insertion rather than the "−" sign. For example, 1997^1998insG instead of 1997–1998insG.
- The designation of both deleterious mutations in the two alleles of a homozygote for a recessive disorder may be designated as [1997G > T+2001A > G] to indicate the substitution in nt 1997 of one allele and in nt 2001 of the other allele of the same gene.
- Analogous to g. or c. for the genomic or cDNA numbering system, p. may be used to distinguish the protein-based nomenclature clearly.
- X may not be the best symbol for a termination codon.

SINGLE-BASE-PAIR SUBSTITUTIONS

Types of Nucleotide Substitutions

A database containing reports of mutations in the coding regions of human genes causing genetic disease, mainly characterized by DNA sequencing, has been maintained by two authors of this chapter (D.N.C. and M.K.). As of April 15, 2000, this database includes 21,591 entries in 1039 genes (this database is referred to as the Human Gene Mutation Database (HGMD[3]) throughout this chapter; http://www.uwcm.ac.uk/uwcm/mg/hgmd0.html). Earlier versions of the HGMD have been published.[4,5] Only one example of each mutation is recorded, owing to the difficulty in determining whether repeated mutations are identical by descent or truly recurrent. Fig. 13-1 illustrates the spectrum of mutations logged in the database. Missense nucleotide substitutions represent the most common type of mutations, accounting for 50 percent of the total entries. Regarding missense mutations,

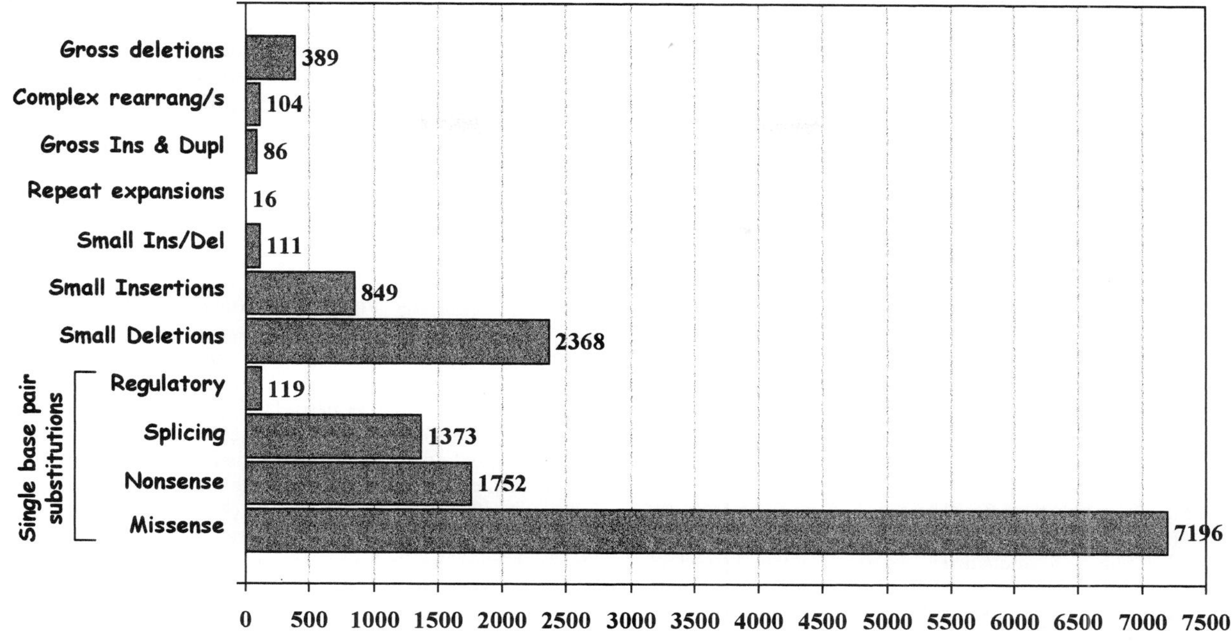

Fig. 13-1. Spectrum of different types of human gene mutations logged in Human Gene Mutation Database as of September 13, 1998 (*http://www.uwcm.ac.uk/uwcm/mg/hgmd0.html*).

evidence for causality comes from one or more of the following sources:

1. Occurrence of the mutation in a region of known structure or function
2. Occurrence of the lesion in an evolutionarily conserved residue
3. Previous independent occurrence of the mutation in an unrelated patient
4. Failure to observe the mutation in a large sample of normal controls
5. Novel appearance and subsequent cosegregation of the gene lesion and disease phenotype through a family pedigree
6. Demonstration that a mutant protein produced *in vitro* possesses the same biochemical properties and characteristics as its *in vivo* counterpart
7. Reversal of the pathological phenotype in the patient/cultured cells by replacement of the mutant gene/protein with its wild-type counterpart.

The spectrum of single-base-pair substitutions logged in the HGMD by November 1997 (the time it was last subjected to an extensive meta-analysis[6]) is summarized in Table 13-2. Mutations occurring in CpG dinucleotides account for 2133 (29.3 percent) of the total. Therefore, they represent a major cause of human genetic disorders (see below). If only CG-to-TG and CG-to-CA transitions (i.e., consistent with methylation-mediated deamination) are considered, this figure falls to 1675 (23 percent). Breakdown of the data by chromosomal location revealed that the proportion of CG-to-TG or CG-to-CA substitutions was significantly higher for autosomal genes (1325/5296 = 25.0 percent) than for X-chromosomal genes (350/1975 = 17.7 percent; $\chi^2 = 43.21$, 1 *df*, $P < 10^{-5}$). In part, this disparity can be explained by a generally more pronounced CpG suppression observed in X-linked genes: the average CpG content was 3.67 percent for the 401 autosomal cDNA sequences provided by the HGMD, and 2.86 percent for the 45 X-chromosomal cDNAs (Student's $t = 2.35$, 444 *df*, $P < 0.01$). Analysis of Table 13-2 yields transversion (T to A or G, A to T or C, G to C or T, C to G or A) and transition (T to C, C to T, G to A, A to G) frequencies of 37.5 percent and 62.5 percent, respectively. There is therefore a highly significant excess of transitions as compared with the expected frequency (33 percent). Most but not

Table 13-2 Spectrum of Single-Base-Pair Substitutions, in the Human Gene Mutation Database

	Nucleotide Resulting from Single-Base-Pair Change				
Initial Nucleotide	**T**	**C**	**A**	**G**	**Total**
T		**654**	271	312	1237
C	**1632** (940)		371	340	2343
A	201	163		**538**	902
G	619	453	**1717** (735)		2789
Total	2452	1270	2359	1190	7271

NOTE: A, adenine; C, cytosine; G, guanine; T, thymidine. **Bold** denotes transitions. Figures in brackets refer to transitions that are CG > TG or CG > CA, respectively. These data were based on 7271 single-base-pair substitutions logged on November 1997.[5]

Table 13-3 Relative Single-Base-Pair Substitution Rates in Human Nuclear Genes Causing Inherited Disease

Original Nucleotide	Substituting Nucleotide			
	T	C	A	G
T	—	1.525	0.374	0.410
C	2.702	—	0.541	0.505
A	0.187	0.268	—	1.127
G	0.521	0.712	3.128	—

NOTE: Relative substitution rates are based on data from the Human Gene Mutation Database and have been corrected for confounding effects as described by Krawczak et al.[5] The estimates are unitless and have been scaled so that the average equals unity.

all of this excess can be attributed to the hypermutability of the CpG dinucleotide. However, even when CpG mutations are removed (36.9 percent of all transitions and 16.8 percent of all transversions) from the analysis, the excess of transitions is still significant (55.8 percent vs 33 percent expected). It is important to point out that mutation frequencies observed in the context of human inherited disease are unlikely to reflect the true underlying rates of mutation occurrence. Since different amino acid substitutions have different effects upon protein structure and function, they have necessarily come to clinical attention (and thus entered the HGMD) with different probabilities. Moreover, codon frequencies differ from one another, implying that different amino acid residues are involved in a mutational event with different prior probabilities. Relative single-base-pair substitution rates corrected for these two confounding factors[6] are presented in Table 13-3. The data in this table confirm the existence of a high rate of C-to-T and G-to-A substitutions (48 percent of total).

DNA Polymerase Fidelity and Single-Nucleotide Substitutions. DNA replication occurs as a result of an accurate, yet error-prone, multistep process. The final accuracy depends on the initial fidelity of the replicative step and the efficiency of subsequent error-correction mechanisms.[7] Since DNA polymerases are involved in replication, recombination, and repair processes (Table 13-4),[8] their base incorporation fidelity is probably a critical factor in determining mutation rates in the cell. To test the hypothesis that nonrandom base misincorporation during DNA replication is a major contributory factor in human mutations, Cooper and Krawczak[5] compared the base substitution rates from Table 13-3 with the *in vitro* measured base substitution error rates (data from studies by Kunkel and Alexander[9] and others) exhibited by vertebrate DNA polymerases α, β, and δ. A significant correlation between these two sets of values was observed for polymerase β but not for polymerases α or δ (Spearman rank correlation coefficient, 0.74; $P < 0.005$). In this comparison, any consideration of the efficacy of the different proofreading and postreplicative mismatch-repair mechanisms was excluded. This is because the purified polymerase preparations used *in vitro* lacked the 3′ to 5′ exonuclease activities thought to be responsible for proofreading *in vivo*. The result obtained for DNA polymerase β is consistent with the postulate that a substantial proportion of the nucleotide substitutions causing human genetic disease are due to misincorporation of bases during DNA replication.

Slipped Mispairing and Single-Nucleotide Substitutions. A mechanistic model for single-base-pair mutagenesis, the slipped-mispairing model,[10] seeks to explain nucleotide misincorporation through transient misalignment of the primer-template caused by looping out of a template base. During replication synthesis, the template strand slips back one base, resulting in the misincorporation of the next nucleotide on the primer strand. After realignment of both primer and template strand, the mismatch may be corrected in favor of the misincorporated base (Fig. 13-2). *Misalignment* or *dislocation* mutagenesis is thought to be mediated by runs of identical bases or by other repetitive DNA sequences in the vicinity. If misincorporation mediated by one-base-pair (1-bp) slippage is important, then a substantial proportion of point mutations should exhibit identity of the newly introduced base to one of the bases flanking the mutation site. Comparison in the HGMD of the observed and expected frequency of this type of mutation revealed that this is indeed the case, but only at certain codon positions.[6] Mutation toward the 5′ flanking nucleotide occurred significantly more often than expected at the second position (642 observed vs 558 expected) but not at the first position (565 observed vs 568 expected) or last position of a codon (167 observed vs 170 expected); mutation toward the 3′ flanking base was significantly favored at the first position (490 observed vs 390 expected) but disfavored at the second position (592 observed vs 659 expected) of a codon. These findings suggest a mechanism of mutation at either position 1 or 2 in the codon (both critical in specifying the encoded amino acid residue) that is biased toward the nucleotide at the other position. Inspection of the genetic code reveals that such a bias invariably serves to avoid the *de novo* introduction of termination codons.

CpG Dinucleotides as Hotspots for Nucleotide Substitutions (Methylation-Mediated Deamination of 5-Methylcytosine)

CpG Distribution in the Vertebrate Genome and Its Origins. In eukaryotic genomes, 5-methylcytosine (5mC) occurs predominantly in CpG dinucleotides, the majority of which appear to be methylated.[11,12] Methylation of cytosine results in a high level of

Table 13-4 Eukaryotic DNA Polymerases

	α	β	γ	δ	ε
Catalytic polypeptide	165 kDa	40 kDa	140 kDa	125 kDa	255 kDa
Associated subunits	70, 58, 48 kDa	None	Unknown	48 kDa	Unknown
Cellular localization	Nuclear	Nuclear	Mitochondrial	Nuclear	Nuclear
Associated activities					
3′ → 5′ Exonuclease	None	None	Yes	Yes	Yes
Primase	Yes	None	None	None	None
Properties					
Processivity	Medium	Low	High	Low	High
Fidelity	High	Low	High	High	High
Major characteristics	Principal replicative DNA polymerase, lagging strand DNA synthesis	Short-patch DNA repair	Mitochondrial DNA polymerase	Leading-strand DNA synthesis	UV-induced repair synthesis

SOURCE: Modified from Wang.[7]

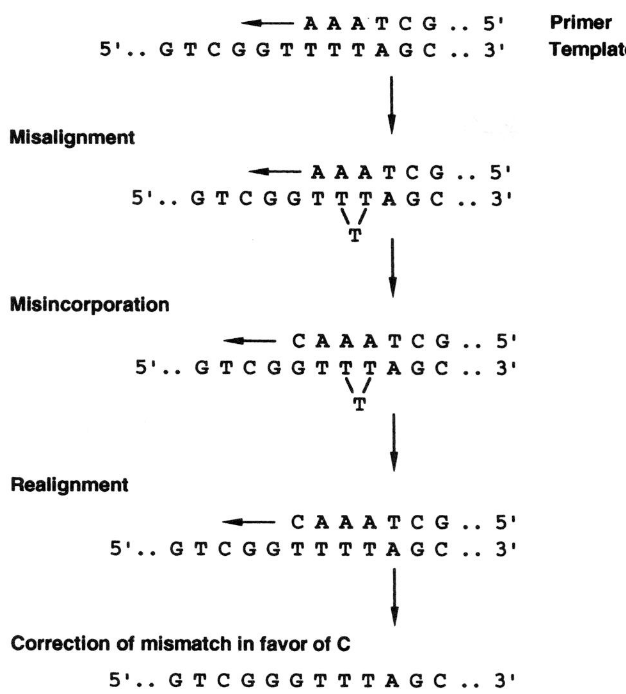

Fig. 13-2. Schematic representation of the slipped-mispairing model for single nucleotide substitutions.

mutation due to the propensity of 5mC to undergo deamination to form thymine (Fig. 13-3). Deamination of 5mC probably occurs with the same frequency as either cytosine or uracil. However, whereas uracil DNA glycosylase activity in eukaryotic cells can recognize and excise uracil, thymine—being a normal DNA base—is thought to be less readily detectable and hence removable by cellular DNA repair mechanisms. One consequence of the hypermutability of 5mC is the paucity of CpG in the genomes of many eukaryotes, the heavily methylated vertebrate genomes exhibiting the most extreme *CpG suppression*.[12] In vertebrate genomes, the frequency of CpG dinucleotides is between 20 and 25 percent of the frequency predicted from observed mononucleotide frequencies.[13,14] The distribution of CpG in the genome is also nonrandom: About 1 percent of the vertebrate genome consists of a fraction that is rich in CpG and that accounts for about 15 percent of all CpG dinucleotides (reviewed by Bird[15]). In contrast to most of the scattered CpG dinucleotides, these *CpG islands* represent unmethylated domains and in many cases appear to coincide with transcribed regions. The evolution of the heavily methylated vertebrate genome has been accompanied by a progressive loss of CpG dinucleotides as a direct consequence of their methylation in the germ line.

The CpG Dinucleotide and Human Genetic Disease. An excess of C-to-T transitions was first reported by Vogel and Röhrborn[16] in a study of the mutations responsible for hemoglobin variants in humans. Further studies confirmed the existence of this phenomenon.[17] Many additional studies in eukaryotes (reviewed by Cooper and Krawczak[5]) have now shown that the CpG dinucleotide is specifically associated with a high frequency of C-to-T and G-to-A transitions. The G-to-A transitions arise as a result of a 5mC-to-T transition on the antisense DNA strand, followed by miscorrection of G to A on the sense strand. A high frequency of polymorphism has also been detected in the human genome by restriction enzymes containing CpG in their recognition sequences.[18] CpG was found by molecular analysis to be a hotspot for mutation first in the factor VIII (F8C) gene[19,20] and subsequently in a wide range of different human genes.[21,22] From the relative dinucleotide mutabilities as estimated by Cooper and Krawczak[5,6] (see below for a description), it follows that the CG-to-TG or CG-to-CA substitutions are approximately 13 times more likely than any other substitution in the CG dinucleotide. This is perhaps an underestimate, since in the HGMD each nucleotide substitution has been logged only once, resulting in the systematic exclusion of multiple independent *de novo* mutations. It has been repeatedly noted in various genes that specific CG-to-TG or CG-to-CA mutations recur independently. For example, the number of CG-to-TG or CG-to-CA mutations in the factor VIII (F8C) gene causing hemophilia A is 25 percent of all different single-nucleotide substitutions, but 48 percent if recurrent mutations are considered (based on 586 F8C point mutations; see Kaufman and Antonarakis[23] and should be http://europium.csc.mrc.ac.uk). The observed frequency of CG-to-TG and CG-to-CA mutation varies between human genes; for example, it is less than 10 percent in the β-globin (HBB) and HPRT genes, but it is greater than 50 percent in the ADA gene. In two studies of the coagulation F8C and F9 genes in which almost all mutations in a given set of patients have been identified, approximately 35 percent of nucleotide substitutions were CG to TG or CG to CA.[24–26] The distribution of CpG mutations within a given gene may also be uniform. For example, 9 of 122 single-base-pair substitutions in exon 7 of the protein C (PROC) gene occur in a CpG; by contrast, none of 13 point mutations reported in exons 5 and 6 are in CpG dinucleotides,[27] although these exons contain a larger number of CpGs. In the assumed absence of a detection bias (see below), variation in CpG mutability is due either to differences in germ-line DNA methylation and/or relative intragenic CpG frequency. Indeed, CpG hypermutability in inherited disease implies that the affected sites are methylated in the germ line and thereby rendered prone to 5mC deamination. That 5mC deamination is directly responsible for mutational events has been evidenced by the fact that several cytosine residues known to have undergone a germ-line mutation

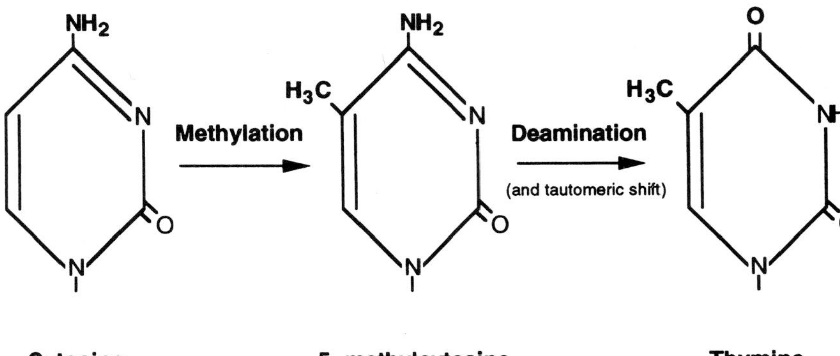

Fig. 13-3. Schematic representation of the molecules for cytosine, 5-methylcytosine, and thymine and the chemical events for the transformation of cytosine to thymine.

Table 13-5 Germ-Line Origin of Mutations in the Clotting Factor IX Gene

	Male	Female	M/F Ratio	*p* Value
All base substitutions	20	16	2.5	4.99×10^{-3}
All deletions	3	11	0.55	NS
Transitions				
At CpG	10	3	6.7	1.65×10^{-3}
Non-CpG	5	4	2.5	NS
Transversions	5	9	1.1	NS
Deletions				
Small (< 50 bp)	1	8	0.25	NS
Large (> 50 bp)	2	3	1.3	NS
Insertions	1	1		
Total	24	28		

NOTE: Modified from Ketterling *et al.*,[30] with the addition of the Kling *et al.*[31] cases. The observed M/F ratio was corrected for the expected 1 : 2 (the expected ratio is $z{:}1 + z$, where z denotes the probability of an X-linked recessive mutation to have at least one affected male descendant. Since $z \leq 1$, the ratio of 1 : 2 is a conservative estimate).

in the low-density-lipoprotein receptor gene (LDLR; hypercholesterolemia) and the tumor protein 53 (TP53) gene (various types of tumor) are indeed methylated in sperm DNA.[28]

The frequency of CG-to-TG or CG-to-CA mutations may differ between male and female germ lines because there is a profound difference in DNA methylation in the germ cells of the two sexes: the oocyte is markedly undermethylated, whereas sperm is heavily methylated.[29,30] Thus, it may be that CG-to-TG or CG-to-CA mutations occur more commonly in male germ cells. Table 13-5 shows the germ-line origin of mutations in the F9 gene. In this data set, there is a sevenfold male excess of transitions at CpG dinucleotides.[31] Pattinson et al[32] have noted differences between ethnic groups in the mutation frequency at specific CpG sites within the F8C gene in a small sample. By contrast, the pattern of germ-line CpG mutation in the F9 gene appeared to be indistinguishable between Asians, mostly of Korean origin, and Caucasians.[33] This finding argues for the absence of population-specific methylation patterns and is consistent with no differences in methylation between individuals from different ethnic backgrounds.[34] In somatic tissues, 5mC deamination also appears to be an important mechanism of single-base-pair substitution.[35,36] Indeed, the relative rate of mitotic cancer-associated CG-to-TG or CG-to-CA transitions observed in the TP53 gene, the most widely mutated gene in human tumorigenesis, is very similar to the overall germ-line rate observed in other human genes.[37] Fig. 13-4 depicts the codon usage in human genes (data from 6,130,940 human codons from GenBank release 107 recorded in http://www.dna.affrc.go.jp/nakamura-bin/showcodon.cgi?species = Homo+sapiens+[gbpri]), together with the relative frequency at which codons are affected by any of the 8604 missense/nonsense recorded in the HGMD on July 14, 1998; http://www.uwcm.ac.uk/uwcm/mg/haha1.html). It is obvious from Fig. 13-4 that codons for Arg and Gly underwent more mutations than expected from codon usage alone in human genes. Although four codons for Arg contain CG dinucleotides, it is less clear why the codons for Gly are hypermutable. They all start with G and could therefore be part of a CG dinucleotide. In addition, they all are GGN, and a nearest neighbor analysis of single-base substitutions (Table 13-6) indicated that a mutated G is often flanked by another G at its 5′ side. To overcome the bias of counting independent mutations only once, we also compared, in Fig. 13-5, the number of recurrent

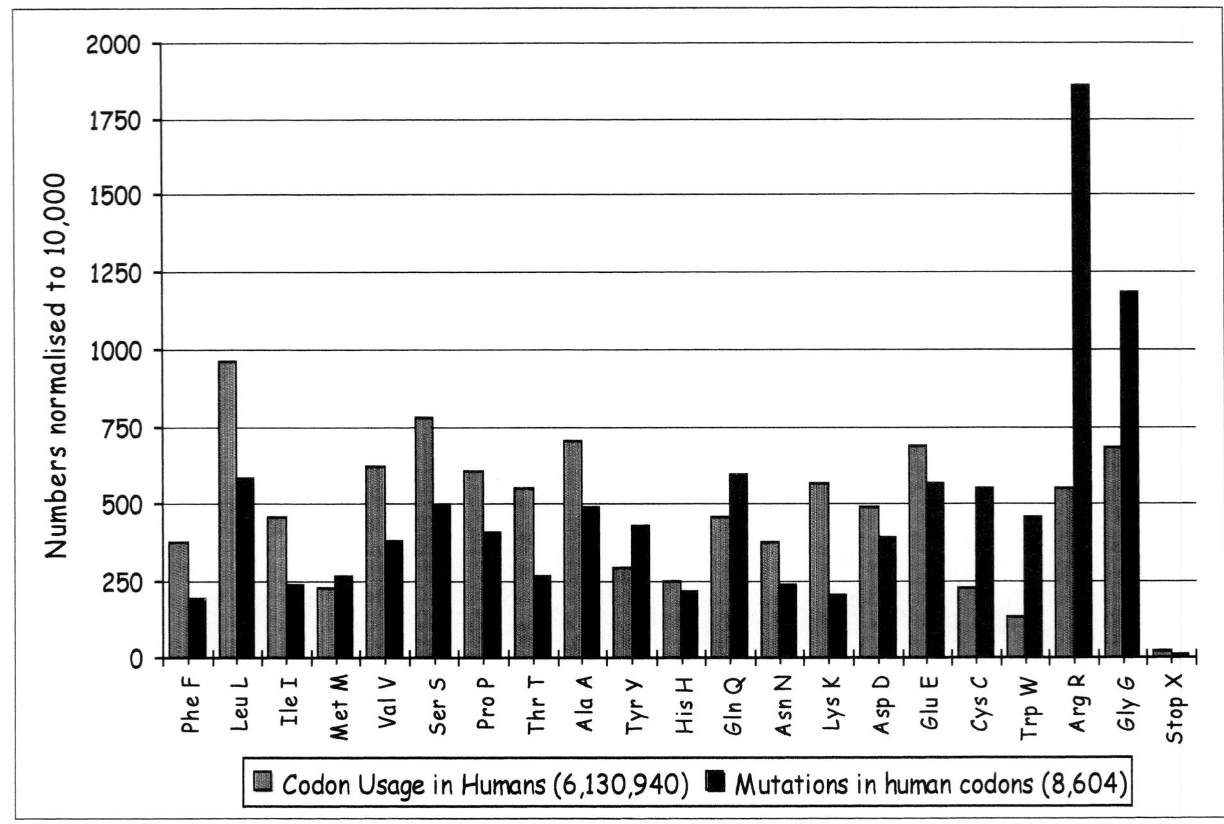

Fig. 13-4. Histogram of codon usage in human genes and mutations found in codons for the various amino acids. The codon usage data are from http://www.dna.affrc.go.jp/nakamura-bin/showcodon.cgi?species=Homo+sapiens+[gbpri] and the mutation data are from http://www.uwcm.ac.uk/uwcm/mg/haha1.html. The values on the *x*-axis were normalized for 10,000.

Table 13-6 Nucleotide Frequencies at the 3′ and 5′ Sides of Point Mutations Causing Human Genetic Disease

(a) Mutated Base	3′ Neighboring Base				
	T	C	A	G	Total
T	202	240	164	631	1237
C	235	354	619	1135 (195)	2343 (1403)
A	311	218	209	164	902
G	493 (374)	613 (457)	732 (547)	951 (676)	2789 (2054)
Total	1241 (1122)	1425 (1269)	1724 (1539)	2881 (1666)	7271 (5596)

(b) 5′ Neighboring Base	Mutated Base				
	T	C	A	G	Total
T	182	509 (314)	161	669	1521 (1326)
C	438	716 (350)	295	998 (263)	2447 (1346)
A	347	519 (355)	173	345	1384 (1220)
G	270	599 (384)	273	777	1919 (1704)
Total	1237	2343 (1403)	902	2789 (2054)	7271 (5596)

NOTE: Figures in parentheses denote observed nearest-neighbor frequencies when CG-to-TG (**a**) and CG-to-CA (**b**) transitions are excluded.

mutations found in different codons of five X-linked genes (F8C, F9, L1CAM, OTC, and BTK) with the codon usage in these five genes. The information included was extracted from the following locus-specific databases: for BTK, http://www.uta.fi/laitokset/imt/bioinfo/BTKbase/ for F8C, http://europium.csc.mrc.ac.uk for F9, http://www.umds.ac.uk/molgen/haemBdatabase.htm; for L1CAM, http://dnalab-www.uia.ac.be/dnalab/l1/#L1CAM mutations; and, for OTC, http://www.peds.umn.edu/otc/. It is again apparent from Fig. 13-5 that codons for Arg are more vulnerable to point mutations, emphasizing the hypermutability of the CG dinucleotide.

Are other mechanisms also responsible for CpG deamination? The suggestion that CpG deamination may result from endogenous

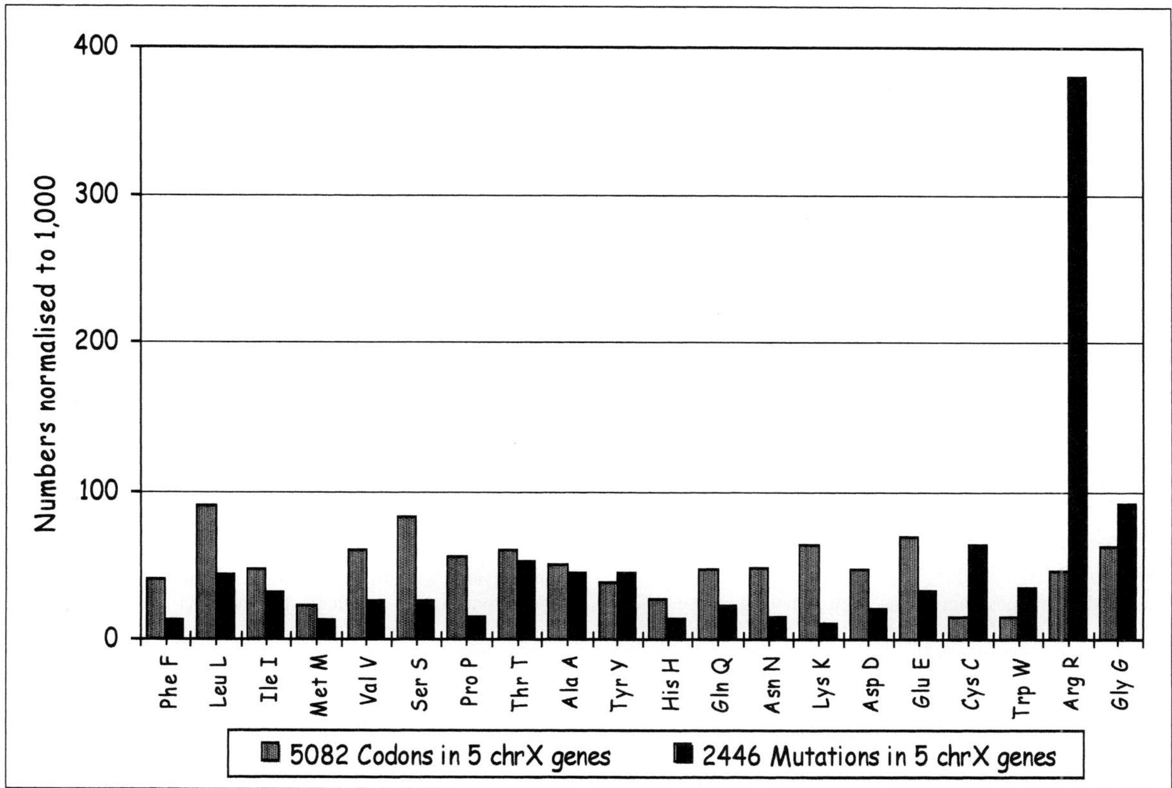

Fig. 13-5. Histogram of the independent recurrent mutations found in codons of five X-linked genes and the occurrence of these codons in these five genes. The genes were F8C, F9, L1CAM, OTC, and BTK. The information for the independent mutations was extracted from the following locus specific databases: for BTK, http://www.helsinki.fi/science/signal/btkbase.html; for F8C, http://146.179.66.63/usr/WWW/WebPages/main.dir/main.htm; for F9, WebPages/database.dir/titlepage.htm; http://dnalab-www.uia.ac.be/dnalab/l1/#L1CAM mutations for L1CAM; and, for OTC, http://www.peds.umn.edu/otc/.

enzymatic activity has been mooted by Steinberg and Gorman,[38] who found that some 70 percent of their (independent) mouse lymphoma cell mutants possessed a specific CGG-to-TGG substitution converting Arg 334 to Trp in the gene-encoding protein-kinase regulatory subunit. In 5 percent of these mutants, a second mutation (CGT to TGT) was found converting Arg 332 to Cys. The co-occurrence of these two mutations at such a high frequency argues for some type of enzymatic mechanism and against two independent methylation-mediated deamination events. Such a mechanism could involve a deaminase, although no such activity has yet been purified. The relevance of the observation to human gene mutation is doubtful, since (1) there are no known examples, including CpG dinucleotides, of pathologic base changes that occur with such a high proportional frequency in humans, and (2) although a very few isolated examples of double mutation have been reported as causes of human genetic disease, these do not involve CpG dinucleotides. Shen et al[39] have reported that DNA methyltransferase is capable of including C-to-T transitions directly in prokaryotes, and the mutation frequency was sensitive to the concentration of the methyl donor, *S*-adenosylmethionine. The importance of this putative deamination mechanism in eukaryotes is at present unclear.

Non-CpG Point-Mutation Hotspots

In an early and not updated analysis, among the 879 point mutations in HGMD not readily explicable by methylation-mediated deamination, a total of 30 codons in 16 different genes were identified as potential *hotspots* for single-base-pair substitutions. These residues were characterized either by a single base being affected by at least two nonidentical substitutions or by mutations affecting two or three nucleotides within that codon. Some trinucleotide and tetranucleotide motifs are significantly overrepresented within 10 bp on either side of the mutation hotspots. These motifs are TTT (17 observed vs 8 expected), CTT (18 vs 8), TGA (23 vs 11), TTG (20 vs 8), CTTT (8 vs 2), TCTT (8 vs 2), and TTTG (11 vs 2). In addition, Cooper and Krawczak[5] screened a region of 10 bp around 219 non-CpG base substitution sites for triplets and quadruplets that occurred at significantly increased frequencies. Only one trinucleotide was found again to occur at a frequency significantly higher than expected: CTT, the topoisomerase-I cleavage site consensus sequence.[40] CTT was observed 36 times in the vicinity of a point mutation, whereas the expected frequency was 20. By contrast, two tetranucleotides were significantly overrepresented at the screened positions. TCGA was observed 17 times (7 expected; this was probably because *Taq*I restriction enzyme was used for detection of the mutations), whereas TGGA was observed 25 times (12 expected). The latter motif fits perfectly with the deletion hotspot consensus sequence drawn up previously for human genes,[41] which, in turn, resembles the putative arrest site for DNA polymerase α.[42] Thus, it may be that the arrest or pausing of the polymerase at the replication fork disposes the replication complex to misincorporation of nucleotides as well as deletions.

A Nearest-Neighbor Analysis of Single-Base-Pair Substitutions

Methylation-mediated deamination as a primary cause of point mutation is characterized by an increased rate of CG-to-TG and CG-to-CA transitions. However, the relative likelihoods of point mutations at other dinucleotides may also vary, as is suggested by the nearest-neighbor frequencies observed in the HGMD (Table 13-6). (Note that each point mutation can be regarded as occurring within two distinct dinucleotides, depending on whether one considers the 5′ or the 3′ neighboring base.) In Table 13-6, considerable differences are apparent with respect to nucleotides occurring adjacent to sites of point mutation. For example, G residues are clearly overrepresented as 3′ flanking nucleotides when T is mutated, and a mutated G is often flanked by another G residue on the 5′ side.

Differences in the phenotypic consequences of specific point mutations, and thus in the likelihood of their coming to clinical attention, introduce a serious bias to the observed spectrum of mutations underlying human disease. In-depth studies of the phenotypic effect of large numbers of different missense mutations in a specific gene are few. One such study for missense mutations in the F9 gene[43] showed that mutations at *generic* residues (amino acid residues conserved in F9 of other mammalian species and in three related serine proteases) would invariably cause disease. Mutations at F9-specific residues (residues conserved in the factor IX of other mammalian species but not in three related serine proteases) were some sixfold less likely to cause disease, whereas mutations at nonconserved residues were 33 times less likely to result in a hemophilia-B phenotype. Bottema et al[43] estimated that 40 percent of all possible missense changes would cause hemophilia B, implying that 60 percent of residues serve merely as *spacers* to maintain the relative position of critical amino acid residues and probably do not fulfill any specific (known) function. Thus, detectable mutations, identified by virtue of their effect on protein structure and function and subsequently on clinical phenotype, appear to be a subset of a rather larger number of mutations, many of which have no clinical effect, at least in the case of hemophilia B. To what extent this finding in hemophilia B (in which <5 percent normal F9 activity must be present to generate a clinically abnormal phenotype) can be extrapolated to other genetic disorders is, however, unclear. Nevertheless, it would seem reasonable to suppose that the phenotypic consequences of a given point mutation are determined by the magnitude of the amino acid exchange as assessed by the resulting structural perturbation of the protein. Thus, specific amino acid substitutions might come to clinical attention more readily, depending on the severity of the resulting phenotype. Several methods have been reported for assessing the relative net effect of a specific amino acid exchange.[44,45] Perhaps the best comparative measure of amino acid relatedness available is that devised by Grantham,[45] who combined the three interdependent properties of composition, polarity, and molecular volume to assign each amino acid pair a mean chemical difference. Krawczak et al[6] devised an iterative multivariate procedure that takes into account the phenotypic consequences of a mutation, measured by means of Grantham's chemical difference between the wild type and mutant amino acid. Over and above the hypermutability of CpG dinucleotides, only a subtle and locally confined influence of the surrounding DNA sequence upon relative single-base-pair substitution rates was observed which extended no further than 2 bp from the substitution site.[6] Maximum-likelihood estimates of relative substitution rates taking the immediate 5′ and 3′ flanking nucleotides into account are summarized in Table 13-7. A steady increase in clinical observation likelihood with increasing chemical difference was also noted. Furthermore, nonsense mutations were found to be more than twice as likely to come to clinical attention as the most extreme missense mutations and three times more likely than the average amino acid change. However, the phenotypic consequences of a given mutation must depend not only on the nature of the amino acid substitution, but also on the location of the substitution within the protein. In general, and with the exception of charged residues, most amino acids that make critical interactions (e.g., disulfide bonds, hydrophobic forces, and hydrogen bonds) are rigid or buried within the protein structure, and their mutational substitution will be profoundly destabilizing.

Strand Difference in Base Substitution Rates

A noteworthy feature of Table 13-7 is that it reveals some asymmetry, suggesting a strand difference for single-base-pair substitutions. For example, the relative rates of CT to CC and AG to GG differ by more than twofold. Since the latter transition is complementary to the former, these two figures should coincide if point mutagenesis were acting similarly on both DNA strands. Estimation of relative substitution rates conditional on both the 5′

Table 13-7 Relative Dinucleotide Mutabilities

	Newly Introduced 5′				Newly Introduced 3′ Base			
d	T	C	A	G	T	C	A	G
TT	—	1.17	0.31	0.36	—	0.71	0.20	0.28
CT	1.17	—	0.31	0.41	—	1.57	0.27	0.43
AT	0.44	0.20	—	2.06	—	1.53	0.40	0.34
GT	0.86	0.71	3.13	—	—	1.17	0.39	0.30
TC	—	0.93	0.37	0.19	2.06	—	0.37	0.56
CC	1.16	—	0.49	0.32	2.54	—	0.39	0.40
AC	0.23	0.37	—	0.95	2.27	—	0.48	0.44
GC	0.48	0.71	2.68	—	2.06	—	0.51	0.32
TA	—	1.19	0.32	0.34	0.16	0.24	—	1.36
CA	1.28	—	0.43	0.42	0.12	0.43	—	1.23
AA	0.14	0.22	—	0.87	0.12	0.16	—	0.92
GA	0.45	0.60	2.82	—	0.24	0.15	—	0.63
TG	—	1.86	0.37	0.52	0.42	0.62	1.84	—
CG	**9.01**	—	0.88	0.90	0.90	1.17	**12.17**	—
AG	0.10	0.19	—	0.60	0.30	0.46	1.38	—
GG	0.46	0.69	3.09	—	0.49	0.54	1.76	—

NOTE: d, Original dinucleotide. Relative substitution rates are unitless and have been scaled so that the average in each half of the table equals unity.

Table 13-8 A Strand Difference in Relative Single-Base-Pair Substitution Rates

Original Substitution	Relative Rate	Watson-Crick Homologue	Relative Rate
GGT > GTT	1.16 ± 0.16	ACC > AAC	0.51 ± 0.08
TGG > TAG	1.64 ± 0.13	CCA > CTA	0.99 ± 0.09
CGG > CAG	13.01 ± 0.88	CCG > CTG	8.35 ± 0.47
CTT > CCT	1.14 ± 0.20	AAG > AGG	0.35 ± 0.10
CTC > CCC	1.20 ± 0.17	GAG > GGG	0.32 ± 0.07
TGC > TCC	0.76 ± 0.13	GCA > GGA	0.19 ± 0.06
CTG > CCG	1.87 ± 0.15	CAG > CGG	0.81 ± 0.13
GGT > GAT	1.79 ± 0.21	ACC > ATC	0.68 ± 0.14
CTG > CAG	0.22 ± 0.04	CAG > CTG	0.03 ± 0.02
CTT > CGT	0.47 ± 0.11	AAG > ACG	0.12 ± 0.04

NOTE: Relative substitution rates (± SD) are unitless and were scaled so that their average, taken over all 192 possible substitution types, is unity. Estimation of standard deviation and significance assessment was by bootstrapping. Only pairs of substitutions are included for which one relative rate estimate was consistently larger than its counterpart in more than 9995 to 10,000 replications of the estimate procedure.

and 3′ flanking nucleotides served to identify 10 pairs of substitutions, complementary to each other, that exhibit the same feature.[6] These are listed in Table 13-8. A strand difference in mutation rates has already been described by Wu and Maeda.[46] By comparison of nonfunctional sequences near the β-globin genes of six primate species, they demonstrated that purine-to-pyrimidine (R-to-Y) transversions occurred approximately 1.5 times more frequently than their pyrimidine-to-purine counterparts. However, complementary transitions were found to occur at equal frequencies. These findings are compatible with the mutational spectrum from the HGMD: R to Y was observed 11 percent more frequently than Y to R, and both T-to-C and A-to-G transitions account for some 10 percent of the mutations in Table 13-2. A slightly different result was obtained for G-to-A transitions, which are 1.4 times more frequent than C-to-T transitions. Nevertheless, Table 13-7 reveals that strand differences in mutation rates depend on the nucleotides flanking the site of mutation. For example, whereas CT to CC is more than 2.5 times more likely than AG to GG, TA is 15 percent more likely to mutate to TG than to CA. A disparity between the likelihoods of CG-to-TG and CG-to-CA transitions is also evident from inspection of Tables 13-7 and 13-8. This observation strongly suggests that, at least within gene coding regions, the two strands are differentially methylated and/or differentially repaired. Holmes et al[47] have demonstrated *in vitro* the existence of a strand-specific correction process in human and *Drosophilia* cells whose efficiency depends on the nature of the mispair. Such differential repair could also account for the observed strand differences in mutation frequency.

Single-Base-Pair Substitutions in Human mRNA Splice Junctions

Single-base-pair substitutions (point mutations) affecting mRNA splicing are nonrandomly distributed, and this nonrandomness can be related to the phenotypic consequences of mutation.[48] Naturally occurring point mutations that affect mRNA splicing fall into four main categories: (1) Mutations within 5′ or 3′ consensus splice sites. Such lesions usually reduce the amount of correctly spliced mature mRNA and/or lead to the utilization of alternative splice sites in the vicinity. This results in the production of mRNAs that either lack a portion of the coding sequence (*exon skipping*) or contain additional sequence of intronic origin (*cryptic splice-site utilization*). (2) Mutations within an intron or exon that may serve to activate cryptic splice sites and lead to the production of aberrant mRNA species. (3) Mutations within a branch-point sequence. (4) Mutations in the introns that may regulate the efficiency of splicing, balance of alternative transcripts, and spliceosome assembly. Our understanding of the mechanism of these latter mutations is poor.

Splice-Junction Mutations Causing Human Genetic Disease

Splicing defects are not an uncommon cause of human genetic disease. The vast majority of known gene lesions that affect splicing are point mutations within 5′ and 3′ splice sites (ss). As shown in Fig. 13-1, the 1373 splicing mutations account for 9.6 percent of the 14363 mutations recorded in the HGMD (as of September 13, 1998). Krawczak et al[48] first collected from the literature (until mid-1991) a total of 101 different examples of point mutation in the vicinity of exon-intron splice junctions of human genes that altered the accuracy or efficiency of mRNA splicing and were responsible for a specific disease phenotype. Since then, the accelerated pace of gene and mutation discovery has greatly enriched our understanding of the importance of different splice signal sequences. Of 1373 different splice-site mutations, 797 (58 percent) affected the 5′ ss (donor splice site), 464 (34 percent) were located in 3′ ss (acceptor splice site), and most of the remaining 112 resulted in the creation of novel splice sites. Fig. 13-6 shows the consensus splice-site sequences of mammalian genes. For both the wild-type and mutated splice sites, *consensus values* (CVs[49]) can be calculated that reflect the similarity of any one splice site to the consensus sequence. A splice site containing the least frequent bases at each position would yield a CV of 0, whereas splice sites containing only the most frequent bases would have a CV of 1. CV for the wild-type splice sites (consensus value for normal [CVN] splice sites) studied were from 0.7 to 1, with a mean of about 0.83 for the 5′ and 3′ ss. Sequences with either extremely small or extremely high CVN were lacking. This finding suggested that splice sites that are less than optimal in terms of their similarity to the consensus sequence are especially prone to the deleterious effects of mutation. Splice sites with an already extremely low degree of similarity would not be further functionally impaired by single-base changes. An analysis was also conducted for the CV of mutated splice sites (CVM[48]). These CVMs were from 0.48 to 0.74 for the 3′ ss and from 0.5 to 0.84 for the 5′ ss. This clearly indicated that mutations at splice-site junctions serve to reduce the similarity to the consensus.

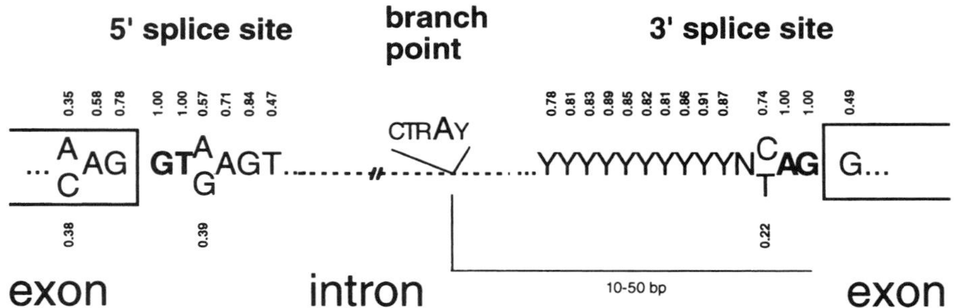

Fig. 13-6. Consensus sequences for the 5′ splice site (ss) (donor site), 3′ ss (acceptor site), and the branch point. Numbers corresponding to the nucleotides represent frequencies of each given nucleotide in the collections of Padget et al[50] and Shapiro and Senapathy.[49]

Location and Spectrum of Splice-Site Mutations

Comparison of the number of mutations in the HGMD reported at particular splice-site positions with their corresponding expectations, based on substitution rates from human gene-coding regions, indicates that point mutations are significantly overrepresented at the invariant positions +1 (observed, 414; expected, 189.5) and +2 (observed, 89; expected, 51.0) of the 5′ ss, and positions −1 (observed, 192; expected 62.8) and −2 (observed, 168; expected, 23.3) of the 3′ ss. Mutations at all other positions within splice sites were underrepresented. Table 13-9 summarizes the observed and expected frequencies of point mutations at different positions in 5′ ss and 3′ ss. Of the 1373 splicing mutations in the HGMD, 414 (30.1 percent) occur at the 5′-ss position +1 and 89 (6.5 percent) at position +2 (http://www.uwcm.ac.uk/uwcm/mg/haha2.html). The majority (58 percent) of the G+1 mutations were to A, and the majority of the T+2 mutations were to C. In the 3′ ss, there are 168 mutations (12 percent) in the invariant A−2, and 192 (14 percent) in the invariant G−1. The majority (53 percent) of the G−1 mutations were to A, and the majority (69 percent) of the A−2 mutations were to G. Therefore, the four invariant nucleotides (of the 24 involved in the splice-site consensus sequences) in the 5′ ss and the 3′ ss represent a total of 863, i.e., 62.8 percent of the splicing mutations. Fig. 13-7 depicts the distribution of mutations within the consensus 5′ ss and 3′ ss logged in the HGMD. It is of interest that a considerable number of mutations have been found in nucleotides +5 and −1 of the consensus 5′ ss, although these positions are not invariant. At position +5 of the 5′ ss, a total of 103 mutations have been reported, whilst, at position −1, a total of 100 mutations have been found (as of September 13, 1998). Table 13-9, however, shows that these numbers are not higher than expected under a model of random mutations.

It appears very likely that the observed nonrandomness of mutation within splice sites is a reflection of relative phenotypic severity (and hence detection bias) rather than any intrinsic difference in the underlying frequency of mutation. The replacement of G residues at positions +1 and +5 of 5′ ss would be predicted to reduce significantly the stability of base pairing of the splice site with the complementary region of U1 small nuclear RNA (snRNA). Binding to U1 snRNA is essential for the pre-mRNA to be folded correctly before cleavage and ligation can occur within the spliceosome. The same argument holds true for the mutations observed at position −1.[51] Only 42 examples of mutations at the +3 and 20 at the +4 positions of 5′ ss, respectively, were noted; the corresponding residues in U1 snRNA are pseudouridines rather than a cytosine. Thus, the spectrum of 5′-ss mutations observed *in vivo* suggests an important role for U1 snRNA binding.

Table 13-9 Observed and Expected Frequencies of Point Mutations at Different Positions in 5′ and 3′ Splice Sites (from the Human Gene Mutation Database, September 13, 1998)

5′ Splice Sites			3′ Splice Sites		
Pos	Obs	Exp	Pos	Obs	Exp
−2	15	84	−6	11	47
−1	100	154	−5	5	57
+1	**414**	**189**	−4	5	48
+2	**89**	**51**	−3	26	45
+3	42	73	−2	**168**	**23**
+4	20	57	−1	**192**	**63**
+5	103	119	−1	4	72
+6	14	68	−2	4	61

NOTE: Pos, position; Obs, observed frequency; Exp, expected frequency.

Mutations Creating Novel Splice Sites

A different category of mutation affecting mRNA splicing is provided by single-base-pair substitutions outside actual splice sites that create novel splice sites that substitute for the wild-type sites. This category may contain more mutations than currently appreciated, because very few sequence data exist for introns as compared with coding regions. A total of 13 mutations creating novel splice sites (13 percent of the 101 splice mutations) were collected in a survey by Krawczak et al;[48] in all but one case, the novel splice site was situated upstream of the original wild-type site. One intriguing finding for mutations creating novel 3′ acceptor splice sites should be noted: All six mutations introduced an A at −2, but never a G at −1. CVs for the activated cryptic splice sites (CVAs) were calculated when possible; in 8 of 12 cases, the CVA was as high as or higher than the wild-type CVN, suggesting that the novel splice sites successfully compete with the wild-type sites for splicing factors. For mutations in the vicinity of 3′ ss, the relative proportion of cryptic splice-site-utilizing mRNA appeared to correlate positively with the CVA/CVN ratio, whereas, at 5′ ss, the distance to the wild-type site may have also played an important role. The current version of the HGMD contains 112 mutations outside the consensus splice sites, and most of them create novel splice sites.

Phenotypic Consequences of Splice-Site Mutation *in Vivo*

The phenotypic consequences of naturally occurring point mutations in the 5′ ss of seven human genes were studied by Talerico and Berget,[52] who observed exon skipping in six cases as compared with only one case (β-globin gene) of cryptic splice-site usage. These initial results suggested that exon skipping might be the preferred *in vivo* phenotype, an assertion confirmed by many subsequent reports. One major mRNA species was usually observed, and this invariably lacked either the exon upstream of the mutated 5′ ss or downstream of the mutated 3′ ss. A detection bias is nevertheless possible, since a single exon-skipped transcript might be easier to detect/identify than a number of less frequent transcripts each resulting from the use of a different cryptic splice site. Several instances of the detection of small amounts of residual

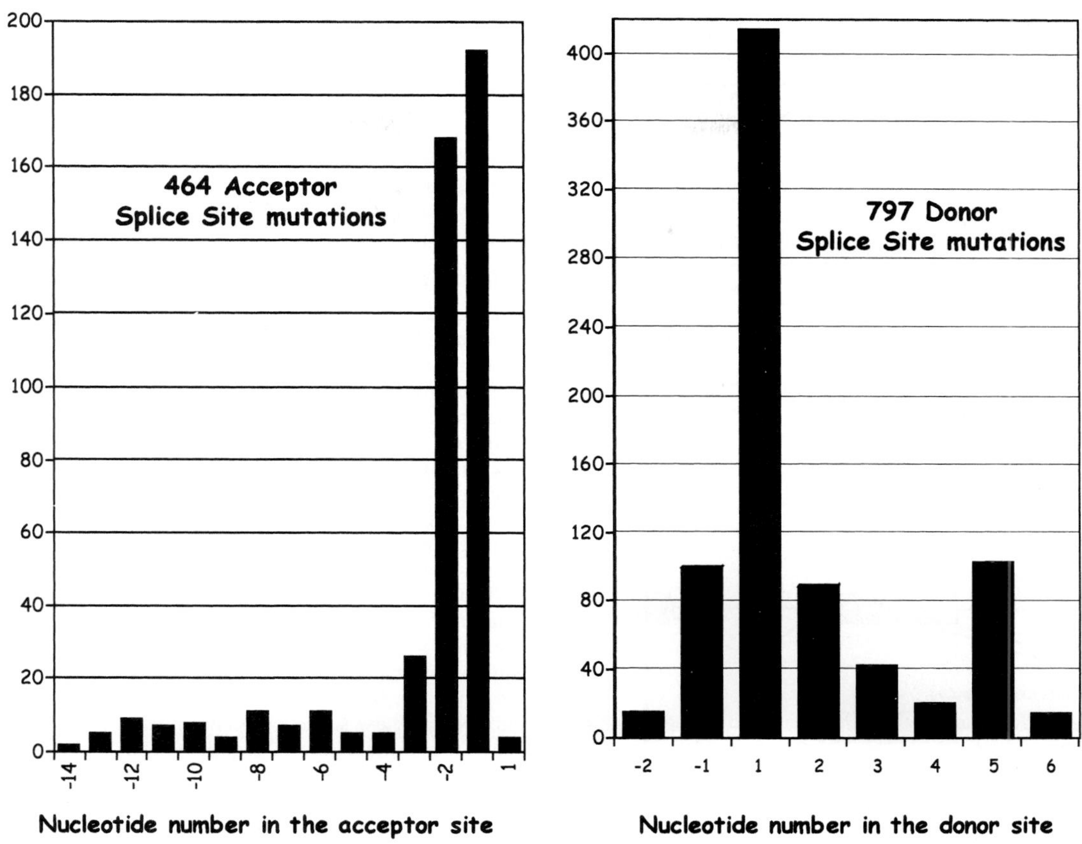

Fig. 13-7. Mutations in the consensus sequences of splice junctions recorded in the Human Gene Mutation Database.

wild-type mRNA from the cells of patients with a 5′-ss defect have also been reported. All these involve the mutation of bases outside the invariant GT dinucleotide, suggesting that normal splicing is still possible in such cases, albeit at greatly reduced efficiency. The choice between exon skipping and cryptic splice-site usage may be visualized merely as a decision about whether to utilize the next available legitimate splice site or the next best, albeit illegitimate, sequence in the immediate vicinity. This choice may be made on the basis of the presence/absence of sites capable of competing with the mutated splice site for splicing factors. Krawczak et al[48] studied the regions both upstream and downstream of their collection of mutations in an attempt to correlate sequence properties with the observed phenotypic consequences of mutation. They presented evidence that, at least for 5′-ss mutations, cryptic splice-site usage is favored under conditions in which a number of such sites are present in the immediate vicinity and exhibit sufficient homology to the splice-site consensus sequence for them to compete successfully with the mutated splice site. Fig. 13-8 schematically represents the consequences of splice mutations with reference to representative examples. In this chapter, exon skipping as a consequence of nonsense mutations in the skipped exon[63,67] is discussed under nonsense mutations.

Mutations within the Pyrimidine Tract

The HGMD contains 69 mutations in the pyrimidine tract of the 3′ ss. Some examples include the steroid 21-hydroxylase B (CYP21B) and HBB genes causing adrenal hyperplasia and β thalassemia, respectively.[68–70] It is not clear how and why these mutations at polypyrimidine tracts exert a pathologic influence on efficient mRNA splicing. It may be that some 3′ ss are more susceptible to the effects of pyrimidine loss than are others by virtue of the relative length of the pyrimidine tract.

Mutations at the Branch Point

An intermediate stage in eukaryotic RNA splicing is the formation of a lariat structure utilizing an A (adenosine) residue approximately 10 to 50 nucleotides from the 3′ ss. A weak consensus sequence, CTRAY, for this branch point has been observed in mammalian genes. After lariat structure formation, the first downstream AG dinucleotide is usually chosen as the acceptor splice site.[71] In a family with X-linked hydrocephalus, an A-to-C mutation 19 nucleotides upstream from a normal splice acceptor site of exon Q of the L1CAM gene on Xq28 segregated with the disease phenotype.[72] The mutation resulted in several RNA species exhibiting exon-Q skipping, insertion of 69 bp due to utilization of a cryptic splice site, or normal splicing. Another example of such mutation was reported in the COL5A1 gene causing Ehlers-Danlos syndrome type II. Affected members from two British families were heterozygous for a T-to-C point mutation in intron 32 (IVS32, −25T > G), causing loss of the 45-bp exon 33 from the mRNA in 60 percent of transcripts of the mutant gene.[73] The mutation lies only 2 bp upstream of a highly conserved adenosine in the consensus branch-site sequence that is required for lariat formation. A similar branch-site point mutation (IVS4, −22T > C) in the LCAT was observed in a family with fish eye disease, a condition characterized by corneal opacities and low plasma high-density-lipoprotein (HDL) cholesterol. The mutation caused intron retention rather than exon skipping.[74] In a patient with erythropoietic protoporphyria, a C-to-T mutation in intron 2 (IVS2, −23C > T) of the ferrochelatase (FECH) gene was found.[75] This mutation was associated with skipping of exon 2.

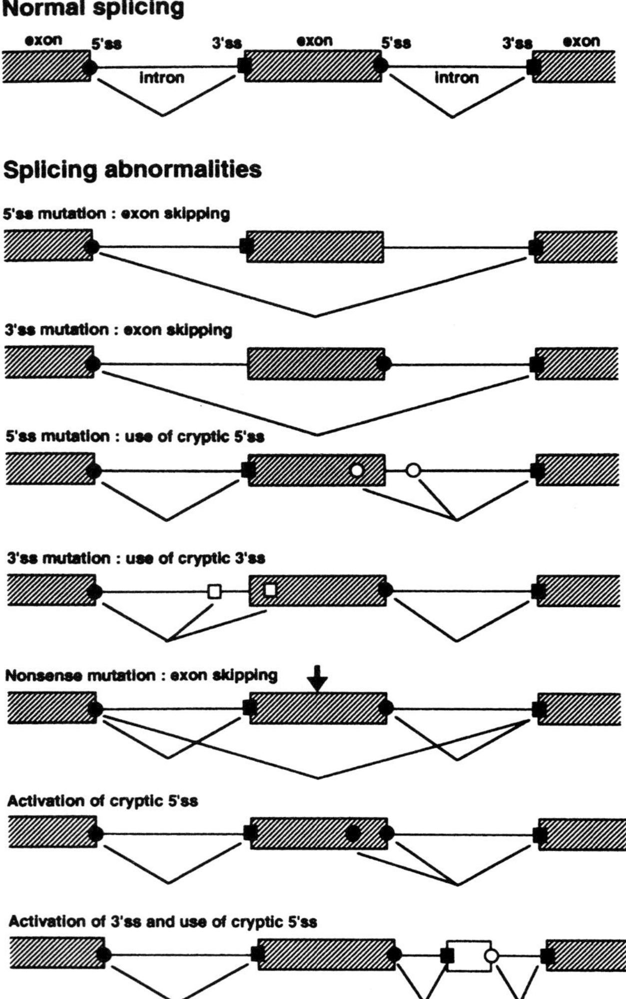

Fig. 13-8. Examples of exon skipping and utilization of cryptic splice sites as a result of mutations in splice sites. *Solid square* and *circle* denote normal or activated 3′ ss and 5′ ss, respectively. *Open square* and *circle* represent cryptic 3′ ss and 5′ ss, respectively. The *arrow* denotes a nonsense mutation. Examples of exon skipping due to 5′ ss mutations are reported in Weil et al,[53,54] Grandchamp et al,[55] Carstens et al,[56] and Wen et al;[57] exon skipping due to 3′ ss mutations is reported in Tromp and Prockop[58] and Dunn et al[59]; use of cryptic 5′ ss due to 5′ ss mutations is reported in Treistman et al[60] and Atweh et al[61]; use of cryptic 3′ ss due to 3′ ss mutations is reported in Carstens et al[56] and Su and Lin[62]; exon skipping due to nonsense mutations is reported in Dietz et al[63]; and activation of cryptic 5′ ss and 3′ ss is reported in Orkin et al,[64] Nakano et al,[65] and Mitchell et al[66]

Mutations in *Alu* Sequences and Creation of a New 5′ Splice Site

The creation of 3′ ss consequent to a point mutation in a member of the *Alu* family of human repetitive elements was noted by Mitchell *et al.*[76] Analysis of the ornithine aminotransferase mRNA of a patient with gyrate atrophy revealed a 142-nucleotide insertion at the junction of exons 3 and 4. The patient possessed a much reduced level (5 percent) of abnormal mRNA in his fibroblasts and an even smaller amount of normal-sized mRNA. An *Alu* sequence is normally present in intron 3 of the ornithine δ-aminotransferase (OAT) gene, 150 bp downstream of exon 3. The patient was homozygous for a C-to-G transversion in the right arm of this *Alu* repeat, which served to create a new 5′ ss. This mutation activated an upstream cryptic 3′ ss (the polyT complement of the *Alu* polyA tail followed by an AG dinucleotide) and a new "exon," containing the majority of the right arm of the *Alu* sequence, was recognized by the splicing apparatus and incorporated into the mRNA. The *splice-mediated insertion* of an *Alu* sequence in reverse orientation may yet prove to be no unusual mechanism of insertional mutagenesis, since *Alu* sequences are interspersed through many coding sequences, the sequence requirements for a functional 3′ ss are far from stringent, and the reverse complement of a consensus *Alu* repeat contains at least two cryptic 3′ ss and several potential 5′ ss.

Other Splicing Mutations

There are certainly several intron sequence motifs, not yet fully recognized, that contribute to the regulation of the splicing mechanism. Mutations for example were detected in IVS3 of the human growth hormone (GH1) gene that affect a novel putative, consensus sequence which also perturb splicing, resulting in exon skipping.[77] These mutations did not occur within the 5′ and 3′ ss or branch consensus sites. The first was a G to A at nt +28 of the second deleted 18 bp (del+28−45) of IVS3 of the human GH1 gene. These mutations segregated with autosomal dominant GH deficiency in both kindreds, and no other allelic GH1 gene changes were detected. Reverse transcriptase-polymerase chain reaction (RT-PCR) amplification showed a $>$10-fold preferred use of alternative splicing. Both mutations were located 28 bp downstream from the 5′ ss, and both perturbed an intronic XGGG repeat similar to that found to regulate mRNA splicing in chicken β-tropomyosin. Binding of heterogeneous nuclear ribonucleoprotein (hnRNP) to these sequences in pre-mRNA transcripts is thought to play an important role in pre-mRNA packaging and transport as well as 5′-ss selection in pre-mRNAs that contain multiple 5′ ss.[77]

In patients with frontotemporal dementia with parkinsonism, three heterozygous mutations in a cluster of 4 nts +13 to +16 of exon 10 of the tau (MAPT) gene were found.[78] All of these mutations destabilized a potential stem-loop structure that is probably involved in regulating the alternative splicing of exon 10. This caused more frequent use of the 5′ ss and an increased proportion of tau transcripts that include exon 10. The increase in exon 10+ mRNA was expected to increase the proportion of tau protein containing four microtubule-binding repeats, which is consistent with the neuropathology described in families with this type of frontotemporal dementia. Mutations in intron regions that regulate the proportion of alternatively spliced exons may therefore be an important mechanism for late-onset phenotypes.

mRNA Processing (Other Than Splicing) and Translation Mutations

Mutations affecting mRNA processing and translation may exert their pathologic effects at any one of the various stages between transcriptional initiation and translation. Mutations other than those affecting mRNA splicing are now described and their phenotypic consequences assessed.

Cap-Site Mutants. The transcription of an mRNA is initiated at the cap site (+1), so named because of the posttranscriptional addition of 7-methylguanine at this position to protect the transcript from exonucleolytic degradation. Wong *et al*[79] described an A-to-C transversion at the cap site in the HBB gene of an Indian patient with β thalassemia. Kozak[80] collated known eukaryotic mRNA sequence data and showed that the cap site is an adenine in 76 percent of cases. A cytosine residue at position 1 was noted in only 6 percent of cases. It is not clear, however, whether it is transcription of the β-globin gene that is severely reduced in the above patient or whether transcriptional initiation occurs efficiently but at a different, incorrect site. In the latter case, the resulting transcript could be either incomplete or unstable.

Mutations in Initiation Codons. There are 59 mutations recorded in the HGMD affecting Met (ATG) translational initiation codons, with a preponderance of M-to-V substitutions.

The consequences for mRNA transcription and translation have not been well studied. It is particularly useful to compare and contrast the two ATG mutations reported in the α_1- and α_2-globin genes, respectively. The α_1-globin gene mutation was associated with a reduction in the steady-state α_1-globin mRNA level to one-fourth normal.[81] The corresponding α_2-globin mRNA level consequent to the α_2-globin gene lesion was similarly reduced to one-third normal.[82] The α_2-globin gene mutation results in a greater reduction in α-globin synthesis and a more severe α-thalassemia phenotype than its α_1-globin counterpart. This is presumably because, in normal individuals, the ratio of α_2 to α_1 mRNA produced from the two genes is 2.6, reflecting the relative importance of the α_2-globin gene in α-globin synthesis. The observed reductions in steady-state mRNA levels are reminiscent of the consequences of nonsense mutations (see below). Mitchell *et al*[66] reported a normal amount of OAT mRNA in Lebanese patients with gyrate atrophy who were homozygous for an initiation codon mutation.

Is the mutant mRNA translated? The answer is likely to be determined by a complex interplay of the different structural features of an mRNA that serve to modulate its translation (reviewed by Kozak[83]). Until fairly recently, it was thought that an AUG codon was an absolute requirement for translational initiation in mammals. However, some exceptions are now known — for example, ACG and CUG (reviewed by Kozak[83]) — indicating that some mutations might be tolerated more than others. The scanning model of translational initiation predicts that the 40S ribosomal subunit initiates at the first AUG codon to be encountered within an acceptable sequence context (GCC A/G CCAUGG is believed to be optimal[83]). Ribosomes may be capable of utilizing mutated AUG codons, albeit with reduced efficiency, or they may be able to initiate translation at the next best available site downstream.[84] The phenotypic consequences of a given ATG mutation are thus likely to depend on the nature of the mutational lesion, the tolerance of the ribosome with respect to translational initiation codon recognition, the presence of alternative downstream ATG codons with flanking translational initiation site consensus sequence, and the functional importance of the absent N-terminal end of the protein.

Creation of a New Initiation Codon. Another type of mutation that interferes with correct initiation is the creation of a cryptic ATG codon (in the context of a favorable Kozak consensus sequence) in the vicinity of the one normally used. An example of this type of lesion is provided by the G-to-A transition at position 122 (relative to the cap site) of the β-globin gene causing β-thalassemia intermedia.[85] This cryptic initiation codon is 26 bp 5′ to the normal ATG codon, and its use would lead to a frameshift and premature termination 36 bp downstream. Although the relative extent of utilization of the two ATG codons in this patient is not known, the comparatively mild clinical phenotype suggests that at least some β-globin is correctly initiated and translated. There are 208 cases in the HGMD for the creation of an ATG (Met) codon, but it is unclear how many of these are then used as aberrant initiation codons.

Mutation in Termination Codons

The first reported example of a mutation in a termination codon was that in the α_2-globin (HBA2) gene causing Hemoglobin Constant Spring ($Hb_{constant\ spring}$), an abnormal hemoglobin that occurs frequently in Southeast Asia.[86,87] The associated α-globin chain is 172 amino acids long, rather than the normal 141 amino acids, as a result of a TAA-to-CAA transition in the termination codon. In this patient, translation extends into the 3′ noncoding region of the α_2-globin mRNA. The resulting mRNA is highly unstable, resulting in low production of hemoglobin in the red cells of heterozygous carriers.[88] Several other mutations are known to occur in the α_2-globin termination codon, and a similar phenotype to $Hb_{constant\ spring}$ is observed.[89] A total of 15 point mutations in the termination codon have been included in the HGMD. Nine of these occur in the TGA, five in the TAA, and one in the TAG termination codons, respectively, of the APRT, ARSB, ATM, CTSK, FGFR3, HBA2, IDUA, PROS1, and AIRE1 genes (see the HGMD). With regard to the distribution of termination codons in mammalian genes, TGA is found in 52 percent, TAA in 27 percent, and TAG in 21 percent of these genes. Elongated proteins may also be generated by a second mechanism — a frameshift mutation close to the natural termination codon that results in the extension of translation until the next available downstream termination codon. A number of examples of this type of lesion are known to cause β thalassemia.[69,90–94] All give rise to an imbalance in α- and β-globin chain synthesis and inclusion-body (containing precipitated α and β chains) formation and are associated with the dominant form of the disease.

Polyadenylation/Cleavage Signal Mutations

All polyadenylated mRNA in higher eukaryotes possess the sequence AAUAAA, or a close homologue, 10 to 30 nucleotides upstream of the polyadenylation site. This motif is thought to play a role in 3′-end formation through endonucleolytic cleavage and polyadenylation of the mRNA transcript. Several single-base-pair substitutions are now known in the cleavage/polyadenylation signal sequences of the α_2- and β-globin genes, and all of these cause a relatively mild form of thalassemia due to the reduction of HbA_2 synthesis to 3 to 5 percent of the normal level. In the β-globin gene mutants, cleavage and polyadenylation at the normal site are markedly reduced but do still occur at < 10 percent of the normal level as judged by both *in vivo* and *in vitro* assays.[95,96] These mutants are characterized by a novel species of β-globin mRNA 1500 nucleotides long and 900 nucleotides larger than the wild-type transcript. This results from the use of an alternative cleavage/polyadenylation site (AATAAAA) 900 bp 3′ to the mutated site; polyadenylation occurs within 15 nucleotides of this cryptic site. This abnormal mRNA may be highly unstable, since it was extremely difficult to isolate. Several other polyadenylated mRNA species up to 2900 bp in length have been reported in an Israeli patient with a polyadenylation site mutation;[97] the β+-thalassemia phenotype exhibited by this patient was consistent with the translation of these extended mRNA species. Outside of the globin genes, a polyadenylation mutation has been described (AATAAC to AGTAAC) in the ARSA gene and causes arylsulfatase pseudodeficiency.[98] An unusual T-to-C substitution causing β-globin gene, 12 bp upstream of the AATAAA polyadenylation signal, has been described in an Irish family.[85] It is thought that this lesion may serve to destabilize the β-globin mRNA.

Nonsense Mutations and Their Effect on mRNA Levels

Nonsense mutations obviously cause premature termination of translation and truncated polypeptides, but these lesions may also exert their effects at the transcriptional level. Benz et al[99] first noticed that some patients with β thalassemia who had nonsense codons in the β-globin gene exhibited very low levels (< 1 percent) of β-globin mRNA in erythrocytes. Subsequently, a considerable number of nonsense or frameshift mutations from a variety of different genes have been shown to be associated with dramatic reductions in the steady-state level of cytoplasmic mRNA. However, this rule is not completely inviolable; a few nonsense mutations are associated with normal levels of cytoplasmic mRNA that appears to be efficiently translated to generate a truncated protein (e.g., low-density lipoprotein receptor [LDLR],[100] apolipoprotein C-II [apo C-II]),[101] and β-globin[102]). Moreover, considerable variation in mRNA levels is apparent between different instances of introduced nonsense codons within the same gene: Thus, measured reticulocyte β-globin mRNA varied from < 1 percent normal in a patient with β thalassemia who had a 1-bp frameshift deletion at codon 44 (Kinniburgh et al[103]) to 15 percent in a patient with a nonsense mutation in codon 17 (Chang and Kan[104]). Brody et al[105] observed that mutations that cause premature termination in the terminal exon of the OAT gene have no effect on mRNA level, but termination in the penultimate exon or earlier is associated with markedly reduced levels of mRNA. Decreased *in vitro* accumulation of cytoplasmic mRNA has been reported to be associated with several nonsense mutations in the β-globin gene but not with missense mutations.[106–110] One potential explanation for the observed effect of nonsense mutations on mRNA metabolism is that mRNA which is incompletely translated is not protected properly from RNase digestion on the ribosome and is therefore likely to exhibit an increased turnover rate. Consistent with this postulate, the β-globin mRNA bearing the codon-44 mutation appears to be highly unstable.[111] Moreover, Daar and Maquat[112] reported that all triosephosphate isomerase I (TPI1) gene nonsense and frameshift mutations tested *in vitro* exhibited a reduced mRNA stability but did not alter the rate of transcription. At least for the β-globin codon 39 mutation, however, the decreased steady-state levels of both nuclear and cytoplasmic mRNA have been shown not to be due to increased mRNA instability in the cytoplasm.[106,107,109]

The mechanism by which an in-frame termination codon results in a decrease in concentration of steady-state cytoplasmic mRNA is not understood. One or more parameters could be affected — the transcription rate, the efficiency of mRNA processing or transport to the cytoplasm, or mRNA stability.[113] Urlaub et al[114] showed that whereas nonsense mutations in the dihydrofolate reductase (DHFR) gene located prior to the final exon resulted in drastically reduced (10- to 20-fold) mRNA levels, nonsense mutations in the last exon of the gene yielded normal levels of DHFR mRNA. Nuclear run-on studies and experiments with the transcriptional inhibitor actinomycin demonstrated that the low mRNA levels resulted neither from a reduced rate of transcription nor from decreased mRNA stability. Similar results were obtained for nonsense mutations artificially introduced into the TPI1 gene and expressed *in vitro*.[115] Urlaub *et al.*[114] proposed two explanatory models that imply some form of coupling between processing and/or transport of the mRNA and translation: (1) Translational translocation model: This model proposes that translation of the mRNA on the ribosome would begin as soon as the mRNA emerged from the nuclear pore and would serve to pull the pre-mRNA physically through the splicing apparatus and through the pores in the nuclear membrane. Nonsense mutations would halt the pulling process, leaving the RNA molecule vulnerable to RNase digestion. However, nonsense mutations occurring in the last exon would not be recognized until the translocation of the mRNA from the nucleus was virtually complete. (2) Nuclear scanning of translation frames model: In this model, pre-mRNA are scanned within the nucleus for nonsense mutations prior to their translocation through the nuclear membrane. Detection of an in-frame termination codon would then result in a slowing of mRNA splicing/translocation. Such a mechanism might be an intrinsic part of the mRNA-splicing process since open-reading-frame recognition could be important for exon definition. The translational translocation model would predict a probability gradient from 5′ to 3′, with a gradually increasing likelihood that an mRNA containing a termination codon would be successfully transported across the nuclear membrane. In support of this hypothesis are the several examples of normal levels of mRNA transcripts derived from genes bearing termination codons in their 3′-most exons (see the OAT example[105]) and the TPI1 and DHFR examples that may imply links between pre-mRNA splicing, mRNA transport, and translation. However, counterexamples, such as the β-globin gene codon-17 and codon-44 nonsense codons quoted above, argue against its validity in all cases, since they are inconsistent with a perfect linear relationship between the relative position of the nonsense mutation and the level of mRNA produced by the mutant allele. The problem with invoking any one model alone is that it cannot adequately explain the inconsistencies observed between studies regarding the possible position effect associated with nonsense mutations *in vivo* and the role of changes in mRNA stability if they occur. In practical terms, the common finding of greatly reduced or absent cytoplasmic mRNA associated with nonsense mutations has important implications for mutation screening. Attempts to obtain mRNA for RT-PCR amplification and DNA sequencing[116,117] may be thwarted in patients with nonsense mutations by a cellular mechanism that links mRNA processing/transport to translation.

Nonsense Mutations and Exon Skipping

Dietz et al[63] and Naylor et al[67] have reported exon skipping in exons that contain nonsense mutations. In a patient with Marfan syndrome, exon B of the fibrillin gene FBN1 that contained a TAT-to-TAG nonsense mutation was completely skipped.[63] The exon skipping was discovered by RT-PCR analysis of fibroblast mRNA. Two additional examples of this phenomenon have been reported by the same authors in the OAT transcripts of patients with gyrate atrophy: exon 6 was skipped when a Trp 178 to Stop mutation was present in this exon; similarly, exon 8 with a Trp 275 to Stop mutation was skipped. The skipping of the exons with nonsense codons in the OAT cases was partial, that is, there were RNA species that contained the nonsense-mutation-containing exons. The authors proposed a mechanism of *reading* pre-mRNA exon sequences in frame either by direct coupling between translation and RNA processing or by a scanning function of ribosome-like molecules in the nucleus. Naylor et al[67] reported similar observations associated with two different nonsense mutations in exons 19 and 22 in the F8C gene in patients with hemophilia A. Partial skipping has been observed with the exon-19 nonsense mutation whereas, in the case of the exon-22 nonsense codon, only PCR products lacking exon 22 were observed. The exon skipping associated with nonsense mutations has been observed in more than 10 disease-related genes in humans. The mechanism that accounts for these observations is unknown.

Dietz and Kendzior,[118] using chimeric constructs in a model *in vivo* expression system, identified premature termination codons as determinants of splice-site selection. Nonsense codon recognition prior to RNA splicing necessitates the ability to read the frame of precursor mRNA in the nucleus. They proposed that maintenance of an open reading frame can serve as an additional level of scrutiny during exon definition.

Regulatory Mutations

Most mutations causing human genetic disease occur in transcribed regions. A different class of molecular lesion is that represented by regulatory mutations. These lesions disrupt the normal processes of gene activation and transcriptional initiation and serve either to increase or decrease the level of mRNA/gene product synthesized rather than altering its nature. The vast majority of regulatory mutations so far described are found in gene promoter regions — the 5′ flanking sequences that contain constitutive promoter elements, enhancers, repressors, the determinants of tissue-specific gene expression, and other regulatory elements. Mutations in the regulatory elements may have several consequences, such as alteration of the amount of mRNA transcript and/or alteration of the developmental expression of a gene. In the majority of regulatory mutations, the mRNA produced is qualitatively normal, and therefore mutation detection methods based on RT-PCR will fail to recognize these lesions. On the other hand, the detection of mutations in potential unknown regulatory elements may predict the existence of such elements. A total of 119 regulatory mutations have been cataloged in the HGMD. Some representative examples of mutations in regulatory elements in the human genome are discussed below.

Mutations in DNA Motifs in the Immediate 5′ Flanking Sequences. Single-base-pair substitutions that occur in the promoter region 5′ to the β-globin (HBB) gene causing β thalassemia give rise to a moderate reduction in globin synthesis. The known naturally occurring mutations are highly clustered around two regions that have been implicated in the regulation of the human β-globin (HBB) gene. One is a CACCC motif located between −91 and −86 relative to the transcriptional initiation site and the other is the TATA box found at about −30. Mutations have been described in the CACCC motif at positions −92, −90, −88, −87, and −86, and the TATA motif at positions −31, −30, −29, and −28, of the β-globin gene.[60,119–127] Almost all of these mutations are associated with a mild clinical phenotype. The CACCC box binds one or more erythroid-specific nuclear factors involved in the developmental activation of β-globin gene transcription. A −101 mutation occurs in the second upstream CACCC motif between −105 and −101 of the β-globin gene.[128] Matsuda et al[129] have reported a T-to-C transition at position −77 of the δ-globin (HBD) gene in Japanese patients with δ thalassemia. This lesion occurs at the second position of an inverted binding motif (TTATCT) for the DNA-binding protein GATA1. Gel retardation and CAT expression assays demonstrated that this mutation appears to impair δ-globin gene expression by abolishing GATA1 binding to its recognition sequence.

Mutations in *cis*-acting regulatory elements can also increase gene expression. The best examples of such mutations have been observed in hereditary persistence of fetal hemoglobin (HPFH), which is usually a heterozygous condition in which inherited gene lesions cause a marked but variable increase in HbF (α_2 and γ_2) synthesis above the normal adult level of <1 percent. The molecular analysis of HPFH has revealed both deletion and nondeletion forms. The nondeletion form of HPFH is caused by point mutations within the highly homologous promoter regions of the γ-globin genes. There are three examples of mutation at homologous positions in the Aγ- and Gγ-globin genes at positions −114, −175, and −202.[130–135] The −202 mutation occurs within a GGGGCCCC motif reminiscent of the GC box (GGGCGG) that serves as a binding site for the transcription factor Sp1. The T-to-C mutations at −175 occur within an ATGCAAAT motif (−182 to −175) known as the octamer, found in the promoters of genes encoding immunoglobulins, histones, and snRNA. The −175 lesion has been shown to increase promoter activity between 3- and 20-fold in erythroid cells.[136–140] This lesion appears to reduce or abolish the ability of the ubiquitous octamer-binding protein (OTF-1, which is thought to be a repressor of γ-globin gene transcription) to bind at this site[140–143] and alters the binding of GATA1.[136,139–141] Using gel-retardation assays, Fucharoen et al[132] demonstrated that the −114 mutation abolishes the binding of CP1 to the distal CCAAT motif of the Gγ-globin gene, although the lesion does not affect the binding of erythroid-specific factors.

Hemophilia B_{leyden} is an F9 variant characterized by severe childhood hemophilia ameliorated at puberty, probably under the influence of testosterone,[144] and is an example of developmental specificity of regulatory mutations. The amelioration in clinical phenotype is foreshadowed by an increase in plasma F9 activity/antigen values from <1 percent to between 30 and 60 percent normal. Several mutations have been found in positions −20, −6, +6, +8, and +13 relative to the transcriptional initiation site in such patients.[145–153] Reitsma et al[146] noted that the region from −5 to +23 possesses significant homology with the region immediately upstream, from −31 to −6. All mutated sites occur within the region of homology. Crossley and Brownlee[154] demonstrated that the +13 mutation lies within a binding site (+1 to +18) for the CCAAT/enhancer-binding protein (C/EBP) and serves to abolish binding of C/EBP to this site. Other transcription factors have been shown to bind in the −32 to +23 region.[155] Hirosawa et al[149] demonstrated that mutations at −20 and −6 were associated with lowered expression of the F9 gene and that restoration of expression in a concentration-dependent fashion was observed on treatment of the cultured cells with androgen. Crossley et al[155] found that an AGCTCAGCTTGTACT motif between −36 and −22, with strong homology to the androgen-response element (ARE) consensus sequence, is functional. It would appear that, before puberty, several transcription factors (including C/EBP, LF-A1/HNF4, and a further protein that binds to the −6 site) are involved in potentiating the expression of the F9 gene. Since mutations interfering with the binding of any of these factors lead to the abolition of F9 gene transcription, these proteins probably act in concert. It is assumed that at puberty, when a testosterone-dependent mechanism mediated by the ARE comes into play, the binding of all three transcription factors ceases to be an absolute requirement for transcription to occur.

Mutations Outside the Immediate 5′ Flanking Sequences. In addition to known mutations in the remote promoter element known as the *locus control region* (LCR; see below), Berg et al[156] have reported a +ATA/−T mutation at −530 upstream the HBB gene that is associated with reduced β-globin synthesis. This lesion reportedly results in a ninefold increase in the binding capacity of BP1, a protein that may therefore possess the properties of a repressor. In two families with X-linked dominant Charcot-Marie-Tooth neuropathy, a T-to-G transversion at position −528 and a C-to-T transition at position −458 to the ATG start codon of the connexin 32 gene (GJB1) have been found.[157] The first mutation is located in the nerve-specific GJB1 promoter just upstream of the transcription start site, whereas the second is located in the 5′ untranslated region (UTR) of the mRNA.

Regulatory mutations have also been reported in the 3′ flanking sequences of genes. A G-to-A transition 69 bp 3′ to the polyadenylation site appears to be responsible for drastically reducing the expression of the δ-globin gene, causing δ thalassemia.[158] The lesion occurs within a motif homologous to the consensus recognition sequence for the erythroid-specific DNA-binding protein GATA1. Gel-retardation assays have shown that the G-to-A transition resulted in an increased binding affinity for GATA1.[158]

Mutation in Remote Promoter Elements. The first indication that mutations at a considerable distance 5′ to the transcriptional initiation site could affect the expression of a downstream gene came from van der Ploeg et al:[159] A >40-kb deletion of the $^{G}\gamma$-, $^{A}\gamma$-, and δ-globin genes was found in a Dutch case of $\gamma\delta\beta$ thalassemia, but this deletion had left the β-globin gene intact, together with at least a 2.5-kb 5′ flanking sequence (Fig. 13-9). The implication was that the removal of sequences far upstream of the β-globin gene had resulted in suppression of its transcriptional activity. Kioussis et al[160] then showed that although the β-globin gene in this patient was identical in sequence to that of the wild type, the surrounding chromatin appeared to be in an inactive conformation as judged by DNase-1 sensitivity and methylation analysis. Curtin et al[161] reported a 90-kb deletion of the β-globin gene cluster in an English patient with $\gamma\delta\beta$ thalassemia; the ε-globin gene and part of the $^{G}\gamma$-globin gene were deleted, but $^{A}\gamma$-, $\psi\beta$-, δ-, and β-globin genes were intact. A deletion more than 25 kb upstream of the β-globin gene therefore served to abolish its expression. Driscoll et al[162] described an important 25-kb deletion in a Hispanic patient with $\gamma\delta\beta$ thalassemia; the deletion was located between 9.5 and 39 kb upstream of the ε-globin gene and included three of the four erythroid cell-specific DNase-1 hypersensitive sites 5′ to the ε-globin gene. All of the globin genes, including the ε-globin gene, remained intact; the β-globin gene, some 60 kb downstream from the 3′ deletion breakpoint, was nevertheless nonfunctional. Grosveld et al[163] showed that DNA containing the four erythroid-specific hypersensitive sites was capable of directing a high level of position-independent β-globin gene expression *in vitro*. The LCR 5′ to the ε-globin gene is thought to organize the β-globin gene cluster into an active chromatin domain and to enhance the transcription of individual globin genes. The Hispanic $\gamma\delta\beta$ thalassemia deletion results in an altered chromatin structure throughout more than 100 kb in the β-globin gene cluster as revealed by a change in the sensitivity to DNase-1 digestion (see

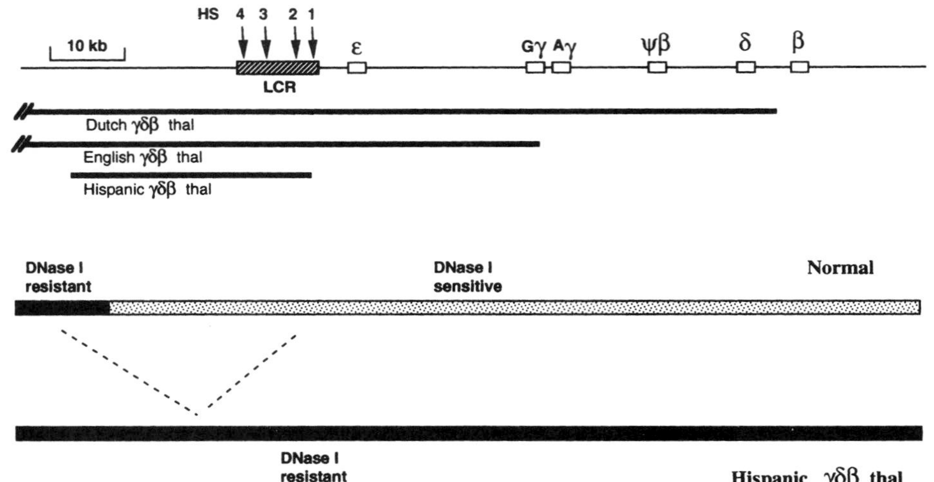

Fig. 13-9. Schematic representation of the deletions in the β-globin gene cluster that eliminate the locus control region (LCR) and result in silencing of the normal β-globin (HBB) gene. The extent of the deletions is shown as *thick black line.* The LCR and its four DNase hypersensitive sequences (HRS) are depicted. The bottom part of the figure shows the conversion of the entire β-globin gene cluster to a DNase I-resistant state as a result of the Hispanic γδ′-thalassemia deletion.

Fig. 13-9). A similar LCR is also present in the α-globin gene cluster at chromosome 16pter-p13.3.[164] Hatton et al[165] reported a 62-kb deletion causing α thalassemia encompassing the embryonic α-like ζ_2-globin gene that left the other genes and pseudogenes of the α-globin gene cluster intact. Though the sequences of the α_1- and α_2-globin genes were found to be normal, they nevertheless appeared to be transcriptionally inactive. Several other examples of similar deletions 5′ to the α-globin gene cluster have now been reported.[166–169] These deletions exhibit an area of overlap between 30 and 50 kb upstream of the α-globin genes. This region contains several DNase-1 hypersensitive sites (two erythroid-specific) and is capable of directing the high-level expression of an α-globin gene both in stably transfected mouse erythroleukemia cells and when integrated into the genomes of transgenic mice.[170,171]

There are also reports of associations of apparently polymorphic variations in the vicinity of certain genes with certain phenotypes. All of these associations require large epidemiologic studies and detailed characterization of the potential regulatory elements to determine whether the polymorphic differences contribute to these phenotypes. For example, there is a G or A polymorphism at position +97 downstream from the termination codon in the 3′ UTR of the prothrombin (*F2*) gene. Eighteen percent of patients with a documented familial history of venous thrombophilia had the A at this position as compared with 1 percent of a group of healthy controls.[172] An association was also found between the presence of the A allele and elevated prothrombin levels. This allele could be therefore used as a risk factor for venous thrombophilia. The polymorphism may either be directly responsible for the association or in linkage disequilibrium with another mutation which in turn is responsible for the observed association.

GENE DELETIONS

Gene deletions have so far been found to be responsible for more than 500 different inherited conditions in humans,[4] and these deletions may be broadly categorized on the basis of the length of DNA deleted. Some deletions consist of only one or a few base pairs, whereas others may span several hundred kilobases. By September 1998, the HGMD contained 2739 gross and small deletions.

Gross Gene Deletions

A total of 400 gross gene deletions have been logged in the HGMD. The nonrandomness of these lesions is apparent at two distinct levels. First, in some X-linked recessive conditions of similar incidence, the frequency of gene deletion does not always correlate with the size and complexity of the underlying gene. For example, some 2.5 to 5 percent of patients with hemophilia A have deletions of the F8C gene (26 exons spanning 186 kb of genomic DNA[173,174]), whereas 84 percent of patients with steroid sulfatase (STS) deficiency possess deletions of the STS genes (10 exons spanning 146 kb of genomic DNA[175]). Second, hotspots for deletion breakpoints have been reported within several human genes, including the Duchenne muscular dystrophy (DMD) gene,[176–179] the GH1 gene,[180,181] the LDLR gene,[182] and the α_1-globin gene.[183] Two main types of recombination events are thought to cause gross gene deletions—homologous unequal recombination, mediated either by related gene sequences or repetitive sequence elements, and nonhomologous recombination involving DNA with minimal sequence homology. Homologous unequal recombination involves the cleavage and rejoining of nonsister chromatids at homologous but nonallelic DNA sequences and generates fusion genes if the recombination breakpoints are intragenic. By contrast, nonhomologous or illegitimate recombination can occur between two sites that show little or minimal sequence homology.

Homologous Unequal Recombination Between Gene Sequences

Homologous recombination describes recombination occurring at meiosis or mitosis between identical or very similar DNA sequences. Homologous unequal recombination involves the recombination at homologous but nonallelic DNA sequences. This type of homologous recombination is thought to be one cause of deletions of the α-globin genes underlying α thalassemia. The α_1- and α_2-globin genes have evolved comparatively recently by gene duplication[184] and are thus virtually identical in sequence. These genes also possess flanking regions of homology (see regions x and z in Fig. 13-10) whose sequence similarity may have been maintained during evolution by gene conversion and unequal crossing-over. These *homology boxes* serve to potentiate homologous unequal recombination through incorrect chromosome alignment at meiosis. Recombinations between homologous x boxes, which are 4.2 kb apart (the *leftward crossover*), have been noted to produce chromosomes with a 4.2-kb deletion and only one α-globin gene[185] and chromosomes with three α-globin genes.[186,187] Recombinations between homologous z boxes that are 3.7 kb apart (the *rightward crossover*) generate chromosomes with a 3.7-kb deletion as well as the reciprocal product chromosomes carrying three α-globin genes.[186] Such recombination events may be common, since their product chromosomes have been reported in many different ethnic groups.[184] In every case, the breakpoints are located within the x or z homology boxes.

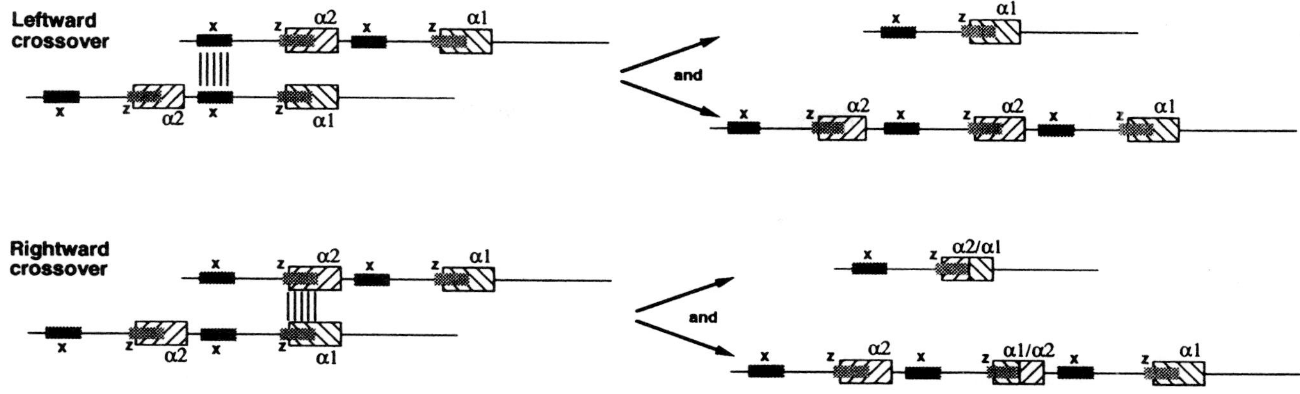

Fig. 13-10. Homologous unequal recombination between the *homology boxes* x and z in the human α-globin gene region. The leftward crossover is due to the misalignment of the x boxes, whereas the rightward crossover is caused by misalignment of the z boxes. The recombination events cause either deletions or duplications as shown.

Homologous Unequal Recombination Between Repetitive Sequence Elements

Recombination with *Alu* Repetitive Elements. Repetitive DNA sequences are thought to cause gene deletions by promoting unequal crossovers. The most abundant repetitive element in the human genome is the *Alu* repeat. There are up to 10^6 copies of *Alu* elements in the human genome, with an average spacing of 4 kb.[188–190] They are about 300 bp long and consist of two similar regions between 120 and 150 bp separated by a short A-rich region. Each *Alu* element is between 70 and 98 percent homologous to the *Alu* consensus sequence. Most of the *Alu* sequences have a polyA tail at their 3′ ends and are flanked by direct repeats (4 to 20 bp). *Alu* sequences are known to contain an internal RNA polymerase-III promoter.[191]

Alu repetitive sequences flanking deletion breakpoints have been noted in many human genetic conditions. *Alu*-sequence-mediated deletions are of essentially three types.

1. Recombination between an *Alu* element and a nonrepetitive DNA sequence that may not possess sequence homology with the *Alu* repeat.
2. Recombination between *Alu* sequences oriented in opposite directions.
3. Recombination between *Alu* sequences oriented in the same direction (Fig. 13-11).

The best examples of the involvement of *Alu* sequences occur in the LDLR and complement component-1 inhibitor (C1I) genes. All but one of the breakpoints associated with five LDLR gene deletions occur within an *Alu* repeat sequence (of which there are a total of 21 within the LDLR gene region). A 5.5-kb deletion[192] involves the formation of a stem-loop structure mediated by inverted repeats on the same DNA strand and derived from oppositely oriented *Alu* sequences in intron 15 and exon 18. A similar mechanism has been postulated for a 5.0-kb LDLR gene deletion[193] but, in this case, while the 3′ breakpoint lies within an *Alu* repeat, the 5′ breakpoint is located in exon 13; two pairs of inverted repeats (10/11 and 7/8 matches) flank the deletion breakpoints and are thought to potentiate the formation of the stem-loop structure. Three other LDLR gene deletions[194–196] are bounded by *Alu* repeats in the same orientation. Here the deletion is proposed to occur by meiotic (or mitotic) recombination between chromosomes misaligned at the highly homologous *Alu* sequences. In the vast majority of cases in which two *Alu* sequences have been implicated in the deletion event, they occur in the same orientation. Therefore, homologous unequal recombination between similarly oriented *Alu* family members, misaligned at meiosis, is probably the most common mechanism of *Alu*-mediated deletion. A clustering of deletion breakpoints within the left arm of *Alu* repeats was first noted by Lehrman et al[197] and has been confirmed on a much larger sample size.[4] However, the reasons for this nonrandomness are less clear. Lehrman et al[197] pointed out that the majority of the left-arm breakpoints lie within the region bounded by the RNA polymerase III promoters A and B and speculated that an open conformation brought about by promoter activity could increase the propensity for recombination to occur. While breakpoints within the right arm of the *Alu* sequence are indeed much less common, Ariga *et al.*[198] have claimed that the breakpoints that do occur within the right arm are invariably located within the region homologous to the sequence between promoters A and B. A similar situation to that found in the LDLR gene pertains in the C1I gene, which possesses a total of 17 *Alu* repeats within a 17-kb region.[199] Deletions and

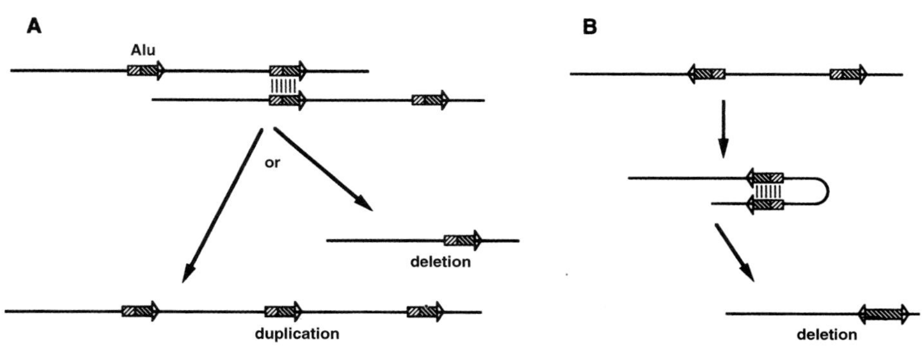

Fig. 13-11. Homologous unequal crossing-over mediated by *Alu* repetitive elements. *Alu*s in the same orientation can mediate unequal crossovers that can cause both deletions and duplications. *Alu*s in the reverse orientation can mediate crossovers via a loop structure that can cause deletions.

partial deletions of the C1I gene appear to account for 15 to 20 percent of the lesions that cause type-1 hereditary angioneurotic edema, and a high proportion of these occur within *Alu* sequences. Clustering of breakpoints is evident; Stoppa-Lyonnet et al[200] have shown that 5/5 deletions/duplications occurred within the first *Alu* sequence element preceding exon 4. However, the breakpoints of these rearrangements were distributed over the entire *Alu* sequence element and were not themselves further clustered.

In contrast to these examples, Henthorn et al[201] collated data on over 30 deletions in the β-globin cluster but noted the presence of *Alu* sequences at only four breakpoints and concluded that the occurrence of deletion breakpoints in *Alu* sequences within the β-globin gene region was not significantly different from that expected by chance alone. However, it could be argued that this was due to the relative paucity of *Alu* sequences (only eight in 60 kb) within the gene cluster. Kornreich et al[202] reached similar conclusions by studying the association between *Alu* sequences and deletion breakpoints in the gene (GLA) encoding α-galactosidase A, a deficiency that causes Fabry disease. Although 12 *Alu* repeats are found in the 12-kb gene region (about 30 percent of the GLA gene comprises *Alu* repeat sequences), deletions were relatively infrequent (only 5 of 130 patients possessed a partial gene deletion); three breakpoints occurred within an *Alu* sequence, and only one resulted from an *Alu*-*Alu* recombination. Finally, no correlation has been found between the locations of deletion breakpoints and *Alu* sequences in the human HPRT gene.[203] The authors suggested that this might be because the truncated 130- to 210-bp *Alu* repeats in the HPRT gene rarely exhibited more than 30-bp sequence identity, much lower than the 200- to 300-bp sequence identity normally required to promote efficient intrachromosomal recombination in mammalian cells.[204]

Recombination Within Non-*Alu* Repeats. Most gene deletions are not mediated by *Alu* repeat sequences. Indeed, although the 66-kb human growth hormone gene cluster contains some 48 *Alu* sequences, these do not appear to be the cause of the high frequency of clustered GH1 gene deletions causing familial growth hormone deficiency.[180] Vnencak-Jones and Phillips[181] studied 10 such patients and showed that in nine the crossovers had occurred within two 99 percent homologous 594-bp regions flanking the GH1 gene. Other types of repetitive sequence element are also thought to mediate homologous unequal recombination. Approximately 90 percent of individuals with ichthyosis have a deletion at their STS gene.[205] Yen et al[206] reported that 24 of 26 patients with an STS deletion had breakpoints clustered within or around a number of low-copy repetitive sequences flanking the STS gene (called *S232-type repeats*), suggesting that the high frequency of deletion at this locus may be due to recombination between these repetitive sequences. In their study of some 30 deletions of the β-globin gene cluster, Henthorn et al[201] noted breakpoints within five long interspersed repeat elements (LINEs). However, this was no higher than random expectation, and thus it is unnecessary to invoke an important role for LINEs in the causation of deletions at this locus. Sequence analysis of deletion breakpoints located within the intron-43 deletion hotspot in the DMD genes of two unrelated DMD patients has revealed the presence of a transposon-like element belonging to the THE-1 family.[207] Finally, the long terminal repeats of the RTVL-H family have been found to mediate homologous unequal recombinations events.[208]

Gene Fusions Caused by Homologous Unequal Recombination. The classic example of a gene fusion is that of hemoglobin Lepore. First reported by Gerald and Diamond,[209] this hemoglobin, which is synthesized in reduced amounts, is an abnormal molecule, with the first 50 to 80 amino acid residues of δ-globin at its N-terminus and the last 60 to 90 amino acid residues of β-globin at its C-terminus. Three different examples of Hb_{LEPORE} have now been described in which the fusion junction occurs at different points.[210–217] The recombination of $Hb_{LEPORE/BOSTON}$ genes has occurred within a 59-bp region of DNA (extending from codon 87 to the 11th nucleotide in intron 2) where the δ- and β-globin gene sequences are almost identical, resulting in the deletion of about 7 kb of intervening DNA.[203] Three haplotypes have been reported for $Hb_{LEPORE/BOSTON}$ chromosomes,[218,219] strongly supporting the view that this gene rearrangement has occurred independently on several different occasions. A similar fusion of $^{A}\gamma$- and β-globin genes due to a 22.5-kb deletion has occurred in Hb_{KENYA}.[220–222] These gene fusions appear to have arisen by homologous unequal recombination during meiosis between one globin gene on one chromosome and a misaligned globin gene on the other chromosome. This mechanism would predict the existence of a second abnormal chromosome; an anti-Lepore fusion gene encoding an N-terminal β-globin fused to C-terminal δ-globin. Consistent with this interpretation, several anti-Lepore hemoglobins have been described.[223–226] Another well-characterized example of the creation of fusion genes by homologous unequal recombination is provided by visual dichromacy (red-green color blindness). The genes involved are those encoding the red (RCP) and green (GCP) visual pigments that are highly homologous and linked in tandem on chromosome Xq28.[227] Several other examples of fusion genes generated by unequal recombination between highly homologous, closely linked genes have also been described: between the cytochrome P_{450} genes CYP11B1 and CYP11B2, causing glucocorticoid-suppressible hyperaldosteronism,[228] between the glucocerebrosidase (GBA) gene and a linked GBA pseudogene causing type-1 Gaucher disease[229] and between the α- and β-myosin heavy-chain genes (MYHCA and MYHCB) causing familial hypertrophic cardiomyopathy.[230] Guioli et al[231] have reported a different mechanism for the generation of a fusion gene in a patient with Kallmann syndrome carrying an X;Y translocation. This translocation resulted from recombination between the Kallmann gene (KALX) on chromosome Xp22.3 and its homologue (KALY) on chromosome Yq11.21. The two sequences possess about 92 percent sequence homology, and the breakpoint occurred within an identical 13-bp region. The KALX/Y fusion gene contained the entire KALX gene except the last exon, but no transcription of the novel gene was detectable.

Nonhomologous Recombination. Nonhomologous (illegitimate) recombination occurs between two sites that show minimal sequence homology. This kind of recombination can explain gross DNA rearrangements, sharing only a few nucleotides at the breakpoints, that are also common in mammalian cells. To account for this type of deletion, we postulate that sequences, originally remote from one another, are brought into close proximity through their attachment to chromosome scaffolding. This would serve to explain the observed periodicities in deletions — for example, the similarity in size but not position of some α- and β-globin gene deletions.[183,232] However, Higgs *et al.*[184] found no association between matrix-associated regions and the deletion breakpoints in either globin gene cluster. Several types of junction have been noted in cases of nonhomologous recombination: *flush junctions* resulting from simple breakage and rejoining;[232] *insertional junctions*, which contain novel nucleotides;[233] and *junctions with limited homology*.[234–236] This last category of junction was first noted by Efstratiadis *et al.*[237] in deletions involving the β-globin gene family. These authors proposed that short (2 to 8 bp) direct repeats flanking deletions were involved in their generation. Since these short regions of homology were not long enough to support meiotic recombination between chromosomes, it was postulated that the deletions arose instead by slipped mispairing during DNA replication. Consistent with this postulate, one direct repeat was usually lost in the deletion event. Woods-Samuels *et al.*[238] noted 2- to 3-bp homologies at the breakpoints of three different deletions in the F8C gene and summarized the sequence features identified at 46 rearrangement junctions from large deletions that have been characterized in the human genome: 48 percent shared 2- to 6-bp homology at the breakpoint junction and, in 22 percent, nucleotides were inserted at the junction. In only 17 percent was the deletion due to *Alu-Alu* recombination.

Gene Conversion. *Gene conversion* is the "modification of one of two alleles by the other."[239] The end result is very similar to that consequent to a double unequal crossing-over event. The difference between the two processes is that the modification of one allele (the target) after gene conversion is nonreciprocal, leaving the other allele (the source) unchanged. Gene conversion has been best studied in yeast.[240] In practice, it is usually not possible to distinguish the two mechanisms of interallelic recombination since, in humans, it would be highly unusual to be able to examine both recombination products. Moreover, the haplotypes created by gene conversion and double unequal crossing-over are expected to be identical. The process of gene conversion may involve the whole or only a part of a gene and can occur either between alleles or between highly homologous but nonallelic sequences. Examples of the latter include the $^{A}\gamma$- and $^{G}\gamma$-globin genes[241–243] and the α_1- and α_2-globin genes.[244] The mechanism underlying gene conversion remains elusive but must entail close physical interaction between the homologous DNA sequences. Gene conversion has been invoked in instances in which it is necessary to account for the association of the same disease-causing mutation with two or more different haplotypes—for example, β^{E}-globin alleles in Southeast Asian populations[245] and the β^{S}-globin mutation in African populations.[246] In the latter example, the β^{S} mutation was found on 16 different haplotypes, which could be subdivided into four groups that could not be derived from each other by less than two crossing-over events. Similarly, Kazazian et al[247] and Pirastu et al[248] invoked gene conversion to explain the spread of the nonsense mutation at codon 39 of the β-globin gene to a considerable number of different haplotypes in Mediterranean β-thalassemia patients. Zhang et al[249] described five different β-globin gene mutations causing β thalassemia that occurred on more than one haplotype in the Chinese population. It was considered unlikely that all cases should have occurred either by recurrent mutation on different haplotypes or through multiple recombination events. Matsuno et al[250] reported that a frameshift mutation at codons 41 and 42 in the β-globin gene occurred in association with two different haplotypes in two ethnically distinct groups: Chinese and Southeast Asians. These authors pointed out that six of seven β-thalassemia mutations known to occur on very different haplotypes were located in a 451-bp region between codon 2 and position 16 of intron 2. Similarly, Powers and Smithies[243] have shown that gene conversion events between the $^{G}\gamma$- and $^{A}\gamma$-globin genes usually involve less than 300-bp long. Matsuno et al[250] also noted the existence of a chi sequence (GCTGGTGG) (known to promote recombination in both *Escherichia coli* and in mouse immunoglobulin genes[251]) at the 5′ end of exon 2 near to the site of the proposed gene conversion. Examples of gene conversion involving the steroid 21-hydroxylase (CYP21B) gene and the closely linked and highly homologous (98 percent) pseudogene have been reported by several investigators.[68,252–256] These events often bring in more than one mutation present in the source sequences. Amor et al[253] noted the presence of six chi-like sequences (GCTGGGG) in the region of the CYP21B gene and pseudogene, which they speculated might play a role in the gene conversion events. Other examples of gene conversion events causing human inherited disorders are that of polycystic kidney disease (PKD1[257]), neutrophil cytosolic factor p47-phox (NCF1, chronic granulomatous disease[258]), immunoglobulin λ-like polypeptide 1 (IGLL1, agammaglobulinemia[259]), GBA (Gaucher disease[260]), von Willebrand factor (VWF[261]), and phosphomannomutase (PMM2[262]). These gene-pseudogene pairs are all closely linked, with the exception of the VWF gene (12p13) and its pseudogene (22q11-q13) and the PMM2 gene (16p13) and its pseudogene (18p). Together, these two exceptions have established a precedent for gene conversion between unlinked loci in the human genome.

Short Gene Deletions

A total of 2368 independent human gene deletions of 20 bp or less (as of September 13, 1998) have been logged in the HGMD (http://www.uwcm.ac.uk/uwcm/mg/haha4.html), which greatly extends earlier versions of the database.[263] This size range was selected because: (1) deletion end points are close enough to permit the study of putative sequence elements involved in the deletion process, (2) deletions arising by mechanisms other than homologous recombination were thought likely to predominate in this size range, and (3) most known short gene deletions have been discovered during DNA-sequencing studies so that the sample is likely to be unbiased. For every deletion, 10 bp of DNA flanking the deletion breakpoints were also noted so as to enable the analysis of the local DNA sequence environment. Excluded are deletions of the mitochondrial genome, which, by virtue of its rapid replication time and own distinct DNA polymerase, may not be directly comparable to deletions occurring within the nuclear genome. The distribution of deletion lengths is presented in Fig. 13-12. In 46 percent (1095 of 2368), the deletion involved only one nucleotide and, in 37 percent (868 of 2368), two to four nucleotides; the remaining deletions of 5 to 20 bp account for 17 percent of these lesions. Approximately 85 percent of the small deletions result in an alteration of the reading frame. Some of the DNA sequences in the HGMD share specific properties that may predispose them to deletion-type mutation. In a study of 1828 deletions, performed in October 1997, significance of these findings was assessed by comparing observations made in the HGMD to results from simulation studies, using 10,000 DNA sequences generated randomly according to codon usage for human genes by Wada et al[264] and to a random sample of 448 human cDNA sequences.

Local DNA Sequence Environment. Mononucleotide frequencies were found to differ from those derived from codon usage data[264] in that nucleotides T and A were overrepresented, whereas C and G were underrepresented. Nucleotides immediately flanking the deletion breakpoints revealed a significant excess of T and deficiency of C residues. A total of 13 codons were overrepresented in frame within the DNA sequences examined: TTT, CTT, CCT, AGT, GGT, TTA, ATA, GTA, TCA, AAA, GAA, AGA, and TAG. Several 3- and 4-bp motifs were found to be significantly overrepresented in a region of 10 bp both upstream and downstream of the deletions, regardless of frame. The most dramatic examples were: TTT (721 observed vs 496 expected), AAA (1072 observed vs 727 expected), AGA (1124 observed vs 879 expected), AAGA (416 observed vs 249 expected), AAAA (346 observed vs 204 expected), AGAA (396 observed vs 255 expected), TTTT (208 observed vs 117 expected), GTAA (119 observed vs 56 expected), TTCT (237 observed vs 150 expected), and TCTT (206 observed vs 132 expected).

Direct Repeats and the Generation of Short Deletions

A variety of different mechanisms for the generation of gene deletions involving the misalignment of short direct repeats have been proposed. Most replication-based models are essentially adaptations of the slipped-mispairing hypothesis proposed by Streisinger et al[265] The basic mechanism is as follows (Fig. 13-13): Two direct repeats, R1 and R2, occur in close proximity to each other with complementary sequences R1′ and R2′ on the other strand. As replication proceeds, the DNA duplex becomes single stranded at the replication fork, enabling illegitimate pairing between R2 and the complementary R1′ sequence. As a result, a single-stranded loop is formed containing the R1 repeat and sequence lying between R1 and R2. DNA repair enzymes may then excise this loop and rejoin the broken ends of the DNA strand. The next round of replication would then generate one deleted and

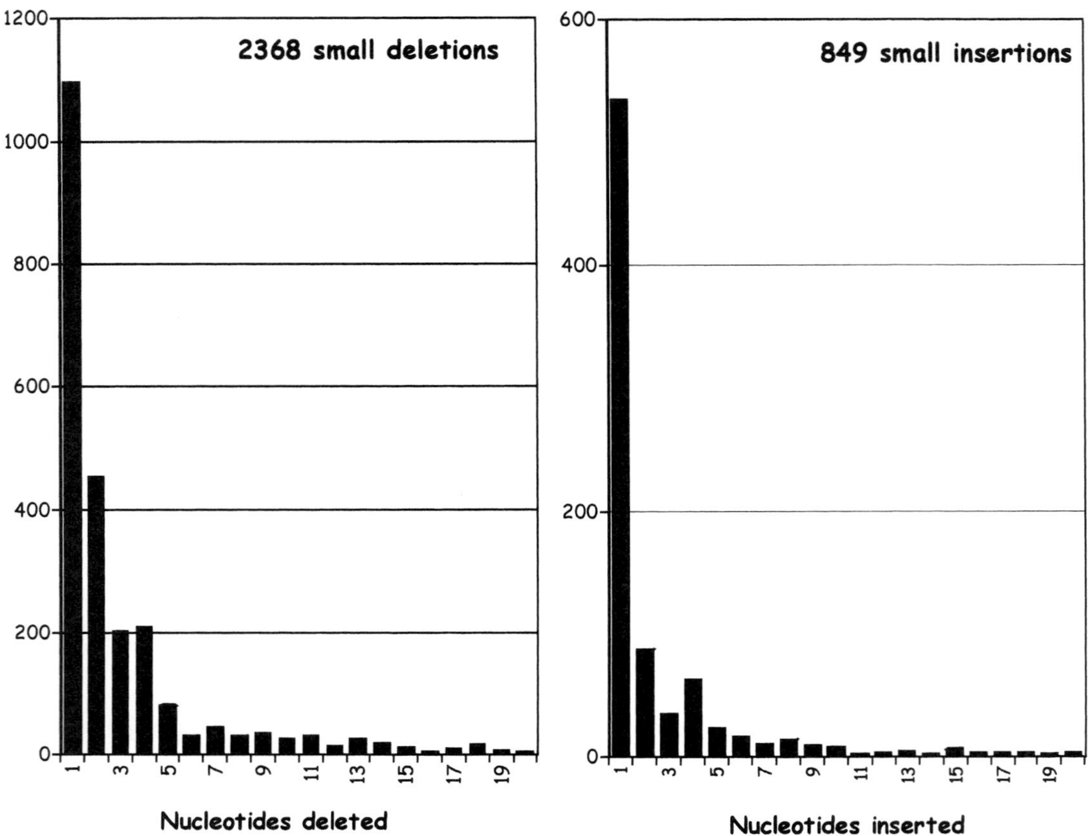

Fig. 13-12. Size distribution of short (<20 bp) human gene deletions and insertions.

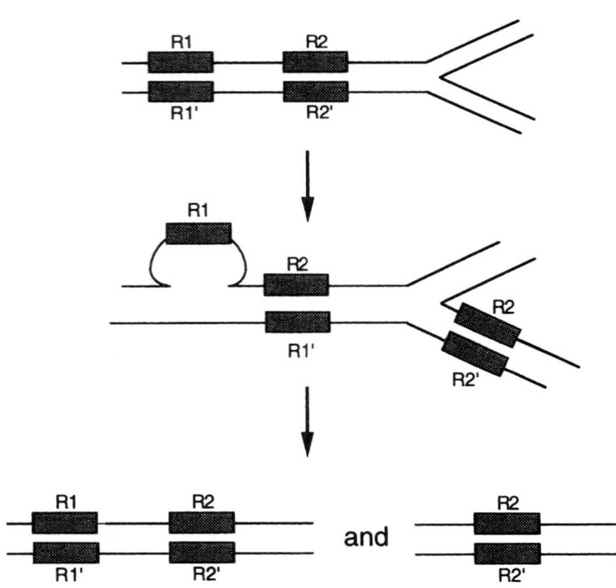

Fig. 13-13. Slipped-mispairing model for the generation of deletions during DNA replication.[237] Top: Double-stranded DNA containing R1 and R2 direct repeats. Middle: Double-stranded DNA becoming single stranded at replication fork and R2 repeat base pairs with complementary R19 repeat producing a single-stranded loop. Bottom: Loop excised and the new double-stranded DNA molecules. One of the two products contains only one of the repeats and lacks the sequences between R1 and R2.

one wild-type duplex. Direct repeats (2 bp or more) could be found flanking and/or overlapping all gene deletions logged in the HGMD. The most frequent length of a direct repeat was 3 bp (793 of 1828; 43.4 percent), while a sizable proportion (869 of 1828; 47.5 percent) were between 4 and 11 bp (Fig. 13-14). The latter occurred more often than expected by chance alone. A strong positive correlation holds between the length of the flanking direct repeats and the amount of DNA deleted, and the likelihood of deletion also appears to increase with the length of the repeat motif. The observations made from the HGMD are thus consistent with the model of slipped mispairing. In accord with the postulate of Efstratiadis et al[237] the deletion of one whole repeat copy plus the sequence between the repeats was observed in 534 (52.7 percent) of 1014 deletions spanning 2 bp or more.

Slipped mispairing can in principle also account for the generation of -1-base frameshift mutations. The production of a frameshift error by these means must involve at least two separate steps: (1) a misalignment occurs within a run of identical bases, followed by (2) further incorporation events that fix the misaligned bases(s). Various lines of evidence from *in vitro* studies now support the validity of this model and demonstrate that deletions/frameshifts can arise during DNA synthesis: (1) Vertebrate polymerases α and β produce many more frameshifts at runs of bases than at nonruns.[9,266] With polβ, hotspots occur predominantly at runs of pyrimidines (particularly TTTT) rather than purines, although this effect is less pronounced with polα. (2) The frequency of frameshift mutations is roughly proportional to the length of the run.[9] (3) The frequency of polβ-dependent frameshift mutation at a run sequence is decreased by experimental interruption of that run.[8] Kunkel and Soni[267] have proposed an alternative mechanism to account for the generation of frameshift

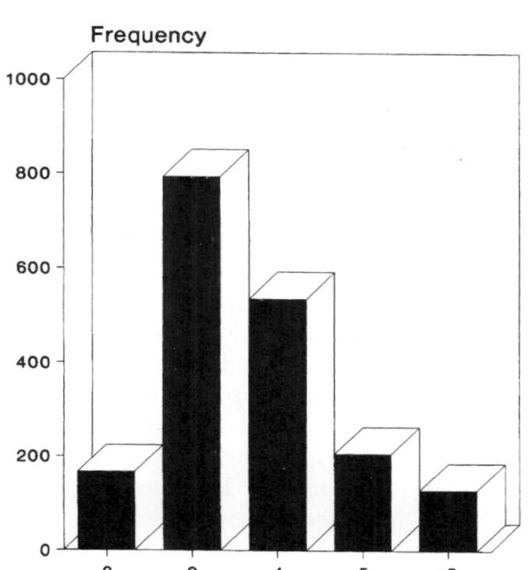

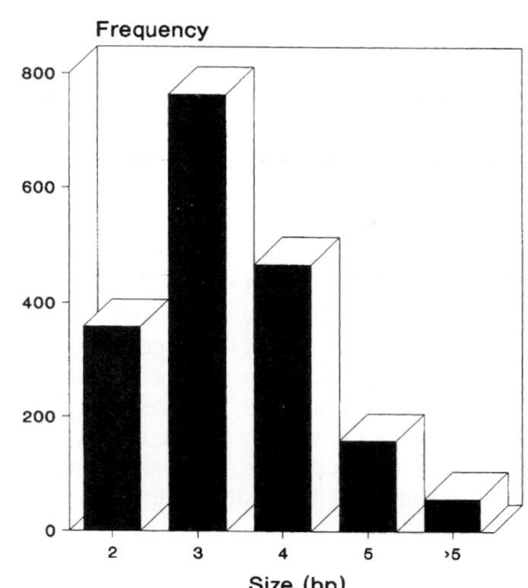

Fig. 13-14. Size distribution of the longest direct (*left*) and inverted (*right*) repeats flanking and/or overlapping short human gene deletions.

mutations at DNA replication: If a misincorporated nucleotide is complementary to the next base 3′, then its translocation to the next position will lead to a frameshift if the misaligned intermediate is rapidly stabilized by further base pairing. Analysis of 814 −1-base frameshifts from the HGMD revealed that the deleted base was identical to one of its neighbors in 500 cases. In addition, 238 deletions overlapped with a run of identical bases of 3 bp or more. Both observations represented a significant excess over expectation. Therefore, a considerable proportion of −1-base frameshift mutations causing human genetic disease may be due to slipped mispairing within runs of identical bases.

Palindromes (Inverted Repeats) and Quasipalindromes in the Vicinity of Short Gene Deletions

Ripley[268] proposed a mechanism of deletion mediated by quasipalindromic (imperfect inverted repeat) sequences. A palindrome possesses self-complementarity within the same DNA strand, which enables this strand to fold back on itself to form a hairpin or cruciform structure. The imperfect self-complementarity of quasipalindromic sequences enables them to form misaligned secondary structures. The nonpalindromic portions of these structures then provide templates for frameshifts and short deletions through the exonucleolytic removal of unpaired bases followed by repair DNA synthesis (Fig. 13-15). This model has been shown to possess predictive value at least in *E. coli*.[269] A search for palindromic sequences that could potentiate the looping out of single-stranded DNA revealed that 1447 of 1828 sequences listed in the HGMD in October 1997 contained at least one pair of inverted repeats of at least 3 bp; these were found to flank or span the deletion in 1387 cases. There were 128 examples of flanking and/or overlapping inverted repeats of at least 6 bp. A typical case was provided by an 8-bp inverted repeat associated with a lactate dehydrogenase B (LDHB) gene deletion;[270] one repeat was completely removed at the 5′ end of the deletion, whereas the other abutted immediately on the 3′ end of the deletion. In general, however, the exact location of the deleted base(s) was not predictable from the location of inverted repeats. Thus, 421 sequences possessed both direct and inverted repeats of 4 bp or longer flanking and/or overlapping the deletion; the presence of the latter may influence the nature of the deletion regardless of whether it occurs through classic mispairing or via the intrarepeat loop mechanism.

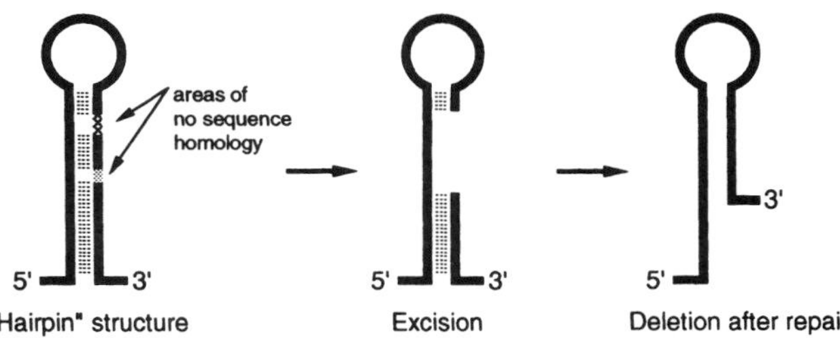

Fig. 13-15. Schematic representation of the excision-repair mechanism for deletions mediated by hairpin structures due to palindrome or quasipalindrome DNA sequences.

Role for Symmetric Elements?

Sequence motifs that possess an axis of internal symmetry (e.g., CTGAAGTC and GGACAGG) and vary in length between 5 and 18 bp, termed *symmetric elements*,[263] were noted in association with 1527 of the 1828 deletions in the HGMD. Symmetric elements spanning 5 bp or more therefore also appear to be overrepresented in the vicinity of short human gene deletions; their potential significance is unclear, however. An example of the presence of symmetric elements near microdeletions is in the case of the BRCA1 gene where the location of such elements at 5 to 7 bp were shown to be at significantly short distances (0 to 10 bp) from deletion breakpoints.[271]

Deletion Hotspots in Human Genes?

By examining the similarities of DNA sequences among deletions, Krawczak and Cooper[263] previously identified a consensus sequence—TG(A/G)(A/G) (T/T) (A/C)—which appears to be common to deletion *hotspots* found in different human genes. This consensus sequence is similar to the core motifs, TGGGG and TGAGC, found in the tandemly repeated immunoglobulin switch (S μ) regions,[272] and to putative arrest sites for polymerase α, which often contain a GAG motif. Indeed, one arrest sitespecifically mentioned by Weaver and DePamphilis [(T/A)GGAG[42]] fits perfectly with the deletion hotspot consensus sequence. The arrest of DNA synthesis at the replication fork may increase the probability of either a slipped-mispairing event or the formation of secondary-structure intermediates potentiated by the presence of inverted repeats or symmetric elements. Monnat et al[203] have sought a variety of sequence motifs in their study of 10 somatic deletions of the human HPRT gene causing Werner syndrome. The same collection of motifs was used for a search of the 1828 deletions and flanking sequences in the HGMD. Only three of these sequence motifs appeared to be overrepresented in the vicinity of short human gene deletions — polypyrimidine runs (C or T) of at least 5 bp, polypurine runs (A or G) of at least 5 bp, and the aforementioned deletion hotspot consensus sequence. Analysis of the precise localization of the deletions logged in the HGMD revealed that 17 codons from seven different genes could be identified as *deletion hotspots* [antithrombin III (AT3) codon 244; cystic fibrosis transmembrane regulator (CFTR) codons 141, 506, 1175, 1200; F8C codon 339; F9 codons 7 and 182; α_2-globin codon 30; β-globin codons 5, 36, 40, 42, 73, 125, and 150; and protein C (PROC) codon 76]. To be classified as a deletion hotspot, the DNA sequence in and around a codon had to be affected by at least two different (and therefore independent) mutations. Either a deletion hotspot consensus-like motif or a run of at least five pyrimidines was found in the vicinity of all these deletion hotspots. That polypyrimidines are significantly associated with deletions is not particularly surprising: Polymerase β-associated deletions occur predominantly in pyrimidine runs and thus, if DNA repair synthesis were a significant cause of frameshift mutation *in vivo*, it would be expected that the mutational spectrum of human gene deletions might show similarities to the polβ-associated mutational spectrum observed *in vitro*. Nevertheless, several differences between these mutational spectra are also apparent. Over 95 percent of polβ-associated frameshift deletions are 1 bp long,[9] whereas only 46.2 percent of the deletions from the HGMD are of this size. Although 988 of the deletions studied in October 1997 included or flanked a pyrimidine run, only 219 (44.9 percent) of these represented losses of a single base pair. This proportion compares with the deletions not associated with pyrimidine runs (595 of 1340; 44.4 percent). Finally, although 76 percent of all nonrun single-base-pair losses *in vitro* involved a G residue, the corresponding figure for human gene mutations was 30.3 percent (i.e., not significantly higher than random expectation).

INSERTIONS

Small Insertions

That insertional mutagenesis might be nonrandom was strongly suggested by the findings of Fearon et al,[273] who reported 10 independent examples of DNA insertion within the same 170-bp intronic region of the *deleted in colorectal carcinoma* (DCC) gene. Currently, 849 small insertions of less than 20 bp are recorded in the HGMD. Figure 13-12 shows the size distribution of these 849 insertions (http://www.uwcm.ac.uk/uwcm/mg/haha5.html). In the majority of cases (63 percent), there is insertion of a single base. Insertions of between 2 and 4 bp represent 22 percent of cases. All other small insertions, i.e., those of 5 to 20 bp, account for 15 percent of such lesions. All mutations interrupt the reading frame of the proteins except for the examples of a three-base insertion in which the novel codons were inserted between existing codons. One of the first such examples was in patients with hereditary elliptocytosis in which the triplet TTG coding for Lys was inserted between codons 147 and 148 in the alpha-spectrin gene (SPTA1)[274] Examples of short insertions leading to human genetic disease have been analyzed previously[41] to determine whether they occur nonrandomly and whether this nonrandomness corresponds to mechanisms of mutagenesis similar to those involved in the generation of short gene deletions.

Insertions due to Slipped Mispairing. In principle, slipped mispairing at the replication fork[237,265] mediated by direct repeats can account for insertion just as for deletion-type mutations: An insertion takes place when the newly synthesized strand disconnects from the primer strand during replication synthesis and slips or folds back so that pairing between different direct-repeat copies becomes possible. If synthesis is resumed so as to stabilize this mispairing, an extra copy plus nucleotide(s) from between the direct repeats is inserted behind the second repeat. Of the insertions considered by Cooper and Krawczak,[41] at least three occurred within runs of the same base while three were duplications of tandemly repeated sequences. The data were, however, too sparse to confirm any relationship with the DNA sequence environment. Nevertheless, pause sites for DNA polymerase a are known to be hotspots for nucleotide insertion.[275]

Insertions Mediated by Inverted Repeats. Analogous to the process of slipped mispairing between direct repeats, the formation of temporary secondary DNA structures may also be mediated by neighboring inverted repeats. In this situation, the newly synthesized DNA strand, instead of annealing to a direct-repeat copy on the primer strand, snaps back and anneals to itself via the two inverted repeats. If DNA synthesis is then resumed, an insertion would result behind the second palindromic copy. Imperfect self-complementarity can also mediate formation of partially misaligned secondary structures.[268] The nonpalindromic portions of these structures may then provide templates for either deletions (by endonucleolytic removal of bases) or putatively insertions (by gap repair). DNA sequences flanking two insertions considered by Cooper and Krawczak[41] contain such quasipalindromes and would correctly predict the insertion of the appropriate base (thymine) at the appropriate site [Leu 100 of the HBD gene and Cys 1146 of the *type-I* $\alpha 1$-collagen (COL1A1) gene].

Insertions Mediated by Symmetric Elements. Inspection of the insertions collated by Cooper and Krawczak[41] reveals that 8 of 20 of these sequences possess symmetric elements overlapping the site of insertion. With one exception, these insertions all represent inverted duplications of sequence motifs derived from either the 5′ or the 3′ end of the symmetric element. This finding is suggestive of a common endogenous mechanism of insertional mutagenesis.

Large Insertions — Retrotransposition

The HGMD contains 86 large insertions and duplications (as of September 13, 1998). To date, the largest "foreign" DNA sequence inserted into a gene is 220 kb into the DMD gene.[276] However, neither the inserted sequence nor the breakpoint junctions have been further characterized. One well-characterized insertion is that of the highly repetitive LINEs into the F8C gene, causing severe hemophilia A.[277] LINEs, which belong to the class of autonomous retrotranposons without long terminal repeats, compose approximately 15 percent of the human genome.[278] The insertion of these elements into exon 14 in the F8C genes of two patients involved the duplication of the target sites, a normal occurrence in such cases[279,280] and consistent with a retrotransposition mechanism. Fig. 13-16 is a schematic representation of retrotransposition. Patient JH-27 of reference 277 was shown to possess a 3785-bp truncated LINE complete with 57-bp polyA tract. The insertion produced a target site duplication of 12 to 15 bp. The LINE in patient JH-28 of reference 277 was slightly shorter (2132 bp) but more complex; one portion of LINE sequence (nts 4020 to 5114) was preceded by another (nts 5115 to 6161) in reverse orientation (3′ to 5′); there was a polyA tail of 77 residues. Dombroski et al[281] have shown that the LINE found in exon 14 of patient JH-27 is an exact but truncated copy of a full-length LINE with open reading frames (ORFs) found at chromosome 22q11.1-q11.2, which, since it is itself flanked by a target-site duplication, may also be the product of a retrotransposition event. Another patient, JH-25, had an insertion of a truncated LINE in intron 10 of the factor VIII gene.[282] The element, which was 681 bp long, had a 66-bp polyA tail and target-site duplication of 13 to 17 bp, and did not cause any abnormality, since it was found in several members of the patient's family, including his normal maternal grandfather (i.e., the mutation in the F8C gene responsible for hemophilia A in this family was not the insertion of the LINE). The involvement of LINEs in insertional mutagenesis has also been reported in other

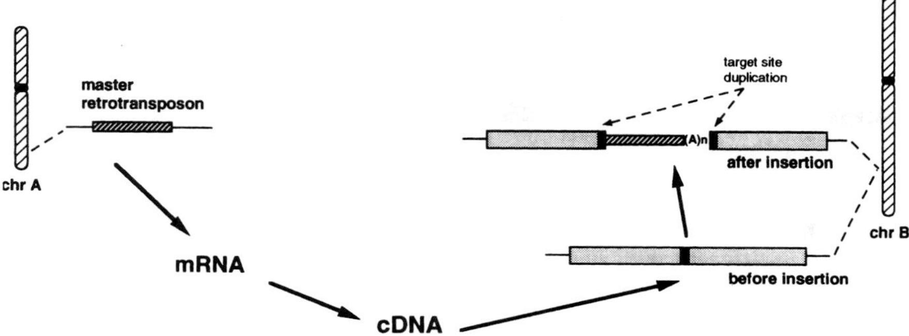

Fig. 13-16. Schematic representation of retrotransposition.

genes causing human disorders such the DMD gene[283] and the adenomatous polyposis of colon (APC) gene in colon carcinoma;[284] in addition, there is an $^{A}\gamma\delta\beta$ thalassemia due to a large deletion in which insertion of about 50 bp from a LINE has been noted,[285] and breast carcinoma where a LINE element was inserted in the MYC gene.[286] Most of the LINEs found retrotransposition events belong to the Ta subset. It seems likely that only full-length LINEs are the source of active mammalian retrotransposition. There are approximately 3000 to 4000 human full-length LINEs, but most of these are inactive because they contain nonsense and frameshift mutations. However, some elements contain two ORFs: ORF1 and ORF2. The ORF1 encodes an RNA-binding protein that is critical for retrotransposition in HeLa cells[287] and also binds specifically to the ORF2-protein product.[288] The ORF2-protein product contains an N-terminal endonuclease domain[289] and a C-terminal reverse transcriptase domain. The proposed mechanism of LINE retrotransposition is as follows:[278] an active LINE is transcribed in the nucleus and is subsequently transported to and translated in the cytoplasm. The two LINE proteins, ORF1 and ORF2, complex with their encoding LINE transcript in ribonucleoprotein particles. The complex is then transported to recipient DNA sequences where target-primed reverse transcription occurs. The new, integrated LINE copy is usually truncated at its 5′ end.

The highly repetitive *Alu*-sequence family has also been shown to be capable of retrotransposition both *in vitro*[290] and *in vivo*. *Alu* elements, which belong to the class of nonautonomous retrotranposons, comprise approximately 10 to 15 percent of the human genome.[278] Insertional inactivation of the NF1 gene by an *Alu* element caused neurofibromatosis type 1, as reported by Wallace *et al.*[291] The insertion, which occurred *de novo*, was localized to intron 5, just 44 bp upstream of exon 33, and resulted in skipping of exon 6. The 320-bp *Alu* repeat was inserted in reverse orientation into a 26-bp stretch of A and T residues. Though the exact mechanism responsible for this interference with splicing is not clear, these findings are consistent with a defect in branch-point recognition. Insertions of *Alu* elements into the human Moloney leukemia virus 12 (MLV 12) oncogene associated with hematopoietic neoplasia B-cell lymphoma,[292] the cholinesterase gene causing acholinesterasemia,[293] the F9 gene causing severe hemophilia B,[294] and the BRCA2 gene in a family with breast cancer[295] have also been reported. The *Alu* element inserted in the MLV12 locus was 308 bp long, contained a polyA tail of 26 residues, and produced an A-rich target-site duplication of 8 bp. The insertion of the 342-bp-long *Alu* element into the cholinesterase gene[293] occurred in an AT-rich region of exon 2. There was a 38-bp-long polyA tail and a target-site duplication of 15 bp. The inserted *Alu* element belonged to the evolutionarily recent subfamily IV. The insertion of the 322-bp-long *Alu* element in the F9 gene[294] occurred in exon 5 and produced a stop codon within the inserted sequence. There was a target-site duplication of 15 bp and a polyA tract of 78 residues. The *de novo* inserted *Alu* sequences in the NF1 and F9 genes both belong to the same subfamily (*Alu* HS), which is the most recent subfamily in the evolution of *Alu* sequences. The mechanism of retrotransposition of *Alu* sequences is unclear, although the ORF2 protein of LINEs may be involved in this event.[278]

The observation that both *Alu* sequences[295] and LINEs[277] exhibit a preference for integration at AT-rich sequences is reminiscent of the AT-rich insertional target sequences of retroviruses.[296,297] Indeed, the two LINE target sites in the F8C gene[277] are 90 percent homologous to a 10-nucleotide motif (GAAGACATAC) present in one of the highly favored retroviral insertion target sequences reported by Shih *et al.*[297]

DUPLICATIONS

The duplication of either whole genes or their constituent exons has played an important role in the evolution of the mammalian genome. However, gene duplication events may also result in disease. The largest duplication reported to date for a single gene is a 400-kb internal duplication of the DMD gene involving exons 13 to 42.[298] Despite this gross alteration in the structure of the gene (and of the resulting protein: about 600 kDa instead of 400 kDa), the patient manifested the relatively mild Becker form of muscular dystrophy. Other gene duplications and partial duplications have been reported, and these vary in size from 45 bp (COL2A1) to 20 kb (HPRT), from a part of an exon (LPL) to an entire gene (HBG2). Usually, the duplicated material exists in tandem with the original sequence, but a particular HPRT gene duplication has been reported by Yang et al[299] that is unusual in that a segment of the gene containing exons 2 and 3 has been placed in the middle of an intron-1 fragment.

One frequent mechanism of gene duplication is homologous unequal recombination. This may take different forms depending on the nature of the DNA sequence at the breakpoints. Thus, homologous unequal recombination in the β-globin gene cluster occurred between the HBG1 and HBG2 genes, whereas in the LDLR gene, it occurred between pairs of *Alu* sequences.[197] In the COL2A1 gene, alignment of two copies of the duplicated exon, in the manner that must have preceded a particular recombination-duplication event, demonstrated 78 percent nucleotide sequence homology around the recombination site.[300] In principle, unequal crossing-over caused by homologous recombination between repetitive sequence elements could lead to either the deletion or the duplication of exons. That the exons found to be duplicated in the C1I[200,301] and COL2A1[300] genes of some patients are deleted in others with deficiencies of these proteins would seem to support this model of mutagenesis. However, other duplication junctions appear to possess little or no homology with each other (e.g., GLA,[202] F8C,[302] and DMD[303,304]). In the lipoprotein lipase (LPL) gene, recombination has occurred between an *Alu* sequence and a region of exon 6, but the sequenced breakpoints exhibited no obvious homology.[305]

One of the best-characterized duplications is in the F8C gene in a family with hemophilia A.[188] The patient had a deletion of 39 kb of exons 23 to 25; however, his normal mother had 23 kb of intron 22 duplicated and reinserted between exons 23 and 24. Since the mother passed on a 39-kb deletion allele to two of her offspring, she must have been a germ-line mosaic for the normal, deletion, and duplication alleles. DNA polymorphism analysis suggested that the deletion and duplication events had occurred on the same chromosome. Gitschier[306] proposed a model in which the duplication had occurred first, either in a grandpaternal gamete or during the mother's early embryogenesis, and the deletion then occurred, probably mediated by the close proximity of the direct repeats, through recombination. The deletion occurred at a pair of CATT sequences normally 39 kb apart in the factor VIII gene. Short repeated sequences are known to mediate recombination events in vertebrate genomes; both $(CAGA)_n$ and $(CAGG)_n$ repeats have been noted in the region of the recombination hotspots found within the murine major histocompatibility gene complex.[307] Several possible topoisomerase-I cleavage sites were noted in the vicinity of the factor VIII gene duplication described by Casula et al[308] Topoisomerase activity has been implicated in several cases of nonhomologous recombination.[40] Other examples of topoisomerase cleavage sites have been reported to be associated with gene duplications;[202,304] potential sites for topoisomerases I and II were found exactly coincident with the breakpoints of a duplication in the dystrophin gene.[304] The significance of these findings remains to be elucidated.

The frequency of gene duplication is difficult to assess on account of the relatively small sample size. As with gene deletions, the frequency of gene duplication is likely to vary dramatically between genes. However, several estimates of the frequency of (partial) gene duplication are available for the dystrophin gene from large studies of patients with Duchenne/Becker muscular dystrophy (DMD/BMD): 6.7 percent,[309] 5.5 percent,[303] and 1.5 percent.[310] Thus, for the DMD gene, a gene for which a disproportionately high rate of large deletions has been reported (>60 percent of total mutations), the duplication frequency is probably 5 to 10 percent of the deletion frequency. A much higher frequency of duplication (uncharacterized and evidenced only by hybridization band intensity) may be found in the CYP21B gene causing 21-hydroxylase deficiency: Haglund-Stengler et al[311] found 11 gene deletions and 9 gene duplications in their study of 43 unrelated patients. However, at other loci, where gene deletions are much less frequent, gene duplications may well be so rare as not to be found. Why are gene duplications usually so much rarer than deletions? One possibility is that deletions are on average more likely to be deleterious and hence more likely to come to clinical attention. This is considered unlikely since with DMD/BMD, for example, it is the maintenance of the reading frame, rather than the nature of the lesion itself, that determines the disease phenotype.[298,303,312,313] A second possibility is that not all mechanisms involved in deletion creation would generate duplications as reciprocal products. Finally, it is possible that duplications are relatively unstable and revert or *decay* to deletions quite rapidly. The F8C partial gene deletion is a case in point. Another example is that of the exon-2+3 duplication in the HPRT gene; cells bearing this gene lesion reverted to wild type in culture through the loss of the duplicated exons.[299,314] Two similar HPRT gene duplications have been reported as spontaneous mutations in the human myeloid leukemia cell line HL60,[314] and these were also found to be highly unstable, exhibiting a reversion rate around 100 times higher than the rate of gene duplication. It would seem therefore that, once duplicated, the enlarged DNA sequence provides the substrate (a premutation) for further rounds of homologous unequal recombination.

Very large duplications also appear to arise from recombination mediated by repeated DNA sequences. Pentao et al[315] have reported that the duplication on chromosome 17p in one patient with Charcot-Marie-Tooth disease type 1A (CMT1A) is a tandem repeat of 1.5 Mb. A repeated element of 17 kb, termed *CMT1A-REP*, flanks the 1.5-Mb CMT1A monomer unit on normal chromosome 17p and was present in an additional copy on the chromosome with the CMT1A duplication. The authors proposed that the CMT1A duplication arose from unequal crossing-over due to misalignment at these CMT1A-REP repeat sequences during meiosis.

INVERSIONS

Inversions appear to be an extremely unusual form of gene mutation. Two examples involving the β-globin gene cluster are presented here: The first is a complex rearrangement of the β-globin gene cluster found in a patient with Indian ${}^{A}\gamma\delta\beta$ thalassemia.[316] Two segments—0.83 kb and 7.46 kb, respectively—were deleted, while the intervening segment was inverted and reintroduced between the ${}^{A}\gamma$- and δ-gene loci. Jennings et al[316] suggested that this mutation may have been made possible by the chromatin-folding pattern of the cluster region bringing the ${}^{A}\gamma$ gene into close proximity with the δ- and β-globin genes. Interestingly, this rearrangement serves to enhance the expression of the upstream fetal ${}^{G}\gamma$ gene. A similar example of an inversion has been reported in the APOA1/C3/A4 gene cluster in a patient with premature atherosclerosis and a deficiency of both APOA1 and APOC3.[317] The inversion was 6 kb long, with breakpoints in exon 4 of the APOA1 gene and intron 1 of the APOC3 gene. This inversion resulted in the reciprocal fusion of portions of the two genes and contains exons 1 to 3 of exon 4 from the APOA1 gene plus exons 2 to 4 and intron 1 from the APOC3 gene; the fusion gene is expressed as a stable mRNA. In the process, however, 9 bp from the APOA1 and 21 bp from the APOC3 gene were deleted. Since *Alu* sequences were also noted in the vicinity of the breakpoints of this inversion, Karathanasis et al[317] speculated that the sequences might be involved in the stabilization of a stem-loop structure prior to the inversion event. A final example of an inversion is provided by a Turkish patient with $\delta\beta^0$ thalassemia and a complex rearrangement of the β-globin gene cluster.[318] The rearrangement consists of a deletion of 11.5 kb, including the β- and δ-globin genes, a second 1.6-kb deletion downstream of the first, and a 7.6-kb inversion of the intervening sequence, including the LINE downstream of the β-globin gene.

Perhaps the most important inversion event is that involving the F8C gene causing severe hemophilia A. The high frequency of the inversion (about 40 percent) in these patients provides an explanation for our initial inability to detect the pathologic lesion in about half of all severe hemophilia-A patients[24] and the impossibility of performing PCR amplification across the exon-22/23 boundary by using cDNA derived from these patients.[67] A CpG island, located within intron 22, acts as a bidirectional promoter for two transcribed genes: F8A and F8B. The F8A gene lacks introns and is transcribed in the opposite direction to the factor VIII gene. Two additional homologues of the F8A gene (the A genes), which are also transcribed, exist about 500 kb upstream of the factor VIII gene. These genes are transcribed in the opposite direction to F8A. It is now known that homologous infrachromosomal recombination occurs between one or other of the upstream A genes and the F8A gene, generating an inversion of the intervening factor VIII gene sequence.[319,320] Such inversions result in the separation of exons 1 to 22 from exons 23 to 26 by some 200 to 500 kb. Most inversions (90 percent) involve the distal of the two A genes; this unique mutational mechanism is estimated to occur with a frequency of 7.2×10^{-6} per gene per gamete per generation (D.S. Millar and D.N. Cooper, unpublished results). An international collaborative effort collected data from a total of 2093 patients with severe hemophilia A;[321] of those, 740 (35 percent) had a type-1 (distal) factor VIII inversion, and 140 (7 percent) showed a type-2 (proximal) inversion. Of 532 mothers of patients with inversions, 98 percent were carriers of the abnormal factor VIII gene. When the maternal grandparental origin was examined, the inversions occurred *de novo* in male germ cells in 69 cases and in female germ cells in 1 case.

Molecular Misreading due to Long Runs of Mononucleotides or Dinucleotides

Long runs of adenines (and perhaps other mononucleotides or dinucleotides) promote a phenomenon called *molecular misreading* by which DNA replication/RNA transcription and/or translation result in erroneous products with different numbers of (A)s from the DNA. Linton et al[322] reported a family with hypobetalipoproteinemia in which the deletion of one C in the A_5CA_3 coding sequence of the APOB gene results in a run of $(A)_8$. The patient, however, did not have a severe disease, because there was some ApoB protein made. This was the result of molecular misreading in which approximately 10 percent of the resulting RNAs contained $(A)_9$ instead of the expected $(A)_8$; this partially restored the reading frame and produced low amounts of normal ApoB. Young et al[323] reported a family with mild to moderately severe hemophilia A with a deletion of one T within the coding A_8TA_2 sequence of the F8C gene. The partial "correction" of the phenotype was due to the restoration of the reading frame because of molecular misreading in which approximately 5 percent of the resulting RNAs contained $(A)_{11}$ instead of the expected $(A)_{10}$. In this family, there was also evidence for ribosomal frameshifting during translation of the mutant RNA. Laken et al[324] reported a T-to-A transversion in the coding A_3TA_4 sequence of the APC gene in 6 percent of Ashkenazi Jews and in about 28 percent of Ashkenazim with a family history of colorectal cancer. Rather than altering the function of the encoded protein, this mutation again creates a small hypermutable region, indirectly causing cancer predisposition because there are many somatic cells in which stretches of $(A)_9$ occur instead of the expected $(A)_8$. The $(A)_9$ results in a frameshifting and truncated dysfunctional APC. The mechanisms of transcriptional slippage during elongation at runs of As or Ts has been documented and studied in *E. coli*.[325] Ribosomal frameshifting has also been studied extensively in model organisms.[326]

Van Leeuwen *et al.*[327] found in neurofibrillary tangles, neuritic plaques, and neuropil threads in the cerebral cortex of Alzheimer and Down syndrome abnormal forms of β-amyloid precursor protein and ubiquitin B. These aberrant proteins were produced because of +1 frameshifting that resulted from a deletion of AG in a sequence GAGAG that occurred in the coding regions of both genes. This dinucleotide deletion was again the result of a molecular misreading during transcription or posttranscriptional editing of RNA.

Expansion of Unstable Repeat Sequences

Since the beginning of this decade, a novel mechanism of mutation has been shown to arise through the instability and expansion of certain trinucleotide and other repeat sequences.[328–330] To date, at least a dozen disorders due to trinucleotide repeat, and one due to 12mer-repeat expansion, have been described[331,332] (see Table 13-10 and Fig. 13-17). This mechanism was first reported as a cause of the fragile X syndrome, one of the most frequent causes of inherited mental retardation, which is associated with the presence of a fragile site on Xq27.3. The FMR1 gene underlying the fragile X syndrome[347–350] was found to contain an ~90-bp CGG repeat sequence in the 5′UTR.[350] A length variation of the trinucleotide repeat in the region was noted[348,349] that appeared to correlate with the expression of the fragile X phenotype. Indeed, the $(CGG)_n$ repeat exhibited copy-number variation of between 6 and 52[351] in normal healthy controls although the majority of individuals possessed between 25 and 35 repeat copies.[333] By contrast, phenotypically normal transmitting males exhibited a repeat copy number of between 60 and 200 (the *premutation*), whereas affected males possessed more than 250 and sometimes in excess of 1000 copies (the *full mutation*[333,352–355]). The instability of both the premutation and the full mutation is further exemplified by the existence of somatic mosaicism for different copy-number alleles in some individuals.[333,356] Alleles with a repeat copy number of <46 exhibit no meiotic instability.[333,352] The premutation represents a small increase in CGG copy number but was not associated with methylation of the gene region or with mental impairment. However, individuals bearing the premutation exhibit a high probability of having either affected children or grandchildren. Expansion of premutations to full mutations only occurs during female meiotic transmission. The probability of repeat expansion correlates with the repeat copy number in the premutation allele.[333] Since the premutation must precede the appearance of the full mutation, all mothers of affected children carried either a full mutation or a premutation; no case of direct conversion of normal copy number to full mutation has been observed.[353] The full mutation was not detected in daughters of normal transmitting males, although small increases in CGG copy number were observed in daughters. All male patients with the fragile X syndrome possessed the full mutation, and all male individuals with the full mutation were mentally retarded. Moreover, 53 percent of females carrying the full mutation also exhibited symptoms of mental retardation. Although the transition from premutation to full mutation was always associated with the expansion of the $(CGG)_n$ repeat, examples of contraction were also observed and were reportedly associated with regression from a full mutation to a premutation.[333,353] Fu et al[333] estimated that about 1 of 500 females in the general population might possess a repeat copy number within the premutation range. In fragile XE mental retardation, the repeat that expands is also a $(CGG)_n$ in the 5′UTR of the FMR2 gene.[334]

The triplet repeats involved in the disorders due to repeat expansions are located in the 5′UTR as in fragile X,[333] the 3′UTR as in myotonic dystrophy,[335] the coding exonic sequences as in Huntington disease,[337] or in an intron as in Friedreich ataxia.[344] The 12mer repeat that is expanded in progressive myoclonus epilepsy type 1 is located in the 5′ flanking region of the CSTB gene.[332] The noncoding repeats could undergo massive expansions to hundreds or thousands copies, which leads to transcriptional suppression. The expansions in coding sequences are less dramatic and result in a gain of function of the abnormal protein that contains longer polyglutamine tracts.

Myotonic dystrophy, which affects approximately 1 in 8000 people, is a progressive disorder of muscle weakness with dominant inheritance and exhibits a unique property termed *anticipation* to denote the earlier onset and increasing severity of the disease in successive generations.[357] It is caused by a $(CTG)_n$ expansion in the 3′UTR of a serine-threonine protein-kinase DMPK.[358–360] The size of the $(CTG)_n$ repeat correlated both with severity and with age of onset; indeed, families in which the severity of the disease had increased in successive generations exhibited a dramatic parallel expansion in repeat copy number. Similarly, infants with severe congenital myotonic dystrophy and their mothers exhibit a greater degree of amplification of CTG repeats than is found in the noncongenital population. In pedigrees exhibiting anticipation, the fragment size increased in successive generations.[335,357,361–363] There are also examples of a contraction rather than an expansion of repeat size,[364] and this may provide an explanation for the incomplete penetrance manifested by myotonic dystrophy. As with the fragile X syndrome, linkage disequilibrium is apparent in heterogeneous populations between myotonic dystrophy and DNA polymorphisms in the vicinity,[359,362] implying either the existence of only one or, at most, a few mutations or that the chromosomal environment predisposes to mutation at the DMPK locus.

In Friedreich ataxia, a recessive disorder, the repeat $(GAA)_n$ is located within an intron of the FRDA1 gene.[344] The age of onset/severity of the phenotype correlates with the size of the repeat.[365] There is a reduction in the amount of frataxin protein (a mitochondrial protein probably involved in cellular iron metabolism) in individuals with abnormal repeat length.[366]

In Huntington disease, spinocerebellar ataxias 1, 2, 3, 6, and 7, dentatorubral-pallidoluysian atrophy, and spinobulbar muscular

Table 13-10 Various Examples of Disorders of Trinucleotide and Other Repeat Expansion

	Disorder	Inheritance	Gene	Chr	OMIM no.	Repeat	Normal	Mutant	Repeat Location	Mutation Type	Parental Gender Bias	Ref.
1	Fragile X syndrome	XLD	FMR1	Xq27.3	309550	CGG	6–52	60–200 premut 230–1000 full mut	5′ UTR	LOF, FraX	Maternal	333
2	Fragile E mental retardation	XLD	FMR2	Xq28	309548	GCC	7–35	130–150 premut 230–750 full mut	5′ UTR	LOF, FraX	ND	334
3	Myotonic dystrophy	AD	DMPK	19q13	160900	CTG	5–37	50–3000	3′ UTR	?Dom negative	Maternal	335
4	Spinobulbar muscular atrophy	XLR	AR	Xq13-21	313700	CAG	11–33	38–66	Coding	COF, LOF	ND	336
5	Huntington disease	AD	HD	4p16.3	143100	CAG	6–39	36–121	Coding	GOF	Paternal	337
6	Dentatrubral-pallidoluysian atrophy	AD	DRPLA	12p13.31	125370	CAG	6–35	51–88	Coding	GOF	Paternal	338
7	Spinocerebellar ataxia 1	AD	SCA1/ATX1	6p23	601556	CAG	6–39	41–81	Coding	GOF	Paternal	339
8	Spinocerebellar ataxia 2	AD	SCA2/ATX2	12q24.1	601517	CAG	14–31	35–64	Coding	GOF	Paternal	340
9	Spinocerebellar ataxia 3	AD	SCA3/MJD1	14q32.1	109150	CAG	12–41	40–84	Coding	GOF	Paternal	341
10	Spinocerebellar ataxia 6/Episodic ataxia type 2	AD	CACNA1A	19p13	601011	CAG	7–18	20–23 EA2 21–27 SCA6	Coding	ND	ND	342
11	Spinocerebellar ataxia 7	AD	SCA7	3p12-13	164500	CAG	7–17	38–130	Coding	GOF	Paternal	343
12	Friedreich ataxia	AR	FRDA1	9q13-21.1	229300	GAA	6–34	80 premut 112–1700 full mut	Intron 1	LOF, FraX	Maternal	344
13	Progressive myoclonus epilepsy 1	AR	CSTB	21q22.3	601145	CCCCGCCCCGCG	2–3	35–80	5′ Flanking	LOF	Paternal	332
14	Synpolydactyly	AD	HOXD13	2q31-q32	142989	$(GCG)_n(GCT)_n(GCA)_n$	15	22–29	Coding	ND	??	345
15	Oculopharyngeal muscular dystrophy	AD	PABP2	14q11.2-q13	602279	GCG	6	7–13	Coding	ND	??	346

Note: Mut, mutation; premut, premutation.

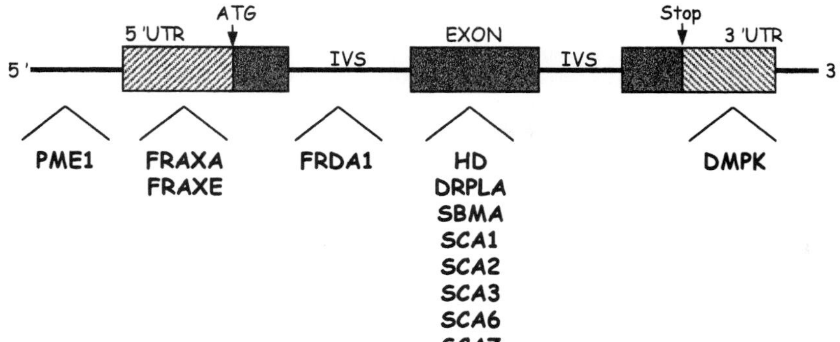

Fig. 13-17. Schematic representation of the location of the different repeat expansions associated with human disorders.

atrophy, the repeat is a $(CAG)_n$ located in the coding regions of the corresponding genes and encodes for polyglutamine.[336,337,339,340–343] The pathophysiology of these neurologic disorders is likely to be due to a gain of function of the abnormal proteins with expanded polyglutamine tracts.[367]

Trinucleotide-repeat expansions are certainly not the only examples of dynamic mutations. Lalioti et al[332] found that the common mutation mechanism in progressive myoclonus epilepsy EPM1 is the expansion of the dodecamer repeat (CCCCGCCCCGCG) in the 5′ flanking region of the CSTB gene. The normal general population contains either two or three copies of this repeat. Alleles with 12 to 17 repeats were also found that were transmitted unstably to offspring. These *premutational* alleles were not connected with a clinical phenotype of EPM1. Abnormal alleles contained between 30 and 75 copies of the 12mer repeat. A marked, cell-specific reduction of CSTB RNA is associated with expanded abnormal alleles. No correlation between number of repeat expansions and age of onset or severity had been found, suggesting a threshold effect of the expansion.[368]

The number of examples of this type of mutation will almost certainly increase and may provide explanations at the molecular level for a variety of intriguing phenomena in human genetics, such as variable expression and multifactorial inheritance.[369]

The following mechanisms could account for repeat instability and expansion: slippage during DNA replication, misalignment with subsequent excision repair, and unequal crossing-over and recombination. The most recently proposed mechanism is that the expansions occur because the triplet repeats form a secondary structure on the 5′ portion of the Okazaki fragments during replication and that may impede the movement of the replication fork. This might in turn result in a double-strand break within the repeat, which could expand during the end joining.[370]

MUTATIONS IN CANCER

A common finding in a diverse array of cancers is genetic instability. Its relationship to tumorigenesis is particularly well understood in hereditary nonpolyposis colon cancer (HNPCC), a syndrome characterized by predisposition to colorectal carcinoma and other cancers of the gastrointestinal and urologic tracts (see Chap. 32). In HNPCC, genetic instability at microsatellite sequences [replication error (RER) positive] has been linked to defects in several mismatch repair (MMR) genes.[371,372] Mutation rates in RER-positive cells are 2 to 3 orders of magnitude higher than in normal RER-negative cells.[371] Multiple mutations are necessary for malignancy, and MMR deficiency greatly speeds the process of accumulating mutations at those loci, which are critical for tumor progression. The target genes of the genome-wide hypermutability evident in MMR-deficient cells are now beginning to be identified. Perhaps the best example is that of the gene encoding the transforming growth factor β (TGFβ) receptor II, which is intimately involved in cellular growth regulation. Colorectal tumors are generally insensitive to the growth-suppressing hormone TGFβ and, in colorectal tumors manifesting microsatellite instability (MI), this insensitivity is almost invariably due to frameshift mutations within a microsatellite sequence (polyadenine tract) embedded within the TGFβR2 gene.[373–375] Similarly, the target sequence of mutations within the transcription factor E2F-4 gene is a $(CAG)_{13}$ trinucleotide repeat within the putative transactivation domain.[376] Thus, mutation-bearing genes that contribute to the development of colorectal neoplasia may be identified firstly through their involvement in the negative regulation of cell growth and secondly on the basis of their containing repetitive sequences that represent likely targets for mutation in RER-positive cells. Some of the mutated genes are directly involved in growth regulation (e.g., APC,[377] E2F4,[376] and IGF2R[378]) or in promoting apoptosis (e.g., BAX[379]) and are therefore likely to play a role in tumor progression. MMR genes may themselves represent mutational targets[380] ("the mutator that mutates the other mutator"), which increases genomic instability still further. Other genes are not involved in these processes (e.g., HPRT[381]) and their mutation merely represent the consequence of a general genome-wide increase in mutability. It should be noted that the instability resulting from the deficiency of a mismatch-repair enzyme is qualitatively different from the instability associated with the triplet-repeat expansion disorders in which the local DNA structure appears to be critical in promoting expansion.[382]

Mutations may predispose individuals to neoplasia directly, but recent findings show that predisposition may also be indirect. A T-to-A transversion at nucleotide 3920 in the APC gene occurs in about 6 percent of Ashkenazi Jews and about 28 percent of Ashkenazim with a family history of colorectal cancer.[383] This lesion is considered unlikely to predispose individuals to cancer directly by altering the function of the encoded protein. Rather, this transversion generates an $(A)_8$ mononucleotide tract from an existing AAATAAAA sequence motif, thereby creating a hypermutable site within the APC coding sequence. The induced instability of this region manifests itself in terms of a high frequency of frameshift insertions in somatic tissues that have probably arisen through DNA slippage during the replication process.

Krawczak et al[37] demonstrated that the bulk of the spectrum of somatic single-base-pair substitutions in the TP53 gene strongly resembles that of their germ-line counterparts seen in other human genes. The latter set of mutations have, however, arisen in a tissue that is usually well protected against exogenous mutagens and carcinogens: the germ cells. Since spectral similarity is strongly suggestive of the involvement of similar mutational mechanisms, it would appear that many TP53 mutations in the soma have arisen directly or indirectly as a consequence of endogenous cellular mechanisms (DNA repair and replication?) rather than through the action of exogenous mutagens. The similarity noted between the cancer-associated mutational spectrum of TP53 and germ-line gene mutations was consistent with the idea that cancer is a critical mediator of negative selection against excessive germ-line mutation. Sommer[384] has speculated that, for such a mediator function to work, there must be a correlation between germ-line and somatic mutation rates. If specific mutations were to occur that enhanced the rates of both germ-line and somatic mutation, a consequent increase in the incidence of cancer before the end of the normal reproductive period would serve to militate against their survival. It follows that TP53 may act as a critical sensor that is built into the genome's molecular warning system and that, through carcinogenesis, kills the individual and saves the species.[384]

REFERENCES

1. Antonarakis SE, and Members of the Nomenclature Working Group: Recommendations for a nomenclature system for human gene mutations. *Hum Mutat* **11**: 1, 1998.
2. Dunnen JT, Antonarakis SE: Mutation nomenclature extensions and suggestions to descrube complex mutations: a discussion. *Hum Mutat* **15**:7–12, 2000.
3. Cooper DN, Ball EV, Krawczak M: The human gene mutation database. *Nucleic Acids Res* **26**:285, 1998.
4. Krawczak M, Cooper DN: The human gene mutation database. *Trends Genet* **13**:121, 1997.
5. Cooper DN, Krawczak M: *Human Gene Mutation*. Oxford, BIOS Scientific, 1993.
6. Krawczak M, Ball EV, Cooper DN: Neighboring nucleotide effects on the rates of germline single base-pair substitution in human genes. *Am J Hum Genet* **63**:474, 1998.
7. Loeb LA, Kunkel TA: Fidelity of DNA synthesis. *Annu Rev Biochem* **52**:429, 1982.
8. Wang TSF: Eukaryotic DNA polymerases. *Annu Rev Biochem* **60**:513, 1991.
9. Kunkel TA, Alexander PS: The base substitution fidelity of eukaryotic DNA polymerases. *J Biol Chem* **261**:160, 1986.
10. Kunkel TA: The mutational specificity of DNA polymerase-β during *in vitro* DNA synthesis. *J Biol Chem* **260**:5787, 1985.
11. Grippo P, Iaccarino M, Parisi E, Scarano E: Methylation of DNA in developing sea urchin embryos. *J Mol Biol* **36**:195, 1968.
12. Cooper DN: Eukaryotic DNA methylation. *Hum Genet* **64**:315, 1983.
13. Bird AP: DNA methylation and the frequency of CpG in animal DNA. *Nucleic Acids Res* **8**:1499, 1980.
14. Nussinov R: Eukaryotic dinucleotide preference rules and their implications for degenerate codon usage. *J Mol Biol* **149**:125, 1981.
15. Bird AP: CpG-rich islands and the function of DNA methylation. *Nature* **321**:209, 1986.
16. Vogel F, Rährborn G: Mutationsvorgänge bei der Entstehung von Hämoglobinvarianten. *Humangenetik* **1**:635, 1965.
17. Vogel F, Kopun M: Higher frequencies of transitions among point mutations. *J Mol Evol* **9**:159, 1977.
18. Barker D, Schäfer M, White R: Restriction sites containing CpG show a higher frequency of polymorphism in human DNA. *Cell* **36**:131, 1984.
19. Youssoufian H, Kazazian HH, Phillips DG, Aronis S, Tsiftis G, Brown VA, Antonarakis SE: Recurrent mutations in hemophilia A give evidence for CpG mutation hotspots. *Nature* **324**:380, 1986.
20. Youssoufian H, Antonarakis SE, Bell W, Griffin AM, Kazazian HH: Nonsense and missense mutations in hemophilia A: Estimate of the relative mutation rate at CG dinucleotides. *Am J Hum Genet* **42**:718, 1988.
21. Green PM, Montandon AJ, Bentley DR, Ljung R, Nilsson IM, Giannelli F: The incidence and distribution of CpG > TpG transitions in the coagulation factor IX gene: A fresh look at CpG mutational hotspots. *Nucleic Acids Res* **18**:3227, 1990.
22. Cooper DN, Krawczak M: Cytosine methylation and the fate of CpG dinucleotides in vertebrate genomes. *Hum Genet* **83**:181, 1989.
23. Kaufman RJ, Antonarakis SE: Structure, biology and genetics of factor VIII, in Hoffman R, Benz EJ, Shattil SJ, Furie B, Cohen HJ, Silberstein LE (eds): *Hematology: Basic Principles and Practice*, 3d ed. New York, Churchill Livingstone, 1999, p 1850.
24. Higuchi M, Kazazian HH, Kasch L, Warran TC, McGinniss MJ, Phillips JA, Kasper C, et al: Molecular characterization of severe hemophilia A suggests that about half the mutations are not within the coding regions and splice junctions of the factor VIII gene. *Proc Natl Acad Sci USA* **88**:7405, 1991.
25. Higuchi M, Antonarakis SE, Kasch L, Oldenburg J, Economou-Petersen E, Olek K, Arai M, et al: Molecular characterization of mild to moderate hemophilia A: Detection of the mutation in 25 of 29 patients by denaturing gradient gel electrophoresis. *Proc Natl Acad Sci USA* **88**:8307, 1991.
26. Koeberl DD, Bottema CDK, Ketterling RP, Lillicrap DP, Sommer SS: Mutations causing hemophilia B: Direct estimate of the underlying rates of spontaneous germ-line transitions, transversions and deletions in a human gene. *Am J Hum Genet* **47**:202, 1990.
27. Reitsma PH, Poort SR, Bernardi F, Gandrille S, Long GL, Sala N, Cooper DN: Protein C deficiency: A database of mutations. *Thromb Haemost* **69**:77, 1993.
28. Rideout WM, Coetzee GA, Olumi AF, Jones PA: 5-Methylcytosine as an endogenous mutagen in the human LDL receptor and p53 genes. *Science* **249**:1288, 1990.
29. Monk M, Boubelik M, Lehnert S: Temporal and regional changes in DNA methylation in the embryonic, extraembryonic and germ lineages during mouse embryo development. *Development* **99**:371, 1987.
30. Driscoll DJ, Migeon BR: Sex differences in methylation of single copy genes in human meiotic germ cells: Implications for X-inactivation, parental imprinting, and origin of CpG mutations. *Somat Cell Mol Genet* **16**:267, 1990.
31. Ketterling RP, Vielhaber E, Bottema CDK, Schaid DJ, Sexauer CL, Sommer SS: Germ-line origin of mutation in families with hemophilia B: The sex ratio varies with the type of mutation. *Am J Hum Genet* **52**:152, 1993.
32. Pattinson JK, Millar DS, Grundy CB, Wieland K, Mibashan RS, Martinowitz U, McVey J, et al: The molecular genetic analysis of hemophilia A: A directed-search strategy for the detection of point mutations in the human factor VIII gene. *Blood* **76**:2242, 1990.
33. Bottema CDK, Ketterling RP, Yoon H-S, Sommer SS: The pattern of factor IX germ-line mutation in Asians is similar to that of Caucasians. *Am J Hum Genet* **47**:835, 1990.
34. Behn-Krappa A, Hölker I, Sandaradura de Silva U, Doerfler W: Patterns of DNA methylation are indistinguishable in different individuals over a wide range of human DNA sequences. *Genomics* **11**:1, 1991.
35. Hollstein M, Sidransky D, Vogelstein B, Harris CC: p53 mutations in human cancer. *Science* **253**:49, 1991.
36. Tornaletti S, Pfeifer GP: Complete and tissue-independent methylation of CpG sites in the p53 gene: Implications for mutations in human cancer. *Oncogene* **10**:1493, 1995.
37. Krawczak M, Smith-Sorensen B, Schmidtke J, Kakkar VV, Cooper DN, Hovig E: The somatic spectrum of cancer-associated single base-pair substitutions in the TP53 gene is determined mainly by endogenous mechanisms of mutation and by selection. *Hum Mutat* **5**:48, 1995.
38. Steinberg RA, Gorman KB: Linked spontaneous CG > TA mutations at CpG sites in the gene for protein kinase regulatory subunit. *Mol Cell Biol* **12**:767, 1992.
39. Shen J-C, Rideout WM, Jones PA: High frequency mutagenesis by a DNA methyltransferase. *Cell* **71**:1073, 1992.
40. Bullock P, Champoux JJ, Botchan M: Association of crossover points with topoisomerase I cleavage sites: A model for non-homologous recombination. *Science* **230**:954, 1985.
41. Cooper DN, Krawczak M: Mechanisms of insertional mutagenesis in human genes causing genetic disease. *Hum Genet* **87**:409, 1991.
42. Weaver DT, DePamphilis ML: Specific sequences in native DNA that arrest synthesis by DNA polymerase α. *J Biol Chem* **257**:2075, 1982.
43. Bottema CDK, Ketterling RP, Li S, Yoon H-P, Phillips JA, Sommer SS: Missense mutations and evolutionary conservation of amino acids: Evidence that many of the amino acids in factor IX function as "spacer" elements. *Am J Hum Genet* **49**:820, 1991.
44. Epstein CJ: Non-randomness of amino-acid changes in the evolution of homologous proteins. *Nature* **215**:355, 1967.
45. Grantham R: Amino acid difference formula to help explain evolution. *Science* **185**:862, 1974.
46. Wu C-I, Maeda N: Inequality in mutation rates of the two strands of DNA. *Nature* **327**:169, 1987.
47. Holmes J, Clark S, Modrich P: Strand-specific mismatch correction in nuclear extracts of human and *Drosophila melanogaster* cell lines. *Proc Natl Acad Sci USA* **87**:5837, 1990.
48. Krawczak M, Reiss J, Cooper DN: The mutational spectrum of single base-pair substitutions in mRNA splice junctions of human genes: Causes and consequences. *Hum Genet* **90**:41, 1992.
49. Shapiro MB, Senapathy P: RNA splice junctions of different classes of eukaryotes: Sequence statistics and functional implications in gene expression. *Nucleic Acids Res* **15**:7155, 1987.

50. Padget RA, Grabowski PJ, Konarska MM, Seiler S, Sharp PA: Splicing of messenger RNA precursors. *Annu Rev Biochem* **55**:1119, 1986.
51. Krainer AR, Maniatis T: Multiple factors including the small nuclear riboproteins U1 and U2 are necessary for the pre-mRNA splicing *in vitro*. *Cell* **42**:725, 1985.
52. Talerico M, Berget SM: Effect of 5′ splice site mutations on splicing of the preceding intron. *Mol Cell Biol* **10**:6299, 1990.
53. Weil D, D'Alessio M, Ramirez F, Eyre DR: Structural and functional characterization of a splicing mutation in the pro-alpha 2(1) collagen gene of an Ehlers-Danlos type VII patient. *J Biol Chem* **265**:16,007, 1990.
54. Weil D, Bernard M, Combates N, Wirtz MK, Hollister DW, Steinmann B, Ramirez F: Identification of a mutation that causes exon skipping during collagen pre-mRNA splicing in an Ehlers-Danlos syndrome variant. *J Biol Chem* **263**:8561, 1988.
55. Grandchamp B, Picat C, de Rooij F, Beaumont C, Wilson P, Deybach JC, Nordmann Y: A point mutation G to A in exon 12 of the PBGD gene results in exon skipping and is responsible for acute intermittent porphyria. *Nucleic Acids Res* **17**:6637, 1989.
56. Carstens RP, Fenton WA, Rosenberg LR: Identification of RNA splicing errors resulting in human ornithine transcarbamylase deficiency. *Am J Hum Genet* **48**:1105, 1991.
57. Wen JK, Osumi T, Hashimoto T, Ogata M: Molecular analysis of human acatalasemia: Identification of a splicing mutation. *J Mol Biol* **211**:383, 1990.
58. Tromp G, Prockop DJ: Single base mutation in the pro-alpha-2(I) collagen gene that causes efficient exon skipping of RNA from exon 27 to exon 29 and synthesis of a shortened but in frame pro-alpha-2(I) chain. *Proc Natl Acad Sci USA* **85**:5254, 1988.
59. Dunn JM, Phillips RA, Zhu X, Becker A, Gallie BL: Mutations in the RB1 gene and their effects on transcription. *Mol Cell Biol* **9**:4596, 1989.
60. Treistman R, Orkin SH, Maniatis T: Specific transcription and RNA splicing defects in five cloned β thalassemia genes. *Nature* **302**:591, 1983.
61. Atweh GF, Wong C, Reed R, Antonarakis SE, Zhu D, Ghosh PK, Maniatis T, et al: A new mutation in IVS1 of the human beta-globin gene causing beta-thalassemia due to abnormal splicing. *Blood* **70**:147, 1987.
62. Su TS, Lin LH: Analysis of a splice acceptor site mutation which produces multiple splicing abnormalities in the human argininosuccinate synthase gene. *J Biol Chem* **265**:19,716, 1990.
63. Dietz HC, Valle D, Francomano CA, Kendzior RJ, Pyeritz RE, Cutting GR: The skipping of consecutive exons *in vivo* induced by nonsense mutations. *Science* **259**:680, 1993.
64. Orkin SH, Kazazian HH, Antonarakis SE, Ostrer H, Goff SC, Sexton JP: Abnormal processing due to the exon mutation of the beta-E-globin gene. *Nature* **300**:768, 1982.
65. Nakano T, Suzuki K: Genetic cause of a juvenile form of Sandhoff disease: Abnormal splicing of beta-hexosaminidase beta chain gene transcript due to a point mutation within intron 12. *J Biol Chem* **264**:5155, 1989.
66. Mitchell GA, Brody LC, Looney J, Steel G, Suchanek M, Dowling C, Kaloustian V der, et al: An initiator codon mutation in ornithine-δ-aminotransferase causing gyrate atrophy of the choroid and retina. *J Clin Invest* **81**:630, 1988.
67. Naylor JA, Green PM, Rizza CR, Giannelli F: Analysis of factor VIII mRNA reveals defects in everyone of 28 hemophilia patients. *Hum Mol Genet* **2**:11, 1993.
68. Higashi Y, Tanae A, Inoue H, Hiromasa T, Fujii-Kariyama Y: Aberrant splicing and missense mutations cause steroid 21-hydroxylase deficiency in humans: Possible gene conversion products. *Proc Natl Acad Sci USA* **85**:7486, 1988.
69. Murru S, Loudianos G, Deiana M, Camaschella C, Sciarratta GV, Agosti S, Parodi MI, et al: Molecular characterization of β-thalassemia intermedia in patients of Italian descent and identification of three novel β-thalassemia mutations. *Blood* **77**:1342, 1991.
70. Beldjord C, Lapoumeroulie C, Pagnier J, Benabadji M, Krishnamoorthy R, Labie D, Bank A: A novel beta-thalassemia gene with a single base mutation in the conversed polypyrimidine sequence at the 3-prime end of IVS2. *Nucleic Acids Res* **16**:4927, 1988.
71. Sharp P: Splicing of messenger RNA precursors. *Science* **235**:767, 1987.
72. Rosenthal A, Jouet M, Kenwrick S: Aberrant splicing of neural cell adhesion molecule L1 mRNA in a family with X-linked hydrocephalus. *Nature Genet* **2**:107, 1992.
73. Burrows NP, Nicholls AC, Richards AJ, Luccarini C, Harrison JB, Yates JR, Pope FM: A point mutation in an intronic branch site results in aberrant splicing of COL5A1 and in Ehlers-Danlos syndrome type II in two British families. *Am J Hum Genet* **63**:390, 1998.
74. Kuivenhoven JA, Weibusch H, Pritchard PH, Funke H, Benne R, Assmann G, Kastelein JJP: An intronic mutation in a lariat branchpoint sequence is a direct cause of an inherited human disorder (fish-eye disease). *J Clin Invest* **98**:358, 1996.
75. Nakahashi Y, Fujita H, Taketani S, Ishida N, Kappas A, Sassa S: The molecular defect of ferrochelatase in a patient with erythropoietic protoporphyria. *Proc Natl Acad Sci USA* **89**:281, 1992.
76. Mitchell GA, Labuda D, Fontaine G, Saudubray JM, Bonnefont JP, Lyonnet S, Brody LC, et al: Splice-mediated insertion of an *Alu* sequence inactivates ornithine δ-aminotransferase: A role for *Alu* elements in human mutation. *Proc Natl Acad Sci USA* **88**:815, 1991.
77. Cogan JD, Prince MA, Lekhakula S, Bundey S, Futrakul A, McCarthy EM, Phillips JA: A novel mechanism of aberrant pre-mRNA splicing in humans. *Hum Mol Genet* **6**:909, 1997.
78. Hutton M, Lendon CL, Rizzu P, Baker M, Froelich S, Houlden H, Pickering-Brown S, et al: Association of missense and 5-prime-splice-site mutations in tau with the inherited dementia FTDP-17. *Nature* **393**:702, 1998.
79. Wong C, Dowling CE, Saiki RK, Higuchi R, Erlich HA, Kazazian HH: Characterization of β-thalassaemia mutations using direct genomic sequencing of amplified single copy DNA. *Nature* **330**:384, 1987.
80. Kozak M: Compilation and analysis of sequences upstream from the translational start site in eukaryotic mRNAs. *Nucleic Acids Res* **12**:857, 1984.
81. Moi P, Cash FE, Liebhaber SA, Cao A, Pirastu M: An initiation codon mutation (AUG to GUG) of the human α_1-globin gene. *J Clin Invest* **80**:1416, 1987.
82. Pirastu M, Saglio G, Chang JC, Cao A, Kan YW: Initiation codon mutation as a cause of a thalassemia. *J Biol Chem* **259**:12,315, 1984.
83. Kozak M: Structural features in eukaryotic mRNAs that modulate the initiation of translation. *J Biol Chem* **266**:19,867, 1991.
84. Neote K, Brown CA, Mahuran DJ, Gravel RA: Translation initiation in the HEXB gene encoding the β-subunit of human β-hexosaminidase. *J Biol Chem* **265**:20,799, 1990.
85. Cai S-P, Eng B, Francombe WH, Olivieri NF, Kendall AG, Waye JS, Chui DHK: Two novel β-thalassemia mutations in the 5′ and 3′ noncoding regions of the β-globin gene. *Blood* **79**:1342, 1992.
86. Clegg JB, Weatherall DJ, Milner PG: Haemoglobin Constant Spring: A chain termination mutant? *Nature* **234**:337, 1971.
87. Milner PF, Clegg JB, Weatherall DJ: Haemoglobin H disease due to a unique haemoglobin variant with an elongated a chain. *Lancet* **1**:729, 1971.
88. Hunt DM, Higgs DR, Winichagoon P, Clegg JB, Weatherall DJ: Haemoglobin Constant Spring has an unstable a chain messenger RNA. *Br J Haematol* **51**:405, 1982.
89. Bunn HF: Mutant hemoglobins having elongated chains. *Hemoglobin* **2**:1, 1978.
90. Beris PH, Miesher PA, Diaz-Chico JC, Hans IS, Kutlar A, Hu H, Wilson HB, Huisman TJH: Inclusion body β-thalassemia trait in a Swiss family is caused by an abnormal hemoglobin (Geneva) with an altered and extended β-chain carboxy terminus due to a modification in codon b114. *Blood* **72**:801, 1988.
91. Ristaldi MS, Pirastu M, Murru S, Casula L, Loudianos G, Cao A, Sciarrata GV, et al: A spontaneous mutation produced a novel elongated β-globin chain structural variant (Hb Agnana) with a thalassemia-like phenotype. *Blood* **75**:1378, 1990.
92. Kazazian HH, Dowling CE, Hurwitz RL, Coleman M, Adams JG: Thalassemia mutations in exon 3 of the β-globin gene often cause a dominant form of thalassemia and show no predilection for malarial-endemic regions of the world. *Am J Hum Genet* **25**(suppl):950, 1989.
93. Fucharoen S, Kobayashi Y, Fucharoen G, Ohba Y, Miyazono K, Fukumaki Y, Takaku F: A single nucleotide deletion in codon 123 of the β-globin gene causes an inclusion body β-thalassaemia trait: A novel elongated globin chain β Makabe. *Br J Haematol* **75**:393, 1990.
94. Thein SL, Hesketh C, Taylor P, Temperley IJ, Hutchinson RM, Old JM, Wood WG, et al: Molecular basis for dominantly inherited inclusion body β-thalassemia. *Proc Natl Acad Sci USA* **87**:3924, 1990.
95. Orkin SH, Cheng T-C, Antonarakis SE, Kazazian HH: Thalassemia due to a mutation in the cleavage-polyadenylation signal of the human β-globin gene. *EMBO J* **4**:453, 1985.
96. Jankovic L, Efremov GD, Petkov G, Kattamis C, George E, Yank K-G, Stoming TA, Huisman THJ: Two novel polyadenylation mutations leading to β^+-thalassaemia. *Br J Haematol* **75**:122, 1990.

97. Rund D, Dowling C, Najjar K, Rachmilewitz EA, Kazazian HH, Oppenheim A: Two mutations in the β-globin polyadenylation signal reveal extended transcripts and new RNA polyadenylation sites. *Proc Natl Acad Sci USA* **89**:4324, 1992.
98. Gieselmann V, Polten A, Kreysing J, von Figura K: Arylsulfatase A pseudodeficiency: Loss of a polyadenylylation signal and *N*-glycosylation site. *Proc Natl Acad Sci USA* **86**:9436, 1989.
99. Benz EJ, Forget BG, Hillman DG, Cohen-Solal M, Pritchard J, Cavallesco C, Prensky W, Housman D: Variability in the amount of β-globin mRNA in β^0-thalassemia. *Cell* **14**:299, 1978.
100. Lehrman MA, Schneider WJ, Brown MS, Davis CG, Elhammer A, Russell DW, Goldstein JL: The Lebanese allele at the low density lipoprotein receptor locus. *J Biol Chem* **262**:401, 1987.
101. Fojo SS, Lohse P, Parrott C, Baggio G, Gabelli C, Thomas F, Hoffman J, Brewer HB: A nonsense mutation in the apolipoprotein C-II Padova gene in a patient with apolipoprotein C-II deficiency. *J Clin Invest* **84**:1215, 1989.
102. Liebhaber SA, Coleman MB, Adams JG, Cash FE, Steinberg MH: Molecular basis for nondeletion α-thalassaemia in American blacks; α_2 116 GAG > UAG. *J Clin Invest* **80**:154, 1987.
103. Kinniburgh AJ, Maquat LE, Schedl T, Rachmilewitz E, Ross J: mRNA-deficient β^0-thalassemia results from a single nucleotide deletion. *Nucleic Acids Res* **10**:5421, 1982.
104. Chang JC, Kan YW: β^0 Thalassemia, a nonsense mutation in man. *Proc Natl Acad Sci USA* **76**:2886, 1979.
105. Brody LC, Mitchell GA, Obie C, Michaud J, Steel G, Fontaine G, Robert MF, et al: Ornithine δ-aminotransferase mutations in gyrate atrophy: Allelic heterogeneity and functional consequences. *J Biol Chem* **267**:3302, 1992.
106. Takeshita K, Forget BG, Scarpa A, Benz EJ: Intranuclear defect in β-globin mRNA accumulation due to a premature translation termination codon. *Blood* **64**:13, 1984.
107. Humphries KR, Ley TJ, Anagnou NP, Baur AW, Nienhuis AW: β^{0-39} Thalassemia gene: A premature termination codon causes β-mRNA deficiency without affecting cytoplasmic β-mRNA stability. *Blood* **64**:23, 1984.
108. Baserga SJ, Benz EJ: Nonsense mutations in the human β-globin gene affect mRNA metabolism. *Proc Natl Acad Sci USA* **85**:2056, 1988.
109. Baserga SJ, Benz EJ: β-Globin nonsense mutation: Deficient accumulation of mRNA occurs despite normal cytoplasmic stability. *Proc Natl Acad Sci USA* **89**:2935, 1992.
110. Atweh GF, Brickner HE, Zhu X-X, Kazazian HH, Forget BG: New amber mutation in a β-thalassemic gene with nonmeasurable levels of mutant messenger RNA *in vivo*. *J Clin Invest* **82**:557, 1988.
111. Maquat LE, Kinniburgh AJ, Rachmilewitz EA, Ross J: Unstable β-globin mRNA in mRNA-deficient β^0-thalassemia. *Cell* **27**:543, 1981.
112. Daar IO, Maquat LE: Premature translation termination mediates triosephosphate isomerase mRNA degradation. *Mol Cell Biol* **8**:802, 1988.
113. Maquat LE: When cells stop making sense: Effects of nonsense codons on RNA metabolism in vertebrate cells. *RNA* **1**:453, 1995.
114. Urlaub G, Mitchell PJ, Ciudad CJ, Chasin LA: Nonsense mutations in the dihydrofolate reductase gene affect RNA processing. *Mol Cell Biol* **9**:2868, 1989.
115. Cheng J, Fogel-Petrovic M, Maquat LE: Translation to near the distal end of the penultimate exon is required for normal levels of spliced triosephosphate isomerase mRNA. *Mol Cell Biol* **10**:5215, 1990.
116. Ploos van Amstel HK, Diepstraten CM, Reitsma PH, Bertina RM: Analysis of platelet protein S mRNA suggests silent alleles as a frequent cause of hereditary protein S deficiency type I. *Thromb Haemost* **65**:808, 1991.
117. Peerlinck K, Eikenboom JCJ, Ploos van Amstel HK, Sangtawesin W, Arnout J, Reitsma PH, Vermylen J, Briet E: A patient with von Willebrand's disease characterized by compound heterozygosity for a substitution of Arg 854 by Gln in the putative factor VIII-binding domain of von Willebrand factor on one allele and very low levels of mRNA from the second allele. *Br J Haematol* **80**:358, 1992.
118. Dietz HC, Kendzior RJ Jr: Maintenance of an open reading frame as an additional level of scrutiny during splice site selection. *Nat Genet* **8**:183, 1994
119. Orkin SH, Antonarakis SE, Kazazian HH: Base substitution at position-88 in a β-thalassemic globin gene: Further evidence for the role of distal promoter element ACACCC. *J Biol Chem* **259**:8679, 1984.
120. Orkin SH, Kazazian HH, Antonarakis SE, Goff SC, Boehm CD, Sexton JP, Waber PG, Giardina PJV: Linkage of β-thalassemia mutations and β-globin polymorphisms with DNA polymorphisms in the human β-globin gene cluster. *Nature* **296**:627, 1982.
121. Antonarakis SE, Orkin SH, Cheng TC, Scott AF, Sexton JP, Trusko SP, Charache S, Kazazian HH: β-Thalassemia in American blacks: Novel mutations in the TATA box and an acceptor splice site. *Proc Natl Acad Sci USA* **81**:1154, 1984.
122. Cai SP, Zhang JZ, Doherty M, Kan YW: A new TATA box mutation detected at prenatal diagnosis for β-thalassemia. *Am J Hum Genet* **45**:112, 1989.
123. Takihara Y, Nakamura T, Yamada H, Takagi Y, Fukumaki Y: A novel mutation in the TATA box in a Japanese patient with β^+ thalassemia. *Blood* **67**:547, 1986.
124. Lin LL, Lin KS, Lin KH, Cheng TY: A novel-34 (C to A) mutant identified in amplified genomic DNA of a Chinese β thalassemia patient. *Am J Hum Genet* **50**:237, 1992.
125. Meloni A, Rosatelli MC, Faa V, Sardu R, Saba L, Murru S, Sciarratta P, et al: Promoter mutations producing mild β-thalassemia in the Italian population. *Br J Haematol* **80**:222, 1992.
126. Faustino P, Osorio-Almeida L, Barbot J, Espirito-Santo D, Goncalves J, Romao L, Martins MC, et al: Novel promoter and splice junction defects add to the genetic, clinical or geographic heterogeneity of β thalassemia in the Portuguese population. *Hum Genet* **89**:573, 1992.
127. Huisman THJ: The β and δ thalassemia repository. *Hemoglobin* **16**:237, 1992.
128. Gonzalez-Rodondo JM, Stoming TA, Kutlar A, Kutlar F, Lanclos KD, Howard EF, Fei YJ, et al: A C to T substitution at nt-101 in a conserved DNA sequence of the promoter region of the β-globin gene is associated with "silent" β thalassemia. *Blood* **73**:1705, 1989.
129. Matsuda M, Sakamoto N, Fukumaki Y: δ-Thalassemia caused by disruption of the site for any erythroid-specific transcription factor, GATA-1, in the δ-globin gene promoter. *Blood* **80**:1347, 1992.
130. Collins FS, Stoeckert CJ, Serjeant GR, Forget BG, Weissman SM: Gγ β^+ HPFH: Cosmid cloning and identification of a specific mutation 5′ to the Gγ gene. *Proc Natl Acad Sci USA* **81**:4894, 1984.
131. Gilman JG, Mishima N, Wen XJ, Kutlar F, Huisman THJ: Upstream promoter mutation associated with a modest elevation of fetal hemoglobin expression in human adults. *Blood* **72**:78, 1988.
132. Fucharoen S, Shimizu K, Fukumaki Y: A novel C > T transition within the distal CCAAT motif of the G-gamma globin gene in the Japanese HPFH: Implication of factor binding in elevated fetal globin expression. *Nucleic Acids Res* **18**:5245, 1990.
133. Stoming TA, Stoming GS, Lanclos KD, Fei YJ, Kutlar F, Huisman THJ: A A-gamma type of nondeletional hereditary persistence of fetal hemoglobin with a T-C mutation at position −175 to the Cap site of the A-gamma globin gene. *Blood* **73**:329, 1989.
134. Oner R, Kutlar F, Gu LH, Huisman THJ: The Georgia type of nondeletion HPFH has a C to T mutation at nucleotide −114 of the Aγ-globin gene. *Blood* **77**:1124, 1991.
135. Ottolenghi S, Nicolis S, Taramelli R, Malgaretti N, Mantovani R, Comi P, Giglioni B, et al: Sardinian Gγ HPFH: A T to C substitution in a conserved octamer sequence in the Gγ promoter. *Blood* **71**:815, 1988.
136. Martin DIK, Tsai S-F, Orkin SH: Increased gamma-globin expression in a nondeletion HPFH mediated by an erythroid-specific DNA-binding factor. *Nature* **338**:435, 1989.
137. Lloyd JA, Lee RF, Lingrel JB: Mutations in two regions upstream of the A gamma globin gene canonical promoter affect gene expression. *Nucleic Acids Res* **17**:4339, 1989.
138. Gumucio DL, Lockwood WK, Weber JL, Saulino AM, Delgrosso K, Surrey S, Schwartz E, et al: The −175 T > C mutation increases promoter strength in erythroid cells: Correlation with evolutionary conservation of binding sites for two trans-acting factors. *Blood* **75**:756, 1990.
139. McDonagh KT, Lin HJ, Lowrey CH, Bodine DM, Nienhuis AW: The upstream region of the human gamma-globin gene promoter: Identification and functional analysis of nuclear protein binding sites. *J Biol Chem* **266**:11,965, 1991.
140. Nicolis S, Ronchi A, Malgaretti N, Mantovani R, Giglioni B, Ottolenghi S: Increased erythroid-specific expression of a mutated HPFH gamma α-globin promoter requires the erythroid factor NFE-1. *Nucleic Acids Res* **17**:5509, 1989.
141. Mantovani R, Malgaretti N, Nicolis S, Ronchi A, Giglioni B, Ottolenghi S: The effects of HPFH mutations in the human gamma α-globin promoter on binding of ubiquitous and erythroid-specific nuclear factors. *Nucleic Acids Res* **16**:7783, 1988.
142. Gumucio DL, Rood KL, Gray TA, Riordan MF, Sartor CI, Collins FS: Nuclear proteins that bind the human gamma-globin gene promoter: Alterations in binding produced by point mutations associated

with hereditary persistence of fetal hemoglobin. *Mol Cell Biol* **8**:5310, 1988.
143. O'Neil D, Kaysen J, Donovan-Peluso M, Castle M, Bank A: Protein-DNA interactions upstream from the human A gamma globin gene. *Nucleic Acids Res* **18**:1977, 1990.
144. Briet E, Bertina RM, van Tilburg NH, Veltkamp JJ: Haemophilia B Leyden: A sex-linked hereditary disorder that improves after puberty. *N Engl J Med* **306**:788, 1982.
145. Reitsma PH, Bertina RM, Ploos van Amstel JK, Riemans A, Briet E: The putative factor IX gene promoter in hemophilia B Leyden. *Blood* **72**:1074, 1988.
146. Reitsma PH, Mandalaki T, Kasper CK, Bertina RM, Briet E: Two novel point mutations correlate with an altered developmental expression of blood coagulation factor IX (hemophilia B Leyden phenotype). *Blood* **73**:743, 1989.
147. Crossley M, Winship P, Brownlee GG: Functional analysis of the normal and an aberrant factor IX promoter, in *Regulation of Liver Gene Expression*. Cold Spring Harbor, NY, Cold Spring Harbor Laboratory, 1989, p 51.
148. Bottema CDK, Koeberl DD, Sommer SS: Direct carrier testing in 14 families with haemophilia B. *Lancet* **2**:526, 1989.
149. Hirosawa S, Fahner JB, Salier J-P, Wu C-T, Lovrien EW, Kurachi K: Structural and functional basis of the developmental regulation of human coagulation factor IX gene: Factor IX Leyden. *Proc Natl Acad Sci USA* **87**:4421, 1990.
150. Crossley M, Winship PR, Austen DEG, Rizza CR, Brownlee GG: A less severe form of haemophilia B Leyden. *Nucleic Acids Res* **18**:4633, 1990.
151. Gispert S, Vidaud M, Vidaud D, Gazengel C, Boneu B, Goossens M: A promoter defect correlates with an abnormal coagulation factor IX gene expression in a French family (hemophilia B Leyden). *Am J Hum Genet* **45**(suppl):A189, 1989.
152. Reijnen MJ, Sladek FM, Bertina RM, Reitsma PH: Disruption of a binding site for hepatocyte nuclear factor 4 results in hemophilia B Leyden. *Proc Natl Acad Sci USA* **89**:6300, 1992.
153. Freedenberg DL, Black B: Altered developmental control of the factor IX gene: A new T to A mutation at position +6 of the FIX gene resulting in hemophilia B Leyden. *Thromb Haemost* **65**:964, 1991.
154. Crossley M, Brownlee GG: Disruption of a C/EBP binding site in the factor IX promoter is associated with haemophilia B. *Nature* **345**:444, 1990.
155. Crossley M, Ludwig M, Stowell KM, De Vos P, Olek K, Brownlee GG: Recovery from hemophilia B Leyden: An androgen-responsive element in the factor IX promoter. *Science* **257**:377, 1992.
156. Berg PE, Mittelman M, Elion J, Labie D, Schechter AN: Increased protein binding to a −350 mutation of the human β-globin gene associated with decreased β-globin synthesis. *Am J Hematol* **36**:42, 1991.
157. Ionasescu VV, Searby C, Ionasescu R, Neuhaus IM, Werner R: Mutations of the noncoding region of the connexin32 gene in X-linked dominant Charcot-Marie-Tooth neuropathy. *Neurology* **47**:541, 1996
158. Moi P, Loudianos G, Lavinha J, Murru S, Cossu P, Casu R, Oggiano L, et al: δ-Thalassemia due to a mutation in an erythroid-specific binding protein sequence 3′ to the δ-globin gene. *Blood* **79**:512, 1992.
159. Van der Ploeg LHT, Konings A, Oort M, Roos D, Bernini L, Flavell RA: Gamma-β-thalassaemia studies showing that deletion of the γ- and δ-genes influences β-globin gene expression in man. *Nature* **283**:637, 1980.
160. Kioussis D, Vanin E, de Lange T, Flavell RA, Grosveld FG: β-Globin gene inactivation by DNA translocation in γ-β-thalassaemia. *Nature* **306**:662, 1983.
161. Curtin P, Pirastu M, Kan YW, Gobert-Jones JA, Stephens AD, Lehmann H: A distant gene deletion affects β-globin gene function in an atypical $\gamma\delta\beta$-thalassemia. *J Clin Invest* **76**:1554, 1985.
162. Driscoll MC, Dobkin CS, Alter BP: $\gamma\delta\beta$-Thalassemia due to a *de novo* mutation deleting the 5′ β-globin gene activation-region hypersensitive sites. *Proc Natl Acad Sci USA* **86**:7470, 1989.
163. Grosveld F, van Assendelft GB, Greaves DR, Kollias G: Position-independent high-level expression of the human β-globin gene in transgenic mice. *Cell* **51**:975, 1989.
164. Jarman AP, Wood WG, Sharpe JA, Gourdon G, Ayyub H, Higgs DR: Characterization of the major regulatory element upstream of the human α-globin gene cluster. *Mol Cell Biol* **11**:4679, 1991.
165. Hatton CSR, Wilkie AOM, Drysdale HC, Wood WG, Vickers MA, Sharpe J, Ayyub H, et al: α-Thalassemia caused by a large (62kb) deletion upstream of the human a globin gene cluster. *Blood* **76**:221, 1990.
166. Wilkie AOM, Lamb J, Harris PC, Finney RD, Higgs DR: A truncated human chromosome 16 associated with α-thalassaemia is stabilized by addition of telomeric repeat (TTAGGG). *Nature* **346**:868, 1990.
167. Romao L, Osorio-Almeida L, Higgs DR, Lavinha J, Liebhaber SA: α-Thalassemia resulting from deletion of regulatory sequences far upstream of the α-globin structural genes. *Blood* **78**:1589, 1991.
168. Romao L, Cash F, Weiss I, Liebhaber S, Pirastu M, Galanello R, Loi A, et al: Human α-globin gene expression is silenced by terminal truncation of chromosome 16p beginning immediately 3′ of the zeta-globin gene. *Hum Genet* **89**:323, 1992.
169. Liebhaber SA, Griese E-U, Weiss I, Cash FE, Ayyub H, Higgs DR, Horst J: Inactivation of human α-globin gene expression by a *de novo* deletion located upstream of the α-globin gene cluster. *Proc Natl Acad Sci USA* **87**:9431, 1990.
170. Higgs DR, Wood WG, Jarman AP, Sharpe J, Lida J, Pretorius IM, Ayyub H: A major positive regulatory region located far upstream of the human α-globin gene locus. *Genes Dev* **4**:1588, 1990.
171. Vyas P, Vickers MA, Simmons DL, Ayyub H, Craddock CF, Higgs DR: *Cis*-acting sequences regulating expression of the human α-globin cluster lie within constitutively open chromatin. *Cell* **69**:781, 1992.
172. Poort SR, Rosendaal FR, Reitsma PH, Bertina RM. A common genetic variation in the 3′-untranslated region of the prothrombin gene is associated with elevated plasma prothrombin levels and an increase in venous thrombosis. *Blood* **88**:3698, 1996.
173. Antonarakis SE, Kazazian HH Jr: The molecular basis of hemophilia A in man. *Trends Genet* **4**:233, 1988.
174. Millar DS, Steinbrecher RA, Wieland K, Grundy CB, Martinowitz U, Krawczak M, Zoll B, et al: The molecular genetic analysis of haemophilia A: Characterization of six partial deletions in the factor VIII gene. *Hum Genet* **86**:219, 1990.
175. Ballabio A, Carrozzo R, Parenti G, Gil A, Zollo M, Persico MG, Gillard E, et al: Molecular heterogeneity of steroid sulfatase deficiency: A multicenter study of 57 unrelated patients at DNA and protein levels. *Genomics* **4**:36, 1989.
176. Forrest SM, Cross GS, Speer A, Gardner-Medwin D, Burn J, Davies KE: Preferential deletion of exons in Duchenne and Becker muscular dystrophies. *Nature* **329**:638, 1987.
177. Forrest SM, Cross GS, Flint T, Speer A, Robson KJH, Davies KE: Further studies of gene deletions that cause Duchenne and Becker muscular dystrophies. *Genomics* **2**:109, 1988.
178. Den Dunnen JT, Bakker E, Klein Breteler EG, Pearson PL, van Ommen GJB: Direct detection of more than 50% of the Duchenne muscular dystrophy mutations by field inversion gels. *Nature* **329**:640, 1987.
179. Wapenaar MC, Kievits T, Hart KA, Abbs S, Blonden LAJ, den Dunnen JT, Grootscholten PM, et al: A deletion hot spot in the Duchenne muscular dystrophy gene. *Genomics* **2**:101, 1988.
180. Vnencak-Jones CL, Phillips JA, Chen EY, Seeburg PH: Molecular basis of human growth hormone deletions. *Proc Natl Acad Sci USA* **85**:5615, 1988.
181. Vnencak-Jones CL, Phillips JA: Hot spots for growth hormone gene deletions in homologous regions outside of *Alu* repeats. *Science* **250**:1745, 1990.
182. Langlois S, Kastelein JJP, Hayden MR: Characterization of six partial deletions in the low density lipoprotein (LDL) receptor gene causing familial hypercholesterolemia (FH). *Am J Hum Genet* **43**:60, 1988.
183. Nicholls RD, Fischel-Ghodsian N, Higgs DR: Recombination at the human α-globin gene cluster: Sequence features and topological constraints. *Cell* **49**:369, 1987.
184. Higgs DR, Vickers MA, Wilkie AOM, Pretorius I-M, Jarman AP, Weatherall DJ: A review of the molecular genetics of the human α-globin gene cluster. *Blood* **73**:1081, 1989.
185. Embury SH, Miller JA, Dozy AM, Kan YW, Chan V, Todd D: Two different molecular organizations account for the single α-globin gene of the α-thalassaemia-2 genotype. *J Clin Invest* **66**:1319, 1980.
186. Trent RJ, Higgs DR, Clegg JB, Weatherall DJ: A new triplicated α-globin gene arrangement in man. *Br J Haematol* **49**:149, 1981.
187. Goossens M, Dozy AM, Embury SH, Zachariades Z, Hadjiminas MG, Stamatoyannopoulos G, Kan YW: Triplicated α-globin loci in humans. *Proc Natl Acad Sci USA* **77**:518, 1980.
188. Hwu HR, Roberts JH, Davidson EH, Britten RJ: Insertion and/or deletion of many repeated DNA sequences in human and higher ape evolution. *Proc Natl Acad Sci USA* **83**:3875, 1986.
189. Moyzis RK, Torney DC, Meyne J, Buckingham JM, Wu JR, Burks C, Sirotkin KM, Goad WG: The distribution of interspersed repetitive DNA sequences in the human genome. *Genomics* **4**:273, 1989.

190. Deininder PL: SINEs: Short interspersed repetitive DNA elements in higher eukaryotes, in Berg DE, Howe MM (eds): *Mobile DNA*. Washington, DC, American Society of Microbiology, 1989, p 619.
191. Jelinek WR, Schmid CW: Repetitive sequences in eukaryotic DNA and their expression. *Annu Rev Biochem* **51**:813, 1982.
192. Lehrman MA, Schneider WJ, Suedhof TF, Brown MS, Goldstein JL, Russell DW: Mutation in LDL receptor: *Alu-Alu* recombination deletes exons encoding transmembrane and cytoplasmic domains. *Science* **227**:140, 1985.
193. Lehrman MA, Russell DW, Goldstein JL, Brown MS: Exon-*Alu* recombination deletes 5 kilobases from the low density lipoprotein receptor gene producing a null phenotype in familial hypercholesterolemia. *Proc Natl Acad Sci USA* **83**:3679, 1986.
194. Hobbs HH, Brown MS, Goldstein JL, Russell DW: Deletion of exon encoding cysteine-rich repeat of low-density lipoprotein receptor alters its binding specificity in a subject with familial hypercholesterolemia. *J Biol Chem* **261**:13,114, 1986.
195. Horsthemke B, Beisiegel U, Dunning A, Havinga JR, Williamson R, Humphries S: Unequal crossing-over between two *Alu*-repetitive DNA sequences in the low-density-lipoprotein-receptor gene. *Eur J Biochem* **164**:77, 1987.
196. Lehrman MA, Russell DW, Goldstein JL, Brown MS: *Alu-Alu* recombination deletes splice acceptor sites and produces secreted low density lipoprotein receptor in a subject with familial hypercholesterolemia. *J Biol Chem* **262**:3354, 1987.
197. Lehrman MA, Goldstein JL, Russell DW, Brown MS: Duplication of seven exons in LDL receptor gene caused by *Alu-Alu* recombination in a subject with familial hypercholesterolemia. *Cell* **48**:827, 1987.
198. Ariga T, Carter PE, Davis AE: Recombinations between *Alu* repeat sequences that result in partial deletions within the C1 inhibitor gene. *Genomics* **8**:607, 1990.
199. Carter PE, Duponchel C, Tosi M, Fothergill JE: Complete nucleotide sequence of the gene for human C1 inhibitor with an unusually high density of *Alu* elements. *Eur J Biochem* **197**:301, 1991.
200. Stoppa-Lyonnet D, Duponchel C, Meo T, Laurent J, Carter PE, Arala-Chaves M, Cohen JHM, et al: Recombination biases in the rearranged C1-inhibitor genes of hereditary angioedema patients. *Am J Hum Genet* **49**:1055, 1991.
201. Henthorn PS, Smithies O, Mager DL: Molecular analysis of deletions in the human β-globin gene cluster: Deletion junctions and locations of breakpoints. *Genomics* **6**:226, 1990.
202. Kornreich R, Bishop DF, Desnick RJ: α-Galactosidase A gene rearrangements causing Fabry disease. *J Biol Chem* **265**:9319, 1990.
203. Monnat RJ, Hackman AFM, Chiaverotti TA: Nucleotide sequence analysis of human hypoxanthine phosphoribosyltransferase (HPRT) gene deletions. *Genomics* **13**:777, 1992.
204. Bollag RJ, Waldman AS, Liskay RM: Homologous recombination in mammalian cells. *Annu Rev Genet* **23**:199, 1989.
205. Shapiro LJ, Yen P, Pomerantz D, Martin E, Rolewic L, Mohandas T: Molecular studies of deletions at the human steroid sulphatase locus. *Proc Natl Acad Sci USA* **86**:8477, 1989.
206. Yen PH, Li X-M, Tsai S-P, Johnson C, Mohandas T, Shapiro LJ: Frequent deletions of the human X chromosome distal short arm result from recombination between low copy repetitive elements. *Cell* **61**:603, 1990.
207. Pizzuti A, Pieretti M, Fenwick RG, Gibbs RA, Caskey CT: A transposon-like element in the deletion-prone region of the dystrophin gene. *Genomics* **13**:594, 1992.
208. Mager DL, Goodchild NL: Homologous recombination between the LTRs of a human retrovirus-like-element causes a 5-kb deletion in two siblings. *Am J Hum Genet* **45**:848, 1989.
209. Gerald PS, Diamond LK: A new hereditary hemoglobinopathy (the Lepore trait) and its interaction with thalassemia trait. *Blood* **13**:835, 1958.
210. Baglioni C: The fusion of two peptide chains in hemoglobin Lepore and its interpretation as a genetic deletion. *Proc Natl Acad Sci USA* **48**:1880, 1962.
211. Barnabus J, Muller CJ: Haemoglobin Lepore Hollandia. *Nature* **194**:931, 1962.
212. Ostertag W, Smith EW: Hemoglobin-Lepore-Baltimore, a third type of a δ, β crossover (δ^{50}, β^{86}). *Eur J Biochem* **10**:371, 1969.
213. Flavell RA, Kooter JW, DeBoer E, Little PFR, Williamson R: Analysis of $\delta\beta$-globin gene in normal and Hb Lepore DNA: Direct determination of gene linkage and intergene distance. *Cell* **15**:25, 1978.
214. Baird M, Schreiner H, Driscoll C, Bank A: Localization of the site of recombination in the formation of the Lepore Boston globin gene. *J Clin Invest* **58**:560, 1981.
215. Mavilio F, Giampaolo A, Care A, Sposi NM, Marinucci M: The $\delta\beta$ crossover region in Lepore Boston hemoglobinopathy is restricted to a 59 base pairs region around the 5′ splice junction of a large globin gene intervening sequence. *Blood* **62**:230, 1983.
216. Chebloune Y, Poncet D, Verdier G: S1-nuclease mapping of the genomic Lepore-Boston DNA demonstrates that the entire large intervening sequence of the fusion gene is of β-type. *Biochem Biophys Res Commun* **120**:116, 1984.
217. Metzenberg AB, Wurzer G, Huisman TH, Smithies O: Homology requirements for unequal crossing over in humans. *Genetics* **128**:143, 1991.
218. Lanclos KD, Patterson J, Eframov GD, Wong SC, Villegas A, Ojwang PJ, Wilson JB, et al: Characterization of chromosomes with hybrid genes for Hb Lepore-Washington, Hb Lepore-Baltimore, Hb P-Nilotic, and Hb Kenya. *Hum Genet* **77**:40, 1987.
219. Fioretti G, de Angioletti M, Masciangelo F, Lacerra G, Scarallo A, de Bonis C, Pagano L, et al: Origin heterogeneity of Hb Lepore-Boston gene in Italy. *Am J Hum Genet* **50**:781, 1992.
220. Huisman THJ, Wrightstone RN, Wilson JB, Schroeder WA, Kendall AG: Hemoglobin Kenya, the product of a fusion of gamma and β polypeptide chains. *Arch Biochem Biophys* **153**:850, 1972.
221. Kendall AG, Ojwang PJ, Schroeder WA, Huisman THJ: Hemoglobin Kenya, the product of a $\gamma\beta$ fusion gene: Studies of the family. *Am J Hum Genet* **25**:548, 1973.
222. Ojwang PJ, Nakatsuji T, Gardiner MB, Reese AL, Gilman JG, Huisman THJ: Gene deletion as the molecular basis for the Kenya-$^{G}\gamma$-HPFH condition. *Hemoglobin* **7**:115, 1983.
223. Lehmann H, Charlesworth D: Observations on hemoglobin P (Congo type). *Biochem J* **119**:43, 1970.
224. Badr FM, Lorkin PA, Lehmann H: Haemoglobin P-Nilotic: Containing β-δ chain. *Nature* **242**:107, 1973.
225. Honig GR, Mason RG, Tremaine LM, Vida LN: Unbalanced globin chain synthesis by Hb Lincoln Park (anti-Lepore) reticulocytes. *Am J Hematol* **5**:335, 1978.
226. Honig GR, Shamsuddin M, Mason RG, Vida LN: Hemoglobin Lincoln Park: A $\beta\delta$ fusion (anti-Lepore) variant with an amino acid deletion in the δ chain-derived segment. *Proc Natl Acad Sci USA* **75**:1475, 1978.
227. Nathans J, Piantanida TP, Eddy RL, Shows TB, Hogness DS: Molecular genetics of inherited variation in human color vision. *Science* **232**:203, 1986.
228. Pascoe L, Curnow KM, Slutsker L, Connell JMC, Speiser PW, New MI, White PC: Glucocorticoid-suppressible hyperaldosteronism results from hybrid genes created by unequal crossovers between CYP11B1 and CYP11B2. *Proc Natl Acad Sci USA* **89**:8327, 1992.
229. Zimran A, Sorge J, Gross E, Kubitz M, West C, Beutler E: A glucocerebrosidase fusion gene in Gaucher disease. *J Clin Invest* **85**:219, 1990.
230. Tanigawa G, Jarcho JA, Kass S, Solomon SD, Vosberg H-P, Seidman JG, Seidman CE: A molecular basis for familial hypertrophic cardiomyopathy: An α/β cardiac myosin heavy chain hybrid gene. *Cell* **62**:991, 1990.
231. Guioli S, Incerti B, Zanaria E, Bardoni B, Franco B, Taylor K, Ballabio A, Camerino G: Kallmann syndrome due to a translocation resulting in an X/Y fusion gene. *Nature Genetics* **1**:337, 1992.
232. Vanin EF, Henthorn PS, Kioussis D, Grosveld F, Smithies O: Unexpected relationships between four large deletions in the human β-globin gene cluster. *Cell* **35**:701, 1983.
233. Piccoli SP, Caimi PG, Cole MD: A conserved sequence at c-myc oncogene chromosomal translocation breakpoints in plasmacytomas. *Nature* **310**:327, 1984.
234. Roth DB, Porter TN, Wilson JH: Mechanisms of nonhomologous recombination in mammalian cells. *Mol Cell Biol* **5**:2599, 1985.
235. Roth DB, Wilson JH: Nonhomologous recombination in mammalian cells: Role for short sequence homologies in the joining reaction. *Mol Cell Biol* **6**:4295, 1986.
236. Gilman JG: The 12.6 kilobase DNA deletion in Dutch β^{0}-thalassaemia. *Br J Haematol* **67**:369, 1987.
237. Efstratiadis A, Posakony JW, Maniatis T, Lawn RM, O'Connell C, Spritz RA, DeRiel JK, et al: The structure and evolution of the human β-globin gene family. *Cell* **21**:653, 1980.
238. Woods-Samuels P, Kazazian HH, Antonarakis SE: Nonhomologous recombination on the human genome: Deletions in the human factor VIII gene. *Genomics* **10**:94, 1991.
239. Vogel F, Motulsky AG: *Human Genetics: Problems and Approaches*, 2d ed. Berlin, Springer-Verlag, 1986.

240. Nagylaki T, Petes TD: Intrachromosomal gene conversion and the maintenance of sequence homogeneity among repeated genes. *Genetics* **100**:315, 1982.
241. Shen S, Slightom JL, Smithies O: A history of the human fetal globin gene duplication. *Cell* **26**:191, 1981.
242. Stoeckert CJ, Collins FS, Weissman S: Human fetal globin DNA sequences suggest novel conversion event. *Nucleic Acids Res* **12**:4469, 1984.
243. Powers PA, Smithies O: Short gene conversion in the human fetal globin gene region: A by-product of chromosome pairing during meiosis? *Genetics* **112**:343, 1986.
244. Liebhaber SA, Goossens M, Kan YW: Homology and concerted evolution at the α_1 and α_2 loci of human α-globin. *Nature* **290**:26, 1981.
245. Antonarakis SE, Orkin SH, Kazazian HH, Goff SC, Boehm CD, Waber PG, Sexton JP, et al: Evidence for multiple origins of the β^E-globin gene in Southeast Asia. *Proc Natl Acad Sci USA* **79**:6608, 1982.
246. Antonarakis SE, Boehm CD, Serjeant GR, Theisen CE, Dover GJ, Kazazian HH: Origin of the β^S-globin gene in blacks: The contribution of recurrent mutation or gene conversion or both. *Proc Natl Acad Sci USA* **81**:853, 1984.
247. Kazazian HH, Orkin SH, Markham AF, Chapman CR, Youssoufian H, Waber PG: Quantification of the close association between DNA haplotypes and specific β-thalassaemia mutations in Mediterraneans. *Nature* **310**:152, 1984.
248. Pirastu M, Galanello R, Doherty MA, Tuveri T, Cao A, Kan YW: The same β-globin gene mutation is present on nine different β-thalassaemia chromosomes in a Sardinian population. *Proc Natl Acad Sci USA* **84**:2882, 1987.
249. Zhang J-Z, Cai S-P, He X, Lin H-X, Lin H-J, Huang Z-G, Chehab FF, Kan YW: Molecular basis of β-thalassaemia in South China. *Hum Genet* **78**:37, 1988.
250. Matsuno Y, Yamashiro Y, Yamamoto K, Hattori Y, Yamamoto K, Ohba Y, Miyaji T: A possible example of gene conversion with a common β-thalassaemia mutation and Chi sequence present in the β-globin gene. *Hum Genet* **88**:357, 1992.
251. Smith GR: Chi hotspots of generalized recombination. *Cell* **34**:709, 1983.
252. Harada F, Kimura A, Iwanaga T, Shimozawa K, Yata J, Sasazuki T: Gene conversion-like events cause steroid 21-hydroxylase deficiency in congenital adrenal hyperplasia. *Proc Natl Acad Sci USA* **84**:8091, 1987.
253. Amor M, Parker KL, Gloverman H, New MI, White PC: Mutation in the CYP21B gene (Ile > Asn) causes steroid 21-hydroxylase deficiency. *Proc Natl Acad Sci USA* **85**:1600, 1988.
254. Morel Y, David M, Forest MG, Betuel H, Hauptman G, Andre J, Bertrand J, Miller WL: Gene conversions and rearrangements cause discordance between inheritance of forms of 21-hydroxylase deficiency and HLA types. *J Clin Endocrinol Metab* **68**:592, 1989.
255. Urabe K, Kimura A, Harada F, Iwanaga T, Sasazuki T: Gene conversion in steroid 210-hydroxylase genes. *Am J Hum Genet* **46**:1178, 1990.
256. Tusie-Luna MT, White PC: Gene conversions and unequal crossovers between CYP21 (steroid 21-hydroxylase gene) and CYP21P involve different mechanisms. *Proc Natl Acad Sci USA* **92**:10,796, 1995.
257. Watnick TJ, Gandolph MA, Weber H, Neumann HP, Germino GG: Gene conversion is a likely cause of mutation in PKD1. *Hum Mol Genet* **7**:1239, 1998.
258. Gorlach A, Lee PL, Roesler J, Hopkins PJ, Christensen B, Green ED, Chanock SJ, Curnutte JT: A p47-phox pseudogene carries the most common mutation causing p47-phox-deficient chronic granulomatous disease. *J Clin Invest* **100**:1907, 1997.
259. Minegishi Y, Coustan-Smith E, Wang YH, Cooper MD, Campana D, Conley ME: Mutations in the human lambda5/14.1 gene result in B cell deficiency and agammaglobulinemia. *J Exp Med* **187**:71, 1998.
260. Eyal N, Wilder S, Horowitz M: Prevalent and rare mutations among Gaucher patients. *Gene* **96**:277, 1990.
261. Eikenboom JC, Vink T, Briet E, Sixma JJ, Reitsma PH: Multiple substitutions in the von Willebrand factor gene that mimic the pseudogene sequence. *Proc Natl Acad Sci USA* **91**:2221, 1994.
262. Schollen E, Pardon E, Heykants L, Renard J, Doggett NA, Callen DF, Cassiman JJ, Matthijs G: Comparative analysis of the phosphomannomutase genes PMM1, PMM2 and PMM2psi: The sequence variation in the processed pseudogene is a reflection of the mutations found in the functional gene. *Hum Mol Genet* **7**:157, 1998.
263. Krawczak M, Cooper DN: Gene deletions causing human genetic disease: Mechanisms of mutagenesis and the role of the local DNA sequence environment. *Hum Genet* **86**:425, 1991.
264. Wada K, Wada Y, Doi H, Ishibashi F, Gojobori T, Ikemura T: Codon usage tabulated from the GenBank genetic sequence data. *Nucleic Acids Res* **19**(suppl):1981, 1991.
265. Streisinger G, Okada Y, Emrich J, Newton J, Tsugita A, Terzaghi E, Inouye M: Frameshift mutations and the genetic code. *Cold Spring Harb Symp Quant Biol* **31**:77, 1966.
266. Kunkel TA: The mutational specificity of DNA polymerases α and γ during *in vitro* DNA synthesis. *J Biol Chem* **260**:12,866, 1985.
267. Kunkel TA, Soni A: Mutagenesis by transient misalignment. *J Biol Chem* **263**:14,784, 1988.
268. Ripley LS: Model for the participation of quasi-palindromic DNA sequences in frameshift mutation. *Proc Natl Acad Sci USA* **79**:4128, 1982.
269. DeBoer JG, Ripley LS: Demonstration of the production of frameshift and base-substitution mutations by quasi-palindromic sequences. *Proc Natl Acad Sci USA* **81**:5528, 1984.
270. Maekawa M, Sudo K, Kanno T, Li SS-L: Molecular characterization of genetic mutation in human lactate dehydrogenase A(M) deficiency. *Biochem Biophys Res Commun* **168**:677, 1990.
271. Schmucker B, Krawczak M: Meiotic microdeletion breakpoints in the BRCA1 gene are significantly associated with symmetric DNA-sequence elements. *Am J Hum Genet* **61**:1454, 1997.
272. Gritzmacher CA: Molecular aspects of heavy-chain class switching. *Crit Rev Immunol* **9**:173, 1989.
273. Fearon ER, Cho KR, Nigro JM, Kern SE, Simons JW, Ruppert JM, Hamilton SR, et al: Identification of a chromosome 18q gene that is altered in colorectal cancers. *Science* **247**:49, 1990.
274. Roux AF, Morle F, Guetarni D, Colonna P, Sahr K, Forget BG, Delaunay J, Godet J: Molecular basis of Sp alpha I/65 hereditary elliptocytosis in North Africa: Insertion of a TTG triplet between codons 147 and 149 in the alpha-spectrin gene from five unrelated families. *Blood* **73**:2196, 1989.
275. Fry M, Loeb LA: A DNA polymerase α pause site is a hotspot for nucleotide misinsertion. *Proc Natl Acad Sci USA* **89**:763, 1992.
276. Bettecken T, Müller CR: Identification of a 220 kb insertion into the Duchenne gene in a family with an atypical course of muscular dystrophy. *Genomics* **4**:592, 1989.
277. Kazazian HH, Wong C, Youssoufian H, Scott AF, Phillips DG, Antonarakis SE: Haemophilia A resulting from *de novo* insertion of L1 sequences represents a novel mechanism for mutation in man. *Nature* **332**:164, 1988.
278. Kazazian HH Jr, Moran JV: The impact of L1 retrotransposons on the human genome. *Nat Genet* **19**:19, 1998.
279. Weiner AM, Deininger PL, Efstratiadis A: Nonviral retroposons: Genes, pseudogenes and transposable elements generated by the reverse flow of genetic information. *Annu Rev Biochem* **55**:631, 1986.
280. Fanning TG, Singer MF: LINE-1: A mammalian transposable element. *Biochim Biophys Acta* **910**:203, 1987.
281. Dombroski BA, Mathias SL, Nanthakumar E, Scott AF, Kazazian HH: Isolation of an active human transposable element. *Science* **254**:1805, 1991.
282. Woods-Samuels P, Wong C, Mathias SL, Scott AF, Kazazian HH, Antonarakis SE: Characterization of a non-deleterious L1 insertion in an intron of the human factor VIII gene and evidence for open reading frame in functional L1 elements. *Genomics* **4**:290, 1989.
283. Holmes SE, Dombroski BA, Krebs CM, Boehm CD, Kazazian HH Jr: A new retrotransposable human L1 element from the LRE2 locus on chromosome 1q produces a chimaeric insertion. *Nat Genet* **7**:143, 1994.
284. Miki Y, Nishisho I, Horii A, Miyoshi Y, Utsunomiya J, Kinzler KW, Vogelstein B, Nakamura Y: Disruption of the APC gene by a retrotransposal insertion of L1 sequence in a colon cancer. *Cancer Res* **52**:643, 1992.
285. Mager DL, Henthorn PS, Smithies O: A Chinese $^G\gamma + {}^A\gamma\delta\beta^{00\text{thalassaemia}}$ deletion: Comparison to other deletions in the human β-globin gene cluster and sequence analysis of the breakpoints. *Nucleic Acids Res* **13**:6559, 1985.
286. Morse J, Rothberg PG, South VJ, Spandorfer JM, Astrin SM: Insertional mutagenesis of the myc locus by a LINE-1 sequence in a human breast carcinoma. *Nature* **333**:87, 1988.
287. Moran JV, Holmes SE, Naas TP, DeBerardinis RJ, Boeke JD, Kazazian HH Jr: High frequency retrotransposition in cultured mammalian cells. *Cell* **87**:917, 1996.
288. Hohjoh H, Singer MF: Cytoplasmic ribonucleoprotein complexes containing human LINE-1 protein and RNA. *EMBO J* **15**:630, 1996.
289. Feng Q, Moran JV, Kazazian HH Jr, Boeke JD: Human L1 retrotransposon encodes a conserved endonuclease required for retrotransposition. *Cell* **87**:905, 1996.

290. Lin CS, Goldthwait DA, Samols D: Identification of *Alu* transposition in human lung carcinoma cells. *Cell* **54**:153, 1988.
291. Wallace MR, Andersen LB, Saulino AM, Gregory PE, Glover TW, Collins FS: A *de novo Alu* insertion results in neurofibromatosis type 1. *Nature* **353**:864, 1991.
292. Economou-Pachnis A, Tsichlis PN: Insertion of an *Alu* SINE in the human homologue of the MIvi-2 locus. *Nucleic Acids Res* **13**:8379, 1985.
293. Muratani K, Hada T, Yamamoto Y, Kaneko T, Shigeto Y, Ohree T, Furuyama J, Higashino K: Inactivation of the cholinesterase gene by *Alu* insertion: Possible mechanism for the human gene transposition. *Proc Natl Acad Sci USA* **88**:11,315, 1991.
294. Vidaud D, Vidaud M, Bahnak BR, Siguret V, Sanchez SG, Laurian Y, Meyer D, et al: Hemophilia B due to a *de novo* insertion of a human-specific *Alu* subfamily member within the coding region of the factor IX gene. *Eur J Hum Genet* **1**:30, 1993.
295. Kariya Y, Kato K, Hayashizaki Y, Himeno S, Tarui S, Matsubara K: Revision of consensus sequence of human *Alu* repeats: A review. *Gene* **53**:1, 1987.
295. Miki Y, Katagiri T, Kasumi F, Yoshimoto T, Nakamura Y: Mutation analysis in the BRCA2 gene in primary breast cancers. *Nat Genet* **13**:245, 1996.
296. Umlauf SW, Cox MM: The functional significance of DNA sequence structure in a site-specific genetic recombination reaction. *EMBO J* **7**:1845, 1988.
297. Shih C-C, Stoye JP, Coffin JM: Highly preferred targets for retrovirus integration. *Cell* **53**:531, 1988.
298. Angelini C, Beggs AH, Hoffman EP, Fanin M, Kunkel LM: Enormous dystrophin in a patient with Becker muscular dystrophy. *Neurology* **40**:808, 1990.
299. Yang TP, Stout JT, Konecki DS, Patel PI, Alford RL, Caskey CT: Spontaneous reversion of novel Lesch-Nyhan mutation by HPRT gene rearrangement. *Somat Cell Mol Genet* **14**:293, 1988.
300. Tiller GE, Rimoin DL, Murray LW, Cohn DH: Tandem duplication within a type II collagen gene (COL2A1) exon in an individual with spondyloepiphyseal dysplasia. *Proc Natl Acad Sci USA* **87**:3889, 1990.
301. Stoppa-Lyonnet D, Carter PE, Meo T, Tosi M: Clusters of intragenic *Alu* repeats predispose the human C1 inhibitor locus to deleterious rearrangements. *Proc Natl Acad Sci USA* **87**:1551, 1990.
302. Murru S, Casula L, Pecorara M, Mori P, Cao A, Pirastu M: Illegitimate recombination produced a duplication within the FVIII gene in a patient with mild hemophilia A. *Genomics* **7**:115, 1990.
303. Hu X, Ray PN, Murphy EG, Thompson MW, Worton RG: Duplicational mutation at the Duchenne muscular dystrophy locus: Its frequency, distribution, origin and phenotype/genotype correlation. *Am J Hum Genet* **46**:682, 1990.
304. Hu X, Ray PN, Worton RG: Mechanisms of tandem duplication in the Duchenne muscular dystrophy gene include both homologous and nonhomologous intrachromosomal recombination. *EMBO J* **10**:2471, 1991.
305. Devlin RH, Deeb S, Brunzell J, Hayden MR: Partial gene duplication involving exon-*Alu* interchange results in lipoprotein lipase deficiency. *Am J Hum Genet* **46**:112, 1990.
306. Gitschier J: Maternal duplication associated with gene deletion in sporadic hemophilia. *Am J Hum Genet* **43**:274, 1988.
307. Steinmetz M, Uematsu Y, Lindahl KF: Hotspots of homologous recombination in mammalian genomes. *Trends Genet* **3**:7, 1987.
308. Casula L, Murru S, Pecorara M, Ristaldi MS, Restagno G, Mancuso G, Morfini M, et al: Recurrent mutations and three novel rearrangements in the factor VIII gene of hemophilia A patients of Italian descent. *Blood* **75**:662, 1990.
309. Den Dunnen JT, Grootsscholten PM, Bakker E, Blonden LAJ, Ginjaar HB, Wapenaar MC, van Paassen HMB, et al: Topography of the Duchenne muscular dystrophy (DMD) gene: FIGE and cDNA analysis of 194 cases reveals 115 deletions and 13 duplications. *Am J Hum Genet* **45**:835, 1989.
310. Cooke A, Lanyon WG, Wilcox DE, Dornan ES, Kataki A, Gillard EF, McWhinnie AJM, et al: Analysis of Scottish Duchenne and Becker muscular dystrophy families with dystrophin cDNA probes. *J Med Genet* **27**:292, 1990.
311. Haglund-Stengler R, Ritzen EM, Luthman H: 21-Hydroxy lase deficiency: Disease-causing mutations categorized by densitometry of 21-hydroxylase-specific deoxyribonucleic acid fragments. *J Clin Endocrinol Metab* **70**:43, 1990.
312. Hu X, Worton RG: Partial gene duplication as a cause of human disease. *Hum Mutat* **1**:3, 1992.
313. Roberts RG, Barby TFM, Manners E, Bobrow M, Bentley DR: Direct detection of dystrophin gene rearrangements by analysis of dystrophin mRNA in peripheral blood lymphocytes. *Am J Hum Genet* **49**:298, 1991.
314. Monnat RJ, Chiaverotti TA, Hackmann AFM, Maresh GA: Molecular structure and genetic stability of human hypoxanthine phosphoribosyltransferase (HPRT) gene duplications. *Genomics* **13**:788, 1992.
315. Pentao L, Wise CA, Chinault AC, Patel PI, Lupski JR: Charcot-Marie-Tooth type 1A duplication appears to arise from recombination at repeat sequences flanking the 1.5 Mb monomer unit. *Nat Genet* **2**:292, 1992.
316. Jennings MW, Jones RW, Wood WG, Weatherall DJ: Analysis of an inversion within the human β-globin gene cluster. *Nucleic Acids Res* **13**:2897, 1985.
317. Karathanasis SK, Ferris E, Haddad IA: DNA inversion within the apolipoproteins AI/CIII/AIV-encoding gene cluster of certain patients with premature atherosclerosis. *Proc Natl Acad Sci USA* **84**:7198, 1987.
318. Kulozik AE, Bellan-Koch A, Kohne E, Kleihauer E: A deletion/inversion rearrangement of the β-globin gene cluster in a Turkish family with $\delta\beta$-thalassemia intermedia. *Blood* **79**:2455, 1992.
319. Lakich D, Kazazian HH, Antonarakis SE, Gitschier J: Inversions of the factor VIII gene as a common cause of severe hemophilia A. *Nat Genet* **5**:236, 1993.
320. Naylor J, Brinke A, Hassock S, Green PM, Giannelli F: Characteristic mRNA abnormality found in half the patients with severe haemophilia A is due to large DNA inversions. *Hum Mol Genet* **2**:1773, 1993.
321. Antonarakis SE, Rossiter JP, Young M, Horst J, de Moerloose P, Sommer SS, Ketterling RP, et al: Factor VIII gene inversions in severe hemophilia A: Results of an international consortium study. *Blood* **86**:2206, 1995.
322. Linton MF, Pierotti V, Young SG: Reading-frame restoration with an apolipoprotein B gene frameshift mutation. *Proc Natl Acad Sci USA* **89**:11,431, 1992.
323. Young M, Inaba H, Hoyer LW, Higuchi M, Kazazian HH Jr, Antonarakis SE: Partial correction of a severe molecular defect in hemophilia A, because of errors during expression of the factor VIII gene. *Am J Hum Genet* **60**:565, 1997.
324. Laken SJ, Petersen GM, Gruber SB, Oddoux C, Ostrer H, Giardiello FM, Hamilton SR, et al: Familial colorectal cancer in Ashkenazim due to a hypermutable tract in APC. *Nat Genet* **17**:79, 1997.
325. Wagner LA, Weiss RB, Driscoll R, Dunn DS, Gesteland RF: Transcriptional slippage occurs during elongation at runs of adenine or thymine in *Escherichia coli*. *Nucleic Acids Res* **18**:3529, 1990.
326. Jacks T, Varmus HE: Expression of the Rous sarcoma virus pol gene by ribosomal frameshifting. *Science* **230**:1237, 1985.
327. Van Leeuwen FW, de Kleijn DP, van den Hurk HH, Neubauer A, Sonnemans MA, Sluijs JA, Koycu S, et al: Frameshift mutants of beta amyloid precursor protein and ubiquitin-B in Alzheimer's and Down patients. *Science* **279**:242, 1998.
328. Caskey CT, Pizzuti A, Fu Y-H, Fenwick RG, Nelson DL: Triplet repeat mutations in human disease. *Science* **256**:784, 1992.
329. Rousseau F, Heitz D, Mandel J-L: The unstable and methylatable mutations causing the fragile X syndrome. *Hum Mutat* **1**:91, 1992.
330. Mandel J-L: Questions of expansion. *Nat Genet* **4**:8, 1993.
331. Wilmot GR, Warren ST: A new mutational basis for disease, in Wells RD, Warren ST (eds): *Genetic Instabilities and Hereditary Neurological Disorders*. New York, Academic Press, 1998, p 3.
332. Lalioti MD, Scott HS, Buresi C, Rossier C, Bottani A, Morris MA, Malafosse A, Antonarakis SE: Dodecamer repeat expansion in cystatin B gene in progressive myoclonus epilepsy. *Nature* **386**:847, 1997.
333. Fu Y-H, Kuhl DPA, Pizzuti A, Pieretti M, Sutcliffe JS, Richards S, Verkerk AJMH, et al: Variation of the CGG repeat at the fragile X site results in genetic instability: Resolution of Sherman paradox. *Cell* **67**:1047, 1991.
334. Knight SJL, Flannery AV, Hirst MC, Campbell L, Christodoulou Z, Phelps SR, Pointon J, et al: Trinucleotide repeat amplification and hypermethylation of a CpG island in FRAXE mental retardation. *Cell* **74**:127, 1993.
335. Brook JD, McCurrach ME, Harley HG, Buckler AJ, Church D, Aburatani H, Hunter K, et al: Molecular basis of myotonic dystrophy: Expansion of a trinucleotide (CTG) repeat at the 3′ end of a transcript encoding a protein kinase family member. *Cell* **68**:799, 1992.
336. La Spada AR, Wilson EM, Lubahn DB, Harding AE, Fischbeck KH: Androgen receptor gene mutations in X-linked spinal muscular atrophy. *Nature* **352**:77, 1991.

337. Huntington's Disease Collaborative Research Group: A novel gene containing a trinucleotide repeat that is expanded and unstable on Huntington's disease chromosomes. *Cell* **72**:971, 1993.
338. Koide R, Ikeuchi T, Onodera O, Tanaka H, Igarashi S, Endo K, Takahashi H, et al: Unstable expansion of CAG repeat in hereditary dentatorubral-pallidoluysian atrophy (DRPLA). *Nat Genet* **6**:9, 1994.
339. Orr HT, Chung MY, Banfi S, Kwiatkowski TJ, Servadio A, Beaudet AL, McCall AE, et al: Expansion of an unstable trinucleotide CAG repeat in spinocerebellar ataxia type 1. *Nat Genet* **4**:221, 1993.
340. Sanpei K, Takano H, Igarashi S, Sato T, Oyake M, Sasaki H, Wakisaka A, et al: Identification of the spinocerebellar ataxia type 2 gene using a direct identification of repeat expansion and cloning technique, DIRECT. *Nat Genet* **14**:277, 1996.
341. Kawaguchi Y, Okamoto T, Taniwaki M, Aizawa M, Inoue M, Katayama S, Kawakami H, et al: CAG expansions in a novel gene for Machado-Joseph disease at chromosome 14q32.1. *Nat Genet* **8**:221, 1994.
342. Zhuchenko O, Bailey J, Bonnen P, Ashizawa T, Stockton DW, Amos C, Dobyns WB, et al: Autosomal dominant cerebellar ataxia (SCA6) associated with small polyglutamine expansions in the alpha(1A)-voltage-dependent calcium channel. *Nat Genet* **15**:62, 1997.
343. David G, Abbas N, Stevanin G, Durr A, Yvert G, Cancel G, Weber C, et al: Cloning of the SCA7 gene reveals a highly unstable CAG repeat expansion. *Nat Genet* **17**:65, 1997.
344. Campuzano V, Montermini L, Molto MD, Pianese L, Cossée M, Cavalcanti F, Monros E, et al: Friedreich's ataxia: Autosomal recessive disease caused by an intronic GAA triplet repeat expansion. *Science* **271**:1423, 1996.
345. Muragaki Y, Mundlos S, Upton J, Olsen BR: Altered growth and branching patterns in synpolydactyly caused by mutations in HOXD13. *Science* **272**:548, 1996.
346. Brais B, Bouchard J-P, Xie Y-G, Rochefort DL, Chretien N, Tome FMS, Lafreniere RG, et al: Short GCG expansions in the PABP2 gene cause oculopharyngeal muscular dystrophy. *Nat Genet* **18**:164, 1998.
347. Pieretti M, Zhang R, Fu Y-H, Warren ST, Oostra BA, Caskey CT, Nelson DL: Absence of expression of the FMR-1 gene in fragile X syndrome. *Cell* **66**:817, 1991.
348. Oberlé I, Rousseau F, Heitz D, Kretz C, Devys D, Hanauer A, Bouú J, et al: Instability of a 550 base pair DNA segment and abnormal methylation in fragile X syndrome. *Science* **252**:1097, 1991.
349. Yu S, Pritchard M, Kremer E, Lynch M, Nancarrow J, Baker E, Holman K, et al: Fragile X genotype characterized by an unstable region of DNA. *Science* **252**:1179, 1991.
350. Verkerk AJMH, Pieretti M, Sutcliffe JS, Fu Y-H, Kuhl DPA, Pizzuti A, Reiner O, et al: Identification of a gene (FMR-1) containing a CGG repeat coincident with a breakpoint cluster region exhibiting length variation in fragile X syndrome. *Cell* **65**:905, 1991.
351. Kremer EJ, Pritchard M, Lynch M, Yu S, Holman K, Baker E, Warren ST, et al: Mapping of DNA instability at the fragile X to a trinucleotide repeat sequence p(CCG)n. *Science* **252**:1711, 1991.
352. Rousseau F, Heitz D, Biancalana V, Blumenfeld S, Kretz C, Boué J, Tommerup N, et al: Direct diagnosis by DNA analysis of the fragile X syndrome of mental retardation. *N Engl J Med* **325**:1673, 1991.
353. Hirst M, Knight S, Davies K, Cross G, Ocraft K, Raeburn S, Heeger S, et al: Prenatal diagnosis of fragile X syndrome. *Lancet* **338**:956, 1991.
354. Dobkin CS, Ding X-H, Jenkins EC, Krawczak MS, Brown WT, Goonewardena P, Willner WT, et al: Prenatal diagnosis of fragile X syndrome. *Lancet* **338**:957, 1991.
355. Pergolizzi RG, Erster SH, Goonewardena P, Brown WT: Detection of full fragile X mutation. *Lancet* **339**:271, 1992.
356. Yu S, Mulley J, Loesch D, Turner G, Donnelly A, Gedeon A, Hillen D, et al: Fragile-X syndrome: Unique genetics of the heritable unstable element. *Am J Hum Genet* **50**:968, 1992.
357. Harper PS, Harley HG, Reardon W, Shaw DJ: Anticipation in myotonic dystrophy: New light on an old problem. *Am J Hum Genet* **51**:10, 1992.
358. Harley HG, Brook JD, Rundel SA, Crow S, Reardon W, Buckler AJ, Harper PS, et al: Expansion of an unstable DNA region and phenotypic variation in myotonic dystrophy. *Nature* **355**:545, 1992.
359. Harley HG, Rundle SA, Reardon W, Myring J, Crow S, Brook JD, Harper PS, Shaw DJ: Unstable DNA sequence in myotonic dystrophy. *Lancet* **339**:1125, 1992.
360. Buxton J, Shelbourne P, Davies J, Jones C, van Tongeren T, Aslanidis C, de Jong P, et al: Detection of an unstable fragment of DNA specific to individuals with myotonic dystrophy. *Nature* **355**:547, 1992.
361. Fu Y-H, Pizzuti A, Fenwick RG, King J, Rajnarayan S, Dunne PW, Dubel J, et al: An unstable triplet repeat in a gene related to myotonic muscular dystrophy. *Science* **255**:1256, 1992.
362. Mahadevan M, Tsilfidis C, Sabourin L, Shutler G, Amemiya C, Jansen G, Neville C, et al: Myotonic dystrophy mutation: An unstable CTG repeat in the 3′ untranslated region of the gene. *Science* **255**:1253, 1992.
363. Tsilfidis C, Mackenzie AE, Mrttler G, Barcel3/4 J, Korneluk RG: Correlation between CTG trinucleotide repeat length and frequency of severe congenital myotonic dystrophy. *Nat Genet* **1**:192, 1992.
364. Shelbourne P, Winquist R, Kunert E, Davies J, Leisti J, Thiele H, Bachmann H, et al: Unstable DNA may be responsible for the incomplete penetrance of the myotonic dystrophy phenotype. *Hum Mol Genet* **1**:467, 1992.
365. Filla A, de Michele G, Cavalcanti F, Pianese L, Monticelli A, Campanella G, Cocozza S: The relationship between trinucleotide (GAA) repeat length and clinical features in Friedreich ataxia. *Am J Hum Genet* **59**:554, 1996.
366. Koutnikova H, Campuzano V, Foury F, Dolle P, Cazzalini O, Koenig M: Studies of human, mouse and yeast homologues indicate a mitochondrial function for frataxin. *Nat Genet* **16**:345, 1997.
367. Goldberg YP, Nicholson DW, Rasper DM, Kalchman MA, Koide HB, Graham RK, Bromm M, et al: Cleavage of huntingtin by apopain, a proapoptotic cysteine protease, is modulated by the polyglutamine tract. *Nat Genet* **13**:442, 1996.
368. Lalioti MD, Scott HS, Genton P, Grid D, Ouazzani R, M'Rabet A, Ibrahim S, et al: A PCR amplification method reveals instability of the dodecamer repeat in progressive myoclonus epilepsy (EPM1) and no correlation between the size of the repeat and age at onset. *Am J Hum Genet* **62**:842, 1998.
369. Sutherland GR, Haan EA, Kremer E, Lynch M, Pritchard M, Yu S, Richards RI: Hereditary unstable DNA: A new explanation for some old genetic questions? *Lancet* **338**:289, 1991.
370. Gordenin DA, Kunkel TA, Resnick MA: Repeat expansion: All in a flap? *Nat Genet* **16**:116, 1997.
371. Kinzler KW, Vogelstein B: Lessons from hereditary colorectal cancer. *Cell* **87**:159, 1996.
372. Papadopoulos N, Lindblom A: Molecular basis of HNPCC: Mutations of MMR genes. *Hum Mutat* **10**:89, 1997.
373. Markowitz S, et al: Inactivation of the type II TGF-beta receptor in colon cancer cells with microsatellite instability. *Science* **268**:1336, 1995.
374. Lu S-L, et al: Mutations of the transforming growth factor-beta type II receptor gene and genomic instability in hereditary nonpolyposis colorectal cancer. *Biochem Biophys Res Commun* **216**:452, 1995.
375. Parsons R, et al: Microsatellite instability and mutations of the transforming growth factor beta type II receptor gene in colorectal cancer. *Cancer Res* **55**:5548, 1995.
376. Yoshitaka T, et al: Mutations of E2F-4 trinucleotide repeats in colorectal cancer with microsatellite instability. *Biochem Biophys Res Commun* **227**:553, 1996.
377. Huang J, et al: APC mutations in colorectal tumors with mismatch repair deficiency. *Proc Natl Acad Sci USA* **93**:9049, 1996.
378. Souza RF, et al: Microsatellite instability in the insulin-like growth factor II receptor gene in gastrointestinal tumors. *Nat Genet* **14**:255, 1996.
379. Rampino N, et al: Somatic frameshift mutations in the BAX gene in colon cancers of the microsatellite mutator phenotype. *Science* **275**:967, 1997.
380. Perucho M: Microsatellite instability: The mutator that mutates the other mutator. *Nature Med* **2**:630, 1996.
381. Eshleman JR, et al: Increased mutation rate at the hprt locus accompanies microsatellite instability in colon cancer. *Oncogene* **10**:33, 1995.
382. Goellner GM, et al: Different mechanisms underlie DNA instability in Huntington disease and colorectal cancer. *Am J Hum Genet* **60**:879, 1997.
383. Laken SJ, et al: Familial colorectal cancer in Ashkenazim due to a hypermutable tract in APC. *Nat Genet* **17**:79, 1997.
384. Sommer S: Does cancer kill the individual and save the species? *Hum Mutat* **3**:166, 1994.

CHAPTER 14

Mouse Models of Human Genetic Disorders

William J. Craigen

1. **The mouse, as a prototypical mammal, has been the subject of systematic experimental investigation for the last century. An ever-enlarging number of mouse mutations exist that provide models for human genetic disorders, and the mouse has become an increasingly important tool for dissecting the molecular basis of common acquired disease states. The most frequently used approaches to modifying the mouse genome are microinjection of purified DNA and homologous recombination in embryonic stem cells.**
2. **The laboratory mouse provides a number of advantages as an experimental system. It is small and hence inexpensive to keep under well-controlled environmental conditions. Mice produce abundant offspring following a short gestation, allowing for large sample sizes, and there exist numerous inbred strains available for selective breeding strategies. The mouse shares many metabolic and developmental pathways with humans, and there are syntenic relationships over much of its genome that correspond to those of humans. Numerous reagents exist for gene mapping and identification, and because of historic interests, there are frequently multiple alleles at a given locus. Complex genetic interactions can be examined using selected compound alleles, double mutations, and strain-specific modifiers. Genetic mechanisms such as haploinsufficiency,[1] digenic inheritance,[2] and imprinting,[3,4] can be experimentally dissected in the mouse.**
3. **Mice can also be used as recipients for human tissues such as bone marrow, and can be genetically "humanized" via the introduction of human alleles, whether disease associated or conferring disease resistance. This may represent single genes or more recently large regions of DNA, and even chromosomal fragments. The development of standardized behavioral testing and an ever-expanding understanding of mouse behavior has provided a means for defining the genetic and molecular basis of learning and memory, an increasingly achievable goal for the future. The mouse is also a unique resource for the development of phenotype driven genetic screens for mutant genes when mutagenesis is coupled to a standardized battery of assessments such as behavioral, sensory, biochemical, and physiological testing.**

Genetically defined mice may serve three purposes: as an experimental system for delineating normal development and biologic function; as a model system for analyzing the molecular basis for human disorders; and a means for testing preclinical therapeutic strategies or treatments. As an experimental organism, the mouse has been the subject of systematic study for almost a century. For experimental purposes, the mouse offers these advantages: small size, a short generation time, numerous offspring, complex behavior, and well-delineated biochemical and developmental pathways. Numerous genetic disorders of humans are also found in the mouse, and with the advent of experimental techniques capable of manipulating the mouse genome, virtually any genotypic equivalent of humans can be introduced into the mouse. Whether a spontaneous, viral, radiation, or chemically induced mutation, or, more recently, as a result of recombinant DNA approaches, these models of mammalian biology, in conjunction with advances in genetic and physical mapping of the mouse genome, have had a major impact on biomedical research, drug development, and the biologic sciences in general. This chapter reviews the existing mouse models of human single gene disorders.

HISTORICAL

The mouse has existed in a commensal relationship with humans for thousands of years. This relationship began in the Asian subcontinent, and as grain cultivation developed the mouse flourished due to its enormous reproductive capacity and ability to adapt to virtually any environment. The word *mouse* is derived from the Sanskrit *mush* (coming from the verb meaning *to steal*). The Egyptians of the Third Dynasty deified the cat, Bastet, in recognition of the cat's task in keeping rodents in check. In contrast, the mouse was deified in 1500 BC as Apollo smintheus, the mouse god of the Greek island of Tenedos. This is represented on coins minted from the time, with Apollo smintheus keeping mice on the nape of his neck.[5]

Chinese culture also has a long history of friendly relations with the mouse. Albino mice were used in religious ceremonies by Chinese priests thousands of years ago, and up until the present time every twelfth year is known as the year of the mouse (*shu nian*). In Japan, the mouse was portrayed as the messenger for the god of wealth, Daikoku. The Japanese were likely the first to maintain mutant strains of mice; fancy mice with multicolored coats and waltzing mice (those with vestibular dysfunction and twirling behavior) being represented in Japanese prints as early as 80 BC.[5]

As an experimental model organism, William Harvey (1578–1657) used the mouse in the study of comparative anatomy of vertebrates. Joseph Priestly (1733–1804), credited with discovering oxygen, used mice to demonstrate that plants in a sealed cylinder evolve oxygen that could sustain a respiring animal. Similarly, Antoine Lavoisier (1743–1794) used the mouse for studying the physiology of respiration.

Mouse fanciers of the eighteenth century bred mice primarily for unusual coat colors, and mutant mice with heritable traits such as *albino*, *pink-eyed dilution*, *chinchilla*, and *spotting* were identified and collected. Mice with these traits were given names such as creamy buffs, ruby eyed yellows, and white English sables, and were highly valued by collectors. A number of these strains serve as the basis for the modern laboratory mouse, now known to

A list of standard abbreviations is located immediately preceding the index in each volume. Additional abbreviations used in this chapter include: (ES) cells = embryonic stem cells; MGD = mouse genome database; RC = recombinant congenic; RI = recombinant inbred.

be primarily a mixture of *M. m. domesticus* and *M. m. musculus* subspecies.[6]

With the rediscovery of Mendel's laws of inheritance at the beginning of the twentieth century, biologists sought model organisms with which to test their validity. Bateson (1903) in England and Cuenot (1908) in France recognized that the quantitative variation in coat color found in fancy mice was a suitable tool to test Mendel's laws. William Castle at the Bussey Institute of Harvard University also recognized the value of the mouse and is credited, along with his many students, with developing modern inbred mouse strains. Clarence Cook Little, later the first director of The Jackson Laboratory, developed the first inbred strain DBA (d = *dilute*, b = *brown*, a = *nonagouti*). A major source of mice in these early experiments was the farm of Ms. Abbie Lathrop of Granbee, Massachusetts, an amateur animal breeder who, in collaboration with Leo Loeb at the University of Pennsylvania, provided early insights into the relationship of inbreeding and the development of mammary cancer in the mouse. Breeding experiments at the time, and for a number of decades to follow, were primarily designed to address the genetic component of cancer. The need for highly inbred strains of mice was recognized and exploited by a number of founding mouse geneticists for use in cancer experiments. These studies involved the use of serially transplanted tumors in the mouse and were designed to address the issues of transplant acceptance or rejection, in addition to the generation of inbred strains with varying susceptibility to spontaneous solid tumors or hematologic malignancies. Inbred strains are generated by carrying out at least 20 consecutive generations of brother/sister matings, and today the number of inbred strains approaches 500. In the 1940s, George Snell, while working at The Jackson Laboratory, developed several different strategies for inbreeding, giving rise to what was later termed congenic strains. These breeding strategies were designed to isolate specific loci that influence the acceptance of transplanted tissues by transferring a chromosomal segment carrying an identifiable locus from one inbred strain to a derivative strain via 10 or more successive backcross matings, selecting for the donor chromosome segment at each generation by use of a phenotypic trait, locus, or specific mutation.

An additional type of inbred strain known as a recombinant inbred (RI) strain was later developed. These strains are created by crossing two inbred strains of mice and then systematically inbreeding randomly selected pairs of the F2 generation. Genes from the initial inbred strains randomly assort and segregate, and thus become fixed in various combinations in the subsequent RI lines. RI strains have been useful in the study of polygenic disorders where multiple loci associated with the disease phenotypes partially segregate in the derivative RI lines. Another breeding strategy that is designed to more rapidly isolate loci of interest is termed recombinant congenic (RC) strains. To generate these strains, a limited number of backcrosses are carried out between a donor and recipient strain, followed by brother-sister matings. In this fashion, the individual strains carry a smaller fraction of the donor genome than that of RI stains, improving the likelihood that donor disease loci will be isolated from each other in the individual RC strains. The shortcomings common to these strategies is the time required to create the inbred stains, the limited number of strains that can be created, and the few family members of each resulting new strain.

The genealogy of inbred strains was recently summarized[7] and is available in tabular and poster form via the Internet (http://genetics.nature.com/mouse/). The rules and guidelines for gene nomenclature and a compilation of variant strains of mice is available in hard copy.[8]

MUTAGENESIS

Detailed reviews of prior strategies for mouse mutagenesis are available,[9,10] along with more recent mutagenesis strategies that take advantage of advances in chromosomal engineering.[11,12] A brief overview is provided here. In the early years of the twentieth century, only spontaneously arising mutations were available to investigators. These rare, visually identifiable mutations were the basis for the first linkage map in the mouse, consisting of two traits: *albino* and *pink-eyed dilution.*[13] Early investigators depended on spontaneous mutation rates in the mouse, which vary from 1 in 20,000 to 1 in 100,000 mutations per locus, and in the early years of mouse experimentation, the fear was voiced that all possible mutations had been identified.[5] Some of the earliest mutagenesis experiments involved the injection of carcinogens into high- and low-susceptibility strains of mice in order to induce additional somatic mutations and hence tumors. Subsequently, ionizing radiation, in the form of x-rays, gamma rays, or neutrons, were used to induce heritable mutations. Additionally, chemical mutagenesis with a variety of compounds has been performed using several breeding strategies. Ionizing radiation typically causes double-strand breaks in chromosomes, leading to deletions, translocations, and other large-scale chromosomal rearrangements. The frequency of mutations arising from ionizing radiation varies with the dosage and frequency of radiation exposure. Similarly, because wild-type breeder males are typically the recipients of the mutagen, mutations induced by chemicals depend on the specific chemical used, the dose, and the timing of mutagenesis with regard to male reproductive development. Chemical mutagenesis commonly leads to point mutations or other small DNA lesions, depending upon the nature of the mutagen and timing of administration.

Historically, two groups have carried large-scale mutagenesis programs; the Medical Research Council Radiobiological Research Unit at Harwell, England, and the Oak Ridge National Laboratory at Oak Ridge, Tennessee. The specific locus test, first developed at Oak Ridge National Laboratory and described in 1951, was used to analyze both the frequency of mutations at specific loci and the types of mutations. Seven loci were selected based upon fully penetrant recessive mutant phenotypes that are easily identifiable, not lethal, and do not interfere with fertility in the homozygous state. Typically, a mutagenized male mouse was mated to females that harbored homozygous recessive alleles at the seven test loci. The loci employed were *agouti* (*a*) *brown* (*b*; presently termed Tyrp1) *albino* (*c*; Tyr), *dilute* (*d*; Myo5a), *short ear* (*se*; Bmp5), *pink-eyed dilution* (*p*), and *piebald spotting* (*s*; Ednrb). Using this test system, the frequency of mutations at each locus could be determined based upon the appearance of the phenotype(s) in the offspring of the mutagenized male. In addition, this led to the generation of a large series of experimentally useful alleles at each locus.

More recent advances in mutagenesis involve the use of recombinant DNA techniques. Although other approaches such as viral mutagenesis and gene trapping have been used to create mutant strains,[14] two DNA-based general strategies have been widely exploited: transgenesis via injected DNA and homologous recombination in embryonic stem cells.[15] These approaches are shown schematically in Fig. 14-1.

The injection of purified recombinant DNA into the male pronucleus of fertilized oocytes can lead to the efficient incorporation of the DNA into the somatic tissues and germ line of the mouse. With the availability of enormous numbers of gene sequences in the form of expressed sequences tags (currently greater than 350,000 exist from the mouse[16]), in the near future virtually all genes in the form of cDNAs will be available for introduction into the mouse. Usually multiple copies of the introduced DNA sequences integrate randomly, often inducing rearrangements of host DNA at the integration site. In this manner, a large number of gene sequences have been introduced into the mouse, typically leading to the expression of normal or mutant proteins. Furthermore, insertional mutagenesis may be associated with the integration event, leading to a variety of phenotypes incidental to the injected DNA. These insertional mutations can lead to significant prenatal lethality in the resulting recombinant strains, generally as an autosomal recessive trait.

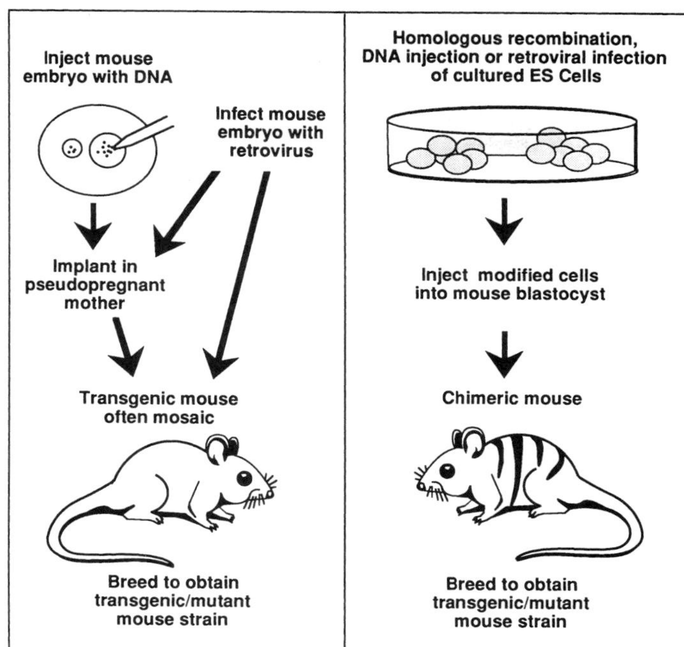

Fig. 14-1 Various strategies for producing transgenic and mutant mice. DNA can be injected into the male pronucleus of fertilized mouse eggs, followed by implantation in pseudopregnant mothers. Mouse embryos can be infected with retroviruses in vivo or in vitro. Transgenic mice may be mosaic, but the transgene can be recovered in nonmosaic form in the offspring of these mice. These strategies are depicted on the left. On the right, cultured embryonic stem (ES) cells can be modified by homologous or nonhomologous recombination or by retroviral infection. The modified cells can be selected and injected into a mouse blastocyst to produce a chimeric mouse, with subsequent recovery of the mutation in the germ line of the offspring of the chimeric mouse. (*From Beaudet AL: Harrison's Principles of Internal Medicine, 12th ed. New York, McGraw-Hill, 1994, p 349. Used by permission.*)

Additional benefits of microinjected DNA include multiple copies of the gene in question, alternatively regulated gene expression under the control of heterologous transcriptional control elements, the introduction of dominant negative or gain of function mutations, and, more recently, the introduction of large DNA fragments such as those contained within bacterial or yeast artificial chromosomes (BACs and YACs) or bacteriophage P1 clones. This latter approach has the benefit of potentially containing regulatory elements that are distant from the coding region of the gene, and the copy number of the introduced large fragment is typically lower. The use of large DNA fragments can also be valuable in localizing specific genes by complementing a mutant mouse phenotype by use of ever-smaller fragments derived from a candidate region. This approach to gene identification takes advantage of the numerous YAC, BAC, and cosmid contigs that have been developed throughout the mouse and human genomes. Furthermore, microcell-mediated chromosome transfer of transmissible human chromosome fragments into mice has been reported, further increasing the size of the human sequences that can be propagated in the mouse.[17]

Finally, microinjection techniques also allow for the cross-species expression of various genes and transcriptional control elements, thus allowing for the identification and analysis of evolutionary conserved genomic elements. For example, the appropriate induction of a *Drosophila* enhancer element in the central nervous system of transgenic mice reflects the remarkable conservation of transcriptional control elements across the animal kingdom.[18]

However, there are potentially significant limitations to this approach in the analysis of gene expression or the generation of disease models. Frequently, the introduced DNA lacks important transcriptional regulatory elements that may be located at a considerable distance from the coding region of the gene in question. This may lead to ectopic expression of the gene, low or excessively high levels of gene transcription, or simply unregulated gene expression. Integration into a transcriptionally silent locus may block expression, or positional effects at the integration site may perturb the expression of surrounding host genes.

The development of homologous recombination in mouse embryonic stem cells (ES cells) represents a major advance in the ability to manipulate the mouse genome. This technology, frequently termed gene knockouts or gene targeting, has revolutionized the ability of mouse biologists to create accurate models of human disease in a rapid and reproducible fashion. A number of reviews of the experimental details of this general approach are available.[19–21] The desired mutation is first created via homologous recombination in ES cells using positive and negative drug selection. Upon injection into blastocytes or aggregation with dissociated morulae, the modified ES cells potentially contribute to all cell lineages in the resulting chimeric mice. All types of mutations can potentially be introduced in this manner, including loss-of-function, dominant-negative, or gain-of-function alleles. These may represent deletions, specific point mutations, or, more recently, complex chromosomal rearrangements such as balanced or unbalanced translocations, large deletions, duplications, or inversions.[22,23] When genetically modified ES cells are incorporated into the germ line of the chimeric mouse, the mutant allele can then be transmitted to subsequent offspring in a Mendelian fashion. More recently, to overcome induced lethality or address tissue-specific expression, the use of conditional alleles via the introduction of recombination elements into a locus, for example, the loxP sites recognized by the Cre DNA recombinase of bacteriophage P1, has been achieved.[24] Using tissue-specific expression of Cre an investigator can specifically modify or eliminate the expression of a gene in specific tissues or at selected times during development or postnatal life. An alternative approach to understanding gene function is to introduce subtly altered genes back into the native genomic locus, an approach frequently referred to as a *knockin*. In this manner, an investigator can replace a gene with its homologue, introduce a specific point mutation, place a reporter gene into the locus of interest, or generate chimeric gene products that incorporate elements of one gene with another.

Incorporation of the ES cell genome in the germ cells of the chimera is typically monitored by transmission of a coat-color phenotype to offspring. A commonly used ES cell strain is the 129/Sv strain that contains the wild-type alleles of the *albino* (*c*), *pink-eyed dilution* (*p*), and *agouti* (*a*) coat-color loci. The recipient blastocysts, typically C57BL/6, carry a recessive (*a/a,* black) coat color, and thus any agouti pups produced by chimeric mice are derived from the microinjected ES cells. For autosomal loci, 50 percent of agouti pups will carry the allele of interest. Because the strain background may have significant effects on the observed phenotype, backcrossing the mutagenized strain to other inbred strains is frequently carried out.

Several instructive examples of significant background effects have been observed. For example, upon introduction of a null mutation at the transforming growth factor β 1 locus, the phenotype was noted to vary considerably with the strain background, from peri-implantation to juvenile lethality. The strain-specific background effect provides an opportunity to identify modifier loci, and in this case, a significant modifier has been mapped to mouse chromosome 5.[25] A similar effect has been identified in conjunction with a mutation at the adenomatous polyposis coli (*Apc*) locus, originally identified in a chemical mutagenesis screen as *Min* (multiple intestinal neoplasias) due to chronic anemia from intestinal blood loss.[26] Selective breeding in association with linkage mapping has identified a locus *Mom1* (modifier of *Min*) that quantitatively influences the number of tumors observed in the original strain. The modifier, more correctly a quantitative trait locus, has been mapped and identified by positional cloning strategies, and encodes a secreted phospholipase (Pla2g2a).[27] This general strategy promises to identify numerous genes that determine genetic contributions to the severity of disease.

Although a large number of mouse models of human genetic disease have been and undoubtedly will continue to be generated, to date the majority of targeted mutations are null alleles, generally due to the deletion of significant portions of the gene of interest. Mutations identified in humans and those that arise spontaneously in the mouse are often missense mutations, frequently with different genetic behavior and mechanisms of action than that of null alleles. However, increasingly, particular specific mutations have been introduced into the mouse genome, often with the desired effect of recapitulating the pathogenetic mechanisms observed in humans. An informative example is that of achondroplasia, where the pathologic mutation of humans is almost invariably a single missense mutation at a CpG dinucleotide. In contrast, the initial mutation introduced into the mouse FGFR3 locus via gene targeting was a loss-of-function deletion that leads to an overgrowth phenotype in the mouse, reflecting the lack of the growth suppressing effect of FGFR3 in long-bone growth. When the specific human mutation was introduced into the mouse, leading to inappropriate activation of the receptor and a gain-of-function effect, the resulting mice were dwarfed, with histologic features seen in humans with achondroplasia.[28]

The accuracy of mouse models of human disease is dependent on many factors, including similarity of the pathway in question, biomechanical factors, the time line of pathology, and the sensitivity of the mouse to the introduced perturbation; for example, the behavioral effects on the mouse of a gene mutation that leads to mild mental retardation in humans may be quite subtle. An additional issue that has only recently been addressed is the conservation of developmental gene expression, both temporal and spatial, in part due to the limited availability of human embryos for comparison. Examples of significant differences in developmental gene expression have recently been described,[29] suggesting there may be considerable differences in development that may significantly affect the conclusions that can be drawn from cross-species comparisons. This should not be surprising, in that despite the remarkable sequence conservation of many developmentally critical genes, all of mouse embryonic development is compressed into a 21-day gestation, in contrast to the 270-day gestation of humans.

The following sections review selected examples of mouse mutations that provide insights into mechanisms of inherited diseases, the strengths and weaknesses of using the mouse as a model system, and possible future directions in the use of the mouse. The reader is provided a more comprehensive, although likely not exhaustive, list of mouse models in Table 14-1, along with the corresponding MIM number, the approved designation for the corresponding mouse locus, and representative references. Models of polygenic disorders have been reviewed elsewhere.[30] Useful Internet sites are listed in Table 14-2.

INTERMEDIARY METABOLISM

The understanding of carbohydrate metabolism, particularly glucose metabolism, has been advanced significantly by the use of mouse models. Selectively bred strains such as the nonobese diabetic mouse (*nod*), in conjunction with subsequent recombinant inbred strains, have been used to identify a large number of loci contributing to this mouse model of insulin dependent diabetes.[31] In addition to specifically engineered mice, spontaneously arising mouse models with monogenic traits such as the *obese* (*ob*) or *diabetic* (*db*) mouse, caused by mutation of the leptin gene and its receptor, respectively, have similarly provided enormous insights into neurohormonal regulation of body mass and appetite. The identification of these genes led to successful searches for humans with similar genetic lesions.[32,33] Targeted disruption of the insulin receptor (Chap 68) leads to a mouse with features similar to humans heterozygous for insulin receptor mutations.[34] Mice harboring a mutation at the hexokinase type 4 (glucokinase) locus (Chap. 67) recapitulate many features found in humans with maturity onset with diabetes of the young (MODY2).[35] Likewise, humans with mutations in the glucose transporter GLUT2 suffer from the autosomal recessive disorder Fanconi-Bickel syndrome, exhibiting fasting hypoglycemia and postprandial hyperglycemia,[36] features observed in the comparable mouse model,[37] in which an alternative route of hepatic glucose release independent of GLUT2 has been demonstrated.[38] A mouse model of glycogen storage disease type 1A (Chap. 71) due to a targeted null mutation at the glucose-6-phosphatase locus provides an excellent model for the human disease, with the mouse exhibiting fasting hypoglycemia, hyperlipidemia, and glycogen storage.[39] Similarly, a mouse model of Pompe disease (GSD type 2), exhibits accumulation of glycogen from birth, along with cardiomyopathy and electrocardiographic abnormalities similar to those seen in affected humans; however, unlike humans with infantile Pompe disease (Chap. 135), the mouse survives to adulthood.[40] The results of mutations in a number of genes involved in glucose metabolism, many without human counterparts, have recently been summarized.[41]

A mouse model of classic galactosemia has been generated by gene targeting and exhibits several biochemical features seen in the human condition (Chap. 72), including elevated galactose and galactose-1-phosphate concentrations in blood and tissues, yet does not demonstrate the pathologic disturbances seen in humans. Specifically, there is no hepatic dysfunction, renal tubular dysfunction, or cataract formation.[42] The galactosemic mouse provides an example of subtle differences in metabolic pathways between mice and humans. This may be in part due to reduced activity of aldose reductase and a failure to accumulate galactitol in the mouse.

Mouse models of disorders of amino acid metabolism abound. A number of mouse strains exhibiting hyperphenylalaninemia (Chap. 77) have been recovered from chemical mutagenesis screens.[43] Several alleles at the phenylalanine hydroxylase locus have been identified, ranging in severity from mild to severe hyperphenylalaninemia[44,45] These mouse models have served as excellent model systems to develop enzyme[46] and gene replacement therapy,[47] and, in addition, have been useful as a model for cardiovascular defects associated with maternal hyperphenylalaninemia.[48] Abnormalities in neurotransmitter receptors observed in affected mice may in part explain the mental retardation associated with untreated disease.[49] Likewise, hyperphenylalaninemia associated with a defect in biopterin metabolism (Chap. 78), specifically GTP cyclohydrolase 1 activity, has been identified following a chemical mutagenesis screen.[50] This mouse potentially provides both a recessive model for "malignant" PKU and a dominant model for dopa-responsive dystonia.[51]

Table 14-1 Mouse Models of Human Genetic Disorders

Human disease	MIM #	Enzyme deficiency/ gene name	Mouse gene symbol	Mouse model*	Reference
		DISORDERS OF CARBOHYDRATE METABOLISM			
Fanconi-Bickel syndrome	227810	GLUT2; Glucose transporter	*Slc2a2*	K	38
Galactosemia	230400	Galactose 1 phosphate uridyltransferase	*Galt*	K	42
Glycogen storage disease IA	232200	Glucose 6 phosphatase	*C6pc*	K	39
Glycogen storage disease II (Pompe disease)	232300	Acid alpha glucosidase	*Gaa*	K	40, 268
Hyperglycerolemia	307030	Glycerol kinase	*Gyk*	K	63
Leprechaunism	246200	Insulin receptor	*Insr*	K	34
Maturity onset diabetes of the young type 2	125851	Glucokinase	*Gck*	K	35
Maturity onset diabetes of the young type 3	600496	Hepatocyte nuclear factor-1-alpha	*Tcf1*	K	269
Muscle glycogenosis, X-linked	311870	Phosphorylase kinase, alpha subunit	*Phk*	S	270
Peroxisome proliferator-activated receptor gamma deficiency	601487	Peroxisome proliferator-activated receptor gamma (PPAR γ)	*Pparg*	K	271, 272
Persistant hyperinsulinemic hypoglycemia of infancy	601820	KIR6.2; inwardly rectifying K^+ channel	*Kcnj11*	K	273
		DISORDERS OF AMINO ACID METABOLISM			
Alkaptonuria	203500	Homogentisate 1,2-dioxygenase	*Hgd^{aku}*	C	274, 275
Argininosuccinic aciduria	207900	Argininosuccinate lyase	*Asl*	K	
Carbamoylphosphate synthetase deficiency	237300	Carbamoylphosphate synthetase I	*Cps1*	K	59
Citrullinemia	215700	Argininosuccinate synthetase	*Ass1*	K	62
Dihydrolipoamide dehydrogenase deficiency	246900	Dihydrolipoamide dehydrogenase (E3)	*Dtd*	K	64
Hartnup disorder	234500	Neutral amino acid transport	*Hph2*	C	276, 277
Hereditary progressive dystonia with marked diurnal variation; PKU, atypical severe	128230; 233910	GTP cyclohydrolase I	*Hphl*	C	51, 50
Homocystinuria	236200	Cystathionine beta-synthase	*Cbs*	K	278
3-Hydroxy-3-methylglutaryl CoA lyase deficiency	246450	3-Hydroxy-3-methylglutaryl CoA lyase	*Hmgcl*	K	66
Hyperprolinemia type 1	239500	Proline dehydrogenase	*Prodh*	C	56
Hyperprolinemia and Gyrate atrophy	258870	Ornithine aminotransferase	*Oat*	K	57
OTC deficiency	311250	Ornithine transcarbamylase	*Otc^{spf}*	S	60, 279
Phenylketonuria	261600	Phenylalanine hydroxylase	*Pah*	C	44, 45, 47, 48
Tyrosinemia, type I	276700	Fumarylacetoacetate hydroxylase	*Fah*	K, R	52–54
Tyrosinemia type III	276710	hydroxyphenylpyruvate dioxygenase	*Hpd*	C	55
		DISORDERS OF BETA OXIDATION			
LCAD deficiency	201460	Long chain acylCoA dehydrogenase	*Acadl*	K	280
Primary carnitine deficiency	212140	Octn2 carnitine transporter	*Slc22a5*	S	69
SCAD deficiency	201470	Short chain acylCoA dehydrogenase	*Acads*	S	67
		DISORDERS OF LYSOSOMAL FUNCTION			
Aspartylglucosaminuria	208400	Aspartylglucosaminidase	*Aga*	K	104
Fabry disease	301500	Alpha galactosidase A	*Ags*	K	91
Galactosialidosis	256540	Protective protein for beta galactosidase and neuraminidase	*Ppgb*	K	94

(Continued on next page)

Table 14-1 (Continued)

Human disease	MIM #	Enzyme deficiency/ gene name	Mouse gene symbol	Mouse model*	Reference
Gaucher disease	230800	Glucocerebrosidase	*Gba*	K	88
G_{M1} gangliosidosis	230500	Beta Galactosidase	*Bgl*	K	93
Hurler Syndrome (MPS I)	252800	Alpha L-iduronidase	*Idua*	K	102
Krabbe disease	245200	Galactocerebrosidase	*Galc^{twi}*	S	96
Mannosidosis, alpha B	248500	Alpha mannosidase, lysosomal	*Man2b1*	K	90
Maroteaux-Lamy (MPS VI)	253200	Arylsulfatase B	*As1*	K	103
Metachromatic leukodystrophy	250100	Arylsulfatase A	*As2*	K	89
Neimann-Pick disease	257200	Acid Sphingomyelinase	*Smpd1*	K	87, 281
Neimann-Pick type C	257220	NPC1	*Npc1*	S	97
Sandhoff disease	268800	Hexosaminidase B	*Hexb*	K	85
Sialidosis	256550	Neuraminidase	*Neul*	S	98, 282
Sly disease (MPS VIII)	253220	Beta glucuronidase	*Gus^{mps}*	S	99, 100, 283
Tay-Sachs disease	272800	Hexosaminidase A	*Hexa*	K	84, 85
Tay-Sachs, AB Variant	272750	Hexosaminidase activator	*Gm2a*	K	86
Wolman disease/cholesterol ester storage disease	278000	Acid lipase	*Lip1*	K	95
		DISORDERS OF PURINE METABOLISM			
2,8-Dihydroxyadenine urolithiasis	102600	Adenine phosphoribosyl transferase	*Aprt*	K	75
Lesch-Nyhan syndrome	308000	Hypoxanthine guanine phosphoribosyl transferase	*Hprt*	K	73
		DISORDERS OF PEROXISOMAL FUNCTION			
Adrenal leukodystrophy	300100	ALDP	*Aldgh*	K	111, 284
Zellweger/cerebrohepatorenal syndrome	214100 170993	PXR1, PEX2	*Pxr1, Pxmp3*	K, K	109, 110
		DISORDERS OF NEURAL CREST			
Congenital central hypoventilation syndrome	209880	Ret proto-oncogene; Endothelin3; GDNF	*Ret, Edn3, Gdnf*	K	285, 286
Hirschprung disease	142623	Ret proto-oncogene; Endothelin converting enzyme 1	*Ret Ecel*	K	285, 287
Hirschprung disease; Waardenburg-Shah syndrome	142623; 277580	Endothelin receptor type B	*Endnrb^{s}*	C, K, R, S	288
Piebald trait	172800	Kit oncogene	*Kit^{w}*	C, R, S	289
Red hair color	266300	Melanocortin 1 receptor	*Mclr^{e}*	S	290, 291
Waardenburg-Shah syndrome	277580	Endothelin3	*Edn3^{ls}*	K, S	292
Waardenburg syndrome type 1 Klein-Waardenburg syndrome	193500 148820	Paired box gene 3 (Pax3)	*Pax3^{sp}*	R, S	293
Waardenburg syndrome type 2	193510	Microphthalmia-associated transcription factor	*Mitf^{mi}*	C, R, Tl, S	294
		DISORDERS OF HEARING AND VISION			
Aniridia type II	106210	Paired box gene 6 (Pax6)	*Pax6*	C, R, S	295
Autosomal recessive retinitis pigmentosa	180072	Phosphodiesterase, cGMP, rod receptor, beta	*Pdeb^{rdl}*	S	296
Branchio-oto-renal syndrome	113650	Eyes absent 1 homologue (Eya1)	Eya1	S	297
Cataract, Coppock-like	123660	Gamma E crystallin, pseudogene activation	*Cryge^{l}*	S, R	298
Cataract, congenital cerulean type 2	601547	Beta B2 crystallin	*Crybb2^{Phil}*	S	299
Cataract, zonular pulverulent 1	116200	gap junction protein alpha-8 connexin-50	*Gja8*	K	300
Cataract, zonular pulverulent 3	601885	gap junction protein alpha-3 connexin-46	*Gja3*	K	301
Choroideremia, X linked	303100	RAB geranylgeranyl transferase, component A	*Chm*	K	302
Cone-rod dystrophy 2	120970	CRX; cone-rod homeobox containing transcription factor	*Crx*	K	303

Table 14-1 (Continued)

Human disease	MIM #	Enzyme deficiency/ gene name	Mouse gene symbol	Mouse model*	Reference
Deafness, conductive, with stapes fixation (DFN3)	304400	POU3F4, POU domain transcription factor	*Pou3f4*	K	304
Deafness, neurosensory, autosomal dominant (DFNA13)	601868	Procollagen type XI, alpha 2	*Col11a2*	K	305
Deafness neurosensory, autosomal dominant (DFNA15)	602459	Pou4F3, POU domain transcription factor	*Pou4f3*	K	306
Deafness, neurosensory, autosomal recessive (DFNB1); autosomal dominant (DFNA3)	220290; 601544	gap junction protein beta-2; connexin-26	*Gjb2*	K	307
Deafness, neurosensory, autosomal recessive (DFNB3)	600316	Myosin XV	$Myol5^{sh2}$	S	308
Jervell and Lange-Nielsen syndrome	220400	KCNE1, potassium channel (also long QT syndrome)	*Kcne1*	K	309
Norrie disease	310600	Norrin	*Nd*	K	310
Oculocutaneous albinism type I	203100	Tyrosinase	Tyr^{c}	C, R, S, TE	311
Oculocutaneous albinism type II	203200	Pink-eyed dilution	*p*	C, R, S	312
Oculocutaneous albinism type III	203290	Tyrosinase related protein	$Typl^{b}$	C, R, S	313, 314
Optic nerve coloboma w/renal disease	120330	Paired box gene 2 (Pax2)	$Pax2^{Krd}$	TI	315, 316
Retinal degeneration, slow	179605	Peripherin 2	$Prph2^{Rd2}$	S	317
Retinitis pigmentosa-4	180380	Rhodopsin	*Rho*	K, TE	318, 319
Stargardt disease	248200	ATP-binding cassette transporter, Retina-specific; ABCR	*Abc10*	K	320
Usher syndrome type IB; DFNB2; DBNA11	276903; 600060; 601317	Myosin VIIA	$Myo7a^{sh1}$	C, S	321
		DISORDERS OF SKIN			
Atrichia with papular lesions, Alopecia universalis congenita	209500; 203655	Hairless, mouse homologue Zinc finger transcription factor	*Hr*	S	322, 323
Bullous erythroderma ichthyosiformis congenita	113800	Keratin complex-1, acidic, gene 10	*Krt1-10*	K, TE	324
Ectodermal dysplasia, X-linked	305100	Ectodysplasin-A (ED1) (Tabby)	Eda^{Ta}	S	191
Ectodermal dysplasia, autosomal (ED3)	129490	Tumor necrosis factor receptor homologue (Downless)	$Edar^{Dl}$	S	192, 193
Epidermolysis bullosa simplex	148066	Keratin complex-1, acidic, gene 14	*Krt1-14*	K, TE	325, 326
Epidermolysis bullosa simplex-limb girdle muscular dystrophy	226670	Plectin	*Plec1*	K	327
Hermansky-Pudlak syndrome	203300; 603401	Hps1; beta-3A-adaptin	*Ep* $Ap3b1^{pe}$	S, S	328–331
Nonepidermolytic palmoplantar keratoderma, Pachyonychia congenita	148067	Keratin complex-1, acidic, gene 16	*Krt1-16*	TE	332
Pilomatricoma	116806	Beta catenin	*Catnb*	K, TE	333–335
		DISORDERS OF SKELETON AND CONNECTIVE TISSUES			
Achondroplasia; Hypochondroplasia; Thanatophoric dwarfism	134934	Fibroblast growth factor receptor 3	*Fgfr3*	K	28, 220
Acrocephalopolysyndactyly type V (Pfeiffer syndrome)	101600	Fibroblast growth factor receptor 1	*Fgfr1*	K	336, 337
Chondrodysplasia punctata, X-linked dominant	302960	delta 8-delta 7 sterol isomerase (tattered)	*Td*	R	338
Cleidocranial dysplasia	119600	Core binding factor 1 (CBFA1)	*Cbfa1*	R	339, 340
Craniosynostosis type 2	123101	Homeo box; msh-like 2	*Msx2*	TE	341
Crouzon syndrome	123500	Fibroblast growth factor receptor 2	*Fgfr2*	K	342
Ehlers-Danlos type 1	130000	Procollagen type 5, Alpha 2	*Col5a2*	K	343
Elhers-Danlos type IV	130050	Procollagen type 3, Alpha 1	*Col3a1*	K	344

(Continued on next page)

Table 14-1 (Continued)

Human disease	MIM #	Enzyme deficiency/ gene name	Mouse gene symbol	Mouse model*	Reference
Greig cephalopolysyndactyly syndrome; Pallister-Hall syndrome	175700; 146510	GLI-Kruppel family member 3; GLI3 (extra toes)	*Gli3*^{Xt}	R, S	345–347
Hand-foot-genital syndrome	140000	Homeobox A13	*Hoxa13*^{hd}	S	348
Hypophosphatasia	171760	Alkaline phosphatase-2, liver	*Akp*^{2}	K	349
Keutel syndrome	245150	Matrix gamma-carboxyglutamate (Gla) protein	*Mglap*	K	350
Limb-mammary syndrome; Ectodactyly, ectodermal dysplasia, clefting (EEC)	603543	Tumor protein p63; p53 homologue (KET)	*Ket*	K	351
Marfan syndrome	154700	Fibrillin	*Fbn1*^{Tsk}	S	222, 352–354
Multiple epiphyseal dysplasia 2	600204	Procollagen type 9, Alpha 1	*Col9a1*	K, TE	355
Nail patella syndrome	161200	LIM homeodomain protein LMX1B	*Lmx1b*	K	356, 357
Oligodontia, autosomal dominant	313500; 167416	Paired box gene 9 (Pax9)	*Pax9*	K	358, 359
Osteopetrosis with renal tubular acidosis/Marble brain disease	259730	Carbonic anhydrase type II	*Car2*	C	360, 361
Osteogenesis imperfecta; Elhers-Danlos type VII	130060; 166200	Procollagen type 1, Alpha 1	*Colal*^{Mov13}	K, R, TE	221, 362
Osteogenesis imperfecta; Ehlers-Danlos type VII	130060; 166200	Procollagen type 1, Alpha 2	*Colla2*^{oim}	S	363
Pycnodysostosis	265800	Cathepsin K	*Ctsk*	K	364
Saethre-Chotzen Syndrome	101400	TWIST; bHLH transcription factor	*Twist*	K	365
Schmid metaphyseal chondrodysplasia	156500	Procollagen type 10, Alpha 1	*Col10a1*	K, TE	366
Split hand/foot malformation (SHFM3)	600095	Dactylin; ubiquitin ligase subunit	*Dac*	S	367
Spondyloepimetaphyseal dysplasia, pakistani type	603005	ATPSK2; sulfurylase/kinase	*Papss2*^{bm}	S	368
Spondyloepiphyseal dysplasia; Achondrogenesis type 2; Spondyloepimetaphyseal dysplasia	183900; 200610; 184250	Procollagen type 2, Alpha 1	*Col2a1*	K, TE	369, 370
Stickler syndrome type II	184840	Procollagen type 11, Alpha 1	*Col11a1*^{cho}	K, S	371
Syndactyly type II	186000	Homeobox D13	*Hoxd13*	S	372, 373
X-linked hypophosphatemia	307800	Phosphate regulating endopeptidase homologue	*Hyp1*	R	374
DISORDERS OF BLOOD ELEMENTS					
Acute intermittent porphyria	176000	Porphobilinogen deaminase	*Pbgd*	K	126, 127
Afibrinogenemia	202400	Fibrinogen-alpha, -beta or -gamma	*Fga* *Fgb Fgg*	K	375
Agranulocytosis, infantile genetic (Kostmann disease)	202700	Granulocyte colony stimulating factor receptor	*Csf3r*	K	376, 377
Alpha-thalassemia	141800	Hemoglobin alpha gene cluster	*Hba*	C, K, R	378
Autoimmune lymphoproliferative syndrome	134637	Fas antigen	*Fas*^{Lpr}	S	209, 210, 379
Beta-thalassemia	141900	Hemoglobin beta gene cluster	*Hbb*	C, K	380
Chediak-Higashi syndrome	214500	Lysosomal trafficking regulator	*Lyst*^{bg}	S	207
Chronic granulomatous disease, X-linked	306400	Cytochrome b-245, beta polypeptide	*Cybb*	K	204
Chronic granulomatous disease, autosomal recessive	233700	Neutrophil cytosolic factor 1; P47-Phox	*Ncf1*	K	205, 381
Colton blood group deficiency	110450	Aquaporin 1; water channel	*Aqp1*	K	216, 217
Complement component 1q deficiency	120550	C1q alpha subunit	*C1q*	K	382
Complement component 2 deficiency	217000	C2	*C2*	K	383
Complement component 3 deficiency	120700	C3	*C3*	K	384
Complement component 4 deficiency	120820	C4	*C4*	K	385

Table 14-1 (Continued)

Human disease	MIM #	Enzyme deficiency/ gene name	Mouse gene symbol	Mouse model*	Reference
Complement component 5 deficiency	120900	C5	*C5*	S	386
Complement component 8 deficiency type II	120960	C8, beta subunit	*C8b*	S	387
Complement component properdin factor B deficiency	138470	Factor B; Bf C3 proactivator	*H2-Bf*	K	383
Elliptocytosis-2	130600	Alpha-spectrin-1, erythroid	*Spna1^{sph}*	TI, S	388
Elliptocytosis-3	182870	Beta-spectin-1	*Spnb1^{ia}*	S	389
Erythropoietin protoporphyria	177000	Ferrochelatase	*Fech^{mIPas}*	C	124, 125
Erythropoietin receptor deficiency	133171	Erythropoietin receptor	*Epor*	K	390, 391
Factor II deficiency	176930	Factor II, prothrombin	*F2*	K	392
Factor V deficiency	227400	Factor V	*F5*	K	393
Factor VII deficiency	227500	Factor VII	*F7*	K	394
Factor XI deficiency	264900	Factor XI, plasma thromboplastin antecedent	*F11*	K	395
Familial atypical mycobacteriosis	209950	Interferon gamma receptor 1	*Ifngr*	K	396
Glanzmann thrombasthenia Type B	273800	Beta3-Integrin	*Itgb3*	K	397
Griscelli syndrome	214450	Myosin VA (*Dilute* locus)	*Myo5a*	S	398
Hemophilia A	306700	Coagulation factor VIII	*F8*	K	163, 399
Hemophilia B	306900	Coagulation factor IX	*F9*	K	400
Hereditary hemolytic anemia	177070	Erythrocyte protein band 4.2	*Epb4.2^{Pa}*	S	401
Hereditary spherocytosis	182900	Ankyrin 1, erythroid	*Ank1^{nb}*	S	168
Hyper-IgM immunodeficiency; common variable immunodeficiency	308230	CD40 ligand	*Cd401*	K	196, 197
Leukocyte adhesion deficiency, Type 1	116920	Beta 2-Integrin	*Itgb2*	K	402
Paroxysmal nocturnal hemoglobinuria	311770	Phosphotidylinositol glycan A	*Piga*	K	403
Plasminogen deficiency	173350	Plasminogen	*Plg*	K	404–406
Pyruvate kinase deficiency/Nonspherocytic hemolytic anemia	266200	Erythrocyte pyruvate kinase	*Pklr*	S	172, 407
Severe combined immunodeficiency	102700	Adenosine deaminase	*Ada*	K	80
Severe combined immunodeficiency, X-linked	300400	IL-2 receptor gamma chain	*I12rg*	K	201
Severe combined immunodeficiency, T-cell negative	600802	Janus kinase3; Jak3 protein kinase of STATs; Zeta chain associated protein 70 (ZAP70)	*Jak3*	K	408
Severe combined immunodeficiency, T-cell negative, NK positive	146661	IL-7 receptor alpha chain	*Il7r*	K	200, 409
Severe combined immunodeficiency, B-cell negative; Omenn syndrome	601457 603554	Recombination activating gene-1 (or 2)	*Rag1 Rag2*	K	410
Severe combined immunodeficiency, bare lymphocyte syndrome	209920	C2TA or RFX5; transcriptional factors of MHC class II expression	*C2ta*	K	411
Sickle cell anemia	141900	Hemoglobin beta gene cluster	*Hbb*	K + TE	176, 412
T-cell immunodeficiency, alopecia and nail dystrophy	601705	Winged helix nude (WHN); transcription factor	*Hfh11^{nu}*	S	Nature 398: 473, 1999; Nature 372: 103, 1994.
Thrombomodulin deficiency	188040	Thrombomodulin	*Thbd*	K	413, 414
Von Willebrand factor deficiency	193400	Von Willebrand factor	*Vwf*	S, K	165
Wiskott-Aldrich syndrome	301000	Wiskott-Aldrich syndrome protein (WASP)	*Wasp*	S	415
X-Linked agammaglobulinemia	300300	Bruton agammaglobulinemia tyrosine kinase	*Btk*	S, K	195

(Continued on next page)

Table 14-1 (Continued)

Human disease	MIM #	Enzyme deficiency/ gene name	Mouse gene symbol	Mouse model*	Reference
		DISORDERS OF LIPOPROTEIN METABOLISM			
Abetalipoproteinemia	200100	Microsomal triglyceride transfer protein	*Mttp*	K	116, 117
Apolipoprotein(a)	152200	Lipoprotein(a), Lp(a)	none	TE	416
Familial hypercholesterolemia	143890	Low density lipoprotein receptor	*Ldlr*	K, TE	417
Familial combined hyperlipidemia	144250	Unknown	*Hyplip 1*	S	418, 419
Hypoalphalipoproteinemia	107680	Apolipoprotein AI	*Apoa1*	K, TE	420
Hypobetalipoproteinemia	107730	Apolipoprotein B	*Apob*	K, TE	421, 422
Hepatic lipase deficiency	151670	Hepatic lipase	*Hpl*	K, TE	120, 423
Hyperlipoproteinemia type 1	238600	Lipoprotein lipase	*Lpl*	K, TE	119, 424
Hyperlipoproteinemia type III	107741	Apolipoprotein E	*Apoe*	K, TE	114, 256
Lecithin:cholesterol acyltransferase deficiency; Fish eye disease	245900	Lecithin:cholesterol acyltransferase	*Lcat*	K	121
		DISORDERS OF METAL METABOLISM			
Hereditary hemochromatosis	235200	HFE; HLA class 1 protein	*Hfe*	K	128
Menkes syndrome; Occipital horn syndrome	304150; 309400	ATPase, copper transporting, alpha polypeptide	$Atp7a^{Mo}$	C, R, S	129, 425, 426
Wilson Disease	277900	ATPase, copper transporting, beta polypeptide	$Atp7b^{tx}$	S	130
		NEUROMUSCULAR DISORDERS			
Congenital muscular dystrophy	156225	Laminin, alpha 2; Merosin	$Lama2^{dy}$	S	427–430
Dystrophia myotonica; myotonic dystrophy	160900	Dystrophin myotonica kinase, B15 (MDPK)	*Dm15*	K, TE	242, 243, 431
Fragile X syndrome	309550	Fragile X mental retardation syndrome 1	*Fmr1*	K	432
Hypokalemic periodic paralysis	170400	Calcium channel, L type, k 1A3 subunit	$Cana1s^{mdg}$	S	433
Kok disease, Hyperekplexia	149400	Glycine receptor, alpha 1 subunit	$Glra1^{spd}$	S	434, 435
Hyperthermia of anesthesia	145600	Ryanodine receptor 1, skeletal muscle	*Ryr1*	K	436
Limb-girdle muscular dystrophy type 2C	253700	Gamma sarcoglycan	*Sgcg*	K	437
Limb-gridle muscular dystrophy type 2D	600119	Alpha sarcoglycan	*Sgca*	K	438
Muscular dystrophy, Duchenne and Becker types	310200	Dystrophin, muscular dystrophy	Dma^{mdx}	C, S	439, 440
Myokymia with periodic ataxia	160120	KCNA1, voltage gated potassium channel	*Kcna1*	K	441
		NEURODEGENERATIVE DISORDERS			
Alzheimer disease	104300	Amyloid beta precursor protein; Presenilin 1 and Presenilin 2	*App* *Psen1* *Psen2*	K, TE	253, 442– 446
Amyloidosis V, amyloid cranial neuropathy with lattice corneal dystrophy	105120	Gelsolin	*Gsn*	K	447
Amyotrophic lateral sclerosis	162230	Neurofilament protein, heavy subunit	*Nfh*	TE	448, 449
Amyotrophic lateral sclerosis	105400	Superoxide dismutase-1, soluble	*Sod1*	K, TE	450
Ataxia telangiectasia	208900	Ataxia telangiectasia	*Atm*	K	451, 452
Charcot-Marie-Tooth neuropathy type 1A; hereditary neuropathy with liability to pressure palsy	118220; 162550	Peripheral myelin protein, 22 kDa	*Pmp22*	K, TE	453, 454
Charcot-Marie-Tooth neuropathy, type 1B, Dejerine-Sottas syndrome	118200 145900	Myelin protein zero	*Mpz*	K	455
Charcot-Marie-Tooth peroneal muscular atrophy, X-linked	302800	Gap junction protein beta 1; Connexin-32	*Gjb1*	K	456

Table 14-1 (Continued)

Human disease	MIM #	Enzyme deficiency/ gene name	Mouse gene symbol	Mouse model*	Reference
Congenital hypomyelinating neuropathy	129010	Krox20/EGR2 Transcription factor	*Egr2*	K	457
Congenital insensitivity to pain with anhidrosis	256800	NTRK1; neurotrophin receptor 1 (TrkA)	*Ntrk1*	K	458
Dentatorubral-pallidoluysian atrophy (DRPLA)	125370	Atrophin-1	*Drpla*	TE	459
Dopamine beta hydroxylase deficiency	223360	Dopamine beta hydroxylase	*Dbh*	K	460
Epilepsy, progressive myoclonus 1 (EPM1)	254800	Cystatin B	*Cstb*	K	461
Epilepsy, progressive with mental retardation	600143	CLN8	*mnd*	S	462
Familial fatal insomnia; Creutzfeldt-Jakob and Gerstmann-Straussler disease	176640	Prion protein	*Prnp*	K, TE	463–465
Familial hemiplegic migraine, Episodic ataxia type 2, Spinocerebellar ataxia type 6	141500; 108500; 183086	CNCNA1A, voltage dependent calcium channel	*Cacnala*	S	466
Huntington disease	143100	Huntingtin, IT15, Huntington disease gene homologue	*Hdh*	K, TE	467–472
Lissencephaly, isolated	601545	LIS1, platelet activating factor acetylhydrolase	*Pafah1b1*	K	473
Machado-Joseph disease	109150	Ataxin 3	*Mjd1*	TE	474
Monoamine oxidase A deficiency	309850	Monoamine oxidase A	*Maoa*	TI	475, 476
Neuronal ceroid lipofuscinosis, late infantile variant, CLN6	601780	Unknown	*Nclf*	S	477
Neuronal ceroid lipofuscinosis, juvenile, CLN3	204200	CLN3	*Cln3*	K	478, 479
Pelizaeus-Merzbacher disease; spastic paraplegia type 2	312080; 312920	Proteolipid protein	Plp^{jp}	K, TE, S	480
Spinal muscular atrophy 1	253300	Survival motor neuron 1 gene	*Smn*	K, TE	481, 482
Spinocerebellar ataxia type 1	164400	Ataxin-1	*Scal*	TE, K	483, 484
Tyrosine hydroxylase deficiency	191290	Tyrosine hydroxylase	*Th*	K	485
		HERITABLE CANCERS			
Adenomatous polyposis of the colon	175100	Adenomatous polyposis coli protein	Apc^{min}	C, K	486
Basal cell nevus syndrome (Gorlin syndrome)	109400	Patched, Drosophila homologue	*Ptch*	K	487
Bloom Syndrome	210900	BLM; RecQ helicase homologue	*Blm*	K	488
Breast cancer type 1	114480	Breast cancer 1 protein	*Brca1*	K	489
Breast cancer type 2	600185	Breast cancer 2 protein	*Brca2*	K	490
Cowden Syndrome; Bannayan-Zonana syndrome; Lhermitte-Duclos disease	158350; 153480	PTEN (phosphatase and tensin homologue)	*Pten*	K	491
Familial colon cancer, nonpolyposis type 1	120435	MutS (E. coli) homologue 2	*Msh2*	K	492, 493
Familial colon cancer, nonpolyposis type 2	120436	MutL (E. coli) homologue 1	*Mlh1*	K	494
Familial colon cancer, nonpolyposis type 3	600259	Postmeiotic segregation	*Pms2*	K	495
Familial retinoblastoma	180200	Retinoblastoma-1	*Rb1*	K	496
Fanconi anemia group C	227645	FAC	*Fancc*	K	497
Li-Fraumeni syndrome	151623	Transformation-related protein 53	*Trp53*	K, TE	498, 499
Malignant melanoma	155600	Cyclin dependent kinase inhibitor 2a; p161NK4a	*Cdkn2a*	K	500
Neurofibromatosis type I	162200	Neurofibromin	*Nf1*	K	501
Neurofibromatosis type II	101000	Merlin/Schwannomin	*Nf2*	K	502
Nijmegen breakage syndrome	251260	P95/Nibrin; RAD50 homologue	*Rad50*	K	503
Multiple endocrine neoplasia type 2; familial medullary thyroid carcinoma	171400 155240	Receptor tyrosine kinase	*Ret*	TE	504

(Continued on next page)

Table 14-1 (Continued)

Human disease	MIM #	Enzyme deficiency/ gene name	Mouse gene symbol	Mouse model*	Reference
Tuberous sclerosis	191092	Tuberin (TSC2)	*Tsc2*	K	505, 506
von Hippel-Lindau syndrome	193300	VHL protein	*Vhlh*	K	507
Werner syndrome	277700	WRN; RecQ helicase homologue	*Wrn*	K	508
Wilms tumor; Denys-Drash syndrome	194070; 194080	Wilms tumor homologue (WT1)	*Wt1*	K	509
Xeroderma pigmentosum group A	278700	XPA	*Xpa*	K	510
Xeroderma pigmentosum group C	278720	XPC	*Xpc*	K	511
Xeroderma pigmentosum group D; Trichothiodystrophy	278730	XPD	*Xpd*	K	512
Xeroderma pigmentosum group G	278780	XPG	*Xpg*	K	513
		DISORDERS OF ENDOCRINE FUNCTION			
Amyloidosis I, hyperthyroxinemia	176300	Transthyretin	*Ttr*	K	514–516
Apparent mineralocorticoid excess	218030	11 beta-hydroxysteroid dehydrogenase type 2	*Hsd11b2*	K	517
Aromatase deficiency	107910	Aromatase	*Cyp19*	K	147
Combined pituitary hormone deficiency	601538 173110	Prophet of Pit-1 (PROP1) Pit-1 (POU1F1)	$Prop1^{df}$ $pit1^{dw}$	S S	154, 518
Congenital adrenal hyperplasia	201910	21 hydroxylase	*Cyp21a1*	S	138, 139
Congenital lipoid adrenal hyperplasia	201710	Steroidogenic acute regulatory protein	*Star*	K	140
Deleted in azoospermia	400003	DAZ; RNA binding protein	*Dazl*	K	519
Dosage sensitive sex reversal/Adrenal hypoplasia congenita	300018; 300200	Dax1; transcription factor	*Ahch*	K	520
Estrogen resistance	133430	Estrogen receptor	*Esr*	K	521
Familial hypocalciuric hypercalcemia; neonatal severe hyperparathyroidism	145980; 239200	Calcium-sensing receptor	*Casr*	K	522
Follicle stimulating hormone, beta chain, deficiency	136530	Follicle stimulating hormone, beta chain	*Fshb*	K	523
Gitelman syndrome	263800	Thiazide sensitive Na/Cl cotransporter	*Slc12a3*	K	524
Glucocorticoid receptor deficiency	138040	Glucocorticoid receptor	*Grl1*	K, TE	525
Generalized resistance to thyroid hormone	188570	Thyroid hormone receptor, beta subunit	*Thrb*	S	526
Gonadal dysgenesis, XY female type, swyer syndrome	306100	SRY	*Tdy*	S	527
Gonadotropin releasing hormone deficiency	152760	Gonadotropin releasing hormone	$Gnrh^{hpg}$	S	528
Growth hormone deficiency	139191	Growth hormone releasing hormone receptor	$Ghrhr^{ht}$	S	156, 529, 530
Laron dwarfism	262500	Growth hormone receptor	*Ghbp*	K	158, 159
Obesity (autosomal dominant)	155541	Melanocortin-4 receptor	*Mc4r*	K	531–533
Obesity (autosomal recessive)	164160; 601007	Leptin; Leptin receptor	Lep^{ob} $Lepr^{db}$	S S	32,33,133
Pro-opiomelanocortin deficiency	176830	Pro-opiomelanocortin (POMC)	*Pomc*	K	534
Pseudohypoaldosteronism type 1, autosomal recessive	264350	Alpha subunit epithelial sodium transporter (ENaC)	*Scnnla*	K	535
Pseudohypoaldosteronism type 1, autosomal dominant	177735	Mineralocorticoid receptor	*Mlr*	K	152, 536
Pseudohypoparathyroidism type Ia	103580	Gsalpha; hormone signal transduction	*Gnas*	K	160–162
Septo-optic dysplasia	182230	Hesx1; paired-like homeobox protein	*Hesxl*	K	537
Steroidogenic factor-1 deficiency	184757	SF1; Fushi Tarazu factor, Drosophila homologue	*Ftzf1*	K	538

Table 14-1 (Continued)

Human disease	MIM #	Enzyme deficiency/ gene name	Mouse gene symbol	Mouse model*	Reference
Testicular feminization syndrome, Spinal and bulbar muscular atrophy (Kennedy disease)	313700; 313200	Androgen receptor	*Ar*^{Tfm}	S, TE	143–145
Unresponsiveness to thyrotropin	275200	Thyroid stimulating hormone receptor	*Tshr*^{hyt}	S	135
Vitamin D-resistant rickets with end-organ unresponsiveness	277440	Vitamin D receptor	*Vdr*	K	148, 149
		DEVELOPMENTAL DISORDERS			
Alagille syndrome	118450	Jagged-1; Notch ligand	*Jag1*	K	539
Angelman syndrome	105830	Ubiquitin conjugating enzyme E3A	*Ube3a*	K	250
Beckwith-Weidemann syndrome	130650	p57KIP2; cyclin-dependent kinase inhibitor	*Cdknlc*	K	540
Coffin-Lowry syndrome	303600	Rsk2; protein kinase	*Li*	R	541
CRASH syndrome	308840	Neural cell adhesion molecule L1	*L1cam*	K	542
Holoprosencephaly type 3	142945	Sonic Hedgehog	*Shh*	K	543
Oculocerebrorenal syndrome of Lowe	309000	Phosphatidylinositol 4,5-bisphosphate 5-phosphatase	*Ocrl*	K	237
Prader-Willi syndrome	176270	SNPRN-UBE3A deletion		K	544
Rubinstein-Taybi syndrome	180849	Creb binding protein; Transcriptional co-activator	*Crebbp*	K	545
Simpson dysmorphia syndrome	312870	Glypican 3	*Gpc3*	K	546
		DISORDERS OF CARDIOVASCULAR FUNCTION			
Cardiomyopathy, dilated II; Desmin related myopathy	125660; 601419	Desmin, intermediate filament	*Des*	K	547–549
Familial hypertrophic cardiomyopathy	192600; 160781; 160790; 115197; 115196	Beta cardiac myosin heavy chain (equivalent to the rodent alpha); Cardiac myosin light chain 2; Cardiac myosinch light chain 3; Cardiac troponin T2; Myosin binding protein C; Alpha tropomyosin	*Myhca* *Mylc2b* *Mylc* *Tnnt2* *Mybpc3* *Tpml*	K, TE	227, 228, 230, 232, 233, 550
Familial hypertrophic cardiomyopathy with WPW	600858, 191044	Troponin I, cardiac	*Tnni3*	K	231, 551
Hereditary hemorrhagic telangiectasia of Osler-Weber-Rendu	187300	Endoglin	*Eng*	K	552
Supravalvar aortic stenosis	185500	Elastin hemizygosity	*Eln*	K	553, 554
		DISORDERS OF HEPATIC FUNCTION			
Cholestasis, progressive familial intraheptic type 3	602347	Multiple drug resistance P-glycoprotein (MDR3)	*Mdr2*	K	555
		DISORDERS OF PULMONARY FUNCTION			
Alpha-I antitrypsin deficiency	107400	Alpha-I-antitrypsin; serine protease inhibitor	*Spil*	TE	556, 557
Cystic fibrosis	219700	Cystic fibrosis transmembrane conductance regulator homologue	*Cftr*	K	212, 213, 215, 558
Pulmonary alveolar proteinosis	265120	Surfactant protein B or GM-CSF receptor beta	*Sftpb* *Csf2rbl*	K	559–561
		DISORDERS OF RENAL STRUCTURES			
Alport syndrome, autosomal recessive	203780	Procollagen type 4, Alpha 3 and Alpha 4	*Col4a3* *Col4a4*	K, TI	562, 563
Polycystic kidney disease, autosomal dominant	173900	Polycystin-1 Polycystin-2	*Pkd1* *Pkd2*	K, K	564, 565
Polycystic kidney disease, autosomal recessive	263200	Unknown	*Pcy* *Cpk*	S	566, 567

*S = spontaneous mutation; C = chemical mutagenesis; K = knockout; TE/TI = transgenic expression or insertion; R = radiation-induced mutation. Specific alleles are indicated by superscript where relevant.

Table 14-2 Internet Resources for Mouse Research*

The Transgenic/Targeted Mutation Database(TBASE)	www.jax.org/tbase/
Database of Gene Knockouts	www.bioscience.org/knockout/knochome.htm
BioMedNet Mouse Knockout Database	http://biomednet.com/db/mkmd
UCD Medpath Transgenic Mouse Searcher 2.0	http://pathology.ucdavis.edu/tgmice/firststop.html
Transgenic Systems for Mutation Analysis — BigBlue and MutaMouse	http://eden.ceh.uvic.ca/bigblue.htm
Biology of the Mammary Gland Database	http://mammary.nih.gov/tools/molecular/tet/slides/tetop-SV40T_html
Skarnes Laboratory Resource of Gene Trap Insertions	http://socrates.berkeley.edu/~skarnes/resource.html
The Genome Database (GDB)	http://gdbwww.gdb.org
Online Mendelian Inheritance in Man (OMIM)	www3.ncbi.nlm.nih.gov/omim
The Mouse Genome Database (MGD)	www.informatics.jax.org/
The Encyclopedia of the Mouse Genome	www.informatics.jax.org/mgihome/encyclopedia/ecyclo.shtml
Induced Mutant Resources of the Jackson Laboratory (IMR)	http://lena.jax.org/resources/documents/imr/
The Portable Dictionary of the Mouse Genome	www.nervenet.or/main/dictionary.html
Genetic and Physical Maps of the Mouse Genome (MIT)	www-genome.wi.mit.edu/cgi-bin/mouse/index
The European Collaborative Interspecific Mouse Backcross (EUCIB)	www.hgmp.mrc.ac.uk/MBx/MBxHomepage.html
The Mouse Atlas Project	http://genex.hgu.mrc.ac.uk/
Gene Expression Database (GXD)	www.informatics.jax.org/menus/expression_menu.shtml
NCBI Human/Mouse Homology Relationships	www3.ncbi.nlm.nih.gov/Homology/
The Dysmorphic Human-Mouse Homology Database	www.hgmp.mrc.ac.uk/DHMHD/dysmorph.html
Whole Mouse Catalog	www.rodentia.com/WMC/
European Mouse Mutant Archive (EMMA)	www.emma,rm.cnr.it
MRC Chromosome Atlas Maps	www.mgu.har.mrc.ac.uk/genelist/atlasmaps.html
Trans-NIH Mouse Initiative	www.nih.gov/science/models/mouse/
NCBI Unigene: Mus musculus	www.ncbi.nlm.nih.gov/UniGene/Mm.Home.html
Online Mendelian Inheritance in Animals (OMIA)	www.angis.su.oz.au/Databases/BIRX/omia/omia_form.html
NetVet and the Electronic Zoo	http://netvet.wustl.edu/rodents.htm
Table of gene expression in the developing ear for multiple species	www.ihr.mrc.ac.uk/hereditary/genetable/index.html

*All active as of September 2000.

Hypertyrosinemia is also found in the mouse. The x-ray-induced lethal albino mouse derives its lethal phenotype from the concomitant loss of fumarylacetoacetate hydrolase as one component of a chromosomal deletion.[52,53] Lethality is also observed in the targeted disruption of the fumarylacetoacetate hydrolase locus that corresponds to tyrosinemia type 1 (Chap. 79). This engineered strain has proven an excellent model for gene replacement therapy and hepatic regeneration via hepatocyte transfer.[54] Similarly, a deficiency of hydroxyphenyl dioxygenase provides a model for a tyrosinemia type 3.[55]

The hyperprolinemic mouse (Pro/Re) provides a model for a deficiency of proline dehydrogenase (Chap. 81). In the homozygous state these animals exhibit a deficit in sensory-motor gating, accompanied by perturbations of regional brain neurochemistry. It has been speculated that this animal serves as a model for the psychiatric and behavioral phenotypes seen in some patients with velocardiofacial syndrome and the associated deletion of chromosome 22q11,[56] because the gene encoding proline dehydrogenase maps within the deletion interval.

The deficiency of ornithine aminotransferase (OAT) in humans leads to hyperornithinemia and a progressive retinal degeneration termed gyrate atrophy (Chap. 83). Targeted disruption of the *Oat* locus in the mouse leads to hyperornithinemia and hypoargininemia, and is associated with postnatal lethality that can be rescued by use of arginine supplementation until weaning. This suggests that in the newborn period OAT normally contributes ornithine to the arginine pool necessary for rapid protein synthesis, unlike in the adult where its absence leads to ornithine accumulation. Following arginine therapy, the mice subsequently develop a retinal degeneration comparable to that seen in humans.[57] The *Oat*-deficient mouse has also been used to demonstrate that the use of an arginine-restricted diet in adult mice prevents hyperornithinemia and retinal degeneration.[58]

Disorders of the urea cycle (Chap. 85) are well represented in the mouse. Carbamoylphosphate synthetase deficiency is comparably severe in humans and the mouse, leading to postnatal death from hyperammonemia.[59] In contrast, two spontaneous mouse models of ornithine transcarbamylase (OTC) deficiency, identified because of delayed maturation of fur (*sparse fur* and *ash*), stand as models for partial ornithine transcarbamylase deficiency.[60] These mouse strains have been the subject of considerable investigation as a model for OTC gene replacement therapy.[61] Deficiency of either argininosuccinate synthetase[62] or argininosuccinate lyase (VR Sutton and WJ Craigen, unpublished observations) by gene targeting leads to perinatal lethality comparable to that seen in humans with severe forms of these disorders. The contributions of these enzymes to the citrulline-nitric oxide pathway remain to be determined.

An interesting contrast in phenotypes is seen with mutations at the glycerol kinase (*Gyk*) locus. This X-linked trait in humans has broad phenotypic variability, ranging from asymptomatic adult males identified by the finding of pseudohypertriglyceridemia to critically ill newborns (Chap. 97). This variability is in part due to variability in the types of observed mutations, with some patients harboring large chromosomal deletions that may include the Duchenne muscular dystrophy locus and/or the adrenal hypoplasia congenita locus, and others with missense mutations in the glycerol kinase gene. In the mouse a null allele similar to that seen in humans carrying a deletion of this locus is uniformly lethal, with the mice exhibiting abnormal triglyceride synthesis, autonomous glucocorticoid synthesis, and altered gluconeogenesis.[63] The mouse should provide the means to examine the pathogenesis of the disorder in a tissue-specific manner, and will likely shed light on the relationship between glycerol and glucose metabolism.

Many of more common organic acidurias found in humans have not yet been generated in the mouse, in part because of the deleterious effects on development these disorders impose. For example, lipoamide dehydrogenase (E3) is a subunit of three distinct dehydrogenases: α-ketoglutarate, pyruvate, and branched chain ketoacid. Humans lacking E3 activity survive to term and exhibit signs and symptoms of the three enzyme-complex deficiencies during infancy, typically with elevations of lactate and branched chain amino acids. In contrast, E3 deficiency in the mouse leads to embryonic lethality,[64] perhaps reflecting the effects of homozygosity for a null allele, a genotype not yet reported in humans.[65] Similarly, 3-hydroxy-3-methylglutaryl CoA lyase deficiency (Chap. 93) in the mouse exhibits perigastrulation lethality, in contrast to the postnatal phenotype observed in humans.[66]

Interestingly, it was demonstrated that the inbred strain BALB/c lacks short chain acyl-CoA dehydrogenase (SCAD) activity,[67] with histologic and biochemical parameters consistent with the human condition (Chap. 101), yet the mice appear to exhibit no symptoms of the disorder. Primary carnitine deficiency in humans affects fatty acid β oxidation, typically presenting in early childhood with hypoglycemia and/or cardiomyopathy. The disorder was recently demonstrated to be caused by a deficiency of a plasma membrane carnitine transporter (OCTN2).[68] A mouse model previously termed Juvenile Visceral Steatosis (*Jvs)* was recently shown to be deficient for the mouse *Octn2* transporter.[69]

Although disorders of the mitochondrial respiratory chain are quite frequent in humans (Chap. 104), there is, to date, limited availability of mouse models of these disorders, in part due to the paucity of genotypic data in humans with Mendelian mitochondrial disorders. Additionally, because a significant fraction of patients harbor heteroplasmic mitochondrial DNA mutations, the inability to manipulate the mitochondrial genome in vivo constitutes a major hurdle in developing accurate animal models. Recently, studies of strain-specific heteroplasmy[70] and the introduction of heteroplasmic deleterious mutations into the mitochondrial genome[71] were described, the former providing insights into tissue-specific mitochondrial DNA segregation and the latter being a model for mitochondrial DNA point mutations. Thus, this area holds considerable promise. Although there is not yet a human equivalent, an excellent model for mitochondrial DNA depletion exists via the use of a conditional knockout of the mitochondrial transcription factor A. This has led to the generation of cardiac-specific mitochondrial DNA depletion by use of tissue-specific Cre expression.[72] The resulting phenotype of dilated cardiomyopathy and atrioventricular block reflects the importance of mitochondrial function in cardiac function. It can be expected that future efforts will be directed towards providing mouse models for specific mitochondrial DNA mutations, other disorders of nuclear and mitochondrial genome communication, and disorders of nuclear-encoded respiratory chain elements.

Several examples of disorders in purine metabolism exist in the mouse. Targeted disruption of the hypoxanthine-guanine phosphoribosyltransferase (HPRT) gene was an early metabolic model, generating a mutant mouse based on the ability to carry out in vitro selection for loss of HPRT activity in ES cells. Unlike the severe neurologic phenotype observed in humans with Lesch-Nyhan syndrome (Chap. 107), there is no significant disability observed in the mouse,[73] despite a reduction of striatal tyrosine hydroxylase activity and dopamine content.[74] In contrast, deficiency of adenosine phosphoribosyltransferase (APRT; Chap. 108) leads to the development of adenine-rich renal stones and progressive renal failure in the mouse, similar to the clinical features observed in humans.[75] There is conflicting information about mice deficient for both HPRT and APRT. It has been reported that HPRT-deficient mice administered an inhibitor of APRT developed self-injurious behavior.[73] In contrast, HPRT mice bred to APRT-deficient mice, leading to doubly deficient animals, have been reported with no significant neurologic morbidity.[76] The lack of urate oxidase activity in humans and some other primates is in contrast to activity present in rodents and a variety of other mammals. Mice engineered to be deficient in urate oxidase exhibit a severe nephropathic hyperuricemia.[77] Because mice do not accumulate uric acid in the absence of HPRT, the lack of a neurologic phenotype suggests that elevate concentrations of uric acid is important aspect to the pathogenesis. Despite the lack of a clear phenotype, HPRT-deficient mice have been useful in dissecting the requirements for the purine salvage pathway and transgenic mice in identifying tissue-specific transcriptional control elements.[78]

In another example of differences in purine metabolism between humans and mice, gene targeting of the adenosine deaminase (ADA) locus in the mouse leads to prenatal lethality,[79,80] in contrast to the postnatal immunodeficiency observed in the humans (Chap. 109). The mouse phenotype is due to a high placental requirement for ADA that is not present in humans, and ADA-deficient mice have been rescued by transgenic expression of ADA solely in the placenta using a placenta-specific transcription control element.[81,82] These animals can thus survive prenatal disease, allowing the development of a progressive lung disease that may be related to excessive stimulation of adenosine receptors in the lung,[83] yet can be maintained to adulthood by the provision of weekly injections of polyethylene glycol-conjugated purified enzyme, originally developed for the treatment of ADA-deficient humans. Low doses are sufficient to correct the pulmonary insufficiency, whereas a tenfold greater dose is needed to alleviate the immunodeficiency, in which toxicity is related to accumulated deoxyadenosine (RE Kellems, personal communication).

Lysosomal storage disorders are a heterogeneous group of inborn errors (Chaps. 134 to 154). A number of mouse models of lysosomal storage, primarily those with engineered mutations, have provided considerable insights into the similarities and differences in mouse and human metabolism. In general, deficiency states in the mouse parallel those observed in humans, with a particularly striking exception. Mice lacking the α subunit of β-hexosaminidase exhibit histologic features of Tay-Sachs disease (G_{M2} gangliosidosis), but otherwise are without any overt clinical manifestations.[84] This difference appears to be due primarily to altered substrate specificity of mouse sialidase that allows for the alternative degradation of ganglioside G_{M2} to G_{A2}, which can then be metabolized by β-hexosaminidase B.[85] In contrast, deficiency for the β subunit of β-hexosaminidase (Sandhoff disease) or G_{M2} activator protein leads to progressive neurologic disease in the mouse.[85,86] Mice with gene-targeted deficiencies of acid sphingomyelinase,[87] glucocerebrosidase,[88] arylsulfatase A,[89] α-mannosidase,[90] α-galactosidase A,[91] sphingolipid activator protein,[92] β-galactosidase,[93] neuraminidase/β-galactosidase protective protein,[94] and acid lipase[95] all exhibit phenotypes similar to those observed in humans. Likewise, spontaneously occurring mutations in galactocerebrosidase (Krabbe disease),[96] NPC1,[97] sialidase,[98] and β-glucuronidase[99] have been studied extensively and provide excellent models of the human disorder, and thus are the primary means for testing novel therapeutic interventions (e.g., references 100 and 101). Mouse models for other mucopolysaccharidoses, in addition to type VII, include MPSI (Hurler disease, α-iduronidase)[102] and MPSVI (Maroteaux-Lamy disease, arylsulfatase B).[103] Finally, a mouse model for aspartylglycosaminuria has been recorded with features compatible with those seen in the human disease.[104]

Mice have provided an important experimental model for a novel treatment approach to glycosphingolipidoses termed substrate deprivation. Use of the imino sugar *N*-butyldeoxynojirimycin leads to depletion of glycosphingolipids in cultured cells and animals by inhibiting the ceramide-specific glucosyltransferase that catalyzes the first step in glycosphingolipid biosynthesis. The long-term treatment of wild-type mice leads to a 50 percent reduction in the amount of glycosphingolipids, without overt pathology.[105] More recently, it was shown that treatment of a mouse model of Sandhoff disease beginning at 3 to 6 weeks of age leads to prolonged survival, delayed onset of symptoms, and reduced accumulation of the glycosphingolipids G_{M2} and G_{A2} in brain and liver.[106] A similar reduction in the accumulation of G_{M2} has been demonstrated in the asymptomatic Tay-Sachs mouse.[107] This approach to treatment holds considerable promise and is currently in human clinical trials. A genetic approach to the same strategy has been attempted in the mouse model of Krabbe disease (the *twitcher* mouse), in which the investigators introduced one null allele for the galactosylceramide synthase gene into *twitcher* mice, and examined the accumulation of galactosylceramide in the brain.[108] A one-third reduction in the amount of galactosylceramide was observed, in addition to histologic improvement and a modest increase in survival, further supporting the substrate deprivation approach to therapy. The availability of these mouse models of lysosomal storage disorders provides the means for understanding the pathophysiology of each disease, the testing of novel therapies, and the ability to address the problems of tissue compartmentalization,

With the recent identification of a number of genes associated with peroxisomal disorders, the mouse will undoubtedly provide insights into the pathophysiology peroxisomal biogenesis disorders. To date, the disruption of peroxisome targeting receptor PXR1[109] and the peroxisome assembly factor PEX2[110] leads to severe clinical consequences with postnatal lethality and biochemical and morphologic features of Zellweger syndrome, closely paralleling the human disorders (Chaps. 129 to 131). In contrast, mice deficient for the gene associated with X-linked adrenoleukodystrophy, despite biochemical similarities to the human disease, fail to develop neurodegeneration or histologic evidence of demyelination by 12 months of age.[111]

DISORDERS OF LIPOPROTEIN METABOLISM

Although the mouse is naturally resistant to atherosclerosis, it has become a favorite subject for the study of lipoprotein metabolism. This is based on the ability to manipulate the mouse genome, breed multiple combinations of genetic alterations onto otherwise uniform genetic backgrounds, feed very defined diets, and perform experimental manipulations in a reasonable time frame.[112] With the deletion of key mouse genes and/or introduction of human apolipoprotein genes, in conjunction with a fat-enriched diet, atherogenesis can be induced within the life span of the mouse.

Historically, atherosclerosis susceptible and resistant inbred strains were identified by dietary manipulation.[113] The first engineered mouse that exhibited hypercholesterolemia was achieved by disrupting the mouse apolipoprotein E gene.[114] Wild-type mice maintained on mouse chow exhibit cholesterol levels of 60 to 100 mg/dl, mainly in the form of HDL. In the absence of apolipoprotein E, the total cholesterol rises to approximately 500 mg/dl while maintained on regular mouse chow. When placed on a "Western diet" chow the cholesterol level rises to approximately 2000 mg/dl and atherosclerosis develops rapidly. Interestingly, replacement of the mouse apoE gene with that of humans fails to protect mice against an atherogenic diet despite similar levels of expression, providing a note of caution concerning the interpretation of results following the introduction of human genes into the mouse.[115]

Gene targeting has also demonstrated an essential function in the mouse of microsomal triglyceride transfer protein (MTTP), the gene responsible for abetalipoproteinemia in humans (Chap. 115). In the mouse, complete loss of MTTP leads to embryonic lethality, hence this does not provide a good model for the human disorder.[116] However, conditional knockout of MTTP with loss of liver-specific expression does demonstrate plasma lipid profiles comparable to those observed in affected humans.[117] Similarly, a more subtle gene targeting of the apoB locus with the introduction of a truncating mutation leads to a lipoprotein phenotype comparable to that seen in humans with hypobetalipoproteinemia.[118]

Unlike humans, loss of lipoprotein lipase in the mouse leads to neonatal death in the homozygous state. This is likely due to the accumulation of triglyceride in pulmonary capillaries,[119] a feature not known to occur to a pathologic extent in humans (Chap. 117). In contrast, loss of hepatic-specific lipoprotein lipase gene in the mouse leads to a mild lipid phenotype with modest elevations of plasma lipids associated with increased amounts of HDL, implying that hepatic-specific lipoprotein lipase plays a greater role in HDL remodeling than in degradation of triglyceride rich particles.[120] Similarly, deletion of the lecithin-cholesterol acyltransferase (LCAT) gene has only modest phenotypic effects in the mouse, with HDL-specific hypertriglyceridemia, and reduced levels of total HDL cholesterol.[121] To date, these mice have not been reported to develop renal disease or corneal opacities observed in a subset of humans (Chap. 118). However, overexpression of human apoA-II in mice leads to a lipoprotein phenotype similar to that seen in humans with fish-eye disease, and these mice accumulate unesterified cholesterol in the cornea.[122]

Using a combination of transgenic and knockout mice, several interesting models of human polygenic lipid disorders have been created. A model of familial combined hyperlipidemia has been generated by crossing transgenic mice carrying the human apoC-III and cholesterol ester transfer protein (CETP) genes to mice lacking the LDL receptor. This combination of gene additions and deletions leads to increased amounts of VLDL and IDL, and parallels the lipoprotein profile seen in humans with familial combined hyperlipidemia.[123] Thus, the combination of the insertion of human transgenes and deletion of mouse genes has provided a broad array of mouse models of Mendelian and multifactorial disorders found in humans.

DISORDERS OF HEME SYNTHESIS

To date, two disorders of heme biosynthesis have been modeled in the mouse. A chemically induced mutation of the ferrochelatase gene was identified following mutagenesis with *N*-ethyl-*N*-nitrosourea.[124,125] Homozygous deficient animals exhibit anemia, sun sensitivity, and liver disease, while heterozygous mice, unlike some humans, have no obvious phenotype. Porphobilinogen deaminase deficiency in the mouse stands as an excellent model for acute intermittent porphyria. Homozygous deficient mice have features akin to those seen in humans, including increased δ-aminolevulinic acid synthetase activity and excretion of δ-aminolevulinic acid following treatment with phenobarbital.[126] Histopathologically, the mice exhibit an axonal neuropathy and muscular atrophy,[127] although similar to ferrochelatase deficiency in the mouse and in contrast to humans (Chap. 124), the phenotype is limited to homozygous mice.

DISORDERS OF METALS

Heredity hemochromatosis is one of the most common autosomal recessive disorders of humans and is associated with missense substitutions within a gene encoding a major histocompatibility complex class I-like protein (Chap. 127). A homozygous null mutation in the mouse similarly leads to rapid iron overload and suggests that loss of function of the hemochromatosis gene product leads to the disorder.[128]

Models of disorders of copper metabolism (Chap. 126) are provided by the *toxic milk* mutant and the various of alleles of the *mottled* mutant, the former analogous to the human autosomal recessive disorder Wilson disease and the latter to the X-linked disorder Menkes disease/occipital horn syndrome.[129] A missense mutation in the ABC-type copper transporter (ATP7B) leads to an accumulation of copper in the *toxic milk* mouse.[130]

At least 16 alleles of the *mottled* locus have been described, with graded effects varying from prenatal lethality to abnormalities in the color and texture of the coat in hemizygous animals. As in humans with Menkes disease, copper accumulates in the intestine of affected animals and is not transported to other organs. Based on a combination of gene targeting and breeding experiments, an interesting interaction with a metallothionein locus has been identified. Metallothioneins, low-molecular-weight proteins that bind copper and other metals, are not essential for viability in the mouse. However, most animals with mutations at both the metallothionein and *mottled* loci do not survive embryogenesis, including females who are heterozygous for a particular *mottled* allele.[131] Death of *mottled* heterozygous females was attributed to X inactivation of the paternal allele in extraembryonic tissues. Based on these results, it has been suggested that metallothioneins protect the embryo from excessive copper accumulation in the absence of the *mottled* gene product, suggesting that autosomal modifiers exist that may influence the severity of Menkes disease.

DISORDERS OF ENDOCRINE FUNCTION

The recent characterization of neurohormonal mediators of energy intake and basal metabolic rate has led to the identification of several single-gene disorders of energy homeostasis. Instrumental in identifying these loci was the characterization of several mouse models of extreme obesity (Chap. 157). Studies of the *obese* (*ob/ob*) mouse established the existence of a secreted regulator of body mass. Positional cloning of the *ob* gene identified the leptin protein as an important metabolic regulator secreted by adipocytes.[132] Children with severe, early onset obesity have been identified with protein truncating mutations in the leptin gene,[32] confirming an important role for leptin in the regulation of energy use in humans. Similarly, the *diabetic (db/db)* mouse serves as an excellent example of a single-gene model of human obesity and obesity-related diabetes. Using a candidate gene approach, the *db* locus was shown to encode the leptin receptor, with the *db* mouse harboring a splice mutation leading to a premature protein truncation of the intracellular signaling domain.[133] A similar truncating mutation has been reported in humans with early onset obesity.[33] Much as the *ob* and *db* mice exhibit hypercortisolism, abnormal glucose metabolism, and hypogonadism, humans with leptin-receptor mutations also exhibit no pubertal development and abnormal growth hormone and thyrotropin secretion. Based on studies in the *ob* and *db* mice, where the loss of leptin function leads to increased bone density in the face of hypogonadism (and prior to the onset of obesity), an additional role for leptin in the regulation of bone density via hypothalamic signaling underlines the importance of leptin in mammalian physiology.[134]

Sporadic congenital hypothyroidism is a common disorder of humans, the etiology of which remains poorly understood (Chap. 158). The autosomal recessive hypothyroid (*hyt/hyt*) mouse has served as an excellent model for the human disorder. Based on studies of this mouse considerable insights have been made concerning the role of thyroid hormone in number of organ systems, particularly the brain. Abnormalities of cytoskeletal components, synaptogenesis, and neuronal process outgrowth have been demonstrated in affected mice, providing insights into the possible mechanisms of mental retardation in hypothyroidism.[135] The molecular basis for the hypothyroid mouse is a missense mutation of the G-protein-linked receptor for thyroid-stimulating hormone (TSH), leading to a loss of function.[136] More recently, humans with congenital hypothyroidism have been investigated and shown to harbor mutations in TSH receptor (Chap. 158), confirming this candidate gene as one cause of human congenital hypothyroidism.[137]

Generalized resistance to thyroid hormone is a dominant disorder of humans typically associated with point mutations in the ligand-binding domain of the thyroid receptor β subunit. An inexact model of this disorder has been generated by disruption of the thyroid receptor β gene in the mouse.[137] In contrast to humans, the mouse phenotype exhibits autosomal recessive inheritance, but has allowed investigators to determine the role of thyroid hormone receptor β subunit in mediating the effects of thyroid hormone.

Several mouse models of human adrenal gland disorders exist (Chap. 159). As in humans, the enzyme steroid 21-hydroxylase resides within the major histocompatibility complex of the mouse, the H-2 complex. One recombinant H-2 haplotype has been identified and shown to harbor a deletion of complement component C4 and one of the two genes for 21-hydroxylase.[138] Homozygosity for the deletion leads to early postnatal death in the mouse, with histologic changes in the adrenal gland similar to those seen in affected humans.[139] Similarly, targeted disruption of the steroidogenic acute regulatory protein (StAR) provides an excellent model for lipoid adrenal hypoplasia congenita. The protein is involved in the translocation of cholesterol from the cytoplasm to the inner mitochondrial membrane and is required for normal steroidogenesis. As is seen in humans, StAR-deficient mice of either chromosomal sex have female external genitalia and die within days from adrenal insufficiency. Differences in the accumulation of lipid in testes and ovary suggest that sex-specific differences in StAR regulation of steroidogenesis exist.[140]

The androgen-resistance syndromes (Chaps. 160 and 161) reflect either an absence of steroid 5 α-reductase 2 or androgen receptor dysfunction. To date, no mouse model for 5 α-reductase 2 has been described, although targeted mutation of the 5 α-reductase 1 enzyme has been reported and has helped define the function of this enzyme in gestation and parturition. Maternal enzyme deficiency leads to a partial embryonic lethality in mid-gestation associated with excess estrogen formation, and can be rescued by the administration of an estrogen receptor antagonist.[141] In addition, there is a defect in prepartum cervical ripening, demonstrating the importance of cervical progesterone catabolism in parturition.[142]

To date, only a single androgen receptor mutation, leading to testicular feminization, has been described in the mouse.[143] However, microinjected transgenes carrying expanded glutamine tracts within the androgen receptor have been used to model trinucleotide repeat instability seen in spinobulbar muscular atrophy (Kennedy disease) with inconsistent results[144,145] and no apparent phenotype.

Estrogen deficiency has also been reported in both males and females deficient in aromatase cytochrome P450. In human females, deficiency of aromatase activity leads to in utero virilization and primary amenorrhea in association with hyperandrogenism. Aromatase deficiency in men leads to continued linear bone growth and an associated delayed bone age beyond puberty, implying an important role for estrogen in male bone metabolism.[146] Similarly, disruption of the aromatase locus in the mouse leads to underdeveloped external genitalia in association with a preovulatory follicular arrest and hypoplasia of mammary glands. In aromatase-deficient male mice, testosterone levels are increased, as are serum levels of FSH and LH, but male reproduction appears unaffected.[147]

Several other hormone receptors of the steroid supergene family cause human genetic disorders and have been mutated in the mouse. Targeted disruption of the vitamin D receptor in the mouse leads to a phenotype similar to that observed in humans (Chap. 165), including hyperparathyroidism, rickets, osteomalacia, and alopecia. However, an additional feature found in the mouse is that of uterine hypoplasia and impaired folliculogenesis, indicating that the vitamin D receptor has a role in the both bone metabolism and female reproduction, a feature previously not recognized in humans.[148] Dietary therapy of calcium homeostasis corrects the bone and parathyroid abnormalities, but fails to reverse the alopecia, implying that hair development has a direct requirement for the vitamin D receptor unrelated to calcium homeostasis.[149]

While mutations at the glucocorticoid receptor and mineralocorticoid receptor loci have been reported in the heterozygous state in humans, to date analysis in the mouse has focused primarily on homozygous loss of function mutations. While most mice deficient for the glucocorticoid receptor die soon after birth, those that do survive have been subjected to behavioral testing. Interestingly, glucocorticoid receptor-deficient mice exhibit spatial learning deficits, invoking either a developmental effect or a role for the receptor in long-term spatial memory formation,[150] and providing a potential target for therapeutic drug development. Mineralocorticoid receptor-deficient mice die within 10 days of birth, with all of the biochemical hallmarks of pseudohypoaldosteronism: hyperkalemia, hyponatremia, and increased concentrations of renin, aldosterone, and angiotensin II. Heterozygous mice exhibit a subtle but discernible phenotype with abnormal fractional excretion of sodium. No changes in protein or mRNA levels of hormone-sensitive sodium channels or sodium/potassium transporters were observed in deficient mice, implying that sodium resorption is not regulated by transcriptional control of these transporters but by other as yet unidentified mechanisms.[151,152]

Disorders of somatic growth are well studied in the mouse (Chap. 162). Given the readily apparent phenotype, a series of dwarf mice have been studied for a number of decades, including the Ames dwarf (*df*), the Little dwarf (*lit*), and the Snell dwarf (*dw*) mouse. The Snell dwarf carries a mutation of the Pit-1 paired-like homeodomain transcription factor that is necessary for normal pituitary cell lineage.[153] The Ames dwarf is caused by a mutation in the Prop-1 (Prophet of Pit-1) transcription factor.[154] A number of clustered mutations have been described in the human Prop-1 gene,[155] whereas Pit-1 mutations appear quite rare. Prop-1-deficient mice fail to activate Pit-1 gene expression, implying there is a cascade of tissue-specific transcription factors necessary for determination and differentiation of pituitary cell lineages. The Little dwarf mouse is an autosomal recessive disorder as a consequence of a point mutation in the growth hormone releasing hormone receptor (GHRHR).[156] Humans carrying mutations in GHRHR have a very similar phenotype, with proportionate dwarfing due to recessive point mutations.[157] Finally, patients with Laron syndrome harbor mutations in the growth hormone receptor and exhibit postnatal growth retardation and proportionate dwarfism.[158] Targeted disruption of the growth hormone receptor in the mouse leads to a similar phenotype, with postnatal growth retardation and markedly decreased serum insulin-like growth factor 1 and serum growth hormone concentrations.[159] These various mouse models of functional growth hormone deficiency have been extremely valuable in determining the pathophysiology of these disorders.

The disorder Albright hereditary osteodystrophy is an autosomal dominant disorder of short stature, skeletal defects, intellectual deficits, and obesity (Chap. 164). It has been associated with heterozygous inactivating mutations of the heterotrimeric G protein α subunit ($G_{s\alpha}$) involved in signal transduction of multiple cell surface receptors to adenylyl cyclase. Maternal inheritance of the disorder in humans has implied a parent of origin effect, with the GNAS1 locus being imprinted. Targeted disruption of the *Gnas1* gene in the mouse confirms the imprinted nature of the locus, with parathyroid hormone resistance seen in offspring bearing a mutated maternal allele, but not those bearing a mutated paternal allele. This parent of origin effect is tissue-specific, with imprinting observed in renal cortex, (the site of parathyroid hormone action), but not renal medulla, the site of ACTH action.[160] More recently, it was shown in the mouse that three distinct transcripts arise from the same transcription unit due to alternative promoter utilization. Most tissues express the $G_{s\alpha}$; however, two other proteins, XlαS and NESP55, are, respectively, paternally and maternally expressed from the same locus in a tissue-restricted pattern. None of the three proteins share a common coding region.[161,162] Thus, remarkable transcriptional regulation contributes to the phenotypic complexity of this disorder, with the ability to carefully exam tissue specificity and carry out selective breeding in the mouse advancing the subject immensely.

DISORDERS OF HEMOSTASIS

Although other species such as the dog provide valuable models of human disorders of hemostasis (Chaps. 169 to 183), the mouse, for historic and practical reasons, remains an exceptional model system. Mice carrying disrupted coagulation factor VIII and factor IX genes have been used primarily as models for gene-replacement therapy. Adenovirus and adeno-associated virus-based vectors have demonstrated long-term correction in clotting parameters in these mouse models.[163,164]

Considerable insight was recently gained into the normal metabolism of von Willebrand factor, based on gene targeting[165] and studies of strain-specific variation in von Willebrand factor levels. The RIIIS/J mouse harbors a dominant modifier locus leading to low plasma levels of von Willebrand factor. It has recently been shown that abnormal tissue distribution of the enzyme *N*-acetylgalactosaminyltransferase, leading to inappropriate expression of this enzyme in endothelial cells, results in incomplete posttranslational modification and rapid clearance of von Willebrand factor from the blood. This effect can be mimicked by the ectopic expression of the *N*-acetylgalactosaminyltransferase gene via transgenic expression from an endothelial cell promoter, confirming the molecular basis for this modifier.[166] The identification of similar modifiers promises to provide both insights into the basic mechanisms of protein metabolism and potential therapeutic targets.

Hemolytic anemias have been studied in the mouse for almost a century, typically in association with coat-color change phenotypes.[167] The normoblastosis (*nb/nb*) mouse carries a mutation in the cytoskeletal associated protein ankyrin,[168] whereas the spherocytosis (*sph/sph*) mouse is deficient in the cytoskeletal protein α-spectrin.[169] These mice serve as models for hereditary elliptocytosis and spherocytosis, respectively (Chap. 183), and have been useful in the determining red cell membrane fragility characteristics in these disorders,[170] along with demonstrating reduced susceptibility to malarial disease.[171] Various red blood cell glycolytic defects have also been described in the mouse, including red blood cell pyruvate kinase deficiency,[172] although to date glucose-6-phosphate dehydrogenase deficiency has not been identified in the mouse. Gene-targeting experiments in mouse ES cells demonstrate that the glucose-6-phosphate dehydrogenase locus confers marked sensitivity to oxidative stress, suggesting that total loss of function may be lethal.[173]

The generation of several models of human thalassemias has been described;[174] the generation of an accurate mouse model for sickle cell anemia, however, has been challenging because of the complex transcriptional regulatory elements required for the coordinate expression of various globin proteins. Deletion of the mouse α and β globin loci by gene targeting followed by substitution with human β S globin transgene has previously been used to construct a mouse model sickle cell disease.[175] A more recent improvement on this strategy has been to introduce the human β S globin locus on a large yeast artificial chromosome. The resulting mice were then bred to mice harboring a murine β globin deletion, followed by breeding with transgenic mice carrying human α globin locus on a murine α globin deletion background. The resulting "humanized" mice demonstrate appropriate developmental expression of the human β globin locus and silencing of the γ globin locus, and exhibit the hallmarks of sickle cell anemia, including microcytic anemia, red blood cell sickling, and reticulocytosis.[176] However, there remain differences in overall globin regulation, reflected in high prenatal lethality, with a tenfold reduction in the frequency of the desired genotype, suggested to be a consequence of in utero sickling.

DISORDERS OF NEURAL CREST CELLS

The neural crest lineage contributes to numerous organ systems, including the skin, sensory organs, the enteric nervous system, endocrine glands, cardiac tissues, and bone elements. Given the essential role of melanocytes in pigmentation, disorders of the neural crest frequently have outwardly visible phenotypes such as albinism that make their identification obvious and cause considerable morbidity to those affected. A number of historically important mutations in the mouse contribute to this category, and increasingly gene targeting has provided additional mutations where spontaneous mutations are lacking. The chromosomal locations of the mouse mutations were used to predict the chromosomal locations of several disorders of pigmentation in humans.[177] In addition, the use of pigmentation to easily mark and follow the generation of transgenic or knockout mice has been described.[178,179]

Hirschsprung disease represents an excellent example of genetic complexity, exhibiting both locus heterogeneity and multigenic effects. Hirschsprung disease is a neuronal dysplasia of the hindgut with an incidence of about 1 in 5000 births. It may be found as an isolated defect or in conjunction with pigmentary defects (Shah-Waardenburg syndrome), and children with Down syndrome are at a significantly increased risk for the condition. The absence of intrinsic ganglion cells in the myenteric and submucosal plexuses along varying lengths of the gastrointestinal tract is a hallmark of the disease. Because enteric neurons are derived from the neural crest, Hirschsprung disease is regarded as a neurocristopathy. Based on a skewed sex ratio (M/F = 4/1) and an increased risk to relatives, Hirschsprung disease has historically been viewed as a sex-modified multifactorial disorder. Segregation analysis has suggested an incompletely penetrant dominant inheritance in Hirschsprung disease families with aganglionosis extending beyond the sigmoid colon. Mutations in the RET receptor oncogene account for approximately 50 percent and 15 to 20 percent of familial and sporadic Hirschsprung disease patients, respectively. RET mutations are also found in rare families segregating both multiple endocrine neoplasia 2 and Hirschsprung disease (Chaps. 42 and 251). The RET gene codes for a transmembrane tyrosine kinase that is a subunit of a multimeric complex, which acts as a receptor for four structurally related secreted proteins: artemin, the glial cell line-derived neurotrophic factor (GDNF), neurturin, and persephin. GDNF-deficient mice exhibit congenital intestinal aganglionosis and renal agenesis, a phenotype very similar to the *Ret*-deficient mouse.

Unlike humans, the phenotype in *Ret*- and GDNF-deficient mice is recessive. In contrast to patients with multiple endocrine neoplasia 2, the majority of Hirschsprung disease mutations result either in reduced dosage of the RET protein or in the loss of RET function. However, the penetrance of RET mutations is only 50 to 70 percent, is gender-dependent, and varies with the segment length of aganglionosis, implicating additional modifier genes in familial Hirschsprung disease, one of which has been mapped to chromosome 9q31.[180] In addition to the RET gene, mutations in the endothelin receptor-B, endothelin-converting enzyme-1, and endothelin-3 gene have also been found in familial Hirschsprung disease, while mutations in endothelin receptor-B, endothelin-3 gene, and Sox10[181] are found in Waardenburg-Shah syndrome. These findings parallel the mutation spectrum seen in *piebald lethal* (endothelin receptor-B) and *lethal spotted* (endothelin-3) strains of mice that have phenotypic similarities to the human condition. In addition, the autosomal dominant *Dom* mouse exhibits aganglionosis and hypopigmentation similar to that of Waardenburg-Shah syndrome. Much as Shah-Waardenburg syndrome patients with equivalent mutations show phenotypic variability,[182] the *Dom* mouse exhibits similar variability. *Dom* mice harbor a mutation in Sox10.[183] Using *Dom* congenic lines to segregate loci that modify the neural crest defects, increased hypopigmentation of *Dom* animals has been observed in association with a C3HeB/FeJLe-*a/a* locus.[184] Linkage analysis localized the pigmentation modifier of the *Dom* phenotype to mouse chromosome 10, in close proximity to a modifier of hypopigmentation for the *piebald* mouse. Finally, the introduction of β-galactosidase reporter genes into neural crest cells of mice has made it possible to visualize and study the fate of enteric neuroblasts.[185] Thus, the combination of linkage and mutation studies in humans and breeding and mutagenesis experiments in the mouse have revealed remarkable insights into a genetically complex developmental pathway.

DISORDERS OF HEARING AND VISION

Considerable anatomic and functional similarities in hearing and vision exist between humans and mice, making the mouse an attractive model system for deafness and visual impairment. This section focuses on examples of deafness where mouse studies have been particularly informative. The inner ear provides for two important sensory functions: a vestibular system for orientation in space and an auditory system for hearing. Much of the recent advances in the structural development of the inner ear, the formation and maintenance of neuronal innervation, and delineation of the causes for heritable human deafness has relied on studies of the mouse. Because many genes important for the formation of inner ear structures likely have other roles in development, the use of human mutations in understanding the basic developmental program of the inner ear is likely to be unrewarding. For example, the recent demonstration that the *Math1* gene is essential to the formation of the inner ear hair cells depended on the availability of a *Math1*-deficient mouse model.[186]

Up to one-third of aged humans have a disorder of hearing and or balance, and profound deafness affects 1 in 1000 newborns (Chap. 254). Deafness is typically divided into syndromic and nonsyndromic forms, with the latter constituting about 70 percent of deafness, the majority of which are autosomal recessive. There is tremendous genetic heterogeneity in deafness, with 27 loci known to cause nonsyndromic autosomal dominant deafness, 26 loci leading to autosomal recessive deafness, and 5 X-linked loci (G Van Camp, RJH Smith. Hereditary Hearing Loss Home Page: http://dnalab-www.uia.ac.be/dnalab/hhh/). In the mouse, vestibular dysfunction is often readily apparent by shaker/waltzer behavior, and over 70 loci are associated with hearing deficits (MGD). Numerous spontaneous mutations involved in the development or maintenance of hearing and/or balance have been identified in the mouse, and recently the molecular bases for a number of these have been reported that have corresponding mutations in humans.[187–189] Both locus heterogeneity and genetic pleiotropy are demonstrated repeatedly with these phenotypes. For example, several unconventional myosins are found throughout the vestibular and cochlear hair cells and are involved in electromechanical transduction. To date, two myosins have been identified that when defective cause deafness. Mutations in the unconventional myosin MYO7A may cause syndromic deafness in the blindness-deafness disorder Usher 1b, or may cause autosomal recessive (DFNB2) or dominant (DFNA11) isolated deafness. In addition to the inner ear, MYO7A is also expressed in ciliated nasal epithelia, sperm, and photoreceptor cells, thus accounting for the additional clinical features seen in Usher syndrome. A large number of different mutations in MYO7A have been reported in humans,[190] giving distinct phenotypes that in part reflect the differing tissue sensitivities to different mutations. Similarly, the *Shaker-1* mouse has several allelic variants of *Myo7a* leading to variation in hair cell development, stereociliary organization, and differing electrophysiological responsiveness.

With the availability of EST clones specifically isolated from human fetal cochlear tissue (http://hearing.bwh.harvard.edu/cochlearcdnalibrary.htm) and similar Web-based resources available in the mouse (www.ihr.mrc.ac.uk/hereditary/genetable/index.html), a more complete understanding of the developmental and morbid aspects of the ear can be anticipated.

DISORDERS OF SKIN

Several classic mouse models of ectodermal dysplasias have provided fascinating insights into the molecular basis for the equivalent human diseases and into the nature of developmental mechanisms at work in the formation of skin appendages. Ectodermal dysplasias are a remarkably heterogenous group of disorders characterized by involvement of nails, hair, teeth, and/or sweat glands, with over 150 distinct disorders recognized. The most common is the X-linked hypohidrotic ectodermal dysplasia, now known to be caused by mutations at the ectodysplasin locus, encoding a transmembrane protein containing an internal collagen-like domain that is believed to mediate self-assembly into a trimeric protein that undergoes regulated cleavage from the cell surface. The mouse model of X-linked hypohidrotic ectodermal dysplasia is the *Tabby* mouse,[191] while an autosomal locus demonstrating an indistinguishable ectodermal phenotype is the

Downless mouse, in which both recessive and dominant alleles have been identified.

Recently, the *Downless* locus was characterized at a molecular level using YAC-mediated complementation of a *Downless* allele that had previously been generated by transgenic insertional mutagenesis.[192] The predicted protein, termed Edar (ectodermal dysplasia receptor), is homologous to members of the tumor necrosis factor receptor superfamily of proteins known to bind trimeric ligands. Mutations of the human Edar gene in families with both autosomal dominant and recessive forms of ectodermal dysplasia have been described.[193] Based on the sequence similarity to known signaling proteins, the patterning of hair follicles during embryogenesis appears to require signaling by ectodysplasin through Edar. In addition, in the absence of Edar, expression of other mediators of follicle placode formation are perturbed. Bone morphogenetic protein 4 and sonic hedgehog, members of the transforming growth factor β superfamily of secreted signaling proteins, fail to be appropriately expressed in the absence of Edar, indicating that Edar is an upstream inducer of these factors during the normal formation of embryonic skin appendages. Because ectodysplasin is uniformly expressed in embryonic dermis, a mechanism must exist for the restricted induction of hair follicle placodes, and it has been speculated that this pathway uses lateral inhibition to localize developmental signals, where Edar is expressed within placode cells and absent in surrounding dermal cells. The uniform expression of activators and inhibitors of differentiation, in this case ectodysplasin and perhaps BMP4, leads to oscillating peaks and troughs of expression, providing a means to localize ligand and receptor interactions and thus allowing for the focal expression of developmental programs.[194] Because *Tabby* and *Downless* lack primary hair follicles but exhibit secondary follicles that arise later in development, other pathways exist for induction of the secondary follicles.

Use of the mouse for these studies takes advantage of the significant conservation in developmental programs shared between mice and humans, and should provide not only a clear understanding of the pathologic state in humans, but also the evolutionary history of dermal appendages, from scales to feathers and fur.

DISORDERS OF IMMUNE SYSTEM

Human genetic disorders of the immune system have been extensively modeled in the mouse, and comparable phenotypes are typically observed. Examples of disorders of humoral immunity that are modeled in the mouse include X-linked agammaglobulinemia due to either spontaneous or targeted mutation at the Bruton agammaglobulinemia tyrosine kinase locus,[195] and hyper-IgM immunodeficiency created by targeted disruption of the CD40 ligand.[196] Deficiency of CD40 ligand is characterized by a block in immunoglobulin isotype switching, in addition to defects in cell-mediated immunity. The mouse model has been very instructive in demonstrating that gene-replacement therapy using DNA sequences that are not subject to the exquisite in vivo regulation that normally controls endogenous gene expression leads to unexpected complications. Low-level constitutive expression of the CD40 ligand transgene via a retroviral vector initially corrects the humoral and cellular immune deficiency in the mice; however, over time, the majority of mice subjected to gene-replacement therapy develop T-cell lymphoproliferative disorders, including T-cell lymphoblastic lymphomas.[197] The benefits of having an appropriate mouse model prior to introducing similar therapies in humans are clear.

Several models of severe combined immunodeficiency (SCID) exist in the mouse, including, amongst others, adenosine deaminase, recombination activating gene-1 (Rag1) and recombination activating gene-2 (Rag2),[198,199] IL-7 receptor α chain,[200] and IL-2 receptor γ subunit[201] deficiency, each with a corresponding human disorder (Chap. 185). The classic *Scid* mouse carries a mutation in the DNA-dependent protein kinase catalytic subunit that is a member of the phosphatidylinositol 3-kinase superfamily, and functions in DNA double-strand break repair and V(D)J recombination pathways. *Scid* mice have been used in many facets of biomedical research, including tumor biology, development of the immune system, and transplantation biology. *Scid* mice are used as an in vivo model for various infectious diseases; and have been shown to support reconstituted normal and pathologic human hematopoietic differentiation.[202] More recently, an interesting application of *Scid* mice is that of a recipient of human myoblasts containing mitochondria harboring pathologic mitochondrial genomes,[203] providing an in vivo model of mitochondrial disease. Interestingly, despite widespread use of this mouse in biomedical research, to date no human genotypic equivalent has been reported.

The chronic granulomatous diseases, both X-linked and autosomal recessive, typify disorders of neutrophil function. Chronic granulomatous disease is caused by mutations in subunits of phagocyte NADPH oxidase involved in the formation of superoxide and related reactive species (Chap. 189). The disorder is one of recurrent life-threatening bacterial and fungal infections, along with granuloma formation. Gene targeting has been used to generate two models of chronic granulomatous disease; deficiency of the X-linked 91-kDa β subunit of NADPH oxidase[204] and the P47-*phox*-deficient autosomal recessive disorder.[205] Both models lack superoxide production and demonstrate increased susceptibility to bacterial and fungal infections, along with abnormal inflammatory responses. Gene therapy using a retroviral vector has been shown to enhance survival in P47-*phox*-deficient mice following challenge with a pathogen.[206]

The spontaneous mouse mutation *beige* was instrumental in identifying the gene mutated in Chediak-Higashi syndrome, based on comparative mapping studies in mice and humans. Both affected patients and *beige* mice exhibit impaired immune function, hypopigmentation, and large cytoplasmic inclusions. Positional cloning of the mouse gene, lysosomal trafficking regulator (*Lyst*) was instrumental in the identification of mutations in its human counterpart.[207] Similarly, leukocyte adhesion deficiency due to mutations in the integrin β-2 gene has been modeled in the mouse. In addition to developing features of the disorder seen in humans (Chap. 188), backcrossing of the mutant integrin β-2 gene onto the inbred strain PL/J gives rise to a mouse with the histologic features of human psoriasis, apparently due to a small number of modifier loci.[208]

Autoimmune syndromes involve abnormal immune self-tolerance. Two spontaneous mutations in the mouse, lymphoproliferation (*lpr*) and generalized lymphoproliferative disease (*gld*), result in lymphoid enlargement in association with autoimmune vasculitis and immune complex glomerulonephritis. *Lpr* results from the mutations in the tumor necrosis factor receptor family member Fas, while *gld* is caused by mutation of the Fas ligand.[209] Humans with autoimmune lymphoproliferative syndrome have recently been shown to harbor mutations at the Fas locus; yet, in concert with the observation of strain-specific modifiers of the mouse phenotype, some members of families with known Fas mutations may have no clinical features of the disorder,[210] implying the existence of modifier loci in both mouse and man.

DISORDERS OF TRANSPORTERS AND CHANNELS

One of the best-studied ion channel disorders of humans is cystic fibrosis (Chap. 201), caused by mutations at the cystic fibrosis transmembrane conductance regulator locus (CFTR). Several distinct mouse models have been generated for cystic fibrosis by gene targeting, leading to both hypomorphic and null mutations.[211,212] Mice bearing a null mutation die of intestinal obstruction soon after birth, thus not allowing for the development of pathologic features seen in most affected humans. However, hypomorphic mutations in the mouse avoid this complication and provide investigators older mice that may develop complications seen in the majority of humans, such as lung colonization with opportunistic bacteria.[213,214] Of particular interest is the identification of a single modifier of the CFTR phenotype in the mouse. Rozmahel and colleagues[215] noted improved survival in mice backcrossed to the outbred strain CD1 or the inbred strains C57Bl/6J or BALB/cJ, but not the DBA/2J or 129/Sv strains. A higher fraction of animals survived weaning on the permissive background, whereas perinatal lethality was observed on the nonpermissive background. The prolonged survival phenotype was then used to localize an unlinked modifier to mouse chromosome 7. Whole-cell patch-clamp studies of intestinal crypt cells provided evidence for the presence of a calcium-activated chloride conductance channel in the long-term survivors that may account for their improved survival. The identification of the relevant modifier locus may contribute to a better understanding of the intestinal pathophysiology of cystic fibrosis, in addition to additional avenues for therapeutic intervention.

The aquaporin family of order-transport proteins provides an interesting example of the utility of mouse mutations. At least six aquaporin family members are expressed in the mammalian kidney. Mutations in the aquaporin-1 gene were identified in rare humans who lack the Colton blood group antigen.[216] Despite the presence of the aquaporin-1 protein in the apical and basolateral membranes of the renal proximal tubules and descending loop of Henle, no obvious kidney dysfunction was seen in these patients. However, detailed studies of aquaporin-1-deficient mice have demonstrated decreased proximal tubule transepithelial water permeability and ineffective fluid absorption.[217] Similarly, pulmonary capillary osmotic water permeability is reduced more than tenfold in aquaporin-1-deficient mice.[218] These studies in kidney and lung tissues demonstrate that water movement in tissues is transcellular and not via interstitial spaces. Mutations in the aquaporin-2 gene in humans leads to autosomal recessive diabetes insipidus.[219] The generation of aquaporin-2-deficient mice and gene targeting of the other aquaporin family members should provide considerable insight into the role of this highly conserved gene family in mammalian physiology. These studies also demonstrate the value of applying classic physiology preparations to genetically altered mice, bringing together historically disparate disciplines.

DISORDERS OF BONE AND CARTILAGE

The mouse as a model system has made significant contributions to the study of skeletal elements, with over 200 loci affecting skeletal development (www.informatics.jax.org/searches/marker_form.shtml). Many mutations affecting embryonic patterning, skeletal growth, and biomechanical properties of bone have been observed, in part due to the visually apparent phenotypes they engender and the historic interest in the human counterparts. Of particular interest are the skeletal dysplasias of humans, of which there are greater than 200 (http://external.csmc.edu/genetics/skeldys/nomenclature.html). As an example, targeted mutation of fibroblast growth factor receptor 3 (FGFR3) has been instrumental in understanding the normal function of FGFR3 and in explaining the pathogenesis of achondroplasia, thanatophoric dysplasia, and hypochondroplasia (Chap. 210). The inhibitory function of FGFR3 on chondrocyte proliferation is revealed by the generation of a loss-of-function mutation in the mouse that leads to long-bone overgrowth and deafness.[220] The morphologic and histopathologic equivalent of achondroplasia has subsequently been introduced into the mouse by means of a knock-in of the specific point mutation (G380R) found in the majority of humans, providing experimental confirmation of the gain of function nature of this mutation.[28]

Similarly, the pathologic mechanisms that give rise to the variable severity observed in humans with osteogenesis imperfecta (Chap. 205) can be reproduced in the mouse, such that mice heterozygous for a null allele at the *Col1a1* locus due to insertion of a retrovirus have a mild phenotype, whereas a strain constructed by the introduction of a missense mutation leading to a dominant negative allele exhibits perinatal lethality, features that parallel the phenotypes observed in humans with similar mutations.[221]

A large number of mutations in collagens and other components of the extracellular matrix now exist in the mouse and allow investigators to explore the interactions of normal and mutant loci. One such interaction has been studied in the dominant mouse mutation *tight skin* (*Tsk*), which arose spontaneously as a consequence of a tandem duplication at the fibrillin locus and leads to subcutaneous hyperplasia, overgrowth of cartilage and bone, emphysema-like lung changes, and autoimmune disease.[222] The introduction of the *Tsk* mutation into mice deficient for Col5a2 leads to progeny without subcutaneous hyperplasia or autoimmune antibodies,[223] reflecting the in vivo interactions of these proteins within the extracellular matrix.

DISORDERS OF THE CARDIOVASCULAR SYSTEM

Use of the mouse in cardiovascular research has gained momentum in recent years, with the benefits of gene manipulation outweighing the limitations of size. Cardiac anomalies or circulatory insufficiency are frequent causes of in utero lethality in mutations exhibiting embryonic lethality.[224] Although for the most part equivalent human diseases have not yet been recognized, a number of genes have been identified that when defective give rise to defects in early cardiogenesis, cardiac looping, and/or cellular interactions that lead to structural defects.[225] One of the better studied areas is that of hypertrophic cardiomyopathy. A number of models of heritable cardiomyopathies (Chap. 213) are now available for the majority of human disease entities,[226] including mice expressing mutant proteins or lacking elements of the sarcomeric contractile apparatus, such as myosin heavy chain α,[227] the essential and regulatory myosin light chains,[228,229] cardiac troponin T2,[230] cardiac troponin I,[231] α tropomyosin,[232] and myosin-binding protein C.[233] The availability of these mutation-bearing mice has led to the development of a variety of physiological techniques in order to identify the phenotypes at the whole organ and whole animal levels. While techniques for exploring aspects of cardiovascular function are well developed for larger animal models, modifications for the small size of the mouse heart and for the rapid cardiac cycle has proven a challenge, bringing together the skills of the molecular biologist with those of physiologists and cardiologists.[234]

In a particularly fascinating finding, application of chromosome engineering to the mouse chromosomal region closely corresponding to the typical human microdeletion of chromosome 22q13 associated with velocardiofacial/DiGeorge syndrome (Chap. 65) leads to a cardiac phenotype with reduced penetrance, with a frequency of about 25 percent, as is observed in humans with the equivalent deletion.[235] Complementation of the defect by a chromosome bearing a duplication of the deleted region demonstrated that the disorder reflects a dosage effect and is not due to breakpoint disruption of a specific gene. The generation of large-scale deletions via Cre recombinase should allow for the modeling of numerous microdeletions and contiguous gene syndromes in the mouse. The benefits of selective breeding strategies and the availability of tissues at all developmental stages offers insights into the pathogenesis of these disorders at a level of detail that is not otherwise available.

DEVELOPMENTAL DISORDERS

Developmental disorders refers to a diverse group of human disorders that at a minimum reflect abnormal embryonic development. Many of the disorders reviewed in this chapter exhibit developmental defects but typically fall into an obvious organ system category, whereas this group of disorders corresponds to clinically distinguishable syndromes that at a molecular level have only recently been defined. The relevant gene products include, amongst others, secreted signaling factors, cell-surface receptors, signal transduction intermediates, cell-cycle regulators, and transcriptional coactivators.

An interesting example of the differences that may exist between mice and humans that effect the accuracy of a mouse model is the gene defect in the oculocerebrorenal syndrome of Lowe, an X-linked recessive human genetic disorder characterized by congenital cataracts, mental retardation, and renal tubular dysfunction (Chap. 252). The causative gene encodes a phosphatidylinositol 4,5-bisphosphate 5-phosphatase that has been localized to the *trans*-Golgi complex and on the surface of lysosomes. Because the lipid phosphatidylinositol 4,5-bisphosphate is required for vesicle trafficking from lysosomes, it has been postulated that there is a defect in lysosomal enzyme trafficking,[236] although the pathogenesis of the clinical phenotype remains unknown. Male mice deficient for the mouse orthologue of OCRL1 have been generated by gene targeting, but do not develop congenital cataracts, renal tubular dysfunction, or any semblance of the neurologic abnormalities seen in affected humans. Because a paralogous autosomal gene exists in the mouse with inositol polyphosphate 5-phosphatase activity (*Inpp5b*), it was suggested that *Ocrl1* deficiency is complemented in mice by *Inpp5b*.[237] To test this hypothesis, mice deficient in *Inpp5b* were also generated by gene targeting. *Inpp5b*-deficient mice are viable and lack any features of Lowe syndrome, although testicular degeneration in males is seen in adulthood. Following mating of *Ocrl1*- and *Inpp5b*-deficient mice, no live born mice or embryos lacking both enzymes were identified, suggesting that *Ocrl1* and *Inpp5b* have overlapping functions in mice but that similar complementation does not occur in humans.

NEUROMUSCULAR DISORDERS

An ever-increasing number of mutations in structural and regulatory elements of the neuromuscular system have been identified in the mouse or selectively generated by gene targeting. In particular, many of the muscular dystrophies found in humans (Chap. 216) have also been observed or created in the mouse, and these mice have been used in defining the pathophysiology of these disorders and in the initial application of gene therapy to neuromuscular disease. Some of the first human muscular dystrophies to have a corresponding locus in the mouse include Duchenne muscular dystrophy and congenital muscular dystrophy. The original *mdx* mouse carries a nonsense mutation within the dystrophin locus, while the dystrophia muscularis (*dy*) mouse serves as a model for congenital muscular dystrophy due to a mutation at the laminin α-2 (merosin) locus, the latter being the most common disease locus in humans with congenital muscular dystrophy. Both proteins are components of the dystrophin-glycoprotein complex, yet lead to distinct forms of muscular dystrophy. In order to understand the effect of loss of each protein on sarcolemmal integrity, Evans blue, a low-molecular-weight molecule that in wild-type animals does not enter skeletal muscle fibers has been used as a measure of membrane integrity. Disruption of the sarcolemma allows influx of the dye. *Mdx* mice exhibit significant Evans blue accumulation in skeletal muscle fibers, whereas merosin-deficient mice show little Evans blue accumulation.[238] This suggests that although the primary defects originate in two components associated with the same protein complex, the pathogenic mechanisms in congenital muscular dystrophy differ from those of Duchenne muscular dystrophy. Thus, each model provides an improved understanding of the disease mechanisms at work in these disorders. In addition, these models have also been the focus of therapeutic efforts using myoblast transplantation,[239,240] and viral and liposome-mediated gene transfer.[241]

Other muscular dystrophies also have mouse equivalents that have contributed to understanding the pathophysiology of the disorders. For example, myotonic dystrophy in humans is caused by a trinucleotide repeat (CTG) expansion within the 3′ untranslated region of the myotonic dystrophy protein kinase (Chap. 217). Mutations engineered into the mouse causing loss of function of the protein kinase fail to accurately recapitulate the human phenotype,[242,243] stimulating investigators to seek out alternative explanations for the pathophysiology of the disorder. This has led to the more appealing hypothesis that the triplet repeat element interferes with muscle-specific alternative splicing by providing a binding site for tissue-specific splicing factors.[244]

Mutations in a variety of ion channel genes can also give rise to neuromuscular phenotypes such as myokymia, periodic paralysis, hyperthermia, and hyperekplexia, each with a corresponding human disorder (Chap. 205). Spontaneous and engineered mutations in channel protein loci exist for each disorder, whether a sodium, potassium, calcium, or chloride channel, and this area has recently been well summarized.[245]

NEURODEGENERATIVE DISORDERS

Neurodegenerative disorders encompass a broad spectrum of diseases with variability in the age of onset, initial signs and symptoms, and pathologic findings. A variety of mouse models exist for a large number of human disorders.[246] Of particular interest is the modeling of disorders of triplet repeat instability. These diseases include the spinocerebellar ataxias (SCAs), Kennedy disease, Huntington disease, myotonic dystrophy, and fragile X syndrome, with the pathogenesis of each disorder being either formation of toxic polyglutamine expansions, suppression of transcription, or perturbation of tissue-specific splicing.[247] It appears that fundamental differences in the stability of these repeated sequences exist between humans and mice. For example, the introduction of repeat lengths that correspond to premutation alleles in humans, with the expectation of high frequency instability in humans, confers only modest instability within the genome of the mouse. However, as the repeat element is lengthened instability is increasingly observed, and in the case of the SCA disorders and Huntington disease,[248] neurologic phenotypes can be observed. Several conclusions have been drawn from these early attempts at modeling triplet repeat disorders in the mouse: expansions and contractions can been seen in the mouse, albeit typically small changes; somatic instability increases with age and varies between tissues; positional effects within the genome influence instability; and parent of original effects can be observed.[249] These differences in stability may reflect the fidelity of replication proof-reading or other fundamental aspects of DNA repair in the mouse.

Selective interbreeding of mutant strains can be quite informative, an excellent example being that of an allele of SCA1 harboring an expanded polyglutamine tract and a disrupted gene encoding the E6-AP ubiquitin-protein ligase subunit previously associated with Angelman syndrome.[250] In the presence of an expanded polyglutamine protein (ataxin-1), aggregates of ubiquitin-positive nuclear inclusions are found that alter the proteasome distribution in affected neurons. Because mutant ataxin-1 is degraded by the ubiquitin-proteasome pathway, cerebellar Purkinje cells that express mutant ataxin-1 but not a ubiquitin-protein ligase have significantly fewer nuclear inclusions. However, instead of ameliorating disease pathogenesis, the Purkinje cell pathology is markedly worse than that of mice bearing mutant ataxin-1 alone. Hence, it was concluded that nuclear inclusions per se are not necessary to induce neurodegeneration, but rather, impaired proteasomal degradation of mutant ataxin-1 likely contributes to the pathogenesis of SCA1.

Similarly, the modeling of the heritable forms of Alzheimer disease (Chap. 234) using a combination of transgene expression and gene targeting has provided novel insights into the developmental roles played by the relevant genes,[251,252] the pathogenesis of histologic abnormalities, and the necessity of additional interacting genetic loci. For Alzheimer disease, an accurate mouse model should exhibit evidence of memory loss and behavioral deficits, along with age-dependent accumulation of beta-amyloid plaques and neurofibrillary tangles leading to neuronal cell death.

In addition, these changes need to be observable within the life span of a mouse in order to be useful. With the identification of loci such as the presenilins and amyloid precursor protein that contribute to monogenic early onset disease in a small fraction of humans, the disorder can be recapitulated in the mouse within its life span. The accumulation of β amyloid deposits in mouse brain has been observed by overexpression of human mutant alleles of the amyloid precursor protein.[253] In contrast, mice bearing mutant alleles of the presenilin genes show increased production of the pathologic Aβ-42 peptide, but do not form β amyloid deposits unless mutant alleles of the amyloid precursor protein are also overproduced.[254,255] Additional loci that confer disease susceptibility, such as apolipoprotein E,[256] have been studied in the mouse using a combination of gene targeting and transgenic strategies. ApoE is highly expressed in glia of the central nervous system and it has been hypothesized that apoE modulates the conversion of amyloid from a soluble to a fibrillar form that becomes deposited in diffuse, neuritic and cerebrovascular plaques. Interestingly, mice lacking apoE but harboring a mutant amyloid precursor protein exhibit reduced amyloid deposition.[257] Furthermore, expression of the human apoE alleles using a glial-specific promoter, including the E4 allele that is a risk factor for development of Alzheimer disease in humans, imparts resistance to β amyloid deposition beyond that observed in apoE-deficient mice.[258] The reason for this remains to be established, but may reflect species-specific differences in binding to the apoE receptor, and thus clearance of β amyloid protein in the central nervous system.

It has been concluded from studies of amyloid precursor protein and presenilin modified mice that behavioral deficits occur before β amyloid protein deposition,[259] reflecting the more subtle functional changes that precede histologic evidence of disease and implying that optimal therapy will need to precede the development of histologically defined disease. In addition, β amyloid deposition in the brain appears to be directed by region-specific factors,[260] hence understanding those local factors that confer resistance to plaque formation will be of importance. These and future modified mice should be instrumental in arriving at novel therapeutic strategies that impede or reverse disease progression.

HERITABLE CANCERS

The mouse has a rich history in the study of cancer biology, with the original inbred strains providing necessary resources for serial transplantation of solid tumors and enhanced or reduced cancer susceptibility. More recently, the mouse has contributed substantially in understanding the roles of cancer-associated genes in normal development. The advantages of the mouse include the ability to examine gene actions on a uniform genetic background, control environmental contributions to tumorigenesis, and reduce the confounding effects of somatic mutations. Moreover, the ability to combine mutant loci within a single strain of mice allows an exploration of the interactions and cooperativity that exist between genes. Both dominantly acting mutant oncogenes and recessive tumor-suppressor genes can be readily manipulated in the mouse, the former typically by microinjection of a transgene into the male pronucleus of fertilized oocytes and the latter by gene targeting in embryonic stem cells. By using tissue-specific transcription control elements tumor formation can be targeted to virtually any organ or tissue type, with the transforming nature of the oncogene allowing for the formation of a tumor or other forms of cancer within a reasonably short time frame.

Gene disruption by homologous recombination provides heterozygous animal models for human familial cancer syndromes such as hereditary nonpolyposis colon cancer (HNPCC), familial adenomatous polyposis, Li-Fraumeni syndrome, and Cowden syndrome. Although these models often faithfully reproduce the disease states seen in humans (Chaps. 36 to 48), not uncommonly there are distinct differences. For example, a null allele at the retinoblastoma locus (*Rb1*) in the heterozygous state does not lead to retinoblastomas in the mouse; instead, it leads to pituitary adenomas. Similarly, loss-of-function alleles of BRCA1 or BRCA2 do not lead to breast tumors in the mouse, perhaps reflecting differences in life span, DNA repair pathways, or genomic stability.[261] Targeted disruption of the neurofibromatous genes *Nf1* or *Nf2* in the heterozygous state fail to give rise to neurofibromas or pigmented macules evident in affected humans, although other tumors seen in humans with NF1 such as pheochromocytomas are observed at a high frequency in heterozygous mice. Neurofibromas can be observed in chimeric mice generated by the introduction of *Nf1*(−/−) ES cells, but unlike humans, the neurofibromas do not arise from peripheral Schwann cells.[262] Mice homozygous for either *Nf1* or *Nf2* null alleles die during gestation (although at distinctly different ages), a reflection of the developmental roles of these loci. In experiments that are only approachable in the mouse, double heterozygotes at the *Nf2* and *p53* loci, which both reside on mouse chromosome 11, have been created with the mutant alleles either in *cis* or *trans*.[263] Although the frequency of tumors is greatly enhanced in the *cis* configuration, when in *trans* there is still an increase in tumor formation in comparison to mice bearing a single mutant allele, reflecting the genetic interactions that occur between these two loci.

While the majority of heritable cancer syndromes in humans represent recessive tumor-suppressor genes, a significant exception is the dominant RET receptor oncogene. Activating mutations of RET lead to multiple endocrine neoplasia 2, a multiorgan system disorder characterized by the development of pheochromocytomas, medullary thyroid carcinomas, and, in a subset of patients, ganglioneuromas. Germ line missense mutations affecting one of five cysteines located in the juxtamembrane domain of the RET receptor are responsible for the majority of human cases. Occasional families have both multiple endocrine neoplasia 2 and Hirschsprung disease, a congenital aganglionosis of the hindgut, segregating within the family. The variability in the observed phenotype in humans has been explained at a molecular level by the demonstration that although all the cysteine substitutions lead to disulfide mediated homodimerization and activation of the receptor, different mutations may also affect the transfer of the receptor to the cell surface. Hence haploinsufficiency may be a concomitant mechanism in some family members with Hirschsprung disease as a consequence of the same mutation.[264] In contrast, loss-of-function mutations in the mouse gives rise only to recessive Hirschsprung disease, with no discernible phenotype in heterozygotes, and the additional feature of renal agenesis, which is not observed in humans. These differences suggest that the same tissues in humans and mice may differ in the response to RET signaling or the amount of RET protein present. Additionally, introduction of these mutations into the mouse by oocyte microinjection leads to development of tumors in a variety of tissues, depending on the transcription control elements used to express the transgene, providing in vivo models for selective tumors such as medullary thyroid carcinoma.[265]

A variety of explanations have been offered for the observed differences between mice and humans in tumor type and frequency. It may reflect species-specific differences in genomic stability, with mechanisms leading to loss of heterozygosity being more pronounced in one species than the other. Another possibility is that growth control pathways may be subtly different between species, much as is seen in certain pathways of intermediary metabolism, or that immune surveillance for transformed cells differs between species. Since the mouse is considerably smaller and shorter lived, perhaps differences in the number of target cells or the life span account in part for the different behaviors. Finally, because many mutant mouse strains develop lymphomas and sarcomas, it has been suggested that this reflects the use of C57BL/6 inbred mice in generating knockout lines, a strain known for its susceptibility to these malignancies.[261,266]

CONCLUSION

In summary, the mouse has made remarkable contributions to the well being of humans and to our understanding of animal biology. It is a certainty that gene targeting will generate numerous additional mutations where the gene of interest is known. However, random mutagenesis will likely provide an increasing number of models of human disease where the gene is not known, the phenotype only occurring on a permissive or sensitized genetic background, or the phenotype occurring only with a specific genotype. This approach to mutagenesis has been termed phenotype-driven mutagenesis,[267] in contrast to the genotype-driven mutagenesis that employs gene targeting or transgenic approaches. Although daunting in scale, chemical mutagenesis for dominant or recessive traits offers the prospect of uncovering numerous as yet unidentified disease-causing genes, providing multiple alleles at a locus, and determining the molecular basis of modifier loci. This approach is increasingly attractive as high throughput approaches to phenotype testing paradigms, genetic mapping, and DNA sequencing are integrated into an overall gene discovery program.

With the inherent advantages of the mouse as an experimental organism, the mouse will remain the primary focus of geneticists for years to come, and because of its malleable genome, the mouse will increasingly enter into the realm of physiologists and biochemists, as our understanding of the mammalian genome moves from one of structure to one of function.

REFERENCES

1. Nutt SL, Busslinger M: Monoallelic expression of Pax5: A paradigm for the haploinsufficiency of mammalian Pax genes? *Biol Chem* **380**:601, 1999.
2. Helwig U, Imai K, Schmahl W, Thomas BE, Varnum DS, Nadeau JH, Balling R: Interaction between undulated and Patch leads to an extreme form of spina bifida in double-mutant mice. *Nat Genet* **11**:60, 1995.
3. Reik W, Walter J: Imprinting mechanisms in mammals. *Curr Opin Genet Dev* **8**:154, 1998.
4. Cattanach BM, Beechey CV: Autosomal and X-chromosome imprinting. *Dev Suppl* 63, 1990.
5. Morse HC: *History, Genetics, and Wild Mice*. New York, Academic Press, 1981.
6. Silver LM: *Mouse Genetics*. Oxford, Oxford University Press, 1995.
7. Beck JA, Lloyd S, Hafezparast M, Lennon-Pierce M, Eppig JT, Festing MF, Fisher EM: Genealogies of mouse inbred strains. *Nat Genet* **24**:23, 2000.
8. Lyon M, Rastan, S, Brown, SDM: *Genetic Variants and Strains of the Laboratory Mouse*, 3d ed. Oxford, Oxford University Press, 1996.
9. Russell LB, Matter BE: Whole-mammal mutagenicity tests: Evaluation of five methods. *Mutat Res* **75**:279, 1980.
10. Flaherty L: Generation, identification, and recovery of mouse mutations. *Methods* **14**:107, 1998.
11. Justice MJ, Zheng B, Woychik RP, Bradley A: Using targeted large deletions and high-efficiency *N*-ethyl-*N*-nitrosourea mutagenesis for functional analyses of the mammalian genome. *Methods* **13**:423, 1997.
12. Justice MJ, Noveroske JK, Weber JS, Zheng B, Bradley A: Mouse ENU mutagenesis. *Hum Mol Genet* **8**:1955, 1999.
13. Haldane JBS, Sprunt AD, Haldane NM: Reduplication in mice. *J Genet* **5**:133, 1915.
14. Friedrich G, Soriano P: Insertional mutagenesis by retroviruses and promoter traps in embryonic stem cells. *Methods Enzymol* **225**:681, 1993.
15. Hogan B, Beddington R, Constantini F, Lacy E: *Manipulating the Mouse Embyro: A Laboratory Manual*, 2nd ed. Cold Spring Harbor, Cold Spring Harbor Laboratory, 1994.
16. Marra M, Hillier L, Kucaba T, Allen M, Barstead R, Beck C, Blistain A, Bonaldo M, Bowers Y, Bowles L, Cardenas M, Chamberlain A, Chappell J, Clifton S, Favello A, Geisel S, Gibbons M, Harvey N, Hill F, Jackson Y, Kohn S, Lennon G, Mardis E, Martin J, Waterston R, et al: An encyclopedia of mouse genes. *Nat Genet* **21**:191, 1999.
17. Tomizuka K, Shinohara T, Yoshida H, Uejima H, Ohguma A, Tanaka S, Sato K, Oshimura M, Ishida I: Double *trans*-chromosomic mice: Maintenance of two individual human chromosome fragments containing Ig heavy and kappa loci and expression of fully human antibodies. *Proc Natl Acad Sci U S A* **97**:722, 2000.
18. Rincon-Limas DE, Lu CH, Canal I, Calleja M, Rodriguez-Esteban C, Izpisua-Belmonte JC, Botas J: Conservation of the expression and function of apterous orthologs in *Drosophila* and mammals. *Proc Natl Acad Sci U S A* **96**:2165, 1999.
19. Ramirez-Solis R, Davis AC, Bradley A: Gene targeting in embryonic stem cells. *Methods Enzymol* **225**:855, 1993.
20. Stewart CL: Production of chimeras between embryonic stem cells and embryos. *Methods Enzymol* **225**:823, 1993.
21. Angrand PO, Daigle N, van der Hoeven F, Scholer HR, Stewart AF: Simplified generation of targeting constructs using ET recombination. *Nucleic Acids Res* **27**:e16, 1999.
22. Ramirez-Solis R, Liu P, Bradley A: Chromosome engineering in mice. *Nature* **378**:720, 1995.
23. Zheng B, Sage M, Cai WW, Thompson DM, Tavsanli BC, Cheah YC, Bradley A: Engineering a mouse balancer chromosome. *Nat Genet* **22**:375, 1999.
24. Sauer B: Inducible gene targeting in mice using the Cre/lox system. *Methods* **14**:381, 1998.
25. Bonyadi M, Rusholme SA, Cousins FM, Su HC, Biron CA, Farrall M, Akhurst RJ: Mapping of a major genetic modifier of embryonic lethality in TGF beta 1 knockout mice. *Nat Genet* **15**:207, 1997.
26. Dietrich WF, Lander ES, Smith JS, Moser AR, Gould KA, Luongo C, Borenstein N, Dove W: Genetic identification of Mom-1, a major modifier locus affecting Min-induced intestinal neoplasia in the mouse. *Cell* **75**:631, 1993.
27. Cormier RT, Hong KH, Halberg RB, Hawkins TL, Richardson P, Mulherkar R, Dove WF, Lander ES: Secretory phospholipase Pla2g2a confers resistance to intestinal tumorigenesis. *Nat Genet* **17**:88, 1997.
28. Wang Y, Spatz MK, Kannan K, Hayk H, Avivi A, Gorivodsky M, Pines M, Yayon A, Lonai P, Givol D: A mouse model for achondroplasia produced by targeting fibroblast growth factor receptor 3. *Proc Natl Acad Sci U S A* **96**:4455, 1999.
29. Fougerousse F, Bullen P, Herasse M, Lindsay S, Richard I, Wilson D, Suel L, Durand M, Robson S, Abitbol M, Beckmann JS, Strachan T: Human-mouse differences in the embryonic expression patterns of developmental control genes and disease genes. *Hum Mol Genet* **9**:165, 2000.
30. Bedell MA, Largaespada DA, Jenkins NA, Copeland NG: Mouse models of human disease. Part II: Recent progress and future directions. *Genes Dev* **11**:11, 1997.
31. Wicker LS, Todd JA, Peterson LB: Genetic control of autoimmune diabetes in the NOD mouse. *Annu Rev Immunol* **13**:179, 1995.
32. Montague CT, Farooqi IS, Whitehead JP, Soos MA, Rau H, Wareham NJ, Sewter CP, Digby JE, Mohammed SN, Hurst JA, Cheetham CH, Earley AR, Barnett AH, Prins JB, O'Rahilly S: Congenital leptin deficiency is associated with severe early onset obesity in humans. *Nature* **387**:903, 1997.
33. Clement K, Vaisse C, Lahlou N, Cabrol S, Pelloux V, Cassuto D, Gourmelen M, Dina C, Chambaz J, Lacorte JM, Basdevant A, Bougneres P, Lebouc Y, Froguel P, Guy-Grand B: A mutation in the human leptin receptor gene causes obesity and pituitary dysfunction. *Nature* **392**:398, 1998.
34. Joshi RL, Lamothe B, Cordonnier N, Mesbah K, Monthioux E, Jami J, Bucchini D: Targeted disruption of the insulin receptor gene in the mouse results in neonatal lethality. *Embo J* **15**:1542, 1996.
35. Bali D, Svetlanov A, Lee HW, Fusco-DeMane D, Leiser M, Li B, Barzilai N, Surana M, Hou H, Fleischer N, et al: Animal model for maturity-onset diabetes of the young generated by disruption of the mouse glucokinase gene. *J Biol Chem* **270**:21464, 1995.
36. Santer R, Schneppenheim R, Dombrowski A, Gotze H, Steinmann B, Schaub J: Mutations in GLUT2, the gene for the liver-type glucose transporter, in patients with Fanconi-Bickel syndrome. *Nat Genet* **17**:324, 1997.
37. Guillam MT, Hummler E, Schaerer E, Yeh JI, Birnbaum MJ, Beermann F, Schmidt A, Deriaz N, Thorens B, Wu JY: Early diabetes and abnormal postnatal pancreatic islet development in mice lacking Glut-2. *Nat Genet* **17**:327, 1997.
38. Guillam MT, Burcelin R, Thorens B: Normal hepatic glucose production in the absence of GLUT2 reveals an alternative pathway for glucose release from hepatocytes. *Proc Natl Acad Sci U S A* **95**:12317, 1998.
39. Lei KJ, Chen H, Pan CJ, Ward JM, Mosinger B Jr, Lee EJ, Westphal H, Mansfield BC, Chou JY: Glucose-6-phosphatase dependent substrate transport in the glycogen storage disease type-1a mouse. *Nat Genet* **13**:203, 1996.

40. Bijvoet AG, van de Kamp EH, Kroos MA, Ding JH, Yang BZ, Visser P, Bakker CE, Verbeet MP, Oostra BA, Reuser AJ, van der Ploeg AT: Generalized glycogen storage and cardiomegaly in a knockout mouse model of Pompe disease. *Hum Mol Genet* **7**:53, 1998.
41. Lamothe B, Baudry A, Desbois P, Lamotte L, Bucchini D, De Meyts P, Joshi RL: Genetic engineering in mice: Impact on insulin signalling and action. *Biochem J* **335**:193, 1998.
42. Leslie ND, Yager KL, McNamara PD, Segal S: A mouse model of galactose-1-phosphate uridyl transferase deficiency. *Biochem Mol Med* **59**:7, 1996.
43. Scriver CR, Eisensmith RC, Woo SL, Kaufman S: The hyperphenylalaninemias of man and mouse. *Annu Rev Genet* **28**:141, 1994.
44. McDonald JD, Charlton CK: Characterization of mutations at the mouse phenylalanine hydroxylase locus. *Genomics* **39**:402, 1997.
45. McDonald JD, Bode VC, Dove WF, Shedlovsky A: Pahhph-5: A mouse mutant deficient in phenylalanine hydroxylase. *Proc Natl Acad Sci U S A* **87**:1965, 1990.
46. Safos S, Chang TM: Enzyme replacement therapy in ENU2 phenylketonuric mice using oral microencapsulated phenylalanine ammonia-lyase: A preliminary report. *Artif Cells Blood Substit Immobil Biotechnol* **23**:681, 1995.
47. Fang B, Eisensmith RC, Li XH, Finegold MJ, Shedlovsky A, Dove W, Woo SL: Gene therapy for phenylketonuria: Phenotypic correction in a genetically deficient mouse model by adenovirus-mediated hepatic gene transfer. *Gene Ther* **1**:247, 1994.
48. McDonald JD, Dyer CA, Gailis L, Kirby ML: Cardiovascular defects among the progeny of mouse phenylketonuria females. *Pediatr Res* **42**:103, 1997.
49. Hommes FA: Loss of neurotransmitter receptors by hyperphenylalaninemia in the HPH-5 mouse brain. *Acta Paediatr Suppl* **407**:120, 1994.
50. Gutlich M, Ziegler I, Witter K, Hemmens B, Hultner L, McDonald JD, Werner T, Rodl W, Bacher A: Molecular characterization of HPH-1: A mouse mutant deficient in GTP cyclohydrolase I activity. *Biochem Biophys Res Commun* **203**:1675, 1994.
51. Ichinose H, Ohye T, Matsuda Y, Hori T, Blau N, Burlina A, Rouse B, Matalon R, Fujita K, Nagatsu T: Characterization of mouse and human GTP cyclohydrolase I genes. Mutations in patients with GTP cyclohydrolase I deficiency. *J Biol Chem* **270**:10062, 1995.
52. Klebig ML, Russell LB, Rinchik EM: Murine fumarylacetoacetate hydrolase (Fah) gene is disrupted by a neonatally lethal albino deletion that defines the hepatocyte-specific developmental regulation 1 (hsdr-1) locus. *Proc Natl Acad Sci U S A* **89**:1363, 1992.
53. Grompe M, al-Dhalimy M, Finegold M, Ou CN, Burlingame T, Kennaway NG, Soriano P: Loss of fumarylacetoacetate hydrolase is responsible for the neonatal hepatic dysfunction phenotype of lethal albino mice. *Genes Dev* **7**:2298, 1993.
54. Overturf K, Al-Dhalimy M, Tanguay R, Brantly M, Ou CN, Finegold M, Grompe M: Hepatocytes corrected by gene therapy are selected in vivo in a murine model of hereditary tyrosinaemia type. *Nat Genet* **12**:266, 1996.
55. Endo F, Awata H, Katoh H, Matsuda I: A nonsense mutation in the 4-hydroxyphenylpyruvic acid dioxygenase gene (Hpd) causes skipping of the constitutive exon and hypertyrosinemia in mouse strain III. *Genomics* **25**:164, 1995.
56. Gogos JA, Santha M, Takacs Z, Beck KD, Luine V, Lucas LR, Nadler JV, Karayiorgou M: The gene encoding proline dehydrogenase modulates sensorimotor gating in mice. *Nat Genet* **21**:434, 1999.
57. Wang T, Lawler AM, Steel G, Sipila I, Milam AH, Valle D: Mice lacking ornithine-delta-aminotransferase have paradoxical neonatal hypoornithinaemia and retinal degeneration. *Nat Genet* **11**:185, 1995.
58. Wang T, Steel G, Milam AH, Valle D: Correction of ornithine accumulation prevents retinal degeneration in a mouse model of gyrate atrophy of the choroid and retina. *Proc Natl Acad Sci U S A* **97**:1224, 2000.
59. Schofield JP, Cox TM, Caskey CT, Wakamiya M: Mice deficient in the urea-cycle enzyme, carbamoyl phosphate synthetase I, die during the early neonatal period from hyperammonemia. *Hepatology* **29**:181, 1999.
60. Veres G, Gibbs RA, Scherer SE, Caskey CT: The molecular basis of the sparse fur mouse mutation. *Science* **237**:415, 1987.
61. Ye X, Robinson MB, Batshaw ML, Furth EE, Smith I, Wilson JM: Prolonged metabolic correction in adult ornithine transcarbamylase-deficient mice with adenoviral vectors. *J Biol Chem* **271**:3639, 1996.
62. Patejunas G, Bradley A, Beaudet AL, O'Brien WE: Generation of a mouse model for citrullinemia by targeted disruption of the argininosuccinate synthetase gene. *Somat Cell Mol Genet* **20**:55, 1994.
63. Huq AH, Lovell RS, Ou CN, Beaudet AL, Craigen WJ: X-linked glycerol kinase deficiency in the mouse leads to growth retardation, altered fat metabolism, autonomous glucocorticoid secretion and neonatal death. *Hum Mol Genet* **6**:1803, 1997.
64. Johnson MT, Yang HS, Magnuson T, Patel MS: Targeted disruption of the murine dihydrolipoamide dehydrogenase gene (Dld) results in perigastrulation lethality. *Proc Natl Acad Sci U S A* **94**:14512, 1997.
65. Hong YS, Kerr DS, Craigen WJ, Tan J, Pan Y, Lusk M, Patel MS: Identification of two mutations in a compound heterozygous child with dihydrolipoamide dehydrogenase deficiency. *Hum Mol Genet* **5**:1925, 1996.
66. Wang SP, Marth JD, Oligny LL, Vachon M, Robert MF, Ashmarina L, Mitchell GA: 3-Hydroxy-3-methylglutaryl-CoA lyase (HL): Gene targeting causes prenatal lethality in HL-deficient mice. *Hum Mol Genet* **7**:2057, 1998.
67. Hinsdale ME, Hamm DA, Wood PA: Effects of short-chain acyl-CoA dehydrogenase deficiency on development expression of metabolic enzyme genes in the mouse. *Biochem Mol Med* **57**:106, 1996.
68. Nezu J, Tamai I, Oku A, Ohashi R, Yabuuchi H, Hashimoto N, Nikaido H, Sai Y, Koizumi A, Shoji Y, Takada G, Matsuishi T, Yoshino M, Kato H, Ohura T, Tsujimoto G, Hayakawa J, Shimane M, Tsuji A: Primary systemic carnitine deficiency is caused by mutations in a gene encoding sodium ion-dependent carnitine transporter. *Nat Genet* **21**:91, 1999.
69. Lu K, Nishimori H, Nakamura Y, Shima K, Kuwajima M: A missense mutation of mouse OCTN2, a sodium-dependent carnitine cotransporter, in the juvenile visceral steatosis mouse. *Biochem Biophys Res Commun* **252**:590, 1998.
70. Jenuth JP, Peterson AC, Shoubridge EA: Tissue-specific selection for different mtDNA genotypes in heteroplasmic mice. *Nat Genet* **16**:93, 1997.
71. Marchington DR, Barlow D, Poulton J: Transmitochondrial mice carrying resistance to chloramphenicol on mitochondrial DNA: Developing the first mouse model of mitochondrial DNA disease. *Nat Med* **5**:957, 1999.
72. Wang J, Wilhelmsson H, Graff C, Li H, Oldfors A, Rustin P, Bruning JC, Kahn CR, Clayton DA, Barsh GS, Thoren P, Larsson NG: Dilated cardiomyopathy and atrioventricular conduction blocks induced by heart-specific inactivation of mitochondrial DNA gene expression. *Nat Genet* **21**:133, 1999.
73. Wu CL, Melton DW: Production of a model for Lesch-Nyhan syndrome in hypoxanthine phosphoribosyltransferase-deficient mice. *Nat Genet* **3**:235, 1993.
74. Jinnah HA, Wojcik BE, Hunt M, Narang N, Lee KY, Goldstein M, Wamsley JK, Langlais PJ, Friedmann T: Dopamine deficiency in a genetic mouse model of Lesch-Nyhan disease. *J Neurosci* **14**:1164, 1994.
75. Engle SJ, Stockelman MG, Chen J, Boivin G, Yum MN, Davies PM, Ying MY, Sahota A, Simmonds HA, Stambrook PJ, Tischfield JA: Adenine phosphoribosyltransferase-deficient mice develop 2,8- dihydroxyadenine nephrolithiasis. *Proc Natl Acad Sci U S A* **93**:5307, 1996.
76. Engle SJ, Womer DE, Davies PM, Boivin G, Sahota A, Simmonds HA, Stambrook PJ, Tischfield JA: HPRT-APRT-deficient mice are not a model for Lesch-Nyhan syndrome. *Hum Mol Genet* **5**:1607, 1996.
77. Wu X, Wakamiya M, Vaishnav S, Geske R, Montgomery C Jr, Jones P, Bradley A, Caskey CT: Hyperuricemia and urate nephropathy in urate oxidase-deficient mice. *Proc Natl Acad Sci U S A* **91**:742, 1994.
78. Rincon-Limas DE, Geske RS, Xue JJ, Hsu CY, Overbeek PA, Patel PI: 5′-Flanking sequences of the human HPRT gene direct neuronal expression in the brain of transgenic mice. *J Neurosci Res* **38**:259, 1994.
79. Wakamiya M, Blackburn MR, Jurecic R, McArthur MJ, Geske RS, Cartwright J Jr, Mitani K, Vaishnav S, Belmont JW, Kellems RE, et al: Disruption of the adenosine deaminase gene causes hepatocellular impairment and perinatal lethality in mice. *Proc Natl Acad Sci U S A* **92**:3673, 1995.
80. Migchielsen AA, Breuer ML, van Roon MA, te Riele H, Zurcher C, Ossendorp F, Toutain S, Hershfield MS, Berns A, Valerio D: Adenosine-deaminase-deficient mice die perinatally and exhibit liver-cell degeneration, atelectasis and small intestinal cell death. *Nat Genet* **10**:279, 1995.
81. Blackburn MR, Wakamiya M, Caskey CT, Kellems RE: Tissue-specific rescue suggests that placental adenosine deaminase is important for fetal development in mice. *J Biol Chem* **270**:23891, 1995.

82. Blackburn MR, Knudsen TB, Kellems RE: Genetically engineered mice demonstrate that adenosine deaminase is essential for early postimplantation development. *Development* **124**:3089, 1997.
83. Blackburn MR, Datta SK, Kellems RE: Adenosine deaminase-deficient mice generated using a two-stage genetic engineering strategy exhibit a combined immunodeficiency. *J Biol Chem* **273**:5093, 1998.
84. Yamanaka S, Johnson MD, Grinberg A, Westphal H, Crawley JN, Taniike M, Suzuki K, Proia RL: Targeted disruption of the Hexa gene results in mice with biochemical and pathologic features of Tay-Sachs disease. *Proc Natl Acad Sci U S A* **91**:9975, 1994.
85. Sango K, Yamanaka S, Hoffmann A, Okuda Y, Grinberg A, Westphal H, McDonald MP, Crawley JN, Sandhoff K, Suzuki K, et al: Mouse models of Tay-Sachs and Sandhoff diseases differ in neurologic phenotype and ganglioside metabolism. *Nat Genet* **11**:170, 1995.
86. Liu Y, Hoffmann A, Grinberg A, Westphal H, McDonald MP, Miller KM, Crawley JN, Sandhoff K, Suzuki K, Proia RL: Mouse model of G_{M2} activator deficiency manifests cerebellar pathology and motor impairment. *Proc Natl Acad Sci U S A* **94**:8138, 1997.
87. Horinouchi K, Erlich S, Perl DP, Ferlinz K, Bisgaier CL, Sandhoff K, Desnick RJ, Stewart CL, Schuchman EH: Acid sphingomyelinase deficient mice: A model of types A and B Niemann-Pick disease. *Nat Genet* **10**:288, 1995.
88. Tybulewicz VL, Tremblay ML, LaMarca ME, Willemsen R, Stubblefield BK, Winfield S, Zablocka B, Sidransky E, Martin BM, Huang SP, et al: Animal model of Gaucher's disease from targeted disruption of the mouse glucocerebrosidase gene. *Nature* **357**:407, 1992.
89. Hess B, Saftig P, Hartmann D, Coenen R, Lullmann-Rauch R, Goebel HH, Evers M, von Figura K, D'Hooge R, Nagels G, De Deyn P, Peters C, Gieselmann V: Phenotype of arylsulfatase A-deficient mice: Relationship to human metachromatic leukodystrophy. *Proc Natl Acad Sci U S A* **93**:14821, 1996.
90. Stinchi S, Lullmann-Rauch R, Hartmann D, Coenen R, Beccari T, Orlacchio A, Figura K, Saftig P: Targeted disruption of the lysosomal alpha-mannosidase gene results in mice resembling a mild form of human alpha-mannosidosis. *Hum Mol Genet* **8**:1365, 1999.
91. Ohshima T, Murray GJ, Swaim WD, Longenecker G, Quirk JM, Cardarelli CO, Sugimoto Y, Pastan I, Gottesman MM, Brady RO, Kulkarni AB: Alpha-galactosidase A deficient mice: A model of Fabry disease. *Proc Natl Acad Sci U S A* **94**:2540, 1997.
92. Fujita N, Suzuki K, Vanier MT, Popko B, Maeda N, Klein A, Henseler M, Sandhoff K, Nakayasu H: Targeted disruption of the mouse sphingolipid activator protein gene: A complex phenotype, including severe leukodystrophy and widespread storage of multiple sphingolipids. *Hum Mol Genet* **5**:711, 1996.
93. Hahn CN, del Pilar Martin M, Schroder M, Vanier MT, Hara Y, Suzuki K, d'Azzo A: Generalized CNS disease and massive G_{M1}-ganglioside accumulation in mice defective in lysosomal acid beta-galactosidase. *Hum Mol Genet* **6**:205, 1997.
94. Zhou XY, Morreau H, Rottier R, Davis D, Bonten E, Gillemans N, Wenger D, Grosveld FG, Doherty P, Suzuki K, et al: Mouse model for the lysosomal disorder galactosialidosis and correction of the phenotype with overexpressing erythroid precursor cells. *Genes Dev* **9**:2623, 1995.
95. Du H, Duanmu M, Witte D, Grabowski GA: Targeted disruption of the mouse lysosomal acid lipase gene: Long-term survival with massive cholesteryl ester and triglyceride storage. *Hum Mol Genet* **7**:1347, 1998.
96. Suzuki K: The twitcher mouse: A model for Krabbe disease and for experimental therapies. *Brain Pathol* **5**:249, 1995.
97. Loftus SK, Morris JA, Carstea ED, Gu JZ, Cummings C, Brown A, Ellison J, Ohno K, Rosenfeld MA, Tagle DA, Pentchev PG, Pavan WJ: Murine model of Niemann-Pick C disease: Mutation in a cholesterol homeostasis gene. *Science* **277**:232, 1997.
98. Rottier RJ, Bonten E, d'Azzo A: A point mutation in the neu-1 locus causes the neuraminidase defect in the SM/J mouse. *Hum Mol Genet* **7**:313, 1998.
99. Sands MS, Birkenmeier EH: A single-base-pair deletion in the beta-glucuronidase gene accounts for the phenotype of murine mucopolysaccharidosis type VII. *Proc Natl Acad Sci U S A* **90**:6567, 1993.
100. Li T, Davidson BL: Phenotype correction in retinal pigment epithelium in murine mucopolysaccharidosis VII by adenovirus-mediated gene transfer. *Proc Natl Acad Sci U S A* **92**:7700, 1995.
101. Marechal V, Naffakh N, Danos O, Heard JM: Disappearance of lysosomal storage in spleen and liver of mucopolysaccharidosis VII mice after transplantation of genetically modified bone marrow cells. *Blood* **82**:1358, 1993.
102. Clarke LA, Russell CS, Pownall S, Warrington CL, Borowski A, Dimmick JE, Toone J, Jirik FR: Murine mucopolysaccharidosis type I: Targeted disruption of the murine alpha-l-iduronidase gene. *Hum Mol Genet* **6**:503, 1997.
103. Evers M, Saftig P, Schmidt P, Hafner A, McLoghlin DB, Schmahl W, Hess B, von Figura K, Peters C: Targeted disruption of the arylsulfatase B gene results in mice resembling the phenotype of mucopolysaccharidosis VI. *Proc Natl Acad Sci U S A* **93**:8214, 1996.
104. Jalanko A, Tenhunen K, McKinney CE, LaMarca ME, Rapola J, Autti T, Joensuu R, Manninen T, Sipila I, Ikonen S, Riekkinen P Jr, Ginns EI, Peltonen L: Mice with an aspartylglucosaminuria mutation similar to humans replicate the pathophysiology in patients. *Hum Mol Genet* **7**:265, 1998.
105. Platt FM, Reinkensmeier G, Dwek RA, Butters TD: Extensive glycosphingolipid depletion in the liver and lymphoid organs of mice treated with *N*-butyldeoxynojirimycin. *J Biol Chem* **272**:19365, 1997.
106. Jeyakumar M, Butters TD, Cortina-Borja M, Hunnam V, Proia RL, Perry VH, Dwek RA, Platt FM: Delayed symptom onset and increased life expectancy in Sandhoff disease mice treated with *N*-butyldeoxynojirimycin. *Proc Natl Acad Sci U S A* **96**:6388, 1999.
107. Platt FM, Neises GR, Reinkensmeier G, Townsend MJ, Perry VH, Proia RL, Winchester B, Dwek RA, Butters TD: Prevention of lysosomal storage in Tay-Sachs mice treated with *N*- butyldeoxynojirimycin. *Science* **276**:428, 1997.
108. Ezoe T, Vanier MT, Oya Y, Popko B, Tohyama J, Matsuda J, Suzuki K: Twitcher mice with only a single active galactosylceramide synthase gene exhibit clearly detectable but therapeutically minor phenotypic improvements. *J Neurosci Res* **59**:179, 2000.
109. Baes M, Gressens P, Baumgart E, Carmeliet P, Casteels M, Fransen M, Evrard P, Fahimi D, Declercq PE, Collen D, van Veldhoven PP, Mannaerts GP: A mouse model for Zellweger syndrome. *Nat Genet* **17**:49, 1997.
110. Faust PL, Hatten ME: Targeted deletion of the PEX2 peroxisome assembly gene in mice provides a model for Zellweger syndrome, a human neuronal migration disorder. *J Cell Biol* **139**:1293, 1997.
111. Kobayashi T, Shinnoh N, Kondo A, Yamada T: Adrenoleukodystrophy protein-deficient mice represent abnormality of very long chain fatty acid metabolism. *Biochem Biophys Res Commun* **232**:631, 1997.
112. Breslow JL: Mouse models of atherosclerosis. *Science* **272**:685, 1996.
113. Paigen B, Plump AS, Rubin EM: The mouse as a model for human cardiovascular disease and hyperlipidemia. *Curr Opin Lipidol* **5**:258, 1994.
114. Plump AS, Breslow JL: Apolipoprotein E and the apolipoprotein E-deficient mouse. *Annu Rev Nutr* **15**:495, 1995.
115. Sullivan PM, Mezdour H, Aratani Y, Knouff C, Najib J, Reddick RL, Quarfordt SH, Maeda N: Targeted replacement of the mouse apolipoprotein E gene with the common human APOE3 allele enhances diet-induced hypercholesterolemia and atherosclerosis. *J Biol Chem* **272**:17972, 1997.
116. Raabe M, Flynn LM, Zlot CH, Wong JS, Veniant MM, Hamilton RL, Young SG: Knockout of the abetalipoproteinemia gene in mice: Reduced lipoprotein secretion in heterozygotes and embryonic lethality in homozygotes. *Proc Natl Acad Sci U S A* **95**:8686, 1998.
117. Raabe M, Veniant MM, Sullivan MA, Zlot CH, Bjorkegren J, Nielsen LB, Wong JS, Hamilton RL, Young SG: Analysis of the role of microsomal triglyceride transfer protein in the liver of tissue-specific knockout mice. *J Clin Invest* **103**:1287, 1999.
118. Kim E, Ambroziak P, Veniant MM, Hamilton RL, Young SG: A gene-targeted mouse model for familial hypobetalipoproteinemia. Low levels of apolipoprotein B mRNA in association with a nonsense mutation in exon 26 of the apolipoprotein B gene. *J Biol Chem* **273**:33977, 1998.
119. Weinstock PH, Bisgaier CL, Aalto-Setala K, Radner H, Ramakrishnan R, Levak-Frank S, Essenburg AD, Zechner R, Breslow JL: Severe hypertriglyceridemia, reduced high density lipoprotein, and neonatal death in lipoprotein lipase knockout mice. Mild hypertriglyceridemia with impaired very-low-density lipoprotein clearance in heterozygotes. *J Clin Invest* **96**:2555, 1995.
120. Homanics GE, de Silva HV, Osada J, Zhang SH, Wong H, Borensztajn J, Maeda N: Mild dyslipidemia in mice following targeted inactivation of the hepatic lipase gene. *J Biol Chem* **270**:2974, 1995.
121. Sakai N, Vaisman BL, Koch CA, Hoyt RF Jr, Meyn SM, Talley GD, Paiz JA, Brewer HB Jr, Santamarina-Fojo S: Targeted disruption of the mouse lecithin:cholesterol acyltransferase (LCAT) gene. Generation of a new animal model for human LCAT deficiency. *J Biol Chem* **272**:7506, 1997.

122. Julve-Gil J, Ruiz-Perez E, Casaroli-Marano RP, Marzal-Casacuberta A, Escola-Gil JC, Gonzalez-Sastre F, Blanco-Vaca F: Free cholesterol deposition in the cornea of human apolipoprotein A-II transgenic mice with functional lecithin: cholesterol acyltransferase deficiency. *Metabolism* **48**:415, 1999.
123. Masucci-Magoulas L, Goldberg IJ, Bisgaier CL, Serajuddin H, Francone OL, Breslow JL, Tall AR: A mouse model with features of familial combined hyperlipidemia. *Science* **275**:391, 1997.
124. Boulechfar S, Lamoril J, Montagutelli X, Guenet JL, Deybach JC, Nordmann Y, Dailey H, Grandchamp B, de Verneuil H: Ferrochelatase structural mutant (Fechm1Pas) in the house mouse. *Genomics* **16**:645, 1993.
125. Tutois S, Montagutelli X, Da Silva V, Jouault H, Rouyer-Fessard P, Leroy-Viard K, Guenet JL, Nordmann Y, Beuzard Y, Deybach JC: Erythropoietic protoporphyria in the house mouse. A recessive inherited ferrochelatase deficiency with anemia, photosensitivity, and liver disease. *J Clin Invest* **88**:1730, 1991.
126. Lindberg RL, Porcher C, Grandchamp B, Ledermann B, Burki K, Brandner S, Aguzzi A, Meyer UA: Porphobilinogen deaminase deficiency in mice causes a neuropathy resembling that of human hepatic porphyria. *Nat Genet* **12**:195, 1996.
127. Lindberg RL, Martini R, Baumgartner M, Erne B, Borg J, Zielasek J, Ricker K, Steck A, Toyka KV, Meyer UA: Motor neuropathy in porphobilinogen deaminase-deficient mice imitates the peripheral neuropathy of human acute porphyria. *J Clin Invest* **103**:1127, 1999.
128. Zhou XY, Tomatsu S, Fleming RE, Parkkila S, Waheed A, Jiang J, Fei Y, Brunt EM, Ruddy DA, Prass CE, Schatzman RC, O'Neill R, Britton RS, Bacon BR, Sly WS: HFE gene knockout produces mouse model of hereditary hemochromatosis. *Proc Natl Acad Sci U S A* **95**:2492, 1998.
129. Levinson B, Vulpe C, Elder B, Martin C, Verley F, Packman S, Gitschier J: The mottled gene is the mouse homologue of the Menkes disease gene. *Nat Genet* **6**:369, 1994.
130. Theophilos MB, Cox DW, Mercer JF: The toxic milk mouse is a murine model of Wilson disease. *Hum Mol Genet* **5**:1619, 1996.
131. Kelly EJ, Palmiter RD: A murine model of Menkes disease reveals a physiological function of metallothionein. *Nat Genet* **13**:219, 1996.
132. Zhang Y, Proenca R, Maffei M, Barone M, Leopold L, Friedman JM: Positional cloning of the mouse obese gene and its human homologue. *Nature* **372**:425, 1994.
133. Lee GH, Proenca R, Montez JM, Carroll KM, Darvishzadeh JG, Lee JI, Friedman JM: Abnormal splicing of the leptin receptor in diabetic mice. *Nature* **379**:632, 1996.
134. Ducy P, Amling M, Takeda S, Priemel M, Schilling AF, Beil FT, Shen J, Vinson C, Rueger JM, Karsenty G: Leptin inhibits bone formation through a hypothalamic relay: A central control of bone mass. *Cell* **100**:197, 2000.
135. Biesiada E, Adams PM, Shanklin DR, Bloom GS, Stein SA: Biology of the congenitally hypothyroid *hyt/hyt* mouse. *Adv Neuroimmunol* **6**:309, 1996.
136. Stein SA, Oates EL, Hall CR, Grumbles RM, Fernandez LM, Taylor NA, Puett D, Jin S: Identification of a point mutation in the thyrotropin receptor of the *hyt/hyt* hypothyroid mouse. *Mol Endocrinol* **8**:129, 1994.
137. Biebermann H, Schoneberg T, Krude H, Schultz G, Gudermann T, Gruters A: Mutations of the human thyrotropin receptor gene causing thyroid hypoplasia and persistent congenital hypothyroidism. *J Clin Endocrinol Metab* **82**:3471, 1997.
138. Gotoh H, Sagai T, Hata J, Shiroishi T, Moriwaki K: Steroid 21-hydroxylase deficiency in mice. *Endocrinology* **123**:1923, 1988.
139. Bornstein SR, Tajima T, Eisenhofer G, Haidan A, Aguilera G: Adrenomedullary function is severely impaired in 21-hydroxylase-deficient mice. *FASEB J* **13**:1185, 1999.
140. Caron KM, Soo SC, Parker KL: Targeted disruption of StAR provides novel insights into congenital adrenal hyperplasia. *Endocr Res* **24**:827, 1998.
141. Mahendroo MS, Cala KM, Landrum DP, Russell DW: Fetal death in mice lacking 5 alpha-reductase type 1 caused by estrogen excess. *Mol Endocrinol* **11**:917, 1997.
142. Mahendroo MS, Porter A, Russell DW, Word RA: The parturition defect in steroid 5 alpha-reductase type 1 knockout mice is due to impaired cervical ripening. *Mol Endocrinol* **13**:981, 1999.
143. Gaspar ML, Meo T, Bourgarel P, Guenet JL, Tosi M: A single base deletion in the Tfm androgen receptor gene creates a short-lived messenger RNA that directs internal translation initiation. *Proc Natl Acad Sci U S A* **88**:8606, 1991.
144. La Spada AR, Peterson KR, Meadows SA, McClain ME, Jeng G, Chmelar RS, Haugen HA, Chen K, Singer MJ, Moore D, Trask BJ, Fischbeck KH, Clegg CH, McKnight GS: Androgen receptor YAC transgenic mice carrying CAG 45 alleles show trinucleotide repeat instability. *Hum Mol Genet* **7**:959, 1998.
145. Bingham PM, Scott MO, Wang S, McPhaul MJ, Wilson EM, Garbern JY, Merry DE, Fischbeck KH: Stability of an expanded trinucleotide repeat in the androgen receptor gene in transgenic mice. *Nat Genet* **9**:191, 1995.
146. Simpson ER, Zhao Y, Agarwal VR, Michael MD, Bulun SE, Hinshelwood MM, Graham-Lorence S, Sun T, Fisher CR, Qin K, Mendelson CR: Aromatase expression in health and disease. *Recent Prog Horm Res* **52**:185, 1997.
147. Fisher CR, Graves KH, Parlow AF, Simpson ER: Characterization of mice deficient in aromatase (ArKO) because of targeted disruption of the cyp19 gene. *Proc Natl Acad Sci U S A* **95**:6965, 1998.
148. Yoshizawa T, Handa Y, Uematsu Y, Takeda S, Sekine K, Yoshihara Y, Kawakami T, Arioka K, Sato H, Uchiyama Y, Masushige S, Fukamizu A, Matsumoto T, Kato S: Mice lacking the vitamin D receptor exhibit impaired bone formation, uterine hypoplasia and growth retardation after weaning. *Nat Genet* **16**:391, 1997.
149. Li YC, Amling M, Pirro AE, Priemel M, Meuse J, Baron R, Delling G, Demay MB: Normalization of mineral ion homeostasis by dietary means prevents hyperparathyroidism, rickets, and osteomalacia, but not alopecia in vitamin D receptor-ablated mice. *Endocrinology* **139**:4391, 1998.
150. Oitzl MS, de Kloet ER, Joels M, Schmid W, Cole TJ: Spatial learning deficits in mice with a targeted glucocorticoid receptor gene disruption. *Eur J Neurosci* **9**:2284, 1997.
151. Hubert C, Gasc JM, Berger S, Schutz G, Corvol P: Effects of mineralocorticoid receptor gene disruption on the components of the renin-angiotensin system in 8-day-old mice. *Mol Endocrinol* **13**:297, 1999.
152. Berger S, Bleich M, Schmid W, Cole TJ, Peters J, Watanabe H, Kriz W, Warth R, Greger R, Schutz G: Mineralocorticoid receptor knockout mice: pathophysiology of Na+ metabolism. *Proc Natl Acad Sci U S A* **95**:9424, 1998.
153. Li S, Crenshaw EBd, Rawson EJ, Simmons DM, Swanson LW, Rosenfeld MG: Dwarf locus mutants lacking three pituitary cell types result from mutations in the POU-domain gene pit-1. *Nature* **347**:528, 1990.
154. Sornson MW, Wu W, Dasen JS, Flynn SE, Norman DJ, O'Connell SM, Gukovsky I, Carriere C, Ryan AK, Miller AP, Zuo L, Gleiberman AS, Andersen B, Beamer WG, Rosenfeld MG: Pituitary lineage determination by the Prophet of Pit-1 homeodomain factor defective in Ames dwarfism. *Nature* **384**:327, 1996.
155. Deladoey J, Fluck C, Buyukgebiz A, Kuhlmann BV, Eble A, Hindmarsh PC, Wu W, Mullis PE: "Hot spot" in the PROP1 gene responsible for combined pituitary hormone deficiency. *J Clin Endocrinol Metab* **84**:1645, 1999.
156. Godfrey P, Rahal JO, Beamer WG, Copeland NG, Jenkins NA, Mayo KE: GHRH receptor of little mice contains a missense mutation in the extracellular domain that disrupts receptor function. *Nat Genet* **4**:227, 1993.
157. Maheshwari HG, Silverman BL, Dupuis J, Baumann G: Phenotype and genetic analysis of a syndrome caused by an inactivating mutation in the growth hormone-releasing hormone receptor: Dwarfism of Sindh. *J Clin Endocrinol Metab* **83**:4065, 1998.
158. Amselem S, Sobrier ML, Duquesnoy P, Rappaport R, Postel-Vinay MC, Gourmelen M, Dallapiccola B, Goossens M: Recurrent nonsense mutations in the growth hormone receptor from patients with Laron dwarfism. *J Clin Invest* **87**:1098, 1991.
159. Zhou Y, Xu BC, Maheshwari HG, He L, Reed M, Lozykowski M, Okada S, Cataldo L, Coschigamo K, Wagner TE, Baumann G, Kopchick JJ: A mammalian model for Laron syndrome produced by targeted disruption of the mouse growth hormone receptor/binding protein gene (the Laron mouse). *Proc Natl Acad Sci U S A* **94**:13215, 1997.
160. Yu S, Yu D, Lee E, Eckhaus M, Lee R, Corria Z, Accili D, Westphal H, Weinstein LS: Variable and tissue-specific hormone resistance in heterotrimeric Gs protein alpha-subunit (Gsalpha) knockout mice is due to tissue-specific imprinting of the Gsalpha gene. *Proc Natl Acad Sci U S A* **95**:8715, 1998.
161. Peters J, Wroe SF, Wells CA, Miller HJ, Bodle D, Beechey CV, Williamson CM, Kelsey G: A cluster of oppositely imprinted transcripts at the Gnas locus in the distal imprinting region of mouse chromosome 2. *Proc Natl Acad Sci U S A* **96**:3830, 1999.
162. Hayward BE, Moran V, Strain L, Bonthron DT: Bidirectional imprinting of a single gene: GNAS1 encodes maternally, paternally,

and biallelically derived proteins. *Proc Natl Acad Sci U S A* **95**:15475, 1998.

163. Connelly S, Andrews JL, Gallo AM, Kayda DB, Qian J, Hoyer L, Kadan MJ, Gorziglia MI, Trapnell BC, McClelland A, Kaleko M: Sustained phenotypic correction of murine hemophilia A by in vivo gene therapy. *Blood* **91**:3273, 1998.
164. Wang L, Takabe K, Bidlingmaier SM, Ill CR, Verma IM: Sustained correction of bleeding disorder in hemophilia B mice by gene therapy. *Proc Natl Acad Sci U S A* **96**:3906, 1999.
165. Denis C, Methia N, Frenette PS, Rayburn H, Ullman-Cullere M, Hynes RO, Wagner DD: A mouse model of severe von Willebrand disease: Defects in hemostasis and thrombosis. *Proc Natl Acad Sci U S A* **95**:9524, 1998.
166. Mohlke KL, Purkayastha AA, Westrick RJ, Smith PL, Petryniak B, Lowe JB, Ginsburg D: Mvwf, a dominant modifier of murine von Willebrand factor, results from altered lineage-specific expression of a glycosyltransferase. *Cell* **96**:111, 1999.
167. Jackson IJ: Molecular and developmental genetics of mouse coat color. *Annu Rev Genet* **28**:189, 1994.
168. White RA, Birkenmeier CS, Lux SE, Barker JE: Ankyrin and the hemolytic anemia mutation, nb, map to mouse chromosome 8: Presence of the nb allele is associated with a truncated erythrocyte ankyrin. *Proc Natl Acad Sci U S A* **87**:3117, 1990.
169. Bodine DMT, Birkenmeier CS, Barker JE: Spectrin deficient inherited hemolytic anemias in the mouse: Characterization by spectrin synthesis and mRNA activity in reticulocytes. *Cell* **37**:721, 1984.
170. Joiner CH, Franco RS, Jiang M, Franco MS, Barker JE, Lux SE: Increased cation permeability in mutant mouse red blood cells with defective membrane skeletons. *Blood* **86**:4307, 1995.
171. Shear HL, Roth EF Jr, Ng C, Nagel RL: Resistance to malaria in ankyrin and spectrin deficient mice. *Br J Haematol* **78**:555, 1991.
172. Kanno H, Morimoto M, Fujii H, Tsujimura T, Asai H, Noguchi T, Kitamura Y, Miwa S: Primary structure of murine red blood cell-type pyruvate kinase (PK) and molecular characterization of PK deficiency identified in the CBA strain. *Blood* **86**:3205, 1995.
173. Pandolfi PP, Sonati F, Rivi R, Mason P, Grosveld F, Luzzatto L: Targeted disruption of the housekeeping gene encoding glucose 6-phosphate dehydrogenase (G6PD): G6PD is dispensable for pentose synthesis but essential for defense against oxidative stress. *EMBO J* **14**:5209, 1995.
174. Paszty C: Transgenic and gene knockout mouse models of sickle cell anemia and the thalassemias. *Curr Opin Hematol* **4**:88, 1997.
175. Ryan TM, Ciavatta DJ, Townes TM: Knockout-transgenic mouse model of sickle cell disease. *Science* **278**:873, 1997.
176. Chang JC, Lu R, Lin C, Xu SM, Kan YW, Porcu S, Carlson E, Kitamura M, Yang S, Flebbe-Rehwaldt L, Gaensler KM: Transgenic knockout mice exclusively expressing human hemoglobin S after transfer of a 240-kb beta-globin yeast artificial chromosome: A mouse model of sickle cell anemia. *Proc Natl Acad Sci U S A* **95**:14886, 1998.
177. Asher JH Jr, Friedman TB: Mouse and hamster mutants as models for Waardenburg syndromes in humans. *J Med Genet* **27**:618, 1990.
178. Overbeek PA, Aguilar-Cordova E, Hanten G, Schaffner DL, Patel P, Lebovitz RM, Lieberman MW: Coinjection strategy for visual identification of transgenic mice. *Transgenic Res* **1**:31, 1991.
179. Zheng B, Mills AA, Bradley A: A system for rapid generation of coat color-tagged knockouts and defined chromosomal rearrangements in mice. *Nucleic Acids Res* **27**:2354, 1999.
180. Bolk S, Pelet A, Hofstra RM, Angrist M, Salomon R, Croaker D, Buys CH, Lyonnet S, Chakravarti A: A human model for multigenic inheritance: phenotypic expression in Hirschsprung disease requires both the RET gene and a new 9q31 locus. *Proc Natl Acad Sci U S A* **97**:268, 2000.
181. Pingault V, Bondurand N, Kuhlbrodt K, Goerich DE, Prehu MO, Puliti A, Herbarth B, Hermans-Borgmeyer I, Legius E, Matthijs G, Amiel J, Lyonnet S, Ceccherini I, Romeo G, Smith JC, Read AP, Wegner M, Goossens M: SOX10 mutations in patients with Waardenburg-Hirschsprung disease. *Nat Genet* **18**:171, 1998.
182. Syrris P, Carter ND, Patton MA: Novel nonsense mutation of the endothelin-B receptor gene in a family with Waardenburg-Hirschsprung disease. *Am J Med Genet* **87**:69, 1999.
183. Herbarth B, Pingault V, Bondurand N, Kuhlbrodt K, Hermans-Borgmeyer I, Puliti A, Lemort N, Goossens M, Wegner M: Mutation of the Sry-related Sox10 gene in Dominant megacolon, a mouse model for human Hirschsprung disease. *Proc Natl Acad Sci U S A* **95**:5161, 1998.
184. Southard-Smith EM, Angrist M, Ellison JS, Agarwala R, Baxevanis AD, Chakravarti A, Pavan WJ: The Sox10(Dom) mouse: Modeling the genetic variation of Waardenburg- Shah (WS4) syndrome. *Genome Res* **9**:215, 1999.
185. Yamauchi Y, Abe K, Mantani A, Hitoshi Y, Suzuki M, Osuzu F, Kuratani S, Yamamura K: A novel transgenic technique that allows specific marking of the neural crest cell lineage in mice. *Dev Biol* **212**:191, 1999.
186. Bermingham NA, Hassan BA, Price SD, Vollrath MA, Ben-Arie N, Eatock RA, Bellen HJ, Lysakowski A, Zoghbi HY: Math1: An essential gene for the generation of inner ear hair cells. *Science* **284**:1837, 1999.
187. Fekete DM: Development of the vertebrate ear: Insights from knockouts and mutants. *Trends Neurosci* **22**:263, 1999.
188. White TW, Paul DL: Genetic diseases and gene knockouts reveal diverse connexin functions. *Annu Rev Physiol* **61**:283, 1999.
189. Fritzsch B, Beisel K: Development and maintenance of ear innervation and function: lessons from mutations in mouse and man. *Am J Hum Genet* **63**:1263, 1998.
190. Liu XZ, Hope C, Walsh J, Newton V, Ke XM, Liang CY, Xu LR, Zhou JM, Trump D, Steel KP, Bundey S, Brown SD: Mutations in the myosin VIIA gene cause a wide phenotypic spectrum, including atypical Usher syndrome. *Am J Hum Genet* **63**:909, 1998.
191. Ferguson BM, Brockdorff N, Formstone E, Ngyuen T, Kronmiller JE, Zonana J: Cloning of Tabby, the murine homolog of the human EDA gene: Evidence for a membrane-associated protein with a short collagenous domain. *Hum Mol Genet* **6**:1589, 1997.
192. Headon DJ, Overbeek PA: Involvement of a novel TNF receptor homologue in hair follicle induction. *Nat Genet* **22**:370, 1999.
193. Monreal AW, Ferguson BM, Headon DJ, Street SL, Overbeek PA, Zonana J: Mutations in the human homologue of mouse dl cause autosomal recessive and dominant hypohidrotic ectodermal dysplasia. *Nat Genet* **22**:366, 1999.
194. Barsh G: Of ancient tales and hairless tails. *Nat Genet* **22**:315, 1999.
195. Khan WN, Alt FW, Gerstein RM, Malynn BA, Larsson I, Rathbun G, Davidson L, Muller S, Kantor AB, Herzenberg LA, et al: Defective B cell development and function in Btk-deficient mice. *Immunity* **3**:283, 1995.
196. Renshaw BR, Fanslow WC, 3rd, Armitage RJ, Campbell KA, Liggitt D, Wright B, Davison BL, Maliszewski CR: Humoral immune responses in CD40 ligand-deficient mice. *J Exp Med* **180**:1889, 1994.
197. Brown MP, Topham DJ, Sangster MY, Zhao J, Flynn KJ, Surman SL, Woodland DL, Doherty PC, Farr AG, Pattengale PK, Brenner MK: Thymic lymphoproliferative disease after successful correction of CD40 ligand deficiency by gene transfer in mice. *Nat Med* **4**:1253, 1998.
198. Mombaerts P, Iacomini J, Johnson RS, Herrup K, Tonegawa S, Papaioannou VE: RAG-1-deficient mice have no mature B and T lymphocytes. *Cell* **68**:869, 1992.
199. Shinkai Y, Rathbun G, Lam KP, Oltz EM, Stewart V, Mendelsohn M, Charron J, Datta M, Young F, Stall AM, et al: RAG-2-deficient mice lack mature lymphocytes owing to inability to initiate V(D)J rearrangement. *Cell* **68**:855, 1992.
200. Maki K, Sunaga S, Komagata Y, Kodaira Y, Mabuchi A, Karasuyama H, Yokomuro K, Miyazaki JI, Ikuta K: Interleukin 7 receptor-deficient mice lack gamma delta T cells. *Proc Natl Acad Sci U S A* **93**:7172, 1996.
201. DiSanto JP, Muller W, Guy-Grand D, Fischer A, Rajewsky K: Lymphoid development in mice with a targeted deletion of the interleukin 2 receptor gamma chain. *Proc Natl Acad Sci U S A* **92**:377, 1995.
202. Leblond V, Autran B, Cesbron JY: The SCID mouse mutant: Definition and potential use as a model for immune and hematological disorders. *Hematol Cell Ther* **39**:213, 1997.
203. Clark KM, Watt DJ, Lightowlers RN, Johnson MA, Relvas JB, Taanman JW, Turnbull DM: SCID mice containing muscle with human mitochondrial DNA mutations. An animal model for mitochondrial DNA defects. *J Clin Invest* **102**:2090, 1998.
204. Pollock JD, Williams DA, Gifford MA, Li LL, Du X, Fisherman J, Orkin SH, Doerschuk CM, Dinauer MC: Mouse model of X-linked chronic granulomatous disease, an inherited defect in phagocyte superoxide production. *Nat Genet* **9**:202, 1995.
205. Jackson SH, Gallin JI, Holland SM: The p47phox mouse knockout model of chronic granulomatous disease. *J Exp Med* **182**:751, 1995.
206. Malech HL: Progress in gene therapy for chronic granulomatous disease. *J Infect Dis* **179(Suppl 2)**:S318, 1999.
207. Barbosa MD, Nguyen QA, Tchernev VT, Ashley JA, Detter JC, Blaydes SM, Brandt SJ, Chotai D, Hodgman C, Solari RC, Lovett M,

Kingsmore SF: Identification of the homologous beige and Chediak-Higashi syndrome genes. *Nature* **382**:262, 1996.

208. Bullard DC, Scharffetter-Kochanek K, McArthur MJ, Chosay JG, McBride ME, Montgomery CA, Beaudet AL: A polygenic mouse model of psoriasiform skin disease in CD18-deficient mice. *Proc Natl Acad Sci U S A* **93**:2116, 1996.
209. Takahashi T, Tanaka M, Brannan CI, Jenkins NA, Copeland NG, Suda T, Nagata S: Generalized lymphoproliferative disease in mice, caused by a point mutation in the Fas ligand. *Cell* **76**:969, 1994.
210. Fisher GH, Rosenberg FJ, Straus SE, Dale JK, Middleton LA, Lin AY, Strober W, Lenardo MJ, Puck JM: Dominant interfering Fas gene mutations impair apoptosis in a human autoimmune lymphoproliferative syndrome. *Cell* **81**:935, 1995.
211. Grubb BR, Boucher RC: Pathophysiology of gene-targeted mouse models for cystic fibrosis. *Physiol Rev* **79**:S193, 1999.
212. van Doorninck JH, French PJ, Verbeek E, Peters RH, Morreau H, Bijman J, Scholte BJ: A mouse model for the cystic fibrosis delta F508 mutation. *EMBO J* **14**:4403, 1995.
213. Delaney SJ, Alton EW, Smith SN, Lunn DP, Farley R, Lovelock PK, Thomson SA, Hume DA, Lamb D, Porteous DJ, Dorin JR, Wainwright BJ: Cystic fibrosis mice carrying the missense mutation G551D replicate human genotype-phenotype correlations. *EMBO J* **15**:955, 1996.
214. Cowley EA, Wang CG, Gosselin D, Radzioch D, Eidelman DH: Mucociliary clearance in cystic fibrosis knockout mice infected with Pseudomonas aeruginosa. *Eur Respir J* **10**:2312, 1997.
215. Rozmahel R, Wilschanski M, Matin A, Plyte S, Oliver M, Auerbach W, Moore A, Forstner J, Durie P, Nadeau J, Bear C, Tsui LC: Modulation of disease severity in cystic fibrosis transmembrane conductance regulator deficient mice by a secondary genetic factor. *Nat Genet* **12**:280, 1996.
216. Preston GM, Smith BL, Zeidel ML, Moulds JJ, Agre P: Mutations in aquaporin-1 in phenotypically normal humans without functional CHIP water channels. *Science* **265**:1585, 1994.
217. Ma T, Yang B, Gillespie A, Carlson EJ, Epstein CJ, Verkman AS: Severely impaired urinary concentrating ability in transgenic mice lacking aquaporin-1 water channels. *J Biol Chem* **273**:4296, 1998.
218. Bai C, Fukuda N, Song Y, Ma T, Matthay MA, Verkman AS: Lung fluid transport in aquaporin-1 and aquaporin-4 knockout mice. *J Clin Invest* **103**:555, 1999.
219. van Lieburg AF, Verdijk MA, Knoers VV, van Essen AJ, Proesmans W, Mallmann R, Monnens LA, van Oost BA, van Os CH, Deen PM: Patients with autosomal nephrogenic diabetes insipidus homozygous for mutations in the aquaporin 2 water-channel gene. *Am J Hum Genet* **55**:648, 1994.
220. Colvin JS, Bohne BA, Harding GW, McEwen DG, Ornitz DM: Skeletal overgrowth and deafness in mice lacking fibroblast growth factor receptor 3. *Nat Genet* **12**:390, 1996.
221. Stacey A, Bateman J, Choi T, Mascara T, Cole W, Jaenisch R: Perinatal lethal osteogenesis imperfecta in transgenic mice bearing an engineered mutant pro-alpha 1(I) collagen gene. *Nature* **332**:131, 1988.
222. Siracusa LD, McGrath R, Ma Q, Moskow JJ, Manne J, Christner PJ, Buchberg AM, Jimenez SA: A tandem duplication within the fibrillin 1 gene is associated with the mouse tight skin mutation. *Genome Res* **6**:300, 1996.
223. Phelps RG, Murai C, Saito S, Hatakeyama A, Andrikopoulos K, Kasturi KN, Bona CA: Effect of targeted mutation in collagen V alpha 2 gene on development of cutaneous hyperplasia in tight skin mice. *Mol Med* **4**:356, 1998.
224. Copp AJ: Death before birth: Clues from gene knockouts and mutations. *Trends Genet* **11**:87, 1995.
225. Belmont JW: Recent progress in the molecular genetics of congenital heart defects. *Clin Genet* **54**:11, 1998.
226. Redwood CS, Moolman-Smook JC, Watkins H: Properties of mutant contractile proteins that cause hypertrophic cardiomyopathy. *Cardiovasc Res* **44**:20, 1999.
227. Geisterfer-Lowrance AA, Christe M, Conner DA, Ingwall JS, Schoen FJ, Seidman CE, Seidman JG: A mouse model of familial hypertrophic cardiomyopathy. *Science* **272**:731, 1996.
228. Chen J, Kubalak SW, Minamisawa S, Price RL, Becker KD, Hickey R, Ross J Jr, Chien KR: Selective requirement of myosin light chain 2v in embryonic heart function. *J Biol Chem* **273**:1252, 1998.
229. James J, Osinska H, Hewett TE, Kimball T, Klevitsky R, Witt S, Hall DG, Gulick J, Robbins J: Transgenic over-expression of a motor protein at high levels results in severe cardiac pathology. *Transgenic Res* **8**:9, 1999.
230. Tardiff JC, Hewett TE, Palmer BM, Olsson C, Factor SM, Moore RL, Robbins J, Leinwand LA: Cardiac troponin T mutations result in allele-specific phenotypes in a mouse model for hypertrophic cardiomyopathy. *J Clin Invest* **104**:469, 1999.
231. Huang X, Pi Y, Lee KJ, Henkel AS, Gregg RG, Powers PA, Walker JW: Cardiac troponin I gene knockout: A mouse model of myocardial troponin I deficiency. *Circ Res* **84**:1, 1999.
232. Blanchard EM, Iizuka K, Christe M, Conner DA, Geisterfer-Lowrance A, Schoen FJ, Maughan DW, Seidman CE, Seidman JG: Targeted ablation of the murine alpha-tropomyosin gene. *Circ Res* **81**:1005, 1997.
233. McConnell BK, Jones KA, Fatkin D, Arroyo LH, Lee RT, Aristizabal O, Turnbull DH, Georgakopoulos D, Kass D, Bond M, Niimura H, Schoen FJ, Conner D, Fischman DH, Seidman CE, Seidman JG: Dilated cardiomyopathy in homozygous myosin-binding protein-C mutant mice. *J Clin Invest* **104**:1235, 1999.
234. James JF, Hewett TE, Robbins J: Cardiac physiology in transgenic mice. *Circ Res* **82**:407, 1998.
235. Lindsay EA, Botta A, Jurecic V, Carattini-Rivera S, Cheah YC, Rosenblatt HM, Bradley A, Baldini A: Congenital heart disease in mice deficient for the DiGeorge syndrome region. *Nature* **401**:379, 1999.
236. Ungewickell AJ, Majerus PW: Increased levels of plasma lysosomal enzymes in patients with Lowe syndrome. *Proc Natl Acad Sci U S A* **96**:13342, 1999.
237. Janne PA, Suchy SF, Bernard D, MacDonald M, Crawley J, Grinberg A, Wynshaw-Boris A, Westphal H, Nussbaum RL: Functional overlap between murine Inpp5b and Ocrl1 may explain why deficiency of the murine ortholog for OCRL1 does not cause Lowe syndrome in mice. *J Clin Invest* **101**:2042, 1998.
238. Straub V, Rafael JA, Chamberlain JS, Campbell KP: Animal models for muscular dystrophy show different patterns of sarcolemmal disruption. *J Cell Biol* **139**:375, 1997.
239. Vilquin JT, Guerette B, Puymirat J, Yaffe D, Tome FM, Fardeau M, Fiszman M, Schwartz K, Tremblay JP: Myoblast transplantations lead to the expression of the laminin alpha 2 chain in normal and dystrophic (dy/dy) mouse muscles. *Gene Ther* **6**:792, 1999.
240. Moisset PA, Gagnon Y, Karpati G, Tremblay JP: Expression of human dystrophin following the transplantation of genetically modified mdx myoblasts. *Gene Ther* **5**:1340, 1998.
241. Baranov A, Glazkov P, Kiselev A, Ostapenko O, Mikhailov V, Ivaschenko T, Sabetsky V, Baranov V: Local and distant transfection of mdx muscle fibers with dystrophin and LacZ genes delivered in vivo by synthetic microspheres. *Gene Ther* **6**:1406, 1999.
242. Reddy S, Smith DB, Rich MM, Leferovich JM, Reilly P, Davis BM, Tran K, Rayburn H, Bronson R, Cros D, Balice-Gordon RJ, Housman D: Mice lacking the myotonic dystrophy protein kinase develop a late onset progressive myopathy. *Nat Genet* **13**:325, 1996.
243. Berul CI, Maguire CT, Aronovitz MJ, Greenwood J, Miller C, Gehrmann J, Housman D, Mendelsohn ME, Reddy S: DMPK dosage alterations result in atrioventricular conduction abnormalities in a mouse myotonic dystrophy model. *J Clin Invest* **103**:R1, 1999.
244. Philips AV, Timchenko LT, Cooper TA: Disruption of splicing regulated by a CUG-binding protein in myotonic dystrophy. *Science* **280**:737, 1998.
245. Cooper EC, Jan LY: Ion channel genes and human neurological disease: Recent progress, prospects, and challenges. *Proc Natl Acad Sci U S A* **96**:4759, 1999.
246. Price DL, Sisodia SS, Borchelt DR: Genetic neurodegenerative diseases: The human illness and transgenic models. *Science* **282**:1079, 1998.
247. Brice A: Unstable mutations and neurodegenerative disorders. *J Neurol* **245**:505, 1998.
248. Lavedan C, Grabczyk E, Usdin K, Nussbaum RL: Long uninterrupted CGG repeats within the first exon of the human FMR1 gene are not intrinsically unstable in transgenic mice. *Genomics* **50**:229, 1998.
249. Korneluk RG, Narang MA: Anticipating anticipation. *Nat Genet* **15**:119, 1997.
250. Jiang YH, Armstrong D, Albrecht U, Atkins CM, Noebels JL, Eichele G, Sweatt JD, Beaudet AL: Mutation of the Angelman ubiquitin ligase in mice causes increased cytoplasmic p53 and deficits of contextual learning and long-term potentiation. *Neuron* **21**:799, 1998.
251. Donoviel DB, Hadjantonakis AK, Ikeda M, Zheng H, Hyslop PS, Bernstein A: Mice lacking both presenilin genes exhibit early embryonic patterning defects. *Genes Dev* **13**:2801, 1999.
252. Price DL, Tanzi RE, Borchelt DR, Sisodia SS: Alzheimer's disease: Genetic studies and transgenic models. *Annu Rev Genet* **32**:461, 1998.

253. Games D, Adams D, Alessandrini R, Barbour R, Berthelette P, Blackwell C, Carr T, Clemens J, Donaldson T, Gillespie F, et al: Alzheimer-type neuropathology in transgenic mice overexpressing V717F beta-amyloid precursor protein. *Nature* **373**:523, 1995.
254. Holcomb L, Gordon MN, McGowan E, Yu X, Benkovic S, Jantzen P, Wright K, Saad I, Mueller R, Morgan D, Sanders S, Zehr C, O'Campo K, Hardy J, Prada CM, Eckman C, Younkin S, Hsiao K, Duff K: Accelerated Alzheimer-type phenotype in transgenic mice carrying both mutant amyloid precursor protein and presenilin 1 transgenes. *Nat Med* **4**:97, 1998.
255. Borchelt DR, Ratovitski T, van Lare J, Lee MK, Gonzales V, Jenkins NA, Copeland NG, Price DL, Sisodia SS: Accelerated amyloid deposition in the brains of transgenic mice coexpressing mutant presenilin 1 and amyloid precursor proteins. *Neuron* **19**:939, 1997.
256. Masliah E, Mallory M, Ge N, Alford M, Veinbergs I, Roses AD: Neurodegeneration in the central nervous system of apoE-deficient mice. *Exp Neurol* **136**:107, 1995.
257. Bales KR, Verina T, Dodel RC, Du Y, Altstiel L, Bender M, Hyslop P, Johnstone EM, Little SP, Cummins DJ, Piccardo P, Ghetti B, Paul SM: Lack of apolipoprotein E dramatically reduces amyloid beta-peptide deposition. *Nat Genet* **17**:263, 1997.
258. Holtzman DM, Bales KR, Wu S, Bhat P, Parsadanian M, Fagan AM, Chang LK, Sun Y, Paul SM: Expression of human apolipoprotein E reduces amyloid-beta deposition in a mouse model of Alzheimer's disease. *J Clin Invest* **103**:R15, 1999.
259. Holcomb LA, Gordon MN, Jantzen P, Hsiao K, Duff K, Morgan D: Behavioral changes in transgenic mice expressing both amyloid precursor protein and presenilin-1 mutations: Lack of association with amyloid deposits. *Behav Genet* **29**:177, 1999.
260. Johnson-Wood K, Lee M, Motter R, Hu K, Gordon G, Barbour R, Khan K, Gordon M, Tan H, Games D, Lieberburg I, Schenk D, Seubert P, McConlogue L: Amyloid precursor protein processing and a beta42 deposition in a transgenic mouse model of Alzheimer disease. *Proc Natl Acad Sci U S A* **94**:1550, 1997.
261. Ghebranious N, Donehower LA: Mouse models in tumor suppression. *Oncogene* **17**:3385, 1998.
262. Cichowski K, Shih TS, Jacks T: Nf1 gene targeting: Toward models and mechanisms. *Semin Cancer Biol* **7**:291, 1996.
263. McClatchey AI, Saotome I, Mercer K, Crowley D, Gusella JF, Bronson RT, Jacks T: Mice heterozygous for a mutation at the Nf2 tumor suppressor locus develop a range of highly metastatic tumors. *Genes Dev* **12**:1121, 1998.
264. Chappuis-Flament S, Pasini A, De Vita G, Segouffin-Cariou C, Fusco A, Attie T, Lenoir GM, Santoro M, Billaud M: Dual effect on the RET receptor of MEN 2 mutations affecting specific extracytoplasmic cysteines. *Oncogene* **17**:2851, 1998.
265. Michiels FM, Chappuis S, Caillou B, Pasini A, Talbot M, Monier R, Lenoir GM, Feunteun J, Billaud M: Development of medullary thyroid carcinoma in transgenic mice expressing the RET proto-oncogene altered by a multiple endocrine neoplasia type 2A mutation. *Proc Natl Acad Sci U S A* **94**:3330, 1997.
266. Jacks T: Tumor suppressor gene mutations in mice. *Annu Rev Genet* **30**:603, 1996.
267. Brown SD: Mouse models of genetic disease: New approaches, new paradigms. *J Inherit Metab Dis* **21**:532, 1998.
268. Raben N, Nagaraju K, Lee E, Kessler P, Byrne B, Lee L, LaMarca M, King C, Ward J, Sauer B, Plotz P: Targeted disruption of the acid alpha-glucosidase gene in mice causes an illness with critical features of both infantile and adult human glycogen storage disease type II. *J Biol Chem* **273**:19086, 1998.
269. Dukes ID, Sreenan S, Roe MW, Levisetti M, Zhou YP, Ostrega D, Bell GI, Pontoglio M, Yaniv M, Philipson L, Polonsky KS: Defective pancreatic beta-cell glycolytic signaling in hepatocyte nuclear factor-1alpha-deficient mice. *J Biol Chem* **273**:24457, 1998.
270. Schneider A, Davidson JJ, Wullrich A, Kilimann MW: Phosphorylase kinase deficiency in I-strain mice is associated with a frameshift mutation in the alpha subunit muscle isoform. *Nat Genet* **5**:381, 1993.
271. Kubota N, Terauchi Y, Miki H, Tamemoto H, Yamauchi T, Komeda K, Satoh S, Nakano R, Ishii C, Sugiyama T, Eto K, Tsubamoto Y, Okuno A, Murakami K, Sekihara H, Hasegawa G, Naito M, Toyoshima Y, Tanaka S, Shiota K, Kitamura T, Fujita T, Ezaki O, Aizawa S, Kadowaki T, et al: PPAR gamma mediates high-fat diet-induced adipocyte hypertrophy and insulin resistance. *Mol Cell* **4**:597, 1999.
272. Barroso I, Gurnell M, Crowley VE, Agostini M, Schwabe JW, Soos MA, Maslen GL, Williams TD, Lewis H, Schafer AJ, Chatterjee VK, O'Rahilly S: Dominant negative mutations in human PPARgamma associated with severe insulin resistance, diabetes mellitus and hypertension. *Nature* **402**:880, 1999.
273. Miki T, Nagashima K, Tashiro F, Kotake K, Yoshitomi H, Tamamoto A, Gonoi T, Iwanaga T, Miyazaki J, Seino S: Defective insulin secretion and enhanced insulin action in KATP channel-deficient mice. *Proc Natl Acad Sci U S A* **95**:10402, 1998.
274. Montagutelli X, Lalouette A, Coude M, Kamoun P, Forest M, Guenet JL: aku, a mutation of the mouse homologous to human alkaptonuria, maps to chromosome 16. *Genomics* **19**:9, 1994.
275. Manning K, Fernandez-Canon JM, Montagutelli X, Grompe M: Identification of the mutation in the alkaptonuria mouse model. Mutations in brief no. 216. Online. *Hum Mutat* **13**:171, 1999.
276. Symula DJ, Shedlovsky A, Guillery EN, Dove WF: A candidate mouse model for Hartnup disorder deficient in neutral amino acid transport. *Mamm Genome* **8**:102, 1997.
277. Symula DJ, Shedlovsky A, Dove WF: Genetic mapping of hph2, a mutation affecting amino acid transport in the mouse. *Mamm Genome* **8**:98, 1997.
278. Watanabe M, Osada J, Aratani Y, Kluckman K, Reddick R, Malinow MR, Maeda N: Mice deficient in cystathionine beta-synthase: Animal models for mild and severe homocyst(e)inemia. *Proc Natl Acad Sci U S A* **92**:1585, 1995.
279. Jones SN, Grompe M, Munir I, Veres G, Craigen WJ, Caskey CT: Ectopic correction of ornithine transcarbamylase deficiency in sparse fur mice. *J Biol Chem* **265**:14684, 1990.
280. Kurtz DM, Rinaldo P, Rhead WJ, Tian L, Millington DS, Vockley J, Hamm DA, Brix AE, Lindsey JR, Pinkert CA, O'Brien WE, Wood PA: Targeted disruption of mouse long-chain acyl-CoA dehydrogenase gene reveals crucial roles for fatty acid oxidation. *Proc Natl Acad Sci U S A* **95**:15592, 1998.
281. Otterbach B, Stoffel W: Acid sphingomyelinase-deficient mice mimic the neurovisceral form of human lysosomal storage disease (Niemann-Pick disease). *Cell* **81**:1053, 1995.
282. Potier M, Lu Shun Yan D, Womack JE: Neuraminidase deficiency in the mouse. *FEBS Lett* **108**:345, 1979.
283. Moullier P, Bohl D, Heard JM, Danos O: Correction of lysosomal storage in the liver and spleen of MPS VII mice by implantation of genetically modified skin fibroblasts. *Nat Genet* **4**:154, 1993.
284. Lu JF, Lawler AM, Watkins PA, Powers JM, Moser AB, Moser HW, Smith KD: A mouse model for X-linked adrenoleukodystrophy. *Proc Natl Acad Sci U S A* **94**:9366, 1997.
285. Schuchardt A, D'Agati V, Larsson-Blomberg L, Costantini F, Pachnis V: Defects in the kidney and enteric nervous system of mice lacking the tyrosine kinase receptor Ret. *Nature* **367**:380, 1994.
286. Moore MW, Klein RD, Farinas I, Sauer H, Armanini M, Phillips H, Reichardt LF, Ryan AM, Carver-Moore K, Rosenthal A: Renal and neuronal abnormalities in mice lacking GDNF. *Nature* **382**:76, 1996.
287. Yanagisawa H, Yanagisawa M, Kapur RP, Richardson JA, Williams SC, Clouthier DE, de Wit D, Emoto N, Hammer RE: Dual genetic pathways of endothelin-mediated intercellular signaling revealed by targeted disruption of endothelin converting enzyme-1 gene. *Development* **125**:825, 1998.
288. Hosoda K, Hammer RE, Richardson JA, Baynash AG, Cheung JC, Giaid A, Yanagisawa M: Targeted and natural (piebald-lethal) mutations of endothelin-B receptor gene produce megacolon associated with spotted coat color in mice. *Cell* **79**:1267, 1994.
289. Ezoe K, Holmes SA, Ho L, Bennett CP, Bolognia JL, Brueton L, Burn J, Falabella R, Gatto EM, Ishii N, et al: Novel mutations and deletions of the KIT (steel factor receptor) gene in human piebaldism. *Am J Hum Genet* **56**:58, 1995.
290. Schioth HB, Phillips SR, Rudzish R, Birch-Machin MA, Wikberg JE, Rees JL: Loss of function mutations of the human melanocortin 1 receptor are common and are associated with red hair. *Biochem Biophys Res Commun* **260**:488, 1999.
291. Robbins LS, Nadeau JH, Johnson KR, Kelly MA, Roselli-Rehfuss L, Baack E, Mountjoy KG, Cone RD: Pigmentation phenotypes of variant extension locus alleles result from point mutations that alter MSH receptor function. *Cell* **72**:827, 1993.
292. Baynash AG, Hosoda K, Giaid A, Richardson JA, Emoto N, Hammer RE, Yanagisawa M: Interaction of endothelin-3 with endothelin-B receptor is essential for development of epidermal melanocytes and enteric neurons. *Cell* **79**:1277, 1994.
293. Tassabehji M, Newton VE, Leverton K, Turnbull K, Seemanova E, Kunze J, Sperling K, Strachan T, Read AP: PAX3 gene structure and mutations: close analogies between Waardenburg syndrome and the Splotch mouse. *Hum Mol Genet* **3**:1069, 1994.

294. Jackson IJ, Raymond S: Manifestations of microphthalmia. *Nat Genet* **8**:209, 1994.
295. Hanson IM, Fletcher JM, Jordan T, Brown A, Taylor D, Adams RJ, Punnett HH, van Heyningen V: Mutations at the PAX6 locus are found in heterogeneous anterior segment malformations including Peters' anomaly. *Nat Genet* **6**:168, 1994.
296. Bowes C, Li T, Danciger M, Baxter LC, Applebury ML, Farber DB: Retinal degeneration in the rd mouse is caused by a defect in the beta subunit of rod cGMP-phosphodiesterase. *Nature* **347**:677, 1990.
297. Johnson KR, Cook SA, Erway LC, Matthews AN, Sanford LP, Paradies NE, Friedman RA: Inner ear and kidney anomalies caused by IAP insertion in an intron of the Eya1 gene in a mouse model of BOR syndrome. *Hum Mol Genet* **8**:645, 1999.
298. Brakenhoff RH, Henskens HA, van Rossum MW, Lubsen NH, Schoenmakers JG: Activation of the gamma E-crystallin pseudogene in the human hereditary Coppock-like cataract. *Hum Mol Genet* **3**:279, 1994.
299. Chambers C, Russell P: Deletion mutation in an eye lens beta-crystallin. An animal model for inherited cataracts. *J Biol Chem* **266**:6742, 1991.
300. White TW, Goodenough DA, Paul DL: Targeted ablation of connexin 50 in mice results in microphthalmia and zonular pulverulent cataracts. *J Cell Biol* **143**:815, 1998.
301. Gong X, Agopian K, Kumar NM, Gilula NB: Genetic factors influence cataract formation in alpha 3 connexin knockout mice. *Dev Genet* **24**:27, 1999.
302. van den Hurk JA, Hendriks W, van de Pol DJ, Oerlemans F, Jaissle G, Ruther K, Kohler K, Hartmann J, Zrenner E, van Bokhoven H, Wieringa B, Ropers HH, Cremers FP: Mouse choroideremia gene mutation causes photoreceptor cell degeneration and is not transmitted through the female germline. *Hum Mol Genet* **6**:851, 1997.
303. Furukawa T, Morrow EM, Li T, Davis FC, Cepko CL: Retinopathy and attenuated circadian entrainment in Crx-deficient mice. *Nat Genet* **23**:466, 1999.
304. Phippard D, Lu L, Lee D, Saunders JC, Crenshaw EB 3rd: Targeted mutagenesis of the POU-domain gene Brn4/Pou3f4 causes developmental defects in the inner ear. *J Neurosci* **19**:5980, 1999.
305. McGuirt WT, Prasad SD, Griffith AJ, Kunst HP, Green GE, Shpargel KB, Runge C, Huybrechts C, Mueller RF, Lynch E, King MC, Brunner HG, Cremers CW, Takanosu M, Li SW, Arita M, Mayne R, Prockop DJ, Van Camp G, Smith RJ: Mutations in COL11A2 cause non-syndromic hearing loss (DFNA13). *Nat Genet* **23**:413, 1999.
306. Erkman L, McEvilly RJ, Luo L, Ryan AK, Hooshmand F, O'Connell SM, Keithley EM, Rapaport DH, Ryan AF, Rosenfeld MG: Role of transcription factors Brn-3.1 and Brn-3.2 in auditory and visual system development. *Nature* **381**:603, 1996.
307. Gabriel HD, Jung D, Butzler C, Temme A, Traub O, Winterhager E, Willecke K: Transplacental uptake of glucose is decreased in embryonic lethal connexin26-deficient mice. *J Cell Biol* **140**:1453, 1998.
308. Probst FJ, Fridell RA, Raphael Y, Saunders TL, Wang A, Liang Y, Morell RJ, Touchman JW, Lyons RH, Noben-Trauth K, Friedman TB, Camper SA: Correction of deafness in shaker-2 mice by an unconventional myosin in a BAC transgene. *Science* **280**:1444, 1998.
309. Charpentier F, Merot J, Riochet D, Le Marec H, Escande D: Adult KCNE1-knockout mice exhibit a mild cardiac cellular phenotype. *Biochem Biophys Res Commun* **251**:806, 1998.
310. Berger W, van de Pol D, Bachner D, Oerlemans F, Winkens H, Hameister H, Wieringa B, Hendriks W, Ropers HH: An animal model for Norrie disease (ND): Gene targeting of the mouse ND gene. *Hum Mol Genet* **5**:51, 1996.
311. Beermann F, Ruppert S, Hummler E, Bosch FX, Muller G, Ruther U, Schutz G: Rescue of the albino phenotype by introduction of a functional tyrosinase gene into mice. *EMBO J* **9**:2819, 1990.
312. Rosemblat S, Durham-Pierre D, Gardner JM, Nakatsu Y, Brilliant MH, Orlow SJ: Identification of a melanosomal membrane protein encoded by the pink-eyed dilution (type II oculocutaneous albinism) gene. *Proc Natl Acad Sci U S A* **91**:12071, 1994.
313. Rinchik EM, Bell JA, Hunsicker PR, Friedman JM, Jackson IJ, Russell LB: Molecular genetics of the brown (b)-locus region of mouse chromosome 4. I. Origin and molecular mapping of radiation- and chemical-induced lethal brown deletions. *Genetics* **137**:845, 1994.
314. Oetting WS, King RA: Molecular basis of albinism: Mutations and polymorphisms of pigmentation genes associated with albinism. *Hum Mutat* **13**:99, 1999.
315. Keller SA, Jones JM, Boyle A, Barrow LL, Killen PD, Green DG, Kapousta NV, Hitchcock PF, Swank RT, Meisler MH: Kidney and retinal defects (Krd), a transgene-induced mutation with a deletion of mouse chromosome 19 that includes the Pax2 locus. *Genomics* **23**:309, 1994.
316. Sanyanusin P, Schimmenti LA, McNoe LA, Ward TA, Pierpont ME, Sullivan MJ, Dobyns WB, Eccles MR: Mutation of the PAX2 gene in a family with optic nerve colobomas, renal anomalies and vesicoureteral reflux. *Nat Genet* **9**:358, 1995.
317. Ma J, Norton JC, Allen AC, Burns JB, Hasel KW, Burns JL, Sutcliffe JG, Travis GH: Retinal degeneration slow (rds) in mouse results from simple insertion of a t haplotype-specific element into protein-coding exon II. *Genomics* **28**:212, 1995.
318. McNally N, Kenna P, Humphries MM, Hobson AH, Khan NW, Bush RA, Sieving PA, Humphries P, Farrar GJ: Structural and functional rescue of murine rod photoreceptors by human rhodopsin transgene. *Hum Mol Genet* **8**:1309, 1999.
319. Humphries MM, Rancourt D, Farrar GJ, Kenna P, Hazel M, Bush RA, Sieving PA, Sheils DM, McNally N, Creighton P, Erven A, Boros A, Gulya K, Capecchi MR, Humphries P: Retinopathy induced in mice by targeted disruption of the rhodopsin gene. *Nat Genet* **15**:216, 1997.
320. Weng J, Mata NL, Azarian SM, Tzekov RT, Birch DG, Travis GH: Insights into the function of Rim protein in photoreceptors and etiology of Stargardt's disease from the phenotype in abcr knockout mice. *Cell* **98**:13, 1999.
321. Weil D, Blanchard S, Kaplan J, Guilford P, Gibson F, Walsh J, Mburu P, Varela A, Levilliers J, Weston MD, et al: Defective myosin VIIA gene responsible for Usher syndrome type 1B. *Nature* **374**:60, 1995.
322. Ahmad W, Faiyaz ul Haque M, Brancolini V, Tsou HC, ul Haque S, Lam H, Aita VM, Owen J, deBlaquiere M, Frank J, Cserhalmi-Friedman PB, Leask A, McGrath JA, Peacocke M, Ahmad M, Ott J, Christiano AM: Alopecia universalis associated with a mutation in the human hairless gene. *Science* **279**:720, 1998.
323. Stoye JP, Fenner S, Greenoak GE, Moran C, Coffin JM: Role of endogenous retroviruses as mutagens: The hairless mutation of mice. *Cell* **54**:383, 1988.
324. Porter RM, Leitgeb S, Melton DW, Swensson O, Eady RA, Magin TM: Gene targeting at the mouse cytokeratin 10 locus: Severe skin fragility and changes of cytokeratin expression in the epidermis. *J Cell Biol* **132**:925, 1996.
325. Lloyd C, Yu QC, Cheng J, Turksen K, Degenstein L, Hutton E, Fuchs E: The basal keratin network of stratified squamous epithelia: Defining K15 function in the absence of K14. *J Cell Biol* **129**:1329, 1995.
326. Coulombe PA, Hutton ME, Letai A, Hebert A, Paller AS, Fuchs E: Point mutations in human keratin 14 genes of epidermolysis bullosa simplex patients: Genetic and functional analyses. *Cell* **66**:1301, 1991.
327. Andra K, Lassmann H, Bittner R, Shorny S, Fassler R, Propst F, Wiche G: Targeted inactivation of plectin reveals essential function in maintaining the integrity of skin, muscle, and heart cytoarchitecture. *Genes Dev* **11**:3143, 1997.
328. Dell'Angelica EC, Shotelersuk V, Aguilar RC, Gahl WA, Bonifacino JS: Altered trafficking of lysosomal proteins in Hermansky-Pudlak syndrome due to mutations in the beta 3A subunit of the AP-3 adaptor. *Mol Cell* **3**:11, 1999.
329. Feng L, Seymour AB, Jiang S, To A, Peden AA, Novak EK, Zhen L, Rusiniak ME, Eicher EM, Robinson MS, Gorin MB, Swank RT: The beta3A subunit gene (Ap3b1) of the AP-3 adaptor complex is altered in the mouse hypopigmentation mutant pearl, a model for Hermansky-Pudlak syndrome and night blindness. *Hum Mol Genet* **8**:323, 1999.
330. Feng GH, Bailin T, Oh J, Spritz RA: Mouse pale ear (ep) is homologous to human Hermansky-Pudlak syndrome and contains a rare "AT-AC" intron. *Hum Mol Genet* **6**:793, 1997.
331. Oh J, Ho L, Ala-Mello S, Amato D, Armstrong L, Bellucci S, Carakushansky G, Ellis JP, Fong CT, Green JS, Heon E, Legius E, Levin AV, Nieuwenhuis HK, Pinckers A, Tamura N, Whiteford ML, Yamasaki H, Spritz RA: Mutation analysis of patients with Hermansky-Pudlak syndrome: A frameshift hot spot in the HPS gene and apparent locus heterogeneity. *Am J Hum Genet* **62**:593, 1998.
332. Takahashi K, Folmer J, Coulombe PA: Increased expression of keratin 16 causes anomalies in cytoarchitecture and keratinization in transgenic mouse skin. *J Cell Biol* **127**:505, 1994.
333. Harada N, Tamai Y, Ishikawa T, Sauer B, Takaku K, Oshima M, Taketo MM: Intestinal polyposis in mice with a dominant stable mutation of the beta-catenin gene. *EMBO J* **18**:5931, 1999.
334. Gat U, DasGupta R, Degenstein L, Fuchs E: De Novo hair follicle morphogenesis and hair tumors in mice expressing a truncated beta-catenin in skin. *Cell* **95**:605, 1998.

335. Chan EF, Gat U, McNiff JM, Fuchs E: A common human skin tumour is caused by activating mutations in beta-catenin. *Nat Genet* **21**:410, 1999.
336. Xu X, Weinstein M, Li C, Deng C: Fibroblast growth factor receptors (FGFRs) and their roles in limb development. *Cell Tissue Res* **296**:33, 1999.
337. Partanen J, Schwartz L, Rossant J: Opposite phenotypes of hypomorphic and Y766 phosphorylation site mutations reveal a function for Fgfr1 in anteroposterior patterning of mouse embryos. *Genes Dev* **12**:2332, 1998.
338. Derry JM, Gormally E, Means GD, Zhao W, Meindl A, Kelley RI, Boyd Y, Herman GE: Mutations in a delta 8-delta 7 sterol isomerase in the tattered mouse and X-linked dominant chondrodysplasia punctata. *Nat Genet* **22**:286, 1999.
339. Otto F, Thornell AP, Crompton T, Denzel A, Gilmour KC, Rosewell IR, Stamp GW, Beddington RS, Mundlos S, Olsen BR, Selby PB, Owen MJ: Cbfa1, a candidate gene for cleidocranial dysplasia syndrome, is essential for osteoblast differentiation and bone development. *Cell* **89**:765, 1997.
340. Lee B, Thirunavukkarasu K, Zhou L, Pastore L, Baldini A, Hecht J, Geoffroy V, Ducy P, Karsenty G: Missense mutations abolishing DNA binding of the osteoblast-specific transcription factor OSF2/CBFA1 in cleidocranial dysplasia. *Nat Genet* **16**:307, 1997.
341. Liu YH, Kundu R, Wu L, Luo W, Ignelzi MA Jr, Snead ML, Maxson RE Jr: Premature suture closure and ectopic cranial bone in mice expressing Msx2 transgenes in the developing skull. *Proc Natl Acad Sci U S A* **92**:6137, 1995.
342. Xu X, Weinstein M, Li C, Naski M, Cohen RI, Ornitz DM, Leder P, Deng C: Fibroblast growth factor receptor 2 (FGFR2)-mediated reciprocal regulation loop between FGF8 and FGF10 is essential for limb induction. *Development* **125**:753, 1998.
343. Andrikopoulos K, Liu X, Keene DR, Jaenisch R, Ramirez F: Targeted mutation in the col5a2 gene reveals a regulatory role for type V collagen during matrix assembly. *Nat Genet* **9**:31, 1995.
344. Liu X, Wu H, Byrne M, Krane S, Jaenisch R: Type III collagen is crucial for collagen I fibrillogenesis and for normal cardiovascular development. *Proc Natl Acad Sci U S A* **94**:1852, 1997.
345. Vortkamp A, Gessler M, Grzeschik KH: GLI3 zinc-finger gene interrupted by translocations in Greig syndrome families. *Nature* **352**:539, 1991.
346. Thien H, Ruther U: The mouse mutation Pdn (Polydactyly Nagoya) is caused by the integration of a retrotransposon into the Gli3 gene. *Mamm Genome* **10**:205, 1999.
347. Hui CC, Joyner AL: A mouse model of greig cephalopolysyndactyly syndrome: The extra-toes J mutation contains an intragenic deletion of the Gli3 gene. *Nat Genet* **3**:241, 1993.
348. Mortlock DP, Innis JW: Mutation of HOXA13 in hand-foot-genital syndrome. *Nat Genet* **15**:179, 1997.
349. Waymire KG, Mahuren JD, Jaje JM, Guilarte TR, Coburn SP, MacGregor GR: Mice lacking tissue non-specific alkaline phosphatase die from seizures due to defective metabolism of vitamin B-6. *Nat Genet* **11**:45, 1995.
350. Munroe PB, Olgunturk RO, Fryns JP, Van Maldergem L, Ziereisen F, Yuksel B, Gardiner RM, Chung E: Mutations in the gene encoding the human matrix Gla protein cause Keutel syndrome. *Nat Genet* **21**:142, 1999.
351. Celli J, Duijf P, Hamel BC, Bamshad M, Kramer B, Smits AP, Newbury-Ecob R, Hennekam RC, Van Buggenhout G, van Haeringen A, Woods CG, van Essen AJ, de Waal R, Vriend G, Haber DA, Yang A, McKeon F, Brunner HG, van Bokhoven H: Heterozygous germline mutations in the p53 homolog p63 are the cause of EEC syndrome. *Cell* **99**:143, 1999.
352. Bona CA, Murai C, Casares S, Kasturi K, Nishimura H, Honjo T, Matsuda F: Structure of the mutant fibrillin-1 gene in the tight skin (TSK) mouse. *DNA Res* **4**:267, 1997.
353. Kielty CM, Raghunath M, Siracusa LD, Sherratt MJ, Peters R, Shuttleworth CA, Jimenez SA: The tight skin mouse: Demonstration of mutant fibrillin-1 production and assembly into abnormal microfibrils. *J Cell Biol* **140**:1159, 1998.
354. Pereira L, Andrikopoulos K, Tian J, Lee SY, Keene DR, Ono R, Reinhardt DP, Sakai LY, Biery NJ, Bunton T, Dietz HC, Ramirez F: Targetting of the gene encoding fibrillin-1 recapitulates the vascular aspect of Marfan syndrome. *Nat Genet* **17**:218, 1997.
355. Nakata K, Ono K, Miyazaki J, Olsen BR, Muragaki Y, Adachi E, Yamamura K, Kimura T: Osteoarthritis associated with mild chondrodysplasia in transgenic mice expressing alpha 1(IX) collagen chains with a central deletion. *Proc Natl Acad Sci U S A* **90**:2870, 1993.
356. Chen H, Lun Y, Ovchinnikov D, Kokubo H, Oberg KC, Pepicelli CV, Gan L, Lee B, Johnson RL: Limb and kidney defects in Lmx1b mutant mice suggest an involvement of LMX1B in human nail patella syndrome. *Nat Genet* **19**:51, 1998.
357. Dreyer SD, Zhou G, Baldini A, Winterpacht A, Zabel B, Cole W, Johnson RL, Lee B: Mutations in LMX1B cause abnormal skeletal patterning and renal dysplasia in nail patella syndrome. *Nat Genet* **19**:47, 1998.
358. Peters H, Neubuser A, Kratochwil K, Balling R: Pax9-deficient mice lack pharyngeal pouch derivatives and teeth and exhibit craniofacial and limb abnormalities. *Genes Dev* **12**:2735, 1998.
359. Stockton DW, Das P, Goldenberg M, D'Souza RN, Patel PI: Mutation of PAX9 is associated with oligodontia. *Nat Genet* **24**:18, 2000.
360. Lewis SE, Erickson RP, Barnett LB, Venta PJ, Tashian RE: *N*-ethyl-*N*-nitrosourea-induced null mutation at the mouse Car-2 locus: An animal model for human carbonic anhydrase II deficiency syndrome. *Proc Natl Acad Sci U S A* **85**:1962, 1988.
361. Lai LW, Chan DM, Erickson RP, Hsu SJ, Lien YH: Correction of renal tubular acidosis in carbonic anhydrase II-deficient mice with gene therapy. *J Clin Invest* **101**:1320, 1998.
362. Liu X, Wu H, Byrne M, Jeffrey J, Krane S, Jaenisch R: A targeted mutation at the known collagenase cleavage site in mouse type I collagen impairs tissue remodeling. *J Cell Biol* **130**:227, 1995.
363. Chipman SD, Sweet HO, McBride DJ Jr, Davisson MT, Marks SC Jr, Shuldiner AR, Wenstrup RJ, Rowe DW, Shapiro JR: Defective pro alpha 2(I) collagen synthesis in a recessive mutation in mice: A model of human osteogenesis imperfecta. *Proc Natl Acad Sci U S A* **90**:1701, 1993.
364. Saftig P, Hunziker E, Wehmeyer O, Jones S, Boyde A, Rommerskirch W, Moritz JD, Schu P, von Figura K: Impaired osteoclastic bone resorption leads to osteopetrosis in cathepsin-K-deficient mice. *Proc Natl Acad Sci U S A* **95**:13453, 1998.
365. Bourgeois P, Bolcato-Bellemin AL, Danse JM, Bloch-Zupan A, Yoshiba K, Stoetzel C, Perrin-Schmitt F: The variable expressivity and incomplete penetrance of the twist-null heterozygous mouse phenotype resemble those of human Saethre-Chotzen syndrome. *Hum Mol Genet* **7**:945, 1998.
366. Chan D, Jacenko O: Phenotypic and biochemical consequences of collagen X mutations in mice and humans. *Matrix Biol* **17**:169, 1998.
367. Sidow A, Bulotsky MS, Kerrebrock AW, Birren BW, Altshuler D, Jaenisch R, Johnson KR, Lander ES: A novel member of the F-box/WD40 gene family, encoding dactylin, is disrupted in the mouse dactylaplasia mutant. *Nat Genet* **23**:104, 1999.
368. ul-Haque MF, King LM, Krakow D, Cantor RM, Rusiniak ME, Swank RT, Superti-Furga A, Haque S, Abbas H, Ahmad W, Ahmad M, Cohn DH: Mutations in orthologous genes in human spondyloepimetaphyseal dysplasia and the brachymorphic mouse. *Nat Genet* **20**:157, 1998.
369. Li SW, Prockop DJ, Helminen H, Fassler R, Lapvetelainen T, Kiraly K, Peltarri A, Arokoski J, Lui H, Arita M, et al: Transgenic mice with targeted inactivation of the Col2 alpha 1 gene for collagen II develop a skeleton with membranous and periosteal bone but no endochondral bone. *Genes Dev* **9**:2821, 1995.
370. Hiltunen A, Metsaranta M, Virolainen P, Aro HT, Vuorio E: Retarded chondrogenesis in transgenic mice with a type II collagen defect results in fracture healing abnormalities. *Dev Dyn* **200**:340, 1994.
371. Li Y, Lacerda DA, Warman ML, Beier DR, Yoshioka H, Ninomiya Y, Oxford JT, Morris NP, Andrikopoulos K, Ramirez F, et al: A fibrillar collagen gene, Col11a1, is essential for skeletal morphogenesis. *Cell* **80**:423, 1995.
372. Muragaki Y, Mundlos S, Upton J, Olsen BR: Altered growth and branching patterns in synpolydactyly caused by mutations in HOXD13. *Science* **272**:548, 1996.
373. Johnson KR, Sweet HO, Donahue LR, Ward-Bailey P, Bronson RT, Davisson MT: A new spontaneous mouse mutation of Hoxd13 with a polyalanine expansion and phenotype similar to human synpolydactyly. *Hum Mol Genet* **7**:1033, 1998.
374. Wang L, Du L, Ecarot B: Evidence for Phex haploinsufficiency in murine X-linked hypophosphatemia. *Mamm Genome* **10**:385, 1999.
375. Bugge TH, Kombrinck KW, Flick MJ, Daugherty CC, Danton MJ, Degen JL: Loss of fibrinogen rescues mice from the pleiotropic effects of plasminogen deficiency. *Cell* **87**:709, 1996.
376. Hermans MH, Ward AC, Antonissen C, Karis A, Lowenberg B, Touw IP: Perturbed granulopoiesis in mice with a targeted mutation in the granulocyte colony-stimulating factor receptor gene associated with severe chronic neutropenia. *Blood* **92**:32, 1998.
377. McLemore ML, Poursine-Laurent J, Link DC: Increased granulocyte colony-stimulating factor responsiveness but normal resting granulo-

poiesis in mice carrying a targeted granulocyte colony-stimulating factor receptor mutation derived from a patient with severe congenital neutropenia. *J Clin Invest* **102**:483, 1998.

378. Paszty C, Mohandas N, Stevens ME, Loring JF, Liebhaber SA, Brion CM, Rubin EM: Lethal alpha-thalassaemia created by gene targeting in mice and its genetic rescue. *Nat Genet* **11**:33, 1995.
379. Singer GG, Carrera AC, Marshak-Rothstein A, Martinez C, Abbas AK: Apoptosis, Fas and systemic autoimmunity: The MRL-*lpr/lpr* model. *Curr Opin Immunol* **6**:913, 1994.
380. Ciavatta DJ, Ryan TM, Farmer SC, Townes TM: Mouse model of human beta zero thalassemia: Targeted deletion of the mouse beta maj- and beta min-globin genes in embryonic stem cells. *Proc Natl Acad Sci U S A* **92**:9259, 1995.
381. Mardiney M 3rd, Jackson SH, Spratt SK, Li F, Holland SM, Malech HL: Enhanced host defense after gene transfer in the murine p47phox-deficient model of chronic granulomatous disease. *Blood* **89**:2268, 1997.
382. Botto M, Dell'Agnola C, Bygrave AE, Thompson EM, Cook HT, Petry F, Loos M, Pandolfi PP, Walport MJ: Homozygous C1q deficiency causes glomerulonephritis associated with multiple apoptotic bodies. *Nat Genet* **19**:56, 1998.
383. Taylor PR, Nash JT, Theodoridis E, Bygrave AE, Walport MJ, Botto M: A targeted disruption of the murine complement factor B gene resulting in loss of expression of three genes in close proximity, factor B, C2, and D17H6S45. *J Biol Chem* **273**:1699, 1998.
384. Pekna M, Hietala MA, Rosklint T, Betsholtz C, Pekny M: Targeted disruption of the murine gene coding for the third complement component (C3). *Scand J Immunol* **47**:25, 1998.
385. Prodeus AP, Zhou X, Maurer M, Galli SJ, Carroll MC: Impaired mast cell-dependent natural immunity in complement C3-deficient mice. *Nature* **390**:172, 1997.
386. Wetsel RA, Fleischer DT, Haviland DL: Deficiency of the murine fifth complement component (C5). A 2-base pair gene deletion in a 5′-exon. *J Biol Chem* **265**:2435, 1990.
387. Tanaka S, Suzuki T, Sakaizumi M, Harada Y, Matsushima Y, Miyashita N, Fukumori Y, Inai S, Moriwaki K, Yonekawa H: Gene responsible for deficient activity of the beta subunit of C8, the eighth component of complement, is located on mouse chromosome 4. *Immunogenetics* **33**:18, 1991.
388. Grimber G, Galand C, Garbarz M, Mattei MG, Cavard C, Zider A, Blanchet P, Boivin P, Briand P, Dhermy D: Inherited haemolytic anaemia created by insertional inactivation of the alpha-spectrin gene. *Transgenic Res* **1**:268, 1992.
389. Bloom ML, Kaysser TM, Birkenmeier CS, Barker JE: The murine mutation jaundiced is caused by replacement of an arginine with a stop codon in the mRNA encoding the ninth repeat of beta- spectrin. *Proc Natl Acad Sci U S A* **91**:10099, 1994.
390. Lin CS, Lim SK, D'Agati V, Costantini F: Differential effects of an erythropoietin receptor gene disruption on primitive and definitive erythropoiesis. *Genes Dev* **10**:154, 1996.
391. Wu H, Liu X, Jaenisch R, Lodish HF: Generation of committed erythroid BFU-E and CFU-E progenitors does not require erythropoietin or the erythropoietin receptor. *Cell* **83**:59, 1995.
392. Xue J, Wu Q, Westfield LA, Tuley EA, Lu D, Zhang Q, Shim K, Zheng X, Sadler JE: Incomplete embryonic lethality and fatal neonatal hemorrhage caused by prothrombin deficiency in mice. *Proc Natl Acad Sci U S A* **95**:7603, 1998.
393. Cui J, O'Shea KS, Purkayastha A, Saunders TL, Ginsburg D: Fatal haemorrhage and incomplete block to embryogenesis in mice lacking coagulation factor V. *Nature* **384**:66, 1996.
394. Rosen ED, Chan JC, Idusogie E, Clotman F, Vlasuk G, Luther T, Jalbert LR, Albrecht S, Zhong L, Lissens A, Schoonjans L, Moons L, Collen D, Castellino FJ, Carmeliet P: Mice lacking factor VII develop normally but suffer fatal perinatal bleeding. *Nature* **390**:290, 1997.
395. Gailani D, Lasky NM, Broze GJ Jr: A murine model of factor XI deficiency. *Blood Coagul Fibrinolysis* **8**:134, 1997.
396. Kamijo R, Le J, Shapiro D, Havell EA, Huang S, Aguet M, Bosland M, Vilcek J: Mice that lack the interferon-gamma receptor have profoundly altered responses to infection with Bacillus Calmette-Guerin and subsequent challenge with lipopolysaccharide. *J Exp Med* **178**:1435, 1993.
397. Hodivala-Dilke KM, McHugh KP, Tsakiris DA, Rayburn H, Crowley D, Ullman-Cullere M, Ross FP, Coller BS, Teitelbaum S, Hynes RO: Beta3-integrin-deficient mice are a model for Glanzmann thrombasthenia showing placental defects and reduced survival. *J Clin Invest* **103**:229, 1999.
398. Pastural E, Barrat FJ, Dufourcq-Lagelouse R, Certain S, Sanal O, Jabado N, Seger R, Griscelli C, Fischer A, de Saint Basile G: Griscelli disease maps to chromosome 15q21 and is associated with mutations in the myosin-Va gene. *Nat Genet* **16**:289, 1997.
399. Bi L, Lawler AM, Antonarakis SE, High KA, Gearhart JD, Kazazian HH Jr: Targeted disruption of the mouse factor VIII gene produces a model of haemophilia A [Letter]. *Nat Genet* **10**:119, 1995.
400. Lin HF, Maeda N, Smithies O, Straight DL, Stafford DW: A coagulation factor IX-deficient mouse model for human hemophilia B. *Blood* **90**:3962, 1997.
401. White RA, Peters LL, Adkison LR, Korsgren C, Cohen CM, Lux SE: The murine pallid mutation is a platelet storage pool disease associated with the protein 4.2 (pallidin) gene. *Nat Genet* **2**:80, 1992.
402. Wilson RW, Ballantyne CM, Smith CW, Montgomery C, Bradley A, O'Brien WE, Beaudet AL: Gene targeting yields a CD18-mutant mouse for study of inflammation. *J Immunol* **151**:1571, 1993.
403. Keller P, Tremml G, Rosti V, Bessler M: X inactivation and somatic cell selection rescue female mice carrying a Piga-null mutation. *Proc Natl Acad Sci U S A* **96**:7479, 1999.
404. Bugge TH, Flick MJ, Daugherty CC, Degen JL: Plasminogen deficiency causes severe thrombosis but is compatible with development and reproduction. *Genes Dev* **9**:794, 1995.
405. Drew AF, Kaufman AH, Kombrinck KW, Danton MJ, Daugherty CC, Degen JL, Bugge TH: Ligneous conjunctivitis in plasminogen-deficient mice. *Blood* **91**:1616, 1998.
406. Romer J, Bugge TH, Pyke C, Lund LR, Flick MJ, Degen JL, Dano K: Impaired wound healing in mice with a disrupted plasminogen gene. *Nat Med* **2**:287, 1996.
407. Tsujino K, Kanno H, Hashimoto K, Fujii H, Jippo T, Morii E, Lee YM, Asai H, Miwa S, Kitamura Y: Delayed onset of hemolytic anemia in CBA-Pk-1slc/Pk-1slc mice with a point mutation of the gene encoding red blood cell type pyruvate kinase. *Blood* **91**:2169, 1998.
408. Bunting KD, Flynn KJ, Riberdy JM, Doherty PC, Sorrentino BP: Virus-specific immunity after gene therapy in a murine model of severe combined immunodeficiency. *Proc Natl Acad Sci U S A* **96**:232, 1999.
409. Puel A, Ziegler SF, Buckley RH, Leonard WJ: Defective IL7R expression in T(−)B(+)NK(+) severe combined immunodeficiency. *Nat Genet* **20**:394, 1998.
410. Schwarz K, Gauss GH, Ludwig L, Pannicke U, Li Z, Lindner D, Friedrich W, Seger RA, Hansen-Hagge TE, Desiderio S, Lieber MR, Bartram CR: RAG mutations in human B cell-negative SCID. *Science* **274**:97, 1996.
411. Clausen BE, Waldburger JM, Schwenk F, Barras E, Mach B, Rajewsky K, Forster I, Reith W: Residual MHC class II expression on mature dendritic cells and activated B cells in RFX5-deficient mice. *Immunity* **8**:143, 1998.
412. Embury SH, Mohandas N, Paszty C, Cooper P, Cheung AT: In vivo blood flow abnormalities in the transgenic knockout sickle cell mouse. *J Clin Invest* **103**:915, 1999.
413. Weiler-Guettler H, Christie PD, Beeler DL, Healy AM, Hancock WW, Rayburn H, Edelberg JM, Rosenberg RD: A targeted point mutation in thrombomodulin generates viable mice with a prethrombotic state. *J Clin Invest* **101**:1983, 1998.
414. Healy AM, Rayburn HB, Rosenberg RD, Weiler H: Absence of the blood-clotting regulator thrombomodulin causes embryonic lethality in mice before development of a functional cardiovascular system. *Proc Natl Acad Sci U S A* **92**:850, 1995.
415. Snapper SB, Rosen FS, Mizoguchi E, Cohen P, Khan W, Liu CH, Hagemann TL, Kwan SP, Ferrini R, Davidson L, Bhan AK, Alt FW: Wiskott-Aldrich syndrome protein-deficient mice reveal a role for WASP in T but not B cell activation. *Immunity* **9**:81, 1998.
416. Lawn RM, Wade DP, Hammer RE, Chiesa G, Verstuyft JG, Rubin EM: Atherogenesis in transgenic mice expressing human apolipoprotein (a) [see Comments]. *Nature* **360**:670, 1992.
417. Powell-Braxton L, Veniant M, Latvala RD, Hirano KI, Won WB, Ross J, Dybdal N, Zlot CH, Young SG, Davidson NO: A mouse model of human familial hypercholesterolemia: Markedly elevated low-density lipoprotein cholesterol levels and severe atherosclerosis on a low-fat chow diet. *Nat Med* **4**:934, 1998.
418. Castellani LW, Weinreb A, Bodnar J, Goto AM, Doolittle M, Mehrabian M, Demant P, Lusis AJ: Mapping a gene for combined hyperlipidaemia in a mutant mouse strain. *Nat Genet* **18**:374, 1998.
419. Pajukanta P, Nuotio I, Terwilliger JD, Porkka KV, Ylitalo K, Pihlajamaki J, Suomalainen AJ, Syvanen AC, Lehtimaki T, Viikari JS, Laakso M, Taskinen MR, Ehnholm C, Peltonen L: Linkage of familial combined hyperlipidaemia to chromosome 1q21-q23. *Nat Genet* **18**:369, 1998.

420. Plump AS, Erickson SK, Weng W, Partin JS, Breslow JL, Williams DL: Apolipoprotein A-I is required for cholesteryl ester accumulation in steroidogenic cells and for normal adrenal steroid production. *J Clin Invest* **97**:2660, 1996.
421. Farese RV Jr, Ruland SL, Flynn LM, Stokowski RP, Young SG: Knockout of the mouse apolipoprotein B gene results in embryonic lethality in homozygotes and protection against diet-induced hypercholesterolemia in heterozygotes. *Proc Natl Acad Sci U S A* **92**:1774, 1995.
422. Huang LS, Voyiaziakis E, Markenson DF, Sokol KA, Hayek T, Breslow JL: Apo B gene knockout in mice results in embryonic lethality in homozygotes and neural tube defects, male infertility, and reduced HDL cholesterol ester and apo A-I transport rates in heterozygotes. *J Clin Invest* **96**:2152, 1995.
423. Dichek HL, Brecht W, Fan J, Ji ZS, McCormick SP, Akeefe H, Conzo L, Sanan DA, Weisgraber KH, Young SG, Taylor JM, Mahley RW: Overexpression of hepatic lipase in transgenic mice decreases apolipoprotein B-containing and high density lipoproteins. Evidence that hepatic lipase acts as a ligand for lipoprotein uptake. *J Biol Chem* **273**:1896, 1998.
424. Levak-Frank S, Radner H, Walsh A, Stollberger R, Knipping G, Hoefler G, Sattler W, Weinstock PH, Breslow JL, Zechner R: Muscle-specific overexpression of lipoprotein lipase causes a severe myopathy characterized by proliferation of mitochondria and peroxisomes in transgenic mice. *J Clin Invest* **96**:976, 1995.
425. Mercer JF, Grimes A, Ambrosini L, Lockhart P, Paynter JA, Dierick H, Glover TW: Mutations in the murine homologue of the Menkes gene in dappled and blotchy mice. *Nat Genet* **6**:374, 1994.
426. Das S, Levinson B, Vulpe C, Whitney S, Gitschier J, Packman S: Similar splicing mutations of the Menkes/mottled copper-transporting ATPase gene in occipital horn syndrome and the blotchy mouse. *Am J Hum Genet* **56**:570, 1995.
427. Helbling-Leclerc A, Zhang X, Topaloglu H, Cruaud C, Tesson F, Weissenbach J, Tome FM, Schwartz K, Fardeau M, Tryggvason K, et al: Mutations in the laminin alpha 2-chain gene (LAMA2) cause merosin-deficient congenital muscular dystrophy. *Nat Genet* **11**:216, 1995.
428. Miyagoe Y, Hanaoka K, Nonaka I, Hayasaka M, Nabeshima Y, Arahata K, Takeda S: Laminin alpha2 chain-null mutant mice by targeted disruption of the Lama2 gene: A new model of merosin (laminin 2)-deficient congenital muscular dystrophy. *FEBS Lett* **415**:33, 1997.
429. Sunada Y, Bernier SM, Kozak CA, Yamada Y, Campbell KP: Deficiency of merosin in dystrophic dy mice and genetic linkage of laminin M chain gene to dy locus. *J Biol Chem* **269**:13729, 1994.
430. Xu H, Wu XR, Wewer UM, Engvall E: Murine muscular dystrophy caused by a mutation in the laminin alpha 2 (Lama2) gene. *Nat Genet* **8**:297, 1994.
431. Jansen G, Groenen PJ, Bachner D, Jap PH, Coerwinkel M, Oerlemans F, van den Broek W, Gohlsch B, Pette D, Plomp JJ, Molenaar PC, Nederhoff MG, van Echteld CJ, Dekker M, Berns A, Hameister H, Wieringa B: Abnormal myotonic dystrophy protein kinase levels produce only mild myopathy in mice. *Nat Genet* **13**:316, 1996.
432. The Dutch-Belgian Fragile X Consortium: Fmrl knockout mice: A model to study fragile X mental retardation. *Cell* **78**:23, 1994.
433. Ptacek LJ, Tawil R, Griggs RC, Engel AG, Layzer RB, Kwiecinski H, McManis PG, Santiago L, Moore M, Fouad G, et al: Dihydropyridine receptor mutations cause hypokalemic periodic paralysis. *Cell* **77**:863, 1994.
434. Ryan SG, Buckwalter MS, Lynch JW, Handford CA, Segura L, Shiang R, Wasmuth JJ, Camper SA, Schofield P, O'Connell P: A missense mutation in the gene encoding the alpha 1 subunit of the inhibitory glycine receptor in the spasmodic mouse. *Nat Genet* **7**:131, 1994.
435. Shiang R, Ryan SG, Zhu YZ, Hahn AF, O'Connell P, Wasmuth JJ: Mutations in the alpha 1 subunit of the inhibitory glycine receptor cause the dominant neurologic disorder, hyperekplexia. *Nat Genet* **5**:351, 1993.
436. Takeshima H, Iino M, Takekura H, Nishi M, Kuno J, Minowa O, Takano H, Noda T: Excitation-contraction uncoupling and muscular degeneration in mice lacking functional skeletal muscle ryanodine-receptor gene. *Nature* **369**:556, 1994.
437. Hack AA, Ly CT, Jiang F, Clendenin CJ, Sigrist KS, Wollmann RL, McNally EM: Gamma-sarcoglycan deficiency leads to muscle membrane defects and apoptosis independent of dystrophin. *J Cell Biol* **142**:1279, 1998.
438. Duclos F, Straub V, Moore SA, Venzke DP, Hrstka RF, Crosbie RH, Durbeej M, Lebakken CS, Ettinger AJ, van der Meulen J, Holt KH, Lim LE, Sanes JR, Davidson BL, Faulkner JA, Williamson R, Campbell KP: Progressive muscular dystrophy in alpha-sarcoglycan-deficient mice. *J Cell Biol* **142**:1461, 1998.
439. Chapman VM, Miller DR, Armstrong D, Caskey CT: Recovery of induced mutations for X chromosome-linked muscular dystrophy in mice. *Proc Natl Acad Sci U S A* **86**:1292, 1989.
440. Sicinski P, Geng Y, Ryder-Cook AS, Barnard EA, Darlison MG, Barnard PJ: The molecular basis of muscular dystrophy in the mdx mouse: A point mutation. *Science* **244**:1578, 1989.
441. Smart SL, Lopantsev V, Zhang CL, Robbins CA, Wang H, Chiu SY, Schwartzkroin PA, Messing A, Tempel BL: Deletion of the K(V)1.1 potassium channel causes epilepsy in mice. *Neuron* **20**:809, 1998.
442. Moran PM, Higgins LS, Cordell B, Moser PC: Age-related learning deficits in transgenic mice expressing the 751-amino acid isoform of human beta-amyloid precursor protein. *Proc Natl Acad Sci U S A* **92**:5341, 1995.
443. Zheng H, Jiang M, Trumbauer ME, Sirinathsinghji DJ, Hopkins R, Smith DW, Heavens RP, Dawson GR, Boyce S, Conner MW, et al: Beta-amyloid precursor protein-deficient mice show reactive gliosis and decreased locomotor activity. *Cell* **81**:525, 1995.
444. Hsiao KK, Borchelt DR, Olson K, Johannsdottir R, Kitt C, Yunis W, Xu S, Eckman C, Younkin S, Price D, et al: Age-related CNS disorder and early death in transgenic FVB/N mice overexpressing Alzheimer amyloid precursor proteins. *Neuron* **15**:1203, 1995.
445. Oyama F, Sawamura N, Kobayashi K, Morishima-Kawashima M, Kuramochi T, Ito M, Tomita T, Maruyama K, Saido TC, Iwatsubo T, Capell A, Walter J, Grunberg J, Ueyama Y, Haass C, Ihara Y: Mutant presenilin 2 transgenic mouse: Effect on an age-dependent increase of amyloid beta-protein 42 in the brain. *J Neurochem* **71**:313, 1998.
446. Qian S, Jiang P, Guan XM, Singh G, Trumbauer ME, Yu H, Chen HY, Van de Ploeg LH, Zheng H: Mutant human presenilin 1 protects presenilin 1 null mouse against embryonic lethality and elevates Abeta1-42/43 expression. *Neuron* **20**:611, 1998.
447. Witke W, Sharpe AH, Hartwig JH, Azuma T, Stossel TP, Kwiatkowski DJ: Hemostatic, inflammatory, and fibroblast responses are blunted in mice lacking gelsolin. *Cell* **81**:41, 1995.
448. Figlewicz DA, Krizus A, Martinoli MG, Meininger V, Dib M, Rouleau GA, Julien JP: Variants of the heavy neurofilament subunit are associated with the development of amyotrophic lateral sclerosis. *Hum Mol Genet* **3**:1757, 1994.
449. Collard JF, Cote F, Julien JP: Defective axonal transport in a transgenic mouse model of amyotrophic lateral sclerosis. *Nature* **375**:61, 1995.
450. Tu PH, Raju P, Robinson KA, Gurney ME, Trojanowski JQ, Lee VM: Transgenic mice carrying a human mutant superoxide dismutase transgene develop neuronal cytoskeletal pathology resembling human amyotrophic lateral sclerosis lesions. *Proc Natl Acad Sci U S A* **93**:3155, 1996.
451. Barlow C, Hirotsune S, Paylor R, Liyanage M, Eckhaus M, Collins F, Shiloh Y, Crawley JN, Ried T, Tagle D, Wynshaw-Boris A: Atm-deficient mice: A paradigm of ataxia telangiectasia. *Cell* **86**:159, 1996.
452. Barlow C, Eckhaus MA, Schaffer AA, Wynshaw-Boris A: Atm haploinsufficiency results in increased sensitivity to sublethal doses of ionizing radiation in mice. *Nat Genet* **21**:359, 1999.
453. Huxley C, Passage E, Manson A, Putzu G, Figarella-Branger D, Pellissier JF, Fontes M: Construction of a mouse model of Charcot-Marie-Tooth disease type 1A by pronuclear injection of human YAC DNA. *Hum Mol Genet* **5**:563, 1996.
454. Adlkofer K, Martini R, Aguzzi A, Zielasek J, Toyka KV, Suter U: Hypermyelination and demyelinating peripheral neuropathy in Pmp22-deficient mice. *Nat Genet* **11**:274, 1995.
455. Martini R, Zielasek J, Toyka KV, Giese KP, Schachner M: Protein zero (P0)-deficient mice show myelin degeneration in peripheral nerves characteristic of inherited human neuropathies. *Nat Genet* **11**:281, 1995.
456. Scherer SS, Xu YT, Nelles E, Fischbeck K, Willecke K, Bone LJ: Connexin32-null mice develop demyelinating peripheral neuropathy. *Glia* **24**:8, 1998.
457. Schneider-Maunoury S, Topilko P, Seitandou T, Levi G, Cohen-Tannoudji M, Pournin S, Babinet C, Charnay P: Disruption of Krox-20 results in alteration of rhombomeres 3 and 5 in the developing hindbrain. *Cell* **75**:1199, 1993.
458. Smeyne RJ, Klein R, Schnapp A, Long LK, Bryant S, Lewin A, Lira SA, Barbacid M: Severe sensory and sympathetic neuropathies in mice carrying a disrupted Trk/NGF receptor gene. *Nature* **368**:246, 1994.
459. Sato T, Oyake M, Nakamura K, Nakao K, Fukusima Y, Onodera O, Igarashi S, Takano H, Kikugawa K, Ishida Y, Shimohata T, Koide R, Ikeuchi T, Tanaka H, Futamura N, Matsumura R, Takayanagi T, Tanaka F, Sobue G, Komure O, Takahashi M, Sano A, Ichikawa Y,

Goto J, Kanazawa I, et al: Transgenic mice harboring a full-length human mutant DRPLA gene exhibit age-dependent intergenerational and somatic instabilities of CAG repeats comparable with those in DRPLA patients. *Hum Mol Genet* **8**:99, 1999.
460. Thomas SA, Matsumoto AM, Palmiter RD: Noradrenaline is essential for mouse fetal development. *Nature* **374**:643, 1995.
461. Pennacchio LA, Bouley DM, Higgins KM, Scott MP, Noebels JL, Myers RM: Progressive ataxia, myoclonic epilepsy and cerebellar apoptosis in cystatin B-deficient mice. *Nat Genet* **20**:251, 1998.
462. Ranta S, Zhang Y, Ross B, Lonka L, Takkunen E, Messer A, Sharp J, Wheeler R, Kusumi K, Mole S, Liu W, Soares MB, Bonaldo MF, Hirvasniemi A, de la Chapelle A, Gilliam TC, Lehesjoki AE: The neuronal ceroid lipofuscinoses in human EPMR and mnd mutant mice are associated with mutations in CLN8. *Nat Genet* **23**:233, 1999.
463. Collinge J, Palmer MS, Sidle KC, Hill AF, Gowland I, Meads J, Asante E, Bradley R, Doey LJ, Lantos PL: Unaltered susceptibility to BSE in transgenic mice expressing human prion protein. *Nature* **378**:779, 1995.
464. Telling GC, Haga T, Torchia M, Tremblay P, DeArmond SJ, Prusiner SB: Interactions between wild-type and mutant prion proteins modulate neurodegeneration in transgenic mice. *Genes Dev* **10**:1736, 1996.
465. Sakaguchi S, Katamine S, Nishida N, Moriuchi R, Shigematsu K, Sugimoto T, Nakatani A, Kataoka Y, Houtani T, Shirabe S, Okada H, Hasegawa S, Miyamoto T, Noda T: Loss of cerebellar Purkinje cells in aged mice homozygous for a disrupted PrP gene. *Nature* **380**:528, 1996.
466. Fletcher CF, Lutz CM, O'Sullivan TN, Shaughnessy JD Jr, Hawkes R, Frankel WN, Copeland NG, Jenkins NA: Absence epilepsy in tottering mutant mice is associated with calcium channel defects. *Cell* **87**:607, 1996.
467. Shelbourne PF, Killeen N, Hevner RF, Johnston HM, Tecott L, Lewandoski M, Ennis M, Ramirez L, Li Z, Iannicola C, Littman DR, Myers RM: A Huntington's disease CAG expansion at the murine Hdh locus is unstable and associated with behavioural abnormalities in mice. *Hum Mol Genet* **8**:763, 1999.
468. Mangiarini L, Sathasivam K, Mahal A, Mott R, Seller M, Bates GP: Instability of highly expanded CAG repeats in mice transgenic for the Huntington's disease mutation. *Nat Genet* **15**:197, 1997.
469. Nasir J, Floresco SB, O'Kusky JR, Diewert VM, Richman JM, Zeisler J, Borowski A, Marth JD, Phillips AG, Hayden MR: Targeted disruption of the Huntington's disease gene results in embryonic lethality and behavioral and morphological changes in heterozygotes. *Cell* **81**:811, 1995.
470. Zeitlin S, Liu JP, Chapman DL, Papaioannou VE, Efstratiadis A: Increased apoptosis and early embryonic lethality in mice nullizygous for the Huntington's disease gene homologue. *Nat Genet* **11**:155, 1995.
471. Wheeler VC, Auerbach W, White JK, Srinidhi J, Auerbach A, Ryan A, Duyao MP, Vrbanac V, Weaver M, Gusella JF, Joyner AL, MacDonald ME: Length-dependent gametic CAG repeat instability in the Huntington's disease knock-in mouse. *Hum Mol Genet* **8**:115, 1999.
472. Duyao MP, Auerbach AB, Ryan A, Persichetti F, Barnes GT, McNeil SM, Ge P, Vonsattel JP, Gusella JF, Joyner AL, et al: Inactivation of the mouse Huntington's disease gene homolog Hdh. *Science* **269**:407, 1995.
473. Hirotsune S, Fleck MW, Gambello MJ, Bix GJ, Chen A, Clark GD, Ledbetter DH, McBain CJ, Wynshaw-Boris A: Graded reduction of Pafah1b1 (Lis1) activity results in neuronal migration defects and early embryonic lethality. *Nat Genet* **19**:333, 1998.
474. Ikeda H, Yamaguchi M, Sugai S, Aze Y, Narumiya S, Kakizuka A: Expanded polyglutamine in the Machado-Joseph disease protein induces cell death in vitro and in vivo. *Nat Genet* **13**:196, 1996.
475. Cases O, Seif I, Grimsby J, Gaspar P, Chen K, Pournin S, Muller U, Aguet M, Babinet C, Shih JC, et al: Aggressive behavior and altered amounts of brain serotonin and norepinephrine in mice lacking MAOA. *Science* **268**:1763, 1995.
476. Kim JJ, Shih JC, Chen K, Chen L, Bao S, Maren S, Anagnostaras SG, Fanselow MS, De Maeyer E, Seif I, Thompson RF: Selective enhancement of emotional, but not motor, learning in monoamine oxidase A-deficient mice. *Proc Natl Acad Sci U S A* **94**:5929, 1997.
477. Bronson RT, Donahue LR, Johnson KR, Tanner A, Lane PW, Faust JR: Neuronal ceroid lipofuscinosis (nclf), a new disorder of the mouse linked to chromosome 9. *Am J Med Genet* **77**:289, 1998.
478. Greene ND, Bernard DL, Taschner PE, Lake BD, de Vos N, Breuning MH, Gardiner RM, Mole SE, Nussbaum RL, Mitchison HM: A murine model for juvenile NCL: Gene targeting of mouse Cln3. *Mol Genet Metab* **66**:309, 1999.
479. Mitchison HM, Bernard DJ, Greene ND, Cooper JD, Junaid MA, Pullarkat RK, de Vos N, Breuning MH, Owens JW, Mobley WC, Gardiner RM, Lake BD, Taschner PE, Nussbaum RL: Targeted disruption of the cln3 gene provides a mouse model for Batten disease. *Neurobiol Dis* **6**:321, 1999.
480. Griffiths IR, Schneider A, Anderson J, Nave KA: Transgenic and natural mouse models of proteolipid protein (PLP)-related dysmyelination and demyelination. *Brain Pathol* **5**:275, 1995.
481. Schrank B, Gotz R, Gunnersen JM, Ure JM, Toyka KV, Smith AG, Sendtner M: Inactivation of the survival motor neuron gene, a candidate gene for human spinal muscular atrophy, leads to massive cell death in early mouse embryos. *Proc Natl Acad Sci U S A* **94**:9920, 1997.
482. Hsieh-Li HM, Chang JG, Jong YJ, Wu MH, Wang NM, Tsai CH, Li H: A mouse model for spinal muscular atrophy. *Nat Genet* **24**:66, 2000.
483. Burright EN, Clark HB, Servadio A, Matilla T, Feddersen RM, Yunis WS, Duvick LA, Zoghbi HY, Orr HT: SCA1 transgenic mice: A model for neurodegeneration caused by an expanded CAG trinucleotide repeat. *Cell* **82**:937, 1995.
484. Matilla A, Roberson ED, Banfi S, Morales J, Armstrong DL, Burright EN, Orr HT, Sweatt JD, Zoghbi HY, Matzuk MM: Mice lacking ataxin-1 display learning deficits and decreased hippocampal paired-pulse facilitation. *J Neurosci* **18**:5508, 1998.
485. Zhou QY, Palmiter RD: Dopamine-deficient mice are severely hypoactive, adipsic, and aphagic. *Cell* **83**:1197, 1995.
486. Su LK, Kinzler KW, Vogelstein B, Preisinger AC, Moser AR, Luongo C, Gould KA, Dove WF: Multiple intestinal neoplasia caused by a mutation in the murine homolog of the APC gene. *Science* **256**:668, 1992.
487. Hahn H, Wojnowski L, Zimmer AM, Hall J, Miller G, Zimmer A: Rhabdomyosarcomas and radiation hypersensitivity in a mouse model of Gorlin syndrome. *Nat Med* **4**:619, 1998.
488. Chester N, Kuo F, Kozak C, O'Hara CD, Leder P: Stage-specific apoptosis, developmental delay, and embryonic lethality in mice homozygous for a targeted disruption in the murine Bloom's syndrome gene. *Genes Dev* **12**:3382, 1998.
489. Gowen LC, Johnson BL, Latour AM, Sulik KK, Koller BH: Brca1 deficiency results in early embryonic lethality characterized by neuroepithelial abnormalities. *Nat Genet* **12**:191, 1996.
490. Sharan SK, Morimatsu M, Albrecht U, Lim DS, Regel E, Dinh C, Sands A, Eichele G, Hasty P, Bradley A: Embryonic lethality and radiation hypersensitivity mediated by Rad51 in mice lacking Brca2. *Nature* **386**:804, 1997.
491. Di Cristofano A, Pesce B, Cordon-Cardo C, Pandolfi PP: Pten is essential for embryonic development and tumour suppression. *Nat Genet* **19**:348, 1998.
492. de Wind N, Dekker M, Berns A, Radman M, te Riele H: Inactivation of the mouse Msh2 gene results in mismatch repair deficiency, methylation tolerance, hyperrecombination, and predisposition to cancer. *Cell* **82**:321, 1995.
493. Reitmair AH, Schmits R, Ewel A, Bapat B, Redston M, Mitri A, Waterhouse P, Mittrucker HW, Wakeham A, Liu B, et al: MSH2-deficient mice are viable and susceptible to lymphoid tumours. *Nat Genet* **11**:64, 1995.
494. Baker SM, Plug AW, Prolla TA, Bronner CE, Harris AC, Yao X, Christie DM, Monell C, Arnheim N, Bradley A, Ashley T, Liskay RM: Involvement of mouse Mlh1 in DNA mismatch repair and meiotic crossing over. *Nat Genet* **13**:336, 1996.
495. Baker SM, Bronner CE, Zhang L, Plug AW, Robatzek M, Warren G, Elliott EA, Yu J, Ashley T, Arnheim N, et al: Male mice defective in the DNA mismatch repair gene PMS2 exhibit abnormal chromosome synapsis in meiosis. *Cell* **82**:309, 1995.
496. Lee EY, Chang CY, Hu N, Wang YC, Lai CC, Herrup K, Lee WH, Bradley A: Mice deficient for Rb are nonviable and show defects in neurogenesis and haematopoiesis. *Nature* **359**:288, 1992.
497. Whitney MA, Royle G, Low MJ, Kelly MA, Axthelm MK, Reifsteck C, Olson S, Braun RE, Heinrich MC, Rathbun RK, Bagby GC, Grompe M: Germ cell defects and hematopoietic hypersensitivity to gamma-interferon in mice with a targeted disruption of the Fanconi anemia C gene. *Blood* **88**:49, 1996.
498. Harvey M, Vogel H, Morris D, Bradley A, Bernstein A, Donehower LA: A mutant p53 transgene accelerates tumour development in heterozygous but not nullizygous p53-deficient mice. *Nat Genet* **9**:305, 1995.
499. Lavigueur A, Maltby V, Mock D, Rossant J, Pawson T, Bernstein A: High incidence of lung, bone, and lymphoid tumors in transgenic mice

overexpressing mutant alleles of the p53 oncogene. *Mol Cell Biol* **9**:3982, 1989.

500. Serrano M, Lee H, Chin L, Cordon-Cardo C, Beach D, DePinho RA: Role of the INK4a locus in tumor suppression and cell mortality. *Cell* **85**:27, 1996.
501. Brannan CI, Perkins AS, Vogel KS, Ratner N, Nordlund ML, Reid SW, Buchberg AM, Jenkins NA, Parada LF, Copeland NG: Targeted disruption of the neurofibromatosis type-1 gene leads to developmental abnormalities in heart and various neural crest-derived tissues. *Genes Dev* **8**:1019, 1994.
502. McClatchey AI, Saotome I, Ramesh V, Gusella JF, Jacks T: The Nf2 tumor suppressor gene product is essential for extraembryonic development immediately prior to gastrulation. *Genes Dev* **11**:1253, 1997.
503. Luo G, Yao MS, Bender CF, Mills M, Bladl AR, Bradley A, Petrini JH: Disruption of mRad50 causes embryonic stem cell lethality, abnormal embryonic development, and sensitivity to ionizing radiation. *Proc Natl Acad Sci U S A* **96**:7376, 1999.
504. Sweetser DA, Froelick GJ, Matsumoto AM, Kafer KE, Marck B, Palmiter RD, Kapur RP: Ganglioneuromas and renal anomalies are induced by activated RET(MEN2B) in transgenic mice. *Oncogene* **18**:877, 1999.
505. Kobayashi T, Minowa O, Kuno J, Mitani H, Hino O, Noda T: Renal carcinogenesis, hepatic hemangiomatosis, and embryonic lethality caused by a germ-line Tsc2 mutation in mice. *Cancer Res* **59**:1206, 1999.
506. Rennebeck G, Kleymenova EV, Anderson R, Yeung RS, Artzt K, Walker CL: Loss of function of the tuberous sclerosis 2 tumor suppressor gene results in embryonic lethality characterized by disrupted neuroepithelial growth and development. *Proc Natl Acad Sci U S A* **95**:15629, 1998.
507. Gnarra JR, Ward JM, Porter FD, Wagner JR, Devor DE, Grinberg A, Emmert-Buck MR, Westphal H, Klausner RD, Linehan WM: Defective placental vasculogenesis causes embryonic lethality in VHL-deficient mice. *Proc Natl Acad Sci U S A* **94**:9102, 1997.
508. Lebel M, Leder P: A deletion within the murine Werner syndrome helicase induces sensitivity to inhibitors of topoisomerase and loss of cellular proliferative capacity. *Proc Natl Acad Sci U S A* **95**:13097, 1998.
509. Kreidberg JA, Sariola H, Loring JM, Maeda M, Pelletier J, Housman D, Jaenisch R: WT-1 is required for early kidney development. *Cell* **74**:679, 1993.
510. Nakane H, Takeuchi S, Yuba S, Saijo M, Nakatsu Y, Murai H, Nakatsuru Y, Ishikawa T, Hirota S, Kitamura Y, et al: High incidence of ultraviolet-B- or chemical-carcinogen-induced skin tumours in mice lacking the xeroderma pigmentosum group A gene. *Nature* **377**:165, 1995.
511. Sands AT, Abuin A, Sanchez A, Conti CJ, Bradley A: High susceptibility to ultraviolet-induced carcinogenesis in mice lacking XPC. *Nature* **377**:162, 1995.
512. de Boer J, van Steeg H, Berg RJ, Garssen J, de Wit J, van Oostrum CT, Beems RB, van der Horst GT, van Kreijl CF, de Gruijl FR, Bootsma D, Hoeijmakers JH, Weeda G: Mouse model for the DNA repair/basal transcription disorder trichothiodystrophy reveals cancer predisposition. *Cancer Res* **59**:3489, 1999.
513. Harada YN, Shiomi N, Koike M, Ikawa M, Okabe M, Hirota S, Kitamura Y, Kitagawa M, Matsunaga T, Nikaido O, Shiomi T: Postnatal growth failure, short life span, and early onset of cellular senescence and subsequent immortalization in mice lacking the xeroderma pigmentosum group G gene. *Mol Cell Biol* **19**:2366, 1999.
514. Wei S, Episkopou V, Piantedosi R, Maeda S, Shimada K, Gottesman ME, Blaner WS: Studies on the metabolism of retinol and retinol-binding protein in transthyretin-deficient mice produced by homologous recombination. *J Biol Chem* **270**:866, 1995.
515. Wolf G: Retinol transport and metabolism in transthyretin-"knockout" mice. *Nutr Rev* **53**:98, 1995.
516. Palha JA, Episkopou V, Maeda S, Shimada K, Gottesman ME, Saraiva MJ: Thyroid hormone metabolism in a transthyretin-null mouse strain. *J Biol Chem* **269**:33135, 1994.
517. Kotelevtsev Y, Brown RW, Fleming S, Kenyon C, Edwards CR, Seckl JR, Mullins JJ: Hypertension in mice lacking 11beta-hydroxysteroid dehydrogenase type 2. *J Clin Invest* **103**:683, 1999.
518. Radovick S, Nations M, Du Y, Berg LA, Weintraub BD, Wondisford FE: A mutation in the POU-homeodomain of Pit-1 responsible for combined pituitary hormone deficiency. *Science* **257**:1115, 1992.
519. Slee R, Grimes B, Speed RM, Taggart M, Maguire SM, Ross A, McGill NI, Saunders PT, Cooke HJ: A human DAZ transgene confers partial rescue of the mouse Dazl null phenotype. *Proc Natl Acad Sci U S A* **96**:8040, 1999.
520. Yu RN, Ito M, Saunders TL, Camper SA, Jameson JL: Role of Ahch in gonadal development and gametogenesis. *Nat Genet* **20**:353, 1998.
521. Ogawa S, Lubahn DB, Korach KS, Pfaff DW: Behavioral effects of estrogen receptor gene disruption in male mice. *Proc Natl Acad Sci U S A* **94**:1476, 1997.
522. Ho C, Conner DA, Pollak MR, Ladd DJ, Kifor O, Warren HB, Brown EM, Seidman JG, Seidman CE: A mouse model of human familial hypocalciuric hypercalcemia and neonatal severe hyperparathyroidism. *Nat Genet* **11**:389, 1995.
523. Kumar TR, Wang Y, Lu N, Matzuk MM: Follicle-stimulating hormone is required for ovarian follicle maturation but not male fertility. *Nat Genet* **15**:201, 1997.
524. Schultheis PJ, Lorenz JN, Meneton P, Nieman ML, Riddle TM, Flagella M, Duffy JJ, Doetschman T, Miller ML, Shull GE: Phenotype resembling Gitelman's syndrome in mice lacking the apical Na+-Cl− cotransporter of the distal convoluted tubule. *J Biol Chem* **273**:29150, 1998.
525. Reichardt HM, Kaestner KH, Tuckermann J, Kretz O, Wessely O, Bock R, Gass P, Schmid W, Herrlich P, Angel P, Schutz G: DNA binding of the glucocorticoid receptor is not essential for survival. *Cell* **93**:531, 1998.
526. Weiss RE, Murata Y, Cua K, Hayashi Y, Seo H, Refetoff S: Thyroid hormone action on liver, heart, and energy expenditure in thyroid hormone receptor beta-deficient mice. *Endocrinology* **139**:4945, 1998.
527. Lovell-Badge R, Robertson E: XY female mice resulting from a heritable mutation in the primary testis-determining gene, Tdy. *Development* **109**:635, 1990.
528. Mason AJ, Hayflick JS, Zoeller RT, Young WSd, Phillips HS, Nikolics K, Seeburg PH: A deletion truncating the gonadotropin-releasing hormone gene is responsible for hypogonadism in the hpg mouse. *Science* **234**:1366, 1986.
529. Wajnrajch MP, Gertner JM, Harbison MD, Chua SC Jr, Leibel RL: Nonsense mutation in the human growth hormone-releasing hormone receptor causes growth failure analogous to the little (lit) mouse. *Nat Genet* **12**:88, 1996.
530. Lin SC, Lin CR, Gukovsky I, Lusis AJ, Sawchenko PE, Rosenfeld MG: Molecular basis of the little mouse phenotype and implications for cell type-specific growth. *Nature* **364**:208, 1993.
531. Huszar D, Lynch CA, Fairchild-Huntress V, Dunmore JH, Fang Q, Berkemeier LR, Gu W, Kesterson RA, Boston BA, Cone RD, Smith FJ, Campfield LA, Burn P, Lee F: Targeted disruption of the melanocortin-4 receptor results in obesity in mice. *Cell* **88**:131, 1997.
532. Marsh DJ, Hollopeter G, Huszar D, Laufer R, Yagaloff KA, Fisher SL, Burn P, Palmiter RD: Response of melanocortin-4 receptor-deficient mice to anorectic and orexigenic peptides. *Nat Genet* **21**:119, 1999.
533. Yeo GS, Farooqi IS, Aminian S, Halsall DJ, Stanhope RG, O'Rahilly S: A frameshift mutation in MC4R associated with dominantly inherited human obesity. *Nat Genet* **20**:111, 1998.
534. Yaswen L, Diehl N, Brennan MB, Hochgeschwender U: Obesity in the mouse model of pro-opiomelanocortin deficiency responds to peripheral melanocortin. *Nat Med* **5**:1066, 1999.
535. Hummler E, Barker P, Talbot C, Wang Q, Verdumo C, Grubb B, Gatzy J, Burnier M, Horisberger JD, Beermann F, Boucher R, Rossier BC: A mouse model for the renal salt-wasting syndrome pseudohypoaldosteronism. *Proc Natl Acad Sci U S A* **94**:11710, 1997.
536. Geller DS, Rodriguez-Soriano J, Vallo Boado A, Schifter S, Bayer M, Chang SS, Lifton RP: Mutations in the mineralocorticoid receptor gene cause autosomal dominant pseudohypoaldosteronism type I. *Nat Genet* **19**:279, 1998.
537. Dattani MT, Martinez-Barbera JP, Thomas PQ, Brickman JM, Gupta R, Martensson IL, Toresson H, Fox M, Wales JK, Hindmarsh PC, Krauss S, Beddington RS, Robinson IC: Mutations in the homeobox gene HESX1/Hesx1 associated with septo-optic dysplasia in human and mouse. *Nat Genet* **19**:125, 1998.
538. Sadovsky Y, Crawford PA, Woodson KG, Polish JA, Clements MA, Tourtellotte LM, Simburger K, Milbrandt J: Mice deficient in the orphan receptor steroidogenic factor 1 lack adrenal glands and gonads but express P450 side-chain-cleavage enzyme in the placenta and have normal embryonic serum levels of corticosteroids. *Proc Natl Acad Sci U S A* **92**:10939, 1995.
539. Xue Y, Gao X, Lindsell CE, Norton CR, Chang B, Hicks C, Gendron-Maguire M, Rand EB, Weinmaster G, Gridley T: Embryonic lethality

and vascular defects in mice lacking the Notch ligand Jagged1. *Hum Mol Genet* **8**:723, 1999.

540. Zhang P, Liegeois NJ, Wong C, Finegold M, Hou H, Thompson JC, Silverman A, Harper JW, DePinho RA, Elledge SJ: Altered cell differentiation and proliferation in mice lacking p57KIP2 indicates a role in Beckwith-Wiedemann syndrome. *Nature* **387**:151, 1997.
541. Blair HJ, Gormally E, Uwechue IC, Boyd Y: Mouse mutants carrying deletions that remove the genes mutated in Coffin-Lowry syndrome and lactic acidosis. *Hum Mol Genet* **7**:549, 1998.
542. Fransen E, D'Hooge R, Van Camp G, Verhoye M, Sijbers J, Reyniers E, Soriano P, Kamiguchi H, Willemsen R, Koekkoek SK, De Zeeuw CI, De Deyn PP, Van der Linden A, Lemmon V, Kooy RF, Willems PJ: L1 knockout mice show dilated ventricles, vermis hypoplasia and impaired exploration patterns. *Hum Mol Genet* **7**:999, 1998.
543. Litingtung Y, Lei L, Westphal H, Chiang C: Sonic hedgehog is essential to foregut development. *Nat Genet* **20**:58, 1998.
544. Tsai TF, Jiang YH, Bressler J, Armstrong D, Beaudet AL: Paternal deletion from Snrpn to Ube3a in the mouse causes hypotonia, growth retardation and partial lethality and provides evidence for a gene contributing to Prader-Willi syndrome. *Hum Mol Genet* **8**:1357, 1999.
545. Oike Y, Hata A, Mamiya T, Kaname T, Noda Y, Suzuki M, Yasue H, Nabeshima T, Araki K, Yamamura K: Truncated CBP protein leads to classical Rubinstein-Taybi syndrome phenotypes in mice: Implications for a dominant-negative mechanism. *Hum Mol Genet* **8**:387, 1999.
546. Cano-Gauci DF, Song HH, Yang H, McKerlie C, Choo B, Shi W, Pullano R, Piscione TD, Grisaru S, Soon S, Sedlackova L, Tanswell AK, Mak TW, Yeger H, Lockwood GA, Rosenblum ND, Filmus J: Glypican-3-deficient mice exhibit developmental overgrowth and some of the abnormalities typical of Simpson-Golabi-Behmel syndrome. *J Cell Biol* **146**:255, 1999.
547. Munoz-Marmol AM, Strasser G, Isamat M, Coulombe PA, Yang Y, Roca X, Vela E, Mate JL, Coll J, Fernandez-Figueras MT, Navas-Palacios JJ, Ariza A, Fuchs E: A dysfunctional desmin mutation in a patient with severe generalized myopathy. *Proc Natl Acad Sci U S A* **95**:11312, 1998.
548. Goldfarb LG, Park KY, Cervenakova L, Gorokhova S, Lee HS, Vasconcelos O, Nagle JW, Semino-Mora C, Sivakumar K, Dalakas MC: Missense mutations in desmin associated with familial cardiac and skeletal myopathy. *Nat Genet* **19**:402, 1998.
549. Thornell L, Carlsson L, Li Z, Mericskay M, Paulin D: Null mutation in the desmin gene gives rise to a cardiomyopathy. *J Mol Cell Cardiol* **29**:2107, 1997.
550. Fatkin D, Christe ME, Aristizabal O, McConnell BK, Srinivasan S, Schoen FJ, Seidman CE, Turnbull DH, Seidman JG: Neonatal cardiomyopathy in mice homozygous for the Arg403Gln mutation in the alpha cardiac myosin heavy chain gene. *J Clin Invest* **103**:147, 1999.
551. Kimura A, Harada H, Park JE, Nishi H, Satoh M, Takahashi M, Hiroi S, Sasaoka T, Ohbuchi N, Nakamura T, Koyanagi T, Hwang TH, Choo JA, Chung KS, Hasegawa A, Nagai R, Okazaki O, Nakamura H, Matsuzaki M, Sakamoto T, Toshima H, Koga Y, Imaizumi T, Sasazuki T: Mutations in the cardiac troponin I gene associated with hypertrophic cardiomyopathy. *Nat Genet* **16**:379, 1997.
552. Li DY, Sorensen LK, Brooke BS, Urness LD, Davis EC, Taylor DG, Boak BB, Wendel DP: Defective angiogenesis in mice lacking endoglin. *Science* **284**:1534, 1999.
553. Li DY, Faury G, Taylor DG, Davis EC, Boyle WA, Mecham RP, Stenzel P, Boak B, Keating MT: Novel arterial pathology in mice and humans hemizygous for elastin. *J Clin Invest* **102**:1783, 1998.
554. Li DY, Brooke B, Davis EC, Mecham RP, Sorensen LK, Boak BB, Eichwald E, Keating MT: Elastin is an essential determinant of arterial morphogenesis. *Nature* **393**:276, 1998.
555. Voshol PJ, Havinga R, Wolters H, Ottenhoff R, Princen HM, Oude Elferink RP, Groen AK, Kuipers F: Reduced plasma cholesterol and increased fecal sterol loss in multidrug resistance gene 2 P-glycoprotein-deficient mice. *Gastroenterology* **114**:1024, 1998.
556. Dycaico MJ, Grant SG, Felts K, Nichols WS, Geller SA, Hager JH, Pollard AJ, Kohler SW, Short HP, Jirik FR, et al: Neonatal hepatitis induced by alpha 1-antitrypsin: A transgenic mouse model. *Science* **242**:1409, 1988.
557. Carlson JA, Rogers BB, Sifers RN, Finegold MJ, Clift SM, DeMayo FJ, Bullock DW, Woo SL: Accumulation of PiZ alpha 1-antitrypsin causes liver damage in transgenic mice. *J Clin Invest* **83**:1183, 1989.
558. Davidson DJ, Dorin JR, McLachlan G, Ranaldi V, Lamb D, Doherty C, Govan J, Porteous DJ: Lung disease in the cystic fibrosis mouse exposed to bacterial pathogens. *Nat Genet* **9**:351, 1995.
559. Tokieda K, Whitsett JA, Clark JC, Weaver TE, Ikeda K, McConnell KB, Jobe AH, Ikegami M, Iwamoto HS: Pulmonary dysfunction in neonatal SP-B-deficient mice. *Am J Physiol* **273**:L875, 1997.
560. Whitsett JA, Nogee LM, Weaver TE, Horowitz AD: Human surfactant protein B: Structure, function, regulation, and genetic disease. *Physiol Rev* **75**:749, 1995.
561. Robb L, Drinkwater CC, Metcalf D, Li R, Kontgen F, Nicola NA, Begley CG: Hematopoietic and lung abnormalities in mice with a null mutation of the common beta subunit of the receptors for granulocyte-macrophage colony-stimulating factor and interleukins 3 and 5. *Proc Natl Acad Sci U S A* **92**:9565, 1995.
562. Cosgrove D, Meehan DT, Grunkemeyer JA, Kornak JM, Sayers R, Hunter WJ, Samuelson GC: Collagen COL4A3 knockout: A mouse model for autosomal Alport syndrome. *Genes Dev* **10**:2981, 1996.
563. Lu W, Phillips CL, Killen PD, Hlaing T, Harrison WR, Elder FF, Miner JH, Overbeek PA, Meisler MH: Insertional mutation of the collagen genes col4a3 and col4a4 in a mouse model of alport syndrome. *Genomics* **61**:113, 1999.
564. Lu W, Peissel B, Babakhanlou H, Pavlova A, Geng L, Fan X, Larson C, Brent G, Zhou J: Perinatal lethality with kidney and pancreas defects in mice with a targetted Pkd1 mutation. *Nat Genet* **17**:179, 1997.
565. Wu G, Markowitz GS, Li L, D'Agati VD, Factor SM, Geng L, Tibara S, Tuchman J, Cai Y, Hoon Park J, van Adelsberg J, Hou H Jr, Kucherlapati R, Edelmann W, Somlo S: Cardiac defects and renal failure in mice with targeted mutations in pkd2. *Nat Genet* **24**:75, 2000.
566. Simon EA, Cook S, Davisson MT, D'Eustachio P, Guay-Woodford LM: The mouse congenital polycystic kidney (cpk) locus maps within 1.3 cM of the chromosome 12 marker D12Nyu2. *Genomics* **21**:415, 1994.
567. Nagao S, Watanabe T, Ogiso N, Marunouchi T, Takahashi H: Genetic mapping of the polycystic kidney gene, pcy, on mouse chromosome 9. *Biochem Genet* **33**:401, 1995.

CHAPTER 15

Genome Imprinting in Human Disease

Carmen Sapienza ▪ Judith G. Hall

1. **An important challenge for contemporary genetics is to understand the mechanisms underlying those traits and conditions that do not follow traditional patterns of inheritance. Many recent observations demonstrate that the expression of a number of traits in humans, mice, and other organisms depends on which parent transmitted the gene responsible for the trait.**
2. **In both the mouse and the human, inheritance of the entire chromosome complement from only one parent results in developmental failure. The gross morphologic complementarity of the phenotypes yielded by inheriting both sets of chromosomes from the father versus inheriting both sets from the mother suggests that the paternal genetic contribution is important to placental development, while the maternal contribution is essential for development of the embryo proper.**
3. **Inheritance of all or part of individual chromosomes from only one parent may also result in an abnormal phenotype, even if the genes responsible for that phenotype are demonstrably wild-type by both genetic and biochemical criteria. An important mechanism by which such uniparental disomy may be achieved in the human is by the *in utero* reduction of trisomies. Evidence derived from chorionic villus sampling indicates that as many as 1 percent of all pregnancies may carry uniparental disomy for particular chromosomes. Uniparental disomy has been demonstrated in several cases of a number of human diseases, including Beckwith-Wiedemann, Prader-Willi, and Angelman syndromes.**
4. **The mechanism by which differential expression of maternal and paternal genomes is achieved is unknown but there is a strong correlation between parental origin-specific gene expression and differential DNA methylation and chromatin structure. The tendency to find more than one gene to be imprinted in a region tends to argue for some imprinting controls to operate over domains that are larger than a single gene. Recent data also indicate that important biochemical differences between alleles at imprinted loci are manifested as asynchronous replication of the alleles during S phase of the cell cycle. In addition, "antisense" transcripts have been shown to be associated with silenced alleles at several imprinted loci.**
5. **Regardless of the biochemical mechanism by which alleles at imprinted loci are marked as "imprinted," cases of most human disease phenotypes that exhibit a strong parental origin effect may be viewed as having failed to complete one or more steps in the imprinting process. These steps include: (a) erasure of the imprint from the previous generation; (b) establishment of a new imprint that is appropriate to the gender of the individual in which the gametes are being created; (c) transmission of a complete and appropriately imprinted genome to the zygote; (d) stable inheritance of the maternal and paternal imprint through somatic cell division; and (e) proper maintenance and translation of the imprint in those somatic cells in which a parental origin-dependent effect on phenotype is required or observed.***

This chapter presents an overview of the human diseases in which imprinting is thought to be involved, as well as some considerations for genetic counseling when imprinting defects are suspected.

In 1990, one of us prefaced a review on the subject of genome imprinting with the observation that reviews on genome imprinting had consumed far more printer's ink than papers containing experimental data on genome imprinting. This situation has been remedied somewhat, but the remedy has become no less problematic. Before beginning the rewrite of this chapter in March of 1998, a search of the NCBI database using the search terms "imprinting AND human" yielded 822 articles published during the prior five years. Searching the database using only the term "imprinting" returned in excess of 2400 citations. These statistics are, in many ways, a tribute to the importance of the experimental embryological investigations of McGrath and Solter, first published in 1984.[1] These landmark studies fostered the scientific equivalent of a burgeoning cottage industry in which biological scientists of almost every experimental persuasion and subdisciplinary leaning were forced to entertain the basic question, "Is there a parent-of-origin effect in my experiment?"

These statistics also make obvious that the topic has left the realm of the curious and is becoming, if not truly mainstream, at least respectable, at an average of 3.2 papers per week published on imprinting in the human. It is an odd state of affairs, then, that despite such a vigorous assault on the subject, we remain substantially ignorant of the precise molecular mechanism(s) by which parent-of-origin-dependent gene expression is achieved. Although this is due, in large part, to the fact that many of these studies are descriptive (identification of new imprinted genes, genes that may be imprinted in one situation but not another, etc.), it also reflects the difficulty of defining the factors believed to be important or required for the operation of the process.

In this review, we provide some measure of the clinical importance of specific "imprinted diseases," as well as discuss the practical problems associated with diagnosis and genetic counseling in such cases. In addition, we discuss the lines of evidence that suggest a role for genome imprinting in human disease in general, and the historical context within which these lines of evidence were developed. We also summarize the accumulated data on biochemical differences between alleles at imprinted loci.

Given the large number of papers published in the field in the last five years, it would be a disservice to the efforts of all of the investigators involved in genome imprinting research (as well as impossible, in the space allotted) to attempt a litany of the

*Chapter 1, Appendix 1 names all the genes referred to by their symbols (italicized uppercase) in the present chapter.

accomplishments detailed in all 800-odd publications. For this reason, part of this review takes the form of a systems-based categorization of human diseases that exhibit a strong parent-of-origin effect into one or more classes of abnormal phenotypes that result from failure to properly accomplish one or more steps in the imprinting process. Our breakdown of the process into discrete steps has been done mainly on logical grounds, but biochemical correlates of some steps in the process have been identified. This type of classification, "by process," rather than "by disease," results in the inclusion of some diseases in more than one category.

DEFINITIONS AND FUNDAMENTAL QUESTIONS: WHAT IS AN IMPRINTED GENE AND WHAT IS THE IMPRINT?

After the publication of 2400 papers on imprinting during the period 1993–1997, it would seem that such simple questions should have simple and concrete answers. In fact, some investigators would feel no qualms in giving simple, concrete answers to one or both of these questions. This level of confidence on the part of many colleagues has given rise to the strong perception that the answers to these questions are: (a) an imprinted gene is defined by the fact that it is transcribed from only one parent's allele, and (b) the imprint is parental origin-dependent methylation of CpG sites in DNA.

While it is undoubtedly true that autosomal genes transcribed from only one parent's allele are imprinted (at last count 19 such genes have been identified in the human (see reference 2 for a review) and that DNA methylation almost certainly has something to do with the establishment or maintenance of the imprint in mammals,[2,3] a number of important qualifying statements must be attached if the whole truth is to be told.

The Identity of "The Mark" that is Placed on an Imprinted Gene

The biochemical identity of the epigenetic mark that is placed on imprinted genes as a result of passage through male or female gametogenesis is unknown. Although this admission is undoubtedly and unfortunately true, in the absolute sense, we are not completely ignorant of biochemical correlates of the process. There are at least two biochemical characteristics that have been demonstrated to be associated with alleles at imprinted loci and allelic differences in gene expression (see reference 4 for discussion): differential methylation of CpG dinucleotides in DNA and differential chromatin structure, as revealed by allelic differences in DNase I sensitivity and histone acetylation. Both characteristics are heritable through cell division, and both are associated, at least in a correlative way, with regulation of gene expression (for review, see reference 5). These two characteristics may, in fact, be related through common biochemical intermediaries, such as the methyl CpG binding protein MeCP2.[6] Most working hypotheses for the establishment of parental origin-dependent differences between alleles at a locus assume that the mark (the "imprint") is a specific biochemical entity that is placed on one allele (the methylation of certain cytosines in DNA or the deacetylation of particular histones, for example), but not the other, as a result of that allele having passed through gametogenesis in one sex, as opposed to the other. The placement of the mark is thought to be dictated by *cis*-acting elements (that may be composed of DNA sequence features other than primary sequence[7,8]) that direct male or female gametogenesis-specific *trans*-acting factors (particular DNA methyltransferases or histone deacetylases, for example) to operate at these sites. An alternative possibility is that the *cis*-acting elements, themselves, are differentially accessible to the *trans*-acting factors as a result of differences in the chromatin configuration assumed by male versus female germ cells. This "imprint," once established, must then be properly "interpreted" within the context of the transcriptional machinery of an individual cell in order for allele-specific gene expression to occur.[9]

The allele-specific methylation of cytosine in CpG dinucleotides has been a strong candidate for playing a role in the establishment and/or maintenance of the imprint since the first demonstrations of a parental origin effect on the methylation of transgenes in the mouse[10–12] (see reference 13 for a recent review). In part, the strength of this candidacy, relative to that of the candidacy of chromatin structure, has to do with the sheer number of reports in which investigators have demonstrated a difference in methylation pattern between alleles, not only at imprinted loci but also at loci on the X chromosome. In one respect, this numerical advantage is less a proof that CpG methylation is involved in imprinting than proof of the old adage, "When your only tool is a hammer, all problems are nails."

This statement is not intended to denigrate the body of work represented by studies demonstrating parental origin effects on DNA methylation (indeed, one of us has been a coauthor on several papers exploiting this tool[11,14–16]). However, it is worth noting that restriction endonuclease-based assays for allele-specific differences in DNA methylation are much less demanding on the investigator, in terms of both time and types of experimental material required, than assays examining chromatin structure. Many more investigators have the wherewithal and impetus to examine allele-specific differences in DNA methylation than allele-specific differences in the acetylation of histones, for example.

To be fair, the methylation juggernaut has also been driven by success; the experiment is often rewarded by a positive result, otherwise investigators would soon tire of the exercise. However, there are a number of additional data that indicate it is worthwhile to be cautious before concluding that the parental origin-specific methylation of cytosine in DNA is all there is to the establishment of a genome imprint. For example, one common feature of loci at which only one allele is expressed in any given cell (including imprinted genes, genes subject to X-inactivation, and genes subject to monoallelic, but not imprinted, expression) is that the alleles are replicated asynchronously during the S phase of the cell cycle.[7,17,18] Alleles on the inactive X chromosome are replicated late in the S phase, while their counterparts on the active X chromosome are replicated early (reviewed in reference 19). The silenced, paternal allele at the imprinted *IGF2R* locus in the mouse is replicated early in the S phase and the expressed, maternal allele is replicated late.[7] Inhibitors of CpG methylation, such as 5-azacytidine, do not alter this feature of either imprinted or X-linked genes,[20] but trichostatin A (an inhibitor of histone deacetylases 1 and 3) does abolish differential replication timing.[19] On the other hand, allele specific expression of *H19* and *IGF2* is lost in mouse embryos in which both alleles of one of the DNA methyltransferase loci have been replaced by a mutant allele.[21]

One should also note that parental origin effects on gene expression have been described in organisms such as *Drosophila melanogaster,*[22,23] whose genome has no detectable level of DNA methylation. However, templating of chromatin structures that appear heritable through cell division and are either permissive or repressive for gene expression have been observed many times in this organism.[24–27]

Curiously, some investigators who argue that the proof of whether a gene is imprinted in mammals lies in demonstrating that the gene is expressed from one parent's allele do not agree that demonstrating a parent-of-origin effect on gene expression in *Drosophila* conforms to the definition of imprinting. The basis of this contradiction in logic appears to lie in the belief that imprinting occurs only in mammals which is, in turn, based entirely on the observation that parthenogenetic mouse embryos die during development while parthenogenetic *Drosophila* do not. In any case, one should be aware that although the methylation of CpG sites in DNA, in all likelihood, plays some role in the establishment, maintenance, or interpretation of genome imprints, other epigenetic processes are also capable of playing any or all of these roles. Until these processes have been investigated with the same vigor as has DNA methylation, it would be unwise to conclude that we know the biochemical identity of "the mark." This cautionary note takes on added significance in light of the recent and rigorous demonstration of true imprinting effects on the expression of several genes in *Drosophila*.[27a]

"The Mark" Versus its Effect: What Is an Imprinted Gene?

Part of the problem in discussing the epigenetic character that identifies an imprinted gene consists of defining when a gene is imprinted. This issue may seem semantic but is important in several respects.

The first concerns the validity of negative statements on whether a gene or chromosome region is imprinted or not. The *failure* to demonstrate an effect of parental origin on the transcription of a gene, or to demonstrate a gross effect on phenotype when a gene is mutated, does not have the same weight of evidence as the *positive* demonstration of an effect. Because imprinted genes may be allele-specifically transcribed only in some individuals[28–30] in some tissues[31,32] or at some time during development,[32] the ability to detect the imprinting of a gene depends on the individual assayed, the tissue and developmental time at which the assay is done, and the phenotype being assayed. Recent examples that *IGF2R* is imprinted in a minority of individuals,[29] that the *WT1* gene is polymorphic and mosaically imprinted,[33] and that the *UBE3A* gene (a strong candidate for the Angelman syndrome locus) is expressed from both alleles except in the brain, where only the maternal allele is transcribed,[31] serve to illustrate this point.

The problem of tissue and developmental time specificity of imprinting is difficult to address from the standpoint of falsifying the hypothesis that any particular gene is imprinted. Although many early studies gave the impression that imprinting is an all-or-nothing phenomenon,[34] more recent studies indicate quantitative effects due to mosaicism in the expression of imprinted genes.[33,35] This state of affairs drove one colleague attending a recent meeting to push the point to its logical conclusion and to question whether a gene expressed from one parent's allele in one cell for one second was imprinted. Rather than drawing the response he expected (laughter), the question brought up more discussion on the second point, that of the definition of phenotype.

This issue is not very complicated when one's interests are gross anatomical or behavioral differences in phenotype, such as those parental origin-dependent traits elaborated by individuals with Prader-Willi or Angelman syndrome. Almost anyone may recognize these diseases as phenotypes that are outside the range of morphological and/or behavioral variation that are considered normal for human beings. The Angelman and Prader-Willi genes are recognized as imprinted because of the obvious pathology exhibited by individuals who lack an expressed maternal copy of the Angelman gene or an expressed paternal copy of the Prader-Willi gene(s) (see "Chromosomal Deletion Syndromes" later in this chapter). However, that the *SNRPN* (or *Snrpn* in the mouse) gene in the Prader-Willi region, for example, is imprinted *could* have been determined in the absence of any disease phenotype by examining allele-specific gene expression in completely normal individuals. In this case, the imprinting of the gene would have been ascertained through a phenotype that was less obvious than the Prader-Willi disease phenotype; that is, imprinting could be ascertained by the presence or absence of an RT-PCR product from the maternal *SNRPN* allele. The phenotypic assay of allele specific transcription at the *SNRPN* locus may be (and has been, see references 36–38) removed even one step further from the observation of gross differences in phenotype. That particular sites in the silenced maternal *SNRPN* allele are methylated, and those same sites in the expressed paternal allele are unmethylated, may be exploited to distinguish between maternal and paternal alleles. In this case, the phenotype assayed, by one of several methods, is the presence or absence of a methyl group at a particular CpG dinucleotide. Whether the methylation of these particular CpG dinucleotides is or is not "the imprint" is, in this respect, immaterial. This epigenetic difference between maternal and paternal alleles is certainly assayable, using biochemical methods, as a parental origin-dependent difference in phenotype and it may be argued that this locus is imprinted regardless of whether this difference has any consequence for the expression of the allele.

Such laboratory-derived biochemical representations of phenotype are no less valuable as genetic traits in the analysis of imprinting as a process, than the disease resulting from the absence of an expressed paternal copy of the *PWS* gene. Yet, applied in other situations, there is the perception that they are not "real" phenotypes. For example, it has become common practice in the literature to summarize the data on the imprinting of the insulin-like growth factor-2 receptor gene by stating that this gene is imprinted in mice but is not imprinted in humans. What this statement means is that, in humans, initial reports indicated that there was not a "functional" imprint on either *IGF2R* allele because both alleles were expressed in most individuals. There are at least two things wrong with this statement: (a) *IGF2R is* expressed from only the maternal allele in a minority of individuals,[28] and (b) a parental origin specific methylation difference between maternal and paternal alleles is observed in both humans and mice.[7]

Most investigators agree that because *IGF2R* is expressed from only the maternal allele in some individuals, it is almost certain to prove important in elucidating the mechanism by which parental origin-dependent gene expression is achieved. Whether this trait is heritable, and whether it is linked to the *IGF2R* locus, should define what types of *cis* and *trans*-acting factors are important in the establishment and interpretation of the imprint. However, that parental origin-specific methylation differences between *IGF2R* alleles are found in humans in whom there is no allele-specific expression is more likely to be regarded as unimportant because the gene is not "functionally" imprinted. Such an interpretation dismisses the issue of how, if methylation is the imprint, a locus can exhibit differential methylation between alleles but not be imprinted.

Potentially important problems arise with dismissing such issues out-of-hand, not the least of which concerns the functional role of the parental origin-specific mark. For example, in the chapter on imprinting in the last edition of this collection, we described "maternal imprinting" as the silencing of the maternal allele at a locus and "paternal imprinting" as the silencing of the paternal allele.[39] This terminology was introduced and has become commonly used by investigators within the field because the allele that was silenced was generally the allele identified as carrying a parental origin specifically methylated CpG site. However, there are also examples of loci at which the allele carrying the parental origin specifically methylated CpG site is the allele that is expressed.[40,41] Consequently, if methylation is the epigenetic signal that establishes whether an allele is imprinted, that signal cannot simply dictate that an allele be silenced. This issue has become complicated further by the identification of parental origin-specific "antisense" transcripts (or, at least, transcripts from the region that run in the direction opposite the coding sequence) of some imprinted genes such as *IGF2*,[42] *IGF2R*,[43] and *UBE3A*.[44] Is it the expression of the "sense" transcript or expression of the antisense transcript that is imprinted? The matter is entirely unclear, especially if the silencing of one allele is related to antisense transcription. Carrying this line of reasoning a little further, parental origin-specific methylation of alleles is one type of imprint on the allele, regardless of whether these differences result in allele-specific gene expression or a disease phenotype. *All* of these characteristics are, in genetic terms, phenotypes, and the importance of each depends entirely on the question being addressed by the investigator.

GENOME IMPRINTING IN HUMAN DISEASE: A SYSTEMATIC APPROACH

This section summarizes the steps that must occur during the imprinting process, and how errors or failure to complete any one step in the process may result in disease or failure to complete development.

A schematic overview of the imprinting process is presented in Fig. 15-1. The process is divided into five steps based on logical requirements and on experimental evidence that indicates that failure to properly complete a particular step may result in some fraction of cases of a particular disease. Three of the steps (1, 2, and 3) are hypothesized to take place in the germ line during meiosis (up to and including fertilization) and two of the steps (4 and 5) are hypothesized to affect the inheritance and interpretation of the imprint in somatic cells. Overall, most investigators in the field agree with the necessity of properly accomplishing these steps:

A. Erasure of the imprint from the previous generation.
B. Establishment of a new imprint that is appropriate to the gender of the individual in which the gametes are being created.
C. Transmission of a complete and appropriately imprinted genome to the zygote.
D. Stable inheritance of the maternal and paternal imprint through somatic cell division.
E. Proper maintenance and translation of the imprint in those somatic cells in which a parental origin-dependent effect on phenotype is required or observed.

Imprint Erasure and Establishment

Although the genome imprinting pathway (Fig. 15-1) is depicted as circular (with the exception of step E, which gives rise to the somatic cells in which the phenotypic consequences of the imprinting process is observed most frequently), one might be forgiven the notion that the process begins with the advent of gametogenesis. This is because the steps that take place during this period must solve the central problem that accompanies the establishment of a parental origin-dependent mark on the genome: Each individual, regardless of gender, receives a maternally imprinted set of chromosomes from their mother and a paternally imprinted set of chromosomes from their father. In the following generation, that same individual must transmit only maternally imprinted chromosomes (if they are female) or only paternally imprinted chromosomes (if they are male).

This problem may be solved, at the conceptual level, in at least two ways: (a) Imprint erasure and reestablishment may be carried out on the genome as a whole, without regard to the parental origin of any gene in the previous generation; or (b) Because females already carry a maternal imprint on that portion of their genomes inherited from their mothers and males already carry a paternal imprint on that portion of their genomes inherited from their fathers, it is possible that imprint erasure and reestablishment normally operate on only that portion of the genome that is imprinted "incorrectly" in each sex; that is, only paternal imprints from the previous generation are changed during oogenesis and only maternal imprints from the previous generation are changed during spermatogenesis. At present it is not possible to say whether one or the other pathway is more likely to be the general case, and both are included in Fig. 15-1 (step A) as plausible alternatives.

An additional question left unanswered by this model is whether imprint erasure and reestablishment are discrete and independent events. Fig. 15-1 assumes that the eradication of the imprint from the previous generation (step A) is a biochemical procedure that is distinct from that involved in the creation of a new imprint (step B). This is not meant to imply that the two events may not be related or tightly coupled, such as might occur during DNA replication and modification, for example. However, if imprint erasure does occur independently of imprint establishment, then it is formally possible that there is a stage at which all or part of the genome exists in a "naive" state in which neither maternal nor paternal imprints are present. This question may be of importance in animal husbandry, as well as have great relevance in the practice of reproductive medicine.

Transmission of a Complete and Appropriately Imprinted Genome to the Zygote

It is generally agreed that the contribution of appropriately imprinted maternal and paternal genomes to the zygote (step C) is normally required for proper development. Although there may be regions of the genome for which uniparental inheritance is compatible with a normal phenotype, the uniparental inheritance of other regions of the genome results in severe disease phenotype or the death of the developing fetus (see "Specific Disorders Associated with Imprinting" later in this chapter). In addition, derivation of the entire genome from only one parent results in human pathologies similar to those observed when mouse embryos containing only maternal chromosomes or only paternal

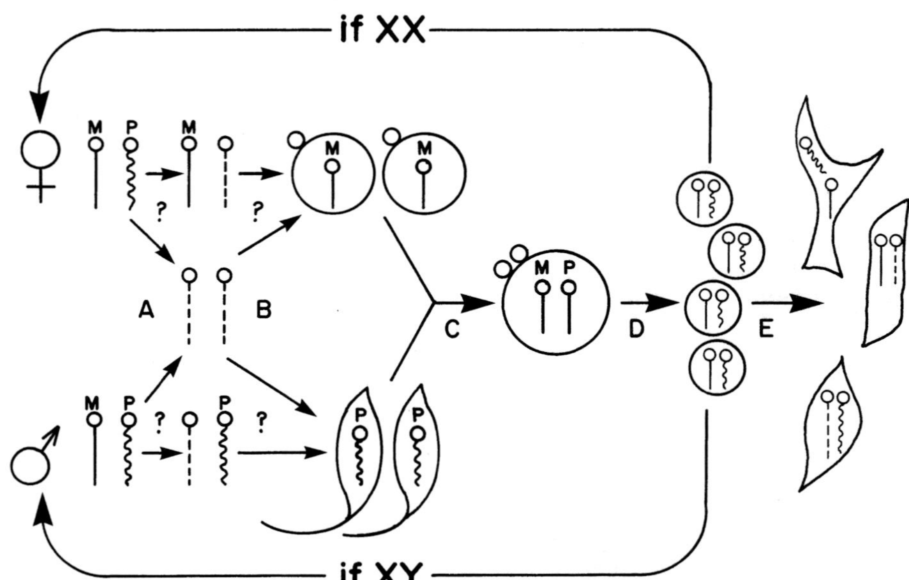

Fig. 15-1 The imprinting cycle. In step *A*, the imprint from the previous generation is erased. Whether all imprints are erased without regard for their imprinted state in the previous generation (maternal or paternal) is unknown (denoted by question marks; see text). In step *B*, a new imprint that is appropriate to the gender of the individual in which the gametes are being created is established. In step *C*, a complete and appropriately imprinted genome is contributed to the zygote. In step *D*, the maternal and paternal imprint is stably inherited through embryogenesis. Those cells that become primordial germ cells reenter the cycle at step *A* at the appropriate time. In step *E*, proper maintenance and translation of the imprint occurs in those differentiated somatic cells in which a parental origin effect on gene expression is observed.

chromosomes are created experimentally. We note that the successful propagation of live and fertile ovine (Dolly) and murine (Cumulina) offspring by transfer of an adult somatic nucleus to an enucleated ovum[45,46] does *not* provide evidence against a developmental requirement for the contribution of appropriately imprinted genomes from each parent (see the following section).

Stable Inheritance of the Maternal and Paternal Imprint Through Somatic Cell Division

Once the zygote has received a properly imprinted set of chromosomes from each parent, the imprint on these chromosomes must be transmitted to daughter cells during embryogenesis (step D). It is possible, and given the epigenetic nature of the imprint, perhaps likely, that not every cell will faithfully inherit the imprint on every gene upon which an imprint was placed. However, it is presumed that most cells have stably inherited the imprint on most genes through cell division throughout embryogenesis because terminally differentiated cells derived from different primary germ layers can be shown, at the very least, to maintain some biochemical characteristics of a parental origin-specific mark. That the imprint is heritable through somatic cell division is likely to account for the successful cloning of Dolly and Cumulina. Presumably, the somatic nucleus used to generate such animals carried a "correct" imprint at all loci for which an imprint is required for successful development.

It also seems likely that at least some aspects of the maternal and paternal imprints have also been maintained in those cells that become primordial germ cells and give rise to the individual's germ line. From the standpoint of the model in Fig. 15-1, however, it is of little consequence whether the imprint is maintained in primordial germ cells and then erased during gametogenesis (Fig. 15-1, as drawn), or whether the imprint is erased from some cells during embryogenesis and these "imprint erased" cells then become primordial germ cells (placing step A between step D and "if XX/if XY").

Proper Maintenance and Translation of the Imprint

The final step in this process (step E) is really a combination of several different processes whose end result is the parental origin-dependent effect on phenotype that is observed. For example, the preferential or exclusive expression of the paternal *IGF2* allele in a population of terminally differentiated cells requires the imprint to have been faithfully transmitted through all of the progenitors of any cell that expresses only the paternal allele. The successful outcome of expressing only the paternal allele also requires that particular postmitotic cell to maintain, for an extended period of time, whatever biochemical structure defines the imprint and to then properly interpret the imprint as an instruction to transcribe only the paternal allele. This step is depicted as uncoupled from the imprint erasure/imprint reestablishment cycle in that the fate of maternal and paternal imprints in the somatic cells in which the parental origin-dependent phenotype is observed does not directly bear on the fate of the imprint in the following generation, although the lability or stability of the imprint may reflect genetic factors that do bear on this fate.[47,48]

The steps involved in the somatic inheritance, maintenance, and translation of the imprint offer great potential for the creation of phenotypic variability between individuals. Errors made at any point in this process may result in failure to demonstrate the parental origin effect that is expected or required to elicit a normal phenotype. The imprint itself may fail to be transmitted from one cell to a daughter cell and to all subsequent daughters of that cell. The imprint itself may fail to be maintained in some fraction of cells in some individuals, or it may be lost or degraded over time as a result of stochastic processes, genetic factors, or environmental factors. In addition, although a cell may have inherited and faithfully maintained an imprint, it may fail to properly interpret the imprint as an instruction to repress or express a particular allele. All of these considerations make it likely that many parental origin-dependent phenotypes that are linked to imprinting will exhibit variable expression and that the variability in phenotype may be traced to different factors in different cases.

HOW ERRORS IN THE IMPRINTING PROCESS CONTRIBUTE TO HUMAN DISEASE

The following sections classify a number of human diseases according to which step in the imprinting process they fail to complete properly. The phenotypic manifestations of these diseases, as well as some discussion of the associated or causal biochemical defects are discussed in the section "Genome Imprinting and Its Relevance to Clinical Genetics" later in this chapter.

Our classification of human diseases according to failure to complete a step in the imprinting pathway begins with step C in Fig. 15-1. Part of the reason to begin with this step is the historical importance of experimental mouse embryology in the discovery of the imprinting process. Although there were a number of earlier reports of parental origin effects on phenotype in several mammalian experimental systems,[49–51] it was not until the investigations of McGrath and Solter in 1984[1,52] that imprinting was recognized to be a requirement for the successful completion of embryogenesis in mammals.

McGrath and Solter performed an experiment that was breathtaking, both in its simplicity of concept and in its technological difficulty (Fig. 15-2). Prior to the first cleavage division of the mouse embryo, the maternal and paternal genetic contributions to the zygote remain physically separate entities and reside in distinct pronuclei. Using a small-bore pipette, these investigators were able to remove the pronucleus containing the paternally derived chromosomes and replace it with a pronucleus containing only maternally derived chromosomes taken from a different zygote. The embryos resulting from this type of microsurgery contain a perfectly diploid genetic complement, with the *proviso* that all chromosomes are maternal in origin. These "gynogenetic" embryos were then transferred to the uterus of a foster mother, where they were able to develop through the preimplantation period and give rise to morphologically normal blastocysts in a large fraction of cases. However, none of these embryos was able to develop to birth[1] and significant postimplantation development occurred in only a small fraction of cases, with a few embryos surviving to the 40-somite stage.[53,54] This result was in marked contrast to the result of the control experiment in which zygotes had their paternal pronucleus removed and replaced by another paternal pronucleus that was taken from a different zygote. These control embryos gave rise to normal mice with high frequency. The reciprocal class of experimental embryos, in which a maternal pronucleus was replaced by a paternal pronucleus (such that the embryo carried two paternal sets of genetic information; an "androgenetic" embryo), also failed to give rise to normal offspring.[1,53] Interestingly, and perhaps significantly, the gross anatomical phenotypes displayed by the best-developed gynogenetic and androgenetic embryos were morphologically complementary. Some gynogenetic embryos had fairly extensive development of many embryonic tissue types, but showed very poor development of extraembryonic tissues.[53,55] A few androgenetic embryos showed extensive development of extraembryonic tissues, but very poor development of the embryo proper (a few developed to the 12-somite stage[53,55]).

The straightforward design of these experiments allows for a simplicity of interpretation rarely encountered in biology: If developmental phenotype is the sole and direct result of genotype, then all three classes of embryos — gynogenotes, androgenotes, and microsurgically reconstituted biparental controls — should develop in the same way and to the same extent because the source

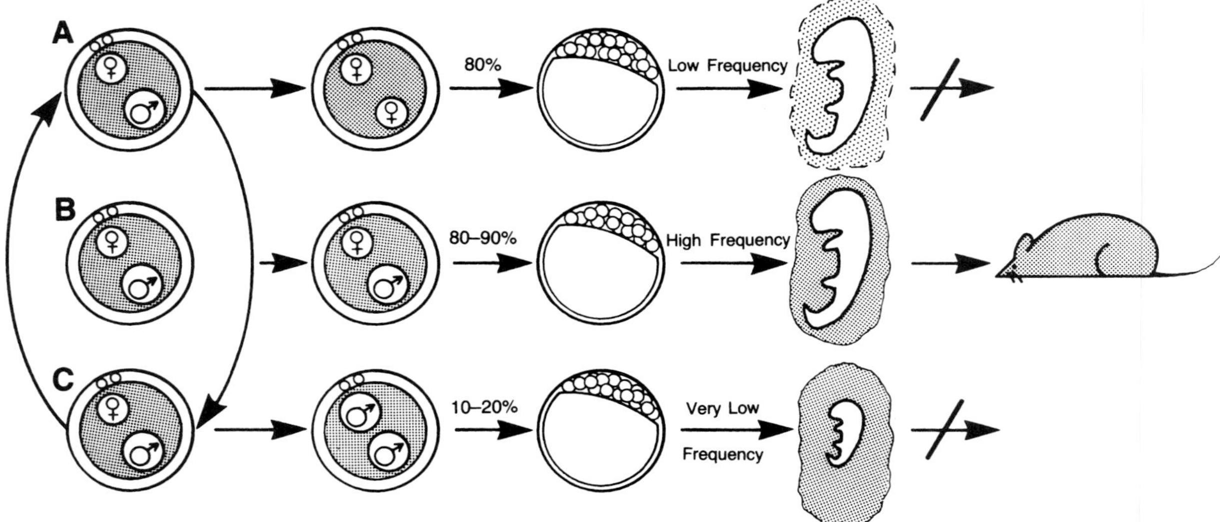

Fig. 15-2 Morphological phenotypes obtained from embryos with: *A.* Two maternal pronuclei (gynogenotes); *B.* Control-operated zygotes (equivalent to normal, fertilized zygotes); and *C.* Embryos with two paternal pronuclei (androgenotes). Rate of successful preimplantation development of gynogenotes and controls to blastocyst stage is nearly equivalent, while androgenotes are much less likely to achieve the blastocyst stage. Neither gynogenotes nor androgenotes develop to term. Some gynogenotes give rise to fairly well-formed fetuses but show scant development of extraembryonic membranes. Androgenotes only rarely develop beyond implantation. The few androgenetic embryos that achieve some measure of postimplantation development have fairly well-developed extraembryonic membranes but the fetuses are very poorly developed.

of the pronuclei was the same in all three cases. That the three types of embryos are not equivalent in developmental potential indicates that the parental origin of the pronuclei plays an important role in development. This implies that maternal and paternal genomes are not equivalent in terms of function, even though they may be equivalent in terms of DNA sequence. This result also indicates that the genomes contributed to the zygote by the male and female parent must be differentially marked, or imprinted, in some way. The imprint affects one or more genes in such a way that failure to inherit an allele at this locus or these loci from both parents results in failure to complete development.

Human Phenotypes Resulting from Improper Contribution of the Imprinted Genome to the Embryo

In humans, phenotypic effects ascribed to the failure to receive a complete and properly imprinted genome have been observed when the missing entity is a single gene, a portion of a chromosome, or the entire genome. Such failures may be a result of parthenogenetic activation of ova, errors of fertilization, or meiotic errors, including chromosome nondisjunction, deletion, or duplication.

The phenotypes most similar to those observed in experimentally created gynogenetic and androgenetic mouse embryos are those of ovarian teratomas and hydatidiform moles. Complete hydatidiform moles are placental neoplasms that contain only paternal chromosomes.[56] Those that arise as the result of fertilization of an anucleate ovum by two sperm may be heterozygous at many different loci. This situation affords the opportunity to examine the expression of imprinted genes under conditions in which both alleles are paternally derived. Interestingly, when allele-specific in situ hybridization is used to assay the expression of *IGF2,* normally expressed from only the paternal allele, some cells express one allele, some express the other, and a few cells express both alleles.[4] These observations indicate that there may be a relationship between the process that gives rise to random monoallelic expression, such as occurs in the mouse at olfactory receptor loci,[17] and monoallelic and parental origin-dependent expression of imprinted genes.

Ovarian teratomas are neoplasms that arise from spontaneously activated ova. They contain only maternal chromosomes,[57] but may differentiate into many different structures and cell types, as do gynogenetic and parthenogenetic mouse embryos (for an interesting perspective on the role of ovarian teratomas in the evolution of imprinting, see reference 58).

The phenotypes exhibited by moles and teratomas are the result of failure to receive any portion of either the maternal (mole) or paternal (teratoma) genome. Other phenotypes result from failure to receive specific portions of the maternal or paternal genome, or inappropriately receiving two copies of the same chromosome region from one parent and none from the other parent (uniparental disomy; see "Uniparental Disomy" later in this chapter). A fraction of cases of Prader-Willi syndrome, Angelman syndrome, and Beckwith-Wiedemann syndrome result from such imbalances in the parental origin-dependent of a chromosome region (see also the section "Genome Imprinting and Its Relevance to Clinical Genetics" later in this chapter).

Prader-Willi and Angelman syndromes are distinct neurobehavioral disorders that result from parental origin-dependent deficiencies of an imprinted gene or genes located at chromosome 15q11-q13. Approximately 60 percent of individuals with Prader-Willi syndrome have cytogenetically detectable deletions of the paternal copy of chromosome 15q11-q13[59] and approximately 60 percent of individuals with Angelman syndrome have cytogenetically detectable deletions of the maternal copy of this chromosome region.[60] An additional, smaller, fraction of cases of both diseases results from uniparental disomy, in which both copies of the same chromosome or chromosome region are inherited from the same parent. When both chromosomes 15 are inherited from the mother (and none from the father), Prader-Willi syndrome results; when both are inherited from the father, Angelman syndrome results.

Uniparental disomy for the paternally derived chromosome 11p is associated with Beckwith-Wiedemann syndrome.[61,62] In addition, deletions and balanced translocations involving chromosome 11p are also found in Beckwith-Wiedemann patients and these segmental aneuploidies also exhibit parental origin dependence (nicely summarized in reference 63).

A very interesting example of a parental origin effect resulting from failure to receive a portion of one parent's genome also points out the importance of carefully defining the phenotype to be examined before eliminating the possibility that a particular chromosome segment may contain an imprinted gene. Individuals with Turner syndrome are sex chromosome aneuploids who are phenotypically female but carry only a single X chromosome. It has been known for many years that some such individuals received their X chromosome from their fathers and others received their X chromosome from their mothers. Because both types of individuals exist and both showed the Turner syndrome phenotype, some investigators argued that this was evidence against the imprinting of any gene on the X chromosome. Although the *Xist* gene, which is involved in X chromosome inactivation, did show imprinting,[64] the developmental time and tissue specificity of the imprint (with expression of only the paternal allele in extraembryonic tissues) did not provide positive data that any X-linked gene exhibited a parental origin effect in embryonic tissue. However, when Turner syndrome patients were stratified according to cognitive ability and social skills, it was found that those individuals who received the X chromosome of their fathers had significantly greater social skills and cognitive ability than those who received their X chromosome from their mothers.[65]

Defects in Which the Imprint Is Not Stably Transmitted, Maintained, or Interpreted

Because many cell divisions may occur between the time at which the properly imprinted genome is contributed to the zygote and the time at which the imprint is designed to result in the expression of only one allele at a locus in a terminally differentiated somatic cell, faithful propagation of the imprint through cell division must occur. If the imprint results in the expression of the allele carrying the mark, then failure to transmit the imprint from one cell to its daughter cell may lead to failure to express either allele at this locus. If the imprint results in the repression of the allele carrying the mark, then failure to transmit the imprint may lead to expression of both alleles at this locus. Anything less than completely faithful replication of the imprint will lead to mosaicism for cells in which the imprint remains and those in which it has been erased or "lost," as is observed in extraembryonic tissue when the cell-specific expression of *MASH2* is examined.[66] When observed in association with abnormal pathology, such events are referred to as "loss of imprinting" or "relaxation of imprinting."[67]

Loss of imprinting appears to be a common event associated with a number of different tumors, but was first described for Wilms tumor (see Chapter 18, "Genomic Imprinting and Cancer," for a more extensive discussion of this topic). True loss of imprinting may be surmised when an individual can be demonstrated to be mosaic for cells that express only one parent's allele, as well as for cells that express both alleles. This has been demonstrated in some cases of Wilms tumor by showing, for example, that tissue taken from the normal kidney adjacent to the tumor maintains the imprint on *IGF2,* while the tumor expresses both alleles of *IGF2*.[67]

Loss of imprinting or relaxation of imprinting has been inferred in a number of other situations, based on the behavior of the population, as a whole. For example, a number of studies report loss of imprinting at *IGF2* and/or *H19* in several different neoplasms,[68] based on the expression of both maternal and paternal alleles in the tumor. However, unless another tissue from the same individual can be shown to maintain the imprint, this observation may be a result of failure to imprint the gene in the first place. There may be specific variant alleles at these loci that are incapable of being imprinted,[69] the individual may lack some *trans*-acting factor associated with the establishment of the imprint, or stochastic or environmental factors may have resulted in the failure to imprint the allele properly. Such distinctions are important because it is possible, and perhaps likely, that this type of imprint failure may be an important factor in predisposing the individual to cancer.[47,48]

Defects in Which the Imprint Fails to Be Erased or Reestablished

Diseases in this category are the result of failure to complete steps A or B in Fig. 15-1. Failure to erase and reestablish an imprint may result in the transmission of an allele that bears the incorrect imprint. For example, if a female transmits an allele that is imprinted as "paternal" at the Angelman syndrome locus, the resulting offspring is predicted to exhibit the disease because neither of the individual's chromosomes will appear to be maternal. Similarly, if a male transmits an allele marked as "maternal" at the Prader-Willi syndrome locus, the resulting offspring is predicted to exhibit the disease because neither of the individual's chromosomes will appear to be paternal. Conceptually, this type of defect may be viewed as an epigenetic form of uniparental disomy.

A number of cases of both Prader-Willi and Angelman syndrome are thought to be the result of such defects.[70] Most of these cases are associated with small deletions in a region of chromosome 15q11 known as "the imprinting center."[71,72] The imprinting center appears to have a bipartite structure that overlaps the *SNRPN* gene. Deletions in exon 1 of the *SNRPN* gene are associated with an inability to switch a maternal imprint to a paternal imprint (resulting in Prader-Willi syndrome), while mutations in the so-called BD exons, located further upstream, are associated with an inability to switch a paternal imprint to a maternal imprint (resulting in Angelman syndrome) (see reference 71 for a review). At the molecular level, these defects are characterized by maternal alleles that appear to have taken on the methylation pattern of paternal alleles and vice versa. A similar phenomenon (imprinting center defects) may be occurring in some cases of Beckwith-Wiedemann syndrome.[72a] Additional data are required, but it appears that maternally derived alleles in the *H19/IGF2* region have methylation and expression patterns that are characteristic of paternal alleles in some nonuniparental disomy cases.

Another indication of defects in the erasure or reestablishment of an imprint at any allele is the observation of "grandparental effects." For example, in the case of "imprinting center mutations" in Prader-Willi and Angelman syndromes, only mutations on the maternal grandpaternal chromosome are predicted to result in Angelman syndrome, whereas mutations on the paternal grandmaternal chromosome are predicted to result in Prader-Willi syndrome.[71,72] Because such imprint switch defects carry the legacy of the previous generation, any bias in the inheritance of grandparental alleles at any locus may indicate the presence of imprinted genes in these regions. A recent example of such a grandparental effect has been observed for the X chromosomes inherited by male offspring in human families that are not affected by any genetic disease.[73]

The discovery that it may be possible for an allele to be neglected by the imprinting process (i.e., come through the germ line essentially unchanged from the previous generation) argues that it may also be possible for an allele that is not normally imprinted to become imprinted. This may occur as a result of a mistake in the recognition of elements required for establishment of the imprint or because genetic events have resulted in the creation of a "neomorphically imprinted" allele.[74] This explanation has been proffered in the case of the familial paraganglioma locus.[75]

Familial paragangliomas are benign head and neck tumors and the disease locus has been mapped to chromosome 11q. Only the offspring of affected or carrier males become affected.[75,76] That the tumors "lose heterozygosity" at loci on chromosome 11q indicates that the responsible gene acts as a tumor-suppressor gene and conforms to the Knudson two-hit model.[75] However, if a tumor suppressor gene is imprinted in all normal individuals, then one might expect a large fraction of the population to exhibit the disease. The fact that this disease is very rare, yet still exhibits a strong parental origin effect, argues that the mutation resulting in familial paraganglioma has transformed this tumor suppressor gene from one that is normally expressed from both alleles to one that is inactivated upon transmission through the male germ line.[75] The nature of such mutations is of great interest in defining the *cis*-acting sequences that are required for establishing an imprint.

The final point considered in this section concerns a tumor that may address the question of whether cells exist in which the imprint has been fully erased. Because testicular germ cell tumors arise from an early germ cell, it may be hypothesized that they arise from cells in which imprint erasure has already occurred. Examination of the expression of a few imprinted genes in such tumors has revealed that many of these tumors express alleles of both *IGF2* and *H19*.[77] It is, therefore, possible that these tumors arise from cells in which imprinting has been erased or lost over some or all of the genome.

GENOME IMPRINTING AND ITS RELEVANCE TO CLINICAL GENETICS

Genomic imprinting is important to understand many clinical disorders and diseases. Imprinted genes are involved in various aspects of growth (intrauterine, postnatal, and cancers), behavior, and placental development. Genomic imprinting effects are observed as clinical disorders when there is a lack of expression of a gene because of deletion, mutation, or deficiency, or when there is overexpression of a gene because of biallelic expression due to duplication, relaxation of imprinting, or loss of imprinting control.

Observations that genomic imprinting may be important in humans have come from (a) hydatidiform moles and ovarian teratomas, which are naturally occurring equivalents of artificially constructed androgenetic and gynegenetic mouse embryos (see the section "How Errors in the Imprinting Process Contribute to Human Disease" earlier in this chapter); (b) triploid phenotypes in which the phenotype differs depending on whether the extra set of chromosomes is contributed by the mother or the father; (c) human chromosomal deletion syndromes (Prader-Willi syndrome and Angelman syndrome), the phenotypes of which differ depending on whether the deletion involves the mother's or the father's chromosome; (d) uniparental disomy in which the phenotype differs depending on which parent has contributed both of the chromosomes; (e) "imprinting center" mutations in Prader-Willi, Angelman, and, perhaps, Beckwith-Wiedemann syndromes; (f) a number of different cancers; (g) X chromosome inactivation; (h) disorders of growth, and; (i) parental origin effects on behavior.

Chromosomal Deletion Syndromes

Prader-Willi syndrome and Angelman syndrome. Prader-Willi syndrome (PWS) and Angelman syndrome (AS) have been studied extensively in relation to genomic imprinting. Although the two syndromes are phenotypically distinct neurobehavioral syndromes, it has become clear that both involve imprinted genes on the long arm of chromosome 15. Both syndromes may be associated with deletions of the same region of chromosome 15 (15q11-q13). In PWS, the deletion is exclusively of the paternally derived chromosome 15, whereas in AS, the deletion is of the maternally derived chromosome 15. This observation suggests that there is a critical region on the paternal chromosome 15 that is required to prevent the Prader-Willi phenotype. Likewise, there is a critical region on the maternal chromosome 15 that must be present in order to prevent Angelman syndrome.[60,70,78]

Prader-Willi syndrome is characterized by hypotonia in the newborn. Failure to thrive may occur without special feeding efforts. However, hyperphagia and obesity develop early in childhood. Affected individuals usually develop small hands and feet; almond-shaped eyes; narrow bitemporal diameter; somewhat long face; mild to moderate developmental delay; hypothalamic hypogonadotrophic hypogonadism; small genitalia; and delayed puberty. Although PWS was recognized more than 40 years ago its relationship to a parent of origin effect was not recognized until the late 1980s.[79] In the early 1980s, a deletion of chromosome 15q11-q13 was recognized in 60 percent of individuals with PWS.[80] Later it was discovered that these deletions were always on the paternally inherited chromosome 15,[59,81] suggesting that there is a critical region on paternal chromosome 15 that must be inherited from the father in order to prevent PWS. Another group of individuals with PWS was recognized as having maternal uniparental disomy of chromosome 15 (two copies of maternal chromosome 15 and no contribution from the father (paternal deficiency)), suggesting that an imprinted gene or genes may be lacking because the paternal chromosome was not inherited.[79] Twenty-five to 30 percent of individuals with PWS have now been recognized to have maternal uniparental disomy of chromosome 15. A small percentage of individuals with PWS have mutations or microdeletions in a region known as the imprinting control region.[82] Molecular studies have revealed that the Prader-Willi critical region has several genes that are expressed only from the paternally inherited chromosome. Among these are *SNRPN* (a developmentally regulated protein component of spliceosome expressed predominantly in neuronal tissue), ZNF127 and FZN 127 (zinc finger proteins), *IPW* (an RNA functional unit[83]), *NDN* (the necdin gene, expressed in differentiating neurons of the brain),[84–87] and two expressed sequence tags (PAR 1 and PAR 5). The distance between these imprinted genes is 1 to 1.5 Mb, which suggests that additional imprinted genes may exist in this critical region. Gunay-Aygun et al. have suggested that there may be phenotypic differences in PWS associated with deletion and PWS associated with uniparental disomy.[88] However, more studies are required to distinguish these subtle variations in these two groups. The paternally deleted region usually contains a gene for pigmentation; as a result, individuals with PWS due to deletions may have fair complexions and blond hair.[89]

Angelman syndrome, also known as "happy puppet syndrome," was first described in 1965. The phenotype is characterized by severe mental retardation; ataxia; seizures; abnormal EEG; very happy disposition; midfacial hypoplasia; and inappropriate outbursts of laughter. Sixty to 70 percent of individuals with AS have been recognized to have a deletion involving maternal chromosome 15q11-q13; about 5 percent have been recognized to have paternal uniparental disomy; and most of the remaining individuals with AS have been found to have mutations within the imprinting control region[90] or the *UBE3A* gene.

UBE3A (a protein that functions in ubiquitination of other proteins) has been localized in the Angelman critical region and been shown to be differentially expressed[90] depending on the parent of origin and the tissue. *UBE3A* has biparental expression in most tissues, but only maternal expression in the brain.[91–93] Therefore, maternal deletion, deficiency, or lack of expression of the maternal allele in the brain is expected to result in the Angelman phenotype. Consistent with this expectation, several patients have been identified who carry mutations in the maternal *UBE3A* allele.[93]

Genes in the PWS/AS critical region have been shown to have parent-specific methylation patterns, parent-specific replication timing patterns, and several control regions that may be involved in differential gene expression.[94] The exact mechanisms of control are not yet understood, but maternal chromosomal abnormalities seem to more often involve improper control of gene expression, whereas the paternal chromosome abnormalities seem to more often involve deficiencies. A specific PCR test based on DNA methylation can be used to identify the parental origin of a particular chromosome.[36,37] Determining the mechanisms leading to Angelman and Prader-Willi syndromes (deletion, chromosomal rearrangements such as translocation, uniparental disomy, or gene control) alterations in a specific case has implications for estimating recurrence risks, for genetic counseling, and for prenatal diagnosis. Higher recurrence risk is associated with mutations involving the imprinting control center or mutations of specific genes, while lowest recurrence risk is associated with uniparental disomy.[95] A recent study suggests that parent of origin-specific DNA methylation analysis at the *SNRPN* locus in amniotic fluid cells and of chorionic villi samples may be useful for prenatal diagnosis when trying to detect imprinting defects.[96]

Individuals with PWS and AS have been noted to have two- to threefold higher levels of plasma γ-aminobutyric acid (GABA) compared to nonretarded moderately obese or retarded nonobese controls.[97] It is speculated that this may be due to an alteration of a subset of postsynaptic GABA receptors leading to reduced sensitivity, with the result that there is a compensatory increase in presynaptic GABA release.[97] The *GABRB3* gene has been localized to the 15q11-q13 region and appears to be imprinted.[96]

Uniparental Disomy

That uniparental disomy could occur was first proposed by Eric Engel in 1980.[98] Uniparental disomy is a situation in which both members of a chromosome pair have been inherited from one parent (maternal deficiency/paternal duplication or vice versa). When two different chromosomes are inherited from one parent, the uniparental disomy is heterodisomy. If identical copies of the same chromosome are inherited, it is called isodisomy. Whole chromosomes or parts of a chromosome can be involved, and an individual may be mosaic for the event; for example, some cells may be trisomic and some may have uniparental disomy. New molecular diagnostic techniques allow us to distinguish between almost any of these possibilities.

Uniparental disomy is surprisingly common and is now known to occur in a number of disorders. The primary mechanism producing uniparental disomy appears to be a "trisomy rescue" after meiotic nondisjunction. Nondisjunction in the first meiotic division results in heterodisomy, whereas nondisjunction in the second meiotic division results in isodisomy. Because of crossing-over during meiosis, there may be isodisomy for only part of a chromosome. Isodisomy may also occur as a result of nondisjunction in a somatic cell; however, this appears to be a relatively rare event.

Ten to 15 percent of all recognized human conceptions might begin as trisomies. However, most trisomic conceptuses are lethal and are miscarried early in pregnancy. The only way that most trisomy conceptions can survive is by loss of one of the three chromosomes, resulting in a disomic cell line. If the parental origin of the loss of a chromosome is random, then this event is expected to lead to uniparental disomy in one-third of surviving cases.

Uniparental disomy has been reported for chromosomes 1,[99] 2,[100] 4,[101] 5,[102] 6,[103–105] 7,[106–110] 8,[111] 9,[112,113] 10,[114] 11,[62,115,116] 13,[117] 14,[118–121] 15,[79,122,123] 16,[124–126] 21,[127] and 22,[128] and the sex chromosomes.[129–131]

Three types of complications and sequelae are seen with uniparental disomy (a) uncovering imprinted genes; (b) producing autosomal recessive disorders; and (c) producing abnormalities related to residual aneuploidy.

Uncovering Imprinted Genes.

Genomic imprinting results in the expression of a gene from only one parent's allele. When uniparental disomy occurs (situation in which both chromosomes come from one parent), if a critical gene is normally expressed from only the missing allele of the other parent, the effects of that imprinted gene may be uncovered. The pioneering work of Cattanach[132] using translocation disomies in mice defined multiple chromosome regions associated with gross phenotypic effects of uniparental disomy. This level of phenotypic screen yielded effects predominantly on growth, behavior, and survival.

Some of the phenotypes observed in the mouse suggested the existence of homologous loci in humans. Thus when two chromosomes 15 are inherited from the mother, the paternally derived Prader-Willi critical region (essential to prevent PWS) are missing, resulting in the PWS phenotype. Conversely, when two chromosomes 15 are inherited from the father, the maternally derived Angelman critical region (essential to prevent AS) are missing, resulting in the AS phenotype. Uniparental disomy for the homologous loci in the mouse produce morphological effects similar to those observed in humans. Thus far, six human chromosome regions that carry imprinted genes and that are homologous to the mouse chromosome regions demonstrated to carry imprinted genes, have been identified; paternal chromosome 6q, maternal chromosome 7q, paternal and maternal chromosome 11p, maternal chromosome 14q, and both maternal and paternal chromosome 15q (Table 15-1).

Such studies have given rise to "imprinting maps" of the mouse and human genomes. While such maps are very useful, they should be interpreted with caution because they are not exclusionary. By this we mean that those regions identified as having some measurable phenotypic effect undoubtedly harbor imprinted genes. However, one cannot draw the opposite conclusion from the negative result. Failure to observe an effect of uniparental disomy on survival, gross morphology, or behavior does not imply that no imprinted genes exist in these regions; it implies only that their absence does not result in any of the

Table 15-1 Imprinted Genes Associated with Human Disease Phenotypes

Gene Symbol	Normally Inactivated Allele	Human Chromosome	Phenotype
IGF2R	Paternal*	6q25-q27	Transient neonatal diabetes mellitus
PEG1/MEST	Maternal	7q32	Russel-Silver syndrome
IGF2	Maternal	11p15	BWS/Wilms
H19	Paternal	11p15	Wilms
P57KIP2	Maternal	11p15	BWS
KVLQT	Maternal	11p15	BWS
?	? Maternal	14q	Precocious puberty/short stature
ZNF127	Paternal	15q11-q13	PWS
FZN127	Paternal	15q11-q13	PWS
IPW	Paternal	15q11-q13	PWS
NDN	Paternal	15q11-q13	PWS
PAR1	Paternal	15q11-q13	PWS
PAR5	Paternal	15q11-q13	PWS
UBE3A	Maternal	15q11-q13	Angelman syndrome

*IGF2R appears to be expressed from only one allele in a minority of individuals.

phenotypes detectable by the screening procedure. For example, the neuronatin gene on mouse chromosome 2 has been shown to be imprinted, but lies outside the region delimited as imprinted by studies using translocation chromosomes.[133] In addition, the recent description of cognitive differences in Turner syndrome individuals carrying a maternal versus a paternal X chromosome (see below) points out the importance of this precaution. In the absence of such tests, one could have concluded that because individuals with Turner syndrome may carry either maternal or paternal X chromosomes, and that females with exclusively maternal X chromosomes have been identified,[130,131] no genes on the X chromosome are imprinted. We now know that at least two genes on the X chromosome, in addition to the cognitive function locus,[65] are imprinted (*Xist*[64] and the choroideremia locus[134]).

Producing Autosomal Recessive Disorders. According to the rules of Mendelian inheritance, a mutant phenotype is expected in one quarter of the offspring when both parents are carriers of a recessive allele at an autosomal locus. When uniparental disomy occurs, it is possible for the offspring to receive both copies of the identical chromosome or chromosomal region (isodisomy) from only one parent. If that chromosome carries the abnormal allele, the autosomal recessive disorder will be manifested in the offspring, even though only one parent is a carrier of the abnormal gene. An autosomal recessive disorder due to uniparental isodisomy was first reported in a female affected with cystic fibrosis.[106] Subsequent to this report, many individuals with recessive disorders as a result of uniparental disomy have been reported (see Table 15-2).

Effects of residual aneuploidy. When trisomy occurs, the extra chromosome is derived from one or the other parent. When a trisomy converts into a disomic cell line, there is a one in three chance that this will result in uniparental disomy. This "trisomy rescue" allows the pregnancy to survive, and allows the fetus to come to term, but puts the fetus at risk both for having uniparental disomy and for having trisomic cells (residual aneuploidy in some tissues). These cells may lead to malformations or dysfunction. They may also subsequently predispose to cancer.

Uniparental disomy should be suspected when chorionic villus sampling or amniocentesis reveals mosaicism. Studies of chorionic villus sampling suggest that at least 2 to 3 percent of pregnancies have some trisomic cells, which suggests that the conception began as trisomy. One-third of trisomy conceptions are predicted to result in uniparental disomy, suggesting that as much as 1 percent of all pregnancies have converted to uniparental disomy. Because many uniparental disomies have phenotypic abnormalities, if mosaicism is detected on prenatal diagnosis, an effort must be made to exclude uniparental disomy, especially with chromosomes 6, 7, 11, 14, and 15.

Because most uniparental disomy results from trisomy rescue and because trisomies are associated with advanced maternal age, it is not surprising that uniparental disomies are associated with advanced maternal age as well. For example, PWS resulting from chromosome 15 deletions is not associated with advanced parental age, but uniparental disomy Prader-Willi is associated with advanced maternal age. Because parents who are carriers of translocations are at a risk for trisomy, they are also at a risk for uniparental disomy, and, consequently, at risk for uncovering the effects of imprinting, producing autosomal recessive disorders, and the effects of residual aneuploidy.

Specific Disorders Associated with Imprinting

Albright Hereditary Osteodystrophy. Albright hereditary osteodystrophy is an autosomal dominant disorder occurring with a variety of phenotypes within the same family. At least two linkage groups have been described. One involves mutations in the human Gs alpha gene (*GNAS1*) which is mapped to chromosome 20q13.11.[135] Depending on which parent transmits the abnormal allele, a different phenotype is produced (i.e., the phenotype is dependent on the parent from whom the mutation is inherited). If the abnormal allele is inherited from the father, a milder phenotype (pseudo-pseudohypoparathyroidism) occurs, in which there is hormone responsiveness. On the other hand, if the abnormal allele is inherited from the mother, a severe hormone-resistant, pseudohypoparathyroidism type 1a develops, which is characterized by seizures, mental retardation, and subcutaneous and intracranial calcification. Both phenotypes can be seen within the same family depending on which parent is transmitting the mutation.[136–138] It is not yet clear whether both Albright hereditary osteodystrophy loci involve parent of origin effects.

Transient neonatal diabetes mellitus. Transient neonatal diabetes mellitus is a rare type of diabetes mellitus that presents in the neonatal period with intrauterine growth retardation. These babies lack insulin in the neonatal period. However, insulin production may start within a few months, and often becomes normal by about age 3 years. This type of transient neonatal diabetes mellitus has been associated with paternal uniparental isodisomy of chromosome 6.[104,139] The gene involved in transient neonatal diabetes mellitus has been localized to chromosome 6q22-q23.[103] Duplications of paternal chromosome 6q have also been associated with transient neonatal diabetes mellitus.[140] The gene for insulin is on chromosome 11 and must have different types of control

Table 15-2 Recessive Disorders Associated with Uniparental Isodisomy

Chromosome	Transmission	Recessive Disorder	Reference
5	Paternal	Spinal muscular atrophy	102
6	Paternal	Complement deficiency	105
7	Maternal	Cystic fibrosis	106
	Maternal	Osteogenesis imperfecta	110
	Paternal	Congenital chloride diarrhea	161
8	Paternal	Lipoprotein lipase deficiency	111
9	Maternal	Cartilage hair hypoplasia	112
11	Maternal	β-Thalassemia	162
13	Paternal	Retinoblastoma	163
14	Maternal	Rod monochromacy	119
15	Maternal	Bloom syndrome	123
16	Paternal	α-Thalassemia	126
	Paternal	Familial Mediterranean fever	125
X	Paternal	Hemophilia	129
	Maternal	Duchenne muscular dystrophy	131

at different times in development and in different tissues (i.e., in utero, in the neonatal period, and in later period). In mice during the embryonic period, only the paternal insulin allele is expressed in the yolk sac, suggesting tissue-specific, time-specific, and parental origin-specific control of alleles at the insulin locus.[141]

Growth Disorders

Growth Retardation. Absence of paternal chromosome 7 (maternal uniparental disomy for chromosome 7) has been associated with intrauterine, as well as postnatal, growth retardation, suggesting that a gene on paternal chromosome 7 is necessary for normal intrauterine and postnatal growth. Maternal uniparental disomy for chromosome 7 has been associated with growth retardation (intrauterine as well as postnatal).[106,107,110] Maternal uniparental disomy for chromosome 7 has also been associated with Russell-Silver syndrome.[109] Russell-Silver syndrome is a growth-retardation syndrome that is characterized by intrauterine and postnatal growth retardation; short stature; normal head size for age; frontal bossing; triangular face; incurved fifth finger; and hemihypertrophy. Hemihypertrophy (one side larger than the other) may reflect mosaicism for uniparental disomy. Ten to 15 percent of individuals with Russell-Silver syndrome may have uniparental disomy for chromosome 7.[109]

In humans, one imprinted gene, *PEG1/MEST,* that is expressed from the paternal allele has been located on chromosome 7 (7q31-q34).[142]

In addition to maternal uniparental disomy for chromosome 7, maternal uniparental disomy for chromosome 2[100] and maternal uniparental disomy for chromosome 16[124] have also been associated with intrauterine growth retardation. However, these reports are associated with residual trisomy mosaicism, which may be responsible for the intrauterine growth retardation.

As mentioned earlier, paternal uniparental disomy for chromosome 6 produces transient neonatal diabetes mellitus as well as intrauterine growth retardation.

Overgrowth Syndromes. The *Beckwith-Wiedemann syndrome* (BWS) is a fetal overgrowth syndrome associated with excessive insulin production (secondary to an enlarged pancreas) and hypoglycemia in the neonatal period. These babies are large for gestational age, have macroglossia and visceromegaly. Omphalocele is often present secondary to visceromegaly. Occasionally, mental retardation is seen and thought to be related to hypoglycemia in the neonatal period. In some patients, visceromegaly may develop postnatally. Recently several genes have been implicated in the Beckwith-Wiedemann phenotype, including *IGF2, H19, p57KIP2,* and *KVLQT1.*[143–145] *KVLQT1* shows tissue-specific imprinting with only paternal expression in most tissues, but biparental expression in the heart.[146]

In individuals with a family history of BWS, the phenotype appears to only occur with maternal transmission.[147] Paternally inherited duplications of 11p15.5 associated with BWS[148] have suggested that a double-dose of paternal alleles, or maternal relaxation of imprinting of these genes, is responsible for BWS in a number of patients, indicating that these genes are imprinted. Comparison of phenotypes of individuals with BWS associated with paternal uniparental disomy p11.5 and of individuals with BWS with normal chromosomes, has revealed that individuals with BWS associated with uniparental disomy tend to have a lower incidence of hypoglycemia, a lower incidence of hemihypertrophy, a lower incidence of facial nevus flammeus, and an increased incidence of learning difficulties compared to BWS with normal chromosomes.[148] Maternally derived inversions and balanced translocations have also been associated with BWS,[149] suggesting that maternal loss of imprinting control (i.e., relaxation and maternal expression) can also be responsible for BWS.

Individuals with BWS have a higher incidence of cancers.[150] Relaxation of imprinting of *IGF2* resulting in biparental expression of *IGF2* is seen in a number of tumors.[151] The risk of recurrence for BWS depends on the genetic rearrangements that produce the disorder. The risk can be as high as 50 percent in complex rearrangements. Hemihypertrophy suggests somatic mosaicism. Discordance of monozygotic female twins suggests somatic loss of control (relaxation) during monozygotic twinning process.

The *Simpson-Golabi-Behmel syndrome* is an X-linked disorder characterized by overgrowth, coarse facies, and anomalies of the skeleton, heart, kidney, gastrointestinal tract, and the central nervous system. Mutations in *GPC3,* a glypican gene, are seen in the Simpson-Golabi-Behmel overgrowth syndrome.[152] The *GPC3* gene is a member of the glypican family of heparin sulfate proteoglycans.[153] The gene codes for a cell-surface receptor proteoglycan that binds insulin-like growth factor 2 and is part of a new class of signaling protein.[154] BWS and Simpson-Golabi-Behmel syndrome have considerable phenotypic overlap and seem to involve a complex pathway of fetal overgrowth. Individuals with Simpson-Golabi-Behmel syndrome are also at risk for developing some types of cancers.[155,156] Suggestions are that fetal macrosomia, low ratio of head to abdominal circumference, and raised maternal serum α-fetoprotein may prove useful markers for prenatal diagnosis of Simpson-Golabi-Behmel syndrome. Postnatal evaluation with α-fetoproteins in Simpson-Golabi-Behmel syndrome and BWS may be an indicator of embryonal tumor.[156]

Hemihypertrophy is seen with BWS and Wilms tumor. This may suggest mosaicism for imprinting of genes involved in growth.

Behavioral disorders. Mouse uniparental disomy studies suggest behavioral abnormalities can be part of imprinting effects. As already discussed, Prader-Willi and Angelman syndrome have distinct behaviors, which appear to be determined by parent of origin. Recent studies in Turner syndrome suggest that there may be genomically imprinted gene(s) on the X chromosome[65] that may influence social functioning and related cognitive abilities. Turner syndrome occurs when there is absence or abnormality of one of the sex chromosomes. Turner syndrome is seen with 45,X karyotypes, ring X chromosomes, X isochromosomes, or terminal deletions involving the X chromosome, or remnants of the Y chromosome, and with mosaicism of any of these. Females with Turner syndrome often have an unusual behavior. They may act immaturely, have a particular spatial perceptual problem, and/or may lack ambition and social skills. Females with Turner syndrome who receive the maintained X chromosome from their father seem to have better social skills as compared to females with Turner syndrome who receive their maintained X chromosome from the mother. This suggests an association of unusual behavior and poor social skills with the loss of the X chromosome contributed by the father. This would also suggest that normal males who can only receive their X chromosome from their mothers are less socially adept because of imprinting of some gene(s) on the X chromosome.[157]

A Role for Folic Acid?

Imprinting is thought to occur during meiosis and involves methylation. One could speculate that if a mother is folic acid deficient between 6 and 12 weeks (the period of embryonic female meiosis), that this might interfere with the normal imprinting process.

When to Suspect Genomic Imprinting

Genomic imprinting is suspected:

1. When pedigree analysis reveals that the disorder is always expressed when transmitted from only the mother or only the father.[158] Both males and females are equally likely to be affected, but the disorder is transmitted only from one parent (mother or father); that is, the transmission is dependent on the sex of the transmitting parent (e.g., BWS is almost always

transmitted by the mother, and glomus tumor is almost always transmitted from the father).

2. In disorders of growth, behavior, and some endocrine disorders as mentioned earlier.
3. When monozygotic female twins are discordant for a particular syndrome, the possibility that an imprinted gene is being expressed must be considered.[159] A number of genomically imprinted disorders have been reported where one of the monozygotic twins is affected, and the other is not affected. There have been several reports of female monozygotic twins discordant for BWS. It has been suggested that genomic imprinting, monozygous twinning, and X inactivation are all related.[160] It is now clear that both genomic imprinting and X inactivation are linked to allelic differences in DNA methylation and chromatin structure. It may be possible that all three are in one way linked to time-specific folic acid deficiency during critical periods because folic acid deficiency has been associated with alteration in methylation and gene expression.
4. When prenatal diagnosis with chorionic villus sampling or amniocentesis reveals mosaicism, the possibility of uniparental disomy and genomic imprinting effects should be considered, and the fetus should be tested accordingly. Placental mosaicism puts the fetus at risk for uniparental disomy and for uncovering complications of uniparental disomy (imprinting, recessive disorders, residual aneuploidy).

Genomic Imprinting and Genetic Counseling

Understanding genomic imprinting is important because there are important implications for diagnosing some genetic disorders. It is also important for giving recurrence risk to families, for counseling families appropriately, and for providing prenatal diagnosis appropriately. Recurrence risks were discussed above. Individuals with specific syndromes involving some imprinted genes (e.g., BWS and Simpson-Golabi-Behmel syndrome) are at a higher risk for developing some types of cancer. These individuals should be counseled appropriately and should be followed accordingly for early detection and treatment. Prenatal diagnosis for PWS and AS is now possible using a specific PCR test.[36,37]

ACKNOWLEDGMENTS

Carmen Sapienza thanks Linda Angeloff Sapienza for her artwork.

REFERENCES

1. McGrath J, Solter D: Completion of mouse embryogenesis requires both the maternal and paternal genomes. *Cell* **37**:179, 1984.
2. Bartolomei MS, Tilghman SM: Genomic imprinting in mammals. *Annu Rev Genet* **31**:493, 1997.
3. Reik W, Walter J: Imprinting mechanisms in mammals. *Curr Opin Genet Dev* **8**:154, 1998.
4. Ohlsson R, Tycko B, Sapienza C: Monoallelic expression: "There can only be one." *Trends Genet* **14**:435, 1998.
5. Wolffe AP, Kurumizaka H: The nucleosome: A powerful regulator of transcription. *Prog Nucleic Acid Res Mol Biol* **61**:379, 1998.
6. Nan X, Ng HH, Johnson CA, Laherty CD, Turner BM, Eisenman RN, Bird A: Transcriptional repression by the methyl-CpG-binding protein MeCP2 involves a histone deacetylase complex. *Nature* **393**:386, 1998.
7. Smrzka OW, Fae I, Stoger R, Kurzbauer R, Fischer GF, Henn T, Weith A, et al.: Conservation of a maternal-specific methylation signal at the human IGF2R locus. *Hum Mol Genet* **4**:1945, 1995.
8. Gabriel JM, Gray TA, Stubbs L, Saitoh S, Ohta T, Nicholls RD: Structure and function correlations at the imprinted mouse snrpn locus. *Mamm Genome* **9**:788, 1998.
9. Latham KE, Doherty AS, Scott CD, Schultz RM: Igf2r and Igf2 gene expression in androgenetic, gynogenetic, and parthenogenetic preimplantation mouse embryos: Absence of regulation by genomic imprinting. *Genes Dev* **8**:290, 1994.
10. Reik W, Collick A, Norris ML, Barton SC, Surani MA: Genomic imprinting determines methylation of parental alleles in transgenic mice. *Nature* **328**:248, 1987.
11. Sapienza C, Peterson AC, Rossant J, Balling R: Degree of methylation of transgenes is dependent on gamete of origin. *Nature* **328**:251, 1987.
12. Swain JL, Stewart TA, Leder P: Parental legacy determines methylation and expression of an autosomal transgene: A molecular mechanism for parental imprinting. *Cell* **50**:719, 1987.
13. Tycko B: DNA methylation in genomic imprinting. *Mutat Res* **386**:131, 1997.
14. Sapienza C, Paquette J, Tran TH, Peterson A: Epigenetic and genetic factors affect transgene methylation imprinting. *Development* **107**:165, 1989.
15. McGowan R, Campbell R, Peterson A, Sapienza C: Cellular mosaicism in the methylation and expression of hemizygous loci in the mouse. *Genes Dev* **3**:1669, 1989.
16. Naumova AK, Olien L, Bird LM, Slamka C, Fonseca M, Verner AE, Wang M, et al.: Transmission-ratio distortion of X chromosomes among male offspring of females with skewed X inactivation. *Dev Genet* **17**:198, 1995.
17. Chess A, Simon I, Cedar H, Axel R: Allelic inactivation regulates olfactory receptor gene expression. *Cell* **78**:823, 1994.
18. Chess A: Expansion of the allelic exclusion principle? *Science* **279**:2067, 1998.
19. Keohane AM, Lavender JS, O'Neill LP, Turner BM: Histone acetylation and X inactivation. *Dev Genet* **22**:65, 1998.
20. Jablonka E, Goitein R, Sperling K, Cedar H, Marcus M: 5-aza-C-induced changes in the time of replication of the X chromosomes of *Microtus agrestis* are followed by non-random reversion to a late pattern of replication. *Chromosoma* **95**:81, 1987.
21. Li E, Beard C, Jaenisch R: Role for DNA methylation in genomic imprinting. *Nature* **366**:362, 1993.
22. Spofford J: Parental control of position-effect variegation. II: Effect of sex of parent contributing white-mottled rearrangement in *Drosophila melanogaster. Genetics* **46**:1151, 1961.
23. Hessler A: A study of parental modification of variegated position effects. *Genetics* **46**:463, 1961.
24. Tartof KD, Henikoff S: Trans-sensing effects from *Drosophila* to humans. *Cell* **65**:201, 1991.
25. Henikoff S: Gene silencing in *Drosophila*. *Curr Top Microbiol Immunol* **197**:193, 1995.
26. Pirrotta V: Chromatin-silencing mechanisms in *Drosophila* maintain patterns of gene expression. *Trends Genet* **13**:314, 1997.
27. Pirrotta V: PcG complexes and chromatin silencing. *Curr Opin Genet Dev* **7**:249, 1997.

27a. Lloyd VK, Sinclair DA, Grigliatti TA: Genomic imprinting and position-effect variegation in *Drosophila melanogaster. Genetics* **151**:1503, 1999.

28. Xu Y, Goodyer CG, Deal C, Polychronakos C: Functional polymorphism in the parental imprinting of the human IGF2R gene. *Biochem Biophys Res Commun* **197**:747, 1993.
29. Giannoukakis N, Deal C, Paquette J, Kukuvitis A, Polychronakos C: Polymorphic functional imprinting of the human IGF2 gene among individuals, in blood cells, is associated with H19 expression. *Biochem Biophys Res Commun* **220**:1014, 1996.
30. Nishiwaki K, Niikawa N, Ishikawa M: Polymorphic and tissue-specific imprinting of the human Wilms tumor gene WT1. *Jpn J Hum Genet* **42**:205, 1997.
31. Rougeulle C, Glatt H, Lalande M: The Angelman syndrome candidate gene, UBE3A/E6-AP, is imprinted in brain. *Nat Genet* **17**:14, 1997.
32. Gould TD, Pfeifer K: Imprinting of mouse Kvlqt1 is developmentally regulated. *Hum Mol Genet* **7**:483, 1998.
33. Jinno Y, Yun K, Nishiwaki K, Kubota T, Ogawa O, Reeve AE, Niikawa N: Mosaic and polymorphic imprinting of the WT1 gene in humans. *Nat Genet* **6**:305, 1994.
34. DeChiara TM, Robertson EJ, Efstratiadis A: Parental imprinting of the mouse insulin-like growth factor II gene. *Cell* **64**:849, 1991.
35. Dao D, Frank D, Qian N, O'Keefe D, Vosatka RJ, Walsh CP, Tycko B: IMPT1, an imprinted gene similar to polyspecific transporter and multi-drug resistance genes. *Hum Mol Genet* **7**:597, 1998.
36. Buchholz T, Jackson J, Smith A: Methylation analysis at three different loci within the imprinted region of chromosome 15q11-13 [letter]. *Am J Med Genet* **72**:117, 1997.
37. Zeschnigk M, Lich C, Buiting K, Doerfler W, Horsthemke B: A single-tube PCR test for the diagnosis of Angelman and Prader-Willi syndrome based on allelic methylation differences at the SNRPN locus. *Eur J Hum Genet* **5**:94, 1997.

38. Kosaki K, McGinniss MJ, Veraksa AN, McGinnis WJ, Jones KL: Prader-Willi and Angelman syndromes: Diagnosis with a bisulfite-treated methylation-specific PCR method. *Am J Med Genet* **73**:308, 1997.
39. Sapienza C, Hall J: Genome imprinting in human disease, in CR Scriver, WS Sly, D Valle (eds): *The Metabolic and Molecular Bases of Inherited Disease*. New York: McGraw-Hill, 1995, p. 437.
40. Sasaki H, Jones PA, Chaillet JR, Ferguson-Smith AC, Barton SC, Reik W, Surani MA: Parental imprinting: Potentially active chromatin of the repressed maternal allele of the mouse insulin-like growth factor II (Igf2) gene. *Genes Dev* **6**:1843, 1992.
41. Stoger R, Kubicka P, Liu CG, Kafri T, Razin A, Cedar H, Barlow DP: Maternal-specific methylation of the imprinted mouse Igf2r locus identifies the expressed locus as carrying the imprinting signal. *Cell* **73**:61, 1993.
42. Moore T, Constancia M, Zubair M, Bailleul B, Feil R, Sasaki H, Reik W: Multiple imprinted sense and antisense transcripts, differential methylation and tandem repeats in a putative imprinting control region upstream of mouse Igf2. *Proc Natl Acad Sci USA* **94**:12509, 1997.
43. Wutz A, Smrzka OW, Schweifer N, Schellander K, Wagner EF, Barlow DP: Imprinted expression of the Igf2r gene depends on an intronic CpG island [see comments]. *Nature* **389**:745, 1997.
44. Rougeulle C, Cardoso C, Fontes M, Colleaux L, Lalande M: An imprinted antisense RNA overlaps UBE3A and a second maternally expressed transcript [letter]. *Nat Genet* **19**:15, 1998.
45. Wilmut I, Schnieke AE, McWhir J, Kind AJ, Campbell KH: Viable offspring derived from fetal and adult mammalian cells [see comments] [published erratum appears in Nature **386**:200, 1997]. *Nature* **385**:810, 1997.
46. Wakayama T, Perry AC, Zuccotti M, Johnson KR, Yanagimachi R: Full-term development of mice from enucleated oocytes injected with cumulus cell nuclei [see comments]. *Nature* **394**:369, 1998.
47. Sapienza C: Genome imprinting, cellular mosaicism and carcinogenesis. *Mol Carcinog* **3**:118, 1990.
48. Cui H HI, Ohlsson R, Hamilton SR, Feinberg AP: Loss of imprinting in normal tissue of colorectal cancer patients with microsatellite instability. *Nature Med* **11**:1276, 1998.
49. Cooper DW: Directed genetic change model for X chromosome inactivation in eutherian mammals. *Nature* **230**:292, 1971.
50. Takagi N, Sasaki M: Preferential inactivation of the paternally derived X chromosome in the extraembryonic membranes of the mouse. *Nature* **256**:640, 1975.
51. Ropers HH, Wolff G, Hitzeroth HW: Preferential X inactivation in human placenta membranes: Is the paternal X inactive in early embryonic development of female mammals? *Hum Genet* **43**:265, 1978.
52. McGrath J, Solter D: Maternal Thp lethality in the mouse is a nuclear, not cytoplasmic, defect. *Nature* **308**:550, 1984.
53. Barton SC, Surani MA, Norris ML: Role of paternal and maternal genomes in mouse development. *Nature* **311**:374, 1984.
54. Surani MA KR, Allen ND, Singh PB, Fundele R, Ferguson-Smith AC, Barton SC: Genome imprinting and development in the mouse. *Development* **89**(suppl):89, 1990.
55. Surani MA, Barton SC, Norris ML: Development of reconstituted mouse eggs suggests imprinting of the genome during gametogenesis. *Nature* **308**:548, 1984.
56. Lawler SD: Genetic studies on hydatidiform moles. *Adv Exp Med Biol* **176**:147, 1984.
57. Linder DMB, Hecht F: Parthenogenetic origin of benign ovarian teratomas. *N Engl J Med* **292**:63, 1975.
58. Varmuza S, Mann M: Genomic imprinting — defusing the ovarian time bomb. *Trends Genet* **10**:118, 1994.
59. Butler MG: Prader-Willi syndrome: Current understanding of cause and diagnosis. *Am J Med Genet* **35**:319, 1990.
60. Knoll JH, Nicholls RD, Magenis RE, Graham JM Jr, Lalande M, Latt SA: Angelman and Prader-Willi syndromes share a common chromosome 15 deletion but differ in parental origin of the deletion. *Am J Med Genet* **32**:285, 1989.
61. Henry I, Bonaiti-Pellie C, Chehensse V, Beldjord C, Schwartz C, Utermann G, Junien C: Uniparental paternal disomy in a genetic cancer-predisposing syndrome. *Nature* **351**:665, 1991.
62. Henry I, Puech A, Riesewijk A, Ahnine L, Mannens M, Beldjord C, Bitoun P, et al.: Somatic mosaicism for partial paternal isodisomy in Wiedemann-Beckwith syndrome: A post-fertilization event. *Eur J Hum Genet* **1**:19, 1993.
63. Mannens M: The Molecular Genetics of Wilms Tumor and Associated Congenital Diseases. Amsterdam: University of Amsterdam, 1991.
64. Kay GF, Barton SC, Surani MA, Rastan S: Imprinting and X chromosome counting mechanisms determine *Xist* expression in early mouse development. *Cell* **77**:639, 1994.
65. Skuse DH, James RS, Bishop DV, Coppin B, Dalton P, Aamodt-Leeper G, Bacarese-Hamilton M, et al.: Evidence from Turner's syndrome of an imprinted X-linked locus affecting cognitive function [see comments]. *Nature* **387**:705, 1997.
66. Guillemot F, Caspary T, Tilghman SM, Copeland NG, Gilbert DJ, Jenkins NA, Anderson DJ, et al.: Genomic imprinting of Mash2, a mouse gene required for trophoblast development. *Nat Genet* **9**:235, 1995.
67. Rainier S, Johnson LA, Dobry CJ, Ping AJ, Grundy PE, Feinberg AP: Relaxation of imprinted genes in human cancer. *Nature* **362**:747, 1993.
68. Zhan S, Shapiro DN, Helman LJ: Loss of imprinting of IGF2 in Ewing's sarcoma. *Oncogene* **11**:2503, 1995.
69. Xu YQ, Grundy P, Polychronakos C: Aberrant imprinting of the insulin-like growth factor II receptor gene in Wilms' tumor. *Oncogene* **14**:1041, 1997.
70. Nicholls RD: New insights reveal complex mechanisms involved in genomic imprinting [editorial; comment]. *Am J Hum Genet* **54**:733, 1994.
71. Ferguson-Smith AC: Imprinting moves to the centre [news; comment]. *Nat Genet* **14**:119, 1996.
72. Dittrich B, Buiting K, Korn B, Rickard S, Buxton J, Saitoh S, Nicholls RD, et al.: Imprint switching on human chromosome 15 may involve alternative transcripts of the SNRPN gene. *Nat Genet* **14**:163, 1996.
72a. Brown KW, Villar AJ, Bickmore W, Clayton-Smith J, Catchpoole D, Maher ER, ReikW: Imprinting mutation in the Beckwith-Wiedemann syndrome leads to biallelic IGF2 expression through an H19-independent pathway. *Hum Mol Genet* **5**:2027, 1996.
73. Naumova AK, Leppert M, Barker DF, Morgan K, Sapienza C: Parental origin-dependent, male offspring-specific transmission-ratio distortion at loci on the human X chromosome. *Am J Hum Genet* **62**:1493, 1998.
74. Nabetani A, Hatada I, Morisaki H, Oshimura M, Mukai T: Mouse U2af1-rs1 is a neomorphic imprinted gene. *Mol Cell Biol* **17**:789, 1997.
75. Baysal BE, Farr JE, Rubinstein WS, Galus RA, Johnson KA, Aston CE, Myers EN, et al.: Fine mapping of an imprinted gene for familial nonchromaffin paragangliomas, on chromosome 11q23. *Am J Hum Genet* **60**:121, 1997.
76. van Schothorst EM, Jansen JC, Bardoel AF, van der Mey AG, James MJ, Sobol H, Weissenbach J, et al.: Confinement of PGL, an imprinted gene causing hereditary paragangliomas, to a 2-cM interval on 11q22-q23 and exclusion of DRD2 and NCAM as candidate genes. *Eur J Hum Genet* **4**:267, 1996.
77. van Gurp RJ, Oosterhuis JW, Kalscheuer V, Mariman EC, Looijenga LH: Biallelic expression of the H19 and IGF2 genes in human testicular germ cell tumors. *J Natl Cancer Inst* **86**:1070, 1994.
78. Magenis RE, Toth-Fejel S, Allen LJ, Black M, Brown MG, Budden S, Cohen R, et al.: Comparison of the 15q deletions in Prader-Willi and Angelman syndromes: Specific regions, extent of deletions, parental origin, and clinical consequences. *Am J Med Genet* **35**:333, 1990.
79. Nicholls RD, Knoll JH, Butler MG, Karam S, Lalande M: Genetic imprinting suggested by maternal heterodisomy in nondeletion Prader-Willi syndrome. *Nature* **342**:281, 1989.
80. Ledbetter DH, Riccardi VM, Airhart SD, Strobel RJ, Keenan BS, Crawford JD: Deletions of chromosome 15 as a cause of the Prader-Willi syndrome. *N Engl J Med* **304**:325, 1981.
81. Robinson WP, Bottani A, Xie YG, Balakrishman J, Binkert F, Machler M, Prader A, et al.: Molecular, cytogenetic, and clinical investigations of Prader-Willi syndrome patients. *Am J Hum Genet* **49**:1219, 1991.
82. Saitoh S, Buiting K, Rogan PK, Buxton JL, Driscoll DJ, Arnemann J, Konig R, et al.: Minimal definition of the imprinting center and fixation of chromosome 15q11-q13 epigenotype by imprinting mutations. *Proc Natl Acad Sci USA* **93**:7811, 1996.
83. Wevrick R, Francke U: An imprinted mouse transcript homologous to the human imprinted in Prader-Willi syndrome (IPW) gene. *Hum Mol Genet* **6**:325, 1997.
84. Watrin F, Roeckel N, Lacroix L, Mignon C, Mattei MG, Disteche C, Muscatelli F: The mouse necdin gene is expressed from the paternal allele only and lies in the 7C region of the mouse chromosome 7, a region of conserved synteny to the human Prader-Willi syndrome region. *Eur J Hum Genet* **5**:324, 1997.
85. Jay P, Rougeulle C, Massacrier A, Moncla A, Mattei MG, Malzac P, Roeckel N, et al.: The human necdin gene, NDN, is maternally imprinted and located in the Prader-Willi syndrome chromosomal region. *Nat Genet* **17**:357, 1997.

86. MacDonald HR, Wevrick R: The necdin gene is deleted in Prader-Willi syndrome and is imprinted in human and mouse. *Hum Mol Genet* **6**:1873, 1997.
87. Mannens M, Wilde A: KVLQT1, the rhythm of imprinting [news; comment]. *Nat Genet* **15**:113, 1997.
88. Gunay-Aygun M, Heeger S, Schwartz S, Cassidy SB: Delayed diagnosis in patients with Prader-Willi syndrome due to maternal uniparental disomy 15. *Am J Med Genet* **71**:106, 1997.
89. Spritz RA, Bailin T, Nicholls RD, Lee ST, Park SK, Mascari MJ, Butler MG: Hypopigmentation in the Prader-Willi syndrome correlates with P gene deletion but not with haplotype of the hemizygous P allele. *Am J Med Genet* **71**:57, 1997.
90. Matsuura T, Sutcliffe JS, Fang P, Galjaard RJ, Jiang YH, Benton CS, Rommens JM, et al.: De novo truncating mutations in E6-AP ubiquitin-protein ligase gene (UBE3A) in Angelman syndrome. *Nat Genet* **15**:74, 1997.
91. Vu TH, Hoffman AR: Imprinting of the Angelman syndrome gene, UBE3A, is restricted to brain [letter]. *Nat Genet* **17**:12, 1997.
92. Donlon T: Fishing out the Angelman syndrome gene [news]. *Nat Med* **3**:281, 1997.
93. Kishino T, Lalande M, Wagstaff J: UBE3A/E6-AP mutations cause Angelman syndrome [published erratum appears in *Nat Genet* **15(4)**:411, 1997]. *Nat Genet* **15**:70, 1997.
94. Glenn CC, Driscoll DJ, Yang TP, Nicholls RD: Genomic imprinting: Potential function and mechanisms revealed by the Prader-Willi and Angelman syndromes. *Mol Hum Reprod* **3**:321, 1997.
95. Burger J, Buiting K, Dittrich B, Gross S, Lich C, Sperling K, Horsthemke B, et al.: Different mechanisms and recurrence risks of imprinting defects in Angelman syndrome. *Am J Hum Genet* **61**:88, 1997.
96. Kubota T, Aradhya S, Macha M, Smith AC, Surh LC, Satish J, Verp MS, et al.: Analysis of parent of origin-specific DNA methylation at SNRPN and PW71 in tissues: Implication for prenatal diagnosis. *J Med Genet* **33**:1011, 1996.
97. Ebert MH, Schmidt DE, Thompson T, Butler MG: Elevated plasma gamma-aminobutyric acid (GABA) levels in individuals with either Prader-Willi syndrome or Angelman syndrome. *J Neuropsychiatry Clin Neurosci* **9**:75, 1997.
98. Engel E: A new genetic concept: uniparental disomy and its potential effect, isodisomy. *Am J Med Genet* **6**:137, 1980.
99. Pulkkinen L, Bullrich F, Czarnecki P, Weiss L, Uitto J: Maternal uniparental disomy of chromosome 1 with reduction to homozygosity of the LAMB3 locus in a patient with Herlitz junctional epidermolysis bullosa. *Am J Hum Genet* **61**:611, 1997.
100. Harrison K, Eisenger K, Anyane-Yeboa K, Brown S: Maternal uniparental disomy of chromosome 2 in a baby with trisomy 2 mosaicism in amniotic fluid culture. *Am J Med Genet* **58**:147, 1995.
101. Lindenbaum RH WC, Norbury CD, Povey S, Rysieck G: An individual with maternal disomy of chromosome 4 and iso (4p) iso (4q) [abstract]. *Am J Hum Genet* **49**:A285, 1991.
102. Brzustowicz LM, Allitto BA, Matseoane D, Theve R, Michaud L, Chatkupt S, Sugarman E, et al.: Paternal isodisomy for chromosome 5 in a child with spinal muscular atrophy. *Am J Hum Genet* **54**:482, 1994.
103. Temple IK, Gardner RJ, Robinson DO, Kibirige MS, Ferguson AW, Baum JD, Barber JC, et al.: Further evidence for an imprinted gene for neonatal diabetes localised to chromosome 6q22-q23. *Hum Mol Genet* **5**:1117, 1996.
104. Abramowicz MJ, Andrien M, Dupont E, Dorchy H, Parma J, Duprez L, Ledley FD, et al.: Isodisomy of chromosome 6 in a newborn with methylmalonic acidemia and agenesis of pancreatic beta cells causing diabetes mellitus. *J Clin Invest* **94**:418, 1994.
105. Welch TR, Beischel LS, Choi E, Balakrishnan K, Bishof NA: Uniparental isodisomy 6 associated with deficiency of the fourth component of complement. *J Clin Invest* **86**:675, 1990.
106. Spence JE, Perciaccante RG, Greig GM, Willard HF, Ledbetter DH, Hejtmancik JF, Pollack MS, et al.: Uniparental disomy as a mechanism for human genetic disease. *Am J Hum Genet* **42**:217, 1988.
107. Voss R B-SE, Vital A, Zlotogora Y, Dogan J, Godfry S, Tikochinski Y: Isodisomy of chromosome 7 in a patient with cystic fibrosis: Could uniparental disomy be common in human. *Am J Hum Genet* **45**:373, 1989.
108. Eggerding FA, Schonberg SA, Chehab FF, Norton ME, Cox VA, Epstein CJ: Uniparental isodisomy for paternal 7p and maternal 7q in a child with growth retardation. *Am J Hum Genet* **55**:253, 1994.
109. Kotzot D, Schmitt S, Bernasconi F, Robinson WP, Lurie IW, Ilyina H, Mehes K, et al.: Uniparental disomy 7 in Silver-Russell syndrome and primordial growth retardation. *Hum Mol Genet* **4**:583, 1995.
110. Spotila LD, Sereda L, Prockop DJ: Partial isodisomy for maternal chromosome 7 and short stature in an individual with a mutation at the COL1A2 locus. *Am J Hum Genet* **51**:1396, 1992.
111. Benlian P, Foubert L, Gagne, Bernard L, De Gennes JL, Langlois S, Robinson W, et al.: Complete paternal isodisomy for chromosome 8 unmasked by lipoprotein lipase deficiency. *Am J Hum Genet* **59**:431, 1996.
112. Sulisalo T, Chapelle A, de la Kaitila I: Uniparental disomy as an explanation of presumptive low penetrance [abstract]. *Am J Hum Genet* **55**:A7, 1994.
113. Wilkinson TA, James RS, Crolla JA, Cockwell AE, Campbell PL, Temple IK: A case of maternal uniparental disomy of chromosome 9 in association with confined placental mosaicism for trisomy 9. *Prenat Diagn* **16**:371, 1996.
114. Jones C, Booth C, Rita D, Jazmines L, Spiro R, McCulloch B, McCaskill C, et al.: Identification of a case of maternal uniparental disomy of chromosome 10 associated with confined placental mosaicism. *Prenat Diagn* **15**:843, 1995.
115. Bischoff FZ, Feldman GL, McCaskill C, Subramanian S, Hughes MR, Shaffer LG: Single cell analysis demonstrating somatic mosaicism involving 11p in a patient with paternal isodisomy and Beckwith-Wiedemann syndrome. *Hum Mol Genet* **4**:395, 1995.
116. Webb A, Beard J, Wright C, Robson S, Wolstenholme J, Goodship J: A case of paternal uniparental disomy for chromosome 11. *Prenat Diagn* **15**:773, 1995.
117. Slater H, Shaw JH, Dawson G, Bankier A, Forrest SM: Maternal uniparental disomy of chromosome 13 in a phenotypically normal child. *J Med Genet* **31**:644, 1994.
118. Healey S PF, Battersby M, Chenevix-Trench G, McGill J: Distinct phenotype in maternal uniparental disomy of chromosome 14. *Am J Med Genet* **51**:147, 1994.
119. Pentao L, Lewis RA, Ledbetter DH, Patel PI, Lupski JR: Maternal uniparental isodisomy of chromosome 14: Association with autosomal recessive rod monochromacy. *Am J Hum Genet* **50**:690, 1992.
120. Papenhausen PR, Mueller OT, Johnson VP, Sutcliffe M, Diamond TM, Kousseff BG: Uniparental isodisomy of chromosome 14 in two cases: An abnormal child and a normal adult [see comments]. *Am J Med Genet* **59**:271, 1995.
121. Tomkins DJ, Roux AF, Waye J, Freeman VC, Cox DW, Whelan DT: Maternal uniparental isodisomy of human chromosome 14 associated with a paternal t(13q14q) and precocious puberty. *Eur J Hum Genet* **4**:153, 1996.
122. Mascari MJ, Gottlieb W, Rogan PK, Butler MG, Waller DA, Armour JA, Jeffreys AJ, et al.: The frequency of uniparental disomy in Prader-Willi syndrome. Implications for molecular diagnosis. *N Engl J Med* **326**:1599, 1992.
123. Woodage T, Prasad M, Dixon JW, Selby RE, Romain DR, Columbano-Green LM, Graham D, et al.: Bloom syndrome and maternal uniparental disomy for chromosome 15. *Am J Hum Genet* **55**:74, 1994.
124. Kalousek DK, Langlois S, Barrett I, Yam I, Wilson DR, Howard-Peebles PN, Johnson MP, et al.: Uniparental disomy for chromosome 16 in humans. *Am J Hum Genet* **52**:8, 1993.
125. Korenstein ARY, Avivi L: Uniparental disomy of chromosome 16 in offspring of Familial Mediterranean Fever patients treated with colchicine [abstract]. *Am J Hum Genet* **55**:A109, 1994.
126. Ngo KY, Lee J, Dixon B, Liu DOWJ: Paternal uniparental isodisomy in a hydrops fetalis alpha thalassemia fetus [abstract]. *Am J Hum Genet* **53**:1207, 1993.
127. Blouin JL, Avramopoulos D, Pangalos C, Antonarakis SE: Normal phenotype with paternal uniparental isodisomy for chromosome 21. *Am J Hum Genet* **53**:1074, 1993.
128. Schinzel AA, Basaran S, Bernasconi F, Karaman B, Yuksel-Apak M, Robinson WP: Maternal uniparental disomy 22 has no impact on the phenotype. *Am J Hum Genet* **54**:21, 1994.
129. Vidaud D VM, Plassa F, Gazengel C, Noel B, Goossens M: Father-to-son transmission of hemophilia A due to uniparental disomy [abstract]. *Am J Hum Genet* **45**:A226, 1989.
130. Schinzel AA, Robinson WP, Binkert F, Torresani T, Werder EA: Exclusively paternal X chromosomes in a girl with short stature. *Hum Genet* **92**:175, 1993.
131. Quan F, Janas J, Toth-Fejel S, Johnson DB, Wolford JK, Popovich BW: Uniparental disomy of the entire X chromosome in a female with Duchenne muscular dystrophy. *Am J Hum Genet* **60**:160, 1997.
132. Cattanach BM, Patrick G, Papworth D, Goodhead DT, Hacker T, Cobb L, Whitehill E: Investigation of lung tumour induction in BALB/cJ mice following paternal X-irradiation. *Int J Radiat Biol* **67**:607, 1995.

133. Williamson CM, Beechey CV, Ball ST, Dutton ER, Cattanach BM, Tease C, Ishino F, et al.: Localisation of the imprinted gene neuronatin, Nnat, confirms and refines the location of a second imprinting region on mouse chromosome 2. *Cytogenet Cell Genet* **81**:73, 1998.
134. van den Hurk JA, Hendriks W, van de Pol DJ, Oerlemans F, Jaissle G, Ruther K, Kohler K, et al.: Mouse choroideremia gene mutation causes photoreceptor cell degeneration and is not transmitted through the female germline. *Hum Mol Genet* **6**:851, 1997.
135. Campbell R, Gosden CM, Bonthron DT: Parental origin of transcription from the human GNAS1 gene. *J Med Genet* **31**:607, 1994.
136. Davies SJ, Hughes HE: Imprinting in Albright's hereditary osteodystrophy. *J Med Genet* **30**:101, 1993.
137. Wilson LC, Oude Luttikhuis ME, Clayton PT, Fraser WD, Trembath RC: Parental origin of Gs alpha gene mutations in Albright's hereditary osteodystrophy. *J Med Genet* **31**:835, 1994.
138. Schuster V, Eschenhagen T, Kruse K, Gierschik P, Kreth HW: Endocrine and molecular biological studies in a German family with Albright hereditary osteodystrophy. *Eur J Pediatr* **152**:185, 1993.
139. Temple IK JR, Crolla JA, Sitch FL, Jacobs PA, Howell WM, Betts P, Baum JD, Shield JPH: An imprinted gene(s) for diabetes? *Nature* **9**:110, 1995.
140. Arthur EI, Zlotogora J, Lerer I, Dagan J, Marks K, Abeliovich D: Transient neonatal diabetes mellitus in a child with invdup (6)(q22q23) of paternal origin. *Eur J Hum Genet* **5**:417, 1997.
141. Giddings SJ, King CD, Harman KW, Flood JF, Carnaghi LR: Allele-specific inactivation of insulin 1 and 2, in the mouse yolk sac, indicates imprinting. *Nat Genet* **6**:310, 1994.
142. Kobayashi S, Kohda T, Miyoshi N, Kuroiwa Y, Aisaka K, Tsutsumi O, Kaneko-Ishino T, et al.: Human PEG1/MEST, an imprinted gene on chromosome 7. *Hum Mol Genet* **6**:781, 1997.
143. Catchpoole D, Lam WW, Valler D, Temple IK, Joyce JA, Reik W, Schofield PN, et al.: Epigenetic modification and uniparental inheritance of H19 in Beckwith- Wiedemann syndrome. *J Med Genet* **34**:353, 1997.
144. Joyce JA, Lam WK, Catchpoole DJ, Jenks P, Reik W, Maher ER, Schofield PN: Imprinting of IGF2 and H19: lack of reciprocity in sporadic Beckwith-Wiedemann syndrome. *Hum Mol Genet* **6**:1543, 1997.
145. O'Keefe D, Dao D, Zhao L, Sanderson R, Warburton D, Weiss L, Anyane-Yeboa K, et al.: Coding mutations in p57KIP2 are present in some cases of Beckwith-Wiedemann syndrome but are rare or absent in Wilms tumors. *Am J Hum Genet* **61**:295, 1997.
146. Lee MP, Hu RJ, Johnson LA, Feinberg AP: Human KVLQT1 gene shows tissue-specific imprinting and encompasses Beckwith-Wiedemann syndrome chromosomal rearrangements. *Nat Genet* **15**:181, 1997.
147. Viljoen D, Ramesar R: Evidence for paternal imprinting in familial Beckwith-Wiedemann syndrome. *J Med Genet* **29**:221, 1992.
148. Slavotinek A, Gaunt L, Donnai D: Paternally inherited duplications of 11p15.5 and Beckwith-Wiedemann syndrome. *J Med Genet* **34**:819, 1997.
149. Weksberg R, Teshima I, Williams BR, Greenberg CR, Pueschel SM, Chernos JE, Fowlow SB, et al.: Molecular characterization of cytogenetic alterations associated with the Beckwith-Wiedemann syndrome (BWS) phenotype refines the localization and suggests the gene for BWS is imprinted. *Hum Mol Genet* **2**:549, 1993.
150. Wiedemann H: Tumors and hypertrophy associated with Wiedemann-Beckwith syndrome. *Eur J Ped* **141**:129, 1983.
151. Versteeg R: Aberrant methylation in cancer [editorial; comment]. *Am J Hum Genet* **60**:751, 1997.
152. Pilia G, Hughes-Benzie RM, MacKenzie A, Baybayan P, Chen EY, Huber R, Neri G, et al.: Mutations in GPC3, a glypican gene, cause the Simpson-Golabi-Behmel overgrowth syndrome. *Nat Genet* **12**:241, 1996.
153. Lindsay S, Ireland M, O'Brien O, Clayton-Smith J, Hurst JA, Mann J, Cole T, et al.: Large scale deletions in the GPC3 gene may account for a minority of cases of Simpson-Golabi-Behmel syndrome. *J Med Genet* **34**:480, 1997.
154. Weksberg R, Squire JA, Templeton DM: Glypicans: A growing trend. *Nat Genet* **12**:225, 1996.
155. Hughes-Benzie RM, Hunter AG, Allanson JE, Mackenzie AE: Simpson-Golabi-Behmel syndrome associated with renal dysplasia and embryonal tumor: Localization of the gene to Xqcen-q21. *Am J Med Genet* **43**:428, 1992.
156. Lapunzina P, Badia I, Galoppo C, De Matteo E, Silberman P, Tello A, Grichener J, et al.: A patient with Simpson-Golabi-Behmel syndrome and hepatocellular carcinoma. *J Med Genet* **35**:153, 1998.
157. McGuffin P, Scourfield J: Human genetics. A father's imprint on his daughter's thinking. *Nature* **387**:652, 1997.
158. Hall J: Genomic imprinting: review and relevance to human diseases. *Am J Hum Genet* **46**:857, 1990.
159. Hall JG, Solehdin F: Genomic imprinting. *Acta Paed Sin* **37**:401, 1996.
160. Lubinsky MS, Hall JG: Genomic imprinting, monozygous twinning, and X inactivation. *Lancet* **337**:1288, 1991.
161. Hoglund P, Holmberg C, de la Chapelle A, Kere J: Paternal isodisomy for chromosome 7 is compatible with normal growth and development in a patient with congenital chloride diarrhea. *Am J Hum Genet* **55**:747, 1994.
162. Beldjord C, Henry I, Bennani C, Vanhaeke D, Labie D: Uniparental disomy: A novel mechanism for thalassemia major [letter]. *Blood* **80**:287, 1992.
163. Cavenee WK, Dryja TP, Phillips RA, Benedict WF, Godbout R, Gallie BL, Murphree AL, et al.: Expression of recessive alleles by chromosomal mechanisms in retinoblastoma. *Nature* **305**:779, 1983.

CHAPTER 16

The Biogenesis of Membranes and Organelles

David D. Sabatini ▪ Milton B. Adesnik

The field of organelle biogenesis has expanded so much in the last few years that it seemed impossible to include a chapter as comprehensive as that found in the last edition of this text without extending the length of the chapter inordinately. Nonetheless, the editors feel that the chapter from the last edition provides an excellent foundation for understanding more recent developments which are now covered throughout the rest of the book where they are relevant to understanding specific diseases of lysosomes, peroxisomes, mitochondria, and membrane receptors. For this reason, we include this chapter from the 7th edition.

1. **The eukaryotic cell is surrounded by a plasma membrane and is characterized by the presence of a nucleus and many cytoplasmic organelles, which are functionally specialized and also delimited by membranes. The nucleus is the site of storage and initial decoding of genomic information. Completion of this decoding, however, requires the translation of mRNA in ribosomes present in the cytoplasm and the delivery of each newly synthesized polypeptide to its site of function. This chapter considers the sorting and targeting processes by which newly synthesized proteins are transferred to their sites of function, which may be in the nucleus, in the cytomatrix that occupies the space between organelles, within a membrane, in the luminal cavity of an organelle, or outside the cell. Many genetic diseases lead to defects in specific organellar functions and, in some cases, this results from faulty protein targeting.**
2. **The plasma membrane and several cytoplasmic organelles, including the ER, Golgi apparatus, secretory granules and vesicles, lysosomes, and endosomes, form an integrated endomembrane system that serves to transfer macromolecules and membrane components from one part of the cell to another, as well as to and from the cell exterior. Many of the proteins of these organelles are synthesized in ribosomes bound to membranes of the ER and are inserted into these membranes, or translocated into the lumen of the ER, during their synthesis. These proteins can then either remain within the ER or be transported along the endomembrane system by a process that involves their incorporation into vesicles. These vesicles are formed by budding from the membrane of a donor compartment and deliver their content by fusing with a membrane of the acceptor compartment. We discuss in detail the mechanisms that: (1) select specific mRNA for translation in ribosomes associated with the ER, (2) determine the transmembrane disposition of integral membrane proteins, (3) mediate the retention of proteins in a specific organelle, or their transport within the endomembrane system, and (4) lead to the production of vesicles in a donor membrane and determine their fusion with a specific acceptor membrane.**
3. **Mitochondria and peroxisomes are organelles that do not communicate with the endomembrane system through vesicular flow and acquire their protein contents by direct uptake of newly synthesized, but not yet fully folded, polypeptides from the cytoplasm. The uptake into mitochondria involves molecular chaperones, as well as receptors on the surface of the organelle, and sorting processes that address the proteins to the various submitochondrial compartments.**

THE ORGANIZATION OF THE EUKARYOTIC CELL

The eukaryotic cell shows an extraordinary degree of organizational complexity. Macromolecular components that carry out different metabolic processes are segregated in distinct subcellular compartments, and these must act in concert to sustain the various cellular functions. The membranes bounding all cellular organelles not only control the passage of substances between the various compartments and the surrounding cytoplasmic matrix, but also provide a framework for the functional integration and assembly of many of the organellar macromolecules into higher-order complexes. This is also true for the *plasma membrane*, which surrounds the entire cell and regulates its interactions with the extracellular milieu.

The presence of a *nucleus*, a compartment limited by a membranous envelope, is the defining feature of the eukaryotic cell. In this compartment, the genome is stored and replicated and the process of decoding the genetic information begins. In the cytoplasm, several membrane-bound organelles form an integrated *endomembrane system* (sometimes referred to as the "vacuolar system,"[1]) which, together with the plasma membrane, is organized for the transfer of macromolecules and membrane components from one part of the cell to another, as well as to and from the cell's exterior. This transport takes place by means of *membrane vesicles*, which bud from one organelle and fuse with another, although in some cases tubular connections may be established that carry material between organelles. The set of

A list of standard abbreviations is located immediately preceding the index in each volume. Additional abbreviations used in this chapter include: BFA = brefeldin A; COP = coat proteins; DAF = decay-accelerating factor; DHFR = dihydrofolate reductase; GAG = glycosaminoglycans; GAP = GTPase activating proteins; GDI = GDP dissociation inhibitors; GDS = GTP dissociation stimulators; GEF = guanine nucleotide exchange protein; GIPL = glycosylinositol phospholipid; IMM = inner mitochondrial membrane; ISG = immature secretory granules; LH = luteinizing hormone; MPP = matrix processing peptidase; MPR = mannose 6-phosphate receptor; NSF = N-ethylmaleimide sensitive factor; OMM = outer mitochondrial membrane; PC = phosphatidylcholine; PDI = protein disulfide isomerase; PE = phosphatidylethanolamine; PI = phosphatidylinositol; PS = phosphatidylserine; REP = rab escort protein; S/A = signal/anchor sequence; SM = sphingomyelin; SNAP = soluble NSF attachment protein; SNAREs = SNAP receptors; SRP = signal recognition particle; TCR = T-cell receptor; TGN = trans-Golgi network; TMD = transmembrane domain; TRAM = translocating chain-associating membrane glycoprotein; TSH = thyroid-stimulating hormone; VLCFA = very long chain fatty acids; VSV = vesicular stomatitis virus; vWF = von Willebrand factor.

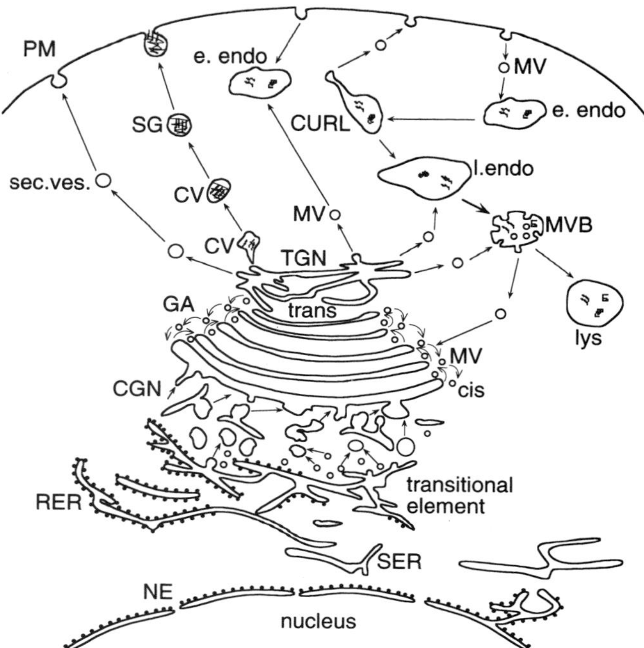

Fig. 16-1 Subcellular compartments that constitute the cellular endomembrane system. The major organelles of the endomembrane system are: the endoplasmic reticulum (ER), with its rough (RER) and smooth (SER) components; the Golgi apparatus (GA); endosomes (endo); lysosomes (lys); secretory vesicles (sec. ves.) and granules (SG); and the plasma membrane (PM). The outer membrane of the nuclear envelope (NE) is studded with ribosomes and is continuous with the rough ER. Transitional elements (TE) are specialized ER cisternae from which membrane vesicles (MV) bud off that deliver materials from the ER to the *cis* region of the Golgi apparatus, possibly by first fusing with each other to form structures that, together with the first (*cis*) Golgi cisterna, constitute the *cis Golgi network* (CGN). Transport across the Golgi apparatus, from the *cis* to the *trans* face, is also mediated by membrane vesicles (MV). The *trans Golgi network* (TGN) is a region in the *trans*-most side of the Golgi apparatus where sorting of proteins destined to distal portions of the endomembrane system takes place. In the TGN, some secretory proteins and plasma membrane proteins are incorporated into secretory vesicles (sec. ves.). Other secretory proteins are packaged into immature secretory granules or condensing vacuoles (CV) that mature into secretory granules (SG). Secretory vesicles and granules release their contents into the extracellular space by *exocytosis*, a process that involves the fusion of their membranes with the plasma membrane. Most secretory vesicles undergo *constitutive exocytosis*, whereas secretory granules undergo *regulated exocytosis* in response to signals received at the plasma membrane. Proteins of the membranes of secretory vesicles or granules are incorporated into the plasma membrane during these exocytic events. In polarized epithelial cells in which the plasma membrane has distinct apical and basolateral domains, two populations of secretory vesicles destined to the two aspects of the cell surface emerge from the TGN. Materials taken into the cell by endocytosis are incorporated into membrane vesicles derived from the plasma membrane and transported to *early endosomes* (e. endo). The endosomal compartment is polymorphic and includes several classes of endosomes that represent stages in their development and their conversion into lysosomes. These include the *CURL* (compartment for uncoupling of receptors from ligands), or sorting endosome, from which membrane vesicles bud to return interiorized receptors to the cell surface, late endosomes (l. endo) and *multivesicular bodies* (MVB), which receive lysosomal hydrolases brought by vesicles derived from the TGN and are converted to *lysosomes* (lys). The interrelationships of the various endosomal compartments and lysosomes are depicted in greater detail in Fig. 16-32. To maintain the characteristic structure and composition of all the organelles of the endomembrane system that communicate with each other by a forward vesicular flow, a retrograde vesicular flow must also take place.

intercommunicating organelles that constitutes the endomembrane system (Fig. 16-1) includes: (1) the *endoplasmic reticulum* (ER), which may be regarded as an extension of the *nuclear envelope* and serves as a major site of protein synthesis and biosynthetic activity; (2) the *Golgi apparatus*, which modifies many of the proteins it receives from the ER and transfers them to other sites in the cell; (3) *secretory vesicles* and *granules*, which contain proteins that have traversed the Golgi apparatus and will be released at the cell surface; (4) *endosomes*, which receive materials taken in from outside the cell within plasma membrane invaginations; and (5) *lysosomes*, which degrade the exogenous material from endosomes as well as endogenous cellular components. Because the luminal cavities of the several membrane-bound compartments of the endomembrane system can communicate with each other and with the extracellular space via transport vesicles or tubular connections, all luminal faces of the membranes in this system can be regarded as topologically equivalent to each other (Fig. 16-2).

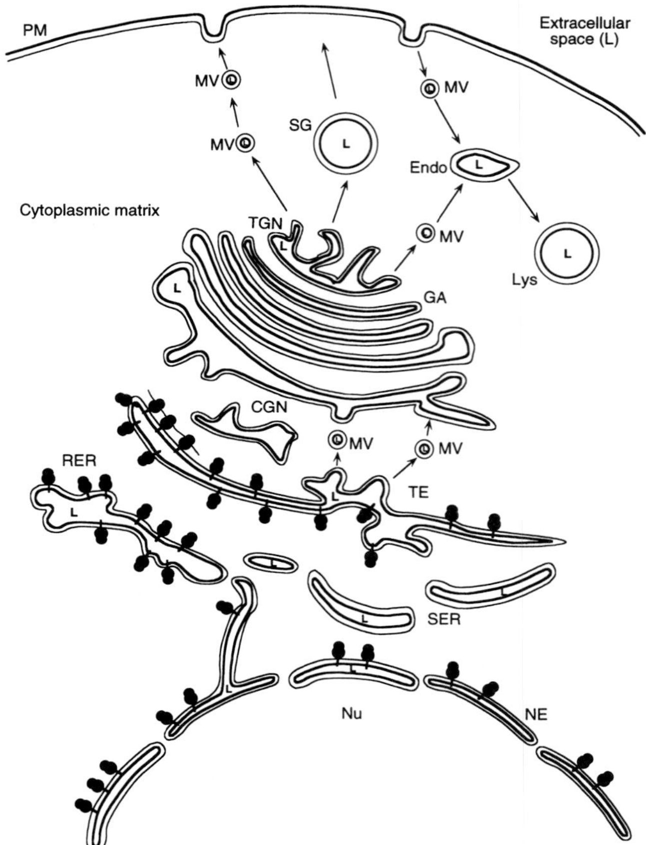

Fig. 16-2 Topologic equivalence of the membrane faces in the different compartments of the cellular endomembrane system. Intracellular traffic mediated by membrane vesicles (MV) first involves the generation of a vesicle from the membrane bounding one compartment by a budding process (also known as fission). The vesicle is then transported through the cytoplasm and its membrane fuses with the membrane of the receiving compartment. During the fusion and fission processes, the integrity of the membrane barrier and the orientation of the luminal (thick line) and cytoplasmic (thin line) membrane faces are maintained. Intracellular transport by membrane vesicles takes place from the ER to the Golgi apparatus, within this organelle, and between it and the plasma membrane. The route that begins with endocytosis also reaches the Golgi apparatus. Therefore, the luminal faces of ER and Golgi membranes are topologically equivalent to the extracellular face of the plasma membrane and the luminal spaces (L) within all components of the endomembrane system are topologically equivalent to each other and to the extracellular space.

Two other membrane-bound organelles that do not directly communicate with the endomembrane system are found in animal cells: (1) *mitochondria*, which generate most of the ATP required to sustain cellular activity, but also play a major role in many other aspects of intermediary metabolism; and (2) *peroxisomes*, in which several oxidative reactions that generate hydrogen peroxide are carried out, as are several important steps in the degradation of long chain fatty acids and in the synthesis of plasmalogens and bile acids.

The portion of the cytoplasm that extends from the nuclear envelope to the plasma membrane and surrounds the membrane-bound organelles is known as the *cytoplasmic matrix* (or *cytomatrix*). It contains filamentous elements such as *microtubules*, *microfilaments*, and *intermediate filaments*, which constitute the *cytoskeleton*. The cytoskeleton serves to organize the cytoplasm and controls the location and movement of the different organelles, and of the cell itself. The cytomatrix also contains *ribosomes* that function in protein synthesis, as well as numerous soluble enzymes that carry out myriad biochemical reactions. Several ribosomes are usually engaged in the translation of a single mRNA molecule, thus forming a *polyribosome* or *polysome*. The term *cytosol* is sometimes applied to the soluble components of the matrix which during cell fractionation are recovered in high-speed supernatants.

Organization of Protein and Lipid Components in Membranes[2-4]

Membranes are lipoprotein structures that consist of amphipathic lipids disposed in a bilayer arrangement and of proteins that penetrate the bilayer or are attached to its surfaces (Fig. 16-3). The most abundant lipid components of membranes are phospholipids, cholesterol, and glycolipids, all of which have their polar groups facing the aqueous environment on the membrane surfaces and their hydrophobic fatty acid chains (in phospholipids and glycolipids), or the sterol ring (in cholesterol), oriented toward the membrane interior. The hydrophobic interior of cellular membranes makes them effective barriers to the passage of highly polar or charged molecules from one compartment to another. The lipid molecules within the bilayer cannot easily flip-flop from one monolayer to the other, but can undergo extensive rotational and lateral translational movements. The resulting membrane fluidity permits the lateral displacement of proteins within the plane of the membrane, which is important in membrane function.

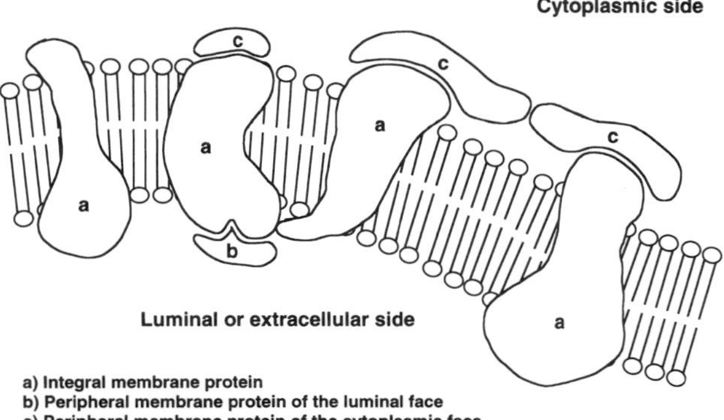

Fig. 16-3 Relationship of integral and peripheral membrane proteins to the membrane phospholipid bilayer. Integral membrane proteins (a) have portions of their mass embedded in the membrane that interact directly with the hydrophobic tails of the phospholipids. Other portions of these proteins are exposed on the cytoplasmic or luminal membrane faces. The extent of exposure on each side of the membrane may vary substantially from one protein to another. Peripheral membrane proteins (b and c) may interact with the exposed portions of integral membrane proteins and are associated with the membrane only by virtue of these interactions. Exposed portions of integral membrane protein molecules may directly interact with each other or may be indirectly linked together via their association with interacting peripheral membrane proteins. On the cytoplasmic face, peripheral membrane proteins may provide a link between integral membrane proteins and the cellular cytoskeleton.

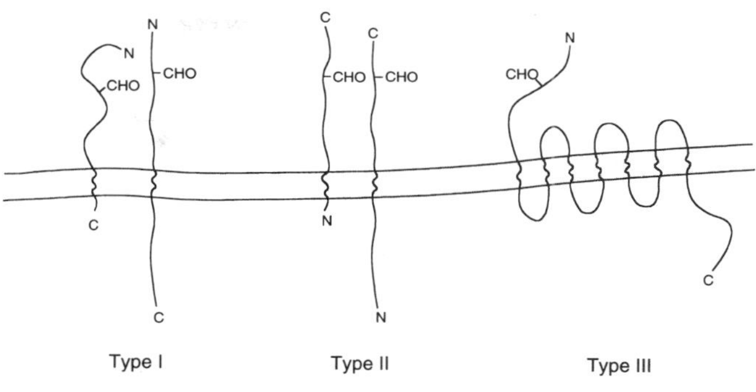

Fig. 16-4 Transmembrane disposition of different types of integral membrane proteins. Types I and II membrane proteins cross the membrane only once. Type I proteins, such as red-cell glycophorin, the LDL and EGF receptors, the heavy chain of the class I histocompatibility antigen, and the viral envelope glycoproteins HA of influenza and G of VSV have their N-termini exposed on the extracellular (or luminal) face of the membrane and their C-termini on the cytoplasmic face. Type II proteins, such as the asialoglycoprotein and transferrin receptors, the sucrase-isomaltase of the intestinal brush border, and the neuraminidase of influenza virus have the opposite transmembrane disposition. In both type I and type II proteins, the length of the segment exposed on each side of the membrane may be very short. Type III membrane proteins, such as rhodopsin, the β-adrenergic receptor, and the anion channel of the red-cell membrane (band 3) cross the membrane several times. Depending on the specific protein, the N- and C-termini may be on either side of the membrane.

Proteins associated with membranes fall into two categories. Those that are embedded in the phospholipid bilayer and, therefore, interact directly with the hydrophobic lipid phase are known as *integral membrane proteins* (see Fig. 16-3). They can only be removed from the membrane by procedures that disrupt the bilayer, such as treatment with detergents. Proteins that do not interact directly with the membrane interior and are bound to the surface of the membrane only via interactions with other proteins or, possibly, with the polar groups of the lipids are known as *peripheral membrane proteins* (see Fig. 16-3). They can be removed from membranes by treatment with mediums of high ionic strength or extreme pH, or that contain chelating or chaotropic agents.

In general, the membrane-embedded portions of integral membrane proteins consist of peptide segments that are rich in hydrophobic amino acids and are approximately 20 amino acids in length, just sufficient to span the thickness of the bilayer in an α-helical configuration. In some cases (see below) proteins are anchored in the membrane solely by a covalently bound lipid moiety. These may be the only integral membrane proteins exposed on only one membrane surface.

Proteins that fully traverse the lipid bilayer may cross the membrane only once and therefore have only one hydrophobic membrane-anchoring domain (Fig. 16-4). This is the case with several well-characterized hormone receptors of the plasma membrane — such as the epidermal growth factor[5,6] (and see ref. 7) and insulin receptors[8,9] (and see ref. 10) — in which the ligand binding portion of the molecule is exposed on the extracellular membrane surface while the signal-transducing domain is located in the cytoplasm. Integral membrane proteins that cross the membrane only once and have portions of their mass exposed on each surface are called *bitopic proteins*.[11] Such proteins have one of two possible transmembrane orientations. *Type I proteins* (see Fig. 16-4) have their C-terminal ends in the cytoplasm and their N-terminal ends exposed on the extracellular surface of the plasma membrane, or on the (topologically equivalent) luminal surface of an organelle within the endomembrane system, such as the ER. *Type II proteins* (see Fig. 16-4) have the reverse disposition, traversing the membrane with an N (cytoplasmic) to C (extracellular or luminal) orientation. As discussed in detail below, the different transmembrane orientations of the two classes of proteins can be explained as a consequence of the mechanism by which polypeptides are inserted into the ER membrane during their synthesis.

Some transmembrane proteins, in particular ion channels, cross the phospholipid bilayer several times (type III or *polytopic proteins*) (see Fig. 16-4), and the N- and C-terminal ends of such proteins may be found on the same or opposite sites of the membrane. The transmembrane domains of these proteins may also be hydrophobic or may be capable of forming *amphipathic helixes*, whose existence within the membrane may be maintained by lateral interactions with other similar helixes within the same polypeptide or within other subunits of a multimeric protein. In the final configuration, a hydrophilic channel is formed by the polar faces of several helixes, which have their hydrophobic faces interacting with the interior of the membrane bilayer.

Many membrane proteins are *glycoproteins* that contain carbohydrate moieties linked to the polypeptide backbone via either N-glycosidic bonds to asparagine residues, or O-glycosidic bonds to serine or threonine residues. Carbohydrate moieties may also be linked to membrane lipids (glycolipids). In all cases, the carbohydrates of membrane components are located only on the extracellular or luminal side of the membrane (see Fig. 16-4). Since the enzymatic system responsible for the formation of N-glycosidic bonds is present only in the ER, only proteins that reside in this organelle or pass through it during their biosynthesis can bear asparagine-linked oligosaccharide chains.

An Overview of Organelle Biogenesis[12-15]

Because of the organizational complexity of eukaryotic cells, the implementation of their genetic programs requires not only the transcription of sets of specific genes and the translation of the resulting messenger RNAs, but also the operation of mechanisms that ensure that the encoded polypeptides are transferred from their sites of synthesis to their sites of function, which may be in the cytomatrix, in a membrane, within a space enclosed by an organellar membrane, or outside the cell.

Aside from a very small number of polypetides that are synthesized on special ribosomes found within mitochondria, the bulk of protein synthesis in mammalian cells takes place in the cytoplasmic matrix — either on ribosomes that appear to be free in the matrix but could be associated with cytoskeletal elements or on ribosomes that during their synthetic activity are attached to the membranes of the ER. The part of the ER to which these ribosomes are attached is called the *rough* ER (RER), on account of the appearance of its cytoplasmic surface in electron micrographs. Portions of the ER devoid of attached ribosomes constitute the *smooth* ER (SER).

As previously noted, the universal structural feature of all cellular membranes is the presence of a phospholipid bilayer with a hydrophobic interior that constitutes a barrier to the passage of polar molecules. In particular, proteins — which normally fold with their charged and polar residues exposed on their surfaces — cannot freely traverse a phospholipid bilayer. Therefore, special mechanisms have evolved that facilitate the incorporation of polypeptides into specific membranes, and when necessary, assist them in their passage across the hydrophobic barrier. In many cases one or more molecular chaperones[16,17] associate with the polypeptide to be incorporated into or to be transported across the membrane and serve to maintain it in a conformation that is compatible with these processes.

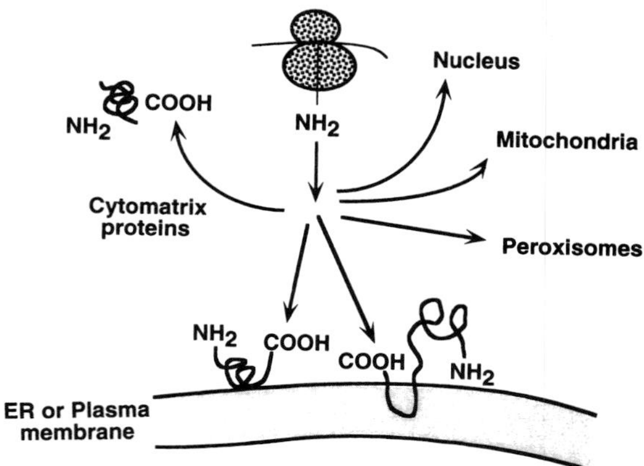

Fig. 16-5 Different fates of polypeptides synthesized on free polysomes. On release from the ribosome, these polypeptides may remain in the cytomatrix (as soluble proteins or as components of the cytoskeleton) or may be posttranslationally incorporated into different organelles.

Proteins destined for the nucleus, mitochondria, or peroxisomes are synthesized in ribosomes that are free in the cytoplasmic matrix, and are directly targeted to their respective organelles (Fig. 16-5). Specific receptors for the newly synthesized organellar proteins are present in the surface of mitochondria and probably also in the surface of peroxisomes. Those receptors must recognize structural features of each polypeptide and participate in a process that leads either to its insertion into the membrane or its translocation across it. The latter process may require the expenditure of energy and entail conformational changes or extensive structural modifications of the polypeptide. Proteins destined to the interior of the nucleus must pass through the nuclear pores of the nuclear envelope.

Some proteins of the ER and of the plasma membrane are also synthesized on free polysomes and become embedded in the membrane only after their synthesis is completed and they are discharged into the cytoplasm (see Fig. 16-5). A similar mechanism could, in principle, also lead to the insertion of proteins in the cytoplasmic surfaces of other organelles.

In contrast to the direct targeting of nuclear, mitochondrial, and peroxisomal proteins to their sites of function, proteins destined for secretion or for incorporation into lysosomes, as well as most proteins of the plasma membrane and the Golgi apparatus, are initially incorporated into the ER, and reach their sites of function by transfer through the cellular endomembrane system. Such proteins, like most proteins of the ER itself, are translocated across or inserted into the ER membrane cotranslationally, that is, during the course of their synthesis in ribosomes bound to the RER membrane (Fig. 16-6). Although these proteins may later undergo extensive posttranslational modifications, it is during or immediately after their synthesis in bound polysomes that they are either transferred to the lumen of the endomembrane system or incorporated into the membrane with a characteristic disposition with respect to the phospholipid bilayer.

After discharge into the ER lumen or incorporation into the ER membrane, proteins synthesized in membrane-bound ribosomes are subjected to *sorting processes*, just beginning to be understood, which ensure that certain polypeptides are retained in the ER while others are transferred to the Golgi apparatus and either remain there or, on exit from this organelle, are transported to lysosomes, secretory vesicles or granules, or the plasma membrane. As already mentioned, transport within the endomembrane system and to and from the plasma membrane is effected by *membrane vesicles* that bud from one organelle, traverse a portion of the cytoplasm, and fuse with another. Throughout this movement, luminal proteins remain segregated within the successive

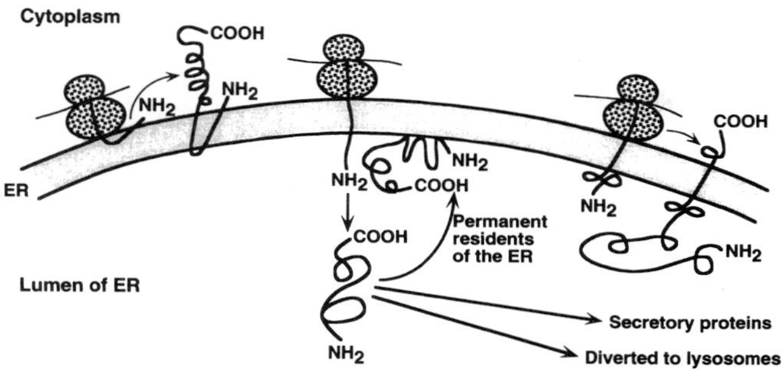

Fig. 16-6 Different fates of polypeptides synthesized in ribosomes bound to the ER membrane. Proteins synthesized in membrane-bound ribosomes are inserted into the ER membranes or translocated into the ER lumen by a process that begins during their synthesis. After their synthesis is completed, these proteins either remain in the ER or are transferred to the membranes or luminal cavities of other organelles within the endomembrane system.

organellar cavities, and membrane proteins retain the characteristic transmembrane disposition that they acquired in the ER.

In the past few years much has been learned about the molecular machinery and intermolecular interactions involved in the formation, targeting, and fusion of the vesicles that mediate interorganellar transport. This has resulted from both the development of in vitro systems that reproduce these phenomena under controlled conditions and from the isolation of yeast mutants defective at specific stages of vesicle formation or consumption. The latter approach has led in many cases to the determination of the biochemical nature and role of the products of the defective genes.

Yeast as a Model Organism to Study Intracellular Protein Trafficking[18,18a]

Although the emphasis in this chapter is on membrane and organelle biogenesis in the mammalian cell, it will frequently be necessary to discuss information on these processes obtained from studies with the yeast *Saccharomyces cerevisiae*. This organism serves as a useful and widely employed model to study fundamental functions of the eukaryotic cell since with yeast one can combine the powerful approach of molecular genetics with physiological and biochemical analyses. Using a variety of elegant but relatively simple selection procedures, a large number of *conditionally lethal* (*temperature-sensitive*) yeast mutants have been identified that, at the nonpermissive temperature, fail to grow because they are defective in various steps along the pathway of protein secretion or in the transport of newly synthesized proteins to a given organelle.

The availability of such mutants has permitted cloning of the respective genes by complementation in which mutant cells are transfected with a wild-type yeast genomic library and transformants containing a plasmid with the gene of interest are selected by virtue of their growth at the restrictive temperature. In addition, the isolation of *extragenic suppressor mutations* has led to the identification of other genes whose products, usually when overexpressed or mutated, can compensate for the defect caused by the original mutation. The products of suppressor genes function in the same pathway and probably interact with the product of the original mutant gene. These and other genetic approaches have facilitated the elucidation of the role of many gene products within the protein targeting and transport machinery of the cell. Moreover, analysis of the sequence of a cloned yeast gene has sometimes revealed the existence of a mammalian homologue and, in some instances, it has even been possible to correct the yeast defect by expressing in the yeast cell a gene encoding the mammalian protein (e.g., ref. 19). Conversely, in some cases, the yeast product has been shown to substitute for the mammalian one in an in vitro transport reaction.[20] Yeast homologues of mammalian proteins involved in transport have also been identified, or cloned, on the basis of their expected sequence homology to known mammalian proteins (e.g., the clathrin heavy and light chains, and the ADP ribosylation factor, *Arf*1p; see ref. 18). Finally, proof that a specific yeast protein whose gene has been cloned is essential can be ascertained from the viability of cells in which the gene has been "knocked out" (disrupted) by homologous recombination procedures, which are easy to carry out in this organism.

Studies on a large set of mutants defective in secretion, designated *sec* mutants,* have illuminated aspects of essentially all steps of transport along the endomembrane system. *Sec* mutants were first recognized because they accumulated precursor forms of exported proteins. It is now clear that some of the corresponding gene products are required for protein insertion into the ER (e.g., *Sec*61p, *Sec*62p, *Sec*63p, *Sec*65p), while others participate in transport from the ER to the Golgi apparatus (e.g., *Sec*12p, *Sec*13p, *Sec*17p, *Sec*18p, *Sec*20p, *Sec*21p, and *Ypt*1p), through the Golgi cisternae (e.g., *Sec*7p, *Sec*14p, *Arf*1p, *Arf*2p), or from the Golgi to the cell surface (e.g., *Sec*2p, *Sec*4p, *Sec*15p). A large number of mutants (*vps*) defective in transport to the vacuole, the yeast equivalent of the mammalian lysosome, are also available, as are mutants in genes (ERD1 and ERD2) required for retention in the ER of proteins that normally reside in this organelle. Other classes of mutants defective in the importation of proteins into the nucleus, mitochondria, or peroxisomes have also been isolated.

GTP-Binding Proteins Control Many Steps along the Secretory Pathway[21-27]

A very important class of yeast genes (e.g., YPT1 and *SEC*4) involved in protein traffic encode proteins that bind and hydrolyze GTP (guanine nucleotide binding proteins). Studies of the corresponding mutants have contributed greatly to focus attention on the role of GTP-binding proteins as "molecular switches" that control the directionality of a wide variety of individual steps in intracellular protein transport.

GTP-binding proteins constitute a superfamily that include the heterotrimeric ($G\alpha\beta\gamma$) *G proteins* that transduce extracellular hormonal and sensory signals into intracellular changes; the protein synthesis elongation factor *EF-Tu*, that delivers aminoacyl-tRNA to the ribosome;[28] the tubulin subunits of microtubules;[29] a large number of low-molecular-weight (20- to 25-kDa) proteins related to the product of the ras oncogene, many of which are now known to be involved in protein transport;[25-27] and subunits of the *signal recognition particle* (SRP) and its *ER membrane receptor* (SR) (see below) that participate in the targeting of nascent polypeptide chains containing insertion signal sequences to the protein translocation apparatus in the ER membrane.[30,31]

The essential feature of GTP-binding proteins, that allows them to serve as molecular switches, is that they have slow or latent GTPase activity and, therefore, can exist in two different conformational states, depending on whether they contain bound GTP or GDP, with the GTP-bound form being referred to as the "active" one. In general, the conformational state of a GTP-binding protein determines its capacity to associate with a downstream effector. In the case of the heterotrimeric G proteins32 ($G\alpha\beta\gamma$) that are coupled to plasma membrane receptors with seven transmembrane domains, such as rhodopsin and the β-adrenergic receptor, activation of the receptor catalyzes the exchange of GDP by GTP in the $G\alpha$ subunit, which in this "activated state" dissociates from the β and γ subunits, and exerts its effect on an effector, such as a channel (e.g., the muscarinic receptor-activated potassium channel) or an enzyme (e.g., phosphodiesterase or adenylcyclase). There are two main types of G proteins that associate with different receptors, those that contain stimulatory α subunits ($Gs\alpha$) and activate the effector and those that contain

*Uppercase letters (e.g., *SEC*4) indicate the wild-type gene and lower-case letters (e.g., *sec*4) the mutant gene. The protein product of the normal gene has only the first letter capitalized and is followed by a lower-case p (e.g., *Sec*4p).

inhibitory α subunits (Giα) and exert the opposite effect. In both cases, the Gα subunit remains active until the switch is turned off by the spontaneous hydrolysis of its bound GTP.[32] Although the best-understood role of heterotrimeric G proteins is in signal transduction at the plasma membrane, evidence has indicated that proteins of this class, not yet fully characterized, are also associated with intracellular membranes and function in regulating various steps of intracellular vesicular transport (see refs. 33 and 34 and our discussion below).

The *ras*-related low-molecular-weight GTP-binding proteins involved in intracellular protein transport, and probably the GTP-binding proteins in the SRP and its cognate receptor (SR) that function in the targeting of newly synthesized polypeptides to the ER (see below), do not appear to control an enzymatic reaction but rather to serve as switches that confer unidirectionality to a sequence of molecular associations. The paradigm for this mode of action is the elongation factor EF-Tu,[22,24,28] which in its GTP-bound or "active" form binds aminoacyl-tRNA in the cytosol, but releases it when GTP hydrolysis takes place (Fig. 16-7). In this case, the molecular switch associated with GTP hydrolysis controls the unidirectional transport of the aminoacyl-tRNA from the site of its charging with the amino acid (the cytosol) to its site of utilization (the ribosome). The cyclic function of EF-Tu requires that the released factor be recharged with GTP by another cytosolic elongation factor, EF-Ts, which functions as a *guanine nucleotide exchange protein*. The EF-Tu GTPase paradigm has served to inspire hypotheses[24–26,35] for the role of small GTP-binding proteins in the vectorial insertion of proteins into the ER, and in the vesicular transport of proteins from one intracellular compartment to another, in which many *ras*-related proteins of the *rab* family have been found to play key regulatory roles.

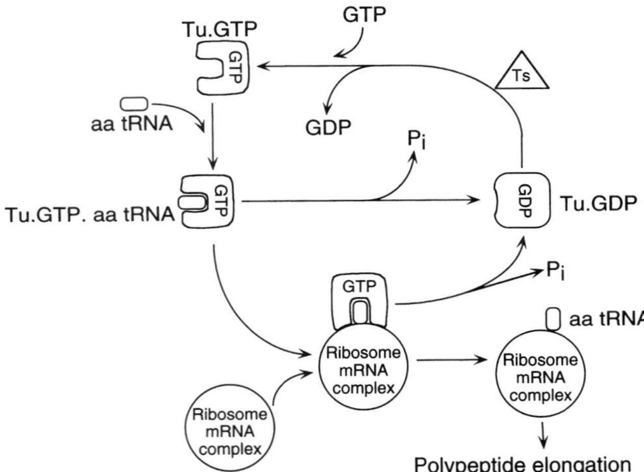

Fig. 16-7 Polypeptide chain elongation factor Tu (EF-Tu) functions as a molecular switch in the delivery of aminoacyl-tRNA to the ribosome. Elongation factor Tu can exist in two different conformations depending on whether it contains bound GTP or GDP. In its active GTP-containing form, Tu binds aminoacyl-tRNA in the cytosol, forming a ternary complex (Tu.GTP.aatRNA). This in turn binds to the A site in a ribosome that is engaged in the translation of a messenger RNA (ribosome-mRNA complex). If the anticodon in the aminoacyl-tRNA does not match the mRNA codon at the A site, the association is weak and nonlasting. In this case, the process of aatRNA delivery to the ribosome is aborted because the ternary complex dissociates from the ribosome before GTP hydrolysis, which is controlled by an internal clock in Tu, takes place. On the other hand, if the mRNA codon at the A site is matched by an anticodon in the cognate tRNA, the association is stable and, therefore, GTP hydrolysis takes place while the ternary complex is bound to the ribosome. Following GTP hydrolysis, which changes the conformation of Tu, Tu.GDP dissociates from the ribosome, leaving the aatRNA bound to the A site, ready for utilization in polypeptide elongation. Elongation factor Ts serves as a guanine nucleotide exchange factor that leads to replacement of the GDP in the inactive form of Tu by GTP.

The low-molecular-weight (20- to 29-kDa) GTP-binding proteins of the *ras* superfamily are divided into several families (*ras, rap, rab, rho, rac, ran*, and *arf*), based on sequence similarities.[36] Many proteins of the *rab* family (for *r*at *b*rain, from which the original DNAs were cloned), of which at least 25 members have now been identified, have been localized to several intracelllular organelles in a variety of cell types and have been shown to be involved in different steps of transport at the endomembrane system (see refs. 26, 26a, and 27 and our discussion below). In some of these processes *arf* proteins (for *A*DP *r*ibosylation *f*actor, the name given to the original member of this family, identified as a cofactor in the cholera toxin-induced ADP ribosylation of Gsα proteins) have also been implicated.

GTP-binding proteins of the *rab* and *ras* families share a common domain structure, which is reflected in their function. In addition to the cysteine-containing C-terminal region that is required for their prenylation and membrane binding (see below), they contain three highly conserved segments that participate in GTP binding and a segment (residues 32 to 40 in the *rab* proteins) known as the *effector domain* (because it corresponds to the effector domain of *ras*, that is, the region on the surface of *ras* that interacts with the protein, called *raf*, that regulates its GTP hydrolysis). Studies with *ras* have shown that its effector domain undergoes a conformational change during the GTP cycle and, therefore, is part of the switch mechanism essential for the function of the protein. Finally, a hypervariable region near the C-terminus of the *rab* proteins appears to determine their specific distribution in different organelles (see refs. 27 and 37). Many different amino acid substitutions in the GTP binding or effector domains of the *ras* protein have been shown to lead to its activation, independently of nucleotide binding,[38] and the same effects are expected to result from similar mutations in other *ras*-related proteins.

With the exception of the *ran* family members, which are nuclear proteins, the different *ras*-related proteins are characterized by specific C- or N-terminal posttranslational modifications that are essential for their function. Thus, proteins in the *ras* and *rho* families are characterized by the C-terminal CAAX sequence motif (where A is an aliphatic residue and X any other amino acid) and *ras* proteins (in which X is M or S) are modified by the addition of a C-15 isoprenoid moiety, farnesyl, to the cysteine residue. The modified proteins then undergo proteolytic removal of the AAX sequence, followed by carboxymethylation of the new C-terminal cysteine residue (see ref. 39). Some of these proteins also undergo palmitoylation (which is a reversible modification) at a neighboring cysteine residue and together these modifications participate in anchoring the proteins to a membrane. Proteins in the *rab* family contain dicysteine motifs near their C-termini (CC, CXC, CCX, CCXX, CCXXX), which receive the C-20 isoprenoid moiety, geranylgeranyl.[40–42] These proteins do not undergo proteolysis, but those with the CXC sequence are carboxymethylated.[43]

In contrast to those in the *ras* and *rab* families, the *arf* proteins are modified only at their N-termini by removal of the initiator methionine and addition of a myristoyl group (a tetradecanoic acyl group) to a glycine residue that immediately follows it.[44] The myristoyl moiety serves as a membrane anchor, but only if the *arf* protein carries bound GTP. An *arf* protein, therefore, cycles on and off a membrane (e.g., a Golgi membrane) during its GTP cycle.[45]

The capacity of *ras*-related GTP-binding proteins to switch between their off (GDP-bound) and on (GTP-bound) states is controlled by a set of regulatory proteins that interact with them (Fig. 16-8). These include (see ref. 25) *GTPase-activating proteins* (GAP) that, when the protein binds to its effector (which may be the GAP itself), increase the GTPase activity up to 100 times (e.g., ref. 46); *guanine nucleotide-exchange proteins* (GEF), also known as *GDP/GTP dissociation stimulators* (GDS), that accelerate the release of GDP, which in the GTP-rich cellular environment promotes the binding of GTP;[47–49] and *GDP dissociation inhibitors* (GDI) that prevent the release of GDP and, at least in

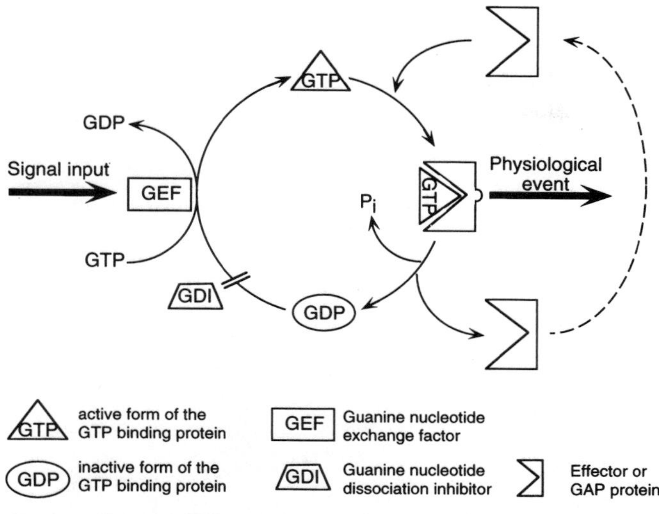

Fig. 16-8 Factors that regulate the activity of GTP-binding proteins of the *ras* superfamily. In the active GTP-containing state (represented by a triangle) the protein binds to the effector that mediates its physiological action. Binding to the effector markedly increases the latent GTPase activity of the GTP-binding protein which, on hydrolysis of GTP, switches its conformation to the GDP-containing inactive state (represented by an oval). In this case, therefore, the effector also functions as a GAP (a GTPase-activating protein) that terminates the physiological action of the GTP-binding protein, but a separate GAP protein may also carry out this function. Conversion of the inactive GTP-binding protein into the active form involves a guanine nucleotide exchange factor (GEF; rectangle) that stimulates the release of GDP, which leads to its replacement by GTP. The GEF may be located in a specific membrane or subcellular structure and its activation may require a signal from an upstream regulator, such as a heterotrimeric G protein, or a protein kinase. A guanine nucleotide dissociation inhibitor (GDI; trapezoid) may also be an important regulator of the activity of a GTP-binding protein by binding to the GDP-containing form and preventing its recharging with GTP. A GDI has been shown to be capable of removing the GDP-containing (inactive) form of a GTP-binding protein from membranes and to form a complex with it. Therefore, it is possible that for *rab* proteins involved in vesicular transport, a GDI may play a role in allowing the cyclic function of the GTP-binding protein by transporting it from the acceptor to the donor membrane.

some cases, after GTP hydrolysis, remove the cognate GTP binding protein from the membrane, or prevent its membrane association.[50,51] GDI proteins may, therefore, maintain in the cytosol a pool of inactive GTP-binding proteins, ready to be activated by GDS proteins that may themselves be membrane-associated. In a plausible scheme (Fig. 16-9), activation of a GTP-binding protein by a specific guanine nucleotide exchange factor (GEF or GDS) located in a donor membrane would trigger the association of the GTP binding with the membrane through its interaction with other membrane proteins, which would promote the formation of a carrier vesicle. On vesicle docking on the correct acceptor membrane GTP hydrolysis would occur, releasing into the cytosol the GTP-binding protein in its GDP state. Docking of the vesicle would be followed by activation of the components of the molecular machinery that leads to membrane fusion.

The involvement of a GTP-binding protein in an intracellular transport process is most easily assessed through the effect on that process of the nonhydrolyzable GTP analogue, GTP-γ-S, which, when bound to a GTP-binding protein, maintains it in the "active" conformation. If a step in the transport process requires this conformation, addition of the analogue should stimulate it. If, on the other hand, the step requires hydrolysis of the bound GTP, it should be inhibited by GTP-γ-S. Of course, hydrolysis of GTP is the step required for the GTP-binding protein to complete a cycle of function and to allow for its reutilization, as well as for the reutilization of the other components to which the protein binds specifically when in the activated state. Therefore, if a transport process—observed in a cell-free system or in permeabilized cells—is regulated by a GTP-binding protein and the result of many cycles of function is being observed, addition of GTP-γ-S should lead to inhibition of transport. Similarly, a GTP-binding protein carrying a mutation that maintains it in the active conformation, after binding to its effector, would not be able to function cyclically. Such a protein would block effector sites and inhibit subsequent cycles in the process, exerting a *dominant negative* effect.

AlF_{3-5} is also a useful reagent that can be used to assess specifically the participation of a heterotrimeric G protein in a cellular process.[52] This complex ion can mimic the γ phosphate of GTP and directly activate the Gα subunit of a G protein that contains bound GDP, but is not able to activate the low-molecular-weight GTP-binding proteins. The specific role of a G protein may also be revealed by the effects of *mastoparan*, a cationic amphiphilic peptide from wasp venon that mimics the polypeptide segment of plasma membrane receptors that interacts with G proteins. This peptide preferentially binds to the C-terminal region of Giα subunits, uncouples them from their receptor, and triggers the replacement of GDP by GTP, thus leading to activation of the inhibitory G protein.

Two toxins capable of catalyzing the ADP ribosylation of Gα subunits, the *pertussis toxin* and *cholera toxin*, have also been very useful in revealing the involvement of a heterotrimeric G protein in a cellular function. The pertussis toxin modifies (by ADP ribosylation) the C-terminal ends of some inhibitory Giα subunits. This uncouples them from the receptors and, by preventing their activation through the GDP-GTP exchange, inhibits their function. The modification induced by pertussis toxin also prevents mastoparan from exerting its effect.[53,54] In contrast, cholera toxin ADP ribosylates the stimulatory Gsα subunits and leads to their constitutive activation.[55]

PROTEIN SYNTHESIS IN THE ROUGH ENDOPLASMIC RETICULUM[11-13,30,31,56-59]

The ER is a complex system of intercommunicating membrane-bound flattened sacs (*cisternae*) and tubules that is present in all eukaryotic cells and in many cases permeates large regions of the cytoplasm. Membranes of the rough portions of the ER contain receptors for ribosomes and for nascent polypeptides, as well as proteins that are involved in the cotranslational incorporation of these polypeptides into the organelle, or in their processing during or soon after their synthesis. In addition, both RER and SER membranes contain enzymatic systems that carry out functions essential to all cells, such as steps in the synthesis of triglycerides, phospholipids, and cholesterol, as well as systems that carry out specialized metabolic or biosynthetic functions and, therefore, are present only in specific cell types.

The RER is most prominent in cells engaged in protein secretion, such as pancreatic acinar and anterior pituitary cells, which synthesize digestive enzymes and polypeptide hormones, respectively; plasma cells, which produce immunoglobulins; and hepatocytes, which manufacture a wide variety of serum proteins. Because the RER plays a major role in the synthesis and assembly of membrane proteins, this organelle is prominent in cells, such as neurons, which maintain greatly expanded plasma membranes.

The degree of development of the SER in different cell types usually reflects the participation of ER membrane enzymes in specialized activities of the cell. Thus, the SER is very well developed in cells of steroid-secreting tissues, where it contains enzymes that catalyze several of the hydroxylation reactions that modify the steroid nucleus. It is also highly developed in skeletal muscle cells, in which it is known as the "sarcoplasmic reticulum," an organelle equipped to sequester calcium ions into its lumen and to release them when the cells are stimulated to contract. In fact, the ER appears to play a major role in the control of cytoplasmic Ca^{2+} levels in almost all cell types.

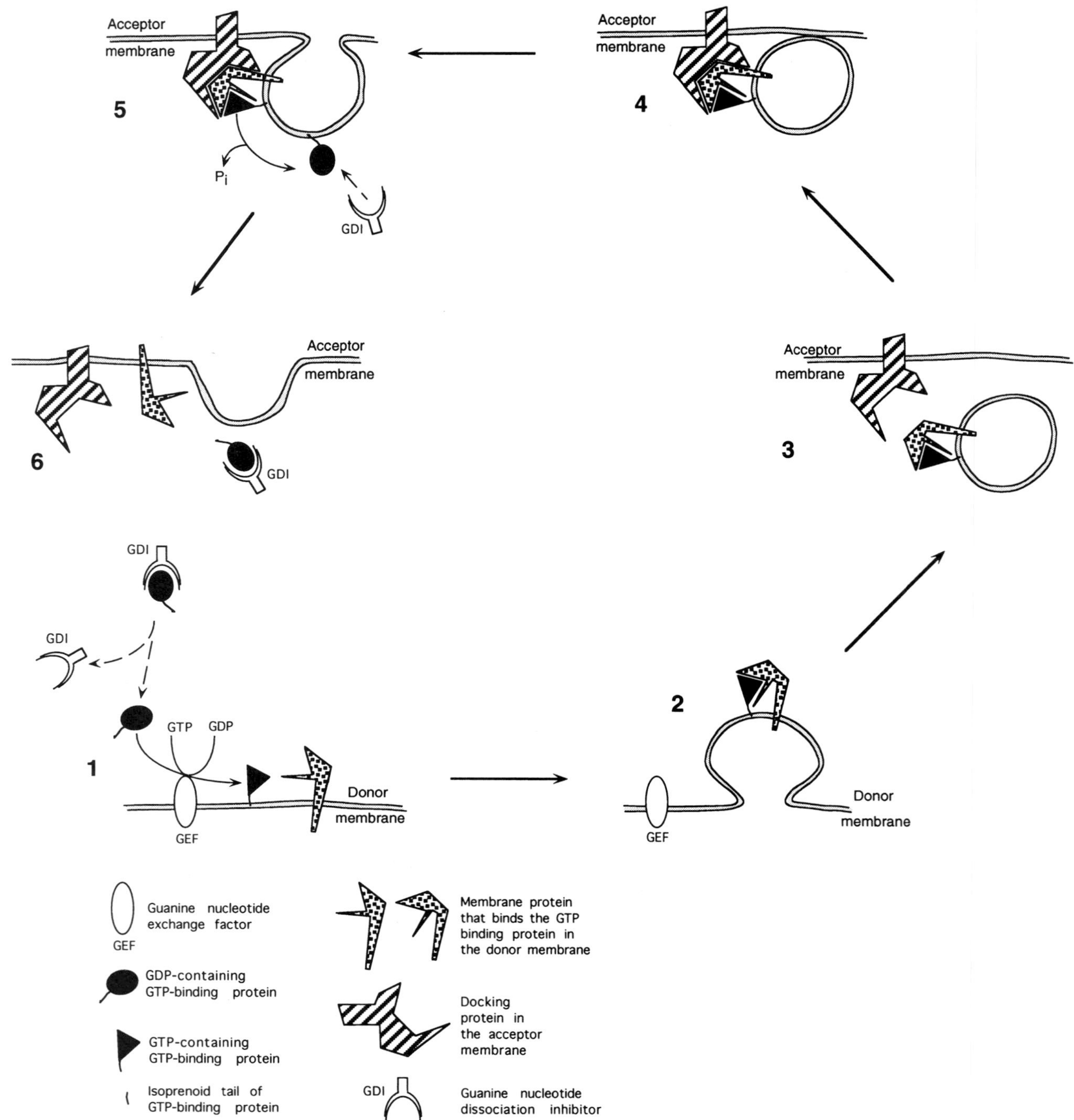

Fig. 16-9 A scheme for the role of a low-molecular-weight GTP-binding protein such as a *rab* protein, in directing the vectorial delivery of a membrane vesicle. In this scheme it is assumed that, in its active form, a *rab* protein promotes vesicle formation in the donor membrane (by a mechanism not depicted) and confers to a membrane protein that becomes incorporated into a forming vesicle the conformation necessary to ensure docking of the vesicle on the correct acceptor membrane. GTP hydrolysis, which is shown as taking place after docking on the acceptor membrane, may play a role in activating the machinery (not depicted) that leads to membrane fusion. (1) A GTP-binding protein (small solid oval with tail) is activated at a donor membrane by a specific guanine nucleotide exchange factor (GEF). The activated GTP-binding protein becomes associated with the membrane via its C-terminal isoprenoid moiety, represented by the tail. (2) The activated form of the GTP-binding protein (filled triangle) interacts with a membrane protein (stippled figure) in the donor membrane that, on changing conformation, is incorporated into a forming vesicle. (3) The free vesicle approaches an acceptor membrane, where a receptor or docking protein (striped figure) is found. (4) Docking of the vesicle on the appropriate acceptor membrane involves the recognition of the membrane protein bearing the GTP-binding protein by the receptor. Therefore, the membrane protein plays a key role in vesicle targeting and, to function in other rounds of transport, must recycle to the donor compartment (in a step that is not depicted). (5) Docking of the vesicle on its receptor promotes GTP hydrolysis, which changes the conformation of the GTP-binding protein and, in some way, activates the membrane fusion machinery (not represented) that completes vesicle delivery. (6) During or after membrane fusion, the transported membrane protein and its receptor, now in the acceptor membrane, dissociate from each other. The GDP-containing form of the GTP-binding protein is shown as being extracted from the acceptor membrane by the action of a GDI (cup-shaped figure), which delivers it back to the GEF in the donor membrane. The role of a GDI in extracting a GTP-binding protein from a membrane has been demonstrated for only one *rab* protein.

Although the membranes of the rough and smooth portions of the ER are continuous, they usually adopt different morphologic configurations within the same cell that must reflect differences in their protein and/or lipid composition. The rough cisternae are frequently arranged in stacks of interconnected flattened disks, whereas the smooth portions usually form an extensive system of thin convoluted tubules. EM of grazing sections of rough cisternae reveal that the ribosomes attached to the membranes form rosettes, hairpins, or spiral patterns, which correspond to membrane-bound polysomes. Individual ribosomes within bound polysomes contact the membrane via their large subunits,[60] which are known to contain the nascent polypeptide chains.

Much information on the biochemical composition and function of the ER has come from the analysis of *rough* and *smooth microsomes*, subcellular fractions derived from rough and smooth portions of the ER, respectively. Extensive fragmentation of the ER takes place during the tissue homogenization that must be carried out before cell fractionation. The broken ER membranes, however, rapidly reseal to form microsomal vesicles that still contain a large part of the luminal content of the intact organelle.[61,62] The rough microsomes retain the ribosomes bound to their membranes and can be separated from the smooth microsomes on the basis of their greater density.

The structural and compositional differences between rough and smooth ER membranes have been best studied in liver cells, where both portions of the organelle are well developed and can be isolated as rough and smooth microsomes, respectively, with high yields and relative purity. Many of the most abundant ER membrane proteins are present in both rough and smooth membranes, but rough microsomes contain several specific membrane polypeptides that are likely to be involved in functions associated with the synthesis and processing of proteins made in bound ribosomes, or with maintaining the characteristic structure of the rough cisternae.[63–65]

Although cellular phospholipids are synthesized in the ER, the phospholipid composition of the ER membranes is not a simple reflection of their biosynthetic capacity. They are rich in phosphatidylcholine (PC), phosphatidylethanolamine (PE), phosphatidylserine (PS), and phosphatidylinositol (PI), but contain very small amounts of sphingomyelin (SM) and cholesterol, which are abundant in the plasma membrane. The fatty acids of ER phospholipids are usually highly unsaturated, which accounts for the high fluidity of the ER membranes (see ref. 4).

Cotranslational Insertion of Polypeptides into ER Membranes: Role of Insertion Signals in Determining the Association with the ER Membranes of Polysomes Synthesizing Specific Proteins

Ribosomes that are part of polysomes found free in the cytoplasmic matrix are structurally and functionally identical to those within polysomes bound to ER membranes.[66,67] Indeed, within the cell, after completion of each polypeptide chain, both polysomal populations may exchange ribosomal subunits.[68] The attachment to the ER membrane of the ribosomes that synthesize secretory, lysosomal, or certain classes of membrane proteins is determined by information contained within the nascent polypeptide chains.[69] Extensive studies with a wide variety of secretory proteins have demonstrated that nascent secretory polypeptides almost invariably contain N-terminal peptide segments that are not present in the mature proteins. These segments serve to determine the attachment of the ribosome bearing the nascent chain to the ER membrane.[70–74] They consist of 15 to 30 amino acid residues and characteristically include a central hydrophobic core of at least eight amino acids (see refs. 75 to 78). Similar N-terminal peptides are found in nascent lysosomal proteins and in many membrane proteins. These peptide segments are known as *transient insertion signals* or *signal sequences* or *presequences*. They serve to trigger the association of the ribosome with the membrane and initiate the complete or partial translocation of the nascent polypeptide through it, but are removed by proteolytic cleavage before synthesis of the polypeptide is completed. The translocation of proteins across the ER membranes initiated by signal sequences (Fig. 16-10) is frequently referred to as the *vectorial discharge of nascent polypeptides*.[79]

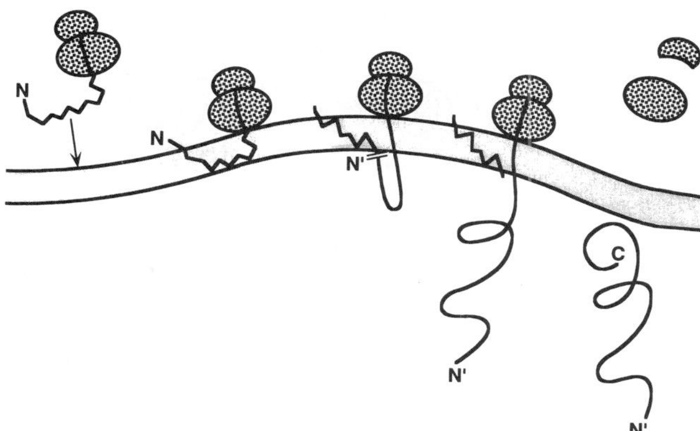

Fig. 16-10 Vectorial discharge of a secretory polypeptide across the ER membrane mediated by a cleavable N-terminal insertion signal. The cotranslational passage of a polypeptide, such as a secretory or lysosomal protein, into the ER lumen is represented in a simplified form that does not include any molecular components of the translocation machinery. The translocation is initiated by an N-terminal signal that is cleaved during the course of polypeptide chain elongation and is completed after polypeptide termination. The signal that has emerged from the ribosome leads to the association of the nascent chain and the ribosome with the membrane. The signal has been drawn as remaining in the membrane after it is cleaved. Its fate, however, has not yet been determined.

Process of Assembly of a Membrane-Bound Polysome (Fig. 16-11)

As is the case with the assembly of a free polysome, the assembly of a membrane-bound polysome begins in the cytoplasm with the binding of a small ribosomal subunit to the 5′ end of the mRNA. After the large ribosomal subunit joins the small subunit at the initiation codon of the mRNA, synthesis of the polypeptide begins. It is only after elongation is in course and the polypeptide is long enough for the signal segment to emerge from the large ribosomal subunit, which normally encloses a 40-amino-acid segment of the nascent chain,[80,81] that the mechanism that leads to translocation begins to operate. This mechanism, illustrated schematically in Fig. 16-11, includes fail-safe features that ensure not only that the nascent polypeptide is inserted into the ER during its synthesis but also that, if insertion cannot take place, synthesis of the polypeptide is halted soon after the signal segment emerges from the ribosome.

The process of targeting the ribosome to the membrane begins with the recognition of the emerging signal by a soluble macromolecular complex, the SRP,[82–91] which consists of six distinct polypeptides and a small RNA molecule (7SL RNA) of approximately 300 nucleotides in length. The SRP interacts not only with the signal but also with the ribosome in such a way as to lead to a temporary block in polypeptide chain elongation. This block is relieved only in a subsequent step, when the SRP binds to its cognate receptor (SR),[87–93] also known as the *docking protein*,[92] which is an integral membrane protein exposed on the cytoplasmic surface of the ER. The pause in translocation caused by SRP ensures that continued growth in the cytoplasm and subsequent folding of the polypeptide, which could prevent insertion in the membrane, do not take place.

RER membranes also contain sites with high affinity for ribosomes, which may be regarded as ribosome receptors.[94] Following docking of the SRP on the membrane, a firm attachment of the ribosome to its receptor takes place, which allows for the coupling of the processes of translation and membrane insertion.

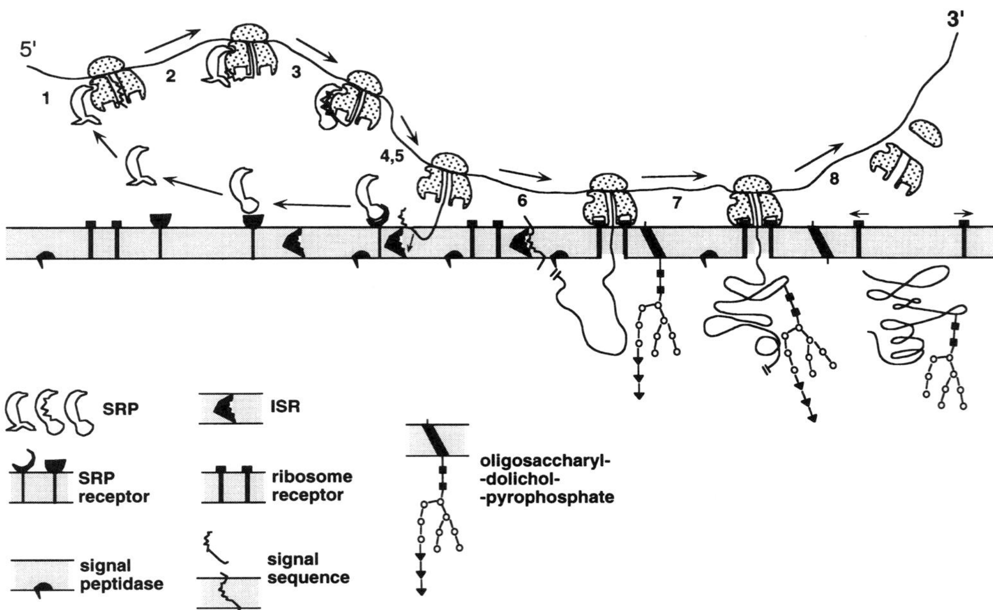

Fig. 16-11 Process of assembly of a membrane-bound polysome and the mechanism for the cotranslational translocation of a nascent polypeptide. An ordered series of molecular recognition events leads to the insertion of a nascent chain in the ER membrane. This involves an initial interaction of SRP with the ribosome (1) and with the emerging signal sequence (2 and 3), followed by binding of SRP to its receptor (4), which in turn leads to release of the SRP from the signal and the ribosome. The latter are then able to bind to their membrane receptors (5 and 6). See the text for the detailed description of the role of the different components of the translocation machinery illustrated in this figure. Note that SRP and its receptor function catalytically and are only transiently associated with the site of translocation. In this figure, only two cotranslational modifications—signal cleavage (6) and core glycosylation (7)—are shown, but several others, such as disulfide exchange and hydroxylation of side chains, are also known to take place cotranslationally. Note that signal cleavage occurs relatively early in translocation so that covalent linkage of the signal to the remainder of the polypeptide is not required for the continuation of translocation. After chain termination (8), it is presumed that the translocation apparatus disassembles and the ribosome detaches from the membrane. Translocation is depicted as taking place through a proteinaceous channel in the membrane, which becomes an extension of a tunnel within the large ribosomal subunit, where the nascent chain is contained.

The exact sequence of events that occurs next is not known, but it is clear that binding of the SRP to its receptor displaces it from the signal and from the ribosome.[95] The signal sequence must then enter the membrane, where it is thought to interact with protein components of a translocation apparatus.[96–100]

Since neither the SRP nor its receptor appear to remain associated with the membrane-bound ribosome at the site of translocation (the number of SRP receptors in the ER membrane is much smaller than the number of active bound ribosomes), the essential role of the SRP/SRP receptor system appears to be simply to target the ribosome and its incipient chain to the ER, without participating in the translocation process itself.

Although it is not yet fully understood how the polypeptide actually traverses the ER membrane, it is clear that an interaction of the nascent chain with membrane proteins is necessary for translocation to occur. Considerable evidence supports a model in which passage of the nascent polypeptide across the hydrophobic barrier within the membrane occurs through the aqueous environment of a proteinaceous channel.[73,79,101–104] The role of the insertion signal would be to open the channel or to trigger its assembly from dispersed membrane protein subunits. The open or assembled state of the channel could be stabilized by the interaction of its components with the large ribosomal subunit, but the channel would be closed or disassembled when the ribosome is released following polypeptide chain termination, or a halt in translocation caused by a stop transfer signal (see below). In alternative models,[105,106] now not in favor (see below), following targeting to the membrane, the insertion signal and the nascent chain would interact directly with the membrane bilayer, and no specific membrane proteins would be required to mediate translocation itself.

It is clear that, in addition to proteins that may participate directly in the translocation process, several membrane enzymes are also located near the site of translocation and are able to interact with the growing chain to modify it as it emerges on the luminal side of the ER membrane. Thus, a *signal peptidase* cleaves off the signal, a *protein oligosaccharyl transferase* links preformed mannose-rich oligosaccharide chains to selected asparagine residues within the nascent polypeptide, and a *protein disulfide isomerase* (PDI) enzyme catalyzes the formation of intramolecular disulfide bonds. These modifications, however, are not required for translocation to occur.

Experimental Analysis of Translocation[107]

The process of cotranslational insertion of nascent polypeptides into ER membranes has been best studied utilizing cell-free systems in which messenger RNAs obtained from natural sources, or produced by in vitro transcription of cloned cDNA templates, are translated in the presence of rough microsomes. The most commonly used translation systems are derived from rabbit reticulocytes or wheat germ, and the most frequently used rough microsomal membranes are obtained from dog pancreas.[108]

When messenger RNA encoding secretory proteins are translated in the absence of membranes, *primary translation products* are obtained, which contain the signal sequences and are devoid of any modifications of their primary structure (Fig. 16-12*Aa*). Such artificial products of in vitro translation, which are generally not produced in vivo, are called *presecretory proteins* or *preproteins*. These are not true precursors of the secretory proteins, since, in vivo, their signals are actually removed before synthesis of the polypeptide is completed. When rough microsomal membranes are present during the in vitro translation, a large fraction of the product synthesized is translocated into the lumen of the microsomes and undergoes signal removal. If the translocated protein does not contain sites for *N*-linked glycosylation, its electrophoretic mobility is greater than that of the primary

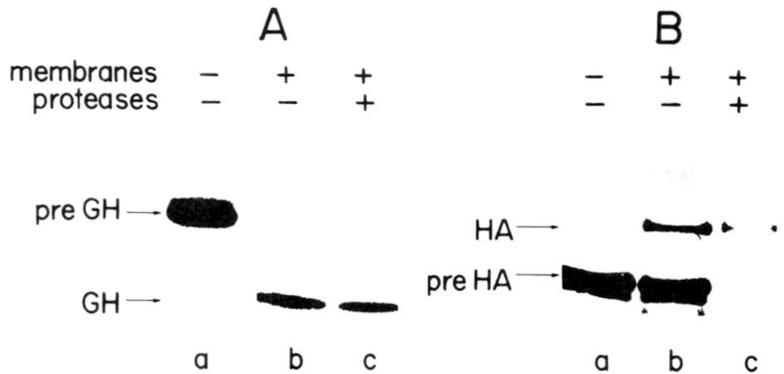

Fig. 16-12 Experimental analysis of the translocation of in vitro synthesized polypeptides: demonstration of signal cleavage, sequestration in the microsomal lumen, and glycosylation. Messenger RNAs encoding pregrowth hormone (*A*) or the hemagglutinin (HA) of influenza virus (*B*) were translated in vitro in the absence (*a*) or presence (*b* and *c*) of dog pancreas microsomal membranes, using a cell-free system for protein synthesis derived from wheat germ. In the absence of microsomal membranes, preproteins containing signal sequences are synthesized (*Aa* and *Ba*). When microsomes are present during translation, a large fraction of the products undergo signal cleavage. For growth hormone, this leads to an increase in electrophoretic mobility (compare *Aa* and *Ab*). In the case of HA, cleavage of the signal is accompanied by core glycosylation and this results in a net increase in mass, which is reflected in a lower electrophoretic mobility (compare *Ba* and *Bb*). In both cases, only the cotranslationlly processed products are translocated into the microsomal lumen since only they, and not the preproteins, are resistant to the degradative action of exogenous proteases (*Ac* and *Bc*). HA is a type I transmembrane glycoprotein, but only a very short segment at its C-terminus (10 amino acids) is exposed on the exterior surface of the microsomes. Therefore, the protease treatment does not lead to a significant reduction in molecular weight and a concomitant increase in its electrophoretic mobility.

translation product (the presecretory protein) by the 2 to 3 kDa that corresponds to the cleaved signal (compare Fig. 16-12*Aa* and *Ab*). The sequestration of the processed polypeptides in the lumen of the microsomes is demonstrated by the fact that they are protected from proteolysis when proteases are added to the reaction mixture after translation is completed (compare Fig. 16-12*Ab* and *Ac*). On the other hand, the presecretory proteins (pre-GH in Fig. 16-12*Ab*), which remain outside the microsomes, are completely digested (Fig. 16-12*Ac*). Destruction of the membranes by detergent solubilization, of course, leads to digestion of the translocated products by the exogenous proteases.

When the messenger RNA utilized for in vitro translation experiments encodes a protein with sites for N glycosylation, translocation of the nascent chain is accompanied by both signal cleavage and addition of N-linked oligosaccharides (see below). In this case, the apparent size of the translocated product, when assessed by gel electrophoresis, may be higher than that of the primary translation product since the contribution of the added oligosaccharide chains may more than compensate for the size reduction resulting from signal cleavage (compare Fig. 16-12*Ba* and *Ab*). On treatment with proteases, only the glycosylated polypeptide remains undigested. The absence of the signal sequence in the translocated glycoproteins becomes apparent when, after dissolution of the microsomal membrane, they are treated with a glycosidase (endoglycosidase H) that removes the oligosaccharide chains (see below).

In vitro translocation experiments of the type just described, with mRNA that encode lysosomal enzymes (most of which are glycoproteins) or type I transmembrane proteins, have demonstrated that these polypeptides also contain transient N-terminal signals that mediate their cotranslational insertion into the ER.

Characterization of Insertion Signals[75–78,109–111]

Insertion signals are necessary to initiate the translocation of nascent polypeptides across the ER membrane. Secretory polypeptides from which the signal is deleted by modification of the corresponding cloned gene can no longer be translocated across ER membranes, in vivo or in vitro. Moreover, in some cases, attachment of a cleavable insertion signal to the N-terminus of a cytosolic protein has been shown to be sufficient to confer on it the capacity to be translocated. Although interaction of the signal with the membrane is necessary to initiate translocation, it is clear that covalent attachment of the signal to the rest of the polypeptide need not be maintained throughout translocation, since signal cleavage generally occurs much before elongation of the nascent chain is completed.[73] However, it is possible that the signal could, even after it is severed from the body of the nascent chain, be necessary for translocation to continue. If this were the case, degradation of the cleaved signal segments by the yet to be discovered *signal peptide peptidase* would occur only after translocation is completed.

Comparison of the amino acid sequences of different insertion signals shows that there is considerable variation in their primary structure. This suggests that general properties of the signals, including conformational features, rather than specific sequence information, are recognized by the various components of the translocation machinery (such as the SRP and the signal peptidase) that interact with the signal. Indeed many random sequences of the human genome that encode peptide segments of relatively high but varying degrees of hydrophobicity were shown to be capable of serving a signal function when linked to the yeast secretory protein invertase, from which the N-terminal signal was removed.[112]

Insertion signals are usually 15 to 30 amino acids in length. Preprotein sequences are conventionally numbered so that the first residue after the cleavage site of the signal is designated +1 and the last residue of the signal is −1. Three segments can be recognized in all cleavable signals[76] (Fig. 16-13): (1) a hydrophobic core (the h-region) 8 to 16 residues in length, which generally ends at residue −6, (2) a hydrophilic N-terminal segment that precedes the core (the n-region) and usually contains, in addition to the positively charged N-terminus, one basic amino acid, (3) an approximately five-residue-long C-terminal segment (the c-region), which defines the cleavage site and usually begins with a helix-breaking glycine or proline residue. In some signals, such as the one in rat growth hormone, the N-terminal segment bears no net charge due to the presence of a negatively charged amino acid residue.

The charges in the n-region of the signal are likely to play a role in initiating the association of the signal with the membrane that triggers the insertion of the nascent polypeptide. Deletion of the n-region from prepropararthyroid hormone does not prevent the elongation arrest caused by SRP or its relief by the SRP receptor, but translocation of the nascent polypeptide is impaired.[113] These observations are in accord with the notion that, as the signal begins to enter the membrane itself, the charges in the n-region associate directly with the polar head groups of the phospholipids.[114,115] If this association is maintained as translocation proceeds, the nascent chain would adopt a loop disposition in the membrane (Fig. 16-14), with its N-terminus on the cytoplasmic face, the hydrophobic core of the signal within the membrane, and the cleavage site on the luminal surface. The formation of this loop would be facilitated by the helix-breaking nature of the residues immediately following the hydrophobic core.

Direct evidence for the loop model has been obtained from an analysis of the behavior of a genetically engineered protein expressed in transfected cells whose N-terminal cleavable insertion signal was extended by the addition of upstream sequences and whose cleavage site was abolished by mutation.[116] Translocation of this protein proceeded normally but, since the signal was not removed, it served as a membrane anchor for the final product, which was a transmembrane protein with the N-terminal extension preceding the signal exposed on the cytoplasmic surface of the ER. The cytoplasmic exposure of the N-terminal extension implies that throughout the course

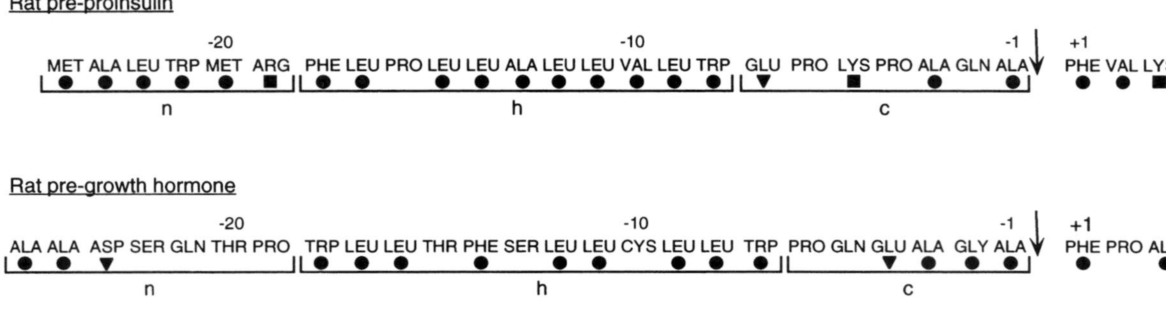

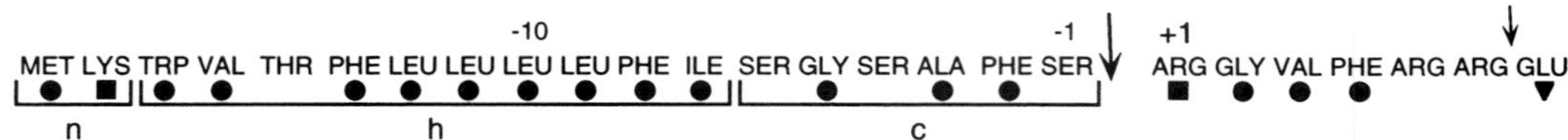

Fig. 16-13 Sequences of transient insertion signals of secretory proteins. The amino acid sequences of the transient insertion signals of numerous proteins are known, and general consensus features for the signals have become apparent. N-terminal segments of the sequences of three presecretory proteins are shown, and the point of cleavage by the signal peptidase is indicated in each case by a downward arrow. The amino acid residue within the signal adjacent to the cleavage site is designated as −1 and the preceding residues in the signal are counted negatively from −1 toward the N-terminus. The three segments in each signal, described in the text, are labelled *n*, *h*, and *c*. Hydrophobic amino acids are marked by solid circles, basic residues by squares, and acidic ones by triangles, all placed beneath the residue abbreviation. The residue designated +1 represents the new N-terminus generated by signal cleavage. In all these cases the −1, −3 rule applies, that is, the −1 position is occupied by a small neutral amino acid (such as Ala, Gly, or Ser) and the −3 position is not occupied by an aromatic, charged, or large and polar residue. In the case of rat pregrowth hormone, the +1 residue corresponds to the N-terminus of the mature protein. In the case of preproinsulin, this residue corresponds to the N-terminus of the β chain of insulin. In the case of preproalbumin, a second cleavage near the N-terminus takes place in the Golgi apparatus, at the site indicated by the arrowhead. This removes a hexapeptide propiece and leaves glutamic acid at the N-terminus of the mature protein.

of translocation the signal was maintained in the loop configuration.

From the analysis of numerous insertion signal sequences, certain rules have emerged that allow the prediction of the site of cleavage of the signal within the sequence of a preprotein with a fair degree of certainty. The −1, −3 rule[77,111,117] states that the −1 position is almost always occupied by small neutral amino acids (such as alanine, glycine, or serine) and that the residue at −3 must not be aromatic (Phe, His, Tyr, Try), charged (Asp, Glu, Lys, Arg), or large and polar (Asn, Gln). It is also apparent that residues

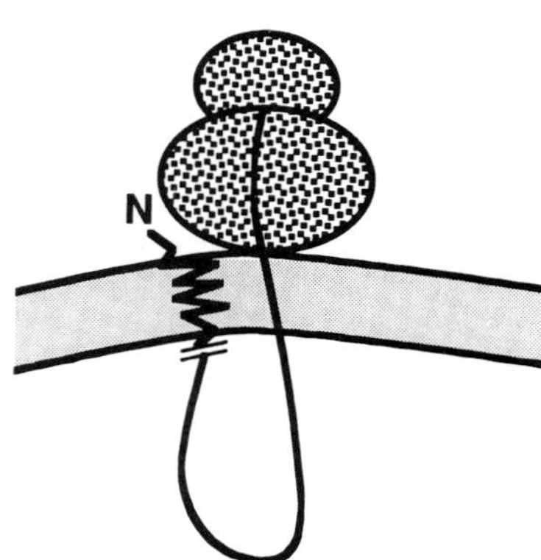

Fig. 16-14 Loop model for the disposition during translocation of the cleavable signal of a polypeptide synthesized in a membrane-bound ribosome. In this model, the extreme N-terminus of the signal remains on the cytoplasmic face of the membrane and the nascent chain has a looped disposition during the initial stages of translocation. In most secretory, lysosomal, and type I transmembrane proteins, the signal is N-terminal and is cleaved during translocation, as depicted in this figure. In type II transmembrane proteins, the signal is not cleaved and the looped configuration would be maintained throughout translocation, until the extreme C-terminus of the polypeptide is released into the lumen.

following the cleavage site may contribute to its recognition by the signal peptidase. Thus, some point mutations, produced by genetic engineering techniques, that affect residues following the cleavage site have been shown to prevent cleavage. A role of the sequence following the cleavage site in determining signal cleavage may account for the fact that some secretory proteins, such as parathyroid hormone and albumin, contain a second transient N-terminal peptide segment, the *propiece*, that is removed from the *proprotein* during or after passage through the Golgi apparatus. In these instances, the N-terminal sequence of the mature protein, which may be important for the function of the protein, might not have permitted cleavage of the signal had it been immediately adjacent to the −1 residue.[118] One function of the propiece could, therefore, be to satisfy the requirements for the creation of a signal peptidase cleavage site in the nascent preprotein.

The conformation that the signal segment attains within the interior of the membrane has not been established. Within a hydrophobic environment, an α-helical conformation would be favored for the core region. However, the core is usually shorter than the approximately 20 amino acid residues that would be required for an α helix to completely span the membrane thickness of 2.5 to 3 nm, whereas in a fully extended configuration a peptide segment of only eight residues could span the membrane. Therefore, it has been suggested[110] that the hydrophobic core of the signal may exist within the membrane partially as an α helix and partially as a fully extended structure. The important role played by the hydrophobicity of the central core of the signal in translocation is apparent from the deleterious effects of mutations in bacterial secretory proteins replacing some of the hydrophobic residues by charged ones, or introducing partial deletions covering core residues.[119,120]

Even though insertion signals are usually removed by cleavage from nascent secretory and lysosomal polypeptides and from many nascent membrane proteins (see below), signal cleavage is not required for translocation. Indeed, one secretory protein, ovalbumin,[121,122] and several viral envelope glycoproteins[123–125] are known to contain signals near their N-termini that mediate translocation, but are not cleaved and are themselves transferred with adjacent portions of the polypeptide into the ER lumen.

Signal Recognition Particle[30,31,58,59]

The SRP plays a central role in selecting ribosomes for binding to the ER and in delivering the nascent chains to a receptor within the membrane. The distribution of SRP within the cell reflects its cyclic participation in these processes. SRP may be found free in the cytoplasm, weakly bound to inactive ribosomes or attached to its receptor in the ER membranes[126] (see Fig. 16-11). The affinity of SRP for ribosomes, however, increases at least 6000 times when the ribosome contains a nascent chain with an exposed signal sequence, to which the SRP also binds.[84]

The most commonly used source of SRP for in vitro studies of its role in translocation is dog pancreas microsomes, from which SRP can be released by treatment with media with high salt concentrations. Indeed, microsomes treated with high levels of salt (KRM) are inactive in translocation unless supplemented with SRP.[82] The pause in translation caused by SRP is best observed when SRP is added to a wheat-germ translation system, which lacks endogenous SRP. In the absence of added microsomes, SRP leads to an effective block in the elongation of nascent proteins that contain a signal peptide, such as preprolactin, but the synthesis of cytosolic proteins, such as globin, proceeds unaffected.[86] In several cases, it has been shown that in the presence of SRP, a ribosome-associated arrested fragment of the preprotein of approximately 80 amino acids accumulates in the translation system. The SRP-mediated arrest of polypeptide chain elongation is relieved by the addition of microsomes to the system, which leads to signal cleavage and translocation,[85,86] or even by the addition of purified SRP receptor.[88]

The SRP obtained from dog pancreas microsomes by washing with a high-salt medium is a particle with a sedimentation efficient of 11S that contains, in addition to the 7SL RNA molecule, six polypeptide chains of molecular weights 9, 14, 19, 54, 68, and 72 kDa.[83,127] The 7SL RNA is an abundant and metabolically stable molecule that contains at its 5′ and 3′ ends sequences of the *Alu* family (one of the most highly repeated families of sequences in the genome) and in its middle region a core segment of 150 nucleotides, termed the S sequence, that is much less frequently repeated.[128] Both protein and RNA components of SRP have been shown to be required for its function. SRP has been disassembled into its RNA and protein components by the removal of Mg^{2+} ions, which normally stabilize its structure, and it has been possible to reassemble a functional particle from the dissociated components.[129] This has allowed studies on the role of the individual proteins on the different aspects of SRP function.[130,131]

It is noteworthy that 7SL RNA from such evolutionarily distant species as *Drosophila melanogaster* and *Xenopus laevis* can replace the canine RNA in the reassembled particles. Reconstitution experiments have shown that the two smallest polypeptides of SRP are required for translational arrest but are not necessary for translocation, which, of course, demonstrates that the arrest in translation is not essential for translocation to occur.[130] In fact, SRP may cause only a slowdown in the translation of certain mRNAs for which arrested peptides have not been detected in the wheat-germ system.

Treatment of SRP with nucleases generates two subparticles that may correspond to domains exerting the functions of SRP.[128] One particle contains the two smallest polypeptides bound to the two ends of the 7SL RNA, and the other the four remaining ones bound to the central region of the RNA.

SRP can be purified by hydrophobic chromatography, which suggests that it interacts with the hydrophobic core of signal sequences. Indeed, replacement of leucine residues in a presecretory protein with β-hydroxyleucine, a polar analogue, abolishes the high-affinity binding of SRP for the ribosome, and hence the translational arrest and subsequent translocation.[85] Moreover, it has been demonstrated that in a ribosome carrying SRP, the nascent chain is in close proximity to the 54-kDa polypeptide of SRP, since the two can be crosslinked through a photoactivatable group incorporated into the nascent chain.[132] In this case, the elongation arrest was maintained after crosslinking and was relieved on binding to the SRP receptor, but translocation could not occur.

Much progress has been made in identifying within the SRP structural domains that carry out its three distinct sequential functions: signal sequence recognition, elongation arrest, and delivery of the nascent chain to the translocation machinery within the ER membrane. The two smaller SRP polypeptides (9 kDa and 14 kDa) form a heterodimer and are required for the elongation arrest to occur, whereas the two largest ones (68 kDa and 72 kDa), which also form a heterodimer, are required for the binding of SRP to its membrane receptor (SR). The 54-kDa polypeptide SRP54 is a GTP-binding protein that contains a putative GTPase segment. Its primary function is in the recognition of the insertion signal in the nascent polypeptide. The C-terminal portion of SRP54 constitutes a methionine-rich "M domain,"[132a–132c] which by itself shows affinity for the signal sequence, although in the native protein this appears to be regulated by the N-terminal "G" domain.[133]

It is noteworthy that genes encoding homologues of the SRP54[133a–135] and of the α subunit of the SRP receptor[135] (also, see below) have been identified in yeast and that, although their deletion leads to poor growth and to the accumulation of precursors of some secretory and membrane proteins in the cytosol, the cells, nevertheless, remain viable. This suggests that another mechanism, independent of SRP, can function in this unicellular eukaryote and effect the translocation of most essential proteins incorporated into the ER. Indeed, the posttranslational translocation of the α-mating factor precursor had previously been observed in yeast, both in vivo and in vitro.[136–138] Evidence has also been presented that "molecular chaperones," encoded by the yeast Ssa1 and Ssa2 genes, facilitate the SRP-independent uptake of the α-factor precursor into the ER.[139,140] Molecular chaperones are members of a family of proteins that mediate the proper folding of other polypeptides and sometimes their assembly into oligomeric complexes.[16] The chaperones involved in posttranslational translocation in the ER belong to the heat-shock hsp70[141] family of proteins and utilize ATP to confer on the polypeptide a conformation compatible with its transport across the membrane. These chaperones have also been shown (see below) to facilitate the uptake of polypeptides into mitochondria.[139,140]

It should be noted that a yeast protein in the lumen of the ER (Kar2p) that can be crosslinked to the nascent chain[142] is also necessary for translocation.[143] Kar2p is the yeast homologue of the mammalian protein Bip (Grp 78), which is a heat-shock protein of the hsp70 family that serves as a molecular chaperone in the lumen of the ER and was first identified as an *immunoglobulin heavy chain binding protein* that functions in the assembly of immunoglobulin molecules.[144,145]

Signal Recognition Particle Receptor or Docking Protein[30,31,59]

The SR is a heterodimeric (SRα, 72 kDa; SRβ, 30 kDa) protein complex exposed on the cytoplasmic surface of the ER membrane, where it receives the SRP bound to a ribosome containing an exposed signal sequence (see Fig. 16-11). This binding displaces the SRP from the ribosome and from the signal and allows the signal to insert into the membrane.[95] The SR is present in the ER in low amounts (0.1 percent of the total membrane protein) and functions catalytically, remaining associated with SRP for only the very brief period required to displace it from the ribosome and to establish the ribosome-membrane junction. These reactions can occur at 0°C in the absence of any polypeptide chain elongation.[95]

The SR has been purified from solubilized rough microsomal membranes by affinity chromatography to immobilized SRP, using the relief of the translation arrest of preprolactin as an assay to detect functional receptor.[87,88] The SR obtained in this manner consists of two subunits, a 69-kDa glycoprotein α subunit and a

30-kDa β subunit.[146] Treatment of rough microsomes with the protease elastase renders the membrane inactive in translocation and leads to the release of a 52-kDa fragment of the α subunit, which can be added back to the proteolyzed membranes at low ionic strength to restore translocation competence.[90,91]

The complete primary structures of the SRP receptor subunits have been derived from the nucleotide sequence of cDNA clones.[31,147] Comparison of the sequence of the α subunit with the N-terminal sequence of the 52-kDa fragment released by proteolysis shows that the protein is anchored to the membrane via a 155-amino-acid N-terminal segment that contains two hydrophobic domains. The portion of the molecule exposed on the cytoplasmic surface contains three extremely hydrophilic regions rich in charged amino acids, with a predominance of basic residues that may interact directly with the 7SL RNA component of the SRP. This portion of the molecule also contains several additional hydrophobic segments that do not interact permanently with the membrane and are probably buried within the protein.

Both the α and β subunits of the SR are GTP-binding proteins and, surprisingly, SRα and the 54-kDa subunit of SRP are sufficiently related in sequence to constitute a new subfamily of GTPases. The exact roles of these three GTPases (SRP54, SRα, and SRβ) have not yet become clear, but most likely, a series of GTP-dependent changes in the conformational states of these proteins controls the sequential macromolecular interactions that

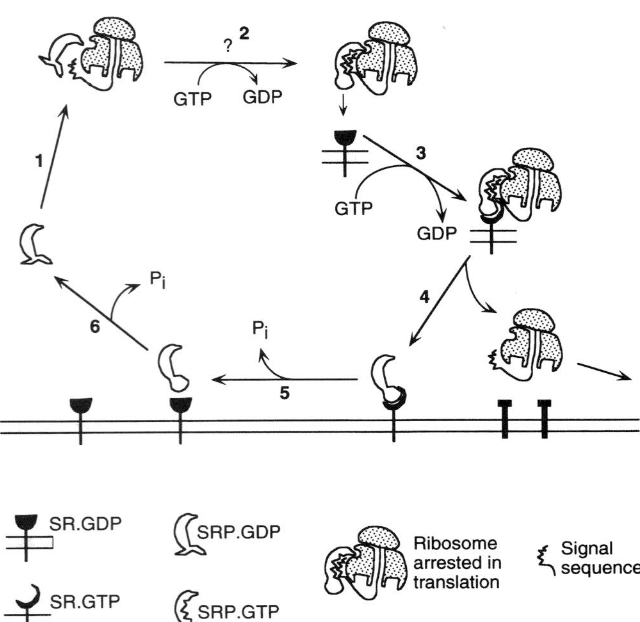

Fig. 16-15 Hypothetical model for the role of GTP hydrolysis cycles within the GTP-binding subunits of SRP and the SRP receptor (SR) in the delivery of a ribosome bearing a nascent polypeptide with a signal sequence to the translocation apparatus in the ER membrane. This tentative scheme assumes that SRP with its 54-kDa subunit (SRP54) containing bound GDP binds to the ribosome, albeit weakly (1), and that binding of the signal sequence that emerges from the ribosome to SRP54 triggers the replacement of GDP for GTP within that protein (2). In this "active conformation" SRP binds more tightly to the ribosome and arrests polypeptide chain elongation. The GTP-containing SRP would also have a higher affinity for SR, which initially has its SRα subunit in the GDP-containing state. The ensuing docking of SRP on SR leads to the exchange of GTP for GDP in SRα (3), which in its "active conformation" in some way causes the release of SRP from the signal sequence and from the ribosome (4). Subsequent interactions of the ribosome and the signal sequence with the ER membrane are not depicted in this figure. The recycling of SRP and SR first involves GTP hydrolysis within SRα (5), which leads to a conformational change in SR that causes it dissociation from SRP and the subsequent hydrolysis of GTP bound to SRP54 (6).

confer directionality to the polypeptide targeting and insertion processes. Using a nonhydrolyzable GTP analogue (GppNHp) it has been established[148] that binding of GTP, but not its hydrolysis, is required for the displacement of the signal sequence from the SRP and for the insertion of the nascent chain into the membrane that takes place after docking on the SR. On the other hand, GTP hydrolysis is required for the dissociation of SRP from the SR,[149] which allows both components to function cyclically. Although it is not known how many and which bound GTP molecules are hydrolyzed in each round of targeting and nascent chain insertion, it has been shown that a mutation in the GTP-binding consensus sequence of the SRα subunit reduces the efficiency of the GTP-dependent insertion of the nascent chain into the membrane and prevents the formation of the stable SRP-SR complex that occurs in the presence of the GppNHp.[150]

Several plausible models can be proposed for the concerted action of the SRP and SR GTP-binding proteins in the targeting and membrane insertion processes. One of these assumes (Fig. 16-15) that binding of ribosome-associated SRP to an emerging signal sequence leads to exchange of GDP for GTP in SRP54 and that in this "active conformation" SRP binds more tightly to the ribosome in a manner that arrests translation. In its active conformation GTP-containing SRP would also have a higher affinity for the SR, to which it binds through its 68- and 72-kDa subunits. Unoccupied SR has at least its α subunit (SRα) in the GDP-bound state and the docking of SRP promotes the exchange of GTP for GDP in this subunit which, in some way, leads to release of the signal sequence from SRP54 and detachment of SRP from the ribosome. These events would not be followed immediately by hydrolysis of the GTP bound to SRP54, or else SRP would rebind to the signal at this point.[149] Hydrolysis of the GTP in the SRα subunit would follow, leading to the dissociation of the SRP-SR complex and release of SRP into the cytosol, where, after hydrolysis of its GTP, it would undergo another cycle of function. It has also been proposed that the GTPase activity of the SRβ subunit, and the accompanying conformational changes, regulate the association of the SR with other components of the translocation machinery in the membrane, to which the nascent chain is delivered after its release from SRP.[150]

Interaction of the Signal Sequence and the Nascent Polypeptide with Membrane Protein Components

After the displacement from the SRP, induced by the SRP receptor, the insertion signal and the nascent chain enter the ER membrane where they interact with protein components (see Fig. 16-11) of a putative translocation machinery, for which the term *translocon apparatus* has been proposed.[58] An association of the nascent chain with membrane proteins was first demonstrated by the observation that partially translocated, incomplete, nascent polypeptides could be removed from the microsomal membrane by treatment with agents, such as urea, that perturb protein-protein interactions but do not remove integral membrane proteins from membranes.[102] Attempts to identify components of the translocation apparatus in the ER membrane have employed crosslinking agents to link a radioactive nascent chain to dog pancreas microsome membrane proteins that are in its close proximity when it traverses the membrane. A 35- to 39-kDa glycoprotein, first thought to be a signal sequence receptor and termed SSRα, was identified in this manner.[96] However, it was later shown that this protein, also termed mp39, can be crosslinked to various other portions of the translocating polypeptide and is therefore unlikely to serve only as a signal sequence receptor.[97] Moreover, although SSRα/mp39 clearly resides in the neighborhood of the site of passage of the nascent chain throughout the course of elongation,[99] this protein does not appear to be necessary for translocation, since translocation-competent microsomes can be reconstituted with detergent extracts from which it was removed.[151] Other microsomal polypeptides have also been crosslinked to nascent chains, including a 34-kDa (imp34) nonglycosylated protein[98] and a 39-kDa multispanning membrane glycoprotein, termed TRAM (translocating chain-associating membrane glycoprotein), that appears to be required for the translocation activity of reconstituted vesicles.[100] TRAM could only be crosslinked to short nascent polypeptide chains, which indicates that it is near the nascent chain only at the beginning of its insertion and that cleavage of the signal sequence may displace it from the passageway in the membrane.

Several translocation-deficient yeast mutants have been identified in genes that encode transmembrane glycoproteins (*Sec*61p, *Sec*62p, *Sec*63p) that are part of a multisubunit complex of the type expected to function in translocation.[152] Of these, *Sec*61p and *Sec*62p could be crosslinked to nascent chains, the latter only when the nascent chains are short.[153] The mammalian homologue of *Sec*61p (40 kDa) has been purified[154] and its sequence, derived from the cloning of its cDNA, reveals that it is likely to have 10 transmembrane domains that contain a number of hydrophobic and charged amino acid residues. *Sec*61p is the major membrane component that can be crosslinked to long nascent chains in both mammalian and yeast cells. This protein is also homologous to the SecYp product of *Escherichia coli* that, together with SecE, are the only two integral membrane proteins required to effect translocation in a system of reconstituted liposomes.[155] Moreover, *Sec*61p becomes tightly associated with ribosomes during the course of translocation. Taken together, these findings raise the strong possibility that *Sec*61p represents a major constituent of the channel through which the nascent chain traverses the membrane.

Further characterization of *Sec*61p, *Sec*62p, and *Sec*63p and other recently identified SEC gene products (*Sec*70p, *Sec*71p, *Sec*72p) whose mutations affect translocation and/or membrane protein integration,[156] and of their mammalian homologues, may soon yield a more complete picture of the molecular assembly that constitutes the translocation apparatus in the ER membrane.

The Signal Peptidase

The signal peptidase activity of microsomes can be demonstrated in detergent solubilized preparations,[157] using as substrates certain completed preproteins synthesized in vitro, such as preprolactin and pregrowth hormone. Most preproteins, however, cannot be processed posttranslationally by microsomal extracts, presumably because they are folded in such a way as to sequester the signal cleavage site. This sequestration of the signal may occur before synthesis of the preprotein is completed, and the incapacity of the masked signals to interact with SRP when this is added late in translation would account for the fact that, beyond a certain length, nascent polypeptides are no longer "translocation-competent."[158]

The solubilized signal peptidase is active only in the presence of phospholipids,[159] and its activity can be inhibited by agents such as chymostatin that inhibit zinc metallopeptidases.[160] Because the peptidase activity cannot be demonstrated without detergent solubilization, and it is not destroyed by proteolysis of intact microsomes,[157,161] it can be concluded that the active site of the signal peptidase is located on the luminal side of the ER membrane (see Fig. 16-11). This location is consistent with the observation that signal cleavage does not take place before the polypeptide attains a minimal length of 70 to 90 residues, which are required to bring the cleavage site to the luminal face of the ER.

A protein complex with signal peptidase activity has been purified from solubilized dog pancreas microsomes.[162] It contains five polypeptide chains of apparent molecular weights ranging from 12 to 25 kDa, one of which is glycosylated. It is likely that only one of these polypeptides carries out the signal cleavage and that the remaining ones participate in other aspects of the translocation process, such as the degradation of the cleaved signal peptide (signal peptide peptidase) or cotranslational modifications of the nascent chain. One or more of the polypeptides in the complex may be part of the channel in the membrane through which translocation is likely to take place. It is noteworthy that neither the SSRα (mp39) nor proteins that have been implicated in ribosome binding (see below) are part of the signal peptidase complex. Two of the protein subunits of the mammalian signal peptidase display substantial sequence homology to the yeast *sec*11 protein,[163] which is also part of a complex with signal peptidase activity[164] and when mutated leads to defective signal cleavage in vivo.[165]

Ribosome Binding Sites on the ER Membrane

After displacement of the SRP by its receptor, binding of the ribosome to the ER membrane takes place (see Fig. 16-11). During the subsequent translocation, the ribosome remains associated with the ER membrane via two types of bonds—one directly linking the large ribosomal subunit and a receptor in the membrane and an indirect link that is provided by the nascent polypeptide chain.[166] The latter is broken on termination of polypeptide growth, or when a prematurely terminated polypeptide is released from the ribosome as a result of the incorporation at the C-terminus of the nascent chain of the chain-terminating peptidyl-tRNA analogue puromycin. Ribosomal subunits can then be detached from the membrane by exposure of the microsomes to mediums of high ionic strength, which disrupt electrostatic interactions between the large ribosomal subunit and its receptor. Ribosomes not containing nascent chains rebind in vitro and at low ionic strengths to rough microsomal membranes stripped of ribosomes but not to other cellular membranes, including those of smooth microsomes.[94,167,168] The number of ribosome binding sites detected by this method is equivalent to the number of ribosomes originally present in the rough microsomes.[169]

The ribosome receptors present in the rough ER contain proteinaceous components, since ribosome binding is abolished by mild proteolysis or heat treatment of the membranes.[94] The specific polypeptides involved in ribosome binding, however, have not been definitively identified. Two transmembrane glycoproteins, *ribophorins I* and *II*, are present only in rough microsomes, are found in amounts stoichiometrically related to the number of ribosomes, and appear to be associated with the binding sites.[63,64,170] These proteins, and only a few other membrane polypeptides, are recovered with the ribosomes when they are sedimented after certain nonionic detergents are used to solubilize the membranes. The proteins recovered in the membrane residue appear to form a two-dimensional network bearing ribosomes. On this basis, it has been proposed[63,64] that ribophorins also play a structural role in the rough ER, providing a scaffolding within the ER membrane that restricts the ribosome binding sites and their associated translocation apparatus to the rough domains and confers on the rough cisternae their characteristic morphology. The cDNAs for both ribophorins have been cloned.[171,172] The primary structure of the polypeptides indicates that both proteins are type I monotopic proteins that cross the membrane only once, and have C-terminal segments of 150 and 70 amino acids, respectively, exposed on the cytoplasmic face of the membrane. It now seems clear that proteins other than the ribophorins must contribute to the ribosome binding sites in the ER membrane, since mild proteolysis that does not appear to cleave the cytoplasmically exposed portions of the ribophorins abolishes the ribosome binding capacity of the membrane.[173,174] Moreover, it has been reported[175] that membrane vesicles that are capable of efficient ribosome binding can be reconstituted from purified lipids and a microsomal protein fraction from which all glycoproteins (including ribophorins) were removed by lectin chromatography. However, a function of the ribophorins associated with translocation has been suggested[176] by the finding that a protein complex consisting of both ribophorins and a 48-kDa polypeptide isolated from microsomal membranes manifests *oligosaccharyl transferase* activity, that is, it catalyzes the transfer of a high-mannose oligosaccharide from a dolichol pyrophosphate donor to asparagine residues in the peptide sequence Asn-X-Ser/Thr. This process (see below) normally occurs as the nascent glycoprotein chain emerges on the luminal side of the ER membrane.

Two other candidate proteins for ribosome receptors, a 34-kDa[177] and a 180-kDa protein,[178] have also been identified, but definitive evidence for their ribosome binding roles is yet to come.

Protein-Conducting Channel in the ER Membrane

It was originally proposed that a transient or permanent aqueous channel through the ER membrane, just under the ribosome, provides a passageway for the nascent polypeptide into the ER lumen. It seems likely that at least some of the ER membrane proteins that have been crosslinked to the nascent polypeptide chain are part of such a channel. Electrophysiological studies[103] of the properties of microsomal membranes fused to planar lipid bilayers have, in fact, demonstrated the existence of large ion-conducting channels in the ER membrane, which appear to be occupied, and therefore occluded, by the nascent polypeptide chain. The conductance of the membrane increased dramatically on addition of puromycin, a drug that releases the nascent chain. The channel also appeared to be stabilized by the bound ribosomes. The conductance was markedly reduced when the ribosomes were detached from the membrane after nascent chain release. Similar electrophysiological studies with *E. coli* plasma membranes — through which translocation in vivo can occur cotranslationally, as well as posttranslationally (i.e., without ribosome binding) — have demonstrated the existence of channels with a conductance comparable to that of those in the mammalian ER in these membranes. In this case, opening (or assembly) of the channels could be triggered by addition of a synthetic signal peptide[104] that appears to function as a physiological ligand for channel opening. These exciting findings provide hope that the full set of molecular components that constitute the prokaryotic and eukaryotic protein conducting channels will be identified within the next few years. The molecular interactions that control channel function may begin to be understood soon thereafter.

Biosynthesis of Membrane Proteins: Role of Insertion and Halt Transfer Signals in Determining Their Transmembrane Disposition[3,11,12,125,179,180]

All membrane glycoproteins and transmembrane proteins that are not contained within mitochondria or peroxisomes are synthesized in ribosomes bound to the RER and are cotranslationally inserted into the ER membrane.

Type I membrane proteins (see Fig. 16-4), which cross the membrane only once and contain their N-termini exposed on the extracellular or luminal surface of the membrane, such as the low-density-lipoprotein (LDL) and EGF receptors, the heavy chain of the histocompatibility antigen, and the much-studied hemagglutinin and G envelope glycoproteins of the influenza and vesicular stomatitis viruses, respectively, are generally synthesized with transient N-terminal insertion signals that are totally equivalent to those in secretory proteins (Fig. 16-16*a*, *b*, and *c*). These signals, via their interaction with SRP, initiate passage of the polypeptides across the membrane and their cleavage results in generation of new N-termini exposed in the lumen of the ER. In contrast to secretory proteins (Fig. 16-16*d*), translocation of a type I membrane polypeptide is interrupted by a highly hydrophobic segment, the *halt-* or *stop-transfer signal*. This sequence constitutes the sole transmembrane segment or *membrane anchoring domain* in the mature protein (Fig. 16-16*e*). The relative lengths of the luminal and cytoplasmic domains of type I polypeptides are determined by the position of the halt-transfer signal within the polypeptide. In rare instances, such as in the envelope glycoproteins of Sindbis[123] and SFV virus,[124] type I proteins contain *uncleaved N-terminal insertion signals* which, after initiating translocation, are themselves translocated and form part of the luminal domain of the mature protein.

Segments that serve as halt-transfer signals consist of approximately 20 hydrophobic or uncharged amino acids, usually followed by several basic residues (Fig. 16-17). The halt-transfer signal must allow for the reutilization of the components of the translocation apparatus in other rounds of translocation. Therefore,

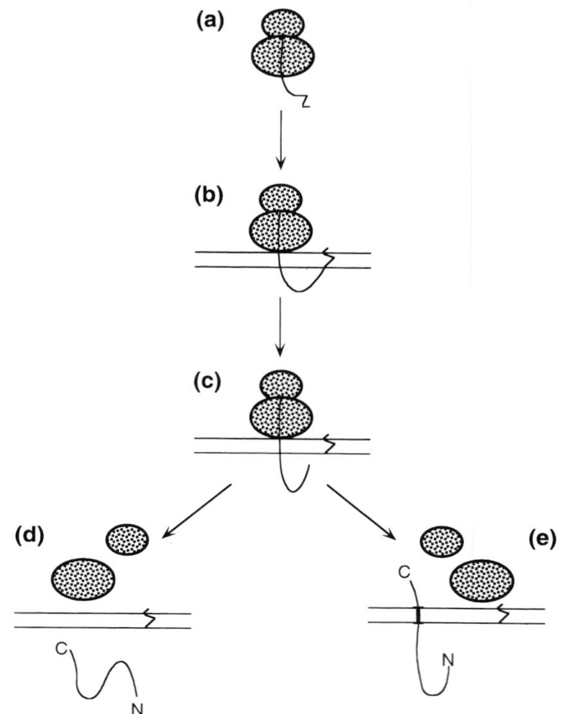

Fig. 16-16 The transmembrane disposition of a type I membrane polypeptide is established by the sequential action of a cleavable N-terminal insertion signal and an interior halt-transfer signal. The early stages of insertion of a type I membrane protein into the ER membrane (*a*, *b*, and *c*) are identical to those of a secretory protein. After signal cleavage takes place, translocation continues until a halt-transfer signal in the interior of the polypeptide reaches the membrane and stops further translocation (*e*). Secretory proteins (*d*) lack signals that stop transfer and, therefore, after completion of synthesis undergo complete vectorial discharge into the lumen of the ER.

if cotranslational translocation occurs through a protein channel, the halt-transfer signal must open this channel laterally or disassemble it to allow for the hydrophobic segment in the signal to become directly associated with the membrane phospholipids and serve as a membrane anchor. In many instances, the halt-transfer segment is located so close to the C-terminus that it must enter the membrane only after synthesis of the polypeptide has been completed and the chain released from the ribosome. In other cases, however, the halt-transfer signal is distant from the C-terminus, and elongation must continue in the cytoplasm after translocation has been halted. It is possible that in these instances the ribosome is dislodged from the membrane by the growing polypeptide chain.

The fact that the presence of the halt-transfer segment is the only feature of type I membrane proteins that distinguishes them from secretory proteins is strikingly demonstrated during B lymphocyte maturation, when the cells shift from the production of a membrane-bound form of IgM to a secretory form with the same antigen specificity.[181,182] This shift simply involves a modification in the processing of the RNA-transcript (primary transcript) from which the μ heavy chain messenger RNA is generated.[183] In pre-B cells, in which the immunoglobulin heavy chain (μ_m) is membrane-bound, the extreme 3′ portion of the coding region of the mRNA encodes the transmembrane and cytoplasmic domains of the polypeptide. At later stages, a different messenger RNA is generated from the same primary transcript. This mRNA encodes a polypeptide (μ_s) that does not contain the membrane-anchoring or cytoplasmic domains of μ_m but contains instead a short segment that includes the cysteine residue that,

Insulin receptor

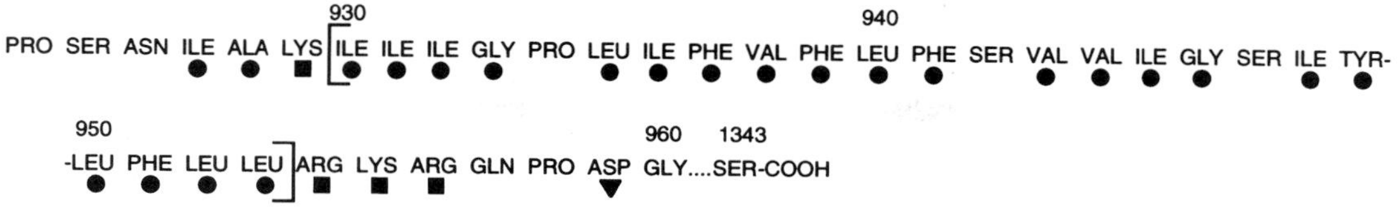

LDL receptor

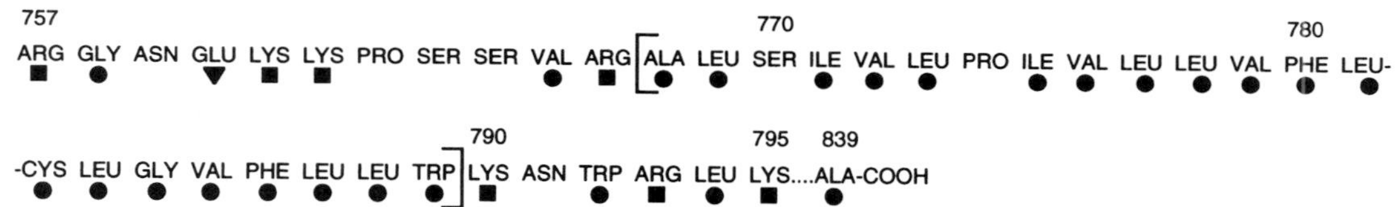

G of VSV

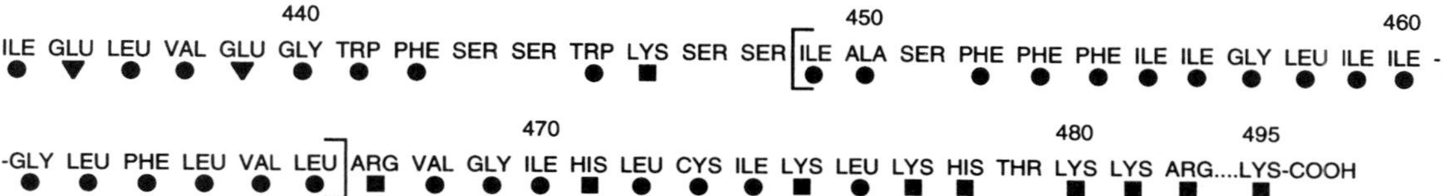

Fig. 16-17 Segments that contain the halt-transfer signal-membrane anchoring domains of type I membrane proteins. The regions of three type I membrane proteins that contain the hydrophobic segments that traverse the phospholipid bilayer in the membrane are presented. The exact borders of the transmembrane domains of these polypeptides have not been determined. Hydrophobic residues are marked with a circle, basic ones with a rectangle, and acidic residues with a triangle. Segments containing long stretches of hydrophobic amino acids uninterrupted by charged residues are enclosed within brackets. Note that these are followed by clusters of basic residues and that they are at varying distances from the C-terminus of the protein. The numbers indicate the positions of the residues within each sequence.

within the pentameric secreted IgM, forms a disulfide bond with the immunoglobulin J chain.

The exclusive role of the hydrophobic halt-transfer signal in maintaining the association of type I proteins with the membrane has been demonstrated experimentally by using genetic engineering techniques to convert membrane proteins into secretory proteins by deleting the region encoding the halt-transfer signal from the mRNA.[184,185] Moreover, in reciprocal experiments, secretory proteins have been converted into type I membrane proteins simply by introducing in them a halt-transfer signal (e.g., ref. 186). Other genetic engineering experiments have shown that 12 to 16 consecutive hydrophobic residues suffice to maintain the anchoring of a type I protein to the membrane[187] and that the charges that follow the hydrophobic segment are not essential for this purpose.[188–191]

The mechanism just described cannot, of course, account for the transmembrane disposition of type II membrane proteins, such as the asialoglycoprotein[191] and transferrin receptors,[192,193] the sucrase-isomaltase of the intestinal brush border,[194] and the neuraminidase of influenza virus.[195–197] These proteins have their C-termini exposed on the outer surface of the membrane and the N-termini on the cytoplasmic side (see Fig. 16-4). The biogenetic origin of the transmembrane disposition of these proteins can be understood, however, in the context of the loop model for the configuration of the signal and the nascent chain during translocation, as depicted in Fig. 16-18. In all these cases, the cotranslational insertion is initiated by a signal within the polypeptide that serves to mediate the translocation of its downstream portions but does not undergo cleavage and remains membrane-associated as the anchoring domain of the mature protein. A signal with these properties is frequently termed a *signal/anchor sequence type II* (S/A type II). The N-terminal portion of the polypeptide that precedes the signal, therefore, remains exposed on the cytoplasmic surface of the membrane. It should be clear that the process of insertion of a type II protein would be identical in all respects to that of a secretory protein, except that the signal does not undergo cleavage and is sufficiently hydrophobic to remain membrane-anchored after polypeptide

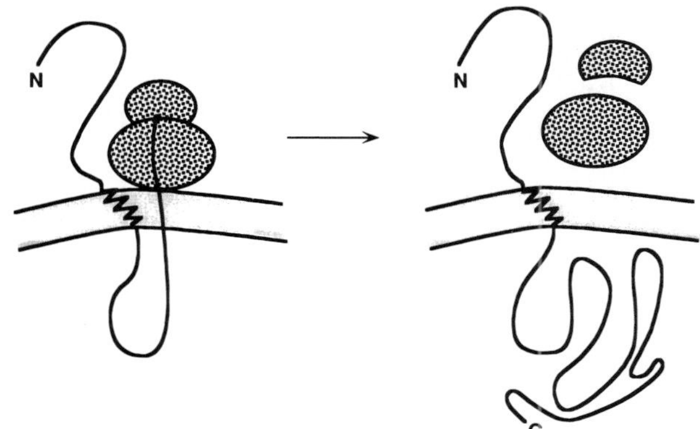

Fig. 16-18 The transmembrane disposition of a type II membrane protein results from the action of a permanent insertion signal that remains as a membrane anchor in the mature protein. The permanent insertion signal that initiates translocation of type II membrane proteins may be near the N-terminus or, as shown in the figure, in the interior of the polypeptide. Insertion begins only after the signal emerges from the ribosome and, therefore, the portion of the polypeptide preceding the signal remains on the cytoplasmic side of the membrane as the signal establishes the looped disposition of the nascent chain within the membrane. The relative lengths of the polypeptide segments on each side of the membrane are determined by the location of the permanent insertion signal within the polypeptide. This type of signal that serves to anchor a type II protein in the membrane is also referred to as a signal/anchor type II sequence (S/A II).

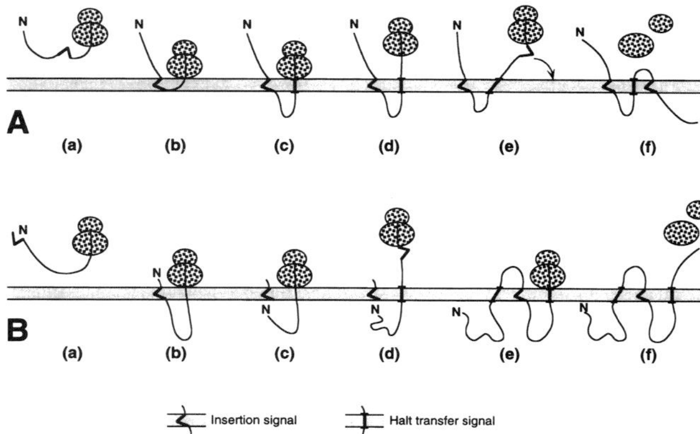

Fig. 16-19 The transmembrane disposition of proteins that traverse the membrane several times can result from the sequential action of a series of alternating insertion and halt-transfer signals. It is presumed that interior insertion signals can reinitiate translocation after this has been interrupted by the action of a preceding halt-transfer signal. Consequently, a series of insertion and halt-transfer signals leads to multiple crossings of the membrane. *A*. The first insertion signal is interior and noncleavable, so that the N-terminus of the protein remains on the cytoplasmic side of the membrane. The last signal is an insertion signal and, therefore, the S-terminal portion of the polypeptide that follows that signal is translocated into the lumen. *B*. The first insertion signal is cleavable and, therefore, the N-terminus of the protein is on the luminal side of the membrane. The last signal is a halt-transfer signal and, therefore, the C-terminus is on the cytoplasmic side. Note that, since elongation of the polypeptide continues after halt transfer, the ribosomes (in *Ad* and *Bd*) have been depicted as being detached from the membrane, until another insertion signal reinitiates translocation and reestablishes their binding to the membrane (*Be*).

chain termination. When the interior insertion signal-membrane anchoring domain of a type II protein is located at some distance from the N-terminal end, it is, of course, necessary that folding of the N-terminal portion does not mask the signal and prevent its interaction with SRP.

Membrane-anchoring domains of type I and type II proteins differ, therefore, not only in their N-to-C orientation within the membrane, but also in that those in type I proteins enter the membrane as part of a translocating polypeptide and serve to arrest translocation, whereas those in type II proteins initiate the membrane insertion process and promote the translocation of following portions of the nascent polypeptide chain.

It should be apparent that a series of alternating insertion and halt-transfer signals within a single polypeptide chain, functioning in succession, could explain the transmembrane disposition of many type III (polytopic) proteins (Fig. 16-19). In these cases, the location of the N-terminus would be determined by whether the first signal is N-terminal and transient (Fig. 16-19*A*) or internal and permanent (Fig. 16-19*B*), and the location of the C-terminus by whether the last signal is an insertion (Fig. 16-19*A*) or a halt-transfer signal (Fig. 16-19*B*). It must be emphasized, however, that the two types of transmembrane domains could be, and frequently are, very similar in their primary structure, which is what determines the stability of their interaction with the phospholipid bilayer. Whether or not a sufficiently hydrophobic segment in a polypeptide functions as an insertion or as a halt-transfer signal could therefore depend on its relative position with respect to other signals within the primary translation product,[198,199] since this determines how the segment is presented to the membrane. If preceded by an insertion signal, cleaved or uncleaved, the hydrophobic segment would enter the membrane directly as it exits the ribosome and, therefore, would halt transfer of a translocating polypeptide. If, on the other hand, the segment is preceded by a halt-transfer signal, it would emerge from the ribosome into the cytoplasm and behave as an insertion signal, promoting the translocation of downstream sequences. The insertion of this type of insertion signal, which emerges from a ribosome already targeted to the membrane, can, however, take place without the requirement for SRP,[200] which highlights that the primary function of SRP is in the initial targeting of a ribosome bearing an appropriate nascent chain to the membrane. It should be noted, however, that the hydrophobicity of a typical cleavable insertion signal, such as that in the hemagglutinin of influenza, may not be sufficient to halt transfer when the signal is paced in the interior of the translocating polypeptide.[201]

Combined Insertion Halt-Transfer Signals in Membrane Proteins

Several membrane proteins have been characterized (such as rhodopsin,[202] the evolutionarily related β_2-adrenergic receptor,[203,204] and the M2 protein encoded in the influenza virus genome[205,206]) that have glycosylated N-terminal segments located on the luminal side of the membrane and yet do not undergo signal removal during their membrane insertion. In the case of rhodopsin, which is a polytopic protein, it has been shown that the first transmembrane segment, which begins 35 residues from the N-terminus, has the capacity to initiate the insertion of the nascent polypeptide into the membrane.[207,208] Although this segment can, therefore, be regarded as an insertion signal, it is clear from the disposition of the polypeptide with respect to the membrane that it must also become a membrane anchor and act to halt translocation of following polypeptide sequences while, paradoxically, promoting the translocation of the preceding portion into the ER lumen, which in fact becomes glycosylated. The first transmembrane domain of rhodopsin is, therefore, a combined insertion-halt-transfer signal whose final orientation in the membrane is that characteristic of the regular halt-transfer signals found in type I monotopic proteins—that is, with the N-terminus in the luminal surface of the membrane. Signals of this type are frequently referred to as *signal/anchor sequences, type I* (S/A type I).

If, as it may be reasonable to assume, the signal in rhodopsin enters the membrane in a loop configuration, which would place the N-terminal portion of the protein in the cytoplasm, then the signal must later reorient to effect the transfer of the preceding peptide segment across the membrane, where its glycosylation occurs. This would lead to the dissipation of the loop and, hence, halt the translocation of amino acids following the signal, which consequently remain on the cytoplasmic side of the membrane (Fig. 16-20*A*). Alternatively, the S/A type I signal may never form a loop within the membrane but on insertion may orient itself in a way that leads to translocation of preceding sequences (Fig. 16-20*B*).

A comparison of the sequences of proteins containing S/A types I and II signals[208] and extensive mutagenesis studies indicate that an important determinant of the behavior of a signal anchor in determining the type II or I disposition is the presence of positive charges in the N-flanking segment of the signal. A prevalence of positive charges tends to retain the N-terminus on the cytoplasmic side of the membrane, and therefore confers to the protein the type II disposition (Fig. 16-20*C*). On the other hand, a prevalence of positive charges on the C-flanking segment of the signal tends to retain that portion of the polypeptide on the cytoplasmic side of the membrane, leading to the type I disposition. Of course, in the case of rhodopsin the other membrane crossings would require the action of a succession of following insertion and halt-transfer signals.

A very-well-characterized S/A type I is that present in the M2 protein encoded by influenza virus, which crosses the membrane only once with a type I transmembrane disposition. This protein lacks a cleavable signal but has a 19-amino-acid hydrophobic sequence preceded by a 24-amino-acid N-terminal ectodomain.[205,206] Replacement of the N-terminal portion of a type II integral membrane protein, comprising its type II signal/anchor, with the N-terminal portion of the M2 protein, comprising its

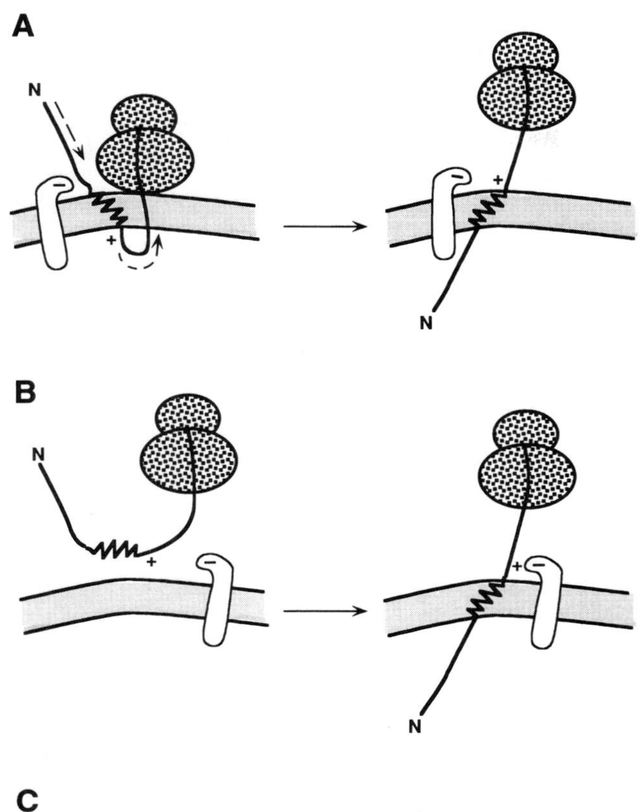

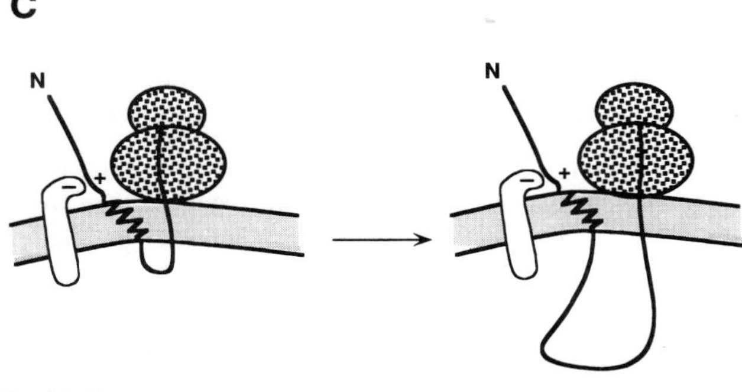

Fig. 16-20 How a combined insertion-halt transfer signal (signal/anchor I) may lead to a type I transmembrane disposition. *A.* The signal is assumed to enter the membrane in the "normal" loop configuration, but because of the absence of positive charges in the N-flanking segment and their presence in the C-flanking segment, it reorients within the membrane to translocate preceding sequences. The dissipation of the loop halts translocation of downstream sequences. *B.* Alternatively, from the early stages of insertion, the prevalence of positive charges in the C-flanking segment of the signal tends to retain that portion of the polypeptide in the cytoplasmic side of the membrane. N-flanking sequences are translocated but, in the absence of a loop, translocation of downstream sequences cannot take place. *C.* A polypeptide with positive charges in the N-flanking segment enters the membrane in a loop configuration, which is maintained throughout translocation, leading to the type II transmembrane disposition.

hydrophobic S/A type I and preceding segment, conferred to the chimeric protein the type I disposition.[209]

Signals with properties similar to those in the M2 protein and in the first transmembrane segment of rhodopsin are also present in several proteins of the ER membrane, such as cytochrome P450[210,211] and its NADPH-dependent reductase,[212] which are synthesized in membrane-bound ribosomes and have uncleaved hydrophobic N-terminal segments, but remain almost completely exposed on the cytoplasmic surface of the ER. In the case of cytochrome P450, the insertion-halt-transfer function (S/A type I) of a segment in the N-terminal portion of this protein has been directly demonstrated by genetic engineering experiments. When linked to the N-terminus of a secretory protein, such as growth hormone, this segment confers on the latter the same disposition with respect to the membrane as that of P450 itself.[210,211,213,214]

Cotranslational Modifications of Polypeptides Synthesized in the ER[215-219]

Glycoproteins are characterized by the presence of oligosaccharide chains that are linked either to nitrogen atoms of asparagine residues or to oxygen atoms of serines and threonines. In collagen, hydroxylysine residues may also bear *O*-linked sugars. The attachment of *N*-linked oligosaccharide chains to proteins takes place during the course of polypeptide chain elongation, while the nascent chains are still traversing the ER membrane (see Fig. 16-11). In this reaction, a preformed oligosaccharide (Glc3Man9GlcNAc2) (Fig. 16-21) is transferred by an *oligosaccharyltransferase* from a membrane-bound dolicholpyrophosphate lipid carrier to asparagine residues in the polypeptide backbone. The active site of this enzyme is located on the luminal face of the ER membrane and recognizes asparagine residues within the triplet sequence Asn-X-Ser/Thr, where X can be any amino acid, except proline or aspartic acid.[220,221] As previously mentioned, oligosaccharyltransferase activity has been found to be associated with a protein complex that contains the two ribophorins and a 48-kDa polypeptide.[176] It was noted that the transmembrane segment of ribophorin I contains a sequence that resembles a proposed recognition sequence for the dolichol moiety of the oligosaccharide donor.

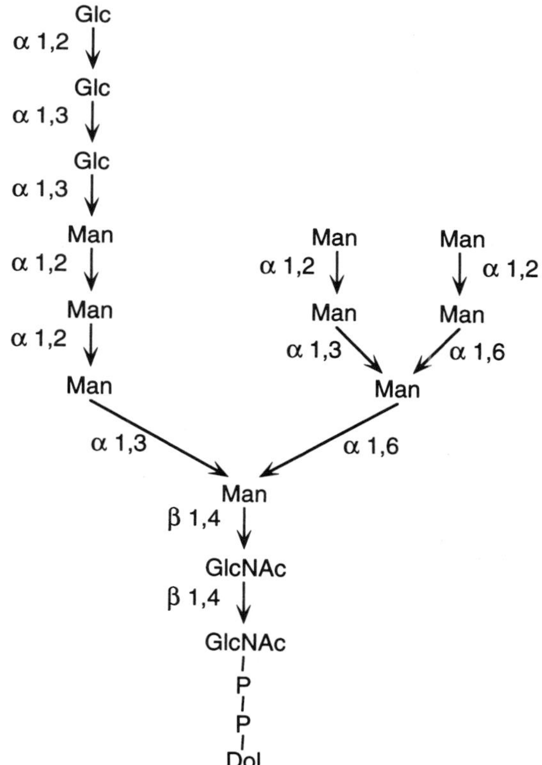

Fig. 16-21 Structure of the lipid-linked oligosaccharide precursor transferred en bloc to nascent glycoproteins. The lipid carrier dolichol pyrophosphate consists of 22 5-carbon isoprene units that are embedded in the ER membrane. After the sugars are added to the lipid carrier, by a series of reactions that are mentioned in the text, the oligosaccharide is transferred en bloc to the nascent polypeptide chain. In this process, the N-acetylglucosamine (GlcNAc) moiety linked to the dolichol pyrophosphate becomes bound to an asparagine residue by an N-glycosidic bond (Glc = glucose; Man = mannose; Dol = dolichol).

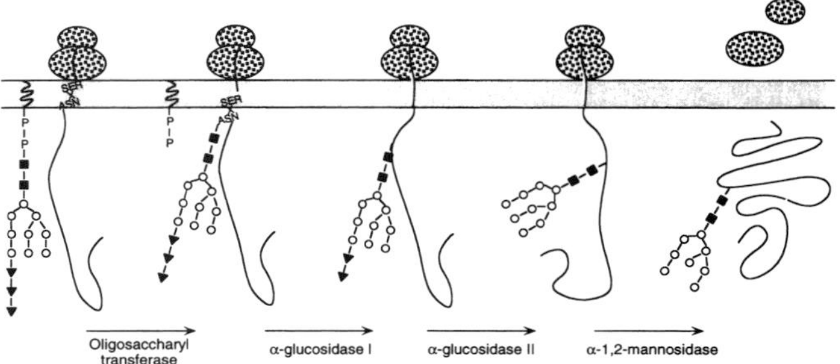

Fig. 16-22 Cotranslational transfer of an N-linked oligosaccharide to a nascent polypeptide and initial trimming in the ER. The oligosaccharyltransferase recognizes the triplet ASN-X-SER in the nascent chain and transfers the high-mannose oligosaccharide from the lipid donor to the asparagine residue. While the polypeptide chain is still growing, α-glucosidases and an α-mannosidase catalyze the sequential removal of the three glucose and one or two mannose residues. Although the glycoprotein is depicted as released into the ER lumen, the same reactions take place during the biosynthesis of membrane glycoproteins in the ER (*based on ref. 217*).

The process by which the oligosaccharide is assembled on the dolichol pyrophosphate carrier involves enzymatic reactions that take place on both sides of the membrane.[218,219] The first seven sugar residues (two GlcNAc and five Man) are transferred directly in a stepwise fashion from the nucleotide sugars UDP-GlcNAc and GDPMan to the membrane-bound dolichol phosphate, which has its acceptor site exposed on the cytoplasmic face of the membrane. It is believed that the resulting intermediate ($Man_5GlcNAc_2$-PPDol) is then reoriented so that its acceptor site is exposed on the luminal side of the membrane where it receives the remaining four mannose and three glucose residues from dolichol phosphate sugars that are formed on the cytoplasmic side but are capable of flipping across the membrane. The synthesis of the oligosaccharide chain on the lipid carrier can be inhibited by the drug *tunicamycin*, which thereby completely prevents the addition of oligosaccharides to asparagine residues.

Only about 30 percent of all the potential asparagine acceptor sites in a polypeptide actually carry oligosaccharide chains.[222] This may reflect the fact that glycosylation can take place only within a narrow window of time during polypeptide chain elongation, after the acceptor asparagine reaches the luminal side of the membrane but before folding of the polypeptide may mask it. In addition, certain asparagine-containing triplet sequences are better acceptors than others, depending on the X residue and the sequences flanking the triplet. Thus, the extent of glycosylation that can be achieved in this narrow window may vary considerably for different potential acceptor sequences.

Soon after its transfer to the polypeptide, and even before the polypeptide is completed,[223] the oligosaccharide chain begins to undergo a trimming process in which the three glucose residues and one or two mannoses are removed (Fig. 16-22). These reactions are catalyzed by α1-2 and α1-3 glucosidases (glucosidases I and II) and by an α1-2 mannosidase, respectively, that are located in the ER membrane and are likely to be closely associated with the translocation apparatus. Oligosaccharides in glycoproteins that reside permanently in the ER, such as the ribophorins[224] or HMG-CoA reductase,[225] or traverse it slowly on their way to the Golgi apparatus, may lose two additional mannose residues in the ER. Oligosaccharides in proteins that are transferred to the Golgi apparatus usually undergo further trimming of mannose residues and the addition of terminal sugars in that organelle.

As a consequence of this biosynthetic pathway, which allows for different degrees of processing of individual oligosaccharides by the ER and Golgi enzymatic enzymes, *N*-linked oligosaccharide chains in the mature glycoproteins fall into three groups (Fig. 16-23). These all share a common *pentasaccharide core structure*,[217] Man-3(Man-6)Manβ1-4GlcNAcβ1-4GlcNAc-Asn, which reflects their derivation from the same high-mannose precursor. One group, the *high-mannose oligosaccharides*, consists of oligosaccharides that generally retain two to six mannose residues linked to the pentasaccharide core. Oligosaccharides in glycoproteins that are permanent residents of the ER belong to this group. A second group consists of *complex oligosaccharides*, in which the core is generally followed by two to four branches that most frequently consist of sialyllactosamine (SA2-3 or 6Galβ1-4GlcNAc) sequences linked to the two outer mannoses of the core. In addition, in complex oligosaccharides, a "bisecting" GlcNAc residue may be bound to the first mannose in the core and a fucose may be linked to the innermost GlcNAc. The outer branches in complex oligosaccharides can vary significantly in length, and in many cases contain fucose residues and polysialic acid chains. A third group of oligosaccharides consists of *hybrid structures* in which one branch retains some of the outer mannose residues characteristic of the high-mannose chains and other branches resemble those in complex oligosaccharides. In hybrid oligosaccharides, the bisecting GlcNAc may also be attached to the first mannose.

High-mannose, but not complex or hybrid, oligosaccharide chains can be removed from glycoproteins by treatment with the enzyme endoglycosidase H,[226,227] which cleaves the core between the two GlcNAc residues. Another endoglycosidase, endo D,[228,229] hydrolyzes the same bond only when the Man residue in the core that is linked by an α1–3 bond to the first mannose is unsubstituted in the 2 position, that is, when the chain has been processed to the $Man_5GlcNAc_2$ species. However, all N-linked oligosaccharides can be removed by treatment with endoglycosidase F.[230] An increase in the electrophoretic mobility of a protein caused by treatment with any one of these enzymes demonstrates the presence of oligosaccharide chains. The acquisition of endo D sensitivity can be used as a criterion to establish the transfer of a newly synthesized glycoprotein from the ER to the *cis* Golgi, where the α1–2 mannosidase I that reduces the number of mannoses to 5 is located. The acquisition of endo H resistance indicates that further progress of the protein through the Golgi apparatus has taken place to sites where the terminal sugars characteristic of complex oligosaccharides are added.

Retention of Resident Proteins in the Endoplasmic Reticulum[231,232]

Whereas most proteins synthesized in membrane-bound ribosomes are transferred to the Golgi apparatus for incorporation into this organelle or for distribution to other sites of the cell, others remain as permanent residents of the ER, where they carry out their functions either as membrane or luminal proteins. The notion was originally suggested,[12] because of its parsimony, that retention of these proteins in the ER is an active process that results from the presence of specific signals (*retention signals*) within the polypeptides that lead them to interact with other components of the ER and prevent them from flowing into the vesicles that carry proteins to the Golgi apparatus. It has long been known (reviewed in ref. 233) that in rodent liver the enzyme β-glucuronidase has a dual localization—being present in lysosomes as well as a peripheral membrane protein in the lumen of the ER—and that a microsomal glycoprotein, egasyn, is responsible for retaining β-glucuronidase in the ER, since the latter is not detected in microsomes from egasyn-deficient mutant animals.[234–236] Moreover, in vivo dissociation of the egasyn-β-glucuronidase complex, induced by organophosphorous compounds, leads to massive and rapid secretion of β-glucuronidase into the plasma.[235] It can, therefore, be concluded that the microsomal β-glucuronidase has a retention signal that mediates its interaction with egasyn. Of course, this raises the question of how egasyn itself is retained in the ER.

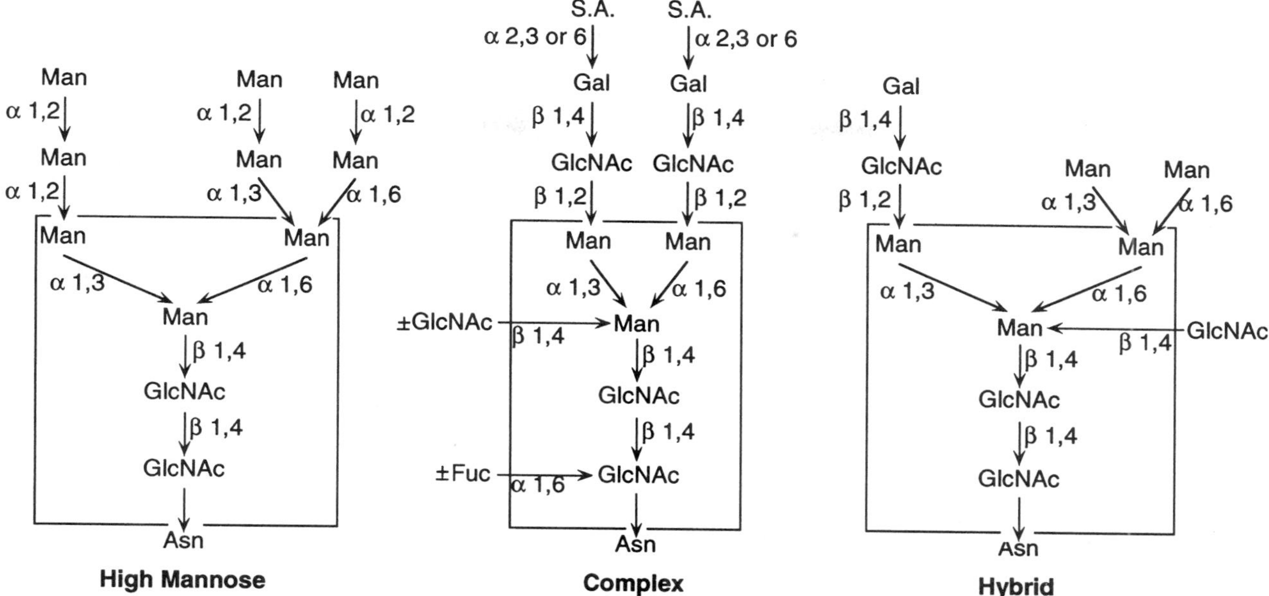

Fig. 16-23 Structures of representative high-mannose, complex, and hybrid oligosaccharides that are *N*-linked to glycoproteins: a common pentasaccharide core is present in all types of chains. The core pentasaccharide structure that is enclosed in the rectangles is present in all *N*-linked oligosaccharide chains. High-mannose oligosaccharides in glycoproteins may have from five to nine mannose units and result from the removal of the glucose residues, as well as of a variable number (zero to four) of mannose residues in the ER and *cis* Golgi from the oligosaccharide originally added to the nascent polypeptide. Some secreted proteins, such as bovine thyroglobulin, contain oligosaccharides with nine mannoses despite their passage through the Golgi apparatus. The oligosaccharides in many proteins that reach the Golgi apparatus undergo further trimming and retain only three of the mannoses and also undergo the addition of terminal sugars to the pentasaccharide core, to form complex oligosaccharide chains. The complex type of oligosaccharide depicted in the figure has only two outer branches, which consist of sialyl-lactosamine sequences (SAα2-3galβ1-4GlcNAc). Other complex oligosaccharides may have additional outer branches, as well as extra sugar residues in the outer chains. In the hybrid oligosaccharide illustrated, only one branch of the original oligosaccharide has been fully trimmed and received terminal sugars. A single purified glycoprotein may show considerable microheterogeneity in its oligosaccharide chains (SA = sialic acid; Gal = galactose; Man = mannose; GlcNAc = N-acetylglucosamine; Fuc = fucose; Asn = asparagine).

The fact that specific information within a protein is not required for it to be exported from the ER and, therefore, proteins that lack retention signals exit from the ER by default is strikingly demonstrated by the observation that β-lactamase, a protein of bacterial origin that could not possibly contain information for passage out of the ER, is secreted when it is synthesized in amphibian oocytes that are microinjected with the corresponding mRNA.[237]

In recent years much evidence has accumulated demonstrating that many luminal proteins of the ER, such as protein disulfide isomerase, microsomal esterases, reticulin and two glucose-regulated proteins (Grp74 and Grp 78 or Bip), and some membrane proteins, are actively concentrated in this organelle by a mechanism that involves a retrieving receptor that, in one or more post-ER compartments, recognizes a signal in the escaped ER proteins and returns them to their site of primary residence. This retention signal consists of a C-terminal tetrapeptide sequence (Lys-Asp-Glu-Leu; KDEL; or a closely related one) that is both necessary and sufficient to cause retention of the protein in the ER, and for which a recycling receptor has been identified.[238–240] For several luminal proteins it has been shown that deletion of the tetrapeptide signal leads to their secretion,[241,242] whereas the addition of the signal to the C-terminus of a secretory protein (lysozyme) leads to its retention in the ER.[242]

The first evidence that proteins containing a KDEL sequence continuously escape from the ER to a *salvage compartment*, which may be an intermediate compartment between the ER and the Golgi apparatus, or the *cis* region of the Golgi apparatus itself (see below), but are returned to the ER, was obtained from the behavior of a chimeric protein consisting of a lysosomal enzyme, cathepsin D, to which a KDEL signal was added.[243] Immunofluorescence studies showed that this protein accumulated in the ER but, nevertheless, it was modified by the enzyme *N*-acetylglucosamine-1-phosphotransferase, which participates in the synthesis of the lysosomal targeting marker, mannose 6-phosphate, and is believed to be located in the *cis* Golgi (see below). Further evidence that resident ER luminal proteins escape from the ER and are retrieved was obtained in yeast. A chimeric protein containing an HDEL C-terminal tetrapeptide (which for certain strains of yeast is functionally equivalent to the mammalian KDEL) also underwent a Golgi-specific glycosylation reaction. However, it did so only if the cells did not carry mutations in the secretory machinery (a *sec* mutation) that made them defective in transport of proteins out of the ER under the experimental conditions used.[244] An elegant selection procedure was devised to identify mutants deficient in the ER retention mechanism.[238] This allowed the cloning of the yeast HDEL receptor gene (ERD2).[238] This in turn led to the subsequent cloning of the cDNA for its human (KDEL binding) counterpart (hERD2).[245] Both the yeast and the mammalian receptors were found to reside primarily in the Golgi apparatus normally,[238–245] as would be expected if the receptors have a "retrieving" rather than a direct "retaining" function. Even more convincing evidence for the recycling function of the receptor came from the demonstration that, in mammalian cells, overexpression of proteins containing the KDEL signal leads to redistribution of the receptor molecules to the ER.[240] This redistribution did not occur when the receptor protein was modified to reduce its affinity for the signal. Interestingly, a C-terminal, luminally exposed, HDEL signal that mediates retention in the ER has also been identified in a yeast transmembrane ER protein, the product of the SEC20 gene.[246] This type II membrane protein, itself, is thought to function in vesicular transport from the ER to the Golgi apparatus and it is, therefore, possible that its receptor-mediated shuttling between these compartments is essential for its function.

The yeast ERD2 gene that encodes the HDEL receptor is essential for growth. Its role in sustaining retrograde transport is apparently essential for maintaining a balance in the bidirectional traffic of membrane constituents between the ER and the Golgi apparatus. Genes that suppress the ERD2 deletion (SED genes) when overexpressed have been identified. One of these (SED5) encodes a 39-kDa protein that is required for ER-to-Golgi transport.[247] This protein has a C-terminal membrane anchor that is largely exposed on the cytoplasmic side of the membrane and has a region of similarity with *syntaxin*, a presynaptic membrane protein that appears to play a role in synaptic vesicle docking at the plasma membrane (see below). The capacity of overexpressed SED5 to suppress the deleterious effect of the ERD2 mutation is likely to be due to an inhibitory effect that it has on anterograde ER-to-Golgi protein flow for a yet unknown reason.

Clearly, the major mechanistic questions about the function of the retrieving KDEL receptor concern what determines that the proteins to be retrieved bind to it in the salvage compartment but are released in the ER. How does the movement of the receptor from one compartment to another take place, and how is the movement regulated? These are related questions, since the binding of the ligand to the receptor in the salvage compartment must somehow trigger its transport back to the ER. It would seem likely that the different environmental conditions in the lumen of the ER and post-ER compartments, such as decreasing Ca^{2+} concentration and pH, play important roles in regulating the association of the receptor and its ligands (Fig. 16-24). In fact, recent in vitro binding studies have demonstrated that optimal binding of the receptor to its ligands occurs at the acid pH (pH 5 to 6) that prevails in the Golgi apparatus, whereas very little binding occurs at pH 7, thought to be characteristic of the ER.[248] It is interesting to note that in some cell types, such as hepatocytes and pancreatic exocrine cells in which the Golgi environment is neutral, a variety of KDEL-containing proteins escape from the ER.[249]

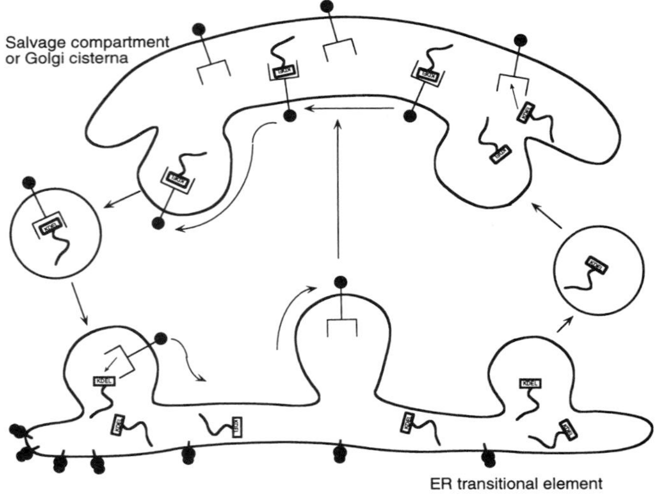

Fig. 16-24 A receptor retrieves escaped ER proteins that contain the KDEL signal from a salvage compartment or from Golgi cisternae. Transmembrane KDEL receptor molecules are normally found in the salvage compartment or Golgi cisternae, where they avidly bind to any escaped luminal ER proteins (right side) that bear the C-terminal KDEL tetrapeptide. The complexes are incorporated into vesicles that bring them back to the ER (left side), where the conditions of neutral pH, and possibly the higher Ca^{2+} concentration, lead to the release of the retrieved proteins from the receptors, which return to their original location (middle budding vesicle in the transitional element).

The retention of most membrane proteins in the ER appears to depend on other types of signals and retention mechanisms. A short cytoplasmic sequence at the C-terminus of the adenovirus membrane glycoprotein E19 is required for its retention in the ER.[250,251] At early times during viral infection, the E19 glycoprotein helps the infected cells to escape from immune surveillance by cytotoxic T lymphocytes. It does so by interacting in the ER with newly synthesized class I major histocompatibility antigen molecules and preventing their transport out of the ER.[252] Similar cytoplasmic C-terminal retention signals have been demonstrated to function in several other ER membrane proteins, including different forms of UDP-glucuronyltransferase, 3-hydroxy-3-methylglutaryl CoA reductase, and a 53-kDa membrane protein of the sarcoplasmic reticulum.[251,253] In all of these cases a *double-lysine motif*, such as XKKXX, KXKXX, or XXKKX, is present at the extreme C-terminus, and addition of one of these sequences to another protein was sufficient to cause its retention in the ER. Moreover, replacement of the lysine at position −3, as well as deletion or addition of even a single amino acid to the C-terminus of the ER protein, abolished the function of the retention signal.[253,254] A study of the subcellular distribution and the posttranslational modifications undergone by chimeric proteins containing the dilysine motif expressed in transfected cells indicated that a retrieving mechanism also contributes to the ER localization of these proteins.[255]

Other ER transmembrane proteins do not contain "double lysine" motifs, and their retention in the organelle appears to be determined by other features of the polypeptides. For example, the C-terminal segments of the cytoplasmic domains of ribophorins I and II and of a 22- to 23-kDa subunit of the signal peptidase do not cause retention of other reporter proteins to which they have been transferred.[253] One plausible mechanism[256] for the retention of these and other components of the translocation apparatus in the ER is their association with other proteins. Their incorporation into the extensive proteinaceous network which exists within the ER membrane and is associated with the ribosome binding sites may prevent entrance of the proteins into the carrier vesicles that emerge from the ER. The formation of multiprotein complexes may also account for the retention in the ER of proteins that have large portions exposed on the cytoplasmic side of the ER membrane, such as cytochrome P_{450} and its reductase, the major components of the microsomal monoxygenase system. Indeed, the formation of multiprotein complexes may be a general mechanism for the retention of proteins within organelles.

Protein Folding, Oligomerization, and Quality Control in the ER[145,257–260a]

In addition to undergoing covalent modifications, polypeptides synthesized in the ER must fold and, in many cases, associate with other subunits to form a mature protein. For both luminal and membrane proteins, these processes must take place in the ER, where conditions are very different from the strongly reducing environment and low calcium concentration of the cytosol. Completion of the folding and assembly processes is necessary for the resulting protein to be transported out of the ER. In this way, the ER exercises quality control on its own products. The fate of the misfolded or unassembled polypeptide subunits is usually degradation within the ER itself,[259,261,262] although in some instances partially assembled polypeptide complexes may leave the ER to be degraded within lysosomes.

The fact that proteins must have a "normal conformation" to be transported out of the ER is most strikingly demonstrated by the behavior of certain multimeric proteins, when their assembly in the ER is perturbed (e.g., ref. 263). Thus, immunoglobulin heavy chains are not transported out of the ER unless the light chains are also present.[264] Similarly, in some cases, the heavy chain of the class I major histocompatibility antigen, which is a type I transmembrane protein, does not exit from the ER unless it becomes associated with β_2-microglobulin.[265,266] Moreover, the formation of a transport-competent MHC class I molecule that on the surface of the cell presents antigenic peptides to cytotoxic T lymphocytes is dependent on its acquisition of the antigenic peptide in the ER. The peptides are generated by proteolysis in the cytosol and are transported into the lumen of the ER by specific transporters (the products of the TAP1 and TAP2 genes) in the ER membrane (see ref. 267). The influenza HA and the VSV G viral envelope glycoproteins must also form oligomers (trimers) in the ER to be transported to the Golgi apparatus.[268–270] Numerous examples also exist of proteins that are normally secreted or transferred to the plasma membrane, but remain in the ER when altered by genetic engineering techniques. The fact that a "normal" conformation that makes the protein "soluble and transportable" is required for exit from the ER would explain the accumulation in this organelle, and the failure to be secreted, of a mutant form of the human serum protein *α_1-antitrypsin*,[271,272] as well as of nonsecreting variants of immunoglobulin chains in certain myelomas.[273] Similarly, many human LDL receptor mutations leading to familial hypercholesterolemia are characterized by the failure of the receptor to be transported out of the ER.[274,275]

The retention in the ER of defective luminal or membrane proteins may not be simply due to their insolubility within the organelle but, at least in some cases, may also be due to their specific recognition by *Bip* (or Grp78),[276] a resident protein of the ER[241] that belongs to the class of molecular chaperones. In B lymphocytes, this 78-kDa protein normally binds to the free heavy chains, or to incompletely assembled immunoglobulin molecules, preventing their premature exit from the ER and, therefore, their secretion from the cell.[144,277] In the *lymphoproliferative heavy chain disease*, in which heavy chains are secreted in the absence of light chains, a deletion mutation in the heavy chain constant region gene that eliminates the CH4 domain of the protein reduces its affinity for Bip.[277] Although Bip was first recognized in pre-B-cell lines that do not yet synthesize light chains,[276,278] its presence has now been demonstrated in many other cell types in which it was found to form complexes with abnormal or incompletely assembled secretory and membrane proteins. Bip is a member of the heat-shock (or stress) family of proteins (hsp), and it accumulates at high levels in the lumen of the ER of cultured fibroblasts when these are subjected to the stress of glucose starvation, or are treated with tunicamycin to prevent *N*-glycosylation.[241] It was originally proposed that by binding to and blocking the transport to the cell surface of abnormally folded polypeptides, Bip may play a role in protecting the organism from the adverse effects that could result from the recognition by the immune system of denatured "self" polypeptides as foreign antigens.[270] On the other hand, as the concept of "molecular chaperone" has evolved, the prevalent view has emerged that, in many instances, the normal function of Bip—rather than to simply prevent exit from the ER—is to stabilize a newly synthesized polypeptide in a form that allows it to achieve its final structure more efficiently, which may require additional folding steps or assembly with other subunits.[17] This is in accord with the fact that the CH1 domain of the immunoglobulin heavy chain, to which Bip binds, is the same portion of the polypeptide that interfaces with the light chain.

Another ER protein that appears to function as a molecular chaperone is an 88-kDa transmembrane protein, *calnexin* (p88),[279] that associates with the MHC class I heavy chain in the ER and may remain associated with it during the formation of the complex with β_2-microglobulin and the antigenic peptide. Binding of the antigenic peptide to MHC molecules may lead to release of the chaperone and export of the complex to the Golgi apparatus.[280,281] The same protein also associates with incompletely assembled T-cell antigen receptors and membrane-bound immunoglobulins.[282]

Protein Degradation in the ER[259,261]

As part of its quality-control function, the ER is capable of carrying out the degradation of many improperly folded or incompletely assembled polypeptides that are retained within it. In addition, the capacity of the ER for protein degradation[283] allows it to play a role in the regulation of some metabolic pathways that utilize ER enzymes, as exemplified by the cholesterol-controlled degradation of HMG-CoA reductase,[284,285] an enzyme whose activity is rate limiting for sterol biosynthesis.

Known substrates for ER degradation include unassembled subunits of the T cell, acetylcholine and asialoglycoprotein receptors, as well as mutant forms of the LDL receptor and of α_1-antitrypsin, the cystic fibrosis transmembrane regulator, and β-hexosaminidase. The degradation of these polypeptides begins soon after their synthesis is completed and proceeds with a half-life of 1 h or less.[259]

The ER degradation system is highly discriminatory with respect to substrate selection. This is best illustrated by studies of the fate of unassembled or partially assembled subunits of the *T-cell receptor* (TCR). This receptor is composed of at least eight (α, β, γ, δ, $\varepsilon 2$, $\zeta 2$) transmembrane polypeptides,[286] which normally form a complex in the ER that is rapidly transported through the Golgi apparatus to the cell surface. In a T-cell hybridoma in which the TCR ζ chains were made in much lower amounts than the other subunits, incomplete multimeric complexes lacking ζ chains were formed and were transported to the Golgi apparatus, but were then diverted to lysosomes for degradation.[287] On the other hand, in a hybridoma in which the δ chains were not synthesized, α chains and α-β disulfide-linked heterodimers were rapidly degraded within the ER itself.[288] Similarly, when individual subunits of the TCR were expressed in transfected fibroblasts,[288,289] the α, β, and δ chains underwent rapid degradation in the ER, although under the same conditions the ζ and ε subunits were stable. Strikingly, the murine γ chain, when expressed by itself, was rapidly degraded, but it was markedly stabilized after it formed a complex with the ε chain.[289]

Studies done primarily with the α chain have attempted to identify the structural features of the isolated TCR subunits that determine their pre-Golgi degradation. The observation[290] that a truncated α chain that consisted only of its luminal domain was retained in the ER but was much more stable than the intact polypeptides, suggested that the transmembrane domain of this polypeptide (this is unusual in that it contains two positively charged amino acids) is responsible for the rapid rate of degradation of the α chain. This hypothesis was substantiated by the finding that transfer of a nine-amino-acid segment of the α-chain transmembrane domain, containing the charged residues, into the transmembrane domain of the *Tac* antigen (the Il-2 receptor) was sufficient to cause retention and rapid degradation of the chimeric protein in the ER. Furthermore, elimination of the charged residues led to escape from the ER of a *Tac* polypeptide containing the TCR α-chain transmembrane domain.[291] These experiments demonstrate that the positively charged residues in the transmembrane domain constitute a critical determinant for the retention and degradation of the α chain in the ER. The availability of this determinant to the degradative system appears to be controlled by the state of assembly of the polypeptide. Thus, association of the α chain with the δ chain, which contains two negatively charged residues in its transmembrane domain, leads to masking of the determinant and to formation of a stable dimeric complex.[292,293] It thus appears that the charged residues have the mutually exclusive roles of targeting the polypeptide for ER degradation or participating in subunit assembly,[294] so that quality control on the assembly process can be exerted by a mechanism that senses the exposure of the charged residues within the ER membrane.

Little is known about the nature of the proteases that carry out the degradation of abnormal or unassembled polypeptides in the ER, or even if the same proteases are involved in the normal turnover of ER resident proteins. The degradative enzymes, however, must be able to function at the high calcium concentration characteristic of the lumen of the ER. Indeed, exposure of cells to calcium ionophores in the presence of EGTA, which leads to the depletion of intracellular Ca^{2+}, inhibited the ER degradation.[256] This observation, together with the finding that calcium depletion accelerated the already rapid degradation of the TCR δ and β chains,[295] indicates that changes in Ca^{2+} concentration alter the susceptibility of the substrates to the proteases. Most likely, ER degradation involves a constellation of enzymes, since the degradation of different substrates has been found to be blocked by protease inhibitors of different specificities.[295,296]

TRANSFER OF PROTEINS FROM THE ER TO THE GOLGI APPARATUS[12,18,56,297–303a]

ER-to-Golgi transport was first demonstrated in pancreatic acinar cells, where the vast majority of the newly synthesized proteins are digestive enzymes to be stored in secretory granules (see ref. 56). Autoradiographic analysis of pulse-labeled slices of pancreatic tissue and cell fractionation studies[304,305] established that the newly synthesized proteins exit from the ER at specialized ER cisternae, known as *transitional elements* or *transitional cisternae,* that are located close to the receiving (*cis*) face of the Golgi apparatus (see Fig. 16-1). Transitional cisternae are partly "rough" and partly "smooth." Nonclathrin-coated coated vesicles and/or tubular elements appear to emerge from their smooth portions. Early cytochemical and immunocytochemical studies demonstrated the presence of specific secretory proteins in the transitional elements and in the vesicles located near the *cis* side of the Golgi apparatus.[306,307] It has therefore been assumed that the tubulovesicular elements seen near the transitional cisternae serve as carriers that transport newly synthesized proteins to the Golgi apparatus.[56] It is now clear, however, that the ER-Golgi interface is a complex region and at least some of the elements that it contains may also be functioning in a retrograde transport that retrieves to the ER constituents that either escaped the organelle or are to be reutilized in new rounds of anterograde transport.

ER-to-Golgi transport is an energy-requiring process and, therefore, can be halted by anoxia or by drugs, such as azide or antimycin, that inhibit respiration, or by inhibitors of oxidative phosphorylation, such as dinitrophenol, oligomycin, or carbonylcyanide *m*-chlorophenylhydrazone (CCCP).[308–313] When the energy supply is exhausted, the proteins accumulate in the transitional elements or in vesicles between them and the *cis* face of the Golgi apparatus.

The kinetics of transport of specific proteins from the ER to the Golgi apparatus have been followed in tissues and in cultured cells by analyzing the acquisition of endo H resistance in polypeptides purified by immunoprecipitation with specific antibodies. Studies with both secretory and integral membrane proteins destined for the cell surface[314–317] have shown that different proteins are transported from the ER to the cell surface at different rates, with half times for transport varying from 10 min to $1\frac{1}{2}$ h. The rate limiting step appears to be passage from the ER to the Golgi apparatus, with transport from this organelle to the cell surface occurring at the same fast rate for all proteins in a given cell. Using cells infected with a temperature-sensitive vesicular stomatitis virus, the transport of the G glycoprotein through the Golgi apparatus has been visualized directly by immunoelectron microscopy. At the nonpermissive temperature, the envelope glycoprotein accumulates in the ER, but within 5 to 10 min after the infected cells are shifted to the permissive temperature,[318,319] it appears in the Golgi cisternae concomitantly with its acquisition of endo H resistance.

Two possible interpretations can be given to the different rates observed for the transport of proteins out of the ER. One is that, in a manner analogous to receptor-mediated endocytosis at the plasma membrane (see below), rapid transport of the proteins requires their interaction with a receptor or carrier in the ER that is incorporated into transport vesicles and that those proteins with highest affinity for the receptor are transported most rapidly. This implies that the transported proteins contain a sorting signal for interaction with the receptor and, hence, that proteins that lack such signals would move at a uniform slow rate, unless they contain a retention signal that completely excludes them from the transport vesicles. In this view, proteins that are transported by default (i.e., lack transport or retention signals) would be free to diffuse in the fluid phase that exists within the luminal cavities of the transporting vesicles and of all the organelles within the endomembrane system and to finally reach the cell surface.[320] A similar default pathway to the plasma membrane could be followed by membrane proteins lacking signals that would be capable of moving by diffusion within the phospholipid bilayers of all the membranes and vesicular carriers that compose the endomembrane system.

In another interpretation, a rapid *bulk flow*, of soluble as well as membrane components, would have its source in the ER and would take place constantly toward the surface of the cell.[320,321] Proteins destined to become permanent residents of the various organelles of the endomembrane system, including the ER itself and the Golgi cisternae, would contain retention signals for local assembly that are recognized by other components of those organelles, with which the newly arrived proteins form oligomeric complexes. In this view, the rate of transport of a protein out of the ER would be determined by the time required for its proper folding, oligomerization and maturation in that organelle. Once secretory, lysosomal, or plasma membrane proteins reach the *trans*-Golgi region, a process that sorts them from each other would take place.

The concept of a rapid bulk flow that begins in the ER is based on studies of the kinetics of uptake and reexport by mammalian cells of simple synthetic peptides that contain an acceptor site for *N*-glycosylation.[320] After entering the cell, these peptides cross the ER membrane, become glycosylated, and reappear in the medium within 10 min. It was thought that after their glycosylation the peptides could no longer cross the membranes of the endomembrane system and, therefore, could exit from the cells only by traversing the entire secretory pathway. Hence, the rapid export of the peptides was taken as reflecting the rapid rate of bulk flow.[320] The validity of this conclusion has been brought into question by experiments showing that the glycosylated peptides do not all exit with the same kinetics from cultured mammalian cells, and that they do not exit at all from Xenopus oocytes, which are capable of secreting almost any secretory protein.[321a] Moreover, studies with yeast indicate that the ER contains an ATP-dependent pump capable of extruding glycosylated peptides directly into the cytosol, from which the peptides could conceivably be secreted from the cells by an equivalent pump present in the plasma membrane.[322]

Insights into ER-to-Golgi Transport Obtained from Studies with Yeast[18,18a,301,302,323]

The study of ER-to-Golgi transport in yeast has been greatly advanced by a combination of biochemical and genetic approaches and has greatly illuminated the equivalent process in mammalian cells. Temperature-sensitive mutations in more than 20 different yeast genes defined by complementation analysis have been obtained that disrupt this transport step at the nonpermissive temperature.[324–327] In most cases, the corresponding wild-type gene could be isolated by complementation and, frequently, extragenic suppressor genes that compensate for the specific mutation when expressed at high levels were identified using libraries constructed in high copy plasmid vectors. At the nonpermissive temperature, mutations in genes involved in ER-to-Golgi transport lead to the expansion of the ER and the accumulation of core-glycosylated forms of secretory protein (e.g., pro-α-factor and invertase) or vacuolar proteins (e.g., carboxypeptidase Y) in this organelle. Many *sec* mutants of this type could be categorized in two classes: those that are defective in vesicle formation (class I; e.g., *sec*12, *sec*13, *sec*16, *sec*23) and those in which vesicles ($\sim$50 nm in diameter) are formed but accumulate within the cell at the nonpermissive temperature (class II; e.g., *sec*17, *sec*18, *sec*22). Apparently, class II mutants have a defect in a subsequent step required for targeting or fusion of the vesicle to the acceptor organelle, the Golgi apparatus.[327]

The assignment of the various mutant strains to one class or the other was facilitated by an *epistasis test*, in which vesicle accumulation was assessed in haploid yeast strains in which two of the mutations were present. This test showed that class I mutations are epistatic with respect to class II, that is, no vesicles accumulated when a mutation in a class I gene was present together with a mutation in a class II gene, and, therefore, that the formation of the vesicles that accumulate at the nonpermissive temperature in the class II mutants depends on the function of class I genes.[327] In addition, the phenomenon of *synthetic lethality* allowed the recognition of genes whose products function in the same step, and may even interact with each other. In such cases, the cells containing both mutations may fail to grow or may secrete at a lower temperature than cells containing either single mutation.[327] In this test, the combination of *sec*17 and *sec*18, as well as five of the six possible pairwise combinations between *sec*12, *sec*13, *sec*16, and *sec*23, exhibited synthetic lethality.

The specific functions of many of the products of the genes involved in vesicle formation and fusion are currently being gleaned from: (1) an analysis of the cloned sequences, (2) the behavior of cell extracts derived from mutants, or depleted of specific gene products, in in vitro assays for overall ER-to-Golgi transport or for the partial steps of vesicle formation or vesicle delivery, (3) the effects in these assays of adding either specific antibodies to purified proteins, or the products themselves of the normal or mutant *SEC* genes, which can be produced in large amounts by recombinant DNA procedures, and (4) the identification and characterization of the gene products of suppressor genes.

The availability of experimental systems that utilize disrupted or perforated yeast or mammalian cells, or cell fractions derived from them, to reconstitute interorganellar transport steps in vitro has permitted the study of the requirements for cytosolic components, as well as of the effects of various impermeant inhibitors, nucleotides, antibodies, peptides, and proteins on transport. The main systems used to investigate ER-to-Golgi transport in yeast employ disrupted spheroplasts[328,329] or microsomal fractions that contain both donor ER and Golgi acceptor membranes.[330] Transport is measured from the extent to which a secretory protein, pro-α-factor, undergoes Golgi-specific outer-chain modifications of its oligosaccharides. ^{35}S-labeled prepro-α-factor is first synthesized in vitro and introduced into the yeast microsomes, or into the ER of permeabilized cells, in a posttranslational translocation reaction (that occurs in yeast and not in mammalian cells). Transport leads to removal of the signal sequence and core glycosylation at three sites within the polypeptide. Vesicular transport from the ER to the Golgi apparatus takes place only when the system is incubated at physiological temperatures in the presence of cytosol and a continuous supply of ATP. With these in vitro systems it has been possible to separate transport into the successive stages of vesicle formation, targeting or docking, and fusion. Indeed, these systems have provided the only direct evidence available for the role of vesicles as mediators of protein transport between organelles.

Much has been learned of the functions of proteins required for vesicle formation in the ER and the intermolecular interactions that take place during this event. Some class I gene products (*sec*12p and *sec*23p) appear to regulate the cyclic function of a low-molecular-weight *ras*-related GTP-binding protein, *Sar1p*, during the process of vesicle formation. Gene cloning and the use of specific antibodies permitted the demonstration that *Sec*12p is a type II integral membrane protein of the ER whose large N-terminal cytoplasmic domain interacts with Sar1p and recruits it from the cytosol.[331] Sar1p was first identified as a suppressor gene product that, when present at high levels, compensates for a mutation in *Sec*12p. Genetic studies showed that it too was necessary for ER-to-Golgi transport.[332] The suppressor effect of Sar1p was also observed in vitro when the protein was added in excess to a transport system containing ER membranes defective in *Sec*12p.[333] It now appears[326] that the exchange of GDP for GTP that leads to the activation of Sar1p is catalyzed by *Sec*12p. This explains why overexpression of Sar1p, with a concomitant increase in the amount of its active GTP-containing form, can compensate for a partial deficiency in *Sec*12p. The GTPase activity of Sar1p is not required for its function in vesicle production, but is required to complete a round of transport, since when the protein is precharged with the nonhydrolyzable analogue GTP-γ-S instead of GTP, it cannot support transport in a Sar1p-depleted extract. The completion of the cycle of GTP utilization by Sar1p seems to involve another class I Sec gene product, *Sec*23p, that, acting as a GAP protein, stimulates the GTPase activity of Sar1p[334] and leads to its release from the vesicle, which now can enter into the targeting phase of vesicular transport in which Ypt1, another low-molecular-weight GTP binding protein, plays a critical role (see below). *Sec*23p is an 85-kDa cytosolic protein that forms a complex with a 105-kDa protein, identified by coimmunoprecipitation and subsequently cloned, now designated *Sec*24p, that is also required for vesicle budding from the ER.[335] Antibodies to the yeast *Sec*23p localize the homologous mammalian protein in exocrine and endocrine pancreatic cells to the cytoplasmic region between the transitional cisternae and the Golgi apparatus,[336] where at least some of the protein appears to be bound to the membranous tubulovesicular elements that characterize that region. The restricted localization of the mammalian homologue of *Sec*23p led to the suggestion that it is associated with an organized structure within the transitional zone of the cell that serves to facilitate vesicular flow from the ER toward the Golgi and permits the efficient reutilization of the protein in many rounds of vesicular transport.

Another class I gene product, *Sec*13p, is also a cytosolic protein (33 kDa) that is peripherally associated with the ER membranes, and is required for vesicle formation and release in vitro.[326] Strikingly, *Sec*13p is normally a component of a very large (700-kDa) cytosolic macromolecular complex, which includes other proteins. When its gene is overexpressed, however, the monomeric form of *Sec*13p that accumulates is also active in a *Sec*13p-dependent vesicle formation assay. The sequence of *Sec*13p consists of a series of repeating polypeptide segments that show homology to a segment that is also repeated in other proteins involved in a variety of cellular processes, including signal transduction (e.g., the β subunit of the heterotrimeric G protein *transducin*) and cell cycle progression. Since *Sec*13p shows synthetic lethal interactions with *Sec*12 and *Sec*23, whose products function in the GTP cycle of Sar1p, it is possible that *Sec*13p also participates in that cycle, either as an upstream regulator at the guanine nucleotide exchange event, as one might expect for a G protein, or as a downstream effector of Sar1p that promotes the budding process itself. If the latter were the case, *Sec*13p could be a component of a coat required for vesicle budding, to promote the assembly of such a coat, to induce the deformation of the donor membrane, or to participate in the membrane fission event that completes the generation of a free vesicle.

Several proteins involved in vesicle docking at the Golgi apparatus have also been studied extensively. One of these is Ypt1p,[337,338] a member of the *rab* family of GTP-binding proteins that shows extensive homology to *Sec*4p, a protein required for vesicle delivery from the Golgi apparatus to the plasma membrane. Ypt1p and *Sec*4p were the first low-molecular-weight GTP-binding proteins shown to have essential functions in protein traffic. From their discovery stems most of our recent knowledge of the role of *rab* family members in vesicular transport. Under restrictive conditions, temperature-sensitive mutants in Ypt1p manifest a defect in ER-to-Golgi transport, both in vivo and in vitro, and vesicles accumulate in the intact cells. In addition, antibodies to Ypt1p block transport in vitro,[339] but do not inhibit vesicle formation.[340] A mammalian homologue of Ypt1p, *rab1a*, has been identified that can functionally replace Ypt1p in a yeast temperature-sensitive strain,[19] and it was shown to be required for ER-to-Golgi transport in a mammalian cell-free system.[341]

It is currently thought that Ypt1p action leads to a loose docking of vesicles on the acceptor membranes, and it is known that other Sec gene products, such as *Sec*18p and *Sec*17p, as well as Ca^{2+}, act subsequently to trigger the fusion step that completes the delivery of the protein to the Golgi apparatus. Ca^{2+} is required for ER-to-Golgi transport in both mammalian cells[342] and yeast,[339] and it is known to act at a late step in this process. That Ypt1p participates in the transport reaction, becoming a vesicle component at a step prior to that requiring Ca^{2+}, is demonstrated by the fact that when the in vitro yeast transport reaction is carried out in the presence of EGTA, completion of transport will occur on the readdition of Ca^{2+}, even in the presence of anti-Ypt1p antibodies that would have blocked transport if added initially.[340]

*Sec*18p is the yeast equivalent of NSF20—an *N*-*e*thyl*m*aleimide (NEM) *s*ensitive *f*actor, originally purified from mammalian tissues,[343] that was first shown to be necessary for intra-Golgi transport and later found to play a widespread role in membrane fusion events in mammalian cells, including ER-to-Golgi transport[344] and endocytic vesicle-endosome fusion.[345] In fact, yeast *Sec*18p could replace NSF in a mammalian transport assay. Studies with the mammalian system have shown that NSF binds to membranes and that this binding is mediated by a *s*oluble *N*SF *a*ttachment *p*rotein (*SNAP*), of which three different gene products, (α, β, and γ SNAP), related in sequence, have been identified.[346] The *Sec*17 yeast gene product is functionally equivalent to the mammalian αSNAP.[347,348]

From a variety of studies carried out in vitro, primarily with mammalian systems, it appears that NSF, which is a tetramer of 76-kDa subunits, serves as a bridge between SNAPs that specifically bind to receptors in the donor and target membranes.[349] Although it has been proposed that NSF plays a direct role in membrane fusion in mammalian intra-Golgi transport, evidence has been obtained that in yeast ER-to-Golgi transport NSF acts after Ypt1p, but before the Ca^{2+}-requiring step that leads to membrane fusion. Thus, when transport is carried out at the permissive temperature, with a lysate from a *Sec*18p temperature-sensitive mutant, in a Ca^{2+}-depleted medium to arrest transport at the Ca^{2+}-sensitive step, fusion will proceed normally when Ca^{2+} is restored, even if the temperature is raised to inactivate *Sec*18p.[340]

The actual vesicles that mediate ER-to-Golgi transport have not yet been purified and characterized biochemically. It is not known what type of coat, if any, they acquire during their formation. However, it has been shown[350] that the *Sec*21 gene product, which is required for ER-to-Golgi transport, is the yeast homologue of γCOP, a subunit of the coat of the non-clathrin-coated vesicles that mediate intra-Golgi transport in mammalian cells (see below). Moreover, as is the case with its mammalian counterpart, *Sec*21p is a subunit of a very large (700- to 800-kDa) complex that in polypeptide composition closely resembles that of the mammalian coatomer (see below). In fact, it has been shown that another polypeptide within the complex containing *Sec*21p is the yeast equivalent of βCOP, the best-characterized subunit of the mammalian coatomer.

Like other members of the ras superfamily of GTP-binding proteins, Ypt1p undergoes prenylation in a cysteine residue at its C-terminus, at which a geranylgeranyl group is added, and it may also undergo palmitoylation at another neighboring cysteine.[351,352] Prenylation allows Ypt1p to become membrane-anchored and is necessary for its activity in transport. Accordingly, a temperature-sensitive mutation (bet2) that inactivates the geranylgeranyl transferase that effects these modifications impairs attachment of Ypt1 to membranes and blocks the delivery of ER-derived transport vesicles to the Golgi apparatus.[353]

Because in yeast many mannose residues are added to glycoproteins on their arrival to the Golgi apparatus, it was possible to use a ^{3}H-mannose suicide technique to isolate conditional lethal mutants that are *b*locked *e*arly in *t*ransport (defining the genes BET1 and BET2) and, therefore, survive incubation at the nonpermissive temperature in medium containing highly radioactive mannose.[325] Other genes that act early in the secretory pathway have been identified as suppressors of the *l*oss of *Y*PT1 (SLY1, SLY2, SLY12, and SLY41) function,[354,355] or suppressors of the bet1 mutation (BOS1, for *b*et *o*ne *s*uppressor; 27 kDa).[356–358] The products of all these genes are involved in ER-to-Golgi transport and, in fact, SLY12 is identical to BET1,[357] and SLY2 to the previously identified SEC22 gene.[359] BOS1 and BET1 are class II genes that are required for vesicle consumption and not for vesicle formation.[325,358] The products of these genes (Bos1p, 27 kDa; Sly12p/Bet1p, 142 amino acids, and Sly2p/*Sec*22p, 214 amino acids) lack insertion signal sequences and are associated with the ER membrane through their hydrophobic C-terminal regions. Therefore, they have most of their masses exposed on the cytoplasmic membrane surface. This disposition, together with the fact that Sly2p/*Sec*22p and Sly12p/Bet1p show sequence similarity to the mammalian synaptic vesicle membrane protein *synaptobrevin* (or *VAMP*)—which is currently thought to play a role as a targeting molecule in the docking of the synaptic vesicle at the presynaptic membrane during neurotransmitter discharge (see refs. 360 and 361)—strongly suggests that the latter two proteins play a role in vesicle docking during ER-to-Golgi transport. It is noteworthy that Sly2p/*Sec*22p and *Ypt*1p, like Bos1p, are components of the transport vesicles that accumulate in an in vitro assay in the absence of acceptor Golgi membranes.[357,362]

Given the role of Ypt1p in targeting, how could it be explained that overexpression of SLY2/SEC22, SLY12/BET1, and SLY41, or a point mutation in the SLY1 gene (Sly1-20 allele) can overcome a complete absence of Ypt1p? It has been suggested[355] that in the case of Sly1-20 this occurs because normally, an activated Ypt1p functions to induce a conformational change in Sly1p, which is mimicked by the mutation. As for Sly2p/*Sec*22p and Sly12p/Bet1p, it is possible that these proteins are normally present in very limiting amounts on the transport vesicles, which, therefore, rely for their efficient docking on the action of Ypt1p. However, when these synaptobrevin-like putative targeting proteins are superabundant, the guiding action of *Ypt*1p may become dispensable for cell viability.

Molecular Interactions that Underlie ER-to-Golgi Transport in Mammalian Cells[18,301,302]

Several systems have been developed that utilize disrupted or detergent-permeabilized cultured cells to reproduce ER-to-Golgi and intra-Golgi transport in vitro under conditions that allow the penetration into the cells of normally impermeant reagents.[363,364] In general, the cells are infected with a temperature-sensitive variant (tsO45) of the vesicular stomatitis virus (VSV) that produces a defective viral envelope glycoprotein (G). At the nonpermissive temperature (37°C), the mutant protein accumulates in the ER, but it rapidly exits toward the Golgi apparatus when the cells are transferred to an environment of 30°C. In these assays, the G protein is metabolically labeled with [^{35}S]methionine prior to permeabilization of the cells, and its passage to the Golgi apparatus is monitored from the extent to which its *N*-linked oligosaccharides are modified by Golgi enzymes. Such modifications can be detected by virtue of the changes in the electrophoretic mobility of the protein caused by digestion with endoglycosidases (endo D, endo H, endo F).

Utilizing semi-intact CHO cells, it was shown that ER-to-*cis*-Golgi transport is a temperature-dependent process that requires cytosolic proteins (including NSF, the NEM-sensitive factor that represents the yeast *Sec*18 homologue), Ca^{2+} ions, and an energy supply, as well as the participation of GTP-binding proteins (*rab*, *arf*, and heterotrimeric G proteins), and the hydrolysis of GTP (e.g., refs. 341, 365, and 366). GTP-γ-S blocks ER-to-Golgi transport when added early during the course of the reaction, which indicates that a critical GTP-binding protein must be charged with GTP during an early phase, possibly during vesicle formation.[364,365]

Three *rab* proteins — *rab*1a, *rab*1b, and *rab*2 — are localized in the ER and Golgi compartments and participate in ER-to-Golgi transport.[341] *Rab*1a and *rab*1b are closely related to each other (92 percent sequence identity) and to the yeast Ypt1p (almost 70 percent identity), which *rab*1a can functionally replace.[19] The addition of specific antibodies that recognize rab1a and *rab*1b has been shown to block in vitro transport, but only if the antibodies are added very soon after transport is allowed to begin. Immunofluorescence studies have shown that antibodies to rab1b block vesicle formation in the ER.[366] Although these findings suggest that the rab proteins complete their function early in transport (as expected if they participate only in vesicle formation), it is possible that they are also active in a later step that can no longer be inhibited by antibodies once these proteins are assembled onto a vesicle. In fact, independent evidence indicates that the *rab*1 proteins interact with their effectors (which leads to GTP hydrolysis) very late, much later than the time at which addition of GTP-γ-S to the system no longer has an effect on transport or the time at which anti-*rab* antibodies no longer are effective (see below).

As may be expected from the role of Ca^{2+} in many membrane fusion events, this ion is also required to complete ER-to-Golgi transport. Thus, chelation of Ca^{2+} with EGTA at any time during the course of the incubation almost instantly and reversibly blocks transport to the Golgi apparatus. The rapid cessation of transport on depletion of Ca^{2+} indicates that Ca^{2+} is required at a very late step in the chain of events that leads to transport. This is also apparent from the finding that after prolonged incubation in EGTA, restoration of Ca^{2+} leads to the rapid resumption and completion of transport, with an initial rate considerably faster than that normally achieved. Moreover, after Ca^{2+} is restored, transport can no longer be inhibited by addition of GTP-γ-S or anti-*rab* antibodies,[367] indicating that GTP and the *rab* proteins have already been incorporated into the transporting machinery. On the other hand, synthetic peptides corresponding to the highly conserved effector domain of the *rab* subfamily of proteins completely block transport, even when added at the time of Ca^{2+} restoration, presumably because they compete with the *rab* proteins for interaction with their as yet unidentified effectors.[367] Thus, this interaction, which may occur on the acceptor membranes, may be one of the last steps in transport.

The cyclic role of *rab*1a, *rab*1b, and *rab*2 in ER-to-Golgi transport is demonstrated by the findings that certain mutations in these proteins designed to maintain them permanently in the active configuration (by amino acid substitutions in the effector or the GTP-binding domains) block ER-to-Golgi transport. This was shown both in cells that express those proteins after transfection with a viral vector,[341] and in an in vitro system to which the purified proteins produced in bacteria are added.[364] These results would be expected if the *rab* proteins unable to hydrolyze GTP remain bound to their effectors, or to other molecules, and prevent their reutilization in new rounds of transport.

In addition to *rab* proteins, GTP-binding proteins of the *arf* and *heterotrimeric G* families also participate in ER-to-Golgi transport as in other interorganellar transport steps in mammalian cells. The *arf* proteins are members of the *ras* superfamily that become membrane-associated through an N-terminal myristate moiety. The yeast protein Arf1p appears to play a role in ER-to-Golgi transport, since ARF shows synthetic lethality with other yeast genes involved in that process, such as YPT1, SEC21, and BET2.[368] The human ARF1 and ARF4 gene products (hARFp) have been shown to be capable of replacing Arf1p in mutant yeast cells.[45] Moreover, synthetic peptides corresponding to the N-terminal region of the human ARF irreversibly inhibited ER-to-Golgi transport in semi-intact cells, apparently by preventing vesicle formation in the ER.[366,369] This is not surprising since studies with in vitro systems that reproduce intra-Golgi transport indicate that an ARF protein is a component of the coatomer-containing coat of the vesicles that mediate that process, and it plays a critical role in triggering the assembly of this coat (see ref. 348). The ARF peptides, however, were also able to inhibit transport when added at a very late stage.[369] This suggests that ARF proteins also participate in late events, such as vesicle docking and fusion.

That heterotrimeric G proteins, like those that function in signal transduction at the plasma membrane, have a role in ER-to-Golgi transport first became apparent from studies that demonstrated strong inhibitory effects of AlF_{3-5}.[342] More recently, export of a viral glycoprotein from the ER, monitored in permeabilized cells using immunofluorescence, was found to be also blocked by the addition of purified $\beta\gamma$ subunits of the G protein, which should bind to free Gα subunits and prevent them from exerting their effects. *Mastoparan*, the cationic peptide that mimics the G protein-binding region of plasma membrane receptors and preferentially activates Giα subunits, also blocked transport.[366] The similar inhibitory effects of the $\beta\gamma$ subunits and mastoparan on transport, despite their opposite actions on Gα subunits, may indicate that heterotrimeric G proteins containing both stimulatory (Gsα) and inhibitory (Giα, or Goα) subunits function in this system and have opposite regulatory effects, as has been reported for the formation of constitutive secretory vesicles in the *trans*-Golgi network (see below and ref. 370).

An additional mechanism that may control vesicular transport between subcellular organelles involves the phosphorylation of specific components by cytosolic protein kinases. Phosphorylation seems to have opposite effects in ER-to-Golgi transport and in transport from the medial Golgi to the *trans*-Golgi network (TGN). Inhibitors of protein phosphatases, such as *okadaic* acid and *microcystin-LR*, blocked ER-to-Golgi transport, both in vivo and in vitro, and this effect was eliminated by treatment with protein kinase antagonists such as *staurosporine* and *H-8*, reagents that, by themselves, do not affect transport.[371] Therefore, the presence of phosphate groups in yet unidentified proteins that participate in ER-to-Golgi transport inhibits this process. It is noteworthy that during mitosis, vesicular transport is inhibited concomitantly with the activation of MPF (mitosis-promoting factor), which is a protein kinase. On the other hand, protein phosphorylation is essential for transport between the medial Golgi and the TGN, since the same protein kinase inhibitors mentioned above completely arrest this process.[364] One can expect that phosphorylation-dephosphorylation events will be found to play a critical role in many vesicular transport processes.

Intermediate Compartment at the ER–Golgi Interface[303,372–374]

The area of cytoplasm between the ER transitional elements and the first (*cis*) cisternae of the Golgi apparatus is rich in tubulovesicular membranous structures. EM images frequently suggest that vesicles or tubules in this region of the cell either bud from or fuse with the adjacent ER or Golgi membranes. The precise interconnections or relationships between these tubulovesicular elements, which are collectively known as the *ER–Golgi intermediate compartment* (ERGIC), and the ER and Golgi have not yet been elucidated. It is known, however, that when cells are incubated at 15°C this compartment greatly expands and that, under these conditions, newly synthesized proteins that are normally transported to the Golgi apparatus, such as the Semliki Forest (SFV) and vesicular stomatitis (VSV) viral envelope glycoproteins, accumulate in it.[375,376] This indicates that the low temperature causes a specific block in transport in this region of the endomembrane system.

Elements of the ER–Golgi intermediate compartment have been regarded as constituting a specialized organelle, since they appear to contain specific resident proteins, most notably a 53-kDa nonglycosylated transmembrane protein (*p53*) which, in some cell types, is also found in the first (*cis*) Golgi cisternae.[377] As expected from a bona fide component of the putative organelle, after incubation of VSV-infected cells at 15°C, p53 colocalizes with the arrested VSV G glycoprotein in the expanded intermediate compartment.[376] A 58-kDa glycoprotein (lacking terminal sugars normally added in the *trans*-Golgi and TGN) found in *cis*-Golgi cisternae is also present in the intermediate-compartment elements,[378] as are *rab*2 and *rab*1p, the two small GTP-binding proteins that play an essential role in ER-to-Golgi vesicular transport.[37,378,379]

It has been possible to isolate from Vero (African green monkey kidney) cells a subcellular fraction that, judging from its content of p53, is highly enriched in elements of the intermediate compartment and is depleted in rough ER and *cis*-Golgi markers.[380] Therefore, much may soon be learned of the biochemical properties of the intermediate compartment. At this moment, however, it is not yet clear if it represents a true, separate, compartment (or organelle) that receives vesicles from ER transitional elements and produces other vesicles that are targeted to the *cis* face of the Golgi apparatus, or if it consists only of expansions of one of the adjacent organelles. One opinion expressed is that it is connected to the ER transitional elements and is therefore part of what would be the equivalent of a *transitional element network* (TEN).[372] Another opinion is that it is continuous with the first *cis*-Golgi cisterna, forming part of a *cis*-Golgi network, or CGN.[232,373,381] Furthermore, the possibility has been suggested that the intermediate compartment is simply a pleomorphic transport intermediate consisting mainly of tubulovesicular membranous elements that are formed by the aggregation and fusion of vesicles that emerge from the transitional elements of the ER or the Golgi apparatus. Such tubulovesicular elements would then coalesce to form the first *cis*-Golgi cisternae.[303,378,379] In this view (Fig. 16-25), only one round of vesicle fission (from the ER) is required for transport to the *cis*-Golgi, but many fusion events would be required to form the *cis*-Golgi network. It has been proposed that because the CGN would be the first way station for traffic that emerges from the ER, it is also likely to be a site of sorting, where elements that are to be returned to the ER are segregated from those that must move along the secretory pathway. For this reason the intermediate compartment has also been termed the *exosome*. This name is intended to reflect a mode of biogenesis and function for the intermediate compartment that would be similar to that of the peripheral endosomal compartment that, as will be discussed later, is viewed by some as resulting from the coalescence and fusion of vesicles formed at the plasma membrane (see below).

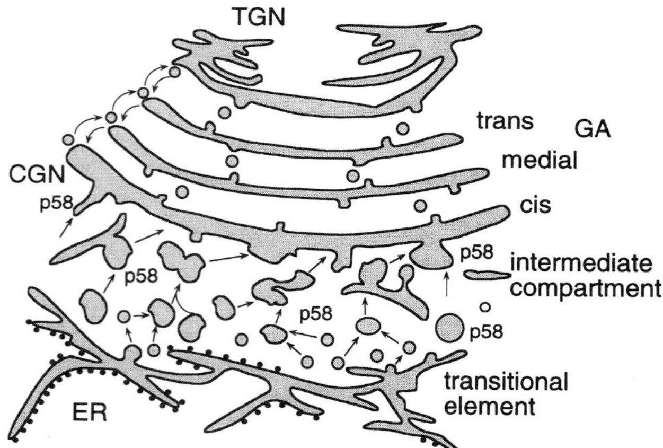

Fig. 16-25 Structure of the ER-Golgi intermediate compartment. Proteins exported from the ER pass through an intermediate compartment that consists of tubulovesicular elements found between the ER transitional elements and the first (*cis*) cisternae of Golgi stacks. In cells incubated at 15°C, the proteins accumulate in this compartment, which also greatly expands at this temperature. The term *cis*-Golgi network (CGN) has also been applied to the intermediate compartment because some of its elements appear to be connected to the *cis*-Golgi cisterna and some proteins (e.g., p58 and p53) of the intermediate compartment are also found in this cisterna. It has been proposed that vesicles that emerge from ER transitional elements fuse with each other to form the elements of the intermediate compartment and that these, in turn, fuse to generate the *cis* cisterna.[303] Specific posttranslational modifications may be carried out in the intermediate compartment, which may also function as a "salvage compartment" in which some proteins that escape the ER are recognized by retrieving receptors. (*Based on Plutner et al.*[386])

Whether the intermediate compartment represents a permanent structure through which proteins pass or consists mainly of transient carriers, its morphologic and biochemical identities seem well established. Functionally, its elements may represent at least one of the *salvage* compartments from which KDEL-containing proteins are recycled back to the ER.[232] The intermediate compartment may also be the site to which certain abnormal proteins, whose degradation begins in the ER, are transported for completion of their degradation at a faster rate.[256] The relationship of the intermediate compartment to a subcompartment of the ER, the *calciosome*,[382] where a Ca^{2+} pump and Ca^{2+} binding proteins are located and where Ca^{2+} ions are stored at high concentrations,[383] has not yet been examined.

It seems that ER transitional cisternae and the intermediate compartment share at least some biochemical properties since the mouse hepatitis coronavirus A59 assembles and specifically buds only at these sites, where, apparently, *N*-acetylgalactosamine residues also become *O*-linked to serines and threonines in the viral glycoprotein.[384] It is possible that protein palmitoylation (see below), which in certain transmembrane proteins modifies cysteine residues located in their cytoplasmic domains, is also a function of the intermediate compartment.[372,385]

Employing the 15°C block and a semi-intact cell system, it has been possible to characterize in VSV-infected cells the requirements for the viral envelope G glycoprotein to enter into and exit from the intermediate compartment.[386] It should be noted that when VSV-infected cells in which pulse-labeled temperature-sensitive G glycoprotein molecules have accumulated in the ER are perforated and incubated for protein transport in vitro, the molecules that emerge from the ER reach the *cis* region of the Golgi apparatus only after a lapse of approximately 10 to 20 min. In contrast, such lag is eliminated if the cells, before perforation, are incubated for 90 min at 15°C. This would be expected if, at the low temperature, vesicles carrying the protein had progressed to the intermediate compartment, even though they may not have undergone the fusion event required to deliver their cargo. In fact, completion of transport after the 15°C block still requires an energy supply, Ca^{2+}, and GTP hydrolysis and is blocked by antibodies to NSF, the factor that is thought to mediate the fusion.

THE GOLGI APPARATUS[18,297,348,373,386a–389]

The Golgi apparatus is a complex organelle that receives both luminal and membrane proteins that are exported from the ER and pass through the intermediate compartment. It effects a wide variety of posttranslational modifications on many of these proteins, including the processing of *N*-linked oligosaccharide chains to complex forms, the *O*-glycosylation of hydroxy amino acid residues, the phosphorylation of mannoses in enzymes destined to lysosomes, the fatty acylation of cysteines, the sulfation of oligosaccharide chains and tyrosine residues in proteins, and the proteolytic processing of many precursor polypeptides. It is also the site of synthesis of glycosaminoglycans (GAG) and sphingolipids. Whereas some of the proteins that reach the Golgi apparatus from the ER remain as permanent residents of its cisternae, others traverse the organelle and are either transported to the cell surface or are segregated within distal elements of the endomembrane system, such as secretory granules or lysosomes.

In secretory cells, and perhaps in all cell types, some membrane proteins that reach the cell surface by exocytosis are retrieved by endocytosis and returned to the Golgi apparatus for reutilization in the packaging of new secretory products.[390–395] The multiple destinations of proteins that emerge from the Golgi apparatus, as well as its participation in the recycling of plasma membrane proteins, make this organelle the cell's center for the distribution and sorting of proteins addressed to various subcellular locations.

Structure and Organization of the Golgi Apparatus[386a,389,396–401]

Characteristically, the Golgi apparatus consists of stacks of three to eight slightly curved, membranous cisternae, or saccules, that are platelike near their centers and dilated toward their rims. Several of these stacks may exist within a single cell, and they may be interconnected.[400–403] A Golgi stack shows a polarized organization with one side, the *cis* face (generally the convex one), oriented toward the ER and the opposite, *trans* face, oriented toward secretory granules or the centrioles. The *cis*-most cisternae is usually fenestrated and connected to the network of tubular and tubulovesicular elements that constitutes the intermediate compartment that transfers materials from the ER to the Golgi apparatus. Together, the intermediate compartment and the *cis* cisterna can be viewed as forming a CGN.

Coated vesicles that are thought to transport proteins from one Golgi cisterna to the next, in a *cis*-to-*trans* direction, are also found near the periphery of the Golgi stacks and may be seen fusing with or budding from the cisternal rims. Vesicles of this type have been generated in vitro, and their coat and the process of its assembly have been extensively characterized (see ref. 348 and discussion below). In certain types of secretory cells, proteins to be packaged in secretory granules first accumulate in the dilated rims of the two or three *trans*-most Golgi cisternae.[386a] In other secretory cells, such as those in pancreatic acini, the concentration of secretory products takes place within separate dilated sacs, known as *condensing vacuoles*, that are adjacent to the trans face of the Golgi and appear to receive material from it by vesicular transport.[304,305]

In its *trans*-most region, the Golgi apparatus extends into a network of tubulovesicular structures that have somewhat thicker membranes and were originally known as GERL,[397,398] but are now generally referred to as the TGN,[388] *trans*-Golgi reticulum,[404] or *transtubular network*.[401] It is in this region of the *trans*-Golgi that many of proteins retrieved from the plasma membrane reach the organelle. Several different types of vesicles are seen near the TGN[388,405] and appear to originate from it. Among these are clathrin-coated vesicles that contain either lysosomal enzymes complexed to the mannose 6-phosphate receptor (see below) or, possibly, secretory proteins destined to be stored in secretory granules. Other vesicles appear to lack a coat (but probably had one when they were formed) and are likely to ferry a constitutive flow of secretory and membrane proteins to the cell surface. In polarized epithelial cells, membrane proteins destined to the two different plasma membrane domains (apical and basolateral) are packed into different vesicles at the TGN.[406–408] The TGN has thus emerged as the major site of sorting for proteins that traverse the endomembrane system.

The polarized organization of the Golgi apparatus is also apparent morphologically from a progressive increase in the thickness of its cisternal membranes, from the *cis* to the *trans* side, seen in EM, and from the intense staining of the *cis* cisternae when cells are incubated for long times with OsO_4.[409] Cytochemically, the *trans*-most cisternae are characterized by a thiamine pyrophosphatase activity[403,410] that is not present in the TGN elements. However, TGN elements do show acid phosphatase activity,[388] presumably reflecting the presence of this hydrolase en route to lysosomes.

The *cis*-, medial, and *trans*-Golgi cisternae represent a series of subcompartments enriched in specific enzymatic activities that sequentially carry out posttranslational modifications on newly synthesized proteins that traverse the organelle unidirectionally. A combination of cytochemical, immunoelectron microscopic, and cell fractionation studies has defined a general pattern of organization within the Golgi apparatus (Fig. 16-26) of the enzymes involved in the processing by *N*-linked oligosaccharide chains (see refs. 411 to 415). The *cis* cisternae contain most of the N-*acetylglucosaminylphosphotransferase* and the N-*acetylglucosamine-1-phospho-diester-α-*N-*acetylglucosaminidase* that add the phosphate marker to the mannose residues of newly synthesized lysosomal hydrolases (see below). An α-mannosidase I, that reduces to five the number of mannose residues in oligosaccharides partially trimmed in the ER, is also found in the *cis* and, possibly, the medial cisternae. As previously mentioned, the presence in a protein of *N*-linked oligosaccharides trimmed to five mannose residues can be detected by their sensitivity to the action of endo D, and this can be used to demonstrate the transport of a glycoprotein to the Golgi apparatus. Medial cisternae contain a number of enzymes, including the N-*acetylglucosaminyltransferase I* that adds the first outer GlcNAc residue in the formation of complex oligosaccharides, the *α-mannosidase II* that is responsible for the removal of the next two mannose residues and hence confers endo H resistance to *N*-linked oligosaccharides, the *transferase II* that adds a second outer GlcNAc, and the *fucosyltransferase* that modifies the innermost GlcNAc. The *glycosyltransferases* that add galactose and sialic acid residues to the regrowing oligosaccharides have been localized mostly to the *trans*-most cisternae and the TGN, respectively.

The general pattern of distribution just described does not imply that Golgi enzymes that carry out successive reactions are totally segregated from each other. Some overlapping in the distribution of enzymatic activities was revealed by the simultaneous immunolocalization of *GlcNAc-transferase I* and *galactosyltransferase*.[416] This showed that, although the bulk of the former enzyme is present in the medial Golgi, substantial amounts are also found in *trans* cisternae. On the other hand, galactosyltransferase is present not only in the *trans* cisternae, but in the TGN as well. Thus, different cisternae may contain characteristic mixtures of enzymes that may even vary with the cell type, and the ordered modification of oligosaccharide chains in glycoproteins may be as much a consequence of the restricted specificity of the various glycosidases and transferases as of their physical segregation in separate compartments. Some authors[373] have advanced the extreme view that the Golgi apparatus is composed of only three compartments — CGN, Golgi stacks, and the TGN. The first and last of these compartments would primarily play a sorting role, while oligosaccharide processing would occur in the Golgi stacks, where the glycosyltransferases and glycosidases would be intermixed.

In addition to the different sets of processing enzymes that they encounter as they move across the Golgi apparatus, newly synthesized proteins confront environments of decreasing pH in their passage from the *cis* cisternae to the TGN. The presence of a *proton pump* has been demonstrated in isolated Golgi fractions.[417] Studies using a probe detectable by immunoelectron microscopy, whose accumulation within membrane-bound compartments is an inverse function of the pH, have revealed that the *trans* cisternae and the TGN are substantially more acidic than the *cis* Golgi cisternae.[418,419] Moreover, secretory vesicles in the *trans*-Golgi region were found to have a low pH, comparable to that of the TGN from which they are derived.

The drug monensin, which is an ionophore that exchanges K^+ ions for protons and thus dissipates pH gradients across membranes,[420,421] inhibits the secretion of many proteins[422] and the passage of viral envelope glycoproteins through the Golgi apparatus. This drug leads to a remarkable swelling of Golgi cisternae, and the movement of the viral glycoproteins through the organelle is halted within the medial region.[423,424] It should be noted that treatment of cells with lysosomotropic drugs (i.e., weak bases such as primaquine, chloroquine, and NH_4Cl), which traverse membranes in their uncharged forms but in their protonated forms accumulate within acidic compartments (raising the intravesicular pH[425,426]), also affects the secretion of many proteins, albeit to different extents for different proteins within a

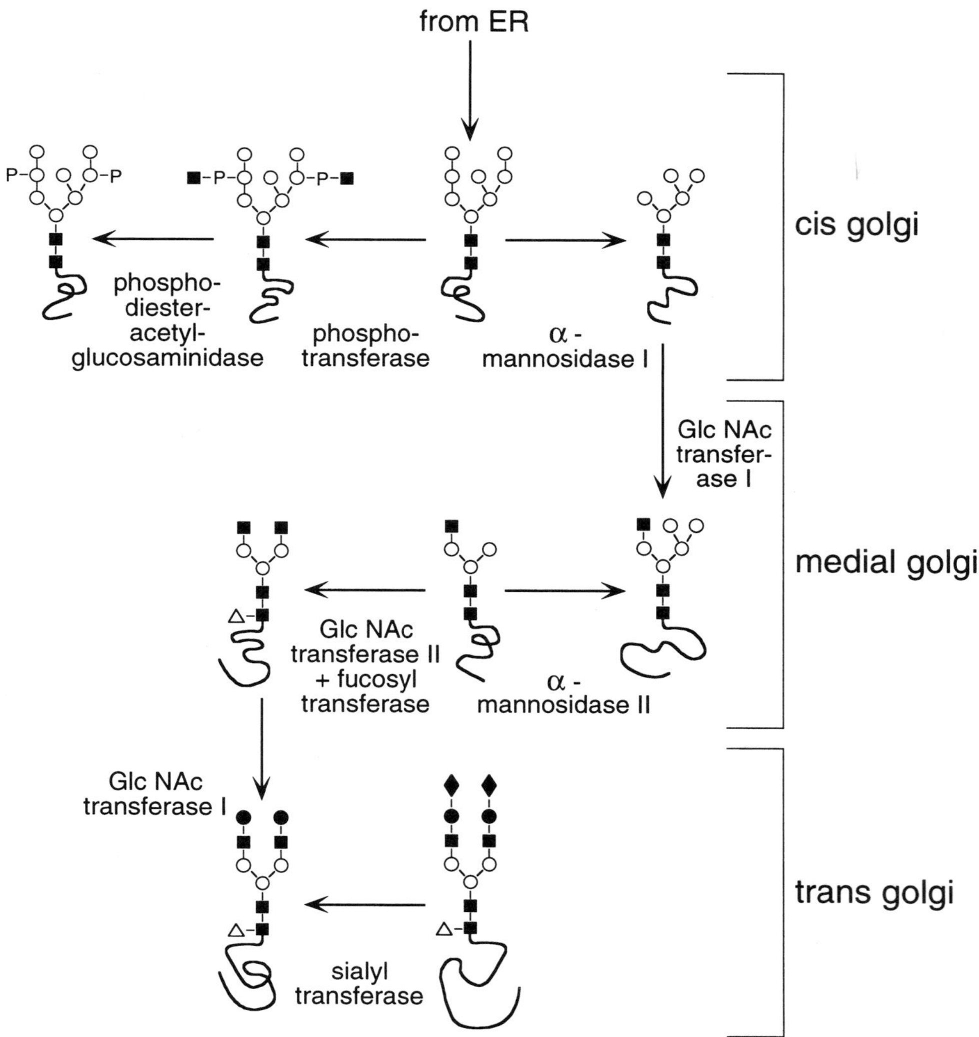

Fig. 16-26 Sequential modifications of oligosaccharide chains as glycoproteins move through the Golgi apparatus. A glycoprotein containing a high-mannose oligosaccharide is transferred from the ER to a *cis*-Golgi cisterna. If the protein is a lysosomal hydrolase, it acquires the mannose 6-phosphate marker by the sequential action of *N*-acetylglucosaminylphosphotransferase (phosphotransferase) and *N*-acetylglucosamine-1-phosphodiester α-*N*-acetylglucosaminidase (phosphodiesterase), as indicated by the leftward arrows. Other polypeptides undergo further removal of the outer mannose residues in the *cis* Golgi by the α-mannosidase I. The products of this reaction are transferred to medial Golgi cisternae, where *N*-acetylglucosaminyltransferase I (transferase I) adds an acetylglucosamine residue to provide the substrate from which the remaining outer mannose residues are removed by the α-mannosidase II. Formation of a complex oligosaccharide begins in medial cisternae by addition of fucosyl residues and is completed in the *trans* Golgi. (*Adapted from Kornfeld and Kornfeld.*[217])

given cell. These drugs appear to act at a late Golgi or post-Golgi stage. In fact, primaquine completely blocks the secretion of albumin from hepatoma cells, leading to its accumulation within vesicles in the *trans* side of the Golgi. It has a lesser effect on the secretion of other proteins, such as transferrin.[427] The acid pH of the Golgi apparatus may actually be required for some proteins to achieve a conformation that allows them to exit from the organelle. Conversely, the aberrant conformation of some abnormal proteins generated using recombinant DNA techniques may be manifested at the acidic pH of Golgi elements, which may account for their accumulation in this organelle.[428]

It has been suggested that a pH gradient may play a role in determining the unidirectional transport of proteins through the Golgi apparatus.[419] It is known that the low pH of endosomes (see below) mediates the dissociation of some ligands from their receptors, which allows for the return of interiorized receptors to the plasma membrane. One could imagine that vesicles that effect the successive transfer of proteins from cisternae to cisternae contain pH-sensitive receptors for these proteins that release their ligands at different pHs, and that this is necessary for the vesicles to return to the cisternae of origin. This idea, however, is not in accord with the notion that transport across the Golgi apparatus is a non-receptor-mediated bulk flow process.

The organization of the Golgi apparatus is dependent on the integrity of the microtubular system: drugs that disassemble microtubules lead to fragmentation of the organelle into dispersed smaller cisternal stacks that remain functional and can reassemble on removal of the microtubule depolymerizing agent.[429,430] This type of fragmentation and preassembly occurs naturally as cells pass through mitosis.[431]

The remarkable effects of the drug *brefeldin* A (BFA) on the endomembrane system have provided insights into the dynamic relationships that exist between the Golgi apparatus on one side and the ER or the endosomal compartment on the other. This fungal metabolite (a macrocyclic lactone synthesized from palmitate), resembling an acyl group, is a powerful inhibitor of ER-to-Golgi transport and of anterograde transport through the Golgi stacks (see refs. 432 and 433). Treatment of cells with BFA leads to the disassembly of the Golgi complex and to the microtubule-dependent retrograde movement of Golgi enzymes into the ER.[434,435] The TGN, however, undergoes fusion with endosomes,[436] and its components do not undergo retrograde transport to the ER.[437] In BFA-treated cells, therefore, resident ER proteins mix with enzymes of the Golgi stacks and may acquire modifications that are characteristic of proteins that normally reach the Golgi apparatus (e.g., refs. 262, 438, and 439).

The retrograde movement of Golgi components to the ER induced by BFA appears to take place via narrow membrane tubules (90 nm in diameter) that do not have an apparent cytoplasmic coat and during the first 10 min of incubation with the drug emerge from swollen Golgi cisternae and extend along microtubules.[435] Although the mechanism for the resorption of Golgi components into the ER is not fully understood, it is likely that this occurs because the drug selectively inhibits the forward transport of proteins from the ER to the Golgi and through this organelle, without blocking the retrograde transport that, presumably, normally retrieves components of the transport machinery that function cyclically. The finding that tubular membrane extensions are prominent soon after BFA is added to cells suggests that such structures may be the normal vehicles for retrograde flow within the Golgi apparatus and from this organelle to the ER. The molecular basis for the inhibitory effects of the drug on anterograde transport through the Golgi is described below.

Signals for the Localization of Resident Proteins in the Golgi Apparatus[440,441]

The critical role that the Golgi apparatus plays in the posttranslational modification and sorting of a wide variety of itinerant as well as resident proteins is dependent on the segregation of the necessary enzymes, such as glycosyltransferases, glycosidases, proteases, and sugar nucleotide transporters, in specific regions of the organelle.

The behavior of chimeric constructs containing portions of Golgi resident proteins linked to segments of reporter proteins that normally completely transverse that organelle has begun to provide information on the location and nature of the signals that determine the localization of the resident proteins, as well as some insight into the mechanisms by which these signals act. Several studies indicate that the transmembrane domains of proteins of the CGN and Golgi stacks are responsible for their localization. This first became apparent[442–444] from the analysis of the M envelope protein of the avian coronavirus infectious bronchitis virus (IBV). This membrane protein accumulates in the CGN/*cis* region of the organelle, leading to budding of the virus into the lumen of the cisternae, from which the viral particles are transported to the plasma membrane within vesicles, in the same manner as a secretory protein.

Necessary and sufficient information for targeting of the M protein to the CGN was found to be contained within the first (N-terminal) of its three transmembrane domains (TMD), which consists of an amphipathic α helix with uncharged polar residues (Asn, Thr, Gln) on one of its faces. When incorporated in a chimeric protein, this α helix was able to confer Golgi localization to proteins normally destined to the plasma membrane, and mutations in its polar residues led to transport of the chimeras to the cell surface. It is noteworthy that the M protein of a murine coronavirus that is targeted to the TGN, rather than the CGN, contains a similar amphipathic helix, but this did not localize a reporter protein to the Golgi.[441] In this case, a cytoplasmic segment of 18 amino acids preceding the TMD may be necessary for Golgi localization, since its deletion caused diversion of the protein to lysosomes.[445] Thus, the different sites of budding within the Golgi of the two coronaviruses seem to be determined by two different types of sorting signals in their M proteins.

Cloning of the cDNA for several endogenous proteins of the Golgi stacks has allowed similar studies on the identification of their localization signals. It is quite striking that all the Golgi stack enzymes whose cDNAs have been cloned—β-1,4-galactosyltransferase (GT); *N*-acetylglucosaminyltransferase (transferase I); α-2,6-sialyltransferase (ST); and α-mannosidase II—have a type II transmembrane disposition in which a short N-terminal cytoplasmic segment is followed by a signal/anchor sequence and a large C-terminal catalytic domain located in the cisternal lumen. For the three transferases, localization signals sufficient for Golgi retention have been found in their transmembrane domains, although flanking sequences were found to enhance the efficiency of retention.[446–453] It has been proposed[440,447] that the function of these signals is to mediate the formation within Golgi membranes of hetero-oligomeric complexes that would include different protein molecules that are to be retained in the same compartment and that such complexes might be stabilized by interactions with other proteins in the luminal and/or cytoplasmic sides of the membranes. As was proposed for the retention of certain proteins in the ER,[256] the inclusion of resident membrane proteins in two-dimensional lattices formed by oligomerization or aggregation would be an effective means of preventing their entrance into the bulk flow carrier vesicles that effect constitutive transport through the organelle. That such a retention mechanism operates in the Golgi is supported by the finding that overexpression of several of the glycosyltransferases leads to their "backup" accumulation in the ER, rather than to their escape to the cell surface.[447,449,451,452] This would be expected if the signals act by mediating oligomerization, which, in principle, could occur in the ER at high enough protein concentrations. On the other hand, if the signals mediate Golgi localization by interacting with retrieving or retaining receptors, saturation of such receptors in overexpressing cells should allow the excess proteins to escape to the cell surface.

In contrast to enzymes of the Golgi stacks, all proteins of the TGN that have been studied (one mammalian and several yeast proteins) have a type I transmembrane disposition and contain localization signals in their cytoplasmic tails. In TGN38, a mammalian protein whose function is not yet known, the signal consists of a short tyrosine-containing segment (YQRL) closely resembling the endocytic signals that mediate the internalization of plasma receptors or lysosomal membrane proteins at the plasma membrane (see below). Indeed, in a chimera, the sorting signal within TGN38 was able to function as an internalization signal in the fraction of molecules that were present in the plasma membrane. Clearly, however, the function of the signal in TGN38 is not limited to triggering internalization since a mutation that changed it to YQDL (the internalization signal in the asialoglycoprotein receptor) did not diminish its endocytotic ability, but markedly reduced its capacity to cause TGN localization.[454] The YQRL signal appears to be recognized by a saturable receptor responsible for the TGN localization of the protein, since the overexpression of chimeric proteins containing the signal led to their accumulation in the plasma membrane and caused the disappearance of the endogenous protein from the TGN. This would be expected if the chimera and the endogenous protein competed for interaction with a saturable receptor.

Critical sorting information was also found to be contained within the cytoplasmic tails of several yeast proteins of the *trans*-Golgi: *Kex1p*, *Kex2p*, and *dipeptidylaminopeptidase* A (DPAP A). These enzymes effect the proteolytic processing of precursor proteins, and comparable enzymes [the furin/PACE (*p*aired basic *a*mino acid residue *c*leaving *e*nzyme)] are present in mammalian cells, probably in the TGN.[454a] Deletion of the cytoplasmic tails of the yeast proteins leads to their default transport to the vacuole.[455–457] In the case of Kex2p, a specific tyrosine residue in the cytoplasmic tail was shown to be essential for Golgi localization.[455] It appears that clathrin, the major structural protein of the coat of vesicles that mediate endocytosis at the plasma membrane and ferry lysosomal enzymes to the incipient lysosome, is involved in retaining Kex2p and DPAP A in the yeast *trans*-Golgi, since a temperature-sensitive mutation in the clathrin heavy chain causes missorting of the proteins to the cell surface at the nonpermissive temperature.[458] This suggests that retention of the proteases in the TGN is mediated by an interaction of their cytoplasmic tails with the adaptor polypeptides that assemble clathrin coats (see below).

Intercisternal Traffic within the Golgi Apparatus[217,297,300,348,373,389]

The sequential passage of a protein across a stack of Golgi cisternae was first strikingly demonstrated in immunoelectron microscopic studies with cells infected with a temperature-sensitive mutant of VSV, in which it is possible to synchronize the transport of the envelope glycoprotein G out of the ER.[318,319] It was clearly shown that the G glycoprotein enters the Golgi apparatus at the *cis* cisterna, traverses the organelle vectorially in approximately 10 min, and exits at the opposite face. When VSV-infected cells are incubated at low temperatures (20°C), large amounts of G glycoprotein accumulate in the TGN, which becomes greatly expanded at this temperature. When the temperature is raised to 32°C, G glycoprotein molecules exit from the TGN toward the plasma membrane within vesicles that are not coated by clathrin.[459]

The demonstration that transfer of newly synthesized proteins through the Golgi stack is a vectorial process involving vesicular carriers that bud from a donor cisterna and fuse with an acceptor one, rather than the flow of proteins along permanent physical connections between cisternae, relied both on cell fusion experiments[460,461] and on in vitro systems in which vectorial transfer between cisternae of different stacks was shown.[348,461a–468] These experiments were possible because of the availability of mutant cell lines defective in some of the oligosaccharide processing enzymes.[469,470] In these cells, the processing of the oligosaccharide chains is arrested at specific points, but the glycoproteins continue to be transferred to the cell surface. Transfer from the cis to medial cisternae was demonstrated when cells deficient in the medial Golgi enzyme GlcNAc transferase I were infected with VSV and fused with wild-type cells.[460] The final mature G glycoprotein produced was shown to carry the normal terminal sugars and therefore had been transferred from the Golgi apparatus of the infected mutant cell to that of the uninfected wild type, where the normal transferase was found. In a similar experiment, transfer from the medial to the *trans* cisternae was inferred from the finding that G glycoprotein molecules synthesized in VSV-infected mutant cells that lacked the *trans*-Golgi enzyme galactosyltransferase were processed to the normal terminally glycosylated form after the infected cells were fused with wild-type cells.[461] The unidirectionality of the transfer between the cisternae within a Golgi stack was demonstrated by the observation, in pulse-chase experiments, that if the cell fusion was carried out after the labeled protein was expected to have passed the appropriate subcompartment in the donor Golgi, processing by the wild-type Golgi apparatus enzyme did not occur.

Biochemical Dissection of Intra-Golgi Transport[18,348,471,472]

The concept that vesicles mediate the intercisternal transfer of proteins in the Golgi apparatus has received its strongest support from experiments in which the transfer of the VSV G protein from the *cis* compartment of one Golgi stack to the medial compartment of another was achieved in a cell-free system. This allowed the isolation of the putative carrier vesicles and their extensive biochemical characterization, including a determination of the requirements for their formation and consumption.[348] However, it has not yet been possible to show that the vesicles, once isolated, have the capacity to deliver their content to acceptor membranes.

The cell-free intra-Golgi transport system utilizes as a donor a Golgi fraction isolated from cells that lack GlcNAc transferase I and that were previously infected with VSV. The acceptor is a Golgi fraction obtained from uninfected wild-type cells.[463,468] Arrival of the G glycoprotein to the acceptor compartment is detected by its acquisition of [^{3}H]*N*-acetylglucosamine residues. In this system, intercisternal transport occurs at physiological temperatures and requires ATP, a cytosolic fraction, and the integrity of proteins that are exposed on the surface of the acceptor membrane and are, therefore, sensitive to proteases.

The kinetics of in vitro intra-Golgi transport show a 7- to 10-min lag before the rate of acquisition of [^{3}H]*N*-acetylglucosamine becomes linear. EM reveals that during this period there is a marked increase in the number of "coated buds" and coated vesicles seen in close proximity to the donor Golgi membranes. Hence, the lag is thought to correspond to the time required for a "donor priming reaction" that leads to the generation of coated vesicles in the donor cisternae. Accordingly, the lag is markedly reduced when the donor Golgi fraction is preincubated with cytosol and ATP in the absence of the acceptor.[461a] The vesicles generated in this reaction appear to represent "bulk flow carriers," in which the cargo molecules are not concentrated and, in fact, are not even necessary for vesicle formation. Thus, the concentration of G glycoprotein in the putative transport vesicles measured by immunoelectron microscopy was found to be very similar to that in the surrounding parental cisternal membranes.[462] Moreover, the formation of the vesicles was not inhibited when the cells from which the donor Golgi was obtained were preincubated for a long time with the protein synthesis inhibitor, *cycloheximide*, which should clear the Golgi cisternae from protein molecules in transit through the organelle. However, *primaquine*, an agent that raises the pH within the Golgi cisterna, completely and irreversibly blocks the formation of vesicles but does not affect the targeting and fusion of the vesicles that were formed before the drug was added. Use of this inhibitor allowed the demonstration that the number of transport-competent vesicles that are present in the in vitro system reaches a maximum after approximately 15 min of incubation.[473]

Before we discuss in detail the sequence of biochemical events that takes place during intercisternal transport, it will be useful to provide a general outline of this process. The formation of a transport vesicle in the donor membrane begins with the assembly of a coat from macromolecular complexes (600 to 700 kDa) called *coatomers* (for *coat protomers*) that are present in the cytosol. The coat is thought to serve as a mechanochemical device that induces the membrane curvature necessary to form a vesicle. The recruitment of coatomers to the Golgi membrane is triggered by the active, GTP-containing form of ARF, a small myristoylated GTP-binding protein that inserts into the membrane and is itself subsequently incorporated into the coat. The coated vesicle that is released from the donor membrane docks on the acceptor membrane and only then does the vesicle shed its coat, in a step that requires the hydrolysis of GTP bound to ARF. Uncoating is followed by fusion of the vesicle membrane to the acceptor membrane — a poorly understood process that requires the activity of NSF,[474] a factor that normally appears to be incorporated into the transport vesicle during its formation at the donor membrane.[473]

The purification of the coated vesicles and the biochemical characterization of their coat became possible after it was observed that addition of the nonhydrolyzable GTP analogue, GTP-γ-S, blocks transport in the cell-free system measured by the incorporation of [^{3}H]GlcNAc into G glycoprotein and leads to the marked accumulation of coated vesicles ($\sim$110 nm in diameter) on the acceptor membranes.[475] This finding provided the first

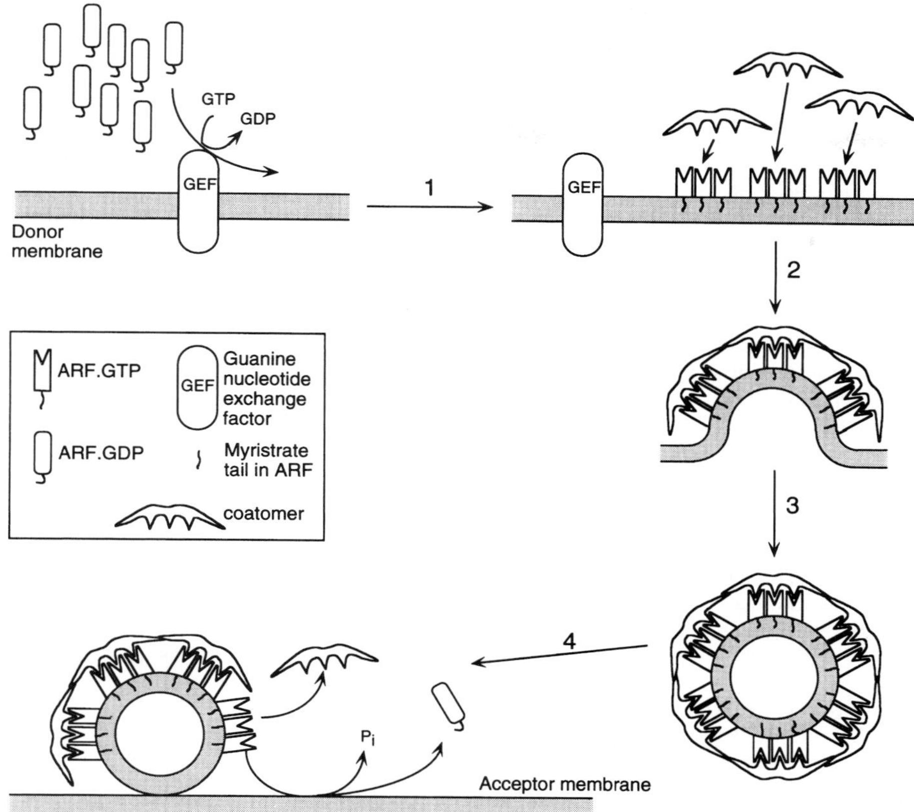

Fig. 16-27 Model for the ARF-mediated assembly of coatomer-coated vesicles in the Golgi apparatus. (1) A guanine nucleotide exchange factor (GEF) in the donor Golgi membrane catalyzes the exchange of GTP for GDP in cytosolic ARF molecules. In their active form these become associated with the membrane through the insertion of their *N*-linked myristate tails in the lipid bilayer. (2) Membrane-associated ARF molecules recruit (perhaps with the assistance of other Golgi membrane proteins, not shown) coatomer complexes from the cytosol. (3) This leads to budding of the coated vesicles, with the ARF molecules incorporated as structural components of the coat in which they are present in the ratio of 3 molecules of ARF per coatomer complex. (4) On docking in the acceptor membrane, by a mechanism not depicted here, coat disassembly is induced by a component of the acceptor membrane that promotes hydrolysis of the GTP bound to ARF. The ARF and coatomers released from the acceptor membrane can then be reutilized in the donor membrane. (*Adapted from Serafini et al.*[481])

indication that GTP-binding proteins are involved in the transport process and that GTP hydrolysis may be required for vesicle uncoating. The accumulated coated vesicles could be removed from the Golgi stacks in a high-salt medium.[476,477] It was thus possible to show that they contain a specific set of polypeptides, with prominent components of $M_r = 170$, 110, 98, and 61 kDa, which are exposed on the vesicle surface and were later called α, β, γ, and δ-COP (for coat proteins), respectively. COP proteins have a peripheral association with the vesicle membrane. In fact, they are found predominantly in the cytosol[478,479] within coatomer complexes that, when purified,[479] were shown to contain two additional polypeptides of 36 and 20 kDa, now designated ε and ζ-COP, respectively.

β-COP was found to be identical[477] to a 110-kDa peripheral membrane protein of the Golgi apparatus that was first identified by immunocytochemistry with a specific monoclonal antibody raised against a Golgi fraction.[480] Immunoelectron microscopy clearly established that β-COP is associated with forming buds in Golgi membranes and with the coated vesicles that accumulate during incubation of the Golgi fraction with GTP-γ-S.[477,478] The sequence of β-COP, deduced from its cloned cDNA,[478] revealed a limited but significant (17 percent) similarity between its N-terminal 450 residues and the corresponding portion of β-adaptin, a component of the coat of clathrin-coated vesicles (see below), suggesting that the two types of coat proteins are evolutionarily derived from a common precursor.

The coated vesicles that accumulate after GTP-γ-S treatment also contain two closely related small (21-kDa) GTP-binding proteins of the *ARF* family that play a critical role in coat assembly. The *N*-myristoylated proteins are present in stoichiometric amounts with respect to the COP polypeptides (three molecules of ARF per β-COP molecule) and, therefore, are also structural components of the coat.[481] In their GDP-bound state, the ARF proteins — first discovered because of their role as cofactors in the cholera toxin-catalyzed ADP ribosylation of the Gα subunits of heterotrimeric G proteins — are found in the cytosol, but are not part of the coatomers. After acquiring GTP, the ARF proteins spontaneously insert through their myristate moiety into phospholipid bilayers.[45] Within the cell, active ARF molecules are associated primarily with Golgi cisternae and Golgi-derived membrane vesicles. Apparently, this is determined by the presence of a specific *guanine nucleotide exchange factor* (GEF) in Golgi cisternae that locally activates ARF molecules and leads to their stable association with the membrane.[482,483] This, in turn, promotes binding of the coatomers[484,485] and their assembly into a coat (Fig. 16-27). In fact, the production of COP-coated vesicles from Golgi cisternae has been achieved in vitro in the absence of any other cytosolic proteins, by the simple addition of coatomers and a recombinant pure myristoylated ARF protein synthesized in *E. coli*.[486] It is noteworthy that vesicle formation requires acyl CoA (supplied experimentally as palmitoyl CoA), and it is believed that this cofactor donates its fatty acid to an unknown acceptor that is activated by acylation.[486a]

Since the active ARF is a key structural component of the vesicle coat, it is expected that hydrolysis of its bound GTP, probably triggered by a GAP protein in the target membrane, will lead to disassembly of the coat. Thus, when ARF is charged with the nonhydrolyzable analogue, GTP-γ-S, transport is blocked[487] and COP-coated vesicles accumulate on the acceptor membranes.[488] It is noteworthy that proteins of the ARF family appear to also play critical roles in other vesicular transport steps, such as ER-to-Golgi transport,[369] and in the formation of clathrin-coated vesicles in the TGN.[489] In fact, recombinant ARF1 stimulates both the binding of coatomers to Golgi membranes and the binding of *AP1 adaptors*, the proteins that promote the assembly of clathrin coats on the Golgi membrane.[489]

A detailed understanding of the molecular interactions involved in the assembly of COP-coated vesicles on Golgi membranes owes much to studies using the drug BFA. In the in vitro system for intra-Golgi transport, BFA inhibited the production of COP-coated vesicles and also led to the formation of extensive tubular interconnections between Golgi cisternae and separate Golgi stacks. Because of these events, even though vesicular transport was interrupted, the processing of the VSV G glycoprotein in donor membranes by enzymes in the acceptor membranes still took place due to the intermixing of Golgi components from adjacent stacks.[490]

It is now clear that BFA acts by inhibiting the assembly of coatomers on Golgi membranes. This was first suggested by the observation that within 30 sec of applying the drug, while the Golgi stacks are still intact, β-COP dissociates from Golgi membranes, but rapidly rebinds to them on removal of the drug.[478,491] Because this effect of BFA was prevented by AlF_{3-5} or by GTP-γ-S (when this analogue was added to permeabilized cells to allow its entrance into the cytoplasm), and because in the absence of the drug these same agents enhanced the association of coatomers (i.e., β-COP) with Golgi membranes,[492] it became obvious that the assembly of the coat is regulated by guanine nucleotide binding proteins and that BFA could act by interrupting the cyclic function of one such protein. In fact, the drug was also shown to cause the rapid and reversible dissociation of ARF from Golgi membranes. Moreover, the in vitro binding of ARF to these membranes is enhanced by GTP-γ-S and inhibited by BFA, when this is added before the nucleotide analogue.[493] In addition, the coatomer binding to Golgi membranes was shown to depend stoichiometrically on the preceding binding of ARF and not to be inhibited by BFA if this was added after ARF was bound.[484,485] Other studies have shown that BFA blocks (possibly indirectly) the GDP-GTP exchange on ARF that is catalyzed by an exchange factor in the Golgi membranes and is required for ARF binding.[482,483] One can therefore conclude that the inhibition of coat assembly caused by the drug is the result of its blocking activation of ARF.

Two facts initially pointed to the possible participation of heterotrimeric G proteins as regulators of intra-Golgi vesicular transport. One is that ARF proteins serve as cofactors for cholera toxin in the ADP ribosylation of Gα subunits and, therefore, are likely to interact with Gα subunits. The other is that AlF_{3-5} (a complex of Al and F) that inactivates Gα subunits but has no effect on low-molecular-weight GTP-binding proteins, such as ARF or *rab* proteins,[52] inhibits transport[475] and stimulates coat assembly.[485] Although the specific G protein(s) involved in intra-Golgi transport have not been identified, it appears that both Gα stimulatory (Gsα) and inhibitory (Giα) subunits are involved in regulating this process. Thus, when added to an in vitro system, purified $\beta\gamma$ subunits — which are expected to capture and block the activity of free α subunits — inhibited the binding of ARF and β-COP to the Golgi membranes that is promoted by the addition of GTP-γ-S.[493] These findings suggested a role for a heterotrimeric G protein as a positive regulator of transport. In addition, a pertussis-toxin-sensitive $G_{i3}\alpha$ inhibitory subunit that could exert a negative control on vesicular transport through the Golgi apparatus has been localized to this organelle in cultured epithelial cells.[494] Overexpression of this subunit in transfected cells was found to retard the constitutive secretion of a basement membrane heparan sulfate proteoglycan, an effect that was suppressed by pretreating the cells with pertussis toxin.[495] The activation of a pertussis-toxin-sensitive G protein by mastoparan has been shown to antagonize the effect of BFA on the β-COP association with Golgi membranes.[496] This indicates that a Gi protein regulates the cycle of β-COP utilization, possibly by inhibiting the budding of vesicles from the donor membranes.

Molecular Machinery for Vesicle Targeting and Fusion[349,361]

The specificity of vesicular transport between different membrane compartments must be based on precise interactions between molecular components characteristic of the donor and acceptor membranes. On the other hand, the universality of vesicle transport processes makes it likely that certain steps that are common to all membrane fission and fusion events are carried out by the same protein machinery, regardless of the specific membranes involved. The paradigm for a protein that participates in multiple targeting processes is NSF, a soluble factor that was first identified as necessary for the completion of an intracisternal transport event in the Golgi apparatus, but is now known to play a role in many other interorganellar transport events.

The observation[497] that intra-Golgi transport was almost completely inhibited by treatment of the Golgi membranes with NEM was the basis for the identification and purification of NSF. This factor is normally associated with Golgi membranes,[343] but can be released from them by incubation in buffers containing ATP, a nucleotide that is also required to stabilize the protein through the purification procedure.[497] As mentioned above, NSF — which is equivalent to the yeast *SEC*18 gene product[20] — is required for vesicular transport between different compartments of the endomembrane system. NSF is a homotetrameric molecule of 76-kDa subunits that contain two putative ATP-binding sites each.[498] The factor manifests a low ATPase activity that appears to be essential for its function in mediating vesicle fusion.[348]

NSF acts late in intra-Golgi transport, after vesicle docking and uncoating. In fact, when in vitro transport is carried out in the absence of NSF and with NEM-treated Golgi fractions, uncoated vesicles accumulate on the acceptor membranes.[474,488] This is in contrast to the effect of the nonhydrolyzable analogue GTP-γ-S, which causes the accumulation of only coated vesicles. That the uncoated vesicles observed after NEM treatment are derived from coated ones, and that NSF acts after uncoating has taken place, was shown by the observation that when NEM-treated Golgi membranes are incubated in the in vitro system in the presence of the GTP-γ-S, only coated vesicles accumulate. Furthermore, the restoration of NSF to an NEM-treated system in which uncoated vesicles were allowed to accumulate led to a substantial completion of transport, even when GTP-γ-S was added. Although these observations indicate that NSF can function even when added late to the transport system, after vesicles have been formed and docked, the factor normally appears to be incorporated into the vesicles during their formation in the donor membrane.[473]

As mentioned in the section on ER-to-Golgi transport, the binding of NSF to Golgi membranes is mediated by SNAPs, which themselves recognize receptors (SNAREs for *SNAP r*eceptors) that are integral components of the membranes. Although SNAREs have not yet been purified from Golgi membranes, it has been possible to purify such proteins from a crude brain membrane fraction.[349] It is now believed that NSF-SNAP-SNARE interactions are required to execute most, if not all, vesicular transport events within the endomembrane system (see refs. 361 and 499). There is indirect evidence for the existence of two types of *SNAP r*eceptors, those (υ-SNAREs) which are found in the membranes of the donor organelle and in the vesicles derived from them and those (t-SNAREs) that are present in the acceptor or target membranes. It has been proposed that during the docking step that precedes membrane fusion complementary SNAREs interact in a process that is facilitated by SNAP and NSF molecules that hold the vesicle (donor) and acceptor (target) membranes together (Fig. 16-28). Fusion would then ensue by a not yet understood process.

Three SNAP polypeptides, α-, β-, and γ-SNAPs (33, 34, and 36 kDa, respectively), were purified from bovine brain cytosol using as an assay their capacity to stimulate the binding of NSF to Golgi membranes.[346,500] The first two SNAPs (α and β) are 83 percent identical in sequence and bind competitively in vitro to the same receptors, although β-SNAP is a protein specific to brain tissue.[501] γ-SNAP binds to a different site and acts synergistically with α-SNAP in stimulating transport.[502] α-SNAP is the mammalian equivalent of the yeast *Sec*17 gene product required for ER-to-Golgi transport in yeast[347] and it, but not β- or γ-SNAP, can restore the capacity of a *sec*17 yeast mutant cytosol to support intra-Golgi transport in a mammalian in vitro system.[346]

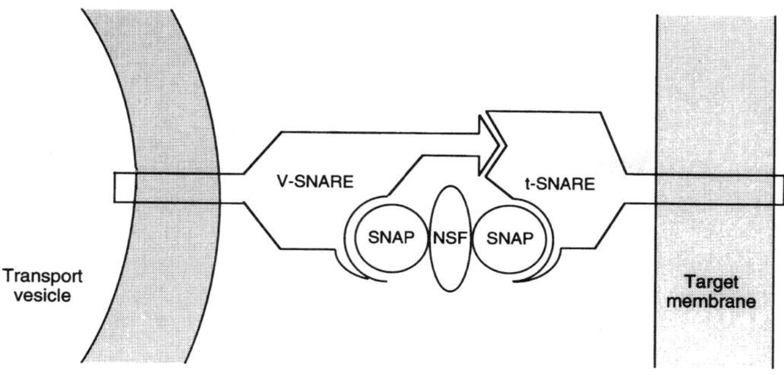

Fig. 16-28 Interactions between complementary SNAREs may determine the specificity of vesicle targeting to an acceptor membrane. SNAREs are integral membrane proteins that, in general, appear to be inserted in the membrane through their C-terminal ends and have most of their mass exposed on the cytoplasmic surface of the membrane. Complementary SNAREs are thought to be present in both the transport vesicles (v-SNARE), which acquire them during vesicle formation in the donor membrane, and in the acceptor membranes (t-SNARE), to which the vesicles are targeted.[349] SNAP proteins bound to SNAREs are capable of binding NSF in the presence of ATP. In this scheme, SNAREs are presumed to be bivalent, having one site that binds to a SNAP and another that is specific for a complementary SNARE. Vesicle docking would then involve an NSF-mediated interaction between SNAPs bound to a v-SNARE and to a t-SNARE, as well as the direct specific interaction between the SNAREs themselves. The sequence of events that follows and leads to membrane fusion is not known. A *rab* protein may also be involved in the targeting and/or triggering of membrane fusion, but at this time the functional relationship between *rab* proteins and SNAREs is obscure. Nevertheless, hydrolysis of ATP (in NSF) and GTP (in a *rab* protein) are likely to follow the interaction between complementary SNAREs.

NSF binds stably to SNAPs only after the latter are bound to their membrane receptors. NSF-SNAP-SNARE complexes formed on intact Golgi membranes can be isolated after detergent treatment but can also be formed when detergent extracts containing SNAREs are mixed with SNAPs and NSF.[503] The complexes (which have a sedimentation coefficient of 20S) contain γ-SNAP and α- or β-SNAP as alternative subunits. NSF must contain bound ATP to assemble into these complexes. When ATP hydrolysis (which occurs in the presence of Mg^2 even at 0°C) is allowed to take place, the particles disassemble and NSF is released. The 20S complexes, however, are stable in the absence of Mg^{2+} or when the nonhydrolyzable ATP analogue ATP-γ-S is present. These properties, together with the availability of recombinant SNAPs and a functionally active form of NSF containing an epitope tag at its C-terminus, for which an antibody is available, have allowed the purification of the SNAP receptors from detergent extracts of crude brain membrane fractions. NSF-SNAP-SNARE complexes formed in the presence of ATP-γ-S were recovered through the binding of the epitope tag on NSF to an immobilized antibody. Subsequent addition of ATP-Mg^{2+} led to the specific elution of the SNAP bound to their SNARE.[349]

Four different brain SNARE polypeptides were obtained in this manner and recognized as previously known proteins on the basis of partial peptide sequence data. Two of these are the closely related proteins, *syntaxins A* and *B*, that are anchored to the plasma membrane through their hydrophobic C-terminal peptide segments and are thought to be involved in the docking of synaptic vesicles near the voltage-gated calcium channels in the presynaptic membrane (see ref. 360). Of the other two SNARE obtained, one (VAMP, also known as *synaptobrevin*-2) is an 18-kDa integral membrane protein of the synaptic vesicle that is also anchored to the surface of the vesicle by a C-terminal hydrophobic domain.[504] The other is a protein named (coincidentally) *SNAP25*, (for *s*ynaptosome-*a*ssociated *p*rotein of 25 kDa), whose exact location has not been determined, although it is found in the presynaptic terminal of neurons.

As previously noted in our discussion of ER-to-Golgi transport in yeast, the synaptic vesicle membrane protein VAMP/synaptobrevin shows significant sequence similarity to the yeast proteins *Sly*12p*Bet*1p and *Sly*2p/*Sec*22p, which are required for transport between the ER and Golgi apparatus, with the latter protein actually becoming incorporated into the transport vesicles. Evidence has indicated that VAMP/synaptobrevin is even more closely related to a yeast gene (SNC2) product that is localized to post-Golgi vesicles and is required for Golgi-to-plasma-membrane transport.[361] Syntaxins are related to three yeast proteins required for vesicular transport: *Sed*5p, a multicopy suppressor of the loss of the *Erd*2p, the carrier that retrieves ER proteins with the HDEL C-terminal signal; *Pep*12p, a protein required for targeting to the yeast vacuole; and the product of SSO1, a multicopy suppressor of a mutation in Sec1p, a protein required for transport to the plasma membrane (see ref. 361). These similarities suggest that the machinery responsible for the regulated secretion of neurotransmitter at the synaptic ending may have evolved from the primitive machinery that mediated constitutive vesicle delivery across the endomembrane system and to the plasma membrane.

SORTING OF PROTEINS THAT EXIT FROM THE GOLGI APPARATUS: SECRETORY PATHWAYS IN EUKARYOTIC CELLS[56,505–507]

Proteins that traverse the Golgi apparatus and reach the TGN must be sorted into membrane-bounded carriers (vesicles or granules, see below) that transport them to their ultimate destination, which may be in the extracellular space, in a specific plasma membrane domain, or in endosomes or lysosomes. Many proteins destined for delivery to the plasma membrane or to be secreted from the cell are transported directly from the Golgi apparatus to the cell surface by a population of vesicles that continuously emerge from the TGN. On exocytosis, the membrane proteins of these vesicles become incorporated into the plasma membrane and the luminal content proteins are discharged into the extracellular medium. This is the basis for the so-called *constitutive* or *nonregulated secretion* of proteins. The continuous discharge that takes place during this process can be contrasted with the *regulated secretion* of proteins and other products (see below) that takes place in many specialized cells. Regulated secretion requires the prior concentration and storage of secretory products into *secretory granules* or *vesicles* that release their content into the extracellular space only when an appropriate stimulus leads to fusion of the granule membrane with the plasma membrane.

Constitutive secretion is a generalized function of all cells. It represents the mechanism by which hepatocytes secrete a wide variety of serum proteins into the blood, fibroblasts secrete collagen and other components of the extracellular matrix, and plasma cells secrete immunoglobulins. The regulated secretory pathway, on the other hand, is utilized by many exocrine and endocrine cells, which must respond quickly to physiological stimulation with a burst of secretory activity. For example, digestive enzymes are stored within zymogen granules of pancreatic acinar cells and, on stimulation by a secretagogue, are released on the apical surfaces of the cells, which confront the acinar lumen, after which they are transported to the intestine. Similarly, distinct cell types in the anterior pituitary gland store specific hormones that are released by exocytosis when the cells are stimulated by the appropriate hypothalamic releasing hormones. In addition, the extended processes of some neurosecretory cells, such as those that constitute the neurohypophysis, are packed with large amounts of secretory granules that are formed in the Golgi apparatus of hypothalamic neurons, and are transferred to the nerve terminals where exocytosis takes place. Many physiological mechanisms rely on unicellular glands — such as mast cells, blood granulocytes, and platelets — that also store their secretory products within granules and discharge their content at the cell surface after appropriate stimulation.

Release of neurotransmitters from neurons represents an important example of regulated secretion. In these cells, two types of secretory vesicles whose contents are released in a regulated fashion are produced.[508] One consists of *large dense core vesicles* (LDCV), which contain peptide neurotransmitters derived from proteins synthesized in the ER. These vesicles are formed in the TGN and are equivalent to the secretory granules of other secretory cells. The other type consists of *synaptic vesicles* (SV), which are highly homogeneous in size (50 nm), lack a dense core, and secrete nonpeptide neurotransmitters on stimulation of the neuron. Synaptic vesicles are clustered near their release sites at nerve endings and undergo repeated cycles of exocytosis and endocytosis within the nerve terminal, where they are refilled with the neurotransmitters.[507,509]

The exocytotic event required for regulated secretion results from the activation of a signal-transducing mechanism that involves either the interaction of a ligand with a plasma membrane receptor or the arrival of a nerve stimulus that opens ion channels. By a variety of mechanisms, these events lead to a transient rise in the cytoplasmic concentration of a "secondary messenger," such as Ca^{2+}, cAMP, or a phosphoinositide (see ref. 510). In a process that is still not well understood, this leads to fusion of the membrane of the secretory vesicle or granule with the plasma membrane.

Biogenesis of Secretory Granules[511–514a]

Secretory granules (SG) are membrane-bound structures that contain a dense core in which the secretory material is highly concentrated. In some granules, the dense core is a stable structure that remains intact even when the membrane is removed after isolation of the granules by cell fractionation.[515,516] The size and shape of a secretory granule is generally characteristic of the products that are stored in it. Frequently, different cell types can be identified by the morphologic characteristics of their granules, as in the pituitary, endocrine pancreas, and blood granulocyte populations.

Many cells capable of regulated secretion are specialized for the production of one major secretory protein (e.g., pituitary thyrotrophs) or of several polypeptides that are derived from a single precursor (e.g., proopiomelanocortin in pituitary corticotrophs). Other cells, such as those in the exocrine pancreas, store within a single type of granule a variety of independently produced secretory proteins[517–521] that are released together on stimulation. However, some endocrine cells, such as the pituitary gonadotrophs, are able to store two different polypeptide hormones (i.e., LH and FSH) in separate granules, which may be easily identified by their different sizes.[522] It is reasonable to assume that in gonadotrophs this segregation is important to allow for the differential release of each hormone at different periods of the menstrual cycle. In the somatomammotrophs of the bovine anterior pituitary, three major types of granules are formed: one contains primarily prolactin, another growth hormone, and a third granins (see below) together with luteinizing hormone (LH) and thyroid-stimulating hormone (TSH).[523,524] In human neutrophils, which also segregate different sets of secretory products into distinct granule types[525–527] (e.g., azurophilic, specific, and secretory gelatinase-containing granules), different stimuli may lead to the differential release of the content of each type of granule.[527]

Studies with pancreatic exocrine[528–530] and endocrine[531] cells and with cultured tumor cell lines[532] have shown that both the constitutive and regulated pathways can operate in a single cell and that different products are channeled preferentially to each pathway. For example, AtT-20 cells (a line of rat pituitary origin) form secretory granules that contain ACTH and other derivatives of POMC. On stimulation with 8-Br-cAMP, they release their granule contents by exocytosis. Although these cells are used as a model to study secretion, the segregation of POMC to the secretory granules is not very efficient. More than two-thirds of the newly synthesized POMC is also steadily released by the constitutive pathway. On the other hand, laminin, a component of the extracellular matrix, is secreted from the same cells essentially exclusively by the constitutive route.[533] A truncated secretory version of the VSV G glycoprotein, synthesized in AtT-20 cells transfected with the appropriate gene,[534] is also excluded from the regulated pathway.

These observations suggest that proteins incorporated into secretory granules contain specific information that leads to their segregation from the constitutively secreted polypeptides which follow different pathways to the surface. In fact, other endocrine or exocrine products, such as proinsulin,[535] growth hormone,[534] and trypsinogen,[533] when synthesized in transfected AtT-20 cells, are as effectively incorporated into granules as the endogenous derivatives of POMC. Similar findings have been made with GH_3 cells, a growth hormone-producing cell line, which after transfection with a gene encoding proparathyroid hormone (pPTH) incorporate this polypeptide in the same granules in which growth hormone is packaged.[536] Since proteins such as these that normally follow the regulated pathway are secreted constitutively when expressed in cells that do not form granules,[537] one can conclude that proteins packaged into granules have common features that can be decoded only by a sorting machinery specific to cells capable of regulated secretion. The notion that constitutively secreted proteins do not contain specific sorting information but specific signals are required for the incorporation of proteins into the granules is supported by the finding that a chimeric polypeptide consisting of the entire truncated secretory form of the VSV G protein (which by itself is secreted constitutively) linked to the C-terminus of human growth hormone is effectively incorporated into granules when synthesized in transfected AtT-20 cells.[538]

As previously noted, many proteins that are stored in secretory granules are synthesized as larger precursors (*proproteins*) that are proteolytically processed intracellularly, either in the TGN or after sorting to *immature secretory granules* (ISG). Processing involves removal of an N-terminal (e.g., proparathyroid hormone or prosomatostatin) or even interior (e.g., proinsulin) propeptide segment (see ref. 514). In some cases, such as that of prosomatostatin, the N-terminal propeptide sequence (82 amino acids) is sufficient to target a reporter polypeptide to storage granules.[539,540] This is perhaps not surprising for prosomatostatin, since its propeptide constitutes the bulk of the precursor, the hormone consisting of only 16 amino acids. In contrast, the interior C peptide (34 amino acids long) of proinsulin that links the B and A chains can be replaced with an unrelated sequence without affecting the targeting of the prohormone.[541] Similarly, the N-terminal propeptide of trypsinogen, which is normally removed from the protein after its secretion, is not required for packaging into granules.[542]

Studies on the targeting of *von Willebrand factor* (vWf) to *Weibel-Palade bodies*, specialized secretory granules characteristic of endothelial cells, have been of particular interest (see ref. 543) because they suggest that this protein contains information that leads to its segregation, not only from constitutively secreted proteins, but also from other proteins that are packaged into granules. Weibel-Palade bodies are approximately 0.1 µm wide and 1 to 4 µm long and are characterized by the presence of a core structure consisting of a bundle of long narrow tubules that appear to be composed, at least in part, of the vWf itself. This is a very large protein (2050 amino acids) derived from a proprotein that dimerizes through disulfide bonds in the ER and undergoes removal of a large N-terminal propeptide segment (741 amino acids) at the time at which it also undergoes multimerization in the TGN and storage in the specialized granules. In cultured endothelial cells, only the large multimers of vWf (10 to 20×10^6 daltons) are stored in the Weibel-Palade bodies. Smaller ones are secreted constitutively.[544] When the vWf is synthesized in transfected cells that carry out regulated secretion, such as the POMC-producing AtT-20 cells or the rat insulinoma RIN5F cell line, the factor is incorporated into newly formed Weibel-Palade body-like structures and not into the secretory granules characteristic of the host cell.[545] Moreover, it was found that the vWf-containing Weibel-Palade-like granules did not form in transfected cell lines that do not carry out regulated secretion, such as Chinese hamster ovary (CHO), monkey kidney (COS), and 3T3 mouse fibroblast cells, even though some of these cells cleave the propeptide and form high-molecular-weight multimers.[545] This suggests that assembly of the storage granule characteristic of endothelial cells requires, in addition to vWf, one or more components that are involved in the formation of secretory granules in other cell types, but does not require components specific to the endothelial cells. In another study,[546] however, Weibel-Palade-like bodies were found to form in transfected CV-1 cells — which are the parental line of COS cells and are not known to carry out regulated secretion. This led to the suggestion that a critical concentration of vWf in the TGN is the only factor required for granule formation and that components of a preexisting regulated secretion pathway are not necessary. Nevertheless, it should be noted that it has not been shown that some components of the regulated secretory machinery are not present in CV-1 cells.

It is interesting that the large propeptide of vWf, which is normally secreted as a noncovalently linked dimer together with the multimers of vWf, is required for storage of the factor in Weibel-Palade-like bodies formed *de novo* in transfected AtT-20 and RIN cells. In itself, however, the propeptide is not sufficient to induce formation of the storage organelle, but its coexpression with the mature vWf (lacking its prosequence) leads to incorporation of both noncovalently-linked molecules into newly formed Weibel-Palade bodies.[546] It can be concluded that the formation of a condensed multimeric form of vWf, for which the propeptide is required, is a key step in the biogenesis of the Weibel-Palade bodies. A study of the effects of specific mutations and deletions indicates, however, that the formation of disulfide bonds between vWf subunits is not necessary for packaging in the bodies.[545,547] On the other hand, the acidic pH that prevails in the *trans* region of the Golgi apparatus is required, since Weibel-Palade bodies do not form in cultured endothelial cells when these are incubated with weak bases that dissipate the acidic pH of intracellular organelles.[548]

Mechanisms for the Sorting of Proteins into Secretory Granules[511–513,548a]

The sorting processes responsible for the formation of secretory granules begin to take place in the *trans* region of the Golgi apparatus and in the TGN. In some cell types that carry out regulated secretion, the condensation of secretory material that leads to the formation of the core of a secretory granule is first detected in the dilated rims of the *trans*-Golgi cisternae (see ref. 386a). In other cell types they first appear in regions of the TGN. The large *condensing vacuoles* that in pancreatic exocrine cells and in other cell types accumulate secretory material may also be specialized regions of the *trans*-Golgi network that ultimately bud off to form an immature secretory granule. In fact, immature granules and condensing vacuoles have many of the properties of the TGN, such as the presence of acid phosphatase, the capacity to carry out the sulfation of tyrosine residues and of oligosaccharides (see ref. 511), and the presence of patches of clathrin on their surfaces.[516] After the dense core aggregate begins to form in the TGN, the process of granule formation continues, with its envelopment by a membrane and the subsequent budding of an *immature secretory granule* (ISG). This undergoes a maturation process in which further condensation of the content occurs and excess membrane is removed. The cytoplasmic surface of the ISG membrane often possesses a patchy clathrin coat.[549] It is not known if this is involved in the formation of the granule, perhaps by inducing its budding from the TGN, or if it is utilized to form coated vesicles that remove from the immature granule membrane and content proteins with other destinations. Indeed, the ISG appears to be a sorting compartment. In pancreatic islet β cells, it may be the site where the C peptide cleaved from proinsulin is diverted into vesicles that bud off from the immature granule and release it constitutively at the cell surface.[550] In some cells the maturation of immature granules involves their fusion with each other to form larger granules from which excess membrane must be removed. In other cell types, maturation involves solely condensation of the core and membrane removal and yields a smaller granule.

It was originally thought that the concentration of secretory material needed to form the core of immature granules in the TGN is effected by membrane-bound pH-sensitive receptors. These would ferry their ligands to regions of the Golgi complex that contain a proton pump capable of generating the acidic medium required to release the ligands. In this *active sorting model* (see ref. 511) receptors would then recycle to more proximal regions of the Golgi apparatus to bind additional ligand molecules. Much support has been obtained, however, for an alternative *passive sorting model* (Fig. 16-29) for the segregation of proteins in secretory granules. This model does not require the participation of receptors to effect the segregation, but simply involves the spontaneous aggregation of the protein molecules to be stored within the same granule. Such an aggregation would require a high concentration of the proteins and would be triggered by the conditions that prevail in the TGN and *trans* region of the Golgi apparatus (i.e., a mildly acidic pH and a high Ca^{2+} concentration). In some cells, the incorporation of proteins into aggregates may also require the presence of specific granule matrix components such as the granins. These (e.g., *chromogranin A*,[551] *chromogranin B/secretogranin I*, and *secretogranin II*[552]) are a family of acidic proteins that are present in secretory granules of many different types of endocrine cells and neurons, where they are stored and released together with cell type-specific peptide hormones and neuropeptides.[553] In vitro, under the conditions that prevail in the TGN, the granins form aggregates that effectively exclude constitutively secreted proteins such as immunoglobulin.[554,555] The Ca^{2+}-induced aggregation of granins is likely to be a consequence of their high content of acidic residues, which bind the divalent cation (see ref. 553).

The process that sorts regulated secretory proteins from constitutive proteins in neuroendocrine cells has been studied extensively using as a model PC12 cells, a line derived from a rat pheochromocytoma. In these cells, the granins undergo sulfation of tyrosine residues in the *trans*-Golgi,[556] where constitutively secreted proteoglycans are sulfated in their carbohydrates.[557] It is, therefore, possible to label selectively with $[^{35}S]SO_4^{2+}$ both types of proteins as they reach the TGN. This allowed the demonstration that the aggregation of the granins is determined by the environmental conditions in the TGN. Thus, the proteins could be extracted from detergent-permeabilized TGN-derived vesicles only when these were incubated in a medium of neutral pH that lacks Ca^{2+}, whereas the constitutively secreted free glycosaminoglycan molecules could be extracted even in Ca^{2+}-containing acidic mediums.[558] In accordance with these findings, the packaging of secretogranin II into the granules of PC12 cells was markedly reduced when the cells were incubated with chloroquine or NH_4Cl. These agents, which are known to neutralize the pH of acidic intracellular organelles, led to the constitutive secretion of a large fraction of the newly synthesized granins.[554]

The aggregation-mediated sorting model easily explains the formation of different secretory granule populations within the same cell, as a result of homophilic interactions (e.g., granules containing either prolactin or growth hormone in somatomammotrophs) or heterophilic interactions, (e.g., granules containing LH, TSH, and granins). The observation that different proteins may be segregated within the core of a single granule — as is sometimes the case with prolactin and growth hormone in the bovine somatomammotrophs[559] and glucagon and glycentin[560] in the α granules of pancreatic islet cells — could be explained by the envelopment of separate aggregates into one immature granule in

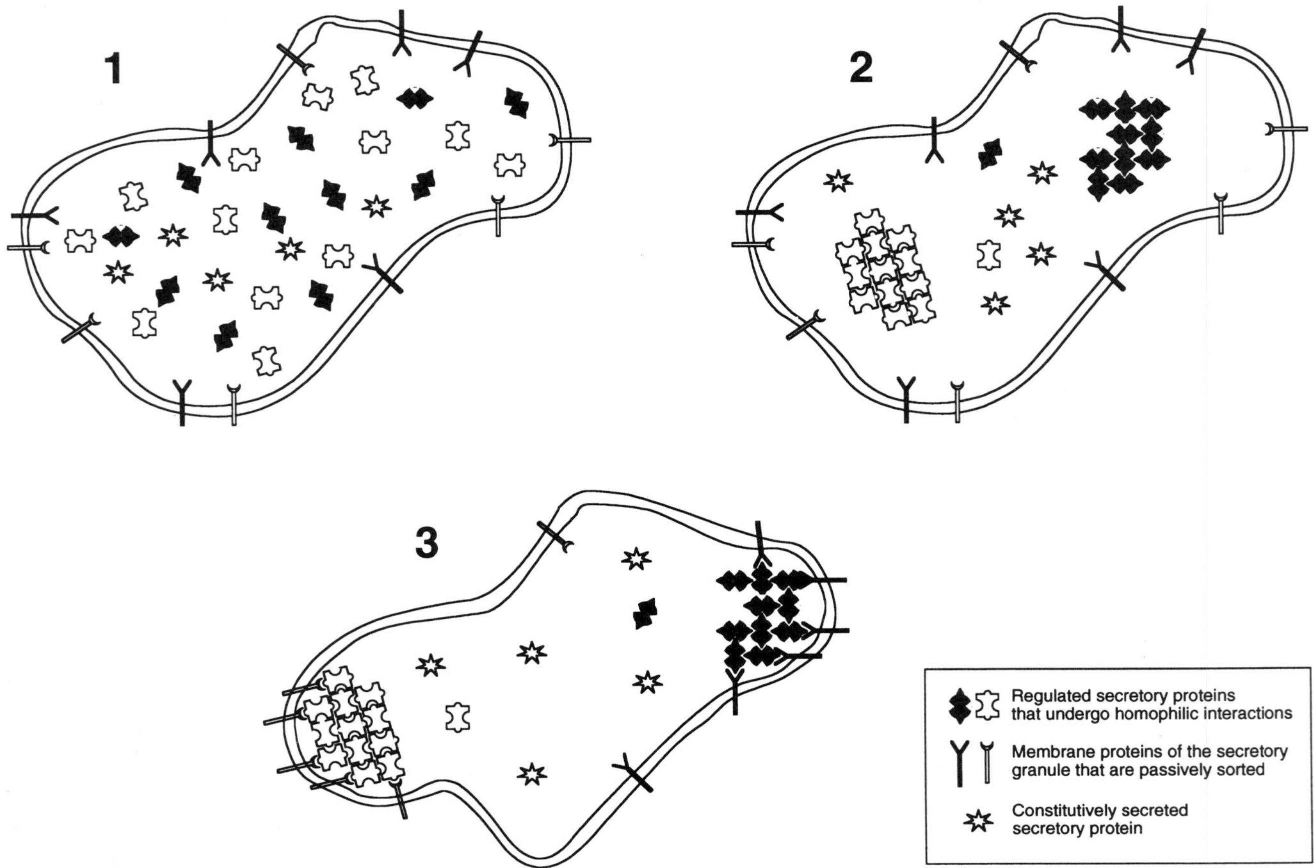

Fig. 16-29 Aggregation-mediated passive sorting of secretory and membrane proteins during the biogenesis of a secretory granule in the TGN. (1) The luminal contents of a TGN cisterna is depicted as consisting of a mixture of secretory proteins. One type (stars) is secreted constitutively, without being incorporated into secretory granules. (2) The two other types are capable of homophilic interactions and undergo self-aggregation in the milieu of the TGN. (3) Some integral membrane proteins of the TGN that are destined to become part of the secretory granule membrane bind specifically to one or the other aggregate. The clustering of these membrane proteins generates a granule membrane with a specific protein composition. In some cases (not shown) self-aggregating luminal proteins also exist in a membrane-bound form and the homophilic interaction between the soluble and the membrane-bound proteins leads to sorting of the secretory and membrane proteins into an immature granule. In other cases, two or more different types of luminal proteins undergo coaggregation, although only one type of protein may interact directly with membrane components.

the TGN, or by the fusion of two different immature granules with each other. The cocondensation of many different proteins in pancreatic acinar cells required to form a zymogen granule would involve extensive heterophilic interactions.

After secretory protein aggregation, the next step in granule formation is the acquisition of a specific membrane. One mechanism by which this can occur is suggested by the finding that certain abundant granule content proteins, such as chromogranin B in PC12 cells, are also present in small amounts in a form tightly associated with the granule membrane.[561] Through homophilic interactions with the luminal aggregate these membrane-associated forms would lead to the membrane envelopment of the developing core, largely excluding nonaggregating constitutive proteins (see Fig. 16-29). A similar homophilic membrane-core interaction may take place during the development of chromaffin granules, in which dopamine-β-hydroxylase exists not only as a content protein but also as a type II membrane protein, anchored to the membrane by its uncleaved signal sequence.[562]

The sorting of membrane proteins to secretory granules has also become amenable to analysis with the identification of several specific proteins of granule membranes. P-selectin is a membrane protein specific to Weibel-Palade bodies of endothelial cells and α granules of platelets. This protein has a type I disposition and its 23 amino acid cytoplasmic C-terminal tail is necessary and sufficient for its sorting to the granules.[563] However, the signal in this tail operates only in cells that assemble regulated secretory granules and the protein is constitutively transported to the plasma membrane in other cell types.[563,564] The presence of a sorting signal in the cytoplasmic domain suggests that it is recognized by cytoplasmic components of a sorting machinery, such as the adaptor or coat proteins that mediate the assembly of clathrin-coated vesicles (see below). Peptidylglycine α-amidating monooxygenase (PAM) is another membrane protein whose cytoplasmic domain contains sorting information for secretory granules.[565] Deletion of this portion of the protein abolishes its targeting to granules, although a truncated form that lacks both the transmembrane and cytoplasmic domains is sorted to secretory granules.[566] It would seem, therefore, that the truncated soluble PAM is sorted by coaggregation with other endogenous regulated secreting proteins, but that this cannot take place when the protein is membrane-anchored. GP2 is a pancreatic zymogen granule membrane protein anchored in the membrane by a glycosylphosphatidylinositol moiety (GPI). Therefore, this protein lacks transmembrane and cytoplasmic domains, but like many luminal proteins, such as the granins, undergoes aggregation, which probably accounts for its sorting to the granule membrane.[548a,567] As will be mentioned below, GPI-linked proteins can be released from membranes by cleavage of their lipid anchor, and after detachment from the membrane, GP2 forms aggregates under TGN conditions.[568]

Biochemical Requirements for the Formation of Constitutive and Regulated Secretory Vesicles in the TGN

The formation of constitutive and regulated secretory vesicles in the TGN resembles in its biochemical requirements the generation of vesicles in other compartments of the endomembrane system. Using a postnuclear supernatant fraction from PC12 cells pulse-labeled with $[^{35}S]SO_4^{2-}$, it has been possible to reproduce in vitro the formation of two distinct populations of vesicles from the TGN. One corresponds to constitutive secretory vesicles that contain heparan sulfate proteoglycan, and another to immature secretory granules containing secretogranin II. The two types of vesicles could be separated by centrifugation. Their production requires an energy supply and the hydrolysis of GTP within a GTP-binding protein, since it was inhibited to a significant extent by the GTP analogue GTP-γ-S.[569] In addition, both in vivo and in vitro studies demonstrated that BFA also inhibits the formation of both types of vesicles in the TGN.[570,571] Since in other systems (see above) this drug blocks vesicle formation by inhibiting the ARF-dependent association of coat proteins with donor membranes, it seems very likely that a similar coat protein-membrane association takes place during the assembly of secretory vesicles in the TGN even though the biochemical nature of the coat remains to be elucidated.

The production of both types of secretory vesicles in the TGN is controlled by heterotrimeric G proteins of the Gi/Go and Gs classes. The involvement of an inhibitory (Giα) G protein became apparent from the findings that AlF_{3-5} suppressed vesicle formation in vitro, while highly purified $\beta\gamma$ subunits, which should block the function of a Gα, stimulated it.[572] Moreover, treatment with mastoparan — the peptide that mimics an activated G protein-coupled receptor and preferentially activates Giα — inhibited cell-free vesicle formation in vitro. This effect was abolished by pertussis toxin pretreatment of the cells, which inactivates Giα. As expected from these effects, treatment of the cells with the toxin alone increased the subsequent in vitro formation of both constitutive secretory vesicles and secretory granules. Evidence that a stimulatory Gsα exerts a positive control in vesicle formation in the TGN came from the observation that pretreatment of the cells with cholera toxin, which activates Gsα by inhibiting its GTPase activity, increases the production of vesicles and immature secretory granules in a subsequent in vitro incubation. Under these conditions, activation of the inhibitory Gi/Go subunits not affected by the toxin, by the addition of GTP-γ-S or AlF_{3-5}, counteracted the stimulatory effect of cholera toxin.[370] Based on these data, a hypothetical scheme has been proposed for the role of both inhibitory and stimulatory G proteins in the formation of secretory vesicles that is shown in Fig. 16-30.

These findings indicate that a highly complex regulatory mechanism operates in the TGN to control vesicle formation. The identification of receptor-like molecules that presumably lead to

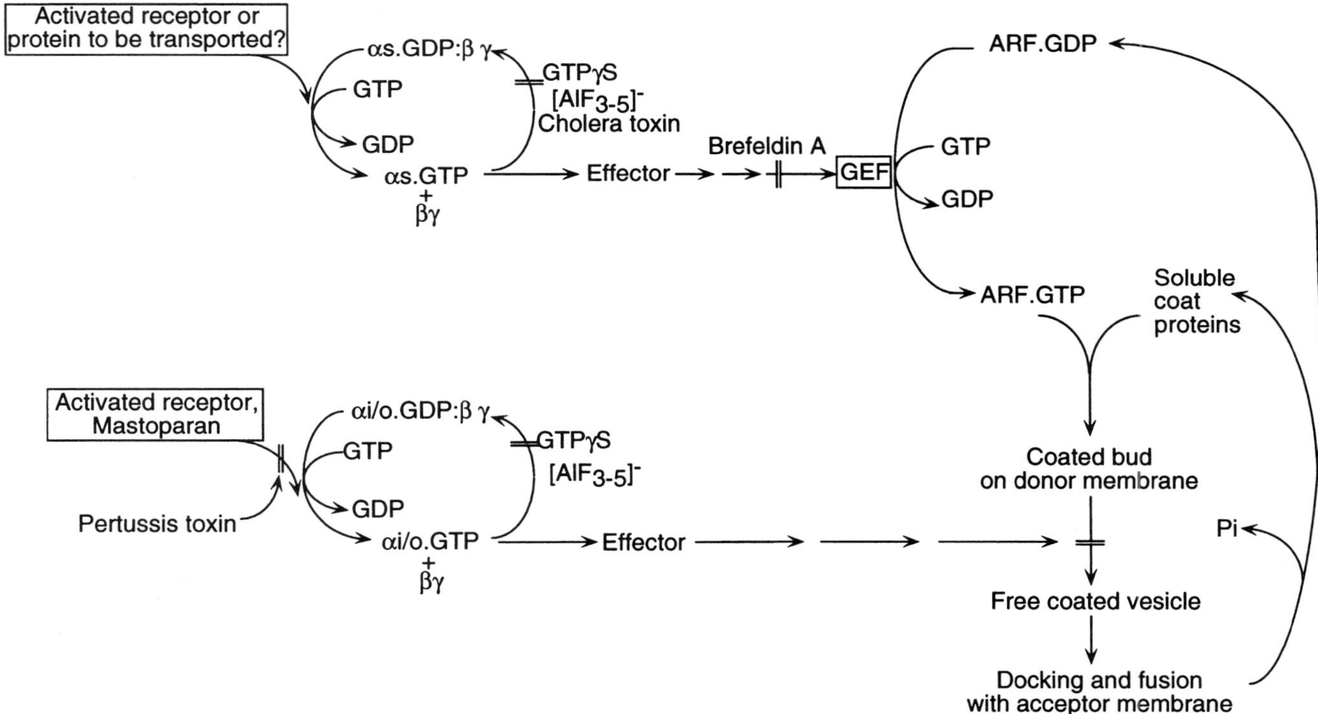

Fig. 16-30 Both stimulatory (Gsα) and inhibitory (Giα/Goα) heterotrimeric G proteins control the production of secretory vesicles in the TGN. This scheme (based on Bauerfeind and Huttner[513]) depicts the formation of a secretory vesicle in the TGN as requiring the activated form of an ARF protein and the recruitment of soluble coat proteins to form a coated bud in the donor membrane (right side of the figure). The activation of ARF depends on the function of a guanine nucleotide exchange protein (GEF), which is controlled either directly by a heterotrimeric G protein of the Gsα type (*top left*), or through an effector regulated by such a G protein. The budding of the coated vesicle from the donor membrane is depicted as being inhibited by the action of an activated G protein of the Giα/Goα class (*bottom*). The stimulatory G protein may be controlled by an intracellular receptor that recognizes a protein to be transported, or by the protein to be transported itself. The effect of cholera toxin is to maintain the Gsα in the active configuration that stimulates coated bud formation and, hence, vesicle release. BFA prevents the activation of the GEF that is necessary for the activation of ARF and, hence, blocks coated bud formation. However, the precise site of action of BFA in the pathway that links the activation of the Gsα to that of the GEF is not known. The inhibitory effect of mastoparan (which is abrogated by pertussis toxin) on vesicle formation suggests that the inhibitory G protein (Giα/Goα) is linked to an intracellular receptor-like molecule that controls its action. Because AlF_{3-5} (which stimulates both Gsα and Giα/Goα) inhibits vesicle formation, it is assumed that the inhibitory G protein acts at a later step (e.g., vesicle fission) than the stimulatory G protein.

GDP-GTP exchange in the Gα subunits and identification of the effectors controlled by these subunits is essential for understanding these processes. As previously mentioned, Gsα appears to promote COP-coated vesicle formation within the Golgi stacks by stimulating GDP-GTP exchange on ARF. It may have a similar role in the TGN, although the specific coat proteins have yet to be identified. The mechanism by which the Giα suppresses vesicle production in the TGN is unknown, but one possibility is that it acts to prevent fission of vesicles with a fully assembled coat.[513]

COVALENT LINKAGE OF LIPIDS TO PROTEINS[39,573–578]

Many proteins synthesized in free and in bound polysomes contain lipid moieties covalently linked to their polypeptide backbones. In some cases, the lipid moiety serves as the sole membrane anchor for a polypeptide that lacks a hydrophobic segment. In others, a polypeptide bearing a permanent lipid anchor carries out a cyclic function that requires attachment and detachment from the membrane. In still other proteins, the lipid only reinforces a membrane anchorage mediated by a hydrophobic segment of the polypeptide. Finally, some proteins bearing lipids do not associate with membranes and remain in the cytoplasm or are secreted from the cell.

Lipid-modified proteins participate in a diverse array of cellular processes including signal transduction and growth regulation, intracellular vesicular transport and protein sorting, cell adhesion, and cytoskeletal organization.

N-Myristoylation of Proteins[39,575,579]

Certain proteins synthesized in free polysomes have the 14-carbon saturated fatty acid chain, *myristate*, bound through an amide linkage to the α amino group of an N-terminal glycine. Examples include: (1) the catalytic subunit of the cAMP-dependent protein kinase, (2) NADH cytochrome-*b*5 reductase, (3) the phosphoprotein phosphatase calcineurin, (4) the Goα subunit of heterotrimeric G proteins, (5) the small GTP-binding ARF proteins, which play a critical role in vesicular transport, and (6) a number of oncogene products, including the transforming protein of the Rous sarcoma virus ($p60^{v\text{-}src}$) and its corresponding cellular protooncogene ($p60^{c\text{-}src}$). *N*-myristoylation of these proteins is a cotranslational process. Following proteolytic removal of the initiator methionine by an independent activity, the enzyme *myristoyl CoA:protein* N-*myristoyltransferase* (NMT) transfers a myristoyl group from myristoyl CoA to the glycine residue exposed at the new N-terminus of the nascent chain.[580] The amino acid sequence following the myristoylated glycine varies significantly in different proteins, but it is clear that a short peptide sequence at the N-terminus determines the modification. In the case of $p60^{v\text{-}src}$, the signal recognized by the NMT is wholly contained within the first 14 residues of the protein.[581] A comprehensive analysis of the N-terminal sequences of chimeric polypeptides containing normal and mutated N-terminal portions of the vaccinia virus LIR protein indicated that the first 5 amino acid residues (GAAAS) represent a minimum sequence required for myristoylation of LIR. When the first 12 amino acids were included, myristoylation was as effective as in the natural protein.[582]

In the case of the $p60^{v\text{-}src}$, myristoylation leads to the association of the protein with the inner (cytoplasmic) face of the plasma membrane. This association is an absolute requirement for the transforming activity of the oncogene product.[583,584] Similarly, the lipid-mediated association of NADH cytochrome b_5 reductase with the cytoplasmic face of the ER membrane[585] is required for the function of this enzyme in the electron transport chain that effects fatty acid desaturation in the ER. It is not yet clear what factors determine the association of different myristoylated proteins with different membranes. It seems likely that specific interactions with other membrane proteins facilitate the incorporation of the acylated polypeptide into a given organelle. In the case of the Src protein, targeting to the plasma membrane appears to be mediated by a specific receptor that binds to the myristoylated N-terminal region of the protein.[586] It is clear that, at least in some cases, portions other than the myristoylated N-terminal region are required to maintain the association of a protein with the membrane. For example, the catalytic subunit of the cAMP-dependent protein kinase is found associated with the regulatory subunit on the cytoplasmic face of the plasma membrane, but is released into the cytoplasm when activated by cAMP.[587] Similarly, the ARF protein—whose myristoylation is essential for its function in generating Golgi vesicles—binds to the Golgi membranes only when it contains bound GTP.[45]

C-Terminal Addition of Glycolipid Anchors to Plasma Membrane Proteins[576–578,588–590a]

Many membrane proteins have been identified as being anchored to the outer leaflet of the plasma membrane lipid bilayer by a glycosylinositolphospholipid (GIPL) moiety (also referred to as GPI or PIG) which is linked via a phosphorylethanolamine in an amide linkage to the C-terminus of the polypeptide (Fig. 16-31). These proteins can usually be released from the cell surface by

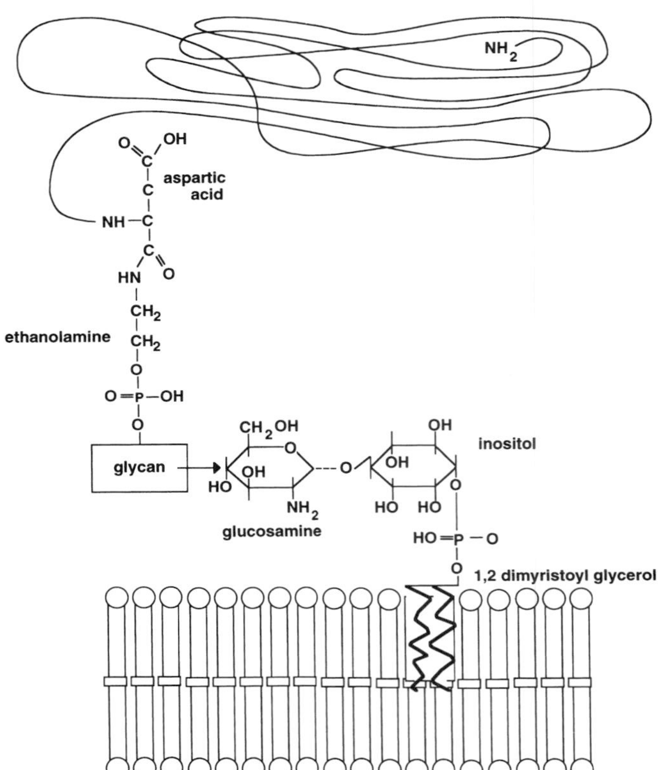

Fig. 16-31 Anchorage of proteins to membranes via a glycosyl phosphatidyl inositol (GIPL or GPI) moiety. A glycan that contains a core structure consisting of Man α1-2 Man α1-6 Man α1-4 GlcN is linked by a phosphodiester bond from the 6-carbon of the first mannose residue to an ethanolamine, which is in turn linked in an amide bond to the C-terminal amino acid in the polypeptide. The glycan is also linked through the glucosamine residue, that is unsubstituted in its amino group, by an α1-4 linkage to the myoinositol residue in phosphatidylinositol. Insertion of the fatty acid chains in the phospholipid bilayer serves to anchor the protein in the membrane. The core glycan may have a variety of substituents, such as a branched chain of galactose residues linked to the second mannose, which, alternatively, may bear a second phosphoethanolanine. Other sugars, such as additional mannoses, *N*-acetylgalactosamine, or sialic acid, may also be bound to the core. The phosphatidylinositol may carry two acyl groups (one of which may be myristate) and in some cases one acyl and one alkyl group. It is believed that even in a single protein there may be significant variation in the structure and composition of the glycan.

treatment with a phosphoinositol-specific phospholipase C (PIPLC). GIPL-linked proteins include the variant surface glycoprotein (VSG) of African trypanosomes, the placental and intestinal alkaline phosphatases, acetylcholinesterase (AChE), 5′ nucleotidase, the Thy-1 antigen of T lymphocytes, one form of the neural adhesion molecule N-CAM, and the decay-accelerating factor (DAF) that protects host red cells from complement-mediated lysis. The membrane anchor in the GIPL moiety is provided by the fatty acids of a diacylglycerol molecule that is part of the complex glycosylinositolphospholipid. The glycan group within GIPL contains a conserved linear core structure[591,592] that includes three mannoses and a nonacetylated glucosamine (ethanolamine-P-6Manα1-2Manα1-6Manα1-4GlcNα1-6) linked to the inositol. Frequently other groups, such as an additional phosphorylethanolamine, mannose, *N*-acetylgalactosamine, or galactose residues, are linked to the core, and an additional fatty acid may be linked to the inositol.

Proteins that acquire the glycosylphosphatidylinositol moiety (in a process also known as *glypiation*) are synthesized as transmembrane precursors. These are type I membrane proteins that are inserted in the ER by an N-terminal cleavable insertion signal and are anchored in the ER membrane by a short hydrophobic (8 to 20 amino acids) peptide segment at the C-terminus, so that few, if any, residues are exposed on the cytoplasmic surface of the membrane. GIPL addition takes place very soon after completion of translation and insertion of the protein in the ER membrane.[593] The reaction can be considered a transpeptidation in which the transmembrane protein precursor loses the C-terminal segment that served as peptide membrane anchor, while an amide linkage to the ethanolamine in a preformed GIPL anchor unit is established. The presence of preformed glycolipid anchors can be detected in both trypanosomes and murine lymphoma cells. Many of the details of the anchor synthesis have been worked out in these systems.[578,590] The enzyme(s) that removes the hydrophobic peptide anchor from the precursor and replaces it with the lipid anchor has not been identified, and the fate of the cleaved peptide is unknown.

In the case of the DAF protein, in which addition of the GIPL anchor involves removal of the last 17 amino acids, the information that determines this modification has been shown to be contained within the last 37 amino acids of the primary translation product.[594] Detailed mutagenesis studies have shown that, in addition to the C-terminal hydrophobic peptide segment, a critical feature for addition of the GIPL anchor is the presence at a position 10 to 12 residues N-terminal to the beginning of the hydrophobic domain of a pair of small amino acid residues that define the cleavage point in the precursor.[595] Exhaustive mutagenesis of the amino acid residue in alkaline phosphatase to which the GIPL is added demonstrated that, in addition to the natural Asp at that site, only Gly, Ala, Cys, Asn, or Ser are compatible with normal processing of the precursor.[596] These are the same residues that are naturally present at the sites of cleavage in the precursors of other GIPL proteins.[576] The importance of the region that determines the cleavage site is highlighted by the fact that the sequences of the GIPL-linked and transmembrane forms of the chicken cell adhesion protein N-CAM (which are encoded in mRNA generated by alternative splicing of a primary transcript) diverge seven amino acids upstream (toward the N-terminus) of the site of GPI addition.[597] The requirement for the lack of a cytoplasmic C-terminal domain for GIPL-linkage is apparent from the fact that addition of such a domain to the precursor of alkaline phosphatase prevented its processing and resulted in a mature transmembrane protein.[598] Moreover, the sequences of the GIPL-linked and transmembrane forms of the lymphocyte adhesion protein *LFA-3* (whose mRNAs are also generated by alternative splicing of a primary transcript) diverge only at sequences beginning two amino acids from the C-terminal end of the transmembrane domain.[599]

Several possible functions for the anchoring of proteins to the cell surface via the glycosylated phosphoinositides have been proposed. These include an enhanced mobility of the protein within the plane of the bilayer, the possibility of regulating the release of the protein by the action of an extracellular phospholipase C, or even generating the intracellular "messenger" diacylglycerol that could serve to activate a protein kinase C.

A defect in the pathway of GIPL addition is the basis for *paroxysmal nocturnal hemoglobinuria* (PNH), an acquired condition in which the GPI-linked proteins DAF and CD59 are absent from the surface of erythrocytes, which renders them susceptible to complement-mediated hemolysis. PNH is due to a somatic mutation in a pluripotent hematopoietic stem cell[600] that affects a gene for an enzyme that functions in the GIPL synthesis pathway.[601,602] On clonal expansion, the defect is manifested in a large, but variable, fraction of both erythrocytes and leukocytes, which lack GPI-linked proteins.[603–606]

Genetic defects in the synthesis or addition of the GIPL anchor have also been found in murine lymphoma cell lines that do not express surface Thy-1 antigen.[607] These fall in several complementation groups, some of which fail to synthesize the preassembled GIPL anchor due to blocks at different steps in the biosynthetic pathway. Some fail to synthesize dolichol-phosphate-mannose,[578] while others secrete a soluble Thy-1, as expected if cleavage of the precursor protein takes place, but lipid addition does not occur. One of the complementation groups (PIG-A) corresponds to a mutation in the same gene that in humans is defective in PNH.[602]

A diverse set of functions is associated with GPI-linked proteins, including enzymatic activities (e.g., acetylcholinesterase, placental and intestinal alkaline phosphatases, 5′ nucleotidase), a cell-adhesion role (N-CAM; LFA-3, and the carcinoembryonic antigen, CEA), and a receptor function (for the Fc of IgG in the FcγRIII receptors). Surprisingly, despite the absence of cytoplasmic and transmembrane domains, several GPI-linked proteins can, on crosslinking with antibodies, transduce signals that lead to cell proliferation. This suggests that they are associated with other effector molecules in the membrane, such as tyrosine kinases.[608]

A GIPL anchor may confer on a protein properties essential for its function. In trypanosomes, it permits the GIPL-linked VSG molecules to pack closely, forming the protective coat that covers the whole organism. Moreover, the blood stages of the parasites also express a glycosylphosphatidylinositol-specific phospholipase C, which may serve to release the surface glycoprotein from dying parasites, and thus facilitate the neutralization of the host immune response. In fact, the susceptibility of all GIPL-linked proteins to release by specific phospholipases may provide the cells with a means to down-regulate the surface levels of a particular protein. Under certain circumstances, this may cause its secretion (e.g., the GP2 pancreatic secretory granule membrane protein that appears in pancreatic juice).[548a,567]

Proteins with a GIPL anchor are able to diffuse in the plane of the membrane at rates approximately tenfold higher than proteins anchored by peptide domains and can attain rates comparable to those of lipids.[576] Although the significance of this property is not clear, it might provide cells with a means to respond to stimuli by rapidly reorganizing their exposed surfaces (e.g., by forming or dissolving patches). It is noteworthy that GIPL-linked proteins are endocytosed very slowly. As first shown for Thy-1,[609] they appear to be excluded from clathrin-coated pits formed at the plasma membrane. On the other hand, GIPL-linked proteins, such as the folate receptor, are closely packed within caveolae.[610,611]

One very important property of GIPL-linked proteins is that, when expressed in polarized epithelial cells, such as those that line the intestinal mucosa or kidney tubules, they are targeted to and accumulate predominantly in the apical plasma membrane domains of the cells.[612,613] In fact, the presence of a GIPL anchor (such as that of DAF or Thy-1) in a chimeric protein can redirect a basolateral plasma membrane protein (such as the VSV-G or herpes GDI glycoproteins) to the apical surface of the cells.[614,615] In a converse experiment, replacement of the GIPL anchor in alkaline phosphatase by the transmembrane and cytoplasmic domains of the VSV-G addressed the protein to the basolateral surface.[615] Moreover, the GIPL-anchored and transmembrane forms of N-CAM, when expressed in the polarized Madin Darby Canine Kidney (MDCK) cell line of dog kidney origin, were differentially targeted to the apical and basolateral surfaces, respectively.[616]

The sorting mechanism that recognizes GIPL anchors and leads to the apical targeting of proteins that bear them, appears to involve the formation of mixed patches of the anchors with sphingoglycoplids in the TGN. Sphingoglycolipids are synthesized in the Golgi apparatus and, themselves, are concentrated in the outer leaflet of the apical membrane to which they are vectorially delivered from the TGN (see refs. 617 and 618). Evidence has been presented that many GIPL-linked proteins do indeed cluster with glycolipids in the Golgi apparatus to form aggregates that are not extractable with the neutral detergent Triton X-100 at low temperature.[619] This is in accordance with an earlier suggestion that such clusters would be formed in the TGN and be selectively incorporated into vesicles routed to the apical surface.[620] It seems plausible that the sorting of such aggregates involves their recognition by a transmembrane protein that in its cytoplasmic domain would interact with components of the sorting machinery.

C-Terminal Prenylation of Proteins[39,577,621,622]

Two types of prenyl groups, the 15-carbon farnesyl and the 20-carbon geranylgeranyl, are found linked by thioether linkages to cysteine residues at or near the C-terminal end of certain proteins synthesized in free ribosomes. The farnesyl moiety consists of three isoprene units and is transferred to the protein by a farnesyltransferase from farnesylpyrophosphate (FPP), an intermediate in cholesterol biosynthesis. The geranylgeranyl moiety consists of four isoprene units and is delivered by transferases from geranylgeranyl pyrophosphate (GGPP), an intermediate whose only known function is in protein prenylation. Proteins containing the geranylgeranyl group are much more abundant than those containing the farnesyl group. The most prominent of the latter are the *ras* proteins and the nuclear envelope *lamins*. Among the geranylgeranylated proteins are the low-molecular-weight GTP-binding proteins of the *rab* family, which participate in vesicular transport, and the γ subunits of heterotrimeric G proteins. Prenylated proteins with a C-terminal CAAX box (where C is cysteine, A an aliphatic, and X any amino acid) are farnesylated when X is serine or methionine (and perhaps to a limited extent when it is cysteine, alanine, or glutamine) and are geranylgeranylated when X is leucine or phenylalanine.[351,623,624] These prenylation reactions are carried out by heterodimeric *farnesyl (FTase)* and *geranylgeranyl (GGTase I)* transferases that share a common α subunit.[623] The specific prenylation is determined solely by the sequence of the extreme C-terminal tetrapeptide, which when transferred to another protein leads to the expected modification.[625] In fact, appropriate tetrapeptides can serve as specific substrates in vitro for these two prenyl transferases.[351,624]

Prenylation of proteins containing the CAAX motif is followed by two additional modifications: proteolytic removal of the three C-terminal residues, followed by carboxymethylation of the new C-terminal cysteine.[625] In some cases, a palmitate residue is added via a thioester linkage to another cysteine residue just upstream of the CAAX motif.[625] The *rab* proteins contain C-terminal dicysteine motifs in various arrangements (CC, CXC, CCX, CCXX, CCXXX), which are modified by prenylation. A distinct geranylgeranyl transferase (GGTase II) has been identified and purified[626] that adds geranylgeranyl groups to *rab* proteins with the CXC (*rab*3a) and CC (*rab*1a) motifs. Some of these proteins (like *rab*3a) may be geranylgeranylated on both cysteine residues at the C-terminus, although it is not clear if the same enzyme carries out both modifications, and may also undergo carboxymethylation at the C-terminal cysteine.[627] GGTase II does not simply recognize the C-terminal tetrapeptide but also an as yet unidentified sequence in the *rab* proteins that is far from the C-teminus.[628] The capacity of the enzyme to recognize features other than the C-terminus of the substrate can be attributed to the fact that, in addition to α and β subunits, similar but not identical to those of the other transferases, GGTase II also contains an additional subunit (95 kDa) designated *component A*, or *r*ab *e*scort *p*rotein (REP). REP binds the unprenylated *rab*, presents it to the catalytic α,β-subunit complex (component B), and remains bound to the substrate after the reaction, until this is taken up by another protein that interacts with the *rab*.[629,630] REP appears to be encoded by the gene affected in choroideremia (CHM), an X-linked form of retinal degeneration, since the human gene product is very similar (90 percent) to the rat REP.[630] Moreover, lymphoblasts from patients with the disease show a reduced ability to modify *rab3a* and *rab1a* in vitro, and this defect can be compensated for by the addition of purified rat REP.[631] Strikingly, the CM gene product had been noted to be related to the GDI for *rab3a*.[632] This relationship can now be understood since both REP and GDI must recognize a *rab* protein. The gene for another human protein, CHML,[633] that is 76 percent identical to that encoded in the CHM gene and 70 percent identical to REP, has also been identified. It was suggested that that protein represents another REP subunit that confers a different *rab* protein specificity to GGTase.

The prenyl modification has been shown to be critical for the function of many proteins and necessary for their insertion into membranes (see ref. 577). Mutant ras proteins that do not undergo prenylation no longer associate with the plasma membrane and are not transforming. However, substitution of their farnesyl groups with a geranylgeranyl (by altering the C-terminal residue in the primary translation product) does not eliminate the plasma membrane targeting and transforming activity of the v-*ras* oncogene product.[634,635] On the other hand, replacement of the farnesyl group with geranylgeranyl on the normal cellular ras protein leads to the potent growth inhibition of mouse NIH 3T3 cells.[635] Since proteins with the same C-terminal prenylation have different subcellular distributions (e.g., the various *rab* proteins, or the lamins and *ras*), targeting information for specific membranes must be encoded in other parts of the polypeptide. For the ras protein the presence of palmitoyl residues just upstream of the farnesylated C-terminus plays a role in targeting to the plasma membrane. Each *rab* protein has a characteristic distribution in the cell and, in some cases, sequences 30 to 40 residues upstream from the C-terminus have been shown to determine their organellar localization, probably by specific protein-protein interactions.[37] Thus, whereas *rab*2 is normally located in the intermediate compartment between the ER and Golgi, replacement of its C-terminus with a short segment (39 residues) of *rab*5 or *rab*7 led to its relocation to the early or late endosome compartments, the respective natural habitats of the latter two proteins.[37]

Acylation of Proteins through Ester and Thioester Linkages[574,575,636-638]

Many transmembrane polypeptides, such as the envelope glycoproteins of a variety of viruses (e.g., G of VSV, HA of influenza, and E2 of α viruses), and cellular membrane proteins, such as the myelin proteolipid protein, the transferrin, insulin, and β-adrenergic receptors, and the HLA-B histocompatibility antigen contain one or more palmitate moieties linked in a thioester bond to a cysteine residue located within the cytoplasmic segment of the protein, near its membrane-anchoring domain. For the viral glycoproteins, acylation is not required for transport to the cell surface but is necessary for viral assembly and budding.[639]

Palmitoylation is a posttranslational event that, for the viral envelope glycoproteins, has been shown to occur approximately 20 min after synthesis of the polypeptide is completed,[640] and probably takes place in the late ER or intermediate compartment just before transport to the Golgi apparatus, and before the high-mannose *N*-linked oligosaccharides are converted into the complex chains.[641] The incorporation of labeled palmitate into some membrane proteins, such as the transferrin receptor, has been shown to continue even several hours after synthesis of the polypeptide is completed,[642] but this may only represent the turnover of preexisting polypeptide-bound palmitate moieties, which turn over three to four times faster than the protein itself.[642] The β-adrenergic receptor (and probably other G protein-coupled receptors with seven membrane-spanning domains) is also palmitoylated on a conserved cysteine. This modification is believed to be necessary to hold the receptor in a conformation that allows its coupling to the G protein.[643]

The enzyme(s) responsible for the acylation of the membrane polypeptides are not strictly specific for palmitic acid and in some cases it may add myristate, stearate, or oleate residues. Because of the location of the modified amino acid residue, the enzyme must be located on the cytoplasmic side of the membrane and could be the same enzyme that catalyzes the palmitoylation of some cytoplasmic proteins, described above.

Some secretory proteins, such as the gastric mucous glycoproteins and immunoglobulin heavy and light chains, have also been shown to be acylated, the first with palmitate, stearate, or oleate, and the latter with myristate moieties that are probably bound in amide linkages to lysine side chains.[644] Similar linkages also appear to be present in the luminal domains of the α and β subunits of the insulin receptor, which also contains palmitate, probably linked in a thioester bond.[645] The enzymes responsible for the fatty acylation of secretory proteins and luminal domains of membrane proteins have not been characterized, but they must be distinct from the enzyme(s) that add fatty acids to cytosolic proteins and to cytoplasmically exposed cysteine residues of membrane proteins.

Many proteins synthesized in free polysomes, such as the H-*ras* oncogene product, which is also prenylated, carry a palmitic acid moiety linked to a cysteine near the C-terminus of the protein.[646] The presence of the fatty acid is required for the membrane association and full transforming activity of the ras protein,[647] which functions in signal transduction from tyrosine kinase receptors at the plasma membrane. Ankyrin, a red-cell cytoskeleton protein, also carries palmitate residues,[648] but the association of this polypeptide with the membrane is a peripheral one and is mediated by a high-affinity binding to the anion transporter (band III) in the membrane.[649]

ENDOCYTOSIS AND THE BIOGENESIS OF LYSOSOMES[1,633-650a]

Lysosomes are membrane-bound cytoplasmic organelles that contain a wide variety of hydrolytic enzymes that function at an acidic pH and together are capable of digesting essentially all types of biologic macromolecules. Both extracellular materials that are taken into the cell by *endocytosis* and intracellular components that undergo *autophagy* are broken down within lysosomes to their elementary constituents. These may then be transferred across the organellar membrane to the cytosol for further degradation or for reutilization in the synthesis of new macromolecules. A cell may contain several hundred lysosomes, and these may be quite variable in their size, shape, and morphologic appearance. This heterogeneity reflects the character of the material being digested within the lysosomes, as well as the various stages in the process of digestion that may be taking place. Some lysosomes may contain recently ingested materials whose origin is easily recognizable, while others, known as *residual bodies*, may contain only undigested remnants.*

The term *endocytosis* refers to a variety of cellular processes that lead to the interiorization of extracellular material. The essential feature of endocytosis is that extracellular fluid or solid particles become surrounded by a portion of the cell plasma membrane that ultimately pinches off from the cell surface to form a membrane-bound cytoplasmic compartment.

The term *phagocytosis* is reserved for the internalizaton of large particles, such as bacteria, protozoa, cellular debris, carbon or silica grains, etc. In general, this process involves the formation of cytoplasmic extensions or pseudopodia that completely surround the particle being ingested to produce a *phagosome*, which later acquires lysosomal enzymes to become a *phagolysosome* in which digestion takes place. The process of phagocytosis requires the reorganization of a network of actin microfilaments located immediately beneath the plasma membrane and, therefore, can be inhibited by the drug cytochalasin D,[664] which interferes with microfilament function. In multicellular organisms, phagocytosis is an activity reserved to "professional phagocytes," such as macrophages and polymorphonuclear leukocytes. Specific proteins in the plasma membrane of these cells serve as receptors which recognize ligands on the surface of the particle being taken in.[665] For example, a receptor in the plasma membrane of macrophages mediates the phagocytic uptake of opsonized bacteria by binding to the Fc portion of specific antibodies that recognize bacterial surface antigens.

Receptor-mediated endocytosis (see ref. 654) is an important mechanism for the efficient uptake of extracellular substances—such as hormones, growth factors, and nutrient-carrier proteins—capable of binding to specific cell surface receptors that mediate their internalization (Fig. 16-32). The receptor-ligand complexes are concentrated in small invaginations of the plasma membrane known as *coated pits*, because of their appearance on EM. The coat covering the region of the pit is composed primarily of *clathrin*,[666] a protein that consists of heavy (approximately 190 kDa) and light (23 to 27 kDa) chains, and a set of *adaptor* or *assembly proteins* (see below). The adaptor proteins facilitate the formation of a clathrin lattice on the cytoplasmic surface of the membrane, and this brings about the clustering of receptors in the coated pits. The pinching off of the pits into the cytoplasm generates *coated vesicles*[667] that contain the receptors and their associated ligands and are completely surrounded by a cage composed of clathrin and its associated proteins (see ref. 657).

In receptor-mediated endocytosis, interaction of the ligands with their specific receptors markedly increases the efficiency of their uptake, since they are actually concentrated on the surface of the cell before being taken in. This process is responsible for the cellular uptake of some nutrients, such as vitamin B_{12} bound to transcobalamin II, cholesterol incorporated in LDL particles, and iron within transferrin molecules. After they bind to the cell-surface receptors that mediate their function, polypeptide hormones and growth factors, such as insulin or EGF, are also interiorized in coated vesicles. This leads to the removal of the hormones and factors from the extracellular fluid. It also provides a means to modulate the capacity of the cell to respond to these agents that control cellular metabolism and proliferation, since it reduces the number of receptors available at the cell surface (i.e., *down-regulation*). Some receptors internalized by endocytosis, such as the EGF receptor, are normally distributed over the surface of the cell[668,669] and move to, or from, coated pits only after binding their ligands. Others, such as the LDL receptor, are continuously concentrated in coated pits, and internalized whether or not they contain a bound ligand.[670]

During the course of receptor-mediated endocytosis, solutes, such as albumin or horseradish peroxidase, that are present in the extracellular fluid but are not bound to specific receptors are also taken in and remain dissolved in the lumen of the endocytic vesicles. The intake of extracellular fluid, and of substances dissolved in it, which takes place continuously in this manner and occurs in all cells, is known as *fluid-phase endocytosis* or *pinocytosis*. Kinetically, this is characterized by a strictly linear

*Lysosomes have been defined as membrane-bound vacuoles rich in lysosomal hydrolases. The term *primary lysosome* was used to designate lysosomes that have not yet acquired the substrate for digestion, and the term *secondary lysosome* for those that have received these substrates subsequent to endocytosis or autophagy.[1] Primary lysosomes are prominent in polymorphonuclear leukocytes, where they are represented by the azurophilic granules.[306] In most other cells (see below), the term *primary lysosomes* can at best only be applied to the small vesicles containing mannose 6-phosphate receptor molecules (see below) that carry newly synthesized hydrolases from the Golgi apparatus (or the TGN) to endosomes that are undergoing transformation into lysosomes.

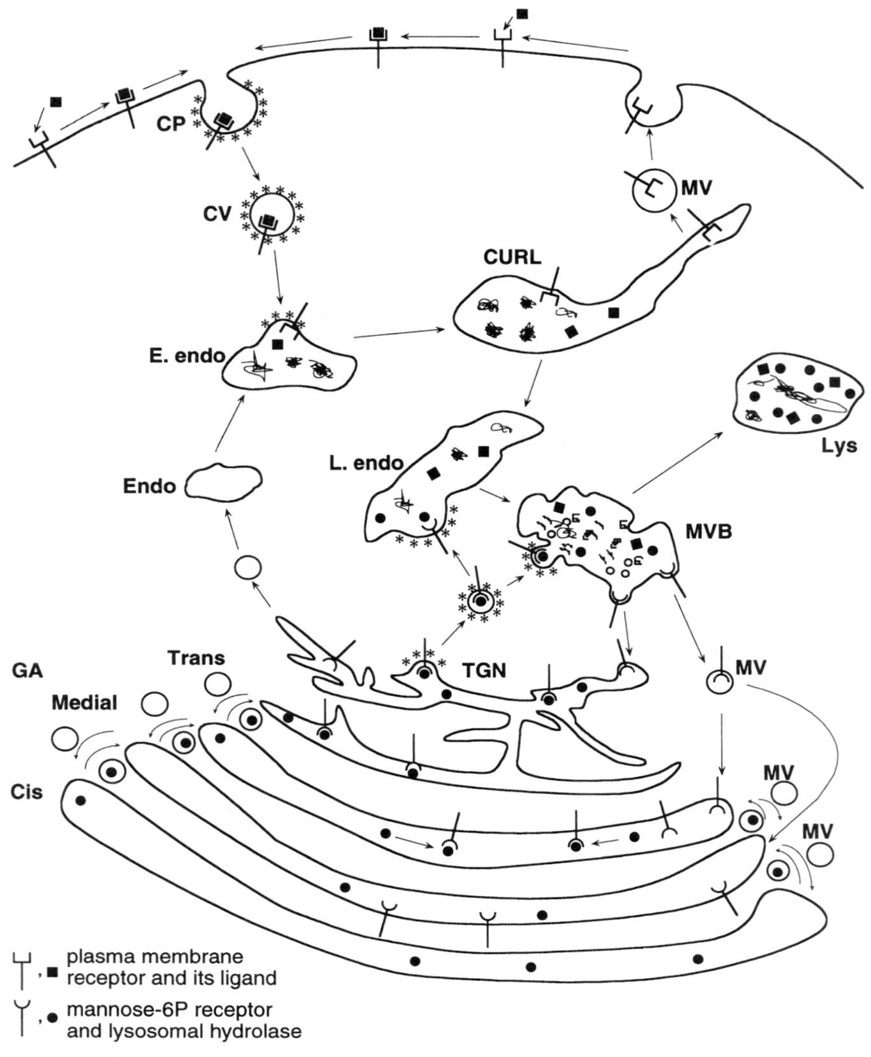

Fig. 16-32 Receptor-mediated endocytosis, membrane recycling, and biogenesis of lysosomes. After binding to its ligand (▪) at the cell surface, a plasma membrane receptor is concentrated in a clathrin-coated pit (CP), which pinches off into the cytoplasm to form a coated vesicle (CV). The coated vesicle becomes at least partially uncoated (not shown) and fuses with an early endosome (E. endo) and, at the low pH in this compartment, the receptor releases its ligand into the endosomal lumen. The endosome itself is originally formed by vesicles that budded from the TGN. Within the endosomal membrane, the receptors become segregated to a region where they become incorporated into membrane vesicles (MV) that bud and return to the cell surface. The endosomal compartment from which receptors return to the cell surface is labeled CURL. Endosomes containing the endocytosed material are further remodeled by acquisition of lysosomal hydrolases (•), which are transported to these late endosomes (L. endo) from the TGN in coated vesicles containing mannose 6-phosphate receptors. The membranes of many late endosomes show numerous invaginations and interiorized vesicles, which accounts for their designation as multivesicular bodies (MVB). These organelles are defined not only by their morphologic appearance but also by the presence within them of lysosomal hydrolases, the mannose 6-phosphate receptor, and endocytosed material. Since the mannose 6-phosphate receptor is absent from the mature lysosome, the final step in the conversion of an endosome to a lysosome (Lys) is the return of the receptor in membrane vesicles (MV) to the TGN and the Golgi apparatus. Conversion of a prelysosome into a lysosome also involves the acquisition of specific lysosomal membrane proteins that may be directly delivered in the same coated vesicles that carry the mannose 6-phosphate receptors and their associated hydrolases, or may first reach the cell surface and then be brought to the developing lysosome via the endosomal compartment.

dependency on the concentration of the solute taken in. In contrast, receptor-mediated endocytosis can be saturated and shows typical Michaelis-Menten kinetics. Pinocytosis may also be carried out, independent of receptor-mediated endocytosis, by vesicles that are not coated by clathrin (see below).

Signals for Endocytosis via Clathrin-Coated Vesicles[671,672]

Immunocytochemical studies first showed that while certain plasma membrane proteins are selectively incorporated into clathrin-coated pits, others are excluded from them.[609] The recognition that a mutation in the cytoplasmic tail of the human LDL receptor eliminated its capacity to cluster in coated pits and, hence, to undergo endocytosis[673,674] not only provided evidence for the role of the cytoplasmic domain of the receptor in determining its endocytic behavior, but also pointed to the role of a specific tyrosine residue in this domain as a critical component of an *endocytic signal* (or *interiorization signal*) required for the clustering of receptors in clathrin-coated pits.

Studies on the effects of specific mutations on the endocytic capacity of the LDL,[675] MPR300,[676] MPR46 kDa,[677] and transferrin receptors,[678] as well as of acid phosphatase,[679,679a] a lysosomal membrane protein that reaches the plasma membrane, have shown that endocytic signals consist of short peptide segments (four to six amino acids in length) that contain at least one aromatic residue and are located near, but not immediately adjacent to, the membrane. In the human LDL receptor, the endocytic signal consists of the sequence FDNPVY,* but comparative studies with other species and mutagenesis studies have shown that the motif NPXY contains sufficient information for clustering this receptor in a coated pit.[675] In the transferrin receptor, which is a type II membrane protein and therefore has an N-terminal cytoplasmic domain, the endocytic signal has the sequence YXRF. However, this could be replaced by the endocytic signal from various other receptors, such as the poly IG and mannose 6-phosphate/insulin-like growth factor II (Man-6-P/IGFII) receptors, both of which are type I membrane proteins.[680] The most characteristic feature of an endocytic signal appears to be its capacity to self-determine the formation of a *tight turn* within the three-dimensional conformation of the polypeptide.[678] MRI determinations of the solution structure of peptides encompassing the endocytic signals in the LDL receptor[681] and the lysosomal acid phosphatase[682] have shown that the peptides by themselves adopt the tight-turn configuration.

The cyclic function of the cation-independent 300-kDa Man-6-P/IGFII receptor (MPR300), a protein that reaches the plasma membrane, requires that it be incorporated into two types of clathrin-coated vesicles, first in those that form in the TGN and second in those that mediate its interiorization at the plasma membrane. This requires the presence in the cytoplasmic domain of the MPR300 of two clustering signals, which have been identified by mutagenesis studies.[683–685] The one functioning at the plasma membrane has the sequence YKYSKV and is located 24 to 29 residues from the membrane, whereas the one functioning in the TGN includes the C-terminal four amino acids (LLHV), as well as a sequence that at least partly overlaps with the internalization signal that functions at the plasma membrane.[685]

The identification of the sequences that serve as internalization signals in the cytoplasmic domains of proteins incorporated into clathrin-coated pits has made it possible to demonstrate that these signals are recognized by the adaptor proteins that mediate the assembly of the clathrin coat[657] (Fig. 16-33). Coat proteins can be released from purified preparations of clathrin-coated vesicles and separated chromatographically into clathrin "*triskelions*" and two additional distinct tetrameric protein complexes, HA1 (or AP1) and HA2 (or AP2). The latter were originally designated *assembly proteins* because of their capacity to promote clathrin assembly into cage structures in vitro.[686] The triskelions, which are three-legged hexameric complexes consisting of three heavy and three light clathrin chains, serve as subunits that undergo higher-order assembly into the clathrin lattice that forms on the cytoplasmic face of the plasma membrane (Fig. 16-34). Each of the adaptors (Fig. 16-35) contains two specific polypeptides of approximately 100 kDa, called *adaptins* (α and β in HA2 and γ and β in HA1), and two other smaller polypeptides (AP50 and AP17 in HA2, and AP47 and AP19 in HA1). Immunocytochemical studies with antibodies specific for the α and γ subunits of the different adaptor complexes indicate that the HA1 adaptor, which in clathrin-coated vesicles from brain is much less abundant than the HA2, is a component of the coat of vesicles that form in the TGN. The HA2 adaptor is derived from the coat of the endocytic vesicles that form in the plasma membrane.[687–689] EM analysis indicates that, when assembled in vitro, the adaptors form an inner layer beneath the clathrin cage, as expected if in native coated vesicles they interact directly with the membrane.[690,691] Adaptor proteins interact specifically with the endocytic signals in the cytoplasmic tails of receptor polypeptides[692] and also with the clathrin molecules (see Fig. 16-33). Thus, the adaptors cause the clustering of receptors in coated pits and facilitate the formation of the clathrin lattice. The capacity of the adaptors to bind specifically to endocytic signals was demonstrated in affinity chromatography experiments that employed as immobilized ligands fusion proteins containing the cytoplasmic tails of the LDL receptor or the MPR300. These

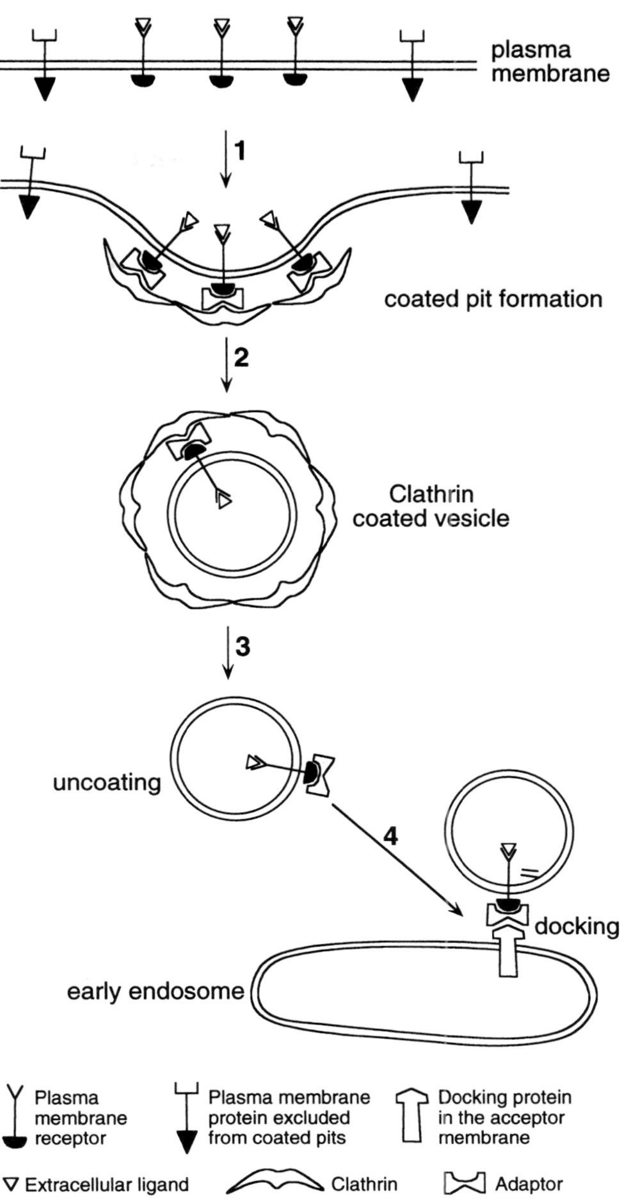

Fig. 16-33 Formation of a clathrin-coated vesicle at the plasma membrane: the role of adaptors in receptor clustering and clathrin coat assembly. (1) Plasma membrane molecules (which may be receptors bearing a ligand in their extracellular domains) that contain endocytic signals (solid semicircles) in their cytoplasmic tails interact via these signals with AP2 adaptor molecules that in turn bind the clathrin triskelions that assemble into the lattice that forms the coat of a coated pit. (2) On complete assembly of the coat, a clathrin-coated vesicle buds into the cytoplasm. For simplicity, only one adaptor-receptor complex is represented in the vesicle. (3) The vesicle undergoes uncoating, probably catalyzed by an uncoating ATPase. (4) In this scheme it is presumed that, after uncoating, an adaptor, which remains bound to the vesicle membrane, recognizes a docking protein in the acceptor membrane of an early endosome. After docking, a molecular machinery whose nature is not yet fully understood (not depicted here) will lead to fusion of the uncoated vesicle membrane with that of the acceptor compartment.

*The single-letter amino acid code is used to represent the amino acids in these sequences. In this code, A is alanine; C, cysteine; D, aspartic acid; E, glutamic acid; F, phenylalanine; G, glycine; H, histidine; I, isoleucine; K, lysine; L, leucine; M, methionine; N, asparagine; P, proline; Q, glutamine; R, arginine; S, serine; T, threonine; V, valine; W, tryptophan; and Y, tyrosine; X corresponds to any amino acid.

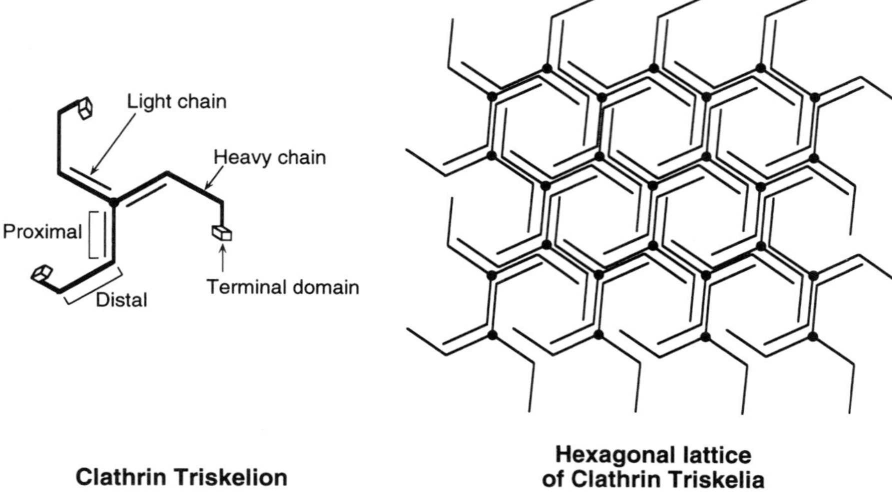

Fig. 16-34 Structure of a clathrin triskelion and of the hexagonal lattice into which it assembles. A clathrin triskelion is a three-legged hexameric complex consisting of three heavy and three light chains. Each heavy chain has a proximal C-terminal segment that interacts with the light chain, a middle region, and a compact globular N-terminal domain that is flexible and bends toward the membrane. The light chains are oriented with their C-terminal ends toward the center of the triskelion. A planar lattice of clathrin consists of hexagons that on each side contain elements of four triskelions. To form the closed cage that surrounds a coated vesicle some of the hexagons must rearrange to form pentagons. (*Adapted from Pearse and Robinson.*[657])

experiments showed that HA1 complexes bind only to the MPR300, whereas HA2 bind to both.[692] In addition, competition studies showed that replacement of the two tyrosine residues within the cytoplasmic domain of the MPR300 eliminated its capacity to compete for binding of HA1 to the wild-type MPR300 receptor, but not for the binding of HA2 to that receptor. Questions now being investigated relate to the targeting and recycling of the adaptors. Why does the HA2 adaptor released after the uncoating of an endocytic vesicle not bind to the MPR in the TGN? Conversely, what prevents the binding of the HA1 adaptor to the plasma membrane? The development of cell-free systems in which coated vesicles are formed from immobilized plasma membrane fragments[693] should help in the identification of the protein factors and small molecules, such as GTP, that regulate the endocytic process and confer specificity and directionality to it.

Endosomal Compartment[651]

Soon after pinching off from the plasma membrane, coated vesicles lose their clathrin coat, as they fuse with membrane-bound tubulovesicular organelles known as *endosomes*,* to which they transfer the material adsorbed at the cell surface. An uncoating ATPase (which corresponds to the heat-shock protein hsp70) has been identified[694] that removes clathrin from coated vesicles in vitro. However, an uncoating role for this protein in vivo has not yet been demonstrated. It is possible that the adaptors, which are not removed from the membrane by this ATPase,[657] play a role in mediating the docking of the vesicle on the endosome or its fusion with the endosomal membrane.

Biochemical studies[695] indicate that endosomes contain a distinct set of membrane proteins and, therefore, do not simply result from the fusion of coated vesicles with each other. The biochemical individuality of endosomes must reflect their biogenetic derivation, at least in part, from other intracellular, presumably Golgi-derived, vesicles (see Fig. 16-32). Endosomes contain a membrane-associated ATPase that concentrates protons and acidifies the lumen of the organelle.[660,696–699] Soon after entering endosomes located near the plasma membrane (designated *early endosomes*), many ligands are dissociated from their receptors because of the acidic pH[698] and are released into the endosomal lumen.[651,699] The receptors are then segregated to a tubular region of the endosomal membrane from which vesicles pinch off that return the receptors to the cell surface to participate in further rounds of endocytosis (see Fig. 16-32). An endosome with these features has been referred to as CURL, for *c*ompartment of *u*ncoupling of *r*eceptors and *l*igands.[700,701] The ligands released in the endosome and, in some cases, nondissociated receptor-ligand complexes, can subsequently undergo intralysosomal digestion. The early endosome is, therefore, a functionally complex compartment in which sorting steps control the flow of material into deeper endosomes and lysosomes and its return to the cell surface. When endocytosis is allowed to proceed in cells incubated at temperatures between 16 and 20°C, transfer of the endocytosed material to deeper, late endosomes and lysosomes is inhibited. Temperature-shift experiments proved useful to study the various elements that compose the endosomal compartment and the pathway by which endocytosed material reaches the lysosome.

The two main classes of endosomes (*early endosomes* and *late endosomes*) differ not only in their morphologic appearance, cellular location, and time at which they acquire the endocytosed marker, but also in their biochemical composition and density (which has allowed their separation by centrifugation in Percoll gradients). They differ also in their relative acidity, which is higher in deeper endosomes. Two main discordant views are currently held with respect to the functional and biogenetic relationships between the two kinds of endosomes (see ref. 651). One postulates that both types of endosomes are stable structures, i.e., distinct organelles (see ref. 702). In this view, the early or *sorting endosome* would generate two types of vesicles, one that returns receptors to the plasma membrane and another that delivers the endocytosed material to the late endosome, from which it would reach the lysosome. The other view (see ref. 703) is that early endosomes, after returning receptors to the plasma membrane, undergo a "maturation process" in which they are gradually transformed into late endosomes. Subsequently, these would be transformed into lysosomes by acquiring the necessary complement of lysosomal hydrolases and membrane proteins brought to them by clathrin-coated vesicles (see Fig. 16-32) that originate from the *trans* Golgi region or TGN.[651,704,705] The presence of lysosomal hydrolases in multivesicular bodies, which are endosomes that contain invaginated membrane tubules or vesicles, suggests that these represent a transition stage in the conversion of an early endosome into a lysosome (see Fig. 16-32). However, according to the view that early and late endosomes are preexisting stable compartments, the *mutivesicular bodies* would be vehicles that transport endocytosed material from the early to the late endosomal compartment.[702]

It has been argued that the protein compositional differences that have been detected between early and late endosomes represent evidence for the stable character of the two endosomal compartments.[695] Such differences, however, could simply reflect the presence of passenger proteins transiently associated with these structures. Nevertheless, the functional distinctiveness of the

*The term *receptosome* has also been proposed to designate this structure (see ref. 652).

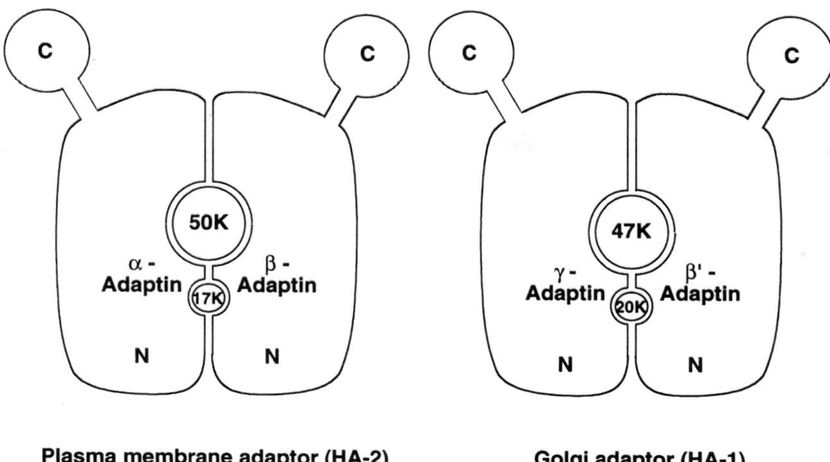

Fig. 16-35 Schematic representation of the oligomeric structures of adaptors. The HA1 and HA2 adaptors that mediate clathrin-coat assembly in the *trans*-Golgi apparatus or the plasma membrane, respectively, are both tetrameric proteins. Freeze-etch EM of the HA2 adaptor shows that it resembles a head with two small protruding ears derived from the C-terminal domains of the adaptins, as depicted. Proteolytic digestion removes the ears as 30-kDa C-terminal fragments of the adaptins, and the remaining complex becomes inactive in promoting coat assembly. It has been suggested that the ears contain the sites that recognize the endocytic signals in plasma membrane proteins or the sorting signal in the mannose 6-phosphate receptor. The ears are linked to the head by flexible hinges that are rich in proline and glycine residues and contain protease sensitive sites. (*From Pearse and Robinson.*[657] *Used by permission.*)

two endosomal compartments is clear. In vitro studies (see ref. 706) have shown that early endosomes can fuse with each other, but not with late endosomes.[707] This fusion appears to be regulated by the low-molecular-weight GTP-binding protein, *rab*5, which is exclusively associated with early endosomes and does not associate with late endosomes even in cells overexpressing it.[708] Conversely, another GTP-binding protein, *rab*7, appears to be exclusively associated with late endosomes (see ref. 27).

Biosynthesis of Lysosomal Enzymes[653,655,656,662,709–711a]

The biogenesis of lysosomes is a complex process that requires that specific sets of soluble hydrolases and membrane proteins, which are synthesized in the ER, be segregated from proteins with other subcellular destinations and be transferred to developing or preexisting lysosomes. Much progress has been made toward an understanding of the mechanism by which the newly synthesized hydrolases are sorted from secretory proteins. Clues as to the nature of the signals that ensure the incorporation of specific proteins into the lysosomal membrane have also begun to emerge.

With rare exceptions, lysosomal enzymes are glycoproteins that contain *N*-linked and sometimes *O*-linked oligosaccharide chains. Like secretory glycoproteins, lysosomal enzymes are synthesized by membrane-bound ribosomes in the ER, and their nascent ribosome-associated chains contain cleavable N-terminal insertion signals that lead to the cotranslational passage of the polypeptides into the lumen of the ER.[712–714] Translocation through the ER membrane is accompanied by the acquisition of *N*-linked high-mannose oligosaccharide chains and cleavage of the signal sequence. These processes are indistinguishable from those that take place during the early stages of the biosynthesis of secretory glycoproteins.[712,713,715] Subsequently, however, the lysosomal polypeptides undergo modifications that confer on some of their oligosaccharide chains the *lysosomal marker*, a mannose 6-phosphate (Man-6-P) residue. The Man-6-P distinguishes lysosomal from secretory glycoproteins and is responsible for addressing the former to their lysosomal destination (see below). The incorporation of a phosphate group at the C-6 position of some mannose residues is the result of two sequential reactions (see Fig. 16-26) that are catalyzed by enzymes that appear to be concentrated in the *cis* region of the Golgi apparatus.[413] The first step is the transfer by a *phosphotransferase* of *N*-acetylglucosaminyl-1-phosphate from UDP-N-acetylglucosamine to the C-6 hydroxyl group of a mannose residue in a partially trimmed high-mannose oligosaccharide. This results in the formation of a phosphodiester bond linking the mannose to the *N*-acetylglucosamine.[716,717] In the second reaction, a specific *phosphodiesterase* removes the *N*-acetylglucosamine residue and thus uncovers the phosphate on the modified mannose residue.[718–720] A defect in the first enzyme in this modification pathway occurs in patients with I-cell disease (mucolipidosis II)[721–727] or pseudo-Hurler polydystrophy.[722–726,728] It is responsible for the secretion of nonphosphorylated hydrolases from cultured fibroblasts derived from these patients, and for the high levels of hydrolases in the patients' sera.

The specificity of the *UDPGlcNAc:lysosomal enzyme N-acetyl-glucosamine-1-phosphotransferase* for some features of the lysosomal polypeptides is the key factor responsible for addition of the lysosomal marker only to those polypeptides destined for lysosomes. Partially purified transferase preparations modify the C-6 position of mannose residues present in lysosomal enzymes much more efficiently (lower K_m) than those in the isolated high-mannose oligosaccharide chains or in the monomeric sugar α-methylmannoside.[716,717] Mannose residues in nonlysosomal glycoproteins are phosphorylated no more effectively than α-methylmannoside.[716,717] The transferase recognizes a specific feature of the lysosomal polypeptide and positions the acceptor oligosaccharide chain in proximity to the enzyme's active site that modifies the mannose residue. Deglycosylated hydrolases are specific inhibitors of the transferase when other lysosomal enzymes are used as acceptors but not when α-methylmannoside is the acceptor.[729] The amino acid sequences of many lysosomal hydrolases have been determined from the nucleotide sequences of cDNA clones, but no significant similarity between the primary sequences can be recognized (e.g., refs. 730 to 737).

Because most lysosomal hydrolases contain several oligosaccharide chains, and mannose phosphorylation takes place on more than one of these chains, the transferase appears to recognize a global structural feature of each protein rather than a localized domain around each oligosaccharide chain. In some cases of mucolipidosis III, the phosphotransferase appears to be defective only in its ability to recognize the lysosomal enzymes as substrates at physiological concentrations (μM), but is unaffected in its capacity to phosphorylate the α-methylmannoside at concentrations near its K_m (200 m*M*).[728]

The phosphorylation of mannose residues in some of the oligosaccharide chains in lysosomal hydrolases does not prevent the processing of other chains, or branches of the same chain, by the set of trimming enzymes and glycosyltransferases that are present in the Golgi apparatus. Thus, the nonphosphorylated chain can become complex oligosaccharides containing *N*-acetylglucosaminyl, galactosyl, and sialyl residues that are characteristic of many secretory proteins.[738–741]

The analysis of chimeric proteins formed between different portions of two highly homologous aspartyl proteases, the lysosomal enzyme cathepsin and the secretory protein pepsinogen, has thrown light on the structural features that constitute the signal for mannose phosphorylation in cathepsin D. The three-dimensional structure of pepsinogen has been determined and it indicates that the N- and C-terminal halves of these proteins are contained in two distinct lobes within each molecule. It was shown that two noncontinuous segments in the C-terminal lobe of cathepsin D (amino acids 188 to 230, and in particular Lys 203, and amino acids 265 to 292) are necessary and sufficient for the phosphorylation of the oligosaccharides in this protein.[742–744] The three-dimensional structure of pepsinogen indicates that the two polypeptide segments that form the phosphotransferase recognition site are closely apposed on the surface of cathepsin D and hence constitute a single site. Nevertheless, the presence of several other segments within the N-terminal lobe of cathepsin D enhanced the phosphorylation of the oligosaccharide in pepsinogen-cathepsin D chimeras and may be part of an extended recognition signal.[744–746] Experiments with chimeras containing artificial glycosylation sites demonstrated that recognition of a lysosomal hydrolase by the phosphotransferase can lead to the modification of oligosaccharides linked at many different residues within the molecule, although those closest to the recognition determinant are preferentially phosphorylated.[745]

Studies with cultured cells indicate that a fraction of newly synthesized phosphorylated hydrolases is normally secreted into the medium (see refs. 713 and 747). The presence of some lysosomal hydrolases in serum and urine also suggests that some cells in the intact organism normally secrete lysosomal hydrolases.[748] Some of the secreted molecules contain the Man-6-P marker, as well as complex oligosaccharide chains. Some hydrolases that reach the lysosome also acquire terminal sugars during their passage through the *trans*-Golgi cisterna, but sugars are later lost within the lysosome. The phosphate group itself is also removed from mature enzymes by lysosomal phosphatases.

Lysosomal hydrolases also undergo a maturation process that involves one or more proteolytic cleavage steps. These cleavages either reduce the molecular weight by loss of a C-terminal segment, as is the case with β-glucuronidase, or generate, by two successive cleavages, two polypeptides from a single precursor, as is the case with cathepsin D.[713,749,750] Lysosomal enzymes secreted when the lysosomal marker is not added, as in I-cell disease, or in normal cells in which glycosylation is prevented by treatment of cells with tunicamycin, do not undergo proteolytic processing.[713,751] Most of the proteolytic modifications of lysosomal enzymes take place in the lysosome itself.[752]

The Man-6-P Marker and the Targeting of Lysosomal Hydrolases to Lysosomes

The study of I-cell disease fibroblasts played an important role in the discovery of the Man-6-P lysosomal marker and of the receptors that recognize it and effect the segregation of newly synthesized hydrolases to the lysosomes. It was originally observed that cultured fibroblasts from patients with I-cell disease are deficient in lysosomal hydrolases and that the medium in which these cells are cultured contains higher levels of the hydrolase activities than the mediums from cultures of normal fibroblasts.[753] It was subsequently demonstrated that lysosomal hydrolases secreted by normal fibroblasts can be taken up by both normal cells and cells from patients with I-cell disease, whereas the enzymes secreted by the defective cells could not be taken up by either cell type.[747] The uptake of normal enzymes was shown to be mediated by a saturable receptor that recognizes these proteins. These observations showed that in I-cell disease, the enzymes themselves are defective — not the cellular apparatus that leads to their incorporation into lysosomes. It was, therefore, proposed[747] that the defect in I-cell disease is in the inability of the cells to equip newly synthesized enzymes with the marker necessary for their interiorization by receptor-mediated endocytosis. The crucial marker present in the oligosaccharide chains of secreted enzymes recognized by the receptor was later shown to be the Man-6-P residue.[754]

The ability of certain cells to take up exogenous lysosomal hydrolases reflects the presence of the Man-6-P receptor in their plasma membrane. However, it is now well established that most of the receptor molecules are located in intracellular membranes and that, in fact, only a small proportion of the cellular complement of receptors is present at the cell surface.[755–757]

Although in cultured fibroblasts the Man-6-P marker is necessary for the targeting of many, if not all, newly synthesized lysosomal hydrolases to lysosomes, alternative mechanisms must operate in other cell types. Thus, hepatocytes, Kupffer cells, and leukocytes from patients with I-cell disease contain nearly normal levels of some lysosomal enzymes, despite their deficiency in phosphotransferase activity.[758] In addition, some hydrolases, such as acid phosphatase and β-glucocerebrosidase, are present at normal levels in fibroblasts of patients with I-cell disease.[759] Acid phosphatase is synthesized as a transmembrane protein and is released from the membrane by proteolytic cleavage after it reaches the lysosome.[679,760] Glucocerebrosidase lacks a Man-6-P marker. In human hepatoma cells, HepG2, its precursor becomes membrane-associated by an unknown mechanism soon after it leaves the ER.[761] A similar membrane association that is independent of the Man-6-P marker was found for the precursor of cathepsin D, which normally contains the marker. Thus, membrane association may represent an important step in an alternative pathway for the delivery of these enzymes to lysosomes.[761]

A sorting signal within the polypeptide rather than in an oligosaccharide chain[762,763] operates in yeast to address digestive enzymes, such as procarboxypeptidase Y, to the vacuole, an organelle analogous to the lysosome. Mutational studies on chimeric proteins indicated that only the first 10 amino acids of procarboxypeptidase Y are required to determine its vacuolar localization.[764] In recent years more than 40 genes (vacuolar protein sorting genes, VPS) have been identified (see refs. 765 and 766) that play essential roles in targeting proteins to the yeast vacuole. The properties of some of these gene products indicate that vacuolar targeting in yeast may be regulated by protein phosphorylation and phosphatidylinositol signaling events (see ref. 767).

Man-6-P Receptors[662,711a,768]

Two different types of Man-6-P receptor (MPR) molecules have been purified by affinity chromatography of solubilized cellular membranes on matrixes containing immobilized ligands. They differ in their binding properties and divalent cation requirements for ligand binding. The first receptor that was identified (referred to as MPRCI, MPR300, or Man-6-P/IGFII receptor) is a 275- to 300-kDa glycoprotein that does not require cations to bind ligand.[769] Subsequently, it was discovered to be identical with the receptor for insulin-like growth factor II (IGFII), although the two ligands bind at different sites (e.g., ref. 770). Specific antibodies to the Man-6-P/IGFII receptor have allowed studies of its subcellular distribution and of the pathway it follows in sorting and transport.[701,704,771–778] The amino acid sequence of this receptor, deduced from the cDNA clone,[779] revealed that it is a type I transmembrane glycoprotein that has a small segment of 17 kDa exposed on the cytoplasmic side of the membrane.[780] The luminal domain of the receptor, where the ligand binding site(s) is found, is composed of 15 homologous segments, each of approximately 145 amino acids in length. The amount of Man-6-P/IGFII receptor present on the cell surface varies with the cell type, but most of this receptor is found in intracellular membranes. By immunocytochemistry, the receptor has been shown to be present in coated vesicles, endosomes, and Golgi membranes, but not in mature lysosomes (see below). The lysosomal sorting role of the MPR300 has been directly demonstrated by gene transfer experiments. Expression of the transfected receptor cDNA in certain cell lines that lack it and normally secrete large amounts of lysosomal enzymes restored the efficient delivery of these enzymes to lysosomes and also conferred on the cells the capacity to take up exogenous hydrolases containing the Man-6-P marker.[781,782]

The second Man-6-P receptor (MPRCD or MPR46) is a 46-kDa glycoprotein that in bovine and murine (but not human tissues) requires divalent cations, particularly Mn^{2+}. It requires a somewhat more acidic pH (6.3) for ligand binding than the larger receptor, which has high affinity for the phosphorylated ligand at neutral pH.[783,784] The amino acid sequence of the 46-kDa receptor, derived from a cDNA clone,[785–786a] shows that it is also a type I transmembrane protein, with a cytoplasmic domain of 69 residues and a luminal domain that shows homology to the repeated segments within the luminal domain of the Man-6-P/IGFII receptor. In particular, significant similarity is found within a pentadecapeptide, limited by cysteine residues, that is also present in all the repeating domains of the large receptor. The discovery of the 46-kDa MPR resulted from the observation that the cell lines that lack the large MPR receptor[787] are still capable of sorting some of their lysosomal hydrolases (with approximately 40 percent efficiency). These cells were found to be incapable of taking up the exogenous lysosomal hydrolases when these were administered under the conditions usually employed, which do not satisfy the cation and pH requirements for binding to the MPR46. Moreover, expression of high levels of MPR46 in these cells, after transfection with the appropriate cDNA, only slightly increased their capacity to take up exogenous hydrolases in neutral medium.[788,789] The MPR46 may well play a role in mediating secretion of lysosomal enzymes, since overexpression of this receptor in cells that contain the MPR300 induces the appearance of large amounts of newly synthesized hydrolases in the medium.[790]

The critical function of the receptors that allows them to selectively transfer lysosomal enzymes bearing the Man-6-P marker to developing lysosomes is the pH dependence of their affinity for the ligands. At neutral or slightly acidic pH, the receptors bind strongly to phosphomannose-containing oligosaccharides or lysosomal hydrolases bearing the marker. However, they release these ligands quantitatively at the strong acid pH characteristic of endosomes or lysosomes.[741,784,789] To explain the fact that the MPR300 is highly efficient in targeting hydrolases to lysosomes, whereas MPR46 leads to secretion of its ligands, it was suggested that the former releases its ligands in deeper endosomal compartments, whereas the latter releases them in early endosomes from which the enzymes can more easily exit from the cell.[790]

Binding of hydrolases to the receptors requires removal of the GlcNac group that initially covers the phosphate group on the C-6 of the mannose residue,[741,789] and high-affinity binding requires the presence of at least two Man-6-P residues in the same molecule, although not necessarily on the same oligosaccharide chain.[784,791,792] Lysosomal hydrolases of the slime mold *Dictyostelium discoideum* bind effectively to their receptor, even though their Man-6-P residues are covered by methyl groups.[793] However, only the MPR300 is capable of recognizing Man-6-P residues bearing this modification.[787]

Delivery of Hydrolases to Incipient Lysosomes

As previously noted, the enzymes that synthesize the Man-6-P marker are located in the *cis* region of the Golgi apparatus and, in principle, the hydrolases could be engaged by the MPR as soon as they are modified. Indeed, in some cell types, such as pancreatic, hepatic, and epididymal, the MPR300 is most concentrated in *cis*-Golgi cisternae.[772,794] In other cell types, however, it is most abundant in the *trans*-Golgi region, TGN, and endosomes.[795] The steady state distribution of MPR46 also varies with the cell type,[796,797] but in all cases studied to date the MPR receptors are absent from mature lysosomes.[704,771–776,778] There is now a consensus that the occupied receptors emerge from the Golgi apparatus in the TGN (Figs. 16-32 and 16-36), where HA1 adaptors must recognize targeting signals in the cytoplasmic domain of the receptors, and mediate their incorporation into clathrin-coated vesicles in which lysosomal enzyme precursors have been found.[798–800] After uncoating, these vesicles then must fuse with endosomal structures that represent intermediates in the formation of lysosomes. As a result of the low pH[704,772,773,778,799,800] in the endosomal compartment, the ligand would then dissociate from the receptor, which would recycle to the TGN and occasionally reach the cell surface.

Immunocytochemical studies on the distribution of the MPR300, lysosomal hydrolases, and membrane proteins, and of endocytosed markers at different times after internalization, have indicated that various types of endosomes may serve as acceptors for the vesicles that deliver the hydrolases during the biogenesis of a lysosome. Some investigators[795] reported that the vast majority of MPR300 molecules are located in a deep endosome compartment that contains lysosomal membrane proteins and hydrolases, but is inaccessible to endocytic markers during incubation at 20°C. This *prelysosome* or intermediate compartment, therefore, has the properties of a deep endosome from which a lysosome could be generated by continued delivery of hydrolases and membrane proteins, followed by retrieval of all MPR molecules. Other investigators[801,802] have found substantial amounts of MPR and some lysosomal enzymes even in early endosomes, which, at 37°C, rapidly acquire endocytic markers, but can even be labeled with them after longer incubations at 18.5°C. These observations are consistent with the maturation model for lysosome biogenesis that involves the progressive transformation of early endosomes to late endosomes and finally into lysosomes.

There is some controversy over whether movement of the receptor from the Golgi apparatus to the receiving endosome takes place only if the receptor is occupied by a ligand, or whether the receptor moves constitutively. One group has reported that receptors accumulate in Golgi membranes and that endosomes are depleted of receptors when cells are treated with tunicamycin,[773] a drug that blocks core glycosylation in the ER and therefore prevents the acquisition of the Man-6-P marker by the newly synthesized hydrolases. The same group also observed that when dissociation of the receptors from their ligands is prevented by administration of lysosomotropic drugs, such as chloroquine or NH_4Cl, that concentrate in the lumen of acidic compartments and raise their pH, the receptors accumulate in endosomes.[773,778] These authors showed that, under these conditions, the failure of the receptor to return to the Golgi apparatus results from its inability to release the ligand and not from the altered pH of the endosome. When cells treated with chloroquine were incubated with Man-6-P, which enters the endosome compartment by fluid-phase pinocytosis, this competing ligand led to dissociation of the complex, which in turn was followed by reappearance of the receptor in Golgi membranes.[778] However, other investigators[803,804] have concluded that the receptor recycles constitutively, i.e., even in the absence of the ligand. It was observed that the level of receptor in the endosome was not significantly reduced when the synthesis of new lysosomal hydrolases was blocked by the protein synthesis inhibitor cycloheximide. The failure of the Man-6-P receptor-ligand complexes to dissociate at the altered pH of the endosomes in cells treated with lysosomotropic drugs accounts for the original finding[805] that secretion of lysosomal enzymes is increased under these conditions, since all the receptors remain occupied and, therefore, inaccessible to the newly synthesized hydrolases.

In addition to undergoing recycling between the Golgi apparatus and prelysosomal endosomes, receptor molecules also recycle through the plasma membrane, where the presence of variable but relatively small amounts (approximately 10 percent) of receptor has been demonstrated in many cell types (see ref. 699). Experiments in which surface receptors were desialylated by treatment with neuraminidase, to follow their rate of resialylation by the TGN sialyl transferase, indicate that after internalization by endocytosis, surface MPR receptors reach the TGN, with a half-time of approximately 3 h.[806] The presence of surface receptors and their recycling, as well as the significant levels of lysosomal hydrolases found in normal serum, suggest that secretion and uptake of lysosomal enzymes is a physiological process. Indeed, there are conditions in which the secretion of enzymes from some cells and their uptake by others correct a genetic defect. Thus, in

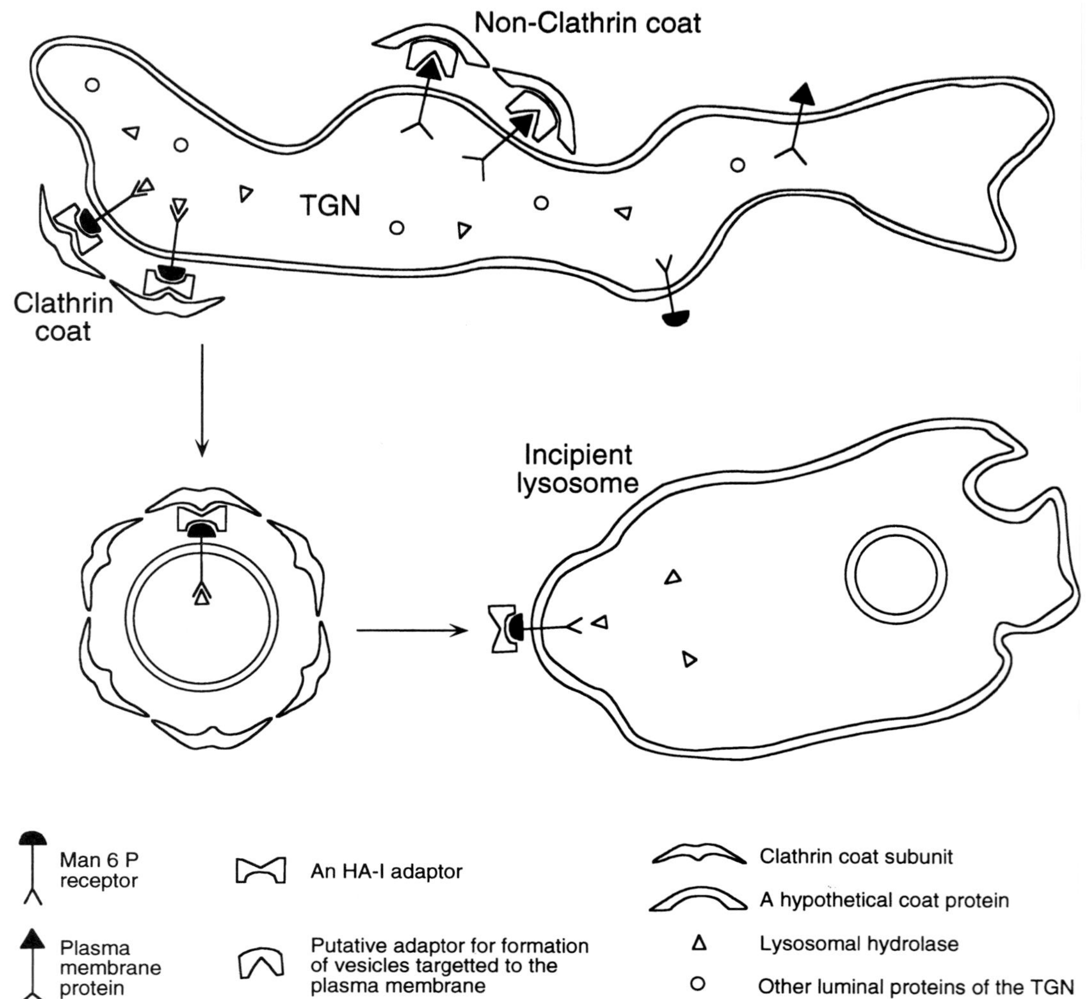

Fig. 16-36 Sorting of lysosomal hydrolases in the TGN: HA1 adaptor-mediated incorporation of Man-6-P receptors into clathrin-coated vesicles. In the TGN, lysosomal hydrolases bind to the luminal domain of Man-6-P receptors. The latter molecules contain sorting signals in their cytoplasmic segments, which are recognized by the HA1 adaptors. This recognition leads to segregation of the receptors to clathrin-coated vesicles that assemble in a manner similar to that described in Fig. 16-33. The clathrin-coated vesicle delivers its contents to an incipient lysosome, with which it fuses. The recognition mechanism responsible for the targeted delivery of the vesicle to the endosome is not known. The figure also depicts the sorting of a plasma membrane protein that in the TGN is incorporated into a vesicle containing a nonclathrin coat.

female carriers of Hunter disease, an X-linked lysosomal disorder that is characterized by a deficiency in iduronate sulfatase, cells that cannot synthesize the normal enzyme because of inactivation of the normal X chromosome appear to be phenotypically normal. Presumably this is the result of cross-feeding by cells in which only the affected X chromosome was inactivated.[807]

Lysosomal Membrane[808,809]

The lysosomal membrane serves as a selective permeability barrier between the lysosomal lumen and the cytoplasm. It is equipped with carriers and transport systems that control the passage of substances between both compartments and with a proton pump that creates the acidic environment necessary for intralysosomal digestion. The lysosomal membrane prevents the egress of macromolecules brought into the lysosome by endocytosis or autophagy and allows the escape of only the end products of their digestion. The amino acids, dipeptides, nucleosides, small monomeric sugars, phosphate or sulfate ions, and other molecules released from lysosomes by active or passive transport may be utilized for biosynthetic reactions in the cytoplasm. Certain nutrients such as cholesterol, released from cholesterol esters brought into lysosomes by endocytosis of LDL particles,[274,810] and cobalamin (vitamin B_{12}), taken up complexed to transcobalamin II,[811,812] are delivered to the cytoplasm by transport through the lysosomal membrane.

Several carrier-mediated transport systems specific for cystine,[813–818] cationic amino acids,[819,820] small neutral amino acids,[821] or tyrosine and other bulky neutral amino acids[822] have been identified in the lysosomal membrane. In the recessively inherited disease *nephropathic cystinosis*, a defect in the carrier that mediates the transport of cystine leads to the accumulation of large amounts of this disulfide amino acid within the lysosome.[813–815,817] Although cystine accumulates within the lysosomal compartment, it could not exist in the cytoplasm, where strongly reducing conditions prevail. The therapeutic administration of the aminothiol cysteamine reduces the accumulation of cystine through the formation within the lysosome of the mixed disulfide of cysteine and cysteamine, which behaves as a lysine analogue and is recognized by the system that transports cationic amino acids.[814,823] Certain compounds such as the acidotropic amines, chloroquine and primaquine, as well as amino acid esters, dipeptides, and oligopeptides (particularly if rich in hydrophobic amino acids) traverse the lysosomal membrane from the cytoplasm to the luminal side. The protonated amines, as well as the free amino acids generated by hydrolysis of the ester and peptide bonds, accumulate within the lysosomes and exit only slowly through the lysosomal membrane. Monosaccharides seem to cross the lysosomal membrane by facilitated diffusion, and a carrier has been identified that mediates the transfer of sialic acid. This carrier appears to be defective in Salla disease,[824,825] in which an intralysosomal accumulation of sialic acid occurs.

A membrane-associated enzyme, *acetyl CoA: α-glycosaminide* N-*acetyltransferase*, transfers acetyl groups from acetyl CoA in the cytoplasm to acceptor glucosamine moieties linked in terminal α linkages to heparan sulfate molecules within the lysosome.[826] The acetylation on heparan sulfate appears to be necessary for its degradation. A deficiency in the transferase produces the Sanfilippo C syndrome,[827] resulting from intralysosomal accumulation of heparan sulfate.

There is a proton pump in the lysosomal membrane that creates and maintains an acid environment (pH 5) within the lysosomal lumen (see refs. 828 and 829). The pump utilizes cytoplasmic ATP, is believed to function in an electrogenic manner,[830–832a] and operates most effectively in the presence of chloride ions, which also accumulate in the lysosomal lumen. In its sensitivity to inhibitors,[830,831] the lysosomal pump strongly resembles other ATPases (known as vacuolar ATPases) that have been identified in the ER,[832a] the Golgi apparatus,[417] and endocytic and secretory vesicles (see refs. 829 and 833). These proton ATPases are responsible for the progressive acidification of the lumen of the organelles that constitute the endomembrane system and are selectively inhibited by the macrolide antibiotic *bafilomycin* A_1.[834] The vacuolar pumps are insensitive to oligomycin, azide, N,N′-dicyclohexylcarbodiimide (DCCC) and other inhibitors that block the function of the mitochondrial F_0F_1 ATPase, and to vanadate, which inhibits the E_1E_2 phosphoenzyme-type ATPases (such as the Na^+/K^+-ATPase of the plasma membrane). On the other hand, levels of the sulfhydryl reagent NEM that inhibit the function of vacuolar ATPases do not affect the other ion-motive enzymes (the F_0F_1 and E_1E_2 ATPases).

The luminal surface of the lysosomal membrane is thought to be protected from the attack of lysosome hydrolases by complex oligosaccharides rich in poly-*N*-acetyllactosamines bearing sialic acid, which appear to be characteristic of lysosomal membrane glycoproteins (see below). Acting as immobilized polyanions, the sialic acid moieties may also play an important role in establishing a Donnan potential for protons that contributes to the internal low pH of lysosomes.[835]

Very little is known of the cytoplasmic surface of the lysosomal membrane, although it must possess receptors that mediate the fusion of lysosomes with other lysosomes or with phagosomes or endosomes to which lysosomal enzymes must be made available. This surface must also interact with the cytoskeletal elements responsible for lysosomal movement.[836,837] A lysosomal membrane protein has been purified that binds to preassembled microtubules and may participate in this process.[838]

Through protein purification[839–841] and the use of polyclonal and monoclonal antibodies prepared against lysosomal membranes,[842–847] several lysosomal membrane proteins have been identified. These have received various names, such as lysosomal associated membrane proteins (*lamp*), lysosomal integral membrane proteins (*limp*), lysosomal glycoproteins (*lgp*), and lysosomal endosomal plasma membrane proteins (*lep 100* and *endolin*), corresponding to their organellar derivation. Immunocytochemical methods indicate that these proteins colocalize with cytoplasmic structures identified as lysosomes because of their content of lysosomal hydrolases and their capacity to accumulate the dye acridine orange.[848] Although their function remains unknown, these proteins have become useful models to study the biosynthesis of the lysosomal membrane. Some of the proteins identified appear to represent equivalent gene products in different species (e.g., human lamp 1 = mouse limp 3 = rat lgp 120 = chicken lep 100; human lamp 2 = mouse limp 4 = rat lgp 110; lamp 3 = CD63). All of them are glycoproteins rich in *N*-linked oligosaccharides, most of which are of the complex type and are, therefore, initially synthesized in the ER and modified in the Golgi apparatus. The oligosaccharides represent up to 65 percent of the mass of the individual proteins, and the lamp molecules bear the bulk of the cellular complement of poly-*N*-acetyllactosamines [(Galβ1-4 GlcNAcβ1-3)$_n$], which are composed of *N*-acetyllactosamine repeats in the side chains of the *N*-linked oligosaccharides. These oligosaccharides usually carry added carbohydrate structures, such as the blood group antigen sialyl Le^x (NeuNAcα2-3Galβ1-4,(Fucα1-3)GlcNαc).[849] Some lysosomal membrane proteins are found in significant amounts only in mature or developing lysosomes and are absent from endosomes or the plasma membrane,[842–844] whereas others appear to undergo a constant circulation through the three compartments.[846]

The complex oligosaccharide chains in lysosomal membrane proteins are likely to play a role in protecting the exposed portions of the polypeptides from the attack of lysosomal proteases, since in tunicamycin-treated cells the proteins have shorter-than-normal half-lives.[847] Lamp 1 and lamp 2 are so abundant that their oligosaccharides may completely coat the luminal side of the membrane and thus serve as an effective barrier to the hydrolases.

It has been suggested that in cells capable of the exocytic discharge of lysosome-like granules (such as cytotoxic lymphocytes, platelets, and phagocytes) the lysosomal membrane proteins incorporated into the plasma membrane serve to protect the cell from the noxious effect of the released content enzymes.[809] The lamp molecules that appear on the surface of granulocytes and monocytes that discharge their granules in inflammatory sites also may provide exposed sialyl Le^x oligosaccharides that serve as ligands recognized by cell-adhesion molecules such as ELAM-1 and GMP-140 (P selectin), of endothelial cells and platelets, respectively (see ref. 809). In fact, since a small proportion of lysosomal membrane proteins are normally present in the plasma membrane (see below) their adhesive properties may contribute to normal cell-cell interactions.

Transport of Membrane Proteins to the Lysosome

Evidence indicates that unlike the situation with the lysosomal hydrolases, the sorting of lysosomal membrane proteins to the lysosome is not mediated by an oligosaccharide bearing the Man-6-P marker.[845,847,849a,850] Thus, the membrane-associated enzymes β-glucocerebrosidase and acetyl-CoA α-D-glycosaminide *N*-acetyltransferase are present at normal levels in I-cell disease fibroblasts. The former enzyme has been directly shown not to be phosphorylated in normal cells.[851] Moreover, the oligosaccharides of some of the previously mentioned purified lysosomal membrane proteins identified with antibodies to the lysosomal membrane do not appear to contain phosphate groups. In pulse labeling and cell fractionation experiments with tunicamycin-treated cultured cells, some of the newly synthesized membrane proteins are, nevertheless, transported to the lysosome with rapid kinetics.[845] Under the same conditions, the lysosomal hydrolases lacking *N*-linked oligosaccharides are secreted. Therefore, the transport of membrane proteins to lysosomes does not seem to be coupled obligatorily to the transport of lysosomal hydrolases, which takes place via the Man-6-P receptor and is interrupted after tunicamycin treatment.

Several studies in which the fate of altered lysosomal membrane proteins or chimeric polypeptides containing segments of lysosomal membrane proteins were examined in transfected cells have demonstrated that the signals that target those proteins to the lysosome are contained within their short cytoplasmic domains.[679,852–855] Human lamp 1 and the equivalent rat lgp 120 contain a glycine^7, tyrosine^8 (G^7Y^8) motif in their 11 amino acid cytoplasmic tails. This motif is also present in lamp 2 and 3, as well as — in an almost equivalent position — in the precursor of the lysosomal acid phosphatase (LAP), a transmembrane protein with a slightly longer cytoplasmic tail (19 amino acids). These proteins are normally present at low levels in the plasma membrane, from which they are removed by rapid endocytosis.

Mutation of the single tyrosine within the G^7Y^8 motif led to the accumulation of the proteins in the plasma membrane,[679,852,853,855] as expected from the abolition of the tyrosine-containing endocytic signal, which is similar to that present in the transferrin and LDL receptors. These observations are consistent with a pathway for delivery of membrane proteins to lysosomes that involves two steps: first, their direct transfer from the TGN to the plasma membrane, and second, their internalization into endosomes and appearance in lysosomes. Indeed, several analyses of the kinetics of delivery of lysosomal membrane proteins to lysosomes and determinations of their transient appearance at the plasma membrane have provided evidence for this indirect pathway.[854,856–858] This mechanism of delivery would require that the interiorization signals that trigger endocytosis of the lysosomal membrane protein have the added feature of favoring transfer of those proteins from early endosomes to deeper endosomes and lysosomes, although a certain fraction of the interiorized molecules would constantly recycle from endosomes to the cell surface. The studies on the effect of mutations within the cytoplasmic domain of lysosomal membrane proteins, and of appropriate chimeric transmembrane proteins, established that this domain contains a motif that is necessary and sufficient for targeting the proteins to lysosomes.[852,854]

An alternative view for the pathway of delivery of lysosomal membrane proteins to lysosomes is that, like the lysosomal hydrolases, the bulk of the membrane proteins are sorted in the TGN from proteins with other destinations and transferred directly to the developing lysosome. Support for this view was obtained from labeling and cell fractionation experiments showing that newly synthesized membrane proteins appear in lysosomes with kinetics so rapid as to make it unlikely that a major fraction of such proteins first reaches the cell surface to then undergo interiorization, a step which proceeds with relatively slow kinetics.[859] It currently appears that both the direct and indirect routes may be utilized with different efficiencies in different cell types and, possibly, at different steps of cell differentiation.[855,860] One study indicates that the machinery that effects the direct delivery of membrane proteins from the TGN to lysosomes can be easily saturated. The membrane proteins that are synthesized in excess of its capacity take the indirect route. It was observed that mutation of either glycine^7 or tyrosine^8 within the cytoplasmic domain of lgp 120 abolished direct transfer of the protein from the TGN to lysosomes and led to the delivery of the mutants to the cell surface. However, whereas the mutant lacking tyrosine^8 was unable to reach the lysosome by either the direct or indirect route and therefore accumulated at the cell surface, the mutant lacking glycine^7 lost only the capacity to follow the direct route. This mutant, therefore, appeared only transiently at the cell surface and followed the indirect route to reach the lysosome.[855]

Potocytosis[658,861–864]

Recently, the existence of a process, termed *potocytosis*, has been recognized[865] that may effect the uptake of small molecules and ions into cells within flask-shaped plasma membrane invaginations called *caveolae*. These structures are prominent in fibroblasts and endothelial cells but are also found in many other cell types. Although in endothelial cells they are involved in transcytosis,[866] perhaps through the fusion of caveolae emerging from opposite sides of the cell, it is not yet clear if caveolae actually pinch off from the plasma membrane or always remain connected to the cell surface.

Caveolae appear to function as specialized sites for the concentration, uptake, and perhaps storage of small molecules that serve as ligands for GIPL-linked plasma membrane receptors. Indeed, it has been proposed[861,862] that small molecules and ions are brought to caveolae by specific plasma membrane receptors (e.g., the folate receptor), carrier proteins, or enzymes that, like 5′ nucleotidase, are GIPL-linked (see below). The release of the ligands within the caveolae would create a high local concentration of small molecules and ions, sufficient to drive their transport into the cytoplasm. It is possible, for example, that in this manner potocytosis is responsible for the uptake of adenosine, which would be released into caveolae by the action of 5′-nucleotidase on AMP, a nucleotide that cannot traverse the plasma membrane. Potocytosis may also be important[867] in the transport across the capillary endothelium of the thyroid hormone, thyroxine, which in serum is bound to the carrier protein transthyretin. This carrier has been found to enter the caveolae of endothelial cells, where it would release its ligand without ever reaching the pericapillary space. Free thyroxine, however, would diffuse into the cytoplasm of the endothelium and across its plasma membrane to the perivascular space.

The most striking structural feature of caveolae is that they contain clusters of GIPL-anchored proteins, such as the receptor for folate and the enzymes 5′-nucleotidase and alkaline phosphatase. More than 80 percent of the plasma membrane content of these proteins appears to be immobilized in clusters within caveolae,[611] and studies with GIPL-linked proteins indicate that, although the unclustered and clustered fractions appear to be in dynamic equilibrium, only the mobile molecules can be interiorized in clathrin-coated vesicles, probably because they associate with other transmembrane receptors. The formation of the clusters of GIPL-linked proteins and the integrity of the caveolae appear to require the presence of cholesterol in the membrane, since manipulations that decrease the concentration of this sterol disperse the GIPL-linked proteins, disassemble the caveolae, and inhibit the uptake of folate that is mediated by its lipid-anchored receptor.[868]

The cytoplasmic face of caveolae is covered by a distinct striated coat that was shown to contain a 22-kDa integral membrane protein, now named *caveolin*,[865] previously identified as a substrate of the *v-src* tyrosine kinase in virally transformed cells. In this regard, it is striking that GPI-linked proteins in the plasma membrane seem to be associated in some way with tyrosine kinases, such as p56lck and p59fyn, and that antibodies to the GPI-linked proteins are able to trigger T-cell activation.

Caveolin is also identical to VIP-21,[869] which was found to be an integral membrane component of TGN-derived vesicles thought to be involved in transport of proteins to the apical surface of polarized epithelial cells.[870] As previously mentioned, in these cells GIPL-linked proteins and sphingolipids cluster together in the TGN to be delivered to the apical surface, where GIPL-linked proteins are known to accumulate preferentially. It is therefore conceivable that there is a mechanistic relationship between the association of caveolin with GIPL-linked proteins in caveolae and in the apically targeted vesicles.

MITOCHONDRIAL BIOGENESIS[870a–880]

Mitochondria are cytoplasmic organelles that carry out cellular respiration and generate most of the ATP that fuels the activities of the cell. They contain a vast array of enzymes that may vary with the cell type, reflecting their central role in various aspects of metabolism. Mitochondria are also capable of storing and releasing calcium ions, and it is thought that this enables them to serve, together with the ER, as regulators of cytoplasmic calcium levels.

Structurally, mitochondria are characterized by the presence of two concentric lipoprotein membranes and two internal compartments (Fig. 16-37). The *outer mitochondrial membrane* (OMM) completely surrounds the organelle, and all molecules entering or leaving the mitochondrion must pass through it. The *inner mitochondrial membrane* (IMM) is separated from the outer by an *intermembrane space* and encloses the major intramitochondrial compartment, known as the *matrix* space or stroma. The surface area of the inner membrane is greatly increased by the presence of numerous infoldings, known as *cristae*, that vary in number and configuration depending on the type of cell and its physiological state. Regions of close contact between the inner and outer mitochondrial membranes are frequently observed, and

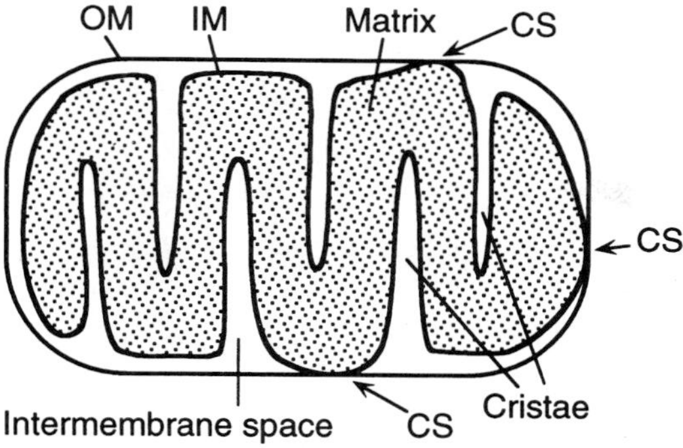

Fig. 16-37 Mitochondrial subcompartments. A mitochondrion contains two concentric membranes, an inner (IM) and an outer one (OM), separated by an intermembrane space. The matrix represents the space completely surrounded by the inner membrane. Contact sites (CS) between the two membranes (marked by arrows) appear to be the sites for the incorporation into the organelle of polypeptides synthesized in the cytoplasm. The cristae are represented by platelike invaginations of the inner membrane but may adopt other configurations. See the text for the characteristic protein contents of the various mitochondrial subcompartments.

importation of proteins into the organelle is known to take place at these "contact" sites.[881–887]

Specific mitochondrial proteins are found in each one of the four submitochondrial compartments (i.e., the two membranes and the intermembrane and matrix spaces). The outer membrane has a relatively low protein content and is characterized by large amounts of the transmembrane protein "porin," which forms channels through which ions and small molecules can pass freely.[888] It also contains receptors for protein import (see below), monoamine oxidase, and, in some cell types such as hepatocytes, cytochrome b5 and cytochrome b5 reductase, proteins that have corresponding, but not identical, counterparts in the ER.

In contrast to the OMM, the IMM is impermeable to small molecules and contains specialized transport systems, such as the ATP-ADP carrier or translocator and transporters for phosphate, carnitine esters, pyruvate, malate, and glycerol phosphate. Most importantly, this membrane contains the components of the electron transport chain that receives electrons generated by dehydrogenation of the citric acid cycle substrates. It also contains the ATP synthase (F1F0-ATPase) that carries out oxidative phosphorylation (see ref. 870a).

The intermembrane space contains enzymes, such as myokinase (adenylate kinase), which functions to equilibrate ATP and AMP with ADP. These enzymes can be released relatively easily from isolated mitochondria by osmotic shock or sonication. The mitochondrial matrix houses enzymes of the citric acid cycle, the pyruvate dehydrogenase complex, and the enzymatic system that carries out the β-oxidation of fatty acids. In the hepatocyte, the matrix is also the site of some of the enzymes of the urea cycle.

The mitochondrial membranes contain both peripheral and integral proteins, and each membrane polypeptide has a characteristic disposition relative to the phospholipid bilayer. For example, cytochrome oxidase, a protein that consists of several subunits and serves as the terminal member of the electron transport chain that carries out the reduction of oxygen, is an integral component of the inner membrane and is exposed on both sides of this membrane. On the other hand, cytochrome *c*, which delivers electrons to cytochrome oxidase, is a peripheral membrane protein reversibly bound to a portion of cytochrome oxidase exposed on the outer face of the inner membrane. The ATP synthase that is driven by a proton gradient to effect ATP synthesis is also a complex protein that in yeast contains nine subunits. Four of these form the F_0, or stalk portion of the complex, which is embedded in the inner membrane. The other subunits (α, β, γ, δ, ε) form a round particle, the F_1 ATPase (with the composition $\alpha_3\beta_3\gamma\delta\varepsilon$), which protrudes into the matrix space and is held onto the membrane by the stalk (see ref. 870a, for organization of components of the electron transport chain).

Mitochondria are the only organelles of mammalian cells that possess a separate genome and the enzymatic machinery necessary for its replication and expression.[871] The mitochondrial genes are contained in a circular double-stranded DNA molecule that in the human consists of 16,569 nucleotide pairs whose sequence has been determined[889] (see Chaps. 104 and 105).

The mitochondrial DNA encodes the ribosomal RNA of the mitochondrial ribosomes, as well as 22 different transfer RNA molecules. Although mitochondria contain at least several hundred different polypeptides, only 13 of these are encoded in the organellar genome and are synthesized within the mitochondria. These include some, but not all, of the subunits of the cytochrome oxidase and of the ATPase, as well as subunits of the coenzyme QH_2-cytochrome *c* reductase, another member of the electron transfer chain. The mitochondrially synthesized polypeptides contain hydrophobic segments and are, in general, components of the inner membrane. Almost all other mitochondrial proteins, including the remaining subunits of the ATPase and cytochrome oxidase, are encoded in nuclear genes and are synthesized outside the mitochondria. They are subsequently taken up into the organelle and sorted into one of the four submitochondrial compartments.

Incorporation of Proteins into Mitochondria (Fig. 16-38)

Much has been learned about this process from studies carried out with yeast and Neurospora. These unicellular eukaryotic organisms are suitable for both genetic analysis and in vivo pulse-chase experiments in which the precursors of polypeptides destined to mitochondria can be identified. The study of protein transfer into mitochondria has also made rapid progress because it has been possible to reproduce this phenomenon in vitro by adding polypeptides synthesized in cell-free systems to isolated mitochondria obtained from either unicellular organisms or cells of higher animals.

Mitochondrial proteins encoded in the nuclear genome are synthesized in polyribosomes that are not bound to ER membranes. Most, but not all, proteins destined to the interior of the mitochondrion are synthesized as larger precursors containing N-terminal extensions or *presequences* (20 to 80 amino acids long) that are removed by intramitochondrial proteases,[890] whose function is essential for normal mitochondrial biogenesis.[891] Each presequence contains an addressing or *targeting signal* that is responsible for the incorporation of the polypeptide into the organelle. The presequence may also contain a sorting or *localization signal* downstream from the targeting signal that determines the intramitochondrial location of the polypeptide. In the absence of a localization signal, the targeting signal within the presequence directs the polypeptide across both the inner and outer mitochondrial membranes into the matrix (Fig. 16-38*A*).[892–895] The localization signal, which in some cases is present within the sequence of the mature protein, may arrest translocation of the polypeptide through the outer (Fig. 16-38*B*) or the inner membrane (Figs. 16-38*D* and 16-38*F*) or, after the protein reaches the matrix, may direct its re-export through the inner membrane toward the intermembrane space (Fig. 16-38*C* and 16-38*E*).

Proteins of the outer mitochondrial membrane are synthesized without cleavable presequences and, therefore, must contain permanent targeting signals. These include porin,[896] the MAS70 protein that functions as an import receptor for a subclass of mitochondrial proteins,[897–899] some proteins of the interior mitochondrial subcompartments (such as cytochrome *c* of the intermembrane space),[901,902] and the ADP-ATP translocator of the inner membrane.[902]

The insertion of outer membrane polypeptides into the membrane and the passage of apocytochrome *c* into the intermembrane space are processes that appear to occur spontaneously,

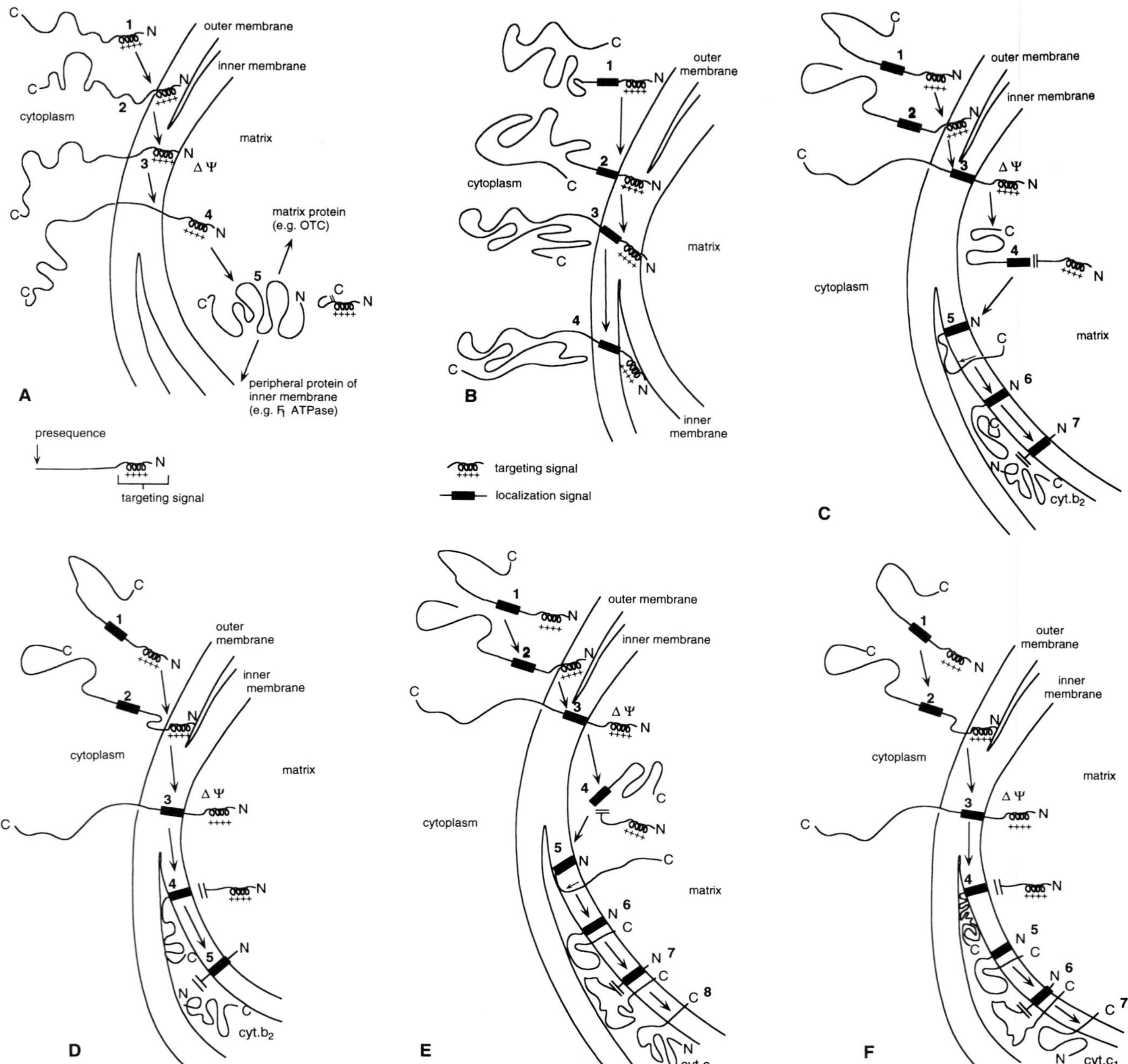

Fig. 16-38 Pathways for the incorporation of polypeptides into mitochondria. *A.* Incorporation of matrix proteins. A targeting signal located within a cleavable presequence at the N-terminus of the polypeptide (1) leads first to the association of the polypeptide first with the outer membrane (2) and then, in the presence of a transmembrane potential (3), to the passage of the polypeptide into the matrix through a point of contact between the two membranes. In an intermediate stage (4), parts of the polypeptide have reached the matrix while others are still exposed on the mitochondrial surface. The presequence is removed by a matrix metalloprotease and (5) the final product may remain in the matrix (as is the case with ornithine transcarbamylase; OTC) or become peripherally associated with the inner membrane (as is the case with the β subunit of the F_1 ATPase). *B.* Incorporation of a protein into the outer membrane. The polypeptide contains an N-terminal targeting signal that is immediately followed by a localization signal (1). As in *A*, the targeting signal leads to association of the polypeptide with the outer membrane (2), but the localization signal prevents passage through the inner membrane at the contact point (3 and 4). The localization signal is a hydrophobic segment similar to the halt-transfer signal of type I membrane proteins. In the figure, the targeting signal of the mature protein is depicted as exposed in the intermembrane space, but this has not been shown and the part of the protein that forms an amphipathic helix may also be embedded in the outer membrane. The model is based on experimental data obtained for a 70-kDa outer membrane protein (OMP). *C* and *D.* Two alternative pathways for the incorporation of a protein (such as cytochrome b_2) into the intermembrane space. *C.* In this case, the targeting signal leads to complete translocation of the polypeptide into the matrix, where it is cleaved by the metalloprotease (1 to 4). This exposes a hydrophobic localization signal which serves as an insertion signal to mediate translocation of the polypeptide across the inner membrane from the matrix to the intermembrane space (4 to 6). The protein is discharged into the intermembrane space as a result of cleavage of the localization-insertion signal by a second protease, which is located on the outer surface of the inner membrane (7). *D.* In this model, the localization signal serves to halt transfer of the polypeptide across the inner membrane (4), which is initiated by the targeting signal (1 to 3). The polypeptide is discharged into the intermembrane space after cleavage by the second protease (5), as in *C. E* and *F.* Alternative pathways for the incorporation into mitochondria of a protein, such as cytochrome c_1, which is associated with the inner membrane but is largely exposed in the intermembrane space. *E.* The mechanism operates as in *C*, but translocation from the matrix into the intermembrane space is halted (7) before completion by a segment located near the C-terminus of the protein. *F.* As in *D*, the localization signal halts translocation into the matrix (4). Before cleavage by the second protease (6), however, the C-terminal region of the polypeptide inserts into the inner membrane (5). (*Based in part on ref. 873.*)

without the requirement of energy.[903–906] The uptake of other polypeptides into the inner mitochondrial compartments (i.e., matrix, inner membrane, and in some cases, the intermembrane space), is an energy-dependent process that requires not only the availability of ATP, but also the existence of an electrochemical potential across the inner membrane (i.e., an energized inner membrane). Thus, uptake of such polypeptides is blocked by the addition of respiratory inhibitors, uncouplers of oxidative phosphorylation, or the ionophore valinomycin, which eliminates the membrane potential by allowing for the equilibration of the K^+ ion concentrations on both sides of the inner membrane.[907–910]

Signals for Targeting of Proteins to Mitochondria[911]

The cleavable presequences within precursors of mitochondrial proteins generally contain at or near the N-terminal region a segment that is rich in basic and hydroxylated amino acids and usually lack acidic amino acids and extensive stretches of hydrophobic residues.[911,912] In mediums of low polarity, or on insertion into lipid bilayers, these segments appear to be able to form amphipathic helixes, which contain positively charged or polar residues on one side of the helix and hydrophobic residues on the other.[912,913] The structure of the mitochondrial presequences is, therefore, fundamentally different from that of the signal sequences characteristic of polypeptides synthesized in the ER.

The presence within the presequences of targeting signals for incorporation of the polypeptides into mitochondria was established by experiments that employed recombinant DNA methods to link the presequences, or portions thereof, to segments of other polypeptides that are not normally targeted to the mitochondria. Thus, when gene segments encoding the presequences of the yeast cytochrome oxidase subunit IV,[914,915] alcohol dehydrogenase III,[892] or rat liver ornithine transcarbamylase (OTC)[916,917] were fused with a DNA sequence encoding dihydrofolate reductase (DHFR), a cytosolic enzyme, the resulting chimeric polypeptides were incorporated into mitochondria, both in vivo and in vitro. Experiments of this type showed that, although the presequence (i.e., the cleaved segment) of the yeast cytochrome oxidase subunit IV is 25 residues in length, only its first 12 amino acids serve as the targeting signal and are required for incorporation of the chimera into the mitochondrial matrix. Proteolytic removal of the shortened presequence, however, did not take place.[915] The efficacy of shortened presequences of only 9 to 12 amino acids in length has also been demonstrated for other mitochondrial proteins, such as δ-aminolevulinate synthase.[918] The crucial role of presequences in determining the uptake of mitochondrial proteins is highlighted by the existence of a natural mutation in a patient with *methylmalonic acidemia* in which a short, apparently N-terminal, deletion within the precursor of methylmalonyl CoA mutase prevents the incorporation of the enzyme into the mitochondria.[919]

The targeting sequences need not always be located at the extreme N-terminus of the precursor polypeptide. In OTC, which contains a 32-residue cleavable presequence, residues 8 to 23 were found to be essential for uptake.[917,920] However, the function of a targeting signal requires that it remain exposed when the polypeptide folds in the cytoplasm after being discharged from the ribosome. Thus, the cytosolic protein DHFR contains a cryptic targeting signal located between residues 26 to 85,[921] but this signal does not normally operate to bring the polypeptide into the mitochondria, apparently because it is "masked" in the folded protein. However, when the first 85 residues of DHFR are linked to the N-terminus of an intact DHFR sequence, or to subunit IV of cytochrome oxidase lacking its own targeting sequence, the normally cryptic signal becomes exposed and the chimeric polypeptides are efficiently incorporated into mitochondria.[921]

Receptors for the Uptake of Proteins into Mitochondria (Fig. 16-39)

With the exception of cytochrome *c*,[922] polypeptides to be incorporated into mitochondria are recognized by receptors present in the OMM.[903,907,923–926] Under appropriate experimental

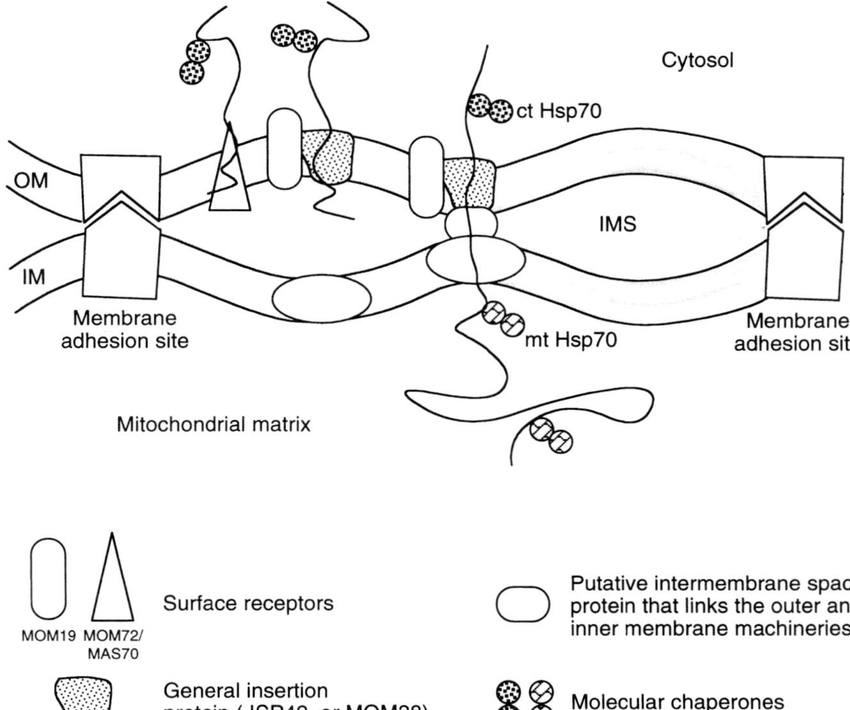

Fig. 16-39 Organization of the translocation machineries in the outer and inner mitochondrial membranes. The scheme (based on Pfanner et al.[878]) represents a region of a mitochondrion where translocation of a polypeptide from the cytosol into the matrix is taking place. This region is shown as flanked by putative adhesion sites that bring the outer (OM) and inner (IM) membranes close to each other. Polypeptides to be incorporated into mitochondria are recognized by one of the two types of outer membrane receptor proteins (MOM19 or MOM72/MAS70). The MOM19, which functions in the translocation of a wide variety of polypeptides, is always associated with the general insertion protein (ISP42 in yeast, or MOM38 in Neurospora) that represents the major component of the translocation machinery of the outer membrane and, therefore, transfers the polypeptide directly to it. The translocation of a polypeptide bound to MOM72/MAS70 requires that this receptor undergoes lateral displacement in the membrane to become associated with the complex of MOM19 and the general insertion site (MOM38 or ISP42). Insertion of the translocating polypeptide into the translocation machinery of the inner membrane leads to coupling of the two machineries, although this may require the function of an intermembrane space protein (IMS). The role of both cytoplasmic (ctHsp70) and mitochondrial (mtHsp70) chaperones is explained in Fig. 16-40.

conditions (e.g., inhibition of polypeptide chain elongation) polysomes synthesizing certain mitochondrial proteins are recovered selectively with sedimentable mitochondria.[927] This suggests that interaction of precursors of mitochondrial proteins with their receptors within the cell may take place before their synthesis is completed. The presence of proteinaceous receptors on the mitochondrial surface for precursors of mitochondrial proteins was first inferred from the observation that the in vitro binding and uptake of precursors is nearly completely abolished by brief treatment of intact mitochondria with low concentrations of proteases.[901,903,907,928] Since several hundred different polypeptides must be imported into the mitochondria, separate receptors for each mitochondrial polypeptide seemed highly improbable. In fact, studies have shown that there are two major types of receptors on the mitochondrial surface, which recognize different sets of proteins. The existence of more than one type of receptor was initially suggested by observations that the addition of a synthetic presequence peptide[929] or of a purified unfolded mitochondrial protein[901,904] to an in vitro uptake system, or mild protease treatment of the mitochondria,[925] selectively blocked the incorporation of some precursors but not others into the organelle.

Following the demonstration that precursors of mitochondrial proteins bind with high affinity and in a saturable manner to protease-sensitive sites on the mitochondrial surface,[925,928,930,931] antibodies were prepared to many purified outer membrane polypeptides. These were examined for their capacity to block the importation of precursor proteins. Two distinct receptor proteins with different specificities were identified. One of these — the yeast MAS70 protein (70 kDa),[898] equivalent to the Neurospora MOM72 (72 kDa)[899,932] — was shown to function in the uptake of the ATP-ADP carrier (an inner membrane protein that contains noncleavable internal targeting signals). Antibodies to this receptor could coprecipitate, from detergent-treated mitochondria, ATP-ADP carrier molecules that had been bound to the organelle before lysis together with the antigen.[932] MAS70, however, is not essential for mitochondrial import. A null mutation in the corresponding yeast gene was not lethal,[933] although it decreased the rate of import of many mitochondrial precursor proteins in vivo.[898]

Antibodies to the second receptor, MOM19, a 19-kDa outer membrane protein of Neurospora,[934] selectively impaired the uptake of precursors that contain cleavable N-terminal targeting sequences, a process that was not inhibited by antibodies to MOM72. MOM19 appears to be a master receptor of broad specificity. It appears to be capable of mediating the uptake of all precursors containing cleavable presequences, regardless of the mitochondrial subcompartment to which they are destined.[934] This receptor is also capable of mediating the uptake of the ATP-ADP carrier when MOM72 is absent or incapacitated, albeit at low efficiency.[899] Surprisingly, different parts of MOM19 may interact with different precursor proteins. Treatment of mitochondria with elastase, a protease that impairs the uptake of many precursors and converts MOM19 to a 17-kDa membrane-associated fragment,[934] did not abolish the import into the matrix of the precursor of the β subunit of the F_1-F_0 ATPase,[925,931] a protein that contains an N-terminal cleavable signal.

A putative third import receptor is a 32-kDa protein with affinity for the targeting signals in mitochondrial presequences. It was identified in yeast mitochondria from its binding to anti-idiotypic antibodies prepared using a synthetic presequence peptide.[935] As in the case of MOM72, antibodies against this membrane protein inhibited the uptake of several mitochondrial precursors and were capable of precipitating from detergent-treated mitochondria complexes containing the antigen associated with precursors that had been previously bound to the organellar surface. A null mutation that eliminated the 32-kDa protein was not lethal, indicating that it too, like the MOM72 receptor, is functionally redundant. The unexpected finding that the 32-kDa protein is identical in amino acid sequence to the phosphate carrier, a protein that functions in the inner mitochondrial membrane, has raised questions about its physiological role in mitochondrial protein import.[936]

Immunolabeling studies indicate that both the MOM19 and MOM72 receptors are distributed throughout the mitochondrial surface, although MOM19 is slightly more concentrated, and MOM72 much more so, at regions of contact between the IMM and OMM.[932,934] This suggests that the import receptors may accept precursor proteins throughout the organellar surface but subsequently carry them by lateral displacement to the sites of contact between the two membranes, where translocation takes place.

Common Import Sites Effect the Translocation of Many Proteins across the Outer Membrane

Following their binding to the surface receptors, whether MOM19 or MOM72/MAS70, precursors of mitochondrial proteins are transferred to common translocation sites, variously called channels, pores, or *general insertion protein* (GIP), which effect their insertion into the outer membrane, rendering them resistant to the attack of exogenous proteases. The existence of these common import sites is strikingly demonstrated by the fact that porin — a major outer membrane protein that does not compete with the ATP-ADP carrier for binding to a surface receptor — does, however, compete with it in an assay in which, after the precursors are bound to mitochondria at low temperature, their importation is allowed to take place during a subsequent incubation at 25°C.[931]

Considerable insight into the process of import was obtained after it became possible to interrupt and arrest the translocation of precursors before its completion.[883,884,887,937] This could be achieved by lowering the temperature or the ATP levels in the system or by sterically blocking traversal of the outer membrane, either by preventing the unfolding of the C-terminal domain of a translocating protein, or by binding antibodies to its C-terminal region. Under the latter conditions, blocked translocation intermediates were detected that spanned both membranes, as indicated by the fact that their N-terminal targeting signals had already been cleaved by the matrix peptidase, while the C-termini remained exposed on the surface of the mitochondria, accessible to exogenous proteases and secondary antibodies.

Translocation intermediates trapped in the state in which they traverse both membranes appear to be contained within hydrophilic proteinaceous channels, since they can be extracted from mitochondria by treatment with protein denaturants, such as solutions of urea or of alkaline pH, that do not remove integral membrane proteins from phospholipid bilayers.[938] A yeast outer membrane protein, designated ISP42 (import site protein of 42 kDa), is a likely component of the importation site in the outer membrane since it could be photochemically crosslinked to a modified trapped precursor.[939] ISP42, whose sequence was derived from the cloned gene,[940] is essential for cell viability since disruption of the gene was lethal in haploid yeast strains. Moreover, a reduced expression of this protein was found to lead to the accumulation of mitochondrial precursors in the cytoplasm.[940]

The Neurospora homologue of ISP42, called MOM38, was identified as a component of a macromolecular complex that can be recovered from digitonin-treated mitochondria by immunoprecipitation with anti-MOM19 antibodies.[941] Strikingly, this complex also contains MOM72, as well as several other membrane proteins. In fact, it was also possible to demonstrate that the ATP-ADP carrier, which on the mitochondrial surface is recognized by MOM72, is also recovered in the complex immunoprecipitated with anti-MOM19 antibodies when trapped at the general insertion site. That MOM38 is a major component of the general insertion site is supported by the finding that in intact mitochondria this protein, and no other component of the complex immunoprecipitable with MOM19 antibodies, has the same sensitivity to exogenous proteases as the general insertion site measured in a functional assay.[941]

Organization of the Translocation Machinery (see Fig. 16-39)

It appears that mitochondria contain equimolar amounts of the receptors, MOM19 and MOM72, and of the import site protein, MOM38, and that all MOM19 molecules are complexed with MOM38, whereas only a fraction (approximately 50 percent) of MOM72 molecules are in such complexes.[941] The stoichiometry suggests that precursor proteins recognized by MOM19 are directly transferred to the site of translocation, whereas those, like the ATP-ADP carrier, that bind to MOM72 would have to move laterally in the membrane to become associated with the MOM38/ISP42 component of the general insertion site.

Insertion of a translocating polypeptide into the IMM has been found to require the presence of a potential across this membrane. However, once insertion into the inner membrane has taken place, completion of translocation through it can proceed without maintenance of the transmembrane potential,[942] requiring only ATP within the matrix to support the activity of molecular chaperones (see below) that apparently pull the translocating polypeptide inward.[943–946]

Given the positively charged nature of the N-terminal targeting signal present in many protein precursors and the inside negative character of the transmembrane potential, it seems possible that insertion into the inner membrane is the result of an electrophoretic effect that leads to the correct positioning of the positively charged signal with respect to the membrane, or activates a charged transmembrane component that effects the insertion.[877] In any case, insertion into the inner membrane is thought to lead to the coupling of independent distinct passageways in the two membranes, which become linked by the translocating polypeptide (see Fig. 16-39).[874,878,910,947,948] Immunoelectron microscopy revealed[884] that trapped translocating polypeptides containing a blocked C-terminus primarily accumulate at translocation contact sites. It has been estimated, from biochemical measurements of the number of trapped polypeptides at saturation, that there are a few thousand active translocation sites in each mitochondrion.[885]

The components of the inner membrane that contribute to the passageway have not yet been identified. Still, it is clear that a separate functional passageway exists in that membrane that is independent of its coupling to the outer membrane (see Fig. 16-39). Thus, when translocation sites of intact mitochondria are jammed by arrested translocating polypeptides, or are destroyed with proteases, removal of the outer membrane to produce mitoplasts leads to the exposure of new importation sites. These sites in the inner membrane are capable of accepting mitochondrial precursors in a process that is dependent on the membrane potential and on ATP hydrolysis, but is not inhibited by antibodies to the outer membrane receptors.[949,950]

The translocation machinery in the outer membrane can also function independently, when not dynamically coupled to the inner membrane. Thus, in the absence of the transmembrane potential, cytochrome *c* heme lyase can be completely translocated across the outer membrane to reach its destination in the intermembrane space, where it is inaccessible to exogenous proteases, unless the outer membrane is removed.[951] Similarly, when its import is carried out in the absence of a transmembrane potential, the ATP-ADP carrier reaches the intermembrane space, even though it is not inserted in the inner membrane.[952]

Role of Molecular Chaperones in the Import of Proteins into Mitochondria[17] (Fig. 16-40)

The import into mitochondria of precursor polypeptides released from free polysomes into the cytosol requires that they be kept in a "transport competent" state in which their targeting signals can be recognized by the receptors in the mitochondrial surface. In addition, for most precursor proteins, spontaneous folding into the "tight conformation" of the mature protein must be prevented. To be able to cross the mitochondrial membranes, the precursor must be capable of undergoing unfolding. Maintaining the unfolded state is the function of molecular chaperones that bind the newly synthesized mitochondria polypeptides in the cytosol (Fig. 16-40).

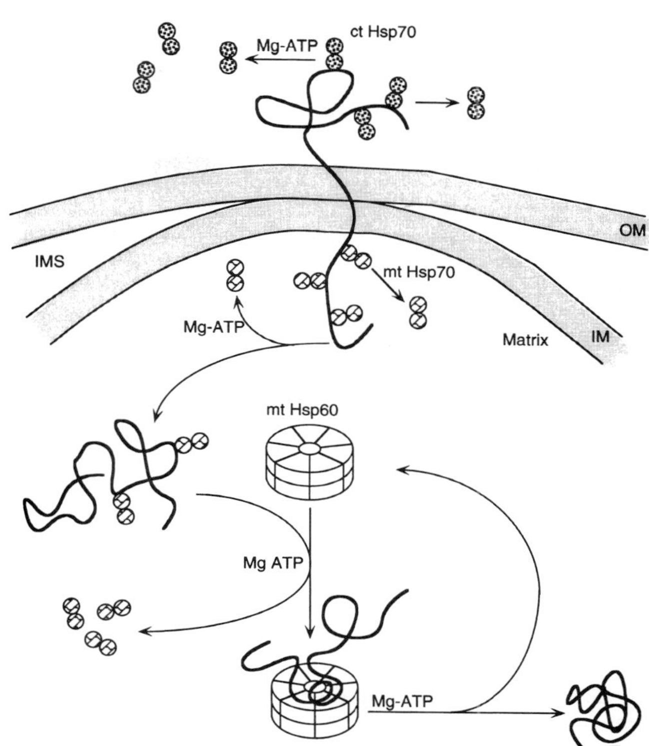

Fig. 16-40 Role of molecular chaperones in the importation of polypeptides into the mitochondrial matrix. Recently synthesized cytoplasmic polypeptides are kept in a loosely folded conformation by cytosolic Hsp70 molecules. In this scheme the polypeptide is represented in the course of translocation through both membranes, and components of the translocation and signal processing machinery other than the chaperones are not shown. As the polypeptide emerges into the matrix it is received by mt-Hsp70 chaperones that apparently pull inward to complete translocation. Dissociation of both the cytoplasmic and matrix chaperones from the polypeptide requires Mg-ATP. Once inside the mitochondrion, the polypeptide is transferred to the mitochondrial tetradecameric chaperonin Hsp60, which completes folding and oligomeric assembly of matrix polypeptides and releases them in a process that requires ATP hydrolysis. OM and IM = outer and inner mitochondrial membranes, respectively; IMS = intermembrane space. (*Adapted from Hartl and Martin.*[17])

The need to prevent folding of a protein to allow its import into mitochondria first became apparent from the observation that a fusion protein containing a mitochondrial targeting signal attached to the cytosolic protein DHFR could not be taken up into the mitochondria in the presence of methotrexate, a ligand that binds to DHFR and stabilizes it in a tightly folded conformation.[953] The methotrexate does not mask the presequence, since the protein still binds to the mitochondrial surface in the presence of this analogue but it is not translocated across the membrane. The block in import reflects the inability of the mitochondrial import apparatus to unfold the tightly folded DHFR on the mitochondrial surface. DHFR has been a convenient probe to follow the state of folding of a protein during its translocation into the mitochondrial matrix since the folded polypeptide is resistant to proteases, which digest the unfolded protein. This property of DHFR is manifested even in chimeras containing DHFR linked to the presequence of a mitochondrial protein, such as subunit IV of cytochrome oxidase, or cytochrome b_2. This has allowed the demonstration that during the uptake of such chimeras (in the absence of the ligand), DHFR undergoes unfolding on the mitochondrial surface and refolds after entering the matrix.[937]

Cytosolic factors with "antifolding" activity, that also prevent the improper aggregation of incompletely folded polypeptides, were in fact identified originally by their capacity to stimulate mitochondrial uptake of precursors in in vitro systems. One group of such antifolding factors comprises the *molecular chaperones* known as *ct-hsp70* (cytosolic heat-shock protein of 70 kDa)—a subset of the heat-shock family of proteins. The expression of many proteins in this family is induced by stress conditions, such as heat shock or glucose starvation, that lead to the partial denaturation (or misfolding) of many proteins within the cell. The ct-hsp70 proteins, however, are constitutively expressed at substantial levels in normal cells, in which they bind to newly synthesized polypeptides and play a role in ensuring their proper folding and oligomerization. Ct-hsp70 proteins are required for the viability of yeast cells, and their role in the uptake of mitochondrial proteins is shown by the fact that, when their levels are decreased by genetic manipulation, the uncleaved precursors of those proteins accumulate in the cytosol.[139] Release of the ct-hsp70 chaperones from the polypeptide precursor to which they bind appears to occur concomitantly with its translocation and requires ATP hydrolysis (see Fig. 16-40), which explains the necessity of extramitochondrial ATP for mitochondrial protein import.[937,954–958] Thus, mitochondrial protein precursors that are first unfolded by treatment with denaturants can be subsequently imported into mitochondria without the need of extramitochondrial ATP.[958,959]

Other cytosolic proteins, not members of the heat-shock family, have been identified that also stimulate the in vitro uptake of mitochondrial polypeptides. One of these isolated from reticulocyte lysate, and named *presequence binding factor* (PBF), was shown to bind to the presequence of OTC and may serve as a chaperone maintaining its translocation competence.[960] A different factor isolated from the reticulocyte lysate that binds to the presequence of ornithine aminotransferase (OAT) is believed to play a role in targeting. Antibodies to this factor blocked the binding to the mitochondrial surface and uptake into the organelle of two different precursor polypeptides.[961]

The insertion of a polypeptide into the inner membrane requires a transmembrane potential ($\Delta\psi$). Its subsequent translocation into the matrix is dependent[944] on the function of another molecular chaperone, *mt-hsp70*, a mitochondrial 70-kDa heat-shock protein (analogous to the bacterial Dnak protein) in the matrix that binds to the entering polypeptide (see Fig. 16-40).[946] A yeast temperature-sensitive mt-hsp70 has been obtained (SSC1) in which, at the nonpermissive temperature, the passage of precursor proteins into the mitochondrial matrix is arrested at translocation contact sites.[944] It appears that during normal translocation several mt-hsp70 molecules within the matrix bind successively to a single emerging translocating polypeptide (see Fig. 16-40). The energy of this interaction is thought to pull the polypeptide into the matrix, causing the unfolding of C-terminal portions that may remain exposed on the mitochondrial surface.[17] That mt-hsp70 plays a role in the unfolding of precursors is indicated by the fact that mitochondria containing a defective mt-hsp70 are still able to take up precursors in vitro if these precursors are previously unfolded by urea denaturation.[944] However, such precursors do not refold properly within the mutant mitochondria, indicating that mt-hsp70 also functions in the refolding of polypeptides after their importation. As is the case with ct-hsp70, the release of mt-hsp70 molecules from the translocating polypeptide requires the hydrolysis of ATP. In the absence of this nucleotide, the chaperonin molecules in the matrix remain bound to the polypeptides, which do not fold into the mature conformations.

Imported polypeptides released from mt-hsp70 are transferred to a second heat-shock protein within the matrix, the chaperonin *hsp60* (see Fig. 16-40), which is analogous to a bacterial chaperonin, GroEL, that functions in the assembly of bacteriophage capsids. Like GroEL, hsp60 is a large oligomer that consists of 14 60-kDa subunits arranged in two superimposed seven-member rings.[17] Hsp60 is not required for translocation itself, but carries out the ATP-dependent folding of matrix polypeptides and, when necessary, their oligomeric assembly. Therefore, it is necessary for yeast viability.[962,963] The capacity of mt-hsp60 to promote the assembly of oligomeric proteins is markedly stimulated by a matrix cochaperonin, *hsp10*, that is analogous to the bacterial protein GroES and promotes the ATPase activity of hsp60.[964] The precursors of both mitochondrial chaperonins mt-hsp70 and hsp60 contain matrix targeting signals that are removed by the matrix peptidase. It is interesting to note that assembly of the hsp60 tetradecamers themselves requires the function of hsp60 molecules already present in the matrix.[963]

Proteolytic Removal of Matrix Targeting Sequences

A *matrix processing peptidase* (MPP) whose activity depends on divalent cations such as Mn^{2+} and Zn^{2+}[890,965] removes the matrix targeting signals within the presequences of mitochondrial precursors. This enzyme usually cleaves the precursor at a site located two amino acids downstream of an arginine residue.[966–969] The matrix peptidase consists of two components.[967–969] One (approximately 55 kDa; known as MPP in *Neurospora crassa* and MAS2/MIF2 in *Saccharomyces cerevisiae*), now designated MPPα, has intrinsic peptidase activity[971] and the other, MPPβ (52 kDa, originally called processing enhancing protein or PEP in *N. crassa* and MAS1/MIF1 in *S. cerevisiae*), binds directly to the presequence,[972] markedly enhancing the activity of MPPα. Both components are essential for viability in yeast.[969] It has been shown in Neurospora that they too are synthesized as precursors, whose presequences are removed in the matrix by the action of the mature MPP.[971] The two components of the matrix peptidase are members of the same gene family, and MPPβ is identical (in Neurospora) or highly homologous (in yeast) to subunit 1 of the bc1 complex (complex III or ubiquinone-cytochrome *c* reductase) of the respiratory chain.[973] In Neurospora, therefore, MPPβ is a bifunctional protein bound to the matrix face of the inner membrane.

Many matrix targeting sequences undergo two proteolytic cleavages within the matrix.[966] Examples include the precursors of OTC, malate dehydrogenase, cytochrome oxidase subunit IV, and the Fe/S subunit of the bc_1 complex. In these cases, the first cleavage, effected by the MPP, creates an intermediate form of the precursor from which a second peptide, generally eight amino acids in length, is subsequently removed by a second specific matrix enzyme, the *mitochondrial intermediate peptidase* (MIP),[974] that has not yet been fully characterized. It has been suggested that the existence in the precursors of these proteins of an octapeptide segment between the two cleavage sites allows for the presence in the mature proteins of N-terminal sequences that would have been incompatible with efficient cleavage by the matrix processing protease. Presequences, such as those in cytochrome peroxidase and cytochromes b_2 and c_1, that in addition to a matrix targeting signal contain a sorting or mitochondrial localization signal that directs the protein to the intermembrane space (see below), undergo removal of these signals by a third mitochondrial peptidase, which is located on the outer face of the inner membrane (see below).

Mechanisms for Submitochondrial Localization of Proteins

Insertion of Proteins into the Matrix. A current view of the pathway followed by mitochondrial polypeptides containing targeting signals to reach the matrix is schematically represented in Fig. 16-38*A*. The N-terminal targeting signal within the presequence first binds to a receptor on the mitochondrial surface (not represented in the figure). This recognition step may occur anywhere on the surface of the organelle, but subsequent steps in import take place only at contact sites, where the inner and outer membranes are closely apposed.[883–887] At these sites the targeting signal inserts in the inner membrane in a process which requires a transmembrane potential ($\Delta\psi$) and leads to the translocation of the signal across this membrane. Cleavage of the signal by a matrix metalloprotease[890] then takes place, but this step is not required for the completion of translocation.[915] Intermediate stages in the uptake process, in which the polypeptide is exposed both within the matrix and on the surface of the mitochondria, have been observed in experiments in which the completion of translocation of the β subunit of the Neurospora F_1 ATPase was interrupted by carrying out the import at low temperatures.[883] These experiments have also shown that after insertion into the inner membrane has been initiated, completion of translocation does not require the transmembrane potential.

Insertion of Proteins into the Outer Mitochondrial Membrane (Fig. 16-38*B*). Proteins destined to the OMM are synthesized without cleavable presequences and, as expected, their uptake does not require an energized inner membrane. It appears that a variety of mechanisms are used to effect the incorporation of different proteins into the OMM. The MOM19 receptor, which is anchored in the outer membrane by an N-terminal hydrophobic sequence, is targeted to the mitochondria independently of protease-accessible surface receptors. This receptor protein appears to assemble directly with the general insertion protein MOM38[975] since antibodies to MOM38 block its incorporation into mitochondria. MOM38 itself contains no obvious hydrophobic segment that could serve as a transmembrane domain.[941] The mechanism for its association with the outer membrane remains obscure. On the other hand, newly synthesized porin[931,932] molecules of Neurospora bind to the MOM19 master receptor, from which they must be transferred to the general insertion site (MOM38) before entering the phospholipid bilayer of the outer membrane.

The MAS70 outer membrane receptor of yeast mitochondria contains an N-terminal, noncleavable, targeting signal. The first 12 residues of this protein, when linked to another polypeptide, were capable of targeting the chimera to the mitochondrial matrix.[893] The outer membrane localization of MAS70, however, is determined by a hydrophobic segment that immediately follows the targeting signal and exerts its function by halting transfer of the polypeptide across the outer membrane, preventing its insertion into the inner membrane, as depicted in Fig. 16-38*B*. When the hydrophobic segment was shortened or deleted, the resulting modified polypeptide was translocated into the matrix.[897,976]

An unusual mechanism seems to explain the incorporation of bovine monoamine oxidase B into the outer mitochondrial membrane. For insertion, this protein must first be coupled in an ATP-dependent reaction to ubiquitin,[977] a 76-amino-acid polypeptide that is generally linked to lysine residues in proteins to mark the proteins for degradation.[978]

Import of Proteins into the Intermembrane Space (Fig. 16-38*C* to 16-38*F*). Several different routes are used to transport newly synthesized polypeptides to the intermembrane space. The import of apocytochrome *c* occurs by a unique pathway.[979] It does not require a protease-sensitive surface receptor,[922] ATP, or a transmembrane potential. This protein, which lacks a cleavable signal,[901] inserts directly into the phospholipid bilayer[980] of the outer membrane. Its sequestration in the intermembrane space is a consequence of its covalent linkage to heme, catalyzed by cytochrome *c* heme lyase.[924,981,982] When heme addition is blocked, translocation of apocytochrome *c* is arrested with the polypeptide spanning the outer membrane so that a portion remains exposed to proteases on the mitochondrial surface, while another is tightly bound to the heme lyase in the intermembrane space.[926] The heme lyase itself, which also lacks a cleavable signal, follows a second import pathway that requires neither ATP hydrolysis nor an energized inner membrane, but involves the general import machinery of the outer membrane that includes the MOM19–MOM38 receptor complex.[951]

An indirect third route to reach the intermembrane space is followed by some proteins of the inner membrane, such as the iron/sulfur protein of the cytochrome bc_1 complex[983] and, probably, subunit IV of cytochrome oxidase.[914] The precursors of these proteins are first transported to the mitochondrial matrix, where their matrix targeting presequences are removed by the two-step cleavage process that involves two different matrix proteases. The presequences do not contain distinct submitochondrial localization signals, and the mature proteins do not become integrated into the phospholipid bilayer of the inner membrane, but rather assemble directly into the multisubunit complexes of that membrane in which they function. In an unknown manner, this assembly leads to their traversal of the inner membrane and their appearance in the intermembrane space. When cleavage of their presequences is inhibited by chelating agents, these proteins accumulate in the matrix.[983]

Other proteins that are free in the intermembrane space (such as cytochrome *c* peroxidase[984] and cytochrome b_2[985,986]) or are attached to the outer face of the inner membrane (such as cytochrome c_1[987]) are synthesized with long bipartite cleavable presequences that contain distinct targeting and localization signals.[894] These presequences are cleaved off in two steps.[988–990] The first is carried out by the matrix metalloprotease, which removes the N-terminal matrix targeting signal. The second cleavage, which removes the localization signal, is carried out by an enzyme (called inner membrane protease 1) that is located on the outer face of the inner membrane and, in contrast to the matrix protease, is resistant to chelating agents.[989,991,992] The localization signals within the presequences of these proteins consist of approximately 20-amino-acid-long hydrophobic segments flanked by basic residues.[985–987]

Two alternative possibilities (Fig. 16-38*C* to 16-38*F*) for the mode of action of the localization signals in cytochromes b_2 and *c* have been proposed. Supporting evidence, often directly contradictory, has been provided for both mechanisms.[877,880] In one view (Fig. 16-38*D* and 16-38*F*), the hydrophobic segment in the localization signal acts as a cleavable halt-transfer signal that stops translocation of the polypeptide as it traverses the inner membrane.[892,895] In the other view (Fig. 16-38*C* and 16-38*E*), after the polypeptide is translocated into the matrix and the matrix targeting signal is removed, the localization signal serves as a cleavable insertion signal (equivalent to the signal sequence of eukaryotic secretory proteins or to the leader peptide of bacterial secretory proteins) that initiates re-export of the polypeptide from the matrix to the intermembrane space.[993] The latter mechanism has been designated a "conservative sorting mechanism"[994] because the re-export step is analogous to the export of proteins from bacteria, which are believed to be the evolutionary ancestors of mitochondria. The two alternative mechanisms are both consistent with the observation that the incorporation of cytochrome b_2 into the intermembrane space takes place in two stages.[988,989] The first, leading to cleavage of the targeting signal by the matrix protease, requires an electrochemical gradient across the inner membrane. The second, which leads to discharge into the intermembrane space and proteolytic removal of the remainder of the presequences on the outer face of the inner membrane, does not require an energized inner membrane. Proponents of both views agree that during the uptake of cytochromes b_2 and c_1 into mitochondria, intermediate precursors are generated that are anchored in the inner membrane by the hydrophobic segments within the localization signals, but are largely exposed on the intermembrane space.[988,989] From these precursors, the released mature proteins are generated by the second cleavage. In the case of cytochrome b_2 (Fig. 16-38*C* and 16-38*D*) and the cytochrome *c* peroxidase, the mature proteins remain free in the intermembrane space. On the other hand, cytochrome c_1 (Fig. 16-38*E* and 16-38*F*) becomes associated with the outer face of the inner membrane, probably via the insertion of a second hydrophobic segment near its C-terminus.[987,995]

The conflicting evidence supporting both models relates to whether (1) the intermediate forms of cytochromes b_2 and c_1 that still contain their localization signals but have lost their matrix targeting signals are at any time found soluble within the mitochondrial matrix; (2) the hsp60 matrix chaperonin that binds to polypeptides that enter the matrix is required for the proteins to achieve their normal disposition in the intermembrane space, as judged by the cleavage of their localization signals; and (3) cleavage of the localization signal can still take place in the absence of intramitochondrial ATP, which would be expected to prevent translocation of the polypeptide into the matrix.

Sorting of Proteins to the Inner Mitochondrial Membrane. The inner mitochondrial membrane contains several large hetero-oligomeric protein complexes that carry out electron transport (complexes I to IV) and ATP synthesis (complex V or ATP synthase, or F_1F_0 ATPase), as well as an ATP-ADP translocator. Some of the polypeptide subunits of these complexes are encoded in the mitochondrial genome. For example, in human cells, 7 of the 39 polypeptides of complex I (NADH: ubiquinone oxido-reductase), 1 (cytochrome *b*) of the 10 in complex III, 3 of the 13 in complex IV (cytochrome oxidase), and 2 of the 12 polypeptides of the ATP synthase are synthesized by ribosomes in the mitochondrial matrix and directly incorporated into the membrane, where they assemble with the other subunits. There is at least one species difference. Subunit 9 of the ATPase is encoded in the mitochondrial genome in yeast, but is encoded in the nucleus in Neurospora and human cells.

From a biogenetic perspective, proteins peripherally associated with the inner face of the inner mitochondrial membrane, such as the β subunit of the F_1F_0 ATPase, can be regarded as matrix proteins. After undergoing cleavage of their presequences, these polypeptides become part of multimeric complexes that include subunits that are integral components of the inner membrane. Some of these integral membrane polypeptides are synthesized in mitochondrial ribosomes and are directly inserted into the membrane, in which they are anchored by their hydrophobic segments. However, several integral membrane polypeptides of the inner membrane that contain transmembrane hydrophobic segments are synthesized in cytoplasmic ribosomes. This is the case with the ADP-ATP translocator[902] and with subunit 9 of the F_0 ATPase.[996,997] In Neurospora the latter protein undergoes complete translocation into the matrix, before insertion into the inner membrane as an integral membrane protein.[994] On the other hand, the ADP-ATP translocator — which is the major polypeptide of the inner membrane, in which it is anchored by three membrane-spanning helixes[998] — is synthesized without a cleavable presequence,[902] and is never discharged into the matrix. Rather, after binding to the MOM72/MAS70 outer membrane receptor and being transferred to the general import site, the ATP-ADP translocator appears to enter the phospholipid bilayer of the inner membrane directly. This polypeptide is directed to the mitochondria by a segment that is not at its extreme N-terminus. Thus, chimeric polypeptides containing the first 111 (but not just the first 72) residues of the yeast translocator linked to β-galactosidase bind to the outer membrane MAS70 receptor and are incorporated into the organelle in an ATP-dependent process, becoming resistant to exogenous proteases.[902,999] The chimeric polypeptide with the first 111 (N-terminal) residues of the translocator precursor, however, does not become incorporated to the inner membrane in a form that is resistant to alkali extraction. This requires the presence of downstream helical portions of the protein and occurs only in the presence of an energized inner membrane.[956,999,1000] As expected for insertion of a protein that does not enter the matrix, intramitochondrial ATP and the hsp60 chaperonin are not required for the insertion of the ATP-ADP carrier into the inner membrane.

BIOGENESIS OF PEROXISOMES[1001-1010a]

Peroxisomes are small membrane-bound organelles that are present in all eukaryotic cells (see Chap. 129). They carry out oxidative reactions that generate hydrogen peroxide and contain the hemoprotein enzyme catalase, which breaks down this reactive product (see ref. 1001). The set of oxidative enzymes present in mammalian peroxisomes varies with the species and the tissue source. In addition to the enzymes that carry out β-oxidation of fatty acids (see below), they include D-amino acid oxidase, urate oxidase, oxalate oxidase, L-α-hydroxyacid oxidases, and other oxidases with specific substrates. Peroxisomal catalase may catalyze the direct decomposition of H_2O_2, to generate H_2O and O_2 from two molecules of H_2O_2, or act peroxidatically, if appropriate substrates for oxidation, such as methanol, ethanol, formate, and nitrites are available. It has been estimated[1001] that approximately 20 percent of the oxygen consumed by rat liver is used for peroxisomal respiration.

Peroxisomes were first recognized on EM as small dense bodies (microbodies) surrounded by a single membrane and containing a dense granular matrix. They are easily identified histochemically by virtue of the peroxidative activity of catalase which, during incubation with diaminobenzidine, generates an electron-dense, polymerized product. Histochemical use of this reaction demonstrated that all cells contain small peroxisomes (0.1 to 0.2 μm; microperoxisomes) and that only some cell types, such as hepatocytes and kidney tubule cells, contain large peroxisomes.[1011,1012] In many species, peroxisomes are also characterized morphologically by a crystalline core that is composed of the enzyme urate oxidase (uricase). This enzyme, which functions in the purine degradative pathway to oxidize uric acid to allantoin, is not present in humans and in other higher primates.

Although peroxisomes appear as round, ovoid, pear-, or dumbbell-shaped individual bodies in thin tissue sections examined by transmission EM, three-dimensional reconstructions from serial sections indicate that many peroxisomes are interconnected to form an extended network.[1013] The variable appearance of this *peroxisomal reticulum*[1014] suggests that it is a dynamic structure that undergoes constant remodeling involving membrane fusion and fission events.

Peroxisomes and lysosomes have similar sedimentation properties. In early cell fractionation studies, they were recovered together in what was designated a "light mitochondrial fraction." In later work it was possible to separate the two organelles by injecting the animals shortly before sacrifice with the detergent Triton WX-1339. This is taken into lysosomes, which become significantly lighter and can be separated from peroxisomes by isopycnic centrifugation.[1015] More recently, methods using sedimentation in metrizamide gradients have yielded highly purified peroxisomes from the livers of untreated animals.[1016,1017] Such fractions have allowed rigorous biochemical characterization of the organelle, as well as in vitro studies on its biogenesis.

Both mitochondria and peroxisomes play important roles in the metabolism of fatty acids that are taken into the cell or released from the triglycerides that are stored in cytoplasmic fat droplets. The degradation of fatty acids takes place by β-oxidation, which requires their prior activation by an acyl CoA synthetase and involves the successive removal of acetyl groups from their carboxyl ends. It is believed that the peroxisomal β-oxidation system is responsible for the oxidation of very long chain fatty acids (VLCFA) and that the shortened products generated from VLCFA in the peroxisome may be efficiently degraded in mitochondria. Acyl CoA synthetases that accept long chain fatty acids are associated with the cytoplasmic face of mitochondria, the ER, and peroxisomes. Enzymes that utilize VLCFA, such as C24:0 and C26:0, are also present in peroxisomes and in the ER, but have not been found in mitochondria.[1018,1019] The acyl CoA synthetase that activates VLCFA in peroxisomes, but not that in the ER, has been found to be deficient in *X-linked adrenoleukodystrophy*, a condition in which VLCFA accumulate in tissues and plasma[1020,1021] (see Chap. 131). The mechanism by which acyl CoA esters are transported across the peroxisomal membrane has not been elucidated. High levels of the peroxisomal β-oxidation system are induced by various hypolipidemic agents, such as clofibrate,[1022] that also lead to an increase in the number of peroxisomes.[1023]

The mitochondrial and peroxisomal β-oxidation systems carry out similar biochemical reactions but employ different enzymatic components.[1022,1024] The peroxisomal system consists of three enzymes that carry out four distinct reactions (see refs. 1008 and 1025). The first reaction is catalyzed by *acyl CoA oxidase*, an FAD-containing enzyme that uses molecular oxygen and generates H_2O_2 as a product. The second and third reactions in peroxisomal β-oxidation are carried out by a single *bifunctional protein* that has enoyl CoA hydratase and β-hydroxyacyl CoA dehydrogenase activities. The final reaction involves the cleavage of 3-ketoacyl CoA by *3-ketoacyl CoA thiolase* to yield acetyl CoA and a saturated acyl CoA that has two fewer carbons than the original substrate.

Rat liver peroxisomes appear to contain two acyl CoA oxidases[1026] and two 3-ketoacyl CoA thiolases,[1027] and only one of each of these is inducible by clofibrate. The two acyl oxidases are apparently encoded in mRNAs generated by differential splicing from the primary transcript of the same gene,[1026] but it has been shown that the two thiolases are derived from two different genes.[1027] A carnitine acyltransferase is contained in peroxisomes that may generate carnitine esters from the acetyl, propionyl, and other acyl CoA products of β-oxidation that are to be transferred to the mitochondria.[1028]

Important steps in the synthesis of bile acids also take place in peroxisomes (see ref. 1029). These organelles carry out the conversion, by β-oxidation, of 3-α, 7-α, 12-α-trihydroxy-5β-cholestanoic acid (THCA) into cholic acid and of 3-α, 7-α, dihydroxy-5β-cholestanoic acid into chenodeoxycholic acid.[1030,1031] The role of peroxisomal enzymes in bile acid synthesis accounts for the accumulation of THCA and various of its polar metabolites in the serum and bile of patients with *Zellweger syndrome* (see below), a genetic disease in which morphologically distinct peroxisomes are absent in hepatocytes[1032] (see Chap. 129).

Peroxisomes also contain enzymes of the acyl-dihydroxyacetone phosphate (DHAP) pathway (DHAP acyltransferase, alkyl-DHAP synthase, and acyl/alkyl-DHAP oxidoreductase) that catalyze the initial steps in the biosynthesis of glycerol-ether lipids (plasmalogens) (see refs. 1008 and 1033). Both the β-oxidation enzymes[1034,1035] and the glycerol-ether lipid biosynthetic enzymes[1036] are markedly diminished in patients with the Zellweger syndrome, consistent with the notion that peroxisomes represent the primary site of plasmalogen synthesis.

The enzyme alanine : glyoxylate aminotransferase (AGT), that catalyzes the conversion of glyoxylate into glycine, which can then be utilized in gluconeogenesis, is present in human liver only within peroxisomes. The absence of this peroxisomal enzyme leads to the overproduction of oxalate from glyoxylate that characterizes primary hyperoxaluria type I[1037] (see Chap. 133). In certain tissues of other animals AGT is present exclusively in mitochondria, or in both mitochondria and peroxisomes. It is striking that in rat liver the mitochondrial and peroxisomal forms of AGT are encoded by mRNA molecules transcribed from different initiation sites of the same gene,[1038] and that in humans a mutation in the AGT gene has been identified that leads to the mistargeting of the enzyme to mitochondria.[1039,1040] It was proposed that a polymorphism for this gene normally exists in the human population so that in some individuals the mitochondrial targeting signal is present in the protein but is not functional because it is overridden by the presence of the peroxisomal targeting signal in the same polypeptide. A mutation that abolishes the latter signal would then lead to mistargeting to the mitochondria.

The intriguing finding has been made by immunoelectron microscopy and cell fractionation that HMG-CoA reductase, the key enzyme of the cholesterol biosynthetic pathway whose major site of function is in the ER membrane, is also present, albeit in an unglycosylated state, in the peroxisomal matrix.[1041,1042] Moreover, it has been reported that the specific activity of HMG-CoA reductase in the peroxisomal fraction increases markedly after the administration of cholestyramine, a treatment that also raises the levels of the microsomal enzyme, albeit to a lesser extent. A mechanism that addresses some HMG-CoA molecules to peroxisomes would require either elimination of their signal for cotranslational insertion in the ER or an abrogation of its function.

Synthesis of Peroxisomal Proteins and Their Incorporation into the Organelle

It is now well established that both matrix proteins and integral proteins of the peroxisomal membrane are synthesized in free polysomes, discharged into the cytosol, and incorporated posttranslationally into the organelle. Early in vivo studies on the biosynthesis of rat liver catalase first demonstrated that, immediately after synthesis, catalase polypeptides[1043,1044] appear in the cytosol and are only subsequently taken up into the peroxisomes, without passage through the ER. Incorporation of the heme and tetramerization of the polypeptide into the mature form of the hemoprotein were shown to take place after uptake into the organelle.[1044] Subsequently, it was demonstrated directly that several enzymes of the peroxisomal matrix, including urate oxidase,[1045] catalase,[1045] and the three proteins involved in β-oxidation,[1046–1048] are synthesized on free polysomes (see Chap. 129).

The posttranslational incorporation into isolated peroxisomes of catalase and fatty acyl CoA oxidase synthesized in mRNA-dependent cell-free systems has been reconstituted in vitro, and found not to proceed at 0°C and to require cytosol and ATP hydrolysis.[1049] A peroxisomal integral membrane protein (22 kDa) of unknown function has also been synthesized in vitro and shown to assemble into the peroxisomal membrane posttranslationally, as indicated by its pattern of resistance to exogenous proteases.[1050] The uptake of the matrix proteins into mammalian peroxisomes could be dissected into two stages: binding of the protein to the surface of the organelle, which takes place at 0°C and does not consume energy; and transport across the membrane, which occurs at 37°C and requires ATP.[1051] The translocation step did not appear to be driven by a transmembrane potential, since it proceeded in the presence of proton ionophores, such as CCCP. On the other hand, studies with the methylotropic yeast *Candida boidinii* (see below) suggested that in this organism the translocation step requires a transmembrane potential, since it was inhibited by CCCP.[1052] This ionophore, however, is known to cause a depletion of cellular ATP through its action on mitochondria.

It appears that two main mechanisms, involving two different types of peroxisomal targeting signals (PTS), effect the uptake of proteins into the peroxisomal matrix. With few exceptions (see below) the import of peroxisomal enzymes into the organelle is not accompanied by the removal of cleavable presequences. Indeed, the major mechanism for uptake into peroxisomes of the polypeptides released from free polysomes involves the recognition of a C-terminal tripeptide, which can serve as a PTS in organisms as evolutionarily diverse as fungi, plants, insects, and mammals. It was first shown[1053] that luciferase, the firefly enzyme which is normally present in the lantern organ of the insect, is incorporated into peroxisomes when synthesized in transfected cultured monkey kidney cells. This demonstrated the extraordinary degree of evolutionary conservation of the mechanism that effects the sorting of peroxisomal proteins. A study of the distribution of chimeric constructs containing portions of the luciferase polypeptide linked to reporter polypeptides[1054] revealed that a C-terminal segment of luciferase, comprising the last 12 amino acids, was sufficient to ensure targeting to peroxisomes. Similarly, C-terminal segments of human catalase, D-amino acid oxidase, rat acyl CoA oxidase, and the bifunctional rat enoyl CoA-hydratase-β-OH-acyl CoA dehydrogenase served as peroxisomal targeting signals when linked to the C-termini of nonperoxisomal reporter proteins.[1055,1056] All these proteins contain the conserved C-terminal tripeptide sequences SKL or SHL, and site-directed mutagenesis studies demonstrated that the consensus tripeptide motif (Ser/Ala/Cys)-(Lys/Arg/His)-Leu could function as a targeting signal.[1057] It appears that this PTS tripeptide must be present at the extreme C-terminus of the polypeptide, since the addition of even one or two C-terminal residues to a polypeptide containing it eliminated its activity. On the other hand, in human catalase a C-terminal 27-amino-acid segment that contains an internal SHL sequence could serve as a targeting signal when linked to a reporter protein.[1055]

Immunoblot analysis suggests that many peroxisomal proteins contain the SKL sequence. A specific antibody for this tripeptide recognized a substantial fraction of the protein bands representing the set of peroxisomal proteins.[1057a] The sorting capacity of the exposed SKL signal has been dramatically demonstrated by the observation that serum albumin, when crosslinked to a short synthetic peptide containing the SKL sequence and microinjected into cells, localizes to peroxisomes. Moreover, it was found that co-injection of a synthetic peptide containing the SKL signal with luciferase suppresses the incorporation of this protein into peroxisomes,[1057b] suggesting that the import system is saturable.

The second mechanism for peroxisomal import involves the recognition of an N-terminal signal that is cleaved off within the organelle. Signals of this type are present in the two very closely related forms of the peroxisomal 3-ketoacyl CoA thiolase. The newly synthesized thiolases contain either 36-(thiolase A) or 26-(thiolase B) amino-acid-long cleavable segments, which differ only in the presence of 10 extra amino acids at the N-terminus of thiolase A. In the case of thiolase B, the first 11 amino acids were shown to be sufficient for peroxisomal targeting. It seems likely that the same segment serves as the targeting signal in thiolase A,[1058] even though it is not present at the extreme N-terminus. As will be discussed below, analysis of the import of peroxisomal proteins in cells from patients with generalized peroxisomal defects, as well as with a variety of yeast mutants, has established that the two types of signals present in peroxisomal proteins are decoded by different molecular machineries. Further studies with Zellweger fibroblasts indicate that cleavage of the N-terminal signals in the thiolase is not required for peroxisomal uptake of this enzyme.

Another peroxisomal matrix protein, the *nonspecific lipid transport protein* (nsLTP), also known as *sterol carrier protein* 2, or SCP-2, is also synthesized with a cleavable N-terminal sequence, but this segment of the polypeptide (20 amino acids) may not be necessary for import into the organelle since the protein also contains a C-terminal targeting tripeptide.[1059] The acyl CoA oxidase that carries out the first step in β-oxidation also undergoes cleavage within the peroxisome, but the two segments produced remain associated in the mature enzyme.[1060]

More than 10 proteins have been identified as specific components of the peroxisomal membrane in several species (see refs. 1008 and 1009). These include the acyl CoA synthetase (76-kDa) exposed on the cytoplasmic face of the membrane, a 69-/70-kDa ATP-binding protein that may be involved in transport across the membrane, and a pore-forming protein (22 kDa). The sequences of five peroxisomal membrane proteins have been determined from cDNA clones and only one of them, which is a methanol-induced protein (pmp20) of *Candida boidinii*, contains the C-terminal peroxisomal targeting signal.[1061] None of the membrane proteins so far identified is glycosylated. Direct evidence has been obtained that three of the major membrane proteins are synthesized in free polysomes and do not undergo posttranslational proteolytic processing.[1062–1064]

Several genetic diseases have been recognized in which the biogenesis of the peroxisome is impaired (see Chap. 129). In some conditions, such as the *Zellweger cerebrohepatorenal syndrome, neonatal adrenoleukodystrophy, infantile Refsum disease*, and *hyperpipecolic acidemia*, known as generalized peroxisomal disorders (see refs. 1065 and 1066), normal peroxisomes appear to be absent or markedly reduced in number, and the patients show metabolic defects in all the major biosynthetic peroxisomal pathways. In particular, they fail to synthesize ether lipids, do not β-oxidize very long chain fatty acids, and accumulate bile acid precursors. The generalized disorders are likely to be manifestations of single defects in peroxisomal components that are essential for normal assembly of the organelle. Thus, fibroblasts from patients with Zellweger syndrome, or with the infantile form of Refsum disease, appear to synthesize peroxisomal enzymes at normal rates, but many of them undergo rapid degradation. Some matrix enzymes, such as catalase, D-amino acid oxidase, L-α-hydroxyacid oxidase, and alanine:glyoxylate amino transferase (AGT), have been found to be localized in the cytosol of Zellweger cells rather than in membrane-bound structures.[1034]

Immunocytochemical and immunoblot analysis using antibodies against several different proteins of the peroxisomal membrane have shown that fibroblasts from Zellweger patients contain abnormal membrane structures of low isopycnic density, which were designated "peroxisomal ghosts."[1067–1069] The ghosts contain uncleaved precursors of the 3-keto-acyl CoA thiolase[1035,1070,1071] and acyl CoA oxidase, as well as residual DHAP acyltransferase activity (DHAPAT).[1071] Thus, Zellweger fibroblasts appear to be capable of assembling a peroxisomal membrane but to be defective in a component of the machinery that effects the import of some, but not all, proteins of the peroxisomal matrix. As a result, the development of the organelle is incomplete. Since the uptake of the thiolase precursor into the peroxisome is mediated by a mechanism that recognizes an N-terminal signal in the protein and not by the more common one that recognizes a C-terminal SKL tripeptide, one can surmise that the Zellweger defect is in a specific component required only to import proteins with the C-terminal targeting signal. This conclusion is supported by the observation that contrary to the case with normal fibroblasts, albumin molecules crosslinked to the tripeptide signal, when microinjected into Zellweger fibroblasts, fail to localize to peroxisomes.[1057b] The fact that in Zellweger fibroblasts the thiolase and the acyl CoA oxidase were taken up but not cleaved[1071] further suggests that the processing protease(s) is itself incorporated into the peroxisome by the mechanism that recognizes the tripeptide C-terminal signal. Further evidence that the import machineries that recognize C- or N-terminal signals operate independently of each other was provided by the isolation of yeast mutants in which, of all tested peroxisomal enzymes, only the thiolase was not imported and by the finding that this defect could not be corrected by introducing into the cells the thiolase wild-type gene.[1072]

Extensive complementation analysis carried out by pairwise fusion of cultured fibroblasts from Zellweger, infantile Refsum disease, or neonatal adrenoleukodystrophy patients followed by measurements of the reappearance of peroxisomal functions has defined eight complementation groups,[1073,1074] demonstrating that mutations in as many different genes can all result in generalized peroxisomal defects. It was also shown that in the heterokaryons resulting from the fusions, previously mistargeted matrix enzymes were rapidly incorporated into preexisting peroxisomal ghosts.

A somatic-cell genetics approach has also been used to generate, identify, and characterize mutants defective in peroxisomal assembly with characteristics similar to Zellweger fibroblasts from permanent Chinese hamster ovary cell (CHO) lines.[1075,1076] The gene affected in one mutant was identified after transfection with a normal rat cDNA expression library, and the cDNA that corrected the defect found to encode a 35-kDa polypeptide of the peroxisomal membrane that was designated *peroxisomal assembly factor 1 (PAF1)*.[1077] This cDNA, as well as its human homologue, were shown to be also capable of correcting the peroxisomal biogenesis defect in fibroblasts from a particular Zellweger patient.[1078]

In other peroxisomal defects, such as acatalasemia,[1079] X-linked adrenoleukodystrophy,[1080] and hyperoxaluria type I,[1037] specific mutations lead to deficiencies in single enzymatic activities, but peroxisomes are present and appear normal in other functions. Although the pseudo-Zellweger or Zellweger-like syndrome[1081] displays some of the biochemical defects of Zellweger syndrome, this condition appears to result from a deficiency in 3-ketoacyl thiolase. In these patients, plasmalogen synthesis is normal but both long chain fatty acids and intermediates in bile acid synthesis accumulate, indicating that a single metabolic step involving the thiolase is common to both pathways.[1082]

Studies on peroxisome biogenesis in yeast, in which the synthesis of peroxisomal enzymes can be induced under conditions that also markedly increase the number of peroxisomes, have been particularly informative. Thus, in *C. boidinii*, peroxisomes are hardly detectable when the cells are grown on glucose. However, within 15 h after they are transferred to a medium containing methanol they occupy 20 to 80 percent of the cytoplasmic volume.[1083] This induction leads to a marked accumulation of peroxisomal enzymes and particularly of two enzymes involved in the early steps of methanol metabolism—alcohol oxidase,[1084] a homo-octamer flavin-containing enzyme, and dihydroxyacetone synthase.[1085] Peroxisomal function is also required for growth of *S. cereviseae* on fatty acids which induce peroxisomal proliferation, such as oleate. Screening for *S. cereviseae* mutants unable to grow on oleate led to the isolation of mutants defective in peroxisomal assembly (*pas mutants*).[1072] The mutants fall into 18 complementation groups. Of the many PAS genes cloned, one (PAS1) encodes a hydrophobic protein that contains two consensus sequences for ATP binding and shows striking sequence similarity to the *Sec*18 gene product, which is the yeast homologue of the mammalian NSF, a protein required for many vesicle fusion events that take place during vesicular transport along the endomembrane pathway (see above). Of the other PAS genes, PAS2 appears to be related to the ubiquitin conjugating enzymes, and PAS3 appears to be an integral membrane protein of undetermined subcellular distribution. The complete characterization of the PAS mutants and the identification of the corresponding mammalian orthologous genes is bound to provide a much better understanding of the complex process of peroxisome biogenesis.

Future studies on peroxisome biogenesis are likely to focus on the mechanism for the uptake of proteins into the organelle and on the identification of receptors, transporters, and soluble factors, including chaperonins, that participate in this process.

REFERENCES

1. Steinman RM, Mellman I, Muller WA, Cohn ZA: Endocytosis and the recycling of plasma membrane. *J Cell Biol* **96**:1, 1983.
2. Singer SJ: The fluid mosaic model of membrane structure, in Abrahamsson S, Pascher I (eds): *Structure of Biological Membranes*. New York, Plenum, 1976, p 443.
3. Singer SJ: The structure and insertion of integral proteins in membranes. *Annu Rev Cell Biol* **6**:247, 1990.
4. Van Meer G: Lipid traffic in animal cells. *Annu Rev Cell Biol* **5**:247, 1989.
5. Ullrich A, Coussens L, Hayflick JS, Dull TJ, Gray A, Tam AW, Lee J, Yarden Y, Libermann TA, Schlessinger J, Downward J, Mayes ELV, Whittle N, Waterfield MD, Seeburg PH: Human epidermal growth factor receptor cDNA sequence and aberrant expression of the amplified gene in A431 epidermoid carcinoma cells. *Nature* **309**:418, 1984.
6. Downward J, Yarden Y, Mayes E, Scrace G, Totty N, Stockwell P, Ullrich A, Schlessinger J, Waterfield MD: Close similarity of epidermal growth factor receptor and v-erb B oncogene protein sequences. *Nature* **307**:521, 1984.
7. Gill GN, Bertics PJ, Santon JB: Epidermal growth factor and its receptor. *Mol Cell Endocrinol* **51**:169, 1987.
8. Ullrich A, Bell JR, Chen EY, Herrera R, Petruzzelli LM, Dull TJ, Gray A, Coussens L, Liao Y-C, Tsubokawa M, Mason A, Seeburg PH, Grunfeld C, Rosen OM, Ramachandran J: Human insulin receptor and its relationship to the tyrosine kinase family of oncogenes. *Nature* **313**:756, 1985.
9. Ebina Y, Ellis L, Jarnagin K, Edery M, Graf L, Clauser E, Ou J-H, Masiarz F, Kan YW, Goldfine ID, Roth RA, Rutter WJ: The human insulin receptor cDNA: The structural basis for hormone-activated transmembrane signalling. *Cell* **40**:747, 1985.
10. Rosen OM: After insulin binds. *Science* **237**:1452, 1987.
11. Blobel G: Intracellular protein topogenesis. *Proc Natl Acad Sci U S A* **77**:1496, 1980.
12. Sabatini DD, Kreibich G, Morimoto T, Adesnik M: Mechanisms for incorporation of proteins in membranes and organelles. *J Cell Biol* **92**:1, 1982.
13. Rapoport TA: Transport of proteins across the endoplasmic reticulum membrane. *Science* **258**:91, 1992.
14. Steer CJ, Hanover JA (eds): *Intracellular Traffic of Proteins*. London, Cambridge University Press, 1991.
15. Loh YP (ed): *Mechanisms of Intracellular Trafficking and Processing of Proproteins*. Boca Raton, FL, CRC Press, 1993.
16. Ellis JR, Van Der Vies SM: Molecular chaperones. *Annu Rev Biochem* **60**:321, 1991.
17. Hartl FU, Martin J: Protein folding in the cell: The role of molecular chaperones Hsp70 and Hsp60. *Annu Rev Biophys Biomol Struct* **21**:293, 1992.
18. Pryer NK, Wuestehube LJ, Schekman R: Vesicle-mediated protein sorting. *Annu Rev Biochem* **61**:471, 1992.

18a. Franzusoff A: Beauty and the yeast: Compartmental organization of the secretory pathway. *Semin Cell Biol* **3**:309, 1992.

19. Haubruck H, Prange R, Vorgias C, Gallwitz D: The ras-related mouse ypt1 protein can functionally replace the YPT1 gene product in yeast. *EMBO J* **8**:1427, 1989.
20. Wilson DW, Wilcox CA, Flynn GC, Chen E, Huang WJ, Henzel WJ, Block MR, Ullrich A, Rothman JE: Fusion protein required for vesicle-mediated transport in both mammalian cells and yeast. *Nature* **339**:355, 1989.
21. Gilman AG: G proteins: Transducers of receptor-generated signals. *Annu Rev Biochem* **56**:615, 1987.
22. Kaziro Y, Itoh H, Hozasa T, Nakafuka M, Saton T: Structure and function of signal-transducing GTP-binding proteins. *Annu Rev Biochem* **60**:349, 1991.
23. Bourne HR, Sanders DA, McCormick F: The GTPase superfamily: Conserved structure and molecular mechanism. *Nature* **349**:117, 1991.
24. Bourne HR: Do GTPases direct membrane traffic in secretion? *Cell* **53**:669, 1988.
25. Goud B, McCaffrey M: Small GTP-binding proteins and their role in transport. *Curr Opin Cell Biol* **3**:626, 1991.
26. Gruenberg J, Clague MJ: Regulation of intracellular membrane transport. *Curr Opin Cell Biol* **4**:593, 1992.

26a. Balch WE: Small GTP-binding proteins in vesicular transport. *Trends Biochem Sci* **15**:473, 1990.

26b. Pfeffer SR: GTP-binding proteins in intracellular transport. *Trends Cell Biol* **2**:41, 1992.

27. Zerial M, Stenmark H: Rab GTPases in vesicular transport. *Curr Opin Cell Biol* **5**:613, 1993.
28. Thompson RC: EFTu provides an internal kinetic standard for translational accuracy. *TIBS* **13**:91, 1988.
29. Gelfand VI, Bershadsky AD: Microtubules dynamics: Mechanism, regulation, and function. *Annu Rev Cell Biol* **7**:93, 1991.
30. Gilmore R: The protein translocation apparatus of the rough endoplasmic reticulum, its associated proteins, and the mechanism of translocation. *Curr Opin Cell Biol* **3**:580, 1991.
31. Nunnari J, Walter P: Protein targeting to and translocation across the membrane of the endoplasmic reticulum. *Curr Opin Cell Biol* **4**:573, 1992.
32. Stryer L, Bourne HR: G proteins: A family of signal transducers. *Annu Rev Cell Biol* **2**:391, 1986.
33. Barr FA, Leyte A, Huttner WB: Trimeric G proteins and vesicle formation. *Trends Cell Biol* **2**:91, 1992.
34. Balch WE: From G minor to G major. Tantalizing evidence is accumulating that trimeric G proteins play a much greater part than expected in signaling vesicle transport in endocytic and exocytic secretory pathways. *Curr Biol* **2**:157, 1992.
35. Gravotta D, Adesnik M, Sabatini DD: Transport of influenza HA from the trans-Golgi network to the apical surface of MDCK cells permeabilized in their basolateral plasma membranes: Energy dependence and involvement of GTP-binding proteins. *J Cell Biol* **111**:2893, 1990.
36. Kahn RA, Der CJ, Bokoch GM: The *ras* superfamily of GTP-binding proteins: Guidelines on nomenclature. *FASEB J* **6**:2512, 1992.
37. Chavrier P, Gorvel J-P, Stelzer E, Simons K, Gruenberg J, Zerial M: Hypervariable C-terminal domain of rab proteins acts as a targeting signal. *Nature* **353**:769, 1991.

38. Barbacid M: *ras* genes. *Annu Rev Biochem* **56**:779, 1987.
39. Chow M, Der CJ, Buss JE: Structure and biological effects of lipid modifications on proteins. *Curr Opin Cell Biol* **4**:629, 1992.
40. Khosravi-Far R, Lutz RJ, Cox AD, Conroy L, Bourne JR, Sinensky M, Balch WE, Buss JE, Der CJ: Isoprenoid modification of rab proteins terminating in CC or CSC motifs. *Proc Natl Acad Sci U S A* **88**:6264, 1991.
41. Kinsella BT, Maltese WA: rab GTP-binding proteins with three different carboxyl-terminal cysteine motifs are modified in vivo by 20-carbon isoprenoids. *J Biol Chem* **267**:3940, 1992.
42. Seabra MC, Golstein JL, Sudhof TC, Brown MS: Rab geranylgeranyl transferase. *J Biol Chem* **267**:14497, 1992.
43. Newman CMH, Giannakouros T, Hancock JF, Fawell EH, Armstrong J, Magee AI: Post-translational processing of Schizosaccharomyces pombe YPT proteins. *J Biol Chem* **267**:11329, 1992.
44. Kahn RA, Goddard C, Newkirk M: Chemical and immunological characterization of the 21-kDa ADP-ribosylation factor of adenylation cyclase. *J Biol Chem* **263**:8282, 1988.
45. Kahn RA, Kern FG, Clark J, Gelmann EP, Rulka C: Human ADP-ribosylation factors: A functionally conserved family of GTP-binding proteins. *J Biol Chem* **266**:2606, 1991.
46. Burstein ES, Linko-Stentz K, Lu Z, Macara IG: Regulation of the GTPase activity of the ras-like protein $p25^{rab3A}$. *J Biol Chem* **266**:2689, 1991.
47. Kaibuchi K, Mizuno T, Fujioka H, Yamamoto T, Kishi K, Fukumoto Y, Hori Y, Takai Y: Molecular cloning of the cDNA for stimulatory GDP/GTP exchange protein for smg p21s (ras p21-like small GTP-binding proteins) and characterization of stimulatory GDP/GTP exchange protein. *Mol Cell Biol* **11**:2873, 1991.
48. Moya M, Roberts D, Novick P: DSS4-1 is a dominant suppressor of *sec*4–8 that encodes a nucleotide exchange protein that aids *Sec*4p function. *Nature* **361**:460, 1993.
49. Burton J, Roberts D, Montaldi M, Novick P, De Camilli P: A mammalian guanine-nucleotide-releasing protein enhances function of yeast secretory protein Sec4. *Nature* **361**:464, 1993.
50. Arki S, Kikuchi A, Hata Y, Isomura M, Takai Y: Regulation of reversible binding of *smg*p25A, a ras p21-like GTP-binding protein, to synaptic plasma membranes and vesicles by its specific regulatory protein, GDP dissociation inhibitor. *J Biol Chem* **265**:13007, 1990.
51. Sasaki T, Kikuchi A, Araki S, Hata Y, Isomura M, Kuroda S, Takai Y: Purification and characterization from bovine brain cytosol of a protein that inhibits the dissociation of GDP from and the subsequent binding of GTP to *smg* p25A, a ras p21-like GTP-binding protein. *J Biol Chem* **265**:2333, 1990.
52. Kahn RA: Fluoride is not an activator of the smaller (20–25 kDa) GTP-binding proteins. *J Biol Chem* **266**:15595, 1991.
53. Ross EM: Signal sorting and amplification through G protein-coupled receptors. *Neuron* **3**:141, 1989.
54. Weingarten R, Ransnäs L, Mueller H, Sklar LA, Bokoch GM: Mastoparan interacts with the carboxy terminus of the a subunit of Gi. *J Biol Chem* **265**:11044, 1990.
55. Kahn RA, Gilman AG: The protein cofactor necessary for ADP-ribosylation of G_s by cholera toxin is itself a GTP binding. *J Biol Chem* **261**:7906, 1986.
56. Palade G: Intracellular aspects of the process of protein synthesis. *Science* **189**:347, 1975.
57. Rapoport TA: Protein transport across the endoplasmic reticulum membrane: Facts, models, mysteries. *FASEB J* **5**:2792, 1991.
58. Walter P, Lingappa VR: Mechanism of protein translocation across the endoplasmic reticulum membrane. *Annu Rev Cell Biol* **2**:499, 1986.
59. Skach WR, Lingappa VR: Intracellular trafficking of pre-(pro) proteins across RER membranes, in Loh YP (ed): *Mechanisms of Intracellular Trafficking and Processing of Proproteins*. Boca Raton, FL, CRC Press, 1993, p 19.
60. Sabatini DD, Tashiro Y, Palade GE: On the attachment of ribosomes to microsomal membranes. *J Mol Biol* **19**:503, 1966.
61. Kreibich G, Debey P, Sabatini DD: Selective release of content from microsomal vesicles without membrane disassembly. I. Permeability changes induced by low detergent concentrations. *J Cell Biol* **58**:436, 1973.
62. Kreibich G, Sabatini DD: Selective release of content from microsomal vesicles without membrane disassembly. II. Electrophoretic and immunological characterization of microsomal subfractions. *J Cell Biol* **61**:789, 1974.
63. Kreibich G, Ulrich BL, Sabatini DD: Proteins of rough microsomal membranes related to ribosome binding. I. Identification of ribophorins I and II, membrane proteins characteristic of rough microsomes. *J Cell Biol* **77**:464, 1978.
64. Kreibich G, Freienstein CM, Pereyra BN, Ulrich BL, Sabatini DD: Proteins of rough microsomal membranes related to ribosome binding. II. Cross-linking of bound ribosomes to the specific membrane proteins exposed at the binding sites. *J Cell Biol* **77**:488, 1978.
65. Hortsch M, Meyer DI: Immunochemical analysis of rough and smooth microsomes from rat liver. Segregation of docking protein in rough membranes. *Eur J Biochem* **150**:559, 1985.
66. Lewis JA, Sabatini DD: Accessibility of proteins in rat liver-free and membrane-bound ribosomes to lactoperoxidase-catalyzed iodination. *J Biol Chem* **252**:5547, 1977.
67. Lewis JA, Sabatini DD: Proteins of rat liver free and membrane-bound ribosomes: Modification of two large subunit proteins by a factor detached from ribosomes at high ionic strength. *Biochim Biophys Acta* **478**:33, 1977.
68. Borgese D, Blobel G, Sabatini DD: In vitro exchange of ribosomal subunits between free and membrane-bound ribosomes. *J Mol Biol* **74**:415, 1973.
69. Blobel G, Sabatini DD: Ribosome-membrane interaction in eukaryotic cells, in Manson LA (ed): *Biomembranes*. New York, Plenum, 1971, vol 2, p 193.
70. Milstein C, Brownlee GG, Harrison TM, Mathews MB: A possible precursor of immunoglobulin light chains. *Nature New Biol* **239**:117, 1972.
71. Swan D, Aviv H, Leder P: Purification and properties of biologically active messenger RNA for a myeloma light chain. *Proc Natl Acad Sci U S A* **69**:1967, 1972.
72. Schechter I: Biologically and chemically pure mRNA coding for a mouse immunoglobulin L-chain prepared with the aid of antibodies and immobilized oligothymidine. *Proc Natl Acad Sci U S A* **70**:2256, 1973.
73. Blobel G, Dobberstein B: Transfer of proteins across membranes. I. Presence of proteolytically processed and unprocessed nascent immunoglobulin light chains on membrane-bound ribosomes of murine myeloma. *J Cell Biol* **67**:835, 1975.
74. Blobel G, Dobberstein B: Transfer of proteins across membranes. II. Reconstitution of functional rought microsomes from heterologous components. *J Cell Biol* **67**:852, 1975.
75. Perlman D, Halvorson HO: A putative signal peptidase recognition site and sequence in eukaryotic and prokaryotic signal peptides. *J Mol Biol* **167**:391, 1983.
76. Von Heijne G: Signal sequences: The limits of variation. *J Mol Biol* **184**:99, 1985.
77. Von Heijne G: Towards a comparative anatomy of N-terminal topogenic protein sequences. *J Mol Biol* **189**:239, 1986.
78. Watson MEE: Compilation of published signal sequences. *Nucleic Acids Res* **12**:5145, 1984.
79. Redman CM, Sabatini DD: Vectorial discharge of peptides released by puromycin from attached ribosomes. *Proc Natl Acad Sci U S A* **56**:608, 1966.
80. Malkin LI, Rich A: Partial resistance of nascent polypeptide chains to proteolytic digestion due to ribosomal shielding. *J Mol Biol* **26**:329, 1967.
81. Blobel G, Sabatini DD: Controlled proteolysis of nascent polypeptides in rat liver cell fractions. I. Location of the polypeptides within ribosomes. *J Cell Biol* **45**:130, 1970.
82. Warren G, Dobberstein B: Protein transfer across microsomal membranes reassembled from separated membrane components. *Nature* **273**:569, 1978.
83. Walter P, Blobel G: Purification of a membrane-associated protein complex required for protein translocation across the endoplasmic reticulum. *Proc Natl Acad Sci U S A* **77**:7112, 1980.
84. Walter P, Ibrahimi I, Blobel G: Translocation of proteins across the endoplasmic reticulum. I. Signal recognition protein (SRP) binds to in vitro assembled polysomes synthesizing secretory proteins. *J Cell Biol* **91**:545, 1981.
85. Walter P, Blobel G: Translocation of proteins across the endoplasmic reticulum. II. Signal recognition protein (SRP) mediates the selected binding to microsomal membranes of in-vitro-assembled polysomes synthesizing secretory proteins. *J Cell Biol* **91**:551, 1981.
86. Walter P, Blobel G: Translocation of proteins across the endoplasmic reticulum. III. Signal recognition protein (SRP) causes signal sequence-dependent and site-specific arrest of chain elongation that is released by microsomal membranes. *J Cell Biol* **91**:557, 1981.

87. Gilmore R, Blobel G, Walter P: Protein translocation across the endoplasmic reticulum. I. Detection in the microsomal membrane of a receptor for a signal recognition particle. *J Cell Biol* **95**:463, 1982.
88. Gilmore R, Walter P, Blobel G: Protein translocation across the endoplasmic reticulum. II. Isolation and characterization of the signal recognition particle receptor. *J Cell Biol* **95**:477, 1982.
89. Walter P, Gilmore R, Blobel G: Protein translocation across the endoplasmic reticulum. *Cell* **38**:5, 1984.
90. Meyer DI, Dobberstein B: Identification and characterization of a membrane component essential for the translocation of proteins across the membrane of the endoplasmic reticulum. *J Cell Biol* **87**:503, 1980.
91. Meyer DI, Dobberstein B: A membrane component essential for vectorial translocation of nascent proteins across the endoplasmic reticulum: Requirements for its extraction and reassociation with the membrane. *J Cell Biol* **87**:498, 1980.
92. Meyer DI, Krause E, Dobberstein B: Secretory protein translocation across membranes—The role of the "Docking Protein." *Nature* **297**:647, 1982.
93. Meyer DI, Louvard D, Dobberstein B: Characterization of molecules involved in protein translocation using specific antibodies. *J Cell Biol* **92**:579, 1982.
94. Borgese N, Mok W, Kreibich G, Sabatini DD: Ribosomal-membrane interaction: In vitro binding of ribosomes to microsomal membranes. *J Mol Biol* **88**:559, 1974.
95. Gilmore R, Blobel G: Transient involvement of signal recognition particle and its receptor in the microsomal membrane prior to protein translocation. *Cell* **35**:677, 1983.
96. Wiedman M, Kurzchalia TV, Hartmann E, Rapoport TA: A signal sequence receptor in the endoplasmic reticulum membrane. *Nature* **328**:830, 1987.
97. Krieg UC, Johnson AE, Walter P: Protein translocation across the endoplasmic reticulum membrane: Identification by photocross-linking of a 39-kD integral membrane glycoprotein as part of a putative translocation tunnel. *J Cell Biol* **109**:2033, 1989.
98. Kellaris KV, Bowen S, Gilmore R: ER translocation intermediates are adjacent to a nonglycosylated 34-kD integral membrane protein. *J Cell Biol* **114**:21, 1991.
99. Thrift RN, Andrews DW, Walter P, Johnson AE: A nascent membrane protein is located adjacent to ER membrane proteins throughout its integration and translation. *J Cell Biol* **112**:809, 1991.
100. Gorlich D, Hartmann E, Prehn S, Rapoport TA: A protein of the endoplasmic reticulum involved early in polypeptide translocation. *Nature* **357**:47, 1992.
101. Sabatini DD, Blobel G: Controlled proteolysis of nascent polypeptides in rat liver cell fractions II. Location of the polypeptides in rough microsomes. *J Cell Biol* **45**:146, 1970.
102. Gilmore R, Blobel G: Translocation of secretory proteins across the microsomal membrane occurs through an environment accessible to aqueous perturbants. *Cell* **42**:497, 1985.
103. Simon SM, Blobel G: A protein-conducting channel in the endoplasmic reticulum. *Cell* **65**:371, 1991.
104. Simon SM, Blobel G: Signal peptides open protein-conducting channels in *E. coli*. *Cell* **69**:677, 1992.
105. Von Heijne G, Blomberg C: Trans-membrane translocation of proteins (the direct transfer model). *Eur J Biochem* **97**:175, 1973.
106. Engelman DM, Steitz TA: The spontaneous insertion of proteins into and across membranes: The helical hairpin hypothesis. *Cell* **23**:411, 1981.
107. Fleischer S, Fleischer B (eds): Membrane biogenesis: Assembly and targeting. *Methods Enzymol* **96**:1, 1983.
108. Scheele G: Methods for the study of protein translocation across the RER membrane using the reticulocyte lysate translation system and canine pancreatic microsomal membranes. *Methods Enzymol* **96**:94, 1983.
109. Von Heijne G: How signal sequences maintain cleavage specificity. *J Mol Biol* **173**:243, 1984.
110. Von Heijne G: Structural and thermodynamic aspects of the transfer of proteins into and across membranes, in Knauf PA, Cook JS (eds): *Current Topics in Membranes and Transport*. New York, Academic Press, 1985, vol 24, p 151.
111. Von Heijne G: A new method for predicting signal sequence cleavage sites. *Nucleic Acids Res* **14**:4683, 1986.
112. Kaiser CA, Preuss D, Grisafi P, Botstein D: Many random sequences functionally replace the secretion signal sequence of yeast invertase. *Science* **235**:312, 1987.
113. Szczesna-Skorupa E, Mead DA, Kemper B: Mutations in the NH_2-terminal domain of the signal peptide of preproparathyroid hormone inhibit translocation without affecting interaction with signal recognition particle. *J Biol Chem* **262**:8896, 1987.
114. Inouye M, Halegoua S: Secretion and membrane localization of proteins in *Escherichia coli*. *CRC Crit Rev Biochem* **7**:339, 1980.
115. Inouye S, Soberon X, Franceschini T, Nakamura K, Itakura K, Inouye M: Role of positive charge on the amino-terminal region of the signal peptide in protein secretion across the membrane. *Proc Natl Acad Sci U S A* **79**:3438, 1982.
116. Shaw AS, Rottier PJM, Rose JK: Evidence for the loop model of signal-sequence insertion into the endoplasmic reticulum. *Proc Natl Acad Sci U S A* **85**:7592, 1988.
117. Von Heijne G: Patterns of amino acids near signal sequence cleavage sites. *Eur J Biochem* **133**:17, 1983.
118. Wiren KM, Freeman MW, Potts JT Jr, Kronenberg HM: Preproparathryoid hormone: A model for analyzing the secretory pathway. *Recent Prog Horm Res* **42**:641, 1986.
119. Emr SD, Silhavy TJ: Molecular components of the signal sequences that function in the initiation of protein export. *J Cell Biol* **95**:689, 1982.
120. Bedouelle H, Bassford PJ Jr, Fowler AV, Zabin I, Beckwith J, Hofnung M: Mutations which alter the function of the signal of the maltose binding protein *Escherichia coli*. *Nature* **285**:78, 1980.
121. Meek RL, Walsh K, Palmiter RD: The signal sequence of ovalbumin is located near the NH_2-terminus. *J Biol Chem* **257**:12245, 1982.
122. Tabe L, Krieg P, Strachan R, Jackson D, Wallis E, Colman A: Segregation of mutant ovalbumins and ovalbumin-globin fusion proteins in Xenopus oocytes. Identification of an ovalbumin signal sequence. *J Mol Biol* **180**:645, 1984.
123. Bonatti S, Blobel G: Absence of a cleavable signal sequence in Sindbis virus glycoproteins PE2. *J Biol Chem* **254**:12261, 1979.
124. Garoff H, Frischauf AM, Simons K, Lehrach H, Delius H: Nucleotide sequence of cDNA coding for Semliki Forest Virus membrane glycoproteins. *Nature* **288**:236, 1980.
125. Garoff H: Using recombinant DNA techniques to study protein targeting in the eucaryotic cell. *Annu Rev Cell Biol* **1**:403, 1983.
126. Walter P, Blobel G: Subcellular distribution of signal recognition particle and 7SL-RNA determined with polypeptide-specific antibodies and complementary DNA probe. *J Cell Biol* **97**:1693, 1983.
127. Walter P, Blobel G: Signal recognition particles contains 7S RNA essential for protein translocation across the endoplasmic reticulum. *Nature* **299**:691, 1982.
128. Gundelfinger ED, Krause E, Melli M, Dobberstein B: The organization of the 7SL RNA in the signal recognition particle. *Nucleic Acids Res* **11**:7363, 1983.
129. Walter P, Blobel G: Disassembly and reconstitution of signal recognition particle. *Cell* **34**:525, 1983.
130. Siegel V, Walter P: Elongation arrest is not a prerequisite for secretory protein translocation across the microsomal membrane. *J Cell Biol* **100**:1913, 1985.
131. Siegel V, Walter P: Each of the activities of signal recognition particle (SRP) is contained within a distinct domain: Analysis of biochemical mutants of SRP. *Cell* **52**:39, 1988.
132. Wiedmann M, Kurzchalia TV, Bielka H, Rapoport TA: Direct probing of the interaction between the signal sequence of nascent preprolactin and the signal recognition particle by specific cross-linking. *J Cell Biol* **104**:201, 1987.
132a. Berstein HD, Poritz MA, Strub K, Hoben PJ, Brenner S, Walter P: Model for signal sequence recognition from amino-acid sequence of 54K subunit of signal recognition particle. *Nature* **340**:482, 1989.
132b. Zopf D, Bernstein HD, Johnson AE, Walter P: The methionine-rich domain of the 54kd protein subunit of the signal recognition particle contains an RNA binding site and can be crosslinked to a signal sequence. *EMBO J* **9**:4511, 1990.
132c. High S, Dobberstein B: The signal sequence interacts with the methionine-rich domain of the 54-kD protein of signal recognition particle. *J Cell Biol* **113**:229, 1991.
133. Lutcke H, High S, Romisch H, Ashford AJ, Dobberstein B: The methionine-rich domain of the 54 kDa subunit of signal recognition particle is sufficient for the interaction with signal sequence. *EMBO J* **11**:1543, 1992.
133a. Hann BC, Walter P: The signal recognition particle in S. cerevisiae. *Cell* **67**:131, 1991.
134. Amaya Y, Nakano A, Ito K, Mori M: Isolation of a yeast gene, SRH1 that encodes a homologue of the 54K subunit of mammalian signal recognition particle. *J Biochem* **107**:457, 1990.

135. Ogg SC, Poritz MA, Walter P: Signal recognition particle receptor is important for cell growth and protein secretion in Saccharomyces cerevisiae. *Mol Cell Biol* **3**:895, 1992.
136. Hansen W, Garcia PD, Walter P: In vitro protein translocation across the yeast endoplasmic reticulum: ATP-dependent post-translational translocation of the prepro-a factor. *Cell* **45**:397, 1986.
137. Rothblatt JA, Meyer DI: Secretion in yeast: Translocation and glycosylation of prepro-a factor in vitro can occur via ATP-dependent post-translational mechanism. *EMBO J* **5**:1031, 1986.
138. Rothblatt JA, Deshaies RJ, Sanders SJ, Daum G, Schekman R: Multiple genes are required for proper insertion of secretory proteins into the endoplasmic reticulum in yeast. *J Cell Biol* **72**:61, 1989.
139. Deshaies RJ, Koch BD, Werner WM, Craig EA, Schekman R: A subfamily of stress proteins facilitates translocation of secretory and mitochondrial precursor polypeptides. *Nature* **332**:800, 1988.
140. Chirico WJ, Waters MG, Blobel G: 70K heat shock related proteins stimulate protein translocation into microsomes. *Nature* **332**:805, 1988.
141. Lindquist S, Craig EA: The heat-shock proteins. *Annu Rev Genet* **22**:631, 1988.
142. Sanders SL, Whitfield KM, Vogel JP, Ross MD, Schekman RW: *Sec*61p and BiP directly facilitate polypeptide translocation into the ER. *Cell* **69**:353, 1992.
143. Vogel JP, Misra LM, Rose MD: Loss of Bip/GRP78 function blocks translocation of secretory proteins in yeast. *J Cell Biol* **110**:1885,1990.
144. Bole DG, Hendershot LM, Kearney JF: Posttranslational association of immunoglobulin heavy chain binding protein with nascent heavy chains in nonsecreting and secreting hybridomas. *J Cell Biol* **102**:1558, 1986.
145. Gething MJ, Sambrook J: Transport and assembly processes in the endoplasmic reticulum. *Semin Cell Biol* **1**:65, 1990.
146. Tajima S, Lauffer L, Rath VL, Walter P: The signal recognition particle receptor is a complex that contains two distinct polypeptide chains. *J Cell Biol* **103**:1167, 1986.
147. Lauffer L, Garcia PD, Harkins RN, Coussens L, Ullrich A, Walter P: Topology of signal recognition particle receptor in endoplasmic reticulum membrane. *Nature* **318**:334, 1985.
148. Connolly T, Collins P, Gilmore R: The signal recognition particle receptor mediates the GTP-dependent displacement of SRP from the signal sequence of the nascent polypeptides. *Cell* **57**:599, 1989.
149. Connolly T, Rapiejko PJ, Gilmore R: Requirement of GTP hydrolysis for dissociation of the signal recognition particle from its receptor. *Science* **252**:1171, 1991.
150. Rapiejko PJ, Gilmore R: Protein translocation across the ER requires a functional GTP binding site in the alpha subunit of the signal recognition particle receptor. *J Cell Biol* **117**:493, 1992.
151. Migliaccio G, Nicchitta CV, Blobel G: The signal sequence receptor, unlike the signal recognition particle receptor, is not essential for protein translocation. *J Cell Biol* **117**:15, 1992.
152. Deshaies RJ, Sanders BL, Feldheim DA, Schekman R: Assembly of yeast Sec proteins involved in translocation into the endoplasmic reticulum into a membrane-bound multisubunit complex. *Nature* **349**:806, 1991.
153. Musch A, Wiedmann M, Rapport TA: Yeast Sec proteins interact with polypeptides traversing the endoplasmic reticulum membrane. *Cell* **69**:343, 1992.
154. Görlich D, Prehn S, Hartmann E, Kalies K-U, Rapoport TA: A mammalian homolog of SEC61p and SECYp is associated with ribosomes and nascent polypeptides during translocation. *Cell* **71**:489, 1992.
155. Brundage L, Hendrick JP, Schiebel E, Driessen AJM, Wickner W: The purified E. coli integral membrane protein SecY/E is sufficient for reconstitution of Sec/A-dependent precursor protein translocation. *Cell* **62**:649, 1990.
156. Green N, Fang H, Walter P: Mutants in three novel complementation groups inhibit membrane protein insertion into and soluble protein translocation across the endoplasmic reticulum membrane of Saccharomyces cerevisiae. *J Cell Biol* **116**:597, 1992.
157. Jackson RC, Blobel G: Post-translational cleavage of presecretory proteins with an extract of rough microsomes from dog pancreas containing signal peptidase activity. *Proc Natl Acad Sci U S A* **74**:5598, 1977.
158. Rothman JE, Lodish HF: Synchronized transmembrane insertion and glycosylation of a nascent membrane protein. *Nature* **269**:775, 1977.
159. Jackson RC, White WR: Phospholipid is required for the processing of presecretory proteins by detergent-solubilized canine pancreatic signal peptidase. *J Biol Chem* **256**:2545, 1981.
160. Mumford RA, Strauss AW, Powers JC, Pierzchala PA, Nishino N, Zimmerman M: A zinc metalloendopeptidase associated with dog pancreatic membranes. *J Cell Biol* **255**:2227, 1980.
161. Walter P, Jackson RC, Marcus MM, Lingappa VR, Blobel G: Tryptic dissection and reconstitution of translocation activity for nascent presecretory proteins across microsomal membranes. *Proc Natl Acad Sci U S A* **76**:1795, 1979.
162. Evans EA, Gilmore R, Blobel G: Purification of the microsomal signal peptidase as a complex. *Proc Natl Acad Sci U S A* **83**:581, 1986.
163. Shelness GS, Blobel G: Two subunits of the canine signal peptidase complex are homologous to yeast Sec11 protein. *J Biol Chem* **265**:9512, 1990.
164. Yadeau JT, Klein C, Blobel B: Yeast signal peptidase contains a glycoprotein and the *Sec11* gene product. *Proc Natl Acad Sci U S A* **88**:517, 1991.
165. Bohni PC, Deshaies J, Schekman RW: SECII is required for signal peptide processing and yeast cell growth. *J Cell Biol* **106**:1035, 1988.
166. Adelman MR, Sabatini DD, Blobel G: Ribosome-membrane interaction: Non-destructive disassembly of rat liver rough microsomes into ribosomal and microsomal components. *J Cell Biol* **56**:206, 1973.
167. Sabatini DD, Ojakian G, Lande MA, Lewis J, Mok W, Adesnik M, Kreibich G: Structural and functional aspects of the protein synthesizing apparatus in the rough endoplasmic reticulum, in Meints RS, Davies E (eds): *Control Mechanisms in Development*. New York, Plenum, 1975, p 151.
168. Kreibich G, Bar-Nun S, Czako-Graham M, Mok W, Nack E, Okada Y, Rosenfeld MG, Sabatini DD: The role of free and membrane-bound polysomes in organelle biogenesis, in Bucher T, Sebald W, Weiss H (eds): *Biological Chemistry of Organelle Formation*. 31, Colloquium der Gesellschaft fur Biologische Chemie 14-19, Mosbach/Baden, Berlin, Springer-Verlag, 1980, p 147.
169. Amar-Costesec A, Todd JA, Kreibich G: Segregation of the polypeptide translocation apparatus to regions of the endoplasmic reticulum containing ribophorins and ribosomes. I. Functional tests on rat liver microsomal subfractions. *J Cell Biol* **99**:2247, 1984.
170. Kreibich G, Marcantonio EE, Sabatini DD: Ribophorins I and II: Membrane proteins characteristic of the rough endoplasmic reticulum. *Methods Enzymol* **96**:520, 1983.
171. Harnik-Ort V, Prakash K, Colman DR, Rosenfeld MG, Adesnik M, Sabatini DD, Kreibich G: Isolation and characterization of cDNA clones for rat ribophorin I: Complete coding sequence and in vitro synthesis and insertion of the encoded product into endoplasmic reticulum membranes. *J Cell Biol* **104**:885, 1987.
172. Crimaudo C, Hortsch M, Gausepohl H, Meyer DI: Human ribophorins I and II: The primary structure and membrane topology of two highly conserved rough endoplasmic reticulum-specific glycoproteins. *EMBO J* **6**:75, 1987.
173. Todd JA, Sabatini DD, Kreibich G: An 83 Kd polypeptide is a component of the protein translocation apparatus of the rough endoplasmic reticulum. *J Cell Biol* **99**:2a, 1984.
174. Hortsch M, Avossa D, Meyer DI: Characterization of secretory protein translocation: Ribosome-membrane interaction in endoplasmic reticulum. *J Cell Biol* **103**:241, 1986.
175. Yoshida M, Tondokoro N, Asano Y, Mirusawa K, Yamagishi R, Morigome T, Sugano H: Studies on membrane proteins involved in ribosome binding on the rough endoplasmic reticulum. Ribophorins have no ribosome-binding activity. *Biochem J* **245**:611, 1987.
176. Kelleher EJ, Kreibich G, Gilmore R: Oligosaccharyltransferase activity is associated with a protein complex composed of ribophorins I and II and a 48 kd protein. *Cell* **69**:55, 1992.
177. Tazawa S, Unuma M, Tondokoro N, Asano Y, Ohsumi T, Ichimura T, Sugano H: Identification of a membrane protein responsible for ribosome binding in rought microsomal membranes. *J Biochem* **1099**:89, 1991.
178. Savitz AJ, Meyer DI: Identification of a ribosome receptor in the rough endoplasmic reticulum. *Nature* **346**:540, 1990.
179. Rapoport TA: Protein translocation across and integration into membranes. *CRC Crit Rev Biochem* **20**:73, 1986.
180. Wickner WT, Lodish HF: Multiple mechanisms of protein insertion into and across membranes. *Science* **230**:400, 1985.

181. Alt FW, Bothwell ALM, Knapp M, Siden E, Mather E, Koshland M, Baltimore D: Synthesis of secreted and membrane-bound immunoglobulin Mu heavy chains is directed by mRNAs that differ at their 3′ ends. *Cell* **20**:293, 1980.
182. Rogers J, Early P, Carter C, Calame K, Bond M, Hood K, Wall R: Two mRNAs with different 3′ ends encode membrane-bound and secreted forms of immunoglobulin Mu chain. *Cell* **20**:303, 1980.
183. Early P, Rogers J, Davis M, Calame K, Bond M, Wall R, Hood L: Two mRNAs can be produced from a single immunoglobulin u gene by alternative RNA processing pathways. *Cell* **20**:313, 1980.
184. Gething M-J, Sambrook J: Construction of influenza haemagglutinin genes that code for intracellular and secreted forms of the protein. *Nature* **300**:598, 1982.
185. Rose JK, Bergmann JE: Expression from cloned cDNA of cell-surface secreted forms of the glycoprotein of vesicular stomatitis virus in eucaryotic cells. *Cell* **30**:753, 1982.
186. Rizzolo LJ, Finidori J, Gonzalez A, Arpin M, Ivanov IE, Adesnik M, Sabatini DD: Biosynthesis and intracellular sorting of growth hormone-viral envelope glycoprotein hybrids. *J Cell Biol* **101**:1351, 1985.
187. Adams GA, Rose JK: Incorporation of a charged amino acid into the membrane-spanning domain blocks cell-surface transport but not membrane anchoring of a viral glycoprotein. *Mol Cell Biol* **5**:14442, 1985.
188. Cutler DF, Garoff H: Mutants of the membrane-binding region of Semliki Forest Virus E2 protein. I. Cell surface transport and fusogenic activity. *J Cell Biol* **102**:889, 1986.
189. Cutler DF, Melancon P, Garoff H: Mutants of the membrane-binding region of Semliki Forest Virus E2 protein. II. Topology and membrane binding. *J Cell Biol* **102**:902, 1986.
190. Zuniga MC, Hood LE: Clonal variation in cell surface display of an H-2 protein lacking a cytoplasmic tail. *J Cell Biol* **102**:1, 1986.
191. Spiess M, Lodish HF: An internal signal sequence: The aisaloglycoprotein receptor membrane anchor. *Cell* **44**:177, 1986.
192. Schneider C, Owen MJ, Banville D, Williams JG: Primary structure of human transferrin receptor deduced from the mRNA sequence. *Nature* **311**:675, 1984.
193. Zerial M, Melancon P, Schneider C, Garoff H: The transmembrane segment of the human transferrin receptor functions as a signal peptide. *EMBO J* **5**:1543, 1986.
194. Hunziker W, Spiess M, Semenza G, Lodish HF: The sucrase-isomaltase complex: Primary structure, membrane-orientation, and evolution of a stalked, intrinsic brush border protein. *Cell* **46**:227, 1986.
195. Blok J, Ear GM, Laver WG, Ward CW, Lilley GG, Woods EF, Roxburgh CM, Inglis AS: Studies on the size, chemical composition and partial sequence of the neuraminidase (NA) from type A influenza virus shows that the N-terminal region of the NA is not processed and serves to anchor the NA in the viral membrane. *Virology* **119**:109, 1982.
196. Fields SG, Winter G, Brownlee GG: Structure of the neuraminidase gene in human influenza virus. *Nature* **290**:213, 1981.
197. Bos TJ, Davis AR, Nayak DP: NH2-terminal hydrophobic region of influenza virus neuraminidase provides the signal function in translocation. *Proc Natl Acad Sci U S A* **81**:2327, 1984.
198. Mize NK, Andrews DW, Lingappa VR: A stop transfer sequence recognizes receptors for nascent chain translocation across the endoplasmic reticulum membrane. *Cell* **47**:711, 1986.
199. Zerial M, Huylebroeck D, Garoff H: Foreign transmembrane peptides replacing the internal signal sequence of transferrin receptor allow its translocation and membrane binding. *Cell* **48**:147, 1987.
200. Wessells HP, Spiess M: Insertion of a multispanning membrane protein occurs sequentially and requires only one signal sequence. *Cell* **55**:61, 1988.
201. Finidori J, Rizzolo L, Gonzalez A, Kreibch G, Adesnik M, Sabatini DD: The influenza haemagglutinin insertion signal is not cleaved and does not halt translocation when presented to the endoplasmic reticulum membrane as part of a translocating polypeptide. *J Cell Biol* **104**:1705, 1987.
202. Nathans J, Hogness DS: Isolation, sequence analysis, and intron-exon arrangement of the gene encoding bovine rhodopsin. *Cell* **34**:807, 1983.
203. Dixon RAF, Kobilka BK, Strader DJ, Benovic JL, Dohlman HG, Frielle T, Bolanowski MA, Bennett CD, Rands E, Diehl RE, Mumford RA, Slater EE, Sigal IS, Caron MG, Lefkowitz RJ, Strader CD: Cloning of the gene and cDNA for mammalian β-adrenergic receptor and homology with rhodopsin. *Nature* **321**:75, 1986.
204. Yarden Y, Rodriguez H, Wong SK-F, Brandt DR, May DC, Burnier J, Harkins RN, Chen EY, Ramachandran J, Ullrich A, Ross EM: The avian β-adrenergic receptor: Primary structure and membrane topology. *Proc Natl Acad Sci U S A* **83**:6795, 1986.
205. Lamb RA, Zebedee S, Richardson CD: Influenza virus M2 protein is an integral membrane protein expressed on the infected-cell surface. *Cell* **40**:627, 1985.
206. Parks GD, Lamb RA: Topology of eukaryotic type II membrane proteins: Importance of N-terminal positively charged residues flanking the hydrophobic domain. *Cell* **64**:777, 1991.
207. Friedlander M, Blobel G: Bovine opsin has more than one signal sequence. *Nature* **318**:338, 1985.
208. Audigier Y, Friedlander M, Blobel G: Multiple topogenic sequences in bovine opsin. *Proc Natl Acad Sci U S A* **84**:5783, 1987.
208a. Hartmann E, Rapoport TA, Lodish HF: Predicting the orientation of eukaryotic membrane spanning proteins. *Proc Natl Acad Sci U S A* **86**:5786, 1989.
209. Parks GD, Hull D, Lamb RA: Transposition of domains between the M2 and HN viral membrane proteins results in polypeptides which can adopt more than one membrane orientation. *J Cell Biol* **109**:2023, 1989.
210. Sakaguchi M, Mihara K, Sato R: A short amino-terminal segment of microsomal cytochrome P-450 functions both as an insertion signal and as a stop transfer sequence. *EMBO J* **6**:2425, 1987.
211. Monier S, Van Luc P, Kreibich G, Sabatini DD, Adesnik M: Signals for the incorporation and orientation of cytochrome P450 in the ER membrane. *J Cell Biol* **107**:457, 1988.
212. Porter TD, Kasper CB: Coding nucleotide sequence of rat NADPH-cytochrome P-450 oxidoreductase cDNA and identification of flavin-binding domains. *Proc Natl Acad Sci U S A* **82**:973, 1985.
213. Szczesna-Skorupa E, Browne N, Mead D, Kemper B: Positive charges at the NH_2 terminus convert the membrane-anchor signal peptide of cytochrome P-450 to a secretory signal peptide. *Proc Natl Acad Sci U S A* **85**:738, 1988.
214. Sato T, Sakaguchi M, Mihara K, Omura T: The amino-terminal structures that determine topological orientation of cytochrome P-450 in microsomal membrane. *EMBO J* **9**:2391, 1990.
215. Lennarz WJ (ed): *Biochemistry of Glycoproteins and Proteoglycans*. New York, Plenum, 1980.
216. Hubbard SC, Ivatt RJ: Synthesis and processing of asparagine-linked oligosaccharides. *Annu Rev Biochem* **50**:555, 1981.
217. Kornfeld R, Kornfeld S: Assembly of asparagine-linked oligosaccharides. *Annu Rev Biochem* **54**:664, 1985.
218. Hirschberg CB, Snider MD: Topography of glycosylation in the rough endoplasmic reticulum and Golgi apparatus. *Annu Rev Biochem* **56**:63, 1987.
219. Abeijon C, Hirschberg CB: Topography of glycosylation reactions in the endoplasmic reticulum. *TIBS* **17**:32, 1992.
219a. Hart GW: Glycosylation. *Curr Opin Cell Biol* 4:1017, 1992.
220. Marshall RD: The nature and metabolism of the carbohydrate-peptide linkages of glycoproteins. *Biochem Soc Symp* **40**:17, 1974.
221. Struck DK, Lennarz WJ: The function of saccharide-lipids in synthesis of glycoproteins, in Lennarz W (ed): *The Biochemistry of Glcyoproteins and Proteoglycans*. New York, Plenum, 1980, p 35.
222. Kronquist KE, Lennarz WJ: Enzymatic conversions of proteins to glycoproteins by lipid-linked saccharides: A study of potential exogenous acceptor proteins. *J Supramol Struct* **8**:51, 1978.
223. Atkinson PH, Lee JT: Co-translational excision of alpha-glucose and alpha-mannose in nascent vesicular stomatitis virus G protein. *J Cell Biol* **98**:2245, 1984.
224. Rosenfeld MG, Marcantonio EE, Hakimi J, Ort VM, Atkinson PH, Sabatini DD, Kreibich G: Biosynthesis and processing of ribophorins in the endoplasmic reticulum. *J Cell Biol* **99**:1076, 1984.
225. Liscum L, Cummings RD, Anderson RG, Demartino GN, Goldstein JL, Brown MS: 3-Hydroxy-3-methyglutaryl-CoA reductase: A transmembrane glycoprotein of the endoplasmic reticulum with N-linked "high-mannose" oligosaccharides. *Proc Natl Acad Sci U S A* **80**:7165, 1983.
226. Tarentino AL, Maley F: Purification and properties of an endo-β-N-acetylglucosaminidase from Streptomyces griseus. *J Biol Chem* **249**:811, 1974.
227. Tarentino AL, Plummer TH, Maley F: The release of intact oligosaccharides form specific glycoproteins by endo-β-N-acetylglucosaminidase H. *J Biol Chem* **249**:818, 1974.
228. Muramatsu T, Atkinson PH, Nathenson SG, Ceccarini C: Cell-surface glycopeptides: Growth-dependent changes in the carbohydrate-peptide linkage region. *J Mol Biol* **80**:781, 1973.

229. Mizuochi T, Amano J, Kobata A: New evidence of the substrate specificity of endo-β1-N-acetylglucosamindase D. *J Biochem (Tokyo)* **95**:1209, 1984.
230. Plummer TH, Elder JH, Alexander S, Phelan AW, Tarnetino AL: Demonstration of peptide: N-glycosidase F activity in endo-β-N-acetylglucosaminidase F preparations. *J Biol Chem* **259**:10700, 1984.
231. Pelham HRB: Control of protein exit from the endoplasmic reticulum. *Annu Rev Cell Biol* **5**:1, 1989.
232. Pelham HRB: Recycling of proteins between the endoplasmic reticulum and Golgi complex. *Curr Opin Cell Biol* **3**:585, 1991.
233. Lusis AG, Paigen K: Mechanisms involved in the intracellular localization of mouse glucuronidase, in Ratazzi MC, Scandelius JG, Whitt JS (eds): *Isozymes: Current Topics in Biological and Medical Research.* New York, Alan R. Liss, 1977, vol 2, p 63.
234. Swank RT, Paigen K: Biochemical and genetic evidence for a macromolecular β-glucuronidase complex in microsomal membranes. *J Mol Biol* **77**:371, 1973.
235. Medda S, Stevens AM, Swank RT: Involvement of the esterase active site of egasyn in compartmentalization of β-glucuronidase within the endoplasmic reticulum. *Cell* **50**:301, 1987.
236. Medda S, Takeuchi K, Devore-Cartes D, Von Deimling O, Heymann E, Swank RT: An accessory protein identical to mouse egasyn is complexed with rat microsomal β-glucuronidase and is identical to rat esterase-3. *J Biol Chem* **262**:7248, 1987.
237. Wiedmann M, Huth A, Rapoport TA: Xenopus oocytes can secrete bacterial beta-lactamase. *Nature* **309**:637, 1984.
238. Semenza JC, Hardwick KG, Dean N, Pelham HRB: ERD2, a yeast gene required for the receptor-mediated retrieval of luminal ER proteins from the secretory pathway. *Cell* **61**:1349, 1990.
239. Lewis MJ, Sweet DJ, Pelham HR: The ERD2 gene determines the specificity of the luminal ER protein retention system. *Cell* **61**:1359, 1990.
240. Lewis MJ, Pelham HR: Ligand-induced redistribution of a human KDEL receptor from the Golgi complex to the endoplasmic reticulum. *Cell* **68**:353, 1992.
241. Munro S, Pelham HRB: An hsp70-like protein in the ER: Identity with the 78 kD glucose-regulated protein and immunoglobulin heavy chain-binding protein. *Cell* **46**:291, 1986.
242. Munro S, Pelham HRB: A C-terminal signal prevents secretion of luminal ER proteins. *Cell* **48**:899, 1987.
243. Pelham HRB: Evidence that luminal ER proteins are sorted from secreted proteins in a post-ER compartment. *EMBO J* **7**:913, 1988.
244. Dean N, Pelham HRB: Recycling of proteins from the Golgi compartment to the ER in yeast. *J Cell Biol* **111**:369, 1990.
245. Lewis MJ, Pelham HR: A human homologue of the yeast HDEL receptor. *Nature* **348**:162, 1990.
246. Sweet DJ, Pelham HR: The saccharomyces cerevisiae SEC20 gene encodes a membrane glycoprotein which is sorted by the HDEL retrieval system. *EMBO J* **11**:423, 1992.
247. Hardwick KG, Pelham HRB: SED5 encodes a 39-kD integral membrane protein required for vesicular transport between the ER and the Golgi complex. *J Cell Biol* **119**:513, 1992.
248. Wilson DW, Lewis MJ, Pelham HRB: pH-dependent binding of KDEL to its receptor in vitro. *J Biol Chem* **268**:7465, 1993.
249. Takemoto H, Yoshimori T, Yamamoto A, Miyata Y, Yakara I, Inoue K, Tashiro Y: Heavy chain binding protein (BiP/GRP78) and endoplasmin are exported from the endoplasmic reticulum in rat exocrine pancreatic cells, similar to protein disulfide-isomerase. *Arch Biochem Biophys* **296**:129, 1992.
250. Paabo S, Bhat BM, Wold WSM, Peterson PA: A short sequence in the COOH-terminus makes an adenovirus membrane glycoprotein a resident of the endoplasmic reticulum. *Cell* **50**:311, 1987.
251. Nilsson T, Jackson M, Peterson PA: Short cytoplasmic sequences serve as retention signals for transmembrane proteins in the endoplasmic reticulum. *Cell* **58**:707, 1989.
252. Severinsson L, Peterson PA: Abrogation of cell surface expression of human class I transplantation antigens by an adenovirus protein in Xenopus laevis oocytes. *J Cell Biol* **101**:540, 1985.
253. Jackson MR, Nilsson T, Peterson PA: Identification of a consensus motif for retention of transmembrane proteins in the endoplasmic reticulum. *EMBO J* **9**:3153, 1990.
254. Shin J, Dunbrack RL Jr, Lee S, Strominger JL: Signals for retention of transmembrane proteins in the endoplasmic reticulum studied with CD4 truncation mutants. *Proc Natl Acad Sci U S A* **88**:1918, 1991.
255. Jackson MR, Nilsson T, Peterson PA: Retrieval of transmembrane proteins to the endoplasmic reticulum. *J Cell Biol* **121**:317, 1993.
256. Tsao YS, Ivessa NE, Adesnik M, Sabatini DD, Kreibich G: Carboxy terminally truncated forms of ribophorin I are degraded in pre-Golgi compartments by a calcium-dependent process. *J Cell Biol* **116**:57, 1992.
257. Rose JK, Doms RW: Regulation of protein export from the endoplasmic reticulum. *Annu Rev Cell Biol* **4**:257, 1988.
258. Hurtley SM, Helenius A: Protein oligomerization in the endoplasmic reticulum. *Annu Rev Cell Biol* **5**:277, 1989.
259. Bonifacino JS, Lippincott-Schwartz J: Degradatation of proteins within the endoplasmic reticulum. *Curr Opin Cell Biol* **3**:592, 1991.
260. Gething M-J, Sambrook J: Protein folding in the cell. *Nature* **355**:33, 1992.
260a. Helenius A, Marquardt T, Braakman I: The endoplasmic reticulum as a protein-folding compartment. *Trends Cell Biol* **2**:227, 1992.
261. Klausner RD, Sitia R: Protein degradation in the endoplasmic reticulum. *Cell* **62**:611, 1990.
262. Ivessa NE, De Lemos-Chiarandini C, Tsao Y-S, Takatsuki A, Adesnik M, Sabatini DD, Kreibich G: O-glycosylation of intact and truncated ribophorins in brefeldin A-treated cells: Newly synthesized intact ribophorins are only transiently accessible to the relocated glycosyltransferases. *J Cell Biol* **117**:949, 1992.
263. Carlin BE, Merlie JP: Assembly of multisubunit membrane proteins, in Strauss AW, Boime I, Kreil G (eds): *Protein Compartmentalization.* New York, Springer-Verlag, 1986, p 71.
264. Mains PE, Sibley CH: The requirement of light chain for the surface deposition of the heavy chain of immunoglobulin M. *J Biol Chem* **258**:5027, 1982.
265. Sege K, Rask L, Peterson PA: Role of β_2-microglobulin in the intracellular processing of HLA antigens. *Biochemistry* **20**:4523, 1981.
266. Severinsson L, Peterson PA: β_2-microglobulin induces intracellular transport of human class I transplantation antigen heavy chains in Xenopus laevis oocytes. *J Cell Biol* **99**:226, 1984.
267. Harding CV, Geuze HJ: Antigen processing and intracellular traffic of antigens and MHC molecules. *Curr Opin Cell Biol* **5**:596, 1993.
268. Kreis TE, Lodish HF: Oligomerization is essential for transport of vesicular stomatitis viral glycoprotein to the cell surface. *Cell* **46**:929, 1986.
269. Copeland CS, Dorns RW, Bolzau EM, Webster RG, Helenius A: Assembly of influenza hemagglutinin trimers and its role in intracellular transport. *J Cell Biol* **103**:1179, 1986.
270. Gething M-J, McCammon K, Sambrook J: Expression of wild type and mutant forms of influenza haemagglutinin: The role of folding and intracellular transport. *Cell* **46**:939, 1986.
271. Perlmutter DH, Kay RM, Cole FS, Rossing TH, Van Thiel D, Colten HR: The cellular defect in α_1-proteinase inhibitor (α_1-PI) deficiency is expressed in human monocytes and in Xenopus oocytes injected with human liver mRNa. *Proc Natl Acad Sci U S A* **82**:6918, 1985.
272. Lomas DA, Evans DLI, Finch JT, Carrell RW: The mechanism of Z α_1-antitrypsin accumulation in the liver. *Nature* **357**:605, 1992.
273. Mosmann TR, Williamson AR: Structural mutations in a mouse immunoglobulin light chain resulting in the failure to be secreted. *Cell* **20**:283, 1980.
274. Brown MS, Goldstein JL: A receptor-mediated pathway for cholesterol homeostasis. *Science* **232**:34, 1986.
275. Esser V, Russell DW: Transport-deficient mutations in the low density lipoprotein receptor. Alterations in the cysteine-rich and cysteine-poor regions of the protein block intracellular transport. *J Biol Chem* **263**:13276, 1988.
276. Haas IG, Wabl M: Immunoglobulin heavy chain binding protein. *Nature* **306**:387, 1983.
277. Hendershot L, Bole D, Kohler G, Kearney JF: Assembly and secretion of heavy chains that do not associate posttranslationally with immunoglobulin heavy chain-binding proteins. *J Cell Biol* **104**:761, 1987.
278. Morrison SL, Scharff MD: Heavy chain-producing variants of a mouse myeloma cell line. *J Immunol* **114**:655, 1975.
279. Ahluwalia N, Bergeron JJ, Wada I, Degen E, Williams DB: The p88 molecular chaperone is identical to the endoplasmic reticulum membrane protein, calnexin. *J Biol Chem* **267**:10914, 1992.
280. Degen E, Williams DB: Participation of a novel 88-kD protein in the biogenesis of murine class I histocompatibility molecules. *J Cell Biol* **112**:1099, 1991.

281. Neefjes JJ, Schumacher TNM, Ploegh HL: Assembly and intracellular transport of major histocompatability complex molecules. *Curr Opin Cell Biol* **3**:601, 1991.

282. Hochstenbach F, David V, Watkins S, Brenner MB: Endoplasmic reticulum resident protein of 90 kilodaltons associates with the T- and B-cell antigen receptors and major histocompatibility complex antigens during their assembly. *Proc Natl Acad Sci U S A* **89**:4734, 1992.

283. Lippincott-Schwartz J, Bonifacino JS, Yuan LC, Klausner RD: Degradation from the endoplasmic reticulum: Disposing of newly synthesized proteins. *Cell* **54**:209, 1988.

284. Faust JR, Luskey KL, Chin DJ, Goldstein JL, Brown MS: Regulation of synthesis and degradation of 3-hydroxy-3-methylglutaryl-coenzyme A reductase by low-density lipoprotein and 25-hydroxycholesterol in UT-1 cells. *Proc Natl Acad Sci U S A* **79**:5205, 1982.

285. Jingami H, Brown MS, Goldstein JL, Anderson RG, Luskey KL: Partial deletion of membrane-bound domain of 3-hydroxy-3-methylglutaryl coenzyme A reductase eliminates sterol-enhanced degradation and prevents formation of crystalloid endoplasmic reticulum. *J Cell Biol* **104**:1693, 1987.

286. De La Hera A, Muller U, Olsson C, Isaaz S, Tunnacliffe A: Structure of the T cell antigen receptor (TCR): Two CD3 epsilon subunits in a functional TCR/CD3 complex. *J Exp Med* **173**:7, 1991.

287. Sussman JJ, Bonifacino JB, Lippincott-Schwartz J, Weissman AM, Saito T, Klausner RD, Ashwell JD: Failure to synthesize the T cell CD3-rate chain: Structure and function of a partial T cell receptor complex. *Cell* **52**:85, 1988.

288. Bonifacino JS, Suzuki CM, Lippincott-Schwartz J, Weissman AM, Klausner RD: Pre-Golgi degradation of newly synthesized T-cell antigen receptor chains: Intrinsic sensitivity and the role of subunit assembly. *J Cell Biol* **109**:73, 1989.

289. Wileman T, Carson BR, Concino M, Ahmed A, Terhorst C: The gamma and epsilon subunits of the CD3 complex inhibit pre-Golgi degradation of newly synthesized T cell antigen receptors. *J Cell Biol* **110**:973, 1990.

290. Bonifacino JS, Suzuki CM, Klausner RD: A peptide sequence confers retention and rapid degradation in the endoplasmic reticulum. *Science* **247**:79, 1990.

291. Bonifacino JS, Cosson P, Klausner RD: Colocalized transmembrane determinants for ER degradation and subunit assembly explain the intracellular fate of TCR chains. *Cell* **63**:503, 1990.

292. Manolios N, Bonifacino JS, Klausner RD: Transmembrane helical interactions and the assembly of the T cell receptor complex. *Science* **249**:274, 1990.

293. Bonifacino JS, Cosson P, Shah N, Klausner RD: Role of potentially charged transmembrane residues in targeting proteins for retention and degradation within the endoplasmic reticulum. *EMBO J* **10**:2783, 1991.

294. Cosson P, Lankford SP, Bonifacino JS, Klausner RD: Membrane protein association by potential intramembrane charge pairs. *Nature* **351**:414, 1991.

295. Wileman T, Kane LP, Carson BR, Terhorst C: Depletion of cellular calcium accelerates protein degradation in the endoplasmic reticulum. *J Biol Chem* **266**:4500, 1991.

296. Wikstrom L, Lodish HF: Nonlysosomal, pre-Golgi degradation of unassembled asialoglycoprotein receptor subunits: A TLCK- and TPCK-sensitive cleavage within the ER. *J Cell Biol* **113**:997, 1991.

297. Farquhar MG: Progress in unraveling pathways of Golgi traffic. *Annu Rev Cell Biol* **1**:447, 1985.

298. Pelham HRB: Speculations on the functions of the major heat shock and glucose-regulated proteins. *Cell* **46**:959, 1986.

299. Rothman JE: Protein sorting by selective retention by ER and Golgi stack. *Cell* **50**:521, 1987.

300. Pfeffer SR, Rothman JE: Biosynthetic protein transport and sorting by the endoplasmic reticulum and Golgi. *Annu Rev Biochem* **56**:829, 1987.

301. Balch WE: Biochemistry of interorganelle transport. *J Biol Chem* **264**:16965, 1989.

302. Balch WE: Molecular dissection of early stages of the eukaryotic secretory pathway. *Curr Opin Cell Biol* **2**:634, 1990.

303. Saraste J, Kuismanen E: Pathways of protein sorting and membrane traffic between the rough endoplasmic reticulum and the Golgi complex. *Semin Cell Biol* **3**:343, 1992.

303a. Kaiser C: Protein transport from the endoplasmic reticulum to the Golgi apparatus, in Peng Loh Y (ed): *Mechanisms of Intracellular Trafficking and Processing of Proproteins*. Boca Raton, FL, CRC Press, 1993, p 79.

304. Jamieson JD, Palade GE: Intracellular transport of secretory proteins in the pancreatic exocrine cell. I. Role of the peripheral elements of the Golgi complex. *J Cell Biol* **34**:577, 1967.

305. Jamieson JD, Palade GE: Intracellular transport of secretory proteins in the pancreatic exocrine cell. II. Transport to condensing vacuoles and zymogen granules. *J Cell Biol* **34**:597, 1967.

306. Bainton DF, Farquhar MG: Segregation and packaging of granule enzymes in eosinophilic leukocytes. *J Cell Biol* **45**:54, 1970.

307. Geuze JJ, Slot JW, Tokuyasu KT, Goedemans WEM, Griffith JM: Immunocytochemical localization of amylase and chymotrypsinogen in the exocrine pancreatic cell with special attention to the Golgi complex. *J Cell Biol* **82**:697, 1979.

308. Jamieson JD, Palade GE: Intracellular transport of secretory proteins in the pancreatic exocrine cell. IV. Metabolic requirements. *J Cell Biol* **39**:589, 1968.

309. Tartakoff A, Vassalli P: Plasma cell immunoglobulin secretion: Arrest is accompanied by alterations of the Golgi complex. *J Exp Med* **146**:1332, 1977.

310. Godelaine D, Spiro MJ, Spiro RG: Processing of the carbohydrate units of thyroglobulin. *J Biol Chem* **256**:10161, 1981.

311. Balch WE, Keller DS: ATP-coupled transport of vesicular stomatitis virus G protein: Functional boundaries of secretory compartments. *J Cell Biol* **261**:14681, 1986.

312. Balch WE, Keller DS: ATP-coupled transport of vesicular stomatitis virus G protein: Functional boundaries of secretory compartments. *J Biol Chem* **261**:14690, 1986.

313. Tartakoff AM: Temperature and energy dependence of secretory protein transport in the exocrine pancreas. *EMBO J* **5**:1477, 1986.

314. Lodish HF, Kong N, Snider M, Strous GJAM: Hepatoma secretory proteins migrate from the rough endoplasmic reticulum to Golgi at characteristic rates. *Nature* **304**:80, 1983.

315. Fitting T, Kabat D: Evidence for a glycoprotein "signal" involved in transport between subcellular organelles: Two membrane glycoproteins encoded by murine Leukemia virus reach the cell surface at different rates. *J Biol Chem* **257**:14011, 1982.

316. Fries E, Gustafsson L, Peterson PA: Four secretory proteins synthesized by hepatocytes are transported from endoplasmic reticulum to Golgi complex at different rates. *EMBO J* **3**:147, 1984.

317. Scheele G, Tartakoff A: Exit of nonglycosylated secretory proteins from the rough endoplasmic reticulum is asynchronous in the exocrine pancreas. *J Biol Chem* **260**:926, 1985.

318. Bergmann JE, Tokuyasu KT, Singer SJ: Passage of an integral membrane protein, the vesicular stomatitis virus glycoprotein, through the Golgi apparatus en route to the plasma membrane. *Proc Natl Acad Sci U S A* **78**:1746, 1981.

319. Bergmann JE, Singer SJ: Immuno-electron icroscopic studies of the intracellular transport of the membrane glycoprotein (G) of vesicular stomatitis virus in infected chinese hamster ovary cells. *J Cell Biol* **97**:1777, 1983.

320. Wieland FT, Gleason ML, Serafini TA, Rothman JE: The rate of bulk flow from the endoplasmic reticulum to the cell surface. *Cell* **50**:289, 1987.

321. Helms JB, Kaarrenbauer A, Wirtz KWA, Rothman JE, Wieland FT: Reconstitution of steps in the constitutive secretory pathway in permeabilized cells. *J Biol Chem* **265**:20027, 1990.

321a. Geetha-Habib M, Park HR, Lennarz WJ: In vivo N-glycosylation and fate of Asn-X-Ser/Thr tripeptides. *J Biol Chem* **265**:13655, 1990.

322. Romisch K, Schekman R: Distinct processes mediate glycoprotein and glycopeptide export from the endoplasmic reticulum in Saccharomyces cerevisiae. *Proc Natl Acad Sci U S A* **89**:7227, 1992.

323. Schekman R: Genetic and biochemical analysis of vesicular traffic in yeast. *Curr Opin Cell Biol* **4**:587, 1992.

324. Novick P, Field C, Schekman R: Identification of 23 complementation groups required for post-translational events in the yeast secretory pathway. *Cell* **21**:205, 1980.

325. Newman AP, Ferro-Novick S: Characterization of new mutants in the early part of the yeast secretory pathway isolated by a [^{3}H]mannose suicide selection. *J Cell Biol* **105**:1587, 1987.

326. Pryer NK, Salama NR, Schekman R, Kaiser CA: Cytosolic *Sec*13p complex is required for vesicle formation from the endoplasmic reticulum in vitro. *J Cell Biol* **120**:865, 1993.

327. Kaiser CA, Schekman R: Distinct sets of SEC genes govern transport vesicle formation and fusion early in the secretory pathway. *Cell* **61**:723, 1990.

328. Baker D, Hicke L, Rexach M, Schleyer M, Schekman R: Reconstitution of SEC gene product-dependent intercompartmental protein transport. *Cell* **54**:335, 1988.
329. Groesch ME, Guendalina R, Ferro-Novick S: Reconstitution of endoplasmic reticulum to golgi transport in yeast: In vitro assay to characterize secretory mutants and functional transport vesicles. *Methods Enzymol* **219**:137, 1992.
330. Wuestehube LJ, Schekman RW: Reconstitution of transport from endoplasmic reticulum to Golgi complex using endoplasmic reticulum-enriched membrane fraction from yeast. *Methods Enzymol* **219**:124, 1992.
331. Nakano A, Muramatsu M: A novel GTP-binding protein, Sar1p, is involved in transport from the endoplasmic reticulum to the Golgi apparatus. *J Cell Biol* **109**:2677, 1989.
332. Nakano A, Brade D, Schekman R: A membrane glycoprotein, *sec*12p, required for protein transport from the endoplasmic reticulum to the Golgi apparatus in yeast. *J Cell Biol* **107**:851, 1988.
333. Barlowe C, D'Enfert C, Schekman R: Purification and characterization of SAR1p, a small GTP-binding protein required for transport vesicle formation from the endoplasmic reticulum. *J Biol Chem* **268**:873, 1993.
334. Yoshihisa T, Barlowe C, Schekman R: Requirement for a GTPase-activating protein in vesicle budding from the endoplasmic reticulum. *Science* **259**:1466, 1993.
335. Hicke L, Yoshihisa T, Schekman R: Sec23p and a novel 105-kDa protein function as a multimeric complex to promote vesicle budding and protein transport from the endoplasmic reticulum. *Mol Biol Cell* **3**:667, 1992.
336. Orci L, Ravazzola M, Meda P, Holcomb C, Moore H-P, Hicke L, Schekman R: Mammalian Sec23p homologue is restricted to the endoplasmic reticulum transitional cytoplasm. *Proc Natl Acad Sci U S A* **88**:8611, 1991.
337. Schmitt HD, Puzicha M, Gallwitz G: Study of a temperature-sensitive mutant of the ras-related *YPT1* gene product in yeast suggests a role in the regulation of intracellular calcium. *Cell* **53**:636, 1988.
338. Segev N, Mulholland J, Botstein D: The yeast GTP-binding YPT1 protein and a mammalian counterpart are associated with the secretion machinery. *Cell* **52**:915, 1986.
339. Baker D, Wuestehube L, Schekman R, Botstein D, Segev N: GTP-binding Ypt1 protein and Ca^{2+} function independently in a cell-free protein transport reaction. *Proc Natl Acad Sci U S A* **87**:355, 1990.
340. Rexach MF, Schekman RW: Distinct biochemical requirements for the budding, targeting, and fusion of ER-derived transport vesicles. *J Cell Biol* **114**:219, 1991.
341. Tisdale EJ, Bourne JR, Khosravi-Far R, Der CJ, Balch WE: GTP-binding mutants of Rab1 and Rab2 are potent inhibitors of vesicular transport from the endoplasmic reticulum to the Golgi complex. *J Cell Biol* **119**:749, 1992.
342. Beckers CJM, Balch WE: Calcium and GTP: Essential components in vesicular trafficking between the endoplasmic reticulum and Golgi apparatus. *J Cell Biol* **108**:1245, 1989.
343. Block MR, Glick BS, Wilcox CA, Wieland FT, Rothman JE: Purification of an N-ethylmaleimide-sensitive protein catalyzing vesicular transport. *Proc Natl Acad Sci U S A* **85**:7852, 1988.
344. Beckers CJM, Block MR, Glick BS, Rothman JE, Balch WE: Vesicular transport between the endoplasmic reticulum and the Golgi stack requires the NEM-sensitive fusion protein. *Nature* **339**:3977, 1989.
345. Diaz R, Mayorga LS, Weidman PJ, Rothman JE, Stahl PD: Vesicle fusion following receptor-mediated endocytosis requires a protein active in Golgi transport. *Nature* **339**:398, 1989.
346. Clary DO, Griff IC, Rothman EJ: SNAPs, a family of NSF attachment proteins involved in intracellular membrane fusion in animals and yeast. *Cell* **61**:709, 1990.
347. Griff IC, Schekman R, Rothman JE, Kaiser CA: The yeast *SEC17* gene product is functionally equivalent to mammalian a-SNAP protein. *J Biol Chem* **267**:12106, 1992.
348. Rothman JE, Orci L: Molecular dissection of the secretory pathway. *Nature* **355**:409, 1992.
349. Sollner T, Whiteheart SW, Brunner M, Erdjument-Bromage H, Geromanos S, Tempst P, Rothman JE: SNAP receptors implicated in vesicle targeting and fusion. *Nature* **362**:318, 1993.
350. Hosobuchi M, Kries T, Schekman R: SEC21 is a gene required for ER to Golgi protein transport that encodes a subunit of a yeast coatomer. *Nature* **355**:409, 1992.
351. Moores SL, Schaber MD, Mosser SD, Rands E, O'Hara MB, Garsky VM, Marshall MS, Pompliano DL, Gibbs JB: Sequence dependence of protein isoprenylation. *J Biol Chem* **266**:14603, 1991.
352. Molenaar CMT, Prange R, Gallwitz D: A carboxyl-terminal cysteine residue is required for palmitic acid binding and biological activity of the *ras*-related yeast YPT1 protein. *EMBO J* **7**:971, 1988.
353. Rossi G, Jiang Y, Newman AP, Ferro-Novick S: Dependence of Ypt1 and sec4 membrane attachment on Bet2. *Nature* **351**:158, 1991.
354. Dascher C, Ossig R, Gallwitz D, Schmitt HD: Identification and structure of four yeast genes (*SLY*) that are able to suppress the functional loss of *YPT1*, a member of the *RAS* superfamily. *Mol Cell Biol* **11**:872, 1991.
355. Ossig R, Dascher C, Trepte H-H, Schmitt HD, Gallwitz D: The yeast *SLY* gene products, suppressors of defects in the essential GTP-binding Ypt1 protein, may act in endoplasmic reticulum-to-Golgi transport. *Mol Cell Biol* **11**:2980, 1991.
356. Newman AP, Shim J, Ferro-Novick S: BETI, BOSI, and SEC22 are members of a group of interlacing yeast genes required for transport from the endoplasmic reticulum to the Golgi complex. *Mol Cell Biol* **10**:3405, 1990.
357. Newman AP, Groesch ME, Ferro-Novick S: Bos1p, a membrane protein required for ER to Golgi transport in yeast, co-purifies with the carrier vesicles and with Bet1p and the ER membrane. *EMBO J* **11**:3609, 1992.
358. Shim J, Newman AP, Ferro-Novick S: The *BOS1* gene encodes an essential 27-kD putative membrane protein that is required for vesicular transport from the ER to the Golgi complex in yeast. *J Cell Biol* **113**:55, 1991.
359. Newman AP, Graf J, Mancini P, Rossi G, Lian JP, Ferro-Novick S: *SEC22* and *SLY2* are identical [Letter]. *Mol Cell Biol* **12**:3663, 1992.
360. Bennett MK, Calakos N, Scheller RH: Syntaxin: A synaptic protein implicated in docking of synaptic vesicles at presynaptic active zones. *Science* **257**:255, 1992.
361. Bennett MK, Scheller RH: The molecular machinery for secretion is conserved from yeast to neurons. *Proc Natl Acad Sci U S A* **90**:2559, 1993.
362. Lian JP, Ferro-Novick S: Bos1p, an integral membrane protein of the endoplasmic reticulum to Golgi transport vesicles, is required for their fusion competence. *Cell* **73**:735, 1993.
363. Schwaninger R, Plutner H, Davidson S, Pind S, Balch WE: Transport of protein between the endoplasmic reticulum and Golgi compartments in semiintact cells. *Methods Enzymol* **219**:110, 1992.
364. Davidson HW, Balch WE: Differential inhibition of multiple vesicular transport steps between the endoplasmic reticulum and trans Golgi network. *J Biol Chem* **268**:4216, 1993.
365. Beckers CJM, Plutner H, Davidson HW, Balch WE: Sequential intermediates in the transport of protein between the endoplasmic reticulum and the Golgi. *J Biol Chem* **265**:18298, 1990.
366. Schwaninger R, Plutner H, Bokoch GM, Balch WE: Multiple GTP-binding proteins regulate vesicular transport from the ER to Golgi membranes. *J Cell Biol* **119**:1077, 1992.
367. Plutner H, Schwaninger R, Pind S, Balch WE: Synthetic peptides of the rab effector domain inhibit vesicular transport through the secretory pathway. *EMBO J* **9**:2375, 1990.
368. Stearns T, Willingham MC, Botstein D, Kahn RA: ADP-ribosylation factor functionally and physically associated with the Golgi complex. *Proc Natl Acad Sci U S A* **87**:1238, 1990.
369. Balch WE, Kahn RA, Schwaninger R: ADP-ribosylation factor is required for vesicular trafficking between the endoplasmic reticulum and the *cis*-Golgi compartment. *J Biol Chem* **267**:13053, 1992.
370. Leyte A, Barr FA, Kehlenbach RH, Wieland BH: Multiple trimeric G-proteins on the trans-Golgi network exert stimulatory and inhibitory effects on secretory vesicle formation. *EMBO J* **11**:4795, 1992.
371. Davidson HW, McGowan CH, Balch WE: Evidence for the regulation of exocyte transport by protein phosphorylation. *J Cell Biol* **116**:1343, 1992.
372. Hauri HP, Schweizer A: The endoplasmic reticulum-Golgi intermediate compartment. *Curr Opin Cell Biol* **4**:600, 1992.
373. Mellman I, Simons K: The Golgi complex: In vitro veritas? *Cell* **68**:829, 1992.
374. Lippincott-Schwartz J: Bidirectional membrane traffic between the endoplasmic reticulum and Golgi apparatus. *Trends Cell Biol* **3**:81, 1993.
375. Saraste J, Kuismanen E: Pre- and post-Golgi vacuoles operate in the transport of Semliki Forest virus membrane glycoprotenis to the cell surface. *Cell* **38**:535, 1984.

376. Schweizer A, Fransen JA, Matter K, Kreis TE, Ginsel L, Hauri HP: Identification of an intermediate compartment involved in protein transport from endoplasmic reticulum to Golgi apparatus. *Eur J Cell Biol* **53**:185, 1990.
377. Schweizer A, Fransen JA, Bachi T, Ginsel L, Hauri HP: Identification, by a monoclonal antibody, of a 53-kd protein associated with a tubo-vesicular compartment at the *cis*-side of the Golgi apparatus. *J Cell Biol* **107**:1643, 1988.
378. Saraste J, Svensson K: Distribution of the intermediate elements operating in ER to Golgi transport. *J Cell Sci* **100**:415, 1991.
378a. Chavrier P, Parton RG, Hauri HP, Simons K, Zerial M: Localization of low molecular weight GTP binding proteins to exocytic and endocytic compartments. *Cell* **62**:317, 1990.
379. Plutner H, Cox AD, Pind S, Khosravi FR, Bourne JR, Schwaninger R, Der CJ, Balch WE: Rab1b regulates vesicular transport between the endoplasmic reticulum and successive Golgi compartments. *J Cell Biol* **115**:31, 1991.
380. Schweizer A, Matter K, Ketcham CM, Hauri HP: The isolated ER-Golgi intermediate compartment exhibits properties that are different from ER and cis-Golgi. *J Cell Biol* **113**:45, 1991.
381. Duden R, Allan V, Kreis T: Involvement of β-COP in membrane traffic through the Golgi complex. *Trends Cell Biol* **1**:14, 1991.
382. Hashimoto S, Bruno B, Lew DP, Pozzan T, Volpe P, Meldolesi J: Immunocytochemistry of calciosomes in liver and pancreas. *J Cell Biol* **107**:2523, 1988.
383. Villa A, Podini P, Clegg DG, Pozzan T, Meldolesi J: Intracellular Ca^{2+} stores in chicken Purkinje neurons: Differential distribution of the low affinity-high capacity Ca^{2+} binding protein, calsequestrin, of Ca^{2+} ATPase and of the ER lumenal protein, Bip. *J Cell Biol* **113**:779, 1991.
384. Tooze SA, Tooze J, Warren G: Site of addition of N-acetyl-galactosamine to the Ei glycoprotein of mouse hepatitis virus-A59. *J Cell Biol* **106**:1475, 1988.
385. Rizzolo J, Kornfeld R: Post-translational protein modification in the endoplasmic reticulum. Demonstration of fatty acylase and deoxymannojirimycin-sensitive alpha-mannosidase activities. *J Biol Chem* **263**:9520, 1988.
386. Plutner H, Davidson HW, Saraste J, Balch WE: Morphological analysis of protein transport from the ER to Golgi membranes in digitonin-permeabilized cells: Role of the P58 containing compartment. *J Cell Biol* **119**:1097, 1992.
386a. Farquhar MG, Palade GE: The Golgi apparatus (complex)-(1954)-(1981)—From artifact to center stage. *J Cell Biol* **91**:77s, 1981.
387. Tartakoff AM: The confined function model of the Golgi complex: Center for ordered processing of biosynthetic products of the rough endoplasmic reticulum. *Int Rev Cytol* **85**:221, 1983.
388. Griffiths G, Simons K: The trans Golgi network: Sorting at the exit site of the Golgi complex. *Science* **234**:438, 1986.
389. Farquhar MG: Protein traffic through the Golgi complex, in Steer CJ, Hanover JA (eds): *Intracellular Trafficking in Proteins*. Cambridge, Cambridge University Press, 1991, p 431.
390. Herzog V, Farquhar MG: Luminal membrane retrieved after exocytosis reaches most Golgi cisternae in secretory cells. *Proc Natl Acad Sci U S A* **74**:5073, 1977.
391. Farquhar MG: Recovery of surface membrane in anterior pituitary cells. Variations in traffic detected with anionic and cationic ferritin. *J Cell Biol* **77**:R35, 1978.
392. Farquhar MG: Membrane recycling in secretory cells: Implications for traffic of products and specialized membranes within the Golgi complex. *Methods Cell Biol* **23**:399, 1981.
393. Farquhar MG: Membrane recycling in secretory cells: Pathways to the Golgi complex. *Ciba Found Symp* **92**:157, 1982.
394. Farquhar MG: Multiple pathways of exocytosis, endocytosis and membrane recycling: Validation of a Golgi route. *Fed Proc* **42**:2407, 1983.
395. Patzak A, Winkler H: Exocytotic exposure and recycling of membrane antigens of chromaffin granules: Ultrastructural evaluation after immunolabeling. *J Cell Biol* **102**:510, 1986.
396. Dalton AJ, Felix MD: Cytologic and cytochemical characteristics of the Golgi substance of epithelial cells of the epididymis—in situ, in homogenates and after isolation. *Am J Anat* **94**:171, 1954.
397. Novikoff AB: GERL, its form and function in neurons of rat spinal ganglia. *Biol Bull* **127**:358, 1964.
398. Novikoff AB: The endoplasmic reticulum: A cytochemist's view (a review). *Proc Natl Acad Sci U S A* **73**:2781, 1976.
399. Mollenhauer HH, Morre DJ: Structural compartmentation of the cytosol: Zones of exclusion, zones of adhesion, cytoskeletal and intercisternal elements. *Subcell Biochem* **5**:327, 1978.
400. Rambourg A, Clermont Y: Three-dimensional electron microscopy: Structure of the Golgi apparatus. *Eur J Cell Biol* **51**:189, 1990.
401. Rambourg A, Clermont Y, Hermo L: Three dimensional architecture of the Golgi apparatus in Sertoli cells of the rat. *Am J Anat* **159**:455, 1979.
402. Rambourg A, Clermont Y, Hermo L: Three dimensional structure of the Golgi apparatus. *Methods Cell Biol* **23**:155, 1981.
403. Novikoff AB, Novikoff PM: Cytochemical contributions to differentiating GERL from the Golgi apaparatus. *Histochem J* **9**:525, 1977.
404. Willingham MC, Pastan IH: Endocytosis and exocytosis: Current concepts of vesicle traffic in animals cells. *Int Rev Cytol* **92**:51, 1984.
405. Orci L, Ravazzola M, Amherdt M, Perrrelet A, Powell SK, Quinn DL, Moore HH: The trans-most cisternae of the Golgi complex: A compartment for sorting of secretory and plasma membrane proteins. *Cell* **51**:1039, 1987.
406. Rindler MJ, Ivanov IE, Plesken H, Rodriguez-Boulan E, Sabatini DD: Viral glycoproteins destined for apical or basolateral plasma membrane domains traverse the same Golgi apparatus during their intracellular transport in doubly infected madin-darby canine kidney cells. *J Cell Biol* **98**:1304, 1984.
407. Wandinger-Ness A, Bennett MK, Antony C, Simons K: Distinct transport vesicles mediate the delivery of plasma membrane proteins to the apical and basolateral domains of MDCK cells. *J Cell Biol* **111**:987, 1987.
408. Rodriguez-Boulan E, Powell SK: Polarity of epithelial and neuronal cells. *Annu Rev Cell Biol* **8**:395, 1992.
409. Friend DS, Murray MJ: Osmium impregnation of the Golgi apparatus. *Am J Anat* **117**:135, 1965.
410. Novikoff AB, Goldfischer S: Nucleoside diphosphatase activity in the Golgi apapratus and its usefulness for cytological studies. *Proc Natl Acad Sci U S A* **47**:802, 1961.
411. Dunphy WG, Fries E, Urbani LJ, Rothman JE: Early and late functions associated with the Golgi apparatus reside in distinct compartments. *Proc Natl Acad Sci U S A* **78**:7453, 1981.
412. Roth J, Berger EJ: Immunocytochemical localization of galactosyl-transferase in HeLa cells: Codistribution with thiamine pyrophosphatase in trans-Golgi cisternae. *J Cell Biol* **93**:223, 1982.
413. Goldberg DE, Kornfeld S: Evidence for extensive subcellular organization of asparagine-linked oligosaccharide processing and lysosomal enzyme phosphorylation. *J Biol Chem* **258**:3159, 1983.
414. Dunphy WG, Rothman JE: Compartmentalization of asparagine-linked oligosaccharide processing in the Golgi apparatus. *J Cell Biol* **97**:270, 1983.
415. Dunphy W, Rothman JE: Attachment of terminal N-acetlyglucosamine to asparagine-linked oligosaccharides occurs in central cisternae of the Golgi stack. *Cell* **40**:463, 1985.
416. Nilsson T, Pypaert M, Hoe ME, Slusarewicz P, Berger EG, Warren G: Overlapping distribution of two glycosyltransferases in the Golgi apparatus of HeLa cells. *J Cell Biol* **120**:5, 1993.
417. Glickman J, Croen K, Kelly S, Al-Awqati Q: Golgi membranes contain an electrogenic H^+ pump in parallel to a chloride conductance. *J Cell Biol* **97**:1303, 1983.
418. Anderson RGW, Falck JR, Goldstein JL, Brown MS: Visualization of acidic organelles in intact cells by electronmicroscopy. *Proc Natl Acad Sci U S A* **81**:4838, 1984.
419. Anderson RGW, Pathak RK: Vesicles and cisternae in the trans Golgi apparatus of human fibroblasts are acidic compartments. *Cell* **40**:535, 1985.
420. Pressman PC: Biological applications of ionophores. *Annu Rev Biochem* **45**:501, 1976.
421. Ledger PW, Tanzer ML: Monensin—A perturbant of cellular physiology. *Trends Biochem Sci* **9**:313, 1984.
422. Tartakoff AM: Perturbation of vesicular traffic with the carboxylic ionophore monensin. *Cell* **32**:1026, 1983.
423. Strous GJAM, Willemsen R, Van Kerkhof P, Slot GW, Geuze HJ, Lodish HF: Vesicular stomatitis virus glycoprotein, albumin, and transferrin are transported to the cell surface via the same Golgi vesicles. *J Cell Biol* **97**:1815, 1983.
424. Griffiths G, Quinn P, Warren G: Dissection of the Golgi complex. I. Monensin inhibits the transport of viral membrane proteins from medial to trans Golgi cisternae in baby hamster kidney cells infected with Semliki forest virus. *J Cell Biol* **96**:835, 1983.
425. Ohkuma S, Poole B: Fluorescence probe measurement of the intralysosomal pH in living cells and the perturbation of pH by various agents. *Proc Natl Acad Sci U S A* **75**:3327, 1978.

426. Ohkuma S, Poole B: Cytoplasmic vacuolation of mouse peritoneal macrophages and the uptake into lysosomes of weakly basic substances. *J Cell Biol* **90**:656, 1981.
427. Strous GJAM, Dumaine A, Zijderhand-Bleekemolen JE, Slot JW, Schwartz AL: Effect of lysosomotropic amines on the secretory pathway and on the recycling of the asialoglycoprotein receptor in human hepatoma cells. *J Cell Biol* **101**:531, 1985.
428. Guan J-L, Rose JK: Conversion of a secretory protein into a transmembrane protein results in its transport to the Golgi complex but not to the cell surface. *Cell* **37**:779, 1984.
429. Thyberg K, Moskalewski S: Microtubules and the organization of the Golgi complex. *Exp Cell Res* **159**:1, 1985.
430. Ho WC, Allan VJ, Van Meer G, Berger EG, Kreis TE: Reclustering of scattered Golgi elements along microtubules. *Eur J Cell Biol* **48**:250, 1989.
431. Lucocq JM, Berger EG, Warren G: Mitotic Golgi fragments in HeLA cells and their role in the reassembly pathway. *J Cell Biol* **109**:463, 1989.
432. Klausner RD, Donaldson JG, Lippincott-Schwartz J: Brefeldin A: Insights into the control of membrane traffic and organelle structure. *J Cell Biol* **116**:1071, 1992.
433. Fujiwara T, Oda K, Yokota S, Takatsuki A, Ikehara Y: Brefeldin A causes disassembly of the Golgi complex and accumulation of secretory proteins in the endoplasmic reticulum. *J Biol Chem* **263**:18545, 1988.
434. Lippincott-Schwartz J, Yuan LC, Bonifacino JS, Klausner RD: Rapid redistribution of Golgi proteins into the ER in cells treated with Brefeldin A: Evidence for membrane cycling from Golgi to ER. *Cell* **56**:801, 1989.
435. Lippincott-Schwartz J, Donaldson JG, Schweizer A, Berger EG, Hauri H-P, Yuan LC, Klausner RD: Microtubule-dependent retrograde transport of proteins into the ER in the presence of Brefeldin A suggests an ER recycling pathway. *Cell* **60**:821, 1990.
436. Wool SA, Park JE, Brown WJ: Brefeldin A causes a microtubule-mediated fusion of the trans-Golgi network and early endosomes. *Cell* **67**:591, 1991.
437. Chege NW, Pfeffer SR: Compartmentation of the Golgi complex: Brefeldin A distinguishes trans-Golgi cisternae from the trans-Golgi network. *J Cell Biol* **111**:893, 1990.
438. Doms RW, Russ G, Yewdell JW: Brefeldin A redistributes resident and itinerant Golgi proteins to the endoplasmic reticulum. *J Cell Biol* **109**:61, 1989.
439. Ulmer JB, Palade GE: Effects of Brefeldin A on the processing of viral envelope glycoproteins in murine eyrthroleukemia cells. *J Biol Chem* **266**:9173, 1991.
440. Machamer CE: Golgi retention signals: Do membranes hold the key? *Trends Cell Biol* **1**:141, 1991.
441. Machamer CE: Targeting and retention of Golgi membrane protein. *Curr Opin Cell Biol* **5**:606, 1993.
442. Machamer CE, Rose JK: A specific transmembrane domain of a coronavirus E1 glycoprotein is required for its retention in the Golgi region. *J Cell Biol* **105**:1205, 1987.
443. Machamer CE, Mentone SA, Rose JK, Farquhar MG: The E1 glycoprotein of an avian coronavirus is targeted to the cis Golgi complex. *Proc Natl Acad Sci U S A* **87**:6944, 1990.
444. Swift AM, Machamer CE: A Golgi retention signal in a membrane-spanning domain of coronavirus E1 protein. *J Cell Biol* **115**:19, 1991.
445. Armstrong J, Patel S: The Golgi sorting domain of coronavirus E1 protein. *J Cell Sci* **98**:567, 1991.
446. Shaper JH, Shaper NL: Enzymes associated with glycosylation. *Curr Opin Struct Biol* **2**:7012, 1992.
447. Nilsson T, Lucocq JM, Mackay D, Warren G: The membrane spanning domain of β-1,4-galactosyltransferase specifies trans Golgi localization. *EMBO J* **10**:3567, 1991.
448. Aoki D, Lee N, Yamaguchi N, Dubois C, Fukuda MN: Golgi retention of a trans-Golgi membrane protein, galactosyltransferase, requires cysteine and histidine residues within the membrane-anchoring domain. *Proc Natl Acad Sci U S A* **89**:4319, 1992.
449. Russo RN, Shaper NL, Taatjes DJ, Shaper JH: β1-4-galactosyltransferase: A short NH_2-terminal fragment that includes the cytoplasmic and transmembrane domain is sufficient for Golgi retention. *J Biol Chem* **267**:9241, 1992.
450. Teasdale RK, D'Agostaro G, Gleason PA: The signal for Golgi retention of bovine β1,2-galactosyltransferase is in the transmembrane domain. *J Biol Chem* **267**:4084, 1992.
451. Munro S: Sequences within and adjacent to the transmembrane segment of α-2,6-sialyltransferase specify Golgi retention. *EMBO J* **10**:3577, 1991.
452. Colley KJ, Lee EU, Paulson JC: The signal anchor and stem regions of the β-galactoside α2,6-sialyltransferase may each act to localize the enzyme to the Golgi apparatus. *J Biol Chem* **267**:7784, 1992.
453. Wong SH, Low SH, Hong W: The 17-residue transmembrane domain of β-galactoside α2,6-sialyltransferase is sufficient for Golgi retention. *J Cell Biol* **117**:245, 1992.
454. Humphrey JS, Peters PJ, Yuan LC, Bonifacino JS: Localization of TGN38 to the trans-Golgi network: Involvement of a cytoplasmic tyrosine-containing sequence. *J Cell Biol* **120**:1123, 1993.
454a. Barr PJ: Mammalian subtilisins: The long-sought dibasic processing endoproteases. *Cell* **66**:1, 1991.
455. Wilcox CA, Redding K, Wright R, Fuller RS: Mutation of a tyrosine localization signal in the cytosolic tail of yeast Kex2 protease disrupts Golgi retention and results in default transport to the vacuole. *Mol Biol Cell* **3**:1353, 1992.
456. Cooper A, Bussey H: Yeast Kex1p is a Golgi-associated membrane protein: Deletions in a cytoplasmic targeting domain result in mislocalization to the vacuolar membrane. *J Cell Biol* **119**:1459, 1992.
457. Roberts CJ, Nothwehr SF, Stevens TH: Membrane protein sorting in the yeast secretory pathway: Evidence that the vacuole may be the default compartment. *J Cell Biol* **119**:69, 1992.
458. Seeger M, Payne GS: Selective and immediate effects of clathrin heavy chain mutations on Golgi membrane protein retention in *Saccharomyces cerevesiae*. *J Cell Biol* **118**:531, 1992.
459. Griffiths G, Pfeiffer S, Simons K, Matlin K: Exit of newly synthesized membrane proteins from trans cisternae of the Golgi complex to the plasma membrane. *J Cell Biol* **101**:949, 1985.
460. Rothman JE, Urbani LJ, Brands R: Transport of protein between cytoplasmic membranes of fused cells: Correspondence to processes reconstituted in a cell-free system. *J Cell Biol* **99**:248, 1984.
461. Rothman JE, Miller RL, Urbani LJ: Intercompartmental transport in the Golgi complex is a dissociative process: Facile transfer of membrane protein between two Golgi populations. *J Cell Biol* **99**:260, 1984.
461a. Balch WE, Glick BS, Rothman JE: Sequential intermediates in the pathway of intercompartmental transport in a cell-free system. *Cell* **39**:525, 1984.
462. Orci L, Glick BS, Rothman JE: A new type of coated vesicular carrier that appears not to contain clathrin: Its possible role in protein transport within the Golgi stack. *Cell* **46**:171, 1986.
463. Balch WE, Dunphy WG, Braell WA, Rothman JE: Reconstitution of the transport of proteins between successive compartments of the Golgi measured by the coupled incorporation of N-acetyl glucosamine. *Cell* **39**:405, 1984.
464. Braell WA, Bach WE, Dobberstein DC, Rothman JE: The glycoprotein that is transported between successive compartments of the Golgi in a cell-free system resides in stacks of cisternae. *Cell* **39**:511, 1984.
465. Wattenberg BW, Balch WE, Rothman JE: A novel prefusion complex formed during protein transport between Golgi cisternae in a cell-free system. *J Biol Chem* **261**:2202, 1986.
466. Wattenberg BW, Rothman JE: Multiple cytosolic components promote intra-Golgi protein transport. Resolution of a protein acting at a late stage, prior to membrane fusion. *J Biol Chem* **261**:2208, 1986.
467. Dunphy WG, Pfeffer SR, Clary DL, Wattenberg BW, Glick BS, Rothman JE: Yeast and mammals utilize similar cytosolic components to drive protein transport through the Golgi complex. *Proc Natl Acad Sci U S A* **83**:1622, 1986.
468. Beckers CJM, Rothman JE: Transport between Golgi cisternae. *Methods Enzymol* **219**:5, 1992.
469. Gottlieb C, Baenziger J, Kornfeld S: Deficient uridine diphosphatase-N-acetylglucosamine glycoprotein N-acetylglucosamine tranferase activity in a clone of chinese hamster ovary cells with altered surface glycoproteins. *J Biol Chem* **250**:3303, 1975.
470. Briles EB, Li E, Kornfeld S: Isolation of wheat germ agglutinin resistant clones of chinese hamster ovary cells deficient in membrane sialic acid and galactose. *J Biol Chem* **252**:1106, 1977.
471. Melancon P, Franzusoff A, Howell KE: Vesicle budding: Insights from cell-free assay. *Trends Cell Biol* **1**:165, 1991.
472. Sztul ES, Melancon P, Howell KE: Targeting and fusion in vesicular transport. *Trends Cell Biol* **2**:381, 1992.

473. Wattenberg BW, Raub TJ, Hiebsch RR, Weidman PJ: The activity of Golgi transport vesicles depends on the presence of the N-ethylmaleimide-sensitive factor (NSF) and a soluble NSF attachment protein (aSNAP) during vesicle formation. *J Cell Biol* **118**:1321, 1992.
474. Malhotra V, Orci L, Glick BS, Block MR, Rothman JE: Role of an N-ethylmaleimide-sensitive transport component in promoting fusion of transport vesicles with cisternae of the Golgi stack. *Cell* **54**:221, 1988.
475. Melancon P, Glick BS, Malhotra V, Weidman PJ, Serafini T, Gleason ML, Orci L, Rothman JE: Involvement of GTP-binding "G" proteins in transport through the Golgi stack. *Cell* **51**:1053, 1987.
476. Malhotra V, Serafini T, Orci L, Shepherd JC, Rothman JE: Purification of a novel class of coated vesicles mediating biosynthetic protein transport through the Golgi stack. *Cell* **58**:329, 1989.
477. Serafini T, Stenbeck G, Brecht A, Lottspeich F, Orci L, Rothman JE, Wieland FT: A coat subunit of Golgi-derived non-clathrin-coated vesicles with homology to the clathrin-coated vesicle coat protein β-adaptin. *Nature* **349**:215, 1991.
478. Duden R, Griffiths G, Frank R, Argos P, Kreis TE: β-COP, a 110 kd protein associated with non-clathrin-coated vesicles and the Golgi complex, shows homology to β-adaptin. *Cell* **64**:649, 1991.
479. Waters MG, Serafini T, Rothman JE: "Coatomer": A cytosolic protein complex containing subunits of non-clathrin-coated Golgi transport vesicles. *Nature* **349**:248, 1991.
480. Allan VJ, Kreis TE: A microtubule-binding protein associated with membranes of the Golgi apparatus. *J Cell Biol* **103**:2229, 1986.
481. Serafini T, Orci L, Amherdt M, Brunner M, Kahn RA, Rothman JE: ADP-ribosylation factor is a subunit of the coat of Golgi-derived COP-coated vesicles: A novel role for a GTP-binding protein. *Cell* **67**:239, 1991.
482. Helms JB, Rothman JE: Inhibition by Brefeldin A of a Golgi membrane enzyme that catalyzed exchange of guanine nucleotide bound to ARF. *Nature* **360**:352, 1992.
483. Donaldson JG, Finazzi D, Klausner RD: Brefeldin A inhibits Golgi membrane-catalysed exchange of guanine nucleotide onto ARF protein. *Nature* **360**:350, 1992.
484. Palmer DJ, Helms B, Beckers CJM, Orci L, Rothman JE: Binding of coatomer to Golgi membranes requires ADP-ribosylation factor. *J Biol Chem* **268**:12083, 1993.
485. Donaldson JG, Cassel D, Kahn RA, Klausner RD: ADP-ribosylation factor, a small GTP-binding protein, is required for binding of the coatomer protein β-COP to Golgi membranes. *Proc Natl Acad Sci U S A* **89**:6408, 1992.
486. Orci L, Palmer DJ, Amherdt M, Rothman JE: Coated vesicle assembly in the Golgi requires only coatomer and ARF proteins from the cytosol. *Nature* **364**:732, 1993.
486a. Pfanner N, Orci L, Glick BS, Amherdt M, Arden SR, Malhotra V, Rothman JE: Fatty acyl-coenzyme A is required for budding of transport vesicles from Golgi cisternae. *Cell* **59**:95, 1989.
487. Taylor TC, Kahn RA, Melancon P: Two distinct members of the ADP-ribosylation factor family of GTP-binding proteins regulate cell-free intra-Golgi transport. *Cell* **80**:69, 1992.
488. Orci L, Malhotra V, Amherdt M, Serafini T, Rothman JE: Dissection of a single round of vesicular transport: Sequential intermediates for intercisternal movement in the Golgi stacks. *Cell* **56**:357, 1989.
489. Stamnes MA, Rothman JE: The binding of AP-1 clathrin adaptor particles to Golgi membranes requires ADP-ribosylation factor, a small GTP-binding protein. *Cell* **73**:999, 1993.
490. Orci L, Tagaya M, Amherdt M, Perrelet A, Donaldson JG, Lippincott-Schwartz J, Klausner RD, Rothman JE: Brefeldin A, a drug that blocks secretion prevents the assembly of non-clathrin-coated buds on Golgi cisternae. *Cell* **64**:1183, 1991.
491. Donaldson JG, Lippincott-Schwartz J, Bloom GS, Kreis TE, Klausner RD: Dissociation of a 110-kD peripheral membrane protein from the Golgi apparatus is an early event in Brefeldin A action. *J Cell Biol* **111**:2295, 1990.
492. Donaldson JG, Lippincott-Schwartz J, Klausner RD: Guanine nucleotides modulate the effects of Brefeldin A in semipermeable cells: Regulation of the association of a 110-kD peripheral membrane protein with the Golgi apparatus. *J Cell Biol* **112**:579, 1991.
493. Donaldson JG, Kahn RA, Lippincott-Schwartz J, Klausner RD: Binding of ARF and β-COP to Golgi membranes: Possible regulation by a trimeric G protein. *Science* **254**:1197, 1991.
494. Ercolani L, Stow JL, Boyle JF, Holtzman EJ, Lin H, Grove JR, Ausiello DA: Membrane localization of the pertussis toxin-sensitive G-protein subunits α_{i-2} and α_{i-3} and expression of a metallothionein-α_{i-2} fusion gene in LLC-PK_1 cells. *Proc Natl Acad Sci U S A* **87**:4635, 1990.
495. Stow JL, De Almeida JB, Narula N, Holtzman EJ, Ercolani L, Ausiello DA: A heterotrimeric G protein, $G\alpha_{i-3}$, on Golgi membranes regulates the secretion of a heparan sulfate proteoglycan in LLC-PK_1 epithelial cells. *J Cell Biol* **114**:1113, 1991.
496. Ktistakis NT, Linder ME, Roth MG: Action of brefeldin A blocked by activation of a pertussis-toxin-sensitive G protein. *Nature* **356**:344, 1992.
497. Glick BS, Rothman JE: Possible role for fatty acyl-coenzyme A in intracellular protein transport. *Nature* **326**:309, 1987.
498. Tagaya M, Wilson DW, Brunner M, Arango N, Rothman JE: Domain structure of an N-ethylmaleimide-sensitive fusion protein involved in vesicular transport. *J Biol Chem* **268**:2662, 1993.
499. Warren G: Bridging the gap. *Nature* **362**:297, 1993.
500. Clary DO, Rothman JE: Purification of three related peripheral membrane proteins needed for vesicular transport. *J Biol Chem* **265**:10109, 1990.
501. Whiteheart SW, Griff IC, Brunner M, Clary DO, Mayer T, Buhrow SA, Rothman JE: SNAP family of NSF attachment proteins includes a brain-specific isoform. *Nature* **362**:353, 1993.
502. Whiteheart SW, Brunner M, Wilson DW, Widemann M, Rothman JE: Soluble N-ethylmaleimide-sensitive fusion attachment proteins (SNAPs) bind to a multi-SNAP receptor complex in Golgi membranes. *J Biol Chem* **267**:12239, 1992.
503. Wilson DW, Whiteheart SW, Wiedmann M, Brunner M, Rothman JE: A multi subunit particle implicated in membrane fusion. *J Cell Biol* **117**:531, 1992.
504. Baumert M, Maycox PR, Navone F, De Camilli P, Jahn R: Synaptobrevin: An integral membrane protein of 18,000 daltons present in small synaptic vesicles of rat brain. *EMBO J* **8**:379, 1989.
505. Kelly RB: Pathways of protein secretion in eukaryotes. *Science* **230**:25, 1985.
506. Burgess TL, Kelly RB: Constitutive and regulated secretion of proteins. *Annu Rev Cell Biol* **3**:243, 1987.
507. De Camilli P, Jahn R: Pathways to regulated exocytosis in neurons. *Annu Rev Physiol* **52**:625, 1990.
508. Matteoli M, De Camilli P: Molecular mechanisms in neurotransmitter release. *Curr Opin Neurobiol* **1**:91, 1993.
509. Sudoff TC, Jahn R: Proteins of synaptic vesicles involved in exocytosis and membrane recycling. *Neuron* **6**:665, 1991.
510. Delisle RC, Williams JAA: Regulation of membrane fusion in secretory exocytosis. *Annu Rev Physiol* **48**:225, 1986.
511. Arvan P, Castle D: Protein sorting and secretion granule formation in regulated secretory cells. *Trends Cell Biol* **2**:327, 1992.
512. Tooze SA, Chanat E, Tooze J, Huttner WB: Secretory granule formation, in Peng Loh Y (ed): *Mechanisms of Intracellular Trafficking and Processing of Proproteins*. Boca Raton, FL, CRC Press, 1993, p 157.
513. Bauerfeind R, Huttner WB: Biogenesis of constitutive secretory vesicles, secretory granules and synaptic vesicles. *Curr Opin Cell Biol* **5**:628, 1993.
514. Shields S, Danoff A: Prohormone processing: The role of propeptides in intracellular sorting, precursor processing and secretion, Peng Loh Y (ed): *Mechanisms of Intracellular Trafficking and Processing of Proproteins*. Boca Raton, FL, CRC Press, 1993, pp 131–155.
514a. Tooze SA, Stinchcombe JE: Biogenesis of secretory granules. *Semin Cell Biol* **3**:357, 1992.
515. Anderson P, Slorach SA, Uvnas B: Sequential exocytosis of storage granules during antigen-induced histamine release from sensitized rat mast cells in vitro. An electronmicroscopic stúdy. *Acta Physiol Scand* **88**:359, 1973.
516. Tooze J, Tooze Z: Clathrin-coated vesicular tranport of secretory proteins during the formation of ACTH-containing secretory granules in AtT-20 cells. *J Cell Biol* **103**:839, 1986.
517. Bendayan M, Roth J, Perrelet A, Orci L: Quantitative immunocytochemical localization of pancreatic secretory proteins in subcellular compartments of the rat acinar cell. *J Histochem Cytochem* **28**:149, 1980.
518. Mroz EA, Lechene C: Pancreatic zymogen granules differ markedly in protein composition. *Science* **232**:871, 1986.
519. Giannattasio G, Zanni A, Rosa P, Meldolesi J, Margolis RK, Margolis RU: Molecular organization of prolactin granules. III.

Intracellular transport of sulfated glycosaminoglycans and glycoproteins of the bovine prolactin granule matrix. *J Cell Biol* **86**:260, 1980.

520. Slaby F, Farquhar MG: Characterization of rat somatotroph and mammotroph secretory granules: Presence of sulfated molecules. *Mol Cell Endocrinol* **18**:33, 1980.
521. Zannini A, Giannattasio G, Nussdorfer G, Margolis RK, Margolis RU, Meldolesi J: Molecular organization of prolactin granules II. Characterization of glucosoaminoglycans and glycoproteins of the bovine prolactin granule matrix. *J Cell Biol* **86**:260, 1980.
522. Inoue K, Kurosumi K: Ultrastructural immunocytochemical localization of LH and FSH in the pituitary of the untreated male rat. *Cell Tissue Res* **235**:77, 1984.
523. Hashimoto S, Fumagalli G, Zanini A, Meldolesi J: Sorting of three secretory proteins to distinct secretory granules in acidophilic cells of cow anterior pituitary. *J Cell Biol* **105**:1579, 1987.
524. Bassetti M, Huttner WB, Zanini A, Rosa P: Co-localization of secretogranins/chromogranins with thyrotropin and luteinizing hormone in secretory granules of cow anterior pituitary. *J Histochem Cytochem* **38**:1353, 1990.
525. Bainton DF, Farquhar MG: Differences in enzyme content of specific granules of PMN leukocytes. I. Histochemical staining of bone marrow smears. *J Cell Biol* **39**:286, 1968.
526. Bainton DF, Farquhar MG: Differences in enzyme content of specific granules of PMN leukocytes. I. Histochemical staining of bone marrow smears. *J Cell Biol* **39**:299, 1968.
527. Lew PD, Monod A, Waldvogel FA, Dewald B, Baggiolini M, Porzan T: Quantitative analysis of the cytosolic free calcium dependency of exocytosis from the subcellular compartments in intact human neutrophils. *J Cell Biol* **102**:2197, 1986.
528. Beaudoin AR, Vachereau A, St Jean P: Evidence that amylase is released from two distinct pools of secretory proteins in the pancreas. *Biochim Biophys Acta* **757**:302, 1983.
529. Beaudoin AR, St Jean P, Vachereau A: Asynchronism between amylase secretion and packaging in the zymogen granules of pig pancreas. *Pancreas* **1**:2, 1986.
530. Arvan P, Castle JD: Phasic release of newly synthesized secretory proteins in the unstimulated rat exocrine pancreas. *J Cell Biol* **104**:243, 1987.
531. Rhodes CJ, Halban PA: Newly synthesized proinsulin-insulin as well as stored insulin are released from pancreatic B cells uniquely by a regulated non constitutive pathway. *J Cell Biol* **105**:145, 1987.
532. Gumbiner B, Kelly RB: Two distinct intracellular pathways transport secretory and membrane glycoproteins to the surface of the pituitary tumor cells. *Cell* **28**:51, 1982.
533. Burgess TL, Craik CS, Kelly RB: The exocrine protein trypsinogen is targeted into the secretory granules of an endocrine cell line. Studies by gene transfer. *J Cell Biol* **101**:639, 1985.
534. Moore HPH, Kelly RB: Secretory protein targeting in a pituitary cell line: Differential transport of foreign secretory proteins to distinct secretory pathways. *J Cell Biol* **101**:1773, 1985.
535. Moore HPH, Walker MD, Lee F, Kelly RB: Expressing a human proinsulin cDNA in a mouse ACTH-secreting cell. Intracellular storage, proteolytic processing and secretion on stimulation. *Cell* **35**:531, 1983.
536. Hellerman JG, Cone RC, Potts JT Jr, Rich A, Mulligan RC, Kronenberg HM: Secretion of human parathyroid hormone from rat pituitary cells infected with a recombinant retrovirus encoding preproparathyroid hormone. *Proc Natl Acad Sci U S A* **81**:5340, 1984.
537. Gonzalez A, Rizzolo L, Rindler M, Adesnik M, Sabatini DD, Gottlieb T: Nonpolarized secretion of truncated forms of the influenza hemagglutinin and the vesicular stomatitis virus G protein from MDCK cells. *Proc Natl Acad Sci U S A* **84**:3738, 1987.
538. Moore HPH, Kelly RB: Rerouting of a secretory protein by fusion with human hormone sequences. *Nature* **321**:443, 1986.
539. Stoller TJ, Shields D: The propeptide of preprosomatostatin mediates intracellular transport and secretion of α-globin from mammalian cells. *J Cell Biol* **108**:1647, 1989.
540. Sevarino KA, Stork P, Ventimiglia R, Mandel G, Goodman RH: Amino-terminal sequences of prosomatostatin direct intracellular targeting but not processing specificity. *Cell* **57**:11, 1989.
541. Powell SK, Orci L, Craik CS, Moore H-PH: Efficient targeting to storage granules of human proinsulins with altered propeptide domain. *J Cell Biol* **106**:1843, 1988.
542. Burgess TL, Craik CS, Matsuuchi L, Kelly RB: In vitro mutagenesis of pretrypsinogen: The role of the amino terminus in intracellular protein targeting to secretory granules. *J Cell Biol* **105**:659, 1987.
543. Wagner DD: Cell biology of von Willebrand factor. *Annu Rev Cell Biol* **6**:217, 1990.
544. Sporn LA, Marder J, Wagner DD: Inducible secretion of large, biologically potent von Willebrand factor multimers. *Cell* **46**:185, 1986.
545. Wagner DD, Saffaripour S, Bonfanti R, Sadler JE, Cramer EM, Chapman B, Mayadas TN: Induction of specific storage organelles by Von Willebrand factor propolypeptide. *Cell* **64**:403, 1991.
546. Voorberg J, Fontijn R, Calafat J, Janssen H, van Mourik JA, Pannekoek H: Biogenesis of Von Willebrand factor-containing organelles in heterologous transfected CV-1 cells. *EMBO J* **12**:749, 1993.
547. Mayadas TN, Wagner DD: Vicinal cysteines in the prosequence play a role in von Willebrand factor multimer assembly. *Proc Natl Acad Sci U S A* **89**:3531, 1992.
548. Wagner DD, Mayadas T, Marder VJ: Initial glycosylation and acidic pH in the Golgi apparatus are required for multimerization of Von Willebrand factor. *J Cell Biol* **102**:1320, 1986.

548a. Rindler MJ: Biogenesis of storage granules and vesicles. *Cur Opin Cell Biol* **4**:616, 1992.

549. Tooze SA, Flatmark T, Tooze J, Huttner WB: Characterization of the immature secretory granule, an intermediate in granule biogenesis. *J Cell Biol* **115**:1491, 1991.
550. Kuliawat R, Arvan P: Protein targeting via the "Constitutive-like" secretory pathway in isolated pancreatic islets: Passive sorting in the immature granule compartment. *J Cell Biol* **118**:521, 1992 .
551. O'Connor DT, Frigon RP: Chromogranin A, the major catecholamine storage vesicle soluble protein. *J Biol Chem* **259**:3237, 1984.
552. Rosa P, Hille A, Lee RWH, Zanini A, De Camilli P, Huttner WB: Secretogranins I and II: Two tyrosine-sulfated secretory proteins common to a variety of cells secreting peptides by the regulated pathway. *J Cell Biol* **101**:1999, 1985.
553. Huttner WB, Gerdes H-H, Rosa P: The granin (chromogranin-secretogranin) family. *Trends Biochem Sci* **16**:27, 1991.
554. Gerdes H-H, Rosa P, Phillips E, Baeuerle PA, Frank R, Argos P, Huttner WB: The primary structure of human secretogranin II, a widespread tyrosine-sulfated secretory granule protein that exhibits low pH and calcium-induced aggregation. *J Biol Chem* **264**:12009, 1989.
555. Gorr S-U, Shioi J, Cohn DV: Interaction of calcium with porcine adrenal chromogranin A (secretory protein-I) and chromogranin B (secretogranin I). *Am J Physiol* **257**:E247, 1989.
556. Baeuerle PA, Huttner WB: Tyrosine sulfation is a *trans*-Golgi-specific protein modification. *J Cell Biol* **105**:2655, 1987.
557. Kimura JH, Lohmander LS, Hascall VC: Studies on the biosynthesis of cartilage proteoglycan in a model system of cultured chondrocytes from the swarm rat chondrosarcoma. *J Cell Biochem* **26**:261, 1984.
558. Chanat E, Huttner WB: Milieu-induced selective aggregation of regulated secretory proteins in the trans-Golgi network. *J Cell Biol* **115**:1505, 1991.
559. Fumagalli G, Zanini A: In cow anterior pituitary, growth hormone and prolactin can be packed in separate granules of the same cell. *J Cell Biol* **100**:2019, 1985.
560. Ravazzola M, Orci L: Glucagon and glicentin immunoreactivity are topologically segregated in the alpha granule of the human pancreatic A cell. *Nature* **284**:66, 1980.
561. Pimplikar SW, Huttner WB: Chromogranin B (secretogranin I), a secretory protein of the regulated pathway, is also present in a tightly membrane-associated form in PC12 cells. *J Biol Chem* **267**:4110, 1992.
562. Taljanidisz J, Stewart L, Smith AJ, Klinman JP: Structure of bovine adrenal dopamine β-monooxygenase, as deduced from cDNA and protein sequencing: Evidence that the membrane-bound form of the enzyme is anchored by an uncleaved signal peptide. *Biochemistry* **28**:10054, 1989.
563. Disdier M, Morrissey JH, Fugate RD, Bainton DF, McEver RP: Cytoplasmic domain of P-selectin (CD62) contains the signal for sorting into the regulated secretory pathway. *Mol Biol Cell* **3**:309, 1992.
564. Koedam JA, Craamer EM, Briend E, Furie B, Furie BC, Wagner DD: P-selectin, a granule membrane protein of platelets and endothelila cells, follows the regulated secretory pathway in AtT-20 cells. *J Cell Biol* **116**:617, 1992.
565. Milgram SL, Mains RE, Eipper BA: COOH-terminal signals mediate the trafficking of a peptide processing enzyme in endocrine cells. *J Cell Biol* **121**:23, 1993.

566. Milgram SL, Johnson RC, Mains RE: Expression of individual forms of peptidylglycine α-amidating monooxygenase in AtT-20 cells: Endoproteolytic processing and routing to secretory granules. *J Cell Biol* **117**:717, 1992.
567. Rindler MJ, Hoops TC: The pancreatic membrane protein GP-2 localizes specifically to secretory granules and is shed into the pancreatic juice as a protein aggregate. *Eur J Cell Biol* **53**:154, 1990.
568. Fukuoka S-I, Freedman SD, Yu H, Sukhatme VP, Scheele GA: GP-2/THP gene family encodes self-binding glycosylphosphatidylinositol-anchored proteins in apical secretory compartments of pancreas and kidney. *Proc Natl Acad Sci U S A* **89**:1189, 1992.
569. Tooze SA, Weiss U, Huttner WB: Requirement for GTP hydrolysis in the formation of secretory vesicles. *Nature* **347**:207, 1990.
570. Rosa P, Barr FA, Stinchcombe JC, Binacchi C, Huttner WB: Brefeldin A inhibits the formation of constitutive secretory vesicles and immature secretory granules for the trans-Golgi network. *Eur J Cell Biol* **59**:265, 1992.
571. Miller SG, Carnell L, Moore H-PH: Post-Golgi membrane traffic: Brefeldin A inhibits export from distal Golgi compartments to the cell surface but not recycling. *J Cell Biol* **118**:267, 1992.
572. Barr FA, Leyte A, Mollner S, Pfeuffer T, Tooze SA, Huttner WB: Trimeric G-proteins of the *trans*-Golgi network are involved in the formation of constitutive secretory vesicles and immature secretory granules. *FEBS Lett* **294**:239, 1991.
573. Schlesinger MJ (ed): *Lipid Modifications of Proteins*. Boca Raton, FL, CRC Press, 1993.
574. Sefton BM, Buss JE: The covalent modification of eukaryotic proteins by lipids. *J Cell Biol* **104**:1449, 1987.
575. Towler DA, Gordon JI: The biology and enzymology of eukaryotic protein acylation. *Annu Rev Biochem* **57**:69, 1988.
576. Cross GAM: Glycolipid anchoring of plasma membrane proteins. *Annu Rev Cell Biol* **6**:1, 1990.
577. Maltese WA: Posttranslational modification of proteins by isoprenoids in mammalian cells. *FASEB J* **4**:3319, 1990.
578. Tartakoff AM, Singh N: How to make a glycoinositol phospholipid anchor. *Trends Biochem Sci* **17**:470, 1992.
579. Gordon JI, Duronio RJ, Rudnick DA, Adams SP, Gokel GW: Protein N-myristoylation. *J Biol Chem* **266**:8647, 1991.
580. Wilcox C, Hu JS, Olson EN: Acylation of proteins with myristic acid occurs cotranslationally. *Science* **238**:1275, 1987.
581. Pellman D, Garber EA, Cross FR, Hanafusa H: An N-terminal peptide from p60src can direct myristylation and plasma membrane localization when fused to heterologous proteins. *Nature* **314**:374, 1985.
582. Ravanello MP, Franke CA, Hruby DE: An NH2-terminal peptide from the vaccinia virus L1R protein directs the myristylation and virion envelope localization of a heterologous fusion protein. *J Biol Chem* **268**:7585, 1993.
583. Cross FR, Garber EA, Pellman D, Hanafusa H: A short sequence in the $p60^{src}$ N terminus is required for $p60^{src}$ myristylation and membrane association and for cell transformation. *Mol Cell Biol* **4**:1834, 1984.
584. Kamps MP, Buss JE, Sefton BM: Rous sarcoma virus transforming protein lacking myristic acid phosphorylates most known polypeptide substrates without inducing transformation. *Cell* **45**:105, 1986.
585. Ozols J, Carr SA, Strittmatter P: Identification of the NH2-terminal blocking group of NADH-cytochrome b5 reductase as myristic acid and the complete amino acid sequence of the membrane binding domain. *J Biol Chem* **259**:13349, 1984.
586. Resh MD, Ling H-P: Identification of a 32K plasma membrane protein that binds to the myristylated amino-terminal sequence of $p60^{v\text{-}src}$. *Nature* **346**:84, 1990.
587. Lohmann SM, Walter U: Regulation of the cellular and subcellular concentrations and distribution of cyclic nucleotide-dependent protein kinases. *Adv Cyclic Nucleotide Protein Phosphoryl Res* **18**:63, 1984.
588. Cross GAM: Eukaryotic protein modification and membrane attachment via phosphatidyl inositol. *Cell* **48**:179, 1987.
589. Low MG, Saltiel AR: Structural and functional roles of glycosylphosphatidylinositol in membranes. *Science* **239**:268, 1988.
590. Thomas JR, Dwek RA, Rademacher TW: Structure, biosynthesis, and function of glycosylphosphatidylinositols. *Biochemistry* **29**:5413, 1990.
590a. Brown DA: Interactions between GPI-anchored proteins and membrane lipids. *Trends Cell Biol* **2**:338, 1992.
591. Homans SW, Ferguson MAJ, Dwek RA, Rademacher TW, Anand R, Williams AF: Complete structure of the glycosyl phosphatidylinositol membrane anchor of rat brain Thy-1 glycoprotein. *Nature* **333**:269, 1988.
592. Homans SW, Edge CJ, Ferguson MAJ, Dwek RA, Rademacher TW: Solution structure of the glycosylphosphatidylinositol membrane anchor glycan of trypanosoma brucei variant surface glycoprotein. *Biochemistry* **28**:2881, 1989.
593. Bangs JD, Girald D, Krakow JL, Hart GW, Englund PT: Rapid processing of the carboxyl terminus of a trypanosome variant surface glycoprotein. *Proc Natl Acad Sci U S A* **82**:3207, 1985.
594. Caras IW, Weddell GN, Davitz MA, Nussenzweig V, Martin DW: Signal for the attachment of a phospholipid membrane anchor in Decay Accelerating Factor. *Science* **238**:1280, 1987.
595. Moran P, Caras IW: A nonfunctional sequence converted to a signal for glycophosphatidylinositol membrane anchor attachment. *J Cell Biol* **115**:329, 1991.
596. Micanovic R, Gerber LD, Berger J, Kodukula K, Udenfriend B: Selectivity of the cleavage/attachment site of phosphatidylinositol-glycan-anchored membrane proteins determined by site-specific mutagenesis at Asp-484 of placental alkaline phosphatase. *Proc Natl Acad Sci U S A* **87**:157, 1990.
597. Barthels D, Santoni M-J, Wille W, Ruppert C, Chaix J-C, Hirsch M-R, Fontecilla-Camps JC, Goridis C: Isolation and nucleotide sequence of mouse NCAM cDNA that codes for a Mr 79 000 polypeptide without a membrane-spanning region. *EMBO J* **6**:907, 1987.
598. Berger J, Micanovic R, Greenspan RJ, Udenfriend S: Conversion of placental akaline phosphatase from a phosphatidylinositol-glycan-anchored protein to an integral transmembrane protein. *Proc Natl Acad Sci U S A* **86**:1457, 1989.
599. Wallner BP, Frey AZ, Tizard R, Mattaliano RJ, Hession C, Sanders ME, Dustin ML, Springer TA: Primary structure of lymphocyte function-associated antigen 3 (LFA-3): The ligand of the T lymphocyte CD2 glycoprotein. *J Exp Med* **166**:923, 1987.
600. Rosse WF: Paroxysmal nocturnal hemoglobinuria: The biochemical defects and the clinical syndrome. *Blood Rev* **3**:192, 1989.
601. Takahashi M, Takeda J, Hirose S, Hyman R, Inoue N, Miyata T, Ueda E, Kitani T, Medof ME, Kinoshita T: Deficient biosynthesis of N-acetylglucosaminyl-phosphatidylinositol, the first intermediate of glycosyl phosphatidylinositol anchor biosynthesis, in cell lines established from patients with paroxysmal nocturnal hemoglobinuria. *J Exp Med* **177**:517, 1993.
602. Takeda J, Miyata T, Kawagoe K, Lida Y, Endo Y, Fujita T, Takahashi M, Kitani T, Kinoshita T: Deficiency of the GPI anchor caused by a somatic mutation of the PIG-A gene in paroxysmal nocturnal hemoglobinuria. *Cell* **73**:703, 1993.
603. Chow F-L, Hall SE, Rosse WF, Telen MJ: Separation of the acetylcholinesterase-deficient red cells in paroxysmal nocturnal hemoglobinuria. *Blood* **67**:893, 1986.
604. Medof ME, Gottlieb A, Kinoshita T, Hall S, Silber R, Nussenzweig V, Rosse WF: Relationship between decay acceleration factor deficiency, diminished acetyl cholinesterase activity, and defective terminal complement pathway restriction in paroxysmal nocturnal hemoglobinuria erythrocytes. *J Clin Invest* **80**:165, 1987.
605. Selvaraj P, Dustin ML, Silber R, Low MG, Springer TA: Deficiency of lymphocyte function-associated antigen 3 (LFA-3) in paroxysmal nocturnal hemoglobinuria. *J Exp Med* **166**:1011, 1987.
606. Selvaraj P, Rosse WF, Silber R, Springer TA: The major Fc receptor in blood has a phosphatidylinositol anchor and is deficient in paroxysmal nocturnal haemoglobinuria. *Nature* **333**:565, 1988.
607. Hyman R: Cell-surface-antigen mutants of haematopoietic cells. Tools to study differentiation, biosynthesis and function. *Biochem J* **225**:27, 1985.
608. Stefanova I, Horejsi V, Ansotegui IJ, Knapp W, Stockinger H: GPI-anchored cell-surface molecules complexed to protein tyroisine kinases. *Science* **254**:1016, 1991.
609. Brestcher MS, Thomson JN, Pearse BMF: Coated pits acts as molecular filters. *Proc Natl Acad Sci U S A* **77**:4156, 1980.
610. Rothberg KG, Ying Y, Kolhouse JF, Kamen BA, Anderson RGW: The glycophospholipid-linked folate receptor internalizes folate without entering the clathrin-coated pit endocytic pathway. *J Cell Biol* **110**:637, 1990.
611. Ying YS, Anderson RGW, Rothberg KG: Each caveola contains multiple glycosyl-phosphatidylinositol-anchored membrane proteins. *Cold Spring Harb Symp Quant Biol* **57**:593, 1992.
612. Lisanti MP, Sargiacomo M, Graeve L, Saltiel AR, Rodriguez-Boulan E: Polarized apical distribution of glycosyl-phosphatidylinositol-

anchored proteins in a renal epithelial cell line. *Proc Natl Acad Sci U S A* **85**:9557, 1988.
613. Lisanti MP, Le Bivic A, Saltiel AR, Rodriguez-Boulan E: Preferred apical distribution of glycosyl-phosphatidylinositol (GPI) anchored proteins: A highly conserved feature of the polarized epithelial cell phenotype. *J Membr Biol* **113**:155, 1990.
614. Lisanti MP, Caras IW, Davitz MA, Rodriguez-Boulan E: A glycophospholipid membrane anchor acts as an apical targeting signal in polarized epithelial cells. *J Cell Biol* **109**:2145, 1989.
615. Brown DA, Crise B, Rose JK: Mechanism of membrane anchoring affects polarized expression of two proteins in MDCK cells. *Science* **245**:1499, 1989.
616. Powell SK, Cunningham BA, Edelman GM, Rodriguez-Boulan E: Targeting of transmembrane and GPI-anchored forms of N-CAM to opposite domains of a polarized epithelial cell. *Nature* **353**:76, 1991.
617. Van Meer G, Burger KNJ: Sphingolipid trafficking — sorted out? *Trends Cell Biol* **2**:332, 1992.
618. Van't Hof W, Van Meer G: Generation of lipid polarity in intestinal epithelial (Caco-2) cells: Sphingolipid synthesis in the Golgi complex and sorting before vesicular traffic to the plasma membrane. *J Cell Biol* **111**:977, 1990.
619. Brown DA, Rose JK: Sorting of GPI-anchored proteins to glycolipid-enriched membrane subdomains during transport to the apical cell surface. *Cell* **68**:533, 1992.
620. Van Meer G, Simons K: Lipid polarity and sorting in epithelial cells. *J Cell Biochem* **36**:51, 1988.
621. Magee T, Newman C: The role of lipid anchors for small G proteins in membrane trafficking. *Trends Cell Biol* **2**:318, 1992.
622. Sinensky M, Lutz RJ: The prenylation of proteins. *Bioessays* **14**:25, 1992.
623. Seabra MC, Reiss Y, Casey PJ, Brown MS, Goldstein JL: Protein farnesyltransferase and geranylgeranyltransferase share a common α subunit. *Cell* **65**:429, 1991.
624. Reiss Y, Stradley SJ, Gierasch LM, Brown MS, Goldstein JL: Sequence requirement for peptide recognition by rat brain p21^{ras} protein farnesyltransferase. *Proc Natl Acad Sci U S A* **88**:732, 1991.
625. Hancock JF, Magee AI, Childs JE, Marshall CJ: All ras proteins are polyisoprenylated but only some are palmitoylated. *Cell* **57**:1167, 1989.
626. Horiuchi H, Kawata M, Katayama M, Yoshida Y, Musha T, Ando S, Takai Y: A novel prenyltransferase for a small GTP-binding protein having a C-terminal Cys-Ala-Cys structure. *J Biol Chem* **266**:16981, 1991.
627. Farnsworth CC, Kawata M, Yoshida Y, Takai Y, Gelb MH, Glomset JA: C terminus of the small GTP-binding protein smg p25A contain two geranylgeranylated cysteine residues and a methyl ester. *Proc Natl Acad Sci U S A* **88**:6196, 1991.
628. Sebra MC, Brown MS, Slaughter CA, Südhof TC, Goldstein JL: Purification of component A of Rab geranylgeranyl transferase: Possible identity with the choroideremia gene product. *Cell* **70**:1049, 1992.
629. Seabra MC, Goldstein JL, Sudhof TC, Brown MS: Rab geranylgeranyl transferase. *J Biol Chem* **267**:14497, 1992.
630. Andres DA, Seabra MC, Brown MS, Armstrong SA, Smeland TE, Cremers FPM, Goldstein JL: cDNA cloning of component A of rab geranylgeranyl transferase and demonstration of its role as a rab escort protein. *Cell* **73**:1091, 1993.
631. Seabra MC, Brown MS, Goldstein JL: Retinal degeneration in choroideremia: Deficiency of rab geranylgeranyl transferase. *Science* **259**:377, 1993.
632. Fodor E: Analysis of choroideraemia gene. *Nature* **351**:614, 1991.
633. Cremers FPM, Molloy CM, Van De Pol DJR, Van Den Hurk JAJM, Bach I, Geurts Van Kessel AHM, Ropers H-H: An autosomal homologue of the choroideremia gene colocalizes with the usher syndrome type II locus on the distal part of chromosome 1q. *Hum Mol Genet* **1**:71, 1992.
634. Hancock JF, Cadwallader K, Paterson H, Marshall CJ: A CAAX or a CAAL motif and a second signal are sufficient for plasma membrane targeting of ras proteins. *EMBO J* **10**:4033, 1991.
635. Cox AD, Hisaka MM, Buss JE, Der CJ: Specific isoprenoid modification is required for function of normal, but not oncogenic, ras protein. *Mol Cell Biol* **12**:2606, 1992.
636. Schlesinger MJ, Veit M, Schmidt MFG: Palmitoylation of cellular and viral proteins, in Schlesinger MJ (ed): *Lipid Modifications of Proteins*. Boca Raton, FL, CRC Press, 1993, p 1.
637. Olson EN: Structure, function and biosynthesis of fatty acid-acetylated proteins, in Strauss AW, Boime I, Kreil G (eds): *Protein Compartmentalization*. New York, Springer-Verlag, 1986, p 87.
638. McIlhinney RAJ: The fats of life: The importance and function of protein acylation. *TIBS* **15**:387, 1990.
639. Schlesinger MJ, Malfer C: Cerulenin blocks fatty acid acylation of glycoproteins and inhibits vesicular stomatitis and sindbis virus particle formation. *J Biol Chem* **257**:9887, 1982.
640. Schmidt MFG, Schlesinger MJ: Relation of fatty acid attachment to the translation and maturation of vesicular stomatitis and Sindbis virus membrane glycoproteins. *J Biol Chem* **255**:3334, 1980.
641. Berger M, Schmidt MFG: Protein fatty acyltransferase is located in the rough endoplasmic reticulum. *FEBS Lett* **187**:289, 1985.
642. Omari MB, Trowbridge IS: Biosynthesis of the human transferrin receptor in cultured cells. *J Biol Chem* **256**:12888, 1981.
643. O'Dowd BF, Hnatowich M, Caron MG, Lefkowitz RJ, Bouvier M: Palmitoylation of the human β2-adrenergic receptor. *J Biol Chem* **264**:7564, 1989.
644. Pillai S, Baltimore D: Myristylation and post-translational acquisition of hydrophobicity by the membrane immunoglobulin heavy chain polypeptide in B lymphocytes. *Proc Natl Acad Sci U S A* **84**:7654, 1987.
645. Hedo JA, Collier E, Watkinson A: Myristyl and palmityl acylation of the insulin receptor. *J Biol Chem* **262**:954, 1987.
646. Buss JE, Sefton BM: Direct identification of palmitic acid as the lipid attached to p21 ras. *Mol Cell Biol* **6**:116, 1986.
647. Willumsen BM, Norris K, Papageorge AG, Hubbert NL, Lowry DR: Harvey murine sarcoma virus p21^{ras} protein: Biological and biochemical significance of the cysteine nearest the carboxy terminus. *EMBO J* **3**:2581, 1984.
648. Staufenbiel M, Lazarides E: Ankyrin is fatty acid acylated in erythrocytes. *Proc Natl Acad Sci U S A* **83**:318, 1986.
649. Bennett V: The membrane skeleton of human erythrocytes and its implications for more complex cells. *Annu Rev Biochem* **54**:273, 1985.
650. De Duve C: Lysosomes revisited. *Eur J Biochem* **137**:391, 1983.
651. Helenius A, Mellman I, Wall D, Hubbard A: Endosomes. *Trends Biochem Sci* **8**:245, 1983.
652. Pastan IH, Willingham MC: Receptor-mediated endocytosis: Coated pits, receptosomes and the Golgi. *Trends Biochem Sci* **8**:250, 1983.
653. Dingle JT, Dean RT, Sly W: *Lysosomes in Biology and Pathology*. Amsterdam, Elsevier, 1984, vol 7.
654. Goldstein JL, Brown MS, Anderson RGW, Russell DW, Schneider WJ: Receptor-mediated endocytosis: Concepts emerging from the LDL receptor system. *Annu Rev Cell Biol* **1**:1, 1985.
655. Von Figura K, Hasilik A: Lysosomal enzymes and their receptors. *Annu Rev Biochem* **55**:167, 1986.
656. Kornfeld S, Mellman I: The biogenesis of lysosomes. *Annu Rev Cell Biol* **5**:482, 1989.
657. Pearse BMF, Robinson MS: Clathrin, adaptors, and sorting. *Annu Rev Cell Biol* **6**:151, 1990.
658. Anderson RGW: Molecular motors that shape endocytic membrane, in Steer CJ, Hanover JA (eds): *Intracellular Trafficking of Proteins*. Cambridge, Cambridge University Press, 1991, p 13.
659. Steer CJ, Heuser J: Clathrin and coated vesicles: Critical determinants of intracellular trafficking, in Steer CJ, Hanover J, eds: *Intracellular Trafficking of Proteins*. Cambridge, Cambridge University Press, 1991, p 157.
660. Maxfield FR, Yamashiro DJ: Aciditication of organelles and the intracellular sorting of proteins during endocytosis, in Steer CJ, Hanover JA (eds): *Intracellular Trafficking of Proteins*. Cambridge, Cambridge University Press, 1991, p 157.
661. Courtoy PJ: Dissection of endosomes, in Steer CJ, Hanover JA (eds): *Intracellular Trafficking of Proteins*. Cambridge, Cambridge University Press, 1991, p 103.
662. Kornfeld S: Structure and function of mannose-6-phosphate/insulin-like growth factor II receptors. *Annu Rev Biochem* **1**:307, 1992.
663. Holtzman E: *Lysosomes*. New York, Plenum, 1992.
663a. Robinson MS: Adaptins. *Trends Cell Biol* **2**:293, 1992.
664. Wang E, Michl J, Pfeffer LM, Silverstein SC, Tamm I: Interferon suppresses pinocytosis but stimulates phagocytosis in mouse peritoneal macrophages: Related changes in cytoskeletal organization. *J Cell Biol* **98**:1328, 1984.
665. Silverstein SC, Michl J, Sung S-SJ: Phagocytosis, in Silverstein SC (ed): *Transport of Macromolecules in Cellular Systems*. Berlin, Dahlem Konferenzen, 1978, p 245.

666. Pearse BMF: Clathrin: A unique protein associated with intracellular transport of membrane by coated vesicles. *Proc Natl Acad Sci U S A* **73**:1255, 1976.
667. Roth TF, Porter KR: Yolk protein uptake in the ooctye of the mosquito Aedes aegypti L. *J Cell Biol* **20**:313, 1964.
668. Schlesinger J: The mechanism and role of hormone-induced clustering of membrane receptors. *Trends Biochem Sci* **5**:210, 1980.
669. Dunn WA, Hubbard AL: Receptor-mediated endocytosis of epidermal growth factor by hepatocytes in the perfused rat liver: Ligand and receptor dynamics. *J Cell Biol* **98**:2148, 1984.
670. Anderson RGW, Brown MS, Beisiegel U, Goldstein JL: Surface distribution and recycling of the LDL receptor as visualized by anti-receptor antibodies. *J Cell Biol* **93**:523, 1982.
671. Vaux D: The structure of an endocytosis signal. *Trends Cell Biol* **2**:189, 1992.
672. Trowbridge IS: Endocytosis and signals for internalization. *Curr Opin Cell Biol* **3**:634, 1991.
673. Davis CG, Lehrman MA, Russel DW, Anderson RGW, Brown MS, Goldstein JL: The J.D. mutation in familiar hypercholesterolemia: Amino acid substitution on cytoplasmic domain impedes internalization of LDL receptors. *Cell* **45**:15, 1986.
674. Davis CG, van Driel IR, Russell DW, Brown MS, Goldstein JL: The low-density lipoprotein receptor. Identification of amino acids in cytoplasmic domain required for rapid endocytosis. *J Biol Chem* **262**:4075, 1987.
675. Chen W-J, Goldstein JL, Brown MS: NPXY, a sequence often found in cytoplasmic tails, is required for coated pit-mediated internalization of the low density lipoprotein receptor. *J Biol Chem* **265**:3116, 1990.
676. Canfield WM, Johnson KF, Ye RD, Gregory W, Kornfeld S: Localization of the signal for rapid internalization of the bovine cation-independent mannose-6-phosphate/insulin-like growth factor-II. *J Biol Chem* **266**:5682, 1991.
677. Johnson KF, Chan W, Kornfeld S: Cation-dependent mannose-6-phosphate receptor contains two internalization signals in its cytoplasmic domain. *Proc Nat Acad Sci U S A* **87**:10010, 1990.
678. Collawn JF, Stangel M, Kuhn LA, Esekogwu V, Jing S, Trowbridge IS, Tainer JA: Transferrin receptor internalization sequence YXRF implicates a tight turn as the structural recognition motif for endocytosis. *Cell* **63**:1061, 1990.
679. Peters C, Braun M, Weber B, Wendland M, Schmidt B, Pohlmann R, Waheed A, von Figura K: Targeting of a lysosomal membrane protein: A tyrosine-containing endocytosis signal in the cytoplasmic tail of lysosomal acid phosphatase is necessary and sufficient for targeting to lysosomes. *EMBO J* **9**:3497, 1990.
679a. Lehmann LE, Eberle W, Krull S, Prill V, Schmidt B, Sander C, von Figura K, Peters C: The internalization signal in the cytoplasmic tail of lysosomal acid phosphatase consists of the hexapeptide PBYRHV. *EMBO J* **11**:4391, 1992.
680. Collawn JF, Kuhn LA, Liu L-FS, Tainer JA, Trowbridge IS: Transplanted LDL and mannose-6-phosphate receptor internalization signals promote high-efficiency endocytosis of the transferrin receptor. *EMBO J* **10**:3247, 1991.
681. Bansal A, Gierasch LM: The NPXY internalization signal of the LDL receptor adopts a reverse-turn conformation. *Cell* **67**:1195, 1991.
682. Eberle W, Sander C, Klaus W, Schmidt B, von Figura K, Peters C: The essential tyrosine of the internalization signal in lysosomal acid phosphatase is part of a β turn. *Cell* **67**:1203, 1991.
683. Jadot M, Canfield WM, Gregory W, Kornfeld S: Characterization of the signal for rapid internalization of the bovine mannose-6-phosphate/insulin-like growth factor-II receptor. *J Biol Chem* **267**:11069, 1992.
684. Johnson KF, Kornfeld S: His-Leu-Leu sequence near the carboxyl terminus of the cytoplasmic domain of the cation-dependent mannose-6-phosphate receptor is necessary for the lysosomal enzyme sorting function. *J Biol Chem* **267**:17110, 1992.
685. Johnson KF, Kornfeld S: The cytoplasmic tail of the mannose-6-phosphate-insulin-like growth factor II receptor has two signals for lysosomal enzyme sorting in the Golgi. *J Cell Biol* **119**:249, 1992.
686. Keen JH, Willingham MC, Pastan IH: Clathrin-coated vesicles: Isolation, dissociation and factor-dependent reassociation of clathrin baskets. *Cell* **16**:303, 1979.
687. Robinson MS: 100-kD coated vesicle proteins: Molecular heterogeneity and intracellular distribution and factor-dependent reassociation of clathrin baskets. *J Cell Biol* **104**:887, 1987.
688. Ahle S, Mann A, Eichelsbacher U, Ungewickell E: Structural relationships between clathrin assembly proteins from the Golgi and the plasma membrane. *EMBO J* **7**:919, 1988.
689. Morris SA, Ahle S, Ungewickell E: Clathrin coated vesicles. *Curr Opin Cell Biol* **1**:684, 1989.
690. Vigers GPA, Crowther RA, Pearse BMF: Three-dimensional structure of clathrin cages in ice. *EMBO J* **5**:529, 1986.
691. Vigers GPA, Crowther RA, Pearse BMF: Location of 100 kD-50kD accessory proteins in clathrin coats. *EMBO J* **5**:279, 1986.
692. Glickman JN, Conibear E, Pearse BMF: Specificity of binding of clathrin adaptors to signals on the mannose-6-phosphate/insulin-like growth factor II receptor. *EMBO J* **8**:1041, 1989.
693. Lin HC, Moore MS, Sanan DA, Anderson RGW: Reconstitution of clathrin-coated pit binding from plasma membranes. *J Cell Biol* **114**:881, 1992.
694. Schlossman DM, Schmid SL, Braell WA, Rothman JE: An enzyme that removes clathrin coats: Purification of an uncoating ATPase. *J Cell Biol* **99**:723, 1984.
695. Schmid SL, Fuchs R, Male P, Mellman I: Two distinct subpopulations of endosomes involved in membrane recycling and transport to lysosomes. *Cell* **52**:73, 1988.
696. Tycko B, Maxfield FR: Rapid acidification of endocytic vesicles containing alpha-2-macroglobulin. *Cell* **228**:643, 1982.
697. Yamashiro DJ, Maxfield FR: Acidification of endocytic compartments and the intracellular pathways of ligands and receptors. *J Cell Biochem* **26**:231, 1984.
698. Di Paola M, Maxfield FR: Conformational changes in the receptors for epidermal growth factor and asialoglycoprotein induced by the mildly acidic pH found in endocytic vesicles. *J Biol Chem* **259**:9164, 1984.
699. Brown MS, Anderson RGW, Goldstein JL: Recycling receptors: The round trip itinerary of a migrant membrane protein. *Cell* **32**:663, 1983.
700. Geuze HJ, Slot JW, Strous GJAM, Lodish HF, Schwartz AL: Intracellular site of asialoglycoprotein receptor-ligand uncoupling: Double-label immunoelectron microscopy during receptor-mediated endocytosis. *Cell* **32**:277, 1983.
701. Geuze HJ, Slot JW, Strous GJAM, Peppard J, Von Figura K, Hasilik A, Schwartz AL: Intracellular receptor sorting during endocytosis: Comparative immunoelectronmicroscopy of multiple receptors in rat liver. *Cell* **37**:195, 1984.
702. Griffiths G, Gruenberg J: The arguments for preexisting early and late endosomes. *Trends Cell Biol* **1**:5, 1991.
703. Murphy RF: Maturation models for endosome and lysosome biogenesis. *Trends Cell Biol* **1**:77, 1991.
704. Brown WJ, Farquhar MG: The mannose-6-phosphate receptor for lysosomal enzymes is concentrated in cis Golgi cisternae. *Cell* **36**:295, 1984.
705. Griffiths G, Hoflack B, Simons K, Mellman I, Kornfeld S: The mannose 6-phosphate receptor and the biogenesis of lysosomes. *Cell* **52**:329, 1988.
706. Gruenberg J, Howell K: Membrane traffic in endocytosis: Insights from cell-free assays. *Annu Rev Cell Biol* **5**:453, 1989.
707. Bomsel M, Parton R, Kuznetsov SA, Schroer TA, Gruenberg J: Microtubule- and motor-dependent fusion in vitro between apical and basolateral endocytic vesicles from MDCK cells. *Cell* **62**:719, 1990.
708. Gorvel J-P, Chavrier P, Zerial M, Gruenberg J: rab5 controls early endosome fusion *in vitro*. *Cell* **64**:915, 1991.
709. Kornfeld S: Trafficking of lysosomal enzymes. *FASEB J* **1**:462, 1987.
710. Kornfeld S: Lysosomal enzyme targeting. *Biochem Soc Trans* **18**:367, 1990.
711. Von Figura K: Molecular recognition and targeting of lysosomal proteins. *Curr Opin Cell Biol* **3**:642, 1991.
711a. Gabel CA: Posttranslational processing and intracellular transport of newly synthesized lysosomal enzymes, in Loh YP (ed): *Mechanisms of Intracellular Trafficking and Processing of Proproteins*. Boca Raton, FL, CRC Press, 1993, p 103.
712. Erickson AH, Blobel G: Early events in the biosynthesis of the lysosomal enzyme cathepsin D. *J Biol Chem* **254**:1171, 1979.
713. Rosenfeld MG, Kreibich G, Popov D, Kato K, Sabatini DD: Biosynthesis of lysosomal hydrolases: Their synthesis in bound polysomes and the role of co- and post-translational processing in determining their subcellular distribution. *J Cell Biol* **93**:135, 1982.
714. Proia R, Neufeld EF: Synthesis of β-hexosaminidase in cell-free translation and in intact fibroblasts: An insoluble precursor alpha

chain in a rare form of Tay Sachs disease. *Proc Natl Acad Sci U S A* **79**:6360, 1982.

715. Erickson AH, Walter P, Blobel G: Translocation of a lysosomal enzyme across the microsomal membrane requires the signal recognition particle. *Biochem Biophys Res Commun* **115**:275, 1983.
716. Reitman ML, Kornfeld S: Lysosomal enzyme targeting. N-acetylglucosaminylphosphotransferase selectively phosphorylates native lysosomal enzymes. *J Biol Chem* **256**:11977, 1981.
717. Waheed A, Hasilik A, Von Figura K: UDP-N-acetylglucosamine: Lysosomal enzyme precursor N-acetylglucosamine-1-phosphotransferase: Partial purification and characterization of the rat liver Golgi enzyme. *J Biol Chem* **257**:12322, 1982.
718. Varki A, Kornfeld S: Identification of a rat liver alpha-N-acetylglucosaminyl phosphodiesterase capable of removing "blocking" alpha-N-acetylglucosamine residues from phosphorylated high mannose oligosaccharides of lysosomal enzymes. *J Biol Chem* **255**:8398, 1980.
719. Varki A, Kornfeld S: Purification and characterization of rat liver alpha-N-acetylglucosaminyl phosphodiesterase. *J Biol Chem* **256**:9937, 1981.
720. Waheed A, Hasilik A, Von Figura K: Processing of the phosphorylated recognition marker in lysosomal enzymes: Characterization and partial purification of the microsomal alpha-N-acetylglucosaminyl phosphodiesterase. *J Biol Chem* **256**:5717, 1981.
721. Hasilik A, Waheed A, Von Figura K: Enzymatic phosphorylation of lysosomal enzymes in the presence of UDP-N-acetylglucosamine. Absence of the activity in I-cell fibroblasts. *Biochem Biophys Res Commun* **98**:761, 1981.
722. Reitman ML, Varki A, Kornfeld S: Fibroblasts from patients with I-cell disease and pseudo-Hurler polydystrophy are deficient in uridine 5′-diphosphate-N-acetylglucosamine: Glycoprotien N-acetylglucosaminyl-phosphotransferase activities. *J Clin Invest* **67**:1574, 1981.
723. Varki AP, Reitman ML, Vannier A, Kornfeld S, Grubb JH, Sly WS: Demonstration of the heterozygous state of I-cell disease and pseudo-Hurler polydystrophy by assay of N-acetylglucosaminylphosphotransferase in white blood cells and fibroblasts. *Am J Hum Genet* **34**:717, 1982.
724. Mueller OT, Honey NK, Little LE, Miller AL, Shows TB: Mucolipidosis II and III. The genetic relationships between two disorders of lysosomal enzyme biosynthesis. *J Clin Invest* **72**:1016, 1983.
725. Lang L, Takahashi T, Tang J, Kornfeld S: Lysosomal enzyme phosphorylation in human fibroblasts: Kinetic parameters offer a biochemical rationale for two distinct defects in the UDP-GlcNAc: Lysosomal enzyme precursor N-acetylglucosamine 1-phosphotransferase. *J Clin Invest* **76**:2191, 1985.
726. Ben-Yoseph Y, Pack BA, Mitchell DA, Elwell DG, Potier M, Melancon SB, Nadler HL: Characterization of the mutant N-acetylglucosaminyl-phosphotransferase in I-cell disease and pseudo-Hurler polydystrophy. Complementation analysis and kinetic studies. *Enzyme* **35**:106, 1986.
727. Waheed A, Pohlman R, Hasilik A, Von Figura K, Van Elsen A, Leroy JG: Deficiency of UDP-N-acetylglucosamine: Lysosomal enzyme N-acetylglucosamine 1-phosphotransferase in organs of I-cell patients. *Biochem Biophys Res Commun* **105**:1052, 1982.
728. Varki AP, Reitman ML, Kornfeld S: Identification of a variant of mucolipidosis III (pseudo Hurler polydystrophy): A catalytically active N-acetylglucosaminylphosphotransferase that fails to phosphorylate lysosomal enzymes. *Proc Natl Acad Sci U S A* **78**:7773, 1981.
729. Lang L, Reitman ML, Tang J, Roberts RM, Kornfeld S: Lysosomal enzyme phosphorylation. Recognition of a protein-dependent determinant allows specific phosphorylation of oligosaccharides present on lysosomal enzymes. *J Biol Chem* **259**:14663, 1984.
730. Faust PL, Kornfeld S, Chirgwin JM: Cloning and sequence analysis of cDNA for human cathepsin D. *Proc Natl Acad Sci U S A* **82**:4910, 1985.
731. Fukushima H, De Wet J, O'Brien JS: Molecular cloning of a cDNA for human alpha-fucosidase. *Proc Natl Acad Sci U S A* **82**:1262, 1985.
732. Myerowitz R, Piekarz R, Neufeld EF, Shows TB, Susuki K: Human β-hexosaminidase alpha chain: Coding sequence and homology with β chain. *Proc Natl Acad Sci U S A* **82**:7830, 1985.
733. Bishop DF, Calhoun PH, Bernstein HS, Hantzopoulos P, Quinn M, Desnick RJ: Human alpha galactosidase A: Nucleotide sequence of a cDNA clone encoding the mature enzyme. *Proc Natl Acad Sci U S A* **83**:4859, 1986.
734. Chan SJ, Segundo BS, McCormick MB, Steiner DF: Nucleotide and predicted amino acid sequences of cloned human and mouse preprocathepsin B cDNAs. *Proc Natl Acad Sci U S A* **83**:772, 1986.
735. Fong D, Calhoun DH, Hsieh WT, Lee B, Wells RD: Isolation of a cDNA clone for the human lysosomal proteinase cathepsin D. *Proc Natl Acad Sci U S A* **83**:2909, 1986.
736. Nishimura Y, Rosenfeld MG, Kreibich G, Gubler V, Sabatini DD, Adesnik M, Andy R: Nucleotide sequence of rat preputial gland β-glucuronidase cDNA and in vitro insertion of its encoded polypeptide into microsomal membranes. *Proc Natl Acad Sci U S A* **83**:7292, 1986.
737. Oshima A, Kyle JW, Miller RD, Hoffmann JW, Powell PP, Grubb JH, Sly WS, Tropak M, Guise KS, Gravel RA: Cloning, sequencing, and expression of cDNA for human β-glucuronidase. *Proc Natl Acad Sci U S A* **89**:685, 1987.
738. Hasilik A, Klein U, Waheed A, Strecker G, Von Figura K: Phosphorylated oligosaccharides in lysosomal enzymes: Identification of alpha-N-acetylglucosamine (1) phospho (6) mannose diester groups. *Proc Natl Acad Sci U S A* **77**:7074, 1980.
739. Hasilik A, Von Figura K: Oligosaccharides in lysosomal enzymes: Distribution of high-mannose and complex oligosaccharides in cathepsin D and β-hexosaminidase. *Eur J Biochem* **121**:125, 1981.
740. Gieselman V, Pohlmann R, Hasilik A, Von Figura K: Biosynthesis and transport of cathepsin D in cultured human fibroblasts. *J Cell Biol* **97**:1, 1983.
741. Varki AP, Kornfeld S: The spectrum of anionic oligosaccharides released by endo-β-N-acetylglucosaminidase H from glycoproteins. Structural studies and interactions with the phosphomannosyl receptor. *J Biol Chem* **258**:2808, 1983.
742. Baranski TJ, Faust PL, Kornfeld S: Generation of a lysosomal enzyme targeting signal in the secretory protein pepsinogen. *Cell* **63**:281, 1990.
743. Baranski TJ, Koelsch B, Hartsuck JA, Kornfeld S: Mapping and molecular modeling of a recognition domain for lysosomal enzyme targeting. *J Biol Chem* **266**:23365, 1991.
744. Baranski TJ, Cantor AB, Kornfeld S: Lysosomal enzyme phosphorylation I. Protein recognition determinants in both lobes of procathepsin D mediates its interaction with UDP-GlcNAc:lysosomal enzyme N-acetylglucosamine-1-phosphotransferase. *J Biol Chem* **267**:23342, 1992.
745. Cantor AB, Kornfeld S: Phosphorylation of Asn-linked oligosaccharides located at novel sites on the lysosomal enzyme cathepsin D. *J Biol Chem* **267**:23357, 1992.
746. Cantor AB, Baranski TJ, Kornfeld B: Lysosomal enzyme phosphorylation. II. Protein recognition determinants in either lobe of procathepsin D are sufficient for phosphorylation of both the amino and carboxyl lobe oligosaccharides. *J Biol Chem* **267**:23349, 1992.
747. Hickmann S, Neufeld EF: A hypothesis for I-cell disease: Defective hydrolases that do not enter lysosomes. *Biochem Biophys Res Commun* **49**:992, 1972.
748. Zuhlsdorf M, Imort M, Hasilik A, Von Figura K: Molecular forms of β-hexosaminidase and cathepsin D in serum and urine of healthy subjects and patients with elevated activity of lysosomal enzymes. *Biochem J* **213**:733, 1983.
749. Erickson AH, Blobel G: Carboxyl-terminal proteolytic processing during biosynthesis of the lysosomal enzymes β-glucuronidase and cathepsin D. *Biochemistry* **22**:5201, 1983.
750. Hasilik A, Von Figura K: Processing of lysosomal enzymes in fibroblasts, in Dingle JT, Dean RT, Sly W (eds): *Lysosomes in Biology and Pathology.* Amsterdam, Elsevier, 1984, vol 7, p 3.
751. Von Figura K, Rey M, Prinz R, Voss B, Ullrich K: Effect of tunicamycin on transport of lysosomal enzymes in cultured skin fibroblasts. *Eur J Biochem* **101**:103, 1979.
752. Hasilik A, Neufeld EF: Biosynthesis of lysosomal enzymes in fibroblasts: Phosphorylation of mannose residues. *J Biol Chem* **255**:4946, 1980.
753. Wiesmann UN, Lightbody J, Vassella F, Herschkowitz NN: Multiple lysosomal enzyme deficiency due to enzyme leakage? *N Engl J Med* **284**:109, 1971.
754. Kaplan A, Achord DT, Sly WS: Phosphohexosyl components of a lysosomal enzyme are recognized by pinocytosis receptors on human fibroblasts. *Proc Natl Acad Sci U S A* **74**:2026, 1977.

755. Rome LH, Weissmann B, Neufeld EF: Direct demonstration of binding of a lysosomal enzyme, alpha-L-iduronidase, to receptors on cultured fibroblasts. *Proc Natl Acad Sci U S A* **76**:2331, 1979.
756. Fischer HD, Gonzalez-Noriega A, Sly WS: β-glucuronidase binding to human fibroblast membrane receptors. *J Biol Chem* **255**:5069, 1980.
757. Sly WS, Fischer HD: The phosphomannosyl recognition system for intracellular and intercellular transport of lysosomal enzymes. *J Cell Biochem* **18**:67, 1982.
758. Owada M, Neufeld EF: Is there a mechanism for introducing acid hydrolases into liver lysosomes that is independent of mannose 6-phosphate recognition? Evidence from I cell disease. *Biochem Biophys Res Commun* **105**:814, 1982.
759. Miller AL, Kress BC, Stein R, Kinnon C, Kern H, Schneider JA, Harms E: Properties of N-acetyl-β-D-hexosaminidase from isolated normal and I-cell lysosomes. *J Biol Chem* **256**:9352, 1981.
760. Lemansky P, Gieselmann V, Hasilik A, Von Figura K: Synthesis and transport of lysosomal acid phosphatase in normal and I-cell fibroblasts. *J Biol Chem* **260**:9023, 1985.
761. Rijnboutt S, Aerts HMFG, Geuze HJ, Tager JM, Strous GJ: Mannose 6-phosphate-independent membrane association of cathepsin D, glucocerebrosidase, and sphingolipid-activating protein in HepG2 cells. *J Biol Chem* **266**:4862, 1991.
762. Schwaiger M, Hasilik A, Von Figura K, Wiemken A, Tanner W: Carbohydrate-free carboxypeptidase Y is transferred into the lysosomal-like yeast vacuole. *Biochem Biophys Res Commun* **104**:950, 1982.
763. Johnson LM, Bankaitis VA, Emr SD: Distinct sequence determinants direct intracellular sorting and modification of a yeast vacuolar protease. *Cell* **48**:875, 1987.
764. Valls LA, Hunter CP, Rothman GH, Stevens TH: Protein sorting in yeast: The localization determinant of yeast vacuolar carboxypeptidase Y resides in the propeptide. *Cell* **48**:887, 1987.
765. Klionsky DJ, Herman PK, Emr SD: The fungal vacuole: Composition, function, and biogenesis. *Microbiol Rev* **54**:266, 1990.
766. Stack JH, Emr SD: Genetics and biochemical studies of protein sorting of the yeast vasicle. *Curr Opin Cell Biol* **5**:641, 1993.
767. Herman PK, Stack JH, Emr SD: An essential role for a protein and lipid kinase complex in secretory protein sorting. *Trends Cell Biol* **2**:363, 1992.
768. Pfeffer SR: Targeting of proteins to the lysosomes. *Curr Top Microbiol Immunol* **170**:43, 1991.
769. Sahagian GG, Distler J, Jourdian GW: Characterization of membrane-associated receptor from bovine liver that binds phosphomannosyl residues of bovine testicular β-galactosidase. *Proc Natl Acad Sci U S A* **78**:4289, 1981.
770. MacDonald RG, Pfeffer SR, Coussens L, Tepper MA, Brocklebank CM, Mole JE, Anderson JK, Chen E, Czech MP, Ullrich A: A single receptor binds both insulin-like growth factor II and mannose-6-phosphate. *Science* **239**:1134, 1988.
771. Willingham MC, Pastan IH, Sahagian GG, Jourdian GW, Neufeld EF: Morphologic study of the internalization of a lysosomal enzyme by the mannose-6-phosphate receptor in cultured chinese hamster ovary cells. *Proc Natl Acad Sci U S A* **78**:6967, 1981.
772. Brown WJ, Farquhar MG: Accumulation of coated vesicles bearing mannose 6-phosphate receptors for lysosomal enzymes in the Golgi region of I-cell fibroblasts. *Proc Natl Acad Sci U S A* **81**:5135, 1984.
773. Brown WJ, Constantinescu E, Farquhar MG: Redistribution of mannose-6-phosphate receptors induced by tunicamycin and chloroquine. *J Cell Biol* **99**:320, 1984.
774. Geuze HG, Slot JW, Strous GJAM, Hasilik A, Von Figura K: Ultrastructural localization of the mannose-6-phosphate receptor in rat liver. *J Cell Biol* **98**:2047, 1984.
775. Geuze HJ, Slot JW, Strous GJ, Luzio JP, Schwartz AL: A cycloheximide-resistant pool of receptors for asialoglycoproteins and mannose 6-phosphate residues in the Golgi complex of hepatocytes. *EMBO J* **3**:2677, 1984.
776. Geuze HJ, Slot JW, Strous GJAM, Hasilik A, Von Figura K: Possible pathways for lysosomal enzyme delivery. *J Cell Biol* **101**:2253, 1985.
777. Pfeffer SR: Mannose 6-phosphate receptors and their role in targeting proteins to lysosomes. *J Membr Biol* **103**:7, 1988.
778. Brown WJ, Goodhouse J, Farquhar MG: Mannose-6-phosphate receptor for lysosomal enzymes cycle between the Golgi complex and endosomes. *J Cell Biol* **103**:1235, 1986.
779. Lobel P, Dahms NM, Breitmeyer J, Chirgwin JM, Kornfeld S: Cloning of the bovine 215-kDa cation-independent mannose 6-phosphate receptor. *Proc Natl Acad Sci U S A* **84**:2233, 1987.
780. Sahagian GG, Steer CJ: Transmembrane orientation of the mannose-6-phosphate receptor in isolated clathrin-coated vesicles. *J Biol Chem* **260**:9838, 1985.
781. Kyle JW, Nolan CM, Oshima A, Sly WS: Expression of human cation-independent mannose 6-phosphate receptor cDNA in receptor-negative mouse P388D1, cells following gene transfer. *J Biol Chem* **263**:16230, 1988.
782. Lobel P, Fujimoto K, Ye RO, Griffiths B, Kornfeld S: Mutations in the cytoplasmic domain of the 275 kd mannose 6-phosphate receptor differentially alter lysosomal enzyme sorting and endocytosis. *Cell* **57**:787, 1989.
783. Hoflack B, Kornfeld S: Purification and characterization of a cation-dependent mannose 6-phosphate receptor from murine P388D1 macrophages and bovine liver. *J Biol Chem* **260**:12008, 1985.
784. Hoflack B, Fujimoto K, Kornfeld S: The interaction of phosphorylated oligosaccharides and lysosomal enzymes with bovine liver cation-dependent mannose-6-phosphate receptor. *J Biol Chem* **262**:123, 1987.
785. Dahms NM, Lobel P, Breitmeyer J, Chirgwin JM, Kornfeld S: 46 kD mannose 6-phosphate receptor: Cloning, expression, and homology to the 215 kD mannose 6-phosphate receptor. *Cell* **50**:181, 1987.
786. Pohlmann R, Nagel G, Schmidt B, Stein M, Lorkowski G, Krentler C, Cully J, Meyer HE, Grzeschik K-H, Mersmann G, Hasilik A, Von Figura K: Cloning of a cDNA encoding the human cation-dependent mannose 6-phosphate-specific receptor. *Proc Natl Acad Sci U S A* **84**:5575, 1987.
786a. Ma Z, Grubb JH, Sly WS: Cloning sequencing, and functional characterization of the murine 46-kDa mannose 6-phosphate receptor. *J Biol Chem* **266**:10589, 1991.
787. Hoflack B, Kornfeld S: Lysosomal enzyme binding to mouse $P388D_1$ macrophage membranes lacking the 215-kDa mannose 6-phosphate receptor: Evidence for the existence of a second mannose 6-phosphate receptor. *Proc Natl Acad Sci U S A* **82**:4428, 1985.
788. Watanabe H, Grubb JH, Sly WS: The overexpressed human 46-kDa mannose 6-phosphate receptor mediates endocytosis and sorting of β-glucuronidase. *Proc Natl Acad Sci U S A* **87**:8036, 1990.
789. Fischer HD, Creek KE, Sly WS: Binding of phosphorylated oligosaccharides to immobilized phosphomannosyl receptors. *J Biol Chem* **257**:9938, 1982.
790. Chao HH-J, Waheed A, Pohlmann R, Hille A, von Figura K: Mannose 6-phosphate receptor dependent secretion of lysosomal enzymes. *EMBO J* **9**:3507, 1990.
791. Natowicz M, Hallett DW, Frier C, Chi M, Schlesinger PH, Baenziger JU: Recognition and receptor-mediated uptake of phosphorylated high mannose-type oligosaccharides by cultured human fibroblasts. *J Cell Biol* **96**:915, 1983.
792. Talkad V, Sly WS: Human β-glucuronidase pinocytosis and binding to the immobilized phosphomannosyl receptor: Effects of treatment of the enzyme with alpha-N-acetylglucosaminyl phosphodiesterase. *J Biol Chem* **258**:7345, 1983.
793. Gabel CA, Costello CE, Reinhold VN, Kurz L, Kornfeld S: Identification of methylphosphomannosyl residues as components of the high mannose oliosaccharides of *Dictyostelium discoideum* glycoproteins. *J Biol Chem* **259**:13762, 1984.
794. Brown WJ, Farquhar MG: The distribution of 215-kilodalton mannose 6-phosphate receptors within cis (heavy) and trans (light) Golgi subfractions varies in different cell types. *Proc Natl Acad Sci U S A* **84**:9001, 1987.
795. Griffiths B, Hoflack B, Simons K, Mellman I, Kornfeld S: The mannose 6-phosphate receptor and the biogenesis of lysosomes. *Cell* **52**:329, 1988.
796. Bleekemolen JE, Stein M, Von Figura K, Slot JW, Geuze HJ: The two mannose 6-phosphate receptors have almost identical subcellular distributions in U937 monocytes. *Eur J Cell Biol* **47**:366, 1988.
797. Matovcik LM, Goodhouse J, Farquhar MG: The recycling itinerary of the 46 kDa mannose 6-phosphate receptor—Golgi to late endosomes—coincides with that of the 215 kDa M6PR. *Eur J Cell Biol* **53**:203, 1990.
798. Campbell CH, Rome LH: Coated vesicles from rat liver and calf brain contain lysosomal enzyme bound to mannose 6-phosphate receptors. *J Biol Chem* **258**:13347, 1983.
799. Schulze-Lohoff E, Hasilik A, Von Figura K: Cathepsin D precursor in clathrin-coated organelles form human fibroblasts. *J Cell Biol* **101**:824, 1985.

800. Lemansky P, Hasilik A, Von Figura K, Helmy S, Fishman J, Fine RE, Kedersha NL, Rome LH: Lysosomal enzyme precursors in coated vesicles derived from the exocytic and endocytic pathways. *J Cell Biol* **104**:1743, 1987.
801. Geuze HJ, Stoorvogel W, Storus GJ, Slot JW, Bleekemolen JE, Mellman I: Sorting of mannose 6-phosphate receptors and lysosomal membrane proteins in endocytic vesicles. *J Cell Biol* **107**:2491, 1988.
802. Croze E, Ivan IE, Kreibich G, Adesnik M, Sabatini DD, Rosenfeld M: Endolyn-78, a membrane glycoprotein present in morphologically diverse components of the endosomal and lysosomal compartments: Implications for lysosome biogenesis. *J Cell Biol* **108**:1597, 1989.
803. Pfeffer SR: The endosomal concentration of a mannose-6-phosphate receptor is unchanged in the absence of ligand synthesis. *J Cell Biol* **105**:229, 1987.
804. Braulke T, Gartung C, Hasilik A, Von Figura K: Is movement of mannose 6-phosphate-specific receptor triggered by binding of lysosomal enzymes? *J Cell Biol* **104**:1735, 1987.
805. Gonzalez-Noriega A, Grubb JH, Talkad V, Sly WS: Chloroquine inhibits lysosomal enzyme pinocytosis and enhances lysosomal enzyme secretion by impairing receptor recycling. *J Cell Biol* **85**:839, 1980.
806. Duncan JR, Kornfeld S: Intracellular movement of two mannose 6-phosphate receptors: Return to the Golgi apparatus. *J Cell Biol* **106**:617, 1988.
807. Migeon BR, Sprenkle JA, Libaers I, Scott JF, Neufeld EF: X-linked Hunter syndrome: The heterozygous phenotype in cell culture. *Am J Hum Genet* **29**:448, 1977.
808. Lloyd JB, Forster S: The lysosomal membrane. *Trends Biochem Sci* **11**:129, 1986.
809. Fukuda M: Lysosomal membrane glycoproteins: Structure, biosynthesis, and intracellular trafficking. *J Biol Chem* **266**:21327, 1991.
810. Brown MS, Goldstein JL: Receptor-mediated control of cholesterol metabolism. *Science* **191**:150, 1976.
811. Youngdahl-Turner P, Mellman IS, Allen RH, Rosenberg LE: Protein-mediated vitamin uptake. Adsorptive endocytosis of the transcobalamin II-cobalamin complex by cultured human fibroblasts. *Exp Cell Res* **118**:127, 1979.
812. Rosenblatt DS, Hosack A, Matiaszuk NV, Cooper BA, LaFramboise R: Defect in vitamin B_{12} release from lysosomes: Newly described inborn error of vitamin B_{12} metabolism. *Science* **228**:1319, 1985.
813. Gahl WA, Bashan N, Tietze F, Bernardini I, Schulman JD: Cystine transport is defective in isolated leukocyte lysosomes from patients with cystinosis. *Science* **217**:1263, 1982.
814. Gahl WA, Tietze F, Bashan N, Steinherz R, Schulman JD: Defective cystine exodus from isolated lysosome-rich fractions of cystinotic leucocytes. *J Biol Chem* **257**:9570, 1982.
815. Jonas AJ, Greene AA, Smith ML, Schneider JA: Cystine accumulation and loss in normal, heterozygous, and cystinotic fibroblasts. *Proc Natl Acad Sci U S A* **79**:4442, 1982.
816. Jonas AJ, Smith ML, Allison WS, Laikind PK, Greene AA, Schneider JA: Proton-translocating ATPase and lysosomal cystine transport. *J Biol Chem* **258**:11727, 1983.
817. Gahl WA, Tietze F, Bashan N, Bernardini I, Raiford D, Schulman JD: Characteristics of cystine counter-transport in normal and cystinotic lysosome-rich leukocyte granular fractions. *Biochem J* **216**:393, 1983.
818. Jonas AJ, Symons LJ, Speller RJ: Polyamines stimulate lysosomal cystine transport. *J Biol Chem* **262**:16391, 1987.
819. Pisoni RL, Thoene JG, Christensen HN: Detection and characterization of carrier-mediated cationic amino acid transport in lysosomes of normal and cystinotic human fibroblasts. *J Biol Chem* **260**:4791, 1985.
820. Pisoni RL, Thoene JG, Lemons RM, Christensen HN: Important differences in cationic amino acid transport by lysosomal system c and system y^+ of the human fibroblast. *J Biol Chem* **262**:15011, 1987.
821. Pisoni RL, Flickinger KS, Thoene JG, Christensen HN: Characterization of carrier-mediated transport systems for small neutral amino acids in human fibroblast lysosomes. *J Biol Chem* **262**:6010, 1987.
822. Bernar J, Tietze F, Kohn LD, Bernardini I, Harper GS, Grollman EF, Gahl WA: Characteristics of a lysosomal membrane transport system for tyrosine and other neutral amino acids in rat thyroid cells. *J Biol Chem* **261**:17107, 1986.
823. Thoene JG, Oshima RG, Crawhall JC, Olson DL, Schneider JA: Intracellular cystine depletion by aminothiols in vitro and in vivo. *J Clin Invest* **58**:180, 1976.
824. Renlund M, Kovanen PT, Ravio KO, Oula P, Gahmberg CG, Ehnholm C: Studies on the defect underlying the lysosomal storage of sialic acid in Salla disease. *J Clin Invest* **77**:568, 1986.
825. Renlund M, Titze F, Gahl WA: Defective sialic acid egress from isolated fibroblast lysosomes of patients with Salla disease. *Science* **232**:759, 1986.
826. Bame KJ, Rome LH: Acetyl coenzyme A: Alpha-glucosaminide N-acetyltransferase. Evidence for a transmembrane acetylation mechanism. *J Biol Chem* **260**:11293, 1985.
827. Klein U, Kresse H, Von Figura K: Sanfilippo syndrome type C: Deficiency of acetyl-CoA: Alpha-glucosaminide N-acetyltransferase in skin fibroblasts. *Proc Natl Acad Sci U S A* **75**:5185, 1978.
828. Reeves JP: The mechanism of lysosomal acidification, in Dingle JT, Dean RT, Sly WS (eds): *Lysosomes in Biology and Pathology.* Amsterdam, Elsevier, 1984, vol 7, p 175.
829. Mellman I, Fuchs R, Helenius A: Acidification of the endocytic and exocytic pathways. *Annu Rev Biochem* **55**:663, 1986.
830. Ohkuma S, Moriyama Y, Takano T: Identification and characterization of a proton pump in lysosomes by fluorescein isothiocyanate-dextran fluorescence. *Proc Natl Acad Sci U S A* **79**:2758, 1982.
831. Harikumar P, Reeves JP: The lysosomal proton pump is electrogenic. *J Biol Chem* **258**:10403, 1983.
832. D'Souza MP, Ambudker SV, August JT, Maloney PC: Reconstitution of the lysosomal proton pump. *Proc Natl Acad Sci U S A* **84**:6980, 1987.
832a. Rees-Jones R, Al-Awqati Q: Proton-translocating adenosinetriphosphatase in rough and smooth microsomes from rat liver. *Biochemistry* **23**:2236, 1984.
833. Rudnick G: ATP-driven H^+ pumping into intracellular organelles. *Annu Rev Physiol* **48**:403, 1986.
834. Bowman EJ, Siebers A, Altendorf K: Bafilomycins: A class of inhibitors of membrane ATPases from microorganisms, animal cells, and plant cells. *Proc Natl Acad Sci U S A* **85**:7972, 1988.
835. Reijngoud D-J, Tager JM: The permeability of the lysosomal membrane. *Biochim Biophys Acta* **272**:419, 1977.
836. Mehrabian M, Bame KJ, Rome LH: Interaction of rat liver lysosomal membranes with actin. *J Cell Biol* **99**:680, 1984.
837. Collot M, Louvard D, Singer SJ: Lysosomes are associated with microtubules and not with intermediate filaments in cultured fibroblasts. *Proc Natl Acad Sci U S A* **81**:788, 1984.
838. Mithieux G, Rousset B: Identification of a lysosome membrane protein which could mediate ATP-dependent stable association of lysosomes to microtubules. *J Biol Chem* **265**:4664, 1989.
839. Burnside J, Schneider DL: Characterization of the membrane proteins of rat liver lysosomes. Composition, enzyme activities and turnover. *Biochem J* **204**:525, 1982.
840. Ohsumi Y, Ishikawa T, Kato M: A rapid and simplified method for the preparation of lysosomal membranes from rat liver. *J Biochem* **93**:547, 1982.
841. Carlsson SR, Roth J, Piller F, Fukuda M: Isolation and characterization of human lysosomal membrane glycoproteins, h-lamp-1 and h-lamp-2. *J Biol Chem* **263**:18911, 1988.
842. Chen JW, Murphy TL, Willingham MC, Pastan I, August JT: Identification of two lysosomal membrane glycoproteins. *J Cell Biol* **101**:85, 1985.
843. Chen JW, Pan W, D'Souza MP, August JT: Lysosome-associated membrane proteins: Characterization of LAMP-1 of macrophage P388 and mouse embryo 3T3 cultured cells. *Arch Biochem Biophys* **239**:574, 1985.
844. Lewis V, Green JA, Marsh M, Vihko P, Helenius A, Mellman I: Glycoproteins of the lysosomal membrane. *J Cell Biol* **100**:1839, 1985.
845. Lippincott-Schwartz J, Fambrough DM: Lysosomal membrane dynamics: Structure and interorganellar movement of a major lysosomal membrane glycoprotein. *J Cell Biol* **102**:1593, 1986.
846. Lippincott-Schwartz J, Fambrough DM: Cycling of the integral membrane glycoprotein, LEP100, between plasma membrane and lysosomes: Kinetic and morphological analysis. *Cell* **49**:669, 1987.
847. Barriocanal JG, Bonifacino JS, Yuan L, Sandoval IV: Biosynthesis, glycosylation, movement through the Golgi system, and transport to lysosomes by an N-linked carbohydrate-independent mechanism of three lysosomal integral membrane proteins. *J Biol Chem* **261**:16755, 1986.
848. Moriyama Y, Takano T, Ohkuma S: Acridine orange as a fluorescent probe for lysosomal proton pump. *J Biochem (Tokyo)* **92**:1333, 1982.

849. Fukuda M: Cell surface glycoconjugates as onco-differentiation markers in hematopoietic cells. *Biochim Biophys Acta* **780**:119, 1985.

849a. D'Souza MP, August JT: A kinetic analysis of biosynthesis and localization of a lysosome-associated membrane glycoprotein. *Arch Biochem Biophys* **249**:522, 1986.

850. Granger BL, Green SA, Gabel CA, Howe CL, Mellman I, Helenius A: Characterization and cloning of Igp110, a lysosomal membrane glycoprotein from mouse and rat cells. *J Biol Chem* **265**:12036, 1990.

851. Erickson AH, Ginns EI, Barranger JA: Biosynthesis of the lysosomal enzyme glucocerebrosidase. *J Biol Chem* **260**:14319, 1985.

852. Williams MA, Fukuda M: Accumulation of membrane glycoproteins in lysosomes requires a tyrosine residue at a particular position in the cytoplasmic tail. *J Cell Biol* **111**:955, 1990.

853. Hunziker W, Harter C, Matter K, Mellman I: Basolateral sorting in MDCK cells requires a distinct cytoplasmic domain determinant. *Cell* **66**:907, 1991.

854. Mathews PM, Martinie JB, Fambrough DM: The pathway and targeting signal for delivery of the integral membrane glycoprotein LEP100 to lysosomes. *J Cell Biol* **118**:1027, 1992.

855. Harter C, Mellman I: Transport of the lysosomal membrane glycoprotein Igp120 (Igp-A) to lysosomes does not require appearance on the plasma membrane. *J Cell Biol* **117**:311, 1992.

856. Waheed A, Gottschalk S, Hille A, Krentler C, Pohlmann R, Braulke T, Hauser H, Geuze H, von Figura K: Human lysosomal acid phosphatase is transported as a transmembrane protein to lysosomes in transfected baby hamster kidney cells. *EMBO J* **7**:2351, 1981.

857. Braun M, Waheed A, Von Figura K: Lysosomal acid phosphatase is transported to lysosomes via the cell surface. *EMBO J* **8**:3633, 1989.

858. Nabi IR, Le Bivic A, Fambrough D, Rodriguez-Boulan E: An endogenous MDCK lysosomal membrane glycoprotein is targeted basolaterally before delivery to lysosomes. *J Cell Biol* **115**:1573, 1991.

859. Green SA, Zimmer K-P, Griffiths G, Mellman I: Kinetics of intracellular transport and sorting of lysosomal membrane and plasma membrane proteins. *J Cell Biol* **105**:1227, 1987.

860. Carlsson SR, Fukuda M: The lysosomal membrane glycoprotein lamp-1 is transported to lysosomes by two alternative pathways. *Arch Biochem Biophys* **296**:630, 1992.

861. Anderson RGW, Kamen BA, Rothberg KG, Lacey SW: Potocytosis: Sequestration and transport of small molecules by caveolae. *Science* **255**:410, 1992.

862. Anderson RGW: Potocytosis of small molecules and ions by caveolae. *Trends Cell Biol* **3**:69, 1993.

863. Van Deurs B, Holm PK, Sandvig K, Hansen SH: Are caveolae involved in clathrin-independent endocytosis? *Trends Cell Biol* **3**:249, 1993.

864. Anderson RGW: Plasmalemmal caveolae and GPI anchored membrane proteins. *Curr Opin Cell Biol* **5**:647, 1993.

865. Rothberg KG, Heuser JE, Donzell WC, Ying YS, Gienney JR, Anderson RG: Caveolin, a protein component of caveolae membrane coats. *Cell* **68**:673, 1992.

866. Simionescu N: Cellular aspects of transcapillary exchange. *Physiol Rev* **63**:1536, 1983.

867. Heltianu C, Dobrula L, Anthoe F, Simionescu M: Evidence for thyroxine transport by the lung and heart capillary endothelium. *Microvasc Res* **37**:188, 1989.

868. Chang W-J, Rothberg KG, Kamen BA, Anderson RGW: Lowering the cholesterol content of MA104 all inhibits receptor-mediated transport of folate. *J Cell Biol* **118**:63, 1992.

869. Glenney JR: The sequence of human caveolin reveals identity with VIP21, a component of transport vesicles. *FEBS Lett* **314**:45, 1992.

870. Kurzchalia TV, Dupree P, Parton RG, Kellner R, Virta H, Lehnert M, Simons K: VIP21, a 21-kD membrane protein is an integral component of Trans-Golgi-Network-Derived transport vesicles. *J Cell Biol* **118**:1003, 1992.

870a. Hatefi Y: The mitochondrial electron transport and oxidative phosphorylation system. *Annu Rev Biochem* **54**:1015, 1985.

871. Attardi G, Schatz G: Biogenesis of mitochondria. *Annu Rev Cell Biol* **4**:289, 1988.

872. Pfanner N, Neupert W: The mitochondrial protein import apparatus. *Annu Rev Biochem* **59**:331, 1990.

873. Douglas MG, Smagula CS, Chen W-J: Mitochondrial import of proteins, in Steer CJ, Hanover JA (eds): *Intracellular Trafficking of Proteins*. Cambridge, Cambridge University Press, 1991, p 658.

874. Glick B, Wachter C, Schatz G: Protein import into mitochondria: Two systems acting in tandem? *Trends Cell Biol* **1**:99, 1991.

875. Glick B, Schatz G: Import of proteins into mitochondria. *Annu Rev Genet* **25**:21, 1991.

876. Wallace DC: Diseases of the mitochondrial DNA. *Annu Rev Biochem* **61**:1175, 1992.

877. Wienhues U, Neupert W: Protein translocation across mitochondrial membranes. *Bioessays* **14**:17, 1992.

878. Pfanner N, Rassow J, van der Klei IJ, Neupert W: A dynamic model of the mitochondrial protein import machinery. *Cell* **68**:999, 1992.

879. Bolotin-Fukuhara M, Grivell LA: Genetic approaches to the study of mitochondrial biogenesis in yeast. *Antonie Van Leeuwenhoek* **62**:131, 1992.

880. Glick BS, Beasley EM, Schatz G: Protein sorting in mitochondria. *TIBS* **17**:453, 1992.

881. Kellems R, Allison V, Butow R: Cytoplasmic type 80S ribosomes associated with yeast mitochondria. II. Evidence for the association of cytoplasmic ribosomes with the outer mitochondrial membrane in situ. *J Biol Chem* **249**:3297, 1974.

882. Kellems RE, Allison VF, Butow RA: Cytoplasmic type 80S ribosomes associated with yeast mitochondria. IV. Attachment of ribosomes to the outer membrane of isolated mitochondria. *J Cell Biol* **65**:1, 1975.

883. Schleyer M, Neupert W: Transport of proteins into mitochondria: Translocational intermediates spanning contact sites between outer and inner membranes. *Cell* **43**:339, 1985.

884. Schwaiger M, Herzog V, Neupert W: Characterization of translocation contact sites involved in the import of mitochondrial protein. *J Cell Biol* **105**:235, 1987.

885. Vestweber D, Schatz G: A chimeric mitochondrial precursor protein with internal disulfide bridges blocks import of authentic precursors into mitochondria and allows quantitation of import sites. *J Cell Biol* **107**:2037, 1988.

886. Rassow J, Guiard B, Wienhues U, Herzog V, Hartl F-U, Neupert W: Translocation arrest by reversible folding of a precursor protein imported into mitochondria. A means to quantitate translocation contact sites. *J Cell Biol* **109**:1421, 1989.

887. Pon L, Moll T, Vestweber D, Marshallsay B, Schatz G: Protein import into mitochondria: ATP-dependent protein translocation activity in a submitochondrial fraction enriched in membrane contact sites and specific proteins. *J Cell Biol* **109**:2603, 1989.

888. Benz R: Porin from bacterial and mitochondrial outer membranes. *CRC Crit Rev Biochem* **19**:145, 1985.

889. Anderson S, Bankier AT, Barrell BG, De Bruijn MHL, Coulson AR, Drouin J, Eperon IC, Nierlich DP, Roe BA, Sanger SF, Schreir PH, Smith AJH, Staden R, Young IG: Sequence and organization of the human mitochondrial genome. *Nature* **290**:457, 1981.

890. Bohni P, Daum G, Schatz G: Import of proteins into mitochondria. Partial purification of a matrix-located protease involved in cleavage of mitochondrial precursor polypeptides. *J Biol Chem* **258**:4937, 1983.

891. Yaffe MP, Ohta S, Schatz G: A yeast mutant temperature-sensitive for mitochondrial assembly is deficient in a mitochondrial protease activity that cleaves imported precursor polypeptides. *EMBO J* **4**:2069, 1985.

892. Van Loon APGM, Brandli AW, Schatz G: The presequences of two imported mitochondrial proteins contain information for intracellular and intramitochondrial sorting. *Cell* **44**:801, 1986.

893. Hurt EC, Muller U, Schatz G: The first twelve amino acids of a yeast mitochondrial outer membrane protein can direct a nuclear-encoded cytochrome oxidase subunit to the mitochondrial inner membrane. *EMBO J* **4**:3509, 1985.

894. Van Loon APGM, Brandli AW, Pesolt-Hurt B, Blank D, Schatz G: Transport of proteins to the mitochondrial intermembrane space: The "matrix-targeting" and the "sorting" domain in the cytochrome c1 presequence. *EMBO J* **6**:2433, 1987.

895. Van Loon APGm, Schatz G: Transport of protein to the mitochondrial inter-membrane space: The "sorting" domain of the cytochrome c_1 presequence is a stop-transfer sequence specific for the mitochondrial inner membrane. *EMBO J* **6**:2441, 1987.

896. Mihara K, Sato R: Molecular cloning and sequencing of cDNA for yeast porin, an outer mitochondrial membrane protein: A search for targeting signal in the primary structure. *EMBO J* **4**:769, 1985.

897. Hase T, Muller U, Riesman H, Schatz G: A 70-kd protein of the yeast mitochondrial outer membrane is targeted and anchored via its extreme amino terminus. *EMBO J* **3**:3157, 1984.

898. Hines V, Brandt A, Griffiths G, Horstmann H, Brutsch H, Schatz G: Protein import into yeast mitochondria is accelerated by the outer membrane protein MAS70. *EMBO J* **9**:3191, 1990.

899. Steger HF, Sollner T, Kiebler M, Dietmeier KA, Pfaller R, Trulzsch KS, Tropschug M, Neupert W, Pfanner N: Import of ADP/ATP carrier into mitochondria: Two receptors act in parallel. *J Cell Biol* **111**:2353, 1990.

900. Zimmerman R, Paluch U, Neupert W: Cell-free synthesis of cytochrome c. *FEBS Lett* **108**:141, 1979.

901. Matsuura A, Arpin M, Hammum E, Margoliash E, Sabatini DD, Morimoto T: *In vitro* synthesis and posttranslational uptake of cytochrome c into apocytochrome *c*. *Proc Natl Acad Sci U S A* **78**:4368, 1981.

902. Adrian GS, McCammon MT, Montgomery DL, Douglas MG: Sequences required for delivery and localization of the ADP/ATP translocator to the mitochondrial inner membrane. *Mol Cell Biol* **6**:626, 1986.

903. Gasser S, Schatz G: Import of proteins into mitochondria. In vitro studies on the biogenesis of the outer membrane. *J Biol Chem* **258**:3427, 1983.

904. Zimmermann R, Hennig B, Neupert W: Different transport pathways of individual precursor proteins in mitochondria. *Eur J Biochem* **116**:455, 1981.

905. Mihara K, Blobel G, Sato R: In vitro synthesis and integration into mitochondria of porin, a major protein of the outer mitochondrial membrane of *Saccharomyces cerevisiae*. *Proc Natl Acad Sci U S A* **79**:7102, 1982.

906. Frietag H, Janes M, Neupert W: Biosynthesis of mitochondrial porin and insertion into the outer mitochondrial membrane of *Neurospora crassa*. *Eur J Biochem* **126**:197, 1982.

907. Zwizinski C, Schleyer M, Neupert W: Transfer of proteins into mitochondria. Precursor to the ADP/ATP carrier binds to receptor sites on isolated mitochondria. *J Biol Chem* **258**:4071, 1983.

908. Nelson N, Schatz G: Energy-dependent processing of cytoplasmically made precursors to mitochondrial proteins. *Proc Natl Acad Sci U S A* **76**:4365, 1979.

909. Zimmerman R, Neupert W: Transport of proteins into mitochondria. Posttranslational transfer of ADP/ATP carrier into mitochondria in vitro. *Eur J Biochem* **109**:217, 1980.

910. Schleyer M, Schmidt B, Neupert W: Requirement of a membrane potential for the posttranslational transfer of proteins into mitochondria. *Eur J Biochem* **125**:109, 1982.

910a. Reid GA, Schatz G: Import of proteins into mitrochondria. Yeast cells grown in the presence of carbonyl cyanide m-chlorophenylhydrazone accumulate massive amounts of some mitochondrial precursor polypeptides. *J Biol Chem* **257**:13056, 1982.

911. Roise D, Schatz G: Mitochondrial presequences. *J Biol Chem* **263**:4509, 1988.

912. Von Heijne G: Mitochondrial targeting sequences may form amphiphilic helices. *EMBO J* **5**:1335, 1986.

913. Roise D, Horvath SJ, Tomich JM, Richards JH, Schatz G: A chemically synthesized pre-sequence of an imported mitochondrial protein can form an amphiphilic helix and perturb natural and artificial phospholipid bilayers. *EMBO J* **5**:1327, 1986.

914. Hurt EC, Pesold-Hurt B, Schatz G: The amino-terminal region of an imported mitochondrial precursor polypeptide can direct cytoplasmic dihydrofolate reductase into the mitochondrial matrix. *EMBO J* **3**:3149, 1984.

915. Hurt EC, Pesold-Hurt B, Suda K, Oppliger W, Schatz G: The first twelve amino acids (less than half of the pre-sequence) of an imported mitochondrial protein can direct mouse cytosolic dihydrofolate reductase into the yeast mitochondrial matrix. *EMBO J* **4**:2061, 1985.

916. Horwich AL, Kalousek F, Mellman I, Rosenberg LE: A leader peptide is sufficient to direct mitochondrial import of a chimeric protein. *EMBO J* **4**:1129, 1985.

917. Horwich AL, Kalousek F, Fenton WA, Pollock RA, Rosenberg LE: Targeting of pre-ornithine transcarbamylase to mitochondria: Definition of critical regions and residues in the leader peptide. *Cell* **44**:451, 1986.

918. Keng T, Alani E, Guarente L: The nine amino-terminal residues of delta-aminolevulinate synthase direct β-galactosidase into the mitochondrial matrix. *Mol Cell Biol* **6**:355, 1986.

919. Fenton WA, Hack AM, Kraus JP, Rosenberg LE: Immunochemical studies of fibroblasts from patients with methymalonyl-CoA mutase apoenzyme deficiency: Detection of a mutation interfering with mitochondrial import. *Proc Natl Acad Sci U S A* **84**:1421, 1987.

920. Horwich AL, Kalousek F, Fenton WA, Furtak K, Pollock RA, Rosenberg LE: The ornithine transcarbamylase leader peptide directs mitochondrial import through both its midportion structure and net positive charge. *J Cell Biol* **105**:669, 1987.

921. Hurt EC, Schatz G: A cytosolic protein contains a cryptic mitochondrial targeting signal. *Nature* **325**:499, 1987.

922. Nicholson DW, Hergersberg C, Neupert W: Role of cytochrome c heme lyase in the import of cytochrome c into mitochondria. *J Biol Chem* **263**:19034, 1988.

923. Hay R, Bohni P, Gasser S: How mitochondria import proteins. *Biochim Biophys Acta* **779**:65, 1984.

924. Korb H, Neupert W: Biogenesis of cytochrome c in Neurospora crassa. Synthesis of apocytochrome c, transfer to mitochondria and conversion to holocytochrome c. *Eur J Biochem* **91**:609, 1978.

925. Zwizinski C, Schleyer M, Neupert W: Proteinaceous receptors for the import of mitochondrial precursors. *J Biol Chem* **259**:7850, 1984.

926. Hennig B, Koehler H, Neupert W: Receptor sites involved in posttranslational transport of apocytochrome c into mitochondria: Specificity, affinity, and number of sites. *Proc Natl Acad Sci U S A* **80**:4963, 1983.

927. Suissa M, Schatz G: Import of proteins into mitochondria. Translatable mRNAs for imported mitochondrial proteins are present in free as well as mitochondria-bound cytoplasmic polysomes. *J Biol Chem* **257**:13048, 1982.

928. Riezman H, Hay R, Witte C, Nelson N, Schatz G: Yeast mitochondrial outer membrane specifically binds cytoplasmically-synthesized precursors of mitochondrial proteins. *EMBO J* **2**:1113, 1983.

929. Gillespie LL, Argan C, Taneja AT, hodges RS, Freeman KB, Shore GC: A synthetic signal peptide blocks import of precursor proteins destined for the mitochondrial inner membrane or matrix. *J Biol Chem* **260**:16045, 1985.

930. Pfaller R, Neupert W: High-affinity binding sites involved in the import of porin into mitochondria. *EMBO J* **6**:2635, 1987.

931. Pfaller R, Steger HF, Rassow J, Pfanner N, Neupert W: Import pathways of precursor proteins into mitochondria: Multiple receptor sites are followed by a common membrane insertion site. *J Cell Biol* **107**:2483, 1988.

932. Söllner T, Pfaller R, Griffiths G, Pfanner N, Neupert W: A mitochondrial import receptor for the ADP/ATP carrier. *Cell* **62**:107, 1990.

933. Riezman H, Hase T, Van Loon APGM, Grivell LA, Suda K, Schatz G: Import of proteins into mitochondria: A 70 kilodalton outer membrane protein with a large carboxy-terminal deletion is still tranported to the outer membrane. *EMBO J* **2**:2161, 1983.

934. Söllner T, Griffiths G, Pfaller R, Pfanner N, Neupert W: MOM19, an import receptor for mitochondrial precursor proteins. *Cell* **59**:1061, 1989.

935. Pain D, Murakami H, Blobel G: Identification of a receptor for protein import into mitochondria. *Nature* **347**:444, 1990.

936. Meyer DI: Mimics—or gimmicks? *Nature* **347**:424, 1990.

937. Pfanner N, Rassow J, Guiard B, Söllner T, Hartl F-U, Neupert W: Energy requirements for unfolding and membrane translocation of precursor proteins during import into mitochondria. *J Biol Chem* **265**:16324, 1990.

938. Pfanner N, Hartl F-U, Guiard B, Neupert W: Mitochondrial precursor proteins are imported through a hydrophilic membrane environment. *Eur J Biochem* **169**:289, 1987.

939. Vestweber D, Brunner J, Baker A, Schatz G: A 42K outer-membrane protein is a component of the yeast mitochondrial protein import site. *Nature* **341**:205, 1989.

940. Baker KP, Schaniel A, Vestweber D, Schatz G: A yeast mitochondrial outer membrane protein essential for protein import and cell viability. *Nature* **348**:605, 1990.

941. Kiebler M, Pfaller R, Sollner T, Griffiths G, Horstmann H, Pfanner N, Neupert W: Identification of a mitochondrial receptor complex required for recognition and membrane insertion of precursor protein. *Nature* **348**:610, 1990.

942. Eilers M, Hwang S, Schatz G: Unfolding and refolding of a purified precursor protein during import into isolated mitochondria. *EMBO J* **7**:1139, 1988.

943. Hwang ST, Schatz G: Translocation of proteins across the mitochondrial inner membrane, but not into the outer membrane, requires nucleoside triphosphates in the matrix. *Proc Natl Acad Sci U S A* **86**:8432, 1989.

944. Kang P-J, Ostermann J, Shilling J, Neupert W, Craig EA, Pfanner N: Requirement for hsp70 in the mitochondrial matrix for translocation and folding of precursor proteins. *Nature* **348**:137, 1990.
945. Neupert W, Hartl F-U, Craig EA, Pfanner N: How do polypeptides cross the mitochondrial membranes. *Cell* **63**:447, 1990.
946. Scherer PE, Krieg UC, Hwang ST, Vestweber D, Schatz G: A precursor protein partly translocated into yeast mitochondria is bound to a 70 kd mitochondrial stress protein. *EMBO J* **9**:4315, 1990.
947. Gasser SM, Daum G, Schatz G: Import of proteins into mitochondria. *J Biol Chem* **257**:13034, 1982.
948. Kolansky DM, Conboy JG, Fenton WA, Rosenberg LE: Energy-dependent translocation of the precursor of ornithine transcarbamylase by isolated rat liver mitochondria. *J Biol Chem* **257**:8467, 1982.
949. Hwang S, Jascur T, Vestweber D, Pon L, Schatz G: Disrupted yeast mitochondria can import precursor proteins directly through their inner membrane. *J Cell Biol* **109**:487, 1989.
950. Ohba M, Schatz G: Disruption of the outer membrane restores protein import to trypsin-treated yeast mitochondria. *EMBO J* **6**:2117, 1987.
951. Lill R, Stuart RA, Drygas ME, Nargang FE, Neupert W: Import of cytochrome c heme lyase into mitochondria: A novel pathway into the intermembrane space. *EMBO J* **11**:449, 1992.
952. Rassow J, Pfanner N: Mitochondrial preproteins en route from the outer membrane to the inner membrane are exposed to the intermembrane space. *FEBS Lett* **293**:85, 1991.
953. Eilers M, Schatz G: Binding of a specific ligand inhibits import of a purified precursor protein into mitochondria. *Nature* **322**:228, 1986.
954. Chen W-J, Douglas MG: Phosphodiester bond cleavage outside mitochondria is required for the completion of protein import into the mitochondrial matrix. *Cell* **49**:651, 1987.
955. Eilers M, Oppliger W, Schatz G: Both ATP and an energized inner membrane are required to import a purified precursor protein into mitochondria. *EMBO J* **6**:1073, 1987.
956. Pfanner N, Tropschug M, Neupert W: Mitochondrial protein import: Nucleoside triphosphates are involved in conferring import-competence to precursors. *Cell* **49**:815, 1987.
957. Verner K, Schatz G: Import of an incompletely folded precursor protein into isolated mitochondria requires an energized inner membrane, but no added ATP. *EMBO J* **6**:2449, 1987.
958. Pfanner N, Pfaller R, Kleene R, Ito M, Tropschug M, Neupert W: Role of mitochondrial protein import. *J Biol Chem* **263**:4049, 1988.
959. Ostermann J, Horwich AL, Neupert W, Hartl F-U: Protein folding in mitochondria requires complex formation with hsp60 and ATP hydrolysis. *Nature* **341**:125, 1989.
960. Murakami K, Mori M: Purified presequence binding factor (PBF) forms an import-competent complex with a purified mitochondrial precursor protein. *EMBO J* **9**:3201, 1990.
961. Ono H, Tuboi S: Purification and identification of a cytosolic factor required for import of precursors of mitochondrial proteins into mitochondria. *Arch Biochem Biophys* **280**:299, 1990.
962. Cheng MY, Hartl F-U, Martin J, Pollock RA, Kalousek F, Neupert W, Hallberg EM, Hallberg RL, Horwich A: Mitochondrial heat-shock protein hsp60 is essential for assembly of proteins imported into yeast mitochondria. *Nature* **337**:620, 1989.
963. Cheng MY, Hartl F-U, Horwich AL: The mitochondrial chaperonin hsp60 is required for its own assembly. *Nature* **348**:455, 1990.
964. Hartman DJ, Hoogenraad NJ, Condron R, Høj PB: Identification of a mammalian 10-kDa heat shock protein, a mitochondrial chaperonin 10 homologue essential for assisted folding of trimeric ornithine transcarbamoylase in vitro. *Proc Natl Acad Sci U S A* **89**:3394, 1992.
965. Yang M, Geli V, Oppliger W, Suda K, James P, Schatz G: The MAS-encoded processing protease of yeast mitochondria. *J Biol Chem* **266**:6416, 1991.
966. Hendrick JP, Hodges PE, Rosenberg LE: Survey of amino-terminal proteolytic cleavage sites in mitochondrial precursor proteins: Leader peptides cleaved by two matrix proteases share a three-amino acid motif. *Proc Natl Acad Sci U S A* **86**:4056, 1989.
967. Hawlitschek G, Schneider H, Schmidt B, Tropschug M, Hartl F-U, Neupert W: Mitochondrial protein import: Identification of processing peptidase and of PEP, a processing enhancing protein. *Cell* **53**:795, 1988.
968. Ou W-J, Okazaki H, Omura T: Purification and characterization of a processing protease from rat liver mitochondria. *EMBO J* **8**:2605, 1989.
969. Yang M, Jensen RE, Yaffe MP, Oppliger W, Schatz G: Import of proteins into yeast mitochondria: The purified matrix processing protease contains two subunits which are encoded by the nuclear MAS1 and MAS2 genes. *EMBO J* **7**:3857, 1988.
970. Stuart RA, Lill R, Neupert W: Sorting out mitochondrial proteins. *Trends Cell Biol* **3**:135, 1993.
971. Schneider H, Arretz M, Wachter E, Neupert W: Matrix processing peptidase of mitochondria. *J Biol Chem* **265**:9881, 1990.
972. Yang M, Geli V, Oppliger W, Suda K, James P, Schatz G: The MAS-encoded processing protease of yeast mitochondria. *J Biol Chem* **266**:6416, 1991.
973. Schulte U, Arretz M, Schneider H, Tropschug M, Wachter E, Neupert W, Weiss H: A family of mitochondrial proteins involved in bioenergetics and biogenesis. *Nature* **339**:147, 1989.
974. Kalousek F, Hendrick JP, Rosenberg LE: Two mitochondrial matrix proteases act sequentially in the processing of mammalian matrix enzymes. *Proc Natl Acad Sci U S A* **85**:7536, 1988.
975. Schneider H, Sollner T, Dietmeier K, Eckerskorn C, Lottspeich F, Trulzsch B, Neupert W, Pfanner N: Targeting of the master receptor MOM19 to mitochondria. *Science* **254**:1659, 1991.
976. Nakai M, Hase T, Matsubara H: Precise determination of the mitochondrial import signal contained in a 70 kDa protein of yeast mitochondrial outer membrane. *J Biochem* **105**:513, 1989.
977. Zhaung Z, McCauley R: Ubiquitin is involved in the in vitro insertion of monoamine oxidase B into mitochondrial outer membranes. *J Biol Chem* **264**:14594, 1989.
978. Rechsteiner M: Ubiquitin-mediated pathways for intracellular proteolysis. *Annu Rev Cell Biol* **3**:1, 1987.
979. Stuart RA, Neupert W: Apocytochrome c: An exceptional mitochondrial precursor protein using an exceptional import pathway. *Biochimie* **72**:115, 1990.
980. Dumont ME, Richards FM: Insertion of Apocytochrome c into lipid vesicles. *J Biol Chem* **259**:4147, 1984.
981. Nicolson DN, Neupert W: Import of cytochrome c into mitochondria: Reduction of heme, mediated by NADH and flavin nucleotides, is obligatory for its covalent linkage to apocytochrome c. *Proc Natl Acad Sci U S A* **86**:4340, 1989.
982. Dumont ME, Ernst JF, Sherman F: Coupling of heme attachment to import of cytochrome c into yeast mitochondria. *J Biol Chem* **263**:15928, 1988.
983. Hartl F-U, Schmidt B, Wachter E, Weiss H, Neupert W: Transport into mitochondria and intramitochondrial sorting of the Fe/S protein of ubiquinol-cytochrome c reductase. *Cell* **47**:939, 1986.
984. Kaput J, Goltz S, Blobel G: Nucleotide sequence of the yeast nuclear gene for cytochrome c peroxidase precursor. Functional implications of the pre sequence for protein transport into mitochondria. *J Biol Chem* **257**:15054, 1982.
985. Schwarz E, Seytter T, Guiard B, Neupert W: Targeting of cytochrome b2 into the mitochondrial intermembrane space: Specific recognition of the sorting signal. *EMBO J* **12**:2295, 1993.
986. Guiard B: Structure, expression and regulation of a nuclear gene encoding a mitochondrial protein: The yeast L(+)-lactate cytochrome c oxido-reductase (cytochrome b_2). *EMBO J* **3**:3157, 1985.
987. Sadler I, Suda K, Schatz G, Kaudewitz F, Haid A: Sequencing of the nuclear gene for the yeast cytochrome c_1 precursor reveals an unusually complex amino-terminal presequence. *EMBO J* **3**:2137, 1984.
988. Reid GA Yonetani T, Schatz G: Import of proteins into mitochondria. Import and maturation of the mitochondrial intermembrane space enzymes cytochrome b2 and cytochrome c peroxidase in intact yeast cells. *J Biol Chem* **257**:13068, 1982.
989. Daum G, Gasser SM, Schatz G: Import of proteins into mitochondria. Energy-dependent, two-step processing of the intermembrane space enzyme cytochrome b_2 by isolated yeast mitochondria. *J Biol Chem* **257**:13075, 1982.
990. Ohashi A, Gibson J, Gregor R, Schatz G: Import of proteins into mitochondria. The precursor of cytochrome c_1 is processed in two steps, one of them heme dependent. *J Biol Chem* **257**:13042, 1982.
991. Schneider A, Behrens M, Scherer P, Pratje E, Michaelis G, Schatz G: Inner membrane protease I, an enzyme mediating intramitochondrial protein sorting in yeast. *EMBO J* **10**:247, 1991.
992. Behrens M, Michaelis G, Pratje E: Mitochondrial inner membrane protease 1 of Saccharomyces cerevisiae shows sequence similarity to the *Escherichia coli* leader peptidase. *Mol Genet* **228**:167, 1991.
993. Hartl F-U, Ostermann J, Guiard B, Neupert W: Successive translocation into and out of the mitochondrial matrix: Targeting of proteins to the intermembrane space by a bipartite signal peptide. *Cell* **51**:1027, 1987.

994. Mahlke K, Pfanner N, Martin J, Horwich AL, Hartl F-U, Neupert W: Sorting pathways of mitochondrial inner membrane proteins. *Eur J Biochem* **192**:551, 1990.
995. Li Y, Leonard K, Weiss H: Membrane-bound and water-soluble cytochrome c_1 from Neurospora mitochondria. *Eur J Biochem* **116**:199, 1981.
996. Zwizinski C, Neupert W: Precursor proteins are transported into mitochondria in the absence of proteolytic cleavage of the additional sequences. *J Biol Chem* **258**:13340, 1983.
997. Viebrock A, Perz A, Sebald W: The imported preprotein of the proteolipid subunit of the mitochondrial ATP synthase from *Neurospora crassa*. Molecular cloning and sequencing of the mRNA. *EMBO J* **5**:565, 1982.
998. Klingenberg M: Molecular aspects of the adenine nucleotide carrier from mitochondria. *Arch Biochem Biophys* **270**:1, 1989.
999. Smagula C, Douglas MG: Mitochondrial import of the ADP/ATP carrier protein in Saccharomyces cerevisiae. *J Biol Chem* **263**:6783, 1988.
1000. Pfanner N, Neupert W: Distinct steps in the import of ADP/ATP carrier into mitochondria. *J Biol Chem* **262**:7528, 1987.
1001. De Duve C, Baudhuin P: Peroxisomes (microbodies and related particles). *Physiol Rev* **46**:323, 1966.
1002. Tolbert NE: Metabolic pathways in peroxisomes and glyoxysomes. *Annu Rev Biochem* **50**:133, 1981.
1003. Kindl H: The biosynthesis of microbodies (peroxisomes, glyoxysomes). *Int Rev Cytol* **80**:193, 1982.
1004. Kindl H, Lazarow PB (eds): Peroxisomes and glyoxysomes. *Ann N Y Acad Sci* **386**:1, 1982.
1005. Borst P: Animal peroxisomes (microbodies), lipid biosynthesis and the Zellweger syndrome. *Trends Biochem* **8**:269, 1983.
1006. Lazarow PB, Fujiki Y: Biogenesis of peroxisomes. *Annu Rev Cell Biol* **1**:489, 1985.
1007. Lazarow PB: The role of peroxisomes in mammalian cellular metabolism. *J Inherit Metab Dis* **10(Suppl)**:11, 1987.
1008. Van Den Bosch H, Schutgens RB, Wanders RJ, Tager JM: Biochemistry of peroxisomes. *Annu Rev Biochem* **61**:157, 1992.
1009. De Hoop MJ, Holtman WL, Ab B: Import of proteins into peroxisomes and other microbodies. *Biochem J* **286**:647, 1992.
1010. Subramani S: Targeting of proteins into the peroxisomal matrix. *J Membr Biol* **125**:99, 1992.
1010a. Lazarow PB: Genetic approaches to studying peroxisome biogenesis. *Trends Cell Biol* **3**:89, 1993.
1011. Novikoff PM, Novikoff AB: Peroxisomes in absorptive cells of mammalian small intestine. *J Cell Biol* **53**:532, 1972.
1012. Novikoff PM, Novikoff AB, Quintana N, Davis C: Studies on microperoxisomes. III. Observations on human and rat hepatocytes. *J Histochem Cytochem* **21**:540, 1973.
1013. Gorgas K: Peroxisomes in sebaceous glands. V. Complex peroxisomes in the mouse preputial gland: Serial sectioning and three-dimensional reconstruction studies. *Anat Embryol* **169**:261, 1984.
1014. Lazarow PB, Shio H, Robbi M: Biogenesis of peroxisomes and the peroxisome reticulum hypothesis, in Bucher T, Sebald W, Weiss H (eds): *Biological Chemistry of Organelle Formation,* 31st Colloquium der Gesellschaft für Biologische Chemie in Mosbach/Baden. New York, Springer-Verlag, 1980, p 187.
1015. Leighton F, Poole B, Beaufay H, Baudhuin P, Coffey JW, Fowler S, De Duve C: The large-scale separation of peroxisomes, mitochondria, and lysosomes from the livers of rats injected with Triton WR-1339: Improved isolation procedures, automated analysis, biochemical and morphological properties of fractions. *J Cell Biol* **37**:482, 1968.
1016. Wattiaux R, Wattiaux-De Coninck S, Ronveaux-Dupal MF, Dubois F: Isolation of rat liver lysosomes by isopycnic centrifugation in a metrizamide gradient. *J Cell Biol* **78**:349, 1978.
1017. Bronfman M, Inestrosa NC, Leighton F: Fatty acid oxidation by human liver peroxisomes. *Biochem Biophys Res Commun* **88**:1030, 1979.
1018. Wanders RJA, Von Roermund CWT, Van Wijland MJA, Chutgens RBH, Heikoop J, Van Den Bosch H, Schram AW, Tager JM: Peroxisomal fatty acid β-oxidation in relation to the accumulation of very long chain fatty acids in cultured skin fibroblasts form patients with Zellweger syndrome and other peroxisomal disorders. *J Clin Invest* **80**:1778, 1987.
1019. Singh H, Derwas N, Poulos A: Very long chain fatty acid β-oxidation by rat liver mitochondria and peroxisomes. *Arch Biochem Biophys* **259**:382, 1987.
1020. Wanders RJA, Van Roermund CWT, Van Wijland MJA, Schutgens RBH, Van Den Bosch H, Schram AW, Tager JM: Direct demonstration that the deficient oxidation of very long chain fatty acids in X-linked adrenoleukodystrophy is due to an impaired ability of peroxisomes to activate very long chain fatty acids. *Biochem Biophys Res Commun* **153**:618, 1988.
1021. Lazo O, Contreras M, Hashmi M, Stanley W, Irazu C, Singh I: Peroxisomal lignoceroyl-CoA ligase deficiency in childhood adrenoleukodystrophy and adrenomyeloneuropathy. *Proc Natl Acad Sci U S A* **85**:7647, 1988.
1022. Lazarow PB, De Duve C: A fatty acyl-CoA oxidizing system in rat liver peroxisomes; enhancement by clofibrate, a hypolipidemic drug. *Proc Natl Acad Sci U S A* **73**:2043, 1976.
1023. Svoboda DJ, Azarnoff DL: Response of hepatic microbodies to a hypolipidemic agent, ethyl chlorophenoxyisobutyrate (CPIB). *J Cell Biol* **30**:442, 1966.
1024. Lazarow PB: Rat liver peroxisomes catalyze the β-oxidation of fatty acids. *J Biol Chem* **253**:1522, 1978.
1025. Hashimoto T: Individual peroxisomal β-oxidation enzymes. *Ann N Y Acad Sci* **386**:5, 1982.
1026. Osumi T, Ishii N, Miyazawa S, Hashimoto T: Isolation and structural characterization of the rat acyl-CoA oxidase gene. *J Biol Chem* **262**:8138, 1987.
1027. Hijikata M, Jin-Kun W, Osumi T, Hashimoto T: Rat peroxisomal 3-ketoacyl-CoA thiolase gene. *J Biol Chem* **265**:4600, 1990.
1028. Farrell SO, Bieber LL: Carnitine octanoyltransferase of mouse liver peroxisomes: Properties and effect of hypolipidemic drugs. *Arch Biochem Biophys* **222**:123, 1983.
1029. Clayton PT: Inborn errors of bile acid metabolism. *J Inherit Metab Dis* **14**:478, 1991.
1030. Bjorkhem I, Kase BF, Pedersen JI: Role of peroxisomes in the biosynthesis of bile acids. *Scand J Clin Lab Invest* **177**:23, 1985.
1031. Kase BF, Prydz K, Bjorkhem I, Pedersen JI: In vitro formation of bile acids from di- and trihydroxy-5β-cholestanoic acid in human liver peroxisomes. *Biochim Biophys Acta* **877**:37, 1986.
1032. Goldfischer S, Moore CL, Johnson AB, Spiro AJ, Valsamis MP, Wisniewski HK, Ritch RH, Norton WT, Rapin I, Gartner LM: Peroxisomal and mitochondrial defects in the cerebro-hepato-renal syndrome. *Science* **182**:62, 1973.
1033. Hajra AK, Bishop JE: Glycerolipid biosynthesis in peroxisomes via the acyldihydroxyacetone phosphate pathway. *Ann N Y Acad Sci* **386**:170, 1982.
1034. Lazarow PB, Black V, Shio H, Fujiki Y, Hajra AK, Datta NS, Bangaru B, Dancis J: Zellweger syndrome: Biochemical and morphological studies on two patients treated with clofibrate. *J Pediatr Res* **19**:1356, 1985.
1035. Schram AW, Strijland A, Hashimoto T, Wanders RJA, Schutgens RBH, Van Den Bosch H, Tager JM: Biosynthesis and maturation of peroxisomal β-oxidation enzymes in fibroblasts in relation to the Zellweger syndrome and infantile Refsum disease. *Proc Natl Acad Sci U S A* **83**:6158, 1986.
1036. Datta NS, Wilson GN, Hajra AK: Deficiency of enzymes catalyzing the biosynthesis of glycerol-ether lipids in Zellweger syndrome. A new category of metabolic disease involving the absence of peroxisomes. *N Engl J Med* **17**:1080, 1984.
1037. Danpure CJ, Jennings PR: Alanine:glyoxylate and serine:pyruvate aminotransferases in primary hyperoxaluria type 1. *Biochem Soc Trans* **14**:1059, 1986.
1038. Oda T, Funai T, Ichiyama A: Generation from a single gene of two mRNAs that encode the mitochondrial and peroxisomal serine:pyruvate aminotransferase of rat liver. *J Biol Chem* **265**:7513, 1990.
1039. Danpure CJ, Cooper PJ, Wise PJ, Jennings PR: An enzyme trafficking defect in two patients with primary hyperoxaluria type I: Peroxisomal alanine/glyoxylate aminotransferase rerouted to mitochondria. *J Cell Biol* **108**:1345, 1989.
1040. Purdue PE, Takada Y, Danpure CJ: Identification of mutations associated with peroxisome-to-mitochondria mistargeting of alanine-glyoxylate aminotransferase in primary hyperoxaluria type I. *J Cell Biol* **111**:2341, 1990.
1041. Keller GA, Barton MC, Shapiro DJ, Singer SJ: 3-Hydroxy-3-methylglutaryl coenzyme A reductase is present in peroxisomes in normal rat liver cells. *Proc Natl Acad Sci U S A* **82**:770, 1985.
1042. Keller GA, Pazirandeh M, Krisans S: 3-Hydroxy-methylglutaryl coenzyme A reductase localization in rat liver peroxisomes and microsomes of control and cholestyramine-treated animals: Quantitative biochemical and immunoelectron microscopical analyses. *J Cell Biol* **103**:875, 1986.

1043. Redman CM, Grab DJ, Irukulla R: The intracellular pathway of newly formed rat liver catalase. *Arch Biochem Biophys* **152**:496, 1972.

1044. Lazarow PB, De Duve C: The synthesis and turnover of rat liver peroxisomes. V. Intracellular pathway of catalase synthesis. *J Cell Biol* **59**:507, 1973.

1045. Goldman BM, Blobel G: Biogenesis of peroxisomes: Intracellular site of synthesis of catalase and uricase. *Proc Natl Acad Sci U S A* **75**:5066, 1978.

1046. Rachubinski RA, Fujiki Y, Mortensen RM, Lazarow PB: Acyl-CoA oxidase and hydratase-dehydrogenase, two enzymes of the peroxisomal β-oxidation system, are synthesized on free polysomes of clofibrate-treated rat liver. *J Cell Biol* **99**:2241, 1984.

1047. Miura S, Mori M, Takiguchi M, Tatibana M, Furuta S, Miyazawa S, Hashimoto T: Biosynthesis and intracellular transport of enzymes of peroxisomal β-oxidation. *J Biol Chem* **259**:6397, 1984.

1048. Fujiki Y, Rachubinski RA, Mortensen RM, Lazarow PB: Synthesis of 3-ketoacyl-CoA thiolase of rat liver peroxisomes on free polyribosomes as a larger precursor. Induction of thiolase mRNA activity by clofibrate. *Biochem J* **226**:697, 1985.

1049. Fujiki Y, Lazarow PB: Post-translational import of fatty acyl-CoA oxidase and catalase into peroxisomes of rat liver in vitro. *J Biol Chem* **260**:5603, 1985.

1050. Fujiki Y, Kasuya I, Mori H: Import of a 22-kDa peroxisomal integral membrane protein into peroxisomes in vitro. *Agric Biol Chem* **53**:591, 1989.

1051. Imanaka T, Small GM, Lazarow PB: Translocation of acyl-CoA oxidase into peroxisomes requires ATP hydrolysis but not a membrane potential. *J Cell Biol* **105**:2915, 1987.

1052. Bellion E, Goodman JM: Proton ionophores prevent assembly of a peroxisomal protein. *Cell* **48**:165, 1987.

1053. Keller GA, Gould S, Deluca M, Subramani S: Firefly luciferase is targeted to peroxisomes in mammalian cells. *Proc Natl Acad Sci U S A* **84**:3264, 1987.

1054. Gould SJ, Keller GA, Subramani S: Identification of a peroxisomal targeting signal at the carboxy terminus of firefly luciferase. *J Cell Biol* **105**:2923, 1987.

1055. Gould SJ, Keller G-A, Subramani S: Identification of peroxisomal targeting signals located at the carboxy terminus of four peroxisomal proteins. *J Cell Biol* **107**:897, 1988.

1056. Miyazawa S, Osumi T, Hashimoto K, Ohno K, Miura S, Fujiki Y: Peroxisome targeting signal of rat liver acyl-coenzyme A oxydase resides at the carboxy terminus. *Mol Cell Biol* **9**:83, 1989.

1057. Gould SJ, Keller G-A, Hosken N, Wilkinson J, Subramani S: A conserved tripeptide sorts proteins to peroxisomes. *J Cell Biol* **108**:1657, 1989.

1057a. Gould SJ, Krisans S, Keller G-A, Subramani S: Antibodies directed against the peroxisomal targeting signal of firefly luciferase recognize multiple mammalian peroxisomal proteins. *J Cell Biol* **110**:27, 1990.

1057b. Walton PA, Gould SJ, Feramisco JR, Subramani S: Transport of microinjected proteins into peroxisomes of mammalian cells: Inability of Zellweger cell lines to import proteins with the SKL tripeptide peroxisomal targeting signal. *Mol Cell Biol* **12**:531, 1992.

1058. Swinkels BW, Gould SJ, Bodnar AG, Rachubinski RA, Subramani S: A novel, cleavable peroxisomal targeting signal at the amino-terminus of the rat 3-ketoacyl-CoA thiolase. *EMBO J* **10**:3255, 1991.

1059. Mori T, Tsukamoto T, Mori H, Tashiro Y, Fujiki Y: Molecular cloning and deduced amino acid sequence of nonspecific lipid transfer protein (sterol carrier protein 2) of rat liver: A higher molecular mass (60 kDa) protein contains the primary sequence of nonspecific lipid transfer as its C-terminal part. *Proc Natl Acad Sci U S A* **88**:4338, 1991.

1060. Osumi T, Hashimoto T, Ui N: Purification and properties of Acyl-CoA oxidase from rat liver. *J Biochem* **87**:1735, 1980.

1061. Garrard LJ, Goodman JM: Two genes encode the major membrane-associated protein of methanol-induced peroxisomes from *Candida boidinii*. *J Biol Chem* **264**:13929, 1989.

1062. Fujiki Y, Rachubinski RA, Lazarow PB: Synthesis of a major integral membrane polypeptide of rat liver peroxisomes on free polysomes. *Proc Natl Acad Sci U S A* **81**:7127, 1984.

1063. Koster A, Heisig M, Heinrich PC, Just WW: In vitro synthesis of peroxisomal membrane polypeptides. *Biochem Biophys Res Commun* **137**:626, 1986.

1064. Suzuki Y, Orii T, Takiguchi M, Mori M, Hijikata M, Hashimoto T: Biosynthesis of membrane polypeptides of rat liver peroxisomes. *J Biochem (Tokyo)* **101**:491, 1987.

1065. Moser HW: New approaches in peroxisomal disorders. *Dev Neurosci* **9**:1, 1987.

1066. Schutgens RBH, Wanders RJA, Heymans HSA, Schram AW, Tager JM, Schrakamp G, Van Den Bosch H: Zellweger syndrome: Biochemical procedures in diagnosis, prevention and treatment. *J Inherit Metab Dis* **10**:33, 1987.

1067. Lazarow PB, Fujiki Y, Small GM, Watkins P, Moser H: Presence of the peroxisomal 22-kDa integral membrane protein in the liver of a person lacking recognizable peroxisomes (Zellweger syndrome). *Proc Natl Acad Sci U S A* **83**:9193, 1986.

1068. Santos MJ, Imanaka T, Shio H, Lazarow PB: Peroxisomal integral membrane proteins in control and Zellweger fibroblasts. *J Biol Chem* **263**:10502, 1988.

1069. Santos MJ, Imanaka T, Shio H, Small GM, Lazarow PB: Peroxisomal membrane ghosts in Zellweger syndrome — aberrant organelle assembly. *Science* **239**:1536, 1988.

1070. Balfe A, Hoefler G, Chen WW, Watkins PA: Aberrant subcellular localization of peroxisomal 3-ketoacyl-CoA thiolase in the Zellweger syndrome and rhinzomelic chondrodysplasia punctata. *Pediatr Res* **27**:304, 1990.

1071. Van Roermund CWT, Brul S, Tager JM, Schutgens RBH, Wanders RJA: Acyl-CoA oxidase, peroxisomal thiolase and dihydroxyacetone phosphate acyltransferase: Aberrant subcellular localization in Zellweger syndrome. *J Inherit Metab Dis* **14**:152, 1991.

1072. Kunau W-H, Hartig A: Peroxisome biogenesis in Saccharomyces cerevisiae. *Antonie Van Leeuwenhoek* **62**:63, 1992.

1073. Brul S, Westerveld A, Strijland A, Wanders RJA, Schram AW, Heymans HSA, Schutgens RBH, van den Bosch H, Tager JM: Genetic heterogeneity in the cerebrohepatorenal (Zellweger) syndrome and other inherited disorders with a generalized impairment of peroxisomal functions. *J Clin Invest* **81**:1710, 1988.

1074. Yajima S, Yasuyuki S, Shimozawa N, Yamaguchi S, Orii T, Fujiki Y, Osumi T, Hashimoto T, Moser HW: Complementation study of peroxisome-deficient disorders by immunofluorescence staining and characterization of fused cells. *Hum Genet* **88**:491, 1992.

1075. Zoeller RA, Allen L-AH, Santos MJ, Lazarow PB, Hashimoto T, Tartakoff AM, Raetz CRH: Chinese hamster ovary cell mutants defective in peroxisome biogenesis. *J Biol Chem* **264**:21872, 1989.

1076. Tsukamoto T, Yokota S, Fujiki Y: Isolation and characterization of Chinese hamster ovary cell mutants defective in assembly of peroxisomes. *J Cell Biol* **110**:651, 1990.

1077. Tsukamoto T, Miura S, Fujiki Y: Restoration by a 35K membrane protein of peroxisome assembly in a peroxisome-deficient mammalian cell mutant. *Nature* **350**:77, 1991.

1078. Shimozawa N, Tsukamoto T, Suzuki Y, Orii T, Shirayoshi Y, Mori T, Fujiki Y: A human gene responsible for Zellweger syndrome that affects peroxisome assembly. *Science* **255**:1132, 1992.

1079. Schroeder WT, Saunders GF: Localization of the human catalase and apolipoprotein A-I genes to chromosome 11. *Cytogenet Cell Genet* **44**:231, 1987.

1080. Hashmi M, Stanley W, Singh I: Lignoceroyl-CoASH ligase-enzyme defect in fatty acid beta-oxidation system in X-linked childhood adrenoleukodystrophy. *FEBS Lett* **196**:247, 1986.

1081. Goldfischer SL, Collins J, Rapin I, Neumann P, Neglia W, Spiro AJ, Ishii T, Roels F, Vamecq J, Van Hoof F: Pseudo-Zellweger syndrome: Deficiencies in several peroxisomal oxidative activities. *J Pediatr* **108**:25, 1986.

1082. Schram AW, Goldfischer S, Van Roermund CWT, Brouwer-Kelder EM, Collins J, Hashimoto T, Heymans HSA, Van Den Bosch H, Schutgens RBH, Tager JM, Wanders RJA: Human peroxisomal 3-oxoacyl-coenzyme A thiolase deficiency. *Proc Natl Acad Sci U S A* **84**:2494, 1987.

1083. Veenhuis M, Van Dijken JP, Harder W: The significance of peroxisomes in the metabolism of one-carbon compounds in yeasts. *Adv Microb Physiol* **24**:1, 1983.

1084. Roggenkamp R, Sahm H, Hinkelman W, Wagner F: Alcohol oxidase and catalase in peroxisomal methanol-grown *Candida boidinii*. *Eur J Biochem* **59**:231, 1975.

1085. Goodman JM: Dihydroxyacetone synthase is an abundant constituent of the methanol-induced peroxisome of Candida boidini. *J Biol Chem* **260**:7108, 1985.

PART 4

CANCER

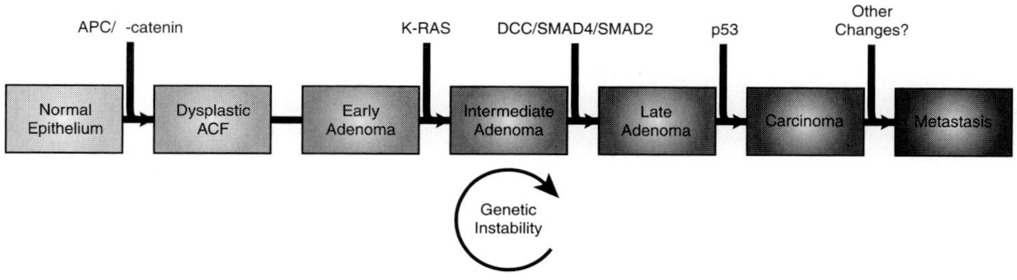

CHAPTER 17

Introduction to Cancer Genetics Chapters

Kenneth W. Kinzler ■ Bert Vogelstein

When the first edition of this book was published in 1960, chapters on cancer were neither numerous nor prominent. Although it was realized that some rare kindreds were prone to neoplasia, it was not known whether genes played a significant role in the common forms of cancer. Moreover, the biochemical and physiological bases of tumorigenesis were so poorly understood that it would have been impossible to write anything relating genes to cancer that was not speculative.

This has now changed dramatically, due to the revolution in cancer research that has occurred in the last two decades. If this revolution were to be summarized in a single sentence, that sentence would be "Cancer is, in essence, a genetic disease." Although cancer is complex, and environmental and nongenetic factors clearly play a role at many stages of the neoplastic process, the tremendous progress made in understanding tumorigenesis is in large part due to the discovery of the genes that, when mutated, lead to cancer. The eighth edition of this book pays tribute to this revolution by including over 40 chapters describing the genetics and biochemical basis of cancers of various organs.

The genetics of cancer are clearly more complex than most of the other diseases described in this book. In this introductory chapter we attempt to answer some basic questions about this topic that hopefully will help put the chapters on cancer in perspective and explain their organization.

HOW IS CANCER DIFFERENT FROM OTHER GENETIC DISEASES?

The simplest genetic diseases (e.g., Duchenne muscular dystrophy; see Chap. 216) are caused by inherited mutations in a single gene that are necessary and sufficient to determine the phenotype (Fig. 17-1). This phenotype generally can be predicted from knowledge of the precise mutation, and modifying genes or environmental influences often play little role. More complex are certain diseases in which single defective genes can predispose patients to pathologic conditions, but the defective gene itself is not sufficient to guarantee the onset of clinically manifest disease. For example, patients who inherit defective low density lipoprotein receptor encoding genes are prone to atherosclerosis, but environmental influences, particularly dietary lipids, play a large role in determining the severity of disease (see Chap. 120).

Certain cancers display an obvious hereditary influence, but like atherosclerosis, the defective inherited gene is itself not sufficient for the development of cancer. Cancers only become manifest following accumulation of additional somatic mutations. These occur either as a result of the imperfection of the DNA copying apparatus ($\sim 10^{-10}$ mutations per base pair per somatic cell generation) or through DNA damage caused by environmental mutagens.

DO CANCERS OCCUR ONLY IN PATIENTS WHO INHERIT A DEFECTIVE CANCER GENE?

It is estimated that only a small fraction (0.1 to 10 percent, depending on the cancer type) of the total cancers in the Western world occur in patients with a hereditary mutation. However, one of the cardinal principles of modern cancer research is that the same genes cause both inherited and sporadic (noninherited) forms of the same tumor type (Fig. 17-2). This principle, first enunciated by Knudson, is well illustrated by retinoblastomas in children (see Chap. 36) and kidney cancers (see Chap. 41) and colorectal tumors in adults (see Chap. 48). For example, approximately 0.5 percent of colorectal cancer patients inherit a defective *APC* gene from one of their parents. This inherited mutation is not sufficient to initiate tumorigenesis. However, every cell of the colon from such patients is "at risk" for acquiring a second mutation, and two mutations of the right type are believed to be sufficient for initiation. The great majority of colorectal cancer patients (>99 percent of the total) do not inherit a mutant *APC* gene. However, these sporadic cases also require *APC* mutations to begin the tumorigenic process. In these sporadic cases, the *APC* mutations occur somatically in isolated colorectal epithelial cells. The number of colorectal epithelial cells with *APC* mutations is therefore several orders of magnitude less in the sporadic cases than in the inherited cases, in which every cell has an *APC* mutation. Accordingly, patients with the hereditary mutations often develop multiple tumors instead of single, isolated tumors, and patients with the familial form of the disease develop tumors at an earlier age than the sporadic patients.

What is the "second mutation," alluded to above, that initiates clinically apparent neoplasia in both the hereditary and sporadic types of tumors? In most known examples, the second mutation is believed to result in inactivation of the wild-type allele inherited from the unaffected parent. As described below, genes that, when mutated, lead to cancer predisposition normally suppress tumorigenesis. If one allele of such a gene (e.g., *APC*) is mutated in the germ line, then the cell still has the product of the wild-type allele as a backup. If a somatic mutation of the wild-type allele occurs, however, then the resulting cell will have no functional suppressor gene product remaining and will begin to proliferate abnormally (*clonal expansion*). One of the cells in the proliferating clone is then likely to accumulate another mutation, resulting in further loss of growth control. Through gradual clonal expansion, a tumor will evolve, with each successive mutation providing a further growth advantage, allowing its progeny to continue to replicate in microenvironments inhibitory to the growth of cells with fewer mutations.

A list of standard abbreviations is located immediately preceding the index in each volume. Nonstandard abbreviations used in this chapter include: LOH = loss of heterozygosity.

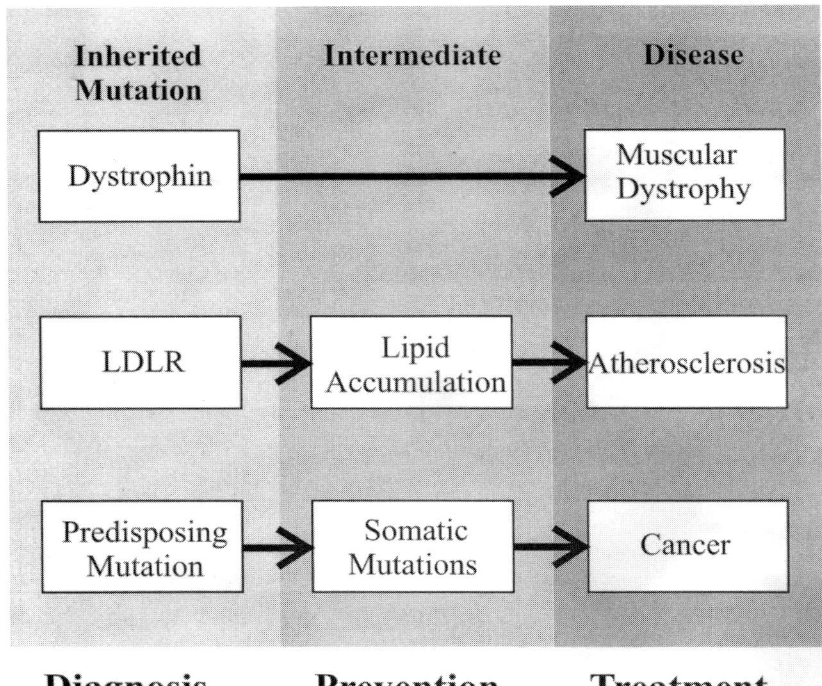

Fig. 17-1 Comparison of genetic diseases. Three types of genetic diseases, of increasing complexity, are illustrated (*Reprinted by permission from Kinzler KW and Vogelstein B: Lessons from hereditary colon cancer Cell 87:161, 1996; copyright 1996 by Cell Press.*)

ARE THE DNA ALTERATIONS IN CANCER DIFFERENT FROM THOSE IN OTHER GENETICALLY DETERMINED DISEASES?

Five different types of genetic alterations have been observed in tumor cells:

1. *Subtle alterations.* Small deletions, insertions, and single base-pair substitutions occur in cancers just as they do in other hereditary diseases (see Chap. 13).
2. *Chromosome number changes.* Somatic losses or gains of chromosomes are often observed in cancers. Although such aneuploidy is occasionally a cause of other inherited diseases (e.g., Down syndrome), the degree of aneuploidy is much more extensive in cancers than ever observed in the phenotypically normal cells of mammals. Most cancers are aneuploid, with chromosome numbers ranging from subdiploid to supratetraploid. Molecular studies have shown that the aneuploidy observed in karyotypic studies actually underestimates the extent of gross chromosomal changes in cancer cells. Even

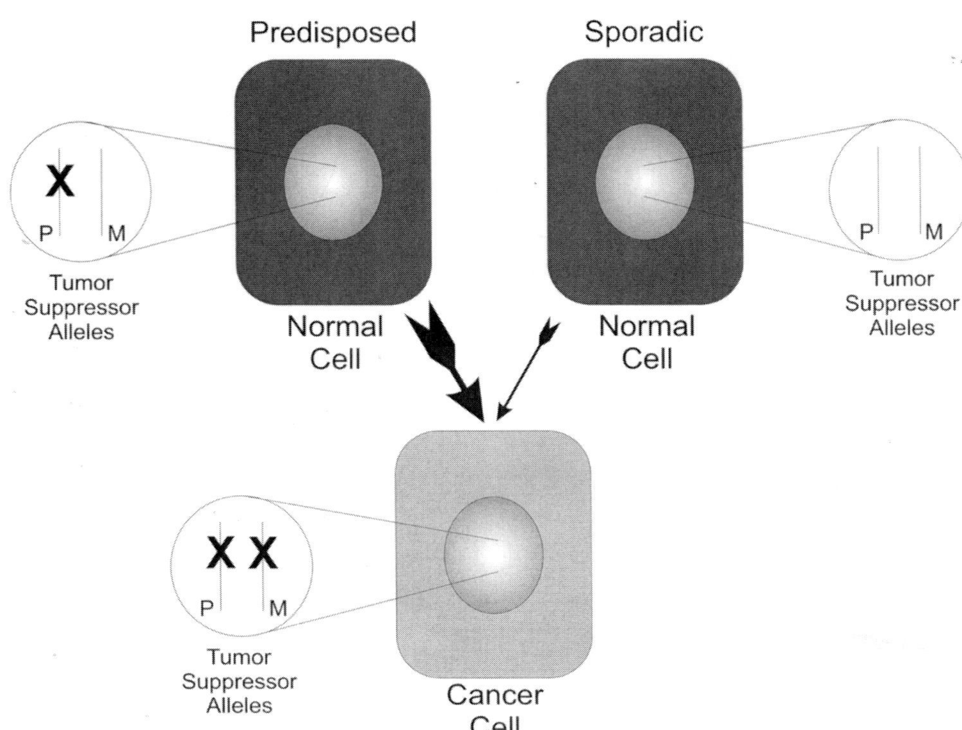

Fig. 17-2 Tumor suppressor gene inactivation. Tumor suppressor gene mutations are thought to initiate many forms of cancer. Both alleles of the tumor suppressor gene must be inactivated for a tumor to form. In familial cancer predisposition syndromes, a mutant allele of a suppressor gene is inherited and is present in every cell. However, tumors are not initiated until the second allele (inherited from the unaffected parent) is inactivated in a somatic cell. In nonfamilial cases, the inactivation of both alleles occurs through somatic mutations. The end result is the same: no functional suppressor gene, leading to tumor initiation.

when cancer cells appear to have two normal copies of a chromosome by karyotype, molecular analyses reveal that both chromosomes often are from the same parent. Thus, instead of one maternal and one paternal chromosome 17 per cell, the cancer cell may have no maternal chromosome 17 and two paternal chromosomes 17. This *loss of heterozygosity* (LOH) often affects more than half the chromosomes in an individual cancer cell. LOH provides an efficient way for the cell to inactivate genes. For example, consider a cell containing two copies of chromosome 5, one with a mutation of a chromosome 5 tumor suppressor gene and the other with a wild-type allele of this gene. The wild-type copy of the gene often will prevent the cell from abnormal proliferation. If the chromosome containing this wild-type allele is lost, then the cell will be left with only the mutant copy of the suppressor gene, and a selective growth advantage will accrue. Such LOH events occur at much higher rates (10^{-5} per generation) than subtle mutations ($\sim 10^{-7}$ per gene per generation), affording the cancer cell a powerful means of ridding itself of wild-type growth-constraining genes. LOH generally occurs through loss of an entire chromosome or through mitotic recombination. Whole chromosome losses are often associated with a duplication of the remaining chromosome, thus making this event invisible by karyotypic methods but detectable by molecular analyses using DNA polymorphisms as probes. Mitotic recombinations generally can be observed only through molecular analyses.

3. *Chromosome translocations.* Balanced and unbalanced translocations are observed frequently in cancers, where they occur by somatic rather than germ-line mutation. In common cancers of epithelial origin (e.g., breast, colon, prostate, stomach), the translocations appear to be random, with no specific breakpoints at the chromosomal or molecular levels. In contrast, leukemias and lymphomas generally contain characteristic translocations that appear to determine many of the biological properties of the neoplasms. For example, acute promyelocytic leukemias virtually always contain a t(15;17) translocation resulting in the fusion of a *Retinoic Acid Receptor* gene on chromosome 17 with the *PML* gene on chromosome 15, and chronic myelogenous leukemias always contain a t(9;22) translocation resulting in fusion of the *abl* oncogene on chromosome 9 with the *BCR* gene on chromosome 22 (see Chap. 19 and 20).
4. *Amplifications.* These alterations are only observed in neoplastic cells in humans and are defined by a five- to hundredfold multiplication of a small region of the chromosome (0.3 to 10 Mb). Gene amplifications generally are observed only in advanced neoplasms. The "amplicons" contain one or more genes whose expression can endow the cell with enhanced proliferative activity, and the higher expression of these genes through an increased copy number is obviously advantageous for the cancer cell (see Chap. 21).
5. *Exogenous sequences.* Certain human cancers are associated with tumor viruses, which contribute genes that result in abnormal cell growth. Representative examples are cervical cancers (see Chap. 53), Burkitt's lymphomas (see Chap. 19), hepatocellular carcinomas (see Chap. 59), and T-cell leukemias (associated with retroviruses). These exogenously introduced genes can best be considered as another class of mutations that contributes to oncogenesis. Like the other mutations described earlier, no exogenous viral gene is sufficient for tumorigenesis. Such viral oncogenes often initiate the tumorigenic process, however, just as defective tumor suppressor genes initiate the process in the many tumors not associated with viral infection.

WHAT GENES ARE MUTATED IN CANCERS?

Two classes of genes are involved in cancer formation. The first class, comprised of oncogenes and tumor suppressor genes, directly controls cellular proliferation. These genes do this by controlling either the rate of cell birth (see Chap. 23) or the rate of cell death (see Chap. 24). Although tumorigenesis largely has been thought of as caused by increases in the rate of cell birth, it is now recognized that tumor expansion represents an imbalance between cell birth and cell death. In normal tissues, cell birth precisely equals cell death, resulting in homeostasis. Defects in either of these processes can result in net growth, perceived as tumorigenesis.

Oncogenes are like the accelerator of an automobile; they normally result in increased cell birth or decreased cell death when expressed (see Chap. 25). A mutation in an oncogene is tantamount to having the cell's "accelerator" pinned to the floor: Cell proliferation continues even when the cell's surrounding environment is giving it clear signals to stop. Mutations in oncogenes include subtle mutations, which change their structure and make them constitutively active, or mutations that increase their expression to levels higher than observed in normal cells.

Continuing with this analogy, tumor suppressor genes are the "brakes" of the cell, normally functioning to inhibit cell growth (see Chap. 26). Just as do automobiles, each cell type has more than one "brake," each of which can be activated under appropriate microenvironmental stimuli. It is only when several of the cell's "brakes" and "accelerators" are rendered dysfunctional through mutation that the cell spins entirely out of control, and cancer ensues.

The second class of genes (caretaker genes) does not control cell growth directly but instead controls the rate of mutation. Cells with defective caretaker genes acquire mutations in all genes, including oncogenes and tumor suppressor genes, at an elevated rate. This higher rate leads to accelerated tumorigenesis. The fact that patients (and cells) with defective caretaker genes are cancer-prone provides one of the most cogent pieces of evidence that mutations in DNA lie at the heart of the neoplastic process.

IS CANCER A SINGLE DISEASE?

Tumors can best be defined as diseases in which a single cell acquires the ability to proliferate abnormally, resulting in an accumulation of progeny. *Cancers* are those tumors which have acquired the ability to invade through surrounding normal tissues. The most advanced form of this invasive process is metastasis, a state in which cancer cells escape from their original location, travel by hematogenous or lymphogenous channels, and take up residence in distant sites. The only difference between a malignant tumor (a.k.a. cancer) and a benign tumor is the capacity of the former to invade. Both benign and malignant tumors can achieve large sizes, but benign tumors are circumscribed and therefore generally can be removed surgically. Malignant tumors often have invaded surrounding or distant tissues prior to their detection, precluding surgical excision of the entire tumor cell population. It is the ability of cancers to destroy other tissues through invasion that makes them lethal.

There are as many tumor types as there are cell types in the human body. Cancers thus represent not a single disease but a group of heterogeneous diseases that share certain biological properties (in particular, clonal cell growth and invasive ability). Cancers can be classified in various ways. Most common cancers of adults are carcinomas, representing cancers derived from epithelial cells. Leukemias and lymphomas are derived from blood-forming cells and lymphoid cells, respectively. Sarcomas are derived from mesenchymal tissues. Melanomas are derived from melanocytes, and retinoblastomas, neuroblastomas, and glioblastomas are derived from stem cells of the retina, neurons, and glia, respectively.

Twenty years ago it could not have been predicted that all these different cancers share common molecular pathogeneses in addition to common biological properties. The cancer research revolution has demonstrated that they do: All result from defects in oncogenes and tumor suppressor genes. Each specific cancer arises through characteristic mutations in specific genes. Although dozens of human oncogenes and tumor suppressor genes have

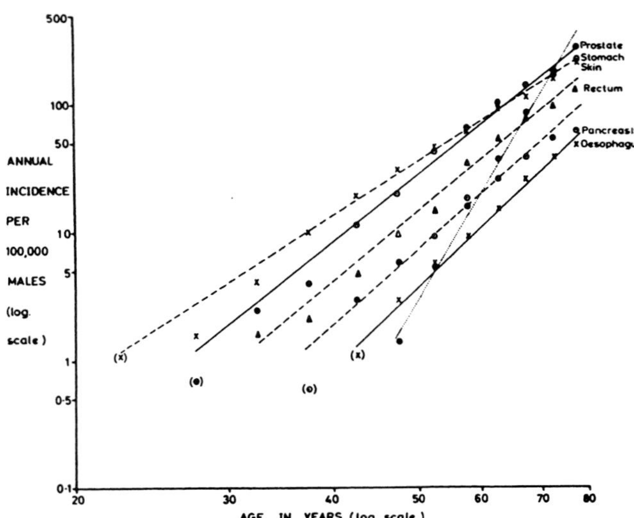

Fig. 17-3 Cancer incidence versus age. The log of the incidence rate and the log of age have a linear relationship, with the incidence increasing dramatically (103- to 107-fold) with age (*Reprinted by permission from Miller DG: On the nature of susceptibility to cancer. The presidential address. Cancer 46:1307,1980; copyright 1980 by the American Cancer Society.*)

been described in the literature, these genes' products appear to converge on a relatively small number of growth-controlling pathways. In some cases, the same gene is involved in multiple cancers. For example, *p53* mutations commonly occur in cancers of the brain, colon, breast, stomach, bladder, and pancreas. In other cases, a defective gene appears to be associated with a single tumor type, such as the *WT1* gene in childhood kidney cancers (see Chap. 38).

HOW MANY MUTATIONS ARE REQUIRED FOR CANCER FORMATION?

Epidemiologic investigations long ago revealed that the incidence of cancer increased exponentially with age (Fig. 17-3). Detailed analysis of age versus incidence curves is consistent with the idea that three to seven mutations are required for full development of cancers. This estimate is consistent with molecular analyses of cancers, in which it is not unusual to observe mutations of four or five different genes. It is generally thought that benign tumors, the precursors of cancers, require fewer mutations (perhaps just two mutations to initiate a small neoplasm). As tumor cells accumulate additional mutations, the resulting clonal expansion causes tumor progression, with progressively larger and more dangerous neoplasms evolving. *Solid tumors* (i.e., those of solid organs such as the colon, bladder, brain, and breast) appear to require a greater number of mutations for their development than *liquid tumors* (i.e., leukemias and lymphomas). The smaller number of mutations required for leukemias may explain the shorter lag time following an initial mutagenic insult. For example, following explosion of the atomic bombs in Japan, leukemias began to appear within a few years, whereas an increased incidence of solid tumors was not evident until at least a decade later.

ORGANIZATION OF THE CANCER CHAPTERS IN THIS BOOK

It is obvious from the preceding that there are numerous interconnections between the principles underlying cancer genetics and that any organization of chapters on cancer is arbitrary. For didactic purposes, however, the chapters are organized into four categories:

The first set of chapters (Chap. 18–22) focuses on basic concepts in cancer genetics.

The second set of chapters (Chap. 23–26) is concerned with control of the cell cycle

The third set of chapters (Chap. 26–49) is devoted to cancers in which heritable mutations of predisposing genes have been identified. These have been divided (see Chap. 27 for additional detail) into those syndromes in which the responsible gene leads to increased mutation rates (caretaker genes) and those in which the responsible gene directly controls cell birth or cell death (gatekeeper genes).

The fourth set (Chap. 50–60) includes chapters on cancers in which heritable predisposing mutations leading to well-defined predisposition syndromes have not been identified. The chapters in this section largely emphasize somatic mutations.

Although this organization necessitates a bit of redundancy, it is hoped that the organization will satisfy those who are searching for information on specific tumor types, those who are interested primarily in specific genes, and those who are interested in acquiring a basic general knowledge of cancer genetics.

CHAPTER 18

Genomic Imprinting and Cancer

Andrew P. Feinberg

1. **Genomic imprinting is an epigenetic modification of a specific parental allele of a gene, or the chromosome on which it resides, in the gamete or zygote leading to differential expression of the two alleles of the gene in somatic cells of the offspring.**
2. **Evidence for genomic imprinting in normal development derives from studies over many years of the whole genome, specific chromosomal regions, and individual imprinted loci. There is now an intense search for an ever-increasing list of imprinted genes that are involved in many different types of cellular processes.**
3. **Genomic imprinting challenges two assumptions of Mendelian genetics applied to human disease: that the maternal and paternal alleles of a gene are equivalent and that two functional copies of a gene always are associated with health. Imprinted genes probably account for many examples of developmental malformations in humans.**
4. **Hydatidiform moles and complete ovarian teratomas, the genome of each of which is derived from a single parental origin, show that an imbalance of maternal and paternal genome equivalents leads to neoplastic growth.**
5. **Several chromosomes show parental origin-specific alterations in cancer, including losses of heterozygosity in Wilms tumor and in acute myelocytic leukemia and gene amplification in neuroblastoma.**
6. **Beckwith-Wiedemann syndrome, a disorder of prenatal overgrowth and cancer, sometimes involves parental origin-specific germ-line chromosomal rearrangements and uniparental disomy.**
7. **Loss of imprinting (LOI) is a recently discovered alteration in cancer that involves loss of parental origin-specific gene expression. LOI may include activation of the normally silent copy of growth-promoting genes and/or silencing of the normally transcribed copy of tumor suppressor genes. These changes can involve a switch of a maternal chromosome to a paternal epigenotype.**
8. **There is a rapidly increasing number of examples of genes and tumors that show LOI. Genes include *IGF2, H19,* and *p57*^{KIP2}. Tumors include Wilms tumor; hepatoblastoma; rhabdomyosarcoma; Ewing sarcoma; uterine, cervical, esophageal, prostate, lung, and colon cancer; choriocarcinoma; and germ-cell tumors. Thus LOI is one of the most common alterations in human cancer.**
9. **Normal genomic imprinting is maintained in part by parental origin-specific, tissue-independent DNA methylation of cytosine within CpG islands, regions rich in CpG dinucleotides. Tumors with LOI show abnormal methylation of these CpG islands.**
10. **Normal genomic imprinting should be viewed as a developmental process rather than as a single event. Thus a combination of both *cis*-acting and *trans*-acting signals is likely to be important in the establishment and maintenance of normal genomic imprinting, and disruption of these same factors can be expected to play a role in LOI in cancer.**
11. **Since normal imprinting is reversible, LOI also may be reversible and amenable to novel therapeutic approaches, such as modification with 5-aza-2′-deoxycytidine, an inhibitor of DNA methylation.**

A list of standard abbreviations is located immediately preceding the index in each volume. Nonstandard abbreviations used in this chapter include: PEV = position effect variegation; UPD = uniparental disomy; PWS = Prader-Willi syndrome; AS = Angleman syndrome; LOH = loss of heterozygosity; BWS = Beckwith-Wiedemann syndrome; WT = Wilms tumor; LOI = loss of imprinting.

Genomic imprinting is an epigenetic modification of a specific parental allele of a gene, or the chromosome on which it resides, in the gamete or zygote leading to differential expression of the two alleles of the gene in somatic cells of the offspring. Alterations of genomic imprinting recently have been identified in human cancers. These alterations have generated a great deal of excitement because they appear to occur commonly in both childhood and adult malignancies, lead to altered expression of growth regulatory genes, and represent potentially reversible changes. Thus they may lead to novel forms of therapy for cancer. This chapter presents the experimental foundations on which these recent discoveries have been made, a summary of our current knowledge (which is evolving rapidly), and prospects for future discovery and application.

TYPES OF EPIGENETIC INHERITANCE

Genomic imprinting is a form of epigenetic inheritance, which is a modification of the genome, heritable by cell progeny, that does not involve a change in DNA sequence. Generally, epigenetic inheritance leads to apparently non-Mendelian properties of the gene, such as modification by the other allele or a change from one generation to the next. Examples in *Drosophila* include transvection at the bithorax locus, or pairing-dependent gene expression caused by *trans*-sensing of alleles.[1] The mechanism of transvection is unknown, although interaction between homologous chromosomes appears to influence expression levels from both chromosomes.[2] A second example of epigenetic inheritance is paramutation in plants, a heritable alteration of one allele caused by a second allele of the same gene on the other chromosome.[3]

A third example of epigenetic inheritance is position-effect variegation (PEV) in *Drosophila.* This involves, for example, the spreading of condensed heterochromatin into adjacent euchromatin at sites of chromosomal rearrangement near the white locus;

this leads to variably colored eyes. Two striking features of PEV are the variability of suppression caused by the heterochromatin, leading to very high apparent pseudomutation rates, and the long distances (several megabases) over which PEV can act.[4] Some of the *trans*-acting factors that mediate PEV appear to be involved in the formation or stabilization of heterochromatin.[5,6] Thus their homologues in mammalian cells may be important in understanding genomic imprinting.

An additional example of epigenetic inheritance, similar to PEV but acting over a much shorter distance (several kilobases), is telomere silencing in yeast, caused by the proximity of a gene to telomere sequences. Factors that mediate telomere silencing also are known, and in some cases mammalian homologues have been identified.[7] Two underlying themes of the various forms of epigenetic inheritance are that they appear to involve changes to chromatin and that they act over a distance larger than that of a single gene.

GENOMIC IMPRINTING IN NORMAL DEVELOPMENT

Evidence for genomic imprinting originated from study of the whole genome, then progressed to studies of individual chromosomes and chromosomal regions, and finally led to identification of specific imprinted genes. The definition of genomic imprinting was first introduced by Helen Crouse in 1960 in her studies of the insect *Sciara,* which preferentially sheds paternal chromosomes during development.[8] In the first sentence of this chapter, a modification of Crouse's original definition is used to reflect the modern emphasis on transcriptional regulation. A striking example of possible whole-genome imprinting is the difference between the mule and the hinny. The mule is a cross of a maternal horse and paternal donkey. It is much larger and quite dissimilar to the hinny, which is the reciprocal cross. Of course, there are other alternative explanations for this phenotypic difference, such as mitochondrial inheritance or differing *in utero* environments.

A whole-genome clue to the existence of genomic imprinting in humans derives from the observation of spontaneously aborted triploid human embryos, which show different histopathology depending on whether the excess of chromosomes is paternal or maternal. Embryos with two maternal genome equivalents and one paternal genome equivalent lead to cystic placentas, a large fetus with malformations, and occasionally a term pregnancy. In contrast, embryos with two paternal genome equivalents and one maternal genome equivalent show marked growth retardation and die *in utero*.

Formal proof for imprinting at the level of the genome was offered by Solter and colleagues, who performed pronuclear transplantation experiments in which a maternal pronucleus was replaced with a second paternal pronucleus, or vice versa.[9] *Androgenotes,* defined as containing a normal chromosome number that is entirely of paternal origin, show mainly extraembryonic tissue. In contrast, *gynogenotes,* whose chromosomes are entirely of maternal origin, show mostly embryonic tissue. Thus it appears that the paternal genome equivalent is comparatively more responsible for placental development, and the maternal genome equivalent is comparatively more responsible for embryo development.

Evidence for imprinting of discrete portions of the genome began with studies of X inactivation. This imprinting was first shown by analyzing *PGK* allele expression in mice heterozygous for a polymorphism in the phosphoglycerate kinase gene, detected as an electrophoretic variant in the protein. Although the X chromosome shows random inactivation in embryonic tissues, this is not the case in extraembryonic tissues, which show preferential inactivation of the paternal X chromosome.[10]

The beginning of our understanding of which autosomes undergo genomic imprinting came from studies over many years by Cattanach and colleagues of mice with germ-line chromosomal translocations.[11] When these mice are bred, there is a high frequency of nondisjunction, leading to both paternal and maternal uniparental disomy (UPD) beyond the translocation breakpoint, depending on which parent harbors the translocation. The phenotypes of these animals provide an estimate that 15 percent of the genome is imprinted.[11] Studies of UPD in mice also suggest that when imprinting occurs, an excess of the paternal genome, coupled with maternal loss, leads to prenatal overgrowth, and an excess of the maternal genome leads to decreased growth. Other phenotypes of UPD include embryonic lethality and behavioral disorders.[11] This work provided a critical clue toward identifying imprinted loci in mouse and, by synteny mapping, in humans. UPD studies have shown that imprinting resides at the level of genes and/or chromosomal regions. However, UPD studies have several inherent limitations. The phenotype by which animals are scored is relatively insensitive. The technique used is also relatively nonspecific, in that there may be only a single imprinted gene within the entire chromosomal region that shows UPD.

The first example of a specific imprinted gene was discovered fortuitously by Swain and colleagues, and it did not involve an endogenous gene. It was noted that a C-*myc* transgene fused to an immunoglobulin enhancer was expressed in some tissues only when inherited from the father. When inherited from the mother, the transgene was transcriptionally silent. In addition, the silent maternally inherited copy was methylated.[12] There are now several examples of transgenes that show parental origin-specific methylation, but transcriptional silencing is less common.[13]

The first example of an imprinted endogenous gene also was discovered fortuitously when DeChiara and colleagues disrupted the insulin-like growth factor II (*IGF2*) gene in knockout experiments.[14] When the disrupted allele was inherited from the father, the animals were runted, but there was no phenotype when the disrupted allele was inherited from the mother. When female mice with the disrupted allele themselves had offspring, those animals were of normal size. *In situ* hybridization and RNase protection experiments confirmed that there was no *IGF2*

Table 18-1 Imprinted Genes in Mouse or Humans

Gene	Expression
ASCL2/Mash2	Maternal
GABA receptor	Paternal and Maternal
GNAS Isoforms	Paternal
GRB10	Maternal
Grf1	Paternal
H19	Maternal
IGF2	Paternal
IGF2R	Maternal
Impact	Paternal
INS1	Paternal
Insulin	Paternal
IPW	Paternal
K_VLQT1	Maternal
Mas	Paternal
Necdin	Paternal
$P57^{KIP2}$	Maternal
PAR-1	Paternal
PAR-5	Paternal
PAR-SN	Paternal
Peg1	Paternal
Peg3	Paternal
SNRPN	Paternal
TSSC3/IPL	Maternal
TSSC5/IMPT1	Maternal
U2afbp-rs	Paternal
UBE3A/E6-AP	Maternal
WT1	Maternal
XIST	Paternal
ZNF127	Paternal

expression in tissues with a disrupted paternal allele. Thus these experiments clearly showed that *IGF2* is imprinted and expressed normally only from the paternal allele.[14] However, *IGF2* is biparentally expressed in two neural tissues, the choroid plexus and the leptomeninges, since animals with a disrupted paternal allele nevertheless expressed the gene in these tissues.[14] These were milestone studies because they showed that genomic imprinting affects normal endogenous genes and also that imprinting is subject to tissue-specific regulation. Recent years have provided more direct approaches to identifying novel imprinted genes.[15] These include positional cloning efforts aimed at identifying imprinted genes near other known imprinted genes, techniques for comparing gene expression in parthenogenetic embryos to that of normal embryos,[16] and restriction landmark genome scanning,[17] which exploits a principle introduced many years ago, to analyze clonality in tumors, and involves a search for DNA methylation near a polymorphic site for which the individual is heterozygous.[18] Approximately 30 imprinted genes have been discovered, although many more are likely to exist. A current inventory (at this writing) of imprinted genes in mouse and humans, which are not necessarily concordant, is provided in Table 18-1. One of the most interesting features of genomic imprinting is that it affects many different cellular processes, including intercellular signaling, RNA processing, and cell cycle control.

GENOMIC IMPRINTING IN HUMAN DISEASE

Two assumptions of Mendelian genetics applied to human disease are that the maternal allele is equivalent to the paternal allele and that two working copies of the gene are associated with normal function. Genomic imprinting challenges the first of these assumptions, since it is a form of epigenetic inheritance that causes parental origin-specific differential gene expression. As will be described later, abnormal imprinting in cancer challenges the second assumption, because loss of imprinting causing biallelic expression of some genes may be a mechanism underlying carcinogenesis.

The literature of the 1970s and 1980s is rich in presumed examples of human genetic disorders that exhibit genomic imprinting. These reports were based primarily on pedigree studies of autosomal dominant disorders that showed parental origin-specific disease penetrance. These disease loci also often show disease anticipation; namely, the phenotype becomes progressively worse from one generation to the next. Although both of these phenomena were ascribed to genomic imprinting,[19] later studies based on molecular cloning of the responsible genes revealed that genomic imprinting often was not the mechanism after all. The classical example is fragile X syndrome, a common cause of mental retardation, which is caused by a trinucleotide repeat expansion.[20,21] This expansion undergoes preferential enlargement in the maternal germ line, accounting for differential disease penetrance as well as anticipation. However, expression is controlled by the length of the repeat and not imprinting per se.[22] Thus parent-of-origin effects may or may not be owing to genomic imprinting. This is not to fault the older studies, since the definition of genomic imprinting itself has evolved somewhat to refer to modification causing parental allele-specific expression rather than any parental allele-specific modification.

Two examples of true imprinted human disease loci are in close proximity on chromosome 15. Their loss causes Prader-Willi syndrome (PWS) or Angelman syndrome (AS). Both involve mental retardation, and PWS also causes obesity, and AS involves gross motor disturbances. Each disorder can be caused by uniparental disomy, PWS by maternal UPD and AS by paternal UPD.[23,24] Similarly, PWS can be caused by intrachromosomal deletions of the paternal chromosome and AS by deletions of the maternal chromosome.[25,26] PWS can be caused by deletions in the small nuclear ribonucleoprotein polypeptide N (*SNRPN*) gene.[27] It has been shown recently that a mutation affecting the splicing of an untranslated upstream exon of *SNRPN* also may lead to AS, as well as abnormal imprinting of other loci.[28] Thus, on chromosome 15, abnormalities of a single gene can affect imprinting of a genomic region and disrupt multiple disease-causing genes, the phenotype depending on the parental origin of the mutated gene. Recently, mutations in *UBE3A*, a ubiquitin protein ligase, also were found in AS patients.[29]

Despite the relative paucity of known human imprinted disease genes, there are probably many more yet to be identified. This seems clear because UPD for specific chromosomes is often associated with multiple congenital anomalies.[30] Chromosomes that likely show this phenomenon include 2, 6, 7, 11, 14, 15, 16, 20, and X.[30] Again, the discovery of these potential imprinted disease-causing regions has been fortuitous, as has much of our knowledge of imprinting. For example, the first such example of UPD pointing the way to an imprinted chromosome was the discovery of a cystic fibrosis patient for whom only the mother was the carrier.[31] Molecular analysis showed that the genotype of the offspring was not owing to gonadal mosaicism but rather to maternal UPD in the offspring. The child also had short stature and possibly Russell-Silver syndrome. This observation indicated that there is at least one imprinted locus on chromosome 7 and that the patient suffered from a deficiency of one or more genes normally expressed only from the paternal allele or duplication of genes normally expressed only from the maternal allele.[31] Not all chromosomes appear to contain disease-related imprinted loci, however, since UPD of chromosomes 4, 5, 9, 10, 13, 21, and 22 has not been associated with birth defects.[30]

INDIRECT EVIDENCE FOR GENOMIC IMPRINTING IN HUMAN CANCER

As in the study of normal genomic imprinting, the idea of a role for genomic imprinting in cancer followed a similar progression of clues regarding whole-genome imprinting, involvement of individual chromosomal regions, and finally imprinting at specific loci. The earliest clues suggesting that genomic imprinting is important in cancer were the whole-genome examples of hydatidiform mole and complete ovarian teratoma. Hydatidiform mole, a malignant tumor of extraembryonic tissue, is caused by an androgenetic embryo arising from two paternal genome equivalents and no maternal genome equivalent.[32] This can be caused by dispermy and loss of the maternal complement or by duplication of the paternal genome and loss of the maternal equivalent. Conversely, complete ovarian teratoma, which is a very curious benign tumor that includes differentiated hair, adipose tissue, and even teeth, arises from a parthenogenetic embryo, with two maternal genome equivalents and no paternal equivalent.[33] Parthenogenesis (literally "virgin birth") is a specialized type of gynogenesis, and it specifically refers to the absence of fertilization and arises within the ovary. These two tumors, although rare, offer two important general lessons for understanding the role of imprinting in cancer. One is that it takes not only 46 chromosomes to create a normal embryo but also a balance of maternal and paternal chromosomes; a relative imbalance of paternal to maternal genetic contributions leads to neoplastic growth. The second lesson is that when there is such an imbalance, the type of neoplasm differs depending on whether there is a maternal or paternal genomic excess.

Another tumor that appears to show imprinting effects is familial paraganglioma, or glomus tumor. In all cases, the transmitting parent is the father.[34] The responsible gene has been localized recently to 11q22.3-q23.34

Chromosomal region-specific evidence for a role for imprinting in cancer followed from an observation several years ago involving loss of heterozygosity (LOH) in Wilms tumor. It had been known already that this most common solid tumor of childhood undergoes LOH of chromosome 11 and that the specifically involved region is 11p15.[35] Schroeder and colleagues noted that in each of five nonfamilial cases with LOH, it was always the maternal allele that was lost.[36] In a binomial distribution, five is the minimum number

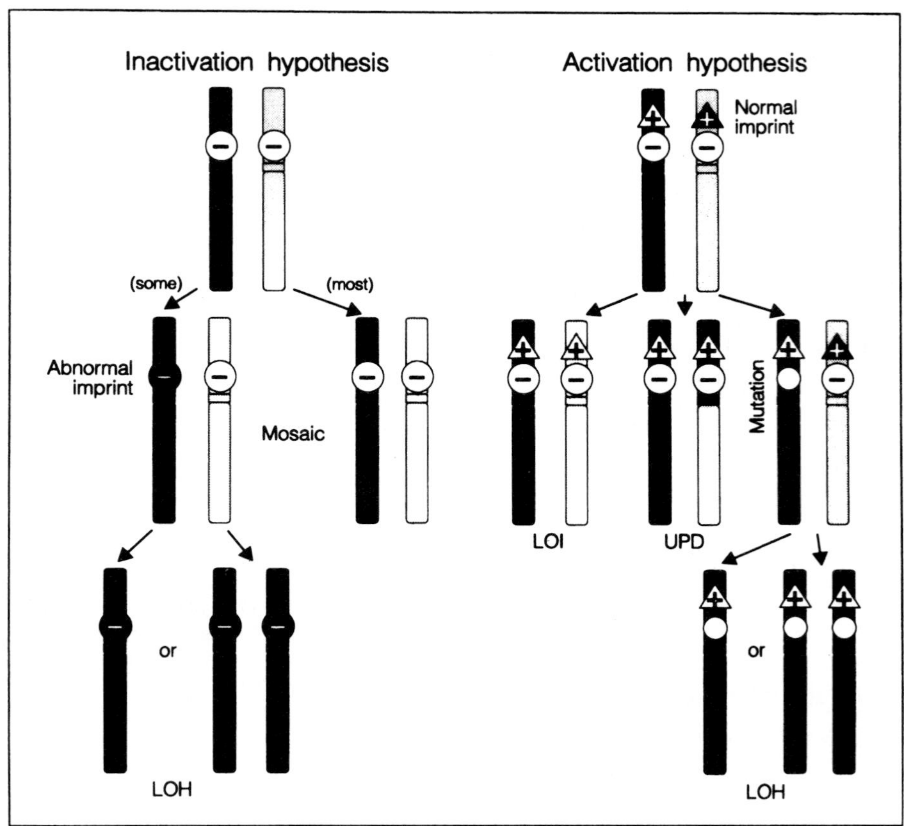

Fig. 18-1 Contrasting hypotheses of genomic imprinting in cancer. The inactivation hypothesis involves loss of expression of a tumor suppressor gene. The paternal allele is inactivated by imprinting, which displays somatic mosaicism (accounting for unilateral tumors), followed by LOH of the maternal allele (arbitrarily shown here affecting the whole chromosome). The activation hypothesis involves normal imprinting of a growth-promoting gene. Overexpression can arise from LOI of the maternal allele or UPD of the paternal allele. LOH of a distinct tumor suppressor gene would be deleterious to cell growth if it involved the transcriptionally active paternal allele of the growth-promoting gene. Alternatively, both models may be correct, with LOI and LOH leading to epigenetic silencing of a tumor suppressor gene and LOI also leading to abnormal activation of a normally silent growth-promoting gene. Dark shading, paternal chromosome; light shading, maternal chromosome, tumor suppressor gene, growth-promoting gene. (*Reprinted from Feinberg AP: Genomic imprinting and gene activation in cancer. Nature Genet 4:110–113, 1993, with permission.*)

required for statistical significance. Unfortunately, the word *imprinting* did not appear anywhere in this important paper, which stimulated a great deal of speculation and study in the following years.

Sapienza and colleagues confirmed and extended this observation to other so-called embryonal tumors of childhood, all of which involve the development of malignancy within what pathologists believe is fetal tissue that is abnormally residual after birth. Examples include hepatoblastoma and rhabdomyosarcoma.[37] They proposed a model in which imprinting is involved in cancer through epigenetic silencing of a tumor suppressor gene (Fig. 18-1). According to this model, a tumor suppressor gene on 11p15 is imprinted and epigenetically silenced on the paternal allele, accounting for the fact that LOH is seen only on the maternal allele (see Fig. 18-1). After all, LOH of the paternal allele would be inconsequential because the locus is silenced normally.[37]

However, Sapienza and colleagues also pointed out a paradox in this logic. If the locus is normally imprinted and epigenetically silenced, then everyone would have only one functional copy of the gene at birth, and then the locus would behave epidemiologically as if it had undergone a germ-line mutation of a tumor suppressor locus following Knudson's two-hit model of carcinogenesis. According to this model, patients with germ-line mutations show bilateral tumors occurring at an earlier age of onset than patients with sporadically occurring tumors, which require two sequential events to take place within a given somatic cell lineage. Thus, Sapienza and colleagues reasoned, epigenetic silencing of a tumor suppressor could not be present in all cells of the body because the tumors, such as Wilms tumor (WT), with preferential LOH of the maternal allele are for the most part late-arising unilateral tumors. On the other hand, imprinting must take place no later than the zygote stage while there is still a topologic distinction between the two parental genome equivalents. Therefore, Sapienza and colleagues proposed the following solution to this conundrum: In some individuals during germ-line development or fertilization, aberrant imprinting occurs, preferentially affecting the paternally inherited chromosome. According to this model, imprinting is subsequently erased during development, but not completely, leaving a mosaic pattern of imprinting in various tissues. Thus the imprint would no longer behave as the first hit of a two-hit Knudsonian locus[37,38] (see Fig. 18-1). One puzzle with this model is that it still proposes a relatively large number of cells with this epigenetic alteration, and thus the tumors may appear at an intermediate stage of frequency and age. However, parental origin-specific LOH appears to occur in quite ordinary late-occurring tumors. Furthermore, at least some tumors should not show aberrant imprinting as the first hit, but all tumors show preferential loss of the maternal allele.

There are now several examples of tumor types that show preferential LOH. Most of these involve the maternal chromosome, but not all do. For example, acute myelogenous leukemia (AML) involves preferential loss of the paternal chromosome 7.[39] A summary of chromosome-specific LOH is presented in Table 18-2. However, in the study of human genetic disorders, one must

Table 18-2 Preferential Chromosomal Alterations in Cancer That Likely Involve Imprinted Genes

Cancer	Chromosome	Alteration	Allele
Wilms tumor	11p	LOH	Maternal
Rhabdomyosarcoma	11p	LOH	Maternal
Osteosarcoma	13q	LOH	Maternal
Acute myelocytic leukemia	7q	LOH	Paternal
Neuroblastoma	1p	LOH	Maternal
Hepatoblastoma	1q	LOH	Paternal
Neuroblastoma	2	Amplification	Paternal

be careful not to assume that parent-of-origin effects are owing to genomic imprinting. For example, bilateral retinoblastoma shows preferential loss of the maternal allele. However, this is owing simply to the higher mutation rate of the paternal gamete rather than imprinting, since the *RB* gene is not imprinted.[40]

Preferential involvement of a specific parental chromosome also applies to other types of chromosomal abnormalities in cancer. For example, Haas and colleagues reported preferential involvement of paternal chromosome 9 and maternal chromosome 22 in the Philadelphia chromosome translocation of chronic myelogenous leukemia based on a cytogenetic polymorphism.[41] However, subsequent studies have not shown imprinting of the rearranged *BCR* and *ABL* genes, and molecular studies have not confirmed preferential parental origin of those chromosomes.[42–44]

Other types of parental origin-specific chromosome alterations have withstood the test of time. For example, the N-*myc* gene on chromosome 2 shows preferential amplification of the paternal allele in neuroblastoma.[45] Preferential LOH of the maternal allele of chromosome 1 in neuroblastoma initially was observed by some investigators and not by others.[45,46] However, this controversy was resolved when it was found that advanced tumors, showing N-*myc* amplification, also show preferential LOH of maternal chromosome 1, whereas earlier-stage tumors without N-*myc* amplification do not.[47] Thus genetic disturbances involving imprinted genes in a given type of cancer may involve multiple chromosomes concurrently. This idea of abnormal imprinting affecting multiple chromosomes is a provocative one for which there are other data. For example, Sapienza has found transmission ratio distortion, concordance of 13q loss, and isochromosome 6 of the same parental origin in retinoblastoma, again consistent with a mechanism of generalized disturbance of imprinting in embryogenesis leading to increased cancer risk.[48]

Despite these intriguing observations of diverse tumors, suggesting a role for genomic imprinting in cancer, direct proof for such a role awaited the discovery of specific imprinted human genes and their altered imprinting in cancer. The guidepost toward these genes was the hereditary disorder Beckwith-Wiedemann syndrome.

BECKWITH-WIEDEMANN SYNDROME

Beckwith-Wiedemann syndrome (BWS) is a disorder of prenatal overgrowth and cancer transmitted as an autosomal dominant trait, although most cases arise sporadically. It is reported to affect 1 in 15,000 children, although the frequency may be much higher because close scrutiny of families of BWS patients often shows subtly affected siblings or parents and the phenotype abates with increasing age of the patient.[49,50] Its cardinal features are macroglossia or enlargement of the tongue, macrosomia caused by prenatal overgrowth throughout gestation, abdominal wall defects (including diastasis recti and umbilical hernia), omphalocele, and craniofacial dysmorphism (including facial nevus flameus, ear pits and creases, prominent occiput, maxillary hypoplasia, widened nasal bridge, high arched palate, and occasionally mild microcephaly). In addition, BWS typically presents with neonatal hypoglycemia, caused in part by overproduction of IGF2.[49,50]

The frequency of embryonal tumors in BWS children is approximately 20 percent, a 1000-fold increase over that of the general population.[51,52] These include WT, hepatoblastoma, rhabdomyosarcoma, and adrenocortical carcinoma.[51,52] In addition, the same organs show dysplastic changes, including adrenal cytomegaly and cysts, nephromegaly with prominent lobulation and nephrogenic rests, hepatomegaly, splenomegaly, and hyperplasia of the islets of Langerhans.[49–52]

A clue to a role for genomic imprinting is increased disease penetrance when BWS is inherited from the mother.[53] As noted earlier, parent-of-origin effects may or may not represent genomic imprinting. However, the tumors these children develop show preferential loss of maternal 11p15, as noted earlier, suggesting that an imprinted locus could cause BWS and also be involved in sporadically occurring tumors.[36,37] Genetic linkage analysis showed that BWS localizes to 11p15, consistent with this idea, and not to 11p13, to which the *WT1* gene had been localized.[54,55]

Further support for the idea that imprinting is involved in BWS came from study of rare chromosomal translocations or inversions affecting approximately 1 percent of BWS patients. About half these rearrangements are balanced, and by analogy with other human genetic disorders, these balanced rearrangements are likely to disrupt the coding sequence of a BWS gene. All the balanced rearrangements have involved the maternally derived chromosome 11.[56,57] The simplest explanation is that the rearrangements are disrupting expression of a maternally expressed gene. Indeed, there are several families in which multiple individuals within the same kindred harbor the same chromosomal rearrangement, but only those inheriting the rearrangement from the mother were affected with BWS.[56,57] The other type of chromosomal rearrangement seen in BWS patients involves unbalanced translocations or duplications. All of these have shown an excess of the paternally derived chromosome.[56] Thus both paternal duplication and maternal rearrangement of chromosome 11 can lead to BWS.

More direct evidence for genomic imprinting of 11p15 in BWS came from studies of Junien and colleagues showing that some patients with BWS have paternal UPD involving a region extending from the β-globin locus to the *ras* gene.[58] This is a very large area of at least 10 Mb and thus does not provide precise localization of an imprinted gene, but it provided an important foundation for later studies of imprinted loci on this chromosome. Curiously, all the patients with UPD are mosaic for this abnormality.[59] Thus it occurs postzygotically and is presumably an early embryonic lethal when present in the zygote.

Paternal UPD causes both duplication of the paternal allele and loss of the maternal allele of the involved genes. Thus UPD by itself is consistent either with loss of function of a gene normally expressed on the maternal chromosome or duplication of a gene normally expressed from the paternal chromosome. The balanced maternal chromosomal rearrangements in other patients could represent loss of function of a maternally expressed gene or, alternatively, disruption of an imprinting control center, a hypothetical *cis*-acting signal that establishes the original imprinting pattern in the germ line. This disruption could lead to abnormal activation of a gene or genes normally silent on the maternal chromosome and thus functional duplication of a gene normally expressed from the paternal chromosome. Evidence for this idea derives from the fact that the balanced chromosomal rearrangements, looked at as a group, span a very large region, >3 Mb, larger than would be expected for a single locus.[57] However, they are clustered into two distinct regions, each of which could conceivably represent a single large gene.[57] The unbalanced paternal chromosome duplications, however, are difficult to explain other than by a mechanism of increased dosage (doubling) of a gene or genes normally expressed only from the paternal chromosome. Of course, BWS may involve both duplication of paternally expressed genes and loss of maternally expressed genes. The identification of genes involved in BWS followed from the discovery of imprinted genes in human 11p15 and is described in the next section.

IMPRINTED GENES ON 11p15 AND LOSS OF IMPRINTING IN CANCER

The first human gene shown to be imprinted at the molecular level was *IGF2,* which was examined because of its localization to 11p15, for the reasons discussed in the preceding section and because it was known to be imprinted in the mouse. In order to test the hypothesis that *IGF2* is imprinted, it was necessary to reverse transcribe (RT) the gene from RNA in a tissue that expresses it, and then polymerase chain reaction (PCR) amplify the cDNA products. If this RT-PCR is performed on an individual heterozygous for a transcribed polymorphism (i.e., a polymorphic site is present within an exon), then one can determine whether one or both alleles are expressed. If only one allele is expressed, then one can determine if it is maternal or paternal by examining parental genomic DNA samples. In this manner, the *IGF2* gene was found to be normally imprinted, with preferential expression of the paternal allele (Fig. 18-2), as in the mouse.[60–63] In mouse, *H19,* a gene within 100 kb of *IGF2* that encodes an untranslated RNA of unclear function, is oppositely imprinted, with preferential expression of the maternal allele.[64] This gene also was tested for imprinting in humans and was found to be imprinted as well, with preferential expression of the maternal allele.[60,65]

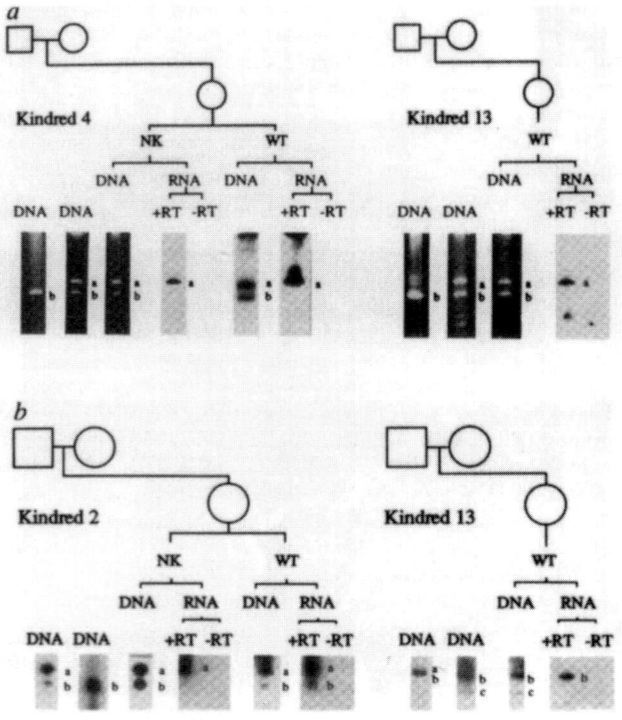

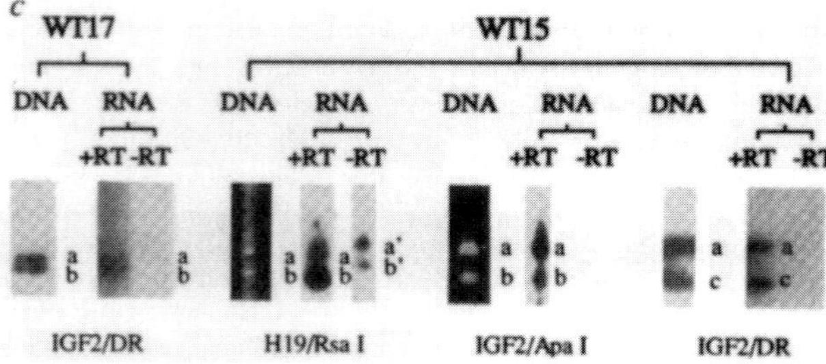

Fig. 18-2 Imprinting of *H19* and *IGF2* genes and loss of imprinting in cancer. *A.* Maternal monoallelic expression of *H19* in normal kidney (NK) and Wilms tumor (WT). Both NK and WT of patient 4 and WT of patient 13 show monoallelic expression of the maternal allele. *B.* Paternal monoallelic expression of *IGF2* in normal kidney. Kindred 2 was analyzed using an ApaI polymorphism and kindred 13 using a dinucleotide repeat (DR) polymorphism. *C.* Biallelic expression of *H19* and *IGF2* in Wilms tumors. WT17 was analyzed using the IGF2/DR polymorphism and shows biallelic expression. WT15 was informative for all three polymorphisms. Both *H19* and *IGF2* show biallelic expression, as does the WT from patient 2 (see *B*). A single DNA-contaminated RNA sample from patient 15 was deliberately included to illustrate the larger-sized fragments (a′,b′) resulting from amplification of genomic sequences. (*Reprinted from Rainier S, Johnson LA, Dobry CJ, Ping AJ, Grundy PE, Feinberg AP: Relaxation of imprinted genes in human cancer.* Nature *362:747–749, 1993, with permission.*)

Examination of RNA from WT led to a surprising discovery. Not one, but both *IGF2* alleles were expressed in 70 percent of Wilms tumors.[60,62] In addition, in 30 percent of cases, both alleles of *H19* were expressed[60] (see Fig. 18-2). The term for this novel genetic alteration in cancer is *loss of imprinting* (LOI), which simply means loss of preferential parental origin-specific gene expression and can involve either abnormal expression of the normally silent allele, leading to biallelic expression, or silencing of the normally expressed allele, leading to epigenetic silencing of the locus.[60,66,67] Thus, in addition to the epigenetic silencing suggested earlier by Sapienza and colleagues (see Fig. 18-1), abnormal imprinting in cancer can lead to activation of normally silent alleles of growth-promoting genes[37,38,60,66,67] (see Fig. 18-1).

Subsequently, a large number of additional tumor types have been shown to undergo LOI. At first, LOI was found in other childhood tumors, such as hepatoblastoma, rhabdomyosarcoma, and Ewing sarcoma.[68–71] LOI of *IGF2* and *H19* also have now been found in many adult tumors, including uterine, cervical, esophageal, prostate, lung, and colon cancer, choriocarcinoma, and germ-cell tumors.[72–78] Thus LOI is one of the most common alterations in human cancer. These data are summarized in Table 18-3.

Care must be used in interpreting evidence of biallelic expression of *IGF2* as LOI, since *IGF2* is normally expressed from both alleles of the adult, or P1, promoter.[79] Nevertheless, abnormal imprinting and biallelic expression from the fetal promoters (P2 to P4) has been demonstrated for most of the tumors described earlier.[69,71,72,80] Finally, LOI of *IGF2* has been described in BWS, albeit in a relatively small percentage of patients.[81,82] Additional patients with large stature and WT but not BWS per se also show LOI of *IGF2.*[83]

A third imprinted gene on chromosome 11p15 is $p57^{KIP2}$, encoding a cyclin-dependent kinase (CDK) inhibitor related to $p21^{WAF1/Cip1}$, a target of p53.[84,85] It was mapped to 11p15 and

Table 18-3 Cancers That Show Loss of Imprinting (LOI)

Tumor Type	Gene
Wilms tumor	IGF2, H19, $p57^{KIP2}$
Rhabdomyosarcoma	IGF2
Hepatoblastoma	IGF2
Bladder	IGF2, H19
Cervical	IGF2, H19
Prostate	IGF2
Testicular	IGF2, H19
Esophageal	H19
Breast	IGF2
Choriocarcinoma	IGF2, H19
Ovarian	IGF2
Colorectal	IGF2

found to be localized within 40 kb of a group of BWS balanced germ-line chromosomal rearrangement breakpoints, in contrast to *IGF2* and *H19,* which are located telomeric to these breakpoints.[57,84] Nevertheless, its chromosomal location suggested that it also may be imprinted and play a role in tumors that show LOH of 11p15. Human $p57^{KIP2}$ was indeed found to be imprinted with preferential expression from the maternal allele.[86] $p57^{KIP2}$ also shows abnormal imprinting and epigenetic silencing in some tumors and in BWS patients.[87] Subsequently, nonsense mutations have been described in BWS, but the frequency is quite low, only 5 percent.[88,89] Interestingly, BWS can arise from $p57^{KIP2}$ mutations transmitted from the father, although with less severity than those transmitted from the mother.[89] Thus the phenotype must in part involve haploinsufficiency of the gene in tissues in which it is not normally imprinted, as well as loss of function in tissues where it is imprinted.[89] This observation is the converse of that made for *UBE3A,* which is mutated at high frequency in AS but is not imprinted in most tissues[29]; yet it must be imprinted in some because it shows UPD effects.

Two additional imprinted 11p15 genes have been identified recently. *TSSC3/IPL* is a maternally expressed homologue of mouse *TDAG51,* which activates Fas and FasL, leading to apoptosis of T lymphocytes.[145,146] TSSC5/IMPT/BWR1C is a putative transmembrane protein that is weakly homologous to bacterial transporter proteins.[147–149] Mutations in *TSSC5* were identified recently in WT and lung cancer[147], suggesting that it may correspond to the long-sought *WT2* gene on 11p15.

A gene spanning a cluster of BWS balanced germ-line chromosomal rearrangement breakpoints has been identified recently as K_VLQT1.[131] This gene, which also causes the autosomal dominant cardiac arrhythmia long QT syndrome, spans at least 350 kb and also shows genomic imprinting, with preferential expression of the maternal allele.[131] In addition, the gene undergoes alternative splicing at the 5′ end, which involves an untranslated upstream sequence, similar to that observed upstream of the *SNRPN* gene.[131] Thus K_VLQT1 may be involved in imprint control similar to the function ascribed to *SNRPN* on chromosome 15. Interestingly, K_VLQT1 is not imprinted in the heart, explaining the lack of parent-of-origin effect in long QT syndrome but marked parent-of-origin effect in translocation-associated BWS.[131]

Finally, a novel antisense transcript, termed LIT1 (Long Intronic Transcript 1), has been identified within K_VLQT1.[147] LIT1 is at least 60 kb in size and appears to be unspliced and untranslated. LIT1 is expressed from the paternal allele, in contrast to K_VLQT1, which is expressed from the maternal allele.[147] Remarkably, LIT1 undergoes LOI in most patients with BWS.[147]

How can such diverse genetic alterations lead to BWS? One possibility is that some of the genes involved, e.g., *IGF2,* $p57^{KIP2}$, and K_VLQT1, all are part of the same biochemical pathway. A second possibility is that one or more of these genes may be coordinately regulated as part of a large genomic region of multiple imprinted genes. LIT1 is an intriguing candidate for such a *cis*-acting regulatory role. A summary of genetic alterations in BWS is presented in Table 18-4.

Table 18-4 Genetic Alterations in Beckwith-Wiedemann Syndrome

Genetic Alteration	Allele
Balanced germ-line chromosomal translocations and inversions	Maternal
Unbalanced germ-line chromosomal translocations and duplications	Paternal
Uniparental disomy	Paternal
Loss of imprinting of IGF2	Maternal
Loss of imprinting of $p57^{KIP2}$	Maternal
Mutation of $p57^{KIP2}$	Maternal
Imprint-specific methylation switch (increased)	Maternal
Gene rearrangement	Maternal
Loss of imprinting of LIT1	Maternal

One of the most intriguing recent observations of LOI in cancer was in the normal tissues of colon cancer patients. LOI was found in 12 of 27 informative colorectal cancer patients (44 percent), in the matched normal mucosa of the same patients, and in all four available blood samples from these patients. The colonic mucosa of noncancer patients showed LOI in 2 of 16 informative cases (12 percent) and in 2 of 15 blood samples (13 percent).[150] It is not yet known whether LOI arose in normal tissue before or coincident with LOI in the tumors, but either way, LOI may become a useful new diagnostic or prognostic marker for cancer. In this regard, most patients with microsatellite instability in their tumors showed LOI in the cancer and normal colon, and consistent with this observation, the LOI patients were significantly younger than the non-LOI patients.[150]

THE EFFECTS OF LOI ON GENE EXPRESSION AND TUMOR CELL GROWTH

Since the time of Laennec, it has been known that cancers lose properties of their normal cellular counterparts and gain properties of other types of cells or developmental stages.[90] One of the most intriguing aspects of LOI is that it may help to explain the abnormal gene expression patterns that are responsible for these characteristics.

Quantitative assays of gene expression in WTs with LOI reveal the following: *IGF2* expression is increased approximately twofold, *H19* expression is lost, and $p57^{KIP2}$ expression is lost.[81] This is true even for tumors that show biallelic expression of *H19.*[87] What appears to take place in tumors with LOI is that the maternal chromosome switches to a paternal epigenotype, affecting several genes over a several hundred kilobase domain. Thus the maternal copy of *IGF2* is expressed, hence biallelic expression. Conversely, the maternal alleles of *H19* and $p57^{KIP2}$ are epigenetically silenced as on the paternal chromosome, leading to little or no detectable expression of these genes overall.[81,91]

These observations suggest a unified model of LOI in some cancers, such as WT, which explains epigenetic silencing of tumor suppressor genes as well as activation of normally silent alleles of growth-promoting genes. According to this model, LOI involves a switch in the epigenotype of a chromosomal region in the case of WT from maternal to paternal.[81,91] Thus *IGF2* shows biallelic expression, and *H19* undergoes epigenetic silencing. However, this model is not meant to be universal. For example, not all tumors show a switch in expression of all three genes, *IGF2, H19,* and $p57^{KIP2}$. Hepatoblastoma shows LOI of *IGF2,* but tumors with biallelic expression of *IGF2* do not necessarily undergo epigenetic silencing of *H19.*[68,69]

What is the biologic effect of these changes in gene expression caused by altered genomic imprinting? IGF2 is an important autocrine and paracrine growth factor.[92–99] Its mitogenic effects are mediated by signaling through the IGF1 receptor.[99] This is clearly an important pathway in cancer because blocking IGF2 at the IGF1 receptor inhibits tumor cell growth and is even the basis of an experimental therapeutic trial.[99–102] In addition, somatic mutations in the *IGF2* receptor gene, which is a metabolic sink for IGF2, have been found in hepatocellular carcinoma, further supporting the idea that signaling by IGF2 is an important mitogenic growth pathway.[103]

Direct evidence for a causative role of insulin-like growth factor II in tumor progression comes from studies of mice harboring an SV40 T-antigen transgene under the control of a rat insulin promoter, known as *RIP-Tag mice.* These animals develop insulinomas at high frequency, and the tumors evolve through sequential stages of tumor progression.[104] When the *RIP-Tag* transgene is bred into a background of mice with homozygously knocked out *IGF2* genes, they still develop tumors, but the tumors are arrested at a stage of benign neoplasia.[105] However, when the *RIP-Tag* transgene is bred into a heterozygous *IGF2* knockout background, in which only the paternal allele has been disrupted, the maternal allele undergoes LOI and the tumors progress through malignancy, but the tumors are smaller.[106] Finally, when the maternal allele is knocked out, the tumors still show LOI, in that the neogene is now expressed from the disrupted allele.[106] Thus LOI is a necessary step in tumor progression in this system. This model also provides a clue to one possible effect of LOI. Tumor cells in which *IGF2* has been homozygously knocked out show increased apoptosis, which is overcome by introduction into them of an *IGF2* expression construct.[105] Thus LOI may be one of the factors that allows tumors to escape the apoptosis caused by other carcinogenic mutations.

H19 is an untranslated RNA that accounts for a significant fraction (3 percent) of embryonic mRNA,[107] but significance remains unclear. An *H19* transgene was reported to be an embryonic lethal, but the lethality was caused by a small insertion in the transgene used to mark it.[108,109] An *H19* expression construct caused suppression of growth in soft agar of WT cells into which it was introduced.[110] However, *H19* maps outside the 11p15 region shown to suppress tumor growth in genetic complementation experiments.[111]

The effect of LOI on $p57^{KIP2}$ may be as important as that of *IGF2* and *H19.* Most or all WTs tumors undergo epigenetic silencing of $p57^{KIP2}$.[87] In some tumors, this appears to be caused by abnormal imprinting. The same effect is seen in tumors with LOH, since the normally expressed maternal allele is lost.[87] Thus $p57^{KIP2}$ may represent an imprinted tumor gene in which epigenetic silencing is the primary carcinogenic event. Indeed, this may turn out to be the first tumor gene in which epigenetic silencing is the only carcinogenic event, if mutations in nonfamilial tumors continue not to be found.

POSSIBLE MECHANISMS OF NORMAL IMPRINTING AND LOSS OF IMPRINTING IN CANCER

DNA Methylation

Cytosine DNA methylation is a covalent modification of DNA in which a methyl group is transferred from *S*-adenosyl methionine to the C-5 position of cytosine by cytosine (DNA-5)-methyltransferase (referred to as *DNA methyltransferase*). DNA methylation occurs almost exclusively at CpG dinucleotides.[112] The pattern of DNA methylation is heritable by somatic cells and maintained after DNA replication by DNA methyltransferase, which has a 100-fold greater affinity for hemimethylated DNA (i.e., parent strand methylated, daughter strand unmethylated) than for unmethylated DNA.[112] However, developing cells in the gamete and embryo undergo dramatic shifts in DNA methylation, which involve both loss of methylation and *de novo* methylation.[112] It is not known what mechanism establishes the original pattern of DNA methylation.

There are two classes of cytosine DNA methylation in the genome. The first occurs throughout the body of genes that show tissue-specific expression, with methylation generally associated with gene silencing. This type of DNA methylation can occur both before and after the changes in gene expression, so they are not necessarily the cause of altered gene expression during development. Rather, they may help to "lock in" a given pattern of gene expression.[112,113]

The second class of normal cytosine methylation involves CpG islands, regions rich in CpG dinucleotides. CpG islands are almost always unmethylated in normal cells, and they are usually within the promoter or first exon of housekeeping genes.[114] However, an important exception is CpG islands on the inactive X chromosome, which are methylated. Thus CpG island methylation, unlike non-CpG island methylation, is thought to be involved in epigenetic silencing in general and marking of the inactive X chromosome in particular.[115]

Several recent discoveries suggest a role for DNA methylation in the control of genomic imprinting. First, some imprinted genes in mice, such as *H19,* show parental origin-specific, tissue-independent methylation of CpG islands. For example, the paternal CpG island in *H19* is methylated and the maternal allele unmethylated, in tissues that express the gene as well as those which do not.[116,117] Thus this methylation represents an imprinting mark on the paternal chromosome and is not secondary to changes in gene expression. Second, knockout mice deficient in DNA methyltransferase and exhibiting widespread genome hypomethylation do not show allele-specific methylation of the *H19* CpG island and exhibit biallelic expression of *H19* and loss of expression of *IGF2.*[118] Similar parental origin-specific methylation also has been observed for a CpG island in the first intron of the maternally inherited, expressed allele of the *IGF2* receptor gene (*IGF2R*).[119] Methyltransferase-deficient knockout mice show loss of methylation of *IGF2R* and epigenetic silencing of the gene.[118]

Widespread alterations in DNA methylation in human tumors were discovered 15 years ago.[120] This remains the most commonly found alteration in human cancer, albeit an epigenetic one, and it occurs ubiquitously in both benign and malignant neoplasms.[121] The precise role of these changes has remained unclear, although both decreased and increased methylation has been found at specific sites in tumors, with an overall decrease in quantitative DNA methylation.[122–124]

Recent work using an experimental mouse model system also supports a role for DNA methylation in cancer. "Min" mice carry a mutation for the adenomatous polyposis coli (*APC*) gene and thereby develop colon tumors. When bred to knockout mice deficient in DNA methyltransferase, Min mice are partially protected from the development of tumors, suggesting that cytosine DNA methylation is involved in tumorigenesis.[125] Consistent with this idea, when these mice are treated with 5-azacytidine, a specific inhibitor of DNA methylation, the incidence of tumors is markedly reduced.[125] Of course, in this model system, decreased methylation may simply protect the animals from methylcytosine-to-thymine transition mutations.[125] Decreased methylation also may or may not be linked to genomic imprinting, which has not yet been examined in the Min mouse system, but the studies reinforce the link between altered DNA methylation and cancer.

DNA Methylation and LOI

In humans as in mice, the paternal allele of a CpG island in the *H19* gene and its promoter is normally methylated, and the maternal allele is unmethylated.[81,116,117] Thus CpG island methylation represents an imprint-specific mark on the paternal chromosome. Because tumors with LOI of *IGF2* showed reduced expression of *H19,* and because normal imprinting of *H19* is associated with methylation of the paternal allele, the methylation pattern of *H19* has been examined in tumors with LOI. In all cases showing LOI of *IGF2,* the *H19* promoter exhibits 90 to 100 percent methylation at the sites normally unmethylated on the maternally inherited allele.[81,91] Thus the maternal allele has acquired a paternal pattern of methylation. This is consistent with the fact that the *IGF2* gene on the same (maternally derived) chromosome is expressed in these tumors, as occurs normally only on the paternally derived chromosome. In contrast, tumors without LOI of *IGF2* show no change in the methylation of *H19,* indicating that these changes are related to abnormal imprinting and not malignancy per se.[81,91] The same alterations in methylation of the maternal allele of *H19* are found in BWS patients with LOI of *IGF2,* indicating that LOI can precede the development of malignancy and not arise secondarily.[81,126,127] These observations are consistent with the model presented earlier of a switch in parental epigenotype. According to this model, LOI, at least in WT, involves a switch of the maternal chromosome to a paternal epigenotype, with activation of the maternal *H19* allele, silencing of the maternal *IGF2* allele, silencing of the maternal $p57^{KIP2}$ allele, and methylation of the maternal *H19* allele, as on the paternal chromosome.

What is the mechanism of altered DNA methylation in cancer? One mechanism that has been proposed is increased DNA methyltransferase expression itself.[128] Based on a quantitative RT-PCR assay, a 20-fold increase in DNA methyltransferase expression was reported in human colon tumors compared with matched normal mucosa, as well as a 400-fold increase in cancer over the normal mucosa of unaffected patients.[128] However, other RT-PCR experiments showed a more modest change.[129] Furthermore, a sensitive and specific RNase protection assay (RPA) found only a 1.8- to 2.5-fold increase in MTase mRNA.[130] This small difference disappeared entirely when histone H4 was used as an internal control, as a measure of nonspecific tumor cell proliferation. Thus the mechanism of altered methylation and genomic imprinting does not involve the known DNA methyltransferase enzyme itself.[130]

Disruption of an Imprinting Control Center

A second potential mechanism of LOI may involve disruption of an imprinting control center on chromosome 11, similar to that recently described for the PWS/AS region of chromosome 15.[28] A cluster of five BWS balanced germ-line chromosomal rearrangement breakpoints lies between $p57^{KIP2}$ on the centromeric side and *IGF2* and *H19* on the telomeric side.[57] Thus disruption of a gene spanning this region could cause abnormal imprinting, as well as BWS and/or cancer, at least when inherited through the germ line. A gene spanning a cluster of BWS-balanced germ-line chromosome rearrangement breakpoints has been identified recently as K_VLQT1.[131] This gene spans at least 350 kb, shows genomic imprinting, and undergoes alternative splicing, similar to that observed upstream of the *SNRPN* gene.[130] Thus this gene may be involved in imprint control similar to the function ascribed to *SNRPN* on chromosome 15.

Other Possible Factors Causing LOI

Clues to other potential mechanisms for LOI come from consideration of the factors thought to be important in establishment and maintenance of normal genomic imprinting in mouse and of other forms of epigenetic inheritance in other species, discussed in the opening section of this chapter. One example is the loss of trans-acting factors, which are thought to help maintain a normal pattern of imprinting after it is established in the germ line. *Trans*-acting modifiers of imprinting are likely to exist, since imprinting of transgenes is host strain-dependent.[132] The human homologues of such genes might thus act as tumor suppressor genes.

Another potential mechanism of imprinting that may be disrupted in cancer involves histone deacetylation, which is linked to X inactivation in mammals and to telomere silencing in yeast.[133,134] Trichostatin A, a histone deacetylase inhibitor, may disrupt normal genomic imprinting.[135,136] Genes for both histone acetylase and histone deacetylase have been isolated recently.[137,138] In addition, telomere silencing in yeast also involves the action of specific genes, e.g., *SIR1* to *SIR4*, at least one of which has a homologue in mammals.[7] Similarly, some examples of gene silencing in mammals may resemble position-effect variegation in *Drosophila*, a form of position-dependent epigenetic silencing.[139] Finally, imprinted loci on maternal and paternal chromosomes may interact during DNA replication. Chromosomal regions harboring imprinted genes replicate synchronously.[140] Furthermore, the two parental homologues of some imprinted genes show nonrandom proximity in late S-phase,[141] suggesting some form of chromosomal crosstalk, as has been observed for epigenetic silencing in *Drosophila*.[142] Although the mechanism of imprinting remains unknown, analysis of tumor cells with altered imprinting should provide an additional tool in unraveling this mystery.

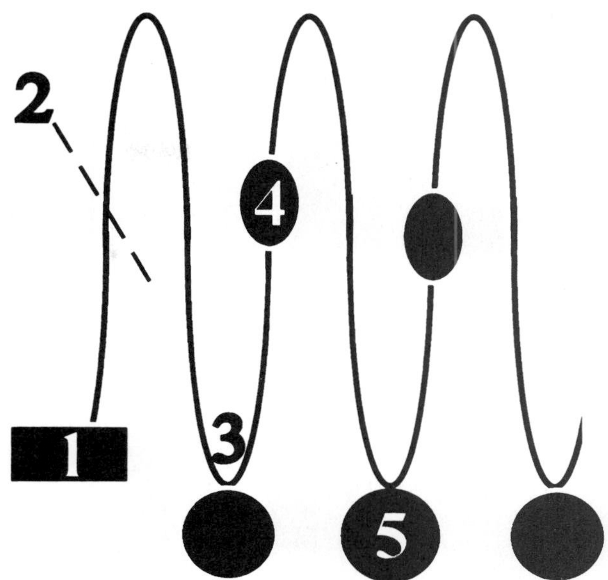

Fig. 18-3 A model of genomic imprinting as a developmental process, at which disturbances of several points may lead to loss of imprinting in cancer. An imprint organizing center (*rectangle*) exerts a long-range *cis*-acting influence on *IGF2* and other imprinted genes (*oval*) via alterations in chromatin structure (represented as DNA loops). This imprint-organizing center establishes the imprinting mark as maternal or paternal. This effect is propagated outward during development similar to the organizing center on the X chromosome. Imprinting is maintained in part by allele-specific methylation of CpG islands, as well as by interactions with *trans*-acting proteins (*circle*). According to this model, loss of imprinting could arise by any of several mechanisms (numbered in the figure): (1) deletion or mutation in the imprint organizing center itself, which would lead to a failure of parental origin-specific switching in the germ line, (2) separation of the imprint-organizing center from the imprinted target genes, as seen in BWS germ-line chromosomal rearrangement cases, (3) abnormal methylation of CpG islands, (4) local mutation of regulatory sequences controlling the target imprinted genes themselves, or (5) loss of or mutations in genes for trans-acting factors that maintain normal imprinting. (*Modified from Feinberg AP, Kalikin LM, Johnson LA, Thompson JS: Loss of imprinting in human cancer.* Cold Spring Harbor Symp Quant Biol *59:357–364, 1994, with permission.*)

In considering these diverse factors that could disrupt imprinting, it is important to view normal genomic imprinting as a developmental process rather than as a single event (Fig. 18-3). In addition to an initial mark on the chromosome, an imprinting signal likely propagates along the chromosome, similar to propagation of a signal along the inactive X chromosome. Furthermore, specific genes show tissue-specific imprinting, and the timing of silencing varies from gene to gene during early embryonic development. Thus a combination of both *cis*-acting and *trans*-acting signals is likely to be important in the establishment and maintenance of normal genomic imprinting, and disruption of these same factors can be expected to play a role in LOI in cancer (see Fig. 18-3). It is also important to note that genomic imprinting normally is erased in primordial germ cells during embryonic development, and thus the aberrant expression in tumors, of factors involved in normal imprint erasure, also could cause loss of imprinting.

IMPLICATIONS FOR CANCER TREATMENT

One of the most exciting aspects of the study of LOI in human cancer is that it is potentially reversible, given that normal imprinting involves epigenetic modifications and that imprinting is normally reversible. A recent experiment suggests that this idea shows some promise.[143] Because tumors with LOI show

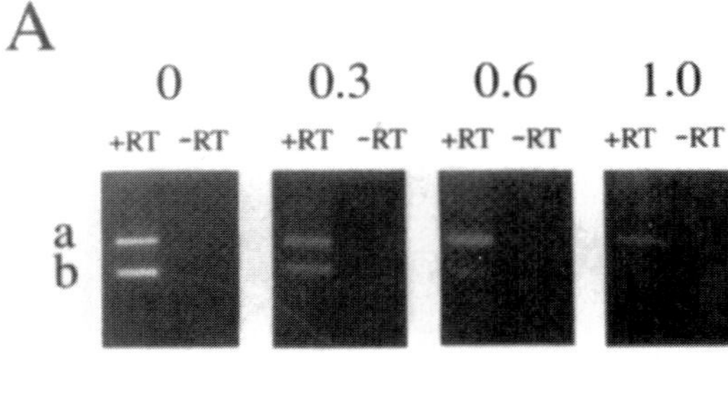

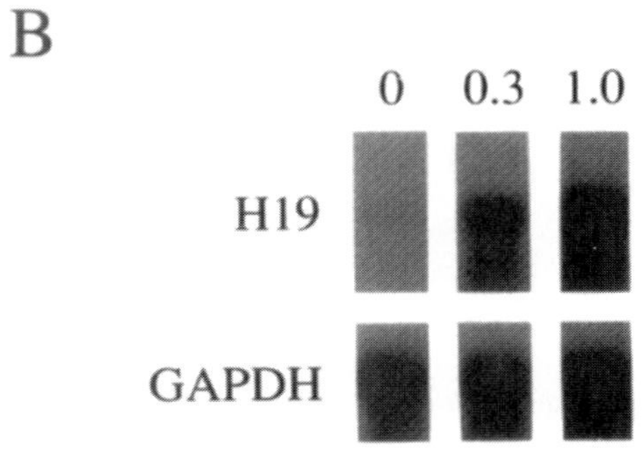

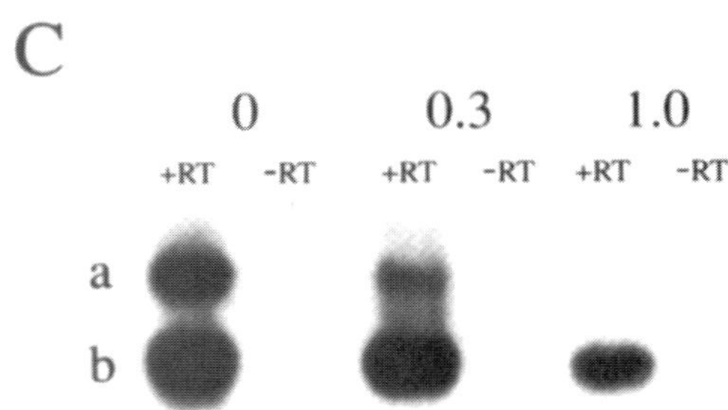

Fig. 18-4 Switch to preferential allelic expression of *IGF2* by 5-aza-2′-deoxycytidine (5-azaCdR) treatment of tumor cells with LOI. RT-PCR was performed on total RNA extracted from JEG-3 choriocarcinoma cells after a single 24-h treatment with 0, 0.3, 0.6, or 1.0 mM 5-azaCdR (indicated). Alternating lanes represent simultaneous experiments with and without reverse transcriptase. PCR products were digested with Apa I. The a and b alleles are 236 and 173 bp, respectively. (*Reprinted from Barletta JM, Rainier S, Feinberg AP: Reversal of loss of imprinting in tumor cells by 5-aza-2′-deoxycytidine.* Cancer Res *57:48–50, 1997, with permission.*)

increased methylation of the *H19* CpG island, LOI may be reversed with an inhibitor of DNA methylation, 5-aza-2′-deoxycytidine (5-azaCdR). Two tumor cell lines exhibiting LOI were treated with 5-azaCdR for 24 hours (1 cell division) at concentrations chosen to maximize methylation-related biologic effects. Treatment with increasing doses of 5-azaCdR led to unequal expression of the two *IGF2* alleles in both cell lines (Fig. 18-4). The cells switched from equal expression of the two alleles to predominant expression of the allele represented by the upper uncut band lacking the Apa I polymorphic site, and this effect was nonrandom and specific to one allele. Similarly, 5-azaCdR-treated tumor cells showed a marked increase in *H19* expression similar to that seen in normally imprinted cells. In addition to this reactivation of overall *H19* expression, *H19* also switched from biallelic to monoallelic expression, again consistent with restoration of normal imprinting. Finally, methylation of the imprint-specific CpG island in *H19* switched from virtually complete methylation to the expected pattern of single-allele methylation.[143] In this experiment, since parental DNA was unavailable, the reestablishment of a normal imprinting pattern could have been due either to a switch of the abnormally imprinted maternal chromosome back to a normal epigenotype. It also could have been due to allele switching, in which the maternal chromosome remained paternally imprinted, but the paternal chromosome switched, to a maternal epigenotype.[143]

Nevertheless, these results are surprising and encouraging because 5-azaCdR may have been expected to show a nonspecific effect on both alleles, similar to that seen in methyltransferase-deficient knockout mice.[118] The fact that 5-azaCdR exerted a specific effect on one chromosome indicates that some imprint-specific information is still retained in tumor cells that show LOI. It further suggests that 5-azaCdR, or drugs with similar effects, may prove useful in the treatment of tumors with LOI, either alone or in conjunction with other agents, and that other strategies for intervention in the pathways regulating genomic imprinting also eventually may be exploited in the design of novel cancer treatments.

ACKNOWLEDGMENT

This work was supported by NIH Grant CA65145.

REFERENCES

1. Tartof KD, Henikoff S: Trans-sensing effects from *Drosophila* to humans. *Cell* **65**:201, 1991.
2. Goldsborough AS, Kornberg TB: Reduction of transcription by homologue asynapsis in *Drosophila* imaginal discs. *Nature* **381**:807, 1996.
3. Patterson GI, Thorpe CJ, Chandler VL: Paramutation, an allelic interaction, is associated with a stable and heritable reduction of transcription of the maze b regulatory gene. *Genetics* **135**:881, 1993.
4. Tartof KD, Bremer M: Mechanisms for the construction and developmental control of heterochromatin formation and imprinted chromosome domains. *Development* **(suppl)**:35, 1990.
5. Tschiersch B, Hofmann A, Krauss V, Dorn R, Korge G, Reuter G: The protein encoded by the *Drosophila* position-effect variegation suppressor gene Su(var)3-9 combines domains of antagonistic regulators of homeotic gene complexes. *EMBO J* **13**:3822, 1994.
6. Gerasimova TI, Gdula DA, Gerasimov DV, Simonova O, Corces VG: A *Drosophila* protein that imparts directionality on a chromatin insulator is an enhancer of position-effect variegation. *Cell* **82**:587, 1995.
7. Brachmann CB, Sherman JM, Devine SE, Cameron EE, Pillus L, Boeke JD: The SIR2 gene family, conserved from bacteria to humans, functions in silencing, cell cycle progression, and chromosome stability. *Genes Dev* **9**:2888, 1995.
8. Crouse H: The controlling element in sex chromosome behavior in Sciara. *Genetics* **45**:1425, 1960.
9. McGrath J, Solter D: Completion of mouse embryogenesis requires both the maternal and paternal genomes. *Cell* **37**:179, 1984.
10. Harper MI, Fosten M, Monk M: Preferential paternal X inactivation in extraembryonic tissues of early mouse embryos. *J Embryol Exp Morphol* **67**:127, 1982.
11. Cattanach BM, Beechey CV: Autosomal and X-chromosome imprinting. *Development* **(suppl)**:63, 1990.
12. Swain JL, Stewart TA, Leder P: Parental legacy determines methylation and expression of an autosomal transgene: A molecular mechanism for parental imprinting. *Cell* **50**:719, 1987.
13. Sapienza C, Paquete J, Tran TH, Peterson A: Epigenetic and genetic factors affect transgene methylation imprinting. *Development* **107**:165, 1989.
14. DeChiara TM, Robertson EJ, Efstratiadis A: Parental imprinting of the mouse insulin-like growth factor-2 gene. *Cell* **64**:849, 1991.
15. Barlow DP, Stoger R, Herrmann BG, Saito K, Schweifer N: The mouse insulin-like growth factor type-2 receptor is imprinted and closely linked to the Tme locus. *Nature* **349**:84, 1991.
16. Kuroiwa Y, Kaneko-Ishino T, Kagitani F, Kohda T, Li L.-L, Tada M, et al: Peg3 imprinted gene on proximal chromosome 7 encodes for a zinc finger protein. *Nature Genet* **12**:186, 1996.
17. Nagai H, Pongliktmongkol M, Kim YS, Yoshikawa H, Matsubara K: Cloning of Not I-cleaved genomic DNA fragments appearing as spots in 2D gel electrophoresis. *Biochem Biophys Res Commun* **213**:258, 1995.

18. Vogelstein B, Fearon ER, Hamilton SR, Feinberg AP: Use of restriction fragment length polymorphisms to determine the clonal origin of human tumors. *Science* **227**:642, 1985.
19. Laird CD: Proposed mechanism of inheritance and expression of the human fragile-X syndrome of mental retardation. *Genetics* **117**:587, 1987.
20. Oberle I, Rousseau F, Heitz D, Kretz C, Devys D, Hanauer A, Boue J, Bertheas MF, Mandel JL: Instability of a 550-base pair DNA segment and abnormal methylation in fragile X syndrome. *Science* **252**:1097, 1991.
21. Fu Y, Kuhl DPA, Pizzuti A, Pieretti M, Sutcliffe JS, Richards S, et al: Variation of the CGG repeat at the fragile X site results in genetic instability: Resolution of the Sherman paradox. *Cell* **67**:1047, 1991.
22. Feng Y, Zhang F, Lokey LK, Chastain JL, Lakkis L, Eberhart D, et al: Translational suppression by trinucleotide repeat expansion at FMR1. *Science* **268**:731, 1995.
23. Nicholls RD, Knoll JHM, Butler MG, Karam S, Lalande M: Genetic imprinting suggested by maternal heterodisomy in nondeletion Prader-Willi syndrome. *Nature* **342**:281, 1989.
24. Knoll JHM, Nicholls RD, Magenis RE, Glatt K, Graham JM Jr, Kaplan L, et al: Angelman syndrome: Three molecular classes identified with chromosome 15q11q13-specific DNA markers. *Am J Hum Genet* **47**:149, 1990.
25. Knoll JH, Nicholls RD, Magenis RE, Graham JM Jr, Lalande M, Latt SA: Angelman and Prader-Willi syndromes share a common chromosome 15 deletion but differ in parental origin of the deletion. *Am J Med Genet* **32**:285, 1989.
26. Mattei MG, Souiah N, Mattei JF: Chromosome 15 anomalies and the Prader-Willi syndrome: Cytogenetic analysis. *Hum Genet* **66**:313, 1984.
27. Nicholls RD: Genomic imprinting and candidate genes in the Prader-Willi and Angelman syndromes. *Curr Opin Genet Dev* **3**:445, 1993.
28. Dittrich B, Buiting K, Korn B, Rickard S, Buxton J, Saitoh S, et al: Imprint switching on human chromosome 15 may involve alternative transcripts of the SNRPN gene. *Nature Genet* **14**:163, 1996.
29. Kishino T, Lalande M, Wagstaff J: UBE3A E6-AP mutations causing Angelman syndrome. *Nature Genet* **15**:70, 1997.
30. Ledbetter DH, Engel E: Uniparental disomy in humans: Development of an imprinting map and its implications for prenatal diagnosis. *Hum Mol Genet* **4**:1757, 1995.
31. Spence JE, Perciaccante RG, Greig GM, Willard HF, Ledbetter DH, Hejtmancik JF, et al: Uniparental disomy as a mechanism for human genetic disease. *Am J Hum Genet* **42**:217, 1988.
32. Kajii T, Ohama K: Androgenetic origin of hydatidiform mole. *Nature* **268**:633, 1977.
33. Linder D, McCaw B, Kaiser X, Hecht F: Parthenogenetic origin of benign ovarian teratomas. *N Engl J Med* **292**:63, 1975.
34. Heutink P, van Schothorst EM, van der Mey AG, Bardoel A, Breedveld G, Pertijs J, et al: Further localization of the gene for hereditary paragangliomas and evidence for linkage in unrelated families. *Eur J Hum Genet* **2**:148, 1994.
35. Reeve AE, Sih SA, Raizis AM, Feinberg AP: Loss of allelic heterozygosity at a second locus on chromosome 11 in sporadic Wilms' tumor cells. *Mol Cell Biol* **9**:1799, 1989.
36. Schroeder W, Chao L, Dao D, Strong L, Pathak S, Riccardi V, et al: Nonrandom loss of maternal chromosome 11 alleles in Wilms tumors. *Am J Hum Genet* **40**:413, 1987.
37. Scrable H, Cavenee W, Ghavimi F, Lovell M, Morgan K, Sapienza C: A model for embryonal rhabdomyosarcoma tumorigenesis that involves genome imprinting. *Proc Natl Acad Sci USA* **86**:7480, 1989.
38. Peterson K, Sapienza C: Imprinting the genome: Imprinted genes, imprinting genes, and a hypothesis for their interaction. *Annu Rev Genet* **27**:7, 1993.
39. Katz F, Webb D, Gibbons B, Reeves B, McMahon C, Chessells J, et al: Possible evidence for genomic imprinting in childhood acute myeloblastic leukaemia associated with monosomy for chromosome 7. *Br J Haematol* **80**:332, 1992.
40. Zhu X, Dunn JM, Phillips RA, Goddard AD, Paton KE, Becker A, et al: Preferential germline mutation of the paternal allele in retinoblastoma. *Nature* **340**:312, 1989.
41. Haas OA, Argyriou-Tirita A, Lion T: Parental origin of chromosomes involved in the translocation t(9;22). *Nature* **359**:414, 1992.
42. Riggins GJ, Zhang F, Warren ST: Lack of imprinting of BCR. *Nature Genet* **6**:226, 1994.
43. Melo JV, Yan XH, Diamond J, Goldman JM: Lack of imprinting of the ABL gene. *Nature Genet* **8**:318, 1994.
44. Melo JV, Yan XH, Diamond J, Goldman JM: Balanced parental contribution to the ABL component of the BCR-ABL gene in chronic myeloid leukemia. *Leukemia* **9**:734, 1995.
45. Cheng JM, Hiemstra JL, Schneider SS, Naumova A, Cheung NV, Cohn SL, et al: Preferential amplification of the paternal allele of the N-myc gene in human neuroblastomas. *Nature Genet* **4**:187, 1993.
46. Caron H, van Sluis P, van Hoeve M, de Kraker J, Bras J, Slater R, et al: Allelic loss of chromosome 1p36 in neuroblastoma is of preferential maternal origin and correlates with N-myc amplification. *Nature Genet* **4**:191, 1993.
47. Caron H, Peter M, van Sluis P, Speleman F, de Kraker J, Laureys G, et al: Evidence for two tumor suppressor loci on chromosomal bands 1p35-36 involved in neuroblastoma: One probably imprinted, another associated with N-myc amplification. *Hum Mol Genet* **4**:535, 1995.
48. Naumova A, Hansen M, Strong L, Jones PA, Hadjistilianou D, Mastrangelo D, et al: Concordance between parental origin of chromosome 13q loss and chromosome 6p duplication in sporadic retinoblastoma. *Am J Hum Genet* **54**:274, 1994.
49. Engstrom W, Lindham S, Schofield P: Wiedemann-Beckwith syndrome. *Eur J Pediatr* **147**:450, 1988.
50. Pettenati MJ, Haines JL, Higgins RR, Wappner RS, Palmer CG, Weaver DD: Wiedemann-Beckwith syndrome: Presentation of clinical and cytogenetic data on 22 new cases and review of the literature. *Hum Genet* **74**:143, 1986.
51. Wiedemann HR: Tumours and hemihypertrophy associated with Wiedemann-Beckwith syndrome. *Eur J Pediatr* **141**:129, 1983.
52. Elias ER, DeBaun MR, Feinberg AP: Beckwith-Wiedemann syndrome, in Jameson JL (ed): *Textbook of Molecular Medicine*. Cambridge, Blackwell Scientific, in press.
53. Viljoen D, Ramesar R: Evidence for paternal imprinting in familial Beckwith-Wiedemann syndrome. *J Med Genet* **29**:221, 1992.
54. Ping AJ, Reeve AE, Law DJ, Young MR, Boehnke M, Feinberg AP: Genetic linkage of Beckwith-Wiedemann syndrome to 11p15. *Am J Hum Genet* **44**:720, 1989.
55. Koufos A, Grundy P, Morgan K, Aleck KA, Hadro T, Lampkin BC, et al: Familial Wiedemann-Beckwith syndrome and a second Wilms tumor locus both map to 11p15. *Am J Hum Genet* **44**:711, 1989.
56. Mannens M, Hoovers JMN, Redeker E, Verjaal M, Feinberg AP, Little P, et al: Parental imprinting of human chromosome region 11p15 involved in the Beckwith-Wiedemann syndrome and various human neoplasia. *Eur J Hum Genet* **2**:3, 1994.
57. Hoovers JMN, Kalikin LM, Johnson LA, Alders M, Redeker B, Law DJ, et al: Multiple genetic loci within 11p15 defined by Beckwith-Wiedemann syndrome: Rearrangement breakpoints and subchromosomal transferable fragments. *Proc Natl Acad Sci USA* **92**:12456, 1995.
58. Henry I, Bonaiti-Pellie C, Chehensse V, Beldjord C, Schwartz C, Utermann G, Junien C: Uniparental paternal disomy in a genetic cancer-predisposing syndrome. *Nature* **351**:609, 1991.
59. Henry I, Peuch A, Riesewijk A, Ahnine L, Mannens M, Beldjord C, et al: Somatic mosaicism for partial paternal isodisomy in Wiedemann-Beckwith syndrome: A post-fertilization event. *Eur J Hum Genet* **1**:19, 1993.
60. Rainier S, Johnson LA, Dobry CJ, Ping AJ, Grundy PE, Feinberg AP: Relaxation of imprinted genes in human cancer. *Nature* **362**:747, 1993.
61. Ohlsson R, Nystrom A, Pfeifer-Ohlsson S, Tohonen V, Hedborg F, Schofield P, et al: IGF2 is parentally imprinted during human embryogenesis and in the Beckwith-Wiedemann syndrome. *Nature Genet* **4**:94, 1993.
62. Ogawa O, Eccles MR, Szeto J, McNoe LA, Yun K, Maw MA, et al: Relaxation of insulin-like growth factor II gene imprinting implicated in Wilms' tumour. *Nature* **362**:749, 1993.
63. Giannoukakis N, Deal C, Paquette J, Goodyer CG, Polychronakos C: Parental genomic imprinting of the human IGF2 gene. *Nature Genet* **4**:98,1993.
64. Bartolomei M, Zemel S, Tilghman SM: Parental imprinting of the mouse H19 gene. *Nature* **351**:153,1991.
65. Zhang Y, Shields T, Crenshaw T, Hao Y, Moulton T, Tycko B: Imprinting of human H19: Allele-specific CpG methylation, loss of the active allele in Wilms tumor, and potential for somatic allele switching. *Am J Hum Genet* **53**:113, 1993.
66. Feinberg AP: Genomic imprinting and gene activation in cancer. *Nature Genet* **4**:110,1993.
67. Feinberg AP, Rainier S, DeBaun MR: Genomic imprinting, DNA methylation, and cancer. *J Natl Cancer Inst Monogr* **17**:21, 1995.
68. Rainier S, Dobry CJ, Feinberg AP: Loss of imprinting in hepatoblastoma. *Cancer Res* **55**:1836, 1995.

69. Li X, Adam G, Cui H, Sandstedt B, Ohlsson R, Ekstrom TJ: Expression, promoter usage and parental imprinting status of insulin-like growth factor II (IGF2) in human hepatoblastoma: Uncoupling of IGF2 and H19 imprinting. *Oncogene* **11**:221, 1995.
70. Zhan SL, Shapiro DN, Helman LJ: Activation of an imprinted allele of the insulin-like growth factor II gene implicated in rhabdomyosarcoma. *J Clin Invest* **94**:445, 1994.
71. Zhan SL, Shapiro DN, Helman LJ: Loss of imprinting of IGF2 in Ewing's sarcoma. *Oncogene* **11**:2503, 1995.
72. Vu TH, Yballe C, Boonyanit S, Hoffman AR: Insulin-like growth factor II in uterine smooth-muscle tumors: Maintenance of genomic imprinting in leiomyomata and loss of imprinting in leiomyosarcomata. *J Clin Endocrinol Metab* **80**:1670, 1995.
73. Doucrasy S, Barrois M, Fogel S, Ahomadegbe JC, Stehelin D, Coll J, et al: High incidence of loss of heterozygosity and abnormal imprinting of H19 and IGF2 genes in invasive cervical carcinomas: Uncoupling of H19 and IGF2 expression and biallelic hypomethylation of H19. *Oncogene* **12**:423, 1996.
74. Hibi K, Nakamura H, Hirai A, Fujikake Y, Kasai Y, Akiyama S, et al: Loss of H19 imprinting in esophageal cancer. *Cancer Res* **56**:480, 1996.
75. Jarrard DF, Bussemakers MJG, Bova GS, Isaacs WB Regional loss of imprinting of the insulin-like growth factor II gene occurs in human prostate tissues. *Clin Cancer Res* **1**:1471, 1995.
76. Kondo M, Suzuki H, Ueda R, Osada H, Takagi K, Takahashi T, et al: Frequent loss of imprinting of the H19 gene is often associated with its overexpression in human lung cancers. *Oncogene* **10**:1193, 1995.
77. Hashomoto K, Azuma C, Koyama M, Ohashi K, Kamiura S, Nobunaga T, et al: Loss of imprinting in choriocarcinoma. *Nature Genet* **9**:109, 1995.
78. Van Gurp RJHLM, Oosterhuis JW, Kalscheuer V, Mariman ECM, Looijenga LHJ: Biallelic expression of the H19 and IGF2 genes in human testicular germ cell tumors. *J Natl Cancer Inst* **86**:1070, 1994.
79. Vu TH, Hoffman AR: Promoter-specific imprinting of the human insulin-like growth factor-II gene. *Nature* **371**:714, 1994.
80. Zhan S, Shapiro D, Zhan S, Zhang L, Hirschfeld S, Elassal J, et al: Concordant loss of imprinting of the human insulin-like growth factor II gene promoters in cancer. *J Biol Chem* **270**:27983, 1995.
81. Steenman MJC, Rainier S, Dobry CJ, Grundy P, Horon IL, Feinberg AP: Loss of imprinting of IGF2 is linked to reduced expression and abnormal methylation of H19 in Wilms' tumor. *Nature Genet* **7**: 433, 1994.
82. Weksberg R, Shen DR, Fei YL, Song QL, Squire J: Disruption of insulin-like growth factor 2 imprinting in Beckwith-Weidemann syndrome. *Nature Genet* **5**:143, 1993.
83. Ogawa O, Becroft DM, Morison IM, Eccles MR, Skeen JE, Mauger DE, et al: Constitutional relaxation of insulin-like growth factor II gene imprinting associated with Wilms' tumour and gigantism. *Nature Genet* **5**:408, 1993.
84. Matsuoka S, Edwards MC, Bai C, Parker S, Zhang P, Baldini A, et al: p57/KIP2, a structurally distinct member of the p21/CIP1 Cdk inhibitor family, is a candidate tumor suppressor gene. *Genes Dev* **9**:650, 1995.
85. Lee M-H, Reynisdottir I, Massague J: Cloning of p57/KIP2, a clini-dependent kinase inhibitor with unique domain structure and tissue distribution. *Genes Dev* **9**:639, 1995.
86. Matsuoka S, Thompson JS, Edwards MC, Barletta JM, Grundy P, Kalikin LM, et al: Imprinting of the gene encoding a human cyclin-dependent kinase inhibitor, p57KIP2, on chromosome 11p15. *Proc Natl Acad Sci USA* **93**:3026, 1996.
87. Thompson JS, Reese KJ, DeBaun MR, Perlman EJ, Feinberg AP: Reduced expression of the cyclin-dependent kinase inhibitor p57KIP2 in Wilms tumor. *Cancer Res* **56**:5723, 1996.
88. Hatada H, Ohashi Y, Fukushima Y, Kaneko M, Inoue Y, Komoto A, et al: An imprinted gene p57KIP2 is mutated in Beckwith-Wiedemann syndrome. *Nature Genet* **14**:171, 1996.
89. Lee MP, DeBaun M, Randhawa G, Reichard BA, Elledge SJ, Feinberg AP: Low frequency of p57KIP2 mutations in Beckwith-Wiedemann syndrome. *Am J Hum Genet* **61**:304, 1997.
90. Pitot HC: Fundamentals of Oncology. New York, Marcel Deckker, 1981.
91. Moulton T, Crenshaw T, Hao Y, Moosikasuwan J, Lin N, Dembitzer F, et al: Epigenetic lesions at the H19 locus in Wilms' tumour patients. *Nature Genet* **7**:440, 1994.
92. Lahm H, Suardet L, Laurent PL, Fischer JR, Ceyhan A, Givel J-C, et al: Growth regulation and co-stimulation of human colorectal cancer cell lines by insulin-like growth factor I, II and transforming growth factor a. *Br J Cancer* **65**:341, 1992.
93. Gelato MC, Vassalotti J: Insulin-like growth factor-II: Possible local growth factor in pheochromocytoma. *J Clin Endocrinol Metab* **71**:1168, 1990.
94. El-Badry OM, Minniti C, Kohn EC, Houghton PJ, Daughaday WH, Helman LJ: Insulin-like growth factor II acts as an autocrine growth and motility factor in human rhabdomyosarcoma tumors. *Cell Growth Diff* **1**:325, 1990.
95. Yee D, Cullen KJ, Paik S, Perdue JF, Hampton B, Schwartz A, et al: Insulin-like growth factor II mRNA expression in human breast cancer. *Cancer Res* **48**:6691, 1988.
96. Lamonerie T, Lavialle C, Haddada H, Brison O: IGF-2 autocrine stimulation in tumorigenic clones of a human colon-carcinoma cell line. *Int J Cancer* **61**:587, 1995.
97. Pommier GJ, Garrouste FL, El Atiq F, Roccabianca M, Marvaldi JL, Remacle-Bonnet MM: Potential autocrine role of insulin-like growth factor II during suramin-induced differentiation of HT29-D4 human colonic adenocarcinoma cell line. *Cancer Res* **52**:3182, 1992.
98. Leventhal PS, Randolph AE, Vesbit TE, Schenone A, Windebank A, Feldman EL: Insulin-like growth factor-II as a paracrine growth factor in human neuroblastoma cells. *Exp Cell Res* **221**:179, 1995.
99. Osborne CK, Coronado EB, Kitten LJ, Arteaga CI, Fuqua SA, Ramasharma K, et al: Insulin-like growth factor-II (IGF-II): A potential autocrine/paracrine growth factor for human breast cancer acting via the IGF-I receptor. *Mol Endocrinol* **3**:1701, 1989.
100. Osborne CK, Clemmons DR, Arteaga CL: Regulation of breast cancer growth by insulin-like growth factors. *J Steroid Biochem Molec Biol* **37**:805, 1990.
101. Vincent TS, Hazen-Martin DJ, Garvin AJ: Inhibition of insulin-like growth factor II autocrine growth of Wilms tumor by suramin in vitro and in vivo. *Cancer Letts* **103**:49, 1996.
102. Miglietta L, Barreca A, Repetto L, Costantini M, Rosso R, Boccardo F: Suramin and serum insulin-like growth factor levels in metastatic cancer patients. *Anticancer Res* **13**:2473, 1993.
103. De Souza AT, Hankins GR, Washington MK, Orton TC, Jirtle RL: M6P/IGF2R gene is mutated in human hepatocellular carcinomas with loss of heterozygosity. *Nature Genet* **11**:447, 1995.
104. Hanahan D: Heritable formation of pancreatic B-cell tumors in transgenic mice expressing recombinant insulin/simian virus 40 oncogones. *Nature* **315**:115, 1985.
105. Christofori G, Naik P, Hanahan D: A second signal supplied by insulin-like growth factor II in oncogene-induced tumorigenesis. *Nature* **369**:414, 1994.
106. Christofori G, Naik P, Hanahan D: Deregulation of both imprinted and expressed alleles of the insulin-like growth factor 2 gene during B-cell tumorigenesis. *Nature Genet* **10**:196, 1995.
107. Brannan CI, Dees EC, Ingram RS, Tilghman SM: The product of the H19 gene may function as an RNA. *Mol Cell Biol* **10**:28, 1990.
108. Brunkow ME, Tilghman SM: Ectopic expression of the H19 gene in mice causes prenatal lethality. *Genes Dev* **5**:1092, 1991.
109. Pfeifer K, Leighton P, Tilghman SM: The structural H19 gene is required for its own imprinting. *Proc Natl Acad Sci USA* **93**:13876, 1996.
110. Hao Y, Crenshaw T, Moulton T, Newcomb E, Tycko B: Tumor-suppressor activity of H19 RNA. *Nature* **365**:764, 1993.
111. Koi M, Johnson LA, Kalikin LM, Little PFR, Nakamura Y, Feinberg AP: Tumor cell growth arrest caused by subchromosomal transferable DNA fragments from human chromosome 11. *Science* **260**:361, 1993.
112. Cedar H, Razin A: DNA methylation and development. *Biochim Biophys Acta* **1049**:1, 1990.
113. Riggs AD: DNA methylation and cell memory. *Cell Biophys* **15**:1, 1989.
114. Bird AP: CpG-rich islands and the function of DNA methylation. *Nature* **321**:209, 1986.
115. Riggs AD, Pfeifer GP: X-chromosome inactivation and cell memory. *Trends Genet* **8**:169, 1992.
116. Ferguson-Smith AC, Sasaki H, Cattanach BM, Surani MA: Parental-origin-specific epigenetic modification of the mouse H19 gene. *Nature* **362**:751, 1993.
117. Bartolomei M, Webber AL, Brunkow ME, Tilghman SM: Epigenetic mechanisms underlying the imprinting of the mouse H19 gene. *Genes Dev* **7**:1663, 1993.
118. Li E, Beard C, Jaenisch R: Role for DNA methylation in genomic imprinting. *Nature* **366**:362, 1993.
119. Stoger R, Kubicka P, Liu C-G, Kafri T, Razin A, Cedar H, et al: Maternal-specific methylation of the imprinted mouse IGF2 locus identifies the expressed locus as carrying the imprinting signal. *Cell* **73**:61, 1993.

120. Feinberg AP, Vogelstein B: Hypomethylation distinguishes genes of some human cancers from their normal counterparts. *Nature* **301**:89, 1983.
121. Goelz SE, Vogelstein B, Hamilton SR, Feinberg AP: Hypomethylation of DNA from benign and malignant human colon neoplasms. *Science* **228**:187, 1985.
122. Feinberg AP, Gehrke CW, Kuo KC, Ehrlich M: Reduced genomic 5-methylcytosine content in human colonic neoplasia. *Cancer Res* **48**:1159, 1988.
123. Feinberg AP: Alterations in DNA methylation in colorectal polyps and cancer. *Prog Clin Biol Res* **279**:309, 1988.
124. Jones PA, Buckley JD: The role of DNA methylation in cancer. *Adv Cancer Res* **54**:1, 1990.
125. Laird PW, Jackson-Grusby L, Fazeli A, Dickinson SL, Jung WE, Li E, et al: Suppression of intestinal neoplasia by DNA hypomethylation. *Cell* **81**:197, 1995.
126. Reik W, Brown KW, Slatter RE, Sartori P, Elliott M, Maher ER: Allelic methylation of H19 and IGF2 in the Beckwith-Wiedemann syndrome. *Hum Mol Genet* **3**:1297, 1995.
127. Reik W, Brown KW, Schneid H, Bouc YL, Bickmore W, Maher ER: Imprinting mutations in the Beckwith-Wiedemann syndrome suggested by an altered imprinting pattern in the IGF2-H19 domain. *Hum Mol Genet* **4**:2379, 1995.
128. El-Deiry WS, Nelkin BD, Celano P, Yen RC, Falco JP, Hamilton SR, et al: High expression of the DNA methyltransferase gene characterizes human neoplastic cells and progression stages of colon cancer. *Proc Natl Acad Sci USA* **88**:3470, 1991.
129. Schmutte C, Yang AS, Nugyen TT, Beart RB, Jones PA: Mechanisms for the involvement of DNA methylation in colon cancer. *Cancer Res* **56**:2375, 1996.
130. Lee PJ, Washer LL, Law DJ, Boland CR, Horon IL, Feinberg AP: Limited upregulation of DNA methyltransferase in human colon cancer reflecting increased cell proliferation. *Proc Natl Acad Sci USA* **93**:10366, 1996.
131. Lee MP, Hu R-J, Johnson LA, Feinberg AP: Human KVLQT1 gene shows tissue-specific imprinting and encompasses Beckwith-Wiedemann syndrome chromosomal rearrangements. *Nature Genet* **15**:181, 1997.
132. Allen ND, Norris ML, Surani MA: Epigenetic control of transgene expression and imprinting by genotype-specific modifiers. *Cell* **61**:353, 1990.
133. Wolffe AP: Inheritance of chromatin states. *Dev Genet* **15**:463, 1994.
134. Thompson JS, Ling X, Grunstein M: Histone H3 amino terminus is required for telomeric and silent mating. *Nature* **369**:245, 1994.
135. Yoshida M, Kijima M, Akita M, Beppu T: Potent and specific inhibition of mammalian histone deacetylase both in vivo and in vitro by trichostatin A. *J Biol Chem* **265**:17174, 1990.
136. Efstratiadis A: Parental imprinting of autosomal mammalian genes. *Curr Opin Genet Dev* **4**:265, 1994.
137. Brownell JE, Zhou J, Ranalli T, Kobayashi R, Edmondson DG, Roth SY, et al: Tetrahymena histone acetyltransferase A: A homolog to yeast gcn5p linking histone acetylation to gene activation. *Cell* **84**:843, 1996.
138. Taunton J, Hassig CA, Schreiber SL: A mammalian histone deacetylase related to the yeast transcriptional regulator rpd3p. *Science* **272**:408, 1996.
139. Walters MC, Magis W, Fiering S, Eidemiller J, Scalzo D, Groudine M, et al: Transcriptional enhancers act in cis to suppress position-effect variegation. *Genes Dev* **10**:185, 1996.
140. Kitsberg D, Selig S, Brandeis M, Simon I, Keshet I, Driscoll DJ, et al: Allele-specific replication timing of imprinted gene regions. *Nature* **364**:459, 1993.
141. LaSalle JM, Lalande M: Homologous association of oppositely imprinted chromosomal domains. *Science* **272**:725, 1996.
142. Tatof KD, Henikoff S: Trans-sensing effects from *Drosophila* to humans. *Cell* **65**:201, 1991.
143. Barletta JM, Rainier S, Feinberg AP: Reversal of loss of imprinting in tumor cells by 5-aza-2′-deoxycytidine. *Cancer Res* **57**:48, 1997.
144. Feinberg AP, Kalikin LM, Johnson LA, Thompson JS: Loss of imprinting in human cancer. *Cold Spring Harbor Symp Quant Biol* **59**:357, 1994.
145. Lee MP, Feinberg AP: Genomic imprinting of a human apoptosis gene homologue, TSSC3. *Cancer Res* **58**:1052, 1998.
146. Qian N, Frank D, O'Keefe D, Dao D, Zhao L, Yuan L, Wang Q, et al: The IPL gene on chromosome 11p15.5 is imprinted in human and mice and is similar to TDAG51, implicated in Fas expression and apoptosis. *Hum Mol Genet* **6**:2021, 1997.
147. Lee MP, DeBaun MR, Mitsuya K, Galonek HL, Brandenburg S, Oshimura M, Feinberg AP: Loss of imprinting of a paternally expressed transcript, with antisense orientation to K_VLQT1, occurs frequently in Beckwith-Wiedemann syndrome and is independent of IGF2 imprinting. *Proc Natl Acad Sci USA* **96**:5203, 1999.
148. Dao D, Frank D, Qian N, O'Keefe D, Vosatka RJ, Walsh CP, Tycko B: IMPT1, an imprinted gene similar to polyspecific transporter and multi-drug resistance genes. *Hum Mol Genet* **7**:597, 1998.
149. Schwienbacher C, Sabbioni S, Campi M, Veronese A, Bernardi G, Menegatti A, Hatada I, et al: Transcriptional map of 170-kb region at chromosome 11p15.5: identification and mutational analysis of the BWR1A gene reveals the presence of mutations in tumor samples. *Proc Natl Acad Sci USA* **95**:3873, 1998.
150. Cui H, Horon IL, Ohlsson R, Hamilton SR, Feinberg AP: Loss of Imprinting in normal tissue of colorectal cancer patients with microsatellite instability. *Nature Med* **4**:1276, 1998.

CHAPTER 19

Genes Altered by Chromosomal Translocations in Leukemias and Lymphomas

A. Thomas Look

1. **Somatically acquired chromosomal translocations activate proto-oncogenes in the hematopoietic cells of both children and adults. This mechanism of gene dysregulation contributes to well over 50 percent of all leukemias that have been characterized cytogenetically and molecularly and to a substantial proportion of lymphomas, notably the Burkitt, large-cell, and follicular types.**
2. **In most instances, chromosomal translocations fuse sequences of a transcription factor or receptor tyrosine kinase gene to those of a normally unrelated gene, resulting in a chimeric protein with oncogenic properties. Repositioning of transcriptional control genes to the vicinity of highly active promoter/enhancer elements, such as those associated with immunoglobulin or T-cell receptor genes, is a second mechanism by which chromosomal translocations induce malignancy.**
3. **The vast majority of translocation-induced leukemias and lymphomas are restricted to cells of a single lineage arrested at a particular stage of development, indicating that the disrupted genes regulate vital processes limited to a subset of committed hematopoietic progenitors. Occasionally, as exemplified by leukemias arising from *MLL* gene abnormalities, more than one lineage or developmental stage is affected, suggesting the involvement of genes active in pluripotent or bipotent stem cells.**
4. **The number of fusion genes with diagnostic and prognostic relevance is increasing rapidly. The hybrid mRNAs produced by these novel structures provide specific molecular probes for identifying affected patients who cannot be diagnosed readily by conventional means or who require chemotherapy tailored to the risk conferred by a particular genetic lesion.**
5. **Studies in murine models, in which specific genes are mutated and homozygously inactivated in "knockout" mice or overexpressed in transgenic mice, have contributed new insights into the essential roles that are played in normal development and oncogenesis by genes discovered because of their proximity to the breakpoints of chromosomal translocations in the human leukemias and lymphomas.**

A list of standard abbreviations is located immediately preceding the index in each volume. Nonstandard abbreviations used in this chapter include: bHLH = basic region/helix-loop-helix; bZIP = basic region/leucine zipper; ALL = acute lymphoblastic leukemia; AML = acute myeloid leukemia; DIC = disseminated intravascular coagilation; CMML = chronic myelomonocytic leukemia; APML = acute promyelocytic leukemia; CML = chronic myeloid leukemia; MDS = myelodysplastic syndrome.

The concept that cancer cells contain genetic information not found in normal cells has provided the impetus for molecular approaches to cancer research. A pivotal step in this progress was the realization that gross chromosomal changes — such as translocations, deletions, inversions and amplifications — can perturb genes intimately involved in carcinogenesis.[1–3] Thus a major concern over the past two decades has been the identification of consistent chromosomal abnormalities in specific types of tumor cells, the isolation of genes affected by these changes, and the elucidation of their mechanisms of action and clinical correlations. A surprising dividend of this venture, aided by technology that permits one to create homozygous null animals by inactivating individual genes (e.g., "knockout" mice), has been the discovery of proteins that not only promote cancer but also have essential functions in normal cell development as well.[4]

Specific reciprocal translocations perhaps are the best example of how cytogenetic changes pave the way for cancer induction and spread. These nonheritable abnormalities occur in a high percentage of hematologic cancers — both leukemias and lymphomas — where they disrupt signaling pathways that enhance cell survival.[4–7] Their actions can directly activate occult proto-oncogenes or, more commonly, create cell type-specific fusion proteins that contain elements of one or more transcription factors.[5,8] It is intriguing that many of the genes involved in translocation-mediated fusions have close homologues in genes controlling embryogenesis in *Drosophila* and other invertebrates, underscoring their faithful conservation in nature and their relevance to programs of early cell development.[9–11] Unfortunately, the downstream genetic programs controlled by the various transcription factors affected by chromosomal translocations are largely unknown, so interrelationships between transcription networks and leukemogenesis remain to be assessed.

The medical benefits gained from analysis of chromosomal translocations in the leukemias and lymphomas are still modest. One of the difficulties is that fusion proteins typically are localized to the cell nucleus, making them inaccessible to most available therapies, requiring instead the introduction of therapeutic molecules into the cell. Nonetheless, the chimeric RNA and DNA of these lesions provide highly specific targets for molecular assays that can resolve interpretive ambiguities created by conventional diagnostic or cell classification methods.[12] One emerging application is the use of polymerase chain reaction-(PCR)-based techniques to detect chimeric RNA in residual leukemia cells.[13] Other applications include the detection of specific high-risk genetic lesions, such as the *E2A-PBX1, MLL-AF4,* and *BCR-ABL* fusion genes, to ensure that patients are assigned to sufficiently aggressive treatment programs.[7,14]

This chapter summarizes the molecular consequences of translocations in the human leukemias and lymphomas. Emphasis is placed on disease types with the highest frequencies of productive rearrangements and on those (often rare) types in which study of molecular aberrations has revealed novel principles of pathogenesis.

DYSREGULATION OF TRANSCRIPTIONAL CONTROL GENES

The majority of transcription factors that are altered by chromosomal translocations in the leukemias and lymphomas (Table 19-1) can be classified into four major types on the basis of recurring structural elements within their DNA- and protein-binding domains: basic region/helix-loop-helix (bHLH), basic region/leucine zipper (bZIP), zinc finger, and homeodomain.[6,8,15] Other less common but still functionally significant motifs include A-T hook, Ets-like, Runt homology, and cysteine-rich (LIM). In some cases, a transcription factor gene is rearranged to a site adjacent to a T-cell receptor (*TCR*) or immunoglobulin (*Ig*) locus, resulting in dysregulated expression of the proto-oncogenic sequences. A second, perhaps more common mechanism involves chromosomal rearrangements that fuse transcriptional control genes into functional chimeras. Such fusions are important because they give rise to novel proteins capable of interacting with DNA and other regulatory elements in ways that usurp normal cellular control mechanisms.[6]

The diversity of transcription factor proto-oncogenes implicated in the human leukemias and lymphoma is striking, although increasingly their essential functions can be traced to a fundamental step in cell growth, development, or survival.[8] Currently, more than 10 transcriptional control genes have been shown to play critical roles in normal hematopoiesis (Fig. 19-1). Some of these factors are lineage-specific, whereas others operate early in hematopoietic development, before lineage commitment. Still others are widely expressed but perform unique functions in a limited number of blood cell types, ostensibly by interacting with lineage-restricted proteins.[4] Of major pathobiologic importance, many transcription factors that control blood cell differentiation are targets for productive rearrangement by translocations in the leukemias and lymphomas, reinforcing their roles as master regulators of hematopoietic cell development. In the following sections I summarize how chromosomal translocations modify transcription factors to generate malignant cells within the hematopoietic system.

Acute Lymphoblastic Leukemias and Non-Hodgkin Lymphomas

The frequency distributions of the various molecular abnormalities mediated by chromosomal translocations are shown diagrammatically in Figs. 19-2 and 19-3, with key associations given in Tables 19-1 and 19-2.

***MYC* Activation in Burkitt Lymphoma and B-Cell Leukemia.** In Burkitt lymphoma and B-cell leukemia, arising in surface Ig-positive "virgin" B lymphoblasts with moderately abundant, vacuolated cytoplasm, the principal genetic change is a juxtapositioning of the *MYC* proto-oncogene next to the *Ig* heavy-chain gene as a result of the t(8;14)(q24;q32).[16–18] *MYC* is a prototypic bHLH/leucine zipper transcription factor whose rearrangement from chromosome 8 to a site near strong *Ig* enhancer elements on chromosome 14 leads to dysregulated expression of the *MYC* oncoprotein. In most instances, the t(8;14) is responsible for inappropriate activation of *MYC;* however, two variants of this rearrangement can produce the same effect, except that they move *Igκ* and *Igλ* light chain genes from chromosome 2 and 22, respectively, to the *MYC* locus on chromosome 8.[19–24] The *MYC* gene often acquires point mutations in its coding or regulatory regions, probably as a result of somatic mutation that occurs after translocation,[25–28] which in some cases encodes proteins that are unable to interact with the *Rb*-related gene *p107*.[29]

A leading question since the discovery of *MYC* activation in Burkitt lymphoma/B-cell leukemia has been: How does the MYC oncoprotein transform B lymphocytes? The answer seems to lie in the effects of *MYC* dysregulation on a transcriptional network comprising at least three other factors, each also harboring bHLH/leucine zipper domains. In this cascade, MYC is able to dimerize with the MAX protein,[30,31] which can bind to DNA, to itself

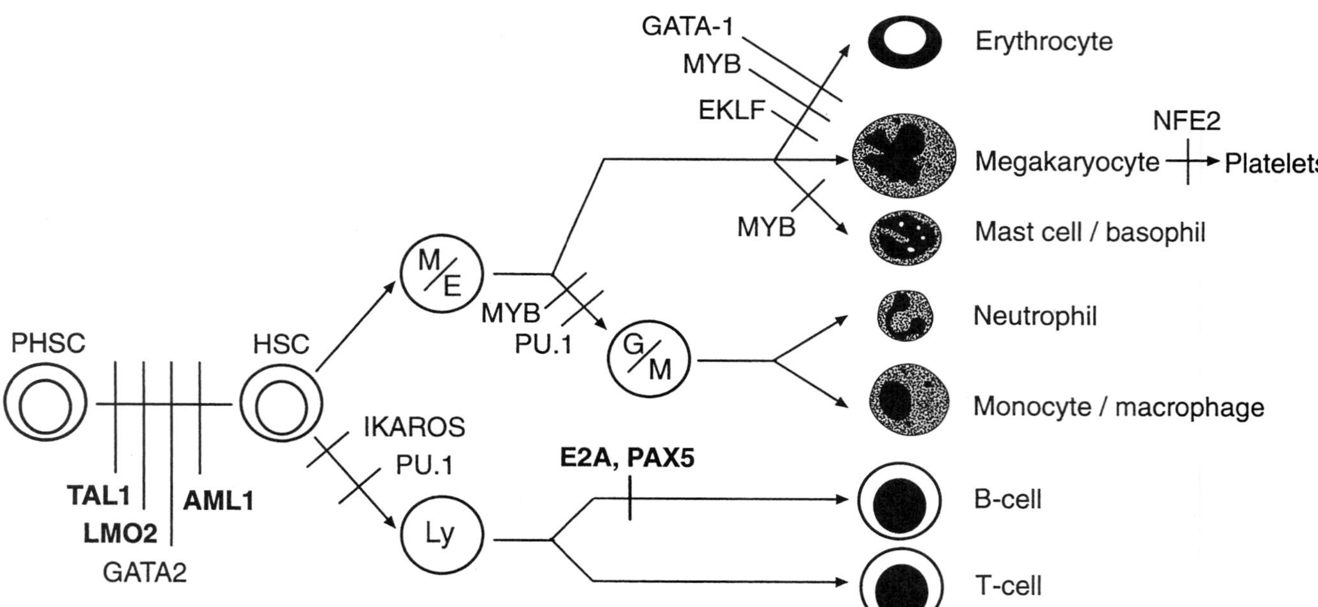

Fig. 19-1 Schematic diagram showing the relative stages at which transcription factors exert their influence on hematopoietic development. Only proteins whose activities have been demonstrated in knockout mice are shown. Factors serving as targets of chromosomal translocations in the leukemias and lymphomas are indicated in boldface type. Note that transcription factor targets can be lineage specific (E2A) or uncommitted to a particular differentiation pathway (AML1). HSC, hematopoietic stem cell; M/E, myeloid/erythroid progenitor; Ly, lymphoid progenitor; G/M, granulocyte/macrophage progenitor. (*Adapted from Shivdasani and Orkin.*[4] Used with permission).

Table 19-1 Transcriptional Control Genes Dysregulated by Chromosomal Translocations that Contribute to Human Leukemias and Lymphomas

Disease	Chromosomal Abnormality	Activated	Mechanism of Activation	Predominate Structural Feature*	Invertebrate Homologue[†]	References
Lymphoid Leukemia/Lymphoma						
B-cell ALL/Burkitt	t(8;14)(q24;q32)	*MYC*	Relocation to *IgH* locus	bHLHzip		16–18
Lymphoma	t(2;8)(p12;q24)	*MYC*	Relocation to IgL locus	bHLHzip		19, 20, 22, 24
	t(8;22)(q24;q11)	*MYC*	Relocation to IgL locus	bHLHzip		21, 23
Pre-B-cell All	t(1;19)(q23;p13)	*E2A-PBX1*	Gene fusion	Homeodomain (PBX1)	*exd* (D), *ceh-20* (C)	130, 131
Pro-B-cell ALL	t(17;19)(q22;p13)	*E2A-HLF*	Gene fusion	bZIP (HLF)	*giant* (D), *ces-2* (C)	178, 179
Pro-B-cell ALL	t(12;21)(p13;q22)	*TEL-AML1*	Gene fusion	Runt homology (AML1)	*runt* (D)	197–201
T-cell ALL	t(8;14)(q24;q11)	*MYC*	Relocation to *TCRα/δ* locus	bHLHzip		51–53
	t(7;19)(q35;p13)	*LYL1*	Relocation to *TCRβ* locus	HLH		48
	t(1;14)(p32;q11)	*TAL1*	Relocation to *TCRα/δ* locus	bHLH		45–47
	t(7;9)(q35;q34)	*TAL2*	Relocation to *TCRβ* locus	bHLH		47
	t(11;14)(p15;q11)	*LMO1 (RBTN1)*	Relocation to *TCRα/δ* locus	Cysteine-rich		77, 78
	t(11;14)(p13;q11)	*LMO2 (RBTN2)*	Relocation to *TCRα/β* locus	Cysteine-rich		79, 80
	t(7;11)(q35;p13)	*LMO2 (RBTN2)*	Relocation to *TCRβ* locus	Cysteine-rich		
	t(10;14)(q24;q11)	*HOX11*	Relocation to *TCRα/δ* locus	Homeodomain		97–100
	t(7;10)(q35;q24)	*HOX11*	Relocation to *TCRβ* locus	Homeodomain		
Diffuse B-cell lymphoma	t(3;14)(q27;q32)	*BCL6*	Relocation to *IgH* locus	Zinc finger	*tramtrack* (D)	212–215
(large cell)	t(3;4)(q27;p11)	*BCL6*	Relocation to *TTF* locus	Zinc finger	*tramtrack* (D)	213, 537
B-CLL	t(14;19)(q32;q13)	*BCL3*	Relocation to *IgH* locus	IκB homology		538–540
B-cell lymphoma	t(10;14)(q24;q32)	*LYT10*	Relocation to *IgH* locus	Rel homology	*dorsal* (D)	541
Lymphoplasmacytoid B-cell lymphoma	t(9;14)(p13;q32)	*PAX5*	Relocation to *IgH* locus	Paired homeobox	*Paired* (D)	542
Myeloid Leukemia						
AML (granulocytic)	t(8;21)(q22;q22)	*AML1-ETO*	Gene fusion	Runt homology (AML1)	*runt* (D)	226–228, 543
Myelodysplasia	t(3;21)(q26;q22)	*AML1-EAP*	Gene fusion	Runt homology (AML1)	*runt* (D)	231
CML (blast crisis)	t(3;21)(q26;q22)	*AML1-EVI1*	Gene fusion	Runt homology (AML1)	*runt* (D)	230
AML (undifferentiated)	t(3;v)(q26;v)	*EVI1*	Aberrant expression	Zinc finger	*evil* (D)	322, 323
AML (myelomonocytic)	inv(16)(p13;q22)	*CBFβ-MYH11*	Gene fusion	Complex with AML1 (CBFβ)		251
AML (promyelocytic)	t(15;17)(q21;q21)	*PML-RARα*	Gene fusion	Zinc finger (RARα)		268–272
AML (promyelocytic)	t(11;17)(q23;q21)	*PLZF-RARα*	Gene fusion	Zinc finger (RARα)		292
AML (promyelocytic)	t(5;17)(q32;q12)	*NPM-RARα*	Gene fusion	Zinc finger (RARα)		290
AML (promyelocytic)	t(11;17)(q13;q21)	*Nν*MA–RARα	Gene fusion	Zinc finger (RARα)		291
AML	t(16;21)(p11;q22)	*FUS-ERG*	Gene fusion	Ets-like (ERG)		544
AML	t(12;22)(p13;q11)	*TEL-MN1*	Gene fusion	Ets-like (TEL)		545
Myelodysplasia	t(3;12)(q26;p13)	*TEL-EVI1*	Gene fusion	Zinc finger (EVI1) Ets-like (TEL)	*evi1* (D)	546
AML (myelomonocytic)	t(8;16)(p11;p13)	*MOZ-CBP*	Gene fusion	Zinc finger (MOZ) CREB-binding protein (CBP)	*Pointed* (D)	547
AML (myelomonocytic)	inv(8)(p11;q13)	*MOZ-TIFZ*	Gene fusion	Zinc finger (MOZ) Nuclear receptor coactivator (TIFZ)		548

(Continued on next page)

Table 19-1 (continued)

Disease	Chromosomal Abnormality	Activated	Mechanism of Activation	Predominate Structural Feature*	Invertebrate Homologue[†]	References
Mixed-Lineage Leukemias[‡]						
Pro-B-cell ALL	t(4;11)(q21;q23)	*MLL-AF4*	Gene fusion	A–T hook (MLL)	*trithorax* (D)	342, 344, 345
AML (monocytic)	t(9;11)(q21;q23)	*MLL-AF9*	Gene fusion	A–T hook (MLL)	*trithorax* (D)	363
ALL/AML	t(11;19)(q23;p13.3)	*MLL-ENL*	Gene fusion	A–T hook (MLL)	*trithorax* (D)	341, 355, 363
AML	t(11;19)(q23;p13.1)	*MLL-ELL*	Gene fusion	A–T hook (MLL)	*trithorax* (D)	355, 356
AML	t(1;11)(q21;q23)	*MLL-AF1Q*	Gene fusion	A–T hook (MLL)	*trithorax* (D)	366
AML	t(1;11)(1p32;q23)	*MLL-AF1P*	Gene fusion	A–T hook (MLL)	*trithorax* (D)	549
AML	t(6;11)(q27;q23)	*MLL-AF6*	Gene fusion	A–T hook (MLL)	*trithorax* (D)	389
AML	t(6;11)(q12;q23)	*MLL-AF6QZ1*	Gene fusion	A–T hook (MLL)	*trithorax* (D)	550
AML	t(10;11)(p12;q23)	*MLL-AF10*	Gene fusion	A–T hook (MLL)	*trithorax* (D)	551
AML	t(11;17)(q23;q21)	*MLL-AF17*	Gene fusion	A–T hook (MLL)	*trithorax* (D)	552
AML	t(X;11)(q13;q23)	*MLL-AFX1*	Gene fusion	A–T hook (MLL)	*trithorax* (D)	553
AMML/CMML	t(11;16)(q23;p13)	*MLL-CBP*	Gene fusion	A–T hook (MLL)	*trithorax* (D)	554, 555

Abbreviations: AML, acute myeloid leukemia; ALL, acute lymphoblastic leukemia; CML, chronic myelogenous leukemia; CMML, chronic myelomonocytic leukemia; bHLHzip, basic region/helix-loop-helix/leucine zipper domain; bZIP, basic region/leucine zipper domain.

*Based on analysis of DNA-binding/protein interaction domain. For gene fusions, the partner contributing this structural feature is given in parentheses.

[†]Organism type is shown in parenthesis: D = *Drosophila;* C = *C. Elegans.*

[‡]Only the predominate lineage is given for *MLL* gene rearrangements.

Table 19-2 **Tyrosine Kinase and Other Genes Dysregulated by Chromosomal Translocations in Human Leukemias and Lymphomas**

Disease	Chromosomal Abnormality	Activated Gene	Mechanism of Activation	Predominate Structural Feature*	Invertebrate Homologue†	References
Tyrosine Kinases						
CMML	t(5;12)(q33;p13)	*TEL-PDGFRβ*	Gene fusion	Tyrosine kinase (PDGFRB)		443
Pre-B-ALL	t(9;12)(p24;p13)	*TEL-JAK2*	Gene fusion	Tyrosine kinase (JAK2)	*Hopscotch* (D)	556, 557
T-cell ALL	t(9;12)(p24;p13)	*TEL-AK2*	Gene fusion	Tyrosine kinase (JAK2)	*Hopscotch* (D)	
CML (atypical)	t(9;12;14)	*TEL-JAK2*	Gene fusion	Tyrosine kinase (JAK2)	*Hopscotch* (D)	
CMML	t(5;7)(q33;q11.2)	*HIPI-PDGFβR*	Gene fusion	Tyrosine kinase (PDGFβR) Huntington interactin protein (HIP1)		558
AML	t(5;14)(q33;q32)	*CEV14-PDGFβR*	Gene fusion	Tyrosine kinase (PDGFβR)		559
AML	t(9;12;14)(q34;p13;q22)	*TEL-ABL*	Gene fusion	Tyrosine kinase (ABL)	*abl* (D)	203, 442
Anaplastic large-cell lymphoma	t(2;5)(p23;q35)	*NPM-ALK*	Gene fusion	Tyrosine kinase (ALK)		457
CML	t(9;22)(q34;q11)	*BCR-ABL*	Gene fusion	Tyrosine kinase (ABL)	*abl* (D)	407, 413, 416, 417
ALL	t(9;22)(q34;q11)	*BCR-ABL*	Gene fusion	Tyrosine kinase (ABL)	*abl* (D)	422–424
T-cell ALL	t(1;7)(p34;q34)	*LCK*	Reloaction to *TCRβ* locus	Tyrosine kinase		560–562
Other Genes						
Centrocytic B-cell lymphoma	t(11;14)(q13;q32)	*Cyclin D1*	Relocation to *IgH* locus	G1 cyclin		493, 494, 499–502
Follicular B cell lymphoma	t(14;18)(q32;q21)	*BCL2*	Relocation to *IgH* locus	Antiapoptotic domain	*ced-9* (C)	517–520
AML	t(6;9)(p23;q34)	*DEK-CAN*	Gene fusion	Nucleoporin (CAN)		563
AML	t(9;9)(q34;q34)	*SET-CAN*	Gene fusion	Nucleoporin (CAN)		528
AML	t(7;11)(p15;p15)	*NUP98-HOXA9*	Gene fusion	Nucleoporin (NUP98)		529, 530
AML	t(3;5)(q35;q35)	*NPM-MLF1*	Gene fusion	Nucleolar shuttle protein (NPM)		535
AML	t(10;11)(p13;q14)	*CALM-AF10*	Gene fusion	Clathrin assembly (CLM)	*Cezf* (C)	564
T-cell PLL	t(x;14)(q28;q11)	*C6.1B*	Relocation to *TCRα/δ* locus	Unknown		565
T-cell ALL	t(7;9)(q34;q34)	*TAN1*	Relocation to *TCRβ* locus	EGF cysteine repeats	*Notch* (D), *lin-12* (C)	566
Pre-B-cell ALL	t(5;14)(q31;q32)	*IL-3*	Relocation to *IgH* locus	Growth factor		567, 568
T-cell lymphoma	t(4;16)(q26;p13)	*IL2-BCM*	Gene fusion	Growth factor		569
T-cell PLL	t(14;14)(q11;q32)	*TCL1*	Relocation to *TCRα/δ* locus	Unknown		570
	inv(14)(q11;q32)	*TCL1*	Relocation to *TCRα/δ* locus	Unknown		
	t(7;14)(q35;q32)	*TCL1*	Relocation to *TCRβ* locus	Unknown		
T-cell PLL	t(X;14)(q28;q11)	*MTCP1*	Relocation to *TCRα/δ* locus	Unknown		571, 572
B-cell lymphoma	t(11;14)(q23;q32)	*RCK*	Relocation to *IgH* locus	Helicase/translation initiation factor		573

Abbreviations: AML, acute myeloid leukemia; ALL, acute lymphoblastic leukemia; CML, chronic myelogenous leukemia; CMML, chronic myelomonocytic leukemia; T-cell PLL, T-cell prolymphocytic leukemia.

*For gene fusions, the partner contributing this structural feature is given in parentheses.

†Organism type is shown in parenthesis: D = *Drosophila*; C = *C. Elegans*.

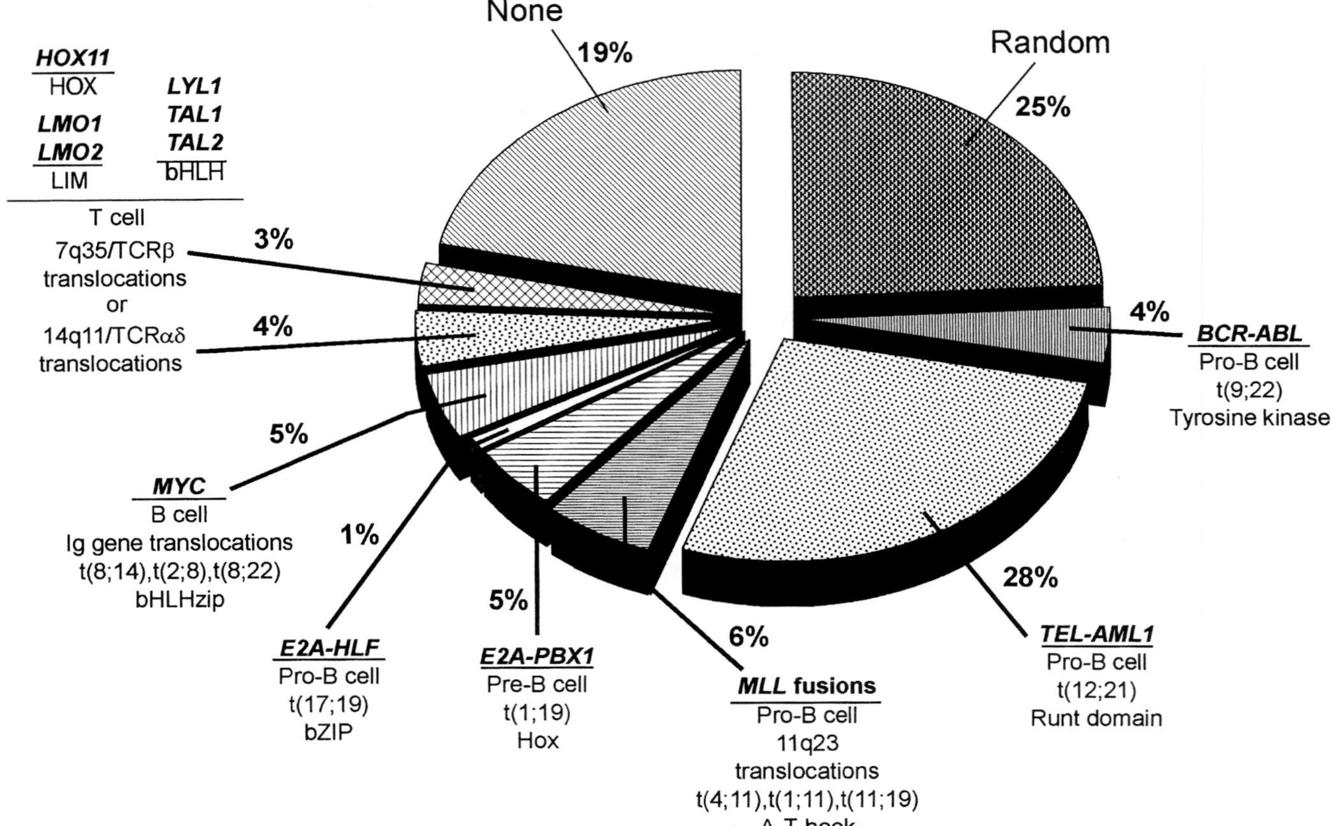

Fig. 19-2 Distribution of translocation-generated fusion genes among the commonly recognized immunologic subtypes of ALL in children and young adults. Key domains for DNA binding and protein-protein interaction of transcription factors are shown in boldface type; an exception is the tyrosine kinase domain indicated for BCR-ABL. The section labeled *random* refers to sporadic rearrangements that have so far been observed only in leukemic cells from single cases. (*Adapted from Look.*[211] *Used with permission*).

(MAX/MAX homodimers), and to the MAD and MXI-1 family of transcription factors.[32,33] Since MYC/MAX heterodimers activate gene expression,[30,31] whereas MAD/MAX heterodimers act as trans-repressors through an association with a protein called SIN3,[34,35] and since MYC and MAD have equal affinities for MAX,[36,37] increased expression of MYC in B lymphocytes is thought to disrupt the equilibrium of MAX heterodimers, leading to untimely activation of responder genes and ultimately to malignant transformation.[38] Experimental support for this hypothesis comes from the induction of B-cell neoplasms in transgenic mice carrying the *MYC* oncogene driven by an *Ig* gene enhancer.[39,40] An activated *MYC* gene also induces tumorigenic conversion when it is introduced in vitro into B lymphoblasts infected with human Epstein-Barr virus.[41] More recent observations implicate the ornithine decarboxylase gene,[42] the *CDC25* cell-cycle phosphatase gene,[43] and the *ARF* tumor suppressor gene[44] as relevant transcriptional targets of MYC/MAX heterodimers.

***bHLH, LIM,* and *HOX11* Genes.** The role of transcription factors as the preferred targets of chromosomal translocations extends to the T-cell lymphomas and acute leukemias, in which the chromosomal breakpoints consistently appear near enhancers included in the *TCR β* locus on chromosome 7, band q34, or the *α/δ* locus on chromosome 14, band q11. Highly active in committed T-cell progenitors, these enhancers stimulate the expression of strategically translocated transcription factors that regulate early hematopoietic cell development or the development of other lineages but are not normally expressed in T lymphoid cells (see Table 19-1). Notable examples include the *bHLH* genes, *TAL1/SCL,*[45–47] *TAL2/SCL2,*[47] and *LYL1,*[48] one of which is essential for the development of all blood cell lineages (*TAL1/SCL*).[4,49,50] The more distantly related *MYC* bHLH/ZIP protein is dysregulated in T-cell[51–53] as well as B-cell lymphomas and leukemias.

When rearranged near enhancers within the *TCR β* locus on chromosome 7, band q34, or the *α/δ* chain locus on chromosome 14, band q11, these regulatory genes become active, and their protein products are thought to bind inappropriately to the promoter/enhancer elements of upstream target genes. The *TAL1* gene, for example, is activated by the t(1;14) or by an intragenic deletion on the 5′ side of the gene that places it under the regulation of the promoter of a gene called *SIL*[54–58]; these rearrangements affect up to one-fourth of all cases of childhood T-cell leukemias and lymphomas.[59,60] Since the TAL1 protein can dimerize with the E2A protein through its bHLH domain to form DNA-binding complexes,[61] and with the LMO2 protein (see below),[61–65] its ectopic expression in T cells bearing the t(1;14) or activating deletions may aberrantly activate specific sets of target genes that are normally quiescent in T-lineage progenitors. It is also possible that TAL1 acts by repressing E2A activity during T-cell development, because E2A/TAL1 heterodimers are inactive as transcriptional trans-activators.[66,67]

Interestingly, TAL1 has emerged as an essential regulator of very early stages of hematopoietic development.[68] Within the hematopoietic system, TAL1 expression is restricted to myeloid and erythroid progenitor cells, megakaryocytes, and mast cells,[69–71] and as noted previously, it is not expressed by normal T lymphocytes or their progenitors.[72] Gene targeting experiments initially showed that mouse embryos lacking a functional *Tal1* gene were devoid of embryonic red blood cells and died at embryonic days 9 to 10.5 of anemia.[49,50] Additional studies of

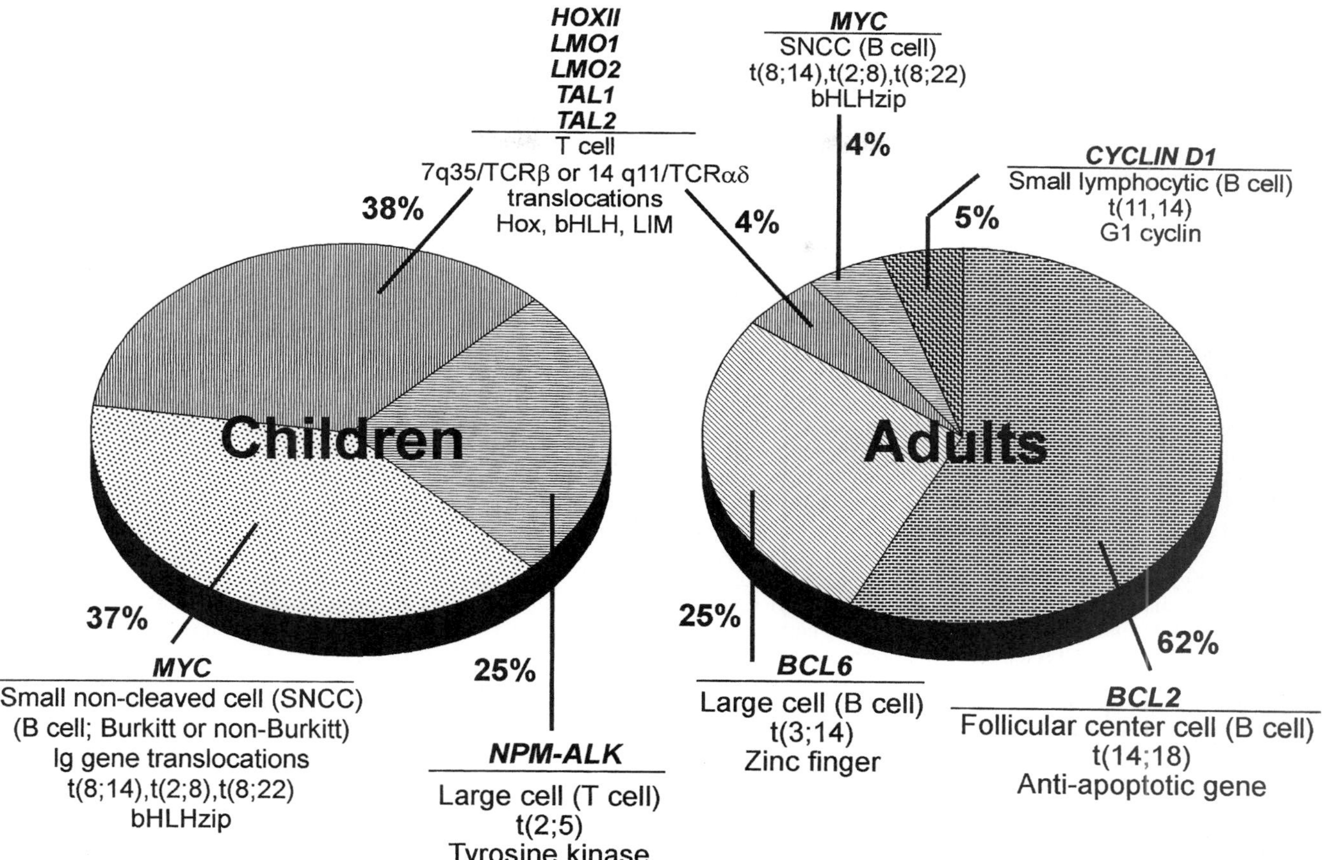

Fig. 19-3 Distribution of histologic subtypes of non-Hodgkin lymphoma in children and adults. Chromosomal translocations and affected genes that occur in a significant fraction (but not all) of the cases within each subtype are shown. (*Adapted from Sandlund, Downing, and Crist.*[574] *Used with permission*).

hematopoietic precursors generated by in vitro differentiation of *Tal* −/− embryonic stem cells, and by assessing the contribution of these cells in vivo to the hematopoietic systems of chimeric mice, have shown that *Tal1* is required for the generation of all hematopoietic cell lineages, including T lymphocytes, suggesting that it plays an essential role in early hematopoietic development, either at the level of mesoderm induction or in maintaining the viability of multipotential hematopoietic progenitors.[68] It would not be surprising if Tal1 were involved in a network of regulatory factors responsible for induction of the hematopoietic lineage, in view of the similar roles of related bHLH proteins as master regulators of mesodermal cell fate, such as those of the MyoD family (MyoD, Myf-5, MRF4, and myogenin),[73,74] which, like the Tal1 protein, form heterocomplexes with the E12/E47 products of the *E2A* gene. An interesting zebrafish mutant cloche affects both blood and endothelial differentiation,[75] and recent microinjection studies suggest that *SCL* acts downstream of cloche to specify hematopoietic and vascular differentiation.[76]

Other types of regulatory genes can be rearranged near *TCR* loci, including those encoding the LMO1 and LMO2 (for cysteine-rich *LIM*-domain *o*nly) proteins (also known as RBTN1/TTG1 and RBTN2/TTG2).[77–80] Although T-cells normally lack expression of either protein, LMO1 is expressed in a segmental and developmentally regulated pattern in the central nervous system,[78] and LMO2 is coexpressed with Tal1 in several lineages, notably in erythroid and other hematopoietic progenitors.[81] Both LMO1 and LMO2 possess zinc finger-like structures in their LIM domains[82] but lack the homeobox DNA-binding domains common to other transcription factors in this family, suggesting that the LIM domain functions in protein-protein rather than protein-DNA interactions. In fact, LMO2 is coexpressed with TAL1 in several cell lineages, including erythroid progenitors,[81] and these two proteins interact to form a transcriptional complex,[64,83] both in erythroid cells and in human and murine T-cell leukemias induced by these gene products.[64,65,83] The functional relevance of this complex in normal development is exemplified by the fact that gene targeting experiments in mice, in which null mutations were introduced into *Lmo2,* yielded the same phenotype as those described earlier for *Tal1,* indicating that functional complexes are required for normal primitive erythropoiesis and likely the formation of all hematopoietic lineages.[68,81,84,85] Additional studies have expanded this complex to include GATA1,[86] a zinc-finger transcription factor that is also required for erythroid cell development,[87] E2A bHLH proteins, and the newly identified LIM-binding protein Ldb1/NLL, suggesting that oligomeric DNA-binding complexes containing LMO2 play important roles in hematopoiesis.[88] Moreover, both LMO1 and LMO2 induce thymic lymphomas in transgenic mice whose thymocytes express these genes under the control of T-cell-specific or ubiquitously expressed promoters.[89–93] Although it is controversial whether *TAL1* is able to induce T-cell lymphomas in mice on its own,[94,95] it has been shown to shorten the time to development of T-cell lymphomas induced by LMO2 in a double transgenic system, apparently recapitulating the cooperativity that the these two proteins exhibit as components of multimeric transcriptional regulatory complexes in human T-cell tumors.[64,65,96]

HOX11 is an example of a different type of developmental gene that is inappropriately placed under the control of *TCR* loci. Located on chromosome 10, band q24,[97–100] this gene encodes a homeodomain transcription factor that can bind DNA and transactivate specific target genes.[101] It is most closely related to *Hlx,* a recently described murine homeobox gene expressed in specific hematopoietic cell lineages and during mouse embryogenesis,[102] and is distantly related to the *Antennapedia* homeobox genes of *Drosophila,* which regulate segment-specific gene expression along the anteroposterior axis of the fly embryo.[103] A very specific homeotic role of *Hox11* in mammalian development was demonstrated by homozygous disruption of this gene, which blocked the formation of the spleen in otherwise normal mice.[104] In the mouse, Hox11 is normally expressed in specific regions of the branchial arches and ectoderm of the pharyngeal pouches of the developing hindbrain, as well as from a single site corresponding to the splanchnic mesoderm beginning at embryonic day 11.5.[104] Because the nervous system develops normally in these mice, the roles of Hox11 proteins in branchial arch and hindbrain structures appear to be compensated for by other transcription factors expressed by these cells; however, the role of Hox11 in cellular organization at the site of splenic development is absolutely essential for the genesis of this organ. Further studies have shown that the splenic anlage actually develops normally in *Hox11 −/−* mice but that the developing spleen cells undergo apoptosis, suggesting that Hox11 normally acts to promote the survival of splenic precursors during organogenesis.[105] In contrast to *Lmo2* and *Tal1,* which have important roles in hematopoietic cell development, Hox11 proteins are not normally expressed in lymphoid and other types of hematopoietic cells, and hematopoietic cells are not affected by loss-of-function mutations in this gene, except in circulating erythrocytes with asplenia-related Howell-Jolly bodies.

Activation of *HOX11* by chromosomal translocations, either the t(10;14)(q24;q11) or the t(7;10)(q35;q24), in developing T cells is thought to interfere with normal regulatory cascades, thereby promoting malignant transformation. The primary oncogenic importance of aberrant expression of Hox11 in the developing thymus has been demonstrated in transgenic mice, in which this protein was redirected to the thymus, where it was associated with the development of T-cell lymphoma/leukemia at high frequencies.[106] HOX11 has been shown to act as an activator of gene expression, and this activity has been shown to depend on the N-terminal 50 amino acids of the protein.[107] In addition, HOX11 interacts directly with phosphatases that normally regulate a G2-phase cell cycle checkpoint, suggesting that overexpression of this protein in T-cell progenitors may cause accelerated entry into mitosis.[108]

***E2A* Fusion Genes.** The *E2A* gene was cloned by virtue of the fact that it encodes a protein (E12) that binds to the κE2 regulatory site of the *Ig κ* light chain gene promoter.[109] It was subsequently shown to encode three differentially spliced products, E12, E47, and E2-5, each of which belongs to the bHLH family of transcriptional regulatory proteins.[109–113] The bHLH domain is comprised of a basic region responsible for sequence-specific DNA binding followed by a structural domain consisting of two amphipathic helices separated by a loop region of variable length (thus helix-loop-helix), that is responsible for homo- and heterodimerization.[109,110] The bHLH family of proteins includes the *daughterless Drosophila* gene[114,115] and members of the MyoD family of myogenic proteins.[73,74] DNA-binding by E2A is mediated by either homodimers or heterodimers with other bHLH proteins, with the precise binding specificity to variations of the so-called E-box sequence motif determined by the dimerization partners of each complex.[116] Recent structural analysis has supported experimental observations regarding the conformations of homo- and heterodimers formed by the E2A bHLH domains.[117] In addition, the N-terminal sequences of E2A that are included in leukemogenic fusion proteins (Fig. 19-4) have been shown to contain two discrete transcriptional activation domains, called AD1 and AD2,[112,118,119] the latter of which is also referred to as a *loop-helix (LH) activation domain.*

In most tissues, E2A heterodimerizes with tissue-specific bHLH family members to coordinate gene expression during development.[110,120] These binding partners include TAL/SCL and LYL1 family members, which heterodimerize with E2A[62,121,122] and are themselves dysregulated in T-cell lymphomas/leukemias and aberrantly expressed as a result of translocations involving the *TCR* gene loci.[45–47] In B cells, however, E2A is able to bind E-box sequences as a homodimeric complex,[120,123] apparently due to stabilization of the complex through an intermolecular disulfide bond, which is disrupted in non-B cells.[124] The importance of E2A proteins in B-cell development is indicated by the fact that homozygous mutant mice lacking functional E2A proteins have arrested B-cell development at an early stage.[125,126] Mice deficient in E2A not only lack pro-B cells but also show defects in T-cell development and acquire T-cell malignancies, suggesting that loss of function of E2A may contribute to leukemogenesis in T cells, in addition to its role as a component of heterodimeric complexes with other bHLH proteins.[127,128]

E2A-PBX1. The *E2A* gene participates in two fusion events with major biologic and clinical implications in acute lymphoblastic leukemia (ALL). The first results from the t(1;19)(q23;p13) chromosomal translocation, which rearranges and joins the *E2A* gene within chromosome band 19p13.3 to the *PBX1* gene from chromosome 1, creating an *E2A-PBX1* chimera on the derivative chromosome 19[129–131] (see Fig. 19-2). Because the breakpoints in the *E2A* gene consistently interrupt the ~3.5-kb intron between exons 13 and 14, the encoded E2A fusion partner invariably consists of the N-terminal two-thirds of the molecule, which includes two transcriptional activation domains (AD1 and AD2), but not the bHLH DNA-binding/protein-interaction domain.[130–132] The PBX1 segment makes up for this deficit by providing a homeodomain motif of ~60 amino acids that enables the E2A-PBX1 chimera to function as a transcription factor, driven by the potent E2A trans-activating domains.[133–137]

An understanding of the likely oncogenic contribution of the PBX1 fusion partner requires insight into the normal function of PBX proteins. These transcription factors are the mammalian homologues of the *Drosophila* protein extradenticle.[138,139] Mutations in the *exd* gene cause homeotic transformations, changes in which one body segment of the fly is transformed to resemble another segment.[140,141] Thus the extradenticle protein may function as an obligatory cofactor in selector gene activity by forming complexes with major homeotic fly proteins of the Antennapedia and Bithorax clusters, termed *Hom,* which then bind to DNA.[142–145] In view of the close sequence homology shared by extradenticle and PBX proteins, it is perhaps not surprising that the latter interact with specific human homologues of the Hom family, called *HOX proteins,* to determine the target genes recognized by PBX1.[142,144,146,147,147–155]

Given that E2A-PBX1 carries the transcriptional activation domains of E2A and the homeodomain of PBX1, how does the chimera induce malignant transformation? When Kamps and Baltimore[156] infected bone marrow progenitors with retroviruses encoding E2A-PBX1, they reproducibly induced acute myeloid leukemia (AML) in mice repopulated with these progenitors. These myeloid leukemia cells could proliferate for extended periods without maturation so long as they received granulocyte-macrophage colony-stimulating factor (GM-CSF).[157] In the absence of growth factor, the cells died rapidly. These observations are consistent with the block of differentiation characteristic of lymphoid cells carrying the t(1;19) in cases of ALL[158,159] and with arrested T-cell development in lymphomas of *E2A-PBX1* transgenic mice.[160] Thus a major effect of the chimera may be to arrest hematopoietic and lymphoid progenitors at particular stages of development.

Additional studies with cell transformation assays have established the specific E2A-PBX1 domains required for malignant conversion.[161] When either of the two transactivation domains of E2A are abolished, there is a loss or reduction of

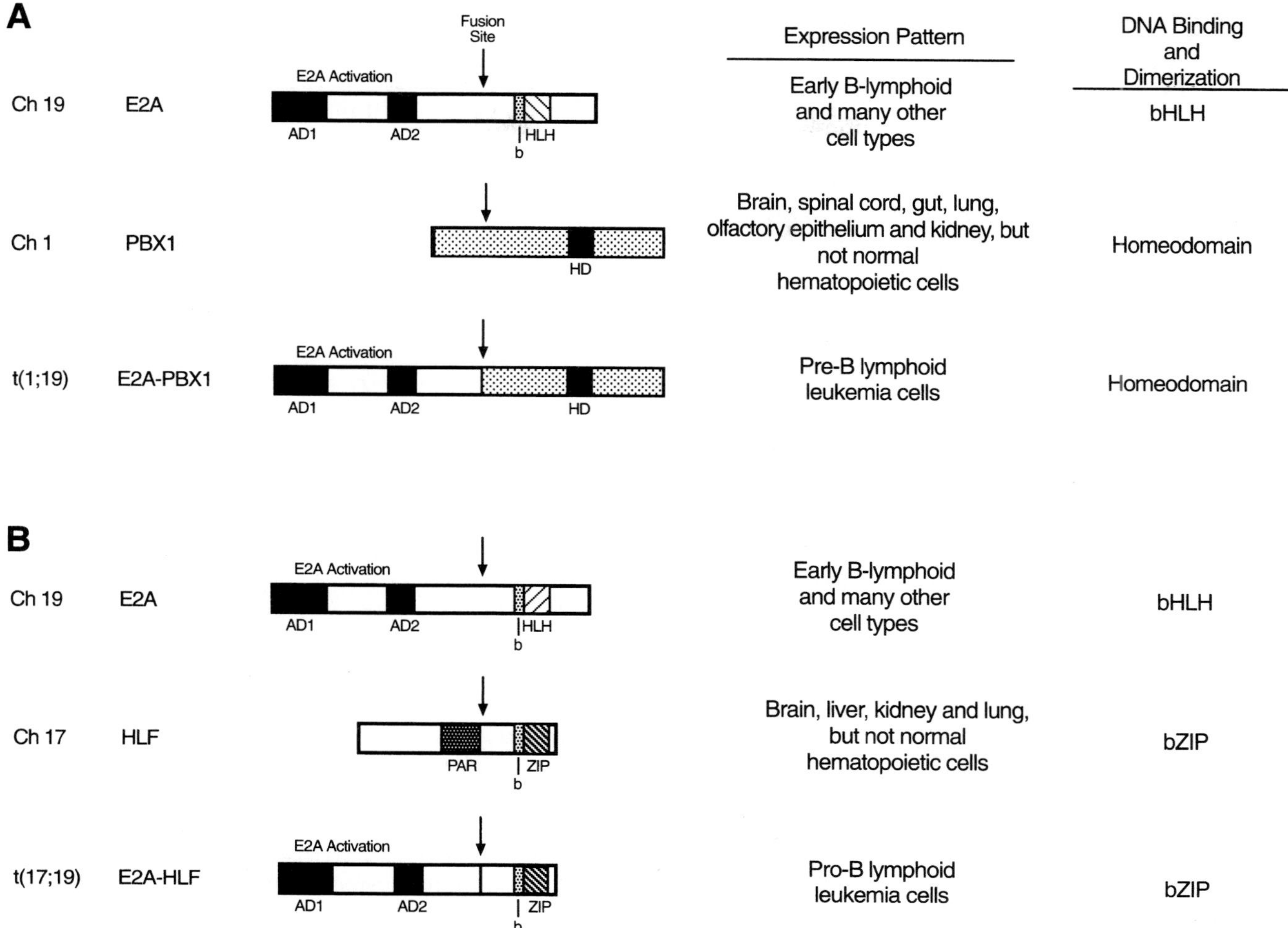

Fig. 19-4 Comparison of the structural features of two major E2A fusion proteins. The E2A portions of the chimeras are identical, retaining both the AD1 and AD2 transcriptional activation domains. The PBX1 fusion partner retains its DNA- and protein-binding domain (homeodomain), as does HLF (bZIP), providing a mechanism for recognition and activation of downstream target genes. Despite the normally wide distribution of E2A and the lack of normal expression of the HLF and PBX1 transcription factors in hematopoietic cells, the two chimeras act specifically on B-cell precursors. HD, homeodomain; bZIP, basic leucine zipper; bHLH, basic helix-loop-helix; Ch, chromosome.

transforming activity. The shortest PBX1 sequence required for oncogenesis includes the homeodomain and its immediately C-terminal 25 amino acids, which also are needed for interaction with specific HOX proteins.[146,162] Unexpectedly, mutant proteins with deletion of the homeodomain and retention of the adjacent flanking region transformed NIH-3T3 cells and induced lymphomas in transgenic mice as efficiently as the full-length chimera.[161,162] Other investigators have confirmed the dispensibility of sequence-specific DNA binding for transformation of fibroblasts while showing that the PBX1 homeodomain is essential for efficient arrest of myeloid cell differentiation.[163] These observations suggest that interaction with members of the HOX family of proteins is sufficient to target the E2A-PBX1 fusion protein to downstream target genes with critical functions in cell transformation but not those which interfere with normal differentiation programs.[161,163] Recent studies have implicated members of related homeodomain families, including Meis1 and pKnox1, as important binding partners and potentially important functional modulators of PBX and HOX proteins.[164–166] Interestingly, these proteins interact through a region of PBX1 that is disrupted in the E2A-PBX1 chimera, suggesting its transforming potential may be augmented by loss of Meis-Knox interactions, which normally may influence target gene recognition, transcriptional properties, or nuclear import of PBX1.[164,165] *E2A-PBX1* is one of the most common fusion genes in children with ALL, occurring in 20 to 25 percent of cases with a pre-B immunophenotype (defined by cytoplasmic but not surface expression of *Ig* genes).[158,167,168] It is also detected in adults with ALL, as well as occasional cases of pro-B-cell ALL, AML, T-cell ALL, and lymphoma.[14,167–176] Patients with pre-B ALL and the t(1;19) tend to have elevated leukocytes at diagnosis and central nervous system leukemia.[14,167,168] Aside from the adverse impact of these features, the *E2A-PBX1* fusion gene was shown to be independently associated with a poor prognosis,[167] although in recent years intensive chemotherapy has improved clinical outcome significantly in these patients.[168] A prudent clinical management strategy for patients with pre-B ALL is to consider the *E2A-PBX1* fusion gene a high-risk biologic feature that warrants an aggressive approach to therapy. Otherwise, these patients may be undertreated with consequent rapid development of drug-resistant disease.

E2A-HLF. A second *E2A* fusion gene is created by the t(17;19)(q21-q22;13) rearrangement,[177] which joins *E2A* to the *HLF* gene within chromosome band 17q21-22[178,179] (see Fig. 19-2). The breakpoint of this translocation consistently leaves the same portion of *HLF* in the chimeric gene but affects either intron 12 or 13 within *E2A*. The resulting hybrid protein is therefore termed *type I* (intron 13 breakpoint) or *type II* (intron 12 breakpoint),[180] although these structural distinctions do not appear to affect the DNA-binding and transcriptional regulatory properties of E2A-HLF.[181]

The HLF (hepatic leukemia factor) component of the chimera is a novel bZIP transcription factor within the PAR subfamily of proteins (defined by a proline- and acidic amino acid—rich domain).[182–185] HLF recently has been shown to encode two proteins from alternatively spliced transcripts that are regulated by different promoters.[186] One isoform is abundant in brain, liver, and kidney, whereas the other is restricted to hepatocytes; these proteins accumulate with different circadian patterns in the liver and have distinct promoter preferences in trans-activation experiments. Very little is known about the normal function of the PAR proteins, including HLF, but their structural similarity with the CES-2 bZIP protein that orchestrates the death of sertoninergic nerve cells in the developing worm *Caenorhabditis elegans* suggests a regulatory role in cell survival,[187–189] as indicated by the mechanism of E2A-HLF oncogenic activity, described below.

The E2A-HLF fusion product retains the entire DNA-binding/protein-protein interaction domain of HLF, as well as the two N-terminal transactivation domains of E2A.[179,180] In leukemic lymphoblasts, the chimeric protein appears to bind DNA as a homodimer,[190,191] as one might predict given the absence of detectable levels of the known normal PAR proteins in hematopoietic precursors. Like E2A-PBX1, the E2A-HLF oncoprotein can transform NIH-3T3 cells, depending on the integrity of the HLF leucine zipper and the E2A transcriptional activation domains.[192] It also induces lymphoid tumors in transgenic mice.[193] However, E2A-PBX1 induces apoptosis in hematopoietic cells through a p53-independent mechanism that requires the DNA-binding homeodomain of PBX1,[194] which is the direct opposite of the effect of the conditional expression of E2A-HLF.

Analysis of the effects of E2A-HLF on cell survival has provided important insight into how E2A-HLF might take control of immature lymphoid cells. When introduced into leukemic cells carrying the t(17;19), a dominant-negative form of E2A-HLF blocked the usual action of the intact chimera, and as a result, the malignant cells underwent apoptosis.[187] By contrast, the dominant-negative mutant had no effect on apoptotic events in leukemic cells without the t(17;19), suggesting that E2A-HLF may increase the number of developing lymphocytes by preventing their suicide.[187] The homology between HLF and the CES-2 protein of *C. elegans,*[188] which functions early in a genetically controlled cell death pathway, suggests that a comparable pathway operates in human B lymphoblasts and is usurped by E2A-HLF to give rise to ALL.[187] In this model (Fig. 19-5), E2A-HLF activates a downstream target gene that is normally repressed by a CES-2-like protein so that cell survival rather than cell death signals ensue. Thus the leukemogenic activity of E2A-HLF may operate through an evolutionarily conserved pathway that determines the sensitivity of specific lymphoid cells to apoptotic stimuli.

The t(17;19) defines a subset (0.5 to 1 percent) of ALL patients with a pro-B immunophenotype.[177] In several reports this rearrangement was linked to disseminated intravascular coagulation (DIC) and hypercalcemia at initial diagnosis.[177,179,180,195,196] Although the rarity of t(17;19)-positive ALL has hampered efforts to assess its prognostic significance, each of seven patients with molecularly identified *E2A-HLF* fusion died of leukemia despite their enrollment on contemporary treatment protocols.[180,190,195,196] Drug resistance in this type of leukemia may be augmented by the role of E2A-HLF in preventing accelerated apoptosis from therapy-induced DNA damage as well as growth factor deprivation.[187]

***TEL-AML1* Fusion Gene.** Generally considered a target of chromosomal translocations in myeloid cells, the *AML1* gene is joined to a second transcriptional control gene, called *TEL,* as a result of the t(12;21) in cases of B-lineage ALL.[197–201] Although rarely detected by routine karyotyping (because the telomeric segments of 12p and 21q appear similar in banded metaphase preparations), the t(12;21) rearrangement is apparent by fluorescence in situ hybridization in approximately one-fourth of children with ALL, making *TEL-AML1* the most common genetic abnormality in the lymphoid leukemias.[199] The *TEL-AML1* fusion product consists of the bHLH domain of *TEL* linked to virtually the entire coding region of *AML1,* including the DNA- and protein-binding domain, which bears close amino acid identity to the Runt protein of *Drosophila.* The exact role of the TEL-AML1 oncoprotein in cell transformation remains unclear, but emerging data suggest that the primary effect relates to a compromise of AML1 transcriptional activity,[202] which is required for normal hematopoiesis (see the section in this chapter on the involvement of the AML1-CBFβ complex in the acute myeloid leukemias).

The *TEL* gene is also involved in multiple other fusion genes associated with chronic myelomonocytic leukemia (CMML) (*TEL-PDGFRβ*), AML (*TEL-MN1, TEL-ABL, TEL-EVI1*), and ALL (*TEL-JAK2*) (see Tables 19-1 and 19-2). *TEL* harbors a 65-amino acid helix-loop-helix dimerization motif that is conserved in a subset of the ETS family of proteins, and this region appears to an essential requirement for constitutive tyrosine kinase and transforming activity of the activity of the TEL-PDGFRβ and TEL-ABL fusion proteins.[203–205] TEL-AML1 also appears to dimerize with itself and with normal TEL proteins in the cell, and there is often associated loss of the normal *TEL* allele in leukemias with *TEL-AML1* fusion genes, suggesting that loss of function may contribute to oncogenicity.[204,206] *Tel* has been homozygously disrupted in mice through gene targeting, and interestingly, the *Tel*-deficient mice die at approximately embryonic day 11 with defective yolk sac angiogenesis and intraembryonic apoptosis of mesenchymal and neural cells.[207]

The *TEL-AML1* fusion gene is associated with a superior treatment outcome in patients with B-lineage ALL, and relapse-free survival has approached 90 percent on several different therapeutic regimens.[204,206,208–210] For example, in a recent trial, children with *TEL* gene rearrangements (primarily *TEL-AML1*) had a 5-year event-free survival probability of 91 $\pm$ 5 percent (SE) compared with 64 $\pm$ 5 percent for those with *TEL* in a germ-line configuration.[208] The prognostic strength of *TEL* rearrangement (usually as a *TEL-AML1* fusion gene) was independent of recognized good-risk features in ALL with B-lineage markers, such as the presenting leukocyte count and hyperdiploidy. Indeed, molecular detection of the *TEL-AML1* fusion gene is the first genetic assay to allow a good-risk subset of patients to be dissected from the otherwise high-risk "pseudodiploid" subset of ALL patients.[211] Thus *TEL-AML1* has been added to the list of genetic abnormalities requiring recognition early in the disease course (Table 19-3).

***BCL6* Activation in Diffuse Large-Cell Lymphoma.** The t(3;14)(q27;q32) and related translocations affect the long arm of chromosome 3 in diffuse large cell lymphomas of the B-cell lineage, leading to the discovery of the *BCL6* proto-oncogene, whose expression is altered in at least 30 percent of these malignancies, the vast majority of which occur in adults.[212–215] *BCL6* encodes a transcription factor containing six zinc-finger DNA-binding motifs near the C-terminus and a POZ regulatory domain near the N-terminus. It is related to the PLZF protein that is fused to RARα as a result of the t(11;17) translocation of acute promyelocytic leukemia. (The postulated developmental roles of highly conserved zinc-finger proteins with POZ domains are discussed in the PLZF section of this chapter.) Like the *AML1-CBFβ* complex in the myeloid cell lineage, but unlike most genes whose expression is altered by translocation to the vicinity of the *Ig* or *TCR* genes, *BCL6* is normally expressed and developmentally regulated in cells of the same lineage in which it is linked to transformation, the B lymphocytes.[216,217] The BCL6 protein is detected in cells of the lymph node germinal center, a region in which antigen-primed B cells normally undergo transformation into either memory B cells or immunoblasts destined to become plasma cells or die as a result of apoptosis.[218] Because BCL6 is

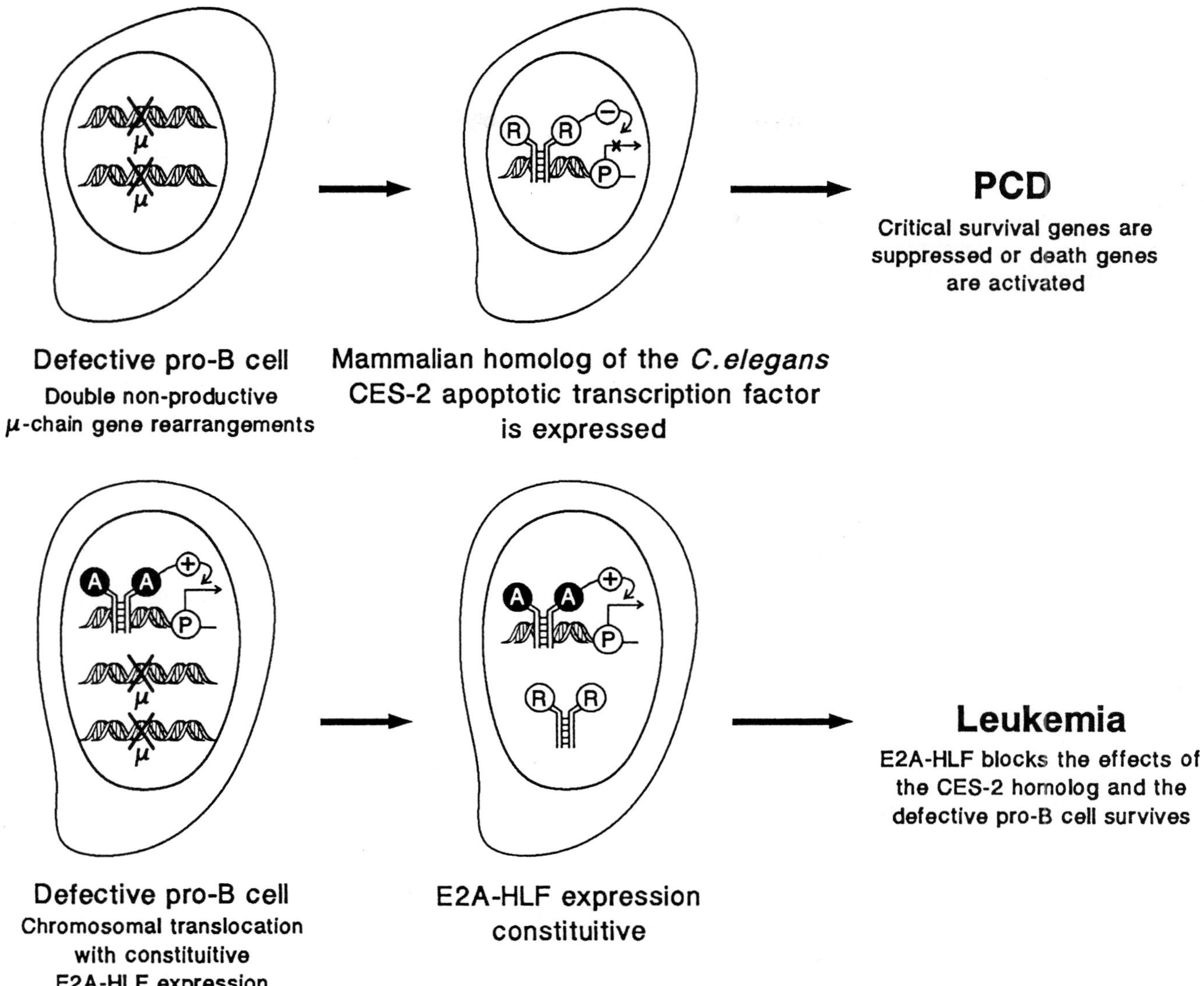
PCD
Critical survival genes are suppressed or death genes are activated
Defective pro-B cell
Double non-productive μ-chain gene rearrangements
Mammalian homolog of the C.elegans CES-2 apoptotic transcription factor is expressed
Leukemia
E2A-HLF blocks the effects of the CES-2 homolog and the defective pro-B cell survives
Defective pro-B cell
Chromosomal translocation with constituitive E2A-HLF expression
E2A-HLF expression constituitive

Fig. 19-5 A proposed model for the anti-apoptotic role of E2A-HLF in leukemogenesis. Leukemic cells with the t(17;19) undergo programmed cell death when E2A-HLF is inhibited through a dominant negative mechanism, suggesting that the primary effect of the hybrid oncoprotein is to prolong cell survival rather than to accelerate cell growth.[187] The close homology of the HLF bZIP domain to that of the CES-2 cell death-specification protein of the nematode *C. elegans*[188] suggests that E2A-HLF may contribute to leukemogenesis by binding to the promoters of target genes normally regulated by a mammalian ortholog of the CES-2 protein, which causes defective pro-B cells to undergo apoptosis. According to this model, E2A-HLF may activate target gene expression in contrast to the proposed repressor effects of CES-2, leading to aberrant survival through an evolutionarily conserved pathway that regulates programmed cell death during B-lymphoid cell development.

Table 19-3 Clinical Risk Assignment in the Childhood Leukemias by Genetic Classification of the Malignant Cells

Abnormality (Risk)	Method of Detection	Treatment
Hyperdiploidy, ≥53 chromosomes (good risk)	DNA flow cytometry	Antimetabolite therapy emphasizing high-dose methotrexate
TEL-AML1 fusion human gene due to t(12;21) (good risk)	RNA PCR to detect *TEL-AML1* fusion transcripts	Antimetabolite therapy emphasizing high-dose methotrexate
E2A-PBX1 fusion gene due to t(1;19) (intermediate risk)	RNA PCR to detect *E2A-PBX1* fusion transcripts	Intensified chemotherapy with alkylating agents and topoisomerase inhibitors
MLL fusion gene due to 11q23 rearrangements and *E2A-HLF* due to t(17;19) (high risk)	RNA PCR to detect *MLL* and *E2A-HLF* fusion transcripts	Experimental forms of intensified chemotherapy or bone marrow transplantation
BCR-ABL fusion gene due to t(9;22), with high leukocyte count (ultra-high risk)	RNA PCR to detect *BCR-ABL* fusion transcripts	Bone marrow transplantation in first remission

normally down-regulated before B cells exit from the germinal center, a reasonable hypothesis is that activated B lymphoblasts constitutively expressing BCL6 are unable to develop normally and instead replicate clonally with the considerable proliferative capacity of a large-cell lymphoma of activated B-lymphocyte origin.[219] This interpretation is supported by the fact that most *BCL6* rearrangements occur within the 5′-noncoding first exon or the first intron of the gene and result in dysregulation of expression of a structurally intact BCL6 protein.[220]

In addition to gene rearrangement mediated by chromosomal translocation, somatic point mutations of the 5′ regulatory regions of the *BCL6* gene have been identified at high frequency in both the diffuse large cell and the follicular lymphomas of B-cell origin, suggesting that dysregulated expression of BCL6 may be linked casually to malignant transformation in high percentages of lymphoid tumors of these pathologic subtypes.[221] Rearrangements of the *BCL6* gene have been shown to have distinct clinicopathologic correlates within the adult diffuse large-cell lymphomas, occurring primarily in extranodal tumors that have not spread to the bone marrow. Importantly, they independently identify a subset of patients with a favorable prognosis.[222]

Acute Myeloid Leukemias

The distribution of gene rearrangements due to chromosomal translocations in AMLs of children and adolescents is shown in Fig. 19-6.

Gene Rearrangements Affecting the *AML1-CBFβ* Complex. The AML1/CBFβ transcription factor complex (Fig. 19-7) is the most frequent target of chromosomal translocations in the human leukemias, in that one of these linked proteins is expressed as an oncogenic chimera in as many as one-third of both ALL and AML patients. This regulatory complex, termed *CBF* because of its identity as a core binding factor (also known as *PEBP2*),[223] consists of a DNA-binding subunit, AML1 (also called *CBFα2* or *PEBP2αB*), and CBFβ (also called *PEBP2β*), a subunit that does not bind DNA independently but rather heterodimerizes with AML1 or one of its closely related family members.[224,225] Chromosomal translocations that modify the AML1/CBFβ complex in myeloid cells include the t(8;21), which generates *AML1-ETO*,[226–229] and the t(3;21), which gives rise to *AML-EVI1, AML-EAP*, or *AML1-MDS1*.[230,231]

The sequence-specific DNA-binding and protein-protein interaction properties of CBF fusion proteins are provided by a large domain within AML1,[232] showing approximately 70 percent homology with the *Drosophila* Runt and Lozenge proteins. The *Drosophila* AML1 homologues participate in several developmental processes, including sex determination, segmentation and neurogenesis (Runt), and determination of photoreceptor identity during eye development (Lozenge). The sequence element recognized by AML1 is TGTGGT,[232] an enhancer core motif that serves as a regulatory element in several viral enhancers, as well as genes whose products are involved in the regulation of hematopoiesis, such as IL-3, GM-CSF, CSF-1, myeloperoxidase, and the TCR receptors.[224,233–240] The binding affinity of AML1 is markedly increased through its heterodimerization with CBFβ, an interaction also mediated through the *runt* homology domain.[232]

The *Aml1* gene was inactivated recently in the germ line of mice by homologous recombination and shown to be essential for definitive hematopoiesis of all lineages.[241,242] Homozygous null

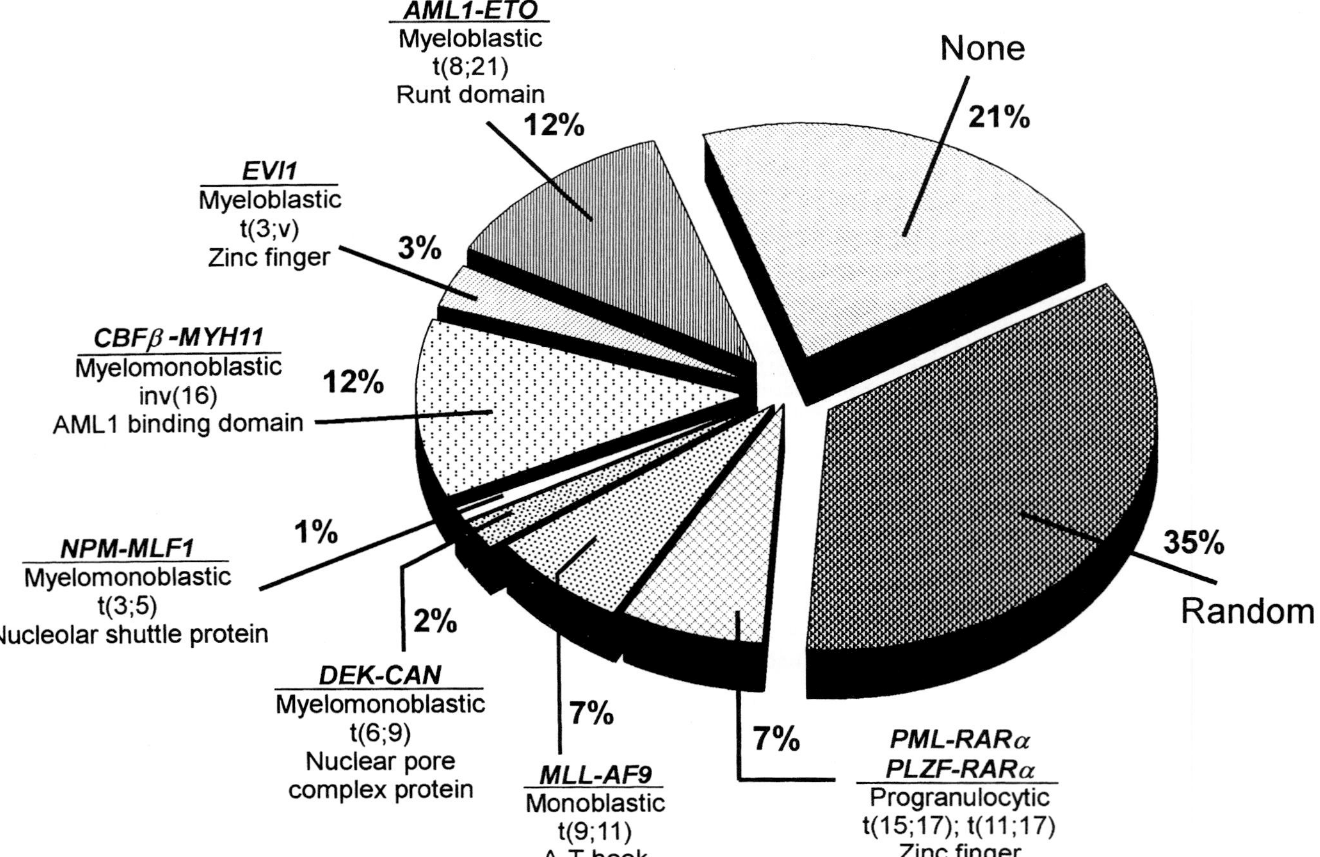

Fig. 19-6 Distribution of translocation-generated fusion genes among the various morphologic subtypes of AML in children and young adults. The section labeled *random* refers to sporadic rearrangements that have so far been observed only in the leukemic cells from single cases. Key domains for DNA binding and protein-protein interaction are given for transcription factors or the type of gene affected for nontranscription factors.

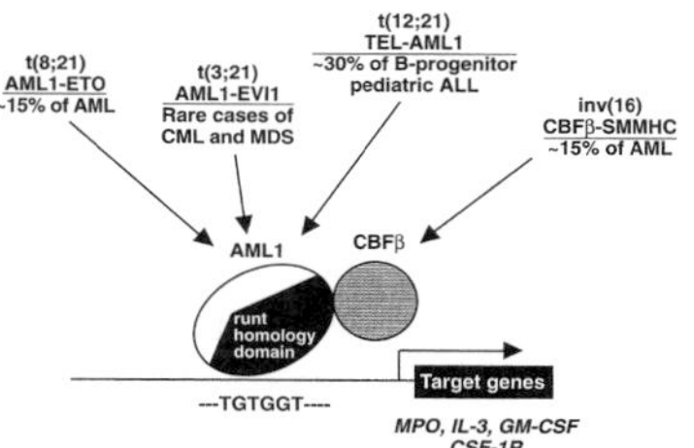

Fig. 19-7 Molecular consequences of chromosomal rearrangements that modify the AML1/CBFβ transcription factor complex, the most frequent target of reciprocal translocations in the human leukemias. In the majority of cases, the structural alteration disrupts the AML1 DNA-binding partner of this complex but not CBFβ, whereas in cases with the inv(16), only the latter protein is affected. The lack of lineage specificity for genetic lesions involving AML1 can be appreciated from the very early site of action of this gene in normal hematopoiesis (see Fig. 19-1), but the molecular basis for the phenotype specificity of each fusion gene in the transformation of myeloid or lymphoid progenitors remains unknown. CML, chronic myeloid leukemia; MDS, myelodysplastic syndrome; AML, acute myeloid leukemia; ALL, acute lymphoblastic leukemia. (*Adapted from Shurtleff et al.*[199] *Used with permission*).

animals display normal morphogenesis and yolk sac-derived erythropoiesis but die between embryonic days 11.5 and 12.5 because of CNS hemorrhage, postulated to be caused by a lack of platelets and possibly potentiated by abnormalities of CNS capillary endothelium.[242] Inactivation of the *Cbfβ* gene in the mouse germ line produced similar effects in homozygous null mice, indicating that CBFβ is required for AML1 function in vivo.[243] From these observations it appears that the AML1/CBFβ complex is an essential regulator of genes required for normal hematopoietic cell development. Hence chromosomal rearrangements that target this complex may interfere with its function in ways that produce arrested differentiation and eventually fully transformed leukemias of specific cell lineages.

The t(8;21), resulting in expression of the AML1-ETO oncoprotein, is the most frequent chromosomal abnormality in the myeloid leukemias of both children and adults; it is found most often in myeloblasts with evidence of granulocytic differentiation (M2 designation by the French-American-British classification system). The fusion protein, which retains the runt homology domain of AML1 and its ability to interact with CBFβ and the core enhancer DNA sequence element, appears to interfere with AML1-mediated transcriptional activation.[232,244] In fact, the C-terminal portion of ETO that is fused in frame with AML1 sequences has been shown to dominantly repress the expression of promoters normally activated by AML1.[240,245,246] The role of ETO in transcriptional repression appears to be directly linked to the ability of sequences included in the fusion protein to recruit the nuclear corepressors N-CoR and mSIN3.[247,248] These proteins assemble in a complex with histone deacetylase, which results in nucleosome assembly and the silencing of gene expression.[249] Thus a biochemical mechanism has been identified that sheds light on the ability of the oncogenic AML1-ETO fusion protein to dominantly oppose the activity of AML1 in the regulation of genes essential for normal myeloid cell development.

The combinatorial versatility of the *AML1* locus is demonstrated by its fusion with sequences from either the *EVI1* gene in t(3;21)-positive chronic myeloid leukemia in blast crisis[230] or to either the *EAP* (Epstein-Barr virus RNA-associated protein) or *MDS1* genes in myelodysplastic syndrome.[231] *EAP* and *MDS1* are located in a region adjacent to *EVI1* on the long arm of chromosome 3 and are often included with *EVI1* in transcripts resulting from these rearrangements.[250] Inclusion of both the Runt-homologous DNA-binding/dimerization domain of AML1 and the zinc-finger DNA-binding domains of EVI1 in the AML1-EVI1 chimeric protein affords ample opportunity for aberrant regulation of target genes.

The CBFβ subunit is involved in another major chromosomal rearrangement in AML, the inversion 16, which affects 15 to 18 percent of AML patients, principally those with myelomonocytic differentiation and increased bone marrow eosinophils (M4-Eo designation in the French-American-British system). This rearrangement joins most of the *CBFβ* gene to the C-terminus of the heavy chain gene of smooth muscle myosin (*MYHII,* also known as *SMMHC*), resulting in formation of a CBFβ-MYH11 protein.[251] Significantly, the fusion protein retains the domain of CBFβ that mediates heterodimerization with AML1.[252,253]

Murine models to study the effects of CBFβ-MYHII on hematopoietic cell development have been produced by inserting the human MYHII cDNA in-frame into the mouse *Cbfb* gene through homologous recombination to "knock in" the fused gene.[254] Similar experiments generated mice in which the *Aml1-ETO* fusion gene has been reconstructed by introducing the appropriate segment of the *ETO* gene into the mouse *Aml1* genomic locus.[255,256] Mouse embryos harboring one allele of *Cbfb-MYHII* or *Aml1-ETO* in the germ line developed CNS hemorrhages at embryologic days 12.5 to 13.5, similar to mice with homozygous loss of *Aml1* or *Cbfb,* indicating that these chimeric proteins dominantly interfere with essential functions of the Aml1/Cbfb complex. Mice expressing Cbfb-MYHII had impairment of primitive as well as definitive hematopoiesis, however, suggesting an additional activity of this fusion protein during hematopoietic cell development.[254] In addition, cells from the fetal livers of embryos expressing the *Aml1-ETO* fusion contained dysplastic multilineage hematopoietic progenitors that had an abnormally high self-renewal capacity and could be established as cell lines in vitro.[255,256] Since both AML1 and CBFβ normally are required for definitive hematopoiesis, the oncogenicity of their respective fusion proteins may stem from disruption of a transcriptional regulatory complex producing arrested myeloid cell differentiation; however, the basis for the phenotypic specificity of leukemias resulting from various types of AML1 and CBFb fusion proteins is unknown (see Fig. 19-7). The available data imply unique activities for each chimeric protein, possibly including gain-of-function as well as loss-of-function effects, as well as global interference with the role of the heterodimeric complex.

Although AML therapy has improved during the past decade, this disease remains extremely difficult to treat with chemotherapy alone, and much of the improvement in survival has arisen from advances in hematopoietic stem cell transplantation. Clinical studies have now demonstrated, however, that the presence of either the *AML1-ETO* or *CBFβ-MYH11* fusion genes in leukemic blast cells at diagnosis will identify patients with a relatively favorable prognosis, especially when treatment consists of intensive chemotherapy including high-dose cytarabine.[12,257–263] The clinical impact of this favorable association with therapeutic outcome is enhanced by the high relative frequency of fusion genes involving the CBF complex in the overall patient population with AML, which approaches approximately one-third of newly diagnosed children and adults with this disease. Molecular analysis of samples taken after the initiation of therapy also has led to the rather surprising finding that both the *AML1-ETO* and the *CBFβ-MYH11* fusion mRNAs can persist in the bone marrow and peripheral blood of AML patients in long-term remission following chemotherapy or bone marrow transplantation.[264–267] These observations illustrate the impact that a more comprehensive understanding of the genetic basis of acute leukemia is having an on clinical management and highlight the need for further work to explain the mechanisms that underlie the intriguing correlations that are emerging between molecular findings and therapeutic response.

Retinoic Acid Receptor Rearrangements

PML-RARα. Dysregulated chimeric transcription factors, which induce differentiation arrest at specific stages of development in the myeloid leukemias, offer a new class of intracellular targets for therapeutic attempts to promote differentiation of these leukemias in vivo so that they lose their proliferative capacity. A major example is the fusion product generated by the t(15;17)(q21;q11-22) in acute promyelocytic leukemia (APML), which links critical ligand- and DNA-binding sequences of the retinoic acid receptor-α gene (*RARα*) on chromosome 17 to sequences of the *PML* gene on chromosome 15.[268–273] In its unaltered form, the RARα protein binds to the retinoic acid ligand through a defined ligand-binding domain and to DNA through a separate zinc-finger region as a heterodimer with retinoid X receptor protein.[274] PML proteins, which also possess zinc-finger motifs, are normally located in novel macromolecular nuclear organelles, called *PML oncogenic domains* (PODs), that include at least three other proteins.[275–277] These nuclear bodies are preferential targets of proteins expressed by DNA tumor viruses[278–280] and are up-regulated in activated inflammatory mononuclear cells and by interferon.[281–283] The PML-RARα fusion proteins disrupt these subnuclear structures, causing normal PML, RXR, and other nuclear proteins to disperse in an abnormal microparticulate pattern.[275–277] The fusion proteins interfere with normal myeloid cell development, possibly through adverse effects on assembly of the PODs that contain PML, and dominant inhibitory effects as a homodimeric complex with normal retinoid receptor and peroxisome-proliferator pathways,[284–287] leading to arrested differentiation in the promyelocyte stage. PML-RARα also has been shown to have antiapoptotic activity and to result in cell survival under conditions of growth factor deprivation, which may contribute to its leukemogenic activity.[285,288,289]

***PLZF-RARα*, *NPM-RARα*, and *NUMA-RARα*.** Three variant translocations have been identified in AML that unequivocally implicate RARα in leukemias arrested at the promyelocyte stage of differentiation, since both fusion proteins involve the retinoid and DNA-binding domains of this nuclear receptor. Very little is known about the NPM-RARα or NuMA-RARα fusion proteins, which have been identified only in rare patients.[290,291] NPM-RARα links RARα in-frame to N-terminal sequences of nucleophosmin (NPM), a nucleolar shuttle protein that is also involved in NPM-ALK fusion proteins in large-cell lymphoma and NPM-MLF1 in AML, while the NuMA-RARα fusion protein represents a similar in-frame fusion with a protein involved in the nuclear mitotic apparatus.

PLZF-RARα was first recognized several years ago,[292] with subsequent structural and functional studies of PLZF providing intriguing insights into the potential mechanism of action. PLZF is a transcription factor containing nine C-terminal zinc-finger motifs related to those of the Krüppel *Drosophila* segmentation protein and containing an N-terminal POZ (poxvirus and zinc-finger) protein-protein interaction domain.[293] This domain inhibits the binding of transcription factors, including RARα, to DNA when linked in cis, suggesting that PLZF-RARα may act by sequestering RXR or other retinoid receptors within inactive multimeric complexes.[293–296] PLZF is expressed in multiple tissues during development, including elevated expression at Rhombomeric boundaries in the vertebrate hindbrain.[297] It is also expressed by early hematopoietic progenitors with a punctate nuclear distribution and is down-regulated during myeloid cell differentiation.[298] These findings, combined with studies showing heterodimerization of PLZF-RARα with normal PLZF through the POZ domain,[295] suggest that normal PLZF also may play a role in normal hematopoietic cell differentiation, one that is inhibited by the fusion protein. Five additional cases of APML with t(11;17)-mediated expression of PLZF-RARα fusion proteins have been reported,[299] indicating that these patients share a proclivity with PML-RARα patients to develop life-threatening DIC.

The Histone Deacetylase Complex and Its Role in APML. Recent studies have provided an attractive model to explain the mechanism through which the PML-RARα and PLZF-RARα fusion proteins contribute to dsyregulated gene expression in APML. In the absence of ligand, RARs have been shown to repress the expression of target genes. The mechanism involves the recruitment of the NCOR and SMRT corepressors, which in turn mediate the assembly of an histone deacetylase complex that has the ability to silence gene expression.[300–305] The PML-RARα fusion protein retains its ability to interact with the RAR corepressors and block transcription in the absence of ligand. However, unlike normal RAR proteins, which release the repressor complex and function as activators of gene expression in response to physiological concentrations of retinoids, the fusion protein remains in a repressor complex and aberrantly blocks target gene expression.[306–310] Studies in the presence of higher levels of retinoids also have helped explain the responsiveness of APMLs harboring *PML-RARα* fusion genes to ATRA. Pharmacologic dosages of ATRA overcome the association of PML-RARα with the histone deacetylase complex and allow the recruitment of coactivators, resulting in the activation of expression of critical target genes and the induction of growth arrest with granulocytic differentiation within the malignant clone.[311–314] These findings provide a mechanistic rationale for use of ATRA acid in patients with APML, which had been shown already to be effective in empirically initiated trials.[311,313,315–317] In response to pharmacologic doses of this compound, PML and its associated proteins are reorganized into normal-appearing nuclear PODs, with subsequent maturation of the leukemic cells into differentiated myeloid cells with limited life-spans in the circulation. Resistance to ATRA as a single agent generally develops within 3 to 4 months, but its role in the remission induction phase of APML therapy has been established, and clinical trials combining ATRA with cytotoxic chemotherapy have led to improved survival of patients whose promyeloblasts express the PML-RARα fusion protein.[316,317]

Biochemical analysis of the association of histone deacetylase complexes formed with PLZF-RARα fusion proteins also has provided an explanation for the clinical observation that all-trans retinoic acid differentiation therapy is not effective in inducing remissions in patients with this variant RARα fusion protein. The mechanism of transformation appears to be quite similar, in that PLZF-RARα proteins heterodimerize with RXR and form repressor complexes that block target gene expression in a fashion unresponsive to physiological retinoid levels.[300–305] However, the POZ domain of the PLZF portion of the fusion protein independently recruits the SMRT and NCOR nuclear corepressors, in complexes that are not disrupted in the presence of high levels of ATRA. Thus the presence of a second ATRA-unresponsive histone deacetylase complex formed by the PLZF fusion partner provides an explanation for the lack of sensitivity of leukemias harboring this fusion protein to treatment with a ligand that specifically overcomes repression mediated through the RARα moiety of the fusion protein.

Mouse Models of APML. The oncogenic properties of PML-RARα have been studied in transgenic mouse models in which expression of the fusion protein is driven by CD11b or cathepsin G regulatory sequences.[318–320] Mice expressing PML-RARα driven by the cathepsin G promoter develop a myeloproliferative disorder, and 25 to 30 percent of the mice develop AML after a relatively long latency period of 6 to 15 months of age.[307,319,320] By contrast, PLZF-RARα was much more active when its expression was driven by the same promoter, inducing leukemia in all the mice from two lines followed for the same time period, and leukemias in the mice were refractory to pharmacologic dosages of retinoic acid, recapitulating the resistance of human PLZF-RARα leukemias to ATRA therapy.[307] A transformation model, based on retroviral transduction of the *PML-RARα* gene into hematopoietic progenitor cells of chickens also has been used to demonstrate leukemogenicity.[321]

***EVI1* Gene Activation.** In some cases of AML with high platelet counts, the inv(3)(q21;q26.2) or the t(3;3)(q21;q26.2) moves promoter/enhancer sequences from one site on chromosome 3 into the *EVI1* locus on the same chromosome,[322,323] leading to increased gene expression. The same effect is produced in murine myeloid leukemias by insertional mutagenesis.[324] The EVI1 protein binds to promoter/enhancer sequences containing the GATA sequence motif and may act by interfering with regulatory signals normally mediated by the GATA family of hematopoietic transcriptional regulators.[325–328] The normal function of EVI1 is unknown, although its tissue distribution (oocytes and kidney cells) and its dominant interfering effect on normal myelopoiesis would suggest an important developmental role in regulatory pathways that interface between proliferation and differentiation.

Acute Mixed-Lineage Leukemias: *MLL* Fusion Genes

An extraordinarily diverse group of chromosomal translocations, deletions, and inversions affect chromosome band 11q23. In contrast to the lineage specificity of many other nonrandom rearrangements, these abnormalities occur in both lymphoid and myeloid leukemias (7 to 10 percent of ALL patients, 5 to 6 percent of AML) and in a high percentage of the so-called mixed-lineage leukemias, defined by expression of markers of more than one hematopoietic cell lineage.[329–331] Leukemias with 11q23 translocations also account for a high percentage of acute leukemias in infants less than 1 year of age (80 and 45 percent of infants with ALL and AML, respectively).[332–337] Perhaps the most striking association is the presence of 11q23 translocations in as many as 85 percent of secondary leukemias in patients treated with topoisomerase II inhibitors.[338,339] Taken together, these examples of phenotypic diversity suggest that 11q23 genetic abnormalities mediate the transformation of multipotential hematopoietic stem cells, which give rise to leukemias in which the myeloid or lymphoid progenitors are blocked at various stages of development.

Molecular Biology of *MLL*. Cloning of the gene most often affected by 11q23 abnormalities fulfilled expectations based on phenotypic, cytogenetic, and clinical studies. Many of the breakpoints that occur within the 11q23 locus interrupt the mixed-lineage leukemia gene (*MLL*, also called *HRX*, *ALL-1*, and *HTRX1*), which encodes a large protein of 3968 amino acids with a predicted molecular mass of 431 kDa.[340–345] Most intriguing with regard to function are three regions of homology with the *Drosophila trithorax* (*trx*) gene, two associated with central zinc-finger domains and the third with a 210-amino acid C-terminal region of 61 percent identity called the *SET* (*S*uvar3-9, *E*nhancer of zeste, *T*rithoroax) domain.[341,342,346–348] *Trithorax* is a master homeotic gene regulator that positively regulates the actions of a wide spectrum of homeotic (*Hom*) genes in the *Antennapedia* and *Bithorax* complexes of the fly and is required throughout embryogenesis for normal development of the head, thorax, and abdomen.[341–344,349]

The N-terminal region of the MLL protein contains three A-T hook domains, first identified in the so-called HMG (high mobility group) proteins, which are thought to help establish chromatin structure[350] and to bind in the minor groove to DNA segments rich in A and T residues. The intervening region between the A-T hooks and the zinc-finger domains includes a 47-amino acid region of homology with the noncatalytic domains of mammalian DNA methyltransferase (MT), an enzyme that acts on the hemimethylated substrate produced after DNA replication to maintain the methylation pattern of cytosine residues in the genomes of somatic cells.[351] Two additional domains have been defined based on their ability to affect transcriptional control, a trans-repression domain overlapping the MT-homology region and a trans-activation domain in the region C-terminus to the zinc fingers.[352] The SET domain has been shown to mediate interactions with Sbf1, a protein related to dual specificity phosphatases but which lacks a functional catalytic domain.[353] Interestingly, enforced expression of Sbf1 mediates transformation of NIH-3T3 fibroblasts and primary cultures of B-cell progenitors, suggesting that it functions as a SET domain-dependent positive regulator of growth-inducing kinase signaling pathways.[354]

***MLL* Fusion Genes.** Translocation breakpoints within the *MLL* gene occur exclusively in an 8.5-kb region located between exons 5 and 11 and join *MLL* sequences with genes from numerous other chromosomes to form a large fusion gene (Fig. 19-8). The resulting chimeric proteins, encoded on the derivative 11 chromosome, include the N-terminal half of MLL, with its A-T hook minor groove DNA-binding motifs, the MT-homology domain, and all or part of the associated transcriptional-repression domain.[341,342] Another consistent feature of MLL fusion proteins is the absence of the two zinc-finger regions and the Trithorax homology regions normally located in the C-terminal half of the protein.

In contrast to the similar regions of *MLL* affected by 11q23 rearrangements, an array of structurally diverse protein partners contributes amino acid segments to the MLL fusion proteins found in ALL, AML, and the mixed-lineage leukemias. Twelve of the genes fused to *MLL* by 11q23 translocations have now been cloned and sequenced (see Table 19-1), making it possible to examine their products for functional motifs that might provide clues to the mechanisms leading to the formation of active transforming proteins. At the time of its cloning, each of these fusion partners was a previously unidentified gene with unknown function. The ELL protein (also known as *MEN*) was cloned originally as an MLL fusion partner in translocations involving chromosome subband 19p13.1.[355,356] In an exciting development, the same protein was independently purified as an elongation factor that increases the catalytic rate of RNA polymerase II transcription.[357] This association seems unlikely to be circumstantial, in that ELL has a close functional analogue called *elongin* (SIII), the transcription elongation factor that is also regulated by the von Hippel-Lindau (VHL) tumor suppressor.[358–361] Many questions remain to be answered before the functional significance of the MLL-ELL fusion is known; for example, is the MLL-ELL fusion protein (which contains almost all the ELL coding sequences, fused in-frame to the usual N-terminal segment of MLL) still active as an elongation accelerator? Is ELL subject to regulation by proteins analogous to VHL? If so, does fusion with MLL block this interaction and remove ELL from positive or negative physiological control? And perhaps most important, which genes are controlled in their expression by ELL, and how do they affect cell physiology? Although the full significance of the functional identity of this MLL fusion partner is still unknown, recognition of ELL emphasizes the potentially important roles of such proteins in chimeric constructs, particularly the potential of the chimeras to interfere with the normal roles and regulation of the fusion partner proteins, in addition to their possible inhibitory effects on the normal function of MLL itself.

Another intriguing development in research on *MLL* fusion genes has been the realization that the identity of the fusion partner may determine the phenotypic specificity of the chimera in hematopoietic stem cell transformation. For example, *ENL*, the partner gene on subband 19p13.3, is frequently involved in translocations affecting both ALL (especially in infants and children) and AML,[362] whereas ELL is restricted to *de novo* and therapy-related cases of AML[355] and is rare in children.[362] ENL is one of three related fusion partners, which include *AF-4* on chromosome band 4q21, involved in the frequent 4;11 translocations found in ALL, and *AF-9* on band 9p22, the gene affected by the 9;11 translocation important in both primary and secondary acute monocytic leukemias of children and adults. Each of these proteins appears to contribute domains with similar structural attributes to chimeric proteins,[341,342,345,363–365] in that they contain nuclear localization signals and regions rich in serine and proline that may function as transcriptional trans-activation domains.[363,365] In support of this possibility, ENL was shown to trans-activate reporter gene expression in mammalian cells and

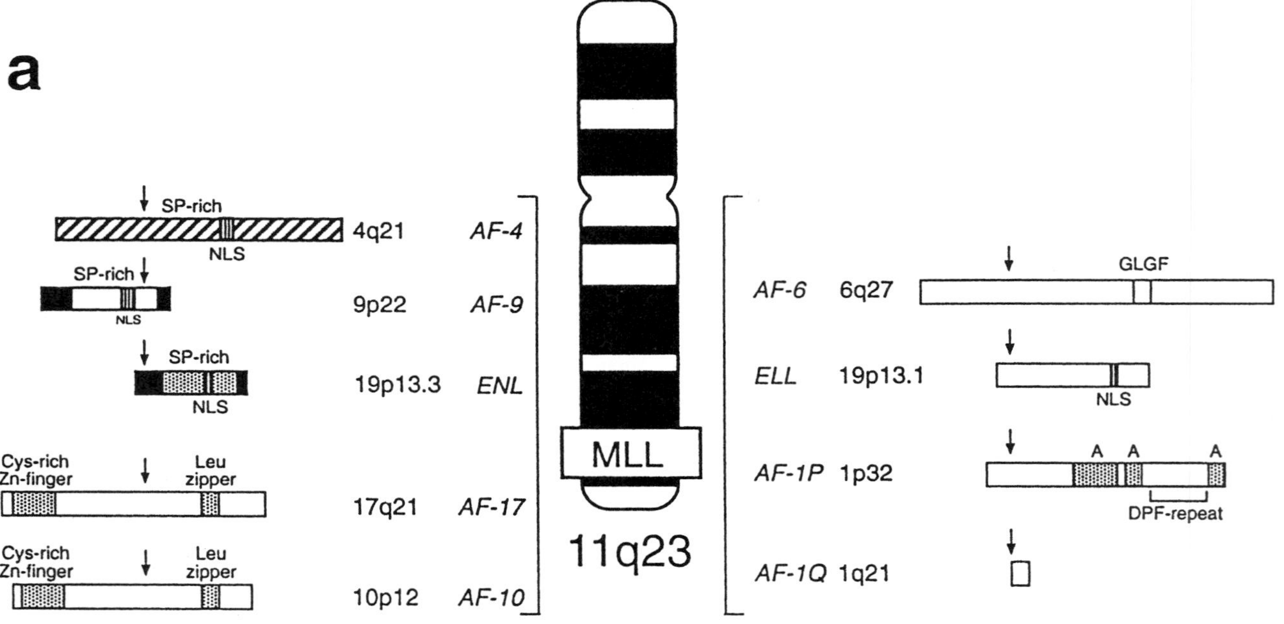

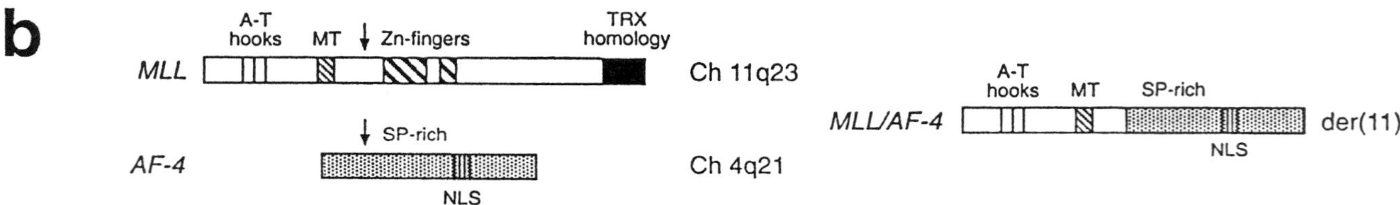

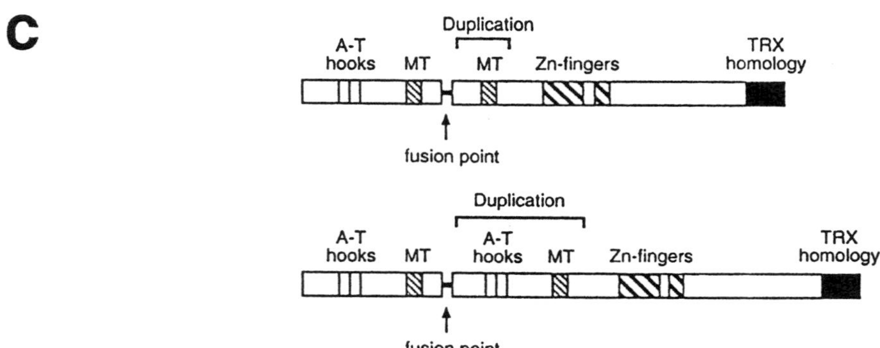

Fig. 19-8 The *MLL* gene and some of its fusion partners. The first three genes shown on the left of the ideogram (*A*) are rich in serine and proline (SP) and contain nuclear localization signals (NLSs), whereas the next two are notable for a cysteine-rich zinc-finger domain and a leucine zipper motif. The AF6 protein contains a novel glycine-leucine-glycine-phenylalanine (GLGF) domain, and AF1P is distinguished by three acidic (A) regions, together with an amino acid repeat motif (aspartic acid-proline-phenylalanine (DPF). AFIQ contributes only a minimal part of its 9-kDa total mass to its fusion with MLL, suggesting that truncation of MLL may itself contribute to leukemogenesis. Regions on the right of the breakpoints (*arrows*) are retained in the fusion product. Of the four major structural elements of *MLL* (*B*), only the A-T hook and mammalian DNA methyltransferase domains are retained in the chimeric proteins. AML cases have been identified recently with "self fusion" rearrangements (*C*), which fuse the same N-terminal *MLL* sequences with duplicated regions of the *MLL* gene. (*Adapted from Downing and Look.*[575] *Used with permission*).

yeast,[365] through the C-terminal serine- and proline-rich region of homology between ENL and AF-9, which is included in the chimeric proteins.

Some *MLL* partner genes appear to contribute functional domains to the chimeric proteins, whereas others truncate *MLL* in ways that may interfere with its normal function. *AF-10* and *AF-17,* potential examples of the first mechanism, are involved in the t(10;11)(p12;q23) and t(11;17)(q23;q21) and contain leucine zipper motifs near their C-termini and cysteine-rich zinc-finger motifs near their N-termini. These structural elements are retained in the oncogenic fusion proteins and may provide dimerization motifs with functional significance. The alternative model is best represented by the *AF1q* gene involved in the t(1;11)(q21;q23). This 9-kDa protein lacks homology to any known protein sequence,[366] and the minimal contribution of its sequences to the uniformly involved MLL N-terminal region implies that loss of MLL function through haploinsufficiency or dominant-negative interference may contribute to leukemogenesis. This interpretation is reinforced by several patients with AML who have lacked 11q23 translocations but have contained partial internal duplications of *MLL* linking the intact gene to a duplication of its N-terminal region.[367,368] In these rearrangements, a region beyond the A-T hook and methyltransferase domains is internally duplicated in-frame with the remainder of the coding sequences (see Fig. 19-4). Thus the partially duplicated *MLL* gene product contains the N-terminal A-T hooks and methyltransferase domains separated from the zinc-finger motifs, indicating that dissociation of N-terminal domains of MLL from regulatory C-terminal regions is a general structural feature of oncogenic MLL fusion proteins.

***Mll, Mll-AF9,* and *MLL-ENL* in Animal Models.** In *Drosophila,* the *MLL* homologue *trx* is a member of a large family of trithorax group proteins that have a positive role in the maintenance of cell-type specific patterns of *HOM-C* gene expression, apparently acting through epigenetic mechanisms that establish and sustain a receptive chromatin configuration.[369] Inactivation of the murine *Mll* gene in the germ line by homologous recombination has suggested that it has a similar function during normal mammalian development.[347,370] Complete loss of *Mll* was lethal during embryogenesis, with the embryos lacking detectable expression of the major *Hox* genes tested, consistent with the requirement for *trx* in maintenance of *HOM-C* gene expression in *Drosophila.* Interestingly, mice lacking function of one *Mll* allele showed a phenotype resulting from haploinsufficiency, with hematopoietic abnormalities that included anemia, thrombopenia and reduced numbers of B cells, bidirectional homeotic transformations of the axial skeleton, and sternal abnormalities. Skeletal abnormalities appeared to be due to shifts in the normal pattern of major *Hox* gene expression, due to inadequate *Mll* gene dosage, so that the hematopoietic cell phenotype may have resulted from a similar mechanism, based on studies that implicate mammalian *Hox* genes in blood cell development.[7,371–376] More recent studies have documented decreased numbers of yolk sac-derived CFU-GEMM, CFU-M, and BFU-E colonies in *Mll*-null embryos.[377] Overall, the results in *Mll*-deficient mice suggest a dual role for 11q23 translocations in human leukemogenesis, including both a gain-of-function effect mediated by the fusion oncogene and simultaneous effects on hematopoietic cell development from haploinsufficiency due to the loss of one normal *MLL* allele.[347]

The leukemogenicity of the *MLL-AF9* fusion gene was demonstrated recently in an animal model by generating this fusion oncogene in embryonic stem (ES) cells and using them to generate chimeric mice.[378] Although ES cells containing the *Mll-AF9* fusion gene gave rise to cells of all lineages in chimeric animals and the cells of numerous tissues expressed the fusion gene, the only tumors to develop in the mice were AMLs, reinforcing the association of this fusion gene with human AML. It also appeared that the fusion gene contributed an early growth advantage to progenitors within the myeloid lineage, because circulating myeloid cells derived from the targeted ES cells were a prominent component of this cell compartment in most of the *Mll-AF9* chimeras from the time of birth. This effect was not observed in mice generated from an ES cell line modified to express a truncated and epitope-tagged *Mll* allele, implying that the disordered growth advantage imparted to myeloid cells did not arise from *Mll* haploinsufficiency but rather from expression of the *Mll-Af9* fusion protein. Although leukemia induction was highly efficient in this model, the latency period ranged from 4 to 12 or more months, implying that additional mutations affecting other oncogenes or tumor suppressors must occur before a fully transformed leukemic clone can emerge.[378]

A retroviral gene transfer assay has been used successfully to document the oncogenic capacity of MLL-ENL (also known as HRX-ENL) by showing its activity in the immortalization and leukemic transformation of myelomonocytic progenitors in mice.[379] Detailed structure-function analysis has indicated that the DNA-binding motifs of MLL are required for the full transforming activity of the fusion protein, including the methyltransferase and A-T hook domains.[380] Within the ENL sequences of the fusion protein, the C-terminal 84 amino acids of ENL, which comprise two helical structures highly conserved with AF9, are both necessary and sufficient for transformation. These structures were shown to function as transcriptional activators, suggesting that the fusion protein acts to dysregulate the expression of target genes that contribute to transformation within the myeloid lineage.

Origins of Therapy-Related AML. *MLL*-associated translocations are a prominent feature of leukemias in patients treated with the epipodophyllotoxins,[338,339,381] but the basis for this association remains uncertain. An intriguing correlation has emerged from analysis of 130 breakpoints by restriction mapping and more than a dozen by genomic DNA sequencing analyses in cases of *de novo* or therapy-related leukemias with 11q23 translocations affecting the *MLL* gene.[382–387] That is, the centromeric portion of the 8.5-kb genomic MLL breakpoint cluster region consistently showed the largest number of breakpoints in cases of *de novo* leukemias, whereas the telomeric portion contained the majority of breakpoints found in therapy-related cases.[386,387] Scaffold attachment sites have been mapped in the vicinity of these breakpoint regions, as well as high-affinity topoisomerase II cleavage sites, which may influence the distribution of breakpoints.[386]

With regard to the molecular mechanisms involved in the origin of 11q23 translocations in *de novo* and secondary AML, studies to date have focused on (1) recombination within Alu repeats, (2) involvement of V-D-J recombinase enzymes in B-lymphoid progenitors, and (3) the possible role of topoisomerase II inhibitors acting to promote breaks at consensus cleavage sites for this enzyme, which would serve as substrates for recombination events leading to *MLL* translocations in the therapy-related leukemias. The first two possibilities have gained credible support,[368,382,383,385,388] but they do not explain the majority of cases.[382,389]

An intriguing mechanism of genetic recombination involves cleavage by topoisomerase II, as suggested by the frequent identification of *MLL* rearrangements in therapy-related cases of AML of patients treated with agents that inhibit this enzyme.[338,339,381] Antineoplastic drugs with this property include both the epipodophyllotoxin and anthracycline classes of drugs. AML linked to these agents tends to appear as an acute leukemia without a myelodysplastic phase within 6 to 24 months after diagnosis of the primary malignancy, in contrast to the longer latency periods and frequent myelodysplastic prodromes of secondary AML induced by alkylating agents. AML arising after treatment with a topoisomerase inhibitor typically has monoblastic or myelomonoblastic morphology,[338,339,381,390–392] suggesting that the target cell is a myeloid progenitor cell stimulated to enter cell division by chemotherapy-induced neutropenia.

Topoisomerase II catalyzes a two-step reaction involving both double-stranded DNA cleavage and strand relaxation and religation.[393] Both the epipodophyllotoxins and the anthracyclines stabilize the DNA-topoisomerase II complex after cleavage, resulting in the accumulation of double-strand DNA breaks, which are prime substrates for nonhomologous recombination.[394,395] Analysis of several 11q23 translocations has identified topoisomerase II consensus binding sites adjacent to chromosomal breakpoints.[385] Other cases of therapy-related AML lack topoisomerase II-binding sites adjacent to the breakpoints, so additional 11q23 translocation junctions will need to be analyzed before the frequency and importance of this mechanism can be fully assessed.[382,386]

Aside from factors predisposing to nonhomologous recombination, how could topoisomerase inhibitors preferentially induce AML with characteristic MLL fusion proteins? The rapid development of these secondary leukemias suggests a collaborative mechanism in which both the drug and the fusion protein act synergistically to accelerate the multistep process leading to AML. A model incorporating the known effects of the epipodophyllotoxins on G2-phase cell cycle checkpoint control and topoisomerase II activity is shown in Fig. 19-9. These compounds arrest cycling cells in G2 phase, and most committed myeloid progenitors harboring epipodophyllotoxin-induced DNA breaks are likely targeted to undergo apoptosis, based on the degree of neutropenia that accompanies a typical course of therapy with these agents (see Fig. 19-9, top panel). Normal myeloid progenitors arrested in G2 occasionally survive, however, with double-strand DNA breaks at the sites of topoisomerase II integration. As these lesions are repaired, some of the breaks are joined by nonhomologous recombination and result in chromosomal rearrangements. The myeloid progenitors with 11q23 translocations producing in-frame *MLL* fusion genes begin to proliferate because of a proliferative advantage conferred by the hybrid MLL protein and growth factors produced in response to epipodophyllotoxin-induced neutropenia. According to this model, MLL fusion proteins may exacerbate this process by relaxing cell cycle checkpoints normally activated by the presence of the integrated topoisomerase II:drug complex, leading to attenuated apoptosis and increased survival of cells with genetic damage at other loci (see Fig. 19-9, bottom panel). In the face of repetitive epipodophyllotoxin treatment, this could lead to the acquisition of additional genetic lesions affecting oncogenes or tumor suppressors in the expanding clone that already expresses an MLL fusion protein, with rapid progression of a multistep process culminating in overt AML.

The exceedingly high frequency of 11q23 translocations associated with infant leukemias suggests a further mechanism that could lead to *MLL* gene rearrangement and biologically active chimeric proteins. A number of pairs of infant twins have been shown to have identical *MLL* gene rearrangements.[396,397] In some cases, the leukemias had identical *Ig* gene rearrangements, consistent with transformation of a common progenitor cell that had completed V-D-J recombination. In other cases the *Ig* rearrangements differed between twin leukemias, suggesting that transformation occurred before *Ig* gene recombination and that the leukemic clones had evolved independently. Nonetheless, the identification of identical *MLL* rearrangements at the DNA sequence level in each twin indicates that the leukemic clone arose in one infant and spread through the placenta to the other sibling. The documentation of *MLL* rearrangements in utero and the high frequency of 11q23 translocations in infant leukemias (approaching 80 percent of ALL patients and 50 percent of AML patients) suggest that pluripotent progenitor cells with self-renewal capacity are in a proliferative state in the developing bone marrow, rendering them uniquely susceptible to transformation by chimeric MLL oncoproteins. This susceptibility may be related to patterns of gene expression or epigenetic changes in chromatin configuration that are found in subsets of progenitors that are expanding to populate the hematopoietic system during infancy.

Myeloid progenitors similarly susceptible to the transforming effects of chimeric MLL proteins or prone to productive *MLL*

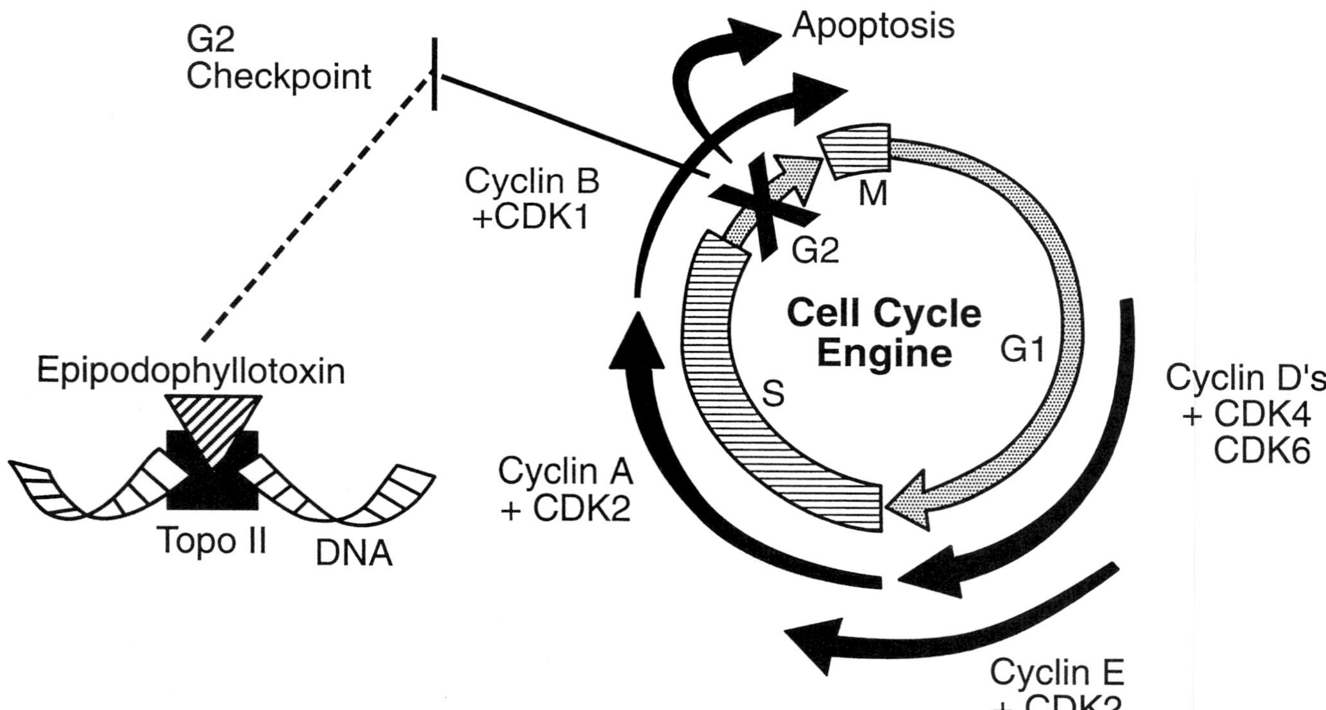

Fig. 19-9 Model accounting for the mechanisms linking epipodophyllotoxin therapy, MLL fusion proteins, cell cycle progression, and the relaxation of cell cycle checkpoints, leading to reduced levels of apoptosis in myeloid progenitor cells after genotoxic chemotherapy (hence increased survival of cells with damaged DNA). The accelerated acquisition of additional genetic lesions in clonogenic preleukemic cells eventually culminates in overt myeloid leukemia. See text for further explanation. (*Adapted from Downing and Look.*[575] *Used with permission*).

rearrangements may be reactivated in patients undergoing therapy with epipodophyllotoxins, accounting for the rapid onset of secondary AML in children and adults treated with these agents. We have recently identified altered transcripts for the p27KIP1 cell cycle kinase inhibitor in leukemias expressing MLL-AF4[398] and have shown that MLL-AF4 induces cell cycle arrest in cell lines when its expression is driven by a conditional promoter,[399] suggesting that hematopoietic stem cells may need to have the capacity to bypass negative cell cycle effects of this fusion protein before they become susceptible to malignant transformation. Moreover, the short latency period between *MLL* rearrangement and overt leukemia following 11q23 translocations in infants and after epipodophyllotoxin therapy suggests that MLL fusion proteins themselves predispose susceptible hematopoietic progenitors to undergo secondary mutations necessary for the development of a fully transformed leukemic clone.

ONCOGENIC ACTIVATION OF TYROSINE KINASES

Cellular tyrosine kinase gene products serve as growth factor receptors or intracellular signal transducers and can be aberrantly activated through a variety of mechanisms, including truncation of the ligand-binding domain of growth factor receptors, loss or replacement of C-terminal regulatory tyrosine residues, and point mutations within intact molecules.[400] In the leukemias and lymphomas, chromosomal translocations produce tyrosine kinase gene fusions that are quite specific for lymphoid progenitor cells of particular lineages and phenotypes. In two instances, the N-terminal sequence of a functionally unrelated protein is fused to a truncated receptor tyrosine kinase. Such kinases normally occupy a proximal position in the transduction of extracellular signals required for cell proliferation, differentiation, and other biologic events that determine cell fate. When activated by growth factors, these transmembrane proteins phosphorylate themselves as well as their substrates, triggering multiple biochemical regulatory cascades. Critical steps in this process are dimerization of two adjacent receptors to initiate signal transduction and phosphorylation of high affinity-binding sites for the SH2 (*S*rc *h*omology) domains of GRB2 and other specific cytoplasmic signaling molecules that convert RAS proteins to their GTP-bound forms (reviewed in ref. 401).

The chimeric proteins resulting from receptor tyrosine kinase fusions invariably lack ligand-binding domains and may lack transmembrane domains, yet they clearly function as oncogenic proteins. The mechanism(s) responsible for constitutive activation of a tyrosine kinase in the absence of growth factor binding appear to be related to shuttling of the chimera to a new cellular location[402] and to constitutive activation due to dimerization stimulated by sequences within the nonkinase fusion partner, such as a leucine zipper motif.[403] Thus hybrid proteins with aberrantly activated tyrosine kinase domains represent a novel product of chromosomal rearrangements, further demonstrating the versatility of genetic mechanisms that transform hematopoietic cells.

ABL Fusion Genes in Chronic and Acute Leukemias

The Philadelphia chromosome, produced by a (9;22)(q34;q11) translocation, was first identified in patients with chronic myeloid leukemia (CML) and later shown to occur in 3 to 5 percent of children and 30 to 40 percent of adults with ALL.[404–406] This translocation results in a *BCR-ABL* chimeric tyrosine kinase oncogene, which contains sequences from the *BCR* gene upstream of the second exon of the *ABL* proto-oncogene.[407–412] Thus t(9;22) breakpoints on the distal tip of the long arm of chromosome 9 occur in the first intron of the *ABL* proto-oncogene, which spans a distance of more than 100 kb upstream of sequences encoding the tyrosine kinase domain.[413–415] By contrast, the breakpoints on chromosome 22 are confined to a 5.8-kb region of genomic DNA known as the *major breakpoint cluster region* (M-bcr),[416] which lies within *BCR*, a gene that encodes a 160-kDa phosphoprotein.[416,417] The 8.5-kb fusion transcript found in CML encodes a 210-kDa hybrid protein that is activated as a tyrosine-specific protein kinase, as is the *v-abl* protein product.[418–421]

Although routine karyotyping does not distinguish between the t(9;22) in CML and ALL, molecular analysis of the *BCR* and *ABL* proto-oncogenes, which are rearranged in both diseases, has revealed differences that apparently mediate the phenotype specificity of these oncogenic fusion kinases.[422–424] In ALL, the rearrangement produces a shorter fusion transcript (6.5 to 7.0 kb) and hybrid protein (185 to 190 kDa) than are generated by the *BCR-ABL* fusion gene in CML[422–424] (Fig. 19-10). The differences are due to unique breakpoints on chromosome 22 in ALL patients that do not lie within the 5.8-kb region of *BCR* that contains the breakpoints in CML. Instead, they are contained within a second minor breakpoint cluster region (M-bcr) located further upstream within the *BCR* gene.[425–427] The ALL fusion protein includes N-terminal *BCR* amino acids but lacks the internal residues that are found in the CML fusion proteins near the *BCR-ABL* junction.

The N-terminal sequences of *ABL* are removed in oncogenic forms of the gene and replaced by the Moloney virus *gag* gene in the case of *v-abl*[428–430] and with *BCR* sequences in the *BCR-ABL* fusion gene of CML and ALL.[418–421] The products of both the *v-abl* and the *BCR-ABL* fusion genes can transform primary hematopoietic cells in vitro, providing a model system for analysis of oncogenic mechanisms.[431]

Both the P185 and P210 BCR-ABL proteins also can induce a CML-like syndrome in vivo in mice when they are expressed in hematopoietic progenitors.[432–435] Mechanistic studies of these fusion proteins have shown that RAS signaling is essential for transformation and that multiple alternative means, including the adapters GRB2, SHC, and CRKL, are used to couple the activated ABL kinase to RAS, resulting in activation of Jun kinase.[436–438] Oncogenic signaling by BCR-ABL also has been shown to involve the cell cycle-regulated genes *MYC* and *cyclin D1*[439,440] and to constitutively activate the transcriptional signal transducer STAT5.[441] The emerging picture is one of multiple signaling pathways that are activated to mediate leukemic transformation by BCR-ABL; hence selective complementation of defective mutant fusion proteins should allow the identification of genetic pathways that are involved in BCR-ABL-mediated hematopoietic cell transformation.[436]

A new mechanism of ABL activation in human leukemia involves a fusion between the Ets transcription factor TEL and the catalytic domain of ABL; the product of this union has been identified in two cases of acute leukemia, one myeloid and the other lymphoid.[203,442] The TEL-ABL fusion kinase resembles the TEL-PDGFβR protein previously described in association with a t(5;12) chromosomal translocation in CML.[443] As with TEL-PDGFβR, the DNA-binding domain of TEL is not incorporated into the chimeric structure. Recently, the TEL-ABL protein was shown to be a constitutively activated kinase located in the cytoskeleton, whose activity depends on oligomerization mediated through a helix-loop-helix domain in the N-terminus of TEL.[203]

Progress also has been made in clarifying the normal role of the ABL kinase. Studies in mice rendered *Abl* deficient by homologous recombination indicate that Abl is not required for embryogenesis; however, mice without this protein develop a wasting syndrome and die shortly after birth.[444,445] In contrast to the BCR-ABL proteins, which are cytoplasmic, normal ABL is a nuclear kinase, whose activity is tightly regulated in vivo.[446] Recent evidence suggests that the kinase is activated by DNA-damaging agents and that it mediates growth arrest in a p53-dependent fashion.[447–450,450,451] Although the precise function of ABL is not known, the available evidence suggests that it regulates pathways that mediate cell cycle arrest after genotoxic damage. It is fascinating that this kinase, which in many ways has functions reminiscent of a tumor suppressor, can be subverted through chromosomal translocation to function in an entirely different

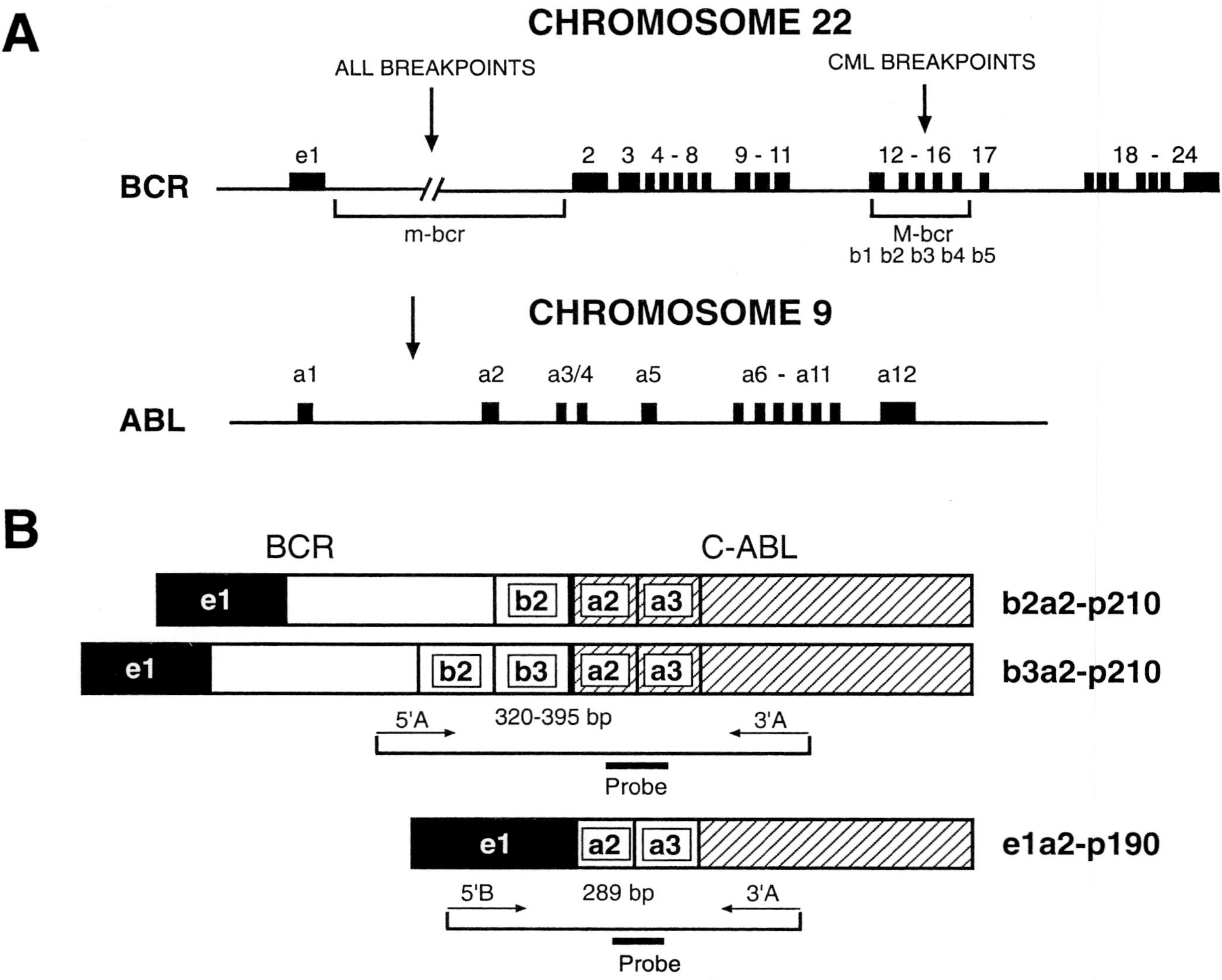

Fig. 19-10 Genomic structure of *BCR* locus on chromosome 22. Breakpoints in chronic myelogenous leukemia (CML) occur primarily in the more 3′ M-bcr region, while those in acute lymphoblastic leukemia (ALL) occur primarily in the m-bcr region. The two common BCR-ABL fusion proteins resulting from M-bcr-type breakpoints are 210 kDa (p210) in size and contain the *BCR* distal exons b1 and b2, with or without b3. By contrast, breakpoints in m-bcr result in a fusion protein of 190 kDa (p190) that contains only the first *BCR* exon, e1. Both the p210 and p190 fusion proteins contain the same portion of ABL. (*Adapted from Okuda, Fisher, and Downing.*[13] *Used with permission*).

cytoplasmic compartment and presumably through different substrates in the malignant transformation of hematopoietic progenitors.

The exceedingly poor prognosis of ALL patients with the Philadelphia chromosome has been attributed to transformation of a primitive hematopoietic stem cell that is inaccessible to most forms of chemotherapy.[406,452–454] Long-term responses (probable cures) have been induced in a subset of children with ALL who have low white blood cell counts at diagnosis, using intensive early-phase chemotherapy, followed by repetitive treatment with pairs of non-cross-resistant drugs.[455] For most patients with BCR-ABL-positive ALL, however, the recommended strategy is allogeneic bone marrow transplantation in first remission, which is also the only known curative approach for CML.[456]

NPM-ALK In Large-Cell Lymphoma

Large-cell lymphomas constitute approximately one-fourth of the non-Hodgkin lymphomas that develop in children and adolescents. In a subset of these tumors, a t(2;5) chromosomal translocation links N-terminal sequences encoded by the ubiquitously expressed nucleophosmin (*NPM*) gene on chromosome 5q35 to the catalytic domain of a previously unidentified tyrosine kinase gene on chromosome 2p23, now termed *ALK* (for *a*naplastic *l*ymphoma *k*inase).[457] The NPM phosphoprotein, which shuttles between the nucleolus and the cytoplasm,[458,459] consists of a putative metal binding site, two acidic amino acid clusters, and two nuclear localization signals.[460] NPM is highly phosphorylated during mitosis and serves as a substrate for CDC2.[461] NPM has been shown to bind to RNA, DNA, the HIV Rev protein, transcription factor YY1, and nucleolar protein p120[461–466] and is thought to play a role in ribosomal assembly, but its specific function remains undefined.

The *ALK* gene product, a tyrosine kinase receptor of 1620 amino acids, shows greatest amino acid identity with members of the insulin receptor subfamily, leukocyte tyrosine kinase in particular (64 percent).[457] Very little is know about the normal function of ALK, with the exception that its murine homologue is exclusively expressed in cells of the central and peripheral nervous systems.[467,468]

The NPM-ALK chimera retains 117 amino acids from NPM and 563 from ALK. In contrast to the cell surface localization of native ALK receptors, immunofluorescence studies with Cos cells have documented both cytoplasmic and nuclear expression of the NPM-ALK chimera.[469,470] The available evidence indicates that the NPM fusion segment contributes an active promoter that drives expression of the ALK kinase domain and a dimerization domain that stimulates its constitutive activation, leading to lymphomagenesis. The transforming potential of NPM-ALK has been demonstrated in NIH-3T3 cells[469,471] and in mice reconstituted with bone marrow cells bearing the chimeric gene.[472] In the latter study, half the animals developed clonal B-lineage large-cell lymphomas that arose in the mesenteric lymph nodes and metastasized to the lungs and kidneys. Experiments with NPM-ALK mutants have established that dimerization mediated by the NPM segment is required to activate the truncated ALK tyrosine kinase for cell transformation and indicate that interactions between ALK and the GRB2 substrate also may be necessary.[469,471]

Discovery of the *NPM-ALK* fusion gene has definite clinical implications. With the availability of ALK-specific antibodies for immunodiagnosis, it is now apparent that a broad morphologic spectrum of large-cell lymphomas expresses the activated chimeric NPM-ALK kinase.[473–476] Other useful assay techniques for this fusion gene include DNA- or RNA-based polymerase chain reaction (PCR) techniques[477,478] and fluorescence *in situ* hybridization assays with interphase cells.[479] Studies to examine the clinical outcome of patients with lymphomas expressing NPM-ALK have demonstrated a favorable prognosis, approaching an 80 percent 5-year survival.[480–482]

In addition to the classic t(2;5), ALK has now been shown to be activated through variant chromosomal rearrangements, including the t(1;2)(q25;p23) and an inv(2)(p23q35), although the presumptive fusion partners remain to be identified.[470,483] In addition, a rare subset of high-risk B-lineage large-cell lymphomas has been described in which the malignant cells express the full-length ALK kinase through an unknown mechanism but clearly lack the t(2;5) chromosomal translocation.[484]

TEL-PDGFRβ in CMML

An attractive hypothesis is that leukemias and lymphomas develop through an accumulation of multiple genetic changes, which eventually give rise to clonal, neoplastic growth. The transition from normal hematopoiesis to myelodysplastic syndrome (MDS) and then to overt AML affords a model in which one might establish the requirement for serial somatic mutations in the genesis of myeloid leukemia.[485] A possible paradigm for the early events in AML pathogenesis was provided by discovery of the t(5;12)(q33;p13) chromosomal translocation in CMML, an MDS subtype characterized by abnormal clonal myeloid cell proliferation and progression to AML.

The t(5;12) produces a fusion transcript in which the tyrosine kinase and transmembrane domains of the platelet-derived growth factor receptor β gene (*PDGFRβ*) on chromosome 5 are linked to a novel *Ets*-like gene (*TEL*) on chromosome 12. The prominent structural features of normal PDGFRβ receptors include five Ig-like extracellular loops and an interrupted intracellular tyrosine kinase domain.[486] This kinase participates in a signal transduction pathway that has a major effect on cell proliferation.[487] Mutated components of the PDGFRβ-related pathway, such as RAS, clearly have transforming potential, as does the PDGFRβ ligand, whose overexpression is associated with a myeloproliferative syndrome in mice.[488]

As emphasized in the preceding section on *AML1* gene fusion, *TEL* is a member of the *Ets* gene family and thus specifies a DNA-binding protein that recognizes the consensus motif C/A GGA A/T.[489] The distinct N-terminal HLH domain of TEL is essential for full transactivating function but probably does not bind DNA directly.[490] By analogy to other transcription factors, such as E2A, MYC, and MYOD, this HLH domain may be involved in protein-protein interactions.[203]

In t(5;12)-induced gene fusion, only the N-terminal HLH domain of *TEL* is incorporated into the chimeric product, which therefore lacks a legitimate DNA-binding domain. How, then, does the TEL-PDGFRβ protein induce CMML? An obvious model is that the retained TEL HLH domain leads to dimerization (hence activation) of the PDGFRβ kinase. Another possibility, raised by retention of the PDGFRβ transmembrane domain, is that the TEL 5′ region acts as a ligand-binding domain by responding to an unknown cognate binding protein. Finally, PDGFRβ may be moved to a new location in the cell, perhaps the nucleus, through localization signals provided by TEL-binding proteins. Displacement to the nucleus could result in phosphorylation of bound transcription factors with consequent aberrant activation of critical downstream targets. Each of these models has been reviewed in detail.[491]

It therefore appears that *TEL-PDGFRβ* fusion is a pivotal early genetic change in the development of CMML. Patients who progress from this MDS subtype to AML often show numerous additional cytogenetic changes, suggesting that malignant progression results from sequential acquisition of new mutations. Identification of the t(5;12) fusion product thus represents an advance in understanding how one form of MDS predisposes to acute leukemia. A variant t(5;12) translocation, the t(10;12)(q24;p13), also may generate a novel *TEL* fusion gene associated with refractory anemia, eosinophilia in the bone marrow, and increasing monocytosis.[492]

OTHER MECHANISMS OF TRANSFORMATION MEDIATED BY CHROMOSOMAL TRANSLOCATIONS

CYCLIN D1 Activation in Mantle Cell Lymphoma

The t(11;14)(q13;q34) was one of the first chromosomal translocations to be dissected molecularly, based on the realization that the breakpoint on chromosome 14 occurred within the *IgH* gene and use of a probe from this gene to isolate DNA from the so-called *BCL1* region on the long arm of chromosome 11.[493,494] Although additional tumors were identified with breakpoints in this region, it initially proved difficult to identify a proto-oncogene whose expression was altered by the translocation.[495–498] This search has now ended with the identification of the gene encoding cyclin D1 (*CCND1*), located 110 kb distal to the original *BCL1* breakpoint.[499–502] Evidence that *CCND1* is the proto-oncogene targeted by the t(11;14) includes the facts that it is the closest gene to the breakpoint cluster region on chromosome 11 and that the majority of tumors with this translocation aberrantly express this cell cycle regulatory protein (for a recent review, see ref. 503). Cyclin D1 is a member of a family of D-type cyclins that act in concert with their catalytic partners, the cyclin-dependent kinases (CDK4 and CDK6), to initiate the phosphorylation of the retinoblastoma protein, pRB, thus coupling growth factor-induced mitogenic signals to the biochemical machinery of the cell cycle (reviewed in ref. 504). B cells normally express two other cyclin D family members, cyclins D2 and D3, but not cyclin D1, so cyclin D1 expression is abnormally induced in this lineage by the translocation, presumably reflecting the influence of the B-cell-specific *IgH* gene enhancer from chromosome 14. The coding region of cyclin D1 is not altered by these translocations,[501,505,506] the breakpoints of which are often 100 kb or more from the gene itself, implying that uncoupling of cyclin D1 expression from mitogenic signals that would normally regulate the levels of cyclin D2 and D3 provides a constitutive proliferative stimulus.[507] Presumably, small lymphocytes in the mantle zone of the lymph node that harbor this translocation and aberrantly express cyclin D1 are unable to exit the cell cycle on cue and thus are unable to differentiate into Ig-secreting plasma cells.[508]

As molecular probes have become available, first for the *BCL1* locus and more recently to identify expression of the cyclin D1 mRNA and protein, it has been possible to clarify the pathologic diagnosis of B-cell lymphomas harboring the t(11;14). These tumors previously were called *mantle-cell* or *diffuse small cleaved-cell lymphomas,* but the term *mantle-cell lymphoma* now has been uniformly adopted by international agreement.[508–510] Comprising about 5 percent of lymphomas overall, these tumors occur primarily in elderly men, are of intermediate grade, and do not respond well to available therapies. It is now clear that virtually all mantle-cell lymphomas harbor the t(11;14) and express cyclin D1, rendering newly available monoclonal antibodies that recognize this protein especially valuable as immunohistochemical reagents for more accurate diagnosis of this important subset of B-cell malignancies.[511–514]

BCL2 in Follicular Lymphoma

The *BCL2* proto-oncogene was discovered through analysis of genes that are dysregulated by the t(14;18), which is the most common chromosomal translocation among human lymphoid malignancies. The t(14;18) is found in more than 80 percent of follicular center cell lymphomas, a common and generally indolent type of B-cell lymphoma that occurs almost exclusively in adults, and in approximately 20 percent of diffuse adult B-cell lymphomas.[515,516] Molecular analysis of the breakpoints of the 14;18 translocation identified *BCL2* as the gene on chromosome 18 that is overexpressed due to its translocation into the *IgH* locus on chromosome 14.[517–520] Functional studies revealed that BCL2 defines a new class of proto-oncogene products that act to prolong cell survival rather than having more typical effects on cell differentiation or proliferation.[521–523] It has since been learned that BCL2 is a member of a large family of highly conserved proteins that either inhibit or promote apoptosis (reviewed in ref. 524), extending down the phylogenetic tree to the CED-9 protein, which inhibits programmed cell death in *C. elegans.*[525] This interesting family of proteins is discussed further in a separate chapter in this volume (see Chap. 24).

Nuclear Pore Genes in AML

Three translocations in acute myeloid leukemia have been shown to involve nuclear pore genes, the t(6;9) and a cryptic t(9;9) or inv(9) producing the *DEK-CAN* and *SET-CAN* fusion genes[526–528] and the t(7;11) producing a *NUP98-HOXA9* chimera.[529,530] The first of these to be cloned was *DEK-CAN,* which is found in children and young adults with myeloid or myelomonocytic AML (M1, M2, or M4 according to the French-American-British classification). A chimeric DEK-CAN protein is produced, comprising nearly the entire DEK protein fused to the C-terminal two-thirds of the CAN protein.[526,527] A SET-CAN fusion protein was identified subsequently in leukemic cells from a single patient,[528] indicating a central role for CAN amino acids in the transforming capacity of these proteins, since identical portions of CAN were retained in each of the oncogenic hybrids. Insight into the normal role of CAN came when a component of the nuclear pore complex, called *NUP214,* was independently purified and shown to be identical to CAN.[531] CAN was shown to be localized to the nuclear pore by immunofluorescence microscopy; by contrast, DEK-CAN proved to be exclusively nuclear, even though the fusion protein retains the nucleoporin-specific FXFG repeats that are thought to mediate protein-protein interactions important for nuclear transport.[532] The essential role of normal CAN in nuclear transport has been proven through studies of embryos in which the gene was inactivated by homologous recombination,[533] and two cellular proteins have been shown to bind to CAN, of which one, a 112-kDa protein, also interacts with the nucleoporin-specific repeat of DEK-CAN and SET-CAN, suggesting that it might play a role in transformation.[534]

The nucleoporin connection recently has become even more intriguing with the cloning of the t(7;11) fusion gene, which encodes a hybrid protein containing the characteristic FXFG repeat region of another member of the nucleoporin complex, NUP98, fused in-frame to the homeobox domain of the major HOX protein HOXA9.[529,530] A current research focus is to determine whether the nucleoporin repeat regions allow these fusion proteins to interfere with protein or RNA transport across the nuclear membrane, resulting in a novel mechanistic contribution to the transformation of myeloid progenitors.[532–534] Alternatively, the presence of the HOXA9 homeodomain in the more recently identified NUP98-HOXA9 fusion protein raises the possibility that these hybrid proteins could interfere with the transcriptional regulation of genes important for myeloid cell development. According to this scenario, the nucleoporin partner primarily may contribute a protein-protein interaction and effector region to the fusion protein, with domains mediating interaction with DNA prompter/enhancer sequences coming from the other partners in these fusions. This would certainly be a plausible mechanism of transformation for the NUP98-HOXA9 fusion protein, because of the emerging evidence that the major HOX proteins contribute to hematopoietic development,[7,371–376] as already discussed in the section on MLL fusion proteins and the role of mammalian Mll and *Drosophila* trithorax in *HOX* and *Hom* gene regulation.[347]

Nucleolar *NPM-MLF1* Gene in AML

Another translocation specific for hematopoietic neoplasia is the t(3;5)(q25.1;q34), which occurs in a subset of MDSs and AMLs. We recently demonstrated that the t(3;5) interrupts the *NPM* gene, encoding a nucleolar shuttle protein, which is also interrupted by the t(2;5) in large-cell lymphoma and the t(5;17) in APML.[290,528] In the t(3;5), the N-terminal portion of NPM is fused in-frame to sequences of a novel gene on chromosome 3 that we have named *myelodysplasia/myeloid leukemia factor 1.*[535] This *MLF1* gene, which is not expressed by mature blood cells, encodes a cytoplasmic protein containing no identifiable structural motifs. The NPM-MLF1 fusion protein trafficks intracellularly under the direction of its NPM amino acid sequences, in that it is predominantly localized within the nucleolus of leukemic cells.[535] These features of MLF1 and NPM-MLF1 suggest that the t(3;5) may contribute to the development of AML through a previously unrecognized mechanism. Current efforts are directed toward the biochemical and biologic characterization of these proteins, as well as that of *MLF2,*[536] an *MLF1*-related gene that we have identified recently.

FUTURE DIRECTIONS

What has been learned about the transforming roles of transcription factors in leukemias and lymphomas? First is the requirement for proto-oncogene activation, usually by chromosomal rearrangement (through reciprocal translocations, inversions, deletions, or tandem duplications), in which the candidate gene comes to lie in the vicinity of a *TCR* or *Ig* gene or is fused with a second gene to form a chimeric protein that may retain many of the key functions of the original factor. Post-activation regulatory events remain largely unknown, although the array of factors so far identified suggests an extraordinarily diverse set of interactions. For example, heterodimerization with other proteins, as in the formation of MYC/MAX, AML1/CBFβ, TAL1/LMO2, or PBX1/HOX complexes, greatly increases the complexity of interactions between oncogenic proteins and transcriptional regulatory networks.

The key to understanding the oncogenic effects of transcription factors lies in the nature of the genes they regulate. Since the majority of these oncoproteins are ectopically expressed, one might predict that they alter the expression of tightly regulated gene programs in normal hematopoietic progenitors. Almost certainly examples will be found in which interaction of these proteins with downstream target genes either activates or represses developmental programs that are normally required only at critical times in the life cycle of the progenitor cell. In some instances, the positive or negative effects of oncogenic transcription factors are probably mediated directly through binding to enhancer sequences in target gene promoters; however, in other cases these proteins may transform cells indirectly, by binding to other transcriptional regulatory proteins and targeting them to nonfunctional or newly functional complexes.

Thus the main challenge for the future is to identify the gene programs controlled by the various transcription factors activated by chromosomal rearrangements. Equally important will be the task of delineating subsequent interactive processes within transcriptional regulatory cascades. This is likely to be even more difficult than deciphering the molecular mechanisms regulating *Drosophila* embryogenesis because of the greater complexity of experimental embryology and genetic analysis in vertebrate model systems. Clues to the normal roles of key gene products will continue to be provided by murine models, in which individual proto-oncogenes are targeted for inactivation by homologous recombination. The oncogenic targets of these proteins in leukemias and lymphomas may still be difficult to decipher because chromosomal translocations often mediate aberrant expression of genes in hematopoietic cells, either as inappropriately expressed intact proteins or as chimeric proteins that contain regulatory subunits from two different proteins.

With increased knowledge of the regulatory networks affected by oncogenic transcription factors, it may be possible to develop new therapeutic strategies for human malignancies, similar to those employing all-*trans*-retinoic acid for the treatment of APML. Indeed, if a fusion protein is crucial to malignant growth, one could alter the disease course by interfering with any of the multiple steps in protein synthesis and action, including oncogene transcription, RNA processing and translation, and DNA or protein-protein interactions. Fused transcription factors would appear ideal for these types of intervention because they represent true chimeras that occur only in rare types of malignant cells. A clear advantage of this approach, which depends on a detailed understanding of the mechanisms underlying each hybrid factor's transforming properties, would be the reduced likelihood of toxicity to normal cells or the development of resistant mutants, by comparison with currently available methods of cancer therapy.

Finally, it is important to realize that aberrant activation of proto-oncogenes by chromosomal translocations is but one event in the multistep process of carcinogenesis. Future molecular research into the leukemias and lymphomas undoubtedly will uncover an array of inactivating mutations affecting tumor suppressors, which act synergistically with proto-oncogenes activated by genetic rearrangement and are required for full expression of malignant phenotypes in hematopoietic cells.

ACKNOWLEDGMENTS

I would like to thank John Gilbert for editorial review and critical comments. This work was supported in part by NIH Grants CA-59571, CA-21765, CA-20180, and CA-71907 and by the American Lebanese Syrian Associated Charities (ALSAC).

REFERENCES

1. Bishop JM: The molecular genetics of cancer. *Science* **235**:305, 1987.
2. Solomon E, Borrow J, Goddard AD: Chromosome aberrations and cancer. *Science* **254**:1153, 1991.
3. Rowley JD: Molecular cytogenetics: Rosetta stone for understanding cancer. Twenty-ninth G. H. A. Clowes Memorial Award Lecture. *Cancer Res* **50**:3816, 1990.
4. Shivdasani RA, Orkin SH: The transcriptional control of hematopoiesis. *Blood* **87**:4025, 1996.
5. Rabbitts TH: Chromosomal translocations in human cancer. *Nature* **372**:143, 1994.
6. Look AT: Oncogenic role of "master" transcription factors in human leukemias and sarcomas: A developmental model, in Vande Woude G (ed): *Advances in Cancer Research.* San Diego, Academic Press, 1995, p. 25.
7. Look AT: Oncogenic transcription factors in the human acute leukemias. *Science* **278**:1059, 1997.
8. Rabbitts TH: Translocations, master genes, and differences between the origins of acute and chronic leukemias. *Cell* **67**:641, 1991.
9. Nusslein-Volhard C, Wieschaus E: Mutations affecting segment number and polarity in *Drosophila. Nature* **287**:795, 1980.
10. Nusslein-Volhard C, Frohnhofer HG, Lehmann R: Determination of anteroposterior polarity in *Drosophila. Science* **238**:1675, 1987.
11. Levine MS, Harding KW: Drosophila: The zygotic contribution, in Glover DM, Hames BD (eds): *Genes and Embryos.* New York, IRL Press, 1989, p. 39.
12. Rowley JD, Aster JC, Sklar J: The clinical applications of new DNA diagnostic technology on the management of cancer patients. *JAMA* **270**:2331, 1993.
13. Okuda T, Fisher R, Downing JR: Molecular diagnostics in pediatric acute lymphoblastic leukemia. *Mol Diagn* **1**:139, 1996.
14. Pui C-H: Childhood leukemias. *N Engl J Med* **332**:1618, 1995.
15. Papavassiliou AG: Molecular medicine transcription factors. *N Engl J Med* **332**:45, 1995.
16. Dalla-Favera R, Bregni M, Erikson J, Patterson D, Gallo RC, Croce CM: Human c-myc oncogene is located on the region of chromosome 8 that is translocated in Burkitt lymphoma cells. *Proc Natl Acad Sci USA* **79**:7824, 1982.
17. Taub R, Kirsch I, Morton C, Lenoir G, Swan D, Tronick S, Aaronson S, Leder P: Translocation of the C-myc gene into the immunoglobulin heavy chain locus in human Burkitt lymphoma and murine plasmacytoma cell. *Proc Natl Acad Sci USA* **79**:7837, 1982.
18. Adams JM, Gerondakis S, Webb E, et al: Cellular myc oncogene is altered by chromosome translocation to an immunoglobulin locus in murine plasmacytomas and is rearranged similarly in Burkitt lymphomas. *Proc Natl Acad Sci USA* **80**:1982, 1983.
19. Emanuel BS, Selden JR, Chaganti RSK, et al: The 2p breakpoint of a 2;8 translocation in Burkitt lymphoma interrups the V kappa locus. *Proc Natl Acad Sci USA* **81**:2444, 1984.
20. Erikson J, Nishikura K, ar-Rushdi A, et al: Translocation of an immunoglobulin kappa locus to a region 3′ of an unrearranged c-myc oncogene enhances c-myc transcription. *Proc Natl Acad Sci USA* **80**:7581, 1983.
21. Hollis GF, Mitchell KF, Battey J, et al: A variant translocation places the lambda immunoglobulin genes 3′ to the c-myc oncogene in Burkitt's lymphoma. *Nature* **307**:752, 1984.
22. Rappold GA, Hameister H, Cremer T, et al: C-myc and immunoglobulin kappa light chain constant genes are on the 8q+ chromosome of three Burkitt lymphoma lines with t(2;8) translocations. *EMBO J* **3**:2951, 1984.
23. Croce CM, Thierfelder W, Erikson J, Nishikura K, Finan J, Lenoir GM, Nowell PC: Transcriptional activation of an unrearranged and untranslocated c-myc oncogene by translocation of a C lambda locus in Burkitt. *Proc Natl Acad Sci USA* **80**:6922, 1983.
24. Taub R, Kelly K, Battey J, Latt S, Lenoir GM, Tantravahi U, Tu Z, Leder P: A novel alteration in the structure of an activated c-myc gene in a variant t(2;8) Burkitt lymphoma. *Cell* **37**:511, 1984.
25. Rabbitts TH, Hamlyn PH, Baer R: Altered nucleotide sequences of a translocated c-myc gene in Burkitt lymphoma. *Nature* **306**:760, 1983.
26. Pelicci PG, Knowles DM 2, Magrath I, Dalla-Favera R, Knowles DM: Chromosomal breakpoints and structural alterations of the c-myc locus differ in endemic and sporadic forms of Burkitt lymphoma. *Proc Natl Acad Sci USA* **83**:2984, 1986.
27. Taub R, Moulding C, Battey J, Murphy W, Vasicek T, Lenoir GM, Leder P: Activation and somatic mutation of the translocated c-myc gene in burkitt lymphoma cells. *Cell* **36**:339, 1984.
28. Bhatia K, Spangler G, Gaidano G, Hamdy N, Dalla-Favera R, Magrath I: Mutations in the coding region of c-myc occur frequently in acquired immunodeficiency syndrome-associated lymphomas. *Blood* **84**:883, 1994.
29. Gu W, Bhatia K, Magrath IT, Dang CV, Dalla-Favera R: Binding and suppression of the myc transciptionsl activation domain by p107. *Science* **264**:251, 1994.
30. Blackwood EM, Eisenman RN: Max: A helix-loop-helix zipper protein that forms a sequence- specific DNA-binding complex with Myc. *Science* **251**:1211, 1991.
31. Prendergast GC, Lawe D, Ziff EB: Association of Myn, the murine homolog of Max, with c-Myc stimulates methylation-sensitive DNA binding and Ras cotransformation. *Cell* **65**:395, 1991.
32. Ayer DE, Kretzner L, Eisenman RN: Mad: A heterodimeric partner for Max that antagonizes Myc transcriptional activity. *Cell* **72**:211, 1993.
33. Zervos AS, Gyuris J, Brent R: Mxi1, a protein that specifically interacts with Max to bind Myc-Mas recognition sites. *Cell* **72**:223, 1993.
34. Ayer DE, Lawrence QA, Eisenman RN: Mad-Max transcriptional repression is mediated by ternary complex formation with mammalian homologs of yeast repressor Sin3. *Cell* **80**:767, 1995.

35. Schreiber-Agus N, Chin L, Chen K, Torres R, Rao G, Guida P, Skoultchi AI, DePinho RA: An amino-terminal domain of Mxi1 mediates anti-Myc oncogenic activity and interacts with a homolog of the yeast transcriptional repressor SIN3. *Cell* **80**:777, 1995.
36. Ayer DE, Eisenman RN: A switch from Myc:Max to Mad:Max heterocomplexes accompanies monocyte/macrophage differentiation. *Genes Dev* **7**:2110, 1993.
37. Larsson LG, Pettersson M, Oberg F, Nilsson K, Luscher B: Expression of mad, mxi1, max and c-myc during induced differentiation of hematopoietic cells: Opposite regulation of mad and c-myc. *Oncogene* **9**:1247, 1994.
38. Amati B, Brooks MW, Levy N, Littlewood TD, Evan GI, Land H: Oncogenic activity of the c-Myc protein requires dimerization with Max. *Cell* **72**:233, 1993.
39. Adams JM, Harris AW, Pinkert CA, Corcoran LM, Alexander WS, Cory S, Palmiter RD, Brinster RL: The c-myc oncogene driven by immunoglobulin enhancers induces lymphoid malignancy in transgenic mice. *Nature* **318**:533, 1985.
40. Langdon WY, Harris AW, Cory S, Adams JM: The C-myc oncogene perturbs B lymphocyte development in Emu-myc transgenic mice. *Cell* **47**:11, 1986.
41. Lombardi L, Newcomb EW, Dalla-Favera R: Pathogenesis of Burkitt lymphoma: Expression of an activated c-myc oncogene causes the tumorigenic conversion of EBV-infected human B lymphoblasts. *Cell* **49**:161, 1987.
42. Packham G, Cleveland JL: c-Myc and apoptosis. *Biochim Biophys Acta* **1242**:11, 1995.
43. Galaktionov K, Chen X, Beach D: Cdc25 cell-cycle phosphatase as a target of c-myc. *Nature* **382**:511, 1996.
44. Zindy F, Eischen CM, Randle DH, Kamijo T, Cleveland JL, Sherr CJ, Roussel MF: MYC signaling via the ARF tumor suppressor regulates p53-dependent apoptosis and immortalization. *Genes Dev* **12**:2424, 1998.
45. Begley CG, Aplan PD, Davey MP, Nakahara K, Tchorz K, Kurtzberg J, Hershfield MS, Haynes BF, Cohen DI, Waldmann TA, et al: Chromosomal translocation in a human leukemic stem-cell line disrupts the T-cell antigen receptor delta-chain diversity region and results in a previously unreported fusion transcript. *Proc Natl Acad Sci USA* **86**:2031, 1989.
46. Chen Q, Cheng JT, Tasi LH, Schneider N, Buchanan G, Carroll A, Crist W, Ozanne B, Siciliano MJ, Baer R: The tal gene undergoes chromosome translocation in T cell leukemia and potentially encodes a helix-loop-helix protein. *EMBO J* **9**:415, 1990.
47. Xia Y, Brown L, Yang CY, Tsan JT, Siciliano MJ, Espinosa R, III, Le Beau MM, Baer RJ: TAL2, a helix-loop-helix gene activated by the (7;9)(q34;q32) translocation in human T-cell leukemia. *Proc Natl Acad Sci USA* **88**:11416, 1991.
48. Mellentin JD, Smith SD, Cleary ML: Lyl-l, a novel gene altered by chromosomal translocation in T-cell leukemia, codes for a protein with a helix-loop-helix DNA binding motif. *Cell* **58**:77, 1989.
49. Shivdasani RA, Mayer EL, Orkin SH: Absence of blood formation in mice lacking the T-cell leukaemia oncoprotein tal-1/SCL. *Nature* **373**:432, 1995.
50. Robb L, Lyons I, Li R, Hartley L, Kontgen F, Harvey RP, Metcalf D, Begley CG: Absence of yolk sac hematopoiesis from mice with a targeted disruption of the scl gene. *Proc Natl Acad Sci USA* **92**:7075, 1995.
51. Finger LR, Harvey RC, Moore RC, Showe LC, Croce CM: A common mechanism of chromosomal translocation in T- and B-cell neoplasia. *Science* **234**:982, 1986.
52. McKeithan TW, Shima EA, Le Beau MM, Minowada J, Rowley JD, Diaz MO: Molecular cloning of the breakpoint junction of a human chromosomal 8;14 translocation involving the T-cell receptor alpha-chain gene and sequences on the 3′ side of MYC. *Proc Natl Acad Sci USA* **83**:6636, 1986.
53. Shima EA, Le Beau MM, McKeithan TW, Minowada J, Showe LC, Mak TW, Minden MD, Rowley JD, Diaz MO: Gene encoding the alpha chain of the T-cell receptor is moved immediately downstream of c-myc in a chromosomal 8;14 translocation in a cell line from a human T-cell leukemia. *Proc Natl Acad Sci USA* **83**:3439, 1986.
54. Brown L, Cheng JT, Chen Q, Siciliano MJ, Crist W, Buchanan G, Baer R: Site-specific recombination of the tal-1 gene is a common occurrence in human T cell leukemia. *EMBO J* **9**:3343, 1990.
55. Aplan PD, Lombardi DP, Kirsch IR: Structural characterization of SIL, a gene frequently disrupted in T-cell acute lymphoblastic leukemia. *Mol Cell Biol* **11**:5462, 1991.
56. Aplan PD, Lombardi DP, Reaman GH, Sather HN, Hammond GD, Kirsch IR: Involvement of the putative hematopoietic transcription factor SCL in T-cell acute lymphoblastic leukemia. *Blood* **79**:1327, 1992.
57. Bernard O, Lecointe N, Jonveaux P, Souyri M, Mauchauffe M, Berger R, Larsen CJ, Mathieu-Mahul D: Two site-specific deletions and t(1;14) translocation restricted to human T-cell acute leukemias disrupt the 5′ part of the tal-1 gene. *Oncogene* **6**:1477, 1991.
58. Breit TM, Mol EJ, Wolvers-Tettero IL, Ludwig WD, van Wering ER, van Dongen JJ: Site-specific deletions involving the tal-1 and sil genes are restricted to cells of the T cell receptor alpha/beta lineage: T cell receptor delta gene deletion mechanism affects multiple genes. *J Exp Med* **177**:965, 1993.
59. Baer R: TAL1, TAL2, and LYL1: a family of basic helix-loop-helix proteins implicated in T cell acute leukaemia. *Semin Cancer Biol* **4**:341, 1993.
60. Bash RO, Hall S, Timmons CF, Crist WM, Amylon M, Smith RG, Baer R: Does activation of the TAL1 gene occur in a majority of patients with T-cell acute lymphoblastic leukemia? A pediatric oncology group study. *Blood* **86**:666, 1995.
61. Hsu H-L, Cheng J-T, Chen Q, Baer R: Enhancer-binding activity of the tal-1 oncoprotein in association with the E47/E12 helix-loop-helix proteins. *Mol Cell Biol* **11**:3037, 1991.
62. Hsu HL, Huang L, Tsan JT, Funk W, Wright WE, Hu JS, Kingston RE, Baer R: Preferred sequences for DNA recognition by the TAL1 helix-loop-helix proteins. *Mol Cell Biol* **14**:1256, 1994.
63. Hsu HL, Wadman I, Baer R: Formation of in vivo complexes between the TAL1 and E2A polypeptides of leukemic T cells. *Proc Natl Acad Sci USA* **91**:3181, 1994.
64. Wadman I, Li J, Bash RO, Forster A, Osada H, Rabbitts TH, Baer R: Specific in vivo association between the bHLH and LIM proteins implicated in human T cell leukemia. *EMBO J* **13**:4831, 1994.
65. Larson RC, Lavenir I, Larson TA, Baer R, Warren AJ, Wadman I, Nottage K, Rabbitts TH: Protein dimerization between Lmo2 (Rbtn2) and Tal1 alters thymocyte development and potentiates T cell tumorigenesis in transgenic mice. *EMBO J* **15**:1021, 1996.
66. Voronova AF, Lee F: The E2A and tal-1 helix-loop-helix proteins associate in vivo and are modulated by Id proteins during interleukin 6-induced myeloid differentiation. *Proc Natl Acad Sci USA* **91**:5952, 1994.
67. Hsu HL, Wadman I, Tsan JT, Baer R: Positive and negative transcriptional control by the TAL1 helix-loop-helix protein. *Proc Natl Acad Sci USA* **91**:5947, 1994.
68. Porcher C, Swat W, Rockwell K, Fujiwara Y, Alt FW, Orkin SH: The T cell leukemia oncoprotein SCL/tal-1 is essential for development of all hematopoietic lineages. *Cell* **86**:47, 1996.
69. Green AR, Salvaris E, Begley CG: Erythroid expression of the "helix-loop-helix" gene, SCL. *Oncogene* **6**:475, 1991.
70. Kallianpur AR, Jordan JE, Brandt SJ: The SCL/TAL-1 gene is expressed in progenitors of both the hematopoietic and vascular systems during embryogenesis. *Blood* **83**:1200, 1994.
71. Mouthon MA, Bernard O, Mitjavila MT, Romeo PH, Vainchenker W, Mathieu-Mahul D: Expression of tal-1 and GATA-binding proteins during human hematopoiesis. *Blood* **81**:647, 1993.
72. Visvader J, Begley CG, Adams JM: Differential expression of the LYL, SCL and E2A helix-loop-helix genes within the hemopoietic system. *Oncogene* **6**:187, 1991.
73. Weintraub H: The MyoD family and myogenesis: Redundancy, networks, and thresholds. *Cell* **75**:1241, 1993.
74. Buckingham M: Molecular biology of muscle development. *Cell* **78**:15, 1994.
75. Stainier DY, Weinstein BM, Detrich HW, Zon LI, Fishman MC: Cloche, an early acting zebrafish gene, is required by both the endothelial and hematopoietic lineages. *Development* **121**:3141, 1995.
76. Liao EC, Paw BH, Oates AC, Pratt SJ, Postlethwait JH, Zon LI: SCL/Tal-1 transcription factor acts downstream of cloche to specify hematopoietic and vascular progenitors in zebrafish. *Genes Dev* **12**:621, 1998.
77. McGuire EA, Hockett RD, Pollock KM, Bartholdi MF, O'Brien SJ, Korsmeyer SJ: The t(11;14)(p15;q11) in a T-cell acute lymphoblastic leukemia cell line activates multiple transcripts, including ttg-1, a gene encoding a potential zinc finger protein. *Mol Cell Biol* **9**:2124, 1989.
78. Greenberg JM, Boehm T, Sofroniew MV, Keynes RJ, Barton SC, Norris ML, Surani MA, Spillantini MG, Rabbits TH: Segmental and developmental regulation of a presumptive T-cell oncogene in the central nervous system. *Nature* **344**:158, 1990.

79. Boehm T, Foroni L, Kaneko Y, Perutz MF, Rabbitts TH: The rhombotin family of cysteine-rich LIM-domain oncogenes: distinct members are involved in T-cell translocations to human chromosomes 11p15 and 11p13. *Proc Natl Acad Sci USA* **88**:4367, 1991.
80. Royer-Pokora B, Loos U, Ludwig WD: TTG-2, a new gene encoding a cysteine-rich protein with the LIM motif, is overexpressed in acute T-cell leukaemia with the t(11;14)(p13;q11). *Oncogene* **6**:1887, 1991.
81. Warren AJ, Colledge WH, Carlton MBL, Evans MJ, Smith AJH, Rabbitts TH: The oncogenic cysteine-rich LIM domain protein Rbtn2 is essential for erythroid development. *Cell* **78**:45, 1994.
82. Perez-Alvarado GC, et al: Structure of the carboxy-terminal LIM domain from the cysteine rich protein CRP. *Nature Struct Biol* **1**:388, 1994.
83. Valge-Archer VE, Osada H, Warren AJ, Forster A, Li J, Baer R, Rabbitts TH: The LIM protein RBTN2 and the basic helix-loop-helix protein TAL1 are present in a complex in erythroid cells. *Proc Natl Acad Sci USA* **91**:8617, 1994.
84. Robb L, Elwood NJ, Elefanty AG, Kontgen F, Li R, Barnett LD, Begley CG: The SCL gene product is required for the generation of all hematopoietic lineages in the adult mouse. *EMBO J* **15**:4123, 1996.
85. Yamada Y, Warren AJ, Dobson C, Forster A, Pannell R, Rabbitts TH: The T cell leukemia LIM protein Lmo2 is necessary for adult mouse hematopoiesis. *Proc Natl Acad Sci USA* **95**:3890, 1998.
86. Osada H, Grutz G, Axelson H, Forster A, Rabbitts TH: Association of erythroid transcription factors: Complexes involving the LIM protein RBTN2 and the zinc-finger protein GATA1. *Proc Natl Acad Sci USA* **92**:9585, 1995.
87. Pevny L, Simon MC, Robertson E, Klein WH, Tsai SF, D'Agati V, Orkin SH, Costantini F: Erythroid differentiation in chimaeric mice blocked by a targeted mutation in the gene for transcription factor GATA-1. *Nature* **349**:257, 1991.
88. Wadman IA, Osada H, Grutz GG, Agulnick AD, Westphal H, Forster A, Rabbitts TH: The LIM-only protein Lmo2 is a bridging molecule assembling an erythroid, DNA-binding complex which includes the TAL1, E47, GATA-1 and Ldb1/NLI proteins. *EMBO J* **16**:3145, 1997.
89. McGuire EA, Rintoul CE, Sclar GM, Korsmeyer SJ: Thymic overexpression of Ttg-1 in transgenic mice results in T-cell acute lymphoblastic leukemia/lymphoma. *Mol Cell Biol* **12**:4186, 1992.
90. Larson RC, Fisch P, Larson TA, Lavenir I, Langford T, King G, Rabbitts TH: T cell tumours of disparate phenotype in mice transgenic for Rbtn-2. *Oncogene* **9**:3675, 1994.
91. Larson RC, Osada H, Larson TA, Lavenir I, Rabbitts TH: The oncogenic LIM protein Rbtn2 causes thymic developmental aberrations that precede malignancy in transgenic mice. *Oncogene* **11**:853, 1995.
92. Fisch P, Boehm T, Lavenir I, Larson T, Arno J, Forster A, Rabbitts TH: T-cell acute lymphoblastic lymphoma induced in transgenic mice by the RBTN1 and RBTN2 LIM-domain genes. *Oncogene* **7**:2389, 1992.
93. Neale GA, Rehg JE, Goorha RM: Ectopic expression of rhombotin-2 causes selective expansion of CD4-CD8-lymphocytes in the thymus and T-cell tumors in transgenic mice. *Blood* **86**:3060, 1995.
94. Robb L, Rasko JE, Bath ML, Strasser A, Begley CG: Scl, a gene frequently activated in human T cell leukaemia, does not induce lymphomas in transgenic mice. *Oncogene* **10**:205, 1995.
95. Kelliher MA, Seldin DC, Leder P: TAL-1 induces T cell acute lymphoblastic leukemia accelerated by casein kinase IIalpha. *EMBO J* **15**:5160, 1996.
96. Rabbitts TH: LMO T-cell translocation oncogenes typify genes activated by chromosomal translocations that alter transcription and developmental processes. *Genes Dev* **12**:2651, 1998.
97. Hatano M, Roberts CW, Minden M, Crist WM, Korsmeyer SJ: Deregulation of a homeobox gene, HOX11, by the t(10;14) in T cell leukemia. *Science* **253**:79, 1991.
98. Kennedy MA, Gonzalez Sarmiento R, Kees UR, Lampert F, Dear N, Boehm T, Rabbitts TH: HOX11, a homeobox-containing T-cell oncogene on human chromosome 10q24. *Proc Natl Acad Sci USA* **88**:8900, 1991.
99. Lu M, Gong ZY, Shen WF, Ho AD: The tcl-3 proto-oncogene altered by chromosomal translocation in T-cell leukemia codes for a homeobox protein. *EMBO J* **10**:2905, 1991.
100. Dube ID, Kamel Reid S, Yuan CC, Lu M, Wu X, Corpus G, Raimondi SC, Crist WM, Carroll AJ, Minowada J, Baker JB: A novel human homeobox gene lies at the chromosome 10 breakpoint in lymphoid neoplasias with chromosomal translocation t(10;14). *Blood* **78**:2996, 1991.
101. Dear TN, Sanchez Garcia I, Rabbitts TH: The HOX11 gene encodes a DNA-binding nuclear transcription factor belonging to a distinct family of homeobox genes. *Proc Natl Acad Sci USA* **90**:4431, 1993.
102. Allen JD, Lints T, Jenkins NA, Copeland NG, Strasser A, Harvey RP, Adams JM: Novel murine homeobox gene on chromosome 1 expressed in specific hematopoietic lineages and during embryogenesis. *Genes Dev* **5**:509, 1991.
103. McGinnis W, Krumlauf R: Homeobox genes and axial patterning. *Cell* **68**:283, 1992.
104. Roberts CWM, Shutter JR, Korsmeyer SJ: Hox11 controls the genesis of the spleen. *Nature* **368**:747, 1994.
105. Dear TN, Colledge WH, Carlton MB, Lavenir I, Larson T, Smith AJ, Warren AJ, Evans MJ, Sofroniew MV, Rabbitts TH: The Hox11 gene is essential for cell survival during spleen development. *Development* **121**:2909, 1995.
106. Hatano M, Roberts CWM, Kawabe T, Shutter J, Korsmeyer SJ: Cell cycle progression, cell death and T cell lymphoma in HOX11 transgenic mice (abstract). *Blood* **80**:355a, 1992.
107. Masson N, Greene WK, Rabbitts TH: Optimal activation of an endogenous gene by HOX11 requires the NH2-terminal 50 amino acids. *Mol Cell Biol* **18**:3502, 1998.
108. Kawabe T, Muslin AJ, Korsmeyer SJ: HOX11 interacts with protein phosphatases PP2A and PP1 and disrupts a G2/M cell-cycle checkpoint. *Nature* **385**:454, 1997.
109. Murre C, McCaw PS, Baltimore D: A new DNA binding and dimerization motif in immunoglobulin enhancer binding, daughterless, MyoD, and myc proteins. *Cell* **56**:777, 1989.
110. Murre C, McCaw PS, Vaessin H, Caudy M, Jan LY, Cabrera CV, Buskin JN, Hauschka SD, Lassar AB, Weintraub H, Baltimore D: Interactions between heterologous helix-loop-helix proteins generate complexes that bind specifically to a common DNA sequence. *Cell* **58**:537, 1989.
111. Sun XH, Baltimore D: An inhibitory domain of E12 transcription factor prevents DNA binding in E12 homodimers but not in E12 heterodimers. *Cell* **64**:459, 1991.
112. Henthorn P, Kiledjian M, Kadesch T: Two distinct transcription factors that bind the immunoglobulin enhancer E5/E2 motif. *Science* **247**:467, 1990.
113. Henthorn P, McCarrick Walmsley R, Kadesch T: Sequence of the cDNA encoding ITF-1, a positive-acting transcription factor. *Nucleic Acids Res* **18**:677, 1990.
114. Cronmiller C, Schedl P, Cline TY: Molecular characterization of daughterless, a *Drosophila* sex determination gene with multiple roles in development. *Genes Dev* **2**:1666, 1988.
115. Caudy M, Vassin H, Brand M, Tuma R, Jan LY, Jan YN: Daughterless, a *Drosophila* gene essential for both neurogenesis and sex determination, has sequence similarities to myc and the achaete-scute complex. *Cell* **55**:1061, 1988.
116. Blackwell TK, Weintraub H: Differences and similarities in DNA-binding preferences of MyoD and E2A protein complexes revealed by binding site selection. *Science* **250**:1104, 1990.
117. Ellenberger T, Fass D, Arnaud M, Harrison SC: Crystal structure of transcription factor E47: E-box recognition by a basic region helix-loop-helix dimer. *Genes Dev* **8**:970, 1994.
118. Aronheim A, Shiran R, Rosen A, Walker MD: The E2A gene product contains two separable and functionally distinct transcription activation domains. *Proc Natl Acad Sci USA* **90**:8063, 1993.
119. Quong MW, Massari ME, Zwart R, Murre C: A new transcriptional-activation motif restricted to a class of helix-loop-helix proteins is functionally conserved in both yeast and mammalian cells. *Mol Cell Biol* **13**:792, 1993.
120. Lassar AB, Davis RL, Wright WE, Kadesch T, Murre C, Voronova A, Baltimore D, Weintraub H: Functional activity of myogenic HLH proteins requires hetero-oligomerization with E12/E47-like proteins in vivo. *Cell* **66**:305, 1991.
121. Xia Y, Hwang LH, Cobb MH, Baer RJ: Products of the TAL2, oncogene in leukemic T cells: bHLH phosphoproteins with DNA-binding activity. *Oncogene* **9**:1437, 1994.
122. Miyamoto A, Cui X, Naumovski L, Cleary ML: Helix-loop-helix proteins LYL1 and E2a form heterodimeric complexes with distinctive DNA-binding properties in hematolymphoid cells. *Mol Cell Biol* **16**:2394, 1996.
123. Bain G, Gruenwald S, Murre C: E2A and E2-2 are subunits of B-cell-specific E2-box DNA-binding proteins. *Mol Cell Biol* **13**:3522, 1993.
124. Benezra R: An intermolecular disulfide bond stabilizes E2A homodimers and is required for DNA binding at physiological temperatures. *Cell* **79**:1057, 1994.

125. Bain G, Robanus Maandag EC, Izon DJ, Amsen D, Kruisbeek AM, Weintraub BC, Krop I, Schlissel MS, Feeney AJ, van Roon M, van der Valk M, te Riele HPJ, Berns A, Murre C: E2A proteins are required for proper B-cell development and initiation of immunoglobulin gene rearrangements. *Cell* **79**:885, 1994.
126. Zhuang Y, Soriano P, Weintraub H: The helix-loop-helix gene E2A is required for B-cell formation. *Cell* **79**:875, 1994.
127. Bain G, Engel I, Maandag EC, te Riele HPJ, Voland JR, Sharp LL, Chun J, Huey B, Pinkel D, Murre C: E2A deficiency leads to abnormalities in $\alpha\beta$ T-cell development and to rapid development of T-cell lymphomas. *Mol Cell Biol* **17**:4782, 1997.
128. Yan W, Young AZ, Soares VC, Kelley R, Benezra R, Zhuang Y: High incidence of T-cell tumors in E2A-null mice and E2A/Id1 double-knockout mice. *Mol Cell Biol* **17**:7317, 1997.
129. Mellentin JD, Murre C, Donlon TA, McCaw PS, Smith SD, Carroll AJ, McDonald ME, Baltimore D, Cleary ML: The gene for enhancer binding proteins E12/E47 lies at the t(1;19) breakpoint in acute leukemias. *Science* **246**:379, 1989.
130. Kamps MP, Murre C, Sun XH, Baltimore D: A new homeobox gene contributes the DNA binding domain of the t(1;19) translocation protein in pre-B ALL. *Cell* **60**:547, 1990.
131. Nourse J, Mellentin JD, Galili N, Wilkinson J, Stanbridge E, Smith SD, Cleary ML: Chromosomal translocation t(1;19) results in synthesis of a homeobox fusion mRNA that codes for a potential chimeric transcription factor. *Cell* **60**:535, 1990.
132. Mellentin JD, Nourse J, Hunger SP, Smith SD, Cleary ML: Molecular analysis of the t(1;19) breakpoint cluster region in pre-B cell acute lymphoblastic leukemias. *Genes Chromosomes Cancer* **2**:239, 1990.
133. McGinnis W, Levine MS, Hafen E, Kuroiwa A, Gehring WJ: A conserved DNA sequence in homoeotic genes of the *Drosophila* Antennapedia and Bithorax complexes. *Nature* **308**:428, 1984.
134. Scott MP, Weiner AJ: Structural relationships among genes that control development: sequence homology between the Antennapedia, Ultrabithorax, and fushi tarazu loci of *Drosophila. Proc Natl Acad Sci USA* **81**:4115, 1984.
135. Van Dijk MA, Voorhoeve PM, Murre C: Pbx1 is converted into a transcriptional activator upon acquiring the N-terminal region of E2A in pre-B-cell acute lymphoblastoid leukemia. *Proc Natl Acad Sci USA* **90**:6061, 1993.
136. LeBrun DL, Cleary ML: Fusion with E2A alters the transcriptional properties of the homeodomain protein PBX1 in t(1;19) leukemias. *Oncogene* **9**:1641, 1994.
137. Lu Q, Wright DD, Kamps MP: Fusion with E2A converts the Pbx1 homeodomain protein into a constitutive transcriptional activator in human leukemias carrying the t(1;19) translocation. *Mol Cell Biol* **14**:3938, 1994.
138. Flegel WA, Singson AW, Margolis JS, Bang AG, Posakony JW, Murre C: Dpbx, a new homeobox gene closely related to the human proto-oncogene pbx1 molecular structure and developmental expression. *Mech Dev* **41**:155, 1993.
139. Rauskolb C, Peifer M, Weischaus E: Extradenticle, a regulator of homeotic gene activity, is a homolog of the homeobox-containing human proto-oncogene pbx1. *Cell* **74**:1101, 1993.
140. Weischaus E, Nusslein Volhard C, Jurgens G: Mutations affecting the pattern of the larval cuticle in *Drosophila* melanogaster: III. Zygotic loci on the X chromosome and the fourth chromosome. *Arch Dev Biol* **193**:267, 1984.
141. Peifer M, Wieschaus E: Mutations in the *Drosophila* gene extradenticle affect the way specific homeo domain proteins regulate segmental identity. *Genes Dev* **4**:1209, 1990.
142. Chan S-K, Jaffe L, Capovilla M, Botas J, Mann RS: The DNA binding specificity of ultrabithorax is modulated by cooperative interactions with extradenticle, another homeoprotein. *Cell* **78**:603, 1994.
143. Rauskolb C, Wieschaus E: Coordinate regulation of downstream genes by extradenticle and the homeotic selector proteins. *EMBO J* **13**:3561, 1994.
144. Van Dijk MA, Murre C: Extradenticle raises the DNA binding specificity of homeotic selector gene products. *Cell* **78**:617, 1994.
145. Johnson FB, Parker E, Krasnow MA: Extradenticle protein is a selective cofactor for the *Drosophila* homeotics: Role of the homeodomain and YPWM amino acid motif in the interaction. *Proc Natl Acad Sci USA* **92**:739, 1995.
146. Chang CP, Shen WF, Rozenfeld S, Lawrence HJ, Largman C, Cleary ML: Pbx proteins display hexapeptide-dependent cooperative DNA binding with a subset of Hox proteins. *Genes Dev* **9**:663, 1995.
147. Lu Q, Kamps MP: Structural determinants within Pbx1 that mediate cooperative DNA binding with pentapeptide-containing hox proteins: Proposal for a model of a Pbx1-Hox-DNA complex. *Mol Cell Biol* **16**:1632, 1996.
148. Neuteboom ST, Peltenburg LT, Van Dijk MA, Murre C: The hexapeptide LFPWMR in Hoxb-8 is required for cooperative DNA binding with Pbx1 and Pbx2 proteins. *Proc Natl Acad Sci USA* **92**:9166, 1995.
149. Van Dijk MA, Peltenburg LT, Murre C: Hox gene products modulate the DNA binding activity of Pbx1 and Pbx2. *Mech Dev* **52**:99, 1995.
150. Lu Q, Knoepfler PS, Scheele J, Wright DD, Kamps MP: Both Pbx1 and E2A-Pbx1 bind the DNA motif ATCAATCAA cooperatively with the products of multiple murine Hox genes, some of which are themselves oncogenes. *Mol Cell Biol* **15**:3786, 1995.
151. Knoepfler PS, Kamps MP: The pentapeptide motif of Hox proteins is required for cooperative DNA binding with Pbx1, physically contacts Pbx1, and enhances DNA binding by Pbx1. *Mol Cell Biol* **15**:5811, 1995.
152. Knoepfler PS, Kamps MP: The highest affinity DNA element bound by Pbx complexes in t(1;19) leukemic cells fails to mediate cooperative DNA-binding or cooperative transactivation by E2a-Pbx1 and class I Hox proteins: Evidence for selective targetting of E2a-Pbx1 to a subset of Pbx-recognition elements. *Oncogene* **14**:2521, 1997.
153. Lu Q, Kamps MP: Heterodimerization of Hox proteins with Pbx1 and oncoprotein E2a-Pbx1 generates unique DNA-binding specifities at nucleotides predicted to contact the N-terminal arm of the Hox homeodomain: Demonstration of Hox-dependent targeting of E2a-Pbx1 in vivo. *Oncogene* **14**:75, 1997.
154. Knoepfler PS, Lu Q, Kamps MP: Pbx1-Hox heterodimers bind DNA on inseparable half-sites that permit intrinsic DNA binding specificity of the Hox partner at nucleotides 3′ to a TAAT motif. *Nucleic Acids Res* **24**:2288, 1996.
155. Chang CP, Brocchieri L, Shen WF, Largman C, Cleary ML: Pbx modulation of Hox homeodomain amino-terminal arms establishes different DNA-binding specificities across the Hox locus. *Mol Cell Biol* **16**:1734, 1996.
156. Kamps MP, Baltimore D: E2A-Pbx1, the t(1;19) translocation protein of human pre-B-cell acute lymphocytic leukemia, causes acute myeloid leukemia in mice. *Mol Cell Biol* **13**:351, 1993.
157. Kamps MP, Wright DD: Oncoprotein E2A-Pbx1 immortalizes a myeloid progenitor in primary marrow cultures without abrogating its factor-dependence. *Oncogene* **9**:3159, 1994.
158. Privitera E, Kamps MP, Hayashi Y, Inaba T, Shapiro LH, Raimondi SC, Behm F, Hendershot L, Carroll AJ, Baltimore D, Look AT: Different molecular consequences of the 1;19 chromosomal translocation in childhood B-cell precursor acute lymphoblastic leukemia. *Blood* **79**:1781, 1992.
159. Borowitz MJ, Hunger SP, Carroll AJ, Shuster JJ, Pullen DJ, Steuber PJ, Cleary ML: Predictability of the t(1;19)(q23;p13) from surface antigen phenotype: Implications for screening cases of childhood ALL for molecular analysis. A Pediatric Oncology Group study. *Blood* **82**:1086, 1993.
160. Dedera DA, Waller EK, LeBrun DP, Sen-Majumdar A, Stevens ME, Barsh GS, Cleary ML: Chimeric homeobox gene E2A-PBX1 induces proliferation, apoptosis, and malignant lymphomas in transgenic mice. *Cell* **74**:833, 1993.
161. Monica K, LeBrun DP, Dedera DA, Brown R, Cleary ML: Transformation properties of the E2A-PBX1 chimeric oncoprotein: Fusion with E2A is essential, but the PBX1 homeodomain is dispensable. *Mol Cell Biol* **14**:8304, 1994.
162. Chang CP, de Vivo I, Cleary ML: The Hox cooperativity motif of the chimeric oncoprotein E2a-Pbx1 is necessary and sufficient for oncogenesis. *Mol Cell Biol* **17**:81, 1997.
163. Kamps MP, Wright DD, Lu Q: DNA-binding by oncoprotein E2a-Pbx1 is important for blocking differentiation but dispensable for fibroblast transformation. *Oncogene* **12**:19, 1996.
164. Chang CP, Jacobs Y, Nakamura T, Jenkins NA, Copeland NG, Cleary ML: Meis proteins are major in vivo DNA binding partners for wild-type but not chimeric Pbx proteins. *Mol Cell Biol* **17**:5679, 1997.
165. Knoepfler PS, Calvo KR, Chen H, Antonarakis SE, Kamps MP: Meis1 and pKnox1 bind DNA cooperatively with Pbx1 utilizing an interaction surface disrupted in oncoprotein E2a-Pbx1. *Proc Natl Acad Sci USA* **94**:14553, 1997.
166. Shen WF, Montgomery J, Rozenfeld S, Lawrence HJ, Buchberg A, Largman C: A subset of the Hox homeodomain proteins stabilize Meis protein-DNA binding. *Mol Cell Biol* **17**:6664, 1997.

167. Crist WM, Carroll AJ, Shuster JJ, Behm FG, Whitehead M, Vietti TJ, Look AT, Mahoney D, Ragab A, Pullen DJ, et al: Poor prognosis of children with pre-B acute lymphoblastic leukemia is associated with the t(1;19)(q23;p13). A Pediatric Oncology Group study. *Blood* **76**:117, 1990.
168. Raimondi SC, Behm FG, Roberson PK, Pui C-H, Williams DL, Crist WM, Look AT, Rivera GK: Cytogenetics of pre-B-cell acute lymphoblastic leukemia with emphasis on prognostic implications of the t(1;19). *J Clin Oncol* **8**:1380, 1990.
169. Williams DL, Look AT, Melvin SL, Roberson PK, Dahl G, Flake T, Stass S: New chromosomal translocations correlate with specific immunophenotypes of childhood acute lymphoblastic leukemia. *Cell* **36**:101, 1984.
170. Michael PM, Levin MD, Garson OM: Translocation 1;19: A new cytogenetic abnormality in acute lymphocytic leukemia. *Cancer Genet Cytogenet* **12**:333, 1984.
171. Miyamoto K, Tomita N, Ishii A, Nonaka H, Kondo T, Tanaka T, Kitajima K: Chromosome abnormalities of leukemia cells in adult patients with T-cell leukemia. *J Natl Cancer Inst* **73**:353, 1984.
172. Yamada T, Craig JM, Hawkins JM, Janossy G, Secker-Walker LM: Molecular investigation of 19p13 in standard and variant translocations: The E12 probe recognizes the 19p13 breakpoint in cases with t(1;19) and acute leukemia other than pre-B immunophenotype. *Leukemia* **5**:36, 1991.
173. Secker-Walker LM, Berger R, Fenaux P, Lai JL, Nelken B, Garson M, Michael PM, Hagemeijer A, Harrison CJ, Kaneko Y, Rubin CM: Prognostic significance of the balanced t(1;19) and unbalanced der(19)t(1;19) translocations in acute lymphoblastic leukemia. *Leukemia* **6**:363, 1992.
174. Ohno H, Inoue T, Akasaka T, Okumura A, Miyanishi S, Ohashi I, Kikuchi M, Masuya M, Amano H, Imanaka T, Ohno Y: Acute lymphoblastic leukemia associated with a t(1;19)(q23;p13) in an adult. *Intern Med* **32**:584, 1993.
175. Vagner-Capodano AM, Mozziconacci MJ, Zattara-Cannoni H, Guitard AM, Thuret I, Michel G: t(1;19) in a M4-ANLL. *Cancer Genet Cytogenet* **73**:86, 1994.
176. Wlodarska I, Stul M, DeWolf-Peeters C, Verhoef G, Mecucci C, Cassiman JJ, Van den Berghe H: t(1;19) without detectable E2A rearrangements in two t(14;18)-positive lymphoma/leukemia cases. *Genes Chromosomes Cancer* **10**:171, 1994.
177. Raimondi SC, Privitera E, Williams DL, Look AT, Behm F, Rivera GK, Crist WM, Pui C-H: New recurring chromosomal translocations in childhood acute lymphoblastic leukemia. *Blood* **77**:2016, 1991.
178. Hunger SP, Ohyashiki K, Toyama K, Cleary ML: Hlf, a novel hepatic bZIP protein, shows altered DNA-binding properties following fusion to E2A in t(17;19) acute lymphoblastic leukemia. *Genes Dev* **6**:1608, 1992.
179. Inaba T, Roberts WM, Shapiro LH, Jolly KW, Raimondi SC, Smith SD, Look AT: Fusion of the leucine zipper gene HLF to the E2A gene in human acute B-lineage leukemia. *Science* **257**:531, 1992.
180. Hunger SP, Devaraj PE, Foroni L, Secker-Walker LM, Cleary ML: Two types of genomic rearrangements create alternative E2A-HLF fusion proteins in t(17;19)-ALL. *Blood* **83**:2261, 1994.
181. Hunger SP, Brown R, Cleary ML: DNA-binding and transcriptional regulatory properties of hepatic leukemia factor (HLF) and the t(17;19) acute lymphoblastic leukemia chimera E2A-HLF. *Mol Cell Biol* **14**:5986, 1994.
182. Landschulz WH, Johnson PF, McKnight SL: The leucine zipper: A hypothetical structure common to a new class of DNA binding proteins. *Science* **240**:1559, 1988.
183. O'Shea EK, Klemm JD, Kim PS, Alber T: X-ray structure of the GCN4 leucine zipper, a two-stranded, parallel coiled coil. *Science* **254**:539, 1991.
184. Ellenberger TE, Brandl CJ, Struhl K, Harrison SC: The GCN4 basic region leucine zipper binds DNA as a dimer of uninterrupted alpha helices: Crystal structure of the protein-DNA complex. *Cell* **71**:1223, 1992.
185. Drolet DW, Scully KM, Simmons DM, Wegner M, Chu KT, Swanson LW, Rosenfeld MG: TEF, a transcription factor expressed specifically in the anterior pituitary during embryogenesis, defines a new class of leucine zipper proteins. *Genes Dev* **5**:1739, 1991.
186. Falvey E, Fleury Olela F, Schibler U: The rat hepatic leukemia factor (HLF) gene encodes two transcriptional activators with distinct circadian rhythms, tissue distributions and target preferences. *EMBO J* **14**:4307, 1995.
187. Inaba T, Inukai T, Yoshihara T, Seyschab H, Ashmun RA, Canman CE, Laken SJ, Kastan MB, Look AT: Reversal of apoptosis by the leukaemia-associated E2A-HLF chimaeric transcription factor. *Nature* **382**:541, 1996.
188. Metzstein MM, Hengartner MO, Tsung N, Ellis RE, Horvitz HR: Transcriptional regulator of programmed cell death encoded by *Caenorhabditis elegans* gene ces-2. *Nature* **382**:545, 1996.
189. Thompson CB: A fate worse than death. *Nature* **382**:492, 1996.
190. Inaba T, Shapiro LH, Funabiki T, Sinclair AE, Jones BG, Ashmun RA, Look AT: DNA-binding specificity and trans-activating potential of the leukemia-associated E2A-hepatic leukemia factor fusion protein. *Mol Cell Biol* **14**:3403, 1994.
191. Vinson CR, Hai T, Boyd SM: Dimerization specificity of the leucine zipper-containing bZIP motif on DNA binding: Prediction and rational design. *Genes Dev* **7**:1047, 1993.
192. Yoshihara T, Inaba T, Shapiro LH, Kato J, Look AT: E2A-HLF-mediated cell transformation requires both the trans-activation domain of E2A and the leucine zipper dimerization domain of HLF. *Mol Cell Biol* **15**:3247, 1995.
193. Hunger SP: Chromosomal translocations involving the E2A gene in acute lymphoblastic leukemia: Clinical features and molecular pathogenesis. *Blood* **87**:1211, 1996.
194. Smith KS, Jacobs Y, Chang CP, Cleary ML: Chimeric oncoprotein E2a-Pbx1 induces apoptosis of hematopoietic cells by a p53-independent mechanism that is suppressed by Bcl-2. *Oncogene* **14**:2917, 1997.
195. Devaraj PE, Foroni L, Sekhar M, Butler T, Wright F, Mehta A, Samson D, Prentice HG, Hoffbrand AV, Secker-Walker LM: E2A/HLF fusion cDNAs and the use of RT-PCR for the detection of minimal residual disease in t(17;19)(q22;p13) acute lymphoblastic leukemia. *Leukemia* **8**:1131, 1994.
196. Ohyashiki K, Fujieda H, Miyauchi J, Ohyashiki JH, Tauchi T, Saito M, Nakazawa S, Abe K, Yamamoto K, Clark SC, et al: Establishment of a novel heterotransplantable acute lymphoblastic leukemia cell line with a t(17;19) chromosomal translocation the growth of which is inhibited by interleukin-3. *Leukemia* **5**:322, 1991.
197. Golub TR, Barker GF, Bohlander SK, Hiebert SW, Ward DC, Bray-Ward P, Morgan E, Raimondi SC, Rowley JD, Gilliland DG: Fusion of the TEL gene on 12p13 to the AML1 gene on 21q22 in acute lymphoblastic leukemia. *Proc Natl Acad Sci USA* **92**:4917, 1995.
198. Romana SP, Mauchauffe M, Le Coniat M, Chumakov I, Le Paslier D, Berger R, Bernard OA: The t(12;21) of acute lymphoblastic leukemia results in a tel- AML1 gene fusion. *Blood* **85**:3662, 1995.
199. Shurtleff SA, Buijs A, Behm FG, Rubnitz JE, Raimondi SC, Hancock ML, Chan GC, Pui CH, Grosveld G, Downing JR: TEL/AML1 fusion resulting from a cryptic t(12;21) is the most common genetic lesion in pediatric ALL and defines a subgroup of patients with an excellent prognosis. *Leukemia* **9**:1985, 1995.
200. Romana SP, Poirel H, Leconiat M, Flexor MA, Mauchauffe M, Jonveaux P, Macintyre EA, Berger R, Bernard OA: High frequency of t(12;21) in childhood B-lineage acute lymphoblastic leukemia. *Blood* **86**:4263, 1995.
201. Liang D-C, Chou T-B, Chen J-S, Shurtleff SA, Rubnitz JE, Downing JR, Pui C-H, Shih L-Y: High incidence of TEL/AML1 fusion resulting from a cryptic t(12;21) in childhood B-lineage acute lymphoblastic leukemia in Taiwan. *Leukemia* **10**:991, 1996.
202. Hiebert SW, Sun W, Davis JN, Golub T, Shurtleff S, Buijs A, Downing JR, Grosveld G, Roussel MF, Gilliland DG, Lenny N, Meyers S: The t(12;21) translocation converts AML-1B from an activator to a repressor of transcription. *Mol Cell Biology* 16:1349, 1996.
203. Golub TR, Goga A, Barker GF, Afar DE, McLaughlin J, Bohlander SK, Rowley JD, Witte ON, Gilliland DG: Oligomerization of the ABL tyrosine kinase by the Ets protein TEL in human leukemia. *Mol Cell Biol* **16**:4107, 1996.
204. Golub TR, Barker GF, Stegmaier K, Gilliland DG: The TEL gene contributes to the pathogenesis of myeloid and lymphoid leukemias by diverse molecular genetic mechanisms. *Curr Top Microbiol Immunol* **220**:67, 1997.
205. Jousset C, Carron C, Boureux A, et al: A domain of TEL conserved in a subset of ETS proteins defines a specific oligomerizaton interface essential to the mitogenic properties of the TEL-PDGFRβ oncoprotein. *EMBO J* **16**:69, 1997.
206. McLean TW, Ringold S, Neuberg D, Stegmaier K, Tantravahi R, Ritz J, Koeffler HP, Takeuchi S, Janssen JW, Seriu T, Bartram CR, Sallan SE, Gilliland DG, Golub TR: TEL/AML-1 dimerizes and is associated with a favorable outcome in childhood acute lymphoblastic leukemia. *Blood* **88**:4252, 1996.

207. Wang LC, Kuo F, Fujiwara Y, Gilliland DG, Golub TR, Orkin SH: Yolk sac angiogenic defect and intra-embryonic apoptosis in mice lacking the Ets-related factor TEL. *EMBO J* **16**:4374, 1997.
208. Rubnitz JE, Downing JR, Pui C-H, Shurtleff SA, Raimondi SC, Evans WE, Head DR, Crist WM, Rivera GK, Hancock ML, Boyett JM, Buijs A, Grosveld G, Behm FG: TEL gene rearrangement in acute lymphoblastic leukemia: A new genetic marker with prognostic significance. *J Clin Oncol* **15**:1150, 1997.
209. Rubnitz JE, Shuster JJ, Land VJ, Link MP, Pullen DJ, Camitta BM, Pui CH, Downing JR, Behm FG: Case-control study suggests a favorable impact of TEL rearrangement in patients with B-lineage acute lymphoblastic leukemia treated with antimetabolite-based therapy. A Pediatric Oncology Group study. *Blood* **89**:1143, 1997.
210. Borkhardt A, Cazzaniga G, Viehmann S, Valsecchi MG, Ludwig WD, Burci L, Mangioni S, Schrappe M, Riehm H, Lampert F, Basso G, Masera G, Harbott J, Biondi A: Incidence and clinical relevance of TEL/AML1 fusion genes in children with acute lymphoblastic leukemia enrolled in the German and Italian multicenter therapy trials. *Blood* **90**:571, 1997.
211. Look AT: Pathobiology of the acute lymphoid leukemia cell, in Hoffman R (ed): *Hematology*, 2d ed. New York, Churchill-Livingstone, 1995, p. 1047.
212. Ye BH, Rao PH, Chaganti RS, Dalla-Favera R: Cloning of bcl-6, the locus involved in chromosome translocations affecting band 3q27 in B-cell lymphoma. *Cancer Res* **53**:2732, 1993.
213. Kerckaert JP, Deweindt C, Tilly H, Quief S, Lecocq G, Bastard C: LAZ-3, a novel zinc-finger encoding gene, is disrupted by recurring chromosome 3q27 translocations in human lymphomas. *Nature Genet* **5**:66, 1993.
214. Miki T, Kawamata N, Hirosawa S, Aoki N: Gene involved in the 3q27 translocation associated with B-cell lymphoma, BCL5, encodes a Kruppel-like zinc-finger protein. *Blood* **83**:26, 1994.
215. Ye BH, Lista F, Lo Coco F, Knowles DM, Offit K, Chaganti RS, Dalla-Favera R: Alterations of a zinc finger-encoding gene, BCL-6, in diffuse large-cell lymphoma. *Science* **262**:747, 1993.
216. Cattoretti G, Chang CC, Cechova K, Zhang J, Ye BH, Falini B, Louie DC, Offit K, Chaganti RS, Dalla-Favera R: BCL-6 protein is expressed in germinal-center B cells. *Blood* **86**:45, 1995.
217. Flenghi L, Ye BH, Fizzotti M, Bigerna B, Cattoretti G, Venturi S, Pacini R, Pileri S, Lo Coco F, Pescarmona E, et al: A specific monoclonal antibody (PG-B6) detects expression of the BCL-6 protein in germinal center B cells. *Am J Pathol* **147**:405, 1995.
218. McLennan ICM: Germinal centers. *Annu Rev Immunol* **12**:117, 1994.
219. Dalla-Favera R, Ye BH, Cattoretti G, Lo Coco F, Chang C-C, Zhang J, Migliazza A, Cechova K, Niu H, Chaganti S, Chen W, Louie DC, Offit K, Chaganti RSK: BCL-6 in diffuse large-cell lymphomas, in De Vita VT, Hellman S, Rosenberg SA (eds): *Important Advances in Oncology*. Philadelphia, Lippincott-Raven, 1996, p. 139.
220. Ye BH, Chaganti S, Chang CC, Niu H, Corradini P, Chaganti RS, Dalla-Favera R: Chromosomal translocations cause deregulated BCL6 expression by promoter substitution in B cell lymphoma. *EMBO J* **14**:6209, 1995.
221. Migliazza A, Martinotti S, Chen W, Fusco C, Ye BH, Knowles DM, Offit K, Chaganti RS, Dalla-Favera R: Frequent somatic hypermutation of the 5′ noncoding region of the BCL6 gene in B-cell lymphoma. *Proc Natl Acad Sci USA* **92**:12520, 1995.
222. Offit K, Lo Coco F, Louie DC, Parsa NZ, Leung D, Portlock C, Ye BH, Lista F, Filippa DA, Rosenbaum A, Ladanyi M, Jhanwar S, Dalla-Favera R, Chaganti RSK: Rearrangement of the BCL-6 gene as a prognostic marker in diffuse large-cell lymphoma. *N Engl J Med* **331**:74, 1994.
223. Speck NA, Stacy T: A new transcription factor family associated with human leukemias. *Crit Rev Eukaryotic Gene Express* **5**:337, 1995.
224. Wang S, Wang Q, Crute BE, Melnikova IN, Keller SR, Speck NA: Cloning and characterization of subunits of the T-cell receptor and murine leukemia virus enhancer core-binding factor. *EMBO J* **13**:3324, 1993.
225. Ogawa E, Inuzuka M, Maruyama M, Satake M, Naito-Fujimoto M, Ito Y, Shigesada K: Molecular cloning and characterization of PEBP2β, the heterodimeric partner of a novel *Drosophila* runt-related DNA binding protein PEBP2α. *Virol* **194**:314, 1993.
226. Miyoshi H, Shimizu K, Kozu T, Maseki N, Kaneko Y, Ohki M: t(8;21) breakpoints on chromosome 21 in acute myeloid leukemia are clustered within a limited region of a single gene, AML1. *Proc Natl Acad Sci USA* **88**:10431, 1991.
227. Gao J, Erickson P, Gardiner K, Le Beau MM, Diaz MO, Patterson D, Rowley JD, Drabkin HA: Isolation of a yeast artificial chromosome spanning the 8;21 translocation breakpoint t(8;21)(q22;q22.3) in acute myelogenous leukemia. *Proc Natl Acad Sci USA* **88**:4882, 1991.
228. Erickson P, Gao J, Chang KS, Look T, Whisenant E, Raimondi S, Lasher R, Trujillo J, Rowley J, Drabkin H: Identification of breakpoints in t(8;21) acute myelogenous leukemia and isolation of a fusion transcript. AML1/ETO, with similarity to *Drosophila* segmentation gene, runt. *Blood* **80**:1825, 1992.
229. Nisson PE, Watkins PC, Sacchi N: Transcriptionally active chimeric gene derived from the fusion of the AML1 gene and a novel gene on chromosome 8 in t(8;21) leukemic cells. *Cancer Genet Cytogenet* **63**:81, 1992.
230. Mitani K, Ogawa S, Tanaka T, Miyoshi H, Kurokawa M, Mano H, Yazaki Y, Ohki M, Hirai H: Generation of the AML1-EVI-1 fusion gene in the t(3;21)(q26;q22) causes blastic crisis in chronic myelocytic leukemia. *EMBO J* **13**:504, 1994.
231. Nucifora G, Begy CR, Erickson P, Drabkin HA, Rowley JD: The 3;21 translocation in myelodysplasia results in a fusion transcript between the AML1 gene and the gene for EAP, a highly conserved protein associated with the Epstein-Barr virus small RNA EBER 1. *Proc Natl Acad Sci USA* **90**:7784, 1993.
232. Meyers S, Downing JR, Hiebert SW: Identification of AML-1 and the (8;21) translocation protein (AML-1/ETO) as sequence specific DNA binding proteins: The runt homology domain is required for DNA binding and protein-protein interactions. *Mol Cell Biol* **13**:6336, 1993.
233. Nuchprayoon I, Meyers S, Scott LM, Suzow J, Hiebert S, Friedman AD: PEBP2/CBF, the murine homolog of the human myeloid AML1 and PEBP2 beta/CBF beta proto-oncoproteins, regulates the murine myeloperoxidase and neutrophil elastase genes in immature myeloid cells. *Mol Cell Biol* **14**:5558, 1994.
234. Takahashi A, Satake M, Yamaguchi-Iwai Y, Bae SC, Lu J, Maruyama M, Zhang YW, Oka H, Arai N, Arai K, et al: Positive and negative regulation of granulocyte-macrophage colony-stimulating factor promoter activity by AML1-related transcription factor, PEBP2. *Blood* **86**:607, 1995.
235. Wotton D, Ghysdael J, Wang S, Speck NA, Owen MJ: Cooperative binding of Ets-1 and core binding factor to DNA. *Mol Cell Biol* **14**:840, 1994.
236. Hernandez-Munain C, Krangel MS: c-Myb and core-binding factor/PEBP2 display functional synergy but bind independently to adjacent sites in the T-cell receptor delta enhancer. *Mol Cell Biol* **15**:3090, 1995.
237. Manley NR, O Connell M, Sun W, Speck NA, Hopkins N: Two factors that bind to highly conserved sequences in mammalian type C retroviral enhancers. *J Virol* **67**:1967, 1993.
238. Sun W, O Connell M, Speck NA: Characterization of a protein that binds multiple sequences in mammalian type C retrovirus enhancers. *J Virol* **67**:1976, 1993.
239. Sun W, Graves BJ, Speck NA: Transactivation of the Moloney murine leukemia virus and T-cell receptor beta-chain enhancers by cbf and ets requires intact binding sites for both proteins. *J Virol* **69**:4941, 1995.
240. Frank R, Zhang J, Uchida H, Meyers S, Hiebert SW, Nimer SD: The AML1/ETO fusion protein blocks transactivation of the GM-CSF promoter by AML1B. *Oncogene* **11**:2667, 1995.
241. Okuda T, van Deursen J, Hiebert SW, Grosveld G, Downing JR: AML1, the target of multiple chromosomal translocations in human leukemia, is essential for normal fetal liver hematopoiesis. *Cell* **84**:321, 1996.
242. Wang Q, Stacy T, Binder M, Marin-Padilla M, Sharpe AH, Speck NA: Disruption of the Cbfa2 gene causes necrosis and hemorrhaging in the central nervous system and blocks definitive hematopoiesis. *Proc Natl Acad Sci USA* **93**:3444, 1996.
243. Wang Q, Stacy T, Miller JD, Lewis AF, Gu T-L, Huang X, Bushweller JH, Bories J-C, Alt FW, Ryan G, Liu PP, Wynshaw-Boris A, Binder M, Marin-Padilla M, Sharpe AH, Speck NA: The CBFβ subunit is essential for CBFα2 (AML1) function in vivo. *Cell* **87**:697, 1996.
244. Meyers S, Lenny N, Hiebert SW: The t(8;21) fusion protein interferes with AML-1B-dependent transcriptional activation. *Mol Cell Biol* **15**:1974, 1995.
245. Meyers S, Lenny N, Hiebert SW: The t(8;21) fusion protein interferes with AML-1B-dependent transcriptional activation. *Mol Cell Biol* **15**:1974, 1995.
246. Westendorf JJ, Yamamoto CM, Lenny N, Downing JR, Selsted ME, Hiebert SW: The t(8;21) fusion product, AML-1-ETO, associates with C/EBP-alpha, inhibits C/EBP-alpha-dependent transcription, and blocks granulocytic differentiation. *Mol Cell Biol* **18**:322, 1998.
247. Wang J, Hoshino TRRL, Kajigaya S, Liu JM: Novel human nuclear receptor co-repressor: cloning and identification as a binding partner for the ETO proto-oncoprotein (abstract). *Blood* **90**:244a, 1998.

248. Lutterbach B, Westendorf JJ, Linggi B, Patten A, Moniwa M, Davie JR, Huynh KD, Bardwell VJ, Lavinsky RM, Rosenfeld MG, Glass C, Seto E, Hiebert SW: ETO, a target of the t(8;21) in acute leukemia, interacts with the N-COR and mSin3 co-repressors. *Mol Cell Biol* (in press).
249. Grunstein M: Histone acetylation in chromatin structure and transcription. *Nature* **389**:349, 1997.
250. Nucifora G, Rowley JD: AML1 and the 8;21 and 3;21 translocations in acute and chronic myeloid leukemia. *Blood* **86**:1, 1995.
251. Liu P, Tarle SA, Hajra A, Claxton DF, Marlton P, Freedman M, Siciliano MJ, Collins FS: Fusion between transcription factor CBFβ/PEBP2β and a myosin heavy chain in acute myeloid leukemia. *Science* **261**:1041, 1993.
252. Shurtleff SA, Meyers S, Hiebert SW, et al: Heterogeneity in CBF beta.MYH11 fusion messages encoded by the inv(16)(p13q22)and the t(16;16)(p13;q22) in acute myelogenous leukemia. *Blood* **85**:3695, 1995.
253. Viswanatha DS, Chen I, Liu PP, Slovak ML, Rankin C, Head DR, Willman CL: Characterization and use of an antibody detecting the CBFβ-SMMHC fusion protein in inv(16)/t(16:16)-associated acute myeloid leukemias. *Blood* **91**:1882, 1998.
254. Castilla LH, Wijmenga C, Wang Q, Stacy T, Speck NA, Eckhaus M, Marin-Padilla M, Collins FS, Wynshaw-Boris A, Liu PP: Failure of embryonic hematopoiesis and lethal hemorrhages in mouse embryos heterozygous for a knocked-in leukemia gene CBFB-MYH11. *Cell* **87**:687, 1996.
255. Yergeau DA, Hetherington CJ, Wang Q, et al: Embryonic lethality and impairment of haematopoiesis in mice heterozygous for an AML-ETO fusion gene. *Nature Genet* **15**:303, 1997.
256. Okuda T, Cai Z, Yang S, et al: Expression of a knocked-in AML1-ETO leukemia gene inhibits the estabalishment of normal definitive hematopoiesis and directly generates dysplastic hematopoietic progenitors. *Blood* **91**:3134, 1998.
257. Martinez-Climent JA, Lane NJ, Rubin CM, Morgan E, Johnstone HS, Mick R, Murphy SB, Vardiman JW, Larson RA, Lebeau MM, Rowley JD: Clinical and prognostic significance of chromosomal abnormalities in childhood acute myeloid leukemia de novo. *Leukemia* **9**:95, 1995.
258. Mrozek K, Heinonen K, de la Chapelle A, Bloomfield CD: Clinical significance of cytogenetics in acute myeloid leukemia. *Semin Oncol* **24**:17, 1997.
259. Berger R, Bernheim A, Ochoa-Noguera ME, Daniel MT, Valensi F, Sigaux F, Flandrin G, Boiron M: Prognostic significance of chromosomal abnormalities in acute nonlymphocytic leukemia: A study of 343 patients. *Cancer Genet Cytogenet* **28**:293, 1987.
260. Samuels BL, Larson RA, Le Beau MM, Daly KM, Bitter MA, Vardiman JW, Barker CM, Rowley JD, Golomb HM: Specific chromosomal abnormalities in acute nonlymphocytic leukemia correlate with drug susceptibility in vivo. *Leukemia* **2**:79, 1988.
261. Keating MJ, Smith TL, Kantarjian H, Cork A, Walters R, Trujillo JM, McCredie KB, Gehan EA, Freireich EJ: Cytogenetic pattern in acute myelogenous leukemia: A major reproducible determinant of outcome. *Leukemia* **2**:403, 1988.
262. Fenaux P, Preudhomme C, Lai JL, Morel P, Beuscart R, Bauters F: Cytogenetics and their prognostic value in de novo acute myeloid leukaemia: A report on 283 cases. *Br J Haematol* **73**:61, 1989.
263. Dastugue N, Payen C, Lafage-Pochitaloff M: Prognostic significance of karyotype in de novo adult acute myeloid leukemia. The BGMT group. *Leukemia* **9**:1491, 1995.
264. Nucifora G, Larson RA, Rowley JD: Persistence of the 8;21 translocation in patients with acute myeloid leukemia type M2 in long-term remission. *Blood* **82**:712, 1993.
265. Miyamoto T, Nagafuji K, Akashi K, Harada M, Kyo T, Akashi T, Takenaka K, Mizuno S, Gondo H, Okamura T, Dohy H, Niho Y: Persistence of multipotent progenitors expressing AML1/ETO transcripts in long-term remission patients with t(8;21) acute myelogenous leukemia. *Blood* **87**:4789, 1996.
266. Tobal K, Johnson PR, Saunders MJ, Yin JA: Detection of CBFB/MYH11 transcripts in patients with inversion and other abnormalities of chromosome 16 at presentation and remission. *Br J Haematol* **91**:104, 1995.
267. Jurlander J, Caligiuri MA, Ruutu T, Baer MR, Strout MP, Oberkircher AR, Hoffmann L, Ball ED, Frei-Lahr DA, Christiansen NP, Block AM, Knuutila S, Herzig GP, Bloomfield CD: Persistence of the AML1/ETO fusion transcript in patients treated with allogeneic bone marrow transplantation for t(8;21) leukemia. *Blood* **88**:2183, 1996.
268. de The H, Chomienne C, Lanotte M, Degos L, Dejean A: The t(15;17) translocation of acute promyelocytic leukaemia fuses the retinoic acid receptor alpha gene to a novel transcribed locus. *Nature* **347**:558, 1990.
269. Borrow J, Goddard AD, Sheer D, Solomon E: Molecular analysis of acute promyelocytic leukemia breakpoint cluster region on chromosome 17. *Science* **249**:1577, 1990.
270. Longo L, Pandolfi PP, Biondi A, Rambaldi A, Mencarelli A, Lo Coco F, Diverio D, Pegoraro L, Avanzi G, Tabilio A, et al: Rearrangements and aberrant expression of the retinoic acid receptor alpha gene in acute promyelocytic leukemias. *J Exp Med* **172**:1571, 1990.
271. de The H, Lavau C, Marchio A, Chomienne C, Degos L, Dejean A: The PML-RARα fusion mRNA generated by the t(15;17) translocation in acute promyelocytic leukemia encodes a functionally altered RAR. *Cell* **66**:675, 1991.
272. Kakizuka A, Miller WH Jr, Umesono K, Warrell RP Jr, Frankel SR, Murty VV, Dmitrovsky E, Evans RM: Chromosomal translocation t(15;17) in human acute promyelocytic leukemia fuses RARα with a novel putative transcription factor, PML. *Cell* **66**:663, 1991.
273. Kastner P, Perez A, Lutz Y, Rochette-Egly C, Gaub MP, Durand B, Lanotte M, Berger R, Chambon P: Structure, localization and transcriptional properties of two classes of retinoic acid receptor alpha fusion proteins in acute promyelocytic leukemia (APL): Structural similarities with a new family of oncoproteins. *EMBO J* **11**:629, 1992.
274. Perez A, Kastner P, Sethi S, Lutz Y, Reibel C, Chambon P: PMLRAR homodimers: Distinct DNA binding properties and heteromeric interactions with RXR. *EMBO J* **12**:3171, 1993.
275. Dyck JA, Maul GG, Miller WH Jr, Chen JD, Kakizuka A, Evans RM: A novel macromolecular structure is a target of the promyelocyte-retinoic acid receptor oncoprotein. *Cell* **76**:333, 1994.
276. Weis K, Rambaud S, Lavau C, Jansen J, Carvalho T, Carmo-Fonseca M, Lamond A, Dejean A: Retinoic acid regulates aberrant nuclear localization of PML-RAR alpha in acute promyelocytic leukemia cells. *Cell* **76**:345, 1994.
277. Koken MH, Puvion Dutilleul F, Guillemin MC, Viron A, Linares-Cruz G, Stuurman N, de Jong L, Szostecki C, Calvo F, Chomienne C, Degos L, Puvion E, The HD: The t(15;17) translocation alters a nuclear body in retinoic acid-reversible fashion. *EMBO J* **13**:1073, 1994.
278. Carvalho T, Seeler JS, Ohman K, Jordan P, Pettersson U, Akusjarvi G, Carmo-Fonseca M, Dejean A: Targeting of adenovirus E1A and E4-ORF3 proteins to nuclear matrix-associated PML bodies. *J Cell Biol* **131**:45, 1995.
279. Doucas V, Ishov AM, Romo A, Juguilon H, Weitzman MD, Evans RM, Maul GG: Adenovirus replication is coupled with the dynamic properties of the PML nuclear structure. *Genes Dev* **10**:196, 1996.
280. Everett RD, Maul GG: HSV-1 IE protein Vmw110 causes redistribution of PML. *EMBO J* **13**:5062, 1994.
281. Terris B, Baldin V, Dubois S, Degott C, Flejou JF, Henin D, Dejean A: PML nuclear bodies are general targets for inflammation and cell proliferation. *Cancer Res* **55**:1590, 1995.
282. Lavau C, Marchio A, Fagioli M, Jansen J, Falini B, Lebon P, Grosveld F, Pandolfi PP, Pelicci PG, Dejean A: The acute promyelocytic leukaemia-associated PML gene is induced by interferon. *Oncogene* **11**:871, 1995.
283. Nason-Burchenal K, Gandini D, Botto M, Allopenna J, Seale JR, Cross NC, Goldman JM, Dmitrovsky E, Pandolfi PP: Interferon augments PML and PML/RARalpha expression in normal myeloid and acute promyelocytic cells and cooperates with all-trans-retinoic acid to induce maturation of a retinoid resistant promyelocytic cell line. *Blood* (in press).
284. Jansen JH, Mahfoudi A, Rambaud S, Lavau C, Wahli W, Dejean A: Multimeric complexes of the PML-retinoic acid receptor alpha fusion protein in acute promyelocytic leukemia cells and interference with retinoid and peroxisome-proliferator signaling pathways. *Proc Natl Acad Sci USA* **92**:7401, 1995.
285. Grignani F, Ferrucci PF, Testa U, Talamo G, Fagioli M, Alcalay M, Mencarelli A, Peschle C, Nicoletti I, Pelicci PG: The acute promyelocytic leukemia-specific PML-RARa fusion protein inhibits differentiation and promotes survival of myeloid precursor cells. *Cell* **74**:423, 1993.
286. Grignani F, Testa U, Fagioli M, Barberi T, Masciulli R, Mariani G, Peschle C, Pelicci PG: Promyelocytic leukemia-specific PML-retinoic acid alpha receptor fusion protein interferes with erythroid differentiation of human erythroleukemia K562 cells. *Cancer Res* **55**:440, 1995.
287. Testa U, Grignani F, Barberi T, Fagioli M, Masciulli R, Ferrucci PF, Seripa D, Camagna A, Alcalay M, Pelicci PG, et al: PML/RAR alpha+ U937 mutant and NB4 cell lines: Retinoic acid restores the monocytic differentiation response to vitamin D3. *Cancer Res* **54**:4508, 1994.

288. Fu S, Consoli U, Hanania EG, Zu Z, Claxton DF, Andreeff M, Deisseroth AB: PML/RAα, a fusion protein in acute promyelocytic leukemia, prevents growth factor withdrawal-induced apoptosis in TF-1 cells. *Clin Cancer Res* **1**:583, 1995.

289. Rogaia D, Grignani Fr, Grignani F, Nicoletti I, Pelicci PG: The acute promyelocytic leukemia-specific PML/RARα fusion protein reduces the frequency of commitment to apoptosis upon growth factor deprivation of GM-CSF-dependent myeloid cells. *Leukemia* **9**:1467, 1995.

290. Redner RL, Rush EA, Faas S, Rudert WA, Corey SJ: The t(5;17) variant of acute promyelocytic leukemia expresses a nucleophosmin-retinoic acid receptor fusion. *Blood* **87**:882, 1996.

291. Wells RA, Catzavelos C, Kamel-Reid S: Fusion of retinoic acid receptor α to NuMA, the nuclear mitotic apparatus protein, by a variant translocation in acute promyelocytic leukaemia. *Nature Genet* **17**:109, 1997.

292. Chen Z, Brand N, Chen A, Chen S-J, Tong J-H, Wang Z-Y, Waxman S, Zelent A: Fusion between a novel Krüppel-like zinc finger gene and the retinoic acid receptor-α locus due to a variant t(11;17) translocation associated with acute promyelocytic leukaemia. *EMBO J* **12**:1161, 1993.

293. Bardwell VJ, Treisman R: The POZ domain: A conserved protein-protein interaction motif. *Genes Dev* **8**:1664, 1994.

294. Chen Z, Guidez F, Rousselot P, Agadir A, Chen S-J, Wang Z-Y, Degos L, Zelent A, Waxman S, Chomienne C: PLZF-RARα fusion proteins generated from the variant t(11:17)(q23;q21) translocation in acaute promyelocytic leukemia inhibit ligand-dependent transactivation of wild-type retinoic acid receptors. *Proc Natl Acad Sci USA* **91**:1178, 1994.

295. Dong S, Zhu J, Reid A, Strutt P, Guidez F, Zhong HJ, Wang ZY, Licht J, Waxman S, Chomienne C, Chen Z, Zelent A, Chen SJ: Amino-terminal protein-protein interaction motif (POZ-domain) is responsible for activities of the promyelocytic leukemia zinc finger-retinoic acid receptor-alpha fusion protein. *Proc Natl Acad Sci USA* **93**:3624, 1996.

296. Licht JD, Shaknovich R, English MA, Melnick A, Li JY, Reddy JC, Dong S, Chen SJ, Zelent A, Waxman S: Reduced and altered DNA-binding and transcriptional properties of the PLZF-retinoic acid receptor-alpha chimera generated in t(11;17)-associated acute promyelocytic leukemia. *Oncogene* **12**:323, 1996.

297. Cook M, Gould A, Brand N, Davies J, Strutt P, Shaknovich R, Licht J, Waxman S, Chen Z, Gluecksohn-Waelsch S, Krumlauf R, Zelent A: Expression of the zinc-finger gene PLZF at rhombomere boundaries in the vertebrate hindbrain. *Proc Natl Acad Sci USA* **92**:2249, 1995.

298. Reid A, Gould A, Brand N, Cook M, Strutt P, Li J, Licht J, Waxman S, Krumlauf R, Zelent A: Leukemia translocation gene, PLZF, is expressed with a speckled nuclear pattern in early hematopoietic progenitors. *Blood* **86**:4544, 1995.

299. Licht JD, Chomienne C, Goy A, Chen A, Scott AA, Head DR, Michaux JL, Wu Y, DeBlasio A, Miller WH Jr, et al: Clinical and molecular characterization of a rare syndrome of acute promyelocytic leukemia associated with translocation (11;17). *Blood* **85**:1083, 1995.

300. Horlein AJ, Naar AM, Heinzel T, Torchia J, Gloss B, Kurokawa R, Ryan A, Kamei Y, Soderstrom M, Glass CK: Ligand-independent repression by the thyroid hormone receptor mediated by a nuclear receptor co-repressor. *Nature* **377**:397, 1995.

301. Kurokawa R, Soderstrom M, Horlein AJ, Halachmi S, Brown M, Rosenfeld MG, Glass CK: Polarity-specific activities of retinoic acid receptors determined by a co-repressor. *Nature* **377**:451, 1995.

302. Alland L, Muhle R, Hou HJ, Potes J, Chin L, Schreiber-Agus N, DePinho RA: Role for N-CoR and histone deacetylase in Sin3-mediated transcriptional repression. *Nature* **387**:49, 1997.

303. Heinzel T, Lavinsky RM, Mullen TM, Soderstrom M, Laherty CD, Torchia J, Yang WM, Brard G, Ngo SD, Davie JR, Seto E, Eisenman RN, Rose DW, Glass CK, Rosenfeld MG: A complex containing N-CoR, mSin3 and histone deacetylase mediates transcriptional repression. *Nature* **387**:43, 1997.

304. Nagy L, Kao HY, Chakravarti D, Lin RJ, Hassig CA, Ayer DE, Schreiber SL, Evans RM: Nuclear receptor repression mediated by a complex containing SMRT, mSin3A, and histone deacetylase. *Cell* **89**:373, 1997.

305. Chen JD, Evans RM: A transcriptional co-repressor that interacts with nuclear hormone receptors. *Nature* **377**:454, 1995.

306. Lin RJ, Nagy L, Inoue S, Shao W, Miller WHJ, Evans RM: Role of the histone deacetylase complex in acute promyelocytic leukaemia. *Nature* **391**:811, 1998.

307. He LZ, Guidez F, Triboli C, Peruzzi D, Ruthardt M, Zelent A, Pandolfi PP: Distinct interactions of PML-RARα and PLZF-RARα with co-repressors determine differential responses to RA in APL. *Nature Genet* **18**:126, 1998.

308. Grignani F, De Matteis S, Nervi C, Tomassoni L, Gelmetti V, Cioce M, Fanelli M, Ruthardt M, Ferrara FF, Zamir I, Seiser C, Lazar MA, Minucci S, Pelicci PG: Fusion proteins of the retinoic acid receptor-alpha recruit histone deacetylase in promyelocytic leukaemia. *Nature* **391**:815, 1998.

309. Hong S-YDG, Wong C-W, Dejean A, Privalsky ML: SMRT corepressor interacts with PAZF and with the PML-retinoic acid receptor α (RARα) and PLZF-RARα oncoproteins associated with acute promyelocytic leukemia. *Proc Natl Acad Sci USA* **94**:9028, 1997.

310. Guidez F, Ivins S, Zhu J, Soderstrom M, Waxman S, Zelent A: Reduced retinoic acid-sensitivities of nuclear receptor corepressor binding to PML- and PLZF-RARα underlie molecular pathogenesis and treatment of acute promyelocytic leukemia. *Blood* **91**:2634, 1998.

311. Huang ME, Ye YC, Chen SR, Chai JR, Lu JX, Zhoa L, Gu LJ, Wang ZY: Use of all-trans retinoic acid in the treatment of acute promyelocytic leukemia. *Blood* **72**:567, 1988.

312. Castaigne S, Chomienne C, Daniel MT, Ballerini P, Berger R, Fenaux P, Degos L: All-trans retinoic acid as a differentiation therapy for acute promyelocytic leukemia: I. Clinical results. *Blood* **76**:1704, 1990.

313. Warrell RP Jr, Frankel SR, Miller WH Jr, Scheinberg DA, Itri LM, Hittelman WN, Vyas R, Andreeff M, Tafuri A, Jakubowski A, Gabrilove J, Gordon MS, Dimitrovsky E: Differentiation therapy of acute promyelocytic leukemia with tretinoin (all-*trans*-retinoic acid). *N Engl J Med* **324**:1385, 1991.

314. Sun GL, Yang RR, Chen SJ, Gu LJ, Xie WY, Zhang FQ, Li XS, Zhong DH, Cai JR, Chen Z, Wang ZY, Lu JX, Huang LA, Qian ZC, Yu HQ, Wang YL: Treatment of APL with all-trans retinoic acid: A report of five-year experience. *Chin J Cancer* **11**:125, 1993.

315. Chen ZX, Xue YQ, Zhang R, Tao RF, Xia XM, Li C, Wang W, Zu WY, Yao XZ, Ling BJ: A clinical and experimental study on all-*trans* retinoic acid-treated acute promyelocytic leukemia patients. *Blood* **78**:1413, 1991.

316. Warrell RP Jr, Maslak P, Eardley A, Heller G, Miller WH Jr, Frankel SR: Treatment of acute promyelocytic leukemia with all-trans retinoic acid: An update of the New York experience. *Leukemia* **8**:929, 1994.

317. Fenaux P, Chastang C, Chomienne C, Degos L: All transretinoic acid (ATRA) in combination with chemotherapy improves survival in newly diagnosed acute promyelocytic leukemia (APL). *Lancet* **343**:1033, 1994.

318. Early E, Moore MA, Kakizuka A, Nason-Burchenal K, Martin P, Evans RM, Dmitrovsky E: Transgenic expression of PML/RARα impairs myelopoiesis. *Proc Natl Acad Sci USA* **93**:7900, 1996.

319. Grisolano JL, Wesselschmidt RL, Ley TJ: Altered myeloid development and acute leukemia in transgenic mice expressing PML-RARα under control of cathepsin G regulatory sequences. *Blood* **89**:376, 1997.

320. He LZ, Triboli C, Rivi R, Peruzzi D, Pelicci PG, Soares V, Cattoretti G, Pandolfi PP: Acute leukemia with promyelocytic features in PML/RARα transgenic mice. *Proc Natl Acad Sci USA* **94**:5302, 1997.

321. Altabef M, Garcia M, Lavaue C, Bae S-C, Dejean A, Samarut J: A retrovirus carrying the promyelocyte-retinoic acid receptor PML-RARalpha fusion gene transforms haematopoietic progenitors in vitro and induces acute leukaemias. *EMBO J* **15**:2707, 1996.

322. Morishita K, Parganas E, Bartholomew C, Sacchi N, Valentine MB, Raimondi SC, Le Beau MM, Ihle JN: The human Evi-1 gene is located on chromosome 3q24-q28 but is not rearranged in three cases of acute nonlymphocytic leukemias containing t(3;5)(q25;q34) translocations. *Oncogene Res* **5**:221, 1990.

323. Morishita K, Parganas E, Willman CL, Whittaker MH, Drabkin H, Oval J, Taetle R, Ihle JN: Activation of Evi-1 gene expression in human acute myelogenous leukemias by translocations spanning 300–400 kb on chromosome 3q26. *Proc Natl Acad Sci USA* **89**:3937, 1992.

324. Morishita K, Parker DS, Mucenski ML, Jenkins NA, Copeland NG, Ihle JN: Retroviral activation of a novel gene encoding a zinc finger protein in IL-3-dependent myeloid leukemia cell lines. *Cell* **54**:831, 1988.

325. Delwel R, Funabiki T, Kreider BL, Morishita K, Ihle JN: Four of the seven zinc fingers of the Evi-1 myeloid-transforming gene are required for sequence-specific binding to GA(C/T)AAGA(T/C)AAGATAA. *Mol Cell Biol* **13**:4291, 1993.

326. Perkins AS, Fishel R, Jenkins NA, Copeland NG: Evi-1, a murine zinc finger proto-oncogene, encodes a sequence-specific DNA-binding protein. *Mol Cell Biol* **11**:2665, 1991.

327. Funabiki T, Kreider BL, Ihle JN: The carboxyl domain of zinc fingers of the Evi-1 myleoid transforming gene binds a consensus sequence of GAAGATGAG. *Oncogene* **9**:1575, 1994.
328. Kreider BL, Orkin SH, Ihle JN: Loss of erythropoietin responsiveness in erythroid progenitors due to expression of the Evi-1 myeloid-transforming gene. *Proc Natl Acad Sci USA* **90**:6454, 1993.
329. Mitelman F: *Catalog of Chromosome Aberrations in Cancer.* New York, Wiley-Liss, 1994.
330. Raimondi SC, Kalwinsky DK, Hayashi Y, Behm FG, Mirro J Jr, Williams DL: Cytogenetics of childhood acute nonlymphocytic leukemia. *Cancer Genet Cytogenet* **40**:13, 1989.
331. Raimondi SC: Current status of cytogenetic research in childhood acute lymphoblastic leukemia. *Blood* **81**:2237, 1993.
332. Pui C-H, Frankel LS, Carroll AJ, Raimondi SC, Shuster JJ, Head DR, Crist WM, Land VJ, Pullen DJ, Steuber CP, Behm FG, Borowitz MJ: Clinical characteristics and treatment outcome of childhood acute lymphoblastic leukemia with the t(4;11) (q21:q23): A collaborative study of 40 cases. *Blood* **77**:440, 1991.
333. Kaneko Y, Maseki N, Takasaki M, Sakurai T, Hayashi Y, Nakazawa S, Mori T, Sakurai M, Takeda T, Shikano T, Hiroshi Y: Clinical and hematologic characteristics in acute leukemia with 11q23 transloca-tions. *Blood* **67**:484, 1986.
334. Heerema NA, Arthur DC, Sather H, Albo V, Feusner J, Lange BJ, Steinherz PG, Zeltzer P, Hammond D, Reaman GH: Cytogenetic features of infants less than 12 months of age at diagnosis of acute lymphoblastic leukemia: Impact of the 11q23 breakpoint on outcome. A Report of the Childrens Cancer Group. *Blood* **83**:2274, 1994.
335. Pui CH, Kane JR, Crist WM: Biology and treatment of infant leukemias. *Leukemia* **9**:762, 1995.
336. Chen CS, Sorensen PH, Domer PH, Reaman GH, Korsmeyer SJ, Heerema NA, Hammond GD, Kersey JH: Molecular rearrangements on chromosome 11q23 predominate in infant acute lymphoblastic leukemia and are associated with specific biologic variables and poor outcome. *Blood* **81**:2386, 1993.
337. Chen C-S, Sorensen PHB, Domer PH, Reaman GH, Korsmeyer SJ, Heerema NA, Hammond GD, Kersey JH: Molecular rearrangements on chromosome 11q23 predominate in infant acute lymphoblastic leukemia and are associated with specific biologic variables and poor outcome. *Blood* **81**:2386, 1993.
338. Pui C-H, Behm FG, Raimondi SC, Dodge RK, George SL, Rivera GK, Mirro J, Kalwinsky DK, Dahl GV, Murphy SB, Crist WM, Williams DL: Secondary acute myeloid leukemia in children treated for acute lymphoid leukemia. *N Engl J Med* **321**:136, 1989.
339. DeVore R, Whitlock J, Hainsworth JD, Johnson DH: Therapy-related acute nonlymphocytic leukemia with monocytic features and rearran-gement of chromosome 11q. *Ann Intern Med* **110**:740, 1989.
340. Ziemin-van der Poel S, McCabe NR, Gill HJ, Espinosa R, Patel Y, Harden A, Rubinelli P, Smith SD, Lebeau MM, Rowley JD, Diaz MO: Identification of a gene, MLL, that spans the breakpoint in 11q23 translocations associated with human leukemias. *Proc Natl Acad Sci USA* **88**:10735, 1991.
341. Tkachuk DC, Kohler S, Cleary ML: Involvement of a homolog of *Drosophila* trithorax by 11q23 chromosomal translocations in acute leukemias. *Cell* **71**:691, 1992.
342. Gu Y, Nakamura T, Alder H, Prasad R, Canaani O, Cimino G, Croce CM, Cananni E: The t(4;11) chromosome translocation of human acute leukemias fuses the ALL-1 gene, related to *Drosophila* trithorax, to the AF-4 gene. *Cell* **71**:701, 1992.
343. Djabali M, Selleri L, Parry P, Bower M, Young BD, Evans G: A trithorax-like gene is interrupted by chromosome 11q23 translocations in acute leukemias. *Nature Genet* **2**:113, 1992.
344. Domer PH, Fakharzadeh SS, Chen CS, Jockel J, Johansen L, Silverman GA, Kersey JH, Korsmeyer SJ: Acute mixed-lineage leukemia t(4;11)(q21;q23) generates an MLL-AF4 fusion product. *Proc Natl Acad Sci USA* **90**:7884, 1993.
345. Morrissey J, Tkachuk DC, Milatovich A, Francke U, Link M, Cleary ML: A serine/proline-rich protein is fused to HRX in t(4;11) acute leukemias. *Blood* **81**:1124, 1993.
346. Jones RS, Gelbart WM: The *Drosophila* polycomb-group gene enhancer of zeste contains a region with sequence similarity to trithorax. *Mol Cell Biol* **13**:6357, 1993.
347. Yu BD, Hess JL, Horning SE, Brown GA, Korsmeyer SJ: Altered Hox expression and segmental identity in Mll-mutant mice. *Nature* **378**:505, 1995.
348. Simon J: Locking in stable states of gene expression: Transcriptional control during *Drosophila* development. *Curr Opin Cell Biol* **7**:376, 1995.
349. Mazo AM, Huang DH, Mozer BA, Dawid IB: The trithorax gene, a trans-acting regulator of the bithorax-complex in *Drosophila,* encodes a protein with zinc-binding domains. *Proc Natl Acad Sci USA* **87**:2112, 1990.
350. Reeves R, Nissen MS: The A-T-DNA-binding domain of mammalian high mobility group I chromosomal proteins. *J Biol Chem* **265**:8573, 1990.
351. Ma Q, Alder H, Nelson KK, Chatterjee D, Gu Y, Nakamura T, Canaani E, Croce CM, Siracusa LD, Buchberg AM: Analysis of the murine ALL-1 gene reveals conserved domains with human ALL-1 and identified a motif shared with DNA methyltransferases. *Proc Natl Acad Sci USA* **90**:6350, 1993.
352. Zeleznik-Le NJ, Harden AM, Rowley JD: 11q23 translocations split the "AT-hook" cruciform DNA-binding region and the transcriptional repression domain from the activation domain of the mixed-lineage leukemia (MLL) gene. *Proc Natl Acad Sci USA* **91**:10610, 1994.
353. Cui X, de Vivo I, Slany R, Miyamoto A, Firestein R, Cleary ML: Association of SET domain and myotubularin-related proteins modulates growth control. *Nature Genet* **18**:331, 1998.
354. de Vivo I, Cui X, Domen J, Cleary ML: Growth stimulation of primary B cell precursors by the anti-phosphatase Sbf1. *Proc Natl Acad Sci USA* **95**:9471, 1998.
355. Thirman MJ, Levitan DA, Kobayashi H, Simon MC, Rowley JD: Cloning of ELL, a gene that fuses to MLL in a t(11;19)(q23;p13.1) in acute myeloid leukemia. *Proc Natl Acad Sci USA* **91**:12110, 1994.
356. Mitani K, Kanda Y, Ogawa S, Tanaka T, Inazawa J, Yazaki Y, Hirai H: Cloning of several species of MLL/MEN chimeric cDNAs in myeloid leukemia with t(11;19)(q23;p13.1) translocation. *Blood* **85**:2017, 1995.
357. Shilatifard A, Lane WS, Jackson KW, Conaway RC, Conaway JW: An RNA polymerase II elongation factor encoded by the human ELL gene. *Science* **271**:1873, 1996.
358. Duan DR, Humphrey JS, Chen DY, Weng Y, Sukegawa J, Lee S, Gnarra JR, Linehan WM, Klausner RD: Characterization of the VHL tumor suppressor gene product: Localization, complex formation, and the effect of natural inactivating mutations. *Proc Natl Acad Sci USA* **92**:6459, 1995.
359. Duan DR, Pause A, Burgess WH, Aso T, Chen YT, Garrett KP, Conaway RC, Conaway JW, Linehan WM, Klausner RD: Inhibiton of transcription elongation by the VHL tumor suppressor protein. *Science* **269**:1402, 1995.
360. Aso T, Lane WS, Conaway JW, Conaway RC: Elongin (SIII): A multisubunit regulator of elongation by RNA polymerase II. *Science* **269**:1439, 1995.
361. Kibel A, Iliopoulos O, DeCaprio JA, Kaelin WG Jr: Binding of the von Hippel-Lindau tumor suppressor protein to elongin B and C. *Science* **269**:1444, 1995.
362. Rubnitz JE, Behm FG, Curcio-Brint AM, Pinheiro RP, Carroll AJ, Raimondi SC, Shurtleff SA, Downing JR: Molecular analysis of t(11;19) breakpoints in childhood acute leukemias. *Blood* **87**:4804, 1996.
363. Nakamura T, Alder H, Gu Y, Prasad R, Canaani O, Kamada N, Gale RP, Lange B, Crist WM, Nowell PC: Genes on chromosomes 4, 9, and 19 involved in 11q23 abnormalities in acute leukemia share sequence homology and/or common motifs. *Proc Natl Acad Sci USA* **90**:4631, 1993.
364. Chen CS, Hilden JM, Frestedt J, Domer PH, Moore R, Korsmeyer SJ, Kersey JH: The chromosome 4q21 gene (AF-4/FEL) is widely expressed in normal tissues and shows breakpoint diversity in t(4;11)(q21;q23) acute leukemia. *Blood* **82**:1080, 1993.
365. Rubnitz JE, Morrissey J, Savage PA, Cleary ML: ENL, the gene fused with HRX in t(11;19) leukemias, encodes a nuclear protein with transcriptional activation potential in lymphoid and myeloid cells. *Blood* **84**:1747, 1994.
366. Tse W, Zhu W, Chen HS, Cohen A: A novel gene, AF1q, fused to MLL in t(1;11)(q21;q23), is specifically expressed in leukemic and immature hematopoietic cells. *Blood* **85**:650, 1995.
367. Schichman SA, Caligiuri MA, Gu Y, Strout MP, Canaani E, Bloomfield CD, Croce CM: ALL-1 partial duplication in acute leukemia. *Proc Natl Acad Sci USA* **91**:6236, 1994.
368. Schichman SA, Caligiuri MA, Strout MP, Carter SL, Gu Y, Canaani E, Bloomfield CD, Croce CM: ALL-1 tandem duplication in acute myeloid leukemia with a normal karyotype involves homologous recombination between Alu elements. *Cancer Res* **54**:4277, 1994.
369. Schumacher A, Magnuson T: Murine polycomb- and trithorax-group genes regulate homeotic pathways and beyond. *Trends Genet* **13**:167, 1997.

370. Yu BD, Hanson R, Hess JL, Horning SE, Korsmeyer SJ: MLL, a mammalian trithorax-group gene, functions as a transcriptional maintenance factor in morphogenesis. *Proc Natl Acad Sci USA* **95**:1998.
371. Sauvageau G, Lansdorp PM, Eaves CJ, Hogge DE, Dragowska WH, Reid DS, Largman C, Lawrence HJ, Humphries RK: Differential expression of homeobox genes in functionally distinct CD34+ subpopulations of human bone marrow cells. *Proc Natl Acad Sci USA* **91**:12223, 1994.
372. Lawrence HJ, Largman C: Homeobox genes in normal hematopoiesis and leukemia. *Blood* **80**:2445, 1992.
373. Lawrence HJ, Sauvageau G, Ahmadi N, Lopez AR, Lebeau MM, Link M, Humphries K, Largman C: Stage- and lineage-specific expression of the HOXA10 homeobox gene in normal and leukemic hematopoietic cells. *Exp Hematol* **23**:1160, 1995.
374. Sauvageau G, Thorsteinsdottir U, Hough MR, Hugo P, Lawrence HJ, Largman C, Humphries RK: Overexpression of HOXB3 in hematopoietic cells causes defective lymphoid development and progressive myeloproliferation. *Immunity* **6**:13, 1997.
375. Sauvageau G, Thorsteinsdottir U, Eaves CJ, Lawrence HJ, Largman C, Lansdorp PM, Humphries RK: Overexpression of HOXB4 in hematopoietic cells causes the selective expansion of more primitive populations in vitro and in vivo. *Genes Dev* **9**:1753, 1995.
376. Thorsteinsdottir U, Sauvageau G, Hough MR, Dragowska W, Lansdorp PM, Lawrence HJ, Largman C, Humphries RK: Overexpression of HOXA10 in murine hematopoietic cells perturbs both myeloid and lymphoid differentiation and leads to acute myeloid leukemia. *Mol Cell Biol* **17**:495, 1997.
377. Hess JL, Yu BD, Li B, Hanson R, Korsmeyer SJ: Defects in yolk sac hematopoiesis in Mll-null embryos. *Blood* **90**:1799, 1997.
378. Corral J, Lavenir I, Impey H, Warren AJ, Forster A, Larson TA, Bell S, McKenzie AN, King G, Rabbitts TH: An MLL-AF9 fusion gene made by homologous recombination causes acute leukemia in chimeric mice: A method to create fusion oncogenes. *Cell* **85**:853, 1996.
379. Lavau C, Szilvassy SJ, Slany R, Cleary ML: Immortalization and leukemic transformation of a myelomonocytic precursor by retrovirally transduced HRX-ENL. *EMBO J* **16**:4426, 1997.
380. Slany RK, Lavau C, Cleary ML: The oncogenic capacity of HRX-ENL requires the transcriptional transactivation activity of ENL and the DNA binding motifs of HRX. *Mol Cell Biol* **18**:122, 1998.
381. Pui C-H, Ribeiro RC, Hancock ML, Rivera GK, Evans WE, Raimondi SC, Head DR, Behm FG, Mahmoud MH, Sandlund JT, Crist WM: Acute myeloid leukemia in children treated with epipodophyllotoxins for acute lymphoblastic leukemia. *N Engl J Med* **325**:1682, 1991.
382. Gu Y, Alder H, Nakamura T, Schichman SA, Prasad R, Canaani O, Saito H, Croce CM, Canaani E: Sequence analysis of the breakpoint cluster region in the ALL-1 gene involved in acute leukemia. *Cancer Res* **54**:2327, 1994.
383. Gu Y, Cimino G, Alder H, Nakamura T, Prasad R, Canaani O, Moir DT, Jones C, Nowell PC, Croce C M: The t(4;11)(q21;q23) chromosome translocations in acute leukemias involve the VDJ recombinase. *Proc Natl Acad Sci USA* **89**:10464, 1992.
384. Felix CA, Winick NJ, Negrini M, Bowman WP, Croce CM, Lange BJ: Common region of ALL-1 gene disrupted in epipodophyllotoxin-related secondary acute myeloid leukemia. *Cancer Res* **53**:2954, 1993.
385. Negrini M, Felix CA, Martin C, Lange BJ, Nakamura T, Canaani E, Croce CM: Potential topoisomerase II DNA-binding sites at the breakpoints of a t(9;11) chromosome translocation in acute myeloid leukemia. *Cancer Res* **53**:4489, 1993.
386. Strissel Broeker PL, Super HG, Thirman MJ, Pomykala H, Yonebayashi Y, Tanabe S, Zeleznik-Le N, Rowley JD: Distribution of 11q23 breakpoints within the MLL breakpoint cluster region in de novo acute leukemia and in treatment-related acute myeloid leukemia: Correlation with scaffold attachment regions and topoisomerase II consensus binding sites. *Blood* **87**:1912, 1996.
387. Domer PH, Head DR, Renganathan N, Raimondi SC, Yang E, Atlas M: Molecular analysis of 13 cases of MLL/11q23 secondary acute leukemia and identification of topoisomerase II consensus-binding sequences near the chromosomal breakpoint of a secondary leukemia with the t(4;11). *Leukemia* **9**:1305, 1995.
388. Bernard OA, Berger R: Molecular basis of 11q23 rearrangements in hematopoietic malignant proliferations. *Genes Chromosomes Cancer* **13**:75, 1995.
389. Prasad R, Gu Y, Alder H, Nakamura T, Canaani O, Saito H, Huebner K, Gale RP, Nowell PC, Kuriyama K, Miyazaki Y, Croce CM, Canaani E: Cloning of the ALL-1 fusion partner, the AF-6 gene, involved in acute myeloid leukemias with the t(6;11) chromosome translocation. *Cancer Res* **53**:5624, 1993.
390. Super HJG, McCabe NR, Thirman MJ, Larson RA, Lebeau MM, Pedersen-Bjergaard J, Philip P, Diaz MO, Rowley JD: Rearrangements of the MLL gene in therapy-related acute myeloid leukemia in patients previously treated with agents targeting DNA-topoisomerase II. *Blood* **81**:3705, 1993.
391. Hunger SP, Tkachuk DC, Amylon MD, Link MP, Carroll AJ, Welborn JL, Willman CL, Cleary ML: HRX involvement in de novo and secondary leukemias with diverse chromosome 11q23 abnormalities. *Blood* **81**:3197, 1993.
392. Bower M, Parry P, Carter M, Lillington DM, Amess J, Lister TA, Evans G, Young BD: Prevalence and clinical correlations of MLL gene rearrangements in AML-M4/5. *Blood* **84**:3776, 1994.
393. Wang JC: DNA topoisomerases. *Annu Rev Biochem* **54**:665, 1985.
394. Bae YS, Kawasaki I, Ikeda H, Liu LF: Illegitimate recombination mediated by calf thymus DNA topoisomerase II in vitro. *Proc Natl Acad Sci USA* **85**:2076, 1988.
395. Sperry AO, Blasquez VC, Garrard WT: Dysfunction of chromosomal loop attachment sites: Illegitimate recombination linked to matrix association regions and topoisomerase II. *Proc Natl Acad Sci USA* **86**:5497, 1989.
396. Ford AM, Ridge SA, Cabrera ME, Mahmoud H, Steel CM, Chan LC, Greaves M: In utero rearrangements in the trithorax-related oncogene in infant leukaemias. *Nature* 363:358, 1993.
397. Super HJG, Rothberg PG, Kobayashi H, Freeman AI, Diaz MO, Rowley JD: Clonal, nonconstitutional rearrangements of the MLL gene in infant twins with acute lymphoblastic leukemia: In utero chromosome rearrangement of 11q23. *Blood* **83**:641, 1994.
398. Fujioka K, Caslini C, Jones BG, Komuro H, Naeve CW, Look AT: Aberrant p27Kip1 transcripts identified in human leukemias expressing the MLL-AF4 fusion protein. *Blood* **88**:356a, 1996.
399. Caslini C, Murti KG, Ashmun D, Domer PH, Korsmeyer SJ, Boer JM, Grosveld GC, Look AT: Subcellular localization and cell cycle effects of the MLL-AF4 fusion oncoprotein. *Blood* **88**:557a, 1996.
400. Schlessinger J, Ullrich A: Growth factor signaling by receptor tyrosine kinases. *Neuron* **9**:383, 1992.
401. Schlessinger J: How receptor tyrosine kinases activate Ras. *Trends Biochem Sci* **18**:273, 1993.
402. Greco A, Pierotti MA, Bongarzone I, Pagliardini S, Lanzi C, Della Porta G: TRK-T1 is a novel oncogene formed by the fusion of TPR and TRK genes in human papillary thyroid carcinomas. *Oncogene* **7**:237, 1992.
403. Rodrigues GA, Park M: Dimerization mediated through a leucine zipper activates the oncogenic potential of the met receptor tyrosine kinase. *Mol Cell Biol* **13**:6711, 1993.
404. Anonymous: Chromosomal abnormalities and their clinical significance in acute lymphoblastic leukemia: Third International Workshop on Chromosomes in Leukemia. *Cancer Res* **43**:868, 1983.
405. Rowley JD: Biological implications of consistent chromosome rearrangements in leukemia and lymphoma. *Cancer Res* **44**:3159, 1984.
406. Ribeiro RC, Abromowitch M, Raimondi SC, et al: Clinical and biologic hallmarks of the Philadelphia chromosome in childhood acute lymphoblastic leukemia. *Blood* **70**:948, 1987.
407. Bartram CR, de Klein A, Hagemeijer A, van Agthoven T, Geurts van Kessel A, Bootsma D, Grosveld G, Ferguson-Smith MA, Davies T, Stone M, et al: Translocation of c-abl oncogene correlates with the presence of a Philadelphia chromosome in chronic myelocytic leukaemia. *Nature* **306**:277, 1983.
408. Gale RP, Canaani E: An 8-kilobase abl RNA transcript in chronic myelogenous leukemia. *Proc Natl Acad Sci USA* **81**:5648, 1984.
409. Collins SJ, Kubonishi I, Miyoshi I, Groudine MT: Altered transcription of the c-abl oncogene in K562 and other chronic myelogenous leukemia cells. *Science* **225**:72, 1984.
410. Stam K, Heisterkamp N, Grosveld G, de Klein A, Verna RS, Coleman M, Dosik H, Groffen J: Evidence of a new chimeric bcr/c-abl mRNA in patients with chronic myelocytic leukemia and the Philadelphia chromosome. *N Engl J Med* **313**:1429, 1985.
411. Canaani E, Gale RP, Steiner-Saltz D, et al: Altered transcription of an oncogene in chronic myeloid leukemia. *Lancet* **1**:593, 1984.
412. Shtivelman E, Lifshitz B, Gale RP, Canaani E: Fused transcript of abl and bcr genes in chronic myelogenous leukemia. *Nature* **315**:550, 1985.
413. Heisterkamp N, Stephenson JR, Groffen J, et al: Localization of the c-abl oncogene adjacent to a translocation breakpoint in chronic myelocytic leukaemia. *Nature* **306**:239, 1983.
414. Leibowitz D, Schaefer Rego K, Popenoe DW, et al: Variable breakpoints on the Philadelphia chromosome in chronic myelogenous leukemia. *Blood* **66**:243, 1985.

415. Grosveld G, Verwoerd T, van Agthoven T, de Klein A, Ramachandran KL, Heisterkamp N, Stam K, Groffen J: The chronic myelocytic cell line K562 contains a breakpoint in bcr and produces a chimeric bcr/c-abl transcript. *Mol Cell Biol* **6**:607, 1986.
416. Groffen J, Stephenson JR, Heisterkamp N, et al: Philadelphia chromosomal breakpoints are clustered within a limited region, bcr, on chromosome 22. *Cell* **36**:93, 1984.
417. Heisterkamp N, Stam K, Groffen J, et al: Structural organization of the bcr gene and its role in Ph1 translocation. *Nature* **315**:758, 1985.
418. Kloetzer W, Kurzrock R, Smith L, Talpaz M, Spiller M, Gutterman J, Arlinghaus R: The human cellular abl gene product in the chronic myelogenous leukemia cell line K562 has an associated tyrosine protein kinase activity. *Virology* **140**:230, 1985.
419. Konopka JB, Watanabe SM, Witte ON: An alteration of the human c-abl protein in K562 leukemia cells unmasks associated tyrosine kinase activity. *Cell* **37**:1935, 1984.
420. Konopka JB, Watanabe SM, Singer JW, et al: Cell lines and clinical isolates derived from Ph1-positive chronic myelogenous leukemia patients express c-abl proteins with a common structural alteration. *Proc Natl Acad Sci USA* **82**:1810, 1985.
421. Naldini L, Stacchini A, Cirillo DM, Aglietta M, Gavosto F, Comoglio PM: Phosphotyrosine antibodies identify the p210 c-abl tyrosine kinase and proteins phosphorylated on tyrosine in human chronic myelogenous leukemia cells. *Mol Cell Biol* **6**:1803, 1986.
422. Chan LC, Karhi KK, Rayter SI, et al: A novel abl protein expressed in Philadelphia chromosome-positive acute lymphoblastic leukaemia. *Nature* **325**:635, 1987.
423. Clark SS, McLaughlin J, Crist WM, et al: Unique forms of the abl tyrosine kinase distinguish Ph1-positive CML from Ph1-positive ALL. *Science* **235**:85, 1987.
424. Kurzrock R, Shtalrid M, Romero P, et al: A novel c-abl protein product in Philadelphia-positive acute lymphoblastic leukemia. *Nature* **325**:631, 1987.
425. Hermans A, Heisterkamp N, von Linden M, van Baal S, Meijer D, van der Plas D, Wiedemann LM, Groffen J, Bootsma D, Grosveld G: Unique fusion of bcr and c-abl genes in Philadelphia chromosome positive acute lymphoblastic leukemia. *Cell* **51**:33, 1987.
426. Walker LC, Ganesan TS, Dhut S, Gibbons B, Lister TA, Rothbard J, Young BD: Novel chimaeric protein expressed in Philadelphia positive acute lymphoblastic leukemia. *Nature* **329**:851, 1987.
427. Fainstein E, Marcelle C, Rosener A, Canaani E, Gale RP, Dreazen O, Smith SD, Croce CM: A new fused transcript in Philadelphia chromosome positive acute lymphocytic leukemia. *Nature* **330**:386, 1987.
428. Witte ON, Ponticelli A, Gifford A, et al: Phosphorylation of the Abelson murine leukemia virus transforming protein. *J Virol* **39**:870, 1981.
429. Reynolds FH Jr, Oroszlan S, Stephenson JR: Abelson urine leukemia virus p120: identification and characterization of tyrosine phosphorylation sites. *J Virol* **44**:1097, 1982.
430. Srinivasan A, Dunn CY, Yuasa Y, Devare SG, Reddy EP, Aaronson SA: Abelson murine leukemia virus: structural requirements for transforming gene function. *Proc Natl Acad Sci USA* **79**:5508, 1982.
431. Daley GQ, McLaughlin J, Witte ON, Baltimore D: The CML-specific P210 bcr/abl protein, unlike v-abl, does not transform NIH/3T3 fibroblasts. *Science* **237**:532, 1987.
432. Daley GQ, Baltimore D: Transformation of an interleukin 3-dependent hematopoietic cell line by the chronic myelogenous leukemia-specific P210bcr/abl protein. *Proc Natl Acad Sci USA* **85**:9312, 1988.
433. Elefanty AG, Hariharan IK, Cory S: bcr-abl, the hallmark of chronic myeloid leukaemia in man, induces multiple haemopoietic neoplasms in mice. *EMBO J* **9**:1069, 1990.
434. Gishizky ML, Johnson White J, Witte ON: Efficient transplantation of BCR-ABL-induced chronic myelogenous leukemia-like syndrome in mice. *Proc Natl Acad Sci USA* **90**:3755, 1993.
435. Kelliher M, Knott A, McLaughlin J, Witte ON, Rosenberg N: Differences in oncogenic potency but not target cell specificity distinguish the two forms of the BCR/ABL oncogene. *Mol Cell Biol* **11**:4710, 1991.
436. Goga A, McLaughlin J, Afar DE, Saffran DC, Witte ON: Alternative signals to RAS for hematopietic transformation by the BCR-ABL oncogene. *Cell* **82**:981, 1995.
437. Senechal K, Halpern J, Sawyers CL: The CRKL adaptor protein transforms fibroblasts and functions in transformation by the BCR-ABL oncogene. *J Biol Chem* (in press).
438. Raitano AB, Halpern JR, Hambuch TM, Sawyers CL: The Bcr-Abl leukemia oncogene activates Jun kinase and requires Jun for transformation. *Proc Natl Acad Sci USA* **92**:11746, 1995.
439. Afar DE, Goga A, McLaughlin J, Witte ON, Sawyers CL: Differential complementation of Bcr-Abl point mutants with c-Myc. *Science* **264**:424, 1994.
440. Afar DE, McLaughlin J, Sherr CJ, Witte ON, Roussel MF: Signaling by ABL oncogenes through cyclin D1. *Proc Natl Acad Sci USA* **92**:9540, 1995.
441. Shuai K, Halpern J, ten Hoeve J, Rao X, Sawyers CL: Constitutive activation of STAT5 by the BCR-ABL oncogene in chronic myelogenous leukemia. *Oncogene* **13**:247, 1996.
442. Papadopoulos P, Ridge SA, Boucher CA, Stocking C, Wiedemann LM: The novel activation of ABL by fusion to an ets-related gene, TEL. *Cancer Res* **55**:34, 1995.
443. Golub TR, Barker GF, Lovett M, Gilliland DG: Fusion of PDGF receptor beta to a novel ets-like gene, tel, in chronic myelomonocytic leukemia with t(5;12) chromosomal translocation. *Cell* **77**:307, 1994.
444. Tybulewicz VL, Crawford CE, Jackson PK, Bronson RT, Mulligan RC: Neonatal lethality and lymphopenia in mice with a homozygous disruption of the c-abl proto-oncogene. *Cell* **65**:1153, 1991.
445. Schwartzberg PL, Stall AM, Hardin JD, Bowdish KS, Humaran T, Boast S, Harbison ML, Robertson EJ, Goff SP: Mice homozygous for the ablm1 mutation show poor viability and depletion of selected B and T cell populations. *Cell* **65**:1165, 1991.
446. Van Etten RA, Jackson P, Baltimore D: The mouse type IV c-abl gene product is a nuclear protein, and activation of transforming ability is associated with cytoplasmic localization. *Cell* **58**:669, 1989.
447. Kharbanda S, Ren R, Pandey P, Shafman TD, Feller SM, Weichselbaum RR, Kufe DW: Activation of the c-Abl tyrosine kinase in the stress response to DNA- damaging agents. *Nature* **376**:785, 1995.
448. Sawyers CL, McLaughlin J, Goga A, Havlik M, Witte O: The nuclear tyrosine kinase c-Abl negatively regulates cell growth. *Cell* **77**:121, 1994.
449. Mattioni T, Jackson PK, Bchini-Hooft van Huijsduijnen O, Picard D: Cell cycle arrest by tyrosine kinase Abl involves altered early mitogenic response. *Oncogene* **10**:1325, 1995.
450. Goga A, Liu X, Hambuch TM, Senechal K, Major E, Berk AJ, Witte ON, Sawyers CL: p53 dependent growth suppression by the c-Abl nuclear tyrosine kinase. *Oncogene* **11**:791, 1995.
451. Yuan Z-M, Huang Y, Whang Y, Sawyers C, Weichselbaum R, Kharbanda S, Kufe D: Role for the c-ABL tyrosine kinase in the growth arrest response to DNA damage. *Nature* **382**:272, 1996.
452. Bloomfield CD, Goldman AL, Berger AR, et al: Chromosomal abnormalities identify high-risk and low-risk patients with acute lymphoblastic leukemia. *Blood* **67**:415, 1986.
453. Jain K, Arlin Z, Mertelsmann R, et al: Philadelphia chromosome and terminal transferase-positive acute leukemia: Similarity of terminal phase of chronic myelogenous leukemia and de novo acute presentation. *J Clin Oncol* **1**:669, 1983.
454. Williams DL, Harber J, Murphy SB, et al: Chromosomal translocation play a unique role in influencing prognosis in childhood acute lymphoblastic leukemia. *Blood* **68**:205, 1986.
455. Roberts WM, Rivera GK, Raimondi SC, Santana VM, Sandlund JT, Crist WM, Pui CH: Intensive chemotherapy for Philadelphia-chromosome-positiveacute lymphoblastic leukaemia. *Lancet* **343**:331, 1994.
456. Thomas ED, Clift RA: Indications for marrow transplantation in chronic myelogenous leukemia. *Blood* **73**:861, 1989.
457. Morris SW, Kirstein MN, Valentine MB, Dittmer KG, Shapiro DN, Saltman DL, Look AT: Fusion of a kinase gene, ALK, to a nucleolar protein gene, NPM, in non-Hodgkin's lymphoma. *Science* **263**:1281, 1994.
458. Borer RA, Lehner CF, Eppenberger HM, Nigg EA: Major nucleolar proteins shuttle between nucleus and cytoplasm. *Cell* **56**:379, 1989.
459. Szebeni A, Herrera JE, Olson MO: Interaction of nucleolar protein B23 with peptides related to nuclear localization signals. *Biochemistry* **34**:8037, 1995.
460. Chan W-Y, Liu QR, Borjigin J, Busch H, Rennert OM, Tease LA, Chan P-K: Characterization of the cDNA encoding human nucleophosmin and studies of its role in normal and abnormal growth. *Biochemistry* **28**:1033, 1989.
461. Peter M, Nakagawa J, Doree M, Labbe JC, Nigg EA: Identification of major nucleolar proteins as candidate mitotic substrates of cdc2 kinase. *Cell* **60**:791, 1990.
462. Dumbar TS, Gentry GA, Olson MOJ: Interaction of nucleolar phosphoprotein B23 with nucleic acids. *Biochemistry* **28**:9495, 1989.
463. Fankhauser C, Izaurralde E, Adachi Y, Wingfield P, Laemmli UK: Specific complex of human immunodeficiency virus type 1 rev and

nucleolar B23 proteins: Dissociation by the Rev response element. *Mol Cell Biol* **11**:2567, 1991.

464. Feuerstein N, Mond JJ, Kinchington PR, Hickey R, Karjalainen Lindsberg ML, Hay I, Ruyechan WT: Evidence for DNA binding activity of numatrin (B23), a cell cycle-regulated nuclear matrix protein. *Biochim Biophys Acta* **1087**:127, 1990.
465. Inouye CJ, Seto E: Relief of YY1-induced transcriptional repression by protein-protein interaction with the nucleolar phosphoprotein B23. *J Biol Chem* **269**:6506, 1994.
466. Valdez BC, Perlaky L, Henning D, Saijo Y, Chan PH, Busch H: Identification of the nuclear and nucleolar localization signals of the protein p120. *J Biol Chem* **269**:23776, 1994.
467. Morris SW, Naeve C, Mathew P, James PL, Kirstein MN, Cui X, Witte DP: ALK, the chromosome 2 gene locus altered by the t(2;5) in non-Hodgkin's lymphoma, encodes a neural receptor tyrosine kinase that is highly related to leukocyte tyrosine kinase (LTK). *Oncogene* **14**:2175, 1997.
468. Iwahara T, Fujimoto J, Wen D, Cupples R, Bucay N, Arakawa T, Mori S, Ratzkin B, Yamamoto T: Molecular characterization of ALK, a receptor tyrosine kinase expressed specifically in the nervous system. *Oncogene* **14**:439, 1997.
469. Bischof D, Pulford K, Mason DY, Morris SW: Role of the nucleophosmin (NPM) portion of the non-Hodgkin's lymphoma-associated NPM-anaplastic lymphoma kinase fusion protein in oncogenesis. *Mol Cell Biol* **17**:2312, 1997.
470. Mason DY, Pulford KAF, Bischof D, Kuefer MU, Butler LH, Lamant L, Delsol G, Morris SW: Nucleolar localization of the nucleophosmin-anaplastic lymphoma kinase is not required for malignant transformation. *Cancer Res* **58**:1057, 1998.
471. Fujimoto J, Shiota M, Iwahara T, Seki N, Satoh H, Mori S, Yamamoto T: Characterization of the transforming activity of p80, a hyperphosphorylated protein in a Ki-1 lymphoma cell line with chromosomal translocation t(2;5). *Proc Natl Acad Sci USA* **93**:4181, 1996.
472. Kuefer MU, Look AT, Pulford K, Behm FG, Pattengale PK, Mason DY, Morris SW: Retrovirus-mediated gene transfer of NPM-ALK causes lymphoid malignancy in mice. *Blood* **90**:2901, 1997.
473. Pulford K, Lamant L, Morris SW, Butler LH, Wood KM, Stroud D, Delsol G, Mason DY: Detection of anaplastic lymphoma kinase ALK and nucleolar protein nucleophosmin NPM-ALK proteins in normal and neoplastic cells with the monoclonal antibody ALK1. *Blood* **89**:1394, 1997.
474. Benharroch D, Meguerian Bedoyan Z, Lamant L, Amin C, Brugieres L, Terrier-Lacombe MJ, Haralambieva E, Pulford K, Pileri S, Morris SW, Mason DY, Delsol G: ALK-positive lymphoma: A single disease with a broad spectrum of morphology. *Blood* **91**:2076, 1998.
475. Falini B, Bigerna B, Fizzotti M, Pulford K, Pileri SA, Delsol G, Carbone A, Paulli M, Magrini U, Menestrina F, Giardini R, Pilotti S, Mezzelani A, Ugolini B, Billi M, Pucciarini A, Pacini R, Peliccci P-G, Flenghi L: ALK expression defines a distinct group of T/Null lymphomas ("ALK lymphomas") with a wide morphological spectrum. *Am J Pathol* **153**:875, 1998.
476. Pittaluga S, Wiodarska I, Pulford K, Campo E, Morris SW, Van den Berghe H, De Wolf-Peeters C: The monoclonal antibody ALK1 identifies a distinct morphological subtype of anaplastic large cell lymphoma associated with 2p23/ALK rearrangements. *Am J Pathol* **151**:343, 1997.
477. Sarris AH, Luthra R, Cabanillas F, Morris SW, Pugh WC: Genomic DNA amplification and the detection of t(2;5)(p23;q35) in lymphoid neoplasms. *Leuk Lymphoma* **29**:507, 1998.
478. Downing JR, Shurtleff SA, Zielenska M, Curcio-Brint AM, Behm FG, Head DR, Sandlund JT, Weisenburger DD, Kossakowska AE, Thorner P, Lorenzanz A, Ladanyi M, Morris SW: Molecular detection of the (2;5) translocation of non-Hodgkin's lymphoma by reverse transcriptase-polymerase chain reaction. *Blood* **85**:3416, 1995.
479. Mathew P, Sanger WG, Weisenburger DD, Valentine M, Valentine V, Pickering D, Higgins C, Hess M, Cui X, Srivastava DK, Morris SW: Detection of the t(2;5)(p23;q35) and NPM-ALK fusion in non-Hodgkin's lymphoma by two-color fluorescence in situ hybridization. *Blood* **89**:1678, 1996.
480. Shiota M, Nakamura S, Ichinohasama R, Abe M, Akagi T, Takeshita M, Mori N, Fujimoto J, Miyauchi J, Mikata A, Nanba K, Takami T, Yamabe H, Takano Y, Izumo T, Nagatani T, Mohri N, Nasu K, Satoh H, Katano H, Yamamoto T, Mori S: Anaplastic large cell lymphomas expressing the novel chimeric protein p80NPM/ALK: A distinct clinicopathologic entity. *Blood* **86**:1954, 1995.
481. Hutchison RE, Banki K, Shuster JJ, Barrett D, Dieck C, Berard CW, Murphy SB, Link MP, Pick TE, Laver J, Schwenn M, Mathew P, Morris SW: Use of an anti-ALK antibody in the characterization of anaplastic large-cell lymphoma of childhood. *Ann Oncol* **8(suppl 1)**:37, 1997.
482. Gascoyne RD, Aoun P, Wu D, Chhanabhai M, Skinnider BF, Pulford KAF, Mason DY, Greiner TC, Morris SW, Connors JM, Vose JM, Viswanatha DS, Coldman A, Weisenburger DD: Prognostic significance of ALK protein expression in adults with anaplastic large cell lymphoma. *Blood* (in press).
483. Wlodarska I, De Wolf-Peeters C, Falini B, Verhoef G, Morris SW, Hagemeijer A, Van den Berghe H: The cryptic inv(2)(p23q35) defines a new molecular genetic subtype of ALK-positive ALCL. *Blood* (in press).
484. Delsol G, Lamant L, Mariame B, Pulford K, Dastugue N, Brousset P, Rigal-Huguet F, Saati TA, Cerretti DP, Morris SW, Mason DY: A new subtype of large B-cell lymphoma expressing the ALK kinase and lacking the 2;5 translocation. *Blood* **89**:1483, 1997.
485. Koeffler HP: Myelodysplastic syndromes. *Hematol Oncol Clin North Am* **6**:485, 1992.
486. Yarden Y, Escobedo JA, Kuang WJ, Yang-Feng TL, Daniel TO, Tremble PM, Chen EY, Ando ME, Harkins RN, Francke U, et al: Structure of the receptor for platelet-derived growth factor helps define a family of closely related growth factor receptors. *Nature* **323**:226, 1986.
487. Satoh T, Fantl WJ, Escobedo JA, Williams LT, Kaziro Y: Platelet-derived growth factor receptor mediates activation of ras through different signaling pathways in different cell types. *Mol Cell Biol* **13**:3706, 1993.
488. Yan XQ, Brady G, Iscove NN: Overexpression of PDGF-B in murine hematopoietic cells induces a lethal myeloproliferative syndrome in vivo. *Oncogene* **9**:163, 1994.
489. Nye JA, Petersen JM, Gunther CV, Jonsen MD, Graves BJ: Interaction of murine ets-1 with GGA-binding sites establishes the ETS domain as a new DNA-binding motif. *Genes Dev* **6**:975, 1992.
490. Rao VN, Ohno T, Prasad DD, Bhattacharya G, Reddy ES: Analysis of the DNA-binding and transcriptional activation functions of human Fli-1 protein. *Oncogene* **8**:2167, 1993.
491. Sawyers CL, Denny CT: Chronic myelomonocytic leukemia: Tel-a-kinase what Ets all about. *Cell* **77**:171, 1994.
492. Wlodarska I, Mecucci C, Marynen P, Guo C, Franckx D, La Starza R, Aventin A, Bosly A, Martelli MF, Cassiman JJ, et al: TEL gene is involved in myelodysplastic syndromes with either the typical t(5;12)(q33;p13) translocation or its variant t(10; 12)(q24;p13). *Blood* **85**:2848, 1995.
493. Erikson J, Finan J, Tsujimoto Y, Nowell PC, Croce CM: The chromosome 14 breakpoint in neoplastic B cells with the t(11;14) translocation involves the immunoglobulin heavy chain locus. *Proc Natl Acad Sci USA* **81**:4144, 1984.
494. Tsujimoto Y, Yunis J, Onorato-Showe L, Erikson J, Nowell PC, Croce CM: Molecular cloning of the chromosomal breakpoint of B-cell lymphomas and leukemias with the t(11;14) chromosome translocation. *Science* **224**:1403, 1984.
495. Tsujimoto Y, Jaffe E, Cossman J, Gorham J, Nowell PC, Croce CM: Clustering of breakpoints on chromosome 11 in human B-cell neoplasms with the t(11;14) chromosome translocation. *Nature* **315**:340, 1985.
496. Louie E, Tsujimoto Y, Heubner K, Croce C: *Am J Hum Genet* **41(suppl)**:31, 1987.
497. Rabbitts PH, Douglas J, Fischer P, Nacheva E, Karpas A, Catovsky D, Melo JV, Baer R, Stinson MA, Rabbitts TH: Chromosome abnormalities at 11q13 in B cell tumours. *Oncogene* **3**:99, 1988.
498. Meeker TC, Grimaldi JC, O'Rourke R, Louie E, Juliusson G, Einhorn S: An additional breakpoint region in the BCL-1 locus associated with the t(11;14)(q13;q32) translocation of B-lymphocytic malignancy. *Blood* **74**:1801, 1989.
499. Lammie GA, Fantl V, Smith R, Schuuring E, Brookes S, Michalides R, Dickson C, Arnold A, Peters G: D11S287, a putative oncogene on chromosome 11q13, is amplified and expressed in squamous cell and mammary carcinomas and linked to BCL-1. *Oncogene* **6**:439, 1991.
500. Rosenberg CL, Wong E, Petty EM, Bale AE, Tsujimoto Y, Harris NL, Arnold A: PRAD1, a candidate BCL1 oncogene: Mapping and expression in centrocytic lymphoma. *Proc Natl Acad Sci USA* **88**:9638, 1991.
501. Withers DA, Harvey RC, Faust JB, Melnyk O, Carey K, Meeker TC: Characterization of a candidate bcl-1 gene. *Mol Cell Biol* **11**:4846, 1991.
502. Brookes S, Lammie GA, Schuuring E, Dickson C, Peters G: Linkage map of a region of human chromosome band 11q13 amplified in

breast and squamous cell tumors. *Genes Chromosomes Cancer* **4**:290, 1992.

503. Hall M, Peters G: Genetic alterations of cyclins, cyclin-dependent kinases, and Cdk inhibitors in human cancer, in Vande Woude GF, Klein G (eds): *Advances in Cancer Research*. San Diego, Academic Press, 1996, p. 67.
504. Sherr CJ: Mammalian G1 cyclins. *Cell* **73**:1059, 1993.
505. Rosenberg CL, Motokura T, Kronenberg HM, Arnold A: Coding sequence of the overexpressed transcript of the putative oncogene PRAD1/cyclin D1 in two primary human tumors. *Oncogene* **8**:519, 1993.
506. Rimokh R, Berger F, Bastard C, Klein B, French M, Archimbaud E, Rouault JP, Santa Lucia B, Duret L, Vuillaume M, et al: Rearrangement of CCND1 (BCL1/PRAD1) 3′ untranslated region in mantle-cell lymphomas and t(11q13)-associated leukemias. *Blood* **83**:3689, 1994.
507. Lukas J, Jadayel D, Bartkova J, Nacheva E, Dyer MJ, Strauss M, Bartek J: BCL-1/cyclin D1 oncoprotein oscillates and subverts the G1 phase control in B-cell neoplasms carrying the t(11;14) translocation. *Oncogene* **9**:2159, 1994.
508. Banks PM, Chan J, Cleary ML, Delsol G, De Wolf-Peeters C, Gatter K, Grogan TM, Harris NL, Isaacson PG, Jaffe ES, et al: Mantle cell lymphoma: A proposal for unification of morphologic, immunologic, and molecular data. *Am J Surg Pathol* **16**:637, 1992.
509. Shivdasani RA, Hess JL, Skarin AT, Pinkus GS: Intermediate lymphocytic lymphoma: Clinical and pathologic features of a recently characterized subtype of non-Hodgkin's lymphoma. *J Clin Oncol* **11**:802, 1993.
510. Harris NL, Jaffe ES, Stein H, Banks PM, Chan JKC, Cleary ML, Delsol G, De Wolf-Peeters C, Falini B, Gatter KC, Grogan TM, Isaacson PG, Knowles DM, Mason DY, Muller-Hermelink H-K, Pileri SA, Piris MA, Ralfkiaer E, Warnke RA: A revised European-American classification of lymphoid neoplasms: A proposal from the International Lymphoma Study Group. *Blood* **84**:1361, 1994.
511. Banno S, Yoshikawa K, Nakamura S, Yamamoto K, Seito T, Nitta M, Takahashi T, Ueda R, Seto M: Monoclonal antibody against PRAD1/cyclin D1 stains nuclei of tumor cells with translocation or amplification at BCL-1 locus. *Jpn J Cancer Res* **85**:918, 1994.
512. de Boer CJ, van Krieken JH, Kluin-Nelemans HC, Kluin PM, Schuuring E: Cyclin D1 messenger RNA overexpression as a marker for mantle cell lymphoma. *Oncogene* **10**:1833, 1995.
513. Nakamura S, Seto M, Banno S, Suzuki S, Koshikawa T, Kitoh K, Kagami Y, Ogura M, Yatabe Y, Kojima M, et al: Immunohistochemical analysis of cyclin D1 protein in hematopoietic neoplasms with special reference to mantle cell lymphoma. *Jpn J Cancer Res* **85**:1270, 1994.
514. Yang WI, Zukerberg LR, Motokura T, Arnold A, Harris NL: Cyclin D1 (Bcl-1, PRAD1) protein expression in low-grade B-cell lymphomas and reactive hyperplasia. *Am J Pathol* **145**:86, 1994.
515. Fukuhara S, Rowley JD, Variakojis D, Golomb HM: Chromosome abnormalities in poorly differentiated lymphocytic lymphoma. *Cancer Res* **39**:3119, 1979.
516. Yunis JJ, Frizzera G, Oken MM, McKenna J, Theologides A, Arnesen M: Multiple recurrent genomic defects in follicular lymphoma. A possible model for cancer. *N Engl J Med* **316**:79, 1987.
517. Tsujimoto Y, Gorham J, Cossman J, Jaffe E, Croce CM: The t(14;18) chromosome translocations involved in B-cell neoplasms result from mistakes in VDJ joining. *Science* **229**:1390, 1985.
518. Bakhshi A, Jensen JP, Goldman P, Wright JJ, McBride OW, Epstein AL, Korsmeyer SJ: Cloning the chromosomal breakpoint of t(14;18) human lymphomas: clustering around JH on chromosome 14 and near a transcriptional unit on 18. *Cell* **41**:899, 1985.
519. Cleary ML, Sklar J: Nucleotide sequence of a t(14;18) chromosomal breakpoint in follicular lymphoma and demonstration of a breakpoint-cluster region near a transcriptionally active locus on chromosome 18. *Proc Natl Acad Sci USA* **82**:7439, 1985.
520. Cleary ML, Smith SD, Sklar J: Cloning and structural analysis of cDNAs for bcl-2 and a hybrid bcl-2/immunoglobulin transcript resulting from the t(14;18) translocation. *Cell* **47**:19, 1986.
521. Vaux DL, Cory S, Adams JM: Bcl-2 gene promotes haemopoietic cell survival and cooperates with c-myc to immortalize pre-B cells. *Nature* **335**:440, 1988.
522. Nunez G, London L, Hockenbery D, Alexander M, McKearn JP, Korsmeyer SJ: Deregulated Bcl-2 gene expression selectively prolongs survival of growth factor-deprived hemopoietic cell lines. *J Immunol* **144**:3602, 1990.
523. Korsmeyer SJ: Bcl-2 initiates a new category of oncogenes: Regulators of cell death. *Blood* **80**:879, 1992.
524. Yang E, Korsmeyer SJ: Molecular thanatopsis: A discourse on the BCL2 family and cell death. *Blood* **88**:386, 1996.
525. Hengartner MO, Horvitz HR: *C. elegans* cell survival gene ced-9 encodes a functional homolog of the mammalian proto-oncogene bcl-2. *Cell* **76**:665, 1994.
526. von Lindern M, Poustka A, Lerach H, Grosveld G: The (6;9) chromosome translocation, associated with a specific subtype of acute nonlymphocytic leukemia, leads to aberrant transcription of a target gene on 9q34. *Mol Cell Biol* **10**:4016, 1990.
527. von Lindern M, van Baal S, Wiegant J, Raap A, Hagemeijer A, Grosveld G: Can, a putative oncogene associated with myeloid leukemogenesis, may be activated by fusion of its 3′ half to different genes: characterization of the set gene. *Mol Cell Biol* **12**:3346, 1992.
528. von Lindern M, Breems D, van Baal S, Adriaansen H, Grosveld G: Characterization of the translocation breakpoint sequences of two DEK-CAN fusion genes present in t(6;9) acute myeloid leukemia and a SET-CAN fusion gene found in a case of acute undifferentiated leukemia. *Genes Chromosomes Cancer* **5**:227, 1992.
529. Borrow J, Shearman AM, Stanton VP Jr, Becher R, Collins T, Williams AJ, Dube I, Katz F, Kwong YL, Morris C, Ohyashiki K, Toyama K, Rowley J, Housman DE: The t(7;11)(p15;p15) translocation in acute myeloid leukaemia fuses the genes for nucleoporin NUP98 and class I homeoprotein HOXA9. *Nature Genet* **12**:159, 1996.
530. Nakamura T, Largaespada DA, Lee MP, Johnson LA, Ohyashiki K, Toyama K, Chen SJ, Willman CL, Chen IM, Feinberg AP, Jenkins NA, Copeland NG, Shaughnessy JD Jr: Fusion of the nucleoporin gene NUP98 to HOXA9 by the chromosome translocation t(7;11)(p15;p15) in human myeloid leukaemia. *Nature Genet* **12**:154, 1996.
531. Kraemer D, Wozniak RW, Blobel G, Radu A: The human CAN protein, a putative oncogene product associated with myeloid leukemogenesis, is a nuclear pore complex protein that faces the cytoplasm. *Proc Natl Acad Sci USA* **91**:1519, 1994.
532. Fornerod M, Boer J, van Baal S, Jaegle M, von Lindern M, Murti KG, Davis D, Bonten J, Buijs A, Grosveld G: Relocation of the carboxyterminal part of CAN from the nuclear envelope to the nucleus as a result of leukemia-specific chromosome rearrangements. *Oncogene* **10**:1739, 1995.
533. van Deursen J, Boer J, Kasper L, Grosveld G: G2 arrest and impaired nucleocytoplasmic transport in mouse embryos lacking the proto-oncogene CAN/Nup214. *EMBO J* **15**:5574, 1996.
534. Fornerod M, Boer J, van Baal S, Morreau H, Grosveld G: Interaction of cellular proteins with the leukemia specific fusion proteins DEK-CAN amd SET-CAN and their normal counterpart, the nucleoporin CAN. *Oncogene* **13**:1801, 1996.
535. Yoneda-Kato N, Look AT, Kirstein MN, Valentine MB, Raimondi SC, Cohen KJ, Carroll AJ, Morris SW: The t(3;5)(q25.1;q34) of myelodysplastic syndrome and acute myeloid leukemia produces a novel fusion gene, NPM-MLF1. *Oncogene* **12**:265, 1996.
536. Kuefer MU, Look AT, Williams DC, Valentine V, Naeve CW, Behm FG, Mullersman JE, Yoneda-Kato N, Montgomery K, Kucherlapati R, Morris SW: cDNA cloning, tissue distribution, and chromosomal localization of myelodysplasia/myeloid leukemia factor 2 (MLF2). *Genomics* **35**:392, 1996.
537. Dallery E, Galiegue Zouitina S, Collyn-d'Hooghe M, Quief S, Denis C, Hildebrand MP, Lantoine D, Deweindt C, Tilly H, Bastard C, et al: TTF, a gene encoding a novel small G protein, fuses to the lymphoma-associated LAZ3 gene by t(3;4) chromosomal translocation. *Oncogene* **10**:2171, 1995.
538. Ohno H, Takimoto G, McKeithan TW: The candidate proto-oncogene bcl-3 is related to genes implicated in cell lineage determination and cell cycle control. *Cell* **60**:991, 1990.
539. Wulczyn FG, Naumann M, Scheidereit C: Candidate proto-oncogene bcl-3 encodes a subunit-specific inhibitor of transcription factor NF-kappa B. *Nature* **358**:597, 1992.
540. Kerr LD, Duckett CS, Wamsley P, Zhang Q, Chiao P, Nabel G, McKeithan TW, Baeuerle PA, Verma IM: The proto-oncogene bcl-3 encodes an I kappa B protein. *Genes Dev* **6**:2352, 1992.
541. Neri A, Chang CC, Lombardi L, Salina M, Corradini P, Maiolo AT, Chaganti RS, Dalla-Favera R: B cell lymphoma-associated chromosomal translocation involves candidate oncogene lyt-10, homologous to NF-kappa B p50. *Cell* **67**:1075, 1991.
542. Iida S, Rao PH, Nallasivam P, Hibshoosh H, Butler M, Louie DC, Dyomin V, Ohno H, Chaganti RSK, Dalla-Favera R: The t(9;14)(p13;q32) chromosomal translocation associated with lymphoplasmacytoid lymphoma involves the PAX-5 gene. *Blood* **88**:4110, 1996.

543. Shimizu K, Miyoshi H, Kozu T, Nagata J, Enomoto K, Maseki N, Kaneko Y, Ohki M: Consistent disruption of the AML1 gene occurs within a single intron in the t(8;21) chromosomal translocation. *Cancer Res* **52**:6945, 1992.
544. Ichikawa H, Shimizu K, Hayashi Y, Ohki M: An RNA-binding protein gene, TLS/FUS, is fused to ERG in human myeloid leukemia with t(16;21) chromosomal translocation. *Cancer Res* **54**:2865, 1994.
545. Buijs A, Sherr S, van Baal S, van Bezouw S, van der Plas D, Geurts van Kessel A, Riegman P, Lekanne Deprez R, Zwarthoff E, Hagemeijer A, et al: Translocation (12;22) (p13;q11) in myeloproliferative disorders results in fusion of the ETS-like TEL gene on 12p13 to the MN1 gene on 22q11 [published erratum appears in *Oncogene* **11(4)**:809, 1995]. *Oncogene* **10**:1511, 1995.
546. Peeters P, Wlodarska I, Baens M, Criel A, Selleslag D, Hagemeier A, Van den Berghe H, Marynen P: Fusion of ETV6 to MDS1/EV11 as a result of t(3;12)(q26;p13) in myeloproliferative disorders. *Cancer Res* **57**:564, 1997.
547. Borrow J, Stanton VP Jr, Andresen JM, Becher R, Behm FG, Chaganti RS, Civin CI, Disteche C, Dube I, Frischauf AM, Horsman D, Mitelman F, Volinia S, Watmore AE, Housman DE: The translocation t(8;16)(p11;p13) of acute myeloid leukaemia fuses a putative acetyltransferase to the CREB-binding protein. *Nature Genet* **14**:33, 1996.
548. Carapeti M, Aguiar RC, Goldman JM, Cross NC: A novel fusion between MOZ and the nuclear receptor coactivator TIF2 in acute myeloid leukemia. *Blood* **91**:3127, 1998.
549. Bernard OA, Mauchauffe M, Mecucci C, Van den Berghe H, Berger R: A novel gene, AF-1p, fused to HRX in t(1;11)(p32;q23), is not related to AF-4, AF-9 nor ENL. *Oncogene* **9**:1039, 1994.
550. Hillion J, Leconiat M, Jonveaux P, Berger R, Bernard OA: AF6q21, a novel partner of the MLL gene in t(6;11)(q21;q23), defines a forkhead transcriptional factor subfamily. *Blood* **90**:3714, 1997.
551. Chaplin T, Ayton P, Bernard OA, Saha V, Della Valle V, Hillion J, Gregorini A, Lillington D, Berger R, Young BD: A novel class of zinc finger/leucine zipper genes identified from the molecular cloning of the t(10;11) translocation in acute leukemia. *Blood* **85**:1435, 1995.
552. Prasad R, Leshkowitz D, Gu Y, Alder H, Nakamura T, Saito H, Huebner K, Berger R, Croce CM, Canaani E: Leucine-zipper dimerization motif encoded by the AF17 gene fused to ALL-1 (MLL) in acute leukemia. *Proc Natl Acad Sci USA* **91**:8107, 1994.
553. Parry P, Wei Y, Evans G: Cloning and characterization of the t(X;11) breakpoint from a leukemic cell line identify a new member of the forkhead gene family. *Genes Chromosomes Cancer* **11**:79, 1994.
554. Taki T, Sako M, Tsuchida M, Hayashi Y: The t(11;16)(q23;p13) translocation in myelodysplastic syndrome fuses the MLL gene to the CBP gene. *Blood* **89**:3945, 1997.
555. Rowley JD, Reshmi S, Sobulo O, Musvee T, Anastasi J, Raimondi S, Schneider NR, Barredo JC, Cantu ES, Schlegelberger B, Behm F, Doggett NA, Borrow J, Zeleznik-Le N: All patients with the T(11;16)(q23;p13.3) that involves MLL and CBP have treatment-related hematologic disorders. *Blood* **90**:535, 1997.
556. Peeters P, Raynoud SD, Cools J, Wlodarska I, Grosgeorge J, Philip P, Monpoux F, Van Rompey L, Baens M, Van den Berghe H, Marynen P: Fusion of TEL, the ETS variant gene 6 (ETV6) to the receptor-associated kinase JAK2 as a result of t(9;12) in a lymphoid and t(9;15;12) in a myeloid leukemia. *Blood* **90**:2535, 1997.
557. Lachronique V, Boureux A, Della Valle V, Poirel H, Tran Quang C, Mauchauffe M, Berthou C, Lessard M, Berger R, Ghysdael J, Bernard OA: A TEL-JAK2 fusion protein with constitutive kinase activity in human leukemia. *Science* **278**:1309, 1997.
558. Ross TS, Bernard OA, Berger R, Gilliland DG: Fusion of Huntington interacting protein 1 to platelet-derived growth factor β receptor (PDGFβR) in chronic myelomonocytic leukemia with t(5;7)(q33;q11.2). *Blood* **91**:4419, 1998.
559. Abe A, Emi N, Mitsune T, Hiroshi T, Marunouchi T, Hidehiko S: Fusion of the platelet-derived growth factor receptor beta to a novel gene CEV14 in acute myelogenous leukemia after clonal evolution. *Blood* **90**:1997.
560. Tycko B, Smith SD, Sklar J: Chromosomal translocations joining LCK and TCRB loci in human T cell leukemia. *J Exp Med* **174**:867, 1991.
561. Burnett RC, David JC, Harden AM, Le Beau MM, Rowley JD, Diaz MO: The LCK gene is involved in the t(1;7)(p34;q34) in the T-cell acute lymphoblastic leukemia derived cell line, HSB-2. *Genes Chromosomes Cancer* **3**:461, 1991.
562. Wright DD, Sefton BM, Kamps MP: Oncogenic activation of the Lck protein accompanies translocation of the LCK gene in the human HSB2 T-cell leukemia. *Mol Cell Biol* **14**:2429, 1994.
563. von Lindern M, Fornerod M, van Baal S, Jaegle M, de Wit T, Buijs A, Grosveld G: The translocation (6;9), associated with a specific subtype of acute myeloid leukemia, results in the fusion of two genes, dek and can, and the expression of a chimeric, leukemia-specific dek-can mRNA. *Mol Cell Biol* **12**:1687, 1992.
564. Dreyling MH, Martinez Climent JA, Zheng M, Mao J, Rowley JD, Bohlander SK: The t(10;11)(p13;q14) in the U937 cell line results in the fusion of the AF10 gene and CALM, encoding a new member of the AP-3 clathrin assembly protein family. *Proc Natl Acad Sci USA* **93**:4804, 1996.
565. Fisch P, Forster A, Sherrington PD, Dyer MJ, Rabbitts TH: The chromosomal translocation t(X;14)(q28;q11) in T-cell pro-lymphocytic leukaemia breaks within one gene and activates another. *Oncogene* **8**:3271, 1993.
566. Ellisen LW, Bird J, West DC, Soreng AL, Reynolds TC, Smith SD, Sklar J: TAN-1, the human homolog of the *Drosophila* notch gene, is broken by chromosomal translocations in T lymphoblastic neoplasms. *Cell* **66**:649, 1991.
567. Grimaldi JC, Meeker TC: The t(5;14) chromosomal translocation in a case of acute lymphocytic leukemia joins the interleukin-3 gene to the immunoglobulin heavy chain gene. *Blood* **73**:2081, 1989.
568. Meeker TC, Hardy D, Willman C, Hogan T, Abrams J: Activation of the interleukin-3 gene by chromosome translocation in acute lymphocytic leukemia with eosinophilia. *Blood* **76**:285, 1990.
569. Laabi Y, Gras MP, Carbonnel F, Brouet JC, Berger R, Larsen CJ, Tsapis A: A new gene, BCM, on chromosome 16 is fused to the interleukin 2 gene by a t(4;16)(q26;p13) translocation in a malignant T cell lymphoma. *EMBO J* **11**:3897, 1992.
570. Virgilio L, Lazzeri C, Bichi R, Nibu K, Narducci MG, Russo G, Rothstein JL, Croce CM: Deregulated expression of TCL1 causes T cell leukemia in mice. *Proc Natl Acad Sci USA* **95**:3885, 1998.
571. Madani A, Choukroun V, Soulier J, Cacheux V, Claisse JF, Valensi F, Daliphard S, Cazin B, Levy V, Leblond V, Daniel MT, Sigaux F, Stern MH: Expression of p13MTCP1 is restricted to mature T-cell proliferations with t(X;14) translocations. *Blood* **87**:1923, 1996.
572. Gritti C, Choukroun V, Soulier J, Madani A, Dastot H, Leblond V, Radford-Weiss I, Valensi F, Varet B, Sigaux F, Stern MH: Alternative origin of p13MTCP1-encoding transcripts in mature T-cell proliferations with t(X;14) translocations. *Oncogene* **15**:1329, 1997.
573. Seto M, Yamamoto K, Takahashi T, Ueda R: Cloning and expression of a murine cDNA homologous to the human RCK/P54, a lymphoma-linked chromosomal translocation junction gene on 11q23. *Gene* **166**:293, 1995.
574. Sandlund JT, Downing JR, Crist WM: Non-Hodgkins's lymphoma in childhood. *N Engl J Med* **334**:1238, 1996.
575. Downing JR, Look AT: MLL fusion genes in the 11q23 acute leukemias, in Freireich EJ, Kantarjian H (eds): *Leukemia: Advances in Research and Treatment*. Boston, Kluwer Academic Publishers, 1995, p. 73.

CHAPTER 20

Chromosome Alterations in Human Solid Tumors

Paul S. Meltzer ▪ Anne Kallioniemi ▪ Jeffrey M. Trent

1. Recurring sites of chromosome change represent the byproducts of molecular events that participate in the generation or progression of human cancers. Chromosome abnormalities in patients with hematopoietic cancers have proven to be of diagnostic and prognostic value, and the molecular defects for many have been described (see Chap. 19). Despite solid tumors being exceedingly more common than the blood-borne cancers of man, and their significantly greater contribution to morbidity and mortality relative to hematologic neoplasms, less is known about chromosome changes and their clinical and biologic importance in solid tumors. Nevertheless, significant information is accumulating on recurring chromosome alterations in solid tumors including the molecular dissection of recurring breakpoints in many malignancies.

2. The pattern of chromosome alterations in human solid tumors is decidedly nonrandom. Solid tumors tend to demonstrate multiple clonal structural and numeric chromosome rearrangements and databases are being developed to describe new karyotypic abnormalities in the context of tumor histopathology.

3. General categories of structural chromosome rearrangements in human solid tumors include chromosome translocations, deletions, inversions and changes associated with increases in DNA sequence copy number (double minutes [dmin]; and homogeneously staining regions [HSRs]).

4. Tumor-specific chromosome rearrangements have been identified in human solid tumors. Chromosome alterations in many common cancers are described.

5. Human sarcomas represent a paradigm for molecular dissection of human solid tumors. Tumor-specific chromosome translocations have been described and characterized at the molecular level for several sarcomas including Ewing's sarcoma, alveolar rhabdomyosarcoma, synovial sarcoma, myxoid liposarcoma, and soft tissue clear-cell sarcoma. In general, these translocations juxtapose segments of two genes, which can give rise to a chimeric fusion transcript. Two closely related genes *EWS* (on chromosome 22q12) and *FUS* (on chromosome 16p11) have been demonstrated to participate in tumor-specific translocations in several sarcomas. In each case, *EWS* or *FUS* acquires a DNA-binding domain from the translocation partner chromosome. These tumor-specific chimeric oncoproteins have transcription factor activity, and it appears that they contribute to malignant transformation by leading to dysregulated gene expression.

6. Numerous benign neoplasms, such as lipoma and leiomyoma, exhibit translocations involving members of the HMGI family of DNA-binding proteins. Multiple-partner genes are involved with one of the two HMGI genes in various tumors. The disturbance of HMGI protein function appears to have a profound effect on the proliferation of mesenchymal cells in multiple lineages, yet these tumors do not become malignant.

7. The clinical value of chromosome rearrangements in the common solid tumors of adults is largely indeterminate. Recent advances and the development of new technical approaches for analysis of complex changes in solid tumors suggest that further insights into chromosome rearrangements (and the genes dysregulated by them) may increase clinical utility.

It is now recognized that most human cancers (including solid tumors) display recurring chromosome abnormalities. However, questions remain in most cases as to their exact biologic significance. How do chromosomal changes relate to changes in expression of important genes (including oncogenes)? What is the significance of a recurring cytogenetic alteration when viewed against a background of other (often multiple) genetic alterations? What clinical significance, if any, do specific cytogenetic abnormalities have for solid tumors? These questions have been the focus of intense study over the past decade and our recognition and recently our molecular understanding of chromosome abnormalities is providing significant insights into neoplasms in general and solid tumors particularly.

Significant progress has been made in tumor cytogenetics in recent years. For example, prior to 1981 there were only 1800 cases of malignancies with abnormal chromosomes reported in all of the world's literature, and <3 percent were from solid tumors. By the end of 1994, there were $>22{,}000$ published cases of neoplasms with abnormal karyotypes, and 27 percent of those were from solid tumors. Knowledge within this area has continued and through June of 1996, 26,523 cases, including 215 balanced and 1588 unbalanced recurrent aberrations, were identified among 75 different neoplastic disorders. This data is regularly updated by Prof. Felix Mitelman, and is available by CD-ROM,[1] or on the World Wide Web (www.ncbi.nlm.nih.gov/CCAP/NG/).

With this explosion in our knowledge of human chromosome alterations in neoplasia, has come the widespread acceptance of the clinical value of chromosome analysis in studies of human hematologic cancers. Specifically, chromosome analysis of malignant cells from patients with hematopoietic cancers provides diagnostic and equally importantly prognostic information independent of other laboratory and clinical feature of disease (see Chap. 24).[2–4] Despite solid tumors representing almost 95 percent of the cancers of humankind, far less is known about chromosome changes and especially their clinical importance in solid tumors. This chapter focuses on features of solid tumor cytogenetics that can be related to our understanding of the biologic and hopefully clinical utility of this information.

Two excellent books by Heim and Mitelman,[3] and Sandberg,[2] survey the field of cancer cytogenetics and provide in-depth descriptions of chromosome changes by histopathologic subtype. There is also a useful (but didactic) description of all published cytogenetic changes in the reported literature, which may be of interest for those who seek a listings of all chromosome changes, in the *Catalog of Chromosome Aberrations in Cancer.*[1] Finally, Thompson provides a comprehensive manual related to methodology for analysis of solid tumors.[5] The interested reader is referred to these sources for in-depth information on techniques as well as detailed karyotypic information on any given tumor type.

GENERAL ASPECTS OF CHROMOSOME CHANGE IN SOLID TUMORS

The diversity of structural chromosome alterations across the spectrum of human cancers is enormous and increasing rapidly. The central dogma underlying the study of chromosomes in cancer is that karyotypic changes are nonrandom, and thus are distributed erratically throughout the human genome. Specific chromosome bands are preferentially involved in rearrangements in different neoplasms, and increasingly, the underlying molecular defects are being understood. Examination of the nonrandom nature of chromosome alterations has led to the identification of >200 recurring chromosome changes in >70 neoplastic disorders (including now many benign proliferations).[1] Every human chromosome, with the exception of the Y chromosome, can be included in some form of neoplasia-associated alteration.

Methodology and Clonality

Technical obstacles are frequently responsible for the relative paucity of cytogenetic information from solid tumor samples. These obstacles include difficulties in sample disaggregation, cell viability due to necrosis of biopsy samples, contamination of samples with normal cells, and the complexity of most tumors (especially carcinomas) that frequently display a heterogeneous pattern of chromosome change. In most solid tumors, the time of clinical manifestation and removal of the tumor mass is thought to occur at a point considerably distant from cellular transformation, resulting in the generation of significant chromosomal rearrangement and imbalances. From a technical point of view, this means that in some solid tumors no two karyotypes from the same specimen may be identical, and that as few as one or as many as 100 chromosome rearrangements may be described within a single karyotype. To confuse matters even more, there is evidence that at least some tumors may arise from multiple stem cells or diverge soon after appearance of an initiating transformation event and then undergo clonal expansion of cell populations with unrelated karyotypes (i.e., they may be "polyclonal" in origin).[6–9] However, even with these complex karyotypes and heterogeneous tumor cell populations it has been possible to describe certain chromosomal abnormalities that are germinal to the development of a given tumor type. *Primary chromosome aberrations* are frequently found as the sole karyotypic abnormality in a neoplastic cell, and reflect their presumed causal role in cellular transformation. *Secondary chromosome aberrations* are thought to be important in tumor progression, do not appear alone, but nevertheless display nonrandom features with distribution patterns that are frequently tumor-type dependent. It is believed that the features of genetic instability, divergence, and heterogeneity observed in most solid tumors, represent significant genetic obstacles to effective patient treatment through "Darwinian" selection of genetically rearranged cells with proliferative (or therapy resistance) advantage.

Despite the difficulty in analyzing solid tumors cytogenetically, there is overwhelming information that most cancers are monoclonal (and thus all cells of a tumor share genetic characteristics of the original transformed cells), and therefore cancer is heritable at the cellular level.[9] This discovery, which was initially based largely on cytogenetic evidence, has been a major factor in reaching the conclusion that changes in DNA sequences of individual cells are responsible for malignant changes in those cells.

Terminology

As described previously, the results of tumor chromosome studies are complex and challenging to summarize. The range of chromosome counts may be quite wide, for example, from hypodiploid (e.g., <46 chromosomes/cell) to hypertetraploid (>96 chromosomes), and it is not uncommon to find more than one modal number. It is also generally true that, even when karyotyping cells with the same number of chromosomes, no two karyotypes from the same specimen are completely identical in all numeric as well as structural abnormalities observed. Consequently the field ordinarily describes the *clonal changes* that are evident and that make up a composite karyotype interpretation of the specimen. A numeric abnormality is said to be clonal if a missing chromosome is observed in at least three karyotypes, and an extra chromosome is found in at least two, while a clonal structural abnormality is described if it is found in two or more cells. Karyotypic anomalies, which are found in a majority of cells from a tumor, are said to represent the *stemline* population, while those abnormalities that are found in a small proportion of karyotypes are said to represent a *sideline* population. Multiple sidelines may (and usually do) exist in the same tumor sample. Many of the problems associated with describing complex karyotypes and multiple sidelines have been addressed by international convention according an International System of Cytogenetic Nomenclature (ISCN)[10] and all descriptions of cancer (and constitutional) karyotypic are written in accordance with the ISCN recommendations. Table 20-1 gives representative examples of abbreviations utilized in chromosome nomenclature of solid tumors.

RECURRING CHROMOSOME ALTERATIONS IN HUMAN SOLID TUMORS

General Findings

Although it has been difficult to obtain information on chromosome alterations in solid tumors, nonetheless, many recurring cytogenetic alterations have been described and a summary of nonrandom chromosomal abnormalities is presented in Table 20-2. Representative examples of chromosome rearrangements in human solid tumors are documented in banded cells from two different cancers (Figs. 20-1 and 20-2). Examples of the utility of

Table 20-1 Chromosome Nomenclature

A–G	Chromosome groups
1–22	Autosome numbers
X, Y	Sex chromosomes
/	Diagonal line indicates *mosaicism*, e.g., 46/47 designates a mosaic with 46-chromosome and 47-chromosome cell lines
p	Short arm of chromosome, "petite"
q	Long arm of chromosome
del	Deletion
der	Derivative of chromosome
dup	Duplication
I	Isochromosome
ins	Insertion
inv	Inversion
r	Ring chromsome
t	Translocation
ter	Terminal (may also be written as pter or qter)
+ or −	Placed *before* the chromosome number, these symbols indicate addition (+) or loss (−) of a whole chromosome; e.g., +21 indicates an extra chromosome 21, as in Down syndrome. Placed *after* the chromosome number, these symbols indicate gain or loss of a chromosome part; e.g., 5p− indicates loss of part of the short arm of chromosome 5, as in cri-du-chat syndrome.

From Gelehrter and Collins.[199] Used with permission.

Table 20-2 Recurring Karyotypic Abnormalities in Human Solid Tumors*

Tumor type	Karyotype abnormalities and other findings
Malignant	
Bladder (transitional cell carcinoma)	**+7; del(10)(q22–q24); del(21)(q22)**; del(21)(q22); del and t of 1q21; i(5p); −9; i(11q); del and t of 11p11–q11; del, t, and dup of 13q14
Brain, rhabdoid tumor	−22
Breast (adenocarcinoma)	del(1)p11–p13; del(3)q11–13; del(5q); **−17; i(1q); der(16)t(1;16)(q10;p10); del(1)(q11–q12); del(3)(p12–p13p41–p21); del(6)(q21–q22); +7; +18; +20**; del and t of 1p11–p13; t of 1q21–q23; 3q11–q13, 7q32–q36, and 11q13–q14; dup of 11q13–q14; dmins; hsrs
Colon (adenocarcinoma)	**+7; +20**; i(1q); inv and t of 1p11–q11; i(7q); I(8q); +7; t of 7p11–q11; +8; +12; del of 12q; i(17q); t of 17p11–q11; del of 17p; −18; dmins
Ewing's sarcoma	**t(11;22)(q24;q12)**; t(1;16)(q11;q11.1) +8
Extraskeletal myxoid chondrosarcoma	**−Y; t(9;22)(q22;q12)**
Fibrosarcoma	**−Y**
Giant cell tumors	**+8**; telomeric fusions of 11p15, 13p, 15p, 18p, 19p, 21p; fus(14p;21p); fus(15p;21p)
Glioma[†]	**+7; −10; −22; −X; +X; −Y**; del(22)(q11–q13); del or t of 9
Hepatoblastoma	gain of 2q
Kidney (renal cell carcinoma)	**del(3)(p14–p21); del(3)(p11–p14); t(3;5)(p13;q22); −3; +7; −8; +10; −Y**; t(3;8)(p14;q24), t(3;11) (p13–p14;p15); i(5p); del(6)(q21–q23)
Kidney (papillary carcinoma)	+7; +17; **t(X;1)(p11;q21)**
Larynx (squamous cell carcinoma)	**−Y**
Liposarcoma (myxoid)	**t(12;16)(q13;p11)**
Lung (adenocarcinoma)	**del(3)(p14p23); +7**
Lung (small cell carcinoma)	**del(3)(p14p23); +7**; del of 5q, 6, 9p, 13q, 17p
Lung (squamous cell carcinoma)	**+7**
Fibrous histiocytoma	**−Y**
Melanoma, cutaneous	t(1;6)(q11–q21; q11–q13); t(1;19)(q11;q13); t of 1q11–q12 that yield 1q gain; del and t of 1p11–q12; i(6p); t of 6p11–q11 that yields 6p gain; other t of 6q11–q13; t of 7q11; +7; del and t 9p
Melanoma, uveal	−3; partial del of 3; +8; i(8q)
Meningioma	**−22; +22; −Y; del(22)(q11–q13)**
Mesothelioma	del, t, dup, or inv of 3p21–p23
Nasopharynx (squamous cell carcinoma)	**−Y**
Neuroblastoma	**del(1)(p32–p36)**; t which yield del of 1p32–p36; der(1)t(1;17)(p36;?); dmins
Ovary (carcinoma)	**+12, +7, +8, −X**; del(6q15–q23), del(3) (p21–p10); +3; +5; loss of 1p; gain of 1q; t(1;17)(p36;?); dmins; hsrs; hsrs of 19q13.1–q13.2, t(6;14)(q21;q24)
Primitive neuroectodermal tumors	i(17q)
Prostate (carcinoma)	**del(10)(q24), +7, −Y**, del(7q)
Retinoblastoma	**i(6p); del(13)(q14.1q14.1)**
Rhabdomyosarcoma (alveolar)	**t(2;13)(q37;q14); t(1;13)(p36;q14)**
Salivary gland (carcinoma)	**del(6)(q22–q25); +8; −Y**
Skin (basal cell carcinoma)	**t(9;16)(q22;p13)**
Oral (squamous cell carcinoma)	**+7**
Synovial sarcoma	**t(X;18)(p11;q11)**
Germ cell tumors (seminoma, teratoma)	i(12p); other structural abnormalities which yield 12p gain
Thyroid (adenocarcinoma)	**inv(10)(q11q21)**
Uterus (adenocarcinoma)	**+10**; i(1q); del or t of 1q21; del(6) (q21)

Table 20-2 (Continued)

Tumor type	Karyotype abnormalities and other findings
Wilms' tumor	**del(11)(p13p13); del(11)(p15p15)**; i(1q); t(1;16)(q10;q10)
Benign	
Barrett's esophagus	**−Y**
Breast fibroadenoma	der(1;16)(q10;p10), del(3p)
Colon (adenoma)	+7; **+8; +12; del of 12q, del(1)(p36)**
Giant cell tumor	**+8**
Kidney (adenoma)	− Y, +7, +17
Lipoma	**t(1;12)(p33−p34;q13−q15); t(2;12) (p22−p23;q13−q15); t(3;12)(q27−q28;q13−q15); t(5;12)(q33;q13−q15); t(11;12)(q13;q13−q15); del(12)(q13q15); t(12;21)(q13−q15;q21); del(13)(q12−q22)**
Lung (hamartoma)	**t(6;14)(p21;q24)**
Neuorepithelioma	**t(11;12)(q24;q12)**
Neurinoma	**−22; −Y**
Orbital fibroma	**t(X;2)(q26;q33)**
Ovary (adenoma)	**+12**
Ovary (fibroma)	**+12**
Ovary (thecoma)	**+12**
Salivary gland (pleomorphic adenoma)	**t(1;8)(p22;q12); t(3;8)(p21;q12); t(6;8)(p21−p22;q12); t(8;13)(p23;q13−q14); del(8)(q12q21−q22); t(8;9)(q12;p22); t(9;12)(p21−p24;q13−q15); inv(12)(p13q13)**
Thyroid adenoma	**+5, +7, +12, structural abnormalities of 19q**
Uterus (leiomyoma)	**r(1)(p11−p36q11−q14); t(2;12) (q35−q37;q14); del(7)(q21−q22q31−q32); t(12;14)(q14−q15;q23−q24); +12; other translocations of 12q13−q15; structural abnormalities with 1p36 and 6p21 breakpoints**

†Includes glioma, anaplastic glioma, glioblastoma, astrocytoma, oligodendroglioma, and ependymoma. **Primary karyotype changes are in boldface type**, secondary changes are in normal type. Generic structural alterations are given by ISCN abbreviations (e.g., del for deletions; t for translocations; inv for inversions; dup for duplications) to shorten text (see Table 20-1 and Thompson[5]).

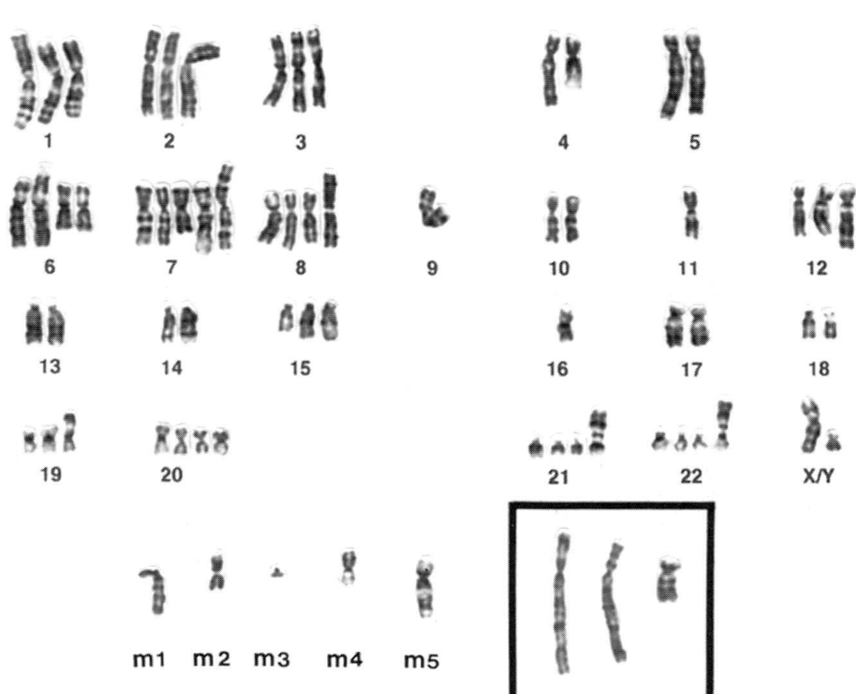

Fig. 20-1 Representative G-banded karyotype from a human malignant melanoma demonstrating numerous structural and numeric alterations. The bottom of the figure illustrates marker (m) chromosomes that represent chromosomes rearranged beyond recognition of their normal component chromosome(s). ***(From Kamb A, Gruis NA, Weaver-Feldhaus J, et al.[98] Used by permission of the publisher.)***

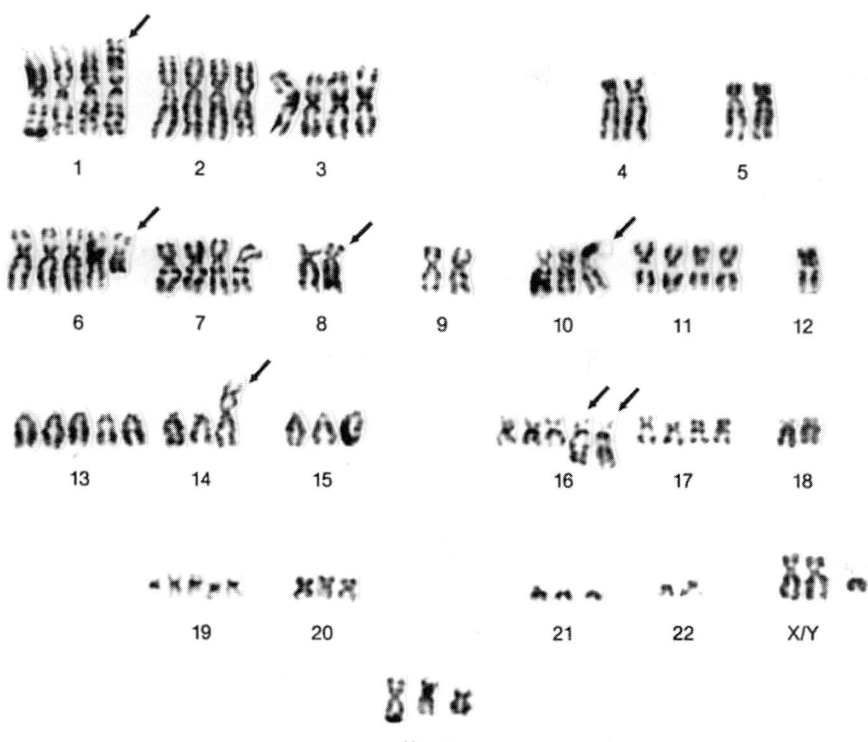

Fig. 20-2 Representative G-banded karyotype from a malignant metastatic colon adenocarcinoma demonstrating numerous structural (arrows) and numeric alterations, as well as unidentifiable marker chromosomes (Umars).

fluorescence *in situ* hybridization (FISH) as a powerful approach to identify either the entire or specific regions of all human chromosomes (Fig. 20-3), and for analysis of complex rearrangements (Fig. 20-4) are provided. More detailed information on these cancers is provided in other chapters. The application of a new technology for independently identifying all chromosomes (termed SKY) has significant potential for elucidating previously unknown chromosomal rearrangements (Fig. 20-3).[11] After a brief discussion of generic classes of chromosome rearrangements, short summaries of recurring chromosome alterations of selected cancers are provided. A detailed description of human sarcomas is presented to highlight the significant and unique (to solid tumors) molecular characterization of these cancers.

Generally, abnormalities of chromosome 1 are nearly universal, and the high frequency of alterations in the majority of solid tumors has led to the suggestion that these changes represent a frequent event in the progression, but not the genesis, of various cancers. In general the reports of clinical relevance have been limited to studies in neuroblastoma where deletion of 1p correlates with specific oncogene (NMYC) amplification (see Chap. 60).[12,13] In addition to structural alterations of chromosome 1, gain of chromosome 7 is one of the most common abnormalities in epithelial tumors and has been identified as a primary karyotype abnormality in a number of tumors.[1,14–18]

Cytologic Evidence of Gene Amplification

Another frequent category of chromosome alteration in solid tumors characterizes a clinically important mechanism for activation of oncogene overexpression — DNA sequence amplification (see Chap. 26). This increase in DNA sequence copy number change often results in cytologically recognizable chromosome alterations referred to as either homogeneously staining regions (HSRs), if integrated within chromosomes, or double minutes (dmin), if extrachromosomal in nature (Fig. 20-5). Figures 20-6 and 20-7 illustrate the use of fluorescence in situ hybridization (FISH) technologies and chromosome microdissection combined to identify changes in DNA copy number recognizable within a tumor, as well as providing specific examples of HSRs and dmin in human breast and ovarian cancer.

Comparative Genomic Hybridization (CGH)

Copy number changes of individual genes and loci, as well as chromosomes and chromosomal subregions, are characteristic of human cancer, especially solid tumors. Conventional cytogenetic studies of solid tumors are sometimes difficult, because metaphases are often impossible to obtain, and genomic instability and clonal heterogeneity make data interpretation difficult. Comparative genomic hybridization (CGH) was developed to allow genome-wide screening of DNA sequence copy number aberrations in cancer (Figs. 20-8 and 20-9).[19,20] Applications of CGH in cancer genetics include characterization of recurrent unbalanced genomic rearrangements, defining novel genes involved in copy number alterations, analysis of progression and clonal evolution of cancer, as well as subclassification and prognostic evaluation of cancer. In this respect, CGH studies have already substantially contributed to our understanding of cancer biology.

CGH has most often been applied to the identification of common clonal chromosomal aberrations in cancer. When CGH data from several studies are combined, consistent patterns of nonrandom genetic aberrations emerge. Some of these changes appear to be common to various kinds of malignant tumors, while others are more tumor-specific. For example, gains of chromosomal regions 1q, 3q, and 8q, as well as losses of 8p, 13q, 16q, and 17p, are common to a number of tumor types, such as breast, ovarian, prostate, renal, and bladder cancer.[21,22] Other alterations, such as 12p and Xp gains in testicular cancer, 13q gain and 9q loss in bladder cancer, 14q loss in renal cancer, and Xp loss in ovarian cancer are more tumor-specific and may reflect the unique pathways of cancer development in different organs.

CGH has also played an important role in pinpointing putative locations of cancer genes, especially at chromosomal sites undergoing DNA amplification. There are several examples of genes whose amplification in cancer were discovered based on leads from CGH analysis. In most cases, the amplification target gene was identified based on candidate genes previously localized

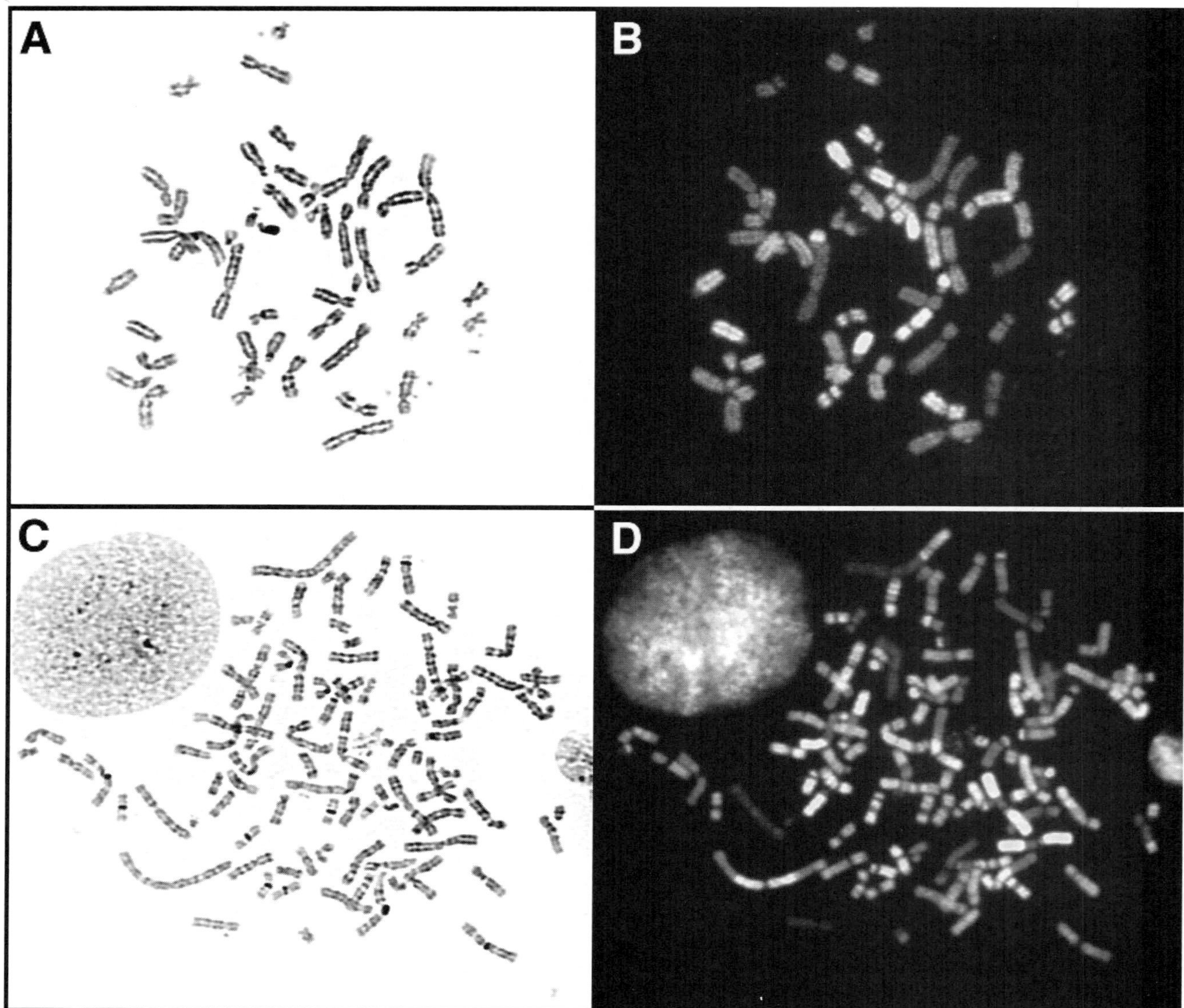

Fig. 20-3 Illustration of a G-banded normal metaphase cell (*A*) and the spectral karyotyping (SKY) of the same cell (*B*) performed following the simultaneous hybridization of 24 combinatorially labeled chromosome painting probes (Schröck et al. Multicolor spectral karyotyping of human chromosomes. *Science* 273:494, 1996). The resulting spectral analysis assigns a unique color to each of the 24 human chromosomes. This is contrasted to the G-banding of a tumor metaphase cell (*C*) and the identical cell following SKY (*D*). In addition to an increase in chromosome number, the combination of colors along the length of a single chromosome in the tumor cell documents extensive interchromosomal rearrangement.

to the region of involvement indicated by CGH. The androgen receptor (AR) (at Xq11-q12) was found to be amplified in recurrent prostate cancer after androgen deprivation therapy.[23] Other CGH studies have implicated amplification of oncogenes whose activation in cancer was previously known to occur by chromosomal translocations only. Such examples include amplification of the REL proto-oncogene (at 2p14-p15) in non-Hodgkin lymphomas,[24,25] BCL2 (at 18q21.3) in recurrent B-cell lymphomas,[26] and PAX7-FKHR fusion gene (fusing 1p36 and 13q14) in alveolar rhabdomyosarcoma.[27] Finally, a common site of amplification in breast and other cancers is at 20q. Several groups have identified novel genes that are involved in this amplification. These include the AIB1 gene, a steroid receptor coactivator,[28] BTAK, a serine/threonine kinase,[29] ZNF217, a transcription factor,[30] and NABC1 gene of unknown function,[30] all of which have been identified as amplified and overexpressed in breast cancers.

Overall, it is likely that many additional examples of novel gene amplifications in cancer are likely to emerge in future studies. The clinical significance of such novel amplified genes needs to be evaluated in large patient materials. The recently developed tissue microarray technology provides a valuable tool for high-throughput molecular profiling of large panels of uncultured tumor specimens.[31,28] This technology can be applied to rapid copy number and expression analyses of several genes in hundreds of tumors in different stages of the disease (Fig. 20-10).

The ability of CGH to evaluate archival tumor tissues makes it especially suitable to the analysis of clonal evolution of cancer progression. Analysis of genetic changes in tumors at different stages, such as premalignant lesions, in situ carcinoma and invasive cancer, may highlight aberrations involved in these specific steps of tumor progression.[32–34] CGH results are particularly informative when clonal relationships between two cancer specimens taken from the same patient are available for analysis.[35] For example, genetic changes that are not found in primary tumors, but do occur in their metastases are informative in

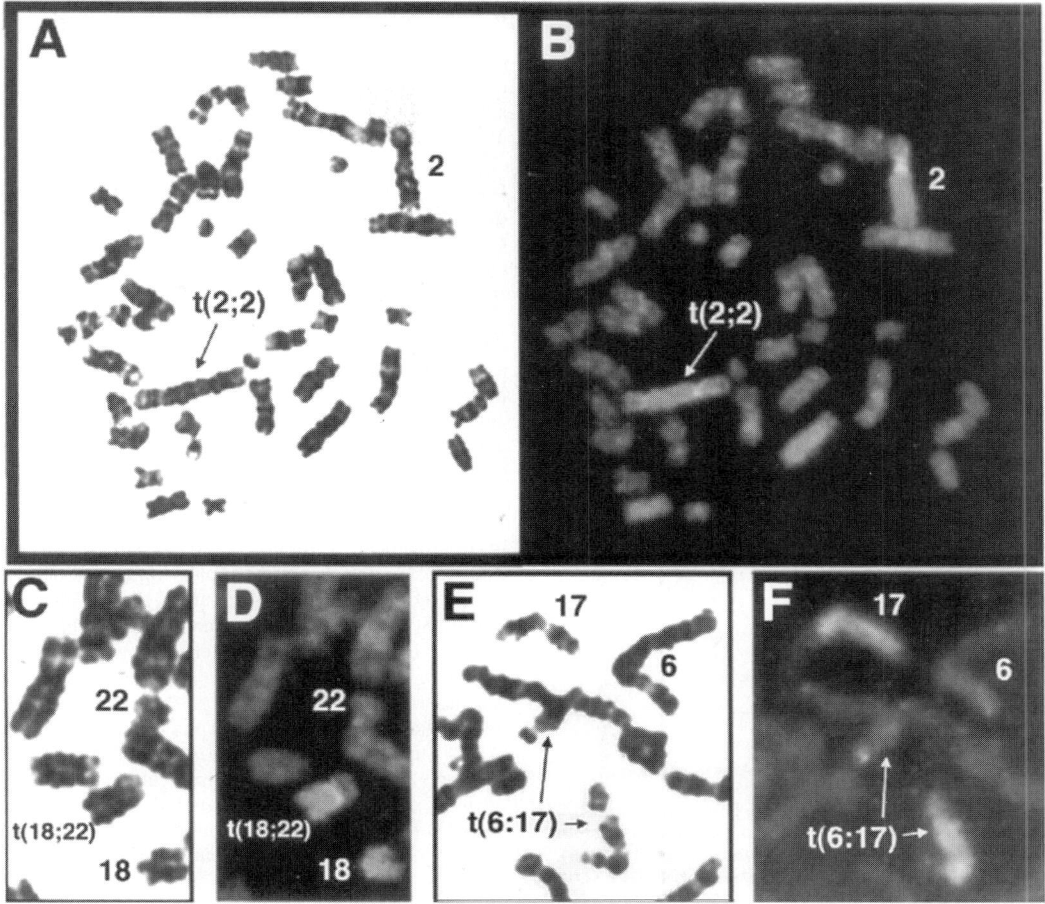

Fig. 20-4 Illustration of the application of fluorescent *in situ* hybridization (FISH) to detect complex chromosome rearrangements in malignancy. In this case, a cancer with three different translocations [t(2;2); t(18;22); and t(6;17)] were studied using probes specific for the long and short arm or each involved chromosome. *A*, G-banded metaphase. *B*, The identical metaphase as *A*, hybridized with fluorescent probes for the long arm and short arm of chromosome 2. A normal copy of chromosome 2 and a rearranged chromosome 2 (arrow) was observed. *C* and *D* represent detection of reciprocal translocations between chromosomes 18 and 22 (C/D) and 6 and 17 (E/F). In both cases, a partial G-banded metaphase is shown on the left, FISH using probes specific for each involved chromosome arm is shown on the right. (*From Guan X-Y, Zhang H, Bittner ML, Jiang Y, Meltzer PS, Trent JM.*[117] *Used by permission of the publisher.*)

pinpointing genetic changes and genes with important roles in the metastatic progression.

The following sections briefly overview several of the major tumor types for which significant cytogenetic information is available.

Transitional Cell Carcinoma (TCC) of the Bladder. Among the first cytogenetic studies to demonstrate the clinical importance of cytogenetic results in a human solid tumor were reports characterizing the propensity for recurrence of bladder tumors with cytogenetic abnormalities.[36,37] Long-term follow-up demonstrated that patients with abnormal karyotypes had a greater rate of tumor recurrence than patients with normal karyotypes (measured as the presence of detectable gross structural rearrangements). More recent studies corroborate these data and in general patients with diploid tumors appear to have a more favorable outcomes than patients with a mix of diploid and hyperdiploid, or hyperdiploid tumors.[38]

Chromosomes most frequently altered in this tumor type[2,3,39–45] include +7, del(10)(q22–24), and del(21)(q22). Other consistent chromosome alterations are also listed in Table 20-2. Another recurring change characterizing bladder cancers is loss of one copy of chromosome 9 (termed monosomy 9).[44,45] These results have been confirmed by loss of heterozygosity (LOH) studies, and appear to suggest that an initiating genetic defect in bladder tumors is associated with deletion of 9p.[44,45]

Brain Tumors. In this brief section, we do not attempt to stratify chromosome alterations into the numerous histologic subtypes of brain (and particularly glial) tumors. In general across all subtypes of brain cancer, several examples of recurring chromosome alteration have been observed. These alterations include trisomy 7, monosomy 10, monosomy 22 or del(22)(q11-q13), and loss of one or both sex chromosomes.[2,3,46–49] Cytologic evidence of gene amplification (especially dmin) are found in up to 50 percent of brain tumors[46,47,49] and initial observation of these changes dates back over three decades.[46] Finally, cytogenetic analysis has defined a minimal region of deletion in glial tumors, 10q25, as a likely site of a tumor suppresser gene important to the development of this malignancy.[48]

Breast Carcinoma. Numerous studies defining the chromosome changes in breast carcinoma have been published recently and the interested reader is referred to these for further detailed information.[1–3,50–58] Briefly, among the most frequent changes in breast carcinomas are the loss of chromosome 17 in primary tumors[55] and the amplification in metastatic tumors of the band region on 17 (q13), which encodes the HER-2/neu oncogene.[59,60] More commonly, structural alterations of chromosomes 1, 3, 7,

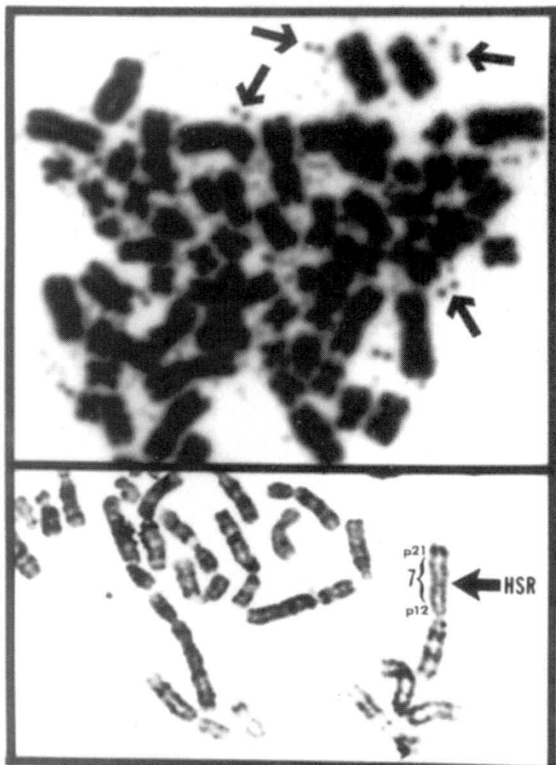

Fig. 20-5 Cytologic evidence of DNA sequence (gene) amplification. Top, example of tumor cell metaphase stained with Giemsa stain and displaying multiple copies of double minutes (dmin) (arrows). Bottom, example of a tumor cell metaphase G-banded and displaying a homogeneously staining region (hsr) involving the short arm of chromosome 7 (arrow).

and 11 are the most frequently structurally altered.[1–3,49–58] As is true for brain cancers, another important feature of breast carcinomas is the common occurrence of gene amplification, most frequently detectable as HSRs in metastatic tumors. As mentioned previously, amplification of the HER-2/*neu* oncogene[59,60] is most characteristic, followed by the recent recognition of amplification of a gene(s) on the long arm of chromosome 20.[50,52,53,61,62]

Karyotypic changes in breast cancer not surprisingly increase in frequency in metastatic tumors in contrast to changes recognized in primary tumors.[50,51,63,64] The most common numeric changes in primary tumors include loss of 17, loss of 19, and gain of chromosome 7, while the chromosomes most frequently structurally altered are chromosomes 1 and 6. Both primary and metastatic lesions often demonstrate overrepresentation of 6p and 1q, frequently with loss of 1p and 6q.[50,51,65]. Although common in both primary and metastatic disease, chromosome 1 alterations are even more frequent in metastatic disease. These data have led to the suggestion that a permissive phenotype for generalized genomic instability may be associated with the transition to metastatic disease.[51]

Colon Cancer. Colon cancer is the paradigm in solid tumors demonstrating associated chromosomal (and now defined genetic) changes associated with disease predisposition, initiation, and progression (see Chap. 48).[1–3,66] Initially, cytogenetic studies were particularly useful in defining the association of altered with disease progression; therefore, it is not surprising that the most frequent chromosomal alterations include both the loss of chromosome 5 and structural rearrangements that frequently involve chromosomes 1 and 6 (usually 1p21-q11 and 6q13-q16). Overall, overrepresentation of 1q, 6p, 8q and chromosomes 7 and 13 is observed while underrepresentation of chromosomes 17, 18, and 15 and 5 are most common.[1–3,67–72] In contrast to breast cancers, studies comparing primary to metastatic samples show a similar overall frequency and distribution of chromosome alterations.

Renal Cell Carcinoma (RCC). Nonpapillary renal cell carcinoma (RCC) is the most common form of adult kidney cancer; and cytogenetic analysis has revealed several recurring sites of chromosome change, including structural alterations of chromosome 3 (particularly 3p11-p14), and the numeric changes +7, −8, +10, and −Y.[1–3,73–77] The deletion of 3p either as a simple deletion or by translocation has strongly suggested the presence of a predisposing gene to 3p25–36. The autosomal dominant disorder von Hippel-Lindau disease is associated with renal cell carcinoma alone or in combination with other phenotypic abnormalities, and this gene has recently been identified and characterized (see Chap. 41.)

Lung Cancer. The overwhelming number of cytogenetic studies in lung cancer have characterized small cell lung carcinoma (SCLC).[1–3,78–81] The most typical finding is del(3)(p14p23); and LOH and other biologic studies have suggested a gene(s) important in SCLC etiology maps to 3p21-p22. SCLC, as many other solid tumors, is characterized by gain of chromosome 7, which has been reported as a sole or primary change in lung carcinomas, as well as a change frequently observed in adjacent normal lung tissue.[15] Other secondary changes include loss of 5q, 6, 9p, 13q, 17p and 9p.[1–3] As is true of breast and brain tumors, cytologic evidence of gene amplification (principally in the form of dmin) have been observed frequently in SCLC and have been shown most frequently to involve amplification of the MYC and RAS oncogene families (particularly L-MYC) (see Chaps. 21 and 58.)

In non-small cell lung carcinomas, deletions of 3p and 5q are also the most common finding although the frequency of 3 loss is significantly less.[80,82,83] In general, these tumors have complex karyotypes, which show loss of 3p, 5q, 8p, Y, 5p, 10p, and gain of 1q, 3q, and 7q.[1–3,82,83]

Malignant Melanoma. Several recent studies of the chromosomes in malignant melanoma have been reported. Briefly, the chromosomes most often involved in both structural and numeric abnormalities are 1, 6, 7, 9, 10, and 11.[1–3,84–89] Figure 20-11 provides an example of the distribution of breakpoints involved in structural alteration from 158 cases of melanoma.[84] Translocations or deletions of the long arm of chromosome 6 (6p11-q12) are very common in this disorder;[90,91] and recently it was recognized that apparent simple deletions in this disorder in fact represented cryptic translocations where the telomere of another chromosome was "captured" to stabilize the breakage event.[92] Importantly, LOH and biologic evidence also exists to indicate that a gene(s) on chromosome 6 is implicated in the control of tumorigenicity in this disorder.[93–95]

Abnormalities of chromosome 1 are exceedingly frequent, involving most often the pericentromeric region 1p12-q12.[1–3,85] The net effect of these abnormalities is usually loss of 1p segments coupled with overrepresentation of 1q, a finding common in many solid tumors. Finally, several studies have suggested a familial predisposition for a subset of malignant melanomas, with suggested linkage to 1p[96] and, more importantly, the identification of a hereditary melanoma gene on 9p (see Chap. 44).[97–99] Mutations in the *P16/CDCK2N* gene appear responsible for only a subset of patients with familial melanoma (approximately 25 percent). Numerous studies, including work in our laboratory are underway to identify additional genes associated with familial melanoma. Regions of chromosome alteration may help pinpoint the location of genes important in susceptibility to this disease.

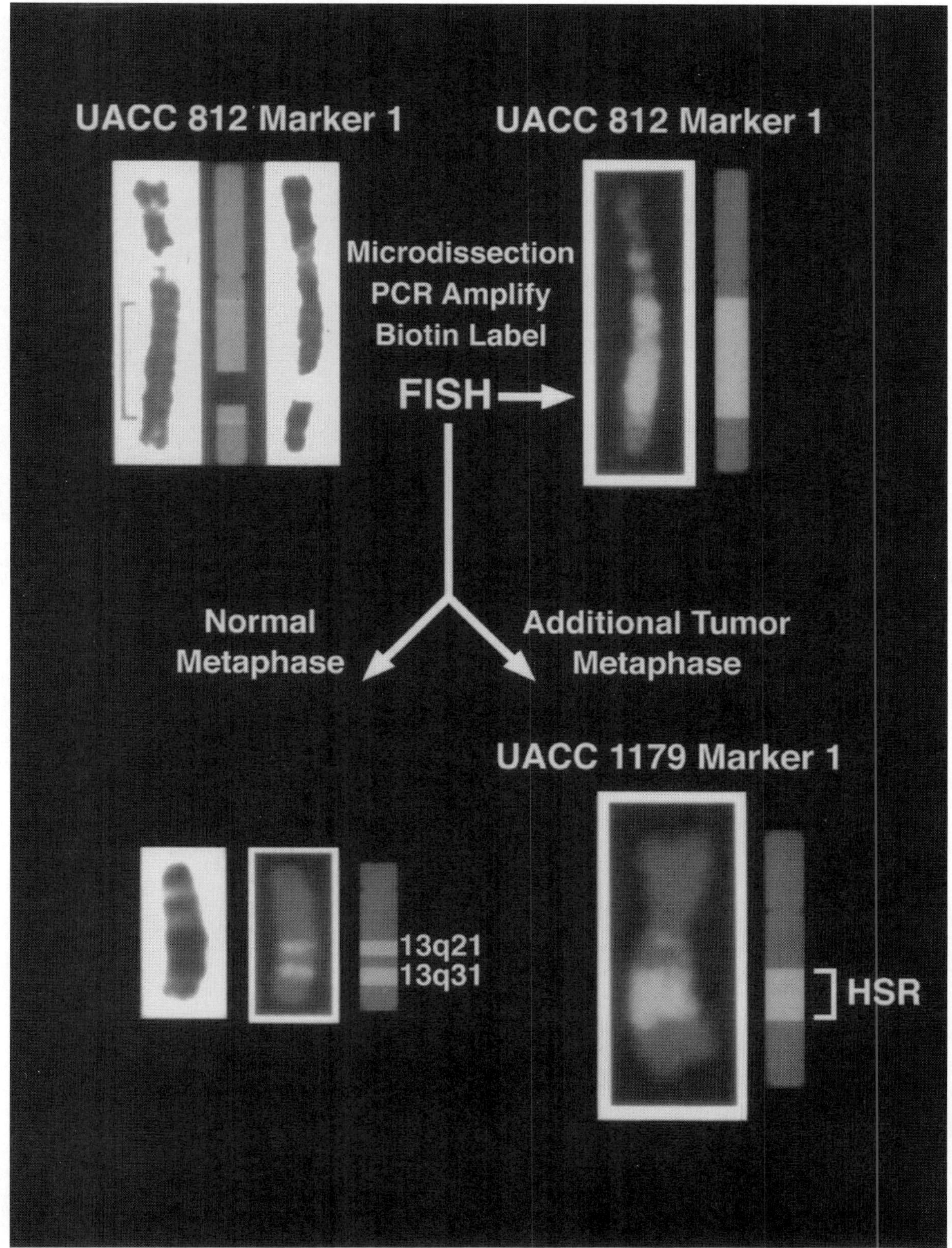

Fig. 20-6 Diagrammatic representation of the detection and characterization of hsrs from human breast cancers by chromosome microdissection (see reference 118). Upper left, G-banded hsr-bearing Marker 1 (left) from case UACC812. Microdissection (right) through the hsr of Marker 1. Upper right, after PCR amplification and biotin labeling of the dissected DNA, the PCR product is purified and hybridized by FISH back to Marker 1 to confirm that the dissection product hybridized to the hsr (bracket). Lower left, the same microdissection probe for the hsr was used to identify the location in the normal cells of the amplified sequences. Results indicated specific hybridization to the two regions of one chromosome (13q21 and 13q31): left, G-banded chromosome 13; right, identical chromosome following hybridization with the hsr probe. Lower right, the same microdissection FISH hsr probe used to hybridize to additional breast tumor cases to determine the commonality of 13q amplification. A representative example of an hsr encoding 13q amplified sequences I presented from case UACC1179 Marker 1. (*From Zhang J, Cui P, Glatfelter AA, Cummings LM, Meltzer PS, Trent JM.*[119] *Used by permission of the publisher.*)

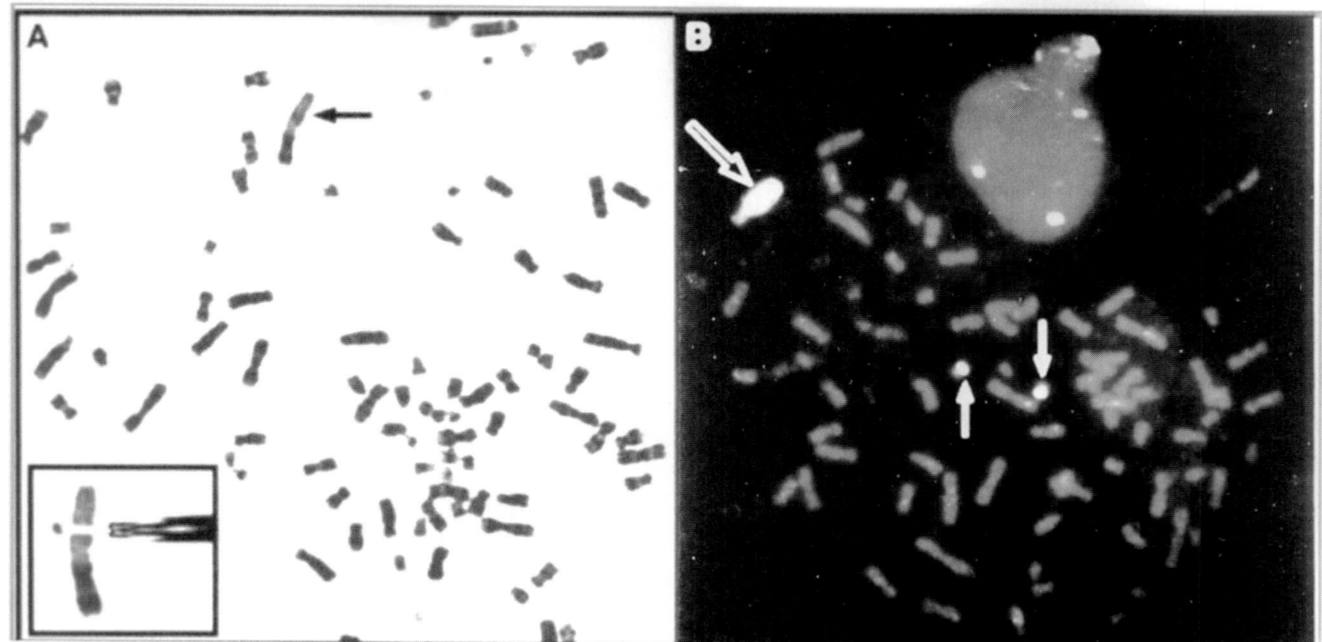

Fig. 20-7 Dissection of a fragment of a homogeneously staining region (hsr) from a human ovarian carcinoma. *A*, G-banded tumor metaphase (insert shows the dissection through the hsr to isolate DNA from the amplified region for use as a FISH probe). *B*, the same case as *A* after FISH illustrating the hsr (thick arrow) and the normal single copy region amplified in this tumor (19q13). (*From Guan X-Y, Cargile CB, Anzick SL, et al.*[110] *Used by permission of the publisher.*)

Studies from our laboratory have demonstrated that a recurring translocation t(1;6)(q11–21;q11–13) has been observed in a number of melanoma cases,[90] and Fig. 20-12 provides an example of this translocation. This figure also provides an illustration of the dissection of the translocation breakpoint (a starting point for positional cloning studies). Translocation of chromosome 1 segments to chromosomes 19 and 11 have also been reported to occur in a nonrandom fashion.[100,101] Evidence of gene amplification (HSRs) has been identified in melanomas, but the frequency is very low.[102]

Neuroblastoma. Deletion of part of the long arm of chromosome 1 (resulting in net loss of 1p32–p36) is the principal change recognized in this pediatric neoplasm.[1–3,11,12] Loss of this chromosomal segment appears often to be followed by amplification of the oncogene *N-MYC,* which is accompanied by recognition of HSRs or dmin in some clinical samples (see Chap. 21 for additional information).

Ovarian Carcinoma. Descriptive cytogenetics in ovarian carcinoma has been difficult because of the complexity of the clonal

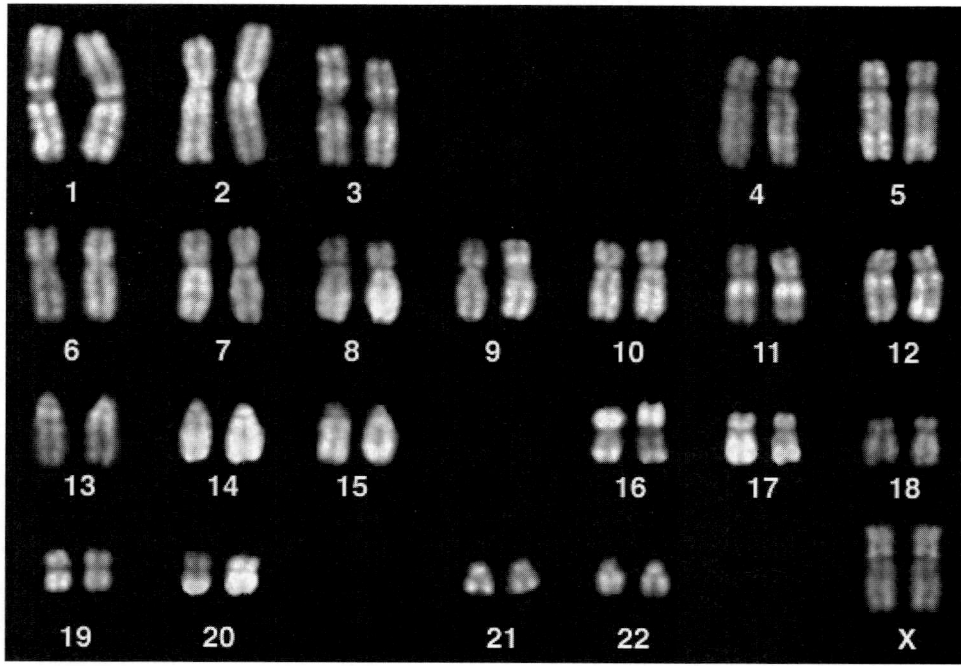

Fig. 20-8 An example of CGH analysis of a breast cancer specimen. Numerous genetic changes in the tumor DNA are visualized as color changes on metaphase chromosomes. Chromosomal regions that appear green reflect DNA gains and amplifications (e.g., 3p14, 8q, 11q13, 12q12–q13, 13q, 17q22–q24, and 20q13) and those that are red, DNA losses and deletions (e.g., 1p21–p31, 4, 8p, 9p, 11p, 11q14-qter, 13q14-qter, 16q12–q21, 18, and X). (*From Heim S, Mitelman F.*[3] *Used by permission of the publisher.*)

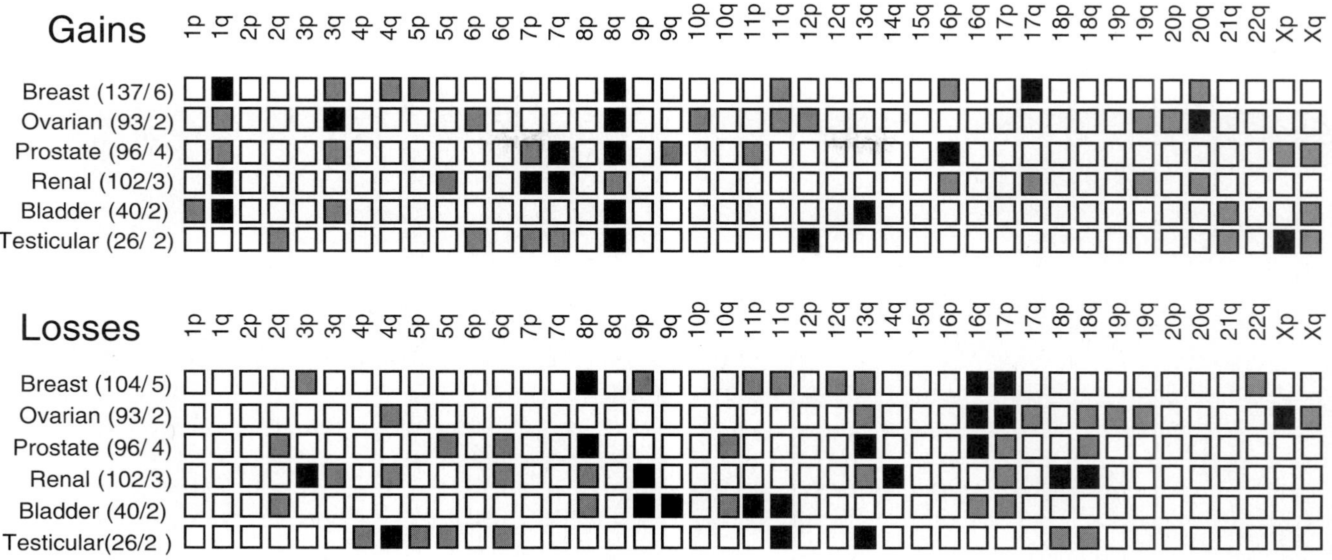

Fig. 20-9 An overview of the most common gains and losses reported in the published CGH studies of selected genital and urological tumors (the references to the original studies can be obtained from www.nhgri.nih.gov/DIR/LCG/CGH). The number of tumors analyzed and the number of studies evaluated for each tumor type are indicated in parenthesis. The black squares (■) indicate the three most-common changes to a particular tumor type, and the gray squares (■) the next most-common regions of involvement. Approximately 10 of the most common changes were indicated for each tumor type. The criterion for selecting the most common changes was not only the frequency, but the systematic presence of the change in independent studies. Distinct patterns of losses and gains are seen for each tumor type, whereas some genetic changes are common to several tumor types. (*From Heim S, Mitelman F.*[3] *Used by permission of the publisher.*)

changes characteristic of this tumor. More so than any other carcinoma, highly fragmented chromosomes, quadriradials, telomeric fusions, and complexly rearranged chromosomes are frequently found.[2,3] Nevertheless, recurring sites of chromosome change have been described, including deletions in the region 6q15–21, and translocation of chromosome 6 with chromosome 14, t(6;14)(q21;q24).[103,104] Although deletion or translocation of chromosome 6 has not been described as the sole primary change, the loss of 6q remains the most frequent abnormality described in this tumor to date. The most frequentchromosome alterations in ovarian cancer are loss of genetic material for several regions including 3p, 6q, 11p, 17q, and 17p13.[1–3,105–107] Cytologic evidence of gene amplification in the forms of HSRs and dmins and molecular evidence for specific amplification (e.g., *KRAS* oncogene) have been seen in several studies.[108–111]

Testicular Germ Cell Tumors. Histopathologic classification of testicular germ cell tumors is based upon the contribution of embryonic (embryonal carcinoma, immature and mature teratomas) or extraembryonic tissues (yolk sac tumors and choriocarcinomas), or combinations of both. Of the published cytogenetic studies of germ cell tumors isochromosomes for 12p, {i(12p)} are the most common and earliest recognizable chromosome change.[1–3,112–114] Structural alterations involving the short arm of chromosome 12 have also been reported but the net change is usually results in an increase relative to the diploid copy number of 12p while decreasing the relative copy number of 12q. This information has been suggested to play a clinically useful role in discriminating patient outcome[115] but the true clinical utility is currently indeterminate.

CHROMOSOME ALTERATIONS AND THE MOLECULAR PATHOGENESIS OF HUMAN SARCOMAS

Although the promise has long been realized, that cytogenetic anomalies might serve as signposts to identify the genes that play critical roles in oncogenesis for numerous leukemias, only recently have translocations in solid tumors yielded to molecular analysis. The common epithelial malignancies of adults lack recurrent tumor-specific chromosome translocations that have been characterized at the molecular level. However, several tumor-specific translocations of sarcomas have now been analyzed in this fashion Table 20-3). In addition, specific genes are now recognized to be the targets of chromosome change in benign tumors. Certain themes have emerged from the study of these rearrangements, which are well illustrated by the genetic abnormalities present in Ewing's sarcoma and alterations of related genes in other cancers.

Chromosome Translocations in Ewing's Sarcoma

Specific chromosome translocations have been characterized in detail in several sarcomas, including alveolar rhabdomyosarcoma and synovial sarcoma, but Ewing's sarcoma presents the most intriguing example for detailed discussion because of the many ramifications arising from molecular analysis of this cancer.[120–122] Ewing's sarcoma is a rare, highly malignant tumor of children and young adults, which can occur in diverse anatomic sites but most frequently arises in bone. The cell of origin is uncertain, and it can be difficult to distinguish morphologically from other so-called "small round blue cell tumors," which include virtually all the solid tumors of childhood in their undifferentiated form.[123] This difficulty helped to fuel interest in the observation that a reciprocal translocation t(11:22)(q24;q12) is present in most cases of Ewing's sarcoma.[124–125] The existence of a recurrent translocation suggested that this rearrangement probably involved genes that were directly related to the pathogenesis of Ewing's sarcoma. In fact, molecular characterization of the t(11:22) has provided strong support for this proposal. Positional cloning techniques revealed that the t(11;22) results in the juxtaposition of sequences from the *FLI1* gene on chromosome 11 and the *EWS* gene on chromosome 22.[126] Although both the der(22) and der(11) might produce fusion transcripts, loss of the der(11) in some tumors and expression analysis strongly implicate the der(22) as the site of the critical rearrangement. The chromosome breakpoints on chromosomes 11 and 22 occur within introns of these genes, and lead to the generation of a chimeric gene in which the 5′ portion of

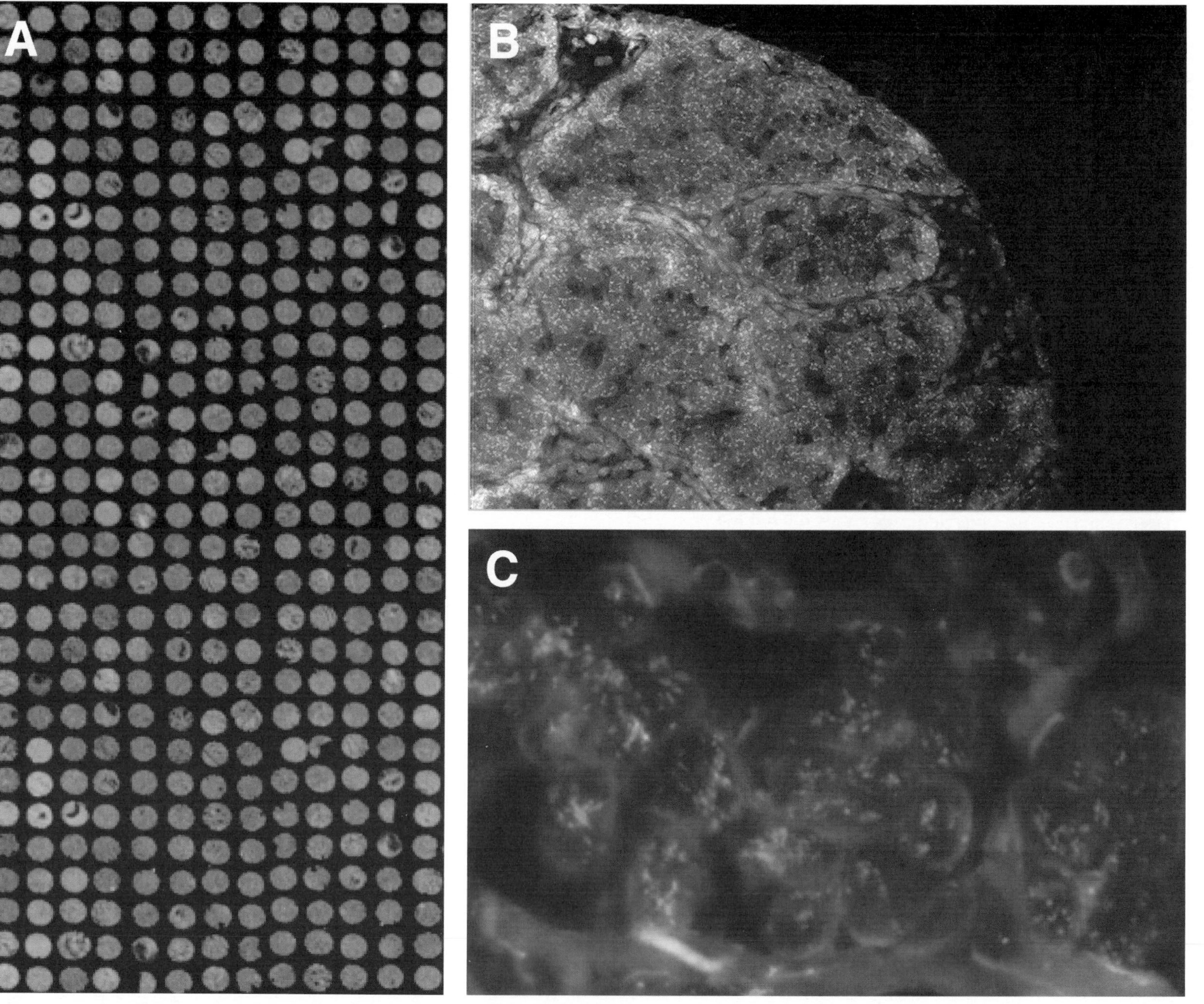

Fig. 20-10 Detection of androgen receptor (AR) amplification in prostate cancer by FISH on sections of a prostate tissue microarray. *A*) overview of a tissue microarray section containing hundreds of different tumor samples (Ø 0.6 mm, each). ×3. *B* and *C*, AR amplification with many clustered AR gene signals (red) and a few centromere X signals (green). B, ×200; C, ×1000. See Color Plate 1.

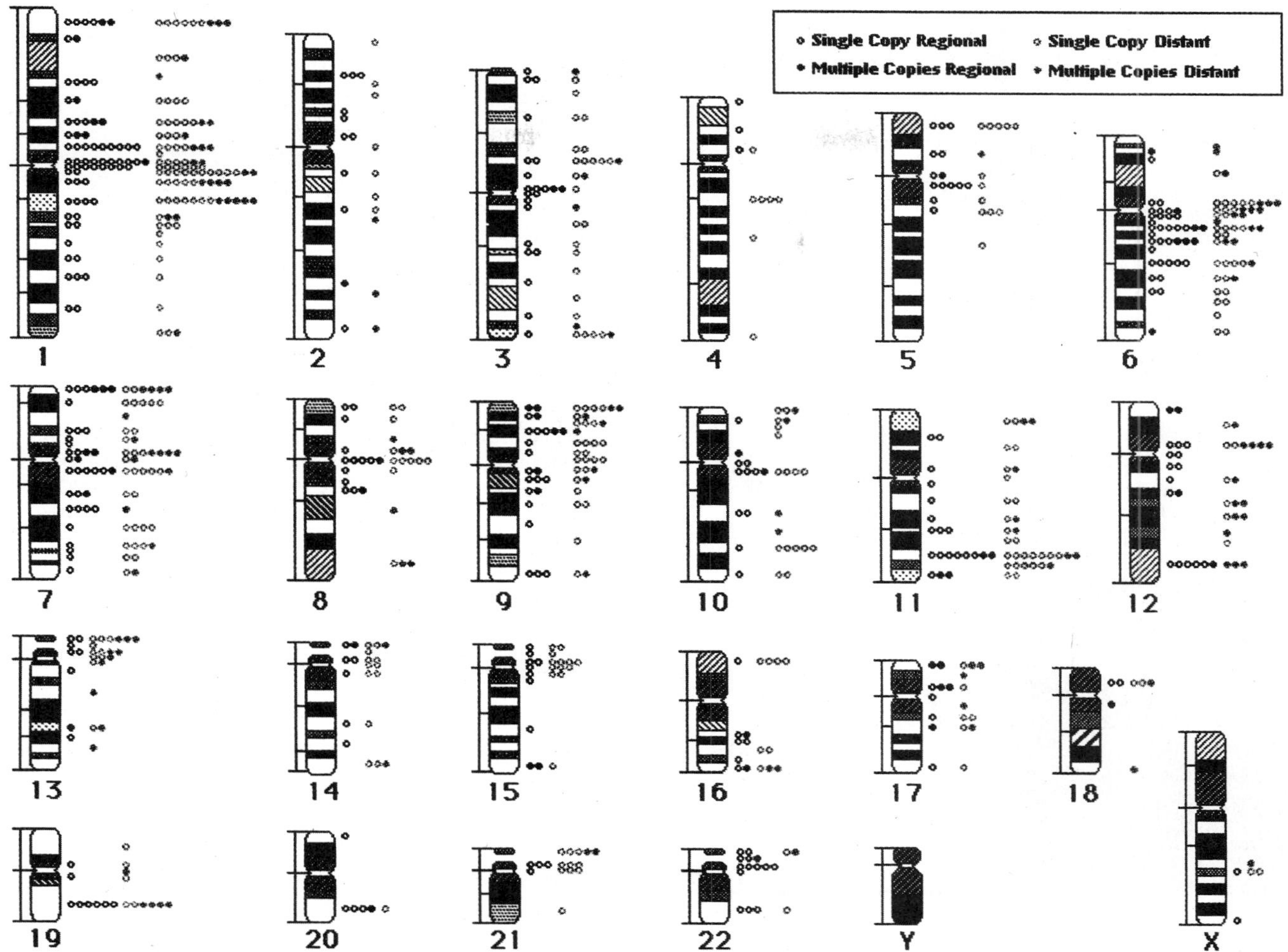

Fig. 20-11 Chromosomal breakpoints identified in clonal structural abnormalities from 158 cases of metastatic melanoma. Dark circles are from cases with tumor limited to the region of surgical dissection, light circles represent cases from patients with disseminated disease at the time of tumor biopsy. (*From Thompson FH, Emerson J, Olson S, et al.*[84] *Used by permission of the publisher.*)

EWS is fused in frame to 3′ sequences from *FLI1* (Figs. 20-13 and 20-14).[127]

Characterization of these genes revealed that *FLI1* has a 97 percent identity with a murine gene (*FLi1* first described as a target of oncogenic retroviral integration on mouse chromosome 9 in a region that is syntenic to human chromosome 11.[128] Sequence analysis demonstrates that *FLI1* is a member of the ETS family of transcription factors that contain a characteristic DNA-binding motif, the ETS domain.[129] The *ETS-1* protooncogene itself was originally defined by the presence of ETS-related sequences in the E26 avian leukosis virus.[130] The 656 amino acid protein encoded by *EWS* was novel but contained a putative RNA-binding domain. Analysis of the genomic structure of *EWS* demonstrated that the gene is composed of 17 exons distributed over approximately 40 kb.[131] The first seven exons encode a repetitive polypeptide with the consensus sequence SYGQQS. This is followed by a hinge region encoded by exons 8 to 10, while the candidate RNA-binding domain is encoded in exons 11 to 13.

The breakpoints in the t(11;22) vary from case to case, but always lead to replacement of the RNA-binding domain of *EWS* by the DNA-binding domain of *FLI1* (Figs. 20-13 and 20-14).[127] The resultant fusion protein would be predicted to have the properties of a transcription factor with a transcriptional activation domain contributed by *EWS* and a DNA-binding domain contributed by *FLI1*. A considerable body of experimental evidence has accumulated to support this interpretation.[134–138] The EWS/FLI1 fusion protein is localized in the nucleus and retains the DNA-binding specificity of FLI1. Reporter gene assays also demonstrate that it is a potent transcriptional activator, and unlike FLI1 it is able to transform NIH 3T3 cells. The *EWS* sequences clearly confer transcriptional activating function. Because the transforming properties of *EWS* cannot be replaced by other strong transcriptional activation domains, they are likely to provide important protein interaction and regulatory functions.[139]

Important observations have emerged as additional cases of Ewing's sarcoma have been characterized. Although the *EWS* gene is consistently involved in every instance, variant translocation partners for *EWS* have been identified in a subset of cases. The most common alternative to *FLI1* is *ERG*, a gene that maps on chromosome 21q22. ERG is also a member of the ETS family of transcription factors. In a manner quite comparable to the *EWS/FLI1* translocation, the *EWS/ERG* fusion transfers the *ERG* DNA-binding domain to the *EWS* transcriptional activating domain.[127,140] A third variant translocation involves *EWS* with an *ETV1* gene on chromosome 7p22.[141] *ETV1* is yet another member of the ETS family, further emphasizing the importance of the ETS DNA-binding domain contributed to the fusion proteins by each of these three transcription factors. Finally, a fourth variant translocation, t(17:22)(q21;q12) has been described that joins the transactivation domain of *EWS* with a fourth member of the ETS family, the

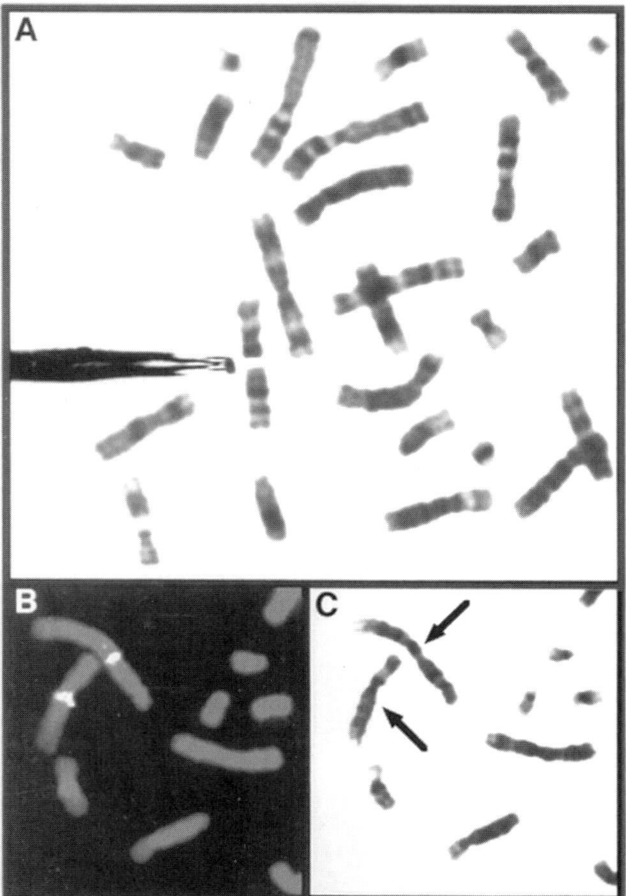

Fig. 20-12 Cytogenetic characterization of a chromosome translocation from a metastatic melanoma. *A*, G-banded tumor metaphase demonstrating a translocation between chromosomes 1 and 6 [t(1;6)(q21;q14)]. Dissection of the chromosomal breakpoint is performed with a glass needle targeted to the translocation breakpoint. *B*, FISH analysis of the dissected material hybridized to a normal human metaphase cell showing chromosome regions involved in the translocation between chromosomes 1 and 6. *C*, the identical cell as *B*, G-banded to confirm the specific chromosomal regions. (*From Zhang J, Cui P, Glatfelter AA, Cummings LM, Meltzer PS, Trent JM.*[119] *Used by permission of the publisher.*)

adenovirus E1A enhancer-binding protein (*ETV4*).[142] *ETV4* is known to activate transcription of matrix metalloproteinase genes, thus potentially linking the*EWS/ETV4* fusion protein with the invasive properties of the tumor.

Diagnostic Implications

Ewing's sarcoma can be difficult to distinguish from other cancers that are morphologically similar. This difficulty has led to an examination of the diagnostic importance of the t(11:22). This is well illustrated by consideration of another diagnostic entity, described variously as primitive neuroepithelioma (PN) or peripheral primitive neuroectodermal tumor of childhood (PNET). These tumors are clinically similar to Ewing's sarcoma, though they occur most often in extraosseus sites during adolescence. However, unlike Ewing's sarcoma, PN consistently expresses ultrastructural features of neural differentiation and is therefore felt to be of neural origin. Although PN can be distinguished from Ewing's sarcoma in this basis, it is now recognized that the t(11:22) is also found in PN.[143,144] The presence of the same underlying molecular genetic alteration

Table 20-3 Chromosome Translocations in Sarcomas

Tumor	Translocation	Genes
Ewing' sarcoma	t(11;22)(q24;q12)	EWS/FLI-1
	t(21;22)(q22;q12)	EWS/ERG
	t(7;22)(p22;q12)	EWS/ETV1
	t(17;22)(q21;q12)	EWS/ETV4
Malignant melanoma (clear cell sarcoma) of the soft parts	t(12;22)(q13;q12)	EWS/ATF1
Dermatofibrosarcoma protuberans	t(17;22)(q22;q13)	COL1A1/PDGFB
Desmoplastic small round cell tumor	t(11;22)(q13;q12)	EWS/WT1
Extraskeletal myxoid chondrasarcoma	t(9;22)(q22;q12)	EWS/TEC
Infantile fibrosarcoma	t(12;15)(p12;q25)	ETV6/NTRK3
Myxoid liposarcoma	t(12;16)(q13;p11)	FUS/CHOP
	t(12;22)(q13;12)	EWS/CHOP
Alveolar rhabdomyosarcoma	t(2;13)(q35;q14)	PAX3/FKHR
	t(1;13)(p36;q14)	PAX7/FKHR
Synovial sarcoma	t(X;18)(p11;q11)	SYT/SSX

suggests that these disorders must be very closely related if not identical. Some pathologists now consider these cancers as part of an as yet incompletely defined Ewing's sarcoma group of peripheral neuroectodermal tumors, all of which are linked by the presence of the t(11:22).[145] In fact, because it is possible to determine the presence of the *EWS/FLI1* fusion gene by either RT-PCR or interphase FISH, it is likely that testing for the presence of this molecular aberration will become part of the routine characterization of these tumors.[146–152] However, the presence of *EWS/FLI1* transcripts in a few tumors with myogenic or biphenotypic features suggests that molecular characterization will supplement, rather than replace, traditional tumor markers.[153] Nonetheless, because of its pathogenic role, the presence of the t(11:22) may ultimately prove more important than markers of cell differentiation, especially if therapies are developed that are directed at the pathways triggered by the *EWS/FLI1* transcription factor.[154] The question also arises as to whether the variant *EWS* translocations within Ewing's sarcoma have different clinical behavior. Currently available data suggest an advantage for patients with *EWS/FLI1* fusions occurring after exon 7 of *EWS* relative to the other variants.[155–157] It will be of interest to define the molecular basis for this effect, which may arise from subtle functional differences in the variant fusion proteins. As illustrated by the following examples, rearrangements involving the *EWS* gene are not confined to Ewing's sarcoma.

***EWS* rearrangements in other sarcomas.** A rare tumor of young adults called malignant melanoma of the soft parts, or clear cell sarcoma, is characterized by a tumor-specific translocation t(12;22)(q13:q12).[158,159] This tumor, which exhibits some neuroectodermal features, most frequently occurs in the tendons and aponeuroses. Molecular characterization of the t(12;22) has revealed that this rearrangement also involves the *EWS* gene, which in this instance gives rise to a chimeric protein carrying sequences from the ATF-1 gene on chromosome 12q13.[160–161] Again in parallel with the t(11:22), ATF-1, a transcription factor in the bZIP family, contributes its DNA-binding domain to the fusion protein.[162,163]

EWS contributes to yet another tumor-specific translocation, the t(11;22)(p13:q12) observed in desmoplastic small round cell tumor.[164,165] This is a tumor that occurs primarily in the abdomen

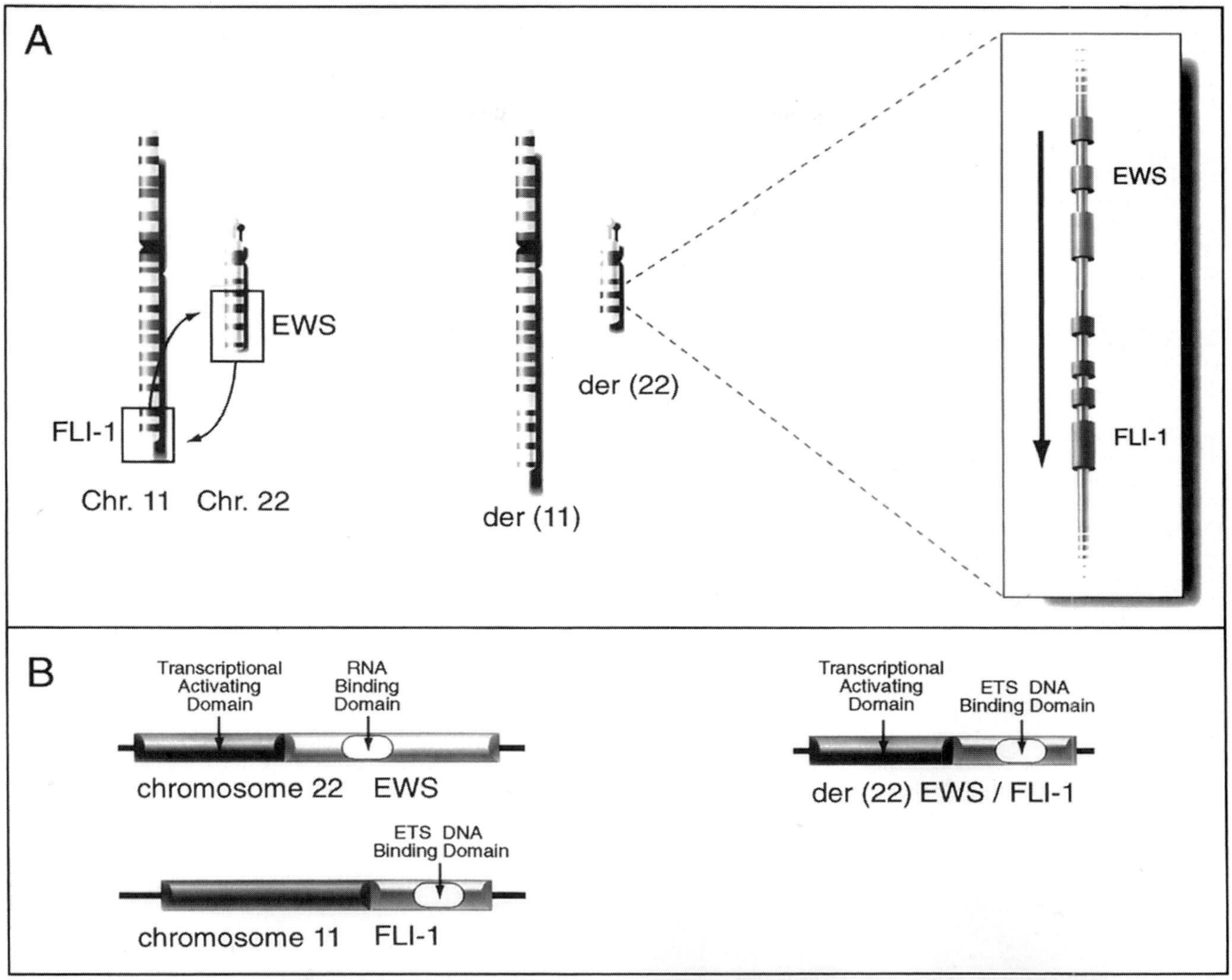

A

EWS

FLI-1

Chr. 11 Chr. 22

der (22)

der (11)

EWS

FLI-1

B

Transcriptional Activating Domain

RNA Binding Domain

chromosome 22 EWS

ETS DNA Binding Domain

chromosome 11 FLI-1

Transcriptional Activating Domain

ETS DNA Binding Domain

der (22) EWS / FLI-1

Fig. 20-13 ***A*, Translocation of sequences from chromosome 11 to chromosome 22 creates a fusion protein derived from the *EWS* and *FLI1* genes in Ewing's sarcoma. In the diagram on the far right, the arrow indicates the direction of transcription, and exons are represented by enlarged areas. *B*, The fusion protein contains transcriptional activating sequences from the N-terminal portion of *EWS* joined to the ETS DNA-binding domain of *FLI-1*.**

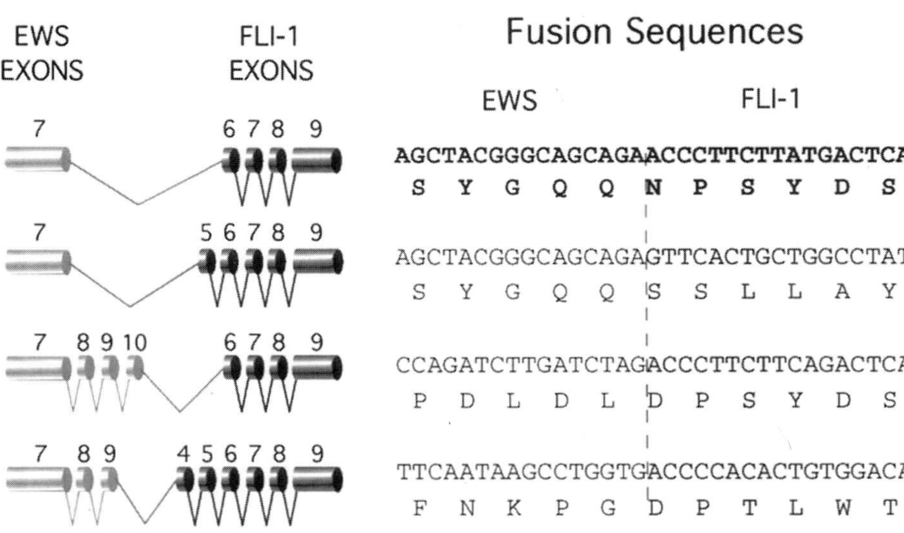

Fig. 20-14 Representative fusion transcripts identified by Zucman et al.[127] illustrating their variability. The most frequent type joins exon 7 of EWS to exon 6 of FLI-1. All of the variants replace the RNA-binding domain of *EWS* with the ETS DNA-binding domain of *FLI-1*.

of adolescent males or in association with other serosal surfaces.[166,167] In this disorder *EWS* forms a chimeric protein with WT-1.[168–171] Remarkably, *WT-1* is the Wilms Tumor gene, which was identified as the target of constitutional deletion in the Wilms tumor-aniridia syndrome.[172] *WT-1*, like the other *EWS* partners is a transcription factor, and the *EWS/WT-1* fusion once again pairs the *EWS* transcriptional activation domain with the zinc finger DNA-binding domain of *WT-1*.

Involvement of *EWS* has been extended to myxoid chondrosarcoma, which exhibits a specific chromosomal translocation t(9;22)(q22–31;q11–12). This rearrangement links *EWS* with almost the entire coding sequence of *CHN*, a member of the steroid hormone receptor superfamily.[173–174] The involvement of *EWS* with multiple partners in so many different sarcomas is remarkable, but even more impressive when one considers *FUS*, a homolog of *EWS*, which is also involved in tumor-specific rearrangements.

An *EWS* homolog also participates in sarcoma translocations. Myxoid liposarcoma (MLPS) is characterized by a t(12;16)(q13;p11).[175] This rearrangement gives rise to a chimeric transcription factor derived from the *CHOP* gene on chromosome 12 and a gene that has been called either *FUS* (for fusion) or *TLS* (for translocated in liposarcoma) on chromosome 16.[176–178] Remarkably, the *FUS/TLS* gene closely resembles the *EWS* gene and contains the same functional domains. *CHOP* is a transcription factor of the C/EBPβ family, and is normally induced in response to starvation or stress stimuli.[179] Heterodimers formed between CHOP and C/EBPβ have reduced DNA-binding activity, and CHOP therefore appears to be a negative regulator.[180–183] However, in the FUS/CHOP chimera the bZIP domain does confer DNA-binding activity. Remarkably, cases of MLPS have now been described that contain *EWS*/CHOP fusions, further emphasizing the functional similarities of *EWS* and *FUS/TLS* as well as the specificity of CHOP for MLPS.[184]

Several conclusions seem inevitable upon consideration of the range of tumors that exhibit rearrangements of either *EWS* or FUS/TLS. These molecular abnormalities appear to be essential to the pathogenesis of the tumors in which they occur. Because all the fusion proteins described above are transcription factors, perturbation of the normal pattern of gene expression must be critical to the malignant transformation of normal precursor cells. Because the occurrence of these translocations is in itself most likely a random event, the emergence of a translocation-bearing tumor clone presumably reflects both the lineage specificity and the oncogenic potency of that specific chimeric transcription factor. The precise reasons for the predominant rearrangement of ETS family genes in Ewing's sarcoma or *CHOP* in myxoid liposarcoma remain to be elucidated, but presumably they relate to the underlying program of gene expression required for the differentiation of the various mesenchymal cell lineages. Elucidation of the detailed downstream biochemical effects of the oncogenic chimeric transcription factors is an important current focus of research. In addition, it should be emphasized that sarcomas bearing chimeric transcription factors are likely to contain additional genetic alterations, such as p53 mutation, which are important to the evolution of the clinically evident malignant tumor.[185,186] However, based on their high incidence in tumors of a given type, it is likely that the translocations that characterize these tumors occur early in their evolution and create a fundamental disturbance of cell function essential to the tumorigenic process.

Rearrangements of the HMGI-C gene in benign tumors. Tumor-specific translocations are not limited to malignant tumors. Benign tumors, notably lipoma and leiomyoma, may be karyotypically abnormal. Rearrangements of chromosome 12q14–q15 have been among the most frequent abnormalities observed in these tumors.[187–189] Diverse partner chromosomes have been observed linked to 12q14–q15 in various tumors. In addition to lipoma and leiomyoma, rearrangements of the 12q14–q15 region have also been observed in pulmonary chondroid hamartoma, pleomorphic adenomas of the salivary gland, endometrial polyps, and a variety of benign tumors of mesenchymal origin.[190–192] The frequent appearance of the 12q breakpoint strongly suggested that a pathogenically important gene resided at that location, a suspicion borne out when the *HMGI-C* gene was mapped to the site of these breakpoints in both leiomyoma and lipoma.[193,194] *HMGI-C* is the human homolog of the murine pygmy gene and is a member of the HMGI family of small nuclear proteins, including *HMGI-C* and *HMGI(Y)*, which are characterized by the presence of a DNA-binding domain called the AT hook that binds to the minor groove of AT-rich DNA and induces DNA bending.[195] The HMGI-C protein consists of only 109 amino acids encoded by five exons with the three AT hook domains being encoded by the first three exons. The third intron is large (140 kb) and is the site of the translocations that fuse sequences from almost every chromosome to the AT hook domains of *HMGI-C*.[194] HMGI proteins have not been shown to have intrinsic transcription factor activity, but appear to function as accessory factors promoting the binding of other proteins to DNA.[196] In addition, HMGI-C is induced in NIH3T3 cells as a delayed early-response gene suggesting a possible connection between HMGI-C and cell cycle progression. The precise biochemical effects of the fusion proteins have not been established, and the multiple-partner genes have not yet been fully characterized. In one case (a lipoma with a t(3:12)), the partner gene contains two tandem LIM motifs, sequences that are known to function as protein interaction domains.[193,194] The second gene in the HMGI family, HMG-I(Y), maps to chromosome 6p21, and variant translocations in benign tumors may involve this gene instead of HMGI-C.[197,198]

The HMGI family translocations present both parallels and sharp contrasts to those involving the *EWS* gene family. Both categories of translocation involve chimeric DNA-binding proteins that most likely exert their oncogenic effects by perturbing normal gene expression. In both cases, a critical domain is provided by either member of a two-gene family. In the case of HMGI, this is a DNA-binding domain, while in the case of *EWS*, it is the transcriptional activating domain. The benign behavior of tumors with HMGI translocations contrasts with the highly malignant properties of tumors with *EWS* translocations. Benign lipomas and leiomyomas do not appear to evolve into malignant tumors. It is not at all clear how the HMGI-C translocations confer proliferative capacity without a tendency to accumulate further genetic alterations that would promote malignant progression. Comparison of the biochemical consequences of these two categories of translocation is likely to prove important in defining the molecular features that distinguish malignant tumors from their benign counterparts.

CONCLUSION

This brief review of the current progress in identifying recurring sites of chromosome change in human solid tumors, reveals that, despite methodological difficulties, a recurring and decidedly nonrandom pattern of chromosome alterations has clearly emerged. It appears likely that as additional cases of solid tumors are cytogenetically examined, the stratification of some specific histopathologic subtypes will be possible, and this may facilitate diagnostic (and possibly prognostic) analysis.

At present the clinical utility of chromosome analysis in solid tumors is largely indeterminate. However, the pinpointing of regions of the genome that are characteristically altered in solid tumors has been, and will continue to be, of significant benefit in targeting future molecular (and hopefully mechanistic) investigations. Continued study of the basic genetics of solid tumors appears a particularly fruitful avenue to continue, as it assuredly will add to our understanding of the causation, progression, and ultimately the control of these disorders.

ACKNOWLEDGMENT

We want to acknowledge the excellent graphic assistance of Darryl Leja, NHGRI, NIH. Also, we thank Drs. Felix Mitelman and Robert Jenkins for their review of recurring chromosomal alterations.

REFERENCES

1. Mitelman F: *Catalog of Chromosome Aberrations in Cancer, '98: Version 1*. New York, Wiley-Liss, 1998.
2. Sandberg AA: *The Chromosomes in Human Cancer and Leukemia*, 2nd ed. New York, Elsevier Science, 1990.
3. Heim S, Mitelman F: *Cancer Cytogenetics. Chromosomal and Molecular Genetic Aberrations of Tumor Cells*, 2nd ed. New York, Wiley-Liss, 1995.
4. de Klein A, Guerts van Kessel A, Grosveld G, et al.: A cellular oncogene is translocated to the Philadelphia chromosome in chronic myelocytic leukaemia. *Nature* **300**:765, 1982.
5. Thompson FH: Cytogenetic methodological approaches and findings in human solid tumors in Barch MJ (ed): *The ACT Cytogenetics Laboratory Manual*, 2nd ed. New York, Raven Press, 1996, p 451.
6. Yang JM, Thompson FH, Knox SM, Dalton WS, Salmon SE, Trent JM: Polyclonal origin of a primary breast carcinoma demonstrated by serial cytogenetic studies of a patient with a history of osteosarcoma [Abstract]. *Cancer Genet Cytogenet* **66**:153, 1993.
7. Pandis N, Heim S, Bardi G, Idvall I, Mandahl N, Mitelman F: Chromosome analysis of 20 breast carcinomas: Cytogenetic multiclonality and karyotypic-pathologic correlations. *Genes Chromosomes Cancer* **6**:51, 1993.
8. Heim S, Caron M, Jin Y, Mandahl N, Mitelman F: Genetic convergence during serial in vitro passage of a polyclonal squamous cell carcinoma. *Cytogenet Cell Genet* **52**:133, 1989.
9. Nowell PC: Tumors as clonal proliferation. *Virchows Arch B Cell Path* **29**:145, 1978.
10. Mitelman F (ed): *ISCN (1995): An International System for Human Cytogenetic Nomenclature*. Basel, S. Karger, 1995.
11. Schrock E, du Manoir S, Veldman T, Schoell B, Wienberg J, Ferguson-Smith MA, Ning Y, Ledbetter DH, Bar-Am I, Soenksen D, Garini Y, Ried T: Multicolor spectral karyotyping of human chromosomes. *Science* **273**:494, 1996
12. Christiansen H, Schestag J, Christiansen NM, Grzeschik K-H, Lampert F: Clinical impact of chromosome 1 aberrations in neuroblastoma: A metaphase and interphase cytogenetic study. *Genes Chromosomes Cancer* **5**:141, 1992.
13. Caron H, van Sluis P, Van Hoeve M, et al.: Allelic loss of chromosome 1p36 in neuroblastoma is of preferential maternal origin and correlates with N-myc amplification. *Nat Genet* **4**:187, 1993.
14. Trent J, Meyskens FL, Salmon SE, et al.: Relation of cytogenetic abnormalities and clinical outcome in metastatic melanoma,. *N Engl J Med* **322**:1508, 1990.
15. Korc M, Meltzer P, Trent J: Enhanced expression of epidermal growth factor receptor correlates with alterations of chromosome 7 in human pancreatic cancer. *Proc Natl Acad Sci U S A* **83**:5141, 1986.
16. Aly MS, Dal Cin P, Van de Voorde W, et al.: Chromosome abnormalities in benign prostatic hyperplasia. *Genes Chromosomes Cancer* **9**:227, 1994.
17. Arps S, Rodewald A, Schmalenberger B, Carl P, Bressel M, Kastendieck H: Cytogenetic survey of 32 cancers of the prostate. *Cancer Genet Cytogenet* **66**:93, 1993.
18. Herrmann ME, Lalley PA: Significance of trisomy 7 in thyroid tumors. *Cancer Genet Cytogenet* **62**:144, 1992.
19. Kallioniemi A, Kallioniemi O-P, Sudar D, Rutovitz D, Gray JW, Waldman F, Pinkel D: Comparative genomic hybridization: A powerful new method for cytogenetic analysis of solid tumors. *Science* **258**:818, 1992.
20. Du Manoir S, Speicher MR, Joos S, Schröck E, Popp S, Dohner H, Kovacs G, Robert-Nicoud M, Lichter P, Cremer T: Detection of complete and partial chromosome gains and losses by comparative genomic hybridization. *Hum Genet* **90**:590, 1993.
21. Forozan F, Karhu R, Kononen J, Kallioniemi A, Kallioniemi O-P: Genome screening by comparative genomic hybridization. *TIG* **13**:405, 1997.
22. Knuutila S, Björkqvist A-M, Autio K, Tarkkanen M, Wolf M, Monni O, Szymanska J, Larramendy ML, Tapper J, Pere H, El-Rifai W, Hemmer S, Wasenius V-M, Vidgren V, Zhu Y: DNA copy number amplifications in human neoplasms. *Am J Pathol* **152**:1107, 1998.
23. Visakorpi T, Kallioniemi A, Syvänen A-C, Hyytinen E, Karhu R, Tammela T, Isola JJ, Kallioniemi O-P: Genetic changes in primary and recurrent prostate cancer by comparative genomic hybridization. *Cancer Res* **55**:342, 1995.
24. Houldsworth J, Mathew S, Rao PH, Dyomina K, Louie DC, Parsa N, Offit K, Chaganti RS: REL proto-oncogene is frequently amplified in extranodal diffuse large cell lymphoma. *Blood* **87**:25, 1996.
25. Joos S, Otano-Joos MI, Ziegler S, Bruderlein S, du Manoir S, Bentz M, Moller P, Lichter P: Primary mediastinal (thymic) B-cell lymphoma is characterized by gains of chromosomal material including 9p and amplification of the REL gene. *Blood* **87**:1571, 1996.
26. Monni O, Joensuu H, Franssila K, Knuutila S: DNA copy number changes in diffuse large B-cell lymphoma—Comparative genomic hybridization study. *Blood* **87**:5269, 1996.
27. Weber-Hall S, McManus A, Anderson J, Nojima T, Abe S, Pritchard-Jones K, Shipley J: Novel formation and amplification of the PAX7-FKHR fusion gene in a case of alveolar rhabdomyosarcoma. *Genes Chromosomes Cancer* **17**:7, 1996.
28. Anzick SL, Kononen J, Walker RL, Azorsa DO, Tanner MM, Guan XY, Sauter G, Kallioniemi OP, Trent JM, Meltzer PS: AIB1, a steroid receptor coactivator amplified in breast and ovarian cancer. *Science* **277**:965, 1997
29. Sen S, Zhou H, White RA: A putative serine/threonine kinase encoding gene BTAK on chromosome 20q13 is amplified and overexpressed in human breast cancer cell lines. *Oncogene* **14**:2195, 1997.
30. Collins C, Rommens JM, Kowbel D, Godfrey T, Tanner M, Hwang SI, Polikoff D, Nonet G, Cochran J, Myambo K, Jay KE, Froula J, Cloutier T, Kuo WL, Yaswen P, Dairkee S, Giovanola J, Hutchinson GB, Isola J, Kallioniemi OP, Palazzolo M, Martin C, Ericsson C, Pinkel D, Gray JW: Positional cloning of ZNF217 and NABC1: Genes amplified at 20q13.2 and overexpressed in breast carcinoma. *Proc Natl Acad Sci U S A* **95**:8703, 1998.
31. Kononen J, Bubendorf L, Kallioniemi A, Bärlund M, Schraml P, Leighton S, Torhorst J, Mihatsch MJ, Sauter G, Kallioniemi O-P: Tissue microarrays for high-throughput molecular profiling of tumor specimens. *Nat Med* **4**:844, 1998.
32. Bubendorf L, Kononen J, Koivisto P, Schraml P, Moch H, Gasser TC, Willi N, Mihatsch MJ, Sauter G, Kallioniemi OP: Survey of gene amplifications during prostate cancer progression by high-throughput fluorescence in situ hybridization on tissue microarrays. *Cancer Res* **59**(4):803, 1999.
33. Heselmeyer K, Schröck E, du Manoir S, Blegen H, Shah K, Steinbeck R, Auer G, Ried T: Gain of chromosome 3q defines the transition from severe dysplasia to invasive carcinoma of the uterine cervix. *Proc Natl Acad Sci U S A* **93**:479, 1996.
34. Kuukasjärvi T, Karhu R, Tanner M, Kähkönen M, Schaffer A, Nupponen N, Pennanen S, Kallioniemi A, Kallioniemi OP, Isola J: Genetic heterogeneity and clonal evolution underlying development of asynchronous metastasis in human breast cancer. *Cancer Res* **57**:1597, 1997.
35. Gronwald J, Storkel S, Holtgreve-Grez H, Hadaczek P, Brinkschmidt C, Jauch A, Lubinski J, Cremer T: Comparison of DNA gains and losses in primary renal clear cell carcinomas and metastatic sties: Importance of 1q and 3p copy number changes in metastatic events. *Cancer Res* **57**:481, 1997.
36. Falor WH: Chromosomes in noninvasive papillary carcinoma of the bladder. *JAMA* **216**:791, 1971.
37. Falor WH, Ward RM: Prognosis in early carcinoma of the bladder based on chromosomal analysis. *J Urol* **199**:44, 1978.
38. Schapers RFM, Smeets AWGB, Pauwels RPE, Van Den Brandt PA, Bosman FT: Cytogenetic analysis in transitional cell carcinoma of the bladder. *Br J Urol* **72**:887, 1993.
39. Wang M-R, Perissel B, Taillandier J, et al.: Nonrandom changes of chromosome 10 in bladder cancer—Detection by FISH to interphase nuclei. *Cancer Genet Cytogenet* **73**:8, 1994.
40. Atkin NB, Baker MC: Cytogenetic study of ten carcinomas of the bladder: Involvement of chromosomes 1 and 11. *Cancer Genet Cytogenet* **15**:253, 1985.
41. Gibas Z, Prout GR, Connolly JG, Pontes JE, Sandberg AA: Nonrandom chromosomal changes in transitional cell carcinoma of the bladder. *Cancer Res* **44**:1257, 1984.
42. Gibas Z, Prout GR, Pontes JE, Connolly JG, Sandberg AA: A possible specific chromosome change in transitional cell carcinoma of the bladder. *Cancer Genet Cytogenet* **19**:229, 1986.

43. Poddighe PJ, Ramaekers FCS, Smeets AWGB, Vooijs GP, Hopman AHN: Structural chromosome 1 aberrations in transitional cell carcinoma of the bladder: Interphase cytogenetics combining a centromeric, telomeric, and library DNA probe. *Cancer Res* **52**:4929, 1992.
44. Cairns P, Shaw ME, Knowles MA: Initiation of bladder cancer may involve deletion of a tumour-suppressor gene on chromosome 9. *Oncogene* **8**:1083, 1993
45. Miyao N, Tsai YC, Lerner SP, et al.: Role of chromosome 9 in human bladder cancer. *Cancer Res* **53**:4066, 1993.
46. Lubs HA, Salmon JH: The chromosomal complement of human solid tumors, II. Karyotypes of glial tumors. *J Neurosurg* **22**:160, 1965.
47. Magnani I, Guerneri S, Pollo B, et al.: Increasing complexity of the karyotype in 50 human gliomas. *Cancer Genet Cytogenet* **75**:77, 1994.
48. Rasheed BKA, McLendon RE, Friedman HS, et al.: Chromosome 10 deletion mapping in human gliomas: A common deletion region in10q25. *Oncogene* **10**:2243, 1995.
49. Reifenberger G, Reifenberger J, Ichimura K, Meltzer PS, Collins PV: Amplification of multiple genes from chromosomal region 12q13-14 in human malignant gliomas: Preliminary mapping of the amplicons shows preferential involvement of CDK4, SAS, and MDM2. *Cancer Res* **54**:4299, 1994.
50. Thompson F, Emerson J, Dalton WS, et al.: Clonal chromosome abnormalities in human breast carcinomas I: 28 cases with primary disease. *Genes Chromosomes Cancer* **7**:185, 1993.
51. Trent J, Yang J-M, Emerson J, et al.: Clonal chromosome abnormalities in human breast carcinomas II: 34 cases with metastatic disease. *Genes Chromosomes Cancer* **7**:194, 1993.
52. Tanner MM, Tirkkonen M, Kallioniemi A, et al.: Increased copy number at 20q13 in breast cancer: Defining the critical region and exclusion of candidate genes. *Cancer Res* **54**:4257, 1994.
53. Adelaide J, Penault-Llorca F, Dib A, Yarden Y, Jacquemier J, Birnbaum D: The heregulin gene can be included in the 8p12 amplification unit in human breast cancer. *Genes Chromosomes Cancer* **11**:66, 1994.
54. Almeida A, Muleris M, Dutrillaux B, Malfoy B: The insulin-like growth factor I receptor gene is the target for the 15q26 amplicon in breast cancer. *Genes Chromosomes Cancer* **11**:63, 1994.
55. Nagai MA, Yamamoto L, Salaorni S, et al.: Detailed deletion mapping of chromosome segment 17q12-21 in sporadic breast tumours. *Genes Chromosomes Cancer* **11**:58, 1994.
56. Bieche I, Champeme M-H, Lidereau R: Loss and gain of distinct regions of chromosome 1q in primary breast cancer. *Clin Cancer Res* **1**:123, 1995.
57. Pandis N, Jin Y, Gorunova L, et al.: Chromosome analysis of 97 primary breast carcinomas: Identification of eight karyotypic subgroups. *Genes Chromosomes Cancer* **12**:173, 1995.
58. Hoggard N, Brintnell B, Howell A, Weissenbach J, Varley J: Allelic imbalance on chromosome 1 in human breast cancer. II. Microsatellite repeat analysis. *Genes Chromosomes Cancer* **12**:24, 1995.
59. Slamon DJ, Clark GM, Wong SG, Levin WJ, Ullrich A, McGuire WL: Human breast cancer: Correlation of relapse and survival with amplification of the HER-2/neu oncogene. *Science* **235**:177, 1987.
60. Slamon DJ, Godolphin W, Jones LA, et al.: Studies of the HER-2/neu proto-oncogene in human breast and ovarian cancer. *Science* **244**:707, 1989.
61. Tanner MM, Tirkkonen M, Kallioniemi A, Isola J, Kuukasjärvi T, Collins C, Kowbel D, Guan X-Y, Trent J, Gray JW, Meltzer P, Kallioniemi O-P: Independent amplification and frequent co-amplification of three nonsyntenic regions on the long arm of chromosome 20 in human breast cancer. *Cancer Res* **56**:3441, 1996.
62. Guan X-Y, Xu J, Anzick SL, Zhang H, Trent JM, Meltzer PS: Hybrid selection of transcribed sequences from microdissected DNA: Isolation of genes within an amplified region at 20q11–q13.2 in breast cancer. *Cancer Res* **56**:3446, 1996.
63. Trent J: Cytogenetic and molecular biologic alterations in human breast cancer: A review. *Breast Cancer Res Treat* **5**:221, 1985.
64. Trent JM, Yang J-M, Thompson FH, Leibovitz A, Villar H, Dalton WS: Chromosome alterations in human breast cancer, in: Sluyser M (ed): *Oncogenes and Hormones in Breast Cancer.* Chichester, Ellis Horwood, 1987, p 142.
65. Devilee P, van Vliet M, van Sloun P, et al.: Allotype of human breast carcinoma. A second major site for loss of heterozygosity is on chromosome 6. *Oncogene* **6**:1705, 1991.
66. Vogelstein B, Fearon ER, Hamilton SR, et al.: Genetic alterations during colorectal-tumor development. *N Engl J Med* **319**:525, 1988.
67. Muleris M, Zafrani B, Validire P, Girodet J, Salmon R-J, Dutrillaux B: Cytogenetic study of 30 colorectal adenomas. *Cancer Genet Cytogenet* **74**:104, 1994.
68. Muleris M, Salmon RJ, Zafrani B, Girodet J, Dutrillaux B: Consistent deficiencies of chromosome 18 and of the short arm of chromosome 17 in eleven cases of human large bowel cancer: A possible recessive determinism. *Ann Genet* **28**:206, 1985.
69. Muleris M, Salmon R-J, Dutrillaux B: Chromosome study demonstrating the clonal evolution and metastatic origin of a metachronous colorectal carcinoma. *Int J Cancer* **38**:167, 1986.
70. Thompson FH, Liu Y, Alberts D, Taetle R, Trent JM: Cytogenetic findings in 51 colorectal carcinomas: correlations with sample site [Abstract]. *Am J Hum Genet* **53**:376, 1993.
71. Muleris M, Salmon R-J, Dutrillaux A-M, et al.: Characteristic chromosomal imbalances in 18 near-diploid colorectal tumors. *Cancer Genet Cytogenet* **29**:298, 1987.
72. Bomme L, Bardi G, Pandis N, Fenger C, Kronborg O, Heim S: Clonal karyotypic abnormalities in colorectal adenomas: Clues to the early genetic events in the adenoma-carcinoma sequence. *Genes Chromosomes Cancer* **10**:190, 1994.
73. Berger CS, Sandberg AA, Todd IAD, et al.: Chromosome in kidney, ureter, and bladder cancer. *Cancer Genet Cytogenet* **23**:1, 1986.
74. Kovacs G, Szucs S, De Reise W, Baumbartel H: Specific chromosome aberration in human renal cell carcinoma. *Int J Cancer* **40**:171, 1987.
75. Pathak S, Strong LC, Ferrell RE, Trindade A: Familial renal cell carcinoma with a 3;11 chromosome translocation limited to tumor cells. *Science* **217**:939, 1982.
76. Yoshida MA, Ohyashiki K, Ochi H, et al.: Rearrangement of chromosome 3 in renal cell carcinoma. *Cancer Genet Cytogenet* **19**:351, 1986.
77. Henn W, Zwergel T, Wullich B, Thonnes M, Zang KD, Seitz G: Bilateral multicentric papillary renal tumors with heteroclonal origin based on tissue-specific karyotype instability. *Cancer* **72**:1315, 1993.
78. Rey JA, Bello MJ, de Campos JM, Kusak ME, Moreno S, Benitez J: Deletion 3p in two lung adenocarcinomas metastatic to the brain. *Cancer Genet Cytogenet* **25**:355, 1987.
79. Levin NA, Brzoska P, Gupta N, Gray JW, Christman MF: Identification of frequent novel genetic alterations in small cell lung carcinoma. *Cancer Res* **54**:5086, 1994.
80. Hosoe S, Ueno K, Shigedo Y, et al.: A frequent deletion of chromosome 5q21 in advanced small cell and non-small cell carcinoma of the lung. *Cancer Res* **54**:1787, 1994.
81. Johansson M, Karauzum SB, Dietrich C, et al.: Karyotypic abnormalities in adenocarcinomas of the lung. *Int J Oncol* **5**:17, 1994.
82. Siegfried JM, Hunt JD, Zhou J-Y, Keller SM, Testa JR: Cytogenetic abnormalities in non-small cell lung carcinoma: Similarity of findings in conventional and feeder cell layer cultures. *Genes Chromosomes Cancer* **6**:30, 1993.
83. Siegfried JM, Ellison DJ, Resau JH, Miura I, Testa JR: Correlation of modal chromosome number of cultured non-small cell lung carcinomas with DNA index of solid tumor tissue. *Cancer Res* **51**:3267, 1991.
84. Thompson FH, Emerson J, Olson S, et al.: Cytogenetics in 158 patients with regional or disseminated melanoma: Subset analysis of near diploid and simple karyotypes. *Cancer Genet Cytogenet* **83**:93, 1995.
85. Morse HG, Moore GE, Ortiz LM, Gonzalez R, Robinson WA: Malignant melanoma: From subcutaneous nodule to brain metastasis. *Cancer Genet Cytogenet* **72**:16, 1994.
86. Morse HG, Moore GE: Cytogenetic homogeneity in eight independent sites in a case of malignant melanoma. *Cancer Genet Cytogenet* **69**:108, 1993.
87. Parmiter AH, Nowell PC: Cytogenetics of melanocytic tumors. *J Invest Dermatol* **100**:254S, 1993.
88. Grammatico P, Catricala C, Potenza C, et al.: Cytogenetic findings in 20 melanomas. *Melanoma Res* **3**:169, 1993.
89. Ozisik YY, Meloni AM, Altungoz O, et al.: Cytogenetic findings in 21 malignant melanomas. *Cancer Genet Cytogenet* **77**:69, 1994.
90. Trent JM, Thompson FH, Meyskens FL: Identification of a recurring translocation site involving chromosome 6 in human malignant melanoma. *Cancer Res* **49**:420, 1989.
91. Guan X-Y, Cao J, Meltzer PS, Trent J: Rapid generation of region-specific genomic clones by chromosome microdissection: Isolation of DNA from a region frequently deleted in malignant melanoma. *Genomics* **14**:680, 1992.
92. Meltzer PS, Guan X-Y, Trent JM: Telomere capture stabilizes chromosome breakage. *Nat Genet* **4**:252, 1993.

93. Millikin D, Meese E, Vogelstein B, Trent J: Loss of heterozygosity for loci on the long arm of chromosome 6 in human malignant melanoma. *Cancer Res* **51**:5449, 1991.
94. Trent JM, Stanbridge EJ, McBride HL, et al.: Tumorigenicity in human melanoma cell lines controlled by introduction of human chromosome 6. *Science* **247**:568, 1990.
95. Su YA, Ray ME, Lin T, Seidel NE, Bodine DM, Meltzer PS, Trent JM: Reversion of Monochromosome-mediated suppression of tumorigenicity in malignant melanoma by retroviral transduction. *Cancer Res* **56**:3186, 1996.
96. Goldstein AM, Dracopoli NC, Ho EC, et al.: Further evidence for a locus for cutaneous malignant melanoma-dysplastic nevus (CMM/DN) on chromosome 1p, and evidence for genetic heterogeneity. *Am J Hum Genet* **52**:537, 1993.
97. Cannon-Albright LA, Goldgar DE, Meyer LJ, et al.: Assignment of a locus for familial melanoma, MLM, to chromosome 9p13-p22. *Science* **258**:1148, 1992.
98. Kamb A, Gruis NA, Weaver-Feldhaus J, et al.: A cell-cycle regulator potentially involved in genesis of many tumor types. *Science* **264**:436, 1994.
99. Goldstein AM, Dracopoli NC, Engelstein M, Fraser MC, Clark WH Jr, Tucker MA: Linkage of cutaneous malignant melanoma/dysplastic nevi to chromosome 9p, and evidence for genetic heterogeneity. *Am J Hum Genet* **54**:489, 1994.
100. Morse HG, Gonzalez R, Moore GE, Robinson WA: Preferential chromosome 11q and/or 17q aberrations in short-term cultures of metastatic melanoma in resections from human brain. *Cancer Genet Cytogenet* **64**:118, 1992.
101. Parmiter AH, Balaban G, Herlyn M, Clark WH, Nowell PC: A t(1;19) chromosome translocation in three cases of human malignant melanoma. *Cancer Res* **46**:1526, 1986.
102. Zhang J, Trent JM, Meltzer PS: Rapid isolation and characterization of amplified DNA by chromosome microdissection: Identification of IGF1R amplification in malignant melanoma. *Oncogene* **8**:2827, 1993.
103. Wake N, Hreshchyshyn MM, Piver SM, Matsui S, Sandberg AA: Specific cytogenetic changes in ovarian cancer involving chromosomes 6 and 14. *Cancer Res* **40**:4512, 1980.
104. Trent JM: Prevalence and Clinical Significance of Cytogenetic Abnormalities in Human Ovarian Cancer. Boston, MA, Nijhoff, 1985.
105. Lee JH, Kavanagh JJ, Wildrick DM, Wharton JT, Blick M: Frequent loss of heterozygosity on chromosome 6q, 11, and 17 in human ovarian carcinomas. *Cancer Res* **50**:2724, 1990.
106. Thompson FH, Emerson J, Alberts D, et al.: Clonal chromosome abnormalities in 54 cases of ovarian carcinoma. *Cancer Genet Cytogenet* **73**:33, 1994.
107. Taetle R, Aickin M, Panda L, Emerson J, Roe D, Thompson F, Davis J, Trent J, Alberts D: Chromosome abnormalities in ovarian adenocarcinoma I. Non-random chromosome abnormalities from 244 cases. *Genes Chromosomes Cancer* (**25**:46, 1999.
108. Guan X-Y, Alberts D, Burgess AC, Thompson FH, Trent JM: Chromosomal analysis of 90 cases of ovarian carcinomas [Abstract]. *Cancer Genet Cytogenet* **41**:291, 1989.
109. Filmus J, Trent JM, Pullano R, Buick RN: A cell line from a human ovarian carcinoma with amplification of the K-ras gene. *Cancer Res* **46**:5179, 1986.
110. Guan X-Y, Cargile CB, Anzick SL, et al.: Chromosome microdissection identifies cryptic sites of DNA sequence amplification in human ovarian carcinoma. *Cancer Res* 1995(**55**:3380, 1999.
111. Sasano H, Garrett CT, Wilkinson DS, Silverberg S, Comerford J, Hyde J: Proto-oncogene amplification in human ovarian neoplasms. *Hum Pathol* **21**:382, 1990.
112. Gibas Z, Prout GR, Pontes JE, Sandberg AA: Chromosome changes in germ cell tumors of the testis. *Cancer Genet Cytogenet* **19**:245, 1986.
113. Oosterhuis JW, de Jong B, Cornelisse CJ, et al.: Karyotyping and DNA flow cytometry of mature residual teratoma after intensive chemotherapy of disseminated nonseminomatous germ cell tumor of the testis: A report of two cases. *Cancer Genet Cytogenet* **22**:149, 1986.
114. Speicher MR, Jauch A, Walt H, et al.: Correlation of microscopic phenotype with genotype in a formalin-fixed, paraffin-embedded testicular germ cell tumor with universal DNA amplification, comparative genomic hybridization, and interphase cytogenetics. *Am J Pathol* **146**:1332, 1995.
115. Bosl GJ, Dmitrovsky E, Reuter VE, et al.: Isochromosome of chromosome 12: Clinically useful marker for male germ cell tumors. *J Natl Cancer Inst* **81**:1874, 1989.
116. Bani MR, Rak J, Adachi D, Wiltshire R, Trent JM, Kerbel RS, Ben-David Y: Multiple features of advanced melanoma recapitulated in tumorigenic variants of early stage (radial growth phase) human melanoma cell lines: Evidence for a dominant phenotype. *J Can Res* **56**:3075, 1996.
117. Guan X-Y, Zhang H, Bittner ML, Jiang Y, Meltzer PS, Trent JM: Rapid generation of human chromosome arm painting probes (CAPs) by chromosome microdissection. *Nat Genet* **12**:10, 1996.
118. Guan, X-Y, Meltzer PS, Dalton WS, Trent JM: Identification of cryptic sites of DNA sequence amplification in human breast cancer by chromosome microdissection. *Nat Genet* **8**:155, 1994.
119. Zhang J, Cui P, Glatfelter AA, Cummings LM, Meltzer PS, Trent JM: Microdissection based cloning of a translocation breakpoint in a human malignant melanoma. *Cancer Res* **55**:4640, 1995.
120. Clark J, Rocques PJ, Crew AJ, Gill S, Shipley J, Chan AM, Gusterson BA, Cooper CS: Identification of novel genes, SYT and SSX, involved in the t(X;18)(p11.2;q11.2) translocation found in human synovial sarcoma. *Nat Genet* **7**:502, 1994.
121. Shapiro DN, Sublett JE, Li B, Downing JR, Naeve CW: Fusion of PAX3 to a member of the forkhead family of transcription factors in human alveolar rhabdomyosarcoma. *Cancer Res* **53**:5108, 1993.
122. Barr FG, Galili N, Holick J, Biegel JA, Rovera G, Emanuel BS: Rearrangement of the PAX3 paired box gene in the paediatric solid tumour alveolar rhabdomyosarcoma. *Nat Genet* **3**:113, 1993.
123. Horowitz ME, Malaner MM, Woo SY, Hicks MJ: Ewing's Sarcoma family of tumors, in Pizzo PA, Poplack DG (eds): *Principles and Practice of Pediatric Oncology*. Philadelphia, JB Lippincott, 1997, 831.
124. Turc-Carel C, Philip I, Berger MP, Philip T, Lenoir GM: Chromosome study of Ewing's sarcoma (ES) cell lines. Consistency of a reciprocal translocation t(11;22)(q24;q12). *Cancer Genet Cytogenet* **12**:1, 1984.
125. Turc-Carel C, Aurias A, Mugneret F, Lizard S, Sidaner I, Volk C, Thiery JP, Olschwang S, Philip I, Berger MP, et al.: Chromosomes in Ewing's sarcoma. I. An evaluation of 85 cases of remarkable consistency of t(11;22)(q24;q12). *Cancer Genet Cytogenet* **32**:229, 1988.
126. Delattre O, Zucman J, Plougastel B, Desmaze C, Melot T, Peter M, Kovar H, Joubert I, de Jong P, Rouleau G, et al.: Gene fusion with an ETS DNA-binding domain caused by chromosome translocation in human tumours. *Nature* **359**:162, 1992.
127. Zucman J, Melot T, Desmaze C, Ghysdael J, Plougastel B, Peter M, Zucker JM, Triche TJ, Sheer D, Turc CC, et al.: Combinatorial generation of variable fusion proteins in the Ewing family of tumours. *Embo J* **12**:4481, 1993.
128. Ben-David Y, Giddens EB, Letwin K, Bernstein A: Erythroleukemia induction by Friend murine leukemia virus: Insertional activation of a new member of the ets gene family, Fli-1, closely linked to c-ets-1. *Genes Dev* **5**:908, 1991.
129. Seth A, Ascione R, Fisher RJ, Mavrothalassitis GJ, Bhat NK, Papas TS: The ets gene family. *Cell Growth Diff* **3**:327, 1992.
130. Watson DK, McWilliams-Smith MJ, Nunn MF, Duesberg PH, O'Brien SJ, Papas TS: The ets sequence from the transforming gene of avian erythroblastosis virus, E26, has unique domains on human chromosomes 11 and 21: both loci are transcriptionally active. *Proc Nat Acad Sci U S A* **82**:7294, 1985.
131. Plougastel B, Zucman J, Peter M, Thomas G, Delattre O: Genomic structure of the EWS gene and its relationship to EWSR1, a site of tumor-associated chromosome translocation. *Genomics* **18**:609, 1993.
132. Ohno T, Rao VN, Reddy ES: EWS/Fli-1 chimeric protein is a transcriptional activator. *Cancer Res* **53**:5859, 1993.
133. Rao VN, Ohno T, Prasad DD, Bhattacharya G, Reddy ES: Analysis of the DNA-binding and transcriptional activation functions of human Fli-1 protein. *Oncogene* **8**:2167, 1993.
134. Mao X, Miesfeldt S, Yang H, Leiden JM, Thompson CB: The FLI-1 and chimeric EWS-FLI-1 oncoproteins display similar DNA binding specificities. *J Biol Chem* **269**:18216, 1994.
135. Lessnick SL, Braun BS, Denny CT, May WA: Multiple domains mediate transformation by the Ewing's sarcoma EWS/FLI-1 fusion gene. *Oncogene* **10**:423, 1995.
136. Bailly RA, Bosselut R, Zucman J, Cormier F, Delattre O, Roussel M, Thomas G, Ghysdael J: DNA-binding and transcriptional activation properties of the EWS-FLI-1 fusion protein resulting from the t(11;22) translocation in Ewing sarcoma. *Mol Cell Biol* **14**:3230, 1994.
137. Magnaghi-Jaulin L, Masutani H, Robin P, Lipinski M, Harel-Bellan A: SRE elements are binding sites for the fusion protein EWS-FLI-1. *Nucleic Acids Res* **24**:1052, 1996.

138. Braun BS, Frieden R, Lessnick SL, May WA, Denny CT: Identification of target genes for the Ewing's sarcoma EWS/FLI fusion protein by representational difference analysis. *Mol Cell Biol* **15**:4623, 1995.
139. Zinszner H, Albalat R, Ron D: A novel effector domain from the RNA-binding protein TLS or EWS is required for oncogenic transformation by CHOP. *Genes Dev* **8**:2513, 1994.
140. Sorensen PH, Lessnick SL, Lopez-Terrada D, Liu XF, Triche TJ, Denny CT: A second Ewing's sarcoma translocation, t(21;22), fuses the EWS gene to another ETS-family transcription factor, ERG. *Nat Genet* **6**:146, 1994.
141. Jeon IS, Davis JN, Braun BS, Sublett JE, Roussel MF, Denny CT, Shapiro DN: A variant Ewing's sarcoma translocation (7;22) fuses the EWS gene to the ETS gene ETV1. *Oncogene* **10**:1229, 1995.
142. Urano F, Umezawa A, Hong W, Kikuchi H, Hata J: A novel chimera gene between EWS and E1A-F, encoding the adenovirus E1A enhancer-binding protein, in extraosseous Ewing's sarcoma. *Biochem Biophys Res Commun* **219**:608, 1996.
143. Stephenson CF, Bridge JA, Sandberg AA: Cytogenetic and pathologic aspects of Ewing's sarcoma and neuroectodermal tumors. *Hum Pathol* **23**:1270, 1992.
144. Giovannini M, Biegel JA, Serra M, Wang JY, Wei YH, Nycum L, Emanuel BS, Evans GA: EWS-erg and EWS-Fli1 fusion transcripts in Ewing's sarcoma and primitive neuroectodermal tumors with variant translocations. *J Clin Invest* **94**:489, 1994.
145. Delattre O, Zucman J, Melot T, Garau XS, Zucker JM, Lenoir GM, Ambros PF, Sheer D, Turc-Carel C, Triche TJ, et al.: The Ewing family of tumors — A subgroup of small-round-cell tumors defined by specific chimeric transcripts. *N Engl J Med* **331**:294, 1994.
146. Desmaze C, Zucman J, Delattre O, Melot T, Thomas G, Aurias A: Interphase molecular cytogenetics of Ewing's sarcoma and peripheral neuroepithelioma t(11;22) with flanking and overlapping cosmid probes. *Cancer Genet Cytogenet* **74**:13, 1994.
147. Selleri L, Giovannini M, Romo A, Zucman J, Delattre O, Thomas G, Evans GA: Cloning of the entire FLI1 gene, disrupted by the Ewing's sarcoma translocation breakpoint on 11q24, in a yeast artificial chromosome. *Cytogenet Cell Genet* **67**:129, 1994.
148. Sorensen PH, Liu XF, Delattre O, Rowland JM, Biggs CA, Thomas G, Triche TJ: Reverse transcriptase PCR amplification of EWS/FLI-1 fusion transcripts as a diagnostic test for peripheral primitive neuroectodermal tumors of childhood. *Diagn Mol Pathol* **2**:147, 1993.
149. Ladanyi M, Lewis R, Garin-Chesa P, Rettig WJ, Huvos AG, Healey JH, Jhanwar SC: EWS rearrangement in Ewing's sarcoma and peripheral neuroectodermal tumor. Molecular detection and correlation with cytogenetic analysis and MIC2 expression. *Diagn Mol Pathol* **2**:141, 1993.
150. Ida K, Kobayashi S, Taki T, Hanada R, Bessho F, Yamamori S, Sugimoto T, Ohki M, Hayashi Y: EWS-FLI-1 and EWS-ERG chimeric mRNAs in Ewing's sarcoma and primitive neuroectodermal tumor. *Int J Cancer* **63**:500, 1995.
151. Scotlandi K, Serra M, Manara MC, Benini S, Sarti M, Maurici D, Lollini PL, Picci P, Bertoni F, Baldini N: Immunostaining of the p30/32MIC2 antigen and molecular detection of EWS rearrangements for the diagnosis of Ewing's sarcoma and peripheral neuroectodermal tumor. *Hum Pathol* **27**:408, 1996.
152. Downing JR, Head DR, Parham DM, Douglass EC, Hulshof MG, Link MP, Motroni TA, Grier HE, Curcio BA, Shapiro DN: Detection of the (11;22)(q24;q12) translocation of Ewing's sarcoma and peripheral neuroectodermal tumor by reverse transcription polymerase chain reaction. *Am J Pathol* **143**:1294, 1993.
153. Sorensen PH, Shimada H, Liu XF, Lim JF, Thomas G, Triche TJ: Biphenotypic sarcomas with myogenic and neural differentiation express the Ewing's sarcoma EWS/FLI1 fusion gene. *Cancer Res* **55**:1385, 1995.
154. Ouchida M, Ohno T, Fujimura Y, Rao VN, Reddy ES: Loss of tumorigenicity of Ewing's sarcoma cells expressing antisense RNA to EWS-fusion transcripts. *Oncogene* **11**:1049, 1995.
155. Zoubek A, Pfleiderer C, Salzer-Kuntschik M, Amann G, Windhager R, Fink FM, Koscielniak E, Delattre O, Strehl S, Ambros PF, et al.: Variability of EWS chimaeric transcripts in Ewing tumours: A comparison of clinical and molecular data. *Br J Cancer* **70**:908, 1994.
156. Zoubek A, Dockhorn-Dworniczak B, Delattre O, Christiansen H, Niggli F, Gatterer-Menz I, Smith TL, Jurgens H, Gadner H, Kovar H: Does expression of different EWS chimeric transcripts define clinically distinct risk groups of Ewing tumor patients? *J Clin Oncol* **14**:1245, 1996.
157. de Alava E, Kawai A, Healey JH, Fligman I, Meyers PA, Huvos AG, Gerald WL, Jhanwar SC, Argani P, Antonescu CR, et al.: EWS-FLI1 fusion transcript structure is an independent determinant of prognosis in Ewing's sarcoma. *J Clin Oncol* **16**:2895, 1998.
158. Stenman G, Kindblom LG, Angervall L: Reciprocal translocation t(12;22)(q13;q13) in clear-cell sarcoma of tendons and aponeuroses. *Genes Chromosomes Cancer* **4**:122, 1992.
159. Mrozek K, Karakousis CP, Perez MC, Bloomfield CD: Translocation t(12;22)(q13;q12.2–12.3) in a clear cell sarcoma of tendons and aponeuroses. *Genes Chromosomes Cancer* **6**:249, 1993.
160. Zucman J, Delattre O, Desmaze C, Epstein AL, Stenman G, Speleman F, Fletchers CD, Aurias A, Thomas G: EWS and ATF-1 gene fusion induced by t(12;22) translocation in malignant melanoma of soft parts. *Nat Genet* **4**:341, 1993.
161. Fujimura Y, Ohno T, Siddique H, Lee L, Rao VN, Reddy ES: The EWS-ATF-1 gene involved in malignant melanoma of soft parts with t(12;22) chromosome translocation, encodes a constitutive transcriptional activator. *Oncogene* **12**:159, 1996.
162. Vallejo M, Ron D, Miller CP, Habener JF: C/ATF, a member of the activating transcription factor family of DNA-binding proteins, dimerizes with CAAT/enhancer-binding proteins and directs their binding to cAMP response elements. *Proc Natl Acad Sci U S A* **90**:4679, 1993.
163. Brown AD, Lopez-Terrada D, Denny C, Lee KA: Promoters containing ATF-binding sites are de-regulated in cells that express the EWS/ATF1 oncogene. *Oncogene* **10**:1749, 1995.
164. Rodriguez E, Sreekantaiah C, Gerald W, Reuter VE, Motzer RJ, Chaganti RS: A recurring translocation, t(11;22)(p13;q11.2), characterizes intra-abdominal desmoplastic small round-cell tumors. *Cancer Genet Cytogenet* **69**:17, 1993.
165. Biegel JA, Conard K, Brooks JJ: Translocation (11;22)(p13;q12): Primary change in intra-abdominal desmoplastic small round cell tumor. *Genes Chromosomes Cancer* **7**:119, 1993.
166. Wills EJ: Peritoneal desmoplastic small round cell tumors with divergent differentiation: A review. *Ultrastruct Pathol* **17**:295, 1993.
167. Parkash V, Gerald WL, Parma A, Miettinen M, Rosai J: Desmoplastic small round cell tumor of the pleura. *Am J Surg Pathol* **19**:659, 1995.
168. Ladanyi M, Gerald W: Fusion of the EWS and WT1 genes in the desmoplastic small round cell tumor. *Cancer Res* **54**:2837, 1994.
169. Brodie SG, Stocker SJ, Wardlaw JC, Duncan MH, McConnell TS, Feddersen RM, Williams TM: EWS and WT-1 gene fusion in desmoplastic small round cell tumor of the abdomen. *Hum Pathol* **26**:1370, 1995.
170. Gerald WL, Rosai J, Ladanyi M: Characterization of the genomic breakpoint and chimeric transcripts in the EWS-WT1 gene fusion of desmoplastic small round cell tumor. *Proc Natl Acad Sci U S A* **92**:1028, 1995.
171. de Alava E, Ladanyi M, Rosai J, Gerald WL: Detection of chimeric transcripts in desmoplastic small round cell tumor and related developmental tumors by reverse transcriptase polymerase chain reaction. A specific diagnostic assay. *Am J Pathol* **147**:1584, 1995.
172. Call KM, Glaser T, Ito CY, Buckler AJ, Pelletier J, Haber DA, Rose EA, Kral A, Yeger H, Lewis WH, Jones C, Housman DE: Isolation and characterization of a zinc finger polypeptide gene at the human chromosome 11 Wilms' tumor locus. *Cell* **60**:509, 1990.
173. Clark J, Benjamin H, Gill S, Sidhar S, Goodwin G, Crew J, Gusterson BA, Shipley J, Cooper CS: Fusion of the EWS gene to CHN, a member of the steroid/thyroid receptor gene superfamily, in a human myxoid chondrosarcoma. *Oncogene* **12**:229, 1996.
174. Gill S, McManus AP, Crew AJ, Benjamin H, Sheer D, Gusterson BA, Pinkerton CR, Patel K, Cooper CS, Shipley JM: Fusion of the EWS gene to a DNA segment from 9q22–31 in a human myxoid chondrosarcoma. *Genes Chromosomes Cancer* **12**:307, 1995.
175. Limon J, Turc-Carel C, Dal Cin P, Rao U, Sandberg AA: Recurrent chromosome translocations in liposarcoma. *Cancer Genet Cytogenet* **22**:93, 1986.
176. Aman P, Ron D, Mandahl N, Fioretos T, Heim S, Arheden K, Willen H, Rydholm A, Mitelman F: Rearrangement of the transcription factor gene CHOP in myxoid liposarcomas with t(12;16)(q13;p11). *Genes Chromosom Cancer* **5**:278, 1992.
177. Crozat A, Aman P, Mandahl N, Ron D: Fusion of CHOP to a novel RNA-binding protein in human myxoid liposarcoma. *Nature* **363**:640, 1993.
178. Rabbitts TH, Forster A, Larson R, Nathan P: Fusion of the dominant negative transcription regulator CHOP with a novel gene FUS by translocation t(12;16) in malignant liposarcoma. *Nat Genet* **4**:175, 1993.

179. Ron D, Habener JF: CHOP, a novel developmentally regulated nuclear protein that dimerizes with transcription factors C/EBP and LAP and functions as a dominant-negative inhibitor of gene transcription. *Genes Dev* **6**:439, 1992.

180. Batchvarova N, Wang XZ, Ron D: Inhibition of adipogenesis by the stress-induced protein CHOP (Gadd153). *Embo J* **14**:4654, 1995.

181. Ubeda M, Wang XZ, Zinszner H, Wu I, Habener JF, Ron D: Stress-induced binding of the transcriptional factor CHOP to a novel DNA control element. *Mol Cell Biol* **16**:1479, 1996.

182. Wang XZ, Ron D: Stress-induced phosphorylation and activation of the transcription factor CHOP (GADD153) by p38 MAP Kinase. *Science* **272**:1347, 1996.

183. Barone MV, Crozat A, Tabaee A, Philipson L, Ron D: CHOP (GADD153) and its oncogenic variant, TLS-CHOP, have opposing effects on the induction of G1/S arrest. *Genes Dev* **8**:453, 1994.

184. Panagopoulos I, Hoglund M, Mertens F, Mandahl N, Mitelman F, Aman P: Fusion of the EWS and CHOP genes in myxoid liposarcoma. *Oncogene* **12**:489, 1996.

185. Komuro H, Hayashi Y, Kawamura M, Hayashi K, Kaneko Y, Kamoshita S, Hanada R, Yamamoto K, Hongo T, Yamada M, et al.: Mutations of the p53 gene are involved in Ewing's sarcomas but not in neuroblastomas. *Cancer Res* **53**:5284, 1993.

186. Hamelin R, Zucman J, Melot T, Delattre O, Thomas G: p53 mutations in human tumors with chimeric EWS/FLI-1 genes. *Int J Cancer* **57**:336, 1994.

187. Sreekantaiah C, Leong SP, Karakousis CP, McGee DL, Rappaport WD, Villar HV, Neal D, Fleming S, Wankel A, Herrington PN, et al.: Cytogenetic profile of 109 lipomas. *Cancer Res* **51**:422, 1991.

188. Mrozek K, Karakousis CP, Bloomfield CD: Chromosome 12 breakpoints are cytogenetically different in benign and malignant lipogenic tumors: localization of breakpoints in lipoma to 12q15 and in myxoid liposarcoma to 12q13.3. *Cancer Res* **53**:1670, 1993.

189. Heim S, Mandahl N, Kristoffersson U, Mitelman F, Rooser B, Rydholm A, Willen H: Reciprocal translocation t(3;12)(q27;q13) in lipoma. *Cancer Genet Cytogenet* **23**:301, 1986.

190. Sreekantaiah C, Sandberg AA: Clustering of aberrations to specific chromosome regions in benign neoplasms. *Int J Cancer* **48**:194, 1991.

191. Kazmierczak B, Rosigkeit J, Wanschura S, Meyer-Bolte K, Van de Ven WJ, Kayser K, Krieghoff B, Kastendiek H, Bartnitzke S, Bullerdiek J: HMGI-C rearrangements as the molecular basis for the majority of pulmonary chondroid hamartomas: a survey of 30 tumors. *Oncogene* **12**:515, 1996.

192. Wanschura S, Kazmierczak B, Pohnke Y, Meyer-Bolte K, Bartnitzke S, Van de Ven WJ, Bullerdiek J: Transcriptional activation of HMGI-C in three pulmonary hamartomas each with a der(14)t(12;14) as the sole cytogenetic abnormality. *Cancer Lett* **102**:17, 1996.

193. Ashar HR, Fejzo MS, Tkachenko A, Zhou X, Fletcher JA, Weremowicz S, Morton CC, Chada K: Disruption of the architectural factor HMGI-C: DNA-binding AT hook motifs fused in lipomas to distinct transcriptional regulatory domains. *Cell* **82**:57, 1995.

194. Schoenmakers EF, Wanschura S, Mols R, Bullerdiek J, Van den Berghe H, Van de Ven WJ: Recurrent rearrangements in the high mobility group protein gene, HMGI-C, in benign mesenchymal tumours. *Nat Genet* **10**:436, 1995.

195. Zhou X, Benson KF, Ashar HR, Chada K: Mutation responsible for the mouse pygmy phenotype in the developmentally regulated factor HMGI-C. *Nature* **376**:771, 1995

196. Chau KY, Patel UA, Lee KL, Lam HY, Crane-Robinson C: The gene for the human architectural transcription factor HMGI-C consists of five exons each coding for a distinct functional element. *Nucleic Acids Res* **23**:4262, 1995.

197. Friedmann M, Holth LT, Zoghbi HY, Reeves R: Organization, inducible-expression and chromosome localization of the human HMG-I(Y) nonhistone protein gene. *Nucleic Acids Res* **21**:4259, 1993.

198. Xiao S, Lux ML, Reeves R, Hidson TJ, Fletcher JA: HMGI(Y) activation by chromosome 6p21 rearrangements in multilineage mesenchymal cells from pulmonary hamartoma. *Am J Pathol* **150**:901, 1997.

199. Gelehrter TD, Collins FS: *Principles of Medical Genetics*. Baltimore, MD, Williams & Wilkins, 1990..

CHAPTER 21

Gene Amplification in Human Cancers: Biological and Clinical Significance

Michael D. Hogarty ▪ Garrett M. Brodeur

1. Gene amplification is a frequent genetic abnormality in human cancer cells and consists of multiple extra copies of a subchromosomal region of DNA (amplicon). Amplification can be manifested cytogenetically as extrachromosomal double-minute chromosomes (dmins) or as chromosomally integrated homogeneously staining regions (HSRs).

2. Several mechanisms have been proposed to explain the development of gene amplification. These have been based primarily on *in vitro* systems in which there is selection for drug resistance, so the mechanisms involved in *de novo* oncogene amplification may be different. Nevertheless, for gene amplification to occur, it may be necessary to have loss of cell cycle control, DNA damage or instability, and a stimulus to progress through the cell cycle.

3. The size of the amplicon can vary from several hundred to several thousand kilobases. The amplified DNA appears to be in a head-to-tail conformation, and the germ line configuration is largely retained, with relatively few genetic rearrangements. In most cases, only a single expressed gene is consistently amplified, but in other cases, two or more genes from a given chromosomal region may confer a selective advantage, either individually or in concert.

4. Amplification of the *MYCN* oncogene occurs in 20 to 25 percent of all neuroblastomas. *MYCN* amplification is strongly associated with advanced stages of disease and a poor outcome. Currently, the presence of *MYCN* amplification is used to identify patients at high risk who need the most intensive treatment.

5. Amplification of several different genetic regions, especially 11q13 or 12q14, is found in many common types of cancer, including carcinomas of the breast, ovary, lung, head and neck, and gastrointestinal tract. The clinical significance of these findings is somewhat controversial, but in some patients, gene amplification may be associated with a more aggressive tumor behavior and a worse outcome.

6. The most common types of genes amplified are oncogenes and drug-resistance genes. Oncogenes, however, account for the vast majority of genes amplified in human cancers. The most common oncogenes amplified are members of the *MYC* family, the *RAS* family, the *EGFR* family, the *FGF* family, and genes involved in cell cycle regulation (*CCND1, CCNE, MDM2, CDK4*).

7. The mechanisms whereby oncogene amplification confers a selective advantage vary depending on the gene, but include overexpression of (a) a transcription factor (*MYC* family) favoring continued proliferation; (b) a signal transduction molecule (*RAS* family), growth factor, or receptor (*EGFR, FGF* families), that mimicks constitutive growth factor stimulation; or (c) cell-cycle regulatory genes (*CCND1, CCNE, MDM2, CDK4*) that lead to loss of cell-cycle control.

8. There are several methods of detecting gene amplification that vary in their difficulty or the need to know the gene (or genes) likely to be amplified. These methods include (a) conventional cytogenetics; (b) Southern blotting; (c) quantitative PCR; (d) fluorescence *in situ* hybridization (FISH); (e) comparative genomic hybridization (CGH); and (f) microarray technology.

INTRODUCTION

Cytogenetically visible rearrangements in human cancer cells fall into three general categories: (a) deletions with a net loss of genetic material; (b) translocations with transposition of genetic material, but no net loss or gain; and (c) gene amplification with a net gain of a specific chromosomal region. Deletions are thought to represent loss of a suppressor gene, whereas translocations and gene amplification generally represent activation of a proto-oncogene. Translocations could result in inactivation of a suppressor gene, but this appears to be a rare event. Gene amplification also can involve drug-resistance genes or other genes that confer a selective advantage when overexpressed. For the purposes of this chapter, gene amplification refers to an increase in copy number (more than six copies per diploid genome) of a specific, subchromosomal region (generally 1 to 2 mb or less). It is not used to refer to numerical gain (generally three to four copies per diploid genome) of whole chromosomes, chromosome arms, or very large chromosomal regions.

Gene amplification usually is apparent cytogenetically, either as extrachromosomal double-minute chromatin bodies, or as chromosomally integrated, homogeneously staining regions. If the copy number is low (e.g., 5 to 10 copies per cell), if the size of the amplified unit (amplicon) is small, or if the karyotype is extremely complex, gene amplification may not be evident by conventional cytogenetics. However, several different molecular approaches have been developed that allow reliable detection of gene amplification in interphase nuclei or from small amounts of tumor DNA (see below). In general, the latter techniques presuppose that the gene (or genes) that might be amplified is known.

Gene amplification almost always results in the overexpression of one or more genes contained in the amplicon. Usually there is a single gene that appears to be the "target" of the gene amplification, but some amplified units may contain two or more genes that could theoretically confer a selective advantage. Furthermore, in some cancers, two or more discrete regions may be amplified. However, in the majority of cases, only a single genetic region is amplified in a given tumor.

Theoretically, the amplification and consequent overexpression of a number of genes could confer a selective advantage on a cancer cell. In practice, the majority of examples that have been studied involve oncogenes or drug-resistance genes. This chapter concentrates on genes that are amplified in a substantial percentage (at least 10 percent) of primary tumors that have been extensively studied (at least 50 cases examined). We discuss *MYCN* amplification in neuroblastomas in detail to illustrate certain points, because it is the most consistent and most extensively studied example of oncogene amplification in a human tumor. However, amplification of the regions 11q13 and 12q14 are also discussed. For the sake of completeness, we discuss amplification of drug-resistance genes in human cancers, but they do not fulfill the criteria for inclusion discussed above.

AMPLIFICATION OF DRUG-RESISTANCE GENES

Culturing mammalian cells under conditions of incrementally increasing concentrations of a cytotoxic drug can lead to amplification of the gene encoding the protein which is the target of that drug.[1] This has suggested the possibility that human cancer cells may become resistant to chemotherapy by amplifying certain genes,[2] such as the dihydrofolate reductase (*DHFR*) gene in methotrexate-resistance, or the multidrug-resistance genes (*MDR1, MRP*) in tumors simultaneously resistant to multiple unrelated chemotherapeutic agents.[3–6] Indeed, there are several reports of human tumor cells that amplified the *DHFR* gene and became resistant to methotrexate.[7–10] However, this occurred in only a few cases, and only after prolonged clinical treatment, so the frequency with which it occurs does not meet our criteria for inclusion in this review. Furthermore, no reports of *MDR1* or *MRP* amplification have been reported in human tumors *in vivo*.[11] Thus, gene amplification appears to be a fairly rare mechanism for the development of drug resistance in humans.

AMPLIFICATION OF ONCOGENES

There are an increasing number of reports of human tumors and cell lines demonstrating amplification of proto-oncogenes. A cataloging of every reported tumor or cell line that has been shown to amplify an oncogene or related genes is beyond the scope of this chapter. Rather, we focus on examples of gene amplification in primary tumors that occur with substantial prevalence (more than 10 percent). The inclusion of cell-line studies would bias these data, because established cell lines in many systems show a higher prevalence of gene amplification than their primary tumor counterparts. For instance, amplification of *MYCN* and *ERBB1* (*EGFR*) are found in ~80 percent of cell lines established from neuroblastomas and head and neck squamous cell carcinomas respectively, whereas they are amplified in ~25 percent and in 10 percent of primary tumor specimens.[12–14]

Many different malignancies have been demonstrated to amplify a variety of oncogenes. These include neuroblastoma, breast and ovarian carcinoma, small cell lung carcinoma (SCLC), and head and neck squamous-cell carcinoma (HNSCC). In these malignancies, the prevalence of gene amplification ranges from 20 to 50 percent (see Table 21-1), often with amplification correlating with an aggressive phenotype (such as with advanced stage or decreased overall survival). In additional malignancies, such as sarcomas, hepatocellular carcinomas, malignant gliomas, and cervical, endometrial, and gastrointestinal cancers, data are accumulating that implicate gene amplification in their pathogenesis or progression as well (Table 21-1).

Genes amplified in human cancers are thought to confer a growth advantage to a clone, analogous to amplification *in vitro* of drug-resistance genes under certain selective external pressures. Genes frequently amplified in cancer tissues include members of the *MYC* (*MYC, MYCN, MYCL*) and *RAS* (*HRAS, KRAS, NRAS*) families of proto-oncogenes, growth factor receptors (*ERBB*-1 and -2, *FGFR*-1 and -2, *MET*), and genes that are involved in cell-cycle regulation (*CCND1, CCNE, MDM2, CDK4*), in addition to other miscellaneous genes (*AKT2, MYB*) (Table 21-2).

Activation of oncogenes is a common mechanism of tumorigenesis, and may occur by point mutation, translocation,

Table 21-1 Recurrent Oncogene Amplification in Human Cancers

Tumor Type	Gene Amplified	Frequency (%)	References
Breast cancer	MYC	20	18, 19, 22, 146
	ERBB2 (EGFR2)	20	18, 19, 22
	CCND1 (Cyclin D1)	15–20	19, 21, 22
	FGFR1	12	22, 24, 56
	FGFR2	12	56
Cervical cancer	MYC	25–50	147
	ERBB2	20	148
Colorectal cancer	HRAS	29	69
	KRAS	22	69
	MYB	15–20	70
Esophageal cancer	MYC	38	149
	CCND1 (Cyclin D1)	25	102
	MDM2	13	150
Gastric cancer	CCNE (Cyclin E)	15	21, 66
	KRAS	10	67
	MET	10	68
Glioblastoma	ERBB1 (EGFR)	33–50	151, 152
	CDK4	15	153
Head and neck cancer	CCND1 (Cyclin D1)	50	14, 72
	ERBB1 (EGFR)	10	14
	MYC	7–10	14, 109
Hepatocellular cancer	CCND1 (Cyclin D1)	13	103, 104
Neuroblastoma	MYCN	20–25	12, 13
Ovarian cancer	MYC	20–30	154, 155
	ERBB2 (EGFR2)	15–30	58, 59
	AKT2	12	60
Sarcoma	MDM2	10–30	110, 111, 150
	CDK4	11	109
Small cell lung cancer	MYC	15–20	62, 63

Table 21-2 Oncogenes Amplified in Human Cancers

Gene Amplified	Locus	Tumors
AKT2	19q13.2	Ovarian cancer
CCND1 (Cyclin D1)	11q13.3	HNSCC, esophageal, breast, HCC
CCNE (Cyclin E)	19q12	Gastric cancer
CDK4	12q14	Sarcoma, glioblastoma
ERBB1 (EGFR)	7p12	Glioblastoma, HNSCC
ERBB2 (EGFR2)	17q11.2-q12	Breast, ovarian, cervical cancer
FGFR1	8p11.1-p11.2	Breast cancer
FGFR2	10q25.3-q26	Breast cancer
HRAS	11p15.5	Colorectal cancer
KRAS	12p13	Colorectal, gastric cancer
MDM2	12q14	Soft tissue sarcomas, osteosarcoma, esophageal cancer
MET	7q31	Gastric cancer
MYB	6q23.3-q24	Colorectal cancer
MYC	8q24.12-q24.13	Ovarian, breast, SCLC, HNSCC, esophageal, cervical cancer
MYCN	2p24.3	Neuroblastoma

or amplification. In many of the malignancies studied to date, amplification of an oncogene is strongly associated with advanced stages of disease and with a poor outcome. In neuroblastoma, for example, *MYCN* amplification is associated with rapid disease progression independent of patient age and stage.[15–17] In other malignancies, however, the presence of amplification does not maintain significance as an independent variable for outcome when stage and histology are considered. In breast cancer, many studies have correlated the presence of ERBB2 (HER-2/*neu*) amplification with clinical parameters such as high stage and grade, lymph node involvement, large tumor size, and steroid hormone-receptor absence.[18,19] In multivariate analysis controlling for the above clinical data, the presence of ERBB2 amplification does not always predict a poor outcome. It remains to be determined, in this instance, whether oncogene amplification is a consequence of aggressive, deregulated cell proliferation and the resulting genomic instability, or if it is an early cellular event that is causative of the more aggressive clinical phenotype.

An amplicon may harbor multiple candidate genes and it may be difficult to determine a putative oncogene target among these. In fact, several genes may act in concert to determine the phenotype arising as a consequence of the amplification event. One widely studied region of amplification is the 11q13 region, amplified in breast and other carcinomas. This amplicon may contain *CCND1* (*Cyclin D1*), *FGF3* (*INT2*), *FGF4* (*HST*), *EMS1, GARP,* or a subset of these genes. Though investigators have implicated *CCND1* based on amplification prevalence and expression patterns in the amplified tumors,[20,21] it now appears likely that multiple genes from this region may be the targets of amplification events, as no single gene is invariably present on all amplicons.[22] Other examples include the 12q14 amplicon in the region of *MDM2, GLI, SAS, CDK4,* and 8p11 with *FGFR1, PLAT,* and others.[23,24] Likewise, it is possible to exploit the presence of amplified domains to discover potential oncogenes. Amplified DNA fragments can be cloned and mapped within the genome. From the amplified domain, new genes may be sought to explain the biologic significance of the amplification, as well as to elucidate their function in normal cells.[20,25] An example is the recently cloned and characterized AIB1 at 20q13, a steroid receptor co-activator which is amplified in ~6 to 10 percent of primary breast cancers.[26]

The prevalence of gene amplification in different tumors, as well as the biologic and clinical significance of amplifying particular genes, is discussed below, with particular emphasis on the role of *MYCN* amplification in neuroblastoma. Tumors that are presented in detail elsewhere in this volume are discussed briefly.

MYCN Amplification in Neuroblastomas

Neuroblastomas are tumors of the peripheral nervous system that are found almost exclusively in children. The peak age at diagnosis is 22 months, and it is rare after 10 years of age. Neuroblastomas often are localized and have a less aggressive behavior in infants, but they are frequently metastatic and have a poor prognosis in older children. The reason for this apparent discrepancy was unclear initially. However, cytogenetic and molecular analysis of these tumors has identified characteristic differences that allow these tumors to be subclassified into three groups that are distinct in terms of biologic features and clinical behavior (see Chap. 60). The feature that characterizes the most aggressive subset of neuroblastomas is amplification of the *MYCN* oncogene.

Cytogenetic examination of neuroblastomas reveals that a substantial number have either dmins, or HSRs, or both in subpopulations of cells. These two abnormalities are cytogenetic manifestations of gene amplification. Dmins are the predominant form of amplified DNA in primary tumors, but dmins and HSRs are found with about equal frequency in neuroblastoma cell lines.[12,13] Indeed, dmins and/or HSRs occur in about 90 percent of neuroblastoma cell lines, but in only 25 percent of primary tumors. Evidence suggests that this represents selection *in vitro* for cell lines derived from tumors that have pre-existing dmins or HSRs, and there is no evidence to date that these abnormalities develop with time in culture, at least in neuroblastomas. It is unclear why HSRs are a more common form of amplified DNA in established cell lines than in primary tumors.

Although cytogenetic analysis of human neuroblastomas frequently has revealed dmins or HSRs in primary tumors and cell lines,[12,13] the nature of the amplified sequences was not known initially. Evidence for amplification of genes associated with drug resistance was sought, but none was found. However, a study was undertaken to determine if a proto-oncogene was amplified in a panel of neuroblastoma cell lines. An oncogene related to the viral oncogene v-*myc,* but distinct from *MYC,* was amplified in the majority of neuroblastoma cell lines tested.[27] The amplified *MYCN* sequence was mapped to the HSRs on different chromosomes in neuroblastoma cell lines, but the normal single-copy locus was mapped to the distal short arm of chromosome 2.[28] Thus, the *MYCN* locus was amplified in neuroblastomas regardless of whether they had dmins or an HSR, and regardless of the chromosomal location of the HSR.

In collaboration with others, we studied primary tumors from untreated patients to determine if *MYCN* amplification occurred. In the initial analysis of 63 primary tumors, amplification ranging from 3- to 300-fold per haploid genome was found in 24 tumors (38 percent).[15] All cases with *MYCN* amplification in this initial study came from patients with advanced stages of disease. The progression-free survival of these patients was analyzed according to the stage of disease and *MYCN* copy number.[17] *MYCN* amplification clearly was associated with rapid tumor progression and a poor outcome, independent of the stage of the tumor.

Table 21-3 Correlation of *MYCN* Copy Number with Stage and Survival in 3,000 Neuroblastomas

Stage at Diagnosis	*MYCN* Amplification	3-yr. Survival (%)
Benign ganglioneuromas	0/64 (0%)	100
Low stages (1, 2)	31/772 (4%)	90
Stage 4-S	15/190 (8%)	80
Advanced stages (3, 4)	612/1974 (31%)	30
TOTAL	658/3000 (22%)	50

These studies have been extended to over 3000 patients with neuroblastoma enrolled in protocols of the Children's Cancer Group (CCG) and the Pediatric Oncology Group (POG) (Table 21-3).[13,16] It is now clear that among patients with less advanced stages of disease, which is traditionally associated with a good prognosis, a minority (5 to 10 percent) have tumors with *MYCN* amplification.[13,16] Our data indicate that virtually all of these patients are destined to have rapid tumor progression and a poor outcome, similar to their counterparts with advanced stages of disease. Over 30 percent of patients with more advanced tumor stages had *MYCN* amplification, and they also had an expectedly poor outcome. Our finding that *MYCN* amplification is associated with poor outcome regardless of the clinical stage of tumor is supported by independent studies from Japan and Europe.[29–35]

We analyzed the *MYCN* copy number in multiple simultaneous or consecutive samples of neuroblastoma tissue from 60 patients[36] to determine whether the presence or absence of *MYCN* was consistent in different tumor samples from a given patient, or if single-copy tumors ever developed amplification at the time of recurrence. Interestingly, we found a consistent pattern of *MYCN* copy number (either amplified or unamplified) in different tumor samples taken from an individual patient, either simultaneously or consecutively.[36] These studies have been extended to over 150 patients with similar results.[37] This suggests that *MYCN* amplification is an intrinsic biologic property of a subset of neuroblastomas. Tumors that develop *MYCN* amplification generally do so by the time of diagnosis, and cases of neuroblastoma with a single copy (per haploid genome) of *MYCN* at diagnosis rarely develop amplification subsequently.

Twenty-five to 30 percent of the children with neuroblastoma have *MYCN* amplification in their tumors, and virtually all of these children have rapidly progressive and fatal disease. However, there is controversy as to whether high levels of *MYCN* expression in single-copy tumors identify a subset with a particularly poor outcome.[38–43] Differences may depend on whether mRNA or protein expression was measured, as well as other details of the population studied or methods of analysis. Thus, it is still possible that activation of *MYCN* by mechanisms other than amplification or overexpression may play an important role. In addition, it is likely that activation of other oncogenes, deletion of specific suppressor genes, or other genetic lesions may contribute to the poor clinical outcome in these patients.

We sought evidence for amplification of other oncogenes, including *MYC, RAS, HRAS, KRAS, EGFR1, EGFR2, SIS, SRC, MYB, FOS,* and *ETS* in neuroblastomas, but found none.[13] However, there are at least six examples of neuroblastoma cell lines or primary tumors that amplify regions that are remote from the *MYCN* locus at 2p24. These include amplification of genes from 2p22 and 2p13 in the IMR-32 cell line,[44] as well as co-amplification of *MYCN* and *MDM2* (from 12q13) in the NGP, TR-14, and LS cell lines.[23,45,46] Finally, there is one report of co-amplification of *MYCN* and *MYCL* in a neuroblastoma cell line,[47] and this has been seen in at least one primary tumor as well (GM Brodeur, unpublished observations, 1988). These findings indicate that more than one locus can be amplified, but no neuroblastoma has been shown to amplify another gene that did not also amplify *MYCN.*

The presence of *MYCN* amplification in human neuroblastomas has been shown to correlate strongly with advanced clinical stage and poor prognosis.[13,15,17,31,38,41–43] Our recent studies[48] showed that 1p LOH is very common in tumors with *MYCN* amplification ($p < 0.001$).[12,13] Both *MYCN* amplification and deletion of 1p (as detected by cytogenetic or molecular analysis) appear strongly correlated with a poor clinical outcome and with each other, but it is not yet clear if they are independent prognostic variables.[49–55] Nevertheless, they appear to characterize a genetically distinct subset of very aggressive neuroblastomas.

Our data, which shows the consistency of *MYCN* copy number over time,[36] suggests that *MYCN* amplification is an intrinsic biologic property of a subset of tumors, so it must occur relatively early in these cases. Because patients with *MYCN* amplification represent a subset of patients with 1p deletion, we suspect that the 1p deletion may precede the development of amplification. Both of these genetic findings are uncommon in the tumors of infants less than 1 year of age, a group in which the overall prognosis of neuroblastoma is much better than their older counterparts. These results suggest at least two possibilities: either all neuroblastomas begin as tumors with a more favorable genotype and phenotype, and some evolve into more aggressive tumors with adverse genetic features over time, or there are at least two different subsets of neuroblastoma, and the more aggressive tumors generally occur in children over 1 year of age. Our data and that of other investigators are more consistent with the latter explanation.[13,16,48,51]

Oncogene Amplification in Other Cancers

Breast cancer. Breast cancer is the single most common cancer occurring in women, and represents a genetically heterogeneous disease with frequent amplification of oncogenes and allelic deletions.[18] *MYC, ERBB2,* and *CCND1* (Cyclin D1) are the most frequently amplified genes in breast cancer, each occurring in 10 to 20 percent of cases. Genes of the fibroblast growth factor receptor family (*FGFR1* and *FGFR2*) are also amplified in another 12 percent of cases each, although it is not clear that their expression is increased above baseline (see Table 21-1).[24,56] Many studies have attempted to correlate the presence of a particular amplified gene with outcome or other clinical prognostic factors with contradictory results. Although there is support for the notion that amplification is a late event in the multistep pathogenesis of breast cancer,[18,57] a more recent study has correlated amplification of certain genes or chromosomal regions with distinct breast cancer phenotypes.[22] Amplification of 12q13-q15 (containing *MDM2, CDK4, SAS,* and/or *GLI*) and 20q13 (containing the recently cloned *AIB1*) each occur in fewer than 10 percent of primary tumors.[22,26]

Ovarian cancer. In ovarian cancer, amplification of *ERBB2* and *MYC* are found in 15 to 30 percent of samples.[58,59] *ERBB2* or *MYC* amplification tends to occur in advanced stages of disease and is seen infrequently in early invasive or borderline ovarian epithelial tumors,[58] again implying that these are late genetic events. *AKT2* is a protein serine/threonine kinase with homology to v-*akt,* a viral oncogene that can cause lymphomas in mice. *AKT2* is amplified independently of *MYC* or *ERBB2* in ~12 percent of ovarian cancers and also correlates with invasiveness.[60] Though amplification of *NRAS* and *KRAS* are seen infrequently in ovarian cancers, there is some evidence that these events occur earlier based on their prevalence in low-stage disease, but this remains speculative.[61]

Lung cancer. Lung cancer is one of the most common fatal malignancies and its incidence is increasing in both men and women. Small cell lung carcinoma makes up ~25% of cases and has a distinct clinical course with a propensity for early metastasis. The *MYC* proto-oncogenes are the only genes amplified in a significant number of small cell lung carcinomas (15 to 20 percent of cases), although cell lines derived from SCLC specimens more frequently have gene amplification.[14,62,63] The majority of these cases involve *MYC,* with amplification of *MYCN* and *MYCL* also occurring.[62,63] However, to date, co-amplification of multiple *MYC* family genes has not been described in SCLC specimens. It is possible that the propensity of SCLC cell lines to amplify *MYC* *in vitro* illustrates this cancer's underlying genetic instability and virulent phenotype.

Although no genes that are frequently amplified in non-SCLC have been identified, a region of amplification at 3q26 has been demonstrated by CGH and reverse chromosome painting in ~40 percent of specimens evaluated.[64,65] The gene target(s) of this amplification remain unknown.

Gastrointestinal cancers. A diverse group of genetic alterations occur in gastrointestinal cancers, involving mutation or deletion of tumor-suppressor genes and DNA repair genes, in addition to amplification of oncogenes. Amplification of *MYC, MDM2,* and *CCND1* occur frequently in esophageal squamous cell carcinoma, the latter being almost uniformly amplified in metastatic disease and correlating with clinical and pathologic staging.[66] In contrast, a plethora of genetic alterations occur in gastric cancer, many presumed to induce cell proliferation via induction of growth factor production or increased growth factor receptor expression, but amplification does not occur commonly. These genetic alterations differ in poorly differentiated and well-differentiated gastric cancers, and *KRAS* or *CCNE* are each amplified in 10 to 15 percent of cases.[21,66,67] Though *MET* is amplified in >10 percent of cases in some series, it is generally not amplified to high copy number.[68]

In colorectal cancers, cytogenetic evidence for gene amplification has long existed in the form of dmins, but with no clear candidate genes. In some series, *MYB, HRAS,* and *KRAS* amplification has been found, but in the majority of colorectal cancers, none of the known oncogenes have been amplified in a significant proportion of cases.[69,70] *MYC* may be amplified in up to 10 percent of tumors, however the level of amplification is often low (two- to five-fold) and the gene is more often overexpressed in the absence of gene amplification, possibly through alterations in *APC*-mediated repression.[71]

HNSCC, other cancers. In HNSCCs, amplification of the 11q13 locus with *CCND1* occurs frequently, while *MYC* and *ERBB1* amplification are also seen.[14,72] These findings are particularly germane in that current clinical prognostic factors are poor for HNSCC and molecular data may in the future become of significant predictive importance. In still other malignancies, gene amplification has been shown to be a prominent feature. In glioblastoma, hepatocellular carcinoma, cervical cancer, and soft tissue sarcomas, the role of oncogene amplification is being elucidated as advanced molecular analyses of these malignancies become more prevalent (see Table 21-1).

MECHANISMS OF GENE AMPLIFICATION

The precise mechanism by which gene amplification occurs in human cancers is not known with certainty.[73] Some information can be obtained by studying amplification of drug-resistance genes in cells grown *in vitro* under selective pressure. However, these systems generally involve the rapid selection for resistance to an antimetabolite or other toxic compound, so it is not clear that these model systems will provide relevant information. It is more likely that the selective pressures that lead to amplification of a gene that provides a growth advantage *in vivo* are not as profound, so the mechanisms leading to gene amplification may be quite different.

Experimentally, it appears that several types of genetic abnormality are required to allow gene amplification to take place. First, there must be loss of cell-cycle control. This occurs frequently by mutation or inactivation of p53 in human tumors,[74,75] but other mechanisms must also be possible, such as overexpression of cyclin D1 (*CCND1*),[76,77] in cells that lack p53 abnormalities. Second, DNA damage or instability must be present. This can be a result of DNA-damaging agents, or due to mutations in genes such as p53 that affect DNA stability and repair.[78,79] Finally, there needs to be some stimulus to progress through the cell cycle. This can occur as a result of oncogene activation, such as *MYC* overexpression, growth factor/receptor activation, or other mechanisms.[80] The order in which these occur may not be important, but the result is that cells progress through the cell cycle with damaged DNA and are unable to pause for proper repair. The consequence is that gross rearrangements can occur, leading to amplification, deletion, or translocation of genes, with resultant oncogene activation or suppressor gene loss (Fig. 21-1).

Unfortunately, no model system exists for selection of oncogene activation in human tumors. This makes it difficult to draw firm conclusions about early events in the amplification process, so only the end-point of gene amplification can be studied. Some information can be obtained by structural analysis of the amplified unit, as well as by analysis of the genomic configuration of the locus that was amplified. In the majority of cases, the initial form of amplified DNA seen in human cancers is the extrachromosomal dmins. These structures lack centromeres or kinetochores, and they apparently segregate randomly in the two daughter cells after cell division. To remain stable, it is likely that dmins are closed circular molecules. Experimental data supporting this hypothesis have come from the study of amplified units involving the *MYCN* gene in human neuroblastomas, as well as other systems.

Several models have been proposed to explain the development of genomic amplification of specific chromosomal regions. These include the overreplication (onionskin) model, the chromosomal breakage/deletion plus episome formation model, and the duplication and crossing-over model. These models were based on the analysis of genomic rearrangements that followed the rapid, stepwise selection of resistance to a particular drug. None of these models are perfectly consistent with what is known about the structure of DNA in tumors with spontaneous amplification of regions containing oncogenes, such as the *MYCN* oncogene in human neuroblastomas, but some insights can be gained.

Amler and colleagues[81,82] used pulsed-field gel electrophoresis (PFGE) to study the restriction pattern of *MYCN* amplicons, using infrequently cutting enzymes and probes around the *MYCN* gene. These studies led to the conclusion that the amplicons were arranged in tandem, head-to-tail arrays in the HSRs, and that most of the amplicons had a consistent restriction pattern (there was relatively little rearrangement). These conclusions were supported by Schneider and colleagues[83] who cloned a representative amplified domain into yeast artificial chromosomes (YACs) from a cell line with 300 copies of *MYCN* per cell as dmins. They showed that the amplicons in dmins were organized in a head-to-tail, apparently circular, arrangement. Structural rearrangements relative to the normal locus were consistently identified, but there was general preservation of the germ line genomic structure. Finally, Corvi and coworkers[84] showed that the germ line copy of *MYCN* was apparently intact on both homologs of chromosome 2, so that models based on deletion of this locus would not explain the process.

Based on the overreplication model, the resolution of this complex structure would result in considerable rearrangement of the amplified sequences relative to the germ line configuration. There should be a mixture of head-to-head, tail-to-tail, and head-to-tail configurations of the DNA in different or adjacent amplicons. Also, a gradient of amplification would be seen, with the highest level of amplification near the gene that is the presumed target of amplification, with decreasing amplification further away from the amplification epicenter. However, the PFGE data by Amler[81] and YAC-cloning data by Schneider[83] are inconsistent with this model, even though some variation from the germ line pattern was detected by both approaches.

The duplication plus crossing over model would suggest that relatively intact copies of the amplicon would occur *in situ* on a given chromosome, leading to an HSR at the site of the normal

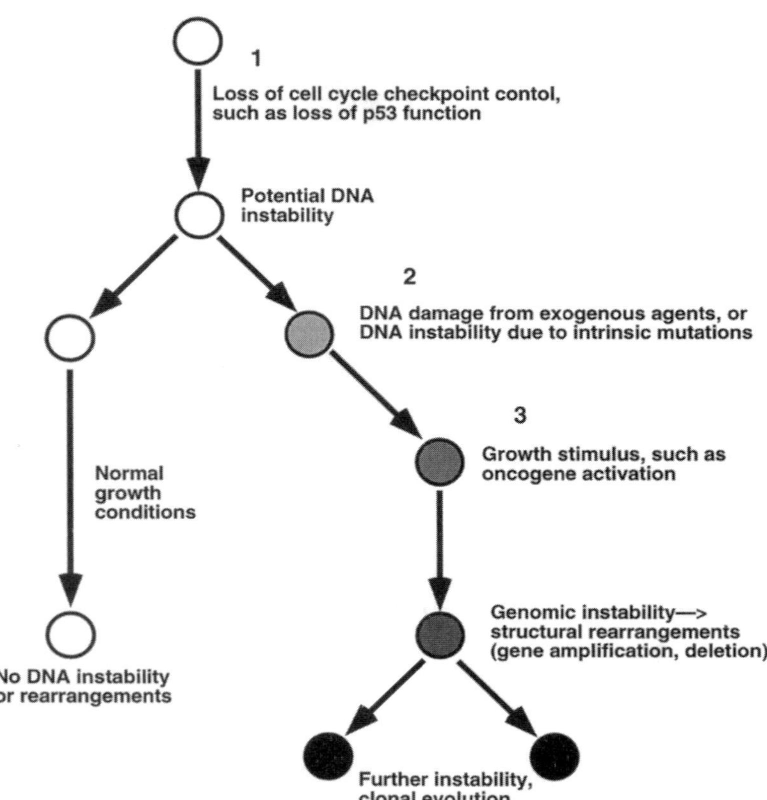

Fig. 21-1 Hypothetical process of gene amplification in mammalian cells. It appears that several types of genetic abnormality are required to allow gene amplification to take place. First, there needs to be loss of cell cycle control. Second, some mechanism of DNA damage or instability must occur. Finally, there needs to be some stimulus to progress through the cell cycle. The events do not need to occur in this order, but the result is that cells progress through the cell cycle with damaged DNA are unable to pause for proper repair. The net result is that gross genetic rearrangements can occur, leading to amplification or other genetic rearrangements.

gene. However, the most common form of amplified DNA is the extrachromosomal dmins, and the chromosomal locations of HSRs representing amplification of *MYCN* in neuroblastomas occur almost everywhere except at the normal chromosomal location of *MYCN* at 2p24.[85] Thus, this model does not seem applicable to what happens when *MYCN* becomes amplified in human neuroblastomas, or perhaps to amplification of oncogenes in general.

However, duplication of the *MYCN* locus has been observed in a few neuroblastoma cell lines that lack true amplification.[86] This may either represent a precursor to amplification of this locus, or an alternate mechanism of *MYCN* activation. Furthermore, amplification of the *MDM2* locus has been seen in a few neuroblastoma cell lines in conjunction with *MYCN* amplification.[23,45,46] In most of these cases, the amplified DNA is in the form of an HSR located at the normal site of *MDM2*. Thus, amplification of this locus may occur by a different mechanism than that involved in *MYCN* amplification.

Finally, the chromosomal breakage/deletion plus episome formation model suggests that one germ line copy of the amplified region is deleted, but this was not detected in the five cell lines studied by Corvi[84] or the cell line studied by Kanda[87] and Shiloh.[44,88] One study by Hunt and Tereba[89] did suggest that one germ line copy of *MYCN* was deleted from a homolog in one cell line by segregating the homologs into separate somatic cell hybrids, but this is inconsistent with data from at least six other cell lines studied by FISH. This suggests that the apparent deletion may have occurred during the formation of the somatic cell hybrids, or that there may be different mechanisms by which *MYCN* amplification can occur.

In summary, none of these models, which are derived primarily from the study of amplification of drug-resistance genes, fully explains the *de novo* amplification of oncogenes in human tumors *in vivo*. It seems likely that a variation of the DNA breakage plus episome formation model without deletion of the normal locus is applicable. Given the apparent retention of the normal parental copies of the amplified region, it is likely that duplication of the amplified region occurs, followed by excision and circularization to form a dmin. Then the copy number increases by unequal segregation of the replicated minutes, providing a selective advantage to the daughter cell with the largest number of dmins, until maximal advantage is achieved. The *in situ* duplication of this locus identified by Corvi and colleagues[86] may represent an initial step in this process. Also, this mechanism may explain the apparent *in situ* amplification of the *MDM2* locus seen in a few neuroblastoma cell lines with HSRs at 12q14.

Further study will be required to elucidate the precise mechanisms involved, but this will be difficult until a model system for *de novo* oncogene amplification can be found. Nevertheless, the study of drug resistance in mammalian cells suggests that several discrete steps are likely to be involved in the process, including loss of cell-cycle control, DNA instability, and a growth-promoting stimulus. Given the infrequency of p53 mutations in neuroblastomas, some alternative mechanism for loss of cell cycle control and DNA instability must be involved.

STRUCTURAL ANALYSIS OF AMPLICONS

Amplification of the *MYCN* Locus at 2p24

Estimates of the size of the amplified domain around the *MYCN* proto-oncogene in neuroblastomas have ranged from 300 kb to 3000 kb, based on physical, chemical, and electrophoretic measurements of the amplified DNA.[85] However, most approaches to map the size of the amplified domain have been indirect. An attempt was made to clone and map the amplified domain around *MYCN* in a representative neuroblastoma cell line NGP using cosmid and lambda vectors.[90,91] Only 140 kb of contiguous DNA around the *MYCN* locus could be mapped, but a number of additional amplified clones were identified that were not contained in the 140 kb contiguous region. The entire 140 kb contiguous locus was amplified in a panel of 12 primary neuroblastomas with *MYCN* amplification, whereas the non-contiguous fragments were amplified in subsets of them.[91] These data indicate that, although each tumor had a relatively unique pattern of amplified DNA fragments, there was a core region that was consistently amplified in different tumors.

Amler and Schwab[81] have analyzed the amplified domain of a series of neuroblastoma cell lines with *MYCN* amplification, most in the form of chromosomally integrated HSRs. They analyzed the amplified domain by pulsed-field gel electrophoresis and hybridization with DNA probes that represent the 5′ and 3′ ends of the *MYCN* gene. They confirmed the heterogeneity of size of the amplified domain seen in different neuroblastomas demonstrated by earlier studies.[44,88,90,91] They also concluded that most amplified regions of DNA consisted of multiple tandem arrays of DNA segments that were several hundred kilobases in size, and that *MYCN* was at or near the center of the amplified units. Rearrangements were more commonly found in the cell lines with HSRs and with higher *MYCN* copy number (greater than 50 to 100 copies/haploid genome).

To determine the size and structural organization of this region in different tumors and cell lines, as well as the core region that is consistently amplified, we analyzed the amplified domain in human neuroblastomas. Because of the large size of the domain, we used the YAC-cloning vector system.[92] Twenty YACs that contained segments of the amplified domain from a representative neuroblastoma cell line were identified, which could be arranged in a contiguous linear map of ~1.2 Mb.[83,93] In general, the YAC clones were consistent with the germ line configuration of the region, but some rearrangements were identified. Our data also indicated that the core of the domain amplified in different tumors was no more than 130 kb, and that the amplicons of one tumor deleted about half of this core.[94] Although it remains possible that there may be other genes near *MYCN* whose expression is important in mediating the aggressive phenotype associated with *MYCN* amplification, our data suggest that *MYCN* is the primary target of amplification in neuroblastomas (Fig. 21-2).

The closest expressed sequence mapping near *MYCN* is the *DDX1* gene. This gene is an RNA helicase that may play a role in mRNA processing or stability. The *DDX1* gene was found because of its co-amplification with *MYCN* in a retinoblastoma cell line.[95] It also appears to be co-amplified in 50 to 60 percent of neuroblastomas, but it does not appear to be amplified independent of the *MYCN* locus.[96–100] The *DDX1* gene has been mapped about 300 kb 5′ and telomeric of *MYCN*, but in the same transcriptional orientation (Fig. 21-2).[97,98,100] Recent evidence suggests that tumors that co-amplify *MYCN* and *DDX1* may be more aggressive than those amplifying *MYCN* alone.[99] Also, transfection of the NIH3T3 mouse fibroblast line with *DDX1* appears to confer properties of transformation, suggesting that amplification and overexpression of *DDX1* may contribute to a more aggressive phenotype.[101]

Amplification of the 11q13 Locus

The 11q13 region contains a number of genes that are potential targets of the amplification that occurs in HNSCCs, breast carcinomas, hepatocellular carcinomas, and selected other tumors.[14,19,21,22,72,102–104] The genes in this region and representative amplicons are shown in Fig. 21-3. The majority of amplicons involve the *CCND1, FGF3* (INT2), and *FGF4* (HST) genes. However, some involve only regions proximal or distal to this, without involving *CCND1, FGF3,* or *FGF4,* so there may be multiple targets of amplification in this region. However, it is likely that amplification of *CCDN1* is the most important contributor to the malignant phenotypes, because *FGF3* and *FGF4* expression is generally low or absent.[105]

Amplification of the 12q14 Locus

The 12q14 region also contains a number of genes that are potential targets of the amplification seen in bone and soft tissue sarcomas, glioblastoma, esophageal cancer, and selected other tumors.[22,106–111] The genes in this region and representative amplicons are shown in Fig. 21-4. The majority of amplicons involve *SAS, CDK4,* and *MDM2.* However, some involve only *SAS* and *CDK4,* whereas others involve only *MDM2,* so there may be at least two target regions of amplification. Interestingly, for sarcomas, the amplification of one or the other region appears to correlate with particular histologic subtypes.[112]

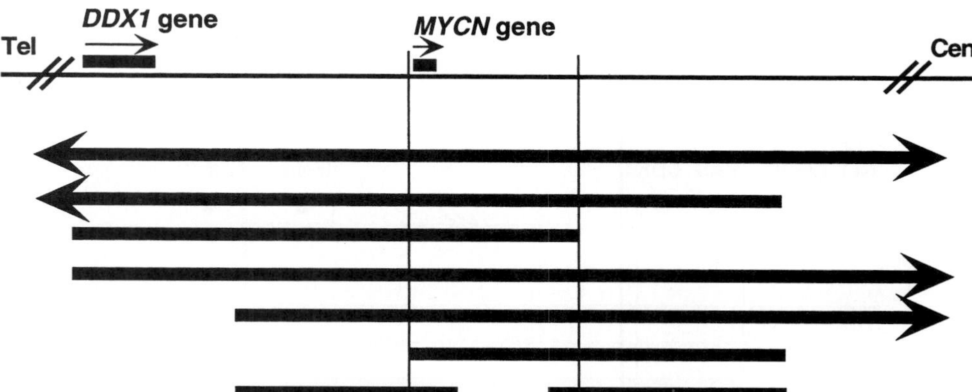

Fig. 21-2 Patterns of *MYCN* amplification at 2p24. Shown at the top is the region of 2p24 containing the *MYCN* and *DDX1* genes. *DDX1* is about 300 kb telomeric of *MYCN,* but both are in the same transcriptional orientation. *MYCN* is amplified in about 22 percent of neuroblastomas, as well as a minority of retinoblastomas, medulloblastomas, small cell lung cancers, and selected other tumors. Shown below are broad lines indicating the extent of amplicons in different tumors. The patterns shown are representative of those seen in human neuroblastomas.[94] Some extend for over a megabase, but all involve the *MYCN* proto-oncogene. About 50 to 60 percent also include the *DDX1* gene, which is overexpressed in these cases, but no tumors amplify *DDX1* unless *MYCN* is also amplified. The core domain that is consistently amplified in all neuroblastomas with *MYCN* amplification is about 130 kb in length. However, one tumor deletes about half of this region, while retaining the *MYCN* gene. Thus, it appears that *MYCN* is the major focus of amplification of this region in neuroblastomas. Nevertheless, recent evidence suggests that overexpression of *DDX1* also has transforming effects, so that co-amplification of both genes may lead to more aggressive tumors than amplification of *MYCN* alone.

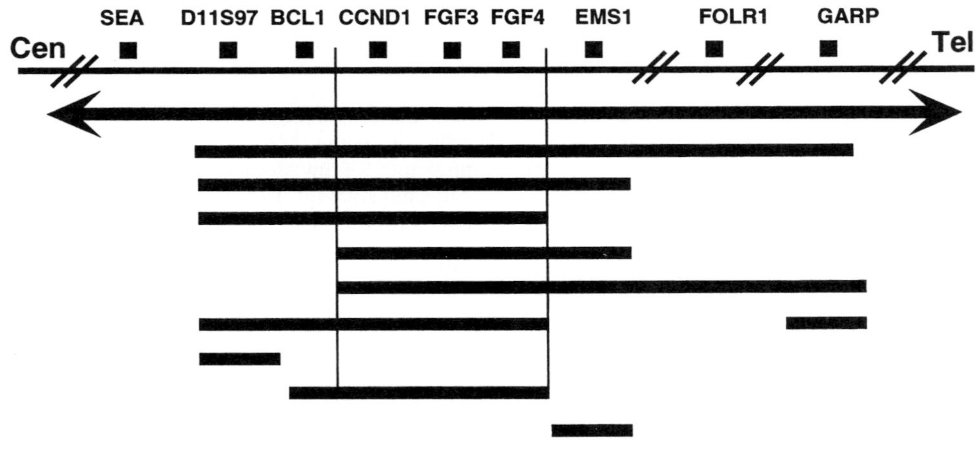

Fig. 21-3 Patterns of 11q13 amplification. Shown at the top is the region of 11q13, which contains a number of genes that are potential targets of the amplification. This region is amplified in head and neck squamous cell carcinomas, breast carcinomas, hepatocellular carcinomas, and selected other tumors. Shown below are broad lines indicating the extent of amplicons in different tumors. The patterns shown are representative of different patterns described in human breast cancers.[22] Some extend over the entire region, but no single gene is consistently amplified in all cases. The majority of amplicons include the *CCND1, FGF3* (INT2), and *FGF4* (HST) genes. However, some include only regions proximal or distal to this, without involving *CCND1, FGF3,* or *FGF4,* so there may be multiple targets of amplification in this region. Furthermore, it is unclear if amplification of *CCDN1, FGF3, FGF4,* or some combination thereof is essential to confer a selective advantage.

BIOLOGICAL SIGNIFICANCE OF GENE AMPLIFICATION

Presumably, the mechanism by which gene amplification confers a selective advantage on the cancer cells is by overexpression of the gene or genes contained within the amplicon. In general, this overexpression is proportional to the increase in copy number, but there is not an absolute correlation. The overexpression of the gene or genes may cause malignant transformation or may alter the cell phenotype by conferring some advantage in cell proliferation or survival. We review briefly what is known about the likely consequences of overexpressing the most frequently amplified genes in human cancers: the *MYC* family, the *RAS* family, the *ERBB* and *FGFR* families, and the cell-cycle control genes, including the cyclins and *MDM2*.

MYC Family Amplification

The structure of the Myc family proteins consists of a transactivating domain at the N-terminal third of the protein, followed by a basic region, helix-loop-helix, and leucine zipper domain (B-HLH-Zip). These proteins are thought to activate transcription by binding to a hexanucleotide motif CACGTG known as an E-box. However, they do not bind well as monomers or as homodimers, but rather as heterodimers with another B-HLH-Zip protein known as Max.[113] This protein lacks a

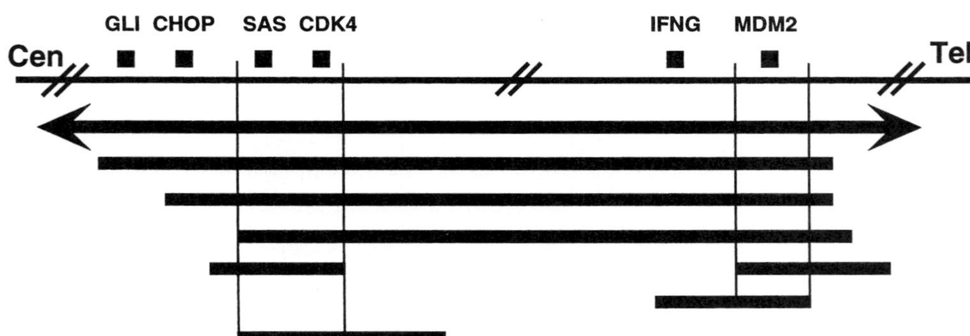

Fig. 21-4 Patterns of 12q14 amplification. Shown at the top is the region of 12q14, which contains a number of genes that are potential targets of the amplification. This region is amplified in bone and soft tissue sarcomas, glioblastoma, esophageal cancer, and selected other tumors. Shown below are broad lines indicating the extent of amplicons in different tumors. The patterns shown are representative of different patterns described in human breast cancers and sarcomas.[22,106–108] Some extend over the entire region, but no single gene is consistently amplified in all cases. The majority of amplicons involve *SAS, CDK4,* and *MDM2.* However, some involve only *SAS* and *CDK4,* whereas others involve only *MDM2,* so there may be at least two target regions of amplification.

transcriptional activation domain, and it can form homodimers that are thought to be transcriptionally repressive.[114–118] Thus, in a state of Max excess, Max homodimers predominate, and transcription is repressed. Conversely, when Myc (or MycN) are expressed at higher levels, Myc-Max heterodimers predominate, resulting in transcriptional activation of Myc target genes, which, to date, remain poorly characterized.[119] Nevertheless, the consequence is progression through the cell cycle and proliferation of the cell population.

Myc oncoproteins have a short half-life (20 to 30 min), so once transcription and translation cease, the levels of Myc fall rapidly, and Max-Max transcriptional repression predominates. However, in tumors that amplify *MYC, MYCN* or *MYCL,* the level of amplification is usually ten- to one hundredfold (or more), with corresponding overexpression of the oncoprotein.[38,41–43,63] This leads to very high steady-state levels of Myc, even when it is not being actively transcribed. This, in turn, presumably favors a state of proliferation, with less likelihood that the cell will enter G0 and become quiescent. This is presumably the selective advantage conferred by overexpressing this family of genes.

RAS Family Amplification

RAS genes encode proteins known as G proteins, which participate in the signaling cascade initiated by the activation of tyrosine kinase receptors or other signaling intermediates. *RAS* activation by specific base-pair mutations or overexpression by amplification leads to enhanced signal transduction through the RAF-1 serine-threonine kinase, the early response kinases (ERK1 and ERK2), and the subsequent induction of transcription of immediate-early genes (e.g., FOS, JUN).[120–122]

The amplification and overexpression of *RAS* genes leads to constitutive signal transduction, mimicking the effects of continual activation of a growth factor receptor, such as EGFR or PDGFR.[120–125] This, in turn, leads to continuous cell proliferation. However, the cellular background is very important, because in certain cellular milieus (such as neural cells), the predominant receptor tyrosine kinase may be signaling differentiation and not proliferation. Activation or overexpression of *RAS* in this context would lead to differentiation of the cell, which would not promote the proliferation of tumor cells.[120–122,125] This may explain why RAS activation is rare in neural tumors, whereas it is one of the most common types of oncogene activation in many other tumor types.[123–125]

Amplification of the *ERBB* and *FGFR* Family

Amplification and overexpression of genes for growth factors or their receptors, such as those of the *EGF/EGFR (ERBB)* and *FGF/FGFR* families, occur in a number of human cancers.[24,56,58] The ERBB and FGF receptors are transmembrane tyrosine kinases, which are involved in cell proliferation. After specific ligand binding, signal transduction occurs through phosphorylation of the SH2 domains of cytoplasmic proteins associated with the receptor. Activation of the Ras-GTP pathway frequently occurs. Kinase activation also leads to PKC phosphorylation, serine/threonine phosphorylations, and changes in phosphatidyl inositol metabolism, with the end result being modulation of specific genes necessary for proliferation.[126,127]

Gastric cancer expresses a number of growth factors and receptors including EGF, TGF-α, ERBB2 and FGFR2.[66,128] EGF is synthesized as a transmembrane precursor, and a secreted protein is released by proteolytic cleavage. It has been shown to enhance growth of cells from most epithelial tumors,[129] and in gastric cancer, EGF expression is associated with poor outcome.[128] Human gastric cancers that possess both EGF and EGFR (or ERBB2) simultaneously have a greater degree of local invasion and lymph node metastasis, further suggesting autocrine stimulation. Additionally, high levels of expression of growth factor receptor alone may result in autophosphorylation and signaling, even in the absence of ligand. Constitutive activation of these growth factor-signaling pathways are a common motif in oncogenesis.[126,127] Amplification and overexpression of either ligand or receptor may cause growth stimulation in an autocrine or paracrine fashion in the appropriate cellular setting and contribute to malignant behavior.

Amplification of the Genes Encoding Regulators of the Cell Cycle

Cells of most higher organisms maintain a stringent "checkpoint control" over progression from G1 into S phase and subsequent cell division. Early in G1, cells are dependent on mitogenic stimuli, but at a certain point a switch to intrinsic cell-cycle machinery occurs with a reduced requirement for growth factor stimuli, apparently ensuring an ordered completion of the cell division cycle. This switch-point is mediated in part by the D-type cyclins, although many proteins may also play important roles as both positive and negative regulators. These proteins include (but are not limited to) other cyclins, cyclin-dependent kinases (cdk), and their inhibitors (cdki). Activation of G1-S cyclins (*CCND1* and *CCNE*) occurs via growth factor signals that induce Cyclin D1 phosphorylation. Activated Cyclins D and E, in association with their predominant cyclin-dependent kinases CDK4 and CDK2, then sequentially phosphorylate the RB protein. This causes the release of E2F from pRB, which activates transcription of genes involved in cell proliferation.[130,131]

Overexpression of *CCND1, CCNE,* or *CDK4* presumably results in a growth advantage for cells by tipping the balance in favor of G1-S transition rather than quiescence. Likewise, overexpression of *MDM2* could have similar effects. MDM2 protein binds p53, a potent cell-cycle inhibitor. By blocking p53-mediated transcriptional activation of cyclin-dependent kinase inhibitors such as p21, cells are more likely to enter S phase.[130,131] This loss of checkpoint control fails to allow time for repair of DNA damage caused by a multitude of insults, such as ionizing radiation, drugs, and cellular toxins, or mutations in DNA repair genes.

METHODS OF DETECTING GENE AMPLIFICATION

A variety of techniques may be used to detect gene amplification.[132] Each technique has its advantages and disadvantages in terms of the amount of tumor tissue or DNA needed, the ease of performing the technique; its sensitivity in detecting low levels of amplification; the size of the amplified unit; and whether the locus (or loci) are known that are likely to be amplified in a given tumor type. The techniques include conventional cytogenetics; Southern analysis; fluorescence *in situ* hybridization (FISH); semiquantitative PCR; comparative genomic hybridization (CGH); and microarray analysis.

Cytogenetic Analysis

Cytogenetic analysis is a labor-intensive technique that is dependent on analyzing dividing cells in the tumor tissue or during adaptation to growth in short-term culture. As a result, it is unsuccessful in the majority of solid tumors and a substantial number of leukemias. The detection of HSRs or dmins provides evidence for gene amplification in the culture, although small HSRs or dmins may escape detection. Also, it is impossible to know with certainty which gene or chromosomal region is amplified. This is a useful technique when investigating a new tumor type, but is not the most efficient or sensitive approach once it is known which gene or genes are likely to be amplified.

Southern Analysis

Southern analysis is the gold standard against which other techniques are compared. This technique relies on the preparation of DNA from tumor tissue that is relatively free of contaminating normal tissue. The DNA is digested with a restriction enzyme, electrophoresed on an agarose gel, blotted to a membrane, and hybridized with a radioactive probe corresponding to the gene or genomic region thought to be amplified.[15,36] This technique is rather labor intensive, and it generally requires 5 to 10 μg of DNA. Frequently, an internal control gene is also hybridized so the intensity of the band of interest can be normalized by quantitative densitometry. However, this technique can miss a small percentage of amplified cells in an unamplified population (such as the bone marrow or a lymph node). Slot blotting is a variation on this technique that requires no digestion, only 1 μg of DNA, and it is easily subjected to densitometric analysis, but low levels of amplification also can be missed.

Fluorescence *In Situ* Hybridization (FISH)

The FISH technique is probably the most efficient and popular technique for the detection of DNA amplification if the gene (or genes) of interest are known.[133,134] It requires only a small amount of tumor tissue, usually a "touch prep" or "cytospin" of several thousand cells on a slide. It can even be done on paraffin-embedded tissue.[134] Hybridization to interphase nuclei takes place overnight under a coverslip, and the results can be interpreted within 24 to 48 h. This technique can also distinguish a small percentage of amplified tumor cells in a population of normal or nonamplified tumor cells, if a counterstain to visualize the "positive" cells is implemented. It may be necessary to utilize a control probe for the centromere or opposite arm of the same chromosome, in order to distinguish between low-level amplification and polysomy for the particular chromosome. However, because this approach requires a fluorescence microscope and sophisticated imaging equipment, and because the probes may be expensive to purchase commercially, FISH is not the ideal approach for all laboratories.

An interesting variation on this technique has been developed whereby amplicons are microdissected and used as FISH hybridization probes to determine the chromosomal origin.[135] This "micro-FISH" approach allows the chromosomal origin of dmins or HSRs to be determined in a single hybridization without knowing a priori the genetic region that is amplified. Indeed, this approach can also identify amplification of previously unsuspected chromosomal regions. However, in addition to the technical demands of FISH, this approach also requires both successful metaphase preparation, with identification of dmins or HSRs, and the ability to perform microdissection and preparation of a microclone library. Therefore, this method is primarily suited for research laboratories.

Semiquantitative PCR

The PCR technique has advantages that might be applied to the detection of genomic amplification in small amounts of tumor DNA.[136–139] As long as the number of cycles of amplification is carefully controlled, and an internal control gene is used for normalization, it is possible to semiquantitatively amplify a given gene or DNA sequence and distinguish the normal copy number from multiple extra copies. Although some claim to detect as low as twofold amplification, generally five- to tenfold amplification is the limit of detection of this technique on primary tumor samples.[136–139]

Comparative Genomic Hybridization (CGH)

This is one of the newest of the approaches to the detection of genomic amplification.[140–142] This approach has the advantage of conventional cytogenetics in that the whole genome is surveyed, not just one or a few specific genomic regions that are known or suspected to be amplified in a given tumor type. Also, because the chromosomal location of the amplified region is known, the likely gene amplified is frequently apparent from past experience. Tumor metaphases are not needed, and only a small amount of DNA is required. However, this approach requires a sophisticated fluorescence microscope and image-capturing capability, as well as software to analyze the data obtained. Furthermore, very small amplicons or low levels of amplification may be missed, and it cannot detect translocations.

Microarray Analysis

DNA microarray technology relies on hybridization just as Southern blotting, FISH, and CGH do. Using this approach, multiple cDNAs, or genomic regions, are "spotted" on a solid-phase support, which may be a glass slide or microchip. Probing with a labeled DNA mixture obtained from tumor samples allows for detection of amplified genomic regions.[143] Comparing data obtained using microarrays and quantitative hybridization has yielded a very good correlation. This technique has the capability to allow high-throughput, although at a substantial cost. The information content requires significant image processing and may not be available in most centers. Commercial development of microarrays containing genomic regions of interest (i.e., those regions with amplification in a particular tumor system) may allow this technology to supplant CGH as the next-generation method of high-resolution genome scanning. Other applications of microarray technology are for analysis of patterns of gene expression,[144] or even analysis of complex genes for mutations.[145]

SUMMARY AND CONCLUSIONS

Gene amplification in human cells is a phenomenon that appears to be restricted to tumor cells. In the majority of cases in which the amplified genomic region has been identified, the target of the amplification appears to be an oncogene, usually of the *MYC, RAS*, or *ERBB* family. A variety of other genes have been shown to be amplified in small numbers of cases, or in tumor-derived cell lines, but the above-mentioned families are found the most consistently. Examples of amplification of genes conferring drug resistance have been found in certain cancers at relapse, but this does not appear to be a common mechanism by which cancer cells become drug resistant *in vivo*.

The mechanism by which amplification of oncogenes in humans occurs is unknown, and it may be different for individual loci. In the majority of cases, however, it probably involves the duplication of a large chromosomal region, followed by deletion and circularization to form an extrachromosomal dmin. Then there is accumulation of these dmins by uneven segregation into the daughter cells during mitosis, until maximal advantage is achieved. This is presumably a consequence of the overexpression of a gene (or genes) on the amplicon that confers the selective advantage. The region amplified may be quite large, from 100 kb to several megabases. However, the region that is consistently amplified may contain little more than the single gene suspected of providing a growth or survival advantage.

The identification of oncogene amplification in certain human cancers provides some insight into the pathogenesis of these diseases. Indeed, in some tumor systems, oncogene amplification had been associated with a greater likelihood of invasion, metastasis, and a poor outcome. Thus, the identification of oncogene amplification in human cancers may have some prognostic value. Ultimately, it may be possible to develop novel therapeutic approaches that target the amplified oncogene or the overexpressed oncoprotein. This approach may be particularly attractive if the amplified gene is mutated or chimeric, allowing the development of selective biological reagents or targeted gene therapy approaches.

ACKNOWLEDGMENTS

This work was supported in part by National Institutes of Health grant RO1-CA-39771.

REFERENCES

1. Schimke RT: Gene amplification in cultured cells. *J Biol Chem* **263**:5989, 1988.
2. Sobrero A, Bertino JR: Clinical aspects of drug resistance. *Cancer Surv* **5**:93, 1986.

3. Pastan I, Gottesman M: Multiple-drug resistance in human cancer. *N Engl J Med* **316**:1388, 1987.
4. Chin JE, Soffir R, Noonan KE, Choi K, Roninson IB: Structure and expression of the human MDR (P-glycoprotein) gene family. *Mol Cell Biol* **9**:3808, 1989.
5. Ling V: P-glycoprotein and resistance to anticancer drugs. *Cancer* **69**:2603, 1992.
6. Grant CE, Valdimarsson G, Hipfner DR, Almquist KC, Cole SPC, Deeley RG: Overexpression of multidrug resistance-associated protein (MRP) increases resistance to natural product drugs. *Cancer Res* **54**:357, 1994.
7. Curt GA, Carney DN, Cowan K, Jolivet J, Bailey BD, Drake JC, Kao-Shan CS, Minna JD, Chabner BA: Unstable methotrexate resistance in human small-cell carcinoma associated with double minute chromosomes. *N Engl J Med* **308**:199, 1983.
8. Horns RCJ, Dower WJ, Schimke RT: Gene amplification in a leukemic patient treated with methotrexate. *J Clin Oncol* **2**:2, 1984.
9. Trent JM, Buick RN, Olson S, Horns RCJ, Schimke RT: Cytologic evidence for gene amplification in methotrexate-resistant cells obtained from a patient with ovarian adenocarcinoma. *J Clin Oncol* **2**:8, 1984.
10. Carman MD, Schornagel JH, Rivest RS, Srimatkandada S, Portlock CS, Duffy T, Bertino JR: Resistance to methotrexate due to gene amplification in a patient with acute leukemia. *J Clin Oncol* **2**:16, 1984.
11. Merkel DE, Fuqua SAW, Tandon AK, Hill SM, Buzdar AU, McGuire WL: Electrophoretic analysis of 248 clinical breast cancer specimens for P-glycoprotein overexpression or gene amplification. *J Clin Oncol* **7**:1129, 1989.
12. Brodeur GM, Green AA, Hayes FA, Williams KJ, Williams DL, Tsiatis AA: Cytogenetic features of human neuroblastomas and cell lines. *Cancer Res* **41**:4678, 1981.
13. Brodeur GM, Fong CT: Molecular biology and genetics of human neuroblastoma. *Cancer Genet Cytogenet* **41**:153, 1989.
14. Leonard JH, Kearsley JH, Chenevix-Trench G, Hayward NK: Analysis of gene amplification in head-and-neck squamous-cell carcinomas. *Int J Cancer* **48**:511, 1991.
15. Brodeur GM, Seeger RC, Schwab M, Varmus HE, Bishop JM: Amplification of N-myc in untreated human neuroblastomas correlates with advanced disease stage. *Science* **224**:1121, 1984.
16. Brodeur GM: Neuroblastoma — Clinical applications of molecular parameters. *Brain Pathol* **1**:47, 1990.
17. Seeger RC, Brodeur GM, Sather H, Dalton A, Siegel SE, Wong KY, Hammond D: Association of multiple copies of the N-myc oncogene with rapid progression of neuroblastomas. *N Engl J Med* **313**:1111, 1985.
18. Garcia I, Dietrich PY, Aapro M, Vauthier G, Vadas L, Engel E: Genetic alterations of c-myc, c-erbB-2, and c-HA-ras proto-oncogenes and clinical associations in human breast carcinomas. *Cancer Res* **49**:6675, 1989.
19. Berns EM, Klijn JG, van Staveren IL, Portengen H, Noordegraaf E, Foekens JA: Prevalence of amplification of the oncogenes c-myc, HER2/neu, and int-2 in one thousand human breast tumours: Correlation with steroid receptors. *Eur J Cancer* **28**:697, 1992.
20. Schuuring E: The involvement of the chromosome 11q13 region in human malignancies: *Cyclin D1* and *EMS1* are two new candidate oncogenes — A review. *Gene* **159**:83, 1995.
21. Karlseder J, Zeillinger R, Schneeberger C, Czerwenka K, Speiser P, Kubista E, Birnbaum D, Gaudray P, Theillet C: Patterns of DNA amplification at band q13 of chromosome 11 in human breast cancer. *Genes Chromosom Cancer* **9**:42, 1994.
22. Courjal F, Cuny M, Simony-Lafontaine J, Louason G, Speiser P, Zeillinger R, Rodriguez C, Theillet C: Mapping of DNA amplifications at 15 chromosomal localizations in 1857 breast tumors: Definition of phenotypic groups. *Cancer Res* **57**:4360, 1997.
23. Van Roy N, Forus A, Myklebost O, Cheng NC, Versteeg R, Speleman F: Identification of two distinct chromosome 12-derived amplification units in neuroblastoma cell line NGP. *Cancer Genet Cytogenet* **82**:151, 1995.
24. Theillet C, Adelaide J, Louason G, Bonnet-Dorion F, Jacquemier J, Adnane J, Longy M, Katsaros D, Sismondi P, Gaudray P, Birnbaum D: FGFRI and PLAT genes and DNA amplification at 8p12 in breast and ovarian cancers. *Genes Chromosom Cancer* **7**:219, 1993.
25. Shiloh Y, Mor O, Manor A, Bar-Am I, Rotman G, Eubanks J, Gutman M, Ranzani GN, Houldsworth J, Evans G, Aviv L: DNA sequences amplified in cancer cells: An interface between tumor biology and human genome analysis. *Mutat Res* **276**:329, 1992.
26. Anzick SL, Kononen J, Walker RL, Azorsa DO, Tanner MM, Guan XY, Sauter G, Kallioniemi OP, Trent JM, Meltzer PS: AIB1, a steroid receptor coactivator amplified in breast and ovarian cancer. *Science* **277**:965, 1997.
27. Schwab M, Alitalo K, Klempnauer KH, Varmus HE, Bishop JM, Gilbert F, Brodeur G, Goldstein M, Trent JM: Amplified DNA with limited homology to myc cellular oncogene is shared by human neuroblastoma cell lines and a neuroblastoma tumour. *Nature* **305**:245, 1983.
28. Schwab M, Varmus HE, Bishop JM, Grzeschik KH, Naylor SL, Sakaguchi AY, Brodeur G, Trent J: Chromosome localization in normal human cells and neuroblastomas of a gene related to c-myc. *Nature* **308**:288, 1984.
29. Tsuda T, Obara M, Hirano H, Gotoh S, Kubomura S, Higashi K, Kuroiwa A, Nakagawara A, Nagahara N, Shimizu K: Analysis of N-myc amplification in relation to disease stage and histologic types in human neuroblastomas. *Cancer* **60**:820, 1987.
30. Rubie H, Hartmann O, Michon J, Frappaz D, Coze C, Chastagner P, Baranzelli MC, Plantaz D, Avet-Loiseau H, Benard J, Delattre O, Favrot M, Peyroulet MC, Thyss A, Perel Y, Bergeron C, Coubon-Collet B, Vannier J-P, Lemerle J, Sommelet D: N-Myc gene amplification is a major prognostic factor in localized neuroblastoma: Results of the French NBL 90 study. *J Clin Oncol* **15**:1171, 1997.
31. Nakagawara A, Ikeda K, Tsuda T, Higashi K, Okabe T: Amplification of N-myc oncogene in stage II and IVS neuroblastomas may be a prognostic indicator. *J Pediatr Surg* **22**:415, 1987.
32. Tonini GP, Boni L, Pession A, Rogers D, Iolascon A, Basso G, Cordero di Montezemolo L, Casale F, De Bernardi B: MYCN oncogene amplification in neuroblastoma is associated with worse prognosis, except in stage 4s: The Italian experience with 295 children. *J Clin Oncol* **15**:85, 1997.
33. Matthay KK, Perez C, Seeger RC, Brodeur GM, Shimada H, Atkinson JB, Black CT, Gerbing R, Haase GM, Stram DO, Swift P, Lukens JN: Successful treatment of stage III neuroblastoma based on prospective biologic staging: A Children's Cancer Group study. *J Clin Oncol* **16**:1256, 1998.
34. Katzenstein HM, Bowman LC, Brodeur GM, Thorner PS, Joshi VV, Smith EI, Look AT, Rowe ST, Nash MB, Holbrook T, Alvarado C, Rao PV, Castleberry RP, Cohn SL: Prognostic significance of age, MYCN oncogene amplification, tumor cell ploidy, and histology in 110 infants with stage D(s) neuroblastoma: The Pediatric Oncology Group experience — A Pediatric Oncology Group study. *J Clin Oncol* **16**:2007, 1998.
35. Kaneko M, Nishihira H, Mugishima H, Ohnuma N, Nakada K, Kawa K, Fukuzawa M, Suita S, Seray Y, Tsuchida Y: Stratification of treatment of stage 4 neuroblastoma patients based on N-myc amplification status. Study Group of Japan for treatment of advanced neuroblastoma, Tokyo, Japan. *Med Pediatr Oncol* **31**:1, 1998.
36. Brodeur GM, Hayes FA, Green AA, Casper JT, Wasson J, Wallach S, Seeger RC: Consistent N-myc copy number in simultaneous or consecutive neuroblastoma samples from sixty individual patients. *Cancer Res* **47**:4248, 1987.
37. Brodeur GM, Maris JM, Yamashiro DJ, Hogarty MD, White PS: Biology and genetics of human neuroblastomas. *J Pediatr Hematol Oncol* **19**:93, 1997.
38. Bartram CR, Berthold F: Amplification and expression of the N-myc gene in neuroblastoma. *Eur J Pediatr* **146**:162, 1987.
39. Bordow SB, Norris MD, Haber PS, Marshall GM, Haber M: Prognostic significance of MYCN oncogene expression in childhood neuroblastoma. *J Clin Oncol* **16**:3286, 1998.
40. Chan H, Gallic B, DeBoer G, Haddad G, Dimitroulakos J, Ikegaki N, Yeger H, Ling V: MYCN protein as a predictor of neuroblastoma prognosis. Annual Meeting of the American Society of Clinical Oncology **16**:513a, 1997.
41. Nisen PD, Waber PG, Rich MA, Pierce S, Garvin JRJ, Gilbert F, Lanzkowsky P: N-myc oncogene RNA expression in neuroblastoma. *J Natl Cancer Inst* **80**:1633, 1988.
42. Seeger RC, Wada R, Brodeur GM, Moss TJ, Bjork RL, Sousa L, Slamon DJ: Expression of N-myc by neuroblastomas with one or multiple copies of the oncogene. *Progr Clin Biol Res* **271**:41, 1988.
43. Slavc I, Ellenbogen R, Jung W-H, Vawter GF, Kretschmar C, Grier H, Korf BR: myc gene amplification and expression in primary human neuroblastoma. *Cancer Res* **50**:1459, 1990.
44. Shiloh Y, Shipley J, Brodeur GM, Bruns G, Korf B, Donlon T, Schreck RR, Seeger R, Sakai K, Latt SA: Differential amplification, assembly and relocation of multiple DNA sequences in human neuroblastomas and neuroblastoma cell lines. *Proc Natl Acad Sci USA* **82**:3761, 1985.

45. Corvi R, Savelyeva L, Breit S, Wenzel A, Handgretinger R, Barak J, Oren M, Amler L, Schwab M: Non-syntenic amplification of MDM2 and MYCN in human neuroblastoma. *Oncogene* **10**:1081, 1995.
46. Corvi R, Savelyeva L, Amler L, Handgetinger R, Schwab M: Cytogenetic evolution of MYCN and MDM2 amplification in the neuroblastoma LS tumor and its cell line. *Eur J Cancer* **31A**:520, 1995.
47. Jinbo T, Iwamura Y, Kaneko M, Sawaguchi S: Coamplification of the L-myc and N-myc oncogenes in a neuroblastoma cell line. *Jpn J Cancer Res* **80**:299, 1989.
48. Fong CT, Dracopoli NC, White PS, Merrill PT, Griffith RC, Housman DE, Brodeur GM: Loss of heterozygosity for chromosome 1p in human neuroblastomas: Correlation with N-myc amplification. *Proc Natl Acad Sci USA* **86**:3753, 1989.
49. Kaneko Y, Kanda N, Maseki N, Sakurai M, Tsuchida Y, Takeda T, Okabe I, Sakurai M: Different karyotypic patterns in early and advanced stage neuroblastomas. *Cancer Res* **47**:311, 1987.
50. Christiansen H, Lampert F: Tumour karyotype discriminates between good and bad prognostic outcome in neuroblastoma. *Br J Cancer* **57**:121, 1988.
51. Hayashi Y, Kanda N, Inaba T, Hanada R, Nagahara N, Muchi H, Yamamoto K: Cytogenetic findings and prognosis in neuroblastoma with emphasis on marker chromosome 1. *Cancer* **63**:126, 1989.
52. Maris JM, White PS, Beltinger CP, Sulman EP, Castleberry RP, Shuster JJ, Look AT, Brodeur GM: Significance of chromosome 1p loss of heterozygosity in neuroblastomas. *Cancer Res* **55**:4664, 1995.
53. Martinsson T, Shoberg P-M, Hedborg F, Kogner P: Deletion of chromosome 1p loci and microsatellite instability in neuroblastomas analyzed with short-tandem repeat polymorphisms. *Cancer Res* **55**:5681, 1995.
54. Gehring M, Berthold F, Edler L, Schwab M, Amler LC: The 1p deletion is not a reliable marker for the prognosis of patients with neuroblastoma. *Cancer Res* **55**:5366, 1995.
55. Caron H, van Sluis P, de Kraker J, Bokkerink J, Egeler M, Laureys G, Slater R, Westerveld A, Voute PA, Versteeg R: Allelic loss of chromosome 1p as a predictor of unfavorable outcome in patients with neuroblastoma. *N Engl J Med* **334**:225, 1996.
56. Adnane J, Gaudray P, Dionne CA, Crumley G, Jaye M, Schlessinger J, Jeanteur P, Birnbaum D, Theillet C: BEK and FLG, two receptors to members of the FGF family, are amplified in subsets of human breast cancers. *Oncogene* **6**:659, 1991.
57. Brison O: Gene amplification and tumor progression. *Biochim Biophys Acta* **1155**:25, 1993.
58. Fajac A, Benard J, Lhomme C, Rey A, Duvillard P, Rochard F, Bernaudin JF, Riou G: c-erbB2 gene amplification and protein expression in ovarian epithelial tumors: Evaluation of their respective prognostic significance by multivariate analysis. *Int J Cancer* **64**:146, 1995.
59. Zhang GL, Zu KL, Yu SY: Amplification of C-erB2 gene in ovarian cancer. *Chung Hua Fu Chan Ko Tsa Chih* **29**:401, 1994.
60. Bellacosa A, de Feo D, Godwin AK, Bell DW, Cheng JQ, Altomare DA, Wan M, Dubeau L, Scambia G, Masciullo V, Ferrandina G, Bennedetti Panici P, Mancuso S, Neri G, Testa JR: Molecular alterations of the AKT2 oncogene in ovarian and breast carcinomas. *Int J Cancer* **64**:280, 1995.
61. Bian M, Fan Q, Huang S: Amplification of proto-oncogenes C-myc, C-N-ras, C-Ki-ras, C-erbB2 in ovarian carcinoma [abstract]. *Chung Hua Fu Chan Ko Tsa Chih* **30**:406, 1995.
62. Chiba W, Sawai S, Hanawa T, Ishida H, Matsui T, Kosaba S, Watanabe S, Hatakenaka R, Matsubara Y, Funatsu T, et al: Correlation between DNA content and amplification of oncogenes (c-myc, L-myc, c-erbB-2) and correlation with prognosis in 143 cases of resected lung cancer. *Gan To Kagaku Ryoho* **20**:824, 1993.
63. Brennan J, O'Connor T, Makuch RW, Simmons AM, Russell E, Linnoila RI, Phelps RM, Gazdar AF, Ihde DC, Johnson BE: myc family DNA amplification in 107 tumors and tumor cell lines from patients with small cell lung cancer treated with different combination chemotherapy regimens. *Cancer Res* **51**:1708, 1991.
64. Brass N, Racz A, Heckel D, Remberger K, Sybrecht GW, Meese EU: Amplification of the genes BCHE and SLC2A2 in 40% of squamous cell carcinoma of the lung. *Cancer Res* **57**:2290, 1997.
65. Balsara BR, Sonoda G, du Manoir S, Siegfried JM, Gabrielson E, Testa JR: Comparative genomic hybridization analysis detects frequent, often high-level, overrepresentation of DNA sequences at 3q, 5p, 7p, and 8q in human non-small cell lung carcinomas. *Cancer Res* **57**:2116, 1997.
66. Tahara E: Genetic alterations in human gastrointestinal cancers, the application to molecular diagnosis. *Cancer* **75**:1410, 1994.
67. Ranzani GN, Pellegata NS, Previdere C, Saragoni A, Vio A, Maltoni M, Amadori D: Heterogeneous proto-oncogene amplification correlates with tumor progression and presence of metastases in gastric cancer patients. *Cancer Res* **50**:7811, 1990.
68. Tsugawa K, Yonemura Y, Hirono Y, Fushida S, Kaji M, Miwa K, Miyazaki I, Yamamoto H: Amplification of the c-met, c-erbB-2 and epidermal growth factor receptor gene in human gastric cancers: Correlation to clinical features. *Oncology* **55**:475, 1998.
69. Salhab N, Jones DJ, Bos JL, Kinsella A, Schofield PF: Detection of ras gene alterations and ras proteins in colorectal cancer. *Dis Colon Rectum* **32**:659, 1989.
70. Greco C, Gandolfo GM, Mattei F, Gradilone A, Alvino S, Pastore LI, Casale V, Casole P, Grassi A, Cianciulli AM: Detection of C-myb genetic alterations and mutant p53 serum protein in patients with benign and malignant colon lesions. *Anticancer Res* **14**:1433, 1994.
71. Tong-Chuan H, Sparks AB, Rago C, Hermeking H, Zawel L, da Costa LT, Morin PJ, Vogelstein B, Kinzler KW: Identification of c-*MYC* as a target of the APC pathway. *Science* **281**:1509, 1998.
72. Merritt WD, Weissler MC, Turk BF, Gilmer TM: Oncogene amplification in squamous cell carcinoma of the head and neck. *Arch Otolaryngol Head Neck Surg* **116**:1394, 1990.
73. Kellems RE (ed): *Gene Amplification in Mammalian Cells*. New York: Marcel Dekker, Inc., 1993.
74. Livingstone LR, White A, Sprouse J, Livanos E, Jacks T, Tlsty TD: Altered cell cycle arrest and gene amplification potential accompany loss of wild-type p53. *Cell* **70**:923, 1992.
75. Yin Y, Tainsky MA, Bischoff FZ, Strong LC, Wahl GM: Wild-type p53 restores cell cycle control and inhibits gene amplification in cells with mutant p53 alleles. *Cell* **70**:937, 1992.
76. Asano K, Sakamoto H, Sasaki H, Ochiya T, Yoshida T, Ohishi Y, Machida T, Kakizoe T, Sugimura T, Terada M: Tumorigenicity and gene amplification potentials of cyclin D1-overexpressing NIH3T3 cells. *Biochem Biophys Res Commun* **217**:1169, 1995.
77. Zhou P, Jiang W, Weghorst CM, Weinstein IB: Overexpression of Cyclin D1 enhances gene amplification. *Cancer Res* **56**:36, 1996.
78. Tlsty TD: Genomic instability and its role in neoplasia. *Curr Top Microbiol Immunol* **221**:37, 1997.
79. Wahl GM, Linke SP, Paulson TG, Huang LC: Maintaining genetic stability through TP53 mediated checkpoint control. *Cancer Surv* **29**:183, 1997.
80. Paulson TG, Almasan A, Brody LL, Wahl GM: Gene amplification in a p53-deficient cell line requires cell cycle progression under conditions that generate DNA breakage. *Mol Cell Biol* **18**:3089, 1998.
81. Amler LC, Schwab M: Amplified N-myc in human neuroblastoma cells is often arranged as clustered tandem repeats of differently recombined DNA. *Mol Cell Biol* **9**:4903, 1989.
82. Amler LC, Schwab M: Multiple amplicons of discrete sizes encompassing N-myc in neuroblastoma cells evolve through differential recombination from a large precursor DNA. *Oncogene* **7**:807, 1992.
83. Schneider SS, Hiemstra JL, Zehnbauer BA, Taillon-Miller P, Le Paslier D, Vogelstein B, Brodeur GM: Isolation and structural analysis of a 1.2-megabase N-myc amplicon from a human neuroblastoma. *Mol Cell Biol* **12**:5563, 1992.
84. Corvi R, Amler LC, Savelyeva L, Gehring M, Schwab M: MYCN is retained in single copy at chromosome 2 band p23-24 during amplification in human neuroblastoma cells. *Proc Natl Acad Sci USA* **91**:5523, 1994.
85. Brodeur GM, Seeger RC: Gene amplification in human neuroblastomas: Basic mechanisms and clinical implications. *Cancer Genet Cytogenet* **19**:101, 1986.
86. Corvi R, Savelyeva L, Schwab M: Duplication of N-MYC at its resident site 2p24 may be a mechanism of activation alternative to amplification in human neuroblastoma cells. *Cancer Res* **55**:3471, 1995.
87. Kanda N, Schreck R, Alt F, Bruns G, Baltimore D, Latt S: Isolation of amplified DNA sequences from IMR-32 human neuroblastoma cells: Facilitation by fluorescence-activated flow sorting of metaphase chromosomes. *Proc Natl Acad Sci USA* **80**:4069, 1983.
88. Shiloh Y, Korf B, Kohl NE, Sakai K, Brodeur GM, Harris P, Kanda N, Seeger RC, Alt F, Latt SA: Amplification and rearrangement of DNA sequences from the chromosomal region 2p24 in human neuroblastomas. *Cancer Res* **46**:5297, 1986.
89. Hunt JD, Valentine M, Tereba A: Excision of N-myc from chromosome 2 in human neuroblastoma cells containing amplified N-myc sequences. *Mol Cell Biol* **10**:823, 1990.
90. Kinzler KW, Zehnbauer BA, Brodeur GM, Seeger RC, Trent JM, Meltzer PS, Vogelstein B: Amplification units containing human N-myc and c-myc genes. *Proc Natl Acad Sci USA* **83**:1031, 1986.

91. Zehnbauer BA, Small D, Brodeur GM, Seeger R, Vogelstein B: Characterization of N-myc amplification units in human neuroblastoma cells. *Mol Cell Biol* **8**:522, 1988.
92. Schneider SS, Zehnbauer BA, Vogelstein B, Brodeur GM: Yeast artificial chromosome (YAC) vector cloning of the *MYCN* amplified domain in human neuroblastomas. *Progr Clin Biol Res* **366**:71, 1991.
93. Reiter JL, Kuroda H, White PS, Schneider-Thabet SS, Taillon-Miller P, Brodeur GM: Physical mapping of the normal and amplified *MYCN* locus. *Genomics,* Submitted, 1999.
94. Reiter JL, Brodeur GM: High-resolution mapping of a 130-kb core region of the MYCN amplicon in neuroblastomas. *Genomics* **32**:97, 1996.
95. Godbout R, Squire J: Amplification of a DEAD box protein in retinoblastoma cell lines. *Proc Natl Acad Sci USA* **90**:7578, 1993.
96. Squire JA, Thorner PS, Weitzman S, Maggi JD, Dirks P, Doyle J, Hale M, Godbout R: Co-amplification of *MYCN* and a DEAD box gene (*DDX1*) in primary neuroblastoma. *Oncogene* **10**:1417, 1995.
97. Noguchi T, Akiyama K, Yokoyama M, Kanda N, Matsunaga T, Nishi Y: Amplification of a DEAD box gene (*DDX1*) with the *MYCN* gene in neuroblastomas as a result of cosegregation of sequences flanking the *MYCN* locus. *Genes Chrom Cancer* **15**:129, 1996.
98. Amler LC, Shurmann J, Schwab M: The DDX1 gene maps within 400 kbp 5′ to MYCN and is frequently coamplified in human neuroblastoma. *Genes Chrom Cancer* **15**:134, 1996.
99. George RE, Kenyon RM, McGuckin AG, Malcolm AJ, Pearson AD, Lunec J: Investigation of co-amplification of the candidate genes ornithine decarboxylase, ribonucleotide reductase, syndecan-1 and a DEAD box gene, DDX1, with N-myc in neuroblastoma. United Kingdom Children's Cancer Study Group. *Oncogene* **12**:1583, 1996.
100. Kuroda H, White PS, Sulman EP, Manohar CF, Reiter JL, Cohn SL, Brodeur GM: Physical mapping of the DDX1 gene 340 kb 5′ of MYCN. *Oncogene* **13**:156, 1996.
101. George RE, Thomas H, McGuckin AG, Angus B, Pearson AD, Lunec J: The DDX1 gene which is frequently co-amplified with MYCN in neuroblastoma is itself oncogenic. *Med Pediatr Oncol* (In press), 2000.
102. Jiang W, Kahn SM, Tomita N, Zhang YL, Lu SH, Weinstein IB: Amplification and expression of the human cyclin D gene in esophageal cancer. *Cancer Res* **52**:2980, 1992.
103. Nishida N, Fukuda Y, Komeda T, Kita R, Sando T, Furukawa M, Amenomori M, Shibagaki I, Nakao K, Ikenaga M: Amplification and overexpression of the cyclin D1 gene in aggressive human hepatocellular carcinoma. *Cancer Res* **54**:3107, 1994.
104. Zhang YJ, Jiang W, Chen CJ, Lee CS, Kahn SM, Santella RM, Weinstein IB: Amplification and overexpression of cyclin D1 in human hepatocellular carcinoma. *Biochem Biophys Res Commun* **196**:1010, 1993.
105. Gaudray P, Szepetowski P, Escot C, Birnbaum D, Theillet C: DNA amplification at 11q13 in human cancer: From complexity to perplexity. *Mutat Res* **276**:317, 1992.
106. Berner J-M, Forus A, Elkahloun A, Meltzer PS, Fodstad Ø, Myklebost O: Separate amplified regions encompassing CDK4 and MDM2 in human sarcomas. *Genes Chrom Cancer* **17**:254, 1996.
107. Elkahloun AG, Bittner M, Hoskins K, Gemmill R, Meltzer PS: Molecular cytogenetic characterization and physical mapping of 12q13-15 amplification in human cancers. *Genes Chrom Cancer* **17**:205, 1996.
108. Reifenberger G, Ichimura K, Reifenberger J, Elkahloun AG, Meltzer PS, Collins VP: Refined mapping of 12q13-15 amplicons in human malignant gliomas suggests CDK4/SAS an MDM2 as independent amplification targets. *Cancer Res* **56**:5141, 1996.
109. Maelandsmo GM, Berner JM, Florenes VA, Forus A, Hovig E, Fodstad Ø, Myklebost O: Homozygous deletion frequency and expression levels of the CDKN2 gene in human sarcomas—relationship to amplification and mRNA levels of CDK4 and CCND1. *Br J Cancer* **72**:393, 1995.
110. Leach FS, Tokino T, Meltzer P, Burrell M, Oliner JD, Smith S, Hill DE, Sidransky D, Kinzler KW, Vogelstein B: p53 mutation and MDM2 amplification in human soft tissue sarcomas. *Cancer Res* **53**:2231, 1993.
111. Florenes VA, Maelandsmo GM, Forus A, Andreassen A, Myklebost O, Fodstad Ø: MDM2 gene amplification and transcript levels in human sarcomas: relationship to TP53 gene status [see comments]. *J Natl Cancer Inst* **86**:1297, 1994.
112. Kanoe H, Nakayama T, Murakami H, Hosaka T, Yamamoto H, Nakashima Y, Tsuboyama T, Nakamura T, Sasaki MS, Toguchida J: Amplification of the CDK4 gene in sarcomas: Tumor specificity and relationship with the RB gene mutation. *Anticancer Res* **18**:2317, 1998.
113. Blackwood EM, Eisenman RN: Max: a helix-loop-helix zipper protein that forms a sequence-specific DNA-binding complex with Myc. *Science* **251**:1211, 1991.
114. Makela TP, Koskinen P, Vastrik I, Alitalo K: Alternative forms of Max as enhancers or suppressors of Myc-Ras cotransformation. *Science* **256**:373, 1992.
115. Reddy CD, Dasgupta P, Saikumar P, Dudek H, Rauscher FJ III, Reddy EP: Mutational analysis of Max: Role of basic, helix-loop-helix/leucine zipper domains in DNA binding, dimerization and regulation of Myc-mediated transcriptional activation. *Oncogene* **7**:2085, 1992.
116. Kretzner L, Blackwood EM, Eisenman RN: Myc and Max proteins possess distinct transcriptional activities. *Nature* **359**:426, 1992.
117. Amati B, Dalton S, Brooks MW, Littlewood TD, Evan GI, Land H: Transcriptional activation by the human c-Myc oncoprotein in yeast requires interaction with Max. *Nature* **359**:423, 1992.
118. Amati B, Brooks MW, Levy N, Littlewood TD, Evan GI, Land H: Oncogenic activity of the c-Myc protein requires dimerization with Max. *Cell* **72**:233, 1993.
119. Grandori C, Eisenman RN: Myc target genes. *Trends Biochem Sci* **22**:177, 1997.
120. Bar-Sagi D: Ras proteins: Biological effects and biochemical targets [review]. *Anticancer Res* **9**:1427, 1989.
121. Hall A: The cellular functions of small GTP-binding proteins. *Science* **249**:635, 1990.
122. Medema RH, Boss JL: The role of p21ras in receptor tyrosine kinase signaling. *Crit Rev Oncogenes* **4**:615, 1993.
123. Marshall CJ: The ras oncogenes. *J Cell Sci (Suppl)* **10**:157, 1988.
124. Field JK, Spandidos DA: The role of ras and myc oncogenes in human solid tumours and their relevance in diagnosis and prognosis [review]. *Anticancer Res* **10**:1, 1990.
125. Bos JL: Ras oncogenes in human cancer: A review. *Cancer Res* **49**:4682, 1989.
126. Bishop JM: Molecular themes in oncogenesis. *Cell* **64**:235, 1991.
127. Ullrich A, Schlessinger J: Signal transduction by receptors with tyrosine kinase activity. *Cell* **61**:203, 1990.
128. Tokunaga A, Masahiko O, Okuda T, Teramoto T, Fujita I, Mizutani T, Keyama T, Yoshiyuki T, Nishi K, Matsukura N: Clinical significance of epidermal growth factor (EGF), EGF receptor, and c-erbB-2 in human gastric cancer. *Cancer* (Suppl) **75**:1418, 1995.
129. Hamburger AW, White CP, Brown RW: Effect of epidermal growth factor on proliferation of human tumor cells in soft agar. *J Natl Cancer Inst* **67**:825, 1981.
130. Hartwell L: Defects in a cell cycle checkpoint may be responsible for the genomic instability of cancer cells. *Cell* **71**:543, 1992.
131. Sherr CJ: Mammalian G1 cyclins. *Cell* **73**:1059, 1993.
132. Wasson JC, Brodeur GM: Molecular analysis of gene amplification in tumors, in NC Dracopoli, JL Haines, BR Korf, DT Moir, CC Morton, CE Seidman, JG Seidman, DR Smith (eds): *Current Protocols in Human Genetics*. New York: Greene Publishing and John Wiley & Sons, 1994, p. 10.5.1.
133. Shapiro DN, Valentine MB, Rowe ST, Sinclair AE, Sublett JE, Roberts WM, Look AT: Detection of N-myc gene amplification by fluorescence in situ hybridization. Diagnostic utility for neuroblastoma. *Am J Pathol* **142**:1339, 1993.
134. Misra DN, Dickman PS, Yunis EJ: Fluorescence in situ hybridization (FISH) detection of MYCN oncogene amplification in neuroblastoma using paraffin-embedded tissues. *Diag Mol Pathol* **4**:128, 1995.
135. Guan X-Y, Meltzer PS, Dalton WS, Trent JM: Identification of cryptic sites of DNA sequence amplification in human breast cancer by chromosome microdissection. *Nature Genet* **8**:155, 1994.
136. Crabbe DC, Peters J, Seeger RC: Rapid detection of MYCN gene amplification in neuroblastomas using the polymerase chain reaction. *Diag Mol Pathol* **1**:229, 1992.
137. Gilbert J, Norris MD, Haber M, Kavallaris M, Marshall GM, Stewart BW: Determination of N-myc gene amplification in neuroblastoma by differential polymerase chain reaction. *Mol Cell Probes* **7**:227, 1993.
138. Huddart SN, Mann JR, McGukin AG, Corbett R: MYCN amplification by differential PCR. *Pediatr Hematol Oncol* **10**:31, 1993.
139. Boerner S, Squire J, Thorner P, McKenna G, Zielenska M: Assessment of MYCN amplification in neuroblastoma biopsies by differential polymerase chain reaction. *Pediatr Pathol* **14**:823, 1994.
140. Kallioniemi A, Kallioniemi O-P, Sudar D, Rutovitz D, Gray JW, Waldman F, Pinkel D: Comparative genomic hybridization for molecular cytogenetic analysis of solid tumors. *Science* **258**:818, 1992.

141. Kallioniemi A, Kallioniemi O-P, Piper J, Tanner M, Stokke T, Chen L, Smith HS, Pinkel D, Gray JW, Waldman FM: Detection and mapping of amplified DNA sequences in breast cancer by comparative genomic hybridization. *Proc Natl Acad Sci USA* **91**:2156, 1994.
142. Ried T, Peterson I, Holtgreve-Grez H, Speicher MR, Schrock E, du Manoir S, Cremer T: Mapping of multiple DNA gains and losses in primary small cell lung carcinomas by comparative genomic hybridization. *Cancer Res* **54**:1801, 1994.
143. Shalon D, Smith SJ, Brown PO: DNA microarray system for analyzing complex DNA samples using two-color fluorescent probe hybridization. *Genome Res* **6**:639, 1996.
144. DeRisi J, Penland L, Brown PO, Bittner ML, Meltzer PS, Ray M, Chen Y, Su YA, Trent JM: Use of a cDNA microarray to analyse gene expression patterns in human cancer. *Nature Genet* **14**:457, 1996.
145. Hacia JG, Brody LC, Chee MS, Fodor SPA, Collins FS: Detection of heterozygous mutations in BRCA1 using high-density oligonucleotide arrays and two-colour fluorescence analysis. *Nature Genet* **14**:441, 1996.
146. Bieche I, Champeme MH, Lidereau R: A tumor suppressor gene on chromosome 1p32-pter controls the amplification of MYC family genes in breast cancer. *Cancer Res* **54**:4274, 1994.
147. Ocadiz R, Sauceda R, Cruz M, Graef AM, Gariglio P: High correlation between molecular alterations of the c-myc oncogene and carcinoma of the uterine cervix. *Cancer Res* **47**:4173, 1987.
148. Mitra AB, Murty VV, Pratap M, Sodhani P, Chaganti RS: ERBB2 (HER2/neu) oncogene is frequently amplified in squamous cell carcinoma of the uterine cervix. *Cancer Res* **54**:637, 1994.
149. He J, Zhang RG, Zhu D: Clinical significance of c-myc gene in esophageal squamous cell carcinoma. *Chung Hua I Hsueh Tsa Chih* **75**:94, 1995.
150. Momand J, Jung D, Wilczynski S, Niland J: The MDM2 gene amplification database. *Nucleic Acids Res* **26**:3453, 1998.
151. Torp SH, Helseth E, Ryan L, Stolan S, Dalen A, Unsgaard G: Amplification of the epidermal growth factor receptor gene in human gliomas. *Anticancer Res* **11**:2095, 1991.
152. Bigner SH, Wong AJ, Mark J, Muhlbaier LH, Kinzler KW, Vogelstein B, Bigner DD: Relationship between gene amplification and chromosomal deviations in malignant human gliomas. *Cancer Genet Cytogenet* **29**:165, 1987.
153. Galanis E, Buckner J, Kimmel D, Jenkins R, Alderete B, O'Fallon J, Wang CH, Scheithauer BW, James CD: Gene amplification as a prognostic factor in primary and secondary high-grade malignant gliomas. *Int J Oncol* **13**:717, 1998.
154. Baker VV, Borst MP, Dixon D, Hatch KD, Shingleton HM, Miller D: c-myc amplification in ovarian cancer. *Gynecol Oncol* **38**:340, 1990.
155. Bast RCJ, Boyer CM, Jacobs I, Xu FJ, Wu S, Wiener J, Kohler M, Berchuck A: Cell growth regulation in epithelial ovarian cancer. *Cancer* **71**:1597, 1993.

CHAPTER 22

Tumor Genome Instability

Daniel P. Cahill ▪ Christoph Lengauer

Genetic instability has long been recognized as a cardinal feature of neoplasia.[1,2] However, the causal role of genetic instability in the formation of cancer has only more recently been studied. Accumulating evidence has strengthened the proposal that genetic instability is required early during tumor progression. Instability drives mutations in oncogenes and tumor suppressor genes, providing the tumor cell with a selective growth advantage.[3] While numerous oncogenes and tumor suppressor genes have been identified in the last 20 years, the molecular details underlying genetic instability are just now being revealed.

The clearest molecular evidence for the genetic instability hypothesis comes from the elucidation of the genes causing hereditary nonpolyposis colon cancer (HNPCC). Patients with HNPCC have an increased risk of tumor development over the course of their lifetime but do not display the widespread changes in the at-risk tissue cellular architecture characteristic of other inherited tumor syndromes, for instance, the thousands of polyps in familial adenomatous polyposis (FAP). Instead, they typically develop a single advanced primary tumor at an atypically young age (see Chap. 32 on HNPCC).

Indeed, the tissue specificity is even more of a mystery upon consideration of the underlying genetic defect in these patients. They inherit a mutation in one of the mismatch repair (MMR) genes, such as *MSH2, MLH1, PMS1, PMS2,* or *GTBP(MSH6)*.[4–11] Unlike classical tumor suppressor genes such as *p53* or *Rb*, the MMR genes do not directly affect the growth or death of a tumor cell.[12] Experimentally, this distinction can be seen upon reintroduction of a MMR gene into a tumor cell that has two mutant copies. In contrast to reintroduction of a classical tumor suppressor, there is no effect on the tumor cell growth or death.[13]

Instead, the loss of MMR genes imbues these tumors with an elevated nucleotide mutation rate — 2 to 3 orders of magnitude higher than normal cells or MMR-proficient cancers of the same cell type[14–16]. Thus, there is an increased rate of mutation at oncogene and tumor suppressor loci throughout the tumor cell genome. This link between isolated cellular genetic instability and organism-wide tumorigenesis is strong evidence for the genetic instability hypothesis, as sequence instability alone is able to drive the autosomal dominant inheritance of colorectal neoplasia in these families (Fig. 22-1).

Defects of another major DNA repair system have been documented in tumors as well. Nucleotide-excision repair (NER) is responsible for repairing damage caused by many exogenous mutagens.[17] Mutations in one of several different NER genes result in xeroderma pigmentosum and related disorders. Patients with these autosomal recessive, inherited diseases develop numerous skin tumors in sun-exposed areas (see also Chap. 28 on xeroderma pigmentosum).[18,19] Surprisingly, skin tumors represent the major tumor type to which patients with NER defects are susceptible, and the incidence of internal cancers in these patients is not raised to the same degree[20–22]. The simplest explanation for these results is that ultraviolet light is the major mutagen that results in NER-correctable DNA damage to which humans are exposed (Fig. 22-1).[20–22]

However, there is a more pervasive genomic abnormality of sporadic tumors. Virtually all epithelial solid tumors have structural and numeric chromosome variation — they are aneuploid.[23] The only exceptions are, strikingly, the MMR deficient tumors, which remain diploid throughout tumor progression. Such observations have led to the suggestion that cancers require instability either at the sequence level or at the chromosomal level, but not generally at both levels.[24] This logic would posit that one form of instability is sufficient to drive tumorigenesis. Consistent with this hypothesis, aneuploidy can be found in the earliest neoplastic lesions, such as benign adenomas of the colon, and the accumulation of aneuploid cells is a classic finding in advanced stages of tumorigenesis.[25–28]

Recent analysis has shown that cancer cell aneuploidy is a reflection of an underlying chromosomal instability (CIN).[29] Quantitative studies of aneuploid tumor cell divisions have demonstrated that the chromosomal abnormalities in these cells are the result of an intrinsic segregation instability.[30] This observation gave rise to the proposal that CIN could be considered the primary class of instability required for neoplastic progression in the majority of tumors.

The causes of CIN underlying the widespread aneuploid phenotype are just beginning to be investigated. One theory posits that karyotypic instability in cancer is a truism; it is a natural side effect of the malignant transformation process, driven by the preceding mutations in growth-controlling oncogenes and tumor suppressor genes such as *ras* or *p53*.

However, the existence of karyotypically stable MMR-deficient tumors argues against a causal role for classical oncogenes and tumor suppressors in the CIN phenotype. These tumors have mutations in the same oncogenes and tumor suppressor genes as CIN tumors, and have similar stage-specific growth and progression characteristics, but are not aneuploid. These cases prove that the mutant genes driving advanced neoplastic progression do not inevitability generate or require aneuploidy.

At the other end of the spectrum, a different theory proposes that aneuploidy is not caused by specific genetic alterations but instead results from the altered cellular architecture that ensues whenever an abnormal chromosome complement is present within cells. Thus, a chance abnormal division in an otherwise normal cell gives rise to a karyotypically abnormal daughter cell with a selective growth advantage compared to its neighbors. The abnormal number of chromosomes in this cell destabilizes the segregation machinery, auto-catalyzing chromosome missegregation and further aneuploidy. Aneuploidy begets aneuploidy.[31]

There is some recent evidence to support an alternative to these hypotheses. Perhaps aneuploid tumors sustain an early mutational event in a chromosome stability gene that drives chromosomal instability (Fig. 22-1). In some tumors, CIN has been proposed to be driven by mutations in mitotic checkpoint genes.[30,32,33] For the

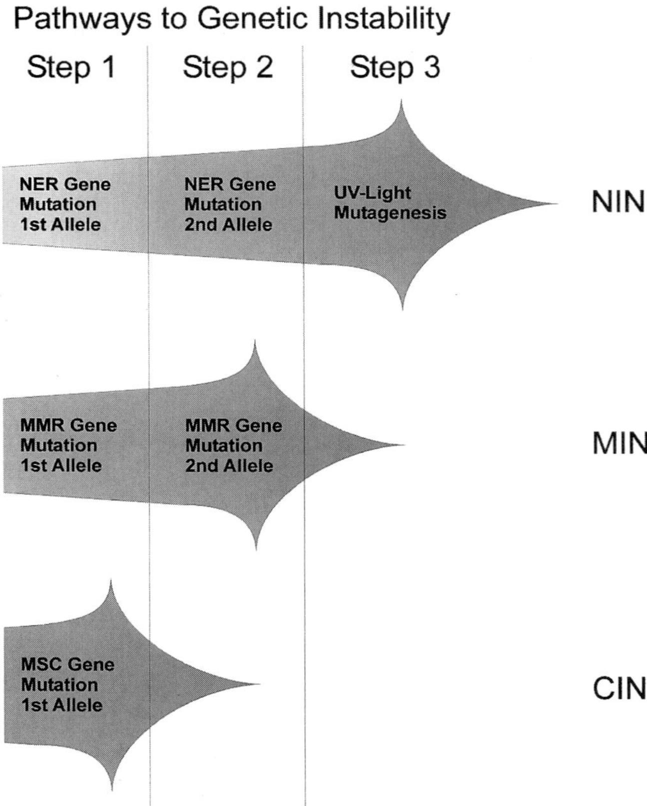

Fig. 22-1 Pathways to genetic instability. Different types of genetic instability require a different number of mutational "hits" in order to engender the respective instability phenotype. In a heterozygote with one defective nucleotide excision repair (NER) allele (step 1), inactivation of the normal allele (step 2) does not immediately lead to mutations. It additionally requires exposure to an environmental agent (i.e., ultraviolet light) (step 3) to create large numbers of mutations (NER-related instability; NIN). In contrast, in a heterozygote with one defective mismatch repair (MMR) allele (step 1), all that is required to begin to develop mutations at a high rate (microsatellite instability; MIN) is the inactivation of the normal allele inherited from the unaffected parent (step 2). Cell fusion and other experiments suggest that chromosomal instability (CIN) can have a dominant quality.[29] One example of a gene that can be mutated in a dominant negative manner to cause CIN is *hBub1*, a component of the mitotic spindle checkpoint (MSC).[30] It apparently requires only a single mutational "hit" of such a gene to engender the CIN phenotype.

majority of tumors, however, the molecular basis of CIN is not known yet. This is an area of active investigation. Many of the known inherited tumor suppressor genes seem to play an important role in genome stability but their mechanistic relationship to genome instability is poorly understood (see chapters 29, 30, 47 and 37 on *ATM*, *BLM*, *BRCA1*/*BRCA2* and *p53*, respectively). It will be interesting to see how many instability genes can be shown to be altered in sporadic cancers.

REFERENCES

1. Loeb LA: Mutator phenotype may be required for multistage carcinogenesis. *Cancer Res* **51**:3075, 1991.
2. Hartwell L: Defects in a cell cycle checkpoint may be responsible for the genomic instability of cancer cells. *Cell* **71**:543, 1992.
3. Lengauer C, Kinzler KW, Vogelstein B: Genetic instabilities in human cancers. *Nature* **396**:643, 1998.
4. Modrich P: Mismatch repair, genetic stability and tumour avoidance. *Philos Trans R Soc Lond B Biol Sci* **347**:89, 1995.
5. Kunkel TA: DNA-mismatch repair. The intricacies of eukaryotic spell-checking. *Curr Biol* **5**:1091, 1995.
6. Peltomaki P, de la Chapelle A: Mutations predisposing to hereditary nonpolyposis colorectal cancer. *Adv Cancer Res* **71**:93, 1997.
7. Sia EA, Jinks-Robertson S, Petes TD: Genetic control of microsatellite stability. *Mutat Res* **383**:61, 1997.
8. Fishel R, Lescoe MK, Rao MR, et al.: The human mutator gene homolog MSH2 and its association with hereditary nonpolyposis colon cancer. *Cell* **75**:1027, 1993.
9. Leach FS, Nicolaides NC, Papadopoulos N, et al.: Mutations of a mutS homolog in hereditary nonpolyposis colorectal cancer. *Cell* **75**:1215, 1993.
10. Bronner CE, Baker SM, Morrison PT, et al.: Mutation in the DNA mismatch repair gene homologue hMLH1 is associated with hereditary non-polyposis colon cancer. *Nature* **368**:258, 1994.
11. Papadopoulos N, Nicolaides NC, Wei YF, et al.: Mutation of a mutL homolog in hereditary colon cancer. *Science* **263**:1625, 1994.
12. Kinzler KW, Vogelstein B: Cancer-susceptibility genes. Gatekeepers and caretakers. *Nature* **386**:761, 1997.
13. Koi M, Umar A, Chauhan DP, et al.: Human chromosome 3 corrects mismatch repair deficiency and microsatellite instability and reduces N-methyl-N′-nitro-N-nitrosoguanidine tolerance in colon tumor cells with homozygous hMLH1 mutation. *Cancer Res* **54**:4308, 1994.
14. Parsons R, Li GM, Longley MJ, et al.: Hypermutability and mismatch repair deficiency in RER+ tumor cells. *Cell* **75**:1227, 1993.
15. Bhattacharyya NP, Skandalis A, Ganesh A, Groden J, Meuth M: Mutator phenotypes in human colorectal carcinoma cell lines. *Proc Natl Acad Sci U S A* **91**:6319, 1994.
16. Eshleman JR, Lang EZ, Bowerfind GK, et al.: Increased mutation rate at the hprt locus accompanies microsatellite instability in colon cancer. *Oncogene* **10**:33, 1995.
17. Wood RD: DNA repair in eukaryotes. *Annu Rev Biochem* **65**:135, 1996.
18. De Weerd-Kastelein EA, Keijzer W, Bootsma D: Genetic heterogeneity of xeroderma pigmentosum demonstrated by somatic cell hybridization. *Nat New Biol* **238**:80, 1972.
19. Bootsma D, Kraemer KH, Cleaver JE, Hoeijmakers JHJ: Nucleotide excision repair syndromes: xeroderma pigmentosum, Cockayne syndrome, and trichothiodystrophy, in Kinzler KW, Vogelstein B, (eds): *The Genetic Basis of Human Cancer*. New York, McGraw-Hill, 1998, p 245–274.
20. Cairns J: The origin of human cancers. *Nature* **289**:353, 1981.
21. Feinberg AP, Coffey DS: Organ site specificity for cancer in chromosomal instability disorders. *Cancer Res* **42**:3252, 1982.
22. Kraemer KH, Lee MM, Scotto J: DNA repair protects against cutaneous and internal neoplasia: evidence from xeroderma pigmentosum. *Carcinogenesis* **5**:511, 1984.
23. Mitelman F: *Catalog of Chromosome Aberrations in Cancer*. Wiley-Liss, 1991.
24. Cahill DP, Kinzler KW, Vogelstein B, Lengauer C: Genetic instability and darwinian selection in tumours. *Trends Cell Biol* **9**:M57, 1999.
25. Auer GU, Heselmeyer KM, Steinbeck RG, Munck-Wikland E, Zetterberg AD: The relationship between aneuploidy and p53 overexpression during genesis of colorectal adenocarcinoma. *Virchows Arch* **424**:343, 1994.
26. Bardi G, Parada LA, Bomme L, et al.: Cytogenetic comparisons of synchronous carcinomas and polyps in patients with colorectal cancer. *Br J Cancer* **76**:765, 1997.
27. Silverstein MJ: *Ductal Carcinoma in Situ of the Breast*. Baltimore, Williams & Wilkins, 1997.
28. Bomme L, Bardi G, Pandis N, Fenger C, Kronborg O, Heim S: Cytogenetic analysis of colorectal adenomas: karyotypic comparisons of synchronous tumors. *Cancer Genet Cytogenet* **106**:66, 1998.
29. Lengauer C, Kinzler KW, Vogelstein B: Genetic instability in colorectal cancers. *Nature* **386**:623, 1997.
30. Cahill DP, Lengauer C, Yu J, et al.: Mutations of mitotic checkpoint genes in human cancers. *Nature* **392**:300, 1998.
31. Duesberg P, Rausch C, Rasnick D, Hehlmann R: Genetic instability of cancer cells is proportional to their degree of aneuploidy. *Proc Natl Acad Sci U S A* **95**:13692, 1998.
32. Li Y, Benezra R: Identification of a human mitotic checkpoint gene: hsMAD2. *Science* **274**:246, 1996.
33. Jin DY, Spencer F, Jeang KT: Human T cell leukemia virus type 1 oncoprotein Tax targets the human mitotic checkpoint protein MAD1. *Cell* **93**:81, 1998.

CHAPTER 23

Cell Cycle Control: An Overview

Bruce E. Clurman ▪ James M. Roberts

INTRODUCTION

The process of cell reproduction is known as the cell cycle.[1–3] Usually the cell cycle produces two progeny, or daughter cells, that closely resemble their parent and who are themselves capable of repeating the process. For this to occur, three things are necessary: replication of the genome; a doubling of cell mass (where cell mass refers generally to all cellular components other than chromosomes); and a precise segregation of chromosomes plus a more or less equal distribution of other cell components to the daughter cells. The execution of these events divides the cell cycle into four phases: chromosomes are replicated during S (synthetic) phase; cell constituents are segregated to daughter cells during M (mitotic) phase; and two G (gap) phases intervene between S and M. G1 precedes S phase, and G2 precedes mitosis (Fig. 23-1). Thus, chromosome replication and segregation are confined to discrete intervals of the cell cycle, whereas the third essential component of cell reproduction — growth — occurs continuously in G1, S, G2, and M. It is during G1 and G2 that cells typically respond to the proliferative and antiproliferative signals that determine whether the cell cycle ought to proceed (signals such as growth factors and cytokines). In this way, the cell cycle has the option of stopping within G1 and G2 without interrupting the critical and precarious events of chromosome replication and chromosome segregation.

Faithful reproduction of the cell requires that these events be coordinated with one another. Thus, mitosis ordinarily waits until all chromosomes have been replicated and the cell has doubled in size. However, there are specialized cell cycles where these processes are uncoupled from one another (Fig. 23-2). Repeated S phases with no intervening M phases, known as endocycles, result in the increased chromosome ploidy that is seen in megakaryocytes. Conversely, the basic cell-cycle logic of meiosis is the execution of two sequential M phases without an S phase. A third important variation is seen in the cleavage cycles that occur after fertilization of amphibian eggs. Amphibian eggs are huge cells, which, after fertilization, undergo extremely rapid cell cycles consisting of alternating S and M phases with no cell growth. After approximately 12 cleavage cycles, the embryo consists of 4000 cells, each containing a full complement of genetic material, and each now reduced to the size of a typical somatic cell.[4,5]

These simple examples show that each of the component processes of the cell cycle — growth, chromosome replication, and mitosis — can occur independently of the others. Because cell reproduction could not occur if these processes were executed in random order, there need to be mechanisms for establishing and enforcing the normal sequence of events. This chapter describes the molecules that control progression through the cell cycle, and illustrates how their activities are linked together to orchestrate the orderly process of cell reproduction. Based on these ideas, we suggest that cancer may be a disease of the cell cycle, a hypothesis that is elaborated on in subsequent chapters.

ORIGINS OF MODERN CELL CYCLE BIOLOGY

The current revolution in our understanding of cell-cycle control owes its origins to yeast genetics and amphibian reproductive cell physiology. It was through these seemingly independent lines of investigation that we came to grasp the fundamental logic of the program that controls cell reproduction, identified the genes and molecules responsible for this program, and learned how these molecules are integrated into pathways that have been evolutionarily conserved from yeast to humans.

The yeasts *Saccharomyces cerevisiae* and *Schizosaccharomyces pombe* have been favorites of cell-cycle research since the pioneering studies of Lee Hartwell and Paul Nurse.[6,7] The power of yeast as a model experimental system is in its facile genetics. It is possible to readily isolate mutations that impair the execution of specific biological processes, such as the events of the cell cycle. Identification of the mutated gene provides information about the proteins required for the execution of that biologic pathway. Of special utility are conditional mutations, because they effect the activity of the encoded protein product only under specific restrictive conditions, elevated temperatures for example. Cells harboring conditional mutations can be first collected and propagated by growth under permissive conditions, and the consequences of the mutation then determined by shifting growth to restrictive conditions.

S. cerevisiae is known as budding yeast, because it reproduces by forming a bud that grows to become the daughter cell. The regular pattern of bud development provides convenient morphologic landmarks that can be used to assemble a temporal map of the cell cycle.[8] Thus, an unbudded cell is in G1, a small bud first emerges coincident with initiation of S phase, and a cell with a large bud is in G2/M. Hartwell isolated a large group of genes required for progression through the cell cycle by identifying conditional mutations that caused a cell population to arrest with a uniform morphology (e.g., all unbudded cells). Because the morphology of a yeast cell defines its position within the cell cycle, each mutant presumably had a position-specific defect in the operation of a cell cycle event. He called these cdc mutations (for "cell division cycle").[9] Thus, some cdc mutants were defective in G1-specific events (and arrested as unbudded cells), others in S phase (small-budded cells), and yet others in events that take place in G2/M (large-budded cells). Further analysis of nuclear morphology and the state of the mitotic spindle gave additional information about the specific processes affected by each mutation. In this way, Hartwell successfully identified the vast majority of genes responsible for regulating the eukaryotic cell cycle.[10]

The characterization of cdc mutations revealed a major principle of cell cycle regulation — that the orderly execution of cell cycle events resulted from a series of dependent relationships in which the completion of one event is required for the beginning of the next.[9] For instance, a cell with a mutation in a gene required

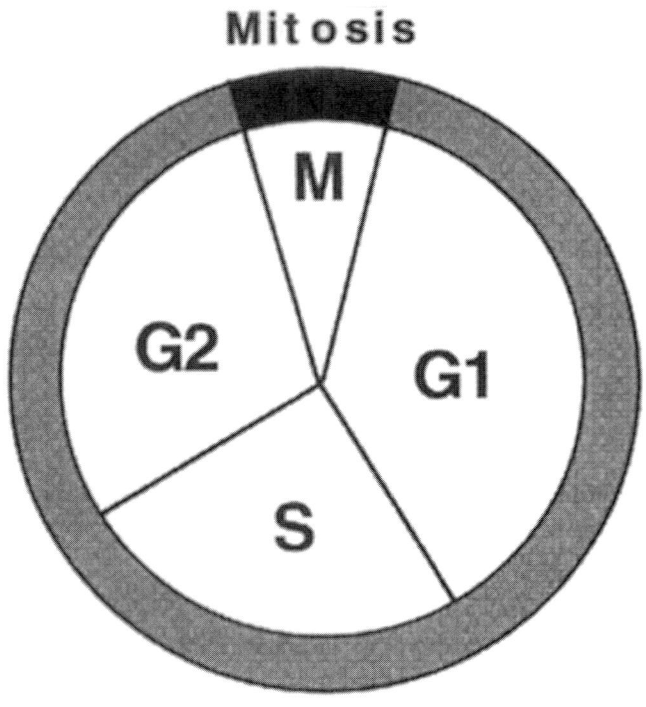

Fig. 23-1 The four phases of the cell cycle. Interphase is composed of S (synthesis) phase, during which time DNA replication occurs, and two G (gap) phases, during which cells respond to various proliferative and antiproliferative stimuli and cell growth occurs. Chromosomes and cellular contents are than distributed to two daughter cells during M (mitosis) phase, and the resulting progeny re-enter the cell cycle in G1.

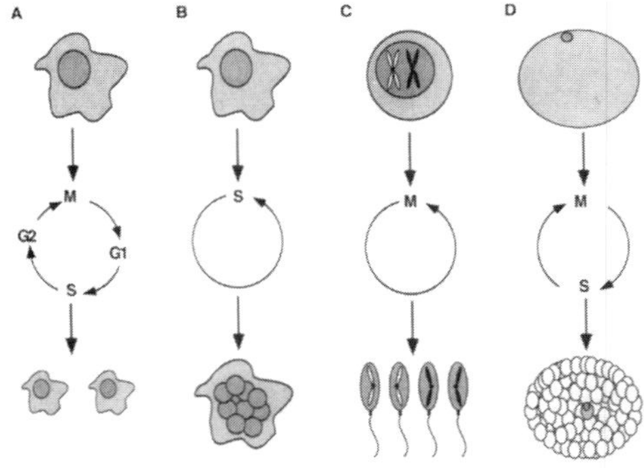

Fig. 23-2 Specialized cell cycles. A, A normal cell cycle is depicted in which a cell gives rise to two identical daughter cells. B, During megakaryopoiesis, promegakaryocytes undergo repeated rounds of DNA replication in the absence of mitosis (endoreduplication), resulting in polyploid megakaryocytes with a DNA content greater than their progenitors. C, In meiosis, two successive cell divisions after DNA replication result in four haploid daughter cells. D, Amphibian eggs undergo 12 rapid cell cycles consisting of alternating S and M phases. No cell growth occurs during these cycles, and the large egg cell is subdivided into approximately 4000 cells, each containing a normal complement of chromosomes.

for DNA replication stops its cell cycle in S phase and does not inappropriately try to begin mitosis (even though it should be capable of doing so). Initially, these dependencies were thought to reflect underlying biochemical pathways in which the product of one event was an essential substrate for the next. Hence, only after an upstream event occurred correctly would the substrates for the next event become available. This is one way to insure that cell cycle events were not executed in random order. The idea that the cell cycle is organized by dependent relationships is still considered one of the most important in cell-cycle biology, but the explanation for dependencies has changed and is discussed shortly.

A particularly important set of dependent pathways is initiated at the transition from G1 into S phase; this is called cell-cycle START.[11] Uniquely at START, the yeast cell senses the external and internal signals that control its proliferation, including mating pheromone, nutrients, and cell size (Fig. 23-3).[12–14] The yeast cell responds by initiating (or failing to initiate) the three parallel pathways required for reproduction of the cell — bud emergence, DNA replication, and spindle pole body duplication (the spindle pole body being the yeast equivalent of the centrosome of the mitotic spindle). The coordinate regulation of these three parallel-reproductive pathways indicates that completion of START represents the commitment of the cell to complete the entire program of events required for cell reproduction. Thus, genes required for START must play pivotal roles in the control of cell proliferation, and among the handful of START-specific genes, the CDC28 gene has gained particular prominence.[6,15,16] Analogous to START, the R POINT (restriction point) in mammalian cells defines a transition within G1 after which completion of the remainder of the cell cycle becomes independent of extracellular mitogens.

In contrast to the budding yeast cell cycle, during which cell growth and cell division are linked in G1 at START, in *S. pombe* (known also as fission yeast), these processes are usually coordinated at the transition between G2 and mitosis.[17] Paul Nurse identified cdc mutants in *S. pombe* that were unable to undergo the G2/M transition and one mutant, called cdc2, received special attention.[18–20] First, CDC2 is required twice during the fission yeast cell cycle, once at the G2/M transition and again at the G1/S transition (where a back-up size control exists). Second, certain dominantly acting mutations of cdc2 caused cells to shorten the length of G2, enter mitosis too quickly, and, consequently, become smaller than normal (known as a "wee" phenotype). This suggests that CDC2 activity is rate limiting for the onset of mitosis. The budding yeast CDC28 gene and the *S. pombe* CDC2 gene are homologs of one another.[17,19] Although CDC28 was first identified through its role at G1/S and cdc2 by its role at G2/M, it is now known that these proteins are required at the G1/S and at G2/M transitions in both types of yeast.[17,21,22] Because of these experiments, CDC2/CDC28 emerged as a key regulator of the cell cycle.

Complementing these genetic analyses of the yeast cell cycle were studies on the meiotic maturation of amphibian eggs. These physiological studies led to the discovery of a natural regulator of cell-cycle progression, an activity named MPF (maturation

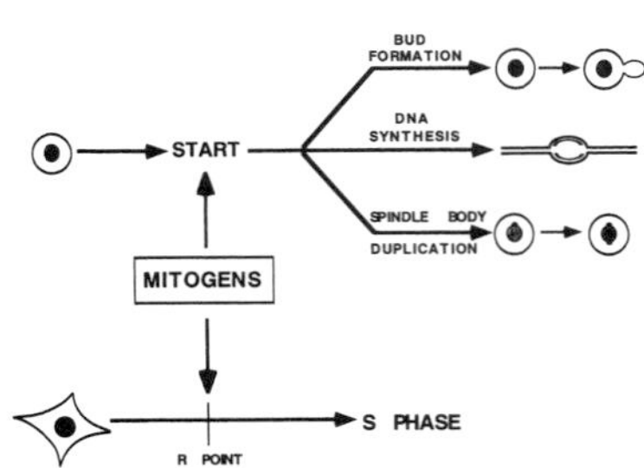

Fig. 23-3 START and the R (restriction) POINT define G1 transitions after which cell cycle progression becomes mitogen independent. At START, budding yeast initiate three independent processes required for cell duplication: bud emergence, DNA synthesis, and spindle-body duplication. A variety of mitogenic and antimitogenic signals determine if cells traverse START, after which cell cycle progression no longer depends upon these stimuli. At the analogous R POINT in mammalian cells, S-phase entry is no longer mitogen dependent. The biochemical bases of START and the R-POINT are discussed in the text.

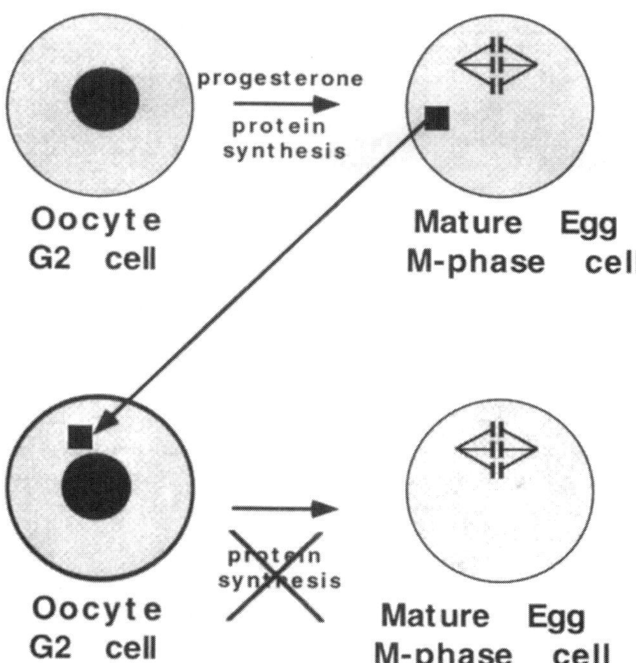

Fig. 23-4 MPF stimulates mitosis in G2-oocytes. As described in the text, injection of cytoplasm extract from an M-phase amphibian egg is sufficient to induce maturation of the recipient egg in the absence of progesterone or protein synthesis.

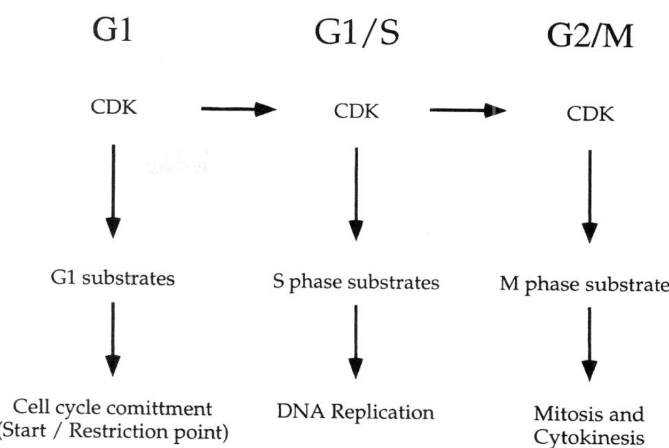

Fig. 23-5 The cdc2 cycle. The enzymatic activity of cdc2 and related kinases (cdks) drives each of the key cell cycle transitions.

promoting factor).[23–25] Amphibians produce mature eggs in response to the hormone progesterone, which induces immature oocytes to emerge from a prolonged arrest in G2 and resume the meiotic cell cycle. The progesterone-stimulated oocyte completes the reductive meiotic divisions and eventually pauses again in metaphase of meiosis II, but now as a mature egg awaiting fertilization. In other words, oocyte maturation requires cell-cycle progression from G2 of meiosis I to metaphase of meiosis II, and is under the control of MPF. Indeed, injection of MPF isolated from a mature egg into the cytoplasm of an immature oocyte is sufficient to initiate meiotic maturation independently of any hormonal trigger (Fig. 23-4). Furthermore, MPF activity is not restricted to meiosis. MPF activity oscillates during each mitotic cycle, being high in M phase and low in interphase.[24,26,27] This indicates that MPF is a fundamental component of cell-cycle regulation in all cell cycles, mitotic as well as meiotic.

Remarkably, MPF activity will continue to oscillate even in enucleated cells.[28] Because MPF activity can oscillate independently of nuclear events, it has been proposed that the MPF cycle might be an autonomous mitotic clock, and that state of the clock (the "time of day") determines which cell cycle event occurs.[26,28,29] Thus, high MPF activity would permit entry into mitosis, and low MPF activity would permit cells to enter S phase. This model supplanted the earlier idea that the obligate order of cell cycle events might simply be established by substrate-product-type relationships. However, the notion of a mitotic clock would then require the existence of additional feedback controls to keep the clock entrained to actual progress through the cell cycle; the clock must stop if essential cell cycle events do not occur. These feedback controls do exist, and are known as checkpoints.[30]

Perhaps the most far-reaching advance in the cell-cycle field in the last 15 years has been the demonstration that cell-cycle controls are evolutionarily conserved.[31,32] This first became evident when it was discovered that the CDC2 and CDC28 genes in fission and budding yeast encode homologous proteins,[17] now known as the CDC2 protein kinase. Furthermore, gene transfer experiments show that the human CDC2 gene can complement mutations in the yeast CDC2 gene.[33] This was reinforced 6 years later when MPF was purified (initially from *Xenopus,* and later from other vertebrates), and its catalytic subunit was shown to be a homolog of CDC2.[34–38] These observations set the stage for our current paradigm of eukaryotic cell cycle control, which in its simplest form depicts the cell cycle as a CDC2 cycle (Fig. 23-5).[39] Thus, in organisms ranging from yeast to humans, the catalytic activity of CDC2 and related kinases is required for each of the major transitions within the cell cycle—from G1 into S, and from G2 into M.[40–46]

CDK REGULATION

In budding and fission yeast, the highly regulated action of a single kinase subunit (cdc28 or cdc2, respectively) drives the cell cycle forward.[47] In higher eukaryotes, cell-cycle control is more complex, and several proteins homologous to cdc2 (termed the cyclin-dependent kinases or cdks) have been identified.[48] Cyclin-dependent kinases are protein kinases that vary in size between 30 and 40 kb and share greater than 40 percent sequence identity. In addition to amino acid homology, cdks share many functional and regulatory features with yeast cdc2/28.[49,50] Almost all cdks require association with protein subunits called cyclins to become active kinases. Cdks also contain conserved amino acid residues that modulate kinase activity when phosphorylated or dephosphorylated. Additionally, specific regulatory molecules that bind and inhibit cdk subunits inhibit cdk activity. Each of these regulatory mechanisms is discussed in detail below. Remarkably, while differences among organisms do exist, this multi-tiered regulatory system has been conserved from yeast to humans.

Each phase of the cell cycle is characterized by a unique pattern of cdk activity (Fig. 23-6).[51–53] In mammalian cells, eight cdks have been identified, and most are active (and required) only in specific phases of the cell cycle. Progression through G1 phase depends upon the activities of cdk2, cdk3, cdk4, and cdk6. The recently described cdk8 protein also may function primarily in G1, and may be involved in transcriptional regulation. Cdk2 and cdc2 are active in S-phase, and cdc2 kinase activity also governs mitotic entry and exit. In distinction to its kindred, cdk5 does not appear to be intimately involved in cell-cycle progression, but may, instead, play a role in the developing nervous system, where it associates with the non-cyclin activator p35.[54,55]

Cyclins: Activating Subunits of CDK Enzymes

Monomeric cdk subunits are essentially devoid of enzymatic activity, and kinase activation requires the association of cdks with cyclins.[49] An active cdk is thus a heterodimeric enzyme consisting of regulatory (cyclin) and enzymatic (cdk) subunits. The cyclins are a group of related proteins that contain a conserved region of homology (the cyclin box) and are usually expressed in a cell cycle specific fashion. Cyclin expression is rate-limiting for cdk

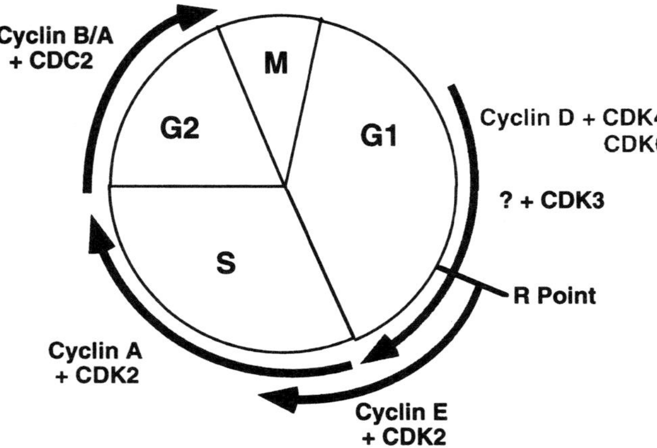

Fig. 23-6 Patterns of cyclin-cdk activity during the mammalian cell cycle. The expression patterns of the key mammalian cyclins is superimposed upon the cell cycle, along with their respective cdk partners. The approximate position of the R POINT is shown (adapted from Sherr[51]).

activation, and control of cyclin expression is a fundamental mechanism underlying cdk periodicity. In general, cyclin levels are determined by both transcriptional control and regulated proteolysis by the ubiquitin-proteosome system.

The recently solved crystal structure of cyclin A bound to cdk2 reveals that cyclins activate cdks in at least two ways. Cyclin binding induces conformational changes in the cdk that first reorients the configuration of the ATP phosphate groups to facilitate phosphotransfer to protein substrates, and second moves the T-loop of the cdk out of a position that would otherwise block entry of protein substrates into the active site (Fig. 23-7).[56,57]

The specificity of cdk action at different times in the cell cycle is in large part determined by its particular cyclin subunit. This functional diversity of cyclins was first established in the yeast *S. cerevisiae* where specific cyclins have been identified that are required for G1, S phase, and mitosis. Budding yeast express three functionally redundant G1 cyclins (cln1, cln2, and cln3), which are required for passage through START.[58–62] While differences between the cln genes have been described, mutant yeast cells with mutated cln alleles can still enter S phase as long as one of these three genes remains functional. Transcription of cln1 and cln2 is controlled by the Swi4/Swi6 transcription factor,[63–65] and cln activity positively reinforces further cln expression.[66–68] Thus, cln1 and cln2 mRNAs rise during G1, reaching peak levels around START.

Once START has been traversed, cln activity is no longer required for subsequent cell-cycle progression. Instead, other cyclins associate with and activate cdc28 during other phases of the cell cycle. Complexes containing cdc28 and the cyclins clb5 and clb6 are required for S phase,[69,70] and the four B-type cyclins, clb1 to clb4 are required for mitosis.[71]

START marks a point of transition in the yeast cell cycle where G1 cyclin expression ends and mitotic cyclin expression begins. This transition comes about because these two classes of cyclin modulate each other's expression. Cln/cdc28 kinase activity directly increases the expression of the clb genes, and conversely clb-cdc28 kinase activity represses cln expression.[72] Not only do G1 cyclins promote the expression of the genes for mitotic cyclins but, as described below, they also increase the stability and functional activity of clb proteins. Furthermore, the cln proteins themselves are rapidly degraded after START. This is discussed below in the section on cell-cycle regulated proteolysis. Together, these controls insure ordered progression through the cell cycle by establishing alternating periods of the cell cycle where either G1 or mitotic cyclins are expressed and functionally active.

Mammalian cyclins C, D1, and E were first identified in a screen for mammalian genes that could complement yeast cyclin mutations.[73–75] At the same time Cyclin D1 was identified by two other approaches — as a mitogen-responsive gene in a macrophage cell line[76] and as a gene located at a chromosome inversion breakpoint in a parathyroid tumor (and in this guise was originally named PRAD1).[77] A dozen mammalian cyclin genes have been identified that are both structurally and functionally homologous to yeast cyclins.[51,52] Like the yeast cyclins, many of these molecules exhibit cell-cycle-dependent periodicity in their expression and activity (Fig. 23-6).

The primary mammalian G1 cyclins are the D-type cyclins and cyclin E. These cyclins associate with the cdk-4/6, and cdk2 subunits, respectively. There are three D-type cyclins (D1, D2, and D3), which are expressed in a cell-type specific fashion.[51,52,78] The G1 role of the D-type cyclins is revealed by their pattern of expression and by their functional properties. Cyclin D expression begins in early G1 when quiescent cells are stimulated to reenter the cell cycle, and cyclin D expression remains at high levels as long as mitogens are present. In other words, the expression of these labile proteins ($t_{\frac{1}{2}} < 20$ min) is not intrinsically periodic, but instead depends upon the presence of cell-type specific mitogens. Inhibition of cyclin D1 function blocks the cell cycle in G1, demonstrating the necessity of cyclin D for the cell cycle.[79,80] Also, enforced overexpression of cyclin D1 shortens the G1 phase of the cell cycle, and partially diminishes the mitogen requirement for cell proliferation, demonstrating that cyclin D1 levels are limiting for G1 progression.[80,81]

Cyclin E activity is also required in G1, although probably somewhat after cyclin D activity.[81–83] Cyclin E protein expression peaks at the G1-S boundary, and then decays as S-phase progresses.[82,84,85] Determinants of cyclin E periodicity include both transcriptional control by E2F and regulated proteolysis (see below). Overexpression of cyclin E results in G1 contraction and decreased mitogen requirements,[81,86] and cyclin E kinase activity is required for S-phase entry.[82,83] Activation of cyclin D and cyclin E-associated kinases may biochemically constitute the restriction point, the mammalian equivalent of START control in yeast.

Later cell-cycle transitions are governed by the cyclin A and cyclin B proteins. Cyclin A associates with both the cdk2 and cdc2 subunits, and cyclin A kinase activity is required at the start of S phase and at the G2-M transition.[87–89] Cyclin B associates with cdc2, and, like the yeast clb proteins, cyclin B-cdc2 kinase activity regulates both mitotic entry and exit.[90]

The cyclin H protein associates with cdk7, and this heterodimer constitutes the cdk-activating kinase (CAK).[91] CAK is also a component of the human transcription factor TFIIH, and is capable of phosphorylating the carboxy-terminal domain (CTD) of RNA polymerase II. Cyclin C is classed as a G1 cyclin, although its role is not yet defined.[73] Cyclin C has recently been shown to associate with cdk8, and cyclin C-cdk8 complexes also have RNA polymerase II CTD kinase activity, although they do not co-purify with TFIIH.[92] Phosphorylation of the CTD by cyclin-cdk complexes may couple cell-cycle events to the cellular transcriptional machinery.

Comparatively little is known about the remaining cyclins that have been identified to date, including cyclins F, G and I. Cyclin F is the largest cyclin, with a molecular weight of 87, and is most closely related to cyclins A and B. Cyclin F mRNA peaks in G2 and cyclin F protein accumulates in interphase and is destroyed during mitosis.[93] Cyclin G mRNA does not fluctuate in a cell cycle-dependent fashion, but is induced by both the p53 protein and growth stimulation of quiescent cells.[94] The cyclin I protein is expressed most highly in post-mitotic tissues, including muscle and neurons, and may have a unique regulatory role.[95]

CDK Regulation by Phosphorylation and Dephosphorylation

In addition to cyclin binding, phosphorylation and dephosphorylation of conserved cdk residues provides another important level of control over kinase activity.[49] Cdks can be either activated or inactivated by phosphorylation (Fig. 23-8). The site of activating

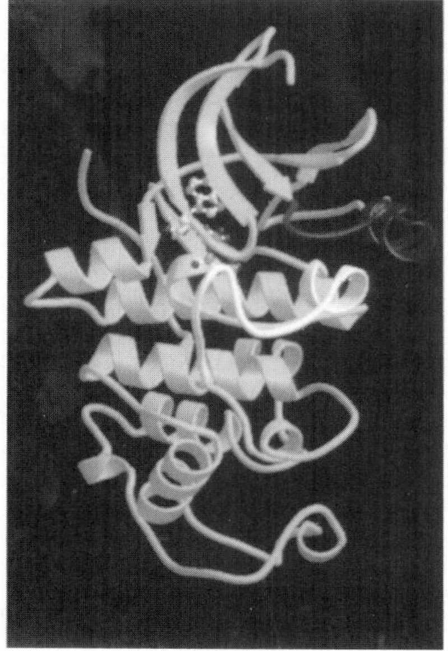

A

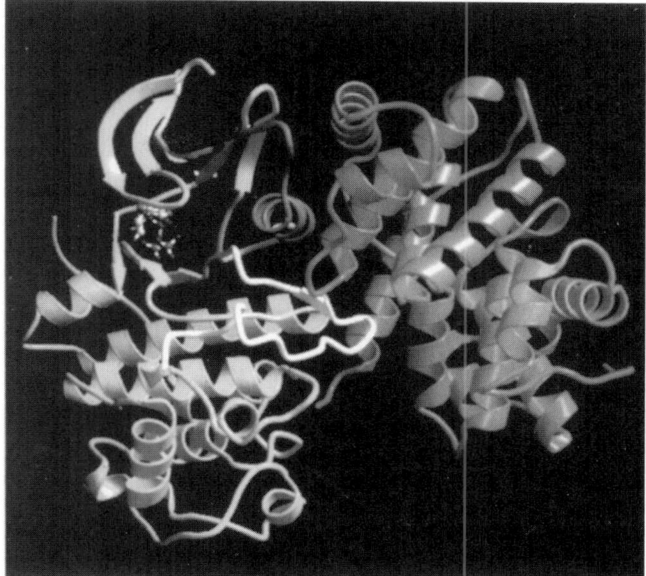

B

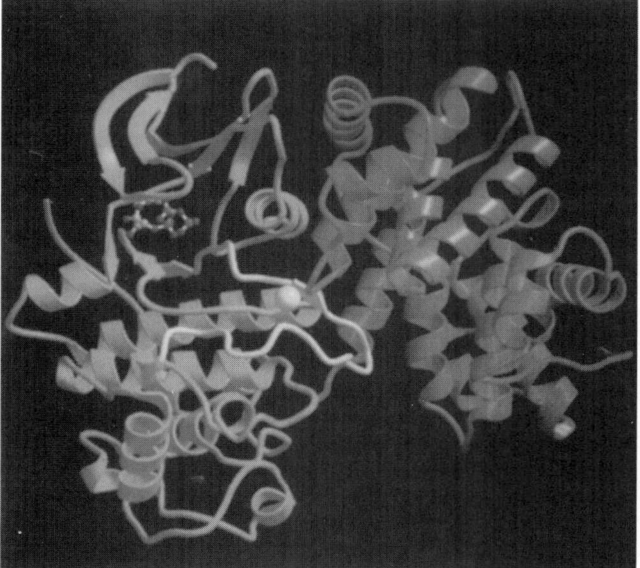

C

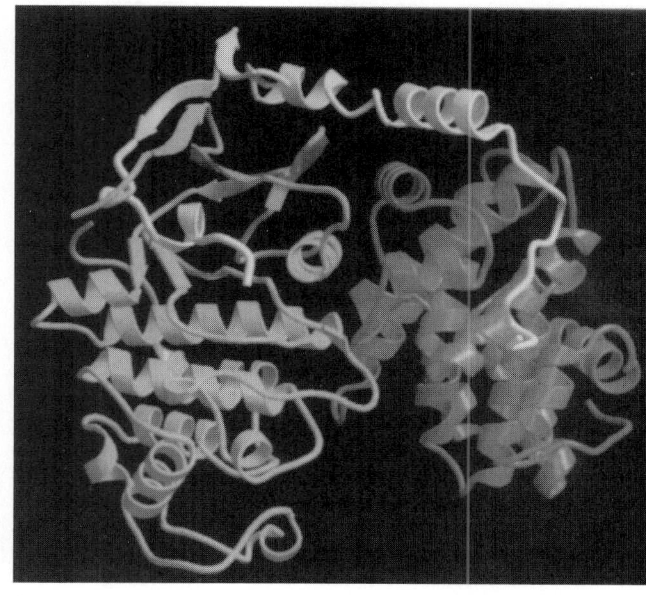

D

Fig. 23-7 Crystal structure of cdk2, cyclin A-cdk2, and cyclin A-cdk2-p27 complexes. A, The structure of monomeric cdk2. The T-loop is indicated in yellow, and the PSTAIRE motif in red. An ATP molecule in indicated within the active site. B, The structure of cdk2 bound to an amino-terminal truncated version of cyclin A. Cyclin binding re-orients the PSTAIRE helix and moves the T-loop, resulting in the re-positioning of ATP-phosphate groups within the complex and allowing substrate accessibility to the active site. C, The structure of cdk-activating kinase (CAK)-phosphorylated cyclin A bound to cdk2. The yellow ball indicates the position of thr160 within the T-loop. D, The structure of a ternary complex of the amino terminus of p27 bound to cyclin A -cdk2. Separate domains of P27 interact with both cyclin A and cdk2. The structure of this complex reveals that p27 inhibits cdk activity by distorting the structure of the active site, and by binding within the catalytic cleft and preventing ATP binding.

phosphorylation is a conserved threonine residue in the so-called "T-loop" (e.g., threonine 161 in cdc2, threonine 160 in cdk2).[56] The binding of cyclin to the cdk, and phosphorylation of this residues together move the T-loop away from the catalytic cleft of the enzyme, thereby providing access to protein substrates.[96] Thr160 is phosphorylated by CAK (cyclin H-cdk7), and this phosphorylation is required for cdk activation.[97–100] CAK activity, however, is neither cell-cycle regulated nor limiting, and the major determinant of Thr160 phosphorylation is probably cyclin binding.[91]

Cdks can also be phosphorylated on a specific amino-terminal tyrosine residue (e.g., tyrosine 15 in cdc2 and cdk2). Tyrosine phosphorylated cdk2 is catalytically inactive, even if it is phosphorylated on the activating threonine within the T-loop.[98,100–103] The kinases that phosphorylate tyr15 are evolutionarily conserved and are known as the wee1 and mik1 kinases.[104–107] Conversely, dephosphorylation of tyrosine by the cdc25 phosphatase activates the cdk.[108–112] Regulation of wee1 and cdc25 is complex,[113,114] but the bottom-line is that the relative activities of these enzymes set a threshold for cdk activation and

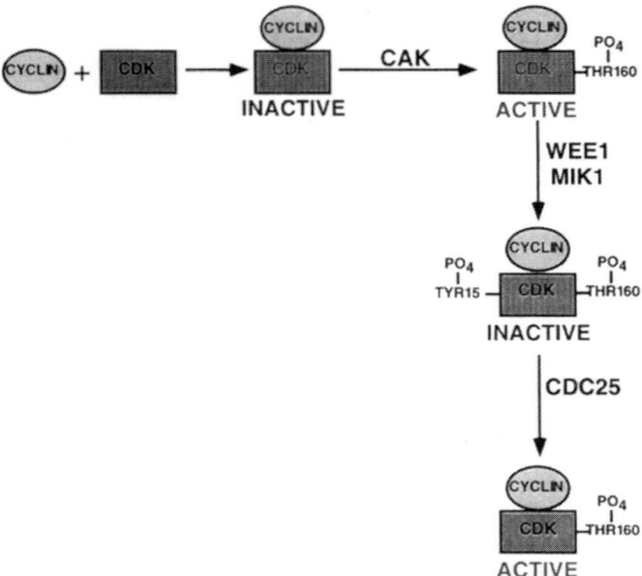

Fig. 23-8 CDK regulation by cyclin binding and cdk phosphorylation. As described in the text, activation of cdks requires cyclin binding and cdk phosphorylation at thr160 by the cdk-activating kinase (CAK). Subsequent phosphorylation of Tyr15 by the wee1 and mik1 kinases and dephosphorylation by cdc25 phosphatases further regulates kinase activity.

determine mitotic entry. Three mammalian cdc25 homologues have been identified (cdc25a, cdc25b, and cdc25c), and each may have a unique cell-cycle role.[115,116] Cdc25a is active in G1 and may be induced by raf-dependent pathways.[117]

CKIs: Inhibitory Subunits of CDK Enzymes

All organisms express proteins that directly bind to and inhibit cdk activity.[118,119] These cdk-inhibitors (CKIs) provide another important strategy by which cdk activity is regulated in response to diverse stimuli. In budding yeast, two kinds of inhibitors have been described. One type is inducible and links the cell cycle to extracellular signals; the other type is an intrinsic component of the mitotic cycle. The best example of the first type of CKI is the FAR1 protein. Mating pheromones induce FAR1, a protein that binds to and inhibits the cln-cdc28 kinase and thereby causes the yeast cell cycle to arrest at START. Another important CDK inhibitor in budding yeast is Sic1, but it is a constitutive element in the mitotic clock and is not known to be induced by extrinsic proliferative signals.[120,121] At the conclusion of each mitosis, Sic1 protein levels rise, inhibiting the clb-cdc28 kinases and facilitating the transition from anaphase to the next G1. Sic1 protein remains at high levels during G1 until activation of the cln-cdc28 kinases at START induce its degradation. This is one mechanism that links activation of the S-phase clb-cdc28 kinases to passage through START.

Mammalian cells express two classes of CKIs that are distinguished by their cdk targets: the Cip/Kip family of CKI's are universal cdk inhibitors, whereas the INK4 proteins are specific cdk4/6 inhibitors (Fig. 23-9).[118] The Cip/Kip family consists of three members: p21, p27, and p57. Overexpression of these molecules causes a G1 arrest in cultured cells, and they are able to inhibit most cyclin-cdk complexes *in vitro*. These molecules bind to assembled cyclin-cdk complexes much more avidly than to monomeric cdk or cyclin subunits. p21 was first identified as a component of cyclin-CDK complexes in proliferating cells[123] and as a protein induced as cells *in vitro* became senescent.[124] Shortly thereafter, it was cloned by a number of independent approaches.[125–128] The p21 protein contains two functional domains, an amino terminal cdk interaction region that is sufficient for cdk inhibition, and a carboxy-terminal region that binds PCNA, a processivity factor associated with DNA polymerase delta.[129–131]

Two biological roles have been suggested for p21.[118,122] The first is in contributing to the cell-cycle arrest that occurs in cells with damaged DNA.[127] This is discussed in greater detail below. Additionally, p21 has been suggested as a facilitator of withdrawal from the cell cycle in cells undergoing terminal differentiation.[132,133]

The CKI p27Kip1 is structurally related to p21Cip1.[134,135] p21 and p27 share significant amino terminal homology within the cdk inhibitory domain, but p27 does not contain the PCNA interaction region. p27 is not a p53 response gene, but p27 levels respond instead to a variety of extracellular mitogenic and antimitogenic signals.[118] In general, p27 levels are high in nondividing cells and low in proliferating cells. The regulation of p27 is complex, with transcriptional, translational and post-translational mechanisms all implicated in different biological contexts.[136]

The mechanism of cdk inhibition by p27 has been clarified by the crystal structure of p27 bound to cyclin A-cdk2 (Fig. 23-7).[96] In the ternary p27-cyclin A-cdk2 complex, separate domains in p27 interacts with the cyclin and the cdk. Although p27 does not significantly alter the structure of the cyclin, it may bind to a site on the cyclin that the cyclin would ordinarily use for interactions with protein substrates. In this way, p27 might inhibit phosphorylation of physiologically important substrates without inhibiting the catalytic activity of the cdk enzyme. In addition, p27 does have dramatic effects on cdk structure. p27 disrupts the structure of the N-terminal lobe of the cdk, widening and distorting the ATP-binding site. In fact, p27 itself inserts into the catalytic cleft and directly interacts with the amino acids that would bind ATP. This would completely prevent cdk-binding of ATP and completely inhibit catalytic activity.

Less is known about p57, the most recently isolated family member that was cloned by virtue of its homology with p27.[137,138] Both the amino and carboxy-terminal domains of p57 are related to p27. Compared with p27, however, p57 expression is relatively restricted to terminally differentiated tissues.

The INK4 family of CKIs includes four structurally related proteins (p15, p16, p18, p19), each of which contains four ankyrin repeats.[118] The first member of this family to be identified, p16, was found to be associated with cdk4 in transformed cells,[138] and subsequently fingered as a candidate tumor suppressor in familial melanoma.[139,140] INK4 proteins bind to monomeric cdk4/6 subunits, preventing their association with D-type cyclins, and

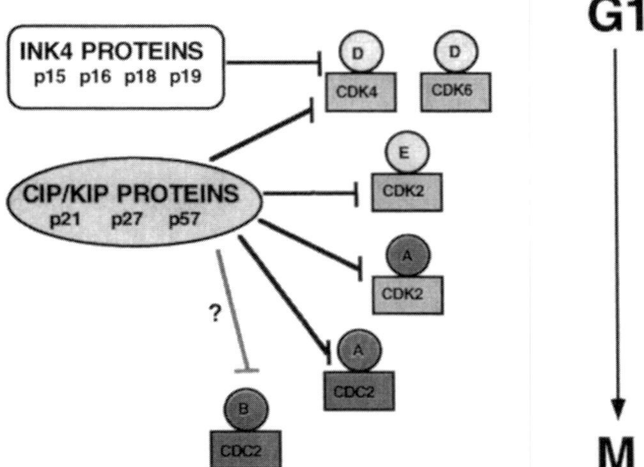

Fig. 23-9 Mammalian CDK-inhibitors are classed by their cyclin-cdk targets. The Cip/Kip proteins (p21, p27, p57) are universal cdk inhibitors that inactivate all cyclin-cdk complexes (with the possible exception of cyclin B-cdc2). In contrast, the INK4 proteins (p15, p16, p18, p19) specifically bind and inhibit only cdk4/6, and cyclin D-cdk4/6 complexes.

INK4 proteins can also inhibit the activity of cyclin D-cdk4/6 complexes. The other INK4 proteins are expressed ubiquitously in mouse tissues and cultured cells, and the expression of p19 does oscillate with the cell cycle.[141,142] While p15 is involved in the anti-proliferative response to TGF-B, the physiological roles of the INK4 protein remain unknown. The frequent deletions of p15 and p16 in primary tumors and the high spontaneous tumor rate in p16-deficient mice indicate that these proteins play a critical role in maintaining normal growth control.[143]

CDK SUBSTRATES

Cdks promote progression through the cell cycle by phosphorylating a group of protein substrates.[53] However, compared with the enormous amount of data concerning cdk regulation, relatively little is known about cdk substrates. The most thoroughly characterized cdk substrates are cell-cycle regulatory proteins themselves. For example, in budding yeast, phosphorylation of p40sic1 by the cln-cdc28 kinase leads to its ubiquitin-mediated proteolysis and progression from G1 to S phase.[120,121] In fact, a yeast strain lacking all cln genes is viable if p40sic1 is also mutated, which suggests that phosphorylation of this CKI is a key function of the cln proteins in promoting cell cycle progression.[144]

A critical regulator of cell-cycle progression in higher eukaryotes, including humans, is the Rb protein. The importance of Rb in cell-cycle control became evident as a result of three separate seminal observations.[145] First, the oncogenic proteins encoded by a variety of DNA tumor viruses (e.g., SV40, adenovirus, and papillomavirus) all bind to the Rb protein.[146–148] Second, the Rb gene is mutated in the germ line in patients suffering hereditary retinoblastoma, and is frequently mutated in tumor cells in patients who develop spontaneous tumors.[149–151] Third, the Rb protein undergoes cell-cycle dependent phosphorylation during G1, and this modifies its interaction with an essential transcription factor known as E2F.[152–156] E2F transcription factors are heterodimeric proteins composed of one E2F subunit and one DP subunit that regulate the transcription of many genes required in S-phase.[157–159] There are five known E2F subunits, which are designated E2F1 to E2F5, and three known DP subunits, which are designated DP1 to DP3. When complexed with Rb, E2F is inactive or it may be a transcriptional repressor, and the cell cycle arrests in the absence of these needed gene products. E2F sequestration is regulated by the phosphorylation state of Rb; unphosphorylated Rb avidly binds E2F while hyperphosphorylated does not. As cells progress through G1, Rb is progressively phosphorylated at multiple sites, ultimately releasing E2F. Viral oncoproteins specifically bind to the unphosphorylated form of Rb, and in doing so automatically release E2F from its Rb-bound inactive state.

The kinases that phosphorylate Rb are the cdks. The pRb protein contains eight consensus cdk-phosphorylation sites, and cyclin D-, E-, and A-cdk complexes have Rb kinase activity *in vitro* and *in vivo*.[160–163] Cyclin D-cdk4 complexes bind stably to Rb, and once Rb is phosphorylated, this complex disassembles.[164] Cyclin D-cdk4/6 and cyclin E-cdk2 complexes probably cooperate to phosphorylate and inactivate Rb during G1. The observation that cyclin D function is dispensable in cells with mutant Rb alleles suggests that pRb phosphorylation is the critical means by which D-type cyclins promote G1 progression.[165–167] Phosphorylation of Rb by cyclin E-cdk2 may also be required prior to S-phase entry, but cyclin E is essential for cell-cycle progression in Rb-mutant cells, demonstrating that other substrates of cyclin E-cdk2 must also exist.[82]

Rb is one member of a family of structurally related "pocket" proteins, which includes p107, p130, and Rb itself.[167] All the pocket proteins bind to members of the E2F family of transcription factors and phosphorylation of these proteins by cyclin-cdk complexes liberates E2F, removing some constraints on cell proliferation. However, neither p107 nor p130 are tumor suppressors, and their function during the cell cycle is poorly understood.

E2F activity is essential for the G1-S transition, but it must also be inactivated for the ensuing S-phase to progress normally.[170,171] E2F/DP heterodimers form stable complexes with cyclin A-cdk2, and phosphorylation of a specific DP residue by cyclin A-cdk2 suppresses E2F DNA-binding. Thus, G1 cyclins activate E2F via Rb phosphorylation, and cyclin A-cdk2 directly inactivates E2F through DP phosphorylation. In this way, sequentially acting cyclin-cdk complexes first initiate and then extinguish E2F activity, causing a pulse of E2F-dependent gene transcription at the G1 to S phase transition.

The elucidation of cdk substrates clearly remains incomplete.[172] For instance, it is thought that proteins directly involved in the initiation of DNA replication will be phosphorylated and activated by cdks at the start of S phase,[173] although not a single such protein has been identified. Almost as short is the list of cdk substrates during mitosis. The first identified mitotic cdk substrates were the nuclear lamins.[174,175] The nuclear lamina is a structure composed of intermediate filament proteins that depolymerizes at the onset of mitosis. The polymerization of lamins is regulated by phosphorylation, and lamins have been shown to be substrates for cyclin B-cdc2. Phosphorylation of lamins promotes their disassembly, and it has been proposed cyclin B-cdc2 lamin kinase activity is responsible for the breakdown of the nuclear lamina at mitosis. Cdc2 kinase activity is also required for assembly of the mitotic spindle.[176] The human Eg5 protein is a kinesin-related motor protein that is needed to build a bipolar spindle. The localization of Eg5 to the spindle apparatus is dependent on phosphorylation at thr927, and this residue is phosphorylated by cyclin B-cdc2. Inhibition of Eg5 function results in a mitotic block, and one mechanism by which cyclin B-cdc2 promotes mitosis is likely to involve Eg5 phosphorylation.

PROTEOLYSIS IN CELL-CYCLE REGULATION

A basic feature of the cell cycle is that its transitions are irreversible. Anaphase cells, for instance, cannot regress to metaphase, nor can S phase cells reverse course and go back to G1. This is accomplished by a cycle of protein destruction that complements the periodic activation of cyclin/cdk complexes. In general, protein destruction eliminates both proteins that have been used in the preceding phase of the cell cycle and proteins that would inhibit progression into the next cell cycle phase.[177] The net effect is to cause the cell cycle to move irreversibly forward.

The paradigm for periodic protein degradation during the cell cycle is the destruction of cyclin B during mitosis (Fig. 23-10).[35,178] The abundance of cyclin B protein oscillates during each cell division cycle, being highest as cells enter mitosis and disappearing after chromosome disjunction has occurred at the metaphase to anaphase transition.[179] This is caused by changes in the rate of its degradation. Many short-lived proteins, including cyclin B, are degraded in the proteosome, a 26S complex that contains multiple proteolytic enzymes and that specifically recognizes and degrades ubiquitinated proteins.[180] Conjugation of a protein to ubiquitin is the signal for its delivery to the proteosome, and this is accomplished in a multistep reaction in which ubiquitin is ultimately transferred through a thiol-ester linkage to lysine side-chains of the target protein.[181,182] Ubiquitin, a 76-amino acid protein, is first attached through its carboxy terminus to an ubiquitin-activating enzyme called E1, in an ATP-dependent reaction. The E1-bound ubiquitin is then transferred to one of a family of carrier proteins called E2, or ubiquitin-conjugating enzymes, which can then transfer ubiquitin to target proteins. Most eukaryotes are thought to have a single E1 gene, but multiple E2 genes (at least 12 in budding yeast). Each of the E2 enzymes recognizes and transfers ubiquitin to only particular proteins, thereby imposing some degree of selectivity on the process of ubiquitin-dependent proteolysis. Further selectivity arises because conjugation of some proteins to ubiquitin requires

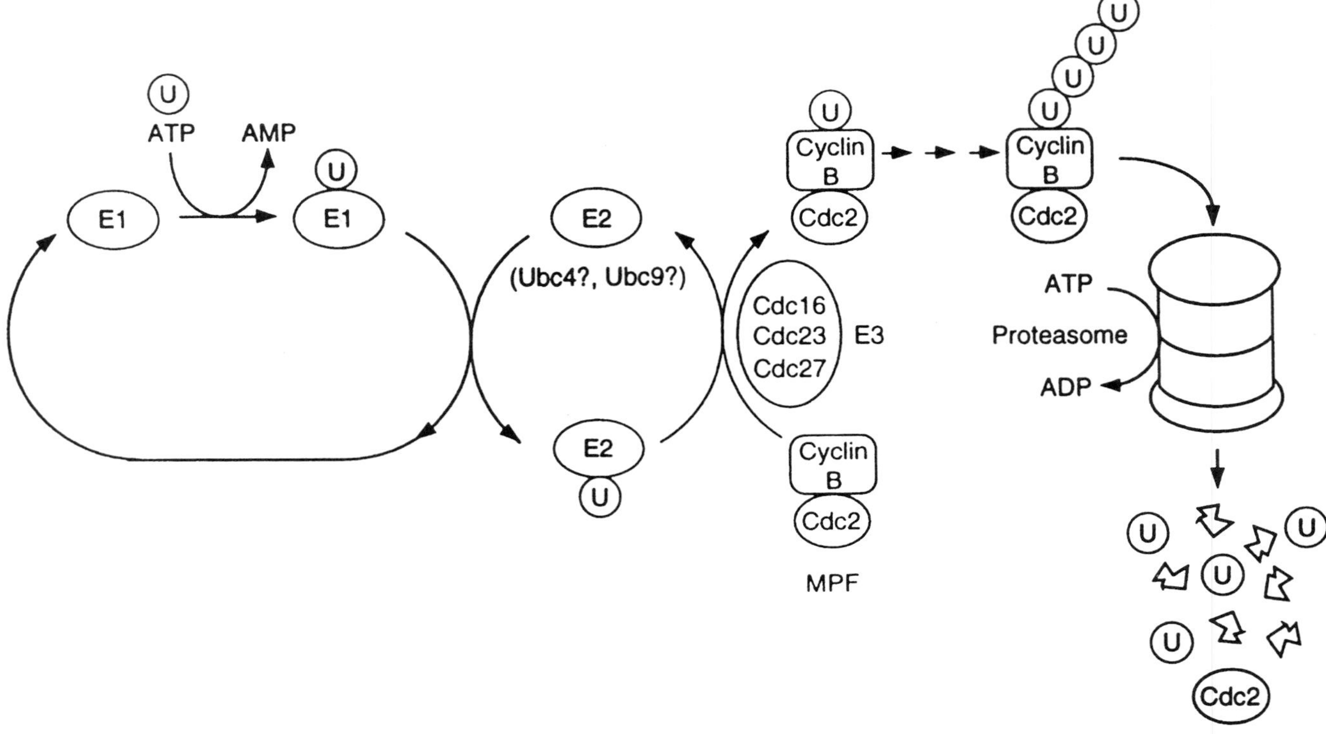

Fig. 23-10 The biochemistry of cyclin destruction. See text for details (reprinted from Murray 1995[190] with permission).

collaboration between an E2 and an E3 enzyme, which is called ubiquitin ligases.

The E2 and E3 enzymes choose proteins for ubiquitination by recognizing specific amino acids motifs.[183] A few types of motifs have been identified, each presumably recognized by certain E2 or E2/E3 combinations. The particular ubiquitination motif within cyclin B is called the cyclin destruction box.[184] A mutant version of cyclin B lacking the destruction box (called cyclin BΔdb) is not conjugated to ubiquitin during mitosis and is not degraded.[185] Consequently, cyclin BΔdb/cdc2 (and its MPF activity) remains active, and the cell cycle becomes blocked in mitosis.[186–188] This important experiment demonstrates that destruction of cyclin B is required for inactivation of cdc2 and MPF activity in anaphase cells, and that inactivation of cdc2 is required for mitosis to be completed. Therefore, just as synthesis of cyclin B is required for a cell to enter mitosis, the destruction of cyclin B is required for a cell to exit mitosis and begin a new cell cycle.[189] Cyclin A also has a destruction box and is degraded in mitosis at about the same time as cyclin B.[190]

The ubiquitination of cyclin B is controlled by an E3-like activity called the anaphase-promoting complex, or APC.[191] As its name implies, the APC is required not only in anaphase for the destruction of cyclin B, but also earlier in mitosis at metaphase to promote the transition into anaphase.[192] It is thought that at the metaphase to anaphase transition the APC is required for the targeted ubiqutination and proteolysis of a protein necessary for cohesion between sister chromatids on the metaphase plate. The APC has been characterized both genetically and biochemically, and shown to be a 20S particle comprising at least three proteins: cdc16, cdc23, and cdc27 (which were originally discovered by Hartwell in the cdc screen described above).[191,193–195]

The activity of the APC is regulated during the cell cycle.[177] The ability of the APC to ubiquitinate B-type cyclins is turned on during mitosis and turned off in G1, leading directly to the periodic accumulation and destruction of these cyclins.[195–197] In this way, the duration of APC activity defines the interval in the cell cycle where the levels of B-type cyclins are kept low; this is a key element in establishing the G1 phase of the cell cycle. Conversely, inactivation of the APC is required for accumulation of S-phase cyclins, like clb5 and clb6 in yeast, and probably cyclin A in mammalian cells, and is, therefore, a prerequisite for entry into S phase. Thus, cyclin/cdks and the APC are complementary activities that work in parallel to control major transitions within the cell cycle. The mechanisms regulating the APC are incompletely understood, but it seems as though APC activity is directly coupled to cyclin/cdk activity. First, during mitosis it is thought that cyclin B/cdc2 initiates the pathway leading to its own destruction by phosphorylating and activating the APC.[177,196] Second, once activated in mitosis the APC remains active until late in G1, when it is inactivated by G1 cyclin/cdk activity.[196] In yeast, this occurs coincidentally with START, and in mammalian cells, it may be one of the events that leads to cell-cycle commitment at the restriction point.

Protein destruction also controls the abundance of the cyclins and CKIs that regulate entry into S phase. Cyclin E in mammalian cells,[198,199] and the G1 cyclins in yeast (the cln proteins),[200–202] are both degraded by ubiquitin-dependent proteolysis. In both cases, phosphorylation of the cyclin triggers its ubiquitination, which is a common theme in regulated protein turnover.[203–205] Often, phosphorylation of a protein is the end result of a signal transduction pathway, and can be used to allow recognition of proteins by E2 and E3 ubiquitin-conjugating enzymes. In the case of cyclin E and the cln proteins, the cyclins are directly phosphorylated by their associated cdks. Thus, cyclin E/cdk2 activity is inherently self-limited, because cdk2 activity initiates the pathway leading to cyclin E destruction. In essence, this is similar to the control of A and B-type cyclin turnover by the APC, because in each instance cyclin degradation is initiated by cdk activity.

Cdk inhibitor levels are also regulated during G1 by proteolysis. In mammalian cells, the cdk inhibitor p27Kip1 is eliminated from cells after mitogenic stimulation by the ubiquitin-proteosome pathway;[206] in budding yeast, the cdk inhibitor p40Sic1 is regulated in a similar manner.[121,144] In fact, biochemical reconstitution of sic1 turnover *in vitro* has led to the identification of an E3 complex that may rival the importance of the APC in cell-cycle control. The sic1 E3 complex is composed of three proteins, skp1, cdc53, and cdc4.[206a,d–f] The skp1-cdc53-cdc4 complex specifically recognizes and promotes the ubiquitination of phosphorylated sic1 in the presence of cdc34 (an E2) and E1. In addition to sic1, the skp1-cdc53-cdc4 complex also functions as an E3 for the *S. cervesiae* cdk inhibitor far1.[206b]

The components of this E3 complex are members of protein families: cdc4 belongs to a large group of proteins defined by a region of homology called an F-box,[206e,f] and cdc53 belongs to the family of proteins termed cullins.[208] Substitution of different family members within the E3 complex can have dramatic affects on its activity. When other F-box proteins replace cdc4, the substrate specificity of the E3 complex can change. For example, substituting Grr1 for cdc4 confers binding to phosphorylated cln1 and cln2, rather than to sic1, while the met30 F-box protein is involved in repression of genes that regulate methionine synthesis.[206d,e] In recognition of its combinatorial nature, this E3 has been named the SCF complex (Skp-Cullin-F-box). The vast number of SCF complexes that may form through interactions between these protein families may regulate the ubiquitination of a large number of cellular proteins. Numerous human homologs of SCF proteins have been identified, and complexes constraining cyclin A, cul1, and p45skp2 have been observed, which suggests that SCF-like complexes can form.[206c] Thus, this pathway for cell-cycle regulated proteolysis during G1 appears to have been evolutionarily conserved, although E3-like activities of these proteins in mammalian cells has not yet been described.

MOLECULAR BASES OF CELL-CYCLE PHYSIOLOGY

Mitogenic and antimitogenic signals control cell proliferation by starting and stopping the cell cycle, but cells respond differently to these signals at different times in the cell cycle.[209] Immediately after mitosis, cells enter a portion of G1 where the continued presence of mitogenic signals (or the absence of antimitogenic signals) is required for continued progression through the remainder of G1 and into S phase. However, at a fixed point in G1, the cell cycle becomes refractory to these signals, and cell division will be completed even if mitogens are absent or antimitogens are present.[210] The restriction point is defined as the end of the mitogen-responsive portion of G1 (or the moment of transition to mitogen independence), and it reflects the execution of the fundamental proliferative decision made by the cell.[211,212] It has been shown that tumor cells characteristically lose restriction point control over cell-cycle progression (they become constitutively mitogen-independent), highlighting the importance of this pathway in the normal regulation of cell proliferation.[213] The restriction point is physiologically analogous to START in the yeast cell cycle, and shares many of its molecular components. Thus, the requirement for cdc28 at START is paralleled by a requirement for cdks in restriction point control.[214]

Mitogenic and antimitogenic signals control the cell cycle in G1 because they control the activity of the cyclins and cdks that are required for progression through G1. Growth factors and cell-substratum interactions are among the best-studied mitogenic signals, and DNA damage and TGF-β are among the best-studied antimitogenic signals. All of these proliferative signals alter the activity of essential G1 cyclin-cdk complexes and bring about either continued cell-cycle progression or cell-cycle arrest.

Mitogenic growth factors have pleiotropic effects on cell cycle proteins that stimulate progression through G1 and entry into S phase.[213,215,216] They increase expression of G1 cyclins, decrease expression of cdk inhibitors, and promote assembly of G1 cyclin-cdk complexes. Growth factors increase expression of all three cyclins needed for entry into S phase—cyclin D (1, 2, and 3), cyclin E and cyclin A—at least in part by increasing transcription of their respective genes. Cyclin D1 transcription has been shown

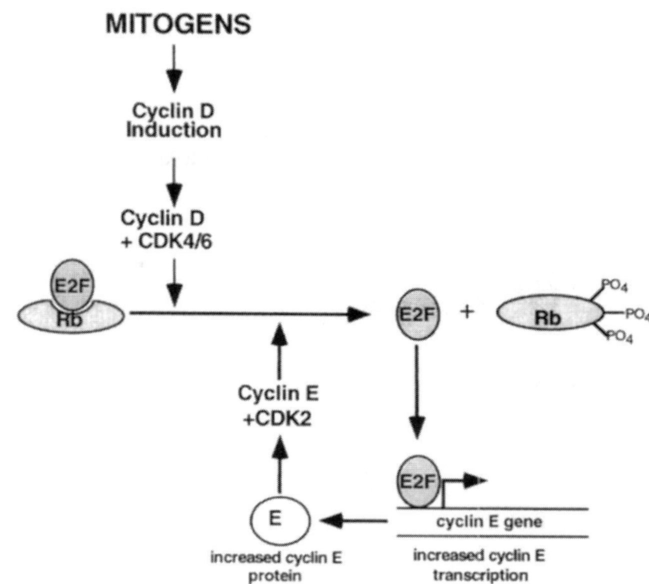

Fig. 23-11 A positive feedback loop reinforces cyclin E transcription. As described in the text, phosphorylation of Rb by cyclin D and cyclin E-associated kinases liberates E2F, which then stimulates cyclin E transcription. Increased cyclin E-cdk2 kinase activity then results in more Rb-phosphorylation, and greater E2F activity. Establishment of this feedback loop renders Rb-phosphorylation mitogen-independent, and may be an important component of the R-point.

to be under the control of at least two growth-factor-modulated signal transduction pathways—the c-myc and ras pathways.[217–219] The biochemical pathways linking c-myc and cyclin D1 transcription are not well defined, but the effects of ras on cyclin D1 transcription appear to be mediated by the MAP kinase pathway.[219] Cyclin D1 transcription begins early in G1, and is followed by an increase in cyclin E gene expression. Cyclin E is one of a large group of genes, which includes DNA polymerase alpha, thymidine kinase, PCNA, dihydrofolate reductase, and many others, that is required for cell proliferation and whose transcription is under control of E2F.[152–159] The induction of cyclin E gene transcription by E2F establishes a positive feedback loop for increasing cyclin E expression (Fig. 23-11).[220] In this pathway, cyclin E-cdk2 phosphorylates Rb, releasing E2F from its Rb-bound inactive state. The free E2F promotes cyclin E gene expression, resulting in increased amounts of cyclin E-cdk2 activity, increasing Rb phosphorylation, and so on. This suggests an interesting and important physiological linkage between cyclin D and cyclin E during the mitogenic response to growth factors. Cyclin D expression is directly elevated by mitogenic growth factors, and this initiates the pathway of Rb phosphorylation and E2F-dependent gene expression. Once initiated, however, Rb phosphorylation can be maintained independently of cyclin D (and, hence, independently of mitogenic growth factors) via the autonomous feedback loop linking Rb to cyclin E. Thus, growth factors are required, through cyclin D, to start the program of E2F-dependent gene expression. These growth factors become dispensable once cyclin E-cdk2 becomes activated and substitutes for cyclin D-cdk4 in phosphorylating Rb. Inherent in this scheme is a transition from a mitogen-dependent to mitogen-independent route for maintaining Rb phosphorylation, and it may be one molecular pathway underlying commitment to cell-cycle progression at the restriction point. Cyclin A transcription also increases in growth factor-stimulated cells just prior to entry into S phase,[51] but the pathways controlling cyclin A transcription are not well understood.

The cdk inhibitor p27Kip1 is another key element in the cell-cycle response to mitogenic growth factors. p27 is required for

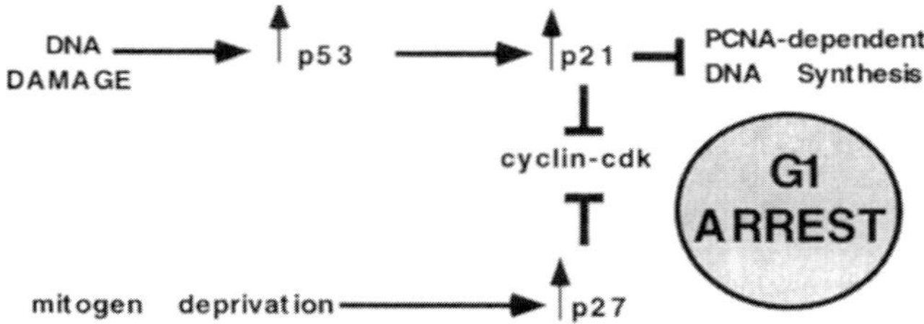

Fig. 23-12 Induction of Cip/Kip proteins by anti-proliferative stimuli imposes a G1 arrest. The p21 and p27 proteins respond to different physiological signals. In the example depicted, DNA damage results in p53 induction and increased p21 transcription, which lead to elevated levels p21 protein and a G1 arrest via cdk inhibition. In addition, p21 inhibits DNA synthesis through the processivity factor PCNA. Similarly, mitogen-deprivation induces p27 expression and cell cycle arrest via cdk inhibition.

cells to stop dividing on schedule when growth factors are withdrawn.[221] p27 is expressed at very low levels in proliferating cells, but its expression greatly increases in cells starved for essential mitogenic growth factors.[222–224] Under these conditions, p27 binds to and inactivates cyclin-cdk complexes and causes the cell cycle to stop (Fig. 23-12). If cells do not make p27, their exit from the cell cycle is delayed, and they will continue to proliferate in the absence of growth factors.[222] Indeed, mice engineered to contain a homozygous deletion of the p27 gene grow twice as fast as control mice, and have increased numbers of cell in all lineages.[225] Conversely, high levels of p27 are sufficient to prevent cell proliferation; therefore, mitogenic stimulation of non-dividing cells requires the elimination of p27.[232] Both control of p27 mRNA translation rate[136] and control of p27 proteolysis by the ubiquitin-proteosome pathway[206] have been implicated in modulating p27 protein levels in response to mitogenic growth factors.

A third mechanism by which growth factors promote cell cycle progression is through assembly of cyclin-cdk complexes. Cyclin D-cdk4 complexes cannot assemble from their individual subunits in growth factor-starved nondividing cells.[226] An assembly factor is induced by growth factors, although its molecular identity is not yet established.

The proliferative response of a cell to environmental signals depends equally on its interactions with soluble extracellular growth factors and on more local interactions with neighboring cells and with the extracellular matrix. Appropriate interactions between specific cell surface receptors (most often the integrin family of proteins) and the extracellular matrix are absolutely required for cell proliferation, a phenomenon known as anchorage-dependence. In fact, loss of anchorage-dependence is the single property of transformed cells that most closely correlates with their ability to form tumors in animals. The effect of cell anchorage on cell-cycle progression, like the effect of growth factors, occurs during G1. Cell anchorage is required for transcription and translation of cyclin D1, for activation of the cyclin E-cdk2 kinase, and for transcription of cyclin A.[227,228] Anchorage regulates cyclin E-cdk2 activity by controlling the levels of the p21 and p27 cdk inhibitors. Therefore, cell anchorage controls the expression and/or activity of all three cyclin/cdk complexes required for the G1/S transition. Cell anchorage and growth factors jointly regulate the cell cycle by modulating the activity of the cyclins and cdks required for G1 and entry into S phase.

The antiproliferative action of agents like TGF-β,[229–234] cyclic-AMP,[235] and DNA damage[125–128,236–238] can also be understood in terms of their effects on cell-cycle proteins. The TGF-β family of cytokines regulates diverse cellular responses, including cell proliferation, cell differentiation, and cell death.[239] The antimitogenic action of TGF-β is a paradigm for the inhibition of cell proliferation by extracellular agents. The active form of TGF-β is a disulfide-linked protein dimer, which, like other members of this cytokine family, signals by bridging together type I and type II receptor serine/threonine kinases on the cell surface. The signal from the heterodimeric type I and type II receptor complex is transduced to the nucleus by a member of the Smad family of nuclear phosphoproteins. The Smad proteins are thought to be transcription factors that promote expression of genes required for the biologic effects of TGF-β or related cytokines. Mutations in DPC4, a member of the Smad protein family located on chromosome 18q21, have been detected in half of all pancreatic cancers,[240] and this may reflect a role for this protein in transmitting an antimitogenic TGF-β-like signal in pancreatic cells. Ultimately, the TGF-β signal has a plethora of effects on cell-cycle proteins, which together impose a tight blockade on progression through G1. TGF-β blocks the activation of cyclin D-cdk4 complexes by inducing expression of the cdk inhibitor p15[232,241] and by inhibiting translation of cdk4 mRNA.[242] TGF-β also blocks activation of cyclin E-cdk2 in some cases by directly inducing p21 and p27, and in other cases by indirectly by promoting the redistribution of p27 from cyclin D-cdk4 complexes to cyclin E-cdk2.[232,233] The biochemical pathways that link activation of the Smad proteins to these diverse effects on cell-cycle proteins have not been determined.

Normal cells will not replicate a damaged chromosome. Instead, cells pause in G1 to repair the DNA lesion, thereby avoiding duplication of a damaged DNA template and preventing the propagation of genetic misinformation to daughter cells. The p53 tumor-suppressor protein controls this DNA damage response.[243,244] The p53 protein is stabilized in cells containing damaged chromosomal DNA; however, it is not understood how DNA damage is detected by the cell nor how this results in decreased turnover of the p53 protein.[245] p53 is a transcriptional transactivator and up-regulation of p53 leads to increased expression of p53-responsive genes.[246–248] Among these genes is one encoding the cdk inhibitor p21Cip1,[127] and p21 protein levels rise in cells with damaged DNA (Fig. 23-12).[238] Consequently, as p53 levels rise, G1 cyclin-cdk complexes contain elevated amounts of p21 and are inactivated. Additionally, p21 binds to and inactivates the DNA polymerase cofactor PCNA, which contributes to the G1/S phase arrest.[129,130] However, p21 does not inhibit the repair functions of PCNA, which allows DNA repair to continue at the same time DNA replication is blocked.[249] Mice containing an engineered homozygous deletion of the p21 gene are viable, but cells taken from these mice have a defective cell-cycle response to DNA damage.[236,237]

CELL-CYCLE CHECKPOINTS

Cells are usually produced only when a new one is needed.[250] Normal cells are periodically recruited into (or released from) the proliferating state by extracellular signals, and this is mediated by activation (or inactivation) of cell-cycle proteins. Tumor cells, in contrast, proliferate when normal cells would not. Current data show that many, and possibly all, cancer cells contain mutations in cell-cycle regulatory proteins, perhaps partly explaining their unregulated proliferation.[251–256] In particular, one or another element in the Rb regulatory pathway, including p16, cyclin D, cdk4, E2F, or Rb itself, may be mutated in almost 100 percent of human tumors (Fig. 23-13).[251–261] Altered expression of other cell-cycle regulatory proteins is also commonly observed (i.e., cyclin E and p27), but often this occurs by mechanisms other than gene mutation.[262–265]

Although mutations in cell-cycle proteins may directly stimulate proliferation, other considerations suggest that these changes are not sufficient to explain the origin of tumorigenic cells. Epidemiologic, molecular, and genetic evidence all suggest that multiple mutations are required to transform a normal cell into a tumor cell.[266–268] But simple calculations show that at normal mutation rates it is very unlikely for a cell with more than two or three mutations to arise within the lifetime of a typical person. This has suggested that increased genetic mutation rates must be a prerequisite for the evolution of malignant cells, and has given rise

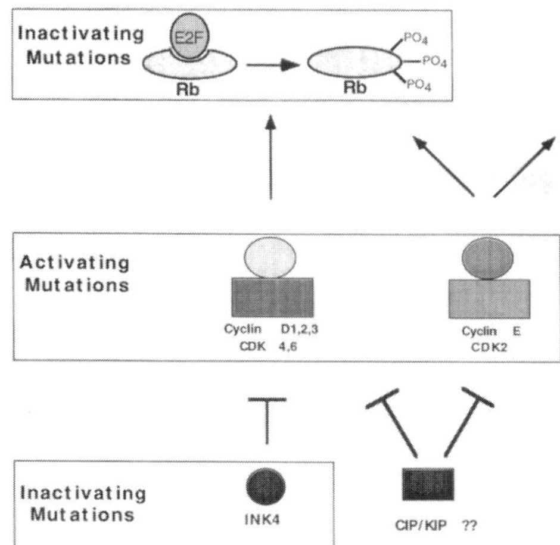

Fig. 23-13 The cyclin D-Rb pathway is frequently mutated in human tumors. Mutations that have been detected in human cancers include both inactivating (recessive) mutations in Rb and the INK4 proteins, and activating (dominant) mutations in the cyclin genes. All result in the deregulation of this pathway.

to the idea that the defining characteristic of a tumor cell may be genetic instability.[269–272] The frequent occurrence in tumor cells of aneuploidy, DNA translocations, DNA deletions, DNA amplifications, and other genetic abnormalities may be a direct manifestation of their genetic instability.

The critical question, therefore, is what controls the genetic stability of a cell? Of course, the accuracy of the enzymes that replicate and segregate chromosomes is largely responsible for the faithful propagation of genetic information. But despite their great fidelity, these enzymes have an intrinsic, spontaneous error rate. Additionally, exogenous agents, such as chemical mutagens, can further elevate the frequency of errors. Therefore, to reduce the accumulation of genetic mistakes normal cells also continually monitor the success of DNA replication and mitosis, and bring the cell cycle to a halt if these do not occur correctly. Once active proliferation is suspended, the cell shifts from duplicating genetic information to repairing it, and only resumes proliferation once the mistakes have been corrected. Checkpoints are the pathways that make progression through the cell cycle dependent on the accurate execution of specific cell-cycle events.[30,269] More specifically, they are the biochemical links between the cyclin-cdk cycle and the macromolecular events of the cell division cycle, such as DNA replication and mitosis.

Checkpoints were first identified experimentally by Weinert and Hartwell in a landmark paper describing the cell-cycle response to DNA damage.[273] DNA damage causes the yeast cell cycle to pause in G2, allowing time for repair enzymes to correct the lesions, thereby preventing the cell from attempting to segregate broken chromosomes during mitosis. It was shown that the RAD9 gene controls this pause in G2, but not because the RAD9 gene was directly involved in the repair process itself. Instead, it was shown that RAD9 is part of a surveillance mechanism, and that activation of the RAD9 pathway by DNA damage prevents cyclin-cdk activity from driving a cell into mitosis.

The molecular mechanism of the DNA damage checkpoint in G2 is beginning to be understood, and it is thought to involve tyrosine phosphorylation and catalytic inactivation of cdc2.[274–278] In cells containing damaged DNA, cdc2 remains inactive because an inhibitory phosphate on tyrosine 15 is not removed.[279–282] The enzyme that ordinarily dephosphorylates tyrosine 15 is the cdc25C phosphatase, but in cells arrested in G2 by the DNA damage checkpoint, this does not happen. The pivotal event in this checkpoint pathway appears to be phosphorylation of cdc25C on serine 216. When cdc25C is phosphorylated on serine 216, it binds to proteins in the 14-3-3 family, and becomes sequestered in a functionally inactive state. Chk1 is the protein kinase responsible for phosphorylating cdc25C on serine 216, and Chk1 is required for the DNA damage checkpoint.[283–286] It is still not understood how Chk1 is activated by DNA damage, but it is possible that this involves a signal transmitted from damaged DNA to Chk1 by the ATM tumor suppressor protein.[279,287]

Subsequent to the discovery of RAD9 a large number of other genes were identified in yeast that together define an intricate network of pathways that make cell-cycle progression dependent on the faithful duplication of chromosomes during S phase.[288,289] A different, but equally robust, set of pathways checks for the proper attachment of chromosomes to the mitotic spindle, and delays mitosis if this has not occurred correctly.[290,291] This checkpoint is triggered by the absence of spindle-induced tension on kinetochores.[292] Once this checkpoint is triggered, it initiates a MAP kinase-dependent pathway[293] that delays the programmed destruction of mitotic cyclins and prevents the initiation of anaphase. It is likely that this pathway modulates activation of the APC, the mitotic proteolytic machinery. Mutations in these checkpoint genes (the MAD and BUB genes) elevate rates of chromosome nondisjunction. Other less well-defined checkpoint pathways are thought to monitor cell growth, cytokinesis, and centrosome duplication, and to prevent cell-cycle progression should those events be executed incorrectly.

Normal cells use cell-cycle checkpoints as fail-safe mechanisms to avoid the accumulation of genomic errors during cell division. Inactivation of checkpoint pathways is thought to underlie the genetic instability seen in tumor cells. Thus, many tumor suppressor genes might be part of checkpoint pathways, and inactivation of these genes could contribute to the clonal evolution of cancer cells by allowing the accumulation of genomic errors that would normally have resulted in either cycle arrest (and repair) or cell death. Perhaps the best example is the p53 gene, the most commonly mutated gene in human tumors.[245,246,252,255,294] p53 governs the G1 checkpoint in human cells that prevents cells from entering S phase and replicating a damaged chromosome. Also, the gene mutated in the cancer-prone syndrome ataxia-telangiectasia is thought to be required for coordinating cell-cycle progression with the repair of DNA damage during S and G2.[295,296] Human homologs of various yeast checkpoint genes are now being characterized, and their relevance to genetic instability in tumor cells will soon be determined.

In conclusion, the process of tumorigenesis may begin with changes in cell-cycle regulation. Mutations in cell-cycle proteins contribute to tumorigenesis in two ways. The first is to promote cell proliferation directly by allowing the cell to override or bypass controls that ordinarily restrict proliferation. The second is to cause the cell to ignore internal "alarms" that signal the presence of errors in the duplication and segregation of genetic information. This results in genetic instability and sets the stage for evolution of malignant cells. For these reasons, cancer can be thought of as a disease of the cell cycle.

REFERENCES

1. Prescott DM: *Reproduction of Eukaryotic Cells*. New York: Academic Press, 1976.
2. Murray A, Hunt T: *The Cell Cycle: An Introduction*, 1st ed. New York: WH Freeman, 1993.
3. Mitchison JM: *The Biology of the Cell Cycle*. London: Cambridge University Press, 1971.
4. Edgar B: Diversification of cell cycle controls in developing embryos. *Curr Opin Cell Biol* **7**:815, 1995.
5. Alberts B, Bray D, Lewis J, Raff M, Roberts K, Watson J: *Molecular Biology of the Cell*. New York: Garland, 1989.
6. Hartwell L: Twenty-five years of cell cycle genetics. *Genetics* **129**:975, 1991.
7. Nurse P: Universal control mechanism regulating onset of M-phase. *Nature* **344**:503, 1990.

8. Hartwell L, Culotti J, Pringle J, Reid B: Genetic control of the cell division cycle in yeast. *Science* **183**:46, 1974.
9. Hartwell L, Mortimer K, Culotti J, Culotti M: Genetic control of the cell division cycle in yeast: V. Genetic analysis of cdc mutants. *Genetics* **74**:267, 1973.
10. Pringle JR, Hartwell LH: The Saccharomyces cerevisiae cell cycle, in Strathern JN, Jones EW, Broach JR (eds): *The Molecular Biology of the Yeast Saccharomyces*. New York: Cold Spring Harbor Laboratory Press, 1981, p. 97.
11. Cross F: Starting the cell cycle: What's the point? *Curr Opin Cell Biol* **7**:790, 1995.
12. Reid B, Hartwell L: Regulation of mating in the cell cycle of Saccharomyces cerevisiae. *J Cell Biol* **75**:355, 1977.
13. Hartwell LH, Unger MW: Unequal division in Saccharomyces cerevisiae and its implications for the control of cell division. *J Cell Biol* **75**:422, 1977.
14. Johnston G, Pringle J, Hartwell L: Coordination of growth with cell division in the yeast S. cerevisiae. *Exp Cell Res* **105**:79, 1977.
15. Nasymth K: Control of the yeast cell cycle by the Cdc28 protein kinase. *Curr Opin Cell Biol* **5**:166, 1993.
16. Lorincz AT, Reed SI: Primary structure homology between the product of the yeast cell cycle control gene CDC28 and vertebrate oncogenes. *Nature* **307**:183, 1984.
17. Nurse P: Genetic control of cell size at cell division in yeast. *Nature* **256**:457, 1975.
18. Hindley J, Phear GA: Sequence of the cell division gene cdc2 from Schizosaccharomyces pombe: Pattern of splicing and homology to protein kinases. *Gene* **31**:129, 1984.
19. Nurse P, Bisset Y: Gene required in G1 for commitment to cell cycle and in G2 for control of mitosis in fission yeast. *Nature* **292**:558, 1981.
20. Beach D, Durkacz B, Nurse P: Functionally homologous cell cycle control genes in fission yeast and budding yeast. *Nature* **300**:706, 1982.
21. Reed SI, Wittenberg C: Mitotic role for the CDC28 protein kinase of S. cerevisae. *Proc Natl Acad Sci U S A* **87**:5697, 1990.
22. Piggot JR, Rai R, Carter BLA: A bifunctional gene product involved in two phases of the yeast cell cycle. *Nature* **298**:391, 1982.
23. Masui H, Markert CL: Cytoplasmic control of nuclear behaviour during meiotic maturation of frog oocytes. *J Exp Zool* **117**:129, 1971.
24. Wasserman WJ, Smith LD: The cyclic behaviour of a cytoplasmic factor controlling nuclear membrane breakdown. *J Cell Biol* **78**:R15, 1978.
25. Reynhout JK, Smith LD: Studies on the appearance and nature of a maturation-inducing factor in the cytoplasm of amphibian oocytes exposed to progesterone. *Dev Biol* **38**:394, 1974.
26. Newport J, Kirschner M: Regulation of the cell cycle during early Xenopus development. *Cell* **37**:731, 1984.
27. Nelkin B, Nichols C, Vogelstein B: Protein factor(s) from mitotic CHO cells induce meiotic maturation in Xenopus Laevis oocytes. *FEBS Lett* **109**:233, 1980.
28. Hara K, Tydeman P, Kirschner M: A cytoplasmic clock with the same period as the division cycle in Xenopus eggs. *Proc Natl Acad Sci U S A* **77**:462, 1980.
29. Murray A, Kirschner MW: Dominoes and clocks: The union of two views of the cell cycle. *Science* **246**:614, 1989.
30. Hartwell L, Weinert T: Checkpoints: Controls that ensure the order of cell cycle events. *Science* **246**:629, 1989.
31. Cross F, Roberts J, Weintraub H: Simple and complex cell cycles. *Ann Rev Cell Biol* **5**:341, 1989.
32. Nurse P: Universal control mechanism regulating onset of M-phase. *Nature* **344**:503, 1990.
33. Lee MG, Nurse P: Complementation used to clone a human homologue of the fission yeast cell cycle control gene cdc2. *Nature* **327**:31, 1987.
34. Gautier J, Norbury C, Lohka M, Nurse P, Maller JL: Purified maturation-promoting factor contains the product of a Xenopus homolog of the fission yeast cell cycle control gene cdc2+. *Cell* **54**:433, 1988.
35. Hunt T: Maturation promoting factor, cyclin and the control of M-phase. *Curr Opin Cell Biol* **1**:268, 1989.
36. Labbe JC, Picard A, Peaucellier G, Cavadore JC, Nurse P, Doree M: Purification of MPF from starfish: Identification as the H1 histone kinase p34 cdc2 and a possible mechanism for its periodic activation. *Cell* **57**:253, 1989.
37. Labbe JC, Lee MG, Nurse P, Picard A, Doree M: Activation at M-phase of a protein kinase encoded by a starfish homologue of the cell cycle gene Cdc2. *Nature* **335**:251, 1988.
38. Dunphy WG, Brizuela L, Beach D, Newport J: The Xenopus cdc2 protein is a component of MPF, a cytoplasmic regulator of mitosis. *Cell* **54**:423, 1988.
39. Murray A: The cell cycle as a cdc2 cycle. *Nature* **342**:14, 1989.
40. Riabowol K, Draetta G, Brizuela L, Vandre D, Beach D: The cdc2 kinase is a nuclear protein that is essential for mitosis in mammalian cells. *Cell* **57**:393, 1989.
41. D'Urso G, Marraccino RL, Marshak DR, Roberts JM: Cell cycle control of DNA replication by a homologue from human cells of the p34-cdc2 protein kinase. *Science* **250**:786, 1990.
42. Th'ng JPH, Wright PS, Hamaguchi J, Lee MG, Norbury CJ, Nurse P, Bradbury EM: The FT210 cell line is a mouse G2 phase mutant with a temperature-sensitive CDC2 gene product. *Cell* **63**:313, 1990.
43. Tsai LE, Lees E, Faha B, Harlow E, Riabowol K: The cdk2 kinase is required for the G1 to S transition in mammalian cells. *Oncogene* **8**:1593, 1993.
44. Fang F, Newport J: Evidence that the G1-S and G2-M transitions are controlled by different cdc2 proteins in higher eukaryotes. *Cell* **66**:731, 1991.
45. Furakawa Y, Piwnica-Worms H, Ernst TJ, Kanakura Y, Griffin JD: Cdc2 gene expression at the to S transition in human T lymphocytes. *Science* **250**:805, 1990.
46. Lamb N, Fernandez A, Watrin A, Labbe J, Cavadore J: Microinjection of the p34cdc2 kinase induces marked changes in cell shape, cytoskeletal organization and chromatin structure in mammalian fibroblasts. *Cell* **60**:151, 1990.
47. Nasymth K: Control of the yeast cell cycle by the Cdc28 protein kinase. *Curr Opin Cell Biol* **5**:166, 1993.
48. Myerson M, Enders GH, Wu C, Su L, Gorka C, Nelson C, Harlow E, Tsai L: The human cdc2 kinase family. *EMBO J* **11**:2909, 1992.
49. Morgan D: Principles of cdk regulation. *Nature* **374**:131, 1995.
50. Lees E: Cyclin-dependent kinase regulation. *Curr Opin Cell Biol* **7**:773, 1995.
51. Sherr C: Mammalian G1 cyclins. *Cell* **73**:1059, 1993.
52. Sherr C: G1 phase progression: Cycling on cue. *Cell* **79**:551, 1994.
53. van den Heuval S, Harlow E: Distinct roles for cyclin-dependent kinases in cell cycle control. *Science* **262**:2050, 1994.
54. Tsai L, Delalle I, Caviness V, Chae T, Harlow E: p35, a neuro-specific regulatory subunit of the cdk5 kinase. *Nature* **371**:419, 1994.
55. Nikoklic M, Dudek H, Kwon Y, Ramos Y, Tsai LH: The cdk5/p35 kinase is essential for neurite outgrowth during neuronal differentiation. *Genes Dev* **8**:816, 1996.
56. De Bondt HL, Rosenblatt J, Jarncarik J, Jones H, Morgan D, Kim S: Crystal structure of the cyclin-dependent kinase 2. *Nature* **363**:595, 1993.
57. Jeffrey PD, Russo AA, Polyak K, Gibbs E, Hurwitz J, Massague J, Paveltich NP: Crystal Structure of a cyclin A-cdk2 complex at 2.3A: Mechanism of cdk activation by cyclins. *Nature* **376**:313, 1995.
58. Cross F: DAF1, a mutant gene affecting size control, pheromone arrest, and cell cycle kinetics of Saccharomyces cerevisiae. *Mol Cell Biol* **8**:4675, 1988.
59. Cross F: Cell cycle arrest caused by CLN gene deficiency in Saccharomyces cerevisiae resembles START-1 arrest and is independent of the mating-pheromone signaling pathway. *Mol Cell Biol* **10**:6482, 1990.
60. Richardson H, Wittenberg C, Cross F, Reed S: An essential G1 function for cyclin-like proteins in yeast. *Cell* **59**:1127, 1989.
61. Hadwiger J, Wittenberg C, Richardson H, Lopes M, Reed S: A family of cyclin homologs that control the G1 phase in yeast. *Proc Natl Acad Sci U S A* **86**:6255, 1989.
62. Wittenberg C, Sugimoto K, Reed SI: G1-specific cyclins of S. cerevisiae: Cell cycle periodicity, regulation by mating pheromone, and association with the p34-CDC28 protein kinase. *Cell* **62**:225, 1990.
63. Koch C, Nasmyth K: Cell cycle regulated transcription in yeast. *Curr Opin Cell Biol* **6**:451, 1994.
64. Koch C, Moll T, Neuberg M, Ahorn H, Nasmyth K: A role for the transcription factors Mbp1 and Swi4 in progression from G1 to S phase. *Science* **261**:1551, 1993.
65. Dirick L, Moll T, Auer H, Nasmyth K: A central role for SWI6 in modulating cell cycle START-specific transcription in yeast. *Nature* **357**:508, 1992.
66. Dirick L, Nasmyth K: Positive feedback in the activation of G1 cyclins in yeast. *Nature* **351**:754, 1991.
67. Cross FR, Tinkelenberg H: A potential positive feedback loop controlling CLN1 and CLN2 gene expression at the start of the yeast cell cycle. *Cell* **65**:875, 1992.

68. Dirick L, Bohm T, Nasmyth K: Roles and regulation of cln-cdc28 kinases at the start of the cell cycle of Saccharomyces cerevisiae. *EMBO J* **14**:4803, 1995.
69. Schwob E, Nasmyth K: CLB5 and CLB6, a new pair of B cyclins involved in S phase and mitotic spindle formation in S. cerevisiae. *Genes Dev* **7**:1160, 1993.
70. Epstein C, Cross F: CLB5: A novel B cyclin from budding yeast with a role in S phase. *Genes Dev* **6**:1695, 1992.
71. Fitch I, Dahmann C, Surana U, Amon A, Nasmyth K, Goetch L, Byers B, Futcher B: Characterization of four B-type cyclin genes of the budding yeast Saccharomyces cerevisiae. *Mol Biol Cell* **3**:805, 1992.
72. Amon A, Tyers M, Futcher B, Nasmyth K: Mechanisms that help the yeast cell cycle clock tick: G2 cyclins transcriptionally activate their own synthesis and repress G1 cyclins. *Cell* **74**:993, 1993.
73. Lew DJ, Dulic V, Reed SI: Isolation of three novel human cyclins by rescue of G1 cyclin (cln) function in yeast. *Cell* **66**:1197, 1991.
74. Koff A, Cross F, Fisher A, Schumacher J, Leguelle K, Philippe M, Roberts JM: Human cyclin E, a new cyclin that interacts with two members of the CDC2 gene family. *Cell* **66**:1217, 1991.
75. Xiong Y, Connolly T, Futcher B, Beach D: Human D-type cyclin. *Cell* **65**:691, 1991.
76. Matsushime H, Roussel M, Ashmun R, Sherr CJ: Colony-stimulating Factor 1 regulates novel cyclins during the G1 phase of the cell cycle. *Cell* **65**:701, 1991.
77. Motokura T, Bloom T, Kim HG, Juppner H, Ruderman JV, Kronenberg HM, Arnold A: A BCL1-linked candidate oncogene which is rearranged in parathyroid tumors encodes a novel cyclin. *Nature* **350**:512, 1991.
78. Sherr C, Kato J, Quell D, Matsuoka M, Roussel M: D-type cyclins and their cyclin-dependent kinases: G1 phase integrators of the mitogenic response. *Cold Spring Harbor Symp Quant Biol* **49**:11, 1994.
79. Baldin V, Lukas J, Marcotte MJ, Pagano M, Draetta G: Cyclin D1 is a nuclear protein required for cell cycle progression in G1. *Genes Dev* **7**:812, 1993.
80. Quelle DE, Ashmun RA, Shurtleff SA, Kato J, Bar-Sagi D, Roussel MF, Sherr CJ: Overexpression of mouse D-type cyclins accelerates G1 phase in rodent fibroblasts. *Genes Dev* **7**:1559, 1993.
81. Resnitzky D, Gossen M, Bujard H, Reed SI: Acceleration of the G1/S phase transition by expression of cyclin D1 and E with an inducible system. *Mol Cell Biol* **14**:1669, 1994.
82. Ohtsubo M, Theodoras AM, Schumacher J, Roberts JM, Pagano M: Human cyclin E: A nuclear protein essential for the G1 to S phase transition. *Mol Cell Biol* **15**:2612, 1995.
83. Knoblich J, Sauer K, Jones L, Richardson H, Saint R, Lehner C: Cyclin E controls S phase progression and its down-regulation during Drosophila embryogenesis is required for the arrest of cell proliferation. *Cell* **77**:107, 1994.
84. Koff A, Giordano A, Desai D, Yamashita K, Harper JW, Elledge S, Nishimoto T, Morgan DO, Franza R, Roberts JM: Formation and activation of a cyclin E/CDK2 complex during the G1 phase of the human cell cycle. *Science* **257**:1689, 1992.
85. Dulic V, Lees E, Reed SI: Association of human cyclin E with a periodic G1-S phase protein kinase. *Science* **257**:1958, 1992.
86. Ohtsubo M, Roberts JM: Cyclin-dependent regulation of G1 in mammalian fibroblasts. *Science* **259**:1908, 1993.
87. Pagano M, Pepperkok P, Verde F, Ansorge W, Draetta G: Cyclin A is required at two points in the human cell cycle. *EMBO J* **11**:961, 1992.
88. Giordano A, Whyte P, Harlow E, Franza BR Jr, Beach D, Draetta G: A 60-kd cdc2-associated polypeptide complexes with the E1A proteins in adenovirus-infected cells. *Cell* **58**:981, 1989.
89. Girard F, Strausfeld U, Fernandez A, Lamb N: Cyclin A is required for the onset of DNA replication in mammalian fibroblasts. *Cell* **67**:1169, 1991.
90. Pines J, Hunter T: Isolation of a human cyclin cDNA: Evidence for cyclin mRNA and protein regulation in the cell cycle and for interaction with p34-cdc2. *Cell* **58**:833, 1989.
91. Nigg E: Cyclin-dependent kinase 7: At the crossroads of transcription, DNA repair and cell cycle control. *Curr Opin Cell Biol* **8**:312, 1996.
92. Tassan JP, Jaquenoud M, Leopold P, Schultz SJ, Nigg EA: Identification of human cyclin-dependent kinase 8, a putative protein kinase partner for cyclin C. *Proc Natl Acad Sci U S A* **92**:8871, 1995.
93. Bai C, Richman R, Elledge SJ: Human cyclin F. *EMBO J* **13**:6087, 1994.
94. Okamoto K, Beach D: Cyclin G is a transcriptional target of the p53 tumor suppressor. *EMBO J* **13**:4816, 1994.
95. Nakamura T, Sanolawa R, Saski Y, Ayusawa D, Oishi M, Mori N: Cyclin I: A new cyclin encoded by a gene isolated from human brain. *Exp Cell Res* **221**:534, 1995.
96. Russo crystal structure.
97. Solomon MJ: The function(s) of CAK, the p34cdc2 activating kinase. *Trends Biochem Sci* **19**:496, 1994.
98. Soloman M, Glotzer M, Lee T, Phillippe M, Kirschner M: Cyclin activation of p34-cdc2. *Cell* **63**:1013, 1990.
99. Solomon MJ, Lee T, Kirschner M: Role of phosphorylation in p34 CDC2 activation: Identification of an activating kinase. *Mol Biol Cell* 3:13, 1991.
100. Solomon MJ, Harper JW, Shuttleworth J: CAK, the p34 CDC2 activating kinase, contains a protein identical or closely related to p40 MO15. *EMBO J* **12**:3133, 1993.
101. Gould KL, Nurse P: Tyrosine phosphorylation of the fission yeast Cdc2+ protein kinase regulates entry into mitosis. *Nature* **342**:39, 1989.
102. Moreneo S, Hayles J, Nurse P: Regulation of p34-cdc2 protein kinase during mitosis. *Cell* **58**:361, 1989.
103. Simanis V, Nurse P: The cell cycle control gene cdc2+ of fission yeast encodes a protein kinase potentially regulated by phosphorylation. *Cell* **45**:261, 1986.
104. Heald R, McLoughlin M, McKeon F: Human wee1 maintains mitotic timing by protecting the nucleus from cytoplasmically activated Cdc2 kinase. *Cell* **74**:463, 1993.
105. Igarashi M, Nagata A, Jinno S, Suto K, Okayama H: Wee1+-like gene in human cells. *Nature* **353**:80, 1991.
106. Lundgren D, Walworth N, Booher R, Dembski M, Kirschner M, Beach D: mik1 and wee1 cooperate in the inhibitory tyrosine phosphorylation of cdc2. *Cell* **64**:1111, 1991.
107. Russell P, Nurse P: Negative regulation of mitosis by wee1+, a gene encoding a protein kinase homolog. *Cell* **49**:559, 1987.
108. Russell P, Nurse P: cdc25+ functions as an inducer in the mitotic control of fission yeast. *Cell* **45**:145, 1986.
109. Sadhu K, Reed S, Richardson H, Russell P: Human homolog of fission yeast cdc25 mitotic inducer is predominantly expressed in G2. *Proc Natl Acad Sci U S A* **87**:5139, 1990.
110. Kumagai A, Dunphy W: The Cdc25 protein controls tyrosine dephosphorylation of the Cdc2 protein in a cell free system. *Cell* **64**:903, 1991.
111. Sebastian B, Kakizuka A, Hunter T: Cdc25 activation of cyclin-dependent kinase by dephosphorylation of threonine-14 and tyrosine 15. *Proc Natl Acad Sci U S A* **90**:3521, 1993.
112. Strausfield V, Labbe JC, Fesquat O, Cavadore JC, Picard A, Sadhu A, Russell P, Durec M: Dephosphorylation and activation of a p34cdc2/cyclin B complex in vitro by human cdc25 protein. *Nature* **35**:242, 1991.
113. Atherton-Fessler S, Hannig G, Piwnica-Worms H: Reversible tyrosine phosphorylation and cell cycle control. *Semin Cell Biol* **4**:433, 1993.
114. Dunphy W: The decision to enter mitosis. *Trends Cell Biol* **4**:202, 1994.
115. Jinno S, Suto K, Nagata A, Igarashi M, Kanaoka Y, Nojima H, Okayama H: Cdc25A is a novel phosphatase functioning early in the cell cycle. *EMBO J* **13**:1549, 1994.
116. Hoffmann I, Draetta G, Karsenti E: Activation of the phosphatase activity of human cdc25A by a cdk2-cyclin E dependent phosphorylation at the G1/S transition. *EMBO J* **13**:4302, 1994.
117. Galaktionov K, Jessus C, Beach D: Raf1 interaction with Cdc25 phosphatase ties mitogenic signal transduction to cell cycle activation. *Genes Dev* **9**:1046, 1995.
118. Sherr C, Roberts J: Inhibitors of mammalian G1 cyclin-dependent kinases. *Genes Dev* **9**:1149, 1995.
119. Peter M, Herskowitz I: Joining the complex: Cyclin-dependent kinase inhibitory proteins and cell cycle. *Cell* **79**:181, 1994.
120. Mendenhall M: An inhibitor of p34 CDC28 protein kinase activity from Saccharomyces cerevisiae. *Science* **259**:216, 1993.
121. Schwob E, Bohm T, Mendenhall M, Nasmyth K: The B-type cyclins kinase inhibitor p40sic1 controls the G1 to S phase transition in S. cerevisiae. *Cell* **79**:233, 1994.
122. Elledge S, Harper W: Cdk inhibitors: on the threshold of checkpoints and development. *Curr Opin Cell Biol* **6**:847, 1994.
123. Xiong Y, Zhang H, Beach D: Subunit rearrangement of the cyclin-dependent kinases is associated with cellular transformation. *Genes Dev* **7**:1572, 1993.
124. Noda A, Ning Y, Venable S, Pereira-Smith O, Smith J: Cloning of senescent cell-derived inhibitors of DNA synthesis using an expression screen. *Exp Cell Res* **211**:90, 1994.

125. Harper JW, Adami GR, Wei N, Keyomarsi K, Elledge SJ: The p21 cdk-interacting protein cip1 is a potent inhibitor of G1 cyclin-dependent Kinases. *Cell* **75**:805, 1993.
126. Xiong Y, Hannon G, Zhang H, Casso D, Kobayashi R, Beach D: p21 is a universal inhibitor of cyclin kinases. *Nature* **366**:701, 1993.
127. El-Deiry WS, Tokino T, Velculescu VE, Levy DB, Parsons R, Trent JM, Lin D, Mercer WE, Kinzler KW, Vogelstein B: WAF1, a potential mediator of p53 tumor suppression. *Cell* **75**:817, 1993.
128. Gu Y, Turek C, Morgan D: Inhibition of CDK2 activity in vivo by an associated 20K regulatory subunit. *Nature* **366**:707, 1993.
129. Waga S, Hannon G, Beach D, Stillman B: The p21 inhibitor of cyclin-dependent kinases controls DNA replication by interaction with PCNA. *Nature* **369**:574, 1994.
130. Flores-Rozas H, Kelman Z, Dean F, Pan Z, Harper JW, Elledge S, O'Donnell M, Hurwitz J: CDK-interacting protein 1 directly binds with proliferating cell nuclear antigen and inhibits DNA replication catalyzed by the DNA polymerase and holoenzyme. *Proc Natl Acad Sci U S A* **91**:8655, 1994.
131. Luo Y, Hurwitz J, Massague J: Cell-cycle inhibition by independent CDK and CPNA binding domains in p21Cip1. *Nature* **375**:159, 1995.
132. Halevy O, Novitch B, Spicer D, Skapek S, Rhee J, Hannon G, Beach D, Lasser A: Correlation of terminal cell cycle arrest of skeletal muscle with induction of p21 by MyoD. *Science* **267**:1018, 1995.
133. Parker S, Eichele G, Zhang P, Rawls A, Sands A, Bradley A, Olson E, Harper JW, Elledge S: p53-independent expression of p21Cip1 in muscle and other terminally differentiating cells. *Science* **267**:1024, 1995.
134. Polyak K, Lee MH, Erdjument-Bromage H, Koff A, Roberts JM, Tempst P, Massague J: Cloning of p27 kip1 a cyclin-dependent kinase inhibitor and a potential mediator of extracellular antimitogenic signals. *Cell* **78**:59, 1994.
135. Toyoshima H, Hunter T: p27, a novel inhibitor of G1-cyclin-cdk protein kinase activity, is related to p21. *Cell* **78**:67, 1994.
136. Hengst L, Reed SI: Translational control of p27Kip1 accumulation during the cell cycle. *Science* **271**:1861, 1996.
137. Lee M, Reynisdottir I, Massague J: Cloning of p57Kip2, a cyclin-dependent kinase inhibitor with unique domain structure and tissue distribution. *Genes Dev* **9**:639, 1995.
138. Matsuoka S, Edwards M, Bai C, Parker S, Zhang P, Baldini A, Harper JW, Elledge S: p57Kip2, a structurally distinct member of the p21Cip1 cdk inhibitor family, is a candidate tumor suppressor gene. *Genes Dev* **9**:650, 1995.
138a. Serrano M, Hannon GJ, Beach D: A new regulatory motif in cell-cycle control causing specific inhibition of cyclin D-Cdk4. *Nature* **366**:704, 1993.
139. Sheaff R, Roberts J: Lessons in p16 from phylum Falconium. *Curr Biol* **5**:28, 1995.
140. Kamb A: Role of a cell cycle regulator in hereditary and sporadic cancer. *Cold Spring Harbor Symp Quant Biol* **49**:39, 1994.
141. Quelle DE, Ashmun RA, Hannon GJ, Rehberger PA, Trono D, Richter KH, Walker C, Beach D, Sherr CJ, Serrano M: Cloning and characterization of murine p16INK4a and p15INK4b genes. *Oncogene* **11**:635, 1995.
142. Hirai H, Roussel MF, Kato JY, Ashmun RA, Sherr CJ: Novel INK4 proteins, p19 and p18, are specific inhibitors of the cyclin D-dependent kinases CDK4 and CDK6. *Mol Cell Biol* **15**:2672, 1995.
143. Serrano M, Lee H, Chin L, Cordon-Cardo C, Beach D, DePinho RA: Role of the INK4a locus in tumor suppression and cell mortality. *Cell* **85**:27, 1996.
144. Schneider B, Yang Y, Futcher B: Linkage of replication to start by the CDK inhibitor sic1. *Science* **272**:560, 1996.
145. Weinberg RA: The retinoblastoma protein and cell cycle control. *Cell* **81**:323, 1995.
146. Dyson N, Howley PM, Munger K, Harlow E: The human papilloma virus-16 E7 oncoprotein is able to bind to the retinoblastoma gene product. *Science* **243**:934, 1989.
147. Whyte P, Williamson NM, Harlow E: Cellular targets for transformation by the adenovirus E1A proteins. *Cell* **56**:67, 1989.
148. Whyte P, Buchkovich KJ, Horowitz JM, Friend SH, Raybuck M, Weinberg RA, Harlow E: Association between an oncogene and an anti-oncogene: The adenovirus E1A proteins bind to the retinoblastoma gene product. *Nature* **334**:124, 1988.
149. Friend SH, Horowitz JM, Gerber MR, Wang XF, Bogenmann E, Li FP, Weinberg RA: Deletions of a DNA sequence in retinoblastomas and mesenchymal tumors: Organization of the sequence and its encoded protein. *Proc Natl Acad Sci U S A* **84**:9059, 1987.
150. Friend SH, Bernards R, Rogelj S, Weinberg RA, Rapaport JM, Albert DM, Dryja TP: A human DNA segment with properties of the gene that predisposes to retinoblastoma and osteosarcoma. *Nature* **323**:643, 1986.
151. Horowitz JM, Park S, Bogenmann E, Cheng J, Yandell DW, Kaye FJ, Minna JD, Dryja TP, Weinberg RA: Frequent inactivation of the retinoblastoma anti-oncogene is restricted to a subset of human tumor cells. *Proc Natl Acad Sci U S A* **87**:2775, 1990.
152. Buchkovich K, Duffy LA, Harlow E: The retinoblastoma protein is phosphorylated during specific phases of the cell cycle. *Cell* **58**:1097, 1989.
153. Mittnacht S, Lees JA, Desai D, Harlow E, Morgan DO, Weinberg RA: Distinct sub-populations of the retinoblastoma protein show a distinct pattern of phosphorylation. *EMBO J* **13**:118, 1994.
154. Nevins J: E2F: A link between the Rb tumor suppressor protein and viral oncoproteins. *Science* **258**:424, 1992.
155. Sherr CJ: The ins and outs of Rb: Coupling gene expression to the cell cycle clock. *Trends Cell Biol* **4**:15, 1994.
156. Lees JA, Saito M, Vidal M, Valentine M, Look T, Harlow E, Dyson N, Helin K: The retinoblastoma protein binds to a family of E2F transcription factors. *Mol Cell Biol* **13**:7813, 1993.
157. Kaelin WG Jr, Krek W, Sellers WR, DeCaprio JA, Ajchenbaum F, Fuchs CS, Chittenden T, Li Y, Farnham PJ, Blanar MA, Livingston DM, Flemington EK: Expression cloning of a cDNA encoding a retinoblastoma-binding protein with E2F-like properties. *Cell* **70**:351, 1992.
158. Helin K, Lees JA, Vidal M, Dyson N, Harlow E, Fattaey A: A cDNA encoding a pRB-binding protein with properties of the transcription factor E2F. *Cell* **70**:337, 1992.
159. Wu CL, Zukerberg LR, Ngwu C, Harlow E, Lees JA: In vivo association of E2F and DP family proteins. *Mol Cell Biol* **15**:2536, 1995.
160. Lees JA, Buchkovich KJ, Marshak DR, Anderson CW, Harlow E: The retinoblastoma protein is phosphorylated on multiple sites by human cdc2. *EMBO J* **10**:4279, 1991.
161. Dowdy S, Hinds P, Lovic K, Reed S, Arnold A, Weinberg RA: Physical interaction of the retinoblastoma protein with human D cyclins. *Cell* **73**:499, 1993.
162. Ewen M, Sluss K, Sherr CJ, Livingston M, Matsushime H, Kato JY, Livingston DM: Functional interactions of the retinoblastoma protein with mammalian D-type cyclins. *Cell* **73**:487, 1993.
163. Hinds P, Mittnacht S, Dulic V, Arnold A, Reed S, Weinberg R: Regulation of retinoblastoma protein functions by ectopic expression of human cyclins. *Cell* **70**:993, 1992.
164. Kato JY, Matsushime H, Hiebert S, Ewen M, Sherr C: Direct binding of cyclin D to the retinoblastoma gene product and pRb phosphorylation by the cyclin D-dependent kinase, cdk4. *Genes Dev* **7**:331, 1993.
165. Bates S, Parry D, Bonetta L, Vousden K, Dickson C, Peters G: Absence of cyclin D/Cdk complexes in cells lacking functional retinoblastoma protein. *Oncogene* **9**:1633, 1994.
166. Lukas J, Parry D, Aagaard L, Mann DJ, Bartkova J, Strauss M, Peters G, Bartek J: Retinoblastoma-protein-dependent cell-cycle inhibition by the tumour suppressor p16. *Nature* **375**:503, 1995.
167. Lukas J, Bartkova J, Rohde M, Strauss M, Bartek J: Cyclin D1 is dispensable for G1 control in retinoblastoma gene-deficient cells independently of cdk4 activity. *Mol Cell Biol* **15**:2600, 1995.
168. Zhu L, Enders GH, Wu CL, Starz MA, Moberg KH, Lees JA, Dyson N, Harlow E: Growth suppression by members of the retinoblastoma protein family. *Cold Spring Harbor Symp Quantit Biol* **59**:75, 1994.
169. Bandara L, Adamczewski J, Hunt T LaThanghe N: Cyclin A and the retinoblastoma gene product complex with a common transcription factor. *Nature* **352**:249, 1991.
170. Shirodkar S, Ewen M, DeCaprio J, Morgan J, Livingston D, Chittenden T: The transcription factor E2F interacts with the retinoblastoma product and a p107-cyclin A complex in a cell cycle regulated manner. *Cell* **68**:157, 1992.
170a. Dynlacht B, Flores O, Lees J Harlow E: Differential regulation of E2F transactivation by cyclin/cdk2 complexes. *Genes Dev* **8**:1772, 1994.
171. Krek W, Ewen M, Shirodkar S, Arany Z, Kaelin W, Livingston D: Negative regulation of the growth-promoting transcription factor E2F-1 by a stably bound cyclin A-dependent protein kinase. *Cell* **78**:161, 1994.
172. Nigg EA: Targets of cyclin-dependent protein kinases. *Curr Opin Cell Biol* **5**:187, 1993.
173. Heichman K, Roberts JM: Rules to replicate by. *Cell* **79**:1, 1994.
174. Nigg EA: Assembly-disassembly of the nuclear lamina. *Curr Opin Cell Biol* **4**:105, 1992.

175. Heald R, McKeon F: Mutations of phosphorylation sites in lamin A that prevent nuclear lamina disassembly in mitosis. *Cell* **61**:579, 1990.
176. Blangy A, Lane HA, d'Herin P, Harper M, Kress M, Nigg EA: Phosphorylation by p34cdc2 regulates spindle association of human Eg5, a kinesin-related motor essential for bipolar spindle formation in vivo. *Cell* **83**:1159, 1995.
177. Deshaies R: The self-destructive personality of a cell cycle in transition. *Curr Opin Cell Biol* **7**:781, 1995.
178. Maller J: Mitotic control. *Curr Opin Cell Biol* **3**:269, 1991.
179. Evans T, Rosenthal E, Youngblom J, Distel D, Hunt T: Cyclin: A protein specified by maternal mRNA in sea urchin eggs that is destroyed at each cleavage division. *Cell* **33**:389, 1983.
180. Ciechanover A: The ubiquitin-proteosome proteolytic pathway. *Cell* **79**:13, 1994.
181. Hochstrasser M: Ubiquitin, proteosomes, and the regulation of intracellular protein degradation. *Curr Opin Cell Biol* **7**:215, 1995.
182. Jentsch S, Schlenker S: Selective protein degradation: A journey's end within the proteosome. *Cell* **82**:881, 1995.
183. Rogers S, Wells R, Rechsteiner M: Amino acid sequences common to rapidly degraded proteins: The PEST hypothesis. *Science* **234**:364, 1986.
184. Glotzer M, Murray A, Kirschner M: Cyclin is degraded by the ubiquitin pathway. *Nature* **349**:132, 1991.
185. Murray AW, Solomon MJ, Kirschner MW: The role of cyclin synthesis and degradation in the control of maturation promoting factor activity. *Nature* **339**:280, 1989.
186. Ghiara JB, Richardson HE, Sugimoto K, Henze M, Lew DJ, Wittenberg C, Reed SI: A cyclin B homolog in S. cerevisiae: Chronic activation of the CDC28 protein kinase by cyclin prevents exit from mitosis. *Cell* **65**:163, 1991.
187. Surana U, Robitsch H, Price C, Schuster T, Fitch I, Futcher AB, Nasmyth K: The role of CDC28 and cyclins during mitosis in the budding yeast S. cerevisiae. *Cell* **65**:145, 1991.
188. King RW, Jackson P, Kirschner MW: Mitosis in transition. *Cell* **79**:563, 1994.
189. Juca FC, Shibuya EK, Dohrmann EE, Ruderman JV: Both cyclin AΔ60 and BΔ97 are stable and arrest cells im M phase but only cyclin BΔ97 turns on cyclin destruction. *EMBO J* **10**:4311, 1991.
190. Murray AW: Cyclin ubiquitination: The destructive end of mitosis. *Cell* **81**:149, 1995.
191. King R, Peters J, Tugendreich S, Rolfe M, Hieter P, Kirschner M: A 20S complex containing cdc27 and cdc16 catalyzes the mitosis-specific conjugation of ubiquitin to cyclin B. *Cell* **81**:279, 1995.
192. Holloway SL, Glotzer M, King RW, Murray AW: Anaphase is initiated by proteolysis rather than by the inactivation of maturation-promoting factor. *Cell* **73**:1393, 1993.
193. Sudakin V, Ganoth D, Dahan A, Heller H, Hershko J, Luca F, Ruderman J, Hershko A: The cyclosome, a large complex containing cyclin-selective ubiquitin ligase activity, targets cyclins for destruction at the end of mitosis. *Mol Biol Cell* **6**:185, 1995.
194. Irniger S, Piatti S, Michaelis C, Nasmyth K: Genes involved in sister chromatid separation are needed for B-type cyclin proteolysis in budding yeast. *Cell* **81**:269, 1995.
195. Seufert W, Futcher B, Jentsch S: Role of a ubiquitin-conjugating enzyme in degradation of S-phase and M-phase cyclins. *Nature* **373**:78, 1995.
196. Felix M, Labbe J, Doree M, Hunt T, Karsenti E: Triggering of cyclin degradation in interphase extracts of amphibian eggs by cdc2 kinase. *Nature* **346**:379, 1990.
197. Amon A, Irniger S, Nasmyth K: Closing the cell cycle circle in yeast: G2 cyclin proteolysis initiated at mitosis persists until the activation of G1 cyclins in the next cell cycle. *Cell* **77**:1037, 1994.
198. Clurman BE, Sheaff RJ, Thress K, Groudine M, Roberts JM: Turnover of cyclin E by the ubiquitin-proteosome pathway is regulated by CDK2 binding and cyclin phosphorylation. *Genes Dev* **10**:1979, 1996.
199. Won K, Reed S: Activation of cyclin E/CDK2 is coupled to site-specific autophosphorylation and ubiquitin-dependent degradation of cyclin E. *EMBO J* **15**:4182, 1996.
200. Lanker S, Valdivieso M, Wittenberg C: Rapid degradation of the G1 cyclin cln2 induced by CDK-dependent phosphorylation. *Science* **271**:1597, 1996.
201. Tyers M, Tokiwa G, Nash R, Futcher B: The cln2-cdc28 kinase complex of S. cerevisiae is regulated by proteolysis and phosphorylation. *EMBO J* **11**:1773, 1992.
202. Yaglom J, Linskens M, Sadis S, Rubin D, Futcher B, Finley D: p34Cdc28-mediated control of cln3 degradation. *Mol Cell Biol* **15**:731, 1995.
203. Chen Z, Hagler J, Palombella V, Melandri F, Scherer D, Ballard D, Maniatis T: Signal-induced site-specific phosphorylation targets IkBa to the ubiquitin-proteosome pathway. *Genes Dev* **9**:1586, 1995.
204. Treier M, Staszewski L, Bohmann D: Ubiquitin-dependent c-Jun degradation in vivo is mediated by the G domain. *Cell* **78**:787, 1994.
205. Willems AR, Lanker S, Patton EF, Craig KL, Nason TF, Kobayashi R, Wittenberg C, Tyers M: Cdc53 targets phosphorylated G1 cyclins for degradation by the ubiquitin proteolytic pathway. *Cell* **86**:453, 1996.
206. Pagano M, Tam SW, Theodoras A, Beer-Romero P, Del Sal G, Chau V, Yew R, Draetta G, Rolfe M: Role of the ubiquitin proteosome pathway in regulating abundance of the cyclin-dependent kinase inhibitor p27. *Science* **269**:682, 1995.
206a. Feldman RM, Correll CC, Kaplan KB, Deshaies RJ: A complex of Cdc4p, Skp1p, and Cdc53p/cullin catalyzes ubiquitination of the phosphorylated CDK inhibitor Sic1p. *Cell* **91**:221, 1997.
206b. Henchoz S, Chi Y, Catarin B, Herskowitz I, Deshaies RJ, Peter M: Phosphorylation- and ubiquitin-dependent degradation of the cyclin-dependent kinase inhibitor Far1p in budding yeast. *Genes Dev* **11**:3046, 1997.
206c. Lisztwan J, Marti A, Sutterluty H, Gstaiger M, Wirbelauer C, Krek W: Association of human CUL-1 and ubiquitin-conjugating enzyme CDC34 with the F-box protein p45(SKP2): Evidence for evolutionary conservation in the subunit composition of the CDC34-SCF pathway. *EMBO J* **17**:368, 1998.
206d. Patton EE, Willems AR, Sa D, Kuras L, Thomas D, Craig KL, Tyers M: Cdc53 is a scaffold protein for multiple Cdc34/Skp1/F-box protein complexes that regulate cell division and methionine biosynthesis in yeast. *Genes Dev* **12**:692, 1998.
206e. Skowyra D, Craig KL, Tyers M, Elledge SJ, Harper JW: F-box proteins are receptors that recruit phosphorylated substrates to the SCF ubiquitin-ligase complex. *Cell* **91**:209, 1997.
206f. Verma R, Feldman RM, Deshaies RJ: SIC1 is ubiquitinated in vitro by a pathway that requires CDC4, CDC34, and cyclin/CDK activities. *Mol Biol Cell* **8**:1427, 1997.
206g. Bai C, Sen P, Hofmann K, Ma L, Goebl M, Harper JW, Elledge SJ: SKP1 connects cell cycle regulators to the ubiquitin proteolysis machinery through a novel motif, the F-box. *Cell* **86**:263, 1996.
207. Plon S, Leppig KA, Do HN, Groudine M: Cloning of the human homolog of the CDC34 cell cycle gene by complementation in yeast. *Proc Natl Acad Sci U S A* **90**:10484, 1993.
208. Kipreos E, Lander L, Wing J, He WW, Hedgecock E: cul-1 is required for cell cycle exit in C. elegans and identifies a novel gene family. *Cell* **85**:829, 1996.
209. Baserga R: The biology of cell reproduction. Cambridge, MA: Harvard University Press, 1985.
210. Zetterberg A, Larson O: Kinetic analysis of regulatory events in G1 leading to proliferation of quiescence of Swiss 3T3 cells. *Proc Natl Acad Sci U S A* **82**:5365, 1985.
211. Pardee AB: A restriction point for control of normal animal cell proliferation. *Proc Natl Acad Sci U S A* **71**:1286, 1974.
212. Zetterberg A: Control of mammalian cell proliferation. *Curr Opin Cell Biol* **2**:296, 1990.
213. Pardee AB: G1 events and regulation of cell proliferation. *Science* **246**:603, 1989.
214. Zetterberg A, Larsson O, Wiman K: What is the restriction point? *Curr Opin Cell Biol* **7**:835, 1995.
215. Chao M: Growth factor signaling: Where is the specificity? *Cell* **68**:995, 1992.
216. Cantley L, Auger K, Carpenter C, Duckworth B, Graziani A, Kapeller R, Soltoff S: Oncogenes and signal transduction. *Cell* **64**:281, 1991.
217. Winston JT, Pledger WJ: Growth factor regulation of cyclin D1 mRNA expression through protein synthesis-dependent and -independent mechanisms. *Mol Biol Cell* **4**:1133, 1993.
218. Roussel MF, Theodoras AM, Pagano M, Sherr CJ: Rescue of defective mitogenic signaling by D-type cyclins. *Proc Natl Acad Sci U S A* **92**:6837, 1995.
219. Albanese C, Johnson J, Watanabe G, Eklund N, Vu D, Arnold A, Pestell R: Transforming p21ras mutants and c-Ets-2 activate the cyclin D1 promoter through distinguishable regions. *J Biol Chem* **270**:23589, 1995.
220. Hatakeyama M, Herrera R, Makela T, Dowdy S, Jacks T, Weinberg R: The cancer cell and the cell cycle clock. *Cold Spring Harbor Symp Quant Biol* **59**:1, 1994.
221. Roberts JM, Koff A, Polyak K, Firpo E, Collins S, Ohtsubo M, Massague J: Cyclins, cdks, and cyclin kinase inhibitors. *Cold Spring Harbor Symp Quant Biol* **59**:31, 1994.

222. Coats S, Flannagan WM, Nourse J, Roberts J: Requirement of p27Kip1 for restriction point control of the fibroblast cell cycle. *Science* **272**:877, 1996.
223. Nourse J, Firpo E, Flanagan M, Meyerson M, Polyak K, Lee MH, Massague J, Crabtree G, Roberts J: IL-2 mediated elimination of the p27kip1 cyclin-cdk kinase inhibitor prevented by rapamycin. *Nature* **372**:570, 1994.
224. Firpo EJ, Koff A, Solomon M, Roberts J: Inactivation of a cdk2 inhibitor during interleukin-2-induced proliferation of human T lymphocytes. *Mol Cell Biol* **14**:4889, 1994.
225. Fero ML, Rivkin M, Tasch M, Porter P, Carow CE, Firpo E, Polyak K, Tsai L, Broudy V, Perlmutter RM, Kaushansky K, Roberts JM: A syndrome of multi-organ hyperplasia with features of gigantism, tumorigenesis and female sterility in p27 kip1-deficient mice. *Cell* **85**:733, 1996.
226. Matsushime H, Quelle D, Shurtleff S, Shibuya M, Sherr C, Kato JY: D-type cyclin-dependent kinase activity in mammalian cells. *Mol Cell Biol* **14**:2066, 1994.
227. Guadagno T, Ohtsubo M, Roberts J, Assoian R: A link between cyclin A expression and adhesion-dependent cell cycle progression. *Science* **262**:1572, 1993.
228. Zhu X, Ohtsubo M, Bohmer RM, Roberts JM, Assoian R: Adhesion-dependent cell cycle progression linked to the expression of cyclin D1 activation of cyclin E-cdk2 and phosphorylation of the retinoblastoma protein. *J Cell Biol* **133**:391, 1996.
229. Draetta G, Loef E: Transforming growth factor β1 inhibition of p34cdc2 phosphorylation and histone H1 kinase activity is associated with G1/S-phase growth arrest. *Mol Cell Biol* **11**:1185, 1991.
230. Koff A, Ohtsuki M, Polyack K, Roberts J, Massague J: Negative regulation of G1 in mammalian cells: Inhibition of cyclin E-dependent kinase by TGF-beta. *Science* **260**:536, 1993.
231. Laiho M, DeCaprio J, Ludlow J, Livingston D, Massague J: Growth inhibition by TGF-β linked to suppression of retinoblastoma protein phosphorylation. *Cell* **62**:175, 1990.
232. Reynisdottir I, Polyak K, Iavarone A, Massague J: Kip/Cip and INK4 cdk inhibitors cooperate to induce cell cycle arrest in response to TGF-beta. *Genes Dev* **9**:1831, 1995.
233. Slingerland J, Hengst L, Pan C, Alexander D, Stampfer M, Reed S: A novel inhibitor of cyclin-cdk activity detected in transforming growth factor B-arrested epithelial cells. *Mol Cell Biol* **14**:3683, 1994.
234. Polyak K, Kato J, Solomon M, Sherr C, Massaque J, Roberts J, Koff A: p27kip1, a cyclin-cdk inhibitor, links transforming growth factor beta and contact inhibition to cell cycle arrest. *Genes Dev* **8**:9, 1994.
235. Kato JM, Matsuoka M, Polyak K, Massague J, Sherr CJ: Cyclic AMP-induced G1 phase arrest mediated by an inhibitor (p27Kip1) of cyclin-dependent kinase-4 activation. *Cell* **79**:487, 1994.
236. Brugarolas J, Chandrasekaran C, Gordon J, Beach D, Jacks T, Hannon G: Radiation-induced cell cycle arrest compromised by p21 deficiency. *Nature* **377**:552, 1995.
237. Deng C, Zhang P, Harper JW, Elledge S, Leder P: Mice lacking p21Cip1/Waf1 undergo normal development but are defective in G1 checkpoint control. *Cell* **82**:675, 1995.
238. Dulic V, Kaufman W, Wilson S, Tlsty T, Lees E, Harper JW, Elledge S, Reed S: p53-dependent inhibition of cyclin-dependent kinase activities in human fibroblasts during radiation-induced G1 arrest. *Cell* **76**:1013, 1994.
239. Massague J: TGF-beta signaling: Receptors, transducers, and mad proteins. *Cell* **85**:947, 1996.
240. Hahn S, Schutte M, Hoque A, Moskaluk C, da Costa L, Rozenblum E, Weinstein C, Fischer A, Hruban R, Kern S: *Science* **271**:350, 1996.
241. Hannon G, Beach D: p15Ink4b is a potential effector of cell cycle arrest by TGF-beta. *Nature* **371**:257, 1994.
242. Ewen M, Sluss H, Whitehouse L, Livingston D: Cdk4 modulation by TGF-β leads to cell cycle arrest. *Cell* **74**:1009, 1993.
243. Kuerbitz S, Plunkett B, Walsh W, Kastan M: Wild-type p53 is a cell cycle checkpoint determinant following irradiation. *Proc Natl Acad Sci U S A* **82**:7491, 1992.
244. Kastan M, Onyekwere O, Sidransky D, Vogelsein B, Craig R: Participation of p53 protein in the cellular response to DNA damage. *Cancer Res* **51**:6304, 1991.
245. Lane D: p53, guardian of the genome. *Nature* **358**:15, 1992.
246. Vogelstein B, Kinzler K: p53 function and dysfunction. *Cell* **70**:523, 1992.
247. Fields S, Jang S: Presence of a potent transcription activating sequence in the p53 protein. *Science* **249**:1046, 1990.
248. Kern S, Kinzler K, Bruskin A, Jarosz D, Friedman P, Prives C, Vogelstein B: Identification of p53 as a sequence specific DNA binding protein. *Science* **252**:1708, 1992.
249. Li R, Waga S, Hannon G, Beach D, Stillman B: Differential effects by the p21 cdk inhibitor on PCNA dependent DNA replication and DNA repair. *Nature* **371**:534, 1994.
250. Raff M: Size control: The regulation of cell numbers in animal development. *Cell* **86**:173, 1996.
251. Clurman BE, Roberts JM: Cell cycle and cancer. *J Natl Cancer Inst* **87**:1499, 1995.
252. Harlow E: An introduction to the puzzle. *Cold Spring Harbor Symp Quant Biol* **59**:709, 1994.
253. Hunter TJ, Pines J: Cyclins and cancer. *Cell* **66**:1071, 1991.
254. Morgan D: Cell cycle control in neoplastic cells. *Curr Opin Genet Dev* **2**:33, 1992.
255. Hall M, Peters G: Genetic alterations of cyclins, cyclin-dependent kinases and Cdk inhibitor's in human cancer *Adv Cancer Res* **68**:67, 1996.
256. Sherr C: Cancer cell cycles. *Science* **274**:1672, 1996.
257. Jiang WY, Zhang Y, Kahn SM, Hollstein M, Santella M, Lu S, Harris CC, Montesano R, Weinstein IB: Altered expression of the cyclin D1 and retinoblastoma genes in human esophageal cancer. *Proc Natl Acad Sci U S A* **90**:9026, 1993.
258. Lee E, To H, Shew J, Bookstein R, Scully P, Lee WH: Inactivation of the retinoblastoma susceptibility gene in human breast cancers. *Science* **241**:218, 1988.
259. Mori T, Miura K, Aoki T, Nishihira T, Mori S, Nakamura Y: Frequent somatic mutation of the MTS1/CDK4I (multiple tumor suppressor/cyclin-dependent kinase 4 inhibitor) gene in esophageal squamous cell carcinoma. *Cancer Res* **54**:3396, 1994.
260. Kamb A, Gruis NA, Weaver-Feldhaus J, Liu Q, Harshman K, Tavtigian SV, Stockert E, Day III RS, Johnson BE, Skolnick MH: A cell cycle regulator potentially involved in genesis of many tumor types. *Science* **264**:436, 1994.
261. Sheaff R, Roberts J: Lessons in p16 from phylum Falconium. *Curr Biol* **5**:28, 1995.
262. Kawamata N, Morosetti R, Miller S, Park D, Spirin K, Nakamaki T, Takeuchi S, Hatta Y, Simpson J, Wilcyznski S, et al: Molecular analysis of the cyclin dependent kinase inhibitor gene p27/Kip1 in human malignancies. *Cancer Res* **55**:2266, 1995.
263. Keyomarsi K, O'Leary N, Molnar G, Lees E, Fingert H, Pardee A: Cyclin E, a potential prognostic marker for breast cancer. *Cancer Res* **54**:380, 1994.
264. Pietenpol J, Bohlander S, Sato Y, Papadoupolos B, Liu C, Friedman B, Trask B, Roberts J, Kinzler K, Rowley J, Vogelstein B: Assignment of the human p27Kip1 gene to 12p13 and its analysis in leukemias. *Cancer Res* **55**:1206, 1995.
265. Ponce-Castenada M, Lee M, Latres E, Polyak K, Lacombe L, Montgomery K, Mathew S, Krauter K, Sheinfeld J, Massague J, et al: p27Kip1: chromosomal mapping to 12p12-12p13.1 and absence of mutations in human tumors. *Cancer Res* **55**:1211, 1995.
266. Fearon E, Vogelstein B: A genetic model for colorectal tumorigenesis. *Cell* **61**:759, 1990.
267. Loeb L: Mutator phenotype may be required for multistage tumorigenesis. *Cancer Res* **54**:4590, 1990.
268. Knudson AG: Genetics of human cancer. *Annu Rev Genet* **20**:231, 1986.
269. Hartwell L, Weinert T, Kadyk L, Garvik B: Cell cycle checkpoint, genomic integrity, and cancer. *Cold Spring Harbor Symp Quant Biol* **59**:259, 1994.
270. Tlsty T, White A, Livanos E, Sage M, Roelofs H, Briot A, Poulose B: Genomic integrity and the genetics of cancer. *Cold Spring Harbor Symp Quant Biol* **59**:265, 1994.
271. Schimke R, Sherwood S, Hill A, Johnston R: Overreplication and recombination of DNA in higher eukaryotes: Potential consequences and biological implications. *Proc Natl Acad Sci U S A* **83**:2157, 1986.
272. Nowell PC: The clonal evolution of tumor cell populations. *Science* **194**:23, 1976.
273. Weinert T, Hartwell L: The RAD9 gene controls the cell cycle response to DNA damage in Saccharomyces cerevisiae. *Science* **241**:317, 1989.
274. Dasso M, Newport J: Completion of DNA replication is monitored by a feedback system that controls the initiation of mitosis in vitro: Studies in Xenopus. *Cell* **61**:811, 1990.
275. Enoch T, Nurse P: Mutation of fission yeast cell cycle control genes abolishes dependence of mitosis on DNA replication. *Cell* **60**:665, 1990.

276. Rowley R, Hudson J, Young P: The wee1 protein kinase is required for radiation-induced mitotic delay. *Nature* **356**:353, 1992.
277. Smythe C, Newport J: Coupling of mitosis to the completion of S phase in Xenopus occurs via modulation of the tyrosine kinase that phosphorylates p34 CDC2. *Cell* **68**:787, 1992.
278. Walworth N, Davey S, Beach D: Fission yeast chk1 protein kinase links the rad checkpoint pathway to cdc2. *Nature* **363**:368, 1993.
279. Nurse P: Checkpoint pathways come of age. *Cell* **91**:865, 1997.
280. Enoch T, Gould KL, Nurse P: Mitotic checkpoint control in fission yeast. *Cold Spring Harbor Symp Quant Biol* **56**:409, 1991.
281. Rhind N, Furnari B, Russell P: Cdc2 tyrosine phosphorylation is required for the DNA damage checkpoint in fission yeast. *Genes Dev* **11**:504, 1997.
282. Rhind N, Russell P: Tyrosine phosphorylation of cdc2 is required for the replication checkpoint in Schizosaccharomyces pombe. *Mol Cell Biol* **18**:3782, 1998.
283. Hermeking H, Lengauer C, Polyak K, et al: 14-3-3 sigma is a p53-regulated inhibitor of G2/M progression. *Mol Cell* **1**:3, 1997.
284. Sanchez Y, Wong C, Thoma RS, et al: Conservation of the Chk1 checkpoint pathway in mammals: Linkage of DNA damage to cdk regulation through cdc25 [see comments]. *Science* **277**:1497, 1997.
285. Peng CY, Graves PR, Thoma RS, et al: Mitotic and G2 checkpoint control: Regulation of 14-3-3 protein binding by phosphorylation of Cdc25C on serine-216 [see comments]. *Science* **277**:1501, 1997.
286. O'Connell MJ, Raleigh JM, Verkade HM, et al: Chk1 is a wee1 kinase in the G2 DNA damage checkpoint inhibiting cdc2 by Y15 phosphorylation. *EMBO J* **16**:545, 1997.
287. Flaggs G, Plug AW, Dunks KM, et al: Atm-dependent interactions of a mammalian chk1 homolog with meiotic chromosomes. *Curr Biol* **7**:977, 1997.
288. Murray AW: The genetics of cell cycle checkpoints. *Curr Op in Genet Dev* **5**:5, 1995.
289. Sanchez Y, Elledge S: Stopped for repairs. *Bioessays* **17**:545, 1995.
290. Li R, Murray A: Feedback control of mitosis in budding yeast. *Cell* **66**:519, 1991.
291. Hoyt A, Totis L, Roberts BT: S. cerevisiae genes required for cell cycle arrest in response to loss of microtubule function. *Cell* **66**:507, 1991.
292. Murray AW: Tense spindles can relax. *Nature* **373**:560, 1995.
293. Minshull J, Sun H, Tonks N, Murray AW: A MAP kinase-dependent spindle assembly checkpoint in Xenopus egg extracts. *Cell* **79**:475, 1994.
294. Lin J, Wu X, Chen J, Chang A, Levine AJ: Functions of the p53 protein in growth regulation and tumor suppression. *Cold Spring Harbor Symp Quant Biol* **59**:215, 1994.
295. Barlow C, Hirotsune S, Paylor R, Liyanage M, Eckhaus M, Collins F, Shiloh Y, Crawley J, Ried T, Tagle D, Wynshaw-Boris A: Atm-deficient mice: a paradigm of ataxia telangectasia. *Cell* **85**:159, 1996.
296. Meyn MS: Ataxia-telangiectasia and cellular responses to DNA damage. *Cancer Res* **55**:5991, 1995.

CHAPTER 24

Apoptosis and Cancer

Charles M. Rudin ▪ Craig B. Thompson

1. **Apoptosis is a descriptive term for the phenotype of cells undergoing programmed cell death. Apoptosis is a critical component of development and homeostasis in multicellular eukaryotic organisms. Apoptotic cell death can be distinguished from necrotic cell death by several criteria, including characteristic morphology and a minimal inflammatory reaction.**
2. **The Bcl-2 family of proteins plays a central role in apoptotic control and is conserved evolutionarily. The realization that Bcl-2 functions to prevent apoptosis defined a new category of oncogene: the antiapoptotic gene. Apoptotic regulation is dependent on the relative balance of opposing Bcl-2 family members. Those family members may function by regulating homeostasis between key intracellular organelles and the cytoplasm.**
3. **The caspases are evolutionarily conserved proteases that function as important mediators of apoptosis. Control of caspase activity is dependent on proteolytic processing of cytoplasmic proenzymes. Some of these proteases have autocatalytic potential. The critical downstream targets of caspase family proteolysis have not been fully defined.**
4. **Many cell surface receptors, including the tumor necrosis factor receptor (TNFR) family, have been shown to modify the apoptotic sensitivity of cells. Different members of the TNFR family can promote or inhibit apoptosis. An apoptotic signaling pathway from some of these receptors has been traced by direct protein–protein interaction from receptor engagement to caspase activation.**
5. **Cellular and viral oncogenes that stimulate proliferation are strong inducers of apoptosis. This induction is probably dependent on cell cycle checkpoints (tumor suppressor gene products) that detect abnormally replicating cells and trigger apoptosis. Inhibition of apoptosis therefore is frequently an essential step in the process of oncogenesis.**
6. **Anticancer therapies induce apoptosis in sensitive cells. Inhibition of apoptosis is a major mechanism of chemotherapeutic resistance. Chemotherapy may accelerate the mutagenesis rate and promote aneuploidy of tumors in which apoptosis has been suppressed. New therapies directed at modifying apoptotic signaling pathways may be helpful in circumventing these problems.**

The term *programmed cell death* refers to the induction of cell death by a regulated pathway inherent to the cell. It can be contrasted with necrotic cell death, which is traumatic and depends on factors entirely external to the cell. *Apoptosis* (from the Greek for "falling leaves") is a descriptive term that was used originally to describe the characteristic phenotype of cells that die in the absence of evident trauma. The apoptotic phenotype has been found to be so ubiquitous among cells undergoing programmed cell death that the terms are now used interchangeably. Wyllie and colleagues in the early 1970s were among the first to observe and record a phenotype of dying cells that appeared to be conserved among widely disparate cell types and was distinct in many respects from necrotic cell death.[1,2] These initial descriptive studies spawned an enormous field of inquiry with direct implications for many problematic areas of medicine, including neurodevelopmental and neurodegenerative diseases, infection, autoimmunity, and cancer.[3–7]

The study of apoptosis has had an important impact on the understanding of organismal growth and differentiation. The characteristic features of the process are conserved widely among multicellular eukaryotes.[8,9] The capacity to initiate an apoptotic pathway appears to be a shared feature of all the cells of the body, including rapidly cycling populations such as leukocytes and long-lived cells such as neurons. Apoptosis plays a crucial role in development, permitting the necessary elimination of surplus cells in the formation of many complex organs, including the brain.[10]

Several morphologic features of apoptotic cells distinguish them from cells that die in response to trauma or hypoxia.[2] Necrotic cell death is characterized by cell swelling and gross disruption of organelles and the cell membrane. Apoptotic cell death is characterized by cell contraction, blebbing of the cytoplasmic membrane, dense condensation of the nucleus, and a pathognomonic autodigestion of the genome into fragments that correspond in size to multiples of the amount of DNA found in individual nucleosomes. If electrophoresed through an agarose gel, DNA from an apoptotic cell therefore can be displayed as a ladder, with rungs corresponding to cleavage between one, two, or multiple nucleosome elements (Fig. 24-1).

Traumatic cell death leads to leakage of intracellular contents and the generation of a potent inflammatory response that depends on multiple cytokines and pyrogens. This response may be critical to confining infection as well as to wound healing and scar formation. In contrast, apoptotic cell death does not lead to uncontrolled cytokine release or the generation of a significant inflammatory response. Apoptotic cell remnants typically are recognized and engulfed by adjacent cells (frequently by cells that are not part of the phagocytic macrophage-monocyte system) prior to breakdown of the cellular membrane and release of intracellular contents.[11–13] The ability to delete cells in an immunologically silent manner may be of central importance in permitting the natural turnover and remodeling of tissues without risking autoimmune disease.

Homeostasis in any cell population requires a balance between the processes of cell proliferation and cell death (Fig. 24-2). Accumulation of abnormal numbers of a clonally related population of cells (i.e., a neoplasm) can result from either uncontrolled proliferation or inhibition of cell death. The regulatory mechanisms that control cell proliferation clearly are extensive and have been the primary focus of research on carcinogenesis for many years. Recently, it has become apparent that the mechanisms of programmed cell death also are tightly regulated, highly responsive to extracellular signals, and similarly integral to the inhibition of carcinogenesis. This chapter outlines the known mechanisms that regulate cell death and some of the implications of dysregulated cell death on carcinogenesis and chemotherapeutic resistance.

A list of standard abbreviations is located immediately preceding the index in each volume. Nonstandard abbreviations used in this chapter include: TNFR = tumor necrosis factor receptor; TRAF = TNF receptor-associated factor; IAP = inhibitor of apoptosis.

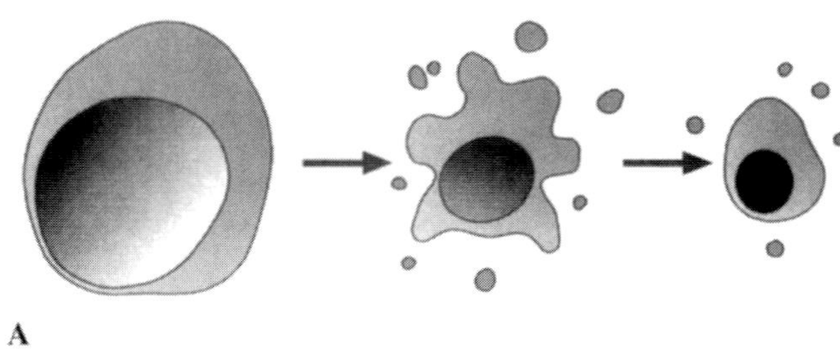

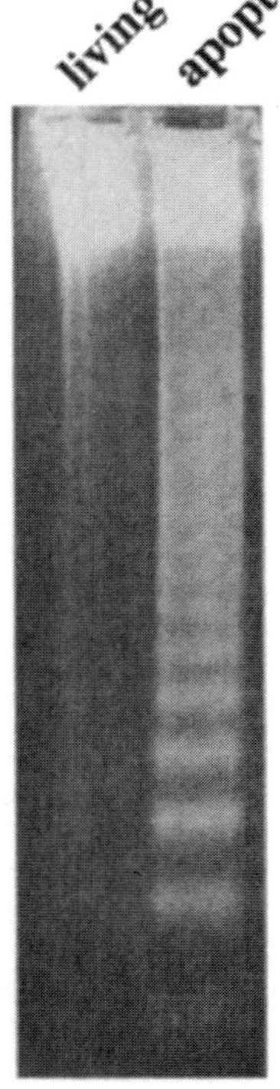

Fig. 24-1 Characteristic cellular changes of apoptosis. *A.* Typical morphologic changes of apoptosis are shown, including blebbing of the cytoplasmic membrane, cell contraction, and marked condensation of the nucleus. Importantly, cytoplasmic contents are not spilled into the extracellular space. *B.* Agarose gel electrophoresis of genomic DNA from apoptotic cells. A pathognomonic laddering of DNA fragments in approximately 200-base pair increments is seen, corresponding to the amount of DNA contained within individual nucleosomes. The cells are murine lymph node cells after 0 h (living) and 48 h (apoptotic) in culture.

BCL-2 AND THE ORIGINS OF THE STUDY OF APOPTOSIS AND CANCER

The *bcl-2* gene (for B-cell lymphoma/leukemia-2) initially was identified as the gene on chromosome 18q21 at the breakpoint of the t(14;18) chromosomal translocation found in the majority of B-cell follicular lymphomas[14–17] (Fig. 24-3). This genomic rearrangement juxtaposes the *bcl-2* gene with the immunoglobulin heavy chain gene enhancer, leading to marked up-regulation and constitutive expression of Bcl-2 in lymphoid cells. The Bcl-2 coding sequence is not altered by this translocation.

The role of Bcl-2 in oncogenesis remained obscure for several years after its discovery. Unlike all previously identified oncogenes, overexpression of the *bcl-2* gene did not increase the proliferative potential of cells in any of the commonly used assays for oncogenic transformation, which depend on a modulation of the growth rate of the transfected cell. The failure to induce rampant growth correlates with the phenotype of most follicular lymphomas, which have an indolent, slowly progressive natural history, have low proliferative indices, and retain many of the phenotypic characteristics of nontransformed lymphocytes.[18]

The first association between Bcl-2 and inhibition of cell death was made in 1988.[19] Stable *bcl-2* transformants of a cell line dependent on the growth factor interleukin-3 (IL-3) were found to survive for prolonged periods after withdrawal of IL-3, much longer than the parental cell line lacking the upregulated *bcl-2* gene. In addition, Bcl-2 was shown to cooperate with a more traditional oncoprotein, c-myc, to immortalize pre-B cells (see below). Bcl-2 subsequently has been found to be a potent inhibitor of apoptosis in a wide variety of experimental systems.[20]

The discovery of the function of Bcl-2 challenged the prevailing view of carcinogenesis and defined a new category of oncogene.[21] Research on oncogenesis had focused largely on the mechanisms regulating cell proliferation: Cancer was thought to arise from the products of abnormally expressed genes driving cell replication (oncogenes) or failing to inhibit cell replication (tumor suppressor genes). Bcl-2, which is overexpressed by the most common chromosomal rearrangement in lymphoid malignancy, was found to have no direct effect on replication but caused a failure to die. This realization implied for the first time that alteration of either side of the homeostatic balance could contribute not only to cell accumulation but also to carcinogenesis. Subsequent work by many groups has confirmed the carcinogenic potential of antiapoptotic gene dysregulation and has led to a broader view of the types of genetic alterations that contribute to cancer.

To place the effects of apoptotic dysregulation in cancer cells in context, the next section summarizes the current understanding of the mechanisms that regulate apoptosis in normal cells.

THE CENTRAL APOPTOTIC PATHWAY

C. elegans and the Evolutionary Conservation of Apoptotic Regulators

The striking morphologic similarity between disparate cell types undergoing apoptosis suggests that the underlying molecular processes may be similar.[22] Many of the features of this central apoptotic control system have been defined, and the outline of this pathway provides insight into potential mechanisms for viral and cellular oncogenic transformation.

Many of the critical factors involved in the control of apoptosis were first defined in the nematode *Caenorhabditis elegans.* Every cell division and cell death event in the normal pathway of *C. elegans* development is known, and this developmental pathway follows a determined, predictable program.[23] All 131 programmed cell death events in the developing worm depend on the normal function of three proteins: CED-3, CED-4, and CED-9. Loss of CED-3 or CED-4 function or a gain-of-function mutation of the CED-9 protein will lead to complete abrogation of cell death in *C. elegans* development.[24,25] Loss of CED-9 function leads to increased apoptotic cell death.[25] CED-9 appears to function by

Table 24-1 Mammalian Bcl-2-Related Proteins

Antiapoptotic	Proapoptotic	BH-3 Proteins (Inhibit Antiapoptotic Function)
Bcl-2	Bcl-x_S	Bad
Bcl-x_L	Bax	Bid
Mcl-1	Bak	Bik
Bcl-w	Mtd/Bok	Hrk
A-1		Bim
		Blk

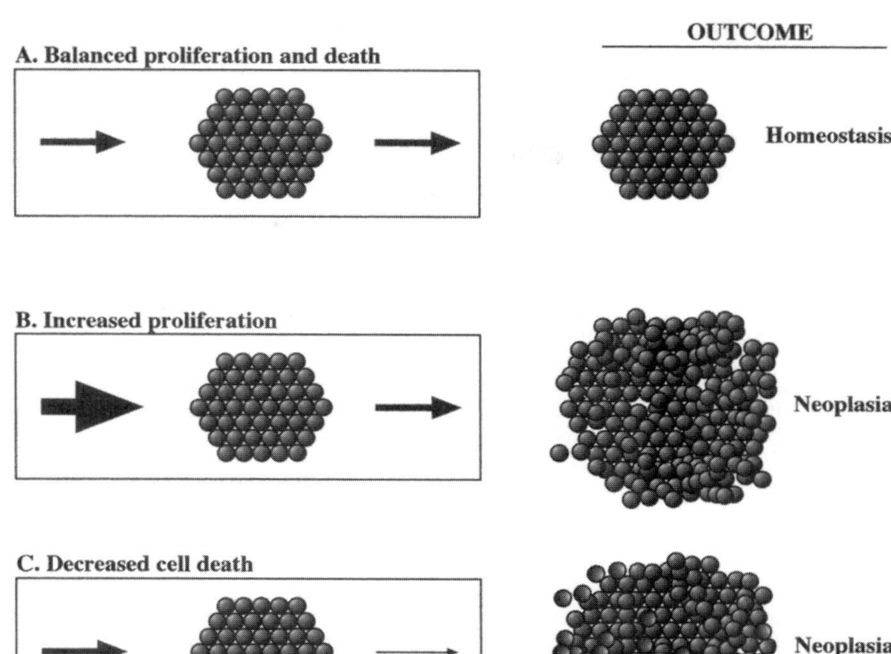

Fig. 24-2 Dysregulation of either side of the homeostatic balance can lead to neoplasia. *A.* A population of cells in homeostatic balance replicates and dies at equal rates. Mutations that result in either an increase in the proliferative rate (*B*) or a decrease in the death rate (*C*) can lead to the accumulation of clonally related cells.

suppressing inappropriate activity of CED-3 and CED-4.[26] CED-4 interacts with CED-3 to facilitate its activation to a protease capable of generating an apoptotic phenotype.[27–31]

Strong evolutionary pressures would be expected to preserve the mechanisms involved in a process as fundamental to the organism as the control of cell death. Many of the proteins central to apoptotic control indeed have been highly conserved, from the roundworm to the human (Fig. 24-4). CED-9 is highly homologous to mammalian Bcl-2.[32,33] Bcl-2 expression in *C. elegans* mimics a CED-9 gain of function and can partially revert a CED-9 loss-of-function mutant. A mammalian homologue of CED-4, Apaf-1, recently was identified and appears to function as a signal transducer between Bcl-2 family members and CED-3-related molecules.[34] CED-3 was found by database searching to be related to the mammalian interleukin-1β converting enzyme, now known as *caspase 1*.[35] As discussed below, caspases have been found to play a central role in the effector phase of apoptosis.

The Bcl-2 Family

Bcl-2 overexpression is capable of inhibiting cell death in response to many disparate apoptotic signals, suggesting that it acts at the convergence of many apoptotic pathways. Bcl-2 has been found to be one of a family of related proteins, several members of which appear to play important positive and negative roles in the control of apoptosis (Table 24-1). Antiapoptotic factors including Bcl-2, Bcl-x_L, and Mcl-1 have been found to be overexpressed in several tumor types. Members of the Bcl-2 family have been found to form both homo- and heterodimers, and the relative balance of

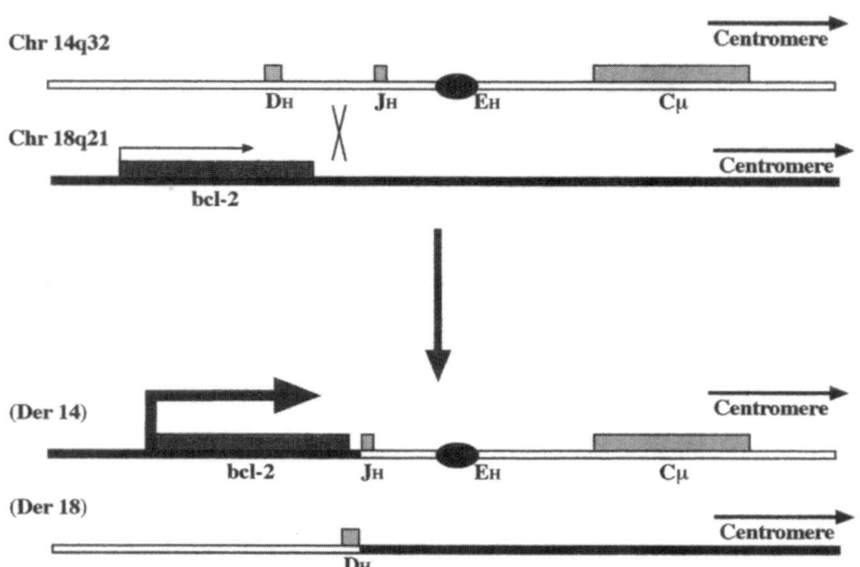

Fig. 24-3 The t(14;18) translocation characteristic of follicular lymphomas. Exons of the immunoglobulin heavy chain gene are represented by light boxes, the *bcl-2* gene by a dark box, and the heavy chain enhancer by a black oval. The translocation involves sites in the immunoglobulin heavy chain locus that normally are involved in the rearrangements necessary to generate a functional heavy chain gene and probably occurs in the pre-B-cell stage. The breakpoint in the *bcl-2* gene frequently is in the 3′ untranslated region and thus does not affect the coding sequence.

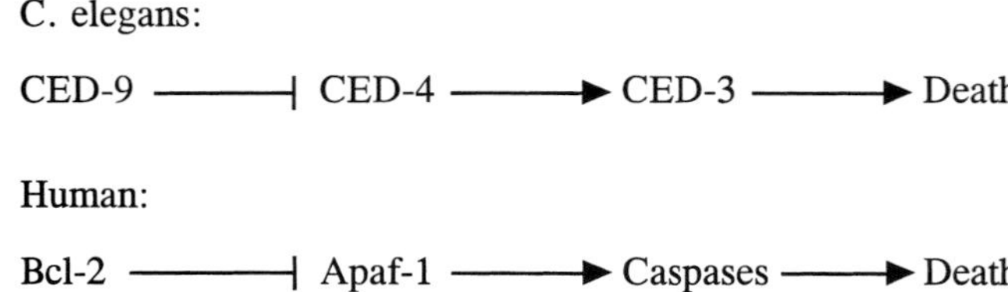

Fig. 24-4 Critical components of apoptotic regulation have been evolutionarily conserved.

antiapoptotic and proapoptotic members in these complexes may be a critical determinant of apoptotic sensitivity.[43]

Bcl-2 family members can be divided into three categories: antiapoptotic factors such as Bcl-2 that inhibit cell death, proapoptotic factors that when overexpressed trigger cell death, and factors that while not intrinsically proapoptotic nevertheless can bind to and inhibit the function of antiapoptotic factors. Members of the third category typically share only a limited homology with the other family members, in a domain known as BH-3.[44]

The mechanism of action of Bcl-2 family members has not been determined, although several important insights have been established. The structure of Bcl-x_L has been determined by x-ray crystallography and nuclear magnetic resonance (NMR) spectroscopy.[45] The molecular structure of Bcl-x_L surprisingly was found to be similar to that of members of the colicin family of bacterial proteins. Colicins are proteins secreted by bacteria that form pores in the surface membranes of other bacterial strains, causing cell death.[46] The relevance of this unexpected structural link between families of proteins involved in mammalian and bacterial cell death is currently unclear.

Bcl-2 appears to be localized to the nuclear endoplasmic reticular and outer mitochondrial membranes.[47–49] Commitment to apoptotic cell death has been associated with loss of mitochondrial membrane potential, and this membrane potential gradient can be maintained by Bcl-2 overexpression.[50–54] Many of the characteristic nuclear changes of apoptosis can be induced by the addition of dATP and cytochrome c to cytoplasmic extracts in vitro.[55] Since cytochrome c normally is tightly sequestered within mitochondria, Bcl-2 family members may function by directly controlling mitochondrial membrane permeability.[56] Indeed, recent observations indicate that Bcl-2 and Bcl-x_L inhibit, whereas the proapoptotic family member Bax promotes, cytochrome c release from the mitochondrial intermembrane space.[56–59]

Antiapoptotic family members also may function by complexing with and inactivating factors that would otherwise trigger caspase activation. As described earlier, in *C. elegans* CED-9 has been found to interact directly with CED-4; this interaction in turn prevents CED-4 from activating the cysteine protease CED-3.[27,28] Bcl-x_L similarly can interact with the mammalian CED-4 homologue Apaf-1, and this interaction may play a role in the inhibition of Apaf-1 activation of downstream caspases.[34,62,63]

The Caspase Family

Another group of proteins that has been implicated strongly in the central apoptotic pathway are the caspases (*c*ysteine proteases with *asp*artic acid specificity).[64,65] Unlike the Bcl-2 family, which appears to modulate apoptotic threshold without participating directly involved in cellular autodigestion, caspase activity has been associated closely with the apoptotic morphology of the dying cell. The family has at least 13 members, which can be subgrouped on the basis of similarity and target specificity[65–69] (Table 24-2). Overexpression of most caspases has been shown to trigger apoptosis in cell lines, although not all appear to be involved in physiological apoptosis. A central role for this family of proteases in the process of apoptosis in mammalian cells has been suggested by studies showing that specific inhibitors of caspases can prevent cell death, or at least an apoptotic morphology, in response to many of the known triggers of programmed cell death.[70,71] These inhibitors include viral products such as p35 and crmA (see below) as well as synthetic oligopeptides that occupy and block the protease activity site.

Regulation of caspase activity may occur on several levels. All the caspases are synthesized as larger inactive proenzymes that must undergo proteolytic processing to the active enzymatic forms.[72] The cleavage sites in these proenzymes are consistent with processing by caspases themselves. High local concentrations of some caspases may be sufficient to permit autocatalysis and activation.[73] The processing sites of some family members appear more likely to be target sites for other caspases, suggesting a sequential cascade of protease activation. Initial activation of a caspase may generate a rapidly and irreversibly amplified signal by initiating autocatalysis as well as triggering activation of downstream proteases. An additional layer of regulation may derive from alternate mRNA splicing. At least four of the caspase genes encode truncated forms as well as full-length proteases.[74–77] These truncated proteins may down-regulate protease activity by directly inhibiting the active proteases or by binding and stabilizing the proenzyme forms.

Among the caspase family, caspase 9 has been most clearly implicated in the central pathway of apoptotic induction (Fig. 24-5). Caspase 9, along with cytochrome c and Apaf-1, was identified as a factor required for induction of apoptotic events in a cell-free system.[55,61] Apaf-1 interacts with and activates caspase 9, which can then process other caspases, including caspase 3.[61] Caspase 3, in turn, has been found to be integrally involved in the generation of apoptotic nuclear morphology (condensation and DNA degradation).[78]

Many potential downstream targets with caspase cleavage sites have been identified and together may elucidate some of the mechanisms underlying apoptotic physiology. Among the defined caspase substrates are proteins involved in nuclear and cytoplasmic structure (e.g., nuclear lamins, actin), signal transduction (e.g., c-Abl, Raf-1, NF-κB p65 and p50), cell cycle control (e.g., MDM-2, Rb), genomic repair and integrity (e.g., poly-ADP ribose polymerase (PARP), DNA-dependent protein kinase), and apoptotic regulation (Bcl-x_L, Bcl-2).[79–93] Nevertheless, clear definition of the roles and relative importance of the various caspases and their downstream targets has been difficult. For example, PARP can be processed by caspase 3, 8, or 9 and has been used as a marker for the nuclear changes associated with apoptosis.[77,92,93] However, PARP cleavage is neither necessary nor sufficient for apoptosis.[94,95]

CELL SURFACE SIGNALS AFFECTING APOPTOSIS

Survival of most cells in the body is highly dependent on their environment. Cells removed from their in vivo context frequently undergo rapid apoptotic cell death. This suggests that in their natural context many cells continuously receive extracellular signals that result in increased apoptotic resistance.[9] These survival signals may be generated by direct cell–cell contact or by locally diffused soluble factors. Externally derived factors that may increase or decrease apoptotic sensitivity include growth factors, cytokines, interleukins, glucocorticoids, androgens, estrogens, and neurotransmitters. The cell membrane receptors that affect apoptotic sensitivity and the resulting intracellular signaling pathways initiated by engagement of these receptors are being studied intensively.

One critical family of cell surface receptors that affect apoptotic sensitivity is composed of proteins related to the tumor necrosis factor receptors (TNFRs).[96] The family includes the two receptors for TNF (TNFR1 and TNFR2) and at least 10 other related receptors. All TNFR family members have related cysteine-rich extracellular domains, each of which interacts with one of a family of TNF-related signaling proteins. The intracellular domains of these receptors differ widely, suggesting that different signaling pathways may be initiated by engagement

Table 24-2 Mammalian Caspase Subfamilies Grouped by Substrate Specificity

Group 1	Group 2	Group 3
Caspase 1 (ICE)	Caspase 2 (ICH-1/NEDD-2)	Caspase 6 (Mch2)
Caspase 4 (ICE rel II/ICH-2/TX)	Caspase 3 (CPP32/Yama/Apopain)	Caspase 8 (FLICE/MACH/Mch5)
Caspase 5 (ICE rel III/TY)	Caspase 7 (ICE-LAP3/Mch3/CMH-1)	Caspase 9 (ICE-LAP6/Mch6)
Caspase 11 (ICH-3)		Caspase 10 (FLICE2/Mch4)
Caspase 12		
Caspase 13 (ERICE)		

of each receptor. Different family members are capable of producing opposing signals, and in fact, engagement of a single receptor may have different effects in different contexts. In many experimental systems, engagement of some family members (e.g., Fas, TNFR1) promotes apoptosis, whereas engagement of others (e.g., CD30, CD40, TNFR2) promotes survival (Fig. 24-6).

Proapoptotic Signaling

The proapoptotic receptors Fas and TNFR1 share a related sequence in their C-terminal cytoplasmic tails known as the *death domain.* Three cytoplasmic proteins have been isolated on the basis of their ability to associate with these receptors.[97–99] These proteins-RIP, TRADD, and FADD—all contain death domains responsible for association with the receptor tails. RIP and FADD associate most strongly with Fas, and TRADD binds to TNFR1. Overexpression of any of these proteins can initiate apoptosis.

FADD contains a unique N-terminal effector domain that is required for apoptotic induction. In contrast, apoptotic signaling by RIP and TRADD depends only on the death domains, suggesting that these proteins may function primarily by recruitment of FADD or similar effector proteins to an activated receptor. TRADD serves as a link between TNFR1 engagement and multiple downstream signaling pathways.[99–101] The TNFR1-TRADD complex engages TRAF2 (see below), leading to NF-κB and c-Jun N-terminal kinase (JNK) activation, and also recruits FADD through association of death domains. Mutation of the FADD effector domain blocks TNFR1-mediated apoptosis; although the association between FADD and TNFR1 may be predominantly indirect (i.e., through TRADD), FADD is integral to apoptotic signaling from TNFR1.

FADD has been shown to recruit the unprocessed precursor of caspase 8 to the activated Fas receptor.[102,103] Caspase 8 binds FADD through a portion of the prodomain homologous to the effector domain of FADD. Mutation within the protease domain of caspase 8 blocks apoptosis in response to engagement of either Fas or TNFR1, suggesting that caspase 8 may be a component of both receptor complexes.[73] Procaspase 8 recruitment to such complexes leads to proteolytic processing; activated caspase 8 may then initiate a cascade of caspase activation, leading to apoptosis. This recruitment of a caspase directly to the receptor complex may explain why apoptotic induction by engagement of Fas is, in some contexts, relatively resistant to modulation by Bcl-2.

Antiapoptotic Signaling

Other members of the TNFR family of cell surface receptors mediate signals that increase the apoptotic threshold of a cell. These receptors, including TNFR2, CD30, and CD40, interact with a family of related intracellular proteins known as *TNF receptor-associated factors* (TRAFs). TRAF2, TRAF3, and TRAF5 have similar binding specificities for sites in the

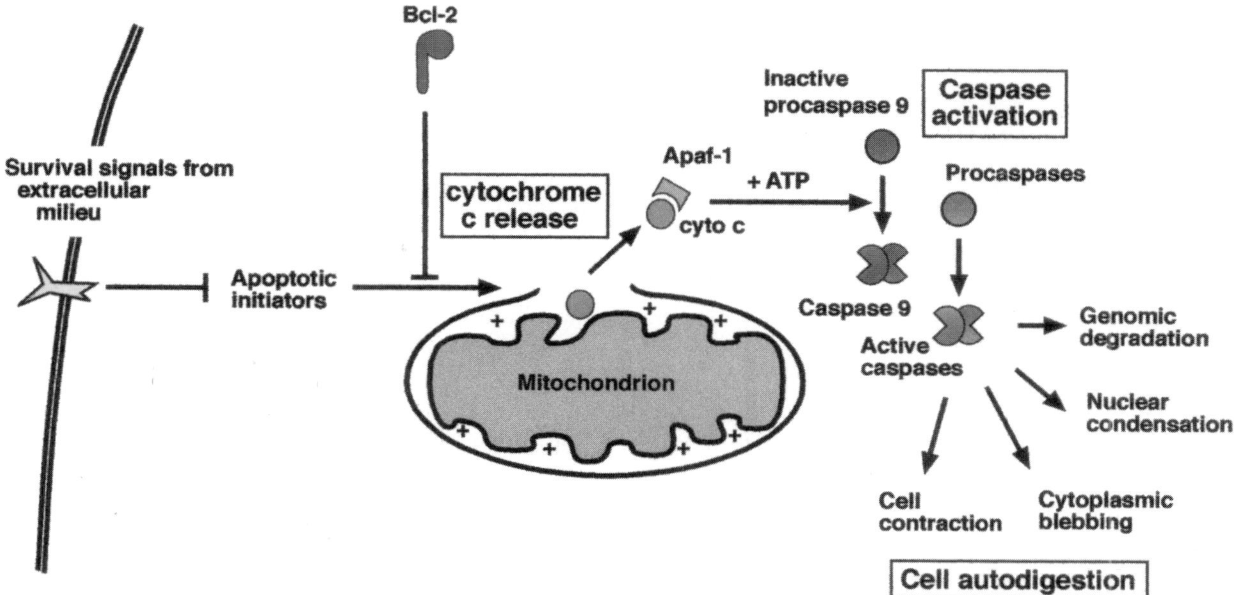

Fig. 24-5 A hypothetical model of the central apoptotic pathway. Initiation of apoptosis is held in check by survival signals received by cell surface receptors. Removal of the cell from its in vivo context or blockade of these survival signals allows induction of the apoptotic pathway, resulting in loss of mitochondrial outer membrane integrity and cytochrome c release. Cytosolic cytochrome c interacts with Apaf-1, which in the presence of ATP leads to caspase 9 processing and activation. This initiates a cascade of caspase activation, and ultimately in the characteristic morphologic changes of apoptosis. Bcl-2 and Bcl-x$_L$ reside in the mitochondrial outer membrane and can inhibit cytochrome c release. Other important apoptotic initiators include cell surface receptor-mediated cell death signals, DNA damage, cell cycle dysregulation, and metabolic alterations.

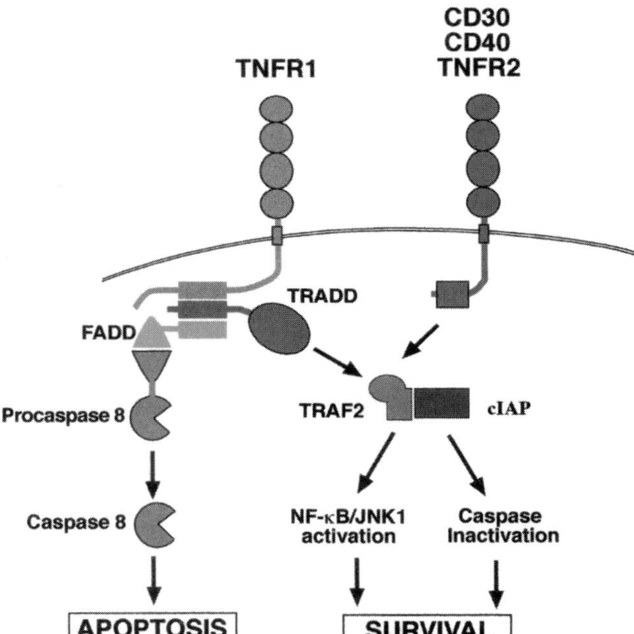

Fig. 24-6 Signaling complexes associated with representatives of the TNFR family. Receptor engagement by extracellular ligand promotes receptor multimerization and initiates formation of the schematically depicted complexes. The cytoplasmic tail of TNFR1 contains a region known as the death domain that interacts with a related domain of TRADD. TRADD serves as a signaling intermediary for both pro- and antiapoptotic pathways through recruitment of additional signaling molecules as shown. The phenotypic result of TNFR1 engagement therefore may be dependent on the relative availability of various second messengers. Signaling through engagement of TNFR2, CD30, or CD40 is also context-dependent. A common pathway for these three receptors is shown: TRAF2 engagement promotes survival through induction of both NF-κB and JNK1 activity and by interaction with the cIAP proteins may lead to inhibition of caspase activity.

cytoplasmic domains of the TNFR2, CD30, and CD40 receptors.[104–111] TRAF1 has been shown to bind directly only to CD30 but forms indirect associations with other receptors through heterodimerization with TRAF2.[104,110] TRAF6 was defined initially as a factor involved in IL-1 receptor signaling but also associates with the cytoplasmic tail of CD40 at a site distinct from the other TRAFs.[112,113]

TRAF proteins associate with multiple sites in the TNFR family cytoplasmic tails and, despite similar binding specificities, may result in distinct biologic responses. NF-κB activation has been associated with increased resistance to apoptosis in several cellular contexts. TRAF2 has been shown to activate NF-κB, whereas TRAF3 may suppress NF-κB activity either directly or by inhibition of TRAF2 function.[114]

The association between TRAF binding and antiapoptotic signaling by these receptors is primarily correlative. The intracellular domains of the TNFR family of proteins are remarkably dissimilar, suggesting that proteins other than the TRAFs are involved in the signaling complexes. The effects of ligand binding to these receptors probably depend on many variables, including the relative numbers of (potentially competing) receptors, the particular set of intracellular second messengers available to associate with these receptors, and the downstream targets present in a given cell.

The TRAF4 protein is unique among the TRAFs in that it has not been reported in association with any cell surface receptors but rather appears to be localized to the nucleus.[115] This factor was identified initially in a screen for proteins overexpressed in metastatic breast cancer, and high-level expression has been reported subsequently in several breast cancer cell lines.[116] The function of this factor is unknown.

VIRAL MIMICRY AND APOPTOTIC INHIBITION

Apoptosis is an important defense against many types of viral infection. Cell suicide in response to viral infection may both inhibit successful viral replication in lytic infections and defend against viral transformation. Viruses have adapted methods to suppress apoptosis in the host that provide insight into the critical components of apoptotic regulation. Several viral proteins that regulate TNF-related signal transduction, inhibit caspase activity, or mimic Bcl-2 activity have been identified. The fact that viruses specifically target these pathways to prevent host cell death underscores their central importance in the regulation of cell survival.

Recently, a family of four mammalian proteins related to the baculovirus inhibitor of apoptosis (IAP) was identified.[117–122] Baculoviruses are small DNA viruses that infect insect cells. Baculoviral IAP inhibits apoptosis in mammalian as well as in insect cells, again demonstrating the evolutionary conservation of apoptotic pathways. Two IAP-related mammalian proteins, cIAP-1 and cIAP-2, were identified as proteins associating with the TNFR2-TRAF2-TRAF1 complex. A third IAP-related protein, ILP, has been shown to be a potent inhibitor of apoptosis when it is overexpressed in mammalian cells, whereas mutations in the fourth, NAIP, have been implicated in the pathogenesis of the neurodegenerative disorder spinal muscular atrophy. The binding properties of the various IAP-related proteins are distinct, and their relative roles in signaling pathways inhibiting apoptosis have not been fully characterized. They may constitute an important link between TNFR family member ligand binding and antiapoptotic effect.

Baculovirus encodes another potent inhibitor of apoptosis, p35, that functions as a specific inhibitor of caspases.[117] The cowpox crmA protein, although unrelated, has a similar function.[123] Mammalian proteins related to these potent and specific inhibitors have not been identified.

A number of viruses encode Bcl-2 homologues, including Epstein-Barr virus (EBV), African swine fever virus, and adenovirus.[124–126] The adenovirus homologue E1B 19kDa has low sequence similarity to Bcl-2 but was used as a probe to identify three novel proteins that also interact with Bcl-2.[124] These proteins may play important roles in the regulation and/or function of Bcl-2, and the low sequence conservation may help define functional domains of Bcl-2.

EBV has been linked causally to infectious mononucleosis, Burkitt lymphoma, nasopharyngeal carcinoma, AIDS-related lymphomas, and posttransplant lymphoproliferative disorder.[127] One of the necessary components of EBV transformation is the latent membrane protein LMP1. LMP1 is a transmembrane protein that may function in part by mimicking an occupied TNFR-related antiapoptotic receptor.[105] LMP-1 has been found to interact with TRAF proteins and to activate NF-κB; this pathway has been implicated in the pathogenesis of some EBV-positive lymphomas.[128] LMP-1 also has been reported to up-regulate endogenous Bcl-2.[129] BHRF1, an EBV-encoded Bcl-2 homologue, is not expressed in viral latency and therefore is unlikely to play a role in viral transformation; however, this protein may be critical in preventing premature host cell death in the lytic cycle of the virus.

ONCOGENES AND APOPTOTIC INDUCTION

A cell may acquire mutations in any of a variety of known oncogenes that in theory would confer a growth advantage to that cell. To prevent the development of neoplasia, the body must have potent mechanisms by which to inactivate such cells. Immune surveillance may play a role in detecting such transformants, but recent evidence suggests that apoptosis plays a much more critical role: the outgrowth of such potential tumor cells may be prevented by the induction of a suicide response within a premalignant cell. The isolated up-regulation of many oncogenes has been demonstrated to result in host cell apoptosis. Overexpression of Bcl-2 or Bcl-x_L has been found to accelerate carcinogenesis, perhaps by facilitating the acquisition of mutations leading to overexpression of dominant oncogenes.[130]

Cellular Oncogenes

The proto-oncogene that has been most clearly associated with apoptotic induction is c-*myc*. The c-*myc* gene encodes a transcription factor that is up-regulated in many transformed cells and induces rapid cell proliferation.[131] However, isolated c-*myc* overexpression results in apoptosis.[19,132–134] Concomitant overexpression of the *bcl-2* gene prevents apoptosis, resulting in an immortalized, transformed phenotype.[19,134] Overexpression of both c-*myc* and *bcl-2* in lymphocytes of transgenic mice results in synergistic tumorigenesis, generating lymphoid tumors much more rapidly than either transgene alone. c-*myc*-induced apoptosis in fibroblasts can be prevented by cytokines such as insulin-like growth factor I and by high-serum growth conditions.[135]

Two models of c-*myc* function have been proposed to explain these findings[135] (Fig. 24-7). The *conflict model* proposes that c-*myc* generates a purely growth-promoting signal. Under favorable conditions, this leads to cell proliferation, but under adverse conditions, a conflict between proliferative and inhibitory signals is generated, resulting in the triggering of apoptosis. The *dual-signal model* proposes that c-*myc* concurrently generates both proliferative and apoptotic signals. Proliferation then requires the suppression of apoptosis either by cytokine signaling or by expression of antiapoptotic genes such as *bcl-2*.

The t(1;19) chromosomal translocation associated with childhood pre-B-cell leukemia generates a chimeric E2A-PBX1 transcription factor. Transgenic mice with this fusion gene under

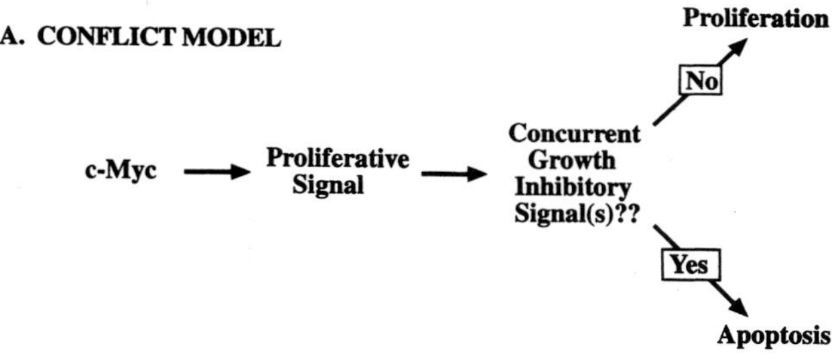

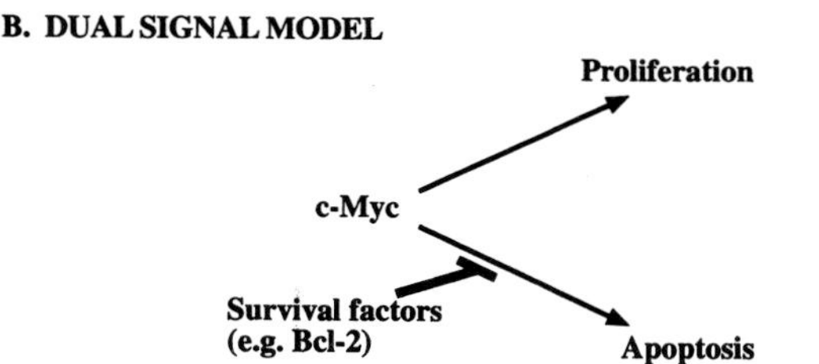

Fig. 24-7 Two models of the signaling pathways of c-*myc*. *A.* The conflict model proposes that c-*myc* generates a purely proliferative signal. Under unfavorable growth conditions, the cell produces inhibitory factors to prevent proliferation. This conflict of opposing signals affecting cell cycle progression results in an apoptotic response. Under favorable growth conditions, no conflict arises, and the cell proliferates. *B.* The dual signal model proposes that c-*myc* generates two signals, one proliferative and the other apoptotic. Proliferation in response to c-*myc* expression depends on suppression of the apoptotic response by survival signals. These signals may be generated by growth factors or antiapoptotic gene up-regulation.

lymphocyte-specific expression demonstrate increased numbers of cycling lymphocyte precursors but also widespread apoptosis in the same populations, resulting in greatly diminished numbers of lymphocytes.[136] All animals died of malignant leukemia/lymphoma within 5 months, presumably because of the outgrowth of cells that acquire secondary mutation(s) that prevent apoptosis.

Viral Oncogenes

Several viral oncogenes also provide insight into the association of oncogene expression with apoptosis. Human papillomavirus has been implicated as a causative agent in cervical carcinoma and other anogenital cancers. Oncogenic papillomaviruses encode a protein, E7, that inactivates the retinoblastoma gene product and is a potent stimulant of cell cycle progression.[137] E7 expression alone causes rapid induction of the cellular *p53* gene (which is involved in cell cycle regulation and apoptotic induction; see below), resulting in apoptotic cell death. These viruses encode a second protein, E6, which binds to and inactivates p53, preventing cell death and thus permitting oncogenic transformation. E7 also induces apoptosis by a p53-independent pathway that is poorly understood; E6 has been shown to be similarly effective in circumventing this p53-independent apoptosis in p53-negative cells.[138]

Adenovirus E1A is another oncogenic protein that induces rapid cell proliferation in transfected cells. Like papillomavirus E7 protein, the adenovirus E1A protein alone is not transforming, because it strongly triggers apoptosis.[139] Viral oncogenes depend on the concurrent expression of the *E1B* gene, which encodes two factors that may both help circumvent apoptosis. E1B 19kDa encodes a Bcl-2 homologue, and E1B 55kDa binds to and inactivates p53.[124,140]

Tumor Suppressor Genes

Tumor suppressor gene function has been found to be much more strongly linked to apoptosis than had been imagined initially. Tumor suppressors, such as p53 and the retinoblastoma gene product pRb, participate in cell cycle regulation and can inhibit proliferation by causing stage-specific cell cycle arrests. These cell cycle arrests are known as *checkpoints*.[141] In yeast, cell cycle checkpoints are thought to function to permit the repair of DNA damage and to ensure integrity of the genome before cell cycle progression. In mammalian cells, in addition to inhibiting the cell cycle progression of abnormal cells, a more important function of checkpoints may be to trigger apoptosis to delete potentially abnormal cells from the body.

p53 is the most commonly mutated gene in human malignancy, and germ-line heterozygous mutation (the Li-Fraumeni syndrome) is associated with high rates of tumorigenesis in many tissues.[142] The p53 protein is a sequence-specific transcription factor that normally is present at very low levels but is up-regulated rapidly by DNA damage or viral infection. p53 induction in response to DNA damage causes a G1-specific cell cycle arrest.[143]

The association between p53 and apoptosis has been demonstrated in vivo and in vitro. Transfection of wild-type p53 into p53-negative tumors results in apoptosis in both solid tumors and hematologic malignancies.[144,145] Loss of p53 in the evolution of experimentally induced tumors of the choroid plexus correlates directly with loss of apoptosis in vivo.[146] Thymocytes from mice with homozygous p53 inactivation demonstrate greatly increased resistance to apoptosis in response to gamma radiation and chemotherapeutic agents.[147,148]

How p53 activation triggers apoptosis is unknown. p53 has been shown to directly up-regulate the transcription of *bax*, a proapoptotic member of the *bcl-2* gene family.[149] However, Bax-deficient mice carry out p53-dependent apoptosis normally, implying that Bax regulation cannot be the primary mechanism of p53-dependent apoptotic signaling.[150] The mechanism of apoptosis induction by p53 may be indirect; strong inhibition of cell cycle progression in a cell primed for proliferation may generate a dichotomy of signals, resulting in activation of a default suicide pathway as proposed in the conflict model for c-*myc* (see Fig. 24-6).

The retinoblastoma gene product pRb also functions as a cell cycle regulator and is inactivated in many human tumors.[151] The pRb protein interacts with at least three members of the E2F family of transcription factors, inhibiting E2F activity and preventing entry into S phase of the cell cycle. Phosphorylation of pRb by cyclin-dependent kinases 4 and 6 releases the E2F factors, permitting E2F-mediated transcriptional regulation and S-phase entry.

Mutation of one *Rb* allele in mice or humans increases the likelihood of tumorigenesis in many tissues. Homozygous inactivation of the *Rb* gene in mice is embryonic lethal, causing massive apoptosis in the brain.[152,153] Again in analogy to c-*myc,* dysregulation of the controls on cell cycle progression by *Rb* inactivation generates not only rapid proliferation but also concurrent apoptotic induction.

The Link Between Proliferative Signals and Apoptosis

In the examples of cellular and viral oncogenes discussed earlier, a surprisingly tight association was found between oncogenic proliferative signals and the triggering of apoptosis. Studies of c-*myc* variants have been unsuccessful in separating the proliferative and apoptotic signals generated by this protein.[132,154] The same regions of c-*myc* that are essential for proliferation are essential for apoptosis. Incremental increases in c-*myc* expression cause parallel increases in both proliferative and apoptotic signals. Both signals are equally dependent on c-*myc* binding to its partner, Max. This unanticipated feature of oncogene activation suggests a fundamental mechanism for avoiding malignant transformation. Gene expression that generates potent proliferative signals may coordinately increase the apoptotic susceptibility of the cell, resulting in cell death unless strong antiapoptotic signals are present. A major function of cell cycle regulatory pathways may be to inextricably link proliferative induction to increased apoptotic sensitivity.

APOPTOSIS AND THE MULTIHIT MODEL OF ONCOGENESIS

The *multihit model* of oncogenesis holds that multiple genetic mutations must occur within a single cell to produce fully malignant transformation. The fact that many potentially oncogenic mutations trigger apoptosis suggests that mutations that inhibit apoptotic control are necessary for tumor cells to grow to sufficient mass to cause problems for the host. In order for the c-*myc* gene to be transforming, a prior event must have occurred to prevent apoptotic induction. *Rb* inactivation alone may promote p53-dependent cell death rather than tumorigenesis unless apoptosis in inhibited. Activation of oncogenes and inactivation of tumor suppressor genes may be insufficient to promote significant expansion of tumor cells without the tumor cell also acquiring defects in its ability to undergo apoptosis. Mutations in genes that affect apoptosis also may be central to the ability of tumor cells to metastasize. Metastatic cells must survive in the absence of many of the survival signals their normal counterparts receive from the extracellular milieu (see Fig. 24-4).

Mutation of apoptotic control genes without secondary mutations in growth regulatory genes similarly is insufficient for tumorigenesis. The characteristic t(14;18) translocation of the *bcl-2* gene has been detected at a low frequency in normal lymphoid hyperplasia in response to infection.[155] The rearrangement has been reported to be detectable by PCR in the peripheral blood of up to 55 percent of the population, and the frequency of the rearrangement increases with age.[156] Cells carrying the translocation may represent a long-lived premalignant population that has the potential to progress to lymphoma with the accumulation of additional mutations.

Inactivation of p53 is unique in eliminating an important negative regulatory control on proliferation while making the cell more resistant to apoptosis in response to aberrant replication. The double-edged effect of p53 inactivation may explain why this mutation is seen frequently in a wide array of human malignancies and also why p53 inactivation is such a frequent target of early gene expression by oncogenic viruses.

APOPTOSIS AND CANCER THERAPY

Chemotherapeutic Resistance

One of the most important problems that arise in cancer patients undergoing treatment is the development of tumors with multidrug resistance. This can arise *de novo* but is especially prevalent in previously treated patients. The multidrug resistance phenotype can be explained in a minority of cases by up-regulation of the *mdr-1* gene, which encodes a cell membrane pump that can expel a defined collection of antineoplastic agents.[157] A more general mechanism of multidrug resistance has been elucidated that involves apoptosis control.

Traditionally, tumoricidal radiation and chemotherapy were thought to function by causing irreparable metabolic or physical damage to cancer cells, resulting in cell necrosis. However, studies of cells killed by radiation and any of a wide variety of antineoplastic agents have demonstrated that these modalities induce typical apoptotic changes in the cells.[158] Cells exposed to chemotherapy are not passively killed by the drug. Instead, most cells appear to die because intracellular surveillance mechanisms recognize the alterations of normal cell physiology caused by chemotherapy and induce apoptosis. These observations suggest that a major mechanism for chemotherapeutic resistance in tumors may result from the inhibition of apoptosis.

Studies of tumor cell lines in vitro as well as tumors arising *in vivo* have demonstrated the relevance of this idea. Overexpression of Bcl-2 or Bcl-x_L can increase tumor resistance to multiple chemotherapeutic agents and radiation.[159–164] Agents that have been tested in such assays represent essentially all major categories of antineoplastic drugs, including antimetabolites, anthracyclines, DNA crosslinking agents, topoisomerase inhibitors, and mitotic spindle inhibitors. Cells overexpressing Bcl-x_L that are exposed to chemotherapeutic agents arrest at the characteristic cell cycle stages where individual drugs are known to have their effects.[164] Subsequent removal of the chemotherapeutic agents from the media permits cell cycle progression and proliferation, confirming the viability of the treated cells. High levels of endogenous Bcl-x_L expression have been reported in tumor cells after exposure of those cells to chemotherapy. Bcl-x_L and Bcl-2 expression in neuroblastoma decreases apoptotic sensitivity to chemotherapy.[161,165] High-level Bcl-2 expression has been correlated with chemotherapeutic resistance in acute myeloid leukemia.[166,167]

Inactivation of p53 similarly has been associated with increased chemotherapeutic resistance, perhaps by the loss of p53-dependent apoptosis.[168] p53-independent mechanisms also can detect DNA damage, cause cell cycle arrest, and initiate apoptosis. Chemotherapeutic mutagens or radiation causes cell cycle arrest and apoptosis in tumors of p53-negative mice.[169] Expression of antiapoptotic control genes therefore may be a more potent mechanism of chemotherapeutic resistance than p53 inactivation.

Antiapoptotic Gene Expression and Mutation Rate

Overexpression of antiapoptotic genes in cancer cells abrogates a major protective mechanism against the expansion of cells that demonstrate abnormal cell cycle progression. Cells that suffer abnormal mitosis, chromosome loss, or major genomic mutation normally are prevented from attempting replication by cell cycle checkpoints that trigger apoptotic cell death. Up-regulation of antiapoptotic gene expression permits the survival and propagation of such mutant cells and thus would be expected to greatly augment the rate of accumulation of genetic errors. Since inhibition of apoptosis appears to be a common step in oncogenesis, this mechanism could explain the high degree of chromosomal instability characteristic of cancer cells.

Cancer treatments may further accelerate mutagenesis. DNA-damaging chemotherapeutic agents and radiation are inherently mutagenic. Cells exposed to high levels of these mutagens are killed unless apoptotic pathways are blocked. Antiapoptotic gene expression therefore may promote tumor evolution by allowing the propagation of chemotherapy-induced mutations.

Inhibition of apoptosis in cells exposed to chemotherapeutic agents may promote chromosomal aberrations. An example of this type of derangement is seen in cells exposed to vincristine or nocodazole, agents that inhibit mitotic spindle formation.[170] These agents induce cell cycle arrest and apoptosis in tumor cells. Cells overexpressing Bcl-x_L arrest but do not die in response to these agents and on drug removal begin to proliferate without completing mitosis, thus becoming polyploid. Loss of appropriate response to aberrant mitoses is thought to play an important role in the chromosomal instability characteristic of most advanced malignancies.[171]

Rational Cancer Treatment Design

As described here, apoptotic regulation has been found to be a critical determinant of tumorigenesis and the therapeutic responsiveness of tumors. One of the challenges that is only beginning to be addressed is the translation of this new perspective on cancer biology into meaningful changes in clinical practice. As the associations between patient outcome and the activity of various antiapoptotic genes become clearer, screening of tumors for the expression of apoptotic regulatory genes may help define prognostic categories and influence treatment decisions.

More fundamentally, the study of apoptotic mechanisms affected by malignancy offers an opportunity for the consideration of entirely new approaches to the treatment of cancer. The unexpected finding that most successful anticancer treatments, including radiotherapy, chemotherapy, and hormonal modulation, function by apoptotic induction has generated increasing interest in therapies specifically targeted to apoptotic pathways. Such treatment may have much less nonspecific toxicity than do traditional antineoplastic agents. Pilot studies of anti-Bcl-2 antibodies and antisense *bcl-2* oligonucleotides as anticancer agents are ongoing.[172,173] Disruption of LMP-1 signaling pathways could play an important role in the treatment of EBV-associated malignancies and lymphoproliferative disorders. Modification of apoptotic pathways by influencing the activity or accessibility of cell surface receptors has not been fully explored. Therapy designed to stimulate apoptosis in target cells may play an increasingly central role in the treatment of cancer.

CONCLUSIONS

A great deal of information about the regulation of apoptosis at the molecular level has been acquired in the years since its initial phenotypic description. In mammalian cells, although many levels of apoptotic regulation have been defined, much of the control appears to be concentrated in a central pathway consisting of highly evolutionarily conserved regulatory proteins. Determination of the apoptotic threshold of a cell depends on interactions between positive and negative signaling elements in this central apoptotic pathway. A number of external conditions, including the presence of growth factors, cytokines, and the membrane proteins of neighboring cells, influence the balance of the central apoptotic regulators through multiple cell surface receptors and intracellular signaling pathways.

The control of apoptosis is integral to many aspects of cancer biology. Apoptosis serves as an essential mechanism to prevent the proliferation of cells with potentially transforming mutations. As a corollary, inhibition of apoptosis may lead to the accumulation of cells with a higher mutation rate, thus accelerating malignant transformation. Cell cycle checkpoint controls play a critical role in detecting aberrant cells and initiating apoptosis. Viral and cellular oncoproteins, by driving cell cycle progression, often are strong inducers of apoptosis. Most antineoplastic therapies function by triggering apoptosis in sensitive cells. Resistance to treatment can result from specific inhibition of apoptotic signaling. Apoptotic inhibition in tumor cells exposed to chemotherapy or radiation may increase mutation rate and hasten tumor evolution.

The study of apoptosis has not had a dramatic effect on clinical practice in oncology. However, the conceptual changes that have derived from apoptosis research have potentially wide clinical ramifications. We can look forward to many more trials of cancer therapy based on the modification of the controlling pathways of apoptotic regulation.

REFERENCES

1. Kerr JFR, Wyllie AH, Currie AR: Apoptosis: A basic biological phenomenon with wide-ranging implications in tissue kinetics. *Br J Cancer* **26**:239,1972.
2. Wyllie AH, Kerr JFR, Currie AR: Cell death: The significance of apoptosis. *Int Rev Cytol* **68**:251, 1980.
3. Thompson CB: Apoptosis in the pathogenesis and treatment of disease. *Science* **267**:1456, 1995.
4. Gougeon M-L, Montagnier L: Apoptosis in AIDS. *Science* **260**:1269, 1993.
5. Mountz JD, Wu J, Cheng J, Zhou T: Autoimmune disease: A problem of defective apoptosis. *Arthritis Rheum* **37**:1415, 1994.
6. Margolis RL, Chuang D-M, Post RM: Programmed cell death: Implications for neuropsychiatric disorders. *Biol Psychiatry* **35**:946, 1994.
7. Harrington EA, Fanidi A, Evan GI: Oncogenes and cell death. *Curr Opin Genet Dev* **4**:120, 1994.
8. Ellis RE, Yan J, Horvitz HR: Mechanism and function of cell death. *Annu Rev Cell Biol* **7**:663, 1991.
9. Raff MC: Social controls on cell survival and cell death. *Nature* **356**:397, 1992.
10. Oppenheim RW: Cell death during development of the nervous system. *Annu Rev Neurosci* **14**:453, 1991.
11. Fadok VA, Voelker DR, Campbell PA, Cohen JJ, Bratton DL, Henson PM: Exposure of phosphatidylserine on the surface of apoptotic lymphocytes triggers specific recognition and removal by macrophages. *J Immunol* **148**:2207, 1992.
12. Fadok VA, Savill JS, Haslett C, Bratton DL, Doherty DE, Campbell PA, Henson PM: Different populations of macrophages use either the vitronectin receptor or the phosphatidylserine receptor to recognize and remove apoptotic cells. *J Immunol* **149**:4029, 1992.
13. Hall SE, Savill JS, Henson PM, Haslett C: Apoptic neutrophils are phagocytosed by fibroblasts with participation of the fibroblast vitronectin receptor and involvement of a mannose/fructose-specific lactin. *J Immunol* **153**:3218, 1994.
14. Tsujimoto Y, Finger LR, Yunis J, Nowell PC, Croce CM: Cloning of the chromosome breakpoint of neoplastic B cells with the t(14;18) chromosome translocation. *Science* **226**:1097, 1984.
15. Tsujimoto Y, Gorman J, Cossman J, Jaffe E, Croce CM: The t(14;18) chromosome translocations involved in B-cell neoplasms result from mistakes in VDJ joining. *Science* **229**:1390, 1985.
16. Bakhshi A, Jensen JP, Goldman P, Wright JJ, McBride OW, Epstein AL, Korsmeyer SJ: Cloning the chromosomal breakpoint of t(14;18) human lymphomas: Clustering around JH on chromosome 14 and near a transcriptional unit on 18. *Cell* **41**:889, 1985.
17. Cleary ML, Sklar J: Nucleotide sequence of a t(14;18) chromosomal breakpoint in follicular lymphoma and demonstration of a breakpoint cluster region near a transcriptionally active locus on chromosome 18. *Proc Natl Acad Sci USA* **82**:7439, 1985.
18. Longo DL, DeVita VT, Jaffe ES, Mauch P, Urba WJ: Lymphocytic lymphomas, in DeVita VT, Hellman S, Rosenberg SA (eds): *Cancer: Principles and Practice of Oncology*, 4th ed.Philadelphia, Lippincott, 1993.
19. Vaux DL, Cory S, Adams JM: Bcl-2 gene promotes haemopoietic cell survival and co-operates with c-Myc to immortalize pre-B cells. *Nature* **335**:440, 1988.
20. Yang E, Korsmeyer SJ: Molecular thanatopsis: A discourse on the BCL2 family and cell death. *Blood* **88**:386, 1996.
21. Korsmeyer SJ: Bcl-2 initiates a new category of oncogenes: Regulators of cell death. *Blood* **80**:879, 1992.

22. Arends MJ, Wyllie AH: Apoptosis: Mechanisms and roles in pathology. *Int Rev Exp Pathol* **32**:223, 1991.
23. Horvitz HR, Shaham S, Hengartner MO: The genetics of programmed cell death in the nematode *Caenorhabditis elegans*. *Cold Spring Harbor Symp Quant Biol* **59**:377, 1994.
24. Ellis RE, Horvitz HR: Genetic control of programmed cell death in the nematode *C.* elegans. *Cell* **44**:817, 1986.
25. Hengartner MO, Ellis RE, Horvitz HR: Caenorhabditis elegans gene ced-9 protects cells from programmed cell death. *Nature* **356**:494, 1992.
26. Shaham S, Horvitz HR: Developing *Caenorhabditis elegans* neurons may contain both cell-death protective and killer activities. *Gene Dev* **10**:578, 1996.
27. Wu D, Wallen HD, Nunez G: Interaction and regulation of subcellular localization of CED-4 by CED-9. *Science* **275**:1126, 1997.
28. Chinnauyan AR, O'Rourke K, Lane BR, Dixit VM: Interaction of CED-4 with CED-3 and CED-9: a molecular framework for cell death. *Science* **275**:1122, 1997.
29. Seshagiri S, Miller LK: *Caenorhabditis elegans* CED-4 stimulates CED-3 processing and CED-3-induced apoptosis. *Curr Biol* **7**:455, 1997.
30. Chinnauyan AR, Shaudhary D, O'Rourke K, Koonin EV, Dixit VM: Role of CED-4 in the activation of CED-3. *Nature* **388**:728, 1997.
31. Irmler M, Hofmann K, Vaux D, Tschopp J: Direct physical interaction between the *Caenorhabditis elegans* "death proteins" CED-3 and CED-4. *FEBS Lett* **406**:189, 1997.
32. Hengartner MO, Horvitz HR: *C.* elegans cell survival gene ced-9 encodes a functional homolog of the mammalian proto-oncogene bcl-2. *Cell* **76**:665, 1994.
33. Vaux DL, Weissman IL, Kim SK: Prevention of programmed cell death in *Caenorhabditis elegans* by human bcl-2. *Science* **258**:1955, 1992.
34. Zou H, Benzel WJ, Liu X, Lutschg A, Wang X: Apaf-1, a human protein homologous to *C.* elegans CED-4, participates in cytochrome c-dependent activation of caspase-3. *Cell* **90**:405, 1997.
35. Yan J, Shahm S, Ledoux S, Ellis HM, Horvitz HR: The *C.* elegans cell death gene ced-3 encodes a protein similar to mammalian interleukin-1β-converting enzyme. *Cell* **75**:641, 1993.
36. Boise LH, Gonzalez-Garcia M, Postema CE, Ding L, Lindsten T, Turka LA, Mao X, Nunes G, Thompson CB: bcl-x, a bcl-2-related gene that functions as a dominant regulator of apoptotic cell death. *Cell* **74**:597, 1993.
37. Oltvai ZN, Milliman CL, Korsmeyer SJ: Bcl-2 heterodimerizes in vivo with a conserved homolog, Bax, that accelerates programmed cell death. *Cell* **74**:609, 1993.
38. Sedlak TW, Oltvai ZN, Yang E, Wang K, Boise LH, Thompson CB, Korsmeyer SJ: Multiple Bcl-2 family members demonstrate selective dimerizations with Bax. *Proc Natl Acad Sci USA* **92**:7834, 1995.
39. Farrow SN, White JHM, Martinou I, Raven T, Pun K-T, Grinham CJ, Martinou J-C, Brown R: Cloning of a bcl-2 homologue by interaction with adenovirus E1B 19K. *Nature* **374**:731, 1995.
40. Chittenden T, Harrington EA, O'Connor R, Flemington C, Lutz RJ, Evan GI, Guild BC: Induction of apoptosis by the Bcl-2 homologue Bak. *Nature* **374**:733, 1995.
41. Kiefer MC, Brauer MJ, Powers VC, Wu JJ, Umansky SR, Tomei LD, Barr PJ: Modulation of apoptosis by the widely distributed Bcl-2 homologue Bak. *Nature* **374**:736, 1995.
42. Yang E, Zha J, Jockel J, Boise LH, Thompson CB, Korsmeyer SJ: Bad, a heterodimeric partner for Bcl-x_L and Bcl-2, displaces Bax and promotes cell death. *Cell* **80**:285, 1995.
43. Sato T, Hanada M, Bodrug S, Irie S, Iwama N, Boise LH, Thompson CB, Golemis E, Fong L, Wang H-G, Reed JC: Interactions among members of the Bcl-2 protein family analyzed with a yeast two-hybrid system. *Proc Natl Acad Sci USA* **91**:9238, 1994.
44. Kelekar A, Thompson CB: Bcl-2 family proteins: The role of the BH3 domain in apoptosis. *Trends Cell Biol* **8**:324, 1998.
45. Muchmore SW, Sattler M, Liang H, Meadows RP, Harlan JE, Yoon HS, Nettesheim D, Chang B, Thompson CB, Wong S, Ng S-C, Fesik SW: X-ray and NMR structure of human Bcl-x_L, an inhibitor of programmed cell death. *Nature* **381**:335, 1996.
46. Cramer WA, Heymann JB, Schendel SL, Deriy BN, Cohen FS, Elkins PA, Stauffacher CB: Structure-function of the channel-forming colicins. *Annu Rev Biophys Biomol Struct* **24**:611, 1995.
47. Monoghan P, Robertson D, Amos T, Dyer M, Mason D, Greaves M: Ultrastructural localizations of Bcl-2 protein. *J Histochem Cytochem* **40**:1819, 1992.
48. Krajewski S, Tanaka S, Takayama S, Schibler MJ, Fenton W, Reed JC: Investigation of the subcellular distribution of the bcl-2 oncoprotein: Residence in the nuclear envelope, endoplasmic reticulum, and outer mitochondrial membranes. *Cancer Res* **53**:4701, 1993.
49. Nguyen M, Miller DG, Yong VW, Korsmeyer SJ, Shore GC: Targeting of Bcl-2 to the mitochondrial outer membrane by a COOH-terminal signal anchor sequence. *J Biol Chem* **268**:25265, 1993.
50. Zamzami N, Marchetti P, Castedo M, Zanin C, Vayssiüre J-L, Petit PX, Kroemer G: Reduction in mitochondrial potential constitutes an early irreversible step of programmed lymphocyte death in vivo. *J Exp Med* **181**:1661, 1995.
51. Castedo M, Hirsch T, Susin SA, Zamzami N, Marchetti P, Macho A, Kroemer G: Sequential acquisition of mitochondrion and plasma membrane alterations during early lymphocyte apoptosis. *J Immunol* **157**:512, 1996.
52. Green DR, Reed JC: Mitochondria and apoptosis. *Science* **281**:1309, 1998.
53. Zamzami N, Marchetti P, Castedo M, Decaudin D, Macho A, Hirsch T, Susin SA, Petit PX, Mignotte B, Kroemer G: Sequential reduction of mitochondrial transmembrane potential and generation of reactive oxygen species in early programmed cell death. *J Exp Med* **182**:367, 1996.
54. Zamzami N, Susin SA, Marchetti P, Hirsh T, Gomez-Monterrey I, Castedo M, Kroemer G: Mitochondrial control of nuclear apoptosis. *J Exp Med* **183**:1533, 1996.
55. Liu X, Kim CN, Yang J, Jemmerson R, Wang X: Induction of apoptotic program in cell-free extracts: Requirement for dATP and cytochrome c. *Cell* **86**:147, 1996.
56. Vander Heiden MG, Chandel NS, Williamson EK, Schumacker PT, Thompson CB: Bcl-x_L regulates the membrane potential and volume homeostasis of mitochondria. *Cell* **9**:627, 1997.
57. Yang J, Liu X, Bhalla K, Kim CN, Ibrado AM, Cai J, Peng TI, Jones DP, Wang X: Prevention of apoptosis by Bcl-2: Release of cytochrome c from mitochondria blocked. *Science* **275**:1129, 1997.
58. Kluck RM, Bossy-Wetzel E, Green DR, Newmeyer DD: The release of cytochrome c from mitochondria: A primary site for Bcl-2 regulation of apoptosis. *Science* **275**:1132, 1997.
59. Rosse T, Olivier R, Monney L, Rager M, Conus S, Fellay I, Jansen B, Borner C: Bcl-2 prolongs cell survival after Bax-induced release of cytochrome c. *Nature* **391**:496, 1998.
60. Huang DC, Adams JM, Cory S: The conserved N-terminal BH4 domain of Bcl-2 homologues is essential for inhibition of apoptosis and interaction with CED-4. *EMBO J* **17**:1029, 1998.
61. Li P, Nijhawan D, Budihardjo I, Srinivasula SM, Ahmad M, Alnemri ES, Wang X: Cytochrome c and dATP-dependent formation of Apaf-1/caspase-9 complex initiates an apoptotic protease cascade. *Cell* **91**:479, 1997.
62. Hu Y, Benedict MA, Wu D, Inohara N, Nunez G: Bcl-x_L interacts with Apaf-1 and inhibits Apaf-1-dependent caspase-9 activation. *Proc Natl Acad Sci USA* **95**:4386, 1998.
63. Pan G, O'Rourke K, Dixit VM: Caspase-9, Bcl-x_L, and Apaf-1 form a ternary complex. *J Biol Chem* **273**:5841, 1998.
64. AkES, Livingston DJ, Nicholson DW, Salvesen G, Thornberry NA, Wong WW, Yuan J: Human ICE/CED-3 protease nomenclature. *Cell* **87**:171, 1996.
65. Nicholson, DW, Thornberry NA: Caspases: Killer proteases. *TIBS* **22**:299, 1997.
66. Talanian RV, Quinlan C, Trautz S, Hackett MC, Mankovich JA, Banach D, Ghayur T, Brady KD, Wong WW: Substrate specificities of caspase family proteases. *J Biol Chem* **272**:9677, 1997.
67. Van de Craen M, Vandenabeele P, Declercq W, Van den Brande I, Van Loo G, Molemans F, Schotte P, Van Criekinge W, Beyaert R, Fiers W: Characterization of seven murine caspase family members. *FEBS Lett* **403**:61, 1997.
68. Vincenz C, Dixit VM: Fas-associated death domain protein interleukin-1 beta-converting enzyme 2 (FLICE2), an ICE/Ced-3 homologue, is proximally involved in CD95- and p55-mediated death signaling. *J Biol Chem* **272**:6578, 1997.
69. Humke EW, Dixit VM: ERICE, a novel FLICE-activatable caspase. *J Biol Chem* **272**:15702, 1998.
70. Miura M, Zhu H, Rotello R, Hartwieg EA, Yuan J: Induction of apoptosis in fibroblasts by IL-1βconverting enzyme, a mammalian homolog of the *C.* elegans cell death gene ced-3. *Cell* **75**:653, 1993.
71. Rabizadeh S, LaCount DJ, Friesen, PD, Bredesen DE: Expression of the baculovirus p35 gene inhibits mammalian neuronal cell death. *J Neurochem* **61**:2318, 1993.
72. Duan H, Chinnaiyan AM, Hudson PL, Wing JP, He WW, Dixit VM: ICE-LAP3, a novel mammalian homologue of the *Caenorhabditis*

elegans cell death protein CED-3, is activated during Fas- and tumor necrosis factor-induced apoptosis. *J Biol Chem* **369**:621, 1996.
73. Walker NP, Talanian RV, Brady KD, Dang LC, Bump NJ, Ferenz CR, Franklin S, Ghayur T, Hackett MC, Hammill LD, Herzog L, Hugunin M, Houy W, Mankovich JA, McGuiness L, Orlewicz E, Paskind M, Pratt CA, Reis P, Summani A, Terranova M, Welch JP, Xiong L, Moller A, Tracey DE, Kamen R, Wong WW: Crystal structure of the cysteine protease interleukin-1 beta-converting enzyme: A (p20/p10)2 homodimer. *Cell* **78**:343, 1995.
74. Alnemri ES, Fernandes-Alnemri T, Litwack G: Cloning and expression of four novel isoforms of human interleukin-1 beta converting enzyme with different apoptotic activities. *J Biol Chem* **270**:4312, 1995.
75. Wang L, Miura M, Bergeron L, Zhu H, Yuan J: Ich-1, an Ice/ced-3-related gene, encodes both positive and negative regulators of programmed cell death. *Cell* **78**:739, 1994.
76. Fernandes-Alnemri T, Litwack G, Alnemri ES: Mch2, a new member of the apoptotic CED-3/ICE cysteine protease gene family. *Cancer Res* **55**:2737, 1995.
77. Duan H, Orth K, Chinnaiyan AM, Poirier GG, Froelich CJ, He W-W, Dixit VM: ICE-LAP6, a novel member of the ICE/Ced-3 gene family, is activated by the cytotoxic T cell protease granzyme B. *J Biol Chem* **271**:16720, 1996.
78. Woo M, Hakem R, Soengas MS, Duncan GS, Shahinian A, Kagi D, Hakem A, McCurrach M, Khoo W, Kaufman SA, Senaldi G, Howard T, Lowe SW, Mak TW: Essential contribution of caspase 3/CPP32 to apoptosis and its associated nuclear changes. *Genes Dev* **12**:806, 1998.
79. Fraser A, Evan G: A license to kill. *Cell* **85**:781, 1996.
80. Nagata S: Apoptosis by death factor. *Cell* **88**:355, 1997.
81. Rao L, Perez D, White E: Lamin proteolysis facilitates nuclear events during apoptosis. *J Cell Biol* **135**:1441, 1996.
82. Kayalor C, Ord T, Testa P, Zhong L, Bredsen DE: Cleavage of actin by interleukin 1β-converting enzyme to reverse DNase I inhibition. *Proc Natl Acad Sci USA* **93**:2234, 1996.
83. Widmann C, Gibson S, Johnson GL: Caspase-dependent cleavage of signaling proteins during apoptosis: A turn-off mechanism for anti-apoptotic signals. *J Biol Chem* **273**:7141, 1998.
84. Ravi R, Bedi A, Fuchs EJ, Bedi A: CD95 (Fas)-induced caspase-mediated proteolysis of NF-κB. *Cancer Res* **58**:882, 1998.
85. Chen L, Marechal V, Moreau J, Levine AJ, Chen J: Proteolytic cleavage of the mdm2 oncoprotein during apoptosis. *J Biol Chem* **272**:22966, 1997.
86. Tan X, Martin SJ, Green DR, Wang JYJ: Degradation of retinoblastoma protein in tumor necrosis factor- and CD95-induced cell death. *J Biol Chem* **272**:9613, 1997.
87. Janicke RU, Walker PA, Lin XY, Porter AG: Specific cleavage of the retinoblastoma protein by an ICE-like protease in apoptosis. *EMBO J* **15**:6969, 1996.
88. Casciola-Rosen L, Nicholson DW, Chong T, Rowan KR, Thornberry NA, Miller DK, Rosen A: Apopain/CPP32 cleaves proteins that are essential for cellular repair: A fundamental principle of apoptotic death. *J Exp Med* **183**:1957, 1996.
89. Cheng EH, Kirsch DG, Clem RJ, Ravi R, Kastan MB, Bedi A, Ueno K, Hardwick JM: Conversion of Bcl-2 to a Bax-like death effector by caspases. *Science* **278**:1966, 1997.
90. Clem RJ, Cheng EH, Karp CL, Kirsch DG, Ueno K, Takahashi A, Kastan MB, Griffin DE, Earnshaw WC, Veliuona MA, Hardwick JM: Modulation of cell death by Bcl-x_L through caspase interaction. *Proc Natl Acad Sci USA* **95**:554, 1998.
91. Lazebnik YA, Kaufmann SH, Disnoyers S, Poirer GG, Earnshaw WC: Cleavage of poly(ADP-ribose) polymerase by a proteinase with properties like ICE. *Nature* **371**:346, 1994.
92. Nicholson DW, Ali A, Thornberry NA, Vaillancourt JP, Ding CK, Gallant M, Gareau Y, Griffin PR, Labelle M, Lazebnik YA, Munday NA, Raju SM, Smulson ME, Yamin T-T, Yu VL, Miller DK: Identification and inhibition of the ICE/CED-3 protease necessary for mammalian apoptosis. *Nature* **376**:37, 1995.
93. Tewari M, Quan LT, O'Rourke K, Desnoyers S, Zeng Z, Beidler DR, Poirier GG, Salvesen GS, Dixit VM: Yama/CPP32 beta, a mammalian homolog of CED-3, is a CrmA-inhibitable protease that cleaves the death substrate poly(ADP-ribose) polymerase. *Cell* **81**:801, 1995.
94. Wang Z-Q, Auer B, Stingle L, Berghammer H, Haidacher D, Schweiger M, Wagner EF: Mice lacking ADPRT and poly(ADP-ribosyl)ation develop normally but are susceptible to skin disease. *Gene Dev* **9**:509, 1995.
95. Boise LH, Thompson CB: Bcl-x_L can inhibit apoptosis in cells that have undergone Fas-induced protease activation. *Proc Natl Acad Sci USA* **94**:3759, 1997.
96. Bazzoni F, Beutler B: The tumor necrosis factor ligand and receptor families. *N Engl J Med* **334**:1717, 1996.
97. Chinnaiyan AM, O'Rourke K, Tewari M, Dixit VM: FADD, a novel death domain-containing protein, interacts with the death domain of Fas and initiates apoptosis. *Cell* **81**:505, 1995.
98. Stanger BZ, Leder P, Lee T, Kim E, Seed B: RIP: A novel protein containing a death domain that interacts with FAS/Apo-1 (CD95) in yeast and causes cell death. *Cell* **81**:513, 1995.
99. Hsu H, Xiong J, Goeddel DV: The TNF receptor 1-associated protein TRADD signals cell death and NF-κB activation. *Cell* **81**:495, 1995.
100. Hsu H, Shu H-B, Pan M-G, Goeddel DV: TRADD-TRAF2 and TRADD-FADD interactions define two distinct TNF receptor 1 signal transduction pathways. *Cell* **84**:299, 1996.
101. Liu Z-G, Hsu H, Goeddel DV, Karin M: Dissection of TNF receptor 1 effector functions: JNK activation is not linked to apoptosis while NF-κB activation prevents cell death. *Cell* **87**:565. 1996.
102. Boldin MP, Goncharov TM, Goltsev YV, Wallach D: Involvement of MACH, a novel MORT/FADD-interacting protease, in Fas/APO-1- and TNF receptor-induced cell death. *Cell* **85**:803, 1996.
103. Muzio M, Chinnaiyan AM, Kischkel FC, O'Rourke K, Shevchenko A, Ni J, Scaffidi C, Bretz JD, Zhang M, Gentz R, Mann M, Krammer PH, Peter ME, Dixit VM: FLICE, a novel FADD-homologous ICE/CED-3-like protease, is recruited to the CD95 (Fas/Apo-1) death-inducing signaling complex. *Cell* **85**:817, 1996.
104. Rothe M, Wong SC, Henzel WJ, Goeddel DV: A novel family of putative signal transducers associated with cytoplasmic domain of the 75 kDa tumor necrosis factor receptor family. *Cell* **78**:681, 1994.
105. Mosialos G, Birkenbach M, Yalamanchili R, VanArsdale T, Ware C, Kieff E: The Epstein-Barr virus transforming protein LMP1 engages signaling proteins for the tumor necrosis factor receptor family. *Cell* **80**:389, 1995.
106. Chang G, Cleary AM, Ye Z, Hong DI, Lederman S, Baltimore D: Involvement of CRAF1, a relative of TRAF, in CD40 signaling. *Science* **267**:1494, 1995.
107. Hu HM, O'Rourke K, Boguski MS, Dixit VM: A novel RING finger protein interacts with the cytoplasmic domain of CD40. *J Biol Chem* **269**:30069, 1994.
108. Sato T, Irie S, Reed JC: A novel member of the TRAF family of putative signal transducing proteins binds to the cytoplasmic domain of CD40. *FEBS Lett* **358**:113, 1995.
109. Nakano H, Oshima H, Chung W, Williams-Abbott L, Ware CF, Yagita H, Okumura K: TRAF5, an activator of NF-κB and putative signal transducer for the lymphotoxin-β receptor. *J Biol Chem* **271**:14661, 1996.
110. Gedrich RW, Gilfillan MC, Duckett CS, VanDongen JL, Thompson CB: CD30 contains two binding sites with different specificities for members of the tumor necrosis factor receptor-associated factor family of signal transducing proteins. *J Biol Chem* **271**:12852, 1996.
111. Ishida T, Tojo T, Aoki T, Kobayashi N, Ohishi T, Watanabe T, Yamamoto T, Inoue J-I: TRAF5, a novel tumor necrosis factor receptor-associated factor family protein, mediates CD40 signaling. *Proc Natl Acad Sci USA* **93**:9437, 1996.
112. Cao Z, Xiong J, Takeuchi M, Kurama T, Goeddel: TRAF6 is a signal transducer for interleukin-1. *Nature* **383**:443, 1996.
113. Ishida T, Mizuchima S-I, Azuma S, Kobayashi N, Tojo T, Suzuki K, Aizawa S, Watanabe T, Mosalios G, Kieff E, Yamamoto T, Inoue J-I: Identification of TRAF6, a novel tumor necrosis factor receptor-associated factor protein that mediates signaling from an amino-terminal domain of the CD40 cytoplasmic region. *J Biol Chem* **271**:28745, 1996.
114. Rothe M, Sarma V, Dixit VM, Goeddel DV: TRAF2-mediated activation of NF-κB by TNF receptor 2 and CD40. *Science* **269**:1424, 1995.
115. Regnier CH, Tomasetto C, Moog-Lutz C, Chenard M-P, Wendling C, Basset P, Rio MC: Presence of a new conserved domain in CART1, a novel member of the tumor necrosis factor receptor-associated protein family, which is expressed in breast carcinoma. *J Biol Chem* **270**:25715, 1995.
116. Masson R, Regnier CH, Chenard MP, Wendling C, Mattei M-G, Tomasetto C, Rio M-C: Tumor necrosis factor receptor associated factor 4 (TRAF4) expression pattern during mouse development. *Mech Dev* **71**:187, 1998.
117. Clem RJ, Miller LK: Control of programmed cell death by the baculovirus genes p34 and iap. *Mol Cell Biol* **14**:5212, 1994.
118. Roy N, Mahadevan MS, McLean M, Shutler G, Yaraghi Z, Farahani R, Baird S, Besner-Johnston A, Lefebvre C, Kang X, Salih M, Aubry H, Tamai K, Guan X, Ioannou P, Crawford TO, de Jong PJ, Surh L,

Ikeda J-E, Korneluk RG, MacKenzie A: The gene for neuronal apoptosis inhibitory protein is partially deleted in individuals with spinal muscular atrophy. *Cell* **80**:167, 1995.

119. Rothe M, Pan M-G, Henzel WJ, Ayres TM, Goeddel DV: The TNFR2-TRAF signaling complex contains two novel proteins related to baculoviral inhibitor of apoptosis proteins. *Cell* **83**:1243, 1995.
120. Duckett CS, Nava VE, Gedrich RW, Clem RJ, VanDongen JL, Gilfillan MC, Shiels H, Hardwick JM, Thompson CB: A conserved family of cellular genes related to the baculovirus iap gene and encoding apoptosis inhibitors. *EMBO J* **15**:2685, 1996
121. Liston P, Roy N, Tamai K, Lefebvre C, Baird S, Cherton-Horvat G, Farahani R, McLean M, Ikeda JE, MacKenzie A, Korneluk RG: Suppression of apoptosis in mammalian cells by NAIP and a related family of IAP genes. *Nature* **379**:349, 1996.
122. Uren AG, Pakusch M, Hawkins CH, Puls KL, Vaux DL: Cloning and expression of apoptosis inhibitory protein homologs that function to inhibit apoptosis and/or bind tumor necrosis factor receptor-associated factors. *Proc Natl Acad Sci USA* **93**:4974, 1996.
123. Ray CA, Black RA, Kronheim SR, Greenstreet TA, Sleath PR, Salvesen GS, Pickup DJ: Viral inhibition of inflammation: Cowpox virus encodes an inhibitor of the interleukin-1β-converting enzyme. *Cell* **69**:597, 1992.
124. Boyd JM, Malstron S, Subramanian T, Venkatesh LK, Schaeper U, Elangovan B, Sa-Eipper C, Chinnadurai G: Adenovirus E1B 19 kDa and Bcl-2 proteins interact with a common set of cellular proteins. *Cell* **79**:341, 1994.
125. Henderson S, Huen D, Rowe M, Dawson C, Johnson G, Rickson A: Epstein-Barr virus-coded BHRF1 protein, a viral homologue of Bcl-2, protects human B cells from programmed cell death. *Proc Natl Acad Sci USA* **90**:8479, 1993.
126. Nielan JG, Lu Z, Afonzo L, Kutish GF, Sussman MD, Rock DL: An African swine fever virus gene with similarity to the proto-oncogene bcl-2 and the Epstein-Barr virus gene BHRF1. *J Virol* **67**:4391, 1993.
127. Liebowitz D, Kieff E: Epstein-Barr virus, in Roizman B, Whitley RJ, Lopez C (eds): *The Human Herpesviruses*. New York, Raven Press, 1993, p. 107.
128. Liebowitz D: Epstein-Barr virus and a cellular signaling pathway in lymphomas from immunosuppressed patients. *N Engl J Med* **338**:1413, 1998.
129. Henderson S, Rowe M, Gregory C, Croom-Carter D, Wang F, Longnecker R, Kieff E, Rickinson A: Induction of Bcl-2 expression by Epstein-Barr virus latent membrane protein 1 protects infected B cells from programmed cell death. *Cell* **65**:1107, 1991.
130. Pena J, Rudin CM, Thompson CB: A Bcl-x_L transgene promotes malignant conversion of chemically initiated skin papillomas. *Cancer Res* **58**:2111, 1998.
131. Evan G, Littlewood T: The role of c-Myc in cell growth. *Curr Opin Genet Dev* **3**:44, 1993.
132. Evan G, Wyllie A, Gilbert C, Littlewood T, Brooks M, Waters C, Penn L, Hancock D: Induction of apoptosis in fibroblasts by c-Myc protein. *Cell* **63**:119, 1992.
133. Langdon WY, Harris AW, Cory S: Growth of E mu-myc transgenic B-lymphoid cells in vitro and their evolution toward autonomy. *Oncogene Res* **3**:271, 1988.
134. Bissonnette RP, Echeverri F, Mahboubi A, Green DR: Apoptotic cell death induced by c-Myc is inhibited by bcl-2. *Nature* **359**:552, 1992.
135. Harrington EA, Bennett MR, Fanidi A, Evan GI: c-Myc-induced apoptosis in fibroblasts is inhibited by specific cytokines. *EMBO J* **13**:3286, 1994.
136. Dedera D, Waller E, LeBrun D, Sen-Majumdar A, Stevens M, Barsh G, Cleary M: Chimeric homeobox gene E2A-PBX1 induces proliferation, apoptosis and malignant lymphomas in transgenic mice. *Cell* **74**:833, 1993.
137. Tommasino M, Crawford L: Human papillomavirus E6 and E7: Proteins which deregulate the cell cycle. *Bioessays* **17**:509, 1995.
138. Pan H, Griep AE: Temporally distinct patterns of p53-dependent and p53-independent apoptosis during mouse lens development. *Gene Dev* **9**:2157, 1995.
139. Rao L, Debbas M, Sabbatini P, Hockenberry D, Korsmeyer S, White E: The adenovirus E1A proteins induce apoptosis, which is inhibited by the E1B 19-kDa and Bcl-2 proteins. *Proc Natl Acad Sci USA* **89**:7742, 1992.
140. Yew PR, Berk AJ: Inhibition of p53 transactivation required for transformation by adenovirus early 1B protein. *Nature* **357**:82, 1992.
141. Murray AW: The genetics of cell cycle checkpoints. *Curr Opin Genet Dev* **5**:5, 1995.
142. Vogelstein B: Cancer: A deadly inheritance. *Nature* **348**:681, 1990.
143. Kuerbitz SJ, Plunkett BS, Walsh WV, Kastan MB: Wild-type p53 is a cell cycle checkpoint determinant following irradiation. *Proc Natl Acad Sci USA* **89**:7491, 1992.
144. Shaw P, Bovey R, Tardy S, Sahli R, Sordat B, Costa J: Induction of apoptosis by wild-type p53 in a human colon tumor-derived cell line. *Proc Natl Acad Sci USA* **89**:4495, 1992.
145. Yonish-Rouach E, Resnitzky D, Lotem J, Sachs L, Kimchi A, Oren M: Wild-type p53 induces apoptosis of myeloid leukaemic cells that is inhibited by interleukin-6. *Nature* **352**:345, 1991.
146. Symonds H, Krall L, Remington L, Saenz-Robles M, Lowe S, Jacks T, Van Dyke T: p53-dependent apoptosis suppresses tumor growth and progression in vivo. *Cell* **78**:703, 1994.
147. Lowe SW, Schmitt EM, Smith SW, Osborne BA, Jacks T: p53 is required for radiation-induced apoptosis in mouse thymocytes. *Nature* **362**:847, 1993.
148. Clarke AR, Purdie CA, Harrison DJ, Morris RG, Bird CC, Hooper ML, Wyllie AH: Thymocyte apoptosis induced by p53-dependent and independent pathways. *Nature* **362**:849, 1993.
149. Miyashita T, Krajewski S, Krajewska M, Wang HG, Lin HK, Liebermann DA, Hoffman B, Reed JC: Tumor suppressor p53 is regulator of bcl-2 and bax gene expression in vitro and in vivo. *Oncogene* **9**:1799, 1994.
150. Knudson CM, Tung KSK, Tourtellote WG, Brown GAJ, Korsmeyer SJ: Bax-deficient mice with lymphoid hyperplasia and male germ cell death. *Science* **270**:96, 1995.
151. Riley DJ, Lee EY-HP, Lee W-H: The retinoblastoma protein: More than a tumor suppressor. *Annu Rev Cell Biol* **10**:1, 1994.
152. Lee EY-HP, Chang C-Y, Hu N, Wang Y-CJ, Lai C-C, Herrup K, Lee W-H, Bradley A: Mice deficient for Rb are nonviable and show defects in neurogenesis and haematopoiesis. *Nature* **359**:288, 1992.
153. Jacks T, Fazeli A, Schmitt EM, Bronson RT, Goodell MA, Weinberg RA: Effects of an Rb mutation in the mouse. *Nature* **359**:295, 1992.
154. Amati B, Littlewood T, Evan G, Land H: The c-Myc protein induces cell cycle progression and apoptosis through dimerisation with Max. *EMBO J* **12**:5083, 1994.
155. Limpens J, de Jong D, van Krieken JH, Price CG, Young BD, van Ommen GJ, Kluin PM: Bcl-2/JH rearrangements in benign lymphoid tissues with follicular hyperplasia. *Oncogene* **6**:2271, 1991.
156. Liu Y, Hernandez AM, Shibata D, Cortopossi GA: BCL2 translocation frequency rises with age in humans. *Proc Natl Acad Sci USA* **91**:8910, 1994.
157. Gottesman MM, Pastan I: Biochemistry of multidrug resistance mediated by the multidrug transporter. *Annu Rev Biochem* **62**:385, 1993.
158. Lowe SW, Ruley HE, Jacks T, Housman DE: p53-dependent apoptosis modulates the cytotoxicity of anticancer agents. *Cell* **74**:957, 1993.
159. Miyashita T, Reed JC: bcl-2 gene transfer increases relative resistance of S49:1 and WEHI7.2 lymphoid cells to cell death and DNA fragmentation induced by glucocorticoids and multiple chemotherapeutic drugs. *Cancer Res* **52**:5407, 1992.
160. Walton MI, Whysong D, O'Connor PM, Hockenberry D, Korsmeyer SJ, Kohn KW: Constitutive expression of human bcl-2 modulates nitrogen mustard and camptothecin induced apoptosis. *Cancer Res* **53**:1853, 1993.
161. Dole M, Nunez G, Merchant AK, Maybaum J, Rode CK, Bloch CA, Castle VP: Bcl-2 inhibits chemotherapy-induced apoptosis in neuroblastoma. *Cancer Res* **54**:3253, 1994.
162. Fisher TC, Milner AE, Gregory CD, Jackman AL, Aherne GW, Hartley JA, Dive C, Hickman JA: bcl-2 modulation of apoptosis induced by anticancer drugs: Resistance to thymidylate stress is independent of classical resistance pathways. *Cancer Res* **53**:3321, 1993.
163. Miyashita T, Reed JC: Bcl-2 oncoprotein blocks chemotherapy-induced apoptosis in a human leukemia cell line. *Blood* **81**:151, 1993.
164. Minn AJ, Rudin CM, Boise LH, Thompson CB: Expression of Bcl-x_L can confer a multidrug resistance phenotype. *Blood* **86**:1903, 1995.
165. Dole MG, Jasty R, Cooper MJ, Thompson CB, Nunez G, Castle VP: Bcl-x_L is expressed in neuroblastoma cells and modulates chemotherapy-induced apoptosis. *Cancer Res* **55**:2576, 1995.
166. Lotem J, Sachs L: Regulation by bcl-2, c-Myc, and p53 of susceptibility to induction of apoptosis by heat shock and cancer chemotherapy compounds in differentiation-competent and -defective myeloid leukemic cells. *Cell Growth Diff* **4**:41, 1993.
167. Campos L, Rouault J-P, Sabido O, Oriol P, Roubi N, Vasselon C, Archimbaud E, Magaud J-P, Guyotat D: High expression of bcl-2 protein in acute myeloid leukemia cells is associated with poor response to chemotherapy. *Blood* **81**:3091, 1993.

168. Lowe SW, Bodis S, McClatchey A, Remington L, Ruley HE, Fisher DE, Housman DE, Jacks T: p53 status and the efficacy of cancer therapy in vivo. *Science* **266**:807, 1994.
169. Strasser A, Harris AW, Jacks T, Cory S: DNA damage can induce apoptosis in proliferating lymphoid cells via p53-independent mechanisms inhibitable by Bcl-2. *Cell* **79**:329, 1994.
170. Minn, AJ, Boise LH, Thompson CB: Expression of Bcl-x_L and loss of p53 can cooperate to overcome a cell cycle checkpoint induced by mitotic spindle damage. *Gene Dev* **10**:2621, 1996.
171. Cahill DP, Lengauer C, Yu J, Riggins GJ, Willson JKV, Markowitz SD, Kinsler KW, Vogelstein B: Mutations of mitotic checkpoint genes in human cancers. *Nature* **392**:300, 1998.
172. Webb A, Cunningham D, Cotter F, Clark PA, di Stefano F, Ross P, Corbo M, Dziewanowska Z: BCL-2 antisense therapy in patients with non-Hodgkin lymphoma. *Lancet* **349**:1137, 1997.
173. Piche A, Grim J, Rancourt C, Gomez-Navarro J, Reed JC, Curiel DT: Modulation of Bcl-2 protein levels by an intracellular anti-Bcl-2 single-chain antibody increases drug-induced cytotoxicity in the breast cancer cell line MCF-7. *Cancer Res* **58**:2134, 1998.

CHAPTER 25

Oncogenes

Morag Park

1. **Oncogenes are altered forms of normal cellular genes called proto-oncogenes. In human cancers, proto-oncogenes are frequently located adjacent to chromosomal breakpoints and are targets for mutation. The products of proto-oncogenes are highly conserved in evolution and serve to regulate the cascade of events that maintains the ordered progression through the cell cycle, cell division, and differentiation. In the cancer cell, this ordered progression is partially lost when one or more of the components of this pathway are altered.**
2. **The control of normal cell growth and differentiation is mediated by the interaction of growth factors and cytokines with their membrane-bound receptors. This event triggers a cascade of intracellular biochemical signals that eventually results in the activation and repression of various genes. Proto-oncogene products have been shown to function at critical steps in these pathways and include proteins such as extracellular cytokines and growth factors, transmembrane growth factor receptors, cytoplasmic proteins that act to transmit the signal to the nucleus, and nuclear proteins that include transcription factors and proteins involved in the control of DNA replication.**
3. **Accumulating evidence suggests that the activation of several oncogenes and the inactivation of several growth-suppressor genes are necessary for acquisition of a complete neoplastic phenotype. It has been possible from experimental studies to subdivide oncogenes into several groups. One class of genes rescues cells from senescence and programmed cell death; they act as immortalizing genes that block cell differentiation. A second class of genes reduces growth factor requirements and induces changes in cell shape that result in a continuous proliferative response that is no longer regulated.**
4. **The use of transgenic mice is providing a powerful experimental approach to investigate the role of oncogenes in cancer. Oncogene expression can be directed to specific tissues, where a role for the oncogene in tumor formation in those tissues can be evaluated. Although transgenic mouse strains carrying a single oncogene generally show an increased incidence of neoplasia, oncogene expression usually precedes tumor formation by many months, and the tumors that result are frequently clonal, implying that other events are necessary. Examination of the secondary events in tumors from oncogene-bearing transgenic mice has confirmed the conclusions derived from in vitro studies and has identified new oncogenes. By crossing two strains of oncogene-bearing mice, the consequence of multiple oncogenes on tumor incidence can be studied in a host capable of mounting a physiological response.**

In the past 15 years, the study of oncogenes has considerably advanced our understanding of the molecular mechanisms leading to cancer. The application of techniques from many cancer research disciplines has led to the discovery of both dominantly acting transforming genes and of tumor-suppressor genes. The dominant transforming genes, collectively called *oncogenes*, are altered forms of normal cellular genes called *proto-oncogenes*. Proto-oncogenes are highly conserved in evolution, and their products are important regulators of normal cell growth and differentiation from primitive eukaryotes to humans. They are localized throughout the cell and regulate the cascade of events that serve to maintain the ordered progression through the cell cycle, cell division, or the differentiated state of the cell. The function of these genes is discussed later, but sites of their activity are represented conceptually in Fig. 25-1. In the normal cell, interaction of growth factors and cytokines with specific membrane receptors triggers a cascade of intracellular biochemical signals that result in the expression and repression of various genes. In a cancer cell, this ordered progression is partially lost when one or more of the components of this pathway becomes altered as an oncogene. Mutations that alter the structure, levels, or sites of expression of the gene products in this pathway have been shown to activate their oncogenic potential.

Just as the growth-promoting proto-oncogenes are thought to regulate the proliferation of normal cells, the actions of tumor-suppressor genes function normally to constrain cell growth. Genetic lesions that inactivate tumor-suppressor genes therefore free the cell from the growth constraints imposed by these genes. The end result of oncogene activation or suppressor gene inactivation is deregulated cell growth. Increasing evidence suggests that the acquisition of multiple sequential alterations involving both oncogenes and tumor-suppressor genes is generally required for the progression from the normal to a fully malignant phenotype. This review focuses on the identification, mechanisms of activation, and function of the oncogene/proto-oncogene class of growth regulators; tumor-suppressor genes are discussed in Chapter 26.

DISCOVERY OF ONCOGENES

The majority of oncogenes were initially isolated as altered forms of proto-oncogenes acquired (transduced) by RNA tumor viruses (v-*onc*). In 1909, Payton Rous discovered that transplantable sarcomas in chickens could be induced by a cell-free agent. The transforming agent was a retrovirus that had transduced part of a normal cellular gene called *src* (*sar*coma). The virally transduced *src* gene (v-*src*) was altered by mutation compared with its cellular counterpart (c-*src*), rendering it constitutively activated. This discovery demonstrated that our cells harbor genes that, when abnormally activated, are capable of inducing tumorigenesis.[1,2] In the last 20 years, over 30 retroviruses have been isolated that induce tumors with short latency, each containing a different oncogene, and their transduced oncogenes have been shown to

A list of standard abbreviations is located immediately preceding the index in each volume. Additional abbreviations used in this chapter include: bcr = breakpoint cluster region, or gene at 22q11 involved in translocations producing the Philadelphia chromosome; CML = chronic myelogenous leukemia; c-*onc* = cellular oncogene; CSF-1R = macrophage colony-stimulating factor-1 receptor; EGFR = epidermal growth factor receptor; *env* = retroviral gene encoding protein components of the virion nucleoprotein core; LTR = long terminal repeat sequences encoding retroviral transcriptional control elements; MMTV = mouse mammary tumor virus; PDGFR = platelet-derived growth factor receptor; Ph = Philadelphia chromosome; *pol* = retroviral gene encoding reverse transcriptase; TGF = transforming growth factor; v-*onc* = viral oncogene.

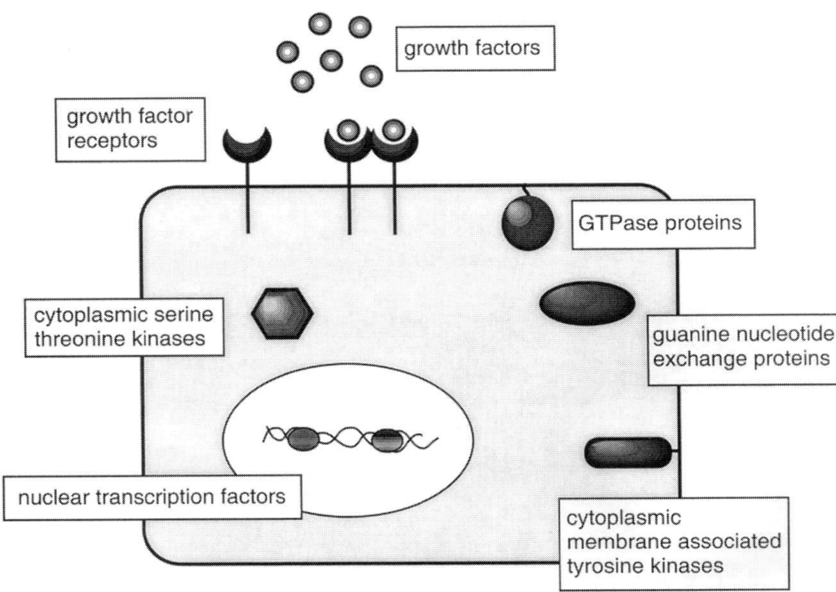

Fig. 25-1 Schematic representation of the cellular compartments where oncogene or proto-oncogene products are localized. These compartments include growth factors, transmembrane growth factor receptors, nonintegral membrane-associated proteins of the *src* tyrosine kinase gene family, *ras* GTPase gene family, guanine nucleotide exchange proteins plus serine threonine kinase oncoproteins localized in the cytoplasm, and nuclear transcription factors.

have critical roles in cell transformation (Fig. 25-2).[3,4] Although retroviruses have not been shown to be etiologic agents involved in human cancer, they have provided useful insights into oncogene research. In addition to the acutely transforming retroviruses, slowly transforming retroviruses do not carry oncogenes but induce tumors by integrating themselves adjacent to a cellular gene and altering its transcriptional regulation (Fig. 25-2).[5] The presence of a provirus integrated in the same region of the cellular genome in independently derived tumors of the same histologic type has enabled investigators to identify new cellular genes that can be activated in specific tumor lineages. Following this strategy, many novel oncogenes have been discovered. An examination of human tumors by a variety of methods has revealed that many of the v-*onc* genes are also altered in human tumors.

DETECTION OF ONCOGENES IN HUMAN TUMORS

Evidence for a genetic role in cancer comes from multiple sources. Many of the cancer-prone syndromes, such as Fanconi syndrome, Bloom syndrome, and ataxia telangiectasia, show greatly increased chromosome instability.[6] Studies of colon cancer have shown that many cancers have accumulated multiple chromosome deletions and mutations.[7] The recent identification of the bacterial *mut*S and *mut*L DNA mismatch repair genes as genetic lesions that predispose individuals to colon cancer further supports the role of mutation in the generation of cancer.[8,9] To identify oncogenes in human tumors, several strategies have been developed. Oncogenes in human tumors were initially identified using DNA transfection techniques. The discovery that oncogenes are frequently activated by chromosomal translocations, however, has stimulated the isolation of genes that map to the breakpoints of nonrandom chromosomal rearrangement present in human tumors, as a method to identify new candidate oncogenes.

Detection of Oncogenes by DNA Transfection

The DNA transfection assay was developed to study and identify the transforming genes of RNA or DNA tumor viruses.[10] The cells used as recipients in most transfection experiments are NIH3T3 cells, which are mouse fibroblasts in origin and are maintained as contact-inhibited, nontumorigenic cell lines. Transformation of these cells by gene transfer is monitored by changes in cell morphology in culture and loss of contact inhibition, where cells overgrow the monolayer and form focal areas of dense layers termed *foci*,[11] or by a modification of this technique in which the cells that have acquired transforming genes produce tumors in nude mice[12] (Fig. 25-3).

To assay for transforming genes, genomic DNA, prepared from human tumors or tumor cell lines, is transferred to recipient cells. Transfer of DNA-containing activated oncogenes will occasionally give rise to foci of morphologically altered cells that have tumorigenic properties. Foci or tumors thus obtained contain cells that are transformed as a result of incorporating human DNA containing an activated oncogene. Human repetitive DNA sequences located in the vicinity of the oncogene can be distinguished from mouse sequences and can be used to clone and isolate molecularly the DNA segment responsible for transformation of the NIH3T3 cells[13,14] (Fig. 25-3). Many of the human transforming genes identified in this manner are related to the *ras* family of oncogenes (Table 25-1). For instance, the transforming genes of a human bladder and lung carcinoma were shown to be homologous to the *ras* genes previously identified in the acute transforming retroviruses of the Harvey and Kirsten sarcoma viruses and were designated c-H-*ras* and c-K-*ras*,[15] respectively. In addition, a third *ras* gene family member was initially identified in a human neuroblastoma tumor cell line and human promyelocytic leukemia cell line and was designated N-*ras* (Table 25-1).[16]

Ras genes in human tumors have been shown to be activated by single point mutations predominantly involving codons 12, 13, and 61 (reviewed by Barbacid, 1987[17]). Although these mutations activate each of the *ras* genes as an oncogene in vitro, there is clear selectivity with regard to which *ras* homologue is mutationally activated in a given human cancer. Approximately 50 percent of colorectal cancers, 95 percent of pancreatic cancers, and 30 percent of lung adenocarcinomas harbor mutant Ki-*ras* genes, but mutant Ha-*ras* or N-*ras* genes are rarely detected in these cancers.[18] Similarly, about 25 percent of acute myelogenous leukemias and myelodysplastic syndromes contain mutant N-*ras* genes, but mutant Ha-*ras* and Ki-*ras* genes are rarely found. Moreover, mutant Ha-*ras* genes are rarely found in human tumors.[19] In most other tumor types (e.g., cancers of the breast, prostate, stomach, bladder, liver, and brain), however, *ras* mutations do not occur often, if at all. As *RAS* genes are ubiquitously expressed and presumably have similar functions in all cells, the basis for this tissue specificity is not understood.

Gene transfer studies have also led to the identification of a growing number of transforming genes that are not members of the *ras* gene family and that have not been previously identified in a

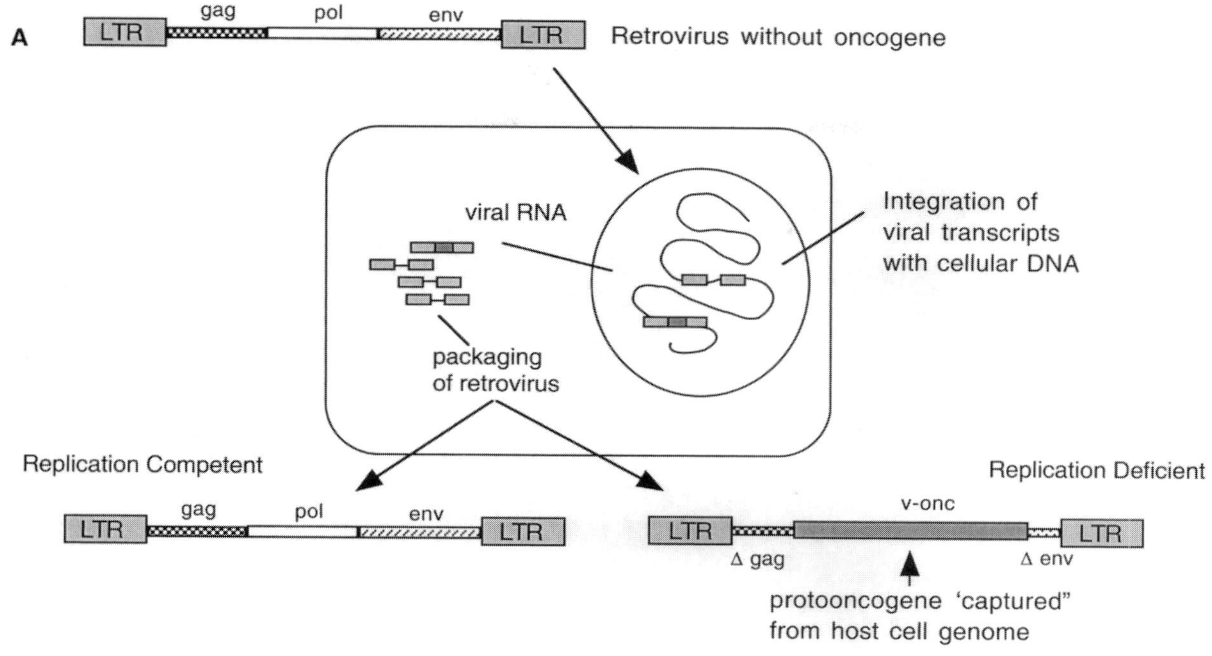

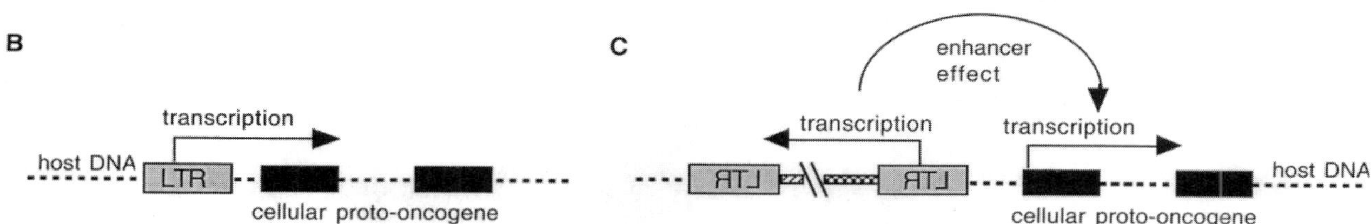

Fig. 25-2 Schematic representation of mechanisms of activation of a host gene by insertion of a provirus and the general structure of leukemia and leukosis and acute transforming retroviral genomes. A: Genome of a nondefective leukemia or leukosis retrovirus, infection of host cell, and integration into the host genome. The *gag* region encodes the internal structural proteins of the virion, the *pol* region encodes the virion RNA-dependent DNA polymerase (reverse transcriptase), and the *env* region encodes the proteins found on the surface of the virion envelope. LTR is the long terminal repeat that appears at each end of the integrated linear DNA forms. Within the LTR region are DNA sequences, which define the initiation site for RNA transcription and at the 3′ end encode a poly A addition site where the viral RNA polyadenylation occurs and transcription enhancer sequences that result in the production of high levels of transcripts. The LTR elements provide all of the necessary functions for eukaryotic transcription to take place and for the provirus to express genomic viral RNA. B and C: Two different configurations of inserted proviral DNA. Replication competent and replication defective viruses are produced. The genome of a replication-defective acute transforming retrovirus containing v-*onc* sequences is shown. Although substantial portions of *gag*, *pol*, and/or *env* may be deleted in acute transforming retroviruses, they still retain the terminal noncoding LTR regions. B: Insertion of a proviral LTR upstream of the first coding exon as observed with c-*myc*. This insertion results in a transcript that no longer contains sequences that regulate c-*myc* expression levels. The protein-coding domains (exons) of the normal host gene are in *solid black rectangles*. C: Integration of an intact provirus upstream (or downstream) from, for example, the *int 1* or *int 2* genes. This form of integration may not alter the gene product but generally results in increased transcription of that gene promoted by the transcriptional enhancing activity of the retroviral LTR.

retrovirus. These include multiple receptor tyrosine kinases (the *neu*, *met*, *trk*, *mas*, *erb*B-2/*HER2*, and *ret*), growth factors (*hst* and KS3 oncogenes), exchange factors that activate members of the Rho GTPase family, and multiple transcription factors (Table 25-1).

Identification of Oncogenes at Chromosomal Breakpoints

The chromosomal location of cellular proto-oncogenes determined by in situ hybridization has led to the identification of several proto-oncogenes at or near chromosomal translocation breakpoints.[20,21] In general, structural rearrangements that juxtapose two different chromosomal regions are thought to contain dominant transforming genes, whereas deletions or monosomies are thought to be the sites of recessive tumor-suppressor genes.

Recurrent tumor-specific chromosome translocations were first identified in cytogenetic analyses of leukemias and myelodysplasias and are considered to be involved in tumor development.[22,23] The tumor-specific chromosome abnormalities of leukemias and lymphomas are usually somatically acquired alterations. In some tumor types such as chronic myelogenous leukemia, the same translocations consistently appear, supporting the hypothesis that these events are a prerequisite for tumor induction. Where it has been possible to characterize and molecularly isolate the genes adjacent to translocation breakpoints, candidate genes implicated in tumor initiation and progression have been identified (Table 25-2). These alterations are discussed in more detail in other chapters.

In many cases, breaks occur within a gene on each of the participating chromosomes, resulting in the formation of a

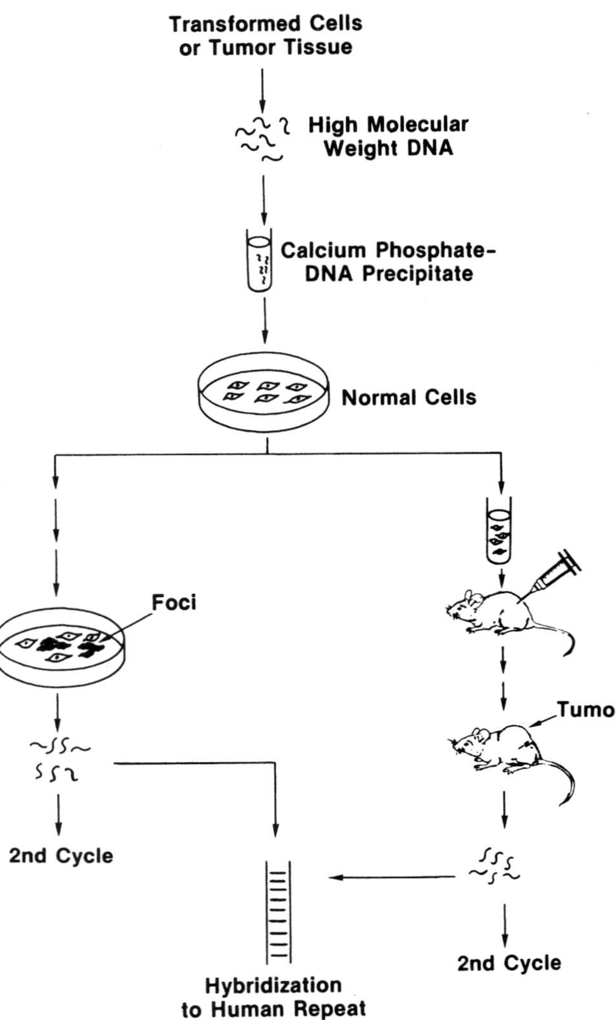

Fig. 25-3 NIH3T3 DNA transfection and/or transformation assay. High molecular weight DNA prepared from transformed cell or tumor DNA is precipitated with calcium phosphate and added to nontransformed mouse NIH3T3 cells. These cells are then assayed for tumor production in nude mice or are assayed for the appearance of foci. DNA is prepared from either primary foci or tumors and is subjected to a second cycle of transfection to facilitate the loss of additional nontransforming sequences that are transferred with the transforming gene. After several cycles of transfection, the majority of the foreign DNA in the focus or tumor corresponds to the transforming gene and can be isolated by recombinant DNA technology.

chimeric gene that encodes a fusion protein. An example of this includes chronic myelogenous leukemia (CML), which is a pluripotent stem cell disease characterized by the presence of a consistent translocation. The Philadelphia (Ph) chromosome translocation between chromosomes 9 and 22, t(9;22)(q34;qll)[24] is present in the leukemic cells of at least 95 percent of all CML patients.[25] The proto-oncogene c-*abl*, which is the normal cellular homologue of the oncogene v-*abl* of Abelson murine leukemic virus (A-MuLV) (Table 25-1) is translocated from chromosome 9, band q34, into the *bcr* gene on chromosome 22 at band q11.[26,27] This gives rise to a chimeric gene expressing a fusion protein containing the N-terminus derived from the Bcr protein and the C-terminus derived from the Abl protein (Fig. 25-4). The resulting chimeric protein has increased catalytic activity when compared with the normal protein and will transform cells in culture.[24]

Although many translocations give rise to a new protein, some, such as those involving the c-*MYC* and immunoglobulin genes on the chromosome translocations 2:14, 8:14, and 22:14 observed in lymphomas, result in altered regulation of the *MYC* gene (reviewed by Stanton et al, 1983[26]). Normally, the expression of this gene is tightly regulated, but, in cells where the translocation has occurred, the gene is constitutively expressed.

As a consequence of technical improvements, cytogenetic abnormalities have now been identified in solid tumors (reviewed by Cooper, 1996[27]). Such rearrangements are found in a high proportion of tumors, suggesting that they could provide much needed markers for use in diagnosis of sarcoma types. In addition to chromosomal rearrangements, frequent chromosomal abnormalities documented in solid tumors involve amplification or deletion of specific chromosomal regions.

Proto-oncogene Amplification

Cellular proto-oncogenes have been found in multiple copies in various tumors and transformed cell lines. The amplified proto-oncogene copies can occur in homogeneously staining chromosomal regions or double-minute chromosomes.[28,29] Oncogene amplification has also been observed by hybridization techniques in tumor cells in the absence of microscopic chromosomal changes. The mechanism of gene amplification is not fully understood, but illegitimate DNA replication occurring more than once during a single cell cycle could account for the increase in multiple segments (amplification units) of DNA from 200 to 2000 kb in size.[30]

All amplified proto-oncogenes express high levels of the corresponding RNA and protein and do not appear to be rearranged. The amplification unit containing the proto-oncogene DNA can be at a site distant from its normal locus as a heterogeneously staining region. The c-*MYC* gene was the first proto-oncogene shown to be amplified. In the promyelocytic leukemia cell line HL60, as well as in the primary tumor, 8 to 30 copies of c-*MYC* per cell were detected.[31,32] Other proto-oncogenes, including c-*MYB*, c-*erb*B (epidermal growth factor receptor or EGFR), *HER*-2 (also called c-*erb*B2 and corresponds to *neu* in the rat), and c-*MYC* family members, have also been shown to be amplified in certain tumors or tumor cell lines (Table 25-3). The presence of multiple copies of proto-oncogenes in tumor cells has been associated with poor prognosis. N-*MYC*, which was first identified as an amplified gene in a human neuroblastoma, is present in multiple copies in 40 percent of neuroblastomas, and its amplification correlates with more advanced stages of the disease.[33,34] Amplification of members of the *MYC* gene family (c-*MYC*, N-*MYC*, and L-*MYC*) in small-cell lung carcinomas also appears to be associated with the more malignant stages of the tumor.[35] The amplified proto-oncogene is frequently tumor specific; for example, N-*MYC* or c-*MYC* may be associated with the progression of neuroblastomas and small-cell lung carcinoma cells, the EGFR (c-*erb*B) gene has been found to be amplified in glioblastomas and several squamous carcinomas,[36,37] and the related *HER*-2 gene is often found amplified in adenocarcinomas[38] and in advanced, hormone-independent mammary tumors with a poor prognosis.[39,40] This suggests that increased expression of these proto-oncogenes plays a role in the development and progression of these tumors.

FUNCTIONS AND MECHANISMS OF ACTIVATION OF PROTO-ONCOGENE PRODUCTS

Conservation of Proto-oncogenes

Homologues of proto-oncogenes have been found in all multicellular animals studied thus far, and their widespread distribution in nature indicates that their protein products have essential

Table 25-1 Oncogenes

Oncogene	Lesion	Neoplasm	Proto-Oncogene
Growth factors			
v-sis		Glioma/fibrosarcoma	B-chain PDGF
int 2	Proviral insertion	Mammary carcinoma	Member of FGF family
KS3	DNA transfection	Kaposi sarcoma	Member of FGF family
HST	DNA transfection	Stomach carcinoma	Member of FGF family
int-l	Proviral insertion	Mammary carcinoma	Possible growth factor
Receptors lacking protein kinase activity			
mas	DNA transfection	Mammary carcinoma	Angiotensin receptor
Tyrosine kinases: integral membrane proteins, growth factor receptors			
*EGFR**	Amplification	Squamous cell carcinoma	Protein kinase (tyr) EGFR
v-fms		Sarcoma	Protein kinase (tyr) CSF-1R
v-kit		Sarcoma	Protein kinase (tyr) stem cell factor R
v-ros		Sarcoma	Protein kinase (tyr)
MET	Rearrangement	MNNG-treated human osteocarcinoma cell line	Protein kinase (tyr) HGF/SFR
TRK	Rearrangement	Colon carcinoma	Protein kinase (tyr) NGFR
NEU	Point mutation	Neuroblastoma	Protein kinase (tyr)
	Amplification	Carcinoma of breast	
RET	Rearrangement	Carcinoma of thyroid Men 2A, Men 2B	Protein kinase (tyr) GDNFR
Tyrosine kinases: membrane associated			
*SRC**		Colon carcinoma	Protein kinase (tyr)
v-yes		Sarcoma	Protein kinase (tyr)
v-fgr		Sarcoma	Protein kinase (tyr)
v-fps		Sarcoma	Protein kinase (tyr)
v-fes		Sarcoma	Protein kinase (tyr)
*BCR/ABL**	Chromosome translocation	Chronic myelogenous leukemia	Protein kinase (tyr)
Membrane-associated G proteins			
*H-RAS**	Point mutation	Colon, lung, pancreas carcinoma	GTPase
*K-RAS**	Point mutation	Acute myelogenous leukemia thyroid carcinoma, melanoma	GTPase
N-RAS	Point mutation	Carcinoma, melanoma	GTPase
gsp	Point mutation	Carcinoma of thyroid	$G_6\alpha$
gip	Point mutation	Ovary, adrenal carcinoma	$G_1\alpha$
GEF family of proteins			
Dbl	Rearrangement	Diffuse B-cell lymphoma	GEF for Rho and Cdc42Hs
Ost		Osteosarcomas	GEF for RhoA and Cdc42Hs
Tiam-1	Metastatic and oncogenic	T lymphoma	GEF for Rac and Cdc42Hs
Vay	Rearrangement	Hematopoietic cells	GEF for Ras?
Lbc	Oncogenic	Myeloid leukemias	GEF for Rho
Serine/threonine kinases: cytoplasmic			
v-mos		Sarcoma	Protein kinase (ser/thr)
v-raf		Sarcoma	Protein kinase (ser/thr)
pim-1	Proviral insertion	T-cell lymphoma	Protein kinase (ser/thr)
Cytoplasmic regulators			
v-crk			SH-2/SH-3 adaptor
Nuclear protein family			
v-myc		Carcinoma myelocytomatosis	Transcription factor
N-MYC	Gene amplification	Neuroblastoma; lung carcinoma	Transcription factor
L-MYC	Gene amplification	Carcinoma of lung	Transcription factor
v-myb		Myeloblastosis	Transcription factor
v-fos		Osteosarcoma	Transcription factor API
v-jun		Sarcoma	Transcrption factor API
v-ski		Carcinoma	Transcription factor
v-rel		Lymphatic leukemia	Mutant NFκB
v-ets		Myeloblastosis	Transcription factor
v-erbA		Erythroblastosis	Mutant thioredoxine receptor

ABBREVIATIONS: CSF-1R = macrophage colony-stimulating factor-1 receptor; EGFR = epidermal growth factor receptor; FGF = fibroblast growth factor; GEF = guanine nucleotide exchange factor; GDNF = glial derived neurotropic factor; HGF/SF = hepatic growth factor/scatter factor; NGF = Nerve growth factor; PDGF = platelet-derived growth factor.

Table 25-2 Molecularly Characterized Neoplastic Rearrangements

Affected Gene	Translocation	Disease	Protein Type
Gene fusions			
c-ABL (9q34)	t(9;22) (q34;q11)	Chronic myelogenous leukemia and acute leukemia	Tyrosine kinase activated by B-cell receptor
BCR (22q11)			
PBX-1 (1q23)	t(1;19)(q23;p13.3)	Acute pre-B-cell leukemia	Homeodomain
E2A (19p13.3)			HLH
PML (15q21)	t(15;17) (q21;q11-22)	Acute myeloid leukemia	Zn finger
RAR (17q21)			
CAN (6p23)	t(6;9) (p23;q34)	Acute myeloid leukemia	No homology
DEK (9q34)			
REL	ins(2;12)	Non-Hodgkin lymphoma	NF-κB family
NRG	(p13;p11.2-14)		No homology
Oncogenes Juxtaposed with immunoglobulin loci			
c-*MYC*	t(8;14) (q24;q32) t(2;8) (p12;q24) t(8;22) (q24;q11)	Burkitt lymphoma, BL-ALL	HLH domain
BCL1 (PRADI?)	t(11;14) (q13;q32)	B-cell chronic lymphocyte leukemia	PRADI-G1 cyclin
BCL-2	t(14;18) (q32;21)	Follicular lymphoma	Inner mitochondrial membrane
BCL-3	t(14;19) (q32;q13.1)	Chronic B-cell leukemia	CDC10 motif
IL-3	t(5;14) (q31;q32)	Acute pre-B-cell leukemia	Growth factor
Oncogenes juxtaposed with T-cell receptor loci			
c-*MYC*	t(8;14) (q24;q11)	Acute T-cell leukemia	HLH domain
LYL-1	t(7;19) (q35;p13)	Acute T-cell leukemia	HLH domain
TAL-1/*SCL*/*TCL*-5)	t(1;14) (p32;q11)	Acute T-cell leukemia	HLH domain
TAL-2	t(7;9) (q35;q34)	Acute T-cell leukemia	HLH domain
Rhombotin 1/Ttg-1	t(11;14) (p15;q11)	Acute T-cell leukemia	LIM domain
Rhombotin 2/Ttg-2	t(11;14) (p13;q11) t(7;11) (q35;p13)	Acute T-cell leukemia	LIM domain
HOX-11	t(10;14) (q24;q11) t(7;10) (q35;q24)	Acute T-cell leukemia	Homeodomain
TAN-1	t(7;9) (q34;q34.3)	Acute T-cell leukemia	Notch homologue
Gene fusions in sarcomas			
FLI1, EWS	t(11;22) (q24;q12)	Ewing sarcoma	Ets transcription factor family
ERG, EWS	t(21;22) (q22;q12)	Ewing sarcoma	Ets transcription factor family
ATV1, EWS	t(7;21) (p22;q12)	Ewing sarcoma	Ets transcription factor family
ATF1, EWS	t(12;22) (q13;q12)	Soft tissue clear cell sarcoma	Transcription factor
CHN, EWS	t(9;22) (q22-31;q12)	Myxoid chondrosarcoma	Steroid receptor family
WT1, EWS	t(11;22) (p13;q12)	Desmoplastic small round cell tumor	Wilm tumor gene
SSX1, SSX2, SYT	t(X;18) (p11.2;q11.2)	Synovial sarcoma	HLH domain
PAX3, EKHR	t(2;13) (q37;q14)	Alveolar	Homeobox homologue
PAX7, EKHR	t(1;13) (q36;q14)	Rhabdomyosarcoma	Homeobox homologue
CHOP, TLS	t(12;16) (q13;p11)	Myxoid liposarcoma	Transcription factor
var, HMGI-C	t(var;12) (var;q13-15)	Lipomas	HMG DNA-binding protein
HMGI-C, ?	t(12;14) (q13-15)	Leiomomas	HMG DNA-binding protein
Oncogenes juxtaposed with other loci			
PTH deregulates *PRADI*	inv(11)(p15;q13)	Parathyroid adenoma	PRADI-GI cyclin
BTGI deregulates *MYC*	t(8;12)(q24;q22)	B-cell chronic lymphocytic leukemia	MYC-HLH domain

ABBREVIATIONS: HLH = helix-loop-helix structural domain; zn = zinc; HMG = high mobility group.

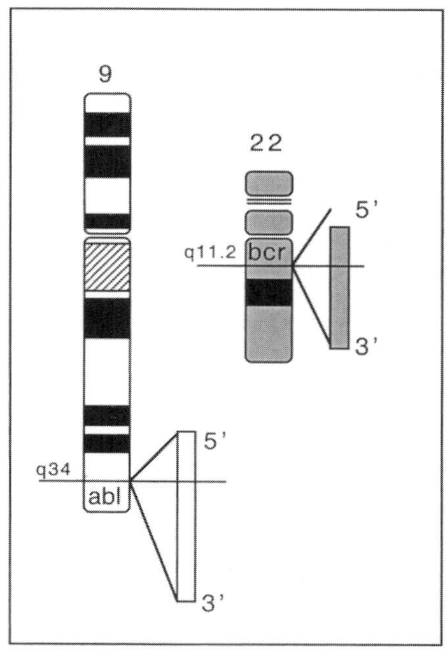

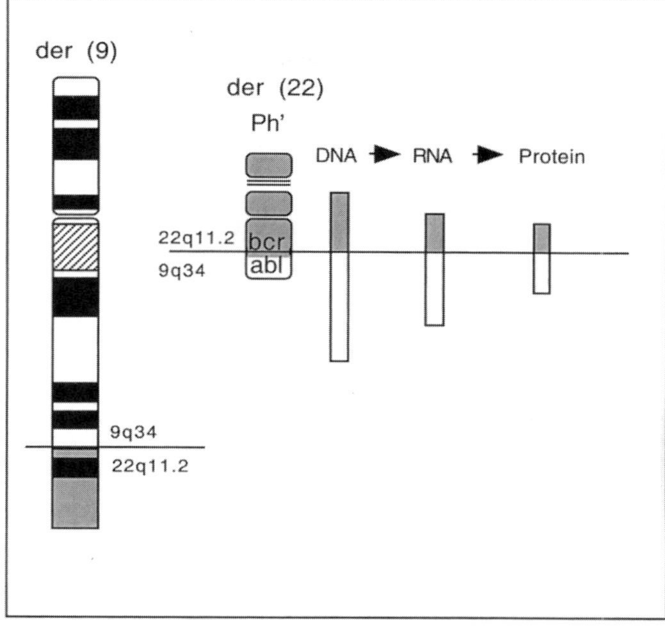

Fig. 25-4 Schematic representation of the chromosomes involved in the generation of the Philadelphia chromosome observed in more than 95 percent of chronic myelogenous leukemia (CML). A schematic presentation of the normal chromosomes 9 and 22, and of the chromosome translocations 9q+ and 22q− are shown. The c-*ABL* proto-oncogene on the distal tip of chromosome 9q34 is translocated into the *BCR* locus on chromosome 22q11.2. This generates a chimeric gene that expresses a chimeric *BCR-ABL* messenger RNA and fusion protein.

biologic roles. The more highly conserved domains of the protein are probably those that have a crucial structural and/or functional role, and characterization of their normal biochemical properties will provide insight into the contribution that an activated oncogene has to cell transformation. Understanding the mechanism of activation of each oncogene requires characterization of the proto-oncogene, a comparison of the changes that have occurred, and systematic testing of changes influencing the transforming potential.

There are essentially only three biochemical mechanisms by which proto-oncogenes act. One mechanism involves phosphorylation of proteins on serine, threonine, or tyrosine residues.[41] Proteins of this class transfer phosphate groups from adenosine triphosphate (ATP) to the side chain of tyrosine, serine, or threonine residues. Phosphorylation serves two basic purposes in signal transduction. In many instances, it changes the conformation and activates the enzymatic kinase activity of the protein. Secondly, phosphorylation of tyrosine residues generates docking sites that recruit target proteins, which the activated kinase may phosphorylate. Thus, phosphorylation acts to potentiate signal transmission through the generation of complexes of signal-transducing molecules at specific sites in the cell where they are required to act. For example, activation of the catalytic activity of a receptor tyrosine kinase by its ligand leads to the formation of a complex of signaling proteins at the plasma membrane where the receptor is localized.

The second mechanism by which genes act to transmit signals is by GTPases.[42] The prototype for this class of proteins is the *ras* gene family. In a similar manner to the kinase gene family, Ras proteins function as molecular switches that are turned of and on via a regulated GDP/GTP cycle. Ras proteins have been implicated as key intermediates that relay the signal from upstream tyrosine kinases to downstream serine-threonine kinase pathways. Some of the conventional heterotrimeric G proteins can also transform cells when altered.[43,44] The third mechanism involves proteins that are localized in the nucleus. A large variety of proteins that control progress through the cell cycle and gene expression are encoded by proto-oncogenes, some of which may also be involved in DNA replication.[45,46] Thus, the relaxation of requirements of transformed cells for growth factors could be mediated by an activated oncogene at multiple levels of the signal transduction pathway.

Table 25-3 Examples of Cellular Proto-Oncogenes Amplified in Human Tumors

Tumor	Oncogene	Amplification
Small-cell lung cancer	c-*myc*	Up to 80×
	N-*myc*	Up to 50×
	L-*myc*	Up to 20×
Neuroblastomas	N-*myc*	Up to 250×
Glioblastomas	c-*erb*B1 (EGFR)	Up to 50×
Mammary carcinoma	c-*erb*B2 (HER2)	Up to 30×
	c-*myc*	Up to 50×
	Cyclin D1	Up to 30×

ABBREVIATION: EGFR = endothelial growth factor receptor.

Growth Factors

Growth factors are responsible for stimulating cells in a resting or G0 stage to enter the cell cycle. This mitogenic response occurs in two phases: a quiescent cell is stimulated to proceed into the G1 phase of the cell cycle by *competence factors* and then becomes committed to DNA synthesis by *progression factors* (Fig. 25-5).[47] Successful transition through the G1 phase requires sustained growth factor stimulation over a period of several hours. This is followed by a critical phase where the presence of a progression factor such as insulin growth factor I is required in addition to the

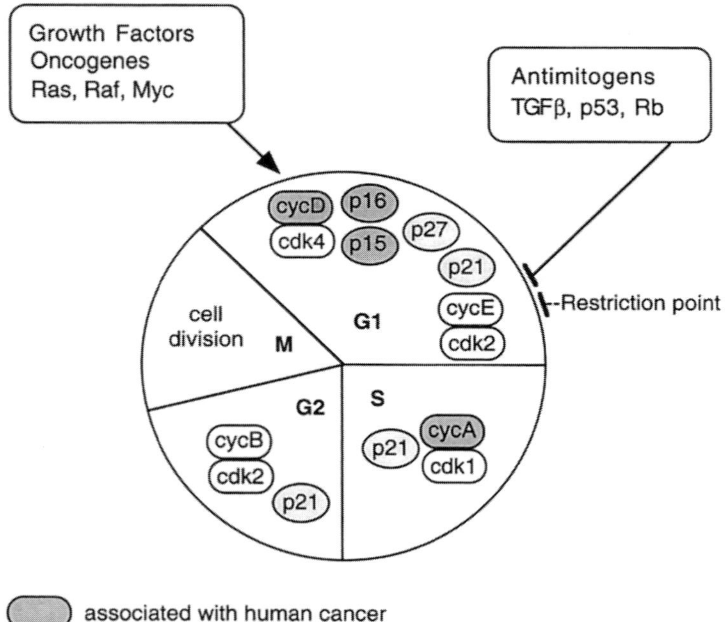

Fig. 25-5 Combinatorial interactions of cyclins and cyclin-dependent kinases (cdks) during the cell cycle. Progression from G0 through the restriction point in G1 requires the continued presence of growth factors. This requirement is overcome by oncogenes, such as Myc, Ras, or Raf, or tyrosine kinases. Progression through G1 can be blocked by antimitogens, TGFβ, or the p53 or Rb tumor-suppressor genes. Cyclins D and E in complexes with cdks are required for progression through G1 and entry into S phase. Cyclins A and B form complexes with cdk2 later in the cell cycle and are involved in progression from G2 to M. The activity of cyclin-D complexes can be inhibited by p15 and p16, thus preventing the advance of the cell from G1 to S. Other inhibitors of cyclin-dependent kinases, p21 and p27, can act throughout the cell cycle. Cyclins and inhibitors found altered in human cancers are shown in grey.

growth factor for successful progression through the cell cycle. This dual signal requirement may prevent accidental triggering of quiescent cells into the cell cycle by transient exposure to mitogenic growth factors. In some cell types, the absence of growth factor stimulation causes the rapid onset of programmed cell death (apoptosis).[48] Therefore, inappropriate expression of a growth factor may result in a constant stimulation of cell growth in addition to a block in cell differentiation.

There is now much evidence to support a role for growth factors and their receptors in the development of human malignancies. The first direct correlation of an oncogene with a growth factor was revealed from a computer-assisted comparison that showed that the amino acid sequence of the v-*sis* oncogene product was highly related to the B chain of platelet-derived growth factor (PDGF) (Table 25-1).[49] PDGF is released from platelets during clotting and is recognized as an important serum mitogen required for mesenchymal cell growth in culture. Connective tissue tumors such as sarcomas and glioblastomas have been shown to express PDGF, whereas their normal tissue counterparts did not.[50] Thus, in an autocrine fashion, the sarcoma and glial tumor cells appear to synthesize the mitogen to which they are normally responsive. On the other hand, no genetic alterations of the PDGF gene have yet been observed that would explain this synthesis. Until the mechanism underlying the expression of PDGF is clarified, it will be difficult to know whether this expression is a cause or an effect of neoplastic growth.

Int-2, whose expression is activated by mouse mammary tumor virus (MMTV) proviral insertion in mouse mammary carcinomas, the *KS3* oncogene identified in a Kaposi sarcomas, and *HST*, a transforming gene identified in a human stomach cancer by DNA transfection, are members of the basic or acidic fibroblast growth factor (FGF) family of related peptide mitogens. Basic FGFs are expressed by human melanoma cell lines but not by normal melanocytes that are dependent on bFGF to proliferate.[51,52] Similarly, transforming growth factor α (TGFα) is frequently produced by carcinomas that express high levels of the EGFR and appears to function as an autocrine in this system through stimulation of the EGFR.[53] Because many ligands and their receptors are not yet characterized, the contribution of autocrine growth stimulatory loops to human malignancies may be greater than is presently appreciated.

Growth Factor Receptors

Oncogenes derived from growth factor receptors confer on the cells the ability to bypass the growth factor requirement, rendering cells growth factor independent. By far, the largest number of receptor-derived oncoproteins are derived from growth factor receptors that have tyrosine kinase activity.

Tyrosine Protein Kinases. More than 40 different protein tyrosine kinases have been identified (Table 25-1).[54] These kinases are subdivided into two main categories: those, such as the EGFR, spanning the plasma membrane and those located in the cytoplasm, many of which are associated with the plasma membrane, such as c-Src (Fig. 25-6). All of the protein tyrosine kinases have sequence homology over a region of approximately 300 amino acids that has been defined as the *catalytic kinase domain*[55] (Fig. 25-6). This domain is responsible for catalyzing the transfer of the phosphate group of ATP to tyrosine residues during trans- and autophosphorylation. This kinase domain is also homologous to the Raf, ERK, and Mos protein members, which have phosphorylation specificity for serine and threonine.[56,57] Phosphorylation on tyrosine is a rare event in normal cells and accounts for only 0.05 percent of all protein phosphorylation, but tyrosine kinases regulate key events in signal transduction pathways that control cell shape and growth.[58]

Growth Factor Receptor Tyrosine Kinases. Many growth factors mediate their effects by means of receptors with tyrosine kinase activity. These receptors have an extracellular ligand-binding domain, a single transmembrane domain, and an intracellular catalytic domain responsible for transducing the signal[59] (Fig. 25-6). Binding of growth factors to cell surface receptors results in receptor dimerization and activation of their intrinsic tyrosine kinase, leading to intermolecular phosphorylation of each receptor on specific tyrosine residues.[60] This results in the recruitment of signaling molecules containing Src homology 2 (SH2) domains,[61] which recognize, in a sequence specific manner, short peptide segments containing phosphotyrosine within activated receptors[62–64] (Fig. 25-7). These include proteins with enzymatic activity, such as phospholipase Cγ (PLCγ), phosphatidylinositol 3-kinase (PI3K), and the GTPase-activating protein for p21Ras (p120GAP), and proteins that lack enzyme activity and function as adaptor proteins, such as Grb2. Collectively, they act to

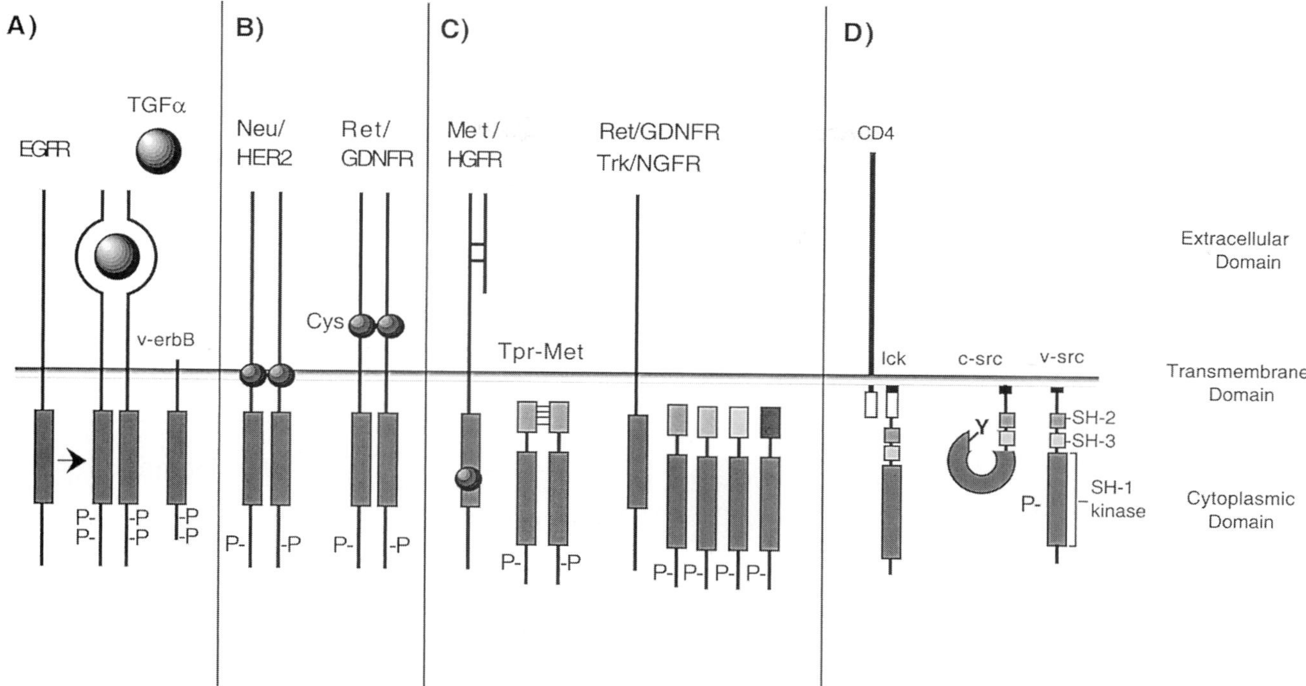

Fig. 25-6 Schematic comparison of structural features of cell surface growth factor receptor tyrosine kinases and membrane-associated tyrosine kinase oncogene products. The cytoplasmic tyrosine kinase domain is represented in grey (*src* homology 1 or SH-1), and SH-2 and SH-3 domains are indicated. A: Ligand binding to the epidermal growth factor receptor (EGFR) promotes receptor dimerization, activation of the kinase, and transphosphorylation of the receptor cytoplasmic domain on tyrosine residues, which then interact with SH-2 domain containing substrates and elicit an intracellular signal. The N- and C-terminal deletions, in addition to point mutations within critical domains of the molecule, that activate v-*erb*B are illustrated. Autocrine production of TGFβ in cells that express the EGFR results in constitutive activation of the EGFR. B: A single point mutation in the transmembrane domain of the *Neu/HER2* oncogene product is sufficient for ligand-independent activation. This mutation promotes receptor dimerization and kinase activation in the absence of ligand. Similarly, the loss of a single cysteine residue in the extracellular domain of the Ret receptor in multiple endocrine neoplasia type-2A syndrome results in a constitutively activated receptor. This mutation frees a cysteine residue that is normally involved in intrareceptor disulphide bond formation and enhances receptor dimerization presumably by the formation of intermolecular disulphide bonds promoting constitutive activation of the receptor catalytic activity. C: The gene rearrangements that activate the Met and Trk and Ret receptor-derived oncogene products. The majority of receptor oncogenes activated by gene rearrangement are fused with a protein domain capable of protein-protein interaction and thus mediate dimerization and constitutive activation of the kinase in the absence of ligand. D: The complex formed between CD4 and the Src family kinase Lck. The protein domains through which Lck and CD4 interact are represented as *open boxes* in these molecules. The c-Src kinase is maintained in an inactive conformation through the interaction of a negative regulatory phosphotyrosine residue in the C-terminus of c-Src with the Src SH-2 domain. The v-*src* oncogene is generated following deletion of this negative regulatory C-terminal tyrosine residue such that the kinase is now in an unconstrained conformation and is constitutively active. Following activation of many growth factor receptor tyrosine kinases, the c-Src SH-2 domain interacts with a phosphorylated tyrosine residue on the receptor with a greater affinity than its C-terminal phosphotyrosine residue (see Fig. 25-8). This relieves the negative regulation of c-Src and activates the kinase. EGF = epidermal growth factor; HGF/SF = hepatocyte growth factor-scatter factor; NGF = nerve growth factor; GDNF = glial cell derived nerve growth factor, TGFβ = transforming growth factor β.

transmit signals that mediate the pleiotrophic responses to growth factors (reviewed in Pawson, 1995[65] and Hunter, 2000[66]). PLCγ hydrolyzes phosphoinositols and thereby generates diacylglycerol and inositol-3-phosphate. PI3K phosphorylates phosphoinositides and generates putative second messengers for cytoskeletal rearrangements and cellular trafficking. By contrast, Grb2 lacks enzymatic activity and contains only SH2 and SH3 domains. SH3 domains also function as protein-protein interaction motifs and recognize proline-rich domains in other proteins.[67] Grb2 serves as an adaptor that binds to phosphotyrosines in activated receptors via its SH2 domain and recruits the Ras nucleotide exchange factors Son of sevenless (mSos-1 and mSos-2) to the receptor via its SH3 domain. Sos catalyzes exchange of GDP bound to Ras for GTP and is considered to be the most important step in Ras activation.[68,69] These proteins, through a series of protein-protein interactions, in part mediated through SH2 domains and SH3 domains, form signaling complexes downstream of receptor tyrosine kinases (reviewed by Pawson & Saxton, 1999[70]). Many of these signaling complexes regulate the activity of serine/threonine kinases, which in turn regulate through phosphorylation the activity of transcription factors. A generalized scheme for receptor signaling is presented in Figure 25-7.

A number of oncogenes encode mutant forms of receptor tyrosine kinases. These include receptors for known factors, such as the epidermal growth factor receptor (EGFR) (v-*erb*B), colony-stimulating factor-1 receptor (CSF-1R) (v-*fms*), hepatocyte growth/scatter factor receptor (*met*), nerve growth factor receptor (*trk*), stem cell factor receptor (SCFR) (*kit*), neuroregulin receptor (Neu/HER2), glial derived neurotopic factor (GDNF) receptor (*ret*), and receptor-like proteins with unknown ligands (*ros*) (Table 25-1). In the receptor-related oncogenes so far examined, the structural changes that activate the transforming potential appear to deregulate the receptor kinase activity, and these oncoproteins transform by delivering a continuous ligand-independent signal (reviewed by Rodrigves & Park, 1994).[71] Receptors isolated as retrovirally transduced oncogenes, such as *v-erb*B (EGFR), v-*fms* (CSF-1R), and v-*kit* (SCFR) (Table 25-1), frequently sustain deletions of the extracellular ligand-binding domain in combination with other structural alterations, such as C-terminal deletions or mutations that remove negative regulatory

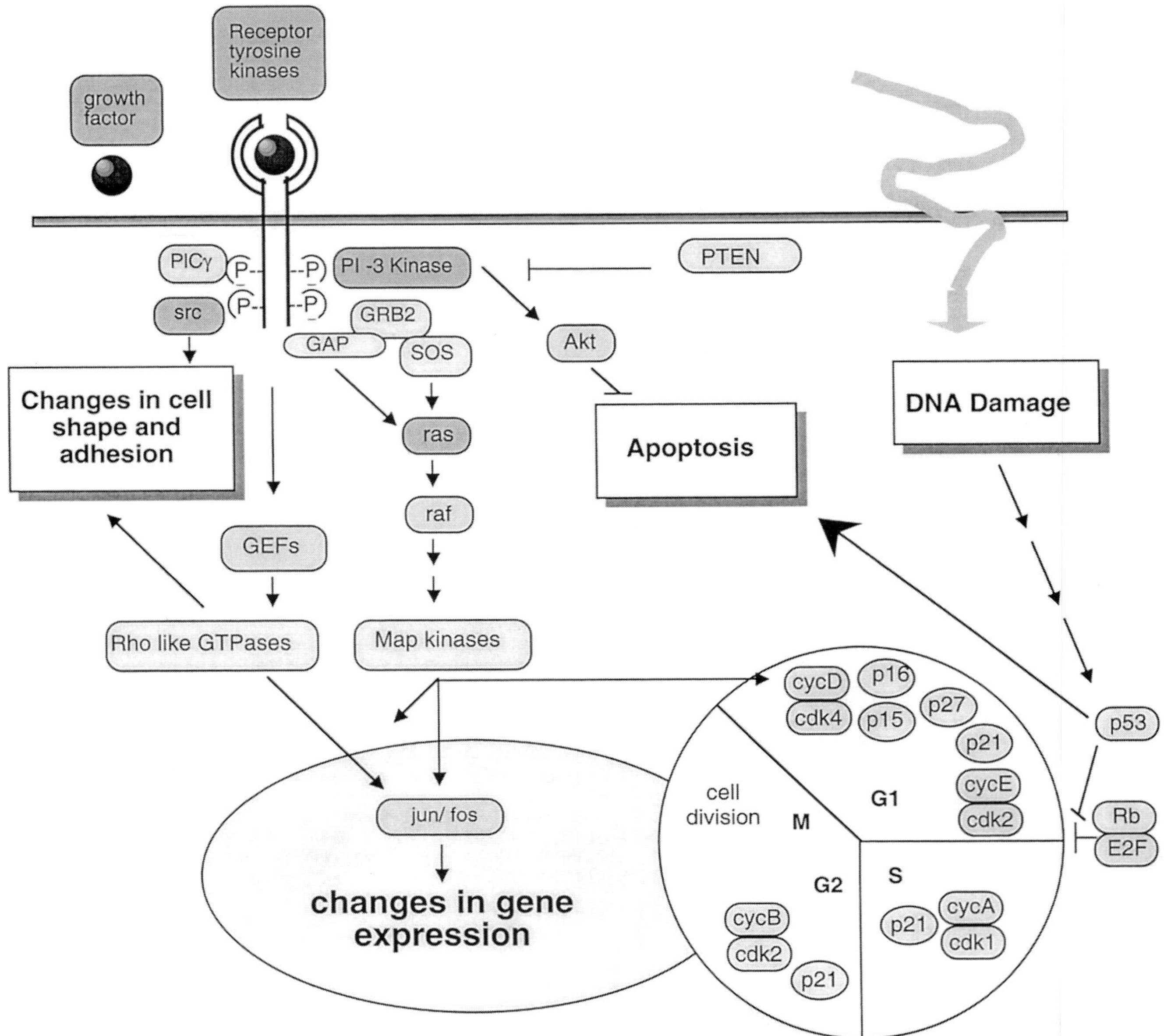

Fig. 25-7 Substrates and mitogenic signaling for receptor tyrosine kinases (RTKs). Activation of receptor tyrosine kinases by the binding of growth factors stimulates cross phosphorylation of their kinase domains. Substrates containing SH-2 domains bind to phosphorylated tyrosine residues on activated receptors. Substrates shown to directly interact with and become activated by or phosphorylated by RTKs; GAP (GTPase-activating protein), PLCγ (phospholipase Cγ), PI-3 kinase (phosphatidylinositol 3′ kinase), and Src (tyrosine kinase) are represented. The Grb2 adaptor protein that lacks enzymatic activity acts as a bridge to translocate the Sos guanine nucleotide exchange protein to the plasma membrane, where it stimulates the exchange of GDP for GTP, activating the Ras protein (see in detail in Fig. 25-8). Activation of Ras translocates the serine threonine kinase Raf to membrane, where it is activated by an unknown mechanism. Activated Raf then activates kinases of the MAP kinase pathway that stimulate the phosphorylation of transcription factors and expression of the *fos* and *jun* transcription factors. Secondary responses involve the breakdown of phosphatidylinositol 4,5 *bis*-phosphate into diacylglycerol (DAG) and inositol triphosphate (InsP3), which stimulate protein kinase C and calcium release, respectively. Components of the signal transduction pathway that have been identified as oncogenes are shown in grey.

domains and render the receptor catalytically active in the absence of ligand.[71])

Mutations that promote ligand-independent dimerization represent a general mechanism for oncogenic activation of receptor tyrosine kinases. A single point mutation in the transmembrane domain of the Neu/HER2 oncogene product is sufficient for ligand-independent activation. This mutation promotes receptor dimerization and kinase activation in the absence of ligand[72,73] (Fig. 25-6). Similarly, the loss of a single cysteine residue in the extracellular domain of the Ret receptor in multiple endocrine neoplasia type 2A syndrome results in a constitutively activated receptor. This mutation frees a cysteine residue that is normally involved in intrareceptor disulphide bond formation and enhances receptor dimerization by the formation of intermolecular disulphide bonds promoting constitutive activation of the receptor catalytic activity.[74,75] A similar mechanism has been demonstrated for the activation of the Neu/HER2 receptor in experimentally induced mammary neoplasias.[76] Alternatively, activation of the

Ret receptor in multiple endocrine neoplasia type 2B occurs by a single point mutation in the kinase domain that increases the basal kinase activity and alters the substrate specificity of the receptor, thus altering the signal transduction pathways activated by the receptor.[77,78]

A growing class of receptor tyrosine kinase oncogenes in human tumors, including *TRK*, *MET*, *RET*, and the platelet-derived growth factor receptor (*PDGFR*), are also rendered constitutively active following genomic rearrangements that juxtapose novel sequences derived from unrelated loci with the kinase domain of the receptor (Fig 25-7).[79] The majority of receptor oncogenes activated by gene rearrangement are fused with a protein domain capable of protein-protein interaction and thus mediate dimerization and constitutive activation of the kinase in the absence of ligand.[71] Receptor fusion oncogenes involving *RET* and *TRK* have been detected in papillary thyroid carcinomas.[80–82] In these tumors, both *RET* (10q11.2)[83] and *TRK* (1q21)[83] are rearranged with loci from the same chromosome, such as H4-*ret* (D10S170, Ptc) 10q21[83] and tropomyosin or tpr/trk (1q21-31).[84] Thus, small intrachromosomal deletions or inversions that are not readily detected cytogenetically may be a common event in the oncogenic activation of these receptor kinases in human tumors.

In addition to structural rearrangements, growth factor receptors are frequently amplified and overexpressed in human tumors. The EGFR is overexpressed in squamous cell carcinomas and gliomas,[36,37] Neu/HER2 in adenocarcinomas of the breast stomach and ovary,[38–40] *MET* (hepatocyte growth factor receptor, HGFR) in human stomach and some colon carcinomas,[85,86] and *bek*, a member of the FGFR family, in human stomach carcinomas[87] (Table 25-4).

Nonreceptor Protein Tyrosine Kinases. The protein products of v-*src*, v-*fes*, v-*fps*, v-*fgr*, v-*yes*, and *lck* are associated with the plasma membrane but are not transmembrane proteins (Fig. 25-6 and Table 25-1). Many of these proteins have a myristilated N-terminal glycine residue that promotes association with the plasma membrane. The cytoplasmic tyrosine protein kinase domain is in the C-terminus of the protein, and all of the tyrosine kinase oncogene proteins are homologous in this region. The *src* subfamily has additional regions of homology not found in the receptor family. These regions include two additional domains named *src* homology 2 and 3 (SH-2 and SH-3) (with SH-1 defined as the kinase domain) (Fig. 25-6).[88] As already discussed, the *src* homology 2 domain is highly conserved in proteins involved in signal transduction and recognizes phosphotyrosine residues, whereas the SH3 domain recognizes proline-rich motifs present in signaling proteins and cytoskeletal proteins.

Association of *src* family kinases with the plasma membrane is essential for their transforming activity. Mutation of the myristoylation signal in these proteins abolishes membrane association and transforming activity, indicating that their signal must be initiated at the plasma membrane, perhaps through interaction with other membrane-bound proteins.[56,89] Oncogenic activation of *src*-like kinases as retrovirally transduced oncoproteins occurs through the acquisition of point mutations and/or deletion of negative regulatory protein domains located at the C-terminus. These alterations generate oncoproteins that phosphorylate cellular proteins on tyrosine residues in an unregulated fashion and thus deliver a continuous, rather than a regulated, signal. The *src* or other *src*-like kinases are essential components of mitogenic signaling pathways downstream from receptor tyrosine kinases.[90] Moreover, *src* kinase activity is activated by receptor tyrosine kinases,[91] suggesting that *src* or *src*-like kinases would be activated in tumors where receptor tyrosine kinases are deregulated. Indeed, activation of c-*src* has been observed in mammary tumors in transgenic mice induced by an oncogenic Neu/HER2 receptor.[92]

The *abl* tyrosine kinase constitutes a separate family of nonreceptor tyrosine kinases that are localized to both the nucleus and the cytoplasm. The Bcr-Abl product has been implicated in the pathogenesis of greater than 95 percent of CML. In a manner similar to receptor fusion oncoproteins, Bcr mediates oligomerization of Bcr-Abl, promoting constitutive activation of the Abl kinase[93] and association with downstream signaling molecules. Moreover, the Bcr-Abl oncoproteins are excluded from the nucleus, which may also prevent interactions with substrates that act to regulate cell growth negatively.[94]

Cytoplasmic Adaptor Proteins. The discovery that some oncogenes encode adaptor proteins that lack contain only SH2 and SH3 domains but lack any catalytic activity has enabled a more complete understanding of the role of these proteins in signal transduction. For example, the v-*crk* oncogene product[95] contains only SH2 and SH3 domains but causes an increase in tyrosine phosphorylated proteins in the cell.[96] Crk and other SH-2/SH-3 domain-containing adaptor proteins bind to phosphorylated tyrosine residues on activated receptor tyrosine kinases or other proteins via their SH2 domains and bind to other proteins via their SH3 domains. In this manner, they bring together heteromeric protein complexes that allow the subsequent phosphorylation of proteins in this complex by the kinase.[97,98] This phosphorylation event, in addition to dephosphorylation events, acts as a mechanism to relay the signal from the cell surface to the nucleus.

Proteins with GTPase Activity. The role of proteins with GTPase activity in tumorigenesis was first identified through the discovery of the *ras* oncogenes that encode a previously unknown form of GTPase. Three *ras* gene family members designated c-Ha-*ras*, c-Ki-*ras*, and N-*ras* involved in malignant transformation have been identified by their presence in rapidly transforming retroviruses and by DNA transfection. In normal cells, members of the *ras* family have been highly conserved throughout evolution and encode cytoplasmic proteins of 21,000 daltons (p21*ras*).[99] Ras proteins are posttranslationally targeted to the plasma membrane through a highly conserved sequence at their N- and C-termini. Membrane association is essential for function of Ras proteins. Certain domains in the Ras proteins are homologous to the subunit of trimeric G proteins, in regions involved in guanine nucleotide binding, and Ras proteins have been shown to bind guanine nucleotides (GTP and GDP).[99] The model proposed for the p21Ras proto-oncogene product is that it exists in equilibrium between two conformations: active, with GTP bound; and inactive, with GDP bound (Fig. 25-8).

In the past 10 years, components of signal transduction pathways have been elucidated and place Ras as a crucial regulator of cell shape, motility, and growth downstream from growth factor receptors (Fig. 25-7). Activation of Ras is coupled to ligand stimulation of growth factor receptors and is mediated by a guanine nucleotide exchange factor (GEF) (Sos). In the case of receptor tyrosine kinases, activation of Ras is mediated by binding of the Grb2 adaptor molecule via its SH2 domain to a specific phosphorylated tyrosine residue on the receptor. Grb2 pulls along the Sos protein, thus localizing it to the plasma membrane where its substrate Ras is localized. Sos then stimulates the exchange of GDP for GTP on Ras, converting Ras from an inactive to an active form[100,101] able to interact with an effector/substrate molecule(s)[102] (Fig. 25-8). Conversely, the inactivation of Ras is mediated in part by the intrinsic GTPase activity of Ras. Usually this activity is low; however, the GTPase activity is stimulated by a GTPase-activating protein GAP, which converts the active GTP-bound form of Ras into the inactive GDP-bound form.[103–105] GAP also contains an SH2 domain and is recruited by activated receptor tyrosine kinases to the plasma membrane.

The activation and inactivation of Ras proteins are carefully orchestrated. The conversion of Ras to the GTP-bound state enables it to interact with other proteins that function as downstream effectors for Ras. One effector for Ras is the serine-threonine kinase Raf. Activation of Ras recruits the Raf kinase to the membrane where it is activated. In turn, Raf activates a linear

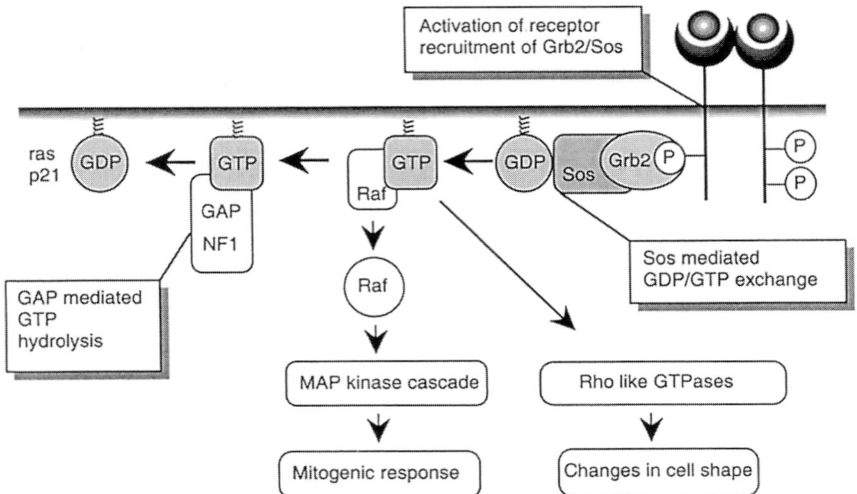

Fig. 25-8 Model for regulation of the Ras p21 product and for the GTPase-activating protein (GAP) as a downstream effector and regulator of *ras* activity. Ras is localized to the inner aspect of the plasma membrane. The alternating relaxed (GDP bound) and activated (GTP bound) states of the p21 Ras protein are shown in normal cells. Conversion of GDP- to GTP-bound forms is the rate-limiting step. Binding of the Grb2 adaptor protein to a specific tyrosine-phosphorylated residue on an activated (growth factor stimulated) receptor tyrosine kinase translocates the Sos guanine nucleotide exchange factor to the plasma membrane, where it stimulates the exchange of GDP for GTP on Ras. Activation of Ras alters its conformation and enables it to interact with and recruit the Raf serine-threonine kinase to the membrane where it becomes activated by an unknown (not Ras) mechanism. Activation of Raf activates the downstream MAP kinase signaling pathway involved in the mitogenic response. In addition, activation of Ras stimulates changes in cell shape and motility mediated through Rho-like GTPase proteins that are part of the Ras superfamily of small GTPase proteins. Inactivation of Ras is in part controlled by the intrinsic intrinsic Ras GTPase, catalyzed by GTPase-activating proteins (GAP and NF1). Oncogenic p21 Ras proteins with mutations at amino acid positions 12, 13, 59, or 61 remain in their active GTP-bound states and constitutively activate downstream signaling pathways.

signaling pathway involving a series of mitogen activated protein (MAP) kinases that culminates in the expression and activation of transcription factors Fos and Jun (Fig. 25-7). These in turn form the AP1 transcription factor that induces transcription of the c-*MYC* transcription factor, which in turn regulates genes whose products control cell cycle progression, culminating in one round of DNA replication and cell division.

The Raf protein kinase was independently isolated as a retrovirally transduced oncoprotein *v-raf* (Table 25-1). Inhibition of the Raf signaling pathway by specific inhibitors or through the use of dominant negatively interfering mutants[106] blocks transformation of fibroblasts in culture by an oncogenic Ras protein. In addition to Raf, transformation of cells by an oncogenic Ras also requires the activity of members of the Rho family of GTPases: Rho and Rac.[107,108] Members of the Rho family of GTPases are involved in rearrangements in the actin cytoskeleton and are thought to regulate the morphologic changes in cell shape associated with transformation of cells by Ras.[109,110]

The *RAS* oncogenes have been identified in a variety of tumors. As discussed previously, the oncogenic forms of Ras differ from their normal counterparts by mutations that result in amino acid substitutions at positions 12, 13, or 61 in the phosphate-binding domain of the protein (reviewed by Barbacid[111]). These oncogenic Ras proteins are locked in their active GTP-bound state through an increased exchange of GDP for GTP or through an inability to interact with or be dephosphorylated by GAPs.[112,113] They therefore have a reduced requirement for GDP/GTP exchange factors and no longer require activation by the Sos exchange factor.

Multiple GAP proteins that function to switch the Ras signal off have been identified. The p120 GAP and neurofibromin (NF1) were the first to be discovered. The p120 GAP appears to control the response of Ras to growth factor stimulation, whereas NF1 appears to control basal Ras activity.[114,115] In humans, loss of the GAP protein NF1 results in the disease neurofibromatosis type 1. Aspects of the disease can be explained in terms of elevated Ras-GTP and are thought to be the result of the loss of neurofibromin GAP activity.[116,117]

GTPase Exchange Factors

Support for Rho-like GTPases in cell transformation and tumorigenesis is also provided by the discovery that multiple independently isolated oncogenes act as exchange factors for Rho-type GTP-binding proteins. Dbl, Vav, Ect-2, Ost, Tiam, Lbc, Lfc, and Dbs were discovered by gene transfer methods by virtue of their ability to transform fibroblasts in culture[118] (Table 25-1). Tiam-1, which appears to directly influence the invasive capacity of T-lymphoma cells, was identified adjacent to a proviral insertion site in retrovirally induced invasive T-lymphoma varients.[119] The *DBL* oncogene was the first member of this family to be identified.[120] Amino acid sequence analysis revealed that Dbl shared homology with a yeast cell division cycle protein Cdc 24, which is an exchange protein for a yeast Rho-like small GTP-binding protein.[120] The homology was restricted to the domain of Cdc24 responsible for the GEF activity, and this result led to the discovery that Dbl is an exchange factor for a mammalian Rho-like protein (Cdc42).[121] All of the oncogenic exchange proteins for small GTP-binding proteins that have been identified, contain a similar domain that is now referred to as a Dbl homology domain. The Dbl domain is essential for the transforming activity of this class of oncogenes, suggesting that their exchange activity for Rho-like GTP-binding proteins is essential for transformation. A full characterization of the mechanism of oncogenic activation of this family of oncoproteins has not been achieved, but the deletion of N-terminal sequences of Dbl or Vav result in oncogenic activation.[122,123] These deletions may remove a negative regulatory domain that normally acts to regulate the GEF activities of these proteins. The current thinking is that Dbl and related proteins activate Rho-like GTP-binding proteins that play important roles in mediating various cytoskeletal reorganizations in cells. Unlike the signaling cascade in which the Ras GEF Sos participates, which binds to the adaptor protein Grb2 and translocates Sos to cell surface receptor tyrosine kinases to activate Ras in response to growth factors, the signaling complexes coupling Dbl-like GEFs to upstream components remain elusive.

Dbl-like GEFs act as exchange factors for members of the Rho family of small GTPases. These proteins are structurally related to the Ras family of GTPases. Members of the Rho family of small GTPases Rho, Rac, and Cdc42 are important regulators of the actin cytoskeleton. Microinjection of activated proteins into serum-starved fibroblasts demonstrates that Rho stimulates the organization of actin stress fibers, Rac stimulates the formation of lamellipodia, and Cdc42 induces filopodial formation.[124] Because of their effects on motile cytoskeletal structures, it is not hard to envision that inappropriate activation of Rho family of GTPases during tumorigenesis could affect whether a cell maintains a differentiated morphology or acquires a motile, invasive phenotype.

Cytoplasmic Serine-Threonine Protein Kinases

The serine-threonine kinases studied so far are soluble cytoplasmic proteins. This class includes the Mos, Cot, Pim-1, and Raf oncogenes in addition to protein kinase C (PKC) (Table 25-1). Oncogenic forms of the v-*raf* serine kinase have lost N-terminal regulatory sequences that lead to constitutive activation of the kinase activity and mitogenic MAP kinase pathway (Fig. 25-7). Phosphorylation of the c-Raf protein kinase is normally tightly regulated. Raf kinase activity is rapidly elevated when resting cells are stimulated by mitogens[125] (Fig. 25-7) or by another member of the serine-threonine kinase family, PKC. Several tumor promoters act via stimulation of the PKC family[126] and mediate activation of the Raf signaling pathway. Although a mutant form of PKCα has been detected as an oncogene and although overexpression of PKC can affect the growth of cells in culture,[127] mutant PKC enzymes are rare in human cancers.

Nuclear Protein Family

The products of oncogenes and proto-oncogenes localized to the nucleus are directly implicated in the control of gene expression involved in cellular proliferation and differentiation. Many of these have been shown to act as transcription factors and appear to be constitutively activated forms of their normal cellular counterparts (reviewed by Lewin, 1991[128]). For example, a complex between c-Jun[129] and c-Fos[130] corresponds to the mammalian transcription factor AP-l, which interacts following phorbol ester treatment or serum stimulation of cells with specific promoter elements to stimulate gene transcription.[131,132] The oncogenic Jun and Fos transcription factors carry mutations that lead to loss of negative regulatory elements, and these factors are now constitutively active.[133] In addition to loss of negative regulatory domains, some oncogenic transcription factors lose positive effector domains, resulting in *dominant negative* proteins that appear to prevent expression of genes required for cell differentiation.[134]

Since many nuclear oncogenes have been implicated in *trans*-activating and/or *trans*-repressing gene expression, it is possible that alteration of these genes either directly (activated c-*myc*, v-*jun*, or v-*erb*A) or indirectly (e.g., induction of their expression by an activated growth factor receptor) may lead to an imbalance in the delicate network of gene expression that regulates cell differentiation and growth control. Consistent with the hypothesis that nuclear oncogenes have central roles in events involved in cellular proliferation, the proto-oncogene forms of these genes are normally expressed in a variety of cell types during proliferation and have RNA and protein products with short half-lives. Because of the lability of the RNA and protein products, changes in transcription could lead to relatively rapid fluctuations in the steady-state levels of RNA and protein.[133] For example, c-*fos* and c-*myc* are expressed in replicating cells, but their expression is negligible in quiescent cells or during terminal differentiation.[134,135] When quiescent murine fibroblasts are stimulated with serum or growth factors to enter the Gl phase of growth, a transient increase in the levels of c-*myc*, c-*fos*, c-*jun*, and c-*myb* is observed (Fig. 25-5).[133–135] It is now accepted that these proto-oncogenes are required for cells to transit from a resting state (G0) to a state in which proliferation can proceed (Gl) (c-*fos*, c-*jun*, and c-*myc*) and to traverse specific points in the cell cycle.

The retroviruses that have transduced *myc*, *myb*, and *fos* express these genes in infected cells at levels higher than their cellular counterparts and in a nonregulated manner. Similarly, the amplification of the c-*MYC* locus in human tumors or the rearranged c-*MYC* locus in Burkitt lymphomas is no longer subjected to control, and these genes are expressed constitutively. Thus, the unregulated and/or ectopic expression of these genes in a differentiated cell substitutes for the growth factor requirement for quiescent cells to enter G1 and provides a constant proliferative signal in the absence of growth factors.

The identification of new oncogenes and tumor-suppressor genes can lead to the delineation of new signaling pathways involved in cancer. The recent dissection of the function of the adenomatous polyposis coli tumor suppressor and β-catenin has identified a critical role for these proteins in tumorigenesis. β-Catenin is found in two distinct multiprotein complexes in the cell. One complex located at the plasma membrane couples cadherins (calcium-dependent adhesion molecules) with the actin cytoskeleton, stabilizing cell-cell adhesion.[136] The other complex, which contains the adenomatosis polyposis coli (APC) protein, a serine-threonine kinase (glycogen synthase kinase 3β), and another protein called Axin, targets β-catenin for degradation.[137,138] In the absence of functional APC, β-catenin is not degraded and free β-catenin acts to enhance transcription through its interaction with a transcription factor: LEF1/TCF. This process is normally regulated by extracellular signals. Mutations in the APC gene that cause loss of function are found in multiple human tumors, thus stabilizing β-catenin and enhancing transcription.[139] Defects in the APC gene are responsible for inherited and sporadic forms of colon cancer and may account for up to 80 percent of the cancers in this tissue, implicating β-catenin-dependent signals as a key event in colon carcinogenesis.[140] Recently, mutations have also been identified in β-catenin that prevent its degradation induced by a wild-type APC protein.[141–143] These have been identified in human melanomas, hepatocellular carcinomas, cancers of the uterine and ovarian endometrium, and a small subset of colon cancers. Where studied, mutations in β-catenin and APC are mutually exclusive (reviewed by Polakis, 1999[144]). The APC gene is targeted for mutation in human colon cancer far more frequently than is β-catenin. This might relate to the specific dietary or environmental insults that give rise to these mutations. In contrast in experimentally induced intestinal tumors induced in rats, the majority contained mutations in β-catenin but not APC.[145] Once activated, β-catenin can constitutively interact with multiple different targets, thus sending persistent signals that override normal cell growth control. Activation of gene transcription through LEF/TCF is probably involved in the cancer process, as the proto-oncogene *myc* has recently been identified as one of the targets of the APC pathway.[146]

In addition to protein kinases acting as signal relays important for the control of cell growth and tumorigenesis, lipid kinases have emerged as controlling many cellular processes.[147,148] One subfamily of lipid kinases include phosphoinositide 3-kinases (PI3′K), which catalyze the addition of a phosphate molecule specifically to the 3-position of the inositol ring of phosphoinositides.[149] Phosphatidylinositol 3,4,5-phosphate acts as a ligand for some proteins that contain a phospholipid-binding PH domain.[150] One of these is a serine-threonine kinase (PDK1) that activates the Akt kinase.[151] Activation of Akt results in the phosphorylation of multiple proteins, some of which act to suppress apoptosis[152] whereas others stimulate a mitogenic response (Fig. 25-7).[153] Notably, the PI3′K and Akt gene β were identified as retroviral oncoproteins and the P13′K gene is amplified in human ovarian cancer.[154] In addition to enzymes that phosphorylate lipids, an enzyme called PTEN was recently identified that dephosphorylates PI-3,4,5. This acts to antagonize the activity of PI3′K, and loss of a functional PTEN gene has been demonstrated in multiple human tumors (reviewed by Cantley & Neel, 1999[154]).

COOPERATION BETWEEN ONCOGENES

Accumulating evidence suggests that the products of proto-oncogenes and growth-suppressor genes function in both common and parallel signaling pathways (reviewed by Weinberg, 1989[155]). The activation of cooperating oncogenes and the inactivation of growth-suppressor genes appear necessary for a complete neoplastic phenotype. Several events are required to influence aspects of the transformed phenotype: for example, cell shape, invasiveness, and anchorage-independent growth, in addition to blocking cell differentiation and driving a cell constantly through uncontrolled cell division. Transformation causes cells to acquire anchorage and/or serum independence, suggesting that oncogenes that cause anchorage-independent growth represent signaling molecules downstream from integrin-mediated adhesive events, whereas oncogenes causing serum independence are part of growth factor signaling pathways, and oncogenes inducing both are part of convergent pathways.[156]

Oncogenes and the Cell Cycle

The signals from the oncogenes described above converge on a control apparatus: the cell cycle clock that controls cell proliferation. The genomic changes and mutations observed in tumor cells are now considered to be the result of defects in checkpoints that control the cell cycle in response to DNA damage, defects in DNA replication, or chromosome attachment to the spindle (reviewed by Hartwell & Weinert, 1989[157]).

There are many regulated decision points required for a cell to progress through the cell cycle, and it is now clear that many of these are targets for oncogene action. Based on studies on yeasts and the conserved nature of the cell cycle components, the eukaryotic cell cycle is believed to be regulated at two major decision points: a point in G1 when a cell becomes committed to DNA synthesis and the G2 mitosis (M) boundary (Fig. 25-5) (reviewed by Murray, 1992[158]).

Many cells in vivo are in a quiescent state (G0) with unduplicated DNA. Growth-inhibitory signals are provided by soluble factors such as TGFβ, cell-to-cell contacts, and adhesion to extracellular matrix components,[159,160] whereas growth stimulatory signals are provided by growth factors. The balance between growth-inhibitory signals and growth stimulatory signals forces cells to make a decision to enter G1 and initiate cell division.[161] At a checkpoint in late G1 (the *restriction point*),[162] a cell decides whether the signals received are suitable for growth and progresses through G1 into S phase (Fig 25-5).

The transition through the restriction point in late G1 represents a critical point where a cell decides between continued proliferation and escape from the cell cycle. In recent years, it has become clear that the deregulation of this transition is critical to malignant growth. Cancer cells escape growth inhibition in several ways. One mechanism involves the activation of growth-promoting genes, growth factors, receptors, *RAS* genes, or nuclear oncoproteins that allow the cell to progress through G1, whereas a second mechanism involves the loss of receptors for growth-inhibitory genes such as TGFβ.[162] Once at the restriction point at the end of G1, the entry into S phase is governed through the activation of cyclin-dependent kinases. The G1 cyclins (D and E types) regulate the G1/S boundary, whereas mitotic cyclins (A and B types) regulate the G2/M transition (Fig. 25-5). Alterations in cyclins can cause transformation. Cyclin D1 was identified as the oncogene product of *PRAD1*, a gene rearranged in human parathyroid carcinomas[163] and expressed at high levels,[164] and as the product of the *bcl1* oncogene, a proviral integration site.[165] Cyclin D1 is amplified and its mRNA overexpressed in many tumor types.[166] Moreover, mice carrying a cyclin D1 transgene under the control of a mammary-specific promoter develop mammary hyperplasia and adenocarcinoma,[206] whereas overexpression of cyclin D1 and c-*myc* in lymphoid cells of transgenic mice gives rise to lymphomas.[168,169]

The control of the G1-S checkpoint is regulated by the phosphorylation of the tumor-suppressor gene product Rb by cyclin D- and E-dependent kinases.[170] Phosphorylated Rb is unable to form complexes with E2F-type transcription factors, which are then free to induce transcription of S-phase-specific genes.[171] Regulation of this checkpoint is lost by several mechanisms. One involves the overexpression of cyclin D. Others involve the loss of function of the tumor-suppressor gene *Rb*, such that it no longer interacts with E2F, or loss of function of inhibitors of cyclin D (p16, p15).[172–174] Thus, the functional inactivation of *Rb* obtained either through the deregulated expression of cyclin D1, inactivation of inhibitors of cyclin D1 (p16, p15), or mutation in the *Rb* gene results in the loss of a cell cycle checkpoint and is thought to be an obligatory step for tumorigenesis.

The product of c-*mos*, a serine-threonine kinase, is also implicated in cell cycle control. It activates serine kinases of the MAP kinase family and is implicated in the reorganization of microtubules that lead to formation of the spindle pole during meiosis in oocytes.[175] The aberrant expression of *mos* in somatic cells leads to cells with 4N DNA content, possibly through interference with the assembly and positioning of the mitotic spindle.[176] Such an event could provide a mechanism for genetic instability that leads to the polyploid DNA content frequently observed in tumor cells.

Oncogenes and Cell Death

Whether in a normal tissue or in a tumor, the balance between cell death and proliferation governs the accumulation of cells. There is now evidence that induced suicide (apoptosis) is a major mechanism for the elimination of cells with DNA damage or an aberrant cell cycle, i.e., cells that are precursors for neoplastic changes. In contrast to *necrosis*, which represents a pathologic response to severe cellular injury, *apoptosis* is a cell's normal response to physiological signals or lack thereof (reviewed by Kerr & Harmon, 1996[177]). Apoptosis is an active process. Internucleosomal cleavage of DNA is a feature of apoptosis, and the resulting DNA ladder is used as an assay for apoptosis. Apoptotic cells can also be detected in tumors, either cytologically or by using molecular assays on tissue sections. Thus, cell death probably accounts for the slow growth rate of some tumors.

Some dominant oncogenes have been shown to exhibit a surprising biologic property: the ability to induce apoptosis. The c-*myc* proto-oncogene, whose expression is altered or deregulated in a large percentage of tumors, can promote apoptosis as well as proliferation.[178,179] Many cytokines are both survival and proliferation signals, suggesting that their receptors transduce signals that stimulate proliferation and entry into the cell cycle as well as inhibiting apoptosis. Thus, a mechanism coupling cell proliferation with apoptosis would provide a safety net for any proliferating cell when stimulated by a mitogen, or a mutation (amplified *myc*) would spontaneously induce cell death when it exhausted available cytokines (Fig 25-9).

Many of the signals that monitor the state of the cell in response to these distinct physiological signals converge on the p53 protein, which then signals the cell cycle clock to shut down until the problem, such as DNA damage is corrected, or alternatively will initiate cell death through apoptosis. The p53 tumor-suppressor gene (reviewed by Lane, 1992 Donehower & Bradley, 1993[180,181]) encodes a transcription factor that regulates the expression of proteins that negatively regulate the cyclin-dependent kinases required for cell cycle progression (reviewed by Hunter, 1993[182]). Thus, if induction of apoptosis were an automatic response to oncogene activation, then an increase in cell number would depend on active suppression of apoptosis.[183] This can be achieved through loss or mutation of p53, a frequent event in human cancers, where cells that sustain DNA damage or oncogene activation no longer trigger apoptosis.[180] Alternatively, the deregulated expression of the *bcl-2* oncogene mediates

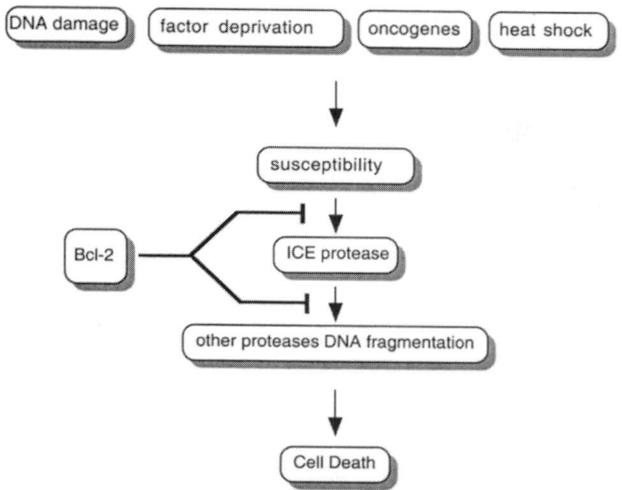

Fig. 25-9 Model for regulation of apoptosis by Bcl-2. Apoptosis is triggered by many agents, including DNA damage, factor deprivation, and oncogene activation (e.g., Myc and stress, such as heat shock). The ability of Bcl-2 to inhibit cell death caused by many different agents argues for the involvement of Bcl-2 in a final common pathway. This involves an ICE-like cysteine protease. Bcl-2 may suppress apoptosis by either preventing cleavage and activation of the cysteine protease proenzyme, interfering with proteolytic activity, or sequestering a target protein.

antiapoptotic effects and specifically blocks the ability of c-*myc* to induce apoptosis.[184,185]

The *Bcl*-2 oncogene was found at the junction of the chromosome 14;18 translocation in follicular lymphoma[186] (Table 25-1) and encodes a membrane-associated protein that is found in the endoplasmic reticulum and nuclear and outer mitochondrial membranes.[187] Although *BCL*-2 activation alone is not sufficient for follicular lymphoma formation, *BCL*-2 translocations appear to lead to cell immortalization and suggest an initiating role for *BCL*-2 in the etiology of tumors through prolonged cell survival. Bcl-2 is a member of a growing family of proteins that have been conserved throughout evolution and inhibits p53-mediated apoptosis induced by growth factor deprivation, deregulated *myc*, or genotoxic agents.[187,188] Since Bcl-2 can inhibit apoptosis induced by a wide variety of agents, the step regulated by Bcl-2 was thought to lie within a common final pathway. Indeed, Bcl-2 proteins inhibit the action of ICE-like proteases that trigger apoptosis (Fig 25-9).[189]

Experimental Evidence for Cooperating Oncogenes

It has been possible to subdivide the oncogenes further into two groups based on their phenotypes in DNA transfection assays performed in embryo fibroblast cells that have a finite life in culture. One class of genes rescues embryo fibroblasts from senescence, thus allowing cells to be continuously maintained in culture (*immortalization*), whereas the second class morphologically alters the rescued cells and renders them tumorigenic (*transformation*).[190–192] It was subsequently discovered that many of the oncogenes could be assigned to either the immortalization group or the transformation group. Furthermore, members of the immortalization group act synergistically with members of the transformation group to transform embryo fibroblasts; for example, foci of transformed cells appear when embryo fibroblasts are transfected with both v-H-*ras* and v-*myc* oncogenes.[190–191] The v-*myc* oncogene rescues cells from senescence and therefore belongs to the immortalization-complementation group, which includes the *myc* gene family and nuclear transcription factors *fos* and *jun* (Table 25-4). In this assay, the v-*ras* gene morphologically transforms immortalized embryo fibroblasts and belongs to the transformation-complementation group.

NIH3T3 cells have properties similar to those of embryo fibroblast cells immortalized with a member(s) of the first complementation group, and therefore these cells are particularly useful in DNA transfection assays for identifying genes of the second complementation group (e.g., *ras*). In general, the protein products of the members of the first group are found in the nucleus and do not generally alter cell morphology or anchorage requirements but appear to immortalize cells. Conversely, products of the second group are found in the cytoplasm and, in most cases, are associated with the cytoplasmic side of the plasma membrane. These oncoproteins can reduce growth factor requirements, induce cell shape changes, and lead to anchorage-independent cell growth, but do not immortalize cells (reviewed in Hunter, 1997[193]).

TRANSGENIC MOUSE MODELS FOR CANCER

Compelling evidence for oncogene cooperation has also come from studies of transgenic mice.[194,195] Specific genes (*transgenes*) are introduced into the germ line of mice by microinjection of recombinant DNA into the male pronucleus of fertilized eggs. Progeny from implanted transgenic embryos are scored for the presence of the transgene by analysis of DNA extracted from the tail of the newborn animal. In this system, the action of activated oncogenes can be assessed in a host capable of mounting a physiological response to tumor formation.

Transgenic mouse strains carrying a single oncogene under the transcriptional control of ubiquitous promoter elements or tissue-specific promoter elements from heterologous genes generally show a strongly enhanced level of neoplasia or hyperplasia, but this frequently occurs only in specific tissues and not in all tissues expressing the oncogene. In many cases, oncogene expression precedes tumor formation by many months. Long latencies and variable penetrance may be observed; frequently, the tumors that do arise are both rare and clonal, inferring that other events are necessary.[197] Retroviruses carrying a single oncogene give rise to tumors, but this occurs largely through virus spread that recruits surrounding cells into forming a polyclonal tumor. Although chronic myelogenous leukemia may be initiated solely by Bcr-Abl expression, its chronic phase may actually represent a preneoplastic syndrome. In general, there is little evidence to support the concept that in vivo expression of a single oncogene can induce polyclonal tumors (reviewed by Frost et al, 1995[196]).

Tumor-prone transgenic mice provide insight into oncogene collaboration. Known or putative oncogenes can be tested for their ability to accelerate tumorigenesis. When two strains of oncogene-bearing mice are crossed, the tumor incidence is often greatly accelerated and increased. Moreover, an effective way to screen for many genes that can collaborate with the transgene is provided by insertional mutagenesis with a retrovirus that lacks an oncogene (Fig. 25-2). These viruses promote tumorigenesis by chance integration next to a cellular gene, altering its transcription. Consequently, sites of integration common to several tumors are used to identify genes that have contributed to the neoplastic process.

Studies with retroviruses and transgenic mice have identified eight genes that can cooperate with *myc* to transform lymphoid cells. In mice bearing a *myc* gene coupled to an immunoglobulin heavy-chain enhancer (Eu), constructed to mimic the translocations that occur in Burkitt lymphoma, B-lymphoid tumors invariably develop.[198] Tumor onset takes place randomly, however, and tumors are monoclonal in nature. Despite its proliferative signal, the deregulated expression of *myc* was not sufficient for full neoplastic transformation, and both the pre-B and B cells died rapidly if deprived of growth factors in culture. Thus, additional oncogenic mutations that can collaborate with the transgene are required. Doubly transgenic progeny from Eu-*myc* and Eu-N-*ras* mice rapidly developed B-cell tumors.[199] Thus, *myc* and *ras* are effective partners in leukomagenesis as well as other tumor types. In addition to *ras*, *myc* synergizes with the *raf* and *pim*-1 serine-threonine kinases in addition to the *abl* tyrosine kinase, the antiapoptotic gene *Bcl*-2, the transcription factor *bmi*-1, as well as mutations in the tumor-suppressor gene *p53*. Mutations in different genes are thought to provide complementary functions. For example, *myc* seems to prevent cells from becoming quiescent by overcoming the G1-S checkpoint, whereas *Bcl-2* blocks apoptosis induced by expression of *myc* and others; for example, *ras*, *raf*, or *pim*-1 may decrease growth factor requirements.

The synergistic action of expression of v-Ha-*ras* and c-*myc* constructs also induces breast cancer when the transgenes are expressed in breast epithelia by using the mouse mammary tumor virus (MMTV) promoter/enhancer.[200] In all cases, however, tumors arise as clonal outgrowths, and nonmalignant cells expressing both oncogenes predominate. Moreover, *RAS* mutations are rare in human breast cancers. Instead, at least three proto-oncogenes have been implicated in human breast carcinogenesis. These include Myc, the HER2/Neu receptor tyrosine kinase, and Cyclin D1, each of which has been found amplified and overexpressed in human mammary tumors.[201,202] Similar transgenetic models for breast cancer have been made involving *myc*, *HER2/neu*, and cyclin D1 under the MMTV or whey acid protein promoter/enhancer.[203–206] Female transgenic mice from each of these systems develop mammary tumors, although it is apparent that events in addition to the transgene are usually required for tumor development.

TARGETING SIGNAL TRANSDUCTION PATHWAYS AS A METHOD FOR THERAPY

The high correlation of the clinical pattern of CML with the Phl chromosome and expression of the chimeric Bcr-Abl protein argue for a role of the *BCR-ABL* gene in the development of CML. Other cellular oncogenes have been implicated in the development of human neoplasia. The *HER*2 gene is amplified in mammary carcinomas with poor prognosis, and the *EGFR* (c-*erb*B) and c-*MYB* genes have been found to be amplified and overexpressed in certain tumors. The expression of the growth factor c-*sis* (B-chain PDGF) is increased in some human sarcoma and glioblastoma cell lines and tumors and may function as an autocrine for these tumors.

A major goal of new antitumor therapies involves interrupting the constitutive signals that drive tumor cell growth. The goal is to introduce agents that specifically turn off the signaling pathway(s) in a given tumor type. Signaling pathways can be inhibited by a variety of reagents, including small peptide-based mimics, antibodies, DNA encoding dominant negative proteins, antisense RNA, and target-specific RNA ribozymes. Most of the efforts to generate novel drugs aimed at signal transduction pathways are aimed at designing small molecules that act as specific inhibitors of enzymatic activity or protein-protein interactions interrupting the ability of docking proteins to interact with their receptor. Intensive efforts have therefore been invested in generating inhibitors of protein tyrosine kinase activity, and highly selective blockers have been synthesized.[207,208] Specific blockers for the EGFR have been shown to block the growth of solid tumors overexpressing EGFR,[209,210,211] although none of these studies reported complete eradication of the tumor. However, antibodies against the HER2/Neu receptor and EGF receptor are already in clinical trials as a treatment for breast cancer,[212] and cancers that overexpress the EGF receptor.[213] Complete tumor eradication was achieved in a JAK-2 kinase-driven pre-B-cell acute lymphoblastic leukemia model using an inhibitor of the JAK-2 kinase.[214] More importantly, no toxic side effects were observed. Specificity in these systems is, however, dependent on either the restricted expression of the oncogene primarily to tumor tissue, such as Jak-2, or an apparent decrease in the redundancy of growth factor-driven signaling pathways observed in human tumors.

Other targets are designed to inhibit proteins such as Ras and cyclin-dependent kinases that are involved in many mitogenic pathways. Specific inhibitors of cyclin-dependent kinases induce cell cycle arrest in the G1-S phase boundary of the cell cycle. Moreover, the frequency with which *ras* genes are activated in human tumors, and that gene's role as an important signal transducer for signals from protein tyrosine kinases, make it an ideal target for inhibitors. One effective strategy is based on the requirement of the Ras protein to first attach to the inner surface of the plasma membrane by linking to an isoprenyl group (farnesyl). A number of small molecules have been developed to inhibit this process in vivo,[215] and some of these inhibit the growth of Ras-transformed cells in vitro; however, the central nature of Ras action in normal cellular signaling pathways requires that inhibitors target only mutant Ras or Ras in tumor cells. Other strategies have been designed to interfere with the interaction of Ras with exchange proteins required for its activation. Other techniques involve gene therapy that is designed to introduce into tumor cells genes encoding dominant negative inhibitors of ras that produce a mutant protein that incorporates into and blocks the signaling pathway. Although these strategies have been used successfully in tumor cells in vitro, this approach awaits further development as a suitable anticancer therapy. As every tumor is usually driven by multiple signaling pathways, a combination of strategies may be essential for complete suppression of tumor growth. Considering that oncogenes were discovered only 20 years ago, the pace of recent developments in the molecular nature of their action has opened the gate to the ability to design specific inhibitors for each of these products.

SUMMARY

It is now accepted that cancer is a multistep process and that activation of oncogenes is involved in at least some steps of this pathway. Although the link between oncogene activation and initiation or progression of human cancer is complex, several oncogenes in human cancers have been identified. Thus, alterations to proto-oncogenes have been implicated in the genesis of human and animal tumors. The same rearrangements and mutations involving genes already identified by retroviral transduction have been found repeatedly in human and animal tumors. Clearly, the link between oncogene activation and development of human cancer is complex, but the discovery of oncogenes has provided a new method, particularly in hematologic malignancies, and now for sarcomas, for tumor diagnosis. Having sufficient information about the structure and function of the proteins encoded by dominant oncogenes will enable the design of specific inhibitors for each oncogene product and should ultimately lead to the development of new treatments for neoplastic disease.

REFERENCES

1. Stehlin D, Varmus HE, Bishop JM, Vogt PK: DNA related to the transforming gene(s) of avian sarcoma viruses is present in normal avian DNA. *Nature* **260**:170, 1976.
2. Temin HM: On the origin of genes for neoplasia: Clowes Memorial Lecture. *Cancer Res* **34**:2835, 1974.
3. Bishop JM: Enemies within: The genesis of retrovirus oncogenes. *Cell* **23**:5, 1982.
4. Aaronson SA: Growth factors and cancer. *Science* **254**:1146, 1991.
5. Hunter T, Karin M: The regulation of transcription by phosphorylation. *Cell* **70**:375, 1992.
6. Hanawalt PC, Sarasin A: Cancer-prone hereditary diseases with DNA processing abnormalities. *Trends Genet* **2**:124, 1986.
7. Vogelstein B, Fearon ER, Scott EK, Hamilton SR, Preisinger AC, Nakamura Y, White R: Allelotype of colorectal carcinomas. *Science* **244**:207, 1989.
8. Leach FSC, Nicolaides NC, Papadopoulos N, Liu B, Jen J, Parsons R, Peltomaki P, Sistonen P, Aaltonen LA, Nystrom-hahti M et al.: Mutations of a mutS homolog in hereditary non-polyposis colorectal cancer. *Cell* **75**:1215–25, 1993.

9. Fishel R, Lescoe MK, Rao MR, Copeland NG, Jenkins NA, Garber J, Kane M, Kolodner R: The human mutator gene homolog MSH2 and its association with hereditary nonpolyposis colon cancer. *Cell* **75**:1027, 1993 [erratum appears in *Cell* **77**:167, 1994].
10. Graham FL, Van der Eb AJ: A new technique for the assay of infectivity of human adenovirus 5 DNA. *J Virol* **52**:456, 1973.
11. Shih C, Weinberg RA: Isolation of a transforming sequence from a human bladder carcinoma cell line. *Cell* **29**:161, 1982.
12. Blair DG, Cooper CS, Oskarsson MK, Eader LA, Vande Woude G: New method for detecting cellular transforming genes. *Science* **218**:1122, 1982.
13. Goldfarb MP, Shimizu K, Perucho M, Wigler M: Isolation and preliminary characterization of a human transforming gene from T24 bladder carcinoma cells. *Nature* **296**:404, 1982.
14. Pulciani S, Santos E, Lauver AV, Long LK, Aaronson SA, Barbacid M: Oncogenes in solid human tumours. *Nature* **300**:539, 1982.
15. Parada LP, Tabin CJ, Shih C, Weinberg RA: Human EJ bladder carcinoma oncogene is homologue of Harvey sarcoma virus *ras* gene. *Nature* **297**:474, 1982.
16. Perucho M, Goldfarb MP, Shimizu K, Lama C, Pogh J, Wigler M: Human-tumor-derived cell lines contain common and different transforming genes. *Cell* **27**:467, 1981.
17. Barbacid M: *ras* Genes. *Annu Rev Biochem* **56**:779, 1987.
18. Bos JL: *ras* Oncogenes in human cancer: A review. Cancer Res **49**:4682, 1989 [erratum appears in *Cancer Res* **50**:1352, 1990].
19. Ahuja HG, Foti A, Bar-Eli M, Cline MJ: The pattern of mutational involvement of *RAS* genes in human hematologic malignancies determined by DNA amplification and direct sequencing. *Blood* **75**:1684, 1990.
20. Rowley JD: The critical role of chromosome translocations in human leukemias [Review, 94 references]. *Annu Rev Genet* **32**:495, 1998.
21. Rabbitts TH: Perspective: Chromosomal translocations can affect genes controlling gene expression and differentiation. Why are these functions targeted? [Review, 41 references]. *J Pathol* **187**:39, 1999.
22. Nowell PC, Rowley JD, Knudson AG Jr: Cancer genetics, cytogenetics: Defining the enemy within. *Nature Med* **4**:1107, 1998.
23. De Klein A, Van Kessel AG, Grosveld G, Bartram CR, Hagemeijer A, Bootsma D, Spurr NK, Heisterkamp N, Groffen J, Stephenson JR: Cellular oncogene is translocated to the Philadelphia chromosome in chronic myelocytic leukaemia. *Nature* **300**:765, 1982.
24. Wang JYJ: Abl tyrosine kinase in signal transduction and cell-cycle regulation. *Curr Opin Genet Dev* **3**:35, 1993.
25. Spencer CA, Groudine M: Control of c-*myc* regulation in normal and neoplastic cells. *Adv Cancer Res* **56**:1, 1991.
26. Stanton LW, Watt R, Marcu KB: Translocation, breakage and truncated transcripts of c-*myc* oncogene in murine plasmacytomas. *Nature* **303**:401, 1983.
27. Cooper CS: Translocations in solid tumours. *Curr Opin Genet Dev* **6**:71, 1996.
28. Alitalo K, Schwab M, Lin CC, Varmus HE, Bishop JM: Homogeneously staining chromosomal regions contain amplified copies of an abundantly expressed cellular oncogene (c-*myc*) in malignant neuroendocrine cells from a human colon carcinoma. *Proc Natl Acad Sci USA* **80**:1707, 1983.
29. Schwab M, Alitalo K, Klempnauer K-H, Varmus HE, Bishop JM, Gilbert F, Brodeur GM, Goldstein M, Trent J: Amplified DNA with limited homology to *myc* cellular oncogene is shared by human neuroblastoma cell lines and a neuroblastoma tumour. *Nature* **305**:245, 1983.
30. Schwab M: Oncogene amplification in solid tumors [Review, 46 references]. *Semin Cancer Biol* **9**:319, 1999.
31. Collins S, Groudine M: Amplification of endogenous *myc*-related DNA sequences in a human myeloid leukaemia cell line. *Nature* **298**:679, 1982.
32. Dalla-Favera R, Wong-Staal F, Gallo RC: *onc* Gene amplification in promyelocytic leukaemia cell line HL-60 and primary leukaemic cells of the same patient. *Nature* **299**:61, 1982.
33. Brodeur GM, Seeger RC, Schwab M, Varmus HE, Bishop JM: Amplification of N-*myc* in untreated human neuroblastomas correlates with advanced disease stage. *Science* **224**:1121, 1984.
34. Little CD, Nau MM, Carney DN, Gazdar AF, Minna JD: Amplification and expression of the c-*myc* oncogene in human lung cancer cell lines. *Nature* **306**:194, 1983.
35. Nau MM, Brooks BJ, Battey J, Sausville E, Gazdar AF, Kirsch IR, McBride OW, Bertness V, Hollis GF, Minna JD: L-*myc*, a new *myc*-related gene amplified and expressed in human small lung cancer. *Nature* **318**:69, 1984.
36. Yamamoto T, Kamat N, Kawano H, Shimizu S, Kuroki T, Toyoshima K, Rikimaru K, Nomura N, Ishizaki R, Pastan I, Gamou S, Shimizu N: High incidence of amplification of the epidermal growth factor receptor gene in human squamous carcinoma cell lines. *Cancer Res* **46**:414, 1986.
37. Reissmann PT, Koga H, Figlin RA, Holmes EC, Slamon DJ: Amplification and overexpression of the cyclin D1 and epidermal growth factor receptor genes in non-small-cell lung cancer. Lung Cancer Study Group. *J Cancer Res Clin Oncol* **125**:61, 1999.
38. Yokota J, Terada M, Toyoshima K, Sugimura T, Yamato T, Battifora H, Cline MJ: Amplification of the c-*erb*B-2 oncogene in human adenocarcinomas *in vivo*. *Lancet* **1**:765, 1986.
39. Zhou D, Battifora H, Yokota J, Yamamoto T, Cline MJ: Association of multiple copies of the C-*erb*B-2 oncogene with spread of breast cancer. *Cancer Res* **47**:6123, 1987.
40. Pegram MD, Pauletti G, Slamon DJ: *HER*-2/neu as a predictive marker of response to breast cancer therapy [Review, 39 references]. *Breast Cancer Res Treat* **52**:65, 1998.
41. Bishop JM: Molecular themes in oncogenesis. *Cell* **64**:235, 1991.
42. Bourne HR, Sanders DA, McCormick F: The GTPase superfamily: I. A conserved switch for diverse cell functions. *Nature* **348**:125, 1990.
43. Reuther GW, Der CJ: The Ras branch of small GTPases: Ras family members don't fall far from the tree [Review, 83 references]. *Curr Opin Cell Biol* **12**:157, 2000.
44. Medema RH, Bos JL: The role of p21ras in receptor tyrosine kinase signaling. *Crit Rev Oncogenesis* **4**:615, 1993.
45. Hunter T: Braking the cycle. *Cell* **75**:839, 1993.
46. Treisman R: Ternary complex factors: Growth factor regulated transcriptional activators. *Curr Opin Genet Dev* **4**:96, 1994.
47. Aaronson SA: Growth factors and cancer. *Science* **254**:1146, 1991.
48. Harrington EA, Fanidi A, Evan GI: Oncogenes and cell death. *Curr Opin Genet Dev* **4**:120, 1994.
49. Waterfield MD, Scrace GT, Whittle N, Stroobant P, Johnsson A, Wasteson A, Westermark B, Heldin CH, Huang JS, Deuel TF: Platelet-derived growth factor is structurally related to the putative transforming protein p28 sis of simian sarcoma virus. *Nature* **304**:35, 1983.
50. Shapiro WR, Shapiro JR: Biology and treatment of malignant glioma [Review, 66 references]. *Oncology (Huntington)* **12**:233 [Discussion 240, 246], 1998.
51. Halaban R, Langdon R, Birchall N, Cuomo C, Baird A, Scott G, Moellmann G, McGuire J: Basic fibroblast growth factor from human keratinocytes is a natural mitogen for melanocytes. *J Cell Biol* **107**:1611, 1988.
52. Yayon A, Ma YS, Safran M, Klagsbrun M, Halaban R: Suppression of autocrine cell proliferation and tumorigenesis of human melanoma cells and fibroblast growth factor transformed fibroblasts by a kinase-deficient FGF receptor 1: Evidence for the involvement of Src-family kinases. *Oncogene* **14**:2999, 1997.
53. Hoodless PA, Wrana JL: Mechanism and function of signaling by the TGF beta superfamily [Review, 160 references]. *Curr Top Microbiol Immunol* **228**:235, 1998.
56. Sagata N, Daar I, Oskarsson M, Showalter SD, Vande Woude GF: The product of the MOS proto-oncogene as a candidate initiator for oocyte maturation. *Nature* **245**:643, 1989.
57. Laird AD, Shalloway D: Oncoprotein signalling and mitosis [Review, 126 references]. *Cell Signal* **9**:249, 1997.
58. Hunter T: Protein kinases and phosphatases: The Yin and Yang of protein phosphorylation and signaling. *Cell* **80**:225, 1995.
59. Ullrich A, Schlessinger J: Signal transduction by receptors with tyrosine kinase activity. *Cell* **61**:203, 1990.
60. Schlessinger J, Ullrich A: Growth factor signaling by receptor tyrosine kinases. *Neuron* **9**:383, 1992.
61. Pawson T, Schlessinger J: SH2 and SH3 domains. *Curr Biol* **3**:434, 1993.
62. Cantley LC, Songyang Z: Specificity in protein-tyrosine kinase signaling [Review, 17 references]. *Adv Second Messenger Phosphoprotein Res* **31**:41, 1997.
63. Pawson T: Tyrosine kinases and their interactions with signalling proteins. *Curr Opin Genet Dev* **2**:4, 1992.
64. Fantl WJ, Escobedo JA, Martin GA, Turck CW, Del Rosario M, McCormick F, Williams LT: Distinct phosphotyrosines on a growth factor receptor bind to specific molecules that mediate different signaling pathways. *Cell* **69**:413, 1992.
65. Pawson T: Protein modules and signalling networks. *Nature* **373**:573, 1995.
66. Hunter T: Signaling: 2000 and beyond [Review, 93 references]. *Cell* **100**:113, 2000.

67. Rozakis-Adcock M, Fernley R, Wade J, Pawson T, Bowtell D: The SH2 and SH3 domains of mammalian Grb2 couple the EGF receptor to the Ras activator mSos1. *Nature* **363**:83, 1993.
68. Gale NW, Kaplan S, Lowenstein EJ, Schlessinger J, Bar-Sagi D: Grb2 mediates the EGF-dependent activation of guanine nucleotide exchange on Ras. *Nature* **363**:88, 1993.
69. McCormick F: *ras* GTPase activating protein: Signal transmitter and signal terminator. *Cell* **56**:5, 1989.
70. Pawson T, Saxton TM: Signaling networks: Do all roads lead to the same genes? [Comment] [Review, 21 references]. *Cell* **97**:675, 1999.
71. Rodrigues GA, Park M: Oncogenic activation of tyrosine kinases. *Curr Opin Genet Dev* **4**:15, 1994.
72. Weiner DB, Liu J, Cohen JA, Williams WV, Greene MI: A point mutation in the *neu* oncogene mimics ligand induction of receptor aggregation. *Nature* **339**:230, 1989.
73. Bargmann CI, Hung M-C, Weinberg RA: Multiple independent activations of the *neu* oncogene by a point mutation altering the transmembrane domain of pl85. *Cell* **45**:649, 1986.
74. Asai N, Iwasha T, Matsuyama M, Takahashi M: Mechanism of activation of the *ret* proto-oncogene by multiple endocrine neoplasia 2A mutations. *Mol Cell Biol* **15**:1613, 1995.
75. Saarma M, Sariola H, Pazchnis V: GDNF signalling through the Ret receptor tyrosine kinase. *Nature* **381**:789, 1996.
76. Siegel PM, Dankort DL, Hardy WR, Muller WJ: Novel activating mutations in the *neu* proto-oncogene involved in induction of mammary tumors. *Mol Cell Biol* **14**:7068, 1994.
77. Santoro M, Carlomango F, Romano A, Bottaro DP, Dathan NA, Grieco M, Fusco A, Vecchio G, Matoskova B, Kraus MH, Di Fiore PP: Activation of RET as a dominant transforming gene by germline mutations of MEN 2A and MEN 2B. *Science* **267**:381, 1995.
78. Carlson KM, Dou S, Chi D, Scavarda N, Toshima K, Jackson CE, Wells SA, Goodfellow PJ, Donis-Keller H: Single missense mutation in the tyrosine kinase catalytic domain of the RET proto-oncogene is associated with multiple endocrine neoplasia type 2B. *Proc Natl Acad Sci USA* **91**:1579, 1994.
79. Rodrigues G, Park M: Dimerization mediated by a leucine zipper oncogenically activates the met receptor tyrosine kinase. *Mol Cell Biol* **13**:6711, 1993.
80. Lanzi C, Borrello MG, Bongarzone I, Migliazza A, Fusco A, Grieco M, Santoro M, Gambetta RA, Zunino F, Porta GD, Pierotti MA: Identification of the product of two oncogenic rearranged forms of the RET proto-oncogene in papillary thyroid carcinomas. *Oncogene* **7**:2189, 1992.
81. Greco A, Pierotti MA, Bongarzone I, Pagliardini S, Lanzi C, Della Porta G: *Trk*-t1 is a novel oncogene formed by the fusion of *tpr* and *trk* genes in a human papillary thyroid carcinoma. *Oncogene* **7**:237, 1992.
82. Bounacer A, Wicker R, Caillou B, Cailleux AF, Sarasin A, Schlumberger M, Suarez HG: High prevalence of activating *ret* proto-oncogene rearrangements, in thyroid tumors from patients who had received external radiation. *Oncogene* **15**:1263, 1997.
83. Pierotti MA, Santoro M, Jenkins RB, Sozzi G, Bongarzone I, Grieco M, Monzini N, Miozzo M, Herrmann MA, Fusco A, Hay ID, Della Porta G, Vecchio G: Characterization of an inversion on the long arm of chromosome 10 juxtaposing D10S170 and RET and creating the oncogenic sequence RET/PTC. *Proc Natl Acad Sci USA* **89**:1616, 1992.
84. Martin-Zanca D, Barbacid M, Parada LF: Expression of the *trk* proto-oncogene is restricted to the sensory cranial and spinal ganglia of neural crest origin in mouse development. *Genes Dev* **4**:683, 1990.
85. Yonemura Y, Kaji M, Hirono Y, Fushida S, Tsugawa K, Fujimura T, Miyazaki I, Harada S, Yamamoto H: Correlation between over-expression of c-MET gene and the progression of gastric cancer. *Int J Oncol* **8**:555, 1996.
86. Vande Woude GF, Jeffers M, Cortner J, Alvord G, Tsarfaty I, Resau J: Met-HGF/SF: Tumorigenesis, invasion and metastasis [Review, 40 references]. *Ciba Found Symp* **212**:119 [Discussion 130, 148], 1997.
87. Porter AC, Vaillancourt RR: Tyrosine kinase receptor-activated signal transduction pathways which lead to oncogenesis [Review, 106 references]. *Oncogene* **17**:1343, 1998.
88. Pawson T: Non-catalytic domains of cytoplasmic protein-tyrosine kinases: Regulatory elements in signal transduction. *Oncogene* **3**:491, 1988.
89. Hunter T: Protein kinases and phosphatases: The Yin and Yang of protein phosphorylation and signaling. *Cell* **80**:225, 1995.
90. Twamley-Stein GM, Pepperkok R, Ansorge W, Courtneidge SA: The Src family tyrosine kinases are required for platelet-derived growth factor-mediated signal transduction in NIH 3T3 cells. *Proc Natl Acad Sci USA* **90**:7696, 1993.
91. Kypta RM, Goldberg Y, Ulug ET, Courtneidge SA: Association between the PDGF receptor and members of the src family of tyrosine kinases. *Cell* **62**:481, 1990.
92. Muthuswamy SK, Siegel PM, Dankort DL, Webster MA, Muller WJ: Mammary tumors expressing the *neu* proto-oncogene possess elevated c-Src tyrosine kinase activity. *Mol Cell Biol* **14**:735, 1994.
93. McWhirter JR, Galasso DL, Wang JYJ: A coiled-coil oligomerization domain of *Bcr* is essential for the transforming function of *Bcr-Abl* oncoproteins. *Mol Cell Biol* **13**:7587, 1993.
94. McWhirter JR, Wang JY: Activation of tyrosine kinase and microfilament-binding functions of c-*abl* by *bcr* sequences in *bcr/abl* fusion proteins. *Mol Cell Biol* **11**:1553, 1991.
95. Matsuda M, Mayer BJ, Fukui Y, Hanafusa H: Binding of transforming protein, P47gag-crk, to a broad range of phosphotyrosine-containing proteins. *Science* **248**:1537, 1989.
96. Mayer BJ, Hanafusa H: Association of the v-*crk* oncogene product with phosphotyrosine-containing proteins and protein kinase activity. *Proc Natl Acad Sci USA* **87**:2638, 1990.
97. Pawson T, Scott JD: Signaling through scaffold, anchoring, and adaptor proteins [Review, 72 references]. *Science* **278**:2075, 1997.
98. Pawson T, Saxton TM: Signaling networks: Do all roads lead to the same genes? [Comment] [Review, 21 references]. *Cell* **97**:675, 1999.
99. Barbacid M: *ras* Genes. *Annu Rev Biochem* **56**:779, 1987.
100. Egan SE, Giddings BW, Brooks MW, Buday L, Sizeland AM, Weinberg RA: Association of Sos Ras exchange protein with GRB2 is implicated in tyrosine kinase signal transduction and transformation. *Nature* **363**:45, 1993.
101. Downward J, Riehl R, Wu L, Weinberg RA: Identification of a nucleotide exchange-promoting activity for p21ras. *Proc Natl Acad Sci USA* **87**:5998, 1990.
102. Shields JM, Pruitt K, McFall A, Shaub A, Der CJ: Understanding Ras: "It ain't over 'til it's over" [Review, 55 references]. *Trends Cell Biol* **10**:147, 2000.
103. Trahey M, McCormick F: A cytoplasmic protein stimulates normal N-*ras* p21 GTPase, but does not affect oncogenic mutants. *Science* **238**:542, 1987.
104. Ellis C, Moran M, McCormick F, Pawson T: Phosphorylation of GAP and GAP-associated proteins by transforming and mitogenic tyrosine kinases. *Nature* **343**:377, 1990.
105. Boguski MS, McCormick F: Proteins regulating Ras and its relatives. *Nature* **366**:643, 1993.
106. Dudley DT, Pang L, Decker SJ, Bridges AJ, Saltiel AR: A synthetic inhibitor of the mitogen-activated protein kinase cascade. *Proc Natl Acad Sci USA* **92**:7686, 1995.
107. Qiu RG, Chen J, Kim D, McCormick F, Symons M: An essential role for Rac in Ras transformation. *Nature* **374**:457, 1995.
108. Khosravi-Far RSP, Clark GJ, Kinch MS, Der CJ: Activation of Rac1, RhoA and mitogen activated protein kinases is required for Ras transformation. *Mol Cell Biol* **15**:6443, 1995.
109. Hall A: Rho GTPases and the actin cytoskeleton [Review, 50 references]. *Science* **279**:509, 1998.
110. Nobes CD, Hall A: Rho GTPases control polarity, protrusion, and adhesion during cell movement. *J Cell Biol* **144**:1235, 1999.
111. Levinson AD: Normal and activated *ras* oncogenes and their encoded products. *Trends Genet* **2**:81, 1986.
112. Trahey M, McCormick F: A cytoplasmic protein stimulates normal N-*ras* p21 GTPase, but does not affect oncogenic mutants. *Science* **238**:542, 1987.
113. Clanton DJ, Hattori S, Shih TY: Mutations of the *ras* gene product p21 that abolish guanine nucleotide binding. *Proc Natl Acad Sci USA* **83**:5076, 1986.
114. Boguski MS, McCormick F: Proteins regulating Ras and its relatives. *Nature* **366**:643, 1993.
115. Henkemeyer M, Rossi DJ, Holmyard DP, Puri MC, Mbamalu G, Harpal K, Shih TS, Jacks T, Pawson T: Vascular system defects and neuronal apoptosis in mice lacking Ras GTPase-activating protein. *Nature* **377**:695, 1995.
116. Xu G, O'Connell P, Viskochil D, Cawthon R, Robertson M, Culver M, Dunn D, Stevens J, Gesteland R, White R, Weiss R: The neurofibromatosis type 1 gene encodes a protein related to GAP. *Cell* **62**:599, 1990.
117. Buchberg AM, Cleveland LS, Jenkins NA, Copeland NG: Sequence homology shared by neurofibromatosis type-1 gene and IRA-1 and

IRA-2 negative regulators of the RAS cyclic AMP pathway. *Nature* **347**:291, 1990.

118. Cerione RA, Zheng Y: The *Dbl* family of oncogenes. *Curr Opin Cell Biol* **8**:216, 1996.
119. Habets GGM, Scholtes EHM, Zuydgeest D, Van der Kammen RA, Stam JC, Berns A, Collard JG: Identification of an invasion-inducing gene, *Tiam*-1, that encodes a protein with homology to GDP-GTP exchangers for rho-like proteins. *Cell* **77**:537, 1994.
121. Ron D, Zannini M, Lewis M, Wickner RB, Hunt LT, Graziani G, Tronick SR, Aaronson SA, Eva A: A region of proto-*dbl* essential for its transforming activity shows sequence similarity to a yeast cell-cycle gene, *CDC24*, and the human breakpoint cluster gene, *bcr*. *New Biol* **3**:372, 1991.
120. Eva A, Aaronson SA: Isolation of a new human oncogene from a diffuse B-cell lymphoma. *Nature* **316**:273, 1985.
122. Katzav S: VAV: Captain Hook for signal transduction? *Crit Rev Oncogenesis* **6**:87, 1995.
123. Westwick JK, Lee RJ, Lambert QT, Symons M, Pestell RG, Der CJ, Whitehead IP: Transforming potential of Dbl family proteins correlates with transcription from the cyclin D1 promoter but not with activation of Jun NH2-terminal kinase, p38/Mpk2, serum response factor, or c-Jun. *J Biol Chem* **273**:16,739, 1998.
124. Hall A: Signal transduction pathways regulated by the Rho family of small GTPases [Review, 17 references]. *Br J Cancer* **80**:25, 1999.
125. Morrison DK, Kaplan DR, Rapp U, Roberts TM: Signal transduction from membrane to cytoplasm: Growth factors and membrane-bound oncogene products increase Raf-1 phosphorylation and associated protein kinase activity. *Proc Natl Acad Sci USA* **85**:8855, 1988.
126. Kikkawa U, Kishimoto A, Nishizuka Y: The protein kinase C family: Heterogeneity and its implications. *Annu Rev Biochem* **53**:31, 1989.
127. Housey GM, Johnson MD, Hsiao WLW, O'Brian CA, Murphy JP, Kirschmeier P: Overproduction of protein kinase C causes disordered growth in rat fibroblasts. *Cell* **52**:343, 1988.
128. Lewin B: Oncogenic conversion by regulatory changes in transcription factors. *Cell* **64**:303, 1991.
129. Rauscher III FJ, Cohen DR, Curran T, Bos TJ, Vogt PK, Bohmann D, Tjian R, Franza BR Jr: *Fos*-associated protein p39 is the product of the *jun* proto-oncogene. *Science* **240**:1010, 1988.
130. Bohmann D, Bos TJ, Admon A, Nishimura T, Vogt PK, Tjian R: Human proto-oncogene c-*jun* encodes a DNA binding protein with structural and functional properties of transcription factor AP-I. *Science* **238**:1386, 1987.
131. Distel RJ, Ro H-S, Rosen BS, Groves DL, Spiegelman BM: Nucleoprotein complexes that regulate gene expression in adipocyte differentiation: Direct participation of c-*fos*. *Cell* **49**:835, 1987.
132. Weinberger C, Thompson C, Ong E, Gruold, Evans R: The C-v-*erb*A gene encodes a thyroid hormone receptor. *Nature* **324**:641, 1986.
133. Greenberg ME, Ziff EB: Stimulation of mouse 3T3 cells induces transcription of the c-*fos* oncogene. *Nature* **311**:433, 1984.
134. Luscher B, Eisenman RN: New light on Myc and Myb. Part I. Myc. *Genes Dev* **4**:2025, 1990.
135. Muller R, Bravo R, Burckhardt J, Curran T: Induction of c-*fos* gene and protein by growth factors precedes activation of c-*myc*. *Nature* **312**:716, 1984.
136. Morin PJ: Beta-catenin signaling and cancer [Review, 88 references]. *Bioessays* **21**:1021, 1999.
137. Su LK, Vogelstein B, Kinzler KW: Association of the APC tumor suppressor protein with catenins. *Science* **262**:1734, 1993.
138. Rubinfeld B, Albert I, Porfiri E, Munemitsu S, Polakis P: Loss of beta-catenin regulation by the APC tumor suppressor protein correlates with loss of structure due to common somatic mutations of the gene. *Cancer Res* **57**:4624, 1997.
139. Shih IM, Yu J, He TC, Vogelstein B, Kinzler KW: The beta-catenin binding domain of adenomatous polyposis coli is sufficient for tumor suppression. *Cancer Res* **60**:1671, 2000.
140. Miyoshi Y, Nagase H, Ando H, Horii A, Ichii S, Nakatsuru S, Aoki T, Miki Y, Mori T, Nakamura Y: Somatic mutations of the APC gene in colorectal tumors: Mutation cluster region in the APC gene. *Hum Mol Genet* **1**:229, 1992.
141. Rubinfeld B, Robbins P, El-Gamil M, Albert I, Porfiri E, Polakis P: Stabilization of beta-catenin by genetic defects in melanoma cell lines [see Comments]. *Science* **275**:1790, 1997.
142. Morin PJ, Sparks AB, Korinek V, Barker N, Clevers H, Vogelstein B, Kinzler KW: Activation of beta-catenin-Tcf signaling in colon cancer by mutations in beta-catenin or APC [see Comments]. *Science* **275**:1787, 1997.
143. Takahashi M, Fukuda K, Sugimura T, Wakabayashi K: Beta-catenin is frequently mutated and demonstrates altered cellular location in azoxymethane-induced rat colon tumors. *Cancer Res* **58**:42, 1998.
144. Polakis P: The oncogenic activation of beta-catenin [Review, 71 references]. *Curr Opin Genet Dev* **9**:15, 1999.
145. Dashwood RH, Suzui M, Nakagama H, Sugimura T, Nagao M: High frequency of beta-catenin (ctnnb1) mutations in the colon tumors induced by two heterocyclic amines in the F344 rat. *Cancer Res* **58**:1127, 1998.
146. He TC, Sparks AB, Rago C, Hermeking H, Zawel L, Da Costa LT, Morin PJ, Vogelstein B, Kinzler KW: Identification of c-MYC as a target of the APC pathway [see Comments]. *Science* **281**:1509, 1998.
147. Fruman DA, Meyers RE, Cantley LC: Phosphoinositide kinases [Review, 153 references]. *Annu Rev Biochem* **67**:481, 1998.
148. Leevers SJ, Vanhaesebroeck B, Waterfield MD: Signalling through phosphoinositide 3-kinases: The lipids take centre stage [Review, 54 references]. *Curr Opin Cell Biol* **11**:219, 1999.
149. Vanhaesebroeck B, Leevers SJ, Panayotou G, Waterfield MD: Phosphoinositide 3-kinases: A conserved family of signal transducers [Review, 53 references]. *Trends Biochem Sci* **22**:267, 1997.
150. Fruman DA, Rameh LE, Cantley LC: Phosphoinositide binding domains: Embracing 3-phosphate [Review, 19 references]. *Cell* **97**:817, 1999.
151. Cohen P, Alessi DR, Cross DA: PDK1, one of the missing links in insulin signal transduction? *FEBS Lett* **410**:3, 1997.
152. Franke TF, Kaplan DR, Cantley LC, Toker A: Direct regulation of the *Akt* proto-oncogene product by phosphatidylinositol-3,4-bisphosphate [see Comments]. *Science* **275**:665, 1997.
153. Chang HW, Aoki M, Fruman D, Auger KR, Bellacosa A, Tsichlis PN, Cantley LC, Roberts TM, Vogt PK: Transformation of chicken cells by the gene encoding the catalytic subunit of PI 3-kinase. *Science* **276**:1848, 1997.
154. Cantley LC, Neel BG: New insights into tumor suppression: PTEN suppresses tumor formation by restraining the phosphoinositide 3-kinase/AKT pathway [Review, 76 references]. *Proc Natl Acad Sci USA* **96**:4240, 1999.
155. Weinberg RA: Oncogenes, anti-oncogenes, and the molecular bases of multistep carcinogenesis. *Cancer Res* **49**:3713, 1989.
156. Schwartz MA, Toksoz D, Khosravi-Far R: Transformation by Rho exchange factor oncogenes is mediated by activation of an integrin-dependent pathway. *EMBO J* **15**:6525, 1996.
157. Hartwell LH, Weinert TA: Checkpoints: Controls that ensure the order of cell cycle events. *Science* **246**:629, 1989.
158. Murray AW: Creative blocks: Cell cycle checkpoints and feedback controls. *Nature* **359**:599, 1992.
159. Attisano L, Wrana JL: Mads and Smads in TGF beta signalling [Review, 65 references]. *Curr Opin Cell Biol* **10**:188, 1998.
160. Massague J: TGF-beta signal transduction [Review, 290 references]. *Annu Rev Biochem* **67**:753, 1998.
161. Kimchi A, Wang X-F, Weinberg RA, Cheifetz S, Massagué J: Absence of transforming growth factor-β receptors and growth inhibitory responses in retinoblastoma cells. *Science* **240**:196, 1987.
162. Pardee AB: G1 events and regulation of cell proliferation. *Science* **246**:961, 1989.
163. Motokura T, Bloom T, Jueppner H, Ruderman J, Kronenberg H, Arnold A: A novel cyclin encoded by a *bcl*-1-linked candidate oncogene. *Nature* **350**:12,336, 1991.
164. Motokura T, Bloom T, Kim HG, Juppner H, Ruderman JV, Kronenberg HM, Arnold A: A novel cyclin encoded by a *bcl*1-linked candidate oncogene. *Nature* **350**:512, 1991.
165. Withers D, Harvey R, Faust J, Melnyk O, Carey K, Meeker T: Characterization of a candidate *bcl*-1 gene. *Mol Cell Biol* **11**:4846, 1991.
166. Motokura T, Arnold A: Cyclin D and oncogenesis. *Curr Opin Genet Dev* **3**:5, 1993.
167. Wang TC, Cardiff RD, Zukerberg L, Lees E, Arnold A, Schmidt EV: Mammary hyperplasia and carcinoma in MMTV-cyclin D1 transgenic mice. *Nature* **369**:669, 1994.
168. Bodrug S, Warner B, Bath M, Lindeman G, Harris A, Adams J: Cyclin D1 transgene impedes lymphocyte maturation and collaborates in lymphomagenesis with the *myc* gene. *EMBO J* **13**:2124, 1994.
169. Lovec H, Grzeschiczek A, Kowalski M, Moroy T: Cyclin D1/Bcl-1 cooperates with *myc* genes in the generation of B-cell lymphoma in transgenic mice. *EMBO J* **13**:3487, 1994.
170. Ewen ME: The cell cycle and the retinoblastoma protein family. *Cancer Metastasis Rev* **13**:45, 1994.

171. Nevins JR: E2F: A link between the Rb tumor suppressor protein and viral oncoproteins. *Science* **258**:424, 1992.
172. Hussussian CJ, Struewing JP, Goldstein AM, Higgins PA, Ally DS, Sheahan MD, Clark WHJR, Tucker MA, Dracopol NC: Germline p16 mutations in familial melanoma. *Nature Genet* **8**:15, 1994.
173. Kamb A, Shattuck-Eidens D, Beles R, Liu Q, Gruis NA, Drig W, Hussey C, Tran T, Miki Y, Weaver-Feldhaus J, et al: Analysis of the p16 gene (CDKN2) as a candidate for the chromosome 9p melanoma susceptibility locus. *Nature Genet* **8**:22, 1994.
174. Caldas C, Hanh SA, Da Costa LT, Redston MS, Schutze M, Seymour AB, Weinstein CL, Hruban RH, Yeo CJ, Kern SE: Frequent somatic mutations and homozygous deletions of the p16 (MTS1) gene in pancreatic adenocarcinoma. *Nature* Genet **8**:27, 1994.
175. Zhou R, Oskarsson M, Paules RS, Schulz N, Cleveland D, Vande Woude GF: Ability of the c-*mos* product to associate with and phosphorylate tubulin. *Nature* **350**:671, 1991.
176. Wang XM, Yew N, Peloquin JG, Vande Woude GF, Borisy GG: *Mos* oncogene product associates with kinetochores in mammalian somatic cells and disrupts mitotic progression. *Proc Natl Acad Sci USA* **91**:8329, 1994.
177. Kerr JFR, Harmon BV: Apoptosis: An historical perspective. *Curr Commun Cell Mol Biol* **3**:5, 1996.
178. Askew DS, Ashmun RA, Simmons BC, Cleveland JL: Constitutive c-*myc* expression in an IL-3-dependent myeloid cell line suppresses cell cycle arrest and accelerates apoptosis. *Oncogene* **6**:1915, 1991.
179. Evan GI, Wyllie AH, Gilbert CS, Littlewood TD, Land H, Brooks M, Waters CM, Penn LZ, Hancock DC: Induction of apoptosis in fibroblasts by c-*myc* protein. *Cell* **69**:119, 1992.
180. Lane DP: p53, guardian of the genome. *Nature* **358**:15, 1992.
181. Donehower LA, Bradley A: The tumor suppressor p53. *Biochim Biophys Acta* **1155**:181, 1993.
182. Hunter T: Braking the cycle. *Cell* **75**:839, 1993.
183. Bissonnette R, Echeverri F, Mahboubi A, Green D: Apoptotic cell death induced by c-*myc* is inhibited by *bcl*-2. *Nature* **359**:552, 1992.
184. Fanidi A, Harrington E, Evan G: Co-operative interaction between c-*myc* and *bcl*-2 can block drug-induced apoptosis. *Nature* **359**:554, 1992.
185. Hockenberry D, Nuñez G, Milliman C, Schreiber RD, Korsmeyer S: Bcl-2, an inner mitochondrial membrane protein blocks programmed cell death. *Nature* **348**:334, 1990.
186. Krajewski S, Tanaka S, Takayama S, Schibler M, Fenton W, Reed JC: Investigation of the subcellular distribution of the *Bcl*-2 oncoprotein: Residence in the nuclear envelope, endoplasmic reticulum, and outer mitochondrial membranes. *Cancer Res* **53**:4701, 1993.
187. Vaux DL, Weissman IL, Kim SK: Prevention of programmed cell-death in *Caenorhabditis elegans* by human *bcl*-2. *Science* **258**:1955, 1992.
188. Henderson S, Huen D, Rowe M, Dawson C, Johnson G, Rickinson A: Epstein-Barr virus-coded BHRF1 protein, a viral homolog of *Bcl*-2, protects human B-cells from programmed cell-death. *Proc Natl Acad Sci USA* **90**:8479, 1993.
189. Miura M, Zhu H, Rotello R, Hartwieg EA, Yuan J: Induction of apoptosis in fibroblasts by IL-1 beta-converting enzyme, a mammalian homolog of the *C. elegans* cell death gene *ced*-3. *Cell* **75**:653, 1993.
190. Parada LF, Land H, Weinberg RA, Wolfe D, Rotter V: Cooperation between gene encoding P53 tumour antigen and *ras* in cellular transformation. *Nature* **312**:648, 1984.
191. Yancopolous GD, Nisen PD, Tesfaye A, Kohl NE, Goldfarb MP, Att FW: N-*myc* can cooperate with *ras* to transform normal cells in culture. *Proc Natl Acad Sci USA* **82**:5455, 1983.
192. Eliyahu D, Raz A, Gruss P, Givol D, Oven M: Participation of p53 cellular tumor antigen in transformation of normal embryonic cells. *Nature* **312**:647, 1984.
193. Hunter T: Oncoprotein networks [Review, 126 references]. *Cell* **88**:333, 1997.
194. Hanahan D: Transgenic mice as probes into complex systems. *Science* **246**:1265, 1989.
195. Adams JM, Cory S: Transgenic models of tumor development. *Science* **254**:1161, 1991.
196. Frost P, Hart I, Kerbel RS: Transgenic mice. *Cancer Metastasis Rev* **14**:77, 1995.
197. Quintanilla M, Brown K, Ramsden M, Balmain A: Carcinogen-specific mutation and amplification of Ha-*ras* during mouse skin carcinogenesis. *Nature* **322**:78, 1986.
198. Adams JM, Harris AW, Pinker CA, Corcoran LM, Alexander WS, Cory S, Palmiter RD, Brinster RL: The c-*myc* oncogene driven by immunoglobulin enhancers induces lymphoid malignancy in transgenic mice. *Nature* **318**:533, 1985.
199. Alexander WS, Bernard O, Cory S, Adams JM: Lymphomagenesis in Emu-*myc* transgenic mice can involve *ras* mutations. *Oncogene* **4**:575, 1989.
200. Sinn E, Muller W, Pattengale PK, Tepler I, Wallace R, Leder P: Coexpression of MMTV/v-Ha-*ras* and MMTV/c-*myc* genes in transgenic mice: Synergistic action of oncogenes *in vivo*. *Cell* **49**:465, 1987.
201. Lammie GA, Fantl V, Smith R, Schuuring E, Brookes R, Michalides C, Dickson C, Arnold A, Peters G: D11S287, a putative oncogene on chromosome 11q13, is amplified and expressed in squamous cell and mammary carcinomas and linked to BCL-1. *Oncogene* **6**:439, 1991.
202. Machotka SV, Garrett CT, Schwartz AM, Callahan R: Amplification of the proto-oncogenes *int*-2, c-*erb*B-2, and c-*myc* in human breast cancer. *Clin Chim Acta* **184**:207, 1989.
203. Cardiff RD, Muller WJ: Transgenic models of mammary tumorigenesis. *Cancer Surv* **16**:97, 1993.
204. Andres AC, Bchini O, Schubaur B, Dolder B, LeMeur M, Gerlinger P: H-*ras* induced transformation of mammary epithelium is favoured by increased oncogene expression or by inhibition of mammary regression. *Oncogene* **6**:771, 1991.
205. Wang TC, Cardiff RD, Zukerberg L, Lees E, Arnold A, Schmidt FV: Mammary hyperplasia and carcinoma in MMTV-cyclin D1 transgenic mice. *Nature* **369**:669, 1994.
206. Muller, W. J. Expression of activated oncogenes in the murine mammary gland: Transgenic models for human breast cancer. *Cancer Metastasis Rev* **10**:217, 1991.
207. Levitzki A, Gazit A: Tyrosine kinases inhibition: An approach to drug development. *Science* **267**:1782, 1995.
208. Gibbs JB, Oliff A: Pharmaceutical research in molecular oncology. *Cell* **79**:193, 1994.
209. Fry DW, Kraker AJ, McMichael A, Ambroso LA, Nelson JM, Leopold WR, Connors RW, Bridges AJ: A specific inhibitor of the epidermal growth factor receptor tyrosine kinase. *Science* **9**:1093, 1994.
210. Buchdunger E, Trinks U, Mett H, Regenass U, Muller M, Meyer T, McGlynn E, Pinna LA, Traxler P, Lydon NB: 4,5-Dianilinophthalimide: A protein-tyrosine kinase inhibitor with selectivity for the epidermal growth factor receptor signal transduction pathway and potent in vivo antitumor activity. *Proc Natl Acad Sci USA* **91**:2334, 1994.
211. Vincent PW, Bridges AJ, Dykes DJ, Fry DW, Leopold WR, Patmore SJ, Roberts BJ, Rose S, Sherwood V, Zhou H, Elliott WL: Anticancer efficacy of the irreversible EGFr tyrosine kinase inhibitor PD 0169414 against human tumor xenografts. *Cancer Chemother Pharmacol* **45**:231, 2000.
212. Shepard HM, Lewis GD, Sarup JC, Fendrly BM, Maneval D, Mordenti J, Figari I, Kotts CE, Palladino MAJR, Ullrich A: Monoclonal antibody therapy of human cancer: Taking the *HER*2 protooncogene to the clinic. *J Clin Immunol* **11**:117, 1991.
213. Baselga J, Mendelsohn J: Receptor blockade with monoclonal antibodies as anti-cancer therapy. *Pharmacol Ther* **64**:127, 1994.
214. Meydan N, Grunberger T, Dadi H, Shahar M, Arpaia E, Lapidot Z, Leader S, Freedman M, Cohen A, Gazit A, Roifman CM: Inhibition of recurrent human pre-B acute lymphoblastic leukemia by Jak-2 tyrosine kinase inhibitor. *Nature* **379**:645, 1996.
215. Kohl NE, Omer CA, Conner MW, Anthony NJ, Davide JP, Desolms SJ, Giuliani EA, Gomez RP, Graham SL, Hamilton K, et al: Inhibition of farnesyltransferase induces regression of mammary and salivary carcinoma in *ras* transgenic mice. *Nature Med* **1**:792, 1995.

CHAPTER 26

Tumor-Suppressor Genes

Eric R. Fearon

Cancers arise as the result of an accumulation of inherited and somatic mutations in proto-oncogenes and tumor-suppressor genes. In contrast to the activating mutations that generate oncogenic alleles from proto-oncogenes, tumor-suppressor genes are targeted by loss-of-function mutations in cancer cells. A third class of mutated genes, with a rather more indirect role in cancer initiation and progression, has been identified; namely, the DNA-repair-pathway genes. Their inactivation in cancer is presumed to contribute to the development of mutations in other genes that directly affect cell proliferation and survival, such as the oncogenes and tumor-suppressor genes. Because DNA-repair genes are affected by loss-of-function mutations in cancer, they are often considered to represent a subset of the tumor-suppressor genes.

While a number of relatively straightforward approaches have enabled the identification of oncogenic alleles in cancer, identification of tumor-suppressor genes has proven more difficult. Somatic cell genetic studies provided early evidence that tumorigenicity was a recessive trait in many cancers. Based on such findings, the existence of tumor-suppressor genes was inferred. The somatic cell genetic approaches have provided a means to define specific chromosomal regions containing tumor-suppressor genes, even though few tumor-suppressor genes have been identified using the approaches.

Knudson's epidemiologic studies of retinoblastoma led to a proposal that has subsequently been termed the "two-hit hypothesis." In brief, Knudson proposed that two inactivating mutations were necessary for retinoblastoma development. The first mutation at the retinoblastoma susceptibility locus could be either a germ line or somatic mutation, while the second mutation was always somatic. Knudson's hypothesis not only illustrated the mechanisms through which inherited and somatic mutations might collaborate in tumorigenesis, but it linked the notion of recessive genetic determinants for cancer susceptibility to the findings from the somatic cell genetic studies.

To date, more than 20 tumor-suppressor genes have been localized and identified through various experimental approaches, often employed in concert. The approaches include cytogenetic studies of constitutional chromosomal alterations in cancer patients, linkage analyses to localize genes that predispose to cancer, and loss of heterozygosity (LOH) or allelic loss studies undertaken on matched pairs of normal and cancer tissue.

The authenticity of a tumor-suppressor gene is most clearly established by the identification of inactivating germ line mutations that segregate with cancer predisposition, coupled with the identification of somatic mutations inactivating the wild-type allele in the cancers arising in those with a germ line mutation. Supportive, but less convincing, evidence of a tumor-suppressor role for other genes may be presented, such as the identification of somatic, inactivating mutations in a gene in one or more types of cancer, or its decreased or absent expression in cancers. Largely because of the difficulties in assigning causal significance to any gene solely based on somatic alterations in its sequence and/or expression in cancers, genes not affected by inactivating, germ line mutations are most appropriately considered as candidate tumor-suppressor genes until additional data are available.

Powerful insights into the cellular functions of many tumor-suppressor proteins, such as pRb, p16, p53, and APC, have been obtained. It has become apparent that tumor-suppressor proteins function in a diverse array of signaling pathways and growth regulatory networks. In some cases, the protein products of tumor-suppressor genes and proto-oncogenes function in overlapping regulatory networks. Further studies of tumor-suppressor gene function will advance our understanding of cancer pathogenesis and the basis for the site-specific pattern of cancer often seen in individuals with germ line mutations in tumor-suppressor genes.

INTRODUCTION

Cancers arise, at least in part, as the result of two distinct, but linked, processes. The first process is mutation of cellular genes. The second process, termed clonal selection, promotes outgrowth of variant progeny with increased proliferative and survival properties. Two classes of genes — proto-oncogenes and tumor-suppressor genes — are affected by mutations in cancer cells. Oncogenes are distinguished by their harboring gain-of-function mutations that endow them with increased or novel function. In contrast, tumor-suppressor genes are affected by loss-of-function mutations. A third class of mutated genes with a more indirect role in cancer initiation and progression has been identified; namely, the DNA-repair-pathway genes. Because DNA-repair genes are affected by loss-of-function mutations in cancer, they are often considered to represent a subset of the tumor-suppressor genes. This chapter focuses predominantly on tumor-suppressor genes that appear to have direct effects on growth control. However, brief mention is made of some of the properties of the DNA-repair subset of tumor-suppressor genes. It also should be emphasized that the vast majority of mutations that contribute to the development and behavior of cancer are somatic and present only in the neoplastic cells of the patient. Although only a small subset of the mutations in a cancer cell are present in the germ line, when present, they not only predispose to cancer, but they can also be passed on to future generations. Studies of the mutations that underlie the highly penetrant inherited cancer syndromes have provided some of the most unique and compelling insights into tumor-suppressor genes and their role in cancer.

The relationship between proto-oncogenes and oncogenes and their functions in growth control and apoptosis have been extensively reviewed previously in Chapters 23, 24 and 25. More than 75 different proto-oncogenes have been identified through various experimental strategies.[1,2] In general, proto-oncogenes have critical roles in growth regulation, and their protein products are distributed throughout virtually all subcellular compartments. Point mutation, chromosomal rearrangement, or gene amplification of the proto-oncogene sequences generates the oncogenic variant alleles present in cancer.

The role of DNA-repair genes in cancer is extensively discussed in Chapters 27, 28 and 32. As noted above, the DNA-repair genes comprise a subset of the tumor-suppressor genes because they are affected by loss-of-function mutations in cancer.

Nevertheless, because of certain features they can be distinguished as a unique subset of the tumor-suppressor genes. Specifically, while protein products of many tumor-suppressor genes are likely to be directly involved in regulating cell growth or differentiation, many DNA-repair proteins are likely to have a more passive role in growth, differentiation, and cell survival. Their inactivation in tumor cells leads to the acquisition of a "mutator phenotype," with a resultant increased rate of mutations in other cellular genes. Because the accumulation of mutations in proto-oncogenes and tumor-suppressor genes appears to be rate-determining in tumorigenesis, the process of tumor progression is greatly accelerated by DNA-repair gene inactivation.

As is reviewed in subsequent chapters, enormous progress has been made in the identification of inherited and somatic mutations in tumor-suppressor genes. Therefore, the findings on the prevalence and nature of specific tumor-suppressor gene mutations in various cancer types is not summarized in any detail here. Rather, the primary aims of this chapter are to review the somatic cell, family, and loss of heterozygosity studies that established the existence of tumor suppressor genes; to provide an overview of the identification and function of selected tumor-suppressor genes; and to highlight some critical insights into cancer development provided by study of tumor-suppressor genes.

SOMATIC CELL GENETIC STUDIES

As reviewed in Chap. 25, the identification of oncogenic alleles in human tumors has been greatly facilitated by several of their features, including the prior identification of retroviral (*v-onc*) genes and the molecular cloning and characterization of novel oncogene sequences at translocation breakpoints.[1,2] In addition, the ability of certain oncogenes, such as activated *K-RAS* or *H-RAS* alleles, to generate tumorigenic properties when transferred to nontumorigenic recipient cells not only supports the critical role of oncogene mutations in cell transformation, but provides a straightforward functional approach for the identification of oncogenic alleles.[3–6]

In contrast, the direct identification of tumor-suppressor genes has proven far more difficult. For example, functional strategies for their identification have a number of theoretical and practical problems. Although the successful transfer of a functional copy of a tumor-suppressor gene to a tumor cell might be expected to revert aspects of its phenotype, the identification of such reverted cells in the midst of a background of fully transformed cells has proven to be a particularly arduous experimental task. Hence, the strategies for identification of tumor-suppressor genes and the mutations in these genes in human cancers have been more circuitous. Nevertheless, because somatic cell genetic studies provided early evidence supporting the existence of tumor-suppressor genes, the studies are reviewed here.

Harris and his colleagues were the first to demonstrate that the growth of murine tumor cells in syngeneic animals could be suppressed when the malignant cells were fused to nonmalignant cells.[7,8] However, tumorigenic revertants often arose when the hybrid cells were cultured for extended periods, and chromosome losses were found in the revertants. It was hypothesized, therefore, that malignancy was a recessive trait that could be suppressed in somatic cell hybrids. This proposal was further supported through studies of somatic cell hybrids from other rodent species and man.[8–10] Hybrids retaining both sets of parental chromosomes were suppressed for tumorigenic growth in athymic mice. Furthermore, it was demonstrated that the loss of specific chromosomes, and not simply chromosome loss in general, correlated with reversion. Tumorigenicity could be suppressed even if activated oncogenes, such as mutant *RAS* genes, were expressed in the hybrids.[11] Because the loss of specific chromosomes was associated with tumorigenic reversion, it was suggested that a single chromosome, and perhaps even a single gene, might be sufficient to suppress the tumorigenic growth of human cancer cells in nude mice. To directly test this hypothesis, single chromosomes were transferred from normal cells to cancer cells, using the technique of microcell-mediated chromosome transfer. As predicted, the transfer of specific human chromosomes suppressed the tumorigenic growth properties of various cancer cell lines.[12–17]

Although the tumorigenic phenotype can often be suppressed following single-chromosome transfer or cell fusion, other traits of the parental cancer cells, such as immortality and anchorage-independent growth, may be retained in the hybrids. Consistent with the notion that most malignant tumors arise from multiple genetic alterations, suppression of tumorigenicity might thus represent correction of only one of the alterations. Nevertheless, because the transferred genes suppressed at least some of the phenotypic properties seen in cancer cells, all genes that suppressed neoplastic growth properties in *in vitro* assays or *in vivo* tumor models have often been referred to collectively as tumor-suppressor genes. As is discussed below, this may be an overly broad definition of tumor-suppressor genes.

KNUDSON'S TWO-HIT HYPOTHESIS

Essentially concurrent with the somatic cell studies, Knudson undertook epidemiologic studies of retinoblastoma.[18] Although most cases of retinoblastoma are sporadic, in some families, autosomal dominant inheritance is seen. Knudson found that familial cases were more likely than sporadic cases to develop bilateral or multifocal disease. In addition, Knudson found that the familial and bilateral/multi-focal cases had, in general, an earlier age of onset. Knudson developed a model based largely on these observations.[18] In this model, he hypothesized that two "hits" or mutagenic events were necessary for retinoblastoma development in all cases (Fig. 26-1). In individuals with the inherited form of retinoblastoma, Knudson proposed that the first hit was present in the germ line, and thus in all cells of the body. However, inactivation of one allele of the susceptibility gene was insufficient for tumor formation, and a second somatic mutation was needed. Given the high likelihood of a somatic mutation occurring in at least one retinal cell during eye development, the dominant inheritance pattern of retinoblastoma in some families could be explained. In the non-hereditary form of retinoblastoma, both mutations were somatic and hypothesized to arise within the same

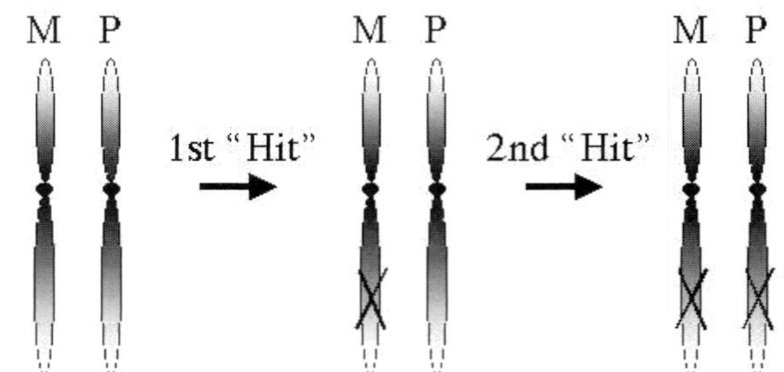

Fig. 26-1 Diagram of the Knudson "two-hit" hypothesis. Knudson proposed that two or more "hits" or mutagenic events were necessary for the development of retinoblastoma and perhaps other tumors. In individuals with inherited retinoblastoma, Knudson proposed the first hit in a retinoblastoma suppressor gene (*RB1*) was present in the germ line, predisposing all developing retinoblasts to cancer ("predisposed cells"). Inactivation of the second *RB1* allele resulted in retinoblastoma development. In the nonhereditary (sporadic) form of retinoblastoma, both *RB1* mutations were somatic. Consistent with retinoblastoma being rare in those who do not carry a germ line *RB1* mutation, there is a low probability that somatic mutations would inactivate both *RB1* in a single developing retinoblast. Knudson's hypothesis illustrated mechanisms through which inherited and somatic genetic changes might collaborate in tumorigenesis, and it postulated a role for recessive genetic determinants in human cancer.

Table 26-1 Germ line and Somatic Mutations in Tumor-Suppressor Genes and Functions of the Tumor-Suppressor Proteins

Gene	Associated Inherited Cancer Syndrome	Cancers With Somatic Mutations	Presumed Function of Protein
RB1	Familial retinoblastoma	Retinoblastoma, osteosarcoma, SCLC, breast, prostate, bladder, pancreas, esophageal, others	Transcriptional regulator; E2F binding
TP53	Li-Fraumeni syndrome	Approx. 50% of all cancers (rare in some types, such as prostate carcinoma and neuroblastoma)	Transcription factor; regulates cell cycle and apoptosis
p16/INK4A	Familial melanoma, familial pancreatic carcinoma	25–30% of many different cancer types (e.g., breast, lung, pancreatic, bladder)	Cyclin-dependent kinase inhibitor (i.e., cdk4 and cdk6)
$p14^{Arf}(p19^{Arf})$	?Familial melanoma?	Approx. 15% of many different cancer types	Regulates Mdm-2 protein stability and hence p53 stability; alternative reading frame of *p16/INK4A* gene
APC	Familial adenomatous polyposis coli (FAP), Gardner syndrome, Turcot syndrome	Colorectal, desmoid tumors	Regulates levels of β-catenin protein in the cytsol; binding to microtubules
WT-1	WAGR, Denys-Drash syndrome	Wilms tumor	Transcription factor
NF-1	Neurofibromatosis type 1	Melanoma, neuroblastoma	p21ras-GTPase
NF-2	Neurofibromatosis type 2	Schwannoma, meningioma, ependymoma	Juxtamembrane link to cytoskeleton
VHL	Von Hippel-Lindau syndrome	Renal (clear cell type), hemangioblastoma	Regulator of protein stability
BRCA1	Inherited breast and ovarian cancer	Ovarian (approx. 10%), rare in breast cancer	DNA repair; complexes with Rad 51 and BRCA2; transcriptional regulation
BRCA2	Inherited breast (both female and male), pancreatic cancer, ?others?	Rare mutations in pancreatic, ?others?	DNA repair; complexes with Rad 51 and BRCA1
MEN-1	Multiple endocrine neoplasia type 1	Parathyroid adenoma, pituitary adenoma, endocrine tumors of the pancreas	Not known
PTCH	Gorlin syndrome, hereditary basal-cell carcinoma syndrome	Basal-cell skin carcinoma, medulloblastoma	Transmembrane receptor for sonic hedgehog factor; negative regulator of smoothened protein
PTEN/MMAC1	Cowden syndrome; sporadic cases of juvenile polyposis syndrome	Glioma, breast, prostate, follicular thyroid, carcinoma, head and neck squamous carcinoma	Phosphoinositide 3-phosphatase; protein tyrosine phosphatase
DPC4	Familial juvenile polyposis syndrome	Pancreatic (approx. 50%), 10–15% of colorectal cancers, rare in others	Transcriptional factor in TGF-β signaling pathway
E-CAD	Familial diffuse-type gastric cancer	Gastric (diffuse type), lobular breast carcinoma, rare in other types (e.g., ovarian)	Cell-cell adhesion molecule
LKB1/STK1	Peutz-Jeghers syndrome	Rare in colorectal, not known in others	Serine/threonine protein kinase
EXT1	Hereditary multiple exostoses	Not known	Glycosyltransferase; heparan sulfate chain elongation
EXT2	Hereditary multiple exostoses	Not known	Glycosyltransferase; heparan sulfate chain elongation
TSC1	Tuberous sclerosis	Not known	Not known; cytoplasmic vesicle localization
TSC2	Tuberous sclerosis	Not known	Putative GTPase-activating protein for Rap1 and rab5; golgi localization
MSH2, MLH1 PMS1, PMS2 MSH6	Hereditary nonpolyposis colorectal cancer	Colorectal, gastric, endometrial	DNA mismatch repair

cell. Although each of the two hits could have been in different genes, Knudson later suggested that both hits might be at the same locus, inactivating both alleles of the retinoblastoma (*RB1*) susceptibility gene. Subsequently, loss of heterozygosity studies and definitive mutational analyses (see below) established this point. The significance of Knudson's hypothesis was two-fold: First, it illustrated the mechanisms through which inherited and somatic genetic changes might collaborate in tumorigenesis. Second, it linked the notion of recessive genetic determinants for human cancer to the somatic cell genetic studies.

APPROACHES TO IDENTIFY TUMOR-SUPPRESSOR GENES

Among the strategies successfully applied to the localization of tumor-suppressor genes are cytogenetic studies to identify constitutional chromosomal alterations in cancer patients; DNA linkage approaches to localize genes involved in inherited predisposition to cancer; and studies of chromosome regions affected by allelic loss (also termed loss of heterozygosity [LOH]) or, in some cases, loss of both alleles (termed homozygous deletion). The approaches ultimately require positional cloning methods to identify and isolate a tumor-suppressor gene from the chromosomal region or the thorough characterization of a positional candidate gene previously mapped to the region. Nevertheless, as summarized in Table 26-1, these strategies have been highly successful in identifying more than 20 tumor-suppressor genes.

Cytogenetic Studies Provide Clues to Tumor-Suppressor Gene Locations

Among the successful approaches to the localization of chromosomal regions that may contain tumor-suppressor genes have been cytogenetic studies carried out on peripheral blood lymphocytes from cancer patients. The rationale for such an approach is that chromosomal deletions, as well as some translocations, might be predicted to inactivate one of the two copies of a tumor-suppressor gene in the affected region. Unfortunately, only a very small subset of cancer patients has constitutional chromosomal deletions or rearrangements detectable by conventional cytogenetic techniques. Nevertheless, when noted, the chromosomal defects have proven extremely valuable for identifying regions likely to contain tumor-suppressor genes.

In upwards of 5 percent of patients with retinoblastoma, cytogenetic studies of peripheral blood lymphocytes or skin fibroblasts have revealed interstitial deletions involving band q14 of chromosome 13.[19] Similarly, some patients with the constellation of findings termed WAGR (for Wilms tumor, aniridia, genitourinary abnormalities, and mental retardation) have been found to have interstitial deletions of chromosome 11p13.[20] Cytogenetic studies of a mentally retarded man with hundreds of adenomatous intestinal polyps and no prior family history of polyposis revealed that the patient had an interstitial deletion involving chromosome 5q, suggesting that mutant alleles of a gene which predisposed to adenomatous polyps might map to chromosome 5q.[21] Furthermore, in some cancer patients, balanced translocations in constitutional cells have been noted, such as those involving chromosome 17q in a very small subset of patients with neurofibromatosis type 1 (NF-1), suggesting the presence of the *NF-1* gene on this chromosome.[22,23]

Linkage Analysis

Recurrent constitutional alterations of specific chromosomal regions in patients with a particular cancer type provide powerful evidence that cancer predisposition genes may reside there. Nevertheless, additional data are required to establish that the predisposition gene functions as a tumor suppressor (see below). Moreover, the identification of a single cancer patient with a constitutional deletion of a particular chromosomal region, such as the patient with the chromosome 5q deletion and polyposis, does not provide definitive proof that a Mendelian cancer predisposition gene maps to the region. In such cases, linkage analysis must be used to document that genetic markers from the implicated chromosomal region co-segregate with the inheritance of the disease phenotype in a number of large, multigenerational kindreds with a specific inherited cancer syndrome.

Localization of cancer predisposition genes for which a candidate chromosomal region has not yet been highlighted by cytogenetic studies can be accomplished using genome-wide linkage scans. Although linkage analysis can pinpoint the location of a cancer predisposition gene to a region much smaller than a chromosomal band, identification of the predisposition gene ultimately requires positional cloning approaches and/or detailed mutational analyses. In several cancer syndromes, including familial polyposis, von Hippel-Lindau syndrome, and neurofibromatosis type 2, further localization and eventual identification of each tumor-suppressor gene was greatly aided through studies of a subset of patients that had interstitial chromosomal deletions, which, while not detectable in conventional cytogenetic analyses, were readily detectable by techniques such as pulsed-field gel electrophoresis.[24–30]

Loss of Heterozygosity Studies

Cytogenetic studies of a subset of patients with retinoblastoma identified deletions involving chromosome band 13q14. Interestingly, in many patients with 13q14 deletions, levels of esterase D, an enzyme of unknown physiological function, were approximately half the levels seen in normal individuals.[31] This finding and further studies of families with inherited retinoblastoma established that the *esterase D* and *RB1* loci were genetically linked.[32] Subsequently, a child with inherited retinoblastoma was found to have esterase D levels approximately one-half of normal, although no chromosome 13 defects were seen in cytogenetic studies of his blood cells and skin fibroblasts.[33] Tumor cells from the patient had no esterase D activity, despite harboring a single copy of chromosome 13 that appeared intact by cytogenetic analysis. To explain the findings, it was proposed that the chromosome 13 retained in the tumor cells had a submicroscopic deletion of both the *esterase D* and *RB1* genes.[33] It was also suggested that cells with a defect in only one *RB1* allele had a normal phenotype. The effect of the predisposing mutation could, however, be unmasked by a second somatic event, such as loss of the chromosome 13 carrying the intact *RB1* gene. This proposal was entirely consistent with Knudson's two-hit hypothesis.

To establish the generality of these observations, others undertook studies of a panel of retinoblastomas using chromosome 13 DNA probes. On comparison of the marker patterns seen in paired normal and tumor samples, LOH or allelic loss of chromosome 13 was seen in greater than 60 percent of the studied tumors.[34] LOH of the 13q region containing the *RB1* locus resulted from various mechanisms (Fig. 26-2). In addition, through the study of inherited cases, it was shown that the *RB1* allele retained in the tumor cells was derived from the affected parent, and that the wild-type *RB1* allele had been lost.[35] These data established that the unmasking of a predisposing mutation at the *RB1* locus, whether the initial mutation had been inherited or had arisen somatically, occurred by the same chromosomal mechanisms.

Genetic analysis of somatically mutated alleles of tumor-suppressor genes can therefore supplement and reinforce information derived from analysis of germ line mutations. For example, LOH was found to target the chromosome 5q region implicated in predisposition to intestinal polyposis in a large fraction of sporadic adenomatous polyps and colorectal cancers.[36,37] Indeed, convincing evidence that a predisposition gene functions as a suppressor gene can be provided by data demonstrating that the chromosome harboring the wild-type allele of the gene is the target of LOH and the mutant allele is specifically retained in tumors. In the vast majority of cases, LOH affects many or all of the markers on the particular chromosomal arm carrying a predisposition and/or tumor-suppressor gene. For this reason, precise localization of a tumor-suppressor gene is rarely achieved by LOH analysis alone.

In addition to LOH affecting particular chromosome regions, a small fraction of cancers have deletions of both parental alleles in the region of a tumor-suppressor gene locus. Such deletion events are often termed homozygous deletions. If they are restricted in their extent, homozygous deletions can be particularly useful for pinpointing the location of a tumor-suppressor gene locus. The identification of homozygous deletions involving chromosome 13q12 and 18q21.1 sequences in certain pancreatic cancers proved instrumental in the localization and subsequent cloning of the *BRCA2* and *DPC4* tumor-suppressor genes, respectively.[38,39] Similarly, the identification of homozygous deletions of chromosome 10q23 sequences in brain, prostate, and breast cancers were critical in the identification of the *PTEN* gene.[40,41]

INSIGHTS INTO RATE-LIMITING MUTATIONS

Multiple mutations in oncogenes and tumor-suppressor genes are present in cancer cells. Distinguishing mutations that underlie cancer initiation from those likely contribute to tumor progression is a critical issue in the cancer genetics field. Most mutations that

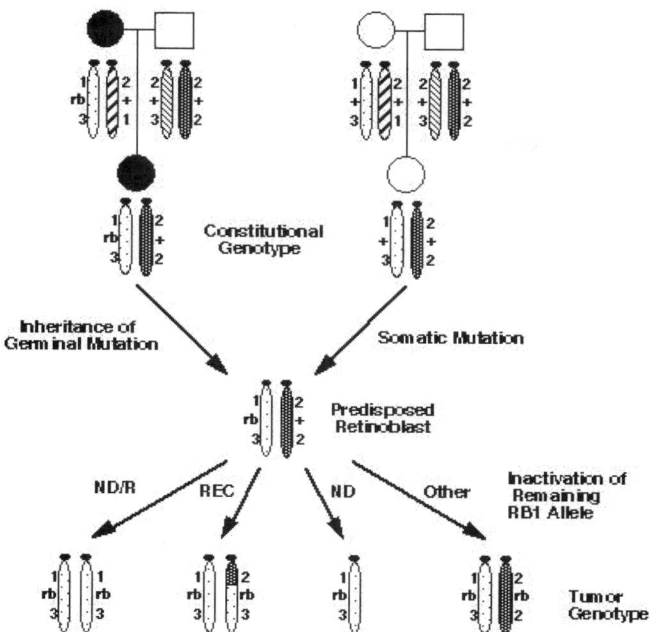

Fig. 26-2 Chromosomal mechanisms result in loss of heterozygosity for alleles at the retinoblastoma predisposition (*RB1*) locus at chromosome band 13q14. In the inherited setting (top left), the affected daughter inherits a mutant *RB1* allele (*rb*) from her affected mother and a normal *RB1* allele (+) from her father (constitutional genotype *rb*/+). DNA polymorphisms can distinguish the two copies of chromosome 13 in her normal cells (polymorphic alleles are designated by a number). Retinoblastoma arises after inactivation of the remaining wild-type *RB1* allele through these mechanisms: chromosome non-disjunction and reduplication of the remaining copy of chromosome 13 (ND/R); mitotic recombination (REC); non-disjunction (ND); and other more localization mutations that inactivate the remaining *RB1* allele (OTHER). In the non-inherited (sporadic) form of the disease, a somatic mutation arises in a developing retinal cell and inactivates one of the *RB1* alleles, and the remaining *RB1* allele is inactivated by one of the mechanisms shown. (Modified with permission from Cavenee W, Koufos A, Hansen M: Recessive mutant genes predisposing to human cancer. Mutat Res 168:3, 1986. The figure corresponds to Fig. 25-3 of Fearon ER: Oncogenes and tumor suppressor genes, in MD Abeloff, JO Armitage, AS Lichter, JE Niederhuber (eds). *Clinical Oncology*. New York: Churchill Livingstone, 1995.)

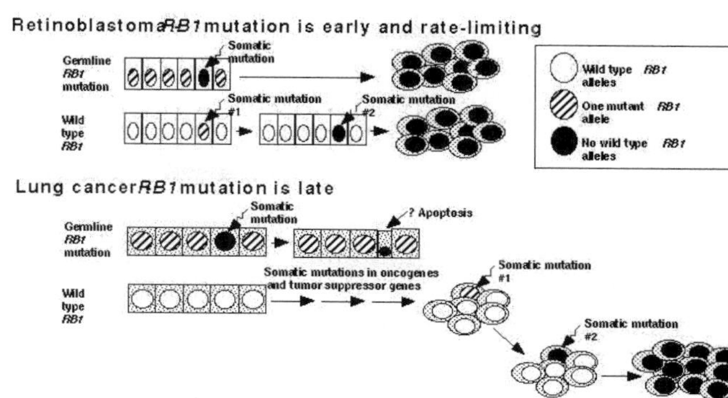

Fig. 26-3 Mutations in the retinoblastoma tumor-suppressor gene (*RB1*) contribute to inherited and sporadic cancers. The figure indicates that cell context affects the contribution of *RB1* mutations to cancer development. In individuals carrying a germ line mutation in one *RB1* allele, somatic inactivation of the remaining normal *RB1* allele is an early and rate-limiting event in retinoblastoma formation. Sporadic forms of retinoblastoma are also dependent on inactivation of both *RB1* alleles. Because somatic inactivation of both *RB1* alleles must occur in a single developing retinoblast before tumor formation can ensue, retinoblastoma is a rare disease in those who do not carry a germ line *RB1* mutation. A rather paradoxical finding is that those who carry a germ line *RB1* mutation are not highly predisposed to other cancer types, such as lung cancer, despite *RB1* mutations being frequently observed in sporadic forms of lung cancer (e.g., small cell lung carcinoma). These observations imply that *RB1* mutations are likely contributors to tumor progression rather than to tumor initiation in most cancer types, other than retinoblastoma and, perhaps, osteosarcoma. Possible explanations are that inactivation of both *RB1* alleles prior to the acquisition of other mutations in oncogenes or tumor-suppressor genes is not associated with any growth advantage, and perhaps *RB1* inactivation may even be associated with induction of apoptosis. (Figure modified with permission from Fig. 1 of Haber DA, Fearon ER: The promise of cancer genetics. *Lancet* 351 (suppl II):1, 1998.)

arise in somatic cells are likely to have little, if any, positive effect on cell growth and survival. In fact, many mutations may have detrimental or even lethal effects. Only a small fraction of mutations are associated with clonal selection, because mutations that promote clonal outgrowth must confer increased proliferative and improved survival properties upon affected cells. Those rare mutations that cause both significant expansion of a variant clone and a marked increase in the risk of malignant conversion of the clone's progeny are said to be "rate-limiting" for cancer development. The low frequency of mutations that can initiate the cancer process in a tissue is a critical bottleneck that presumably blocks or delays development of many cancers until late in adult life. However, after sustaining a rate-limiting mutation and successfully transiting the bottleneck, the generation of a highly expanded population of precancerous cells is essentially assured. Additional somatic mutations then arise in one or more of the precancerous cells and contribute to their progression to frank malignancy.

The role of rate-limiting mutations in cancer development is well illustrated in those individuals who carry inherited mutations in tumor-suppressor genes, such as the *RB1* and *APC* genes. Germ line inactivation of one *RB1* allele is not associated with any adverse effects per se. However, inactivation of the remaining functional *RB1* allele in developing retinoblasts initiates retinoblastoma formation (Fig. 26-3). The likelihood that this second somatic event will occur in one or more developing retinoblasts of an individual with a germ line *RB1* mutation is very high, which explains why inherited retinoblastoma is often a highly penetrant, dominant syndrome, with cancers arising at an early age and often in a bilateral or multifocal pattern. Sporadic cases of retinoblastoma are also critically dependent on *RB1* inactivation (Fig. 26-3). However, in an individual lacking a germ line mutation of *RB1*, the likelihood is very low that both *RB1* alleles will be coincidentally inactivated by somatic mutation in a single, developing retinoblast. This accounts, therefore, for the low prevalence of retinoblastoma in the general population, as well as the disease's more common later onset and its unifocal presentation when it does occur.

Further support for the concept of rate-limiting mutations has been provided through studies of the *APC* gene. Germ line mutation of one *APC* allele in those individuals affected by familial adenomatous polyposis (FAP) predisposes to the development of hundreds to thousands of adenomatous polyps in the colon and rectum, and to a very high risk that one or more carcinomas will arise from the large population of adenomas.[42] In those with FAP, somatic mutation of the remaining wild-type *APC* allele leads to adenoma formation, indicating that the *APC* protein has a critical role in tumor suppression in intestinal epithelial cells. Similar to *RB1* inactivation in retinoblastoma, *APC* pathway inactivation may be a rate-limiting step in essentially all colorectal tumors, because more than 75 percent of sporadic colorectal adenomas and carcinomas have somatic mutations inactivating *APC* function.[42]

TISSUE-SPECIFIC EFFECTS OF GERM LINE MUTATIONS

In general, those individuals carrying a germ line mutation of a specific tumor-suppressor gene are predisposed to a limited spectrum of cancer types. This finding is puzzling for at least tworeasons. First, most tumor-suppressor genes are expressed in many different adult tissues. Second, somatic mutations in certain tumor-suppressor genes are present in a broad spectrum of sporadic cancer types (Table 26-1). With respect to this latter point, children who carry a germ line mutation in the *RB1* gene have a very elevated risk of developing retinoblastoma, and a more modest risk of developing osteosarcoma, but no significantly increased risk of most common cancers. Thus, it is curious that somatic *RB1* mutations have been found and are believed critical in the development of many different cancer types, such as lung, breast, prostate, pancreas, and bladder cancer. Several potential explanations have been offered, and two are considered here. The *RB1* gene may be a primary controlling factor in retinoblast growth regulation, such that its inactivation leads to retinoblastoma. However, in other tissues, including lung or breast epithelial cells, *RB1* may have a less critical or even redundant role in growth control, and its inactivation may not promote neoplastic growth unless other mutations are also present (Fig. 26-3). An alternative, and perhaps equally tenable, proposal is that somatic inactivation of *RB1* may trigger programmed cell death or apoptosis in many cells types, unless other somatic mutations have arisen previously and altered the cell's ability to resist apoptosis following disruption of *RB1* function (Fig. 26-3).

TUMOR-SUPPRESSOR GENE FUNCTION

The protein products of tumor-suppressor genes have been implicated in a diverse array of cellular processes, including cell-cycle control, differentiation, cell-cell adhesion, apoptosis, and maintenance of genomic integrity. The presumed functions of selected tumor suppressor proteins are summarized in Table 26-1. Given the diversity of their functions, have any themes emerged? Yes, some have emerged. Perhaps the principal theme is that the protein products of tumor-suppressor genes often function in conserved signaling pathways. Moreover, in these signaling pathways, individual tumor-suppressor proteins function in concert with the products of other tumor-suppressor genes and proto-oncogenes.

One of the best studied of these regulatory networks is the one in which the *RB1* gene and its protein product pRb function.[43] The pRb protein appears to have an important role in regulating cell-cycle progression, presumably as a result of its ability to silence expression of E2F-target genes, such as those needed for the DNA synthetic (S) phase of the cell cycle. The functional activity of the pRb protein is correlated with its phosphorylation status, and the cyclin D1 protein and cyclin-dependent kinase 4 (cdk4) proteins regulate pRb phosphorylation. The p16 tumor-suppressor protein is a critical regulator of the activity of the cdk4/cyclin D1 complex. As noted above, a subset of sporadic cancers of various types have inactivating mutation in the *RB1* gene. In other cancers, the pRb functional pathway is inactivated as a result of mutations in other components of the pathway.[43] Many cancers that lack *RB1* mutations have inactivating mutations in the p16/INK4A gene. In others that lack *RB1* mutations, such as some breast cancers, gene amplification and overexpression of cyclin D1 is found. In other cancers, such as some glioblastomas and sarcomas, amplification and overexpression of the *CDK4* gene is frequently observed. The net effect of mutations in the pathway is to inactivate pRb function, including its ability to regulate expression of E2F-target genes (Fig. 26-4*A*).

Studies of other tumor-suppressor proteins have also supported the existence of regulatory networks in which tumor-suppressor gene and proto-oncogene protein products function. A critical function of the APC protein is regulation of β-catenin (β-cat) protein stability in the cytosol (Fig. 26-4*B*) (reviewed in reference 44). APC mutations result in increased levels of β-cat in the cell, and constitutive complexing of β-cat with transcription factors of the T-cell factor (Tcf) or lymphoid-enhancer factor (Lef) family, such as Tcf-4. When bound to Tcf/Lef factors, β-cat functions as a

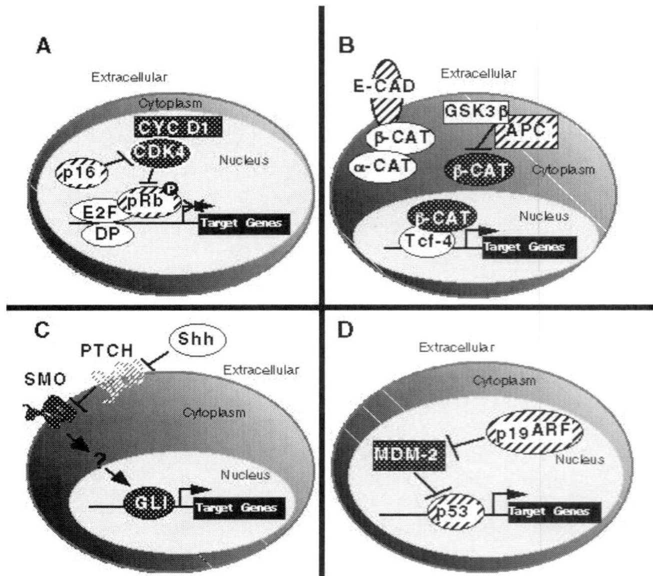

Fig. 26-4 The protein products of tumor-suppressor genes often function in conserved signaling pathways with other tumor-suppressor gene and oncogene protein products. Tumor-suppressor proteins are indicated with striped symbols and oncogene proteins with filled symbols. *A,* The pRb tumor-suppressor pathway. The protein product of the *RB1* gene, pRb, is regulated by phosphorylation. The hyperphosphorylated form of pRb is inactive and unable to bind to E2F and regulate transcription of E2F-target genes. The cyclin D1 (CYC D1) and cyclin-dependent kinase 4 (CDK4) proteins appear to have a critical role in regulating pRb phosphorylation. The p16 protein is a critical inhibitor of the activity of the CYC D1 and CDK4 complex. Inactivating mutations in the pRb or p16 tumor-suppressor proteins or activating mutations (e.g., gene amplification) of CYC D1 or CDK4 are present in the majority of cancers. *B,* The APC and E-cadherin tumor-suppressor pathways. The APC protein, in collaboration with glycogen synthase kinase 3β (GSK3β), has a critical role in regulating β-catein (β-CAT) protein stability in the cell. If APC is inactivated by mutation, or β-CAT is activated by mutation of its N-terminus, β-CAT levels cannot be appropriately regulated. β-CAT complexes with Tcf (T-cell factor) or Lef (lymphoid-enhancer factor) transcription factors, such as Tcf-4, and activates expression of Tcf-target genes (e.g., *c-MYC*). β-CAT also functions in E-cadherin (E-CAD) cell-cell adhesion, linking E-CAD to the cytoskeleton via its interaction with α-catenin (α-CAT). E-CAD functions as a tumor-suppressor gene, although it is not clear that the consequence of E-CAD inactivation is similar to that of APC inactivation; i.e., there are no data to demonstrate that E-CAD and APC function in a shared or common signaling pathway even though both proteins interact with β-CAT. *C,* The patched (*PTCH*) tumor-suppressor pathway. Germ line mutations in the *PTCH* gene are responsible for Gorlin syndrome and hereditary nevoid basal-cell cancer syndrome, in which affected individuals develop large numbers of basal-cell cancers, as well as medulloblastomas. The *PTCH* protein inhibits the activity of the smoothened (*SMO*) protein, and the sonic hedgehog (Shh) factor regulates *PTCH* activity. *SMO* functions to activate expression of the Gli transcription factor. Inactivating mutations in *PTCH,* or activating mutation in *SMO* or Gli, have been found in cancer, and are mutually exclusive. *D,* The p53 tumor-suppressor pathway. p53 functions as a transcription factor and regulates expression of a large number of target genes with roles in cell cycle control and apoptosis (e.g., p21, Bax). p53 protein stability is regulated by the MDM-2 protein, and MDM-2 protein stability is regulated by the p19^{Arf} (also known as p14^{Arf}) protein. Inactivating mutation in p53 are found in upwards of 50 percent of all human cancers. In some cancers, activating mutations in MDM-2 or inactivation of p19^{Arf} appear to have the same net consequence as p53 inactivation. (Figure modified with permission from Fig. 2 of Haber DA, Fearon ER. The promise of cancer genetics. *Lancet* 351 (suppl II):1, 1998.)

transcriptional coactivator, and, in cancers with APC mutations, Tcf transcriptional activity is deregulated. In a subset of the colorectal cancers lacking APC inactivation, activating (oncogenic) mutations in the β-cat protein have been found. These mutations render β-cat resistant to regulation by APC, and the mutant β-cat protein accumulates in the cell and deregulates Tcf transcription. While most Tcf-4-regulated genes remain to be identified, the *c-MYC* gene was recently suggested as a target of the APC/β-cat/Tcf-4 pathway, and mutations in APC or β-cat appear to result in transcriptional activation of *c-MYC*.[45] Other tumor-suppressor gene regulatory networks include the p53/mdm-2/p19^{Arf} and Ptch/Smo/Gli networks (Figs. 26-4*C* and 26-4*D*).

CANDIDATE TUMOR-SUPPRESSOR GENES

The tumor-suppressor genes discussed above and summarized in Table 26-1 are noteworthy in that germ line-inactivating mutations in the genes are associated with inherited predisposition to cancer. The link between germ line mutation and inherited cancer provides incontrovertible evidence of the importance of the genes in tumorigenesis. In addition, as reviewed above, other findings, such as the demonstration of LOH of one allele of a tumor-suppressor gene and somatic mutation of the remaining allele in sporadic tumors, often support a more widespread role for many of the genes in cancer (Table 26-1). While many members of the tumor-suppressor gene class have been definitively linked to inherited cancer syndromes, it seems reasonable to suspect that germ line mutations in a number of tumor-suppressor genes may be associated with quite enigmatic cancer syndromes. Germ line mutations in yet other tumor-suppressor genes may fail entirely to predispose to cancer. Tumor-suppressor genes in this last group might still be frequently inactivated by somatic mutations in cancer. As such, the genes would be presumed to have important roles in cancer development, although their principal role might be in tumor progression rather than initiation. Nevertheless, because the compelling link between germ line mutations and inherited cancer might be lacking for some tumor-suppressor genes, the genes might be initially termed "candidate" tumor-suppressor genes to reflect uncertainties regarding their role in cancer development. Should further genetic and functional data bolster their candidacy, they might then be considered full-fledged tumor-suppressor genes.

Somatic Mutational Analysis as a Primary Approach to Tumor-Suppressor Gene Identification

An approach that has contributed significantly to the identification and characterization of tumor-suppressor genes is allelic loss or LOH studies. Consistent with Knudson's hypothesis, chromosomal regions frequently affected by LOH in one or more cancers have been proposed to contain inactivating mutations in a tumor-suppressor gene(s). For some of the chromosome regions frequently affected by LOH in one or more cancer types, no cancer predisposition genes have been localized to the affected regions. For other chromosome regions, although a tumor-suppressor gene with a role in a particular inherited cancer syndrome might have already been identified in the region, somatic mutations of the gene are rare or absent in sporadic cancers. Chromosomes 1p, 3p, 8p, 10q, 17q, 18q, and 22q are among the regions for which tumor-suppressor genes with important roles in sporadic cancer remain to be fully defined. Studies of candidate tumor-suppressor genes from several chromosome regions frequently affected by LOH in cancer are reviewed below, because the studies suggest that those who would hope to identify tumor-suppressor genes solely from LOH and somatic mutational analyses should proceed with caution.

Allelic losses of 18q are frequent in a number of cancers, including colorectal, pancreatic, gastric, and endometrial cancer.[37,46,47] It has been rather difficult to definitively localize the region(s) on 18q that contain the tumor-suppressor gene(s) solely through LOH analyses, because a large portion of 18q is often lost. However, in pancreatic and colorectal cancers, the common region of LOH appears to include chromosome bands 18q12.3 to 18q21.3. As noted above, the identification of homozygous deletions at chromosome band 18q21.1 in 20 to 25 percent of pancreatic cancers was critical in the identification of the *DPC4* gene.[39] Subsequent studies revealed that *DPC4* encodes a transcription factor that functions in the TGF-β signaling pathway, and DPC4 is somatically mutated in about 50 percent of pancreatic cancers, in 10 to 15 percent of colorectal cancers, and in a small fraction of other cancer types.[48] In addition, the *DPC4* gene has been found to be mutated in the germ line of some patients with juvenile polyposis syndrome (JPS).[49] Those patients with JPS develop benign (hamartomatous) polyps of the intestinal tract and are at increased risk of colorectal and gastric cancer. Thus, because of its role in an inherited cancer syndrome and the sizable cohort of somatic, inactivating mutations found in sporadic pancreatic, colorectal, and gastric cancers, *DPC4* has been definitively established as a tumor-suppressor gene. Nevertheless, *DPC4* is only mutated in a subset of the pancreatic, colorectal, gastric, and other cancers with 18q LOH,[48,50] and the existence of other tumor-suppressor genes on chromosome 18q must be considered, including the *DPC4*-related gene known as *JV18-1/MADR2/SMAD2* and the *DCC* (deleted in colorectal cancer) gene.

Somatic, inactivating mutations in the *SMAD2* gene at 18q12.3 have been found in about 5 percent of colorectal cancers,[51,52] and *SMAD2* mutations are rare or absent in the majority of other cancer types studied.[48,53–56] *DCC* is an enormous gene that spans >1350 kb at 18q21.2, and the gene encodes a large transmembrane protein.[46] Somatic mutations in *DCC* have been detected in only a small subset of cancers,[46] although there are both theoretical and practical difficulties associated with screening for inactivating mutations in a gene the size of *DCC*. In the majority of colorectal cancers and cancer cell lines, *DCC* expression is markedly reduced or absent, consistent with the hypothesis that loss of *DCC* function may contribute to the cancer cell phenotype.[46] Nevertheless, in the majority of cases, the mutational and/or epigenetic mechanisms underlying loss of *DCC* expression remain to be determined. As a result of these uncertainties, it is not clear whether *DCC* inactivation is a causal factor in cancer development or a reflection of the cancer phenotype. Intriguingly, recent studies indicate that the *DCC* protein may induce apoptosis in some cell types, a function perhaps consistent with its possible role as a tumor-suppressor gene in certain cancer types.[57] Perhaps the principal lesson from the studies of chromosome 18q is that at least three different 18q genes that are affected by somatic, inactivating mutations in cancer have already been identified. Such findings illustrate the difficulties that may be encountered in definitive identification of the gene(s) targeted by a common LOH event. Furthermore, the findings with the *SMAD2* and *DCC* genes reinforce the point that, in the absence of other supporting data, such as the identification of germ line mutations in those with a cancer predisposition syndrome, a limited cohort of somatic alterations provides rather weak evidence to implicate any gene in cancer development.

Properties of selected candidate tumor-suppressor genes are summarized in Table 26-2. However, findings on the *MCC* and *FHIT* candidate tumor-suppressor genes are reviewed here to highlight additional problematic issues in the evaluation of candidate tumor-suppressor genes. In the search for the adenomatous polyposis coli (*APC*) gene at chromosome 5q21, a candidate tumor-suppressor gene, termed *MCC* (for mutated in colorectal cancer), was identified prior to the cloning of *APC*.[58] *MCC* was somatically mutated in 5 to 10 percent of colorectal cancers, and the mutations included missense mutations affecting conserved amino acids, splicing mutations, and gross rearrangement of the gene. In large part because the *APC* gene, and not *MCC*, was mutated in the germ line of those with familial polyposis, further studies on *MCC* have lagged. The *MCC* gene may have a role in some colorectal cancers. However, more definitive insights into the role of *MCC* in human cancer await the results of further studies.

The *FHIT* (fragile histidine triad) gene at chromosome 3p14.2 is a controversial candidate tumor-suppressor gene.[59–61] *FHIT* is a very large gene, spanning roughly 1000 kb, although it encodes a small protein of 147 amino acids that appears to function as a

Table 26-2 Selected Candidate Tumor-Suppressor Genes and Their Encoded Proteins

Gene	Cancers with Somatic Mutations	Protein Function	Comments
TGF-β type II R	RER + colorectal and gastric cancer, head and neck, lung, and esophageal squamous cell carcinoma	TGF-β receptor component	Both alleles inactivated in RER+ cancers with mutations; mutations less frequent in non-RER+ cancers; germ line variant allele proposed to be associated with "HNPCC-like" phenotype
BAX	RER+ colorectal	Pro-apoptotic factor	Mutations are heterozygous (1 allele) in the majority of cancers; ?genetically unstable microsatellite tract vs. specific target for inactivation?
FHIT	Lung, cervical, renal, others	Dinucleoside polyphosphate hydrolase	Mutations detected in 5–10% of cancers; majority of mutations affect noncoding sequences; aberrant splicing and reduced RNA and protein levels are common; ?genetically unstable locus vs. specific target for inactivation?
α-CAT	Some prostate and lung, ?others	Links E-cadherin cell-adhesion complex to cytoskeleton	Mutations present in a small fraction of cancers
DCC	Some colorectal, neuroblastoma, male germ cell cancer, gliomas, ?others?	Netrin-1 receptor component; regulates cell migration and apoptosis	Mutations rarely detected; decreased or absent expression is seen in >50% of a variety of cancer types
MADR2/SMAD2	Some colorectal	Transcription factor/signaling molecule in TGF-β pathway	Mutations in <5% of colorectal and other cancers (e.g., gastric)
CDX2	Rare mutations in colorectal	Homeobox transcription factor	Cdx2+/− knockout mice are predisposed to intestinal tumors; decreased Cdx2 protein expression in human and rodent colorectal tumors
MKK4	Rare mutations in pancreas, lung, breast and colorectal; ?others?	Stress- and cytokine-induced protein kinase	
PP2R1B	Lung, colorectal	Subunit of serine/threonine protein phosphatase 2A	Mutations are heterozygous in some cases
MCC	Rare mutations in colorectal	Not known	Mutations in about 5–10% of sporadic colorectal cancers

dinucleoside polyphosphate hydrolase. Somatic mutations at the *FHIT* locus have been identified in a number of different cancer types. However, in most cases, the mutations do not affect *FHIT* coding exons. The most consistent observations are that aberrant *FHIT* transcripts are found in cancer. While most aberrant *FHIT* transcripts appear to arise from alternative splicing and such transcripts have been found at low abundance in normal tissues, in several cancer types, the aberrant transcripts have been correlated with markedly reduced *FHIT* gene and protein expression. Hence, based on the somatic mutations observed at the *FHIT* locus and the aberrant expression of *FHIT* transcripts and protein, *FHIT* has been suggested as a tumor-suppressor gene. Unfortunately, some gaps exist in the data set needed to definitively establish *FHIT* as a tumor-suppressor gene. For instance, germ line mutations in *FHIT* have not yet been clearly linked to a cancer predisposition syndrome. It is also uncertain whether the limited cohort of somatic mutations in *FHIT* is a cause of cancer or a reflection of *FHIT*'s location at a chromosome fragile site. Finally, the relationship of the biochemical action of the *FHIT* protein to its potential tumor suppression function remains to be more clearly established.

In summary, the results obtained thus far in studies of the *SMAD2, DCC, MCC,* and *FHIT* genes indicate that a cautious approach is both reasonable and appropriate for those investigators who hope to rely predominantly on LOH and somatic mutational analyses for identification and evaluation of tumor-suppressor genes.

Other Approaches to Identify Candidate Tumor-Suppressor Genes

Germ line inactivation of the mouse homologues of human tumor-suppressor genes has generated some useful new cancer models. Unfortunately, several mouse models of inherited cancer, including mice with germ line *Rb* and *Nf2* defects, do not manifest the tumor types seen in man, and, in fact, develop tumors not seen in humans with the corresponding defect.[62] Other mouse models, including mice heterozygous for defects in the homologues of the *BRCA1, BRCA2, WT1,* and *VHL* genes, fail to manifest an elevated rate of spontaneous tumors. Nevertheless, it seems reasonable to suggest that another approach for identification of candidate tumor-suppressor genes in human cancer is to carefully consider the tumor predisposition phenotypes seen in mouse "knockout" models. In fact, several knockout models display increased rates of spontaneous tumor development. For instance, gonadal stromal tumors develop in mice homozygous for inactivating mutations in *α-inhibin,* and intestinal adenomas are seen in mice heterozygous for inactivating mutations in the *Cdx2* homeobox gene. Mutations in *α-inhibin* have not been described in man, and somatic mutations in *CDX2* are uncommon in colorectal cancers in man.[63] Thus, it seems likely that mouse knockout models may not always accurately predict the identities of tumor-suppressor genes that are frequently mutated in cancers arising in man. Nonetheless, the mouse models may still be of considerable utility for highlighting potential tumor-suppressor gene signaling pathways, and other genes in the pathway may be frequently mutated in human cancer.

Finally, there are some caveats concerning the premature designation of a gene as a tumor suppressor. An increasing number of genes that have decreased or absent expression in cancers are being discovered. These genes are sometimes termed tumor suppressors based simply on their decreased expression. Similarly, other genes that antagonize the tumorigenic or *in vitro* growth properties of cancer cell lines may be termed tumor suppressors. Undoubtedly, some of these genes may prove critical in growth regulation and may even be targets for loss-of-function mutations in human cancer. However, it should be remembered that the altered expression of many genes in cancers may not result from specific inactivation by mutational mechanisms, but may simply reflect the altered growth properties of cancer cells. Finally, as is the case for the retinoblastoma-related gene termed p107, the p53-related gene known as p73, and the p53 target gene known as *p21/WAF1/CIP1,* some genes may have particularly potent growth suppressive properties in cancer cells, but may be rarely, if ever, mutated in human cancer. In the end, it is the sum total of the mutational and functional data that establish whether a gene has a causal role in tumorigenesis and is appropriately designated as a tumor-suppressor gene.

SUMMARY

There is now compelling evidence to support the importance of tumor-suppressor genes in cancer. Evidence for the existence of tumor-suppressor genes emerged gradually from somatic cell genetic and epidemiologic studies, as well as studies of chromosome losses in tumor cells using cytogenetic and molecular genetic techniques. In the last decade, more than two dozen well-documented tumor-suppressor genes and a number of intriguing candidate tumor-suppressor genes have been identified. The genes are inactivated in the germ line in some cancer patients, and, in such cases, their inactivation strongly predisposes to cancer. Far more frequently, tumor-suppressor genes are inactivated by somatic mutations arising during tumor development. As is reinforced in subsequent chapters, although we have learned much about tumor-suppressor genes, much work remains. A more complete description of tumorigenesis will emerge with the identification of additional tumor-suppressor genes, the detailed characterization of their normal cellular functions, and the elucidation of germ line and somatic mutations that inactivate these genes in human tumors. These findings will provide new insights into cancer pathogenesis, and should prove crucial in improving the management and treatment of patients and families with cancer.

REFERENCES

1. Bishop JM: Molecular themes in oncogenesis. *Cell* **64**:235, 1991.
2. Rabbitts TH: Chromosomal translocations in human cancer. *Nature* **372**:143, 1994.
3. Shih C, Shilo BZ, Goldfarb MP, Dannenberg A, Weinberg RA: Passage of phenotypes of chemically transformed cells via transfection of DNA and chromatin. *Proc Natl Acad Sci USA* **76**:5714, 1979.
4. Parada LF, Tabin CJ, Shih C, Weinberg RA: Human EJ bladder carcinoma oncogene is homologue of Harvey sarcoma virus ras gene. *Nature* **297**:474, 1982.
5. Der CJ, Krontiris TG, Cooper GM: Transforming genes of human bladder and lung carcinoma cell lines are homologous to the ras genes of Harvey and Kirsten sarcoma viruses. *Proc Natl Acad Sci USA* **79**:3637, 1982.
6. Santos E, Tronick SR, Aaronson SA, Pulciani S, Barbacid M: T24 human bladder carcinoma oncogene is an activated form of the normal human homologue of BALB- and Harvey-MSV transforming genes. *Nature* **298**:343, 1982.
7. Ephrussi B, Davidson RL, Weiss MC, Harris H, Klein G: Malignancy of somatic cell hybrids. *Nature* **224**:1314, 1969.
8. Harris H: The analysis of malignancy in cell fusion: the position in 1988. *Can Res* **48**:3302, 1988.
9. Klinger HP: Suppression of tumorigenicity. *Cytogenet Cell Genet* **32**:68, 1982.
10. Stanbridge EJ, Der CJ, Doersen CJ, Nishimi RY, Peehl DM, Weissman BE, Wilkinson JE: Human cell hybrids: analysis of transformation and tumorigenicity. *Science* **215**:252, 1982.
11. Geiser AG, Der CJ, Marshall CJ, Stanbridge EJ: Suppression of tumorigenicity with continued expression of the c-Ha-ras oncogene in EJ bladder carcinoma-human fibroblast hybrid cells. *Proc Natl Acad Sci USA* **83**:5209, 1986.
12. Saxon PJ, Srivatsan ES, Stanbridge EJ: Introduction of human chromosome 11 via microcell transfer controls tumorigenic expression of HeLa cells. *EMBO J* **5**:3461, 1986.
13. Weissman BE, Saxon PJ, Pasquale SR, Jones GR, Geiser AG, Stanbridge EJ: Introduction of a normal human chromosome 11 into a Wilms' tumor cell line controls its tumorigenic expression. *Science* **236**:175, 1987.
14. Shimizu M, Yokota J, Mori N, Shuin T, Shinoda M, Terada M, Oshimura M: Introduction of normal chromosome 3p modulates the tumorigenicity of a human renal cell carcinoma cell line YCR. *Oncogene* **5**:185, 1990.
15. Trent JM, Stanbridge EJ, McBride HL, Meese EU, Casey G, Araujo DE, Witkowski CM, Nagle RB: Tumorigenicity in human melanoma cell lines controlled by introduction of human chromosome 6. *Science* **247**:568, 1990.
16. Oshimura M, Hugoh H, Koi M, Shimizu M, Yamada H, Satoh H, Barrett JC: Transfer of human chromosome 11 suppresses tumorigenicity of some but not all tumor cell lines. *J Cell Biochem* **42**:135, 1990.
17. Tanaka K, Oshimura M, Kikuchi R, Seki M, Hayashi T, Miyaki M: Suppression of tumorigenicity in human colon carcinoma cells by introduction of normal chromosome 5 or 18. *Nature* **349**:340, 1991.
18. Knudson AG: Mutation and cancer: Statistical study of retinoblastoma. *Proc Natl Acad Sci USA* **68**:820, 1971.
19. Francke U: Retinoblastoma and chromosome 13. *Cytogenet Cell Genet* **16**:131, 1976.
20. Francke U, Holmes LB, Atkins L, Riccardi VM: Aniridia-Wilms' tumor association: Evidence for specific deletion of 11p13. *Cytogenet Cell Genet* **24**:185, 1979.
21. Herrera L, Kakati S, Gibas L, Pietrzak E, Sandberg AA: Brief clinical report: Gardner syndrome in a man with an interstitial deletion of 5q. *Am J Med Genet* **25**:473, 1986.
22. Fountain JW, Wallace MR, Bruce MA, Seizinger BR, Menon AG, Gusella JF, Michels VV, Schmidt MA, Dewald GW, Collins FS: Physical mapping of a translocation breakpoint in neurofibromatosis. *Science* **244**:1085, 1989.
23. O'Connell P, Leach R, Cawthon RM, Culver M, Stevens J, Viskochil D, Fournier RE, Rich DC, Ledbetter DH, White R: Two von Recklinghausen neurofibromatosis translocations map within a 600 kb region of 17q11.2. *Science* **244**:1087, 1989.
24. Groden J, Thliveris A, Samowitz W, Carlson M, Gelbert LA, Joslyn G, Stevens J, Spirio L, Robertson M: Identification and characterization of the familial adenomatous polyposis coli gene. *Cell* **66**:589, 1991.
25. Joslyn G, Carlson M, Thliveris A, Albertsen H, Gelbert L, Samowitz W, Groden J, Stevens J, Spirio L, Robertson M: Identification of deletion mutations and three new genes at the familial polyposis locus. *Cell* **66**:601, 1991.
26. Kinzler K, Nilbert M, Su L, Vogelstein B, Bryan T, Levy D, Smith K, Preisinger A, Hedge P, McKechnie D, Rinniear R, Markham A, Groffen J, Boguski M, Altschul S, Horii A, Ando H, Miyoshi Y, Miki Y, Nishisho I, Nakamura Y: Identification of FAP locus genes from chromosome 5q21. *Science* **253**:661, 1991.
27. Nishisho I, Nakamura Y, Miyoshi Y, Miki Y, Ando H, Horii A, Koyama K, Utsunomiya J, Baba S, Hedge P: Mutations of chromosome 5q21 genes in FAP and colorectal cancer patients. *Science* **253**:665, 1991.
28. Latif F, Tory K, Gnarra J, Yao M, Duh FM, Orcutt ML, Stackhouse T, Kuzmin I, Modi W, Geil L, et al: Identification of the von Hippel-Lindau disease tumor suppressor gene. *Science* **260**:1317, 1993.
29. Trofatter JA, MacCollin MM, Rutter JL, Murrell JR, Duyao MP, Parry DM, Eldridge R, Kley N, Menon AG, Pulaski K, et al: A novel moesin-, ezrin-, radixin-like gene is a candidate for the neurofibromatosis 2 tumor suppressor. *Cell* **72**:791, 1993.
30. Rouleau GA, Merel P, Lutchman M, Sanson M, Zucman J, Marineau C, Hoang-Xuan K, Demczuk S, Desmaze C, Plougastel B: Alteration in a new gene encoding a putative membrane-organizing protein causes neuro-fibromatosis type 2. *Nature* **363**:515, 1993.
31. Sparkes RS, Sparkes MC, Wilson MG, Towner JW, Benedict W, Murphree AL, Yunis JJ: Regional assignment of genes for human esterase D and retinoblastoma to chromosome band 13q14. *Science* **208**:1042, 1980.
32. Sparkes RS, Murphree AL, Lingua RW, Sparkes MC, Field LL, Funderburk SJ, Benedict WF: Gene for hereditary retinoblastoma assigned to human chromosome 13 by linkage to esterase D. *Science* **219**:971, 1983.
33. Benedict WF, Murphree AL, Banerjee A, Spina CA, Sparkes MC, Sparkes RS: Patient with 13 chromosome deletion: evidence that the retinoblastoma gene is a recessive cancer gene. *Science* **219**:973, 1983.
34. Cavenee WK, Dryja TP, Phillips RA, Benedict WF, Godbout R, Gallie BL, Murphree AL, Strong LC, White RL: Expression of recessive alleles by chromosomal mechanisms in retinoblastoma. *Nature* **305**:779, 1983.

35. Cavenee WK, Hansen MF, Nordenskjold M, Kock E, Maumenee I, Squire JA, Phillips RA, Gallie BL: Genetic origin of mutations predisposing to retinoblastoma. *Science* **228**:501, 1985.
36. Solomon E, Voss R, Hall V, Bodmer WF, Jass JR, Jeffreys AJ, Lucibello FC, Patel I, Rider SH: Chromosome 5 allele loss in human colorectal carcinomas. *Nature* **328**:616, 1987.
37. Vogelstein B, Fearon ER, Hamilton S, Kern S, Preisinger A, Leppert M, Nakamura Y, White R, Smits A, Bos J: Genetic alterations during colorectal-tumor development. *N Engl J Med* **319**:525, 1988.
38. Schutte M, Rozenblum E, Moskaluk CA, Guan X, Hoque AT, Hahn SA, da Costa LT, de Jong PJ, Kern SE: An integrated high-resolution physical map of the DPC/BRCA2 region at chromosome 13q12. *Can Res* **55**:4570, 1995.
39. Hahn SA, Schutte M, Hoque AT, Moskaluk CA, da Costa LT, Rozenblum E, Fischer A, Yeo CJ, Hruban RH, Kern SE: DPC4, a candidate tumor suppressor gene at human chromosome 18q21.1. *Science* **271**:350, 1996.
40. Li J, Yen C, Liaw D, Podsypanina K, Bose S, Wang SI, Puc J, Miliaresis C, Rodgers L, McCombie R, Bigner SH, Giovanella BC, Ittmann M, Tycko B, Hibshoosh H, Wigler MH, Parsons R: PTEN, a putative protein tyrosine phosphatase gene mutated in human brain, breast, and prostate cancer [see comments]. *Science* **275**:1943, 1997.
41. Steck PA, Pershouse MA, Jasser SA, Yung WK, Lin H, Ligon AH, Langford LA, Baumgard ML, Hattier T, Davis T, Frye C, Hu R, Swedlund B, Teng DH, Tavtigian SV: Identification of a candidate tumour suppressor gene, MMAC1, at chromosome 10q23.3 that is mutated in multiple advanced cancers. *Nat Genet* **15**:356, 1997.
42. Kinzler KW, Vogelstein B: Lessons from hereditary colorectal cancer. *Cell* **87**:159, 1996.
43. Sellers WR, Kaelin WG Jr: Role of the retinoblastoma protein in the pathogenesis of human cancer. *J Clin Onc* **15**:3301, 1997.
44. Clevers H, van de Wetering M: TCF/LEF factor earn their wings. *Trends Genet* **13**:485, 1997.
45. He TC, Sparks AB, Rago C, Hermeking H, Zawel L, da Costa LT, Morin PJ, Vogelstein B, Kinzler KW: Identification of c-MYC as a target of the APC pathway. *Science* **281**:1509, 1998.
46. Cho KR, Fearon ER: DCC—linking tumour suppressor genes and altered cell surface interactions in cancer. *Eur J Cancer* **31A**:1055, 1995.
47. Hahn SA, Seymour AB, Hoque AT, Schutte M, da Costa LT, Redston MS, Caldas C, Weinstein CL, Fischer A, Yeo CJ and others: Allelotype of pancreatic adenocarcinoma using xenograft enrichment. *Can Res* **55**:4670, 1995.
48. Moskaluk CA, Kern SE: Cancer gets Mad: DPC4 and other TGFβ pathway genes in human cancer. *Biochimica et Biophysica Acta* **1288**:M31, 1996.
49. Howe JR, Roth S, Ringold JC, Summers RW, Jarvinen HJ, Tomlinson IP, Houlston RS, Bevan S, Mitros FA, Stone EM: Mutations in the SMAD4/DPC4 gene in juvenile polyposis. *Science* **280**:1086, 1998.
50. Schutte M, Hruban RH, Hedrick L, Cho KR, Nadasdy GM, Weinstein CL, Bova GS, Isaacs WB, Cairns P, Nawroz H, Sidransky D, Casero JRA, Meltzer PS, Hahn SA, Kern SE: *DPC4* gene in various tumor types. *Can Res* **56**:2527, 1996.
51. Riggins GJ, Thiagalingam S, Rozenblum E, Weinstein CL, Kern SE, Hamilton SR, Willson JK, Markowitz SD, Kinzler KW, Vogelstein B: Mad-related genes in the human. *Nature Genet* **13**:347, 1996.
52. Eppert K, Scherer SW, Ozcelik H, Pirone R, Hoodless P, Kim H, Tsui LC, Gallinger S, Andrulis IL, Thomsen GH, Wrana JL, Attisano L: MADR2 maps to 18q21 and encodes a TGFbeta-regulated MAD-related protein that is functionally mutated in colorectal carcinoma. *Cell* **86**:543, 1996.
53. Uchida K, Nagatake M, Osada H, Yatabe Y, Kondo M, Mitsudomi T, Masuda A, Takahashi T: Somatic *in vivo* alterations of the *JV18-1* gene at 18q21 in human lung cancers. *Can Res* **56**:5583, 1996.
54. Maesawa C, Tamura G, Nishizuka S, Iwaya T, Ogasawara S, Ishida K, Sakata K, Sato N, Ikeda K, Kimura Y, Saito K, Satodate R: *MAD*-related genes on 18q21.1, *Smad2* and *Smad4*, are altered infrequently in esophageal squamous cell carcinoma. *Jpn J Can Res* **88**:340, 1997.
55. Kong X-T, Choi SH, Inoue A, Xu F, Chen T, Takita J, Yokota J, Bessho F, Yanagisawa M, Hanada R, Yamamoto K, Hayashi Y: Expression and mutational analysis of the *DCC, DPC4,* and *MADR2/JV18-1* genes in neuroblastoma. *Can Res* **57**:3772, 1997.
56. Ikezoe T, Takeuchi S, Kamioka M, Daibata M, Kubonishi I, Taguchi H, Miyoshi I: Analysis of the Smad2 gene in hematological malignancies. *Leukemia* **12**:94, 1998.
57. Mehlen P, Rabizadeh S, Snipas SJ, Assa-Munt N, Salvesen GS, Bredesen DE: The DCC gene product induces apoptosis by a mechanism requiring receptor proteolysis. *Nature* **395**:801, 1998.
58. Kinzler KW, Nilbert MC, Vogelstein B, Levy DB, Smith KJ, Preisinger AC, Hamilton SRH, Markham A, et al.: Identification of a gene located at chromosome 5q21 that is mutated in colorectal cancers. *Science* **251**:1366, 1991.
59. Sozzi G, Huebner K, Croce CM: FHIT in human cancer. *Adv Can Res* **74**:141-66: 1998.
60. Mao L: Tumor suppressor genes: does FHIT fit? *J Natl Canc Inst* **90**:412, 1998.
61. Le Beau MM, Drabkin H, Glover TW, Gemmill R, Rassool FV, McKeithan TW, Smith DI: An FHIT tumor suppressor gene? *Genes Chrom Canc* **21**:281, 1998.
62. Jacks T: Tumor suppressor gene mutations in mice. *Annu Rev Genet* **30**:603, 1996.
63. Wicking C, Simms LA, Evans T, Walsh M, Chawengsaksophak K, Beck F, Chenevix-Trench G, Young J, Jass J, Leggett B, Wainwright B: CDX2, a human homologue of Drosophila caudal, is mutated in both alleles in a replication error positive colorectal cancer. *Oncogene* **17**:657, 1998.

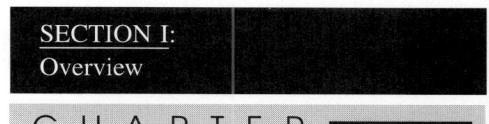

CHAPTER 27

Familial Cancer Syndromes: The Role of Caretakers and Gatekeepers

Kenneth W. Kinzler ▪ Bert Vogelstein

The past decade has witnessed the elucidation of the specific genetic bases of nearly twenty inherited predispositions to cancer. This information not only is yielding immediate practical benefits in the form of genetic testing but also is providing important insights into mechanisms regulating cancer susceptibility.

The inheritance of a predisposition to a sporadic event such as tumor formation has always presented an interesting problem. The complexity of this problem is compounded by studies of the age dependence of cancer incidence and other studies that suggest that multiple genetic changes are required for cancer formation. This prompted Knudson to postulate that individuals with an autosomal dominant cancer susceptibility inherited one genetic alteration that was rate-limiting for tumor formation but that subsequent steps also were required for a tumor to form. Over the years, Knudson's hypothesis has been refined to include the idea that one of the key subsequent steps is a somatic, inactivating mutation of the wild-type allele inherited from the unaffected parent. Knudson's hypotheses have been confirmed abundantly within the last 20 years (e.g., *Rb* in retinoblastoma, Chap. 36; *APC* in colorectal cancer, Chap. 48), and concrete demonstrations of the multiple genetic events required for tumorigenesis have emerged (e.g., colorectal cancer, Chap. 48). The characterization of the genes underlying inherited predispositions to neoplasia also has provided important insights into the nature of tumor suppressor genes.

It appears that most tumor suppressor genes can be broadly divided into two groups, called *gatekeepers* and *caretakers*. Gatekeepers are genes that directly regulate the growth of tumors by inhibiting their growth or by promoting their death. The functions of these genes are rate-limiting for tumor growth, and as a result, both the maternal and paternal copies of these genes must be inactivated for a tumor to develop (Fig. 27-1). In accord with Knudson's hypothesis, predisposed individuals inherit one damaged copy of such a gene and as a result require only one additional mutation for tumor initiation. The identity of gatekeepers varies with each tissue such that inactivation of a given gene leads to specific forms of cancer predisposition. For example, inherited mutations of *APC* lead to colon tumors but not kidney cancers (see Chap. 48), whereas inherited mutations of *VHL* predispose to kidney cancers but not colon cancers (see Chap. 41). Because these gatekeeping genes are rate-limiting for tumor initiation, they must be mutated in sporadic cancers through somatic mutations as well as mutated in the germ line of predisposed individuals.

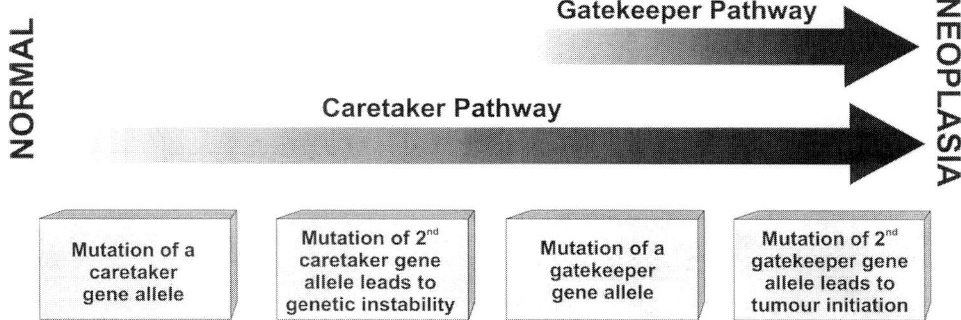

Fig. 27-1 Pathways to neoplasia. Inherited mutation of either a gatekeeper or caretaker can predispose an individual to neoplasia. However, additional genetic changes are required to convert a predisposed cell to a neoplastic cell. In the case of the caretaker pathway, three additional mutations generally are required. However, the genetic instability that follows inactivation of the second caretaker allele accelerates the accumulation of the latter mutations. In the case of the gatekeeper pathway, only one additional mutation (inactivation of the second gatekeeper allele) is required to initiate neoplasia. (Although the concepts depicted in this figure apply to all inherited cancer susceptibilities, variations do occur. For example, inherited mutations of both alleles of a caretaker gene occur in recessively inherited diseases such as xeroderma pigmentosum, and a single dominant negative mutation can substitute for two inactivating mutations of a caretaker gene).

In contrast, inactivation of caretakers does not directly promote growth of tumors. Rather, inactivation of caretakers leads to a genetic instability that only indirectly promotes growth by causing an increased mutation rate. Because numerous mutations are required for the full development of a cancer, inactivation of caretakers, with the consequent increase in genetic instability, can greatly accelerate the development of cancers. Caretaker mutations in the germ line occur in two different forms. In dominantly inherited diseases (e.g., hereditary nonpolypsosis colorectal cancer; see Chap. 32), only one mutant allele of the caretaker is inherited; as with gatekeepers, the remaining allele of the caretaker gene must be mutated for a phenotypic defect (i.e., increased mutation rate) to be realized (see Fig. 27-1). In other cases, both alleles of the gene must be inherited in mutant form to cause susceptibility (e.g., *XP;* see Chap. 28). The targets of the accelerated mutagenesis that occurs in cells with defective caretakers are the gatekeeping tumor suppressor genes, other tumor suppressor genes (whose inactivation can lead to tumor progression), and oncogenes (genes whose activation leads to cancer). Somatic mutations of caretaker genes are only rarely found as initiating events in tumors arising in the general population, presumably because such mutations would still need to be followed by several other mutations in order for a tumor to initiate (see Fig. 27-1).

For the purposes of this book, we have divided cancer susceptibility syndromes into two forms, gatekeepers and caretakers, based on the predominant mechanism underlying the susceptibility. In some cases, the mechanism underlying the susceptibility is not completely characterized, and the assignments were made based on the best current evidence. For example, the *BRCA1* and *BRCA2* genes (see Chap. 47) have been hypothesized to function as caretakers in some studies and as gatekeepers in others; further research will be required to discriminate the true role of these genes in tumor suppression.

CHAPTER 28

Nucleotide Excision Repair Syndromes: Xeroderma Pigmentosum, Cockayne Syndrome, and Trichothiodystrophy*

Dirk Bootsma ▪ Kenneth H. Kraemer
James E. Cleaver ▪ Jan H. J. Hoeijmakers

1. Three rare autosomal recessive syndromes are associated with a nucleotide excision repair (NER) defect: xeroderma pigmentosum (XP), Cockayne syndrome (CS), and the photosensitive form of trichothiodystrophy (TTD). A common denominator of all three conditions is an extreme sensitivity to sunlight. XP patients exhibit in addition to photosensitivity a greater than thousand-fold increased frequency of sunlight-induced skin cancers. Other features include progressive degenerative alterations of the skin and eyes and in some cases accelerated neurologic degeneration due to increased neuronal death. Patients with CS have a combination of sun sensitivity, short stature, severe neurologic abnormalities due to dysmyelination, cataracts, dental caries, a wizened appearance, and a characteristic bird-like facies. They do not display cancer predisposition. The hallmark of TTD is sulfur-deficient brittle hair and nails. Patients also have ichthyosis and many symptoms characteristic of CS. About half of TTD patients are hypersensitive to ultraviolet (UV) light, and they have a NER defect. As in CS, there are no indications for an increased risk of cancer. In addition to the preceding, rare patients showing combined XP-CS symptoms have been described.

2. The NER pathway removes a remarkably wide array of structurally unrelated DNA lesions. Among these are numerous helix-distorting chemical adducts induced by carcinogens such as benz[a]pyrene, as well as cyclobutane pyrimidine dimers (CPD) and [6-4]pyrimidine-pyrimidone photoproducts (6-4PP) produced in human skin by the shortwave UV component of the solar spectrum. This explains why patients with inherited deficiencies in the NER process display marked hypersensitivity to sun exposure. Defective repair also results in genetic instability leading to increased chromosome abnormalities and mutagenesis and in many cases predisposition to cancer. At least two NER subpathways exist: a rapid transcription-coupled repair (TCR) pathway responsible for the efficient elimination of lesions from the transcribed strand of active genes that permits rapid resumption of the vital process of transcription and for some lesions a less efficient global genome repair (GGR) subpathway that surveys the entire genome.

3. Complementation analysis by cell fusion has allowed a further genetic classification of XP, CS, and TTD patients. In XP, seven different complementation groups are distinguished, representing seven distinct defective genes involved in NER in XP: XP-A, -B, -C, -D, -E, -F, and -G. In addition, another class of XP patients (XP variant) appears to be deficient in a gene product that in normal cells permits semiconservative replication of previously damaged sites in the DNA template (postreplication repair). Similarly, complementation analysis has revealed two complementation groups in CS, CS-A and CS-B, and three in TTD, of which two overlap with XP groups: TTD-A, XP-B, and XP-D. Patients with combined XP-CS have been assigned to three XP complementation groups: XP-B, XP-D and XP-G.

4. The NER defect in the cells of most XP and TTD patients is located in the core of the NER mechanism and affects both

*This text is a complete revision of Chapter 148, Xeroderma Pigmentosum and Cockayne Syndrome, in the 7th edition of *Metabolic and Molecular Bases of Inherited Diseases.* Part of this chapter is an updated version of Hoeijmakers JHJ: Human nucleotide excision repair syndromes: Molecular clues to unexpected intricacies, *Eur J Cancer* 30A(13):1912, 1994; used with permission from Elsevier Science, Ltd., The Boulevard, Lanfordlane, Kidlington OX5 1GB, UK.

A list of standard abbreviations is located immediately preceding the index in each volume. Nonstandard abbreviations used in this chapter include: XP = xeroderma pigmentosum; NER = nucleotide excision repair; CS = Cockayne syndrome; TTD = trichothiodystrophy; BER = base escision repair; TCR = transcription-coupled repair; GGR = global genome repair; UDS = unscheduled DNA synthesis; SCE = sister chromatid exchange; UVS = ultraviolet sensitivity; DDB = DNA damage-binding protein; MEFs = mouse embryonal fibroblasts.

transcription-coupled and global genome repair. In XP-C cells the defect is limited to the global genome repair system, whereas in CS only the transcription-coupled repair pathway is impaired.

5. **All XP, CS, and TTD genes, except TTD-A and XP-variant, have been cloned, and their functions in the NER mechanism are known or in the process of being clarified. Disease-causing mutations have been identified in most of the corresponding genes.**
6. **Several of the protein (complexes) involved in NER participate in other DNA transactions as well. All NER genes associated with TTD:XP-B, XP-D, and TTD-A — are simultaneously implicated in basal transcription. The XP-F complex probably has a dual involvement in a mitotic recombination pathway, and later steps in NER are shared with replication. The notion of function sharing has important implications for the clinical consequences of inherited mutations in these NER proteins. It is likely that the symptoms, which are not easy to explain on the basis of an NER defect per se (e.g., the brittle hair and nerve dysmyelination), are caused by subtle insufficiencies in basal transcription.**
7. **Mouse models for NER deficiencies have been generated. They provide excellent tools for understanding the complex relationships between DNA repair defects and clinical consequences.**
8. **Prenatal diagnosis for XP, CS, and TTD is possible if an unequivocal NER defect or the responsible mutations in the family have been demonstrated.**

The development and maintenance of life have critically depended on the evolvement of mechanisms that ensure genetic integrity and stability. DNA, the vital carrier of genetic information, is continually subject to undesired chemical alterations. Numerous environmental or endogenous compounds and various types of radiation, such as x-rays and ultraviolet (UV) light, induce a wide variety of lesions in the bases, sugars, or phosphates that make up the DNA. Obviously, such lesions (adducts, crosslinks, breaks, etc.) interfere with the proper functioning of the genome. An intricate network of single- and multistep DNA repair systems constitutes the main protecting barrier against the deleterious consequences of DNA injury. This is illustrated by the phenotype of inherited defects in one of these repair pathways. Invariably such disorders are associated with a characteristic hypersensitivity to a specific class of genotoxic agents. In addition, the DNA lesions that persist lead to cell malfunctioning and to enhanced mutagenesis because of the higher chance that mistakes are made on replication of a damaged template. Somatic mutagenesis is the initiator and driving force for the multistep process of carcinogenesis. Rare inborn disorders with hallmarks characteristic for repair defects or inadequate response to DNA damage comprise a class of *chromosomal instability syndromes.* Well-known examples are Fanconi anemia, ataxia telangiectasia, and Bloom syndrome, all of which display different manifestations of cancer proneness and increased sensitivity to specific mutagens. The prototype repair disorder, however, is xeroderma pigmentosum (XP), in which a defect in the nucleotide excision repair (NER) pathway underlies the pronounced predisposition to skin cancer and the characteristic photosensitivity of most patients. It clearly highlights the importance of the NER process. In the past decade, impressive progress has been made in unravelling the molecular intricacies of NER; for instance, all seven NER genes involved in XP (named *XP-A* through *XP-G*) have been cloned and their defect analyzed in patients; in addition, the core of the NER process has been reconstituted in vitro from purified components, which has enabled a stepwise dissection of the contribution of the various gene functions.

Genetic analysis of NER mutants and biochemical studies have provided evidence for the involvement of more than 20 gene products in the repair process. As discussed below, these proteins have been conserved to a remarkable degree throughout the over 1.2×10^6 years of eukaryotic evolution, underlining the fundamental importance of this process. This makes it likely that the mode of action of NER in lower eukaryotes, such as the baker's yeast *Saccharomyces cerevisiae,* is probably to a large extent similar to that in humans. On the other hand, clear differences have become apparent with the process in the prokaryotic model organism *Escherichia coli.*

Furthermore, intimate links between NER and other cellular processes have been disclosed, some of which were quite unexpected. Tight coordination of repair and cell cycle regulation exists: On encountering abnormally high levels of damage, a transient arrest in cell cycle progression is introduced before DNA replication or prior to cell division. This gives the repair machinery the opportunity to remove the lesions before they give rise to permanent, potentially catastrophic changes in the genetic material. In addition, connections with recombination, replication, chromatin dynamics, and the basic transcription apparatus have been unveiled.

For all the human NER syndromes and many of the NER genes, bona fide mouse models have been generated. This will be of great importance for clinical studies, for understanding the biologic relevance of the NER system, and for cancer research in general.

In this chapter the present knowledge of consequences of NER deficiency will be discussed. Besides XP, other disorders such as Cockayne syndrome (CS) and the remarkable hair disorder trichothiodystrophy (TTD) will be covered, since both are associated with repair deficiency as well. It will become clear that the relation between the molecular defect and the clinical symptoms appears straightforward in some cases. In other instances there is a beginning of understanding, and a great deal of mystery remains. For a comprehensive review of DNA damage and the intricate network of DNA repair systems in general, the interested reader is referred to Friedberg, Walker, and Siede.[1]

CLINICAL ASPECTS OF XP, CS, AND TTD

Xeroderma Pigmentosum

XP is a rare autosomal recessive disease. Affected patients (homozygotes) have sun sensitivity resulting in progressive degenerative changes of sun-exposed portions of the skin and eyes, often leading to neoplasia. Some XP patients have, in addition, progressive neurologic degeneration.[2] Obligate heterozygotes (parents) generally are asymptomatic.

History. *Xeroderma,* or "parchment skin," was the term given by Moritz Kaposi to the condition he observed in a patient in 1863 and reported in the dermatology textbook he wrote with Ferdinand von Hebra in 1874.[3] In 1882, the term *pigmentosum* was added to emphasize the striking pigmentary abnormalities. Eye involvement, including cloudiness of the cornea, was recognized by Kaposi. In 1883, Neisser reported two brothers with cutaneous XP and neurologic degeneration beginning in the second decade.[4] De Sanctis and Cacchione in 1932 described three siblings with cutaneous XP associated with microcephaly, progressive mental deterioration, dwarfism, and immature sexual development — the DeSanctis-Cacchione syndrome.[5]

Epidemiology. XP has been found in all races worldwide. The frequency is about 1 in 1 million in the United States and Europe[6] but is considerably higher in Japan (1 in 100,000)[7] and North Africa. In a literature survey of more than 800 patients,[2] there were nearly equal numbers of male (54 percent) and female (46 percent) patients. Consanguinity of the patient's parents was reported in 31 percent. Nearly 20 percent of the patients, including a high proportion of Japanese patients, had neurologic abnormalities.

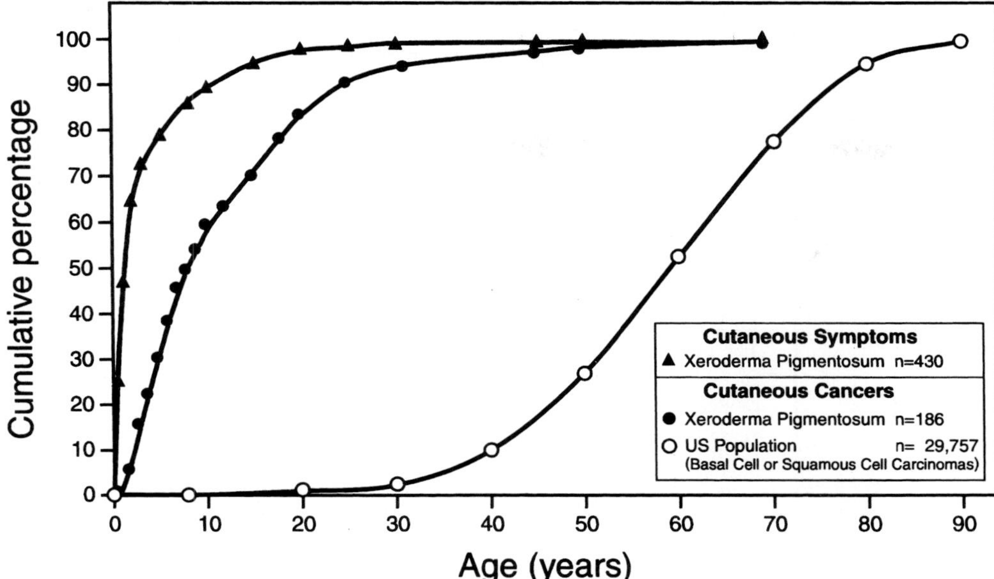

Fig. 28-1 Age at onset of XP symptoms. Age at onset of cutaneous symptoms (generally sun sensitivity or pigmentation) was reported for 430 patients. Age at first skin cancer was reported for 186 patients and is compared with age distribution for 29,757 patients with basal cell carcinoma or squamous cell carcinoma in the U.S. general population. (*From Kraemer et al.*[2] *Used by permission.*)

Symptoms. The median age of onset of symptoms is between 1 and 2 years. In 5 percent of the reported patients, onset of symptoms is delayed until after 14 years[2] (Fig. 28-1). Initial symptoms include abnormal reaction to sun exposure in 19 percent (including severe sunburn with blistering and persistent erythema on minimal sun exposure) (Table 28-1). However, many patients sunburn normally. Freckling occurs by 2 years of age in most of the patients. The cutaneous abnormalities are usually strikingly limited to sun-exposed areas of the body (Fig. 28-2). At an early stage, the skin appears similar to that seen in farmers and sailors after many years of sun exposure: areas of increased pigment alternating with areas of decreased pigment, which display atrophy and telangiectasia. A few patients who exhibit a wide spectrum of characteristic cutaneous and ocular findings have been unambiguously diagnosed as having XP, even though the erythematous response to sun exposure was normal.[6] This may be a distinctive feature of the form of XP known as *variant or pigmented xerodermoid.*[6]

Premalignant actinic keratoses and malignant and benign neoplasms develop.[2] The neoplasms are predominantly basal cell or squamous cell carcinomas (at least 45 percent of patients, many with multiple primary neoplasms) but also include melanomas (5 percent of patients), sarcomas, keratocanthomas, and angiomas. About 90 percent of the basal cell and squamous cell carcinomas occur on the face, head, and neck—the sites of greatest UV exposure. The median age of onset of first skin neoplasm is 8 years, nearly 50 years younger than that in the general population of the United States (see Fig. 28-1). This represents one of the largest reductions in age of onset of neoplasia documented for any recessive human genetic disease. The frequency of basal cell carcinomas, squamous-cell carcinomas, or melanomas of the skin is 2000 times greater than in the general population for patients under 20 years of age.[8] There is an approximate 30-year reduction in survival, with a 70 percent probability of surviving to age 40 years.[2] Many patients die of neoplasia.

Ocular abnormalities include photophobia, which may vary among patients from severe to absent; conjuctivitis of the interpalpebral (sun-exposed) area; ectropion (turning out of the lids) due to atrophy of the skin of the eyelids; exposure keratitis; and benign and malignant neoplasms of the lids, conjunctiva, and limbus (see Table 28-1). The distribution of ocular damage and neoplasms corresponds closely with the sites of UV exposure. The ocular neoplasms involve the anterior portion of the eye (lids, cornea, conjunctiva) almost exclusively. This portion of the eye shields the posterior eye (uveal tract, retina) from UV radiation; visible light is the only radiation that reaches the photosensitive cells of the retina. The frequency of ocular neoplasms is greatly increased in patients under 20 years of age.[6] There is also a great increase in squamous cell carcinoma of the tip of the tongue, another sun-exposed portion of the body.

The 18 percent of XP patients with neurologic abnormalities have a sex ratio, reported age, frequency of ocular abnormalities, and frequency of cutaneous neoplasms similar to those of patients with only skin and eye involvement.[6] The neurologic symptoms vary in age of onset and severity but are characterized by

Table 28-1 Most Common Clinical Features of Xeroderma Pigmentosum

Skin abnormalities (usually limited to sun-exposed sites)
Erythema and bullae (acute sensitivity in infancy)
Freckles
Xerosis (dryness) and scaling
Areas of hyperpigmentation alternating with hyperpigmentation
Telangiectasia
Atrophy
Benign lesion: actinic keratoses, keratocanthomas, angiomas, fibromas
Malignant lesions: basal cell carcinoma, squamous cell carcinoma, melanoma
Ophthalmologic abnormalities (limited to anterior UV-exposed portion of the eye)
Atrophy of lids
Conjunctivitus with photophobia, lacrimation, edema
Corneal abnormalities: keratitis, opacification, impaired vision
Neoplasms of conjunctiva, cornea, and lids
Neurologic manifestations
Microcephaly
Low intelligence
Progressive mental deterioration
Progressive sensorineural deafness
Abnormal motor activity
Hyporeflexia or areflexia
Primary neuronal degeneration

SOURCE: Adapted from Cleaver and Kraemer.[6] Used by permission.

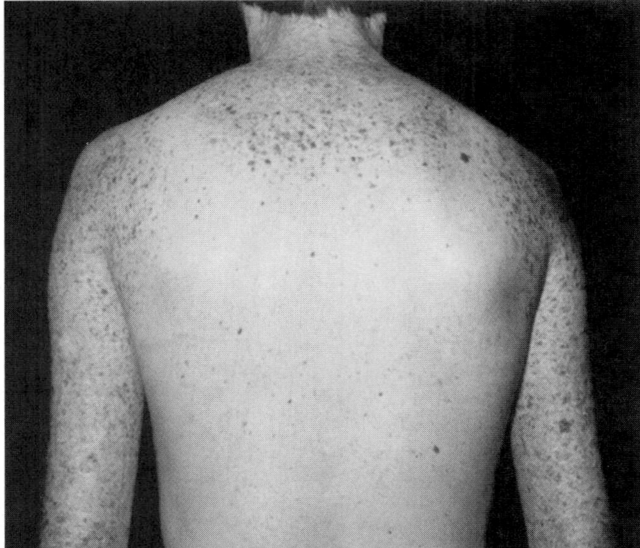

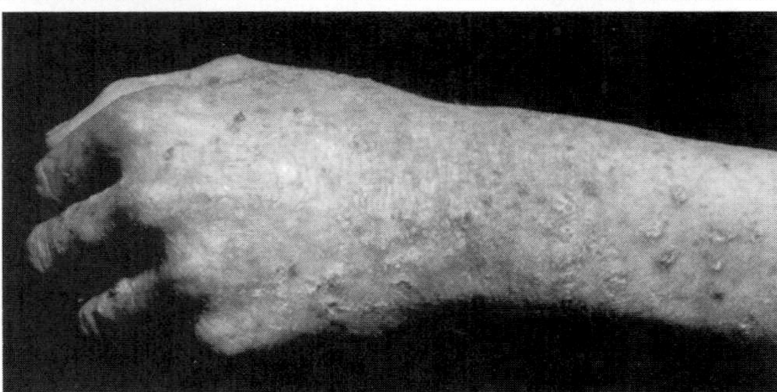

Fig. 28-2 Typical skin abnormalities in an adolescent XP patient (complementation group XP-C). *Top:* Pigmentation abnormalities; freckling and dryness and atrophy visible at the sun-exposed areas of the skin. *Bottom:* Hand of same patient showing actinic keratosis and (pre)malignant lesions. (*Courtesy of Department of Dermatology, Erasmus University, Rotterdam.*)

progressive deterioration[9,10] (see Table 28-1). Diminished deep tendon reflexes and sensorineural deafness are frequent early abnormalities. In some patients, progressive mental retardation becomes evident only in the second decade of life. Patients with the DeSanctis-Cacchione syndrome have neurologic and somatic abnormalities beginning in the first years of life.[5] They have microcephaly, intellectual deterioration with loss of the ability to talk, and increasing spasticity with loss of ability to walk, leading to quadriparesis, in addition to dwarfism and immature sexual development. Among the few autopsies reported, the major finding is a primary neuronal degeneration with loss (or absence) of neurons, particularly in the cerebral cortex and cerebellum, without evidence of a storage process or inflammatory changes.[6] The severity of neurologic disease has been reported to correlate with the degree of sensitivity of cultured skin fibroblasts to UV inhibition of colony-forming ability.[11]

Evidence is presented for an increased risk of neoplasms in non-integumental tissues in individuals with XP.[8] However, more data are required to draw definite conclusions on this point. There are reports of patients with primary brain tumors (including two sarcomas), two with leukemia, two with lung tumors, and patients with gastric carcinomas.[6] Chemical carcinogens are suspected to play a role in these neoplasms, since cultured cells from XP patients are hypersensitive to certain DNA-binding chemical carcinogens that produce damaged DNA that is normally acted on by the NER system. These include benz[a]pyrene derivatives (found in cigarette smoke) and tryptophan pyrolysis products (found in charred food).[6]

Table 28-2 Most Common Clinical Features of Cockayne Syndrome

Growth failure
Decreased height and weight
Decreased head circumference (microcephaly)
Neurologic manifestations
Delayed psychomotor development
Increased muscle tone
Tremor
Limb ataxia/incoordination
Gait abnormality
Hearing loss
Calcification of basal ganglia of brain
Ophthalmologic abnormalities
Cataracts
Optic atrophy/hypoplasia
Pigmentary retinopathy
Dental abnormalities: Caries
Skin abnormalities
Photosensitivity
Thin, dry hair

Cockayne Syndrome

CS is a rare, pleiotropic, autosomal recessive disorder with an extensive variation in symptoms and severity. Patients have cutaneous, neurologic, and somatic abnormalities (Table 28-2). Sun sensitivity of the skin is apparent in about three-fourths of affected individuals. In contrast to XP, CS patients do not have skin cancer predisposition. Since many patients exhibit multiple symptoms of premature aging, CS is also considered one of the progeroid disorders. The average age of death of reported patients is 12 years.

The first report on this condition by Cockayne appeared in 1936[6]: dwarfism with retinal atrophy and deafness. An extensive review, comprising 140 cases, was published by Nance and Berry in 1992.[12] These authors distinguish three clinically different classes of the disease: (1) a classic form (or CSI), which includes the majority of the patients, (2) a severe form (or CSII), characterized by early onset and severe progression of manifestations, and (3) a mild form, typified by late onset and slow progression of symptoms. Classical CS patients (CSI) (Fig. 28-3) show (1) growth failure (short stature), (2) neurodevelopmental and later neurologic dysfunction, (3) cutaneous photosensitivity (with or without thin or dry skin or hair), (4) progressive ocular abnormalities (such as progressive pigmentary retinopathy and/or cataracts), (5) hearing loss, (6) dental caries, and (7) a characteristic physical appearance (cachectic dwarfism, wizened facial appearance: bird-like facies). The last four criteria are more often registered in the older children. For diagnosis of CS in the infant, the presence of the first two criteria and a few of the other five criteria, together with biochemical and cellular evidence (UV sensitivity and DNA repair characteristics of CS in fibroblasts; see below), are required. Pathologic calcifications have been observed in the basal ganglia and at other locations in the central nervous system. Primary dysmyelination is an important feature seen in the nervous system of CS patients, in contrast to primary neuronal degeneration in XP. Often sexual development is impaired. The symptoms described above are much more severe and the onset much earlier in the CSII form of the disease. The characteristic facial and somatic appearance is present within the first 2 years of life. The prognosis is much worse than that of the classic CS patients. Death usually occurs by age 6 or 7. For details on the different forms of CS and further reference to other publications, the reader is referred to the review of Nance and Berry.[12]

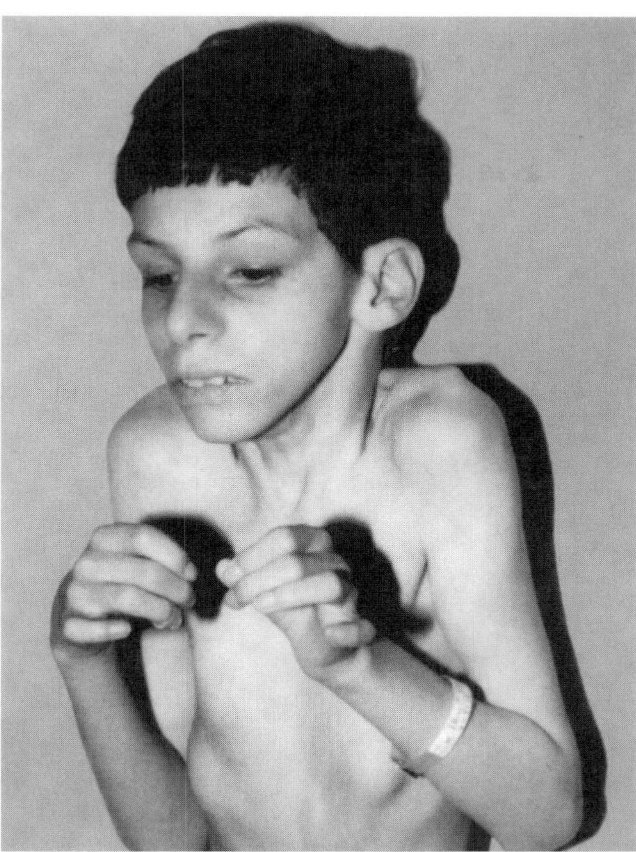

Fig. 28-3 Patient with CS. Growth failure, characteristic wizened facial appearance (bird-like facies), and skeletal deformation are visible. (*Photograph kindly provided by D. Atherton, Hospital for Sick Children, London. From Lehmann.*[13] *Used by permission.*)

Trichothiodystrophy

TTD (sulfur-deficient brittle hair) is a rare autosomal recessive disorder. It represents a specific hair dysplasia associated with a variable range of abnormalities in organs derived from ectoderm and neuroendoderm (Fig. 28-4). About half the patients show photosensitivity of the skin that is due to a defect in NER.

The term *trichothiodystrophy* was introduced by Price in 1979.[14] The clinical hallmark of TTD is sulfur-deficient brittle hair, which is due to a reduced content of a class of matrix hair proteins that provide the hair shaft with its natural strength by crosslinking the keratin filaments. With polarizing light microscopy, a typical tiger tail pattern of the hair is visible. On scanning electron microscopy, the hair is flattened and irregular with longitudinal ridging and often somewhat twisted along the axis. Frequently, fractures are apparent, and the viscoelastic parameters of hair are different from controls.[15] The amino acid composition of the hair proteins is dramatically changed, with a strong reduction in cysteine and to a lesser extent proline, threonine, and serine residues and a concomitant relative increase in aspartic acid, methionine, phenylalanine, alanine, leucine, and lysine.[16] This is due to the strong reduction or complete absence of the class of ultra-high sulfur-rich matrix proteins, up to 30 percent of which are composed of cysteine residues that are involved in disulfide crosslinks. In addition, nails are dystrophic. Cutaneous signs include photosensitivity, ichthyosis, keratosis, erythema, and collodion baby. In many cases the brittle hair is associated with a heterogeneous complex of neuroectodermal abnormalities. Neurologic and developmental impairments within TTD are reminiscent of those found in CS. In a few cases, calcification of basal ganglia and dysmyelination[17–19] have been reported, as has been observed in CS (Table 28-3). Clinical manifestations and their severity vary extensively between TTD individuals. The broad spectrum of symptoms partly explains the confusing nomenclature in the literature for (probably) the same disease.[20,21] *PIBIDS* is an acronym for a specific combination of symptoms: photosensitivity, ichthyosis, brittle hair and nails, impaired intelligence, decreased fertility, and short stature. TTD also encompasses IBIDS, BIDS, and SIBIDS (osteosclerosis and IBIDS). Several other names have been used to describe patients in whom a number of the preceding features are present in combination with brittle hair: Pollitt, Tay, Amish brittle hair, Sabinas, and Marinesco-Sjögren syndromes and ONMR (onychotrichodysplasia, neutropenia, mental retardation). These patients, whether they have TTD or not, do not show photosensitivity and probably do not have a DNA repair defect. A practical classification scheme, based on a checklist of clinical abnormalities associated with TTD, is proposed by Tolmie et al.[19] and may be helpful in diagnosis of TTD patients.

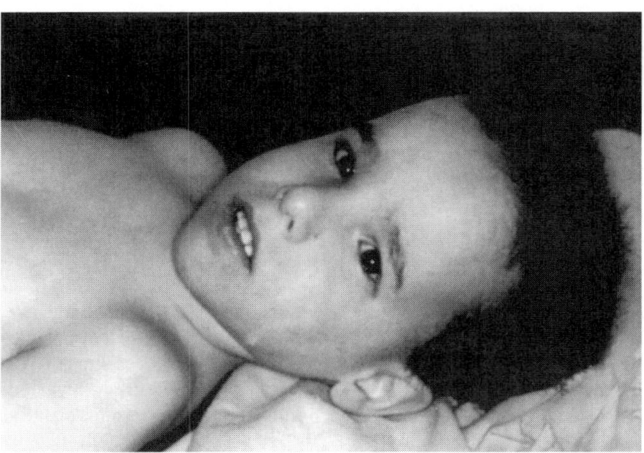

Fig. 28-4 Patient with TTD. Note the brittle hair as one of the crucial features of TTD. (*Photograph kindly provided by A. Sarasin, CNRS, Villejuif, France, and C. Blanchet-Bardon, Hopital Saint-Louis, Paris. From Lehmann.*[13] *Used by permission.*)

Table 28-3 Main Clinical Symptoms of NER Syndromes

Clinical Symptoms	XP	XP-CS	CS	TTD
Photosensitivity	++	++	+*	+*
Abnormal pigmentation	++	+	−	−
Skin cancer	++	+	−	−
Progressive mental degeneration	−/+†	+	+	+
Neuronal loss	−/+†	−	−	−
Neurodysmyelination	−	++	+	+
Wizened facies	−	+	+	+
Growth defect	+/−†	+	+	+
Hypogonadism	−/+	+	+	+
Brittle hair and nails	−	−	−	+
Ichthyosis	−	−	−	+

*Also TTD and CS patients occur without photosensitivity and NER defect.
†These neurologic and growth defects are characteristic features of XP patients with the DeSanctis-Cacchione syndrome.

A TTD patient has been described who lost his hair during an episode of pneumonia.[22] Within a period of a few months, the scalp hair returned. This peculiar phenomenon of hair loss after fever may be indicative of a thermosensitive mutation in the gene responsible for the disorder in these patients (see below).

Xeroderma Pigmentosum-Cockayne Syndrome Complex

A number of patients have been identified with clinical features of both XP and CS.[23–25] These patients had the cutaneous pigmentary and, in most cases, neoplastic features of XP along with the dwarfism, mental retardation, increased reflexes, and retinal degeneration typical of CS. They may correspond with the severe form of CS (CSII).

BIOCHEMICAL AND CELLULAR ASPECTS OF XP, CS, AND TTD

Production of Cellular Damage by Sunlight

Sunlight is the major environmental agent that is involved in many of the clinical symptoms of XP; it does so by damaging cutaneous cells. Understanding the biochemical defects in XP requires knowledge of the way the damaging wavelengths in sunlight are absorbed by macromolecules and the nature of the damage that is produced.

The wavelengths of sunlight reaching the surface of the earth extend into the near-UV region, the shortest detectable being about 290 nm. Shorter-wavelength UV (present in solar radiation in space) is blocked from reaching the ground by ozone and other components of the atmosphere. This lower limit slightly overlaps the upper region of the absorption spectra of nucleic acids and proteins. Energy in this region of overlap is absorbed by macromolecules in the skin, producing harmful effects that include erythema, burns, and actinic carcinogenesis.[26–28] Comparisons between direct sunlight and short-wavelength UV light (254 nm) indicate that sunlight in the midwestern United States is equivalent in germicidal activity to about 0.1 to 0.2 J/m^2 of surface per minute (J/m^{2}min) of 254-nm UV light.[6,] Since normal human cells in culture have a D_{37}* of only about 3 to 5 J/m^2 of radiation at 254 nm, the direct exposure of human proliferating cells to sunlight can result in significant amounts of cell killing.

Radiation at the UV end of the sun's spectrum produces its biologic effects through absorption of quanta in molecules that have unsaturated chemical bonds, such as aromatic amino acids in proteins and purine and pyrimidine components of DNA and RNA. The action spectra for production of DNA damage (pyrimidine photoproducts), cell killing, production of aberrant chromosomes, and induction of unscheduled DNA repair synthesis (i.e., DNA synthesis not associated with the normal cell cycle; see below) are all similar, exhibiting maximum efficiency in wavelengths from 260 to 280 nm. Although there is negligible energy in this region of the sun's spectrum, there is sufficient overlap of the shortest end of the sun's spectrum with the longer-wavelength side of the absorption spectrum of DNA for significant photochemical reaction to occur. Shorter-wavelength UV is absorbed by the outer, nondividing layers of skin cells. An action spectrum of production of DNA damage in human skin shows a peak at about 302 nm.[6]

Two kinds of pyrimidine photoproducts are the most relevant type of damage induced in DNA by absorption of UV light. The most frequent is the cyclobutane pyrimidine dimer (Fig. 28-5). This is formed between adjacent pyrimidines in the same strand of DNA by the formation of two bonds between the 5 positions and between the 6 positions on the pyrimidine rings. An alternative dipyrimidine photoproduct is the [6-4]pyrimidine-pyrimidone product, mainly consisting of 5′TC or 5′CC (see Fig. 28-5), which is formed at lower rates than the cyclobutane dimer but is also important biologically. Various estimates suggest that the [6-4] photoproduct is formed at 10 to 50 percent of the frequency of cyclobutane dimers by low doses of 254-nm light. Numerous biologic effects, such as cell killing, production of chromosome aberrations, mutagenesis, and carcinogenesis, can be attributed to these photoproducts in DNA. Other photoproducts have biologic effects in some circumstances. These include the unstable cytosine

*The D_{37} is the dose required to reduce survival to 0.37 from the initial value of 1.0 and in target theory corresponds to the dose required to produce an average of one lethal hit on the sensitive target of an irradiated organism when the survival curve is exponential.

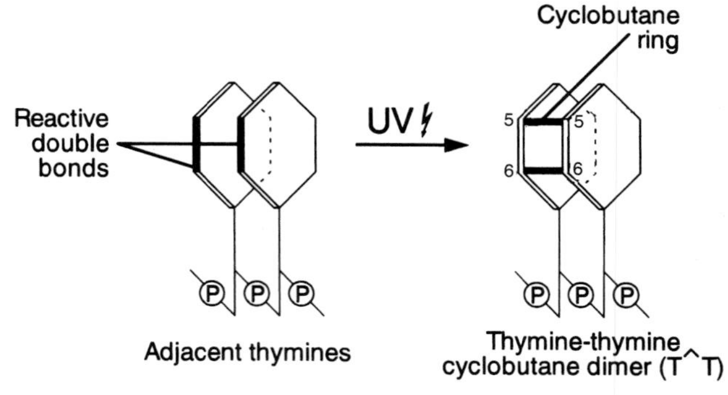

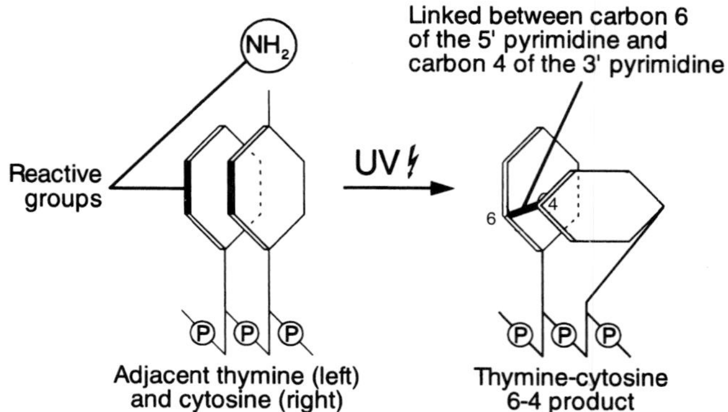

Fig. 28-5 Main UV-induced DNA lesions. ***Top***: **The cyclobutane pyrimidine dimer between adjacent thymines on the same strand of DNA.** ***Bottom***: **[6-4] photoproduct between adjacent thymine and cytosine on same strand of DNA. Particularly the latter results in considerable distortion of the phosphodiester backbone of DNA.**

hydrate, purine photoproducts, and at relatively high doses, locally denatured regions, DNA-protein crosslinks, and single-strand breaks.

Repair of Sunlight-Induced DNA Damage

At least three different biochemical repair systems operate in sunlight-exposed cells to safeguard DNA from permanent damage. These are excision repair, postreplication repair (which is more like a damage-tolerance mechanism), and photoreactivation. These systems have been found in bacteria, yeast, amphibians, fish, rodents, marsupials, and mammals. They are especially important in the skin, where they mend damage to DNA caused by UV light. Some of the repair systems also can mend damage to DNA caused by chemical carcinogens. These systems presumably protect internal tissues against the carcinogenic and mutagenic consequences of exposure to chemicals that damage DNA.

Excision repair is extremely versatile and can mend a large variety of UV light, x-ray, and chemically induced forms of damage to DNA.[6,29] Excision repair may be subdivided into NER and base excision repair (BER). The NER system, which will be discussed in the next section, excises damaged single strands of DNA and replaces them with a new sequence of bases, using as a template for base pairing the intact strand of DNA opposite the original damaged site. BER removes damaged bases, leaving the sugar-phosphate backbone of the DNA intact and creating an AP (apurinic or apyrimidinic) site. This site is subsequently converted into a strand break and repaired by short-patch repair of usually one or a few nucleotides.

Postreplication repair is not a damage-repair pathway per se but a damage-tolerance mechanism that solves the problem the replication machinery faces when it encounters a damage in the template. This poorly defined process has been studied best in *S.*

cerevisiae, where two subpathways have been distinguished.[30] The first is reinitiation of DNA replication at a more downstream location, leaving a gap opposite the lesion. After replication of the complementary strand, the newly copied information is used to fill in the gap in the other strand by recombination. This pathway is in principle error-free. The second subpathway induces translesion DNA replication. However, this process is error-prone and may be the main determinant of all damage-induced mutations. Very little is known about this pathway in mammals, and it is not sure whether it follows the same principal steps in higher species.

The third repair system, photoreactivation, simply reverts the damaged DNA to the normal chemical state without removing or exchanging any material from the DNA. This is accomplished by a single protein, photolyase, carrying two blue-light–harvesting chromophore cofactors that provide the energy for disrupting the dipyrimidine bonds. The photoreactivation system was thought to be specific for one form of damage induced by UV light — the cyclobutane pyrimidine dimer. A [6-4] photoproduct — specific photolyase was observed in *Drosophila* and various other organisms (*Xenopus,* plants) pointing to a widespread occurrence.[31] CPD-photoreactivation has been demonstrated in bacteria, yeast, fish, amphibians, and marsupials, but the existence and importance of this system in human tissue are still controversial.[6] Interestingly, two human genes were identified in the sequence data-base with significant overall homology to the *Drosophila* [6-4]-photolyase but even more to blue-light receptors in plants[31,32] that carry out a variety of blue-light–sensing functions. This renders it unlikely that the human genes are involved in DNA repair.

The NER System

NER is one of the major and most versatile repair mechanisms that operates in the cell. This universal system eliminates a remarkably diverse array of structurally unrelated lesions that range from UV-induced photoproducts (cyclobutane pyrimidine dimers and [6-4] photoproducts) to bulky and small chemical adducts as well as interstrand crosslinks. Thus it is not surprising that the NER process entails multiple steps and involves the concerted action of a number of proteins. The details of this repair mechanism are best understood in the case of the UvrABC system in the bacterium *E. coli.*[33–36] Briefly, at least six distinct steps can be discerned: (1) lesion recognition and (2) lesion demarcation, which involves conformational changes in DNA, are carried out by the UvrA2B complex. (3) A complex of UvrB and UvrC incises the damaged strand on both sides of the lesion at some distance, leaving the nondamaged strand intact. (4) The damage-containing oligomer is removed by the helicase action of UvrD, followed by (5) gap-filling DNA synthesis by DNA polymerase I. The process is completed by (6) the sealing of the new DNA to the preexisting strand by DNA ligase. In principle, this mode of repair is error-free because it uses the nucleotide sequence information of the intact complementary DNA strand.

Although in outline and in concept quite simple, it is becoming increasingly apparent that the scheme of the NER repair mechanism as depicted above for *E. coli* represents a dramatic oversimplification, particularly when extrapolated to eukaryotes. This notion is based on a number of observations.

First, a minimum of two in-part overlapping NER subpathways have been discovered; these are represented schematically in Fig. 28-6. One subpathway, here referred to as *transcription-coupled repair (TCR),* deals with the complication that the vital process of transcription is blocked by lesions in the template. To cope with this urgent problem, TCR takes care for the complete elimination of injury in the transcribed strand of active structural genes.[37,38] This holds particularly for lesions for which repair otherwise would be too slow or inefficient. In this specialized NER subpathway, initial damage detection is thought to be carried out by RNA polymerase II, when it is blocked in front of a lesion. As part of the repair mechanism, the stalled RNA polymerase complex has to be displaced to give the repair machinery access to the injury. The process occurs in *E. coli* and eukaryotes. Another branch of the NER system — here designated *global genome repair (GGR)* — accomplishes removal of lesions in the entire genome. Damage recognition in this repair system is performed by a specific NER protein (complex) and is for many lesions (e.g., CPD lesions) — but not all (e.g., [6-4] photoproducts) — more slow and less efficient when compared with TCR. The efficiency of damage recognition by the GGR system varies strongly from lesion to lesion and also may vary with the chromatin conformation, the location in the genome, and the state of differentiation of the cell. This is not so surprising when one realizes the tremendous task that is faced by this system in continually surveilling the 2 m of DNA double helix in every mammalian nucleus for trace amounts of a diversity of lesions.

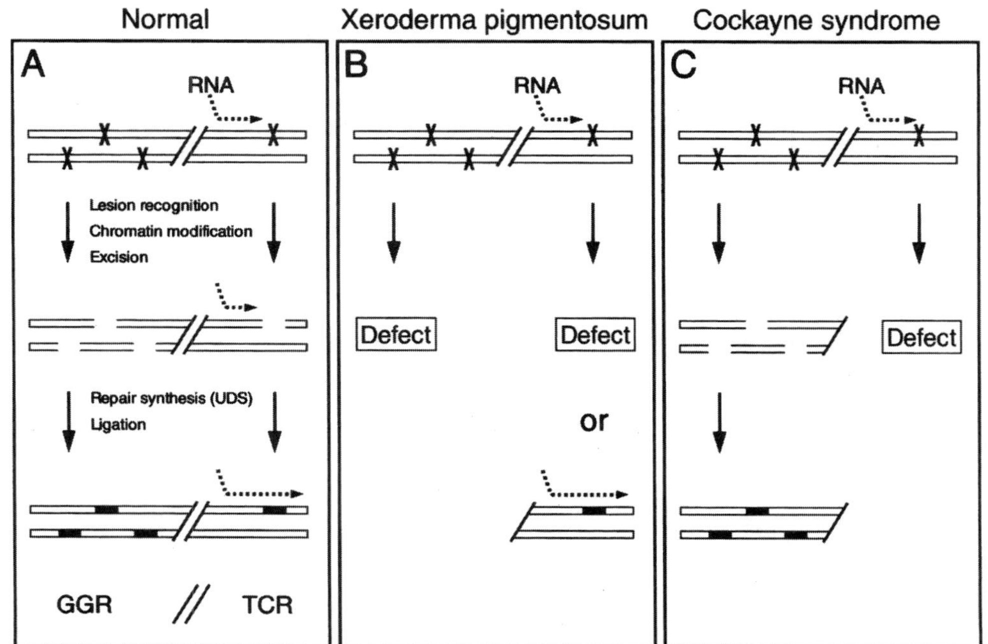

Fig. 28-6 NER pathways and defects in XP and CS. This simplified scheme shows in the left panel (normal cells) the transcription-coupled repair (TCR) pathway (*at right*) that mends lesions in the transcribed strand of active genes, and the global genome repair (GGR) pathway (*at left*) that deals with lesions in the remaining part of the genome. In XP (*center panel*), the genetic defect in most cases affects both mechanisms; in XP complementation group C, only GGR is impaired. In CS (*right panel*) the defect is opposite XP-C; only TCR is deficient.

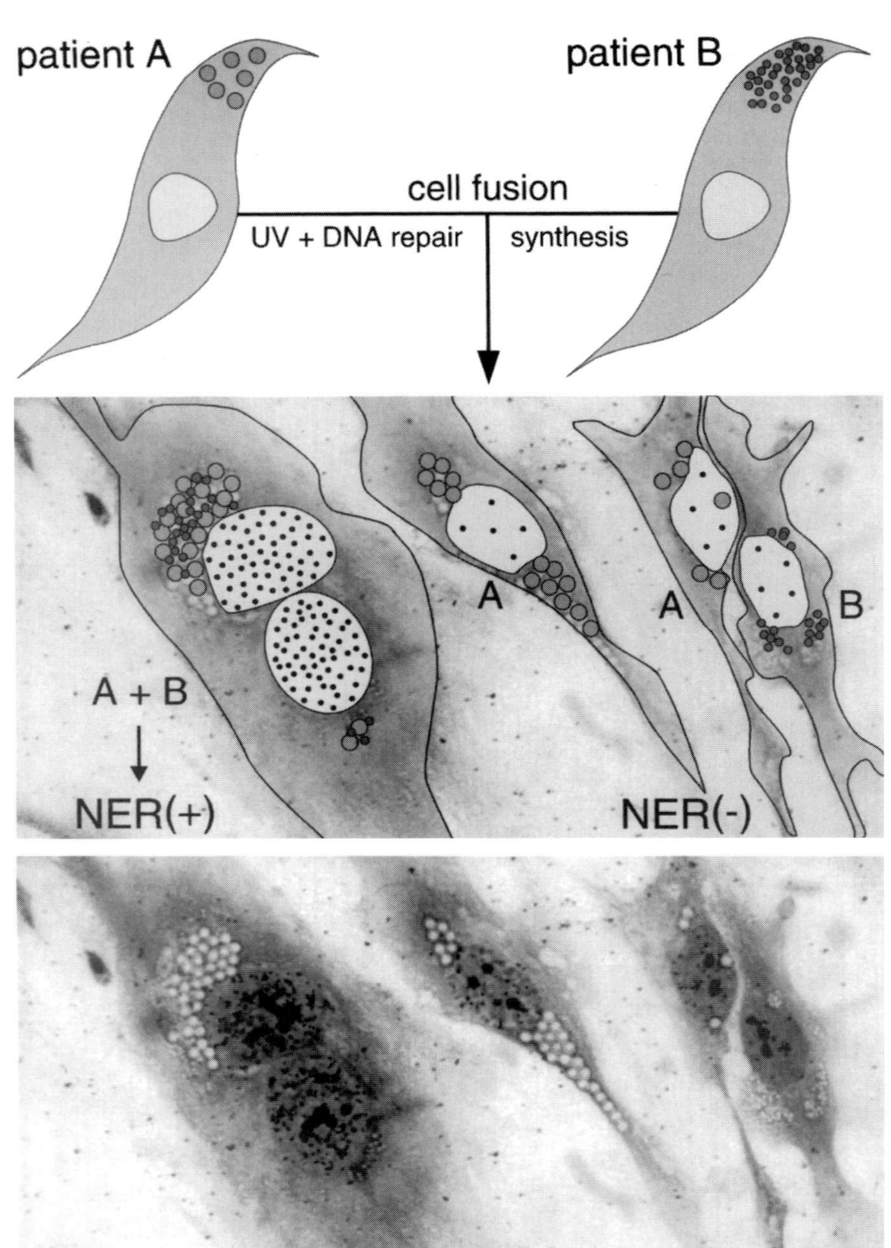

Fig. 28-7 Genetic heterogeneity in XP studied by cell fusion and UV-induced unscheduled DNA synthesis (UDS). ***Top*****: A schematic representation of the micrograph presented at the bottom. Cultured fibroblasts from two unrelated patients (A and B) were fused, exposed to UV light, pulse labeled with [^{3}H]thymidine, fixed, and autoradiographed to visualize DNA repair synthesis (UDS). Cells of patient A are marked with engulfed large latex beads and those of patient B with small beads. This marking enables the identification of the fused cells containing nuclei of both patients (heterokaryons). If the patients are mutated in different DNA repair genes (gene *A* and gene *B*), the heterokaryon will be able to perform normal levels of DNA repair synthesis (UDS is visualized by wild-type levels of autoradiographic grains in the emulsion above the nuclei). In this case patients A and B belong to two different complementation groups. (*From the Department of Cell Biology and Genetics, Erasmus University, Rotterdam, W. Vermeulen and D. Bootsma.*)**

NER is visualized under the microscope by the unscheduled DNA synthesis (UDS) test. Cultured fibroblasts are exposed to UV and briefly (2-3 h) incubated in [^{3}H]thymidine-containing medium. Cells in G1 or G2 phase of the cell cycle become radioactively labeled by the gap-filling DNA-synthesis step of the NER process. Following autoradiography, the repair capacity of these cells can be quantified at the single-cell level. The UDS test has proven to be a powerful tool to measure NER in repair-proficient and -deficient cells (see Figs. 28-7 and 28-11).

NER Activity in XP, CS, and TTD Cells

Defective DNA excision repair in UV-irradiated skin fibroblasts from some XP patients was reported for the first time by Cleaver in 1968[39] and in skin in vivo by Epstein et al.[40] The NER defect in TTD cells was first reported by Stefanini et al.[41] The defect in most XP and TTD cells is reflected by decreased levels of UDS (Fig. 28-7). Measurement of UV-induced UDS is in fact required for a definitive diagnosis of NER-deficient XP and TTD. Different levels of UDS in unrelated XP patients suggested heterogeneity at the molecular level in this syndrome.[42] A number of XP patients have shown a normal response in the UDS test. They have been designated as *XP variants*[43] and were found to have a defect in the ill-defined postreplication repair process.[44] Similarly, various degrees of NER deficiency have been demonstrated among TTD patients, including normal DNA repair in approximately half of patients.[49]

UDS in CS cells is not significantly different from that in normal cells. However, by measuring NER separately in transcribed and nontranscribed strands of specific genes, a technique developed by the group of Hanawalt,[45] Venema et al.[46] have demonstrated deficient repair of the transcribed strand of active genes in CS cells (see Fig. 28-6). The less efficient GGR is still functional. Since TCR makes a relatively small contribution to the total repair synthesis, CS fibroblasts show near-normal levels of UDS. The TCR defect prevents the rapid recovery of RNA synthesis after UV exposure. This delayed recovery of

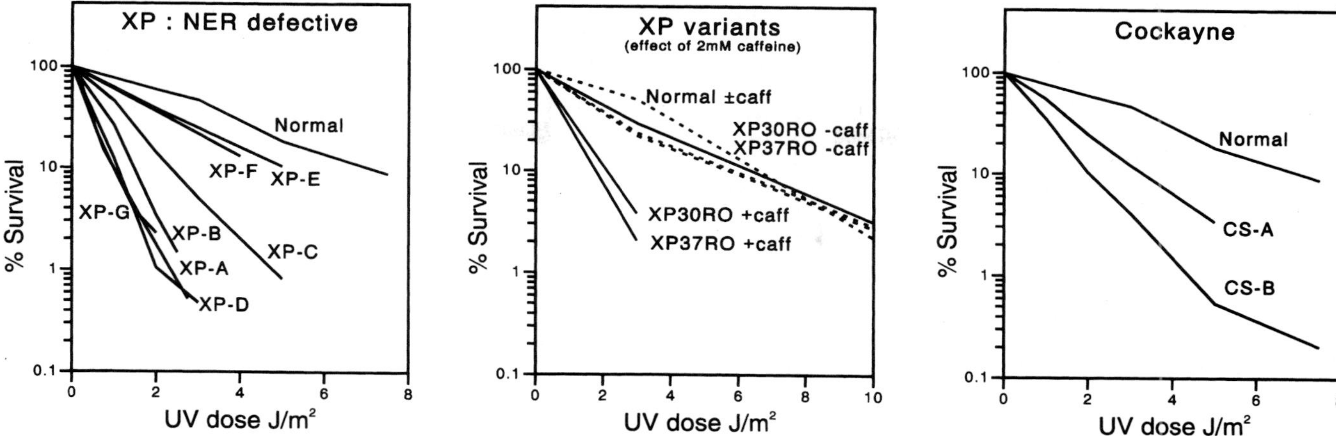

Fig. 28-8 UV-sensitivity of XP and CS cells. (*Left*) XP cells of different complementation groups. (*Center*) XP-variant cells in the presence and absence of caffeine. Caffeine sensitizes XP-variant cells to UV. (*Right*) CS cells. (*From the Department of Cell Biology and Genetics: Raams, Jaspers, and Hoeijmakers.*)

RNA synthesis and also of S-phase DNA synthesis in CS cells following UV exposure is used as a diagnostic criterion of CS[25,47,48] in combination with clinical symptoms.

Colony-Forming Ability of XP, CS, and TTD Cells

The number of cells in culture that can grow into colonies after UV irradiation can be used as an in vitro measurement of sensitivity. Heterogeneity in the response of fibroblasts of unrelated XP patients is evident (Fig. 28-8, left panel). In all cases, NER-deficient XP fibroblasts are more sensitive than normal cells, and those from patients who exhibit neurologic abnormalities are generally the most sensitive.[10]

XP cells are also more sensitive to carcinogenic chemicals creating bulky DNA adducts (including benz[a]pyrene) but are normal in response to DNA methylating agents and, with a few exceptions, to x-rays.[6]

Fibroblasts of XP-variants do not exhibit a significant increase of UV-sensitivity under standard test conditions. A dramatic increase in sensitivity becomes apparent if XP-variant cells are incubated in the presence of caffeine after UV exposure (see Fig. 28-8, middle panel). This effect of caffeine on UV-sensitivity may be used as a diagnostic test that is specific for the XP-variant type and much simpler than the demonstration of a defective post-replication repair.

The delayed recovery of RNA synthesis as a result of the TCR defect in CS cells probably causes the increased sensitivity in CS cells (see Fig. 28-8, right panel). An increasing number of patients have been diagnosed as probable CS cases who do not show photosensitivity.[12] Fibroblasts of these patients do not display increased sensitivity in the colony-formation test. Similar patterns of UV sensitivity are observed with fibroblast cultures of photosensitive and non-photosensitive TTD patients.[49] These non-photosensitive CS and TTD fibroblasts also behave like normal cells in UDS and in DNA- and RNA-synthesis recovery tests. These results suggest that these patients do not have a DNA repair defect and that their clinical symptoms have another cause. (For an explanation, see "Implications for Diagnosis" below.)

CS cells are also sensitive to UV-mimetic carcinogens such as 4NQO and *N*-acetoxy-*N*-2-acetyl-2-aminofluorene but not to monofunctional alkylating agents.[50]

Mutational Events in XP, CS, and TTD Cells

Cultured cells from most XP and CS patients have a normal karyotype. Distinctive spontaneous karyotypic changes characteristic for some diseases with a high cancer incidence, such as ataxia telangiectasia, Fanconi anemia, and Bloom syndrome,[21] are not seen in XP patients.

XP cells show a normal frequency of spontaneous sister chromatid exchanges (SCEs) but a greater than normal frequency after exposure to UV light and most chemical carcinogens.[6] Similarly, XP cells show more chromosome aberrations than normal cells after exposure to UV light and chemical carcinogens.[6]

The frequency with which cells resistant to 6-thioguanine, ouabain, diphtheria toxin, or other toxic chemicals are produced by irradiation with UV light or artificial sunlight or by exposure to chemical carcinogens is greater in all XP cells, including XP-variants, than in normal cells.[6] This implies that the genetic defects in XP cells confer increased mutability. In the XP-variant, the repair system has lost fidelity and so produces a high frequency of mutations. Evidence has been presented for increased transformation to anchorage independence (growth in suspension instead of attached to the bottom of a culture disk, which is considered to represent a step in the direction of neoplastic transformation) after UV irradiation of XP-variant cells compared with normal cells.[51]

Shuttle vector plasmids that are capable of autonomous replication in both mammalian cells and *E. coli* have been used for measuring the frequency and spectrum of mutations following exposure of transfected cells to DNA damage.[6] There were significantly fewer plasmids with tandem or multiple base substitution mutations or with single or tandem transversion mutations after transfection of UV-damaged plasmids in XP cells than in normal cells. With all cell lines, the predominant base substitution mutation was the G-C to A-T transition; i.e., the C mutated to a T. Thus, with these human cells, the major UV photoproduct, the TT cyclobutane dimer, is not the major premutagenic lesion. This finding is consistent with the A rule: a tendency of polymerases to insert adenines opposite noninstructional lesions. Thus insertion of A opposite TT dimers results in the correct pairing, whereas insertion of A opposite a C, involved in cyclobutane dimers and [6-4] photoproducts (see Fig. 28-5), results in G-C to A-T transitions.

UV-damaged viruses and plasmids also have been used as substrates to measure the capacity of NER-deficient cells to repair DNA damage by monitoring the extent of their biologic recovery, e.g., by their ability to propagate in bacterial hosts.[6] The extent of this host-cell reactivation by various cell types often parallels the ability to survive UV damage. Host-cell reactivation assays employing UV-damaged plasmids treated in vitro with CPD-photolyase (which selectively removes cyclobutane dimers) have been used to study repair of different types of photoproducts. While XP-A cells show poor repair of all types of photoproducts, CS cells have faulty repair of cyclobutane dimers but normal repair of non-dimer photoproducts.[52,53]

GENETIC ASPECTS OF XP, CS, AND TTD

Complementation Analysis of NER Deficiency Syndromes

The clinical heterogeneity in XP and the marked differences in cellular expression of the NER defect in terms of unscheduled DNA synthesis in different patients[42] were studied by using a cell fusion assay to investigate genetic heterogeneity in XP.[54] Heterokaryons formed between fibroblasts of different XP patients exposed to UV light either showed normal or nearly normal levels of UDS (i.e., patients complement each other's defects and therefore belong to different complementation groups; see Fig. 28-7) or exhibited the impaired levels of UDS seen in the unfused XP cells (i.e., patients are in the same complementation group). Each complementation group may represent a gene that, if mutated and in homozygous condition, causes XP (intergenic complementation).

A total of seven complementation groups have been identified in NER-deficient XP.[6] In comparison, at least 15 distinct genes involved in NER (the *RAD3* epistasis group) have been identified in *S. cerevisiae*. This difference is probably due to incompatibility of some defects with normal embryonic development.

By using the RNA-synthesis recovery test in cell fusion studies, the patients with CS (in its classic form, without XP features and/or without GGR deficiency) could be assigned to two complementation groups: CS-A and CS-B.[47,55]

The rare patients having the XP-CS complex were found to be members of complementation groups XP-B, -D, and -G.[24] There is also genetic overlap between XP and TTD, although the clinical features are very different. Almost all UV-sensitive TTD patients fall into the XP-D group.[49] Recently, one TTD family was found to belong to XP-B,[56] and a third kindred constitutes a distinct NER-deficient complementation group, TTD-A[41] not (yet) associated with XP.

Thus both genetic heterogeneity within and genetic overlap between all NER disorders is found. A specific subset of XP groups (notably XP-D and XP-B) is associated with extreme variability ranging from XP to CS to TTD. Therefore, these disorders may in fact be considered different manifestations of one heterogeneous clinical continuum.

Characteristics of Complementation Groups

Some of the properties of the XP and TTD complementation groups are summarized in Table 28-4.

XP Group A. Group A usually corresponds to the most severe clinical form of XP, in which there are both skin symptoms and central nervous system (CNS) disorders. Many patients exhibit manifestations from birth or early in life and correspond to the clinical category of the DeSanctis-Cacchione syndrome with progressive neurologic degeneration.[6]

Excision repair is generally very low (< 2 percent of normal) in cells of most XP-A patients, and they are about 10 times more sensitive than normal to killing by UV irradiation or other UV-mimicking carcinogens (see Fig. 28-8). The genetic defect in this group interferes with both TCR and GGR.

There are exceptions to these general characteristics of group A cells. Cells from a British patient without CNS disorders (XP8LO) exhibited about 30 percent of normal cellular excision repair and higher survival after UV than other group A cells.[6] A 35-year-old Egyptian male (XP13CA) had the typical low level of unscheduled synthesis but was neurologically normal, had normal stature, and was fertile. Two other group A patients (XP12BE and XP1LO) also show milder neurologic abnormalities, whereas their cells are less UV sensitive than the majority in group A.[6] In one Italian family, group A siblings exhibited different clinical symptoms; only one had CNS signs.[6] In cell cultures, it appeared that the sibling without CNS disorder had, on average, higher repair due to a subpopulation of cells with normal repair mixed with typical group A cells. Therefore, although group A patients usually have the associated neurologic abnormalities of the DeSanctis-Cacchione syndrome, several are known who are neurologically normal or have less severe neurologic abnormalities.

XP Group B. For many years XP group B consisted only of 1 patient (XP11BE)[23] (Fig. 28-9). This patient died of acute hypertension at age 33. She had small stature, deafness, mental retardation, immature sexual development, premature senility, absence of subcutaneous fat, and optic nerve and retinal pigment degeneration characteristic of CS. She exhibited acute sun sensitivity, ocular changes, and multiple cutaneous malignancy at age 18, all typical of XP.

Two siblings (XP1BA and XP2BA) with mild features of XP and CS were recently assigned to XP-B.[58] Developmental abnormalities are nearly absent in these individuals, and neurologic symptoms became evident only after the second decade of life.[59]

A remarkable clinical variation is observed between these two XP-B families. The two siblings do not display any cutaneous malignancies despite a relatively advanced age for XP of more than 40 years, whereas patient XP11BE had skin tumors at 18

Table 28-4 Properties of XP, CS, and TTD Complementation Groups

Complementation Group	UV sensitivity	Residual UDS*	NER Activity TCR†	NER Activity GGR‡	Relative Frequency§	Skin Cancer	Neurologic Abnormalities	Clinical Phenotype
XP-A	+++	< 5%	–	–	High	+	++	XP
XP-B	++	3–40%	–	–	3 families	+/–	++/+	XP/CS or TTD
XP-C	+	15–30%	+	–	High	+	–	XP
XP-D	++	15–50%	–	–	Intermediate	+/–	++/–	XP, XP/CS or TTD
XP-E	±	50%	?	?	Rare	+/–	–	XP
XP-F	+	15–30%	–	–	Rare	+/–	–/±	XP
XP-G	++	< 5–25%	–	–	Rare	+/–	++/+	XP or XP/CS
TTD-A	+	10%	–	–	1 family	–	+	TTD
CS-A	+	Normal range	–	+	Intermediate	–	++	CS
CS-B	+	Normal range	–	+	High	–	++	CS
XP-V¶	+/±	Normal range	+	+	High	+/–	–	XP

*Unscheduled DNA synthesis, expressed as percentage of repair synthesis in normal cells.
†Transcription coupled repair.
‡Global genome repair.
§The overall frequency of XP is between 10^{-5} to 10^{-6}; less than 500 cases have been classified.
¶XP-variant, defect in post-replication repair, proficient NER.

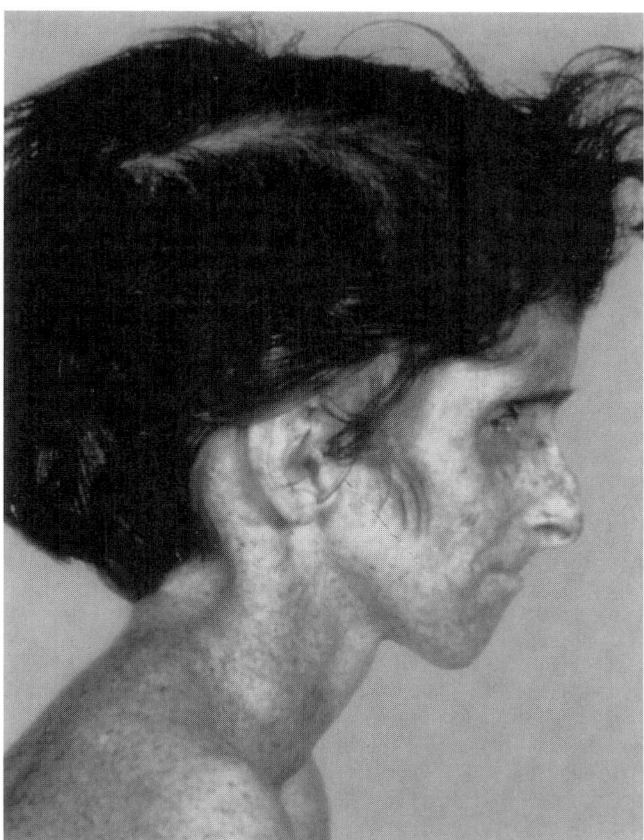

Fig. 28-9 XP patient (XP11BE). This patient, 28 years old, from complementation group B, exhibits skin, ocular, and neurologic characteristics that have been ascribed to both XP and CS. (*From Kraemer.*[57] *Used by permission.*)

years. Nevertheless, the level of UDS representing the repair defect is similar in both families (5–10 percent of NER-proficient cells) and affects both TCR and GGR. A new Slovenian 28 year-old patient with XP and CS features was assigned to this group, having the same residual UDS level (Bohnert, Jaspers, and Bootsma, unpublished observations).

The assignment to XP-B of two siblings (TTD4VI and TTD6VI) with relatively mild clinical features of TTD and moderately impaired NER characteristics (about 40 percent UDS)[56] extends the clinical heterogeneity within this complementation group.

XP Group C. Group C is one of the largest groups and is often referred to as the classic form of XP. The patients usually show only skin and eye disorders. These vary considerably in severity, depending on sun exposure. Patients of over 80 years of age have been diagnosed. Tumors of the tip of the tongue have been observed in several patients. A case of XP-C is presented in Fig. 28-2. The level of UDS varies between 15 and 30 percent of normal, and XP-C cells are less sensitive to killing by UV light and chemical carcinogens than cells from groups A and D (see Fig. 28-8). One characteristic of repair unique to this group is that the repair sites are clustered rather than random[60] due to a selective loss in the capacity to perform GGR in the presence of normal levels of TCR.[61] In this respect, this defect is opposite to the deficiency in the classic form of CS[46] (see Fig. 28-6).

One exceptional patient (XP1MI) exhibited symptoms of XP, systemic lupus erythematosus, microcephaly, and a marginal degree of mental retardation.[62] Cells from this patient had DNA repair levels typical for XP-C but were the most UV-sensitive in group C.[11] Two reported instances of CNS tumors in XP patients — XP106LO and Hawaiian patient XP15BE — are in this group.[6]

XP Group D. This is a very interesting group because of the extensive clinical heterogeneity. Many XP-D patients have skin and neurologic abnormalities like those in group A, although the onset of the CNS disorders may be delayed until the second decade. Patients with a very mild photosensitivity also were found in this group (Jaspers and Bootsma, unpublished observations). In addition to these classic XP patients, almost all the photosensitive TTD patients have been assigned to this complementation group.[49,63] So far no reports on the occurrence of skin cancer within this group of XP-D TTD patients have appeared. Furthermore, five patients with the combined XP-CS complex of varying severity were found to belong to XP group D[6] (Jaspers and Bootsma, unpublished observations). Thus XP-D is a complex group involving diverse clinical syndromes.[64] GGR, measured as UDS, varies from 15 to over 70 percent, with no clear correlation with the clinical severity or type of symptoms. Some evidence suggests that the amount of UDS in the XP and XP-CS cases is higher than expected from the low amount of dimer excision observed in these cells and their sensitivity to cell killing (comparable with XP-A cells; see Fig. 28-8). This is perhaps due to better repair of [6-4] photoproducts in these cells.[6]

XP Group E. Patients in the rare group E exhibit mild skin symptoms and are neurologically normal.[23] The level of excision repair is high (>50 percent of normal), and the level relative to normal cells increases with increasing UV dose. The cells are only slightly more sensitive than normal to UV damage (see Fig. 28-8). Patients have been reported from Europe and Japan. One XP-E patient (XP2RO) died from metastatic tumor of endothelial origin.

XP Group F. Most representatives of group F have been described in Japan.[65] The patients had acute sun sensitivity in infancy but relatively mild symptoms with late onset of skin cancer despite a substantially reduced level of repair. Two patients have been reported with neurologic deficits late in life. Excision repair was 15 to 30 percent of normal but increased to 60 percent with incubation and appears long-lasting. The cells seem to be more defective in repair of damage that occurs at rapid rates and at early times after irradiation such as [6-4] photoproducts.[6] They show an intermediate sensitivity to killing by UV light and a high degree of excision of pyrimidine dimers when measured at late times after irradiation. There was a marked enhancement of UV survival when cells were held in a density-inhibited condition after irradiation.[66]

XP Group G. Until 1996 this rare group comprised only eight patients, all from Europe and Japan,[24,67] but since then, at least seven additional patients have been identified from all continents (Jaspers and Bootsma, unpublished observations). The clinical symptoms vary from mild cutaneous and no neurologic abnormalities to severe dermatologic and neurologic impairment characteristic of XP. So far a skin tumor was reported in only one patient from Japan (XP31KO), which appeared at a relatively late age. UDS and survival levels are usually very low, but significant residual activity was observed in a few (e.g., XP31KO, 25 percent UDS). A rapidly growing subset of patients with very low UDS levels (2 percent or less) displays severe symptoms of CS already at birth; very often XP features do not become manifest (presumably due to continuous hospitalization and early demise). Occasionally, these infants were first thought to have a related disorder such as cerebro-oculofacial syndrome (COFS). The category of XP-CS patients is now in the majority within XP group G, but this may well represent a selection bias over the more standard XP patients, who are genetically scrutinized to a lesser extent. Interestingly, cells from some patients with either XP or XP-CS showed mild cellular hypersensitivity to ionizing radiation and/or hydrogen peroxide.[67,68] This sensitivity, pointing to a possible deficiency in the repair of oxidative radical damage, was suggested (at least partially) to underlie the severe clinical phenotypes in XP-G.[68,69]

XP-Variant. Patients in the variant group have mild to severe skin symptoms and usually have normal CNS functions. The variant form is found worldwide and is a frequently occurring and distinct group, even though it cannot often be identified clinically without cell culture studies. Originally defined as a clinically recognized XP without a defect in excision repair,[23,43] it also was described earlier under the clinical designation *pigmented xerodermoid.*[70] With careful clinical investigation, some patients in this group may be recognized by relatively mild symptoms and the absence of an enhanced erythematous response, but this is insufficient for unambiguous diagnosis, and other XP-variant patients may have severe clinical symptoms.[23]

The high level of mutagenesis with near-normal levels of cell survival after UV irradiation could be interpreted as an indication that the inherited disorder has made XP-variant cells error-prone.[6] The outstanding feature of this form of XP is that after UV irradiation, replication forks appear to stop or to be interrupted during semi-conservative replication at every site of DNA damage.[44] This is interpreted as a defect in postreplication repair.

Whether the variant group is homogeneous or has multiple subgroups is not known, but the clinical heterogeneity is suggestive. The pigmented xerodermoid family of Jung et al.,[70] although biochemically identical to other XP-variants, is unusual because no clinical symptoms were evident until after age 40, and patients lived into their eighties. These mild symptoms contrast with other variant families from comparable environments in whom the disease is quite severe.[6] One attempt at studying complementation between cells from different XP-variant patients indicated a single XP-variant group.[71]

TTD Group A. The cells of one TTD patient (TTD1BR) complemented cells from all seven XP complementation groups and apparently represents a third TTD complementation group (TTD-A) in addition to XP-B and XP-D.[41] This patient, first described in 1982,[72] has typical symptoms of TTD and has been sensitive to sunlight since early childhood. His clinical features are quite distinct from those associated with XP, showing no significant freckling or other pigmentary changes and no skin tumors.[41]

CS Complementation Groups. Complementation analysis has disclosed two groups in the classic form of CS: CS-A and CS-B. CS is clinically heterogeneous. The clinical differentiation among CS individuals, based on the age of onset and severity of the disease (CSI and CSII),[12] does not correlate with these two complementation groups. Clinical variation is further complicated by other syndromes, which resemble many of the traits observed in CS: CAMFAK (cataracts, microcephaly, failure to thrive, kyphoscoliosis) and COFS (cerebro-oculofacial syndrome). Assays of DNA repair have been normal in these syndromes.[12] In addition to these COFS and CAMFAK patients, who usually show no evidence of UV sensitivity,[12] there is an increasing group of other patients without clinical and cellular photosensitivity and with only some or various hallmarks of a CS diagnosis[12,73] (Jaspers and Bootsma, unpublished observations). In the absence of a suitable biochemical marker, the genetic relationship of these patients, as well as the CAMFAK and COFS patients, to CS remains to be established.

Two other patients with a CS-type DNA repair defect, assigned to CS complementation group B, exhibit only XP symptoms.[74] At the other side of the spectrum, there are individuals with clear CS hallmarks (dwarfism, mental retardation, deafness, and peculiar facies) but without a reduced post-UV RNA synthesis recovery and photosensitivity.[73]

UVS Syndrome. Two siblings were described with a sun-sensitive skin but no apparent clinical symptoms of CS or XP.[75] Accordingly, hypersensitivity and irreversible inhibition of transcription were found after UV exposure. The level of UDS was normal, a biochemical pattern grossly reminiscent of CS but also observed in some XP-D patients (Jaspers and Bootsma, unpublished observations). Careful genetic analysis revealed that these siblings belong to a separate category called *ultraviolet sensitive* (UVS) that is different from all XP and CS groups and XP-variants.[76]

These observations strengthen the notion that the syndromes XP, CS, and TTD are closely related biochemically and may be part of a broad clinical continuum.

Genetic Classification of Other Eukaryotic NER Mutants

The clinical and genetic heterogeneity in NER syndromes raised the question of whether the complementation groups represent single gene defects, inherited in a simple Mendelian fashion, or whether more than one genetic locus is involved in each patient.[77] Cloning of the responsible genes would give the answer.

An important first step on the way to cloning repair genes was the isolation of repair-deficient rodent mutant cell lines. Many of these cell lines are of Chinese hamster origin (CHO and V79 cell lines). So far complementation analysis of these UV-sensitive mutants has revealed at least 11 distinct complementation groups.[78,79] The main features are summarized in Table 28-5. The first five groups consist of cell lines that are extremely

Table 28-5 Properties of Rodent NER Complementation Groups

Group	Representative Mutant	Parental Strain*	Sensitivity† UV	Sensitivity† MMC	Incision Deficiency	Correcting Human Gene	XP or CS Equivalent
1	UV20, 43-3B	CHO	++	+++	Yes	*ERCC1*	Not identified
2	UV5, VH-1	CHO/V79	++	+	Yes	*ERCC2*	XP-D
3	UV24, 28-1	CHO	++	+	Yes	*ERCC3*	XP-B
4	UV41	CHO	++	+++	Yes	*ERCC4*	XP-F
5	UV135, Q31	CHO, mouse lymphoma	+(+)	±	Yes	*ERCC5*	XP-G
6	UV61, US46	CHO, mouse lymphoma	+	+	Partial	*ERCC6*	CS-B
7	VB11	V79	+	±	Partial	?	?
8	US31	Mouse lymphoma	+	+	?	*ERCC8*	CS-A
9	CHO4PV	CHO	+	+	Partial	—	?
10	CHO7PV	CHO	+	+	Partial	—	?
11	UVS1	CHO	+/++	+	Yes	*ERCC11*‡	XP-F

* CHO = Chinese hamster ovary.
† +: 2–5×; ++: 5–10×; +++: > 10× wild-type sensitivity; MMC = mitomycin C.
‡ *ERCC11* and *ERCC4* are probably identical.

sensitive to UV and bulky adducts and, in that respect, resemble the XP groups A, B, D, and G. Repair in the few representatives of the remaining groups (except group 11) appears to be only partially disturbed, as in CS-A and CS-B and in XP groups C, E, and F and UVS. A unique characteristic of groups 1 and 4 is their extreme sensitivity to crosslinking agents such as mitomycin C (MMC). This suggests that the NER genes affected in these mutants act in additional systems other than NER or respond to crosslink damage in DNA. Cell fusion studies performed by Thompson[80] showed that human genes could complement the rodent repair defects in these mutant cell lines.

Another relevant class of eukaryotic NER mutants is presented by the *RAD3* epistasis group of bakers yeast *S. cerevisiae.* At least 15 complementation groups have been identified in this category of UV-sensitive yeast mutants (for review, see ref. 36). The versatility of yeast genetics has permitted the cloning of almost all the corresponding genes. The strong parallels with the mammalian system that have emerged in recent years make this organism a relevant paradigm for human NER. As shown below, there is considerable overlap between the yeast and Chinese hamster mutants and the human NER syndromes. This overlap is represented by the sequence homology of DNA repair genes and proteins in yeast, *Drosophila,* and mammals including humans and is based on strong evolutionary conservation of DNA repair mechanisms. It emphasizes the important function of DNA repair in maintaining life.

Cloning of Human NER Genes

Different strategies have been followed to clone human NER genes. A time-consuming but successful procedure has been transfection of genomic DNA from repair-proficient human cells or from a chromosome-specific cosmid library to repair-deficient rodent mutants followed by UV selection of repair-competent, UV-resistant transformants. The correcting gene subsequently can be isolated via standard recombinant DNA techniques. This strategy has resulted in the cloning of the human excision repair cross-complementing (*ERCC*) genes that correct the rodent complementation groups 1 to 6: *ERCC1,*[81] *ERCC2,*[82] *ERCC3,*[83] *ERCC4,*[84] *ERCC5,*[85] and *ERCC6.*[86]

Their possible role in NER syndromes in humans can be investigated by DNA transfection of the cloned genes into cells of the different complementation groups of XP, CS, or TTD. Alternatively, the cDNA or the gene product can be microinjected into the nucleus or cytoplasm of cultured fibroblasts of NER-deficient patients. Introduction of the *ERCC2, ERCC3, ERCC5,* and *ERCC6* genes into human NER-deficient cells alleviated the specific defects in cells from XP-D,[87,88] XP-B,[89] XP-G,[90] and CS-B,[91] respectively. An example is presented in Fig. 28-10.

The cloning of the *XPG* and *CSB* genes nicely demonstrates the unexpected contribution of findings in related and sometimes unrelated fields of research. The serendipitous cloning of the *XPG* gene was based on the screening of a *Xenopus laevis* cDNA expression library with antiserum from a human patient with the autoimmune disease lupus erythematosis by Clarkson and coworkers (Geneva).[90] The isolated full-length frog and corresponding human cDNA turned out to be homologous to the yeast NER gene *RAD2.* The human cDNA was able to correct the defect in cells of an XP-G patient. Independently, the *ERCC5* gene was cloned and also found to be homologous to *RAD2.*[92] Extracts of ERCC5 and XP-G cells appeared both deficient in the same protein.[93] A possible role of the *ERCC6* gene in CS was suggested by an observation of Fryns et al. (Leuven) that a CS patient had a constitutional deletion of a region of chromosome 10 to which we had mapped *ERCC6.*[91,94]

Genomic DNA transfection directly to cultured cells of patients with NER syndromes has, with one notable exception,[95] been unsuccessful. The difficulty of isolating repair-competent transformants after transfection of repair-defective human cells is due to the low amount of DNA that stably integrates in the genome of these cells. Compared with rodent cells, approximately 30- to more than 100-fold less DNA is integrated. This raises the number of cells required to be transfected to generate one genomic transformant containing a specific gene to extremely high levels (depending on gene length, to more than 10^9 cells[96]). Therefore, the one example of successful isolation of an NER gene, the gene defective in XP group A (*XPA*), by Tanaka and coworkers[95] via very large-scale genomic DNA transfection to XP-A cells was a formidable effort. They used an interspecies system (mouse DNA into human cells) to be able to identify and isolate the correcting (mouse) gene. This enabled the cloning of the human counterpart by cross-hybridization.

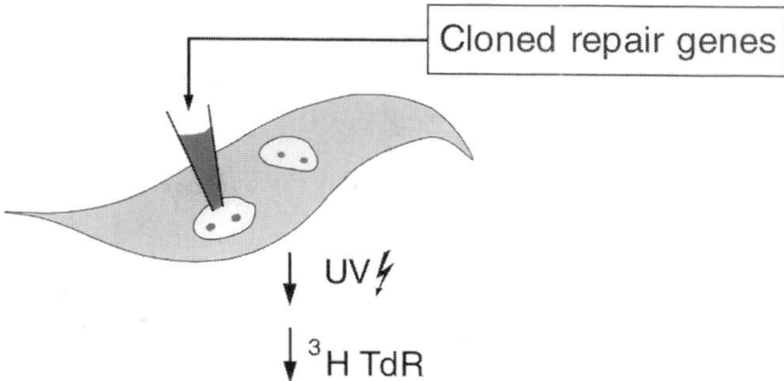

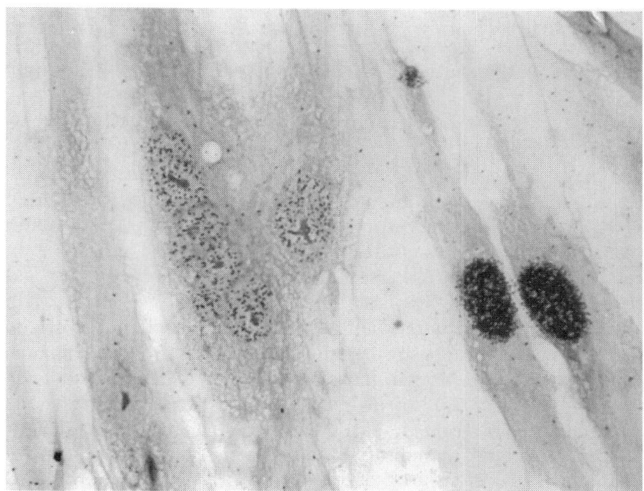

Fig. 28-10 Correction of NER defect in XP-B (XP11BE; see Fig. 28-9) multinuclear cells after microinjection of ERCC3 in one of the nuclei. *Top:* Scheme of microinjection procedure. *Bottom:* DNA repair synthesis (UDS) is corrected to normal levels in the multinucleated cell after introduction of ERCC3 cDNA. The low UDS level of the mononuclear fibroblast (*left*) reflects the NER defect of XP11BE cells. The two heavily labeled fibroblasts at the right were in S phase. (*From the Department of Cell Biology and Genetics, Erasmus University Rotterdam, W. Vermeulen.*)

An alternative transfection approach has been the use of episomally replicating plasmid vectors carrying the Epstein-Barr virus replication origin and the gene for the Epstein-Barr virus nuclear antigen, *EBNA1.* With these vectors containing human cDNAs, the *XPC* gene was cloned by Legerski et al.[97] and the *CSA* gene by the group of Friedberg.[98] Fusion of CS-A cells with the only rodent mutant representing complementation group 8 and transfection of the cloned *CSA* gene in these rodent mutant cells revealed the identity of *CSA* and *ERCC8* (see ref. 99 and Table 28-5).

Sequence homology based on evolutionary conservation has been used for the cloning of several other (human) DNA repair genes in different manners. One method uses nucleotide sequence homology to cross species barriers. Attempts to use cloned yeast

NER genes for the isolation of homologous human sequences by low-stringency cross-hybridization with human DNA libraries has resulted in the cloning of two human genes homologous to *S. cerevisiae RAD6: HHR6A* and *HHR6B.*[100] *RAD6* encodes a protein involved in ubiquitin conjugation and is implicated in postreplication repair and damage-induced mutagenesis. The yeast protein and its two human counterparts may exert their functions by modulating chromatin structure via histone ubiquitination.[101]

Alternatively, sequence conservation may permit the design of degenerate oligonucleotide primers based on conserved domains. These primers can be used for the cloning of homologous sequences by polymerase chain reaction (PCR) amplification. In this manner we have succeeded in cloning a human cDNA with clear homology to the yeast *RAD1* gene.[102] Subsequent transfection and microinjection experiments revealed that this human *RAD1* homologue corrected the DNA repair defects in rodent ERCC 4 and 11 mutants (revealing for the first time intragenic complementation between two rodent complementation groups) and XP-F fibroblasts.[102] Independently, the *ERCC4* gene was cloned by Thompson and collaborators (Livermore) by cosmid DNA transfection.[84]

These types of cloning strategies based on sequence conservation are enhanced by computerized database homology searching using powerful sequence-similarity search algorithms. The wealth of sequence information that is now available and will be even more so in the future as a result of the Human Genome Project and related efforts opens the possibility of identification of mammalian homologues of known relevant genes of lower species. This can be done by critical database screening based on conserved domains. Examples are two human genes homologous to the *S. cerevisiae* NER gene *RAD23: HHR23A* and *HHR23B.*[103] The same procedures also work in the other direction: from human DNA sequences to the isolation of homologues in lower eukaryotes. An example is the cloning of the *S. cerevisiae* counterpart of *CSB (ERCC6): RAD26.*[104]

Another obvious procedure for cloning genes starts with purification of the gene product, followed by designing nucleotide primers on the basis of a partial amino acid sequence obtained by microsequencing of the protein and cloning of the gene by PCR. A gene that may be involved in XP complementation group E was cloned in this manner. The purification and characterization of this DNA damage-binding protein (DDB) were reported by Hwang et al. (see ref. 105 and references therein) and the group of S. Linn.[106,107] Similarly, Hanaoka and collaborators purified the XPC protein (in a complex with another polypeptide that turned out to be HHR23B) and subsequently cloned the cDNAs.[103]

MAMMALIAN NER GENES: THEIR FUNCTION IN THE NER PATHWAY AND ROLE IN NER SYNDROMES

Candidates for the NER genes involved in all seven XP complementation groups have been molecularly cloned, although the gene responsible for XP-E is still uncertain. In addition, the two genes implicated in the classic form of CS have been isolated, and two of the three TTD (photosensitive form) genes have been identified. Futhermore, several human NER genes have been cloned for which no human NER complementation groups are known yet but for which either a rodent mutant or a yeast NER equivalent exists.

Using *in vitro* NER assay systems based on cell-free extracts (developed by the groups of Wood and Sancar[108,109]), several proteins known to be involved in DNA replication also have been demonstrated to participate in the incision and/or DNA synthesis step of the NER pathway. The core of the mammalian NER reaction was reconstituted successfully *in vitro* with (partly) purified components.[110,111] These *in vitro* systems provide valuable tools for studying the function of isolated repair proteins.

Computer-assisted comparison of the predicted amino acid sequence of the encoded proteins with known gene products present in large databases has highlighted a striking functional resemblance with NER proteins of the yeast *RAD3* epistasis group. The extent of similarity suggests a golden rule: For each yeast NER protein there is a counterpart in humans, and vice versa. The conclusion must be that the entire NER mechanism is strongly conserved in all eukaryotes. The primary amino acid sequence also disclosed homology with functional protein domains, such as well-characterized DNA-binding and helix-unwinding sequence motifs. This type of information provided valuable clues to the biochemical activity of the encoded polypeptides. Finally, over-production, purification, and enzymologic characterization have led to the elucidation of functional properties of several of the NER proteins and the identification of intricate complexes. Table 28-6 lists all mammalian NER genes cloned to date and summarizes their main properties.

In the following paragraphs the function of the genes involved in the NER syndromes will be discussed within the context of a model for the NER pathway that is based on currently available evidence, taking into account our still considerable ignorance. A schematic representation of the model for the multistep NER mechanism is depicted in Fig. 28-11.

Four subsequent phases are distinguished:

1. *Damage recognition.* How do cells identify lesions in the DNA? Which proteins are involved, and what is their specificity?
2. *Demarcation of the lesion.* Chromatin and DNA have to be made accessible to enzymes that will remove the damage.
3. *Dual incision.* Nicks have to be made at both sides of the lesion in the damaged strand only.
4. *Postincision events.* The damage-containing oligomer should be removed and the gap filled in by repair DNA synthesis, followed by ligation.

Damage Recognition (XPC-HHR23B, XPA, XPE?) (Fig. 28-11 and Table 28-6)

The first step in NER is expected to be the binding of a damage-recognition factor to the lesion, which enables the association of further repair components. Evidence for involvement of a protein complex composed of XPC and HHR23B in this step was presented by Sugasawa et al.[112] *In vivo*, the XPC protein is stably bound to HHR23B, one of the two human homologues of the yeast repair protein RAD 23.[103] XPC-HHR23B and XPC alone display a similar high affinity for both single- and double-stranded DNA and a preference for UV-damaged DNA.[103,113,114] *In vitro* experiments by Sugasawa et al.[112] revealed that XPC-HHR23B is the first actor in NER and capable of recruiting the rest of the repair machinery to the lesion.

Also XPA and XPE (or DDB) may be involved in damage recognition, since both proteins have a high affinity for UV-damaged DNA.The *XPA* gene specifies a protein with the sequence hallmarks of a DNA-binding Zn21-finger domain.[115] The gene product has been purified, and biochemical evidence confirmed that it is a zinc metalloprotein with affinity for double-stranded (ds) and single-stranded (ss) DNA.[116–118] A marked preference has been found for a number of lesions, including [6-4] photoproducts and Cs-Pt adducts but poor binding to cyclobutane pyrimidine dimers.[116,119] This parallels strikingly the preference of the NER pathway itself and is reminiscent of the lesion-binding spectrum of the *E. coli* UvrA2B complex. However, it also may reflect the limitations of *in vitro* studies, since in these assays the configuration of DNA is different from DNA packed into nuclear chromatin. Using the *in vitro* cell-free NER assay, the XPA product has been functionally assigned to a step in the pre-incision stage of the reaction.[108] These data are consistent with the idea that XPA is implicated in damage recognition. Studies of mutations in *XPA* demonstrated that an intact Zn-finger is indispensable for proper function of the protein.[118,120,121] The *S. cerevisiae* homologue of *XPA* is *RAD14.*[122] *RAD14* also binds preferentially to [6-4] photoproducts and chelates zinc.[123]

Table 28-6 Main Properties of Cloned Human NER Genes

Gene*	Chrom. Location	Size Protein (aa)†	Yeast Homologue	Protein Properties‡
XPA	9q34	273	*RAD14*	Zn^{2+}-finger, binds different types of damaged DNA, transient interaction with ERCC1, RPA and TFIIH(?) complex
XPB(ERCC3)	2q21	782	*RAD25*	3′ → 5′ DNA helicase, subunit of TFIIH, essential for transcription initiation
XPC	3p25.1§	940	*RAD4*	Complexed with HHR23B, strong damage-specific DNA binding, involved in global genome repair only, initiator of global genome repair
XPD(ERCC2)	19q13.2§	760	*RAD3*	5′ → 3′ DNA helicase, subunit of TFIIH, essential for transcription initiation
XPE	11	1140	*Identified*¶	Binds UV-damaged DNA, no causative mutations identified in complex with 48 kD, WD-repeat containing protein
XPF(ERCC4)	16p13.3	~905	*RAD1*	Also identical to ERCC11, complex with ERCC1 makes 5′ incision, Y structure–specific endonuclease, dual function in recombination
XPG(ERCC5)	13q32-33	1186	*RAD2*	Y structure–specific endonuclease, makes 3′ incision
CSA(ERCC8)	5	396	*RAD28*	5 WD-repeats, involved in transcription-coupled repair only
CSB(ERCC6)	10q11-21	1493	*RAD26*	DNA-dependent ATPase (helicase?), involved in transcription-coupled repair only, present in (elongating) RNA polymerase II complex
ERCC1	19q13.2§	297	*RAD10*	Partial homology to UvrC and many nucleases, complex with XPF makes 5′ incision Y structure–specific endonuclease, dual function in recombination
HHR23A	19p13.2	363	*RAD23*	Ubiquitin-like N-terminus, 2 ubiquitin-associated domains
HHR23B	3p25.14§	409	*RAD23*	As HHR23A, fraction of HHR23B complexed with XPC, complex binds ssDNA and is involved in global genome repair only
$p62^{TFIIH}$	11p14-15.1	548	*TFB1*	Subunit of TFIIH, essential for transcription initiation
$p52^{TFIIH}$	6p21.3	513	*TFB2*	Subunit of TFIIH, essential for transcription initiation
$p44^{TFIIH}$	5q1.3	395	*SSL1*	DNA-binding Zn^{2+}-finger, subunit of TFIIH, essential for transcription initiation.
$p34^{TFIIH}$	12	303	*TFB4*	Zn^{2+}-finger, subunit of TFIIH, essential for transcription initiation.

*Not included in this table are the genes for protein involved in the DNA-synthesis step of the NER reaction, such as PCNA, RPA, RF-C, DNA ligase.
† aa: amino acids.
‡ Question marks indicate properties inferred but not proven.
§ The *XPC* and *HHR23B* genes are located on a common 650 kb M1ul fragment; *ERCC1* and *XPD(ERCC2)* are less than 20 kb apart.
¶ A yeast gene encoding a product with clear overall homology to the XPE protein has been identified in the yeast genome database. In addition, a second human gene with significant similarity to XPE has been discovered (van der Spek, Hoeijmakers, unpublished results).

The other potential damage-recognition factor, DDB, was first identified in human cell lysates by specific retention with UV-damaged oligonucleotides.[124] This DDB activity is possibly implicated in XP-E, since it is absent in extracts derived from some, but not all, XP-E patients.[125,126] Microinjection of purified DDB transiently corrects the partial NER defect in XP-E cells that lack the DDB activity.[107] The DDB activity copurified with a heterodimeric complex consisting of 124- and 41-kDa proteins.[106,127] Mutations have been described to occur in the small subunit in DDB-deficient XP-E patients.[128] Structural homologues of the large subunit were found in a database search, including a DDB-like polypeptide in human and yeast (van der Spek and Hoeijmakers, unpublished observations) and *Caenorhabditis elegans.*[129] These gene products probably represent a novel class of DNA-binding proteins. It is tempting to speculate that the relatively mild DNA repair defect in XP-E cells is due to the fact that this second human *XPE*-like gene might be functionally redundant to the original human *XPE* gene. The XP-E correcting factor has a strong preference for binding to DNA containing [6-4] photoproducts but exhibits modest discrimination of cyclobutane pyrimidine dimers and no measurable affinity for psoralen-thymine monoadducts.[130] The striking abundance of the protein in normal cells (in the order of 10^5 copies per cell[106]) suggests that it has an additional function. A general characteristic of NER factors is that they seem to be present only in trace amounts. One possibility is that the XP-E correcting protein assists XPA in detection of some lesions, but direct interaction between these polypeptides has not been demonstrated.

Alternatively, evidence has been presented that XPA can transiently associate with the ERCC1-XPF incision complex by interaction with ERCC1,[131,132] while binding domains for RPA[133,134] and TFIIH[135,136] also have been reported (see below). The network of protein-protein contacts between XPA and other core NER factors suggests that XPA has a central role in coordinating events in NER. The idea that XPA is the NER initiation factor[137] appears to be wrong. The work of Sugasawa et al.[112] demonstrates that XPC acts prior to XPA in vitro and serves to recruit the remainder of the NER machinery to the lesion.

XPC is the sole XP factor that is dispensable for TCR. Detection of the primary lesion in the transcription-coupled NER subpathway might be performed by RNA polymerase II. The transcription machinery probably subjects the DNA to a more rigorous test for intactness than achieved via the standard NER damage-recognition complex. This may explain why lesions that are poorly removed from the genome overall are efficiently eliminated by the TCR mode.

Demarcation of the Lesion (XPB, XPD) (Fig. 28-11 and Table 28-6).

By analogy with the *E. coli* system, it is plausible that after damage detection the DNA and chromatin have to be made accessible for recognition by the incision protein complex(es). This may involve the induction of a strongly kinked, locally unwound — but uniform for all lesions — DNA structure as observed with the UvrA2B complex, which overrides the aberrant lesion-specific conformation. By analogy with the recently described mechanism of action of *E. coli* photoreactivating enzyme, this may involve flipping out of the photoproduct from the DNA axis.[138]

By using *in vitro* repair systems, the groups of Wood[139] and Sancar[140] have shown that once lesions have been recognized, an open DNA complex is found by the coordinating activities of XPC-HHR23B, TFIIH, XPA, and RPA. TFIIH possesses bidirectional DNA unwinding activity and will be discussed in the next

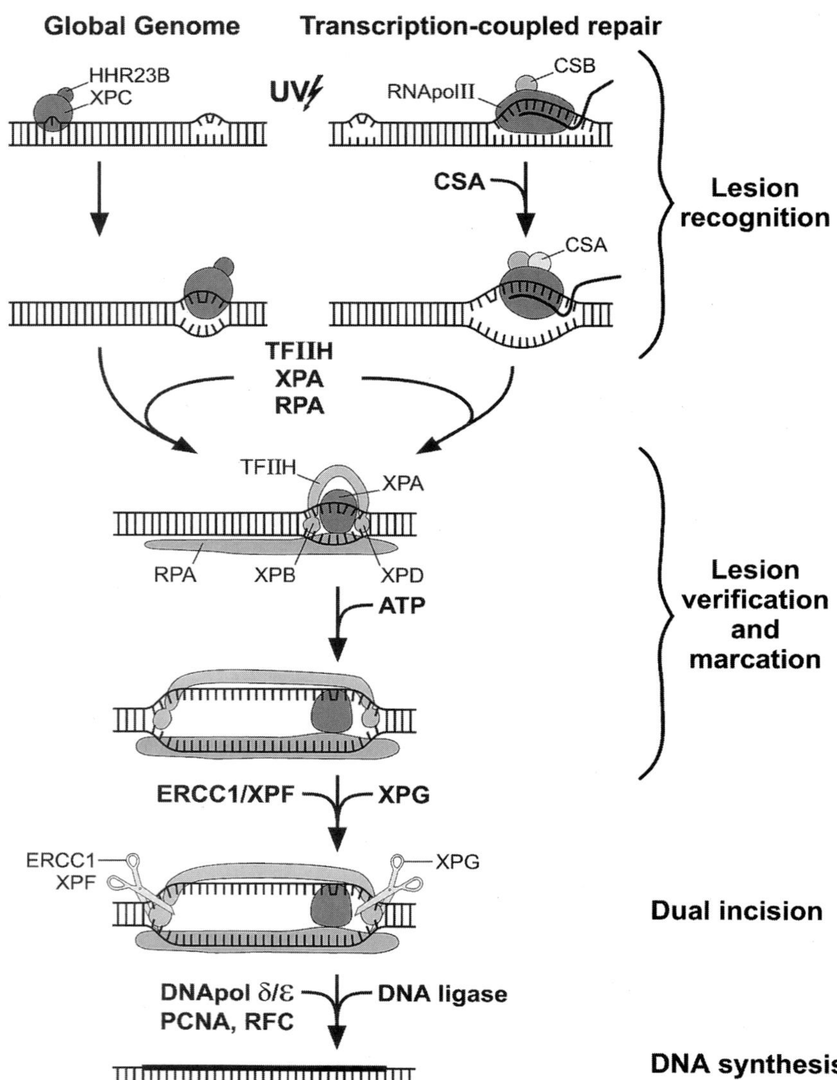

Fig. 28-11 Model for the first steps in the human NER mechanism. I-II: Damage recognition. II-III: Damage demarcation. III-IV: DNA unwinding. IV: Dual incision.

section. The RPA complex is composed of three single-stranded DNA binding proteins. It was found previously to participate in initiation and elongation of DNA replication and already shown to play a role prior or at the incision step in NER.[108,141] RPA may stabilize the unwound intermediate. XPA may account for correct positioning of the pre-incision complex, since it can bind the DNA lesion and interacts with both TFIIH and RPA.[133–135] In addition, XPG seems to stabilize this opened pre-incision complex.[139,140,142]

Both studies of Wood et al. and Sancar et al. indicate a two-step unwinding model with an ATP-dependent TFIIH-mediated initial opening and a subsequent extension of the open complex 5′ away from the lesion.

The Role of the TFIIH Transcription-Repair Complex (Fig. 28-11 and Table 28-6). Many parallels exist between XPD and XPB (and their yeast counterparts RAD3 and RAD25, also known as SSL2).[89] Based on identification of helicase motifs in the primary amino acid sequence Weeda et al.[89] proposed that both proteins form a complex with bidirectional helix-unwinding activity. As apparent below, this early idea has been corroborated in later studies. The notion that null alleles of one or both genes in yeast,[143,144] *Drosophila,*[145] and mouse[146] are inviable indicates that these repair proteins must be involved in an additional process essential for viability. The nature of the latter was elucidated by a surprising discovery made by Egly and coworkers,[147] who were studying transcription initiation, an intricate process involving the concerted action of numerous products (for a review, see ref. 148). A multisubunit component required in a late stage of RNA polymerase II basal transcription initiation is TFIIH, previously also designated BTF2. It is a complex of at least nine polypeptides[149,150] (Table 28-7). The two largest subunits of this basal transcription factor were found to be the repair proteins XPB[147] and XPD.[151,152] Moreover, purified TFIIH corrects the XP-B, XP-D, and TTD-A repair defects *in vivo* as well as *in vitro*,[56,153] indicating the presence of at least three repair proteins in this transcription factor and a striking relationship with NER complementation groups involving TTD.

With the cell-free NER assay it also was shown that TFIIH stimulates NER activity.[153] Since in this assay neither transcription nor translation can occur, this stimulation suggests a direct involvement of TFIIH in the NER reaction. Correcting activities

Table 28-7 Main Properties of Human and Yeast TFIIH Components

Human Gene	Yeast Gene	Features/Function
XPB (ERCC3)	*RAD25/SSL2*	$3' \rightarrow 5'$ helicase
XPD (ERCC2)	*RAD3*	$5' \rightarrow 3'$ helicase
p62	*TFB1*	Unknown
p52	*TFB2*	Unknown
p44	*SSL1*	2 Zn^{2+}-fingers
Mo15/CDK7	*Kin28*	CDK-like kinase
p34	*Scp34*	SSL1-like Zn^{2+}-finger
cyclinH	*cc11*	Homology to cyclins
MAT1	*TFB3*	Ring Zn^{2+}-finger

of XP-B, XP-D, and TTD-A exactly co-elute with transcription and helicase activities of TFIIH.[56,153] NER-competent cell lysates and purified TFIIH fractions can be deprived of repair activity after immunoprecipitation with antibodies directed against some components of TFIIH (anti-XPB, -p62, -p44, -p43; see Table 28-7).[56,154] Furthermore, mutations in the yeast SSL1 and TFB1, yeast homologues of the human TFIIH subunits p44 and p62, give rise to a UV-sensitive phenotype consistent with a function in repair.[155]

These data suggest that the entire transcription initiation factor TFIIH is involved in NER. The dual functionality of the entire TFIIH complex is also evident from recent studies with yeast TFIIH.[156–159] Purified TFIIH displays the following activities and properties: a DNA-dependent ATPase, a protein kinase phosphorylating the C-terminus of the large subunit of RNA polymerase II, and a bidirectional DNA unwinding activity (see ref. 151 and references therein). The latter is due to the XPB ($3' \rightarrow 5'$) and the XPD ($5' \rightarrow 3'$) helicases. In addition, the TFIIH complex is endowed with two proteins (p44 and p34) containing one or more Zn^{2+}-finger domains that likely mediate DNA and/or protein-protein interactions[154] (see Table 28-7). Studies using *in vitro* transcription initiation assays have not fully established the role of TFIIH in transcription initiation. However, several plausible models can be advanced. The bidirectional helicase activity may be required for inducing a specific DNA conformation by locally opening the template[148] for loading RNA polymerase onto the transcribed strand. Alternatively, or in addition, the complex may promote promoter clearance.[160]

What can be the role of the TFIIH complex in NER? Since TFIIH repair mutants show defects in both TCR and GGR (see Table 28-4), the complex probably functions in the core of the NER reaction. Furthermore, it is reasonable to suppose that TFIIH catalyses a similar step in the context of NER and transcription initiation. Thus one of the options is that it induces a melted DNA conformation required for loading a NER incision complex onto the template and/or for altering the DNA conformation around the lesion in a manner similar to UvrA2B. Alternatively, or in addition, this complex may be involved in clearance of the damaged region, possibly including release of the damage-containing oligonucleotide and turnover of repair proteins (see Fig. 28-11).

Dual Incision (ERCC1/XPF Complex, XPG) (Fig. 28-11 and Table 28-5)

Following lesion demarcation, the actual incisions are performed by the structure-specific endonucleases XPG and ERCC1-XPF complex. XPG makes the 3′ incision and ERCC1-XPF the 5′ incision.[102,161,162]

The *XPG* gene is identical to the previously cloned human *ERCC5* gene and homologous to the yeast *RAD2* (see Table 28-6). XPG-mediated incisions always occur in one strand of duplex DNA at the 3′ side of a junction with single-stranded DNA. One single-stranded arm, protruding in either the 3′ or the 5′ direction, is necessary and sufficient for the correct positioning of XPG incisions.[163]

The ERCC1-XPF complex (also containing ERCC4 and ERCC11 correcting activities[164,165]) has a yeast counterpart comprising the RAD1 and the RAD10 protein. The RAD1-RAD10 complex possesses a single-stranded DNA-endonuclease activity that specifically cleaves the 3′ protruding single strand at the transition from a double- to single-strand region,[166–168] leading to the suggestion that this heterodimer makes the 5′ incision. The yeast complex is also implicated in intrachromosomal mitotic recombination.[168–170] Both processes encompass DNA incision as an obligatory step in their reaction mechanism.

In collaboration with Wood et al., we have shown that *ERCC4* and *XPF* (and probably *ERCC11*) are identical. Causative mutations and strongly reduced but still detectable XPF protein levels were identified in XP-F patients.[102] The incisions are made asymmetrically, with the 3′ incision 2 to 8 nucleotides and the 5′ incision 15 to 24 nucleotides away from the lesion, corresponding to the borders of the open complex.[171,173] The exact incision position seems to depend on the type of DNA lesion.[161,173,174] Although incisions occur near synchronously, consensus exists that the 3′ incision precedes the 5′ incision.[175]

Other factors are also required for an efficient excision of damaged DNA. One of them is the single-stranded binding protein complex RPA (see above). It plays a crucial role in nuclease positioning. Each side of the molecule, oriented on single-stranded DNA, interacts with a distinct nuclease. Bound to single-stranded DNA, the 3′ oriented side of RPA interacts with ERCC1-XPF and strongly stimulates its nuclease activity, whereas the 5′ oriented side of RPA does not interact with the complex and blocks ERCC1-XPF-mediated incision. RPA presumably contributes but is not sufficient to confer strand specificity to XPG (de Laat, Hoeijmakers et al., unpublished observations). These findings position RPA to the non-damaged strand of the opened NER intermediate. Given the intimate link between XPG and TFIIH,[176,177] TFIIH is an attractive candidate to be involved in XPG positioning as well.

Postincision Events (Fig. 28-11)

The final stages of the NER reaction should entail release of the damage-containing oligomer, turnover of the bound NER proteins, gap-filling DNA synthesis [used most frequently for assaying NER (UDS)], and sealing of the remaining nick by ligation. At present it is unknown which proteins carry out the first of these steps. Again, the TFIIH complex is a potential candidate because it harbors two helicases that could peel off the damage-containing 28-29-mer. Alternatively, it is possible that the DNA replication machinery carries out this reaction.

Use of the cell-free NER assay has permitted identification of the proliferating cell nuclear antigen (PCNA) as being required for the gap-filling DNA synthesis step.[108,178] PCNA is known to stimulate DNA polymerase delta and/or epsilon in regular DNA replication. The implication of PCNA in this part of the NER reaction mechanism suggests that the repair synthesis itself is mediated by any or both of these polymerases. The final sealing of the new DNA to the preexisting strand is thought to be carried out by DNA ligase I.

It is interesting to note that mutations in the ligase I gene can give rise to a UV-sensitive phenotype.[179] So far only one patient with a ligase I defect has been discovered, but it may well turn out that this individual (designated 46BR) belongs in a new category of NER-deficient patients.

So far we have dealt with steps in the core of the NER reaction. As mentioned earlier, two subpathways have been distinguished in NER: GGR and TCR. Gene functions specific for these subpathways are discussed in the following paragraphs. Finally, as discussed below, instead of a stepwise assembly of individual factors described earlier, evidence has been presented in the analogous yeast system for the existence of a preassembled "repairosome."[158] Furthermore, the preceding tentative model does not incorporate yet the chromatin dynamics that must play a part in vivo.

Steps Specific for the GGR Pathway (XPC) (Table 28-6)

Analysis of mutants has lead to the identification of at least three genes selectively implicated in the repair of the nontranscribed bulk of the genome: *RAD7* and *RAD16* in yeast[180] and *XPC* in humans.[181] The function of the XPC-HHR23B complex in damage recognition was described earlier. The XPC amino acid sequence displays significant homology to the yeast RAD4 protein.[97,103] However, *rad4* null mutants, in contrast to *XPC* mutants, are defective in both NER subpathways.[180] This may reflect a principal difference between mammals and yeast. A notable feature of the HHR23 proteins is the presence of an ubiquitin-like domain in the N-terminus.[103] In some other ubiquitin-fusion proteins this moiety is thought to function as a chaperone, facilitating complex formation. Hence this domain may perform a similar role in assembling the XPC-HHR23B complex. To date, no known human NER syndromes have been associated with the *HHR23B* gene, and a simple explanation might be that the highly homologous HHR23A protein diminished the effect of loss of HHR23B function.

In keeping with the golden rule derived from the striking correspondence between yeast and mammalian NER, it would be expected that human homologues of RAD7 and RAD16 exist and that they participate in the global repair process. The RAD7 sequence does not reveal any clue to its function.[182] The *RAD16* gene, however, encodes a protein containing a special type of DNA-binding Zn^{2+} finger and an extended region with strong homology to a specific subfamily of presumed DNA helicases.[183] Interestingly, CSB, a protein specific for TCR, is also equipped with such domains.[91] A characteristic of other members of this helicase subfamily is that they reside in multiprotein complexes. Genetic evidence in yeast suggests that the complex interacts with chromatin (see ref. 184 and references therein).

In this light, what is the role of these genes? One possibility, suggested elsewhere, is that they are involved in uncoupling essential NER components from the transcription machinery to make them available for GGR,[103] or vice versa when repair is finished, to allow recovery of RNA synthesis. The TFIIH transcription-repair complex is the most logical partner in this option. The CSA and CSB proteins might be involved in this process (see below). On the other hand, the RAD16 protein (complex?) may be implicated in altering chromatin structure required for global genome repair. Obviously, these speculations need to be experimentally investigated.

Steps Specific for TCR (CSA,CSB) (Table 28-6)

Two genes involved in TCR that are defective in CS are *CSA* and *CSB*. The protein sequence of CSA contains the consensus of five WD-repeats.[98] This type of motif is present in many proteins believed to possess a regulatory rather than a catalytic function.[185] Many of these WD-repeat proteins reside in multiprotein complexes. CSA is thought to associate with p44 (a component of TFIIH; see Table 28-7) and with CSB.[98]

CSB is a member of the closely related subfamily of putative DNA/RNA helicases, described earlier, to which RAD16 also belongs. A yeast homologue of this protein was unknown, but the sequence conservation seen for all other eukaryotic NER factors permitted bridging the large evolutionary gap between human and yeast. Like CSB, a yeast disruption mutant, designated *rad26*, displayed a selective defect in TCR.[104] Interestingly, inactivation of this NER subpathway in yeast does not induce a significant UV sensitivity, suggesting that this process is not very important for UV survival in yeast.

Hanawalt and Mellon[38] argued that in order to couple NER to transcription, the stalled RNA polymerase II complex has to retract or dissociate to allow access of repair proteins to the lesion.[186,187] It is possible that defects in this process underlie the total TCR defect in CS cells, implicating CSA and CSB in the release of RNA polymerase II from the damaged site. The role for CSA and CSB, with the latter found to be associated with elongating RNA polymerase II complexes,[186,188,189] is still matter for speculation.[190]

Higher-Order NER Complexes

Although most of the important players in mammalian NER are identified, it is not known yet how these factors assemble on a lesion and how they interact with each other. Several reports appeared in the literature dealing with proposed interactions between NER factors. However, many of these studies are based on associations either in a rather artificial environment (immobilized fusion proteins) or after overexpression in yeast (two-hybrid system). In both systems, transient or low-affinity interactions can be selected, which may not reflect the in vivo situation.

A central role for the XPA protein is likely in view of the very severe NER-deficient phenotype of XP-A cells. Biochemical studies with XPA suggest that this factor serves as an nucleation point in the repair reaction. Interaction of XPA (in addition to that with damaged DNA) has been described with ERCC1,[131,132,191] RPA,[133,134] and TFIIH.[135,136] Binding of both ERCC1 and RPA to XPA has a synergistic effect on the DNA damage-specific binding affinity of XPA.[134,191] RPA is claimed to interact with XPG,[134] whereas XPG and XPC may be associated with TFIIH.[152,177] Several of these assumed interactions depend on isolation conditions,[111] and variable or different results have been obtained by other laboratories.[56,110] Using specific isolation conditions, an NER supercomplex ("repairosome") was purified from yeast cells.[158] The majority of the different yeast NER factors are reported to reside in this "repairosome." However, this isolated complex still lacks some essential factors because it is not active in a reconstituted NER reaction. Also, the amount of each of the NER factors residing in this complex is not known.

Mouse Models for Genetic Defects in NER

Gene targeting by homologous recombination in totipotent embryonal stem (ES) cells permits the generation of mouse mutants in any cloned NER gene. This methodology enables the development of experimental animal models for all types of NER deficiencies and associated syndromes. Genes can be fully inactivated (knockout mutants), but it is also possible to reconstruct specific partially inactivating mutations encountered in patients in the mouse genome. The use of this genetic tool will have a major impact on clinical and fundamental research of the human NER syndromes and cancer in general. First, it will help in understanding the complex ramifications and biologic relevance of NER pathways particularly with respect to understanding the mechanisms of carcinogenesis, neurodegeneration, photoimmunology, and aging. Second, animal models for human NER syndromes will be instrumental for clinical research on these conditions, including diagnosis, prevention, and therapy. Furthermore, it may lead to the discovery of new disorders for NER genes for which no corresponding condition has been identified yet. In addition, it will help in disentangling the intricate genotype-phenotype relationships of CS and TTD. Crossing animals with different genetic lesions will permit the study of synergistic effects with other mechanisms implicated in genetic (in)stability, such as cell cycle control, complementary repair pathways, and apoptosis. Finally, since the NER system targets a very wide spectrum of DNA lesions, mice deficient in this pathway will be a valuable and sensitive model for assessing the genotoxic effect of known and unknown compounds.

The ERCC1 Mouse. The first NER-deficient mouse mutant was generated in the *ERCC1* gene,[192] one of the NER genes for which no parallel human syndrome is yet known.[193] Thus it was not *a priori* evident whether full inactivation of this function would be compatible with life, particularly since both the yeast and rodent mutants provide evidence for a dual involvement of this gene in an additional mitotic recombination repair pathway with unpredictable biologic impact, as noted previously. A functional knockout mutation appeared barely viable; indeed, most ERCC1-deficient embryos die in utero or perinatally, and the few mutants surviving are severely runted and usually die before weaning, i.e., within 4 weeks.[194] Recent evidence indicates that the genetic makeup influences the life span and embryonal death to a considerable extent; maximal life span is extended to several months in a C57B1/6 strain, and mutant embryonal death is postponed to the moment of birth in an FVB background.[194] This indicates that these two types of early death may have different causes. One of the causes of postnatal death is liver malfunction, probably due to increased nuclear aneuploidy. Elevated levels of aneuploid nuclei are also apparent in kidney, and there is ferritin deposition in spleen. Increased levels of p53 are reported in liver, brain, and kidney.[192] Subcutaneous fat is absent. As far as investigated, the neurologic status of the mice seems normal. Several of the preceding clinical features point to premature aging, possibly as a result of accumulation of unremoved endogenous DNA lesions. At the cellular level, replicative senescence is seen as well as increased spontaneous transformation.[194] As expected, mouse embryonal fibroblasts (MEFs) derived from the mutant mice display a total NER defect and are hypersensitive to UV and chemical genotoxins that are substrates of the NER pathway. In addition, there is cellular sensitivity to crosslinking agents, presumably as a consequence of an additional defect in one of the recombination repair pathways. In order to create a milder phenotype, a mouse mutant was designed in which only the very C-terminal 7 amino acids were deleted[194] (ERCC1^{*292}; Fig. 28-12). However, apart from an extended life span to more than 6 months, most of the other features were very similar to those of the full knockout mice, indicating that the very last part of the protein is still important for its biologic functions. The signs of premature senescence observed in the ERCC1$^{2/2}$ suggest that accumulation of unrepaired DNA damage contributes to early aging. The ERCC1^{*292} mice were used in a carcinogenesis experiment. Cutaneous application of dimethylbenz[a]anthracene (DMBA) at a dose easily tolerated by XPA knockout mice (see below) caused death within 3 days, revealing an extreme sensitivity to genotoxins.[195] Apart from the UV sensitivity, the clinical picture is very different from any of the human NER syndromes. The lack of similarity between the mouse and the human NER mutants may, in part, reflect species differences, but the picture also may be compounded by the dual functionality of the ERCC1 protein. In this connection, a comparison of the severe clinical phenotype of ERCC1 mutant mice with that of XPA knockout mice (also harboring a complete NER defect) will be very instructive.

The XPA Mouse. A closer but still partial correspondence to the parallel human disease was noted with a mouse model for XP-A generated independently in two laboratories. Consistent with the human pathology, XPA knockout mice display cutaneous and ocular photosensitivity and a greatly increased susceptibility to UV- and DMBA-induced skin cancer.[195,196] However, in contrast to XP-A patients, knockout mutant mice appear physiologically normal, are fertile, and at the age of 18 months fail to develop the neuropathology characteristic of the human condition. One factor that should be taken into account in this regard is the difference in life span. The accelerated neurodegeneration observed in XP-A human patients is manifested over the course of several years, whereas such a time period cannot be reached in the mouse model. As in the case with ERCC1 in one genetic background, approximately half the XPA-deficient embryos died in the midfetal stage (with signs of anemia),[196] whereas in another background this phenomenon was absent.[195] XPA-deficient MEFs exhibited all parameters of a total NER deficiency. This indicates that the NER phenotype is as predicted and also as observed in ERCC1-deficient mice. The fact that, with respect to the NER defect, XPA and ERCC1 knockout mice are indistinguishable permits a valid comparison between these two phenotypes. Considering the additional function of ERCC1 in a mitotic recombination repair pathway, it is logical to conclude that the extra symptoms registered in the ERCC1-deficient mice, such as liver and kidney aneuploidy, growth retardation, and premature aging, are a consequence of a compromise of this second function.

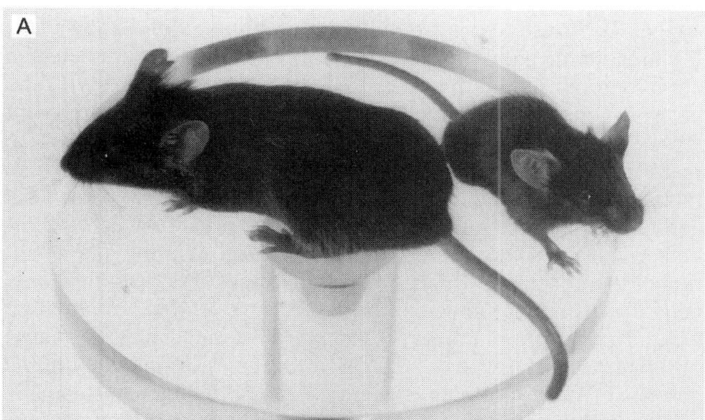

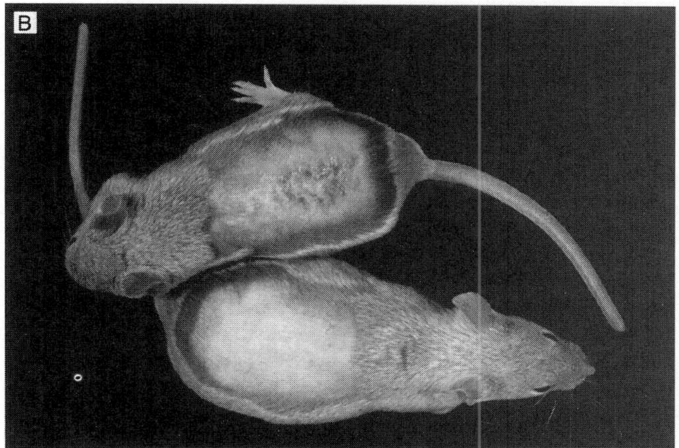

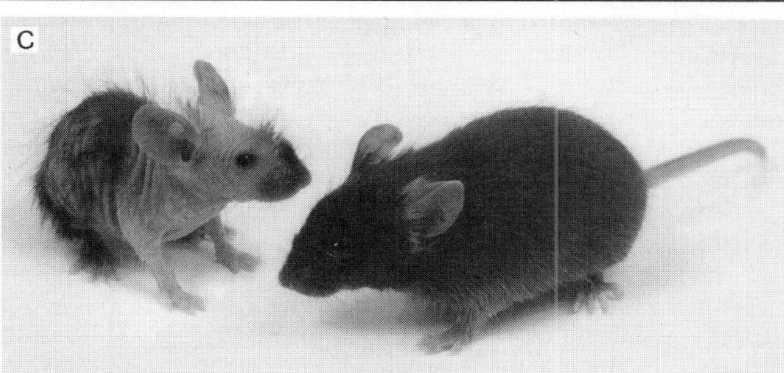

Fig. 28-12 Mouse models of NER syndromes. NER-deficient mice were obtained by targeting mouse embryonic stem cells with a DNA construct containing a mutated NER gene, followed by blastocyst injection and breeding germ-line chimeras. *Top:* ERCC1-mutant mouse showing growth defects (compare the small mutant mouse with its normal litter mate). This mouse is extremely sensitive to ultraviolet light and UV-mimicking agents. *Center:* Homozygous and heterozygous CSB mutant mouse representing a mouse model for CS. The UV-induced erythema on the skin reflects the severe UV sensitivity of this CSB2/2 mouse. *Bottom*: Homozygous TTD mutant showing brittle hair and other characteristic features of TTD. (*From the Department of Cell Biology and Genetics, Erasmus University, Rotterdam; G. Weeda, ERCC1 mouse, B. van der Horst, CSB mouse, and Jan de Boer, TTD mouse.*)

The XPC Mouse. A phenotype very similar to XPA mice is observed in mice carrying an inactivating mutation in the *XPC* gene. As in the case of XP-C patients, a normal development and clear UV hypersensitivity and increased frequency of skin cancer were found.[197]

The CSB Mouse. We have mimicked a mutation of a known CS-B patient in the mouse genome.[198] Analysis of repair parameters in embryonic fibroblasts from the CSB mutant versus wild-type and heterozygous mice showed a specific loss of TCR. In agreement with the human syndrome, CSB-deficient mice are photosensitive (see Fig. 28-12). The other CS-like clinical features observed were mild, such as slightly retarded growth and neurologic (behavioral and motor coordination) abnormalities. Remarkably, when a GGR defect was introduced in CSB-deficient mice, a strong augmentation of the CS phenotype was observed. Such XPC/CSB and XPA/CSB double mutant mice exhibit a very severe growth retardation (75 percent), are unable to walk, and die around day 18. These observations suggest that a CS defect becomes exaggerated in the absence of GGR, pointing to accumulation of endogenous damage as a contributing factor to the CS symptoms.[190] In striking contrast to human CS, CSB-deficient mice appear clearly prone to skin cancer when exposed to UV light or to the chemical carcinogen DMBA.[198] Thus, in the mouse, intact GGR is not sufficient to protect from tumorigenesis. This finding could imply that CS patients may have a hitherto unnoticed cancer predisposition. Alternatively, the species difference in tumorigenesis could be due to the fact that, in humans compared with rodents, the GGR pathway is more potent in eliminating cyclobutane pyrimidine dimers, the major UV-induced lesion.[198]

Mouse Mutants in the TFIIH Subunits XPB and XPD. Like some of the other NER genes, the TFIIH complex has a dual functionality complicating the clinical outcome of a mutation in the genes involved. In the case of TFIIH, the second function entails initiation of basal transcription of all structural genes transcribed by RNA polymerase II. This is one of the most fundamental processes in the cell. Complete inactivation of such a function is most probably lethal, explaining the rarity of mutants in TFIIH genes. We have made knockout mutations in the mouse for both *XPB* and *XPD.* Although heterozygous mice were readily obtained, 2/2 mutants were selectively absent from the offspring. Death occurs at the two-cell stage when embryonal transcription has to start up.[146] This demonstrates that inactivation of these genes is lethal and that this is due to their role in transcription. More subtle mutations had to be made mimicking the phenotype-determining allele in the corresponding human patients. We have generated a mouse model for TTD by using a novel gene targeting strategy (gene-cDNA fusion targeting).[199] Part of the coding region of the mouse *XPD* gene is replaced by the corresponding part of the human cDNA that encodes the point mutation causing the disease in a TTD patient. The mice reflect to a remarkable extent the clinical symptoms of the TTD patient (see Fig. 28-12): brittle hair, developmental abnormalities, UV sensitivity, skin abnormalities, and reduced life span.[199] The same divergence between the CSB patient and the CSB model is observed in the case of TTD: The TTD mice show increased sensitivity to experimental induction of skin cancer by UVB and chemicals, whereas TTD patients do not show elevated cancer incidence (De Boer, Hoeijmakers et al., unpublished results).

IMPLICATIONS FOR DIAGNOSIS AND TREATMENT

Clinical Heterogeneity and Pleiotropy Associated with Mutations in TFIIH

It is clear that the spectrum of diseases linked with mutations in the TFIIH subunits *XPB, XPD,* and *TTDA* is remarkably heterogeneous and pleiotropic. It includes seemingly unrelated symptoms as photosensitivity, predisposition to skin cancer, brittle hair and nails, neurodysmyelination, impaired sexual development, ichthyosis, and dental caries. The rare XP group B consists of only 6 patients: 4 had the XP-CS complex and two had TTD. The more common group D is associated with classic XP, combinations of XP and CS, and TTD[56,58,200] (see Table 28-4). The clinical variability in TTD is also apparent from the fact that at least seven disorders are thought to be identical or closely related to TTD. These include the following syndromes: Pollitt (MIM 275550), Tay (242170), Sabinas (211390), Netherton (256500), ONMR (258360), hair-brain (234050), and the Marinesco-Sjögren (248800) syndromes.[20,21] The occurrence of TTD in three distinct NER-deficient complementation groups argues against a chance association between genetic loci separately involved in NER and in brittle hair. Consistent with the idea that these processes are intimately connected is the recent identification of point mutations in the *XPD* and *XPB* genes in TTD patients[201,202] (Fig. 28-13) and the generation of TTD mice by introducing a specific mutation in the *XPD* gene.[199] The positions of the relatively large number of mapped XPD mutations and the three XPB mutations indicate that mutations resulting in XP, combined XP and CS (XP-CS), or TTD do not overlap (see Fig. 28-13). Therefore, these mutations may interfere with the functions of these genes in a specific manner, resulting in the three different phenotypes.

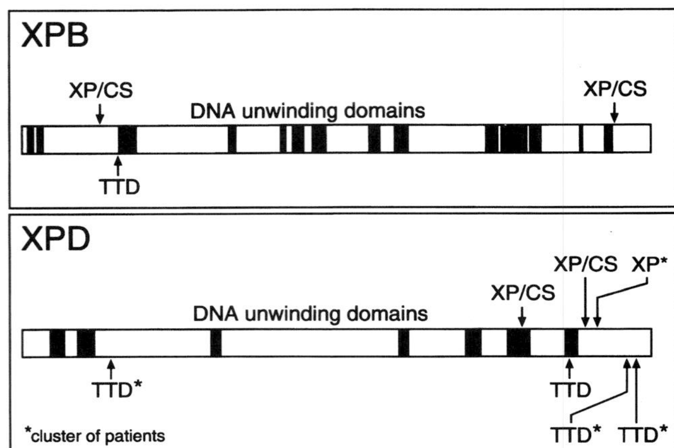

Fig. 28-13 Position of mutations in the *XPB* and *XPD* genes in patients with XP, XP-CS, and TTD. Clusters of different mutations causing TTD or XP were found at specific sites. (*From Broughton*[201] *and unpublished results.*)

The Clinical Features Derived from the NER Defect

In striking contrast to the pleiotropy and clinical heterogeneity selectively associated with XP-B and XP-D, the symptoms seen in the most common XP groups, A (totally deficient in NER) and C (defective in the GGR subpathway) are much more uniform. They involve photosensitivity, pigmentation abnormalities, predisposition to skin cancer, and in the case of XP-A, accelerated neurodegeneration (which is not associated with neurodysmyelination) but no CS and TTD symptoms. The gene products affected in these groups are not vital and therefore do not appear to be essential for basal transcription. This indicates that these forms of XP present the manifestations of a pure NER defect. The fact that XP-C is associated with a strong cancer predisposition suggests that the global genome subpathway is of major importance for preventing mutagenesis and carcinogenesis. This may provide a plausible explanation why, in CS, no significant cancer proneness is observed; CS patients still possess a potent GGR system. The TCR subpathway may be important for cell survival but less relevant for preventing mutagenesis, since it accomplishes — and only for some lesions — more rapid repair in only one of the strands of an active gene.

Evidence for the Involvement of Transcriptional Defects in CS and TTD

Mutations in subunits of the multifunctional and intricate TFIIH are envisioned to have multiple effects. The selective association of TFIIH with the peculiar forms of XP and the dual role of this complex in repair and transcription make it tempting to link the unexpected TTD and CS features with the additional transcription-related function of the NER genes involved. Indeed, it would be highly unlikely that all mutations in subunits of this bifunctional complex would only affect the repair function and leave the inherent transcriptional role entirely intact. This interpretation is supported by the phenotype of a *Drosophila ERCC3* mutant, *haywire*. This mutant displays UV sensitivity, CNS abnormalities, and impaired sexual development, as found in XP-B.[145] Spermatogenesis in *Drosophila* is very sensitive to the level of β_2-tubulin.[203] Mutations in the *Drosophila ERCC3* gene seem to affect β-tubulin expression, causing the male sterility.[145] It is therefore likely that expression of this gene in *Drosophila* (and, by inference, possibly in humans) is particularly sensitive to the level of transcription and thereby to subtle mutations in TFIIH. This could easily explain the immature sexual development found in TTD and CS. Expression of the myelin basic protein is known to be critically dependent on transcription. It has been demonstrated that reduced transcription of the myelin basic protein gene in mice causes neurologic abnormalities.[204] Thus the characteristic neurodysmyelination of CS and TTD[18,205] also may relate to suboptimal transcription of this or other genes involved in myelin sheath formation. Similarly, reduced transcription of genes encoding the class of ultrahigh-sulfur proteins of the hairshaft may account for the observed reduced cysteine content in the brittle hair of TTD patients[20] and TTD mice.[199] Experimental support for this hypothesis was obtained by the finding of reduced transcription of a skin-specific gene in the TTD mouse.[199] A comparable explanation is proposed for the poor enamelation of teeth in CS and TTD. Thus mutations in TFIIH that subtly disturb its transcription function may affect a specific subset of genes whose functioning critically depends on the level or fine-tuning of transcription. It is logical to suppose that strong secondary structures in a promoter requires full unwinding capacity, i.e., a maximally active complex, to permit efficient transcription. Recent studies indicate that the requirement for basal transcription factors may vary from promoter to promoter depending on the sequence around the initiation site, the topologic state of the DNA, and the local chromatin structure.[206] These mechanisms can readily explain the pronounced clinical heterogeneity even within families. Obviously, total inactivation of the transcription is lethal; this is consistent with the observation that deletion mutants of TFIIH subunits in yeast, *Drosophila,* and mice are inviable.[56,146] The narrow window of viable mutations also explains the rarity of these TFIIH-associated diseases.

As noted previously,[207] there are many parallels between CS and TTD, suggesting that they are manifestations of a broad clinical continuum. This is consistent with the finding that mutations in different subunits of the same (TFIIH) complex give rise to a similar set of CS and TTD features. Thus defects in *CSA* and *CSB* as well as *XPG* also may affect basal transcription because they give rise to a comparable phenotype (see also below).

Transcription and Repair/Transcription Syndromes

A tentative model proposed for the etiology of the defects in the conglomerate of CS, TTD, and related disorders is shown in Table 28-8. In this model, mutations in TFIIH subunits inactivating only the NER function result in an XP phenotype as observed in the classic patients of XP group D. If, in addition, the transcription function is subtly affected, the combination of XP and CS features is found. Theoretically, mutations causing a (still viable) transcription problem without NER impairment may be expected as well. Indeed, recently CS (-like) patients without an associated NER defect were identified.[73] This model fits with the observation of specific sites of mutations in XPB and XPD resulting in a XP, XP-CS, or TTD phenotype (see Fig. 28-13).

When CS features are due to mutations that cripple the transcription function of TFIIH, how can the differences between CS and TTD, i.e., the additional presence of brittle hair and nails in TTD, be rationalized? In view of the intrinsic properties of complexes such as TFIIH, it is likely that some mutations also will affect the stability of the complex. In fact, a significant proportion of TFIIH mutations in yeast yield a temperature-sensitive phenotype,[155] pointing to complex instability. It is feasible that such types of mutations also occur among TFIIH patients. As mentioned earlier, an exceptional TTD individual exhibited a reversible sudden, dramatic worsening of the brittleness of the hair formed during an episode of fever.[22] This fits with a human temperature-sensitive TFIIH mutation. Furthermore, it suggests that transcription of the genes for cysteine-rich matrix proteins of hair and nails is affected by TFIIH instability. In other cells, the steady-state levels of TFIIH may be sufficient, because *de novo* synthesis is high enough to cope with the reduced $t_{1/2}$ of the complex. However, the cysteine-rich matrix proteins are one of the last gene products produced in very large quantities in keratinocytes before they die. Thus the hallmark of TTD may be due to a TFIIH stability problem becoming overt in terminally differentiated cells that are exhausted for TFIIH before completion of their differentiation program.

Many TTD patients are not noticeably photosensitive and have normal NER.[73] According to the scheme in Table 28-8, these patients may have a TFIIH transcription and stability problem without concomitant impairment of the NER function of the

Table 28-8 Model for the Relation Between TFIIH Defects and Clinical Features

TFIIH-Related Disorder	NER	TFIIH Funcion* Transcription	Stability	Documented Gene Mutation
XP	−	+	+	*XPD*
XP-CS	−	+/−	+	*XPD, XPB, XPG*†
CS (photosensitive)	+/− ‡	+/−	+	*CSA, CSB*†
CS (nonphotosensitive)§	+	+/−	+	?
TTD (photosensitive)	−	+/−	+/−	*XPD, XPB, TTDA*
TTD (nonphotosensitive)§	+	+/−	+/−	?

* Symbol designation: +, normal repair or transcription function or stability of TFIIH; +/−, partly affected function/stability; −, severely impaired function.

† TFIIH transcription may be indirectly affected by mutations in *XPG, CSA,* and *CSB*. In addition, *XPG* affects total NER; *CSA* and *CSB* affect only transcription-coupled repair.

‡ Only the NER subpathway of transcription-coupled repair is distributed.

§ CS patients without a NER defect have been identified[74] (Jaspers, Kleijer, and Hoeijmakers unpublished observations). There may be many disorders related to nonphotosensitive variants of TTD and CS such as Netherton syndrome, brain-hair syndrome, Pollitt syndrome, etc.

complex. These findings extend the implications to non-repair-defective disorders. Therefore, and in view of the model's pronounced heterogeneity, it is possible that the Sjögren-Larsson (MIM 270200), RUD (308200), ICE (146720), OTD (257960), IFAP (308205), CAM(F)AK (212540), Rothmund-Thomson (268400), KID (242150), and COF syndromes[21,56] also fall within this category. Interestingly, some of these diseases show occurrence of skin cancer.

When the CS features in TTD are due to a basal transcription problem, this also should apply to the other complementation groups with CS patients, i.e., CS-A, CS-B, and XP-G. Although the CSA, CSB, and probably the XPG proteins are not vital and therefore not essential for transcription, they may influence TFIIH functioning indirectly (see Table 28-8). For instance, CSA and CSB could have an auxiliary function for TFIIH in transcription and in transcription-coupled (but not global genome) repair. Some XP-G (XP-CS) patients are more severely affected than XP-A patients,[24] although the latter are, in general, more defective in NER, suggesting that XPG has an additional, nonrepair function. Consistent with these considerations, interactions between TFIIH components and the CS proteins have been claimed.[98,152,177]

In conclusion, these findings provide evidence for the presence of a wide class of disorders that can collectively be called *transcription syndromes*.[207] A prediction from this model is that these patients carry mutations in transcription factors that do not affect the NER process. This explanation introduces a novel concept into human genetics. It can be envisioned that similar phenomena are associated with subtle defects in translation, implying the potential existence of translation syndromes.

Patient Care

Treatment. Treatment of XP, CS, and TTD patients is purely symptomatic. The discovery of the molecular defects in these disorders has not (yet) resulted in specific modalities for treatment.

Treatment of XP patients is a multifaceted process involving early diagnosis, genetic counseling, patient and family education, and regular monitoring of the skin.[208] The diagnosis is suspected in patients with marked sun sensitivity, photophobia, and/or early onset of freckling. Laboratory tests of UV sensitivity of fibroblasts and of excision repair confirm the diagnosis. Genetic counseling is directed toward acquainting the patients and their parents with the inherited aspects of the disease and its rarity, the increased risk for parents (with the 25 percent probability that the disease will appear among subsequent offspring), and the improbability of the patients having affected children.[2,21,209]

Patients should be shielded from sunlight by protective measures, including wearing two layers of clothing, using long hairstyles, wearing broad-brimmed hats and UV-absorbing sunglasses with side shields, and using chemical sunscreens with sun protection factor (SPF) numbers of 15 or higher. Patients should avoid direct exposure to sunlight, especially during the peak UV hours (about 10 A.M. to 3 P.M. in the continental United States) and indirect UV light reflected from snow or water. Window glass and many plastic shields for fluorescent lamps will absorb UV radiation indoors. Known chemical carcinogens such as tobacco smoke should be avoided. Patients and their families should be taught to examine their skin and to recognize and bring to medical attention any lesions suspected to be malignant. Color photographs are often useful for follow-up.

Malignant skin neoplasms are treated as in patients who do not have XP by excision, electrodesiccation, and curettage, cryosurgery, or chemosurgery. XP patients have received x-ray therapy for malignant skin tumors and have had a normal response.[208] Dermabrasion or dermatome shaving has been used in patients with multiple tumors, permitting the epidermis to be repopulated by cells from the hair follicles, which are relatively shielded from sunlight.[208] Total removal of the skin of the face with grafting of skin from sun-shielded areas has been used in extreme cases. Oral retinoids have been shown to prevent new skin cancers in XP patients but have many severe side effects.[210]

Nance and Berry[12] mention several measures that can be taken in management of CS patients, including monitoring of treatable complications of this condition such as hypertension, hearing loss, and dental carries. As in XP, photosensitive CS patients should avoid excessive sun exposure and use sunscreens when outdoors. If the condition is compatible with life into the teens and twenties (in the case of CSI), the neurologic and neurosensory capacities should be assessed periodically. This assessment of intellectual, social, visual, and auditory skills can help in providing appropriate home and school services for the patient. Nance and Berry[12] also recommend physical therapy directed toward preventing contractures and maintaining ambulation in the older patient.

Although little is known about the treatment of TTD patients, the overlap of clinical symptoms in TTD and CS (neurologic and growth defects) indicates comparable management of patients suffering from these diseases.

Prenatal Diagnosis. Since the NER-deficiency syndromes have autosomal recessive inheritance, parents of an affected child face a high risk of recurrence (25 percent) in subsequent pregnancies. Prenatal diagnosis is possible if the deficiency has been demonstrated unequivocally in cultured skin fibroblasts of the index patient.

Early reports of prenatal diagnosis of XP concern the analysis of UDS in cultured amniocytes.[211,212] This approach allows a relatively rapid diagnosis within 1 or 2 weeks after amniocentesis in the sixteenth week, since only a few cells are needed for the autoradiographic assessment of UDS. A much earlier diagnosis is possible, however, by chronic villus sampling (CVS) in the tenth to twelfth weeks of pregnancy. Autoradiographic analysis of the early outgrowths of cells from the villi then allows a first-trimester diagnosis. Successful prenatal diagnoses using chorionic villus cells have been reported for XP and TTD.[22,213,214] The TCR defect in CS can be demonstrated indirectly by measuring the recovery of RNA or DNA synthesis after UV exposure of cultured cells. The reliability of this test for the (postnatal) diagnosis of CS using cultured skin fibroblasts has been shown extensively. Cases of prenatal diagnosis using amniocytes[48] and chorionic villus cells[213] have been reported. Because of the earlier stage of sampling, the use of chronic villus cells may be prefered, but the present experience for CS is very small. Therefore, if initial results on the chorionic villus cells suggest a normal fetus, it may be considered to confirm the diagnosis by amniocentesis. Mutation analysis using DNA from uncultured chorion villi would, in principle, allow reliable and early diagnosis. This requires knowledge of the gene involved and of the mutations in the family. In general, it may not be practical to search for these mutations in these rare diseases unless common mutations are known, as reported for Japanese XP-A patients.[215]

Note added in proof. In 1999 the gene responsible for the variant from of XP has been cloned (Masutani et al.: *Nature* **399**:700, 1999; and Johnson et al.: *Science* **285**:263, 1999).

ACKNOWLEDGMENTS

We are indebted to all members of the DNA repair group of the Medical Genetics Centre South-West Netherlands (MGC) for valuable and stimulating discussions and for providing new information for this chapter. We thank Dr. W. J. Kleijer, Dr. M. F. Niermeijer, and Dr. P. C. Hanawalt for a thoughtful review of the manuscript and Rita Boucke (secretary), Mirko Kuit (photography), Wim Vermeulen, Koos Jaspers, Geert Weeda, Bert van der Horst, Wouter de Laat, and Jan de Boer for their help in preparing this chapter. The research of the MGC group is supported by the Dutch Cancer Society, the Netherlands Organization for Scientific Research (NWO) through the Foundations of Medical Sciences and Chemical Sciences, the Commission of the European Community, and the Louis Jeantet Foundation.

REFERENCES

1. Friedberg EC, Walker GC, Siede W: *DNA Repair and Mutagenesis*. Washington, ASM Press, 1995.
2. Kraemer KH, Lee MM, Scotto J: Xeroderma pigmentosum: Cutaneous, ocular and neurologic abnormalities in 830 published cases. *Arch Dermatol* **123**:241, 1987.
3. von Hebra F, Kaposi M: *On diseases of the Skin, Including the Exanthemata*, vol 3, trans by W. Tay. London, New Sydenham Society, 1874, p 252.
4. Neisser A: Ueber das Xeroderma pigmentosum (Kaposi) lioderma essentialis cum melanosi et telangiectasia. *Viertel Dermatol Syphil* 47, 1883.
5. DeSanctis C, Cacchione A: Lidiozia xerodermica. *Riv Sper Freniatr* **56**:269, 1932.
6. See reference(s) cited in: Cleaver JE, Kraemer KH: Xeroderma pigmentosum and Cockayne syndrome, in Scriver CR, Beaudet AL, Sly WS, Valle D (eds): *The Metabolic and Molecular Bases of Inherited Disease*, 7th ed. New York, McGraw-Hill, 1995, p 4393.
7. Takebe H, Nishigori C, Satoh Y: Genetics and skin cancer of xeroderma pigmentosum in Japan. *Jpn J Cancer Res (Gann)* **78**:1135, 1987.
8. Kraemer KH, Lee MM, Andrews AD, Lambert WC: The role of sunlight and DNA repair in melanoma and non-melanoma skin cancer: The xeroderma pigmentosum paradigm. *Arch Dermatol* **130**:1018, 1994.
9. Mimaki T, Itoh N, Abe J, Tagawa T, Sato K, Yabuuchi H, Takebe H: Neurological manifestations of xeroderma pigmentosum. *Ann Neurol* **20**:70, 1986.
10. Robbins JH, Brumback RA, Mendiones M, Barrett SF, Carl JR, Cho S, Denckla MB, Ganges MB, Gerber LH, Guthrie RA, Meer J, Moshell AN, Polinsky RJ, Ravin PD, Sonies BC, Tarone RE: Neurological disease in xeroderma pigmentosum: Documentation of a late onset type of the juvenile onset form. *Brain* **114**:1335, 1991.
11. Andrews AD, Barrett SF, Robbins JH: Xeroderma pigmentosum neurological abnormalities correlate with colony-forming ability after ultraviolet radiation. *Proc Natl Acad Sci USA* **75**:1984, 1978.
12. Nance MA, Berry SA: Cockayne syndrome: Review of 140 cases. *Am J Med Genet* **42**:68, 1992.
13. Lehmann AR: Nucleotide excision repair and the link with transcription. *Trends Biochem Sci* **20**:402, 1995.
14. Price VH, Odom RB, War WH, Jones FT: Trichothiodystrophy: Sulfur-deficient brittle hair as a marker for a neuroectodermal symptom complex. *Arch Dermatol* **116**:1378, 1980.
15. Tsambaos D, Nikiforidis G, Balas C, Marinoni S: Trichothiodystrophic hair reveals an abnormal pattern of viscoelastic parameters. *Skin Pharmacol* **7**:257, 1994.
16. van Neste DJJ, Gillespie JM, Marshall RC, Taieb A, de Brouwer B: Morphological and biochemical characteristics of trichothiodystrophy-variant hair are maintained after grafting of scalp specimens on to nuce mice. *Br J Dermatol* **128**:384, 1993.
17. Chen E, Cleaver JE, Weber CA, Packman S, Barkovich AJ, Koch TK, Williams ML, Golabi M, Price VH: Trichothiodystrophy: Clinical spectrum, central nervous system imaging, and biochemical characterization of two siblings. *J Invest Dermatol* **103**:154, 1994.
18. Peserico A, Battistella PA, Bertoli P: MRI of a very hereditary ectodermal dysplasia: PIBI(D)S. *Neuroradiology* **34**:316, 1992.
19. Tolmie JL, de Berker D, Dawber R, Galloway C, Gergory DW, Lehmann AR, McClure J, Pollitt JR, Stephenson JPB: Syndromes associated with trichothiodystrophy. *Clin Dysmorphol* **1**:1, 1994.
20. Itin PH, Pittelkow MR: Trichothiodystrophy: Review of sulfur-deficient brittle hair syndromes and association with the ectodermal dysplasias. *J Am Acad Dermatol* **22**:705, 1990.
21. McKusick VA: *Mendelian Inheritance in Man*, 11th ed. Baltimore, Johns Hopkins University Press, 1994.
22. Kleijer WJ, Beemer FA, Boom BW: Intermittent hair loss in a child with PIBI(D)S syndrome and trichothiodystrophy with defective DNA repair—Xeroderma pigmentosum group D. *Am J Med Gen* **52**:227, 1994.
23. Robbins JH, Kraemer KH, Lutzner MA, Festoff BW, Coon HG: Xeroderma pigmentosum: An inherited disease with sun sensitivity, multiple cutaneous neoplasms and abnormal DNA repair. *Ann Intern Med* **80**:221, 1974.
24. Hamel BCJ, Raams A, Schuitema-Dijkstra AR, Simons P, van der Burgt I, Jaspers NGJ, Kleijer WJ: Xeroderma pigmentosum-Cockayne syndrome complex: A further case. *J Med Genet* **33**:607, 1996.
25. Moriwaki SI, Stefanini M, Lehmann AR, Hoeijmakers JHJ, Robbins JH, Rapin I, Botta E, Tanganelli B, Vermeulen W, Broughton BC, Kraemer KH: DNA repair and ultraviolet mutagenesis in cells from a new patient with xeroderma pigmentosum group G and Cockayne syndrome resemble xeroderma pigmentosum cells. *J Invest Dermatol* **107**:647, 1996.
26. Setlow RB: The wavelengths in sunlight effective in producing skin cancer: A theoretical analysis. *Proc Natl Acad Sci USA* **71**:3363, 1974.
27. Epstein JH: Ultraviolet carcinogenesis. *Photophysiology* **5**:235, 1970.
28. Blum HF: *Carcinogenesis by Ultraviolet Light*. Princeton, NJ, Princeton University Press, 1959.
29. Cleaver JE: Repair processes for photochemical damage in mammalian cells, in Lett JT, Adler H, Zelle M (eds): *Advances in Radiation Biology*. New York, Academic Press, 1974, p 1.
30. Lawrence C: The Rad6 DNA repair pathway in *Saccharomyces cerevisiae*: What does it do and how does it do it? *Bioessays* **16**:253, 1994.
31. Todo T, Takemori H, Ryo H, Ihara M, Matsunaga T, Nikaido O, Sato K, Nomura T: A new photoreactivating enzyme that specifically repairs ultraviolet light-induced [6-4] photoproducts. *Nature* **361**:371, 1993.
32. Todo T, Ryo H, Yamamoto K, Toh H, Inui T, Ayaki H, Nomura T, Ikenaga M: Similarity among *Drosophila* [6-4] photolyase, a human photolyase homolog, and the DNA photolyase-blue-light photoreceptor family. *Science* **272**:109, 1996.
33. Sancar A, Sancar GB: DNA repair enzymes. *Annu Rev Biochem* **57**:29, 1988.
34. van Houten B: Nucleotide excision repair in *Escherichia coli*. *Microbiol Rev* **54**:18, 1990.
35. Grossman L, Thiagalingam S: Nucleotide excision repair, a tracking mechanism in search of damage. *J Biol Chem* **268**:16871, 1993.
36. Hoeijmakers JHJ: Nucleotide excision repair: I. From *E. coli* to yeast. *Trends Genet* **9**:173, 1993.
37. Bohr VA: Gene specific DNA repair. *Carcinogenesis* **12**:1983, 1991.
38. Hanawalt P, Mellon I: Stranded in an active gene. *Curr Biol* **3**:67, 1993.
39. Cleaver JE: Defective repair replication of DNA in xeroderma pigmentosum. *Nature* **218**:652, 1968.
40. Epstein JH, Fukuyama K, Reed WB, Epstein WL: Defect in DNA synthesis in skin of patients with xeroderma pigmentosum demonstrated in vivo. *Science* **168**:1477, 1970.
41. Stefanini M, Vermeulen W, Weeda G, Giliani S, Nardo T, Mezzina M, Sarasin A, Harper JL, Arlett CF, Hoeijmakers JHJ, Lehmann AR: A new nucleotide-excision-repair gene associated with the disorder trichothiodystrophy. *Am J Hum Genet* **53**:817, 1993.
42. Bootsma D, Mulder MP, Pot F, Cohen JA: Different inherited levels of DNA repair replication in xeroderma pigmentosum cell strains after exposure to ultraviolet irradiation. *Mutat Res* **9**:507, 1970.
43. Cleaver JE: Xeroderma pigmentosum: Variants with normal DNA repair and normal sensitivity to ultraviolet light. *J Invest Dermatol* **58**:124, 1972.
44. Lehmann AR, Kirk-Bell S, Arlett CF, Paterson MC, Lohman PHM, de Weerd-Kastelein EA, Bootsma D: Xeroderma pigmentosum cells with normal levels of excision repair have a defect in DNA synthesis after UV-irradiation. *Proc Natl Acad Sci USA* **72**:219, 1975.
45. Bohr VA, Smith CA, Okumoto DS, Hanawalt PC: DNA repair in an active gene: removal of pyrimidine dimers from the DHFR gene of CHO cells is much more efficient than in the genome overall. *Cell* **40**:359, 1985.
46. Venema J, Mullenders LHF, Natarajan AT, van Zeeland AA, Mayne LV: The genetic defect in Cockayne syndrome is associated with a defect in repair of UV-induced DNA damage in transcriptionally active DNA. *Proc Natl Acad Sci USA* **87**:4707, 1990.
47. Tanaka K, Kawai K, Kumahara Y, Ikenaga M, Okada Y: Genetic complementation groups in Cockayne syndrome. *Somat Cell Genet* **7**:445, 1981.
48. Lehmann AR, Francis AJ, Gianelli F: Prenatal diagnosis of Cockayne syndrome. *Lancet* **1**:486, 1985.
49. Stefanini M, Lagomarsini P, Giliani S, Nardo T, Botta E, Peserico A, Kleijer WJ, Lehmann AR, Sarasin A: Genetic heterogeneity of the excision repair defect associated with trichothiodystrophy. *Carcinogenesis* **14**:1101, 1993.
50. Wade MH, Chu EHY: Effects of DNA damaging agents on cultured fibroblasts derived from patients with Cockayne syndrome. *Mutat Res* **59**:49, 1979.
51. McCormick JJ, Kately-Kohler S, Watanabe M, Maher VM: Abnormal sensitivity of human fibroblasts from xeroderma pigmentosum variants to transformation to anchorage independence by ultraviolet radiation. *Cancer Res* **46**:489, 1986.

52. Barrett SF, Robbins JH, Tarone RE, Kraemer KH: Defective repair of cyclobutane pyrimidine dimers with normal repair of other DNA photoproducts in a transcriptionally active gene transfected into Cockayne syndrome cells. *Mutat Res* **255**:281, 1991.
53. Parris CN, Kraemer KH: Ultraviolet induced mutations in Cockayne syndrome cells are primarily caused by cyclobutane dimer photoproducts while repair of other photoproducts is normal. *Proc Natl Acad Sci USA* **90**:7260, 1993.
54. de Weerd-Kastelein EA, Keijzer W, Bootsma D: Genetic heterogeneity of xeroderma pigmentosum demonstrated by somatic cell hybridization. *Nature New Biol* **238**:80, 1972.
55. Lehmann AR: Three complementation groups in Cockayne syndrome. *Mutat Res* **106**:347, 1982.
56. Vermeulen W, van Vuuren AJ, Chipoulet M, Schaeffer L, Appeldoorn E, Weeda G, Jaspers NGJ, Priestley A, Arlett CF, Lehmann AR, Stefanini M, Mezzina M, Sarasin A, Bootsma D, Egly J-M, Hoeijmakers JHJ: Three unusual repair deficiencies associated with transcription factor BTF2(TFIIH): Evidence for the existence of a transcription syndrome. *Cold Spring Harbor Symp Quant Biol* **59**:317, 1994.
57. Kraemer KH: Xeroderma pigmentosum, in Demis DJ, McGuire J (eds): *Clinical Dermatology*, vol 4. Philadelphia, Harper & Row, 1980, p 1.
58. Vermeulen W, Scott RJ, Potger S, Muller HJ, Cole J, Arlett CF, Kleijer WJ, Bootsma D, Hoeijmakers JHJ, Weeda G: Clinical heterogeneity within xeroderma pigmentosum associated with mutations in the DNA repair and transcription gene ERCC3. *Am J Hum Genet* **54**:191, 1994.
59. Scott RJ, Itin P, Kleijer WJ, Kolb K, Arlett C, Muller H: Xeroderma pigmentosum-Cockayne syndrome complex in two new patients: Absence of skin tumors despite severe deficiency of DNA excision repair. *J Am Acad Dermatol* **29**:883, 1993.
60. Mansbridge JN, Hanawalt PC: Domain-limited repair of DNA in ultraviolet fibroblasts from xeroderma pigmentosum complementation group C, in Friedberg EC, Bridges BA (eds): *Cellular Responses to DNA Damage*. New York, Alan R Liss, 1983, p 195.
61. Venema J, van Hoffen A, Natarajan AT, van Zeeland AA, Mullenders LHF: The residual repair capacity of xeroderma pigmentosum complementation group C fibroblasts is highly specific for transcriptionally active DNA. *Nucleic Acids Res* **18**:443, 1990.
62. Hananian J, Cleaver JE: Xeroderma pigmentosum exhibiting neurological disorders and systemic lupus erythematosus. *Clin Genet* **17**:39, 1980.
63. Lehmann AR, Arlett CF, Broughton BC, Harcourt SA, Steingrimsdottir H, Stefanini M, Malcolm A, Taylor R, Natarajan AT, Green S: Trichothiodystrophy, a human DNA repair disorder with heterogeneity in the cellular response to ultraviolet light. *Cancer Res* **48**:6090, 1988.
64. Wood RD: Seven genes for three diseases. *Nature* **350**:190, 1991.
65. Arase S, Kozuka T, Tanaka K, Ikenaga M, Takebe H: A sixth complementation group in xeroderma pigmentosum. *Mutat Res* **59**:143, 1979.
66. Nishigori C, Fujiwara H, Uyeno K, Kawaguchi T, Takebe H: Xeroderma pigmentosum patients belonging to complementation group F and efficient liquid recovery of ultraviolet damage. *Photodermatol Photoimmunol Photomed* **8**:146, 1991.
67. Vermeulen W, Jaeken J, Jaspers NGJ, Bootsma D, Hoeijmakers JHJ: Xeroderma pigmentosum complementation group G associated with Cockayne syndrome. *Am J Hum Genet* **53**:185, 1993.
68. Cooper PT, Nouspikel T, Clarkson S, Leadon S: Defective transcription-coupled repair of oxidative base damage in Cockayne syndrome patients from XP group G. *Science* **275**:990, 1997.
69. Nouspikel T, Lalle P, Leadon S, Cooper P, Clarkson S: A common mutational pattern in Cockayne syndrome patients from xeroderma pigmentosum group G: implications for a second XPG function. *Proc Natl Acad Sci USA* **94**:3116, 1997.
70. Jung EG: New form of molecular defect in xeroderma pigmentosum. *Nature* **228**:361, 1970.
71. Jaspers NGJ, Jansen-v.d., Kuilen G, Bootsma D: Complementation analysis of xeroderma pigmentosum variants. *Exp Cell Res* **136**:81, 1981.
72. Jorizzo JL, Atherton DJ, Crounse RG, Wells RS: Ichthyosis, brittle hair, impaired intelligence, decreased fertility and short stature (IBIDS syndrome). *Br J Dermatol* **106**:705, 1982.
73. Lehmann AR, Thompson AF, Harcourt SA, Stefanini M, Norris PG: Cockaynes syndrome: Correlation of clinical features with cellular sensitivity of RNA synthesis to UV irradiation. *J Med Genet* **30**:679, 1993.
74. Itoh T, Cleaver JE, Yamaizumi M: Cockayne syndrome complementation group B associated with xeroderma pigmentosum phenotype. *Hum Genet* **97**:176, 1996.
75. Itoh T, Ono T, Yamaizumi M: A new UV-sensitive syndrome not belonging to any complementation groups of xeroderma pigmentosum or Cockayne syndrome: Siblings showing biochemical characteristics of Cockayne syndrome without typical clinical manifestations. *Mutat Res* **314**:233, 1994.
76. Itoh T, Fujiwara Y, Ono T, Yamaizumi M: UVs syndrome, a new general category of photosensitive disorder with defective DNA repair, is distinct from xeroderma pigmentosum variant and rodent complementation group 1. *Am J Hum Genet* **56**:1267, 1995.
77. Lambert WC, Lambert MW: Co-recessive inheritance: a model for DNA repair, genetic disease and carcinogenesis. *Mutat Res* **145**:227, 1985.
78. Thompson LH, Busch DB, Brookman K, Mooney CL: Genetic diversity of UV-sensitive DNA repair mutants of Chinese hamster ovary cells. *Proc Natl Acad Sci USA* **78**:3734, 1981.
79. Collins AR: Mutant rodent cell lines sensitive to ultraviolet light, ionizing radiation and cross-linking agents: A comprehensive survey of genetic and biochemical characteristics. *Mutat Res* **293**:99, 1993.
80. Thompson LH: Somatic cell genetics approach to dissecting mammalian DNA repair. *Environ Mol Mutagen* **14**:264, 1989.
81. Westerveld A, Hoeijmakers JHJ, van Duin M, de Wit J, Odijk H, Pastink A, Wood RD, Bootsma D: Molecular cloning of a human DNA repair gene. *Nature* **310**:425, 1984.
82. Weber CA, Salazar EP, Stewart SA, Thompson LH: Molecular cloning and biological characterization of a human gene, ERCC2, that corrects the nucleotide excision repair defect in CHO UV5 cells. *Mol Cell Biol* **8**:1137, 1988.
83. Weeda G, van Ham RCA, Masurel R, Westerveld A, Odijk H, de Wit J, Bootsma D, van der Eb AJ, Hoeijmakers JHJ: Molecular cloning and biological characterization of the human excision repair gene ERCC-3. *Mol Cell Biol* **10**:2570, 1990.
84. Thompson LH, Brookman KW, Weber CA, Salazar EP, Reardon JT, Sancar A, Deng Z, Siciliano MJ: Molecular cloning of the human nucleotide-excision-repair gene ERCC4. *Proc Natl Acad Sci USA* **91**:6855, 1994.
85. Mudgett JS, MacInnes MA: Isolation of the functional human excision repair gene ERCC 5 by intercosmid recombination. *Genomics* **8**:623, 1990.
86. Troelstra C, Odijk H, de Wit J, Westerveld A, Thompson LH, Bootsma D, Hoeijmakers JHJ: Molecular cloning of the human DNA excision repair gene ERCC-6. *Mol Cell Biol* **10**:5806, 1990.
87. Weber CA, Thompson LH, Salazar EP: Characterization of ERCC2 and its correction of xeroderma pigmentosum group D, in *Proceedings of the American Association for Cancer Research Special Conference on Cellular Responses to Environmental DNA Damage, Banff, Canada*. December 1, 1991.
88. Flejter WL, McDaniel LD, Johns D, Friedberg EC, Schultz RA: Correction of xeroderma pigmentosum complementation group D mutant cell phenotypes by chromosome and gene transfer: involvement of the human ERCC2 DNA repair gene. *Proc Natl Acad Sci USA* **89**:261, 1992.
89. Weeda G, van Ham RCA, Vermeulen W, Bootsma D, van der Eb AJ, Hoeijmakers JHJ: A presumed DNA helicase encoded by ERCC-3 is involved in the human repair disorders xeroderma pigmentosum and Cockayne syndrome. *Cell* **62**:777, 1990.
90. Scherly D, Nouspikel T, Corlet J, Ucla C, Bairoch A, Clarkson SG: Complementation of the DNA repair defect in xeroderma pigmentosum group G cells by a human cDNA related to yeast RAD2. *Nature* **363**:182, 1993.
91. Troelstra C, van Gool A, de Wit J, Vermeulen W, Bootsma D, Hoeijmakers JHJ: ERCC6, a member of a subfamily of putative helicases, is involved in Cockayne syndrome and preferential repair of active genes. *Cell* **71**:939, 1992.
92. MacInnes MA, Dickson JA, Hernandez RR, Learmont D, Lin GY, Mudgett JS, Park MS, Schauer S, Reynolds RJ, Strniste GF, Yu JY: Human ERCC5 cDNA-cosmid complementation for excision repair and bipartite amino acid domains conserved with RAD proteins of *S. cerevisiae* and *S. pombe*. *Mol Cell Biol* **13**:6393, 1993.
93. O'Donovan A, Wood RD: Identical defects in DNA repair in xeroderma pigmentosum group G and rodent ERCC group 5. *Nature* **363**:185, 1993.
94. Fryns JP, Bulcke J, Verdu P, Carton H, Kleczkowska A, van den Berghe H: Apparent late-onset Cockayne syndrome and interstitial deletion of

the long arm of chromosome 10 [del(10)(q11.23q21.2)]. *Am J Med Genet* **40**:343, 1991.

95. Tanaka K, Satokata I, Ogita Z, Uchida T, Okada Y: Molecular cloning of a mouse DNA repair gene that complements the defect of group A xeroderma pigmentosum. *Proc Natl Acad Sci USA* **86**:5512, 1989.
96. Hoeijmakers JHJ, Odijk H, Westerveld A: Differences between rodent and human cell lines in the amount of integrated DNA after transfection. *Exp Cell Res* **169**:111, 1987.
97. Legerski R, Peterson C: Expression cloning of a human DNA repair gene involved in xeroderma pigmentosum group C. *Nature* **359**:70, 1992.
98. Henning KA, Li L, Iyer N, McDaniel L, Reagan MS, Legerski R, Schultz RA, Stefanini M, Lehmann AR, Mayne LV, Friedberg EC: The Cockayne syndrome group A gene encodes a WD repeat protein that interacts with CSB protein and a subunit of RNA polymerase II TFIIH. *Cell* **82**:555, 1995.
99. Itoh T, Shiomi T, Shiomi N, Harada Y, Wakasugi M, Matsunaga T, Nikaido O, Friedberg EC, Yamaizumi M: Rodent complementation group 8 (ERCC8) corresponds to Cockayne syndrome complementation group A. *Mutat Res* **362**:167, 1996.
100. Koken MH, Reynolds P, Jaspers-Dekker I, Prakash L, Prakash S, Bootsma D, Hoeijmakers JH: Structural and functional conservation of two human homologs of the yeast DNA repair gene RAD6. *Proc Natl Acad Sci USA* **88**:8865, 1991.
101. Jentsch S: The ubiquitin-conjugation system. *Annu Rev Genet* **26**:179, 1992.
102. Sijbers AM, de Laat WL, Ariza RR, Biggerstaff M, Wei YF, Moggs JG, Carter KC, Shell BK, Evans E, de Jong MC, Rademakers S, de Rooij J, Jaspers NGJ, Hoeijmakers JHJ, Wood RD: Xeroderma pigmentosum group F caused by a defect in a structure-specific DNA repair endonuclease. *Cell* **86**:811, 1996.
103. Masutani C, Sugasawa K, Yanagisawa J, Sonoyama T, Ui M, Enomoto T, Takio K, Tanaka K, van der Spek PJ, Bootsma D, Hoeijmakers JHJ, Hanaoka F: Purification and cloning of a nucleotide excision repair complex involving the xeroderma pigmentosum group C protein and a human homolog of yeast RAD23. *EMBO J* **13**:1831, 1994.
104. van Gool AJ, Verhage R, Swagemakers SMA, van de Putte P, Brouwer J, Troelstra C, Bootsma D, Hoeijmakers JHJ: RAD26, the functional S. cerevisiae homolog of the Cockayne syndrome B gene ERCC6. *EMBO J* **13**:5361, 1994.
105. Hwang BJ, Liao JC, Chu G: Isolation of a cDNA encoding a UV-damaged DNA binding factor defective in xeroderma pigmentosum group E cells. *Mutat Res* **362**:105, 1996.
106. Keeney S, Chang GJ, Linn S: Characterization of human DNA damage binding protein implicated in xeroderma pigmentosum E. *J Biol Chem* **268**:21293, 1993.
107. Keeney S, Eker APM, Brody T, Vermeulen W, Bootsma D, Hoeijmakers JHJ, Linn S: Correction of the DNA repair defect in xeroderma pigmentosum group E by injection of a DNA damage-binding protein. *Proc Natl Acad Sci USA* **91**:4053, 1994.
108. Shivji MKK, Kenny MK, Wood RD: Proliferating cell nuclear antigen is required for DNA excision repair. *Cell* **69**:367, 1992.
109. Sibghat-Ullah, Husain I, Carlton W, Sancar A: Human nucleotide excision repair in vitro: Repair of pyrimidine dimers, psoralen and cisplatin adducts by HeLa cell-free extract. *Nucleic Acids Res* **17**:4471, 1989.
110. Aboussekhra A, Biggerstaff M, Shivji MKK, Vilpo JA, Moncollin V, Podust VN, Protic M, Hubscher U, Egly J, Wood RD: Mammalian DNA nucleotide excision repair reconstituted with purified components. *Cell* **80**:859, 1995.
111. Mu D, Park C-H, Matsunaga T, Hsu DS, Reardon JT, Sancar A: Reconstitution of human DNA repair excision nuclease in a highly defined system. *J Biol Chem* **270**:2415, 1995.
112. Sugasawa K, Ng JMY, Masutani C, Iwai S, van der Spek PJ, Eker APM, Hanaoka F, Bootsma D, Hoeijmakers JHJ: Xeroderma pigmentosum group C protein complex is the initiator of global genome nucleotide excision repair. *Mol Cell* **2**: August, 1998.
113. Reardon J, Mu D, Sancar A: Overproduction, purification, and characterization of the XPC subunit of the human DNA repair excision nuclease. *J Biol Chem* **271**:19451, 1996.
114. Shivji MKK, Eker APM, Wood RD: DNA repair defect in xeroderma pigmentosum group C and complementing factor from HeLa cells. *J Biol Chem* **269**:22749, 1994.
115. Tanaka K, Miura N, Satokata I, Miyamoto I, Yoshida MC, Satoh Y, Kondo S, Yasui A, Okayama H, Okada Y: Analysis of a human DNA excision repair gene involved in group A xeroderma pigmentosum and containing a zinc-finger domain. *Nature* **348**:73, 1990.
116. Robins P, Jones CJ, Biggerstaff M, Lindahl T, Wood RD: Complementation of DNA repair in xeroderma pigmentosum group A cell extracts by a protein with affinity for damaged DNA. *EMBO J* **10**:3913, 1991.
117. Eker APM, Vermeulen W, Miura N, Tanaka K, Jaspers NGJ, Hoeijmakers JHJ, Bootsma D: Xeroderma pigmentosum group A correcting protein from calf thymus. *Mutat Res* **274**:211, 1992.
118. Miyamoto I, Miura N, Niwa H, Miyazaki J, Tanaka K: Mutational analysis of the structure and function of the xeroderma pigmentosum group A complementing protein. *J Biol Chem* **267**:12182, 1992.
119. Jones CJ, Wood RD: Preferential binding of the xeroderma pigmentosum group A complementing protein to damaged DNA. *Biochemistry* **32**:12096, 1993.
120. Asahina H, Kuraoka I, Shirakawa M, Morita EH, Miura N, Miyamoto I, Ohtsuka E, Okada Y, Tanaka K: The XPA protein is a zinc metalloprotein with an ability to recognize various kinds of DNA damage. *Mutat Res* **315**:29, 1994.
121. Miura N, Miyamoto I, Asahina H, Satokata I, Tanaka K, Okada Y: Identification and characterization of XPAC protein, the gene product of the human XPAC (xeroderma pigmentosum group A complementing) gene. *J Biol Chem* **266**:19786, 1991.
122. Bankmann M, Prakash L, Prakash S: Yeast RAD14 and human xeroderma pigmentosum group A DNA repair genes encode homologous proteins. *Nature* **355**:555, 1992.
123. Guzder SN, Sung P, Prakash L, Prakash S: Yeast DNA-repair gene RAD14 encodes a zinc metalloprotein with affinity for ultraviolet-damaged DNA. *Proc Natl Acad Sci USA* **90**:5433, 1993.
124. Chu G, Chang E: Xeroderma pigmentosum group E cells lack a nuclear factor that binds to damaged DNA. *Science* **242**:564, 1988.
125. Kataoka H, Fujiwara Y: UV damage-specific DNA protein in xeroderma pigmentosum complementation group E. *Biochem Biophys Res Commun* **175**:1139, 1991.
126. Keeney S. Wein H, Linn S: Biochemical heterogeneity in xeroderma pigmentosum complementation group E. *Mutat Res* **273**:49, 1992.
127. Hwang BJ, Chu G: Purification and characterization of a human protein that binds to damaged DNA. *Biochemistry* **32**:1657, 1993.
128. Nichols AF, Ong P, Linn S: Mutations specific to the xeroderma pigmentosum group E Ddb(—) phenotype. *J Biol Chem* **271**:24317, 1996.
129. Takao M, Abramic M, Moos M, Otrin VR, Wootton JC, Mclenigan M, Levine AS, Protic M: A 127 kDa component of a UV-damaged DNA-binding complex which is defective in some xeroderma pigmentosum group E patients is homologous to a slime mold protein. *Nucleic Acids Res* **21**:4111, 1993.
130. Reardon JT, Nichols AF, Keeney S, Smith CA, Taylor JS, Linn S, Sancar A: Comparative analysis of binding of human damaged DNA-binding protein (XPE) and *Escherichia coli* damage recognition protein (UvrA) to the major ultraviolet photoproducts T[CS]TT[Ts] TT[6-4]T and T[Dewar]T. *J Biol Chem* **268**:21301, 1993.
131. Li L, Elledge SJ, Peterson CA, Bales ES, Legerski RJ: Specific association between the human DNA repair proteins XPA and ERCC1. *Proc Natl Acad Sci USA* **91**:5012, 1994.
132. Park C-H, Sancar A: Formation of a ternary complex by human XPA, ERCC1 and ERCC4(XPF) excision repair proteins. *Proc Natl Acad Sci USA* **91**:5017, 1994.
133. Saijo M, Kuraoka I, Masutani C, Hanaoka F, Tanaka K: Sequential binding of DNA repair proteins RPA and ERCC1 to XPA in vitro. *Nucleic Acids Res* **24**:4719, 1996.
134. He Z, Henricksen LA, Wold MS, Ingles CJ: RPA involvement in the damage and incision step of nucleotide excision repair. *Nature* **374**:566, 1995.
135. Park C-H, Mu D, Reardon JT, Sancar A: The general transcription-repair factor TFIIH is recruited to the excision repair complex by the XPA protein independent of the TFIIE transcription factor. *J Biol Chem* **270**:4896, 1995.
136. Nocentini S, Coin F, Saijo M, Tanaka K, Egly J: DNA damage recognition by XPA protein promotes efficient recruitment of transcription factor II H. *J Biol Chem* **272**:22991, 1997.
137. Bootsma D, Kraemer KH, Cleaver JE, Hoeijmakers JHJ: Nucleotide excision repair syndromes: xeroderma pigmentosum, Cockayne syndrome and trichothiodystrophy, in Vogelstein B, Kinzler KW (eds): *The Genetic Basis of Human Cancer*. New York, McGraw-Hill, 1998, p. 245.
138. Park H-W, Kim S-T, Sancar A, Deisenhofer J: Crystal structure of DNA photolyase from *Escherichia coli*. *Science* **268**:1866, 1995.
139. Evans E, Moggs J, Hwang J, Egly J, Wood R: Mechanisms of open complex and dual incision formation by nucleotide excision repair factors. *EMBO J* **16**:6559, 1997.

140. Mu D, Wakasugi M, Hsu D, Sancar A: Characterization of reaction intermediates of excision repair nuclease. *J Biol Chem* **272**:28971, 1997.
141. Coverley D, Kenny MK, Lane DP, Wood RD: A role for the human single-stranded DNA binding protein HSSB/RPA in an early stage of nucleotide excision repair. *Nucleic Acids Res* **20**:3873, 1992.
142. Wakasugi M, Reardon J, Sancar A: The non-catalytic function of XPG protein during dual incision in human nucleotide excision repair. *J Biol Chem* **272**:16030, 1997.
143. Naumovski L, Friedberg EC: A DNA repair gene required for the incision of damaged DNA is essential for viability in *Saccharomyces cerevisiae*. *Proc Natl Acad Sci USA* **80**:4818, 1983.
144. Park E, Guzder S, Koken MHM, Jaspers-Dekker I, Weeda G, Hoeijmakers JHJ, Prakash S, Prakash L: RAD25, a yeast homolog of human xeroderma pigmentosum group B DNA repair gene is essential for viability. *Proc Natl Acad Sci USA* **89**:11416, 1992.
145. Mounkes LC, Jones RS, Liang B-C, Gelbart W, Fuller MT: A *Drosophila* model for xeroderma pigmentosum and Cockayne syndrome: Haywire encodes the fly homolog of ERCC3, a human excision repair gene. *Cell* **71**:925, 1992.
146. de Boer J, Donker I, de Wit J, Hoeijmakers JHJ, Weeda G: Disruption of the mouse XPD DNA repair/basal transcription gene results in preimplantation lethality. *Cancer Res* **58**:89, 1998.
147. Schaeffer L, Roy R, Humbert S, Moncollin V, Vermeulen W, Hoeijmakers JHJ, Chambon P, Egly J: DNA repair helicase: A component of BTF2 (TFIIH) basic transcription factor. *Science* **260**:58, 1993.
148. Conaway RC, Conaway JW: General initiation factors for RNA polymerase II. *Annu Rev Biochem* **62**:161, 1993.
149. Feaver WJ, Svejstrup JQ, Henry NL, Kornberg RD: Relationship of CDK-activating kinase and RNA polymerase II CTD kinase TFIIH/TFIIK. *Cell* **79**:1103, 1994.
150. Roy R, Adamczewski JP, Seroz T, Vermeulen W, Tassan J-P, Schaeffer L, Nigg EA, Hoeijmakers JHJ, Egly J: The MO15 cell cycle kinase is associated with the TFIIH transcription repair factor. *Cell* **79**:1093, 1994.
151. Schaeffer L, Moncollin V, Roy R, Staub A, Mezzina M, Sarasin A, Weeda G, Hoeijmakers JHJ, Egly JM: The ERCC2/DNA repair protein is associated with the class II BTF2/TFIIH transcription factor. *EMBO J* **13**:2388, 1994.
152. Drapkin R, Reardon JT, Ansari A, Huang JC, Zawel L, Ahn K, Sancar A, Reinberg D: Dual role of TFIIH in DNA excision repair and in transcription by RNA polymerase II. *Nature* **368**:769, 1994.
153. van Vuuren AJ, Vermeulen W, Ma L, Weeda G, Appeldoorn E, Jaspers NGJ, van der Eb AJ, Bootsma D, Hoeijmakers JHJ, Humbert S, Schaeffer L, Egly J-M: Correction of xeroderma pigmentosum repair defect by basal transcription factor BTF2(TFIIH). *EMBO J* **13**:1645, 1994.
154. Humbert S, van Vuuren AJ, Lutz Y, Hoeijmakers JHJ, Egly J-M, Moncollin V: Characterization of p44/SSL1 and p34 subunits of the BTF2/TFIIH transcription/repair factor. *EMBO J* **13**:2393, 1994.
155. Wang Z, Buratowski S, Svejstrup JQ, Feaver WJ, Wu X, Kornberg RD, Donahue TD, Friedberg EC: The yeast TFB1 and SSL1 genes, which encode subunits of transcription factor IIH, are required for nucleotide excision repair and RNA polymerase II transcription. *Mol Cell Biol* **15**:2288, 1995.
156. Feaver WJ, Svejstrup JQ, Bardwell L, Bardwell AJ, Buratowski S, Gulyas KD, Donahue TF, Friedberg EC, Kornberg RD: Dual roles of a multiprotein complex from S. cerevisiae in transcription and DNA repair. *Cell* **75**:1379, 1993.
157. Guzder SN, Sung P, Bailly V, Prakash L, Prakash S: RAD25 is a DNA helicase required for DNA repair and RNA polymerase II transcription. *Nature* **369**:578, 1994.
158. Svejstrup JQ, Want Z, Feaver WJ, Wu X, Bushnell DA, Donahue TF, Friedberg EC, Kornberg RD: Different forms of TFIIH for transcription and DNA repair: holo-TFIIH and a nucleotide excision repairosome. *Cell* **80**:21, 1995.
159. Wang Z, Svejstrup JQ, Feaver WJ, Wu X, Kornberg RD, Friedberg EC: Transcription factor b (TFIIH) is required during nucleotide excision repair in yeast. *Nature* **368**:74, 1994.
160. Okhuma Y: Multiple functions of general transcription factors TFIIE and TFIIH: Possible points of regulation by trans-acting factors. *J Biochem* **122**:481, 1997.
161. Matsunaga T, Mu D, Park C-H, Reardon JT, Sancar A: Human DNA repair excision nuclease: Analysis of the roles of the subunits involved in dual incisions by using anti-XPG and anti-ERCC1 antibodies. *J Biol Chem* **270**:20862, 1995.
162. O'Donovan A, Davies AA, Moggs JG, West SC, Wood RD: XPG endonuclease makes the 3′ incision in human DNA nucleotide excision repair. *Nature* **371**:432, 1994.
163. de Laat WL, Appeldoorn E, Jaspers NGJ, Hoeijmakers JHJ: DNA structural elements required for ERCC1-XPF endonuclease activity. *J Biol Chem* **273**:7835, 1998.
164. van Vuuren AJ, Appeldoorn E, Odijk H, Yasui A, Jaspers NGJ, Bootsma D, Hoeijmakers JHJ: Evidence for a repair enzyme complex involving ERCC1 and complementing activities of ERCC4, ERCC11 and xeroderma pigmentosum group F. *EMBO J* **12**:3693, 1993.
165. Biggerstaff M, Szymkowski DE, Wood RD: Co-correction of ERCC1, ERCC4 and xeroderma pigmentosum group F DNA repair defects in vitro. *EMBO J* **12**:3685, 1993.
166. Bardwell AJ, Bardwell L, Tomkinson AE, Friedberg EC: Specific cleavage of model recombination and repair intermediates by the yeast Rad1-Rad10 DNA endonuclease. *Science* **265**:2082, 1994.
167. Davies AA, Friedberg EC, Tomkinson AE, Wood RD, West SC: Role of the Rad1 and Rad10 proteins in nucleotide excision repair and recombination. *J Biol Chem* **270**:24638, 1995.
168. Fishman-Lobell J, Haber JE: Removal of nonhomologous DNA ends in double-strand break recombination: The role of the yeast ultraviolet repair gene RAD1. *Science* **258**:480, 1992.
169. Saffran WA, Greenberg RB, Thaler MS, Jones MM: Single strand and double strand DNA damage-induced reciprocal recombination in yeast: Dependence on nucleotide excision repair and RAD1 recombination. *Nucleic Acids Res* **22**:2823, 1994.
170. Schiestl RH, Prakash S: RAD10, an excision repair gene of *Saccharomyces cerevisiae* is involved in the RAD1 pathway of mitotic recombination. *Mol Cell Biol* **10**:2485, 1990.
171. Evans E, Fellows J, Coffer A, Wood RD: Open complex formation around a lesion during nucleotide excision repair provides a structure for cleavage by human XPG protein. *EMBO J* **16**:625 1997.
172. Huang JC, Svoboda DL, Reardon JT, Sancar A: Human nucleotide excision nuclease removes thymine dimers from DNA by incising the 22nd phosphodiester bond 5′ and the 6th phosphodiester bond 3′ to the photodimer. *Proc Natl Acad Sci USA* **89**:3664, 1992.
173. Moggs JG, Yarema KJ, Essigmann JM, Wood RD: Analysis of incision sites produced by human cell extracts and purified proteins during nucleotide excision repair of a 1,3- intrastrand d(GpTpG)-cisplatin adduct. *J Biol Chem* **271**:7177,1996.
174. Svoboda DL, Taylor JS, Hearst JE, Sancar A: DNA repair by eukaryotic endonuclease. *J Biol Chem* **268**:1931, 1993.
175. Mu D, Hsu DS, Sancar A: Reaction mechanism of human DNA repair excision nuclease. *J Biol Chem* **271**:8285, 1996.
176. Bardwell AJ, Bardwell L, Iyer N, Svejstrup JQ, Feaver WJ, Kornberg RD, Friedberg EC: Yeast nucleotide excision repair proteins rad2 and rad4 interact with RNA polymerase II basal transcription factor b (TFIIH). *Mol Cell Biol* **14**:3569, 1994.
177. Iyer N, Reagan MS, Wu K-J, Canagarajah B, Friedberg EC: Interactions involving the human RNA polymerase II transcription/nucleotide excision repair complex TFIIH, the nucleotide excision repair protein XPG, and Cockayne syndrome group B (CSB) protein. *Biochemistry* **35**:2157, 1996.
178. Nichols AF, Sancar A: Purification of PCNA as a nucleotide excision repair protein. *Nucleic Acids Res* **20**:2441, 1992.
179. Barnes DE, Tomkinson AE, Lehmann AR, Webster ADB, Lindahl T: Mutations in the DNA ligase 1 gene of an individual with immunodeficiencies and cellular hypersensitivity to DNA-damaging agents. *Cell* **69**:495, 1992.
180. Verhage R, Zeeman A, de Groot N, Gleig F, Bang D, van der Putte P, Brouwer J: The RAD7 and RAD16 genes are essential for repair of non-transcribed DNA in *Saccharomyces cerevisiae*. *Mol Cell Biol* **14**:6135, 1994.
181. Venema J, van Hoffen A, Karcagi V, Natarajan AT, van Zeeland AA, Mullenders LHF: Xeroderma pigmentosum complementation group C cells remove pyrimidine dimers selectively from the transcribed strand of active genes. *Mol Cell Biol* **11**:4128, 1991.
182. Perozzi G, Prakash S: RAD7 of *Saccharomyces cerevisiae*: Transcripts, nucleotide sequence analysis and functional relationship between the RAD7 and RAD23 gene products. *Mol Cell Biol* **6**:1497, 1986.
183. Bang DD, Verhage R, Goosen N, Brouwer J, Putte PVD: Molecular cloning of RAD16, a gene involved in differential repair in *Saccharomyces cerevisiae*. *Nucleic Acids Res* **20**:3925, 1992.
184. Wolffe AP: Switched-on chromatin. *Curr Biol* **4**:525, 1994.
185. Neer EJ, Schmidt CJ, Nambudripad R, Smith TF: The ancient regulatory-protein family of WD-repeat proteins. *Nature* **371**:297, 1994.

186. Selby C, Sancar A: Human transcription-repair coupling factor CSB/ERCC6 is a DNA-stimulatedATPase but is not a helicase and does not disrupt the ternary transcription complex of stalled RNA polymerase II. *J Biol Chem* **272**:1885, 1997.
187. Donahue BH, Yin S, Taylor J-S, Reines D, Hanawalt PC: Transcript cleavage by RNA polymerase II arrested by a cyclobutane pyrimidine dimer in the DNA template. *Proc Natl Acad Sci USA* **91**:8502, 1994.
188. Tantin D, Kansal A, Carey M: Recruitment of the putative transcription-repair coupling factor CSB/ERCC6 to RNA polymerase II elongation complexes. *Mol Cell Biol* **17**:6803, 1997.
189. van Gool A, Citterio E, Rademakers S, van Os R, Vermeulen W, Constantinou A, Egly J, Bootsma D, Hoeijmakers J: The Cockayne syndrome B protein, involved in transcription-coupled DNA repair, resides in a RNA polymerase II-containing complex. *EMBO J* **16**:5955, 1997.
190. van Gool A, van der Horst G, Citterio E, Hoeijmakers J: Cockayne syndrome: Defective repair of transcription? *EMBO J* **16**:4155, 1997.
191. Nagai A, Saijo M, Kuraoka I, Matsuda T, Kodo N, Nakatsu Y, Mimaki T, Mino M, Biggerstaff M, Wood RD, Sijbers A, Hoeijmakers JHJ, Tanaka K: Enhancement of damage-specific DNA binding of XPA by interaction with the ERCC1 DNA repair protein. *Biochem Biophys Res Commun* **211**:960, 1995.
192. McWhir J, Seldridge J, Harrison DJ, Squires S, Melton DW: Mice with DNA repair gene (ERCC-1) deficiency have elevated levels of p53, liver nuclear abnormalities and die before weaning. *Nature Genet* **5**:217, 1993.
193. van Duin M, Vredeveldt G, Mayne LV, Odijk H, Vermeulen W, Klein B, Weeda G, Hoeijmakers JHJ, Bootsma D, Westerveld A: The cloned human DNA excision repair gene ERCC-1 fails to correct xeroderma pigmentosum complementation groups A through I. *Mutat Res* **217**:83, 1989.
194. Weeda G, Donker I, de Wit J, Morreau H. Janssens R, Vissers CJ, Nigg A, van Steeg H, Bootsma D, Hoeijmakers JHJ: Disruption of mouse ERCC1 results in a novel repair syndrome with growth failure, nuclear abnormalities and senescence. *Curr Biol* **7**:427, 1997.
195. Nakane H, Takeuchi S, Yuba S, Saijo M, Nakatsu Y, Ishikawa T, Hirota S, Kitamura Y, Kato Y, Tsunoda Y, Miyauchi H, Horio T, Tokunaga T, Matsunaga T, Nikaido O, Nishimune Y, Okada Y, Tanaka K: High incidence of ultraviolet-B or chemical-carcinogen-induced skin tumours in mice lacking the xeroderma pigmentosum group A gene. *Nature* **377**:165, 1995.
196. de Vries A, van Oostrom CTM, Hofhuis FMA, Dortant PM, Berg RJW, de Gruijl FR, Wester PW, van Kreijl CF, Capel PJA, van Steeg H, Verbeek SJ: Increased susceptibility to ultraviolet-B and carcinogens of mice lacking the DNA excision repair gene XPA. *Nature* **377**:169, 1995.
197. Sands AT, Abuin A, Sanchez A, Conti CJ, Bradley A: High susceptibility to ultraviolet-induced carcinogenesis in mice lacking XPC. *Nature* **377**:162, 1995.
198. van der Horst GTJ, van Steeg H, Berg RJW, van Gool AJ, de Wit J, Weeda G, Morreau H, Beems RB, van Kreijl CF, de Gruijl FR, Bootsma D, Hoeijmakers JHJ: Defective transcription-coupled repair in Cockayne syndrome B mice is associated with skin cancer predisposition. *Cell* **89**:425, 1997.
199. De Boer J, de Wit, van Steeg H, Berg RJW, Morreau H, Visser P, Lehmann AR, Duran M, Hoeijmakers JHJ, Weeda G: A mouse model for the basal transcription/DNA repair syndrome: Trichothiodystrophy. *Mol Cell* **1**:981,1998.
200. Johnson RT, Squires S: The XPD complementation group. Insights into xeroderma pigmentosum, Cockaynes syndrome and trichothiodystrophy. *Mutat Res* **273**:97, 1992.
201. Broughton BC, Steingrimsdottir H, Weber CA, Lehmann AR: Mutations in xeroderma pigmentosum group D DNA repair/transcription gene in patients with trichothiodystrophy. *Nature Genet* **7**:189, 1994.
202. Weeda G, Eveno E, Donker I, Vermeulen W, Chevallier-Lagente O, Taïeb A, Stary A, Hoeijmakers JHJ, Mezzina M, Sarasin A: A mutation in the XPB/ERCC3 DNA repair transcription gene, associated with trichothiodystrophy. *Am J Hum Genet* **60**:320, 1997.
203. Kemphues KJ, Kaufman TC, Raff RA, Raff EC: The testis-specific beta-tubulin subunit in *Drosophila melanogaster* has multiple functions in spermatogenesis. *Cell* **31**:655, 1982.
204. Readhead C, Popko B, Takahashi N, Shine HD, Saavedra RA, Sidman RL, Hood L: Expression of a myelin basic protein gene in transgenic shiverer mice: Correction of the dysmyelinating phenotype. *Cell* **48**:703, 1987.
205. Sasaki K, Tachi N, Shinoda M, Satoh N, Minami R, Ohnishi A: Demyelinating peripheral neuropathy in Cockayne syndrome: A histopathologic and morphometric study. *Brain Dev* **14**:114, 1992.
206. Parvin JD, Sharp PA: DNA topology and a minimum set of basal factors for transcription by RNA polymerase II. *Cell* **73**:533, 1993.
207. Bootsma D, Hoeijmakers JHJ: DNA repair: Engagement with transcription. *Nature* **363**:114, 1993.
208. Kraemer KH, Slor H: Xeroderma pigmentosum. *Clin Dermatol* **3**:33, 1985.
209. Lynch HT, Anderson DE, Smith JL, Howell JB, Krush AJ: Xeroderma pigmentosum, malignant melanoma and congenital ichthyosis. *Arch Dermatol* **96**:625, 1967.
210. Kraemer KH, Digiovanna JJ, Moshell AN, Tarone RE, Peck GL: Prevention of skin cancer with oral 13-cisretinoic acid in xeroderma pigmentosum. *N Engl J Med* **318**:1633, 1988.
211. Ramsay CA, Coltart TM, Blunt S, Pawsey CA, Gianelli F: Prenatal diagnosis of xeroderma pigmentosum: Report of the first successful case. *Lancet* **2**:1109, 1974.
212. Halley DFF, Keijzer W, Jaspers NGJ, Niermeijer MF, Kleijer WJ, Boué A, Bootsma D: Prenatal diagnosis of xeroderma pigmentosum (group C) using assays of unscheduled DNA synthesis and postreplication repair. *Clin Genet* **16**:137, 1979.
213. Cleaver JE, Volpe JPG, Charles WC, Thomas GH: Prenatal diagnosis of xeroderma pigmentosum and Cockayne Syndrome. *Prenatal Diagn* **14**:921, 1994.
214. Sarasin A, Blanchet-Bardon C, Renault G, Lehmann A, Arlett C, Dumez Y: Prenatal diagnosis in a subset of trichothiodystrophy patients defective in DNA repair. *Br J Dermatol* **127**:485, 1992.
215. Matsumoto N, Saito N, Harada N, Tanaka K, Niikawa N: DNA-based prenatal carrier detection for group A xeroderma pigmentosum in a chorionic villus sample. *Prenatal Diagn* **15**:1675, 1995.

CHAPTER 29

Ataxia-Telangiectasia

Richard A. Gatti

1. **The diagnosis of ataxia-telangiectasia (A-T) is based primarily on clinical examination and should include progressive cerebellar ataxia with onset between 1 and 3 years of age. Ocular apraxia is a reliable diagnostic criterion after 3 years of age. Telangiectasias often are manifested several years after the onset of ataxia; the degree of telangiectasia is quite variable from family to family. Serum α-fetoprotein (AFP) is elevated in 95 percent of patients. Magnetic resonance imaging shows a dystrophic cerebellum. Karyotyping, if successful, reveals characteristic translocations involving chromosomes 14q11-12, 14q32, 7q35, and 7p14. Immunodeficiency and cancer, usually lymphoid, are observed in many A-T patients. Most patients have no measurable ATM (A-T mutated) protein in lysates of their cells or cell lines, while a few have small amounts.**
2. **Because A-T patients are radiosensitive, conventional doses of radiation therapy are contraindicated. In all young patients with lymphoid malignancies, an underlying diagnosis of A-T should be considered before one calculates doses of radiation or radiomimetic drugs.**
3. **The incidence of A-T is estimated at 1 per 40,000 live births in the United States. The carrier frequency was estimated at 1 percent; recent molecular studies support this early estimate. In some assays, carriers are indistinguishable from normal individuals. Despite this, female carriers are reported to be at a fivefold increased risk of breast cancer. Carriers may account for 5 percent of all cancer patients in the United States. Carriers are intermediate in their *in vitro* responses to ionizing radiation-induced DNA damage. Whether they are clinically more radiosensitive than normals is not known. Conventional wisdom suggests that exposure of A-T carriers to ionizing radiation should be minimized. However, mammograms are recommended, and the same age-dependent schedule as for noncarriers should be followed. Thus far, attempts to demonstrate an increased frequency of ATM mutations in breast cancer patients have not corroborated earlier epidemiologic observations. Given the lack of convincing data on cancer risks for A-T carriers, it is prudent to advise carriers only that the possibility of an increased cancer risk is still under investigation.**
4. **The ATM gene and gene product(s) are very large: 3056 amino acids, 350 kDa, a 13-kb transcript (and smaller, alternatively spliced products), and 66 exons that cover 150 kb of genomic DNA. ATM is expressed in all organs tested. ATM belongs to a large-molecular-weight family of protein kinases. Delayed or reduced expression of p53 in radiation-damaged A-T cells suggests that ATM interacts with proteins upstream of p53 in sensing double-strand break DNA damage. The ATM gene product also plays a role in gametogenesis, as part of the synaptonemal complex.**
5. **Seventy percent of ATM mutations result in a shortened (truncated) protein. These mutations are found over the entire gene and are best detected by mRNA-based techniques that first translate the mRNA to cDNA by RT-PCR before screening for mutations. The favored RT-PCR-based methods are PTT, REF, SSCP, and direct sequencing. Rapid assays that are DNA-based are being developed for the more common mutations, and for mutations that are common to particular ethnic populations, such as the Amish, Moroccan Jews, Sardinians, Italians, British, Costa Ricans, Norwegians, Poles, Turks, Iranians, and Hispanics.**
6. **Several related syndromes overlap with A-T. Nijmegen Breakage syndrome (NBS) Berlin Breakage syndrome (BBS) share t(7;14) translocations, radiosensitivity, immunodeficiency, and cancer susceptibility with A-T, but these patients do not have ataxia, telangiectasia, or elevated AFP. NBS/BBS patients are microcephalic and mentally retarded and sometimes have syndactyly or anal stenosis. NBS and BBS result from mutations in the same gene, *NBS1*, on chromosome 8q21. AT_{Fresno} combines the A-T and NBS syndromes. AT_{Fresno} patients have ATM mutations. Ninety percent of European NBS/BBS patients carry a 657del5 Slavic mutation. Patients with *hMre11* deficiency share the progressive ataxia, radiosensitivity, and t(7;14) chromosomal aberrations with A-T patients; however they have normal AFP, no telangiectasia, and a milder phenotype.**
7. **A-T is a very pleiotropic syndrome that stems from the defective functioning of a single gene—Purkinje cells degenerate and migrate abnormally in the cerebellum during prenatal development; the thymus remains embryonic; histology of most organs shows variability in nuclear size, i.e., nucleomegaly; and radiation hypersensitivity. The ATM gene product senses double-stranded DNA breaks, probably by phosphorylating pivotal molecules such as p53; when the ATM protein is defective, the signal to arrest the cell cycle is not given and DNA damage does not get properly repaired before the next replication cycle begins. A-T cells have G1, S, and G2/M checkpoint defects. In addition to phosphorylating p53, the ATM protein phosphorylates IkB-α, to release the transcription factor NFkB. It also interacts with RPA, Chk1, Chk2, Rb, c-abl, ATR, MLH1, and Rad51. Thus, by functioning as a hierarchical protein kinase, the ATM protein acts on both cell-cycle signaling and on the processing of double-strand DNA breaks, whether physiological, as in meiotic recombination and gene rearrangements, or nonphysiological double-strand breaks, as in the DNA damage caused by environmental agents.**
8. **Therapy for A-T patients remains restricted mainly to supportive care. Free-radical scavengers are recommended, such as vitamin E, α-lipoic acid, and coenzyme Q10. Daily folic acid may minimize chromosome breakage events. Physical therapy is expremely important to avoid debilitating contractures. Patients with frequent severe infections may require intravenous γ-globulin.**

Now that the ataxia-telangiectasia (A-T) gene has been isolated, it seems more pertinent than ever to carefully review the changes that occur in the various physiological systems that are affected by

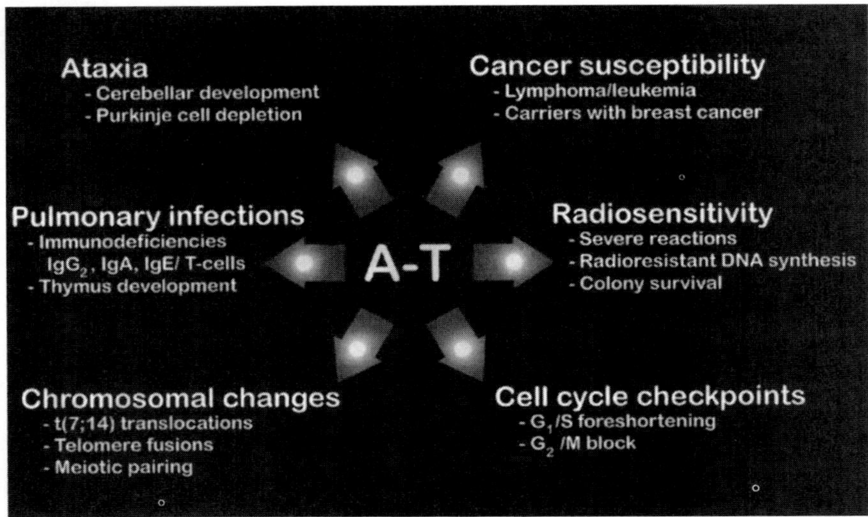

Fig. 29-1 The A-T syndrome.

A-T, trying to relate each facet of the syndrome to the functions of the gene. With the gene in hand, many new and old hypotheses are now testable. While it is clear that the gene functions both in the cytoplasm and in the nucleus, and that elucidating these functions is the present frontier of A-T research, the next frontier will involve translating how mistakes in single cells can misdirect the function and fate of entire cell lineages and result in cerebellar degeneration, thymic dystrophy, and tumor formation.

THE ATAXIA-TELANGIECTASIA SYNDROME

The A-T syndrome varies little from family to family in its late stages.[1–6] Its primary features include (a) progressive gait and truncal ataxia with onset from 1 to 3 years of age; (b) progressively slurred speech; (c) oculomotor apraxia, i.e., an inability to follow an object across the visual fields; (d) oculocutaneous telangiectasia, usually by 6 years of age; (e) elevated serum α-fetoprotein; (f) frequent infections, with accompanying serum and cellular immunodeficiencies; (g) susceptibility to cancer, usually leukemia or lymphoma; (h) hypersensitivity to ionizing radiation, contraindicating the use of conventional doses of radiation therapy for cancer; and (i) reciprocal translocations that involve chromosomes 7 and 14 almost exclusively. Other features include premature aging and endocrine abnormalities. Fig. 29-1 highlights some of the major features of this complex syndrome.

Neurology and Neuropathology

The most obvious and disabling characteristic of the A-T syndrome is the progressive cerebellar ataxia. Shortly after learning to walk, A-T children begin to stagger. By 10 years of age, they are confined to a wheelchair for the remainder of their lives. The ataxia begins as purely truncal but within several years also involves peripheral coordination. Deep tendon reflexes are decreased or absent in older patients; plantar reflexes are upgoing or absent. Slurred speech and oculomotor apraxia are noted early. Both horizontal and vertical saccadic eye movements are affected. Writing is affected by 7 or 8 years of age. Choreoathetosis is found in almost all these patients. Myoclonic jerking and intention tremors are present in about 25 percent. Drooling is a frequent complaint. All teenage A-T patients need help dressing, eating, washing, and using the toilet. The neurologic status of some patients appears to improve between 3 and 7 years of age, and then begins to progress again; this is probably due to the rapid neurologic learning curve of young individuals. Muscle power is normal at first, but wanes with disuse, especially in the legs. Arm strength generally remains. Contractures in fingers and toes are common in older patients, but may be prevented through rigorous exercise.

The typical patient with A-T is of normal intelligence, although slow responses make it difficult to support this by timed IQ testing. Many American and British patients have finished high school with good grades; some have finished college or university. A few seem to be minimally retarded. Most patients have excellent memories.

The most obvious lesion in the central nervous system at postmortem examination is the paucity of Purkinje cells (PCs) in the cerebellum. About 10 years ago, my laboratory wished to determine whether these cells are absent from birth or degenerate afterward. Knowing that basket cells form only around preexisting PCs, we sought to visualize basket cells by Bielschowsky silver-staining. We showed that normal or nearly normal numbers of basket cells were present (Fig. 29-2). We therefore concluded that PC numbers must also have been normal or near normal at birth and degenerated after birth.[7,8]

We also found evidence suggesting that PC migration and arborization are not completely normal.[8] A significant number of ectopic PCs can be found in cerebellar sections from A-T patients from both undermigration and overmigration (Fig. 29-2). PCs make their last cell division at about 13 weeks of gestation and then begin to migrate toward the pial surface. Following the tracts of climbing fibers, they arrive at the single-cell PC layer during the fifth to seventh month of gestation. Thus, this lesion of ectopic PCs would most likely be expressed by the last trimester of pregnancy. This is the earliest known manifestation of the A-T defect.

It remains possible that PCs are not the primary A-T lesion and that the observed PC defects are due to other factors, such as an absence or abnormalities of supporting cells such as basket cells, mossy fibers, parallel fibers, climbing fibers, or glial cells. The frequent presence of choreoathetosis suggests that the basal ganglia, not the cerebellum, are the primary site of neuropathology in A-T. Anterograde or retrograde degeneration of PCs would then occur, with the underlying lesion being either afferent or efferent to the PCs. Becker-Catania, in our laboratory, was able to demonstrate the presence of ATM message in PCs, as well as in cells of the internal and external granular layers and in neurons of the dentate nucleus. ATM mRNA is seen in both healthy and affected tissues (Fig. 29-2). However, because most mutated ATM proteins would be truncated and unstable, the primary site of pathogenesis in the cerebellum remains unclear. This has important implications when considering where to target gene or cell therapy.

Changes also have been noted in the dentate and olivary nuclei. The medulla shows neuroaxonal dystrophy.[9] Degenerative changes are seen in the substantia nigra. Diffuse demyelination in the

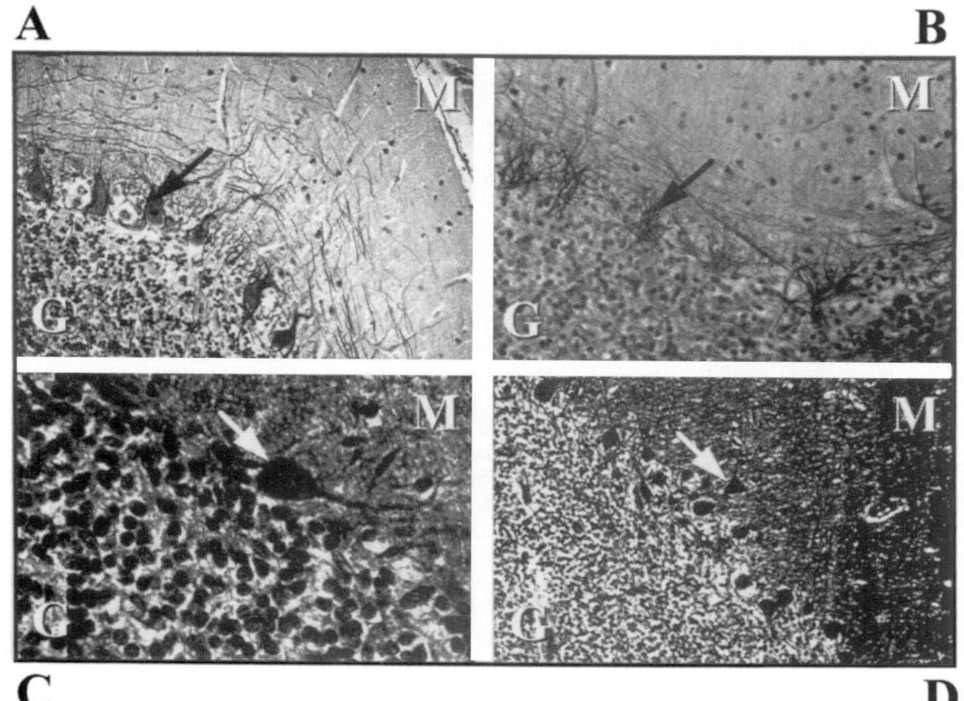

Fig. 29-2 Neuropathology. Photomicrographs of the cerebellum. M—molecular layer; G—granular cell layer. *A,* Bielschovsky stain of normal cerebellum (10×) showing basket cell fibers surrounding Purkinje cells (arrow). *B,* Bielschovsky stain of cerebellum from an A-T patient (10×) showing empty basket cells (arrow) in the Purkinje cell layer. *C, In situ* hybridization with ATM cDNA on normal infant cerebellum (40×) showing a Purkinje cell (arrow) with a positive peroxidase stain for ATM mRNA. *D, In situ* hybridization with ATM cDNA on cerebellum from an A-T patient (20×) showing ectopic (overmigrated) Purkinje cells (arrow) with a positive peroxidase stain for ATM mRNA. (Courtesy of S. Becker-Catania.)

posterior columns of the spinal cord was noted in some of the original autopsies[1] and is a progressive change. For further details of postmortem changes in A-T patients, consult the two lengthy reviews authored by Sedgwick and Boder.[2,5]

Nucleomegaly is a universal finding throughout the organs of A-T patients.[2,5] Nucleomegaly is best seen in organs where nuclear morphology is very regular, such as the hepatic cords and renal tubules. Here it is obvious that the size of the nucleus is extremely variable in A-T tissues, as compared to normal. Some nuclei are very large, hyperchromatic (dark staining), and irregular in shape. Nucleomegaly also is seen in association with normal aging and in viral lesions. Numerous studies, however, have failed to demonstrate virus or viral particles in A-T cells, including Gadjusek's attempt to inoculate primates with brain-tissue extracts from two A-T patients.[5] It is entirely possible that the nucleomegaly seen in A-T tissues results from defective cell-cycle checkpoints that lead to mitotic division without cell replication in random cells. Naeim *et al.*[10] demonstrated polyploidy (4n and 8n) in lymphoblastoid cell lines (LCLs) from A-T patients by flow cytometric cell-cycle analysis.

It was expected that by developing mouse strains in which the *atm* gene was made nonfunctional by one means or another, animal models would become available for dissecting the neuropathology of A-T. Unfortunately, at least five independent *atm* knockouts (atm-/-) have failed to show the severe progressive ataxia seen in A-T patients.[16,169,203,222,223,254,255] This observation limits the application of neuropathology findings in atm-/- mice to patients. Kuljis and Baltimore[254] described changes in the cerebellar cortex when the tissues were examined by electron microscopy. More recently, Borghesani *et al.*[203] described an atmy/y strain that survives beyond 1 year. The mice do not show a progressive ataxia; however, they do show significant changes in Pcs and they manifest motor learning deficits compatible with perturbed cerebellar function. Based on *in vitro* irradiation of yet another atm-/- strain, Herzog *et al.*[256] suggested that inappropriate cell death and apoptosis may underlie the abnormal neurologic development. All of these knockout strains show changes in radiosensitivity, immunologic development, and marked cancer susceptibility.

Telangiectasia

Fig. 29-3 shows a typical pattern of telangiectasia in a 12-year-old patient. Telangiectasias aid in diagnosis. Telangiectasias can be seen on the conjunctiva, as well as on the ears, over the bridge of the nose, in the antecubital fossae, and behind the knees in some patients. Occasional patients have them all over their bodies. Telangiectasias usually do not appear until about 4 to 6 years of age, and although they are a hallmark of the disorder, they sometimes do not become obvious for several years after the onset of ataxia. Elderly individuals without A-T occasionally have similar telangiectasias in many of the same places. Boder felt that telangiectasias appear in response to ultraviolet light exposure; however, that would not explain finding them behind the knee in some patients. About 5 percent of A-T patients never develop prominent telangiectasias. These tend to be patients with milder symptoms. Cafe-au-lait spots are found in almost all A-T patients but are not pathognomonic for just A-T.

Telangiectasias are composed of dilated capillaries. The pattern of these capillaries does not resemble a response to angiogenic factors; instead, it appears to be a response of endothelial cells to a dilatory stimulus. On the other hand, it is still possible that the propensity of A-T patients to develop tumors and form telangiectasias reflects a defective balance between activation of the p53 pathway, apoptosis, angiogenesis, and oxidative stress.[317,325] Van Meir *et al.* have shown that at least one pathway for inhibition of angiogenesis is through p53,[11] and that p53 expression and phosphorylation are reduced in A-T cells (see "Cell-Cycle Aberrations," below). Recent studies of gene

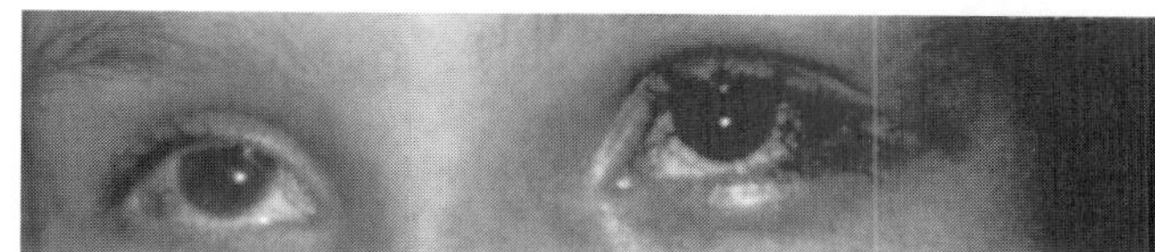

Fig. 29-3 Characteristic telangiectasias over the conjunctiva of a 12-year-old A-T patient.

expression arrays in several laboratories find that unstimulated A-T cells are already in an elevated state of oxidative stress. With rare exceptions,[1,12–15] telangiectasias are not found internally at surgery or at postmortem examination, nor do atm knockout mice manifest internal telangiectasias.[16] Amromin *et al.*[15] noted widely distributed gliovascular nodules in the cerebral white matter and, to a lesser extent, in the brain stem and spinal cord postmortem in a 32-year-old patient. These nodules consisted of dilated capillary loops, many with fibrin thrombi, with perivascular hemorrhages and hemosiderosis, surrounded by demyelinated white matter, reactive gliosis, and numerous atypical astrocytes. These nodules were not seen in the cerebellum and have not been observed in other postmortem examinations of younger patients.

Telangiectasia occasionally develop within the fields of prior radiation therapy, not only in A-T patients or carriers, but in apparently normal persons as well.[289] Telangiectasia are sometimes observed in the parents and sibs of A-T patients and may be a subtle manifestation of heterozygosity and radiosensitivity.

Radiosensitivity *In Vivo* and *In Vitro*

Over the past 30 years, radiation therapists have observed that when A-T patients with cancer are treated with conventional doses of ionizing radiation, they develop life-threatening sequelae characteristic of much higher doses.[17–21] This radiosensitivity can also be demonstrated *in vitro* using fibroblasts or lymphoblasts from A-T homozygotes, which are sensitive to ionizing radiation and to a variety of radiomimetic and free-radical-producing agents.[22,23,111] (Also see the discussion of colony survival assay under "Differential Diagnosis" below.)

Early radiosensitivity assays for A-T measured colony formation efficiency of fibroblasts. Cells are irradiated and then cultured, and the number of colonies that grow are scored after a measured period of incubation. Fibroblasts from A-T heterozygotes form colonies with an efficiency that is intermediate between A-T homozygosity and normal;[22] the same observation can be made using neocarzinostatin.[24] Despite this, colony-forming efficiency is not a reliable way to detect individual heterozygotes.[23–26] Many other methods have been tried to identify A-T heterozygotes, but none are reliable because the normal and heterozygous data sets overlap.[10,27–31] Recently, a "comet" assay has been described for identifying ATM heterozygotes by measuring DNA repair in peripheral blood lymphocytes (BPL) following 3 Gy of irradiation.[315]

Now that genetic testing in families with prior affected patients can identify A-T heterozygotes (carriers) more easily, physicians are confronted with the dilemma of having to advise carriers about the risks of radiation exposure. Unfortunately, there are as yet no clinical studies on which to base such advice. For example, data are lacking on whether the *in vitro* radiosensitivity of heterozygotes has any clinical correlate; i.e., unusual reactions to standard radiologic procedures or increased cancer risk. One can only make the general recommendation that exposure to all types of ionizing radiation be minimized in persons suspected of being A-T carriers, e.g., both parents, remembering as well that two-thirds of the sibs of A-T patients are likely to be carriers. Whether routine dental x-rays should be recommended in A-T patients is also an unresolved issue.

ATM knockout mice that are heterozygous (atm +/–) do not show an abnormal response to total-body irradiation.[16] Some caveats: (a) Only one specific site in the ATM gene was disrupted in each of the knockout mice strains, and (b) knockout mouse models seldom mimic a human disease in all facets of the syndrome. Swift's epidemiologic data suggest that exposure of heterozygotes to myelograms and other diagnostic x-rays may increase their cancer risk.[32] There is also cause for concern about mammograms in female A-T carriers, who appear to be at an increased risk of breast cancer (see below). The recommendation at this writing is that mammograms be continued on the same age-dependent schedule used for noncarriers but that the most up-to-date mammography machines be employed to minimize exposure to only a few rads. The added risk of cancer to such women is only slightly increased (from 1.5 in 100 from annual mammography screening doses in noncarriers to perhaps 2 in 100 in A-T carriers), and this should be compared to a 1 in 9 natural lifetime risk and the 30 percent reduction in mortality from annual mammography screening in women over age 40.[33–35]

Epidemiologic and radiosensitivity studies of A-T family members further suggest that many cancer patients may be receiving the wrong doses of radiotherapy—too much for A-T heterozygotes and too little for noncarriers.[33,34,36] Considering that 5 percent of cancer patients under 46 years of age may be A-T carriers and intermediate in their radiosensitivity,[37] this issue could involve many thousands of patients annually (see "Cancer Susceptibility," below). Some x-ray dosage regimens were first tested empirically on cadres of cancer patients, and if those cadres were to have contained up to 5 percent A-T carriers, one can easily imagine how radiation sequelae might be more apt to appear in the A-T carriers, thereby lowering the "safe" doses defined for everyone else. Once A-T carrier testing can be implemented on a wide scale, these issues may be resolved.

Although radiation damage to DNA has been used for many years as a laboratory tool for characterizing the phenotype of A-T cells, it should be remembered that A-T cells normally are not exposed to irradiation *in vivo.* Thus, the radiosensitivity of A-T cells is largely a laboratory artifact because irradiation damage mimics double-strand DNA breaks and tests the cells' abilities to rejoin these breaks in an orderly fashion. Because the complex A-T syndrome develops quite uniformly in most affected patients, the major substrate for ATM protein must be a naturally-occurring molecule(s) generated by an equally common event that causes double-strand DNA breaks. p53 is a good candidate for the major substrate,[198,199] while oxidative stress and the normal production of DNA-damaging free-radical products of metabolism are good candidates for the commonly-recurring and inciting event.[38,328,329] Although many attempts have been made to demonstrate defective DNA repair in A-T cells, this has not been convincingly defined.[39] Recent observations suggest that it is the *inability* to sense this damage that is defective in A-T cells, not the actual mechanisms of repair.[38,40]

When DNA synthesis of irradiated fibroblasts is measured, A-T homozygotes show a characteristic dose-response curve (Fig. 29-4) that is diagnostic of the disease.[82] This phenomenon is called radioresistant DNA synthesis (RDS) because, unlike normal cells which temporarily halt the synthesis of new DNA after irradiation damage, A-T cells simply continue into S phase of the cell cycle. Later experiments that attempted to complement RDS and other radiomimetic features of A-T cells by transfection found, however, that these phenomena often were dissociated.[6,83] Thus, RDS most likely reflects a cell-cycle checkpoint failure at S phase that is independent of other radiosensitivity phenotypes of A-T cells. Using RDS, heterozygous cells cannot be distinguished from normals.

The shape of the RDS curve (Fig. 29-4) for A-T cells has been insightfully interpreted by Painter[85,86] as having two components, one reflecting replicon initiation and the other reflecting chain elongation. The slope of the curve above 20 Gy determines the second component, and this slope does not differ in normal and A-T fibroblasts. The early component, however, is essentially missing from the A-T curves, suggesting that replicon initiation is quite abnormal. Painter further suggested that while in unirradiated normal cells initiation occurs synchronously at the origins of a cluster of replicons and that in irradiated normal cells damage to one replicon inhibits the entire cluster, in irradiated A-T cells damage to one replicon inhibits only that replicon; i.e., the damage is not sensed or translated to the rest of the cluster, and chain elongation near the growing forks is not curbed. Thus, radiation to A-T cells blocks initiation of individual replicons rather than blocking the initiation of clusters of replicons.[39,85,86] Hand and Gautschi[87] provided evidence that one single-strand break may inactivate the initiation of as many as 100 replicons.

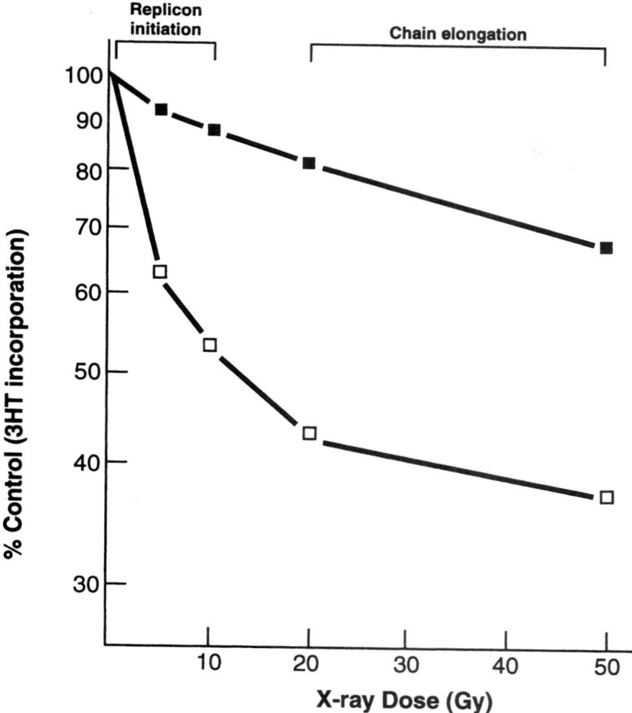

Fig. 29-4 Graph of radioresistant DNA synthesis (RDS) depicting theoretical targets of radiation at increasing doses of radiation. The major defect in A-T (black squares) is seen at very low radiation doses, affecting replicon initiation, while chain elongation appears normal in A-T, as depicted by the normal slope of that portion of the curve.

Although Painter's interpretation of the RDS curve was put forth over 10 years ago, it remains a very attractive hypothesis for explaining one facet of the pathogenesis of A-T. Atomic force microscopy analyses suggest that ATM protein can exist either as a monomer or as a tetramer in the repair of double-strand DNA breaks.[134,200–202,318]

Cancer Susceptibility

During their shortened lifetimes, 38 percent of A-T homozygotes develop a malignancy.[41] This represents a 61- and a 184-fold increase in European-American and African-American patients, respectively. Roughly 85 percent of these malignancies are either leukemia or lymphoma. In younger patients, an acute lymphocytic leukemia is most often of T-cell origin,[42,43] although the pre-B origin common to ALL of childhood (HLADR1, CD101, CD51, and CD191) has also been seen in A-T patients. When leukemia develops in older A-T homozygotes, it is usually an aggressive T-cell leukemia with a morphology similar to that of chronic lymphoblastic leukemia, hence the old name T-CLL;[42–45] T-cell prolymphocytic leukemia (T-PLL) is the equivalent modern nomenclature.[45,46] The leukemic cells often contain a transloca-tion and/or inversion involving the T-cell receptor α-chain gene complex at 14q11-12[47–49] (see discussion of non-leukemic clonal expansions in A-T patients under "Chromosomal Instability," below). Myeloid leukemia is very uncommon in A-T patients. Lymphomas in A-T homozygotes, in contrast to leukemias, are common and are usually B-cell types, although T-cell lymphomas also have been observed. As A-T patients are living longer, more nonlymphoid cancers are being observed. Several of our older patients have developed breast cancer and melanoma. Cancers of the stomach and ovary have been reported.[5,42] When fibroids or leiomyomas are found in A-T females, a special effort should be made by the pathologist to quantitate high-power fields for mitotic figures, because leiomyosarcomas of precocious onset have been reported.[50] For specific lists of other tumor types and frequencies, see references 41, 42, and 44.

A-T heterozygotes are also believed to be cancer-prone.[37] They are not clinically distinguishable from normal individuals. An increased incidence of breast cancer in female A-T heterozygotes has been reported in the United States, England, and Norway.[32,51–53] In the U.S. study, the risk of breast cancer was found to be fivefold higher among the mothers of A-T homozygotes than in a comparable female population.[32,52] Based on this observation, Swift *et al.* estimated that between 8 and 18 percent of all breast cancer patients may be A-T heterozygotes.[37] This would imply that ATM is the most common cancer susceptibility gene in the general population. While the issue is far from settled, many recent genetic studies of breast cancer cohorts have failed to find an increased frequency of mutations in the ATM gene,[54,55,257,258,306,331] with the exceptions of a report of an allelic variant at the ATM locus being associated through a rare HRAS1 allele in a stratified study of 66 sib pairs affected with breast cancer[260] and recent findings be Teraoka *et al.*[305] of 11 ATM mutations in 142 breast cancer patients versus only 1 in 80 controls. They used primarily denaturing high-power liquid chromatography (dHPLC); all mutations detected were of the missense type. Vorechovsky *et al.*[54] looked for ATM mutations in tumor tissue from 38 sporadic breast cancers. They first screened this material by single-stranded conformational polymorphism (SSCP) gels, and then sequenced any regions suspected of harboring mutations. They found no significant mutations. Spurr and coworkers[56] looked for a linkage to BRCA1 and BRCA2 in 63 early onset breast cancer families; 55 percent linked to BRCA1 and 45 percent linked to BRCA2. This implied that none linked to 11q22-23, as Wooster *et al.*[58] and Cortessis *et al.*[57] had reported earlier. However, because the epidemiologic data from A-T families suggested that the breast cancer seen among A-T mothers (who are obligate heterozygotes) peaks in the age group of 45 to 54,[52] and is not an early onset pattern, other studies have screened late-onset or sporadic breast cancers for ATM mutations. Using PTT, FitzGerald *et al.*[55] detected ATM mutations in 2 of 401 women with sporadic early onset breast cancer. They also found mutations in 2 of 202 control samples. Recently, Swift and coworkers[59] again noted an increased incidence of breast cancer in A-T heterozygotes who were identified by haplotyping members of extended A-T families.

The apparent paradox of (a) not finding many ATM mutations in breast cancer cohorts and (b) not finding A-T patients in the families of breast cancer patients with ATM mutations may find resolution in the hypothesis that two types of A-T carriers may exist within the general population, those with nonsense (truncating) mutations and those with missense mutations, and each type of mutation may have a different Phenotype—both in the heterozygous and in the homozygous state. Heterozygous missense mutations might create a dominant negative situation,[330] whereby the defective copy of the ATM protein *binds* to sustrates but cannot *phosphorylate* them, or vice versa. This would create a far more serious situation than a nonsense mutation that would not produce any stable defective protein. Most A-T patients have two truncating mutations. Homozygous missense mutations are extremely uncommon in A-T patients and some could even be lethal. Thus, it is possible that ATM missense carriers are more likely to be cancer prone than ATM nonsense carriers. (This hypothesis is developed further in reference 306.)

Several independent studies of ATM knockout mice have confirmed the extreme cancer susceptibility of atm−/− homozygotes; all atm−/− strains develop massive, widely metastasized malignant thymic lymphomas.[16,169,203,222,223,254,255] Heterozygous animals have not shown tumors, nor has breast cancer been observed in either homozygous or heterozygous animals.

Carter *et al.* reported significant loss of heterozygosity in sporadic breast cancers across chromosome 11q22-23[60] as did others.[267–270,297,298] Although this region includes the ATM gene (at 11q22.3-23.1) and the CHK1 gene (at 11q23.3),[271] it measures 35 cM and probably includes more than 1000 other genes as well. Thus, the contribution of ATM mutations to familial breast cancer appears to be low, with ATM perhaps playing a more important role in a sporadic, low-penetrance form of breast cancer.

The most frequently reported cancers in American A-T heterozygotes are breast, trachea/bronchus/lung, stomach, prostate, melanoma, and gallbladder.[32] In Italy and Costa Rica, gastric cancer has been especially noteworthy. Among 64 A-T parents and grandparents in Costa Rica, half of the 12 cancers reported were gastric cancer.[61] (Costa Rica ranks among the top three countries in the world for stomach cancer in the general population, making it difficult to interpret these observations.) In Italian families, 7 of 20 cancers in grandparents were gastric cancer.[62] Stomach cancer has been reported in homozygotes as well,[42,44] including two families in which both affected sibs developed stomach cancer. Despite this, Morrell *et al.*[41] did not note any increase in stomach cancers in A-T homozygotes.

Other recent observations move the cancer susceptibility association with A-T in new directions. Most individuals who develop T-PLL have ATM mutations in one or both alleles. While it was first thought that these patients represented constitutional A-T heterozygotes, the data are lacking to establish this.[259] Thus, these patients may be at no increased prior risk of cancer but simply develop an ATM mutation somatically. The ATM mutations found in T-PLL cells are mainly missense mutations,[84] unlike the predominantly nonsense mutations found in A-T patients[237]. However, if A-T heterozygotes acquire T-PLL by a second "hit"[84,129] on the ATM gene, this would then suggest that ATM can function as a tumor-suppressor gene, in addition to its growing list of other roles.[264]

Four reports link loss of ATM integrity to an aggressive subgroup of B-cell chronic lymphocytic leukemia (B-CLL) patients.[301–304] Perphas 40 percent of B-CLL patients have 11q deletions or fail to express ATM protein. Here again, where ATM mutations have been identified, they have been mainly missense types. Unfortunately, missense mutations are still very difficult to detect in such a large gene (see below).

A gain of chromosome 3q is present in many cancers, including cervical carcinomas, small cell lung carcinomas, head and neck squamous cell carcinomas, and embryonal rhabdomyosarcomas.[261] When microcell hybrids were transferred into a differentiation-competent myoblast cell line C2C12, the cells exhibited a nondifferentiating phenotype.[262] Selecting 3q candidate genes, ATR (AT- and rad3-related/FRAP-related protein 1) was tested. ATR is a protein kinase with strong homology to ATM.[71,72,233] It was found that forced expression of ATR resulted in a phenocopy of the 3q-containing microcell hybrids. ATR apparently inhibits MyoD, which is a marker for classifying sarcomas as rhabdosarcomas. ATR is thought to share functional overlap with ATM in cell-cycle progression[139,263] and may be phosphorylated by ATM. Like ATM, ATR phosphorylates the Serine 15 position on p53, albeit at a much-reduced level and at a slower rate.[199] Furthermore, overexpression of ATR corrects the defective radiation-induced S-phase checkpoint in A-T cells.[263] (ATR's relationship to ATM is further described in "Chromosomal Instability" below).

Cell-Cycle Aberrations

Important checkpoints monitor the progress of the cell cycle and prevent mutagenic damage to DNA from becoming fixed into future cell generations. The G1 checkpoint prevents replication of a damaged DNA template; the G2 checkpoint prevents segregation of damaged chromosomes.[64] Kastan *et al.*[65,66] showed that A-T cells have a delayed radiation-induced increase in p53, compared to normal cells. p53, dubbed the "guardian of the genome," acts to suppress normal cell-cycle progression at G1 until DNA repairs have been completed. (For reviews pertinent to p53 in A-T cells, see references 38, 40, and 67.) It accomplishes this by binding DNA at sequence-specific sites, thereby transcriptionally activating a signal-transduction cascade. In so doing, p53 functions as a tumor suppressor. Cells from p53 knockout mice, lacking both normal alleles of p53 (p53−/−), fail to observe the G1 checkpoint; they do not experience G1 arrest after irradiation nor do they show neurologic abnormalities, immune defects, or problems with sterility,[40,67,68] as in A-T. The strong association of multiple types of cancer with p53 deficiency[67,74–77] further suggests that involvement of this pathway in apoptosis and in differentiation may help explain the increased frequency of cancer in A-T.

Interestingly, p53−/− mutants are not radiosensitive.[76,78] Thus, yet another mechanism must account for the radiosensitivity of A-T cells. Much work still needs to be done before the role of ATM proteins in intracellular signaling can be fully appreciated. For example, despite much evidence of the inefficiency of G1/S, S, and G2/M checkpoints in A-T cells, holding A-T cells in G0 for up to 7 days does not improve their postirradiation survival,[40] which suggests that even these checkpoint defects may not be the crucial common denominator underlying A-T pathogenesis. Evidence presented by Jung and *et al.*[79,80] using SV40-transformed fibroblasts, implicates the NF-kB and IkB-α proteins in ATM function; the ATM protein appears to phosphorylate IkB-α, thereby activating the transcription factor NF-kB.[81] These findings would also support observations of increased radiation-induced apoptosis in cell lines derived from A-T patients.[40,76,77] However, a recent report by Ashburner *et al.*[324] suggests that the constitutive activation of NFκB reported by Jung *et al.* may be due more to SV40-transformation than to the A-T phenotype. The phosphorylation of replication factor A (RPA) is also delayed in A-T cells after irradiation.[69,265] Three groups have independently shown that the Serine-15 position of p53 is selectively phosphorylated by ATM.[198,199,300] Further, Shafman *et al.*[70] have reported that c-abl binds to an SH_3 domain on the ATM molecule.

Immunodeficiency

At postmortem examination, virtually every A-T homozygote has a small embryonic-like thymus.[12] In the late 1960s, and again in the early 1980s, many attempts were made to characterize the immunodeficiencies of A-T patients.[88] No single, consistent abnormality could be identified in all A-T patients; affected sibs often differ in the degree and profile of their immunodeficiencies. In a review of British patients, Woods and Taylor[89] noted normal immunologic function in 27 of 70 patients. Only 10 percent had severe immunodeficiencies.

When the genomic order of the IGH V, D, J, and H gene subfamilies was first described, we noted that the immunoglobulin (Ig) classes that were most frequently decreased in A-T patients were those with the greatest genomic distances between the variable (V) genes and the respective heavy-chain genes;[90] 60 to 80 percent of A-T homozygotes manifest an IgA, IgE, and/or IgG2 deficiency,[12,88,89–95,121,122] whereas serum levels of IgM, IgG1, and IgG3 are usually normal. This suggests that B cells from these patients have a maturational problem with Ig class switching, perhaps based on a recombinase-related deficiency. On a similar note, an increased proportion of T gamma/delta cells noted in one early study suggested a maturational delay in T cells; however, this was before normal T gamma/delta cell ranges had been clearly defined and has not been generally confirmed. IgM levels are occasionally extremely high (see below), which could be based on a similar defective maturational mechanism that arrests some B cells at the IgM-producing stage. However, when V(D)J recombination was examined in A-T cells, both signal and coding joint formation were normal.[96–98] Approximately half of A-T patients with immunodeficiencies have T-cell deficiencies. CD41/CD45RA1 (naive) T cells are decreased in some patients.[99] Responses to antigens are poor, especially allogeneic antigens.[12,88,100–105] T-cell cytotoxicity to influenza-infected target cells is reduced.[106] T lymphocytes show abnormally fast capping of FITC-labeled concanavalin A.[88] Markedly elevated cyclic AMP levels have been observed in T cells from A-T patients.[88] Neutrophil chemotaxis was reported to be decreased in some studies and normal in others. Similarly, NK cell activity and NK cell levels have been described as normal, decreased, or increased in various studies.[88,107,108,266] Some of these discrepancies no doubt reflect the transient immune status of patients with active infections. Although 91 percent of Costa Rican A-T patients had diminished PHA responses, 65 percent of them had the same mutation; thus, this sample would be skewed against some features and would favor others, and probably has only minimal bearing on patients around the world with other mutations. Further immunologic analyses of this cohort are under way. Knockout ATM mice have many of these same immune defects as A-T patients; T and B cell precursors in thymus and bone marrow, respectively, are present in normal numbers.[169]

Sanal *et al.*[275] have recently described a new form of immunodeficiency in A-T patients. IgG antibody responses to pneumococcal polysaccharide vaccine (serotypes 3, 6A, 7F, 14, 19F, and 23F) were studied in 29 classic A-T patients; in 22 patients (76 percent), no responses were observed. The remaining patients had responses to 1, 2, or 4 serotypes. Zeilin *et al.*[327] support this finding.

Hyper-IgM with Ataxia-Telangiectasia

Elevated serum IgM levels are fairly common in A-T patients,[100,277] arising perhaps as compensation for low IgA, IgE, and IgG2 levels. However, occasional A-T patients with classic symptoms have an extended syndrome that may include very high serum IgM levels, splenomegaly, lymphoadenopathy, neutropenia, thrombocytopenia, hypertension, renal anomalies, and congestive heart failure from high blood viscosity.[109,110] The latter symptoms were somewhat ameliorated by reducing blood volume, and further by splenomegaly. Steroids markedly improved three patients (unpublished, personal experience). The postirradiation colony survival assay (CSA)[111] in six of these families, although not easily quantifiable, suggests a level of radiosensitivity that is intermediate between that seen in normals and that seen in other A-T patients (see "Differential Diagnosis," below). In three families, ATM mutations have already been identified. It is of interest that in three families, the affected sibs were discordant for hyper-IgM.[278–280] Another patient was atypical in that depletion of cerebellar Purkinje cells was not seen, and ATM protein levels were normal.[109] In an Argentine family, the hyper-IgM followed treatment of the immunodeficiency with IVIg.[281] Thus, while hyper-IgM and A-T have been observed together in a number of families, the underlying pathology remains obscure and the observation of discordant sibs in three families suggests that the hyper-IgM represents a somatic, not a genetic, variation. Recently, Rosenblatt *et al.*[296] have provided some evidence that this hyper-IgM may be due to an up-regulation of the CD40 ligand gene.

α-Fetoprotein

Although elevated serum α-fetoprotein (AFP) levels can be very useful in confirming a suspected diagnosis of A-T, 5 to 10 percent of typical A-T patients have normal AFP levels. This is independent of race, sex, or complementation group, and is usually concordant in affected sibs. AFP levels do not increase with patient age.[89] Serum AFP levels still elevated from infancy sometimes can be misleading in children under 2 years of age in whom normal ranges have not been carefully defined by most clinical laboratories. Thus, it is best to avoid using AFP as a diagnostic criterion until after 2 years of age. Other causes of elevated AFP, such as liver disease, familial hyper-AFP[309,310] and the presence of a teratoma, are not likely to confound a diagnosis of A-T. Ishiguro *et al.*[115] showed that the lectin-binding profile of elevated AFPs from A-T patients was most likely of hepatic origin, and although no evidence of liver disease is present at postmortem examination, other liver proteins, such as serum glutamic-pyruvic transaminase (SGPT), serum glutamic-oxalacetic transaminase (SGOT), alkaline phosphatase, and carcinoembryonic antigen, are often increased as well.[90,112]

AFP is thought to have a suppressor effect on the developing immune system and on immune function.[112–114,311,312] The mechanisms by which AFP is elevated in sera of most A-T patients remains unclear but may involve the NFκB/IκBα complex and/or p53, both of which are phosphorylated by ATM.[79,80,98,199,300,313]

With the routine monitoring of AFP in amniotic fluid now in vogue, the question is occasionally asked whether amniotic AFP levels are elevated when the fetus has A-T. AFP levels are very high in all fetuses, peaking at about 13 weeks of gestation.[112] In two cases who had been diagnosed by prenatal testing, and in which a decision had been made by the parents not to terminate the pregnancies, amniotic AFP levels were measured and were within normal ranges. A cord blood AFP was elevated in one of these patients, and remained so over the next 3 years. (In the other patient, cord blood was not tested.) Thus, although the serum AFP level of a fetus is high, there appears to be no extravasation or secretion into the amniotic fluid of A-T-affected fetuses, as occurs in open neural tube defects and Down syndrome.

Chromosomal Instability

A-T homozygotes show nonrandom chromosomal aberrations in lymphocytes, such as translocations and inversions, which preferentially involve chromosomal breakpoints at 14q11, 14q32, 7q35, 7p14, 2p11, and 22q11.[43,117] These aberrations appeared to correlate generally with the regions of the T-cell receptor (TCR-α, β, and γ) and B-cell receptor (IGH, IGK, and IGL) gene complexes. Because these six sites contain the only gene complexes in the genome that are presently known to require site-specific gene rearrangement/recombination before expressing a mature protein, it was logical to examine V(D)J recombination mechanisms in A-T cells. As was noted above, signal and coding joint formation are both normal.[96–98] When we examined the chromosomes of fibroblasts from eight A-T homozygotes, all with typical 7:14 translocations in their lymphocytes, the fibroblast aberrations were totally random.[117,118] Hecht and Hecht studied almost 50,000 amniotic fluid cell metaphases; of 37 translocations in that non-A-T sample, none involved chromosomes 7 and 14.[119] This is intriguing when one considers that, like lymphocytes and lymphoblasts, fibroblasts and amniotic cells express the radiosensitivity defect, suggesting that the radiosensitivity is intrinsic to A-T cells, whereas the chromosome aberrations are secondary to chromosome movement and telomere clustering in the nucleus.[134] Heterozygotes show t(7;14) translocations in lymphocytes, but only in 1 to 2 percent of metaphases.[119]

In some patients, cell clones with the above breakpoints expand,[45,120] sometimes accounting for 100 percent of the lymphocytes that are karyotyped. Despite this, lymphocyte counts remain within the normal range for years thereafter. Some of these clones have been followed for 10 to 20 years by us and others.[48,118] These clones tend to evolve, with subclones adding new rearrangements, such as inv(14;14)(q11;q32), i(8q), and 6q-, in addition to many other smaller clones. Eventually, most such patients develop T-PLL, previously referred to as T-CLL (T-cell chronic lymphoblastic leukemia).[45,46] Affected sibs usually are not concordant for developing such clones, thus again implicating somatic influences superimposed on an A-T genotype.

These clonal expansions have allowed the breakpoint sites to be analyzed by molecular techniques. Three types of patients have been studied: (a) A-T patients with nonleukemic clones, (b) A-T patients with leukemic clones, and (c) non-A-T patients with similar cytogenetic translocations and T-PLL. Thanks to many years of perseverance by Taylor and coworkers[124] in trying to pinpoint the breakpoints of these translocations or inversions, a fascinating story is now emerging that is quite similar to that of myc in Burkitt lymphoma. The A-T expanded clones always juxtapose one of the TCR genes, usually TCRα, with another family of genes located proximal to, but not actually within, the B-cell receptor-gene complexes. The most common and best-studied translocations are those involving 14q11 (TCRα) and a breakpoint cluster region 10 Mb proximal to the IGH locus at 14q32. Within

400 kb, at least 8 such breakpoints have been identified in A-T patients with and without leukemia, and in several non-A-T patients with T-PLL. This region centers on the TCL-1 (T-cell leukemia-1) gene,[123] the 1.3-kb transcript of which is preferentially expressed in immature (and leukemic) B and T cells. Circulating mature T cells do not express this gene. Leukemia cells without the t(14;14) or inv(14;14) clones typically do not express TCL-1.[223]

An occasional A-T patient has a large t(X;14)(q28;q11) clone, including at least two that have developed T-CLL/T-PLL and one without leukemia when last studied.[45] The breakpoints at Xq28 cluster to within a few kilobases in a region of 70 kb proximal to the factor VIII gene. This region contains the genes c6.1A and c6.1B. (The latter gene is believed to be the crucial one in these translocations, because two of the breakpoints fall within the first exon of c6.1B, also known as MTCP1, "mature T-cell proliferation-1."[124–126]) Most interesting, c6.1B has homology with TCL-1 (40 percent identity, 60 percent similarity) and is a mitochondrial protein.[127] TCL-1 and MTCP-1 also share three-dimensional structure. TCL-1 prevents apoptosis and is p53-independent. Because TCRα/TCL-1 translocations do not by themselves cause leukemia, another factor must interact with the protein product or products that result from the translocations. Based on the recent finding that most non-AT patients with T-PLL have ATM mutations in one or both alleles, the ATM protein is a likely candidate for this role.[84] Despite this, leukemia cells from an occasional A-T/T-PLL patient do not show abnormal TCL-1 expression, suggesting that yet other genes are involved in this pathway from clonal expansion to leukemia.

Inherited cytogenetic defects involving translocations or deletions at 11q22-23 have not been observed in A-T homozygotes, even though karyotypes of >500 patients have been examined worldwide. Many cytogenetic reports on children with suspected A-T return with the statement "insufficient metaphases for analysis." This problem occurs because the necessary lymphocyte response to mitogens, such as phytohemagglutinin (PHA), is often weak or delayed in A-T patients, and when cell cultures are harvested routinely at 48 h, few cells are dividing. Harvest results can be improved by using a double-dose of mitogen and harvesting at 72 h or at several time points.

Telomeric fusions are observed frequently in A-T patients, which is a provocative finding considering the strong homology between ATM and the yeast Tel-1 mutant gene.[71] Tumor cells and senescent cells of normal persons can also show such fusions.[133] Pandita *et al.*[130] showed that although the telomeres of A-T cell lines are shorter than normal cells, telomerase activity was normal. Metcalfe *et al.*[135] demonstrated significant telomere shortening in A-T peripheral blood lymphocytes (PBLs). PBLs from 20 A-T patients showed an average loss of 95 ± 23 bp (base pairs) per year of age, compared to a loss of 35 ± 9 bp per year in normals. The preleukemic T-cell clones described above showed an even greater loss of 158 ± 9 bp per year and are especially prone to show telomeric fusions. Recently, as the biochemistry of telomere maintenance is being unravelled,[134] it appears that the Ku70/85 heterodimeric complex is physically bound to telomeres in yeast. Ku protects telomeres from nucleases and recombinases. Cells without Ku do not repair double-strand breaks or perform gene rearrangements for T or B cell maturation; Ku-deficient mutants display telomere shortening. In mammalian cells, Ku is the DNA-binding subunit of a large enzyme, DNA-dependent protein kinase (DNA-PK_{cs}), which is a member of the large-molecular-weight protein kinase family that also includes ATM.[71,72] The Ku complex interacts with the Rad50/Mre11/Xrs2/Brca1 complex for nonhomologous end-joining.[134] Xrs2 (yeast) was recently identified as the human Nijmegen Breakage syndrome protein, nibrin[201,202] (See discussion of "Related Syndromes" below.) The Rad50/Mre11/NBS1 complex, together with Ku and Brca1, is required for the telomerase pathway of end maintenance. The Rad50/Mre11/NBS1/Brca1 complex may be the exonuclease that provides the single-strand substrate required for telomerase

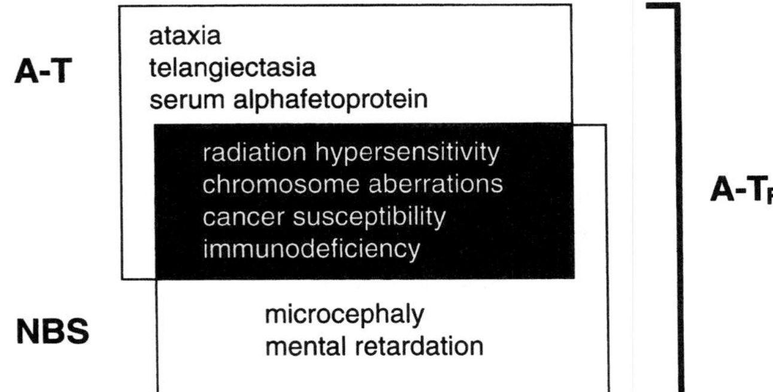

Fig. 29-5 Overlapping A-T and NBS syndromes combine to form the AT_{Fresno} syndrome.

activity. ATM interacts with the Rad50/Mre11/NBS1/Brca1 complex by phosphorylating both Brca1[299] and nibrin.[307] This would explain the overlap of symptoms between A-T and NBS (Fig. 29-5). Patients lacking hMre 11 protein have recently been described and closely resemble A-T patients in that they manifest progressive ataxia, t(7;14) translocations, and radiosensitivity. ATM protein expression is normal; nibrin and Rad50 expression are diminished.[308]

Accelerated telomeric shortening is probably a characteristic of all rapidly dividing A-T cells. It is of further interest that telomeric shortening is associated with senescence of CD282/CD81 T cells in AIDS patients and centenarians.[136] In both situations, this may account for waning T-cell immunity. A similar mechanism might explain the abnormal development and function of the immune system in A-T patients. Thus, the precocious onset of cancers such as basal cell carcinoma,[2] leiomyosarcoma,[50] and T-PLL[124] may reflect the basic propensity of their cells to accelerate telomere shortening and a waning immunity due not so much to poor V(D)J joining but to telomere shortening and senescence. This would also provide a p53-independent, radiation-independent pathway to cancer susceptibility in A-T patients.

When the ATM gene was isolated and sequenced, it was noted to have its strongest homology to the yeast tel1 gene, primarily through sharing a region of PI-3 kinase homology, and secondarily through sharing weak homology with rad3.[137–141] (Reference 141 contains a comprehensive analysis of homologies between kinase, rad3, RH3, and FRB domains.) Absence of tel1 results in telomere shortening. Rad3 is a fission yeast gene containing helicase motifs that is required for G2 arrest after DNA damage.[142,143] Of the large family of genes sharing PI-3 kinase homology with ATM, only tel1, mec1 (another yeast gene), and mei41 (of *Drosophila*) also share some rad3 homology. (The rad3 homology of tel1 is admittedly weak.) A growing body of evidence suggests that tel1, mec1, and ATM perform overlapping functions. Of the three, only mec1 is an essential gene. In yeast, mec1 (mitosis entry checkpoint) is required for regulation of the S/M and G2/M checkpoints,[144] the rate of ongoing S phase in response to damage,[145] and meiotic recombination.[145,146] Cells with mutations in mec1 (also called ESR1 or SAD3) proceed directly to mitosis when DNA replication is inhibited with hydroxyurea and are unable to delay the onset of mitosis (G2/M) on induction of DNA damage.[147] Rad53 is also regulated by MEC1 and Tel1.[147] Although tel1 mutants are not radiosensitive and mec1 mutants are, tel1/mec1 double-mutants somehow synergize to increase the sensitivity to DNA damage from ionizing radiation and radiomimetic drugs.[141] The human homologue of mec1, called ATR (AT-related Rad3-related) or FRP1 (FRAP-related protein), was recently cloned and maps to chromosome 3q22-q24.[141,148] It plays a reciprocal role to ATM on synapsing chromosomes during meiotic recombination,[139] localizing to the nonsynapsed portion of the chromosomes and interacting with Rad51 and BRCA1. RPA and chk1 also colocalize with ATR on late pachynema chromosomes.[271,272] RPA binds to single-stranded DNA, and probably facilitates formation of recombination intermediates.[273,274] (ATR is also discussed under "Cancer Susceptibility" above.)

Complementation Groups

Fusion of fibroblasts from unrelated patients will often correct or "complement" their radiosensitivity, as measured by RDS.[149–151,204] Five complementation groups have been defined (Groups A, C, D, E, and V1).[151] The first four groups are phenotypically identical and can be distinguished from one another only by complementation studies. It was unclear whether these complementation groups represented several distinct A-T genes, perhaps forming part of a common enzymatic pathway or coding for parts of a common multimeric molecule, or, alternatively, whether the complementation groups represented intragenic mutations of a single gene. It was also possible that complementation was a nongenetic phenomenon. In 1988, we localized the gene for A-T Group A (ATA) to chromosome 11q22-23.[152] In 1991, in a collaboration with Shiloh's lab, A-T Group C (ATC) was localized to the same region, also by linkage analysis.[153] Between 1990 and 1994, 26 genes were shown to complement A-T fibroblasts; none were localized to chromosome 11q23.1.[6,40,154,155] No convincing evidence for genetic heterogeneity was ever found in the linkage analysis studies despite such expectations. In 1995, when Savitsky *et al.*[72] identified part of a single gene (ATM), mutations were found for all four major complementation groups. Most interesting is that one homozygous mutation is present in both a Group C patient and a Group E patient, suggesting either that complementation groups in A-T are somewhat artifactual or that assigning patients to complementation groups is somewhat error-prone. To date, no laboratory has confirmed whether the cells from these two patients complement each other. Most likely this reflects that complementation group assignment by fusion of A-T fibroblasts is extremely tedious and that no laboratory has performed such studies since around 1990. Varying chromosomal ploidy between fused (4N) and nonfused (2N) cells also may have accounted for what appeared to be "complementation".

Complementation of A-T cells by gene transfections was a commonly used approach to cloning the gene. Many genes complemented various facets of the radiophenotype. These complementing genes presumably interact in some way with the ATM gene, the protein, or the signal transduction pathway. Some may bypass the ATM block in A-T cells, and they might provide exciting therapeutic opportunities for replacement therapy in A-T patients.[156] Despite the lack of success in cloning the A-T gene by complementation analyses, and the existing confusion about how intragenic mutations might complement, complementation may eventually provide a useful way of identifying functional domains in the ATM molecule.

Genetics

A-T is transmitted as an autosomal recessive disease.[1–6] The incidence of A-T has been estimated at 1 in 40,000 to 100,000 live births, while the gene frequency is believed to be as high as 3 percent of the general population.[4,163] Recent studies of breast cancer in several large populations have provided convincing data in support of an $\approx$1 percent carrier frequency.[55,258,282] All races are affected by A-T. Despite the A-T gene's affecting so many different and apparently unrelated systems, the disease is inherited in each family as a single autosomal recessive gene defect. It is unclear why, in an autosomal recessive disorder, so many of the parents of British, Italian, and American patients are unrelated. This is borne out by the recent finding that most A-T patients worldwide are compound heterozygotes; i.e., they have different paternal and maternal mutations.[72,157] In the rare instances where two patients share a common mutation, their haplotypes usually differ, indicating independent origins for the mutation. The large size of the gene certainly provides a large target for new mutations. Recent studies suggest that gametogenesis is abnormal in ATM knockout mice[16] and that mitotic and meiotic recombination is increased in A-T patients.[76,158] Furthermore, as was discussed above, the ATM gene shares homology with mec1 (yeast) and mei41 (*Drosophila*),[40,141] and both are meiotic-recombination defective mutants.[40,159] Whether this would affect heterozygous parents in A-T families sufficiently to influence the incidence of affected fetuses remains to be clarified. Recombination fractions in A-T families (i.e., in the parents) were normal across a 40 cM range of chromosome 11q22-23.[161]

Claims that "A-T is not always a recessive disorder"[45,160] are misleading and belie the consortium experience of having localized the ATM gene to the proper 400-kb genomic segment using a mathematical model that assumed autosomal recessive inheritance of a single gene and included 176 families. Families that do *not* link to 11q22-23 should be considered to carry mutations in other genes and to likely represent other syndromes. New names will have to be given to such "AT-like" disorders (see "Related Syndromes," below).

The rate of spontaneous mutations is unknown. Of the 176 consortium families, however, all but seven linked to chromosome 11q23.1.[161,162] Follow-up studies have found mutations in the ATM gene in six of these families. (A seventh family may be due to uniparental disomy.) Thus, linkage analyses of 175 families did not detect spontaneous mutations. Using the ratio of 5:176 and a gene frequency estimate of 0.01, mutation rate estimates approximate $1.5-3\times10^{-4}$ percent. This is rather high even for a large gene. Of course, if the ATM gene product really affects gametogenesis,[16,139,169] it may be inappropriate to apply standard genetic algorithms, which are based on the Hardy-Weinberg equilibrium, to the existing epidemiologic data.[163,164] It may also be that some young patients succumb to malignancies before a diagnosis of A-T can be recognized, further skewing the data. Furthermore, recent studies of ATM mutations in A-T patients versus cancer patients from non-AT families suggest that the frequencies of truncating versus missense ATM mutations may differ in the general population (See "Cancer Susceptibility" above).[306]

Endocrine Defects

Very little research has been done on endocrine defects in A-T patients. This may change considering that ATM knockout mice have problems with both spermatogenesis and ovulation.[16,39,169] Gonadal streaks, absent or hypoplastic ovaries, dysgerminomas, and undeveloped fallopian tubes have been observed at postmortem examination in both mice[16] and human patients.[2] Laboratory tests of pituitary function reveal no consistent abnormality.

In stark contrast to the earlier statement that "female hypogonadism with sexual infantilism is found consistently [in A-T patients],"[2,5] most female patients followed by the author have normal menstrual cycles, and although menstruation sometimes starts late, cycles come at regular intervals. There is no other evidence as to whether these patients ovulate normally. Anecdotally, some long-lived female patients may have entered menopause prematurely. Others report very irregular cycles. Most male patients develop normal secondary sex characteristics. Some of these patients can have erections and even ejaculate. Studies of sperm haplotyping on semen from several A-T patients have documented that some actually produce sperm. None have fathered a child. One report of a putative female A-T patient having borne a child is clouded because this woman lived beyond 50 years, which is highly atypical for A-T, and a similarly affected sib demonstrated remarkable dexterity while already in her thirties (she worked in a knitware factory). In contract, female NBS patients manifest very severe endocrine defects, most showing little or no development of secondary sex characteristics and markedly elevated (prepubertal) follicle-stimulating hormone (FSH) and luteinizing hormone (LH) levels.[283]

Some patients develop insulin-resistant diabetes, usually in the late teens. This is characterized by hyperglycemia without glycosuria or ketosis.[165,166] Other forms of diabetes, such as juvenile diabetes mellitus and late-onset diabetes, have been frequently observed among nonaffected members of A-T families. A genetic imprinting model has been considered, but this would not explain the pattern of diabetes in these families. Telomere silencing of subtelomeric genes, such as the insulin gene, might be an alternative hypothesis.[134]

Premature Aging

Many of the chromosomal instability syndromes, such as A-T, Fanconi anemia, xeroderma pigmentosum, and Bloom syndrome, show progeroid features.[167] Young A-T patients often have strands of gray hairs and develop keratoses; precocious basal cell carcinoma has been reported.[2,42] Some of these findings may reflect either premature menarche or the accelerated shortening of telomeres described above[135] (see "Chromosomal Instability"). However, thymic dystrophy and lymphoid depletion are also characteristic of aging and may be secondary to recombination defects during T-cell maturation rather than to telomeric shortening. Autoantibody formation is also found in both aging populations and A-T patients[9,168,170] (see the discussion in reference 170).

Postmortem examinations of older patients show progeric changes, such as neurofibrillary tangles in large neurons of the cerebral cortex, hippocampus, basal ganglia, and spinal cord, similar to those seen in Alzheimer disease.[15] Lipofuscin granules have been found in many neurons, in satellite cells of the dorsal ganglia, and in Schwann cells. Further, Marinesco bodies seen in the pigmented neurons of the substantia nigra in A-T patients are considered signs of precocious aging.[171]

Other Findings

Among Costa Rican families with classical A-T, about 40 percent of patients have clubbing of the fingertips, a finding that is usually associated with poorly oxygenated blood supply. These A-T children do not have cardiac defects. Most, but not all, live in San José, which is 3700 feet above sea level, not high enough to aggravate most cardiac or pulmonary problems. The mutations in these families have all been identified, and the clubbing does not associate with a particular mutation (see "Patient Mutations," below). It is possible that as part of their A-T syndrome these patients also have a pulmonary abnormality that compromises the oxygenation of their blood, such as microscopic arteriovenous fistulas or an anomalous bronchial tree.[197] However, this is purely speculative; at this writing, there is no explanation for the clubbing in Costa Rican A-T patients.[61]

Many of the Costa Rican patients also have hypertrichosis (excessive body hair).[61] This has been noted in other A-T patients as well.[5] Considering the diverse endocrinologic abnormalities that have been described in A-T patients (and in ATM knockout mice), hypertrichosis could reflect a mild hormonal imbalance in some patients.

Swift *et al.*[32] observed a fourfold increase of ischemic heart disease among female A-T carriers. Thus, while heterozygotes are at a 3.2-fold increased mortality risk, only 44 percent and 35 percent of the deaths (men and women, respectively) observed by Swift *et al.* were attributable to cancer; 34 percent and 35 percent of the deaths (men and women, respectively) were attributable to heart disease.

Related Syndromes

The related Nijmegen Breakage syndrome (NBS)[172] and the Berlin Breakage syndrome (BBS),[173] respectively assigned to complementation groups V1 and V2, do not show ataxia and do not link to chromosome 11q23.[162,174,175] These syndromes found their way into the A-T literature because cells from these patients manifest the 7;14 translocations and radioresistant DNA synthesis that are typical of A-T cells. These patients are also cancer susceptible and immunodeficient. Telangiectasias are absent, and the serum AFP level is normal. NBS patients have birdlike facies, microcephaly, and mental retardation (A-T patients typically are not mentally retarded). BBS very closely resembles NBS, and when the NBS1 gene was cloned in 1998, both BBS and NBS patients had mutations in that gene. NBS1 is on chromosome 8q11.[253] The NBS1 protein, nibrin, is absent from cell lysates of both NBS and BBS patients. NBS and BBS are now considered to be a single disorder. Because new evidence suggests that ATM phosphorylates nibrin,[307] in the Rad50/Mre11/nibrin complex, it would follow that the A-T and NBS phenotypes might overlap and that these genes might complement radioresistant synthesis.[151] Why NBS cells complement the radioresistant DNA synthesis of BBS is again a mystery of complementation experiments. Only a handful of BBS patients have been described in the literature. They have most of the signs and symptoms of NBS, with the possible addition to the syndrome of syndactyly, anal atresia, and hypospadias. Most of the reported NBS and BBS families have been of eastern Europe origin and carry the 657del5 mutation.[176–178,283,284]

AT_{Fresno} (AT_F) combines the classical A-T syndrome with NBS (Fig. 29-5).[179] Whenever microcephaly and mental retardation are seen in an otherwise classical A-T patient, diagnosis of AT_F should be suspected. However, because AT_F families link to chromosome 11q23.1 and ATM mutations have been found in four AT_F families, the clinical importance of this diagnostic distinction is presently unclear. Furthermore, the same ATM mutations found in two AT_F families have also been observed in classic A-T patients. If a second modifier gene were involved, it would have to link to the 11q22-23 region as well.

Many other reports describe patients who do not meet all the diagnostic criteria for A-T discussed above.[180–182,189,308,314] Many of these reports describe: (1) very young patients (when the A-T syndrome would not yet be fully expressed), (2) transient ataxias (some possibly infectious), (3) probable A-T patients without telangiectasias,[162,183,184] (4) patients with normal AFP levels, or (5) those with nearly normal immunologic parameters. Recent screening for ATM mutations in such "variant" families in the international consortium (families that were categorically excluded from the linkage analyses so as to avoid contaminating the positional cloning data) suggests that most of these were A-T. In several families with classically affected patients, prominent telangiectasias have been noted in members who do not have ataxia and who do not carry the two affected ATM haplotypes.[162] Some of these persons are bona fide A-T heterozygotes.

Other families have been described with intermediate radiosensitivity, a parameter that is difficult to quantitate; nonetheless, in some hands, this must be considered a quantifiable result that will probably relate in some way to the sites of ATM mutations in those families or to mutations in other genes that link to the 11q22-23 region[308,318] (see "Correlating Phenotypes with Genotypes," below). Undoubtedly, other radiosensitive individuals exist whose symptoms partially overlap the A-T syndrome. It will be interesting to learn whether these patients have leaky ATM mutations or mutations in other genes that interact with the ATM protein.

Differential Diagnosis

The most difficult challenge in making a diagnosis of A-T involves very young patients. The most common misdiagnosis is cerebral palsy, especially when there is a spastic component to the child's movements. With time, however, a diagnosis of A-T becomes clear when the ataxia is notably progressive, eye movements demonstrate poor tracking, and speech becomes slurred. The absence of telangiectasia at this stage should not weigh against a diagnosis of A-T. Family history may be helpful if a prior child exists with similar signs and symptoms and the parents are related. Both factors should certainly raise suspicion about a hereditary disorder, and A-T is the most common hereditary early-onset progressive ataxia. The presence or absence of cancer in the family generally is not helpful, for it can be interpreted in many ways. Laboratory studies should include serum AFP, a cytogenetic search for t(7;14) translocations, *in vitro* radiosensitivity (see below), and an immunologic evaluation. Recent evidence suggests that ATM protein levels in lysates of A-T cells are be very low or absent in most classical patients; these can be measured semi-quantitatively by Western blotting. In those bona fide A-T patients with ATM protein (~20%), the function is assumed to be compromised. This need not be limited to just the p53 kinase function; defects in alternative splicing, DNA binding, or tissue specificity could also have similar phenotypic effects.

Even if some of the above tests are not informative, a diagnosis of A-T may still be valid for these following reasons: (a) The AFP remains normal throughout life in 5 percent of patients. As was discussed above, the serum AFP is occasionally elevated in normal children under 2 years of age, and thus is not a reliable test until after that age. (b) A cytogenetic search for t(7;14) translocations or clones is often unsuccessful in A-T patients because a poor mitogenic response makes it difficult to find enough good-quality metaphases for analysis (see "Chromosomal Instability," above). Even if sufficient metaphases are found, the translocations are sometimes missed. Radiation-induced and bleomycin-induced breakage studies may be helpful, but they seldom contribute to making the diagnosis because of overlap between normal and A-T ranges.[89] (c) The immunologic evaluation is normal in some A-T patients. Whether it becomes progressively more abnormal in older A-T patients is debatable (see "Immunodeficiency," above). The response to allogeneic cells, the mixed lymphocyte response, is quite abnormal in some patients; however, this is a very laborious and costly test that is hard to quantitate without extensive controls and is therefore difficult to justify for strictly clinical purposes.

A MRI (magnetic resonance imaging) of the cerebellum will usually reveal marked dystrophy in children over 4 years of age (Fig. 29-6). Newer techniques for imaging the cerebellum are also being evaluated, such as functional MRI and PET (positron emission tomography) scanning;[231,232] however, both depend heavily on patient cooperation and may not be applicable to very young children. Furthermore, PET scanning uses radioactive tracers, and although the exposure doses are very small, they could theoretically contribute to cancer risk, especially in the bladder where the radioisotope accumulates rapidly during the procedure. When risk-benefit ratios are considered for procedures using ionizing radiation, difficult judgments must be made.

The most dangerous diagnostic situation for a young A-T patient occurs when cancer is the presenting symptom. Fortunately, this does not occur very often. Anecdotally, one child had a cerebellar astrocytoma removed at 27 months of age, but his unsteady gait actually worsened postoperatively. His clinicians were quite concerned and confused by the persistent ataxia until several years later, when the patient's younger sister began to stagger as well and a diagnosis of A-T was made on both children. Because the astrocytoma was totally resectable, no consideration was given to further therapy with chemotherapeutic agents or radiation. The patient died more than 20 years later without any sequelae of the cancer or surgery. Other children have not been so fortunate,[17–19] presenting with a malignancy and receiving conventional doses of irradiation because it was not realized that they were suffering from A-T, only to suffer iatrogenic deaths. The late Dr. Boder claimed that she could make a diagnosis of A-T in any child under 2 years of age. While this is a challenging claim, it is certainly true that most young A-T patients do have at least some suspicious neurologic findings at a very early age. On questioning, mothers sometimes volunteer that they noted head tilting or swaying in these infants (Fig. 29-7). Thus, it is prudent for pediatric oncologists and radiation oncologists to rule out the diagnosis of A-T before treating *any* young child with cancer, either by obtaining a complete history and performing a careful neurologic examination with this in mind, or by obtaining a neurologic consultation as part of the workup.

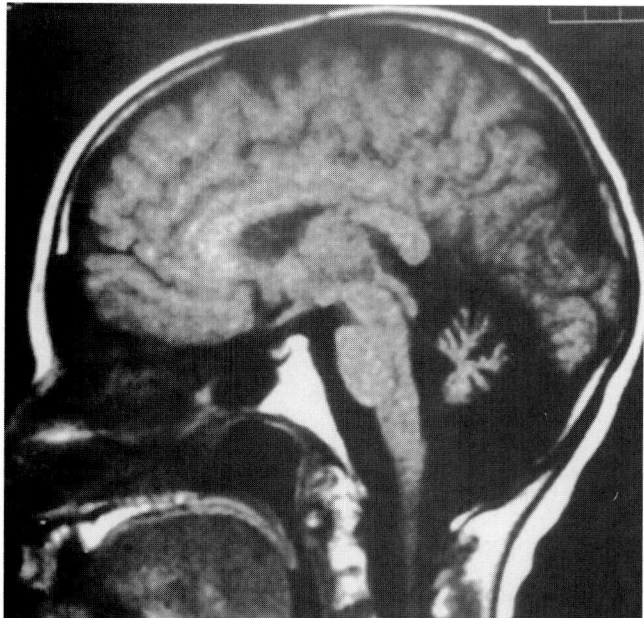

Fig. 29-6 Magnetic resonance imaging of a 6-year-old A-T patient showing markedly reduced size of the cerebellar shadow.

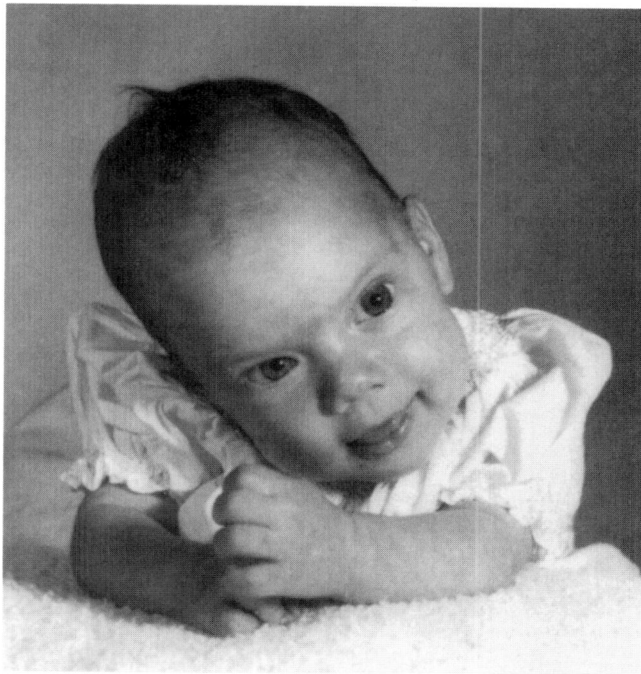

Fig. 29-7 Head-tilting in a 6-month-old infant with A-T. Staggering was not noted until she began to walk.

While the presence of hypersensitivity to ionizing radiation is a laboratory hallmark of the disease, clinical testing for this has not been readily available, primarily because most radiosensitivity assays use fibroblasts, and establishing fibroblasts in A-T patients is painful and labor intensive. With this in mind, Huo *et al.*[111] laboratory established the CSA, a clonogenic assay that evaluates the colony survival fraction of LCLs from patients after the cells have received 1 Gy of ionizing irradiation.[111] From a single 10-ml heparinized blood sample (that should be shipped without refrigeration), cells are transformed with Epstein-Barr virus. Once a stable cell line is established, the cells are plated in two cell concentrations on 96-well tissue culture trays that are irradiated (or not irradiated) and returned to an incubator for 10 days, at which point the number of wells containing colonies larger than 32 cells is scored and compared to the colony survival fractions of normal cells. Unlike other colony survival assays, the CSA conditions were selected so that heterozygotes would score as normals, which allows for more reliable detection of A-T homozygotes (Fig. 29-8). Recently, two referred patients with

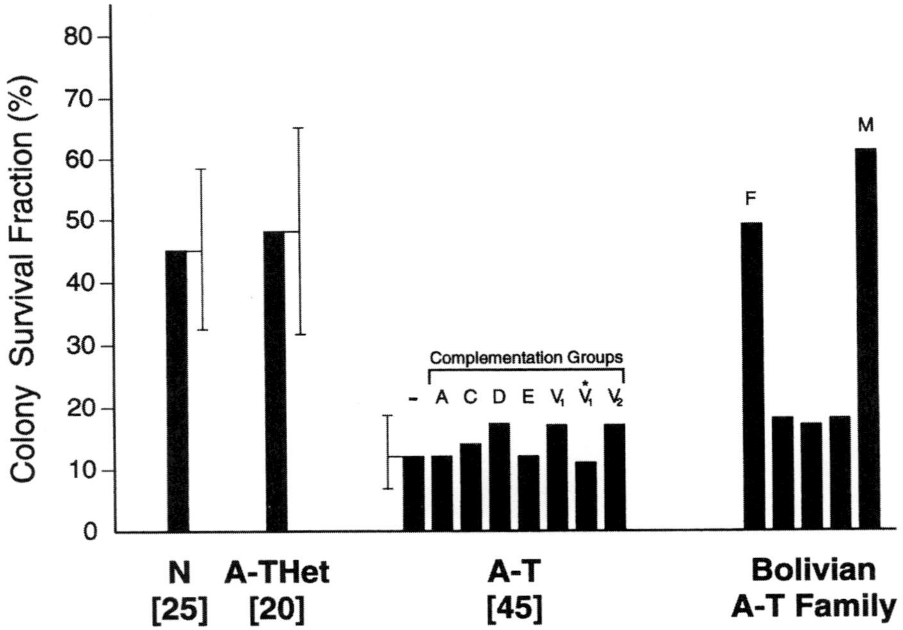

Fig. 29-8 Colony survival assay (CSA) measures radiosensitivity of LCLs from patients with A-T, A-T heterozygotes, normals, and a Bolivian family with three affected children, following 1 Gy of irradiation. Also included are results from patients with NBS (V1), BBS (V2), and AT_F (V1*).

normal CSA results on repeated testing were subsequently found to have the typical (GAA)n expansions of Friedreich ataxia on chromosome 9q13. Although the differential diagnosis between Friedreich ataxia (FRDA) and A-T is usually not difficult — FRDA is a later-onset ataxia (usually around puberty) and most FRDA patients have hypertrophic cardiomyopathy (by ECG testing), whereas A-T patients generally do not have cardiac problems — this experience served to underscore the value of using radiosensitivity to confirm a suspected early diagnosis of A-T. FRDA patients have normal CSA results.[111,185] Patients from all complementation groups, including NBS and BBS, have the same markedly reduced CSA levels. Human Mre11 deficiency patients[308] are also radiosensitive but have not yet been tested by CSA

Abnormal facies other than the slowly developing smile, or masklike expression of many A-T patients, should raise suspicion about other diagnoses. Severe mental retardation and inability to speak at an appropriate age are also uncharacteristic of A-T. Mental retardation is seen more commonly in lower socioeconomic-level families and countries, perhaps because they lack the resources needed to keep A-T patients in the mainstream of family and community life, whereby they must learn to respond to various personal challenges. The absence of oculomotor apraxia by 5 years of age is also strong evidence against the diagnosis of A-T.

Ataxia is common to a variety of other hereditary disorders:[186] (a) as a major feature with progressive ataxia — hMre11 deficiency[308] β-lipoprotein abnormalities selective vitamin E deficiency, hexosaminidase deficiency (GM2), and cholesterolosis; (b) as a major feature with intermittent ataxia — urea-cycle defects, maple syrup urine disease, isovaleric acidosis, 2-hydroxyglutaric aciduria, Hartnup disease, pyruvate dysmetabolism, and mitochondrial disease; and (c) as a minor feature of Niemann-Pick syndrome, metachromatic leukodystrophy, multiple sulfatase deficiency, late-onset globoid cell leukodystrophy, adrenoleukodystrophy, sialidosis type 1, and ceroid lipofuscinosis. The latter can be diagnosed only by biopsy of the conjunctiva or brain. Most of the other listed disorders will show abnormalities in urinary amino acids, lysosomal hydrolases, or very long chain fatty acids. Retinitis pigmentosa, deafness, polyneuropathy, and ataxia characterize Refsum disease.[187] Non-hereditary ataxia may result from an acute infection or from a posterior fossa tumor. (For further information, see reference 5.)

Determining whether a new patient's ataxia has been inherited in a dominant or a recessive manner can aid in distinguishing A-T from olivopontocerebellar atrophy and any of the spinocerebellar ataxias, all of which are dominant disorders. The familial pattern for age at onset of the ataxia is also helpful, because few other familial ataxias present in early childhood as A-T does. While an occasional case of early-onset FRDA might be mistaken for A-T on this basis, neurologic examination will reveal spinal cord ataxia with a positive Romberg sign, and, in the laboratory, homozygosity for a (GAA)n expansion in the first intron of the FRDA gene is easily diagnosed[188,316]; FRDA cells are also not radiosensitive.[111]

Determining whether two mutations exist within the ATM gene of a child suspected of having A-T is the most definitive way of establishing a diagnosis. At this writing such an approach is just becoming feasible (see "Patient Mutations," below). In families of certain ethnic backgrounds, rapid DNA assays can be performed for mutations that are common in that population. By first haplotyping the DNA of a suspected A-T patient in the chromosome 11q22-23 region, previously described haplotypes carrying mutated ATM genes can be identified. However, unless the patient is homozygous for a mutation — which is very unlikely unless the parents are consanguineous — a second mutation must still be sought. This requires a great deal of effort either by mRNA/cDNA/RT-PCR-based screening assays or by a systematic genomic search of the 66 exons of the ATM gene. Even this approach is not 100 percent effective in finding all mutations, because some lie deep within introns and others require analysis of both genomic DNA and mRNA. Eventually, we hope to determine the mutations and affected haplotypes for most A-T families. This database will expedite both the diagnosis of A-T and prenatal diagnosis.

Aicardi *et al.*[189] described a group of 14 patients with a late-onset progressive ataxia, choreoathetosis, and oculomotor apraxia without frequent infections or telangiectasia. The AFP was normal and a search for t(7;14) translocations was negative. Aicardi suggested that these children suffered from "an unusual type of spinocerebellar degeneration," probably not A-T. However, it would be informative to determine whether any of those patients are radiosensitive, for example, by CSA.

Prenatal Diagnosis

With the fine mapping of the ATM gene, a set of highly informative genetic markers was developed that now allows accurate haplotyping within families, with basically 100 percent reliability of the fetus either being affected or not being affected, i.e., less than 1 percent recombination between ATM and the markers used. The finding of only a single A-T gene for all complementation groups also simplifies this diagnostic approach. This is in contrast to earlier attempts to perform prenatal diagnoses by trying to quantitate spontaneous chromosome breakage[89,109–193] (see the discussion in reference 150), assessing radiation-induced chromosomal damage of amniocytes or fetal fibroblasts, or performing RDS, all of which were misleading at one time or another (anonymous oral communications). One hopes that these approaches have by now been abandoned.

Prenatal diagnosis by haplotyping relies on a prior affected child to (a) establish a firm diagnosis of A-T and (b) identify the two affected chromosome 11q23.1 segments (i.e., haplotypes) carrying the ATM gene.[192] Figure 29-9 illustrates haplotyping and how it was possible to determine that the first cousin of an affected patient was not affected. A definitive diagnosis was possible only because a prior affected cousin existed in a consanguineous family. It is of paramount importance that the diagnosis of A-T in the prior affected member be confirmed before attempting haplotyping for prenatal diagnosis. The markers we use today are all within 1 percent recombination of the ATM gene: D11S1817,[194] D11S1819,[194] NS22,[285] D11S2179,[195] and D11S1818.[194] Two of these markers are within the ATM gene itself, thereby circumventing the need for reporting the risk of recombination separating the testing markers from the actual ATM gene. Most of this testing can be performed before conception, i.e., preconceptional testing. Once a DNA sample is available from the fetus, either from growing amniocytes or from a chorionic villous biopsy, the entire haplotyping can be completed within a week. With new "molecular beacons" this will become even more streamlined.[298] Because abortion guidelines vary with the country or state of residence of the mother, we ask for the referring laboratory's deadline for reporting the results of prenatal diagnosis to the family, rather than for the due date or the date of last menses. In keeping with modern guidelines for genetic testing, the results are conveyed to the family by a genetic counselor.

Therapy

No effective therapy exists for halting the progression of the ataxia.[2,5,196] Clinical trials are under way to test the efficacy of myoinositol, *N*-acetylcysteine, and L-dopa on general symptoms. To date, preliminary data have been disappointing. (For a review of other AT-related medications, see reference 196.) Vitamin E has been prescribed by some A-T specialists for years, based on anecedotal information from Dr. Elena Boder.[15] Recent studies suggesting that A-T cells may be in a constant state of increased oxidative stress make it likely that most antioxidants or free-radical scanvengers might counteract some of the progressive neurological deterioration of A-T patients.[38,317,325,326,327] Thus, vitamin E continues to be recommended; α-lipoic acid and coenzyme Q10 may also slow the deterioration. Folic acid may formation further help to minimize chromosomal fragility and the formation of double-strand DNA breaks. All of the above dietary supplements are available without a prescription.

Areas of great concern to the health of A-T patients are pulmonary infections and malignancy. Pulmonary infections usually are due to the normal spectrum of microbes and are treatable by conventional approaches. Opportunistic infections do not occur in A-T patients as they do in patients with other immunodeficiency disorders (with the possible exception of mycobacterium). Malignancies must be treated with great care to avoid conventional doses of radiation therapy or radiomimetic agents. If possible, neurotoxic chemotherapeutic agents should be avoided.

Not all A-T patients manifest frequent pulmonary or sinus infections. Those with chronic bronchiectasis are best treated in the same way as patients with cystic fibrosis: routine chest percussion, postural drainage, and generally aggressive pulmonary hygiene. Periodic pulmonary function studies may assist in monitoring infection-prone patients. In older patients, pulmonary

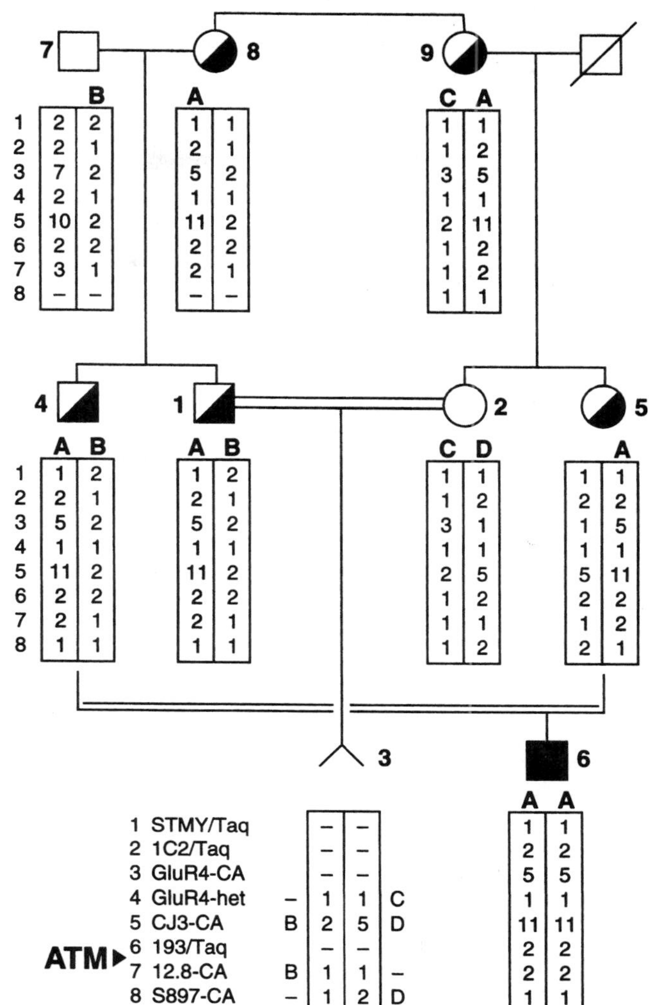

Fig. 29-9 Prenatal testing to determine whether a fetus (3) is affected. By history, two brothers had married two sisters who were their first cousins. One couple (4 and 5) had an affected child (6), prompting the second couple (1 and 2) to seek prenatal testing. However, testing before conception would have identified the mother (2) as a noncarrier, thereby circumventing any further testing on the fetus. Haplotype [A] carries the affected ATM gene. The genetic markers that are currently being used for prenatal testing are given in the text.

infections are the major cause of failing health and death. Increasing bulbar dysfunction may predispose to aspiration pneumonia. In addition to appropriate antibiotics, intravenous γ-globulin every 3 to 4 weeks may reduce the frequency of infections in infection-prone patients. There is some indication that the lungs of A-T patients may not be anatomically normal. Pump *et al.*[197] made a latexlike impression of one lung (using a substance called Vultex moulage [General Latex and Chemicals Ltd., Verdun, Quebec]) from a single A-T patient. They found bronchiectatic changes in many parts of the lung, with saccular dilatations throughout the bronchi.

Perhaps the most effective impact on care that the physician can make is to strongly encourage the parents of young A-T patients to institute an aggressive and engaging physical exercise program aimed at enhancing lung function, preventing contractures, and avoiding positional kyphoscoliosis. Almost all patients who have been denied such care develop severe contractures of the feet and hands. These become apparent in the late teens. An annual assessment by a physical therapist allows this care to be customized.

Speech therapy is also effective, not in arresting the progression of the dysarthria, but in minimizing the frustration felt by the patients when they cannot be understood by peers. Increased social interaction generally improves speech clarity.

Some of the neurologic symptoms, such as ataxia, drooling, and tremors, can be partially relieved by various agents.[196] Buspirone, a serotonergic 5-hydroxytryptophan agonist, is active in some types of cerebellar ataxia.[253] Amantadine improves balance and coordination and minimizes drooling in some patients. Postural tremors may be reduced by baclofen, a GABA inhibitor, or propranolol and other β blockers, while cerebellar tremors and myoclonus may respond to low doses of clonazepam or valproic acid. However, these agents sometimes increase the ataxia, drowsiness, or depression. Methyl scopolamine or propantheline hydrochloride are sometimes effective in reducing drooling. Ligating the salivary ducts can also alleviate drooling. This may also reduce the risk of aspiration pneumonia.

When radiation therapy is planned for treating a malignancy in an A-T patient, doses should be reduced by approximately 30 percent. Some chemotherapeutic agents, especially alkylating agents, probably should also be used in reduced doses. It has been suggested that topoisomerase inhibitors should be avoided. Unfortunately, there is only anecdotal literature on the important and recurring issue of oncologic treatment of A-T patients.

Occasionally, the possibility of bone marrow transplantation arises, usually because a young A-T patient has developed leukemia and has an HLA-compatible sib to serve as a potential donor. Despite several such attempts over the past 20 years, the author is unaware of a single transplant with convincing documentation of long-term engraftment. This could be for several reasons, the most compelling of which is the difficulty of establishing a safe but effective regimen for delivering the marrow-ablating irradiation or chemotherapy for the reasons given above. In general, hyperfractionation of radiation doses would seem prudent under such circumstances if this need were to arise. There is, of course, only a remote possibility that bone marrow transplantation would alter the cerebellar degeneration.[286,287] Hematopoietic stem cell transplantation might reduce the need for complete ablation but probably would also reduce the chances of a full immunologic engraftment. Neural stem cell engraftment may eventually become an important therapeutic alternative.

Many A-T patients have been immunized inadvertently for smallpox, polio, and varicella, with no apparent sequelae. Nevertheless, natural varicella infections are often quite severe. Thus, contrary to the general warning that patients with immunodeficiencies not be given live vaccines, varicella immunization is advisable for patients whose immune status is satisfactory.

Prognosis

Most A-T patients in the United States live well beyond 20 years. Many are now in their thirties. This is a major change from just a few years ago when it was unusual for these patients to live beyond their teenage years. Unfortunately, this is still true in many countries, for reasons that are unknown; however, the improved survival in the United States may be related to better nutrition, better diagnostics, better treatment of pulmonary infections and malignancies, and more aggressive physical therapy. There is hope among A-T investigators that the young children being diagnosed today will benefit from some currently undiscovered therapy before their neurologic status becomes irreversible.

MOLECULAR GENETICS

Our laboratory utilized a large Amish pedigree, that included four branches of the family with living affected members, to localize the ATM gene to 11q22-23 in 1988.[152,205] This family was later assigned by Jaspers and coworkers to complementation group A.[150–151,204] To our initial surprise, when lod scores from all A-T families were added together, regardless of complementation group assignments, the cumulative lod scores increased.[152,206,207] This suggested that either (a) the complementation group genes were all clustered in the 11q22-23 region, (b) most of the families were of similar complementation groups (Groups A and C were thought to include over 80 percent of the typed families), (c) the complementation groups represented intragenic mutations, or (d) complementation typing with A-T fibroblasts did not reflect Mendelian inheritance. In all our subsequent linkage analyses over the next 7 years, we never found any convincing evidence for genetic heterogeneity.[18,206–208] The cloning of a single gene for all complementation groups corroborated these early interpretations.

Subsequent to our initial report localizing the A-T gene to 11q22-23,[152] many reports followed that confirmed and extended that observation.[153,161,162,181,206–221] In the final linkage studies of 169 bona fide families that had been entered into a 9-country consortium, over 40 genetic markers were tested. The location score curve peaked at D11S535 with a lod score of 73. The 2-lod support region containing the A-T locus was a 500-kb interval beginning 150-kb proximal to S384 and ending just short of S1294. If we counted the number of families with recombinants in the candidate region, the same 500-kb region of common overlap

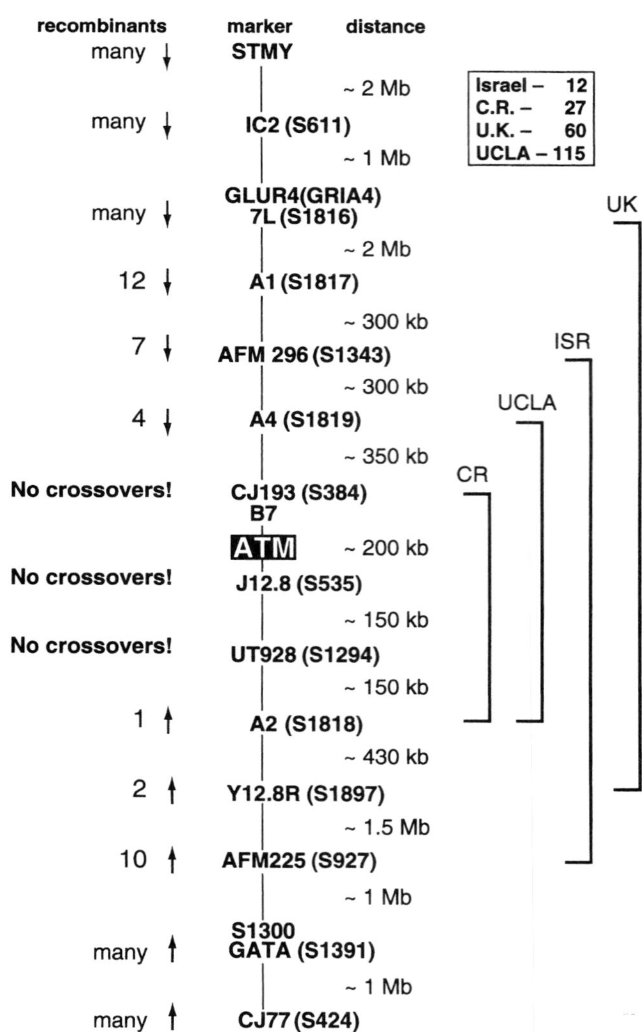

Fig. 29-10 Combined linkage and physical map of 11 cM surrounding the ATM gene. The map is based on the combined linkage analysis of 249 families (59 CEPH and 190 A-T) and pulsed-field gel analyses.[220] Also depicted are the most likely regions for the ATM gene that were based on the number of families from the respective consortium members (see box and brackets at right). On the left, the number of recombinants in the consortium families is given. The position of the ATM gene on this map was added later.

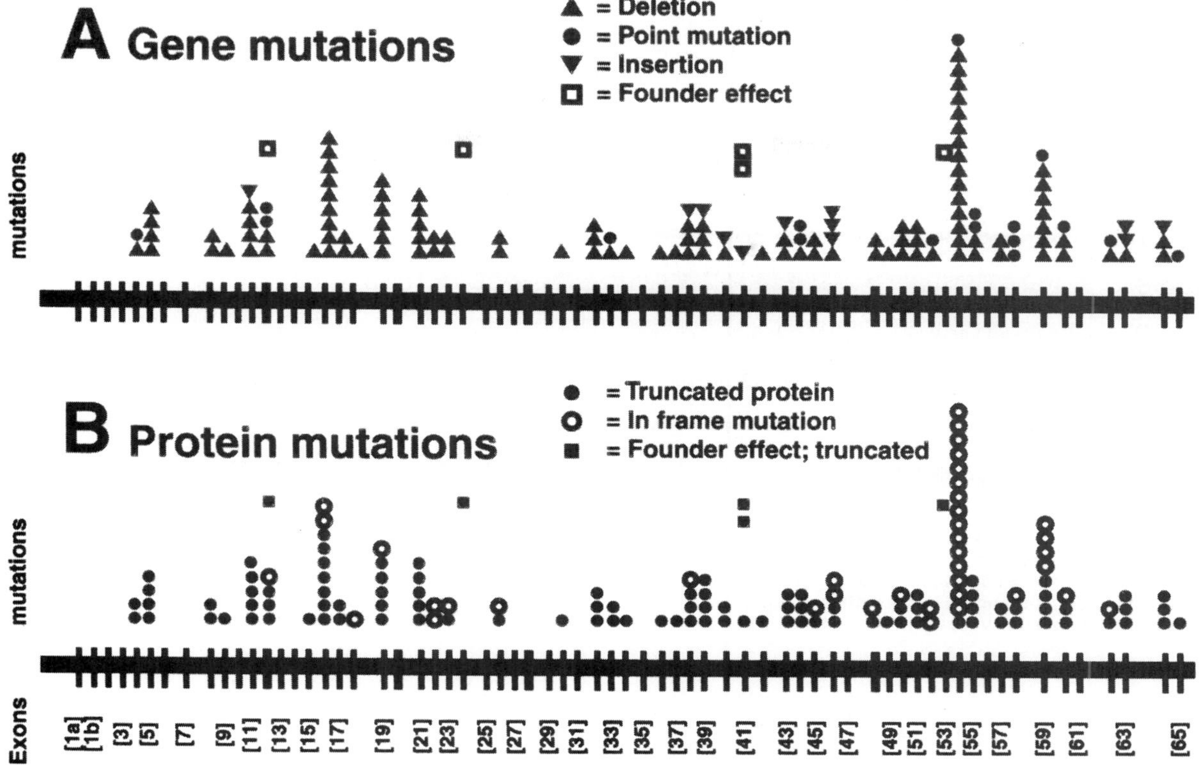

Fig. 29-11 Spectrum of 120 ATM mutations based on studies of cDNA from cells of patients from many countries. *A,* Mutations seen in related (or probably related, because they share haplotypes) families are indicated only once (by boxes) to avoid biasing the distribution. The exact position of many of these mutations will be revised once the genomic mutation sites have been defined. *B,* The majority of mutations result in truncated ATM proteins. (For an updated version of this figure, see Web site: http://www.vmresearch.org/atm.htm.)

could be appreciated. The accuracy of these positional cloning experiments depended heavily on the construction of an accurate genetic map (Fig. 29-10).

From 1993 to 1995, detailed YAC, BAC, and cosmid maps were made of the candidate region by several of the consortium laboratories, and, using these genomic segments, many transcripts from many cDNA libraries were isolated. Five recovery methods were used, including exon trapping,[224] the only method that did not depend on whether the A-T gene was being expressed in any particular library. Each of the recovered transcripts had to be sequenced so that PCR primers could be designed and used to amplify and screen for mutations, using cDNAs from 100 A-T patients as templates for the PCRs. In 1993, several labs found a large transcript, E14/CAND3/NPAT, which was ubiquitously expressed, thus qualifying it as a good candidate A-T gene. Despite very thorough searches of CAND3 for mutations in over 100 A-T patients, using SSCP, heteroduplex analysis (HA), density gradient gel electrophoresis (DGGE), and direct cDNA sequencing, no mutations were found. In 1995, the ATM gene was isolated by the Israeli members of the consortium[72,73] from within the 500-kb region defined by the linkage analyses. E14/CAND3/NPAT was only 544 bp upstream of the initiation site for ATM, oriented in the opposite transcriptional direction and sharing a common promoter.[225–227] Although this gene also contains a kinase domain, its function remains unknown.

The ATM Gene

The ATM gene transcript is 13 kb (9054 nt of ORF), with 66 exons, the largest being exon 12 with 372 nucleotides (nt) (GDB accession numbers U82828, U26455, X91196, U40887-40918, and U33841, as well as the reports of Savitsky *et al.*,[72,140] Rasio *et al.*,[228] Uziel *et al.*,[229] Byrd *et al.*,[225] Vorechovsky *et al.*,[54] Pecker *et al.*,[230] and Platzer *et al.*[251]). It has a molecular weight of 350 and is a member of a family of high-molecular-weight protein kinases.[72,139–141,233] Northern blots reveal expression in all tissues, with several transcripts of 10.5 (fibroblasts), 6.2, and 4.9 kb. Recent studies by Rotman and coworkers[194,319] indicate that a considerable amount of alternative splicing occurs at the 5′ end. The 3′ portion of the gene has strong homology to yeast and mammalian phosphatidylinositol 3-kinases, as well as to DNA-PK. Thus, ATM appears to play a major role as an intracellular signal transducer that gives warning to the cell, via cell-cycle checkpoints, of DNA damage that must be repaired before the next cell division. However, as was discussed above, another role for the ATM protein remains to be elucidated, one that is p53-independent and probably involves replicon initiation and meiotic pairing during gametogenesis. A leucine zipper domain around exon 27 suggests that the ATM protein may form homo- or heterodimers and bind DNA. When this region of the gene was transfected into normal cells, the normal cells developed an A-T phenotype, which suggests a dominant negative effect for the leucine zipper region.[288,330] An SH_3 domain (residues 1373 to 1382) binds c-abl in response to DNA damage.[70]

Patient Mutations

Over 400 mutations in the ATM gene have been identified (Fig. 29-11).[72,157,222,225,234,235,237,252,289,321–323] A Web site has been created for tracking those already published: http://www.vmresearch.org/atm.htm. Intially these laboratories used a variety of screening approaches; restriction endonuclease fingerprinting (REF), SSCP followed by single-strand sequencing, protein truncation testing (PTT), and conformation sensitive gel electrophoresis (CSGE).[157] Each screening approach strongly biases the types of mutations found. Almost all the early work used mRNA

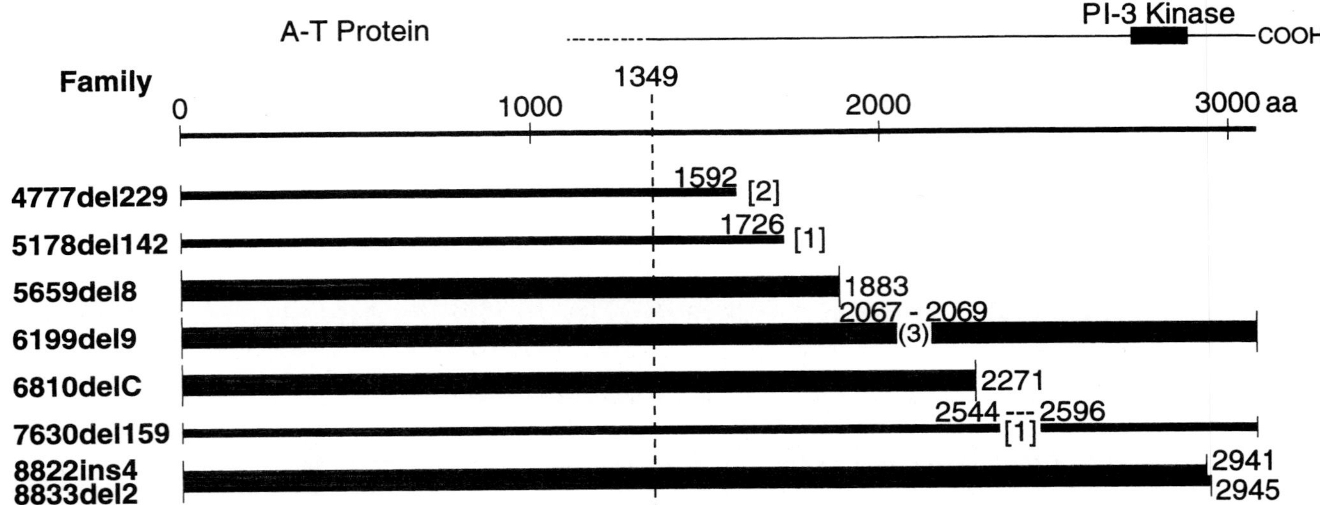

Fig. 29-12 Depiction of theoretical protein truncations based on cDNA and genomic mutations and their relationship to the most conserved portion of the PI-3 kinase domain. Bracketed numbers represent deleted exons; numbers in parentheses represent deleted codons. While most deletions result in truncation of the protein, a few do not create frameshifts, and presumably the protein continues to be translated downstream from the deletion, thereby including the presumably important PI-3 kinase domain. Thick bars represent patients with homozygous mutations. Such patients can now be analyzed for phenotype-genotype correlations (see Table 29-3).

as a template (via reverse transcription of mRNA to cDNA). About 70 percent of ATM mutations result in truncated proteins, most of which affect splice sites;[222,252] these are detected efficiently by PTT, which is still the method of choice if live cells are available as a source of RNA. Platzer *et al.*[251] used dye terminator methodology to directly sequence 27.3 kb of DNA on each of 72 patients; only 50 percent of mutations were detected. A comparative discussion of mutation detection strategies for ATM is beyond the scope of this chapter. (For further details, see references 236 and 237.)

Because the 3′ half of the ATM gene was sequenced first, the distribution of mutations shown in Fig. 29-11 is slightly biased against finding equal numbers of mutations in the 5′ half. Most A-T patients are compound heterozygotes. One potential hotspot (approximately 15 percent of mutations) was identified, in exon 54.[235] Exon 54 is just proximal to the PI-3 kinase homology domain, and, therefore, mutations in this region could be especially important. In screening cDNAs, two types of changes were observed here: c2544del159nt and c2546del9nt, both of which resulted in in-frame deletions in cDNA (for example, see mutation 7630del159nt in Fig. 29-12 which deletes 53 amino acids). (The numbers prefacing a cDNA change indicates the first codon to be affected.) The genomic mutation that causes the 159nt-exon 54 to be skipped during splicing may appear anywhere within that genomic region. For example, three genomic mutations are now known to cause a splicing deletion of exon 54: 7788G > A, 7926A > C, and IVS53-2A > C. (Many of the published cDNA changes have not been updated in the literature with the corresponding genomic mutations.) Further studies of exon 54 similarly indicate that many of the 15 patients from around the world with the 7636del9 (c2547del9) mutation share a common haplotype and they are mainly of Irish-English background.[252,289] Thus, the putative exon 54 hotspot contains at least four different mutations and many of the patients are probably distantly related; i.e., the frequency of the 7636del9 mutation should be counted only once for this lineage.

Because of the marginal effect that the 7636del9 in-frame mutation might have on the predicted protein—i.e., it would delete three amino acids (codons 2547–49)—it could be argued that this represents a polymorphism and not a true mutation. Wright *et al.*[235] addressed this issue by screening 75 parents of CEPH families; no examples of this mutation were found. Lavin *et al.*[320] introduced this mutation into atm−/− cell and it did not restore a normal phenotype, except for a small amount of ATM protein.

Vorechovsky *et al.*[54] found 7 similar unique DNA changes in a group of 38 breast tumors that were not observed in paired blood samples or in an extended sampling of 224 unrelated chromosomes. These are "rare allelic variants" (RAVs). Considering together the prediction that 1 in every 500 bp in the human genome is "mutated," and the 150-kb genomic size of the ATM gene, one would expect to find 300 polymorphic sites within the ATM gene. Those changes that obviously affect coding or splicing regions are mostly mutations, certainly those detected by PTT would truncate the protein.[157,252] However, it has been increasingly difficult to interpret the biological effects of so-called "silent mutations" and "missense mutations," as well as the effects of changes found deep within introns, in cases where RNA is not also available for analysis. A "silent mutation" that leads to a splicing defect is shown in Fig. 29-13. In this example, a genomic 2250G > A mutation does not change the amino acid (AAG and AAA are both lysine codons); however, the cDNA-based PTT indicates that this "silent" mutation results in a more deleterious 126 nt deletion.

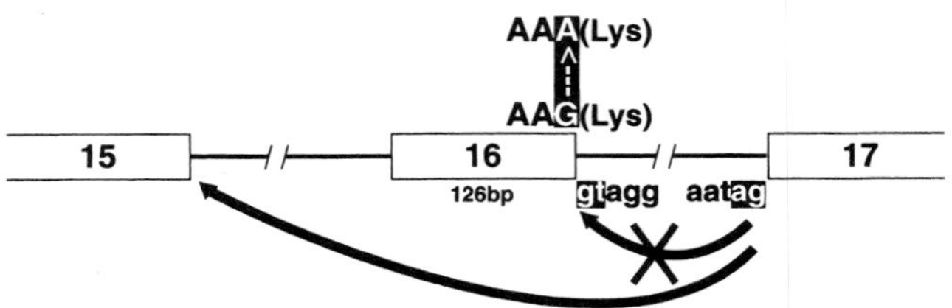

Fig. 29-13 Genomic mutation 2250G > A at the end of exon 16 would not result in a change of the lysine at codon 709. The G > A transition is a "silent mutation." However, protein truncation testing (PTT) demonstrates that this mutation results in a 126-nt deletion in the cDNA. This perturbs the donor splice site of exon 16 and causes the acceptor site to skip upstream to the donor site of exon 15, thereby deleting exon 16. Because the deletion does not result in a frameshift, downstream translation of the truncated protein should not be affected. However, western blotting of lysates from the cells of this patient, failed to show any ATM protein. Thus, what might appear from genomic analysis to be an insignificant mutation is in fact a deleterious one, as evidenced by the characteristic A-T phenotype of two unrelated homozygous patients with this mutation.

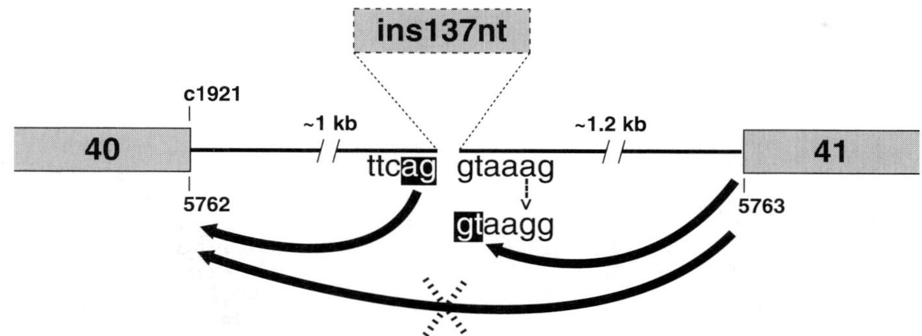

Fig. 29-14 Mutation IVS40+1126A>G inserts an artificial 137-bp exon into the mRNA by creating a new donor splice site 5 nucleotides upstream of the mutation (at IVS40+1122) and taking advantage of an existing potential acceptor splice site further upstream (for further details, see reference 239).

Because the last nucleotide in an exon is a "G" 79 percent of the time,[238] the G > A change most likely disturbs the splice donor site for exon 16 so that the splice acceptor site at exon 17 skips upstream to the next acceptable splice donor site, that of exon 15. This deletes the 126 nt of exon 16, thereby truncating the protein by 42 amino acids. Mutation IVS40 + 1126A > G, described by McConville *et al.*,[239] is an example of how a change deep within intron 40 leads to the formation of a new artifical exon (Fig. 29-14). The expanded mRNA apparently results in a "leaky" mutation that is associated with a somewhat milder phenotype (see "Correlating Phenotypes with Genotypes" below).

Castellvi-Bel *et al.*[323] have detected 10 conventional polymorphisms (Table 29-1) and 2 RAVs (Table 29-2). Udar *et al.*[285] have identified an additional complex microsatellite repeat within the ATM gene. Given the low frequency of RAVs in general populations, they must represent rather recent changes in the genome. Another microsatellite repeat, DNA11S2179 was described by Vanagaite *et al.*[195] Because we have only screened approximately 23 kb (or 15 percent) of the genomic region containing the ATM gene, we would have expected to find about 45 (0.15 × 300) unique DNA changes. Combining the seven RAVs described by Vorechovsky *et al.*[54] with our 34 polymorphisms, this estimate compares favorably with the 41 polymorphisms actually found to date. Undoubtedly, other investigators will find additional DNA changes within introns of the gene that are not mutations; i.e., they do not compromise the integrity of the ATM protein. If large populations of cancer patients are to be screened using only DNA, some significant "mutations" may be misinterpreted as insignificant, and polymorphisms may be mistaken as mutations. Indeed, within the Internet Web site for ATM mutations in A-T homozygotes, [http://www.vmresearch.org/atm.htm], roughly 60 percent of patients have only one allele defined, strongly suggesting that present mutation detection methods do not detect a large proportion of ATM mutations. Perhaps some of these mutations reside in the 3′UT region, a region that has not yet been screened because of the great difficulty of distinguishing mutations from polymorphisms. This limitation will also mask potential genotype-phenotype correlations.

In an almost independent effort to localize the A-T gene without segregation analysis (in the event that meiotic recombination might be increased in A-T—a chromosomal breakage syndrome, after all—and the linkage results might mislead the positional cloning experiments), we utilized a subset of 27 Costa Rican families to track ancestral haplotypes,[223] a form of linkage disequilibrium analysis and "identity by descent" analysis. Even before the cloning of the gene, it was possible to establish that only a single gene was responsible for all of the Costa Rican families by pairing each of the Costa Rican haplotypes with a different one (Fig. 29-15). We further reasoned that the patients carrying

Table 29-1 Common Polymorphisms in the *ATM* Gene

	Allelic frequency (N ∼ 100)
10807A > G	72:28
IVS3−122T > C	55:45
IVS4 + 36insAA	61:39
IVS6 + 70delT	71:29
IVS16−34C > A	75:25
IVS22−77T > C	72:28
IVS24−9delT	86:14
IVS25−15delA	63:37
5557G > A	75:25
IVS48−69insATT	61:39
IVS62−55T > C	69:31

Table 29-2 "Rare Allelic Variants" in the *ATM* Gene

	Allelic frequency (%) (N ∼ 100)
10677G > C	1
10742G > T	0.5
10819G > T	0.5
10948A > G	1
IVS3−300G > A	4
IVS7−28T > C	0.5
IVS8−24del5	1
IVS13−137T > C	1
IVS14−55T > G	5
1986T > C	0.5
IVS20 + 27delT	1
IVS23−76T > C (28% in IRAT)	0
IVS25−35T > A	3
IVS27−65T > C	2
IVS30−54T > C	0.5
4362 A > C	0.5
IVS38−8T > C	6
5793T > C	1
IVS47−11G > T	0.5
IVS49−16T > A	0.5
IVS53 + 34insA	1
IVS60−50delTTAGTT	0.5
IVS62 + 8A > C	2
IVS62−65G > A	0.5

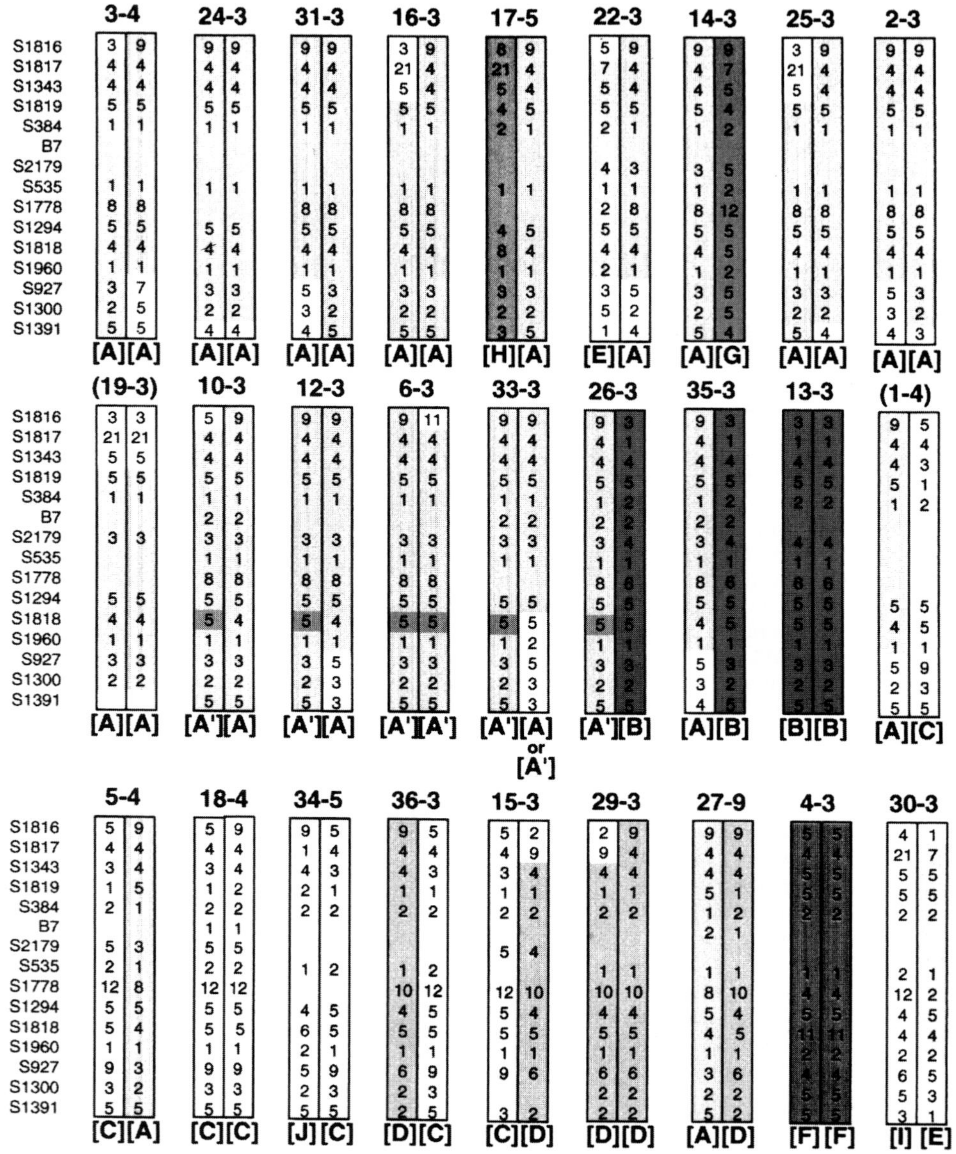

	3-4		24-3		31-3		16-3		17-5		22-3		14-3		25-3		2-3	
S1816	3	9	9	9	9	9	3	9	8	9	5	9	9	9	3	9	9	9
S1817	4	4	4	4	4	4	21	4	21	4	7	4	4	7	21	4	4	4
S1343	4	4	4	4	4	4	5	4	5	4	5	4	4	5	5	4	4	4
S1819	5	5	5	5	5	5	5	5	4	5	5	5	5	4	5	5	5	5
S384	1	1	1	1	1	1	1	1	2	1	2	1	1	2	1	1	1	1
B7																		
S2179											4	3	3	5				
S535	1	1	1	1	1	1	1	1	1	1	1	1	1	2	1	1	1	1
S1778	8	8			8	8	8	8			2	8	8	12	8	8	8	8
S1294	5	5	5	5	5	5	5	5	4	5	5	5	5	5	5	5	5	5
S1818	4	4	4	4	4	4	4	4	8	4	4	4	4	5	4	4	4	4
S1960	1	1	1	1	1	1	1	1	1	1	2	1	1	2	1	1	1	1
S927	3	7	3	3	5	3	3	3	3	3	3	5	3	5	3	3	5	3
S1300	2	5	2	2	3	2	2	2	2	2	5	2	2	5	2	2	3	2
S1391	5	5	4	4	4	5	5	5	3	5	1	4	5	4	5	4	4	3
	[A]	[A]	[A]	[A]	[A]	[A]	[A]	[A]	[H]	[A]	[E]	[A]	[A]	[G]	[A]	[A]	[A]	[A]

	(19-3)		10-3		12-3		6-3		33-3		26-3		35-3		13-3		(1-4)	
S1816	3	3	5	9	9	9	9	11	9	9	9	3	9	3	3	3	9	5
S1817	21	21	4	4	4	4	4	4	4	4	4	1	4	1	1	1	4	4
S1343	5	5	4	4	4	4	4	4	4	4	4	4	4	4	4	4	4	3
S1819	5	5	5	5	5	5	5	5	5	5	5	5	5	5	5	5	5	1
S384	1	1	1	1	1	1	1	1	1	1	1	2	1	2	2	2	1	2
B7			2	2					2	2	2	2	2	2				
S2179	3	3	3	3	3	3	3	3	3	3	3	4	3	4	4	4		
S535			1	1	1	1	1	1	1	1	1	1	1	1	1	1		
S1778			8	8	8	8	8	8			8	6	8	6	6	6		
S1294	5	5	5	5	5	5	5	5	5	5	5	5	5	5	5	5	5	5
S1818	4	4	5	4	5	4	5	5	5	5	5	5	4	5	5	5	4	5
S1960	1	1	1	1	1	1	1	1	1	2	1	1	1	1	1	1	1	1
S927	3	3	3	3	3	5	3	3	3	5	3	3	5	3	3	3	5	9
S1300	2	2	2	2	2	3	2	2	2	3	2	2	3	2	2	2	2	3
S1391			5	5	5	3	5	5	5	3	5	5	4	5	5	5	5	5
	[A]	[A]	[A']	[A]	[A']	[A]	[A']	[A']	[A']	[A] or [A']	[A']	[B]	[A]	[B]	[B]	[B]	[A]	[C]

	5-4		18-4		34-5		36-3		15-3		29-3		27-9		4-3		30-3	
S1816	5	9	5	9	9	5	9	5	5	2	2	9	9	9	5	5	4	1
S1817	4	4	4	4	1	4	4	4	4	9	9	4	4	4	4	4	21	7
S1343	3	4	3	4	4	3	4	3	3	4	4	4	4	4	5	5	5	5
S1819	1	5	1	2	2	1	1	1	1	1	1	1	5	1	5	5	5	5
S384	2	1	2	2	2	2	2	2	2	2	2	2	1	2	2	2	2	2
B7			1	1									2	1				
S2179	5	3	5	5					5	4								
S535	2	1	2	2	1	2	1	2			1	1	1	1	1	1	2	1
S1778	12	8	12	12			10	12	12	10	10	10	8	10	4	4	12	2
S1294	5	5	5	5	4	5	4	5	5	4	4	4	5	4	5	5	4	5
S1818	5	4	5	5	6	5	5	5	5	5	5	5	4	5	11	11	4	4
S1960	1	1	1	1	2	1	1	1	1	1	1	1	1	1	2	2	2	2
S927	9	3	9	9	5	9	6	9	9	6	6	6	3	6	4	4	6	5
S1300	3	2	3	3	2	3	2	3			2	2	2	2	5	5	5	3
S1391	5	5	5	5	5	5	2	5	3	2	2	2	5	2	5	5	3	1
	[C]	[A]	[C]	[C]	[J]	[C]	[D]	[C]	[C]	[D]	[D]	[D]	[A]	[D]	[F]	[F]	[I]	[E]

Fig. 29-15 Haplotyping of 27 Costa Rican A-T patients defined by genotyping with 15 markers across 7 cM flanking the most likely region for the later-cloned ATM gene. The most prominent haplotype, haplotype [A], was found in 19 patients (70 percent), 12 of whom were homozygous for this haplotype. Subsequent studies have confirmed that these patients all carry an identical mutation, as demonstrated by the assay shown in Fig. 29-14. As different descendants of the original carrier inherited haplotype [A], the genomic region that remained associated with the true region of the gene was reduced by random recombination. Thus, "ancestral haplotyping" provided further localization of the gene. Furthermore, by pairing the 10 haplotypes observed in these families, it was possible to predict that a single gene was causing the syndrome (with the exception of haplotype [F], which was never observed paired with another haplotype).

haplotype [A] were carrying the same mutation. We later confirmed this and found that roughly two-thirds of these purportedly "unrelated" families shared the same mutation on the same affected haplotype (haplotype [A] in Fig. 29-15). Inferred (ancestral) recombination events involving this common haplotype in earlier generations also allowed us to further localize the candidate region for the gene. Nine other haplotypes were identified within the Costa Rican population. We have identified the mutations and developed rapid DNA screening tests for seven Costa Rican mutations.[221,252,290] Together, these tests identify >99 percent of ATM mutations in that country. Such rapid screening tests take less than a day to screen hundreds of DNAs (Fig. 29-16). This provides an opportunity to compare the clinical symptoms of multiple patients with the same mutation; indeed, some of the patients are homozygous for this mutation. It also allows >99 percent of A-T carriers to be identified in Costa Rica.

Our laboratory has taken this approach in other ethnic populations as well.[252] A peculiar 3245ATC > TGAT mutation accounts for 55 percent of Norwegian patients[252] and has been traced to a single common ancestor who lived from 1684 to 1755 and had eight children.[293] Despite the appearance of breast cancer in several of the extant branches of this extended family, the frequency of the 3245ATG > TGAT mutation was not increased in Norwegian breast cancer patients from the same region. Rapid screening tests are now available for Amish (1563delAG), Moroccan Jews (103C > T),[291] Sardinian (3894insT), Mennonites (5932G > T), and other genetic isolates. Some of these mutations are represented as boxes in Fig. 29-11 because they are founder-effect defects; i.e., they are common to multiple patients from presumably related families. As can be seen in Table 29-3, also have observed five recurring defects in Polish families that represent 30 percent of Polish A-T patients, four mutations that

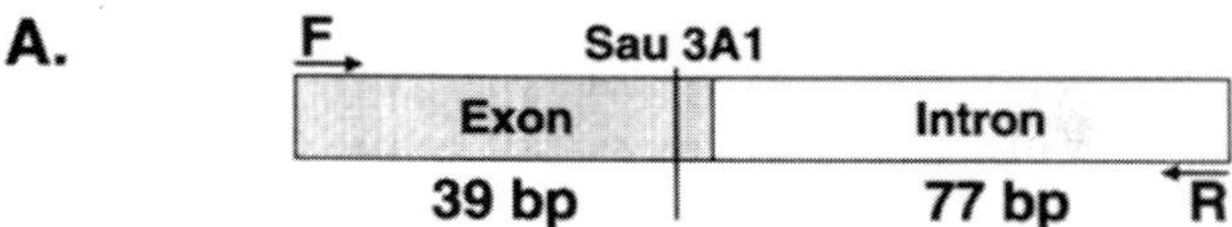

B. **Normal [Sau 3A1]: 39 + 77 bp**
delC: 115

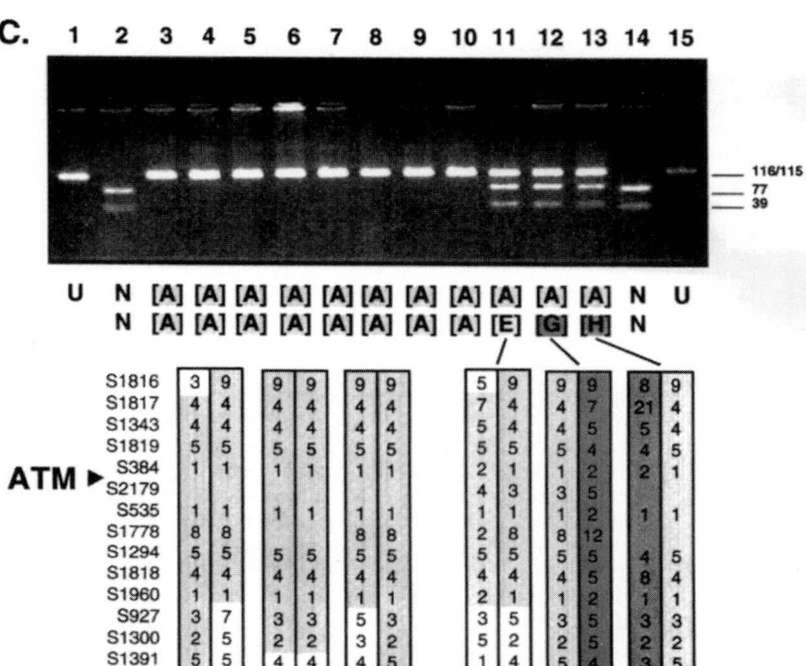

Fig. 29-16 Example of a rapid assay for the Costa Rican haplotype [A] mutation, a deletion of a "C" at position 5908 that destroys a Sau3A1 recognition site. Thus, in haplotype [A] homozygotes, a 115-bp PCR fragment is seen on agarose gels. A 116nt fragment is also seen in compound heterozygotes who carry another ATM mutation as well.

encompass 55 percent of Iranian families, and five mutations that encompass >25 percent of Turkish patients. In the United Kingdom, 11 mutations represent 73 percent of mutations found in A-T patients.[289] In Japan, only two mutations encompass ~50 percent of patients. Founder-effect mutations are also being identified among Hispanic A-T patients by comparing over 100 families from Spain, Brazil, Mexico, Argentina, and Puerto Rico to those of Costa Rica and the United States.

Correlating Phenotypes with Genotypes

Correlating phenotypes with genotypes requires that the mutations of a large number of patients first be defined. Because most nonconsanguineous A-T patients have two distinct mutations, such studies further require that both mutations be defined before the symptoms can be compared. Another major caveat for this aspect of A-T research is that although most patients have two stable forms of mutated ATM mRNA in LCLs and PBLs, as demonstrated by the extensive analyses with RNA-based assays, cells from most patients do not appear to contain any stable ATM protein—even when small deletions occur. This makes it somewhat difficult to conceptualize how specific mutations will affect phenotypes.

Nonetheless, 14 families from the British Midlands were described with "late-onset ataxia" and intermediate radiosensitivity.[219,239] They share a common chromosome 11q23.1 haplotype ("418") that was identified during the positional cloning studies and before the shared phenotype was appreciated. The report describes a very interesting 137-bp insertion into the mRNA (a new exon!) coupled with a point mutation that enhances the efficiency of an abnormal ("cryptic") splice site (see Fig. 29-14). Each patient has a different second mutation, and this has not been defined in all cases. This subset of families could provide interesting insights about phenotype-genotype relationships; however, the "late-onset ataxia" data are not convincingly homogeneous, given in Table 1 of that report[239] as years 8, 3, 3, 3, 5, 2, 2.5, 2.5, 1.8, 12, and 1.5. Considering that the average age at onset is characteristically between 1 and 3 years, only 4 of the 12 patients would qualify as "late-onset". Furthermore, we have a family with three affected siblings who are heterozygous for the same "418" mutation; their ages at onset were 8 months, 18 months, and 3 years. Thus, it is difficult to draw any convincing phenotype/genotype correlations with such mutations unless a substantial number of patients can be identified who are homozygous for that mutation. the McConville *et al.*[239] report lacks a single patient who is homozygous for this mutation. On the other hand, the author's suggestion that a small subset of patients may exist with two "mild" ATM mutations that do not lead to clinically obvious A-T deserves further study.

In collaboration with Sanal and coworkers (unpublished), we have studied a family in which all four sibs are affected with A-T. Because the parents are first cousins, the children are homozygous for their mutation at 6199del9, which deletes three amino acids at codons 2067–2069, well before the region of strongest homology with PI3-K (see Fig. 29-12). Table 29-4 describes the partial phenotypes of these four sibs and gives a preview of phenotype-genotype analyses. Note that this mutation is not associated with infections or immunodeficiencies in this family. The same mutation has not been seen in any other family to date.

Table 29-3 ATM Mutations in Ethnic Populations

Ethnicity	Mutation	Frequency (%)	Rapid assay
Costa Rica			
[A]	5908C≥T	56	Yes
[B]	IVS63del17 kb	7	Yes
[C]	7449G > A(del70)	12	Yes
[D]	4507C > T	12	Yes
[E]	8264del5	4	Yes
[F]	1120C > T	2	Yes
Poland			
[A]	IVS53-2A > C(del 159)	9	Yes
[B]	6095G > A(del89)	7	Yes
[C]	7010delGT	4.5	Yes
[D]	5932G > T(del88)	4.5*	Yes
[E]	5546gelT	4.5	—
Italy			
[A]	7517del4	20	Yes
[B]	3576G > A	7	—
[S1]	3894insT	Sardinia (> 95%)	Yes
[S2]		Sardinia (< 5%)	—
United Kingdom†			
[FM1-11]		73	—
[FM7]	5762ins137	18‡	Yes
[FM10]	7636del9	15§	Yes
North African Jews¶	103C > T	> 99	Yes
Amish	1563delAG	> 99	Yes
Utah Mormon			
[1]	IVS32-12A > G	—	—
[2]	8494C > T	—	—
[3]	IVS62 + 1G > A	—	—
African American			
[1]	IVS16-10T > G	—	—
[2]	2810insCTAG	—	—
[3]	7327C > T	—	—
[4]	7926A > C	—	—
Japan			
[A]	7883del5	25	Yes
[B]	IVS33 + 2T > C	25	—
Norway			
[A]	3245ATC > TGAT	55	Yes
Turkey	5 mutations	31	—
Iran	4 mutations	55	—
Brazil	4 mutations	60	—
Argentina	2 mutations	25	—
Spain	2 mutations	23	—
Amer-Hispanic	2 mutation	15	—

*Also found in Mennonites.
†Based on reference 289
‡Milder phenotype?
§Widely disseminated
¶Based on Reference 291

Another report suggests that patients who have *some* ATM protein in their cell lysates may have milder or variant phenotypes.[294] This remains to be confirmed and depends to some extent on the ability of a laboratory to reliably quanititate the protein levels. In our hands, 81 percent of classic A-T patients (101 of 124) do not have any measurable protein; in the remaining < 19 percent, the protein level is present but almost always reduced.[295]

Table 29-4 Phenotypes of Four Consanguineous Hemozygous Affected Siblings with Mutation 6199del9 [deleted codons 2067–2069 (haplotypes in parentheses)]

	Sib 1	Sib 2	Sib 3	Sib 4
	(AC)	(AC)	(AC)	(AC)
Ataxia onset (year)	1	2.5	2	0.5
Walked unaided until (year)	7	7	9	7
Telangiectasia onset (year)	4	4	2.5	4
Dysarthria onset (year)	2	2.5	2.5	3
Gray hairs	0	0	0	0
Frequent infections	0	0	0	0
Serum immunoglobulins	N	N	N	N
α-fetoprotein (ng/ml)	54	30	16	—

Epilogue

Each of the first eight A-T workshops has painstakingly brought us a little closer to understanding this complex disorder. Summaries were published for most of the workshops,[240–244,292,332] and books were published based on the first,[245] second,[246] fifth,[247] and sixth[248] workshops. The recorded comments and discussions that followed the presentations at the 1984 workshop (ATW2) are still very pertinent to much of today's research.[246]

In 1981 (ATW1), a better phenotype was described in preparation for linkage studies. In 1984 (ATW2), the neurodegenerative nature of A-T was clarified by the presence of basket cell "footprints,"[7,8] and plans for positional cloning continued. By 1987 (ATW3), as part of that approach, many key families around the world had been assigned to complementation groups, primarily through the work of Jaspers and coworkers.[150,151] In 1989 (ATW4), formal presentations and confirmations were made regarding the localization of an A-T gene to chromosome 11q22-23.[152] A higher-resolution map of distal chromosome 11 was already under way,[209,248] taking advantage of the burgeoning new genome projects around the world, such as the CEPH linkage mapping consortium in Paris.[203] However, at that time, most investigators felt that the A-T gene would be cloned not by the slower positional cloning approach but by more direct transfection and complementation experiments. Indeed, a candidate A-T gene (ATDC) isolated by this method was much discussed at ATW5 (1992).[249,250] It was already becoming clear, however, that ATDC was not the true gene, and complementational cloning was potentially misleading. The ATW6 (1994) workshop confirmed both of these conclusions, for by then 26 cDNA clones had been found to complement RDS, radiomimetic sensitivity, or both, but none localized to 11q22-23.[6,63,154,244]

In 1995, the gene was cloned purely by positional cloning.[72] A scientific logjam was broken! Many new investigators entered the field of A-T research to make antibodies, to construct full-length cDNAs, and to develop functional assays. Once again, however, from what was to have been the pinnacle, many new peaks were sighted. ATW7 addressed new mutations, the failure of many investigators to find an increase in the frequency of ATM mutations in breast cancer patients, the pathology of the knockout mice, the molecules with which the ATM protein interacts, and the recent cloning of the NBS1 gene.[202] ATW8[332] brought together > 200 scientists to review the many complex facets of A-T biology, as well as to establish the validity of using p53 phosphorylation at serine 15 as a functional and specific assay for the ATM protein. Three major stumbling blocks still have to be addressed: (a) the lack of a progressive ataxia in the knockout mice, which almost negates this model for unraveling the neuropathology of A-T; (b) the lack of sufficient amounts of purified ATM protein for functional and structural studies; and (c) an effective therapeutic approach.

ACKNOWLEDGMENTS

This chapter is dedicated to Drs. Elena Boder and Robert Sedgwick, both of whom died in 1995 knowing that the ATM gene had finally been cloned. Almost 40 years had elapsed since their seminal observations and descriptions of the A-T syndrome. I thank them for having provided me with almost 30 years of enlightenment on A-T, their encouragement to persevere in the linkage studies, and their insights and efforts in identifying new families for our research.

The positional cloning project was initiated with funding from three major grants between 1984 and 1986 from the Ataxia-Telangiectasia Medical Research Foundation: to Richard Gatti (Los Angeles), to Yosef Shiloh (Tel Aviv), and to N. J. G Jaspers (Rotterdam). For additional support we thank the Department of Energy (ER60548) (1987 to 1999), the American Cancer Society (CD-328), the National Cancer Institute (CA16042), the North Atlantic Treaty Organization (ARW920385), the Ataxia-Telangiectasia Medical Trust-UK, the Ataxia-Telangiectasia Children's Project, the Joseph Drown Foundation, the Andrew Norman Foundation, the Eric Lightner Memorial Fund, and the Harry Ringel Foundation. We acknowledge Ken Lange and his four generations of graduate students in biomathematics for devising new analytic approaches in response to each obstacle we encountered, which ensured constant progress in the positional cloning of the gene. Last and most important, the A-T patients, their families, and the referring immunologists and neurologists must be acknowledged for their continuing cooperation in innumerable blood drawings, skin biopsies, and clinical discussions.

REFERENCES

1. Boder E, Sedgwick RP: Ataxia-telangiectasia: A familial syndrome of progressive cerebellar ataxia, oculocutaneous telangiectasia and frequent pulmonary infection. *Pediatrics* **21**:526, 1958.
2. Sedgwick RP, Boder E: Ataxia-telangiectasia, in Vinken PJ, Bruyn GW (eds): *Handbook of Clinical Neurology*, vol. 14. Amsterdam, North-Holland, 1972, pp 267–339.
3. Boder E: Ataxia-telangi: ectasia: An overview, in Gatti RA, Swift M (eds): *Ataxia-Telangiectasia: Genetics, Neuropathology, and Immunology of a Degenerative Disease of Childhood*. New York, Liss, 1985, pp 1–63.
4. Gatti RA, Boder E, Vinters HV, Sparkes RS, Norman A, Lange K: Ataxia-telangiectasia: An interdisciplinary approach to pathogenesis. *Medicine* **70**:99, 1991.
5. Sedgwick RP, Boder E: Ataxia-telangiectasia, in de Jong JMBV (ed): *Handbook of Clinical Neurology*, vol. 16, *Hereditary Neuropathies and Spinocerebellar Atrophies*. Amsterdam, Elsevier, 1991, pp 347–423.
6. Shiloh Y: Ataxia-telangiectasia: Closer to unraveling the mystery. *Eur J Hum Genet* **3**:116, 1995.
7. Gatti RA, Vinters HV: Cerebellar pathology in ataxia-telangiectasia, in Gatti RA, Swift M (eds): *Ataxia-Telangiectasia: Genetics, Neuropathology, and Immunology of a Degenerative Disease of Childhood*. New York, Liss, 1985, pp 225–232.
8. Vinters HV, Gatti RA, Rakic P: Sequence of cellular events in cerebellar ontogeny relevant to expression of neuronal abnormalities in ataxia-telangiectasia, in Gatti RA, Swift M (eds): *Ataxia-Telangiectasia: Genetics, Neuropathology, and Immunology of a Degenerative Disease of Childhood*. New York, Liss, 1985, pp 233–255.
9. Aguilar MJ, Kamoshita S, Landing BH, Boder E, Sedgwick RP: Pathological observations in ataxia-telangiectasia: A report on 5 cases. *J Neuropathol Exp Neurol* **27**:659, 1968.
10. Naeim A, Repinski C, Huo Y, Hong J-H, Chessa L, Naeim F, Gatti RA: Ataxia-telangiectasia: Flow cytometric cell cycle analysis of lymphoblastoid cell lines in G2/M before and after gamma-irradiation. *Mod Pathol* **7**:587, 1994.
11. Van Meir EG, Polverini PJ, Chazin VR, Su Huang H-J, de Tribolet N, Cavenee WK: Release of an inhibitor of angiogenesis upon induction of wild-type p53 expression in glioblastoma cells. *Nat Genet* **8**:171, 1994.
12. Peterson RD, Kelly WD, Good RA: Ataxia-telangiectasia: Its association with a defective thymus, immunological-deficiency disease, and malignancy. *Lancet* **1**:1189, 1964.
13. Centerwall WR, Miller MM: Ataxia-telangiectasia and sinopulmonary infections: A syndrome of slowly progressive deterioration in childhood. *Am J Dis Child* **95**:385, 1958.

13a. Sourander P, Bonnevier JO, Olsson Y: A case of ataxia-telangiectasia with lesions in the spinal cord. *Acta Neurol Scand* **42**:354, 1966.

14. Thieffry S, Arthuis M, Farkas-Barceton E, Vinh LeT: L'ataxia-telangiectasia: Une observation anatomo-clinique familiale. *Ann Pediatr* **13**:749, 1966.
15. Amromin GD, Boder E, Teplitz R: Ataxia-telangiectasia with a 32-year survival: A clinicopathological report. *J Neuropathol Exp Neurol* **38**:621, 1979.
16. Barlow C, Hirotsune S, Paylor R, Liyanage M, Eckhaus M, Collins F, Shiloh Y, Crawley JN, Tied T, Tagle D, Wynshaw-Boris A: Atm-deficient mice: A paradigm of ataxia-telangiectasia. *Cell* **86**:159, 1996.
17. Gotoff SP, Aminmokri E, Liebner EJ: Ataxia-telangiectasia. Neoplasia, untoward response to x-irradiation, and tuberous sclerosis. *Am J Dis Child* **114**:617, 1967.
18. Morgan JL, Holcomb TM, Morrissey RW: Radiation reaction in ataxia-telangiectasia. *Am J Dis Child* **116**:557, 1968.
19. Cunliffe PN, Mann JR, Cameron AH, Roberts KD, Ward HWC: Radiosensitivity in ataxia-telangiectasia. *Br J Radiol* **48**:374, 1975.
20. Abadir R, Hakami N: Ataxia-telangiectasia with cancer. An indication for reduced radiotherapy and chemotherapy does. *Br J Radiol* **56**:343, 1983.
21. Hart RM, Kimler BR, Evans RG, Park CH: Radiotherapeutic management of medulloblastoma in a pediatric patient with ataxia-telangiectasia. *Int J Radiat Oncol Biol Phys* **13**:1237, 1987.
22. Taylor AMR, Harnden DG, Arlett CF, Harcourt SA, Lehmann AR, Stevens S, Bridges BA: Ataxia-telangiectasia: A human mutation with abnormal radiation sensitivity. *Nature* **258**:427, 1975.
23. Shiloh Y, Tabor E, Becker Y: In vitro phenotype of ataxia-telangiectasia fibroblast strains: Clues to the nature of the "AT DNA lesion" and the molecular defect in AT, in Gatti RA, Swift M (eds): *Ataxia-telangiectasia: Genetics, Neuropathology, and Immunology of a Degenerative Disease of Childhood*. New York, Liss, 1985, pp 111–121.
24. Shiloh Y, Tabor E, Becker Y: The response of ataxia-telangiectasia homozygous and heterozygous skin fibroblasts to neocarzinostatin. *Carcinogenesis* **3**:815, 1982.
25. Paterson MC, Mac Farlane SJ, Gentner NE, Smith BP: Cellular hypersensitivity to chronic gamma-radiation in cultured fibroblasts from ataxia-telangiectasia heterozygotes, in Gatti RA, Swift M (eds): *Ataxia-Telangiectasia: Genetics, Neuropathology, and Immunology of a Degenerative Disease of Childhood*. New York, Liss, 1985, pp 73–87.
26. Weeks DE, Paterson MC, Lange K, Andrais B, Davis RC, Yoder F, Gatti RA: Assessment of chronic gamma radiosensitivity as an in vitro assay for heterozygote identification of ataxia-telangiectasia. *Radiation Res* **128**:90, 1991.
27. Parshad R, Sanford KK, Jones GM, Tarone RE: G2 chromosomal radiosensitivity of ataxia-telangiectasia heterozygotes. *Cancer Genet Cytogenet* **14**:163, 1985.
28. Parshad R, Sanford KK, Jones GM: Chromosomal radiosensitivity during the G2 cell cycle period of skin fibroblasts from individuals with familial cancer. *Proc Natl Acad Sci USA* **82**:5400, 1985.
29. Shiloh Y, Parshad R, Frydman M, Sanford KK, Portnoi S, Ziv Y, Jones GM: G2 chromosomal radiosensitivity in families with ataxia-telangiectasia. *Hum Genet* **84**:15, 1989.
30. Rosin MP, Ochs HD, Gatti RA, Boder E: Heterogeneity of chromosomal breakage levels in epithelial tissue of ataxia-telangiectasia homozygotes and heterozygotes. *Hum Genet* **83**:133, 1989.
31. Scott D, Jones LA, Elyan SAG, Spreadborough A, Cown R, Ribiero G: Identification of A-T heterozygotes, in Gatti RA, Painter RB (eds): *Ataxia-Telangiectasia*. Heidelberg, Springer-Verlag, 1993, pp 101–116.
32. Swift A, Morrell D, Massey RB, Chase CL: Incidence of cancer in 161 families affected by ataxia-telangiectasia. *N Engl J Med* **325**:1831, 1991.
33. Norman A, Kagan AR, Chan SL: The importance of genetics for the optimization of radiation therapy. *Am J Clin Oncol* **11**:84, 1988.
34. Norman A, Withers R: Recommendation about radiation exposure for A-T heterozygotes in Gatti RA, Painter RB (eds): *Ataxia-Telangiectasia*. Heidelberg, Springer-Verlag, 1993, pp 137–142.
35. Law J: Patient dose and risk in mammography. *Brit J Radiol* **64**:360, 1991.

36. Peterson RDA, Funkhouser JD, Tuck-Miller CM, Gatti RA: Cancer susceptibility in ataxia-telangiectasia, in *Leukemia.* New York, Macmillan, 1992, pp 8–13.
37. Swift M, Sholman L, Perry M, Chase C: Malignant neoplasms in the families of patients with ataxia-telangiectasia. *Cancer Res* **36**:209, 1976.
38. Rotman G, Shloh Y: The ATM gene and protein: Possible roles in genome surveillance, checkpoint controls and cellular defense against oxidative stree. *Cancer Surv* **29**:285, 1997.
39. Painter R: Altered DNA synthesis in irradiated and unirradiated ataxia-telangiectasia cells, in Gatti RA, Swift M (eds): *Ataxia-Telangiectasia: Genetics, Neuropathology, and Immunology of a Degenerative Disease of Childhood.* New York, Liss, 1985, pp 89–100.
40. Meyn MS: Ataxia-telangiectasia and cellular responses to DNA damage. *Cancer Res* **55**:5991, 1995.
41. Morrell D, Cromartie E, Swift M: Mortality and cancer incidence in 263 patients with ataxia-telangiectasia. *J Natl Cancer Inst* **77**:89, 1986.
42. Spector BD, Filipovich AH, Perry GS, Kersey JH: Epidemiology of cancer in ataxia-telangiectasia, in Bridges BA, Harnden DG (eds): *Ataxia-Telangiectasia: Cellular and Molecular Link between Cancer, Neuropathology and Immune Deficiency.* New York, Wiley, 1982, pp 103–107.
43. Hecht F, Koler RD, Rigas DA, Dahnke G, Case M, Tisdale V, Miller RW: Leukaemia and lymphocytes in ataxia-telangiectasia. *Lancet* **2**:1193, 1966.
44. Gatti RA, Good RA: Occurrence of malignancy in immunodeficiency diseases. *Cancer* **28**:89, 1971.
45. Taylor AMR, Metcalfe JA, Thick J, Mak Y-F: Leukemia and lymphoma in ataxia-telangiectasia. *Blood* **87**:423, 1996.
46. Foon KA, Gale RP: Is there a T-cell form of chronic lymphocytic leukaemia? *Leukemia* **6**:867, 1992.
47. Hollis RJ, Kennaugh AA, Butterworth SV, Taylor AMR: Growth of chromosomally abnormal T cell clones in ataxia-telangiectasia patients is associated with translocation at 14q11—a model for other T cell neoplasia. *Hum Genet* **76**:389, 1987.
48. Russo G, Isobe M, Gatti RA, Finan J, Batuman O, Huebner K, Nowell PC, Croce CM: Molecular analysis of a t(14;14) translocation in leukemic T-cells of an ataxia-telangiectasia patient. *Proc Natl Acad Sci USA* **86**:602, 1989.
49. Davey MP, Bertness V, Nakahara K, Johnson JP, McBride OW, Waldmann TA, Kirsch IR: Juxtaposition of the T-cell receptor alpha-chain locus (14q11) and a region (14q32) of potential importance in leukemogenesis by a 14;14 translocation in a patients with T-cell chronic lymphocytic leukemia and ataxia-telangiectasia. *Proc Natl Acad Sci USA* **85**:9287, 1988.
50. Gatti RA, Nieberg R, Boder E: Uterine tumors in ataxia-telangiectasia. *Gynecol Oncol* **32**:257, 1989.
51. Pippard EC, Hall AJ, Baker DJP, Bridges BA: Cancer in homozygotes and heterozygotes of ataxia-telangiectasia and xeroderma pigmentosum in Britain. *Cancer Res* **48**:2929, 1988.
52. Swift M, Reitnauer PJ, Morrell D, Chase CL: Breast and other cancers in families with ataxia-telangiectasia. *N Engl J Med* **316**:1289, 1987.
53. Borresen A-L, Andersen TI, Tretli S, Heiberg A, Moller P: Breast cancer and other cancers in Norwegian families with ataxia-telangiectasia. *Genes Chrom Cancer* **2**:339, 1990.
54. Vorechovsky I, Rasio D, Luo L, Monaco C, Hammarstrom L, Webster DB, Zaloudik J, Barbanti-Brodano G, James M, Russo G, Croce CM, Negrini M: The ATM gene and susceptibility to breast cancer: Analysis of 38 breast tumors reveals no evidence for mutation. *Cancer Res* **56**:2726, 1996.
55. FitzGerald MG, Bean JM, Hegde SR, Unsal H, MacDonald DJ, Harkin DP, Finkelstein DM, Isselbacher KJ, Haber DA: Heterozygous ATM mutations do not contribute to early onset of breast cancer. *Nat Genet* **15**:307, 1997.
56. Spurr NK, Kelsell CP, Mavrakis E, Bryant SP, Crockford G, Bishop DT: Genetic heterogeneity in UK breast and ovarian cancer families. *Am J Hum Genet* **S57**:A5, 1995.
57. Cortessis V, Ingles S, Millikan R, Diep A, Gatti RA, Richardson L, Thompson WD, Paganini-Hill A, Sparkes RS, Haile RW: Linkage analysis of DRD2, a marker linked to the ataxia-telangiectasia gene, in 64 families with premenopausal bilateral breast cancer. *Cancer Res* **53**:5083, 1993.
58. Wooster R, Easton DF, Ford D, Mangion J, Ponder BAJ, Peto J, Stratton M: The A-T gene does not make a major contribution to familial breast cancer, in Gatti RA, Painter RB (eds): *Ataxia-Telangiectasia.* Heidelberg, Springer-Verlag, 1993, pp 127–136.
59. Athma P, Rappaport R, Swift M: Molecular genotyping shows that ataxia-telangiectasia heterozygotes are predisposed to breast cancer. *Cancer Genet Cytogenet* **92**:130, 1996.
60. Carter SL, Negrini M, Baffa R, Illum DR, Rosenberg AL, Schwartz GF, Croce CM: Loss of heterozygosity at 11q22-23 in breast cancer. *Cancer Res* **54**:6270, 1994.
61. Porras O, Arguendas O, Arata M, Barrantes M, Gonzalez L, Saenz E: Epidemiology of ataxia-telangiectasia in Costa Rica, in Gatti RA, Painter RB (eds): *Ataxia-Telangiectasia.* Heidelberg, Springer-Verlag, 1993, pp 199–208.
62. Chessa L, Fiorilli M: Epidemiology of ataxia-telangiectasia in Italy, in Gatti RA, Painter RB (eds): *Ataxia-Telangiectasia.* Heidelberg: Springer-Verlag, 1993, pp 191–198.
63. Lohrer HD: Regulation of the cell cycle following DNA damage in normal and ataxia-telangiectasia cells. *Experentia* **52**:316, 1996.
64. Hartwell LH, Weinert TA: Checkpoints: Controls that ensure the order of cell cycle events. *Science* **246**:629, 1989.
65. Kastan MB, Zhan Q, El-Deiry WS, Carrier F, Jacks Y, Walsh WV, Plunkett BS, Vogelstein B, Fornace AJ: A mammalian cell cycle checkpoint pathway utilizing p53 and GADD45 is defective in ataxia-telangiectasia. *Cell* **71**:587, 1992.
66. Kastan MB: Ataxia-telangiectasia: defective in a p53-dependent signal transduction pathway, in Gatti RA, Painter RB (eds): *Ataxia-Telangiectasia.* Heidelberg, Springer-Verlag, 1993, pp 163–173.
67. Donehower LA, Harvey M, Stagle BL, McArthur MJ, Montgomery CA, Butel JS, Bradley A: Mice deficient for p53 are developmentally normal but susceptible to spontaneous tumors. *Nature* **356**:215, 1992.
68. Purdie CA, Harrison DJ, Peter A, Dobbie L, White S, Howie SE, Salter DM, Bird CC, Wyllie AH, Hooper ML: Tumour incidence, spectrum and ploidy in mice with a large deletion in the p53 gene. *Oncogene* **9**:603, 1994.
69. Liu VF, Weaver DT: The ionizing radiation-induced replication protein A phosphorylation response differs between ataxia-telangiectasia and normal human cells. *Mol Cell Biol* **13**:7222, 1993.
70. Shafman T, Khanna KK, Kedar P, Spring K, Kozlov S, Yen T, Hobson K, Gatei M, Zhang N, Watters D, Egerton M, Shiloh Y, Kharbanda S, Kufe D, Lavin MF: Interaction between ATM protein and c-Abl in response to DNA damage. *Nature* **387**:520, 1997.
71. Lavin MF, Khanna KK, Beamish H, Spring K, Watters D, Shiloh Y: Relationship of the ataxia-telangiectasia protein ATM to phosphoinositide 3-kinase. *Trends Biol Sci* **20**:382, 1995.
72. Savisky K, Bar-Shira A, Gilad S, Rotman G, Ziv Y, Vanagaite L, Tagle DA, Smith S, Uziel T, Sfez S, Ashkenazi M, Pecker I, Frydman M, Harnik R, Patanjali SR, Simmons A, Clines GA, Sartiel A, Gatti RA, Chessa L, Sanal O, Lavin MF, Jaspers NGJ, Taylor MR, Arlett CF, Miki T, Weissman SM, Lovett M, Collins FS, Shiloh Y: A single ataxia-telangiectasia gene with a product similar to PI-3 kinase. *Science* **268**:1749, 1995.
73. Nowak R: Discovery of AT gene sparks biomedical research bonanza. *Science* **268**:1700, 1995.
74. Hartwell LH, Kastan MB: Cell cycle control and cancer. *Science* **266**:1821, 1994.
75. Vogelstein B: A deadly inheritance. *Nature* **348**:681, 1990.
76. Meyn MS, Strasfeld L, Allen C: Testing the role of p53 in the expression of genetic instability and apoptosis in ataxia-telangiectasia. *Int J Radiat Biol* **66**:S141, 1994.
77. Lowe SW, Ruley HE, Jacks T, Housman DE: P53-dependent apoptosis modulates the cytotoxicity of anticancer agents. *Cell* **74**:957, 1993.
78. Lee JM, Bernstein A: P53 mutations increase resistance to ionizing radiation. *Proc Natl Acad Sci USA* **90**:5742, 1993.
79. Jung M, Zhang Y, Dritschilo A: Correction of radiation sensitivity in ataxia-telangiectasia cells by a truncated IkB-α. *Science* **268**:1619, 1995.
80. Jung M, Kondratyev A, Lee SA, Dimtchev A, Dritschilo A: ATM gene product phosphorylates IkB-α. *Canc Res* **57**:24, 1997.
81. Thanos D, Maniatis T: NF-kB: A lesson in family values. *Cell* **80**:529, 1995.
82. Painter RB, Young BR: Radiosensitivity in ataxia-telangiectasia: A new explanation. *Proc Natl Acad Sci USA* **77**:7315, 1980.
83. Thacker J: Cellular radiosensitivity in ataxia-telangiectasia. *Int J Radiat Biol* **66**:S87, 1994.
84. Vorechovsky I, Luo L, Dyer MJS, Catovsky D, Amlot PL, Yaxley JC, Foroni L, Hammarstrom L, Webster DB, Yuille MAR: Clustering of missense mutations in the ataxia-telangiectasia gene in a sporadic T-cell leukaemia. *Nat Genet* **17**:96, 1997.
85. Painter RB: Inhibition of mammalian cell DNA synthesis by ionizing radiation. *Int J Radiat Biol* **49**:771, 1986.

86. Painter RB: Radiobiology of ataxia-telangiectasia, in Gatti RA, Painter RB (eds): *Ataxia-Telangiectasia*. Heidelberg, Springer-Verlag, 1993, pp 257–268.
87. Hand R, Gautschi JR: Replication of mammalian DNA in vitro: Evidence for initiation from fiber autoradiography. *J Cell Biol* **82**:485, 1979.
88. Gatti RA, Bick MB, Tam CF, Medici MA, Oxelius V-A, Holland M, Goldstein AL, Boder E: Ataxia-telangiectasia: A multiparameter analysis of eight families. *Clin Immunol Immunopathol* **23**:501, 1982.
89. Woods CG, Taylor AMR: Ataxia-telangiectasia in the British Isles: The clinical and laboratory features of 70 affected individuals. *Q J Med New Series* **298**:169, 1992.
90. Gatti RA: Ataxia-telangiectasia: A neuroendocrine-immune disease? Alternative models of pathogenesis, in Fabris N, Garaci E, Hadden J, Mitchison, NA (eds): *Immunoregulation*. New York, Plenum, 1983, pp 385–398.
91. Thieffry S, Arthuis M, Aicardi J, Lyon G: L'ataxie-telangiectasie. *Rev Neurol* **105**:390, 1961.
92. Oxelius V-A, Berkel AI, Hanson LA: IgG2 deficiency in ataxia-telangiectasia. *N Engl J Med* **306**:515, 1982.
93. Rivat-Peran L. Buriot D, Salier J-P, Rivat C, Dumitresco S-M, Griscelli C: Immunoglobulins in ataxia-telangiectasia: Evidence for IgG4 and IgA2 subclass deficiencies. *Clin Immunol Immunopathol* **20**:99, 1981.
94. Ammann AJ, Cain WA, Ishizaka K, Hong R, Good RA: Immunoglobulin E deficiency in ataxia-telangiectasia. *N Engl J Med* **281**:469, 1969.
95. Polmar SH, Waldmann TA, Balestra ST, Jost M, Terry WD: Immunoglobulin E in immunologic deficiency disease. *J Clin Invest* **51**:326, 1972.
96. Hsieh C-L, Lieber MR: Lymphoid V(D)J recombination: Accessibility and reaction fidelity in normal and ataxia-telangiectasia cells, in Gatti RA, Painter RB (eds): *Ataxia-Telangiectasia*. Heidelberg, Springer-Verlag, 1993, pp 143–154.
97. Hsieh CL, Arlett CF, Lieber MR: V(D)J recombination in ataxia-telangiectasia, Bloom's syndrome and a DNA ligase I-associated immunodeficiency disorder. *J Biol Chem* **268**:20105, 1993.
98. Kirsch IR: V(D)J recombination and ataxia-telangiectasia: A review. *Int J Radiat Biol* **66**:S97, 1994.
99. Paganelli R, Scala E, Scarselli E, Ortolani C, Cossarizza A, Carmini D, Aiuti F, Fiorilli M: Selective deficiency of CD41/CD45RA1 lymphocytes in patients with ataxia-telangiectasia. *J Clin Immunol* **12**:84, 1992.
100. Eisen AH: Delayed hypersensitivity in ataxia-telangiectasia. *N Engl J Med* **272**:801, 1965.
101. Oppenheim JJ, Barlow M, Waldmann TA, Block JB: Impaired in vitro lymphocyte transformation in patients with ataxia-telangiectasia. *Br Med J* **2**:330, 1966.
102. Leiken SI, Bazelon M, Park KH: In vitro lymphocyte transformation in ataxia-telangiectasia. *J Pediatr* **68**:477, 1966.
103. Epstein WL, Fudenberg HH, Reed WB, Boder E, Sedggwick RP: Immunologic studies in ataxia-telangiectasia. *Int Arch Allergy* **30**:15, 1966.
104. Hosking G: Ataxia telangiectasia. *Dev Med Child Neurol* **24**:77, 1982.
105. Waldmann TA, Misiti J, Nelson DL, Kraemer KH: Ataxia-telangiectasia: A multisystem hereditary disease with immunodeficiency, impaired organ maturation, x-ray hypersensitivity, and a high incidence of neoplasia. *Ann Intern Med* **99**:367, 1983.
106. Nelson DL, Biddison WE, Shaw S: Defective in vitro production of influenza virus-specific cytotoxic T lymphocytes in ataxia-telangiectasia. *J Immunol* **130**:2629, 1983.
107. Weaver M, Gatti RA: Lymphocyte subpopulations in ataxia-telangiectasia, in Gatti RA, Swift M (eds): *Ataxia-Telangiectasia: Genetics, Neuropathology, and Immunology of a Degenerative Disease of Childhood*. New York, Liss, 1985, pp 309–314.
108. Peter HH: The origin of human NK cells: An ontogenic model derived from studies in patients with immunodeficiencies. *Blut* **46**:239, 1983.
109. Sanal O, Ersoy F, Tezcan I, Gogus S: Ataxia-telangiectasia presenting as hyper IgM syndrome, in Chapel HM, Levinsky JR, Webster ADB (eds): *Progress in Immune Deficiency*, vol III. London, Royal Society of Medicine, 1991.
110. Thiele EA, Bonilla F, Rosen F, Riviello JI: Ataxia telangiectasia associated with the hyper-IgM syndrome. San Francisco, International Neurology Conference, Sept. 9–11, 1994.
111. Huo YK, Wang Z, Hong J-H, Chessa L, McBride WH, Perlman SL, Gatti RA: Radiosensitivity of ataxia-telangiectasia X-linked agammaglobulinemia and related syndromes. *Cancer Res* **54**:2544, 1994.
112. McFarlin DE, Strober W, Waldmann TA: Ataxia-telangiectasia. *Medicine* **51**:281, 1972.
113. Waldmann TA, McIntire KR: Serum alpha-fetoprotein levels in patients with ataxia-telangiectasia. *Lancet* **2**:112, 1972.
114. Yamashita T, Nakane A, Watanabe T, Miyoshi I, Kasai M: Evidence that alpha-fetoprotein suppresses the immunological function in transgenic mice. *Biochem Biophy Res Commun* **201**:1154, 1994.
115. Ishiguro T, Taketa K, Gatti RA: Tissue of origin of elevated alpha-fetoprotein in ataxia-telangiectasia. *Dis Markers* **4**:293, 1986.
116. Gatti RA, Aurias A, Griscelli C, Sparkes RS: Translocations involving chromosomes 2p and 22q in ataxia-telangiectasia. *Dis Markers* **3**:169, 1985.
117. Kojis TL, Gatti RA, Sparkes RS: The cytogenetics of ataxia-telangiectasia. *Cancer Genet Cytogenet* **56**:143, 1992.
118. Kojis TL, Schreck RR, Gatti RA, Sparkes RS: Tissue specificity of chromosomal rearrangements in ataxia-telangiectasia. *Hum Genet* **83**:337, 1989.
119. Hecht F, Hecht BK: Ataxia-telangiectasia breakpoints in chromosome rearrangements reflect genes important to T and B lymphocytes, in Gatti RA, Swift M (eds): *Ataxia-Telangiectasia: Genetics, Neuropathology, and Immunology of a Degenerative Disease of Childhood*. New York, Liss, 1985, pp 189–195.
120. Hecht F, McCaw BK, Koler RD: Ataxia-telangiectasia — Clonal growth of translocation lymphocytes. *N Engl J Med* **289**:286, 1972.
121. Berkel AI: Studies of IgG subclasses in ataxia-telangiectasia patients. *Monogr Allergy* **29**:100, 1986.
122. Roifman CM, Gelfand EW: Heterogeneity of the immunological deficiency in ataxia-telangiectasia: Absence of a clinical-pathological correlation, in Gatti RA, Swift M (eds): *Ataxia-Telangiectasia: Genetics, Neuropathology, and Immunology of a Degenerative Disease of Childhood*. New York, Liss, 1985, pp 273–285.
123. Virgilio L, Narducci MG, Isobe M, Billips LG, Cooper MD, Croce CM, Russo G: Identification of the TCL1 gene involved in T cell malignancies. *Proc Natl Acad Sci USA* **91**:12530, 1994.
124. Taylor AMR, Lowe PA, Stacey M, Thick J, Campbell L, Beatty D, Biggs P, Formstone CJ: Development of T cell leukaemia in an ataxia-telangiectasia patient following clonal selection in t(X;14) containing lymphocytes. *Leukemia* **6**:961, 1992.
125. Kenwrick S, Llevinson B, Taylor S, Shapiro A, Gitschier J: Isolation and sequence of two genes associated with a CpG island 59 of the factor VIII gene. *Hum Mol Genet* **1**:179, 1992.
126. Soulier J, Madni A, Cacheux V, Rosenwajg M, Sigaux F, Stern M-H: The MTCP-1/c6-1B gene encodes for a cytoplasmic 8kd protein overexpressed in T cell leukaemia bearing a t(X;14) translocation. *Oncogene* **9**:3565, 1994.
127. Madani A, Soulier J, Schmid M, Plichtova R, Lerme F, Gateau-Roesch O, Garnier J-P, Pla M, Sigaux F, Stern M-H: The 8 kd protein of the putative oncogene MTCP-1 is a mitochondrial protein. *Oncogene* **10**:2259, 1995.
128. Fu T, Virgilio L, Narducci MG, Facciano A, Russo G, Croce CM: Characterisation and localisation of the TCL-1 oncogene product. *Cancer Res* **54**:6297, 1994.
129. Knudsen AG: Hereditary cancer, oncogenes, and antioncogenes. *Cancer Res* **45**:1437, 1985.
130. Pandita TK, Pathak S, Geard C: Chromosome and associations, telomeres and telomerase activity in ataxia-telangiectasia cells. *Cytogenet Cell Genet* **71**:86, 1995.
131. Moyzis RK, Buckingham JM, Cram LS, Dani M, Deaven LL, Jones MD, Meyne J, Ratliff RL, Wu J-R: A highly conserved repetitive DNA sequence (TTAGGG)n, present in the telomeres of human chromosomes. *Proc Natl Acad Sci USA* **85**:6622, 1988.
132. Kipling D, Cooke HJ: Beginning or end? Telomere structure, genetics and biology. *Hum Mol Genet* **1**:3, 1992.
133. De Lange T, Shiue L, Myers RM, Cox DR, Naylor SL, Killery AM, Varmus HE: Structure and variability of human chromosome ends. *Mol Cell Biol* **10**:518, 1990.
134. Shore D: Telomeres–Unstickky ends. *Science* **281**:1818, 1998.
135. Metcalfe JA, Parkhill J, Campbell L, Stacey M, Biggs P, Byrd PJ, Taylor AMR: Accelerated telomere shortening in ataxia-telangiectasia. *Nat Genet* **13**:350, 1996.
136. Effros RB, Allsopp R, Chiu C-P, Hausner MA, Hirji K, Wang L, Harley CB, Villeponteau B, West MD, Giorgi JV: Shortened telomeres in the expanded CD28-CD81 cell subset in HIV disease implicate replicative senescence in MIV pathogenesis. *AIDS* **10**:F17, 1996.
137. Enoch T, Norbury C: Cellular responses to DNA damage: Cell cycle checkpoints, apoptosis and the roles of p53 and ATM. *Trends Biol Sci* **20**:426, 1995.

138. Lehmann AR, Carr AM: The ataxia-telangiectasia gene: A link between checkpoint controls, neurodegeneration and cancer. *Trends Genet* **11**:375, 1995.
139. Keegan KS, Holtzmann DA, Plug AW, Christenson ER, Brainerd EE, Flaggs G, Bentley NJ, Taylor EM, Meyn MS, Moss SB, Carr AM, Ashley T, Hoekstra MF: The Atr and Atm protein kinases associate with different sites along meiotically pairing chromosomes. *Genes Dev* **10**:2423, 1996.
140. Savitsky K, Sfez S, Tagle DA, Ziv Y, Sartiel A, Collins FS, Shiloh Y, Rotman G: The complete sequence of the coding region of the ATM gene reveals similarity to cell cycle regulators in different species. *Hum Mol Genet* **4**:2025, 1995.
141. Cimprich KA, Shin TB, Keith CT, Schreiber SL: cDNA cloning and gene mapping of a candidate human cell cycle checkpoint protein. *Proc Natl Acad Sci USA* **93**:2850, 1996.
142. Al-Khodairy F, Carr AM: DNA repair mutants defining G2 checkpoint pathways in Schizosaccharomyces pombe. *EMBO J* **11**:1343, 1992.
143. Seaton BL, Yucel J, Sunnerhagen P, Subramani P: Isolation and characterization of S. pombe rad3 gene involved in the DNA damage and DNA synthesis checkpoints. *Gene* **119**:83, 1992.
144. Weinert TA, Kiser GL, Hartwell LH: Mitotic checkpoint genes in budding yeast and the dependence of mitosis on DNA replication and repair. *Genes Dev* **8**:652, 1994.
145. Paulovich AG, Hartwell LH: A checkpoint regulates the rate of progression through S phase in *S. cerevisiae* in response to DNA damage. *Cell* **82**:841, 1995.
146. Kato R, Ogawa H: An essential gene, ESR1, is required for mitotic cell growth, DNA repair and meiotic recombination in Saccharomyces cerevisiae. *Nucleic Acids Res* **22**:3104, 1994.
147. Sanchez Y, Desany BA, Jones WJ, Liu Q, Wang B, Elledge SJ: Regulation of RAD53 by the ATM-like kinases MEC1 and TEL1 in yeast cell cycle checkpoint pathways. *Science* **271**:357, 1996.
148. Morrow DW, Tagle DA, Shiloh Y, Collins FS, Hieter P: TEL1, an S. cerevisiae homolog of the human gene mutated in ataxia-telangiectasia, is functionally related to the yeast checkpoint gene MEC1. *Cell* **82**:831, 1995.
149. Jaspers NGJ, Bootsma D: Genetic heterogeneity in ataxia-telangiectasia studies by cell fusion. *Proc Natl Acad Sci USA* **79**:2641, 1982.
150. Jaspers NGJ, Painter RB, Paterson MC, Kidson C, Inoue T: Complementation analysis of ataxia-telangiectasia, in Gatti RA, Swift M (eds): *Ataxia-Telangiectasia: Genetics, Neuropathology, and Immunology of a Degenerative Disease of Childhood*. New York, Liss, 1985, pp 147–162.
151. Jaspers NGJ, Gatti RA, Baan C, Linssen PCML, Bootsma D: Genetic complementation analysis of ataxia-telangiectasia and Nijmegen breakage syndrome: A survey of 50 patients. *Cytogenet Cell Genet* **49**:259, 1988.
152. Gatti RA, Berkel I, Boder E, Braedt G, Charmley P, Concannon P, Ersoy F, Foroud T, Jaspers NGJ, Lange K, Lathrop GM, Leppert M, Nakamura Y, O'Connell P, Paterson M, Salser W, Sanal O, Silver J, Sparkes RS, Susi E, Weeks DE, Wei S, White R, Yoder F: Localization of an ataxia-telangiectasia gene to chromosome 11q22-23. *Nature* **336**:577, 1988.
153. Ziv Y, Rotman G, Frydman M, Dagan J, Cohen T, Foroud T, Gatti RA, Shiloh Y: The ATC (ataxia-telangiectasia Group C) locus localizes to chromosome 11q22-q23. *Genomics* **9**:373, 1991.
154. Meyn MS, Lu-Kuo JM, Herzing LBK: Expression cloning of multiple human cDNAs that complement the phenotypic defects of ataxia-telangiectasia Group D fibroblasts. *Am J Hum Genet* **53**:1206, 1993.
155. Gatti RA, Nakamura Y, Nussmeier M, Susi E, Shan W, Grody WW: Informativeness of VNTR genetic markers for detecting chimerism after bone marrow transplantation. *Dis Markers* **7**:105, 1989.
156. Fritz E, Elsea SH, Patel PI, Myen MS: Overexpression of a truncated human topoisomerase III partially corrects multiple aspects of the ataxia-telangiectasia phenotype. *Proc Natl Acad Sci USA* **94**:4538, 1997.
157. Telatar M, Wang Z, Udar N, Liang T, Bernatowska-Matuszkiewicz E, Lavin M, Shiloh Y, Concannon P, Good RA, Gatti RA: Ataxia-telangiectasia: Mutations in ATM cDNA detected by protein-truncation screening. *Am J Hum Genet* **59**:40, 1996.
158. Meyn MS: High spontaneous intrachromosomal recombination rates in ataxia-telangiectasia. *Science* **260**:1327, 1993.
159. Muriel WJ, Lamb JR, Lehmann AR: UV mutation spectra in cell lines from patients with Cockayne's syndrome and ataxia-telangiectasia, using the shuttle vector pZ189. *Mutat Res* **254**:119, 1991.
160. Woods CG, Bunday SE, Taylor AMR: Unusual features in the inheritance of ataxia-telangiectasia. *Hum Genet* **84**:555, 1990.
161. Lange E, Corresen A-L, Chen X, Chessa L, Chiplunkar S, Concannon P, Dandekar S, Gerken S, Lange K, Liang T, McConville C, Polakow J, Porras O, Rotman G, Sanal O, Sheikhavandi S, Shiloh Y, Sobel E, Taylor M, Telatar M, Teraoka S, Tolun A, Udar N, Uhrhammer N, Vanagaite L, Wang Z, Wapelhorst B, Yang H-M, Yang L, Ziv Y, Gatti RA: Localization of an ataxia-telangiectasia gene to a 500-kb interval on chromosome 11q23.1: Linkage analysis of 176 families in an international consortium. *Am J Hum Genet* **57**:112, 1995.
162. Gatti RA, Lange E, Rotman G, Chen S, Uhrhammer N, Liang T, Chiplunkar S, Yang L, Udar N, Dandekar S, Sheikhavandi S, Wang Z, Yang U-M, Polakow J, Elashoff M, Telatar M, Sanal O, Chessa L, McConville C, Taylor M, Shiloh Y, Porras O, Borresen A-L, Wegner R-D, Curry C, Gerken S, Lange K, Concannon P: Genetic haplotyping of ataxia-telangiectasia families localizes the major gene to an 850-kb region on chromosome 11q23.1. *Int J Radiat Biol* **66**:S57, 1994.
163. Swift M, Morrell D, Cromartie E, Chamberlin AR, Skolnick MH, Bishop DT: The incidence and gene frequency of ataxia-telangiectasia in the United States. *Am J Hum Genet* **39**:573, 1986.
164. Swift M: Genetics and epidemiology of ataxia-telangiectasia, in Gatti RA, Swift M (eds): *Ataxia-Telangiectasia: Genetics, Neuropathology, and Immunology of a Degenerative Disease of Childhood*. New York, Liss, 1985, pp 133–144.
165. Barlow MH, McFarlin ED, Schalch DS: An unusual type of diabetes mellitus with marked hyperinsulinism in patients with ataxia telangiectasia. *Clin Res* **13**:530, 1965.
166. Schalch DS, McFarlin DE, Barlow MH: An unusual form of diabetes mellitus in ataxia telangiectasia. *N Engl J Med* **282**:1396, 1970.
167. Gatti RA, Walford RL: Immune function and features of aging in chromosomal instability syndromes, in Segre D, Smith L (eds): *Immunologic Aspects of Aging*. New York, Marcel Dekker, 1981, pp 449–465.
168. Terplan KL, Krauss RF: Histopathologic brain changes in association with ataxia-telangiectasia. *Neurology* **19**:446, 1969.
169. Xu Y, Ashley T, Brainerd EE, Bronson RT, Meyn MS, Baltimore D: Targeted disruption of ATM leads to growth retardation, chromosomal fragmentation during meiosis, immune defect, and thymic lymphoma. *Genes Dev* **10**:2411, 1996.
170. Herndon RM: Selective vulnerability in the nervous system, in Gatti RA, Swift M (eds): *Ataxia-Telangiectasia: Genetics, Neuropathology, and Immunology of a Degenerative Disease of Childhood*. New York, Liss, 1985, pp 257–267.
171. Kamoshita S, Aguilar MJ, Landing BH: Precocious aging in ataxia-telangiectasia: Pathological evidence in the central nervous system, in *Proceedings of the First International Congress of Child Neurology*. Toronto, 1975.
172. Weemaes CMR, Hustinx TWJ, Scheres JMJC, Van Munster PJJ, Bakkeren JAJM, Taalman RDFM: A new chromosomal instability disorder: The Nijmegen breakage syndrome. *Acta Paediatr Scand* **70**:557, 1981.
173. Wegner RD, Metzger M, Hanefeld NG, Jaspers J, Baan C, Magdorf K, Kunze J, Sperling K: A new chromosomal instability disorder confirmed by complementation studies. *Clin Genet* **33**:20, 1988.
174. Stumm M, Seemanova E, Gatti RA, Sperling K, Reis A, Wegner R-D: The ataxia-telangiectasia variant genes 1 and 2 show no linkage to the AT candidate region on chromosome 11q22-23. *Am J Hum Genet* **57**:960, 1995.
175. Saar K, Chrzanowska KH, Stumm M, Jung M, Nurnberg G, Wienker TF, Seemanova E, Wegner R-D, Reis A, Sperling K: The gene for ataxia-telangiectasia-variant (Nijmegen breakage syndrome) maps to a 1 cM interval on chromosome 8q21. *Am J Hum Genet* **60**:605, 1997.
176. Taalman RDFM, Hustinx TWJ, Weemaes CMR, Seemanova E, Schmidt A, Passarge E, Scheres JMJC: Further delineation of the Nijmegen breakage syndrome. *Am J Med Genet* **32**:425, 1989.
177. Burgt I, Chrzanowska K, Smeets D, Weemaes C: Nijmegen breakage syndrome. *J Med Genet* **33**:153, 1996.
178. Chrzanowska KH, Kleijer WJ, Krajewska-Walasek M, Bialecka M, Gutkowska A, Goryluk-Kozakiewicz B, Michalkiewicz J: Eleven Polish patients with microcephaly, immunodeficiency and chromosomal instability: The Nijmegen breakage syndrome. *Am J Med Genet* **57**:462, 1995.
179. Curry CJR, O'Lague P, Tsai J, Hutchinson HT, Jaspers NGJ, Wara D, Gatti RA: AT_{Fresno}: A phenotype linking ataxia-telangiectasia with the Nijmegen breakage syndrome. *Am J Hum Genet* **45**:270, 1989.
180. Gatti RA: Ataxia-telangiectasia: genetic studies, in Griscelli C, Gupta S (eds): *New Concepts in Immunodeficiency*. Chichester, UK, Wiley, 1993, pp 203–229.

181. Lange E, Gatti RA, Sobel E, Concannon P, Lange K: How many A-T genes? in Gatti RA, Painter RB (eds): *Ataxia-Telangiectasia*. Heidelberg, Springer-Verlag, 1993, pp 37–54.
182. Taylor AMR, McConville CM, Woods GW, Byrd PJ, Hernandez D: Clinical and cellular heterogeneity in ataxia-telangiectasia, in Gatti RA, Painter RB (eds): *Ataxia-Telangiectasia*. Heidelberg, Springer-Verlag, 1993, pp 209–233.
183. Maserati E, Ottoline A, Veggiatti P, Lanzi G, Pasquali F: Ataxia without telangiectasia in two sisters with rearrangements of chromosomes 7 and 14. *Clin Genet* **34**:283, 1988.
184. Byrne E, Hallpike JF, Manson JI, Sutherland GR, Thong YH: Progressive multisystem degeneration with IgE deficiency and chromosomal instability. *J Neurol Sci* **66**:307, 1984.
185. Regueiro JR, Porras O, Lavin M, Gatti RA: Ataxia-Telangiectasia. A primary immunodeficiency revisited. *Allergy Immunol Clin North Am,* In press.
186. Harding A: *The Inherited Ataxias and Related Disorders*. London, Churchill Livingstone, 1984.
187. Bird TD: Hereditary motor sensory neuropathies: Charcot-Marie-Tooth syndrome. *Neurol Clin North Am* **7**:9, 1989.
188. Campuzano V, Montermini L, Molto MD, Pianese L, Cossee M, Cavalcanti F, Monros E, Rodius F, Duclos F, Monticelli A, Zara F, Canizares J, Koutnikova H, Bidichandani SI, Gellera C, Brice A, Trouillas P, De Michele G, Filla A, De Frutos, Palau F, Patel PI, Di Donato S, Mandel J-L, Cocozza S, Koenig M, Pandolfo M: Friedreich's ataxia: Autosomal recessive disease cased by an intronic GAA triplet repeat expansion. *Science* **271**:1423, 1996.
189. Aicardi J, Barbosas C, Andermann E, Andermann F, Morcos R, Ghanem Q, Fukuyama Y, Awaya Y, Moe P: Ataxia-ocular motor apraxia: A syndrome mimicking ataxia-telangiectasia. *Ann Neurol* **24**:497, 1988.
190. Jaspers NGJ, van der Kraan M, Linssen PCML, Macek M, Seemanova E, Kleijer WJ: First-trimester prenatal diagnosis of the Nijmegen breakage syndrome and ataxia-telangiectasia using an assay of radioresistant DNA synthesis. *Prenat Diagn* **10**:667, 1990.
191. Gianelli F, Avery JA, Pembrey ME, Blunt S: Prenatal exclusion of ataxia-telangiectasia, in Bridges BA, Harnden DG (eds): *Ataxia-Telangiectasia: Cellular and Molecular Link between Cancer, Neuropathology and Immune Deficiency*. New York, Wiley, 1982, pp 393–407.
192. Gatti RA, Peterson KL, Novak J, Chen X, Yang-Chen L, Liang T, Lange E, Lange K: Prenatal genotyping of ataxia-telangiectasia. *Lancet* **342**:376, 1993.
193. Kleijer WJ, van der Kraan M, Los FJ, Jaspers MGJ: Prenatal diagnosis of ataxia-telangiectasia and Nijmegen breakage syndrome by the assay of radioresistant DNA synthesis. *Int J Radiat Biol* **66**:S167, 1994.
194. Rotman G, Savitski K, Vanagaite L, Bar-Shira A, Ziv Y, Gilad S, Vchenik V, Smith S, Shiloh Y: Physical and genetic mapping at the ATA/ATC locus on chromosome 11q22-23. *Int J Radiat Biol* **66**:S63, 1994.
195. Vanagaite L, James MR, Rotman G, Savitsky K, Var-Shira A, Gilad S, Ziv Y, Uchenik V, Sartiel A, Collins FS, Sheffield VC, Richard CW III, Weissenbach J, Shiloh Y: A high-density microsatellite map of the ataxia telangiectasia locus. *Hum Genet* **95**:451, 1995.
196. Perlman SL: Treatment of ataxia-telangiectasia, in Gatti RA, Painter RB (eds): *Ataxia-Telangiectasia*. Heidelberg, Springer-Verlag, 1993, pp 269–278.
197. Pump KK, Dunn HG, Meuwissen H: A study of the bronchial and vascular structures of a lung from a case of ataxia-telangiectasia. *Dis Chest* **47**:473, 1965.
198. Banin S, Moyal L, Shieh S-Y, Taya Y, Anderson CW, Chessa L, Smorodinsky NI, Prives C, Reiss Y, Shiloh Y, Ziv Y: Enhanced phosphorylation of p53 by ATM in response to DNA damage. *Science* **281**:1675, 1998.
199. Canman CE, Lim D-S, Cimprich KA, Taya Y, Tamai K, Sakaguchi K, Appella E, Kastan MB, Siliciano JD: Activation of the ATM kinase by ionizing radiation and phosphorylation of p53. *Science* **281**:1677, 1998.
200. Hendrickson EA: Insights from model systems: Cell-cycle regulation of mammalian DNA double-strand-break repair. *Am J Hum Genet* **61**:795, 1997.
201. Carney JP, Maser RS, Olivares H, Davis EM, Le Beau M, Yates JR, Hays L, Morgan WF, Petrini JHJ: The hMre11/hRad50 protein complex and Nijmegen breakage syndrome: Linkage of double-strand break repair to the cellular DNA damage response. *Cell* **93**:477, 1998.
202. Varon R, Vissinga C, Platzer M, Cerosaletti KM, Chrzanowska KH, Saar K, Beckmann G, Seemanova E, Cooper PR, Nowak NJ, Stumm M, Weemaes CMR, Gatti RA, Wilson RK, Digweed M, Rosenthal A, Sperling K, Concannon P, Reis A: Nibrin, a novel DNA double-strand break repair protein, is mutated in Nijmegen Breakage Syndrome. *Cell* **93**:467, 1998.
203. Borghesani PR, Alt FA, Bottaro A, Davidson L, Aksoy S, Rathbun GA, Roberts TM, Swat W, Segal RA, Gu Y: Abnormal development of Purkinje cells and lymphocytes in *Atm* mutant mice. *Proc Natl Acad Sci USA* In press.
204. Murnane JP, Painter RB: Complementation of the defects in DNA synthesis in irradiated and unirradiated ataxia-telangiectasia cells. *Proc Natl Acad Sci USA* **79**:1960, 1982.
205. Gatti RA, Shaked R, Wei S, Koyama M, Salser W, Silver J: DNA polymorphism in the human THY-1 gene. *Hum Immunol* **22**:145, 1988.
206. Sanal O, Wei S, Foroud T, Malhotra U, Concannon P, Charmley P, Salser W, Lange K, Gatti RA: Further mapping of an ataxia-telangiectasia locus to the chromosome 11q23 region. *Am J Hum Genet* **47**:860, 1990.
207. Foroud T, Wei S, Ziv Y, Sobel E, Lange E, Chao A, Goradia T, Huo Y, Tolun A, Chessa L, Charmley P, Sanal O, Salman N, Julier C, Lathrop GM, Concannon P, McConville C, Taylor M, Shiloh Y, Lange K, Gatti RA: Localization of an ataxia-telangiectasia locus to a 3-cM interval on chromosome 11q23: Linkage analyses of 111 families by an international consortium. *Am J Hum Genet* **49**:1263, 1991.
208. Sanal O, Lange E, Telatar M, Sobel E, Salazar-Novak J, Ersoy F, Concannon P, Tolun A, Gatti RA: Ataxia-telangiectasia-linkage analysis of chromosome 11q22-23 markers in Turkish families. *FASEB J* **6**:2848, 1992.
209. Charmley P, Foroud T, Wei S, Concannon P, Weeks DE, Lange D, Gatti RA: A primary linkage map of the human chromosome 11q22-23 region. *Genomics* **6**:316, 1990.
210. Charmley P, Nguyen J, Wei S, Gatti RA: Genetic linkage analysis and homology of syntenic relationships of genes located on human chromosome 11q. *Genomics* **10**:608, 1991.
211. Concannon P, Malhotra U, Charmley P, Reynolds J, Lange K, Gatti RA: Ataxia-telangiectasia gene (ATA) on chromosome 11 is distinct from the ETS-1 gene. *Genomics* **46**:789, 1990.
212. Wei S, Rocchi M, Archidiacono N, Sacchi N, Romeo G, Gatti RA: Physical mapping of the human chromosome 11q23 region containing the ataxia-telangiectasia locus. *Cancer Genet Cytogenet* **46**:1, 1990.
213. McConville CM, Byrd PJ, Ambrose HJ, Taylor AMR: Genetic and physical mapping of the ataxia-telangiectasia locus on chromosome 11q22-23. *Int J Radiat Biol* **66**:545, 1994.
214. McConville CM, Formstone CJ, Hernandez D, Thick J, Taylor AMR: Fine mapping of the chromosome 11q22-23 region using PFGE, linkage and haplotype analysis: Localization of the gene for ataxia-telangiectasia to a 5 cM region flanked by NCAM/DRD2 and STMY/CJ52.75, ph2.22. *Nucleic Acids Res* **18**:4334, 1990.
215. McConville C, Woods CG, Farrall M, Metcalfe JA, Taylor AMR: Analysis of 7 polymorphic markers at chromosome 11q22-23 in 35 ataxia-telangiectasia families: Further evidence of linkage. *Hum Genet* **85**:215, 1990.
216. McConville CM, Byrd PJ, Ambrose H, Stankovic T, Ziv Y, Bar-Shira A, Vanagaite L, Rotman G, Shiloh Y, Gillett GT, Riley JH, Taylor AMR: Paired STSs amplified from radiation hybrids, and from associated YACs, identify highly polymorphic loci flanking the ataxia-telangiectasia locus on chromosome 11q22-23. *Hum Mol Genet* **2**:969, 1993.
217. Cornelis F, James M, Cherif D, Tokino T, Davies J, Girault D, Bernard C, Litt M, Berger R, Nakamura Y, Lathrop M, Julier C: Precise localization of a gene responsible for ataxia-telangiectasia on chromosome 11q, in Gatti RA, Painter RB (eds): *Ataxia-Telangiectasia*. Heidelberg, Springer-Verlag, 1993, pp 23–36.
218. Oskato R, Bar-Shira A, Vanagaite L, Ziv Y, Ehrlich S, Rotman G, McConville CM, Chakravarti A, Shiloh Y: Ataxia-telangiectasia: Allelic association with 11q22-23 markers in Moroccan-Jewish patients. *Am J Hum Genet* **53**:A1055, 1993.
219. Taylor AMR, McConville CM, Rotman G, Shiloh Y, Byrd PJ: A haplotype common to intermediate radiosensitivity variants of ataxia-telangiectasia in the UK. *Int J Radiat Biol* **66**:S35, 1994.
220. Uhrhammer N, Concannon P, Huo Y, Nakamura Y, Gatti RA: A pulsed-field gel electrophoresis map in the ataxia-telangiectasia region of chromosome 11q22.3. *Genomics* **20**:278, 1994.
221. Uhrhammer N, Lange E, Porras O, Naeim A, Chen X, Sheikhavandi S, Chiplunkar S, Yang L, Dandekar S, Liang T, Patel N, Udar N, Concannon P, Gerken S, Shiloh Y, Lange K, Gatti RA: Sublocalization of an ataxia-telangiectasia gene distal to D11S384 by ancestral haplotyping in Costa Rican families. *Am J Hum Genet* **57**:103, 1995.

222. Teraoka S, Telatar M, Becker-Catania S, Liang T, Onegut S, Tolun A, Chessa L, Sanal O, Bernatowska E, Gatti RA, Concannon P: Splicing defects in the ataxia-telangiectasia gene, ATM: under lying mutations and phenotypic consequences. *Am J Hum Genet* **64**:1617, 1999.
223. Croce CM: Role of TCL1 and ALL1 in human leukemias and development. *Cancer Res* **59**:177s, 1998.
224. Buckler AJ, Chang DD, Graw SL, Brook JD, Haber DA, Sharp PA, Housman DE: Exon amplification: A strategy to isolate mammalian genes based on RNA splicing. *PNAS* **88**:4005, 1991.
225. Byrd PJ, McConville CM, Cooper P, Parkhill J, Stankovic T, McGuire GM, Thick JA, Taylor AMR: Mutations revealed by sequencing the 59 half of the gene for ataxia-telangiectasia. *Hum Mol Genet* **5**:145, 1996.
226. Imai T, Yamauchi M, Seki N, Sugawara T, Saito T, Matsuda Y, Ito H, Nagase T, Nomua N, Hori T: Identification and characterization of a new gene physically linked to the ATM gene. *Genome Res* 6:439, 1996.
227. Chen X, Yang L, Udar N, Liang T, Uhrhammer N, Xu S, Bay JO, Wang Z, Dandakar U, Chiplunkar S, Klisak I, Telatar M, Yang H, Concannon P, Gatti RA: CAND3: A ubiquitously-expressed gene immediately adjacent and in opposite transcriptional orientation to the ATM gene at 11q23.1. *Mamm Genome* **8**:129, 1997.
228. Rasio D, Negrini M, Croce CM: Genomic organization of the ATM locus involved in ataxia-telangiectasia. *Cancer Res* **55**:6053, 1995.
229. Uziel T, Savitsky K, Platzer M, Ziv Y, Helbitz T, Nehls M, Boehm T, Rosenthal A, Shiloh Y, Rotman G: Genomic organization of the ATM gene. *Genomics* **33**:317, 1996.
230. Pecker I, Avrahan KB, Gilbert DJ, Savitsky K, Rotman G, Harnik R, Fukao T, Schrock E, Hirotsune S, Tagle DA, Collins FS, Wynshow-Boris A, Ried T, Copeland NG, Jenkins NA, Shiloh Y, Ziv Y: Identification and chromosomal localization of atm, the mouse homolog of the ataxia-telangiectasia gene. *Genomics* **35**:39, 1996.
231. Gao J-H, Parsons LM, Bowers JM, Xiong J, Li J, Fox PT: Cerebellum implicated in sensory acquisition and discrimination rather than motor control. *Science* **272**:545, 1996.
232. Barinaga M: The cerebellum: Movement coordinator or much more? [editorial overview]. *Science* **272**:482, 1996.
233. Keith CT, Schreiber SL: PIK-related kinases: DNA repair, recombination, and cell cycle checkpoints. *Science* **270**:50, 1995.
234. Gilad S, Khosravi R, Shkedy D, Uziel T, Ziv Y, Savitsky K, Rotman G, Smith S, Chessa L, Jorgensen TJ, Harnik R, Frydman M, Sanal O, Portnoi S, Goldwicz Z, Jaspers MGJ, Gatti RA, Lenoir G, Lavin M, Tatsumi K, Wegner RD, Shiloh Y, Bar-Shira A: Predominance of null mutation in ataxia-telangiectasia. *Hum Mol Genet* **5**:433, 1996.
235. Wright J, Teraoka S, Onengut S, Tolun A, Gatti RA, Ochs HD, Concannon P: A high frequency of distinct ATM mutations in ataxia-telangiectasia. *Am J Hum Genet* **59**:839, 1996.
236. Forrest S, Cotton R, Landegren U, Southern E: How to find all those mutations. *Nat Genet* **10**:375, 1995.
237. Concannon P, Gatti RA: Diversity of ATM gene mutations detected in patients with ataxia-telangiectasia. *Hum Mutat* **10**:100, 1997.
238. Hawkins JD: *Gene Structure and Expression*, 2d ed. Cambridge, UK, Cambridge University Press, 1991, p 127.
239. McConville CM, Stankovic T, Byrd PJ, McGuire GM, Yao Q-Y, Lennox GG, Taylor AMR:Mutations associated with variant phenotypes in ataxia-telangiectasia. *Am J Hum Genet* **59**:320, 1996.
240. Gatti RA: Ataxia-telangiectasia: Immune dysfunction is one of many defects. *Immunol Today* **5**:121, 1984.
241. Lehmann A, Jaspers NJG, Gatti RA: Ataxia-telangiectasia: Meeting report. *Cancer Res* **47**:4750, 1987.
242. Lehmann AR, Jaspers NGJ, Gatti RA: Meeting report: Fourth International Workshop on Ataxia-Telangiectasia. *Cancer Res* **49**:6162, 1989.
243. Taylor AMR, Jaspers NGJ, Gatti RA: Meeting report: Fifth International Workshop on Ataxia-Telangiectasia. *Cancer Res* **53**:438, 1993.
244. Gatti RA, McConville CM, Taylor AMR: Meeting report. Sixth International Workshop on Ataxia-Telangiectasia. *Cancer Res* **54**:6007, 1994.
245. Bridges BA, Harnden DG (eds): *Ataxia-Telangiectasia: A Cellular and Molecular Link between Cancer, Neuropathology, and Immune Deficiency.* Chichester, UK, Wiley, 1982, p 1–402.
246. Gatti RA, Swift M (eds): *Ataxia-Telangiectasia: Genetics, Neuropathology, and Immunology of a Degenerative Disease of Childhood.* New York, Liss, 1985.
247. Gatti RA, Painter RB (eds): *Ataxia-Telangiectasia*, vol 77. NATO ASI Series. Heidelberg, Springer-Verlag, 1993.
248. Julier C, Nakamura Y, Lathrop M, O'Connell P, Leppert M, Litt M, Mohandas T, Lalouel J-M, White R: Detailed map of the long arm of chromosome 11. *Genomics* **7**:335, 1990.
249. Kapp LN, Painter RB, Yu L-C, van Loon N, Richard CW, James MR, Cox DR, Murnane JP: Cloning of a candidate gene for ataxia-telangiectasia group D. *Am J Hum Genet* **51**:45, 1992.
250. Kapp LN, Murnane JP: Cloning and characterization of a candidate gene for A-T complementation Group D, in Gatti RA, Painter RB (eds): *Ataxia-Telangiectasia*. Heidelberg, Springer-Verlag, 1993, pp 7–22.
251. Platzer M, Rotman G, Bauer D, Uziel T, Savitsky K, Bar-Shira A, Gilad S, Shiloh Y, Rosenthal A: Ataxia-telangiectasia locus: Sequence analysis of 184 kb of human genomic DNA containing the entire ATM gene. *Genome Res* **7**:592, 1997.
252. Telatar M, Teraoka S, Wang Z, Chun HH, Liang T, Castellvi-Bel S, Udar N, Borresen-Dale A-L, Chessa L, Bernatowska-Matuszkiewicz E, Porras O, Watanabe M, Junker A, Concannon P, Gatti RA: Ataxia-telangiectasia: Identification and detection of founder mutations in the ATM gene in ethnic populations. *Am J Hum Genet* **62**:86, 1998.
253. Trouillas P, Xie J, Adeleine P: Buspirone, a serotonergic 5-HT1A agonist, is active in cerebellar ataxia. A new fact in favor of the serotonergic theory of ataxia. *Prog Brain Res* **114**:589, 1997.
254. Kuljis RO, Xu Y, Aguila MC, Baltimore D: Degeneration of neurons, synapses, and neuropil and glial activation in a murine Atm knockout model of ataxia-telangiectasia. *Proc Natl Acad Sci USA* **94**:12688, 1997.
255. Westphal CH, Rowan S, Schmaltz C, Elson A, Fisher DE, Leder P: atm and p53 cooperate in apoptosis and suppression of tumorigenesis, but not in resistance to acute radiation toxicity. *Nat Genetics* **16**:397, 1997.
256. Herzog K-H, Chong MJ, Kapsetaki M, Morgan JI, McKinnon PJ: Requirement for ATM in ionizing radiation-induced cell death in the developing central nervous system. *Science* **280**:1089, 1998.
257. Bay J-O, Grancho M, Pernin D, Presneau N, Rio P, Tchirkov A, Uhrhammer N, Verrelle P, Gatti RA, Bignon Y-J: No evidence for constitutional ATM mutation in breast/gastric cancer families. *Intl J Oncol* **12**:1385, 1998.
258. Chen J, Birksholtz GC, Lindblom P, Rubio C, Lindblom A: The role of ataxia-telangiectasia heterozygotes in familial breast cancer. *Cancer Res* **58**:1376, 1998.
259. Luo L, Lu F-M, Hart S, Foroni L, Rabbani H, Hammarstrom L, Webster ADB, Vorechowsky I: Ataxia-telangiectasia and T-cell leukemias: no evidence for somatic ATM mutation in sporadic T-ALL or for hypermethylation of the ATM-NPAT/E14 bidirectional promoter in T-PLL. *Cancer Res* **58**:2293, 1998.
260. Larson GP, Zhang G, Ding S, Foldenauer K, Udar N, Gatti RA, Neuberg D, Lunetta KL, Ruckdeschel JC, Longmate J, Flanagan S, Krontiris TG: An allelic variant at the ATM locus is implicated in breast cancer susceptibility. *Genet Testing* **1**:165, 1998.
261. Forozan F, Karthu R, Kononen J, Kallionieni A, Kallioniemi OP: Genome screening by comparative genomic hybridization. *Trends Genet* **13**:405, 1997.
262. Smith L, Liu SJ, Goodrich L, Jacobson D, Degnin C, Bentley N, Carr A, Flaggs G, Keegan K, Hoekstra M, Thayer M: Duplication of ATR inhibits MyoD, induces aneuploidy and eliminates radiation-induced G1 arrest. *Nat Genet* **19**:39, 1998.
263. Cliby WA, Roberts CJ, Cimprich KA, Stringer CM, Lamb JR, Schreiber SL, Friend SH: Overexpression of a kinase-inactive ATR protein causes sensitivity of DNA-damaging agents and defects in cell cycle checkpoints. *EMBO J* **17**:159, 1998.
264. Stilgenbauer S, Schaffner C, Litterst A, Liebisch P, Gilad S, Bar-Shira A, James MR, Lichter P, Dohner H: Evidence for ATM as a tumor suppressor gene in T-prolymphocytic leukemia. *Nat Med* **3**:1155, 1997.
265. Hendricksen LA, Carter T, Dutta A, Wold MS: Phosphorylation of human replication protein A by the DNA-dependent protein kinase is involved in the modulation of DNA replication. *Nucleic Acids Res* **24**:3107, 1996.
266. Rivero ME, Porras O, Leiva I, Pacheco A, Regueiro JR: Phenotypical and functional characterization of herpes virus saimiri-immortalized T cells from ataxia-telangiectasia patient [abstract #61]. Clermont-Ferrand, France: Seventh International Workshop on Ataxia-Telangiectasia, November 22–24, 1997.
267. Gabra H, Watson VJE, Taylor KJ, Mackay J, Leonard RC, Steel CM, Porteous DJ, Smyth JF: Definition and refinement of a region of loss of heterozygosity at 11q23.3-q24.3 in epithelial ovarian cancer associated with poor prognosis. *Cancer Res* **56**:950, 1996.
268. Koreth J, Bakkenist CJ, McGee J: Allelic deletions at chromosome 11q22-q23.1 and 11q25-qterm are frequent in sporadic breast but not colorectal cancers. *Oncogene* **14**:431, 1997.
269. Nanashima A, Tagawa Y, Tasutake T, Fujise N, Kashima K, Nakagoe T, Ayabe H: Deletion of chromosome 11 and development of colorectal carcinoma. *Cancer Detect Prev* **21**:7, 1997.

270. Hui AB, Lo KW, Leung SF, Choi PH, Fong Y, Lee JC, Huang DP: Loss of heterozygosity on the long arm of chromosome 11 in nasopharyngeal carcinoma. *Cancer Res* **56**:3225, 1996.
271. Flaggs G, Plug AW, Dunks KM, Mundt KE, Ford JC, Quiggle MRE, Taylor EM, Westphal CH, Ashley T, Hoekstra MF, Carr AM: Atm-dependent interactions of a mammalian Chk1 homolog with meiotic chromosomes. *Curr Biol* **7**:977, 1997.
272. Plug AW, Peters AHFM, Xu Y, Keegan KS, Hoekstra MF, Baltimore D, de Boer P, Ashley T: ATM and RPA in meiotic chromosome synapsis and recombination. *Nat Genet* **17**:457, 1997.
273. Baumann P, Benson FE, West SC: Human Rad51 protein promotes ATP-dependent homologous pairing and strand transfer reactions in vitro. *Cell* **87**:757, 1996.
274. Cox MM, Lehman IR: recA protein-promoted DNA strand exchange: Stable complexes of recA protein and single-stranded DNA formed in the presence of ATP and single-stranded DNA-binding protein. *J Biol Chem* **257**:8523, 1982.
275. Sanal O, Smeets D, Aksoy Y, Beerket AI, Ersoy F, Gariboglu S, Metin A, Ogus H, Weemaes C, Yel L: Heterogenicity in ataxia-telangiectasia: Various laboratory features of 47 patients [abstract #47]. Clermont-Ferrand, France: Seventh International Workshop on Ataxia-Telangiectasia, November 22–24, 1997.
276. Schubert R, Kappenhagen N, Royer N, Zielen S: Ongoing apoptosis of lymphocytes in patients with ataxia-telangiectasia. [abstract #66]. Clermont-Ferrand, France: Seventh International Workshop on Ataxia-Telangiectasia, November 22–24, 1997.
277. Fiorilli M, Businco L, Pandolfi F, Paganelli R, Russo G, Aiuti F: Heterogeneity of immunological abnormalities in ataxia-telangiectasia. *J Clin Immunol* **3**:135, 1983.
278. Porras O: Personal communication. oral 1997
279. Pastorino AC, Almeida AG, Dias MJM, Jacob CMA, Duarte AJS, Grumach AS: Ataxia-telangiectasia. Aspectos clinico-laboratoriasis de 11 pacientes. *Latin American Group for Immunodeficiency meeting*. Sao Paolo, Brazil, Sept 3–5, 1998.
280. Sanal O, Berkel AI, Ersoy F, Tezcan I, Topaloglu H: Clinical variants of ataxia-telangiectasia. In: Ataxia-telangiectasia, in Gatti RA, Painter RB (eds): *Ataxia-Telangiectasia. NATO ASI series*. Berlin, Springer-Verlag, 1993, pp 183–187.
281. Bezrodnik L, Krasovec S, Gaillard MI, Rivas EM: Sindrome de ataxia telangiectasia: presentacion de 9 pacientes. *Latin American Group for Immunodeficiency meeting*. Sao Paolo, Brazil, Sept 3–5, 1998.
282. Vorechovsky I, Luo L, Lindblom A, Negrini M, Webster DB, Croce CM, Hammarstrom L: ATM mutations in cancer families. *Cancer Res* **56**:4130, 1996.
283. Chrzanowska K, Krajewska-Walasek M, Bernatowska E, Kostyk E, Midro AT, Metera M, Bialecka M, Gregorek H, Michalkiewicz J, Brrzeziinska A, Rozynek A: Polish patients with Nijmegen breakage syndrome. *Clinical and genetic studies* [abstract #24]. Clermont-Ferrand France: Seventh International Workshop on Ataxia-Telangiectasia, November 22–24, 1997.
284. Cerosaletti KM, Lange E, Stringham HM, Weemaes CMR, Smeets D, Solder B, Belohradsky BH, Taylor AMR, Marnes P, Elliott A, Komatsu K, Gatti RA, Boehnke M, Concannon P: Fine localization of the Nijmegen breakage syndrome gene to 8q21: Evidence for a common founder haplotype. *Am J Hum Genet* **63**:125, 1998.
285. Udar N, Farzad S, Taj -Q, Bay J-Q, Gatti RA: NS22, a high polymorphic marker with the ATM gene. *Am J Med Genet* **82**:287, 1999.
286. Krivit W, Sung JH, Shapiro EG, Lockman LA: Microglia: The effector cell for reconstitution of the central nervous system following bone marrow transplantation for lysosomal and peroxisomal storage diseases. *Cell Transplant* **4**:385, 1995.
287. Unger ER, Sung JH, Manivel JC, Chenggis ML, Blazar BR, Krivitt W. Male donor-derived cells in the brains of female sex-mismatched bone marrow transplant recipients: A Y-chromosome specific in situ hybridization study. *J Neuropathol Exp Neurol* **52**:460, 1993.
288. Lim DS, Kirsch DG, Lee A, Rhodes N, Gilmer T, Kastan MB: Functional interactions between ATM and adapting proteins [abstract #526]. *AACR Proc* **39**:S77, 1998.
289. Stankovic T, Kidd AMJ, Sutcliffe A, McGuire GM, Robinson P, Weber P, Bedenham T, Bradwell AR, Easton DF, Lennox GG, Haites N, Byrd PJ, Talyor AMR: ATM mutations and phenotypes in ataxia-telangiectasia families in the British Isles: Expression of mutant ATM and the risk of leukemia, lymphoma, and breast cancer. *Am J Hum Genet* **62**:334, 1998.
290. Telatar M, Wang Z, Castellvi-Bel S, Tai L-Q, Sheikhavandi S, Regueiro JG, Porras O, Gatti RA: A model for ATM heterozygote identification in a large population: Four founder-effect ATM mutations identify most of Cost Rican patients with ataxia telangiectasia. *Mol Genet Metab* **64**:36, 1998.
291. Gilad S, Bar-Shira A, Harnik R, Shkedy D, Ziv Y, Shosravi R, Brown K, Vanagaite L, Xu G, Frydman M, Lavin MF, Hill D, Tagle DA, Shiloh Y: Ataxia-telangiectasia: Founder effect among North African Jews. *Hum Mol Genet* **5**:2033, 1996.
292. Uhrhammer N, Bay J-O, Bignon Y-J: Seventh International Workshop on Ataxia-Telangiectasia. *Cancer Res* **58**:3480, 1998.
293. Laake K, Telatar M, Geitvik GA, Hansen RO, Heiberg A, Andresen AM, Gatt RA, Borresen-Dale A-L: Identical mutation in 55% of the ATM alleles in 11 Norwegian AT families: Evidence for a founder effect. *Eur J Hum Genet* **6**:235, 1998.
294. Gilad S, Chessa L, Khosravi R, Russel P, Galanty Y, Piane M, Gatti RA, Jorgensen TJ, Shiloh Y, Bar-Shira A: Genotype-phenotype relationships in ataxia-telangiectasia and variants. *Am J Hum Genet* **62**:551, 1998.
295. Becker-Catania SG, Chen G, Hwang MJ, Wang Z, Sun X, Sanal O, Bernatowska-Matuszkiewicz E, Chessa L, Lee EYH-P, Gatti RA: ATM protein expression, mutations, radiosensitivity and clinical phenotype in 124 ataxia-telangiectasia pateients. Submitted.
296. Rosenblatt HM, Brown B, Parikh N, Jorczak A: Abnormal up-regulation of CD-40 ligand (CD40L) in patients with ataxia-telangiectasia (AT) and elevated serum IGM levels [abstract #5336]. *FASEB J* **12**:A922, 1998.
297. Laake K Odegard A, Andersen Tl, Bukholm lK, Karesen R, Nesland JM, Ottestad L, Shiloh Y, Borresen-Dale A-L: Loss of heterozygosity at 11q23.1 in breast carcinomas: indication for involvement of a gene distal and close to ATM. *Gene Chrom Cancer* **18**:175, 1997.
298. Tyagi S, Bratu DP, Kramer FR: Multicolor molecular beacons for allele discrimination. *Nature Biotech* **16**:49, 1998.
299. Cortez D, Wang Y, Qin J, Elledge SJ: Requirement of ATM-dependent phosphorylation of Brca1 in the DNA damage response to double-strand breaks. *Science* **286**:1162, 1999.
300. Khanna KK, Keating KE, Kozlov S, Scott S, Gatei M, Hobson K, Taya Y, Gabrielli B, Chan D, Less-Miller SP, Lavin MF: ATM associates with and phosphorylates p53: Mapping the region of interaction. *Nat Genet* **20**:398, 1998.
301. Fegen C, Robinson H, Thompson P, Whittaker JA, White D: Karyotypic evolution in CLL: Identification of a new sub-group with deletions of 11q and advanced or progressive disease. *Leukemia* **9**:2003, 1995.
302. Starostik P, Manshouri T, O'Brien S, Freireich E, Kantarjian H, Lerner S, Keating M, Albitar M: The ATM gene is deleted in a subgroup of B-cell chronic lymphocytic leukemia. *Proceedings of the American Society of Hematology, Dec 8-10, 1997, San Diego, Calif.* (abst 396, p 90a).
303. Stankovic T, Weber P, Stewart G, Bedenham T, Byrd PJ, Moss PA, Taylor AM: Inactivation of ataxia telangiectasia mutated gene in B-cell chronic lymphocytic leukaemia. *Lancet* **353**:26, 1999.
304. Bullrich F, Tasio D, Kitada S, Starostik P, Kipps T, Keating M, Albitar M, Reed JC, Croce CM: ATM mutations in B-cell chronic lymphocytic leukemia. *Cancer Res* **59**:2427, 1999.
305. Teraoka SN, Malone KE, Doody D, Ostrander EA, Daling JR, Concannon P: Increased frequency of ATM mutations in breast cancer patients with early-onset disease or positive family history. submitted.
306. Gatti RA, Tward A, Concannon P: Cancer risk in ATM heterozygotes: a model of phenotypic and mechanistic differences between missense and truncating mutations. *Molec Genet Metab* **69**:419, 1999.
307. Zhao S, Yuan FS-S, Weng Y-C, Lin Y-L, Hsu H-C, Lin S-Cj, Gerbino E, Song M-H, Zdzienicka MZ, Gatti RA, Shay J, Ziv Y, Shiloh Y, Lee EY-HP: A functional link between ATM kinase and NBS1 in the DNA damage response. *Nature* In press.
308. Stewart GS, Maser RS, Stankovic T, Bressan Da, Kaplan Ml, Jaspers NGJ, Raams A, Byrd PJ, Petrini JHJ, Taylor AMR: The DNA double-strand break repair gene hMRE11 is mutated in individuals with an ataxia-telangiectasia-like disorder. *Cell* **99**:577, 1999.
309. Greenberg F, Rose E, Alpert E: Hereditary persistence of alpha-fetoprotein. *Gastroenterology* **98**:1083, 1990.
310. McVey JH, Michaelides K, Hansen LP, Ferguson-Smith M, Tilghman S, Krumlauf R, Tuddenham EGD: A G > A substitution in an HNF 1 binding site in the human α-fetoprotein gene is associated with hereditary persistence of α-fetoprotein (HPAFP). *Human Molec Genet* **2**:379, 1993.
311. Murgita RA, Wigzell H: The effects of mouse alpha-fetoprotein on T-cell-dependent and T-cell-independent immune response in vivo. *Scand J Immunol* **5**:1215, 1976.

312. Murgita RA, Anderson LC, Sherman MS: Effects of human alpha-fetoprotein on human B and T lymphocyte proliferation in vitro. *Clin Exp Immunol* **33**:347, 1978.
313. Lee KC, Crowe AJ, Barton MC: P53-mediated repression of alpha-fetoprotein gene expression by specific DNA binding. *Mol Cell Biol* **19**:1279, 1999.
314. Hernandez D, McConville CM, Stacey M, Woods, CG, Brown MM, Shutt P, Rysiecki G, Taylor AMR: A family sowing no evidence of linkage between the ataxia telaphigectasia Taylor AMR: A family showing no evidence of linkage between the ataxia telaphigectasia gene and chromosome 11q22-23. *J Med Genet* **30**:135, 1993.
315. Djozenova CS, Schindler D, Stopper H, Hoehn H, Flentje M, Oppitz U: Identification of ataxia telangiectasia heterozygotes, a cancer-prone population, using the single-cell gel electrophoresis (Comet) assay. *Lab Invest* **79**:699, 1999.
315. Geschwind DH, perlman S, Grody W, Telatar M, Montermini L, pandolfo M, Gatti RA: Friedreich's ataxia GAA repeat expansion in patients with recessive or sporadic ataxia. *Neurology* **49**:1004, 1997.
317. Lavin MF: Radiosensitivity and oxidative signalling in ataxia telangiectasia: An update. *Radiother Oncol* **47**:113, 1998.
318. Smith GCM, Cary RB, Lakin ND, Hann BC, Teo S-H, Chen DJ, Jackson SP: Purification and DNA binding properties of the ataxia-telangiectasia gene product ATM. *Proc Natl Acad Sci USA* **96**:11134, 1999.
319. Savitsky K, Platzer M, Uziel T, Gilad S, Sartiel A, Rosenthal A, Elroy-Stein O, Shiloh Y, Rotman G: Ataxia-telangiectasia: Structural diversity of untranslated sequences suggests complex post-transcription regulation of ATM gene expression. *Nucleic Acids Res* **25**:1678, 1997.
320. Lavin M: Written personal communication. 1999.
321. Broeks A, de Klein A, Floore AN, Muijtjens M, Kleijer WJ, Jaspers NG, van't Veer LJ: ATM germline mutations in classical ataxia-telangiectasia patients in the Dutch population. *Hum Mutat* **12**:330, 1998.
322. Sandoval N, Platzer M, Rosenthal A, Dork T, Bendix R, Skawran B, Stuhrmann M, Wegner R-D, Sperling K, Banin S, Shiloh Y, Baumer A, Mernthaler U, Sennefelder H, Brohm M, Weber BHF, Schindler D: Characterization of ATM gene mutations in 66 ataxia telangiectasia families. *Hum Mol Genet* **8**:69, 1999.
323. Castellvi-Bel S, Sheikhavandi S, Telatar M, Tai L-Q, Hwang M, Wang Z, Yang Z, Cheng R, Gatti RA: New mutations, polymorphisms, and rare variants in the ATM gene detected by a novel strategy. *Hum Mutat* **14**:156, 1999.
324. Ashburner BP, Shackelford RE, Baldwin AS, Paules RS: Lack of involvement of ataxia telangiectasia mutated (ATM) in regulation of nuclear factor-κB (NF-κB) in human diploid fibroblasts. *Cancer Res* **59**:5456, 1999.
325. Reichenback J, Schubert R, Schwan C, Muller K, Bohles HJ, Zielen S: Anti-oxidative capacity in patients with ataxia telangiectasia. *Clin Exp Immunol* **117**:535, 1999.
326. Battisti C, Formichi P, Federico A: Vitamin E serum levels are normal in ataxia telangiectasia (Louis-Bar disease). *J Neurol Sci* 141:114, 1996.
327. Zielen S, Schubert R, Schindler D, Buehring l: Patients with A-T are unable to produce lgG antibodies to pneumococcal polysaccharides. International Workshop on Ataxia-Telangiectasia, Nov 22-24, 1997, Clermont-Ferrand, France (abst 41).
328. Cornforth MW, Bedford JS: On the nature of a defect in cells from individuals with ataxia-telangiectasia. *Science* **227**:1589, 1985.
329. Meyn MS: Ataxia-telanigectasia, cancer and the pathobiology of the ATM gene. *Clin Genet* **55**:289, 1999.
330. Morgan SE, Lovly C, Pandita TK, Shiloh Y, Kastan MB: Fragments of ATM which have dominant-negative or complementing activity. *Mol Cell Biol* 17:2020, 1997.
331. Shafman TD, Levitz S, Nixon AJ, Gibans L-A, Nichols KE, Bell DW, Ishioka C, Isselbacher KJ, Gelman R, Garber J, Harris JR, Haber DA: Prevalence of germline truncating mutations in ATM in women with a second breast cancer after radiation therapy for a contralateral tumor. *Genes Chrom Cancer.* In press.
332. Lavin MF, Concannon P, Gatti RA: Eighth International Workshop on Ataxia-Telangiectasia (ATW8). *Cancer Res* **59**:3845, 1999.

CHAPTER 30

Bloom Syndrome

James German ▪ Nathan A. Ellis

1. **Clinically, Bloom syndrome (BS) features (a) proportional dwarfism, usually accompanied by (b) a sun-sensitive erythematous skin lesion limited to the face and dorsa of the hands and forearms, (c) a characteristic facies and head configuration, and (d) immunodeficiency, often associated with otitis media and pneumonia. (e) Affected males fail to produce spermatozoa, and females although sometimes fertile experience an unusually early cessation of menstrual cycles. (f) Excessive numbers of well-circumscribed areas of dermal hypo- and hyperpigmentation are present. (g) The three major complications are chronic lung disease, diabetes mellitus, and — by far the most important and most frequent — cancer.**
2. **BS is a genetically determined trait that is transmitted in a straightforward autosomal recessive fashion, with mutations at a single locus, *BLM*, being responsible. Various mutations at *BLM* are segregating in human populations, but the same phenotype (BS) is produced by either homozygosity or compound heterozygosity of those so far identified. The mutations are predominantly null alleles, but missense mutations also have been detected. BS is rare in all populations, but in the Ashkenazi Jewish population, one particular mutant allele, a 6-bp deletion and 7-bp insertion that results in premature translation termination, has, through founder effect, reached a relatively high carrier frequency of approximately 1 percent; in 31 percent of all persons with BS, one or both parents are Ashkenazi Jews.**
3. **The genome is abnormally unstable in the somatic cells of persons with BS. Mutations arise spontaneously and accumulate in numbers manyfold greater than normal, including both microscopically visible chromatid gaps, breaks, and rearrangements and mutations at specific loci. Exchanges take place excessively between chromatids, usually at what appear to be homologous sites. One consequence of this hyperrecombinability is the reduction to homozygosity of constitutionally heterozygous loci distal to the points of crossing-over. The hyperrecombinability in persons with BS who are genetic compounds can lead to reversion at *BLM* itself: Crossing-over between two different mutated sites within *BLM* can result in the generation of a functionally normal gene, and thereby correction of the cellular phenotype of the somatic cells that comprise the progeny of the cell in which the recombinational event had occurred.**
4. **Many of the clinical characteristics of BS may be viewed as direct or indirect consequences of the hypermutability. It is postulated to be a major causative factor in BS's small size by way of the induction of factors which either inhibit further cell division or promote cell death. Another major consequence of the hypermutability is proneness to neoplasia; BS more than any other known human state predisposes to the development of cancer of the types and sites that affect the general population, and at unusually early ages. BS thus is the prototype of a class of disease that may be called the somatic mutational disorders.**
5. **Diagnosis of BS is based on clinical observation; the phenotype is striking. Laboratory confirmation ordinarily is by cytogenetic demonstration of the characteristically increased tendency of chromatid exchange to take place. BS is the only condition known that features a greatly increased rate of sister-chromatid exchange (SCE). Blood lymphocytes in short-term culture are suitable for demonstrating this. Under certain circumstances, diagnosis can be confirmed by demonstrating mutation(s) in *BLM*.**
6. **With respect to the clinical management of BS, measures to increase the size have not been found. Protection from the sun, especially during infancy and childhood, is valuable in reducing the severity of the facial skin lesion. Greater than normal surveillance for carcinoma is indicated in persons who reach adulthood; however, because many are the sites and types of neoplasm that may arise, devising a surveillance program in BS is a particularly challenging matter, for both the affected person and the physician.**
7. **The mapping of *BLM* to chromosome band 15q26.1 and its subsequent molecular isolation identified a nuclear protein that contains a 350-amino acid domain consisting of 7 motifs characteristic of DNA and RNA helicases. The helicase domain of the BLM protein is 40 to 45 percent identical to the helicase domain present in the RecQ subfamily of DNA helicases. Although DNA-dependent ATPase and DNA duplex unwinding activities have been demonstrated for several RecQ helicases, including BLM, the nucleic acid substrates these proteins act on in the cell are unknown. Whatever these substrates are, the molecular and genetic evidence implicates the RecQ helicases in the cellular mechanisms that maintain genomic stability. Therefore, the biochemical, molecular, and functional characterization of BLM, a protein not known earlier in mammalian cells, promises to provide fundamental understanding of how stability of the genome is maintained as the zygote expands via the cell-division cycle into the greater than 10^{17} cells that will constitute the normal size adult body.**

Homozygosity or compound mutant heterozygosity at *BLM,* a gene distal on chromosome No. 15, results in a striking phenotype known as Bloom syndrome (BS).[1–5] A constant clinical feature of BS, and one that makes a lasting impression on the observer, is a well-proportioned small size. The additional constant feature, but one not apparent from physical observation of the patient, is instability of the genome; BS somatic cells accumulate more mutations than any other cell type known, apparently at any and every part of the genome. The genomic instability, which is of a characteristic type and which is to some extent recognizable through the microscope as "chromosome breakage,"[6,7] doubtless is responsible for the most important complication of BS, namely cancer. The genomic instability also probably is responsible for there being fewer than a normal number of cells in the tissues and organs of the affected person, hence, the abnormally small size.

BS's rarity explains its obscurity as an entity in clinical medicine; in contrast, the remarkable genomic instability and consequent hypermutability of the BS cell and the dramatic cancer proneness of the affected individual have awarded it prominence among students of mutation, DNA synthesis, DNA repair, and recombination, and among human biologists interested in the developmental consequences of mutation in somatic cells, including the consequences of somatic crossing-over which is greatly increased in BS. This chapter describes the clinical entity and its genetics; summarizes what is known of the hypermutability of BS cells including the microscopically visible chromosome breakage, the feature that first called attention to BS as an important clinical entity and experimental model; and presents its molecular genetics and recently acquired information about the protein encoded by *BLM.*

Diagnosing BS is always a momentous occasion because the physician who identifies a person with BS simultaneously identifies a person who, along with the other few persons alive with this very rare disorder, is at a far greater risk than anyone else of developing one or many of the cancers of the standard sites and types that affect humans, and at an unusually early age. Cancer emerges excessively in BS because throughout intrauterine and postnatal life an excessive number of mutations of various types arise and accumulate in the somatic cells. However, some, possibly most, of the clinical features of BS other than the cancer proneness are also attributable to this genomic instability. Consequently, BS is the prototype of a class of human disease that can be referred to as the *somatic mutational disorders.*[4,8]

Thus, despite BS being exceedingly rare, it takes on inordinate significance in both academic medicine and human biology for two reasons. First, it displays dramatically the clinical consequences of an excessive somatic mutation rate. Any abnormality present in a person with BS, even though it may not be a recognized or constant feature of the syndrome, is brought under suspicion of being etiologically a consequence of mutation, either directly or indirectly. Second, the BS cell and *BLM,* the BS gene, constitute valuable experimental materials in cell biology. It has been clear for a long time that the protein encoded by *BLM* is of pivotal importance in the maintenance of the genomic stability of somatic cells. Now its exact role there can be defined because with the cloning of the gene, molecular reagents have become available to investigate directly the function of the BLM protein.

THE CLINICAL ENTITY

Unreported data held in the files of the 168 persons who comprise the Bloom's Syndrome Registry are the source of most of the information presented here.[9] The Registry is comprised of the vast majority of persons ever diagnosed with BS up to 1991 (when it arbitrarily was closed to new accessions), and as far as can be determined is an unbiased representation of this very rare entity (Table 30-1). The mean age of those alive in the Registry is 21.6 years (range 4 to 46 years), and the mean age at death has been 23.6 years (range < 1 to 49 years). Published clinical information from the Registry about BS, including photographs of affected persons, is found in references 1 to 5.

The predominating and constant clinical features of BS are two (1 and 2 below). Only the first is obvious from physical observation:

1. An overall *small body size* with fairly normal proportioning except for a slightly disproportionately small brain/head accompanied by dolichocephaly. Subcutaneous fatty tissue is disproportionately sparse. The several fetuses whose size has been monitored by sonography have been much smaller than expected for their ages. The mean birthweight for males is 1906 g (range 930 to 3400) and for females 1810 g (range 920 to 2667). The mean adult height for men is 147.5 cm (range 130 to 162), for women 138.6 cm (range 122 to 151) (Fig. 30-1).

2. An enormous *predisposition to cancer,* probably of all cell types and at all sites.

Table 30-1 Composition of the Population in the Bloom's Syndrome Registry

	No.	Age* (yr.) Mean	Range
Persons affected with BS			
Alive	108 (64%)	21.6	4–46
Dead	60 (35%)	23.6	<1–49
Total affected persons	168		
Families			
With 1 affected with BS	116 (83%)		
With 2 affected with BS	22 (16%)		
With 3 affected with BS	0 (0%)		
With 4 affected with BS	2 (1%)		
Total families	140		
Dwelling places of persons			
North America	83		
Europe	41		
Asia Minor	16		
Japan	12		
Meso- & South America	11		
Australia	3		
North Africa	2		
Ethnic origins of families			
European, non-Jewish	66		
Mixed	34**		
German	11		
Italian	9		
Dutch/Flemish	6		
British	5		
Other	4		
Jewish	42		
Ashkenazi***	41		
Non-Ashkenazi	1		
Japanese	10		
South American Mixed	6		
African American	4		
Turkish	4		
Arab Mohammedan	2		
Mexican Mestizo	2		
Gypsy	1		
*Consanguinity*** **			
Non-Jewish	31/105 families		
Ashkenazi Jewish*****	2/35 families		
Non-Ashkenazi Jewish	1/1 families		

NOTE: 114 of the 168 registered persons have been examined personally by at least one registrar, i.e., by the late David Bloom, James German, and, or, Eberhard Passarge.
*Age at present if living; age at death if dead.
**Most non-Jewish United Statesans, Canadians, and Australians are classified "Mixed."
***One or both parents.
****Of the parents of affected individuals.
*****Both parents.

Eleven additional features that may or may not be present in persons with BS and that vary in severity are the following. Ordinarily the presence of several of these serves to distinguish BS from other disorders that feature a striking degree of growth deficiency:

3. A *characteristic facies* (Fig. 30-2). The face is somewhat keel-shaped because of the small narrow cranium, malar hypoplasia, nasal prominence, and small mandible. The ears may be protuberant and unusually prominent.
4. *Hypersensitivity to sunlight* of the areas of the skin ordinarily exposed to the sun during infancy; i.e., the face and the dorsa of the hands and forearms.

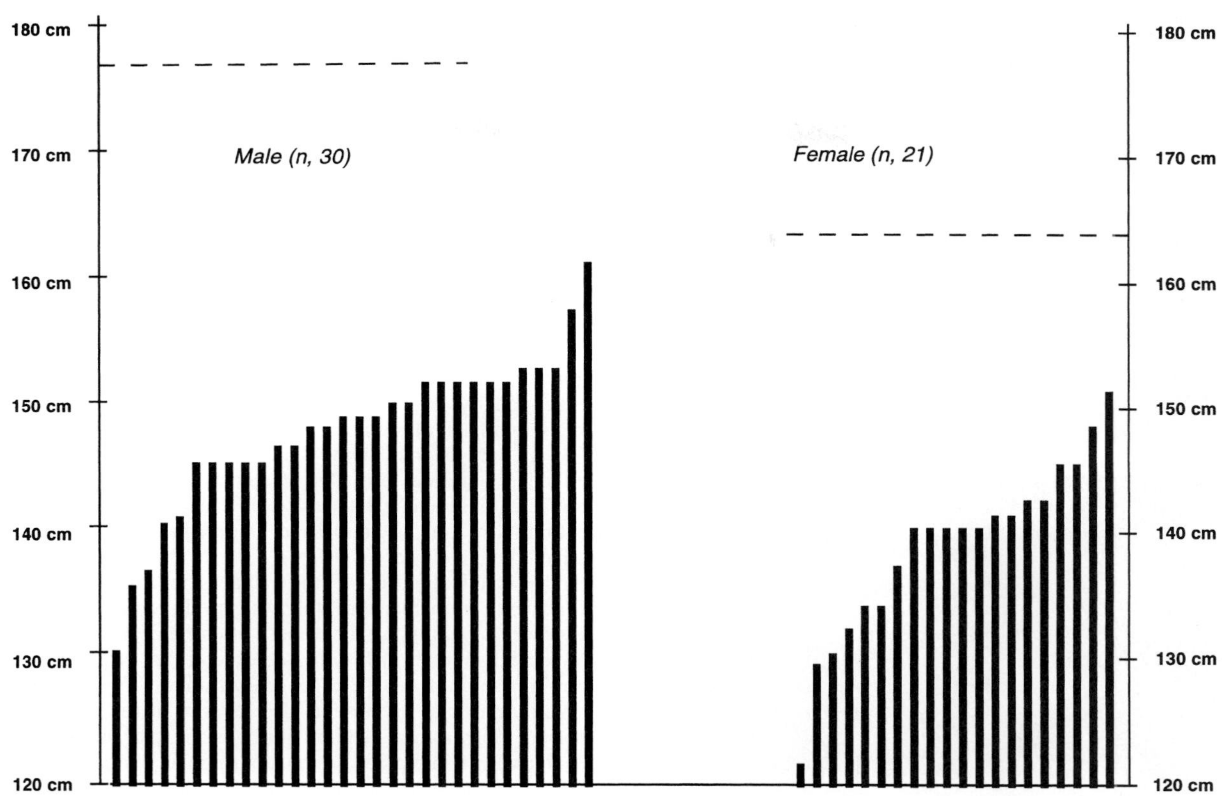

Fig. 30-1 Distribution of known heights (tops of vertical bars) of persons in the Registry who have reached the age of 20 years. (Dashed lines show the means for normal adults.)

5. Patchy areas of *hyper- and hypopigmentation of the skin.*
6. A *characteristic voice,* high-pitched and of a somewhat coarse, squeaky timbre.
7. A variable degree of *vomiting and diarrhea* during infancy, that often rapidly leads to life-threatening dehydration. Their basis is obscure. Also, a large proportion of affected infants and young children show a profound *lack of interest in eating.* The gastrointestinal problems along with the repeated respiratory tract and ear infections make infancy a trying period for many parents of children with BS.
8. *Diabetes mellitus,* as yet neither well characterized clinically nor studied experimentally (Table 30-2). Diabetes has been diagnosed in 20 of the 168 persons in the Registry (11.9 percent), at a mean age of 24.9 years (range 11 to 40 years). Although in many ways the diabetes of BS resembles standard late-onset, non-insulin-dependent diabetes, it has not yet been studied sufficiently to permit such classification; six of the diabetics in the Registry have required insulin therapy, and ketoacidosis has occurred in several.
9. In men, abnormally small testes accompanied by a total *failure of spermatogenesis,* and in women, an abnormally *early cessation of menstruation* accompanied by *reduced fertility.* Nevertheless, three women with BS have given birth to four normal, healthy babies.
10. *Immunodeficiency* of a generalized type, ranging from mild and essentially asymptomatic to severe, manifested by recurrent respiratory tract infections complicated by otitis media and pneumonia.[10] In 20 percent of cases, at least one life-threatening bacterial infection of the respiratory tract that would have led to early death in the preantibiotic era is recorded. Inadequately treated lung infections may lead to bronchiectasis and crippling chronic lung disease that in five instances has been fatal, becoming the second commonest cause of death, next after cancer (Table 30-2). Serious ear infections have occurred in 29 percent of persons with BS, which may decrease auditory acuity. The severe and recurring vomiting and diarrhea of infancy mentioned in 7 above conceivably is caused by bacterial infection, but information concerning this is unavailable. Although also not known to be on an infectious basis, a mild, sometimes recurring, idiopathic hepatitis has been reported in several affected individuals, and evidence of liver toxicity is common when cancer chemotherapy is administered.
11. A slightly excessive incidence of *minor anatomic anomalies,* including mildly anomalous digits, pilonidal dimples, wedges of altered color of the irides, and obstructing anomalies of the urethra, this last being of major clinical importance in several cases.
12. *Restricted intellectual ability.* Intelligence in BS usually is judged (without testing) to be average to low-average. When limitation does exist, it varies widely in degree from minimal to moderately severe. It is impossible to predict early in life whether a person with BS will have some degree of mental deficiency or be quite normal. Although several affected individuals have been frankly deficient mentally, several others have completed college, a few of them obtaining higher degrees. However, even when testing indicates normal intelligence, there tends to be a poorly defined and unexplained learning disability and short attention span. Characteristically this is associated with an inability to develop a normally wide array of interests. From earliest childhood, the person with BS typically exhibits a charming, pleasant personality, but fails to mature from a childlike judgment and gullibility, and (perhaps fortunately, in view of the grim specter of early neoplasia) maintains a seemingly inordinate optimism. Several affected persons have displayed a strikingly poor memory. Although only conjectural, the possible role played by malnutrition early in life, the result of

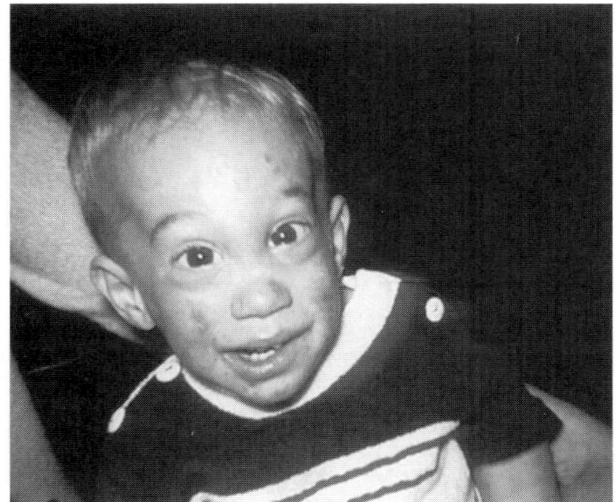

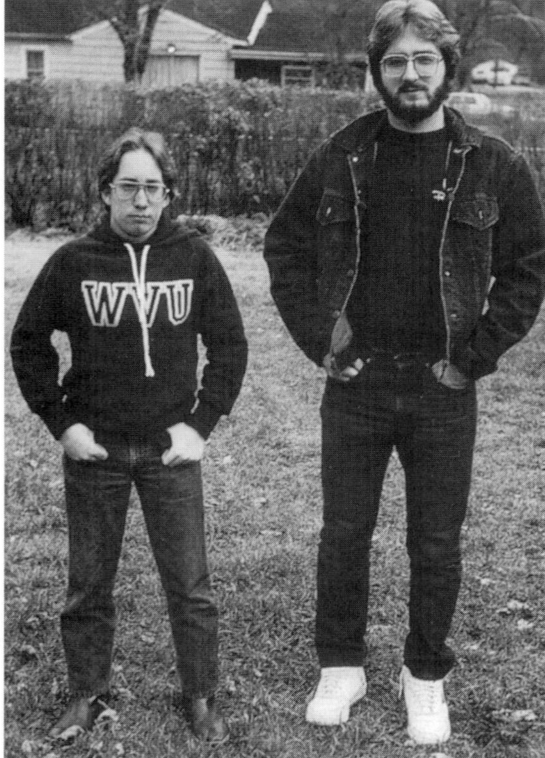

Fig. 30-2 51(KeMc) in the Bloom's Syndrome Registry manifests the major clinical features of BS. His birthweight was 2160 g and his birth length 44.5 cm. He exhibited striking dolichocephaly and hypoplastic malar areas. Within the first year of life, a moderate to severe photosensitive erythematous skin lesion appeared that was limited to the face and hands. He also had a recurring fissure of the lower lip. *A,* 51(KeMc) at about 18 months showing the facial erythematous skin lesion. *B,* On left, 51(KeMc) at age 17, exhibiting small body size (height 147 cm, weight 41 kg) and the photosensitive facial skin lesion, and on right, his unaffected brother at age 19. The unaffected brother is just under 6 feet tall. 51(KeMc), who is healthy at age 27, was successfully treated for acute undifferentiated leukemia at age 12.

the infant's/child's severe lack of interest in eating (mentioned earlier along with the striking paucity of subcutaneous fat), deserves investigation, because, if etiologically significant in the restriction on intellectual maturation, treatment in the form of nonvolitional feeding possibly would be preventive.

13. Any one of an array of seemingly *unrelated clinical entities or features.* Each has occurred in only one or a few individuals, and they are not to be considered part of BS itself. They include hyperlipidemia, congenital thrombocytopenia, chronic idiopathic thrombocytopenic purpura, acanthosis nigricans, mild anemia and in some cases a poorly defined dyserythropoiesis, asthma, psoriatic arthritis, and Legg-Perthes disease.

The Skin in BS

In BS, two unrelated skin lesions coexist:

A Sun-Sensitive Facial Lesion. The clinically more important skin lesion of BS is a sun-sensitive erythema that is limited almost exclusively to the face, usually unassociated with dyspigmentation. The cheeks and nose are the areas most often affected, explaining an early erroneous confusion of BS and lupus. The dorsa of the hands and forearms may be mildly affected. In exceptionally severe cases, the erythema does extend to the ears, sides, and back of the neck, the suprasternal area, and very rarely and in mild degree to the shoulders or upper chest. However, effectively ruling out the diagnosis BS is any prominent erythematous, telangiectatic lesion that affects the trunk, lower extremities, arms, or buttocks, even though the face might also be affected.

The clinical onset of the facial skin lesion usually is as persistent erythema that follows the infant's first significant exposure to sunlight, which most often has been during the first or second summer of life. In one exceptional case, the lesion did not appear until age 12. The sun-sensitive skin lesion varies in severity and may be absent. The severity of the erythema when present ranges from a faint blush during the summertime to a disfiguring, flaming red lesion of irregular distribution over the bridge of the nose, cheeks, and other facial areas. Crying may accentuate what appears on first examination to be a minimal or absent lesion. The lower eyelids often are hyperemic, and atrophy of the lower lid with loss of eyelashes is common. In many cases, blistering, encrustation, and a recurring fissure of the lower lip during summertime become particularly aggravating aspects of the lesion.

The severity and extent of the skin lesion usually is apparent by early childhood. Often parents intuitively protect a child from the sun when they realize that hypersensitivity is present, which may explain the failure of progression in severity at later ages in many cases. Similarly, in sibships with multiple affected children, the rigorous protection from the sun of later-born affecteds is associated with a mild or absent skin lesion. Ordinarily, if there is to be a skin lesion, it makes its appearance during the first two years of life. (It is not congenital, as originally described—"congenital telangiectatic erythema resembling lupus erythematosus in dwarfs."[11]) Although some form of sun sensitivity quite clearly exists early in life in BS, the few objective tests of nonfacial skin that have been carried out by dermatologists have failed either to characterize the defect or even to detect its existence. Furthermore, several adults with BS report that they enjoy sun-bathing and tanning, and that they are unaware of sun hypersensitivity of other than facial skin. However, the lesion in the area that was symptomatic early in life persists, as does its continued accentuation by sun exposure.

Usually, careful examination of the affected area reveals an accompanying telangiectasia, varying in degree from minimal to prominent. It usually is absent during infancy. Even when the erythema is minimal to absent, careful examination often reveals a faint degree of telangiectasia at the margin of the upper lip or about the nose or cheeks. In severe cases, irregular patches of atrophic skin and dyspigmentation accompany the erythema and telangiectasia. In 6 of the 168 registered cases, prominent telangiectasia of the bulbar conjunctiva—as prominent as in the entity ataxia-telangiectasia—has been present, unrelated to the severity of the skin lesion.

The pathogenesis of the sun-sensitive skin lesion of BS is obscure. Histologic study of the characteristic sun-sensitive skin lesion in BS has been made in a few cases, but has contributed

Table 30-2 The Serious Medical Complications in the 168 Persons in the Bloom's Syndrome Registry

	Number of Persons Affected	Death from the Complication	Age at diagnosis (yrs)	
			Mean	Range
Chronic lung disease	7	5		
Diabetes mellitus	20	0	24.9	11–40
Cancer*				
Persons with 1 or >1 primaries	71	50	24.7	2–48
Persons with 2 or >2 primaries	19			
Persons with 3 or >3 primaries	5			
Persons with 4 or >4 primaries	3			
Persons with 5 primaries	2			

*A total of 100 cancers diagnosed, in 71 of the 168 persons in the Registry.

little to an understanding of the pathogenesis; biopsy is not indicated for diagnostic purposes. In males, the lesion is more severe than in females, and relatively greater underdiagnosis of BS itself in females probably contributes to their slight under-representation in the Bloom's Syndrome Registry—93 males versus 75 females.

A Non-Sun-Sensitive Lesion Not Limited to the Face. A second skin abnormality exists in BS, clinically and presumably pathogenetically completely different from the sun-sensitive lesion. It consists of prominent, well-circumscribed areas of hyperpigmentation—the café-au-lait spots of normal people but present in BS in excessive numbers and often quite extensive. In addition, circumscribed areas of hypopigmentation usually are present. These lesions may appear anywhere on the body but are most commonly found on the trunk. The hyperpigmented lesions vary in diameter from a few millimeters to many centimeters, in an occasional person being linear and extending over the back of the thorax. Most often, the several hyperpigmented lesions tend to have similar degrees of brownness, but an occasional spot may be considerably darker than the others. Sometimes the brownish spots, large as well as small, are found in a localized cluster. Well-demarcated hypopigmented areas also are highly characteristic of BS but usually are less conspicuous than the hyperpigmented lesions. Exceptionally, a hypopigmented area can, like a hyper-pigmented one, be extensive, covering an area many centimeters in diameter. In affected individuals of sub-Saharan African ancestry, the hyper- and hypopigmented areas are more prominent than in lighter-complexioned persons, some appearing quite black and others strikingly white. It usually is in early childhood that the pigmentary changes are first noted, rather than in infancy.

Neoplasia[4,12]

At any time in the life of a person with BS a neoplasm is much more likely to appear than in other people of the same age. The four most impressive aspects of the neoplasia proneness of BS are the great frequency with which both benign (not discussed further here) and malignant neoplasia arise, the wide variety of anatomic sites and cellular types, the exceptionally early age at which neoplasms become clinically apparent, and the frequency with which multiple neoplasms arise in one person.

The first 100 cancers that arose in BS after it was recognized as a clinical entity in 1954 are listed in Table 30-3 along with the age ranges at which they were diagnosed. The distribution of sites and types of cancers in BS resembles that in the general population; but, in BS they have arisen at a greatly increased frequency and in the case of the carcinomata and acute myelogenous leukemias decades earlier than expected. The mean age at diagnosis of cancer has been 24.7 years (range 2 to 48 years). It has been responsible for the death of 50 of the 60 persons in the Registry who have died.

Precisely because of this remarkable excess in BS of the cancers that affect other people, BS has been chosen as a model. The study of BS at the cellular, chromosomal, and DNA levels should facilitate the analysis of the changes responsible for the initiation and progression of the generality of human cancer. The hypothesis in such work is that among the changes that take place spontaneously in BS cells are the very ones that are responsible, as in other people, not just for neoplastic transformation but also for progression of a transformed clone into clinical cancer. That is, the changes that arise abnormally frequently in BS cells very probably are the ones responsible for these processes in other people. In BS, these changes take place spontaneously; in others they may also be spontaneous during normal cell metabolism—very possibly this is the usual situation in human cancer—or they may be the effects of environmental mutational agents.

The reader will note that the inherited mutations responsible for the phenotype BS are in a category different from those that arise at the loci mutated in, for example, retinoblastoma, Wilms tumor, and familial polyposis coli. Those cell-proliferation-controlling loci when mutated become so-called cancer genes and can represent one step of many in cancer's initiation and progression. In contrast, homozygosity or compound heterozygosity for mutation(s) at *BLM* constitutes a mutator genotype. In BS cells, the somatic mutations that must occur for clinical cancer to emerge were not inherited through the germ line but are just far more likely to arise spontaneously than in cells of other people because BS is a mutator phenotype. It also is noteworthy that in BS, every cell in the body capable of further division is at the high risk of neoplastic transformation.

Somatic mutation at *BLM* is not itself known to be of significance as a step in either cancer initiation or progression. That a somatic mutation can give rise to a genetically unstable cell lineage that is of etiologic significance in cancer, however, is a concept that derives from the study of sporadic cancer, as well as hereditary nonpolyposis colorectal cancer (HNPCC), and, therefore, the development through somatic mutation of a lineage "with Bloom syndrome" is an interesting theoretical possibility, evidence for which may be sought.

Thus, the basis for the predisposition to cancer in BS doubtless is the remarkably excessive genomic instability featured by BS

Table 30-3 The First 100 Cancers Recorded in the Bloom's Syndrome Registry[12], Showing the Age Groups at Time of Diagnosis

	Age Group					
Class & type	**0–10**	**11–20**	**21–30**	**31–40**	**41–50**	**Total**
Rare tumors* ($n = 5$)						
Medulloblastoma	1					1
Wilms tumor	2					2
Osteogenic sarcoma	1	1				2
Leukemia, acute ($n = 22$)						
Lymphocytic	4	2	1			7
Myelogenous	1	1	3	1		6
Biphenotypic		1		1		2
Other or unspecified	1	3	2	1		7
Lymphoma ($n = 22$)						
Non-Hodgkin	4	6	6	3	1	20
Hodgkin disease		2				2
Carcinoma ($n = 51$)						
Skin		2	3	3		8
Auditory canal, external			1	1		2
Tongue, posterior			1	1	2	4
Esophagus, squamous				3		3
Esophagus, adeno					1	1
Stomach			1	1		2
Colon						
Cecum, ascending			1	2		3
Hepatic flexure transverse		1		2	1	4
Descending, sigmoid, rectum			1	5		6
Tonsil				1		1
Larynx, epiglottis			2	1		3
Lung				1		1
Uterus						
Cervix		1	3			4
Corpus					1	1
Breast			1	5	1	7
Metastatic, primary site unknown			1			1
Totals	14	20	27	32	7	100

*A meningioma was diagnosed at age 9 in one registered individual. Two Wilms tumors and a retinoblastoma diagnosed at 5 months, 22 months, and 2 years of age, respectively, are known to have occurred in children with BS who are known to the Registry, but not officially registered.

cells. The immunodeficiency of BS quite conceivably contributes to the cancer proneness, but its role in progression is difficult to determine because of the major role played by mutation.

GENOMIC INSTABILITY

The enzymatic systems that carry out the fundamental processes of the replication and transmission of the genetic material from generation to generation, of both germ-line and somatic cells, are diverse and complex. To ensure fidelity, these systems incorporate multiple mechanisms to maintain genomic stability, including (a) proofreading capacities of the DNA polymerases and replication machinery; (b) mechanisms that allow the DNA replication complex to idle at damaged DNA in a way that permits repair; (c) mechanisms that allow the bypass of the damaged DNA altogether (trans-lesion synthesis); (d) repair enzymes that recognize damaged DNA and either repair the damage directly or recruit other enzymes to carry that out; (e) proteins that signal to the cell the presence of DNA damage and that prevent the cell's traversing its cycle prior to repair; and (f) systems that package and condense the chromatin and that ensure the proper segregation of the chromosomes at mitosis. These systems maintain genomic stability and act to prevent errors that might lead, on the one hand, to unscheduled cell death or, on the other, to abnormal, unregulated cellular proliferation.

Genetically determined defects in the systems that maintain genomic stability and ensure fidelity of replication have been identified in many model organisms, and also in the human. In human genetics, genomic instability was first recognized through microscopic observation of chromosomal abnormalities — chromosome breakage — in cultured cells from individuals with certain rare syndromes, first BS and then Fanconi anemia, ataxia-telangiectasia, the Nijmegen breakage syndrome, Werner syndrome, and xeroderma pigmentosum (the last only after ultraviolet light irradiation). In all of these syndromes, the cytogenetic abnormalities are accompanied by an increase in the rate of spontaneous somatic mutations and, or, mutagen-induced mutations. This hypermutability provides an explanation for the predisposition to various types of cancers, a feature shared by all these syndromes. These clinical entities, along with several others that lack chromosome breakage (e.g., HNPCC) but that are characterized by some form of genomic instability at the molecular level, fall under the rubric somatic mutational disorders.

BS is the prototypic somatic mutational disorder. When the chromosomes in BS cells that are proliferating in culture but are otherwise untreated are examined microscopically, an abundance of gaps, breaks, and structural rearrangements in the chromosomes is found.[7] However, the difference from normal is quantitative, and similar lesions in the chromosomes are present in untreated cells from other people, just much less frequently. The two most

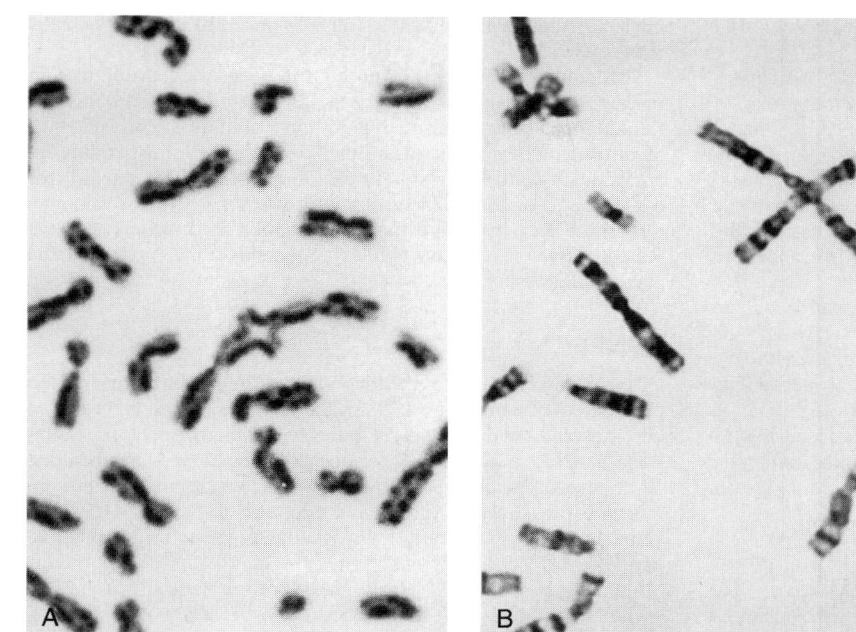

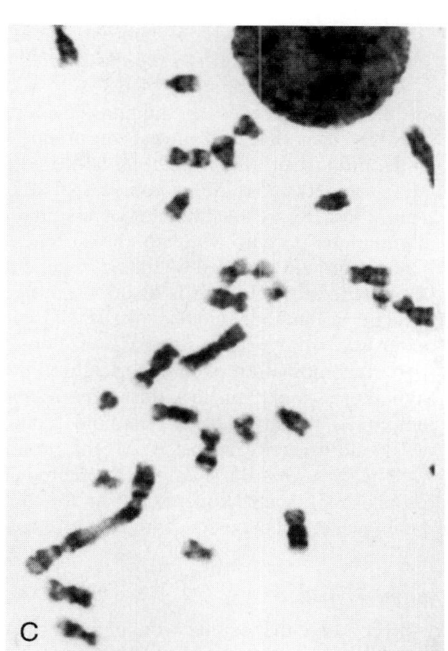

Fig. 30-3 ***A,*** **A portion of a Bloom syndrome lymphocyte metaphase. The cell had been cultured in BrdU-containing medium to make possible the differential staining (light or dark) of sister chromatids; alternating regions of light and dark staining signify exchanges between sister chromatids (SCEs). The number of SCEs in cells from normal persons averages <10/metaphase, whereas BS lymphocytes show (as here) 60 to 90/metaphase or more; a greatly elevated SCE frequency is diagnostic of BS. Also present in this cell is a quadriradial configuration (QR), the result of an interchange between chromatids of the No. 1 chromosomes. QRs affecting homologous regions of the homologous chromosomes are present in approximately 1 percent of BS blood T lymphocytes, but they also are found on rare occasions in cells from healthy persons without BS. Both QRs and SCEs can be induced in normal cells by exposure to certain DNA-damaging agents, as in** ***B;*** **BS cells, already with an elevated constitutional number of such lesions, show an excessive response to such agents.** ***B,*** **G-banded metaphase chromosomes showing a QR, the result of a chromatid interchange at the proximal portions of the long arms of the No. 1 chromosomes. The cell, from a healthy person without BS, had been exposed in vitro to mitomycin C several hours before it entered mitosis. QRs of this type are present in excessive number in untreated cells from persons with BS.** ***C,*** **G-banded metaphase chromosomes of a BS lymphocyte showing a telomere association, presumably the result of a chromatid interchange (equivalent to those that resulted in the QRs in** ***A*** **and** ***B*****) that had taken place near the ends of the short arms of the No. 1 chromosomes. (Reprinted with permission from German J: Bloom syndrome: A mendelian prototype of somatic mutational disease.** ***Medicine*** **72:393, 1993.)**

characteristic cytogenetic abnormalities (1 and 2 below) are the result of a strikingly increased tendency in BS somatic cells for exchange to take place between DNA strands, probably at the time they replicate during the S phase of the cell-division cycle:

1. The exchanges may be between a chromatid of each of the two homologues of a chromosome pair (e.g., between the two Nos. 1 or the two Nos. 19), the points of exchange being at seemingly homologous regions of the chromatids involved. In the mitosis that follows, such an interchange is detectable microscopically as a symmetric, four-armed configuration — a quadriradial, or QR — composed of the pair of chromosomes between which the interchange had taken place (Fig. 30-3). Or,
2. The exchanges may be intrachromosomal, between the two sister chromatids of one chromosome. The consequence of these exchanges also are microscopically visible in appropriately treated cells — SCEs (Fig. 30-3*A*). In cells from non-BS individuals, a mean of fewer than 10 SCEs/metaphase is found; in striking contrast, BS cells characteristically have from 50 to 100 SCEs/metaphase depending on the type of cell examined, but in blood lymphocytes in short-term culture.

Submicroscopic mutations also are increased in BS. BS cells taken directly from the circulating blood can be shown to have a dramatic increase over normal in the number of mutations accumulated at the two loci that have been studied extensively; namely, the locus on the X chromosome that encodes the enzyme HPRT and the glycophorin A locus on chromosome No. 4 that determines the MN blood type (reviewed in references 4 and 13). The types of mutations that have been detected include somatic crossing-over.[14] Other evidence of the genomic instability of BS cells, at least *in vitro,* is excessive mutation at regions of the genome composed of repeat sequences.[15–17]

Explanation for BS's Clinical Features

Again, spontaneous mutations arise more frequently than normal in the genome of a cell that itself is mutant at both of its BS loci. The hypermutability of BS somatic cells exists *in vivo* as well as *in vitro.* The mutations that arise in the somatic cells of a person with BS are of various types and affect many, probably all, regions of the genome. Many of the mutations would be lethal to the cell in which they arise, or by some mechanism would check further cell cycling, resulting in the small but normally proportioned body in BS. The mutations presumably occur in all cell lineages throughout both pre- and postnatal development. By this hypothesis, the various tissues and organs of the person with BS are constituted of fewer cells than normal. (Endocrinologic studies have failed to provide any explanation for the restriction on growth.)

However, among those myriad mutations that are not cell-lethal, some by chance would affect cell-proliferation-controlling and proto-oncogene loci. This hypothesis explains the frequent emergence of neoplasia in different cell types at various anatomic sites in BS (as discussed more extensively earlier).

The basis of the pigmentary disturbance in BS is plausibly explained by heritable mutations that arise during development in somatic cell lineages concerned with the determination of the melanin content of the skin. Somatic crossing-over in particular, which is excessive in BS, is the type of mutation that would explain adjacent, localized hyper- and hypopigmented areas.

These lesions very possibly are equivalent to the "twin spots" of classical experimental *Drosophila* genetics.

Thus, the clinical study of BS is, to a large extent, an analysis of the consequences on human development of mutations of various types that will have been arising excessively in somatic cells throughout life, probably at all regions of the genome and in all tissues. It is possible, of course, that at least some of the clinical features of BS are attributable not to somatic mutation but, in some completely obscure way, to the absence from the cell of the nuclear protein encoded by the *BLM* gene itself (see below), in the same sense that clotting is disturbed in hemophilia.

The immunodeficiency of BS has not been subjected to extensive study, and its basis is obscure. In view of the hyperrecombination phenotype featured by BS cells, a reasonable hypothesis to explain it is that some recombinational mechanism employed normally by lymphoid cell lineages to generate antigenic diversity utilize BLM, the protein that is absent in BS (see below). That BLM adjoins the paired chromosomes in meiotic prophase of spermatogenesis[18] at the time when crossing-over takes place, is consonant with this proposal.

DIAGNOSIS

Any cell type that can be brought into mitosis by the cytogeneticist can be employed to rule a clinical diagnosis of BS in or out. Blood lymphocytes stimulated to enter cell cycling by phytohemagglutinin are the most used, but freshly aspirated bone marrow cells or long-term cultures of skin fibroblasts or of embryonic/fetal cells also can be examined. The two most valuable indicators of BS are (a) the demonstration of the symmetric QR interchange configuration in untreated cells and (b) the greatly increased number of SCEs in cells allowed to pass two cell cycles in medium containing BrdU (Fig. 30-3). BS is the only disorder that features an increased rate of SCE. Therefore, an SCE analysis is indicated in any child or adult with unexplained growth deficiency (i.e., BS should be included in the differential diagnosis), regardless of whether the facial skin lesion characteristic of BS is present.

BS should be considered whenever severe intrauterine growth deficiency is encountered and cannot be explained, especially if the deficiency extends into infancy and childhood. Also, BS might well be considered in small but well-proportioned children or adults with a sun-sensitive, erythematous skin lesion that is limited to the face, even if their growth deficiency is of only moderate degree. Correspondingly, a normal birthweight with a postnatal length/height not less than the third percentile for normals militate strongly against the diagnosis BS.

Although surveys have not yet been done, so that the value of SCE screening is unknown, an SCE analysis will possibly identify persons with BS in unusually small members of the following groups of individuals, even when the characteristic skin lesion is lacking:

1. Persons with excessive numbers of café-au-lait spots, usually accompanied by hypopigmented spots;
2. Persons with unexplained immunodeficiency;
3. Children or adults with an unexplained restriction on intelligence;
4. Persons in whom diabetes mellitus develops later than the usual age of onset of type I and earlier than that of type II;
5. Infertile men with abnormally small testes for which no explanation can be found, and possibly women with an exceptionally early onset of menopause;
6. Children or adults who develop clinical neoplasia.

As stated earlier, it is unknown how valuable a routine SCE analysis would be for unusually small persons who develop cancer but who lack BS's facial lesion; however, in the Registry, 7 of the 71 individuals with BS who have developed cancer were recognized to have BS only at the time or after a cancer was diagnosed. Only then was the significance of their small size, unusual facies, or facial skin lesion recognized by some physicians who knew of BS.

BS doubtless is underdiagnosed. Many cases of it long remain in diagnostic wastebaskets, such as idiopathic intrauterine growth retardation, "primordial dwarfism," and "failure to thrive," until an informed physician requests an SCE analysis. Some patients are erroneously considered to have a rare disorder other than BS; for example, 10 of the 168 persons with proven BS in the Bloom's Syndrome Registry were thought possibly or definitely to have Russell-Silver dwarfism until cytogenetic study provided the correct diagnosis.

GENETICS

Clinical BS is the phenotype that results from the inheritance from each parent of a mutation at *BLM,* the BS gene, which is located in chromosome band 15q26.1.[19] Individuals heterozygous for mutations at *BLM* ("carriers") are normally developed and healthy. With respect to the germ line, however, where the BS protein attaches transiently during meiotic prophase to synapsed chromosome bivalents,[18] the only study available points to an effect of heterozygosity for *BLM* mutation.[20]

Mutation(s) at *BLM* appear to segregate in most if not all human populations, but in all, BS is very rare. Only in Ashkenazi Jews is mutation at *BLM* known to have reached a relatively high frequency; a population survey of BS in Israel in 1971 and 1972 indicated a heterozygote frequency greater than 1 in 120. The recent identification of a 6-bp deletion and 7-bp insertion in exon 10 of *BLM* (see below), referred to as blm^{Ash}, now has permitted a more accurate determination of the frequency of carriers in that major subgroup of Jewry. A survey of New York City Ashkenazi Jews conducted in collaboration with the Department of Medical Genetics of Mt. Sinai Hospital Medical School sets the number at 1 in 107.[21] Other studies have provided similar results.[22–24]

The mutated loci on the two No. 15 chromosomes in any given individual with BS may correctly be suspected to be identical—homozygous—when either that person's parents are consanguineous or the parents both are Ashkenazi Jews. In those two situations, the mutations at *BLM* are usually identical by virtue of their descent from a common ancestor who was a carrier of a BS mutation.[19,25] In addition to homozygosity, however, two unlike mutations sometimes are inherited and are responsible for BS; such individuals are referred to as genetic compounds, or said to have compound heterozygosity. The phenotype BS seems to be the same regardless of whether the mutant *BLM* loci are or are not inherited from a common ancestor. As becomes apparent below, the majority of the many BS-associated mutations at *BLM* are essentially nulls for the encoded protein.

The carrier of a BS mutation ordinarily is identified only after having become the parent of a child with BS. Molecular isolation of *BLM* now does provide another means of heterozygote detection among other relatives of persons with BS, as well as in the population at large.[21,26] The risk of other children with BS is 1 in 4 after an affected child has been born to a union of proven heterozygotes. Pregnancies at risk can be monitored by sonography and cytogenetics, and in families in which the mutation has been analyzed at the molecular level, by molecular haplotyping or by direct determination of whether a mutation is present on one, both, or neither of the No. 15 chromosomes.

MOLECULAR GENETICS OF *BLM*

The chromosome abnormalities observed in BS cells noted earlier pointed to a defect in some fundamental process of DNA metabolism that helps maintain genomic stability. Retarded replication-fork progression and abnormal replicational intermediates, but the absence of defects in known DNA-repair systems, implicated a disturbance of the process of DNA replication itself.[4] Biochemical studies of a number of enzymes that participate in replication and repair did reveal abnormalities in

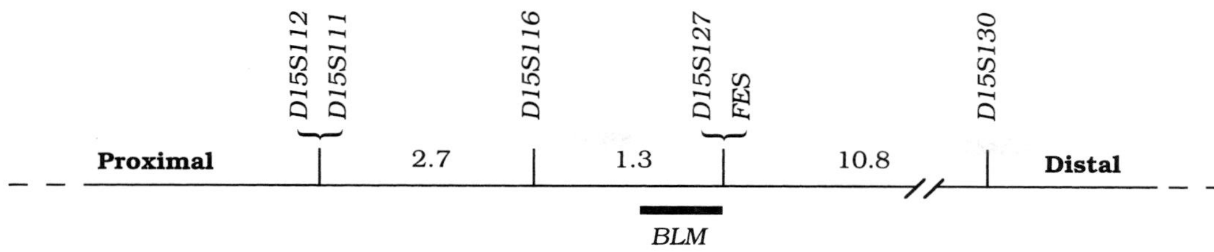

Fig. 30-4 Map positions of six highly polymorphic DNA markers on chromosome 15 linked to *BLM*. The loci shown above the line representing chromosome 15 were employed in homozygosity mapping (genetic map distances in cM). Braced loci have not been separated by recombinational analysis. *FES* and *D15S127* are separated by 30 kb (see Fig. 30-6). The location of *BLM* is represented by the thick line between DNA markers *FES*/*D15S127* and *D15S116*.

the enzymatic activities of DNA ligase I, topoisomerase II in BrdU-treated cells, uracil DNA glycosylase, O^6-methylguanine methyltransferase, N-methylpurine DNA glycosylase, and superoxide dismutase. However, none of these abnormalities, though often demonstrable, identified the primary defect in BS; they appear to be phenotypic consequences of the BS mutation. Because the identification of the primary defect promised to reveal an important element in nucleic acid metabolism, a positional cloning strategy was undertaken to isolate *BLM*—as result of which a previously unknown protein in mammalian cells was identified.[26]

Localization of *BLM* to 15q26.1[19]

A limited amount of evidence from cell hybridization studies had suggested that BS is a single-gene disorder.[27] The first step in the positional cloning effort to isolate the gene was to identify linkages between *BLM* and mapped polymorphic markers. Introduction of a normal human chromosome 15 by microcell-mediated chromosome transfer was shown to correct toward normal the high-SCE phenotype of a BS cell line.[28] Subsequently, homozygosity mapping demonstrated tight linkage between *BLM* and *FES*.[19] *FES* already had been localized by *in situ* hybridization to 15q26.1. Linkage in most of these families was detected thereafter[25] at five additional highly polymorphic DNA markers that flank *FES* (depicted in Fig. 30-4). Thus, homozygosity mapping permitted assignment of *BLM* to a 2-cM interval that includes *FES*.

Founder Effect in Ashkenazi Jews with Bloom Syndrome[3,22]

As mentioned earlier, BS is more common in the Ashkenazi Jewish than in any other known population.[3] Several of the polymorphic microsatellite loci found to be tightly linked to *BLM* by homozygosity mapping were genotyped in affected and unaffected individuals from the Ashkenazi Jewish population. A striking allele association between blm^{Ash} and one of the six alleles at *FES*, specifically allele C3, and between blm^{Ash} and two related alleles of the CA-repeat locus *D15S127* (a locus that is 30 kb proximal to *FES*), specifically alleles 145 bp and 147 bp, was detected in Ashkenazi Jews with BS.[25] (The association of blm^{Ash} with two alleles rather than one at *D15S127* is assumed to result from recurrent mutation at *D15S127*, producing toggling between the 145 and 147 bp alleles.)

This linkage disequilibrium confirmed the linkage results from homozygosity mapping and provided strong support for a founder-effect hypothesis to explain the increased incidence of BS in the Ashkenazim relative to other populations. By one historical model, a chromosome that bore blm^{Ash} in the genome of a postulated "founder" was carried into eastern Europe several centuries ago as the Jews, along with many others, migrated there. Subsequently, blm^{Ash} and its flanking chromosomal segments increased in frequency in the Jews there as result of genetic drift. In other words, today Ashkenazi Jews with BS inherit their mutated *BLM* gene identical by descent from a common ancestor who lived possibly 30 generations ago, making the parents of such individuals distant cousins. Definitive evidence for the founder-effect hypothesis has been obtained by mutational analysis of the mutated *BLM* in the majority of Ashkenazi Jewish persons ever diagnosed BS (presented below).

Evidence for Allelic Heterogeneity at *BLM*[29]

A strikingly elevated SCE rate is uniquely characteristic of BS cells and is present in all cell types examined: mitogen-stimulated blood T and B lymphocytes in short-term culture; Epstein-Barr virus-transformed lymphocytes in long-term culture; cells from the bone marrow in short-term culture; cultured diploid fibroblasts, including fibroblasts from skin, amniotic fluid, chorionic villi, and surgical specimens; and aneuploid SV40-transformed fibroblasts in long-term culture. All persons with BS have high-SCE cells. However, an important, and until recently unexplained, exception was recognized over two decades ago: a small number of blood lymphocytes with a normal SCE rate circulate in the blood in a minority of persons with BS. In these persons, the frequency of low-SCE cells detected in short-term cultures of phytohemagglutinin-stimulated T lymphocytes ranges from under 1 percent to in excess of 50 percent (the highest level recorded in the Registry being 75 percent). The low-SCE cells are functionally normal because cell hybrids formed by a low-SCE BS cell and a high-SCE BS cell have a low-SCE phenotype,[27] just as do cell hybrids formed between a low-SCE cell from a normal person and a high-SCE BS cell.[30]

This enigmatic high-SCE/low-SCE mosaicism was investigated by comparing its incidence in subpopulations of persons with BS sorted according to whether or not *BLM* was known to have been inherited identical by descent. A striking negative correlation emerged:[29] In persons with BS whose parents share a common ancestor, the case in persons born either to consanguineous parents or to two Ashkenazi Jewish parents (approximately half the BS families), a population of low-SCE cells is almost never found; conversely, the mosaicism occurs almost exclusively in persons with BS whose parents are not known to share a common ancestor. Because those who share a common ancestor almost all inherit the identical mutation at *BLM*, the negative correlation was interpreted to mean that emergence of low-SCE cells in BS depends in some way on the pre-existence of compound heterozygosity, i.e., on having two different mutated *BLM* alleles. A corollary to this was that BS is genetically heterogeneous. That multiple mutations are present at *BLM* now has been confirmed by mutational analysis of *BLM* in different persons with BS (below, Table 30-4).

Somatic Intragenic Recombination[31]

The population cytogenetic data just summarized[29] indicated that high-SCE/low-SCE mosaic persons are genetic compounds. The requirement of compound heterozygosity, when considered with the known high rate of homologous recombination taking place in BS somatic cells as compared to normal cells, suggested that a specific form of crossing-over not known to occur in higher organisms, namely, intragenic recombination, explains the mosaicism in some persons with BS. Somatic crossing-over

Table 30-4 Representative BLM Mutations Identified in Persons with Bloom Syndrome (August 31, 1996)[a]

Identification[b]	Ancestry	Zygosity of the Mutation[c]	Nucleotide Change[d]	Protein Change[e]
		Missense mutations		
139(ViKre)[g]	Mixed European	Heterozygous	2015A > G (2089A > G)	Q672R
31(CaDe)[g]	Dutch	Heterozygous	2015A > G (2089A > G)	Q672R
40(DoRoe)	Mixed European	Homozygous	2702G > A (2776G > A)	C901Y[f]
113(DaDem)	Italian	Homozygous	3164G > C (3238G > C)	C1055S
		Nonsense mutations		
97(AsOk)	Japanese	Homozygous	557-559delCAA (631-633)	S186X
112(NaSch)	Mixed European	Heterozygous	814A > T (888A > T)	K272X
98(RoMo)[g]	Mixed European	Heterozygous	1090A > T (1164A > T)	R364X
81(MaGrou)	French Canadian	Homozygous	1784C > A (1858C > A)	S595X
11(IaTh)[g]	Mixed European	Heterozygous	1933C > T (2007C > T)	Q645X
61(DoHop)	Mixed European	Homozygous	1933C > T (2007C > T)	Q645X
NRI(ErBor)[g]	Mixed European	Heterozygous	1933C > T (2007C > T)	Q645X
NR8(KeSol)[g]	Mixed European	Heterozygous	1933C > T (2007C > T)	Q645X
51(KeMc)	Mixed European	Homozygous	2098C > T (2172C > T)	Q700X
		Frameshift mutations		
93(YoYa)	Japanese	Homozygous	1544insA (1618insA)	514+1 > X
15(MaRo)	Ashkenazi Jewish	Homozygous	2207-2212delATCTGAinsTAGATTC[h]	735+4 > X
42(RaFr)	Ashkenazi Jewish	Homozygous	2207-2212delATCTGAinsTAGATTC[h]	735+4 > X
107(MyAsa)	Ashkenazi/Sephardic	Homozygous	2207-2212delATCTGAinsTAGATTC[h]	735+4 > X
NR2(CrSpe)	Ashkenazi Jewish	Homozygous	2207-2212delATCTGAinsTAGATTC[h]	735+4 > X
126(BrNa)	Ashkenazi/Sephardic	Heterozygous	2207-2212delATCTGAinsTAGATTC[h]	735+4 > X
		Exon-skipping mutations		
126(BrNa)	Ashkenazi/Sephardic	Heterozygous	Skips exon 2[i]	[i]
112(NaSch)	Mixed European	Heterozygous	Skips exon 6[j]	362+4 > X
		Exonic deletion		
92(VaBia)	Italian	Homozygous	Skips exons 11 & 12[k]	769+1 > X

[a]Mutation screening reported in this table was carried out on 25 persons with BS from whom cell lines were available. Total RNA was prepared by using Trizol (Gibco BRL). Mutations in the RNA product of BLM were detected by RT-PCR followed by single-stranded conformation polymorphism (SSCP) analysis[26], by an RNase cleavage assay (unpublished observations) marketed by Ambion, or by both techniques. The mutations were then identified by direct sequencing of PCR-amplified cDNA and confirmed by sequencing of the genomic DNA.

[b]Bloom's Syndrome Registry designations. Mutation has gone undetected in only one person with BS of the 25 examined, namely, 140(DrKas). Mutations in four persons from whom a cell line was available are not reported here.

[c]In all persons studied, zygosity of the mutation was confirmed by analysis of the genomic DNA. Similarly, mutations were confirmed in available parents.

[d]Standard nomenclature (from Antonarakis SE: Recomendation for a nomenclature system for human gene mutations. Nomenclature Working Group. *Hum Mutat* 11:1, 1998) has been used to indicate the genetic alteration in the gene. In parentheses, the nucleotide positions are as identified in the *BLM* cDNA H1-5′.[26]

[e]Standard nomenclature has been used to indicate the alteration in the gene product except in the case of frameshift mutation. The effect of a frameshift is shown by first indicating the number of BLM amino acid residues that are incorporated followed by the number of out-of-frame residues that are incorporated until a stop codon is reached (denoted by an X).

[f]This missense mutation formally could be a polymorphism.

[g]In this heterozygote, the other mutated *BLM* allele has yet to be determined or is not reported here.

[h]This mutation also is known as blm^{Ash} and is described as a 6-bp deletion and 7-bp insertion at nucleotide 2281 in the *BLM* cDNA.

[i]An RT-PCR product with a smaller-than-normal size was detected by agarose gel electrophoresis. Sequencing of the abnormal fragment identified a deletion of exon 2, cDNA nucleotides 71 to 172. Sequence analysis of genomic DNA amplified with oligonucleotide primers flanking exon 2 revealed a G-to-T transversion in the 5′ splice site (GT to TT). Splicing out of exon 2 removes the initiator methionine for BLM. Use by the ribosome of the next downstream ATG would result in the generation of a small out-of-frame peptide.

[j]An RT-PCR product with a smaller-than-normal size was detected by agarose gel electrophoresis. Sequencing of the abnormal cDNA fragment identified a deletion of exon 6, nucleotides 1162 to 1294. Sequence analysis of genomic DNA amplified with oligonucleotide primers flanking exon 6 revealed a G-to-A transition in the 3′ splice site (AG to AA). Splicing of exons 5 and 7 results in the addition of 4 out-of-frame amino acids followed by premature termination.

[k]The mutation present in 92 (VaBia) was assigned incorrectly in reference [26] as a G to C at nucleotide position 2596 in the *BLM* cDNA. Subsequently, a deletion of exons 11 and 12—nucleotides 2382 to 2629 in the *BLM* cDNA—was detected by RT-PCR analysis, and its existence was confirmed in genomic DNA by Southern blot analysis and PCR as a 6126-bp deletion confirmed by DNA sequencing. Splicing of exons 10 and 13 results in the addition of 1 out-of-frame amino acid followed by premature termination.

between the paternally derived and the maternally derived mutated sites within *BLM* could generate a functionally wild-type *BLM* that corrects the high-SCE phenotype of a BS cell (Fig. 30-5). By this model, the newly generated, functionally wild-type gene on one chromosome No. 15 can segregate at mitosis with either the non-recombinant chromatid of the other chromosome No. 15—allele losses distal to *BLM* then ensue (i.e., reduction to homozygosity)—or with the recombinant chromatid that now carries a doubly mutant *BLM*—allele losses distal to *BLM* do not ensue.

Evidence supporting the intragenic recombination model was obtained by genotype analysis of 12 loci syntenic with *BLM*—6 proximal and 6 distal to it—in 11 persons who exhibited the high-SCE/low-SCE mosaicism.[31] In 5 of the 11 persons examined, polymorphic loci on chromosome 15q distal to *BLM* that were heterozygous in their high-SCE cells had become homozygous in their low-SCE cells, whereas loci proximal to *BLM* that were heterozygous on 15q had remained heterozygous. In the remaining six persons, loci both proximal and distal to *BLM* that were heterozygous in their high-SCE cells remained heterozygous in their low-SCE cells. These observations indicate that intragenic recombination between the two different mutated alleles at *BLM* is a mechanism that can generate a functionally wild-type *BLM* gene (Fig. 30-5). Thus, the low-SCE lymphocytes present in the blood of mosaic persons can be the progeny of a somatic stem cell in

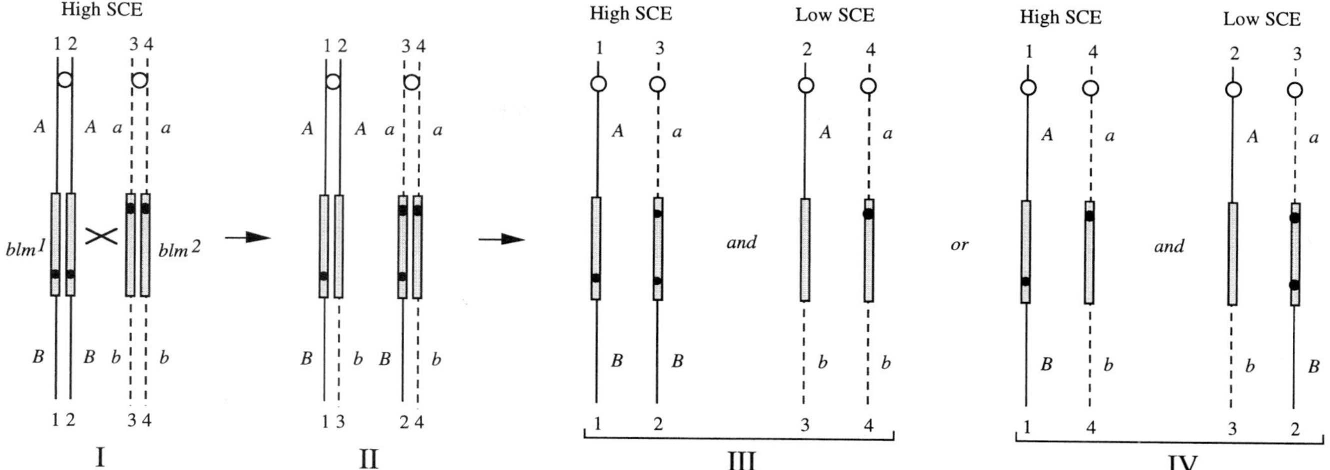

Fig. 30-5 Model to generate a wild-type *BLM* locus via somatic intragenic recombination: *I*, The two pairs of sister chromatids of the homologous chromosome Nos. 15 in a G2 somatic cell of a BS genetic compound (blm^1/blm^2) are numbered 1-1 to 4-4. Each of the two mutations in *BLM* (the hatched rectangle), represented by black dots, one inherited from each parent, is at a different site in the gene. Flanking markers proximal to and distal to the mutated loci are heterozygous *A/a* and *B/b*. *II*, After homologous interchange between chromatids 2-2 and 3-3 at a point between the sites of mutation within *BLM* (the X in *I*), a wild-type gene is reconstituted on chromatid 2-3 that corrects to normal the high-SCE phenotype of BS cells. Simultaneously, the distal marker *b* becomes associated with the wild-type gene on chromatid 2-3. *III* and *IV*, By segregational events at mitosis, two pairs of daughter cells are possible. If chromatids 2-3 and 4-4 co-segregate to the same daughter cell, the distal marker becomes homozygous *b/b* (the diagram on the right side of *III*). On the other hand, if chromatid 2-3 and 3-2 co-segregate, the distal marker remains heterozygous *b/B* (the diagram on the right side of *IV*). The proximal marker remains heterozygous *A/a* in both cases. In the sister cells, segregation of chromatids 1-1 and 3-2 (the diagram on the left side of *III*) or of chromatids 1-1 and 4-4 (the diagram on the left side of *IV*) do not give rise to a low-SCE phenotype. (*Note*: Cells of heterozygous carriers of a mutation at *BLM, viz. blm*/BLM parents of persons with BS, display a low-SCE rate.) (Reprinted with permission from Ellis NA, Lennon DJ, Proytcheva M, Alhadeff B, Henderson EE, German J: Somatic intragenic recombination within the mutated locus *BLM* can correct the high-SCE phenotype of Bloom syndrome cells. *Am J Hum Genet* 57:1019, 1995.)

which such an intragenic recombinational event had occurred. (Other mechanisms that generate high-SCE/low-SCE mosaicism have now also been identified [e.g., back mutation[32]].)

Isolation and Mutational Analysis of *BLM**

The availability of the five low-SCE cell lines just mentioned in which somatic intragenic recombination had led to reduction to homozygosity at loci distal but not proximal to *BLM*[31] provided an efficient strategy to determine the exact location of *BLM*. The objective became to identify (a) the most proximal polymorphic locus that was constitutionally heterozygous and that had been reduced to homozygosity in the five low-SCE cell lines and (b) the most distal polymorphic locus that had remained constitutionally heterozygous in them. *BLM* would have to be in the short interval defined by the reduced and the unreduced, i.e., still heterozygous, markers. The power of this approach, termed *somatic crossover-point* (*SCP*) *mapping,* would be limited only by the density of polymorphic loci available in the immediate vicinity of the gene.

As mentioned earlier, *BLM* had been localized by homozygosity mapping to a 2-cM interval flanking *FES.* A 2-Mb yeast artificial chromosome (YAC) and P1 contig encompassing *FES* was constructed, and the required, closely spaced, polymorphic DNA markers in the contig were identified.[34] *BLM* then was assigned by SCP mapping to an interval in this contig of only 250 kb in size that was bounded by the polymorphic loci *D15S1108* and *D15S127* (Fig. 30-6). Then a cosmid clone (referred to as 905) that was present in the 250-kb interval was used to isolate by direct selection an 849-bp clone from a fibroblast cDNA library. By hybridization and RT-PCR techniques, this cDNA clone, in turn, was used to isolate many additional cDNAs from fibroblast, lymphoblastoid, and HeLa cells. A 4,437-bp cDNA sequence, referred to as H1-5′, was defined that contained a long open reading frame encoding a 1,417 amino acid protein. By Southern blot analysis of genomic DNA and of sequences cloned in YACs, P1s, and cosmids, the H1-5′ sequences hybridized to single-copy sequences spanning about 100 kb of the genome. (The complete genomic sequences of this region are available in the DNA sequence database at the National Center for Biotechnology Information.) A 4.5-kb transcript was identified by Northern blot analysis of total RNAs prepared from various human cells proliferating *in vitro.* Northern analysis of seven lymphoblastoid cell lines derived from seven unrelated persons with BS revealed three cell lines in which the levels of mRNA that hybridized to labeled H1-5′ sequences were five- to tenfold less than those in control normal cell lines. In addition, there was a fourth cell line in which both the mRNA levels were reduced and the length of the mRNA was approximately 200 bp shorter than the normal mRNA molecule. Because it is known that mutations which produce premature translation termination often reduce mRNA stability, the abnormalities in mRNA levels here suggested that the gene encoding these mRNAs was mutated. (Extensive Northern analysis has now been performed on over 30 BS cell lines, and reduced steady-state levels of *BLM* mRNAs are a general result.)

Mutations in the H1-5′ sequences then were sought in persons with BS. Initially, analysis was carried out using RT-PCR and single-stranded conformation polymorphism (SSCP) on RNA from 13 BS lymphoblastoid cell lines. In 10 of the 13 cell lines examined, 7 different mutations were detected. Five of the seven mutations led to premature translation termination, and two were amino acid substitutions at highly conserved residues (see below and Table 30-4). Using additional mutation-searching methods, including an RNAse cleavage assay (marketed by Ambion), the protein truncation test, PCR-restriction enzyme analysis, Southern blot analysis, DNA-HPLC heteroduplex analysis, and DNA

*Work both published (reviewed in reference 33) and in progress in the authors' laboratories is mentioned in this and the subsequent sections of this chapter. Construction of the physical map of the *BLM* region[34] and the identification of mutations in *BLM* by the SSCP analysis[26] were done by collaboration between the laboratory of Joanna Groden (University of Cincinnati) and ours.

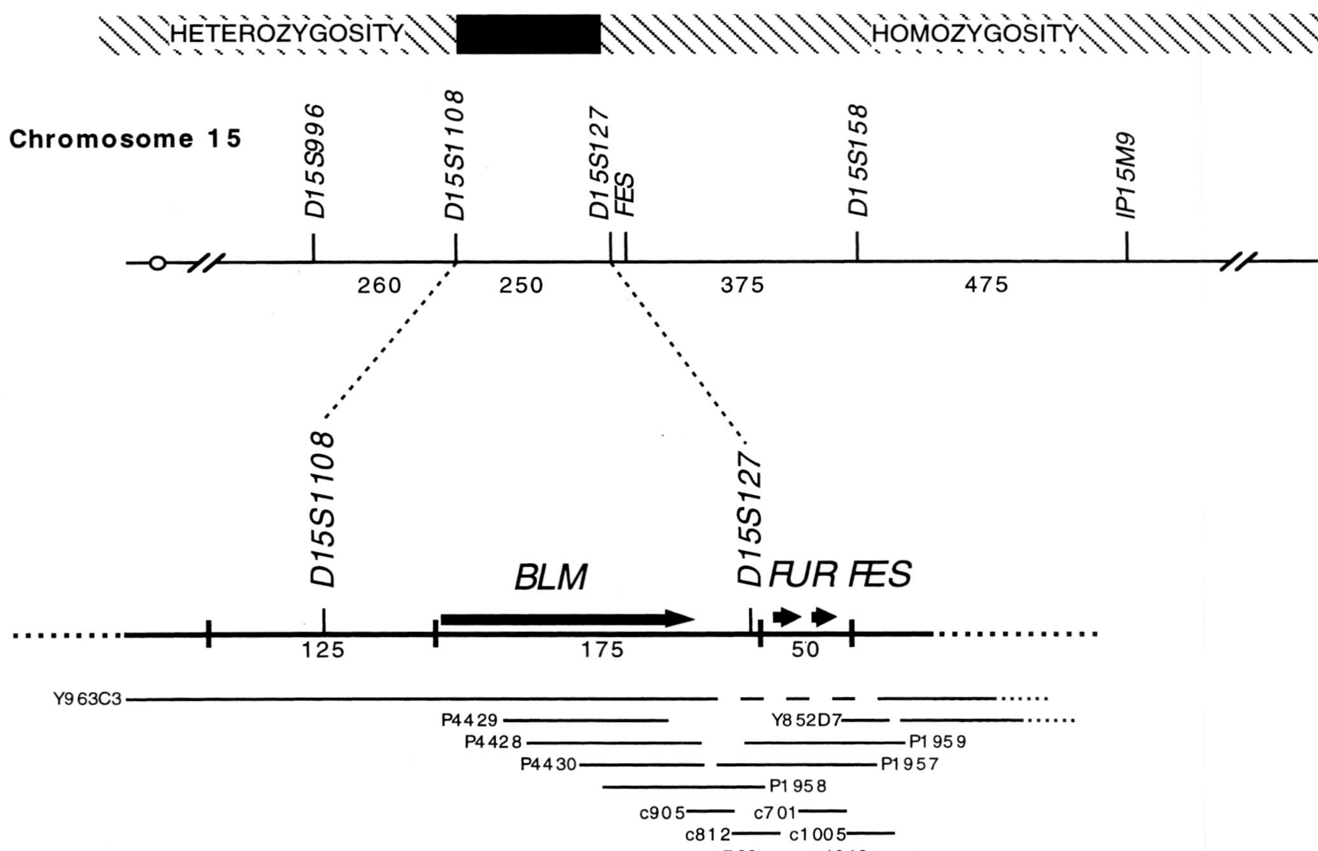

Fig. 30-6 SCP mapping of *BLM*. Genetic map of the *BLM* region of 15q. On the upper horizontal line, the order and distances (shown in kb) between the polymorphic microsatellite loci were estimated by long-range-restriction mapping.[34] The distance between *D15S127* and *FES* (not indicated) was determined to be 30 kb by restriction enzyme mapping of a cosmid contig (see the following). Vertical lines indicate the position of the marker loci, and the circle represents the centromere. The interval between loci *D15S1108* and *D15S127* is expanded below the map. Vertical lines intersecting mark the unmethylated CpG-rich regions identified by long-range restriction mapping, and arrows indicate the direction of transcription of three genes in the region. Certain Yacs, P1s, and cosmids (Y, P, and c, respectively) from the contig are depicted by horizontal lines underneath the map.[34] Dashes on the YAC lines indicate internal deletions. At the top of the figure, the horizontal cross-hatched bar to the right indicates regions distal to *BLM* that had become homozygous. The minimal region to which *BLM* was thus assigned by SCP mapping is represented in black. (Reprinted, slightly modified, with permission from Ellis NA, Groden J, Ye T-Z, Straughen J, Lennon DJ, Ciocci S, Proytcheva M, German J: The Bloom's syndrome gene product is homologous to RecQ helicases. *Cell* 83:655, 1995.)

sequencing, we have identified 48 unique mutations in 108 of 121 persons with BS examined. The mutations listed in Table 30-4 are representative, but eventually a complete report of the mutational analysis will be made. Nine of the 48 mutations are amino acid substitutions made at conserved residues, the alteration of which putatively disturbs the enzymatic activity of the protein (see below); 14 are nonsense mutations; 17 are oligonucleotide insertions or deletions that cause frameshifting and premature translation termination immediately downstream of the mutation; 5 are mutations at splice sites, some of which are known to disturb the proper splicing of the mRNA; and 3 are deletions of 1 or more exons. In the 9 missense alleles, the open reading frame is maintained, but in the remaining 39 mutant alleles the open reading frame is in some way disrupted.

Two unusual examples are these: (a) In one of the exon-skipping mutations, the initiator AUG is not present in the cDNA; the next downstream AUG is out of frame, resulting in failure to produce normal BLM product. (b) In one of the genomic deletions, the last three exons of *BLM* are deleted, resulting in the loss of the polyadenylation-addition signal. Presumably, the RNA polymerase continues to transcribe until it meets with an intergenic sequence that can serve as a polyadenylation-addition signal, or until it transcribes through a downstream gene—one that is transcribed in the same direction as *BLM*—and terminates transcription at the end of that gene. Whatever the effects are of losing the polyadenylation-addition signal, the putative protein could contain no more than 1250 amino acids of BLM. As is discussed below, domains necessary for the proper function and expression of BLM extend at least to amino acid residue 1334; consequently, even if the proteins are expressed from mutant alleles that lack the last 100 or so amino acids, they are predicted to be nonfunctional. As mentioned above, Northern analysis has been performed on over 30 BS cell lines, and the mRNAs from alleles encoding BLM proteins with premature translation termination are expressed at reduced levels. Therefore, the effects of the mutations at *BLM* comprise both alterations in expression at the message level and alterations in protein expression and function.

From the mutation searching, three conclusions are drawn: (a) The discovery of mutations in the H1-5′ sequence in persons with BS proves that the gene that had been isolated is *BLM*. (b) That multiple mutations exist in the gene confirms the allelic heterogeneity at *BLM* predicted from the Registry cytogenetics.[29] (c) The identification of 38 premature-translation-termination mutations, many of which are homozygous in persons with BS, demonstrates that loss of function of the BLM protein is the major underlying cause of the clinical syndrome and that null mutations at *BLM* are not cell-lethal.[26] In addition, because mutations in *BLM* have been detected in nearly all of the persons with BS examined, the clinical entity caused by mutation at *BLM*; BS-causing mutations of loci other than *BLM* either do not exist or are very rare.

During the initial mutational analysis of four persons with Ashkenazi Jewish ancestry, the aforementioned 6-bp deletion and 7-bp insertion mutation at nucleotide 2281 was detected — blm^{Ash}. Fortuitously, this mutation introduces a *Bst*NI site that can be detected by restriction-enzyme digestion in DNA amplified by PCR of both cDNA and genomic DNA.[35] Fifty-eight of 60 chromosomes derived from Ashkenazi Jewish persons with BS that have been examined contain this *Bst*NI site, i.e., transmit this one mutation.[36] This confirms the hypothesis that founder effect is the explanation for the elevated frequency of BS in the Ashkenazi Jewish population.[3] Assay for the *Bst*NI site in genomic DNA samples from all persons with BS available through the Registry has revealed a conspicuous absence of blm^{Ash} from all of the 49 non-Jewish persons with Northern European ancestry examined, as well as from all of the 8 Italians, 8 Japanese, 4 North Americans with African ancestry, 4 Turks, 4 Brazilians, an Argentinean, a Portuguese, a Spaniard, a Persian Jew, a Lebanese, and an Indian.

However — and completely unexpectedly — the blm^{Ash} mutation turned up in five of the seven unrelated persons with BS examined from American families that were of Spanish ancestry.[36] These five persons were born into Catholic families that for many generations have lived in El Salvador, Mexico, or the American Southwest; these families were unaware of Jewish ancestry, although one family reports an oral tradition of these being a distant ancestor of the maternal grandmother of the proposita who was "a Sephardi."

The unexpected finding of blm^{Ash} in only this one particular group of non-Jews supports the following hypothesis:[36] blm^{Ash} was a mutation at *BLM* that was segregating in the Jews of Spain in the fifteenth century, probably at a low frequency as do various *BLM* mutations in many non-Jewish populations today. Sometime during the colonization of the Americas by Spain after the expulsion of the Sephardim in 1492 by Ferdinand and Isabella, a Spanish Jew who had been converted to Christianity, a *converso,* and who by chance was heterozygous for blm^{Ash} migrated to New Spain. This person transmitted blm^{Ash} to his or her descendants. By this hypothesis, two different founder effects pertaining to blm^{Ash} have been identified, the one long-recognized that took place in Eastern Europe and another that took place in New Spain. From the available genetic evidence, the exact historical path(s) of blm^{Ash} into both the Ashkenazim and the Sephardim cannot be delineated. However, our observations in the genetics of BS point to the existence of a common ancestor of, or to admixture between, these two major Jewish populations. More broadly, they are examples of the impact of migration and genetic drift on the formation of human populations.

Eighteen of the 48 mutations identified in persons with BS have recurred in 2 or more unrelated persons. That said, 7 of these 18 mutations have been identified in just 2 unrelated persons, suggesting that the common ancestor to the families transmitting these particular 7 mutations lived relatively recently. In contrast, a nonsense mutation at nucleotide 2007 in the *BLM* cDNA has been found in 17 purportedly unrelated persons of non-Jewish European ancestry (Table 30-4 and our unpublished observations). The survey reveals that in human populations founder effect takes place repeatedly.

MOLECULAR BIOLOGY OF THE BLM PROTEIN

Homology searching of the amino acid sequence databases revealed that the 1,417 amino acid protein encoded by the *BLM* cDNA sequence contains homology to RecQ helicases (Fig. 30-7), a subfamily of DExH box-containing DNA and RNA helicases.[26] The RecQ helicases are member of a much larger group of proteins that contain seven amino acid motifs that are present in most DNA and RNA helicases. Helicases are defined biochemically by two activities: (a) they are DNA- or RNA-dependent ATPases, and (b) with ATP and Mg^{++} as co-factors, they catalyze the unwinding of duplex nucleic acids. Because nucleic acids are predominantly in a duplex form in the cell, helicases are active in all processes in nucleic acid metabolism that require access to single-stranded molecules, namely, DNA replication, DNA repair, recombination, RNA transcription, and protein translation. Given the fact that the BLM protein is a helicase,[37] two questions arise: In which of these many processes does BLM participate? and What are the specific nucleic acid substrates in the cell on which BLM acts? Recent experimental evidence from the study of RecQ family members and BLM has provided some important insights.

The RecQ Gene Family

recQ was isolated as a mutation in *E. coli* that generated resistance to thymineless death and was identified as a member of the RecF pathway of DNA recombination.[38] In appropriately marked bacterial strains, *recQ* mutants are hyporecombinogenic, which strongly suggests that RecQ carries out a step in DNA recombination. When the RecQ protein was purified, it was found to have DNA-dependent ATPase and DNA strand-displacement activities that defined it as a DNA helicase.[39] Together with the RecA and SSB (single-stranded DNA-binding) proteins, RecQ can catalyze both the formation and the dissolution of recombinational intermediates *in vitro.*[40] What might drive the reaction in the cell in one direction or the other is unknown; however, genetic evidence has been presented to suggest that RecQ can inhibit illegitimate recombination.[41] So, in *E. coli,* RecQ could help maintain genomic stability by preventing the formation of duplexes between imperfectly homologous DNA sequences. Also, there is evidence that the RecF pathway operates during DNA replication to maintain and reactivate replication complexes which have stalled, e.g., when they have encountered sites of DNA damage such as cyclopyrimidine dimers.[42] RecQ, as a member of the RecF pathway, could be helping maintain the integrity of the replication complex when fork progression is impeded.

In *Saccharomyces cerevisiae* where the entire genomic DNA sequence is known, there is a single RecQ family member. This gene, *SGS1,* was first identified as a mutation that is a slow-growth suppressor of a cell containing a mutation in its topoisomerase 3 (*TOP3*) gene.[43] *top3* mutants not only proliferate slowly but also have, by measures at several different loci, vastly elevated recombination frequencies; e.g., at the rDNA locus, near telomeres, and in diploids at genes marked by heteroallelic mutations. Suppression of these phenotypes by deletion of *SGS1* suggests that top3p and sgs1p (the proteins) interact physically. Supporting this possibility, *SGS1* was identified by *TOP3* in a yeast two-hybrid screen.[43] In addition to interaction with top3p, sgs1p interacts physically with top2p.[44] Finally, *sgs1/top1* double mutants exhibit a slow-growth phenotype that neither single mutant exhibits.[45] Thus, with the three topoisomerases in yeast, sgs1p has genetic interactions, physical interactions, or both. sgs1p possesses DNA-dependent ATPase and DNA strand-displacement activities.[45]

Mutation in *SGS1* by itself also causes a hyperrecombination phenotype that is milder than that in *TOP3.*[46] In addition, *sgs1* cell-doubling time is increased, and the mutant cells feature increased nondisjunction in both mitosis and meiosis.[44,46] These attributes raise the possibility of a defect in genomic stability. It has been suggested that sgs1p suppresses recombination, for example, in highly repetitive DNA sequences,[43,46] and recent genetic evidence suggests that sgs1p, like RecQ, can inhibit illegitimate recombination.[47] *E. coli* RecQ *in vitro* can enter and unwind a closed circular duplex DNA molecule, and it can stimulate the activity of *E. coli* topoisomerase 3 to catenate such double-stranded molecules.[48] These data suggest that at the very least a functional interaction exists between RecQ and

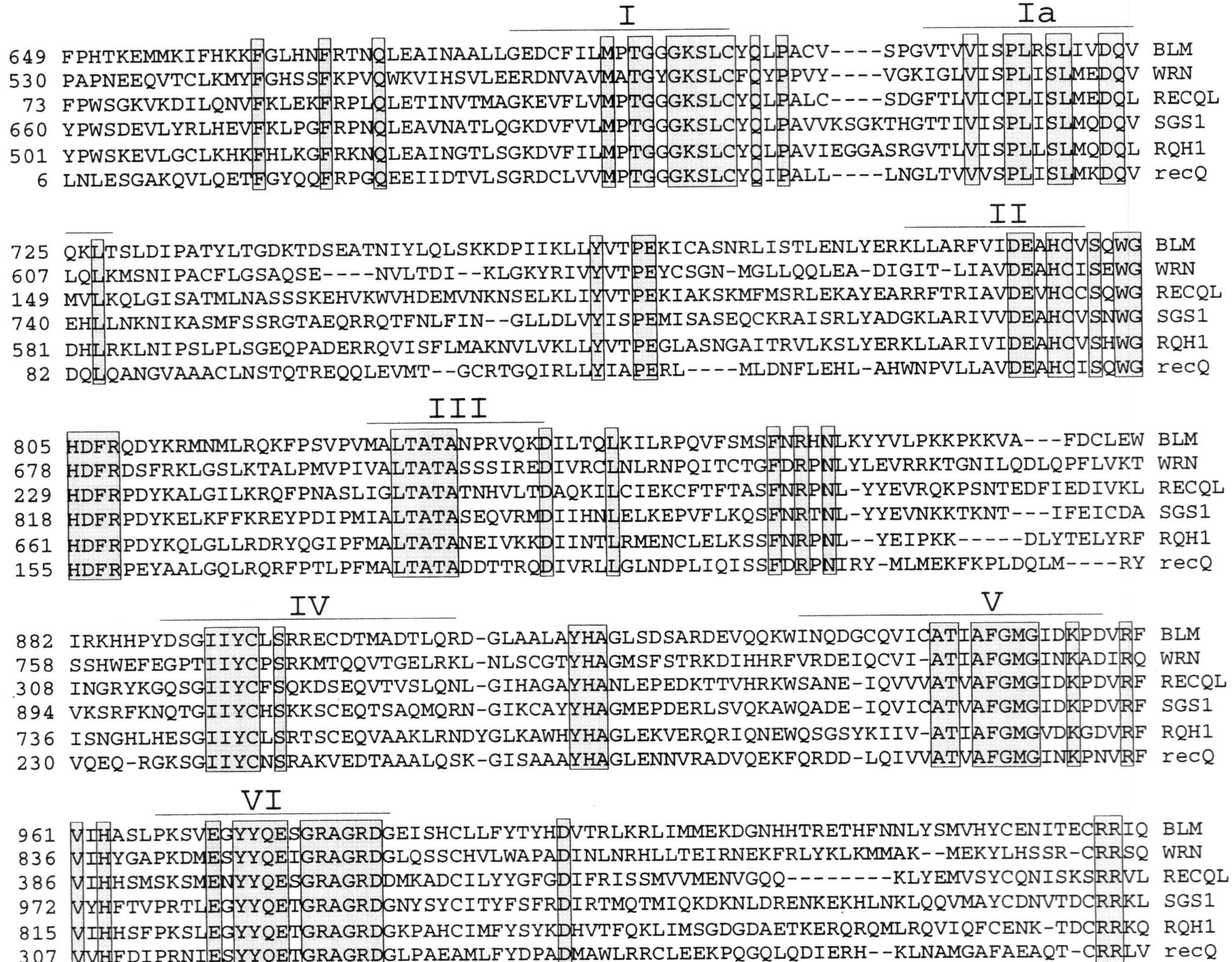

Fig. 30-7 Alignment of the amino acid sequences in the domains containing the seven helicase motifs (I, Ia, II, III, IV, V and VI) of selected RecQ helicases. The Megalign computer program (DNA-Star) performed the sequence alignments. Numbers at left indicate the amino acid positions in each protein, and gene product names are at the right. Identities present in all six selected proteins are boxed. Overlined sequences mark the seven helicase motifs in the helicase domain. The DExH box is in helicase motif II. (Reprinted with permission from Ellis, NA, German J: Molecular genetics of Bloom's syndrome. *Hum Mol Genet* 5:1457, 1996.)

topoisomerase 3 and that potentially the function of the yeast and bacterial RecQ family proteins is highly conserved.

The structure of *S. cerevisiae*'s sgs1p differs from *E. coli*'s RecQ in an important way: RecQ is a 610 amino acid protein with an N-terminal helicase domain (approximately 300 amino acids) and a C-terminal domain of unknown function. These two domains are highly positively charged. Sgs1p, on the other hand, is a 1,447 amino acid protein that, in addition to the helicase and C-terminal domains, contains a highly negatively charged N-terminal domain (approximately 650 amino acids). The regions of sgs1p that interact with topoisomerases have been mapped to this N-terminal domain.[43,44] In its structure, BLM resembles sgs1p in having a highly negatively charged N-terminal domain (650 amino acids) along with positively charged helicase and C-terminal domains. Thus, as with sgs1p, the N-terminal domain of BLM could provide specificity to the function of the helicase by determining BLM's interactions with other proteins.

In *Schizosaccharomyces pombe,* an *SGS1*-like *recQ* gene, referred to as *rqh1+,* is present that was identified by a mutation, *rad12,* that causes hypersensitivity to UV irradiation, and by a second, *hus2,* that caused hypersensitivity to hydroxyurea.[49,50] These mutations also confer hyperrecombination and chromosome-nondisjunction phenotypes similar to those in *S. cerevisiae sgs1.* Molecular genetic evidence points to a function for rqh1+ protein in maintaining replication-fork integrity when DNA damage or fork-progression inhibition occurs during S phase,[49,50] and possibly a function in signaling to the cell-cycle-control machinery.[51] *top3* mutants in *S. pombe* are viable for only a limited number of cells generations, and, like *rqh1* mutants, they exhibit a 'cut' phenotype, which signifies aberrant chromosome segregation. Consistent with a conserved interaction between RecQ family proteins and topoisomerase 3s, *rqh1* mutation suppresses the *top3* lethal phenotype.[52] Such observations support the hypothesis that the RecQ family proteins and topoisomerase 3s together facilitate sister-chromatid separation at the sites of termination of DNA replication.[43,52] The combined genetic and biochemical evidence points to possible roles for RecQ family proteins in three critical processes: the suppression of illegitimate recombination events, the maintenance of replication fork integrity during periods when the complex is stalled, and separation of sister chromatids.

The cloning of *rqh1+* uncovered another feature of the domain structure of the RecQ family. Immediately C-terminal of the central helicase domain, rqh1+ and BLM both contain segment of 200 amino acids that have approximately 20 percent identity, referred to as the C-terminal extended homology region. The other RecQ family members mentioned above contain this region, but in pairwise comparisons, the homology varies both in the number of amino acids and in the percent of identity[53]. Additionally, by homology searching of the protein databases, a second motif was identified as C-terminal of the extended homology region.[54] This motif, called the HRDC (for *h*elicase and *R*NAase*D* *C*-terminal domain), is implicated in DNA binding. Because mutation in the C-terminal extended homology region can destroy helicase activity (see below), and because the HRDC is proposed to act in DNA binding,[54] these regions may play a role in the recognition of specific substrates *in vivo*.

Mammalian cells have a RecQ-like protein consisting of 659 amino acids that is referred to as RECQL1 (also called RECQL). RECQ1 was isolated as a major ATPase of HeLa cells and was shown to have DNA helicase activity.[55,56] The cellular role of RECQ1 is unknown. After *RECQL1* and *BLM*, a third RecQ family member was identified: *WRN*, the gene that when mutated results in Werner syndrome (WS)—defined clinically by premature aging (see Chap. 33)—encodes a 1,432 amino acid product having domain structures similar to that of sgs1p and BLM.[57] WRN is a DNA helicase,[58,59] but, unlike BLM or the other known RecQ helicases, WRN contains a 5′ to 3′ exonuclease activity in its N-terminal domain.[60] This difference in their N-terminal domain structures and functions could explain, in part, why clinical BS bears essentially no resemblance to clinical WS. WS does predispose to certain rare neoplasms, and WS cells exhibit what has been called "variegated translocation mosaicism."[61] Although excessive chromosome breakage as seen in BS is not present, fibroblasts cultured from WS skin grow as clones, with each clonal line marked by a distinctive chromosome translocation.[61,62] WS cells also exhibit an increased frequency of mutations at the only specific locus tested so far, the *HPRT* locus, which are mostly deletions. Thus, the identification of *WRN* may have established a connection between the aging process and the maintenance of genomic stability. Correspondingly, the *sgs1* mutation in yeast gives a premature aging phenotype which is associated with the formation of extrachromosomal rDNA circles.[63,64]

Recently, two additional human RecQ helicase family members, *RECQL4* and *RECQ5*, were identified by searching the cDNA sequence database.[65] A report has been made of mutations in *RECQL4* in persons diagnosed with Rothmund-Thomson syndrome.[66] For *BLM* and *WRN* we know that absence of a normal allele leads to genomic instability. For the three other RecQ members, *RECQL1*, and *RECQL5*, although there is no information to suggest that mutations in them produce viable phenotypes, it is possible that unexplained entities caused by such already are known in clinical medicine.

Structure and Function of the BLM Helicase

Homology to the RecQ helicases strongly suggested that BLM itself is a DNA helicase. To demonstrate that BLM has this activity, however, it was expressed with a C-terminal hexahistidine tag in *S. cerevisiae*, partially purified by nickel-chelation chromatography, and tested in conventional assays for DNA-dependent ATPase and strand-displacement activities.[37,67] BLM can unwind a number of different DNA duplex substrates, but it has a striking preference for G4 DNA (a tetrameric DNA structure that can form between runs of guanines).[68]

In the 108 persons with BS in whom the 48 different mutations have been identified, 4 of the 9 missense mutations identified (above) alter different amino acid residues in the helicase domain. One mutation replaces the glutamine at residue 672 with an arginine (Q672R; see Table 30-4); this glutamine lies 10 amino acid residues N-terminal of the helicase motif I, and it is conserved in all RecQ helicases (see Fig. 30-7). Two mutations have been identified in motif IV, and one at a conserved histidine residue between motifs V and VI (our unpublished observations). We expect that all four of these amino acid substitutions either reduce or destroy BLM's helicase activity. Experimentally, the Q672R mutation has been introduced into a *BLM* cDNA expression construct, mutant BLM produced in yeast, and the partially purified protein assayed for helicase activity; indeed, BLM Q672R protein has reduced DNA-dependent ATPase activity and lacks detectable DNA strand-displacement activity.[67]

In addition to finding mutations inside the helicase domain, a cluster of 5 amino acid substitutions has been found in a 50 amino-acid stretch of the RecQ C-terminal extended homology region (reference 69 and our unpublished observations). The first such mutation that has been studied in some detail replaces a conserved cystine at residue 1055 with a serine (C1055S). This amino acid substitution has been introduced experimentally into the *BLM* cDNA expression construct, the mutant BLM then produced in yeast, and the partially purified protein assayed for helicase activity; the BLM C1055S protein lacks detectable ATPase and DNA strand-displacement activities.[67] A similar result was obtained when this mutation was introduced at the same position of the mouse *Blm* gene.[53] (Mouse and human *BLM* genes are highly conserved throughout this region.) Given the clustering of the amino acid substitutions in this region, we predict that the other mutations in the C-terminal extended homology region have similar effects on BLM's helicase activity. The observation that *BLM* mutations in persons with BS ablate its helicase activity may be interpreted to mean that the helicase activity is indispensable to the protein's normal function.

Antibodies to an N-terminal segment of BLM have been raised in rabbits, and a protein of apparent molecular weight of 180-kDa has been identified by Western blot analysis of fibroblast, lymphoblastoid, and HeLa cells. This 180-kDa molecule is absent from all the BS cell lines homozygous for premature translation-termination mutations that have been examined.[67,70] This indicates that the 180-kDa molecule is BLM, the BS protein. Simultaneously, it demonstrates that anti-BLM antibody is useful for characterizing BLM, for defining its location in the cell, and for identifying proteins with which BLM may interact.

With the BLM antibodies available, it has been possible to introduce a *BLM* cDNA expression construct into BLM-lacking BS cells and to determine whether BLM becomes detectable by Western blot analysis and, or, by cellular immunofluorescence. The normal *BLM* expression construct was transfected into SV40-transformed BS fibroblasts (cell line GM08505). This cell line is derived from a diploid fibroblast line homozygous for blm^{Ash}, and it has the high-SCE phenotype of BS and lacks detectable BLM protein. Transfection of *BLM* restores the 180-kDa BLM molecule to GM08505 cells and concomitantly reduces the SCE rate of these cells from a mean of 58 SCEs per 46 metaphase chromosomes to a mean of 23.[70] The same level of SCE reduction has been observed when normal cells are hybridized to GM08505 cells or when a normal chromosome 15 is introduced into these cells by chromosome-mediated gene transfer,[71] i.e., not completely to the level seen in non-SV40-transformed non-BS fibroblasts. Consequently, the transfected *BLM* cDNA functions in GM08505 cells to reduce SCEs as efficiently as the *BLM* gene when in its normal chromosomal location; similar correction results now have been reported by others.[72]

These complementation experiments have allowed the development of a system for studying structure-function relationships of BLM. Two BS-causing mutations mentioned above—the helicase-negative Q672R and the C1055S amino acid substitutions—were introduced experimentally into the *BLM* cDNA and transfected into GM08505 cells. Although a 180-kDa molecule was detectable by Western analysis after transfection and cloning of the cells, albeit present at levels lower than when normal *BLM* cDNA is transfected, expression of the mutant BLM proteins failed to reduce the high-SCE rate of these cells.[67] Experiments are underway using the transfection system to investigate the effects of small, experimentally produced deletions in the nonhelicase domains and of exchanging homologous domains between other RecQ helicases and BLM, e.g., the N-terminal domain of WRN for that of BLM.

The intracellular localization of BLM has been determined by employing BLM antibodies and the indirect immunofluorescence technique in the study of various BS and non-BS cell lines. BLM protein is present in the nucleus of all cells examined save those from persons with BS. Consistent with BLM's presence in the nucleus, transient transfections of constructs in which amino acids C-terminal of residue 1341 were deleted demonstrated that BLM protein contains a nuclear localization signal (NLS) in its last 100 amino acids. Examination of the sequences there disclosed a bipartite NLS at residues 1334 to 1349 as found in numerous other nuclear proteins (e.g., DNA polymerase α and topoisomerase II).[73] The WRN helicase contains an NLS at a similar location (residues 1370 to 1376).[74]Because the NLSs of BLM and WRN are at the C-termini, premature translation-termination mutations N-terminal of the NLSs render the proteins nonfunctional, via the mutant protein's inability to be moved into the nucleus. Supporting this observation is the finding of a protein-truncating mutation in the *BLM* of a person with BS that encodes a BLM abnormal only in lacking its C-terminal 175 amino acids (our unpublished observation).

The abundance of BLM at different phases of the cell cycle varies strikingly, being at its lowest in early G1. Presently being defined by immunofluorescence microscopy are interesting focal concentrations that BLM makes before and during S and its association with chromatin and nuclear matrix, co-localization with other nuclear proteins or lack thereof, and its representation in various nucleoprotein complexes (e.g., nuclear bodies, DNA replication "centers"). These microscopic observations complemented by appropriate immunoprecipitation and biochemical experiments will eventually define BLM's role(s) in the various mechanisms that require opening of the DNA helix. A knockout of the mouse *Blm* gene has been produced by homologous recombination and embryonic stem cell technology.[75] *Blm* –/– fibroblasts exhibit a high SCE phenotype indicating that the mutation introduced into the mouse gene is a null. The Blm –/– embryos die at day 13.5 developmentally delayed and anemic. A wave of apoptosis occurs in the postimplantation embryo, which provides a possible explanation for the developmental delay observed later in gestation. That the *Blm* null mutation is lethal in mouse, whereas the human *BLM* null (BS) is not, points to some underlying variation during evolution in the requirement for *BLM* or the *RecQ* family genes relative to their physiological function. The development of a mouse model of BS would be desirable in order to permit physiological experimentation.

MANAGEMENT

Growth

A means of increasing growth in BS is unknown—and is not to be found if the correct explanation for the restriction on size is the excessive cell death secondary to the myriad somatic mutations arising throughout development postulated above.

Babies and young children with BS are notoriously poor eaters, and the course ordinarily followed is to set nutritious food before them, supplement it with a multiple vitamin preparation, and just let the child eat as his body dictates through appetite. Coercion to eat is to no avail, and, on the contrary, undue attention from the family would sometimes seem to have undesirable psychological effects. Nonvolitional feeding of infants with BS is under investigation in a few centers, by, for example, surgically placed intragastric feeding tubes, and some promising results are being obtained in the four children so treated. As postulated earlier, if the presently unexplained restriction on learning and the adult onset diabetes are on a nutritional basis, secondary perhaps to disturbed leptin activity, such a simple measure could be valuable in BS.

Growth hormone production when estimated in BS usually is found in the normal to low-normal range. A few affected persons have been treated with growth hormone, usually without much effect. (That a few males with BS have reached five feet or slightly more in height without any specific treatment is unexplained.) Although more information on the possibly beneficial effect of growth hormone with respect to final body size in BS is desirable, reports of cancer that has arisen during or following its administration, including in BS, commonly deter trials.

The Skin

Avoidance of the sun and the regular use of a hat or bonnet and sun-screening ointments control the facial skin lesion of BS best. Especially advisable are measures that limit sun exposure in the first few years of life, judging from the observation that in most cases the severity of the skin lesion appears to be established at that time.

Cancer

Although knowledge of the cancer proneness of BS quite naturally is distressing to an affected family, such knowledge can be life saving. Here, information is withheld from neither affected adults nor the parents of affected children. Families and patients handle this information well if it is presented to them appropriately by the physician or geneticist in charge, i.e., in comprehensible and useful terms. It can be presented in the context of the already great frequency of cancer in the general population, and then supplemented by an explanation of the basis for the inordinate increase and its prematurity in the person with BS. That the risk, although always more than in other people, is relatively much less at the early ages can be emphasized, as well as the shift of type toward carcinoma after adulthood is reached.[12] The potential value such knowledge of the cancer proneness provides to an affected person also can be emphasized, and some idea of practical and effective surveillance programs to be instituted at different ages can be provided. In this way, the physician who makes the diagnosis also, in lieu of treatment in the usual sense, offers a modus operandi.

Until the prognosis of leukemia if diagnosed and treated in its earliest stages can be shown to be better than treatment initiated after the disease becomes symptomatic, periodic hematologic surveillance of children with BS is not recommended. However, for adults with BS, close and long-term contact with an internist or clinic knowledgeable about BS is highly advisable. An unusual degree of attention then will be paid to symptoms that in other persons might properly be ignored but that in BS will permit early diagnosis of carcinoma, where surgical excision still provides the best chance of cure. (Among symptoms and signs that already have led to early diagnosis of cancer in persons in the Registry—sometimes but unfortunately not always life-saving—are these: hoarseness [laryngeal carcinoma]; pain in the side of the throat [posterior lingual carcinoma]; mild dysphagia [esophageal carcinoma]; red blood-staining in the feces [carcinoma of the lower large bowel]; a lump in the breast palpable by the patient; a positive Papanicolaou smear [cervical carcinoma-*in-situ*]; lower abdominal pain [uterine adenocarcinoma]; unexplained recurring abdominal discomfort [pelvic lymphoma; adenocarcinoma of the colon]; intussusception [lymphoma of the small bowel]; and abrupt onset of convulsions [meningioma] or headache [medulloblastoma].) After the age of 20, annual visits with the internist seem advisable with at least annual screening by conventional methods for carcinoma of the breast, cervix, and colon.

In the treatment of the cancers that arise in persons with BS, consideration should be given to the hypersensitivity such persons usually show to many of the DNA-damaging chemicals in standard regimens of therapy. Several persons with BS have shown severe damage or destruction of the bowel mucosa and bone marrow, and this can be lethal. Although specific recommendations of dosage of chemotherapeutic agents in BS cannot be given, doses approximately half the standard dose of the DNA-damaging agents have usually been tolerated, and in several have proven adequate for cure. Ionizing irradiation has been tolerated seemingly normally in the usual dosage.

The "management" of a person with BS is not to be viewed by his physician as of little value just because normal body size cannot be prescribed for nor cancer prevented. Knowledge of the correct diagnosis and an understanding of the condition are of inestimable value to parents of affected persons. Also, the affected individual benefits both physically and emotionally when in the hands of one who knows the correct diagnosis, understands the syndrome itself, and is able to communicate both appropriately and wisely accurate information about it, including its important complications.

CONCLUDING COMMENTS

Since 1960 when its clinical and laboratory investigation began, rare BS has been a source of important, as well as very interesting, biological information, as reviewed here. The new things that can be learned from BS depend to a considerable extent on technical advances. First, experimental laboratory observation of the chromosomes of BS cells supplemented by long-term contact with affected individuals provided *some of the earliest and clearest evidence that chromosome mutation is etiologic in human cancer.* Cytogenetics complemented by molecular biology also showed that somatic crossing-over can take place in mammalian cells. Most recently, recombinant DNA technology applied to the study of BS, still in conjunction with clinical investigation, notably the use in the laboratory of cell lines derived from families about whom reliable clinical and genetic information had been accumulated, has brought to light a protein not previously known to exist in mammalian cells. With the identification of BLM as a protein important in DNA metabolism, but one that is not lethal when absent from the nucleus, the BS cell and the BS gene in themselves become valuable experimental material. Now the nucleic acid enzymologist and molecular biologist can employ them to investigate little understood, if not previously completely obscure, nuclear mechanisms by which the genetic material is manipulated — and manipulated properly if genomic stability is to be maintained. For, a major consequence for the cell of absence from it of the normal functioning of the *BLM* gene product is an unacceptably high rate of mutation, including hyperrecombination. (Definition of the role of BLM in the germ line has just begun, but clinical observations in BS supplemented by some preliminary laboratory information indicate that it is an important one, probably — judging from the cytogenetics of BS somatic cells — concerned with the control of meiotic recombination.)

The identification of BLM coincides temporally with that of other "new" proteins such as WRN (absent in Werner syndrome), ATM (absent or abnormal in ataxia-telangiectasia), nibrin (absent in Nijmegen breakage syndrome), and the Fanconi anemia proteins. All these proteins were introduced into cell biology via intensive investigation in several laboratories of a group of rare, recessively transmitted phenotypes that, although clinically dissimilar, have for heuristic purposes been lumped for the past 30 years as "chromosome-breakage syndromes."[76] The several proteins concerned with DNA repair (some of which deal with transcription as well) that are absent or abnormal in xeroderma pigmentosum, Cockayne syndrome, and trichothiodystrophy are often advantageously grouped with those abnormal in the classic "breakage" syndromes. The continued study of this recently recognized group of proteins will provide increasingly detailed understanding of cellular mechanisms by which stability of the genome is maintained, and quite possibly also will bring to light some previously unrecognized mutational mechanisms.

Some of this information is of direct and immediate value in the clinical management of the disease states themselves. This is fortunate for the affected persons and families, many of whom have become steadfast — essential — partners with the clinical investigators and their colleagues at the laboratory bench, both in accurately defining and then in understanding their conditions. However, in the broader sense, these rare disorders can be viewed as models for the cell biologist to find out new things. Their greatest importance, therefore, is in providing fundamental understanding in an area of biology that until relatively recently had not even been recognized as something to be studied — how the genome of somatic cells is guarded against change, and what the consequences of somatic mutation can be.

REFERENCES

1. German J: Bloom's syndrome. I. Genetical and clinical observations in the first twenty-seven patients. *Am J Hum Genet* **21**:196, 1969.
2. German J: Bloom's syndrome. II. The prototype of genetic disorders predisposing to chromosome instability and cancer, in German J (ed): *Chromosomes and Cancer.* New York: John Wiley, 1974, p 601.
3. German J: Bloom's syndrome. VIII. Review of clinical and genetic aspects, in Goodman RM, Motulsky AG (eds): *Genetic Diseases Among Ashkenazi Jews.* New York: Raven Press, 1979, p 121.
4. German J: Bloom syndrome: A mendelian prototype of somatic mutational disease. *Medicine* **72**:393, 1993.
5. German J: Bloom's syndrome, in Cohen PR, Kurzrock R (eds): *Genodermatoses with Malignant Potential.* Philadelphia: W.B. Saunders, 1995, p 7.
6. German J: Genes which increase chromosomal instability in somatic cells and predispose to cancer, in Steinberg AG, Bearn AG (eds): *Progress in Medical Genetics,* vol. VIII. New York: Grune and Stratton, 1972, p 61.
7. Ray JH, German J: The cytogenetics of the "chromosome-breakage syndromes," in German J (ed): *Chromosome Mutation and Neoplasia.* New York: Alan R. Liss, 1983, p 135.
8. German J: Bloom's syndrome XVII. A genetic disorder that displays the consequences of excessive somatic mutation, in Bonne-Tamir B, Adam A (eds): *Genetic Diversity Among Jews.* New York: Oxford University Press, 1992, p 129.
9. German J, Passarge E: Bloom's syndrome. XIII. Report from the Registry for 1987. *Clin Genet* **35**:57, 1989.
10. German J: The immunodeficiency of Bloom syndrome, in Ochs HD, Smith JCIE, Puck J (eds): *Primary Immunodeficiency Diseases. A Molecular and Genetic Approach.* New York: Oxford University Press, 1999, p 335.
11. Bloom D: Congenital telangiectatic erythema resembling lupus erythematosus in dwarfs. *Am J Dis Child* **88**:754, 1954.
12. German J: Bloom's syndrome. XX. The first 100 cancers. *Cancer Genet Cytogenet* **93**:101, 1997.
13. Tachibana A, Tatsumi K, Masui T, Kato T: Large deletions at the *HPRT* locus associated with the mutator phenotype in a Bloom's syndrome lymphoblastoid cell line. *Mol Carcinog* **17**:41, 1996.
14. Groden J, Nakamura Y, German J: Molecular evidence that homologous recombination occurs in proliferating human somatic cells. *Proc Natl Acad Sci USA* **87**:4315, 1990.
15. Groden J, German J: Bloom's syndrome. XVIII. Hypermutability of a tandem-repeat locus. *Hum Genet* **90**:360, 1992.
16. Foucault F, Buard J, Praz F, Jaulin C, Stoppa-Lyonnet D, Vergnaud G, Amor-Gueret M: Stability of microsatellites and minisatellites in Bloom syndrome, a human syndrome of genetic instability. *Mutat Res* **362**:227, 1996.
17. Kaneko H, Inoue R, Yamada Y, Sukegawa K, Fukao T, Tashita H, Teramoto T, Kasahara K, Takami T, Kondo N: Microsatellite instability in B-cell lymphoma originating from Bloom syndrome. *Int J Cancer* **69**:480, 1996.
18. Walpita D, Plug AW, Neff NF, German J, Ashley T: Bloom syndrome protein (BLM) co-localizes with RPS in meiotic prophase nuclei of mammalian spermatocytes. *Proc Natl Acad Sci USA* **96**:5622, 1999.
19. German J, Roe AM, Leppert M, Ellis NA: Bloom syndrome: An analysis of consanguineous families assigns the locus mutated to chromosome band 15q26.1. *Proc Natl Acad Sci USA* **91**:6669, 1994.
20. Martin RM, Rademaker A, German J: Chromosomal breakage in spermatozoa: A heterozygous effect of the Bloom syndrome mutation. *Am J Hum Genet* **53**:1242, 1994.
21. Li L, Eng C, Desnick B, German J, Ellis NA: Carrier frequency of the Bloom syndrome blm^{Ash} mutation in the Ashkenazi Jewish population. *Mol Genet Metab* **64**:286, 1998.
22. Shahrabani-Gargir L, Shomrat R, Yaron Y, Orr-Urtreger A, Groden J, Legum C: High frequency of a common Bloom syndrome Ashkenazi mutation among Jews of Polish origin. *Genet Test* **2**:293, 1998.

23. Oddoux C, Clayton CM, Nelson HR, Ostrer H: Prevalence of Bloom syndrome heterozygotes among Ashkenazi Jews. *Am J Hum Genet* **64**:1241, 1999.
24. Roa BB, Savino CV, Richards CS: Ashkenazi Jewish population frequency of the Bloom syndrome gene 2281 delta 6ins7 mutation. *Genet Test* **3**:219, 1999.
25. Ellis NA, Roe AM, Kozloski J, Proytcheva M, Falk C, German J: Linkage disequilibrium between the FES, D15S127, and *BLM* loci in Ashkenazi Jews with Bloom syndrome. *Am J Hum Genet* **55**:453, 1994.
26. Ellis NA, Groden J, Ye T-Z, Straughen J, Lennon DJ, Ciocci S, Proytcheva M, German J: The Bloom's syndrome gene product is homologous to RecQ helicases. *Cell* **83**:655, 1995.
27. Weksberg R, Smith C, Anson-Cartwright L, Maloney K: Bloom syndrome: A single complementation group defines patients of diverse ethnic origin. *Am J Hum Genet* **42**:816, 1988.
28. McDaniel LD, Schultz RA: Elevated sister chromatid exchange phenotype of Bloom syndrome cells is complemented by human chromosome 15. *Proc Natl Acad Sci USA* **89**:7968, 1992.
29. German J, Ellis NA, Proytcheva M: Bloom's syndrome. XIX. Cytogenetic and population evidence for genetic heterogeneity. *Clin Genet* **49**:223, 1996.
30. Bryant EM, Hoehn H, Martin GM: Normalization of sister chromatid exchange frequencies in Bloom's syndrome by euploid cell hybridization. *Nature* **279**:795, 1979.
21. Ellis NA, Lennon DJ, Proytcheva M, Alhadeff B, Henderson EE, German J: Somatic intragenic recombination within the mutated locus *BLM* can correct the high-SCE phenotype of Bloom syndrome cells. *Am J Hum Genet* **57**:1019, 1995.
32. Ellis NA, Ciocci S, German J: Back mutation at *BLM* can correct the high-SCE phenotype of Bloom syndrome (BS) cells. *Am J Hum Genet* **63**:A175, 1998.
33. Ellis NA, German J: Molecular genetics of Bloom's syndrome. *Hum Mol Genet* **5**:1457, 1996.
34. Straughen J, Ciocci S, Ye T-Z, Lennon DN, Proytcheva M, Goodfellow P, German J, Ellis NA, Groden J: Physical mapping of the Bloom syndrome region by the identification of YAC and P1 clones from human chromosome 15 band q26.1. *Genomics* **33**:118, 1996.
35. Straughen J, Johnson J, McLaren D, Proytcheva M, Ellis NA, German J, Groden J: A rapid method for detecting the predominant Ashkenazi Jewish mutation in the Bloom's syndrome gene. *Hum Mut* **11**:175, 1998.
36. Ellis NA, Ciocci S, Proytcheva M, Lennon D, Groden J, German J: The Ashkenazi Jewish Bloom syndrome mutation blm^{Ash} is present in non-Jewish Central Americans. *Am J Hum Genet* **63**:1685, 1998.
37. Karow JK, Chakraverty RK, Hickson ID: The Bloom's syndrome gene product is a $3'–5'$ DNA helicase. *J Biol Chem* **272**:30611, 1997.
38. Nakayama H, Nakayama K, Nakayama R, Irino N, Nakayama Y, Hanawalt PC: Isolation and genetic characterization of a thymineless death-resistant mutant of *Escherichia coli* K12: identification of a new mutation (*recQ1*) that blocks the RecF recombination pathway. *Mol Gen Genet* **195**:474, 1984.
39. Umezu K, Nakayama K, Nakayama H: *Escherichia coli* RecQ protein is a DNA helicase. *Proc Natl Acad Sci USA* **87**:5363, 1990.
40. Harmon FG, Kowalczykowski SC: RecQ helicase, in concert with RecA and SSB proteins, initiates and disrupts DNA recombination. *Genes Dev* **12**:1134, 1998.
41. Hanada K, Ukita T, Kohno Y, Saito K, Kato J, Ikeda H: RecQ DNA helicase is a suppressor of illegitimate recombination in *Escherichia coli*. *Proc Natl Acad Sci USA* **94**:3860, 1997.
42. Courcelle J, Carswell-Crumpton C, Hanawalt PC: *recF* and *recR* are required for the resumption of replication at DNA replication forks in *Escherichia coli*. *Proc Natl Acad Sci USA* **94**:3714, 1997.
43. Gangloff S, McDonald JP, Bendixen C, Arthur L, Rothstein R: The yeast type I topoisomerase top3 interacts with Sgs1, a DNA helicase homolog: a potential eukaryotic reverse gyrase. *Mol Cell Biol* **14**:8391, 1994.
44. Watt PM, Louis EJ, Borts RH, Hickson ID: Sgs1: A eukaryotic homolog of *E. coli* RecQ that interacts with topoisomerase II in vivo and is required for faithful chromosome segregation. *Cell* **81**:253, 1995.
45. Lu J, Mullen JR, Brill SJ, Kleff S, Romeo AM, Sternglanz R: Human homologues of yeast helicase. *Nature* **383**:678, 1996.
46. Watt PM, Hickson ID, Borts RH, Louis EJ: SGS1, a homologue of the Bloom's and Werner's syndrome genes, is required for maintenance of genome stability in *Saccharomyces cerevisiae*. *Genetics* **144**:935, 1996.
47. Yamagata K, Kato J, Shimamoto A, Goto M, Furuichi Y, Ikeda H: Bloom's and Werner's syndrome genes suppress hyperrecombination in yeast sgs1 mutant: Implication for genomic instability in human diseases. *Proc Natl Acad Sci USA* **95**:8733, 1998.
48. Harmon FG, DiGate RJ, Kowalczykowski SC: RecQ helicase and topoisomerase III comprise a novel DNA strand passage function: a conserved mechanism for control of DNA recombination. *Mol Cell* **3**:611, 1999.
49. Murray JM, Lindsay HD, Munday CA, Carr AM: Role of *Schizosaccharomyces pombe* RecQ homolog, recombination, and checkpoint genes in UV damage tolerance. *Mol Cell Biol* **17**:6868, 1997.
50. Stewart E, Chapman CR, Al-Khodairy F, Carr AM, Enoch T: rqh1+, a fission yeast gene related to the Bloom's and Werner's syndrome genes, is required for reversible S phase arrest. *Embo J* **16**:2682, 1997.
51. Davey S, Han CS, Ramer SA, Klassen JC, Jacobson A, Eisenberger A, Hopkins KM, Sieberman HB, Freyer GA: Fission yeast rad12+ regulates cell cycle checkpoint control and is homologous to the Bloom's syndrome disease gene. *Mol Cell Biol* **18**:2721, 1998.
52. Goodwin A, Wang SW, Toda T, Norbury C, Hickson I: Topoisomerase III is essential for accurate nuclear division in *Schizosaccharomyces pombe*. *Nucleic Acids Res* **27**:4050, 1999.
53. Bahr A, De Graeve F, Kedinger C, Chatton B: Point mutations causing Bloom's syndrome abolish ATPase and DNA helicase activities of the BLM protein. *Oncogene* **17**:2565, 1998.
54. Morozov V, Mushegian AR, Koonin EV, Bork P: A putative nucleic acid-binding domain in Bloom's and Werner's syndrome helicases. *Trends Biochem Sci* **22**:417, 1997.
55. Puranam KL, Blackshear PJ: Cloning and characterization of *RECQL*, a potential human homologue of the *Escherichia coli* DNA helicase RecQ. *J Biol Chem* **269**:29838, 1994.
56. Seki M, Miyazawa H, Tada S, Yanagisawa J, Yamaoka T, Hoshino S, Ozawa K, Eki T, Nogami M, Okumura K, Taguchi H, Hanaoka H, Enomoto T: Molecular cloning of cDNA encoding human DNA helicase Q1 which has homology to *Escherichia coli* RecQ helicase and localization of the gene at chromosome 12p12. *Nucleic Acids Res* **22**:4566, 1994.
57. Yu C-E, Oshima J, Fu Y-H, Wijsman EM, Hisama F, Alisch R, Matthews S, Nakuro J, Miki T, Ouais S, Martin GM, Mulligan J, Shellenberg GD: Positional cloning of the Werner syndrome gene. *Science* **272**:258, 1996.
58. Gray MD, Shen JC, Kamath-Loeb AS, Blank A, Sopher BL, Martin GM, Oshima J, Soeb SA: The Werner syndrome protein is a DNA helicase. *Nat Genet* **17**:100, 1997.
59. Suzuki N, Shimamoto A, Imamura O, Kuromitsu J, Kitao S, Goto M, Furuichi Y: DNA helicase activity in Werner's syndrome gene product synthesized in a baculovirus system. *Nucleic Acids Res* **25**:2973, 1997.
60. Huang S, Li B, Gray MD, Oshima J, Mian IS, Campisi J: The premature aging syndrome protein, WRN, is a $3' \rightarrow 5'$ exonuclease. *Nat Genet* **20**:114, 1998.
61. Hoehn H, Bryant EM, Au K, Norwood TH, Bowman H, Martin GM: Variegated translocation mosaicism in human skin fibroblast cultures. *Cytogenet Cell Genet* **15**:282, 1975.
62. Schonberg S, Niermeijer MF, Bootsma D, Henderson E, German J: Werner's syndrome: Proliferation in vitro of clones of cells bearing chromosome translocations. *Am J Hum Genet* **36**:387, 1984.
63. Sinclair DA, Mills K, Guarente L: Accelerated aging and nucleolar fragmentation in yeast sgs1 mutants. *Science* **277**:1313, 1997.
64. Sinclair DA, Guarente L: Extrachromosomal rDNA circles—a cause of aging in yeast. *Cell* **91**:1033, 1997.
65. Kitao S, Ohsugi I, Ichikawa K, Goto M, Furuichi Y, Shimamoto A: Cloning of two new human helicase genes of the *RecQ* family: Biological significance of multiple species in higher eukaryotes. *Genomics* **54**:443, 1998.
66. Kitao S, Shimamoto A, Goto M, Miller RW, Smithson WA, Lindor NM, Furuichi Y: Mutations in RECQL4 cause a subset of cases of Rothmund-Thomson syndrome. *Nat genet* **22**:82, 1999.
67. Neff NF, Ellis NA, Ye TZ, Noonan J, Huang K, Proytcheva M, Sanz M: The DNA helicase activity of BLM is necessary for the correction of the genomic instability of Bloom syndrome cells. *Mol Biol Cell* **10**:665, 1999.
68. Sun H, Karow JK, Hickson ID, Maizels N: The Bloom's syndrome helicase unwinds G4 DNA. *J Biol Chem* **273**:27587, 1998.
69. Foucault F, Vaury C, Barakat A, Thibout D, Planchon P, Jaulin C, Praz F, Amor-Guert M: Characterization of a new BLM mutation associated with a topoisomerase II alpha defect in a patient with Bloom's syndrome. *Hum Mol Genet* **6**:1427, 1997.
70. Ellis NA, Proytcheva M, Sanz MM, Ye TZ, German J: Transfection of *BLM* into cultured Bloom syndrome cells reduces the SCE rate toward normal. *Am J Hum Genet* **65**:1368, 1999.

71. McDaniel LD, Schultz RA: Elevated sister chromatid exchange phenotype of Bloom syndrome cells is complemented by human chromosome 15. *Proc Natl Acad Sci USA* **89**:7968, 1992.
72. Giesler T, Baker K, Zhang B, McDaniel LD, Schultz RA: Correction of the Bloom syndrome cellular phenotypes. *Somat Cell Mol Genet* **23**:303, 1997.
73. Kaneko H, Orii KO, Matsui E, Shimozawa N, Fukao T, Matsumoto T, Shimamoto A, Furuichi Y, Hayakawa S, Kasahara K, Kondo N: BLM (the causative gene of Bloom syndrome) protein translocation into the nucleus by a nuclear localization signal. *Biochem Biophys Res Commun* **240**:348, 1997.
74. Matsumoto T, Shimamoto A, Goto M, Furuichi Y: Impaired nuclear localization of defective DNA helicases in Werner syndrome. *Nat Genet* **16**:335, 1997.
75. Chester N, Kuo F, Kozak C, O'Hara CD, Leder P: Stage-specific apoptosis, developmental delay, and embryonic lethality in mice homozygous for a targeted disruption in the murine Bloom's syndrome gene. *Genes Dev* **12**:3382, 1998.
76. German J: Chromosomal breakage syndromes.. *Birth Defects: Original Article Series* **5**:117, 1969.

CHAPTER 31

Fanconi Anemia

Arleen D. Auerbach ▪ Manuel Buchwald ▪ Hans Joenje

1. Fanconi anemia (FA) is an autosomal recessive disorder that is characterized clinically by diverse congenital abnormalities and a predisposition to bone marrow failure and malignancy, particularly acute myelogenous leukemia (AML). FA patients exhibit extreme clinical heterogeneity and may have abnormalities in any major organ system. It is recognized that the FA phenotype is so variable, with considerable overlap with the phenotypes of a variety of genetic and nongenetic diseases, that diagnosis on the basis of clinical manifestations alone is difficult.

2. FA is found in all races and ethnic groups and has been widely reported to have a carrier frequency of 1 in 300. This estimate was based on the incidence of affected individuals before the full spectrum of the FA phenotype was recognized. The true gene frequency is likely to be considerably higher than this; a low estimate would result from an incomplete ascertainment of cases before the widespread application of chromosomal breakage tests for FA diagnosis. Up to 0.5 percent of the general population may be heterozygous at an FA locus.

3. Hypersensitivity of FA cells to the clastogenic (chromosome-breaking) effect of crosslinking agents provides a unique cellular marker for the disorder. This is used as a diagnostic criterion because of the difficulty of diagnosing FA on the basis of clinical manifestations alone. Comparative studies have led to the choice of diepoxybutane (DEB) as the agent most widely used for FA diagnosis. The crosslinking test can be used to identify preanemic patients as well as patients with aplastic anemia or leukemia who may or may not have the physical stigmata associated with FA.

4. The hypersensitivity of FA cells to crosslinking agents has been used to assess complementation in somatic cell hybrids. Complementation groups usually are considered to represent distinct disease genes, and for FA, at least four groups (A, C, D, and G) represent distinct genes. The first FA gene isolated by expression cloning methodology (*FANCC,* alias *FAC*) mapped to chromosome 9q22.3 by *in situ* hybridization. *FANCA* (alias *FAA*) was mapped by linkage of the disease in FA-A families to microsatellite markers positioned close to the telomere of chromosome 16 (16q24.3). *FANCD* (alias *FAD*) was mapped to 3p22-26 by microcell-mediated chromosome transfer. *FANCG* (alias *FAG*) is identical with the previously isolated human gene *XRCC9,* which was mapped to 9p13. Considerable variability in the prevalence of the different complementation groups has been observed among various ethnic groups. Overall, FA-A is the most prevalent group, accounting for 60 to 65 percent of all FA cases.

5. A cDNA expression cloning procedure was adapted and used successfully to clone the gene defective in FA-C cells (*FANCC*). The *FANCC* coding region contains 14 exons and leads to a predicted protein of 558 amino acids. The predicted structure of FANCC does not resemble that of any known protein and has no obvious functional domains. The protein is found primarily in the cytoplasm, although approximately 10 percent is in the nucleus. FANCC appears to play a direct role in protecting cells against the damage produced by crosslinking agents.

6. Homologous recombination in embryonic stem (ES) cells has been used to target the endogenous *Fancc* locus, with the consequent removal of exon 8 or exon 9. These cells have been used to derive strains of mice (*Fancc*$^{-/-}$) in which no active Fancc protein is produced. The mutant mice show the characteristic FA sensitivity to crosslinkers but do not demonstrate any morphologic or hematopoietic phenotypes up to 1 year of age. In addition to the cellular sensitivity, the principal phenotype of *Fancc*$^{-/-}$ mice is decreased fertility of both male and female animals. This phenotype appears to be a more severe version of similar disease-related complications in FA patients.

7. *FANCA* was cloned by two parallel approaches. One was essentially the same as that used to clone *FANCC.* A cDNA clone was identified that corrected the crosslink hypersensitivity of FA-A cells but not that of FA-C cells. *FANCA* also was identified through positional cloning of the 16q24.3 region. The defective gene was identified by fine mapping, contig isolation, and exon trapping. *FANCA* codes for a predicted protein of 1455 amino acids that has no strong homologies to known proteins. On the basis of a predicted nuclear localization signal, the protein may be localized to the nucleus. The gene contains 43 exons spanning approximately 80 kb. More than 70 mutations in *FANCA* have been described worldwide. The heterogeneity of the mutation spectrum and the frequency of intragenic deletions present a considerable challenge for the molecular diagnosis of FA-A.

8. A cDNA representing the FA-G gene *FANCG* was isolated from the same expression library used for the functional cloning of *FANCC* and *FANCA.* The 2.5-kb complementing cDNA was identified as identical to human *XRCC9,* a novel gene defined by its capacity to partially complement the MMC-sensitive Chinese hamster mutant UV40. The encoded FAG/XRCC9 protein has no sequence similarities to any other known protein, including FAA and FAC, and has no functional motifs.

9. Transplantation with hematopoietic stem cells from bone marrow or umbilical cord blood currently offers the only possibility for a cure for bone marrow failure in FA as well as a possible cure for or prevention of leukemia. Recent analyses of HLA-matched sibling transplants show that increased survival is associated with younger age, less severe hematologic disease, and absence of malignant transformation.

Fanconi anemia (FA) is an autosomal recessive disorder that is characterized clinically by diverse congenital abnormalities and a predisposition to bone marrow failure and malignancy, particularly

A list of standard abbreviations is located immediately preceding the index in each volume. Nonstandard abbreviations used in this chapter include: FA = Fanconi anemia; AML = acute myelogenous leukemia; DEB = diepoxybutane; MMC = mitomycin C; MDS = myelodysplastic syndrome; BM = bone marrow.

acute myelogenous leukemia (AML).[1-3] FA patients exhibit extreme clinical heterogeneity and may have abnormalities in any major organ system.[4] Clinical heterogeneity in FA is both interfamilial and intrafamilial; there is a lack of concordance for specific congenital malformations among affected siblings, and even monozygotic twins may exhibit phenotypic heterogeneity.[5] FA cells exhibit an abnormally high level of chromosomal breakage and are hypersensitive to both the cytotoxic and the clastogenic effects of DNA crosslinking agents such as diepoxybutane (DEB) and mitomycin C (MMC).[6-9] The relationship of this DNA instability to the potential for FA patients to develop cancer is unknown.

It is recognized that the FA phenotype is so variable, with considerable overlap with the phenotypes of a variety of genetic and nongenetic diseases, that a correct diagnosis on the basis of clinical manifestations alone is difficult.[10,11] Although the pathophysiology of the syndrome is unknown, diagnosis of FA has been facilitated by the study of DEB-induced chromosomal breakage, which provides a unique marker for the FA genotype.[12-15] This cellular characteristic can be used as a diagnostic test to identify preanemic patients as well as patients with aplastic anemia or leukemia who may or may not have the classic physical stigmata associated with FA.[16]

The clinical variability of FA may be in part dependent on the existence of considerable genetic heterogeneity. A minimum of eight complementation groups have been identified through somatic cell studies, and at least four of these groups (FA-A, FA-C, FA-D, and FA-G) represent independent genetic loci.[17-20] Analysis of patients mutant in the first FA gene to be cloned (*FANCC*) has shown that some of the clinical variability in this group of patients can be accounted for by the different *FANCC* mutations present.[21-23] Further heterogeneity may be attributed to specific genetic events as more of the genes are identified and more patients are analyzed.

Biochemical studies of cells from FA patients have led to a large volume of literature that includes considerable variability in the reproducibility of the results. In hindsight, it can be seen that many of these studies have inadvertently mixed cells from different complementation groups, since the cells under study were not classified.[24] Nevertheless, reproducible phenotypes involving processes that can be explained by defects in DNA repair, oxygen sensitivity, growth factor homeostasis, and cell cycle regulation now are known to be characteristic of FA cells.[25,26] The specific defects in each complementation group are not known.

The procedures for the cloning of FA genes initially exploited the increased sensitivity of FA cells to MMC or DEB. While early studies using genomic DNA were unsuccessful, the use of episomal cDNA libraries led to the identification of *FANCC*, the gene defective in FA patients of group C.[27] A similar approach has led to the identification of *FANCA* and *FANCG*.[28] The *FANCA* gene, which is defective in the majority of FA patients, also was identified by the positional cloning approach.[29] Thus one can expect that during the next few years considerable progress will be made in our understanding of the fundamental defects in FA and their relationship to the development of the FA phenotype. The reader interested in additional material on FA is referred to the book *Fanconi Anemia: Clinial, Cytogenetic and Experimental Aspects*.[30] A chapter on FA in *Aplastic Anemia Acquired and Inherited* offers a comprehensive review of the literature on the clinical aspects of syndrome.[4] Reviews on FA also have been published recently.[24-26,31-34]

CLINICAL ASPECTS ON FA

Historical Perspective

In 1927, Fanconi described a family in which three male children between the ages of 5 and 7 years had pancytopenia and birth defects.[35] On the basis of his observations in this family and others, Fanconi's chief criteria for the diagnosis of FA included pancytopenia, hyperpigmentation, skeletal malformations, small stature, urogenital abnormalities, and familial occurrence. According to Fanconi, Naegeli suggested in 1931 that the term *Fanconi's anemia* be used to describe such patients.[1] Fanconi's observations formed the basis of the chief criteria for the diagnosis of FA for many years. Consideration of FA in the differential diagnosis of a patient manifesting clinical features of the syndrome depends on the clinician's concept of the FA phenotype. Most patients reported in textbooks and in the literature present a clinical picture similar to that of the original patients described by Fanconi. In a study comparing the frequencies of congenital anomalies among FA probands and their affected siblings, Glanz and Fraser observed that there was a significant reduction in the incidence of congenital anomalies among affected siblings compared with probands.[10] Affected siblings with milder phenotypic features were diagnosed after the diagnosis of FA in another affected family member, not because of their phenotypic presentation. In fact, patients with bone marrow failure who completely lacked congenital malformations, who were previously described as having the Estren-Damenshek syndrome, were found in the same sibships as classic FA.[10,36,37] In a survey of black African children with FA and associated congenital malformations, more than 90 percent of diagnoses were delayed until the development of hematologic abnormalities.[38] The delay in diagnosis in the majority of FA patients with congenital malformations indicates the need for an increased awareness among physicians of the clinical features associated with the syndrome.[11] It has been recognized that the FA phenotype is extremely variable and that congenital malformations in FA may involve any of the major organ systems. FA patients may present with *v*ertebral anomalies, *a*nal atresia, *t*racheo*e*sophageal fistula, and *r*adial (*l*imb), *r*enal, and *c*ardiac abnormalities. These abnormalities constitute the *VATER* or *VACTERL* syndrome; thus there is considerable overlap of FA with these syndromes. Other syndromes with phenotypic overlap with FA include Holt-Oram syndrome, thrombocytopenia absent radius (TAR), Baller-Gerold syndrome, velocardiofacial syndrome, Diamond-Blackfan anemia, and dyskeratosis congenita. Abnormalities of the central nervous system, gastrointestinal system, and skeletal system (in addition to radial ray defects) have been added to the FA phenotype.[11]

Incidence

FA is found in all races and ethnic groups and is widely cited as having a carrier frequency of 1 in 300.[2] This estimate was based on the incidence of affected individuals in New York State in 1971, before recognition of the full spectrum of the FA phenotype. The true gene frequency is likely to be considerably higher than this; a low estimate would result from an incomplete ascertainment of cases before the widespread application of DEB testing for FA diagnosis.[13] Up to 0.5 percent of the general population may be heterozygous for the FA gene. Generally applicable methods for carrier screening are not available, since heterozygotes cannot be detected by the DEB test, and DNA methods for carrier screening are not available for FA complementation groups other than FA-C. The frequency of FA varies among ethnic populations; some have a particularly high incidence because of a founder effect. The heterozygote frequency has been estimated at 1 in 100 in South African Afrikaans and 1 in 89 (specifically for the IVS4 mutation in *FANCC*) in individuals of Ashkenazi Jewish descent.[39,40] The incidence of individuals affected with FA also is high in certain ethnic groups, such as Turkish and Saudi Arabian, in which consanguineous marriages are common.

Variable Expressivity

A recent analysis of congenital malformations among siblings with FA revealed that there is both interfamilial and intrafamilial phenotypic variation in the specific types of congenital malformations among affected siblings.[5] Fifty-three sibships composed of 120 siblings were analyzed. Even the two sets of monozygotic

(MZ) twins described in this report were phenotypically discordant. In MZ twin pair 1, the fetuses were examined after pregnancy termination as a result of prenatal diagnosis performed because of the presence of two prior affected siblings in the pedigree. Twin A had a bifid thumb, whereas twin B had no physical stigmata of FA. The proband in this sibship had duodenal atresia, whereas the other affected sibling had no congenital abnormalities. In MZ twin pair 2, 15-year-old girls with FA, twin A had unilateral absence of the radius, bilateral absent thumbs, and an absent right clavicle. Twin B had a bifid right thumb, a hypoplastic left thumb, and an absent left clavicle. However, the analysis showed that the occurrence of malformations among FA siblings is nonrandom; siblings usually were concordant for the presence or absence of multiple congenital malformations. Also, an analysis of hematologic abnormalities in FA demonstrated a concordance in the findings in sibships; the age at detection of hematologic abnormalities in probands and siblings was correlated ($p = 0.006$).[41] To explain the clinical heterogeneity in FA, it has been postulated that the phenotypic features of an affected individual depend on the specific FA mutation, somatic DNA instability, other genes, and environmental factors. Thus FA may be caused by genes that directly or indirectly affect morphogenesis.

DIAGNOSTIC CRITERIA

Crosslinker Hypersensitivity

Diagnosis of FA on the basis of clinical manifestations often is difficult and unreliable owing to the considerable overlap of the FA phenotype with those of a variety of genetic and nongenetic diseases.[42–44] Schroeder *et al.* first suggested the use of spontaneous chromosomal breakage as a cellular market for FA; however, longitudinal studies of chromosome instability in FA patients have shown a wide variation in the frequency of baseline breakage within the same individual, ranging from no breakage to high levels.[6,45] Numerous studies of the sensitivity of FA cells to a variety of DNA crosslinking agents have been performed over the past 27 years.[7,8,12,13,16,46–48] Hypersensitivity of FA cells to the clastogenic (chromosome-breaking) effect of crosslinking agents provides a unique cellular marker for the disorder. Comparative studies have led to the choice of DEB as the agent most widely used for FA diagnosis.[16,49] Extensive experience with the DEB test has demonstrated the sensitivity, specificity, and reproducibility of the results.[13,16] Crosslinker hypersensitivity can be used to identify preanemic patients as well as patients with aplastic anemia or leukemia who may or may not have the physical stigmata associated with FA (Tables 31-1 through 31-6 and Figs. 31-1, 31-2 and 31-3).

Clinical Features

The International Fanconi Anemia Registry. More than 800 cases of FA have been reported in varying detail in the literature, and these cases have been reviewed by Young and Alter.[4] The cases in the literature, particularly those reported before the present decade, were reported when aplastic anemia or leukemia developed in individuals with characteristic physical abnormalities; thus reviews in the literature are biased toward the most severe clinical cases. The literature also contains cases diagnosed on the basis of physical manifestations alone, without confirmation by DEB testing; some of these cases are now known to be misdiagnosed. The International Fanconi Anemia Registry (IFAR) was established at the Rockefeller University in 1982 to collect clinical, genetic, and hematologic information from a large number of FA patients in order to study the full spectrum of clinical features of the disease.[50] The primary source of case material for the IFAR is physician reporting. Once a potential case is identified, an IFAR questionnaire form is completed by the referring physician, and copies of laboratory reports and other patient records are obtained with the consent of the patient or guardian. Diagnosis of FA is confirmed by study of chromosomal breakage induced by DEB or another crosslinking agent. Clinical information from the IFAR has been analyzed for phenotypic features and hematologic abnormalities, and the results have been reported in the literature.[3,11,13,41,51] The purpose of some of these reports was to address the need for earlier diagnosis of FA by increasing the awareness of clinicians of the complete phenotypic spectrum of the syndrome. Currently, there are over 700 patients in the IFAR with a diagnosis of FA confirmed in the United States. Large numbers of subjects and long follow-up make this database unique compared with literature reports. However, there are

Table 31-1 Summary of Major Congenital Malformations Observed in IFAR Patients

Abnormality	All FA Patients (percent)
Radial ray	49.1
Other skeletal	21.6
Renal and urinary tract	33.8
Male genital	19.7
Gastrointestinal	14.3
Heart	13.2
Hearing loss	11.3
Central nervous system	7.7

Table 31-2 Radial Ray Abnormalities in IFAR Patients

Bilateral Radial Ray Defect	Unilateral Radial Ray Defect
Absent radii and thumbs	Absent radius and thumb
Absent radius and bilateral thumb abnormality	Hypoplastic radius and thumb abnormality
Hypoplastic radii and bilateral thumb abnormality	Absent thumb
Bilateral absent thumbs	Hypoplastic thumb
Bilateral hypoplastic thumb	Bifid thumb
Unilateral absent thumb, contralateral abnormal thumb	Other
Unilateral hypoplastic thumb, contralateral abnormal thumb	Other

Table 31-3 Other Skeletal Malformations Reported in IFAR Patients

Abnormality	All FA Patients (percent)
Congenital hip	6.6
Vertebral	3.2
Scoliosis	3.2
Rib	3.0
Clubfoot	1.4
Sacral agenesis (hypoplasia)	1.1
Perthes disease	1.1
Sprengel deformity	1.1
Genu valgum	0.8
Leg length discrepancy	0.5
Kyphosis	0.5
Spina bifida	0.3
Navicular aplasia	0.3
Brachydactyly	0.3
Arachnodactyly	0.3
Metacarpal (other than first)	0.3
Craniosynostosis	0.3
Humeral abnormality	0.3
Short toes	0.3
Upper thoracic spine	0.3

Table 31-4 Gastrointestinal Malformations Reported in IFAR Patients

Abnormality	All FA Patients (percent)
Anorectal	5.1
Duodenal atresia	4.6
Tracheoesophageal fistula	3.5
Esophageal atresia	1.4
Annular pancreas	1.4
Intestinal malrotation	1.1
Intestinal obstruction	1.1
Duodenal web	0.5
Biliary atresia	0.3
Foregut duplication cyst	0.3

potential limitations, such as selective reporting and incompleteness and inaccuracy of data reporting. Approximately 10 percent of the patients were examined at the Rockefeller University Hospital or affiliated institutions, which provides a check on the accuracy of data reporting. Summaries of the phenotypic features and hematologic manifestations of FA presented here are taken from the IFAR. Tables 31-1 through 31-6 and Figs. 31-1 through 31-3 show some of the clinical features manifested by the FA patients examined.

Growth Parameters. FA is associated with abnormal growth parameters both prenatally and postnatally. Short stature is a well-recognized feature of the syndrome; the mean stature of FA patients in the IFAR is near the fifth percentile. However, although patients with FA often are shorter than the general population and shorter than their expected heights, most of these individuals are not extremely short. Weight and head circumference are also often less than the fifth percentile. Some children with FA have reduced growth hormone responsiveness and hypothyroidism, which may further compromise their growth. A significant number of FA patients also exhibit highly elevated levels of insulin with a high insulin-glucose ratio on oral glucose tolerance testing, implying insulin resistance.[52] We suggest endocrine evaluation in all FA children, since correction of growth hormone or thyroid hormone deficiency may improve the final height outcome.

Major Congenital Malformations. In a survey of the clinical findings obtained from the IFAR, a number of congenital malformations associated with FA have been described. A review of these data indicated that the FA phenotype is more variable than was previously recognized. Gastrointestinal, central nervous system, and skeletal malformations in FA patients, previously not included as part of the FA phenotype, were observed.[11] Major congenital malformations reported in IFAR patients are summarized in Tables 31-1 through 31-5. This analysis showed that most FA patients with congenital malformations are not diagnosed until after the onset of hematologic abnormalities; delayed diagnosis may be due to lack of physician awareness of the phenotypic

Table 31-5 Central Nervous System Abnormalities Reported in IFAR Patients

Abnormality	All FA Patients (percent)
Hydrocephalus or ventriculomegaly	4.6
Absent septum pellucidum, corpus callosum	1.4
Neural tube defect	0.8
Migration defect	0.8
Arnold-Chiari malformation	0.5
Moyamoya	0.5
Single ventricle	0.3

Table 31-6 Minor Anomalies and Mild Malformations Reported in IFAR Patients

Abnormality	Specific Types
Skin pigmentation	Café-au-lait spots, hyperpigmentation, hypopigmentation
Eye	Short palpebral fissures (microphthalmia), almond-shaped palpebral fissures, hypertelorism, hypotelorism, epicanthal folds
Nose	Flattened nasal bridge, nasal pit
Ear, minor	Low set, protruding, minor helix abnormality
Oral cavity	Arched palate, geographic tongue, thin upper lip
Face	Triangular face, facial asymmetry, facial flattening
Neck	Webbing of neck, low hairline
Hand	Thenar hypoplasia, clinodactyly of fifth digit, syndactyly of fingers, hyperextensible thumbs, arachnodactyly, contractures
Foot	Syndactyly of toes, wide space between first and second toes, pes planus, hypoplastic toenails
Prominent forehead	
Other	Sacral dimple, frontal hair upsweep, chest asymmetry, pectus excavatum

spectrum of FA. From a developmental standpoint, it is interesting that radial ray abnormalities in FA patients can be bilateral or unilateral (see Table 31-2). Even patients with bilateral abnormalities usually exhibit asymmetry, with their limbs having different specific anomalies[13] (see Table 31-2 and Fig. 31-1).

Minor Malformations. Approximately one-third of FA patients do not manifest congenital malformations[11] (see Fig. 31-2). In these patients the diagnosis of FA generally is made only after a patient presents with clinical symptoms of hematologic dysfunction; the mean age of diagnosis in this group is considerably older than that for FA patients with malformations. FA patients without congenital malformations frequently have alterations in growth parameters, with height, weight, or head circumference below the fifth percentile. Other very common findings in these patients are skin pigmentation abnormalities and/or microphthalmia. Minor anomalies and mild malformations reported among FA patients

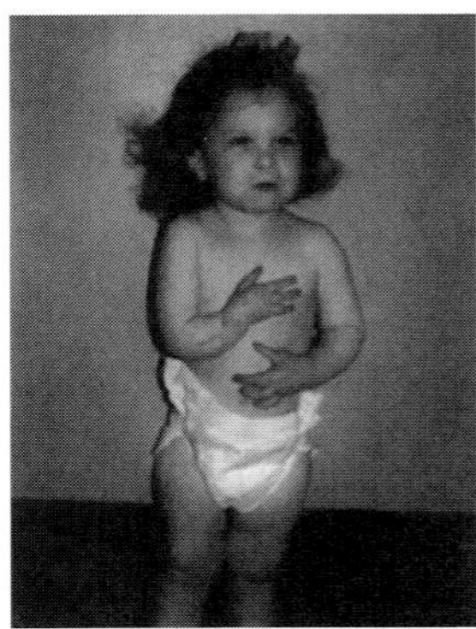

Fig. 31-1 A 2-year-old male of Ashkenazi Jewish ancestry who demonstrates physical features associated with FA. The photograph was taken after surgery on his hands. Before the surgery, the right hand exhibited a hypoplastic radius and absent thumb, whereas the left hand had a hypoplastic thumb. The patient exhibits growth retardation, dysmorphic facial features, microphthalmia, microcephaly, and café-au-lait spots; he also has a kidney abnormality, undescended testes, and a small penis. This patient is homozygous for the IVS4+4 A>T mutation in *FANCC*.

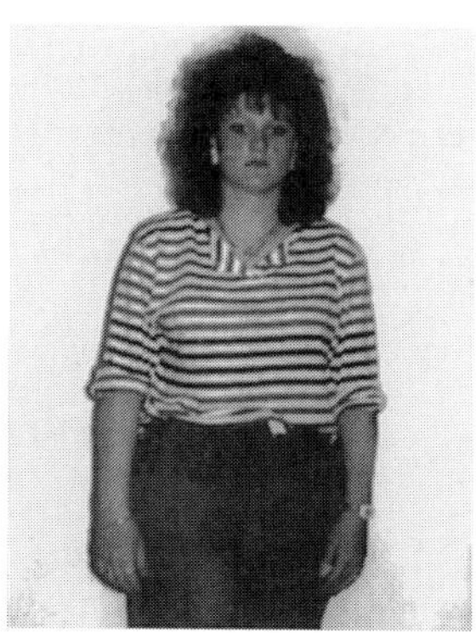

Fig. 31-2 A 17-year-old female with normal phenotypic features. She was diagnosed with FA at age 12 on the basis of hematologic abnormalities and a positive DEB test. She also exhibited short stature and café-au-lait spots. She died at age 21 of AML. This patient is the product of a consanguineous marriage and was homozygous for the Q13X mutation in exon 1 of *FANCC*.

lacking major malformations are listed in Table 31-6.[51] It is noteworthy that many FA patients have distinctive facial characteristics, including microphthalmia and small facial size (see Fig. 31-3). Increased awareness of the facial anomalies as well as the complete spectrum of minor malformations in FA by clinicians should allow an earlier diagnosis to be made in patients without congenital anomalies.

Fertility. Older females have irregular menses, and menopause usually starts during the fourth decade. Fifteen percent of females cited in the literature or reported to the IFAR who reached at least 16 years of age and were not receiving androgen therapy had at least one pregnancy.[4,53] Thus pregnancy can occur in FA, although it often is associated with complications such as progression of bone marrow failure and preeclampsia. Genital malformations and hypoplastic gonads are common findings in males with FA[54] (see Table 31-1). There are extremely few reported cases of affected males having offspring.[55] Results of semen analysis on several males in the IFAR showed abnormal spermatogenesis, with very low sperm counts.

Hematologic Manifestations. An analysis of hematologic data from 388 patients with FA reported to the IFAR showed that hematologic abnormalities were detected in 332 persons at a median age of 7 years (range, birth to 31 years).[41] Actuarial risk of developing a hematologic abnormalities by 40 years of age was 98 percent; actuarial risk of death from hematologic causes was 81 percent by 40 years of age. Initial hematologic findings were diverse; thrombocytopenia associated with an elevated hemoglobin F (HbF) level and macrocytosis usually preceded the onset of anemia or neutropenia. In some cases, patients presented with myelodysplastic syndrome (MDS) or AML without a prior diagnosis of aplastic anemia. Thrombocytopenia and pancytopenia often were associated with decreased bone marrow (BM) cellularity. Actuarial risk of clonal cytogenetic abnormalities during BM failure was 67 percent by 30 years of age. Fifty-nine patients developed MDS and/or AML; actuarial risk of MDS and/or AML by 40 years of age was 52 percent.

In a recent study of genotype-phenotype correlations in FA-C patients, it was shown that the *FANCC* genotype affects clinical outcome and allows division of these patients into three groups: (1) patients with the IVS4 mutation ($n = 26$), (2) patients with at least one exon 14 mutation (R548X or L554P) ($n = 16$), and (3) patients with at least one exon 1 mutation (322delG or Q13X) and no known exon 14 mutation ($n = 17$).[56] Individuals with IVS4 or exon 14 mutations had a significantly earlier onset of hematologic abnormalities and poorer survival compared with exon 1 patients and with the non-FA-C IFAR population. Sixteen of the 59 FA-C patients (27 percent) have developed AML. The incidence of leukemia in each of the FA-C subgroups ranges from 19 to 37 percent. The median age at diagnosis of leukemia is younger in the IVS4 and exon 14 groups compared with the exon 1 group (10.8 and 15.9 years versus 21.9 years). Twenty-eight of the 59 FA-C patients have died. Leukemia was the cause of death in 13 of those 28 (46 percent). Three patients with a history of leukemia have survived; one patient was recently diagnosed, and two are in remission after BM transplantation.

These data indicate an extraordinarily high risk of BM failure and AML in persons with FA and underscore the potential use of FA as a model of BM failure and leukemia development. Recent preliminary data have suggested an increased frequency of *FANCC* sequence variants in children with sporadic AML.[57] Study of a larger series of AML patients and controls, together with analysis of epidemiologic data, is required to substantiate this interesting finding.

Nonhematologic Malignancies. Patients with FA have an increased cancer predisposition. In addition to the extraordinarily high frequency of AML in FA patients (actuarial risk of 52 percent for the development of MDS and/or AML by 40 years of age),[41] FA patients have been reported to exhibit malignancies of a variety of organ systems, most commonly gastrointestinal and

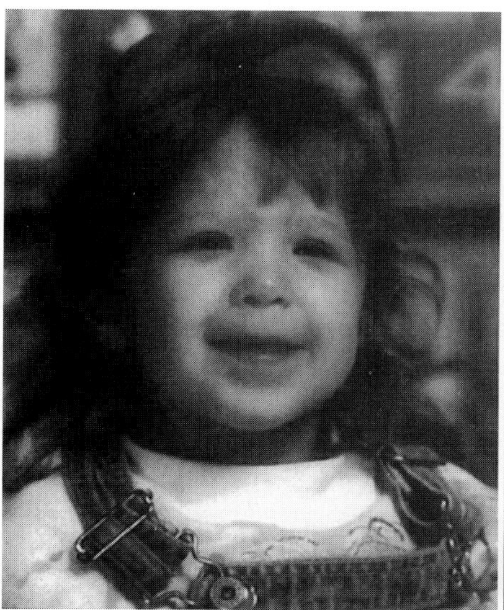

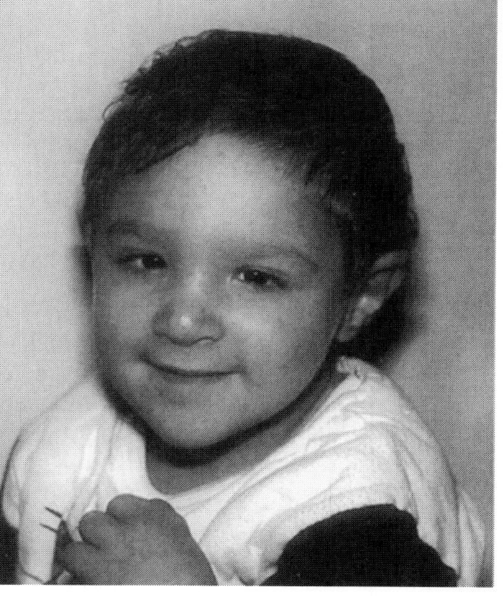

Fig. 31-3 Two unrelated FA patients exhibiting typical facial features of FA. Note microphthalmia and elfinlike facies. These patients are of Ashkenazi Jewish ancestry and are homozygous for the IVS4+4 A>T mutation in FANCC, but similar facial features frequently are seen in genetically diverse FA patients.

Table 31-7 Nonhematologic Malignancies in FA Patients

Type	Specific Variety	No. (n=800)
Oropharygeal	Gingiva, tongue, jaw, mandible, pharynx	17
Gastrointestinal	Esophagus, stomach, anus, colon	13
Gynecologic	Vulva, cervix, breast	9
Central nervous system	Medulloblastoma, astrocytoma	5
Other	Skin, renal, bronchial, lymphoma	6

SOURCE: Adapted from Young NS, Alter BP: Clinical features of Fanconi's anemia, in Young NS, Alter BP (eds): *Aplastic Anemia Acquired and Inherited.* Philadelphia, Saunders, 1994, p 275. Eight hundred patients reported in the literature are reviewed. Cancers exclude leukemia and liver tumors. The latter tumors are associated with androgen therapy.

gynecologic[4,58] (Table 31-7). The high incidence of nonhematologic malignancy in FA patients is especially striking because of the predicted early death from hematologic causes associated with the syndrome (median estimated survival is 23 years; actuarial risk of death from hematologic causes is 81 percent by 40 years of age). Thus patients are unusually young when they develop cancer, and the incidence of malignancy probably would be considerably higher if patients had a longer life expectancy. Most of the nonhematologic tumors in FA patients are squamous cell carcinomas. Liver tumors, mostly hepatocellular carcinomas, are also common in FA. Most of these tumors occur in patients who have been treated with androgen therapy for BM failure. Discontinuation of androgens may lead to resolution of the liver tumors.[4]

GENETIC HETEROGENEITY

Complementation Groups

The hypersensitivity of FA cells to crosslinking agents has been used to assess the complementation of the cellular defect in somatic cell hybrids. Successful complementation is considered indicative of the existence of various genes causing FA, as has been performed previously for xeroderma pigmentosum through the analysis of heterokaryons.[59] The most successful approach has involved the use of Epstein-Barr virus-immortalized lymphoblastoid cell lines. Such studies have revealed an extensive degree of genetic heterogeneity. In the first systematic study, lymphoblastoid cell lines from seven unrelated FA patients were investigated.[18] A HPRT-ouab-resistant derivative of one of these cell lines (HSC72) was used as a universal fusion partner in hybridizations with the other cell lines, allowing selective outgrowth of hybrids in culture medium containing hypoxanthine-aminopterin-thymidine (HAT) plus ouabain. MMC sensitivity versus resistance of the hybrids was used as a criterion for complementation. Two groups of cell lines could be distinguished among the seven studied: three that failed to complement the reference cell line HSC72 in fusion hybrids (termed A) and three that fully complemented the defect (termed B or non-A). The correction of the drug sensitivity phenotype was confirmed by the analysis of both spontaneous and MMC-induced chromosomal breakage.

The three non-A cell lines subsequently were marked with dominant drug resistance markers that were introduced by stable transfection with plasmids conferring hygromycin or neomycin resistance and allowed the selection of fusion hybrids generated from combinations of these cell lines. Since all possible combinations yielded crosslinker-resistant hybrids, each non-A cell line apparently represented a separate complementation group: FA-B, FA-C, and FA-D.[17] This analysis was taken a step further by means of the generation of doubly marked derivatives of the three non-A cell lines and analysis of complementation after fusion with cell lines from another 13 FA patients.[19] All cell lines except one failed to complement only one reference group cell line and therefore could be classified as belonging to an existing group. Mutation screening in four patients who had been assigned to the C group by complementation analysis revealed mutations in *FANCC*, supporting the validity of the complementation analysis. A single cell line (EUFA130) derived from a patient of Turkish ancestry complemented all four existing groups and therefore represented a fifth complementation group, FA-E.[19] Recently, group E, defined as "different from groups A-D,"[60] appeared heterogeneous and could be split up into at least four distinct groups, designated FA-E, FA-F, FA-G and FA-H. Thus at least eight groups are now distinguished.[20]

One Gene per Group?

Complementation groups usually are considered to represent distinct disease genes. However, in another autosomal recessive chromosomal instability disorder, ataxia-telangiectasia, this assumption has not been borne out, since mutations were found in a single gene (*ATM*) in patients previously assigned to four different complementation groups.[61] For FA, however, at least four complementation groups (A, C, D, and G) must represent distinct genes on the basis of their separate positions in the human genetic map. The first FA gene isolated by expression cloning methodology (*FANCC*) mapped to chromosome 9q22.3 by *in situ* hybridization, whereas different map positions were recently established for *FANCA, FANCD,* and *FANCG.* A consortium of investigators used a panel of nine FA families classified as FA-A by complementation analysis to map the *FANCA* locus to 16q24.3.[62] A genomewide search using microsatellite markers led to the initial linkage to D16S520. More refined analysis, including other FA families, led to a lod score of 8.01 at $\theta = 0.00$ to marker D16S305. This finding was independently replicated by the results of a genomewide scan using homozygosity mapping to identify genes causing FA.[63] This study was performed using 23 inbred families from the IFAR. Complementation studies were not performed in these patients, but families known to belong to FA-C were excluded from the family set. Significant genetic heterogeneity ($p = 0.0013$) was shown with marker D16S520 (maximum lod score $= 6.08$; $\alpha = 0.66$). Simultaneous search analysis suggested several additional chromosomal regions that were not the locations for FA-C and FA-D that could account for a small fraction of FA in the family set, but sample size was insufficient to provide statistical significance. Fine genetic mapping using multipoint linkage analysis with a test of heterogeneity showed $Z_{max} = 27.16$, $\theta = 0.00$, $\alpha = 0.73$ at D16S303, the most telomeric marker on chromosome 16q. The mapping panel for this study included 50 multiplex or consanguineous families from the IFAR selected only on the basis of being non-group C.[64]

Microcell-mediated chromosome transfer was used to map the *FANCD* gene to the short arm of chromosome 3, 3p22-26,[65] while the recently cloned group G gene maps to chromosome 9p13. A gene mutated in cell line PD20, the immortalized fibroblast cell line used for the microcell fusion studies that mapped *FANCD* to chromosome 3p, has been isolated by positional cloning.[65a] As this gene has not yet been found mutated in the FA-D reference cell line HSC62, further studies are required to resolve the issue as to whether this is the *FANCD* gene. These data suggest that for FA the one group equals one gene concept does seem to hold up.[66] Results from the complementation studies thus strongly suggest that at least eight distinct genes, when defective, can cause FA.

Relative Prevalence of Complementation Groups

Cell fusion studies are a time-consuming and labor-intensive means of determining the genetic subtype of FA patients. Consequently, only a limited number of patients have been analyzed by functional complementation analysis, and the results may well be biased depending on the different ethnic backgrounds of the patients analyzed. The figures reported in a recent cumulative European-U.S.-Canadian survey based on 47 patients indicate 66 percent to be group A, 4.3 percent to be B, 12.7 percent to be C, 4.3 percent to be D, and 12.7 percent to be E (non-A-D).

Group E now consists of groups E-H; the relative prevalence of these groups is not yet established. Results of a fine mapping study based on a racially and ethnically diverse mapping panel of 50 non-C IFAR families indicated that 73 percent of these families were in group A.[64] This result is based on the fraction of families showing linkage to marker D16S303, the most telomeric marker on chromosome 16q, which is known be very close to the location of *FANCA* on the physical map.[29] Since approximately 15 percent of IFAR patients are in group C, FA-A accounts for about 62 percent of patients in the IFAR.

It is clear that different populations may have widely different pictures. The IVS4+4 A>T splice site mutation in *FANCC* is responsible for most cases of FA in the Ashkenazi Jewish population.[21,22] In a study of over 3000 Jewish individuals, primarily of Ashkenazi descent, the frequency of IVS4 carriers was shown to be 1 in 89.[40] The high carrier frequency of the IVS4 mutation places FA-C in the group of so-called Jewish genetic diseases, which includes Tay-Sachs, Gaucher, and Canavan diseases, among others. With a carrier frequency of more than 1 percent and simple testing available, the IVS4 mutation merits inclusion in the battery of tests routinely provided to the Jewish population. Group C also is relatively prevalent among Dutch patients, mainly exhibiting the exon 1 frameshift 322delG, whereas group A is the prevalent complementation group represented in Italy as well as in the Afrikaans-speaking population of South Africa.[60,62,67] Somatic cell hybidization analysis of 21 consecutively sampled patients, mainly from Germany and The Netherlands, found all eight complementation groups represented. We are virtually ignorant about complementation groups in the relatively large Asian populations, even though FA has been encountered in people of Chinese, Korean, Japanese, and Indian ancestry (Auerbach, unpublished IFAR data). Once the genes for the different complementation groups have been identified, the relative prevalences of the groups in different parts of the world can begin to be estimated through mutation screening methods.

THE BASIC DEFECT IN FA

Defining the basic defect in FA has been complicated by the extensive genetic heterogeneity present in the disease. The bulk of the biochemical literature has been derived from the analysis of unclassified FA cell lines. If the fundamental defect is different in the various complementation groups, this could lead to the inadvertent analysis of two or more basic defects simultaneously. This may explain some of the difficulties encountered by different laboratories in reproducing each other's results. At present, hypotheses to account for the pleiotropic FA phenotype postulate abnormalities in DNA repair, oxygen metabolism, growth factor homeostasis, and cell cycle regulation.[24–26,34]

DNA Repair

FA has been considered a DNA repair disorder in which the defect(s) lie in the repair of DNA crosslinks, thus explaining the increased sensitivity of FA cells to DNA crosslinking agents, hypomutability, and increased frequency of forming deletions.[68–73] Defects in DNA repair would cause abnormal cell replication in hematopoietic, osteogenic, and other cells and would lead to the developmental defects. However, biochemical studies of DNA repair defects in FA cells have been inconclusive or contradictory.[24,25] This may represent the confounding effect of studying cells from different complementation groups or the fact that repair deficiencies may be secondary to the primary (proximate) basic defect. The most convincing evidence for a DNA repair defect is in FA-A, where cell extracts are defective in incising crosslinked DNA and have lower amounts of a protein that binds to interstrand crosslinks.[74,75] In contrast, in FA-C it has been suggested that the defect lies in the initial induction of crosslinks, not in the subsequent repair phase.[76] In a recent study, FA cells exhibited inappropriately elevated levels of homologous recombination activity.[77] Defects in blunt DNA end-joining, which can be corrected by transfection of *FANCC,* have been reported in FA-C.[78] Similarly, defects in double-strand break processing are characteristic of FA-B and FA-D cells.[79] In addition, FA group C and D cells exhibited an elevated frequency of aberrant rearrangements generated during V(D)J recombination, again consistent with excessive degradation of DNA ends during repair of double-strand breaks.[80] Since double-strand breaks are frequently produced during fundamental cellular processess such as replication, repair, and recombination, these studies suggest a mechanism for the elevated chromosomal breakage and deletion proneness in FA.

Oxygen Toxicity

It has been suggested that the FA phenotype may arise from defects in oxygen metabolism.[81] This would explain the sensitivity of the growth of FA cells to ambient oxygen, which is reflected in increased chromosomal aberrations and as accumulation of cells in the G2 phase of the cell cycle.[82–84] The increased sensitivity to oxygen could be due either to increased production of toxic intermediates (e.g., free radicals) or to their decreased removal.[85–87] The sensitivity of FA cells to DNA crosslinking agents may result from aberrant handling of reactive metabolities produced during intracellular activation.[81,88] The increased sensitivity to ambient oxygen also could affect the growth of FA cells *in vivo*, including those in the hematopoietic cell lineages. However, introduction of *FANCC* cDNA into FA-C lymphoblasts does not alter their oxygen sensitivity.[89] This result is consistent with the view that the oxygen sensitivity is a secondary feature of the basic defect, since SV40-transformed FA fibroblasts are not oxygen-sensitive but still retain their hypersensitivity to DNA crosslinkers.[90] The possible involvement of cytochrome P450 in spontaneous and induced chromosomal breaks has been suggested.[91]

Growth Factor Homeostasis

The nearly universal BM failure and the high incidence of congenital malformations in FA patients have led to suggestions that the FA genes function directly in cellular growth and/or differentiation.[26,92,93] Antisense oligonucleotides complementary to FANCC mRNA inhibit the *in vitro* clonal growth of normal erythroid and granulocyte-macrophage progenitor cells, even in the presence of exogenous growth factors.[94] Similarly, peripheral blood CD34+ cells isolated from an FA-C patient and transduced with a recombinant adeno-associated virus containing the FANCC cDNA exhibit a 5- to 10-fold increase in the number of progenitor colonies formed in vitro.[95] FA fibroblasts grow slower and senesce more rapidly than do matched controls and demonstrate ultrastructural and physiological changes characteristic of cells from aged individuals.[9,96,97] The FA gene products may play a role in regulating the levels of growth factors, many of which act in both hematopoiesis and osteogenesis.[98] Addition of interleukin-6 (IL-6) to FA lymphoblast cultures reduces the sensitivity of those cells to MMC and DEB and decreases the number of chromosomal breaks.[99] Increased amounts of tumor necrosis factor-α (TNFα) have been reported in FA cell cultures and in patient serum samples, and anti-TNFα antibodies partially correct the chromosomal fragility of FA cells.[99–101]

Cell Cycle Regulation/Apoptosis

The basic defect may directly cause the known abnormalities of cell cycle regulation seen in FA cells.[102] More specifically, it has been suggested that FA cells may be defective in apoptosis, or programmed cell death, implicated in the G2 arrest and death of cells treated with DNA crosslinking agents.[103,104] The high variability of the FA phenotype, including lack of concordance between identical twins, suggests that the FA gene products may function in a cellular process such as apoptosis.[5] Such a relationship is also implied by the involvement of apoptosis in hematopoiesis and in embryonic development, i.e., formation of the forelimb, which is abnormal in many FA patients.[105,106] The role of FANCC in apoptosis has been investigated by various groups and is discussed in more detail below.

The primary defects in FA probably involve one (or more) of the previously mentioned biologic systems. The FA gene products could function as separate steps in the same pathway (e.g., growth factor homeostasis) or could be in different pathways (e.g., some in DNA repair and others in oxygen metabolism), or all products could be part of a multiprotein complex involved in one pathway (e.g., DNA repair). Each of these models would be expected to lead to a set of similar phenotypes in the various patients.[107] An intriguing recent observation is the elevation of *MxA,* one of the interferon-inducible genes, in cells of four FA complementation groups and its reduction in complemented FA-C cells.[108] This would suggest that the FA subtypes converge onto a final common pathway related to interferon signaling.

IDENTIFICATION OF THE FA GENES

In view of the difficulties in defining the basic defect in FA through biochemical analysis of FA cells, various groups have attempted to clone the defective genes directly. The first approach used to identify the FA genes involved correcting the MMC sensitivity of FA cells by introducing genomic DNA from normal cells (marker rescue) and then isolating the complementing DNA. This procedure has been used to isolate the normal human version of several mutant genes in ultraviolet (UV)- and MMC-sensitive Chinese hamster ovary (CHO) cells.[59] The genes so identified are called *ERCC* (*e*xcision *r*epair *c*ross-*c*omplementing) and are the human homologues of the mutant *CHO* genes. They show similarities to bacterial and yeast repair genes, suggesting their direct role in similar processes in mammalian cells.[109–111] Several *ERCC* genes were shown subsequently to be equivalent to xeroderma pigmentosum genes.[34,112] With respect to FA, partial complementation of the MMC-sensitive phenotype of both FA-A and FA-D cells using mouse DNA was reported, but these initial studies did not lead to the identification of an FA gene.[114–116] To overcome the disadvantages of the preceding method for the cloning of FA genes, a cDNA expression cloning procedure was adapted and used successfully to initially clone the gene defective in FA-C cells (*FANCC*) and, more recently, *FANCA* and *FANCG.*

Cloning of *FANCC*

The cDNA expression system uses the pREP4 vector, based on the regulatory sequences of the Epstein-Barr virus that allow it to function as an episomal shuttle vector between bacterial and human cells.[117] A cDNA library constructed in pREP4 was used to clone a set of cDNAs that specifically complemented the MMC and DEB sensitivity of FA-C cells.[27] After transfection of the cDNA library into HSC536 (FA-C) cells and selection in MMC and/or DEB, the low-molecular-weight DNA was isolated from populations of growing cells. Eight candidate cDNAs were detected in the various pools and were tested individually for their ability to specifically complement the cellular defect of FA-C cells. A set of complementing cDNAs was identified that coded for the same predicted ORF. Alternate forms of the cDNA contain three alternative 3′ UTRs, each terminated by a consensus polyadenylation signal, in combination with one of two 5′ UTRs. The 5′ UTRs reflect the presence of alternative transcriptional start sites spliced to a common downstream exon, since they all possess suitable splice donor sites only at the 3′ end.[27,118,119] The murine, rat, and bovine cDNAs also are characterized by multiple 3′ UTRs.[120,121] Their significance is not known. The FA-C cells used in the selection of the FANCC cDNA carry a mutation predicted to produce an L554P substitution that inactivates the cDNA.[27,122] The second mutant allele of this cell line leads to a deletion of 327 bp that eliminates all putative ATG start codons, leading to a nonfunctional transcript.[123] *FANCC* was localized to 9q22.3 by *in situ* hybridization.[17] The mapping of *FANCC* was confirmed by genetic analysis of known FA-C patients.[21,22] Analysis of these patients led to the identification of frameshift, splicing, amino acid substitutions, and chain termination mutations. In some cases (e.g., IVS4+4 A>T) no protein is detected, whereas in others (e.g., L554P) a protein of normal size is seen.[21,22,124,125] Thus a number of protein modifications lead to the FA phenotype, suggesting that all alterations abrogate *FANCC* function. Figure 31-4 summarizes known mutations and polymorphic sequence variations in *FANCC.* Mutations and polymorphisms in *FANCC* are listed in the Fanconi Anemia Mutation Database at *http://www.rockefeller.edu/fanconi/mutate/.*

Features of *FANCC*

The *FANCC* coding region contains 14 exons and leads to a predicted protein of 558 amino acids.[27] The noncoding 5′ exons, now called −1, −1a, and −1b, have suitable splice signals as their 3′ ends but not at their 5′ ends.[27,118,119] The region upstream of exon −1 has promoter activity in transfection assays using a luciferase reporter gene.[119] All 17 exons have been mapped to phages isolated from a genomic library; the minimum size of *FANCC* is 150 kb, since two introns are not completely defined.[126] The 3′ terminal half of the mouse gene was isolated as a step toward the development of the *Fancc*$^{-/-}$ mouse model; the human and mouse genes are strikingly similar in this region.[127] The mouse ORF shows 79 percent amino acid similarity to the human.[120] The mouse and rat genes have been mapped, the former in close proximity to the flexed-tail locus.[128]

Function of FANCC

The predicted structure of FANCC (and Fancc) does not resemble that of any known protein. The protein is found primarily in the cytoplasm, although approximately 10 percent is in the nucleus.[124,129,130] The predicted ORF codes for a 63-kDa protein

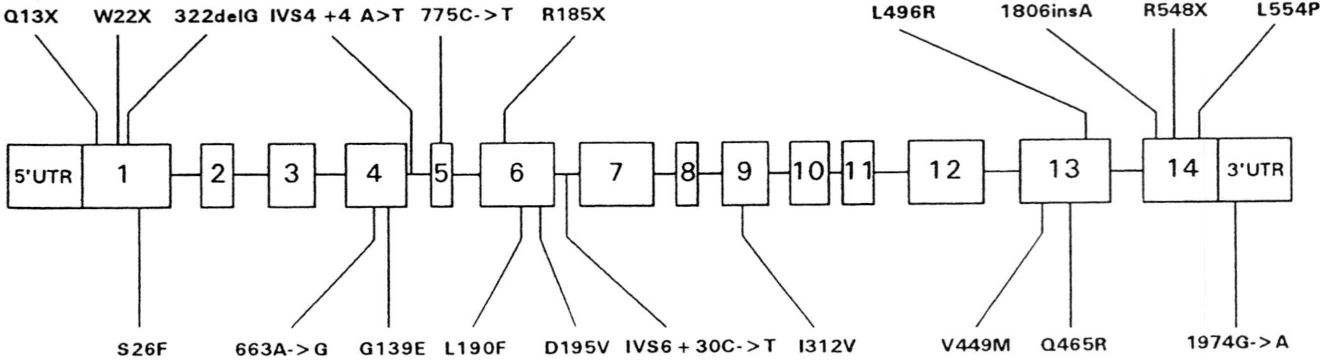

Fig. 31-4 Nucleotide sequence changes in the *FANCC* gene. A schematic diagram of the 14 coding exons of the gene is provided, with the pathogenic mutations shown above and polymorphisms shown below the diagram.[195] *(Data are from Refs. 21, 22, 27, and 195–200.)*

(558 amino acids) with a preponderance of hydrophobic amino acids but no predicted transmembrane domains.[27] No functional motifs have been identified within the protein that could serve as clues to its biologic role.[27] Comparison of the primary sequences of the human, mouse, rat, and bovine proteins does not reveal, apart from putative phosphorylation sites, any obvious regions of higher homology, thus precluding identification of more instructive functional domains.[121] The FA cellular phenotype of increased sensitivity to MMC can be recreated by introducing *FANCC* antisense oligonucleotides into wild-type cells, suggesting that FANCC plays a direct role in protecting cells against the cytotoxic and clastogenic action of this compound.[94]

In vitro transcription and translation of the cDNA produce a protein with an apparent molecular weight of 60 kDa, and a protein of similar size is immunoprecipitated from lymphoblasts or transfected cells using anti-FANCC antibodies.[117,124,129] The predicted protein has no obvious nuclear localization motifs and, as determined by immunofluorescence and subcellular fractionation, appears to be primarily cytoplasmic.[124,129] Targeting of FANCC to the nucleus renders it incapable of correcting the MMC sensitivity of FA-C cells.[76] Immunoprecipitation of FANCC from cell extracts has identified a set of associated cytoplasmic proteins of approximately 70, 50, and 30 kDa.[131] The existence of FANCC-binding proteins is also supported by the fact that overexpression of the L554P mutant protein in normal cells leads to an FA-like phenotype, suggesting that the presence of elevated levels of an inactive mutant protein sequesters other proteins.[125] The 50-kDa protein appears to be an amino truncated form of FANCC that reinitiates at amino acid 55.[23] The molecular chaperone GRP94 binds to FANCC and modulates its intracellular expression.[132]

The cytoplasmic localization of FANCC has led to studies aimed at determining whether the protein has a function in apoptosis. Initial studies have focused on the possible role of FANCC in MMC-mediated apoptosis. Results suggest that FA-C cells may have a generalized defect in apoptosis that is mediated by treatment with MMC or gamma radiation and may involve a failure to induce p53, although conflicting results regarding p53 have been reported.[133–135] Human MO7e and mouse 32D cells expressing FANCC constitutively show a significant delay in cell death compared with the neomycin controls after IL-3 deprivation.[136–138] Thus FANCC appears to play a role in the apoptotic pathway of hematopoietic cells, a role consistent with its cytoplasmic localization as well as its increased expression in hematopoietic precursors. A hypothesis that could explain these observations is that the normal role of FANCC is to modulate the apoptosis that may occur during normal fluctuation of growth factors levels in the marrow microenvironment.[105] More hemopoietic cells will die in FA-C patients than in normal individuals and, with time, will lead to hemopoietic failure. Direct involvement of FANCC in cell cycle regulation has been implied by its direct interaction with a cyclin-dependent kinase (cdc2) which, in turn, regulates G2 progression.[139] However, cell cycle checkpoints do not appear affected in FA-C cells.[140]

Patterns of *FANCC* and *Fancc* Expression

The analysis of gene expression can yield two essential pieces of information about gene function: the sites and levels where the gene functions and the mechanisms that mediate expression. In the case of FA-C, the pleiotropic phenotype of patients and the presence of three putative transcription start sites of the gene point to complex regulation.[27,118,119] Both the human and mouse genes are expressed ubiquitously at low levels in adult tissues.[27,120] Analysis of Fancc expression, using polymerase chain reaction (PCR)-derived cDNA libraries from single hemopoietic cells, shows that higher levels of expression can be detected in less differentiated (multilineage progenitors) than in more differentiated cells (single-lineage progenitors). During mouse embryogenesis, Fancc expression is high in undifferentiated mesenchymal cells 8 to 10 days postconception. Starting at 13 days, expression becomes restricted to regions with rapidly replicating chondro- and osteoprogenitors (e.g., perichondrium), a pattern that persists to later stages (15–19.5 days), except in regions where differentiation has taken place (e.g., hypertrophic chondrocytes of the epiphyseal growth plate). As bone development proceeds, expression is seen in osteogenic and hematopoietic cells in the zone of calcification.[141]

Cloning of *FANCA*

FANCA was cloned by two parallel approaches. One was essentially the same as that used to clone *FANCC*.[27] HSC72 (FA-A) cells were transfected and selected in hygromycin and MMC. A surviving cell population was obtained that exhibited a wild-type level of resistance to MMC and was fully cross-resistant to DEB and *cis*-diamminedichloroplatinum(II). Only one clone was identified that corrected crosslinker hypersensitivity of FA-A cells but not of FA-C cells. Screening of a bacterial artificial chromosome library with the cDNA yielded a positive clone that was used to localize the gene by fluorescence *in situ* hybridization; a signal was observed at the telomere of chromosome 16q, which is the genetic map location established for *FANCA*, thus strengthening the candidacy of this cDNA.[62] To obtain further proof of the identity of the candidate cDNA, cell lines from FA patients classified as FA-A by complementation analysis were screened for mutations in this gene. Various sequence variations were encountered in patients from different ancestral backgrounds; these variations were likely to be pathogenic on the basis of their severity and their segregation with the disease in three informative multiplex families. These data confirmed that the cDNA indeed represented the *FANCA* gene.[28]

The alternative approach used was positional cloning. Subsequent to the mapping of the FA-A locus to 16q24.3, a consortium was established with the objective of cloning the *FANCA* gene as well as a putative breast cancer tumor suppressor gene that maps to the same region of chromosome 16q.[62,63] The candidate region of 16q24.3 was narrowed by further linkage studies and by allelic association analysis. The preliminary physical map of the critical region was developed by screening a gridded chromosome 16 cosmid library with sequence tagged sites and expressed sequence tags. An integrated cosmid contig of about 650 kb was obtained. The cosmids were used for exon trapping and direct selection of cDNAs. Products obtained from the direct selection were used to probe high-density gridded cDNA clones, resulting in the identification of a clone that contained a poly(A) tail and was located at the 3′ end of a candidate gene. An overlapping cDNA clone was then identified; together these two clones gave a combined sequence of 2.3 kb. Exon trapping identified potential additional exons, which were used to extend the sequence by RT-PCR and to screen cDNA libraries for larger clones. One of these was found to be partially deleted in an Italian FA-A patient and was investigated in more detail as a candidate for the *FANCA* gene. Several additional mutations, all of which would be expected to disrupt the function of the protein, were observed in FA-A patients of various ethnic origins.[29] The sequence of this putative *FANCA* cDNA was found to be virtually identical to the cDNA isolated from an expression library, as described previously.

Features of *FANCA*

FANCA has an open reading frame of 4365 bp predicted to encode a protein of 1455 amino acids (~163 kd).[28,29] The gene contains 43 exons ranging from 34 to 188 bp[142] and spans ~80 kb between microsatellites D16S3026 and D16S303.[29] There are no homologies to any known protein that might suggest a function for FAA. Sequence analysis has identified two overlapping nuclear localization signals, as well as a partial leucine-zipper consensus domain, but neither of these domains has yet been demonstrated to be functional.

Over 70 mutations in *FANCA* have been reported worldwide.[28,29,143–148] These include missense, nonsense, splicing, and frameshift mutations, which are widely distributed over the gene. A large number of the mutations are microdeletions/

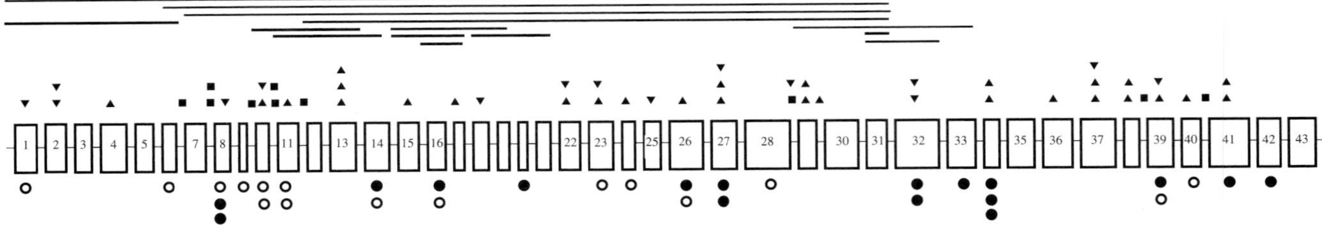

— LARGE DELETION
▲ MICRODELETION / MICROINSERTION
O POLYMORPHISMS IN THE CODING SEQUENCE
● MISSENSE MUTATION
■ SPLICE SITE ALTERATION
▼ NONSENSE MUTATION

Fig. 31-5 Spectrum of ~85 mutations in the *FANCA* gene. A schematic diagram of the 43 coding exons of the gene is provided, with large deletions, microdeletions/microinsertions, and nonsense mutations shown above and missense mutations and polymorphisms in the coding sequence shown below the diagram.[142] (*Data are from Refs. 28, 29, and 143–148.*) Specific mutations and polymorphisms in *FANCA* are listed in the Fanconi Anemia Mutation Database at *http://www.rockefeller.edu/fanconi/mutate/*.

microinsertions associated with short direct repeats or homonucleotide tracts, a type of mutation thought to be generated by a mechanism of slipped-strand mispairing during DNA replication.[143] The sequence CCTG (CAGG), observed to be a hot spot for homologous recombination leading to mutations in a large number of human genes, is found in the vicinity of some mutations in *FANCA*. In addition, the TTC repeat (MboII restriction site) motif, another hot spot for spontaneous deletions, is also associated with microdeletions/microinsertions in *FANCA*.[143] Very few *FANCA* mutations are shared between affected individuals. The two most common mutations, 3788-3790del and 1115-1118del, are carried on about 5 and 2 percent of *FANCA* alleles, respectively.[143] 3788-3790del, a common mutation demonstrating a founder effect in the Brazilian population, appears in a variety of ethnic groups. The mutation spectrum of *FANCA* also includes a variety of large genomic deletions that are difficult to detect by PCR-based screening methods. The presence of numerous *Alu* repeat elements in *FANCA* suggests that *Alu*-mediated recombination might be an important mechanism for the generation of *FANCA* mutations.[146,147] The heterogeneity of the mutation spectrum and the frequency of intragenic deletions make the molecular diagnosis of FA a formidable task. The assignment of complementation group based on screening of FA patients for mutations in *FANCA* will be much less useful than it was for *FANCC*.[21,40,56] A more practical method for initial identification of FA-A patients may be to use retroviral gene transfer into primary T-lymphocytes or lymphoblastoid cell lines, as recently described.[149–151] The subsequent identification of the specific mutations in a family, a step necessary in order to offer rapid prenatal diagnosis and carrier detection as well as genetic counseling, will offer a significant challenge. Mutations and polymorphisms in *FANCA* are listed in the Fanconi Anemia Mutation Database at *http://www.rockefeller.edu/fanconi/mutate/*. Figure 31-5 summarizes the spectrum of known mutations in *FANCA*.

The presence of sequence-specific hypermutable regions in *FANCA* suggests that *FANCA* may have a higher mutation rate than the genes for the other FA complementation groups, which would explain why FA-A accounts for approximately two-thirds of all FA patients.[143] This also raises the possibility that *FANCA* may be susceptible to increased somatic mutation, which would have implications for FA-A heterozygotes. The FA cellular phenotype of genomic instability predisposes FA cells to malignant transformation and a very high cancer incidence in FA patients. The epidemiologic and molecular implications of the hypothesis of increased somatic mutation in *FANCA* increasing the cancer risk of *FANCA* heterozygotes are currently being tested. So far there is no evidence to implicate a mutated *FANCA* gene in breast tumors with loss of heterozygosity at 16q24.3.[152]

Cloning of *FANCG*

A cDNA representing the group G gene, *FANCG,* was recently isolated by expression library transfection of a lymphoblast cell line derived from an FA-G patient.[153] The 2.5-kb complementing cDNA insert was identified as human *XRCC9,* a recently described novel gene defined by its capacity to partially cross-complement the MMC-sensitive Chinese hamster mutant.[154,155]

XRCC9 is localized to chromosome band 9p13,[154] a region reported to harbor a non-A,B,C,D FA gene.[156] Proof that this gene indeed represented the *FANCG* gene came from the presence of pathogenic mutations in four unrelated FA patients. FA-G is the first proven example of a FA complementation group with a counterpart among experimentally obtained hamster cell mutants selected on the basis of sensitivity to DNA damaging agents. The encoded protein has no sequence similarities to any other known protein, including FANCA and FANCC, has no functional motifs, and has no apparent homolog in yeast. Thus *FANCG* is yet another FA gene with an enigmatic function. The recently described partial nuclear localization of *FANCA* and *FANCC* indicates that at least part of the FA pathway is confined to the nucleus.[130,157] Even though the precise functions of the FANCC, FANCA, and FANCG/XRCC9 proteins are elusive so far, they are assumed to operate in concert with at least five additional proteins, i.e., the products from the *FANCB, FANCD, FANCE, FANCF,* and *FANCH* genes.

ANIMAL MODELS FOR FA-C

Mouse models of human disease can be useful in a variety of studies, including the development of novel therapies. Flexed-tailed mice have been considered as possible models for FA-C, since the *f* locus is positioned close to *Fancc*.[128] However, flexed-tail mice do not have an increased sensitivity to MMC.[158] Either the flexed-tail mouse is not mutated at the *Fancc* locus or the mutation is mild. Since no natural mouse mutations in the *Fancc* locus are known, a murine model must be developed experimentally. Homologous recombination in embryonic stem (ES) cells has been used to target the endogenous *Fancc* locus with the consequent removal of exon 8 or exon 9.[159,160] These cells have been used to derive strains of mice (*Fancc*$^{-/-}$) in which no active Fancc protein is produced. The mutant mice show the characteristic FA sensitivity to DNA crosslinking agents but do not demonstrate any morphologic phenotypes or hematopoietic failure to 1 year of age.[161,162]

In addition to the cellular sensitivity to DNA crosslinking agents, the principal phenotype of *Fancc*$^{-/-}$ mice is markedly decreased fertility of both male and female animals.[159,160] This phenotype appears to be a more severe version of similar complications seen in FA patients (see "Fertility" above). Male mice have testicular atrophy, degeneration of seminiferous tubules, low numbers of mature sperm, and epithelial sloughing in the epididymis. These results suggest that *Fancc* plays a role in sperm maturation. Females cannot carry embryos beyond days 9 to 10 of gestation. Analysis of a small number of *Fancc*$^{-/-}$ females shows ovarian hypoplasia and/or abnormal decidua, suggesting that the defect is physiological.

The mild hematologic and morphologic phenotype of *Fancc*$^{-/-}$ mice perhaps is surprising given the abundant levels of *Fancc* expression during embryogenesis, especially in early mesenchyme and zones of endochondral ossification and in early hematopoietic progenitors. On the other hand, treatment of *Fancc*$^{-/-}$ mice with chronic, low doses of MMC leads to profound pancytopenia, detected both by a striking acellularity of the marrow cavity and loss of progenitors in *in vitro* assays, and subsequent death.[163] Hematopoietic progenitor cells from *Fancc*$^{-/-}$mice are hypersensitive to interferon-γ (IFN-γ)[160,163] as well as TNFα and macrophage inflammatory protein-1α, both with respect to growth and apoptosis.[165] Recently, transgenic mice overexpressing human FANCC were created.[166] Experiments with these *FANCC*-transgenic mice implicate FANCC in the regulation of apoptosis mediated by the Fas death receptor. These various studies suggest a role for *FANCC* in bone marrow homeostasis. Thus these FA-C mouse models promise to be useful in helping us understand the *in vivo* role of *FANCC* as well as in testing new therapies.

DIAGNOSIS AND TREATMENT

The DEB Test

The clinical variability in FA is so great that diagnosis must be based on a laboratory test that measures the sensitivity of cells to chromosomal breakage induced by crosslinking agents.[13,16] Comparative studies have led to the choice of DEB as the agent most widely used for FA diagnosis because of reports of false-positive and false-negative diagnoses when other agents are used. It is recommended that patients have a peripheral blood sample tested at birth if they have congenital malformations known to be associated with FA.[11] All siblings of FA patients also should be screened routinely, because a lack of concordance of phenotype in affected siblings makes clinical diagnosis unreliable even within sibships.[5] Peripheral blood is the preferred tissue for the diagnosis of FA, since the sample is easy to obtain and work with and the results of the analysis of crosslinker-induced chromosome breakage can be obtained within 3 to 4 days. Data from DEB testing indicate that there is great variability in the degree of hypersensitivity in FA patients, although there is no overlap with the normal range[13] (Fig. 31-6). Approximately 10 percent of patients with a positive crosslinker test appear to have two populations of lymphocytes; the majority of crosslinker-treated cells examined have no chromosomal breakage, whereas the remainder exhibit the high number of breaks and exchanges typical of FA patients.[13] Interestingly, there is no correlation between the degree of crosslinker hypersensitivity and the presence or absence of birth defects in FA patients.

The chromosomal breakage test also can be applied to the study of fetal cells obtained by chorionic villus sampling (CVS), amniocentesis (AFC), or percutaneous umbilical blood sampling (PUBS).[14,15] Prenatal testing for FA in North American pregnancies with a known 1 in 4 recurrence risk (in couples who have had a previously affected child) tested from 1978 through March 1998 are as follows: 80 CVS, 78 AFC, 158 total (28 FA, 130 normal).[167] These results are consistent with the expected ratio. Results from CVS sometimes are uncertain; in these cases it is recommended that PUBS be performed to clarify the diagnosis. The protocols used for both prenatal and postnatal diagnosis of FA using the DEB test are described in detail in *Current Protocols in Human Genetics*.[168]

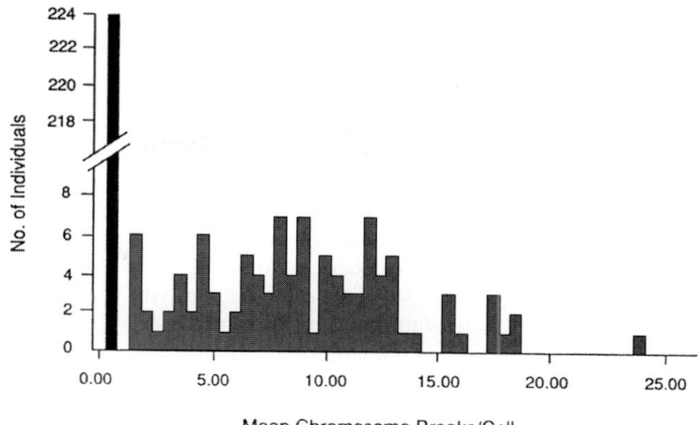

Fig. 31-6 DEB-induced chromosomal breakage in peripheral blood lymphocytes from patients studied at Rockefeller University. Solid bar: 5 DEB-insensitive (non-FA) patients; hatched bars: 5 DEB-sensitive (FA) patients. There is no overlap in the range for the two groups when data are expressed as mean chromosome breaks per cell. Note heterogeneity in the degree of hypersensitivity of FA patients. (*From Auerbach et al.*[13] *Used by permission.*)

Hematologic Mosaicism

Two sets of observations suggest that a proportion of FA patients may exhibit hematologic mosaicism. First, two cell types are occasionally detected in chromosomal breakage tests of cross-linker-treated PHA-stimulated peripheral blood lymphocytes, one demonstrating an FA phenotype and the other demonstrating a normal one.[13,169] In addition, lymphoblastoid cell lines derived from FA patients may be DEB/MMC-resistant.[170] Apparently, in a proportion of blood cells from such mosaic patients the disease phenotype has reverted to normal. The origin of such a reversion in an MMC-resistant lymphoblastoid cell line from a female FA-C patient has been determined recently. This patient was compound heterozygous for two frameshift mutations, one in exon 1 (322delG) and the other in exon 14 (1806insA). Because of mitotic recombination in the phenotypically reverted cells, both mutations are now present in the same allele, whereas the other one has lost its mutation.[171] This phenomenon also has been described in lymphoblast lines from patients with Bloom syndrome and has been correlated with a presumed hyperrecombination phenotype of Bloom syndrome cells.[172] Although the clinical significance of this type of mosaicism in lymphoid cells is unclear, FA patients with sustained mosaicism may benefit from having phenotypically reverted cells. If such an event occurred in a hematopoietic stem cell, it might provide the capability of normal hematopoiesis and ultimately lead to improvement in the patient's hematologic condition. Several examples of patients with mosaicism who had unusually mild or no hematologic symptoms have been seen (Auerbach, unpublished IFAR data).[171] Thus hematopoietic mosaicism may serve as a natural model for gene therapeutic intervention to improve hematopoiesis in FA patients. However, most patients in the IFAR who manifested lymphocyte mosaicism developed severe hematologic disease. Further studies will be necessary to elucidate the diagnostic and clinical implications of mosaicism in FA.

Treatment

Allogeneic hematopoietic cell transplantation using stem cells from BM or umbilical cord blood currently offers the only proven treatment with the potential possibility for a cure for correcting the BM failure in FA patients as well as a possible cure or prevention of leukemia. Nontransplantation treatment strategies include androgen therapy (most commonly oxymetholone initiated at 2 mg/kg/day, which provides improvement in peripheral blood counts in about 50 percent of FA patients treated.[4] However, even patients who exhibit a good initial response to androgens usually become refractory to this treatment in time and eventually require blood cell and platelet transfusions to maintain adequate peripheral blood counts. Complications of androgen therapy include virilization, acne, liver toxicity, and liver tumors. If either of the latter two complications occur, alternative therapies have to be investigated. Treatment with hematopoietic growth factors may provide improvement in white blood counts but generally does not result in significant improvement in red blood cell or platelet counts.[173–175] Granulocyte colony-stimulating factor (G-CSF) treatment was associated with the occurrence of monosomy 7 in the BM of some patients; long-term administration of this drug requires close monitoring for the development of MDS or leukemia. The use of gene therapy for treatment of FA-C currently is under investigation in a phase I clinical trial at the National Institutes of Health.[177] In this approach, hematopoietic progenitor cells from an FA-C patient are collected by aphoresis, transduced *ex vivo* with an retroviral vector containing a normal *FANCC* cDNA, and reinfused into the patient.[176,178] The aim of this approach is to provide hematopoietic reconstitution with a genetically normalized pool of stem cells. Unfortunately, current methods of targeting retroviral vectors to primitive human stem cells are extremely inefficient.[177] There is no evidence of a long-term cure for any genetic disease achieved by this method; thus it seems unlikely that gene therapy will provide a cure for FA in the near future.

Early experience with BM transplantation for FA showed a poor outcome that was primarily due to regimen-related toxicity; the use of a specially designed pretransplant conditioning protocol that considers the hypersensitivity of FA cells to DNA crosslinking agents including cyclophosphamide greatly improved the results of transplantation in patients with an unaffected HLA-identical sibling available as a donor.[179–182] Recent analysis of 151 HLA-matched sibling transplants for FA from the multicenter International Bone Marrow Registry (IBMTR) and 18 HLA-matched sibling transplants for FA from Cincinnati shows that increased survival is associated with younger age, less severe hematologic disease, and absence of malignant transformation.[183,184] However, only 30 to 40 percent of patients in need of therapy have an HLA-matched family donor. Experience has indicated that many families will pursue future pregnancies in hopes of having a nonaffected HLA-matched sibling to provide a source of hematopoietic stem cells for transplantation.[185] Preimplantation diagnosois of unaffected HLA-matched embryos is also being investigated as an option for families in which the FA mutations are known, but no pregnancies have yet been achieved in FA families using this technology. Although the results of unrelated BM transplants are inferior to those using an HLA-matched sibling, such transplants may be the only option for a patient with severe hematologic disease or evidence of malignant transformation.[151,154]

In vitro studies have shown that there are a sufficient number of stem/progenitor cells in cord blood for hematopoietic reconstitution; this has led to the use of umbilical cord blood as an alternative to in place of BM as a source of transplantable stem cells.[186] To test whether umbilical cord blood from an HLA-identical sibling could be used for transplantation, one would first need to harvest the cord blood at the birth of an individual known to be histocompatible and not affected with hematopoietic disease. Cord blood was used successfully for the first time in a clinical trial in 1988 to treat a patient affected with FA.[187,188] Subsequently, the Placental Blood Program was established at the New York Blood Center in 1992 to test the feasibility of using banked placental blood from unrelated donors for transplantation.[189] Since 1988, there have been an estimated 500 related and unrelated donor umbilical cord blood transplants.[190] The results of phase I clinical trials using both matched and mismatched (up to three mismatched antigens with high-resolution typing) unrelated donor umbilical cord blood from the Placental Blood Program for transplantation have shown that this source of transplantable hematopoietic stem cells has a high probability of donor engraftment and a low risk of severe acute graft-versus-host disease.[191,192] Several FA patients were included in these trials. Since most FA patients do not have a matched sibling or unrelated donor from the National Marrow Donor Program (NMDP) or other international BM donor pools, the availability of an alterative source of stem cells for hematopoietic reconstitution may be a breakthrough in the treatment of FA. Although the results of unrelated hematopoietic stem cell transplants are inferior to those using an HLA-matched sibling, such transplants may be the only option for a patient with severe hematologic disease or evidence of malignant transformation.[183,193,194]

ACKNOWLEDGMENTS

We gratefully acknowledge the contribution of the many physicians who referred patients to the IFAR and the students, fellows, and collaborators who have contributed to research in Fanconi anemia. Most of all we acknowledge the fortitude and commitment of patients with FA and their families for their continuous support of FA research.

Work in the laboratory of ADA was supported in part by Grant HL 32987 from the National Institutes of Health, by the Fanconi Anemia Research Fund, Inc. (FARF), and by General Clinical Research Center Grants RR00102 from the National Institutes of Health to the Rockefeller University Hospital and RR-06020 to The New York, Presbyterian Hospital-Weill Medical College of Cornell University. Work in the laboratory of MB was supported by grants from NIH (HL 50131), the Medical Research Council of Canada, the National Cancer Institute of Canada, the Genetic Diseases Network (Canada), and private donations. Work in the laboratory of HJ was supported by the Dutch Cancer Society, the European Cancer Centre, Amsterdam, the Commission of the European Union (Contract PL 931562), and FARF and FA patient support organizations in Italy, France, Germany, and the Netherlands.

REFERENCES

1. Fanconi G: Familial constitutional panmyelocytopathy, Fanconi's anemia (F.A.): I. Clinical aspects. *Semin Hematol* **4**:233, 1967.
2. Swift M: Fanconi's anemia in the genetics of neoplasia. *Nature* **230**:370, 1971.
3. Auerbach AD, Allen RG: Leukemia and preleukemia in Fanconi anemia patients: A review of the literature and report of the International Fanconi Anemia Registry. *Cancer Genet Cytogenet* **51**:1, 1991.
4. Young NS, Alter BP: Clinical features of Fanconi's anemia, in Young NS, Alter BP (eds): *Aplastic Anemia Acquired and Inherited.* Philadelphia, Saunders, 1994, p 275.
5. Giampietro PF, Verlander PC, Maschan A, Davis JG, Auerbach AD: Fanconi anemia: A model for somatic gene mutation during development. *Am J Med Genet* **52**:36, 1994.
6. Schroeder TM, Anschultz F, Knoff A: Spontane Chromosomenaberrationen bei familiarer Panmyelopathie. *Humangenetik* **1**:194, 1964.
7. Sasaki MS, Tonomura A: A high susceptibility of Fanconi's anemia to chromosome breakage by DNA cross-linking agents. *Cancer Res* **33:1829, 1973.**
8. Auerbach AD, Wolman SR: Susceptibility of Fanconi's anaemia fibroblasts to chromosome damage by carcinogens. *Nature* **261**:494, 1976.
9. Weksberg R, Buchwald B, Sargent P, Thompson MW, Siminovitch L: Specific cellular defects in patients with Fanconi anemia. *J Cell Physiol* **101**:311, 1979.
10. Glanz A, Fraser FC: Spectrum of anomalies in Fanconi anaemia. *J Med Genet* **19**:412, 1982.
11. Giampietro PF, Adler-Brecher B, Verlander PC, Pavlakis SG, Davis JG, Auerbach AD: The need for more accurate and timely diagnosis in

Fanconi anemia: A report from the International Fanconi Anemia Registry. *Pediatrics* **91**:1116, 1993.

12. Auerbach AD, Adler B, Chaganti RSK: Prenatal and postnatal diagnosis and carrier detection of Fanconi anemia by a cytogenetic method. *Pediatrics* **67**:128, 1981.
13. Auerbach AD, Rogatko A, Schroeder-Kurth TM: International Fanconi Anemia Registry: Relation of clinical symptoms to diepoxybutane sensitivity. *Blood* **73**:391, 1989.
14. Auerbach AD, Sagi M, Adler B: Fanconi anemia: Prenatal diagnosis in 30 fetuses at risk. *Pediatrics* **76**:794, 1985.
15. Auerbach AD, Zhang M, Ghosh R, Pergament E, Verlinsky Y, Nicholas H, Bot EJ: Clastogen-induced chromosomal breakage as a marker for first trimester prenatal diagnosis of Fanconi anemia. *Hum Genet* **73**:86, 1986.
16. Auerbach AD: Fanconi anemia diagnosis and the diepoxybutane (DEB) test (editorial). *Exp Hematol* **21**:731, 1993.
17. Strathdee CA, Duncan AMV, Buchwald M: Evidence for at least four Fanconi anemia genes including *FACC* on chromosome 9. *Nature Genet* **1**:196, 1992.
18. Buchwald M, Clarke C, Ng J, Duckworth-Rysiecki, Weksberg R: Complementation and gene transfer studies in Fanconi anemia, in Schroeder-Kurth TM, Auerbach AD, Obe G (eds): *Fanconi Anemia: Clinical, Cytogenetic and Experimental Aspects*. Heidelberg, Springer-Verlag, 1989, p 228.
19. Joenje H, Lo Ten Foe, JR, Ostra AB, van Berkel CGM, Rooimans MA, Schroeder-Kurth T, Wagner R-D, et al: Classification of Fanconi anemia patients by complementation analysis: Evidence for a fifth genetic subtype. *Blood* **86**:2156, 1995.
20. Joenje H, Oostra AB, Wijker M, Di Summa F, Van Berkel C, Ebell W, Van Weel M, et al: Evidence for at least eight Fanconi anemia genes. *Am J Hum Genet* **61**:940, 1997.
21. Verlander PC, Lin JD, Udono MU, Zhang Q, Gibson RA, Mathew CG, Auerbach AD: Mutation analysis of the Fanconi anemia gene *FACC*. *Am J Hum Genet* **54**:595, 1994.
22. Whitney MA, Saito H, Jakobs PM, Gibson RA, Moses RE, Grompe MA: A common mutation in the *FACC* gene causes Fanconi anaemia in Ashkenazi-Jewish individuals. *Nature Genet* **4**:202, 1993.
23. Yamashita T, Wu N, Kupfer G, Corless C, Joenje H, Grompe M, D'Andrea AD: The clinical variability of Fanconi anemia (type C) results from expression of an amino terminal truncated Fanconi anemia complementation group C polypeptide with partial activity. *Blood* **87**:4424, 1996.
24. Buchwald M, Moustacchi E: Is Fanconi anemia caused by a defect in the processing of DNA damage? *Mutat Res* **408**:75, 1998.
25. Dos Santos CC, Gavish H, Buchwald M: Fanconi anemia revisited: Old ideas and new advances. *Stem Cell* **12**:142, 1994.
26. Liu JM, Buchwald M, Walsh CE, Young NS: Fanconi anemia and novel strategies for therapy. *Blood* **84**:3995, 1994.
27. Strathdee CA, Gavish H, Shannon W, Buchwald M: Cloning of cDNAs for Fanconi anaemia by functional complementation. *Nature* **356**:763, 1992.
28. Lo Ten Foe, JR, Rooimans MA, Bosnoyan-Collins L, Alon N, Wijker M, Parker L, Lightfoot J, et al: A cDNA for the major Fanconi anemia gene, *FANCA*. *Nature Genet* **14**:320, 1996.
29. The Fanconi Anaemia Breast Cancer Consortium: Positional cloning of the Fanconi anaemia group A gene. *Nature Genet* **14**:324, 1996.
30. Schroeder-Kurth TM, Auerbach AD, Obe G: *Fanconi Anemia: Clinical, Cytogenetic and Experimental Aspects*. Heidelberg, Springer-Verlag, 1989.
31. Joenje H, Mathew C, Gluckman E: Fanconi anemia research: Current status and prospects. *Eur J Cancer* **31A**:268, 1995.
32. D'Andrea A, Grompe M: Molecular biology of Fanconi anemia: Implication for diagnosis and therapy. *Blood* **90**:1725, 1997.
33. D'Apolito M, Zelante L, Savoia A: Molecular basis of Fanconi anemia. *Haematologica* **83**:533, 1998.
34. Auerbach AD, Verlander PC: Disorders of DNA replication and repair. *Curr Opin Pediatr* **9**:600, 1997.
35. Fanconi G: Familaäre infantile perniziosaartige Anämie (pernizioses Blutbild und Konstitution). *Jahrb Kinderh* **117**:257, 1927.
36. Estren S, Dameshek W: Familial hypoplastic anemia of childhood: Report of eight cases in two families with beneficial effect of splenectomy in one case. *Am J Dis Child* **73**:671, 1947.
37. Dallapiccola B, Alimena G, Brinchi V, Isacchi G, Gandini E: Absence of chromosome heterogeneity between classical Fanconi's anemia and the Estren Dameshek type. *Cancer Genet Cytogent* **2**:349, 1980.
38. Macdougall LG, Greeff MC, Rosendorff J, Bernstein R: Fanconi anemia in black African children. *Am J Med Genet* **36**:408, 1990.
39. Rosendorff J, Bernstein R, Macdougall L, Jenkins T: Fanconi anemia: Another disease of unusually high prevalence in the Afrikaans population in South Africa. *Am J Med Genet* **2**:793, 1987.
40. Verlander PC, Kaporis A, Liu Q, Zhang Q, Seligsohn U, Auerbach AD: Carrier frequency of the IVS4+4 A>T mutation of the Fanconi anemia gene *FANCC* in the Ashkenazi Jewish population. *Blood* **86**:4034, 1995.
41. Butturini A, Gale RP, Verlander PC, Adler-Brecher B, Gillio AP, Auerbach AD: Hematologic abnormalities in Fanconi anemia: An International Fanconi Anemia Registry study. *Blood* **84**:1650, 1994.
42. Giampietro PF, Auerbach AD, Elias ER, Gutman A, Zellers N, Davis JD: A new recessive syndrome characterized by increased chromosomal breakage and several features which overlap with Fanconi anemia. *Am J Med Genet* **78**:70, 1998.
43. Poole SR, Smith ACM, Hays T, McGavran L, Auerbach AD: Monozygotic twin girls with congenital malformations resembling Fanconi anemia. *Am J Med Genet* **42**:780, 1992.
44. Milner RGD, Khallour KA, Gibson R, Hajianpour A, Matthew CG: A new autosomal recessive anomaly mimicking Fanconi's anemia phenotype. *Arch Dis Child* **68**:101, 1993.
45. Schroder TM, Tilgen D, Kruger J, Vogel F: Formal genetics of Fanconi's anemia. *Hum Genet* **32**:257, 1976.
46. Schuler D, Kiss A, Fabian F: Chromosomal peculiarities and in vitro examinations in Fanconi's anaemia. *Humangenetik* **7**:314, 1969.
47. Cervenka J, Arthur D, Yasis C: Mitomycin C test for diagnostic differentiation of idiopathic aplastic anemia and Fanconi anemia. *Pediatrics* **67**:119, 1981.
48. Poll EHA, Arwert F, Joenje H, Eriksson AW: Cytogenetic toxicity of antitumor platinum compounds in Fanconi's anemia. *Hum Genet* **61**:228, 1982.
49. Schroeder-Kurth TM, Zhu TH, Hong Y, Westphal I: Variation in cellular sensitivities among Fanconi anemia patients, non-Fanconi anemia patients, their parents and siblings, and control probands, in Schroder-Kurth TM, Auerbach AD, Obe G (eds): *Fanconi Anemia: Clinical, Cytogenetic and Experimental Aspects*. Heidelberg, Springer-Verlag, 1989, p 105.
50. Auerbach AD, Rogatko A, Schroder TM: International Fanconi Anemia Registry (IFAR): First report, in Schroeder TM, Auerbach AD, Obe G (eds): *Fanconi Anemia, Clinical Cytogenetic and Experimental Aspects*. Heidelberg, Springer-Verlag, 1989, p 3.
51. Giampietro PF, Verlander PC, Davis JG, Auerbach AD: Diagnosis of Fanconi anemia in patients without congenital malformations: An International Fanconi Anemia Registry Study. *Am J Med Genet* **68**:58, 1997.
52. Wajnrajch MP, Gertner JM, Huma Z, Popovic J, Lin K, Verlander PC, Batish SD, Giampietro PF, Davis JG, New MI, Auerbach AD: Evaluation of growth and hormonal status in patients referred to the International Fanconi Anemia Registry. *J Pediatrics* In Press, 2000.
53. Alter BP, Frissora CL, Halperin DS, Freedman MH, Chitkara U, Alvarez E, Lynch L, et al: Fanconi's anemia and pregnancy. *Br J Haematol* **77**:410, 1991.
54. Bargman GJ, Shahidi NT, Gilbert EF, Opitz JM: Studies of malformation syndromes of man: XLVII. Disappearance of spermatogonia in the Fanconi anemia syndrome. *Eur J Pediatr* **125**:162, 1977.
55. Liu JM, Auerbach AD, Young NS: Fanconi anemia presenting unexpectedly in an adult kindred with no dysmorphic features. *Am J Med* **91**:555, 1991.
56. Gillio AP, Verlander PC, Batish SD, Giampietro PF, Auerbach AD: Phenotypic consequences of mutations in the Fanconi anemia *FANCC* gene: An International Fanconi Anemia Registry study. *Blood* **90**:58, 1997.
57. Awan A, Taylor GM, Gokhale DA, Dearden SP, Witt A, Stevens RF, Birch JM, et al: Increased frequency of Fanconi anemia group C genetic variants in children with sporadic acute myeloid leukemia. *Blood* **91**:4813, 1998.
58. Alter BP: Fanconi's anemia and malignancies. *Am J Hematol* **53:99, 1996.**
59. Thompson LH: Properties and applications of human DNA repair genes. *Mutat Res* **247**:213, 1991.
60. Joenje H, for EUFAR: Fanconi anemia complementation groups in Germany and the Netherlands. *Hum Genet* **97**:280, 1996.
61. Savitsky K, Bar-Shira A, Gilad S, Rotman G, Ziv Y, Vanagaite L, Tagle DA, et al: A single ataxia telangiectasia gene with a product similar to P1-2 kinase. *Science* **268**:1749, 1995.
62. Pronk JC, Gibson RA, Savoia A, Wijker M, Morgan NV, Melchionda S, Ford D, et al: Localisation of the Fanconi anaemia complementation group A gene to chromosome 16q24.3. *Nature Genet* **11**:338, 1995.

63. Gschwend M, Levran O, Kruglyak L, Ranade K, Verlander PC, Shen S, Faure S, et al: A locus for Fanconi anemia on 16q determined by homozygosity of mapping. *Am J Hum Genet* **59**:377, 1996.
64. Levran O, Fann C, Erlich T, Ott J, Auerbach AD: Linkage analysis of Fanconi anemia: Refinement of the FANCA locus at 16q24.3. *Am J Hum Genet* **59**:A225, 1996.
65. Whitney M, Thayer M, Reifsteck C, Olson S, Smith L, Jakobs PM, Leach R, et al: Microcell mediated chromosome transfer maps the Fanconi anemia group D gene to chromosome 3p. *Nature Genet* **11**:341, 1995.
65a. Timmers CD, Hejna JA, Reifsteck C, Olson SB, Moses RE, Thayer MJ, Grompe M: Positional cloning of the Fanconi anemia complementation group D (*FANCD*) gene. *Am J Hum Genet* **65**(Suppl):A20, 1999.
66. Buchwald M: Complementation groups: One or more per gene? *Nature Genet* **11**:228, 1995.
67. Savoia A, Zatterale A, Del Principe D, Joenje H: Fanconi anemia in Italy: High prevalence of complementation group A in two geographic clusters. *Hum Genet* **97**:599, 1996.
68. Setlow RB: Repair deficient human disorders and cancer. *Nature* **271**:713, 1978.
69. Ishida R, Buchwald M: Susceptibility of Fanconi's anemia lymphoblasts to DNA cross-linking and alkylating agents. *Cancer Res* **42**:4000, 1982.
70. Fujiwara Y, Tatsumi M, Sasaki MS: Cross-link repair in human cells and its possible defect in Fanconi's anemia cells. *J Mol Biol* **113:635, 1977.**
71. Papadopoulo D, Guillouf C, Mohnrenweiser H, Moustacchi E: Hypomutability in Fanconi anemia cells is associated with increased deletion frequency at the HPRT locus. *Proc Natl Acad Sci USA* **87**:8383, 1990.
72. Guillouf C, Laquerbe A, Moustacchi E, Papadopoulo D: Mutagenic processing of psoralen monoadducts differ in normal and Fanconi anemia cells. *Mutagenesis* **8**:355, 1993.
73. Laquerbe A, Moustacchi E, Fuscoe JC, Papadopoulo D: The molecular mechanism underlying formation of deletions in Fanconi anemia cells may involve a site-specific recombination. *Proc Natl Acad Sci USA* **92**:831, 1995.
74. Lambert MW, Tsongalis GJ, Lambert WC, Hang B, Parrish DD: Defective DNA endonuclease activities in Fanconi's anemia, complementation group A, cells. *Mutat Res* **273**:57, 1992.
75. Lambert M, Tsongalis G, Lambert W, Parrish D: Correction of the DNA repair defect in Fanconi anemia complementation groups A and D cells. *Biochem Biophys Res Commun* **230**:587, 1997.
76. Youssoufian H: Cytoplasmic localization of FANCC is essential for the correction of a pre-repair defect in Fanconi anemia group C cells. *J Clin Invest* **97**:2003, 1996.
77. Thyagarajan B, Campbell C: Elevated homologous recombination activity in Fanconi anemia fibroblasts. *J Biol Chem* **272**:23328, 1997.
78. Escarceller M, Buchwald M, Singleton BK, Jeggo PA, Jackson SP, Moustacchi E, Papadopoulo D: Fanconi anemia C gene product plays a role in the fidelity of blunt DNA end-joining. *J Mol Biol* **279**:375, 1998.
79. Escarceller M, Rousset S, Moustacchi E, Papadopoulo D: The fidelity of double strand breaks processing is impaired in complementation groups B and D of Fanconi anemia, a genetic instability sydrome. *Somat Cell Mol Genet* **23**:401, 1997.
80. Smith J, Andrau JC, Kallenbach S, Laquerbe A, Doyen N, Papadopoulo D: Abnormal rearrangements associated with V(D)J recombination in Fanconi anemia. *J Mol Biol* **281**:815, 1998.
81. Joenje H, Gille JJP: Oxygen metabolism and chromosomal breakage, in Schroeder-Kurth TM, Auerbach AD, Obe G (eds): *Fanconi Anemia: Clinical, Cytogenetic and Experimental Aspects*. Berlin, Springer-Verlag, 1989, p 174.
82. Schindler D, Hoehn H: Fanconi anemia mutation causes cellular susceptibility to ambient oxygen. *Am J Human Genet* **43**:429, 1988.
83. Joenje H, Arwert F, Eriksson AW, de Koning J, Oostra AB: Oxygen-dependence of chromosomal aberrations in Fanconi's anemia. *Nature* **290**:142, 1981.
84. Poot M, Gross O, Epe B, Pflaum M, Hoehn H: Cell cycle defect in connection with oxygen and iron sensitivity in Fanconi anemia lymphoblastoid cells. *Exp Cell Res* **222**:262, 1996.
85. Korkina LG, Samochatova EV, Maschan AA, Suslova TB, Cheremisina ZP, Afanasev IB: Release of active oxygen radicals by leukocytes of Fanconi anemia patients. *J Leukoc Biol* **52**:357, 1992.
86. Gille JJP, Wortelboer HM, Joenje H: Antioxidant status of Fanconi anemia fibroblasts. *Hum Genet* **77**:28, 1987.
87. Porfirio B, Ambroso G, Giannella G, Isacchi G, Dallapiccola B: Partial correction of chromosome instability in Fanconi anemia by desferrioxamine. *Hum Genet* **83**:49, 1989.
88. Clarke A, Philpott N, Gordon-Smith E, Rutherford T: The sensitivity of Fanconi anemia group C cells to apoptosis induced by mitomycin C is due to oxygen radical generation, not DNA crosslinking. *Br J Hematol* **96**:240, 1997.
89. Joenje H, Youssoufian H, Kruyt FAE, dos Santos CC, Wevrick R, Buchwald M: Expression of the Fanconi anemia gene *FANCC* in human cell lines: Lack of effect of oxygen tension. *Blood Cells Mol Dis* **21**:182, 1995.
90. Saito H, Hammond AT, Moses RE: Hypersensitivity to oxygen is a uniform and secondary defect in Fanconi anemia cells. *Mutat Res* **294**:255, 1993.
91. Ruppitsch W, Meisslitzer C, Hirsh-Kauffmann M, Schweiger M: The role of oxygen metabolism for the pathological phenotype of Fanconi anemia. *Hum Genet* **99**:710, 1997.
92. Chaganti RSK, Houldsworth J: Fanconi anemia: A pleiotropic mutation with multiple cellular and developmental abnormalities. *Ann Genet* **34**:206, 1991.
93. Rosselli F, Sanceau J, Wietzerbin J, Moustacchi E: Abnormal lymphokine production: A novel feature of the genetic disease Fanconi anemia. *Hum Genet* **89**:42, 1992.
94. Segal GM, Magenis RE, Brown M, Keeble W, Smith TD, Heinrich MC, Bagby GC: Repression of Fanconi anemia gene (FACC) inhibits growth of hematopoietic progenitor cells. *J Clin Invest* **94**:846, 1994.
95. Walsh CE, Nienhuis AW, Samuski RJ, Brown MG, Miller JL, Young NS, Liu JM: Phenotypic correction of Fanconi anemia in human hematopoietic cells with a recombinant adeno-associated virus vector. *J Clin Invest* **94**:1440, 1994.
96. Elmore E, Swift M: Growth of cultured cells from patients with Fanconi anemia. *J Cell Physiol* **87**:229, 1975.
97. Willingale-Theune J, Schweiger M, Hirsh-Kauffman M, Meek AE, Paulin-Levasseur M, Traub P: Ultrastructure of Fanconi anemia fibroblasts. *J Cell Sci* **93**:651, 1989.
98. Centrella M, McCarthy TL, Canalis E: Growth factors and cytokines, in Hall BK (ed): *Bone*, vol 4. Boca Raton, FL, CRC Press, 1992.
99. Bagnara GP, Bonsi L, Strippoli P, Ramenghi U, Timeus F, Bonifazi F, Bonafe M, et al: Production of interleukin 6, leukemia inhibitory factor and granulocyte-macrophage colony stimulating factor by peripheral blood mononuclear cells in Fanconi's anemia. *Stem Cells* **11**(suppl 2): 137, 1993.
100. Rosselli F, Sanceau J, Gluckman E, Wietzerbin J, Moustacchi E: Abnormal lymphokine production: A novel feature of the genetic disease Fanconi anemia: II. In vitro and in vivo spontaneous production of tumor necrosis factor alpha. *Blood* **84**:1216, 1994.
101. Schultz JC, Shahidi NT: Tumor necrosis factor alpha overproduction in Fanconi's anemia. *Am J Hematol* **42**:196, 1993.
102. Kubbies M, Schindler D, Hoehn H, Schinzel A, Rabinovitch PS: Endogenous blockage and delay of the chromosome cycle despite normal recruitment and growth phase explain poor proliferation and frequent endomitosis. *Am J Hum Genet* **37**:1022, 1985.
103. Raff MC: Social controls on cell survival and cell death. *Nature* **356**:397, 1992.
104. Sorensen CM, Barry MA, Eastman A: Analysis of events associated with cell cycle arrest at G2 phase and cell death induced by cisplatin. *J Natl Cancer Inst* **82**:749, 1990.
105. Koury MJ: Programmed cell death (apoptosis) in hematopoiesis. *Exp Hematol* **20**:391, 1992.
106. Jiang H, Kocklar DM: Induction of tissue transglutamine and apoptosis by retinoic acid in the limb bud. *Teratology* **46**:333, 1992.
107. Carreau M, Buchwald M: Fanconi's anemia: What have we learned from cloning the genes? *Mol Med Today* **4**:201, 1998.
108. Li Y, Youssoufian H: MxA overexpression reveals a common genetic link in four Fanconi anemia complementation groups. *J Clin Invest* **100**:2873, 1997.
109. van Duim M, de Wit J, Odjik H, Westerveld A, Yasui A, Koken MHM, Hoeijmakers JHJ, Bootsma D: Molecular characterization of the human excision repair gene ERCC-1: cDNA cloning and amino acid homology with the yeast repair gene RAD6. *Proc Natl Acad Sci USA* **88**:8865, 1991.
110. Westerveld A, Hoeijmakers JHJ, van Duin M, de Wit J, Odjik H, Pastink A, Wood RD, Bootsma D: Molecular cloning of a human DNA repair gene. *Nature* **310**:425, 1984.
111. Weber CA, Salazar EP, Sterwart SA, Thompson LH: Molecular cloning and biological characterization of a human gene, *ERCC2*, that

corrects the nucleotide excision repair defect in CHO UV5 cells. *Mol Cell Biol* **8**:1137, 1988.

112. Wevrick R, Buchwald M: Mammalian DNA-repair genes. *Curr Opin Gen Dev* **3**:470, 1993.
113. Mudgett JS, MacInnes MA: Isolation of the functional human excision repair gene ERCC5 by intercosmid recombination. *Genomics* **8**:623, 1990.
114. Diatloff-Zito C, Rosselli F, Heddle J, Moustacchi E: Partial complementation of the Fanconi anemia defect upon transfection by heterologous DNA. *Hum Genet* **86**:151, 1990.
115. Buchwald M, Clarke C: DNA-mediated transfer of a human gene that confers resistance to mitomycin C. *J Cell Phys* **148**:472, 1991.
116. Diatloff-Zito C, Duchaud E, Viegas-Piquignot E, Fraser D, Moustacchi E: Identification and chromosomal localization of a DNA fragment implicated in the partial correction of the Fanconi anemia group D cellular defect. *Mutat Res* **307**:33, 1994.
117. Groger RK, Morrow DM, Tykocinski ML: Directional antisense and sense cDNA cloning using Epstein-Barr virus episomal expression vectors. *Gene* **81**:285, 1989.
118. Parker L: Analysis of the 5′ end of human *FANCC*. M.Sc. thesis, University of Toronto, 1995.
119. Savoia A, Centra M, Lanzano L, de Cillis GP, Zelante L, Buchwald M: Characterization of the 5′ region of the Fanconi anemia group C gene. *Hum Mol Genet* **4**:1231, 1995.
120. Wevrick R, Clarke CA, Buchwald M: Cloning and analysis of the murine Fanconi anemia group C cDNA. *Hum Mol Genet* **2**:655, 1993.
121. Wong, JCY, Alon N, Buchwald M: Cloning of the bovine and rat Fanconi anemia group C cDNAs. *Mammalian Genome* **8**:522, 1997.
122. Gavish H, dos Santos CC, Buchwald M: Leu554-Pro substitution completely abolishes complementing activity of the Fanconi anemia (FACC) protein. *Hum Mol Genet* **2**:123, 1993.
123. Parker L, dos Santos C, Buchwald M: A mutation (delta 327) in the Fanconi anemia group C gene generates a novel transcript lacking the first two coding exons. *Hum Mutat* Suppl 1:S275, 1998.
124. Yamashita T, Barber DL, Zhu Y, Wu N, D'Andrea AD: The Fanconi anemia polypeptide FACC is localized to the cytoplasm. *Proc Natl Acad Sci USA* **91**:6712, 1994.
125. Youssoufian H, Li Y, Martin ME, Buchwald M: Induction of Fanconi anemia cellular phenotype in human 293 cells by overexpression of a mutant *FANCC* allele. *J Clin Invest* **97**:957, 1996.
126. Savoia A, Centra M, Ianzano L, Zelante Z, Buchwald M: Genomic structure of Fanconi anemia complementation C (*FANCC*) gene polymorphisms. *Mol Cell Probes* **10**:213, 1996.
127. Chen M, Tomkins D, Auerbach W, McKerlie C, Youssoufian H, Liu L, Gan O, Carreau M, Buchwald M: Inactivation of *Fancc* in mice produces inducible chromosomal instability and reduced fertility reminiscent of Fanconi anemia. *Nature Genet* **12**:448, 1996.
128. Wevrick R, Barke JE, Nadeau JH, Szpirer C, Buchwald M: Mapping of the murine and rat *Facc* genes and assessment of flexed-tail as a candidate mouse homolog of Fanconi anemia group C. *Mammal Gen* **4**:440, 1993.
129. Youssoufian H: Localization of Fanconi anemia C protein to the cytoplasm of mammalian cells. *Proc Natl Acad Sci USA* **91**:7975, 1994.
130. Hoatlin ME, Christianson TA, Keeble WW, Hammond AT, Zhi Y, Heinrich MC, Tower PA, Bagby GC: The Fanconi anemia group C gene product is located both in the nucleus and cytoplasm of human cells. *Blood* **91**:1418, 1998.
131. Youssoufian H, Auerbach AD, Verlander PC, Steimle V, Mach B: Identification of cytosolic proteins that bind to the Fanconi anemia polypeptide FACC in vitro: Evidence of a multimeric complex. *J Biol Chem* **270**:9876, 1995.
132. Hoshino T, Wang J, Devetten MP, Iwata N, Kajigawa S, Wise RJ, Liu JM, Youssoufian H: Molecular chaperone GRP94 binds to the Fanconi anemia group C protein and regulates its intracellular expression *Blood* **91**:4379, 1998.
133. Kruyt FA, Dijkmans LM, van den Berg TK, Joenje H: Fanconi anemia genes act to suppress a cross-linker-inducible p53-independent apoptosis pathway in lymphoblast cell lines. *Blood* **87**:938, 1996.
134. Rosselli F, Ridet A, Soussi T, Duchaud E, Alapetite C, Moustacchi E: p53-dependent pathway of radio-induced apoptosis is altered in Fanconi anemia. *Oncogene* **10**:9, 1995.
135. Kupfer GM, D'Andrea AD: The effect of the Fanconi anemia polypeptide, FANCC, upon p53 induction and G2 checkpoint regulation. *Blood* **88**:1019, 1996.
136. Avanzi GC, Lista P, Giovinazzo B, Miniero R, Sagli G, Benetton G, Coda R, et al: Cattoretti G, Pegoraro L: Selective growth response to IL-3 of a human leukaemic cell line with megakaryoblastic features. *Br J Hematol* **69**:359, 1988.
137. Metcalf D: Multi-CSF-dependent colony formation by cells of a murine hematopoietic cell line: Specificity and action of multi-CSF. *Blood* **65**:357, 1985.
138. Cumming RC, Liu JM, Youssoufian H, Buchwald M: Suppression of apoptosis in hematopoietic factor-dependent cell lines by expression of the FANCC gene. *Blood* **88**:4558, 1996.
139. Kupfer GM, Naf D, Suliman A, Pulsipher M, D'Andrea AD: The Fanconi anemia polypeptide, FANCC, binds to the cyclin-dependent kinase cdc2. *Blood* **90**:1047, 1997.
140. Heinrich MC, Hoatlin ME, Zigler AJ, Silvey KV, Bakke AC, Keeble WW, Zhi Y, et al: DNA cross-linker-induced G2/M arrest in group C Fanconi anemia lymphoblasts reflects normal checkpoint function. *Blood* **91**:275, 1998.
141. Krasnoshtein F, Buchwald M: Development expression of the *Fancc* gene correlates with congenital defects in Fanconi anemia patients. *Hum Mol Genet* **5**:85, 1996.
142. Ianzano L, d'Apolitol M, Centra M, Savino M, Levran O, Auerbach AD, Clenton-Jansen A-M, et al: The genomic organization of the Fanconi anemia group A (*FANCA*) gene. *Genomics* **41**:309, 1997.
143. Levran O, Erlich T, Magdalena N, Gregory JJ, Batish SD, Verlander PC, Auerbach AD: Sequence variation in the Fanconi anemia gene *FANCA*. *Proc Natl Acad Sci USA* **94**:13051, 1997.
144. Levran O, Doggett, NA, Auerbach AD: Identification of *Alu*-mediated deletions in the Fanconi anemia gene *FANCA, Hum Mutat* **12**:145, 1998.
145. Savino M, Ianzano L, Strippoli P, Ramenghi U, Arslanian A, Bagnara GP, Joenje H, et al: Mutations of the Fanconi anemia group A gene (*FANCA*) in Italian patients. *Am J Hum Genet* **61**:1246, 1997.
146. Wijker M, Morgan NV, Herterich S, van Berkel CGM, Tipping AJ, Gross HJ, Gille JJP, et al: Heterogeneous spectrum of mutations in the Fanconi anaemia group A gene. *Eur J Hum Genet* **7**:52, 1999.
147. Centra M, Memeo E, d'Apolito M, Savino M, Ianzano L, Notarangelo A, Liu J, et al: Fine exon-intron structure of the Fanconi anemia group A (*FANCA*) gene and characterization of two genomic deletions. *Genomics* **51**:463, 1998.
148. Morgan NM, Tipping AJ, Joenje H, Mathew CG: High frequency of large Intragenic Deletions in the Fanconi anemia group A gene *Am J Hum Genet* **65**:1330, 1999.
149. Hanenberg H, Batish SD, Vieten L, Verlander PC, Williams D, Auerbach AD: Phenotypic correction of primary T cells from patients with Fanconi anemia with retroviral vectors as a diagnostic tool. (submitted).
150. Fu K-L, Lo Ten Foe JR, Joenje H, Rao KW, Liu JM, Walsh C: Functional correction of Fanconi anemia group A hematopoietic cells by retroviral gene transfer. *Blood* **90**:3293, 1997.
151. Pulsipher M, Kupfer GM, Naf D, Suliman A, Lee JS, Jakobs P, Grompe M, et al: Subtyping analysis of Fanconi anemia by immunoblotting and retroviral gene transfer. *Mol Med* **4**:468, 1998.
152. Cleton-Jansen A-M, Moerland EW, Pronk JC, van Berkel C, Apostolou S, Crawford J, Savoia A, Auerbach AD, et al: Mutation analysis of the Fanconi anaemia A gene in breast tumors with loss of heterozygosity at 16q24.3. *Br J Cancer* **79**:1049, 1999.
153. De Winter JP, Waisfisz Q, Rooimans MA, Van Berkel CGM, Bosnoyan-Collins L, Alon N, Carreau M, et al: The Fanconi anemia group G gene is identical with human *XRCC9*. *Nature Genet* **20**:281, 1998.
154. Liu N, Lamerdin JE, Tucker JD, Zhou Z-Q, Walter CA, Albala JS, Busch DB, Thompson LH: The human XRCC9 gene corrects chromosomal instability and mutagen sensitivities in CHO UV40 cells. *Proc Natl Acad Sci USA* **94**:9232, 1997.
155. Busch DB, Zdzienicka MZ, Natarajan AT, Jones NJ, Overkamp WJI, Collins A, Mitchell DL, et al: A CHO mutant, UV40, that is sensitive to diverse mutagens and represents a new complementation group of mitomycin C sensitivity. *Mutat Res* **363**:209, 1996.
156. Saar K, Schindler D, Wegner R-D, Reis A, Wienker F, Hoehn H, Joenje H, et al: Localisation of a Fanconi anaemia gene to chromosome 9p. *Eur J Hum Genet* **6**:501, 1998.
157. Kupfer GM, Naf D, Suliman A, Pulsipher M, D'Andrea AD: The Fanconi anemia proteins, FANCA and FANCC, interact to form a nuclear complex. *Nature Genet* **17**:487, 1997.
158. Urlando C, Krasnoshtein F, Heddle JA, Buchwald M: Assessment of the flexed-tail mouse as a possible model for Fanconi anemia: Analysis of mitomycin C-induced micronuclei. *Mutat Res* **370**:99, 1996.
159. Chen M, Tomkins D, Auerbach W, McKerlie C, Youssoufian H, Liu L, Gan O, et al: Inactivation of *Fancc* in mice produces inducible

chromosomal instability and reduced fertility reminiscent of Fanconi anemia. *Nature Genet* **12**:448, 1996.
160. Whitney MA, Royle G, Low MJ, Kelly MA, Axthelm MK, Reifsteck C, Olson S, et al: Germ cell defects and hematopoietic hypersensitivity to gamma-interferon in mice with a targeted disruption of the Fanconi anemia C gene. *Blood* **88**:49, 1996.
161. Otsuki T, Wang J, Demuth I, Digweed M, Liu J: Assessment of mitomycin C sensitivity in Fanconi anemia complementation group C gene (Fac) knock-out mouse cells. *Int J Hematol* **67**:243, 1998.
162. Tomkins DJ, Care M, Carreau M, Buchwald M: Development and characterization of immortalized fibroblastoid cell lines from an FA(C) mouse model. *Mutat Res* **408**:27, 1998.
163. Carreau M, Gan O, Liu L, Doedens M, McKerlie C, Dick JE, Buchwald M: FAC regulates regeneration of early and commited hematopoietic progenitors after DNA damage. *Blood* **91**:2737, 1998.
164. Rathbun RK, Faulkner GR, Ostroski MH, Christianson TA, Hughes G, Jones G, Cahn R, et al: Inactivation of the Fanconi anemia group C gene augments interferon-gamma-induced apoptotic responses in hematopoietic cells. *Blood* **90**:974, 1997.
165. Haneline LS, Broxmeyer HE, Cooper S, Hangoc G, Carreau M, Buchwald M, Clapp WC: Multiple inhibitory cytokines induce deregulated progenitor growth and apoptosis in hematopoietic cells from *Fancc*$^{-/-}$ mice. *Blood* **91**:4092, 1998.
166. Wang J, Otsuki T, Youssoufian H, Lo Ten Foe J, Kim S, Devetten M, Yu J, et al: Overexpression of the Fanconi anemia group C gene (FAC) protects hematopoietic progenitors from death induced by Fas-mediated apoptosis. *Cancer Res* **58**:3538, 1998.
167. Auerbach AD: Prenatal diagnosis of Fanconi anemia, in New MI (ed.): *Proceedings of the Diagnosis and Treatment of the Unborn Child Conference* Italy, Idelson Publishing Company, 1998 p 27–35.
168. Auerbach AD: Diagnosis of Fanconi anemia by diepoxybutane analysis, in Dracopoli NC, Haines JL, Korf BR, Moir DT, Morton CC, Seidman CE, Seidman JG, Smith DR (eds): *Current Protocols in Human Genetics*. New York, Current Protocols, 1994, p 8.7.1.
169. Kwee ML, Poll EHA, van de Kamp JJP, De Koning H, Eriksson AW, Joenje H: Unusual response to bifunctional alkylating agent in a case of Fanconi anemia. *Hum Genet* **64**:384, 1983.
170. Auerbach AD, Koorse RE, Ghosh R, Venkatraj VS, Zhang M, Chiorazzi N: Complementation studies in Fanconi anemia, in Schroder TM, Auerbach AD, Obe G (eds): *Fanconi Anemia, Clinical, Cytogenetic and Experimental Aspects*. Heidelberg, Springer-Verlag, 1989, p 213.
171. Lo Ten Foe JR, Kwee ML, Rooimans, MA, Oostra AB, Veerman AJP, Pauli RM, Shahidi NT, et al: Somatic mosaicism Fanconi anemia: molecular basis and clinical significance. *Eur J Hum Genet* **5**:137, 1997.
172. Ellis NA, Lennon DJ, Proytcheva M, Alhadeff B, Henderson EE, German J: Somatic intragenic recombination within the mutated locus BLM can correct the high sister-chromatid exchange phenotype of Bloom syndrome cells. *Am J Hum Genet* **57**:994, 1995.
173. Rackoff WR, Orazi A, Robinson CA, et al: Prolonged administration of granulocyte colony-stimulating factor (Filgrastim) to patients with Fanconi anemia: A pilot study. *Blood* **88**:1588, 1996.
174. Guinan EC, Lopez KD, Huhn RD, Felser JM, Nathan DG: Evaluation of granulocyte-macrophage colony-stimulating factor for treatment of pancytopenia in children with Fanconi anemia. *Pediatrics* **124**:144, 1994.
175. Scagni P, Saracco P, Timeus F, Farinasso L, Dall'Aglio M, Bosa EM, Crescenzio N, et al: Use of recombinant granulocyte colony-stimulating factor in Fanconi's anemia. *Haematologica* **83**:432, 1998.
176. Walsh CE, Grompe M, Vanin E, Buchwald M, Young NS, Nienhuis AW, Liu JM: A functionally active retrovirus vector for gene therapy in Fanconi anemia group C. *Blood* **84**:453, 1994.
177. Walsh CE, Mann MM, Emmons RVB, Wang S, Liu JM: Transduction of CD34-enriched human peripheral and umbilical cord blood progenitors using a retroviral vector with the Fanconi anemia group C gene. *J Invest Med* **43**:379, 1995.
178. Liu JM: Gene transfer for the eventual treatment of Fanconi's anemia. *Semin Hematol* **35**:168, 1998.
179. Gluckman E, Devergie A, Schaison G, Bussel A, Berger R, Sohier J, Bernard J: Bone marrow transplantation in Fanconi anemia. *Br J Haematol* **45**:557, 1980.
180. Berger R, Bernheim A, Gluckman E, Gisselbrecht C: In vitro effect of cyclophosphamide metabolites on chromosomes of Fanconi anaemia patients. *Br J Haematol* **45**:565, 1980.
181. Auerbach AD, Adler B, O'Reilly RJ, Kirkpatrick D, Chaganti RSK: Effect of procarbazine and cyclophosphamide on chromosome breakage in Fanconi anemia cells: Relevance to bone marrow transplantation. *Cancer Genet Cytogent* **9**:25, 1983.
182. Gluckman E, Devergie A, Dutreix J: Bone marrow transplantation for Fanconi's anemia, in Schroder-Kurth TM, Auerbach AD, Obe G (eds): *Fanconi Anemia: Clinical, Cytogenetic and Experimental Aspects*. Berlin, Springer-Verlag, 1989, p 60.
183. Gluckman E, Auerbach AD, Horowitz MM, Sobocinski KA, Ash RC, Bortin MM, Butturini A, et al: Bone marrow transplantation for Fanconi anemia. *Blood* **86**:2856, 1995.
184. Kohli-Kumar M, Morris C, DeLaat C, Sambrano J, Masterson M, Mueller R, Shahidi NT, et al: Bone marrow transplantation in Fanconi anemia using matched sibling donors. *Blood* **94**:2050, 1994.
185. Auerbach AD: Umbilical cord blood transplants for genetic disease: Diagnostic and ethical issues in fetal studies. *Blood Cells* **20**:303, 1994.
186. Broxmeyer HE, Douglas GW, Hangoc G, Cooper S, Bard J, English D, Arny M, Boyse EA: Human umbilical cord blood as a potential source of transplantable hematopoietic stem/progenitor cells. *Proc Natl Acad Sci USA* **86**:3828, 1989.
187. Gluckman E, Broxmeyer HE, Auerbach AD, Friedman HS, Douglas GW, Devergie A, Esperou H, et al: Hematopoietic reconstitution in a patient with Fanconi's anemia by means of umbilical-cord blood from an HLA-identical sibling. *N Engl J Med* **321**:1174, 1989.
188. Kohli-Kumar M, Harris RE, Broxmeyer HE, Shahidi N, Auerbach AD, Harris RE: Cord blood transplant in Fanconi anemia. *Br J Haematol* **85**:419, 1993.
189. Rubinstein P, Rosenfield RE, Adamson JW, Stevens CE: Stored placental blood for unrelated bone marrow reconstitution. *Blood* **81**:1679, 1993.
190. Cairo MS, Wagner JE: Placental and/or umbilical cord blood: An alternative source of hematopoietic stem cells for transplantation. *Blood* **90**:4665, 1997.
191. Kurtzberg J, Laughlin M, Graham ML, Smith C, Olson JF, Halperin E, Ciocci G, Carrier C, Stevens CE, Rubinstein P: Placental blood as a source for hematopoietic stem cells for transplantation into unrelated recipients. *N Engl J Med* **335**:157, 1996.
192. Wagner JE, Rosenthal J, Sweetman R, Shu XO, Davies SM, Ramsay NKC, McGlave PB, Sender L, Cairo MS: Successful transplantation of HLA-matched and HLA-mismatched umbilical cord blood from unrelated donors: Analysis of engraftment and acute graft-versus-host disease. *Blood* **88**:795, 1996.
193. Davies SM, Kahn S, Wagner JE, Arthur DC, Auerbach AD, Ramsay NKC, Weisdorf DJ: Unrelated donor bone marrow transplantation for Fanconi anemia. *Bone Marrow Transplant* **17**:43, 1996.
194. Wagner JE, Davies SM, Auerbach AD: Hematopoietic cell transplant in the treatment of Fancoini anemia, in Forman SJ, Blume KG, Thomas, ED (eds), *Hematopoietic Cell Transplantation*, 2d ed. Malden, MA, Blackwell Science, 1998.
195. Gibson RA, Buchwald M, Roberts RG, Mathew CG: Characterization of the exon structure of the Fanconi anemia group C gene by vectorette PCR. *Hum Mol Genet* **2**:35, 1993.
196. Gibson RA, Hajianpoujr A, Murer-Orlando M, Buchwald M, Mathew CG: A nonsense mutation and exon skipping in the Fanconi anemia group C gene. *Hum Mol Genet* **2**:797, 1993.
197. Gibson RA, Morgan NV, Goldstein LH, Pearson IC, Kesterton IP, Foot NJ, Jansen S, et al: Novel mutations and polymorphisms in the Fanconi anemia group C gene. *Hum Mutat* **8**:140, 1996.
198. Lo Ten Foe JR, Rooimans MA, Joenje H, Arwert F: A novel frameshift mutation (1806insA) in exon 14 of the Fanconi anemia C gene, FAC. *Hum Mutat* **7**:264, 1996.
199. Lo Ten Foe JR, Barel MT, Tuss P, Digweed M, Arwert F, Joenje H: Sequence variations in the Fanconi anaemia gene, FAC: pathogenicity of 1806insA and R548X and recognition of D195V as a polymorphic variant. *Hum Genet* **98**:522, 1996.
200. Lo Ten Foe JR, Kruyt FAC, Zweekhorst MBM, Pals G, Gibson RA, Mathew CG, Joenje H, Arwert F: Exon 6 skipping in the Fanconi anemia C gene associated with a nonsense/missense mutation (775C > T) in exon 5. *Hum Mutat* Suppl. 1:S25, 1998.

CHAPTER 32

Hereditary Nonpolyposis Colorectal Cancer (HNPCC)

C. Richard Boland

Colorectal cancer is a fairly common disease of Western populations with a typical onset at about age 70 years. The international epidemiology of this disease suggests that environmental factors, probably dietary, are the most important influences for the high prevalence of this disease in certain countries.[1] Woven into the epidemiologic fabric for colorectal cancer is an important influence of genetic factors. Individuals who have even one first-degree relative with colorectal neoplasia (i.e., either cancers or adenomatous polyps) have an increased risk for these tumors themselves, which will appear earlier in life.[2-4] The familial risk increases when there is more than one family member involved or cancers occur before age 50.[3,4]

The most readily distinguished form of familial risk is the autosomal dominant genetic disease familial adenomatous polyposis (FAP). This disease has a distinctive phenotypic syndrome characterized by a large number of precursor adenomatous polyps in the colon and occurs in about 1 in 10,000 births. This is completely unrelated to the more common autosomal dominant colon cancer syndrome termed *hereditary nonpolyposis colorectal cancer* (HNPCC). HNPCC is due to an inactivating germ-line mutation in one of the DNA mismatch repair (MMR) genes (see below). This disease has no antecedent clinical phenotype until a cancer develops and was a controversial entity until the biologic basis of this disease was discovered in 1993.[5-8] Patients with HNPCC are at increased risk for cancers of the colon, endometrium, small intestine, ovary, stomach, urinary tract, brain, and some other, but not all, epithelial organs.[9-12] The mean age to develop colorectal cancer is in the early to mid-40's; however, many tumors occur in the 20's and even in teenagers. Although population-based surveys have not been completed, HNPCC may be the most common form of familial predisposition to cancer.[13-22] Now that the genetic basis of this disease has been elucidated, and the involvement of non-colonic cancers clearly demonstrated, it may be advised to refer to the disease as "Lynch syndrome" when a germ-line mutation in a DNA MMR gene has been identified in a family, and use "HNPCC" for familial clusters of colon cancer without an identifiable germ-line mutation,

FAMILY HISTORY AND COLORECTAL CANCER

The hereditary aspects of colon cancer are complex. The age-adjusted relative risk of developing colorectal cancer in individuals with one affected first-degree relative is 1.72 compared with those without such a family history. This risk rises to 2.75 when there are two or more affected first-degree relatives, and the relative risk increases as the family history occurs in younger relatives, reaching 5.37 when the affected siblings are between 30 and 44 years of age.[3] Similarly, the relative risk for colorectal cancer is 1.78 for the first-degree relatives of patients with adenomatous polyps. The relative risk of cancer rises to 2.59 when the sibling is less than 60 years old and 3.25 when a sibling and parent are both affected.[4] This modest increase in risk, which worsens with increasing familial involvement and earlier age tumors, cannot be attributed solely to HNPCC. In all likelihood, several genetic risk factors play a partial role, as do dietary and other environmental influences. The challenge in defining HNPCC families has been to recognize the disease in the face of a large background incidence of colorectal cancer and the occasional clusters of sporadic tumors in families.

THE HISTORY OF HNPCC

The historical roots of HNPCC can be traced back to the end of the nineteenth century when a University of Michigan pathologist, A. S. Warthin, recognized a cluster of cancers in the family of his seamstress.[23,24] His patient's family was large and has been reported five times during the twentieth century, serving as the prototype for HNPCC.[25-29] Following this lead, Lynch documented family histories on this and other families, and by the 1970s, it became clear that the medical histories of several large families strongly suggested the involvement of an autosomal dominant disease that gave rise to early-onset cancers with a predisposition for proximal colonic involvement and cancers in certain other organs.[29-32]

Prior to identification of the genes for this disease, ascertainment was limited by the need for large families with a high degree of involvement. Two different subsets of families were identified. *Lynch syndrome I* (or *site-specific familial colorectal cancer*) was attached to those families which only manifested colorectal cancers. *Lynch syndrome II* (or *cancer family syndrome*) was assigned to families that also had tumors of other organs, principally of the female genital tract.[31] Over time, it has emerged that these are not distinct syndromes, but there may be specific mutations that predispose to cancers at extracolonic sites. In fact, one common mutation in *hMLH1* has been reported to result in a greatly reduced frequency of extracolonic tumors.[33]

To cope with the uncertainties surrounding HNPCC, the International Collaborative Group on Hereditary Non-Polyposis Colorectal Cancer convened in 1991 to develop clinical criteria to standardize the study of this disease.[34] The "Amsterdam criteria" are listed in Table 32-1 but appear to be overly restrictive and do not take into account the possibility of later-onset variants, the implications of noncolonic tumors, or the limitations imposed by small family size or incomplete data recovery. Not all HNPCC families, diagnosed genetically, meet the Amsterdam criteria.

HNPCC has attracted interest not only because of its impact in clinical medicine; the genetic basis of this disease has led to the understanding of a unique pathogenetic mechanism for tumor

A list of standard abbreviations is located immediately preceding the index in each volume. Nonstandard abbreviations used in this chapter include: FAP = familial adenomatous polyposis; HNPCC = hereditary nonpolyposis colorectal cancer; MMR = mismatch repair; MSI = microsatellite instability; RER = replicative error; MSS = microsatellite stable.

Table 32-1 Amsterdam Criteria for HNPCC

1. At least three affected relatives with verified colorectal cancer
2. At least one is a first-degree relative of the other two
3. FAP is excluded
4. At least two successive generations affected
5. One colon cancer at < 50 years of age

development. The history surrounding the identification of the HNPCC genes and the unique type of genomic instability associated with these tumors has been reviewed in detail elsewhere.[24,35]

CLINICAL MANIFESTATIONS OF HNPCC

HNPCC is an autosomal dominantly inherited genetic disease characterized by an increased risk for cancers of the colon, rectum, and a number of other organs (Table 32-2). Endometrial cancer is nearly as common as colorectal cancers in some registries[36,37] and is a key component of the HNPCC phenotype. Small intestinal cancers are extremely rare in the general population, but the risk for these is greatly increased in HNPCC patients. These remain unusual tumors even in this setting, but they have an early age of onset (49 years), may present with obstructive symptoms like colorectal tumors, and appear to be associated with a better prognosis than what would be expected in the general population.[38]

Between 60 and 70 percent of colorectal cancers occur proximal to the splenic flexure.[23] There is an increased risk of synchronous and metachronous cancers of the colon, rectum, and other organs. Multiple adenomatous polyps of the colon and microadenomas, such as are seen in FAP, do not occur in HNPCC. Although the incidence of adenomatous polyps may be slightly increased in HNPCC patients,[39,40] this does not entirely explain the greatly increased incidence of carcinomas. It has been suggested that a higher rate of progression from adenoma to carcinoma is the major factor accounting for the cancer predisposition in HNPCC (Table 32-3).

There appears to be no significant increase in risk for cancer of the lung, breast, prostate, bladder, bone marrow, larynx, or brain if one ascertains tumors from clinical collections of families and compares them against population-based estimates.[12] The use of genetic techniques has provided insight into the extracolonic tumors that occur in HNPCC. An excess of gastric cancer occurs in members of affected families, and both intestinal and diffuse-type tumors may be found. The mean age of diagnosis of gastric cancer in these families is 56 years. Not all the gastric cancers have the characteristic hypermutability of HNPCC, so it is not necessarily the case that all of these tumors are attributable to the syndrome.[41] There are anecdotal accounts of early-onset breast cancers in HNPCC kindreds, and the report of convincing genetic evidence for the appearance of an HNPCC-related breast cancer in one case indicates that this tumor may occasionally occur in this setting.[42] Brain cancers, including a wide pathologic spectrum, have been reported to occur in 3.35 percent of a Dutch HNPCC registry.[43] Other tumors occurring with an increased relative risk include urinary tract tumors and ovarian cancer.

The prevalence of HNPCC in the general population is unknown. This is complicated by the fact that there is a 5 to 6 percent lifetime prevalence of colorectal cancer in North America, and it is at least this high in much of western Europe. Various estimates of prevalence have been attempted, as listed in Table 32-4.[15–20,44]. The apparent proportion of families with HNPCC (based on a history of multiple cancers in the family) is approximately 3 to 4 percent of all colorectal cancers (with one remarkable outlier study from Finland[18]). These estimates predict a prevalence of HNPCC in the population of approximately 2 per 1000 persons; however, this is probably an underestimate because of limitations in family size (which limits recognition), historical recall (which is inaccurate), penetrance (which is undetermined), and involvement of organs other than the colon (which have not been considered in these studies). A more realistic estimate for the frequency of HNPCC in the general population may be much higher but is probably less than some estimates that have been as high as 1 per 200.

The diagnosis of HNPCC is made clinically by taking a family history. Even a single first-degree relative who develops a colorectal or endometrial cancer at a very young age raises this possibility. A subset of HNPCC families is easier to recognize by virtue of a constellation of findings that constitute the Muir-Torre variant.[45,46] This syndrome consists of all of the features of HNPCC plus sebaceous gland tumors (adenomas, epitheliomas,

Table 32-2 Estimates of Cancer Risk by Organ Site in HNPCC

Cancer Site	Lifetime Risk	Relative Risk	Median Age
Any cancer by age 70	91% (men), 69% (women)[36]		
Colon or rectum	74% (men), 30% (women)[36]		46 yrs[9]
With *hMLH1* mutations	80%		41 yrs[37]
With *hMSH2* mutations	80%		44 yrs[37]
Endometrium	20% (by age 70)[113]	(vs. 3% risk in the general population)	46 yrs[9]
	42% (by age 70)[36]		
	61% (*hMSH2* mutations)[37]		
	42% (*hMLH1* mutations)[37]		
Stomach		4.1[9]	54 yrs[9]
With *hMLH1* mutations		4.4[37]	
With *hMSH2* mutations		19.3[37]	
Ovaries		3.5[9]	40 yrs[9]
With *hMLH1* mutations		6.4[37]	
With *hMSH2* mutations		8.0[37]	
Small intestine		25[9]	53 yrs[9]
With *hMLH1* mutations		292[37]	
With *hMSH2* mutations		103[37]	
Hepatobiliary system		4.9[9]	66 yrs[9]
Kidney		3.2[9]	66 yrs[9]
Ureter		22	56 yrs[9]
Kidney/ureter (*hMSH2* mutations)		75.3[37]	

Table 32-3 Adenomatous Polyps of the Colon in HNPCC (Clinical Diagnoses of HNPCC)

A. Lanspa et al., Nebraska patients[39]

	HNPCC Patients* (N = 44, Mean Age 42.4)	Control Patients (N = 88, Mean Age 44.4)
Adenomatous polyps	30% (13/44)	11% (10/88)
Proximal colonic adenomas	18% (8/44)	1% (1/88)
Multiple colonic adenomas	20% (9/44)	4% (4/88)

B. Jass et al., New Zealand patients[40]

	HNPCC Patients	Age-Matched Autopsy Controls
Men < 50 years old	30% (3/10)*	5% (2/42)
Women < 50 years old	44% (4/9)†	5% (1/21)
Men 50–69 years old	66% (2/3)	36% (16/44)
Women 50–69 years old	100% (1/1)	12% (1/8)
Men > 70 years old	None available	46% (13/28)
Women > 70 years old	None available	33% (5/15)

*$p = 0.015$ vs. Controls (by χ^2).
†$p = 0.0075$ vs. Controls (by χ^2).

and carcinomas) and keratoacanthomas. The latter is a keratin-filled skin tumor that occurs in sun-exposed areas. Basal and squamous cell carcinomas also occur in Muir-Torre syndrome. Although these skin tumors are unusual manifestations of HNPCC, this diagnosis should be considered in any patient who has more than one skin tumor of this variety. To date, all Muir-Torre syndrome families who have had germ-line mutations identified have been linked to *hMSH2*.[47–49]

The pathologic features of colorectal neoplasms in HNPCC (Fig. 32-1) are somewhat unique.[23,50–52] As mentioned, the tumors occur at early ages, and most are in the proximal colon. Using typical pathologic criteria, 37 percent of colorectal cancers in HNPCC will be classified as poorly differentiated,[23] which would suggest that the tumors will behave aggressively. Contrary to this, colorectal cancers in HNPCC have a better outcome than sporadic tumors matched for stage.[23] Colorectal cancers in HNPCC are significantly more likely to be diploid or near-diploid compared with sporadic tumors.[53,54] In one flow cytometry study, 68 percent of HNPCC cancers were diploid, and 90 percent were diploid or near-diploid with a DNA index less than 1.27.[54] Over 35 percent of colorectal cancers in HNPCC are mucinous carcinomas.[23] HNPCC tumors (as well as other colorectal cancers with the MSI phenotype) are more likely to be exophytic, larger, look poorly differentiated, show focal or predominant mucin production, and show an intense Crohn-like reaction of tumor-infiltrating lymphocytes.[55] The combined pathologic features mentioned above should increase one's suspicion of HNPCC, even if found outside familial clusters of colorectal cancer.

THE HNPCC GENES

hMSH2: The First HNPCC Gene

The discovery of the HNPCC genes is an interesting story of excellent basic science research, fierce competition among several laboratories interested in the problem, and in some instances unusual good fortune.[24] It had been proposed by Loeb in the 1980s that a "hypermutable phenotype" would be necessary to account for all the mutations that seemed to be present in most cancers.[56,57] No mechanism was available to account for this at that time.

In 1993, three laboratories working independently reported that an unusual form of somatic mutation occurred in 12 to 15 percent of colorectal cancers. The mutations were insertions or deletions of simple repetitive elements that make up microsatellite sequences (see below). Each laboratory added to the interpretation. A group led by Perucho used an arbitrarily primed polymerase chain reaction (PCR) looking for genomic amplifications or deletions that might be present in colorectal cancers.[58] Instead, they noted that 12 percent of colorectal cancers harbored somatic deletions that altered the lengths of the microsatellite sequences.

Table 32-4 Prevalence of HNPCC in the Population

Ascertainment Method	Age Limit	Locale	Proportion of Families Estimated to Have HNPCC	Reference
Record search	70	Finland	3.8%	15
Patient recall	None	Italy	3.9%	16
Death certificates	None	UK	4.0%	17
Record search	50	Finland	30.0%	18
Record search	55	Ireland	6.0%	19
Patient recall	50	Canada	3.1%	20
Genetic testing	—	Finland	2%	75

NOTE: All estimates (except ref. 75) are based on family histories (not genetic diagnoses) and required 3 or more family members with colorectal cancer. These are probably underestimates (see text).

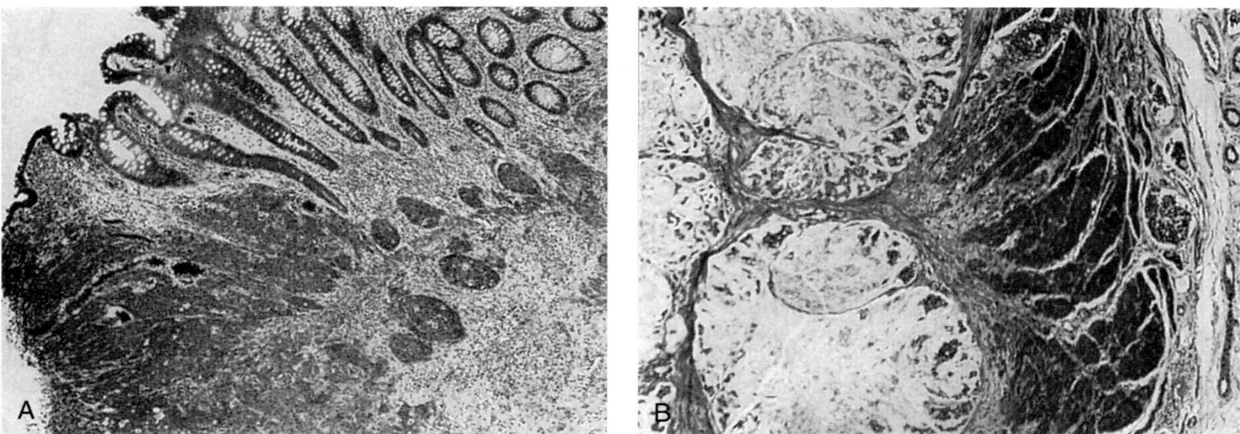

Fig. 32-1 Histopathology of HNPCC. ***A.*** **Poorly differentiated carcinoma without evidence of a glandular formation. The tumor cells have round regular nuclei. Such a tumor would be typically interpreted to be highly aggressive. (*Courtesy of T. Smyrk, M.D., Omaha, Nebraska.*)** ***B.*** **Mucinous adenocarcinoma is characteristic of more than one-third of colon cancers in HNPCC. (*Courtesy of T. Smyrk, M.D., Omaha, Nebraska.*)**

Their approach permitted them to estimate that affected tumors carried more than 10^5 of these types of mutations. They also noted that tumors with these "ubiquitous somatic mutations at simple repetitive sequences" had unique features that distinguished them from most colorectal cancers, and they proposed that this represented a novel form of carcinogenesis.[5]

Another group led by Thibodeau also was looking for genetic losses at tumor suppressor gene loci using PCR-based amplification of microsatellite sequences and recognized that *microsatellite instability* (initially called MIN but, by consensus, now abbreviated MSI[59]) was significantly correlated with tumors of the proximal colon. MSI was inversely related with loss of heterozygosity on chromosomes 5q, 17p, and 18q and positively correlated with improved patient survival. This group proposed that 28 percent of colorectal cancers developed through this unique mechanism of genomic instability.[6]

A third group, representing a multinational collaboration that included Vogelstein in the United States and de la Chapelle in Finland, performed a genome-wide search for a genetic locus of HNPCC. Using two large kindreds, one such locus was mapped to 2p15-16.[7] Microsatellite markers had been used to map the locus. Pursuing the hypothesis that the HNPCC gene would be a tumor suppressor gene, they looked for loss of heterozygosity in the tumors, using the microsatellites as targets. They also found insertion or deletion mutations at the repetitive sequences, which they termed the *replicative error* (RER) *phenotype.*[8] All three groups brought unique insights to bear on the issue, and together they illuminated for the first time the nature of HNPCC and discovered a novel mechanism for carcinogenesis.

The next step forward in solving the HNPCC riddle came unexpectedly from laboratories focused on yeast genetics who had not previously ventured into human genetics, let alone hereditary colon cancer. The characteristic mutational pattern (i.e., MSI) published in the autoradiograms used to resolve the amplified microsatellites by the preceding three groups resembled the mutational pattern seen in bacteria and yeast that had lost genes required for DNA MMR (Fig. 32-2). The microbial DNA MMR systems were complex and involved several genes of the Mut HLS mismatch repair pathway.[60,61] The system, which consists of several proteins working together in a complex, repairs errors in

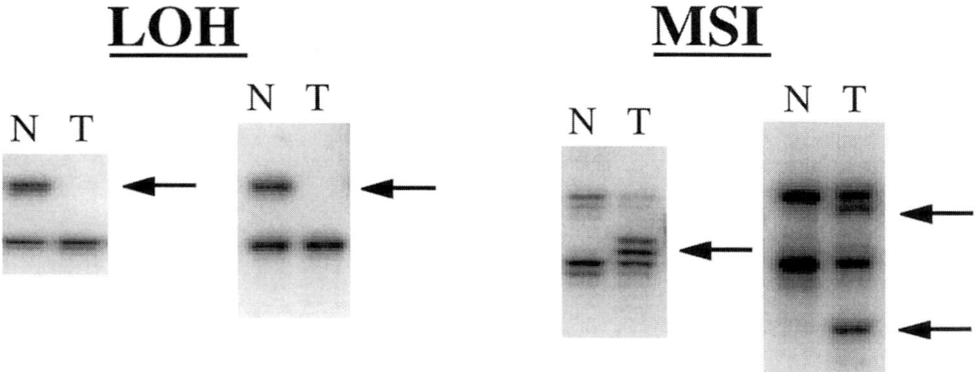

Fig. 32-2 Autoradiogram demonstrating microsatellite instability. A repetitive and polymorphic DNA sequence (microsatellite) is amplified by the polymerase chain reaction (PCR), and the normal tissue (N), if informative, provides two amplicons. On the left are two examples of loss of heterozygosity (LOH), in which one of the PCR products has been deleted from the genome of the tumor tissue (T) and lost from the autoradiogram, as indicated by the arrows. On the right are two examples of microsatellite instability (MSI), in which the length of the PCR product has been altered by an insertion or deletion mutation in the microsatellite sequence and the appearance of new bands on the autoradiogram (*arrows*). In the examples of MSI, residual normal DNA has been amplified along with the DNA from the neoplasm.

Table 32-5 The HNPCC Genes

HNPCC Gene	Chromosomal Location	*E. coli* Homologue	cDNA Size	Genomic Structure	Protein
hMSH2	2p 15-16	*MutS*	2727 bp	16 exons ~73 kb	934 aa's 106 kD
hMSH6	2p 15-16	*MutS*	4245	10 exons	1360 aa's 160 kD
hMLH1	3p 21	*MutL*	2268 bp	19 exons ~58 kb	756 aa's 85 kD
hPMS1	2q 31	*MutL*	2795 bp	—	932 aa's
hPMS2	7p 22[1]	*MutL*	2586 bp	15 exon ~16 kb	862 aa's 96 kD

DNA replication that occur during S phase that result in single-base-pair mismatches or mispaired loops that occur at repetitive sequences such as microsatellites. Strand et al. demonstrated that mutations in three yeast genes involved in DNA MMR (*PMS1, MLH,* and *MSH2*) led to 100- to 700-fold increases in mutations at poly(GT) sequences and, based on what had been reported in colorectal cancer, specifically suggested that these genes might be the loci sought by those studying HNPCC.[62] In a remarkably short period of time, investigating groups led by Kolodner[63] and Vogelstein[64] reported that a human *MutS* homologue (*hMSH2**) could be found on chromosome 2p. Germ-line mutations of this gene in HNPCC families demonstrated that it was responsible for the disease.[64] *hMSH2* was the second homologue found in the human genome related to the bacterial *MutS* or *yMHS* gene. Subsequently, at least 8 human homologues of the *MutS* genes have been found.

The genetics of HNPCC are somewhat complex but follow the paradigms of other tumor suppressor genes. HNPCC is inherited as an autosomal dominant characteristic when an inactivating germ-line mutation occurs in *hMSH2* or certain other DNA MMR genes. Resultingly, every somatic cell carries one inactivated copy and one wild-type copy of the MMR gene. With certain notable exceptions,[65] the phenotype at the cellular level or for the individual is normal but is susceptible to loss of the wild-type allele in a target tissue,[66] which leads to a hypermutable phenotype (MSI). The hypermutable cell then is susceptible to the accumulation of mutations at a greatly accelerated rate, which may then result in clonal expansion and the neoplastic phenotype. Thus a germ-line mutation at *hMSH2* leaves an individual susceptible to the development of hypermutability, which then facilitates the rapid accumulation of other mutations that are permissive of a neoplastic phenotype. There is not yet a suitable explanation for why specific organs are at selective risk to develop cancer. Certain germ-line mutations appear to have a *dominant negative* effect, in which heterozygous cells are themselves hypermutable. In this instance, MMR deficiency may be detected in phenotypically normal cells.[65]

Other HNPCC Genes: *hMLH1, hPMS1, hPMS2,* and *hMSH6*

Shortly after the first HNPCC locus was mapped to 2p, a second HNPCC locus was mapped to 3p in a Scandinavian kindred.[67] Based on the paradigm that led from 2p to *hMSH2,* these same two groups turned their attention to the *MutL* gene of *E. coli* (and the yeast *MutL* homologue). This research led to three human homologues, now termed *hMLH1, hPMS1,* and *hPMS2,* located on 3p, 2q, and 7p, all of which have be linked to HNPCC families.[68–70]

The identification of the DNA MMR genes and their linkage to HNPCC families led to a sharp increase in interest in the field and the identification of numerous families with inactivating germ-line mutations. *hMSH2* and *hMLH1* account for the majority of families with HNPCC and in roughly equal proportions.[71–75] Smaller numbers of families have HNPCC on the basis of mutations and *hPMS2,* and one family has been found with a germ-line mutation in *hPMS1.*[70] A dominant negative germ-line mutation in *hPMS2* has been identified that raises new possibilities for tumor development.[76] Two HNPCC families have been reported who have germ-line mutations in *hMSH6,* a gene that encodes for a protein that heterodimerizes with the hMSH2 protein.[77–79] In each of these families, the cancers had MSI at mono- and di-nucleotide repeat sequences. The genes known to give rise to HNPCC are listed in Table 32-5.

*The *Escherichia coli* gene is called *MutS,* the yeast homologue is called the *MutS homologue* or *yMSH,* and the human homologues are called *hMSH* genes.

Can HNPCC Occur in the Absence of MSI?

A single, somewhat atypical family has been reported that stretches the borders of what constitutes HNPCC. Loss of the DNA MMR system results in a tissue that is hypermutable but not necessarily neoplastic as such. Several genes with potential tumor suppressor activity have been identified that contain repetitive sequences in their coding regions. The first of these to be identified was the type II receptor of transforming growth factor (TGF) β_1 (*TGF*β_1*RII,* or *RII*). Members of a kindred with several cases of colorectal cancer shared an inactivating germ-line mutation in *RII,* and as expected, the tumors lacked MSI. Neither of two mutation-carrying offspring (ages 57 and 48) of an affected individual have developed cancers, and no other tumors have been found in the gene carriers. In one of the colon cancers, loss of heterozygosity was found at the *RII* locus. The clinical implications of this finding remain to be established.[80]

THE CELLULAR AND MOLECULAR BIOLOGY OF HNPCC

It is necessary to become familiar with the DNA MMR system to fully understand the implications of HNPCC. Cancers develop in HNPCC when the DNA MMR system fails. As described, DNA MMR requires the concerted action of several proteins. Loss of any component of the system will inactivate, to some degree, the repair system.

The DNA MMR System

The DNA MMR system is illustrated schematically in Fig. 32-3.[81–84] During the synthesis of a new strand of DNA, many of the replication errors are immediately corrected by the 3′ to 5′ exonuclease activity of DNA polymerase. The combined activities of all the proofreading functions reduce the rate of replication errors to approximately 1 per 10^{12} base pairs. It is estimated that 99.9 percent of the mutations that escaped the proofreading activity of DNA polymerase are repaired by the MMR system, particularly single-base-pair mismatches and "loop outs" of unpaired bases, which tend to occur during reannealing of the new and template strands at repetitive sequences such as

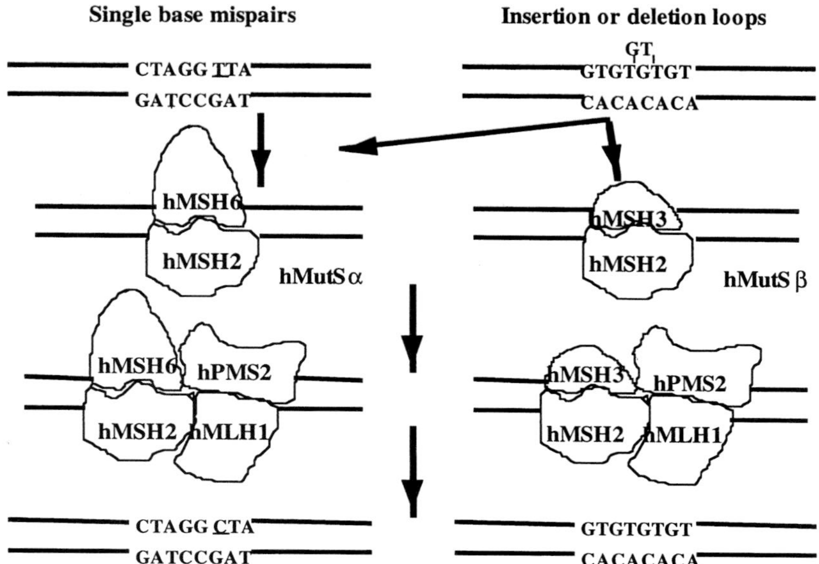

Fig. 32-3 DNA mismatch repair. During new strand synthesis, DNA polymerase may create mismatches, which will deform the newly formed DNA double helix. The newly synthesized strand transiently has gaps. The *hMutSα* complex (made up of *hMSH2* and *hMSH6*) recognizes the mismatch during S or G2 in the cell cycle and binds to it. The *hMHS2-hMSH6* complex has a particular affinity for recognition of single-base-pair mismatches. A second heteroduplex called *hMutSβ*, made up of *hMSH2* and *hMSH3*, has the additional ability to recognize and bind to loop-outs created at misaligned repetitive sequences that may occur at microsatellites. Some overlap may occur in these recognition affinities. There is no evidence for a functional *hMSH2* homoduplex. The *hMutLα* complex (made up of *hMLH1* and *hPMS2*) binds to the DNA mismatch-*hMutSα* complex in order to discriminate the strand containing the error. The role of *hPMS1* is not yet determined. After recognition of the mismatch, the complex accomplishes long patch excision, resynthesis, and ligation.

microsatellites. Commonly affected microsatellite sequences include mononucleotide repeats (such as A_n or G_n) and dinucleotide repeats (such as $\{CA/GT\}_n$).

A newly synthesized mispair will deform the double helix of DNA, creating a physical aberration. The deformed DNA strand is recognized and bound by a complex made up of a heterodimer of hMSH2 and either hMSH6 (initially called the *GT binding protein*, or GTBP)[85] or hMSH3. The hMSH2-hMSH6 heteroduplex is called hMutSα and favors binding to single-base-pair mismatches, and the hMSH2-hMSH3 heteroduplex is called hMutSβ and favors recognition of loop-outs that occur during misalignment of newly synthesized repetitive sequences such as microsatellites.[81–83] The regulation of the individual components of the DNA MMR system is currently not understood.

After the recognition complex binds to a DNA mismatch, the repair system must identify which of the two DNA strands represents the original template and which is the newly synthesized—and therefore erroneous—strand. This is achieved by the recruitment to the complex of a second heterodimer, made up of hMLH1 and hPMS2 (together called hMutLα), which binds to the DNA mispair-hMutSα/β complex; the full complex identifies the newly synthesized DNA strand, perhaps by virtue of gaps that remain between newly synthesized Okazaki segments. In lower organisms, newly synthesized strands are recognized by the transient absence of methylation. It is not known whether this mechanism also participates in the human MMR system. The repair system also requires the activity of several other enzymes, including helicase II, the DNA pol III holoenzyme, DNA ligase, single-stranded DNA-binding protein, and other DNA exonucleases. The DNA MMR system excises the newly synthesized strand from the point of its recognition (presumably the gap) back to the mismatch and then fully resynthesizes it.[60,61,83,84] This process is also known as *long patch excision*, which distinguishes it from another system (*short patch excision*) that repairs different types of DNA abnormalities (see Chap. 28). This process is probably even more complex in humans, and additional components of the system will likely be reported in the future.[86,87]

Understanding the DNA MMR system began with studies in *E. coli* and its Mut HLS system. In yeast, six *MutS* homologues (*yMSH1, yMSH2, yMSH3, yMSH4, yMSH5,* and *yMSH6*) and four *MutL* homologues (*yPMS1, yMLH1, yMLH2,* and *yMLH3*) have been identified.[60,88] *yMSH2-, yPMS1-,* and *yMLH1*-mutant strains of *Saccharomyces cerevisiae* undergo destabilization of microsatellite sequences during replication, as do the *MutL* and *MutS* mutants of *E. coli.* The human DNA MMR system is probably more complex, but at this time, mutations in only five of the involved genes are known to cause Lynch syndrome.

The genomic instability at microsatellite sequences was the initial finding that suggested that DNA MMR was inactivated in HNPCC tumors. The phenotype for cells carrying one mutant and one wild-type DNA MMR gene is normal. A second, somatic event occurs that results in inactivation of the wild-type allele, inactivating the DNA MMR system, which permits a hypermutable phenotype.[66] As mentioned earlier, the hMutS complex has two variants that may serve to add specificity to the recognition of DNA alterations. An issue that remains unclear is whether there is heterogeneity in the hMutLα complex that can further modify the repair system. Several *hPMS2*-related genes have been found on chromosome 7, the function of which remains unknown,[89] and these are potential candidates for additional participants in human DNA MMR.

The *hMSH2* gene encodes a protein with a relative mass of 106,000 that may be found immunohistochemically in the nucleus of a variety of tissues. In the intestinal tract, hMSH2 expression is limited to the replicating compartment of the crypt unit.[90,91] Most benign and malignant colorectal tumors express hMSH2 protein throughout the neoplastic tissue. Tumors from patients with germline mutations in *hMSH2* do not express the protein, consistent with the "two hit" mechanism of gene inactivation.[91] In cultured cells, expression of the hMSH2 protein is regulated based on progression through the cell cycle. Levels remain relatively low in resting cells but are induced when progression through the cell cycle toward mitosis occurs.[92]

Knockout Models

Mice deficient in DNA MMR genes have been developed using knockout techniques. Hemizygous mice (i.e., the equivalent of HNPCC) have an apparently normal phenotype in all the MMR knockout models. Somewhat surprisingly, MSH2-deficient mice have a seemingly normal embryonic development but are at high risk for developing lymphomas at an early age. Nullizygous cells from these animals have a mutator phenotype and are relatively tolerant of methylation damage, and nullizygous animals do not spontaneously develop tumors of the colon or other sites characteristically affected in HNPCC.[93] However, it has been reported that MSH2-deficient mice develop a very high incidence of intestinal neoplasms (mostly small intestinal) if they survive beyond 6 months, that 7 percent develop keratoacanthoma-like skin lesions, and all die by 1 year.[94] Interestingly, 70 percent of the intestinal tumors had inactivation of the *APC* gene.

Mice with knockouts in *MLH1, PMS1,* and *PMS2* have surprisingly few tumors,[95] which may reflect differences in structure of the colorectal tumor suppressor genes between the mice and humans. This explanation is supported by the observation that hypermutability can be found in the tissues of mice deficient in PMS2.[96] Mice nullizygous for *PMS2* (which do not develop intestinal neoplasms) crossed with *Min* mice (which are heterozygous for the mouse equivalent of the *APC* gene) develop more adenomas of the small intestines than do the *Min* mice.[97] These findings underscore the interaction among the genes involved in the development of colorectal cancer.

An *MSH6* knockout mouse has been developed. Cells without MSH6 activity are defective in the repair of single-base-pair mismatches, but repair of insertion/deletion mismatches was not impaired, as one may have predicted based on the yeast model. Nullizygous animals are at greatest risk for lymphomas, rather than colorectal cancers, and these tumors did not demonstrate MSI.[98]

Knockout mice with no *MLH1* genes have the MSI phenotype, have no DNA MMR activity in cell extracts, and are sterile due to defective spermatogenesis.[99,100] MLH1-deficient spermatocytes show numerous prematurely separated chromosomes and meiotic pachytene arrest. Male mice defective at the *PMS2* locus have abnormal chromosome synapses in meiosis and are highly prone to the development of sarcomas and lymphomas.[101] None of the knockout mice or the heterozygotes of these models develop a syndrome that closely resembles HNPCC.

THE PATHOPHYSIOLOGY OF HNPCC TUMORS

Most sporadic colorectal cancers develop through a mechanism that involves loss of relatively large chromosomal segments, which is thought to represent the deletion of wild-type tumor suppressor genes from the nucleus.[102] A proportion of sporadic colorectal cancers (perhaps 15 percent) and nearly all HNPCC-related cancers progress through a different mechanism, with MSI. MSI is inversely correlated with loss of heterozygosity of chromosomes 5q, 17p, and 18q.[6] In sporadic colorectal cancers, over half show mutations in the *K-RAS* oncogene.

What Growth-Controlling Genes Are Altered in HNPCC Cancers?

One of the initial reports indicated that mutations at *K-RAS, APC,* and *p53* were at least as common in HNPCC colon cancers as in sporadic ones.[7] One of the other initial investigations in the area reported that *K-RAS* and *p53* mutations were significantly less frequent in tumors with MSI but did not look for *APC* mutations.[5] The third of these initial groups did not look for point mutations in *APC, K-RAS,* or *p53* but noted an inverse relationship between MSI and loss of heterozygosity at 5q, 17p, and 18q.[6] A failure to microdissect the neoplastic tissue from infiltrating stroma or inflammatory cells (which can be considerable in these tumors) could lead to a systematic underestimate of cancer-associated mutations. This concern notwithstanding, one group has reported an inverse relationship between MSI and *p53* mutations in colon cancer cell lines,[103] and two groups reported a significant reduction in the incidence of mutations in *APC, p53,* and *K-RAS-2* in HNPCC colon cancers.[104,105] Additionally, immunohistochemical detection of the p53 protein in colorectal tissues is a surrogate for point mutations in the gene, since these mutations often stabilize the gene product. There is an inverse relationship between MSI and p53 immunostaining, which supports the contention that *p53* mutations may be less common in colon cancers with MSI.[106] One group has reported that the putative inverse relationship between MSI and *p53* mutations may not obtain in distal colorectal cancers.[107] This area still requires additional clarification.

An analysis of 101 colon cancers led the Vogelstein group to conclude that *APC* mutations were present in colorectal tumors with or without MSI, but that in MSI there was a significant predilection for frameshift mutations at repetitive sequences, particularly in polyadenine tracts.[108] At this point in time, the data suggest that most colorectal neoplasia begins with inactivation of the *APC* gene whether or not the tumor has MSI. However, the genetic events after *APC* inactivation may diverge thereafter depending on the mechanism underlying the genomic instability, which will select for specific genes in multistep tumor progression (Fig. 32-4).

The genomic instability seen at microsatellites in human colorectal neoplasms is an early event and can be found in the adenomatous polyps that serve as precursors to cancer in HNPCC.[109] Although MSI has been described in phenotypically normal human lymphocytes in unusual instances,[65] the mucosa in the colons from most patients with HNPCC does not show this abnormality.[110] The adenomatous polyps associated with sporadic tumors with MSI, or those in HNPCC, also have MSI, unlike sporadic adenomas, which rarely do.[109,111] The proportion of microsatellite loci that are mutated increases with progression from adenoma to carcinoma in both instances.[111,112]

In one series of cancers from patients with HNPCC, 95 percent showed the MSI phenotype, regardless of stage. In contrast, this type of genomic instability was found in only 3 percent of early

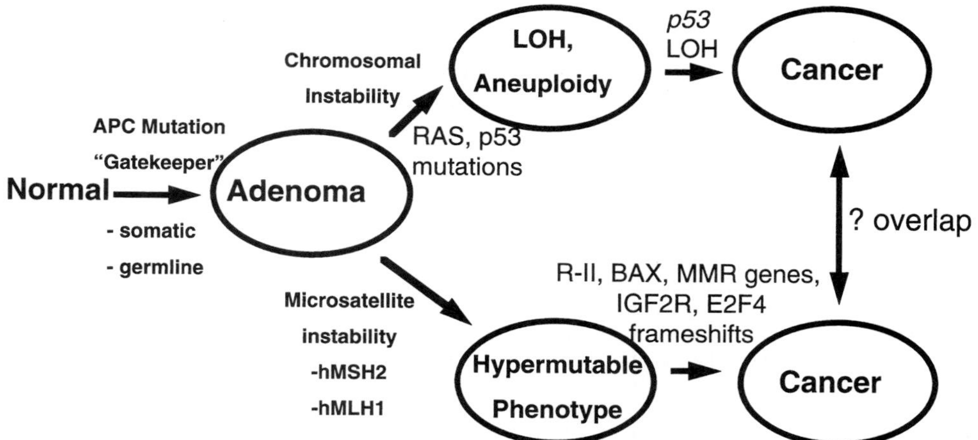

Fig. 32-4 Dual pathways for tumor development. The initial pathway for multistep carcinogenesis is depicted as the "chromosomal instability" at the top and involves LOH at tumor suppressor genes. The lower pathway (MSI) or the "mutator pathway" involves a unique destabilizing mechanism and inactivation of different genes, although both result in cancer. Both pathways may begin with an inactivating mutation at the *APC* locus, but the mutations leading to the lower pathway are those which would be expected with the loss of DNA MMR activity. These very distinct mechanisms lead to a similar pathologic result.

sporadic tumors (i.e., adenomas or intramucosal carcinomas) and 13 to 24 percent of sporadic invasive cancers. MSI has been reported in 35 percent of the liver metastases, suggesting that loss of the MMR system may play a role in tumor progression.[104]

One survey reported that 16 percent of sporadic colorectal cancers and 86 percent of colorectal cancers from HNPCC patients had MSI, including all patients in which a germ-line mutation in *hMSH2* was found. This lesion (i.e., MSI) was present in only 3 percent of 33 sporadic colorectal adenomas but in 57 percent of 14 adenomas associated with HNPCC. In addition, MSI was present in all the extracolonic cancers derived from HNPCC patients.[113] Although MSI has been described in phenotypically normal lymphocytes in patients with certain germ-line mutations in a DNA MMR gene,[65] the normal-appearing mucosa in the colons of patients with HNPCC does not show this abnormality.[110]

MSI in Non-HNPCC Tumors

MSI was first described in colorectal cancers not selected on the basis of a suspicion for HNPCC. Depending on the criteria used, 12 to 28 percent of colorectal cancers have MSI.[5–7] MSI is neither characteristic of colorectal cancer, limited to tumors of this organ, nor limited to HNPCC. MSI can be found in gastric cancers, endometrial cancers, ovarian tumors, urinary bladder tumors, non-small-cell lung cancers, small-cell lung cancers, breast cancers, and other tumors. In some instances, inactivation of a DNA MMR gene can be found, but this is not always the case. In some colon cancers, MSI can be found in association with loss of heterozygosity at one of the DNA MMR gene loci.[66] In the overwhelming majority of instances, there are no germ-line mutations at any of the known HNPCC loci when MSI is found.

As mentioned, a sizable minority of all sporadic colorectal cancers have MSI, and most of these are unrelated to HNPCC. Most of these tumors do not express hMHL1 immunohistochemically.[114,115] The mechanism responsible for silencing the *hMLH1* gene is frequently hypermethylation of promoter sequences in its 5′ upstream regulatory region.[116–119] Treating cultured tumor cells with 5-azacytidine can restore expression of hMLH1.[117–118] Hypermethylation and silencing of the *hMSH2* gene have not been found.[117,119]

Somatic Mutations Unique to Tumors with MSI

The finding of a type of hypermutability that was unrelated to the type of genomic instability seen in sporadic colorectal cancers (i.e., that manifested by widespread loss of heterozygosity) led to speculation that a distinct molecular pathway was responsible for HNPCC and related tumors.[35] An increased rate of mutation at the *hprt* locus was found in colorectal cancer cell lines that had MSI.[120] A recognition that MSI was associated with a disproportionate hypermutability at microsatellite sequences prompted several laboratories to look for repetitive sequences in the coding regions of genes that might be involved in growth control, with the speculation that these sequences would be at increased risk to experience a frameshift in a cell with MSI, resulting in a loss of function for the gene product.

The paradigm of this process was established on the identification of inactivating mutations in the type II transforming growth factor (TGF) β_1 receptor (called *RII*) in colon cancer cells with MSI.[121] TGFβ_1 signaling results in an inhibition of growth in colorectal epithelium.[122] Two repetitive sequences were found in coding regions of *RII*, a $(CA)_3$ and an A_8 sequence. Mutations in *RII* were concentrated on the A_8 sequence in MSI tumors and not found in non-MSI tumors. In each instance, the mutation resulted in loss of the RII transcript expression and a failure of cells to bind or respond to the TGFβ ligand. This is of particular importance because the TGFβ system inhibits the growth of colonic epithelial cells, and loss of this system in tumors with MSI represents a critical escape from growth control. Similar inactivating mutations in the *RII* gene have been found in gastric cancer cell lines and resected gastric carcinoma specimens; the mutations usually occur in a coding polyadenine tract.[123] It appears that inactivating mutations in growth-regulating genes may be a key mechanism by which tumors with MSI become neoplastic. These mutations are not commonly found in adenomas and may represent relatively late events in the multistep progressive neoplastic process in the evolution of a tumor in HNPCC.[124,125]

Table 32-6 Growth Regulatory Genes Mutated in Colorectal Cancers with MSI (Somatic Mutations in HNPCC)

GeneTarget	Repetitive Genetic Sequence	Frequency of Mutation in Colorectal Cancers with MSI or HNPCC	Reference
TGFβ_1 RII	A_8	85–90%(MSI)	121, 123, 124, 125
IGF IIR	G_8	9% of MSI tumors, 1/8 HNPCC tumors	126
Bax	G_8	51–54% (MSI); 52% in HNPCC	127, 130, 131
MSH6	C_8	33% in HNPCC	131
MSH3	A_8	52% in HNPCC	128, 129, 131, 132
E2F4	(CAG)n	65% (MSI)	129, 133
APC	Several	(See text)	108

Additional genes that may be involved in growth control also contain repetitive sequences in coding regions, which puts them at risk for mutation when the DNA MMR system is inactivated. Several of these have been found to be mutated in some proportion of HNPCC tumors, including the insulin-like growth factor II (IGF-II) receptor (which acts "in series" with *RII* in TGFβ signaling), *BAX, hMSH3, hMSH6,* and *E2F4;* the genes and the hypermutable sequences are listed in Table 32-6.[124,126–133] The requirement for involvement of any of these genes in the evolution of a tumor with MSI and the sequence of events involved remains to be determined. Of particular interest, two of the genes are themselves DNA MMR genes: *hMSH3* and *hMSH6.* This raises the possibility of a cascade of events in which a partial loss of DNA MMR activity could lead to mutations in other MMR genes and amplify the genomic instability.[134]

MSI and Resistance to Cytotoxic Drugs. Inactivation of the DNA MMR system is associated with increased resistance to DNA alkylation, which is toxic to wild-type cells.[135] Restoration of the DNA MMR system in a colon cancer cell line defective at the *hMLH1* locus increases sensitivity to alkylation and restores the G2/M cell cycle checkpoint.[136,137] The DNA MMR system also is required for transcription-coupled DNA repair.[138] These findings imply additional growth advantages for tumor cells defective in DNA MMR, since the G2/M checkpoint may be bypassed in these cells, and an additional level of mutation repair is lost. Evidence is accumulating that DNA MMR-defective cells may be relatively resistant to cytotoxic chemotherapy used to treat cancer.[136,137,139–143] Cell lines have been identified that are deficient for each of the major human DNA MMR genes, which provide valuable models for study.[144] All these observations have come from experiments on cultured cells, and the clinical implications of this have not yet been tested on patients.

MSI and Neoplasia in Ulcerative Colitis. MSI is commonly seen in cancers associated with ulcerative colitis, as well as the dysplasias that antedate these tumors.[145] An intronic polymorphism in the *hMSH2* gene is more common in patients who develop colitis-associated neoplasia than in control patients with or without colitis.[146] Moreover, MSI may be found in the non-neoplastic colonic mucosa from patients with chronic ulcerative colitis.[147] It has not yet been confirmed whether inactivation of the DNA MMR system is an essential part of tumor development in chronic inflammation.

Table 32-7 Frequency of Specific Germ-Line Mutations in HNPCC

HNPCC Gene	Frequency/Proportion of Families[64]
hMSH2	31%
hMLH1	33%
hPMS1	Rare (one family)
hPMS2	4%
GTBP (hMSH6)	Rare (a few families)
Undetermined loci	32%

Table 32-8 The Bethesda Guidelines for Testing of Colorectal Tumors for MSI[148]

1. Individuals with cancer in families that meet the Amsterdam criteria
2. Individuals with two HNPCC-related cancers including synchronous and metachronous colorectal cancer or associated extracolonic cancers*
3. Individuals with colorectal cancer and a first-degree relative with colorectal cancer and/or HNPCC-related extracolonic cancer and/or a colorectal adenoma; one of the cancers diagnosed at age less than 45, the adenoma at age less than 40
4. Individuals with colorectal cancer or endometrial cancer diagnosed at age less than 45
5. Individuals with right-sided colorectal cancer with an undifferentiated pattern (solid/cribriform) on histopathology diagnosed at age less than 45†
6. Individuals with signet-ring-cell-type colorectal cancer diagnosed at age less than 45‡
7. Individuals with adenomas diagnosed at age less than 40

*Endometrial, ovarian, gastric, hepatobiliary, small bowel, transitional cell carcinoma of the renal pelvis or ureter.
†*Solid/cribriform* defined as poorly undifferentiated carcinoma composed of irregular solid sheets of large eosinophilic cells and containing small glandlike spaces.
‡Composed of more than 50% signet-ring cells.

THE DIAGNOSIS AND MANAGEMENT OF HNPCC

Identification of the role of the DNA MMR system in the genesis of HNPCC provided a breakthrough in the premorbid diagnosis of the disease. Although many more proteins participate in the DNA MMR system, as a practical issue, two of the genes — *hMSH2* and *hMLH1* — appear to account for most Lynch syndrome diagnoses (Table 32-7). Unfortunately, the nature of the genes and the heterogeneity of the mutational spectrum have limited the clinical practicality of sequencing for germ-line mutations.

Testing for MSI: MSI-H, MSH-L, and MSS

Insight into the pathophysiology and genetic basis of HNPCC has provided multiple strategies for making this diagnosis. It is possible to screen for HNPCC by observing MSI in a tumor specimen. Guidelines for MSI testing were drawn up at a consensus workshop on HNPCC and have been referred to as the *Bethesda guidelines*[148] (Table 32-8). Furthermore, another workshop has led to the identification of a verified panel of consensus microsatellite loci that can ensure uniformity of diagnosis between laboratories.[59] According to these guidelines, five markers are considered to be a suitable panel to determine the presence of MSI. These microsatellite loci include two polyadenine sequences (*BAT25* and *BAT26*) and three dinucleotide repeats (*D2S123, D5S346,* and *D17S250*).

If two or more microsatellite amplifications demonstrate microsatellite instability (compared with normal tissue from that patient), the tumor is called *MSI-H,* for high-frequency MSI. This group of tumors is phenotypically indistinguishable from HNPCC colon cancers, although the sporadic tumors are (by definition) not accompanied by germ-line mutations in a DNA MMR gene. Other markers may be shown to be equally useful, but these markers have been carefully validated, have undergone comparisons between reference laboratories, and are the currently recommended panel for MSI testing.[149,150] If none of five microsatellite markers shows instability, the tumor is considered to be *microsatellite stable* (MSS). The use of additional markers in these tumors is unlikely to be helpful.[149,150] If only one of five markers shows a frameshift mutation, this is termed *MSI-L,* for low-frequency MSI. The MSS and MSI-L tumors share the same phenotypic characteristics, distinct from the MSI-H group. In the case of ambiguous amplifications (or non-informative analyses), additional markers have been suggested, although in most instances five markers are adequate.[59] Some proportion of MSS tumors will show microsatellite instability in a small fraction of tested loci (i.e., < 10 percent) if a very large number is analyzed. The implications of this are not yet clear, and it is not evident that there are any distinctions to be made between the MSS and MSI-L tumor groups, or what *MSI-L* represents.

Screening Populations for HNPCC

Several groups have used methods other than direct sequencing to diagnose HNPCC. A group in the Netherlands used denaturing gradient gel electrophoresis (DGGE) to more rapidly screen for sequence aberrations and found germ-line mutations in *hMSH2* or *hMLH1* in 47 of 184 (26 percent) suspected cancer families based on the history of multiple tumors among relatives.[74] This study recognized the predictive value of including endometrial cancer in the clinical diagnosis of families with HNPCC.

A large clinical study from Finland screened over 500 consecutive colorectal cancers for MSI, and if instability was noted at two or more of seven tested microsatellites, the patient was referred for sequencing of *hMSH2* and *hMLH1.*[75] Using these criteria, 63 of 509 (12 percent) tumors showed MSI, but only 10 of 63 (16 percent) of those with MSI had a germ-line mutation detected, and half of these came from a known founder mutation that is common in Finland. The authors estimated that at least 2 percent of their colorectal cancer patients had HNPCC. This and all other studies are limited to the extent that all the relevant HNPCC genes are known and by the inherent problems in finding all the genetic mechanisms by which these genes might be inactivated.

Making a Definitive Diagnosis of HNPCC

Although 92 percent of HNPCC-associated colon cancers have MSI,[72] only a minority of tumors with MSI come from HNPCC families.[151] Direct sequencing of the DNA MMR genes is a possible strategy to make the diagnosis of HNPCC, but the number of exons involved and the relative absence of "founder mutations" make this clinically impractical. Knowledge of the critical loci for HNPCC makes linkage analysis a possible approach, but multiple affected family members must be available for testing, and the diagnostic power is limited.[152] The large fraction of inactivating germ-line mutations in *hMSH2* that result in a truncated protein suggest that an *in vitro* transcription/translation assay may be clinically useful. This latter approach provided a positive test in about half of patients who met the Amsterdam criteria for HNPCC.[153]

Direct sequencing of the exons in *hMSH2* and *hMLH1* is a direct, if labor-intensive, approach to diagnosis. At this time, the full spectrum of disease-producing germ-line mutations and innocuous polymorphisms has not been catalogued, which may complicate the interpretation of DNA sequence data. Analyses based on harvesting RNA from lymphocytes is complicated by the observation that both *hMSH2* and *hMLH1* may undergo alternative splicing that will generate different messages and proteins, which

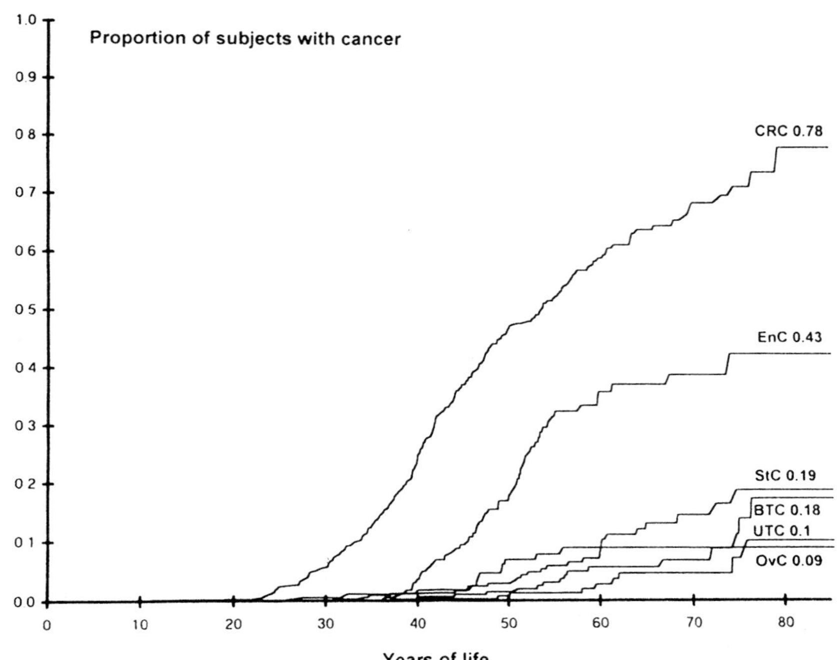

Fig. 32-5 Lifetime risk of different cancers in hereditary nonpolyposis colorectal cancer (HNPCC) syndrome. Lines represent estimates for colorectal cancer (CRC), endometrial cancer (EnC), stomach cancer (StC), biliary tract cancers (BTC), ureteral cancers (UTC), and ovarian cancers (OvC). (*From Aarnio et al.*[161])

may complicate interpretation.[154–156] Unfortunately, the range of germ-line mutations in *hMSH2* and *hMLH1* is wide and includes insertions, deletions, nonsense mutations, and missense mutations.[72] These considerations make screening for a germ-line diagnosis in HNPCC a daunting undertaking. Nonetheless, when a mutation is correctly identified in a family, direct sequencing or *in vitro* transcription/translation will be highly reliable for other at-risk members of that family. In exceptional instances, founder mutations may be responsible for a large proportion of familial colon cancer in a specific geographic region with a relatively immobile population.[157,158]

Several published lists of germ-line mutations are available,[87,159] but an Internet site has been established to catalog and continuously update these mutations (*http://www.nfdht.nl/database/mdbchoice.htm*). This site contains a database for HNPCC pathologic germ-line mutations and intragenic polymorphisms and permits the submission of novel mutations.

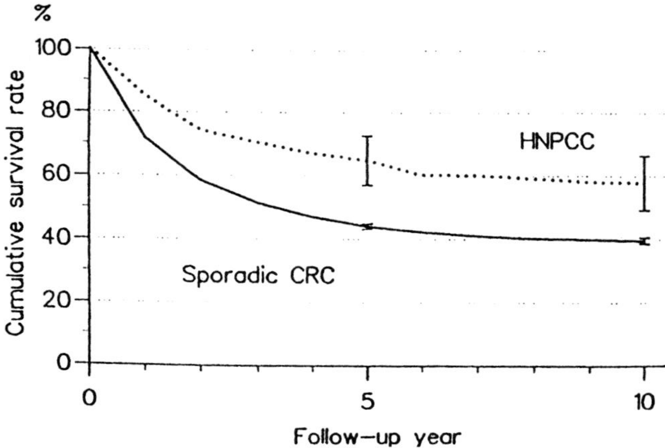

Fig. 32-6 Better survival rates in patients with *MLH1*-associated hereditary colorectal cancer. (*From Sankila et al.*[162] *Used by permission.*)

Finding the germ-line mutation in an individual family has important implications. First, it permits the physician and genetic counselor to increase the certainty with which a diagnosis is made. Half those at risk will be informed that they did not inherit a high risk for cancer, and half will be informed with certainty of their risks, for which a surveillance program should be initiated.

Cancer Risk in HNPCC

The lifetime risk for cancer in HNPCC can only be estimated at this time (see Table 32-2). Cumulative risk for colorectal cancer has been estimated to range from 30 to 78 percent and endometrial cancer from 20 percent[161] to 43 percent for women[161] (Fig. 32-5 and Table 32-2). Patients with HNPCC must be identified because of the extremely high risk for metachronous cancers after successful treatment of the index tumor.[161] Patients with *hMLH1*-associated HNPCC in Finland have a significantly better survival rate when compared with patients with sporadic colorectal cancers[162] (Fig. 32-6). It is not known whether this observation is generally applicable to all *hMLH1* and *hMSH2*-associated HNPCC families.

Management of Patients with HNPCC

Once HNPCC patients are identified, a screening program consisting of colonoscopy or barium enema and sigmoidoscopy significantly reduces the rate of tumor development and death in patients with HNPCC[163] (Fig. 32-7). The observation that a screening program actually lowered the colorectal cancer incidence rates in family members with HNPCC suggests that the adenomatous polyps in this disease may be more prone to malignant transformation than adenomas in the general population and that their removal is an important part of a prevention program. Compared with sporadic cancers, at the time of diagnosis a lower stage of disease is commonly present in HNPCC, significantly fewer distant metastases are present, and survival is significantly better.[164,165] Colorectal lesions (including all adenomas) are detected in as many as 41 percent of asymptomatic patients who are referred for colonoscopy, but compliance with screening is surprisingly difficult.[166] Some reports have suggested that half the adenomas and perhaps as many of the early carcinomas in HNPCC are flat, making them a challenge for the

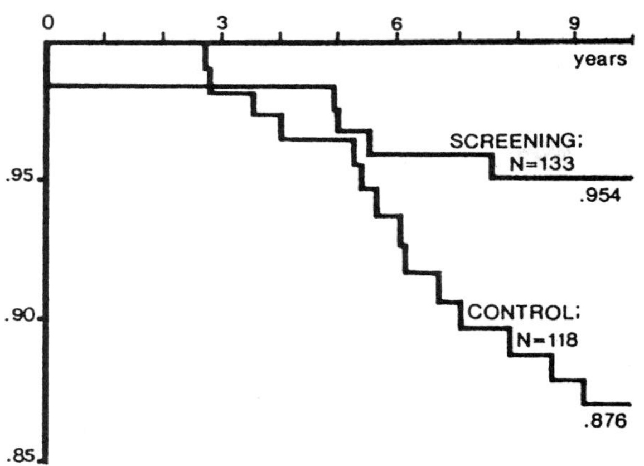

Fig. 32-7 Screening reduces colorectal cancer rate in families with hereditary nonpolyposis colorectal cancer. (*From Jarvinen et al.*[163] Used by permission.)

colonoscopist and very difficult lesions for detection radiographically.[167]

When a young individual (i.e., less than 45 years of age) develops colorectal cancer, this raises the concern that the patient and patient's relatives are at increased risk for HNPCC. One study suggested that the relative risk for colorectal cancer in the close relatives of such patients is increased five-fold and may be even higher for female relatives.[168] MSI is significantly more likely to occur in the colorectal cancers of young patients and can be found in 58 percent of patients under 35 years of age, even when the family history does not suggest HNPCC.[169] Even in such patients, less than half will have detectable germ-line mutations in the known DNA MMR genes.

The following approach might be followed to identify HNPCC. A careful family history should be taken in all patients who develop a cancer. A full pedigree should be drawn, and critical information should include all relatives who develop tumors, the organs affected, the age of first cancer, the occurrence of multiple cancers, and the ages reached by individuals who did not develop cancer. When the Amsterdam criteria are met, HNPCC is very likely. Under these circumstances, the *in vitro* transcription/translation assay for premature truncating mutations in *hMSH2* or *hMLH1* will provide a diagnosis in about half of families.[153] When available, tumor tissue can be valuable. Microsatellite analysis may be performed from paraffin-embedded tissues. Patients with HNPCC are likely to have MSI at multiple loci. If no MSI is found, the likelihood of HNPCC is substantially reduced, since perhaps 5 percent of such cancers lack this. Sporadic colorectal cancers are common, and phenocopies may occur in some families; in this instance, testing for MSI might be helpful. If available, direct sequencing of the DNA MMR genes is the gold standard for diagnosis, but some alterations—particularly missense mutations—may be ambiguous and difficult to interpret.

Although the rodent models suggest that inactivation of each of the DNA MMR genes is associated with a unique phenotype, there is less information of this type in human populations. One study has suggested that minor variations in non-colorectal cancers may be found between *hMSH2* and *hMLH1* families.[170] The Muir-Torre syndrome has been linked only to *hMSH2* mutations thus far.[48,49] Of interest, not all kindreds with the mutations found in some Muir-Torre syndrome families will necessarily develop the characteristic skin tumors.

TREATMENT OF HNPCC

When an HNPCC patient presents with an invasive cancer, the appropriate treatment is to perform a subtotal colectomy with an ileosigmoid or ileorectal anastamosis. The increased risk for tumor development in the rest of the colon mandates aggressive surgical treatment, but the ability to screen the rectum for recurrent disease makes a total proctocolectomy unnecessary. If a patient should present with an invasive rectal cancer, a total proctocolectomy may be required. The risk of rectal cancer in a patient with HNPCC after a rectal-sparing operation is approximately 12 percent at 12 years.[171] One report suggested that patients with *hMHS2* mutations had a 28 percent risk of rectal cancer, compared with an 8 percent risk in *hMLH1* patients.[172] The annual rate of metachronous colorectal cancer for their patients was 2.1 percent for *hMLH1* patients, 1.7 percent for *hMSH2* patients, and 0.33 percent for patients with sporadic cancers. When the diagnosis is known at the time of surgery, it is recommended that the proximal colon be removed, even if it is free of neoplasia, to simplify surveillance and protect the patient against the need for a second laparotomy or a missed diagnosis of a proximal cancer.

Patients who are identified in the presymptomatic stage by genetic testing should be informed that their lifetime risk for colorectal cancer may be as high as 80 to 90 percent and that surveillance colonoscopy every 3 years can significantly reduce morbidity and mortality. The occurrence of "interval cancers" in patients who have undergone surveillance at 2- to 3-year intervals has prompted some to argue for more aggressive surveillance, perhaps on an annual basis, because of the unique natural history of these tumors.[173] Surveillance colonoscopy every 2 to 3 years will increase the patient's life expectancy and is less expensive than waiting for signs or symptoms of a colorectal tumor.[174] A task force report from the Cancer Genetics Studies Consortium has recommended colonoscopy every 1 to 3 years beginning at age 20 to 25 in individuals known to have HNPCC.[175] Screening for endometrial carcinoma should begin at 25 to 35 years of age, but the optimal means of surveillance is not yet certain. There is no consensus on screening for cancer of other organs, since the risks are much lower outside the colon and uterus. Some patients will elect surgical removal of the colon and/or uterus (and perhaps ovaries) when informed of the risks of cancer and the limitations of screening; these decisions will depend on the level of risk the patient is willing to assume and his or her attitude about the screening tests. There is insufficient evidence at this time to estimate the effectiveness of screening tests, and some cautious patients may prefer prophylactic surgery.

The age of onset of tumors can be variable within an HNPCC family, leading to the misperception of a "skipped generation," which should be taken into account when managing families.[176] In the same vein, a retrospective study has indicated that in only 40 percent of patients was a family history available that suggested HNPCC when it was actually encountered.[177] In such families, the presence of a villous adenoma in a young patient should heighten the clinical suspicion for HNPCC, and perhaps such a lesion should be interpreted with the same implications as a cancer.

There are no known medical treatments for patients with HNPCC. Aspirin may play an important protective effect against the development of sporadic colorectal cancer; however, its impact on HNPCC is unknown. No other interventions or dietary modifications have been demonstrated to have a beneficial effect in this disease.

ACKNOWLEDGMENTS

This work was supported by Grant RO1-72851 and The Research Service of the Department of Veterans Affairs.

REFERENCES

1. Boland CR: Neoplasia of the gastrointestinal tract, in Yamada T (ed): *Textbook of Gastroenterology*, vol 24, 2d ed. Philadelphia, Lippincott, 1995, pp 578–595.
2. Cannon-Albright LA, Skolnick MH, Bishop DT, et al: Common inheritance of colonic adenomatous polyps and associated colorectal cancers. *N Engl J Med* **319**:533, 1988.

3. Fuchs CS, Giovannucci EL, Colditz GA, et al: A prospective study of family history and the risk of colorectal cancer. *N Engl J Med* **331**:1669, 1994.
4. Winawer SJ, Zauber AG, Gerdes H, et al: Risk of colorectal cancer in the families of patients with adenomatous polyps. The National Polyp Study Workgroup. *N Engl J Med* **334**:82, 1996.
5. Ionov Y, Peinado MA, Malkhosyan S, et al: Ubiquitous somatic mutations in simple repeated sequences reveal a new mechanism for colonic carcinogenesis. *Nature* **363**:558, 1993.
6. Thibodeau SN, Bren G, Schaid D: Microsatellite instability in cancer of the proximal colon. *Science* **260**:816, 1993.
7. Peltomaki P, Aaltonen LA, Sistonen P, et al: Genetic mapping of a locus predisposing to human colorectal cancer. *Science* **260**:810, 1993.
8. Aaltonen LA, Peltomaki P, Leach FS, et al: Clues to the pathogenesis of familial colorectal cancer. *Science* **260**:812, 1993.
9. Lynch HT, Lanspa S, Smyrk T, Boman B, Watson P, Lynch J: Hereditary nonpolyposis colorectal cancer (Lynch syndromes I & II): Genetics, pathology, natural history, and cancer control, part I. *Cancer Genet Cytogenet* **53**:143, 1991.
10. Lynch HT, Ens J, Lynch JF, et al: Tumor variation in three extended Lynch syndrome II kindreds. *Am J Gastroenterol* **83**:74, 1988.
11. Vasen HFA, Offerhaus GJA, den Hartog Jager FCA, et al: The tumor spectrum in hereditary non-polyposis colorectal cancer: a study of 24 kindreds in the Netherlands. *Int J Cancer* **46**:31, 1990.
12. Watson P, Lynch HT: Extracolonic cancer in hereditary nonpolyposis colorectal cancer. *Cancer* **71**:677, 1993.
13. St. John DJB, McDermott FT, Hopper Jl, et al: Cancer risk in relatives of patients with common colorectal cancer. *Ann Intern Med* **118**:785, 1993.
14. Houlston RS, Murday V, Harocopos C, et al: Screening and genetic counselling for relatives of patients with colorectal cancer in a family cancer clinic. *Br Med J* **301**:18, 1990.
15. Mecklin J-P, Jarvinen JH, Aukee S, et al: Screening for colorectal carcinoma in cancer family syndrome kindreds. *Scand J Gastroenterol* **22**:449, 1987.
16. Ponz de Leon M, Sassatelli R, Sacchetti C, et al: Familial aggregation of tumors in the three year experience of a population-based colorectal cancer registry. *Cancer Res* **49**:4344, 1989.
17. Stephenson BM, Finan PJ, Gascoyne J, et al: Frequency of familial colorectal cancer. *Br J Surg* **78**:1162, 1991.
18. Mecklin J-P: Frequency of hereditary colorectal cancer. *Gastroenterology* **93**:1021, 1987.
19. Kee F, Collins BJ: How prevalent is cancer family syndrome? *Gut* **32**:309, 1991.
20. Westlake PJ, Bryant HE, Huchcroft SA, et al: Frequency of hereditary nonpolyposis colorectal cancer in southern Alberta. *Dig Dis Sci* **36**:1441, 1991.
21. Kee F, Collins BJ: Families at risk of colorectal cancer: who are they? *Gut* **33**:787, 1992.
22. Mecklin J-P, Jarvinen HJ, Peltokallio P: Cancer family syndrome: Genetic analysis of 22 Finnish kindreds. *Gastroenterology* **90**:328, 1986.
23. Lynch HT, Smyrk TC, Watson P, et al: Genetics, natural history, tumor spectrum, and pathology of hereditary nonpolyposis colorectal cancer: An updated review. *Gastroenterology* **104**:1535, 1993.
24. Marra G, Boland CR: Hereditary nonpolyposis colorectal cancer (HNPCC): The syndrome, the genes, and an historical perspective. *J Natl Cancer Inst* **87**:1114, 1995.
25. Warthin AS: Heredity with reference to carcinoma. *Arch Intern Med* **12**:546, 1913.
26. Warthin AS: The further study of a cancer family. *J Cancer Res* **9**:279, 1925.
27. Warthin AS: Heredity of carcinoma in man. *Ann Intern Med* **4**:681, 1931.
28. Hauser IJ, Weller CV: A further report on the cancer family of Warthin. *Am J Cancer* **27**:434, 1936.
29. Lynch HT, Krush AJ: Cancer family "G" revisited: 1895-1970. *Cancer* **27**:1505, 1971.
30. Lynch HT, Shaw MW, Magnuson CW, et al: Hereditary factors in two large midwestern kindreds. *Arch Intern Med* **117**:206, 1966.
31. Boland CR, Troncale FJ: Familial colonic cancer in the absence of antecedent polyposis. *Ann Intern Med* **100**:700, 1984.
32. Boland CR: Familial colonic cancer syndromes. *West J Med* **139**:351, 1983.
33. Jager A, Bisgaard M, Myrhoj T, et al: Reduced frequency of extracolonic cancers in hereditary nonpolyposis colorectal cancer families with monoallelic hMLH1 expression. *Am J Hum Genet* **61**:129, 1997.
34. Vasen HFA, Mecklin J-P, Khan PM, et al: The International Collaborative Group on hereditary non-polyposis colorectal cancer. *Dis Colon Rectum* **34**:424, 1991.
35. Kinzler KW, Vogelstein B: Lessons from hereditary colorectal cancer. *Cell* **87**:159, 1996.
36. Dunlop MG, Farrington SM, Carothers AD, et al: Cancer risk associated with germline DNA mismatch repair gene mutations. *Hum Mol Genet* **6**:105, 1997.
37. Vasen H, Wijnen J, Menko F, et al: Cancer risk in families with hereditary nonpolyposis colorectal cancer diagnosed by mutation analysis. *Gastroenterology* **110**:1020, 1996.
38. Rodriguez-Bigas MA, Vasen H, Lynch H, et al: Characteristics of small bowel carcinoma in hereditary nonpolyposis colorectal carcinoma. *Cancer* **83**:240, 1998.
39. Lanspa ST, Lynch HT, Smyrk TC, et al: Colorectal adenomas in the Lynch syndromes: Results of a colonoscopy screening program. *Gastroenterology* **98**:1117, 1990.
40. Jass JR, Stewart SM: Evolution of hereditary non-polyposis colorectal cancer. *Gut* **33**:783 1992.
41. Aarnio M, Salovaara R, Aaltonen LA, et al: Features of gastric cancer in hereditary non-polyposis colorectal cancer syndrome. *Int J Cancer* **74**:551, 1997.
42. Risinger JI, Barrett JC, Watson P, et al: Molecular genetic evidence of the occurrence of breast cancer as an integral tumor in patients with the hereditary nonpolyposis colorectal carcinoma syndrome. *Cancer* **77**:1836, 1996.
43. Vasen HF, Sanders EA, Taal BG, et al: The risk of brain tumors in hereditary non-polyposis colorectal cancer (HNPCC). *Int J Cancer* **65**:422, 1996.
44. Mecklin J-P, Jarvinen HJ, Aukee S, Elomaa I, Karajalainen K: Screening for colorectal carcinoma in cancer family syndrome kindreds. *Scand J Gastroenterol* **22**:449, 1987.
45. Lynch HT, Lynch PM, Pester J, et al: The cancer family syndrome: Rare cutaneous phenotypic linkage of Torre's syndrome. *Arch Intern Med* **141**:607, 1980.
46. Lynch HT, Fusaro RM, Roberts L, et al: Muir-Torre syndrome in several members of a family with a variant of cancer family syndrome. *Br J Dermatol* **113**:295, 1985.
47. Honchel R, Halling KC, Schaid DJ, et al: Microsatellite instability in Muir-Torre syndrome. *Cancer Res* **54**:1159, 1994.
48. Kolodner RD, Hall NR, Lipford J, et al: Structure of the human MSH2 locus and analysis of two Muir-Torre kindreds for msh2 mutations. *Genomics* **24**:516, 1994.
49. Kruse R, Lamberti C, Wang Y, et al: Is the mismatch repair deficient type of Muir-Torre syndrome confined to mutations in the hMSH2 gene? *Hum Genet* **98**:747, 1996.
50. Kee F, Patterson CC, Collins BJ, et al: Histologic characteristics and outcome of familial non-polyposis colorectal cancer. *Scand J Gastroenterol* **26**:419, 1991.
51. Jass JR, Smyrk TC, Stewart SM, et al: Pathology of hereditary non-polyposis colorectal cancer. *Anticancer Res* **14**:1631, 1994.
52. Mecklin J-P, Sipponen P, Jarvinen HJ: Histopathology of colorectal carcinomas and adenomas in cancer family syndrome. *Dis Colon Rectum* **29**:849, 1986.
53. Frei JV: Hereditary nonpolyposis colorectal cancer (Lynch syndrome): II. Diploid malignancies with prolonged survival. *Cancer* **69**:1108, 1992.
54. Kouri M, Laasonen A, Mecklin J-P, et al: Diploid predominance in hereditary nonpolyposis colorectal carcinoma evaluated by flow cytometry. *Cancer* **65**:1825, 1990.
55. Kim H, Jen J, Vogelstein B, et al: Clinical and pathological characteristics of sporadic colorectal carcinomas with DNA replication errors in microsatellite sequences. *Am J Pathol* **145**:148, 1994.
56. Loeb LA: Mutator phenotype may be required for multistage carcinogenesis. *Cancer Res* **51**:3075, 1991.
57. Loeb LA: Microsatellite instability: Marker of a mutator phenotype in cancer. *Cancer Res* **54**:5059, 1994.
58. Peinado MA, Malkhosyan S, Velazquez, et al: Isolation and characterization of allelic losses and gains in colorectal tumors by arbitrarily primed polymerase chain reaction. *Proc Natl Acad Sci USA* **89**:10065, 1992.
59. Boland CR, Thibodeau SN, Hamilton SR, et al: A National Cancer Institute workshop on microsatellite instability for cancer detection and familial predisposition: Development of international criteria for the determination of microsatellite instability in colorectal cancer. *Cancer Res* (in press).

60. Fishel R, Kolodner RD: Identification of mismatch repair genes and their role in the development of cancer. *Curr Opin Genet Dev* **5**:382, 1995.
61. Kolodner RD: Mismatch repair: mechanisms and relationship to cancer susceptibility. *TIBS* **20**:397, 1995.
62. Strand M, Prolla TA, Liskay RM, Petes TD: Destabilization of tracts of simple repetetive DNA in yeast by mutations affecting DNA mismatch repair. *Nature* **365**:274, 1993.
63. Fishel R, Lescoe MK, Rao MRS, et al: The human mutator gene homolog MSH2 and its association with hereditary nonpolyposis colon cancer. *Cell* **75**:1027, 1993.
64. Leach FS, Nicolaides NC, Papadopoulos N, et al: Mutations of a mutS homolog in hereditary nonpolyposis colorectal cancer. *Cell* **75**:1215, 1993.
65. Parsons R, Li G-M, Longley M, et al: Mismatch repair deficiency in phenotypically normal human cells. *Science* **268**:738, 1995.
66. Hemminki A, Peltomaki P, Mecklin J-K: Loss of the wild type MLH1 gene is a feature of hereditary nonpolyposis colorectal cancer. *Nature Genet* **8**:405, 1994.
67. Lindblom A, Tannergard P, Werelius B, et al: Genetic mapping of a second locus predisposing to hereditary non-polyposis colon cancer. *Nature Genet* **5**:279, 1993.
68. Bronner CE, Baker SM, Morrison PT, et al: Mutation in the DNA mismatch repair gene homologue hMLH1 is associated with hereditary non-polyposis colon cancer. *Nature* **368**:258, 1994.
69. Papadopoulos N, Nicolaides NC, Wei YF, et al: Mutation of a mutL homolog in hereditary colon cancer. *Science* **263**:1625, 1994.
70. Nicolaides NC, Papadopoulos N, Liu B, et al: Mutations of two PMS homologues in hereditary nonpolyposis colon cancer. *Nature* **371**:75, 1994.
71. Liu B, Nicolaides NC, Markowitz S, et al: Mismatch repair gene defects in sporadic colorectal cancers with microsatellite instability. *Nature Genet* **9**:48, 1995.
72. Liu B, Parsons R, Papadopoulos N, et al: Analysis of mismatch repair genes in hereditary non-polyposis colorectal cancer. *Nature Med* **2**:169, 1996.
73. Luce MC, Marra G, Chauhan DP, et al: In vitro transcription/translation assay for the screening of hMLH1 and hMSH2 mutations in familial colon cancer. *Gastroenterology* **109**:1368, 1995.
74. Wijnen JT, Vasen H, Khan PM, et al: Clinical findings with implications for genetic testing in families with clustering of colorectal cancer. *N Engl J Med* **339**:511, 1998.
75. Aaltonen LA, Salovaara R, Kristo P, et al: Incidence of hereditary nonpolyposis colorectal cancer and the feasibility of molecular screening for the disease. *N Engl J Med* **338**:1481, 1998.
76. Nicolaides N, Littman S, Modrich P, et al: A naturally occurring hPMS2 mutation can confer a dominant negative mutator phenotype. *Mol Cell Biol* **18**:1635, 1998.
77. Acharya S, Wilson T, Gradia S, et al: hMSH2 forms specific mispair-binding complexes with hMSH3 and hMSH6. *Proc Natl Acad Sci USA* **93**:13629, 1996.
78. Miyaki M, Konishi M, Tanaka K, et al: Germline mutation of MSH6 as the cause of hereditary nonpolyposis colorectal cancer. *Nature Genet* **17**:271, 1997.
79. Akiyama Y, Sato H, Yamada T, et al: Germ-line mutation of the hMSH6/GTBP gene in an atypical hereditary nonpolyposis colorectal cancer kindred. *Cancer Res* **57**:3920, 1997.
80. Lu SL, Kawabata M, Imamura T, et al: HNPC associated with germline mutation in the TGF-β type II receptor gene. *Nature Genet* **19**:17, 1998.
81. Cooper DL, Lahue RS, Modrich P: Methyl-directed mismatch repair is bidirectional. *J Biol Chem* **268**:11823, 1993.
82. Kunkel TA: Misalignment-mediated DNA synthesis errors. *Biochemistry* **29**:8003, 1990.
83. Modrich P: Mechanisms and biological effects of mismatch repair. *Annu Rev Genet* **25**:229, 1991.
84. Sancar A: DNA repair in humans. *Annu Rev Genet* **29**:69, 1995.
85. Drummond JT, Li G-M, Longley MJ, et al: Isolation of an hMSH2-p160 heterodimer that restores DNA mismatch repair to tumor cells. *Science* **268**:1909, 1995.
86. Umar A, Boyer JC, Kunkel TA: DNA loop repair by human cell extracts. *Science* **266**:814, 1994.
87. Marra G, Boland CR: DNA repair and colorectal cancer. *Gastroenterol Clin North Am* **25(4):755, 1996.**
88. Marsischky GT, Filosi N, Kane MF, et al: Redundancy of *Saccharomyces cerevisiae* MSH3 and MSH6 in MSH2-dependent mismatch repair. *Genes Dev* **10**:407, 1996.
89. Nicolaides NC, Carter KC, Shell BK, et al: Genomic organization of the human PMS2 gene family. *Genomics* **30**:195, 1995.
90. Wilson TM, Ewel A, Duguid JR, et al: Differential cellular expression of the human MSH2 repair enzyme in small and large intestine. *Cancer Res* **55**:5146, 1995.
91. Leach FS, Polyak K, Burrell M, et al: Expression of the human mismatch repair gene hMSH2 in normal and neoplastic tissues. *Cancer Res* **56**:235, 1996.
92. Marra G, Chang CL, Laghi LA, Chauhan DP, Young D, Boland CR: Expression of the human MutS homolog 2 (hMSH2) protein in resting and proliferating cells. *Oncogene* **13**:2189, 1996.
93. de Wind N, Dekker M, Berns A, et al: Inactivation of the mouse Msh2 gene results in mismatch repair deficiency, methylation tolerance, hyperrecombination, and predisposition to cancer. *Cell* **82**:321, 1995.
94. Reitmair AH, Redston M, Cai JC, et al: Spontaneous carcinomas and skin neoplasms in Msh2-deficient mice. *Cancer Res* **56**:3842, 1996.
95. Prolla TA, Baker SM, Harris AC, et al: Tumour susceptibility and spontaneous mutation in mice deficient in Mlh1, Pms1 and Pms2 DNA mismatch repair. *Nature Genet* **18**:276, 1998.
96. Narayanan L, Fritzell JA, Baker SM, et al: Elevated levels of mutation in multiple tissues of mice deficient in the DNA mismatch repair gene Pms2. *Proc Natl Acad Sci USA* **94**:3122, 1997.
97. Baker SM, Harris AC, Tsao JL, et al: Enhanced intestinal adenomatous polyp formation in Pms2; Min Mice. *Cancer Res* **58**:1087, 1998.
98. Edelmann W, Yang K, Umar A, et al: Mutation in the mismatch repair gene Msh6 causes cancer susceptibility. *Cell* **92**:467, 1997.
99. Edelmann W, Cohen PE, Kane M, et al: Meiotic pachytene arrest in MLH1-deficient mice. *Cell* **85**:1125, 1996.
100. Baker SM, Plug AW, Prolla TA, et al: Involvement of mouse Mlh1 in DNA mismatch repair and meiotic crossing over. *Nature Genet* **13**:336, 1996.
101. Baker SM, Bronner CE, Zhang L, et al: Male mice defective in the DNA mismatch repair gene PMS2 exhibit abnormal chromosome synapsis in meiosis. *Cell* **82**:309, 1995.
102. Fearon ER, Vogelstein B: A genetic model for colorectal tumorigenesis. *Cell* **61**:759, 1990.
103. Cottu PH, Muzeau F, Estreicher A, et al: Inverse correlation between RER$^+$ status and p53 mutation in colorectal cancer cell lines. *Oncogene* **13**:2727, 1996.
104. Konishi M, Kikuchi-Yanoshita R, Tanaka K, et al: Molecular nature of colon tumors in hereditary nonpolyposis colon cancer, familial polyposis, and sporadic colon cancer. *Gastroenterology* **111**:307, 1996.
105. Losi L, Ponz de Leon M, Jiricny J, et al: K-ras and p53 mutations in hereditary non-polyposis colorectal cancers. *Int J Cancer* **74**:94, 1997.
106. Kim H, Jen J, Vogelstein B, et al: Clinical and pathological characteristics of sporadic colorectal carcinomas with DNA replication errors in microsatellite sequences. *Am J Pathol* **145**:148, 1994.
107. Ilyas M, Tomlinson IP, Novelli MR, et al: Clinico-pathological features and p53 expression in left-sided sporadic colorectal cancer with and without microsatellite instability. *J Pathol* **179**:370, 1996.
108. Huang J, Papadopoulos N, McKinley AJ, et al: APC mutations in colorectal tumors with mismatch repair deficiency. *Proc Natl Acad Sci USA* **93**:9049, 1996.
109. Shibata D, Peinado MA, Ionov Y, et al: Genomic instability in repeated sequences is an early somatic event in colorectal tumorigenesis that persists after transformation. *Nature Genet* **6**:273, 1994.
110. Willliams GT, Geraghty JM, Campbell F, et al: Normal colonic mucosa in hereditary non-polyposis colorectal cancer shows no generalised increase in somatic mutation. *Br J Cancer* **71**:1077, 1995.
111. Jacoby RF, Marshall DJ, Kailas S, et al: Genetic instability associated with adenoma to carcinoma progression in hereditary colon cancer. *Gastroenterology* **109**:73, 1995.
112. Shibata D, Navidi W, Salovaara R, et al: Somatic microsatellite mutations as molecular tumor clocks. *Nature Med* **2**:676, 1996.
113. Aaltonen LA, Peltomaki P, Mecklin J-P, et al: Replication errors in benign and malignant tumors from hereditary nonpolyposis colorectal cancer patients. *Cancer Res* **54**:1645, 1994.
114. Thibodeau SN, French AJ, Roche PC, et al: Altered expression of hMSH2 and hMLH1 in tumors with microsatellite instability and genetic alterations in mismatch repair genes. *Cancer Res* **56**:4836, 1996.
115. Thibodeau SN, French AJ, Cunningham JM, et al: Microsatellite instability in colorectal cancer: Different mutator phenotypes and the principal involvement of hMLH1. *Cancer Res* **58**:1713, 1998.
116. Kane MF, Loda M, Gaida GM, et al: Methylation of the hMLH1 promoter correlates with lack of expression of hMLH1 in sporadic

colon tumors and mismatch repair-defective human tumor cell lines. *Cancer Res* **57**:808, 1997.
117. Herman JG, Umar A, Polyak K, et al: Incidence and functional consequences of hMLH1 promoter hypermethylation in colorectal carcinoma. *Proc Natl Acad Sci USA* **95**:6870, 1998.
118. Veigl ML, Kasturi L, Olechnowicz J, et al: Biallelic inactivation of hMLH1 by epigenetic gene silencing, a novel mechanism causing human MSI cancers. *Proc Natl Acad Sci USA* **95**:8698, 1998.
119. Cunningham JM, Christensen ER, Tester DJ, et al: Hypermethylation of the hMLH1 promoter in colon cancer with microsatellite instability. *Cancer Res* **58**:3455, 1998.
120. Eshleman JR, Lang EZ, Bowerfind GK, et al: Increased mutation rate at the hprt locus accompanies microsatellite instability in colon cancer. *Oncogene* **10**:33, 1995.
121. Markowitz S, Wang J, Myeroff L, et al: Inactivation of the type II TGF-β receptor in colon cancer cells with microsatellite instability. *Science* **268**:1336, 1995.
122. Alexandrow M, Moses HL: Transforming growth factor β and cell cycle regulation. *Cancer Res* **55**:1452, 1995.
123. Myeroff LL, Parsons R, Kim SJ, et al: A transforming growth factor β receptor type II gene mutation common in colon and gastric but rare in endometrial cancers with microsatellite instability. *Cancer Res* **55**:5545, 1995.
124. Akiyama Y, Iwanaga R, Saitoh K, et al: Transforming growth factor β type II receptor gene muations in adenomas from hereditary nonpolyposis colorectal cancer. *Gastroenterology* **112**:33, 1997.
125. Grady WM, Rajput A, Myeroff L, et al: Mutation of the type II transforming growth factor-β receptor is coincident with the transformation of human colon adenomas to malignant carcinomas. *Cancer Res* **58**:3101, 1998.
126. Souza R, Appel R, Yin J, et al: Microsatellite instability in the insulin-like growth factor II receptor gene in gastrointestinal tumours. *Nature Genet* **14**:255, 1996.
127. Rampino N, Yamamoto H, Ionov Y, et al: Somatic frameshift mutations in the BAX gene in colon cancers of the microsatellite mutator phenotype. *Science* **275**:967, 1997.
128. Akiyama Y, Tsubouchi N, Yuasa Y: Frequent somatic mutations of hMSH3 with reference to microsatellite instability in hereditary nonpolyposis colorectal cancer. *Biochem Biophys Res Commun* **236**:248, 1997.
129. Ikeda M, Orimo H, Moriyama H, et al: Close correlation between mutations of E2F4 and hMSH3 genes in colorectal cancers with microsatellite instability. *Cancer Res* **58**:594, 1998.
130. Yagi OK, Akiyama Y, Nomizu T, et al: Proapoptotic gene BAX is frequently mutated in hereditary nonpolyposis colorectal cancers but not in adenomas. *Gastroenterology* **114**:268, 1998.
131. Yamamoto H, Sawai H, Weber TK, et al: Somatic frameshift mutations in DNA mismatch repair and proapoptosis genes in hereditary nonpolyposis colorectal cancer. *Cancer Res* **58**:997, 1998.
132. Yin J, Kong D, Wang S, et al: Mutation of hMSH3 and hMSH6 mismatch repair genes in genetically unstable human colorectal and gastric carcinomas. *Hum Mutat* **10**:474, 1997.
133. Yoshitaka T, Matsubara N, Ikeda M, et al: Mutations of E2F-4 trinucleotide repeats in colorectal cancer with microsatellite instability. *Biochem Biophys Res Commun* **227**:553, 1996.
134. Perucho M: Microsatellite instability: The mutator that mutates the other mutator. *Nature Med* **2**:630, 1996.
135. White RL, Fox MS: Genetic consequences of transfection with heteroduplex bacteriophage lambda DNA. *Mol Gen Genet* **141**:163, 1975.
136. Koi M, Umar A, Chauhan DP, et al: Human chromosome 3 corrects mismatch repair deficiency and microsatellite instability and reduces *N*-methyl-*N*′nitro-*N*-nitrosoguanidine tolerance in humancolon tumor cells with homozygous hMLH1 mutation. *Cancer Res* **54**:4308, 1994.
137. Hawn MT, Umar A, Carethers JM, et al: Evidence for a connection between the mismatch repair system and the G2 cell cycle checkpoint. *Cancer Res* **55**:3721, 1995.
138. Mellon I, Rajpal DK, Koi M, et al: Transcription-coupled nucleotide excision repair deficiency associated with mutations in human mismatch repair genes. *Science* **272**:557, 1996.
139. Carethers JM, Chauhan DP, Fink D, Nebel S, Bresailer RS, Howell SB, Boland CR: Mismatch repair proficiency and *in vitro* response to 5-fluorouracil. *Gastroenterology* **117**:123, 1999.
140. Aebi S, Kurdi-Haidar B, Gordon R, et al: Loss of DNA mismatch repair in acquired resistance to cisplatin. *Cancer Res* **56**:3087, 1996.
141. Duckett DR, Drummond JT, Murchie AIH, et al: Human MutSa recognizes damaged DNA base pairs containing O^6-methylthymine, or the cisplatin-d(GpG) adduct. *Proc Natl Acad Sci USA* **93**:6443, 1996.
142. Fink D, Nebel S, Norris PS, et al: The effect of different chemotherapeutic agents on the enrichment of DNA mismatch repair-deficient tumour cells. *Br J Cancer* **77**:703, 1998.
143. Aebi S, Kurdi-Haidar B, Gordon R, et al: Loss of DNA mismatch repair in acquired resistance to cisplatin. *Cancer Res* **56**:3087, 1996.
144. Boyer JC, Umar A, Risinger JI, et al: Microsatellite instability, mismatch repair deficiency, and genetic defects in human cancer cell lines. *Cancer Res* **55**:6063, 1995.
145. Suzuki H, Harpaz N, Tarmin L, et al: Microsatellite instability in ulcerative colitis-associated colorectal dysplasias and cancers. *Cancer Res* **54**:4841, 1994.
146. Brentnall TA, Rubin CE, Crispin DA, et al: A germline substitution in the human MSH2 gene is associated with cancer and high grade dysplasia in ulcerative colitis. *Gastroenterology* **109**:151, 1995.
147. Brentnall TA, Crispin DA, Bronner MP, et al: Microsatellite instability is present in non-neoplastic mucosa from patients with longstanding ulcerative colitis. *Cancer Res* **56**:1237, 1996.
148. Rodriguez-Bigas MA, Boland CR, Hamilton SR, et al: A National Cancer Institute workshop on hereditary nonpolyposis colorectal cancer syndrome: Meeting highlights and Bethesda guidelines. *J Natl Cancer Inst* **89**:1758, 1997.
149. Bocker T, Diermann J, Friedl W, et al: Microsatellite instability analysis: A multicenter study for reliability and quality control. *Cancer Res* **57**:4739, 1997.
150. Dietmaier W, Wallinger S, Bocker T, et al: Diagnostic microsatellite instabilty: Definition and correlation with mismatch repair protein expression. *Cancer Res* **57**:4749, 1997.
151. Samowitz WS, Slattery ML, Kerber RA: Microsatellite instability in human colonic cancer is not a useful clinical indicator of familial colorectal cancer. *Gastroenterology* **109**:1765, 1995.
152. Froggatt NJ, Koch J, Davies R, et al: Genetic linkage analysis in hereditary non-polyposis colon cancer syndrome. *J Med Genet* **32**:352, 1995.
153. Luce MC, Marra G, Chauhan DP, et al: In vitro transcription/translation assay for the screening of hMLH1 and hMSH2 mutations in familial colon cancer. *Gastroenterology* **109**:1368, 1995.
154. Hall NR, Taylor GR, Finan PJ, et al: Intron splice acceptor site sequence variation in the hereditary non-polyposis colorectal cancer gene hMSH2. *Eur J Cancer* **30A**:1550, 1994.
155. Charbonnier F, Martin C, Scotte M, et al: Alternative splicing of MLH1 messenger RNA in human normal cells. *Cancer Res* **55**:1839, 1995.
156. Xia L, Shen W, Ritacca F, et al: A truncated hMSH2 transcript occurs as a common variant in the population: Implications for genetic diagnosis. *Cancer Res* **56**:2289, 1996.
157. Lahti MN, Sistonen P, Mecklin JP, et al: Close linkage to chromosome 3p and conservation of ancestral founding haplotype in hereditary nonpolyposis colorectal cancer families. *Proc Natl Acad Sci USA* **91**:6054, 1994.
158. Lahti MN, Kristo P, Nicolaides NC, et al: Founding mutations and Alu-mediated recombination in hereditary colon cancer. *Nature Med* **1**:1203, 1995.
159. Peltomaki P, Vaden H, et al: Mutations predisposing to hereditary nonpolyposis colorectal cancer: Database and results of a collaborative study. *Gastroenterology* **113**:1146, 1997.
160. Watson P, Vasen HFA, Mecklin JP, et al: The risk of endometrial cancer in hereditary nonpolyposis colorectal cancer. *Am J Med* **96**:516, 1994.
161. Aarnio M, Mecklin JP, Aaltonen LA, et al: Life-time risk of different cancers in hereditary nonpolyposis colorectal cancer (HNPCC) syndrome. *Int J Cancer* **64**:430, 1995.
162. Sankila R, Aaltonen LA, Jarvinen HJ, et al: Better survival rates in patients with MLH1-associated hereditary colorectal cancer. *Gastroenterology* **110**:682, 1996.
163. Jarvinen HJ, Mecklin JP, Sistonen P: Screening reduces colorectal cancer rate in families with hereditary nonpolyposis colorectal cancer. *Gastroenterology* **108**:1405, 1995.
164. Watson P, Lin KM, Rodriguez-Bigas MA, et al: Colorectal carcinoma survival among hereditary nonpolyposis colorectal carcinoma family members. *Cancer* **83**:259, 1998.
165. Percesepe A, Benatti P, Roncucci L, et al: Survival analysis in families affected by hereditary nonpolyposis colorectal cancer. *Int J Cancer* **71**:373, 1997.
166. Ponz de Leon M, Casa GD, Benatti P, et al: Frequency and type of colorectal tumors in asymptomatic high-risk individuals in families with hereditary nonpolyposis colorectal cancer. *Cancer Epidemiol Biomark Prevent* **7**:639, 1998.

167. Watanabe T, Muto T, Sawada T, et al: Flat adenoma as a precursor of colorectal carcinoma in hereditary nonpolyposis colorectal carcinoma. *Cancer* **77**:627, 1996.
168. Hall NR, Finan PJ, Ward B, et al: Genetic susceptibility to colorectal cancer in patients under 45 years of age. *Br J Surg* **81**:1485, 1994.
169. Liu B, Farrington SM, Petersen GM, et al: Genetic instability occurs in the majority of young patients with colorectal cancer. *Nature Med* **1**:348, 1995.
170. Vasen HFA, Wijnen JT, Menko FH, et al: Cancer risk in families with hereditary nonpolyposis colorectal cancer diagnosed by mutation analysis. *Gastroenterology* **110**:1020, 1996.
171. Rodriguez-Bigas MA, Vasen HF, Pekka-Mecklin J, et al: Rectal cancer risk in hereditary nonpolyposis colorectal cancer after abdominal colectomy. International Collaborative Group on HNPCC. *Ann Surg* **225**:202, 1997.
172. Lin KM, Shashidharan M, Ternent CA, et al: Colorectal and extracolonic cancer variations in MLH1/MSH2 hereditary nonpolyposis colorectal cancer kindreds and the general population. *Dis Colon Rectum* **41**:428, 1998.
173. Vasen HFA, Nagengast FM, Khan PM: Interval cancers in hereditary non-polyposis colorectal cancer (Lynch syndrome). *Lancet* **345**:1183, 1995.
174. Vasen H, van Ballegooijen M, Buskens E, et al: A cost-effectiveness analysis of colorectal screening of hereditary nonpolyposis colorectal carcinoma gene carriers. *Cancer* **82**:1632, 1998.
175. Burke W, Petersen G, Lynch P, et al: Recommendations for follow-up care of individuals with an inherited predisposition to cancer. *JAMA* **277**:915, 1997.
176. Menko FH, Te Meerman GJ, Sampson JR: Variable age of onset in hereditary nonpolyposis colorectal cancer: Clinical implications. *Gastroenterology* **104**:946, 1993.
177. Mecklin JP, Jarvinen HJ: Clinical features of colorectal carcinoma in cancer family syndrome. *Dis Colon Rectum* **29**:160, 1986.

CHAPTER 33

Werner Syndrome

Gerard D. Schellenberg ▪ Tetsuro Miki
Chang-En Yu ▪ Jun Nakura

1. Werner syndrome (WS) is a rare autosomal recessive disorder that is observed in many different ethnic groups. Prevalence estimates range from 1 in 22,000 to 1 in 1 million. All cases of WS are inherited and result from mutations in a single gene.

2. WS is characterized clinically by the premature appearance of cataracts, scleroderma-like skin pathology, short stature, graying hair and hair loss, and a general appearance of premature aging. More variable features include adult-onset diabetes mellitus, hypogonadism, osteoporosis, osteosclerosis, soft tissue calcification, hyperkeratosis, ulcers on the feet and ankles, premature vascular disease, elevated rates of some neoplasms, a hoarse high-pitched voice, and flat feet. Subjects often appear 20 to 30 years older than their chronologic age, and WS may be a model disease for accelerated aging. The mean age at death is 47 years, with the leading cause being neoplasia, followed by myocardial infarcts and cerebral vascular incidents.

3. WS subjects are at increased risk for a variety of neoplasms. This increased risk results primarily from an increase in non-epithelial-derived cancers and is not an across-the-board elevation in all common cancers. Soft tissue sarcomas, osteosarcomas, melanomas, and thyroid cancer are the predominant forms of cancer.

4. The gene for WS (*WRN*), located on chromosome 8p12, has been cloned and encodes a 1432-amino acid protein (WRNp) that has homology to the super-family of DExH box DNA and RNA helicases; WRNp has the seven motifs found in this class of protein, including the ATP-binding and Mg^{2+}-binding motifs. Outside the helicase domain, WRNp is homologous to an RNase D motif that may indicate a $3' \rightarrow 5'$ proofreading exonuclease activity.

5. Mutations have been identified in the *WRN* gene in all WS subjects studied. All the mutations result in a predicted truncated protein, the result of either a nonsense mutation or mutations leading to a frameshift. One splice-junction mutation is found in 50 to 60 percent of Japanese WS subjects. WS appears to be the result of loss of function of WRNp. No missense WS mutations have been found.

6. *In vitro*, WRNp is a functional $3' \rightarrow 5'$ DNA helicase. The *in vivo* function of WRNp is not known. WS is a genomic instability syndrome with elevated rates of chromosomal translocation and deletions and an elevated somatic cell mutation rate. This mutator phenotype, resulting from the loss of WRNp, could be a defect in an as yet unidentified DNA repair system, a defect in DNA replication initiation, or a defect in some other aspect of DNA metabolism that requires DNA unwinding.

A list of standard abbreviations is located immediately preceding the index in each volume. Nonstandard abbreviations used in this chapter include: WS = Werner syndrome; HA = hyaluronic acid; VTRP = variable transcription repeat; YAC = yeast artificial chromosome.

Werner syndrome (WS) is a rare autosomal recessive disease first described in 1904 by Otto Werner in his doctoral thesis.[1,2] As a medical student in an ophthalmologic clinic, Werner saw a family with two brothers and two sisters, ages 31, 36, 38, and 40 years, with bilateral cataracts, sclerodermal skin changes, hyperkeratosis, and ulcers on the feet and ankles. He observed that one 36-year-old gave "the impression of extreme senility," thus hinting in this early work at the potential connection between WS and accelerated aging.[2] In 1934, Oppenheimer and Kugel[3] extended the description of the disease and gave it the eponym *Werner's syndrome.* Thannhauser, in a classic article published in 1945, described many of the clinical features now associated with WS.[4]

The WS phenotype is complex, age-dependent, and variable (Figs. 33-1 and 33-2). Affected subjects are typically normal throughout childhood and early adolescence, with the only symptoms being growth retardation occurring at or near puberty. Beginning in the second and third decades of life, graying and loss of hair begin, and scleroderma-like changes occur typically on the face, legs, and feet. In the fourth and subsequent decades, WS individuals develop many of the diseases that are common in the elderly, including arteriosclerotic vascular disease, neoplasms, diabetes mellitus, osteoporosis, and bilateral cataracts (for reviews of the clinical features of WS, see refs. 4 through 9). WS individuals often are described as having a "senile" appearance and look 20 to 30 years older than their true chronologic age.

Over the past 20 to 30 years, the biochemistry, cell biology, and genetics of WS have been studied intensively. The vigor with which this disorder has been pursued is not based on its importance to public health, since WS is quite rare. The physical appearance of premature aging and other clinical features led to the proposal that WS is a partial model of accelerated human aging.[10] Parallels between WS and aging are also based on *in vitro* studies of cell growth potential. In fibroblasts from normal subjects, the number of doublings a culture is capable of before senescence occurs is inversely proportional to the age of the donor; cultures from children have a cumulative cell-doubling capacity of approximately 50 divisions, whereas cultures from elderly donors are capable of only 30 to 40 divisions.[7,11] In contrast, WS fibroblasts have a very limited potential for division, with a mean cumulative doubling of only 12.4.[7,12] Thus WS has been studied in the hope that WS also may provide clues to how aging processes contribute to susceptibility to some of the common diseases of old age.

Another feature of WS is an elevated risk for a wide variety of cancers[13] and that WS cells exhibit genomic instability. Genomic instability has been demonstrated both *in vitro* and *in vivo* as an elevated somatic cell mutation rate,[14–17] as well as increased rates of random chromosomal breakage, deletions, and rearrangements.[18–24] A number of other inherited disorders also exhibit the combination of genomic instability and elevated cancer risks (see Chaps. 28, 29, 30, and 32 for discussions of xeroderma pigmentosum, ataxia-telangiectasia, Bloom syndrome, and hereditary nonpolyposis colorectal cancer, respectively). The study of WS and other inherited cancer-susceptibility disorders may provide additional clues to the mechanisms of cancer development.

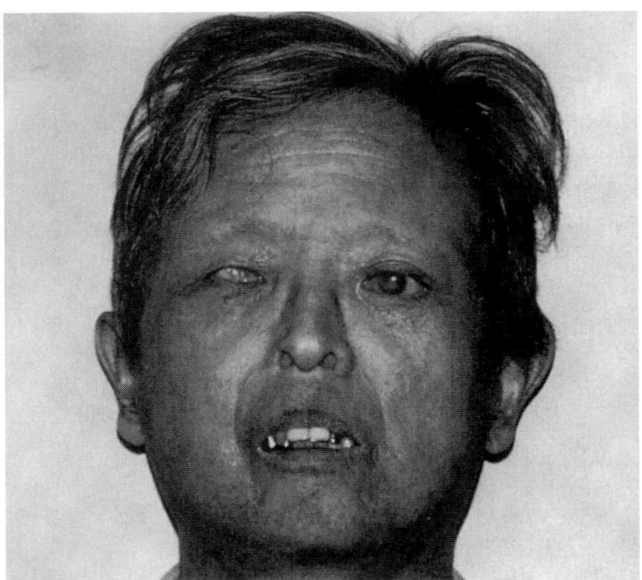

Fig. 33-1 A 51-year-old Japanese WS patient (definite diagnosis by the criteria in Table 33-3) with a known *WRN* mutation. See refs. 3, 4, 6, 38, and 128 for other photographs of WS subjects.

Positional cloning methods have been used to identify the gene responsible for WS[25] (the *WRN* gene). This gene encodes a predicted protein homologous to a superfamily of enzymes termed *helicases* that unwind double-stranded RNA or DNA into single strands. Now that the *WRN* gene has been identified, it should be possible to design experimental approaches to directly address questions concerning the relationship of WS to aging and age-related disease processes.

CLINICAL ASPECTS OF WS

Prevalence

Prevalence estimates for WS are difficult to obtain because the disorder is extremely rare, a fact that makes case finding difficult. Also, since the appearance of the full phenotypic spectrum of WS is not complete until the third and fourth decades of life (average age at diagnosis is 38.7 years[6]), younger subjects may be missed. Two methods have been used to generate prevalence and gene-frequency estimates. The first is case counting in defined populations. This method depends on case identification by community physicians. Since WS is rare and many physicians may not be familiar with the disorder, underdiagnosis may result, and the true prevalence may be underestimated. Also, the number of cases actually identified is typically small, making the estimates inaccurate. The second method for estimating prevalence is based on comparing consanguinity rates in the parents of WS subjects to estimates of consanguinity rates in the general population.[26,27] This method depends on accurate estimates of consanguinity in the general population. Consanguinity rates are difficult to measure and may vary even within an ethnic group or country, depending on whether the cases come from rural or urban settings.[28] Case-counting methods have yielded estimates ranging from 1 in 95,000 to 1 in 455,000 (Table 33-1), corresponding to allele frequencies of 0.0032 and 0.0015, respectively.[5,29] Prevalence estimates based on consanguinity rates range from 1 in 22,000 to 1 in 1 million, corresponding to allele frequencies of 0.0067 and 0.001, respectively.[5,6,29] Now that the gene has been cloned, populations can be screened directly for specific mutations,[25] and direct measurements of carrier frequencies can be obtained. In a preliminary study, 178 Japanese control subjects were screened for the most common Japanese WS mutation (mutation 4 in Table 33-2) by direct DNA sequencing. This mutation appears to account for 50 to 60 percent of all Japanese WS cases. A single heterozygote was identified, yielding an allele frequency of 0.0027 with a 95 percent upper confidence limit of 0.008.[25] Based on a mutation frequency of 60 in Japanese WS cases, the allele frequency in the Japanese population for all WS alleles should be approximately 0.0045. This frequency estimate is within the range of estimates (0.001–0.0067) obtained by the methods described

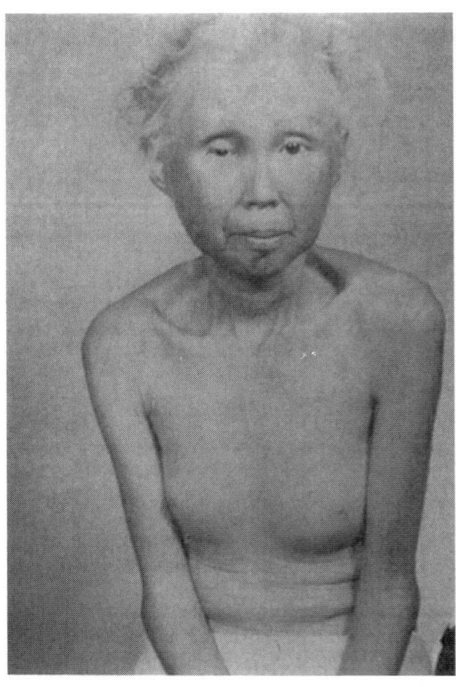

A

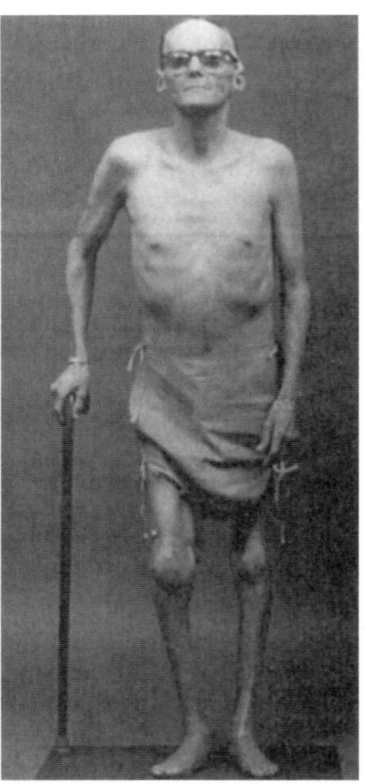

B

Fig. 33-2 *A.* A 48-year-old Japanese woman with WS (case 1 in Epstein et al.[6]). *B.* A 51-year-old Caucasian man with WS. Subject has typical thin limbs with normal trunk with scleroderma-like skin atrophy of the lower legs and feet. *C.* Skin atrophy of the feet and ankles. *D,E.* Ulcers on the ankles.

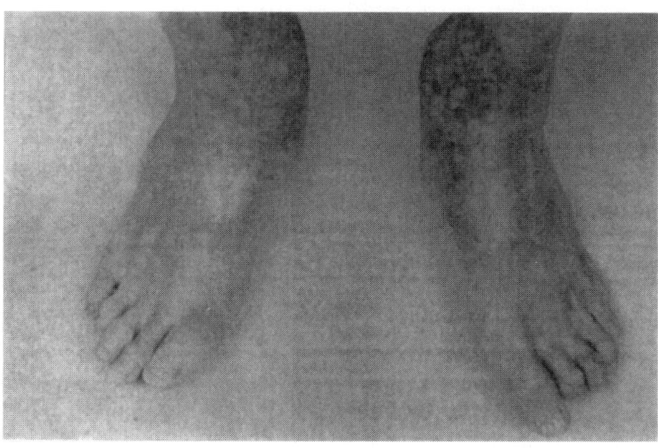

C

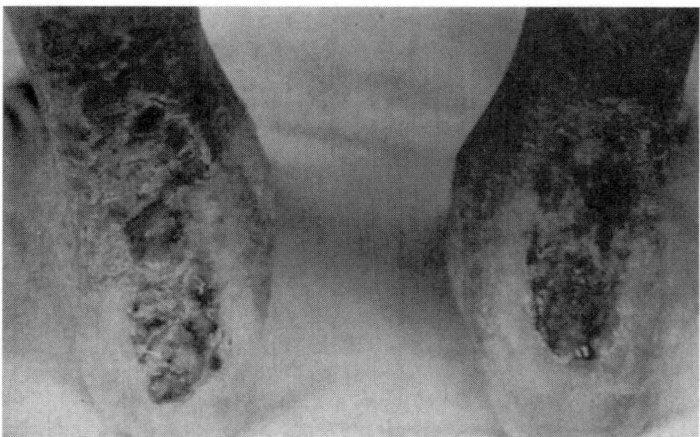

D

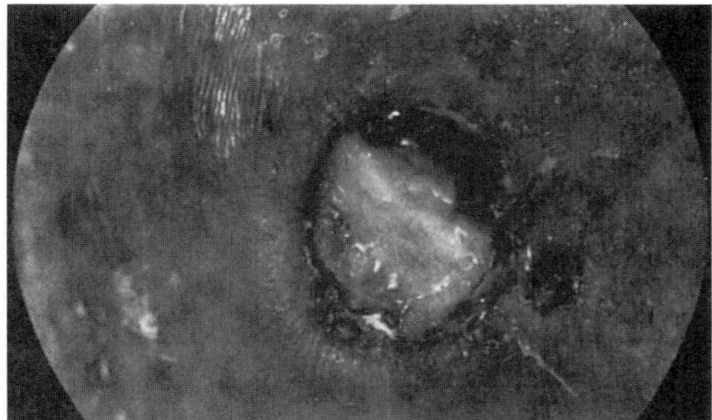

E

Fig. 33-2 (Continued)

above. Additional studies with a larger sample are needed to establish reliable allele frequency estimates for WS mutations.

Fraction of WS That Is Due to Inherited Factors

There is no evidence that WS is genetically or etiologically heterogeneous. The genetic mapping studies discussed below suggest that WS in different ethnic groups is caused by the same locus on chromosome 8.[30–32] Subsequent identification of the gene permitted mutational analysis; to date, mutations in this gene, either in the homozygous state or as compound heterozygotes, have been identified in all the patients studied[25,33–37] (see Table 18-2). Thus all WS appears to be inherited. No WS phenocopies have been documented. The existence of new mutations on a heterozygous background cannot be ruled out. While a subject's environment may influence the expression of various components of the WS phenotype, there is no evidence that there is sporadic WS induced by environmental factors.

Diagnostic Criteria

There are no generally accepted standard diagnostic criteria for WS, although several have been used in research. The clinical picture of WS has been developed from case studies of subjects who are frequently in their thirties or forties. Since an early diagnosis usually is not possible, the onset of features such as growth cessation and graying of the hair is estimated retrospectively, depends on the subject's recollections, and may not be precise. Further, cohorts of WS subjects have not been followed longitudinally until death with subsequent autopsies; thus estimates of late-onset features such as vascular disease, diabetes mellitus, and neoplasms may be low. Estimates of the prevalence of a particular feature can vary considerably. For example, estimates of the percentage of WS patients with vascular disease vary from 25 percent[6] to 100 percent.[29] This variability may reflect the ages of the patient groups studied, different environmental influences (e.g., diet), or differing genetic backgrounds in different ethnic groups. Despite the limitations of the data collected, the clinical description of WS discussed below is remarkably consistent across the large numbers of WS cases that have been described in the literature. The reader is referred to Epstein et al.[6] for an excellent detailed description of the clinical and pathologic findings in a large number of WS subjects.

Two different criteria for diagnosis have been used in research on WS. The criteria used by Nakura et al.[32] (Table 33-3) consist of six primary features found in most WS subjects and an additional nine symptoms found less consistently. A diagnosis of "definite" requires all six cardinal symptoms and two of the less frequent features. "Probable" WS requires the first three cardinal signs and any two others. One limitation of these criteria is that hyaluronic acid analysis is not routinely available. Also, while parental consanguinity is a useful indicator of recessive inheritance, the majority of Caucasian subjects (64 percent[6]) and many Japanese subjects (20–32 percent[38,39]) are not from consanguineous families. Goto and coworkers[5] used a similar set of criteria (Table 33-4), and a diagnosis of WS requires that a subject have three of the four major symptom groups.

Features Found in Most Patients

Cataracts. The most constant feature of WS is cataracts (see Fig. 33-1), which are present in 94 to 100 percent of the subjects[6,7,39] (see Table 33-3). Cataracts typically appear in the third decade of life. In different case-review studies, the observed mean age at appearance was between 23 years[39] and 30 years.[6] Cataracts are usually bilateral, although they may be at different stages of development in each eye, and are typically indistinguishable from those seen in elderly subjects (see ref. 6 for a detailed review of ocular pathologies).

Table 33-1 Estimates of Prevalence Rates for WS

Population	Case-Counting-Based Estimates	Consanguinity-Based Estimates	Reference
Caucasian (Sardinian)	1/95,000 to 1/203,000	1/93,000 to 1/455,000	29
Japanese	1/300,000 to 1/500,000	1/22,000 to 1/370,000	5
Mostly Caucasian		1/45,000 to 1/1,000,000	6

Table 33-2 Summary of *WRN* Mutations

Mutation	Codon	Exon	Type of Mutation	Nucleotide Sequence	Comment	Predicted Protein Length
None	—	—	—	—	—	1432
1	1165	30	Substitution	CAG (Gln) to *T*AG (terminator)	Nonsense	1164
2	1305	33	Substitution	CGA (Arg) to *T*GA (terminator)	Nonsense	1304
3	1230–1273	32	4-bp deletion	ACAG deleted	Deletion/frameshift	1245
4	1047–1078	26	Substitution	tag-GGT to ta*c*-GGT	Substitution at a splice-donor site, exon 26 excluded	1060
A	369	9	Substitution	CGA (Arg) to TGA (terminator)	Nonsense	368
B	889	22	Substitution	CGA (Arg) to TGA (terminator)	Nonsense	888
C	759–816	20	Substitution	GAG-gta to CAG-tta	Substitution at splice-receptor site	760
D	389	9	1-bp deletion	AGAG (Arg) to GAG (Glu)	Frameshift	391
E	697–942	19–23	Deletion (> 15 kb)	—	Genomic deletion	1186
F	1154–1191	30	Deletion of exon 30 from WRN cDNA	—	—	1157
G	1104–1128	28	Deletion of exon 28 from the WRN cDNA	—	—	1138
H	426	10	4-bp insertion	ATCT inserted	Insertion/frameshift	429
I	696	18	105-bp insertion	—	Insertion/frameshift	708
J	697–942	19–23	Deletion of exons 19–23 from the WRN cDNA	—	Deletion/frameshift	704
K	1149	29	1-bp deletion	GAG (Glu) to GGC (Gly)	Deletion/frameshift	1160
L	1154	30		tttgttcagATT to tt*ag*TTCAGATT	Altered splice site, frameshift	1165
M	463	11	Substitution	TAT (Tyr) TAA (terminator)	Nonsense	462
N	168	5	2-bp deletion	AAG (Lys) to GCT (Ala)	Frameshift	176

NOTE: Mutations A–N were not numbered due to different numbers being assigned to different mutations in published descriptions.

Table 33-3 Signs of WS

Feature	Mean Age of Onset (years)	Onset Range (years)	Number of Patients Affected (%)
Cardinal signs			
1. Bilateral cataracts	23–30	10–46	94–100
2. Dermatological pathology (tight skin, atrophic skin, pigmentary alterations, ulceration, hyperkeratosis, regional subcutaneous atrophy), characteristic "bird" facies	23, 25	5–42	86–100
3. Short stature	13	10–20	86–100
4. Consanguinity (3d cousin or greater) or affected sibling	N.A.	N.A.	68
5. Premature graying and/or thinning of scalp hair	20–21	5–42	80–100
6. Positive hyaluronic acid test	N.A.D.	N.A.D	100
Further signs and symptoms			
1. Diabetes mellitus	30–34[6,39]	10–55	44–67*
2. Hypogonadism (secondary sexual underdevelopment, diminished fertility, testicular or ovarian atrophy)	N.A.	N.A.	
3. Osteoporosis	N.A.D.	N.A.D.	33–100
4. Osteosclerosis of distal phalanges of fingers and/or toes (X-ray diagnosis)	N.A.D.	N.A.D.	N.A.D.
5. Soft tissue calcification	N.A.D.	N.A.D.	25–53
6. Premature atherosclerosis (e.g., history of myocardial infarction)	N.A.D.	N.A.D.	25–100
7. Mesenchymal neoplasms, rare neoplasms, or multiple neoplasms	N.A.D.	20–64†	N.A.D.
8. Voice changes (high-pitched squeaky or hoarse voice)	21–27	10–40	50–100
9. Flat feet	N.A.D.	N.A.D.	

NOTE: Diagnostic criteria are reproduced from Nakura et al.[32] (with permission from *Genomics*) and categories are as follows: definite, all cardinal signs, (number 6 when available) and any two others; probable, the first three cardinal signs and any two others; possible, either cataracts or dermatological alterations and any four others; exclusion, onset of signs and symptoms before adolescence (except short stature) or a negative hyaluronic acids test. Data on prevalence estimates of symptoms and onset means are primarily from several case-report summaries.[6,29,39–43] as summarized by Tollefsbol and Cohen[7] and from Goto.[50] N.A.D., no available data; N.A., not applicable.

* Percent affected given includes subjects with impaired glucose tolerance.

† Range given is for all cancers.

Table 33-4 WS Diagnostic Criteria of Goto*

1. Characteristic habitus and stature	Short stature
	Low body weight
	Thin limbs with a stocky trunk
	Beak-shaped nose
2. Premature senescence	Birdlike appearance
	Loss of hair
	Skin hyperpigmentation
	Hoarse voice
	Diffuse arteriosclerosis
	Juvenile bilateral cataracts
	Osteoporosis
3. Scleroderma-like skin changes	Atrophic skin and muscle
	Hyperkeratosis
	Telangiectasia
	Tight skin over the bones of the feet
	Skin ulcers
	Localized calcification
4. Endocrine abnormalities	Diabetes mellitus
	Hypogonadism

*A diagnosis of WS requires three of the four criteria listed in the table.

SOURCE: Adapted from Goto et al.[30] Used by permission.

Dermatologic Pathology. By the second decade of life, most WS subjects have skin with a scleroderma-like appearance. The skin is tight, shiny, and smooth as a result of both dermal atrophy and loss of underlying connective tissue, muscle, and subcutaneous fat tissue.[4,6,38,49] Sites of abnormal skin include the upper and lower limbs; the ankles and feet are particularly severely affected. Atrophy of facial tissues results in the typical "birdlike" appearance with a sharp nose but relatively full cheeks. Hyperkeratosis also occurs, often resulting in ulcers on the feet and ankles. Ulceration can be severe (see Fig. 33-2), causing gangrene; amputation is sometimes required. Other skin abnormalities include general hyperpigmentation, areas of hypopigmentation, telangiectasia (36 percent of subjects), nail deformity (42 percent of subjects), and in general, thin, dry skin.

Stature and Habitus. Short stature is another feature typical of WS and is observed in most subjects (86–100 percent[38,39,50]). In Japanese subjects, males range in height from 137 to 161 cm (mean, 151–153 cm) and females range from 122 to 151 cm (mean, 131.7–144.2 cm). Non-Japanese (primarily Caucasian[6]) subjects are somewhat taller, with reported means of 157 cm (5 ft 1 in) and 146 cm (4 ft 9 $\frac{1}{2}$ in) for males and females, respectively. Growth arrest appears during early adolescence (between 10 and 20 years) and appears to result from the lack of a growth spurt at puberty. The short stature is accompanied by low body weight. While many body features are proportional to the subject's size, a consistent feature is thin limbs with a stocky trunk, which are observed in 76 to 100 percent of the subjects studied.[38,39] Muscle atrophy in the limbs is consistently observed. Despite the short stature, thyroid-stimulating hormone and growth hormone levels appear to be normal in adults.[39]

Graying and Loss of Hair. The hair of WS subjects often begins to turn gray in late adolescence, although gray hair can appear as early as 5 years of age.[6,38,39] This feature is perhaps one of the earliest symptoms (see Table 33-3). With time, the hair often becomes completely white. Loss of scalp and eyebrow hair and loss of eyelashes occur along with graying of the hair. The combination of the sparse gray or white hair and the dermal atrophy described above gives WS subjects the physical appearance of someone 20 to 30 years older than their chronologic age.

Excess Urinary Hyaluronic Acid. Excess hyaluronic acid (HA) in WS subjects' urine has been repeatedly observed.[38–43] Urinary HA was first identified in the analysis of urine for the connective tissue breakdown product, acid glycosaminoglycans. While acid glycosaminoglycan levels were normal, HA was high. HA levels are also elevated in Hutchinson-Gilford syndrome (progeria),[40] another disorder often mentioned as an accelerated aging disorder. HA is absent or is present in low levels in normal subjects.[44]

Features Found in a Subset of Patients

The following signs and symptoms are observed in a subset of patients. As was discussed earlier, the frequencies of some of these features may represent underestimates. In terms of morbidity and mortality, vascular disease and cancers are the most important; cancers, followed by myocardial and cerebrovascular accidents, are the most common causes of premature death (the average age at death for all causes is 47 years[6]).

Hypogonadism. Secondary sexual underdevelopment is a fairly common finding in WS subjects, occurring in 66 percent[39] to 96 percent[29] of the subjects studied. In males, small genitalia and sparse pubic hair are common though not universal. WS women have poorly developed genitalia with small uteruses. In about half the women studied, breasts were small, atrophic, or underdeveloped.[6] Both men and women with hypogonadism have had children, although fertility is reduced. The onset of menses ranges from 9 to 20 years (mean, 13.9 years; $n = 35$). Menstruation frequently ceases prematurely (18–45 years; mean, 33 years) before menopause.[6]

Osteoporosis and Soft Tissue Calcification. Osteoporosis is observed in a subset of WS subjects, often occurring most dramatically in the lower limbs, feet, and ankles and to a lesser extent in the upper limbs and spine. The rest of the trunk and the skull typically show less severe or no osteoporosis. In case series of Japanese and Caucasian subjects who were typically about 40 years of age, 33 to 41 percent of subjects showed evidence of loss of bone mass. The exception to this observed prevalence was a study of WS in Sardinians in which all subjects ($n = 6$) showed osteoporosis.[29] Soft tissue calcification is observed in WS often around the Achilles tendon and the knee and elbow tendons and in the ligaments and tissues surrounding these areas. Soft tissue calcification of the hands and feet was also observed.

Diabetes Mellitus. A diabetic tendency is observed in 44 to 70 percent of WS subjects.[6,7,38,39,45,50] In one study of oral glucose tolerance, 55 percent were categorized as having diabetes mellitus and another 22 percent had impaired glucose tolerance. Fasting glucose levels are elevated in only a subset of patients with abnormal glucose tolerance tests, indicating that in WS, diabetes is mild; symptoms of polyuria, polydipsia, pruritus, and weight loss are rarely found.[6] Hyperglycemia is typically treated by dietary restriction. Complications typical of diabetes (nephropathy, retinopathy, and neuropathy) have not been reported for WS. Since some WS subjects show no diabetic tendencies, factors other than mutations in the *WRN* gene must contribute to the appearance of diabetes in these subjects.

Vascular Disease. Premature generalized vascular disease is a common feature in WS and accounts for 15 percent of the deaths in WS subjects.[50] Between 70 and 90 percent of patients show hypercholesterolemia and hypertriglyceridemia,[9,46,47] and most were classified (WHO criteria) as having type IIb hyperlipidemia. Vascular calcification is observed, most frequently in the legs and feet. Clinical evidence of vascular disease was reported in 25 to 100 percent of WS subjects (average, 42 percent); the symptoms were abnormal electrocardiograms, congestive heart failure, angina, and infarction. In one autopsy series, all the subjects exhibited atherosclerosis beyond that expected for normal individuals of the same age.[6] Calcification of coronary arteries and of the leaflets or rings of the mitral and/or aortic valves occurs in some subjects.

Neoplasia. WS subjects have an elevated risk of developing a wide variety of carcinomas and sarcomas,[6,13,23,48] and malignancies are the leading cause of death (80 percent).[50] The reported case histories of a large number of Japanese and Caucasian WS subjects have been comprehensively reviewed with respect to the prevalence of cancers.[13] In WS patients there was an over-representation of nonepithelial cancer; the ratio of epithelial to nonepithelial cancer was 1:1 versus 10:1 in the general population.[49] The most common cancers in the Japanese WS subjects were soft tissue sarcomas, osteosarcomas, melanomas, and thyroid carcinomas; together these accounted for 57 percent of cancers in WS patients versus 2 percent in the general Japanese population. Conservative estimates based on the incidence rates of these cancers in the general population and an estimated population of 5000 WS subjects in Japan (probably a considerable overestimate) suggest that the incidence of soft tissue sarcomas is at least 20-fold higher in WS patients than in the general Japanese population. Acral lentiginous melanoma of the feet and nasal mucosa, the predominant form of melanoma observed in Japanese WS subjects, is extremely rare in Japan (0.16 cases per 100,000 people per year).[51] The osteosarcomas were also in excess of expected rates, with an unusual age distribution; 12 of the 13 cases observed occurred between the ages of 35 and 64 years, unlike the typical occurrence in the general population, where the incidence of osteosarcomas is highest in late adolescence. The thyroid carcinomas observed included both papillary (8 of 21 cases) and follicular carcinomas (10 of 21 cases). While papillary thyroid carcinomas are relatively common among the Japanese, follicular carcinomas are less common[52,53] and are proportionally in excess in WS subjects. In addition to the cancers mentioned earlier, a strikingly wide spectrum of isolated cases of other carcinomas is observed. Benign meningiomas may be common in WS; in a case series of 147 neoplasias reported by Goto and coworkers,[13] there were 15 benign meningiomas. Whether this represents an elevated frequency among WS patients is not known.

The elevation in cancer incidence in WS is not simply an increase in all forms of neoplasms but rather a selective increase in some relatively rare cancers. Thus WS is not an exact mimic of aging in terms of neoplasms. Conspicuously missing from the spectrum of cancers elevated in WS are some of the common epithelial malignancies, particularly prostate cancer, which in normal populations is very common in elderly men.

Central Nervous System. Early studies suggested that the central nervous system is not affected in most WS subjects.[6,54] However, more recent work with more modern methods and older subjects indicates that by 40 years of age, 40 percent of subjects have brain atrophy, as determined by computed tomographic (CT) and magnetic resonance imaging (MRI) analyses.[50,55] Mild senile dementia was reported in 21 percent of the patients studied.[39] Single cases of extensive cerebral atrophy[55] and a case of spastic paraparesis with polyneuropathy have been reported.[56] Neuropathologic data are limited; initial autopsies of two intellectually normal WS subjects, 51 and 57 years of age, using standard histologic methods, did not reveal Alzheimer disease-type changes (senile plaques or neurofibrillary tangles) typically associated with normal aging.[57] More recently, these same 2 patients were examined using more sensitive silver and immunohistologic methods using antibodies to the Alzheimer Aβ protein and hyperphosphorylated tau, the principal components of Alzheimer-type amyloid and neurofibrillary tangles, respectively. For the older subject, in the temporal and frontal lobes, and in the hippocampus, extensive Aβ deposits were found. The amyloid load was similar to that observed in Alzheimer disease patients and was greater than that observed in aged normal controls.[58] Tau pathology was not significantly different from controls. Additional autopsies of WS patients who die after the age of 40 are needed to determine how severely the brain is affected.

Other Clinical Features of WS. In addition to the symptoms listed above, a subset (percent affected) of WS subjects have the following findings: flat feet (92 percent), irregular teeth (42 percent), hyperreflexia (79 percent), and a hoarse, high-pitched voice (83 percent; mean age of onset 21–27 years) caused by thickening and ulceration of the vocal cords.[4–7,9,38,39,50]

THE WS GENE

Pattern of Inheritance

The first cases of WS reported by Otto Werner in 1904 were familial, and subsequently, numerous pedigrees with multiple affected siblings were described. The parents of WS subjects are rarely affected, although several pedigrees with parent-child WS pairs exist.[5,9] Thannhauser in 1945 suggested that the inheritance of WS is recessive because of the high rate of consanguinity in the families of WS patients.[4] Elevated rates of consanguinity have been observed consistently in studies of both Japanese and Caucasians. Another line of evidence that WS is recessive is provided by segregation analysis. Epstein et al.[6] estimated that the percentage of affected offspring produced by unaffected parents range from 17.9 $\pm$ 2.5 percent to 26.5 $\pm$ 3.2 percent, depending on the method used to correct for ascertainment bias. These estimates are close to the 25 percent value expected for a recessively inherited disease. Thus WS is clearly a recessively inherited disorder, a conclusion subsequently supported by mutational analysis of WS subjects.[25] WS is found equally in both sexes, and there is no birth-order effect.[6]

Genetic Localization of the WS Gene

By the end of the 1980s, extensive *in vitro* biochemical and biologic studies had not revealed the primary defect responsible for WS. Fortunately, genetic mapping methods and resources had been sufficiently developed,[59,60] making localization of disease loci for inherited disorders highly feasible provided that a sufficient number of families could be identified.

The *WRN* locus was localized initially by using a combination of 8 outbred families and 13 consanguineous pedigrees, all from Japan.[30] Markers spanning much of the genome were analyzed by conventional maximum-likelihood methods; markers at 8p11.1-21.1 (Fig. 33-3) showed significant cosegregation with the WS phenotype. This localization was confirmed by homozygosity mapping methods[61,62] using primarily single affected subjects from a series of Japanese consanguineous families.[31] Significant positive-linkage results also were obtained with a panel of nine non-Japanese WS subjects who were primarily Caucasians.[32]

Initial mapping studies placed the *WRN* locus in a broad region from D8S137 to ANK1,[30–32,63,64] an interval spanning 16.6 cM[65,66] (see Fig. 33-3). Assignment of the *WRN* locus to this interval was based both on observed recombinants and on multipoint analysis.[32] Marker D8S339 was the closest marker showing the least recombination with WS. The D8S137-ANK1 interval contained relatively few known genes, which included heregulin (*HRB*), fibroblast growth factor receptor 1 (*FGFR1*), and DNA polymerase-β. *FGFR1* and *HRG* were excluded by recombination events between these genes and WS in affected subjects. The *pol-β* gene was excluded by DNA sequence analysis (no mutations were found[67]) and by radiation hybrid mapping, which placed the gene outside the D8S137-ANK1 region.[66]

High-Resolution Mapping of the *WRN* Gene

Fine mapping of the *WRN* locus became possible when short tandem repeat polymorphism (STRP) markers in linkage disequilibrium with WS were identified.[68] The first marker found that showed linkage disequilibrium with WS was at the glutathione reductase (*GSR*) gene. *GSR* had previously been assigned to

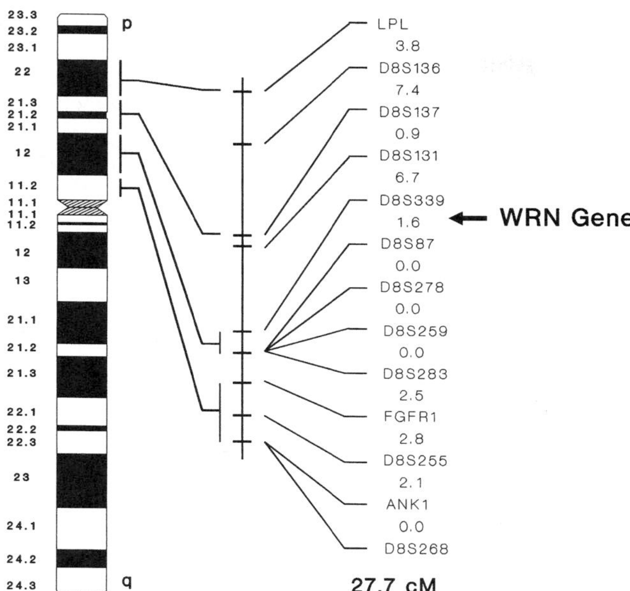

Fig. 33-3 Genetic map of the *WRN* region of chromosome 8. Genetic distances are sex-equal and are given in centimorgans (cM). The total length of the map is given at the bottom. (*From Oshima et al.*[66] *Used by permission.*)

chromosome 8 by somatic cell hybrid mapping but had not been mapped to a specific region of the chromosome. During the process of mapping *GSR* as a candidate gene, two STRP loci were identified in a cosmid clone containing the gene; in a group of 17 Japanese subjects, both STRP's had alleles that were in linkage disequilibrium ($p = 0.0025–0.001$) with the WS gene.[68] Subsequent analysis of other markers in the region demonstrated that D8S339 also was in disequilibrium with *WRN* in the same group of families, an observation confirmed in other studies.[69] *GSR* and D8S339 were subsequently found to be separated by approximately 200 kb (Fig. 33-4). Other markers flanking *GSR* and D8S339, including the clusters D8S131-D8S137 and D8S278-D8S87-D8S259-D8S283, were not in linkage disequilibrium with *WRN*.

To refine the location of the *WRN* gene, chromosome walking methods were used to clone DNA flanking D8S339/*GSR*. A yeast artificial chromosome (YAC) contig was constructed, using *GSR* as a starting point, and the contig was used as a source of cloned DNA for the identification of an additional 18 additional STRP loci[70–72] (see Fig. 33-4). Genotype data from these markers were used in three different approaches in an attempt to narrow the *WRN* region. First, the markers were used to define recombinants in WS pedigrees. Definitive recombinants were identified at D8S2194/D8S2192 and at D8S2186. Second, the markers were tested for linkage disequilibrium to identify the boundaries of the region of linkage disequilibrium. In Japanese kindreds, markers D8S2196 and D8S2162 and many markers in between were in linkage disequilibrium with *WRN*, while D8S2194-D8S2192 and D8S2186 as well as more distant flanking markers (D8S131-D8S137 and D8S278-D8S259-D8S87-D8S283) were not.[73,74] Third, because markers in this region are in disequilibrium with *WRN*, many of the subjects studied are presumed to be descendants of a common ancestor and thus should share a definable common haplotype. The genotype data from markers spanning the region were used to define a common ancestral haplotype and determine where ancestral recombinants had disrupted that haplotype.[68,74] The combined approach using these three methods yielded an interval of approximately 1.2 megabases (Mb) that contained the *WRN* gene.

Positional Cloning of the *WRN* Gene

The *WRN* gene was identified by positional cloning methods,[25] with the effort focused on the 1.2-Mb region indicated by the preceding genetic studies. The YAC contig was converted to P1 clones, which are less prone to deletion and rearrangement artifacts. The P1 clones were used as a source of DNA to identify genes in the region, using exon trapping,[75] cDNA selection methods (hybridization of cDNA libraries to YAC and P1 clones[76]), and DNA sequence analysis (comparison of DNA sequence with the DNA sequence databases of known genes and potential expressed sequence-tagged sites). Each of these methods yielded gene fragments that were then used to isolate full-length cDNA clones for each gene in the *WRN* region. These candidates were screened for mutations by reverse-transcriptase polymerase chain reaction (RT-PCR) methods or direct DNA sequence analysis of genomic DNA. A total of 10 genes were characterized and screened for mutations before the *WRN* gene was identified. These were *GSR*, protein phosphatase 2 catalytic subunit β (*PPP2CB*), general transcription factor IIEβ (*GTF2E2*), a β-tubullin pseudogene 1 (*TUBBP1*), and six previously unidentified genes of unknown function.

The *WRN* gene was identified initially as a match between the genomic DNA of a P1 and 245-bp sequence in the expressed sequence tag database.[25] This short sequence was used to identify a 5.2-kb full-length cDNA clone that encodes a predicted protein of 1432 amino acids. The same gene also was identified by exon trapping. Comparison of the DNA sequence to known genes revealed a striking homology to genes in the super-family of DNA and RNA helicases (Fig. 33-5). Thus WS joins a list of inherited disorders caused by mutations in helicase genes. These disorders are xeroderma pigmentosum, complementation groups B[77] and D (helicases ERCC2 and ERCC3, respectively[78–82]), trichothiodystrophy (ERCC2[83,84]), Cockayne syndrome (helicase ERCC6,[85]), Bloom syndrome,[86] and X chromosome-linked α-thalassemia mental retardation syndrome.[87,88]

WRN Mutations

During initial characterization of the gene, four mutations were identified in the 3′ end[25] (see Table 33-2). Two (mutations 1 and 2) were single-base substitution nonsense mutations that result in truncated proteins of 1164 and 1060 amino acids, respectively, compared with 1432 for the normal protein. Mutation 3 is a 4-bp deletion resulting in a frameshift and a predicted truncated protein. This mutation was observed in a single Syrian family. Mutation 4 is a single base-pair intronic substitution at a splice junction that results in skipping of an exon and a frameshift, producing a truncated protein (see Fig. 33-5). The first four mutations identified were in the 3′ end of the gene, and all leave the helicase consensus domain intact. This bias resulted from the 3′ being available for mutational analysis first. Since the helicase region contains the ATPase region of the protein and presumably is the enzymatic component of the helicase, 3′-truncated proteins could still retain DNA/RNA-unwinding activity.

To screen the middle and the 5′ end of the gene, the genomic structure of *WRN* was determined. The gene consists of 35 exons, with the coding region beginning in the second exon.[33,35] The gene spans at least 100 kb, although the actual size of the gene is unknown. Five additional mutations (A–E, Table 33-2) were identified in the remainder of the gene. Two additional nonsense mutations and a splice-junction mutation were found. Another mutation is a 1-bp deletion that results in a frameshift and a premature stop codon. Mutation E is a large genomic deletion (0.15 kb) that probably occurred by a recombination event between two highly homologous Alu elements that are separated by 15 kb. Two of these mutations result in predicted truncated protein products that do not contain the helicase domains.

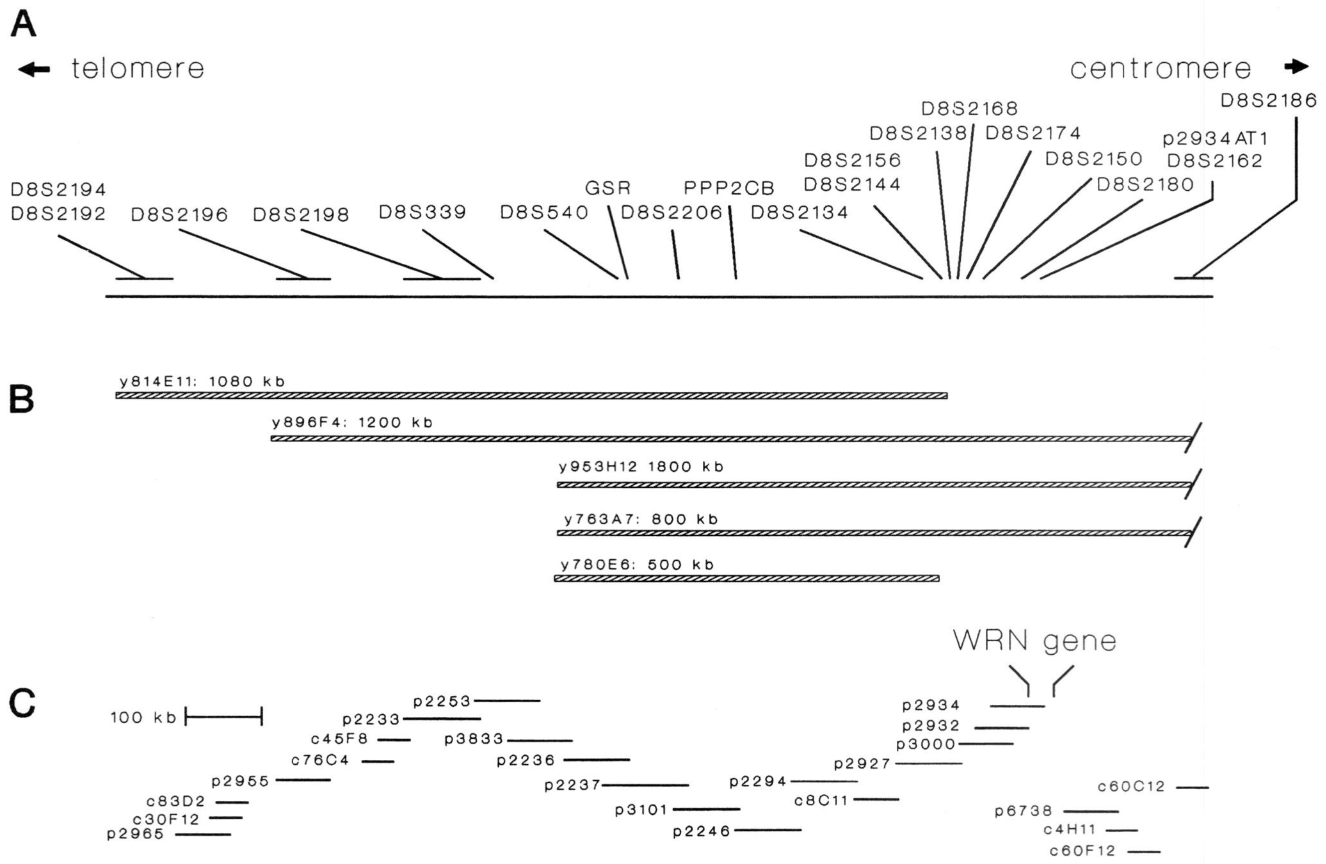

Fig. 33-4 Genetic markers, YACs, P1, and cosmid clones used in the positional cloning of the *WRN* gene. *A.* STRP loci. *B.* YAC clones. *C.* P1 clones (beginning with a *p*) and cosmid clones (beginning with a *c*). The size scale in kilobase units (kb) given in *C* also applies to *A* and *B.* (*Reproduced from Yu et al.*[72] *Used by permission.*)

To date, a total of 19 WS mutations[25,33,35–37] have been identified (see Table 33-2). All mutations, whether point mutations, insertions, or deletions, result in a predicted truncated protein product, and no missense mutations have been identified. The predicted truncated WRN proteins from the different mutations range in length from 176 to 1304 amino acids, with some retaining the helicase domain and others consisting only of the N-terminal end of the protein. Compound heterozygotes exist for a number of different WS mutations. Despite the variety of predicted protein products and combinations of mutant alleles, there is no evidence that the severity of the disease correlates with the type of mutation observed.[35,89] Thus differential phenotype-genotype relationships may be subtle and difficult to detect and will require additional work. Heterozygotes (normal allele/WS mutation) do not appear to manifest any characteristics of WS, and some live past the age of 90. Presently, no other disease has been

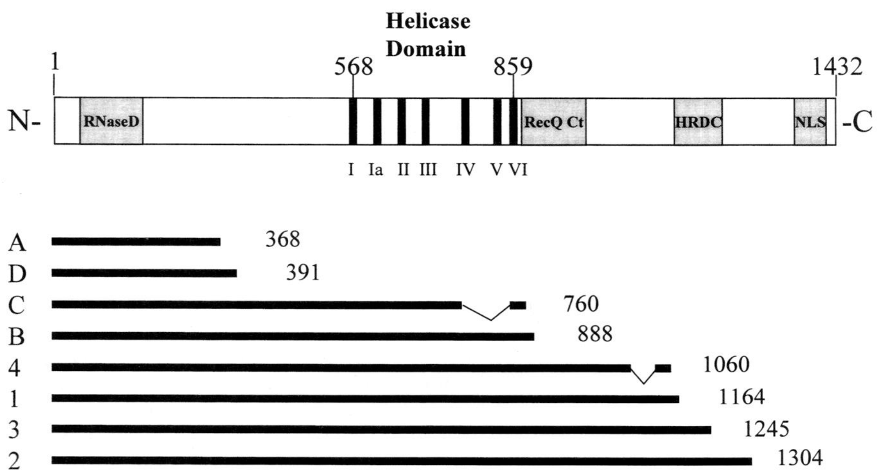

Fig. 33-5 The WS helicase. *A.* Schematic diagram of WRNp with the seven helicase motifs (I–VI) shown as solid bars. *B.* WS mutations: Bars indicate extent of translation of mutated WS alleles. Numbers to the right of the bars indicate the length of the mutated protein product. Breaks indicate skipped exons. All mutations result in production of a truncated protein due to nonsense mutations, frame shift mutations or skipped exons due to splice site mutations or genomic deletions.

associated with *WRN* mutations. In particular, subjects with Hutchinson-Gilford syndrome, a progeroid syndrome with a childhood onset, do not have *WRN* mutations.[90]

Pathogenic Mechanism of *WRN* Mutations

A common mechanism may exist for all *WRN* mutations. WRNp is localized primarily to the nucleus of cells.[91,92] This localization can be demonstrated either by cell fractionation methods or by generating a green-fluorescent protein (GFP) WRN fusion protein with GFP attached to the N-terminus of WRNp.[91] All WS mutations result in predicted truncated proteins that are missing 128 or more amino acids of the C-terminal end (see Table 33-2). When WS mutations are introduced into the GFP-WRNp fusion proteins, truncated proteins are produced that lack the C-terminus. Only the normal fusion protein goes to the nucleus, while all the C-terminus–deficient fusion proteins remain in the cytoplasm. This work shows that the C-terminus of WRN contains a nuclear localization signal that is missing in all WS mutation proteins. Assuming that the biologic function of the WRN protein is in the nucleus, *WRN* mutations keep the protein from reaching the site of its normal function, even if the enzymatic helicase portion of the molecule is intact and functional. Within the nucleus, WRNp may be localized to the nucleolus in human but not in murine cells.[92] This observation is intriguing because the yeast helicase SGS1p, which is partially homologous to WRNp, is also localized in the nucleolus, and mutations in SGS1p shorten life span and result in other age-related phenotypes in yeast.[93]

A second consequence of WS mutations is that the levels of WRN mRNA are reduced in mutation homozygotes to 30 percent compared with normal homozygotes.[94] The reduced levels are presumably due to reduced mRNA stability. In heterozygotes, WRN mRNA is less than the expected 65 percent, suggesting there may be some feedback regulation of transcription, mRNA processing, or mRNA degradation.

Origins of *WRN* Mutations

The existence of common Japanese founders was confirmed by mutational analysis. Among Japanese subjects, 50 to 60 percent had the same mutation (mutation 4).[33,35,89] Most of these subjects had the 141-bp allele at *GSR* that was overrepresented in WS patients compared with controls (frequency, 0.40 and 0.07, respectively) and therefore was responsible for the linkage disequilibrium observed at *GSR*. Further, for two highly polymorphic STRP loci within the *WRN* gene (D8S2162 and p2934AT1; see Fig. 33-4), haplotypes were identical for all mutation 4 carriers tested. In Japanese subjects, a second mutation (mutation A in Table 33-2) is also common in Japanese subjects, with a mutation frequency of 17.5 percent. Haplotype analysis suggests that this mutation is also the result of a common founder.[35] Mutations 2 and A are found in both Japanese and Caucasian subjects. For both mutations, different haplotypes for STRP markers within the *WRN* gene were observed in Caucasian versus Japanese subjects, suggesting an independent origin.[33] However, a common ancient founder cannot be completely ruled out, since intragenic recombination or mutations at the STRP loci cannot be excluded.

In Vitro WRNp Studies

The predicted sequence of WRNp indicates that it is a member of a super-family of DExH box DNA and RNA helicases. These DNA- and RNA-unwinding proteins share a common structure of seven motifs (I, Ia, II, III, IV, V, and VI) ranging in size from approximately 15 to 25 amino acids.[95] Motif I contains a nucleotide-binding site, and motif II has the DExH sequence of a Mg^{2+}-binding site (DEAH in the *WRN* gene); these sites presumably participate in the hydrolysis of ATP that occurs as the enzyme unwinds a double-stranded DNA or RNA helix. WRNp shows homology to these seven motifs in helicases from a wide variety of organisms, including *Escherichia coli* (recQ), *Saccharomyces cerevisiae* (SgS1), *Caenorhabditis elegans* (F18C5C), and humans (RECQL).[25] The region of shared homology is in the center of WRNp, spanning amino acids 540 to 963. The sequences in between the seven motifs are not conserved, although the spacing between motifs is highly conserved. The homology between the predicted protein and other helicases strongly suggests that WRNp is a functional helicase.

Other domains shared with other proteins are more subtle than the helicase homology region. In the N-terminal end, between amino acids 59 and 105, is a domain shared with RNase D (called the *RNase D domain*) that is also found in the $3' \rightarrow 5'$ proofreading exonuclease domain of bacterial DNA polymerase.[96,97] This RNase D domain is not found in SGS1p or in the Bloom syndrome helicase (BLMp). Thus the WRN protein may have an exonuclease activity, although this has not been directly demonstrated. In the C-terminal end, from approximately amino acids 1150 to 1229, is another domain homologous to a different region of RNase D called the *helicase and RNase D C-terminal (HRDC) domain.* HRDC is found in some helicases including reqQ (*E. coli*), SGS1 (yeast), and BLM (human) and in RNases including RNase D (*E. coli*) and a number of eukaryotic homologues.[98] The HDRC domain is not required for helicase or RNase activities because not all helicases or RNases have this domain. The N-terminal end is highly acidic, containing 109 glutamate or aspartate residues, including one segment with 14 amino acids in a stretch of 19S. There is a 27-amino acid tandem repeat sequence beginning at amino acid 424 in the protein. The mouse and rat WRN homologues do not contain this repeat.[99]

The prediction from the WRNp sequence that WRNp is a helicase[25] has been confirmed recently by functional studies.[100–102] WRNp generated in an insect cell-baculovirus system can unwind double-stranded DNA (dsDNA) in an ATP-dependent process, and ATP hydrolysis is dsDNA-dependent. Mutation 4 (see Table 33-2) that has the helicase domain but lacks 372 amino acids from the C-terminus and is missing the HRDC domain still retains helicase activity. However, WRNp with a $^{K}577^{M}$ mutation at a highly conserved amino acid in the helicase I motif does not have helicase activity. The preferred polarity of WRNp helicase activity is $3' \rightarrow 5'$. RNA-DNA heteroduplexes are also unwound but with a lower efficiency than for DNA homoduplexes. As seen with other helicases, DNA unwinding activity is enhanced by the addition of single-strand DNA binding proteins from a number of different sources, with human single-strand binding protein being the most effective.[102]

WRNp and WS

The normal function of WRNp is unknown. It could function to unwind DNA during replication, repair, transcription, or any number of other DNA transactions requiring duplex unwinding. Other helicases function as part of multiprotein complexes. For example, ERCC2 and ERCC3, which are defective in xeroderma pigmentosum, are part of the RNA polymerase II basal transcription factor (TFIIH).[101] ERCC6, the helicase defective in Cockayne syndrome group B subjects, interacts with the product of the CSA gene, which is mutated in Cockayne syndrome group A subjects.[102] CSA in turn interacts with TFIIH. Thus the Cockayne syndrome helicase also may interact with TFIIH. By analogy to these other helicases, WRNp may interact with other proteins in a complex to perform its normal function in DNA metabolism. Since the N-terminal and C-terminal ends of each of these helicases are unique, presumably protein-protein interactions are dependent on the nonhelicase segments of the protein. Isolation of the other proteins that complex with WRNp will be critical to understanding the function of this helicase.

Previous studies of the biology of WS have yielded limited information on the potential function of WRNp. Two different lines of evidence indicate that WS cells have a mutator phenotype. First, both *in vitro* and *in vivo* studies show an elevated mutation rate using the hypoxanthine phosphoribosyltransferase gene as a reporter locus.[14–17] Characterization of the types of mutations that occur in WS cells indicates that the proportion of deletion mutations is higher than expected. These deletions may occur by nonhomologous recombination, since sequences of the deletions are not homologous.[17] The second indication of genomic instability is the elevated rate of random chromosomal rearrangements in WS cells, again observed both *in vitro* and *in vivo*.[18–23]

The WS mutator phenotype could result from defective DNA repair. For xeroderma pigmentosum and Cockayne syndrome, helicase defects result in faulty nucleotide excision repair and strand-specific transcription-coupled repair, respectively. Defective DNA repair in WS cells has been difficult to reproducibly demonstrate. Unscheduled DNA synthesis[105–107] and post-ultraviolet (UV) irradiation cell survival[108] are not defective in WS cells, and there is no increased sensitivity to a variety of DNA-damaging agents, including bleomycin, *cis*-dichlorodiamine platinum, diepoxybutane, isonicotinic acid hydrazide, 1-methyl-3-nitro-1-nitrosoguanidine, hydroxyurea, and methyl methanesulfonate.[107–113] Cells from WS subjects are sensitive to the DNA damaging agent 4-nitro-quinline-1-oxide (4NQO), and cells from heterozygotes have a level of sensitivity intermediate to normal individuals and WS subjects, suggesting a DNA repair defect. WS cell proliferation was more sensitive than normal cells to the topoisomerase I inhibitor camptothecin.[114] For topoisomerase II inhibitors, ellipticine and amsacrine do not differentially affect WS cell proliferation, while both positive and negative results have been reported with etoposide.[112,113] Mismatch repair is normal in Epstein-Barr virus-transformed lymphoblastoid cell lines but may be reduced in SV40-transformed fibroblastoid cell lines, although additional work is needed to confirm this finding.[115] Microsatellite length stability is not reduced,[116] and sister-chromatid exchange, with or without treatment with clastogens, is not elevated in WS cells.[110,118,117] To date, no specific DNA repair system has been associated with the loss of WRNp function.

Other alterations in DNA metabolism have been reported. For DNA synthesis, reduced chain-elongation rates[105] and increased distances between synthesis initiation sites[119,120] have been reported. This reduced rate of DNA synthesis could be responsible for the prolonged S phase observed in WS cells.[119,121] DNA ligation may be abnormal in WS cells.[122,123] While the rate of ligation is not altered, the accuracy of ligation events is reduced, suggesting a possible mechanism for generating mutations. Elevated rates of homologous recombination also have been reported.[124] Whether the WRN helicase defect is directly responsible for any of these alterations in DNA handling remains to be determined. The primary mechanism by which defective helicase mutations give rise to the WS phenotype also remains to be determined.

Model Organisms and WRNp Function

Recent work in model organisms has provided information about the normal function of WRNp. In yeast, the WRNp homologue Sgs1p is a suppressor of illegitimate recombination between nonhomologous or short homologous DNA sequences. In SGS1 loss-of-function mutants, genomic instability and a hyperrecombination occur.[125] The hyperrecombination phenotype can be partially suppressed by either WRNp or BLMp.[126] Thus the genomic instability observed in WS subjects could be due to processes related to illegitimate recombination.

In *Xenopus laevis,* a helicase called FFA-1 for focus-forming activity-1 was identified that is a homologue of WRNp and is required for DNA replication initiation.[127] FFA-1 is an ATP- and dsDNA-dependent helicase. DNA replication is initiated when an ssDNA-binding protein called *replication protein A* and FFA-1 bind to a specific DNA sequence that serves as an origin of replication. The gene for FFA-1 was cloned and shown to encode a 1436-amino acid protein that contains the 7 helicase motifs found in WRNp and other RecQ-type helicases. In addition, unlike Sgs1p, RecQ, and other helicases, FFA-1 is homologous to WRNp across the entire length of protein, not just in the helicase, HRDC, and RNase D domains. FFA-1 is 66 percent similar and 50 percent identical to WRNp. Thus WRNp may be involved in DNA replication initiation, which is consistent with previous work demonstrating altered DNA synthesis in WS cells.[105,119–121] However, WRNp is probably not required for all DNA synthesis because WS mutations most likely result in the complete loss of function of WRNp, and other paralogues must exist in humans that can substitute for WRNp in DNA replication initiation.

RECENT IMPLICATIONS OF IDENTIFICATION OF THE *WRN* GENE FOR DIAGNOSIS

The diagnosis of WS can now potentially be confirmed definitively by mutational analysis of the *WRN* gene; WS subjects should be either homozygous or compound heterozygotes for mutations in this gene. In work to date, mutations have been identified in all subjects studied, including some with diagnoses of "probable" and "possible."[33] The mutational analysis confirms the usefulness of the clinical criteria outlined in Tables 33-3 and 33-4. The principal advantage of mutational analysis is that the diagnosis can be made at a young age, when WS is first suspected. In contrast, the mean age at diagnosis using clinical criteria is 37 years, because in some patients some of the defining symptoms do not develop until the third and fourth decades of life. Screening the *WRN* gene for mutations in Japanese subjects is simplified because one mutation accounts for 60 percent of the WS cases and two others make up an additional 33 percent. In Caucasians, it is not known what the frequencies of the different WS mutations are. Since the gene has 34 coding exons, complete analysis of the entire gene for a subject is expensive. The development of an *in vitro* protein-truncation assay for WS should facilitate mutation detection. Because WS is such a rare disorder, it is unlikely that mutation screening will become universally available.

ACKNOWLEDGMENTS

We thank Thomas D. Bird, Mary T. Ersek, and Raymond J. Monnat for reading the text before publication. We also thank Charles J. Epstein for making some of the photographs available. This work was funded in part by grant RO1 AG12019 (GDS) from the National Institute on Aging. We also thank the WS subjects who participated in the research described here.

REFERENCES

1. Werner CWO: Udber kataract in Verbindung mit Sclerodermie. *Doctoral dissertation*, Kiel, Schmidt & Klarnig, West Germany, 1904.
2. Werner O (trans H Hoehn): On cataract in conjunction with sclerodema. *Adv Exp Med Biol* **190**:1, 1985.
3. Oppenheimer BS, Kugel VH: Werner's syndrome, a heredofamilial disorder with scleroderma, bilateral juvenile cataracts, precocioius graying of the hair and endocrine stigmatization. *Trans Assoc Am Phys* **49**:358, 1934.
4. Thannhauser SJ: Werner's syndrome (progeria of the adult) and Rothmund's syndrome: Two types of closely related heredofamilial atrophic dermatoses with juvenile cataracts and endocrine features: A critical study with five new cases. *Ann Intern Med* **23**:559, 1945.
5. Goto M, Tanimoto K, Horiuchi Y, Sasazuki T: Family analysis of Werner's syndrome: A survey of 42 Japanese families with a review of the literature. *Clin Genet* **19**:8, 1981.
6. Epstein CJ, Martin GM, Schultz A, Motulsky AG: Werner's syndrome: A review of its symptomatology, natural history, pathologic features, genetics, and relationship to the natural aging process. *Medicine* **45**:177, 1966.
7. Tollefsbol TO, Cohen HJ: Werner's syndrome: An underdiagnosed disorder resembling premature aging. *Age* **7**:75, 1984.
8. Jacobson HG, Rifkin H, Zucker D: Werner's syndrome: A clinical entity. *Radiology* **74**:373, 1960.
9. Zucker-Franklin D, Rifkin H, Jacobson HG: Werner's syndrome: An analysis of ten cases. *Geriatrics* **23**:123, 1968.
10. Martin GM: Genetic syndromes in man with potential relevance to the pathobiology of aging. *Birth Defects* **14**:5, 1978.
11. Hayflick L: The limited *in vitro* lifetime of human diploid cell strains. *Exp Cell Res* **37**:614, 1965.

12. Martin GM, Sprague CA, Epstein CJ: Replicative life-span of cultivated human cells. *Lab Invest* **23**:86, 1970.
13. Goto M, Miller RW, Ishikawa Y, Sugano H: Excess of rare cancers in Werner syndrome (adult progeria). *Epidemiol Biomarkers Prevent* **5**:239, 1996.
14. Fukuchi K, Tanaka K, Nakura J, Kumahara Y, Uchida T, Okada Y: Elevated spontaneous mutation rate in SV40 Werner syndrome fibroblast cell lines. *Somat Cell Mol Genet* **11**:303, 1985.
15. Fukuchi K, Martin GM, Monnat RJ: Mutator phenotype of Werner syndrome is characterized by extensive deletions. *Proc Natl Acad Sci USA* **86**:5893, 1989.
16. Fukuchi K, Tanaka K, Kumahara Y, Maramo K, Pride M, Martin GM, Monnet RJ: Increased frequency of 6-thioguanine-resistant peripheral blood lymhocytes in Werner syndrome patients. *Hum Genet* **84**:249, 1990.
17. Monnat RJ, Hackmann AFM, Chiaverotti TA: Nucleotide sequence analysis of human hypoxanthine phosphoribosyltransferase (HPRT) gene deletions. *Genomics* **13**:777, 1992.
18. Hoehn H, Bryant EM, Au K, Norwood TH, Boman H, Martin GM: Variegated translocation mosaicism in human skin fibroblast cultures. *Cytogenet Cell Genet* **15**:282, 1975.
19. Salk D, Hoehn H, Martin GM: Cytogenetics of Werner's syndrome cultured in skin fibroblasts: Variegated translocation mosaicism. *Hum Genet* **62**:16, 1982.
20. Salk D: Werner's syndrome: A review of recent research with an analysis of connective tissue metabolism, growth control of cultured cells, and chromosomal aberrations. *Hum Genet* **62**:1, 1982.
21. Salk D, Au K, Hoehn H, Martin GM: Cytogenetics of Werner's syndrome cultured skin fibroblasts: Variegated translocation mosaicism. *Cytogenet Cell Genet* **30**:92, 1981.
22. Scappaticci S, Cerimele D, Fraccaro M: Clonal structural chromosomal rearrangements in primary fibroblast cultures and in lymphocytes of patients with Werner's syndrome. *Hum Genet* **62**:16, 1982.
23. Salk D, Au K, Hoehn H, Martin GM: Cytogenetic aspects of Werner syndrome. *Adv Exp Med Biol* **190**:541, 1985.
24. Morita K, Nishigori C, Sasaki MS, Matsuyoshi N, Ohta K, Okamoto H, Ikai K, et al: Werner's syndrome: Chromosome analyses of cultured fibroblasts and mitogen-stimulated lymphocytes. *Br J Dermatol* **136**:620, 1997.
25. Yu CE, Oshima J, Fu YH, Wijsman EM, Hisama F, Alisch R, Matthews S, et al: Positional cloning of the Werner's syndrome gene. *Science* **272**:258, 1996.
26. Barrai I, Mi MP, Morton NE, Yasuda N: Estimation of prevalence under incomplete selection. *Am J Hum Genet* **17**:221, 1965.
27. Dahlberg G: Methods for population genetics. *Am J Biol* **25**:90, 1950.
28. Neal JV, Kodani MB, Brewer R, Anderson RC: The incidence of consanguineous matings in Japan: Remarks on the estimation of comparative gene frequencies and the expected rate of induced recessive mutations. *Am J Hum Genet* **1**:156, 1949.
29. Cerimele D, Cotton F, Scappaticci S, Rabbiosi G, Borroni G, Sanna E, Zei G, et al: High prevalence of Werner's syndrome in Sardinia: Description of six patients and estimates of the gene frequency. *Hum Genet* **62**:25, 1982.
30. Goto M, Weber J, Woods K, Drayna D: Genetic linkage of Werner's syndrome to five markers on chromosome 8. *Nature* **355**:735, 1992.
31. Schellenberg GD, Martin GM, Wijsman EM, Nakura J, Miki T, Ogihara T: Homozygosity mapping and Werner's syndrome. *Lancet* **339**:1002, 1992.
32. Nakura J, Wijsman EM, Miki T, Kamino K, Yu CE, Oshima J, Fukuchi K, et al: Homozygosity mapping of the Werner syndrome locus (WRN). *Genomics* **23**:600, 1994.
33. Yu CE, Oshima J, Wijsman EM, Nakura J, Miki T, Puissan C, Matthews S, et al: Werner's syndrome collaborative group: Mutations in the consensus helicase domains of the Werner's syndrome gene. *Am J Hum Genet* **60**:330, 1997.
34. Meisslitzer C, Ruppitsch W, Weirichschwaiger H, Weirich HG, Jabkowsky J, Klein G, Schweiger M, Hirschkauffmann M: Werner syndrome: Characterization of mutations in the WRN gene in an affected family. *Eur J Hum Genet* **5**:364, 1997.
35. Matsumoto T, Imamura O, Yamabe Y, Kuromitsu J, Tokutake Y, Shimamoto A, Suzuki N, Satoh M, Kitao S, Ichikawa K, Kataoka H, Sugawara K, Thomas W, Mason B, Tsuchihashi Z, Drayna D, Sugawara M, Sugimoto M, Furuchi Y, Goto M: Mutation and haplotype analyses of the Werner's syndrome gene based on its genomic structure: Genetic epidemiology in the Japanese population. *Hum Genet* **100**:123 1997.
36. Goto M, Imamura O, Kuromitsu J, Matsumoto T, Yamabe Y, Tokutake Y, Suzuki N, et al: Analysis of helicase gene mutations in Japanese Werner's syndrome. *Hum Genet* **9**:191, 1997.
37. Oshima J, Yu CE, Piussan C, Klein G, Jabkowski J, Balci S, Miki T, et al: Homozygous and compound heterozygous mutations at the Werner syndrome locus. *Hum Mol Genet* **5**:1909, 1996.
38. Goto M, Horiuchi Y, Tanimoto K, Ishii T, Nakashima H: Werner's syndrome: Analysis of 15 cases with a review of the Japanese literature. *J Am Geriatr Soc* **26**:341, 1978.
39. Murata K, Nakashima H: Werner's syndrome: Twenty-four cases with a review of the Japanese medical literature. *J Am Geriatr Soc* **30**:303, 1982.
40. Kieras FJ, Brown WT, Houck GE, Zebrower M: Elevation of urinary hyaluronic acid in Werner's syndrome and progeria. *Biochem Med Metab Biol* **36**:276, 1986.
41. Tokunaga M, Futami T, Wakamatsu E, Endo M, Yosizawa Z: Werner's syndrome as "hyaluronuria." *Clin Chim Acta* **62**:89, 1975.
42. Goto M, Murata K: Urinary excretion of macromolecular acidic glycosaminoglycans in Werner's syndrome. *Clin Chim Acta* **85**:101, 1978.
43. Murata K: Urinary acidic glycosaminoglycans in Werner's syndrome. *Experimentia* **38**:313, 1982.
44. Varada DP, Cifonelli JA, Dorfman A: The acid mucopolysaccharides in normal urine. *Biochem Biophys Acta* **141**:103, 1967.
45. Imura H, Nakao Y, Kuzuya H, Okamoto M, Okamoto M, Yamada K: Clinical, endocrine and metabolic aspects of the Werner syndrome compared with those of normal aging. *Adv Exp Med Biol* **190**:171, 1985.
46. Mori S, Yokote K, Morisaki N, Saito Y, Yoshida S: Inheritable abnormal lipoprotein metabolism in Werner's syndrome similar to familial hypercholesterolemia. *Eur J Clin Invest* **20**:137, 1990.
47. Goto M, Kato Y: Hypercoagulable state indicates an additional risk factor for atherosclerosis in Werner's syndrome. *Thromb Haemost* **73**:576, 1995.
48. Sato K, Goto M, Nishioka K, Arima K, Hori N, Yamashita N, Fujimoto Y, Nanko H, Olwawa K, Ohara K: Werner's syndrome associated with malignancies: Five cases with a survey of case histories in Japan. *Gerontology* **34**:212, 1988.
49. Miller RW, Myers MH: Age distribution of epithelial and non-epithelial cancers. *Lancet* **2**:1250, 1983.
50. Goto M: Hierarchical deterioration of body systems in Werner's syndrome: Implications for normal ageing. *Mech Age Dev* **98**:239, 1997
51. Elwood JM: Epidemiology and control of melanoma in white populations and in Japan. *J Invest Dermatol* **92**:214, 1989.
52. Sampson RJ, Key CR, Buncher CR, Iijima S: Thyroid carcinoma at autopsy in Hiroshima and Nagasaki: I. Prevalence of thyroid cancer at autopsy. *JAMA* **209**:65, 1969.
53. Correa P, Chen VW: Endocrine gland cancer. *Cancer* **75**:338, 1995.
54. Postiglione A, Soricelli A, Covelli EM, Iazzetta N, Ruocco A, Milan G, Santoro L, Alfano B, Brunetti A: Premature aging in Werner's syndrome spares the central nervous system. *Neurobiol Aging* **17**:325, 1996.
55. Kakigi R, Endo C, Neshige R, Kohno H, Kuroda Y: Accelerated aging in the brain in Werner's syndrome. *Neurology* **42**:922, 1992.
56. Umehara F, Abe M, Nagawa M, Izumo S, Arimura K, Matsumuro K, Osame M: Werner's syndrome associated with spastic paraparesis and peripheral neuropathy. *Neurology* **43**:1252, 1993.
57. Sumi SM: Neuropathology of the Werner syndrome. *Adv Exp Med Biol* **190**:215, 1985.
58. Leverenz JB, Yu CE, Schellenberg GD: Aging-associated neuropathology in Werner syndrome. *Acta Neuropathol* **96**:421, 1998.
59. Weissenbach J, Gyapay G, Dib C, Vignal A, Morissette J, Millasseau P, Vaysseix G, Lathrop M: A second generation linkage map of the human genome. *Nature* **359**:794, 1993.
60. NIH/CEPH Collaborative Mapping Group: A comprehensive genetic linkage map of the human genome. *Science* **258**:148, 1992.
61. Lander ES, Botstein D: Homozygosity mapping: A way to map human recessive traits with the DNA of inbred children. *Science* **236**:1567, 1987.
62. Smith CAB: Detection of linkage in human genetics. *J R Stat Soc B* **15**:153, 1953.
63. Ye L, Nakura J, Mitsuda N, Fujioka Y, Kamino K, Ohta T, Jinno Y, Niikawa N, Miki T, Ogihara T: Genetic association between chromosome 8 microsatellite (MS8-134) and Werner syndrome (WRN): Chromosome microdissection and homozygosity mapping. *Genomics* **28**:566, 1995.

64. Thomas W, Rubenstein M, Goto M, Drayna D: A genetic analysis of the Werner syndrome region on human chromosome 8p. *Genomics* **16**:685, 1993.
65. Tomfohrde J, Wood S, Schertzer M, Wagner MJ, Wells DE, Parrish J, Sadler LA, Blanton SH, Daiger SP, Wang ZY, Wilkie PJ, Weber JL: Human chromosome linkage map based on short tandem repeat polymorphisms: Effect of genotyping errors. *Genomics* **14**:144, 1992.
66. Oshima J, Yu CE, Boehnke M, Weber JL, Edelhoff S, Wagner MJ, Wells DE, Wood S, Disteche CM, Martin GM, Schellenberg GD: Integrated mapping analysis of the Werner syndrome region of chromosome 8. *Genomics* **23**:100, 1994.
67. Chang M, Burmer GC, Sweasy J, Loeb LA, Edelhoff S, Disteche CM, Yu CE, Anderson L, Oshima J, Nakura J, Miki T, Kamino K, Ogihara T, Schellenberg GD, Martin GM: Evidence against DNA polymerase beta as a candidate gene for Werner syndrome. *Hum Genet* **93**:507, 1994.
68. Yu C, Oshima J, Goddard KAB, Miki T, Nakura J, Ogihara T, Fraccaro M, Piussan C, Martin GM, Schellenberg GD, Wijsman EM: Linkage disequilibrium and haplotype studies of chromosome 8p 11.1.1 markers and Werner's syndrome. *Am J Hum Genet* **55**:356, 1994.
69. Kihara K, Nakura J, Ye L, Mitsuda N, Kamino K, Zhao Y, Fujioka Y, Miki T, Ogihara T: Carrier detection of Werner's syndrome using a microsatellite that exhibits linkage disequilibrium with the Werner's syndrome locus. *Jpn J Hum Genet* **39**:403, 1994.
70. Ye L, Nakura J, Mitsuda N: A highly polymorphic dinucleotide repeat at the D8S1222 locus. *Jpn J Hum Genet* **40**:287, 1995.
71. Nakura J, Ye L, Kihara K, Yamagata H, Mamino K, Nakamura Y, Miki T, Ogihara T: Two dinucleotide repeat polymorphisms at the D8S1442 and D8S1443 loci. *Jpn J Hum Genet* **40**:281, 1995.
72. Yu CE, Oshima J, Hisama F, Matthews S, Trask BJ, Schellenberg GD: A YAC, P1 and cosmid contig and 17 new polymorphic markers for the Werner's syndrome region at 8p12. *Genomics* **35**:431, 1996.
73. Goddard KAB, Yu CE, Oshima J, Miki T, Nakura J, Piussan C, Martin GM, Schellenberg GD, Wijsman EM: International Werner's syndrome collaborative group: Toward localization of the Werner syndrome gene by linkage disequilibrium and ancestral haplotyping: Lessons learned from analysis of 35 chromosome 8p11.1.1 markers. *Am J Hum Genet* **58**:1286, 1996.
74. Nakura J, Miki T, Ye L, Mitsuda N, Zhao Y, Kihara K, Yu CE, et al: Narrowing the position of the Werner syndrome locus by homozygosity analysis: Extension of homozygosity analysis. *Genomics* **36**:130, 1996.
75. Parimoo S, Kolluri R, Weissman S: cDNA selection from total yeast DNA containing YACs. *Nucleic Acids Res* **21**:4422, 1993.
76. Weeda G, van Ham RCA, Vermeulen W, Bootsma D, van der Eb AJ, Hoeijmakers JHJ: A presumed DNA helicase encoded by ERCC is involved in the human repair disorders xeroderma pigmentosa and Cockayne's syndrome. *Cell* **62**:777, 1990.
77. Broughton BC, Thompson AF, Harcourt SA, Vermeulen W, Hoeijmakers JHJ, Botta E, Stefanini M, King MD, Weber CA, Cole J, Arlett CF, Lehmann AR: Molecular and cellular analysis of the DNA repair defect in a patient in xeroderma pigmentosum complementation group D who has the clinical features of xeroderma pigmentosum and Cockayne syndrome. *Am J Hum Genet* **56**:167, 1995.
78. Flejter WL, McDaniel LD, Johns D, Friedberg EC, Schultz RA: Correction of xeroderma pigmentosum complementation group D mutant cell phenotypes by chromosome and gene transfer: Involvement of the human ERCC2 DNA repair gene. *Proc Natl Acad Sci USA* **89**:261, 1992.
79. Frederick GD, Amirkhan RH, Schultz RA, Friedberg EC: Structural and mutational analysis of the xeroderma pimentosum group D (XPD) gene. *Hum Mol Genet* **3**:1783, 1994.
80. Takayama K, Salazar EP, Broughton BC, Lehmann AR, Sarasin A, Thompson LH, Weber CA: Defects in the DNA repair and transcription gene ERCC2(XPD) in trichothiodystrophy. *Am J Hum Genet* **58**:263, 1996.
81. Sung P, Bailly V, Weber C, Thompson LH, Prakash L, Prakash S: Human xeroderma pigmentosum group D gene encodes a DNA helicase. *Nature* **365**:852, 1993.
82. Broughton BC, Steingrimsdottir H, Weber CA, Lehmann AR: Mutations in the xeroderma pigmentosum group D DNA repair/transcription gene in patients with trichothiodystrophy. *Nature Genet* **7**:189, 1994.
83. Takayama K, Salazar EP, Broughton BC, Lehmann AR, Sarasin A, Thompson LH, Weber CA: Defects in the DNA repair and transcription gene ERCC2(XPD) in trichothiodystrophy. *Am J Hum Genet* **58**:263, 1996.
84. Troelstra C, van Gool A, Wit JD, Vermeulen W, Bootsma D, Hoeijmakers JHJ: ERCC6, a member of a subfamily of putative helicases, is involved in Cockayne's syndrome and preferential repair of active genes. *Cell* **71**:939, 1992.
85. Ellis NA, Groden J, Ye TZ, Straughen J, Lennon DJ, Ciocci S, Proytcheva M, German J: The Bloom's syndrome gene product is homologous to RecQ helicases. *Cell* **83**:655, 1995.
86. Stayton CL, Dabovic B, Gulisano M, Gecz J, Broccoli V, Giovanazzi S, Bossolasco M, Monaco L, Rastan S, Boncinelli EE, Bianchi M, Consalez GG: Cloning and characterization of a new human Xq13 gene, encoding a putative helicase. *Hum Mol Genet* **3**:1957, 1994.
87. Ion A, Telvi L, Chaussain JL, Galacteros F, Valayer J, Fellous M, McElreavey K: A novel mutation in the putative DNA helicase XH2 is responsible for male-to-female sex reversal associated with an atypical form of the ATR syndrome. *Am J Hum Genet* **58**:1185, 1996.
88. Miki T, Nakura J, Ye L, Mitsuda N, Morishima A, Sato N, Kamino K, Ogihara T: Molecular and epidemiological studies of Werner syndrome in the Japanese population. *Mech Age Dev* **98**:255, 1997.
89. Oshima J, Brown WT, Martin GM: No detectable mutations at Werner helicase locus in progeria. *Lancet* **348**:1106, 1996.
90. Matsumoto T, Shimamoto A, Goto M, Furuichi Y: Impaired localization of defective DNA helicases in Werner's syndrome. *Nature Genet* **16**:335, 1997.
91. Marciniak RA, Lombard DB, Johnson FB, Guarente L: Nucleolar localization of the Werner syndrome protein in human cells. *Proc Natl Acad Sci USA* **95**:6887, 1998.
92. Sinclair DA, Mills K, Guatente L: Accelerated aging and nuceolar fragmentation in yeast sgs1 mutants. *Science* **277**:1313, 1997.
93. Yamabe Y, Sugimoto M, Satoh M, Suzuki N, Sugawara M, Goto M, Furuichi Y: Down-regulation of the defective transcripts of the Werner's syndrome gene in the cells of patients. *Biochem Biophys Res Commun* **236**:151, 1997.
94. Gorbalenya AE, Koonin EV, Donchenko AP, Blinov VM: Two related superfamilies of putative helicases involved in replication, repair and expression of DNA and RNA genomes. *Nucleic Acids Res* **17**:4713, 1989.
95. Mushegian AR, Bassett DE, Boguski MS, Bork P, Koonin EV: Positionally cloned human disease genes: patterns of evolutionary conservation and functional motifs. *Proc Natl Acad Sci USA* **94**:5831, 1997.
96. Lombard DB, Guarente L: Cloning the gene for Werner syndrome: A disease with many symptoms of premature aging. *Trends Genet* **12**:283, 1996.
97. Morozov V, Mushegian AR, Koonin EV, Bork P: A putative nucleic acid-binding domain in Bloom's and Werner's syndrome helicases. *TIBS* **22**:417, 1997.
98. Imamura O, Ichikawa K, Yamabe Y, Goto M, Sugawara M, Furuchi Y: Cloning of a mouse homologue of the Werner syndrome gene and assignment to 8A4 by flourescence in situ hybridization. *Genomics* **41**:298, 1997.
99. Gray MD, Shen JC, Kamathloeb AS, Blank A, Sopher BL, Martin GM, Oshima J, Loeb LA: The Werner syndrome protein is a DNA helicase. *Nature Genet* **17**:100, 1997.
100. Suzuki N, Shimamoto A, Imamura O, Kuromitsu J, Kitao S, Goto M, Furuichi Y: DNA helicase activity in Werner's syndrome gene product synthesized in a baculovirus system. *Nucleic Acids Res* **25**:2973, 1997.
101. Shen JC, Gray MD, Oshima J, Loeb LA: Characterization of Werner syndrome protein DNA helicase activity: Directionality, substrate dependence and stimulation by replication protein A. *Nucleic Acids Res* **26**:2879, 1998.
102. Schaeffer L, Roy R, Humbert S, Moncollin V, Vermeulen W, Hoeijmakers JHJ, Chambon P, Egly JM: DNA repair helicase: A component of BTF2 (TFIIH) basic transcription factor. *Science* **260**:58, 1993.
103. Henning KA, Li L, Lyer N, McDaniel LD, Reagan MS, Legerski R, Schultz RA, Stefanini M, Lehmann AR, Mayne LV, Friedberg EC: The Cockayne syndrome group A gene encodes a WD repeat protein that interacts with CBS protein and a subunit of RNA polymerase II TFIIH. *Cell* **82**:555, 1995.
104. Fujiwara Y, Higashikawa T, Tatsumi M: A retarded rate of DNA replication and normal level of DNA repair in Werner's syndrome fibroblast cultures. *J Cell Physiol* **92**:365, 1977.
105. Higashikawa T, Fujiwara Y: Normal level of unscheduled DNA synthesis in Werner's syndrome fibroblasts in culture. *Exp Cell Res* **113**:438, 1978.
106. Stefanini M, Scappaticci S, Lagomarsini P, Borroni G, Berardesca E, Nuzzo F: Chromosome instability in lymphocytes from a patient with

Werner's syndrome is not associated with DNA repair defects. *Mutat Res* **219**:179, 1989.
107. Saito H, Moses RE: Immortalization of Werner syndrome and progeria fibroblasts. *Exp Cell Res* **192**:373, 1991.
108. Arlett CF, Harcourt SA: Survey of radiosensitivity in a variety of human cell strains. *Cancer Res* **40**:926, 1980.
109. Gebhart E, Schnizel M, Ruprecht KW: Cytogenetic studies using various clastogens in two patients with Werner syndrome and control individuals. *Hum Genet* **70**:324, 1985.
110. Gebhart E, Bauer R, Raub U, Schinzel M, Ruprecht KW, Jonas JB: Spontaneous and induced chromosomal instability in Werner syndrome. *Hum Genet* **80**:135, 1988.
111. Okada M, Goto M, Furuichi Y, Sugimoto M: Differential effects of cytotoxic drugs on mortal and immortalized B-lymphoblastoid cell lines from normal and Werner's syndrome patients. *Biol Pharm Bull* **21**:235, 1998.
112. Elli R, Chessa L, Antonelli A, Petrinelli P, Ambra R, Marcucci L: Effects of topoisomerase II inhibition in lymphoblasts from patients with progeroid and "chromosome instability" syndromes. *Cancer Genet Cytogenet* **87**:112, 1996.
113. Ogburn CE, Oshima J, Poot M, Chen R, Hunt KE, Gollahon KA, Rabinovitch PS, Martin GM: An apoptosis-inducing genotoxin differentiates heterozygotic carriers from Werner helicase mutations from wild-type and homozygous mutants. *Hum Genet* **101**:12, 1997.
114. Bennett SE, Umar A, Oshima J, Monnat RJ, Kunkel TA: Mismatch repair in extracts of Werner syndrome cell lines. *Cancer Res* **57**:2956, 1997.
115. Brooks-Wilson AR, Emond MJ, Monnat RJ: Unexpectedly low loss of heterozygosity in genetically unstable Werner syndrome cell lines. *Genes Chrom Cancer* **18**:133, 1997.
116. Melaragno MI, Pagni D, Smith MDC: Cytogenetic aspects of Werner's syndrome lymphocyte cultures. *Mech Age Dev* **78**:117, 1995.
117. Gawkrodger DJ, Priestley GC, Vijayalamix, Ross JA, Narcisi P, Hunter JAA: Werner's syndrome. *Arch Dermatol* **121**:636, 1985.
118. Takeuchi F, Hanaoka F, Goto M, Akaoka I, Hori T, Yamada M, Miyamoto T: Altered frequency of initiation sites of DNA replication in Werner's syndrome cells. *Hum Genet* **60**:365, 1982.
119. Hanaoka F, Takeuchi F, Matsumura T, Goto M, Miyamoto T, Tamada M: Decrease in the average size of replicons in a Werner syndrome cell line by a simian virus 40 infection. *Exp Cell Res* **144**:463, 1983.
120. Poot M, Hoehn H, Runger TM, Martin GM: Impaired S-phase transit of Werner syndrome cells expressed in lymphoblastoid cell lines. *Exp Cell Res* **202**:267, 1992.
121. Runger TM, Sobotta P, Dekant B, Moller K, Bauer C, Kraemer KH: *In vivo* assessment of DNA ligation efficiency and fidelity in cells from patients with Franconi's anemia and other cancer-prone hereditary disorders. *Toxicol Lett* **67**:309, 1993.
122. Runger TM, Bauer C, Dekant B, Moller K, Sobotta P, Czemy C, Poot M, Martin GM: Hypermutable ligation of plasmid DNA ends in cells from patients with Werner syndrome. *J Invest Dermatol* **102**:45, 1994.
123. Cheng RZ, Murano S, Kurz B, Shmookler Reis RJS: Homologous recombination is elevated in some Werner-like syndromes but not during normal or *in vitro* senescence of mammalian cells. *Mutat Res* **237**:259, 1990.
124. Watt PM, Hickson ID, Borts RH, Louis EJ: SGS1, a homologue of the Bloom's and Werner's syndrome genes, is required for maintenance of genome stability in *Saccharomyces cerevisiae*. *Genetics* **144**:935, 1996.
125. Yamagata K, Kato J, Shimamoto A, Goto M, Furuichi Y, Ikeda H: Bloom's and Werner's syndrome genes suppress hyperrecombination in yeast sgs1 mutant: Implication for genomic instability in human diseases. *Proc Natl Acad Sci USA* **95**:8733, 1998.
126. Yan H, Chen C.-Y, Kobayashi R, Newport J: Replication focus-forming activity 1 and the Werner syndrome gene product. *Nature Genet* **19**:375, 1998.
127. Adoue DPF: Werner's syndrome. *N Engl J Med* **337**:977, 1997.

CHAPTER 34

Peutz-Jeghers Syndrome

Lauri A. Aaltonen

1. **The typical features of Peutz-Jeghers syndrome (PJS) are mucocutaneous melanin pigmentation and gastrointestinal polyposis.**
2. **Peutz-Jeghers polyps are hamartomas characterized by a stromal tree-like pattern of smooth muscle tissue.**
3. **PJS patients are predisposed to cancer. An excess of gastrointestinal as well as extraintestinal cancers has been reported in PJS families. The cancer predisposition is less focused than in many other cancer-susceptibility syndromes.**
4. **The major predisposing gene is *LKB1*. *LKB1* mutations are found in most but not all PJS patients. At present it is unclear whether more predisposing loci exist.**
5. **LKB1 is a serine/threonine kinase, but detailed information on its function is at present not available. The germ-line mutations associated with tumorigenesis are usually of an inactivating nature, suggesting a role as a tumor suppressor.**

The syndrome is named after Peutz and Jeghers, the discoverers of the disease. The first report was by Peutz in 1921,[1] followed by work by Jeghers et al. in 1949.[2] The major hallmarks of Peutz-Jeghers syndrome (PJS) are mucocutaneous melanin pigmentation and intestinal hamartomatous polyposis.[3] PJS patients appear to be at increased risk of cancer (Table 34-1). Especially malignant tumors of the gastrointestinal tract, breast, uterine cervix, and ovary may be associated with the disease.[4–6] Benign ovarian (such as granulosa cell tumor, sex cord tumor with annular tubules) and testicular (Sertoli cell tumor) lesions are relatively frequently found in PJS.[3] Since PJS is a rare disorder, considerably more rare than, for example, familial adenomatous polyposis, it has been difficult to evaluate the cancer spectrum and risk levels typical for PJS. Giardiello et al.[4] reported an 18-fold lifetime risk of malignancy in PJS. Boardman et al.[5] reported a similar relative risk for women, but in their study the risk for men was only 6.2. Gastrointestinal cancer and gynecologic malignancies in particular, as well as breast cancer, were associated with PJS in this study.

Germ-line mutations in a serine/threonine kinase gene *LKB1* (also called *STK11*) located on chromosome 19p 13.3 recently have been shown to underlie a major proportion of PJS cases.[7] *LKB1* is believed to act as a tumor suppressor gene,[7,8] and detailed functional analyses are underway to evaluate the role and partners of LKB1 in cell growth control and development.

CLINICAL ASPECTS

Incidence

The incidence of the PJS is difficult to evaluate, since even in countries with a nationwide adenomatous polyposis registry little attention has been paid to hamartomatous polyposis syndromes, and careful registration and evaluation of this group of patients have not been performed. Based on the experience of polyposis registries, PJS is clearly more rare than familial adenomatous polyposis, which is believed to be the most common polyposis syndrome, with a carrier frequency of 1 in 5000 to 10,000 live births.[3] A frequency of 1 in 8300 to 1 in 29,000 live births has been estimated.[9] The relatively frequent complications due to bowel obstruction today can be adequately treated surgically. Thus the syndrome is likely to have a smaller impact on biologic fitness now than some decades ago.

Since the molecular background of the PJS has been revealed recently, it is likely that more attention will be focused on PJS, and more light may be shed on the issue of its incidence. Molecular analyses also may reveal cases that do not fulfill the present diagnostic criteria. One difficulty is that although PJS is considered an autosomal dominant disease, patients frequently lack a PJS family history. Future molecular analyses should reveal the background of such patients, but initial results suggest that germ-line *LKB1* defects also play a role in "sporadic" PJS.[10] Interestingly, *de novo* mutations appear to be frequent in PJS patients without a family history.[11] This may reflect the improved biologic fitness of PJS patients, and PJS in the future may be somewhat more common through this effect.

Diagnostic Criteria and Histologic Features

PJS has two clinical hallmarks: mucocutaneous melanin pigmentation and hamartomatous intestinal polyposis. The pigmentation is most often present in and around the mouth but also on hands and feet and axillary pits.[3] The significance of the pigmentation as a key feature of the syndrome is clear, but the presence of similar melanin spots in up to 15 percent of the normal population hampers the use of this sign in clinical practice.[12] The degree of

Table 34-1 Cancer Cases Reported in Patients with Peutz-Jeghers Syndrome.

Gastrointestinal	
Esophagus	1
Stomach	16
Small intestine	22
Large intestine	26
Pancreas	8
Extraintestinal	
Breast	17
Uterine cervix	10
Ovary	7
Uterus	2
Fallopian tube	1
Testis	1
Prostate	1
Lung	9
Thyroid	2
Leiomyosarcoma	2
Gall bladder	1
Liver	1
Basal cell	1
Osteosarcoma	1
Multiple myeloma	1

SOURCE: Data from Hemminki[6,7] and Boardman et al.[5]

A list of standard abbreviations is located immediately preceding the index in each volume. Nonstandard abbreviations used in this chapter include: PJS = Peutz-Jeghers syndrome; LOH = loss of heterozygosity.

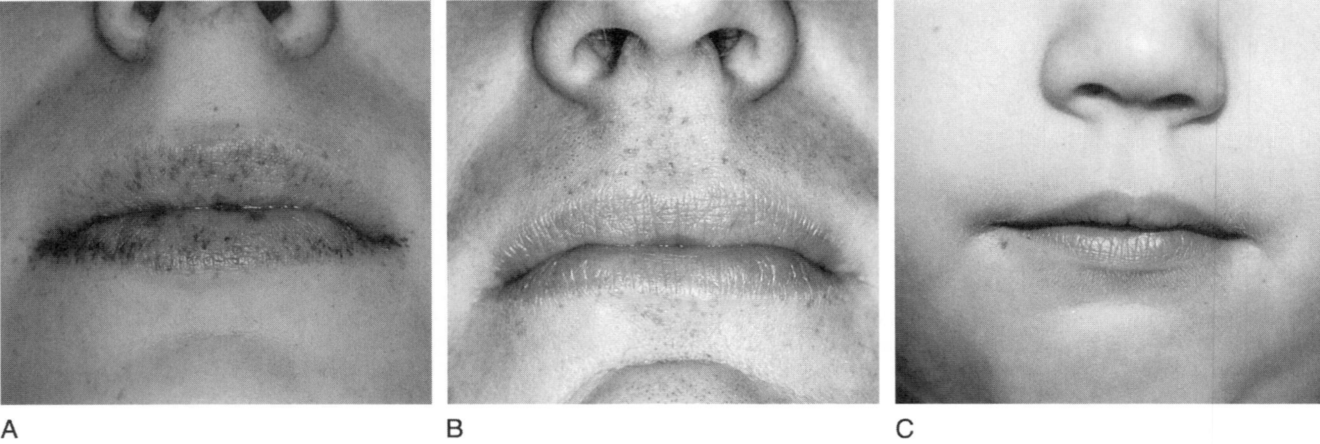

Fig. 34-1 *A.* Typical perioral pigmentation in a Peutz-Jeghers patient. *B, C.* Perioral pigmentation in a 31-year-old patient (B) and his 6-year-old daughter (*C*) illustrates the variation in pigmentation even within a family and the difficulty in relying on pigmentation in PJS diagnostics.

pigmentation varies greatly, even within a family (Fig. 34-1). In a subset of the PJS patients the pigmentation diminishes with age, and some never display it.

The presence of intestinal Peutz-Jeghers polyposis is the diagnostic feature of PJS. Peutz-Jeghers polyps are hamartomatous lesions that have pathognomonic histologic characteristics (Fig. 34-2). In contrast to juvenile polyps, for example, Peutz-Jeghers polyps display a core of a prominent tree-like smooth muscle cell structure that extends into the lamina propria. The overlying folded epithelium contains histologically normal cells without features of neoplasia.[3] The number of polyps in PJS is low as compared with familial adenomatous polyposis and varies greatly from zero to dozens of lesions. A single Peutz-Jeghers polyp without a PJS family history or other features of the syndrome may well be a sporadic lesion. Although the polyps may occur anywhere in the gastrointestinal tract, the small intestine is the most commonly affected part of the bowel. PJS patients commonly also display hyperplastic and adenomatous polyps, but the diagnosis is based on the pathognomonic histology of Peutz-Jeghers polyps. Neoplastic changes sometimes may arise in the Peutz-Jeghers polyps themselves.[13–15]

While it is clear that pigmentation without any other signs of the syndrome is not a good indicator of PJS (see Fig. 34-1) and that, similarily, one Peutz-Jeghers polyp without family history of PJS may be a sporadic lesion, it is less clear how one should evaluate the family members of diagnosed PJS patients. A recent study that identified a locus predisposing to PJS suggested that all individuals carrying the affected haplotype had one of the two cardinal features of PJS.[8] This was slightly unexpected, since PJS-like pigmentation is not rare in the normal population,[12] and many of the relatives displaying pigmentation did not display a prominent polyposis.[8] This emphasizes that pigmentation as evaluated by an experienced physician is a useful clue, but nevertheless, pigmentation as the only sign should be interpreted with caution.

The ultimate diagnostic laboratory test is the detection of a *LKB1* germ-line mutation.[7] The mutations are usually truncating, which facilitates interpretation of the results. When a mutation in a particular family has been detected, the relatives who are willing to undergo genetic testing can be analyzed with reasonable efficiency.

Differential Diagnosis

The different polyposis syndromes have overlapping clinical features. Polyps of mixed histologic subtypes (e.g., adenoma, hyperplastic polyp, hamartoma) are seen relatively commonly in PJS patients, and careful histologic evaluation of the removed lesions is essential. The striking phenotype of familial adenomatous polyposis with typically hundreds or thousands of adenomas is usually easily distinguishable from the other polyposis syndromes including PJS. The two other major hamartomatous polyposis syndromes, Cowden syndrome and juvenile polyposis, are more difficult in this regard. Detection of multiple lesions displaying the pathognomonic polyp core with arborizing smooth muscle pattern forms the basis of the PJS diagnosis. It is still to be determined which number of polyps should be considered

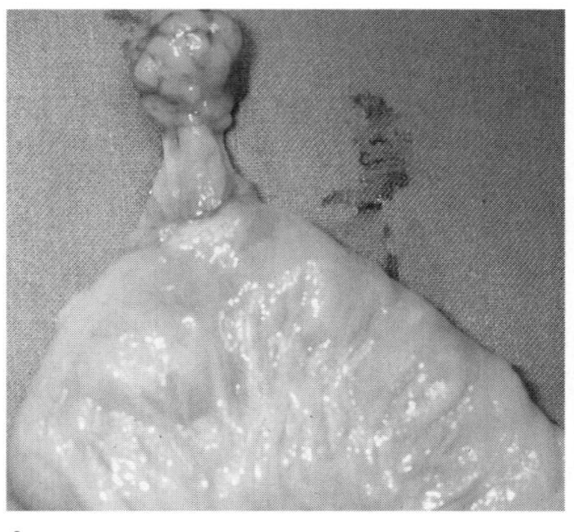

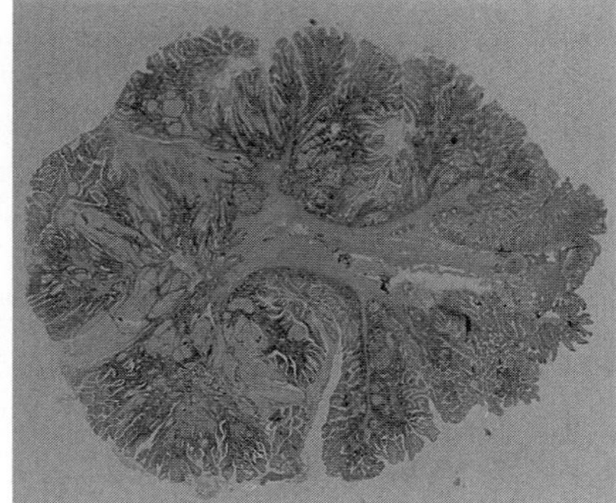

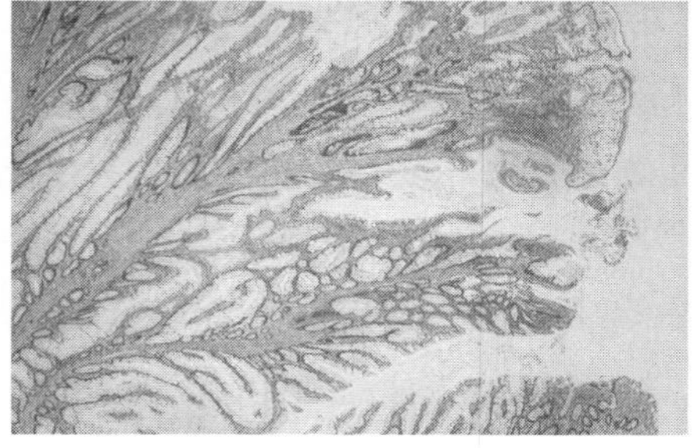

A B C

Fig. 34-2 *A.* A hamartomatous Peutz-Jeghers polyp. *B.* Histologic view of the lesion. *C.* Microscopical view. Note the smooth muscle cell core of the polyp.

suggestive of PJS. The required number also depends on the presence or absence of a family history of PJS. In a patient without any evidence of PJS with one Peutz-Jeghers polyp the finding may well be sporadic. However, if the patient has a family history of PJS, PJS is likely.

GENETIC LOCI

Loci for Hereditary PJS

Few genetic loci have been implicated in PJS. A study by Amos et al.[16] found evidence for linkage on chromosome 1 in a large U.S. kindred, but further genotyping analyses did not support the finding (Amos, personal communication). In 1997, Hemminki et al.[8] used a novel approach to reveal a predisposing locus. Malignant tumors often display multiple genetic alterations that tend to occur during tumor development and in part drive the process. Benign tumors, such as hamartomatous polyps, are likely to harbor many fewer molecular changes. It was hypothesized that by studying multiple polyps from a single Peutz-Jeghers patient, genetic loci associated with early development of these lesions might be revealed. Indeed, the short arm of chromosome 19 appeared to be deleted in some of the polyps. This result was confirmed by microdissection and polymerase chain reaction (PCR) assays; loss of heterozygosity (LOH) experiments using 19p microsatellite markers demonstrated the loss of the wild-type (maternal) chromosome in a subset of the polyp cells. The same markers were used for genetic linkage analysis in a collection of twelve PJS families, and conclusive evidence of linkage was obtained. These experiments showed that a PJS susceptibility gene that is likely to have a tumor suppressor function resided in 19p.[8]

However, not all families display 19p linkage. A small subset of the families has been demonstrated to be incompatible with linkage to 19p,[17] and in one PJS family, evidence of linkage to chromosome 19q has been reported.[18]

Sporadic Tumors and Chromosome 19p

The PJS locus on 19p is not one of the most common targets of chromosomal deletions during sporadic tumor progression. In some tumor types, such as adenoma malignum of the uterine cervix, pancreatic cancer, and chronic myelocytic leukemia, 19p deletions appear to be relatively common.[19–21] Interestingly, adenoma malignum is a rare tumor that appears to be associated with PJS.[6] Avizienyte et al.[22] detected LOH at D19S886 in 13 of 50 (26 percent) colorectal carcinomas. A recent paper by Dong et al.[23] reported LOH at the locus D19S886 and/or D19S883 in 10 of 19 (53 percent) colorectal cancers, but no LOH in 25 informative colorectal adenomas.

MUTATIONS OF SERINE/THREONINE KINASE GENE *LKB1* UNDERLIE PJS

The gene for PJS was identified through positional cloning.[7] The effort was greatly facilitated by the fact that the target area in chromosome 19p determined by linkage results was covered by a physical map.[24] Researchers working at and in collaboration with the Lawrence Livermore National Laboratory had constructed a cosmid contig that soon spanned across the whole region of interest.

After mapping the PJS locus through comparative genomic hybridization[25] and targeted linkage analysis, Hemminki et al.[7] first reduced the target area by creating novel polymorphic microsatellite and biallelic markers and analyzing the families displaying critical recombinations. In this way the area was reduced to 800 kb. Genes and expressed sequence tags that mapped to the region of interest were analyzed for mutations in PJS families using reverse-transcriptase (RT) PCR and sequencing. Since these efforts produced only negative findings, the researchers performed direct cDNA selection experiments to derive novel transcripts that map to the area. Multiple candidate sequences were isolated from this gene-rich area. One of these represented the *LKB1* gene, a previously cloned gene that had not been mapped to a chromosomal locus. The full-length *LKB1* cDNA had been reported in 1996 as a Gen Bank submission by Dr. Nezu.[26]

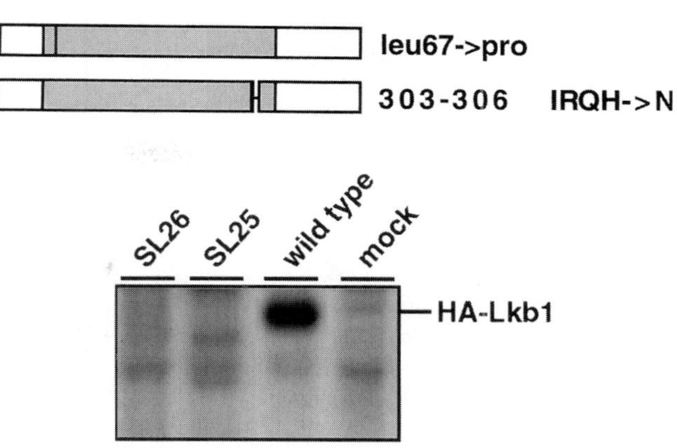

Fig. 34-3 Functional analysis of LKB1 kinase activity. *A.* The mutations in SL25 (missense change, leu67 → pro) and SL 26 (in-frame deletion of 9 bases, 303–306 IRQH → N), respectively. The kinase domain is shown in red. *B.* The results of an autophosphorylation assay. While the wild-type LKB1 is capable of autophosphorylation, the missense mutation in SL25 and the in-frame deletion of 9 bp in SL26 have resulted in a protein that displays no kinase activity.

Mutation analysis of the *LKB1* cDNA soon revealed multiple truncating mutations in PJS patients. Eleven of the 12 patients used in the PJS gene search displayed a mutation. The changes segregated with the disease phenotype and were absent in multiple control individuals.[7] Subsequent work has shown that approximately 60 percent of unselected PJS patients display *LKB1* mutations.[10,12] The difference is likely due to patient selection; the samples used in the initial mutation screen were derived from scrutinized 19p-linked PJS families.

LKB1 encodes a 432-amino-acid protein that through sequence homology was predicted to act as a serine/threonine kinase. The gene appears to be ubiquitously expressed, with especially prominent expression in the pancreas and testis.[7] Mutations in kinase genes had been described in association with hereditary cancer earlier, but this was the first time that inactivating mutations in such a gene were reported. The detailed function of LKB1 remains to be clarified. The gene has no human homologues but is highly homologuous to a *Xenopus* cytoplasmic serine/threonine kinase *XEEK1*.[27] XEEK1 is expressed only during the very first days of embryonic life and may be involved in early development. XEEK1 is capable of autophosphorylation. Recent work has demonstrated that the same is also true for LKB1[10] (Fig. 34-3). It is likely that autophosphorylation is not the main function of the gene, and yeast double-hybrid experiments and other assays should provide further data on how LKB1 is involved in cell growth regulation and which proteins are its substrates and upstream effectors.

Somatic Mutations in *LKB1*

Bignell et al.[28] reported absence of mutations in sporadic breast cancers. Avizienyte et al.[22] studied a set of colonic, testicular, cervical, and lung cancers, as well as sarcomas and myeloma and melanoma cell lines. One missense mutation was found in a testicular cancer as well as in a lung cancer, and one mutation leading to frameshift and truncating protein product was detected in an adenocarcinoma of the uterine cervix (unpublished data). Subsequently, the missense mutation detected in a testicular cancer was shown to in part but not completely abolish the kinase function of the LKB1 protein.[10] Tomlinson et al.[29] reported the absence of *LKB1* mutations in colorectal and ovarian cancers. In contrast to the results of Avizienyte et al. and Tomlinson et al., Dong et al.[23] reported frequent mutations in Korean distal colorectal tumors. This finding is somewhat surprising because previous studies had failed to detect any mutations in colorectal cancers, and germ-line mutations of *LKB1* are usually truncating.[7,12] Park et al.[30] found little evidence of *LKB1* involvement in gastric carcinomas; only 1 of 23 samples displayed a missense mutation. Two of the 23 tumors were reported to display somatic nucleotide changes that did not lead to amino acid substitutions.

To summarize, most reports thus far have found little evidence of somatic mutational inactivation of *LKB1,* although clearly in a few tumor cases somatic inactivation of *LKB1* has been seen. It remains to be clarified whether *LKB1* indeed plays a significant role in sporadic colorectal tumorigenesis. Whether *LKB1* inactivation through epigenetic events such as methylation plays a role in sporadic cancers needs to be clarified. Also, *LKB1* mutations may play a more prominent role in tumor types that have not yet been examined.

Animal Models

Animal models for PJS are not yet available, but multiple research groups are at present working toward a mouse model. *Xenopus Xeek1* mutants also could serve as a model organism. Since the *Xenopus LKB1* homologue *Xeek1* is expressed in early embryos, and since the knockout mice for the other hamartomatous polyposis genes *PTEN*[31] and *Smad4/DPC4*[32] failed to develop, a conditional knockout mouse might serve research better than a conventional knockout animal. The animal models are expected to reveal data on LKB1 function in development as well as tumorigenesis.

IMPLICATIONS FOR DIAGNOSIS

The discoveries on the molecular background of PJS will allow identification of at-risk individuals in a subset of the families. Predictive testing always should be associated with appropriate genetic counseling, and testing should be performed only after obtaining informed consent.

First, the genetic defect in a particular family should be detected through *LKB1* germ-line analysis of a typically affected patient.[7] Since *LKB1* is a relatively small gene, genomic sequencing of the nine coding exons[28] consisting of 1299 nucleotides is recommended. Since no mutation analysis technique is complete, and since locus heterogeneity still is a possibility in PJS, a negative mutation analysis result gives little information. Since the current mutation detection rate in PJS patients in whom no linkage information is available is not much more than 50 percent,[10] the option that the analyses will not reveal a mutation should be explained carefully to the patient before a sample is derived and analyzed. This issue is different, of course, in families segregating a characterized mutation, where unambiguous results can be obtained.

Unlike in Bannayan-Riley-Ruvalcaba syndrome,[33] PJS patients without a family history of the disease often have a *LKB1* germ-line defect, and thus these patients and their relatives also may benefit from molecular analyses.

Most *LKB1* defects appear to be truncating, and interpretation of the mutation analysis result is not problematic in such cases. However, a subset of the changes consists of small in-frame deletions or missense mutations. The autophosphorylation function of LKB1 may in the future provide clues to the functional significance of such *LKB1* variants.[10] If an allele encoded by a particular mutation displays a defect in the autophosphorylation assay, it is likely to be pathogenic. A result indicating normal kinase function would be difficult to interprete, since other functions of LKB1 are not known.

IMPLICATIONS FOR TREATMENT

Accurate diagnosis of PJS is important in view of cancer prevention. The at-risk individuals appear to need surveillance for at least gastrointestinal and gynecologic tumors, as well as breast cancer. The unraveling of the molecular background of the various hamartomatous syndromes may well contribute to the management of patients in the future. Ideally, the molecular analyses could clarify the particular predisposing defect in a patient, and tumor prevention measures could be targeted to the sites at greatest risk. Considering the complex and overlapping clinical features of the hamartomatous polyposis syndromes, molecular methods for exact diagnosis and evaluation of tumor risk would be welcome. However, molecular epidemiologic studies should first characterize the cancer risks associated with the different genetic defects. Owing to the rarity of the syndromes, this can be achieved only through collaborative efforts.

The ultimate goal of the molecular research conducted is to prevent tumors in susceptible individuals through clarifying the exact mechanisms of tumor predisposition.

ACKNOWLEDGMENTS

Drs. Särvinen, Salovaara, and Ylikorkala are acknowledged for providing the figures.

REFERENCES

1. Peutz JL: A very remarkable case of familial polyposis of mucous membrane of intestinal tract and accompanied by peculiar pigmentations of skin and mucous membrane. (in Dutch). *Ned Tijdschr Geneeskd* **10**:134, 1921.
2. Jeghers H, McKusick VA, Katz KH: Generalized intestinal polyposis and melanin spots of the oral mucosa, lips and digits. *N Engl J Med* **241**:992, 1949.
3. Phillips RKS, Spigelman AD, Thomson JPS: *Familial Adenomatous Polyposis and Other Polyposis Syndromes*. London, Edward Arnold, 1994.
4. Giardiello FM, Welsh SB, Hamilton SR, Offerhaus GJ, Gittelsohn AM, Booker SV, Krush AJ, Yardley JH, Luk GD: Increased risk of cancer in the Peutz-Jeghers syndrome. *New Engl J Med* **316**:1511, 1987.
5. Boardman LA, Thibodeau SN, Schaid DJ, Lindor NM, McDonnell SK, Burgart LJ, Ahlquist Da, Podratz KC, Pittelkow M, Hartmann LC: Increased risk for cancer in patients with the Peutz-Jeghers syndrome. *Ann Intern Med* **128**:896, 1998.
6. Hemminki A: Inherited predisposition to gastrointestinal cancer: The molecular backgrounds of Peutz-Jeghers syndrome and hereditary nonpolyposis colorectal cancer. Academic dissertation, University of Helsinki, 1998.
7. Hemminki A, Markie D, Tomlinson I, Avizienyte E, Roth S, Loukola A, Bignell G, Warren W, Aminoff M, Höglund P, Järvinen H, Kristo P, Pelin K, Ridanpää M, Salovaara R, Toro T, Bodmer W, Olschwang S, Olsen AS, Stratton Mr, de la Chapelle A, Aaltonen lA:A serine/threonine kinase gene defective in Peutz-Jeghers syndrome. *Nature* **391**:184, 1998.
8. Hemminki A, Tomlinson I, Markie D, Järvinen H, Sistonen P, Björkqvist A-M, Knuutila S, Salovaara R, Bodmer W, Shibata D, de la Chapelle A, Aaltonen LA: Localization of a susceptibility locus for Peutz-Jeghers syndrome to 19p using comparative genomic hybridization and targeted linkage analysis. *Nature Genet* **15**:87, 1997.
9. Finan MC, Ray MK: Gastrointestinal polyposis syndromes. *Dermatol Clin* **7**:419, 1989.
10. Ylikorkala A, Avizienyte E, Tomlinson IPM, Tiainen M, Roth S, Loukola A, Hemminki A, Johansson M, Sistonen P, Markie D, Neale K, Phillips R, Zauber P, Twama T, Sampson J, Järvinen H, Mäkelä TP, Aaltonen La: Mutations and impaired function of LKB1 in familial and non-familial Peutz-Jeghers syndrome and a sporadic testicular cancer. *Hum Mol Genet* **8**:45, 1999.
11. Westerman AM, Entius MM, Boor PP, Koole R, de Baar E, Offerhaus GJ, Lubinski J, Lindhout D, Halley DJ, de Rooij FW, Wilson JH: Novel Mutations in the LKB1/STK11 gene in Dutch Peutz-Jeghers families. *Hum Mutat* **13**:476, 1999.
12. Westerman AM, Chong YK, Entius MM, Wilson JHP, van Velthuysen, Lindhout D, Offerhaus GJA: The diagnostic value of mucocutaneous

pigmentations in Peutz-Jeghers Syndrome. Abstract book, first joint meeting, ICG-HNPCC & LCPG, 1997, p 23.

13. Hizawa K, Iida M, Matsumoto T, Kohrogi N, Yao T, Fujishima M: Neoplastic transformation arising in Peutz-Jeghers polyposis. *Dis Colon Rectum* **36**:953, 1993.
14. De Facq L, De Sutter J, De Man M, Van der Spek P, Lepoutre L: A case of Peutz-Jeghers syndrome with nasal polyposis, extreme iron deficiency anemia, and hamartoma-adenoma transformation: Management by combined surgical and endoscopic approach. *Am J Gastroenterol* **90**:1330, 1995.
15. Defago MR, Higa AL, Campra JL, Paradelo M, Uehara A, Torres Mazzucchi MH, Videla R: Carcinoma in situ arising in a gastric hamartomatous polyp in a patient with Peutz-Jeghers syndrome. *Endoscopy* **28**:267, 1996.
16. Bali D, Gourley IS, McGarrity TJ, Spencer CA, Howard L, Frazier ML, Lynch PM, Seldin MF, Amos CI: Peutz-Jeghers syndrome maps to chromosome 1p. In American Society of Human Genetics, abstract 1067, 1995.
17. Olschwang S, Markie D, Seal S, Neale K, Phillips R, Cottrell S, Ellis I, Hodgson S, Zauber P, Spigelman A, Iwama T, Loff S, McKeown C, Marchese C, Sampson J, Davies S, Talbot I, Wyke J, Thomas G, Bodmer W, Hemminki A, Avizienyte E, de la Chapelle A, Aaltonen LA, Stratton M, Houlston R, Tomlinson I: Peutz-Jeghers disease: Most families compatible with linkage to 19p13.3, but evidence for a second locus at a different site. *J Med Genet* **35**:42, 1997.
18. Mehenni H, Blouin J-L, Radhakrishna U, Bhardwaj SS, Bhardwaj K, Dixit VB, Richards KF, Bermejo-Fenoll A, Leal AS, Raval RC, Antonarakis SE: Peutz-Jeghers syndrome: Confirmation of linkage to chromosome 19p13.3 and identification of a potential second locus, on 19q13.4. *Am J Hum Genet* **61**:1327, 1997.
19. Lee JY, Dong SM, Kim HS, Kim HS, Kim SY, Na EY, Shin MS, Lee SH, Park WS, Kim KM, Lee YS, Jang JJ, Yoo NJ: A distinct region of chromosome 19p13.3 associated with the sporadic form of adenoma malignum of the uterine cervix. *Cancer Res* **58**:1140, 1998.
20. Hoglund M, Gorunova L, Andren-Sandberg A, Dawiskiba S, Mitelman F, Johansson B: Cytogenetic and fluorescence in situ hybridization analyses of chromosome 19 aberrations in pancreatic carcinomas: Frequent loss of 19p13.3 and gain of 19q13.1-13.2. *Genes Chromosomes Cancer* **21**:8, 1998.
21. Mori N, Morosetti R, Lee S, Spira S, Ben-Yehuda D, Schiller G, Landolfi R, Mizoguchi H, Koeffler HP: Allelotype analysis in the evolution of chronic myelocytic leukemia. *Blood* **90**:2010, 1997.
22. Avizienyte E, Roth S, Loukola A, Hemminki A, Lothe RA, Stenwig AE, Fosså SD, Salovaara R, Aaltonen LA: Somatic mutations in LKB1 are rare in sporadic colorectal and testicular tumors. *Cancer Res* **58**:2087, 1998.
23. Dong SM, Kim KM, Kim SY, Shin MS, Na EY, Lee SH, Park WS, Yoo NJ, Jang JJ, Yoon CY, Kim JW, Kim SY, Yang YM, Kim SH, Kim CS, Lee JY: Frequent somatic mutations in serine threonine kinase 11/Peutz-Jeghers syndrome gene in left-sided colon cancer. *Cancer Res* **58**:3787, 1998.
24. Ashworth LK: An integrated metric physical map of human chromosome 19. *Nature Genet* **11**:422, 1995.
25. Kallioniemi A, Kallioniemi O-P, Sudar D, Rutovitz D, Gray JW, Waldman F, Pinkel D: Comparative genomic hybridization for molecular cytogenetic analysis of solid tumors. *Science* **258**:818, 1992.
26. Nezu J: Molecular cloning of a novel serine/threonine protein kinase expressed in human fetal liver (direct submission to GenBank). In http:// *www.ncbi.nlm.nih.gov/irx/cgi-bin/birx_doc?genbank+65606,* 1996.
27. Su J-Y, Erikson E, Maller JL: Cloning and characterization of a novel serine/threonine protein kinase expressed in early *Xenopus* embryos. *J Biol Chem* **271**:14430, 1996.
28. Bignell GR, Barfoot R, Seal S, Collins N, Warren W, Stratton MR: Low frequency of somatic mutations in the LKB1/Peutz-Jeghers syndrome gene in sporadic breast cancer. *Cancer Res* **58**:1384, 1998.
29. Wang ZJ, Taylor F, Churchman M, Norbury G, Tomlinson I: Genetic pathways of colorectal carcinogenesis rarely involve the PTEN and LKB1 genes outside the inherited hamartoma syndromes. *Am J Pathol* **153**:363, 1998.
30. Park WS, Moon YW, Yang YM, Kim YS, Kim YD, Fuller BG, Vortmeyer AO, Fogt F, Lubensky IA, Zhuang Z: Mutations of the STK11 gene in sporadic gastric carcinoma. *Int J Oncol* **13**:601, 1998.
31. Di Cristofano A, Pesce B, Cordon-Cardo C, Pandolfi PP: Pten is essential for embryonic development and tumor suppression. *Nature Genet* **19**:348, 1997.
32. Takaku K, Oshima M, Miyoshi H, Matsui M, Seldin MF, Taketo MM: Intestinal tumorigenesis in compound mutant mice of both Dpc4 (Smad4) and Apc genes. *Cell* **92**:645, 1998.
33. Carethers JM, Furnari FB, Zigman AF, Lavine JE, Jones MC, Graham GE, Teebi AS, Huang HJ, Ha HT, Chauhan DP, Chang CL, Cavenee WK, Boland CR: Absence of PTEN/MMAC1 germ-line mutations in sporadic Bannayan-Riley-Ruvalcaba syndrome. *Cancer Res* **58**:2724, 1998.

CHAPTER 35

Juvenile Polyposis Syndrome

James R. Howe

1. **Juvenile polyposis (JP) is an autosomal dominant syndrome characterized by multiple hamartomatous polyps of the gastrointestinal (GI) tract. Patients may have juvenile polyps of the stomach, small intestine, and/or colon. The diagnosis of JP is made by having more than five juvenile polyps in the colon, juvenile polyps throughout the GI tract, or one or more juvenile polyps in the setting of a family history of JP. Patients with other genetically distinct syndromes may also have hamartomatous polyps, and these conditions need to be excluded by careful history and physical examination. Due to the association of juvenile polyps with several heterogeneous syndromes, it is likely that there are multiple genes that predispose to JP.**
2. **Approximately 20 to 50 percent of JP cases are familial, with the remainder arising *de novo.* As many as 20 percent of patients may have associated anomalies, which are more common in sporadic cases. Patients with JP are at approximately 50 percent risk for the developing GI cancers, the majority of which are colorectal cancers, but they are also at risk for upper GI cancers.**
3. **The pathologic features of juvenile polyps are dilated, cystic glands, infiltration of the lamina propria by inflammatory cells, and an overabundance of stroma. Larger polyps may also contain adenomatous areas; adenocarcinoma has also been described within juvenile polyps. Although the exact mechanism of carcinogenesis is unclear, it has been suggested that the changes seen in the lamina propria are brought about through *landscaper defects,* where changes in this tissue layer lead to an environment predisposing to neoplastic transformation of the overlying epithelium.**
4. **Loss of heterozygosity studies have revealed a tumor-suppressor locus for JP on chromosome 10q22, with the minimal region of overlap defining a 3-cM region approximately 7 cM centromeric to the *PTEN* gene. Germ line *PTEN* mutations have been described in four unrelated patients with JP, but it is possible that some of these patients had Cowden syndrome.**
5. **A gene for JP has been mapped to chromosome 18q21.1 by genetic linkage analysis, within an interval containing the two tumor-suppressor genes *DCC* and *DPC4 (Smad4).* Germ line mutations in one of these genes, *Smad4,* have been found in 6 of 10 familial and sporadic JP patients. In familial cases, these mutations segregated with the JP phenotype, and all were predicted to cause truncation of the Smad4 protein, resulting in loss of its C-terminus required for oligomerization.**
6. **The *Smad4* gene consists of 11 exons and encodes for 552 amino acids. Smad4 is a common mediator for the transforming growth factor-β, activin, and bone morphogenetic protein signaling pathways. The Smad4 protein associates with other Smad proteins following their phosphorylation by activated receptors, then translocates to the nucleus where it regulates transcription through direct binding to specific DNA sequences. Smad4 is required for differentiation of the mesoderm and visceral endoderm during embryogenesis; transgenic mice with *Smad4* and *Apc* mutations have polyps with stromal proliferation reminiscent of juvenile polyps.**

HISTORY

The first clearly documented juvenile polyp was reported by Diamond in 1939, in a 30-month-old girl with a prolapsing polyp of the rectum. Although Diamond described the polyp as an adenoma, photomicrographs show a juvenile polyp.[1] Helwig gave an excellent pathologic description of juvenile polyps in 1946, and differentiated these "adenomas" in children from those of adults by their showing "foci in which the glandular structures are embedded in a stroma of cellular connective tissue infiltrated with inflammatory cells".[2] Ravitch reported an 18-month-old male who died postoperatively after exploration for an intussusception, and who, at autopsy, was found to have adenomatous polyps from stomach to anus.[3] Review of these photomicrographs reveals that this patient actually had generalized juvenile polyposis. Juvenile polyps later became known as a distinct form of colonic polyps through the work of Horilleno, Eckert, and Ackerman in 1957,[4] and Morson in 1962.[5] McColl and associates coined the term *juvenile polyposis coli* in 1964, to differentiate patients with multiple juvenile polyps from those with either adenomatous polyposis or solitary juvenile polyps.[6] Smilow, Pryor, and Swinton described a clear familial pattern of JP in a three-generation kindred in 1966. They hypothesized an autosomal dominant inheritance, reported one affected family member with colon cancer, and did not believe there was adequate evidence to suggest that juvenile polyps had malignant potential.[7] Veale and coworkers also noted the familial association of juvenile polyps, and described seven cases of JP in four families. Despite 14 other members of these families having developed colorectal cancer, they also did not suggest that juvenile polyps might predispose to malignancy.[8] The conclusions of these groups that JP was a benign condition, albeit complicated in some cases by GI bleeding and congenital anomalies, were supported by previous studies in solitary juvenile polyps. Roth and Helwig followed 60 children (with a mean followup of 6.4 years) and 27 adults (for a mean followup of 10.6 years) diagnosed with juvenile polyps, and found that no cases of GI cancer developed in these patients.[9] For nearly a decade, it was believed that both solitary juvenile polyps and polyps from JP patients were hamartomas with no malignant potential.

In 1975, however, a kindred was described in which 10 family members had JP of the stomach and/or colon, and 11 family members had developed GI carcinoma. The authors believed that the same gene causing JP was also likely to predispose to GI cancer, but they were careful not to suggest that these malignancies developed within juvenile polyps.[10] Since this report, there have been many accounts of GI malignancy developing in patients with JP, including colon cancer,[10–19] stomach cancer,[10,19,20] and pancreatic cancer.[10,21] The risk of developing colorectal cancer in affected family members has been estimated to be from as low as 9 percent[15] to as high as 68 percent,[22] and these patients are also at risk for cancers of the upper GI tract.[23]

Our understanding of the genetics of JP has been confounded somewhat by the association of juvenile polyps with several heterogeneous genetic syndromes. The first suggestion of a chromosomal localization for JP was reported by Jacoby and colleagues as a result of cytogenetic[24] and loss of heterozygosity (LOH) studies[25] in 1997. Howe and associates described the first locus to be identified by genetic linkage analysis in 1998,[26] and JP patients were reported with germ line mutations of two different tumor-suppressor genes in 1998.[27,28]

CLINICAL ASPECTS

Incidence

The incidence of juvenile polyps is considered to be 1 to 2 percent of the population, but the vast majority of these cases are solitary juvenile polyps and not cases of JP. The average age of diagnosis of solitary juvenile polyps is 3 to 5 years, and these polyps are usually sloughed into the stool and do not recur.[4,9] Helwig found incidental juvenile polyps in 5 of 449 autopsies performed on consecutive patients less than 21 years of age.[2] Toccalino and colleagues found 50 cases of juvenile polyps in 4000 pediatric gastroenterologic consultations (1.25 percent) over a 6-year-period in Argentina.[29] Sulser and associates found 3 cases of juvenile polyps in 90 consecutive patients with polyps (all 3 patients were adults: 2 with solitary polyps, and 1 with approximately 100 polyps).[30] Retrepo and coworkers performed autopsies on 508 patients over 10 years of age from Medellin, Colombia, and found 12 cases of juvenile polyps (2.4 percent). This number would have undoubtedly been higher if individuals aged 0 to 10 years were included.[31]

Restrepo and associates also compared the number of adenomatous and hamartomatous GI polyposis patients seen in 763 cases of colonic polyps from Cali and Medellin, Colombia over a 30-year-period. They found 27 cases of JP (most patients having between 25 and 100 polyps), 14 cases of familial adenomatous polyposis (FAP), and 10 patients with Peutz-Jeghers syndrome. Thirteen of 27 JP cases could be traced to 5 families (2 were suggestive of being familial), and in 12 patients, JP appeared to arise *de novo*.[32] Juvenile polyposis was the most common GI polyposis syndrome seen in this population, which has been described in other developing nations, such as Nigeria.[33] In contrast, Burt and colleagues suggested that the incidence of JP is less than Peutz-Jeghers syndrome, which they estimated to be one-tenth as common as FAP.[34] Because FAP has an incidence of 1 in 8000 live births, Burt et al. would place the incidence of JP at approximately 1 in 100,000. The incidence estimates from Restrepo and Burt vary by a factor of 10: Restrepo found JP to be more common than FAP, but could have been biased by the presence of several JP families from a small geographic region or by other factors unique to developing countries. Chevrel and coworkers from France suggested that JP represented 10 percent of cases of GI polyposis, which they reported had an incidence of 1 in 16,000.[35] Because JP is relatively rare and there are no data available from population-based registries, a more reliable estimate of the incidence of JP is not possible.

Diagnostic Criteria

The criteria currently accepted for diagnosing JP were described by Jass and associates in 1978, and are met by patients with (a) more than five juvenile polyps of the colorectum; (b) juvenile polyps throughout the GI tract; or (c) any number of juvenile polyps with a family history of JP.[36] Howe and colleagues have also suggested that members of JP families with either affected offspring or a history of GI cancer should be considered as affected, even in the absence of histologic demonstration of juvenile polyps.[26] In larger pedigrees, it is often found that members of earlier generations have never had endoscopic screening confirming the presence of juvenile polyps, but have died of GI cancer and had affected offspring.[8,23]

It is important to recognize that these criteria define JP of the GI tract, but not necessarily the more narrow definitions of sporadic or familial JP, for they do not take into account the association of JP with other specific and genetically heterogeneous syndromes, including Cowden syndrome (CS; MIM 158350), Bannayan-Ruvalcaba-Riley syndrome (BRR; MIM 153480), Gorlin syndrome (or basal cell nevus syndrome, BCNS; MIM 109400), and hereditary mixed polyposis syndrome (HMPS; MIM 601228). Patients with CS have benign and malignant lesions of the breast, thyroid, skin (trichilemmomas), and mucous membranes; 40 to 60 percent may have hamartomatous intestinal polyps.[37] Nelen and colleagues mapped the gene for CS to 10q22-24,[38] and Liaw and associates identified germ line mutations in the *PTEN* gene.[39] The clinical manifestations of BRR are hamartomatous GI polyposis, macrocephaly, pseudopapilledema, multiple lipomas, and enlarged penis with speckled pigmentation of the glans. Germ line mutations in these patients have also been found in the *PTEN* gene, suggesting that CS and BRR are allelic conditions.[40] Patients with Gorlin syndrome may have multiple basal cell nevi, palmar pits (also seen in CS), medulloblastoma, mental retardation, ophthalmologic anomalies, and multiple skeletal abnormalities. The incidence of hamartomatous GI polyps appears to be low, however, with large reviews by Gorlin,[41] Evans,[42] and Shanley and collaborators making no mention of GI tract involvement.[43] However, there have been case reports of Gorlin syndrome patients with hamartomatous polyps of the stomach.[44,45] This disorder was mapped to chromosome 9q22.3-31,[46] and found to be caused by germ line mutations in the human *PTC* gene.[47,48] To date, only one family has been well documented with HMPS, in which affected family members have atypical juvenile polyps, colonic adenomas, and colorectal carcinoma, with no extracolonic manifestations.[49] Thomas and coworkers mapped the gene for HMPS in this family to chromosome 6q.[50]

Patients with Cronkhite-Canada syndrome (MIM 175500) have acquired, generalized GI polyposis in which gastric polyps are indistinguishable from juvenile polyps in the stomach, but in which colonic polyps tend to be sessile rather than pedunculated.[51] Distinguishing between this syndrome and JP is aided by Cronkhite-Canada being nonfamilial, of adult onset, and accompanied by diffuse pigmentation, alopecia, and onchorotrophia.[52,53] Although the polyps seen in patients with Peutz-Jeghers syndrome (PJS; MIM 175200) are also hamartomatous, they differ from juvenile polyps in that they contain muscle bundles in the head and stalk of the polyps, whereas juvenile polyps do not have this muscle within their expanded lamina propria. Patients with PJS have pigmented lesions on the lips and buccal mucosa, and may have polyps throughout the GI tract, but these are most commonly found in the small intestine.[54] Hemminki and collaborators established linkage of PJS to markers on chromosome 19p13 in 1997,[55] and germ line mutations were identified soon thereafter in the *LKB1* gene.[56]

Because of the overlap of these clinical syndromes involving JP, patients should be classified as having JP if they meet any of the diagnostic criteria suggested by Jass, *and* do not meet the diagnostic criteria for CS, BRR, BCNS, HMPS, or Cronkhite-Canada syndrome. This task may be troublesome in sporadic cases where there is a higher association with other anomalies, and may even be difficult in families with multiple affected members due to incomplete penetrance or variable expression. Eventually, these syndromes will be more accurately classified by the germ line defects responsible for each case.

Subtypes of Juvenile Polyposis

Sachatello categorized JP patients into three groups to highlight differences in phenotype: (a) juvenile polyposis of infancy; (b) juvenile polyposis coli, to designate those with colonic involvement only; and (c) generalized juvenile polyposis.[57] The latter two groups may be somewhat artificial, for even within families with generalized juvenile polyposis, many members may have colonic involvement only. Hizawa and colleagues have suggested a fourth entity, juvenile polyposis of the stomach, based on 3 patients they followed for 1, 7, and 30 years who had not developed polyps outside the stomach.[58] In a large kindred from Iowa originally described by Stemper, Kent, and Summers,[10] long-term followup of 29 affected family members revealed that 27 had juvenile polyps or cancer of the colorectum, while 11 (38 percent) had polyps or cancer of the upper GI tract. However, only 17 patients had endoscopic or radiologic evaluation of the upper GI tract (65 percent of those screened for this component of the disease had upper GI involvement).[23] Therefore, there is variable expression of the extent of GI tract involvement within families with the same germ line defect. Many of the families reported in the literature have either not been screened for upper GI involvement, or have had few members and no long-term follow-up. This makes it difficult to determine whether juvenile polyposis coli, generalized juvenile polyposis, and juvenile polyposis of the stomach are truly discrete entities or result from variable expression of the same genetic defect.

Juvenile polyposis of infancy has a biologic behavior that appears to be somewhat different from these other subgroups. The patient with generalized juvenile polyposis described by Ravitch presented with diarrhea since birth, malnutrition, anemia, edema, and digital clubbing, and died at 18 months of age following operation for intussusception.[3] Soper and Kent described an infant with macrocephaly and no family history of polyposis who had diarrhea from 3 months of age. The infant later developed hypoalbuminemia, rectal prolapse, and intussusception related to polyposis of the small intestine and colon. He died at age 18 months after reoperation for progressive deterioration, although colectomy was not performed.[59] Gourley and coworkers believed that the hypoalbuminemia seen in a similar patient was due to protein-losing enteropathy, based upon the improvement in serum protein levels after removal of 12 juvenile colonic polyps.[60] Sachatello and colleagues reviewed the literature and reported another infant with small and large intestinal JP with a ventricular septal defect, hepatosplenomegaly, hypoalbuminemia, digital clubbing, diarrhea, duplication of the left renal pelvis and ureter, and a bifid uterus and vagina.[57] They proposed a non-sex-linked recessive inheritance because there was no family history of polyposis in these patients. Of the seven patients reviewed, only one survived beyond 2 years of age,[61] perhaps due to early subtotal colonic resection. Sachatello believed that JP of infancy warranted a separate subgroup to highlight the unfavorable prognosis seen in these patients.[57]

Associated Conditions

One unusual condition, which has been described concurrently with JP, is ganglioneuromatous proliferation within polyps. Donnelly, Sieber, and Yunis described a 9-year-old male with sporadic JP who had both juvenile polyps and polyps with ganglioneuromatous proliferation; only one polyp was found with both of these elements present.[62] Weidner, Flanders, and Mitros reported a 16-year-old male with sporadic JP and ganglioneuromatosis of both normal colonic mucosa and within juvenile polyps.[63] Pham and Villanueva gave an account of a 25-year-old with sporadic JP with eight polyps removed over a 1-year-period in which three polyps demonstrated ganglioneuromatous proliferation within the lamina propria.[64] The only familial cases were described in a father and three children with diffuse, polypoid ganglioneuromatosis and epithelial changes resembling JP.[65] None of the patients in these four reports were known to have a family history of MEN2B or neurofibromatosis. Mendelsohn and Diamond believed that the ganglioneuromatous proliferation resulted in the formation of juvenile polyps in their patients, and emphasized that ganglion cells are not normally present within the lamina propria.[65] Whether excess trophic factors are being produced in these polyps causing neural differentiation, or that they result from changes in the same or different genes predisposing to JP, has not been resolved.

The association of JP with features of hereditary hemorrhagic telangiectasia has been depicted as a separate entity (MIM 175050). Cox and colleagues described a mother and daughter with generalized JP, digital clubbing, blanching lesions on the buccal mucosa, and pulmonary arteriovenous malformations. The mother had three normal siblings and a normal son, and there was no family history of either JP or hereditary hemorrhagic telangiectasia.[66] Conte and associates reported a man dying at age 36 of metastatic adenocarcinoma of the colon, pulmonary arteriovenous malformation, hypertrophic pulmonary osteoarthropathy, and digital clubbing. His son and daughter both presented with rectal bleeding and were found to have multiple juvenile polyps in the ileum and colon in their colectomy specimens. They also had pulmonary arteriovenous malformations, hypertrophic pulmonary osteoarthropathy, and digital clubbing.[67] Three similar cases of sporadic JP, digital clubbing, and hypertrophic osteoarthropathy have also been described; two had pulmonary arteriovenous malformations,[68,69] while the other did not.[70] Cox and coworkers suggested that the simultaneous occurrence of these disorders was likely to result from a new autosomal dominant syndrome rather than new mutations in genes predisposing to both hereditary hemorrhagic telangiectasia and JP.[66] Conversely, none of the patients described with hereditary hemorrhagic telangiectasia and germ line mutations of the endoglin gene on 9q33-34,[71,72] or of the activin receptor-like kinase 1 gene from the pericentromeric region of chromosome 12,[73] have been specifically noted to have JP.

The majority of cases of familial JP thus far reported have not had extraintestinal manifestations. Hofting, Pott, and Stolte reviewed 272 JP patients reported in the literature and determined the rate of extraintestinal anomalies to be 11 percent.[74] A similar review of 218 patients (83 familial cases, 73 sporadic, 62 unknown) by Coburn and associates estimated the incidence of congenital malformations to be 15 percent, with reports of 17 cardiothoracic, 12 central nervous system, 8 soft tissue, 5 GI, and 4 genitourinary anomalies.[75] Bussey, Veale, and Morson reported that the incidence of associated congenital anomalies in the 50 patients in the St. Mark's Registry was approximately 20 percent, with the majority occurring in sporadic patients, who accounted for about 75 percent of cases.[76] Because sporadic cases presumably arise through new mutation, these patients are more likely to have deletions or mutations involving more than just the JP gene.

The first description of JP by McColl and colleagues in 1964 reported 11 cases from 8 families, in which 4 sporadic cases had congenital anomalies. One patient had macrocephaly, hypertelorism, and polydactyly; another had intestinal malrotation (transverse colon below the jejunum), cryptorchidism, mild communicating hydrocephalus, and a Meckel's diverticulum with fecal fistula; another had a mesenteric lymphangioma; and the fourth's cecum was found in a subhepatic position and had episodes of acute porphyria.[6,8] In 27 cases of JP from Colombia (15 familial, 12 sporadic), 4 patients (3 familial, 1 sporadic case) had congenital cardiac anomalies. One patient had tetralogy of Fallot and his second cousin had coarctation of the aorta; another patient had subvalvular aortic stenosis and familial congenital lymphedema, and the other had an atrial septal defect.[32] Walpole and Cullity reported a patient with sporadic generalized JP with macrocephaly, cryptorchidism, digital clubbing, and mental retardation, who ultimately died of pancreatic cancer at age 19.[21] Lipper and associates described a patient with sporadic JP and spina bifida.[77] Jarvinen's review of 18 patients in the Finnish

Polyposis Registry revealed one with a ventricular septal defect and another with panhypopituitarism.[78] Watanabe and colleagues reported a brother and sister who were found to have juvenile polyps of the stomach only, whose mother had died at age 37 of metastatic gastric carcinoma. Both children were noted to be of low intelligence and have brown hair (as did their mother, who was of normal intelligence), which is unusual in the Japanese population.[79]

Desai and colleagues studied the anomalies associated with 23 patients considered to have JP, consisting of 17 sporadic cases and 2 members each from 3 families. They suggested that two patients actually had Gorlin syndrome, two had Bannayan-Riley-Ruvalcaba syndrome, and one had associated hereditary hemorrhagic telangiectasia (and two others were suspected but not all diagnostic criteria were present). Extracolonic abnormalities were detected in 17 of 23 (78 percent) patients. Sixteen patients had skeletal abnormalities (13 hypertelorism, 9 macrocephaly, 5 broad hands, 3 digital clubbing, 1 polydactyly, 1 cleft palate), 13 had dermatologic manifestations (5 telangiectasia, 2 penile pigmentation, 2 nevi, 2 freckles, 1 basal cell cancer, 1 skin pits, 1 palmar nodules), 5 had mental retardation (3 also had hydrocephalus), 4 had cryptorchidism, 2 had ventricular septal defects (both closing without intervention), and 1 had an intestinal malrotation.[80] This study was clouded somewhat by the inclusion of patients with other distinct clinical syndromes.

PATHOLOGY

Horilleno, Eckert, and Ackerman performed a comprehensive review of juvenile polyps by examining the pathologic features of 55 cases of nonfamilial colorectal polyps presenting to St. Louis Children's Hospital between 1935 and 1955. Three-fourths were located within the rectum and 15 percent were in the sigmoid colon, which was probably biased by the fact that sigmoidoscopy was the only endoscopic technique available at the time.[4] Seventy-three percent had solitary polyps, and of the 15 children with more than 1 polyp, 10 had 2, 3 had 3, and 2 had more than 3 polyps. Mestre later showed that with colonoscopic evaluation, 53 percent of children had multiple polyps, of which 60 percent were proximal to the sigmoid colon.[81] Grossly, Horilleno noted that 75 percent of the polyps had pedicles, while 25 percent were sessile, and most measured 1 to 1.5 cm in size (range: 0.3 to 4.0 cm). The external surfaces of the polyps were generally smooth, although finely granular, and smaller polyps were friable while larger polyps were firm (Fig. 35-1). Their shape was commonly disclike, or in some cases, spherical or mushroom-shaped. They were gray, brown, or red in color, which was related to the density of connective tissue within them or recent hemorrhage. On gross sectioning, the polyps usually had a central fibrous region and small peripheral cysts filled with mucin; areas of hemorrhage were common.[4]

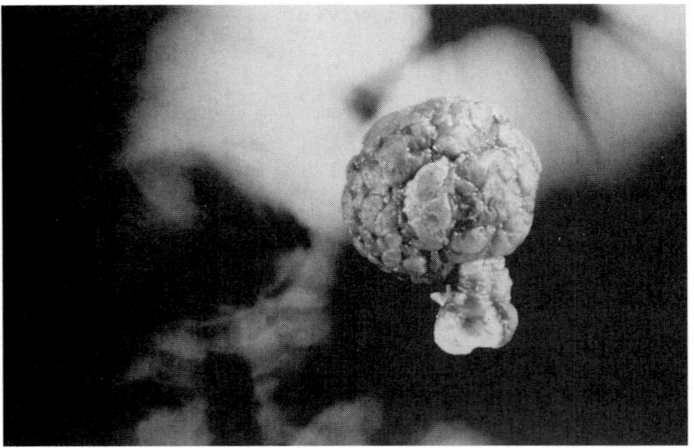

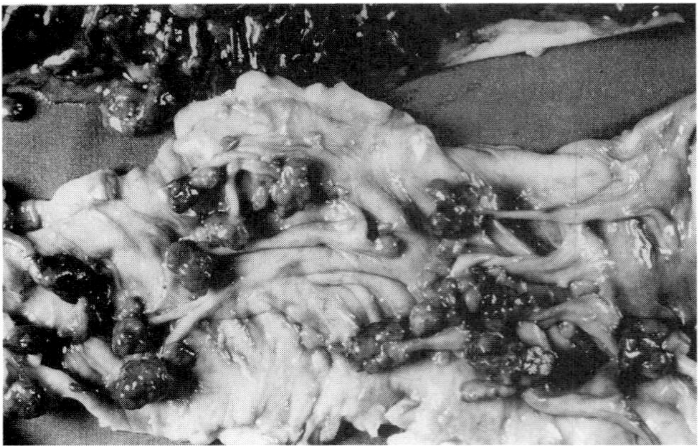

Fig. 35-1 Large juvenile polyp of the ascending colon from a member of the Iowa JP kindred, superimposed the patient's barium enema (above). This polyp was removed endoscopically (photo courtesy of R.W. Summers). Multiple juvenile polyps of the intestine at autopsy in a 20-year-old member of the Iowa JP kindred who died of duodenal cancer (below). Note the hypervascular, bosselated appearance, and pedunculated nature of these polyps.

Microscopically, there are three distinguishing features of juvenile polyps: (a) dilated, cystic spaces lined by glandular epithelium; (b) infiltration by inflammatory cells (lymphocytes, plasma cells, eosinophils, and polymorphonuclear cells); and (c) overabundance of stromal elements all occurring within the lamina propria (Fig. 35-3). These polyps are classified as hamartomatous, to distinguish them from the adenomatous polyps seen in FAP. Hamartomas are defined as abnormal arrangements of tissues that are normally found at a particular site, and hamartomatous intestinal polyps have been divided into the juvenile and Peutz-Jeghers types. Juvenile polyps differ from the polyps seen in Peutz-Jeghers syndrome in that they are devoid of smooth muscle coursing through the stalk and head of the polyps, while the latter have branching of muscular bundles in these regions.[82] Juvenile polyps have also been referred to as "retention polyps" in the past, referring to the cystic glandular spaces filled with mucin.[5] The histologic features of gastric juvenile polyps are similar to those of colonic juvenile polyps, although the lamina propria is usually less inflamed and the cysts are less prominent. Juvenile polyps of the stomach tend to be multiple, diffuse, and less pedunculated than colonic polyps (Fig. 35-2), and can be difficult to differentiate from hyperplastic polyps and those seen in the Cronkhite-Canada syndrome.[51,83]

Another frequent microscopic finding in juvenile polyps is the loss of epithelium at the surface and replacement by fibrin. Based on these findings, Horilleno and associates speculated that juvenile polyps were caused by trauma to the epithelium from feces, resulting in hyperplasia of the mucous glands, inflammation, and deposition of connective tissue. Fibrin could cover these denuded surfaces, sealing the glands and thus creating retention cysts.[4] Roth and Helwig concurred with this theory on the formation of solitary juvenile polyps, and went on to suggest that the polyps develop stalks as they enlarge and are pulled into the fecal stream. They ultimately infarct by twisting on their pedicle, and are sloughed into the stool.[9] Morson believed instead that juvenile polyps were hamartomas of the intestinal mucosa not involving the muscularis mucosae, because of their different appearance relative to inflammatory polyps, their onset in infancy or childhood, and their natural history.[5] Franzin and associates compared the histologic features of 24 juvenile polyps and 27 inflammatory polyps removed from patients with ulcerative colitis, Crohn disease, or after various interventions (such as ureterosigmoidostomy or polypectomy for adenomas). They concluded that these two groups of polyps were very similar, composed of granulation tissue covered by a thin layer of epithelium, and therefore agreed

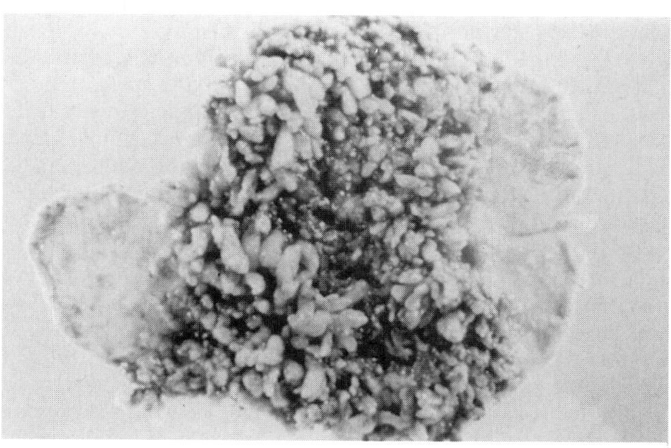

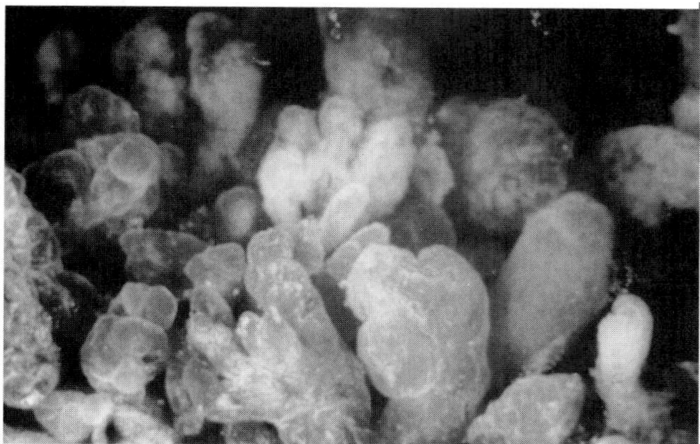

Fig. 35-2 Juvenile polyps of the stomach in a member of the Iowa kindred in a subtotal gastrectomy specimen (above). These polyps are diffuse with some antral sparing. The gastric polyps tend to be thick finger- or leaflike projections and may appear edematous. Unlike the intestinal polyps, they are not usually pedunculated (below; photos courtesy of F.A. Mitros and J.A. Benda).

with the hypothesis of an inflammatory origin for juvenile polyps.[84]

These speculations were based on observations made in solitary juvenile polyps, not in patients meeting the diagnostic criteria for JP. Grossly and microscopically, solitary juvenile polyps are indistinguishable from those in patients with JP. However, the multiplicity of polyps seen in JP patients suggests a germ line defect, while solitary juvenile polyps are likely to arise from two somatic mutations, as Knudson hypothesized in retinoblastoma.[85] Subramony and colleagues looked at normal colonic mucosa and juvenile polyps of various sizes in eight members of a JP family who underwent colectomy. The number of polyps in each specimen varied from 3 to greater than 50, and 6 of 8 specimens also had areas of nodular colonic mucosa. Normal mucosa showed an infiltration of inflammatory cells in the superficial one-third of the lamina propria, with no changes in the glandular elements, but there was significant variability from different areas of the colon. Other areas showed mild abnormalities in the colonic crypts. Foci of nodular colorectal mucosa without discrete polyps had a dense inflammatory infiltrate without surface erosion, which appeared to be the cause of the elevation of the mucosa. Polyps less than 1 cm in size had typical features of juvenile polyps, some with superficial ulceration and granulation tissue. Those 1 to 2.9 cm in size were usually pedunculated, with areas of mild to moderate dysplasia of the glands. Polyps larger than 3 cm were usually mixed (having features of both adenomatous and juvenile polyps) and had moderately dysplastic

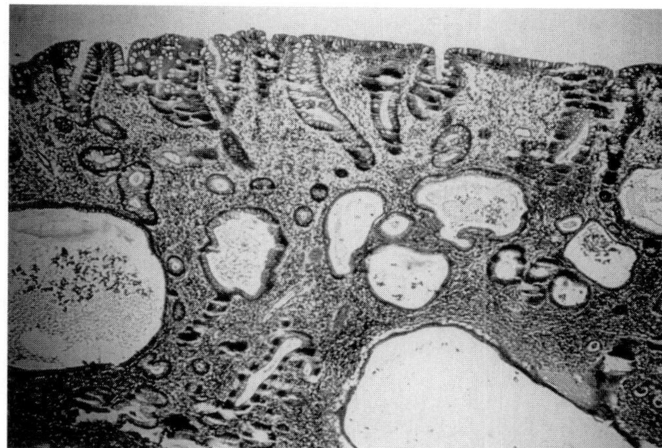

Fig. 35-3 Photomicrograph of a colonic juvenile polyp that demonstrates the characteristic features of cystically dilated glands and strikingly expanded lamina propria with a pronounced inflammatory infiltrate.

epithelium. The largest polyp examined had mixed features of villous adenoma and juvenile polyp, with areas of severe dysplasia, and focal invasive adenocarcinoma in the adenomatous portion of the polyp. The authors concluded that the origin of these polyps was due to an unknown inflammatory stimulus, similar to that proposed for solitary polyps,[4,9] but that they should not be considered as hamartomatous, which implies no malignant potential.[86]

Mechanisms of Neoplastic Transformation in Juvenile Polyps

As discussed above, the belief that juvenile polyps were originally thought to be hamartomas with no malignant potential gradually gave way to the knowledge that patients with juvenile polyps were at increased risk for GI cancer, with numerous reports demonstrating this association. One issue which is less clear is whether juvenile polyps themselves actually develop into adenocarcinoma, or whether patients with JP are predisposed to both juvenile polyps and intestinal cancers, which arise through different precursor lesions. Giardello and colleagues noted that two sporadic and five familial JP patients they studied had adenomatous epithelium within colorectal juvenile polyps.[87] They found 13 similar cases described in the literature, suggesting that juvenile polyps may undergo adenomatous change and thereby be at risk for progression to carcinoma.

To date, there have been two reports of adenocarcinoma developing in a juvenile polyp and three cases of carcinoma *in situ* within juvenile polyps. Liu and associates gave the first description of carcinoma within a juvenile polyp, in a 16-year-old boy with a solitary 4.5-cm juvenile colonic polyp with foci of signet ring carcinoma, capillary-lymphatic invasion, and metastasis to one lymph node.[11] Subramony and colleagues noted a case of invasive adenocarcinoma within adenomatous elements of a mixed villous and juvenile polyp.[86] Longo and coworkers gave an account of a patient with sporadic JP who at age 4 had a juvenile polyp removed with dysplasia, at age 6 with adenomatous changes, and at age 19 with a focus of intramucosal carcinoma in a juvenile polyp.[69] Ramaswamy, Elhosseiny, and Tchertkoff reported a 19-year-old patient who was found to have hundreds of juvenile polyps at total colectomy, some of which displayed adenomatous changes with severe epithelial dysplasia, as well as foci of carcinoma *in situ*.[14] Jones, Hebert, and Trainer reported a 24-year-old man with hematochezia and no family history of polyposis, who had four juvenile polyps removed, three with adenomatous changes, and one showing intramucosal carcinoma.[17] In 1979, Goodman, Yardley, and Milligan hypothesized that juvenile polyps develop from inflamed hyperplastic polyps, which then may develop an adenomatous focus, which becomes progressively dysplastic, and finally undergoes malignant transformation.[12] This view was supported by Grigioni and coworkers, who described a patient similar to that of Goodman et al. with hyperplastic polyps, juvenile polyps, juvenile polyps with adenomatous change, adenomas, and adenocarcinoma.[88] Jass thought that it was unlikely that cancer developed from solitary adenomas in JP. This was based on the fact that of 1032 polyps removed from 80 JP patients, only 21 were adenomas without juvenile features, and that dysplasia was a frequent finding within juvenile polyps.[36]

Kinzler and Vogelstein proposed a new class of cancer susceptibility genes based on the example provided by JP, which they designated as "landscaper" genes. These genes act indirectly, as opposed to gatekeeper and caretaker genes, which regulate cell growth or are involved in DNA-mismatch repair. This model is based on observations that both histologic and genetic changes in juvenile polyps appear to predominantly involve cells in the lamina propria,[25] yet patients with JP are at risk for epithelial malignancies. Kinzler and Vogelstein hypothesized that the germ line defects in JP patients may create an abnormal stromal environment predisposing the overlying epithelium to neoplastic transformation, perhaps through the production of paracrine factors.[89]

Risk of Gastrointestinal Malignancy

Estimates of the risk for developing colorectal or GI cancer in JP patients have varied widely. In a review published in 1984, Jarvinen and Franssila calculated that the risk of colorectal cancer was 9 percent, with 9 cases of colorectal cancer developing in 102 patients with familial and sporadic JP. Thirty-three additional cases of GI cancers in these 19 families were not included because these individuals did not have juvenile polyps documented.[15] Hofting et al.[74] and Coburn et al.[75] reviewed the literature and found a 17 to 18 percent incidence of GI cancer. Examination of 87 JP patients from the St. Mark's polyposis registry revealed 18 (20.7 percent) cases of colorectal cancer.[36] Many patients from these families had undergone colectomy, which probably reduced their risk of developing cancer, and Jass estimated that the cumulative risk of colorectal cancer might be as high as 68 percent by the age of 60 years.[22]

Howe et al. reported the long-term follow-up of the Iowa kindred, which had been first described in 1975,[10] consisting of 117 known members, 29 of whom had been diagnosed with either juvenile polyps or GI cancer.[23] Of these 29 patients, 16 developed GI cancer for an overall incidence of 55 percent. Eleven of these 29 (38 percent) developed colorectal cancer, and 6 (21 percent) had upper GI cancers (4 stomach, 1 duodenum, 1 pancreas). The median age of diagnosis of colorectal cancer was 42.0 years (range: 17.4 to 68.2 years) and 57.6 years (range: 20.8 to 72.8 years) for upper-GI cancer. The definition used for affected differed from previous studies in that family members with a history of GI cancer were also defined as being affected, even in the absence of a histologic diagnosis of juvenile polyps. Many of these individuals had died of advanced cancers in the earlier part of this century, and 12 of the 16 with cancer either also had documented juvenile polyps or had offspring with JP. This paper also reviewed previous reports of 131 familial JP patients from 22 families,[7,8,11–18,20,21,23,32,36,69,79,86–88,90–93] and found 42 cases of colorectal cancer (31.5 percent), 15 of stomach cancer (11.3 percent), and 1 case each of pancreatic and duodenal cancer (0.75 percent). Overall, 58 of these 131 patients (44.4 percent) developed GI cancer, confirming a significant predisposition to cancer in JP.[23]

GENETICS

Pattern of Inheritance

The observation that familial JP was an autosomal dominant disorder in 1966[7,8] has been confirmed over the following decades. Twenty to 50 percent of cases have a family history,[74–76] while the remaining cases presumably arise *de novo* from new mutations, rather than recessive inheritance as hypothesized by Sachatello.[57] The mean age at diagnosis has varied between studies, with Veale estimating it at 4.5 years in sporadic cases and 9.5 years in familial cases.[8] Coburn's review of the literature, including both sporadic and familial cases, found a mean age of diagnosis of 18.5 years,[75] while Howe et al. reported the mean age at presentation to be 30.5 years in the Iowa kindred.[23] The age of diagnosis is clearly influenced by whether patients are detected by screening endoscopy, or whether they present with symptoms, and thus far there have been no reliable prospective or retrospective studies to carefully determine the age of onset. For these reasons, the age-related penetrance in JP is also unknown, but there is evidence to suggest that it is incomplete by middle age. Howe et al. reported that one member of the Iowa kindred inheriting a predisposing germ line mutation was asymptomatic and has had both negative upper and lower endoscopy at the age of 44.5 years.[94] There is variable expression in terms of upper and lower GI polyposis within and between families, and the association of multiple juvenile polyps with a variety of genetic conditions suggest that there is significant genetic heterogeneity, with multiple chromosomal loci influencing the development of these polyps. A slight preponderance of cases in males have been described in some reports (17 of 23 by Desai,[80] 15 of 27 by Restrepo,[32] 80 of 149 by Coburn[75]), but the sex distribution in the Iowa kindred was essentially equal (14 males of 29).[23]

Cytogenetic and Loss of Heterozygosity (LOH) Studies

In 1997, Jacoby and colleagues reported a 4-year-old patient with multiple colonic juvenile polyps, hypoplastic ears, tricuspid insufficiency, widely spaced canthi, and who was < 5th percentile for head circumference, height, and weight. On cytogenetic analysis, this patient was noted to have an interstitial deletion of 10q22.3-q24.1, leading the authors to hypothesize that this region contained a tumor-suppressor gene associated with JP.[24] Based on the findings in this patient, they evaluated this region for LOH in juvenile polyps from 13 unrelated JP patients (5 of whom had less than 5 polyps) and 3 with solitary juvenile polyps. The marker *D10S219* was deleted in 39 of 47 (83 percent) polyps from these 16 patients and the minimal region of overlap of all deletions was an approximately 3-cM region between markers *D10S219* and *D10S1696*. They next performed fluorescent *in situ* hybridization on tissue sections from juvenile polyps using a cosmid clone mapping near this region, and compared the staining in epithelial versus lamina propria cells. They found that 30 of 39 (77 percent) polyps examined had somatic deletions from 10q, predominantly within lymphocytes and macrophages in the lamina propria. These findings suggested the presence of a tumor-suppressor gene predisposing to juvenile polyps on 10q22 (named *JP1*),[25] in the same vicinity as the locus recently mapped for Cowden syndrome.[38]

Linkage Studies

Prior to these reports, linkage studies in familial JP had been limited to one study that had excluded *APC* and *MCC* as the gene for JP in an Australian family.[95] After Jacoby's report of 10q deletions in juvenile polyps, Marsh and associates genotyped 4 microsatellite markers from this region on 47 members of 8 JP families, and were able to exclude linkage of the JP gene by multipoint lod scores less than − 2.0 over the entire putative *JP1* interval. Howe et al. genotyped 43 members (13 affected, 24 at-risk, 6 spouses) of the Iowa kindred using 5 microsatellite markers from this region and also found no evidence for linkage.[26]

In the latter study, markers were also examined from the regions of several genes known to play an important role in either the development of sporadic colorectal cancer or hamartomatous polyps. These included *MSH2* (2p16), *MLH1* (3p21), *MCC, APC*

(5q21-22), *HMPS* (6q21), *JP1, PTEN* (10q22-24), *KRAS2* (12p12), *TP53* (17p13), *DCC* (18q21), and *LKB1* (19p13), as well as *CDKN2* (9q21). No evidence for linkage was found with markers from most of these regions, but linkage was detected with markers from 18q21. Genotyping and linkage analysis with 27 microsatellite markers from 18q21 resulted in lod scores >3.0 with 7 different markers, with a maximum lod score of 5.00 (at $\theta = 0.001$) with the marker *D18S1099*. Haplotype analysis revealed five affected individuals with recombination events, allowing for localization of the JP gene to an 11.9-cM interval between markers *D18S1118* and *D18S487* on 18q21.1.[28] This interval was known to contain two tumor-suppressor genes, *DCC* (deleted in colorectal carcinoma[96]), and *DPC4* (*d*eleted in *p*ancreatic *c*ancer *4,* also known as *Smad4*[97]), and was also known to be commonly deleted in both sporadic colorectal[96] and pancreatic carcinomas.[98] This is the only locus for JP identified by linkage thus far, but efforts continue to identify additional loci for this apparently genetically heterogeneous syndrome.

PTEN Mutations on 10q23

The *PTEN* gene on 10q23 is a tumor-suppressor gene that is frequently mutated in glioblastomas, prostate cancers, and breast cancers, with homology to tyrosine phosphatases and the protein tensin.[99,100] It has also been shown to be the predisposing locus for both CS[39] and BRR[40] (see Chap. 45 for more detail on the *PTEN* gene). There have been two reports describing *PTEN* mutations in JP patients.[27,101] Lynch and colleagues reported a R334X germ line mutation in two members of a family believed to have both CS and JP. The affected father had a history of small intestinal cancer, skin lesions, and macrocephaly, while his affected son also had skin lesions, macrocephaly, and small intestinal and colonic polyps. Eng and Ji have suggested that these patients might be more accurately classified as having CS.[102] Olschwang and associates reported *PTEN* mutations in 3 of 14 patients presenting with GI bleeding and >10 juvenile polyps. One patient had a deletion at codon 232 leading to a premature stop at codon 255, was 74 years of age with upper and lower GI juvenile polyps, had a laryngeal cancer treated by radiotherapy 2 years earlier, and a heterogeneous thyroid nodule. Another patient, 10 years of age with generalized JP (with no extraintestinal manifestations of CS), was found to have a M35R substitution, while a third patient was 14 years old with colonic JP (and no family history of CS or BRR) with a mutation in a splice donor site of exon 6.[27] Eng and Ji believed the first patient was suggestive of having CS, and made the point that CS could not be ruled out in the other two patients (aged 10 and 14 years) because the penetrance is <10 percent below the age of 15 years. These authors cautioned that the diagnosis of JP should be made after exclusion of other syndromes such as CS and BRR, and if *PTEN* mutations were found in these patients, then a high index of suspicion for the diagnosis of CS or BRR should be maintained.[102]

This recommendation was also influenced by two studies in which *PTEN* mutations were not found in JP patients. Riggins and associates sequenced the *PTEN* gene in 11 patients with familial JP and found no mutations.[103] Marsh and coworkers found no *PTEN* mutations in members of 14 JP families and 11 sporadic cases, and concluded that *PTEN* was either not a predisposing gene for JP or that it was only involved in a small group of cases. Furthermore, they raised the possibility that if there were a susceptibility locus on 10q22-24, as suggested by Jacoby,[25] then the 3 cM region as proposed for *JP1* is 7 cM centromeric to the *PTEN* gene.[104] In summary, mutations of *PTEN* or another nearby gene on 10q22-24 may be responsible for a subset of patients with JP, but it is important to rule out CS or BRR in these patients because approximately 80 percent of CS patients and 60 percent of BRR patients have *PTEN* mutations[105] and may also have hamartomatous polyps. Patients with CS need to be followed closely for the development of breast and thyroid neoplasms, while JP patients do not.

Smad4 Mutations on 18q21.1

The finding of linkage to chromosome 18q21.1 in an interval containing two tumor-suppressor genes thought to play a role in the development of GI cancers led us to screen these genes for mutations in affected members of the Iowa JP kindred. After sequencing all 11 exons of *Smad4* and 14 of 29 *DCC* exons, a 4 base-pair (bp) deletion was found in exon 9 of the *Smad4* gene. All 13 affected members of this kindred had this deletion, as did 4 of 26 individuals at-risk, while 7 spouses and 242 control patients did not (Fig. 35-4). The maximum 2-point lod score of this deletion with the JP phenotype in this family was 5.79 at $\theta = 0.00$. This deletion occurred between nucleotides 1372 and 1375 (codons 414 to 416) and resulted in a frameshift, creating a new stop codon at the end of exon 9 (codon 434).[28]

To further study the importance of the *Smad4* gene in JP, all exons were sequenced in eight other unrelated patients. The same 4 bp deletion in exon 9 was also found in affected members of JP families from Mississippi (originally described by Subramony et al.[86]) and Finland.[28] Since this report, an additional Caucasian kindred from Texas has also been found with the same deletion. The sharing of this common deletion from exon 9 raises the possibility that these kindreds may either have a common ancestor or that this region is a mutational hotspot. Genotyping of members of all four families with several markers from 18q21 revealed that there was no shared haplotype between these families for markers closest to the *Smad4* gene, suggesting that this area in exon 9 is indeed more susceptible to mutation.[106]

In the six other unrelated patients studied, four had the wild-type sequence for all exons of the *Smad4* gene. One patient with sporadic generalized JP was found to have a 2 bp deletion at codon 348 of exon 8, which caused a frameshift and stop at codon 350.

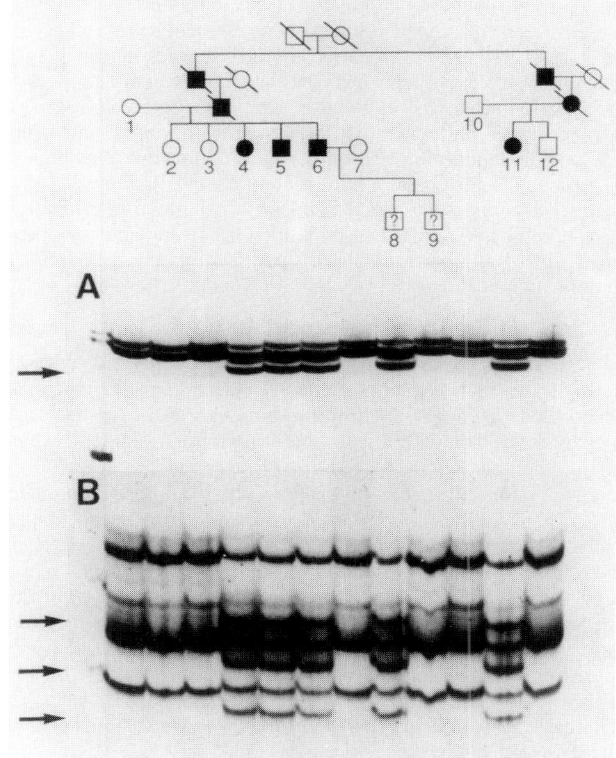

Fig. 35-4 *A* Denaturing and *B* nondenaturing gels of Iowa JP kindred members showing the exon 9 PCR product. Affected individuals 4, 5, 6, and 11, as well as one at-risk (*), all have an extra band (arrow in *A*) on denaturing gels that is produced by the 4-bp deletion. The mutant allele is also seen as a shift by SSCP analysis (arrows in *B*; reproduced from Howe et al.[28] with permission).

Table 35-1 Smad4 Sequencing Results in 10 Unrelated JP Patients

Patient	Type	Codon (exon)	Nucleotide Change	Predicted Effect	Control Pts.
I-13*	Familial	414–416 (9)	4 bp deletion	Frameshift, stop at codon 434	0/242
M-1*	Familial	414–416 (9)	4 bp deletion	Frameshift, stop at codon 434	0/242
T-1*	Familial	414–416 (9)	4 bp deletion	Frameshift, stop at codon 434	0/242
JP 5/1*	Familial	414–416 (9)	4 bp deletion	Frameshift, stop at codon 434	0/242
JP 11/1	Sporadic	348 (8)	2 bp deletion	Frameshift, stop at codon 350	0/101
JP 10/1	Sporadic	229–231 (5)	1 bp insertion	Frameshift, stop at codon 235	0/101
JP 6/1	Sporadic	—	—	—	
JP 4/1	Familial	—	—	—	
JP 1/1	Sporadic‡	—	—	—	
JP 2/13†	Familial	—	—	—	

*Sequence variant segregates with JP phenotype in respective family (13, 5, 5, and 2 affecteds with the mutation in the Iowa, Mississippi, Texas, and JP 5 Finnish kindreds, respectively).
†Multipoint lod score of 1.00 with chromosome 18q21 markers in this family (6 affected, 11 normals).
‡JP 1/1 has a brother with colon cancer but no family members with documented JP (modified and reprinted from Howe et al.[28] by permission).

Another patient with sporadic JP diagnosed at age 6 with 30 to 40 colonic juvenile polyps had a 1 bp insertion between codons 229 and 231 of exon 5. This mutation, which added a guanine to six sequential guanines, caused a frameshift and stop at codon 235.[28] A summary of the results of *Smad4* sequencing in these patients is shown in Table 35-1.

Fraction of Cases due to *Smad4* and *PTEN*

There is little doubt that there is genetic heterogeneity in JP patients, but the degree of this heterogeneity and the number of genes involved remain to be defined. As discussed above, we have found *Smad4* mutations in 60 percent of the familial and sporadic cases thus far examined. However, no evidence for linkage to 18q21 markers has been seen in other JP families, and gel shifts were observed in only 1 of 20 unrelated individuals studied by conformation-sensitive gel electrophoresis of the *Smad4* gene.[107] It would, therefore, appear that the frequency of *Smad4* mutations in JP patients might range from as low as 23 percent to as high as 60 percent. The role of *PTEN* mutations in JP remains to be clarified. Riggins et al.[103] and Marsh et al.[104] found no mutations in 36 sporadic and familial cases, while Olschwang and coworkers found 3 of 14 (21 percent) of their patients had germ line *PTEN* mutations.

The *Smad4* Gene and Human Tumors

Hahn and associates identified a new tumor-suppressor locus by virtue of the fact that approximately 90 percent of pancreatic cancers had deletions of chromosome 18q and 30 percent had homozygous losses within a common interval on 18q21.1, which did not include the *DCC* gene.[98] They found three expressed sequences from this region, one of which showed significant homology to the *Drosophila Mad* (*m*others *a*gainst *d*ecapentaplegic) gene. This gene was named *DPC4* based on its being the fourth deletion locus described in pancreatic cancers, and it encodes for a 552 amino acid protein. Somatic mutations of this gene were found in 6 of 27 pancreatic cancers without homozygous deletions on 18q21, implicating it as a tumor suppressor predisposing to pancreatic cancer.[97] *DPC4* is now referred to as *Smad4,* a nomenclature that combines the terms for the homologous *Mad* genes in *Drosophila melanogaster* and *sma* genes in *Caenorhabditis elegans.*[108]

Subsequent studies have shown that the rates of *Smad4* mutations are modest in other GI tumors, and are distinctly uncommon in extraintestinal tumors. Thiagalingam and coworkers found loss or mutation of *Smad4* in 5 of 18 colorectal carcinoma cell lines exhibiting 18q loss. These tumors were taken from a panel of 55 tumors with 18q loss (out of a total of 100 colorectal tumors), suggesting an overall mutation rate of approximately 15 percent.[109] Tagaki and associates found 5 *Smad4* mutations in 31 primary colorectal cancers, for a total mutation rate of 16 percent.[110] MacGrogan and colleagues found *Smad4* mutations in 4 of 21 (19 percent) primary colorectal carcinomas and cell lines.[111] Hoque and coworkers found LOH on 18q21 and a *Smad4* mutation in one of six (17 percent) colitis-associated colorectal cancers.[112] Lei and collaborators found no mutations of *Smad4* in 10 gastric, 10 esophageal, and 10 colitis-associated colorectal cancers.[113] Powell and coworkers found one case with inactivation of both copies of *Smad4* (one deleted and the other with nonsense mutation at codon 334) in a panel of 35 gastric adenocarcinomas.[114] Hahn and colleagues reported 5 mutations in 32 (16 percent) carcinomas of the biliary tract, even though they only examined exons 8 through 11.[115] Moskaluk and colleagues sequenced the *Smad4* gene from members of 11 families with familial pancreatic cancer (defined as 2 affected first-degree relatives) and found no mutations in these patients. They speculated that this situation could be similar to that seen in Li-Fraumeni syndrome, in which affected family members have germ line mutations of the *p53* gene but do not develop colorectal cancers, while sporadic colorectal cancers have a high rate of *p53* mutation.[116]

Schutte and associates analyzed 64 non-GI tumors (11 prostate, 8 breast, 8 ovary, 7 bladder, 6 hepatocellular carcinoma, 6 lung cancers, 5 head and neck carcinomas, 4 melanomas, 3 osteosarcomas, 3 renal cell carcinomas, 2 glioblastomas, and 1 medulloblastoma) displaying 18q loss for sequence changes in the *Smad4* gene, and found only 2 alterations, 1 in a breast and the other in an ovarian cancer. They concluded that another tumor-suppressor gene from 18q might be involved in the development of these tumors.[117] Kim and coworkers found 2 mutations in head and neck tumors derived from cell lines of 11 patients and 20 primary tumors (6 percent).[118] MacGrogan and collaborators found no mutations in 45 primary and metastatic prostate cancers.[111]

Function of the *Smad4* Gene

The Smad4 protein is the common mediator involved in the transforming growth factor-β (TGF-β), activin, and bone morphogenetic protein (BMP) signal-transduction pathways. Members of the TGF-β superfamily initiate a wide spectrum of effects on a variety of cell types, including cell differentiation, proliferation, and apoptosis.[119,120] Currently, there are eight known *Smad* genes in vertebrates. The Smad2 and Smad3 proteins function as cytoplasmic effectors in the TGF-β and activin pathways. Their counterparts in the BMP pathway are Smad1, Smad5, and possibly Smad9. Smad6 and Smad7 function as inhibitors of all three pathways by binding to type I receptors and interfering with phosphorylation.[120]

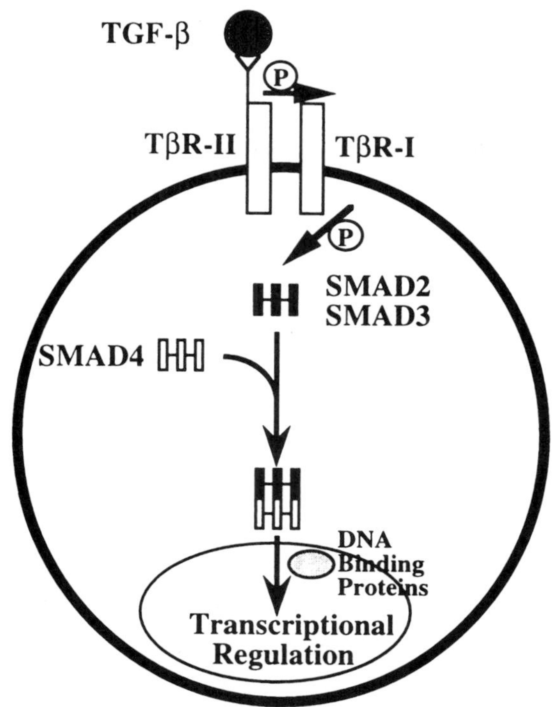

Fig. 35-5 Overview of the TGF-β signaling pathway. TGF-β binds to TβR-II, which then phosphorylates TβR-I, thereby activating it. TβR-I then phosphorylates Smad2 or Smad3, allowing them to form homo-oligomers or hetero-oligomers with Smad4. Hetero-oligomeric complexes of Smad4 with Smad2 or Smad3 associate with DNA-binding proteins. These complexes then bind to sequences in the promoter regions of genes under TGF-β control, regulating their transcription.

An overview of the sequence of proteins involved in the TGF-β signaling pathway is shown in Fig. 35-5. TGF-β binds to plasma membrane serine/threonine kinases, and, specifically, to the type II TGF-β receptor (TβR-II). This then complexes with the type I receptor (TβR-I), causing phosphorylation in a serine- and threonine-rich domain of TβR-I.[121] These activated type I receptors phosphorylate cytoplasmic monomers of Smad2 or Smad3, allowing these to form oligomers and to associate with Smad4 monomers or oligomers.[122,123] Hetero-oligomers of Smad2 or Smad3 and Smad4 then migrate to the nucleus and regulate transcription in conjunction with DNA-binding proteins.[124]

The mechanism by which this transcriptional regulation occurs is just beginning to be understood. Within the nucleus, the Smad4 protein appears to bind directly to DNA,[125] and it has been shown that both Smad3 and Smad4 efficiently bind the 8-bp nucleotide sequence GTCTAGAC.[126] Another sequence that binds Smad3 and Smad4 (AG(C/A)CAGACA, dubbed the "CAGA box") has been described at positions −730, −580, and −280 within the plasminogen activator inhibitor-1 promoter, which is strongly inducible by TGF-β. Experiments cloning CAGA boxes upstream of various promoters resulted in markedly increased responses to TGF-β, and mutations within these sites decreased these responses.[127] The recently identified human DNA-binding protein *hFAST-1* also appears to bind to specific DNA sequences in response to TGF-β in the presence of Smad2 and Smad4.[128] In *Xenopus*, it has been proposed that FAST-1 binds to the C-terminus region of Smad2, and Smad4 stabilizes these proteins by binding to Smad2.[129] This complex appears to be required for transcription of TGF-β and activin target genes, which is achieved by hFAST-1 and Smad4 associating with their sequence-specific binding elements.[128]

The majority of *Smad4* mutations thus far described in human cancers have been between codons 330 and 526,[97,110,117,118] within several highly conserved domains. This C-terminus of *Smad4* is important in the formation of *Smad4* homo-oligomers (initially believed to be homo-trimers), which then form hetero-oligomers with other Smad proteins.[122] Recently, it has been suggested that the majority of intracellular Smad4 is found in the form of monomers rather than homo-trimers, and that Smad4 competes with Smad2 and Smad3 in the formation of hetero-trimer complexes.[123] It has been demonstrated that mutations which disrupt Smad4 homo- and hetero-oligomerization lead to loss of TGF-β superfamily induced signaling pathways.[130] Lagna and associates showed that loss of the terminal 38 amino acids of Smad4 leads to a dominant negative effect on the induction of mesoderm in *Xenopus* embryos by Smad2, and that mutant and wild-type proteins form oligomers which may be responsible for their loss of activity.[131]

Zhou and colleagues constructed heterozygous and homozygous *Smad4* deletions by homologous recombination in the colorectal cancer cell line HCT116, which has a truncating mutation of TβR-II and requires restoration of this gene in order to mediate TGF-β signaling. When TβR-II was reintroduced into these cells, cell lines with heterozygous *Smad4* deletions generated an equal response to TGF-β as cell lines without deletion, while those having homozygous deletions had no signaling. Similar results were observed when an activated TβR-I receptor (TβR-I^{T204D}) was introduced into these cells, or when they were stimulated by the addition of activin. Furthermore, the proliferation of cell lines in which a functional TβR-II gene had been introduced was substantially decreased in the parental cell line, and in those with heterozygous *Smad4* deletions, when placed in medium containing TGF-β. Similar cell lines with homozygous *Smad4* deletions had a significantly lower level of growth inhibition. These results indicated that *Smad4* mutation was a potential mechanism by which tumor cells could escape the antiproliferative effects of TGF-β.[132]

Animal Models

Generation of transgenic mice with heterozygous and homozygous inactivation of *Smad4* has added insight into the role of this gene in embryogenesis and tumor formation. Sirard and colleagues created *Smad4* mutant embryonic stem cells by homologous recombination, using a construct replacing exons 8 and 9 with a neomycin resistance gene. They followed 25 *Smad4* heterozygous mutant (+/−) mice for 11 months, and found no increase in tumors relative to wild-type mice, suggesting that loss of the other allele was necessary for tumor development. *Smad4* homozygous mutant (−/−) mice died *in utero*, predominantly at 7.5 days of embryogenesis. These embryos manifested impaired growth, with poor separation of embryonic and extraembryonic boundaries. Histologic comparison of wild-type and −/− embryos at 6.5 days revealed that −/− embryos had no mesoderm formation, as well as abnormal development of the visceral endoderm. This defect in gastrula formation could be rescued by aggregation with tetraploid embryonic cells, but the resulting embryos had impaired development of anterior structures.[133] Yang and coworkers confirmed these findings using a similar model, and concluded that Smad4 is necessary for epiblast proliferation, egg-cylinder formation, and induction of the mesoderm.[134]

Takaku and associates created transgenic mice by homologous recombination using a construct disrupting the *Smad4* gene within exon 1, and generated compound *Smad4/Apc* mutant mice, taking advantage of the fact that these genes are approximately 30 cM apart on mouse chromosome 18. *Smad4* −/− mutant mice died in utero, while *Smad4* +/− mutants were viable, fertile, and had no histologic abnormalities within their intestines or pancreas relative to wild-type litter mates. Compound $Apc^{\Delta716}$ and *Smad4* heterozygous mutant mice had only about 12 percent of the number of intestinal polyps seen in $Apc^{\Delta716}$ +/− mice, but their average size was larger (1 to 2 mm vs. 0.5 mm). Fifty-three percent also had epidermoid cysts, and 20 percent developed adenocarcinoma of the ampulla of Vater, which was not seen in *Apc* or *Smad4* +/− mice. Intestinal polyps from the compound mutant mice also showed stromal proliferation similar to that observed in juvenile polyps, and an increased incidence of malignant tumors relative to $Apc^{\Delta716}$ +/− mice. Examination of tumor DNA from compound heterozygous mutant mice revealed that adenocarcinomas had lost the wild-type chromosome 18 and reduplicated the compound mutant chromosome.[135] Together, these studies demonstrate that *Smad4* most likely functions as a tumor-suppressor gene, for heterozygous mutants did not display increased numbers of tumors and were phenotypically normal. Furthermore, formation of tumors may require somatic mutations in addition to loss of *Smad4,* as seen in polyps of *cis*-compound *Smad4/APC* mutants, which had histologic changes reminiscent of those seen in JP patients.

Mutations of Other Genes in the TGF-β Pathway

Mutations within the TβR-II gene have been demonstrated in 90 percent of tumors with microsatellite instability, occurring within a 10-bp polyadenine tract of this gene.[136–138] Restoration of functional TβR-II expression in deficient cell lines reduces their tumorigenicity in cell cultures and nude mice.[139] There has been one report of a germ line mutation at codon 315 (T315M) of TβR-II in an hereditary colorectal cancer family without microsatellite instability, which suggests that mutations outside the polyadenine tract in this gene may be another mechanism for the development of colorectal cancer, independent of defects in DNA mismatch-repair.[140]

Smad2 has been mapped to chromosome 18q21.1 approximately 3 Mb centromeric to the *Smad4* gene, appears to be ubiquitously expressed,[141] and consists of 11 exons and 467 amino acids.[142] It may play a role in the development of sporadic colorectal cancers, but mutations within *Smad2* appear to be infrequent in these tumors. Analysis of *Smad2* in 18 colorectal cancer cell lines revealed homozygous loss in one tumor, and a truncated protein in another.[143] Of 66 sporadic colorectal carcinomas, 4 (6 percent) were found with missense mutations in *Smad2.* Adjacent normal mucosa from these patients did not have these mutations, indicating that these events were somatic within the tumors. No germ line mutations of *Smad2* were identified in a panel of 15 patients with a strong family history of colorectal cancer or early age of onset.[142]

Smad3 has been mapped to chromosome 15q21-22,[143] and consists of 9 exons and 424 amino acids.[144] Examination of 167 cancer cell lines (70 colorectal, 22 breast, 22 brain, 15 lung, 12 pancreas, 8 head and neck, 6 ovary, 4 esophagus, 4 stomach, and 4 prostate) by *in vitro* synthesized protein assays for Smad3, found no truncated proteins in any of these tumor lines.[145] Study of the *Smad3* gene in 35 sporadic and 15 HNPCC colorectal cancers revealed no mutations, but 2 of 17 informative tumors showed LOH from this region.[144] These studies suggest that both *Smad2* and *Smad3* may not significantly contribute to colorectal carcinogenesis, but do not address the question as to whether alterations in these genes contribute to the development of hamartomatous polyps.

Currently, little is known about *Smad6* and *Smad7* except that they are inhibitory through their binding to type I receptors, thus interfering with phosphorylation of downstream Smad proteins. They both have high homology to other *Smad* genes in their C-terminus, but appear to lack conserved regions in their amino-terminal domains common to other *Smad* genes.[120,145] *Smad6* encodes a 235 amino acid protein, and has been localized to chromosome 15q21-22, the same region as the *Smad3* gene.[143,145] Smad7 has been shown to inhibit TGF-β signaling by binding to the type I receptor and preventing the phosphorylation of Smad2. A truncated Smad7 protein demonstrated loss of this inhibition.[146] Although it has not yet been demonstrated, it is conceivable that other mutations could lead to stable binding with type I receptors and sustained inhibition of the antiproliferative effects of TGF-β.

IMPLICATIONS FOR DIAGNOSIS AND TREATMENT

Genetic Testing

Genetic testing of at-risk members of JP families has the potential to significantly improve the current method of presymptomatic diagnosis, which consists of periodic upper and lower screening endoscopy. Compliance with this regimen has been poor for insurance reasons, and because it is uncomfortable, relatively expensive, and needs to be repeated every 1 to 3 years.[94] DNA testing would simplify initial screening by requiring a single blood sample, and theoretically would allow noncarriers to avoid repetitive endoscopy. Health care resources could then be focused on the close surveillance of carriers and the early detection of their GI neoplasms.

The major problem with genetic testing for JP is the potential for genetic heterogeneity. As mentioned earlier, patients must be carefully evaluated clinically and pathologically to exclude other conditions associated with hamartomatous polyps, and even then, these associations may go undetected due to incomplete penetrance or variable expression. If the diagnostic criteria for JP are satisfied, then we begin with single-stranded conformational polymorphism (SSCP) and sequencing of all exons of the *Smad4* gene in an affected member of the kindred. If mutations are identified, the sequence changes are examined for their potential biologic significance, and then SSCP or sequencing is used to determine whether these changes are present in other family members. Whether germ line mutations predispose to the JP phenotype is confirmed by its segregation with all affected family members and the absence of similar changes in a large number of control subjects. If no mutations are detected in *Smad4,* then the *PTEN* gene is sequenced in an affected family member. If a mutation is found, then the rest of the family is examined for that exon, and all family members with mutations must be followed closely for the development of GI cancers, as well as for those of the thyroid and breast. If mutations are not found in either *Smad4* or *PTEN* genes, then presymptomatic genetic testing is considered nondiagnostic. These families are then made a part of ongoing linkage studies attempting to identify other loci predisposing to JP.

The small number of mutations reported thus far limit our ability to estimate what percent of JP cases will be detected by sequencing these two genes. As discussed earlier, *Smad4* mutations may be responsible for anywhere from 23 to 60 percent of cases,[28] while *PTEN* mutations may account for 0 to 21 percent of cases.[27,103,104] Other genes will undoubtedly emerge as the search for additional JP loci continues, which will improve our ability to provide genetic testing. The confusion regarding the classification of certain patients with hamartomatous polyposis should also be resolved in the near future, as they are categorized according to the specific germ line mutations present in each individual.

Genetic Counseling and Clinical Management

Genetic counseling should be offered to all JP patients, to make them are aware of the autosomal dominant nature of this syndrome, its spectrum of expression, and the risk for malignancy. Frequently encountered old myths, such as the recommendation to not have children, should be dispelled and replaced by patient education. Indications for screening endoscopy, endoscopic polypectomy, and surgical treatment also need to be discussed. Finally, the current status of genetic testing and the possibility of nondiagnostic results should be explored. The considerable experience with genetic testing for other GI cancer syndromes provides excellent models on which we base our approach for genetic counseling in JP, as reviewed by Petersen and Boyd for FAP[147] and Lynch, Smyrk, and Lynch in HNPCC.[148]

Adult patients found to have germ line mutations in *Smad4* or *PTEN* must be notified that they have inherited an abnormality in a gene predisposing to JP.[149] Patients with positive genetic tests should have upper and lower endoscopy performed at this time to determine whether they currently have polyps, whether these require intervention, and to decide on the interval for future screening. Screening endoscopy should begin in the early second decade in asymptomatic patients, because the earliest age of cancer diagnoses that we have seen have been at 17.4 years for colorectal and 20.5 years for upper GI cancers.[23] Patients who develop symptoms of hematochezia, melena, rectal prolapse, intussusception, or frequent abdominal pain should have baseline endoscopy performed at the time these symptoms are recognized. If endoscopy is negative for polyps, screening should be carried out every 1 to 3 years as long as these patients remain asymptomatic. When polyps are encountered, they should be removed endoscopically to decrease the chance for malignant transformation and to help avoid the bleeding and anemia frequently seen in these patients. These patients should have annual endoscopy until the GI tract is free of polyps, then every 1 to 3 years thereafter. Although some authors have advocated subtotal colectomy in affected patients,[19] this may not be necessary if patients agree to periodic follow-up. Subtotal colectomy or total colectomy with ileoanal pull-through is recommended in patients who are likely to be lost to follow-up, have large polyps that cannot be removed endoscopically, have recurrent episodes of significant GI bleeding or protein-losing enteropathy, or have severe dysplasia or adenocarcinoma on biopsy. The diffuse nature of gastric polyposis makes endoscopic polypectomy impractical, and, therefore, symptomatic patients require subtotal or total gastrectomy.

Patients with nondiagnostic genetic test results should be screened by endoscopy every 3 years while asymptomatic and free of polyps. Patients with negative genetic test results should be screened for colon cancer as recommended for the normal population, and until further experience with these patients accumulates, we also recommend intermittent screening (such as every 5 to 10 years until the age of 50) to guard against the unlikely event of an error in genetic testing. Children should participate in genetic counseling sessions to learn about the condition that runs in their family, but the issue of at what age children should be informed of testing results remains controversial. In FAP, although the vast majority of parents questioned wanted to have their children tested at birth, most did not think they should be told until they were old enough to understand.[150] Accordingly, as long as children remain asymptomatic, it may be best to delay giving the results of genetic testing to patients until they begin screening endoscopy in adolescence. Other important issues to be discussed with families in any genetic testing scenario include how test results could change the patient's insurability, as well as the possibility of detecting nonpaternity. With the current pace of advances in the molecular biology of cancer, we expect that presymptomatic genetic testing will become the important first step in the life-long management of patients with JP.

REFERENCES

1. Diamond M: Adenoma of the rectum in children: Report of a case in a thirty-month-old girl. *Am J Dis Child* **57**:360, 1939.
2. Helwig EB: Adenoma of the large bowel in children. *Am J Dis Child* **72**:1946.
3. Ravitch MM: Polypoid adenomatosis of the entire gastrointestinal tract. *Ann Surg* **128**:283, 1948.
4. Horrilleno EG, Eckert C, Ackerman LV: Polyps of the rectum and colon in children. *Cancer* **10**:1210, 1957.
5. Morson BC: Some peculiarities in the histology of intestinal polyps. *Dis Colon Rectum* **5**:337, 1962.
6. McColl I, Bussey HJR, Veale AMO, Morson BC: Juvenile polyposis coli. *Proc Roy Soc Med* **57**:896, 1964.
7. Smilow PC, Pryor CA, Swinton NW: Juvenile polyposis coli: A report of three patients in three generations of one family. *Dis Colon Rectum* **9**:248, 1966.
8. Veale AMO, McColl I, Bussey HJR, Morson BC: Juvenile polyposis coli. *J Med Genet* **3**:5, 1966.
9. Roth SI, Helwig EB: Juvenile polyps of the colon and rectum. *Cancer* **16**:468, 1963.
10. Stemper TJ, Kent TH, Summers RW: Juvenile polyposis and gastrointestinal carcinoma. *Ann Intern Med* **83**:639, 1975.
11. Liu T-H, Chen M-C, Tseng H-C: Malignant change of juvenile polyp of colon. *Chin Med J* **4**:434, 1978.
12. Goodman ZD, Yardley JH, Milligan FD: Pathogenesis of colonic polyps in multiple juvenile polyposis. *Cancer* **43**:1906, 1979.
13. Rozen P, Baratz M: Familial juvenile colonic polyposis with associated colon cancer. *Cancer* **49**:1500, 1982.
14. Ramaswamy G, Elhosseiny AA, Tchertkoff V: Juvenile polyposis of the colon with atypical adenomatous changes and carcinoma in situ. *Dis Colon Rectum* **27**:393, 1984.
15. Jarvinen HJ, Franssila KO: Familial juvenile polyposis coli: Increased risk of colorectal cancer. *Gut* **25**:792, 1984.
16. Baptist SJ, Sabatini MT: Coexisting juvenile polyps and tubulovillous adenoma of colon with carcinoma in situ: Report of a case. *Hum Pathol* **16**:1061, 1985.
17. Jones MA, Hebert JC, Trainer TD: Juvenile polyp with intramucosal carcinoma. *Arch Path Lab Med* **111**:200, 1987.
18. Bentley E, Chandrasoma P, Radin R, Cohen H: Generalized juvenile polyposis with carcinoma. *Am J Gastroenterol* **84**:1456, 1989.
19. Scott-Conner CEH, Hausmann M, Hall TJ, Skelton DS, Anglin BL, Subramony C: Familial juvenile polyposis: Patterns of recurrence and implications for surgical management. *J Am Coll Surg* **181**:407, 1995.
20. Yoshida T, Haraguchi Y, Tanaka A, Higa A, Daimon Y, Mizuta Y, Tamaki M, et al: A case of generalized juvenile gastrointestinal polyposis associated with gastric carcinoma. *Endoscopy* **20**:33, 1988.
21. Walpole IR, Cullity G: Juvenile polyposis: A case with early presentation and death attributable to adenocarcinoma of the pancreas. *Am J Med Genet* **32**:1, 1989.
22. Jass JR: Juvenile polyposis, in Phillips RKS, Spigelman AD, Thomson JPS (eds). *Familial Adenomatous Polyposis and Other Polyposis Syndromes*. London: Edward Arnold, 1994, p 203.
23. Howe JR, Mitros FA, Summers RW: The risk of gastrointestinal carcinoma in familial juvenile polyposis. *Ann Surg Oncol* **5**:751, 1998.
24. Jacoby RF, Schlack S, Sekhon G, Laxova R: Del(10)(q22.3q24.1) associated with juvenile polyposis. *Am J Med Genet* **70**:361, 1997.
25. Jacoby RF, Schlack S, Cole CE, Skarbek M, Harris C, Meisner LF: A juvenile polyposis tumor suppressor locus at 10q22 is deleted from nonepithelial cells in the lamina propria. *Gastroenterology* **112**:1398, 1997.
26. Howe JR, Ringold JC, Summers RW, Mitros FA, Nishimura DY, Stone EM: A gene for familial juvenile polyposis maps to chromosome 18q21.1. *Am J Hum Genet* **62**:1129, 1998.
27. Olschwang S, Serova-Sinilnikova OM, Lenoir GM, Thomas G: PTEN germ-line mutations in juvenile polyposis coli. *Nat Genet* **18**:12, 1998.
28. Howe JR, Roth S, Ringold JC, Summers RW, Jarvinen HJ, Sistonen P, Tomlinson IPM, et al: Mutations in the SMAD4/DPC4 gene in juvenile polyposis. *Science* **280**:1086, 1998.
29. Toccalino H, Guastavino E, De Pinni F, O'Donnell JC, Williams M: Juvenile polyps of the rectum and colon. *Acta Paediatr* **62**:337, 1973.
30. Sulser H, Deyhle P, Clavadetscher P, Ammann P: Juvenile dickdarmschleimhautpolypen bei erwachsenen. *Schweiz Med Wschr* **106**:107, 1976.
31. Restrepo C, Correa P, Duque E, Cuello C: Polyps in a low-risk colonic cancer population in Colombia, South America. *Dis Colon Rectum* **24**:29, 1981.
32. Restrepo C, Moreno J, Duque E, Cuello C, Amsel J, Correa P: Juvenile colonic polyposis in Colombia. *Dis Colon Rectum* **21**:600, 1978.
33. Williams AO, Prince DL: Intestinal polyps in the Nigerian African. *J Clin Pathol* **28**:367, 1975.
34. Burt RW, Bishop DT, Lynch HT, Rozen P, Winawer SJ: Risk and Surveillance of individuals with heritable factors for colorectal cancer. *Bull WHO* **68**:655, 1993.
35. Chevrel J-P, Amouroux J, Gueraud J-P: Trois cas familiaux de polypose juvenile. *Chirurgie* **101**:708, 1975.
36. Jass JR, Williams CB, Bussey HJR, Morson BC: Juvenile polyposis—A precancerous condition. *Histopathology* **13**:619, 1988.
37. Gentry WC Jr, Eskritt NR, Gorlin RJ: Multiple hamartoma syndrome (Cowden disease). *Arch Dermatol* **109**:521, 1974.
38. Nelen MR, Padberg GW, Peeters EAJ, Lin AY, van den Helm B, Frants RR, Coulon V, et al: Localization of the gene for Cowden disease to chromosome 10q22-23. *Nat Genet* **13**:114, 1996.
39. Liaw D, Marsh DL, Li J, Dahia PLM, Wang SI, Zheng Z, Bose S, et al: Germ line mutations of the PTEN gene in Cowden disease, an inherited breast and thyroid cancer syndrome. *Nat Genet* **16**:64, 1997.

40. Marsh DJ, Dahia PLM, Zheng Z, Liaw D, Parsons R, Gorlin RJ, Eng C: Germline mutations in PTEN are present in Bannayan-Zonana syndrome. *Nat Genet* **16**:333, 1997.
41. Gorlin RJ: Nevoid basal-cell carcinoma syndrome. *Medicine (Baltimore)* **66**:98, 1987.
42. Evans DG, Ladusans EJ, Rimmer S, Burnell LD, Thakker N, Farndon PA: Complications of the naevoid basal cell carcinoma syndrome: Results of a population-based study. *J Med Genet* **30**:460, 1993.
43. Shanley S, Ratcliffe J, Hockey A, Haan E, Oley C, Ravine D, Martin N, et al: Nevoid basal cell carcinoma syndrome: Review of 118 affected individuals. *Am J Med Genet* **50**:282, 1994.
44. Scully RE, Galdabini JJ, McNeely BU: Case records of the Massachusetts General Hospital. Weekly clinicopathological exercises. Case 14-1976. *N Engl J Med* **294**:772, 1976.
45. Schwartz RA: Basal-cell-nevus syndrome and gastrointestinal polyposis. *N Engl J Med* **299**:49, 1978.
46. Farndon PA, Del Mastro RG, Evans DG, Kilpatrick MW: Location of gene for Gorlin syndrome. *Lancet* **339**:581, 1992.
47. Hahn H, Wicking C, Zaphiropoulous PG, Gailani MR, Shanley S, Chidambaram A, Vorechovsky I, et al: Mutations of the human homolog of *Drosophila* patched in the nevoid basal cell carcinoma syndrome. *Cell* **85**:841, 1996.
48. Johnson RL, Rothman AL, Xie J, Goodrich LV, Bare JW, Bonifas JM, Quinn AG, et al: Human homolog of patched, a candidate gene for the basal cell nevus syndrome. *Science* **272**:1668, 1996.
49. Whitelaw SC, Murday VA, Tomlinson IPM, Thomas HJW, Cottrell SE, Ginsberg A, Bukofzer S, et al: Clinical and molecular features of the hereditary mixed polyposis syndrome. *Gastroenterology* **112**:327, 1997.
50. Thomas HJW, Whitelaw SC, Cottrell SE, Murday VA, Tomlinson IPM, Markie D, Jones T, et al: Genetic mapping of the hereditary mixed polyposis syndrome to chromosome 6q. *Am J Hum Genet* **58**:770, 1996.
51. Burke AP, Sobin LH: The pathology of Cronkhite-Canada polyps. A comparison to juvenile polyposis. *Am J Surg Pathol* **13**:940, 1989.
52. Cronkhite LW, Canada WJ: Generalized gastrointestinal polyposis: an unusual syndrome of polyposis, pigmentation, alopecia, and onychatrophia. *N Engl J Med* **252**:1011, 1955.
53. Daniel ES, Ludwig SL, Lewin KJ, Ruprecht RM, Rajacich GM, Schwabe AD: The Cronkhite-Canada syndrome. An analysis of clinical and pathologic features and therapy in 55 patients. *Medicine (Baltimore)* **61**:293, 1982.
54. Spigelman AD, Phillips RKS: Peutz-Jeghers syndrome, in Phillips RKS, Spigelman AD, Thomson JPS (eds). *Familial Adenomatous Polyposis and Other Polyposis Syndromes*. London: Edward Arnold, 1994, p 188.
55. Hemminki A, Tomlinson I, Markie D, Jarvinen H, Sistonen P, Bjorkqvist AM, Knuutila S, et al: Localization of a susceptibility locus for Peutz-Jeghers syndrome to 19p using comparative genomic hybridization and targeted linkage analysis. *Nat Genet* **15**:87, 1997.
56. Hemminki A, Markie D, Tomlinson I, Avizienyte E, Roth S, Loukola A, Bignell G, et al: A serine/threonine kinase gene defective in Peutz-Jeghers syndrome. *Nature* **391**:184, 1998.
57. Sachatello CR, Hahn IL, Carrington CB: Juvenile gastrointestinal polyposis in a female infant: Report of a case and review of the literature of a recently recognized syndrome. *Surgery* **75**:107, 1974.
58. Hizawa K, Iida M, Yao T, Aoyagi K, Fujishima M: Juvenile polyposis of the stomach: Clinicopathological features and its malignant potential. *J Clin Pathol* **50**:771, 1997.
59. Soper RT, Kent TH: Fatal juvenile polyposis of infancy. *Surgery* **69**:692, 1971.
60. Gourley GR, Odell GB, Selkurt J, Morrissey J, Gilbert E: Juvenile polyps associated with protein-losing enteropathy. *Dig Dis Sci* **27**:941, 1982.
61. Ray JE, Heald RJ: Growing up with juvenile gastrointestinal polyposis: report of a case. *Dis Colon Rectum* **14**:375, 1971.
62. Donnelly WH, Sieber WK, Yunis EJ: Polypoid ganglioneurofibromatosis of the large bowel. *Arch Pathol* **87**:537, 1969.
63. Weidner N, Flanders DJ, Mitros FA: Mucosal ganglioneuromatosis associated with multiple colonic polyps. *Am J Surg Pathol* **8**:779, 1984.
64. Pham BN, Villanueva RP: Ganglioneuromatous proliferation associated with juvenile polyposis coli. *Arch Path Lab Med* **113**:91, 1989.
65. Mendelsohn G, Diamond MP: Familial ganglioneuromatous polyposis of the large bowel. Report of a family with associated juvenile polyposis. *Am J Surg Pathol* **8**:515, 1984.
66. Cox KL, Frates RC Jr, Wong A, Gandhi G: Hereditary generalized juvenile polyposis associated with pulmonary arteriovenous malformation. *Gastroenterology* **78**:1566, 1980.
67. Conte WJ, Rotter JI, Schwartz AG, Congleton JE: Hereditary generalized juvenile polyposis, arteriovenous malformations and colonic carcinoma. *Clin Res* **30**:93A, 1982.
68. Baert AL, Casteels-Van Daele M, Broeckx J, Wijndaele L, Wilms G, Eggermont E: Generalized juvenile polyposis with pulmonary arteriovenous malformations and hypertrophic osteoarthropathy. *AJR Am J Roentgenol* **141**:661, 1983.
69. Longo WE, Touloukian RJ, West B, Ballantyne GH: Malignant potential of juvenile polyposis coli. *Dis Colon Rectum* **33**:980, 1990.
70. Simpson EL, Dalinka MK: Association of hypertrophic osteoarthropathy with gastrointestinal polyposis. *AJR Am J Roentgenol* **144**:983, 1985.
71. McAllister KA, Lennon F, Bowles-Biesecker B, McKinnon WC, Helmbold EA, Markel DS, Jackson CE, et al: Genetic heterogeneity in hereditary haemorrhagic telangiectasia: possible correlation with clinical phenotype. *J Med Genet* **31**:927, 1994.
72. McAllister KA, Grogg KM, Johnson DW, Gallione CJ, Baldwin MA, Jackson CE, Helmbold EA, et al: Endoglin, a TGF-beta binding protein of endothelial cells, is the gene for hereditary haemorrhagic telangiectasia type 1. *Nat Genet* **8**:345, 1994.
73. Johnson DW, Berg JN, Baldwin MA, Gallione CJ, Marondel I, Yoon S-J, Stenzel TT, et al: Mutations in the activin receptor-like kinase I gene in hereditary haemorrhagic telangiectasia type 2. *Nat Genet* **13**:189, 1996.
74. Hofting I, Pott G, Stolte M: Das Syndrom der Juvenilen Polyposis. *Leber Magen Darm* **23**:107, 1993.
75. Coburn MC, Pricolo VE, DeLuca FG, Bland KI: Malignant potential in intestinal juvenile polyposis syndromes. *Ann Surg Oncol* **2**:386, 1995.
76. Bussey HJR, Veale AMO, Morson BC: Genetics of gastrointestinal polyposis. *Gastroenterology* **74**:1325, 1978.
77. Lipper S, Kahn LB, Sandler RS, Varma V: Multiple juvenile polyposis: A study of the pathogenesis of juvenile polyps and their relationship to colonic adenomas. *Hum Pathol* **12**:804, 1981.
78. Jarvinen HJ: Juvenile gastrointestinal polyposis. *Probl Gen Surg* **10**:749, 1993.
79. Watanabe A, Nagashima H, Motoi M, Ogawa K: Familial juvenile polyposis of the stomach. *Gastroenterology* **77**:148, 1979.
80. Desai DC, Murday V, Phillips RKS, Neale KF, Milla P, Hodgson SV: A survey of phenotypic features in juvenile polyposis. *J Med Genet* **35**:476, 1998.
81. Mestre JR: The changing pattern of juvenile polyps. *Am J Gastroenterol* **81**:312, 1986.
82. Jass JR: Pathology of polyposis syndromes with special reference to juvenile polyposis, in Utsunomiya J, Lynch HT (eds). *Hereditary Colorectal Cancer*. Tokyo: Springer-Verlag, 1990, p 343.
83. Mitros FA: Personal communication. Sept 1, 1998.
84. Franzin G, Zamboni G, Dina R, Scarpa A, Fratton A: Juvenile and inflammatory polyps of the colon-a histological and histochemical study. *Histopathology* **7**:719, 1983.
85. Knudson AG Jr, Hethcote HW, Brown BW: Mutation and childhood cancer: A probabilistic model for the incidence of retinoblastoma. *Proc Natl Acad Sci U S A* **72**:5116, 1975.
86. Subramony C, Scott-Conner CEH, Skelton D, Hall TJ: Familial juvenile polyposis. Study of a kindred: Evolution of polyps and relationship to gastrointestinal carcinoma. *Am J Clin Pathol* **102**:91, 1994.
87. Giardiello FM, Hamilton SR, Kern SE, Offerhaus GJA, Green PA, Celano P, Krush AJ, et al: Colorectal neoplasia in juvenile polyposis or juvenile polyps. *Arch Dis Child* **66**:971, 1991.
88. Grigioni WF, Alampi G, Martinelli G, Piccaluga A: Atypical juvenile polyposis. *Histopathology* **5**:361, 1981.
89. Kinzler KW, Vogelstein B: Landscaping the cancer terrain. *Science* **280**:1036, 1998.
90. Grotsky HW, Rickert RR, Smith WD, Newsome JF: Familial juvenile polyposis coli: A clinical and pathologic study of a large kindred. *Gastroenterology* **82**:494, 1982.
91. Sassatelli R, Bertoni G, Serra L, Bedogni G, Ponz de Leon M: Generalized juvenile polyposis with mixed pattern and gastric cancer. *Gastroenterology* **104**:910, 1993.
92. Hofting I, Pott G, Schrameyer B, Stolte M: Familiare juvenile polyposis mit vorwiegender magenbeteiligung. *Z Gastroenterol* **31**:480, 1993.
93. Sharma AK, Sharma SS, Mathur P: Familial juvenile polyposis with adenomatous-carcinomatous change. *J Gastroenterol Hepatol* **10**:131, 1995.
94. Howe JR, Ringold JC, Hughes J, Summers RW: Direct genetic testing for *SMAD4* mutations in patients at risk for juvenile polyposis. In preparation. *Surgery* **126**:162, 1999.

95. Leggett BA, Thomas LR, Knight N, Healey S, Chenevix-Trench G, Searle J: Exclusion of APC and MCC as the gene defect in one family with familial juvenile polyposis. *Gastroenterology* **105**:1313, 1993.
96. Fearon ER, Cho KR, Nigro JM, Kern SE, Simons JW, Ruppert JM, Hamilton SR, et al: Identification of a chromosome 18q gene that is altered in colorectal cancers. *Science* **247**:49, 1990.
97. Hahn SA, Shutte M, Shamsul Hoque ATM, Moskaluk CA, da Costa LT, Rozenblum E, Weinstein CL, et al: DPC4, a candidate tumor suppressor gene at human chromosome 18q21.1. *Science* **271**:350, 1996.
98. Hahn SA, Shamsul Hoque ATM, Moskaluk CA, da Costa LT, Scutte M, Rozenblum E, Seymour AB, et al: Homozygous deletion map at 18q21.1 in pancreatic cancer. *Cancer Res* **56**:490, 1996.
99. Li J, Yen C, Liaw D, Podsypanina K, Bose S, Wang SI, Puc J, et al: PTEN, a putative protein tyrosine phosphatase gene mutated in human brain, breast, and prostate cancer. *Science* **275**:1943, 1997.
100. Steck PA, Pershouse MA, Jasser SA, Yung WK, Lin H, Ligon AH, Langford LA, et al: Identification of a candidate tumour suppressor gene, MMAC1, at chromosome 10q23.3 that is mutated in multiple advanced cancers. *Nat Genet* **15**:356, 1997.
101. Lynch ED, Ostermeyer EA, Lee MK, Arena JF, Ji H, Dann JKS, et al: Inherited mutations in PTEN that are associated with breast cancer, Cowden disease, and juvenile polyposis. *Am J Hum Genet* **61**:1254, 1997.
102. Eng C, Ji H: Molecular classification of the inherited hamartoma polyposis syndromes: Clearing the muddied waters. *Am J Hum Genet* **62**:1020, 1998.
103. Riggins GJ, Hamilton SR, Kinzler KW, Vogelstein B: Normal PTEN gene in juvenile polyposis. *NOGO* **1**:1, 1997.
104. Marsh DJ, Roth S, Lunetta KL, Hemminki A, Dahia PLM, Sistonen P, Zheng Z, et al: Exclusion of PTEN and 10q22-24 as the susceptibility locus for juvenile polyposis syndrome. *Cancer Res* **57**:5017, 1997.
105. Marsh DJ, Coulon V, Lunetta KL, Rocca-Serra P, Dahia PL, Zheng Z, Liaw D, et al: Mutation spectrum and genotype-phenotype analyses in Cowden disease and Bannayan-Zonana syndrome, two hamartoma syndromes with germline PTEN mutation. *Hum Mol Genet* **7**:507, 1998.
106. Howe JR, Wagner B, Amos C, Ringold JC, Roth S, Aaltonen LA: Haplotype analysis of a common Smad4 exon 9 deletion in juvenile polyposis families. In preparation.
107. Houlston R, Bevan S, Williams A, et al: Mutations in DPC4 (*Smad4*) cause juvenile polyposis syndrome, but only account for a minority of cases. *Hum Mol Genet* **7**:1907, 1998.
108. Derynck R, Gelbart WM, Harland RM, Heldin CH, Kern SE, Massague J, Melton DA, et al: Nomenclature: vertebrate mediators of TGF-β family signals. *Cell* **87**:173, 1996.
109. Thiagalingam S, Lebauer C, Leach FS, Schutte M, Hahn SA, Overhauser J, Willson SA, et al: Evaluation of candidate tumour suppressor genes on chromosome 18 in colorectal cancers. *Nat Genet* **13**:343, 1996.
110. Takagi Y, Kohmura H, Futamura M, Kida H, Tanemura H, Shimokawa K, Saji S: Somatic alterations of the DPC4 gene in human colorectal cancers in vivo. *Gastroenterology* **111**:1369, 1996.
111. MacGrogan D, Pegram M, Slamon D, Bookstein R: Comparative mutational analysis of DPC4(Smad4) in prostatic and colorectal carcinomas. *Oncogene* **15**:1111, 1997.
112. Hoque ATMS, Hahn SA, Schutte M, Kern SE: DPC4 gene mutation in colitis associated neoplasia. *Gut* **40**:120, 1997.
113. Lei P, Zou T-T, Shi Y-Q, Zhou X, Smolinski KN, Yin J, Souza RF, et al: Infrequent DPC4 gene mutation in esophageal cancer, gastric cancer and ulcerative colitis-associated neoplasms. *Oncogene* **13**:2459, 1996.
114. Powell SM, Harper JC, Hamilton SR, Robinson CR, Cummings OW: Inactivation of Smad4 in gastric carcinomas. *Cancer Res* **57**:4221, 1997.
115. Hahn SA, Bartsch D, Schroers A, Galehdari H, Becker M, Ramaswamy A, Schwarte-Waldhoff I, et al: Mutations of the DPC4/Smad4 gene in biliary tract carcinoma. *Cancer Res* **58**:1124, 1998.
116. Moskaluk CA, Hruban RA, Schutte M, Lietman AS, Smyrk T, Fusaro L, Fusaro R, et al: Genomic sequencing of DPC4 in the analysis of familial pancreatic cancer. *Diagn Mol Pathol* **6**:85, 1997.
117. Schutte M, Hruban RH, Hedrick L, Cho KR, Nadasdy GM, Weinstein CL, Bova GS, et al: DPC4 in various tumor types. *Cancer Res* **56**:2527, 1996.
118. Kim SK, Fan Y, Papadimitrakopoulou V, Clayman G, Hittelman WN, Hong WK, Lotan R, et al: DPC4, a candidate tumor suppressor gene, is altered infrequently in head and neck squamous cell carcinoma. *Cancer Res* **56**:2519, 1996.
119. Massague J: TGFβ signaling: Receptors, transducers, and Mad proteins. *Cell* **85**:947, 1996.
120. Heldin C-H, Miyazono K, Ten Dijke P: TGFβ signaling from cell membrane to nucleus through SMAD proteins. *Nature* **390**:465, 1997.
121. Wrana JL, Attisano L, Wieser R, Ventura F, Massague J: Mechanism of activation of the TGF-beta receptor. *Nature* **370**:341, 1994.
122. Shi Y, Hata A, Lo RS, Massague J, Pavletich NP: A structural basis for mutational inactivation of the tumor suppressor Smad4. *Nature* **388**:87, 1997.
123. Kawabata M, Inoue H, Hanyu A, Imamura T, Miyazono K: Smad protein exist as monomers in vivo and undergo homo- and hetero-oligomerization upon activation by serine/threonine kinase receptors. *EMBO J* **17**:4056, 1998.
124. Liu F, Pouponnot C, Massague J: Dual role of the Smad4/DPC4 tumor suppressor in TGF-β-inducible transcriptional complexes. *Genes Dev* **11**:3157, 1997.
125. Yingling JM, Datto MB, Wong C, Frederick JP, Liberati NT, Wang XF: Tumor suppressor Smad4 is a transforming growth factor beta-inducible DNA binding protein. *Mol Cell Biol* **17**:7019, 1997.
126. Zawel L, Dai JL, Buckhaults P, Zhou S, Kinzler KW, Vogelstein B, Kern SE: Human Smad3 and Smad4 are sequence-specific transcription activators. *Mol Cell* **1**:611, 1998.
127. Dennler S, Itoh S, Vivien D, ten Dijke P, Huet S, Gauthier JM: Direct binding of Smad3 and Smad4 to critical TGF beta-inducible elements in the promoter of human plasminogen activator inhibitor-type 1 gene. *EMBO J* **17**:3091, 1998.
128. Zhou S, Zawel L, Lengauer C, Kinzler KW, Vogelstein B: Characterization of human FAST-1, a TGF-β and activin signal transducer. *Mol Cell* **2**:121, 1998.
129. Chen X, Weisberg E, Fridmacher V, Watanabe M, Naco G, Whitman M: Smad4 and FAST-1 in the assembly of activin-responsive factor. *Nature* **389**:85, 1997.
130. Wu RY, Zhang Y, Feng XH, Derynck R: Heteromeric and homomeric interactions correlate with signaling activity and functional cooperativity of Smad3 and Smad4/DPC4. *Mol Cell Biol* **17**:2521, 1997.
131. Lagna G, Hata A, Hemmati-Brivanlou A, Massague J: Partnership between DPC4 and SMAD proteins in TGF-β signaling pathways. *Nature* **383**:832, 1996.
132. Zhou S, Buckhaults P, Zawel L, Bunz F, Riggins G, Le Dai J, Kern SE, et al: Targeted deletion of Smad4 shows it is required for transforming growth factor beta and activin signaling in colorectal cancer cells. *Proc Natl Acad Sci U S A* **95**:2412, 1998.
133. Sirard C, de la Pompa JL, Elia A, Itie A, Mirtsos C, Cheung A, Hahn S, et al: The tumor suppressor gene Smad4/Dpc4 is required for gastrulation and later for anterior development of the mouse embryo. *Genes Dev* **12**:107, 1998.
134. Yang X, Li C, Xu X, Deng C: The tumor suppressor SMAD4/DPC4 is essential for epiblast proliferation and mesoderm induction in mice. *Proc Natl Acad Sci U S A* **95**:3667, 1998.
135. Takaku K, Oshima M, Miyoshi H, Matsui M, Seldin MF, Taketo MM: Intestinal tumorigenesis in compound mutant mice of both DPC4 (Smad4) and APC genes. *Cell* **92**:645, 1998.
136. Markowitz S, Wang J, Myerhoff L, Parsons R, Sun L, Lutterbaugh J, Fan RS, et al: Inactivation of the type II TGF-β receptor in colon cancer cells with microsatellite instability. *Science* **268**:1336, 1995.
137. Parsons R, Myeroff LL, Liu B, Willson JKV, Markowitz SD, Kinzler KW, Vogelstein B: Microsatellite instability and mutations of the transforming growth factor β type II receptor gene in colorectal cancer. *Cancer Res* **55**:5548, 1995.
138. Samowitz WS, Slattery ML: Transforming growth factor-β receptor type 2 mutations and microsatellite instability in sporadic colorectal adenomas and carcinomas. *Am J Pathol* **151**:33, 1997.
139. Wang J, Sun L, Myeroff L, Wang X, Gentry LE, Yang J, Liang J, et al: Demonstration that mutation of the type II transforming growth factor beta receptor inactivates its tumor suppressor activity in replication error-positive colon carcinoma cells. *J Biol Chem* **270**:22044, 1995.
140. Lu S-L, Kawabata M, Imamura T, Akiyama Y, Nomizu T, Miyazono K, Yuasa Y: HNPCC associated with germline mutation in the TGF-β type II receptor gene. *Nat Genet* **19**:17, 1998.
141. Nakao A, Roijer E, Imamura T, Souchelnytskyi S, Stenman G, Heldin C-H, ten Dijke P: Identification of Smad2, a human Mad-related protein in the transforming growth factor-beta signaling pathway. *J Biol Chem* **272**:2896, 1997.
142. Eppert K, Scherer SW, Ozcelik H, Pirone R, Hoodless P, Kim H, Tsui L-C, et al: MADR2 maps to 18q21 and encodes a TGFB-regulated

MAD-related protein that is functionally mutated in colorectal carcinoma. *Cell* **86**:543, 1996.

143. Riggins GJ, Thiagalingam S, Rozenblum E, Weinstein CL, Kern SE, Hamilton SR, Willson JKV, et al: Mad-related genes in the human. *Nature Genet* **13**:347, 1996.
144. Arai T, Akiyama Y, Okabe S, Ando M, Endo M, Yuasa Y: Genomic structure of the human Smad3 gene and its infrequent alterations in colorectal cancers. *Cancer Lett* **122**:157, 1998.
145. Riggins GJ, Kinzler KW, Vogelstein B, Thiagalingam S: Frequency of Smad gene mutations in human cancers. *Cancer Res* **57**:2578, 1997.
146. Hayashi H, Abdollah S, Qiu Y, Cai J, Xu Y-Y, Grinnell BW, Richardson MA, et al: The MAD-related protein Smad7 associates with the TGF-β receptor and functions as an antagonist of TGF-β signaling. *Cell* **89**:1165, 1997.
147. Petersen GM, Boyd PA: Gene tests and counseling for colorectal cancer risk: Lessons from familial polyposis. *Monogr Natl Cancer Inst* **17**:67, 1995.
148. Lynch HT, Smyrk T, Lynch J: An update of HNPCC (Lynch syndrome). *Cancer Genet Cytogenet* **93**:84, 1997.
149. Pelias MZ: Duty to disclose in medical genetics: A legal perspective. *Am J Med Genet* **39**:347, 1991.
150. Whitelaw S, Northover JM, Hodgson SV: Attitudes to predictive DNA testing in familial adenomatous polyposis. *J Med Genet* **33**:540, 1996.

Retinoblastoma

Irene F. Newsham ▪ Theodora Hadjistilianou
Webster K. Cavenee

1. **Retinoblastoma is the most common intraocular malignancy in children, with a worldwide incidence between 1 in 13,500 and 1 in 25,000 live births. The presenting signs and symptoms include leukokoria, strabismus, low-vision orbital cellulitis, unilateral mydriasis, and heterochromia. The disease can be unifocal or multifocal and unilateral or bilateral. The average age of diagnosis is 12 months for bilateral and 18 months for unilateral cases, and 90 percent of affected individuals are diagnosed before age 3 years. Unusual manifestations of this disease include late onset retinoblastoma, 13q-deletion syndrome, retinoma, trilateral retinoblastoma, and second-site primary tumors, including osteosarcoma, Ewing sarcoma, leukemia, and lymphoma.**
2. **Early diagnosis and treatment are of primary importance in the survival of retinoblastoma patients. A variety of diagnostic approaches are used, including computed tomography (CT), magnetic resonance imaging (MRI), ultrasonography, and fine-needle aspiration biopsy (FNAB). Each has advantages, and when used in combination, they can establish the proper disease classification. Effective methods for the treatment of retinoblastoma tumors include enucleation, external-beam irradiation, episcleral plaques, xenon arc and argon laser photocoagulation, cryotherapy, and chemotherapy. The choice of treatment depends on several factors, such as multifocal or unifocal disease, site and size of the tumor, diffuse or focal vitreous seeding, age at diagnosis, and histopathologic findings.**
3. **Retinoblastoma has served as the prototypic example of a genetic predisposition to cancer. It is estimated that 60 percent of cases are nonhereditary and unilateral, 15 percent are hereditary and unilateral, and 25 percent are hereditary and bilateral. A model encompassing these findings suggests a requirement for as few as two stochastic mutational events for tumor formation. The first of these events can be inherited through the germ line or can be somatically acquired, whereas the second occurs somatically in either case and leads to a tumor that is doubly defective at the retinoblastoma locus. Cytogenetic analyses have demonstrated the involvement of a genetic alteration in a gene for negative growth regulation at chromosome band 13q14. This model has been tested and confirmed using restriction-fragment-length polymorphisms (RFLP) for loci on chromosome 13. These studies have shown that the second wild-type retinoblastoma allele may be lost by several somatic mutational mechanisms, including mitotic nondisjunction with loss of the wild-type chromosome, mitotic nondisjunction with duplication of the mutant chromosome, mitotic recombination between the RB1 locus and the centromere, and other regionalized events, such as deletion and point mutation.**
4. **The 200-kb genomic locus for RB1 has been isolated, and its exon/intron structure has been characterized. Current molecular technology has allowed the identification of a variety of aberrations in this locus in retinoblastoma patients and their tumors at the DNA, RNA, and protein levels. RB1 alterations also have been detected in a variety of clinically related second-site primary tumors and nonrelated tumors, including osteosarcoma, breast carcinoma, and small-cell lung carcinoma. The ability to detect mutations in RB1 coupled with the isolation of polymorphic sequences within the gene locus, has further extended the prenatal risk assessment for this pediatric tumor.**
5. **The RB1 locus is transcribed into a 4.7-kb mRNA with a corresponding protein product of 110 kDa that is ubiquitously expressed in normal human and rat tissues, including brain, kidney, ovary, spleen, liver, placenta, and retina. The $p110^{RB}$ protein is differentially phosphorylated, and the unphosphorylated form is found predominantly in the G1 stage of the cell cycle, with an initial phosphorylation occurring at the G1/S boundary. This protein can be physically complexed with a number of viral and cellular proteins. SV40 large T antigen, adenovirus E1A protein, and papillomavirus E7 protein all contain conserved regions that are required for binding with the $p110^{RB}$ protein. The same regions appear to be necessary for the transforming function of the viral proteins.**
6. **Intracellular proteins whose function are mediated by the retinoblastoma protein have been isolated from complexes formed *in vitro* using pRB "pocket-binding" affinity chromatography columns against different cell lysates. Transcription factors DRTF and E2F have been isolated, and their physical and functional relationships to the retinoblastoma protein have been assessed. Other cellular proteins identified in these complexes include cyclin D1, p16, and the RB-like proteins p107 and p130. Interestingly, the complexing of these factors to $p110^{RB}$ has also been shown to oscillate in a cell cycle-dependent manner, thereby linking the tumor-suppressing function of the retinoblastoma protein with transcriptional regulation.**

CLINICAL ASPECTS AND TREATMENT OF RETINOBLASTOMA

Epidemiology

Retinoblastoma is the most common intraocular malignancy in children. In 1964, Francois[1] reported an incidence varying from 1 in 34,000 to 1 in 14,000 births and noted a steady increase in the frequency of occurrence of the tumor between 1927 and 1960. A number of studies support this finding and indicate a worldwide incidence of 1 in 3500 to 1 in 25,000, with no significant difference between the sexes or races.[2–9] An apparent mortality rate for blacks 2.5 times greater than that for whites has been reported, but seems to be attributable to delays in diagnosis rather than a higher disease incidence.[10] In general, there seems to be little correlation of disease incidence with geographic location. However, in some populations (e.g., Jamaicans, Nigerians, Haitians),[11] apparently higher incidence rates have been observed for what appears to be the unilateral sporadic form of retinoblastoma; this may suggest an environmental modification of the probability of tumor formation.[12]

Presenting Signs and Symptoms

Differential Diagnosis. In the majority of cases, the first sign at presentation is the characteristic cat's-eye reflex, which is usually noted by the child's parents or pediatrician. This white, pink-white, or yellow-white pupillary reflex, termed leukokoria, results from replacement of the vitreous by the tumor or by a tumor growing in the macula[13,14] (Fig. 36-1). Another common symptom, strabismus (exotropia or esotropia), can occur alone when small macular tumors interfere with vision, or can be associated with leukokoria. It is not uncommon to find after an accurate patient history is taken that strabismus occurred some months before leukokoria.

Less frequent presenting signs for retinoblastoma are red, painful eye with secondary glaucoma, low-vision orbital cellulitis, unilateral mydriasis, and heterochromia.[15] Sometimes the tumor can be difficult to differentiate from a variety of simulating lesions, such as persistent hyperplastic primary vitreous, retrolental fibroplasia, Coats disease, *toxocara canis* infection, retinal dysplasia, and chronic retinal detachment.[16,17] In 265 patients with pseudoretinoblastoma, persistent hyperplastic primary vitreous, followed by retrolental fibroplasia and posterior cataract, was the most common simulating condition.[18] Of 136 children with suspected retinoblastoma reported to the Ocular Oncology Service of the Wills Eye Hospital in Philadelphia between 1974 and 1978, 60 had retinoblastoma and 76 had simulating lesions, the most frequent being ocular toxocariasis (26 percent), persistent hyperplastic primary vitreous (20 percent), and Coats disease (16 percent). Despite these complications, most simulating lesions can be distinguished through modern diagnostic methods (described later in this chapter) or after a careful history of the family and the affected child.[16,17,19]

A complete workup for such a patient includes an ophthalmologic examination; a systemic, pediatric, and radiographic evaluation; and, more recently, genetic studies (Table 36-1).[17,19,20] At fundus examination, the disease can be unifocal or multifocal; in bilateral cases, usually one eye is in a more advanced stage, while the contralateral eye has one or more tumor foci (Fig. 36-1*B*). Furthermore, fundus examination of the first-degree relatives may also document the presence of a retinoma or a regressed retinoblastoma and indicate a potential hereditary basis for the tumor.

The average age at diagnosis is 12 months for bilateral retinoblastoma and 18 months for unilateral cases, with 90 percent of the patients diagnosed before age 3. Several factors may influence the time of diagnosis and therapy,[21,22] including (a) ignorance of the revealing signs, (b) difficulty in ophthalmoscopic examination

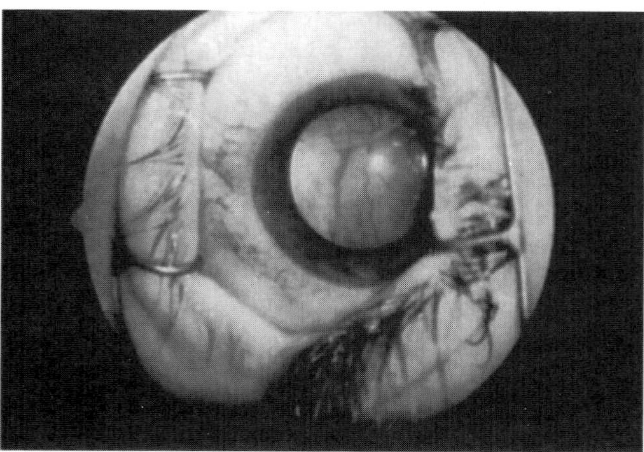

A

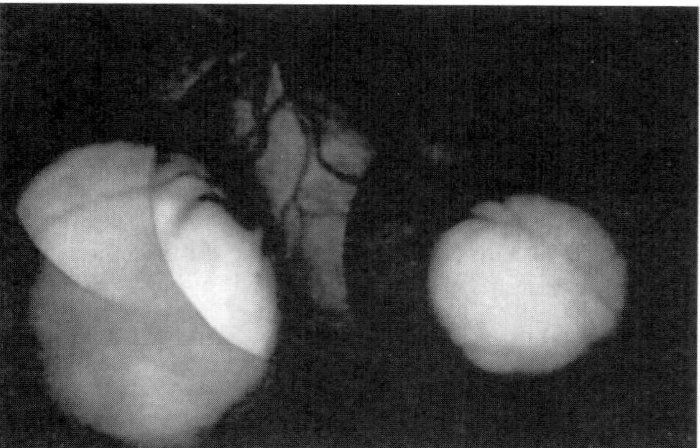

B

Fig. 36-1 Presenting signs of retinoblastoma. *A,* Leukokoria: exophytic retinoblastoma, overlying retinal detachment, clear lens, and visible retinal blood vessels. *B,* Multifocal retinoblastoma. (Courtesy of R. Frezzotti, MD, Director of the Institute of Ophthalmological Sciences, University of Siena, Italy.)

Table 36-1 Clinical and Laboratory Assessment for Retinoblastoma Patients

Ophthalmologic examination
Binocular indirect ophthalmoscopy with scleral indentation (child, parents, siblings, relatives)
Site and dimensions of the tumor(s)
Necrosis, calcification
Degree of vascularization, hemorrhage
Vitreous "seeding"
Retinal detachment
Fundus photography and drawing of the lesion(s)
Slit-lamp examination
Pseudohypopion, hyphema
Corneal and lens transparency
Rubeosis iris
Corneal diameter (buphthalmos)
Pupil, anisocoria
Tonometry
Ecography (calcification, biometry)
Aqueous and vitreous cytology and enzymology—fine-needle aspiration biopsy
Systemic examination
Radiographic examination
Skull x-ray
Computed tomography (orbits and brain with and without contrast enhancement)
Magnetic resonance imaging (orbits and brain)
Pediatric examination
Bone marrow biopsy
Lumbar puncture (cerebrospinal fluid examination)
Serologic tests (toxocara)
Neurologic evaluation
Electroencephalogram
Genetic studies
Esterase D
High-resolution chromosome analysis—karyotyping
DNA analysis of blood and tumor tissues

(age of the patient, level of transparency of the media, full mydriasis, and scleral indentation), (c) socioeconomic situation, (d) unusual clinical manifestations, and (e) multiple consultants.

Unusual Clinical Manifestations

Late Retinoblastoma. It is an exceptional instance when retinoblastoma presents after the age of 7, and the older the child, the more unusual the first signs of the disease. These unusual manifestations include orbital cellulitis and edema of the lids; hypopyon, hyphema, iris heterochromia, and keratitis (anterior segment); and vitreous opacification, retinal cysts, vitreous hemorrhage, and endophthalmitis (posterior segment).[23] Atypical uveitis in an older child, particularly if associated with secondary glaucoma and a poor response to corticosteroids, may be the first manifestation of a late retinoblastoma[24] (Fig. 36-2*A*). Repetitive diagnostic anterior chamber paracentesis may yield negative results.[23] Among 618 cases of retinoblastoma in older children, 41 (6.6 percent) were misdiagnosed as primary ocular inflammations.[25]

Sometimes retinoblastoma can resemble a panophthalmitis, which is frequently seen as a reaction to a necrotic uveal melanoma.[26] Pseudohypopyon as a result of retinoblastoma cells settled in the anterior chamber is another rare sign of the disease (Fig. 36-2*B*). A diffuse, infiltrating retinoblastoma can present with hypopyon or a severe anterior uveitis.[27,28] The term *diffuse infiltrated retinoblastoma* has been used to describe a form of the tumor in which no well-defined exophytic or endophytic mass is evident. This retinoblastoma pattern frequently produces aqueous and vitreous seeding, particularly in older children,[27,29–32] and seems to have a low potential for malignancy, although there is still controversy on this point.[27,28] Furthermore, cystic retinoblastoma, presumably a variant of the diffuse infiltrating type, tends to simulate uveitis and presents with clinically visible cysts.[33,34]

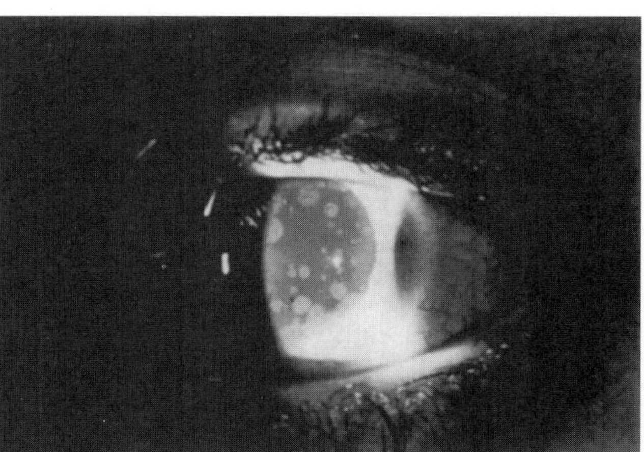

A

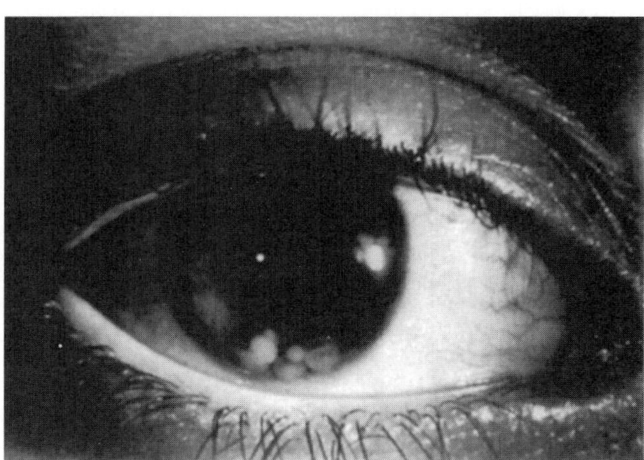

B

Fig. 36-2 Unusual manifestations of retinoblastoma. *A*, Pseudouveitis in retinoblastoma. *B*, Nodules at the pupillary margin and pseudohypopyon caused by a retinoblastoma. (Courtesy of R. Frezzotti, MD, Director of the Institute of Ophthalmological Sciences, University of Siena, Italy.)

Associated Clinical Abnormalities

13q-Deletion Syndrome. The 13q-deletion syndrome includes sporadic retinoblastoma in association with moderate growth and mental retardation, a broad, prominent, nasal bridge, a short nose, ear abnormalities, and muscular hypotonia.[35,36] Niebuhr and Ottosen also reported seven cases of retinoblastoma associated with systemic abnormalities (mental retardation, microcephaly, genital malformations, and ear abnormalities) in a review of 13q deletions and 13 ring chromosomes.[37] Such a karyotypic analysis prompted by the presentation of dysmorphic features can facilitate early detection of a deletion in the long arm of chromosome 13. Subsequent ophthalmoscopic examination can identify the retinoblastoma at an earlier stage.[38]

Retinoma. The term *retinoma* has been used to denote a benign tumor of retinocytic origin. Although the origins of this entity are obscure, it has been proposed that it arises from a mutation in the retinoblastoma susceptibility gene in a well-differentiated retinocyte and leads to a hyperplastic nodule of differentiated cells.[39] Retinomas are composed of apparently benign cells that show photoreceptor differentiation with no evidence of necrosis or mitotic activity, but with numerous rosettes.[40] Characteristically, retinomas have at least two of the following characteristics: irregular translucent retinal mass, calcification, and pigment epithelium migration and proliferation (Fig. 36-3*A*). Histopathologic and immunohistochemical studies suggest that retinomas are primary benign tumors, not regressed retinoblastomas. Malignant transformation of retinomas is quite rare, although some cases have been reported, notably a 7-year-old girl who developed an undifferentiated retinoblastoma 3 years after the diagnosis of a retinoma.[41,42]

Various physiological conditions (including reduced blood supply and necrosis, calcium [as an inhibitor of tumor growth], and host immune defense mechanisms) could be implicated in the spontaneous regression of retinoblastoma (Fig. 36-3*B*). Often, bulbi with intraocular calcification are the final physical embodiment of a spontaneously regressed retinoblastoma.[43] These phthisis bulbi can be attributed to tumor necrosis after ocular ischemia but cannot explain the retinoma, because the vascular supply in these lesions is intact.[44] On the basis of the available data, it appears that the term *regressed retinoblastoma* should be reserved to describe shrunken, calcified, phthisical eyes, whereas retinoma should be used to refer to nonprogressive retinal lesions that are highly associated with retinoblastoma but lack a malignant pattern.[45]

Trilateral Retinoblastoma. Bader and coauthors[46] coined the term *trilateral retinoblastoma* to describe the association between bilateral retinoblastoma and midline brain tumors, usually in the pineal region. Similar observations had been reported by Jensen and Miller[10] and Jakobiec et al.,[47] and had suggested that involvement of the pineal gland (third eye) represents a further point of origin for multicentric retinoblastoma rather than a second primary tumor.[48] In patients with hereditary retinoblastoma, both the pineal and the retina may contain susceptible cells. Because these pineal tumors may be indistinguishable from well-differentiated retinoblastomas, they are also called *ectopic retinoblastomas.*[46] It is possible that pineal tumors have been misinterpreted as intracranial spread of retinoblastoma,[49] whereas the advent of CT scanning and MRI has facilitated more accurate diagnoses. This is clinically important, because an ectopic intracranial retinoblastoma requires adequate therapy to the whole neuraxis,

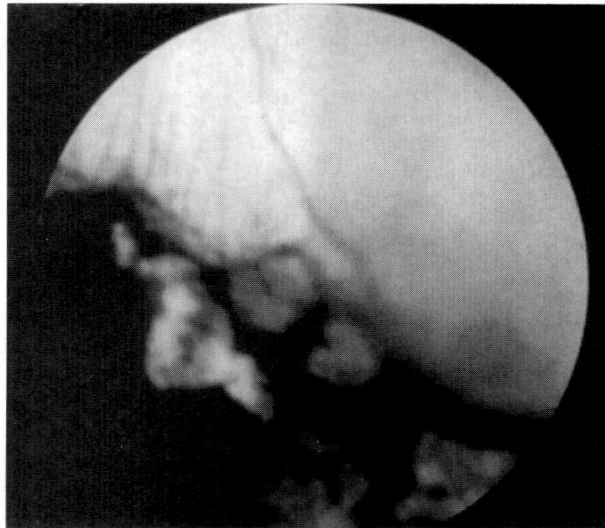

A

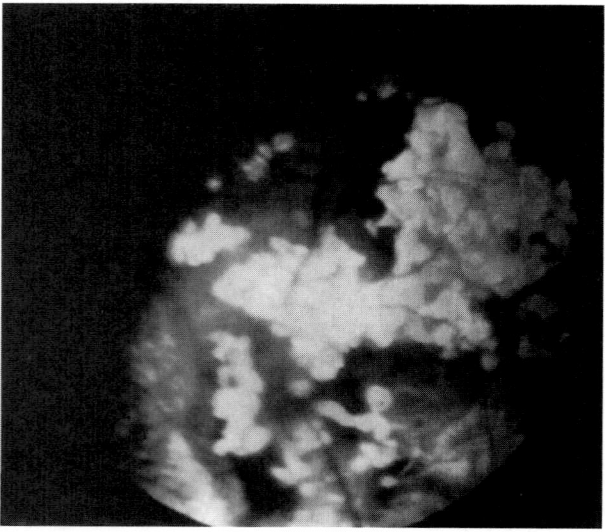

B

Fig. 36-3 Abnormalities associated with retinoblastoma. *A,* Retinoma: translucent retinal mass and pigment epithelium migration and proliferation. *B,* Spontaneously regressed retinoblastoma. (Courtesy of R. Frezzotti, MD, Director of the Institute of Ophthalmological Sciences, University of Siena, Italy.)

as well as high-dose equivalent radiotherapy to the primary tumor. Intrathecal therapy with methotrexate should also be considered.[50]

Second Malignant Tumors. The term *second site primary malignant tumor* refers to nonmetastatic tumors arising in disease-free patients successfully treated for the initial disease. Some of the tumors found in association with retinoblastoma include osteosarcoma, fibrosarcoma, chondrosarcoma, epithelial malignant tumors, Ewing sarcoma, leukemia, lymphoma, melanoma, brain tumors, and pinealoblastoma. These second tumors have been classified into five groups:[51] (a) tumors appearing in the irradiated area; (b) tumors appearing outside and remote from the irradiated area; (c) tumors in patients not receiving radiotherapy; (d) tumors that cannot be characterized as primary or metastases; and (e) tumors appearing in members of retinoblastoma families who are free of retinal tumors.

Reese, Merriam, and Martin[52] reported the first two cases of second tumors in 55 retinoblastoma patients treated with external radiation and surgery. These patients presented with a maxillary sinus sarcoma and a rhabdomyosarcoma of the temporal muscle. A similar case of mixed-cell fibrosarcoma has been reported by Frezzotti and Guerra.[53] A causal relationship between radiation therapy and secondary tumors has been suggested.[54–56] However, from the reported series of cases, two important observations have emerged: (a) The great majority of children in whom second neoplasms developed had suffered bilateral retinoblastoma, and (b) the incidence of second neoplasms in this group of children was similar whether or not they received radiation. These conclusions have been supported by studies that have reported the incidence of second nonocular tumors and analyzed the effect of radiation therapy. Osteogenic sarcomas have been the most common second-site neoplasms in all the published series. Derkinderen,[57] Lueder,[58] Draper,[59] and their colleagues found low rates of development of second tumors and are in agreement that the incidence increases with radiation therapy. Abramson *et al.* reported the incidence of second tumors in patients with hereditary retinoblastoma and found a frequency of 20 percent at 10 years, 50 percent at 20 years, and 90 percent at 30 years after diagnosis.[60] Somewhat lower rates have been recorded by other authors. For example, in a series of 215 bilateral retinoblastomas, second tumors developed in 4.4 percent of the patients during the first 10 years of follow-up, in 18.3 percent after 20 years, and in 26.1 percent after 30 years.[61]

Histopathology

Retinoblastoma occurs either as an intraocular mass between the choroid and the retina (exophytic) or as a bulge from the retina toward vitreous (endophytic). However, most of the advanced tumors examined showed both patterns of growth. Retinoblastoma rarely spreads superficially (1 percent), forming no mass and invading the whole retina (diffuse infiltrating retinoblastoma).

The tumor is histologically characterized by the presence of rosettes and fleurettes, which are believed to represent maturation and differentiation of the neoplastic cells. Rosettes are spherical structures (circular in section) constituted by uniform cuboidal or short columnar cells arranged in an orderly fashion around a small round lumen (Flexner-Wintersteiner rosette) or without any lumen (Homer-Right rosette). The latter type can often be found in other neuroectodermal tumors, such as medulloblastomas. Fleurettes are arranged in the opposite way, with short and thin stromal axes surrounded by fairly differentiated neoplastic cells with the apical part facing the externum, resembling the shape of a flower (Fig. 36-4*A*). Often the tumor appears highly necrotic, with the surviving cells positioned around blood vessels, creating structures called pseudorosettes. Calcified foci can be found in areas of necrosis, as can debris from nucleic acids, giving rise to basophilic vessel walls.[62,63]

A retinoblastoma tumor is capable of spreading outside the bulb through the eye coats, invading the choroid and the sclera. It is the invasion of this highly vascularized choroid that represents an effective vehicle for distant metastasis (Fig. 36-4*B*), and such choroid invasion is directly correlated with a poor prognosis. Invasion also can involve the optic nerve and meningeal space, providing access to the central nervous system. Growth patterns and other histologic parameters (such as pseudorosettes, necrosis, and calcification), although necessary for the identification of the tumor itself, do not seem to offer much information in regard to the prognosis. The degree of differentiation and the number of mitoses show a weak correlation with the prognosis; however, stronger relationships exist with invasion of the choroid and sclera. In particular, progressive invasion of the eye coats, even in the horizontal plane, is highly informative in determining the prognosis.[64,65]

Diagnosis

Because many of the symptoms described above are clearly not specific to retinoblastoma and because early surgical or conservative treatment is of primary importance in the survival of these patients, it is imperative to confirm these impressions by

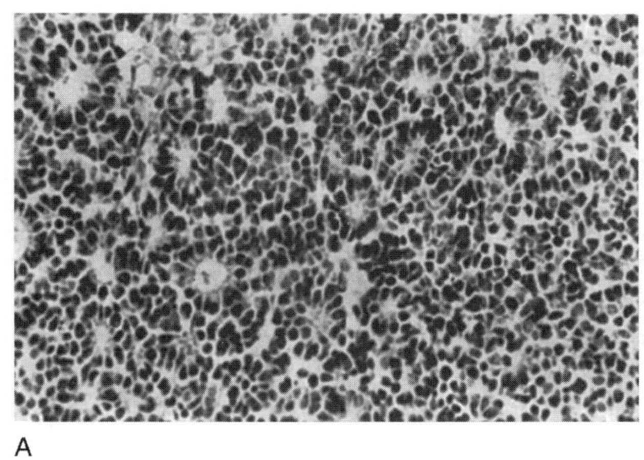

A

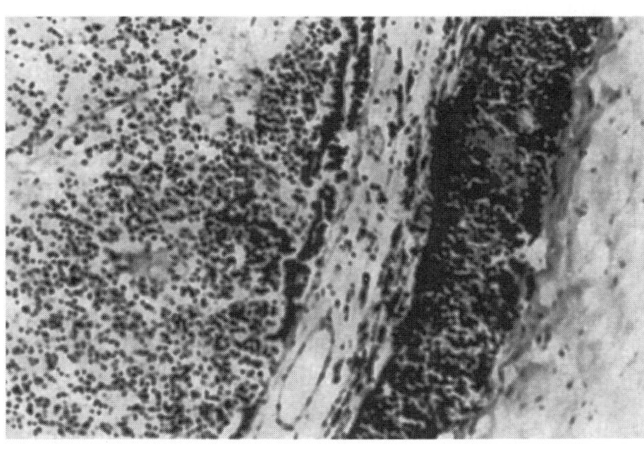

B

Fig. 36-4 Histopathology of retinoblastoma. *A,* A well-differentiated retinoblastoma showing rosettes and fleurettes (hematoxylin-eosin, 100). *B,* Low-differentiated retinoblastoma infiltrating the choroid and sclera (hematoxylin-eosin, 100). (Courtesy of P. Toti, MD, Institute of Anatomic Pathology, University of Siena, Italy.)

examination. There are a variety of diagnostic tools available for this, including CT, MRI, ultrasonography, and FNAB. The application and advantages of each procedure are briefly discussed below.

Computed Tomography and Magnetic Resonance Imaging. CT is a valuable adjunct in the differential diagnosis, staging, and treatment of retinoblastoma.[66,67] Intraocular calcification in children under 3 years of age is highly suggestive of a retinoblastoma. Some studies have reported that the degree of calcification appeared to depend on tumor size, with the smallest tumor showing calcification 8 mm in diameter and 4 mm in thickness[68,69] (Fig. 36-5*A*). However, in children more than 3 years of age confusion may arise from some simulating lesions, including retinal astrocytoma, retrolental fibroplasia, toxocariasis, and optic-nerve-head drusen, which can also produce calcifications.[68–70] Thus, CT is often coupled with MRI to better detect subtle scleral invasion, infiltrative spread along the optic nerve, subarachnoid seeding, or involvement of the central nervous system through direct tumor extension or by metastasis.[71] Furthermore, MRI appears to be more sensitive in the differential diagnosis of lesions simulating retinoblastoma[70,72,73] and in the evaluation of the degree of tumor differentiation.[74]

The role of both CT and MRI in staging and therapy is of great importance in accurately determining extraocular disease such as intracranial metastasis, retrobulbar spread, orbital recurrence, and secondary tumors, and it is often on the basis of these diagnostic results that further treatment (radiotherapy and/or chemotherapy) is planned. Still, subtle optic nerve involvement cannot be predicted reliably.[68] By using CT as a diagnostic tool, Danziger

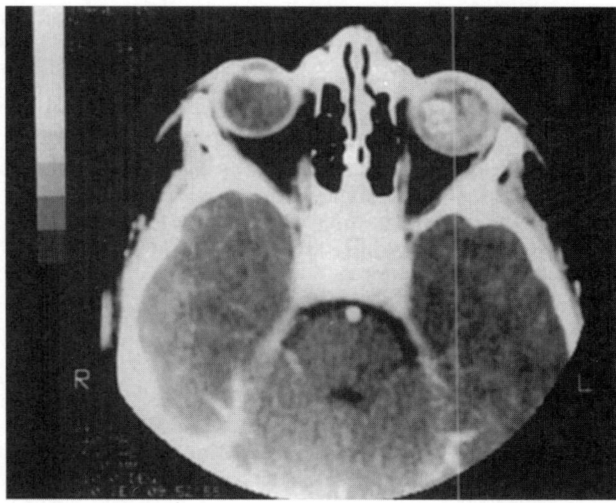

A

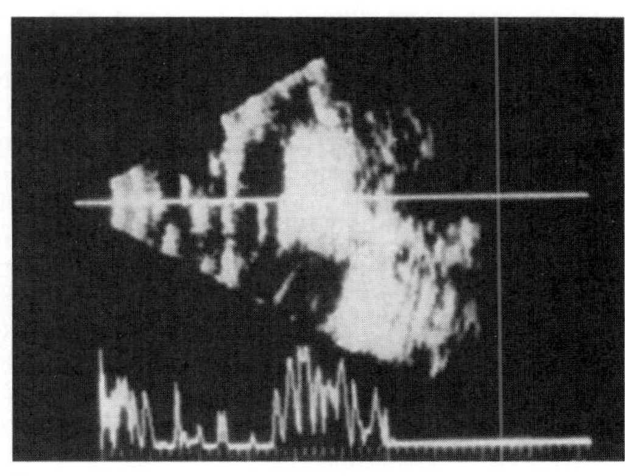

B

Fig. 36-5 Diagnostic tools for retinoblastoma. *A,* CT scan: retinoblastoma filling the whole vitreous cavity with typical calcifications (Courtesy of C. Venturi, MD, Department of Neuroradiology, University of Siena, Italy). *B,* B scan technique. The echogram shows a lesion with an irregular oval shape and dense acoustic tissue. High attenuation of ultrasound is occurring, with the shadowing of the echoes coming from the orbital tissue. The tumor has developed in the vitreous and occupies it almost entirely. (Courtesy of E. Motolese, MD, Institute of Ophthalmological Sciences, University of Siena, Italy.)

and Price[75] proposed the division of retinoblastoma cases into three groups: grade I tumors are high-density masses with calcification in any part of the eyeball; grade II tumors are high-density masses involving the optic nerve and orbital soft tissue but with rare calcifications; and grade III tumors are intracranial or extraorbital high-density masses showing marked contrast enhancement. These classifications further aid in the determination of appropriate therapeutic measures.

Ultrasonography. Ultrasonography is another diagnostic technique that can distinguish the type of growth for retinoblastoma and related tumor types. Endophytic and exophytic growths show variations in the ultrasonographic context of both A and B scanning techniques.

B Scan Technique. In the case of an endophytic growth, the retinoblastoma appears as a single or, more often, a multiple lesion on the retinal plane. The tumors are monolobate or multilobate and have a roundish or irregular oval shape, with dense acoustics and variable homogeneity (Fig. 36-5*B*). A discrete attenuation of the ultrasound occurs, with the shadowing of the echoes coming from the orbital tissue. The attenuation is considerable if, as is often the case, areas of calcification are found inside the tumor mass.[76] The tumor itself may develop within the vitreous chamber and occupy it almost entirely, and, at times, areas of pseudocysts may be found in front of and/or in the context of the neoplastic mass, thus making it difficult to recognize the lesion.[77] Nevertheless, the attenuation of the ultrasound is considerable.

With the exophytic growth, the diagnosis is harder to establish, especially if the tumor is analyzed during the initial stage. It is easily confused with the high echogenic portion of the sclera, while no significant evidence of it appears on the retinal plane. The only significant noticeable sign is a certain attenuation of the ultrasound coming from the orbital tissue, with a display on the echogram that simulates the acoustic shadow of the optic nerve, but does not resemble it in topography and size.[77]

A Scan Technique. In the case of an endophytic tumor growth, a standardized A scan tracing shows an opening peak that appears at high or medium reflectivity but is never maximal. This is the case because the internal retinal surface is considerably compromised and heterogeneous, thus attenuating the contrast that exists at the vitreous-retinal interface level. The opening peak can be maximal, however, if the tumor has an exophytic growth as long as the layer of the limiting internal membrane and the nerve fibers are not disintegrated by the growth of the tumor.[77,78]

In the opposite case, a peak at high reflectivity found during a subsequent checkup may reveal a peritumorous satellite area, even if small and confined, rather than an opening peak of the tumor. The internal structure of the tumor usually appears quite regular at medium-high reflectivity and at medium reflectivity in the case of a retinoblastoma with no calcifications.[77] Vitreous activity with the absence of seeding is minor in retinoblastoma before photocoagulation, while afterward it is possible to find juxtalesional vitreous echoes at medium reflectivity and, sometimes, areas of peritumorous retinal fissions.[79]

Invasion of the sclera entails the loss of its homogeneity as an acoustic interface and causes a decrease in the reflectivity of the closing scleral peak that may be mistaken for the retinal echoes of the same tumor. This represents an important ultrasonographic sign, which can determine the margins and posterior borders of the lesion. In the A and B scanning methods, the calcifications are characteristically evident even when the amplitude appears reduced. Furthermore, suspicion of invasion of the optic nerve is indicated by the presence in the nervous tissue of an ultrasonographic tracing that reproduces the features of a retinoblastoma in an A scan.

Fine-Needle Aspiration Biopsy. The cytologic approach to the study of retinoblastoma has become particularly relevant as the techniques for obtaining tumor material have improved. Specimens from the posterior chamber can be obtained by using vitrectomy techniques in addition to anterior chamber paracentesis for cytologic and enzymologic evaluation of the aqueous. Aqueous and vitreous aspiration for cytologic studies may be useful in differentiating retinoblastoma from the previously described simulating conditions.

The use of fine-needle biopsy in ophthalmology, originally introduced by Schyberg for the diagnosis of orbital tumors, was utilized in the diagnosis of intraocular neoplasms by Jakobiec et al.[80] and extended to the diagnosis of intraocular and extraocular retinoblastoma by Char and Miller.[81] This approach is not recommended as a routine procedure for retinoblastoma and generally is reserved for children who present with unusual manifestations or for differentiating an orbital recurrence of retinoblastoma from a second malignant neoplasm.[81] A limbal approach is used for anterior segment tumors, whereas a via pars plana approach after opening of the conjunctiva, scleral diathermy, and 1.5-mm sclerotomy is used for posterior tumors.[82,83] Complications that may occur with the use of fine-needle biopsy include intraocular hemorrhage, retinal detachment, and recurrence in the orbit or along the intraocular needle tract. Although tumoral-cell seedings within the scleral needle tracks after biopsy are controversial,[84,85] this possibility suggests that fine-needle biopsy be limited to patients who present diagnostic uncertainties. These patients include older children with suspected retinoblastoma and rather atypical findings and children with orbital masses who previously have been treated for retinoblastoma.[86–88]

Therapy

If a retinoblastoma or a related ocular tumor is discovered at an early stage and diagnostic tools have appropriately classified the type, there are several current and effective methods for treatment, including enucleation, external-beam irradiation, episcleral plaques, xenon arc and argon laser photocoagulation, cryotherapy, and chemotherapy. The choice of treatment depends on factors such as (a) multifocal or unifocal disease, (b) site and size of the tumor, (c) diffuse or focal vitreous seeding, (d) age of the child, and (e) histopathologic findings. Therefore, an appropriate therapeutic approach greatly depends on accurate staging of the disease.

Staging and Classification. The most widely used staging system for retinoblastoma, which was proposed by Reese and Ellsworth,[89] is based on the ophthalmoscopic evaluation of the tumor extension and generally is limited to patients with intraocular retinoblastoma. Pratt extended this system to include intraocular and extraocular extension of the disease.[90] Another system is based on an accurate evaluation of the histopathologic findings.[91] Most recently, a pretreatment TNM classification has been introduced that also addresses the importance of visual acuity in addition to patient survival and ocular extension.[92] Table 36-2 presents the different criteria for these classification systems.

Enucleation. Enucleation is the standard treatment in unilateral cases and for the more severely affected eye in bilateral ones. An attempt to save the eye is worthwhile only when there is hope for useful vision and no risk of a systemic prognosis.[93] Generally there are several major indications that call for the nonconservative removal of the diseased eye. These tumor characteristics include (a) a large mass involving more than 50 percent of the retina associated with retinal detachment, (b) a buphthalmic painful eye, (c) a phthisical eye (in bilateral cases), and (d) unsuccessful conservative treatment (radiotherapy with or without chemotherapy and photocoagulation). Regardless of which of the various enucleation techniques is used, the procedure should be performed with the least trauma possible for the patient while avoiding scleral perforation, and at least 10 mm of the optic nerve should be resected.[94] After enucleation, the use of an implant is recommended for both cosmetic reasons and to stimulate orbital growth. Usually a conformer is used for 2 to 3 days directly after surgery, followed by a temporary insert prosthesis (about 1 week after enucleation) after complete healing of the surgical incision.[13]

External Irradiation. Retinoblastoma is a highly radiosensitive tumor, and the first attempt at its treatment with x-rays occurred in 1903.[95] External-beam irradiation, utilizing gamma rays from a linear accelerator, is now the most commonly used treatment for intraocular and orbital disease. This technique is indicated when (a) in unilateral retinoblastoma cases there is a large tumor not involving the macula and optic nerve, (b) in bilateral retinoblastoma cases there are advanced tumors in both eyes, or in the remaining eye when multiple tumors or diffuse vitreous seeding is present, and (c) in orbital tissue, where histopathologic studies of the enucleated eye and optic nerve document an invasion of the optic nerve, scleral invasion, or orbital recurrence.[13]

The goal of external irradiation in retinoblastoma is to sterilize the entire retina and vitreous of malignant cells with the best possible visual prognosis. A dose generally considered to be optimally therapeutic is 4000 rad fractionated into about 20 doses over a 3- to 4-week period. At the Utrecht Retinoblastoma Center, a highly accurate irradiation method has been developed,[96] based on the temporal approach, which ensures precise delivery of a

Table 36-2 Classification Systems for Retinoblastoma

Reese-Ellsworth Classification	Pratt Classification	Standard Classification	TNM Classification
Group I: Very favorable prognosis A: Solitary tumor, less than 4 dd* in size, at or behind the equator B: Multiple tumors, none more than 4 dd in size, at or behind the equator	I: Tumor (unifocal or multifocal) confined to the retina A: Occupying 1 quadrant or less B: Occupying 2 quadrants or less C: Occupying more than 50% of the retinal surface	Stage I: Lesions amenable to local therapy	T1: Tumor or tumors 10 dd or less in largest diameter T1a: Macula not involved T1b: Macula involved
Group II: Favorable prognosis A: Solitary lesion, 4–10 dd at or behind the equator B: Multiple lesions, 4–10 dd at or behind the equator	II: Tumor (unifocal or multifocal) confined to the globe A: With vitreous seeding B: Extending to optic-nerve head C: Extending to choroid D: Extending to choroid and optic-nerve head E: Extending to emissaries	Stage II: Lesions unsuitable for conservative local therapy but still confined to the eye—subdivisions based on histologic assessment of the eye N0: No invasion of the optic nerve N1: Invasion up to or into the lamina cribrosa N2: Invasion beyond the lamina cribrosa resection line free N3: Optic nerve involved up to the resection line C0: No choroidal invasion C1: Superficial involvement of the choroid up to half of its thickness C2: Full-thickness choroidal invasion C3: Scleral invasion, including tumor in the emissary vessels C4: Extrascleral invasion	T2: Tumor or tumors larger than 10 dd involving up to half the retina T2a: Macula not involved T2b: Macula involved
Group III: Doubtful prognosis A: Any lesion anterior to the equator B: Solitary tumor larger than 10 dd behind the equator	III: Extraocular extension of tumor (regional) A: Extending beyond cut end of optic nerve (including subarachnoid extension) B: Extending through sclera into orbital contents C: Extending to choroid and beyond cut end of optic nerve (including subarachnoid extension) D: Extending though sclera into orbital contents and beyond cut end of optic nerve (including subarachnoid extension)	Stage III: Local spread beyond the eye without hematogenous metastases 1: Orbital tumors 2: Preauricular or cervical nodes 3: Central nervous system disease	T3: Tumor or tumors involving more than half the retina
Group IV: Unfavorable prognosis A: Multiple tumors, some larger than 10 dd B: Any lesion extending anteriorly to the ora serrata	IV: Distant metastases A: Extending through optic nerve to brain B: Blood-borne metastases to soft tissue and bone C: Bone-marrow metastases	Stage IV: Hematogenous metastases	T4: Extraretinal or orbital extension T4a: Invasion of optic nerve T4b: Invasion of choroidea, corpus ciliare, iris, or anterior chamber T4c: Scleral involvement T4d: Two or more a–c
Group V: Very unfavorable prognosis A: Massive tumors involving over 50% of the retina B: Vitreous seeding			N: Regional lymph nodes NX: Minimum requirements to assess the regional lymph nodes cannot be met N0: No evidence of regional lymph node involvement N1: Evidence of involvement of regional lymph nodes
			M: Distant metastases M0: No evidence of distant metastases M1: Evidence of distant metastases (can be subdivided according to the organs involved)

*dd denotes disk diameter; one dd = 1.6 mm.

uniform radiation dose to the whole retina or vitreous with maximal sparing of the lens. Accurate positioning of the collimated field is obtained by magnetic fixation of the eye to the beam-defining collimator by a low-vacuum contact lens. Because the eye is fixed in the isocenter of the accelerator, rotation of the gantry directs the beam. Other centers have adopted this technique and have confirmed the extreme precision and sharp-beam profile that can be obtained.[97,98]

Four regression patterns after radiation for retinoblastoma have been described by Reese and Ellsworth[99] and by Buys et al.[101] These patterns are described as follows: type I—characterized by calcification, marked alterations of the retinal pigment epithelium, and the cottage cheese aspect; type II—the tumor is shrunken in size and adopts a gray, translucent appearance (fish flesh); type III—a combination of the patterns seen for types I and II; and type IV—represented by the typical pattern after cobalt-plaque treatment, with complete destruction of the tumor and choroid; the white scar represents the sclera underlying the tumor.

Buys *et al.* found that the most common type of regression at the first evaluation was type III (43.8 percent). However, after a minimum of 7 years, a decrease in this pattern was found (from 43.8 to 36 percent). It was also reported that the type II patterns can turn into any one of the other types over a number of years. Furthermore, a correlation seems to exist between the size of the tumor and the regression pattern.[101]

As with most procedures, complications can arise after external irradiation. They are divided into immediate, usually reversible complications and late, usually irreversible complications. The most severe complications are growth retardation of the orbital region, dry-eye syndrome caused by the reduced or absent lacrimal secretion, radiation cataract, iris atrophy, vascular changes, and retinal exudates (radiation retinopathy).[102]

Episcleral Plaques. The use of radon seed brachytherapy for the conservative treatment of retinoblastoma was introduced in 1929. In 1948, Stallard developed radioactive applicators using radium, and these applications were later modified to use ^{60}Co. Later techniques expanded to include ^{125}Ie, ^{192}Ir, and ^{106}Ru eye plaques, which are now all used routinely in the focal treatment of the disease.[103] Many treatment centers have a preference for ^{125}I

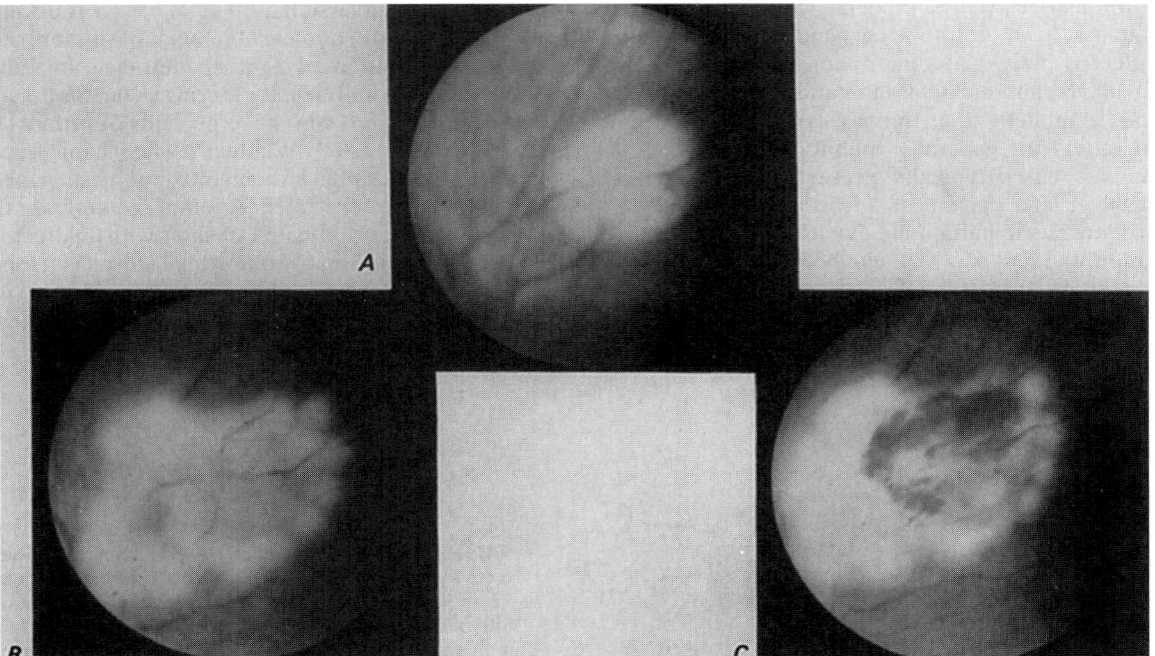

Fig. 36-6 Regression patterns for retinoblastoma after photocoagulation. *A,* A small retinoblastoma. *B,* After indirect xenon-arc photocoagulation. *C,* After direct xenon-arc photocoagulation. (Courtesy of R. Frezzotti, MD, Director of the Institute of Ophthalmological Sciences, University of Siena, Italy.)

plaques because orbital tissues can be shielded with a gold-plaque carrier, ridge plaques can limit the spread of radiation to the nerve and foveal region, and there is less radiation exposure for the patient and the assisting staff.[104] Regardless of the type used, the episcleral plaque technique is highly advantageous compared with other forms of therapy because the procedure time is short while the dose of irradiation is delivered directly to the tumor, minimizing radiation effects to the extraocular structures.

The use of radioactive scleral plaques as a primary treatment is particularly successful for medium-size tumors no greater than 12 mm in diameter and more than 3 mm from the optic disk or macula.[105] Scleral plaques are also useful as a secondary treatment for recurrent or new tumors which are impossible to control using photo- or cryocoagulation. The regression patterns seen after plaque treatment appear to be identical to those described for external-beam irradiation (types I, II, and III). However, a type IV radiation regression pattern characterized by complete destruction of the tumor choroid and all vessels, leaving a white scleral patch, has been observed only after cobalt plaque treatment.[100]

Photocoagulation. In 1955, Meyer-Schwickerath developed a photocoagulation technique using a xenon arc in which retinoblastomas are surrounded by a ring of coagulation placed in the normal retina before the tumor tissue itself is treated.[106] The experience of others[104,107–110] suggests that the success of photocoagulation is due to the destruction of the retinal blood supply, not to its effect on the tumor itself or on the underlying choroid. The best results have occurred with tumors up to 4 to 5 disk diameters in size, with an elevation of 4 diopters,[111,112] although tumors up to 6 or more disk diameters have also been treated successfully in this way.[107,108] Indications, contraindications, and results of photocoagulation appear to be disparate. There are different opinions regarding the size, elevation, site, and clinical conditions in which retinoblastoma should be treated with photocoagulation.[109] Photocoagulation has been suggested as a primary approach for small and moderate retinoblastomas posterior to the equator and for the treatment of recurrent or new tumors after external radiotherapy or radioactive plaques.[108] Photocoagulation is not appropriate when tumors lie directly on the optic nerve or when there is vitreous seeding.

Complications arising from the use of photocoagulation may include occasional retinal hemorrhage; retinal traction; retinal folds; macular distortion; iris damage; corneal edema; and/or cataract (caused by inadvertent iris heating or energy absorption by preexisting opacities). The regression patterns observed after photocoagulation treatment depend on the size and elevation of the tumor (Fig. 36-6). Furthermore, it appears that vascularization of the tumor can influence sensitivity to xenon photocoagulation.[107] After photocoagulation, small tumors appear as a flat avascular pigmented scar. Larger tumors may present marked coarctation, reduced vascularization, and a translucent gray appearance similar to that described as fish flesh. However, both of these regression patterns closely resemble those of types I and II after radiotherapy.

Cryocoagulation. Cryotherapy[113] for retinoblastoma can be used as a primary or supplementary treatment after other conservative therapeutic attempts and can be effective in clinical situations involving new or recurrent tumors after irradiation therapy or in tumors anterior to the equator in eyes that have not been treated.[114] Cryotherapy can be successful on tumors up to 3.5 mm in diameter and 2.0 mm in thickness, but more than one treatment may be necessary.[115]

Vitreous base tumors are very rarely cured with cryocoagulation alone.[116] Localization of the tumor is obtained by indentation with a cryoprobe under indirect ophthalmoscopy. Tumors are frozen with applications of −80°C for 30 to 60 s, and the treatment is typically repeated three times.[117] Cryotherapy destroys the tumor by direct intracellular and intravascular formation of microcrystals. The most frequent complications after cryotherapy are conjunctival and lid edema.

Chemotherapy. To date, chemotherapy has played only a secondary role in the treatment of retinoblastoma, because good control can be achieved with more local treatment. There is also a relative paucity of randomized studies on the efficacy of chemotherapy compared with other therapeutic procedures, and this is further complicated by a lack of suitable markers for the detection of minimal residual disease.[57,59,60,118] The first to use a chemotherapeutic agent in retinoblastoma treatment was Kupfer, who obtained partial regression of a retinal tumor mass by using nitrogen mustard.[119] After this preliminary experience, other antitumor drugs, especially vincristine and cyclophosphamide, were used alone or in combination in several situations, such as in association with radiotherapy for advanced disease[120,121] to reduce the mortality caused by micrometastatic disease[120–127] and with locally advanced disease or distant metastasis.[128–130] Especially in the last group of patients, sequential chemotherapy protocols or courses of intensive chemotherapy followed by autologous bone marrow transplantation have given encouraging results. Despite these achievements, the role of antiblastic chemotherapy in the treatment of retinoblastoma remains controversial, and the only generally accepted indications for it are orbital or metastatic disease, trilateral retinoblastoma, and salvage therapy for relapses in the residual eye. More controversial indications include shrinkage of the neoplastic mass, optic nerve infiltration beyond the lamina cribrosa, and choroidal infiltration (whole thickness and/or ciliary body invasion) with or without optic nerve involvement up to the lamina cribrosa. This mode of therapy still awaits homogeneous staging and therapeutic criteria to evaluate its general efficacy.[131,132]

THE GENETICS OF RETINOBLASTOMA

Retinoblastoma has served as the prototypic example of the genetic predisposition to cancer.[133] Although the majority of tumors occur with no preceding family history, the inherited form of the disease has been extensively documented.[134–136] The familial disease is transmitted, with few exceptions, as a typical Mendelian autosomal dominant trait with virtually full penetrance. It has been estimated from epidemiologic data[137] that about 60 percent of cases are nonhereditary and unilateral, 15 percent are hereditary and unilateral, and 25 percent are hereditary and bilateral.

Although there are examples of apparent nonpenetrance among antecedent or collateral relatives of familial retinoblastoma patients, among descendants of such patients penetrance is nearly complete.[137] There have been a few pedigrees reported in which the disease seems to have truly skipped a generation, in other words being transmitted from grandparent to grandchild via an unaffected parent. Retrospective analysis of families of retinoblastoma probands has yielded several examples of presumed obligate carriers who did not develop the disease. Examination of a number of retinoblastoma pedigrees[15,135–139] showed apparent nonpenetrance in 52 of 128 families either through multiply affected sibships with both parents unaffected or through other affected relatives (such as cousins and aunts) with unaffected intervening relatives. In contrast, when pooled data from published sources were used to determine the segregation ratio among the offspring of familial retinoblastoma patients, it was observed that bilaterally affected parents had 49 percent affected offspring, as is expected for a dominantly inherited disease with complete penetrance, whereas unilaterally affected parents had 42 percent affected offspring, indicating some lack of penetrance.[139] These data were relevant to the proposal of a host resistance model by which heritable resistance factors to a predisposing gene are minimal in bilaterally affected individuals, intermediate in unilaterally affected individuals, and maximal in unaffected carriers.[139]

One proposed model[133,137] encompasses the observations that familial cases are generally multifocal and bilateral, whereas sporadic cases typically present with unilateral unifocal disease of later diagnosis. According to the model, as few as two stochastic mutational events are required for tumor formation, the first of which can be inherited through the germ line (in heritable cases) or can occur somatically in individual retinal cells (in nonheritable cases). The second event occurs somatically in either case and leads to tumor formation in each doubly defective retinal cell. This empirically based hypothesis has been supported by direct experimental scrutiny using molecular genetic approaches.

Cytogenetics

The involvement of genetic alteration in the first step of this pathway of oncogenesis has been supported by cytogenetic analysis which has shown that a small proportion of patients carry a microscopically visible deletion of one chromosome 13 homologue in all their constitutional cells. Since the first such report,[140] more than 30 deletions have been described occurring in a small percentage of retinoblastoma cases;[141–143] the common region of overlap of such deletions is chromosome 13, band q14.[144,145] An example of such a deletion of one constitutional chromosome 13 homologue is illustrated in Fig. 36-7. In the context of the two-hit model, such deletions could act as the first hit and, when they are germinal, could confer the risk of tumor formation in an autosomal dominant manner. Evidence that the same locus is involved in retinoblastoma cases that lack an apparent chromosomal deletion was provided through the demonstration of tight genetic linkage between the retinoblastoma and esterase D loci,[146] the latter being a moderately polymorphic isozymic enzyme whose encoding locus also maps to 13q14.[147]

Furthermore, cytogenetic analysis has provided important information concerning the occasional occurrence of apparent nonpenetrance in some retinoblastoma families. A large kindred has been reported in which unilateral retinoblastoma was transmitted by a number of unaffected individuals. Each affected individual carried the same constitutional deletion involving 13q14, whereas the unaffected carriers had a balanced insertional translocation involving the same region.[148] This and other related reports of chromosomal translocations, inversions, or deletions in transmitting parents[148,150] provide a clear biologic basis for segregation distortion without invoking nonpenetrance. In addition, two reports describe individuals who carry a constitutional

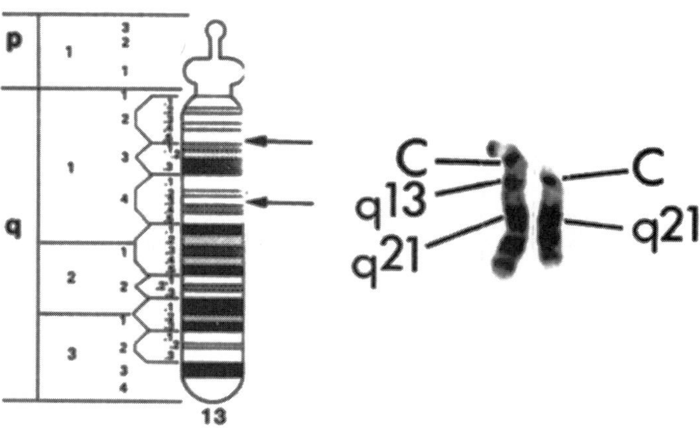

Fig. 36-7 Chromosome 13 deletion in constitutional cells from a patient with retinoblastoma. The idiogram of chromosome 13 to the left indicates the two breakpoints (arrows) of the interstitial deletion. To the right is a G-banded partial karyotype with the normal homologue on the left (centromere, C, bands q13 and q21 indicated) and the deleted homologue on the right (centromere and q21 band indicated). Only one chromosome homologue is altered. Hence, this aberration may represent the first and predisposing event in the child. (Courtesy of David Ledbetter, Baylor College of Medicine, Houston.)

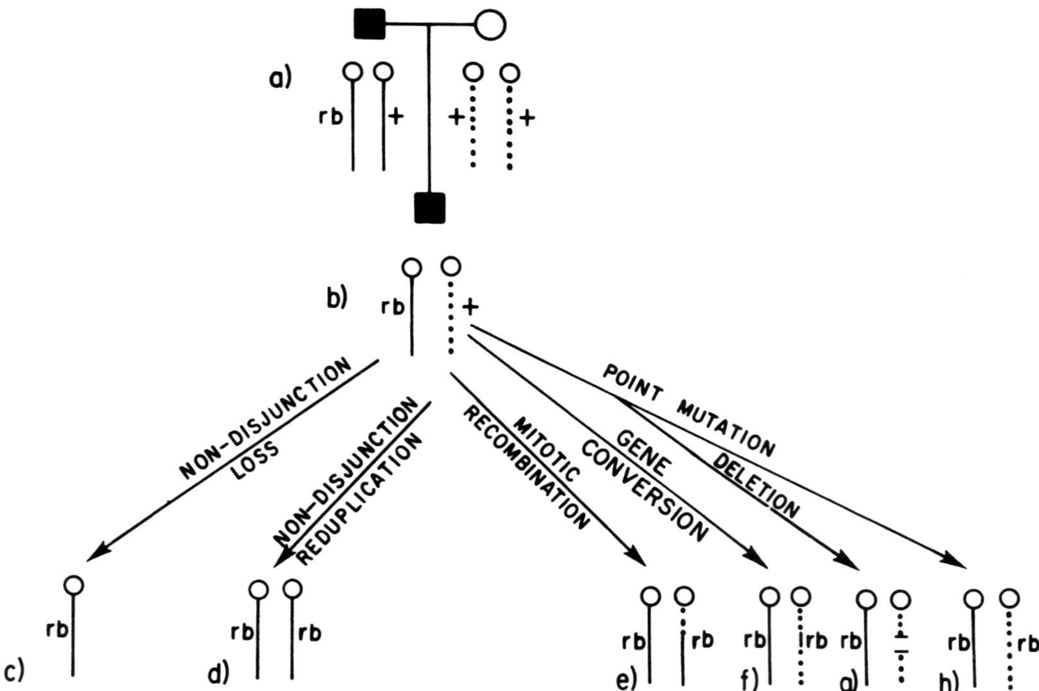

Fig. 36-8 Chromosomal mechanisms that could reveal recessive mutations. In this example, an affected male (a) who carries a recessive defect at the RB1 locus on chromosome 13, designated rb, in all his cells mates with a genotypically wild-type, +, female. One of their children (b) inherits the defective chromosome 13 from his father and so is rb/+ at the RB1 locus in all his cells. A tumor in his retinal cells may develop by eliminating the dominant wild-type allele at the RB1 locus by the mechanisms required to effect the tumor cell genotype shown schematically in c to h. (Reprinted by permission from Cavenee et al., *Nature,* vol. 305, p. 779, copyright 1983, Macmillan Journals, Limited.)

deletion involving 13q14 but have no signs of retinoblastoma at age 5[151] or 25 years.[152] Whether a significant proportion of unaffected carriers can be accounted for by such mechanisms remains to be demonstrated. Another theoretical explanation for isolated multiply affected sibships with unaffected parents is parental mosaicism. Chromosomal mosaicism for deletions involving 13q14 was reported in one series in lymphocytes from 5 to 50 sporadic retinoblastoma patients.[153] In these cases, a significant proportion of retinal cells must have carried the deletion; alternatively, if relatively few retinoblasts carried the deletion, an individual could be at low risk for expressing the disease, but at high risk for its transmission. The increasing resolution of cytogenetic technology and the use of DNA probes for loci in the immediate vicinity of the retinoblastoma locus (gene symbol RB1) have also allowed the detection of more subtle genomic rearrangements that were undetectable previously and have shed light on individuals carrying nonpenetrant mutations in the retinoblastoma susceptibility locus (see below).

The presence of 13q14 deletion in patients without mental retardation or major anomalies,[154] and in familial cases in which transmission might appear to be autosomal dominant,[155] suggests that high-resolution chromosome analysis should be done in all patients with retinoblastoma. When a deletion is found in a proband, parental studies should be considered to rule out deletion, insertional translocation, or mosaicism.

Molecular Genetics

Specific predictions of the nature of the second tumor-eliciting event in the two-step model on oncogenesis[133,137] have been proposed:[156] (a) The autosomal dominant hereditary form of retinoblastoma, in the absence of a gross chromosomal deletion, involves the same genetic locus that is involved in cases showing large deletions of chromosome 13. Thus, the first step in the pathway toward tumorigenesis in these cases is a submicroscopic mutational event at the RB1 locus. (b) The same genetic change that has occurred as a germ-line mutation in hereditary retinoblastoma occurs as a somatic genetic alteration of the RB1 locus in a retinal cell in nonhereditary retinoblastoma. (c) The second step in tumorigenesis in both heritable and nonhereditable retinoblastoma involves somatic alteration of the normal allele at the RB1 locus in such a way that the mutant allele is unmasked. Thus, the first mutation in this process, although it may be inherited as an autosomal dominant trait at the organism level, is in fact a recessive defect in the individual retinal cell.

The model that arises from these considerations is shown in Fig. 36-8. It outlines specific chromosomal mechanisms that should allow phenotypic expression of a recessive germinal mutation of the RB1 locus (Fig. 36-8*A*). This aberration is inherited by an individual who thus carries such a mutation in all somatic as well as germ-line cells (Fig. 36-8*B*). Any additional event that results in homozygosity or hemizygosity for the mutant allele (that is, the RB1 locus is mutant on both chromosome 13 homologues) will result in a tumor clone. Several chromosomal mechanisms can be imagined in this process: (a) mitotic nondisjunction with loss of the wild-type chromosome (Fig. 36-8*C*), resulting in hemizygosity at all loci on chromosome 13; (b) mitotic nondisjunction with duplication of the mutant chromosome (Fig. 36-8*D*), resulting in homozygosity at all loci on the chromosome; (c) mitotic recombination (Fig. 36-8*E*) between the RB1 locus encoding the mutant allele and the centromere, resulting in heterozygosity at loci in the proximal region and homozygosity throughout the rest of the chromosome, including the RB1 locus; and (d) several other more regionalized events such as gene conversion (Fig. 36-8*F*), deletion (Fig. 36-8*G*), or mutation (Fig. 36-8*H*). Both nonheritable and hereditable retinoblastoma could arise through the appearance of homozygosity at the RB1 locus, the difference being two somatic events in the former instance and one germinal event and one somatic event in the latter instance.

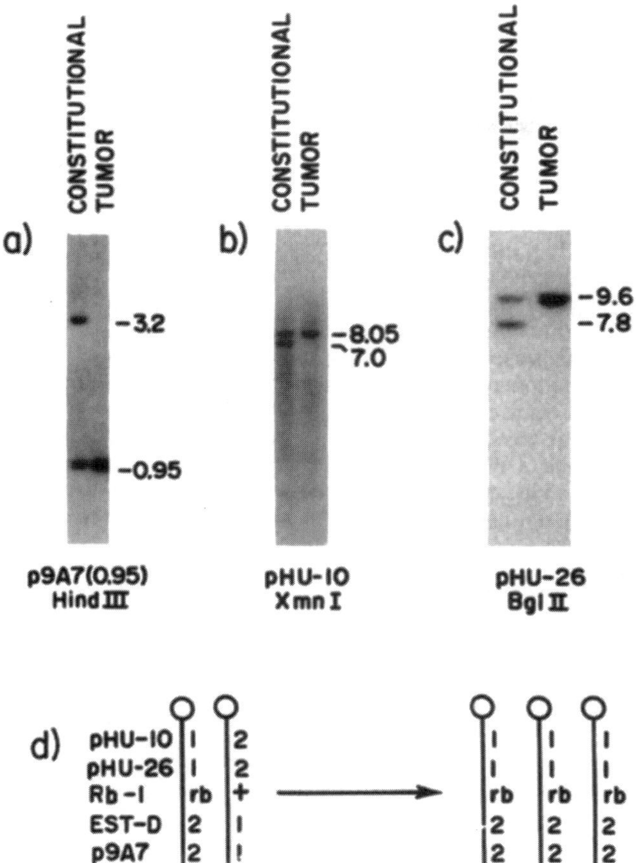

Fig. 36-9 Homozygosity effected by segregation of one chromosome 13 homologue with duplication of the remaining one. *A,* Results obtained when *Hind*III-digested DNA was hybridized to p9A7, which contains an insert homologous to a locus on chromosome 13 mapping between band q22 and the terminus of the long arm. B, The pattern obtained when *Xmn*I-digested DNA was hybridized to the insert fragment derived from the plasmid pHU10, which is homologous to a locus on chromosome 13 mapping between bands q12 and q22. *C,* The pattern obtained when *Bgl*II-digested DNA was hybridized to the insert fragment isolated from the plasmid pHU26, which is homologous to a locus on chromosome 13 mapping between bands q12 and q22. *D,* A diagram incorporating these data with previous analysis of the esterase D alleles present and the karyotype of the two samples from patient Rb-409. (Reprinted by permission from Cavenee et al., *Nature,* vol. 305, p. 780, copyright 1983, Macmillan Journals, Limited.)

The approach that has been taken to examine these hypotheses relies on the variability of DNA sequences among humans, which results in inherited differences in restriction-endonuclease recognition sites. In this approach, segments of the human genome are isolated in recombinant DNA form, and the loci homologous to these probe segments are tested for their encompassing restriction-endonuclease recognition sequences, which vary between unrelated individuals. Two types of such variation have been defined. The first, and most abundant, results from simple base-pair changes within the recognition-site sequence for a particular restriction endonuclease and yields alleles of greater (when the effect of the mutation is loss of a site) or lesser (when the effect of the mutation is gain of a site) length.[157] The second type results from the insertion or deletion of varying numbers of blocks of like DNA sequence into or out of the genomic locus.[158] Practically, the net result is the observation of two alleles at the locus encompassing a site change (presence or absence of the site) or numerous alleles at a locus subject to insertion or deletion of larger segments of DNA, respectively. In either case, however, any given individual will reveal only two alleles at the locus, one from the paternally derived chromosome and one from the maternally derived homologue. In all cases examined to date, these types of markers have been shown to behave in family studies in the manner that would be predicted for simple Mendelian codominant alleles. Recombinant DNA probes for loci mapped along the length of human chromosome 13 have been isolated, characterized,[159,160] and used in multilocus analysis to detect alterations in the somatic genotypes of tumors compared with the germ-line genotype of the individuals harboring these tumors.[156,161,162] A reasonably large series of retinoblastoma cases has been examined in this manner; examples are illustrated in Fig. 36-9 and Fig. 36-10.

Nondisjunction and Duplication. The mechanism depicted in Fig. 36-8*D,* in which, together with the nondisjunctional loss of the wild-type chromosome, the mutant chromosome is duplicated, would be difficult to detect cytogenetically or by quantitation of esterase D activity. However, with the use of codominant DNA markers, these events were detected as a loss of one allele at each informative locus on the chromosome. The patient described in Fig. 36-9 was found to be heterozygous at the ESD locus and showed no visible abnormality of either chromosome 13. An examination of tumor tissue from this individual again showed no abnormalities of chromosome 13 except that in addition to the expected two copies of the chromosome, another copy was present as a translocation involving chromosomes 13 and 14. However, the tumor cells exhibited only one of the two isozymic types of the esterase D enzyme — the allele from the father. It was proposed[163] that this resulted from somatic inactivation of the maternally derived allele of the ESD locus on one homologue of chromosome 13.

Constitutional and tumor cells derived from this patient were tested with seven recombinant DNA probes. Three of the probes revealed heterozygosity in the germ-line tissue: p9A7, which maps in the region 13q22-qter, and pHU26 and pHU10, both of which map in the region 13q12-q22. In each of these cases (Fig. 36-9*A* to *C*), although both codominant alleles were present in the germ line, only one allele at each locus was present in the tumor, and this allele was derived in each case from the chromosome 13 inherited from the father. A reasonable interpretation of these results is diagrammed in Fig. 36-9*D.* Rather than somatic inactivation of the ESD locus on one chromosome 13 homologue, these data are consistent with the complete loss of the entire maternally derived chromosome accompanied by duplication of the paternally derived chromosome. It is likely that this chromosome carried a *de novo* germinal mutation, because the father showed no evidence of retinoblastoma, but the subject was bilaterally affected. It is also possible that one or two of the chromosomes 13 in the tumor were derived by mitotic exchange between the wild-type mutant chromosomes (as diagrammed in Fig. 36-8*E*) so that an original mutant chromosome and a recombinant chromosome (or two) were maintained. If this had happened, the point of interchange must have been proximal to the region detected by the most proximal marker locus, because all the markers, including esterase D (which maps to 13q14), show reduction to homozygosity in the tumor.

Mitotic Recombination. Another possible mechanism by which part of a pair of chromosomes may become homozygous, although not previously observed in humans, is illustrated in Fig. 36-8*E.* A somatic, or mitotic, recombination between the mutant and wild-type chromosome homologues, with subsequent segregation, can result in a cell that maintains heterozygosity at loci proximal to the breakpoint of the recombinational event, but shows homozygosity at loci distal to such a breakpoint. An instance of this mechanism was presented in patient Rb-412.[156] The germ-line cells from this person had been determined to be heterozygous at the ESD locus as well as heterozygous for a quinacrine-staining satellite heteromorphism on the short arm of chromosome 13. An examination of the tumor cells derived from this patient showed the presence of

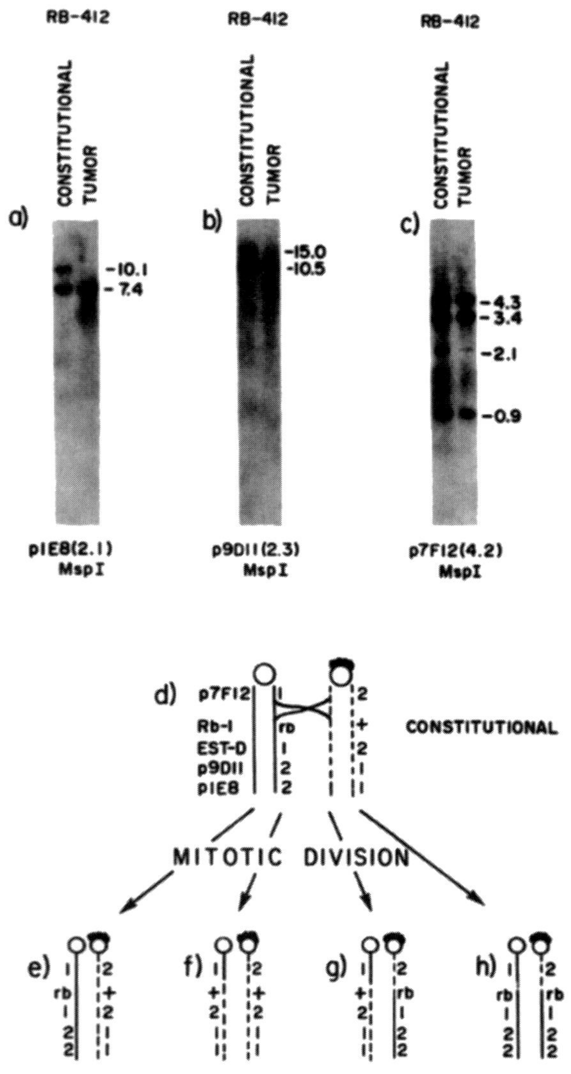

Fig. 36-10 Homozygosity effected by a mitotic recombination event. *A,* The pattern obtained when the hybridization probe was p1E8, which is homologous to a locus on chromosome 13 mapping between band q22 and the terminus of the long arm. *B,* Results obtained when the hybridization probe was p9D11, which is homologous to a locus on chromosome 13 mapping to band q22. *C,* Results obtained with the hybridization probe p7F12, which is homologous to a locus on chromosome 13 mapping between bands q12 and q14. *D,* Diagram showing inferred haplotypes on each chromosome derived from karyology, esterase D determinations, and these data. The cap on the chromosome homologues represented by the dashed lines denotes a fluorescent-staining heterochromatic region. In this figure, the point of crossover must lie between the RB1 and 7F12 loci and is shown occurring between chromatids of the chromosome 13 homologue at the four-strand stage of mitotic chromosome replication. *E–H,* Diagram of the four possible combinations of wild-type and recombinant homologues. Possibilities *E* to *G* result in a phenotypically wild-type cell. The allelic data shown in *H* corresponds to the experimental data and results in homozygosity for the mutant (rb) allele at the RB1 locus. (Reprinted by permission from Cavenee et al., *Nature,* vol. 305, p. 781, copyright 1983, Macmillan Journals, Limited.)

both types of satellite staining, but only one isozymic form of esterase D. A reasonable interpretation of these data[162] was that both chromosomes 13 were present in their entirety in the Rb-412 tumor and that a somatic inactivation of one of the isozymic forms of esterase D had occurred during tumor formation. Alternatively, a mitotic recombination event occurring between the centromere and the ESD locus, as was described above, could generate chromosomes consistent with these results. Germ-line and tumor genotypes of this patient were examined at chromosome 13 loci defined by seven DNA probes (Fig. 36-10). Three of the markers were heterozygous in skin fibroblasts from Rb-412: p1E8, which maps distal to 13q22; p9D11, which maps at 13q22; and p7F12, which maps between the RB1 locus and the centromere. The tumor tissue from this patient showed a loss of one allele at the 9D11 and 1E8 loci, whereas the 7F12 locus remained heterozygous (Fig. 36-10*C*). An interpretation of these results, taken together with the satellite heteromorphism and esterase D data described above, is illustrated in Fig. 36-10*D* and suggests that a recombination event took place between the mutant and wild-type chromosomes 13 in the cell that gave rise to the tumor. The crossover point was between the 7F12 and the RB1 loci, and each locus distal to the RB1 locus became homozygous. Between RB1 and the terminus of the short arm, however, two markers maintained both the maternal and paternal haplotypes.

Data similar to those shown in Figs. 36-9 and 36-10 have been obtained in more than 75 percent of the retinoblastoma tumors examined. They provide experimental support for the proposed recessive model of oncogenesis,[133,137,156] by which predisposing mutations are revealed by elimination of the homologous wild-type locus through chromosomal segregation or recombination rather than simple point mutation. The supposition that it was the chromosome 13 homologue carrying the wild-type RB1 allele that was lost during the process of tumorigenesis was tested by comparing constitutional and tumor genotypes of patients with familial retinoblastoma.

The model described in Fig. 36-8 demands that the chromosomes 13 remaining in the tumors of such children be derived from the affected parent. The analysis[163] of one such case, KS2H, is shown in Fig. 36-11. This child was constitutionally heterozygous at the HU26 locus. His retinoblastoma tumor tissue (Rb-KS2H) showed only the longer allele at this locus. His unaffected parent, KS2C, was constitutionally heterozygous at this locus, while his affected parent, KS2F, was homozygous for the longer allele. Therefore, the proband must have inherited the shorter allele at the locus from his unaffected parent, and it was this chromosome that was lost in the tumor. The chromosome remaining in the tumor was inherited from his affected parent and must be the one carrying the initial predisposing mutation at RB1. In this family, the proband inherited the predisposition to retinoblastoma from his father, KS2F, who had inherited it from his mother, KS2G (Fig. 36-11*B*). He obtained the shorter allele from his unaffected mother and the longer allele from his affected father. It is the latter chromosome that must contain the mutant RB1 locus, and it was this chromosome which was retained in the child's tumor. Corroborating evidence of this interpretation was obtained by examining genotypic combinations at other loci on chromosome 13 in other members of the family. Assignment of the alleles at each of these loci, in combination with those for HU26, and a consideration of the allelic combinations from the grandparents (KS2A, KS2B, and KS2G), parents (KS2C and KS2F), child (KS2H), and child's tumor (Rb-KS2H) made it possible to infer chromosomal haplotypes (Fig. 36-11*B*). The proband (KS2H) inherited a nonrecombinant chromosome from his paternal grandmother (KS2G) through his father (KS2F) and a recombinant chromosome from his mother (KS2C). It appears that the chromosome retained in the tumor (Rb-KS2H) was inherited from his affected grandmother (KS2G) through his affected father (KS2F). In other inherited cases examined, the prediction that the chromosome 13 derived from the affected parent would be retained in the tumor has also been confirmed.

It is noteworthy that although the unmasking of predisposing mutations at the RB1 locus occurs in mechanistically similar ways in sporadic and heritable retinoblastoma patients, only the latter carry the initial mutation in each of their cells. Patients with heritable disease also seem to be at greatly increased risk for the

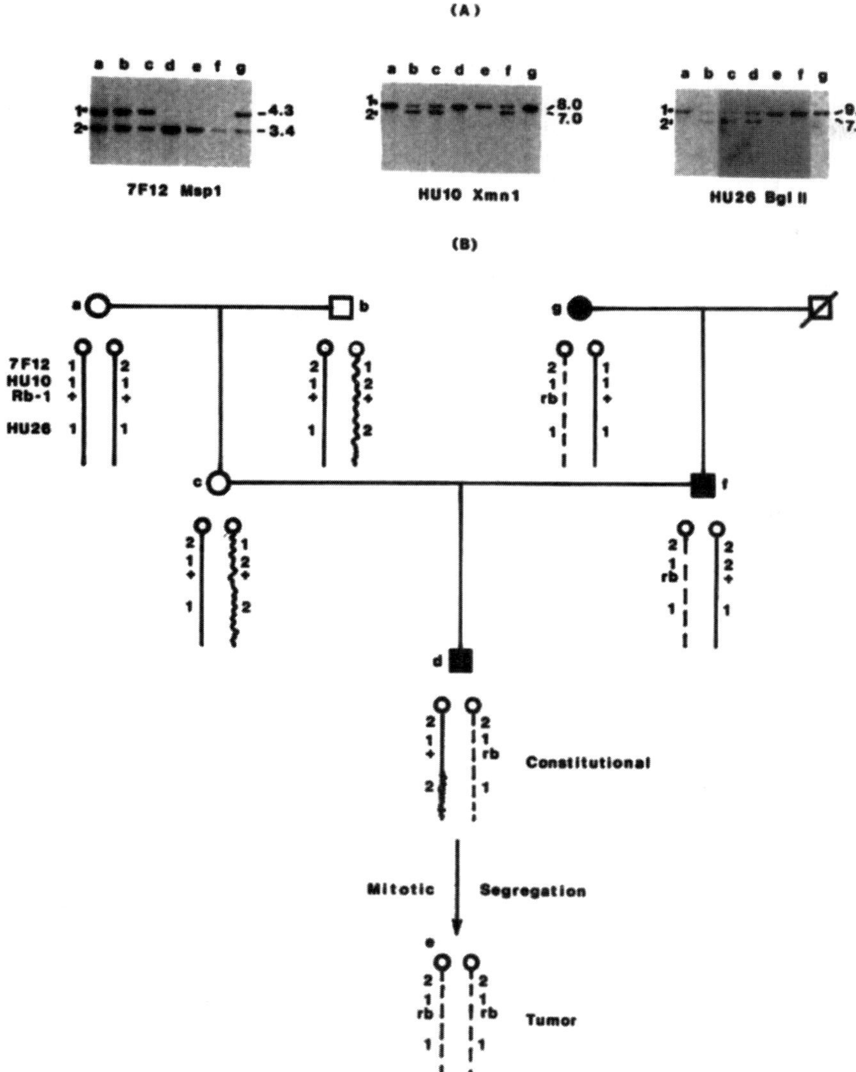

Fig. 36-11 Loss of germ line heterozygosity in a hereditary retinoblastoma tumor. *A,* DNA was isolated from peripheral blood leukocytes from each of the indicated individuals and from a primary tumor biopsy from the proband KS2H. The DNA was digested with the indicated restriction endonucleases, separated by electrophoresis through 0.8% agarose gels, transferred to nylon membranes, and hybridized to the indicated probes homologous to loci on human chromosome 13. The family members are designated: (a) KS2A, (b) KS2B, (c) KS2C, (d) KS2H, (e) Rb-KS2H (tumor), (f) KS2F, and (g) KS2g. *B,* Pedigree Rb-KS2 and inferred chromosome 13 haplotypes at the 7F12, HU10, RB1, and HU26 loci. Filled symbols = individuals with retinoblastoma; dashed line = nonrecombinant chromosome; straight and wavy lines = recombinant chromosome. (Reprinted by permission from Cavenee et al., *Science* 228:501, 26 April 1985, copyright 1985, American Association for the Advancement of Science.)

development of second-site primary tumors, particularly osteogenic sarcoma.[164] A testable corollary of the model outlined above is that this high propensity is not merely fortuitous but is genetically determined by the predisposing RB1 mutation. This notion of pathogenetic causality in the clinical association between these two rare tumor types was tested by determining the constitutional and osteosarcoma genotypes at RFLP loci on chromosome 13. The data indicated that osteosarcomas arising in retinoblastoma patients had become homozygous specifically around the chromosomal region carrying the RB1 locus.[165] Furthermore, the same chromosomal mechanisms eliciting losses of constitutional heterozygosity were observed in sporadic osteosarcomas, suggesting a genetic similarity in pathogenetic causality. These findings are of obvious relevance to the interpretation of human mixed-cancer families, as they suggest differential expression of a single pleiotropic mutation in the etiology of clinically associated cancer of different histologic types.

A likely explanation for the association between retinoblastoma and osteosarcoma is that both tumors arise subsequent to chromosomal mechanisms, which unmask recessive mutations. This may involve either one common locus that is involved in normal regulation of differentiation of both tissues or separate loci that are located closely within chromosome region 13q14. In either case, germ-line deletions of the retinoblastoma locus may also affect the osteosarcoma locus. Deletions are likely to be an important form of predisposing mutations at the RB1 locus, because a considerable fraction of bilateral retinoblastoma patients carry visible constitutional chromosome deletions[141–143] and submicroscopic deletions have been detected by reduction of esterase D activity.[147]

These epidemiologic, genetic, cytogenetic, and molecular genetic studies provided data with which to make specific predictions about the nature of the RB1 locus that have been useful in its molecular isolation. First, any candidate gene should map to the 13q14.1 region of the genome. Second, by analogy with other human diseases, such as Duchenne muscular dystrophy,[166] chronic granulomatous disease,[167] and several of the hemoglobinopathies, at least a proportion of mutations at the RB1 locus should be submicroscopic deletions. Third, a comparison of normal and tumor tissues from heritable cases should show hemizygous aberrancy in the former and homozygous defects in the latter. Fourth, even in the absence of detectable genomic alterations, defects in the mRNA transcribed from the locus or the protein products translated from the mRNA should be detected in tumors.

To provide DNA probes for landmark locations within 13q14, metaphase chromosomes 13 were sorted using a fluorescence-activated cell sorter, and portions of this were used in the derivation of a chromosome-enriched recombinant DNA library.[168] Several unique sequence probes were isolated from this library, and their physical location were determined by *in situ* hybridization to metaphase chromosomes and by determining hybridization dosage in normal cells from retinoblastoma patients with cytogenetically visible deletions of chromosome 13. One such probe, termed H3-8, was localized to the region 13q14.1, thus fulfilling the first criterion listed above.[169] When this probe was used to determine the genomic organization of its cognate locus in retinoblastoma tumors, 2 of 37 showed hybridization patterns consistent with homozygous deletion,[170] thus fulfilling the second criterion. In addition, these deletions were shown to arise either germinally or somatically in bilateral or unilateral disease, respectively,[170] thereby fulfilling the third criterion. The H3-8 probe was used to isolate larger, overlapping segments of DNA, and a unique sequence subfragment of one of these segments was used as a hybridization probe to determine the genomic organization of the approximately 200-kb locus and the transcription pattern of its 4.7-kb mRNA in tumor and normal tissues. Several provocative findings arose. First, deletions that were entirely contained within the locus were observed in some cases. Further characterization of the complete RB1 genomic sequence[171] allowed a rigorous and complete cataloging of the different mutations that affect the gene in retinoblastoma tumors. Simple Southern blot hybridizations have identified submicroscopic deletions involving various regions of the gene in up to 40 percent of tumor tissues or constitutional cells from individuals affected by retinoblastoma.[169,170,172–174] Application of the polymerase chain reaction amplification technique coupled with DNA sequencing and RNase protection assays has increased the proportion of retinoblastomas with measurable RB1 locus alterations by detecting subtle exonic and intronic base changes.[175,176] Figure 36-12 schematically represents some of the characterized retinoblastoma mutations.

Recently, epigenetic mechanisms of mutagenesis involving methylation have also been discovered for RB1. Typical of "housekeeping genes," Rb has a small CpG island that encompasses the promoter region. Fujita and colleagues[177] studied the methylation status of CpGs in the 5′ promoter region of RB1 using methylation-sensitive restriction enzymes. They discovered altered methylation in 9.3 percent (13 of 140) of unilateral sporadic cases, but only 1 percent (1 of 101) of bilateral hereditary tumors. These tumor-associated alterations affected regions as small as the RB1 promoter itself to as large as 5.5 kb extending into the first intron, inhibiting binding of transcription factors and resulting in reduction of Rb expression.[178] Thus, aberrant methylation can act as the functional equivalent of a genetic loss-of-function mutation for Rb. Hypermethylation of promoter regions in other tumor suppressor genes has also been reported, the most notable being p16 on chromosome 9p. p16 is frequently hypermethylated in several cancer lines and also in 20 to 40 percent of primary tumors.[179,180] CpG dinucleotides also occur throughout the coding region of the Rb gene, suggesting that they, too, may be susceptible targets for alteration. In Rb tumors, most

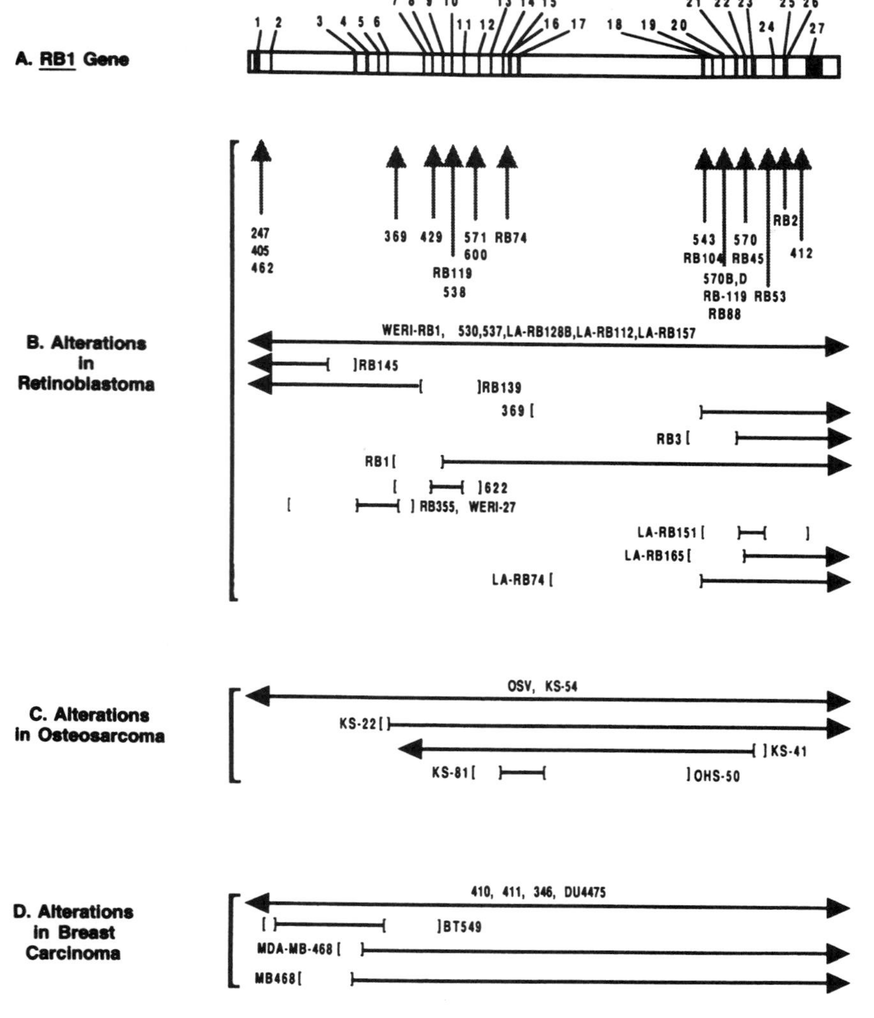

Fig. 36-12 Genomic alteration in the RB1 gene for retinoblastoma and associated tumors. RB1 gene alterations are designated as they appeared in their respective primary references. ↔ = complete deletion of the RB1 locus; [ ]→, ←[ ], and [ ]-[ ] = partial deletion of the RB1 locus, where one or both deletion endpoints occur within the bracketed area in the genomic sequence. Vertical hatched arrows indicate the position of small deletions/point mutations characterized by PCR/DNA sequencing or RNase protection assays. (Reprinted by permission from Gennett and Cavenee, *Brain Pathology* 1:25–32, copyright 1990, ISN Journals.)

common point mutations have been found to be C-to-T transitions, occurring at CGA (arginine) codons. One study determined that as many as 69 percent of the single-base substitutions found in 119 patients occurred at CGA codons and led to premature terminations. Thus, the mutational spectra for Rb suggests methylated CpGs are common and important targets of mutation.[181]

The extensive size of the genomic locus has made complete sequence analysis of RB1 alleles a labor-intensive approach, and so alterations at the transcription level have been pursued to increase the sensitivity of detection of mutations in the locus. When transcription patterns were first analyzed in tumor tissue, no apparent RNA transcript was detected in retinoblastomas or osteosarcomas, although normal-size mRNA was present in retinal cells and several other tissue types (see "Biochemical Characterization of the Retinoblastoma Gene Product" below). These results have been extended by several other groups,[177,178] and transcripts of aberrant size have been identified in tumors previously shown to contain normal genomic structure, thus fulfilling the last criterion listed above. Investigations of RB1 gene alterations at both the DNA and RNA levels cumulatively reveal a strong correlative relationship between lack of the RB1 gene product and the appearance of retinoblastoma tumors. In addition, both DNA and RNA alterations appear to be common in both sporadic and heritable disease, as would be expected from the genetic model discussed earlier.

In addition to cancers such as osteosarcoma, which are clinically related to retinoblastoma, other tumors have been found to have aberrancies of the retinoblastoma gene. The involvement of RB1 in these tumors is inferred from alterations in the gene structure itself or as loss of heterozygosity for DNA markers in the 13q14 region surrounding the RB1 gene. Some examples of such alterations found in osteosarcomas and breast carcinomas are shown in Fig. 36-12. Molecular analysis of small cell lung carcinomas has revealed RB1 structural abnormalities in approximately 15 percent of cases,[179] and loss of heterozygosity for chromosome 13 has been detected in about 25 percent of breast cancers and their derived cell lines analyzed to date.[180,181] A more detailed analysis of the involvement of loss of heterozygosity for chromosome 13 in tumors has been compiled[182] and clearly shows that not all tumors result from direct or indirect alteration of the RB1 locus. However, the cumulative data suggest that RB1 is pleiotropically active, and subsets of tumors may share a common pathogenetic mechanism, which results from unmasking mutations that affect the tumor-suppressing function of RB1.

The observations described above satisfy all the physical criteria for the identity of the RB1 locus as a tumor-suppressor gene. As in all cases of "reverse genetics," however, proof of this requires biochemical and functional analysis. The nature of this gene and the effect its elimination has on oncogenesis rely on the cell biologic and biochemical approaches described below. Its isolation alone, however, constitutes a powerful example of the reverse genetics approach to gene identification through physical and genetic mapping.

Genetic Complementation. The genetic model requiring sequential inactivating mutations and structural evidence in its support suggests that retinoblastoma and its genetically associated tumors arise through loss of function of the RB1 locus. One prediction of this line of reasoning is that the replacement of wild-type RB1 function into cells which lack that function should have normalizing effects on at least parts of the tumorigenic phenotype. This has been directly addressed through the introduction of the wild-type gene into retinoblastoma (the WERI-Rb27 line) and osteosarcoma (the SaOS-2 line) cells through recombinant retroviral vector transfer and assessment of morphology, growth rate, or tumorigenic capability.[183]

Neither type of cell was affected in any capacity after infection by the vector carrying an irrelevant luciferase (Lux) gene. However, after the introduction of the vector carrying the Rb cDNA, two separate morphologies were apparent in the affected populations: One was flattened and greatly enlarged and represented 90 to 95 percent of the population, while the remainder was composed of small cells and mimicked uninfected cells. This suggested that these two RB^+-reconstituted cell lines differed from the RB^- parental lines in their morphology and cell division rates, which correlated with the presence of the expression of wild-type RB. Subcutaneous injection of Lux- and RB^+-reconstituted cells into nude mice resulted in palpable tumors only in those injected with Lux-infected cells, indicating that induction of wild-type $p110^{RB}$ protein expression was capable of suppressing tumorigenicity in both retinoblastomas and osteosarcomas. Similar suppression of tumorigenicity has been demonstrated after the introduction of these retroviral RB^+ vectors into bladder[184] and prostate[185] carcinoma cells, although the effect of reconstituted RB expression on their morphology and growth rate was less dramatic.

There is also evidence that the location of injection may create environments that are more or less suited for tumor growth. In fact, some cancer cells incapable of forming tumors when injected subcutaneously are able to do so when grafted into the anterior chamber of the rodent eye.[186] When retinoblastoma cells used in the retroviral reconstitution experiments were assayed in this site,[187] the malignant WERI-Rb27 parental line formed tumors 40 days after inoculations of 10^3 to 10^4 cells (compared to the 10^7 cells required in subcutaneous injections). Also, 11 of 14 RB^1-reconstituted clones were unable to form tumors. Evaluation of the levels of $pp110^{RB}$ showed that they resulted from the growth of a small fraction of uninfected parental cells such that the tumor cells were unable to express the RB1 protein. All this suggests that $pp110^{RB}$ can function to suppress the tumorigenic phenotype in retinoblastoma cell lines, as predicted by the model.

Other experiments with the breast cancer cell line MDA-468-S4 and retinoblastoma cell lines WERI-RB1 and Y79 have provided less support for the tumor-suppressing ability of $p110^{RB}$.[188] In these studies, expression of exogenous $p110^{RB}$ did not alter growth rate or cloning efficiency in the breast cancer cell line, whereas reintroduction of Rb into both RB cell lines reduced colony formation but had no effect on morphology, growth rate, or tumorigenicity. In clear contrast to the studies described above, the reconstituted retinoblastoma cell line formed intraocular tumors with the same efficiency as did the RB^2 parental cell lines. These tumors, formed in the anterior chamber of the eye, were excised from the mice and expanded in culture. All the tumor cells recovered showed expression of $p110^{RB}$ at levels similar to those of the original parental clones, indicating that tumor formation was not due to loss of function of the transferred RB1 gene. These experiments suggest that tumorigenesis is not deterred by replacement of a normal RB1 allele or expression of RB in homozygously RB-defective cells. Certainly, this confusing situation and the role of $p110^{RB}$ in the tumorigenic process require further exploration.

Prenatal Diagnosis

Advantage has been taken of the increasingly precise molecular elucidation of genomic alterations in retinoblastoma tumors to provide conceptual and methodologic approaches to the assignment of disease risk.[189,190] These methods are either indirect and linkage-based[189] or direct[190] in their detection of genetic defects.

The first approach used polymorphic restriction-fragment-length alleles as linkage markers to deduce genotypes at the RB1 locus in the children of retinoblastoma gene carriers. This method takes advantage of neutral DNA sequence variation in the population, which results in the variable presence of bacterial restriction-endonuclease recognition sites at loci on chromosome 13. This approach had three major limitations. First, most of the loci identified by RFLP[159,160] were genetically distant from the RB1 locus,[191] and, consequently, the reliability of the method was reduced by the occurrence of meiotic recombination. Second, the population frequencies of alleles of these loci were such that only a fraction of families were informative. Third, the method required

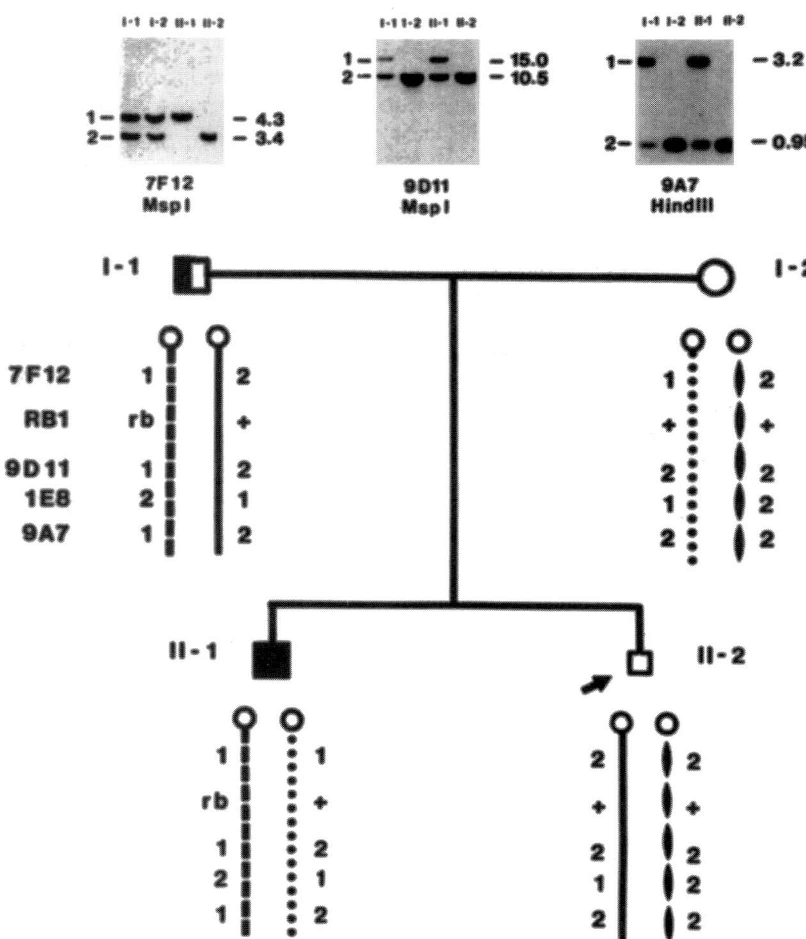

Fig. 36-13 Pedigree of a familial retinoblastoma case that shows no evidence of meiotic recombination. Closed symbols = bilaterally affected family members; half-closed symbols = unilaterally affected members; open symbols = unaffected members. Arrows indicate the family member for whom diagnosis before illness was performed; the indications of the presence or absence of disease are based on subjects' status at their most recent ophthalmic examination. Inferred alleles at the retinoblastoma (RB1) locus are designated rb for a mutant allele and + for a wild-type allele. The circles with vertical lines below them that are shown under each family member symbol represent the member's two constitutional chromosome 13 homologues. The numbers beside each chromosome symbol represent the allelic form of each locus. The vertical order of loci within each family is the same as that shown under the symbol for its I-1 member. The data illustrate the power of information about a first child in discriminating which chromosome a second child has inherited from the affected parent. (Reprinted from Cavenee et al., *New England Journal of Medicine,* vol. 314, pp. 1201–1207, 1986, by permission.)

an affected parent and a first child to define the haplotypic phase. Therefore, analysis was restricted to nuclear families in which informative allelic combinations could be discerned at loci flanking the RB1 locus.

The family described in Fig. 36-13 illustrates how parental haplotypes of chromosome 13 can be deduced through the analysis of the parents and an affected first child. In this example, the first child (II-I) inherited the predisposition for retinoblastoma (Fig. 36-13*B*) and the longer alleles at the 7F12 and 9D11 loci (Fig. 36-13*A*) from his affected father. The fetus (II-2), however, inherited the alternative chromosome 13, which carried the shorter alleles at the 7F12 and 9D11 loci. Because the 7F12 and 9D11 loci flank the RB1 locus at recombination distances of approximately 12 and 30 percent, respectively, the fetus will have inherited the predisposition for retinoblastoma only if two meiotic crossovers occurred between these two loci. The risk estimate for the development of retinoblastoma by this child arises from the conjoint probability of two such crossing-over events. Because the parental haplotype was inferred from the first child, these risk estimates must also consider crossovers in both children, giving a joint probability of 84 percent that retinoblastoma will not develop in the second child. At age 8 years, this child showed no signs of the disease, in accordance with this prediction.

There were several major limitations to this initial approach. First, chromosome 13 haplotypes could not be determined in the carrier parent unless there was either one affected grandparent or one previously affected child, or unless the first unaffected child had passed the age for development of retinoblastoma (which is 7 years or more). Second, there was a chance that gene carriers would remain unaffected because of the somewhat less than absolute penetrance of these predisposing mutations. Third, relatively few and incompletely informative markers for chromosome 13 had been isolated, and these markers were not, for the most part, tightly linked to the RB1 locus. This resulted in risk estimates that were much less precise than desired and allowed only a very few clinical decisions to be based solely on these analyses. Most of these limitations could be minimized if several highly informative and closely linked markers were isolated. The isolation of a cDNA for the closely linked gene esterase D[192,193] allowed an RFLP with better allele frequencies than the protein polymorphism at the same locus. Clearly, the most desirable situation in this regard is the ability to determine the gene defect directly in individual retinoblastoma cases. This is particularly important in counseling families with a single case of bilateral retinoblastoma, because in most instances linkage-based analysis can be used only if there is more than one affected family member. There was a similar need for direct determination of mutations of the RB1 locus in cases of sporadic unilateral retinoblastoma; such patients constitute more than 50 percent of all retinoblastoma cases, and about 10 percent of them carry germ-line mutations.

The isolation of the retinoblastoma susceptibility gene has allowed these goals to be reached, because, as was previously mentioned, the predictive value of RFLP analysis increases in direct proportion to the proximity of informative marker loci to the disease locus. Intragenic polymorphisms are, of course, the best of this class, and so far five independent intragenic RFLPs have been described.[194] Four of these polymorphisms were due to restriction-site alterations for KpnI, XbaI, MboII, and TthIII, and a fifth was due to length variability in the number of tandem repeats of a 50-bp sequence that resulted in eight distinct alleles. The inheritance pattern of these polymorphisms in 13 families with heritable retinoblastoma showed cosegregation of alleles with the disease locus. Furthermore, because of their location within the gene itself, inference errors arising from undetected meiotic recombination within the gene are much reduced in comparison with even the nearest flanking polymorphic probe. As more sequence data have become available, these intragenic polymorphisms have been adapted from standard Southern protocols to PCR amplification methods.[195–197]

These modern approaches to risk assessment may still be complicated somewhat by parental bias in the origin of RB1 mutations. Evidence has been provided that paternal gametogenesis confers a higher mutation rate on the RB1 locus.[198,199] The examination of sporadic bilateral retinoblastoma cases showed that disease arises subsequent to a new germ-line mutation in the paternal allele, followed by somatic alteration or loss of the maternally derived wild-type allele in 13 of 14 cases. In contrast, the examination of sporadic unilateral retinoblastoma tumors showed that only 4 of 10 unilateral tumors retained the allele derived from the father. This suggests that mutations in the RB1 locus occur more commonly during spermatogenesis, or that the paternal chromosome in the early embryo is at a higher risk for mutation. Similar analysis of 13 sporadic osteosarcomas showed that 12 were preferentially mutated in the paternal allele.[200] Considering the clinical association between heritable retinoblastoma and second-site primary tumors such as osteosarcoma, the mechanisms which result in germ-line mutations in retinoblastoma probably are also responsible for producing sporadic related diseases.

Genomic imprinting is one mechanism that might explain the unusual imbalance in mutation and retention of the paternal allele of specific retinoblastomas and related tumors. This is a process, described as epigenetic allele inactivation, that is dependent on the gamete of origin.[201] Imprinted alleles may act as mutated alleles but differ from mutations in the classical sense in that they show a preference for inheritance from only one sex. Consistent with this is the analysis of polymorphic markers on chromosome 13q in parents of patients with sporadic retinoblastoma, which showed that three of three bilateral tumors retained the paternal chromosome (in accordance with previous studies) and that seven of eight unilateral tumors also did so.[202] The discrepancy between the parental biases shown in this report and those discussed above may be explained by the imprinting process being superimposed on the genetic background of the patient.

Although the pattern of inheritance for retinoblastoma suggests 90 percent penetrance,[203] cases of transmitted, nonpenetrant mutations of the RB1 locus have been described (see "Molecular Genetics," above), and these asymptomatic mutations may have an impact on the accuracy of DNA diagnostics. DNA analysis at the level afforded by current technologies offers the possibility of discriminating in unaffected offspring noncarriers from asymptomatic carriers of a nonpenetrant mutation. For example, screening of the RB1 coding structure using exon-by-exon single-stranded conformation polymorphism (SSCP) analysis utilizes the sequence-dependent migration of single-stranded DNA through gel matrices. Such experiments have revealed abnormalities in exon 20, as well as in the promoter region of RB1.[204,205] The former were determined to be single-base changes resulting in amino acid substitutions. The discovery of these alterations suggests that they might serve to reduce the functional efficiency of the retinoblastoma gene product rather than ablate its suppressing ability altogether. It is interesting to note that these studies may suggest the potential existence of different sets of functional mutations in retinoblastoma—and that these groups may, in turn, define differentially functioning regions of the gene product itself. Such predictions require a full characterization of the biochemical role of the retinoblastoma gene product in both normal and tumorigenic cells.

BIOCHEMICAL CHARACTERIZATION OF THE RETINOBLASTOMA GENE PRODUCT

After the documentation of the types of mutations and rearrangements of the RB1 locus in retinoblastomas and other tumors, an understanding of their significance required an understanding of the normal biologic and biochemical function of the protein that locus encoded. The impetus and basis for this was the prior determination of the genomic structure for RB1 and the isolation and sequencing of its 4.7-kb mRNA described above. Analysis of the tissue specificity of RB1 mRNA expression showed ubiquitous presence in normal human and rat tissues, including brain, kidney, ovary, spleen, liver, placenta, and retina. This surprising result was augmented by the demonstration that genomic DNA sequences homologous to human RB1 cDNA were present in a variety of organisms. The sequences were measurably divergent among vertebrates, with homology decreasing as a function of the distance from humans along the evolutionary tree.[177] Thus, although the tumors elicited by inherited mutations of the RB1 locus are relatively narrow in type, its broad tissue expression and species conservation suggested a common and potentially pivotal role in the growth or differentiation of cell types of a variety of ontogenies. Moreover, these observations raise the possibility of interaction of the RB1 gene or its product with others to provide tissue specificity.

The Retinoblastoma Protein

Sequence analysis of an initial cDNA clone provided a great deal of predictive information about the nature and features of the RB1 protein product:[177] it was 816 amino acids in length, had an estimated molecular mass of 94 kDa, and contained 10 dispersed potential glycosylation sites and a leucine zipper (indicated by the presence of periodic leucine residues every seventh position in an alpha helix,[206] which is thought to be important for dimerization of proteins) within exon 20. Furthermore, the region containing amino acids 663 to 716 contains 14 prolines among its 54 residues. Such proline-rich regions have been observed in the nuclear oncogenes, *c-myc* and *c-myb*.[207] The subsequent isolation of several full-length 4.7-kb cDNA clones[172] showed that the initial size estimate of 94 kDa was based on a sequence missing 236 of the 5′-most amino acids, whereas the full-length sequence resulted in a predicted protein of about 110 kDa with the same structural motifs inferred from the first analysis.

Transcriptional analysis of the gene identified three potential sites of initiation at nucleotide positions 11, 144, and 151.[208] Deletion analysis of the 59 RB gene sequences indicated that the region between nucleotides 2154 and 1186 possessed promoter function, with a critical initiating subregion of nucleotides 113 to 1183. Identified enhancer-like sequences included interferon-responsive elements, heat-shock elements, and three Sp1 transcription-factor-binding regions at nucleotides 2291, 176, and 1123.[209]

These transcriptional and translational features led to the suggestion that the RB1 gene product might be a nucleic acid-binding protein that exerts its tumor-suppressor activity through the regulation of transcription of a variety of cellular proteins. In 1987, Lee and coworkers[210] prepared rabbit antiserums against a trpE-RB fusion protein and purified an anti-RB antibody that precipitated a protein of 110,000 to 114,000 daltons. These reagents led to the uncovering of several other interesting features. First, there was no evidence of glycosylation despite such potential sites in the sequence. Second, subcellular fractionation of ^{35}S-methionine-labeled cells into nuclear, cytoplasmic, and membrane fractions, showed that 85 percent of the RB1 protein resided in the nucleus, a location that was further substantiated by immunohistochemical staining with the anti-RB antibody. In fact, the RB protein was shown to be retained on and eluted from single-stranded DNA cellulose columns. Third, when cells were metabolically labeled with ^{32}P-phosphoric acid, the anti-RB antibody immunoprecipitated ^{32}P-labeled protein which was shown to be identical to the RB protein (pp110^{RB}). Finally, analyses of pp110^{RB} expression and its phosphorylation have led to insights into the mechanisms by which it exerts its effects in normal cells and more general ideas about how tumor cells can bypass controls on their proliferation.

Involvement of pp110^{RB} in the Cell Cycle

Phosphorylation of pp110^{RB}. The process of cell proliferation can be subdivided into discrete stages of quiescence (G0), preparation for DNA replication (G1), DNA duplication (S), preparation for mitosis (G2), and actual cell division (M). The traverse of a cell from the G0/G1 through mitosis (M) stages is designated as one cell cycle. Much of what is known about the events that positively and negatively regulate the intricate pathways of this cycle have been deciphered using cell-division cycle (cdc) mutants in yeast.[211] The genetics and biochemistry of these mutants have led to a reasonably detailed view of the complex steps, which, in combination, control the nuclear and cytoplasmic events involved in normal cell proliferation. A great deal of evidence has been accumulated showing that cells of a variety of types require a substantial lag time to progress through a number of substages within G1, regardless of whether the cycling arises from stimulation out of the quiescent G0 stage or from the completion of a previous cell cycle. It is during these substages of G1 that proliferation and cellular differentiation are initiated and controlled, and it appears that the switches for entry into or exit from G1 are the main determinants of postembryonic cell proliferation.[212] Thus, it seems quite reasonable to propose that genes with tumor-suppressor function, such as RB1, may function as negative control elements in the process. Further, it may be that the inactivation of such a gene allows defective cells to traverse the stages of the cell cycle under conditions of growth that would be insufficient for the proliferation of normal cells.[211,213]

One way to achieve functional inactivation of the RB1 gene is to mutate it in such a way that the synthesis of p110^{RB} is reduced, or its degradation is increased. This was tested by determining the steady-state amount of p110^{RB} protein in the different phases of the cell cycle[214] through fluorescent staining of cellular p110^{RB} and DNA in conjunction with flow cytometry. The results showed that the amount of p110^{RB} per cell increased as cells progressed through the cell cycle, such that cells in later G2/M stages immediately before cell division contained approximately twice as much p110^{RB} as cells entering G1. Further, p110^{RB} had an invariant half-life of about 10 h, and pulse labeling of synchronized cells showed that p110^{RB} was synthesized in both quiescent and proliferative phases. These data suggested that the antiproliferative activity of the protein is not regulated in normal cells at the transcriptional level or the translational level.

The first indication that posttranslational modification of the RB protein is involved in cell-cycle control was provided by the uncovering of a correlation in several cell types between cell-cycle stage and the phosphorylation state of the protein.[214,215] Cell lysates prepared from quiescent or cycling cells (human umbilical vein endothelial cells, primary T lymphocytes, cells of a human breast cancer, and HeLa cells) showed an apparent size shift from p110^{RB} in the quiescent cells to pp112–114RB in proliferating cells (Fig. 36-14). Treatment of the latter lysates with potato acid phosphatase reduced the more slowly migrating protein species (p112–p114^{RB}) to the same mobility as the p110^{RB} species, suggesting that the former were actually multiply phosphorylated forms of the latter protein species.

The timing of the p110^{RB} to pp112–114RB transition was concurrent with the initiation of incorporation of radioactive thymidine into cellular DNA. Quantitation of the relative abundance of the higher-molecular-weight phosphorylated proteins to their nascent protein products showed that G1 (resting) cells had a 10:1 p110^{RB}:pp112–114RB ratio while G2/M (cycling) cells had a 1:1 ratio. After mitosis and cell division, the ratio returned to 10:1.[216] Regardless of the enzymatic mechanism involved, it is clear that phase-specific phosphorylation and dephosphorylation

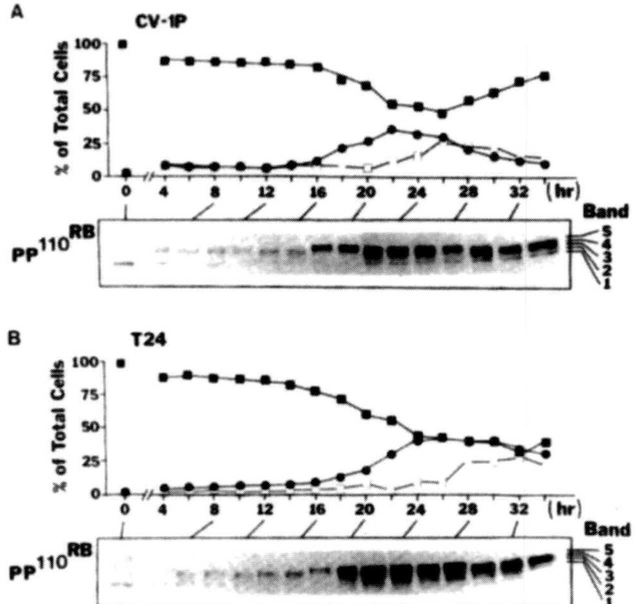

Fig. 36-14 Oscillation of phosphorylation of the p110^{RB} protein during the different stages of the cell cycle. CV-1P cells (*A*) and T24 cells (*B*) were synchronized in G0/G1 by density arrest and then allowed to enter the cell cycle by sparsely replating cells in fresh medium. Equal numbers of cells were seeded into about 50 culture dishes (3×10^6 cells per dish) and were allowed to grow to time points of 18 to 34 h. One entire plate was harvested for each lane on the Western blot. A second batch of dishes (1.5×10^6 cells per dish) was plated 16 h later than the first and was harvested for hours 2 to 16. Again, each lane contained cells from one plate. At 2-h intervals after replating, cells were collected for cell cycle distribution analysis and RB protein determination. The percentage of cells in G1 (filled squares), S (filled circles), and G2/M (open squares) at each indicated time was determined by flow cytometry. RB protein was analyzed by immunoprecipitation followed by immunoblotting; five RB bands could be distinguished. The sudden change in signal intensity in CV-1P and T24 cells is due both to a decrease in the number of cells seeded for hours 2 to 16 and to random variability in the counting of different batches. (Reprinted by permission from Chen et al., *Cell*, vol. 58, pp. 1193–1198, copyright 1989, Cell Press.)

of the RB protein occurs during the cell cycle and proliferation. Mapping tryptic phosphopeptides of the human protein showed that the phosphorylation was on serine and threonine, but not tyrosine residues, which suggests the possibility of cell-cycle regulation by serine/threonine protein kinases.[217] One candidate is cdc2, a protein kinase that is known to be important in yeast at the G1/S and G2/M phases,[218] and which has been isolated in a protein complex that is capable of activating DNA synthesis in G1 cell extracts.[219] Lin *et al.*[217] found that human cdc2 phosphorylates each of the tryptic p110^{RB} phosphopeptides *in vitro* and *in vivo,* and the consensus target sequence for cdc2 phosphorylation[220] (Basic/Polar-Ser/Thr-Pro-X-Basic) occurs eight times within the p110^{RB} protein. Together these studies strongly suggest that human cdc2 is involved in regulating the cell-cycle phosphorylation of p110^{RB} protein. It is also possible that other cdc2-like kinases exist in the cell and play a role in the process as well.

Changes in the phosphorylation state of the RB protein also have been linked to cellular differentiation. Unlike proliferating cells, which actively cycle and divide, terminally differentiated cells cease normal cellular division and are shunted into a G0/G1 quiescent-like state. The effects of the induction of cellular differentiation on the phosphorylation status of p110^{RB} have been analyzed in several leukemic cell lines, which could be induced to differentiate after treatment with phorbol esters or retinoic acid. Monoblastic U937 and HL-60 showed a marked dephosphorylation of p110^{RB} after differentiation,[221,222] and similar treatment of other partially responsive cells led to a coordinate level of p110^{RB} phosphorylation. These experiments have led to several models for the function played by phosphorylation of p110^{RB} in G0/G1.[223] The first is that p110^{RB} regulates a cellular block which prevents exit from G1 by blocking the initiation of DNA synthesis. Phosphorylation of p110^{RB} would render it inactive, thereby releasing the cell from its negative regulation and allowing the cell to progress through a full cell cycle. An alternative model depicts the dephosphorylation of RB as a subcellular event that communicates the precise time for cell cycle exit (i.e., from M to G1/G0). As such, dephosphorylation may be part of a signaling pathway in which intracellular or extracellular factors switch G1 cells into the quiescent stage (G0). One relevant addition to the cell-cycle stage effect of p110^{RB} is the recent demonstration that it undergoes three separate rounds of phosphorylation in T lymphocytes stimulated to proliferate with the mitogen phytohemagglutinin A.[224] The first occurs in middle to late G1, as was described earlier, the second during S phase, and the third in G2/M. Because these modifications occur at different locations on the protein, it is possible that p110^{RB} actually has several different proliferation-controlling functions. The complexity of function that phosphorylation of p110^{RB} produces at the cellular level is further enhanced by more recent demonstrations that this protein can be physically complexed with a number of viral and cellular proteins.

Cyclin D1, p16, and pp110. Recent developments in our understanding of the components of the cell cycle have strengthened the central role the Rb protein plays in growth regulation. One of the most important checkpoints in mammalian cells in late G1, deemed the restriction point, has many positive and negative controllers, including pp110. These key controllers include cyclins (A, D1-3, E, etc.) cyclin-dependent kinases (cdk2, 4, 6, etc.), and cyclin-dependent kinase inhibitors (p16, p15, etc.).[225] At the biochemical level, the kinase complexes of cyclin D1-cdk4 or cdk6 promote progression through late G1 by phosphorylating the retinoblastoma protein product. The Rb phosphorylation described above can be negatively regulated by cdk4/6I or p16INK/CDKN2 (henceforth referred to as p16) (Fig. 36-15). Thus, it appears that the normal biochemical pathway that regulates progression through G1 can be disrupted by

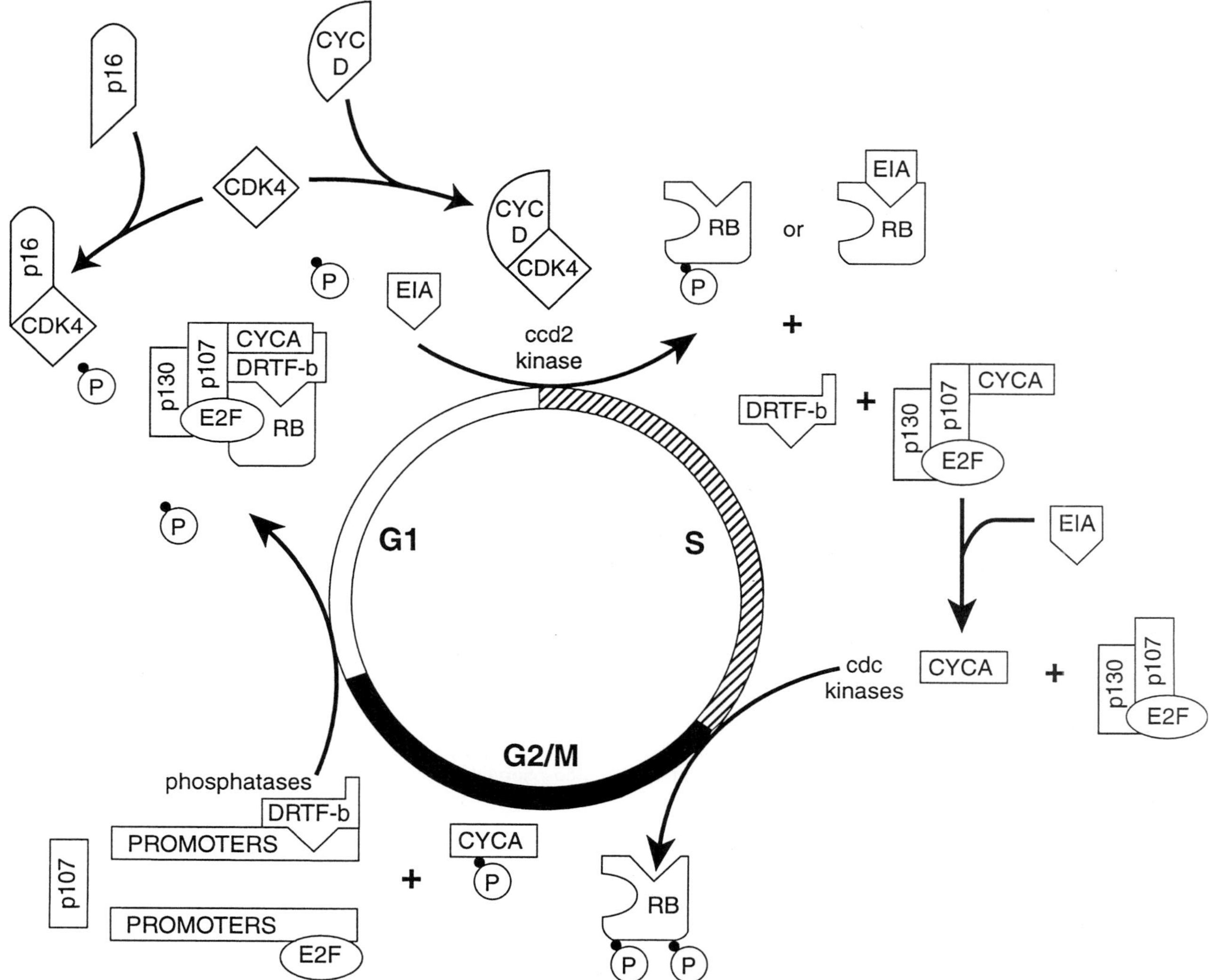

Fig. 36-15 Cell-cycle-dependent binding of cellular proteins to p110^{RB}. The cell-cycle stage-dependent complexing and dissociation of cellular proteins are schematically represented. DRTF and E2F are transcription factors that have been shown to bind to p110^{RB} at the G1 stage of the cell cycle. On phosphorylation of the protein at the G1/S boundary, these transcriptional factors are released from the complex. Phosphorylation of p110^{RB} appears to be controlled by a family of cdc kinases that are active at both the G1/S and G2/M boundaries. E1A has also been shown to bind p110^{RB}, thereby dissociating DRTF and E2F from the G1 complex in much the same manner as occurs when p110^{RB} is phosphorylated. At the completion of the cell cycle, phosphatases dephosphorylate p110^{RB}, thus allowing the protein to sequester E2F and DRTF back into their inactive complexed forms. Cyc A = cyclin A.

abnormalities targeted at any one of these specific components. As discussed at length throughout this chapter, pRb itself can be inactivated by mutation, deletion, methylation, and viral sequestration (see "Viral Oncoproteins," below).

In addition, cell-cycle components such as cyclin D1, whose encoding locus resides at 11q13, can be amplified or rearranged and overexpressed in tumor cells.[225–227] D-type cyclins and their associated cdks (4 and 6) are able to bind to pp110 through an N-terminal LXCXE motif.[228–230] In fact, Rb[230] and E2F[231] are the only known substrates for cycD/cdk4 complexes *in vitro,* and this complex phosphorylates most of the sites *in vivo* on the retinoblastoma protein. Their interaction is strengthened by their apparent involvement in a negative feedback loop where hypophosphorylated Rb seems to stimulate cyclin D1 transcription, and D1 and D1/cdk4 complexes are down-regulated in Rb-deficient cells[231–234] (Fig. 36-15).

Negative regulators active at the G1/S boundary, such as the cdk inhibitors, can also be altered in tumors. One such inhibitor, p16, appears to function normally by down-modulating the phosphorylating activity of its target kinases cdk4[235] and cdk6[236] by binding in competition with cyclin D1. p16 has been found deleted, mutated, or silenced by promoter methylation in a majority of tumor cell lines[237–241] and in a variety of tumors,[242–248] albeit in a much smaller fraction. p16 is elevated in cells that lack functional Rb, suggesting that Rb may suppress p16 expression,[249,250] the reciprocal of what is found for Rb and cyclin D1. This speaks to the positive (cyclin D1) and negative (p16) regulatory roles displayed by each of these cell cycle components and suggests that the pleiotropic tissue specificity of the tumors in which RB1 inactivation occurs may be at the fundamental level of governing cell growth. It further suggests that the cyclin D1-cdk4-p16 pathway operates upstream of pRB, as both the G1-accelerating function of cyclin D1-ckd4 and growth suppression by p16 require functional pRB.

The inverse correlation and reciprocity of function between cell-cycle controllers and Rb are clearly demonstrated in adult small cell lung carcinomas (SCLCs) and non-small cell lung carcinomas (NSCLCs). The Rb gene has been shown to be a common target for somatic mutations.[179] The frequency of absent or aberrant Rb protein expression for SCLC tumors is 90 percent and 15 percent for NSCLC.[251] Several recent studies that have examined the loss of p16 gene expression in these tumor types found a striking inverse correlation. The absence of p16 was a rare event in SCLC,[252,253] with 80 to 100 percent of cell lines and primary tumors displaying a p16+/pRb − phenotype. In contrast, the majority of NSCLCs (67 to 100 percent) analyzed lacked detectable p16 protein, rendering them p16 −/Rb+.[252–254] In one study,[252] cyclin D1 was observed to be overexpressed in most cell lines, suggesting that this alteration may be a common early event in both lung-tumor subtypes. However, this controversial model of the role of cyclin D1 as the earliest mutational event has not been substantiated in other studies examining lung[255] or esophageal carcinomas.[226] Nonetheless, the data clearly demonstrate that the p16-Rb pathway is inactivated in both SCLC and NSCLC at a very high frequency, but that the targets of the inactivating mutational events are distinct, depending on the subtype of lung tumor analyzed.

pp110^{RB} Protein Complexes

Viral Oncoproteins. At about the same time the oscillation of pp110^{RB} phosphorylation within the cell cycle was being uncovered, an unexpected link between this negative growth regulator and the cellular transforming capacities of the viral oncoproteins of polyomaviruses (SV40), adenoviruses (Ad-2 and AD-5), and papillomaviruses (HPV-16) was reported. Each of these DNA tumor viruses encodes a set of proteins, some of which are capable of disrupting the normal regulation of cellular proliferation, leading to *in vitro* transformation of cells and establishment of the tumorigenic phenotype. For example, the E1A protein of oncogenic adenoviruses is capable of immortalizing primary cells and mediating transcription, negatively and positively, for both viral and cellular genes.[256] Furthermore, the E1A of infected cells can be coimmunoprecipitated with a set of host-cell proteins of various molecular weights. The large T oncoprotein of SV40 is a nuclear phosphoprotein of 708 amino acids, which is necessary for cellular transformation by the virus.[257] It typically functions in concert with the SV40 small t protein product, but when expressed at high levels, it can perform all the functions required for transformation. Finally, the protein product of the E7 open-reading frame of human papillomaviruses of types associated with progressive cervical neoplasia is also capable of immortalizing cells *in vitro.*[258] The functional similarities between these oncoproteins are also mirrored to some extent in their amino acid sequences and predicted higher-order structures. For example, deletion and mutation studies have shown that small segments of the SV40 T protein (between residues 105 and 114)[259,260] or the E1A protein (between residues 121 and 139)[261] are required for transforming capacity; these regions are structurally homologous. Comparisons of the amino acid sequences of E7 and E1A revealed a similar relationship between the NH_2 terminus of E7 and the two conserved regions in E1A.[262] These similarities have led to the prediction that these regions may bind cellular proteins that actively participate in and/or cooperate with the transforming properties of large T, E1A, and E7.[206]

Several lines of evidence point to the retinoblastoma gene product as one such cellular protein. As was mentioned above, earlier studies had shown the E1A protein to be complexed with a variety of cellular proteins, and one of these proteins had a molecular mass of about 110 kDa.[263] Using various monoclonal antibodies raised against large T, E1A, and p110^{RB}, as well as polyclonal antibodies raised against E7, *in vitro* immunoprecipitation from cell lysates showed coprecipitation of the p110^{RB} with each of the oncoproteins from a variety of cell lines transformed by viral infection or their normal counterparts.[264–266] The presence of p110^{RB} in these complexes was further confirmed by the demonstration of the expected protein fragments generated by partial proteolysis using staphylococcus V8 protease.

The extent to which these associations represented functional relationships in which both partners are active participants in a common regulatory pathway has also been documented. The analysis of a series of mutant species of large T and E1A proteins revealed that mutations affecting the sequences necessary for transformation also affected the ability of the oncoprotein to form complexes with p110^{RB}.[259,260,265,267] Examples of the effect mutations of large T have on p110^{RB} binding are shown in Fig. 36-16. Because one function of these viral oncoproteins appears to be the creation of a cellular environment that is permissive for DNA synthesis, it may be that one of their modes of action involves sequestration of the antiproliferative p110^{RB}, such that viral infection releases the cell from its negative regulation by RB, allowing it to inappropriately or more frequently enter S phase. An examination of the data derived from immunoprecipitations with large T showed that lysates from ^{32}P-labeled cells contained phosphorylated T but not phosphorylated pp110^{RB}.[268] An RB species did, however, coprecipitate with the anti-T antibody and was shown by densitometric analysis of gel electrophoresis patterns to be p110^{RB}, the unphosphorylated form. This protein species was the only form of p110^{RB} consistently bound to T, even though immunoprecipitation of the same lysates with an anti-RB antibody demonstrated the simultaneous existence of the other phosphorylated forms, that is, p112–114RB. Binding of large T to the unphosphorylated form held true for a stably SV40-transformed derivative of the cells used in the previous experiments, indicating that viral transformation does not alter the overall state of RB protein phosphorylation. These studies also showed that newly synthesized T did not immediately bind to p110^{RB}, and this led to the hypothesis that the structure of T must change in some way to facilitate its successful heterologous binding. In fact, when large T from synchronized ^{35}S-labeled cell

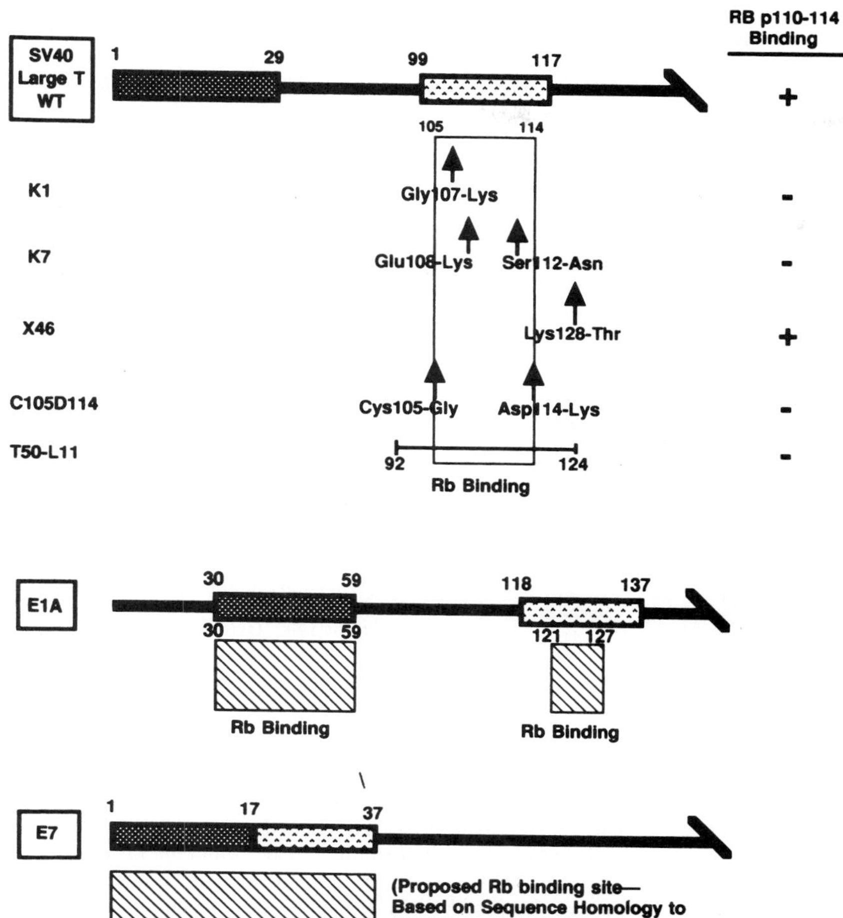

Fig. 36-16 Binding sites for the retinoblastoma protein in SV40 large T antigen, adenovirus E1A, and papillomavirus E7 proteins. The sequences of several SV40 large T mutants are shown with their corresponding p110^{RB}-binding properties; + = T antigen was capable of complexing with the retinoblastoma protein; − = complex formation was abolished by the mutation. Regions in E1A and E7 necessary for binding p110^{RB} assessed by similar mutational analyses are also depicted.

lysates was examined by sucrose gradients, it was determined that newly synthesized large T proteins existed as monomers and over the course of the cell cycle gradually oligomerized;[268] only after oligomerization was the oncoprotein capable of binding to p110^{RB}. This is supported by the SV40 mutant 5080 (Fig. 36-16) that carries a Pro_{584}-Leu substitution, which renders it transformation-deficient[270] and inefficient for oligomerization;[271] it also fails to coprecipitate with the RB protein.[269] It is possible that such oligomer-forming behavior is a process by which large T can bind to more than one protein involved in cellular growth regulation. It is tantalizing to note that regions of E1A and T involved in binding p110^{RB} also interact with at least one cellular protein, p107.[272,273] Whatever the reason for the multiple oncoproteins binding to p110^{RB}, the data together support a model in which the unphosphorylated form of RB (p110^{RB}) is the species active in growth suppression. It follows that binding by E1A, E7, or large T would serve to inactivate the growth suppression normally exerted by pRB. Further, in the absence of viral infection, it is the phosphorylation of the RB protein that serves to override growth suppression and allows cell division to take place.

Retinoblastoma Protein-Binding Sites. Binding of viral oncoproteins to p110^{RB} and the subsequent release of these infected cells from negative growth control suggested that there may be cellular proteins with analogous properties. These proteins might be sequestered by p110^{RB} and be maintained in an inactivated form until phosphorylation of p110^{RB} makes them available for proliferation or transcriptional/translational uses. To determine the regions in the RB gene that are required for binding of the viral oncoproteins and potentially other cellular regulatory proteins, a systematic series of deletion mutants were generated in the p110^{RB} coding regions.[274,275] Polypeptide products generated through *in vitro* protein synthesis systems were analyzed for their ability to bind and coimmunoprecipitate SV40 large T or E1A. The data showed two distinct noncontiguous regions in p110^{RB} necessary for complexing with these oncoproteins; these regions included amino acid residues 393 to 572 and residues 646 to 772. It was further determined that a spacer region of undefined length between these two blocks was required to maintain this binding integrity.

Comparison of these binding regions with many of the naturally occurring RB mutations revealed striking similarities. The mutations displayed in Fig. 36-17 are naturally occurring examples from retinoblastomas, as well as other tumors commonly found to be mutated for RB1 (see the discussion above). Each of these mutants was in some way affected in a region essential for the binding of E1A and large T. The absence of p110^{RB} binding, using mutant proteins of cells from bladder carcinoma,[276] small-cell-lung carcinoma,[277] prostate carcinoma,[278] and osteosarcoma,[279] has been confirmed by *in vitro* immunoprecipitation experiments. This is strong evidence that the regions that normally bind to viral-transforming proteins are also involved in naturally mutated RB proteins in tumorigenic cells.

Cellular-Binding Proteins. The viral oncoprotein-binding data suggested the existence of intracellular proteins whose function is mediated by binding to the RB protein or whose binding mediates the function of the RB protein itself. Several approaches have been

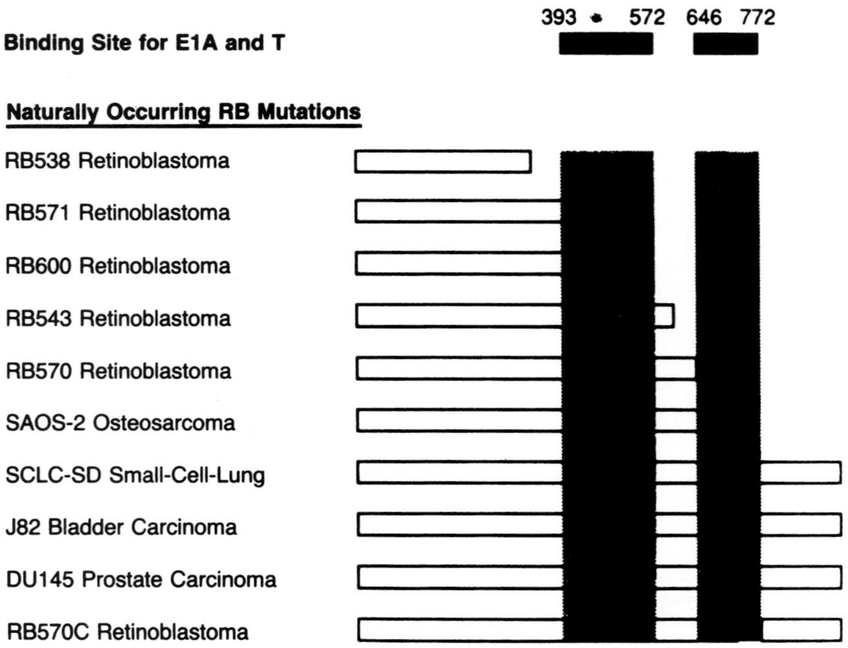

Binding Site for E1A and T — 393 • 572 646 772

Naturally Occurring RB Mutations

RB538 Retinoblastoma
RB571 Retinoblastoma
RB600 Retinoblastoma
RB543 Retinoblastoma
RB570 Retinoblastoma
SAOS-2 Osteosarcoma
SCLC-SD Small-Cell-Lung
J82 Bladder Carcinoma
DU145 Prostate Carcinoma
RB570C Retinoblastoma

Fig. 36-17 Comparison of binding sites of EB to E1A/SV40 T antigen with naturally occurring RB1 mutations. This comparison includes RB1 mutations characterized in retinoblastoma, osteosarcoma, bladder carcinoma, and prostate carcinoma cells. The solid boxes at the top of the figure represent the regions of RB essential for binding to E1A and SV40 T antigen. The stippled regions indicate the positions of the binding regions relative to the RB sequences present in the naturally occurring mutants (open boxes). Amino acid sequences that are essential for binding to E1A and SV40 T are absent in each mutant. (Reprinted by permission from Hu et al., *EMBO J* 9(4):1147–1155, copyright 1990, Oxford University Press.)

used to search for these putative cellular components, and each has been in some way based on complementarity to the viral oncoprotein-binding regions. One line of experimentation involved screening a human lung fibroblast cDNA expression library with a 60-kDa recombinant RB protein. This analysis identified two individual cDNAs—RBP-1 and RBP-2280—whose products bound specifically to antimouse pRB monoclonal antibodies, although neither cross-hybridized with the other. Northern analyses of lung mRNA revealed 5.2- and 4.3-kb transcripts homologous to RBP-1, whereas RBP-2 detected a 6.0-kb transcript. DNA sequencing of these cDNAs indicated no homologies to known protein sequences except that each contained a 10-amino acid motif that mimicked the $p110^{RB}$-binding domain.

A second approach utilized *in vitro* immunoprecipitation techniques. For these experiments, excess free $p110^{RB}$ was added to drive the reaction equilibrium toward complex formation with subsequent coprecipitation of these RB complexes with anti-RB antibodies.[280–281] A 56-kDa pRB fusion protein containing both regions necessary for the binding of T antigen to the C terminus stoichiometrically precipitated a 46-kDa protein from HeLa cells. Competition studies with large T antigen and the addition of p56 kDa RB protein containing deletion/insertion mutations, indicate that this 46-kDa cellular protein is directly associated with the recombinant p56 kDa RB protein through its T-binding domains.

The most successful approach to date for isolating cellular RB complexing proteins involves generating glutathione-S-transferase pRB fusion proteins, which then are used as protein-affinity chromatography agents against different cell lysates. The pRB portion of these proteins contains the minimal conserved region required for binding of SV40 large T and adenovirus E1A oncoproteins. When cellular lysates of the retinoblastoma cell line WERI-Rb27 were passed over affinity columns of fusion proteins that included regions of RB necessary for SV40 T-antigen binding, several cellular proteins, ranging in size from 25 to 146 kDa, were retained.[282] Similar-sized proteins could be separated from extracts of a variety of tumor cell lines. Each of the proteins was found primarily in the cellular nucleus, and at least one, of 68 to 72 kDa, displayed apparently S-phase-dependent binding behavior.

The function of the proteins isolated in each of these ways became clear through analyses of their physical relationship to $p105^{RB}$ and their effect on cellular transcription. DRTF is a sequence-specific transcription factor found in different forms (DRTF-b or DRTF-a) as embryonal carcinoma stem cells differentiate.[283,284] DRTF-b migrates faster than does DRTF-a in band-shift assays, suggesting that the DRTF-b complex is missing one or more protein components found in DRTF-a. To determine whether this transcription factor interacted with the tumor-suppressor RB product $p110^{RB}$, E1A protein was added to cell lysates of the embryonic stem-cell line F9. Using band-shift-binding assays, it was shown that E1A sequestered a protein from the DRTF-a complex, creating the DRTF-b form, an effect dependent on the E1A-conserved regions 1 and 2 that were previously determined to be necessary for transformation. Monoclonal antibodies to RB produced a similar shift from DRTF-a to DRTF-b, leading to the conclusion that $p110^{RB}$ is part of the DRTF transcription complex and providing a link between tumor-suppressor activity and control of gene transcription.

Because E1A affected the complexing of $p110^{RB}$ into DRTF, E1A-associated proteins were analyzed to see if they were part of the same complex. One such protein, cyclin A, like $p110^{RB}$, varies in mass amount during the mitotic phase of the cell cycle. The addition of an anticyclin A antibody to DRTF complexes caused a disruption of the RB-containing DRTF-a complex, but not a disruption of the RB-deficient DRTF-b complex.[285] Furthermore, the RB-deficient DRTF-b complex could complex with $p110^{RB}$ only when cyclin A was added, thus indicating that cyclin A facilitated the sequestering of RB into the DRTF complex. A consideration of the binding characteristics of DRTF, RB, and cyclin A in light of the cell-cycle regulation of the latter two, suggests that DRTF has an important cell-specific role in regulating the transcription of genes whose protein products are required for progression through the cell cycle (Fig. 36-15). Such coordinated behavior could provide a molecular mechanism by which viral and cellular transforming oncoproteins might act in part to sequester RB from DRTF-a. This would have the effect of freeing the transcriptionally active DRTF-b form, which is no longer under the negative regulation of $p110^{RB}$.

These experiments show that Rb probably functions in growth control and differentiation through interactions with a variety of cellular proteins. Other interacting proteins in this category include RIZ286, Myo D287, c-Abl288, MDM2289, and E2F[286–289] (described below). The transcriptional activators hBRG1/hBRM have also been functionally linked with pRB. hBRG1 (human brahma-related gene 1 protein) and its family member hBRM are the mammalian homologues of the yeast SNF2/SWI2 transcriptional activator and the Drosophila brahma protein. These proteins are thought to restructure chromatin and facilitate the function of specific transcription factors. All share a domain that is also found in many nuclear proteins, such as the E1A-binding protein p300.[290] hBRG1 interacts only with hypophosphorylated pp110^{RB} through the same LXCXE motif found in other pRB-interacting proteins described in this chapter.[291] This suggests that these transcriptional activators are rendered nonfunctional in G1 by their association with pRB and are released upon phosphorylation of the retinoblastoma protein.

E2F is another sequence-specific transcription factor that was initially identified as a cellular factor involved in the regulation of the adenovirus early E2 gene by the E1A protein. Using a glutathione-S-transferase protein fused to the 379 to 792 binding domain residues of p110^{RB} and a degenerate mixture of 62-bp DNA oligonucleotides, Chittenden *et al.*[292] attempted to determine whether any pRB pocket-binding cellular protein had sequence-specific DNA-binding activity. After several rounds of enrichment, two oligonucleotides were found to be the major components in the selected population. More than 80 percent of the sequenced oligonucleotides shared a class 1 TTTGGCGGG consensus sequence, while 15 percent contained a class 2 ATTTGCGCGGG consensus sequence. Comparison of these with other known sequence-binding sites uncovered a strong similarity to the binding site of E2F (TTTCGCGC). One interpretation of this study is that E2F binds specifically to the p110^{RB} product. Isolation of two cDNAs encoding E2F or E2F-like proteins (one of which corresponds to RBP-1, as was discussed earlier)[293,294] should provide the reagents needed to test this hypothesis.

Further studies determined that E2F was associated with the unphosphorylated form of p110^{RB} present in the G1 phase of the cell cycle near the G1-S border.[295,296] This behavior is consistent with the recruitment of unphosphorylated p110^{RB} into the DRTF complex and suggests that E2F can play a role in transcription or regulation, either alone or in concert with other proteins in the DRTF factor. Furthermore, as E2F is released upon entry into S phase, it can be found complexed with cyclin A; an E2F-cyclin A complex may be cooperatively released upon phosphorylation of p110^{RB} in the S phase of the cell cycle. The function of the RB/E2F in G1 phase transition is becoming more clearly defined. The complex is active in silencing the E1A promoter when bound to an E2F binding site.[297] In this form, RB/E2F inhibits the function of other promoter elements, such as enhancers, thereby causing transcription to cease. On phosphorylation of p110^{RB} or the addition of E1A, E2F is released and becomes a positive transcriptional element. Thus, positive and negative regulation of transcription is linked not only to E2F but also to the phosphorylation cycle of the retinoblastoma-suppressor gene. All these experiments are consistent with a model in which p110^{RB} controls the transcription of genes that contain E2F sites in their promoters, are cyclically expressed in relation to the cell cycle, and are important for cell proliferation.

RB can also suppress the growth of cells (mass increase), as well as their proliferation. Genes regulated by E2F are transcribed by RNA polymerase (pol) II, suggesting that Rb can specifically control proliferation through E2F. How Rb inhibits cell growth might be explained by the recent discovery that Rb can also regulate transcription by pol I and pol III.[303] These polymerases regulate the synthesis of rRNA and tRNA, and, therefore, their inhibition can repress the level of protein synthesis. As the rate of growth can be shown to be directly proportional to the rate of protein accumulation, Rb regulation of pol I and pol III may be the means by which it regulates cell growth.

pp110^{RB} Protein Family Members. An intriguing aspect of the E2F studies described above is the independent association of E2F with both cyclin A and p110^{RB}, even though neither of the latter two contains known structural similarities. Isolation of p107, a retinoblastoma-like protein, has shed light on this confusing phenomenon.[298] Anti-p107 antibodies precipitated p107 together with a few other cellular proteins, the most abundant being cyclin A and another being E2F. The demonstration that this p107 protein is a component of the E2F-cyclin A complex provided the structural basis for its binding behavior. It appears that p107 mediates the indirect binding of E2F to cyclin A, which explains how E2F can bind the structurally dissimilar p110^{RB} and cyclin A proteins.

Another member of this family of proteins, p130, was recently isolated, increasing the complexity of this growth regulation pathway. p130 shares 50 percent identity with p107 and has homology to pp110^{RB} in the pocket-binding domain.[299] Several studies show that this is the same p130 protein found associated with adenovirus E1A.[300,301] Both p107 and p130 bind to the viral oncoproteins and share the spacer region between the two subunits of the pocket-binding domain. This spacer region mediates their interaction with cyclins A and E.[302,303] Because these pRb-related proteins can bind to E2F,[300] they also exhibit growth-suppressing properties similar to those seen with pRB.[303] Interestingly, p130 has been mapped to the long arm of chromosome 16 in a region known to undergo allelic deletion and translocation in another pediatric cancer, Wilms' tumor.[304–306] This suggests that these Rb-related family members should be studied further for mutations in adult tumors not altered for either Rb or p16, and examined for their potential role as tumor-suppressor genes in the fashion described above for the retinoblastoma gene.

Retinoblastoma Mouse Models

The retinoblastoma genotypes and related phenotypes described throughout this chapter paint a somewhat paradoxical picture of the function of RB1. The p110^{RB} protein seems to play a central role in the regulation of the cell-cycle activity common to all cells, yet germ-line mutations in RB1 predispose individuals to a very specific spectrum of tumors. Thus, it remains unclear whether p110^{RB} serves solely as a barrier against specific tumorigenesis or actually plays an important role in normal cellular development. One approach, which has been undertaken to resolve and define these issues for RB1, involves the generation and analysis of animal models such as homozygous mutant (Rb −/−) knockout or transgenic mice. By creating mouse embryonic stem cell lines manipulated genetically to a null status at the RB1 locus and fusing these cell lines with normal blastocyst-stage mouse embryos, mice heterozygous for the mutant Rb allele (Rb+/−) are generated. These predisposed heterozygous mice can be observed for signs of increased tumor incidence and phenotypic abnormalities as well as backcrossed to generate homozygous Rb −/− progeny whose development and tumor profiles should help define the role RB1 in the normal cell.

Several Rb −/− mice have been engineered with insertional mutations in the regions of exons 3–4[305] and exon 20.[306] Observations of these mice and the progeny of their backcrosses were strikingly similar and unexpected. Most notable was the absence of any retinoblastomas or retinomas in the over 200 Rb+/− mice observed. These mice are genotypically equivalent to humans who inherit a mutated RB1 allele and are inevitably diagnosed, at greater than 90 percent penetrance, with retinoblastoma tumors. This systemic difference is further exemplified by the high incidence of brain tumors[306] and pituitary adenocarcinomas[305] exhibited in these Rb+/− animals after 8 to 10 months of observation. Molecular analysis of these tumors reveals loss of the remaining wild-type Rb allele, providing evidence that the two-hit hypothesis described in this chapter for humans also holds for these heterozygous mouse tissues.

Backcrosses of Rb+/− mice did not produce the expected 25 percent Rb −/− progeny. In fact, these Rb −/− embryos were not viable past approximately 13 days of gestation,[305,306] precluding the ability to study pRb^{110} function in normal development. However, chimeric animals partially composed of Rb-deficient cells were viable and showed a widespread contribution of these mutant cells to all adult tissues and normal development of most tissues, including the retina and erythrocytes.[307] This indicates that Rb function is not required for the differentiation of cells in many adult tissues. When nonviable Rb −/− embryos were examined pathologically, significant defects in the brain and blood-forming tissues were discovered. There was massive cell death in the central nervous system tissues, which was highest in the hindbrain. An apparent block in hepatic erythropoiesis most likely accounts for the observation that 65 to 90 percent of red blood cells remain nucleated.

The results from these mouse models do little to solve the Rb paradox, but they do suggest that there may be fundamental systemic differences in the function of pRb in mouse and human tissues. Despite these discrepancies, it is clear that Rb does not play a critical role in regulating cell division or cell differentiation up to the thirteenth day of gestation of the mouse. One explanation for the lack of retinoblastoma tumors in Rb+/− animals is that the population of susceptible target cells in the relatively small mouse eye is below the threshold required for tumorigenesis to occur. However, retinoblastomas have been observed in transgenic mice expressing SV40 T antigen (see "Viral Oncoprotein," above).[308] Thus, there may be a requirement for additional genetic alterations to occur for retinoblastoma tumors to appear in the mouse. Alternatively, in the absence of Rb expression, a Rb-related protein such as p107 or p130 (see "$pp110^{RB}$ Protein Family Members," above) might provide an analogous function in most tissues, preempting a role for $p110^{RB}$ in tumorigenesis in the mouse.

Rb −/− cells isolated from early viable embryos provide a source for a variety of cell types that can be used to look in more detail at the function of Rb at the cellular level. Most importantly, these cells do not possess the multitude of other genetic lesions present in most human tumor cell genomes that might confuse or mask the precise role the pRb loss plays in tumorigenesis. Preliminary observations on Rb −/− fibroblasts show a shorter G1 phase of the cell cycle and a smaller cell size than in the wild type.[309] In addition, although most cell-cycle-regulated genes analyzed show no temporal or quantitative differences, cyclin E is derepressed earlier in G1 than is the case in wild-type cells. Cyclin E, found associated with cdk2, is one of the components responsible for phosphorylating pRb in late G1.[225] Studies utilizing double heterozygote and/or knockout mice for Rb and E2F support this theory. These studies revealed that the Rb1(−/−); E2F1(−/−) double mutant genotype is lethal, suggesting inactivation of E2F1 is not sufficient to rescue the lethal Rb1(−/−) phenotype.[316] Clearly, E2F deregulation is only one mechanism by which pRb1 functions to regulate cell growth *in vivo*. Further studies utilizing a number of other tissue types as well as cells from doubly Rb and p53 mutant mice[310–313] will no doubt add to our understanding of the role Rb plays in normal cellular function, as well as how it cooperates with other cellular oncogenes and tumor-suppressor genes with which it shares cellular control pathways.

ACKNOWLEDGMENTS

The authors are grateful to Prof. R. Frezzotti for his support and constructive criticisms and Dr. E. Motolese and Dr. G. Addabbo for assistance with sections of this review. Thanks also to Ms. C. Mallia for secretarial assistance. The work cited in this review was partly supported by a National Research Council (Italy) grant on retinoblastoma, #9000111.

REFERENCES

1. Francois J: Recent data on the heredity of retinoblastoma, in Boniuk M (ed): *Ocular and Adnexal Tumors*. St. Louis: Mosby, 1964.
2. Beck K, Jensen OA: Bilateral retinoblastoma in Denmark. *Arch Ophthalmol* **39**:561, 1961.
3. Hemmes GF, Tfsdscar J, Francois J: in Boniuk M (ed): *Ocular and Adnexal Tumors*. St. Louis: Mosby, 1964, p 123.
4. Albert DM, Lahav M, Lesser R, Craft J: Recent observations regarding retinoblastoma. *Trans Ophthal Mol Soc UK* **94**:909, 1974.
5. Berkow RL, Freshman JK: Retinoblastoma in Navajo Indian children. *Am J Dis Child* **137**:137, 1983.
6. Devesa SA: The incidence of retinoblastoma. *Am J Ophthalmol* **80**:263, 1975.
7. Sanders BM, Draper GJ, Kingston JE: Retinoblastoma in Great Britain 1969–80: Incidence, treatment, and survival. *Br J Ophthalmol* **75**:567, 1988.
8. Matsunaga E: Genetic epidemiology of retinoblastoma, in Lynch HP III, Hirayama T (eds): *Genetic Epidemiology of Cancer*. Boca Raton, FL: CRC, 1987, p 119.
9. Mahoney MC, Burnett WS, Majerovics A, Tanenbaum H: The epidemiology of ophthalmic malignancies in New York State. *Ophthalmology* **97**:1143, 1990.
10. Jensen RD, Miller RW: Retinoblastoma: Epidemiologic characteristics. *N Engl J Med* **285**:307, 1971.
11. Bras G, Cole H, Ashmeade-Dyer A, Walter DC: Report on 151 childhood malignancies observed in Jamaica. *J Natl Cancer Inst* **43**:417, 1969.
12. Parkin DM, Stiller CA, Draper GJ, Bieber C: The international incidence of childhood cancer. *Int J Cancer* **42**:511, 1988.
13. Frezzotti R, Bardelli AM, Fois A, Lasorella G, Acquaviva A, Hadjistilianou T, Bernardini C: Retinoblastoma: Terapie conservative del retinoblastoma, in Frezzotti R (ed): *Patologie Clinica e Terapia delle malattie dell' Orbita*. Ralazione 65° Congresso S.O.I., Siena 5–8, 1985, p 405.
14. Senft S, Al-Kaft A, Bergquist G, Jaafar M, Nasr A, Hidayat A, Sackey K, Cothier E: Retinoblastoma: The Saudi Arabian experience. *Ophthalmol Paediatr Genet* **9(2)**:115, 1988.
15. Ellsworth RM: The practical management of retinoblastoma. *Trans Am Ophthalmol Soc* **67**:461, 1969.
16. Francois J: Differential diagnosis of leukocoria in children. *Ann Ophthalmol* **10**:1375, 1978.
17. Shields JA, Augsburger JJ: Current approaches to the diagnosis and management of retinoblastoma. *Surv Ophthalmol* **25**:347, 1981.
18. Howard GM, Ellsworth RM: Differential diagnosis of retinoblastoma: A statistical study of 500 children. *Am J Ophthalmol* **60**:610, 1965.
19. Balmer A, Gailloud CL, Uffer S, Munier F, Pescia G: Retinoblastome et pseudoretinoblastome: Etude diagnostique. *Klin Mbl Augenheilk* **192**:589, 1988.
20. Murphree L, Rother C: Retinoblastoma, in Ryan SR (ed): *Retina*. St. Louis: Mosby, 1989, p 515.
21. Balmer A, Gaillaud C: Retinoblastoma: Diagnosis and treatment. *Dev Ophthalmol* **7**:36, 1983.
22. Haik GB, Siedlecki A, Ellsworth RM, Sturgis-Buckhait L: Documented delays in the diagnosis of retinoblastoma. *Ann Ophthalmol* **17**:731, 1985.
23. Binder PS: Unusual manifestations of retinoblastoma. *Am J Ophthalmol* **77**(5):674, 1974.
24. Richards WW: Retinoblastoma simulating uveitis. *Am J Ophthalmol* **65**(3):427, 1968.
25. Stafford W, Yanoff M, Parnell BL: Retinoblastoma initially misdiagnosed as primary ocular inflammation. *Arch Ophthalmol* **82**:771, 1969.
26. Rozansky VM: A necrotic retinoblastoma simulating panophthalmitis. *Surv Ophthalmol* **9**:381, 1964.
27. Morgan G: Diffuse infiltrating retinoblastoma. *Br J Ophthalmol* **55**:600, 1971.
28. Garner A, Kanski JJ, Kinnear F: Retinoblastoma: Report of a case with minimal retinal involvement but massive anterior segment spread. *Br J Ophthalmol* **71**:858, 1987.
29. Schofield PB: Diffuse infiltrating retinoblastoma. *Br J Ophthalmol* **44**:35, 1960.
30. Nicholson DH, Norton EWD: Diffuse infiltrating retinoblastoma. *Trans Am Ophthalmol Soc* **78**:265, 1980.
31. Shields JA, Shields CL, Eagle RC, Blair CJ: Spontaneous pseudohypopyon secondary to diffuse infiltrating retinoblastoma. *Arch Ophthalmol* **106**:1301, 1988.

32. Shields CL, Shields JA, Shah P: Retinoblastoma in older children. *Ophthalmology* **98**:395, 1991.
33. Ginsberg J, Spaulding A, Asburg T: Cystic retinoblastoma. *Am J Ophthalmol* **80(5)**:930, 1975.
34. Ohnishi Y, Yamana Y, Minei M, Yoshitomi F: Snowball opacity in retinoblastoma. *Jpn J Ophthalmol* **26**:159, 1982.
35. Allderdice PW, Davis JG, Miller OJ: The 13q-deletion syndrome. *Am J Hum Genet* **21**:499, 1969.
36. Francke U, King F: Sporadic bilateral retinoblastoma and 13q-chromosome deletion. *Med Pediatr Oncol* **2**:379, 1976.
37. Niebuhr E, Ottosen J: Ring chromosome D(13) associated with multiple congenital malformations. *Ann Genet* **16**:157, 1973.
38. Seidman DJ, Shields JA, Augsburger JJ, Nelson LB, Lee ML, Sciorra LJ: Early diagnosis of retinoblastoma based on dysmorphic features and karyotype analysis. *Ophthalmology* **94**:663, 1987.
39. Gallie BL, Ellsworth RM, Abramson DH, Phillips RA: Retinoma: Spontaneous regression of retinoblastoma or benign manifestation of the mutation. *Br J Cancer* **45**:513, 1982.
40. Margo C, Hidayat CA, Kopelman J, Zimmerman LE: Retinocytoma: A benign variant of retinoblastoma. *Arch Ophthalmol* **101**:1519, 1983.
41. Eagle RC, Shields JA, Donoso L, Milner RS: Malignant transformation of spontaneously regressed retinoblastoma, retinoma/retinocytoma variant. *Ophthalmology* **96**:1389, 1989.
42. Abramson DH: Retinoma, retinocytoma, and the retinoblastoma gene [editorial]. *Arch Ophthalmol* **101**:1517, 1983.
43. Khodadoust AA, Roozitalab HM, Smith RE, Green WR: Spontaneous regression of retinoblastoma. *Surv Ophthalmol* **21**:467, 1977.
44. Aaby AA, Price RL, Zakov ZN: Spontaneously regressing retinoblastoma, retinoma or retinoblastoma group O. *Am J Ophthalmol* **96**:315, 1983.
45. Gallie BL, Phillips RA, Ellsworth RM, Abramson DH: Significance of retinoma and phthisis bulbi for retinoblastoma. *Ophthalmology* **89**:1393, 1982.
46. Bader JL, Miller RN, Meadows AT, Zimmerman LE, Champion LAA, Voute PA: Trilateral retinoblastoma. *Lancet* **582**:8194, 1980.
47. Jakobiec FA, Tso M, Zimmerman LE, Danis P: Retinoblastoma and intracranial malignancy. *Cancer* **39**:2048, 1977.
48. Dudgeon J, Lee WR: The trilateral retinoblastoma syndrome. *Trans Ophthalmol Soc UK* **103**:523, 1983.
49. Zimmerman LE, Burns RP, Wankum G, Tully R, Esterly JA: Trilateral retinoblastoma: Ectopic intracranial retinoblastoma associated with bilateral retinoblastoma. *Paediatr Ophthalmol Strabismus* **19(6)**:320, 1982.
50. Kingston JE, Plowman PN, Hungerford JL: Ectopic intracranial retinoblastoma in childhood. *Br J Ophthalmol* **69**:742, 1985.
51. Francois J, De Sutter E, Coppieters R, De Bie S: Late extraocular tumors in retinoblastoma survivors. *Ophthalmologica (Basel)* **181**:93, 1980.
52. Reese AB, Merriam GR, Martin HE: Treatment of bilateral retinoblastoma by irradiation and surgery: Report on 15 years results. *Am J Ophthalmol* **32**:175, 1949.
53. Frezzotti R, Guerra R: Sarcoma following irradiated retinoblastoma. *Arch Ophthalmol* **70**:471, 1963.
54. Forrest AW: Tumors following radiation about the eye. *Trans Am Acad Ophthalmol Otolaryngol* **65**:694, 1961.
55. Soloway HB: Radiation induced neoplasms following curative therapy for retinoblastoma. *Cancer* **19**:1984, 1966.
56. Sagerman RH, Cassady R, Tretter P, Ellsworth R: Radiation induced neoplasia following external beam therapy for children with retinoblastoma. *Am J Roentgenol Radium Ther Mucl Med* **105**:529, 1969.
57. Derkinderen DJ, Koten JW, Wolterbeek R, Beemer FA, Tan KE, Den Otter W: Non-ocular cancer in hereditary retinoblastoma survivors and relatives. *Ophthalmic Paediatr Genet* **8**:23, 1987.
58. Leuder GT, Judisch GF, O'Gorman TW: Second non-ocular tumors in survivors of heritable retinoblastoma. *Arch Ophthalmol* **104**:372, 1986.
59. Draper GJ, Sanders BM, Kingston JE: Second primary neoplasms in patients with retinoblastoma. *Br J Cancer* **53**:661, 1986.
60. Abramson DH, Ellsworth RM, Kitchin FD, Tung G: Second non-ocular tumors in retinoblastoma survivors: Are they radiation-induced? *Ophthalmology* **91**:1351, 1984.
61. Roarty JD, McLean IW, Zimmerman LE: Incidence of second neoplasms in patients with bilateral retinoblastoma. *Ophthalmology* **95**:1583, 1988.
62. Sang DN, Albert DM: Retinoblastoma: Clinical and histopathologic features. *Hum Pathol* **13**:133, 1982.
63. Brown DH: The clinicopathology of retinoblastoma. *Am J Ophthalmol* **97**:189, 1984.
64. Tosi P, Cintorino P, Toti V, Ninfo V, Montesco MC, Frezzotti R, Radjistilianou T, Acquaviva A, Barbini P: Histopathological evaluation for the prognosis of retinoblastoma. *Ophthalmic Paediatr Genet* **10**:173, 1987.
65. Kopelman JE, McLean IW, Rosenberg SH: Multivariate analysis of risk factors of metastasis in retinoblastoma treated by enucleation. *Ophthalmology* **94**:371, 1987.
66. Goldberg L, Danziger A: Computer tomographic scanning in the management of retinoblastoma. *Am J Ophthalmol* **84(3)**:380, 1977.
67. De Nicola M, Salvolini V: La risonanza magnetica nucleare e la tomografia assiale computerizzata nel retinoblastoma, in *Tumori Intraoculari. International Symposium Intraocular Tumors*. Palermo, Italy: Medical Books, 1990, p 43.
68. Char DH, Hedges TR, Norman D: Retinoblastoma: CT diagnosis. *Ophthalmology* **91**:1347, 1984.
69. Arrigg PG, Hedges RT, Char DH: Computed tomography in the diagnosis of retinoblastoma. *Br J Ophthalmol* **67**:558, 1983.
70. Mafee MF, Goldberg MF, Greenwald MJ, Schulman J, Malmed A, Flanders AE: Retinoblastoma and simulating lesions: Role of CT and MR imaging. *Radiol Clin North Am* **25**(4):667, 1987.
71. Schulman JA, Peyman G, Mafee MF, Laurence L, Bauman AE, Goldman A: The use of magnetic resonance imaging in the evaluation of retinoblastoma. *J Pediatr Ophthalmol Strabismus* **23**:144, 1986.
72. Mafee MF, Goldberg MF, Cohen SB, Gotsis ED, Safran M, Chekuri L, Raofi B: Magnetic resonance imaging versus computed tomography of leukocoric eyes and use of in vitro proton magnetic resonance spectroscopy of retinoblastoma. *Ophthalmology* **96**:965, 1989.
73. Haik BG, Saint Louis L, Smith ME, Ellsworth RM, Abramson DH, Cahill P, Deck M, Coleman DJ: Magnetic resonance imaging in the evaluation of leukocoria. *Ophthalmology* **92**:1143, 1985.
74. Benhamou E, Borges J, Tso MOM: Magnetic resonance imaging in retinoblastoma and retinocytoma: A case report. *J Paediatr Ophthalmol Strabismus* **26**:276, 1989.
75. Danziger A, Price HI: CT findings in retinoblastoma. *Am J Radiol* **133**:695, 1979.
76. Coleman DJ, Lizzi FC, Jack PL: *Ultrasonography of the Eye and Orbit*. Philadelphia: Lea & Febiger, 1977, p 209.
77. Sampaolesi R, Zacrate J: Errors in the diagnosis of retinoblastoma, in *Ultrasound in Ophthalmology. Proceedings of the 11th S.I.D.U.O. Congress*. Kluwer Academic, 1986, p 189.
78. Ossolning KC: *Proceedings of the 10th Course and Workshop on Clinical Echo-Ophthalmology*. Vienna, December 12–15, 1973.
79. Motolese E, Addabbo G: Diagnosi ecografica delle neoplasie oculari. Atti Convegno interdisciplinare problemi oculari nell'infanzia. Siena 14–15 ottobre, 1988. *Boll Ocul* **68**(5), 1989.
80. Jakobiec FA, Coleman DJ, Chattock A, Smith M: Ultrasonically guided needle biopsy and cytologic diagnosis of solid intraocular tumors. *Ophthalmology* **86**:1662, 1979.
81. Char DH, Miller TR: Fine needle biopsy in retinoblastoma. *Am J Ophthalmol* **97**:686, 1984.
82. Shields JA: Diagnostic approaches to intraocular tumors, in *Diagnosis and Management of Intraocular Tumors*. St. Louis: Mosby, 1983.
83. Midena E, Segato T, Piermarocchi S, Boccato P: Fine-needle aspiration biopsy in ophthalmology. *Surv Ophthalmol* **29**:410, 1985.
84. Augsburger JJ, Shields JA, Folberg R, Lang W, O'Hara BJ, Claricci J: Fine-needle aspiration biopsy in the diagnosis of intraocular cancer. *Ophthalmology* **92**:39, 1985.
85. Karcioglu ZA, Gordon R, Karcioglu G: Tumor seeding in ocular fine-needle aspiration biopsy. *Ophthalmology* **92**:1763, 1985.
86. Frezzotti R, Tosi P, Bardelli AM, Cintorino M, Hadjistilianou T: Cytologic diagnosis of retinoblastoma. *Proceedings I International Symposium on Ophthalmic Cytology*, Parma, Italy, October 9, 1987.
87. Arora R, Betharia SM: Fine-needle aspiration of paediatric orbital tumors. *Orbit* **7(2)**:115, 1988.
88. Frezzotti R, Hadjistilianou T, Greco G, Bartolomei A, Pannini S, Minacci C, Disanto A, Cintorino M: L'agobiopsia (FNAB) nella diagnosi differenziale delle neoplasie oculari ed orbitarie. *Atti LXIX Congresso S.O.I.* Rome, Oct. 12–15, 1989.
89. Reese AM, Ellsworth RM: Management of retinoblastoma. *Ann N Y Acad Sci* **114**:958, 1964.
90. Pratt CB: Management of malignant solid tumors in children. *Pediatr Clin North Am* **19(4)**:1141, 1972.
91. Stannard C, Lipper S, Sealy R, Sevel D: Retinoblastoma: Correlation of invasion of the optic nerve and choroid with prognosis and metastases. *Br J Ophthalmol* **63**:560, 1979.

92. Rosengren B, Monge OR, Flage T: Proposal of new pretreatment clinical TNM-classification of retinoblastoma. *Acta Oncol* **28**(4):547, 1989.
93. Shields JA, Shields CL, Sivalingam V: Decreasing frequency of enucleation in patients with retinoblastoma. *Am J Ophthalmol* **108**:185, 1989.
94. Ellsworth RM: Orbital retinoblastoma. *Trans Am Ophthalmol Soc* **72**:79, 1974.
95. Hilgartner HL: Report of a case of double glioma treated with X-ray. *Tex J Med* **18**:322, 1903.
96. Schipper J: An accurate and simple method for megavoltage radiation therapy of retinoblastoma. *Radiothes Oncol* **1**:31, 1983.
97. Harnett AN, Hungerford J, Lambert G, Hirst A, Darlinson R, Hart B, Trodd TC, Plowman P: Modern lateral external beam (lens sparing) radiotherapy for retinoblastoma. *Ophthalmic Paediatr Genet* **8**(1):53, 1987.
98. McCormick B, Ellsworth RM, Abramson DH: Results of external beam radiation for children with retinoblastoma: A comparison of two techniques. *J Pediatr Ophthalmol* **26**:239, 1989.
99. Reese AB, Ellsworth RM: The evaluation and current concept of retinoblastoma therapy. *Trans Am Acad Ophthalmol Otolaryngol* **67**:164, 1963.
100. Buys RJ, Abramson DH, Ellsworth RM, Haik B: Radiation regression patterns after cobalt plaque insertion for retinoblastoma. *Arch Ophthalmol* **101**:1206, 1983.
101. Abramson DH, Gerardi CM, Ellsworth RM, McCormick B, Sussman D, Turner L: Radiation regression patterns in treated retinoblastoma: 7 to 21 years later. *J Paediatr Ophthalmol Strabismus* **28**(2):108, 1991.
102. MacFaul PA, Bedford MA: Ocular complications after therapeutic irradiation. *Br J Ophthalmol* **54**:237, 1970.
103. Lommatzch PK: Die Anwendung von Betastrahlen mit 106 Ur/106 Rh Applikatoren bei dei Behandlung des Retinoblastomas. *Klin Monatsbl Augenheilkd* **156**:662, 1970.
104. Char DH: Retinoblastoma therapy, in *Clinical Ocular Oncology*. New York: Churchill Livingstone, 1989, p 207.
105. Shields J, Giblin ME, Shields C, Macroe AM, Karlsson V: Episcleral plaque radiotherapy for retinoblastoma. *Ophthalmology* **96**:530, 1989.
106. Meyer-Schwickerath G: The preservation of vision by treatment of intraocular tumors with light coagulation. *Arch Ophthalmol* **66**:458, 1961.
107. Frezzotti R, Hadjistilianou T: Is retinoblastoma vascularization a prognostic factor for xenon photocoagulation and for radiosensitivity? *Orbit* **7**(2):101, 1988.
108. Hadjistilianou T, Greco G, Frezzotti R: Photocoagulation therapy of retinoblastoma. *Orbit* **9(4)**:283, 1990.
109. Abramson DH: The focal treatment of retinoblastoma with emphasis on xenon arc photocoagulation. *Acta Ophthalmol* **67**(suppl 194):6, 1989.
110. Shields JA, Shields CL, Parsons H, Giblin ME: The role of photocoagulation in the management of retinoblastoma. *Arch Ophthalmol* **108**:205, 1990.
111. Hopping W, Meyer-Schwickerath G: Light coagulation treatment in retinoblastoma, in Boniuk M (ed): *Ocular and Adnexal Tumors*. St. Louis: Mosby, 1964.
112. Hopping W, Schmitt G: The treatment of retinoblastoma. *Mod Probl Ophthalmol* **13**:106, 1977.
113. Lincoff H, McLean J, Long R: The cryosurgical treatment of intraocular tumors. *Am J Ophthalmol* **63**:389, 1967.
114. Abramson DH, Ellsworth RM, Rozakis GW: Cryotherapy for retinoblastoma. *Arch Ophthalmol* **100**:1253, 1982.
115. Shields JA, Parson H, Shields CL, Giblin ME: The role of cryotherapy in the management of retinoblastoma. *Am J Ophthalmol* **108**:260, 1989.
116. Molteno ACB, Griffiths JS, Marcus PB, Van Der Watt JJ: Retinoblastoma treated by freezing. *Br J Ophthalmol* **55**:492, 1971.
117. Rubin ML: Cryopexy for retinoblastoma. *Am J Ophthalmol* **66**:870, 1968.
118. White L: The role of chemotherapy in the treatment of retinoblastoma. *Retina* **3**:194, 1983.
119. Kupfer C: Retinoblastoma treated with intravenous nitrogen mustard. *Am J Ophthalmol* **36**:1721, 1953.
120. Haye C, Schlienger B: La chimiotherapie des tumers de la retine. *Bull Mem Soc Franc Ophthalmol* **92**:119, 1980.
121. Zucher JM, Lemercier N, Schlienger P, Marguilis E, Haye C: Chemotherapeutic conservative management in twenty-three patients with locally extended bilateral retinoblastoma. *Eur J Clin Oncol* **10**:1, 1982.
122. Wolff JA, Boesel CP, Dyment PG, Ellsworth RM, Gallie B, Hammond D, Leiken SL, Maurer HS, Tretter PK, Wara WM: Treatment of retinoblastoma. A preliminary report. *Int Cong Series* **570**:364, 1981.
123. Pratt CB: Management of malignant solid tumors in children. *Pediatr Clin North Am* **19**(4):1141, 1972.
124. Howarth C, Meyer D, Hustu O, Johnson WW, Shanks E, Pratt C: Stage-related combined modality treatment of retinoblastoma. *Cancer* **45**:851, 1980.
125. Acquaviva A, Barberi L, Bernardini C, D'Ambrosio A, Lasorella G: Medical therapy in retinoblastoma in children. *J Neurosurg Sci* **26**(1):49, 1982.
126. Zelter M, Gonzales G, Schwartz L, Gallo G, Schvartzman, Damel A, Sackmann MF: Treatment of retinoblastoma: Results obtained from a prospective study of 51 patients. *Cancer* **61**:153, 1988.
127. Akiyama K, Iwasaki M, Amemiya T, Yanai M: Chemotherapy for retinoblastoma. *Ophthalmic Paediatr Genet* **10(2)**:111, 1988.
128. Pratt CB, Kun LE: Response of orbital and central nervous system metastases of retinoblastoma following treatment with cyclophosphamide/doxorubicin. *Pediatr Hematol Oncol* **4**:125, 1987.
129. Hungerford J, Kingston J, Plowman N: Orbital recurrence of retinoblastoma. *Ophthalmic Paediatr Genet* **8**:63, 1987.
130. Saarinen UM, Sariola N, Hovi L: Recurrent disseminated retinoblastoma treated by high-dose chemotherapy, total body irradiation, and autologous bone marrow rescue. *Am J Hematol Oncol* **13**(4):315, 1991.
131. White L: Chemotherapy in retinoblastoma: Current status and future directions. *Am J Pediatr Hematol Oncol* **13**(2):189, 1991.
132. White L: Chemotherapy in retinoblastoma: Where do we go from here? *Ophthalmic Paediatr Genet* **12**(3):115, 1991.
133. Hethcote HW, Knudson AGIR: Model for the incidence of embryonal cancers: Application to retinoblastoma. *Proc Natl Acad Sci U S A* **75**:2453, 1978.
134. Falls HF, Neel JV: Genetics of retinoblastoma. *Arch Ophthalmol* **151**:197, 1951.
135. Schappert-Kimmiiser J, Hemmes GD, Nijiland R: The heredity of retinoblastoma. *Ophthalmologica* **151**:197, 1966.
136. Vogel F: Neue untersuchunger zur genetik des retinoblastoms. *Z Menschl Vereh Konstit Lehre* **34**:205, 1957.
137. Knudson AGJR: Mutation and cancer: Statistical study of retinoblastoma. *Proc Natl Acad Sci U S A* **68**:820, 1971.
138. Macklin MT: A study of retinoblastoma in Ohio. *Am J Hum Genet* **12**:1, 1960.
139. Matsunaga E: Hereditary retinoblastoma: Delayed mutation or host resistance? *Am J Hum Genet* **30**:406, 1978.
140. Lele KP, Penrose LS, Stallard HB: Chromosome deletion in a case of retinoblastoma. *Ann Hum Genet* **27**:171, 1963.
141. Chaum E, Ellsworth RM, Abramsom DH, Haik BG, Kitchin FD, Chaganti RSK: Cytogenetic analysis of retinoblastoma: Evidence for multifocal origin and in vivo gene amplification. *Cytogenet Cell Genet* **38**:82, 1984.
142. Turleau C, de Grouchy U, Chavin-Coi IN F, Junien C, Seger J, Schieinger P, Leblanc A, Haye C: Cytogenetic forms of retinoblastoma: Their incidence in a survey of 66 patients. *Cancer Genet Cytogenet* **16**:321, 1985.
143. Squire J, Gallie BL, Phillips RA: A detailed analysis of chromosomal changes inheritable and non-heritable retinoblastoma. *Hum Genet* **70**:291, 1985.
144. Francke U: Retinoblastoma and chromosome 13. *Cytogenet Cell Genet* **16**:131, 1976.
145. Ward P, Packman S, Loughman W, Sparkes M, Sparkes RS, McMahon A, Gregory T, Ablin A: Location of the retinoblastoma susceptibility gene(s) and the human esterase D locus. *J Med Genet* **21**:92, 1984.
146. Sparkes RS, Murphree AL, Lingua RW, Sparkes MC, Field LL, Funderburk SJ, Benedict WF: Gene for hereditary retinoblastoma assigned to human chromosome 13 by linkage analysis to esterase D. *Science* **219**:971, 1983.
147. Sparkes RS, Sparkes MC, Wilson MG, Towner JW, Benedict WF, Murphree AL, Yunis JJ: Regional assignment of genes for esterase D and retinoblastoma to chromosome band 13q14. *Science* **208**:1042, 1980.
148. Strong LC, Riccardi VM, Ferrell RD, Sparkes RS: Familial retinoblastoma and chromosome 13 deletion transmitted via an insertional translocation. *Science* **213**:1501, 1981.
149. Sparkes RS, Muller H, Klisak I: Retinoblastoma with 13q-chromosomal deletion associated with maternal paracentric inversion of 13q. *Science* **203**:1027, 1979.
150. Riccardi VM, Hittner HM, Francke U, Pippin S, Holmquist GP, Kretzer FL, Ferrell R: Partial triplication and deletion of 13q: Study of

a family presenting with bilateral retinoblastoma. *Clin Genet* **15**:332, 1979.

151. Warburton D, Anyane-Yeboa K, Taterka P: Deletion of 13q14 without retinoblastoma: A case of non-penetrance. *Am J Hum Genet* **39**:A137, 1986.
152. Wilson WG, Carter BT, Conway BP, Atkin JF, Watson BA, Sparkes RS: Variable manifestations of deletion (13)(q14.1-q14.3) in two generations. *Am J Hum Genet* **39**:A47, 1986.
153. Motegi T: High rate of detection of 13q14 deletion mosaicism among retinoblastoma patients (using more extensive methods). *Hum Genet* **61**:95, 1982.
154. Wilson WG, Campochiaro PA, Conway BP, Sudduth KW, Watson BA, Sparkes RS: Deletion (13)(q14.1-q14.3) in two generations: Variability of ocular manifestations and definition of the phenotype. *Am J Med Genet* **28**:675, 1987.
155. Fukushima Y, Kuroki Y, Ito T, Kondo I, Nishigaki I: Familial retinoblastoma (mother and son) with 13q14 deletion. *Hum Genet* **77**:104, 1987.
156. Cavenee WK, Dryja TP, Phillips RA, Benedict WF, Godbout R, Gallie BL, Murphree AL, Strong LC, White RL: Expression of recessive alleles by chromosomal mechanisms in retinoblastoma. *Nature* **305**:779, 1983.
157. Barker D, Schaefer M, White RL: Restriction sites containing CpG show a higher frequency of polymorphism in human DNA. *Cell* **36**:131, 1984.
158. Wyman AR, White RL: A highly polymorphic locus in human DNA. *Proc Natl Acad Sci U S A* **77**:6754, 1980.
159. Cavenee WK, Leach RJ, Mohandas T, Pearson P, White RL: Isolation and regional localization of DNA segments revealing polymorphic loci from human chromosome 13. *Am J Hum Genet* **36**:10, 1984.
160. Dryja TP, Rapaport JM, Weichselbaum R, Bruns GAP: Chromosome 13 restriction fragment length polymorphisms. *Hum Genet* **65**:320, 1984.
161. Dryja TP, Cavenee WK, White RL, Rapaport JM, Peterson R, Albert DM, Bruns GAP: Homozygosity of chromosome 13 in retinoblastoma. *N Engl J Med* **310**:550, 1984.
162. Godbout R, Dryja TP, Squire JA, Gallie BL, Phillips RA: Somatic inactivation of genes on chromosome 13 is a common event in retinoblastoma. *Nature* **304**:550, 1983.
163. Cavenee WK, Hansen MF, Nordenskjold M, Kock E, Maumenee I, Squire JA, Phillips RA, Gallie BL: Genetic origin of mutations predisposing to retinoblastoma. *Science* **228**:501, 1985.
164. Abramson DH, Ellsworth RM, Kitchin FD, Tung G: Second nonocular tumors in retinoblastoma survivors: Are they radiation-induced? *Ophthalmology* **99**:1351, 1984.
165. Hansen MF, Koufos A, Gallie BL, Phillips RA, Fodstad O, Brogger A, Gedde-Dahl T, Cavenee WK: Osteosarcoma and retinoblastoma: A shared chromosomal mechanism revealing recessive predisposition. *Proc Natl Acad Sci U S A* **82**:6216, 1985.
166. Monaco AP, Bertelson CJ, Middlesworth W, Colletti C-A, Aldridge J, Fischbeck KH, Bartlett R, Pericak-Vance MA, Roses AD, Kunkel LM: Detection of deletions spanning the Duchenne muscular dystrophy locus using a tightly linked DNA segment. *Nature* **316**:842, 1985.
167. Royer-Pokora B, Kunkel LM, Monaco AP, Goff SC, Newburger PE, Baehner PL, Cole FS, Curnutte JT, Orkin SH: Cloning the gene for an inherited human disorder—chronic granulomatous disease—on the basis of its chromosomal location. *Nature* **322**:32, 1986.
168. Lalande M, Dryja TP, Schreck RR, Shipley J, Flint A, Latt SA: Isolation of human chromosome 13-specific DNA sequences cloned from flow sorted chromosomes and potentially linked to the retinoblastoma locus. *Cancer Genet Cytogenet* **13**:283, 1984.
169. Lalande M, Donlon T, Petersen RA, Lieberparb R, Manter S, Latt SA: Molecular detection and differentiation of deletions in band 13q14 in human retinoblastoma. *Cancer Genet Cytogenet* **23**:151, 1986.
170. Dryja TP, Rapoport JM, Joyce JM, Petersen RA: Molecular detection of deletions involving band q14 of chromosome 13 in retinoblastomas. *Proc Natl Acad Sci U S A* **83**:7391, 1986.
171. Bookstein R, Lee EY-HP, To H, Young L-J, Sey T, Hayes R, Friedmann T, Lee W-H: Human retinoblastoma susceptibility gene: Genomic organization and analysis of heterozygous intragenic deletion mutants. *Proc Natl Acad Sci U S A* **85**:2210, 1988.
172. Friend SH, Bernards R, Rogelj S, Weinberg RA, Rapoport JM, Albert DM, Dryja TP: A human DNA segment with properties of the gene that predisposes to retinoblastoma and osteosarcoma. *Nature* **323:643, 1986.**
173. Fung Y-KT, Murphree A, Tang A, Qian J, Hinrichs S, Benedict W: Structural evidence for the authenticity of the human retinoblastoma gene. *Science* **236**:1657, 1987.
174. Horsthemke B, Gregor V, Barnert H, Hopping W, Passarge E: Detection of submicroscopic deletions and a DNA polymorphism at the retinoblastoma locus. *Hum Genet* **76**:257, 1987.
175. Dunn J, Phillips R, Zhu X, Becker A, Gallie B: Mutations in the RB1 gene and their effect on transcription. *Mol Cell Biol* **9**:4596, 1989.
176. Yandell D, Campbell T, Dayton S, Petersen R, Walton D, Little J, McConkie-Rosell A, Buckley E, Dryja T: Oncogenic point mutations in the human retinoblastoma gene: Their application to genetic counseling. *N Engl J Med* **321**:1639, 1989.
177. Lee W-H, Bookstein R, Hong F, Young L-J, Shew J-Y, Lee EY-HP: Human retinoblastoma susceptibility gene: Cloning, identification, and sequence. *Science* **235**:1394, 1987.
178. Horowitz J, Park S-H, Bogenmann E, Cheng J-C, Yandell D, Kaye F, Minna J, Dryja T, Weinberg R: Frequent inactivation of the retinoblastoma anti-oncogene is restricted to a subset of human tumor cells. *Proc Natl Acad Sci U S A* **87**:2775, 1990.
179. Harbour J, Lai S-L, Whang-Peng J, Gazdar A, Minna J, Kaye F: Abnormalities in structure and expression of the human retinoblastoma gene in SCLC. *Science* **242**:263, 1988.
180. Tang A, Varley J, Chakroborty S, Murphree A, Fung Y-KT: Structural rearrangement of the retinoblastoma gene in human breast carcinoma. *Science* **242**:263, 1988.
181. Bookstein R, Lee EY-HP, Peccei A, Lee W-H: Human retinoblastoma gene: Long-range mapping and analysis of its deletion in a breast cancer cell line. *Mol Cell Biol* **9**:1628, 1989.
182. Seizinger B, Klinger H, Junien C, Nakamura Y, Lebeau M, Cavenee W, Emanual B, Ponder B, Naylor S, Mitelman R, Louis D, Menon A, Newsham I, Decker J, Laelbing M, Henry IV, Deimling A: Report of the committee on chromosome and gene loss in human neoplasia. *Cytogenet Cell Genet* **58**:1080, 1991.
183. Huang H-JS, Yee J-K, Shew J-Y, Chen P-L, Bookstein R, Friedmann T, Lee EY-HP, Lee W-H: Suppression of the neoplastic phenotype by replacement of the RB gene in human cancer cells. *Science* **242**:1563, 1988.
184. Takahashi R, Hashimoto T, Xu H-J, Matsui T, Mikki T, Bigo-Marshall H, Aaronson S, Benedict W: The retinoblastoma gene functions as a growth and tumor suppressor in human bladder carcinoma cells. *Proc Natl Acad Sci U S A* **88**:5257, 1991.
185. Bookstein R, Shew J-Y, Chen P-L, Scully P, Lee W-H: Suppression of tumorigenicity of human prostate carcinoma cells by replacing a mutated RB gene. *Science* **247**:712, 1990.
186. Niederkorn J, Streilein J, Shaddock J: Deviant immune responses to allogeneic tumors injected intracamerally and subcutaneously in mice. *Invest Ophthalmol Vis Sci* **20**:355, 1981.
187. Madreperla S, Whittum-Hudson J, Prendergast R, Chen P-L, Lee W-H: Intraocular tumor suppression of retinoblastoma gene-reconstituted retinoblastoma cells. *Cancer Res* **51**:6381, 1991.
188. Muncaster M, Cohen B, Phillips R, Gallie B: Failure of RB1 to reverse the malignant phenotype of human tumor cell lines. *Cancer Res* **52**:654, 1992.
189. Cavenee WK, Murphree AL, Shull MS, Benedict WF, Sparkes RS, Kock E, Nordenskjold M: Prediction of familial predisposition to retinoblastoma. *N Engl J Med* **314**:1201, 1986.
190. Horsthemke B, Barnert HJ, Greger V, Passarge E, Hopping W: Early diagnosis in hereditary retinoblastoma by detection of molecular deletions at gene locus. *Lancet* **28**:511, 1987.
191. Leppert M, Cavenee W, Callahan P, Holm T, O'Connell P, Thompson K, Lathrop GM, Lalouel J-M, White R: A primary genetic map of chromosome 13q. *Am J Hum Genet* **39**:425, 1986.
192. Lee EY-HP, Lee WH: Molecular cloning of the human esterase D gene, a genetic marker for retinoblastoma. *Proc Natl Acad Sci U S A* **83**:6337, 1986.
193. Squire J, Dryja TP, Dunn J, Goddard A, Hoffman T, Musarella M, Willard HF, Becker AJ, Gallie BL, Phillips RA: Cloning of the esterase D gene: A polymorphic probe closely linked to the retinoblastoma locus on chromosome 13. *Proc Natl Acad Sci U S A* **83**:6573, 1986.
194. Wiggs J, Nordenskjold M, Yandell D, Rapaport J, Grondin V, Janson M, Werelius B, Peterson R, Craft A, Riedel K, Liberfarb R, Walton D, Wilson W, Dryja TP: Prediction of risk of hereditary retinoblastoma using DNA polymorphisms within the retinoblastoma gene. *N Engl J Med* **318**:151, 1988.
195. Vaughn G, Toguchida J, McGee T, Dryja T: PCR detection of the TthIII 1 RFLP within the retinoblastoma locus by PCR. *Nucleic Acids Res* **18**:4965, 1990.
196. McGee T, Cowley G, Yandell D, Dryja T: Detection of the Xba I RFLP within the retinoblastoma locus by PCR. *Nucleic Acids Res* **18**:207, 1990.

197. Scharf S, Bowcock A, McClure G, Klitz W, Yandell D, Erlich H: Amplification and characterization of the retinoblastoma gene VNTR by PCR. *Am J Hum Genet* **50**:371, 1992.
198. Dryja T, Mukai S, Petersen R, Rapaport J, Walton D, Yandell D: Parental origin of mutations of the retinoblastoma gene. *Nature* **339**:556, 1989.
199. Zhu X, Dunn J, Phillips R, Goddard A, Paton K, Becker A, Gallie B: Preferential germline mutation of the paternal allele in retinoblastoma. *Nature* **340**:313, 1989.
200. Toguchida J, Ishizaki K, Sasaki M, Hakamura Y, Ikenaga M, Kato M, Sugimot M, Kotoura Y, Yamamuro T: Preferential mutation of paternally derived RB gene as the initial event in sporadic osteosarcoma. *Nature* **338**:156, 1989.
201. Sapeinza C: Genome imprinting and dominance modification. *Ann N Y Acad Sci* **564**:24, 1989.
202. Leach R, Magewu N, Buckley J, Benedict W, Rother C, Murphree A, Griegels, Rajewsky M, Jones P: Preferential retention of paternal alleles in human retinoblastoma: Evidence for genomic imprinting. *Cell Growth Diff* **1**:401, 1990.
203. Vogel W: Genetics of retinoblastoma. *Hum Genet* **52**:1, 1979.
204. Onadim Z, Hogg A, Baird P, Cowell J: Oncogenic point mutations in exon 20 of the RB1 gene in families showing incomplete penetrance and mild expression of the retinoblastoma phenotype. *Proc Natl Acad Sci U S A* **89**:6177, 1992.
205. Sakai T, Ohtani N, McGee T, Robbins P, Dryja T: Oncogenic germ-line mutations in Sp1 and ATF sites in the human retinoblastoma gene. *Nature* **353**:83, 1991.
206. Landshulz WH, Johnson PF, McKnight SL: The leucine zipper: A hypothetical structure common to a new class of DNA binding proteins. *Science* **240**:1759, 1988.
207. Patthy L: Evolution of the proteases of blood coagulation and fibrinolysis by assembly from modules. *Cell* **41**:657, 1985.
208. Hong FD, Huang H-JS, To H, Young L-JS, Oro A, Bookstein R, Lee EY-HP, Lee W-H: Structure of the human retinoblastoma gene. *Proc Natl Acad Sci U S A* **86**:5502, 1989.
209. Jones NC, Rigby PWJ, Ziff EB: Trans-acting protein factors and the regulation of eukaryotic transcription: Lessons from studies on DNA tumor viruses. *Gene Dev* **2**:267, 1988.
210. Lee W-H, Shew J-Y, Hong FD, Sery TW, Donoso LA, Young L-J, Bookstein R, Lee EY-HP: The retinoblastoma susceptibility gene encodes a nuclear phosphoprotein associated with DNA binding activity. *Nature* **329**:642, 1987.
211. Cross F, Weintraub H, Roberts J: Simple and complex cell cycles. *Annu Rev Cell Biol* **5**:341, 1989.
212. Pardee AB: G1 events and regulation of cell proliferation. *Science* **246**:605, 1989.
213. Pardee AB: Molecules involved in proliferation of normal and cancer cells: Presidential address. *Cancer Res* **47**:1488, 1987.
214. Mihara K, Cao X-R, Yen A, Chandler S, Driscoll B, Murphree AL, T-ang A, Fung Y-KT: Cell cycle-dependent regulation of phosphorylation of the human retinoblastoma gene product. *Science* **246**:1300, 1989.
215. Decaprio JA, Ludlow JW, Lynch D, Furukawa Y, Griffin J, Liwnica-Worms H, Huang C-M, Livingston DM: The product of the retinoblastoma susceptibility gene has properties of a cell cycle regulatory element. *Cell* **58**:1085, 1989.
216. Buchkovich K, Duffy LA, Harlow E: The retinoblastoma protein is phosphorylated during specific phases of the cell cycle. *Cell* **58**:1097, 1989.
217. Lin BT-Y, Gruenwald S, Morla AO, Lee W-H, Wang JYJ: Retinoblastoma cancer suppressor gene product is a substrate of the cell cycle regulator cdc2 kinase. *EMBO J* **10**:857, 1991.
218. Nurse P, Thuriaux P, Nasmyth K: Genetic control of the cell division cycle in the fission yeast *Schizosaccharomyces pombe*. *Mol Gen Genet* **146**:167, 1976.
219. D'Urso G, Marraccino RL, Marshak DR, Roberts JM: Cell cycle control of DNA replication by a homologue from human cells of the p34c-src protein kinase. *Science* **250**:786, 1990.
220. Shenoy S, Choi J-K, Bagrodia S, Copeland TD, Maller JL, Shalloway D: Purified maturation promoting factor phosphorylates pp60c-src at the sites phosphorylated during fibroblast mitosis. *Cell* **57**:763, 1989.
221. Chen P-L, Scully P, Shew J-Y, Wang JYJ, Lee W-H: Phosphorylation of the retinoblastoma gene product is modulated during the cell cycle and cellular differentiation. *Cell* **58**:1193, 1989.
222. Furukawa Y, Decaprio JA, Freedman A, Kanakura Y, Nakamura M, Ernst TJ, Livingston DM, Griffin JD: Expression and state of phosphorylation of the retinoblastoma susceptibility gene product in cycling and noncycling human hematopoietic cells. *Proc Natl Acad Sci U S A* **87**:2770, 1990.
223. Cooper JA, Whyte P: RB and the cell cycle: Entrance or exit? *Cell* **58**:1009, 1989.
224. Decaprio JA, Furukawa Y, Ajchenbaum F, Griffin JD, Livingston DM: The retinoblastoma-susceptibility gene product becomes phosphorylated in multiple stages during cell cycle entry and progression. *Proc Natl Acad Sci U S A* **89**:1795, 1992.
225. Hunter T, Pines J: Cyclins and cancer: II. Cyclin D and CDK inhibitors come of age. *Cell* **79**:573, 1994.
226. Jinag W, Kahn SM, Tomita N, Zhang Y-J, Lu SH, Weinstein IB: Amplification and expression of the human cyclin D gene in esophageal cancer. *Cancer Res* **52**:2980, 1992.
227. Motokura T, Arnold A: Cyclins and oncogenesis. *Biochim Biophys Acta* **1155**:63, 1993.
228. Dowdy SF, Hinds PW, Louie K, Reed S, Arnold A, Weinberg RA: Physical interaction of the retinoblastoma protein with human D cyclins. *Cell* **73**:499, 1993.
229. Ewen ME, Sluss HK, Sherr CJ, Matshushime H, Kato J, Livingston DM: Functional interactions of the retinoblastoma protein with mammalian D-type cyclins. *Cell* **73**:487, 1993.
230. Kato J, Matsushime H, Hiebert SW, Ewen ME, Sherr CJ: Direct binding of cyclin D to the retinoblastoma gene product (pRb) and pRb phosphorylation by the cyclin D-dependent kinase CDK4. *Genes Dev* **7**:331, 1993.
231. Fagan R, Flint KJ, Jones N: Phosphorylation of E2F-1 modulates its interaction with the retinoblastoma gene product and the adenoviral E4 19-kDa protein. *Cell* **78**:799, 1994.
232. Bates S, Parry D, Bonetta L, Vousden K, Dickson C, Peters G: Absence of cyclin D/cdk complexes in cells lacking functional retinoblastoma protein. *Oncogene* **9**:1633, 1994.
233. Mller H, Lukas J, Schneider A, Warthoe P, Bartek J, Ellers M, Strasu M: Cyclin D1 expression is regulated by the retinoblastoma protein. *Proc Natl Acad Sci U S A* **91**:2945, 1994.
234. Tam SW, Theodoras AM, Shay JW, Draetta GF, Pagano M: Differential expression and regulation of cyclin D1 protein in normal and tumor human cells: Association with Cdk4 is required for cyclin D1 function in G1 progression. *Oncogene* **9**:2663, 1994.
235. Serrano M, Hannon GJ, Beach D: A new regulatory motif in cell-cycle control causing specific inhibition of cyclin D/CDK4. *Nature* **366**:704, 1993.
236. Hannon GI, Beach D: p15INK4B is a potential effector of TGF-B-induced cell cycle arrest. *Nature* **371**:257, 1994.
237. Kamb A, Gruis NA, Weaver-Feldhaus J, Lie Q, Harshman K, Tavtigian SV, Stockert E, Day RSI, Johnson BE, Skolnick MH: A cell cycle regulator potentially involved in genesis of many tumor types. *Science* **264**:436, 1994.
238. Nobori T, Miura K, Wu DJ, Lois A, Takabayashi K, Carson DA: Deletions of the cyclin-dependent kinase-4 inhibitor gene in multiple human cancers. *Nature* **368**:753, 1994.
239. Merlo A, Herman JG, Mao L, Lee DJ, Gabrielson E, Burger PC, Baylin SB, Sidransky D: 59 CpG island methylation is associated with transcriptional silencing of the tumour suppressor p16/CDKN2/ MTS1 in human cancers. *Nat Med* **1:686, 1995.**
240. Costello JF, Berger MS, Huang H-JS, Cavenee WK: Silencing of p16/ CDKN2 expression in human gliomas by methylation and chromatin condensation. *Cancer Res* **56**:2405, 1996.
241. Arap W, Kishikawa R, Furnari FB, Cavenee WK, Huang H-JS: Replacement of the p16/CDKN2 gene suppresses human glioma cell growth. *Cancer Res* **55**:1351, 1995.
242. Bonetta L: Open questions on p16. *Nature* **370**:180, 1994.
243. Cairns P, Mao L, Merlo A, Lee DJ, Schwab D, Eby Y, Tokino K, van der Riet P, Blaugrund JE, Sidransky D: Rates of p16 (MTS1) mutations in primary tumors with 9p loss. *Science* **265**:415, 1994.
244. Kamp A, Liu Q, Harshman K, Tavtigian S: Rates of p16 (MTS1) mutations in primary tumors with 9p loss. *Science* **265**:416, 1994.
245. Spruck CHI, Gonzalex-Sulueta M, Shibata A, Simoneay AR, Lin M-F, Gonzales F, Tsai YC, Jones PA: p16 gene in uncultured tumours. *Nature* **370**:183, 1994.
246. He J, Olson JJ, James CD: Lack of p16INK4 or retinoblastoma protein (pRb) or amplification-associated overexpression of cdk4 is observed in distinct subsets of malignant glial tumors and cell lines. *Cancer Res* **55**:4833, 1995.
247. Mori T, Miura K, Aoki T, Nishihara T, Mori S, Nakamura M: Frequent somatic mutation of MTS1/CDK4 (multiple tumor suppressor/cyclin-dependent kinase 4 inhibitor) gene in esophageal squamous cell carcinoma. *Cancer Res* **54**:3396, 1994.

248. Caldas C, Hahn SA, da Costa LT, Redston MS, Schutte M, Seymour AB, Weinstein CK, Hruban RH, Yeo CJ, Kern SE: Frequent somatic mutations and homozygous deletions of the p16 (MTS1) gene in pancreatic adenocarcinoma. *Nat Genet* **8**:27, 1994.
249. Parry D, Bates S, Mann DJ, Peters G: Lack of cyclin D/Cdk complexes in RB-negative cells correlates with high levels of p16INK4/MTS1 tumour suppressor gene product. *EMBO J* **14**:503, 1995.
250. Li Y, Nichols MA, Shay JW, Xiong Y: Transcriptional repression of the D-type cyclin-dependent linases inhibitor p16 by the retinoblastoma susceptibility gene product, pRb. *Cancer Res* **54**:6078, 1994.
251. Shimizu E, Coxon A, Otterson GA, Steinberg SM, Kratzke RA, Kim YW, Fedorko J, Oie H, Johnson B, Mulsine JL, Minna JD, Gazdar AF, Kaye FJ: RB protein status and clinical correlation from 171 cell lines representing lung cancer, extrapulmonary small cell carcinoma, and mesothelioma. *Oncogene* **9**:2441, 1994.
252. Shapiro GI, Edwards CD, Kobzik L, Godleski J, Richars W, Sugarbaker DJ, Rollins BJ: Reciprocal Rb inactivation and p16INK4 expression in primary lung cancers and cell lines. *Cancer Res* **55**:505, 1995.
253. Otterson GA, Kratzke RA, Coxon A, Kim YW, Kaye FJ: Absence of p16INK4 protein is restricted to the subset of lung cancer lines that retains wild-type RB. *Oncogene* **9**:3375, 1994.
254. Sakaguchi M, Fuji Y, Hirabayashi H, Yoon H-E, Komoto Y, Oue T, Kusafuka T, Okada A, Matsuda H: Inversely correlated expression of p16 and Rb protein in non-small cell lung cancers: An immunohistochemical study. *Int J Cancer* **65**:442, 1996.
255. Schauer IE, Siriwardana S, Langan TA, Sclarani RA: Cyclin Da overexpression vs. retinoblastoma inactivation: Implications for growth control evasion in non-small cell and small cell lung cancer. *Proc Natl Acad Sci U S A* **91**:7827, 1994.
256. Berk A: Adenovirus promoters and E1A transactivation. *Annu Rev Genet* **20**:45, 1986.
257. Livingston DM, Bradley MK: Review: The simian virus 40 large T antigen — A lot packed into a little. *Mol Biol Med* **4**:63, 1987.
258. Zur Hausen H, Schneider A, in Howley PM, Salzman MP (eds): *The Papovaviridae, vol 2: The Papillomaviruses*. New York: Plenum, 1987, pp 245–263.
259. Cherington V, Brown M, Paucha E, St. Louis J, Spiegelman BM, Roberts TM: Separation of simian virus 40 large T-antigen-transforming and origin-binding functions from the ability to block differentiation. *Mol Cell Biol* **8**:1380, 1988.
260. Clayton CE, Murphy D, Lovett M, Rigby PWJ: A fragment of the SV40 T-antigen gene transforms. *Nature* **299**:59, 1982.
261. Whyte P, Ruley HE, Harlow E: Two regions of the adenovirus early region 1A proteins are required for transformation. *J Virol* **62**:257, 1988.
262. Phelps WC, Yee CL, Munger K, Howley PM: The human papilloma type 16 E7 gene encodes transactivation and transformation functions similar to those of adenovirus E1A. *Cell* **53**:539, 1988.
263. Harlow E, Whyte P, Franza BR Jr, Schley C: Association of adenovirus early-region 1A proteins with cellular polypeptides. *Mol Cell Biol* **6**:1579, 1986.
264. Whyte P, Buchkovich KJ, Horowitz JM, Friend SH, Raybuck M, Weinberg RA, Harlow E: Association between an oncogene and an antioncogene: The adenovirus E1A proteins bind to the retinoblastoma gene product. *Nature* **234**:124, 1988.
265. Decaprio JA, Ludlow JW, Figge J, Shew J-Y, Huang C-M, Lee W-H, Marsilio E, Paucha E, Livingston DM: SV40 large tumor antigen forms a specific complex with the product of the retinoblastoma susceptibility gene. *Cell* **54**:275, 1988.
266. Dyson N, Howley PM, Munger K, Harlow E: The human papilloma virus-16 E7 oncoprotein is able to bind to the retinoblastoma gene product. *Science* **243**:934, 1989.
267. Kalderon D, Smith AE: In vitro mutagenesis of a putative DNA binding domain of SV40 large T. *Virology* **139**:109, 1984.
268. Ludlow JW, Decaprio JA, Huang C-M, Lee W-H, Paucha E, Livingston DM: SV40 large T antigen binds preferentially to an underphosphorylated member of the retinoblastoma susceptibility gene product family. *Cell* **56**:57, 1989.
269. Ludlow JW, Shon J, Pipas JM, Livingston DM, Decaprip JA: The retinoblastoma susceptibility gene product undergoes cell cycle-dependent dephosphorylation and binding to and release from SV40 large T. *Cell* **60**:387, 1990.
270. Peden KWC, Srinivasan A, Parber JM, Pipas JM: Mutants with changes within or near a hydrophobic region of simian virus 40 large tumor antigen are defective for binding cellular protein p53. *Virology* **168**:13, 1989.
271. Tack LC, Cartwright CA, Wright JH, Eckhard W, Peden KWC, Srinivasan A, Pipas JM: Properties of a simian virus 40 mutant T antigen substituted in the hydrophobic region: Defective ATP-ase and oligomerization activities and altered phosphorylation accompany an inability to complex with cellular p53. *J Virol* **63**:3362, 1989.
272. Dyson N, Buchovich K, Whyte P, Harlow E: The cellular 107K protein that binds to adenovirus E1A also associates with the large T antigens of SV40 and JC virus. *Cell* **58**:249, 1989.
273. Ewen ME, Ludlow JW, Marsilio E, Decaprio JA, Millikan RC, Cheng SH, Paucha E, Livingston DM: An N-terminal transformation-governing sequence of SV40 large T antigen contributes to the binding of both $p110^{RB}$ and a second cellular protein, p120. *Cell* **58**:257, 1989.
274. Hu Q, Dyson N, Harlow E: The regions of the retinoblastoma protein needed for binding to adenovirus E1A or SV40 large T antigen are common sites for mutations. *EMBO J* **9**(4):1147, 1990.
275. Huang S, Wang N-P, Tseng BY, Lee W-H, Lee EH-YP: Two distinct and frequently mutated regions of retinoblastoma protein are required for binding to SV40 T antigen. *EMBO J* **9**(6):1815, 1990.
276. Horowitz J, Yandell DW, Park S-H, Canning S, Whyte P, Buchkovich K, Harlow E, Weinberg RA, Dryja TP: Point mutational inactivation of the retinoblastoma antioncogene. *Science* **243**:937, 1989.
277. Shew J-Y, Ling N, Yang X, Fodstad O, Lee W-H: Antibodies detecting abnormalities of the retinoblastoma susceptibility gene product ($pp110^{RB}$) in osteosarcomas and synovial sarcomas. *Oncogene Res* **4**:205, 1989.
278. Bookstein R, Shew J-Y, Chen P-L, Scully P, Lee W-H: Suppression of tumorigenicity of human prostate carcinoma cells by replacing a mutated RB gene. *Science* **247**:712, 1990.
279. Shew J-Y, Lin BT-Y, Chen P-L, Tseng BY, Yang-Feng TL, Lee W-H: C-terminal truncation of the retinoblastoma gene product leads to functional inactivation. *Proc Natl Acad Sci U S A* **87**:6, 1990.
280. Defeo-Jones D, Huang PS, Jones RE, Haskell KM, Vuocolo GA, Hanobik MG, Huber HE, Oliff A: Cloning of cDNAs for cellular proteins that bind to the retinoblastoma gene product. *Nature* **352**:251, 1991.
281. Huang S, Lee W-H, Lee EY-HP: A cellular protein that competes with SV40 T antigen for binding to the retinoblastoma gene product. *Nature* **350**:160, 1991.
282. Kaelin WG, Pallas DC, Decaprio JA, Kaye FJ, Livingston DM: Identification of cellular proteins that can interact specifically with the T/E1A-binding region of the retinoblastoma gene product. *Cell* **64**:521, 1991.
283. Partridge JF, Lathangue NB: A developmentally regulated and tissue-dependent transcription factor complexes with the retinoblastoma gene product. *EMBO J* **10**:3819, 1991.
284. Bandara LR, Lathangue NB: Adenovirus E1A prevents the retinoblastoma gene product from complexing with a cellular transcription factor. *Nature* **351**:494, 1991.
285. Bandara LR, Adamczewski JP, Hunt T, Lathangue NB: Cyclin A and the retinoblastoma gene product complex with a common transcription factor. *Nature* **352**:249, 1991.
286. Buyse IM, Shao G, Huang S: The retinoblastoma protein binds to RIZ, a zinc-finger protein that shares an epotope with the adenovirus E1A protein. *Proc Natl Acad Sci U S A* **92**:4467, 1995.
287. Gu W, Schneider JW, Condorelli G, Kaushal S, Mahdavi V, Nadal-Ginard B: Interaction of myogenic factors and the retinoblastoma protein mediates muscle cell commitment and differentiation. *Cell* **72**:309, 1993.
288. Welch PJ, Wang JYJ: Abrogation of retinoblastoma protein function by c-Abl through tyrosine kinase-dependent and -independent mechanisms. *Mol Cell Biol* **15**:5542, 1995.
289. Xiao Z-X, Chen J, Levine AJ, Modjtahedi N, Xing J, Sellers WR, Livingston DM: Interaction between the retinoblastoma protein and the oncoprotein MDM2. *Nature (London)* **375**:694, 1995.
290. Eckner R, Ewen ME, Newsome D, Gerdes M, DeCaprio JA, Lawrence JB, Lingston DM: Molecular cloning and functional analysis of the adenovirus E1A-associated 300-kD protein (p300) reveals a protein with properties of a transcriptional adaptor. *Genes Dev* **8**:869, 1994.
291. Strober BE, Dunaief JL, Sushovan G, Goff SP: Functional interactions between the hBRM/hBRG1 transcriptional activators and the pRB family of proteins. *Mol Cell Biol* **16**:1576, 1996.
292. Chittenden T, Livingston DM, Kaelin WG: The T/E1A-binding domain of the retinoblastoma product can interact selectively with a sequence-specific DNA-binding protein. *Cell* **65**:1073, 1991.
293. Helin K, Lees JA, Vidal M, Dyson N, Harlow E, Fattaey A: A cDNA encoding a pRB-binding protein with properties of the transcription factor E2F. *Cell* **70**:337, 1992.

294. Kaelin WG, Krek W, Sellers WR, Decaprio JA, Ajchenbaum F, Fuchs CS, Chittenden T, Li Y, Farnham PJ, Blanar MA, Livingston DM, Flemington EK: Expression cloning of a cDNA encoding a retinoblastoma-binding protein with E2F-like properties. *Cell* **70**:351, 1992.
295. Chellappan SP, Hiebert S, Mudry JM, Horowitz JM, Nevins JR: The E2F transcription factor is a cellular target for the RB protein. *Cell* **65**:1053, 1991.
296. Bagchi S, Weinmann R, Raychaudhuri P: The retinoblastoma protein copurifies with E2F-I, and E1A-regulated inhibitor of the transcription factor E2F. *Cell* **65**:1063, 1991.
297. Weintraub SJ, Prater CA, Dean DC: Retinoblastoma protein switches the E2F site from positive to negative element. *Nature* **358**:259, 1992.
298. Ewen ME, Xing Y, Lawrence JB, Livingston DM: Molecular cloning, chromosomal mapping, and expression of the cDNA for p107, a retinoblastoma gene product-related protein. *Cell* **66**:1155, 1991.
299. Hannon GJ, Demetrick D, Beach D: Isolation of the Rb-related p130 through its interaction with CDK2 and cyclins. *Genes Dev* **7**:2378, 1993.
300. Cobrinik D, Whyte P, Peeper DS, Jacks T, Weinberg RA: Cell cycle-specific association of E2F with the p130 E1A-binding protein. *Genes Dev* **7**:2392, 1993.
301. Li Y, Graham C, Lacy S, Duncan AMV, Whyte P: The adenovirus E1A-associated 130-kD protein is encoded by a member of the retinoblastoma gene family and physically interacts with cyclins A and E. *Genes Dev* **7**:2366, 1993.
302. Ewen ME, Faha B, Harlow D, Livingston D: Interaction of p107 with cyclin A independent of complex formation with viral oncoproteins. *Science* **255**:85, 1992.
303. Zhu L, van der Heuvel K, Fattaey A, Ewen M, Livingston D, Dyson N, Harlow E: Inhibition of cell proliferation by p107, a relative of the retinoblastoma protein. *Genes Dev* **7**:1111, 1993.
304. Maw MA, Grundy PE, Millow LJ, Eccles MR, Dunn RS, Smith PJ, Feinberg AP, Law DJ, Paterson MC, Telzerow PE: A third Wilms' tumor locus on chromosome 16q. *Cancer Res* **52**:3094, 1992.
305. Slater RM, Mannens MM: Cytogenetics and molecular genetics of Wilms' tumor of childhood. *Cancer Genet Cytogenet* **61**:111, 1992.
306. Newsham I, Röhrborn-Kindler A, Daub D, Cavenee WK: A constitutional BWS-related t(11;16) chromosome translocation occurring in the same region of chromosome 16 implicated in Wilms' tumors. *Gene Chrom Cancer* **12**:1, 1995.
307. Jacks T, Faxeli A, Schmitt EM, Bronson RT, Goodell MA, Weinberg RA: Effects of an Rb mutation in the mouse. *Nature* **359**:295, 1992.
308. Lee EY-HP, Chang CY, Hu N, Wang Y-CJ, Lai C-C, Herrup K, Lee W-H, Bradley A: Mice deficient for Rb are nonviable and show defects in neurogenesis and haematopoiesis. *Nature* **359**:288, 1992.
309. Williams BO, Schmitt EM, Remington L, Bronson RT, Albert DM, Weinberg RA, Jacks T: Extensive contribution of Rb-deficient cells to adult chimeric mice with limited histopathological consequences. *EMBO J* **13**:4251, 1994.
310. Windle JJ, Albert DM, O'Brien JM, Marcus DM, Disteche CM, Bernards, Mellon PL: Retinoblastoma in transgenic mice. *Nature* **343**:665, 1990.
311. Herrera RE, Sah VP, Williams BO, Makela TP, Weinberg RA, Jacks T: Altered cell cycle kinetics, gene expression, and G1 restriction point regulation in Rb-deficient fibroblasts. *Mol Cell Biol* **16**:2402, 1996.
312. Harvey M, Vogel H, Lee EY-HP, Bradley A, Donehower LA: Mice deficient in both p53 and Rb develop tumors primarily of endocrine origin. *Cancer Res* **55**:1146, 1995.
313. Williams BO, Remington L, Albert DM, Mukai S, Bronson RT, Jacks T: Cooperative tumorigenic effects of germline mutations in Rb and p53. *Nat Genet* **7**:480, 1994.

CHAPTER 37

Li-Fraumeni Syndrome

David Malkin

1. The Li-Fraumeni syndrome (LFS) is a rare autosomal dominantly inherited disorder. It is characterized by the diagnosis of bone or soft tissue sarcoma at an early age in an individual who has one first-degree relative with early onset cancer and a second close relative with early onset cancer or sarcoma diagnosed at any age.

2. Families in which the classic phenotype of the syndrome is not expressed completely are termed Li-Fraumeni syndrome-like (LFS-L) and are represented by many different features. Common to all these families is the occurrence of a variety of cancers of a distinct histopathologic type.

3. Germ-line alterations of the *p53* tumor-suppressor gene located on chromosome 17p13 have been observed in the majority of LFS families and in a proportion of LFS-L families. This gene encodes a 53-kDa nuclear phosphoprotein that is composed of 393 amino acids. Genetic alterations primarily result from base-pair substitutions that result in missense mutations. These changes are among the most frequently observed genetic abnormalities in human cancer. Somatic inactivation of *p53* occurs through base-pair substitutions or binding to other cellular proteins or to certain DNA tumor virus proteins.

4. The p53 protein binds specific DNA sequences and appears to be a transcription factor that may regulate the expression of other growth regulatory genes in a positive or negative manner. The antiproliferative effect of wild-type p53 is exerted at a checkpoint control site before G1/S of the cell cycle, with G2/M and the mitotic spindle being other potential targets. p53 mediates apoptosis and plays an important role in modulating the cellular response to DNA damage induced by ultraviolet (UV) irradiation or γ-irradiation and certain chemotherapeutic agents.

5. *p53* mutations are not observed in all classic LFS families. Germ-line *p53* mutations are seen in a small number of patients and families with cancer phenotypes that only superficially resemble LFS. Other mechanisms of *p53* inactivation may occur in some clinical settings, and other genes involved in cell cycle regulation may be altered in *p53* wild-type families.

6. Mouse models of *p53* deficiency have been created. These *p53* knockouts exhibit an increased rate of development of a spectrum of tumors, including lymphomas and sarcomas. Transgenic *p53* mice have been generated that have a tumor phenotype distinct from that of the *p53*-deficient animals. Mice heterozygous for a deleted *p53* allele exhibit an intermediate phenotype in that the rate of tumor formation is slower than that of the *p53*-null animals yet faster than that of wild-type littermates. These mice have been used as *in vivo* models to analyze p53 function and dysfunction in the setting of interventions with chemotherapy, radiation therapy, or teratogenic agents.

7. Predictive genetic testing for carriers of mutant *p53* is available in research settings in a few centers. The interpretation of results with respect to diagnostic capabilities and options for therapeutic intervention is under scrutiny. The value of such screening is tempered by the need to evaluate risk, counseling issues, the need for informed consent, and regulations on testing.

Studies of hereditary cancer clusters have led to the identification of genes critical to both carcinogenesis and normal development. The Li-Fraumeni syndrome (LFS) is a rare familial cancer syndrome that represents the paradigm of human cancer predisposition to multiple childhood and adult onset neoplasms. Before identification of a specific genetic defect that was inherited in a significant proportion of LFS families, it could not be definitely established that such a diverse spectrum of tumors could result from the alteration of a specific gene as a presumptive initiating event. The span of time from the initial clinical description of a family with this constellation of tumors to identification of germ-line alterations of the *p53* tumor-suppressor gene in many families was 20 years. The realization of a genetic link resulted from expertise in classic genetic epidemiology and the molecular biology of sporadic tumorigenesis and in many ways represented the realization of the development of the now burgeoning field of molecular epidemiology. The link between an extremely rare clinical phenotype (LFS) with alterations of perhaps the most commonly altered gene in human cancer (*p53*) points out the value of studying rare genetic phenotypes. These studies have led to a clearer understanding of the role *p53* plays in cell cycle control as well as to a cloudier picture of the way in which the LFS phenotype is derived in the absence of *p53* alterations. The generation of mouse models of deficient *p53* or altered *p53* functions has provided an opportunity to study not only the tumorigenic effects of this genotype but also the potential results of therapeutic, carcinogenic, and teratogenic interventions in tissues harboring an altered *p53* allele.

In addition to expanding our knowledge of cell cycle control, the study of these LFS families formed the early foundations on which recommendations and guidelines could be established to develop and monitor genetic testing programs for predisposition to both early and late onset disease. The models developed for other genetic diseases have been helpful as guides, but the unique imprecise nature of human carcinogenesis and the *p53*-LFS association require complex interactions among several disciplines.

The genetics of LFS and the complex roles of *p53* are still being elucidated. A vast literature has been generated about this gene, and characterizations of its roles in clinical genetics and clinical medicine are relatively early in their development. Future editions of this textbook will continue to clarify the relationship between the LFS phenotype and its variable genotype.

CLINICAL ASPECTS

Historical Perspective

In 1969, Li and Fraumeni reported the results of a retrospective survey of 280 medical records and 418 death certificates of

A list of standard abbreviations is located immediately preceding the index in each volume. Nonstandard abbreviations used in this chapter include: LFS = Li-Fraumeni syndrome; LFS-L = Li-Fraumeni syndrome-like; PCNA = poliferating cell nuclear antigen; ADCC = Adrenocortical carcinoma; ES = embryonic stem

childhood rhabdomyosarcoma patients diagnosed in the United States.[1,2] Five families were identified in whom siblings or cousins had been diagnosed with a childhood sarcoma. A high concentration of cancers of diverse types was observed in the ancestral line of one parent in each family. The most frequent of these cancers were soft tissue sarcomas, early onset breast cancers, and other early onset cancers. In fact, three of the mothers of the index children had developed breast cancer before 30 years of age. Other frequently occurring tumors included acute leukemias, brain tumors, and carcinoma of the lung, pancreas, and skin in first- and second-degree relatives and adrenocortical carcinoma in siblings. By making assumptions about family size, the authors estimated that among this series of childhood probands, considerably fewer than one pair of affected siblings would have been expected by chance. The occurrence of cancer in both a parent and a child in these families suggested the possibility of vertical transmission of an oncogenic agent through generations of genetically susceptible individuals.[1] Although it was implied, inherited predisposition on an exclusively genetic basis was not shown directly.

Within the first few years after these initial reports, several other phenotypically similar families were described in which unusual clusterings of cancers were observed.[3–6] In particular, Lynch and colleagues, in describing these pedigrees, coined the term *SBLA syndrome.* The letters represented what the authors considered the principal component tumors: sarcoma (*S*), breast and brain cancer (*B*), leukemia, lung, and laryngeal cancer (*L*), and adrenocortical carcinoma (*A*).[7] Although this terminology was initially prevalent, the syndrome is now more commonly known as the *Li-Fraumeni syndrome.*

It was suggested from the original reports that the familial occurrence of neoplasms originating at discordant sites might represent a counterpart of the tendency for a single individual to develop multiple primary tumors.[1,2] In fact, subsequent epidemiologic studies have confirmed that the neoplasms in LFS tend to develop in children and young adults, often as multiple primary cancers in affected individuals.[8] These studies also provided evidence to indicate that genetic predisposition is a primary causative factor. A follow-up study of the original four families found that over a 12-year period, 10 of the 31 surviving family members had developed 16 additional cancers, in comparison with less than 1 expected from general population rates.[9] These 16 malignancies were of the same types that had been observed originally and included 5 breast cancers, 4 soft tissue sarcomas, and 2 central nervous system tumors. Even after exclusion of the sarcomas that had arisen in the radiation fields of previous tumors, the remaining number of cancers still represented a significant excess above the expected (12 observed, 0.5 expected). Furthermore, 12 of these 16 cancers (primarily sarcomas and breast carcinomas) occurred in family members who had survived their original cancers. Analysis of 200 affected LFS family members in 24 families demonstrated a relative risk of occurrence of a second neoplasm of 5.3, with a cumulative probability of a second cancer occurrence of 57 percent at 30 years postdiagnosis of a first cancer. Over 70 percent of subsequent cancers were component cancers of LFS. The high frequency of second cancers with the same histopathologic diagnosis as types originally described in these families supported the argument in favor of genetic predisposition.

Defining the Classic LFS

Ascertainment biases have complicated interpretation of the original description and subsequent reports of LFS kindreds. These biases develop from the preferential attention given to the most dramatically affected kindreds, the possibility of chance occurrence of cancer in rare families (phenocopies), the uncertainty of the prevalence of the syndrome in the general population, and uncertainties in defining the spectrum of cancers in the syndrome and ultimately in characterizing the penetrance of the predisposing gene or genes.[10] The first attempt to formulate a "definition" of the syndrome was presented by Li and colleagues

Li-Fraumeni Syndrome "Classic" Pedigree

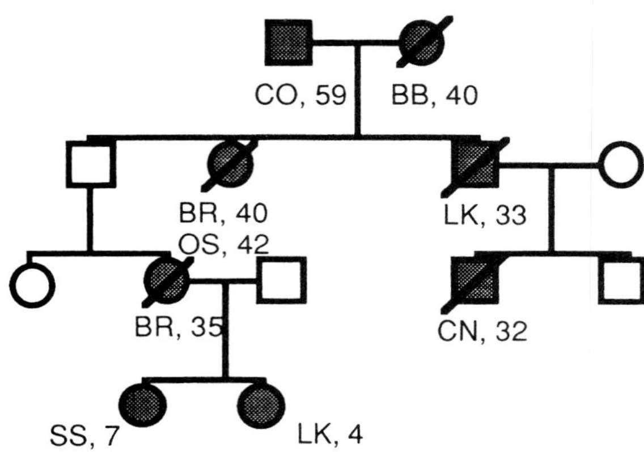

Fig. 37-1 Classic Li-Fraumeni syndrome pedigree. Notable features include the presence of a sarcoma before age 45 years and at least two first-degree relatives with cancer before age 45. In addition, multiple primary tumors occur in an affected member. Note also should be made of the presence of tumors less typical of the component neoplasms of LFS. The pattern of inheritance best fits an autosomal dominant model. BB 5, bilateral breast cancer; BR 5, breast cancer; CN 5, brain tumor; CO 5, colon cancer; LK 5, leukemia; SS 5, soft tissue sarcoma; OS 5, osteosarcoma.

in 1988, based on a prospective analysis of the characteristic component tumors and other detailed information on 24 kindreds.[11] To be eligible for this study, each kindred was required to conform to the following criteria: (1) a bone or soft tissue sarcoma diagnosed under 45 years of age in an individual who was then designated the proband, (2) one first-degree relative of the proband with cancer diagnosed before 45 years of age, and (3) one first- or second-degree relative of the proband in the same lineage with cancer before age 45 years or sarcoma diagnosed at any age.

These criteria have until recently found wide acceptance as a clinical definition of the syndrome, and families that adhere to these criteria have been referred to as having "classic" LFS. Such a family is illustrated in Fig. 37-1. This extensive study revealed continued expression of the dominantly inherited syndrome among young family members. Within the 24 families, 151 blood relatives had developed cancer, and of these cancers, 119 (79 percent) were diagnosed before the age of 45, compared with 10 percent of all cancers in this age range in the general population. Of note, excess occurrences were predominantly confined over time to the six previously described cancer types: breast carcinomas, soft tissue sarcomas, osteosarcomas, leukemias, brain tumors, and adrenocortical carcinomas. Adrenocortical carcinomas were confined to children under 14 years of age. Multiple primary tumors occurred in 15 family members, with the second and subsequent cancers also representing the principal tumor types. The analysis failed to implicate any additional tumors as components of the syndrome. However, subsequent analysis of many families at several major centers as well as in relatively isolated settings has identified cases that resemble the "classic" syndrome yet, in lacking one particular criterion or being associated with other, less frequently observed cancers, fail to meet the most stringent interpretation of the definition.[12–16] Several tumors are now considered to be associated with LFS, including germ-cell tumors,[17] melanoma,[17,18] and prostate and pancreatic cancer.[19] Families with these component tumors have been referred to as *extended LFS.*[20]

Defining LFS-like Families

Several families have been identified which demonstrate the clustering of tumors seen in typical extended LFS families but do not conform to the classic definition. These families have been defined in more than one way, reflecting the confusion arising from the lack of a definitive causative association in all cases. Eeles and colleagues defined *Li-Fraumeni-syndrome-like* (LFS-L) as the clustering of two different tumors seen in extended LFS in individuals who are first- or second-degree relatives with respect to each other and are affected at any age.[20] Birch et al.[16] have suggested that an age restriction of under 60 years be imposed because estimates of age-specific cancer risk in classic LFS are elevated up to but not beyond this point.[10] Further molecular epidemiologic studies are required to clarify the distinction between LFS and LFS-L and to determine the importance of perceived or actual differences.

GENETIC ASPECTS

Classic Genetic Analysis

Williams and Strong[21] and Lustbader et al.[13] performed segregation analyses in hospital-based series of survivors of childhood soft tissue sarcoma patients. Among the first-degree relatives of children in the series, 34 cancers occurred (21 expected), with the excess being predominantly breast cancers and sarcomas diagnosed at a young age. The relatives at the most elevated risk were those of children with soft tissue sarcomas diagnosed at young ages, with sarcomas of embryonal histologic subtype, and with multiple primary sarcomas.[12,19,21] It became evident that the cancer distribution in the families was most compatible with a rare autosomal dominant gene, the gene frequency being equal to 0.00002, or 1 in 50,000. The penetrance was estimated to be almost 50 percent by 30 years and 90 percent by 60 years of age.[21] This point becomes significant for any potential revisions to the original classic definition in that the age limit for tumor occurrence has been increased from 45 years, as established in 1988, to the current 60 years, as recommended by participants in the Third Workshop on Collaborative, Interdisciplinary Studies of *p53* and Li-Fraumeni Syndrome in 1996. The relative risk of developing cancer in children who carried the gene or genes was estimated to be 100 times the background rate. Although the age-specific penetrance was somewhat higher in females, this phenomenon was thought to be due to the occurrence of breast cancer. Maternal and paternal lineages appear to contribute equally to the evidence favoring a dominant gene.[13] These calculations generally have held up to the test of time, even as the genetic etiology of the syndrome has become apparent. Nevertheless, despite the careful phenotypic and statistical study of the syndrome, it became clear that the identification of a defective gene or genes conferring a predisposition in carriers within these families would assist in clarifying the definition of the syndrome.

Searching for an Etiologic "Agent"

Early attempts to isolate the LFS gene or genes were hampered by a variety of factors. The rarity, ambiguity of definition, and infrequent recognition of the syndrome, along with the high mortality among affected family members, significantly reduced the number of available informative tissue and blood samples. Cancers occurring in relatives who were not gene carriers were not histopathologically distinct from cancers in gene carriers. Consistent constitutional karyotypic alterations do not occur in these families, precluding a specific chromosomal site on which to focus a search for the responsible gene. Precancerous conditions such as benign adenomas and associated phenotypic malformations are not characteristic of LFS families and therefore cannot be used to map genes in the same fashion that the presence of aniridia (absence of the iris) was useful in the localization of the Wilms' tumor gene (*WT1*) to chromosome 11p13.[22–24]

Early cytogenetic, immunologic, serologic, and other attempts to determine the biologic basis of LFS were largely uninformative.[25] A report of two families suggested an association of HLA tissue type B12 with the disorder,[6] yet no follow-up of this observation is available. Studies of fibroblast cell lines from affected members of one family showed reduced cell killing by graded doses of ionizing radiation, and apparent activation of the c-*raf*-1 oncogene was reported in one of these lines.[26] However, fibroblasts from other families have demonstrated a normal cytotoxic response.[27] More recently, normal skin fibroblasts derived from affected LFS patients have been shown to exhibit features consistent with immortalization in the absence of stimulation by exogenous oncogenic or viral factors.[28] These features of altered morphology, aneuploidy, anchorage-independent growth, and an extended life span in culture appeared to occur spontaneously.[29] Furthermore, these spontaneously immortalized cells also have been shown to form tumors in nude mice when transformed by an activated Ha-*ras* oncogene,[30] perhaps suggesting that alterations in other genes, including the tumor-suppressor genes, enhance susceptibility to *ras*-induced transformation.

MOLECULAR BIOLOGY OF *p53*

The *p53* Tumor-Suppressor Gene

Comparisons between the frequencies of familial tumors, in particular retinoblastoma and Wilms tumor,[31–33] and their sporadic counterparts led Knudson *et al.*[34] to suggest that the familial forms of some cancers could be explained by the inheritance of constitutional mutations in growth-limiting genes. The resulting inactivation of these genes could facilitate cellular transformation. Inactivations of these growth-limiting, or tumor-suppressor, genes result from mutations in both alleles or a mutation in one allele followed by a loss of or reduction to homozygosity in the second as well as functional or structural alterations of the transcribed message or protein product. Mutant tumor-suppressor genes may be found in either germ cells or somatic cells. In germ cells they arise spontaneously in the gamete or are transmitted from generation to generation within a family.

Alterations of the *p53* tumor-suppressor gene and its encoded protein are the most frequently encountered genetic events in human malignancy.[35–38] The human gene, located on the short arm of human chromosome 17 band 13,[39] is approximately 20 kb in length, yields a 2.8-kb mRNA transcript, and encodes a 53-kDa nuclear phosphoprotein[40] composed of 393 amino acids. The gene contains 11 exons, only the first of which is noncoding. Analysis of the nucleotide and amino acid sequences demonstrates five evolutionarily conserved domains from *Xenopus* to human.[41] Attempts to identify *p53*-like genes in invertebrates such as sea urchins, yeast, and worms have been unsuccessful. The conserved regions are regarded as being essential for the normal function of the wild-type protein. The first conserved domain is contained within the noncoding exon 1; the other four are encompassed by codons 129–146, 171–179, 234–260, and 270–287 in exons 4, 5, 7, and 8, respectively[41] (Fig. 37-2). Several properties of the p53 protein are indicated by the presence of two DNA-binding domains,[42] two SV40 large tumor-antigen (T-Ag) binding sites,[43,44] a nuclear localization signal,[45] an oligomerization domain,[46,47] and several phosphorylation sites.[48]

The p53 protein was identified initially in SV40-transformed cells, where it was thought to be a transformation-specific protein, or tumor antigen, because of its apparent interaction with the large T antigen of the SV40 virus.[40,49] This virus, which is found in monkeys, is a member of the polyomavirus family. These viruses encode viral T-antigen proteins, which are synthesized immediately after infection. The proteins are responsible for the loss of cell growth control that is induced by the virus both *in vitro* and *in vivo*. Transfection assays in rat fibroblast NIH 3T3 cells initially suggested that *p53* was an oncogene because it was capable of immortalizing these cells by itself or of transforming them in conjunction with the *ras* oncogene.[50–52] It was demonstrated subsequently that only mutant forms of p53 conferred these biologic properties, whereas the wild-type protein actually suppressed transformation.[53] Furthermore, it was shown that sequence differences and substantial gene rearrangements occurred in Friend leukemia virus-infected erythroleukemia cells,

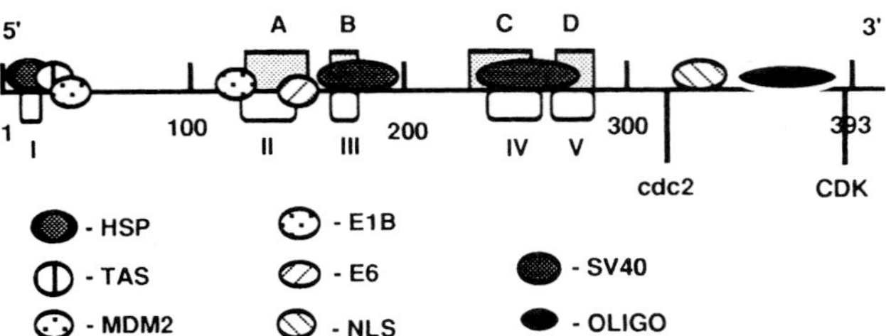

Fig. 37-2 Structural features of the *p53* gene and its encoded protein. The gene encodes a 53-kDa nuclear phosphoprotein. The 393 amino acids are spread over 11 exons. The transcription activation site (TAS), heat shock protein binding site (HSP), SV40 large T antigen binding sites (SV40), nuclear localization signal (NLS), oligomerization domain (OLIGO), and phosphorylation sites (P) all identify potential functional regions. The five evolutionarily conserved domains (HCD I-V) correspond closely to the regions most frequently mutated in sporadic cancer [hotspot regions (HSR A-D)]. Sites of binding of the extracellular E1B 55-kDa protein of adenovirus type 5 (E1B) and the E6 gene product of human papillomavirus types 16 and 18 (E6) are also indicated, as is the position of the MDM2 gene product-binding site (MDM2).

suggesting that an altered form of p53 was involved in the transformation process. Analysis of two colorectal tumors demonstrated allelic deletions of chromosome 17p and expressed high levels of p53 mRNA from the remaining allele. The second allele was shown to harbor a point mutation that changed a valine to alanine at residue 143 in one tumor and changed arginine to histidine at codon 175 in the other.[53a] These observations provided a practical illustration of the Knudson two-hit hypothesis and subsequently were extended by the demonstration of a variety of amino acid substitutions in several different tumor types.[53b] These exciting reports, coupled with the fact that the introduction of wild-type p53 protein blocks the growth of many transformed cells,[54,55] suggest that the normal function of p53 is in fact that of a growth suppressor.[56]

The p53 protein consists of five primary structural regions (see Fig. 37-2). First, an acidic N-terminus acts as a transcriptional activating domain if placed in apposition to DNA through the DNA-binding domain. Second, the internal highly conserved hydrophobic proline-rich region appears to be important in maintaining the overall structural integrity of the protein. Third, the DNA-binding region between amino acid residues 120 and 290 recognizes a DNA sequence motif containing two contiguous or closely spaced monomers 59-(purine)3C(A/T)(A/T)G-(pyrimidine)3-39.[56a,57] Fourth, the highly charged basic region at the C-terminus is required for the formation of homologous p53 tetrameric complexes.[58] Fifth, a nuclear transport sequence spanning codons 316 to 325 aids the protein's localization into the nucleus.[59] p53 is multiply phosphorylated by at least four protein kinases, with two sites being at the N-terminus, which is phosphorylated by a casein kinase I-like enzyme[60] and DNA-dependent protein kinase.[61] The other phosphorylation sites are at the C-terminus, at position 315, phosphorylated by $p34^{cdc2}$ kinase, and CKII at codon 392, phosphorylated by casein kinase II.[62] The latter enzyme phosphorylates many substrates, including both transcription factors and DNA-binding proteins. The casein kinase II site also acts as a binding site for a ribosomal RNA moiety. These structural features all support the cell cycle control role of p53 activity (see below).

The p53 protein binds specific DNA sequences and appears to be a transcription factor that may regulate the expression of other growth regulatory genes in either a positive or negative manner.[63,64] The introduction of wild-type p53 protein into a variety of transformed cell types inhibits their growth, most likely by blocking progression of cells through the cell cycle late in the G1 phase of cell replication at a checkpoint control site before G1/S.[65–68] Recent evidence also suggests that the antiproliferative effect of p53 may involve cell cycle regulation at the G2/M restriction point.[69–72] Cells lacking wild-type p53 display an attenuated G2 checkpoint response. The addition of methylxanthines such as caffeine, which are known to disrupt cell cycle arrest at the G2 checkpoint, leads to increased sensitivity of cultured cells to both radio- and chemotherapy.[73,74] Because cells lacking functional p53 have already lost the ability to arrest in G1, the loss of the G2 checkpoint seems to have an additive effect. This observation implies that p53-negative tumor cells may be more responsive to a combination of DNA-damaging agents and agents that abrogate the G2 checkpoint. As a component of a spindle checkpoint, p53 may ensure the maintenance of diploidy during cell cycle progression.[75] p53 may actively participate in maintaining genomic stability through regulation of centrosome duplication or as a monitor that limits centrosome overproduction.[76] Although p53 may not play a major role in the S-phase recombinational events leading to sister chromatid formation,[77] suggesting that conversion of radiation damage to chromatin lesions is independent of p53, the time to peak levels of chromosomal damage is shorter in p53-deficient cells. This observation is consistent with kinetic differences based on specific p53 genotypes. These kinetic differences also have been observed in p53-deficient LFS-derived lymphocytes.[78]

Other functions of p53 are suggested by experiments demonstrating that reentry of resting cells into the cell cycle can be blocked by the introduction of anti-p53 antibodies or antisense p53 cDNA fragments.[79,80] p53 may potentiate cell differentiation in this manner. Early work suggested that wild-type p53 could be involved in restricting precursor cell populations by mediating apoptosis, or programmed cell death, in the absence of appropriate differentiation or proliferation signals.[81,82] In p53-deficient thymocytes, substantial resistance to apoptotic induction by radiation was observed compared with wild-type littermates.[83,84] These observations were corroborated in solid tumors in nude mice subjected to radiation or chemotherapy.[85] Strikingly, acquired resistance could be induced by repeated low doses of radiation, with acquired *p53* mutations being observed in 50 percent of tumors. The relative degree of radioresistance and apoptosis seems to be cell type-specific, for in colorectal carcinoma cells lines and head and neck squamous cell cancer cell lines lacking functional p53,[86,87] significant differences in response compared with wild-type counterparts could not be demonstrated.

As suggested earlier, cells that either lack *p53* gene expression or overexpress mutant p53 do not exhibit G1 arrest. The fidelity of DNA repair during cell cycle arrest may play a role in the capacity of cells to tolerate radiation injury and therefore have an impact on radiation sensitivity. It has been reported in this context that p53 may play a role in the cellular response to γ-radiation damage, ultraviolet light, or certain chemotherapeutic drugs through inhibition of DNA synthesis[84,85,88–93] after DNA damage and thereby provide a cell cycle "checkpoint."[94,95] This response is particularly effective in the setting of double-strand DNA breaks. The *in vitro* effect has been observed in vivo in SCID mice carrying xenografts treated with either adriamycin or γ-irradiation.[96]

Transcriptional targets of *p53* include *mdm*-2, a gene that is commonly amplified in human sarcomas and is involved in a negative regulatory system that terminates a cell's response to DNA damage.[97,98] Other targets include a cyclin of unknown function called *cyclin G1*[99]; Bax, a promoter of apoptosis[100]; GADD45, a DNA repair protein[101]; and $p21^{CIP1/WAF1}$ a multifunctional regulatory and the best candidate to date for the control of cell cycle arrest.[102–104] The abundant increases in p53 protein expression induced by ionizing radiation lead to the transcription of $p21^{CIP1/WAF1}$. This inhibits cyclin-dependent kinase activity, which is in turn required for entry into S phase and DNA replication. Furthermore, $p21^{CIP1/WAF1}$ also binds and inhibits a subunit of DNA polymerase called *poliferating cell nuclear antigen* (PCNA) directly,[105] thereby blocking DNA replication.

GADD45 is also induced by stresses that arrest cell growth or agents that induce DNA damage. Like p21$^{CIP1/WAF1}$, GADD45 has been shown to bind PCNA to induce excision repair of damaged DNA by a poorly understood mechanism.[106] p53 also binds ERCCC3, an excision repair molecule that recognizes and removes damaged DNA segments.[107] Taken together, these observations suggest that p53 may inhibit DNA replication through p21 while simulating DNA repair through GADD45 or ERCC3 simultaneously.

Structural analysis of the p53 core-DNA co-crystal using x-ray diffraction,[108] as well as the oligomerization domain using multidimensional nuclear magnetic resonance (NMR) spectroscopy,[109,109a] suggests that several highly conserved amino acid residues within the central core form actual contacts at the minor or major grooves of the DNA helix. Furthermore, each monomeric unit of p53 interacts with another subunit; the resulting dimer in turn interacts with another dimer, forming a four-helix bundle or p53 tetramer. It is believed that this cooperative binding greatly facilitates interactions with p53 response elements.[110]

Inactivation of p53 function occurs via several mechanisms. The occurrence of missense mutations, deletions, or nonsense mutations of the gene prevents the protein from oligomerizing and forming tetrameric complexes that can bind specific DNA sequences.[111] In fact, representative mutants from each of the four mutation hotspot regions (see Fig. 37-2.) have been tested for binding to p53-binding sites *in vitro* and for activation of p53-binding site reporter gene expression *in vivo* and *in vitro*. The majority of mutants lose the ability to bind p53-binding sites and therefore cannot activate expression of adjacent reporter genes.[56,112–114] Some mutations alter the conformation of the p53 protein, exposing epitopes that may alter certain functional properties. Because these properties are found in only a fraction of *p53* mutants, they are unlikely to be central to *p53* function. Nevertheless, the possibility remains that subtle genetic changes induce conformational alterations that affect the structure of functionally important domains distant from the mutation sites.[111] The impact of subtle genetic changes to *p53* may be exemplified by recent suggestions that a commonly observed polymorphism may in fact not be functionally neutral. Conformational changes of a mutant molecule also can affect wild-type molecules complexed with the mutant form within tetramers, preventing the complex from binding to DNA and transcriptionally activating reporter genes.[112,114,115] In fact, the vast majority of *p53* mutations are missense in nature,[116] accounting for upward of 85 percent of reported gene alterations. This observation is in stark contrast to many other genes in which variably sized deletions, alterations, or splice site defects are reported.

Inactivation of the p53 protein through binding of other cellular proteins also may prevent normal binding and thus prevent transcriptional activation.[117,118] Some of the DNA tumor virus genes, including SV40 T antigen, the *E1B* gene of adenovirus, and the *E6* gene of human papillomavirus, encode proteins that bind to p53. In cells that coexpress one of these viral oncoproteins along with p53, expression of p53-inducible reporter genes cannot be activated.[118] This inhibition of expression may be critical for viral replication and/or cell transformation. Disruption of normal p53 function also may be altered by alteration of *mdm*-2, a cellular gene that was identified originally by virtue of its amplification in a spontaneously transformed mouse cell line.[97,98,117,119] The Mdm-2 gene product binds to p53, resulting in inhibition of the ability of p53 to transactivate genes adjacent to p53-binding sites. At least in human sarcomas, the amplification of *Mdm*-2 may lead to consequent overexpression of Mdm-2, which probably interferes with p53 activity.[97,120] Finally, p53 interactions with other tumor-suppressor genes have been observed. Interaction with the Wilms' tumor gene (*WT1*) in transfected cells modulates the ability of each protein to transactivate its targets.[121] Coincident mutations in *p53* and the retinoblastoma susceptibility gene (*RB1*) cooperate in transformation of certain cell types in mice.[122,123]

Tumor suppressors frequently have functional and structural cousins. Recent work suggests that p53 belongs to a larger group of related proteins. First, the gene *p73* was discovered to encode a protein sequence similar to that of p53, particularly in the core DNA-binding domain. *p73* is localized to chromosome 1p36.33 in a region frequently deleted in a wide range of tumors including neuroblastoma, breast cancer, melanoma, and hepatocellular carcinoma. Expression of a single copy of the wild-type gene in the absence of mutations of the remaining allele has been observed in several tumor types, although initial speculation that *p73* was a novel tumor suppressor gene that may be imprinted has not been validated. p73 may be functionally similar to p53 in that when overexpressed, it activates transcription of p53-responsive genes (i.e., p21^{CIP1}) and inhibits cell growth in a p53-like manner by inducing apoptosis. In distinction to p53, p73 is not induced following exposure to UV radiation, nor do p73-deficient mice develop cancer. The sequence and functional similarities between p53 and p73 make the latter an obvious candidate to examine both as a potential predisposing gene in wt-p53 LFS and LFS-L families, as well as a modifier of cellular phenotype in *p53*-mutant individuals. It ultimately also will be important to examine whether p73 alterations modify the response of LFS cell lines to DNA-damaging agents. Similarly, isolation of two proteins, p51 and p40, encoded by the alternatively spliced mRNA products of a gene located on chromosome 3q28 offers further opportunities to study functionally and structurally related p53 homologues. Although the p51 sequence more closely resembles that of p73 rather than p53, p51 expression in Saos-2 cells leads to suppression of colony formation, as well as apoptotic cell death and activation of p21^{CIP1}. Somatic mutations of the gene are rare (examined to date in nonsarcomatous tumors including neuroblastoma, brain tumors, and carcinoma of lung, pancreas, liver, breast and colon), suggesting that inactivation of p51 may occur through alternative mechanisms. *p51* and *p73* may serve as back-up genes whose expression is induced by the loss of p53 function, or *p51* and *p73* may provide tumor-suppressor functions in cells lacking p53. The potential for germ-line alterations in genes that are structurally similar to *p53* to play a role in human carcinogenesis in the absence of *p53* alterations is intriguing and an area of intense study.

Therefore, although the precise functions of p53 are not clear, models have been proposed to account for the many observations summarized above.[94,124] In a cell with normal p53, levels of the protein rise in response to DNA damage mediated by pRB1,[125] and the cell arrests before the G1/S transition. At this point, genomic repair or apoptosis ensues, with the mechanism being determined by the transforming oncoprotein or oncoproteins. In cells in which the p53 pathway has been inactivated by gene mutations or by host or viral oncoprotein interactions, G1 arrest does not occur and damaged DNA is replicated. During mitosis, the presence of damaged DNA results in mutation, aneuploidy, mitotic failure, and cell death. p53 alterations are necessary but not sufficient for the ultimate cancer that arises from these malignant clones, since other genetic events are clearly required.

Patient Mutations

Inactivating mutations of the *p53* gene and disruptions of the p53 protein have been associated with some fraction of virtually every sporadically occurring malignancy. Included among these are osteosarcomas,[126] soft tissue sarcomas,[127] rhabdomyosarcomas,[128] leukemias,[129,130] brain tumors,[131] and carcinomas of the lung[132] and breast.[133] Together, these tumors account for more than two-thirds of the cancers in selected series of LFS families[2,11,134] (Fig. 37-3). Transgenic mice that overexpress mutant alleles of the *p53* gene in the presence of two wild-type alleles produce offspring with a high incidence of osteosarcoma, lung adenocarcinoma, lymphoma, and rhabdomyosarcoma.[135]

Based on these observations, five LFS families were studied to determine whether *p53* played any role in the occurrence of cancer in affected family members. Base-pair mutations were identified in

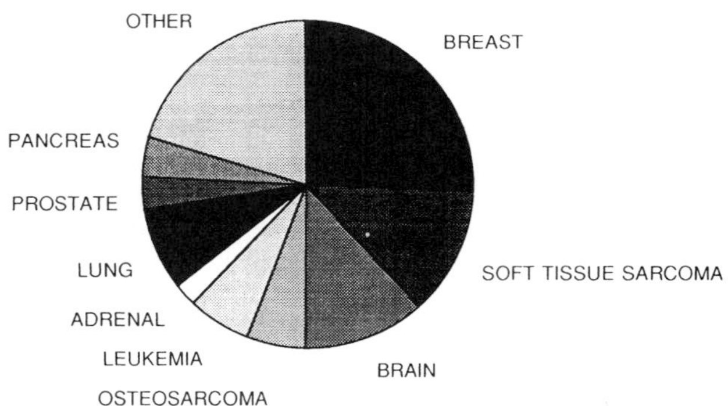

Fig. 37-3 Relative incidence of tumor types by age in 24 Li-Fraumeni syndrome families. The frequencies are confounded by the means of ascertainment, in this case through the proband, who has a sarcoma and who was therefore excluded from the tabulations. (*Adapted from Garber et al.*[10] *Used by permission.*)

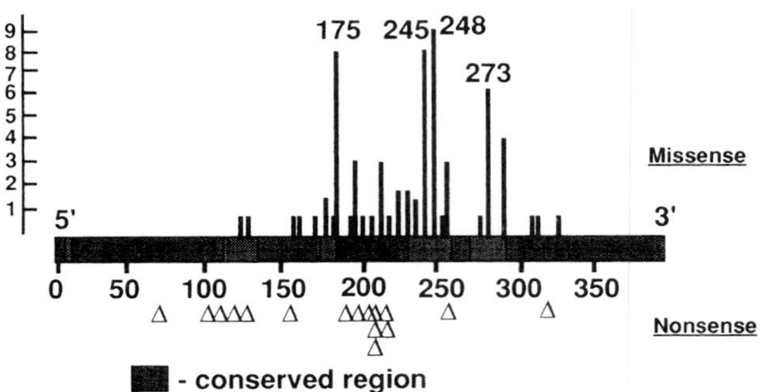

Fig. 37-4 Sites and frequency of reported human germ-line *p53* mutations. The horizontal axis represents the codon number; the vertical axis indicates the number of reported mutations. Missense mutations are designated above the *p53* cartoon, while nonsense mutations are seen below the cartoon. It is noteworthy that the four most frequently cited amino acid residues are at codons 175, 245, 248, and 273—not dissimilar to acquired mutations.

the germ line of affected members in each of the five families studied.[136] These missense mutations were all found within one highly conserved region of the gene, affecting codons 245, 248 (two families), 252, and 258 of the *p53* gene. In fact, subsequent analysis of one of the families revealed the codon 252 change to be artifactual; a 2-bp deletion was identified at codon 184 in exon 5.[137] This observation raises concerns with respect to the application of research technology in gene analysis to the clinical setting, as will be discussed below. Tumors in affected individuals who were tested had lost the remaining wild-type allele.[136] Furthermore, analysis of one of these families, using a highly polymorphic DNA sequence telomeric of *p53,* confirmed the cosegregation of the abnormal *p53* allele with the polymorphism. Unaffected members could be identified as gene carriers, suggesting that they might be at risk of developing cancer at a later date. After this initial report, a sixth classic LFS family was reported with another constitutional mutation in the same region as the previously identified ones.[137] In this family, however, one affected member was not a carrier of the mutant gene, suggesting that the mechanism of tumor formation in this individual did not involve *p53*. The apparent clustering of germ-line *p53* mutations in a short span of 14 codons within a highly conserved domain initially sparked much speculation about its possible significance, with suggestions that germ-line mutations may be restricted and that other mutations may be lethal in this context.[138] However, extensive analysis of other classic LFS families and subsequently several clinical scenarios of LFS-L phenotypes demonstrated the wide spectrum of germ-line *p53* mutations that were not dissimilar to those observed in sporadic tumors (Fig. 37-4).

Several families that fit the operative definition of LFS have been studied. Isolated families with germ-line *p53* mutations have been reported.[139,140] However, one study of eight families from the Manchester registry in England suggested that mutations of the *p53* gene would not be found in all classic LFS families.[141] Only two of these families were shown initially to carry germ-line mutations when only exon 7 was examined. Further analysis of other exons has still demonstrated the apparent absence of mutations within exons 5 to 8 in some of these families.[142] Ongoing studies suggest that not all classic LFS families have detectable germ-line mutations of the *p53* gene. In one quite typical Li-Fraumeni kindred, although no *p53* gene mutations were identified, overexpression of wild-type p53 was observed, suggesting that the biologically or biochemically altered protein yielded a similar phenotype to the mutant gene, perhaps by one of the several mechanisms described above.[143] Subsequent analysis of this family has in fact confirmed the presence of a point mutation. This observation again points out the evolution of technologic improvements in studying the genetics of LFS. Evidence from several studies conducted in the United States, France, and the United Kingdom[16,144,145] suggests that the actual frequency of germ-line *p53* mutations in classic LFS families is somewhere between 50 and 70 percent. In the French series, germ-line *p53* mutations were particularly associated with families in which a young child was affected with rhabdomyosarcoma, while in the U.K. series the mutations appeared to be associated with families that included children with rhabdomyosarcoma and/or adrenocortical carcinoma. It is likely that as the clinical definition is expanded, the rate of germ-line *p53* mutations observed will increase.

The lack of 100 percent concordance between *p53* mutations and the classic phenotype may be explained in several ways. It is possible that post-translational *p53* alterations, as described previously,[143,146] occur more frequently than has been found to date. Recently, mutations outside the most commonly cited hotspot regions have been identified, particularly in the oligomerization domain.[146a] Presumably, more of these types of mutations will be discovered as these regions of the gene are analyzed more extensively. Evidence for endogenous promoter defects leading to aberrant expression of the p53 message has been sought with inconclusive success. Complete *p53* deletion, the effects of modifier genes, or alterations of other genes that may influence the phenotype generated by the presence of a specific germ-line *p53* alteration also have been postulated. Despite these gaps, the high frequency of germ-line *p53* mutations in LFS families and the tight association of tumor formation in p53-deficient mice (see below) confirm a causal association of germ-line *p53* alterations and cancer predisposition.

Patient Mutations: Non-LFS

As DNA screening techniques improved, it became possible to analyze large populations of patients for constitutional abnormalities of the *p53* gene. Several recent studies have demonstrated that certain groups of "high risk" patients and their families carry germ-line *p53* mutations that presumably predispose them to the development of their respective malignancies. Germ-line *p53* mutations may be inherited from a parent who is healthy at the time when cancer is diagnosed in the child. Numerous studies of non-LFS patients and families have helped characterize the genetic heterogeneity of the p53 carrier state.

A striking feature of LFS kindreds is the high frequency, approaching 50 percent, of affected members who develop multiple primary neoplasms.[9] One multicenter study demonstrated germ-line mutations of the *p53* tumor-suppressor gene in leukocyte DNA from 4 of 59 patients (6.8 percent) who had survived second cancers but did not have family histories compatible with LFS.[147] Although one mutation at codon 248 in exon 7 was identical to that previously implicated in LFS,[136] three other mutations at codons 273, 282, and 325 had not been reported previously in the germ line. In addition to implicating codons outside the classically defined conserved regions of the *p53* gene, this study demonstrated the occurrence of germ-line *p53* mutations in patients with cancers not commonly represented among LFS component tumors. These included non-Hodgkin lymphoma, colon and gastric carcinoma, and neuroblastoma. A subsequent analysis of four patients with multifocal osteosarcoma and no family history of cancer demonstrated one apparently *de novo* germ-line *p53* mutation.[148] A similar analysis of patients with multifocal glioma demonstrated a very high frequency of germ-line *p53* mutations, although several of these individuals had family histories consistent with LFS or LFS-L.[148a] This observation suggests that other cancer patients who present with multiple nonfamilial tumors carry germ-line *p53* mutations.

An extensive analysis of 196 patients with malignant sarcomas was reported along with the second tumor study cited earlier.[149] Exons 2 through 11 were screened, thereby encompassing the complete coding region of the gene as well as less frequently evaluated regions. Eight of these 196 (4 percent) harbored germ-line *p53* mutations, and 5 of the 8 mutations were identified in patients from families with a high incidence of cancer. Both missense and nonsense germ-line mutations were found. The nonsense mutations arose as a result of a single-base frameshift mutation involving an insertion in two cases, a two-base deletion in one case, and the direct creation of a stop codon in one case. All occurred in codons outside the conserved domains (codons 71–72, 151–152, and 209–210), and all presumably yield a truncated p53 protein. Novel mutations, as well as the passage of a mutant allele for generations in at least one family, also were observed. In these cases, as in the previously described study, the affected individual presented a history that was not entirely consistent with LFS. This study also confirmed the observation of neutral polymorphisms within the *p53* sequence that must be evaluated carefully to rule out their disease-associated potential. One of these, at codon 213 in exon 6 (a nonconserved region), has been identified frequently in sporadic tumors.[116,127] Finally, this study pointed out the vagaries of the clinical definition of LFS in that one family with definitive germ-line inheritance of *p53* mutations had an excess of gastric carcinoma, a tumor that is thought to be rare in the operative definition of the syndrome. However, this family is from Japan, a country with a significantly higher incidence of gastric carcinoma than exists in North American or European populations. Other factors, both genetic and environmental, may influence the types of tumors that arise in patients who are carriers of the same *p53* germ-line mutations.

Although sarcomas and multiple primary cancers in affected patients constitute the most consistent characteristic features of the LFS phenotype, certain other cancers are also commonly represented. Among these, early onset breast cancer is most frequently encountered. However, little is known about the frequency of germ-line *p53* mutations in breast cancer patients outside families with classic LFS. Using a hydroxylamine mismatch base-pair technique, 5 families with early onset breast cancer were screened for constitutional mutations in all 11 exons of the *p53* gene.[150] No mutations were identified in these families, suggesting that *p53* probably did not play a significant role in the genesis of hereditary early onset breast cancer. These observations are also supported by another study that screened 25 breast cancer families in which no germ-line mutations of the gene were found in exons 5 through 9.[151] Nevertheless, in a third study, 1 of 67 unselected breast cancer patients and 1 of 40 early onset breast cancer patients were found to be carriers of mutant *p53*.[152] The mutation found in the unselected patient was at codon 181 (exon 5). The patient's pedigree showed a strong family history of cancer, although it did not quite fit the classic definition of LFS, since the relative with sarcoma was 47 years old (i.e., older than 45) at the time of diagnosis. In addition, studies of other family members as well as functional studies of the mutant gene suggest that this codon 181 mutation may be functionally silent and may not impart any increased cancer risk.[153] By contrast, the mutation found in the early onset breast cancer patient was at codon 245, a highly conserved amino acid. The identical mutation was identified in the patient's mother, who also had breast cancer. These findings suggest that germ-line *p53* mutations occur rarely in early onset breast cancer outside of LFS families and are corroborated by similar results reported elsewhere.[154] It is clear that other genetic events are responsible for the genesis of this familial cancer clustering. In fact, two genes for early onset hereditary breast cancer have been isolated, *BRCA1* and *BRCA2,* and intense efforts are in progress to fully characterize the mutational spectrum, genotype-phenotype correlation, and clinical implications of these genes. In light of the enormous efforts in characterizing the *BRCA* genes, it must be kept in mind that perhaps 1 percent of familial breast cancer may be due to germ-line *p53* mutations—a not insubstantial frequency.

Initial surveys of patients ascertained solely by the presence of a neoplasm that is a component tumor of LFS have yielded interesting observations. Adrenocortical carcinoma (ADCC) occurs rarely in the pediatric cancer population.[155] However, in LFS kindreds it is not uncommon to encounter at least one affected individual with this tumor.[11,16] Analysis of five patients with ADCC demonstrated inherited germ-line *p53* mutations in three.[156] Each of the families had cancer constellations that were consistent with LFS. In a survey of children with apparently sporadic adrenocortical carcinoma, 3 of 6 (50 percent) harbored germ-line *p53* mutations, and in one the alteration was demonstrated to be inherited from the child's mother, who subsequently developed breast cancer.[157]

Two studies of childhood sarcoma patients confirmed the presence of germ-line *p53* mutations in a small fraction of those who lacked striking family histories of cancer. Among 235 children with osteosarcoma, 7 (3 percent) were found to carry mutations, and 3 of these 7 lacked a family history of cancer.[158] A similar survey of 33 childhood rhabdomyosarcoma patients identified 3 (9 percent) with germ-line *p53* mutations.[159] Although no association between the presence of mutations and histopathologic subtype or tumor grade was noted, it was of interest that the average age at onset of the tumors in children carrying germ-line *p53* mutations was lower than that of children with wild-type *p53* ($p < 0.06$), suggesting that the biologic nature of the tumors may be different.

A screen of primary lymphoblasts from 25 pediatric patients with acute lymphoblastic leukemia identified *p53* mutations in 4, one of whom was shown to harbor the mutation (in exon 8) in the remission marrow, suggesting its germ-line origin.[160] The proband's family history was consistent with LFS. An analysis of primary lymphoblasts in affected members of 10 familial leukemia pedigrees identified two families in which nonhereditary *p53* alterations were present.[161] These included a 2-bp deletion in exon 6 in one and a codon 248 missense mutation in the other. Therefore, although leukemia represents a common component tumor of LFS, it appears that germ-line mutations of *p53* in primary leukemia patients are rare events. However, it is possible that when such alterations do exist in the germ line, they are potentially associated with an increased risk of secondary acute myelogenous leukemia related to prior treatment of the primary cancer with topoisomerase inhibitors.[162]

Most published germ-line *p53* mutations occur in the conserved regions of the gene and are missense in nature. There are no obvious differences in the mutation types or sites between LFS and LFS-L families. Approximately 75 percent are transitions, and the majority of these occur at CpG dinucleotides (Table 37-1). Transversions and occasional base-pair deletions or insertions also have been described. Three examples of intronic mutations have been reported. A novel germ-line *p53* splice-acceptor site mutation was found in a family that closely resembles the breast-ovarian cancer syndrome and in which the

Table 37-1 Types of *p53* Mutations Found in the Germ Line

Mutation	Li-Fraumeni Syndrome, %	Li-Fraumeni Like Syndrome, %
Missense	70	84
Transition	81	67
Transversion	19	33
CpG site	69	4
Nonsense	4	4
Insertion/deletion	26	12

proband had a choroid plexus carcinoma.[163] This mutation, involving a single-base substitution in intron 5, results in deletion of exon 6 and creation of a frameshift leading to a premature stop codon in exon 7 that is thought to yield significant disruptions of the message. Another report identified a point mutation in the splice donor site of intron 4, leading to an aberrant larger transcript that could be detected in both tumor and constitutional DNA.[164] The third example is somewhat more unusual in that the mutation, detected in intron 5, consisted of a deletion of an 11-bp sequence that involved a region of splicing recognition. Like the first example, this deletion resulted in deletion of exon 6 and a premature stop codon in exon 7.[165] All three pedigrees resembled LSF but were more consistent with the LFS-L phenotype.

Whether specific germ-line *p53* mutations are more penetrant and are associated with different cancer phenotypes has not been resolved. Studies of possible correlations between mutation type and cancer phenotype are limited by the relative lack of fully characterized families. Furthermore, the influence of external factors on the development of malignancy in carriers is also unknown. One would expect that exposure to occupational or environmental carcinogens will contribute to the precise determination of cancer type and age at onset. At least superficially, however, it does not appear that the pattern of germ-line alterations of *p53* differs significantly from that of somatic mutations. Perhaps as more genotype-phenotype studies are performed, a distinctive pattern will emerge.

The studies described above clearly demonstrate that patients with germ-line *p53* mutations cannot be identified solely by a review of the family's history of cancer. The method by which the proband was ascertained will influence the frequency of carriers in the study population (Table 37-2). It has been shown that germ-line *p53* mutations may be inherited from a parent who has no clinical evidence of cancer at the time the disease is diagnosed in the child. A tumor may arise in a child before one does in the parent as a result of the presumed stochastic acquisition of one or more additional genetic abnormalities in the cell that give rise to the malignant clone. Multicenter studies are in progress to determine the frequency of germ-line *p53* mutations in patients afflicted with other component tumors of LFS. These, as well as studies of non-LFS cancer-prone families, will help characterize the genetic heterogeneity of the *p53* carrier status.

Table 37-2 Estimated Frequency of Germ-Line *p53* Mutations in Specific Cancer Patients and Families

Clinical Phenotype	Mutation Frequency, %
LFS and ADCC	75–100
LFS	50–85
LFS variant	10–30
Multisite cancer (non-LFS)	0–20
Sporadic ADCC	40–70
Sporadic rhabdomyosarcoma	5–15
Osteosarcoma	1–10
Second neoplasms	5–15
Early onset breast cancer	1

Molecular Genetic Approaches to LFS Patients

As both the biologic and biochemical characteristics of *p53* have been elucidated, it also has been important to attempt to establish the functional significance of germ-line *p53* mutations and the structural features of the corresponding mutant p53 proteins. In addition, before associating a germ-line *p53* mutation with the development of cancer, one must carefully determine its functional significance. In one particularly extensive analysis, seven distinct *p53* mutations identified from LFS families were studied.[153] Oligonucleotide-directed mutagenesis of the *p53* cDNA was performed to generate mutant clones that could then be subcloned into expression vectors for transfection assays. The structural properties of the germ-line *p53* mutants showed a high degree of variability. However, with the exception of one mutant, at codon 181, none of the germ-line mutants retained all the structural features of the wild-type protein. Six of seven missense mutations disrupted the growth inhibitory properties and structure of the wild-type p53 protein. One mutation, at codon 181, was not recognized by the antibody PAb240, which recognizes an epitope specific for a mutant conformation,[166] and did not appear to alter the ability to suppress cell growth when transfected into Saos-2 osteosarcoma cells. Genetic analysis of this mutation demonstrated that it was not always associated with the development of cancer in the family from which it was derived. The mutation was not present in a member of the kindred who had developed two cancers, and the codon 181 mutant gene, not the normal allele, was somatically lost in tumor tissue from a cancer in another relative. It thus became apparent that certain germ-line mutations of *p53* might change the amino acid sequence in a conserved domain yet not be associated with an increased cancer risk.[153]

The functional significance of heterozygous germ-line mutations in members of LFS families also has been examined through the expression of the mutant *p53* allele in normal skin fibroblasts.[167] It was observed that both normal and mutant p53 RNA is expressed at low levels. In contrast to the transfection studies, the normal skin fibroblasts provide a system in which both wild-type and mutant *p53* alleles are naturally expressed at similarly low levels without potentially interfering dosage effects. Based on the studies demonstrating that mutant *p53* may inactivate the transcriptional activity of the wild-type protein, it has been postulated that direct analysis of the transcriptional activity of p53 expressed in fibroblasts or lymphocytes should permit the detection of inactivating germ-line mutations.[168] Using a short-term biologic assay in which p53 cDNA was amplified from cells and cloned into a eukaryotic expression vector that was then transfected with a reporter plasmid for the transcriptional activity of p53 into Saos-2 cells lacking p53, analysis of transcriptional activation could be performed. This assay demonstrated transcriptional activity in two of five and three of five clones from two LFS patients, respectively, indicating the presence of both wild-type and mutant p53 in these cells. The rapidity and apparent sensitivity of this assay suggest that it may be valuable as a functional screen. Yet another functional assay has been described that takes advantage of the fact that plasmids can be generated by homologous recombination *in vivo* in the yeast *S. cerevisiae.*[169] By this method, p53 is tested for its ability to activate transcription from a promoter containing p53-binding sites in these yeast. Cotransformation of a p53 PCR product and a cut promoter-containing plasmid results in repair of the plasmid with the PCR product *in vivo* and constitutive expression of full-length human p53 protein in the yeast. Clones that have repaired the plasmid are selected on media lacking leucine, and subsequent screening for histidine prototrophy identifies colonies that contain transcriptionally active p53.[169] This assay has the advantage of being rapid (less than 5 days) and having few steps, although it does assume that cancer-causing mutations of *p53* are defective in transactivation. Subsequent improvements in the efficiency of this assay have increased the spectrum of mutants, including temperature-sensitive forms that can be functionally evaluated.[170] Nevertheless, even this assay will miss mutant p53 if one considers growth arrest that is not dependent on transcriptional activation as the functional yardstick.

The combined value of appropriate multiple functional assays, standard DNA sequence analysis, and careful evaluation of the inheritance pattern of a potential mutation cannot be overestimated in conferring a significant level of confidence to the clinical relevance of a germ-line *p53* gene sequence alteration with respect to the patient's disease or the risk to unaffected relatives.

Animal Models

Transgenic animals that carry distinct deregulated oncogenes develop tumors that appear to be cell-type-specific. Because of difficulties in studying the effects of the genetic defects and potential interventions in humans, the development of mouse models that reflect the human genotype provides formidable tools with which to study the role of natural germ-line *p53* mutations in carcinogenesis and perhaps to develop treatment regimens. To better study *p53 in vivo*, several mouse models have been created that either lack functional p53 or express dominant-negative mutant alleles that inhibit wild-type p53 function. These animals have been used to study the interactions of p53 with other cell cycle regulatory elements that function in a p53-dependent or -independent manner. Furthermore, studies of both germ-line and somatic alterations in p53 in mice have greatly enhanced our understanding of the pathobiologic role of this gene in carcinogenesis.

The first attempt to determine the *in vivo* role of p53 in neoplasia involved generating *p53* transgenic mice that carry transgenes encoding for a p53 protein that differs from wild-type p53 either by a ^{193}Arg → Pro or by a ^{135}Ala → Val substitution.[135] The transgenes are under the transcriptional control of the endogenous promoter, and the mice carry the normal wild-type *p53* complement. Thus they weakly resemble the human *p53* genotype, although neither mutation has been implicated in LFS. The transgene was expressed in a wide range of tissues, yet tumors (primarily osteosarcomas, lymphomas, and adenocarcinomas of the lung) occur in only 20 percent of the mice, suggesting the presence of intrinsic tissue-specific differences. These mice provided a model with which to analyze the interactions of genetic and environmental factors in influencing cancer predisposition. For example, on infection of the *p53* transgenics with the polycthemia-inducing strain of Friend leukemia virus (FV-P), the animals progressed to the late stage of erythroleukemia more rapidly than did normal mice.[171] In addition, Friend leukemic cell lines derived from the *p53* transgenic mice overproduce mutant p53 protein and demonstrate a high rate of rearrangement of the *ets*-related *Spi*-1 oncogene, as had been reported previously in similar lines derived from nontransgenic animals. Thus p53 appears to play a rate-limiting role in the progression of the disease, with its mutant form present as an early event that accelerates neoplastic transformation. This transgenic model in fact contributed to the hypothesis that the tumor spectrum in LFS may arise from the transmission of a mutant *p53* gene (Fig. 37-5).

Because p53 is implicated in cell cycle control, it was proposed that this protein may be essential for normal embryonic development.[172] Although p53 is virtually ubiquitously expressed in murine tissues, its relatively short half-life of 20 min (wild-type conformation) yields generally low total protein levels. The amount of p53 mRNA expressed in developing mouse embryos reaches a maximum at 9 to 11 days, after which levels fall markedly.[173] Homologous recombination has been used in mouse embryonic stem (ES) cells to derive null alleles of *p53*.[172,174,175] Two models have been developed from the replacement with a neo^{r} cassette of exons 2 through 6 of the gene.[174,175] The third model includes an insertion of a *pol*II promoter-driven neo^{r} cassette into exon 5, together with a deletion of 350 nucleotides of intron 4 and 106 nucleotides of exon 5.[172] None of the $p53^{-/-}$ mice express detectable intact or truncated mRNA or protein. The mutant *p53* allele has been established in the germ line of chimeric mice with mixed inbred (C57Bl/6 3 129/Sv),[172,175] pure 129/Sv,[176] or 129/O1a[174,176] backgrounds. In all these situations, spontaneous development of different tumor types, principally lymphomas and sarcomas, occurred in more than 75 percent of the animals before 6 months of age. In heterozygotes ($p53^{+/-}$), tumor development, predominantly sarcoma, is delayed. Nevertheless, by 18 months of age, approximately 50 percent have developed neoplasms. Interestingly, multiple primary tumors have been noted in approximately 30 percent of the tumor-bearing $p53^{-/-}$ mice. In all mouse backgrounds, virtually none of the $p53^{+/+}$ animals had developed tumors by 18 months of age.

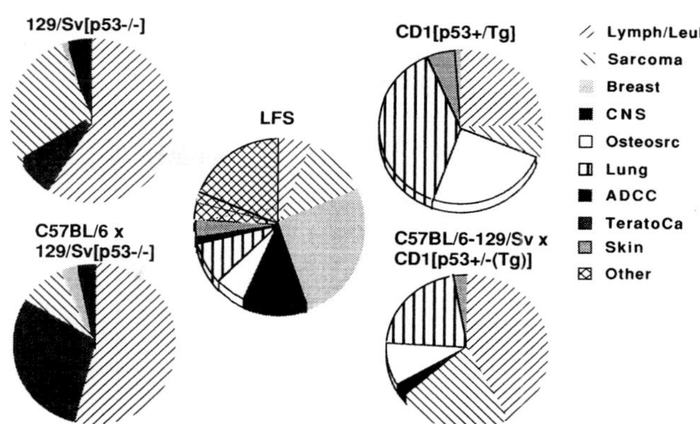

Fig. 37-5 Spectrum of tumors in *p53* mouse models compared with the human LFS phenotype. Not all tumors are represented; rather, those most frequently encountered with the category "other" contain isolated reports within specific mouse models. The particular mouse strain and the *p53* genotype are indicated above each pie.

The importance of genetic background in influencing specific tumor type is best exemplified by the occurrence of unusual cancers, including pineoblastomas and islet-cell tumors, in $p53^{-/-}$ mice crossed with mice heterozygous for an *RB1* mutation in exon 3 of that gene.[122,123] In addition to these unusual tumor phenotypes, these mice had decreased viability and demonstrated other uncharacteristic pathologies, including bronchial epithelial hyperplasia and retinal dysplasia. Interestingly, in this situation the mechanism by which the *RB1* allele was knocked out may be significant in the cancer phenotype that is derived from the intercross. Deletion of exon 20 of *RB1* when crossed with $p53^{-/-}$ animals yields animals with a variety of endocrine tumors, including pituitary adenomas, medullary carcinoma of the thyroid, and parathyroid carcinomas, in addition to the previously mentioned islet-cell tumors.[123] Surprisingly, no pineoblastomas are found. In both intercross models, the accumulation of abnormal genetic events results in an increased rate of tumorigenesis. Thus, as the number of null alleles of each tumor-suppressor gene is increased, the age at onset decreases and the rate of tumorigenesis increases.

The relative lack of strain-to-strain variability in the *p53*-null-induced phenotype suggests that the *p53* genotype is important in dictating phenotype. Evidence from other genetic crosses supports this premise. For example, adenomatous polyposis coli (APC)-mutant (*Min*) mice develop bowel adenomas with malignant potential. This malignant phenotype demonstrates great strain-to-strain variability, and in fact, the development of malignant tumors is accelerated and modified when they are outbred to different genetic backgrounds, in particular to one carrying a modifier of *Min* termed *Mom*-1.[177] It is likely that similar or other variations of the *p53*-null-induced phenotype can be induced in a like manner by the interaction of modifier genes that play a role in the development of p53-induced tumors.

The interaction of genetic events in early embryonic development has been facilitated by the use of *p53*-null animals. As was described earlier, amplification of the *mdm*-2 gene product is thought to represent an alternative mechanism for preventing p53 function in tumor development. Recently, it was shown that Mdm-2-null mice are not viable, being embryonically lethal near the time of implantation.[178] However, when mice heterozygous for *mdm*-2 were crossed with those heterozygous for *p53,* viable progeny homozygous for both *p53* and *mdm*-2 were obtained.[178,179] These observations suggest that a critical *in vivo* function of Mdm-2 is the negative regulation of p53 activity.

Provocative studies have tested whether the tumorigenic activity of a mutant *p53* allele is altered by the presence or absence of wild-type p53 in vivo. Mice carrying the ^{135}Ala → Val mutant transgene were crossed with p53-deficient mice.[180] The mutant p53-Tg accelerated tumor formation in *p53*$^{+/-}$ but not *p53*$^{-/-}$ mice, suggesting that this loss-of-function mutation had a dominant negative effect with respect to tumor incidence and cell growth rates. Although the tumor spectrum was similar in transgenic and nontransgenic mice, the transgenice mice showed a predisposition to lung adenocarcinomas. Thus, a given p53 alteration may have distinct tissue specificity with respect to its tumorigenic potential. It will ultimately be of interest to extend this approach to other alleles that behave differently *in vivo* or *in vitro*. At least one group[181] is trying to establish mouse models to study tumor-derived p53 mutants *in vivo* that would establish a more precise model of LFS and clarify the role played by point mutant forms of altered p53 as distinct from the null genotype.

In some strains, *p53*$^{-/-}$ mice become colonized with pathogens, suggesting that p53 deficiency may be associated with a poorer prognosis after infection with common low-virulence organisms or viruses.[175] In all strains, the *p53*$^{-/-}$ state is compatible with normal murine development, although the yield of *p53*$^{-/-}$ offspring from heterozygous crosses varies from 16.6 to 23 percent.[172,175] This apparent increase in fetal loss has been correlated in part by demonstration of fetal exencephaly in a subset of animals,[182] yet it does not mirror the human counterpart in that fetal loss is not characteristic of human LFS families.[183] This may in fact be related to the fact that humans harboring *p53* mutations are heterozygous, whereas the mice are homozygously deleted of *p53* alleles. Thus the presence of one wild-type *p53* allele in a human may be sufficient to ensure fetal viability.

p53-deficient mice are more sensitive to the effects of certain carcinogenic agents.[184] Mice exposed to dimethylnitrosamine (DMN) developed liver hemangiosarcomas more rapidly than did similarly treated *p53*$^{+/+}$ animals.[184] *p53*$^{-/-}$ mice treated with an initiator, dimethylbenzanthracene (DMBA), and a promoter, 12-*O*-tetradecanoyl-phorbol-13-acetate (TPA), showed a more rapid rate of malignant progression of skin papillomas to carcinomas compared with their *p53*$^{+/+}$ counterparts. These studies help distinguish whether *p53* mutations play rate-limiting or tissue-specific roles in the tumor progression pathway.

p53-deficient mice have been used to evaluate the effects of environmental factors on both tumorigenesis and development. p53-deficient and transgenic mice exposed to sublethal doses of γ-irradiation develop tumors, predominantly sarcomas, earlier than do untreated animals.[92,93] This susceptibility is associated with a twofold increase in the accumulation of radiation-induced double-strand DNA breaks compared with what is seen in *p53*$^{+/+}$ animals. Using *p53*-transgenic mice, it has been demonstrated that the presence of *p53* mutations does not alter the latency period of chronic ultraviolet B-induced squamous cell carcinoma but does significantly increase the number of tumors and the propensity for multiple tumor formation.[185] Although p53 protein was undetectable in the keratinocytes of the untreated mice, it was elevated in 93 percent of skin tumors derived from the treated animals. These studies confirm that p53 prevents the accumulation of cells sustaining radiation-induced or chemically induced DNA damage.

It has been demonstrated that caloric restriction inhibits the development of spontaneous lymphoma in C57BL/6 mice.[186] Such treatment of *p53*$^{-/-}$ mice modulates spontaneous tumorigenesis, delaying the onset of tumor formation by a median of 16 weeks in *ad libitum* fed mice and 25 weeks in calorie-restricted animals.[187] It is thought that dietary perturbations can influence the outcome of a genomic liability such as the accelerated tumorigenesis demonstrated in p53-deficient mice. Given the important role of p53 in cell cycle control, a p53-deficient state would be expected to deregulate the differentiation and development and yield aberrant morphogenesis and embryonic lethality. In fact, studies of the effects of the teratogen and DNA-damaging carcinogen benzo[*a*]pyrene[188] and the anticonvulsant and teratogenic drug phenytoin[189] on pregnant p53-deficient mice demonstrated a two- to fourfold increase in the incidence of *in utero* fetal resorption (death), teratogenicity, and postpartum lethality over *p53*$^{+/+}$ controls. These observations provide substantial support for the embryoprotective role of p53.

The cumulative data from these studies indicate that loss or alterations of *p53* may accelerate prior tumor predisposition, that the rate and spectrum of development of some cancers may be strain-dependent, and that normal murine development is possible even in the absence of p53. Certain similarities exist between the various *p53* mouse models and LFS families in that a p53-related transformation pathway leads to development of a wide spectrum of cancers. Inheritance of one mutant and one wild-type *p53* allele in affected members of LFS families is more analogous to the *p53*$^{+/-}$ or p53-Tg mice that developed tumors at a relatively slower rate. However, none of these animal models presents a completely accurate reflection of the LFS genotype in that the vast majority of documented human germ-line *p53* mutations are missense in nature, with less than 10 percent being nonfunctional. Although the transgenic mice carry point mutations, the ^{135}Ala and ^{193}Arg mutations have not been reported in the human germ line. Although null alleles are valuable tools, their effects reflect the complete absence of gene function, a phenomenon that is not generally observed in the human syndrome. Changes at the nucleotide level would represent a more exact model and are being developed. Finally, although the tumor spectrum in current *p53*-altered mice is highly variable, none of these mice spontaneously mimic the human phenotype in its preponderance of sarcomas and breast cancers, except when the animals are radiated. Furthermore, the lymphomas predominant in mice are seen only rarely in LFS. Although these differences could be species-dependent, it is reasonable to suspect that specific mutations influence tumor development and yield a more accurate human phenotype. This hypothesis is substantiated by the recent studies of *p53*-null crosses exemplifying the *in vivo* role of p53 in distinct pathways of cell cycle control. The *Mdm*-2-null mouse that results in an early embryonic lethal phenotype is rescued by deletion of *p53* in that double-homozygous null mice are viable. A shift in tumor phenotype resulting from cooperativity of mutations is demonstrated in the intercrosses of *Min* mice and p53-deficient mice, highlighting the striking tissue-specific differences in the tumor-suppressor effects of p53.[190] Mice that overexpress a c-*myc* transgene stochastically develop clonal tumors — a relatively low incidence of T-cell lymphomas.[191] Lymphoma development is dramatically accelerated by the synergistic activity of the *p53*-null mutation in intercrosses,[192] while no significant increase in tumor incidence was seen in *myc* mice carrying a single-function *p53* allele. These studies, although making a strong case for the biochemical and functional interactions of *p53* with other genes crucial to tumor formation, also leave the way open to the analysis of similar synergistic effects that might be observed with a spectrum of *p53* point mutations yielding disrupted p53 function rather than the null allele that yields no function whatsoever. The tumors derived from these mice, carrying point mutations, will most closely resemble spontaneous tumors that can be studied for biochemical interactions and response to therapy. It also will be possible to evaluate *in vivo* the effect of coexistence of mutant and wild-type p53 and the functional influence of one on the other.

LABORATORY SCIENCE MEETS CLINICAL PRACTICE

Several important issues exist as a result of the identification of germ-line mutations of the *p53* tumor-suppressor gene in rare cancer-prone families. These include ethical concerns about predictive testing in unaffected members of LFS and LFS-L families, selection of patients to be tested, and selection of practical and accurate laboratory techniques to definitively identify *p53* mutations. In addition, the development of pilot testing programs and evaluation of the roles of interventions based on testing results have to be considered.

For several reasons, *p53* testing is still not believed to be appropriate for the general population, particularly in light of the demonstrably low carrier rate. Even in the general cancer population, the prevalence of germ-line *p53* mutations will be a fraction of 1 percent. Although the sensitivity and specificity of screening methods have improved with the advent of automated DNA sequence analysis and functional assays, both false-positive and false-negative results have been noted.

Even within the high-risk population, problems are apparent. It is unclear why the same germ-line *p53* mutation can give rise to different cancer phenotypes, and it is not clear if in families that do not have classic LFS the cancer risks from *p53* mutation are as high as they are in LFS.[20] Because 85 percent of all missense mutations described in the germ line occur in exons 5, 7, and 8 of the gene, predictive testing must include those regions. However, most centers are now sequencing the entire coding region of *p53* as well as the flanking splice-acceptor sites to increase the likelihood of identifying less common alterations.

Recommendations for multicenter research studies that incorporate a multidisciplinary approach to surveying, screening, and testing were established in 1992[193] and are being updated. These initial recommendations, although specifically addressing *p53* testing in LFS, could be applied to a number of other cancer-predisposition gene testing programs. In fact, both the American Society of Clinical Oncology[194] and the American Society of Human Genetics[195] have developed policy statements that include brief references to *p53* testing. Although the interpretation of who should be tested remains open, certain common recommendations are stated, including the necessity that cancer risk counseling be part of the mission of clinical oncologists, the need for informed consent, formats for regulation of genetic testing, and continued efforts to address research issues.

The component malignancies of LFS are for the most part exceedingly difficult to cure, with the possible exception of early-detected breast cancer, childhood acute lymphoblastic leukemia, and rare germ-cell tumors of the testis. Although the prognosis for component solid tumors improves with earlier stage at diagnosis, only mammography screening for breast cancer has been shown to reduce mortality.[196] Its efficacy under age 50 (the predominant risk in LFS) is disputed. Furthermore, the potential theoretical risk of repeated low-dose radiation from such screening methods to tissue that harbors altered p53 has not been carefully scrutinized in this setting. Chemopreventive trials are under way, but the rarity of the germ-line mutant *p53* carrier state makes studies of these patients impractical.

Despite the many drawbacks of predictive testing for *p53* at this time, the possibility of reducing the marked loss of human potential resulting from the death of a child or young adult makes further pilot research efforts worthwhile. To this end, further studies of the role of p53 in the development of human cancer, the development of more accurate testing techniques, and the development of novel animal models will continue to be important.

REFERENCES

1. Li FP, Fraumeni JF Jr: Soft tissue sarcomas breast cancer and other neoplasms: A familial cancer syndrome? *Ann Intern Med* **71**:747, 1969.
2. Li FP, Fraumeni JF Jr: Rhabdomyosarcoma in children: Epidemiologic study and identification of a familial cancer syndrome. *J Natl Cancer Inst* **43**:1365, 1969.
3. Bottomley RH, Trainer AL, Condit PT: Chromosome studies in a cancer family. *Cancer* **28**:519, 1971.
4. Lynch HT, Krush AJ, Harlan WL, Sharp EA: Association of soft tissue sarcoma, leukemia, and brain tumors in families affected with breast cancer. *Am J Surg* **39**:199, 1973.
5. Blattner WA, McGuire DB, Mulvihill JJ, Lampkin BC, Hananian J, Fraumeni JF Jr: Genealogy of cancer in a family. *JAMA* **241**:259, 1979.
6. Pearson ADJ, Craft AW, Ratcliffe JM, Birch JM, Morris-Jonese PH, Roberts DF: Two families with the Li-Fraumeni cancer family syndrome. *J Med Genet* **19**:362, 1982.
7. Lynch HT, Mulcahy GM, Harris RE, Guirgis HA, Lynch JF: Genetic and pathologic findings in a kindred with hereditary sarcoma, breast cancer, brain tumors, leukemia, lung, laryngeal, and adrenal cortical carcinoma. *Cancer* **41**:2055, 1978.
8. Draper GJ, Sanders BM, Kingston JE: Second primary neoplasms in patients with retinoblastoma. *Br J Cancer* **53**:661, 1986.
9. Li FP, Fraumeni JF Jr: Prospective study of a family cancer syndrome. *JAMA* **247**:2692, 1982.
10. Garber JE, Goldstein AM, Kantor AF, Dreyfus MG, Fraumeni JF Jr, Li FP: Follow-up study of twenty-four families with Li-Fraumeni syndrome. *Cancer Res* **51**:6094, 1991.
11. Li FP, Fraumeni JF Jr, Mulvihill JJ, Blattner WA, Dreyfus MG, Tucker MA, Miller RW: A cancer family syndrome in twenty-four kindreds. *Cancer Res* **48**:5358, 1988.
12. Birch JM, Hartley AL, Blair V, et al: Cancer in the families of children with soft tissue sarcoma. *Cancer* **66**:2239, 1990.
13. Lustbader ED, Williams WR, Bondy ML, Strom S, Strong LC: Segregation analysis of cancer in families of childhood soft-tissue sarcoma patients. *Am J Hum Genet* **51**:344, 1992.
14. Hartley AL, Birch JM, Kelsey AM, Marsden HB, Harris M, Teare MD: Malignant melanoma in families of children with osteosarcoma, chondrosarcoma and adrenal cortical carcinoma. *J Med Genet* **24**:664, 1987.
15. Hartley AL, Birch JM, Tricker K, Wallace SA, Kelsey AM, Harris M, Morris Jones PH: Wilms tumor in the Li-Fraumeni cancer family syndrome. *Cancer Genet Cytogenet* **67**:133, 1993.
16. Birch JM, Hartley AL, Tricker KJ, et al: Prevalence and diversity of constitutional mutations in the p53 gene among 21 Li-Fraumeni families. *Cancer Res* **54**:1298, 1994.
17. Hartley AL, Birch JM, Kelsey AM, Marsden HB, Harris M, Teare MD: Are germ cell tumors part of the Li-Fraumeni cancer family syndrome? *Cancer Genet Cytogenet* **42**:221, 1989.
18. Garber JE, Liepman MK, Gelles EJ, Corson JM, Antman KH: Melanoma and soft tissue sarcoma in seven patients. *Cancer* **66**:2432, 1990.
19. Strong LC, Stine M, Norsted TL: Cancer in survivors of childhood soft tissue sarcoma and their relatives. *J Natl Cancer Inst* **79**:1213, 1987.
20. Eeles RA: Germ line mutations in the p53 gene, in Ponder BAJ, Cavenee WK, Solomon E (eds): *Cancer Surveys,* vol 25: *Genetics and Cancer: A Second Look*. Cold Spring Harbor, NY, Cold Spring Harbor Laboratory Press, 1995, p 101.
21. Williams WR, Strong LC: Genetic epidemiology of soft tissue sarcomas in children, in Muller H, Weber W (eds): *Familial Cancer.* 1st International Research Conference on Familial Cancer. Basel, Karger, 1985, p 151.
22. Call KM, Glaser T, Ito CY, Buckler AJ, Pelletier J, Haber DA, Rose EA, Kral A, Yeger H, Lewis WH, Jones C, Housman DE: Isolation and characterization of a zinc finger polypeptide gene at the human chromosome 11 Wilms tumor locus. *Cell* **60**:509, 1990.
23. Gessler M, Poustka A, Cavenee W, Neve RL, Orkin SH, Bruns GAP: Homozygous deletion in Wilms tumors of a zinc-finger identified by chromosome jumping. *Nature* **343**:774, 1990.
24. Huang A, Campbell CE, Bonetta L, McAndrews-Hill MS, Coppes MJ, Williams BRG: Tissue, developmental, and tumor-specific expression of divergent transcripts in Wilms tumor. *Science* **250**:991, 1990.
25. Li FP: Cancer families: Human models of susceptibility to neoplasia. *Cancer Res* **48**:5381, 1988.

26. Bech-Hansen NT, Sell BM, Lampkin BC, Blattner WA, McKeen EA, Fraumeni JF Jr, Paterson MC: Transmission of in vitro radioresistance in a cancer-prone family. *Lancet* **1**:1135, 1981.
27. Chang EH, Pirollo KF, Zou ZQ, Cheung HY, Lawler EL, Garner R, White E, Bernstein WB, Fraumeni JF Jr, Blattner WA: Oncogenes in radioresistant, noncancerous skin fibroblasts from a cancer-prone family. *Science* **237**:1036, 1987.
28. Little JB, Nove J, Dahlberg WK, Troilo P, Nichols WW, Strong LC: Normal cytotoxic response of skin fibroblasts from patients with Li-Fraumeni cancer syndrome to DNA-damaging agents in vitro. *Cancer Res* **47**:4229, 1987.
29. Bischoff FZ, Strong LC, Yim SO, Pratt DR, Siciliano MJ, Giovanella BC, Tainsky MA: Tumorigenic transformation of spontaneously immortalized fibroblasts from patients with a familial cancer syndrome. *Oncogene* **7**:183, 1991.
30. Bischoff FZ, Yim SO, Pathak S, Grant G, Siciliano MJ, Giovanella BC, Strong LC, Tainsky MA: Spontaneous abnormalities in normal fibroblasts from patients with Li-Fraumeni cancer syndrome: Aneuploidy and immortalization. *Cancer Res* **50**:3234, 1990.
31. Knudson AG: Mutation and cancer: Statistical study of retinoblastoma. *Proc Natl Acad Sci USA* **68**:820, 1971.
32. Knudson AG, Strong LC: Mutation and cancer: A model for Wilms tumor of the kidney. *J Natl Cancer Inst* **48**:313, 1972.
33. Knudson AG, Strong LC, Anderson DE: Hereditary cancer in man. *Prog Med Genet* **9**:13, 1973.
34. Comings DE: A general theory of carcinogenesis. *Proc Natl Acad Sci USA* **70**:3324, 1973.
35. Caron de Fromentel C, Soussi T: TP53 suppressor gene: A model for investigating human mutagenesis. *Gene Chromos Cancer* **4**:1, 1992.
36. Harris CC: p53: At the crossroads of molecular carcinogenesis and risk assessment. *Science* **262**:1980, 1993.
37. Harris CC, Hollstein M: Clinical implications of the p53 tumor suppressor gene. *N Engl J Med* **329**:1318, 1993.
38. Hollstein M, Sidransky D, Vogelstein B, Harris CC: p53 mutations in human cancers. *Science* **253**:49, 1991.
39. McBride OW, Merry D, Givol D: The gene for human p53 cellular tumor antigen is located on chromosome 17 short arm (17p13). *Proc Natl Acad Sci USA* **83**:130, 1986.
40. Lane DP, Crawford LV: T antigen is bound to a host protein in SV40-transformed cells. *Nature* **278**:261, 1979.
41. Soussi T, Caron de Fromentel C, May P: Structural aspects of the p53 protein in relation to gene evolution. *Oncogene* **5**:945, 1990.
42. Foord OS, Bhattacharya P, Reich Z, Rotter V: A DNA binding domain is contained in the C-terminus of wild-type p53 protein. *Nucleic Acids Res* **19**:5191, 1991.
43. Fields S, Jang SK: Presence of a potent transcription activating sequence in the p53 protein. *Science* **249**:1046, 1990.
44. Jenkins JR, Rudge K, Currie GA: Cellular immortalization by a cDNA clone encoding the transformation associated phosphoprotein p53. *Nature* **312**:651, 1984.
45. Addison C, Jenkins JR, Sturzbecher H-W: The p53 nuclear localization signal is structurally linked to a $p34^{cdc2}$ kinase motif. *Oncogene* **5**:423, 1990.
46. Milner J, Medcalf EA: Cotranslation of activated mutant p53 with wild-type drives the wild-type p53 protein into the mutant conformation. *Cell* **65**:765, 1991.
47. Stenger JE, Mayr GA, Mann K, Tegtmeyer P: Formation of stable p53 homotetramers and multiples of tetramers. *Mol Carcinogen* **5**:102, 1992.
48. Meek DW, Eckhart W: Phosphorylation of p53 in normal and simian virus 40-transformed NIH 3T3 cells. *Mol Cell Biol* **8**:461, 1988.
49. Linzer DIH, Levine AJ: Characterization of a 54K dalton cellular antigen present in SV40 transformed cells and uninfected embryonal carcinoma cells. *Cell* **17**:43, 1979.
50. Eliyahu D, Michalovitz D, Eliyahu S, Pinhasi-Kimhi O, Oren M: Wild-type p53 can inhibit oncogene-mediated focus formation. *Proc Natl Acad Sci USA* **86**:8763, 1984.
51. Jenkins JR, Chumakov P, Addison C, Sturzbecher HW, Wode-Evans A: Two distinct regions of the murine p53 primary amino acid sequence are implicated in stable complex formation within simian virus 40 antigen. *J Virol* **62**:3903, 1988.
52. Rovinski B, Benchimol S: Immortalisation of rat embryo fibroblasts by the cellular p53 oncogene. *Oncogene* **2**:445, 1988.
53. Hinds PW, Finlay CA, Levine AJ: Mutation is required to activate the p53 gene for cooperation with the ras oncogene and transformation. *J Virol* **63**:739, 1989.

53a. Baker SJ, Fearon ER, Nigro JM, Hamilton SR, Preisinger AC, Jessup JM, van Tuinen P, Ledbetter DH, Barker DF, Nakamura Y, White R, Vogelstein B: Chromosome 17 deletions and p53 gene mutations in colorectal carcinomas. *Science* **244**:217, 1989.

53b. Nigro JM, Baker SJ, Preisinger AC, Jessup JM, Hostetter R, Cleary K, Bigner SH, Davidson N, Baylin S, Devilee P, Glover T, Collins FS, Weston A, Modali R, Harris CC, Vogelstein B: Mutations in the p53 gene occur in diverse human tumor types. *Nature* **342**:705, 1989.

54. Baker SJ, Markowitz K, Fearon ER, Wilson JKV, Vogelstein B: Suppression of human colorectal carcinoma cell growth by wild-type p53. *Science* **249**:1912, 1990.
55. Diller L, Kassel J, Nelson CE, Gryka MA, Litwack G, Gebhardt MA, Friend SH: p53 functions as a cell cycle control protein in osteosarcomas. *Mol Cell Biol* **10**:5772, 1990.
56. Levine AJ, Momand J, Finlay CA: The p53 tumor suppressor gene. *Nature* **351**:453, 1991.

56a. El-Deiry WS, Kern SE, Pientenpol JA, Kinzler KW, Vogelstein B: Definition of a consensus binding site for p53. *Nature Genet* **1**:45, 1992.

57. Funk WD, Park DT, Karas RH, Wright WE, Shay JW: A transcriptionally active DNA-binding site for p53 protein complexes. *Mol Cell Biol* **12**:2866, 1992.
58. Iwabuchi K, Li B, Bartel P, Fields S: Use of the two-hybrid system to identify the domain of p53 involved in oligomerization. *Oncogene* **8**:1693, 1993.
59. Shaulsky G, Goldfinger N, Ben-Zeev A, Rotter V: Nuclear accumulation of p53 protein is mediated by several nuclear localization signals and plays a role in tumorigenesis. *Mol Cell Biol* **10**:6565, 1990.
60. Milne DM, Palmer RH, Campbell DG, Meek DW: Phosphorylation of the p53 tumor-suppressor protein at three N terminal sites by a novel casein kinase I-like enzyme. *Oncogene* **7**:1316, 1992.
61. Lees-Milner SP, Chen Y, Anderson CW: Human cells contain a DNA-activated protein kinase that phosphorylates simian virus 40 T-antigen, mouse p53, and the human Ku autoantigen. *Mol Cell Biol* **9**:3982, 1990.
62. Meek DW, Simon S, Kikkawa U, Eckhart W: The p53 tumor suppressor proteins is phosphorylated at serine 389 by casein kinase II. *EMBO J* **9**:3253, 1990.
63. Finlay CA, Hinds PW, Levine AJ: The p53 proto-oncogene can act as a suppressor of transformation. *Cell* **57**:1083, 1989.
64. Vogelstein B, Kinzler KW: p53 function and dysfunction. *Cell* **70**:523, 1992.
65. Mercer WE, Shields MT, Lin D, Appella E, Ullrich SJ: Growth suppression induced by wild-type p53 protein is accompanied by selective down-regulation of proliferating cell-nuclear antigen expression. *Proc Natl Acad Sci USA* **88**:1958, 1991.
66. Baker SJ, Markowitz K, Fearon ER, Wilson JKV, Vogelstein B: Suppression of human colorectal carcinoma cell growth by wild-type p53. *Science* **249**:1912, 1990.
67. Diller L, Kassel J, Nelson CE, Gryka MA, Litwack G, Gebhardt MA, Friend SH: p53 functions as a cell cycle control protein in osteosarcomas. *Mol Cell Biol* **10**:5772, 1990.
68. Michalovitz D, Halevy O, Oren M: Conditional inhibition of transformation and of cell proliferation by a temperature-sensitive mutant of p53. *Cell* **62**:671, 1990.
69. Paules RS, Levedakou EN, Wilson SJ, Innes CL, Rhodes N, Tlsty TD, Galloway DA, Donehower LA, Tainsky MA, Kaufmann WK: Defective G2 checkpoint function in cells from individuals with familial cancer syndrome. *Cancer Res* **55**:1763, 1995.
70. Guillof C, Rosselli F, Krisnaraju K, Moustacchi E, Hoffmann B, Liebermann DA: p53 involvement in control of G2 exit of the cell cycle: Role in DNA damage-induced apoptosis. *Oncogene* **10**:2263, 1995.
71. Stewart N, Hicks GG, Paraskevas F, Mowat M: Evidence for a second cell cycle block at G2/M by p53. *Oncogene* **10**:109, 1995.
72. Wang Y, Prives C: Increased and altered DNA binding of human p53 by S and G2/M but not G1 cyclin-dependent kinases. *Nature* **376**:88, 1995.
73. Fan S, Smith MK, Rivet DJ, Duba D, Zhan Q, Kohn K, Fornace AJ, O'Connor PM: Disruption of p53 function sensitizes breast cancer MCF-7 cells to cisplatin and pentoxifylline. *Cancer Res* **55**:1649, 1995.
74. Powell SN, DeFrank JS, Connell P, Eogen M, Preffer F, Dombkowski D, Tang W, Friend S: Differential sensitivity of p53(2) and p53(1) cells to caffeine-induced radiosensitization and override of G2 delay. *Cancer Res* **55**:1643, 1995.

75. Cross SM, Sanchez CA, Morgan CA, Schimke MK, Ramel S, Idzerda RL, Raskind WH, Reid BJ: A p53-dependent mouse spindle checkpoint. *Science* **267**:1353, 1995.
76. Fukasawa K, Choi T, Kuriyama R, Rulong S, Vande Woude GF: Abnormal centrosome amplification in the absence of p53. *Science* **271**:1744, 1996.
77. Bouffler SD, Kemp CJ, Balmain A, Cox R: Spontaneous and ionizing radiation-induced chromosomal abnormalities in p53-deficient mice. *Cancer Res* **5**:3883, 1995.
78. Parshad R, Price FM, Pirollo KF, Chang EH, Sandford KK: Cytogenetic responses to G2 phase X-irradiation in relation to DNA repair and radiosensitivity in cancer prone family with Li-Fraumeni syndrome. *Radiat Res* **136**:236, 1993.
79. Funk WD, Park DT, Karas RH, Wright WE, Shay JW: A transcriptionally active DNA-binding site for p53 protein complexes. *Mol Cell Biol* **12**:2866, 1992.
80. Eliyahu D, Raz A, Gruss P, Givol D, Oren M: Participants of p53 cellular tumor antigen in transformation of normal embryonic cells. *Nature* **312**:646, 1984.
81. Yonish-Rouach E, Resnitzky D, Lotem J, Sachs L, Kimchi A, Oren M: Wild-type p53 induces apoptosis of myeloid leukemic cells that is inhibited by interleukin-6. *Nature* **352**:345, 1991.
82. Shaw P, Bovey R, Tardy S, Sahli R, Sordat B, Costa J: Induction of apoptosis by wild-type p53 in a human colon tumor-derived cell line. *Proc Natl Acad Sci USA* **89**:4495, 1992.
83. Clarke AR, Purdie CA, Harrison DJ, Morris RG, Bird CC, Hooper ML, Wyllie AH: Thymocyte apoptosis induced by p53-dependent and independent pathways. *Nature* **362**:849, 1993.
84. Lowe SW, Schmitt EM, Smith SW, Osborne BA, Jacks T: p53 is required for radiation-induced apoptosis in mouse thymocytes. *Nature* **362**:847, 1993.
85. Lowe SW, Ruley HE, Jacks T, Housman DE: p53-dependent apoptosis modulates the cytotoxicity of anticancer agents. *Cell* **74**:957, 1993.
86. Slichenmeyer WJ, Nelson WG, Slebos RJ, Kastan MB: Loss of a p53-associated G1 checkpoint does not decrease cell survival following DNA damage. *Cancer Res* **53**:4164, 1993.
87. Brachman DG, Beckett M, Graves D, Haraf D, Vokes E, Weichselbaum RR: p53 mutation does not correlate with radiosensitivity in 24 head and neck cancer cell lines. *Cancer Res* **53**:3667, 1993.
88. Maltzman W, Czyzk L: UV irradiation stimulates levels of p53 cellular tumor antigen in nontransformed mouse cells. *Mol Cell Biol* **4**:1689, 1984.
89. Kuerbitz SJ, Beverly SP, Walsh WV, Kastan MB: Wild-type p53 is a cell cycle checkpoint determinant following irradiation. *Proc Natl Acad Sci USA* **89**:7491, 1992.
90. Kastan MB, Onyekwere O, Sidransky D, Vogelstein B, Craig RW: Participation of p53 protein in the cellular response to DNA damage. *Cancer Res* **51**:6304, 1991.
91. Yamaizumi M, Sugano T: UV-induced nuclear accumulation of p53 is evoked through DNA damage of actively transcribed genes independent of the cell cycle. *Oncogene* **9**:2775, 1994.
92. Lee JM, Abrhamson JLA, Kandel R, Donehower LA, Bernstein A: Susceptibility to radiation-carcinogenesis and accumulation of chromosomal breakage in p53-deficient mice. *Oncogene* **9**:3731, 1994.
93. Lee JM, Bernstein A: p53 mutations increase resistance to ionizing radiation. *Proc Natl Acad Sci USA* **90**:5742, 1993.
94. Lane DP: p53, guardian of the genome. *Nature* **358**:15, 1992.
95. Zambetti GP, Levine AJ: A comparison of the biological activities of wild-type and mutant p53. *FASEB J* **7**:855, 1993.
96. Lowe LW, Bodis B, McCarthy A, Remington LH, Ruley E, Fisher D, Housman DE, Jacks T: p53 can determine the efficacy of cancer therapy in vitro. *Science* **266**:807, 1994.
97. Barak Y, Juven T, Haffner R, Oren M: mdm-2 expression is induced by wild-type p53 activity. *EMBO J* **12**:461, 1993.
98. Wu X, Bayle H, Olson D, Levine AJ: The p53-mdm2 autoregulatory feedback loop. *Gene Dev* **7**:1126, 1993.
99. Okamoto K, Beach D: Cyclin G is a transcriptional target of the tumor suppressor protein p53. *EMBO J* **13**:4816, 1994.
100. Myashita T, Reed TC: Tumor suppressor p53 is a direct transcriptional activator of the numan bax gene. *Cell* **80**:293, 1995.
101. Kastan MB, Zhan Q, El-Deiry WS, Carrier F, Jacks T, Walsh WV, Plunkett BS, Vogelstein B, Fornace AJ: A mammalian cell cycle checkpoint pathway utilizing p53 and GADD45 is defective in ataxia-telangiectasia. *Cell* **71**:587, 1992.
102. Harper JW, Adami GR, Wei N, Keyomarsi K, Elledge SJ: The p21 Cdk-interacting protein Cip1 is a potent inhibitor of G1 cyclin-dependent kinases. *Cell* **75**:805, 1993.
103. Xiong Y, Hannon GJ, Zhang H, Casso D, Kobayashi R, Beach D: p21 is a universal inhibitor of cylcin kinases. *Nature* **366**:701, 1993.
104. Gu Y, Turck CW, Morgan DO: Inhibition of CDK2 activity *in vivo* by an associated 20K regulatory subunit. *Nature* **366**:707, 1993.
105. Pines J: p21 inhibits cyclin shock. *Nature* **369**:520, 1994.
106. Smith ML, Chen I-T, Zhan Q, Bae I, Chen C-Y, Glimer TM, Kastan MB, O'Connor PM, Fornace AJ Jr: Interaction of the p53-regulated protein GADD45 with proliferating cell nuclear antigen. *Science* **266**:1376, 1994.
107. Wang XW, Forrester K, Yeh H, Feitelson MA, Gu JR, Harris CC: Hepatitis B virus X protein inhibits p53 sequence-specific DNA binding, transcriptional activity, and association with transcription factor ERCC3. *Proc Natl Acad Sci USA* **91**:2230, 1994.
108. Cho Y, Gorina S, Jeffrey PD, Pavletich NP: Crystal structure of a p53 tumor suppressor-DNA complex: Understanding tumorigenic mutations. *Science* **265**:346, 1994.
109. Clore GM, Omichinski JF, Sakaguchi K, Zambrano N, Sakamoto H, Appella E, Gronenborn AM: High-resolution structure of the oligomerization domain of p53 by multidimensional NMR. *Science* **265**:386, 1994.
109a. Lee W, Harvey TS, Yin Y, Yau P, Litchfield D, Arrowsmith CH: Solution structure of the tetrameric minimum transforming domain of p53. *Struct Biol* **1**:877, 1994.
110. Prives C: How loops, b sheets, and a helices help us to understand p53. *Cell* **78**:543, 1994.
111. Vogelstein B, Kinzler KW: X-rays strike p53 again. *Nature* **370**:174, 1994.
112. Farmer G, Bargonetti J, Zhu H, Friedman P, Prywes R, Prives C: Wild-type p53 activates transcription in vitro. *Nature* **358**:83, 1992.
113. Kern SE, Kinzler KW, Bruskin A, Jarosz D, Friedman P, Prives C, Vogelstein B: Identification of p53 as a sequence-specific DNA-binding protein. *Science* **252**:1708, 1991.
114. Kern SE, Pientenpol JA, Thiagalingam S, Seymour A, Kinzler KW, Vogelstein B: Oncogenic forms of p53 inhibit p53-regulated gene expression. *Science* **256**:827, 1992.
115. Milner J, Medcalf EA: Cotranslation of activated mutant p53 with wild-type p53 protein drives the wild-type p53 protein into the mutant conformation. *Cell* **65**:765, 1991.
116. Cariello NF, Cui L, Beroud C, Soussi T: Database and software for the analysis of mutations in the human p53 gene. *Cancer Res* **54**:4454, 1994.
117. Momand J, Zambetti GP, Olson DC, George D, Levine AJ: The mdm-2 oncogene product forms a complex with the p53 protein and inhibits p53-mediated transactivation. *Cell* **69**:1237, 1992.
118. Sheffner M, Werness BA, Huibregste JM, Levine AJ, Howley PM: The E6 oncoprotein encoded by human papillomavirus types 16 and 18 promotes the degradation of p53. *Cell* **63**:1129, 1990.
119. Fakharzadeh SS, Trusko SP, George DL: Tumorigenic potential associated with enhanced expression of a gene that is amplified in a mouse tumor cell line. *EMBO J* **10**:1565, 1991.
120. Oliner JD, Kinzler KW, Meltzer PS, George DL, Vogelstein B: Amplification of a gene encoding a p53-associated protein in human sarcomas. *Nature* **358**:80, 1992.
121. Maheswaran S, Park S, Bernard A, Morris JF, Rauscher FJ, Hill DE, Haber DA: Physical and functional interaction between WT1 and p53 proteins. *Proc Natl Acad Sci USA* **90**:5100, 1993.
122. Williams BO, Remington L, Albert DM, Mukai S, Bronson RT, Jacks T: Cooperative tumorigenic effects of germ line mutations in Rb and p53 proteins. *Nature Genet* **7**:480, 1994.
123. Harvey M, Vogel H, Lee EYHP, Bradley A, Donehower LA: Mice deficient in both p53 and Rb develop tumors primarily of endocrine origin. *Cancer Res* **55**:1146, 1995.
124. Shimamura A, Fisher DE: p53 in life and death. *Clin Cancer Res* **2**:435, 1996.
125. Hansen R, Reddel R, Braithwaite A: The transforming oncoproteins determine the mechanism by which p53 suppresses cell transformation: pRB-mediated growth arrest or apoptosis. *Oncogene* **11**:2535, 1995.
126. Miller CW, Aslo A, Tsay C, Slamon D, Ishizaki K, Toguchida J: Frequency and structure of p53 rearrangements in human osteosarcoma. *Cancer Res* **50**:7950, 1990.
127. Toguchida J, Yamaguchi T, Ritchie B, Beauchamp RL, Dayton SH, et al: Mutation spectrum of the p53 gene in bone and soft tissue sarcomas. *Cancer Res* **52**:6194, 1992.

128. Felix CA, Kappel CC, Mitsudomi T, Nau MM, Tsokos M, et al: Frequency and diversity of p53 mutations in childhood rhabdomyosarcoma. *Cancer Res* **52**:2243, 1992.
129. Slingerland JM, Minden MD, Benchimol S: Mutation of the p53-gene in human myelogenous leukemia. *Blood* **77**:1500, 1991.
130. Prococimer M, Rotter V: Structure and function of p53 in normal cells and their aberrations in cancer cells: Projection of the hematologic cell lineages. *Blood* **84**:2391, 1994.
131. Mashiyama S, Murakami Y, Yoshimoto T, Sekiya T, Hayashi K: Detection of p53 gene mutations in human brain tumors by single-strand conformation polymorphism analysis of polymerase chain reaction products. *Oncogene* **6**:1313, 1991.
132. Takahashi T, Nan MM, Chiba I, Buchhagen DL, Minna JD: p53: A frequent target for genetic abnormalities in lung cancer. *Science* **246**:491, 1989.
133. Osborne RJ, Merlo GR, Mitsudomi T, Venesio T, Liscia DS, et al: Mutations in the p53 gene in primary human breast cancers. *Cancer Res* **51**:6194, 1991.
134. Malkin D: p53 and the Li-Fraumeni syndrome. *Biochem Biophys Acta* **1198**:197, 1994.
135. Laviguer A, Maltby V, Mock D, Rossant J, Pawson T, Bernstein A: High incidence of lung, bone, and lymphoid tumors in transgenic mice overexpressing mutant alleles of the p53 oncogene. *Mol Cell Biol* **9**:3982, 1989.
136. Malkin D, Li FP, Strong LC, Fraumeni JF Jr, Nelson CE, Kim DH, Kassel J, Gryka MA, Bischoff FZ, Tainsky MA, Friend SH: Germ line p53 mutations ina familial syndrome of breast cancer, sarcomas, and other neoplasms. *Science* **250**:1233, 1990.
137. Malkin D, Friend SH: Correction: A Li-Fraumeni syndrome mutation. *Science* **259**:878, 1993.
137a. Srivastava S, Zou Z, Pirollo K, Blattner W, Chang EH: Germ line transmission of a mutated p53 gene in a cancer-prone family with Li-Fraumeni syndrome. *Nature* **348**:747, 1990.
138. Vogelstein B: A deadly inheritance. *Nature* **348**:681, 1990.
139. Law JC, Strong LC, Chidambaram A, Ferrell RE: A germ line mutation in exon 5 of the p53 gene in an extended cancer family. *Cancer Res* **51**:6385, 1991.
140. Metzger AK, Sheffield VC, Duyk G, Daneshuar L, Edwards MSB, Cogen PH: Identification of a germ line mutation in the p53 gene in a patient with intracranial ependymoma. *Proc Natl Acad Sci USA* **88**:7825, 1991.
141. Santibanez-Koref MF, Birch JM, Hartley AL, Morris-Jones PH, Craft AW, et al: p53 germ line mutations in Li-Fraumeni syndrome. *Lancet* **338**:1490, 1991.
142. Birch JM: Germ line mutations in the p53 tumor suppressor gene: Scientific, clinical and ethical challenges. *Br J Cancer* **66**:424, 1992.
143. Barnes DM, Hanby AM, Gillett CE, Mohammed S, Hodson S, Bobrow LG, Leigh IM, Purkis T, MacGEoch C, Spur AM, Bartek J, Vojtesek B, Picksley SM, Lane DP: Abnormal expression of wild-type p53 protein in normal cells of a cancer family patient. *Lancet* **340**:259, 1992.
144. Frebourg T, Barbier N, Yan Y-X, Garber JE, Dreyfus M, Fraumeni JF Jr, Li FP, Friend SH: Germ line p53 mutations in 15 families with Li-Fraumeni syndrome. *Am J Hum Genet* **56**:608, 1995.
145. Brugieres L, Gardes M, Moutou C, Chompret A, Meresse V, et al: Screening for germ line p53 mutations in children with malignant tumor and a family history of cancer. *Cancer Res* **53**:452, 1993.
146. Birch JM, Heighway J, Teare MD, Kelsey AM, Hartley AL, Tricker KJ, Crowther D, Lane DP, Santibanez-Koref MF: Linkage studies in a Li-Fraumeni family with increased expression of p53 protein but no germ line mutation in p53. *Br J Cancer* **70**:1176, 1994.
146a. Varley JM, McGown G, Thorncroft M, Cochrane S, Morrison P, Woll P, Kelsey AM, Mitchell ELD, Boyle J, Birch JM, Evans DGR: A previously undescribed mutation within the tetramerization domain of TP53 in a family with Li-Fraumeni syndrome. *Oncogene* **12**:2437, 1996.
147. Malkin D, Jolly KW, Barbier N, Look AT, Friend SH, Gebhardt MC, Andersen TI, Borresen A-L, Li FP, Strong LC: Germ line mutations of the p53 tumor suppressor gene in children and young adults with second malignant neoplasms. *N Engl J Med* **326**:1309, 1992.
148. Iavarone A, Mattay KK, Steinkirchner TM, Israel MA: Germ line and somatic p53 gene mutations in multifocal osteogenic sarcoma. *Proc Natl Acad Sci USA* **89**:4207, 1992.
148a. Kyritsis AP, Bondy ML, Xiao M, Berman EL, Cunningham JE, Lee PS, Levin VA, Saya H: Germ line p53 gene mutations in subsets of glioma patients. *J Natl Cancer Inst* **86**:344, 1994.
149. Toguchida J, Yamaguchi T, Dayton SH, Beauchamp RL, Herrera GE, Ishizaki K, Yamamuro T, Meyers PA, Little JB, Sasaki MS, Weichselbaum RR, Yandell DW: Prevalence and spectrum of germ line mutations of the p53 gene among patients with sarcoma. *N Engl J Med* **326**:1301, 1992.
150. Prosser J, Elder PA, Condie A, MacFayden I, Steel CM, Evans HJ: Mutations in p53 do not account for heritable breast cancer: A study in five affected families. *Br J Cancer* **63**:181, 1991.
151. Warren W, Eeles RA, Ponder BAJ, Easton DF, Averill D, Ponder MA, Anderson K, Evans AM, DeMars R, Love R, Dundas S, Stratton MR, Trowbridge P, Cooper CS, Peto J: No evidence for germ line mutations in exons 5-9 of the p53 gene in 25 breast cancer families. *Oncogene* **7**:1043, 1992.
152. Borresen A-L, Andersen TI, Garber J, Barbier N, Thorlacius S, Eyfjord J, Ottestad L, Smith-Sorensen B, Hovig E, Malkin D, Friend SH: Screening for germ line TP53 mutations in breast cancer patients. *Cancer Res* **52**:3234, 1992.
153. Frebourg T, Barbier N, Kassel J, Ng YS, Romero P, Friend SH: A functional screen for germ line p53 mutations based on transcriptional activation. *Cancer Res* **52**:6976, 1992.
154. Sidransky D, Tokino T, Helzlsouer K, Zehnbauer B, Rausch G, Shelton B, Prestigiacomo L, Vogelstein B, Davidson N: Inherited p53 gene mutations in breast cancer. *Cancer Res* **52**:2984, 1992.
155. Loriaux DL, Cutler GB Jr: Diseases of the adrenal glands, in Kohler PO (ed): *Clinical Endocrinology.* New York, Wiley, 1986, p 157.
156. Sameshima Y, Tsunematsu Y, Watanabe S, Tsukamoto T, Kawaha K, et al: Detection of novel germ line p53 mutations in diverse cancer prone families identified by selecting patients with childhood adrenocortical carcinoma. *J Natl Cancer Inst* **84**:703, 1992.
157. Wagner J, Portwine C, Rabin K, Leclerc J-M, Narod SA, Malkin D: High frequency of germ line p53 mutations in childhood adrenocortical cancer. *J Natl Cancer Inst* **86**:1707, 1994.
158. McIntyre JF, Smith-Sorensen B, Friend SH, Kassel J, Borresen A-L, Yan YX, Russo C, Sato J, Barbier N, Miser J, Malkin D, Gebhardt MC: Germline mutations of the p53 tumor suppressor gene in children with osteosarcoma. *J Clin Oncol* **12:925, 1994.**
159. Diller L, Sexsmith E, Gottlieb A, Li FP, Malkin D: Germ line p53 mutations are frequently detected in young children with rhabdomyosarcoma. *J Clin Invest* **95**:1606, 1995.
160. Felix CA, Nau MM, Takahashi T, Mitsudomi T, Chiba I, Poplack DG, Reaman GH, Cole DE, Letterio JJ, Whang-Peng J, Knutsen T, Minna JD: Hereditary and acquired p53 mutations in childhood acute lymphoblastic leukemia. *J Clin Invest* **89**:640, 1992.
161. Felix CA, D'Amico D, Mitsudomi T, Nau MM, Li FP, Fraumeni JF Jr, Cole DE, McCalla J, Reaman GH, Whang-Peng J, Knutsen T, Minna JD, Poplack DG: Absence of hereditary p53 mutations in 10 familial leukemia pedigrees. *J Clin Invest* **90**:653, 1992.
162. Felix CA, Hosler MR, Provisor D, Salhany K, Sexsmith EA, Slater DJ, Cheung NKV, Winick NJ, Strauss EA, Heyn R, Lange BJ, Malkin D: The p53 gene in pediatric therapy-related leukemia and myelodysplasia. *Blood* **10:**4376, 1996.
163. Jolly KW, Malkin D, Douglass EC, Brown TF, Sinclair AE, Look, AT: Splice-site mutation of the p53 gene in a family with hereditary breast-ovarian cancer. *Oncogene* **9**:97, 1994.
164. Warneford SG, Wilton LJ, Townsend ML, Rowe PB, Reddell RR, Dalla-Pozza L, Symonds G: Germ line splicing mutation of the p53 gene in a cancer-prone family. *Cell Growth Differ* **3**:839, 1992.
165. Felix CA, Strauss EA, D'Amico D, Tsokos M, Winter S, Mitsudomi T, Nau MM, Brown DL, Leahey AM, Horowitz ME, Poplack DG, Costin D, Minna JD: A novel germ line p53 splicing mutation in a pediatric patient with a second malignant neoplasm. *Oncogene* **8**:1203, 1993.
166. Gannon JV, Greaves R, Iggo R, Lane DP: Activating mutations in p53 produce common conformation effects: A monoclonal antibody specific for the mutant form. *EMBO J* **9**:1591, 1990.
167. Srivastava S, Tong YA, Devadas K, Zou A-Q, Sykes VW, Chang EW: Detection of both mutant and wild-type p53 protein in normal skin fibroblasts and demonstration of a shared second hit on p53 in diverse tumors from a cancer-prone family with Li-Fraumeni syndrome. *Oncogene* **7**:987, 1992.
168. Frebourg T, Kassel J, Lam KT, Gryka MA, Barbier N, Andersen TI, Borresen A-L, Friend SH: Germ line mutations of the p53 tumor suppressor gene in patients with high risk for cancer inactivate the p53 protein. *Proc Natl Acad Sci USA* **89**:6413, 1992.

169. Ishioka C, Frebourg T, Yan Y-X, Vidal M, Friend SH, Schmidt S, Iggo R: Screening patients for heterozygous p53 mutations using a functional assay in yeast. *Nature Genet* **5**:124, 1993.
170. Flaman JM, Frebourg T, Moreau V, Charbonnier F, Martin C, Chappuis P, Sappino AP, Limacher IM, Bron L, Benhatter J: A simple p53 functional assay for screening cell lines, blood and tumors. *Proc Natl Acad Sci USA* **92**:3963, 1995.
171. Lavigueur A, Bernstein A: p53 transgenic mice: Accelerated erythroleukemia induction by Friend virus. *Oncogene* **6**:2197, 1991.
172. Donehower LA, Harvey M, Slagle BL, McArthur MJ, Montgomery CA, Butel J, Bradley A: Mice deficient for p53 are developmentally normal but susceptible to spontaneous tumors. *Nature* **356**:215, 1992.
173. Rogel A, Popliker M, Webb C, Oren M: p53 cellular tumor antigen: Analysis of mRNA levels in normal cell adult tissues, embryos, and tumors. *Mol Cell Biol* **5**:2851, 1985.
174. Purdie CA, Harrison DJ, Peter A, Dobbie L, White S, Howie SEM, Salter DM, Bird CC, Wyllie AH, Hooper ML, Clarke AR: Tumor incidence, spectrum and ploidy in mice with a large deletion in the p53 gene. *Oncogene* **9**:603, 1994.
175. Jacks T, Remington L, Williams BO, Schmitt EM, Halachmi S, Bronson RT, Weinberg RA: Tumor spectrum analysis in p53 mutant mice. *Current Biol* **4**:1, 1994.
176. Harvey M, McArthur MJ, Montgomery CA Jr, Bradley A, Donehower LA: Genetic background alters the spectrum of tumors that develop in p53-deficient mice. *FASEB J* **7**:849, 1993.
177. Dietrich WF, Lander ES, Smith JS, Moser AR, Gould KA, Luongo C, Borenstein N, Dove W: Genetic identification of Mom-1, a major modifiar locus affecting Min-induced intestinal neoplasia in the mouse. *Cell* **75**:631, 1993.
178. Montes de Oca Luna R, Wagner DS, Lozano G: Rescue of embryonic lethality in mdm-2-deficient mice by deletion of p53. *Nature* **378**:203, 1995.
179. Jones SN, Roe AE, Donehower LA, Bradley A: Rescue of embryonic lethality in Mdm-2-deficient mice by absence of p53. *Nature* **378**:206, 1995.
180. Harvey M, Vogel H, Morris D, Bradley A, Bernstein A, Donehower LA: A mutant p53 transgene accelerates tumor development in heterozygous but not nullizygous p53-deficient mice. *Nature Genet* **9**:305, 1995.
181. Liu G, Montes de Oca Luna R, Lozano G: Establishing mouse models to study tumor derived p53 mutants in vivo: Cancer genetics and tumor suppressor genes. *Cold Spring Harbor Lab Meeting* **172:** 1996.
182. Sah VP, Attardi LD, Mulligan GJ, Williams BO, Bronson RT, Jacks T: A subset of p53-deficient embryos exhibit exencephaly. *Nature Genet* **7**:480, 1994.
183. Hartley AL, Birch JM, Blair V, Kelsey AM, Morris-Jones PH: Fetal loss and infant deaths in families of children with soft-tissue sarcoma. *Int J Cancer* **56**:646, 1994.
184. Harvey M, McArthur MJ, Montgomery CA Jr, Butel JS, Bradley A, Donehower LA: Spontaneous and carcinogen-induced tumorigenesis in p53-deficient mice. *Nature Genet* **5**:225, 1993.
185. Li G, Ho VC, Berean K, Tron VA: Ultraviolet radiation induction of squamous cell carcinomas in p53 transgenic mice. *Cancer Res* **55**:2070, 1995.
186. Koizumi A, Tsudada M, Wada Y, Masuda H, Weindruch R: *J Nutr* **122**:1446, 1992.
187. Hursting SD, Perkins SN, Phang JM: Calorie restriction delays spontaneous tumorigenesis in p53-knockout transgenic mice. *Proc Natl Acad Sci USA* **91**:7036, 1994.
188. Nicol CJ, Harrison ML, Laposa RR, Gimelshtein IL, Wells PG: A teratologic suppressor role for p53 in benzo[a]pyrene-treated transgenic p53-deficient mice. *Nature Genet* **10**:181, 1995.
189. Laposa RR, Chan KC, Wiley MJ, Wells PG: Evidence for DNA damage and teratological suppressor genes in the initiation of and resistance to chemical teratogenesis: phenytoin teratogenicity in p53-deficient mice. *Toxicologist* **15**:161, 1995.
190. Clarke AR, Cummings MC, Harrison DJ: Interaction between murine germ line mutations in p53 and APC predisposes to pancreatic neoplasia but not to increased intestinal malignancy. *Oncogene* **11**:1913, 1995.
191. Stewart M, Cameron E, Campbell M, McFarlane R, Toth S, Lang K et al: Conditional expression and oncogenicity of c-myc linked to a CD2 gene dominant control region. *Int J Cancer* **53**:1023, 1993.
192. Blyth K, Terry A, O'Hara M, Baxter EW, Campbell M, Stewart M, Donehower LA, Onions DE, Neil JC, Cameron ER: Synergy between a human c-myc transgene and p53 null genotype in murine thymic lymphomas: Contrasting effects of homozygous and heterozygous p53 loss. *Oncogene* **10**:1717, 1995.
193. Li FP, Garber JE, Friend SH, Strong LC, Patenaude AF, Juengst ET, Reilly PR, Corea P, Fraumeni JF Jr: Recommendations on predictive testing for germ line p53 mutations among cancer-prone individuals. *J Natl Cancer Inst* **84**:1156, 1992.
194. American Society of Clinical Oncology: Statement of the American Society of Clinical Oncology: Genetic testing for cancer susceptibility. *J Clin Oncol* **14**:1730, 1996.
195. American Society of Human Genetics: Statements of the American Society of Human Genetics on genetic testing for breast and ovarian cancer predisposition. *Am J Hum Genet* **55:**i, 1994.
196. Shapiro S: Determining the efficacy of breast cancer screening. *Cancer* **63**:1873, 1989.

CHAPTER 38

Wilms Tumor

Daniel A. Haber

1. Wilms tumor is a pediatric kidney cancer that can arise sporadically or in children with congenital syndromes conferring genetic susceptibility. In addition, some 10 percent of children with Wilms tumor present with bilateral cancers, evidence of a predisposing genetic lesion.

2. The genetic loci associated with the development of Wilms tumor have been identified by analysis of gross karyotype abnormalities in children with Wilms-associated syndromes, as well as by molecular analyses of DNA losses in tumor specimens. A genetic locus on chromosome 11 band p13 has been linked to Wilms tumor arising in the context of aniridia and abnormalities of genitourinary development (e.g., WAGR syndrome). A second locus on chromosome 11 band p15 is associated with hemihypertrophy (e.g., Beckwith-Wiedemann syndrome) and predisposition to Wilms tumor and other pediatric neoplasms. A third Wilms locus has been mapped recently to chromosome 17q12-21.

3. The *WT1* gene, mapping within the 11p13 genetic locus, was isolated in 1990. It encodes a transcription factor whose expression is strictly developmentally regulated in the normal kidney. Like the fetal kidney cells from which they appear to originate, most Wilms tumors express high levels of WT1 protein. However, in a fraction of Wilms tumors, *WT1* is either deleted or mutated to an inactive form, consistent with its characterization as a tumor suppressor gene. Reintroduction of wild-type WT1 into a Wilms tumor cell line with an aberrant endogenous *WT1* transcript results in inhibition of cell growth.

4. Inactivation of *WT1* in one germ-line allele confers a high degree of susceptibility to Wilms tumor, which is triggered by loss of the second *WT1* allele in somatic tissues. Hemizygosity for *WT1* in the germ line also results in a variable degree of developmental abnormalities in the genitourinary tract, more prominent in males than in females. Moreover, specific point mutations within the DNA-binding domain of *WT1* result in a dominant negative phenotype, characterized by severe abnormalities in sexual and renal development (Denys-Drash syndrome). In the mouse, hemizygous inactivation of *WT1* is not associated with genitourinary defects or tumor predisposition. However, homozygous inactivation of *WT1* leads to failure of renal and gonadal development, as well as to malformations of the heart and diaphragm.

5. The protein encoded by *WT1* belongs to a class of zinc-binding transcription factors, with multiple variants produced by alternative splicing. The four zinc-finger domains of *WT1* recognize GC-rich DNA target sequences, an effect that is modulated by the variable insertion of three amino acids (KTS) between zinc fingers 3 and 4. *WT1* appears to function as a transcriptional repressor, although physiologically relevant target genes remain to be defined. Potential protein interactors include another tumor suppressor gene product, p53, whose function is modulated by WT1. Inducible expression of WT1 in tissue culture cells triggers apoptosis, associated with repression of the epidermal growth factor receptor and induction of the cyclin-dependent kinase inhibitor p21. Dimerization of WT1 may contribute to the dominant negative phenotype displayed by mutants with a disrupted DNA-binding domain. Characterization of the normal pathways involved in *WT1* function and of any potential interactions with other Wilms tumor genes may lead to a better understanding of normal kidney development and tumorigenesis.

Wilms tumor, or nephroblastoma, is a pediatric kidney cancer that can present either as a sporadic case or in the setting of genetic predisposition. Both epidemiologic studies of tumor incidence and early genetic studies pointed to the presence of one or more genes whose loss was associated with tumor development. The isolation of the first of these genes, *WT1,* has led to the discovery of a tumor suppressor gene encoding a transcription factor with a striking kidney-specific pattern of expression. Mutations in *WT1* have been linked both to the formation of Wilms tumor and to a range of developmental abnormalities in genitourinary development. The characterization of this gene and the ongoing search for the other Wilms tumor genes provide a key to understanding the basis of normal kidney development and tumorigenesis.

HISTOLOGY

The histologic characteristics of Wilms tumor are complex, consistent with its classification as a primitive, multilineage malignancy of renal stem cells.[1] The classic description is that of a "triphasic" tumor, including blastemal, epithelial, and stromal components (Fig. 38-1). All these components are thought to be derived from the malignant stem cell, although genetic evidence of shared lineage has not been demonstrated. Wilms tumors can vary in the predominance of one histologic component over the others, and some tumors show evidence of further multilineage differentiation, with the presence of muscle or neural elements. Clinical prognosis does not appear to be affected by the histologic appearance of the tumors, with the exception of anaplastic variants that have a more aggressive course.[2] Tumors with triphasic histology characteristic of Wilms tumor may arise outside the kidney. Such "extrarenal" Wilms tumors have been reported from a number of sites, primarily the pelvis and abdomen.[3] Although Wilms tumor is primarily a cancer of children under 5 years of age, it also has been reported in young adults. The histology of these tumors is similar to that of classic Wilms tumor seen in young children, leading to the suggestion that they arise from a small number of renal stem cells that have persisted into adulthood.

The relationship between Wilms tumor and normal renal development is best illustrated by the persistent nephrogenic rests seen within the normal kidney of children with Wilms tumor.[4,5] These lesions, also called *precursor lesions, persistent metanephric blastema, nephroblastomatosis* or *nodular renal blastema* are comprised of primitive blastemal cells with varying degrees of differentiation. They are usually less than 1 cm in diameter but rarely can become massive, compressing the normal kidney and

A list of standard abbreviations is located immediately preceding the index in each volume.

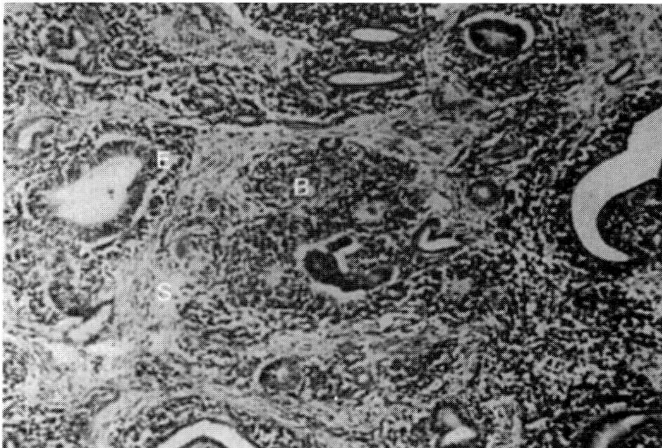

Fig. 38-1 Wilms tumor histology. The classic triphasic histologic pattern includes areas of primitive blastemal cells (B), epithelial cells (E), and stromal cell components (S). Tumors also can contain areas of further differentiation along muscle and rarely neural lineages. Expression of the *WT1* tumor suppressor gene appears restricted to the epithelial and blastemal components of Wilms tumors. (*Photomicrograph, hematoxylin and eosin stain, provided by Dr. Nancy Harris, Department of Pathology, Massachusetts General Hospital, Boston, Massachusetts.*)

easily mistaken for a genuine tumor. Although foci of Wilms tumor can arise within a large nephrogenic rest, the precursor lesions themselves do not appear to be malignant, and some have been shown to regress when followed noninvasively. Nephrogenic rests are present in the normal kidney at birth but are rarely found after 1 year of age. In contrast, virtually all children with genetic susceptibility to Wilms tumor have one or more such lesions within otherwise normal kidney. In these children, nephrogenic rests may represent the effect of a constitutional mutation predisposing to abnormal renal development, the first step toward the formation of Wilms tumor. In support of this notion is the observation that nephrogenic rests located in the periphery of a renal lobe, so-called perilobar rests, are found more frequently in the kidneys of children whose genetic susceptibility to Wilms tumor is associated with the locus on chromosome 11p15. Nephrogenic rests located within the renal lobe, known as intralobar rests, are smaller and less well defined histologically and are seen more commonly in the kidneys of children with evidence of a genetic lesion at the chromosome 11p13 locus.[5] However, even in the absence of genetic predisposition, some 30 percent of children with apparently sporadic Wilms tumor have nephrogenic rests within the normal surrounding kidney. Molecular evidence indicates that these nephrogenic rests harbor the same mutation in *WT1* as that found in the accompanying Wilms tumor, suggesting that both the tumor and the precursor lesion are derived from the same renal stem cell in which the tumor suppressor gene was mutated.[6]

CLINICAL FEATURES

Nephroblastosis was first described in 1899 by a German physician, Max Wilms, as a uniformly fatal cancer of children. With the use of modern multimodality therapy, the treatment of Wilms tumor has advanced dramatically, with a reported cure rate of 90 percent by the National Wilms Tumor Study Group.[7] Wilms tumor usually arises by age 5, with equal incidence between sexes and among different ethnic groups. In children with genetic susceptibility, the age of incidence is usually under 2 years, and frequent screening by renal ultrasound is recommended. The usual presenting feature is that of an abdominal mass, with an adrenal malignancy such as neuroblastoma as the main differential diagnostic consideration. Initial preoperative evaluation is directed at excluding the presence of pulmonary metastases, local spread into the inferior vena cava, or involvement of draining lymph nodes. The surgical management of Wilms tumor calls for skill and experience, requiring resection of the affected kidney, exploration of the inferior vena cava, and lymph node dissection. Of utmost importance is examination of the contralateral kidney for any synchronous tumor. The occurrence of bilateral tumors in some 10 percent of patients is an indication of genetic susceptibility to Wilms tumor, but it cannot be excluded by a negative family history or the absence of associated congenital abnormalities. Most children with bilateral tumors have no prior evidence of genetic risk, and genetic studies to date have indicated that most of these children may harbor *de novo* germ-line mutations.[8,9] In the presence of bilateral Wilms tumors, most surgeons will perform a full nephrectomy on the side with the larger tumor and a partial nephrectomy on the other side, attempting to preserve as much renal function as possible.

Postoperative treatment of Wilms tumor with chemotherapy and radiation therapy is evolving as multi-institutional groups adjust the recommended regimens so as to improve the effectiveness and lower the toxicity of treatment.[10] Most children who fit into favorable prognostic groups based on tumor histology and stage are treated with chemotherapy including actinomycin D and vincristine. Radiation therapy in addition to chemotherapy is reserved for patients with anaplastic tumors or cancers of advanced stage. Wilms tumor appears to be very sensitive to chemotherapy drugs, and even patients with advanced metastatic disease have an excellent cure rate. The incidence of secondary malignancies in children cured of Wilms tumor is low and appears to be treatment-related, consisting primarily of soft tissue sarcomas arising within the radiation field and acute leukemia attributed to the use of alkylating agents and radiation therapy.[11] Genetic predisposition to Wilms tumor is only rarely associated with susceptibility to other tumor types, such as gonadoblastoma in Denys-Drash syndrome or adrenal carcinoma and hepatocellular carcinoma in Beckwith-Wiedemann syndrome. In the absence of such congenital syndromes, the great majority of children treated for Wilms tumor are fertile when they reach reproductive age, and the risk of Wilms tumor arising in their offspring has been found to be very low.[12]

THE KNUDSON MODEL IN WILMS TUMOR

Much of the conceptual basis for the genetic study of tumor suppressor genes was laid by Knudson in a series of epidemiologic studies of retinoblastoma, Wilms tumor, and neuroblastoma.[13–15] These childhood tumors are remarkable in that 10 to 30 percent of affected children present with bilateral or multicentric cancers. Bilateral tumors have an age of onset that is 1 to 2 years earlier than that of unilateral cancers, and in the case of the eye tumor retinoblastoma, they are often associated with a positive family history. By comparing the incidence of unilateral versus bilateral retinoblastomas in patients with a positive family history, Knudson found that the data fit the Poisson distribution for a single rare event. Thus these individuals, who had inherited one genetic mutation, only required one additional "genetic hit" in the target tissues to develop a tumor (Fig. 38-2). Given the number of target cells at risk for the second hit, multiple tumors are common, and they tend to arise early in life. In contrast, in the absence of genetic predisposition, two rare independent events are required for tumor formation, hence a low incidence of tumors, which are unilateral and which present at a later age. In addition to the difference in the mean age of tumor development between inherited and sporadic cases, the rate of decline in the incidence of new tumors is also predicted by the Knudson "two-hit" model. In genetically predisposed individuals, the age of onset declines exponentially, consistent with the exponential rate of differentiation of susceptible nephroblasts. In contrast, in sporadic cases, a more delayed decline in the incidence of new tumors is noted, suggesting that the second genetic lesion depends on the variable timing of the initial mutation.

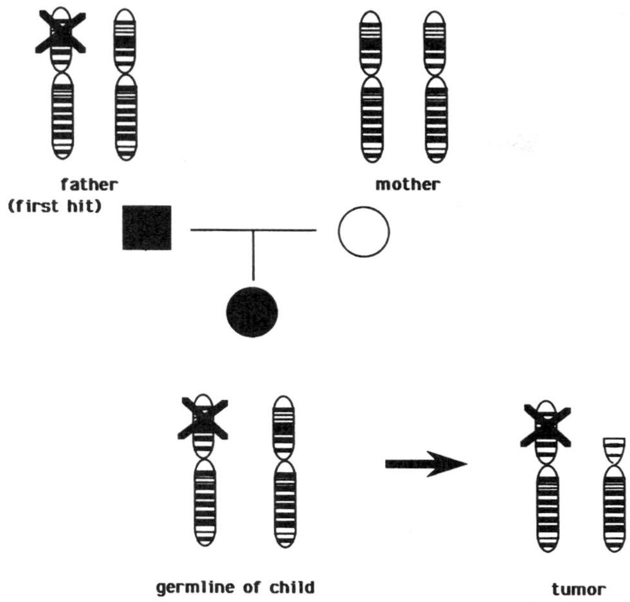

Fig. 38-2 Schematic representation of the Knudson model. Based on epidemiologic analyses of the age of incidence and number of tumors observed in children with genetic predisposition versus those with sporadic tumors, Knudson and Strong[12–14] predicted that two rate-limiting "hits" are required for tumorigenesis. This hypothesis has evolved with the detection of allelic losses in tumors and the concept of recessive oncogenes or tumor suppressor genes.[18,22] Thus a mutation present either in the germ line or in the germ cells of a parent constitutes the first hit. The child born with such a mutation in the germ line requires only one additional hit in the target tissue to trigger tumorigenesis. The relatively high frequency of this second hit explains the early age of onset of tumors and the fact that they are often bilateral. In contrast, a child without a germ-line mutation requires two independent rare events within the target tissue in order to achieve two rate-limiting hits. The low probability of two independent mutations at the same locus explains the later onset of tumors in sporadic cases and the fact that they are unilateral. In most cases of Wilms tumor, the initial hit results from a point mutation or a small deletion within the target tumor suppressor gene, while the second hit consists of a gross chromosomal deletion or non-disjunction event. These large chromosomal events can be identified by the loss of restriction fragment length polymorphisms (RFLP) in the affected locus (so-called loss of heterozygosity), thus providing a clue to the presence of a tumor suppressor gene.

The predictions of the Knudson model were first confirmed by the cloning of the retinoblastoma susceptibility gene, *RB1*.[16–18] Indeed, the two genetic hits represent the inactivation of the two alleles of this tumor suppressor gene.[19–22] The first hit appears to be most commonly a mutation or small deletion that is found in the germ line of predisposed individuals or in somatic tissues in sporadic cases. Loss of the second allele, which represents the second hit, is seen most commonly as a wholesale loss of a chromosome or a chromosomal recombinational event in somatic tissues. Such large chromosomal losses may be more frequent than the initial point mutation but are only tolerated in the heterozygous state, explaining their prevalence as second rather than first hits. They have proven to be of critical importance in molecular mapping studies of tumor suppressor genes such as those responsible for retinoblastoma and Wilms tumor, since the loss of surrounding restriction fragment length polymorphisms (RFLP) points to the presence of a critical genetic locus.[23]

The epidemiology of Wilms tumor shares a number of features with that of retinoblastoma. Bilateral tumors are noted in 5 to 10 percent of patients, and as predicted by the Knudson model, these present at an earlier age than unilateral cases.[14,24,25] However, familial Wilms tumor is rare, estimated at 1 percent of patients. Based on the number of bilateral tumors, the mathematical model proposed by Knudson and Strong predicts that some 30 percent of children have a genetic predisposition to Wilms tumor. In the majority of cases, this genetic susceptibility appears to represent a *de novo* germ-line mutation rather than a transmitted parental gene. In this context, it is of interest that in most Wilms tumors that show allelic DNA losses involving the 11p13 genetic locus, the lost allele (representing the second hit) is of maternal origin. These observations suggest that the initial mutation is likely to occur in the paternal germ cells during spermatogenesis.

Another distinction between retinoblastoma and Wilms tumor is the presence of a phenotype conferred by a single mutated allele. Individuals with a germ-line mutation in *RB1* who fail to develop a tumor during the first few years of life have no detectable ocular abnormalities as adults, suggesting that hemizygosity for *RB1* is phenotypically silent. In contrast, children with hemizygous deletions involving the 11p13 Wilms tumor locus (WAGR syndrome) have developmental abnormalities of the genitourinary tract as well as nephrogenic rests within both kidneys.[26,27] Since nephrogenic rests consist of a proliferation of primitive blastemal cells, their presence may increase the size of the target cell population, thus enhancing the probability of a second genetic hit. The number of genetic lesions important in the development of Wilms tumor may in fact be greater than two. The Knudson model, based on the statistics of "hit kinetics," has proved to be accurate in predicting the number of genetic events that are rate-limiting. However, genetic events that are necessary for malignant transformation but that are more frequent or that are dependent on these initial "hits" will not be detected by such an analysis. At least three genetic loci have been implicated in the initial events in Wilms tumorigenesis, and tumor specimens have been shown to have a number of additional chromosomal abnormalities that may have a role in tumor progression. The isolation of the first of these genes and the characterization of the genetic lesions that contribute to the development of Wilms tumor have provided an initial appreciation for the genetic complexity of this malignancy.[28]

GENETIC LOCI ASSOCIATED WITH WILMS TUMOR

The identification of the major genetic loci associated with the development of Wilms tumor has resulted from studies of both germ-line and tumor material, using karyotype analysis, genetic linkage and molecular genetic studies, as well as clinical observations on patients with congenital abnormalities. Two distinct genetic loci have been mapped to the short arm of chromosome 11 (Table 38-1), while a third locus on chromosome 17q has been implicated in some familial cases.

Chromosome 11p13 Locus

The first linkage of Wilms tumor susceptibility to a chromosomal locus was derived from a clinical observation. In 1964, Miller and coworkers noted a higher than expected incidence of Wilms tumor in children with aniridia, a rare eye abnormality consisting of malformation or absence of the iris.[29] While Wilms tumor arises in 1 in 10,000 children and aniridia occurs in 1 in 70,000 children, aniridia is noted in 1 in 70 children with Wilms tumor, and this tumor develops in 1 in 3 children with aniridia. As would be expected from the Knudson model, children with aniridia who develop a Wilms tumor have a high incidence of bilateral tumors, consistent with the presence of a predisposing germ-line lesion. This lesion is most clearly evident in children with a constellation of symptoms that includes aniridia, developmental abnormalities of the genitourinary tract (such as hypospadias, undescended testes, renal hypoplasia, or ureteral atresia), and mental retardation.[26,27] Children with this so-called WAGR syndrome (an acronym for *W*ilms, *a*nirida, *g*enitourinary defects, mental *r*etardation) were found to have a gross cytogenetic deletion within band 13 of the short arm of chromosome 11[30,31] (Fig. 38-3). This discovery was the first to link a gene conferring susceptibility

Table 38-1 Summary of the Two Major Congenital Syndromes Associated with Increased Susceptibility to Wilms Tumor*

	WAGR Syndrome	Beckwith-Wiedemann Syndrome
Chromosomal locus	11p13	11p15
Tumor suppressor gene	*WT1*	Unknown
Wilms tumor incidence	< 50%	< 5%
Associated features	Aniridia	Macroglossia
	Genitourinary defects	Organomegaly/hemihypertrophy
	Mental retardation	Umbilical hernia
		Neonatal hypoglycemia
		Additional tumors
		Adrenocortical carcinoma
		Hepatoblastoma

*The WAGR syndrome results from a hemizygous chromosomal deletion within the chromosome 11p13 locus, affecting the *WT1* and aniridia genes. Beckwith-Wiedemann syndrome results from an abnormality in the 11p15 locus that may involve gene dosage as well as parental imprinting. The gene responsible for this syndrome and for the associated risk of developing Wilms tumor has not been identified.

to Wilms tumor to a genetic locus. The complex congenital abnormalities of children with WAGR syndrome results from a deletion that affects a number of adjacent genes, a so-called contiguous-gene syndrome (Fig. 38-4). The aniridia locus was distinguished from the Wilms tumor locus by the existence of patients with an 11p13 chromosome translocation who suffered from aniridia without developing Wilms tumor.[32,33] Aniridia is now known to result from a hemizygous deletion of a homeobox gene, *Pax6*.[34] The genitourinary defects associated with WAGR syndrome are variable in their severity and appear to result from hemizygosity for the Wilms tumor gene itself (see below). The etiology of the mental retardation is still unclear.

The involvement of the chromosome 11p13 locus in Wilms tumor development also was evidenced by molecular analysis of tumor specimens. Chromosome abnormalities in Wilms tumor specimens are complex but frequently involve the short arm of chromosome 11.[35–38] More precise molecular studies, involving the use of polymorphic DNA markers, were used to demonstrate loss of heterozygosity on chromosome 11p.[39–42] This represents the loss of gross chromosomal fragments or recombinational events resulting in the loss of the second allele of a putative tumor suppressor gene (the second genetic hit). The loss of heterozygosity at chromosome 11p13 that results from such mechanisms usually extends to the telomere, spanning the 11p15 locus. It therefore can be difficult to distinguish involvement of the two Wilms loci on the short arm of chromosome 11, but cases in which a more limited loss of DNA affects each locus in isolation have confirmed the independence of these two genetic loci.[43,44]

Chromosome 11p15

Like the 11p13 Wilms tumor locus, the 11p15 locus has been implicated both by genetic susceptibility studies and by allelic losses in tumor specimens.[39–46] However, the genetic mechanisms underlying the effects of the 11p15 locus appear to be more complex, involving genomic imprinting and unequal duplication of parental chromosomes. Increased susceptibility to Wilms tumor was noted by Wiedemann and by Beckwith in a syndrome that now bears their name.[47,48] Beckwith-Wiedemann syndrome consists of abnormally enlarged organs, particularly the tongue and abdominal viscera, which can result in an umbilical hernia. Soft tissues also can be enlarged, with one side more affected than the other, resulting in hemihypertrophy of the body. Neonatal hypoglycemia is also evident in more serious cases. Pediatric neoplasms are seen in 7.5 percent of children with Beckwith-Wiedemann syndrome, a far lower incidence than that in patients with WAGR syndrome, and these tumors include adrenocortical carcinoma and hepatoblastoma as well as Wilms tumor. The true penetrance of Beckwith-Wiedemann syndrome is difficult to ascertain, since the different manifestations of the syndrome can be quite variable, often rendering the clinical diagnosis uncertain.[49,50]

The association of Beckwith-Wiedemann syndrome with the chromosome 11p15 locus is based on genetic linkage studies in the rare families in which the condition is inherited,[51,52] as well as gross cytogenetic abnormalities in the germ line of some sporadically affected individuals.[53,54] Abnormal karyotypes in such patients most frequently consist of a duplication of

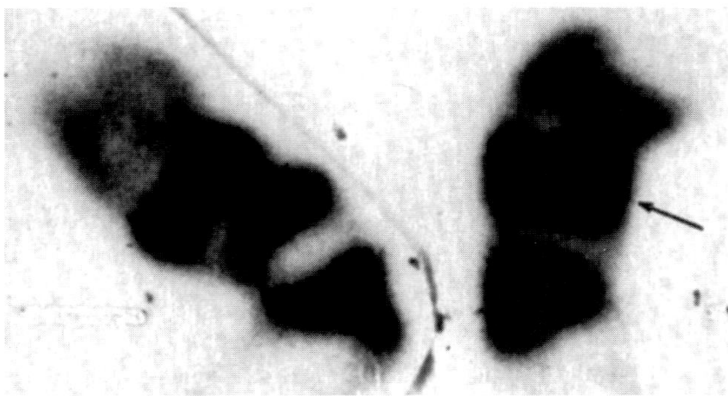

Fig. 38-3 Cytogenetic abnormality in WAGR syndrome. One of the two chromosomes 11 in the germ line of a child with WAGR syndrome contains a deletion within band p13 (arrow). This large hemizygous deletion, encompassing a number of contiguous genes, leads to a 50 percent probability of developing Wilms tumor, abnormal development of the iris (aniridia), abnormalities of genitourinary development, and mental retardation.

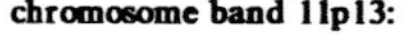

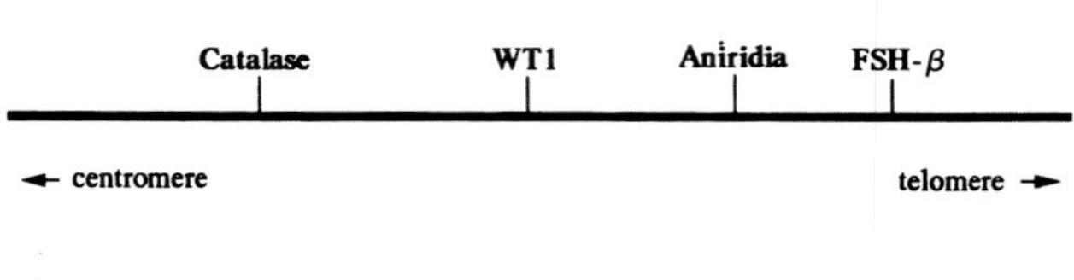

Fig. 38-4 Schematic map of the WAGR region. The 11p13 chromosomal deletion in children with WAGR syndrome is flanked on the centromeric side by the gene encoding catalase and on the telomeric side by the gene for the β subunit of follicle-stimulating hormone. Within the deletion are located the Wilms tumor susceptibility gene *WT1* and the anirida gene.

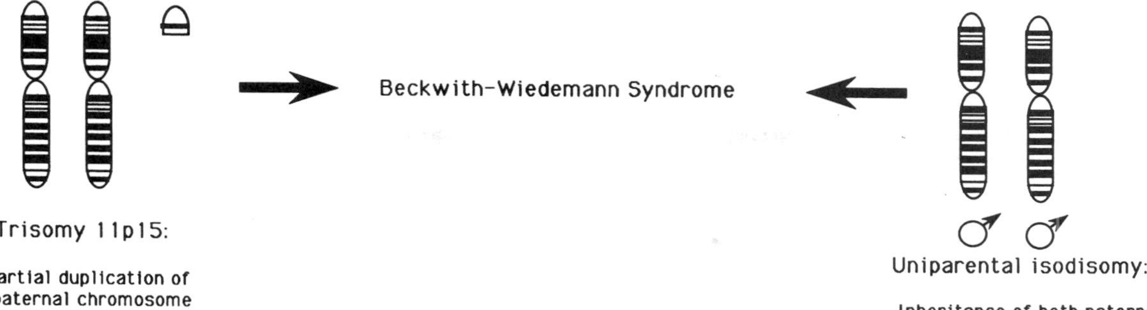

Fig. 38-5 Genetic mechanisms underlying Beckwith-Wiedemann syndrome. Beckwith-Wiedemann syndrome (hemihypertrophy, organomegaly, neonatal hypoglycemia, and susceptibility to Wilms tumor, adrenocortical carcinoma, and hepatoblastoma) can be inherited and has been linked to chromosome 11p15 by studies of large pedigrees. In sporadic cases, gross chromosome abnormalities in the germ line of affected children also have implicated chromosome 11p15 and have suggested that genomic imprinting may play a role in the syndrome. In some cases, RFLP analysis has shown that affected children have inherited two copies of the paternal chromosomes 11 and neither of the maternal chromosomes 11.[57,58] In other cases, a partial duplication of the paternal 11p15 chromosomal fragment results in trisomy for this genetic locus.[52] These observations are consistent with a mechanism whereby the maternal allele is silent or "imprinted" and the syndrome results from the increased gene dosage caused by the presence of two paternal alleles.

chromosome band 11p15, although in two cases a ring chromosome has been reported.[55] The role of genetic imprinting in Beckwith-Wiedemann syndrome is suggested by a number of unusual observations. In the familial syndrome, the disease appears to be more severe when the affected chromosome is transmitted by the mother rather than the father.[56] In contrast, in cases where trisomy for 11p15 is present, the duplicated chromosome is invariably of paternal origin.[57] Finally, molecular studies have shown that in some cases of Beckwith-Wiedemann syndrome, affected children are diploid for 11p15 but have inherited two copies of the paternal chromosome and no maternal chromosome — so-called uniparental isodisomy.[58,59] One possible explanation for these unusual genetic abnormalities may be that they can lead to differences in the dosage of a critically regulated gene (Fig. 38-5). If such a gene were imprinted and expressed only from the paternal allele, duplication of the paternal chromosome, either in the form of uniparental isodisomy or partial 11p15 trisomy, would then lead to a twofold overexpression. In familial transmission of Beckwith-Wiedemann syndrome, a mutation resulting in increased expression of this gene would be expected to have a greater impact if it arose on the imprinted maternal allele than in the already expressed paternal allele.

The Wilms tumor gene at the 11p15 locus remains to be identified, but a number of candidate genes are of particular interest. The insulin-like growth factor II (*IGFII*) gene encodes an embryonic growth factor whose expression in most tissues is derived solely from the paternally derived allele. Inactivation of one allele of *IGFII* in the mouse germ line results in small-sized offspring if the disrupted gene is transmitted by the father but has no effect if transmitted by the mother.[60,61] Thus the organomegaly associated with Beckwith-Wiedemann syndrome could be attributed to the doubling of IGFII expression levels caused by duplication of the actively transcribed paternal allele.[62,63] The potential role of *IGFII* in Beckwith-Wiedemann syndrome is supported by the observation that some affected children show constitutional loss of imprinting of this gene (i.e., expression from both alleles), without evidence of gross chromosomal alterations.[64,65] Furthermore, sporadic Wilms tumors have high expression of IGFII,[66,67] and some tumors also show loss or relaxation of imprinting,[68,69] suggesting that this growth factor also may contribute directly to tumorigenesis. However, two other candidate genes at chromosome 11p15 have been reported recently. The cyclin-dependent kinase inhibitor *p57* is also imprinted,[70] and inactivating mutations in the expressed paternal allele have been detected in the germ line of two children with Beckwith-Wiedemann syndrome.[71] These observations suggest that the overgrowth syndrome may result from loss of growth inhibition by p57, although additional genetic events would presumably be required to explain the chromosomal evidence for increased paternal gene copy number. A third gene at chromosome 11p15, *H19,* also has been implicated in Wilms tumorigenesis. *H19* encodes an abundant transcript lacking an open reading frame, suggesting that it functions as RNA.[72] Transfection studies have shown that it suppresses tumor formation in nude mice without affecting *in vitro* growth properties.[73] Of particular interest is the observation that *H19* and *IGFII* share regulatory sequences, with a reciprocal pattern of imprinting. Thus *H19* is expressed from the maternally derived allele,[72] and expression would be lost in children who inherit two copies of the paternally derived chromosome 11.

The association between the 11p15 chromosomal locus and Wilms tumor is supported by the increased incidence of this tumor in children with Beckwith-Wiedemann syndrome. However, molecular genetic analyses of Wilms tumor specimens have demonstrated allelic losses that affect 11p15 but spare the 11p13 genetic locus.[43,45] These allelic losses are usually indicative of gene deletion or loss-of-function events, which are difficult to reconcile with the apparent increased gene dosage mechanism commonly invoked for Beckwith-Wiedemann syndrome. It is therefore possible that the 11p15 Beckwith-Wiedemann and Wilms tumor locus contains multiple genes, disrupted by different genetic mechanisms. Molecular studies also have suggested that both the 11p13 and 11p15 Wilms tumor genes can contribute to tumorigenesis within the same tumor, based on cases in which distinct allelic losses are seen at both of these loci.[45,74] Unlike the *WT1* gene isolated from the Wilms tumor locus on chromosome 11p13, which appears to be specifically involved in kidney development and tumorigenesis (see below), the putative gene(s) residing at chromosome locus 11p15 has been linked to a number of different tumor types. In addition to adrenocortical carcinoma, Wilms tumor, and hepatoblastoma that are associated with Beckwith-Wiedemann syndrome, somatic allelic losses at 11p15 have been reported in breast cancer, lung cancer, and acute myelogenous leukemia.[75,76]

Familial Wilms Tumor

Familial transmission of susceptibility to Wilms tumor is rare, estimated at less than 1 percent of cases.[14,25] Thus the majority of children with evidence of genetic susceptibility appear to have *de novo* germ-line mutations. The 11p13 Wilms tumor gene *WT1* has been implicated in a few familial cases of children with bilateral tumors or genitourinary defects.[8,9] However, in three large

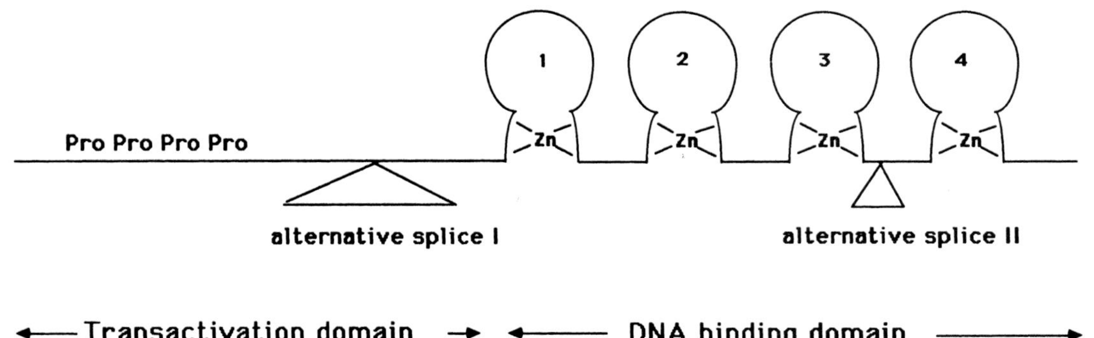

Fig. 38-6 Functional domains of the *WT1* gene product. The predicted polypeptide encoded by *WT1* contains two functional domains: The C-terminus contains four "zinc fingers" of the cysteine-histidine class, which constitute the DNA-binding domain of *WT1*. This domain has a high degree of homology with that of the early growth response gene 1 (EGR1), and it confers a similar DNA-binding specificity. The N-terminus of *WT1* is rich in prolines (Pro) and constitutes the transactivation domain of *WT1*. This domain appears to be capable of suppressing the transcription of genes that are potential targets of WT1. Two alternative splices are variably inserted in the *WT1* transcript, resulting in the presence of four distinct mRNA species. The function of alternative splice I is unknown, while insertion of alternative splice II disrupts the linker between zinc fingers 3 and 4 and alters the DNA-binding specificity of the encoded protein.

pedigrees of familial Wilms tumor, genetic linkage analysis has excluded chromosome 11.[77–79] Recently, analysis of a Canadian Wilms tumor kindred, remarkable for the relatively late onset of tumors and the absence of associated genitourinary defects, has indicated genetic linkage to chromosome 17q12-22.[80]

THE *WT1* GENE AT CHROMOSOME 11p13

Identification and Characterization of *WT1*

The isolation of the 11p13 Wilms tumor gene resulted from the analysis of patients with chromosomal deletions and translocations as well as the generation of human-hamster cell hybrids containing defined segments of chromosome 11p13.[81–86] These studies provided detailed maps of the WAGR region within chromosome 11p13, flanked on the centromeric side by the gene encoding catalase[87,88] and on the telomeric side by the gene for the β subunit of follicle-stimulating hormone[89–92] (see Fig. 38-4). The *WT1* gene was isolated within the smallest region of overlap among chromosomal deletions.[93,94]

WT1 encodes a protein migrating at 55 kDa, with two regions of recognizable homology that indicate it functions as a transcription factor (Fig. 38-6). The C-terminus contains four *zinc-finger domains,* loop structures of amino acids that each contain two regularly spaced cysteines and histidines, bind to zinc ions, and mediate recognition of a specific DNA sequence.[95] The N-terminus of *WT1* is rich in prolines and glutamines, a feature shared by the transactivation domains of some transcription factors.[96] Two alternative splices are present within the *WT1* transcript, resulting in four distinct mRNA species that are expressed in constant proportion to each other.[97] Alternative splice I, inserted within the N-terminus of *WT1,* encodes 17 amino acids including five serines and one threonine, potential sites for protein phosphorylation. Alternative splice II encodes three amino acids (lysine, threonine, serine, or KTS) that disrupt the critical spacing between the third and fourth zinc-finger domains. In the absence of alternative splice II, the *WT1* zinc-finger domains share extensive homology with the early growth response gene (*EGR1,* also known as *NGFIA, Krox 24,* or *Zif 268*)[98] and recognize the *EGR1* DNA-binding consensus sequence.[89] WT1 protein also recognizes a GC-rich sequence,[100,101] and binding-site-selection experiments have identified the sequence 5′-GCGTGGGAGT-3′ as a potential higher-affinity binding site.[102] In transient transfection experiments using promoter reporter constructs, WT1 functions as a repressor of transcription.[103] This effect, combined with the ability of WT1 to bind the GC-rich sequences present in many promoters, has led to the identification of many potential WT1 target genes.[104] These have included *EGR1,*[99] *IGFII,*[105] platelet-derived growth factor-A (*PDGF-A*),[106,107] IGF receptor,[108,109] epidermal growth factor receptor (*EGFR*),[101] c-*myc*, *bcl2,*[110] retinoic acid receptor α,[111] *Pax2,*[112] and transforming growth factor β[113] among many others. However, with the possible exception of *EGFR,*[101] *IGFII,*[114] and *IGFR,*[109] none of these WT1-regulated promoters are correlated with regulation of endogenous genes by WT1. Thus a level of target specificity may be evident with native promoters that is not observed in transient transfection assays. Interpretation of transient transfection experiments is further confounded by evidence that WT1 can function as an activator as well as a repressor of transcription, depending on cellular and promoter context and even on the choice of expression vector.[115–117]

Insertion of alternative splice II (KTS) abolishes binding of WT1 to the GC-rich promoters.[99] An alternative DNA-binding sequence has been proposed,[118] but no potential targets have been identified. The WT1(+KTS) isoform accounts for 80 percent of the cellular WT1 transcript,[97] suggesting that it makes an important contribution to the function of this tumor suppressor. Recently, WT1(+KTS) has been shown to associate with subnuclear clusters, in contrast to WT1(−KTS), which is diffusely localized in the nucleus.[119,120] Colocalization and coimmunoprecipitation studies have suggested that WT1(+KTS) is associated with small nucleoriboproteins (snRNPs), implying a potential role in pre-mRNA splicing.[119] However, the subnuclear clusters containing WT1(+KTS) are distinct from interchromatin granules containing the essential splicing factor SC35, which are thought to constitute assembly sites for the cellular splicing machinery.[120] Thus the identity of WT1-associated subnuclear clusters is uncertain, and the relationship between WT1 and the pre-mRNA splicing machinery remains to be defined. In addition to alternative splicing, WT1 is phosphorylated *in vivo*, although the physiologic consequences of this protein modification are unknown.[121]

Expression of WT1 during Kidney Development

WT1 is normally expressed in a small number of tissues, primarily those of the developing genitourinary tract.[122,123] This expression pattern is in marked contrast to the ubiquitously expressed tumor suppressor genes *RB* and *p53* and may provide insight into the normal role of WT1 in cellular growth and differentiation. In the mouse kidney, WT1 expression is detectable by day 8 of gestation, rising to peak sharply around birth and then rapidly declining to low adult levels by day 17.[123] In humans, WT1 expression has been reported to be high in 20-week kidney and barely detectable in the adult organ.[74] Within the developing kidney, specific structures have been shown by *in situ* RNA hybridization to express WT1, including the condensed mesenchyme, renal vesicle,

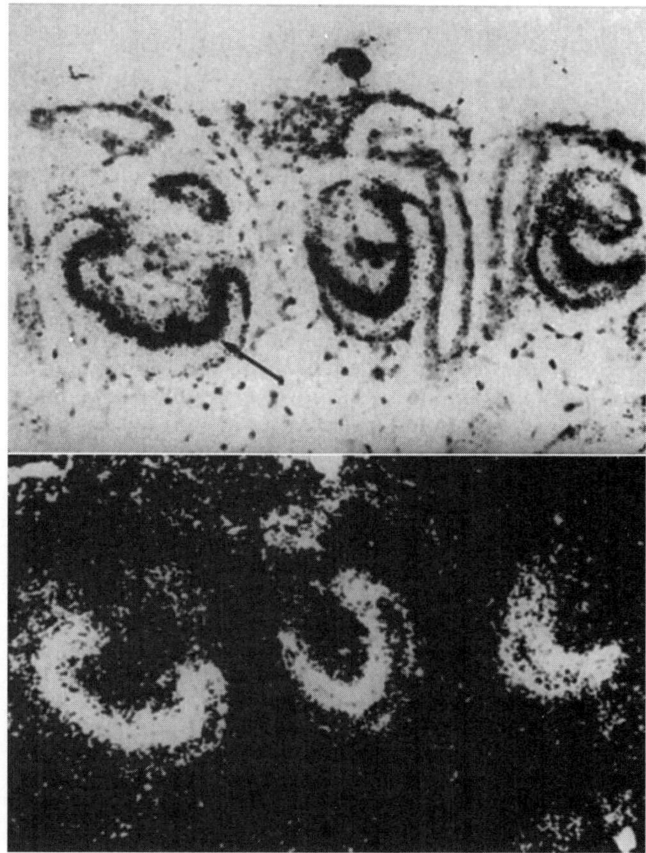

Fig. 38-7 Localization of *WT1* mRNA expression in the developing kidney. Analysis of 20-week human kidney by *in situ* hybridization with the *WT1* probe. Light phase (*upper panel*) and dark phase (*lower panel*) photomicrographs are shown to demonstrate the hybridization signal and the structures within the developing kidney that express *WT1* mRNA. The "S-shaped body" is a precursor of the renal glomerulus, whose inner surface demonstrates high levels of *WT1* mRNA expression (arrow). (*Photomicrograph kindly provided by Dr. Nic Hastie, Medical Research Council, Edinburgh, UK.*)

and glomerular epithelium[122] (Fig. 38-7). The transient expression pattern of WT1 in these early kidney structures is consistent with a gene that is critical during a defined period in normal kidney development (Fig. 38-8). Disruption of this gene by a mutation thus may lead to uncontrolled proliferation of the early renal progenitor cells that are characteristic of Wilms tumor.

WT1 is also expressed in other specific cell types, such as the Sertoli cells of the testis, granulosa cells of the ovary, muscle cells of the uterus, stromal cells of the spleen, and mesothelial cells of the pericardial, pleural, and peritoneal lining.[124–126] The WT1 pattern of expression in these tissues differs from that seen in the kidney, with persistent high levels of expression in adult organs. Expression of WT1 is also noted in acute leukemia cells, although the normal hematopoietic counterparts that express WT1 have not been identified. In addition to Wilms tumors, *WT1* mutations have been reported in mesothelioma and leukemia.[126,127] However, with the exception of one case of gonadoblastoma,[128] individuals with a germ-line *WT1* mutation do not have an increased incidence of tumors from tissues other than kidney. This suggests that the role played by WT1 in these tissues is not rate-limiting for tumorigenesis, as it appears to be in the kidney.[28]

Inactivation of *WT1* in the Germ Line and in Wilms Tumors

Germ-line mutations in one *WT1* allele have been documented in children with bilateral Wilms tumors, consistent with the predictions of Knudson and Strong.[8,9] The germ-line mutation results either from a *de novo* event or, rarely, from familial transmission. Tumor specimens from these children confirm loss of the remaining wild-type *WT1* allele, evidence of the "second hit." However, unlike retinoblastoma, in which the initial germ-line mutation is phenotypically silent, a heterozygous *WT1* mutation in the germ line may result in dramatic developmental abnormalities. Mutations that result in a premature termination result in a phenotype that is similar to that of WAGR patients, bearing a hemizygous deletion of *WT1*.[9] This consists of variable severity of genitourinary abnormalities (undescended testes, abnormal urethral meatus, malformed kidneys) that are more severe in boys than in girls. This observation suggests that *WT1* itself is the gene responsible for the genitourinary defects seen in children with WAGR syndrome. However, children with specific germ-line mutations that affect the *WT1* DNA-binding domains

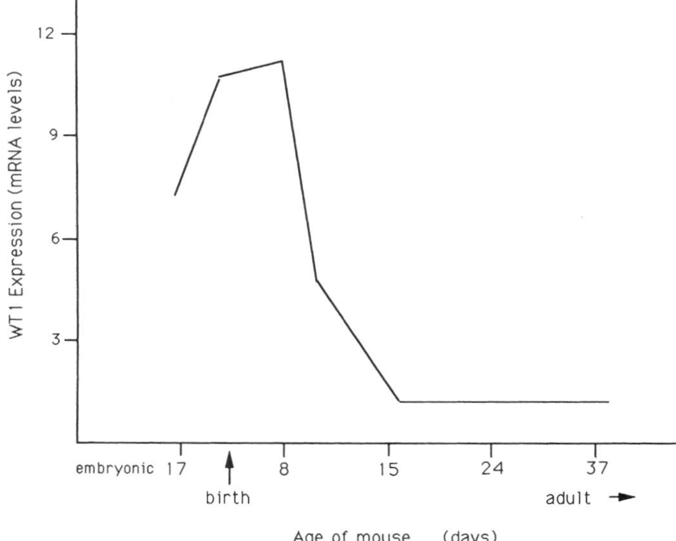

Fig. 38-8 Time course of *WT1* expression in the mouse kidney. Schematic representation of *WT1* mRNA levels in the mouse kidney assayed by Northern blot. *WT1* expression is detectable at the earliest embryonic time point, peaks about the time of birth, and then rapidly declines to adult levels.[95] In human kidney, *WT1* is expressed at high levels at 20 weeks and is no longer detectable in the adult organ.[66,94] Other tissues with high *WT1* mRNA levels, such as the gonads, do not show this dramatic pattern of expression. Instead, *WT1* expression increases during fetal development and remains high in the adult tissue.[96]

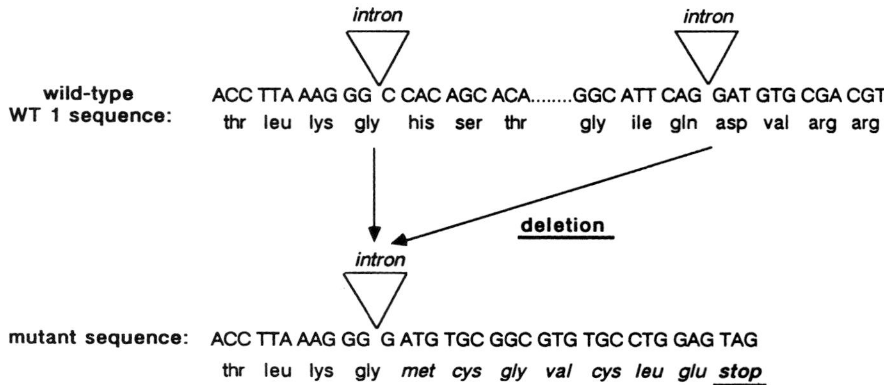

Fig. 38-9 Presence of inactivating mutations within the *WT1* transcript. A subset of Wilms tumors contain inactivated copies of *WT1*, consistent with its characterization as a tumor suppressor gene. Gross deletions of *WT1* appear to be rare, but small internal deletions or mutations can be found by nucleotide sequence analysis using the polymerase chain reaction (PCR). In this example,[7] a fragment of genomic DNA encoding an entire exon (flanked by two introns) has been deleted. The *WT1* transcript in this Wilms tumor is the product of abnormal splicing, joining together the exons on either side of the deletion. The abnormal splice junction results in a frameshift, leading to seven novel amino acids (italics) followed by premature chain termination caused by a stop codon.

develop a far more severe constellation of genitourinary abnormalities known as *Denys-Drash syndrome*.[128] These children have gross abnormalities of sexual development, resulting in pseudohermaphroditism and mesangial sclerosis of the kidney, leading to renal failure within the first years of life. These observations suggest that expression of WT1 proteins with altered DNA-binding domains can exert a "dominant negative" effect that disrupts normal genitourinary development to a far greater extent than simple reduction in gene dosage seen in WAGR syndrome.

Most Wilms tumors express high levels of *WT1* mRNA and protein, consistent with their apparent cells of origin in the fetal kidney. By *in situ* RNA hybridization, *WT1* expression has been localized to the epithelial and blastemal histologic components within the tumor.[122] While in most Wilms tumors the *WT1* transcript appears to be grossly intact, in 10 percent of patients deletions and point mutations within the gene have been identified[74,129–133] (Fig. 38-9). These mutations identify *WT1* as the target of gene inactivation events at the chromosome 11p13 locus and confirm its characterization as a tumor-suppressor gene. The majority of *WT1* mutations reported in Wilms tumors are homozygous, resulting from an initial point mutation in one allele and followed by loss of the second allele through a gross chromosomal event. However, some tumors have been found to express a single mutated *WT1* allele, along with the remaining wild-type allele.[74,131] These observations have suggested that specific types of mutations, particularly those involving the DNA-binding domain of *WT1*, may act as "dominant negative" mutations, in effect suppressing the function of the coexpressed wild-type allele.[134,135] A potential mechanism of action for such dominant negative mutations has been defined *in vitro*. WT1 dimerizes through the N-terminal domain, and mutants with an altered DNA-binding domain abrogate the transactivational properties of wild-type WT1.[120,136,137] These mutants physically associate with subnuclear clusters and recruit transcriptionally active WT1(−KTS), in effect achieving an apparent intranuclear sequestration of the wild-type protein.[120]

In addition to mutational inactivation, unusual mechanisms of disrupting WT1 function contribute to Wilms tumor. An in-frame deletion of *WT1* exon 2, within the transactivation domain, is observed in 10 percent of primary Wilms tumor specimens.[138] This splicing abnormality is not associated with a mutation in flanking exon-intron junctions, but it is observed together with omission of alternative splice II (WT1 exon 5), suggesting a gene-specific abnormality in pre-mRNA processing. The encoded protein, WT1-del2, is a potent transcriptional activator, capable of antagonizing transcriptional repression of promoter reporters by wild-type WT1.[138] Another unusual disruption of *WT1* occurs in a rare pediatric sarcoma, desmoplastic small round cell tumor (DSRT), which is characterized by a chromosomal translocation fusing the potent transactivation domain of the Ewing sarcoma gene *EWS* to zinc fingers 2 to 4 of *WT1*.[139,140] These two transactivating variants of *WT1*, together with two Wilms tumor-associated point mutations that also convert *WT1* into a potent transactivator,[126,141] provide strong genetic evidence for the physiologic importance of transcriptional repression by wild-type WT1. They also raise the possibility that specific target genes might be repressed by wild-type WT1 and induced by these transforming WT1 variants.

In addition to abnormalities in pre-mRNA splicing, RNA editing has been reported in WT1.[142] The altered amino acid, within the transactivation domain of *WT1*, appears to result in a subtle change in transactivational activity. The RNA-edited *WT1* transcripts constitute a fraction of the mRNA in rat kidney, but their role in Wilms tumor development is unknown.

Inactivation of *WT1* in the Mouse and Animal Models of Wilms Tumor

WT1 is highly conserved in the mouse, both in terms of nucleotide conservation and pattern of tissue and developmental expression.[123] However, the genetic consequences of *WT1* inactivation differ between human and mouse, particularly with respect to tumorigenesis. The small eye mouse mutation[143,144] is homologous to the aniridia phenotype in humans and involves the *Pax6* gene on mouse chromosome 2, which is syntenic with human chromosome band 11p13. One variant of the mouse mutation, so-called *Sey/Dey*, includes small eyes, a small body size, and a white belly patch. The *Sey/Dey* mutation results from a hemizygous chromosomal deletion analogous to the WAGR deletion in humans, including hemizygosity for the mouse *WT1* gene.[123,145] Homozygosity for the *Sey/Dey* allele is an embryonic lethal, but heterozygous mice have no detectable abnormalities of genitourinary development, nor do they appear to have an increased risk of renal tumors. These observations have been confirmed in *WT1*-hemizygous mice generated by homologous recombination.[146] This apparent discrepancy between the effect of hemizygosity for *WT1* in mouse and humans raises a number of interesting questions. *WT1* pathways in the mouse may involve greater functional redundancy or genetic safeguards than in humans, conferring protection against malignant transformation in a somatic kidney cell following loss of the remaining wild-type allele. Alternatively, the small number of target cells in the mouse kidney may reduce the probability of the second genetic hit. Finally, an intriguing genetic observation is that the two Wilms tumor loci that share the short arm of human chromosome 11 are separated in the mouse, with 11p13 syntenic with mouse chromosome 2, while 11p15 maps to mouse chromosome 7.[145] Thus, whereas a single chromosomal recombinational event is sufficient to cause loss of both genes in humans, two separate genetic events would be required in the mouse. While the mouse appears to be a reluctant Wilms tumor model, nephroblastomas do arise in the rat. The best studied models are nephroblastomas that arise either spontaneously or following transplacental treatment with the chemical carcinogen *N*-ethylnitrosourea or x-irradiation.[147–149] Point mutations in *WT1* have been observed in some rat nephroblastomas,[150] implying that its inactivation contributes to tumorigenesis.

In contrast to the *WT1*-hemizygous mice, homozygous inactivation of *WT1* has profound developmental consequences. *WT1*-null mice die at embryonic day 11.[146] The precise cause of death is uncertain, but gross cardiac and diaphragmatic defects appear to be implicated. WT1 is expressed in the mesothelial lining of these organs,[125,126] suggesting a potential developmental role. Of particular interest, *WT1*-null mice fail to develop either kidneys or gonads. Developmental arrest in the gonads precedes the sexually undifferentiated stage, implicating WT1 in a very early step in gonadogenesis. The arrest in kidney differentiation precedes the induction of mesoderm by the ureteric bud, and mesenchymal tissue from *WT1*-null mice is resistant to exogenous induction signals.[146] Histologic analysis of nephrogenic tissue from *WT1*-null mice reveals widespread apoptosis of blastemal stem cells. The role of WT1 in kidney development thus appears to involve a survival and potentially a permissive function for differentiating stem cells. The stage of peak WT1 expression that accompanies the differentiation of glomeruli is not reached in *WT1*-null mice, consistent with a developmental arrest at the first developmental stage requiring WT1 expression.

Functional Properties of WT1

Reconstitution of WT1 function in models of kidney differentiation remains to be achieved. However, a number of different functional properties are evident in cultured cell lines. Stable transfection of wild-type WT1 into a Wilms tumor cell line results in growth inhibition.[138] Inducible expression of the WT1(−KTS) isoform triggers apoptosis in osteosarcoma cell lines.[101] This effect is associated with transcriptional repression of the epidermal growth factor receptor (EGFR) and inhibition of endogenous EGFR synthesis, and it is abrogated by constitutive expression of EGFR. Thus, in these cells, inhibition of a growth factor pathway contributes to WT1-mediated cell death. Unlike other transcription factors whose overexpression triggers apoptosis, the ability of WT1 to induce cell death is independent of p53, indicating that it is not the result of conflicting growth-regulating signals but rather a direct effect of WT1.[101] Expression of high levels of WT1 also leads to G1 phase cell cycle arrest.[151] This effect is associated with induction of the cyclin-dependent kinase inhibitor p21, and it is also independent of p53, another tumor suppressor known to induce p21 expression.[152] Increased p21 mRNA expression rapidly follows the inducible expression of WT1 protein, but direct regulation of the p21 promoter by WT1 has not been demonstrated. As in other developmental pathways, the combination of apoptotic signals and p21 induction may contribute to cellular differentiation.[153,154]

In addition to its growth inhibiting properties, WT1 also demonstrates the ability to inhibit apoptosis, specifically that mediated by p53.[155] WT1 and p53 proteins are coimmunoprecipitated from Wilms tumor specimens and developing rat kidney, and expression of WT1 leads to stabilization of wild-type p53 and modulation of its transactivational properties,[116,155] in addition to inhibition of apoptosis. Inhibition of p53-mediated cell death is observed in cells expressing low levels of WT1, consistent with the antiapoptotic role of WT1 in renal stem cells that has been postulated by analysis of *WT1*-null mice. The ability of WT1 to stabilize and partially inactivate p53 is of particular interest, given that the majority of sporadic Wilms tumors contain wild-type WT1 and express high steady-state levels of wild-type p53,[156,157] unlike many tumor types in which p53 is stabilized by inactivating mutations. Mutational inactivation of p53 in Wilms tumor is associated with the rare anaplastic variant,[158] which displays resistance to chemotherapy and an adverse prognosis.

Concluding Remarks

Wilms tumor is a genetically complex embryonic tumor whose histologic appearance is consistent with arrested differentiation of renal stem cells. The identification of the first Wilms tumor suppressor gene, *WT1,* has revealed a transcriptional regulator that is required for early kidney differentiation but whose inactivation, presumably at a later stage of kidney development, results in Wilms tumor. Further characterization of this gene and isolation of additional Wilms tumor genes will provide greater understanding of the link between normal differentiation in the kidney and malignant transformation.

REFERENCES

1. Bennington J, Beckwith J: Tumors of the kidney, renal pelvis and ureter, in *Atlas of Tumor Pathology,* series 2, fascile 12. Washington, DC, Armed Forces Institute of Pathology, 1975.
2. Breslow N, Churchill F, Nesmith B, Thomas P, Beckwith J, Othersen H, D'Angio G: Clinicopathologic features and prognosis for Wilms' tumor patients with metastases at dignosis. *Cancer* **58:**2501, 1986.
3. Coppes M, Wilson P, Weitzman S: Extrarenal Wilms' tumor: Staging, treatment and prognosis. *J Clin Oncol* **9:**167, 1991.
4. Bove K, McAdams A: The nephroblastomatosis complex and its relationship to Wilms' tumor: a clinicopathologic treatise. *Perspect Pediatr Pathol* **3:**185, 1976.
5. Beckwith J, Kiviat N, Bonadio J: Nephrogenic rests, nephroblastomatosis, and the pathogenesis of Wilms' tumor. *Pediatr Pathol* **10:**1, 1989.
6. Park S, Bernard A, Bove K, Sens D, Hazen-Martin D, Garvin A, Haber D: Inactivation of WT1 in nephrogenic rests, genetic precursors to Wilms' tumour. *Nature Genet* **5:**363, 1993.
7. National Wilms Tumor Study Committee: Wilms' tumor: Status report, 1990. *J Clin Oncol* **9:**877, 1990.
8. Huff V, Miwa H, Haber D, Call K, Housman D, Strong L, Saunders G: Evidence for WT1 as a Wilms tumor (WT) gene: Intragenic germinal deletion in bilateral WT. *Am J Hum Genet* **48:**997, 1991.
9. Pelletier J, Bruening W, Li F, Haber D, Glaser T, Housman D: WT1 mutations contribute to abnormal genital system development and hereditary Wilms' tumour. *Nature* **353:**431, 1991.
10. Grundy P, Breslow N, Green D, Sharples K, Evans A, D'Angio G: Prognostic factors for children with recurrent Wilms' tumor: Results from the second and third National Wilms' Tumor Study. *J Clin Oncol* **7:**638, 1989.
11. Bryd R, Levine A: Late treatment of Wilms' tumor, in Pochedly C, Baum ES (eds): *Clinical and Biological Manifestations*, vol 19. New York, Elsevier, 1984, p 347.
12. Li F, Gimbrere K, Gelber R, Sallan S, Flamant F, Green D, Heyn R, Meadows A: Outcome of pregnancy in survivors of Wilms' tumor. *JAMA* **257:**216, 1987.
13. Knudson A: Mutation and cancer: Statistical study of retinoblastoma. *Proc Natl Acad Sci USA* **68:**820, 1971.
14. Knudson A, Strong L: Mutation and cancer: A model for Wilms tumor of the kidney. *J Natl Cancer Inst* **48:**313, 1972.
15. Knudson A, Strong L: Mutation and cancer: Neuroblastoma and pheochromocytoma. *Am J Hum Genet* **24:**514, 1972.
16. Friend S, Bernards R, Rogelj S, Weinberg R, Rapaport J, Albert D, Dryja T: A human DNA segment with properties of the gene that predisposes to retinoblastoma and osteosarcoma. *Nature* **323:**643, 1986.
17. Lee W, Bookstein R, Hong F, Young L, Shew J, Lee E: Human retinoblastoma susceptibility gene: Cloning, identification, and sequence. *Science* **235:**1394, 1987.
18. Fung Y, Murphree A, T'Ang A, Ouian J, Hinrichs S, Benedict W: Structural evidence for the authenticity of the retinoblastoma tumor susceptibility gene. *Science* **236:**1657, 1987.
19. Comings D: A general theory of carcinogenesis. *Proc Natl Acad Sci USA* **70:**3324, 1973.
20. Knudson A: Hereditary cancer, oncogenes, and antioncogenes. *Cancer Res* **45:**1437, 1985.

21. Dunn J, Philips R, Becker A, Gallie B: Identification of germline and somatic mutations affecting the retinoblastoma gene. *Science* **241:**1797, 1988.
22. Yandell D, Campbell T, Dayton S, Petersen R, Walton D, Little J, McConkie-Rosell A, Buckley E, Dryja T: Oncogenic point mutations in the human retinoblastoma gene: Their application to genetic counselling. *N Engl J Med* **321:**1689, 1989.
23. Cavenee W, Dryja T, Phillips R, Benedict W, Godbout R, Gallie B, Murphree A, Strong L, White R: Expression of recessive alleles by chromosomal mechanisms in retinoblastoma. *Nature* **305:**779, 1983.
24. Matsunaga E: Genetics of Wilms' tumor. *Hum Genet* **57:**231, 1981.
25. Cochran W, Froggatt P: Bjilateral nephroblastoma in two sisters. *J Urol* **97:**216, 1967.
26. Pendergrass T: Congenital anomalies in children with Wilms' tumor, a new survey. *Cancer* **37:**403, 1976.
27. Breslow N, Beckwith J: Epidemiological features of Wilms' tumor: Results of the National Wilms' Tumor Study. *J Natl Cancer Inst* **68:**429, 1982.
28. Haber D, Housman D: Rate-limiting steps: The genetics of pediatric cancers. *Cell* **64:**5, 1991.
29. Miller R, Fraumeni J, Manning M: Association of Wilms' tumor with aniridia, hemihypertrophy and other congenital malformations. *N Engl J Med* **270:**922, 1964.
30. Riccardi V, Sujansky E, Smith A, Francke U: Chromosomal imbalance in the aniridia-Wilms' tumor association: 11p interstitial deletion. *Pediatrics* **61:**604, 1978.
31. Francke U, Holmes L, Atkins L, Riccardi V: Aniridia-Wilms' tumor association: Evidence for specific deletion of 11p13. *Cytogenet Cell Genet* **24:**185, 1979.
32. Simola K, Knuutila S, Kaitila I, Pirkola A, Pohja P: Familial aniridia and translocation t(4;11)(q22;p13) without Wilms' tumor. *Hum Genet* **63:**158, 1983.
33. Moore J, Hyman S, Antonarakis S, Mules E, Thomas F: Familial isolated aniridia associated with a translocation involving chromosomes 11 and 22 [t(11;22)(p13;q12.20)]. *Hum Genet* **72:**297, 1986.
34. Ton C, Hirronen M, Miwa H, Weil M, Monaghan P, Jordan T, van Heyningen V, Hastie N, Meigers-Heijboer H, Drechsler M, Royer-Pokora B, Collins F, Swaroop A, Strong LC, Saunders GF: Positional cloning and characterization of a paired box- and homeobox-containing gene from the aniridia region. *Cell* **67:**1059, 1991.
35. Kondo K, Chilcote R, Maurer H, Rowley J: Chromosome abnormalities in tumor cells from patients with sporadic Wilms' tumor. *Cancer Res* **44:**5376, 1984.
36. Douglass E, Wilimas J, Green A, Look A: Abnormalities of chromosomes 1 and 11 in Wilms' tumor. *Cancer Genet Cytogenet* **14:**331, 1985.
37. Solis V, Pritchard J, Cowell J: Cytogenetic changes in Wilms' tumors. *Cancer Genet Cytogenet* **34:**223, 1988.
38. Wang-Wuu S, Soukup S, Bove K, Gotwals B, Lampkin B: Chromosome analysis of 31 Wilms tumors. *Cancer Res* **50:**2786, 1990.
39. Fearon E, Vogelstein B, Feinberg A: Somatic deletion and duplication of genes on chromosome 11 in Wilms' tumours. *Nature* **309:**176, 1984.
40. Koufos A, Hansen M, Lampkin B, Workman M, Copeland N, Jenkins N, Cavenee W: Loss of alleles at loci on human chromosome 11 during genesis of Wilms' tumour. *Nature* **309:**170, 1984.
41. Orkin S, Goldman D, Sallan S: Development of homozygosity for chromosome 11p markers in Wilms' tumour. *Nature* **309:**172, 1984.
42. Reeve A, Housiaux P, Gardner R, Chewing W, Grindley R, Millow L: Loss of a Harvey ras allele in sporadic Wilms' tumour. *Nature* **309:**174, 1984.
43. Mannens M, Slater R, Heyting C, Bliek J, Kraker JD, Coad N, Pagter-Holthuizen P, Pearson P: Molecular nature of genetic changes resulting in loss of heterozygosity for chromosome 11 in Wilms' tumor. *Hum Genet* **81:**41, 1988.
44. Glaser T, Jones C, Douglass E, Housman D: Constitutional and somatic mutations of chromosome 11p in Wilms' tumor. Cold Spring Harbor Lab, Cold Spring Harbor, New York, pp. 253–277, 1989.
45. Henry I, Jeanpierre M, Couillin P, Barichard F, Serre J, Journel H, Lamouroux A, Turleau C, Grouchy J, Junien C: Molecular definition of the 11p15.5 region involved in Beckwith-Wiedemann syndrome and probably in predisposition to adrenocortical carcinoma. *Hum Genet* **81:**273, 1989.
46. Reeve A, Sih S, Raizis A, Feinberg A: Loss of allelic heterozygosity at a second locus on chromosome 11 in sporadic Wilms' tumor cells. *Mol Cell Biol* **9:**1799, 1989.
47. Wiedemann H: Complexe malformatif familial avec hernie ombilicale et macroglossie — Un syndrome nouveau? *J Genet Hum* **13:**223, 1964.
48. Beckwith J: Macroglossia, omphalocele, adrenal cytomegaly, gigantism and hyperplastic visceromegaly. *Birth Defects* **5:**188, 1969.
49. Sotelo-Avila C, Gonzalez-Crussi F, Fowler J: Complete and incomplete forms of Beckwith-Wiedemann syndrome: Their oncogenic potential. *J Pediatr* **96:**47, 1980.
50. Wiedemann H: Tumor and hemihypertrophy associated with Wiedemann-Beckwith's syndrome. *Eur J Pediatr* **141:**129, 1983.
51. Koufos A, Grundy P, Morgan K, Aleck K, Hadro T, Lampkin B, Kalbakji A, Cavenee W: Familial Wiedemann-Beckwith syndrome and a second Wilms' tumor locus both map to 11p15.5. *Am J Hum Genet* **44:**711, 1989.
52. Ping J, Reeve A, Law D, Young M, Boehnke M, Feinberg A: Genetic linkage of Beckwith-Wiedemann syndrome to 11p15. *Am J Hum Genet* **23:**165, 1989.
53. Waziri M, Patil S, Hanson J, Bartley S: Abnormality of chromosome 11 in patients with features of Beckwith-Wiedemann syndrome. *J Pediatr* **102:**873, 1983.
54. Turleau C, Grouchy J, Nihoul-Fekete C, Chavin-Colin F, Junien C: Del 11p13/nephroblastoma without aniridia. *Hum Genet* **67:**455, 1984.
55. Romain D, Gebbie O, Parfitt R, Columbano-Green L, Smythe R, Chapman C, Kerr A: Two cases of ring chromosome 11. *J Med Genet* **20:**380, 1983.
56. Niikawa N, Ishikiriyama S, Takahashi S, Inagawa A, Tonoki H, Ohta Y, Hase N, Kamei T, Kajii T: The Wiedemann-Beckwith syndrome: Pedigree studies on five families with evidence for autosomal dominant inheritance with variable expressivity. *Am J Med Genet* **24:**41, 1986.
57. Brown K, Williams J, Maitland N, Mott M: Genomic imprinting and the Beckwith-Wiedemann syndrome. *Am J Hum Genet* **46:**1000, 1990.
58. Henry I, Bonaiti-Pellie C, Chehensse V, Beldjord C, Schwartz C, Utermann G, Junien C: Uniparental paternal disomy in a genetic cancer-predisposing syndrome. *Nature* **351:**665, 1991.
59. Grundy P, Telzerow P, Haber D, Li F, Paterson M, Garber J: Chromosome 11 uniparental isodisomy in a child with hemihypertrophy and embryonal neoplasms. *Lancet* **338**: 1079, 1992.
60. DeChiara T, Efstradiadis A, Robertson E: A growth-deficiency phenotype in heterozygous mice carrying an insulin-like growth factor II gene disrupted by targeting. *Nature* **345:**78, 1990.
61. DeChiara T, Roberson E, Efstradiatis A: Parental imprinting of the mouse insulin-like growth factor II gene. *Cell* **64:**849, 1991.
62. Giannoukakis N, Deal C, Paquette J, Goodyer C, Polychronakos C: Parental genomic imprinting of the human IGF2 gene. *Nature Genet* **4:**98, 1993.
63. Ohlsson R, Nystrom A, Pfeifer-Ohlsson S, Tohonen V, Hedborg F, Schofield P, Flam F, Ekstrom T: IGF2 is parentally imprinted during human embryogenesis and in the Beckwith-Wiedemann syndrome. *Nature Genet* **4:**94, 1993.
64. Weksberg R, Shen D, Fei Y, Song Q, Squire J: Disruption of insulin-like growth factor 2 imprinting in Beckwith-Wiedemann syndrome. *Nature Genet* **5:**143, 1993.
65. Ogawa O, Becroft D, Morison I, Ecles M, Skeen J, Mauger D, Reeve A: Constitutional relaxation of insulin-like growth factor II gene imprinting associated with Wilms' tumour and gigantism. *Nature Genet* **5:**408, 1993.
66. Reeve A, Eccles M, Wilkins R, Bell G, Millow L: Expression of insulin-like growth factor-II transcripts in Wilms' tumour. *Nature* **317:**258, 1985.
67. Scott J, Cowell J, Roberson M, Priestly L, Wadey R, Hopkins B, Pritchard J, Bell G, Rall L, Graham C, Knott T: Insulin like growth factor-II gene expression in Wilms' tumor and embryonic tissues. *Nature* **317:**260, 1985.
68. Rainier S, Johnson L, Dobry C, Ping A, Grundy P, Feinberg A: Relaxation of imprinted genes in human cancer. *Nature* **362:**747, 1993.
69. Ogawa O, Eccles M, Szeto J, McNoe L, Yun K, Maw M, Smith P, Reeve A: Relaxation of insulin-like growth factor II gene imprinting implicated in Wilms' tumour. *Nature* **362:**749, 1993.
70. Matsuoka S, Thompson J, Edwards M, Barletta J, Grundy P, Kalikin L, Harper J, Elledge S, Feinberg A: Imprinting of the gene encoding a human cyclin-dependent kinase inhibitor, $p57^{KIP2}$, on chromosome 11p15. *Proc Natl Acad Sci USA* **93:**3026, 1996.
71. Hatada I, Ohashi H, Fukushima Y, Kaneko Y, Inoue M, Komoto Y, Okada A, Ohishi S, Nabetani A, Morisaki H, Nakayama M, Niikawa N, Mukai T: An imprinted gene $p57^{KP2}$ is mutated in Beckwith-Wiedemann syndrome. *Nature Genet* **14:**171, 1996.
72. Bartolomei M, Zemel S, Tilghman S: Parental imprinting of the mouse H19 gene. *Nature* **351:**153, 1991.
73. Hao Y, Crenshaw T, Moulton T, Newcomb E, Tycko B: Tumour-suppressor activity of H19 RNA. *Nature* **365:**764, 1993.

74. Haber D, Buckler A, Glaser T, Call K, Pelletier J, Sohn R, Douglass E, Housman D: An internal deletion within an 11p13 zinc finger gene contributes to the development of Wilms' tumor. *Cell* **61:**1257, 1990.
75. Weston A, Willey J, Modali R, Sugimura H, McDowell E, Resau J, Light B, Haugen A, Mann D, Trump B, Harris C: Differential DNA sequence deletions from chromosomes 3, 11, 13, and 17 in squamous-cell carcinoma, large-cell carcinoma and adenocarcinoma of the lung. *Proc Natl Acad Sci USA* **86:**5099, 1989.
76. Ahuja H, Foti A, Zhou D, Cline M: Analysis of proto-oncogenes in acute myeloid leukemia: Loss of heterozygosity for the Ha-ras gene. *Blood* **75:**819, 1990.
77. Huff V, Compton D, Chao L, Strong L, Geiser C, Saunders G: Lack of linkage of familial Wilms' tumour to chromosomal band 11p13. *Nature* **336:**377, 1988.
78. Grundy P, Koufos A, Morgan K, Li F, Meadows A, Cavenee W: Familial predisposition to Wilms' tumour does not map to the short arm of chromosome 11. *Nature* **336:**374, 1988.
79. Schwartz C, Haber D, Stanton V, Strong L, Skolnick M, Housman D: Familial predisposition to Wilms tumor does not segregate with the WT1 gene. *Genomics* **10:**927, 1991.
80. Rahman N, Arbour A, Tonin P, Renshaw J, Pelletier J, Baruchel S, Pritchard-Jones K, Stratton M, Narod S: Evidence for a familial Wilms' tumour gene (FWT1) on chromosome 17q12-21. *Nature Genet* **13:**461, 1996.
81. Glaser T, Jones C, Call K, Lewis W, Bruns G, Junien C, Waziri M, Housman D: Mapping the WAGR region of chromosome 11p: Somatic cell hybrids provide a fine-structure map. *Cytogenet Cell Genet* **46:**620, 1987.
82. Glaser T, Rose E, Morse H, Housman D, Jones C: A panel of irradiation-reduced hybrids selectively retaining human chromosome 11p13: Their structure and use to purify the WAGR gene complex. *Genomics* **6:**48, 1990.
83. Porteous D, Bickmore W, Christie S, Boyd P, Cranston G, Fletcher J, Gosden J, Rout D, Seawright A, Simola K, van Heyningen V, Hastie N: HRAS1 selected chromosome transfer generates markers that colocalize aniridia- and genitourinary dysplasia-associated translocation breakpoints and the Wilms' tumor gene within 11p13. *Proc Natl Acad Sci USA* **84:**5355, 1987.
84. Davis L, Byers M, Fukushima Y, Quin S, Nowak N, Scoggin C, Shows T: Four new DNA markers are assigned to the WAGR region of 11p13: Isolation and regional assignment of 112 chromosome 11 anonymous DNA segments. *Genomics* **3:**264, 1988.
85. Couillin P, Azoulay M, Henry I, Ravise N, Grisard M, Jeanpierre C, Barichard F, Metezeau F, Chandelier J, Lewis W, van Heyningen V, Junien C: Characterization of a panel of somatic cell hybrids for subregional mapping along 11p and within band 11p13. Subdivision of the WAGR complex region. *Hum Genet* **82:**171, 1989.
86. Gessler M, Thomas G, Couillin P, Junien C, McGillvray B, Hayden M, Jaschek G, Bruns G: A deletion map of the WAGR region of chromosome 11. *Am J Hum Genet* **44:**486, 1989.
87. Junien C, Turleau C, Grouchy JD, Said R, Rethore M, Tenconi R, Dufier J: Regional assignment of catalase (CAT) gene to band 11p13: Association with the aniridia-Wilms' tumor-gonadoblastoma (WAGR) complex. *Ann Genet* **23:**165, 1980.
88. van Heyningen V, Boyd P, Seaqright A, Fletcher J, Fantes J, Buckton K, Spowart G, Porteous D, Hill R, Newton M, Hastie N: Molecular analysis of chromosome 11 deletions in aniridia-Wilms' tumor syndrome. *Proc Natl Acad Sci USA* **82:**8592, 1985.
89. Glaser T, Lewis W, Bruns G, Watkins P, Rogler C, Shows T, Powers V, Willard H, Goguen J, Simola K, Housman D: The B-subunit of follicle-stimulating hormone is deleted in patients with aniridia and Wilms' tumour, allowing a further definition of the WAGR locus. *Nature* **321:**882, 1986.
90. Compton D, Weil M, Jones C, Riccardi V, Strong L, Saunders G: Long range physical map of the Wilms' tumor-aniridia region on human chromosome 11. *Cell* **55:**827, 1988.
91. Gessler M, Bruns G: A physical map around the WAGR complex on the short arm of chromosome 11. *Genomics* **5:**43, 1989.
92. Rose E, Glaser T, Jones C, Smith C, Lewis W, Call C, Minden M, Champagne E, Boncetta L, Yeger H, Housman D: Complete physical map of the WAGR region of 11p13 localizes a candidate Wilms' tumor gene. *Cell* **60:**495, 1990.
93. Call K, Glaser T, Ito C, Buckler A, Pelletier J, Haber D, Rose E, Kral A, Yeger H, Lewis W, Jones C, Housman D: Isolation and characterization of a zinc finger polypeptide gene at the human chromosome 11 Wilms' tumor locus. *Cell* **60:**509, 1990.
94. Gessler M, Poustka A, Cavenee W, Neve R, Orkin S, Bruns G: Homozygous deletion in Wilms tumours of a zinc-finger gene identified by chromosome jumping. *Nature* **343:**774, 1990.
95. Evans R, Hollenberg S: Zinc fingers: Gilt by association. *Cell* **52:**1, 1988.
96. Mitchell P, Tijan R: Transcriptional regulation in mammalian cells by sequence-specific DNA binding proteins. *Science* **245:**371, 1989.
97. Haber D, Sohn R, Buckler A, Pelletier J, Call K, Housman D: Alternative splicing and genomic structure of the Wilms tumor gene WT1. *Proc Natl Acad Sci USA* **88:**9618, 1991.
98. Sukhatme V, Cao X, Chang L, Tsai-Morris C, Stamenkovich D, Ferreira P, Cohen D, Edewards S, Shows T, Curran T, LeBeau M, Adamson E: A zinc finger encoding gene coregulated with c-fos during growth and differentiation and after cellular depolarization. *Cell* **53:**37, 1988.
99. Rauscher F, Morris J, Tournay O, Cook D, Curran T: Binding of the Wilms' tumor locus zinc finger protein to the EGR-1 consensus sequence. *Science* **250:**1259, 1990.
100. Wang Z, Qiu Q, Enger K, Deuel T: A second transcriptionally active DNA-binding site for the Wilms tumor gene product, WT1. *Proc Natl Acad Sci USA* **90:**8896, 1993.
101. Englert C, Hou X, Maheswaran S, Bennett P, Ngwu C, Re G, Garvin A, Rosner M, Haber D: WT1 suppresses synthesis of the epidermal growth factor receptor and induces apoptosis. *EMBO J* **14:**4662, 1995.
102. Nakagama H, Heinrich G, Pelletier J, Housman D: Sequence and structural requirements for high-affinity binding by the WT1 gene product. *Mol Cell Biol* **15:**1489, 1995.
103. Madden S, Cook D, Morris J, Gashler A, Sukhatme V, Rauscher F III: Transcriptional repression mediated by the WT1 Wilms tumor gene product. *Science* **253:**1550, 1991.
104. Rauscher F III: The WT1 Wilms tumor gene product: A developmentally regulated transcription factor in the kidney that functions as a tumor suppressor. *FASEB J* **7:**896, 1993.
105. Drummond I, Badden S, Rohwer-Nutter P, Bell G, Sukhatme V, Rauscher F III: Repression of the insulin-like growth factor II gene by the Wilms tumor suppressor WT1. *Science* **257:**674, 1992.
106. Gashler A, Bonthron D, Madden S, Rauscher F III, Collins T, Sukhatme V: Human platelet-derived growth factor A chain is transcriptionally repressed by the Wilms tumor suppressor WT1. *Proc Natl Acad Sci USA* **89:**10984, 1992.
107. Wang Z, Madden S, Deuel T, Rauscher F III: The Wilms' tumor gene product, WT1, represses transcription of the platelet-derived growth factor A-chain gene. *J Biol Chem* **267:**21999, 1992.
108. Werner H, Re G, Drummond I, Sukhatme V, Rauscher F III, Sens D, Garvin A, LeRoith D, Roberts C Jr: Increased expression of the insulin-like growth factor I receptor gene IGF1R in Wilms tumor is correlated with modulation of IGF1R promoter activity by the WT1 Wilms tumor gene product. *Proc Natl Acad Sci USA* **90:**5828, 1993.
109. Werner H, Shen-Orr Z, Rauscher F III, Morris J, Toberts C, LeRoith D: Inhhibition of cellular proliferation by the Wilms' tumor suppressor WT1 is associated with suppression of insulin-like growth factor I receptor gene expression. *Mol Cell Biol* **15:**3516, 1995.
110. Hewitt S, Hamada S, McDonnell T, Rauscher F III, Saunders G: Regulation of the proto-oncogenes bcl-2 and c-myc by the Wilms' tumor suppressor gene WT1. *Cancer Res* **55:**5386, 1995.
111. Goodyer P, Dehbi M, Torban E, Bruening W, Pelletier J: Repression of the retinoic acid receptor-α gene by the Wilms' tumor suppressor gene product, wt1. *Oncogene* **10:**1125, 1995.
112. Ryan G, Steele-Perkins V, Morris J, Rauscher F III: Repression of Pax-2 by WT1 during normal kidney development. *Development* **121:**867, 1995.
113. Dey B, Sukhatme V, Roberts A, Sporn M, Rauscher F III, Kim S: Repression of the transforming growth factor $\beta 1$ gene by the Wilms tumor suppressor WT1 gene product. *Mol Endocrinol* **8:**595, 1994.
114. Nichols K, Re G, Yan Y, Garvin A, Haber D: WT1 induces expression of insulin-like growth factor 2 in Wilms' tumor cells. *Cancer Res* **55:**4540, 1995.
115. Wang Z-Y, Qiu Q-Q, Deuel T: The Wilms' tumor gene product WT1 activates or suppresses transcription through separate functional domains. *J Biol Chem* **268:**9172, 1993.
116. Maheswaran S, Park S, Bernard A, Morris J, Rauscher F III, Hill D, Haber D: Physical and functional interction between WT1 and p53 proteins. *Proc Natl Acad Sci USA* **90:**5100, 1993.
117. Reddy J, Hosono S, Licht J: The transcriptional effect of WT1 is modulated by choice of expression vector. *J Biol Chem* **270:**29976, 1995.

118. Bickmore W, Oghene K, Little M, Seawright A, van Heyningen V, Hastie N: Modulation of DNA binding specificity by alternative splicing of the Wilms tumor wt1 gene transcript. *Science* **257**:235, 1992.
119. Larsson S, Charlieu J, Miyagawa K, Engelkamp D, Rassoutzadegan M, Ross A, Cuzin F, van Heyningen V, Hastie N: Subnuclear localization of WT1 in splicing or transcription factor domains is regulated by alternative splicing. *Cell* **81**:391, 1995.
120. Englert C, Vidal M, Maheswaran S, Ge Y, Ezzell R, Isselbacher K, Haber D: Truncated WT1 mutants alter the subnuclear localization of the wild-type protein. *Proc Natl Acad Sci USA* **92**:11960, 1995.
121. Ye Y, Raychaudhuri B, Gurney A, Campbell C, Williams B: Regulation of WT1 by phosphorylation: inhibition of DNA binding, alteration of transcriptional activity and cellular translocation. *EMBO J* **15**:5606, 1996.
122. Pritchard-Jones K, Fleming S, Davidson D, Bickmore W, Porteous D, Gosden C, Bard J, Buckler A, Pelletier J, Housman D, van Heyningen V, Hastie N: The candidate Wilms' tumour gene is involved in genitourinary development. *Nature* **346**:194, 1990.
123. Buckler A, Pelletier J, Haber D, Glaser T, Housman D: Isolation, characterization, and expression of the murine Wilms' tumor gene (WT1) during kidney development. *Mol Cell Biol* **11**:1707, 1991.
124. Pelletier J, Schalling M, Buckler A, Rogers A, Haber D, Housman D: Expression of the Wilms' tumor gene WT1 in the murine urogenital system. *Genes Dev* **5**:1345, 1991.
125. Armstrong J, Pritchard-Jones K, Bickmore W, Hastie N, Bard J: The expression of the Wilms' tumor gene, WT1, in the developing mammalian embryo. *Mech Dev* **40**:85, 1992.
126. Park S, Schalling M, Bernard A, Maheswaran S, Shipley G, Roberts D, Fletcher J, Shipman R, Rheinwald J, Demetri G, Griffin J, Minden M, Housman D, Haber D: The Wilms tumour gene WT1 is expressed in murine mesoderm-derived tissues and mutated in a human mesothelioma. *Nature Genet* **4**:415, 1993.
127. King-Underwood L, Renshaw J, Pritchard-Jones K: Mutations in the Wilms' tumor gene WT1 in leukemias. *Blood* **87**:2171, 1996.
128. Pelletier J, Bruening W, Kashtan C, Mauer S, Manivel J, Striegel J, Houghton D, Junien C, Habib R, Fouser L, Fine R, Silverman B, Haber D, Housman D: Germline mutations in the Wilms' tumor suppressor gene are associated with abnormal urogenital development in Denys-Drash syndrome. *Cell* **67**:437, 1991.
129. Ton C, Huff V, Call K, Cohn S, Strong L, Housman D, Saunders G: Smallest region of overlap in Wilms' tumor deletions uniquely implicates an 11p13 zinc finger gene as the disease locus. *Genomics* **10**:293, 1991.
130. Cowell J, Wadey R, Haber D, Call K, Housman D, Prichard J: Structural rearrangements of the WT1 gene in Wilms' tumor cells. *Oncogene* **6**:595, 1991.
131. Little M, Prosser J, Condie A, Smith P, van Heyningen V, Hastie N: Zinc finger point mutations within the WT1 gene in Wilms tumor patients. *Proc Natl Acad Sci USA* **89**:4791, 1992.
132. Coppes M, Liefers G, Paul P, Yeger H, Williams B: Homozygous somatic WT1 point mutations in sporadic unilateral Wilms tumor. *Proc Natl Acad Sci USA* **90**:1416, 1993.
133. Varanasi R, Bardeesy N, Gharemani M, Petruzzi M-J, Nowak N, Adam M, Grundy P, Shows T, Pelletier J: Fine structure analysis of the WT1 gene in sporadic Wilms tumors. *Proc Natl Acad Sci USA* **91**:3554, 1994.
134. Herskowitz I: Functional inactivation of genes by dominant negative mutations. *Nature* **329**:219, 1987.
135. Haber D, Timmers H, Pelletier J, Sharp P, Housman D: A dominant mutation in the Wilms tumor gene WT1 cooperates with the viral oncogene E1A in transformation of primary kidney cells. *Proc Natl Acad Sci USA* **89**:6010, 1992.
136. Reddy J, Morris J, Wang J, English M, Haber D, Shi Y, Licht J: WT1-mediated transcriptional activation is inhibited by dominant negative mutant proteins. *J Biol Chem* **270**:10878, 1995.
137. Moffett P, Bruening W, Nakagama H, Bardeesy N, Housman D, Housman D, Pelletier J: Antagonism of WT1 activity by protein self-association. *Proc Natl Acad Sci USA* **92**:11105, 1995.
138. Haber D, Park S, Maheswaran S, Englert C, Re G, Hazen-Martin D, Sens D, Garvin A: WT1-mediated growth suppression of Wilms tumor cells expressing a WT1 splicing variant. *Science* **262**:2057, 1993.
139. Ladanyi M, Gerald W: Fusion of the EWS and WT1 genes in the desmoplastic small round cell tumor. *Cancer Res* **54**:2837, 1994.
140. Gerald W, Rosai J, Ladanyi M: Characterization of the genomic breakpoint and chimeric transcripts in the EWS-WT1 gene fusion of desmoplastic small round cell tumor. *Proc Natl Acad Sci USA* **92**:1028, 1995.
141. Park S, Tomlinson G, Nisen P, Haber D: Altered trans-activational properties of a mutated WT1 gene product in a WAGR-associated Wilms' tumor. *Cancer Res* **53**:4757, 1993.
142. Sharma P, Bowman M, Madden S, Rauscher F III, Sukumar S: RNA editing in the Wilms' tumor susceptibility gene, WT1. *Genes Dev* **8**:720, 1994.
143. Theiler K, Varnum D, Stevens L: Development of Dickie's small eye, a mutation in the house mouse. *Anat Embryol* **155**:81, 1978.
144. Hogan B, Horsburgh G, Cohen J, Hetherington C, Fisher G, Lyon M: Small eyes (Sey): A homozygous lethal mutation on chromosome 2 which affects the differentiation of both lens and nasal placodes in the mouse. *J Embryol Exp Morphol* **97**:95, 1986.
145. Glaser T, Lane J, Housman D: A mouse model of the aniridia-Wilms' tumor deletion syndrome. *Science* **250**:823, 1990.
146. Kreidberg J, Sariola H, Loring J, Maeda M, Pelletier J, Housman D, Jaenisch R: WT1 is required for early kidney development. *Cell* **74**:679, 1993.
147. Hasgekar N, Pendse A, Lalitha V: Rat renal mesenchymal tumor as an experimental model for human congenital mesoblastic nephroma. *Pediatr Pathol* **9**:131, 1989.
148. Ohaki Y: Renal tumors induced transplacentally in the rat by *N*-ethylnitrosourea. *Pediatr Pathol* **9**:19, 1989.
149. Deshpande R, Hasgekar N, Chitale A, Lalitha V: Rat renal mesenchymal tumor as an experimental model for human congenital mesoblastic nephroma: II. Comparative pathology. *Pediatr Pathol* **9**:141, 1989.
150. Sharma P, Bowman M, Yu B, Sukumar S: A rodent model for Wilms tumors: Embryonal kidney neoplasms induced by *N*-nitros-*N*9-methylurea. *Proc Natl Acad Sci USA* **91**:9931, 1994.
151. Kudoh T, Ishidate T, Moriyama M, Toyoshima K, Akiyama T: G1 phase arrest induced by Wilms tumor protein WT1 is abrogated by cyclin/CDK complexes. *Proc Natl Acad Sci USA* **92**:4517, 1995.
152. Englert C, Maheswaran S, Garvin AJ, Kreidberg J, Haber DA: Induction of p21 by the Wilms' tumor suppressor gene WT1. *Cancer Res* **57**:1429–1434, 1970.
153. Sherr C, Roberts R: Inhibitors of mammalian G1 cyclin-dependent kinases. *Genes Dev* **9**:1149, 1995.
154. Wang J, Walsh K: Resistance to apoptosis conferred by cdk inhibitors during myocyte differentiation. *Science* **273**:359, 1996.
155. Maheswaran S, Englert C, Bennett P, Heinrich G, Haber D: The WT1 gene product stabilizes p53 and inhibits p53-mediated apoptosis. *Genes Dev* **9**:2143, 1995.
156. Lemoine N, Hughes C, Cowell J: Aberrant expression of the tumour suppressor gene p53 is very frequent in Wilms' tumours. *J Pathol* **168**:237, 1992.
157. Malkin D, Sexsmith E, Yeger H, Williams B, Coppes M: Mutations of the p53 tumor suppressor gene occur infrequently in Wilms' tumor. *Cancer Res* **54**:2077, 1994.
158. Bardeesy N, Falkoff D, Petruzzi M, Nowak N, Zabel B, Adam M, Aguiar M, Grundy P, Shows T, Pelletier J: Anaplastic Wilms' tumour, a subtype displaying poor prognosis, harbours p53 gene mutations. *Nature Genet* **7**:91, 1994.

CHAPTER 39

Neurofibromatosis 1

David H. Gutmann ▪ Francis S. Collins

1. **Von Recklinghausen neurofibromatosis, or neurofibromatosis type 1 (NF1), is a common autosomal dominant disorder that affects 1 in 3000 individuals. It is characterized clinically by the finding of two or more of the following: café-au-lait spots, neurofibromas, freckling in non-sun-exposed areas, optic glioma, Lisch nodules, distinctive bony lesions, and a first-degree relative with NF1. Less common manifestations include short stature and macrocephaly. NF1 patients also can have learning disabilities, seizures, scoliosis, hypertension, plexiform neurofibromas, or pheochromocytomas.**
2. **There is a high spontaneous mutation rate in NF1, with 30 to 50 percent of cases representing new mutations. Although the penetrance of NF1 is essentially 100 percent, NF1 tends to show variable expressivity in that there is a wide range of clinical severity and complications in patients within the same family, who all presumably carry the same mutation.**
3. **Syndromes related to NF1 include neurofibromatosis type 2 (bilateral vestibular neurofibromatosis), segmental or mosaic NF1, Watson syndrome, and neurofibromatosis 1–Noonan syndrome.**
4. **The gene for NF1 was identified by positional cloning and resides on chromosome 17q11.2. This gene has an open reading frame of 8454 nucleotides and spans approximately 300,000 nucleotides of genomic DNA. The messenger RNA is 11,000 to 13,000 nucleotides and is detectable at varying levels in all tissues examined. Germ-line mutations in the *NF1* gene have been found in affected patients and range from large (megabase) deletions to missense and nonsense mutations.**
5. **The protein product of the *NF1* locus (neurofibromin) is 2818 amino acids and is expressed as a 250-kDa protein in brain, spleen, kidney, testis, and thymus. This protein has structural and functional similarity to a family of GTPase-activating proteins (GAPs) that down-regulate a cellular proto-oncogene, p21-*ras*. *ras* has been implicated in the control of cell growth and differentiation, and the ability of neurofibromin to down-regulate p21-*ras* suggests that the loss of neurofibromin may lead to uncontrolled cell growth or tumor formation. Subcellular localization and biochemical purification experiments have demonstrated that neurofibromin is associated with cytoplasmic microtubules.**
6. **Somatic mutations in the *NF1* gene that result in an absence of neurofibromin expression have been described for a variety of tumor types. Loss of neurofibromin in neurofibrosarcomas derived from NF1 patients results in increased p21-*ras* activation and presumably tumor formation. Neurofibromin expression is also absent in non-NF1 patients' tumors, including metastatic malignant melanomas and neuroblastomas. The loss of neurofibromin in malignancy supports the notion that neurofibromin is a tumor-suppressor gene product.**
7. **The diagnosis of neurofibromatosis 1 is based largely on clinical criteria despite progress in defining the molecular genetics of the disorder. Treatment of patients with NF1 is directed at education and genetic counseling, early detection of malignancy, and surveillance for the appearance of complications of NF1.**

A list of standard abbreviations is located immediately preceding the index in each volume. Nonstandard abbreviations used in this chapter include: NF1 = neurofibromatosis type 1; UBOs = unidentified bright objects; NGF = nerve growth factor; GAPs = GTPase-activating proteins; MAPs = microtubule-associated proteins.

Von Recklinghausen neurofibromatosis, or neurofibromatosis type 1 (NF1), is one of the most common autosomal dominant disorders in humans, afflicting all ethnic groups, both sexes, and all age groups. It is more common than Duchenne muscular dystrophy and Huntington disease combined and has a greater prevalence in the Western world than does cystic fibrosis. Yet NF1 has received far less attention in the public eye and the medical literature than have these other single-gene disorders. Among the multitude of reasons for this decreased visibility, three seem to stand out: (1) The pleiotropic and variable manifestations of NF1 affect many different organ systems and thus lead to the involvement of a multitude of subspecialists in the care of these patients. However, until recently no single specialist or subspecialist had considered NF1 a disease of major concern. Now this role has been taken on by medical geneticists. (2) Until very recently, NF1 lacked a firm biologic basis, and investigations into its pathogenesis were more descriptive than definitive. In the absence of a biologic hypothesis for the basic defect, very little attention was given to this disorder by basic scientists. (3) It is a tragic reality that many patients with NF1 are at least to some degree disfigured. In a society that often values physical beauty more than strength of character, such individuals have been discriminated against, either overtly or subtly, and often have responded by remaining in the background. There have been few poster children for von Recklinghausen neurofibromatosis, no telethons, and very little public sympathy. The learning disabilities suffered by many individuals with NF1 have further inhibited their ability to achieve positions of power, wealth, and influence.

All these circumstances are undergoing a turnaround. The founding of the National Neurofibromatosis Foundation (NNFF) in America in 1978, LINK (Let's Increase Neurofibromatosis Knowledge) in 1982, and the International Neurofibromatosis Association in 1992 signifies a new determination of NF1 sufferers and their families to increase public awareness of the disease, support research, and reach out to each other in support groups. The clinical care of NF patients, previously fragmented and poorly coordinated, has been greatly improved over the past 15 years by the establishment of a large number of NF specialty clinics, which are now present in most major medical centers. The directors of such clinics are usually pediatricians, internists, neurologists, or geneticists, and the clinics offer diagnosis, counseling, and regular evaluation of affected individuals for complications of the disease and coordinated access to subspecialists when the need arises. Such clinics, initially arising out of the pioneering efforts of Vincent Riccardi at Baylor, have provided a wealth of information about the natural history of the disease and corrected a number of misconceptions.

Table 39-1 **Estimates of Prevalence and Mutation Rate of *NF1***

Methods of Study (Year)	Ascertainment	Prevalence	Mutation Rate
Crowe et al. (1956)	Surveys of admissions at general hospital and state mental institutions	1/2500–3000	$1.4–2.6 \times 10^{-4}$
Sergeyev (1975)	Population sample of 16-year-old Russian youths	1/7800	$4.4–4.9 \times 10^{-5}$
Samuelsson and Axelson (1981)	Population-based	1/4600	4.3×10.5^{-5}
Huson et al. (1989)	Population-based	1/2500–4950	$3.1–10.5 \times 10^{-5}$

From the scientific point of view, identification of the *NF1* gene by a positional cloning strategy[1–3] and recognition that the protein product is a participant in p21-*ras*-mediated growth control[4–7] have catapulted NF1 into the scientific spotlight, resulting in the recruitment of a significant number of basic scientists into research on this disorder who previously would not have paid it much mind. Thus the complexion of NF1 has changed dramatically over the past 15 years, and it now seems highly appropriate to include a chapter on this disorder in this textbook.

There are three recent excellent books[8–10] on neurofibromatosis, with particular emphasis on the clinical aspects. No attempt will be made here to duplicate those sources and the wealth of clinical detail they provide; the interested reader is referred to those sources as well as to the classic monograph of Crowe, Schull, and Neel.[11] Furthermore, no coverage of neurofibromatosis type 2 (NF2, formerly referred to as *central neurofibromatosis* or *bilateral vestibular neurofibromatosis*) will be attempted.[12,13]

CLINICAL ASPECTS

Historical Perspective

Scattered descriptions of cases that almost certainly represent NF1, sometimes even including drawings, can be found through many centuries of medical writing.[14,15] While other writers previously had focused on the skin tumors and occasionally had noted the familial nature of the disorder, it was von Recklinghausen in 1882 who gave the disease its first full description, including recognition that the tumors arose from the fibrous tissue surrounding small nerves, leading to his designation of these tumors as *neurofibromas*.[16] The autosomal dominant inheritance pattern was defined early in the twentieth century.[17] A crucial diagnostic element, the iris nodule, was defined by the Viennese ophthalmologist Lisch in 1937,[18] although the true significance and usefulness of this observation have come to general attention only in the past decade.[19,20]

The landmark study of Crowe, Schull, and Neel[11] brought together for the first time all the salient clinical features of NF1, including the high incidence, the high spontaneous mutation rate, the usefulness of the café-au-lait spot as a diagnostic feature, and recognition of the wide range of complications that can occur. Other important large-scale studies of the disease include those of Borberg[21] (followed up 35 years later by Sorenson *et al.*[22]), Carey *et al.*,[23] Riccardi,[9,24] and Huson *et al.*[25–27] While none of these studies is completely devoid of bias of ascertainment, together they provide a wealth of information about this pleiotropic disease.

Incidence

Because NF1 often is not diagnosed at birth, especially if the case is a new mutation, true birth incidence rates are difficult to obtain. Population surveys in the United States,[11] Russia,[28] Denmark,[29] and Wales[26] (Table 39-1) have resulted in an estimate of disease prevalence of approximately 1 in 2500 to 1 in 5000. A lower estimate of 1 in 7800 is provided by the Russian study, but this almost certainly represents an underestimate. When underascertainment and increased mortality are considered, the true birth incidence of NF1 is probably about 1 in 3000. There is no evidence that this frequency varies among ethnic groups. This is expected for a disorder with such a high percentage of spontaneous mutations.

Diagnostic Criteria

Despite opinions to the contrary in the medical literature, the diagnosis of NF1 usually is not difficult or controversial when performed by an experienced clinician. In 1987, the National Institutes of Health (NIH) convened a consensus panel to define diagnostic criteria for NF1, and the list that resulted (Table 39-2) reflects extensive clinical experience and only rarely leads to a false-positive diagnosis.[30] The same panel also set out the distinguishing features between NF1 and NF2 (see below), ending many decades of confusion about these two disorders, which are now known to be completely distinct, both genetically and clinically. Recently, these diagnostic criteria were updated based on a decade of improved clinical and basic science insights.[31]

The diagnostic criteria listed in Table 39-2 do not eliminate the occurrence of certain clinical dilemmas, however. A frequent dilemma is the identification of a child under 4 years of age with six or more café-au-lait spots, no family history, and no other manifestations of NF1. According to the NIH criteria, this is insufficient evidence to make a diagnosis of NF1, but such children must be followed for the appearance of other manifestations. Most of these children will eventually turn out to have NF1 as additional features manifest.

Defining Features Present in Most Patients

Café-au-Lait Spots. The café-au-lait spot (Fig. 39-1), a flat, evenly pigmented macule, usually is not apparent at birth but becomes visible during the first year of life. While up to 25 percent of the normal population will have one to three café-au-lait

Table 39-2 **Diagnostic Criteria for NF1**

Two or more of the following:
- Six or more café-au-lait spots
  - 1.5 cm or larger in postpubertal individuals
  - 0.5 cm or larger in prepubertal individuals
- Two or more neurofibromas of any type or one or more plexiform neurofibromas
- Freckling of armpits or groin
- Optic glioma (tumor of the optic pathway)
- Two or more Lisch nodules (benign iris hamartomas)
- A distinctive bony lesion
  - Dysplasia of the sphenoid bone
  - Dysplasia or thinning of long bone cortex
- First-degree relative with NF1

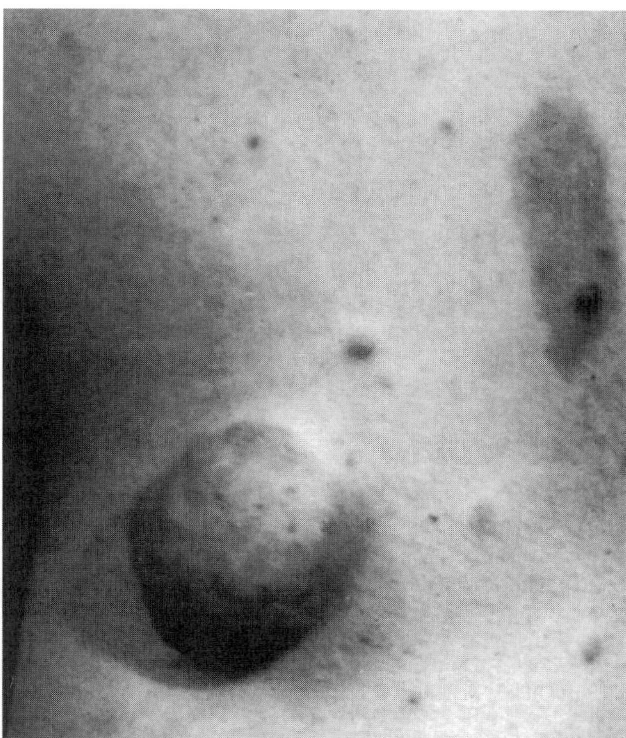

Fig. 39-1 Typical neurofibroma and a café-au-lait spot on the skin of an adult with NF1.

spots,[32] the presence of six or more is highly suspicious for NF1[11] if the size criteria listed in Table 39-2 are closely followed. Melanocytes within a café-au-lait spot have an increased number of macromelanosomes,[33] although this is not diagnostic for NF1. The café-au-lait spots tend to fade in later life and may be difficult or impossible to identify in elderly individuals. Visualization using a Wood's lamp often reveals these macules when they are not discernible on bedside examination.

Peripheral Neurofibromas. Peripheral neurofibromas are soft, fleshy tumors (Figs. 39-1 and 39-2) that are usually not present in childhood but make their appearance slightly before or during adolescence.[9] They tend to increase in size and number with age, although the rate can be extremely variable. Some females affected with NF1 note an increase in the rate of progression during pregnancy, suggesting that these tumors may be hormone-responsive. Pathologically, these lesions arise from cells in the peripheral nerve sheath and are made up of a mixture of cell types, including Schwann cells, fibroblasts, mast cells, and vascular elements.[34]

There are typically two types of neurofibromas: discrete and plexiform. While a discrete neurofibroma arises from a single site along a peripheral nerve as a focal mass with well-defined margins, plexiform neurofibromas usually involve multiple nerve fascicles (see below). A subset of patients can have firmer and sometimes painful neurofibromas along the course of peripheral nerves. These neurofibromas can be quite difficult to manage surgically. Even more challenging are the spinal neurofibromas arising from dorsal nerve roots, which can lead to pain and neurologic compromise. It should be emphasized that dermal neurofibromas are benign tumors without a propensity for malignant transformation.

Freckling. The occurrence of freckles in the axilla, groin, and intertriginous areas was first pointed out by Crowe[35] and is a useful diagnostic feature. Such freckling is not apparent at birth but often appears during childhood. In adults, freckling may be seen in the neck regions or inframammary areas in women. The occurrence of such freckling in the inframammary areas and other skin folds[36] is a curious observation that suggests that these lesions are modulated by the local environment.

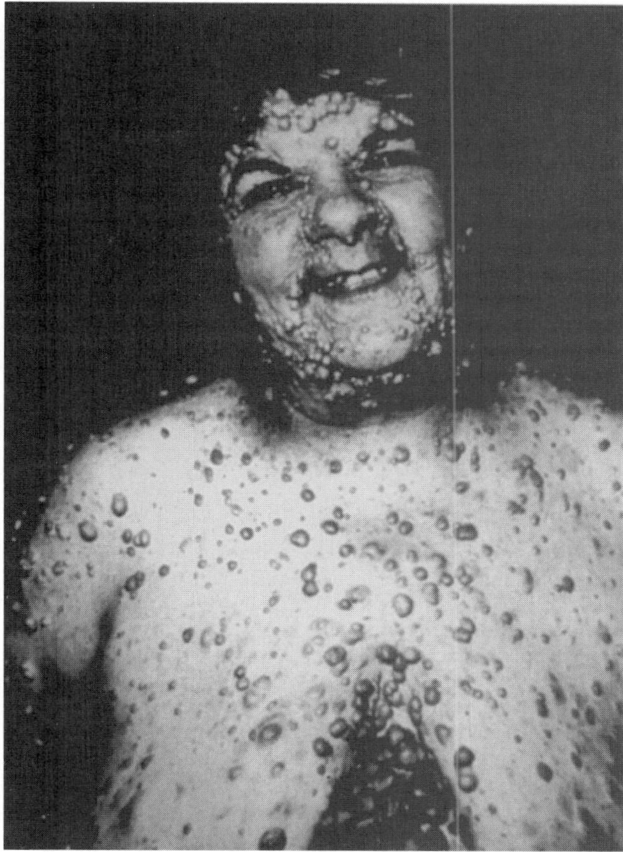

Fig. 39-2 An older individual with NF1, demonstrating extensive involvement on the skin surface with peripheral neurofibromas.

Lisch Nodules. Raised, often pigmented nodules of the iris, pathologically representing hamartomas, are now called *Lisch nodules* (Fig. 39-3) and represent an extremely important diagnostic feature of NF1.[19,20] Like café-au-lait spots and freckling, Lisch nodules never result in significant disease but

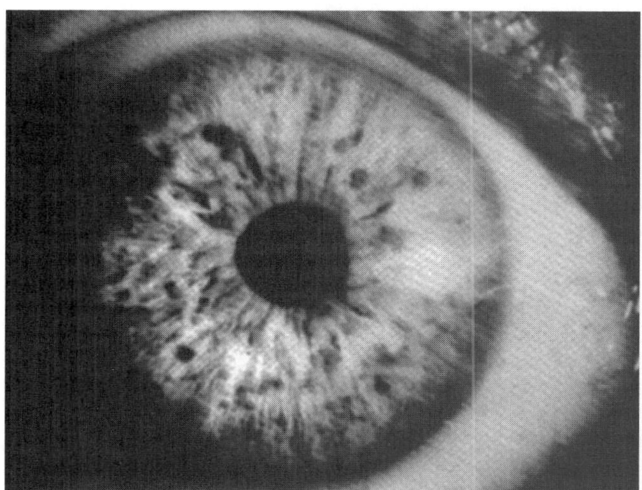

Fig. 39-3 Typical Lisch nodules (hamartomas) of the iris in an adult with NF1.

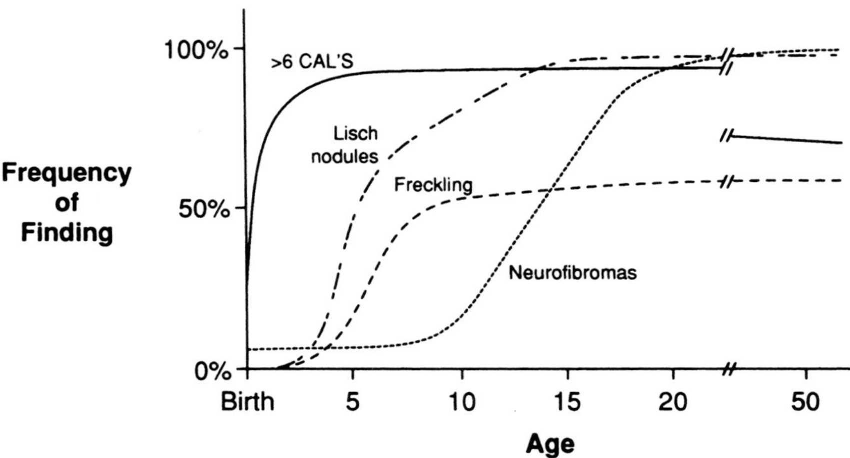

Fig. 39-4 Typical time course of appearance of the major clinical features of NF1. CAL = café-au-lait spots.

can be helpful in establishing the diagnosis. While they can be seen with simple lighting in individuals with light irises, a slit-lamp examination is usually essential to be certain of their presence and to distinguish them from iris nevi. Typically, these lesions are not detected until after 5 years of age.

Time Course

The defining features of NF1 described earlier, while somewhat variable in appearance, tend to follow the pattern shown in Fig. 39-4. As implied by the figure, it is unusual for an individual with NF1 to reach adolescence without having amply satisfied the diagnostic criteria in Table 39-2.

Common but Nondiagnostic and Nonmorbid Features

While not considered specific enough for inclusion in the list of diagnostic criteria, macrocephaly[25] and short stature[24] are common accompaniments of NF1. The macrocephaly reflects concomitant megalencephaly. Careful studies of adult height suggest that individuals with NF1 are on average about 3 inches shorter than predicted by their family backgrounds.[9,25] With both these circumstances, it is important not to overlook other, more significant causes. For instance, aqueductal stenosis leading to hydrocephalus is a known but uncommon complication of NF1 that requires surgical intervention.[37] Similarly, growth failure occasionally can arise as a result of hypothalamic involvement by optic glioma.

Variable but Significant Complications

The defining features of NF1 listed in Table 39-2 are found in most affected patients and, while often associated with significant cosmetic concerns related to neurofibroma growth, usually are not life-threatening. A range of other complications that are quite variable from one patient to the next can be more serious. Approximately one-third of patients with NF1 suffer from one or more of these serious complications during their lifetimes (Fig. 39-5).

Learning Disability. Frank mental retardation (IQ < 70) is uncommon in NF1. Recent molecular information indicates that such patients are much more likely to have the disease because of a large deletion that removes the entire *NF1* gene and considerable flanking DNA.[38] Presumably, other nearby genes are also reduced to hemizygosity by the deletion in these patients and contribute to the retardation.

Although retardation is uncommon, standard IQ testing reveals a downward shift of performance scores by 5 to 10 IQ points in affected individuals.[36] Approximately 40 to 60 percent of all individuals with NF1 have learning disabilities. Analysis of the specific behavioral phenotype in children with NF1 has demonstrated a higher incidence of minor signs of neurologic impairment (motor abnormalities involving balance and gait), lower IQ scores, and poor performance on tasks involving nonverbal learning. In addition, children with NF1 often exhibit areas of increased T_2 signal intensity on magnetic resonance imaging (MRI) of the brain. It has been suggested that children with such areas (unidentified bright objects, or UBOs) have significantly lower

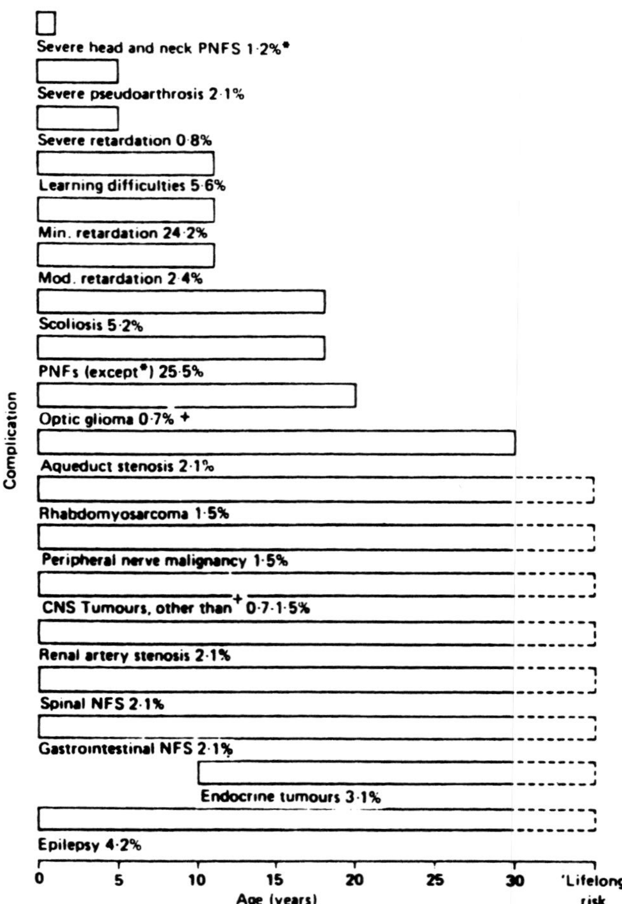

Fig. 39-5 Age range of presentation and frequency of major NF1 complications. PNF = plexiform neurofibroma; NFS = neurofibrosarcoma. (*From Huson et al.*[27] *Used by permission.*)

IQ and language scores, with impaired visual motor integration and coordination.[39] Although this hypothesis is intriguing, it has not been confirmed in all studies examining this association.[40,41] UBOs are seen most commonly in the basal ganglia, cerebellum, brainstem, and subcortical white matter regions. In one pathologic study, these hyperintense foci corresponded to areas of vacuolar and spongiotic change, with fluid-filled vacuoles surrounded by infiltrating astrocytes.[42] Recent studies have demonstrated increased neurofibromin expression in activated astrocytes both *in vivo* and *in vitro*, suggesting that reduced *NF1* gene expression may alter the normal astrogliotic response in the brain.[43,44] Intervention is highly warranted if the preceding problems emerge, and all children with NF1 should be followed closely for developmental progress and subjected to a thorough educational evaluation at age 3 or 4 if there is any indication of significant delay.

Plexiform Neurofibromas. A plexiform neurofibroma is a much more complex, usually congenital (though often not immediately visible) lesion that may diffusely involve nerve, muscle, connective tissue, vascular elements, and overlying skin.[36] Such lesions, which occur in approximately 20 percent of affected individuals, commonly lead to overgrowth of surrounding tissues during childhood and in their most severe form can lead to massive distortion of the face or an extremity (Fig. 39-6). When these lesions occur around the orbit, they are often associated with sphenoid wing dysplasia, and the tumor may extend inside the cranial vault, accompanied by pulsating exophthalmos.[9] Severe plexiform lesions are almost invariably apparent by age 4 or 5, so it is possible to reassure older individuals without plexiform lesions that they are not at significant risk for the development of this particularly troubling and disfiguring complication.

Malignancy. The frequency of malignancy in NF1 is difficult to discern accurately, since most series reflect a referral bias and therefore overestimate the occurrence of this complication.[42] Nonetheless, there is clearly an increased risk of specific cancers in NF1, amounting to perhaps 2 to 5 percent of affected individuals.[9,23,25,29,46]

A particularly aggressive and often fatal malignancy is the neurofibrosarcoma, or malignant peripheral nerve sheath tumor (MPNST), which commonly arises in a plexiform neurofibroma in a young adult. Often the first symptom is pain or rapid growth, which should always prompt rapid investigation in an individual with a plexiform lesion. These malignancies are highly aggressive and metastatic cancers that are relatively resistant to chemotherapy and radiation.[47] Survival remains poor when wide excision or amputation is not possible.

A second strongly associated tumor is optic glioma. MRI scanning of affected children with NF1 has revealed radiographic evidence of optic nerve or optic chiasm enlargement in up to 15 to 20 percent of patients,[48–50] but the vast majority of these patients have normal vision and never become symptomatic. Most of these tumors are detected in children younger than 6 years. A small subgroup, however, presents with progressive visual loss associated with an expanding lesion. Occasionally, optic pathway gliomas can lead to precocious puberty when hypothalamic involvement ensues. While this occurs only in a minority of patients with NF1, all children with NF1 should have regular ophthalmologic evaluations.

While the risk of other malignancies of the nervous system is less impressive, there appears to be a moderately increased risk of central nervous system tumors, especially astrocytomas.[34] Pheochromocytoma is commonly quoted as a complication of NF1 but is in fact quite uncommon in this population.[11,45,46]

Seizures. A seizure disorder will develop in approximately 5 percent of patients with NF1, and the onset can occur at any time.[9] While occasionally a definable intracranial tumor will be found to be at fault, usually no cause can be defined. In this regard, the recent advent of MRI scanning has uncovered MRI inhomogeneities in the brains of many children with NF1 on T_2-weighted images. These UBOs are of uncertain etiology and generally should not be interpreted as clinically significant.[51] There is some evidence that they tend to disappear with age, and it is not correct, on the basis of current evidence, to refer to them as hamartomas.

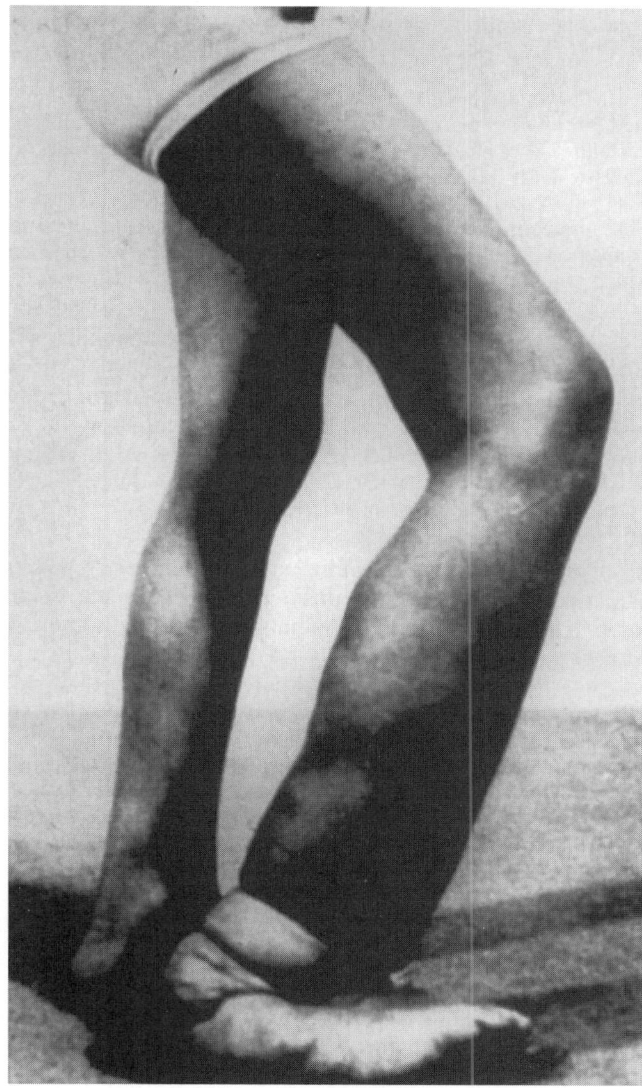

Fig. 39-6 Massive plexiform neurofibroma of the lower extremity in an adolescent with NF1.

Scoliosis. Vertebral defects, including scalloping from dural ectasia,[52] are extremely common in NF1, and approximately 10 percent of affected individuals have scoliosis during late childhood and adolescence.[9] In some instances this can be severe enough to require bracing and/or surgery and may or may not be associated with local neurofibroma formation.

Pseudarthrosis. A peculiar and uncommon complication that defies the classification of NF1 as a disorder purely of the neural crest is the involvement of long bones. This often is noted first as bowing, particularly of the tibia, in young children. This may progress to thinning of the cortex, pathologic fracture, and severe difficulties with nonunion of the fragments. This process may go on to form a pseudarthrosis, or false joint, leaving the limb severely compromised. The pathologic basis of this unusual process is unknown.

Hypertension. Hypertension is extremely common in adults with NF1, affecting perhaps one-third of these patients.[24] In general, this proves to be essential hypertension with no underlying cause, but the new development of hypertension always should raise the possibility of renal artery stenosis, which is particularly common in children,[53] or pheochromocytoma, which occasionally occurs in adults with NF1 (see above).

Miscellaneous Complications. Frequent but less well understood problems associated with neurofibromatosis 1 include headache, which can be bothersome but usually not disabling. The new onset of headache always should trigger evaluation for an intracranial tumor, but many patients experience lifelong stable headache patterns with no identifiable etiology. Generalized itching or itching localized to newly developing neurofibromas is reported by many individuals.[9] Similarly, constipation seems to be a frequent concomitant of the disease, especially in patients who have plexiform neurofibromas in the pelvic area.[54] These complications may interfere with autonomic innervation of the colon and produce both bowel and bladder problems.

GENETIC ASPECTS

Inheritance Pattern

Preiser and Davenport[17] surveyed the literature in 1918 and concluded that approximately 50 percent of the children of individuals affected with NF1 also were afflicted, regardless of sex. They noted numerous examples of male-to-male transmission, concluding that the disease follows an autosomal dominant pattern of inheritance. In 1981, Hall suggested that the sex of the affected parent might have an impact on the severity of the disease,[55,56] a phenomenon we would now ascribe to parental imprinting.[57] In that study, children of affected mothers tended to be slightly more severely affected than did children of affected fathers. Subsequent careful analyses of this issue have failed to confirm this maternal effect,[23,54,55] although a very modest effect would be difficult to exclude with such variability of the disease.[58,59]

Mutation Rate

All large series indicate after careful examination that 30 to 50 percent of patients with NF1 do not have an affected parent.[11,29,59] Such individuals presumably represent spontaneous mutations. With the cloning of the *NF1* gene, several examples have now been documented of *de novo* alterations in the *NF1* gene in such individuals (see below). Given that NF1 is a common disease and that so many of its sufferers have new mutations, one cannot escape the conclusion that the mutation rate for this locus is unusually high. In fact, calculations of this frequency (see Table 39-1) indicate a mutation rate of approximately 10^{-4} per allele per generation. Evidence based on linkage analysis has indicated that the vast majority of new mutations arise from the paternal allele,[60,61] indicating that these mutations apparently occur during spermatogenesis. Whether they are meiotic or mitotic errors has not been determined, although mitotic errors are suggested by the absence of a significant paternal age effect in new mutation cases.

With such a high mutation rate, it would be predicted that the reproductive fitness of individuals with NF1 must be significantly reduced in order for the disease to be present at an equilibrium frequency. The Welsh study[59] found a fitness of 0.31 for affected males and 0.60 for affected females (1.0 is the expected value). A large proportion of the reduced fertility can be attributed to a failure of affected individuals to marry, which presumably reflects the psychosocial consequences of the condition.

Penetrance

The penetrance of NF1 is essentially 100 percent in individuals who have reached adulthood and have been subjected to careful examination by an experienced physician, including a slit-lamp examination. Rare cases of normal parents giving rise to two affected children have been described[62] and could be examples of germ-line mosaicism in one of the parents, although the possibility of independent spontaneous mutations cannot be excluded until molecular studies are carried out in such patients. The importance of careful examination of both parents before giving genetic counseling cannot be overemphasized, however. There are numerous reports of circumstances in which one of the parents was sufficiently mildly affected to be unaware of his or her diagnosis.

Variable Expressivity

NF1 is a classic example of the tendency for autosomal dominant conditions to show variable expressivity, which can at times be dramatic in NF1. Even the more constant defining features of the disease are subject to considerable heterogeneity when considered closely. It has been known for some time that large families with multiple afflicted individuals are likely to demonstrate a wide range of severity and complications, and the variability within a family of significant size is similar to the variability seen in comparisons of different families. This indicates that the specific germ-line mutation at the *NF1* locus does not accurately predict the phenotype in a specific individual, since all affected individuals in the same family carry the same germ-line mutation.

To distinguish between genetic influences and environmental and/or chance influences, Easton and coworkers[63] examined a series of monozygotic twins concordant for NF1 and compared them with other pairs of first-degree affected relatives. There was a significant correlation in the number of café-au-lait spots and neurofibromas between identical twins, with a lower but significant correlation in first-degree relatives and almost no correlation between more distant relatives. This suggests that these features are controlled by other genetic influences but that the specific mutation in the *NF1* gene itself plays a minor role. Optic glioma, scoliosis, epilepsy, and learning disability were concordant in twin pairs, but plexiform neurofibromas were not. Furthermore, there was no indication that the presence of one complication predicted the occurrence of another except for the fact that neurofibrosarcoma has been observed commonly to occur almost exclusively in individuals with plexiform neurofibromas.

Related Syndromes

NF1 has been described in the literature in association with almost every imaginable disorder, but most of these reports appear to represent the coincidental occurrence of two unrelated conditions. A classification scheme proposed by Riccardi and Eichner[9] divides the neurofibromatoses into eight syndromes, but this scheme has not found wide application because of the blurred boundaries between several categories. A full discussion of variant syndromes is beyond the scope of this chapter, but a few of the most relevant conditions will be mentioned.

Neurofibromatosis Type 2. Type 2 neurofibromatosis, formerly designated *central neurofibromatosis* or *bilateral vestibular neurofibromatosis,* is now appreciated to be distinct, both clinically and genetically, from NF1.[64,65] The *NF2* gene has been mapped to chromosome 22 and was identified in 1993.[12,13] Individuals with NF2 often have a small number of café-au-lait spots (rarely more than six) and may have one or two peripheral neurofibromas but usually not more. They occasionally have Lisch nodules.[66] Ophthalmologic evaluation is extremely useful because of the presence of posterior subcapsular cataracts in a sizable proportion of these patients.[67] The hallmark of NF2 is the development of bilateral eighth cranial nerve tumors, properly called *vestibular schwannomas* rather than acoustic neuromas, in 95 percent of these patients by age 30 years.[64] Inheritance is autosomal dominant. Other tumors of cranial and cervical nerve roots are common, and management presents great challenges for neurosurgeons and otolaryngologists. Past statements that acoustic neuroma is a complication of NF1 are almost certainly due to the confusion between these two entities; since more careful definitions of the two disorders have been applied, there has been no indication that individuals with NF1 have an increased risk of eighth cranial nerve tumors compared with the general population. NF2 is much less common than NF1, affecting approximately 1 in 40,000 individuals.

Segmental (Mosaic) NF1. Occasionally individuals are encountered who have features of NF1 limited to one segment of the body.[68] These features may include café-au-lait spots, freckling, and peripheral or plexiform neurofibromas, and Lisch nodules may be seen in an individual who has that segment of the body affected. Such individuals invariably have normal parents but on rare occasions can have a child with classic NF1.[69] There is strong circumstantial evidence that these cases represent somatic mutation of the *NF1* gene early in embryogenesis so that derivatives of that mutant line display the features of NF1. If the mosaicism involves the germ line, the disease can then be transmitted. Recently, germ-line mosaicism for an *NF1* gene mutation was found in a clinically unaffected father of a child with new onset NF1.[70] In addition, somatic mosaicism for an *NF1* gene deletion was detected in an individual with NF1.[71] Analysis of cases of segmental NF1 probably will demonstrate similar somatic mosaicism.

Watson Syndrome. A variant of NF1 that appears to breed true in certain families involves multiple café-au-lait spots, dull intelligence, short stature, pulmonary valvular stenosis, and only a small number of neurofibromas.[72] Reevaluation of these families has indicated that they also have Lisch nodules, further contributing to the blurring of these two phenotypes. In fact, molecular analyses have demonstrated that in at least two families that appear to fall into the category of Watson syndrome, deletions are present in the *NF1* gene. Currently, there appears to be no distinguishing aspect between the deletions causing Watson syndrome and those associated with more classic NF1.

Neurofibromatosis–Noonan Syndrome. The occurrence of features reminiscent of Noonan syndrome in patients with neurofibromatosis 1 has been noted for some time,[73] raising the question of whether these could be overlapping syndromes or even could be due to deletion of adjacent genes. In most of these families, however, individuals with clear-cut Noonan syndrome represent only a proportion of those affected with NF1, and some of the features associated with Noonan syndrome (such as pectus excavatum, mild hypertelorism, and short stature) are frequently observed in NF1.[74] A linkage study of autosomal dominant Noonan syndrome occurring in the absence of NF1 has indicated no linkage to markers in the *NF1* region of chromosome 17, casting into doubt any notion that Noonan syndrome, at least in the aggregate, could be due to a mutation in a gene closely adjacent to *NF1*. At least one family with neurofibromatosis–Noonan syndrome (NFNS) has been found to harbor a deletion in the *NF1* gene, but the fact that very large deletions removing flanking regions on either side of *NF1* do not consistently result in NFNS casts further doubt on the adjacent gene theory. The most appropriate synthesis of the data at the present time indicates that the phenotype of NF1 can include features that overlap with those described in Noonan syndrome, but these disorders are probably genetically distinct.

Spinal Neurofibromatosis. Rare families have been identified with a predominance of spinal tumors and relatively few peripheral neurofibromas. A linkage study has indicated that one such family appears to be linked to NF1, whereas another does not, implying locus heterogeneity for this set of conditions.[75] While this condition underscores the variable expressivity of NF1, spinal neurofibromatosis does not represent a distinct subtype of NF1.

MOLECULAR BIOLOGY OF THE *NF1* GENE

Cloning of the *NF1* Gene

Since no information was available on the structure or function of the *NF1* gene product before the 1980s, the only feasible approach available to identify the gene was positional cloning.[76] The isolation of the gene for von Recklinghausen neurofibromatosis began with an international collaboration to assemble linkage data in families with NF1. By early 1987, this worldwide effort made possible the construction of an exclusion map that narrowed the candidate chromosomes to a handful.[77] Examination of these selected chromosomes with RFLP markers culminated in the establishment of linkage of NF1 to the pericentromeric region of chromosome 17 in the late spring of 1987.[77–80] No linkage disequilibrium was ever found. One of the linked markers was an anonymous probe called pA10-41, and another was the gene for nerve growth factor receptor (17q12-22).[81] The linkage of NF1 with the nerve growth factor (NGF) receptor gene was exciting because of the role of NGF in neural crest tissue development. Further analysis using RFLP markers, however, excluded the NGF receptor gene as a candidate for the *NF1* gene, since numerous crossover events were identified.[82]

An intense genetic mapping effort resulted in the establishment of a multipoint linkage map constructed from data assembled by the NF1 collaborative group (Fig. 39-7). This map represented the outcome of the study of 142 families with over 700 affected individuals and narrowed the distance between flanking probes and the *NF1* gene to 3 cM, or about 3 million bp.[83] Candidate genes in this interval, such as the *erbA1* and *erbB2* proto-oncogenes, were subsequently excluded as candidate genes for NF1 by the identification of recombinants.

The discovery of two patients with NF1 and balanced translocations involving the long arm of chromosome 17 dramatically accelerated the process. These two NF1 patients had reciprocal translocations, one between chromosomes 1p34.3

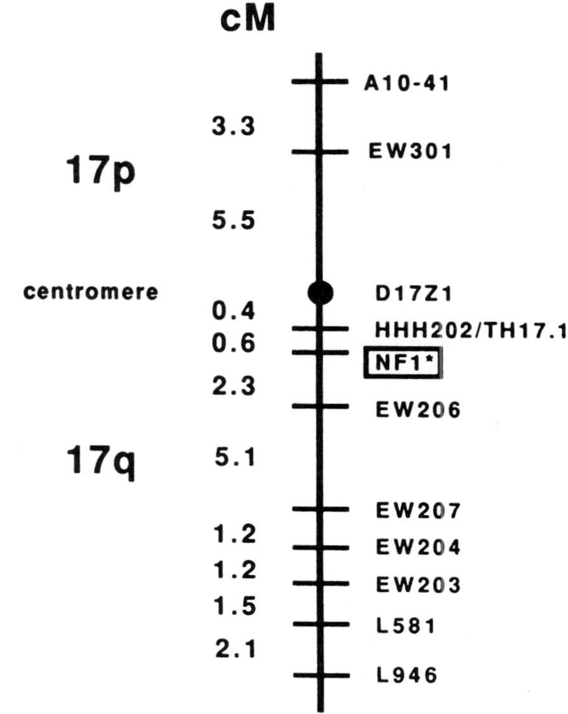

Fig. 39-7 Linkage map for chromosome 17 demonstrating the position of the *NF1* locus relative to other DNA markers linked to the disease. The map distance of the various markers is represented in centimorgans (cM).

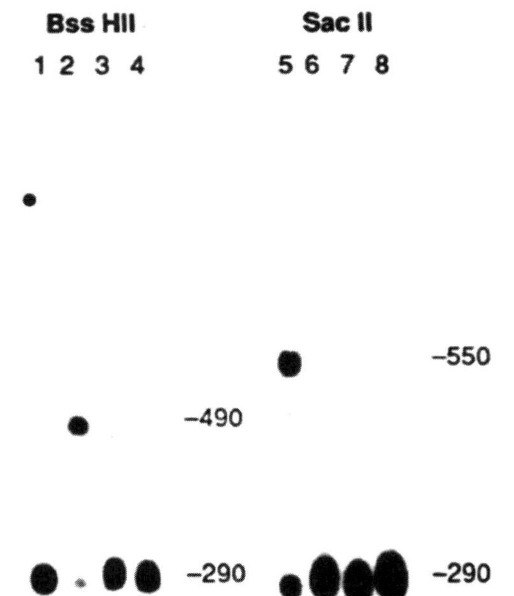

Fig. 39-8 Pulsed-field gel analysis with probe 17L1A in an NF1 patient with [1;17] translocation. Genomic DNA is digested with a rare-cutting restriction enzyme (either BssHII or SacII), separated by pulsed-field gel electrophoresis, and probed with 17L1A. The DNA source in each lane is 1 and 8, patients with NF1; 2 and 5, a patient with a 1;17 translocation has a unique band not seen in the other DNA samples, indicating the presence of a rearrangement of the DNA in the region near the *NF1* gene in this patient. (*Adapted from Fountain et al.*[84] *Used by permission.*)

and 17q11.2 and the other between chromosomes 17q11.2 and 22q11.2.[84-88] Support for the notion that these translocations disrupt the *NF1* gene was provided by the fact that one breakpoint in each of the translocations involved 17q11.2, precisely where the *NF1* gene had been mapped by linkage analysis.

The identification of translocation breakpoints permitted analysis of the genetic region by physical mapping techniques and bridged the gap between linkage mapping and physical mapping.[89] Using restriction enzymes that recognize rare restriction sites in DNA, one could search for an anomalously migrating DNA fragment resulting from the disruption of this region by the translocations. To identify the translocation breakpoints by physical mapping, markers capable of visualizing these areas had to be generated. Using a series of chromosome 17-specific *NotI*-linking clones tested against a somatic cell hybrid mapping panel, a clone termed *17L1A* was identified that detected abnormalities by pulsed-field gel electrophoresis in the 1;17 translocation patient and her affected offspring (Fig. 39-8). The presence of abnormal fragments provided conclusive evidence that the translocation breakpoints map near the 17L1A clone.

The use of cosmid libraries to look for abnormal fragments on pulsed-field gel electrophoresis provided an additional clone, called *1F10,* that detected abnormal fragments in both translocation patients. These two cloned probes were then shown to reside on the same 600-kb DNA fragment and bracketed the two translocations. This narrowed the interval in which the *NF1* gene must reside to 600 kb of DNA.[87] Of interest was the fact that 17L1A represented a CpG island, a hypomethylated region often associated with five regulatory sequences of active genes.

The construction of a physical map of the region around the *NF1* gene laid the groundwork for identifying candidate cDNA transcripts. Using a combination of jump library clones, yeast artificial chromosome probes, and cosmids, candidate cDNA transcripts were identified. Unexpectedly, however, the first candidate gene came from another route: By comparison with a syntenic region on mouse chromosome 11, the mouse *evi2* gene, which is involved in virally induced murine leukemia, was found to map between these two breakpoints.[90-92] Cloning of the human *EVI2A* gene excluded it as a candidate for the *NF1* gene in that neither translocation actually interrupted the gene and no mutations were found in it in other patients with NF1.[93] A second candidate gene, *EVI2B,* similar to *EVI2A,* was identified but also was excluded as a potential candidate.[92] The third candidate gene, *OMGP* (oligodendrocyte myelin glycoprotein), which was exciting because of its almost exclusive expression in Schwann cells and oligodendrocytes, also failed to satisfy the criteria for an *NF1* gene candidate, since no mutations could be identified in this gene in NF1 patients.[94,95]

The fourth candidate gene was much larger and was cloned and shown to be the *NF1* gene in several ways.[1-3] First, the transcript crossed both translocation breakpoints and would therefore be interrupted in these unique NF1 patients.[1-3] Second, more subtle mutations were identified in patients with NF1 that would alter the coding potential of this candidate transcript.[2] These included a patient with a *de novo* 400-nucleotide insertion that produced an abnormally large fragment on Southern blot analysis using the NF1 cDNA as a probe and another patient with a nonsense mutation.[96] These mutations provided conclusive evidence that the correct gene had been found.

The *NF1* gene has an open reading frame of nearly 9 kb and spans approximately 300 kb of genomic DNA[97] (Fig. 39-9). The messenger RNA has been estimated to be 11 to 13 kb and has been detected in all tissues examined by RT-PCR and northern blot analysis. At least 57 exons have been identified, with three additional alternatively spliced exons (see "Identification of NF1 Gene Product" below). The three previous candidate genes were all found embedded in one large intron and were transcribed from the opposite strand from the *NF1* gene.[93] The predicted protein has 2818 amino acids and a molecular weight of 327 kDa.[98] Analysis of the amino acid sequence failed to reveal any nuclear localization signals or transmembrane domains, suggesting that the gene product resides in the cytoplasm. Comparison of the gene with other previously identified coding sequences revealed unexpected sequence similarity between the *NF1* gene product and a family of GTPase-activating proteins (GAPs) (see "Neurofibromin as a GTPase-Activating Protein" below).[4] Analyses of homologous genes from mouse, chicken, hamster, and *Drosophila* species demonstrate striking species conservation and underscore the fundamental importance of this gene.[99-102]

Further analysis of the genomic organization of the *NF1* gene demonstrated that the promoter of this gene resides within a CpG-rich region; this is consistent with the observation that most active eukaryotic gene promoters are contained within CpG islands.[103] During the construction of a yeast artificial chromosome contig containing the entire *NF1* gene, other homologous loci were found by low-stringency hybridization on Southern blot.[104,105] These loci were determined by a hybrid mapping panel and fluorescent *in situ* hybridization to reside on chromosomes 14, 15, and 22. At least two loci were found on chromosome 14. These homologous loci apparently represent unprocessed pseudogenes in that their coding sequences contain frameshift, nonsense, and missense mutations. However, these loci also may represent mutation reservoirs that can be crossed into the *NF1* locus on chromosome 17 by interchromosomal gene conversion. This phenomenon potentially could contribute to the high rate of mutation in NF1.

Patient Mutations

Analysis of NF1 patients for mutations is still in its infancy and is hampered by the large size of the gene. Approximately 20 mutations have been studied in some detail. Five types of *NF1* gene mutations have been described to date in patients with NF1: (1) Translocations have been described in two patients with NF1 and were described earlier in this chapter. These balanced translocations provided some of the first clues to the precise physical location of the *NF1* gene on chromosome 17. (2) Megabase deletions have been reported in patients with NF1.[38]

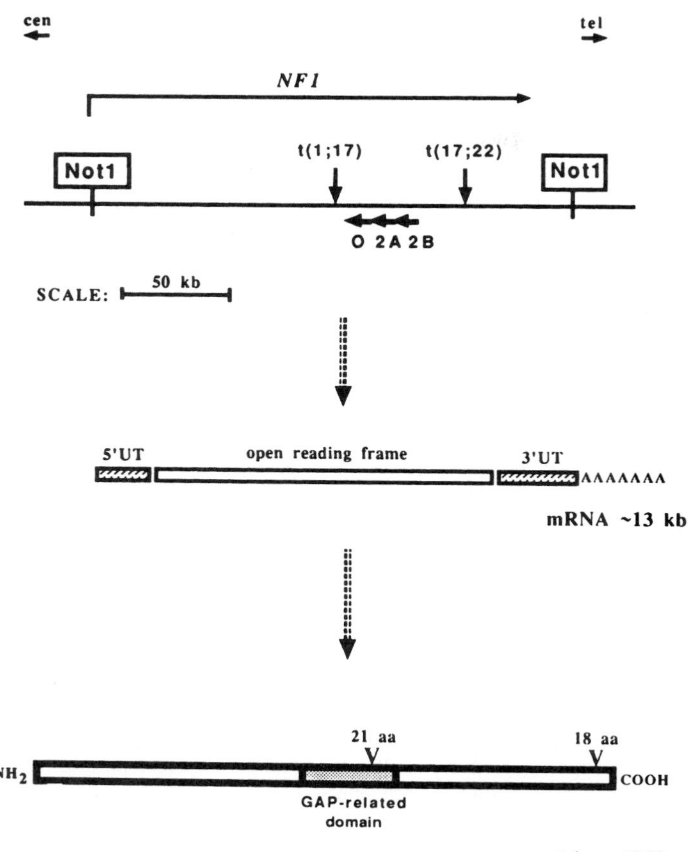

Fig. 39-9 The genetic organization of the *NF1* locus. The genomic structure of the *NF1* locus demonstrates the location of the two NotI restriction sites separated by 1300 kb. The initiation codon is located upstream of the centromeric NotI site and is positioned within a CpG-rich area. The position of the two translocation breakpoints [t(1;17) and t(17;22)] described in two patients with NF1 and their interruption of the *NF1* gene are illustrated. Three genes (O for *OMgP,* 2A for *EVI2A,* and 2B for *EVI2B*) are embedded within one intron on the opposite strand from the *NF1* gene. The mRNA for NF1 is 11 to 13 kb and has an open reading frame of 8454 nucleotides with at least 2 kb of 3′ untranslated sequence. Translation of this open reading frame predicts a protein of 2818 amino acids with an estimated molecular weight of 327 kDa. Sequence similarity between a central 300- to 400-amino-acid region of the *NF1* gene product, neurofibromin, and a family of GTPase-activating proteins (GAPs) is illustrated by the GAP-related domain. The location of the two alternatively spliced isoforms is denoted by the 21-amino-acid insertion into the GAP-related domain and the 18-amino-acid insertion in the C-terminus of neurofibromin.

These deletions extend well beyond the *NF1* gene and may include other genes on chromosome 17q11.2. These patients manifest typical NF1 but also have significant mental retardation. (3) Large internal deletions entirely contained within the *NF1* gene have been reported in patients with NF1. One of these deletions removed 90 kb of DNA encompassing the 5′ portion of the *NF1* gene, while the other deleted 40 kb of NF1 DNA.[106] The phenotypes of these patients were indistinguishable from those of classic NF1 patients. (4) Small rearrangements within the *NF1* gene have been described. One of these rearrangements involved the insertion of a human Alu repeat in the intron between two *NF1* exons, resulting in abnormal mRNA splicing and premature termination of the *NF1* mRNA coding sequence.[96] (5) Many point mutations have been described in patients with NF1.[2] These mutations include the creation of stop codons, missense mutations, and frameshift mutations. One of these missense mutations involves a nonconservative substitution at codon 1423 within the NF1-GAP-related domain (*NF1GRD*).[107] This mutation, when expressed in insect Sf9 cells, results in a reduced ability of the *NF1GRD* to accelerate the hydrolysis of *ras*-GTP and perhaps altered *NF1* gene product, termed *neurofibromin,* function. This mutation also has been observed in anaplastic astrocytomas and colonic adenocarcinomas. Thus far there does not appear to be a hotspot for mutation within the *NF1* gene, since all these mutations are randomly distributed throughout the *NF1* coding sequences.[108] To this end, the phenotypes of patients with all the preceding mutation types (except megabase deletions) are likely to be similar in that they all result in the loss of a functional protein. The fact that mutations all result in a loss of *NF1* protein function is consistent with the notion of *NF1* as a tumor-suppressor gene.

The tumor-suppressor mechanism suggests that loss of both copies of the *NF1* gene would culminate in a transformed or neoplastic phenotype.[109–112] In this hypothesis, affected individuals would inherit one mutated *NF1* gene from their parents (or as a new mutation), but neurofibromas or neurofibrosarcomas would develop only when the second gene became nonfunctional as a result of somatic mutation. This set of events is termed the *Knudson hypothesis* and was first elegantly demonstrated for retinoblastoma.[113,114] In patients with retinoblastoma, all somatic cells contain the germ-line-inherited mutation in one of the retinoblastoma genes. Retinoblastomas arise as a result of loss of the second copy of the retinoblastoma gene in retinal cells.

Occasionally, the second somatic mutation in the tumor can be detected by Southern blot analysis. In white blood cells from patients with NF1, the DNA may be heterozygous for a particular DNA marker polymorphism on chromosome 17, but when tumor cells develop, the remaining wild-type gene is lost, eliminating that particular allele (Fig. 39-10). This is termed *loss of*

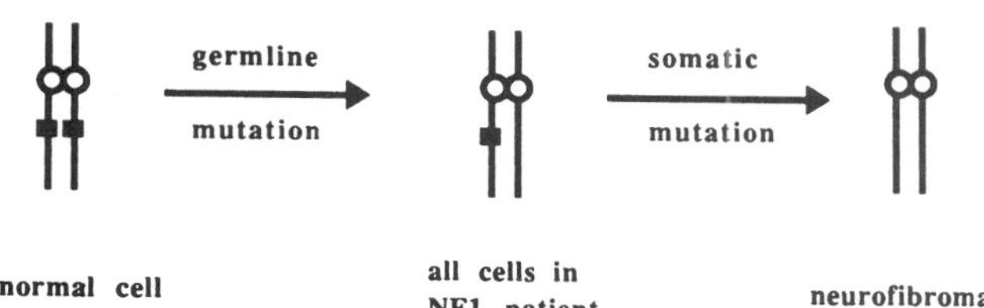

Fig. 39-10 Illustration of loss of heterozygosity in NF1. A given DNA marker polymorphism, denoted by the filled squares, is present in a normal NF1 chromosome 17. A germ-line mutation found in all cells in an NF1 patient would alter the *NF1* gene to result in the loss of one of the DNA markers. Because the patient has one normal chromosome 17 DNA polymorphism and one mutated chromosome 17 DNA polymorphism, the patient is said to be heterozygous with respect to that DNA marker. Mutation of the one remaining normal *NF1* gene in a tumor results in the loss of both copies of the gene and loss of heterozygosity with respect to that DNA marker polymorphism.

heterozygosity and is taken as proof that a second somatic event has occurred that results in the loss of the one remaining functional *NF1* gene. Interpretation of these data for chromosome 17 are confounded by the frequent loss of heterozygosity for markers near the *p53* gene on chromosome 17p as well.[115] Loss of heterozygosity centered at the *NF1* locus has been observed in selected tumors from some patients with NF1, supporting the notion that *NF1* is a tumor-suppressor gene and that the manifestations of the disease result from somatic loss of the second *NF1* gene copy. A tumor in an NF1 patient has been found to display loss of heterozygosity for chromosome 17 markers but in addition demonstrates a large deletion in the *NF1* gene in tumor cell but not white blood cell DNA.[116] This supports the notion that a "second hit" occurs in the *NF1* gene during the development of neurofibrosarcomas in patients with NF1.

Mutations in the *NF1* gene have been described in other tumor types, including malignant melanomas, neuroblastomas, pheochromocytomas, and neurofibrosarcomas.[117,118] Examination of a series of malignant melanoma cell lines derived from metastatic foci demonstrated reduced or absent neurofibromin expression in up to 25 percent of tumors.[119,120] Similar examination of neuroblastomas revealed that *NF1* mRNA and neurofibromin expression is reduced in up to 30 percent of neuroblastomas.[120,121] Similarly, three neurofibrosarcomas derived from NF1 patients demonstrated elevated levels of *ras*-GTP and nearly undetectable levels of neurofibromin, suggesting a relationship between lack of neurofibromin expression and unregulated *ras* activity in these cells (see below).[122,123] Abnormalities at the DNA level have been reported for pheochromocytomas from NF1 patients.[124] Examination of these fresh tumors demonstrated loss of neurofibromin expression in six of six pheochromocytomas as well as one adrenal cortical tumor from patients with NF1.[125] It is likely that examination of other tumors will uncover alterations in neurofibromin expression that are consistent with its proposed role as a tumor-suppressor gene product. Consistent with the proposed role of neurofibromin as a negative growth regulator, tumors from patients with and without NF1 have been examined for alterations in *NF1* gene expression. The hallmark of NF1 is the neurofibroma, a benign tumor composed predominantly of Schwann cells, fibroblasts, and to a lesser extent, mast cells. It has been presumed that the cellular defect in the neurofibroma results from abnormal Schwann cell function secondary to loss of neurofibromin function. Malignancies in NF1 are believed to result from the constitutional inactivation of one *NF1* gene followed by a number of somatic events, including inactivation of the other *NF1* allele. Although loss of the normal allele has been proved for the malignant nerve sheath tumor (neurofibrosarcoma),[116] it had not been evaluated in the etiology of the benign neurofibroma. Recent work has demonstrated loss of heterozygosity in 22 neurofibromas from five unrelated NF1 patients.[126] In eight of these tumors, somatic deletions involving the wild-type *NF1* gene could be demonstrated, indicating that inactivation of the normal *NF1* gene is associated with the development of the neurofibroma. In related studies on Schwann cells derived from the dorsal root ganglia of neurofibromin-deficient mice, abnormalities in Schwann cell proliferation and high levels of activated p21-*ras* were observed, as would be predicted by loss of neurofibromin GAP function.[127] In addition, these neurofibromin-deficient Schwann cells had abnormal proliferative responses to neuronal contact.[128] Additional studies also have demonstrated abnormalities in fibroblasts derived from neurofibromin-deficient mouse embryos.[129] These results collectively suggest that defects in both the Schwann cells and the fibroblasts may contribute to the development of the benign neurofibroma.

Children with NF1 are at increased risk for the development of malignant myeloid disorders. Although myeloid disorders are an uncommon complication of NF1 in childhood, NF1 constitutes as many as 10 percent of the spontaneous cases of myeloid proliferative disorders in children. Examination of bone marrow samples from children with NF1 in whom malignant myeloid disorders developed demonstrated loss of heterozygosity at the *NF1* locus.[130] In each case, the mutant *NF1* allele was inherited from the parent with NF1, and the normal allele was deleted in the myeloid leukemic cells. These results are consistent with the hypothesis that loss of neurofibromin expression predisposes myeloid cells to leukemic transformation. Mice heterozygous for a germ-line *NF1* mutation also develop myeloid leukemias with loss of the wild-type *NF1* allele in the leukemic cells.[131] Analysis of these myeloid leukemic cells with loss of neurofibromin expression demonstrates an exaggerated and prolonged increase in p21-*ras* activation in response to granulocyte macrophage colony stimulating factor (GM-CSF). This increased sensitivity to GM-CSF reflects abnormal p21-*ras* signaling that probably leads to chronic clonal hyperproliferation and malignant transformation. Primary leukemic cells from children with NF1 also show an exaggerated increase in p21-*ras* activity in response to GM-CSF.[132]

Additional support for the hypothesis that neurofibromin functions to suppress growth by regulating *ras* derives from experiments on the ability of one of these neurofibrosarcoma cell lines (ST88-14) to grow in soft agar.[133] Whereas ST88-14 cells form colonies in soft agar, ST88-14 cells treated with pharmacologic agents that block *ras* function fail to grow in soft agar. These results argue that neurofibromin loss leads to increased *ras* activity, which in turn is partly responsible for the abnormal growth properties of these tumor cells.

Animal Models

The search for spontaneous animal models of NF1 was initially disappointing. Three early models of NF1 were reported. In the bicolor damselfish, spontaneous neurofibromas and hyperpigmented spots develop, but the disorder appears to be transmissible, and these tumors tend to be more invasive and malignant than human neurofibromas.[134] One murine model was reported as resulting from the overexpression of the HTLV-I *tat* gene in mice.[135] Neurofibroma-like tumors developed in the offspring. However, other phenotypic features of NF1 were absent, and the neurofibromas lacked Schwann cells, unlike human NF1 neurofibromas. Similarly, the relationship between HTLV-I and human NF1 is unclear, since there is no increased incidence of HTLV-I exposure or infection in NF1 patients.[136] The third model of NF1 was achieved by injecting *N*-nitroso-*N*-ethylurea into pregnant Syrian golden hamsters.[102,137] The progeny develop neurofibromas histologically identical to those observed in NF1 patients, as well as pigmented lesions similar to café-au-lait spots. However, these hamsters also have Wilms tumors and other malignancies not typically seen in NF1 patients. Recently, point mutations in the *neu* proto-oncogene were identified in these hamster tumors. No mutations have been identified to date in the hamster *NF1* gene by Southern or Western blot analysis.[137]

In an effort to develop a mouse model for neurofibromatosis 1, mice were generated that carried a null mutation at the murine *NF1* locus using gene targeting in embryonic stem cells.[138,139] Heterozygous mutant mice containing one mutant *NF1* and one wild-type allele are phenotypically normal without evidence of neurofibromas, pigmentary abnormalities, or Lisch nodules. However, 75 percent of heterozygous mice succumb to tumors within 27 months compared with 15 percent of wild-type animals.[138] In addition to developing the tumor type seen in older wild-type mice, heterozygote *NF1* mice develop certain tumor types characteristic of human NF1. One animal developed a neurofibrosarcoma at 21 months of age, and 12 developed adrenal tumors at 15 to 28 months. Nine of the adrenal tumors were pheochromocytomas. Examination of these tumors demonstrated loss of the wild-type *NF1* allele and evidence of reduction to homozygosity for the *NF1* gene in the tumor DNA. These data support the hypothesis that the loss of *NF1* gene function contributes to the development of tumors.

The breeding of heterozygous knockout animals to yield mice in which both copies of the *NF1* gene were disrupted by homologous recombination (homozygous knockout mice) produced embryos that died *in utero* from generalized tissue edema.[138,139] Examination of the hearts in these mice at embryonic day 12.5 demonstrates a double-outlet right ventricle defect resulting from a failure of the aorta and pulmonary artery to separate. Double-outlet right ventricles have been observed in developing chicks in which the neural crest cells migrating to form elements of the cardiac vasculature are ablated. These results suggest that neurofibromin may be critical for the function of these neural crest–derived cells, although other mechanisms are possible. In addition to the cardiac vessel defect, the skeletal musculature is hypoplastic relative to normal mouse embryos. The existence of a muscle-specific isoform of the *NF1* gene and the observation that neurofibromin expression is increased in skeletal and cardiac muscle during embryonic development argue that neurofibromin also may be critical for normal muscle differentiation.[140,141] Additionally, examination of the sympathetic ganglia in these homozygous mutant mice demonstrates hyperplasia and an increased mitotic index.[142] These neurons also exhibit a reduced requirement for exogenous survival factors (neurotrophins), arguing that loss of neurofibromin may drive some cells to proliferate even in the absence of survival factors. In addition, there may be some genetic cooperativity between NF1 and p53 such that superior cervical ganglia neurons deficient in both neurofibromin and p53 have longer survival in the absence of neurotrophins.[143]

Mice heterozygous for a targeted mutation in the *Nf1* gene ($Nf1^{+/-}$) have been carefully analyzed for features seen in patients with NF1 who also are heterozygous for a mutant *Nf1* allele. $Nf1^{+/-}$ mice demonstrate learning and memory deficits.[144] As observed in people with NF1, these deficits are restricted to specific types of learning (spatial memory but not associative learning), are not fully penetrant, and can be compensated for with extended training.

In *Drosophila,* the *NF1* gene may function in the protein kinase A (PKA) signaling pathway.[145] Targeted disruption of both *Drosophila NF1* genes results in reductions in fly size. Whereas homozygous null $NF1^{-/-}$ mice are embryonic lethal, *Drosophila NF1*-null flies are fertile and viable. Partial rescue of the *Drosophila* mutant phenotype can be obtained with activated PKA. In addition, *Drosophila NF1* is essential for the response to certain polypeptides at the neuromuscular junction in flies.[146]

Identification of the *NF1* Gene Product

The protein product of the *NF1* locus has been identified. Using antibodies generated against fusion proteins and synthetic peptides, a unique 250-kDa protein is identifiable in all cell lines examined.[147–151] This NF1-GAP-related protein was originally termed *NF1GRP* to underscore its relationship to mammalian GAP and the yeast *IRA1* and *IRA2* genes (see below).[4,149] The NNFF consortium agreed to call this protein product *neurofibromin.* This protein was localized to the cytoplasm by differential centrifugation, glycerol gradients, and indirect immunofluorescence.[147,150] The difference between the predicted (327 kDa) and the observed (250 kDa) molecular weights results from anomalous migration in SDS-PAGE, not from posttranslational modifications (DH Gutmann, unpublished results). Expression of the full-length cDNA in insect cells produces a protein that migrates at 250 kDa.[153] Similarly, antibodies directed against both N- and C-terminal epitopes all recognize the same 250-kDa protein.[154]

The tissue distribution of neurofibromin is somewhat controversial in that the mRNA appears to be present at some level in all tissues.[1] Initial examination of whole-cell homogenates from mouse and rat tissues suggested that neurofibromin also was ubiquitously expressed.[149] Subsequent analysis by western blotting, immunoprecipitation, and immunohistochemistry demonstrated that the highest levels of expression are in the brain, spleen, kidney, testis, and thymus[102,148] (DH Gutmann, unpublished data). Immunohistochemical analysis of tissue sections from human and rodent tissues demonstrates prominent nervous system expression of neurofibromin.[102,147,148] Neurofibromin can be detected in the dendritic processes of central nervous system neurons (pyramidal neurons in cortical layers 2 and 5 and cerebellar Purkinje cells), peripheral nervous system neuronal axons, nonmyelinating Schwann cells, oligodendrocytes, and dorsal root ganglia but not astrocytes, microglia, and myelinating Schwann cells.[148,155] Neurofibromin expression is expressed in reactive astrocytes.[156] There does not appear to be abundant expression in adult lung, muscle, intestine, heart, or skin.

The expression of neurofibromin during embryogenesis is being studied in the avian and rodent systems. Preliminary results suggest that neurofibromin is expressed in the developing brain and spinal cord.[100,101] This pattern of expression potentially could account for the described learning disabilities previously unattributable to a purely neural crest–derived tissue disorder. Neurofibromin expression appears to rise dramatically after day 10 of mouse development. In the rat, neurofibromin is ubiquitously expressed from days 10 through 16, after which it becomes increased in spinal cord and brain.[157] At this time, neurofibromin can be found in skeletal muscle, skin, lung, adrenal cortex, and cartilage. By postnatal day 6, the distribution of neurofibromin is identical to that seen in adults. These data, combined with the observation that homozygous mouse *NF1* gene knockouts exhibit developmental arrest and death around embryonic day 13, suggest that events occurring during this time interval depend heavily on the proper expression of neurofibromin. Future studies directed at understanding these events will provide insights into the pathogenesis of NF1.

Neurofibromin as a GTPase-Activating Protein

As mentioned earlier, analysis of the amino acid sequence of the *NF1* gene product revealed sequence similarity between a small portion of the gene and a family of GAPs.[4,158–163] These proteins, both in mammals and in yeast, appear to regulate the GTP state of the cellular p21-*ras* proto-oncogene.[164,165] GAP molecules accelerate the hydrolysis of p21-*ras*-GTP to p21-*ras*-GDP, converting the proto-oncogene from the active form to the inactive form.[162,166] Although the effector of p21-*ras* in mammalian cells is unknown, in yeast, p21-*ras* is important in cAMP regulation.[164,167,168] This sequence similarity was supported by functional studies in mammalian cells and yeast, suggesting that the NF1GRD can act as a GAP molecule *in vitro* and *in vivo*.[5–7,169,170] Recent experiments also have demonstrated that the full-length neurofibromin molecule has GAP-like activity.[122,123,153]

It is exciting to postulate that neurofibromin functions as a tumor-suppressor gene product by down-regulating the normal function of the p21-*ras* proto-oncogene (Fig. 39-11). Previous studies demonstrated that p21-*ras* functions as part of a tyrosine kinase signal transduction pathway involving receptor tyrosine kinases such as epidermal, nerve, and platelet-derived growth factors (EGF, NGF, and PDGF) receptors.[171–173] Support for the involvement of p21-*ras* in such pathways derives from a large number of experiments in a wide variety of signal transduction systems. First, overexpression of the active form of p21-*ras* (v-*ras*) results in neurite extension in a rat pheochromocytoma cell line (PC12) similar to that observed with NGF treatment.[174,175] This effect can be reversed by injecting PC12 cells with antibodies against p21-*ras*.[176] There are conflicting data regarding the existence of a separate p21-*ras*-independent pathway that also culminates in neurite extension.[177] Second, overexpression of activated p21-*ras* can induce morphologic transformation of fibroblast cell lines and unlimited cell proliferation.[178,179] Third, some fibroblast cell lines can be induced to differentiate into adipocytes with overexpression of activated p21-*ras*.[180] Fourth, p21-*ras* is associated with surface immunoglobulin capping as part of a signal transduction (antigen presentation) pathway in B lymphocytes.[181,182]

GAP molecules such as mammalian GAP and the yeast IRA1 and IRA2 proteins may serve to regulate p21-*ras*-mediated growth and differentiation pathways by maintaining p21-*ras* in the

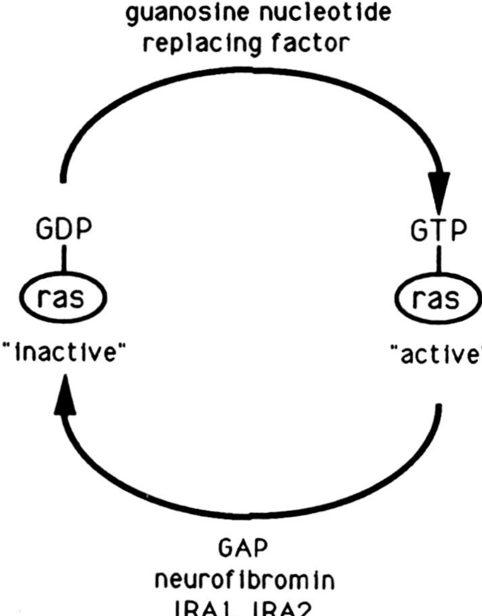

Fig. 39-11 The p21-*ras* cycle of activation and inactivation by GAP-related proteins. p21-*ras* is inactive in the GDP-bound state and is converted to an active GTP-bound state by guanosine nucleotide-replacing proteins that substitute GTP for GDP. Interaction of GAP-like proteins with p21-*ras* accelerates the conversion of p21-*ras*-GTP to p21-*ras*-GDP by increasing the intrinsic GTPase activity of p21-*ras* and converting p21-*ras* to the inactive GDP-bound form. In resting cells, the majority of p21-*ras* is inactive and in the GDP-bound form.

inactive GDP-bound state. This model is supported by studies that demonstrate that stimulation of tyrosine kinase receptors such as the EGF and PDGF receptors results in phosphorylation of mammalian GAP on tyrosine residues and inactivation of its GTPase-activating properties.[172,183,184] This inactivation would lead to increased p21-*ras* in the active GTP-bound state and to unregulated cell proliferation in the case of EGF and PDGF. The role of GAP in NGF receptor signal transduction pathways leading to cell differentiation and neurite extension is less well understood. By analogy, it is appealing to suggest that inactivation of neurofibromin as a result of mutation results in higher levels of p21-*ras*-GTP within affected cells and unlimited cell proliferation, leading to the formation of neurofibromas or neurofibrosarcomas. As was stated previously, examination of three neurofibrosarcomas demonstrated dramatically reduced expression of neurofibromin and elevated p21-*ras*-GTP levels.[122,123] Neurofibromin is phosphorylated on serine and threonine residues in response to EGF and PDGF stimulation but not on tyrosine residues and therefore must involve a pathway distinct from the tyrosine phosphorylation cascade that acts on mammalian GAP.[185,186]

Recent studies have suggested that neurofibromin may suppress cell growth through mechanisms unrelated to *ras* regulation. In NIH3T3 fibroblasts, overexpression of the *NF1* tumor-suppressor gene resulted in a threefold reduction in cell growth without any changes in *ras* activity.[187] Similarly, overexpression of full-length neurofibromin in a human colon carcinoma cell line resulted in reduced tumor growth in nude mice. In these experiments, the growth-suppressor activity of neurofibromin resulted from neurofibromin interfering with *ras* activation of *raf*.[188,189] Finally, *ras* activity can regulate neurofibromin expression.[44] This finding suggests either that neurofibromin is a critical regulator of *ras* in some cells or that neurofibromin may be stimulated by *ras* activation to perform some other function or functions within cells. Further work will be required to distinguish between these nonmutually exclusive possibilities.

Neurofibromin Associates with Cytoplasmic Microtubules

Subcellular localization of neurofibromin demonstrated an association with cytoplasmic microtubules by indirect immunofluorescence and biochemical purification.[150,154,190] Previously described microtubule-associated proteins (MAPs) fall into three classes based on their molecular weights: MAP1 (250 kDa), MAP2 (250 kDa), and tau (35 to 65 kDa).[191–194] Some of these proteins are involved in the stabilization of microtubules through bundling, a process in which the tight association of microtubule filaments is facilitated.[195,196] Other MAP molecules actively promote microtubule movement, and some are involved in microtubule-mediated intracytoplasmic transport.[197] Subpopulations of microtubules are implicated in signal transduction pathways involving neurotransmitters and surface receptors.[198]

Biochemical properties of MAP molecules include GTP and temperature-dependent microtubule association, dissociation from microtubules by ion-exchange chromatography, improved association with taxol treatment, and coimmunoprecipitation with tubulin.[199–204] These properties have been observed with neurofibromin and indicate that there are specific interactions between neurofibromin and microtubules. Studies also have demonstrated that tubulin can partially inhibit the GAP activity of neurofibromin, an effect that is reversed with antitubulin antibodies.[153] In addition, a 20-amino-acid sequence is found in neurofibromin that is shared with two other MAP molecules (MAP2 and tau) and has been reported to be a serine phosphorylation sequence that is important in regulating tau association with microtubules.[150,205] Phosphorylation of tau on that serine residue results in a conformational change and dissociation from the microtubules.

The finding that neurofibromin associates with microtubules does not mean that neurofibromin is a MAP. Intracytoplasmic organelles copurify with microtubules in a manner analogous to MAP molecules, yet these organelles would not be considered MAP molecules because they lack a role in stabilizing or facilitating microtubule-mediated functions. Further examination of the biochemical and physical nature of this association is necessary before neurofibromin can be assigned as a member of the MAP family.

The discovery that neurofibromin is a GAP-like molecule that associates with microtubules suggests several hypotheses to explain its function in cell growth and differentiation (Fig. 39-12). One model, which fits the upstream view of p21-*ras*-GAP interactions, envisions that neurofibromin is regulated by serine/threonine kinases.[206,207] Neurofibromin would be active as a GAP while associated with microtubules, keeping p21-*ras* in the inactive form and inhibiting cell division. After phosphorylation, neurofibromin would dissociate from the microtubules, and its GAP activity would be reduced or altered. Alternatively, neurofibromin could be compartmentalized in the microtubule compartment (perhaps performing some other function) until it is required for the control of p21-*ras*. Phosphorylation of neurofibromin on critical serine residues would release it from the microtubules to interact with p21-*ras*. Support for this alternative model is provided by experiments that have failed to demonstrate any alteration of GAP activity after neurofibromin phosphorylation *in vitro*. Similarly, the interaction of neurofibromin with microtubules may actually reduce its GAP activity, as suggested by recent experiments,[153] and its dissociation from the microtubules may allow neurofibromin to associate with and down-regulate p21-*ras*. Of interest is the finding that the same domain of neurofibromin, the GAP-related domain, is the portion of neurofibromin required for microtubule association, suggesting a direct relationship between neurofibromin, p21-*ras* regulation, and microtubule association.[152,153,208] Further studies have demonstrated the involvement of neurofibromin in a B-lymphocyte signal transduction pathway involving microtubules and p21-*ras*. In this system, neurofibromin and p21-*ras* colocalize during immunoglobulin receptor internalization, and neurofibromin is rapidly

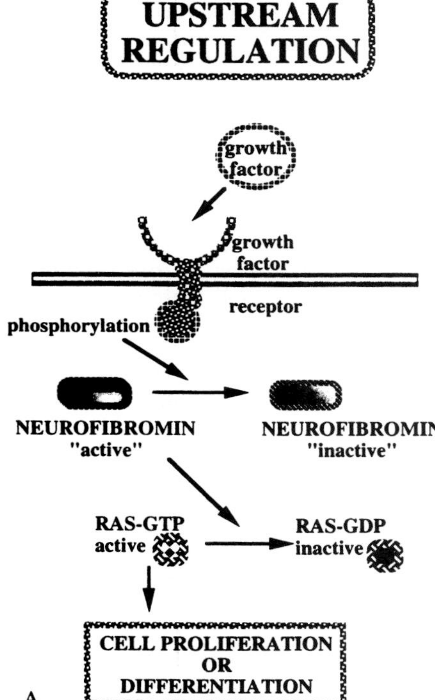

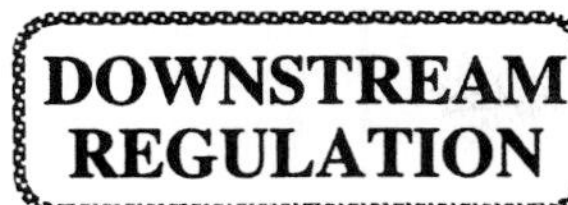

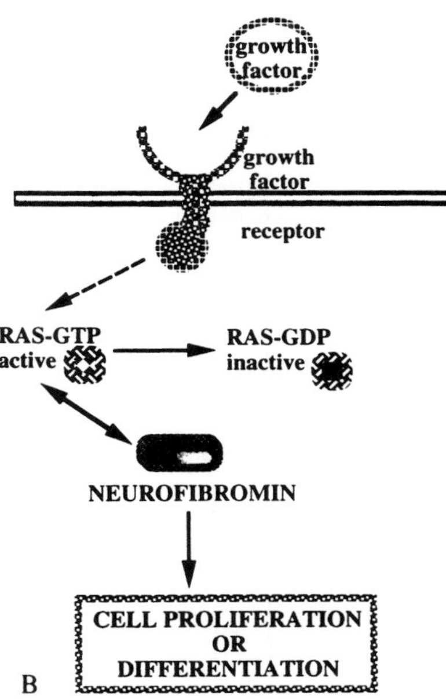

Fig. 39-12 Upstream versus downstream models of p21-*ras*-neurofibromin interactions. *A.* In the upstream model, stimulation of appropriate cells expressing growth factor receptors leads to an inactivation of neurofibromin, perhaps through phosphorylation cascades. Inactivation of neurofibromin releases p21-*ras* from its down-regulation, allowing p21-*ras* to predominate in the active GTP-bound form and signal other intracellular proteins to culminate in cell proliferation or differentiation. *B.* The downstream model on the other hand envisions p21-*ras* as a regulator of neurofibromin and states that it transmits a signal via neurofibromin and p21-*ras* to culminate in cell proliferation or differentiation. For more detail, refer to the text.

phosphorylated.[186] A second model, which falls into the category of a downstream hypothesis for p21-*ras*-GAP interaction, is that neurofibromin is induced by the process of p21-*ras*-GTP to p21-*ras*-GDP conversion to transmit a signal through its influence on microtubule organization. Further investigations will be required to refute or support either of these two nonmutually exclusive hypotheses unequivocally.

Neurofibromin Isoforms

Several isoforms of neurofibromin have been identified that arise from alternative splicing.[2,98] The first inserts 21 amino acids within the NF1GRD. This type 2 isoform is expressed in tissues different from those in which type 1 neurofibromin is expressed and may be regulated by brain-specific differentiation events.[209] It is expressed in many species, including chickens.[210] The type 2 isoform is the predominant mRNA species after week 22 of human fetal development and can be induced in a neuroblastoma cell line by retinoic acid treatment.[209] Similar induction of type 2 neurofibromin expression is observed during Schwann cell differentiations, as reflected by an increase in *NF1* mRNA and neurofibromin levels as well as a switch from type 1 to type 2 *NF1* mRNA in Schwann cells stimulated to differentiate in response to treatments that increase intracellular cAMP.[210,211] In addition, *NF1* isoform expression is altered during mouse embryogenesis, with type 2 *NF1* mRNA expressed before embryonic day 10 and type 1 *NF1* mRNA predominating thereafter.[212] Studies in yeast demonstrate that this isoform also has GAP-like catalytic activity, although moderately reduced from that observed with native type 1 neurofibromin.[210] Whether this isoform can associate with cytoplasmic microtubules is being investigated.

A second, less well-characterized isoform has been identified near the C-terminus of the protein and results from an 18-amino-acid insertion.[2,98] This isoform is detected on the RNA level predominantly in muscle. It is expressed in cardiac muscle (both fetal and adult), skeletal muscle, and some smooth muscle tissues.[213] Little or no expression is found in brain, spleen, or kidney. The expression of an isoform of *NF1* in muscle is intriguing in light of a small number of patients with NF1 and cardiac disease.[214,215] In addition, it was demonstrated recently that neurofibromin expression increases while p21-*ras* activity decreases in myoblasts stimulated to differentiate *in vitro*.[141] Similarly, neurofibromin is transiently expressed in developing myotomes during murine and chick embryonic development.[100,151,157] The relationship between the muscle expression of this isoform and the clinical manifestations of NF1 remains unelucidated.

Recently, an additional isoform of the *NF1* gene was identified that is expressed predominantly in the brain.[216] This alternatively spliced isoform containing exon 9a is enriched in human and rodent cerebral cortex, where its expression correlates with cortical neuron maturation both *in vitro* and *in vivo*.[217] The finding of a brain-specific *NF1* isoform suggests that neurofibromin may play unique roles during central nervous system development.

BIOLOGIC PROPERTIES OF NEUROFIBROMAS

Both plexiform and cutaneous neurofibromas can arise from any nerve throughout the body and at any time, including embryonically. Neurofibromas tend to grow more rapidly during pregnancy and puberty, implying some hormone sensitivity.[218,219] Neurofibromas grow as a mixed population of cells that includes fibroblasts, mast cells, Schwann cells, axons, perineural cells, and endothelial cells.[218–224] The clonal nature of neurofibromas is controversial and has not been resolved conclusively.[225,226]

Neurofibromas have been found to contain mitogens that stimulate Schwann cell and fibroblast proliferation.[227,228] One study using purified Schwann cells from neurofibromas demonstrated that these NF1 Schwann cells promoted angiogenesis and could invade chick chorioallantoic membranes.[229] These results suggest that neurofibroma Schwann cells are intrinsically different from normal Schwann cells. NF1 fibroblasts also have been examined for evidence of abnormal growth characteristics.

Although many of these studies have been difficult to reproduce, it has been suggested that NF1 fibroblasts are more sensitive to ionizing radiation and have an increased rate of transformation by Kirsten murine sarcoma viruses.[230–233]

Diagnosis and Treatment

Conventional Treatment of NF1 Patients. The treatment of patients affected with NF1 often requires the expertise of many medical and surgical subspecialists coordinated by one physician or a team of physicians familiar with NF1.[234] For this reason, we advocate the establishment of neurofibromatosis clinics staffed by physicians who regularly see NF1 patients and are familiar with the diagnosis, management, and complications of the disorder. Closely affiliated with the clinic should be a diverse collection of other physicians and health care providers with subspecialties in given areas of medicine or surgery. These persons include ophthalmologists, neurologists, plastic surgeons, neurosurgeons, otolaryngologists, psychiatrists, social workers, child psychologists, orthopedic surgeons, dermatologists, and oncologists. The role of an NF clinic is not only to provide coordinated care from a centralized caregiver familiar with NF1 but also to provide up-to-date information to patients and their families about the disease through regular communication via NNFF-sponsored newsletters and scientific symposia.

The approach to a new patient suspected of having NF1 involves careful history taking and examination. Before the clinic appointment, it is helpful for a genetic counselor to contact the patient to review the patient's clinical features and family history. Often this phone call will precipitate further investigation on the part of the patient and family members in an attempt to determine which other family members have features consistent with NF1. A careful exploration of the family may uncover relatives with subtle features of NF1; this is particularly true in light of its variable expressivity. Hospital records, autopsy reports, and surgical pathology reports also should be requested.

Once the patient arrives in the clinic, he or she should be examined thoroughly by one of the NF1 physicians. A careful cutaneous examination is performed to look for palpable neurofibromas, axillary or inguinal freckling, and café-au-lait spots. The café-au-lait spots can be better visualized under a Wood lamp. The number of pigmented lesions and their greatest diameters are recorded. An ophthalmologic examination with attention to measurement of visual acuity is important to rule out symptomatic optic glioma. In individuals beyond the age of 7 to 8, inspection of the iris should reveal Lisch nodules, especially in patients with light-colored irises. If Lisch nodules are not appreciated and diagnostic criteria for NF1 have not been met, referral to an opthalmologist for a slit-lamp evaluation is made. During a general physical examination, attention is focused on the detection of any curvature of the spine, especially in young children. Severe cases are referred to an orthopedic surgeon. In addition, inspection of the long bones of the upper and lower extremities is warranted in young children to exclude bowing and thinning of the cortices of these bones and prevent the formation of pseudarthroses. Suspicious bones are examined by plain x-rays, and affected patients are referred to an orthopedic surgeon knowledgeable about the bracing and management of this problem. In children, height, weight, and head circumference are noted during each visit and are charted to evaluate the child's growth curve. Inspection of the face and fingers is done to look for facial dysmorphisms or dermatoglyphics suggestive of disorders besides NF1. In addition, blood pressure should be measured during each visit. We recommend routine general medical appointments spaced 6 months after each visit to the NF1 clinic to allow for blood pressure determinations twice a year. Any abnormal rise in blood pressure always warrants further investigation for renal artery stenosis or pheochromocytoma. Patients should be questioned about headache (location, frequency, and character) and bowel or bladder difficulties to screen for deep neurofibromatous involvement of splanchnic nerves.

A screening neurologic examination should be performed during each visit, with special attention to visual acuity, visual fields, and funduscopic evaluation. We strongly advocate the limited and directed use of brain imaging studies and do not obtain them unless there is a change in the symptoms or in the neurologic examination. The limited use of brain imaging studies is based on the low yield of these studies in detecting asymptomatic lesions that require treatment as well as the high likelihood of finding a high-intensity lesion on T_2-weighted MRI. These high-intensity lesions are sometimes referred to as UBOs and can be seen in upward of 60 percent of these children. Their clinical significance is uncertain, and their detection often raises unnecessary concern on the part of both the family and the physician.

During the evaluation, attention is also paid to the social history. In children, school performance is a good reflection of overall learning ability. Formal evaluation of IQ by the school district is recommended early (age 3 to 4) to identify children with learning disabilities. Early detection and aggressive intervention appear to be beneficial in NF1 patients. We encourage families to communicate regularly with the school and to obtain physical, speech, and occupational therapy as appropriate.

Patients with NF1 are seen on a yearly basis in the clinic, during which time they are educated about new information regarding the disease; a forum is provided for a discussion of their concerns and questions. In addition, patients are monitored for the development of new complications, and new family members are evaluated for signs of NF1. The removal of neurofibromas that are particularly large or cosmetically distressing or that rub on clothing straps is coordinated with a plastic surgeon. Otherwise, we encourage patients not to have multiple neurofibromas removed solely for cosmetic reasons, since they can grow back in these areas after surgery.

An integral part of the diagnosis and care of NF1 patients involves the genetic counselor. In our clinic, genetic counselors explain in detail the pattern of inheritance of NF1 (autosomal dominant), its penetrance (essentially 100 percent by 5 years of age), and its variable expressivity. Education is provided, and common misconceptions regarding the disease are dispelled. The emotional impact of NF1 on the patient as well as the other family members is addressed. Families are also given information about support group resources. Explanations of the natural history of the disorder, its behavior during puberty and pregnancy, and its unpredictability are explored. Prenatal counseling is provided for the parents and siblings of affected patients. Prenatal testing, when appropriate, is offered to families in which linkage analysis is informative (see below).

Molecular Genetic Approaches to NF1 Patients. With the entire *NF1* gene cloned and the protein identified, it is now theoretically possible to study gene mutations in patients with NF1. The approaches taken to screen for mutations involve a combination of DNA, RNA, and protein analysis. However, given the large size of the gene and the heterogeneity of the mutations, the search for causative mutations is quite labor-intensive. In the years since cloning of the full-length *NF1* gene, only a handful of mutations have been characterized owing to the arduous task of screening 60 exons for DNA alterations. Therefore, routine clinical application of DNA analysis in the diagnosis of NF1 is not yet a reality. In families in which the clinical diagnosis is certain, multiple members are affected, and closely linked polymorphic markers are informative, linkage analysis using closely spaced markers or microsatellite repeat sequences remains the most practical application of DNA diagnostics.[235]

It is possible that mutations in different regions and/or domains of the *NF1* gene will produce different phenotypes, as has been demonstrated for mutations within the dystrophin gene. As was true with the dystrophin gene, in which other related but distinct disorders were caused by mutations within the same gene, it is important to study neurologic disorders with abnormalities similar to those found in NF1 for alterations in the *NF1* gene.

To date, it has not been possible to provide diagnostic information by surveying for alterations at the protein level. No anomalously migrating protein species have been observed, as was noted for Becker muscular dystrophy. It appears that all the mutations described so far result in a lack of neurofibromin expression as opposed to a smaller or larger protein product. Theoretically, an assay capable of distinguishing 100 percent levels from 50 percent levels of neurofibromin could detect most affected individuals (since most mutations would be null at the protein level). This requires a level of reliable quantification that has not been achieved, however.

NF1 remains a clinical diagnosis. Using the diagnostic criteria established in the NIH consensus statement, the diagnosis of NF1 can be made confidently in the vast majority of individuals. For selected individuals desiring prenatal diagnosis, genetic testing and counseling can be provided. In families with two or more affected individuals with NF1, linkage analysis can be performed. Recently, a commercial test for *NF1* gene mutations was developed that relies on a protein truncation assay.[236] With this technique, RNA from white blood cells is reverse transcribed and converted into overlapping *NF1* cDNA fragments *in vitro*. Neurofibromin proteins from individuals with NF1 that are larger or smaller than the predicted fragment sizes are then used to direct the search for the underlying *NF1* gene mutation. The advantage of this system is the speed with which mutations potentially can be identified. However, it is unclear at this point whether this test will identify a significant portion of *NF1* gene mutations in individuals with NF1 to warrant more widespread use.

The cloning of the *NF1* gene has opened the door to a more complete understanding of NF1 pathobiology with the eventual goal of designing specific, nonsurgical treatments for affected patients. The finding of elevated p21-*ras*-GTP levels in tumors from NF1 patients suggests that drug therapies directed at up-regulating neurofibromin GAP activity or down-regulating p21-*ras* activity may have a beneficial effect on the growth of neurofibromas. A number of groups have been studying the lipid sensitivity of neurofibromin GAP activity *in vitro* and have found that specific lipids preferentially alter neurofibromin GAP activity as opposed to mammalian p120-GAP catalytic activity.[169,237–239] The discovery of a compound capable of up-regulating or replacing neurofibromin may prove to be a useful therapy in the future.

Similarly, drugs that interfere with p21-*ras* activity, such as pharmaceutical agents that block farnesylation, a reaction necessary for p21-*ras* membrane localization, may have therapeutic potential in NF1.[240–242] Farnesylation-blocking agents have been shown to inhibit the mitogenic effects of growth factors and the tumorigenic properties of neuroblastoma cells. More useful therapies may involve drugs that inhibit farnesyl transferase (the addition of farnesyl groups to the p21-*ras* protein) rather than lovastatin and compactin, which are HMG-CoA reductase inhibitors that block farnesyl synthesis. Further study of these and related drugs may uncover useful therapies for NF1 patients.

ACKNOWLEDGMENTS

We thank the members of our neurofibromatosis research group, past and present, especially Drs. Lone Andersen, Steve Doran, Jane Fountain, R. Todd Geist, Paula Gregory, Douglas Marchuk, Anna Mitchell, Margaret Wallace, and Susan Wilson-Gunn. We also thank our collaborators elsewhere, including Drs. Roymarie Ballester, Dafna Bar-Sagi, Mark Boguski, Gideon Bollag, Dennis Choi, Jeff DeClue, Julian Downward, Ab Guha, Chung Hsu, Tyler Jacks, Richard Jove, David Louis, Douglas Lowy, Frank McCormick, Lynn Rutkowski, Gihan Tennekoon, and Michael Wigler. We also thank numerous members of the NF1 research community for providing preprints of manuscripts and are particularly grateful to Dr. Susan Huson for supplying drafts of several chapters on the clinical manifestations of NF1. Nancy North provided expert assistance in the preparation of this manuscript.

REFERENCES

1. Wallace MR, Marchuk DA, Anderson LB, Letcher R, Odeh HM, Saulino AM, Fountain JW, Brereton A, Nicholson J, Mitchell AL, Brownstein BH, Collins FS: Type 1 neurofibromatosis gene: Identification of a large transcript disrupted in three NF1 patients. *Science* **249**:181, 1990.
2. Cawthon RM, Weiss R, Xu G, Viskochil D, Culver M, Stevens J, Robertson M, Dunn D, Gesteland R, O'Connell P, White R: A major segment of the neurofibromatosis type 1 gene: cDNA sequence, genomic structure, and point mutations. *Cell* **62**:193, 1990.
3. Viskochil D, Buchberg AM, Xu G, Cawthon RM, Stevens J, Wolff RK, Culver M, Carey JC, Copeland NG, Jenkins NA, White R, O'Connell P: Deletions and a translocation interrupt a cloned gene at the neurofibromatosis type 1 locus. *Cell* **62**:187, 1990.
4. Xu G, O'Connell P, Viskochil D, Cawthon R, Robertson M, Culver M, Dunn D, Stevens J, Gesteland R, White R, Weiss R: The neurofibromatosis type 1 gene encodes a protein related to GAP. *Cell* **62**:599, 1990.
5. Xu G, Lin B, Tanaka K, Dunn D, Wood D, Gesteland R, White R, Weiss R, Tamanoi F: The catalytic domain of the neurofibromatosis type 1 gene product stimulates ras GTPase and complements ira mutants of *S. cerevesiae*. *Cell* **63**:835, 1990.
6. Martin GA, Viskochil D, Bollag G, McCabe PC, Crosier WJ, Haubruck H, Conroy L, Clark R, O'Connell P, Cawthon RM, Innis MA, McCormick F: The GAP-related domain of the neurofibromatosis type 1 gene product interacts with ras p21. *Cell* **63**:843, 1990.
7. Ballester R, Marchuk DA, Boguski M, Saulino AM, Letcher R, Wigler M, Collins FS: The *NF1* locus encodes a protein functionally related to mammalian GAP and yeast IRA proteins. *Cell* **63**:851, 1990.
8. Huson SM, Hughes RAC: *The Neurofibromatoses: A Pathogenetic and Clinical Overview.* London, Chapman and Hall, 1994.
9. Friedman J, Gutmann DH, MacCollin M, RiccardiVM: Neurofibromatosis: Phenotype, Natural History and Pathogenesis, 3rd ed. Baltimore, Johns Hopkins University Press, 1999.
10. Korf BR, Carey JC: Molecular genetics of neurofibromatosis, in Rubenstein AE, Korf BR (eds): *Neurofibromatosis: A Handbook for Patients, Families, and Health-Care Professionals*. New York, Thieme, 1990, p 178.
11. Crowe FW, Schull WJ, Neel JV: *A Clinical, Pathological and Genetic Study of Multiple Neurofibromatosis.* Springfield, IL, Charles C Thomas, 1956.
12. Trofatter JA, MacCollin MM, Rutter JL, Murrell JR, Duyao MP, Parry DM, Eldridge R, Kley N, Menon AG, Pulaski K, Haase VH, Ambrose CM, Munroe E, Bove C, Haines JL, Martuzza RL, MacDonald ME, Seizinger DR, Short MP, Buckler AJ, Gusella JF: A novel moesin-, ezrin-, radixin gene is a candidate for the neurofibromatosis 2 tumor suppressor. *Cell* **72**:791, 1993.
13. Rouleau GA, Merel P, Lutchman M, Sanson M, Zucman J, Marineau C, Hoang-Zuan K, Demczuk S, Desmaze C, Plougastel B, Pulst SM, Lenoir G, Bijlsma E, Fashold R, Dumanski J, de Jong P, Parry D, Eldridge R, Aurias A, Delattre O, Thomas G: Alteration in a new gene encoding a putative membrane-organizing protein causes neurofibromatosis type 2. *Nature* **363**:515, 1993.
14. Zanca A: Antique illustrations of neurofibromatosis. *Int J Dermatol* **19**:55, 1980.
15. Hecht F: Recognition of neurofibromatosis before von Recklinghausen. *Neurofibromatosis* **2**:180, 1989.
16. Von Recklinghausen FD: *Ueber die multiplen fibrome der Hautund inhre beziehung zu den multiplen neuromen.* Berlin, Hirschwald, 1882.
17. Preiser SA, Davenport CB: Multiple neurofibromatosis (von Recklinghausen disease) and its inheritance. *Am J Med Sci* **156**:507, 1918.
18. Lisch K: Ueber beteiligung der augen, insbesondere das vorkommen von irisknotchen bei der neurofibromatose (Recklinghausen). *Augenheilkde* **93**:137, 1937.
19. Lewis RA, Riccardi VM: Von Recklinghausen neurofibromatosis: Incidence of iris hamartomata. *Ophthalmology* **88**:348, 1981.
20. Lubs M-LE, Bauer MS, Formas ME, Djokic B: Lisch nodules in neurofibromatosis type 1. *N Engl J Med* **324**:1264, 1991.
21. Borberg A: Clinical and genetic investigations into tuberous sclerosis and Recklinghausen's neurofibromatosis. *Acta Psychiatr Neurol Suppl* **71**:1, 1951.
22. Sorenson SA, Mulvhill JT, Nielsen A: Long-term follow up of von Recklinghausen neurofibromatosis: Survival and malignant neoplasms. *N Engl J Med* **314**:1010, 1986.
23. Carey JC, Laub JM, Hall BD: Penetrance and variability in neurofibromatosis: A genetic study of 60 families. *Birth Defects* **15(5B)**:271, 1979.

24. Riccardi VM: Von Recklinghausen neurofibromatosis. *N Engl J Med* **305**:1617, 1981.
25. Huson SM, Harper PS, Compston DAS: Von Recklinghausen neurofibromatosis: A clinical and population study in south east Wales. *Brain* **111**:1535, 1988.
26. Huson SM, Compston DAS, Harper PS, Clark P: A genetic study of von Recklinghausen neurofibromatosis in south east Wales: I. Prevalence, fitness, mutation rate, and effect of parental transmission on severity. *J Med Genet* **26**:704, 1989.
27. Huson SM, Compston DAS, Harper PS: A genetic study of von Recklinghausen neurofibromatosis in south east Wales: II. Guidelines for genetic counselling. *J Med Genet* **26**:712, 1989.
28. Sergeyev AS: On the mutation rate of neurofibromatosis. *Hum Genet* **28**:129, 1975.
29. Samuelsson B, Axelsson R: Neurofibromatosis: A clinical and genetic study of 96 cases in Gothenburg, Sweden. *Acta Dermatol Venereol Suppl (Stockh)* **95**:67, 1981.
30. NIH Consensus Development Conference: Neurofibromatosis statement. *Arch Neurol* **45**:575, 1988.
31. Gutmann DH, Aylsworth A, Carey JC, Korf B, Marks J Pyertiz RE, Rubunstein A, Viskochil D: The diagnostic evaluation and multidisciplinary management of neurofibromatosis 1 and neurofibromatosis 2. *JAMA* **278**:51, 1997.
32. Burwell RG, James NJ, Johnston DI: Café au lait spots in school children. *Arch Dis Child* **57**:631, 1982.
33. Benedict PH, Szabo G, Fitzpatrick TB, Sinesi SJ: Melanotic macules in Albright syndrome and in neurofibromatosis. *JAMA* **205**:72, 1968.
34. Lott IT, Richardson EP Jr: Neuropathological findings and the biology of neurofibromatosis. *Adv Neurol* **28**:23, 1981.
35. Crowe FW: Axillary freckling as a diagnostic aid in neurofibromatosis. *Ann Intern Med* **61**:1142, 1964.
36. Riccardi VM, Eichner JE: *Neurofibromatosis: Phenotype, Natural History, and Pathogenesis.* Baltimore, Johns Hopkins University Press, 1986.
37. Horwich A, Riccardi VM, Francke V: Brief clinical report: Aqueductal stenosis leading to hydrocephalus, an unusual manifestation of neurofibromatosis. *Am J Med Genet* **14**:577, 1983.
38. Kayes LM, Riccardi VM, Burke W, Bennett RL, Stephens K: Large *de novo* DNA deletion in a patient with sporadic neurofibromatosis, mental retardation and dysmorphism. *J Med Genet* **29**:686, 1992.
39. North K, Joy P, Yuille D, Cocks N, Mobbs E, Hutchiins P, McHugh K, de Silva M: Specific learning disability in children with neurofibromatosis type 1: Significance of MRI abnormalities. *Neurology* **44**:878, 1994.
40. North KK, Riccardi V, Samango-Sprouse C, Ferner R, Moore B, Leguis E, Ratner N, Denckla MG: Cognitive function and academic performance in neurofibromatosis 1: Consensus statement from the NF1 Cognitive Disorders Task Force. *Neurology* **48**:1121, 1997.
41. Moore BD, Slopis JM, Schomer D, Jackson EF, Levy BM: Neuropsychological significance of areas of high signal intensity on brain MRIs of children with neurofibromatosis. *Neurology* **46**:1660, 1996.
42. DiPaolo DP, Zimmerman RA, Rorke LB, Zackai EH, Bilaniuk LT, Yachnis AT: Neurofibromatosis type 1: Pathologic substrate of high signal intensity foci in the brain. *Radiology* **195**:721, 1995.
43. Giordano MJ, Mahadeo DK, He YY, Geist RT, Hsu C, Gutmann DH: Increased expression of the neurofibromatosis 1 (NF1) gene product, neurofibromin, in astrocytes in response to cerebral ischemia. *J Neurosci Res* **43**:246, 1996.
44. Gutmann DH, Giordano MJ, Mahadeo DK, Lau N, Silbergeld D, Guha A: Increased neurofibromatosis 1 gene expression in astrocytic tumors: Positive regulation by p21-*ras*. *Oncogene* **12**:2121, 1996.
45. Brasfield RD, Das Gupta TK: Von Recklinghausen's disease: A clinicopathological study. *Ann Surg* **175**:86, 1972.
46. Hope DG, Mulvhill JJ: Malignancy in neurofibromatosis. *Adv Neurol* **29**:33, 1981.
47. Thomas JE, Piepgras DG, Scheithauer BW, Onofrio BM, Shives TC: Neurogenic tumors of the sciatic nerve: A clinicopathologic study of 35 cases. *Mayo Clin Proc* **58**:640, 1983.
48. Lewis RA, Gerson LP, Axelsson KA, Riccardi VM, Whitford RP: Von Recklinghausen neurofibromatosis: II. Incidence of optic gliomata. *Ophthalmology* **91**:929, 1984.
49. Listernick R, Charrow J, Greewald MJ, Esterly NA: Optic gliomas in children with neurofibromatosis type 1. *J Pediatr* **114**:788, 1989.
50. Listernick R, Louis DN, Packer PJ, Gutmann DH: Optic pathway gliomas in children with neurofibromatosis 1: Consensus statement from the NF1 Optic Pathway Glioma Taskforce. *Ann Neurol* **41**:143, 1997.
51. Duffner PK, Cohen ME, Seidel FG, Shucard DW: The significance of MRI abnormalities in children with neurofibromatosis. *Neurology* **39**:373, 1989.
52. Holt JF: Neurofibromatosis in children. *AJR* **130**:615, 1978.
53. Daniels SR, Loggie JM, McEnery PT, Towbin RB: Clinical spectrum of intrinsic renovascular hypertension in children. *Pediatrics* **80**:698, 1993.
54. Hochberg FH, Dasilva AB, Galdabini J, Richardson EP Jr: Gastrointestinal involvement in von Recklinghausen's neurofibromatosis. *Neurology* **24**:1144, 1974.
55. Hall JG: Possible maternal and hormonal factors in neurofibromatosis. *Adv Neurol* **29**:125, 1981.
56. Miller M, Hall JG: Possible maternal effect on severity of neurofibromatosis. *Lancet* **2**:1071, 1978.
57. Hall JG: Genomic impringing: Review and relevance of genetic diseases. *Am J Hum Genet* **46**:857, 1990.
58. Riccardi VM, Wald JS: Discounting an adverse maternal effect on severity of neurofibromatosis. *Pediatrics* **79**:386, 1987.
59. Huson SM, Clark D, Compston DAS, Harper PS: A genetic study of von Recklinghausen's neurofibromatosis in south east Wales: I. Prevalance, fitness, mutation rate and effect of parental transmission on severity. *J Med Genet* **26**:704, 1989.
60. Jadayel D, Fain P, Upadhyaya M, Ponder MA, Huson SM, Carey J, Fryer A, Mathew CGP, Barker DF, Ponder BAJ: Paternal origin of new mutations in von Recklinghausen neurofibromatosis. *Nature* **343**:558, 1990.
61. Stephens K, Kayes L, Riccardi VM, Rising M, Sybert VP, Pagon RA: Preferential mutation of the neurofibromatosis type 1 gene in paternally-derived chromosomes. *Hum Genet* **88**:279, 1992.
62. Riccardi VM, Lewis RA: Penetrance of von Recklinghausen neurofibromatosis: A distinction between predecessors and descendents. *Am J Hum Genet* **42**:284, 1988.
63. Easton DF, Ponder MA, Huson SM, Ponder BAJ: An analysis of variation in expression of neurofibromatosis (NF) type (NF1): Evidence for modifying genes. *Am J Hum Genet* **53**:305, 1993.
64. Eldridge R: Central neurofibromatosis with bilateral acoustic neuroma. *Adv Neurol* **29**:57, 1981.
65. Martuza RL, Eldridge R: Neurofibromatosis 2 (bilateral acoustic neurofibromatosis). *N Engl J Med* **318**:684, 1988.
66. Charles SJ, Moore AT, Yates JRW, Ferguson-Smith MA: Lisch nodules in neurofibromatosis type 2. *Arch Ophthalmol* **107**:1571, 1989.
67. Kaiser-Kupfer MI, Freidlin V, Datiles MB: The association of posterior capsular lens opacity with bilateral acoustic neuromas in patients with neurofibromatosis. *Arch Ophthalmol* **107**:541, 1989.
68. Trattner A, David M, Hodak E, Ben-David E, Sandbank M: Segmental neurofibromatosis. *J Am Acad Dermatol* **23**:866, 1990.
69. Rubenstein AE, Bader JL, Aron AA, Wallace S: Familial transmission of segmental neurofibromatosis. *Neurology* **33(suppl 2)**:76, 1983.
70. Lazaro C, Ravella A, Gaona A, Volpini V, Estivill X: Neurofibromatosis type 1 due to germline mosaicism in a clinically normal father. *N Engl J Med* **33**:1403, 1994.
71. Colman SD, Rasmussen SA, Ho VT, Abernathy CR, Wallace MR: Somatic mosaicism in a patient with neurofibromatosis type 1. *Am J Hum Genet* **58**:484, 1996.
72. Allanson JE, Upadhyaya M, Watson GH, Parington M, Mackenzie A, MacLeod A, Safarazi M, Broadhead W, Harper PS: Watson syndrome: Is it a subtype of type 1 NF? *J Med Genet* **28**:752, 1991.
73. Opitz JM, Weaver DD:L The neurofibromatosis-Noonan syndrome. *Am J Med Genet* **21**:477, 1985.
74. Stern HJ, Saal HM, Fain PR, Golgar DE, Rosenbaum KN, Barher DF: Clinical reliability of type 1 neurofibromatosis: Is there a NF-Noonan syndrome? *J Med Genet* **29**:184, 1992.
75. Pulst S-M, Riccardi VM, Fain P, Korenberg JR: Familial spinal neurofibromatosis: Clinical and DNA linkage analysis. *Neurology* **41**:1923, 1991.
76. Collins FS: Positional cloning: Let's not call it reverse anymore. *Nature Genet* **1**:3, 1992.
77. Barker D, Wright E, Nguyen K, Cannon L, Fain P, Goldgar D, Bishop DT, Carey J, Kivlin J, Willard H, Nakamura Y, O'Connell P, Leppert M, White RL, Skolnick M: A genomic search for linkage of neurofibromatosis to RFLPs. *J Med Genet* **24**:536, 1987.
78. Diehl SR, Boehnke M, Erickson RP, Baxter AB, Bruce MA, Lieberman JL, Platt DJ, Ploughman LM, Seiler KA, Sweet AM, Collins FS: Linkage analysis of von Recklinghausen neurofibromatosis to DNA markers on chromosome 17. *Genomics* **1**:361, 1987.

79. Seizinger BR, Rouleau GA, Lane AH, Farmer G, Ozelius LJ, Haines JL, Parry DM, Korf BR, Pericak-Vance MA, Faryniarz AG, Hobbs WJ, Iannazzi JA, Roy JC, Menon A, Bader JL, Spence MA, Chao MV, Mulvihill JJ, Roses AD, Martuza RL, Breakefield XO, Conneally PM, Gusella JF: Linkage analysis in von Recklinghausen neurofibromatosis (NF1) with DNA markers for chromosome 17. *Genomics* **1**:346, 1987.
80. Skolnick MH, Ponder B, Seizinger B: Linkage of NF1 to 12 chromosome 17 markers: A summary of eight concurrent reports. *Genomics* **1**:382, 1987.
81. Seizinger BR, Rouleau GA, Ozelius LJ, Lane AH, Faryniarz AG, Chao MV, Huson S, Korf BR, Parry DM, Pericak-Vance MA, Collins FS, Hobbs WJ, Falcone BG, Iannazzi JA, Roy JC, St. George-Hyslop PH, Tanzi RE, Bothwell MA, Upadhyaya M, Harper P, Goldstein AE, Hoover DL, Bader JL, Spence MA, Mulvihill JJ, Aylsworth AS, Vance JM, Rossenwasser GOD, Gaskell PC, Roses AD, Martuza RL, Breakefield XO, Gusella JF: Genetic linkage of von Recklinghausen neurofibromatosis to the nerve growth factor receptor gene. *Cell* **49**:589, 1987.
82. Darby JK, Feder J, Selby M, Riccardi V, Ferrel R, Siao D, Goslin K, Rutter W, Shooter EM, Cavilli-Sforza LL: A discordant sibship analysis between beta-NGF and neurofibromatosis. *Am J Hum Genet* **37**:52, 1985.
83. Goldgar DE, Green P, Parry DM, Mulvihill JJ: Multipoint linkage analysis in neurofibromatosis type 1: An international collaboration. *Am J Hum Genet* **44**:6, 1989.
84. Fountain JW, Wallace MR, Bruce MA, Seizinger BR, Menon AG, Gusella JF, Michels VV, Schmidt MA, Dewald GW, Collins FS: Physical mapping of a translocation breakpoint in neurofibromatosis. *Science* **244**:1085, 1989.
85. Ledbetter DH, Rich DC, O'Connell P, Leppert M, Carey JC: Precise localization of NF1 to 17q11.2 by balanced translocation. *Am J Hum Genet* **44**:20, 1989.
86. Menon AG, Ledbetter DH, Rich DC, Seizinger BR, Rouleau GA, Michels VV, Schmidt MA, Dewald G, DallaTorre CM, Haines JL, Gusella JF: Characterization of a translocation within the von Recklinghausen neurofibromatosis region of chromosome 17. *Genomics* **5**:245, 1989.
87. O'Connell P, Leach R, Cawthon RM, Culver M, Stevens J, Viskochil D, Fournier REK, Rich DC, Ledbetter DH, White R: Two NF1 translocations map within a 600-kilobase segment of 17q11.2. *Science* **244**:1087, 1989.
88. Schmidt MA, Michels VV, Dewald GW: Cases of neurofibromatosis with rearrangements of chromosome 17 involving band 17q11.2. *Am J Med Genet* **28**:771, 1987.
89. Fountain JW, Wallace MR, Brereton AB, O'Connell P, White RL, Rich DC, Ledbetter DH, Leach RJ, Fournier REK, Menon AG, Gusella JF, Barker D, Stephens K, Collins FS: Physical mapping of the von Recklinghausen neurofibromatosis region on chromosome 17. *Am J Hum Genet* **44**:58, 1989.
90. Buchberg AM, Bedigian HG, Taylor BA, Brownell E, Ihle JN, Nagata S, Jenkins NA, Copeland NG: Localization of *evi*-2 to chromosome 11: Linkage to other proto-oncogene and growth factor loci using interspecific backcross mice. *Oncogene Res* **2**:149, 1989.
91. Cawthon RM, Anderson LB, Buchberg AM, Xu G, O'Connell P, Viskochil D, Weiss RB, Wallace MR, Marchuk DA, Culver M, Stevens J, Jenkins NA, Copeland NG, Collins FS, White R: cDNA sequence and genomic structure of *EVI2B*, a gene lying within an intron of the neurofibromatosis type 1 gene. *Genomics* **9**:446, 1991.
92. O'Connell P, Viskochil D, Buchberg AM, Fountain J, Cawthon RM, Culver M, Stevens J, Rich DC, Ledbetter DH, Wallace M, Carey JC, Jenkins NA, Copeland NG, Collins FS, White R: The human homolog of murine evi2 lies between two von Recklinghausen neurofibromatosis translocations. *Genomics* **7**:547, 1990.
93. Cawthon RM, O'Connell P, Buchberg AM, Viskochil D, Weiss RB, Culver M, Stevens J, Jenkins NA, Copeland NG, White R: Identification and characterization of transcripts from the neurofibromatosis 1 region: The sequence and genomic structure of *EVI2* and mapping of other transcripts. *Genomics* **7**:555, 1990.
94. Mikol DD, Gulcher JR, Stefansson K: The oligodendrocyte-myelin glycoprotein belongs to a distinct family of proteins and contains the HNK-1 carbohydrate. *J Cell Biol* **110**:471, 1990.
95. Viskochil D, Cawthon R, O'Connell P, Xu G, Stevens J, Culver M, Carey J, White R: The gene encoding the oligodendrocyte-myelin glycoprotein is embedded within the neurofibromatosis type 1 gene. *Mol Cell Biol* **11**:906, 1991.
96. Wallace MR, Anderson LB, Saulino AM, Gregory P, Glover T, Collins FS: A *de novo* insertion mutation causing neurofibromatosis type 1. *Nature* **353**:864, 1991.
97. Li Y, O'Connell P, Breidenbach HH, Cawthon R, Stevens J, Xu G, Neil S, Robertson M, White R, Viskochil D: Genomic organization of the neurofibromatosis 1 gene (NF1). *Genomics* **25**:9, 1995.
98. Marchuk DA, Saulino AM, Tavakkol R, Swaroop M, Wallace MR, Andersen LB, Mitchell AL, Gutmann DH, Boguski M, Collins FS: cDNA cloning of the type 1 neurofibromatosis gene: Complete sequence of the *NF1* gene product. *Genomics* **11**:931, 1991.
99. Buchberg AM, Cleveland LS, Jenkins NA, Copeland NG: Sequence homology shared by neurofibromatosis type 1 gene and IRA1 and IRA2 negative regulators of the *RAS* cyclic AMP pathway. *Nature* **347**:291, 1990.
100. Kavka AL, Chan SW, Hellen K, Yu H, Gutmann DH, Barabld KF: Expression of avian neurofibromatosis (aNF1) message and protein in neural crest cells (unpublished observation).
101. Stocker KM, Baizer L, Coston T, Sherman L, Ciment G: Regulated expression of neurofibromin in migrating neural crest cells of avian embryos. *J Neurobiol* **27**:535, 1995.
102. Nakamura T, Nemotto T, Arai M, Kasuga T, Gutmann DH, Collins FS, Ishikawa T: Specific expression of the neurofibromatosis type 1 (NF1) gene in hamster Schwann cell. *Am J Pathol* **144**:549, 1994.
103. Bird AP: CpG-rich islands and the function of DNA methylation. *Nature* **321**:209, 1986.
104. Legius E, Marchuk DA, Hall BK, Andersen LB, Wallace MR, Collins FS, Glover TW: NF1-related locus on chromosome 15. *Genomics* **13**:1316, 1993.
105. Marchuk DA, Tavakkol R, Wallace MR, Brownstein BH, Taillon-Miller P, Fong C-T, Legius E, Andersen LB, Glover TW, Collins FS: A yeast artificial chromosome contig encompassing the type 1 neurofibromatosis gene. *Genomics* **13**:372, 1992.
106. Upadhyaya M, Cheryson A, Broadhead W, Fryer A, Shaw DJ, Huson S, Wallace MR, Andersen LB, Marchuk DA, Viskochil D, Black D, O'Connell P, Collins FS, Harper PS: A 90 kb DNA deletion associated with neurofibromatosis type 1. *J Med Genet* **27**:738, 1990.
107. Li Y, Bollag G, Clark R, Stevens J, Conroy L, Fults D, Ward K, Friedman E, Samowitz W, Robertson M, Bradley P, McCormick F, White R, Cawthon R: Somatic mutations in the neurofibromatosis 1 gene in human tumors. *Cell* **69**:275, 1993.
108. Upadhyaya M: Analysis of mutations at the neurofibromatosis 1 (NF1) locus. *Hum Mol Genet* **1**:735, 1992.
109. Marshall CJ: Tumor suppressor genes. *Cell* **64**:313, 1991.
110. Sager R: Tumor suppressor genes: The puzzle and the promise. *Science* **246**:1406, 1989.
111. Weinberg RA: Tumor suppressor genes. *Science* **254**:1138, 1991.
112. Stanbridge EJ: Human tumor suppressor genes. *Annu Rev Genet* **24**:615, 1990.
113. Knudson AG: Mutation and cancer: Statistical study of retinoblastoma. *Proc Natl Acad Sci USA* **68**:820, 1971.
114. Knudson AG: Hereditary cancer, oncogenes, and antioncogenes. *Cancer Res* **45**:1437, 1985.
115. Menon AG, Anderson KM, Riccardi VM, Chung RY, Whaley JM, Yandell DW, Farmer GE, Freiman RM, Lee JK, Li FP, Barker DF, Ledbetter DH, Kleider A, Martuza RL, Gusella JF, Seizinger BR: Chromosome 17p deletions and *p53* gene mutation associated with the formation of malignant neurofibrosarcomas in von Recklinghausen neurofibromatosis. *Proc Natl Acad Sci USA* **87**:5435, 1990.
116. Legius E, Marchuk DA, Collins FS, Glover TW: Somatic depletion of neurofibromatosis type 1 gene in a neurofibrosarcoma supports a tumor suppressor gene hypothesis. *Nature Genet* **3**:122, 1993.
117. Glover TW, Stein CK, Legius E, Andersen LB, Brereton A, Johnson S: Molecular and cytogenetic analysis of tumors in von Recklinghausen neurofibromatosis. *Gene Chrom Cancer* **3**:62, 1991.
118. Seizinger BR: NF1: A prevalent cause of tumorigenesis in human cancers. *Nature Genet* **3**:97, 1993.
119. Andersen LB, Fountain JW, Gutmann DH, Tarle SA, Glover TW, Dracopoli NC, Housman DE, Collins FS: Mutations in the neurofibromatosis 1 gene in sporadic malignant melanomas. *Nature Genet* **3**:118, 1993.
120. Johnson MR, Look AT, DeClue JE, Valentine MB, Lowy DR: Inactivation of the NF1 gene in human melanoma and neuroblastoma cell lines without impaired regulation of GTP-ras. *Proc Natl Acad Sci USA* **90**:5539, 1993.
121. The I, Murthy AE, Hannigan GE, Jacoby LB, Menon AG, Gusella JF, Bernards A: Neurofibromatosis type 1 gene mutations in neuroblastoma. *Nature Genet* **3**:62, 1993.

122. DeClue JE, Papageorge AG, Fletcher J, Diehl SR, Ratner N, Vass WC, Lowy DR: Abnormal regulation of mammalian p21^{ras} contributes to malignant tumor growth in von Recklinghausen (type 1) neurofibromatosis. *Cell* **69**:265, 1992.
123. Basu TN, Gutmann DH, Fletcher JA, Glover TW, Collins FS, Downward J: Aberrant regulation of *ras* proteins in tumor cells from type 1 neurofibromatosis patients. *Nature* **356**:713, 1992.
124. Xu W, Mulligan LM, Ponder MA, Liu L, Smith BA, Mathew CGP, Ponder BAJ: Loss of NF1 alleles in phaeochromocytomas from patients with type 1 neurofibromatosis. *Gene Chrom Cancer* **4**:337, 1992.
125. Gutmann DH, Cole JL, Stone WJ, Ponder BAJ, Collins FS: Loss of neurofibromin in adrenal gland tumors from patients with neurofibromatosis type 1. *Gene Chrom Cancer* **10**:55-58, 1994.
126. Colman SD, Williams CA, Wallace MR: Benign neurofibromas in type 1 neurofibromatosis (NF1) show somatic deletions of the *NF1* gene. *Nature Genet* **11**:90, 1995.
127. Kim HA, Rosenbaum T, Marchionni MA, Ratner N, DeClue JE: Schwann cells from neurofibromin-deficient mice exhibit activation of p21-*ras*, inhibition of cell proliferation and morphological changes. *Oncogene* **11**:324, 1995.
128. Kim HA, Ling B, Ratner N: NF1-deficient mouse Schwann cells are angiogenic and invasive and can be induced to hyperproliferate: Reversion of some phenotypes by an inhibitor of farsenyl protein transferase. *Mol Cell Biol* **17**:862, 1997.
129. Rosenbaum T, Boissy YL, Kombrinck K, Brannan CI, Jenkins NA, Copeland NG, Ratner NA: Neurofibromin-deficient fibroblasts fail to form perineurium in vitro. *Development* **121**:3583, 1995.
130. Shannon KM, O'Connell P, Martin GA, Paderanga D, Olson K, Kinndorf P, McCormick F: Loss of normal *NF1* allele from the bone marrow of children with type 1 neurofibromatosis and malignant myeloid disorders. *New Engl J Med* **330**:597, 1994.
131. Largaespada DA, Brannan CI, Jenkins NA, Copeland NG: NF1 deficiency causes ras-mediated granulocyte/macrophage colony stimulating factor hypersensitivity and chronic myeloid leukemia. *Nature Genet* **12**:137, 1996.
132. Bollag G, Clapp DW, Shih S, Adler F, Zhang YY, Thompson P, Lange BJ, Freedman MH, McCormick F, Jacks T, Shannon K: Loss of *NF1* results in activation of the *Ras* signaling pathway and leads to abberant growth in haematopoietic cells. *Nature Genet* **12**:144, 1996.
133. Yan N, Ricca C, Fletcher J, Glover T, Seizinger BR, Manne V: Farnesyltransferase inhibitors block the neurofibromatosis type 1 (NF1) malignant phenotype. *Cancer Res* **55**:3569, 1995.
134. Schmale MC, Hensley GT, Udey LR: Neurofibromatosis in the bicolor damselfish as a model of von Recklinghausen neurofibromatosis. *Ann NY Acad Sci* **486**:386, 1986.
135. Hinrichs SH, Nerenberg M, Reynolds RK, Khoury G, Jay G: A transgenic mouse model for human neurofibromatosis. *Science* **237**:1340, 1987.
136. Nerenberg MI, Minor T, Nagashima K, Takebayashi K, Akai K, Wiley CA, Riccardi VM: Absence of association of HTLV-1 infection with type 1 neurofibromatosis in the United States or Japan. *Neurology* **41**:1687, 1991.
137. Nakamura T, Hara M, Kasuga T: Transplacental induction of peripheral nervous tumor in the Syrian golden hamster by *N*-nitroso-*N*-ethylurea. *Am J Pathol* **135**:251, 1989.
138. Jacks T, Shih TS, Schmitt EM, Bronson RT, Bernards A, Weinberg RA: Tumor predisposition in mice heterozygous for a targeted mutation in *NF1*. *Nature Genet* **7**:353, 1994.
139. Brannan CI, Perkins AS, Vogel KS, Ratner N, Nordlund ML, Reid SW, Buchberg AM, Jenkins NA, Parada LF, Copeland NG: Targeted disruption of the neurofibromatosis type-1 gene leads to developmental abnormalities in heart and various neural crest-derived tissues. *Gene Dev* **8**:1019, 1994.
140. Gutmann DH, Andersen LB, Cole JL, Swaroop M, Collins FS: An alternatively spliced mRNA in the carboxy terminus of the neurofibromatosis type 1 (NF1) gene is expressed in muscle. *Hum Mol Genet* **2**:989, 1993.
141. Gutmann DH, Cole JL, Collins FS: Modulation of neurofibromatosis type 1 (NF1) gene expression during in vitro myoblast differentiation. *J Neurosci Res* **37**:398, 1994.
142. Vogel KS, Brannan CI, Jenkins NA, Copeland NG, Parada LF: Loss of neurofibromin results in neurotrophin-independent survival of embryonic sensory and sympathetic neurons. *Cell* **82**:733, 1995.
143. Vogel KS, Parada LF: Sympathetic neuron survival and proliferation are prolonged by loss of p53 and neurofibromin. *Mol Cell Neurosci* **11**:19, 1998.
144. Silva AJ, Frankland PW, Marowitz Z, Friedman E, Lazlo G, Cioffi D, Jacks T, Bourtchladze R: A mouse model for the learning and memory deficits associated with neurofibromatosis type 1. *Nature Genet* **15**:281, 1997.
145. The I, Hannigan GE, Cowley GS, Reginald S, Zhong Y, Gusella JF, Hariharan IK, Bernards A: Rescue of a *Drosophila NF1* mutant phenotype by protein kinase A. *Science* **276**:791, 1997.
146. Guo H-F, The I, Hannan F, Bernards A, Zhong Y: Requirement of *Drosophila NF1* for activation of adenylyl cyclase by PACAP38-like neuropeptides. *Science* **276**:795, 1997.
147. DeClue JE, Cohen BD, Lowy DR: Identification and characterization of the neurofibromatosis type 1 protein product. *Proc Natl Acad Sci USA* **88**:9914, 1991.
148. Daston MM, Scrable H, Nordlund M, Sturbaum AK, Nissen LM, Ratner N: The protein product of the neurofibromatosis type 1 gene is expressed at highest abundance in neurons, Schwann cells, and oligodendrocytes. *Neuron* **8**:415, 1992.
149. Gutmann DH, Wood DL, Collins FS: Identification of the neurofibromatosis type 1 gene product. *Proc Natl Acad Sci USA* **88**:9658, 1991.
150. Hattori S, Ohmi N, Makawa M, Hoshino M, Kawakita M, Nakamura S: Antibody against neurofibromatosis type 1 gene product reacts with a triton-insoluble GTPase activating protein ras p21. *Biochem Biophys Res Commun* **177**:83, 1991.
151. Golubic M, Roudebush M, Dobrowolski S, Wolfman A, Stacey DW: Catalytic properties, tissue, and intracellular distribution of the native neurofibromatosis type 1 protein. *Oncogene* **7**:2151, 1992.
152. Gregory PE, Gutmann DH, Boguski M, Mitchell AM, Parks S, Jacks T, Wood DL, Jove R, Collins FS: The neurofibromatosis type 1 gene product, neurofibromin, associates with microtubules. *Somat Cell Mol Genet* **19**:265, 1993.
153. Bollag G, McCormick F, Clark R: Characterization of full-length neurofibromin: Tubulin inhibits *RAS* GAP activity. *EMBO J* **12**:1923, 1993.
154. Gutmann DH, Collins FS: Recent progress toward understanding the molecular biology of von Recklinghausen neurofibromatosis. *Ann Neurol* **31**:555, 1992.
155. Nordlund M, Gu X, Shipley MT, Ratner N: Neurofibromin is enriched in the endoplasmic reticulum of CNS neurons. *Neuroscience* **13**:1588, 1993.
156. Hewett SJ, Choi DW, Gutmann DH: Expression of the neurofibromatosis 1 (NF1) gene in reactive astrocytes in vitro. *Neuroreport* **6**:1565, 1995.
157. Daston MM, Ratner N: Neurofibromin, a predominantly neuronal GTPase activating protein in the adult, is ubiquitously expressed during development. *Dec Dyn* **19**:216, 1993.
158. Tanaka K, Nakafuku M, Satoh T, Marshall MS, Gibbs JB, Matsumoto K, Kaziro Y, Toh-e A: *S. cerevisiae* genes *IRA1* and *IRA2* encode proteins that may be functionally equivalent to mammalian ras GTPase activating protein. *Cell* **60**:803, 1990.
159. Tanaka K, Matsumoto K, Toh-e A: IRA1, an inhibitory regulator of the *RAS*-cyclic AMP pathway in *Saccharomyces cerevisiae*. *Mol Cell Biol* **9**:757, 1989.
160. Tanaka K, Nakafuku M, Tamanoi F, Kaziro Y, Matsumoto K, Toh-e A: *IRA2*, a second gene of *Saccharomyces cerevisiae* that encodes a protein with a domain homologous to mammalian *ras* GTPase-activating protein. *Mol Cell Biol* **10**:4303, 1990.
161. Tanaka K, Lin BK, Wood DR, Tamanoi F: *IRA2*, an upstream negative regulator of *RAS* in yeast, is a *RAS* GTPase-activating protein. *Proc Natl Acad Sci USA* **88**:468, 1991.
162. Trahey M, Wong G, Halenbeck R, Rubinfeld B, Martin GA, Ladner M, Long CM, Crosier WJ, Watt K, Koths K, McCormick F: Molecular cloning of two types of GAP complementary DNA from human placenta. *Science* **242**:1697, 1988.
163. Wang Y, Boguski M, Riggs M, Rodgers L, Wigler M: *Sar1*, a gene from *Schizosaccharomyces pombe* encoding a GAP-like protein that regulates *ras*1. *Cell Regul* **2**:253, 1992.
164. Wigler MH: GAPs is understanding *ras*. *Nature* **346**:696, 1990.
165. Marshall CJ: How does p21 *ras* transform cells? *Trends Genet* **7**:91, 1991.
166. Adari H, Lowy DR, Willumsen BM, Der CJ, McCormick F: Guanosine triphosphatase activating protein (GAP) interacts with the p21 *ras* effector binding domain. *Science* **240**:518, 1988.
167. Mitts MR, Bradshaw-Rouse J, Heideman W: Interactions between adenylate cyclase and the yeast GTPase-activating protein IRA1. *Mol Cell Biol* **11**:4591, 1991.
168. Broach JR: *RAS* genes in *Saccharomyces cerevisiae:* Signal transduction in search of a pathway. *Trends Genet* **7**:28, 1991.

169. Golubic M, Tanaka K, Dobrowolski S, Wood D, Tsai MH, Marshall M, Tamanoi F, Stacey DW: The GTPase stimulatory activity of the neurofibromatosis type 1 and yeast IRA2 proteins are inhibited by arachidonic acid. *EMBO J* **10**:2897, 1991.
170. Weismuller L, Wittinghofer A: Expression of the GTPase activating domain of the neurofibromatosis type 1 (NF1) gene in *Escherichia coli* and the role of the conserved lysine residue. *J Biol Chem* **267**:10207, 1992.
171. Kamata T, Feramisco JR: Epidermal growth factor stimulates guanine nucleotide binding activity and phosphorylation of ras oncogene proteins. *Nature* **310**:147, 1984.
172. Moran MF, Polakis P, McCormick F, Pawson T, Ellis C: Protein-tyrosine kinases regulate the phosphorylation, protein interactions, subcellular distribution, and activity of p21*ras* GTPase-activating protein. *Mol Cell Biol* **11**:1804, 1991.
173. Satoh T, Endo M, Nakafuku M, Akiyama T, Yamamoto T, Kaziro Y: Accumulation of p21 *ras*-GTP in response to stimulation with epidermal growth factor and oncogene products with tyrosine kinase activity. *Proc Natl Acad Sci USA* **87**:7926, 1990.
174. Bar-Sagi D, Feramisco JR: Microinjection of the *ras* oncogene protein into PC12 cells induces morphological differentiation. *Cell* **42**:841, 1985.
175. Noda M, Ko M, Ogura A, Liu D-G, Amano T, Takano T, Ikawa Y: Sarcoma viruses carrying *ras* oncogenes induce differentiation-associated properties in a neuronal cell line. *Nature* **318**:73, 1985.
176. Hagag N, Halegoua S, Viola M: Inhibition of growth factor-induced differentiation of PC12 cells by microinjection of antibody to *ras* p21. *Nature* **319**:680, 1986.
177. Zhang K, Papageorge AG, Lowy DR: Mechanistic aspect of signalling through *ras* in NIH3T3 cells. *Science* **257**:671, 1992.
178. Feramisco JR, Clark R, Wong G, Arnheim N, Milley R, McCormick F: Transient reversion of *ras* oncogene-induced cell transformation by antibodies specific for amino acid 12 of *ras* protein. *Nature* **314**:639, 1985.
179. Feramisco JR, Gross M, Kamata T, Rosenberg M, Sweet RW: Microinjection of the oncogene form of the human H-*ras* (T-24) protein results in rapid proliferation of quiecent cells. *Cell* **38**:109, 1984.
180. Benito M, Porras A, Nebreda AR, Santos E: Differentiation of 3T3-L1 fibroblasts to adipocytes induces by transfection of *ras* oncogenes. *Science* **253**:565, 1991.
181. Graziadei L, Raibowol K, Bar-Sagi D: Co-capping of *ras* proteins with surface immunoglobulins in B lymphocytes. *Nature* **347**:396, 1990.
182. Kaplan S, Bar-Sagi D: Association of p21 *ras* with cellular polypeptides. *J Biol Chem* **266**:18934, 1991.
183. Downward J, Graves JD, Warne PH, Rayter S, Cantrell DA: Stimulation of $p21^{ras}$ upon T-cell activation. *Nature* **346**:719, 1990.
184. Ellis C, Moran M, McCormick F, Pawson T: Phosphorylation of GAP and GAP-associated proteins by transforming and mitogenic tyrosine kinases. *Nature* **343**:377, 1990.
185. Gutmann DH, Basu TN, Gregory PE, Wood DL, Downward J, Collins FS: The role of the neurofibromatosis type 1 (NF1) gene product in growth factor-mediated signal transduction. *Neurology* **42**:A183, 1992.
186. Boyer M, Gutmann DH, Collins F, Bar-Sagi D: Co-capping of neurofibromin, but not GAP, with surface immunoglobulins in B lymphocytes. *Oncogene* **9**:349, 1994.
187. Johnson MR, DeClue JE, Felzmann S, Vass WC, Xu G, White R, Lowy DR: Neurofibromin can inhibit *ras*-dependent growth by a mechanism independent of its GTPase-accelerating function. *Mol Cell Biol* **14**:641, 1994.
188. Li Y, White R: Suppression of a human colon cancer cell line by introduction of an exogenous *NF1* gene. *Cancer Res* **56**:2872, 1996.
189. Clark GJ, Drugan JK, Terrell RS, Bradham C, Der CJ, Bell RM, Campbell S: Peptides containing a consensus *Ras* binding sequence from Raf-1 and the GTPase activating protein NF1 inhibit *Ras* function. *Proc Natl Acad Sci USA* **93**:1577, 1996.
190. Gutmann DH, Gregory PE, Wood DL, Collins FS: The neurofibromatosis type 1 gene product encodes a signal transduction protein which associates with microtubules. *J Cell Biochem* **16B:A143, 1992.**
191. Cleveland DW: Microtubule mapping. *Cell* **60**:701, 1990.
192. Matus A: Microtubule-associated proteins. *Curr Opin Cell Biol* **2**:10, 1990.
193. Olmsted JB: Microtubule-associated proteins. *Annu Rev Cell Biol* **2**:421, 1986.
194. Wiche G: High-MW microtubule-associated proteins: Properties and functions. *Biochem J* **259**:1, 1989.
195. Obar RA, Collins CA, Hammarback JA, Shpetner HS, Vallee RB: Molecular cloning of the microtubule-associated mechanochemical enzyme dynamin reveals homology with a new family of GTP-binding proteins. *Nature* **347**:256, 1990.
196. Shpetner HS, Vallee RB: Identification of dynamin, a novel mechanochemical enzyme that mediates interactions between microtubules. *Cell* **59**:421, 1989.
197. Van der Bliek AM, Meyerowitz EM: Dynamin-like protein encoded by the *Drosophila* shibire gene associated with vesicular traffic. *Nature* **351**:411, 1991.
198. Jasmin BJ, Changeux J-P, Cartaud J: Compartmentalization of cold-stable and acetylated microtubules in the subsynaptic domain of chick skeletal muscle fibre. *Nature* **344**:673, 1990.
199. Vallee RB: A taxol-dependent procedure for the isolation of microtubules and microtubule-associated proteins (MAPs). *J Cell Biol* **92**:435, 1982.
200. Vallee RB: Reversible assembly purification of microtubules without assembly-promoting agents and further purification of tubulin, microtubule-associated proteins, and MAP fragments. *Methods Enzymol* **134**:89, 1986.
201. Vallee RB: Molecular characterization of high molecular weight microtubule-associated proteins: Some answers, many questions. *Cell Motil Cytoskel* **15**:204, 1990.
202. Vallee RB, Bloom GS, Theurkauf WE: Microtubule-associated proteins: Subunits of the cytomatrix. *Cell Biol* **99**:38, 1984.
203. Vallee RB, Collins CA: Purification of microtubules and microtubule-associated proteins from sea urchin eggs and cultured mammalian cells using taxol, and use of exogenous taxol-stabilized brain microtubules for purifying microtubule-associated proteins. *Methods Enzymol* **134**:116, 1986.
204. Collins CA: Reversible assembly purification of taxol-treated microtubules. *Methods Enzymol* **196**:246, 1991.
205. Steiner B, Mandelkow E-M, Biernat J, Gustke N, Meyer HE, Schmidt B, Mieskes G, Soauling HD, Drechsel D, Kirschner MW, Goedert M, Mandelkow E: Phosphorylation of microtubule-associated protein tau: Identification of the site for calcium-calmodulin dependent kinase and relationship with tau phosphorylation in Alzheimer tangles. *EMBO J* **9**:3539, 1990.
206. Hall A: ras and GAP: Who's controlling whom? *Cell* **61**:921, 1990.
207. McCormick F: *ras* GTPase activating protein: Signal transmitter and signal terminator. *Cell* **56**:5, 1989.
208. Mitchell AL, Gutmann DH, Gregory PE, Cole J, Park S, Jove R, Collins FS: Localization of the domain in the neurofibromatosis type 1 protein (neurofibromin) that interacts with microtubules. *Am J Hum Genet* **43**:A62, 1993.
209. Nishi T, Lee PSY, Oka K, Levin VA, Tanase S, Morino Y, Saya H: Differential expression of two types of the neurofibromatosis type 1 (NF1) gene transcripts related to neuronal differentiation. *Oncogene* **6**:1555, 1991.
210. Anderson LB, Ballester R, Marchuk DA, Chang E, Gutmann DH, Saulino AM, Camonis J, Wigner M, Collins FS: A conserved alternative splice in the von Recklinghausen neurofibromatosis (NF1) gene produces two neurofibromin isoforms, both of which have GTPase activating protein ability. *Mol Cell Biol* **13**:487, 1993.
211. Gutmann DH, Tennekoon GI, Cole JL, Collins FS, Rutkowski JL: Modulation of the neurofibromatosis type 1 gene product, neurofibromin, during Schwann cell differentiation. *J Neurosci Res* **36**:216, 1993.
212. Gutmann DH, Cole JL, Collins FS: Expression of the neurofibromatosis type 1 (NF1) gene during mouse embryonic development. *Prog Brain Res* **105**:327, 1995.
213. Gutmann DH, Geist RT, Rose K, Wright DE: Expression of two new protein isoforms of the neurofibromatosis type 1 (NF1) gene product, neurofibromin, in muscle tissues. *Dev Dyn* **202**:302, 1995.
214. Neiman HL, Mena E, Holt JF, Stern AM, Perry BL: Neurofibromatosis and congenital heart disease. *AJR* **122**:146, 1974.
215. Kaufman RL, Hartmann AF, McAlister WH: Congenital heart disease associated with neurofibromatosis. *Birth Defects* **8**:92, 1972.
216. Danglot G, Regnier V, Fauvet D, Vassal G, Kujas M, Bernheim A: Neurofibromatosis 1 (NF1) mRNAs expressed in the central nervous system are differentially spliced in the 59 part of the gene. *Hum Mol Gen* **34**:915-920, 1995.
217. Geist RT, Gutmann DH: Expression of a developmentally-regulated neuron-specific isoform of the neurofibromatosis 1 (NF1) gene. *Neurosci Lett* **211**:85, 1996.
218. Martuza RL, MacLaughlin DT, Ojemann RG: Specific estradiol binding in schwannomas, meningiomas, and neurofibromas. *Neurosurgery* **9**:665, 1981.

219. Riccardi VM: Growth-promoting factors in neurofibroma crude extracts. *Ann NY Acad Sci* **486**:66, 1986.
220. Peltonen J, Aho H, Rinne UK, Penttinen R: Neurofibromatosis tumor and skin cells in culture. *Acta Neuropathol (Berl)* **61**:275, 1983.
221. Peltonen J, Jaakkola S, Lebwohl M, Renvall S, Risteli L, Virtanen I, Uitto J: Cellular differentiation and expression of matrix genes in type 1 neurofibromatosis. *Lab Invest* **59**:760, 1988.
222. Pintar JE, Sonnenfeld KH, Fisher J, Klein RS, Kreider B: Molecular and immunocytochemical studies of neurofibromas and related cell types. *Ann NY Acad Sci* **486**:96, 1986.
223. Krone W, Jirikowski G, Muhleck O, Kling H, Gall H: Cell culture studies on neurofibromatosis (von Recklinghausen): II. Occurrence of glial cells in primary cultures of peripheral neurofibromas. *Hum Genet* **63**:247, 1983.
224. Krone W, Mao R, Muhleck S, Kling H, Fink T: Cell culture studies on neurofibromatosis (von Recklinghausen): Characterization of cells growing from neurofibromas. *Ann NY Acad Sci* **486**:354, 1986.
225. Fialkow PJ, Sagebiel RW, Gartler SM, Rimoin DL: Multiple cell origin of hereditary neurofibromatosis. *N Engl J Med* **284**:298, 1971.
226. Skuse GR, Kosciolek BA, Rowley PT: The neurofibroma in von Recklinghausen neurofibromatosis has a unicellular origin. *Am J Hum Genet* **49**:600, 1991.
227. Pleasure D, Kreider B, Sobue G, Ross AH, Koprowski H, Sonnenfeld KH, Rubenstein AE: Schwann-like cells cultured from human dermal neurofibromas: Immunohistological identification and response to Schwann cell mitogens. *Ann NY Acad Sci* **486**:227, 1986.
228. Ratner N, Lieberman MA, Riccardi VM, Hong D: Mitogen accumulation in von Recklinghausen neurofibromatosis. *Ann Neurol* **27**:298, 1990.
229. Sheela S, Riccardi VM, Ratner N: Angiogenic and invasive properties of neurofibroma Schwann cells. *J Cell Biol* **111**:645, 1990.
230. Bidot-Lopez P, Frankel JW: Enhanced viral transformation of skin fibroblasts from neurofibromatosis patients. *Ann Clin Lab Sci* **13**:27, 1983.
231. Frankel JW, Bidot P, Kopelovich L: Enhanced sensitivity of skin fibroblasts from neurofibromatosis patients to transformation by the Kirsten murine sarcoma virus. *Ann NY Acad Sci* **486**:403, 1986.
232. Kopelovich L, Rich RF: Enchanced radiotolerance to ionizing radiation is correlated with increased cancer proneness of cultured fibroblasts from precursor states in neurofibromatosis patients. *Cancer Genet Cytogenet* **22**:203, 1986.
233. Woods WG, McKenzie B, Letourneau MA, Byrne TD: Sensitivity of cultured skin fibroblasts from patients with neurofibromatosis to DNA-damaging agents. *Ann NY Acad Sci* **486**:336, 1986.
234. Huson SM: Recent developments in the diagnosis and management of neurofibromatosis. *Arch Dis Child* **64**:745, 1989.
235. Andersen LB, Tarle SA, Marchuk DA, Leguis E, Collins FS: A compound nucleotide repeat in the neurofibromatosis (NF1) gene. *Hum Mol Genet* **2**:1083, 1993.
236. Heim RA, Silvermna LM, Farber RA, Kam-Morgan LNW, Luce MC: Screening for truncated NF1 proteins. *Nature Genet* **8**:218, 1994.
237. Tsai M-H, Yu C-L, Stacey DW: A cytoplasmic protein inhibits the GTPase activity of H-*Ras* in a phospholipid-dependent manner. *Science* **250**:982, 1990.
238. Gibbs JB: *Ras* C-terminal processing enzymes: New drug targets? *Cell* **65**:1, 1991.
239. Bollag G, McCormick F: Differential regulation of *ras*GAP and neurofibromatosis gene product activities. *Nature* **351**:576, 1991.
240. Chen W-J, Andres DA, Goldstein JL, Brown MS: Cloning and expression of a cDNA encoding the alpha subunit of rat p21*ras* protein farnesyltransferase. *Proc Natl Acad Sci USA* **88**:11368, 1991.
241. Kinsella BT, Erdman RA, Maltese WA: Posttranslational modification of Ha-*ras* p21 by farnesyl versus geranylgeranyl isoprenoids is determined by the COOH-terminal amino acid. *Proc Natl Acad Sci USA* **88**:8934, 1991.
242. Pitts AF, Winters TR, Green SH: Ras isoprenylation is required for ras-induced but not for NGF-induced neuronal differentiation of PC12 cells. *J Cell Biol* **115**:795, 1991.

CHAPTER 40

Neurofibromatosis 2

Mia MacCollin ▪ James Gusella

1. **Neurofibromatosis 2 (NF2) is an autosomal dominant disorder that affects approximately 1 in 40,000 individuals. It is characterized by the development of bilateral vestibular schwannomas and other histologically benign intracranial, spinal, and peripheral nerve tumors. The only nontumorous manifestations of NF2 are cataract and retinal hamartoma. NF2 is fully penetrant by age 60 years, and half of all cases represent new mutations.**
2. **Syndromes related to NF2 include sporadic unilateral vestibular schwannoma, mosaic inactivation of the NF2 gene, schwannomatosis, and multiple meningiomas. NF2 is genetically and clinically distinct from von Recklinghausen disease or neurofibromatosis 1.**
3. **Positional cloning identified the gene for NF2 on chromosome 22q. It spans 110 kb with 16 constitutive exons and 1 alternatively spliced exon. The NF2 protein product is a member of the protein 4.1 family of cytoskeleton-associated proteins. These proteins play a critical role in maintaining membrane stability and cell shape by connecting integral membrane proteins to the spectrin–actin lattice of the cytoskeleton.**
4. **A large number of germ-line mutations have been detected in NF2 patients, with the majority predicted to result in gross protein truncation. Detection of somatic alterations in NF2-related tumors has supported the hypothesis that the *NF2* gene acts as a true tumor suppressor in both schwannomas and meningiomas. NF2 also appears to play a role in the development of mesothelioma, although this tumor is not seen in patients with NF2.**
5. **Diagnosis of NF2 is currently dependent on clinical criteria, although genetic diagnosis may soon be feasible. Treatment of NF2-related tumors remains largely surgical. Advances in hearing augmentation, such as auditory brainstem implants, may improve the quality of life for many patients.**

CLINICAL ASPECTS

Historical Notes and Nomenclature

In 1822, J.H. Wishart made a case report of an unfortunate 21-year-old man who was found at autopsy to have multiple dural-based tumors, hydrocephalus, and multiple tumors at the skull base, a classic description of what is now recognized as neurofibromatosis 2 (NF2).[1] Seventy years after Wishart's observations, Fredrich Daniel von Recklinghausen published his famous monograph on neurofibromatosis 1 (NF1),[2] and in several subsequent publications the presence of skin and spinal cord tumors in both NF1 and NF2 blurred the distinctions between the disorders. In 1902, Henneberg and Koch recognized a clinically distinct form of NF, which lacked skin alterations typical of von Recklinghausen disease and included "acoustic neuromas."[3] They referred to this distinct disorder as "central neurofibromatosis" in contrast to the peripheral features of von Recklinghausen disease. In 1915, Bassoe and Nuzum described a patient with bilateral cerebellopontine angle tumors and other central nervous system tumors.[4] In 1930, a family with 38 members who had bilateral cerebellopontine angle tumors transmitted in an autosomal dominant fashion was reported, emphasizing the genetic nature of this disorder.[5] Several subsequent works confirmed that the form of NF characterized by bilateral cerebellopontine angle tumors is a disorder distinct from the more common or peripheral form at NF.[6–8] Overlapping clinical features, such as multiple spine and skin tumors, continue to cause confusion between these two diseases.[9]

In 1987, a Consensus Development Conference was held at the National Institutes of Health (NIH) to clarify the various clinical types of NF, and 4 years later a second NIH conference was held to evaluate the clinical aspects of acoustic neuroma.[10,11] As a result of these efforts, formal diagnostic criteria were proposed that have improved diagnostic certainty and allowed clinical and molecular genetic studies of phenotypically homogenous groups of patients. The conferees recommended the adoption of the term neurofibromatosis type 2 (NF2) instead of central, bilateral vestibular, or bilateral acoustic neurofibromatosis. In addition, the term "vestibular schwannoma" was preferred to the previously used "acoustic neuroma," based on the observation that the tumors originate from the vestibular rather than the acoustic branch of the eighth cranial nerve. Finally, the older term "neurilemmoma" has been replaced by "schwannoma," based on work implicating the Schwann cell as the cell of origin in these tumors.[12]

Incidence of Inherited and Sporadic Disease

NF2 is a rare disorder, and because of the wide variety of specialists who manage these patients and because of frequent misdiagnoses, its prevalence is difficult to ascertain. Evans et al. found the incidence at birth to be approximately 1 in 40,000 in a population-based study.[13] This makes NF2 approximately 10 times less common than neurofibromatosis type 1 (NF1), which has an incidence of 1 in 3000.[10] In both this work and that of Parry et al., sporadic versus inherited cases were divided evenly.[13,14] This may reflect a relatively high mutation rate at the *NF2* locus and low reproductive fitness, especially in severely affected patients. Unilateral vestibular schwannoma, unlike NF2, is a very common disorder, with an incidence of about 1 per 100,000 per year.[11] In two large autopsy series, the incidence of occult vestibular schwannoma was even higher (0.82 to 0.87 percent).[15,16] Less than 5 percent of individuals with unilateral vestibular schwannoma eventually develop bilateral disease and NF2.[11,17] Both unilateral vestibular schwannoma and NF2 show no racial, ethnic, or gender predilection.

Diagnostic Criteria

Diagnostic criteria for both NF1 and NF2 have been proposed by the NIH (Table 40-1).[10] Several workers have suggested expansion of these criteria in the hope that diagnosis may be made earlier in patients with multiple features of the disorder but without bilateral vestibular schwannoma.[18,19] Caution must be used in counseling patients on their reproductive and health risks when they do not

A list of standard abbreviations is located immediately preceding the index in each volume. Additional abbreviations used in this chapter include: ERM = ezrin, radixin, moesin; BAER = brain stem auditory evoked response; NF = neurofibromatosis; NIH = National Institutes of Health.

Table 40-1 Diagnostic Criteria for NF2

Bilateral eighth-nerve masses seen with appropriate imaging techniques
or
A first-degree relative with NF2 and unilateral eighth nerve mass or two of the following:
- Neurofibroma
- Meningioma
- Glioma
- Schwannoma
- Juvenile posterior subcapsular lenticular opacity

SOURCE: Adapted from Mulvihill JJ, Parry DM, Sherman JL, Pikus A, Kaiser-Kupfer MI, Eldridge R: NIH conference: Neurofibromatosis 1 (Recklinghausen disease) and neurofibromatosis 2 (bilateral acoustic neurofibromatosis): An update. *Ann Intern Med* 113:39, 1990.

meet the NIH criteria because the more liberal criteria have not been validated clinically. When the NIH criteria are applied strictly, it is rare to find an overlap between NF1 and NF2 in a single patient. Nearly all individuals with NF2 eventually develop bilateral vestibular schwannoma, and this alone is enough to diagnose the disorder. In the presence of other cardinal features of NF2, such as a positive family history, or other NF2-related tumors, the diagnosis may be considered in an individual with unilateral vestibular schwannoma on the presumption that bilateral tumors will appear in time. Because the appearance of all NF2-related tumors increases with age, the diagnosis should be strongly suspected in a child of an affected individual who has any manifestation, including a skin tumor alone.[20]

Major Clinical Features of NF2

Vestibular Schwannoma. The occurrence of bilateral vestibular schwannoma is a nearly universal feature of individuals with NF2, and so the diagnosis of NF2 should be reconsidered in any individual without a positive family history who does not have these tumors. Vestibular tumors originate within the internal auditory canal, where the eighth nerve lies in close proximity to the facial nerve (Fig. 40-1). Initial symptoms include tinnitus, hearing loss, and balance dysfunction. Significant facial palsy is rare even in large tumors and if present should suggest a facial nerve tumor. Disability is often insidious in onset, although occasionally sudden hearing loss may occur, presumably owing to vascular compromise by the tumor. Patients often report difficulty in using the telephone in one ear, or unsteadiness when walking at night or on uneven ground. With time, vestibular tumors extend medially into the cerebellar pontine angle and, if left untreated, cause compression of the brain stem and hydrocephalus. Schwannomas also may develop on other cranial nerves, with sensory nerves more frequently affected than motor nerves.[7,14]

Meningioma. Approximately half of individuals with NF2 develop meningioma (Fig. 40-2).[14,18] Most of these tumors are intracranial; spinal meningioma is not uncommon, and there is a single report of a cutaneous meningioma.[9] There is no site of predilection for meningioma as there is for schwannoma, although meningioma intermixed with schwannoma is a common and incidental finding when the cerebral pontine angle is explored surgically.[21] Because of the multiplicity and slow growth patterns of these tumors, it is often neither possible nor advisable to remove all meningiomas from an NF2 patient. Therapy should be considered when a tumor causes symptoms resulting from compression or development of edema in the adjacent brain. Special attention is needed for meningiomas in the orbit that may compress the optic nerve and result in visual loss, and meningiomas at the skull base that may cause symptoms of cranial neuropathy, brain stem compression, and hydrocephalus.

Spinal Tumors. Two-thirds or more of NF2 patients develop spinal tumors. This can be one of the most devastating and difficult to manage aspects of this disease (Fig. 40-3).[14,22] The most common spinal tumor is a schwannoma, which often originates within the intravertebral canal on the dorsal root and extends both medially and laterally to form a dumbbell shape. This configuration is identical to that of spinal neurofibromas in NF1, and occasionally may cause diagnostic confusion between the two disorders. Less commonly, patients develop meningiomas of the spinal coverings. Intramedullary tumors, such as astrocytoma and ependymoma, are reported to occur in 5 to 10 percent of all NF2 patients,[14,18] although 33 percent of severely affected individuals who underwent complete spinal imaging had evidence of intramedullary cord tumors.[22] Most individuals with spinal cord tumors have multiple tumors (50 percent in the study of Mautner et al.[22]), and there is no site of predilection for either intra- or extramedullary tumor formation. Although ependymoma in patients without NF2 is optimally treated with complete resection and occasionally with radiotherapy and chemotherapy,[23] it is unclear whether ependymoma in NF2 patients warrants aggressive management.

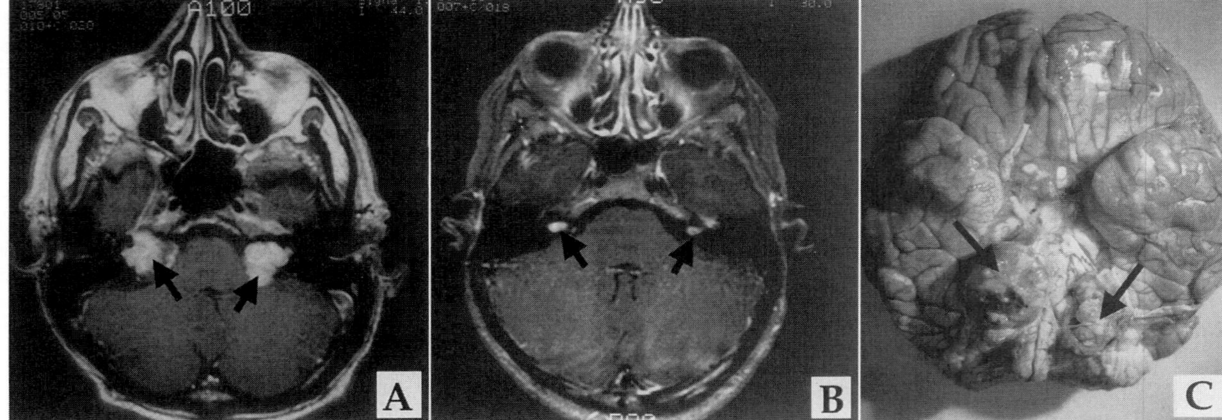

Fig. 40-1. Bilateral vestibular schwannoma. *A,* Axial T1-weighted contrast-enhanced image of the skull base in a 45-year-old man with NF2. Very large multilobulated tumors with extracannicular extension are seen (arrows). *B,* Similar MRI of the patient's presymptomatic adolescent nephew. Small enhancing masses are seen in both internal auditory canals (arrows). *C,* Gross pathologic view of the skull base in an NF2 patient; arrows point to tumors in the cerebellar pontine angles (Photo courtesy of Dr. David Louis, Neuropathology Department, Massachusetts General Hospital.)

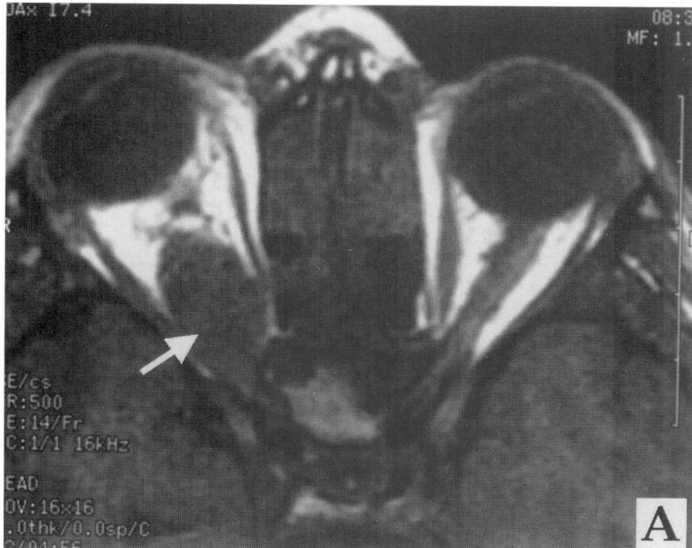

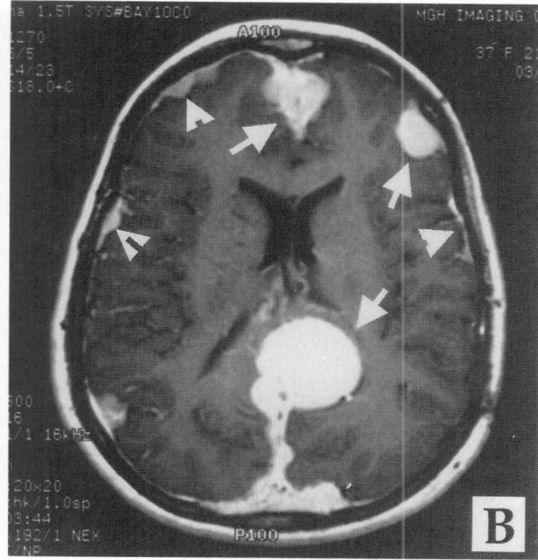

Fig. 40-2. Radiographic appearance of intracranial meningioma in NF2. *A,* Orbital mass in a child with NF2. Orbital tumors in NF2 affected children may be confused with optic glioma; the latter tumor is seen in NF1 but not NF2. T1-weighted MRI. *B,* Multiple discrete lesions (arrows) and diffuse enhancement (arrowheads) suggestive of meningiomatosis in an adult with NF2.

Other Features of NF2. In addition to vestibular schwannoma and spinal schwannoma, NF2 patients are prone to the development of schwannomas along other cranial nerves, in the brachial and lumbar plexuses, and along peripheral nerves. Two-thirds of these patients will develop skin tumors, primarily schwannomas.[14,18,24] Unlike NF1 patients, it is rare for a single patient to develop more than 10 skin tumors.[14,24] There have been several reports of peripheral neuropathy occurring in the context of NF2, although the pathophysiology of this process is unknown.[14,18,25,26]

The ophthalmologic consequences of NF2 are an under-recognized and important aspect of the disease.[27–29] For example, Bouzas et al. studied 54 NF2 patients and found that one-third had decreased visual acuity in one or both eyes, which was directly or indirectly related to the diagnosis.[28] Posterior subcapsular lens opacity progressing to actual cataract is the most common ocular finding (Fig. 40-4). Lens opacities may appear before vestibular schwannoma in at-risk children.[20] Retinal hamartoma and epiretinal membrane are seen in up to one-third of these patients, making indirect ophthalmoscopy mandatory in the evaluation of NF2 patients. Finally, the neuro-ophthalmologic consequences of intracranial and intraorbital tumors may result in decreased visual acuity and diplopia. Because all NF2 patients are also at risk for hearing loss, early recognition of visual impairment from any of these causes is extremely important.

Features not Associated with NF2. Because NF2 is uncommon and because diagnostic confusion continues to exist, it is worth noting several features associated with NF1 that are not increased in the NF2 population. NF2 patients do not have the associated cognitive problems, including mental retardation and learning

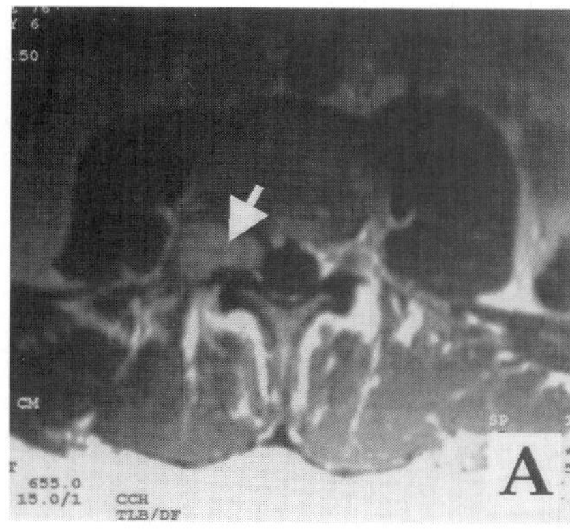

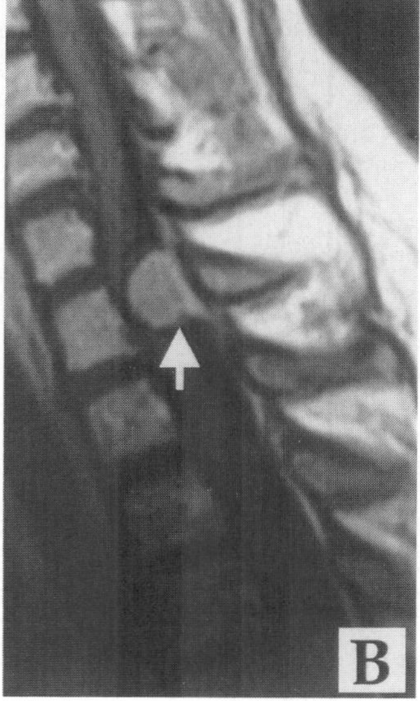

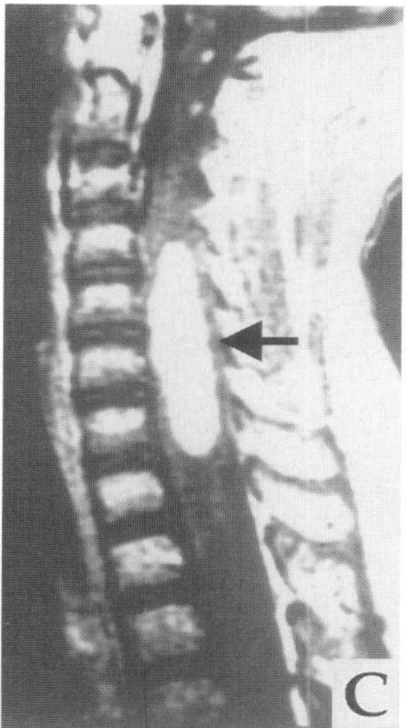

Fig. 40-3. Spinal cord tumors associated with NF2. *A,* Dorsal root schwannoma that has assumed a "dumbbell" configuration (arrow). *B,* Meningioma lying posterior to and displacing the thoracic spinal cord of a child with NF2 (arrow). *C,* Intramedullary cervical spine tumor. Biopsy revealed ependymoma, although the radiographic appearance also is consistent with astrocytoma. T1-weighted contrast enhanced MRIs.

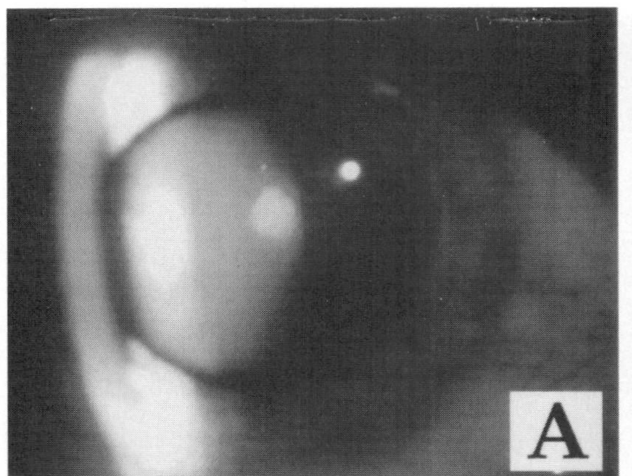

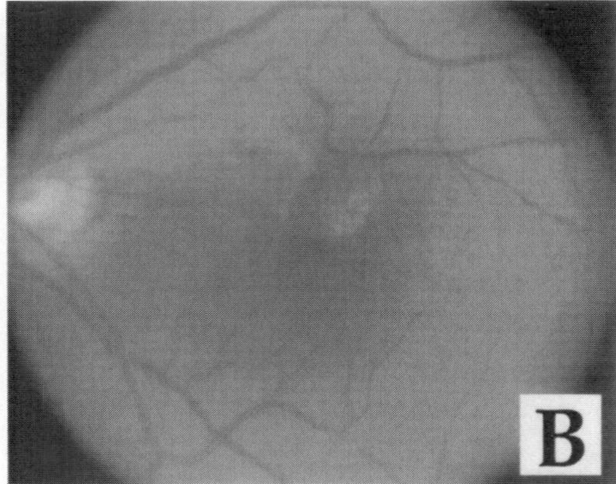

Fig. 40-4. Ocular findings in NF2. *A,* Slit-lamp photograph revealing posterior capsular cataract. *B,* Fundus photograph revealing an epiretinal membrane near the macula. (Courtesy of Dr. Muriel Kaiser, National Eye Institute.)

disability, that NF1 patients have, nor do they have significant numbers of Lisch nodules. The schwannomas of NF2 rarely, if ever, transform to neurofibrosarcomas, and the overall incidence of malignant tumors in the NF2 population is probably not increased over that in the general population. Approximately half of NF2-affected individuals have small numbers of café-au-lait macules.[14,18] Because 10 percent of the general population also has one or two of these macules, this finding has limited diagnostic value.[30,31] NF2 patients do not have significant numbers of café-au-lait macules (six or more over 15 mm in greatest diameter in postpubertal persons), although their skin is more frequently scrutinized, perhaps leading to this misconception.

Clinical Course

In a large population-based study, the average age of the onset of symptoms among NF2 patients was 21 years, with a range of 2 to 52 years.[18] Similar findings were reported by Parry et al., who reported an average age at onset of symptoms of 20 years and a range of 7 to 70 years.[14] Most patients present with symptoms referable to compression of the eighth cranial nerve, including deafness, tinnitus, and balance dysfunction. Other presenting problems may include facial weakness, visual impairment, and painful skin tumors. Headache and seizure are distinctly uncommon modes of presentation. In the case of deafness, the inability to use a phone in one ear is often an important clue, as it is the only test of unilateral hearing that normally occurs in everyday life. Unfortunately, the study of Parry et al. documented an 8-year lag between age at first symptom and diagnosis, underscoring the need for increased clinical recognition of this disorder.[14] Recognition of NF2 in the pediatric population is an especially critical area, as NF2 is classically thought of as an adult disease. Skin tumors and ocular findings, which often are not prominent in an older patient, may be important clues in the pediatric age range.[20]

The clinical course of NF2 is extremely variable and depends on tumor burden, surgical management, and complications. A small number of NF2 patients develop only vestibular schwannoma with disability primarily related to the seventh and eighth cranial nerves. More commonly, patients exhibit a progressive deterioration with loss of hearing, ambulation, and sight along with chronic pain caused by the tumor burden. Although the spectrum of NF2 among affected individuals is quite wide, there is some intrafamilial homogeneity that may be helpful in the counseling and management of patients with a positive family history. The course of NF2 is most likely minimally affected by gender or pregnancy.[32,33]

The average age at death in the NF2 population has been reported to be 36 years; in the same study, actuarial survival after diagnosis was 15 years.[18] It is important to realize that several factors may affect this figure in the near future. Early recognition of the disease, both clinically and by presymptomatic diagnosis of at-risk offspring, allows diagnosis of tumors at an earlier and presumably more surgically approachable stage.[34] Improvements in imaging techniques have allowed the detection of smaller tumors and better preoperative assessment of anatomy.[35] Finally, the advances in surgical techniques described below certainly will improve outcome.[35,36]

Related Syndromes

Unilateral Vestibular Schwannoma. Sporadic unilateral vestibular schwannoma is a common tumor in the general population, accounting for 5 to 10 percent of all intracranial tumors and the vast majority of cerebral pontine angle tumors.[37] Less than 5 percent of individuals with vestibular schwannoma develop bilateral tumors, and the probability of doing so is critically dependent on the age at which the tumor is detected (Fig. 40-5).[17] For those under age 25, the development of a unilateral vestibular schwannoma should prompt a careful evaluation for other features of the disease. Conversely, there is little rationale for screening persons 55 and over with unilateral vestibular schwannoma for NF2. The offspring of persons with unilateral vestibular schwannoma alone do not have an increased incidence of either NF2 or unilateral vestibular schwannoma.

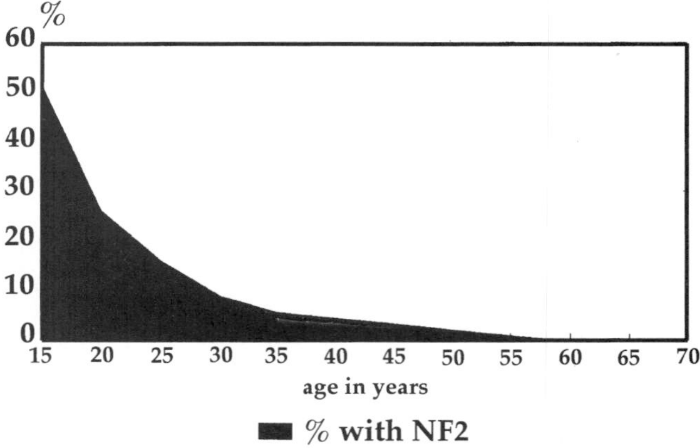

Fig. 40-5. Age-specific risk of having NF2 on presenting with vestibular schwannoma. (From Evans et al.[17] by permission of the author and *The Journal of Laryngology and Otology*.)

Mosaicism in the NF2 Gene. Somatic mosaicism of frameshifting and nonsense mutation has been reported to cause a mild form of sporadic NF2.[38] Other reports of clinically suspected mosaicism have been made in individuals with unilateral vestibular schwannoma and multiple other ipsilateral tumors.[39] A single case of germ-line mosaicism has been reported, resulting in affected sibs carrying an identical *NF2* gene mutation with clinically normal parents in whom the mutation could not be detected in lymphoblast DNA.[40] It remains unclear whether persons with somatic mosaicism carry any genetic risk for bearing affected offspring (i.e., if somatic mosaicism may coexist with germ-line mosaicism).

Recognition of mosaic individuals may be problematic, as they may not have bilateral vestibular schwannomas and genetic analysis in peripheral tissues such as lymphocytes may not reveal the underlying mutation. Mosaicism should be considered in any individual with unilateral vestibular schwannoma and other NF2-related tumors, especially if the tumors are anatomically localized. Molecular genetic analysis of resected tumor material may be a viable alternative to analysis of peripheral tissues for a definitive diagnosis of mosaicism. Germ-line mosaicism for *NF2* mutations appears to be sufficiently rare to make screening of the sibs of an affected individual with normal parents unnecessary.

Schwannomatosis. Schwannomatosis is defined as multiple pathologically proven schwannomas without vestibular schwannoma diagnostic of NF2.[41] Previous terms for this condition have included multiple neurilemmomas, agminated neurilemmomas, multiple schwannomas, and neurilemmomatosis. Schwannomatosis appears to be a clinically distinct entity from NF1 and NF2. Persons with schwannomatosis may develop intracranial, spinal nerve root, or peripheral tumors; like persons with NF2, they do not develop malignancy. In one-third of all reported cases, schwannomatosis patients have had anatomically localized tumors suggestive of segmental disease.[41–43] There are few cases of familial involvement with schwannomatosis; in these rare kindreds autosomal dominant inheritance with highly variable expressivity and incomplete penetrance is seen.[41] Although schwannomatosis appears to be a tumor-suppressor gene syndrome, it is unclear if it is due to an aberration in *NF1*, *NF2*, or an unknown transcript.

Multiple Meningiomas. Although many patients with NF2 develop multiple meningiomas, the appearance of meningiomas rarely predates that of vestibular schwannoma in a single patient. Rare instances of families with multiple meningiomas without vestibular schwannoma segregating as an autosomal dominant trait have been reported.[44] Genetic linkage analysis of one such family showed that the trait segregates separately from the *NF2* gene, implicating a second genetic locus.[45] This result is supported by the data presented below, which implicate a non-NF2 gene in approximately half of all sporadic meningiomas. Multiple meningiomas in a patient without a family history are more commonly due to noncontiguous spread of a single tumor.[46] Presumably, the latter condition carries no genetic risk to offspring. Because sporadic meningioma is classically a tumor of older adults, the finding of a single meningioma in an individual under age 25 years should prompt an evaluation for an underlying genetic condition.[17]

Histopathology

The tumors of NF2 are derived from Schwann cells, meningeal cells, and glial cells, and are histologically benign. Vestibular schwannomas from NF2 patients have several pathologic differences from those that occur sporadically. About 40 percent of vestibular tumors from NF2 patients have a lobular pattern that is uncommon in sporadic tumors.[21] Intermixture of meningioma with vestibular schwannoma in NF2 patients is not uncommon.[21] NF2-associated vestibular schwannomas have been reported to be more invasive of the eighth cranial nerve and to have a higher proportion of dividing cells.[47,48] Less is known about histologic distinctions between nonvestibular tumors in their sporadic and NF2-associated forms. Some workers have reported a predominance of fibroblastic meningioma, although others have found equal numbers of fibroblastic and meningothelial tumors in NF2 patients.[12,49] No histologic differences between glial tumors in NF2 and those in sporadic cases have been reported.[49]

GENETIC ASPECTS OF NF2

Historical Aspects

Early studies on the pathogenetic mechanisms underlying NF2 revealed that NF2-related tumors often lost large stretches of chromosome 22.[50–52] This finding not only suggested that the *NF2* gene is on chromosome 22, but also supported the hypothesis that it is a classic tumor suppressor.[53] In conjunction with these initial investigations on tumors, studies were made of a large NF2-affected kindred by the method of linkage analysis.[54] This genetic linkage approach confirmed the position of *NF2* on chromosome 22 and refined its localization to band 22q12. Further work with tumor material and other affected kindreds narrowed the critical region on chromosome 22 to approximately 6 Mb.[55]

In 1992, a single, affected individual was identified, who, along with her affected daughter, carried a 30-kb deletion recognizable with the probe neurofilament heavy chain and the rare cutting enzyme *NotI* (Fig. 40-6).[55] Taking this patient's deleted region as a target, the transcribed sequences within this area were isolated by using the method of exon trapping. Subsequent identification of cDNA using these exons as probes revealed that the predicted protein carried especially high homology to the 4.1 family of cytoskeletal-associated proteins. Because of this homology, the putative protein product has been named *merlin* (for moezin-ezrin-radixin-like protein); alternatively, schwannomin has been suggested to reflect the role of this protein in the prevention of the development of schwannomas.[56]

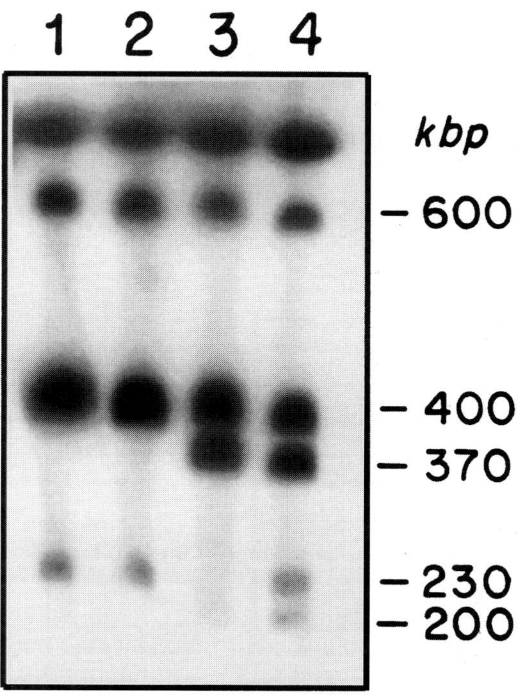

Fig. 40-6. Pulsed-field gel analysis of lymphoblast DNA from NF2 patients. DNA in agarose blocks was digested with the rare cutting restriction enzyme NotI, subjected to electrophoresis, blotted, and hybridized to a radiolabeled neurofilament heavy chain probe. Lane 1: unrelated NF2 patient. Lane 2: unaffected individual. Lane 3: affected daughter. Lane 4: affected mother. (From Trofatter et al.[55] by permission of *Cell*.)

Clinical Genetics

NF2 shows autosomal-dominant transmission with full penetrance by age 60.[14,18] In two studies, a parent of origin effect on severity was observed, with the mean age in paternally inherited cases being 24 years, and that in maternally inherited cases being 18 years.[6,18] Subsequent work has not confirmed this disparity, which may reflect a difference in the reproductive fitness of severely affected males versus females.[14] There is a marked degree of heterogeneity in NF2, and several authors have divided the disease into clinical subtypes. The mild, or Gardner, subtype is characterized by the onset of symptoms in the third decade or later, few associated brain or spinal tumors, and survival into the sixth decade. The severe, or Wishart, subtype involves onset before age 25, rapid clinical progression, multiple intracranial and spinal tumors, and death in the third or fourth decade. The existence of a third subtype (Lee-Abbott) with variable age at hearing loss, cataract, and early age at death has not been confirmed.[14,18,57] The manifestations and clinical subtype of NF2 usually are similar within members of a family.[14,18,38,40] Despite the clinical heterogeneity of NF2, there is no evidence of genetic heterogeneity as is seen in other tumor-suppressor gene syndromes, such as tuberous sclerosis complex.[58] All series have shown that half of affected individuals do not have an affected parent; *de novo* alteration in the *NF2* gene has been documented in several of these individuals.[40,59]

The *NF2* Gene and Protein Product

The *NF2* gene spans 110 kilobases and includes 16 constitutive exons and 1 alternatively spliced exon.[55,56] *NF2* is widely expressed, producing mRNAs in three different size ranges of approximately 7, 4.4, and 2.6 kb.[55,60] Two major alternative forms of the NF2 protein product exist. Isoform 1 is a protein of 595 amino acids produced from exons 1 through 15 and exon 17. The presence of the alternatively spliced exon 16 alters the C-terminus of the protein, replacing 16 amino acids with 11 novel residues in isoform 2. Additional alternative splices predicting other minor species have also been described.[61,62] The *NF2* gene is highly conserved through evolution, as the mouse protein is 98 percent identical to human *NF2*, and the mouse *NF2* gene, which maps to chromosome 11 in a region of synteny conservation with 22q, is similarly alternatively spliced.[63,64]

The NF2 protein product is a member of the protein 4.1 family of cytoskeleton-associated proteins (Fig. 40-7). The proteins of this family include protein 4.1 itself, talin, ezrin, radixin, moesin, and several protein tyrosine phosphatases. All family members have a homologous domain of approximately 270 amino acids at the N-terminus.[65] In the NF2 protein and its close relatives, this domain is followed by a long α-helical segment and a charged C-terminal domain. Protein 4.1, the best-studied member of the family, plays a critical role in maintaining membrane stability and cell shape in the erythrocyte by connecting integral membrane proteins, glycophorin, and the anion channel to be spectrin-actin lattice of the cytoskeleton. Protein 4.1 is the only other family member in which disease-causing mutation is known (hereditary elliptocytosis; Chap. 183).

The ERM proteins, to which the NF2 protein is most closely related, share 70 to 75 percent amino acid identity with each other and are located in actin-rich surface projections such as microvilli, filopodia, membrane ruffles, lamellipodia in migrating cells, neuronal growth cones, and mitotic cleavage furrows. The NF2 protein is 45 to 46 percent identical to the ERMs with a common structural pattern except for the two different charged C-termini produced by alternative splicing. Both isoforms localize preferentially to the motile regions of cultured cells, such as the leading or ruffling edges, where they colocalize with F-actin. Where it has been tested, the NF2 protein does not colocalize with ezrin or moesin, suggesting a membrane-cytoskeleton linker function that is distinguishable from the ERM proteins.[66] A function of the NF2 protein in the motile regions of the cell suggests that schwannomas and meningiomas may form when the appropriate cell loses the ability to accurately regulate cell movement, shape, or communication, leading to a loss of growth control.

Germ-Line Mutations

Several studies aimed at identifying germ-line mutations in typical NF2 patients have been reported.[38,67–69] In at least two studies, exon scanning was shown to detect mutation in two-thirds of patients.[40,59] Small numbers of patients have been reported to have gene deletions detected by Southern blot or flanking microsatellite analysis.[38,55,70–72] A wide variety of mutations have been identified in all *NF2* exons except for exons 16 and 17. The vast majority of the alterations predict truncation of the protein product as a result of the introduction of a stop codon, a frameshift with premature termination, or a splicing alteration, supporting the view that loss of the protein's normal function is crucial to the development of tumors. C to T transitions in CGA codons causing nonsense mutations are an especially common occurrence.[73] Less than 10 percent of detected mutations involve in-frame deletions and missense mutations, which indicates that alteration of particular functional domains can abolish the *NF2* tumor-suppressor activity.[74] No frequent polymorphisms, even in codon wobble positions, have been reported in the *NF2* gene.

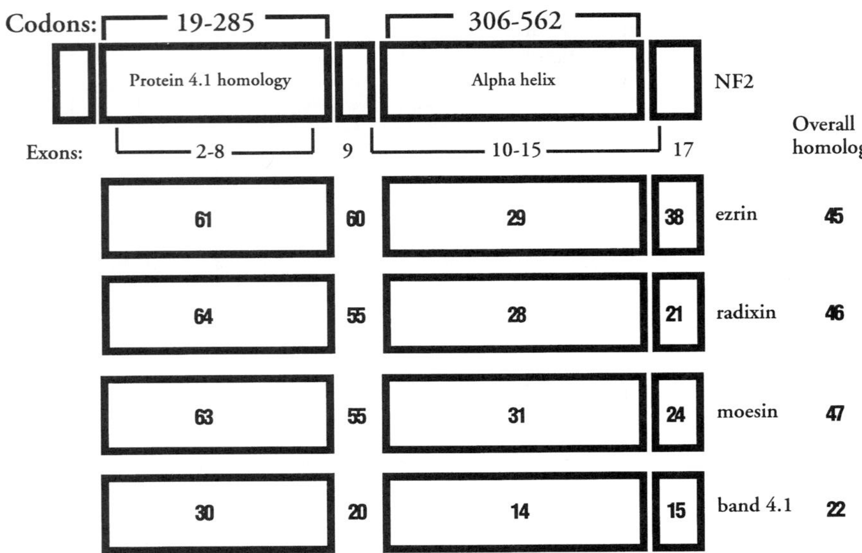

Fig. 40-7. ERM proteins related to NF2. The NF2 protein product is a member of the band 4.1 family of cytoskeletal-associated proteins. This diagram depicts the domain of the NF2 protein, which includes a region of homology in the amino terminal half that defines membership in the protein 4.1 family, an α-helical domain, and a terminus affected by alternative splicing. The percentage amino acid identity with the three most closely related family members ezrin, radixin, and moesin, and with band 4.1 itself is shown within each region. The C-terminus of the ERM proteins contains an actin-binding region not found in the NF2 protein.

A strong effect of the genotype on the resulting phenotype in NF2 is suggested by the clinical observations that intrafamilial homogeneity is marked in NF2. Several studies have supported the hypothesis that the underlying *NF2* gene mutation is predictive of the resulting phenotype when the gross variables of mild versus severe disease is examined.[38,40,55,56,59,67–69,73,75–77] In these studies, a total of 110 independently occurring nonsense and frameshift mutations produced severe disease in 95 cases studied (86 percent), while splice-site mutation produced severe disease in 49 percent of cases and rare nontruncating changes produced severe disease in only 33 percent of cases. Despite studies in other tumor-suppressor genes that have linked position within the gene to specific manifestations, no effect of the position of the mutation has been determined in NF2.

Several studies that present a more detailed analysis of the effects of genotype on phenotype have been reported.[38,40,67,75] Overall, patients with nonsense or frameshift mutations have earlier ages at onset and diagnosis and greater numbers of tumors then any other group of patients. At the other end of the spectrum, families in whom mutations cannot be identified by exon scanning have late ages of onset and diagnosis and a low frequency of nonvestibular tumors.[40] Such families may harbor larger deletions or insertions not identified by the methodologies used in these studies, mutations in introns and untranslated regulatory elements, or mosaicism not detectable in the tissue analyzed. Also of importance to the clinician is that families with splice-site mutation display far more intrafamilial variability than other families,[77] so that caution should be exercised when giving anticipatory guidance to these families. These studies also point out an irony in current *NF2* screening protocols, because patients with mild phenotypes may be more likely to seek molecular diagnostic services than those with severe manifestations, and are the least likely to have identifiable *NF2* gene changes by current techniques.

Somatic Mutations

A number of studies have looked at somatic mutations in the *NF2* gene in resected tumor tissues from both NF2-affected and NF2-unaffected individuals. Mutations found in tumor material but not in normal tissue from the same individual are essential in confirming that *NF2* behaves like other well-documented tumor-suppressor genes.[53] In a study of 38 sporadic and NF2-derived schwannomas, Jacoby et al. found 25 somatic mutations affecting expression of the *merlin* protein.[78] All 25 mutations involved gross truncation with nonsense, frameshift, or splice-site alteration. Deletion was an especially common mechanism of mutation, with over half the mutations (14 of 25) involving the removal of 1 to 34 base pairs. As would be expected, many of these tumors (16 of 38) also showed loss of polymorphic markers on chromosome 22, indicating large deletions of that chromosome. Similar results have been reported in a follow-up study by the same group and by several other groups.[79–85] No differences have been reported between mutations detected in vestibular and nonvestibular tumors, or between tumors derived from NF2 patients and sporadic tumors. These studies support the hypothesis that the *NF2* gene is the major tumor suppressor for schwannoma.

Analysis of meningiomas, the second most common tumor type in NF2, has revealed slightly different results. Wellenreuther et al., in a comprehensive analysis of 70 sporadic meningiomas, identified 43 mutations in 41 tumors.[86] Similar to the results in schwannoma, only 1 of the 43 involved a nontruncating event. Mutational events were much more common in tumors that had lost heterozygosity for chromosome 22, supporting the hypothesis that *NF2* is the meningioma locus on chromosome 22. These authors found that *NF2* mutations occurred much more frequently in specific pathologic subtypes of meningiomas. These and other studies suggest that *NF2* is a tumor suppressor for meningioma but that another protein or proteins not on chromosome 22 may also fill this role.[83,84,87]

Analysis of glial tumors has shown conflicting results. A total of 6 of 15 ependymomas analyzed in two studies carried a mutation in the *NF2* gene.[88,89] No mutations have been found in astrocytic tumors, even those with loss of heterozygosity of chromosome 22 markers.[88,90] Further work is needed to determine if pathologic or anatomic subgroups of glial tumors exist in which the *NF2* gene is more important as a tumor suppressor.

Loss of heterozygosity has also been observed for chromosome 22q markers in many different types of tumors that are not characteristic of NF2. Screening for mutations that affect the *NF2* gene in such tumors has yielded mixed results. Only a handful of putative mutations of the *NF2* gene have been found in malignant melanoma, breast adenocarcinoma, and colon cancer, and none have been seen in ovarian carcinoma or hepatocellular carcinoma.[91–93] A high rate of *NF2* mutation has been detected in malignant mesothelioma, suggesting that loss of *NF2* may be important in the progression of this aggressive mesodermal tumor type.[94,95] Further work is needed to determine what role *NF2* plays in the proliferation of cells beyond those giving rise to the nervous system tumors of NF2.

DIAGNOSIS AND TREATMENT

Diagnosis of NF2 is based on the NIH clinical criteria (Table 40-1). A careful clinical examination with special attention to a dermatologic evaluation, the neurologic symptomatology, and a slit-lamp examination to evaluate possible retinal or lenticular manifestations are mandatory. Initial radiographic evaluation of a patient known or suspected to have NF2 should include a cranial MRI scan with and without gadolinium enhancement. Small intracanalicular tumors may not be seen on standard 5-mm slice thickness through the posterior fossa. Optimal evaluation includes 3-mm cuts overlapping by 1.5 mm on both axial and coronal post-contrast enhancement views through the internal auditory canals.[35] Large vestibular schwannomas (those greater than 2 cm) and meningiomas may be visualized by computer tomography (CT). In general, however, CT is obscured by bony artifact in the region of the internal auditory canal and skull base and cannot substitute for MRI. Audiologic evaluation including brain stem auditory evoked response (BAER) may rarely reveal a functional deficit in a nerve in which no enhancement is visible. BAER also may be useful in defining the baseline functional impact of an otherwise presymptomatic tumor. Spinal MRI may be helpful in defining asymptomatic tumors; it is mandatory in individuals with unexplained neurologic symptoms or signs.

Increasingly, presymptomatic genetic testing may supplant clinical testing for individuals at risk for NF2.[34,96,97] Because NF2 is a fully penetrant disease and because the age of onset shows homogeneity within families, such testing probably is useful only for the children of an at-risk individual. The age at testing depends on the family's attitude toward presymptomatic surgery and the severity of disease in the family. Genetic testing may be done on the basis of linkage when there is more than one affected family member, or on the basis of mutational analysis of a known affected individual. Caution must be exercised when using a founder to phase chromosomes for linkage because of the high incidence of mosaicism in this disorder.[98] Because no mutation can be detected in at least one-third of individuals with typical NF2, mutational analysis is not useful for confirming or excluding a suspected diagnosis in a proband.

Therapy for vestibular schwannoma remains primarily surgical.[35,36,99,100] Close neurologic monitoring is mandatory for determining the timing of surgical intervention. Small vestibular tumors (less than 1.5 cm) that are completely intercanalicular can often be completely resected with preservation of both hearing and facial function.[35,36] Larger tumors probably are best managed expectantly, with debulking or decompression carried out when brain stem compression, or increasing facial and/or hearing function, ensues.[36] Other cranial and spinal tumors, including meningiomas, other cranial nerve schwannomas, and ependymomas, should be monitored for symptomatology. These tumors are very slow growing, and intervention on a minimally functionally active tumor may produce disability years before it would occur otherwise. Facial nerve reconstruction may be very important for patients who find facial palsy more debilitating than hearing loss.[36,101]

Stereotactic radiosurgery, most commonly with the gamma knife, has been offered as an alternative to surgery in selected patients with vestibular schwannomas.[102–104] Radiation therapy for other NF2-associated tumors should be carefully considered because radiation exposure may induce, accelerate, or transform tumors in a patient with an inactivated tumor-suppressor gene. There is currently no medical therapy available for NF2 patients. Various agents, including progesterone inhibitors, and antiangiogenesis factors have shown promising results in cell culture and animal models.[105–107] Management of patients with vestibular tumors should include counseling on the often insidious problems with balance they may encounter. Drowning or near-drowning owing to underwater disorientation is an especially important consideration.[6]

Hearing and speech augmentation and preservation play an important role in the management of NF2 patients. All patients and their families should be referred to audiologists to receive training in optimization of hearing and speech production. Teaching may enhance lip-reading skills, and sign language often may be more effectively acquired before the patient loses hearing. Hearing aids may be helpful early in the course of the disease. Rarely, patients who have had a vascular insult to the cochlea, but who are otherwise without nerve damage, may benefit from a cochlear implant.[108] An alternative technology for placement of a cochlear implant-type electrode proximal to the nerve in the lateral recess of the fourth ventricle recently was developed by the House Ear Institute in Los Angeles.[109,110] Initial results with this device in 24 adult-deafened NF2 patients have been extremely promising.[111]

Resources for Patients with NF2

Diagnosis, evaluation, and treatment of complex patients with NF2 is best done in a neurofibromatosis center that is experienced in the multiple complications and delicate management of this disease.[17,32] Such multidisciplinary clinics are now available in most major medical centers and are accredited by the National Neurofibromatosis Foundation (New York, NY) and Neurofibromatosis, Inc. (Lanthan, MD). Both organizations publish newsletters and maintain a network of local support chapters that are invaluable resources for patient and family education and support.

REFERENCES

1. Wishart JH: Case of tumours in the skull, dura mater, and brain. *Edinburgh Med Surg J* **18**:393, 1822.
2. Crump TT: Translation of case reports in Ueber die multiplen Fibrome der Haut und ihre Beziehung zu den multiplen Neuromen by F.V. Recklinghausen. *Adv Neurol* **29**:259, 1981.
3. Henneberg R, Koch M: Ueber centrale Neurofibromatose und die Geschwulste des Kleinhirnbruckenwinkels (Acusticus-neurome). *Arch Psychiatrie* **36**:251, 1902.
4. Bassoe P, Nuzum F: Report of a case of central and peripheral neurofibromatosis. *J Nerv Ment Dis* **42**:785, 1915.
5. Gardner WJ, Frazier CH: Bilateral acoustic neurofibromas: A clinical study and field survey of a family of five generations with bilateral deafness in thirty-eight members. *Arch Neurol Psychiatr* **23**:266, 1929.
6. Kanter WR, Eldridge R, Fabricant R, Allen JC, Koerber T: Central neurofibromatosis with bilateral acoustic neuroma: Genetic, clinical and biochemical distinctions from peripheral neurofibromatosis. *Neurology* **30**:851, 1980.
7. Martuza RL, Eldridge R: Neurofibromatosis 2 (bilateral acoustic neurofibromatosis). *N Engl J Med* **318**:684, 1988.
8. Riccardi VM: *Neurofibromatosis: Phenotype, Natural History, and Pathogenesis*, 2nd ed. Baltimore: Johns Hopkins University Press, 1992, p 224.
9. Argenyi ZB, Thieberg MD, Hayes CM, Whitaker DC: Primary cutaneous meningioma associated with von Recklinghausen's disease. *J Cutan Pathol* **21**:549, 1994.
10. Mulvihill JJ, Parry DM, Sherman JL, Pikus A, Kaiser-Kupfer MI, Eldridge R: NIH conference: Neurofibromatosis 1 (Recklinghausen disease) and neurofibromatosis 2 (bilateral acoustic neurofibromatosis): An update. *Ann Intern Med* **113**:39, 1990.
11. Eldridge R, Parry DM: Summary: Vestibular schwannoma (acoustic neuroma): Consensus development conference. *Neurosurgery* **30**:961, 1992.
12. Russell D, Rubinstein L: *Pathology of Tumors of the Nervous System*, 5th ed. Baltimore: Williams & Wilkins, 1989.
13. Evans DG, Huson SM, Donnai D, Neary W, Blair V, Teare D, Newton V, Strachan T, Ramsden R, Harris R: A genetic study of type 2 neurofibromatosis in the United Kingdom: I. Prevalence, mutation rate, fitness and confirmation of maternal transmission effect on severity. *J Med Genet* **29**:841, 1992.
14. Parry DM, Eldridge R, Kaiser-Kupfer MI, Bouzas E, Pikus A, Patronas N: Neurofibromatosis 2 (NF2): Clinical characteristics of 63 affected individuals and clinical evidence for heterogeneity. *Am J Med Genet* **52**:450, 1994.
15. Leonard J, Talbot M: Asymptomatic acoustic neurilemoma. *Arch Otolaryngol* **91**:117, 1970.
16. Stewart T, Liland J, Schuknecht H: Occult schwannomas of the vestibular nerve. *Arch Otolaryngol* **101**:91, 1975.
17. Evans DGR, Ramsden R, Huson SM, Harris R, Lye R, King T: Type 2 neurofibromatosis: The need for supraregional care? *J Laryngol Otol* **107**:401, 1993.
18. Evans DGR, Huson SM, Donnai D, Neary W, Blair V, Newton V, Harris R: A clinical study of type 2 neurofibromatosis. *QJM* **304**:603, 1992.
19. Gutmann, DH, Aylsworth, A, Carey, JC, Korf, B, Marks, J, Pyeritz, RE, Rubenstein, A, Viskochil, D. The diagnostic evaluation and multidisciplinary management of neurofibromatosis 1 and neurofibromatosis 2. *JAMA* **278**:51, 1997.
20. Mautner VF, Tatagiba M, Guthoff R, Samii M, Pulst SM: Neurofibromatosis 2 in the pediatric age group. *Neurosurgery* **33**:92, 1993.
21. Sobel R, Wang Y: Vestibular (acoustic) schwannomas: Histological features in neurofibromatosis 2 and in unilateral cases. *J Neuropathol Exp Neurol* **52**:106, 1993.
22. Mautner VF, Tatagiba M, Lindenau M, Funsterer C, Pulst SM, Kluwe L, Zanella F: Spinal tumors in patients with neurofibromatosis type 2: MR imaging study of frequency, multiplicity, and variety. *AJR Am J Roentgenol* **165**:951, 1995.
23. McCormick P, Torres R, Post K, Stein B: Intramedullary ependymoma of the spinal cord. *J Neurosurg* **72**:523, 1990.
24. Mautner VF, Lindenau M, Baser M, Kluwe L, Gottschalk J: Skin abnormalities in neurofibromatosis 2. *Arch Dermatol* **133**:1539, 1997.
25. Thomas PK, King RHM, Chiang TR, Scaravilli F, Sharma AK, Downie AW: Neurofibromatosis neuropathy. *Muscle Nerve* **13**:93, 1990.
26. Kilpatrick T, Hjorth R, Gonzales MF: A case of neurofibromatosis 2 presenting with a mononeuritis multiplex. *J Neurol Neurosurg Psychiatry* **55**:391, 1992.
27. Kaiser-Kupfer M, Freidlin V, Datiles M, Edwards P, Sherman J, Parry D, McCain L, Eldridge R: The association of posterior capsular lens opacities with bilateral acoustic neuromas in patients with neurofibromatosis type 2. *Arch Ophthalmol* **107**:541, 1989.
28. Bouzas E, Parry D, Eldridge R, Kaiser-Kupfer M: Visual impairment in patients with neurofibromatosis 2. *Neurology* **43**:622, 1993.
29. Ragge N, Baser M, Klein J, Nechiporuk A, Sainz J, Pulst SM, Riccardi V: Ocular abnormalities in neurofibromatosis 2. *Am J Ophthalmol* **20**:634, 1995.
30. Crowe FW, Schull WJ: Diagnostic importance of the cafe au lait spot in neurofibromatosis. *Arch Intern Med* **91**:758, 1953.
31. Kopf AW, Levine LJ, Rigel DS, Friedman RJ, Levenstein M: Prevalence of congenital-nevus-like nevi, nevi spili and café au lait spots. *Arch Dermatol* **121**:766, 1985.
32. Short MP, Martuza RL, Huson SM: Neurofibromatosis 2: Clinical features, genetic counselling and management issues, in Huson SM, Hughes RAC (eds): *The Neurofibromatoses: A Pathogenetic and Clinical Overview*. London: Chapman and Hall, 1994, p 414.
33. Evans DG, Blair V, Strachan T, Lye RH, Ramsden RT: Variation of expression of the gene for type 2 neurofibromatosis: Absence of a gender effect on vestibular schwannomas, but confirmation of a preponderance of meningiomas in females. *J Laryng Oto* **109**:830, 1995.

34. Harsh G, MacCollin M, McKenna M, Nadol J, Ojemann R, Short MP: Molecular genetic screening for children at risk of neurofibromatosis 2. *Arch Otolaryngol Head Neck Surg* **121**:590, 1995.
35. Briggs R, Brackmann D, Baser M, Hitselberg W: Comprehensive management of bilateral acoustic neuromas. *Arch Otolaryngol Head Neck Surg* **120**:1307, 1994.
36. Ojemann RG: Management of acoustic neuromas (vestibular schwannomas). *Clin Neurosurg* **40**:489, 1993.
37. Bruce J, Fetell M: Tumors of the skull and cranial nerves, in Rowland LP (ed): *Merritt's Textbook of Neurology*, 9th ed. Baltimore: Williams & Wilkins, 1995, p 320.
38. Evans DGR, Trueman L, Wallace A, Collins S, Strachan T: Genotype/phenotype correlations in type 2 neurofibromatosis (NF2): Evidence for more severe disease associated with truncating mutations. *J Med Genet* **35**:450, 1998.
39. MacCollin MM, Jacoby LB, Jones D, Ojemann R, Feit H, Gusella J: Somatic mosaicism of the neurofibromatosis 2 tumor suppresser gene. *Neurology* **48:**A29, 1997.
40. Parry D, MacCollin M, Kaiser-Kupfer M, Pulaski K, Nicholson HS, Bolesta M, Eldridge R, Gusella J: Germ line mutations in the neurofibromatosis 2 (NF2) gene: Correlations with disease severity and retinal abnormalities. *Am J Hum Genet* **59**:529, 1996.
41. Jacoby LB, Jones D, Davis K, Kronn D, Short MP, Gusella J, MacCollin M: Molecular analysis of the NF2 tumor-suppressor gene in schwannomatosis. *Am J Hum Genet* **61**:1293, 1997.
42. MacCollin M, Woodfin W, Kronn D, Short MP: Schwannomatosis: A clinical and pathologic study. *Neurology* **46**:1072, 1996.
43. Buenger K, Porter N, Dozier S, Wagner R: Localized multiple neurilemmoma of the lower extremity. *Cutis* **51**:36, 1993.
44. Sieb JP, Pulst SM, Buch A: Familial CNS tumors. *J Neurol* **239**:343, 1992.
45. Pulst SM, Rouleau G, Marineau C, Fain P, Sieb J: Familial meningioma is not allelic to neurofibromatosis 2. *Neurology* **43**:2096, 1993.
46. Von Deimling A, Kraus JA, Stangl AP, Wellenreuther R, Lenartz D, Schramm J, Louis DN, Ramesh V, Gusella JF, Wiestler OD: Evidence of subarachnoid spread in the development of multiple meningiomas. *Brain Pathol* **5**:11, 1995.
47. Jaaskelainin J, Paetau A, Pyykko I, Blomstedt G, Palva T, Troupp H: Interface between the facial nerve and large acoustic neurinomas: Immunohistochemical study of the cleavage plane in NF2 and non-NF2 cases. *J Neurosurg* **870**:541, 1993.
48. Aguiar P, Tatagiba M, Samii M, Dankoweit-Timpe E, Ostertag H: The comparison between the growth fraction of bilateral vestibular schwannomas in neurofibromatosis 2 (NF2) and unilateral vestibular schwannomas using the monoclonal antibody MIB 1. *Acta Neurochir (Wien)* **134**:40, 1995.
49. Louis D, Ramesh V, Gusella J: Neuropathology and molecular genetics of neurofibromatosis 2 and related tumors. *Brain Pathol* **5**:163, 1995.
50. Seizinger B, Martuza R, Gusella J: Loss of genes on chromosome 22 in tumorigenesis of human acoustic neuroma. *Nature* **322**:644, 1986.
51. Seizinger B, de la Monte S, Atkins L, Gusella J, Martuza R: Molecular genetic approach to human meningioma: Loss of genes on chromosome 22. *Proc Natl Acad Sci U S A* **68**:820, 1971.
52. Seizinger B, Rouleau G, Ozelius L, Lane LJ, St. George-Hyslop P, Huson S, Gusella J, Martuza R: Common pathogenetic mechanism for three tumor types in bilateral acoustic neurofibromatosis. *Science* **236**:317, 1987.
53. Knudson AG: Mutation and cancer: A statistical study. *Proc Natl Acad Sci U S A* **68**:820, 1971.
54. Rouleau GA, Wertelecki W, Haines JL, Hobbs WJ, Trofatter JA, Seizinger BR, Martuza RL, Superneau DW, Connealy PM, Gusella JF: Genetic linkage of bilateral acoustic neurofibromatosis to a DNA marker on chromosome 22. *Nature* **329**:246, 1987.
55. Trofatter J, MacCollin M, Rutter J, Murrell J, Duyao M, Parry D, Eldridge R, Kley N, Menon A, Pulaski K, Haase V, Ambrose C, Munroe D, Bove C, Haines J, Martuza R, MacDonald M, Seizinger B, Short MP, Buckler A, Gusella J: A novel moesin-, ezrin-, radixin-like gene is a candidate for the neurofibromatosis 2 tumor suppressor. *Cell* **72**:791, 1993.
56. Rouleau G, Merel P, Lutchman M, Sanson M, Zucman J, Marineau C, Hoang-Xuan K, Demczuk S, Desmaze C, Plougastel B, Pulst S, Lenoir G, Bijisma E, Rashold R, Dumanski J, de Jong P, Parry D, Eldridge R, Aurias A, Delattre O, Thomas G: Alteration in a new gene encoding a positive membrane-organizing protein causes neuro-fibromatosis type 2. *Nature* **363**:515, 1993.
57. Lee DK, Abbott ML: Familial central nervous system neoplasia: Case report of a family with von Recklinghausen's neurofibromatosis. *Arch Neurol* **20**:154, 1969.
58. Narod S, Parry D, Parboosingh J, Lenoir G, Ruttledge M, Fischer G, Eldridge R, Martuza R, Frontali M, Haines J, Gusella J, Rouleau G: Neurofibromatosis type 2 appears to be a genetically homogeneous disease. *Am J Hum Genet* **51**:486, 1992.
59. MacCollin M, Ramesh V, Jacoby LB, Louis D, Rubio M, Pulaski K, Trofatter J, Short MP, Bove C, Eldridge R, Parry D, Gusella J: Mutational analysis of patients with neurofibromatosis 2. *Am J Hum Genet* **55**:314, 1994.
60. Gutmann DH, Wright DE, Geist R, Snider W: Expression of the neurofibromatosis 2 (NF2) gene isoforms during rat embryonic development. *Hum Mol Genet* **4**:471, 1995.
61. Pykett M, Murphy M, Harnish P, George D: The neurofibromatosis 2 (NF2) tumor suppressor gene encodes multiple alternatively spliced transcripts. *Hum Mol Genet* **3**:559, 1994.
62. Hitotsumatsu T, Kitamoto T, Iwaki T, Fukui M, Tateishi J: An exon 8 spliced out transcript of the neurofibromatosis 2 gene is constitutively expressed in various human tissues. *J Biochem (Tokyo)* **116**:1205, 1994.
63. Haase V, Trofatter J, MacCollin M, Tarttelin E, Gusella J, Ramesh V: The murine NF2 homologue encodes a highly conserved merlin protein with alternative forms. *Hum Mol Genet* **3**:407, 1994.
64. Hara T, Bianchi A, Seizinger B, Kley N: Molecular cloning and characterization of alternatively spliced transcripts of the mouse neurofibromatosis 2 gene. *Cancer Res* **54**:330, 1994.
65. Arpin M, Algrain M, Louvard D: Membrane-actin microfilament connections: An increasing diversity of players related to band 4.1. *Curr Opin Cell Biol* **6**:136, 1994.
66. Gonzalez-Agosti C, Xu L, Pinney D, Beauchamp R, Hobbs W, Gusella J, Ramesh V: The merlin tumor suppressor localizes preferentially in membrane ruffles. *Oncogene* **13**:1239, 1996.
67. Kluwe L, Bayer S, Baser M, Hazim W, Wolfgang H, Funsterer C, Mautner VF: Identification of NF2 germ-line mutations and comparison with neurofibromatosis 2 phenotypes. *Hum Genet* **98**:534, 1996.
68. Merel P, Hoang-Xuan K, Sanson M, Bijlsma E, Rouleu G, Laurent-Puig P, Pulst S, Baser M, Lenoir G, Sterkers JM, Philippon J, Resche F, Mautner V, Fischer G, Hulsebos T, Aurias A, Delattre O, Thomas G: Screening for germ-line mutations in the NF2 gene. *Genes Chrom Cancer* **12**:117, 1995.
69. Bourn D, Carter S, Mason S, Evans DGR, Strachan T: Germline mutations in the neurofibromatosis type 2 tumour suppressor gene. *Hum Mol Genet* **3**:813, 1994.
70. Watson C, Gaunt L, Evans G, Patel K, Harris R, Strachan T: A disease-associated germline deletion maps the type 2 neurofibromatosis (NF2) gene between the Ewing sarcoma region and the leukaemia inhibitory factor locus. *Hum Mol Genet* **2**:701, 1993.
71. Kluwe L, Pulst S, Koppen J, Matner VP: A 163-bp deletion at the C-terminus of the schwannomin gene associated with variable phenotypes of neurofibromatosis type 2. *Hum Genet* **95**:443, 1995.
72. Sanson M, Marineau C, Desmaze C, Lutchman M, Ruttledge M, Baron C, Narod S, Delattre O, Lenoir G, Thomas G, Aurias A, Rouleau G: Germline deletion in a neurofibromatosis type 2 kindred inactivates the NF2 gene and a candidate meningioma locus. *Hum Mol Genet* **2**:1215, 1993.
73. Sainz J, Figueroa K, Baser M, Mautner VF, Pulst SM: High frequency of nonsense mutations in the NF2 gene caused by C to T transitions in five CGA codons. *Hum Mol Genet* **4**:137, 1995.
74. MacCollin M, Mohney T, Trofatter J, Wertelecki W, Ramesh V, Gusella J: DNA diagnosis of neurofibromatosis 2: Altered coding sequence of the merlin tumor suppressor in an extended pedigree. *JAMA* **270**:2316, 1993.
75. Ruttledge M, Andermann A, Phelan C, Claudio J, Han F, Chretien N, Rangaratnam S, MacCollin M, Short MP, Parry D, Michels V, Riccardi V, Weksberg R, Kitamura K, Bradburn J, Hall B, Propping P, Rouleau G: Type of mutation in the neurofibromatosis type 2 gene (NF2) frequently determines severity of disease. *Am J Hum Genet* **59**:331, 1996.
76. MacCollin M, Braverman N, Viskochil D, Ruttledge M, Davis K, Ojemann R, Gusella J, Parry D: A point mutation associated with a severe phenotype of neurofibromatosis 2. *Ann Neurol* **40**:440, 1996.
77. Kluwe L, MacCollin M, Tatagiba M, Thomas S, Hazim W, Haase W, Mautner VF: Phenotypic variability associated with 14 splice-site mutations in the NF2 gene. *Am J Med Genet* **18**:228, 1998.
78. Jacoby LB, MacCollin M, Louis DN, Mohney T, Rubio MP, Pulaski K, Trofatter J, Kley N, Seizinger B, Ramesh V, Gusella J: Exon scanning

for mutation of the NF2 gene in schwannomas. *Hum Mol Genet* **3**:413, 1994.

79. Jacoby L, MacCollin M, Barone R, Ramesh V, Gusella J: Frequency and distribution of NF2 mutations in schwannomas. *Genes Chromosomes Cancer* **17**:45, 1996.
80. Biljlsma E, Merel P, Bosch A, Westerveld A, Delatre O, Thomas G, Hulsebos T: Analysis of mutations in the SCh gene in schwannomas. *Genes Chromosomes Cancer* **11**:7, 1994.
81. Twist E, Ruttledge M, Rousseau M, Sanson M, Papi L, Merel P, Delattre O, Thomas G, Rouleau G: The neurofibromatosis type 2 gene is inactivated in schwannomas. *Hum Mol Genet* **3**:147, 1994.
82. Sainz J, Huynh D, Figueroa K, Ragge N, Baser M, Pulst SM: Mutations of the neurofibromatosis type 2 gene and lack of the gene product in vestibular schwannomas. *Hum Mol Genet* **3**:885, 1994.
83. Deprez R, Bianchi A, Groen N, Seizinger B, Hagemeijer A, van Drunen E, Bootsma D, Koper J, Avezaat C, Kley N, Zwarthoff E: Frequent NF2 gene transcript mutations in sporadic meningiomas and vestibular schwannomas. *Am J Hum Genet* **54**:1022, 1994.
84. Merel P, Hoang-Xuan K, Sanson M, Moreau-Aubry A, Bijlsma EK, Lazaro C, Moisan JP, Resche F, Nishisho J, Estivill X, Delattre JY, Poisson M, Theillet C, Hulsebos T, Delattre O, Thomas G: Predominant occurrence of somatic mutations of the NF2 gene in meningiomas and schwannomas. *Genes Chromosomes Cancer* **13**:211, 1995.
85. Welling DB, Guida M, Goll F, Pearl DK, Glasscock ME, Pappas DG, Linthicum FH, Rogers D, Prior TW: Mutational spectrum in the neurofibromatosis type 2 gene in sporadic and familial schwannomas. *Hum Genet* **98**:189, 1996.
86. Wellenreuther R, Kraus JA, Lenartz D, Menon AG, Schramm J, Louis DN, Ramesh V, Guesella JF, Wiestler OD, von Deimling A: Analysis of the neurofibromatosis 2 gene reveals molecular variants of meningioma. *Am J Pathol* **146**:827, 1995.
87. Ruttledge M, Sarrazin J, Rangaratnam S, Phelan C, Twist E, Merel P, Delattre O, Thomas G, Nordenskjold M, Collins VP, Dumanski J, Rouleau G: Evidence for the complete inactivation of the NF2 gene in the majority of sporadic meningiomas. *Nat Genet* **6**:180, 1994.
88. Rubio MP, Correa K, Ramesh V, MacCollin M, Jacoby L, von Deimling A, Gusella J, Louis D: Analysis of the neurofibromatosis 2 gene in human ependymomas and astrocytomas. *Cancer Res* **54**:45, 1994.
89. Birch B, Johnson F, Parsa A, Desai R, Yoon J, Lycette C, Li YM, Bruce J: Frequent type 2 neurofibromatosis gene transcript mutations in sporadic intramedullary spinal cord ependymomas. *Neurosurgery* **39**:135, 1996.
90. Hoang-Xuan K, Merel P, Vega F, Hugot JP, Cornu P, Delattre JY, Poisson M, Thomas G, Delattre O: Analysis of the NF2 tumor-suppressor gene and of chromosome 22 deletions in gliomas. *Int J Cancer* **60**:478, 1995.
91. Bianchi A, Hara T, Ramesh V, Gao J, Klein-Szanto AJP, Morin F, Menon A, Trofatter J, Gusella J, Seizinger B, Kley N: Mutations in transcript isoforms of the neurofibromatosis 2 gene in multiple human tumour types. *Nat Genet* **6**:185, 1994.
92. Englefield P, Foulkes W, Campbell I: Loss of heterozygosity on chromosome 22 in ovarian carcinoma is distal to and is not accompanied by mutations in NF2 at 22112. *Br J Cancer* **70**:905, 1994.
93. Kanai Y, Tsuda H, Oda T, Sakamoto M, Hirohashi S: Analysis of the neurofibromatosis 2 gene in human breast and hepatocellular carcinomas. *Jpn J Clin Oncol* **25**:1, 1995.
94. Sekido Y, Pass H, Bader S, Mew D, Christman M, Gazdar A, Minna J: Neurofibromatosis type 2 (NF2) gene is somatically mutated in mesothelioma but not in lung cancer. *Cancer Res* **55**:1227, 1995.
95. Bianchi AB, Mitsunaga SI, Cheng JQ, Klein WM, Jhanwar SC, Seizinger B, Kley N, Klein-Szanto AJ, Testa JR: High frequency of inactivating mutations in the neurofibromatosis type 2 gene (NF2) in primary malignant mesotheliomas. *Proc Natl Acad Sci U S A* **92**:10854, 1995.
96. Sainio M, Strachan T, Blomstedt G, Salonen O, Setala K, Palotie A, Palo J, Pyykoo I, Peltonen L, Jaaskelainen J: Presymptomatic DNA and MRI diagnosis of neurofibromatosis 2 with mild clinical course in an extended pedigree. *Neurology* **45**:1314, 1995.
97. Bijlsma EK, Merel P, Fleury P, van Asperen C, Westerveld A, Delattre O, Thomas G, Hulsebos T: Family with neurofibromatosis type 2 and autosomal dominant hearing loss: Identification of carriers of the mutated NF2 gene. *Hum Genet* **96**:1, 1995.
98. Bijlsma EK, Wallace AJ, Evans DG: Misleading linkage results in an NF2 presymptomatic test owing to mosaicism. *J Med Genet* **34**:934, 1997.
99. Nadol JB Jr, Chiong CM, Ojemann RG, McKenna MJ, Martuza RL, Montgomery WW, Levine RA, Ronner SF, Glynn RJ: Preservation of hearing and facial nerve function in resection of acoustic neuroma. *Laryngoscope* **102**:1153, 1992.
100. Samii M, Matthies C, Tatagiba M: Management of vestibular schwannomas (acoustic neuromas): Auditory and facial nerve function after resection of 120 vestibular schwannomas in patients with neurofibromatosis 2. *Neurosurgery* **40**:696, 1997.
101. Tatagiba M, Matthies C, Samii M: Facial nerve reconstruction in neurofibromatosis 2. *Acta Neurochir (Wien)* **126**:72, 1994.
102. Linskey M, Lunsford D, Flickinger J: Tumor control after stereotactic radiosurgery in neurofibromatosis patients with bilateral acoustic tumors. *Neurosurgery* **31**:829, 1992.
103. Lunsford LD, Linskey M: Stereotactic radiosurgery in the treatment of patients with acoustic tumors. *Otolaryngol Clin North Am* **25**:471, 1992.
104. Ito K, Kurita H, Sugasawa K, Mizuno M, Sasaki T: Analyses of neuro-otological complications after radiosurgery for acoustic neurinomas. *Int J Radiat Oncol Biol Phys* **39**:983, 1997.
105. Lamberts S, Tanghe H, Avezaat C, Braakman R, Wijngaarde R, Koper J, de Jong FH: Mifepristone (RU 486) treatment of meningiomas. *J Neurol Neurosurg Psychiatry* **55**:486, 1992.
106. Takamiya Y, Friedlander R, Brem H, Malick A, Martuza R: Inhibition of angiogenesis and growth of human nerve-sheath tumors by AGM-1470. *J Neurosurg* **78**:470, 1993.
107. Schrell UM, Rittig MG, Anders M, Koch UH, Marschalek R, Kiewewetter F, Fahlbusch, R: Hydroxyurea for treatment of unresectable and recurrent meningiomas. II. Decrease in the size of meningiomas in patients treated with hydroxyurea. *J Neurosurg* **86**:840, 1997.
108. Hoffman R, Kohan D, Cohen N: Cochlear implants in the management of bilateral acoustic neuromas. *Am J Otol* **13**:525, 1992.
109. Brackmann D, Hitselberger W, Nelson R, Moore J, Waring M, Portillo F, Shannon R, Telischi F: Auditory brainstem implant: I. Issues in surgical implantation. *Otolaryngol Head Neck Surg* **108**:624, 1993.
110. Shannon R, Fayad J, Moore J, Lo W, Otto S, Nelson R, O'Leary M: Auditory brainstem implant: II. Postsurgical issues and performance. *Otolaryngol Head Neck Surg* **108**:634, 1993.
111. Otto SR, Shannon RV, Brackmann DE, Hitselberger WE, Staller S, Menapace C: The multichannel auditory brain stem implant: performance in twenty patients. *Otolaryngol Head Neck Surg* **118(3 Pt 1)**:291, 1998.

CHAPTER 41

Renal Carcinoma

W. Marston Linehan ▪ Berton Zbar ▪ D. Richard Klausner

1. Renal carcinoma appears in both a sporadic and a hereditary form. Eighty-five percent of sporadic renal carcinomas are of the clear cell histologic type, 5 to 10 percent are papillary renal carcinoma, and the remainder are less common histologic types such as chromophobe and collecting-duct renal carcinomas.

2. The most well characterized form of hereditary renal carcinoma is von Hippel-Lindau (VHL). VHL is a hereditary cancer syndrome in which affected individuals are at risk to develop tumors in a number of organs, including the kidneys, cerebellum, spine, eye, inner ear, adrenal gland, and pancreas. VHL families are categorized as VHL type I (without pheochromocytoma) or VHL type II (with pheochromocytoma).

3. The *VHL* gene, which has the characteristics of a tumor-suppressor gene, has been identified on the short arm of chromosome 3. The *VHL* gene has three exons and encodes a protein of 213 amino acids. Both copies of the *VHL* gene are inactivated in tumors in VHL patients—mutation in the inherited allele and loss of the wild-type allele. *VHL* gene mutation analysis provides a method for early diagnosis of VHL in asymptomatic individuals or in clinical situations such as hereditary pheochromocytoma where the diagnosis is in doubt. Since VHL manifestations often occur in childhood, testing early in life is recommended so that appropriate intervention can be instituted. There is a marked genotype/phenotype correlation with *VHL* gene mutation and the manifestation of the VHL; VHL type II families are characterized by missense mutations of the *VHL* gene. There is a "hot spot" for VHL type II at a single codon in the 5′ end of exon 3 of the *VHL* gene.

4. Inactivation of both copies of the *VHL* gene is an early event in clear cell renal carcinoma, where a high percentage of *VHL* gene mutations and loss of heterozygosity (LOH) have been detected. *VHL* gene mutations including nucleotide insertions, deletions, substitutions, and nonsense mutations have been found in each of the three exons. Neither *VHL* gene mutation nor *VHL* LOH is found in papillary renal carcinoma. A molecular genetic classification of renal carcinoma, clear cell versus papillary, has been proposed, with clear cell renal carcinoma characterized by *VHL* gene mutation. *VHL* gene mutations have been detected in DNA extracted from formalin-fixed material and tissue aspirates, providing a potentially useful diagnostic tool. Somatic *VHL* gene mutations have been detected in sporadic tumors from other organs affected in VHL, including cerebellar hemangioblastoma and epididymal cystadenoma. With the exception of rare reports, *VHL* is not mutated or implicated in other sporadic cancers.

5. The *VHL* suppressor gene product has begun to be characterized. VHL forms a stable tetramolecular complex with two subunits of the highly conserved heterotrimeric transcription elongation factor elongin (SIII) and an additional protein called Cul-2. Elongin is composed of three subunits: A, B and C. Elongin A is required to inhibit processing of RNA pol II, allowing cell processivity of transcription. Elongin B enhances the assembly of elongin C to either elongin A or VHL. VHL and elongin A compete for binding to B and C via a short shared sequence motif. This sequence, found in the third exon of *VHL*, is highly mutated in both VHL and sporadic renal cell carcinoma (RCC), and these loss-of-function *VHL* mutations are associated with loss of assembly of VHL with the B and C subunits. While VHL can competitively inhibit the assembly of a functional ABC transcription elongation factor, it is not clear that transcription elongation inhibition is the mode of action of VHL. These proteins combine to target other proteins for ubiquitin-mediated degradation, and this observation may provide the best current hint of the biochemical function of the VHL complex. Cul-2, the fourth known component of the VHL complex, is a member of the Cdc53 family of proteins. The VHL-Cul-2 association depends on the integrity of the VHL-elongin B/C heterotrimeric complex. Cul-2 is a cytosolic protein that can be translocated to the nucleus by the VHL protein. The VHL protein has been found both in the nucleus and the cytosol of transiently transfected cells. There is a tightly regulated, cell density-dependent transport of VHL into and/or out of the nucleus. In densely grown cells, the VHL signal is predominantly in the cytoplasm, whereas in sparse cultures, most of the signal is detected in the nucleus. Immunofluorescence studies of mutant VHL protein revealed that the C-terminal region of the VHL protein is required for localization to or retention in the cytosol. In exon 1 deletion mutants, the protein remains predominantly in the cytosol under both sparse and confluent conditions. The VHL protein is required for cell cycle exit on serum withdrawal. RCC cells ($VHL^{-/-}$) fail to exit the cell cycle on serum withdrawal. Reintroduction of the wild-type *VHL* gene restores the ability of the $VHL^{-/-}$ RCC cells to exit the cell cycle. The cyclin-dependent kinase inhibitor p27 has been shown to accumulate on serum withdrawal in the presence of VHL. This is associated with stabilization of the p27 protein.

6. Sporadic clear cell renal carcinomas are characterized by a high degree of neoangiogenesis; angiogenesis is also a striking feature in the clinical manifestations of VHL. Both clear cell renal carcinoma and cerebellar hemangioblastoma are characterized by a marked elevation in expression of vascular endothelial growth factor (VEGF). The increased expression of VEGF is reversed in renal carcinoma cells by reintroduction of the wild-type *VHL* gene. This reversal is blocked by either anoxia or low serum conditions, suggesting that VHL may play a role in the

A list of standard abbreviations is located immediately preceding the index in each volume. Nonstandard abbreviations used in this chapter include: HCRC = hereditary clear cell renal carcinoma; VHL = von Hipple-Lindau; HPRC = hereditary papillary renal carcinoma; LOH = loss of heterozygosity; ELST = endolymphatic sac tumor.

normal regulated induction of angiogenesis. This critical gene is one of the first identified targets of VHL function.

7. **Hereditary papillary renal cell carcinoma (HPRC) is a hereditary cancer syndrome in which affected individuals are at risk to develop bilateral, multifocal papillary renal cell carcinoma. This syndrome, which has an autosomal dominant inheritance pattern, is caused by missense mutations in the tyrosine kinase domain of the *MET* proto-oncogene.**
8. **Familial renal oncocytoma is characterized by a predisposition to develop bilateral, multiple renal oncocytomas in affected family members.**

Renal carcinoma, the most common cancer in the kidney, affects nearly 28,000 Americans annually and is associated with over 12,000 deaths per year.[1] Renal carcinoma, which accounts for approximately 3 percent of adult cancers, most commonly occurs in adults between the ages of 50 and 70; however, it has been reported in children as young as 3 years.[2] Clear cell type (or a variant of clear cell) makes up 80 to 85 percent of renal carcinoma. Little is known about the etiology of renal cancer, although a number of environmental, hormonal, and cellular factors have been studied. Renal carcinoma has been increasing at a rate of approximately 2 percent per year and affects males twice as frequently as females.[3] There is a strong correlation with cigarette smoking and an increased incidence of renal cancer among leather workers and workers exposed to asbestos.[4–7] There is an increased incidence of renal carcinoma in patients with end-stage renal disease, which is particularly notable in patients who have acquired cystic disease.[8,9] The risk of developing renal cell carcinoma for end-stage renal patients with cystic changes on dialysis has been estimated to be 30 times higher than that in the general population.[10] Five to 10 percent of renal carcinoma is of the papillary histologic type.[11,12] The remaining tumors are made up of rare histologic types such as chromophobe and collecting-duct renal carcinoma.

Renal carcinoma occurs in both hereditary and nonhereditary, sporadic forms. Estimates from case-control studies suggest that up to 4 percent of renal carcinoma may be hereditary on the basis of family history.[3] There are three forms of hereditary renal cell carcinoma (Table 41-1). One is hereditary clear cell renal carcinoma (HCRC), in which 50 percent of offspring of an affected individual are likely to develop renal carcinoma.[13,14] A second form of hereditary renal carcinoma is that associated with von Hippel-Lindau (VHL), in which affected individuals develop tumors in a number of organs, including the kidneys.[3,15] A third form of inherited renal carcinoma is hereditary papillary renal carcinoma (HPRC).[16,17] While patients with sporadic renal carcinoma are likely to develop a solitary renal tumor between the ages of 50 and 70, patients with hereditary renal cell carcinoma tend to develop multifocal, early-onset renal carcinoma.[3]

LOCATION OF THE CLEAR CELL RENAL CARCINOMA GENE: CHROMOSOME 3

An initial indication of the location of a renal carcinoma gene came from the studies of Cohen et al.,[13] who in 1979 reported a family with an autosomal dominant inheritance pattern of bilateral, multifocal renal carcinoma. Affected individuals in this kindred were characterized by a balanced germ-line translocation from chromosome 3 to chromosome 8. Subsequently, Pathak[18] reported a renal cell carcinoma family with a chromosome 3 to chromosome 11 translocation. In 1989 Kovaks et al.[19] described a family carrying a constitutional translocation (3;6)(p13;q25.1) in which affected individuals developed multiple, bilateral, early-onset renal carcinoma.

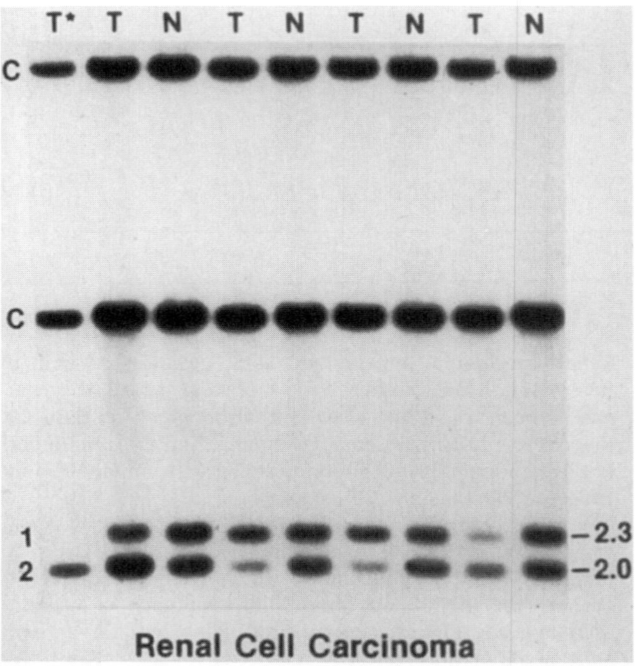

Fig. 41-1 RFLP analysis of sporadic renal cell carcinoma tumors (T) and corresponding normal tissue (N) with a probe for the chromosome 3p DNF 15S2 locus. 1 and 2 indicate the two polymorphic chromosome 3p alleles; C indicates a constant band. The bands on the lower part of the figure represent the 2.3- and 2.0-kb alleles, one of which is lost in the tumors indicated. The residual bands represent the presence of normal lymphocytes; the lane marked T* indicates a renal tumor grown in an immunodeficient mouse. (*From Zbar et al.*[20] *Used with permission.*)

These and other findings led to genetic studies of chromosome 3 in nonhereditary renal cell carcinoma. When renal carcinoma was evaluated for loss of heterozygosity (LOH) on chromosome 3 by RFLP analysis (Fig. 41-1), consistent loss of a segment of the short arm of chromosome 3 was detected in tumor tissue from patients with sporadic, nonhereditary clear cell renal carcinoma.[20–28] Cytogenetic analysis of sporadic renal cell carcinoma confirmed these findings.[23,28–30] Loss of a segment of chromosome 3 was found to be a consistent feature of the common form of renal carcinoma, clear cell renal carcinoma, but not of papillary renal carcinoma.[21,31–34] In a detailed analysis of 60 tumors, Anglard et al.[21] detected LOH in nearly 90 percent of clear cell renal carcinomas and defined by deletion analysis (Fig. 41-2) an area of minimal deletion in the 3p21-26 region of chromosome 3. Since this region was too large to study by conventional cloning methods available at the time, investigators turned to the hereditary form of renal cell carcinoma associated with von Hippel-Lindau to search for the kidney cancer gene.

Table 41-1 Hereditary Forms of Renal Carcinoma

1.	Hereditary clear-cell renal carcinoma	(HCRC)
2.	Von Hippel-Lindau	(VHL)
3.	Hereditary papillary renal carcinoma	(HPRC)

VON HIPPEL-LINDAU

Von Hippel-Lindau (VHL) is a hereditary cancer syndrome in which affected individuals are at risk to develop tumors in a number of organs, including the kidneys. In the early 1860s, reports began to appear from ophthalmologists that described angiomatous lesions of the retina that were associated with blindness and which were associated occasionally with similar cerebellar lesions.[35] In 1894, Collins described angiomas that appeared in the retinas of two siblings.[36] Von Hippel, a German ophthalmologist, first recognized that there was a hereditary

CHROMOSOME 3 DELETION MAP: SPORADIC RENAL CELL CARCINOMA

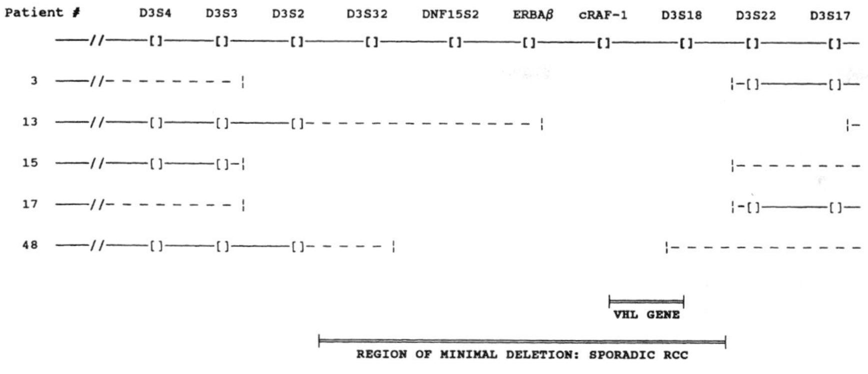

Fig. 41-2 Deletion map showing the area of minimal deletion on chromosome 3p in sporadic renal cell carcinoma. Analysis of the genotypes identified the locus in the telomeric portion of chromosome 3p bounded by the markers *D3S2* and *D3S22* as the region of a potential renal cell carcinoma disease gene. (*From Anglard et al.*[21] *Used with permission.*)

component to the retinal angiomas.[37] The Swedish ophthalmologist Arvid Lindau determined that the retinal angiomas and cerebellar hemangioblastomas together were part of the familial syndrome that bears his name.[38] Although subsequent clinical reports of small families confirmed the association of the retinal angiomas, central nervous system (CNS) hemangioblastomas, renal tumors and cysts, epididymal cystadenomas, pancreatic cysts and tumors, and pheochromocytomas,[35] it was in 1964 that Melmon and Rosen codified the term *von Hippel-Lindau* with the definitive article in which a large family with these diverse manifestations was characterized[39] (Table 41-2).

VHL is estimated to occur in 1 in 36,000 live births; inheritance of the gene follows an autosomal dominant pattern with a penetrance from 80 to 90 percent but with highly varied expressivity.[15] The age of onset of VHL is variable and depends on (1) which asymptomatic lesions are sought and (2) the expression within the family. The retinal angiomas are generally the earliest lesions detected, followed by CNS and spinal hemangiomas. The mean age at diagnosis of retinal hemangiomas is 25 years (range 1–67 years); for CNS hemangioblastoma, it is 30 years (range 11–78 years); and for renal cell carcinoma, the mean age is 37 years (range 16–67 years).[35] In kindreds with pheochromocytoma (VHL type II), pheochromocytoma is often detected before other manifestations and can appear before age 10 years.

Renal Manifestations of VHL

Renal cell carcinoma occurs in 28 to 45 percent of individuals affected with VHL. Affected individuals may develop renal cysts, renal cysts lined with renal cell carcinomas, or solid renal cell carcinomas. Although the renal tumors often are detected when they are small and confined to the kidney, these tumors are malignant and can metastasize (Fig. 41-3). Poston et al.[40] characterized the findings after renal surgery in 161 lesions from 12 patients with VHL and renal cell carcinoma. Pathologic evaluation revealed 45 solid lesions, 41 of which were renal cell carcinoma, and 116 cystic lesions, 25 of which were malignant. Of 66 malignant lesions, 35 (53 percent) contained cells with only clear cell cytologic features; 30 (46 percent) were comprised of predominantly clear cells with scattered granular cells. A single malignant lesion (1.5 percent) was found to have sarcomatoid renal cell carcinoma with clear and granular cells. This study established the clear cell cytologic feature as the primary finding in renal lesions of VHL patients.[40] When Walther et al.[41] examined in detail grossly normal renal parenchyma from 16 VHL patients,

Table 41-2 Von Hippel-Lindau Manifestations

Bilateral, multifocal clear-cell renal carcinoma
Bilateral, multifocal renal cysts
Cerebellar and spinal hemangioblastoma
Endolymphatic sac tumors (ELSTs)
Retinal angioma
Pancreatic cysts, microcystic adenomas, islet-cell tumors
Pheochromocytoma
Epididymal cystadenoma

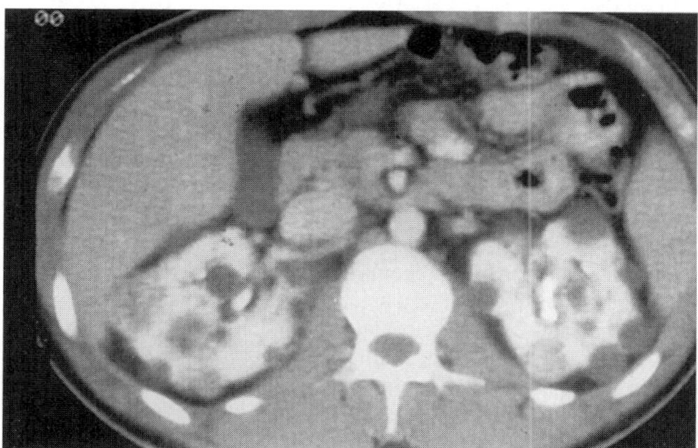

A

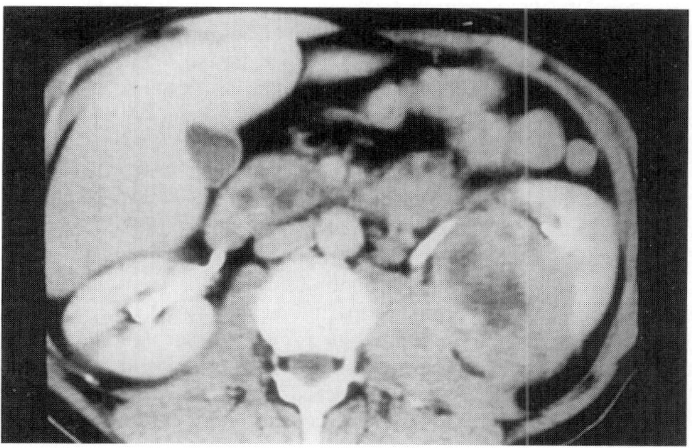

B

Fig. 41-3 *A.* Abdominal CT scan of a VHL patient reveals bilateral multifocal renal carcinomas and cysts. *B.* Abdominal CT scan of a VHL patient reveals a large renal mass, which had spread to the lungs. (*From Linehan et al.*[152] *Used with permission.*)

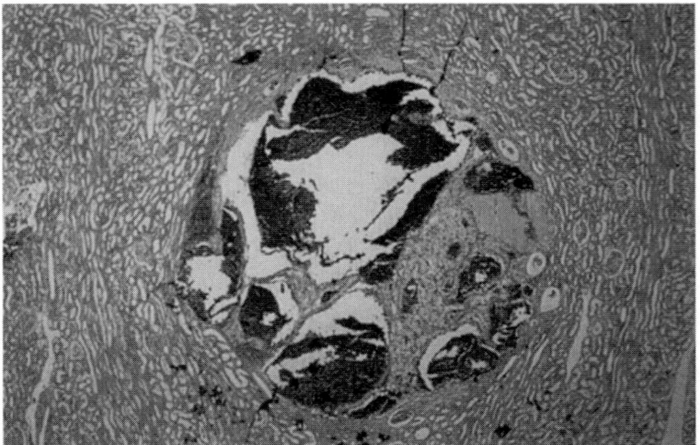

Fig. 41-4 A microscopic focus of renal cell carcinoma detected in grossly "normal" renal tissue from a VHL patient. (*From Linehan et al.*[152] *Used with permission.*)

microscopic renal cystic and solid neoplasms containing only clear cell cytologic features were found (Fig. 41-4). The extrapolated number of lesions in the average kidney, represented at the mean age of 37 years, was estimated as 1100 nonmalignant cysts with a clear cell lining and 600 clear cell neoplasms.[41]

For detection of even small renal lesions in VHL, computed tomographic (CT) scans and ultrasound are the preferred techniques.[35,42,43] Treatment of renal cell carcinoma involves parenchymal sparing surgery whenever possible.[44–48] Intraoperative ultrasound may be used to identify solid as well as cystic lesions to be removed surgically.[49,50] The prevalence of microscopic renal carcinoma makes it likely that tumors will reappear; the goal of surgery is to maintain renal function as long as possible while reducing the risk of metastases. A serial CT study of the natural history of renal lesions in VHL patients revealed that there is a wide variation in the growth rates of the renal lesions.[51] Although clinicians often recommend surgery when the solid renal lesions reach the 2.5- to 3-cm size, the role of surgical resection in the management of VHL-associated renal carcinoma (i.e., whether survival can be extended or quality of life enhanced by aggressive screening and early detection programs) remains to be determined.

Retinal Angioma

Retinal angiomas are often the first manifestation of VHL (Fig. 41-5). Fifty-eight to 60 percent of affected VHL patients will develop these benign vascular tumors of the retina. The histologic pattern of the ocular manifestation is strikingly similar to that of clear cell renal cell carcinoma and cerebellar hemangioblastoma. These tumors can be multifocal, bilateral, and recurrent. While the mean age of diagnosis is reported to be 25 years, these tumors can occur in infants. Although the retinal angiomas are nonmalignant, these tumors can cause glaucoma, cataracts, retinal detachment, and blindness. It is critical that at-risk individuals have a thorough ophthalmologic examination. Ophthalmologic examination often includes tonometry, fluorescein angioscopy, and indirect ophthalmoscopy. Periodic ophthalmologic evaluation is a part of the management of VHL patients. Treatment of retinal angiomas is often by laser therapy. An aggressive approach to screening and treatment of eye lesions in VHL patients often can result in successful long-term preservation of vision. Many clinicians recommend initiation of ophthalmologic screening at an early age (1 year of age) so that preservation of vision can be maintained.[15]

CNS Hemangioblastoma

CNS hemangioblastomas occur in 60 to 65 percent of affected VHL individuals and can cause increased intracranial pressure, obstructive hydrocephalus, hemorrhage, or death. The hemangioblastomas are characterized by three cell types: endothelial cells, stromal cells, and pericytes. These vascular tumors form channels and caverns and can organize into a vascular mural nodule within a fluid-filled cyst. The cells in the CNS tumors are remarkably similar to those seen in the clear cell renal carcinoma as well as epididymal cystadenomas. There is marked hypertrophy of the afferent and efferent vessels in the cerebellar and spinal tumors; the gross appearance of these tumors can be one of a mass of blood vessels. The VHL-associated CNS hemangioblastomas occur most often in the spine and cerebellum as well as in the brainstem at the craniocervical junction. These tumors occasionally occur above the tentorium.[15,52] Hemangioblastoma can occur in the pituitary, although this is an infrequent occurrence. The number of CNS lesions, as well as the number of renal and pancreatic lesions, is often underestimated by radiographic imaging studies.

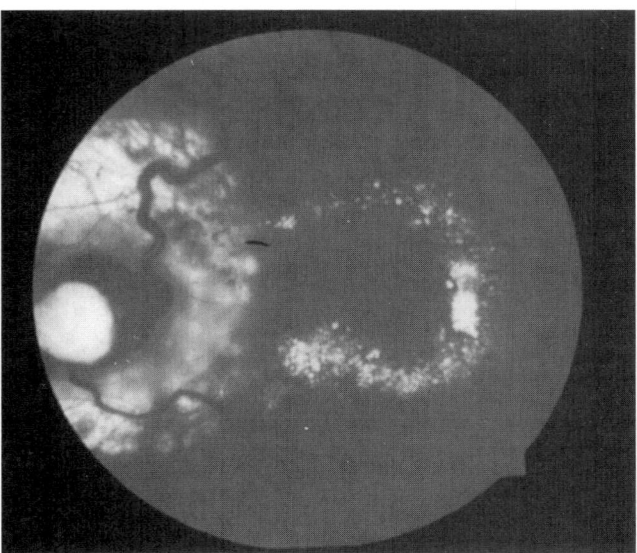

Fig. 41-5 Retinal lesion of a VHL patient showing the hypervascular retinal angioma that characterize VHL. (*From Linehan et al.*[151] *Used with permission.*)

Although the mean age of diagnosis of CNS hemangioblastoma in VHL patients is 29 years, these tumors can occur in children. Symptoms can include headache, nausea, broad-based gait, and vertigo. Signs include papilledema, dysmetria, ataxia, slurred speech, and nystagmus; focal weakness may be an indication of a spinal lesion. Diagnosis of CNS hemangioblastoma is by T_1-weighted magnetic resonance imaging (MRI) of both the head and the spine[15,52] (Fig. 41-6). Treatment is most often by surgical removal. Surgical selection is often complicated in VHL patients. The decision to recommend surgery relates to the size, number, and locations of tumors and the presence of associated findings such as syringomyelia or hydrocephalus. More studies will be needed to determine whether quality of life can be enhanced or survival can be extended by early CNS tumor detection and aggressive genetic and clinical screening programs.[52] Focused radiation therapy with the "gamma knife" is sometimes used, although its role in the management of CNS hemangioblastoma remains to be determined.

The Cell of Origin in Hemangioblastoma

Hemangioblastomas are a mixture of stromal cells and immature vascular cells. The neoplastic cell that forms these tumors is not known. Two advances provide further understanding of VHL hemangioblastomas. First, Lee and Vortmeyer used microdissection to identify which cell type showed loss of heterozygosity in

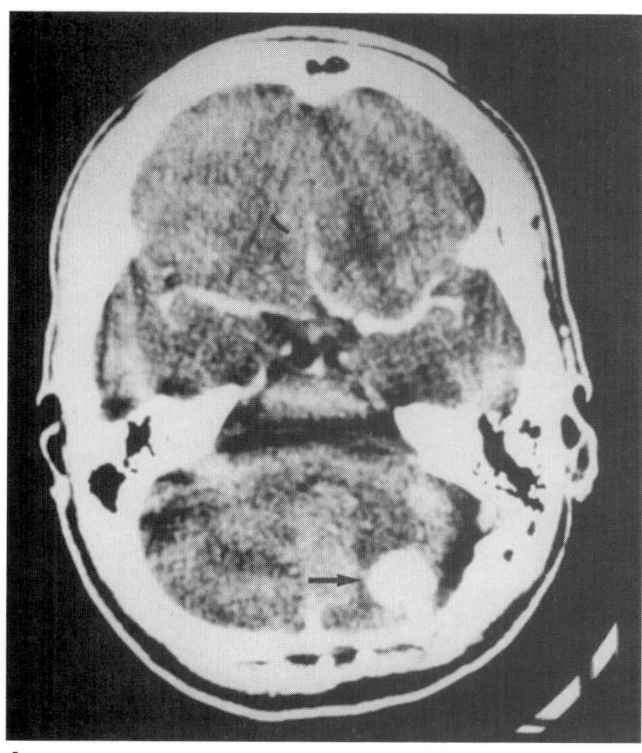

A

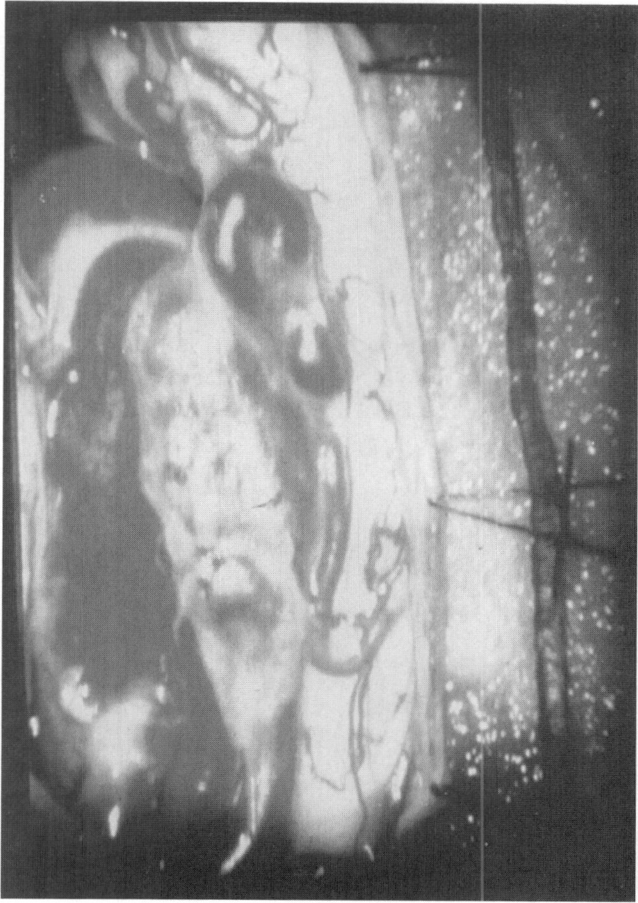

B

Fig. 41-6 ***A.*** **Cerebellar hemangioblastoma detected by an MRI examination.** ***B.*** **Spinal hemangioblastoma revealing the intense hypervascularity of these lesions.** ***(From Linehan et al.[152] Used with permission.)***

sporadic hemangioblastomas.[53,54] Microdissected stromal cells from hemangioblastomas showed LOH with markers on chromosome 3p, suggesting that stromal cells had one of the two "hits" (molecular events) required to produce tumors. It was not possible to isolate the immature vascular cells by microdissection. These results suggest that the stromal cell is the neoplastic cell in hemangioblastomas. Using cultures of mouse embryonic stem cells, a common progenitor that gives rise to both blood cells and vascular endothelial cells has been identified.[55,56] Because this progenitor cell can be grown in culture, it now can be studied in detail. It is possible that the hemangioblast described by Choi et al. may be related to the cell of origin of VHL hemangioblastomas.

Pheochromocytoma

Pheochromocytoma has been reported to occur in 18 percent of VHL patients.[15] There is a marked clustering of pheochromocytoma in certain families, and this is now known as a distinct subtype of VHL, *VHL type II.* The pheochromocytomas can be bilateral, multifocal, and extraadrenal, and they can become malignant. Symptoms of pheochromocytoma in VHL patients include paroxysmal or sustained hypertension, episodic sweating, palpitations, headaches, and anxiety attacks and are due to the release of the catecholamines epinephrine and norepinephrine. Blood pressure can increase to levels that cause fatal cerebral hemorrhage or acute myocardial infarction. Unsuspected pheochromocytoma can be particularly ominous in a patient who has a cerebellar hemangioblastoma, who is pregnant, or who is undergoing surgical resection of a CNS, renal, or pancreatic lesion.

Abdominal CT scanning, which is often performed in the initial screening of VHL patients, frequently provides the initial detection of VHL-associated pheochromocytoma (Fig. 41-7). MRI is a particularly useful method for making the diagnosis. If there is a suspicion that a patient may have an extraadrenal pheochromocytoma,[131] I-MIBG (metaiodobenzylguanidine) scintigraphy may be recommended[57] (Fig. 41-8). The diagnosis of pheochromocytoma is made by demonstration of elevated levels of catecholamines and/or their metabolites in the urine or blood. Evaluation of VHL patients includes measurement of serum and blood catecholamines, most often epinephrine, norepinephrine, and metanephrine. The clonidine suppression and/or glucagon stimulation tests may aid in making the diagnosis of an indeterminate or potentially nonfunctioning adrenal mass lesion.[58,59] The treatment of pheochromocytoma is surgical resection of tumors that are functioning or larger than 5 cm. Treatment of bilateral pheochromocytomas may require surgical removal of both glands. Because removal of both adrenal glands requires that the patient be on lifetime of replacement therapy, some physicians perform partial adrenalectomies to preserve functioning adrenal tissue. While this has the potential advantage of preserving adrenal function, such patients need careful monitoring for recurrent pheochromocytoma. The addition of laparoscopic adrenalectomy has added another potentially less invasive method for management of VHL-associated tumors.[58,60] Detection and treatment of functioning pheochromocytomas are important. Undetected pheochromocytomas are life-threatening and have lead to the death of VHL patients. The role of treatment of occult, nonfunctioning pheochromocytomas is currently under study.

Pancreatic Manifestations of VHL

VHL-associated pancreatic lesions include pancreatic cysts, serous microcystic adenomas, and islet cell tumors (Fig. 41-9). Pancreatic cysts are the most common manifestations, but the frequency

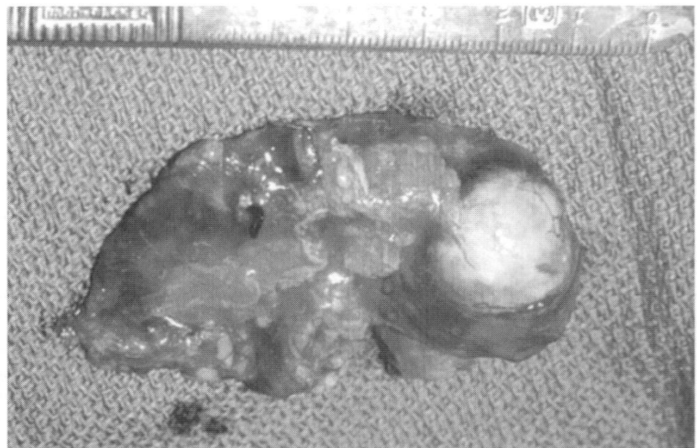

A

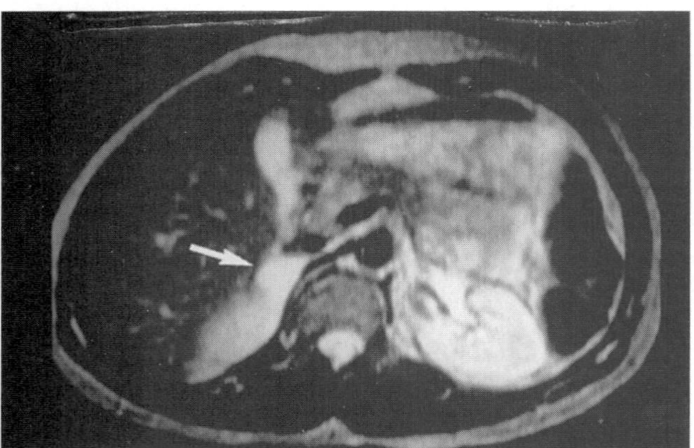

B

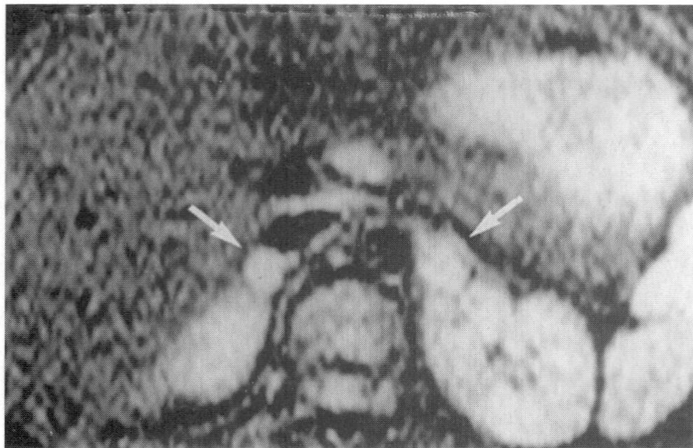

C

Fig. 41-7 ***A.*** **Adrenal gland removed at surgery with a large pheochromocytoma on the left side of the gland.** ***B,C.*** **Abdominal CT scan reveals a solitary, right-sided pheochromocytoma (*B*, middle panel). In another patient, abdominal MRI scan reveals the presence of bilateral pheochromocytomas in a 12-year-old boy (*C*, right panel). (*From Linehan et al.*[152] *Used with permission.*)**

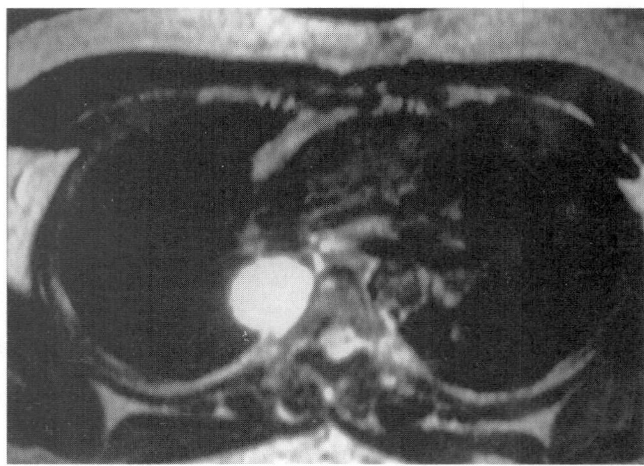

Fig. 41-8 MRI showing an extraadrenal pheochromocytoma. (*From Linehan et al.*[152] Used with permission.)

depends on the individual family being studied. The reported frequency of pancreatic cysts in VHL patients varies from 0 percent in two large families[61,62] to 93 percent in others.[63] Pancreatic cysts usually appear in the 20- to 40-year age group, but they have been detected in patients as young as 15 years of age. The cysts appear throughout the body of the pancreas with no localization to a particular site. Epithelium-lined collections of serous fluid produce the cysts, which vary in size from 7 mm to over 10 cm. Serous cystadenoma (or microcystic adenoma) contains multiple macroscopic and microscopic cysts that are separated by thickened walls of stroma arranged in a stellate pattern with a central nidus, which can be scar-like or calcified.[35] Pancreatic cysts are most often asymptomatic. Symptoms can be caused by biliary obstruction or associated with such diffuse disease that pancreatic insufficiency results and steatorrhea and diarrhea occur. Obstruction is managed by the placement of biliary stents; pancreatic insufficiency, by enzyme replacement. Rarely, cystic enlargement is associated with such local pain or early satiety that percutaneous drainage is required.[35]

Pancreatic islet cell tumors also occur in VHL patients, apparently independently of pancreatic cystic disease. These tumors, of neural origin, are comprised of nests of polygonal cells with vesicular nuclei. Like VHL-associated renal CNS, and retinal tumors, the pancreatic islet cell tumors are markedly vascular. While most grow slowly and are asymptomatic, pancreatic islet cell tumors can grow rapidly or metastasize. Diagnosis of islet cell tumors is by CT scan, where the tumor appears as a characteristically intensely enhancing lesion. Although the standard treatment of growing islet cell tumors is surgical resection, the decision to recommend surgery for the management of VHL-associated islet cell tumors is complicated. While

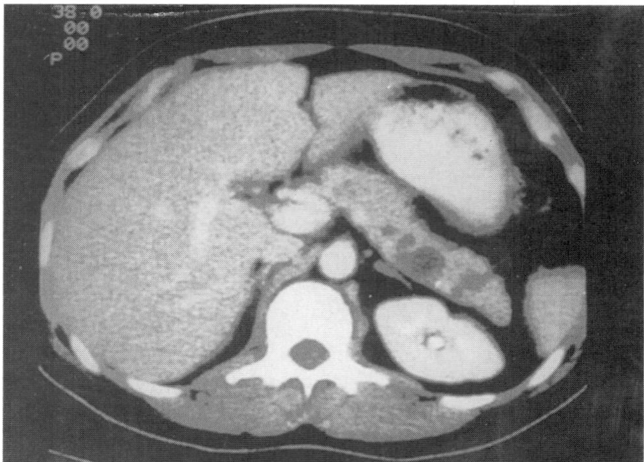

Fig. 41-9 Abdominal imaging reveals pancreatic cysts and islet cell tumors in a VHL patient. (*From Linehan et al.*[152] *Used with permission.*)

advanced islet cell tumors are life-threatening, they can invade locally and metastasize, and the role of surgical resection in prolonging survival and quality of life remains to be determined.

Papillary Cystadenoma of the Epididymis and Broad Ligament

Papillary cystadenomas of the epididymis can be unilateral or bilateral and are present in 10 to 26 percent of affected VHL males. These benign tumors, which can involve the spermatic cord, are found most often in the globus major of the epididymis. The lesions, which are typically 2 to 3 cm in size, can reach 5 cm. The histology of these tumors resembles that of renal and pancreatic cysts and endolymphatic sac tumors. The epididymal cysts are lined by clear cells that contain glycogen and fat with papillary and tubular structures and a surrounding collagenous pseudocapsule.[35] These tumors do not have malignant potential, and treatment is most often conservative. Rarely, a symptomatic epididymal cystadenoma will require surgery. Papillary cystadenomas also may occur in women, in tissue associated with the mesonephric tubules near the ovaries and uterine tubes and in remnants of the longer mesonephric duct, close to the lateral walls of the uterus and vagina.[35,64]

Endolymphatic Sac Tumors

A more recently appreciated manifestation of VHL is the presence of a tumor in the inner ear, an endolymphatic sac tumor (ELST) (Fig. 41-10). Lying between the dura of the posterior fossa, the endolymphatic sac is located at the end of the endolymphatic sac canal.[35] Although the prevalence and clinical characteristics of endolymphatic sac tumors in VHL patients have been characterized only recently,[65] it has been estimated that up to 10 percent of VHL patients may have ELST. ELST is a low-grade malignancy with a papillary histologic growth pattern. Although a metastatic ELST has not been reported, this tumor can invade locally and be associated with hearing damage or facial paresis. Evaluation of VHL patients for ELST involves imaging with high-resolution CT and MRI through the inner ear. Audiologic evaluation is used for assessment of hearing and cochlear function. Significant audiologic abnormalities may be detected in up to 50 percent of VHL patients. The possibility exists that there are two components, one

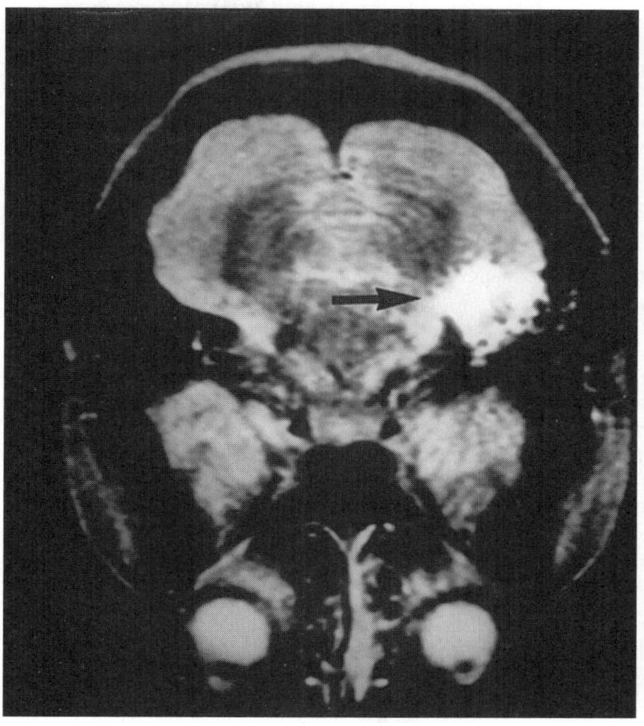

A

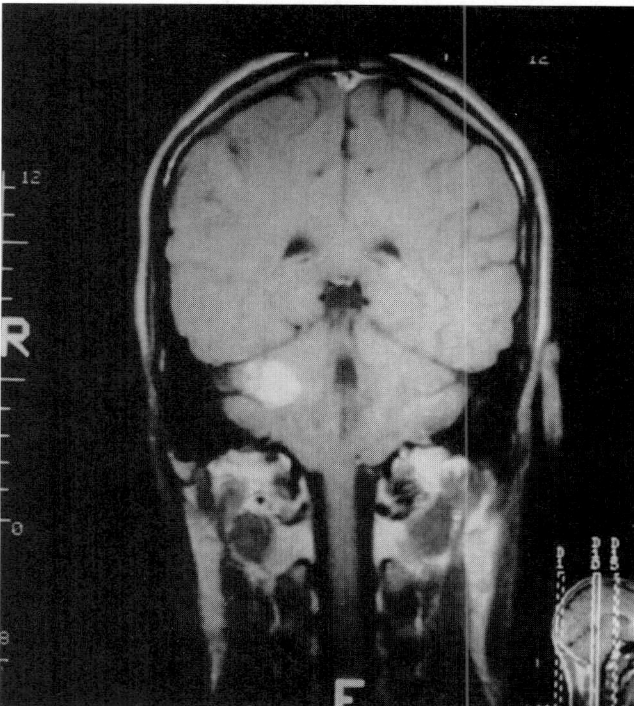

B

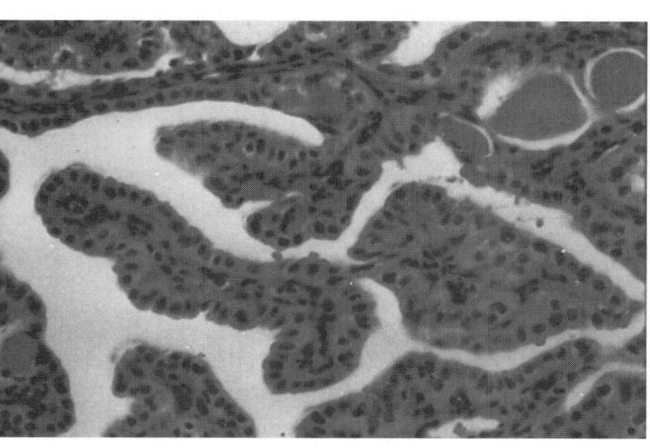

C

Fig. 41-10 Imaging studies reveal endolymphatic sac tumors (ELST) in VHL patients. Histologically, this tumor is a low-grade papillary neoplasm that invades locally but which has low potential to metastasize. (*From Linehan et al.*[152] *Used with permission.*)

neoplastic and the other neurologic, to the otologic manifestations of VHL. It is not known yet if these two aspects of VHL are related. Early detection of the endolymphatic sac tumors is possible with MRI and CT scanning of the internal auditory canal. The role of early surgical intervention to preserve hearing remains to be determined.[35]

THE *VHL* GENE: CHARACTERISTICS OF A TUMOR-SUPPRESSOR GENE

In order to determine if the genetics of VHL fit Knudson's "two hit" hypothesis of a tumor-suppressor gene, Tory et al.[66] evaluated renal cell carcinomas, pheochromocytoma, spinal hemangioblastoma, and cerebellar hemangioblastoma from VHL patients. Multiple renal cell carcinomas, pheochromocytomas, and spinal and cerebellar hemangioblastomas from VHL patients showed loss of the wild-type chromosome 3p allele, demonstrating that both copies of the *VHL* gene were inactivated in VHL tumor tissue.[66] To assess for the earliest abnormalities in renal manifestations of VHL, Lubensky et al.[67] performed detailed analysis of chromosome 3p LOH in microdissected renal lesions from VHL patients by PCR-SSCP analysis (Fig. 41-11). Two benign cysts, five atypical cysts, five microscopic renal cell carcinoma in situ, five single cell-lined cysts, and two microscopic and seven macroscopic renal cell carcinomas were evaluated. Twenty-five of 26 of the renal lesions had (1) nonrandom allelic loss at the *VHL* gene locus with loss of the wild-type allele and (2) retention of the inherited, mutated *VHL* allele.[67] Although clinical, radiologic, and pathologic data have suggested that benign and atypical renal lesions may represent the precursors of renal cell carcinoma in VHL patients, the finding of LOH of the *VHL* gene as an early event suggests that atypical and benign clear cell cysts may represent early stages in the development and progression of renal cell carcinoma in VHL patients.[67]

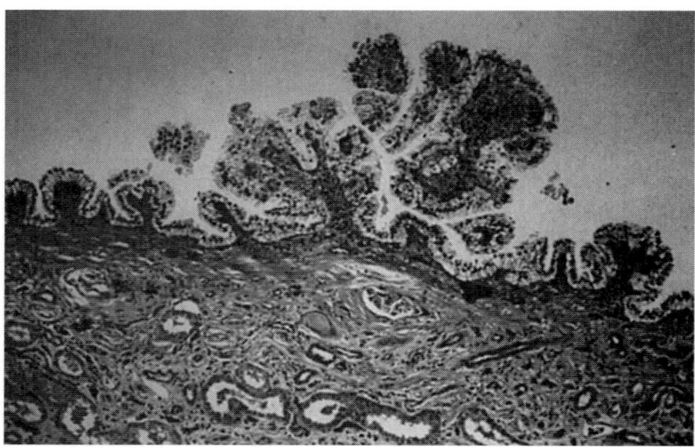

A

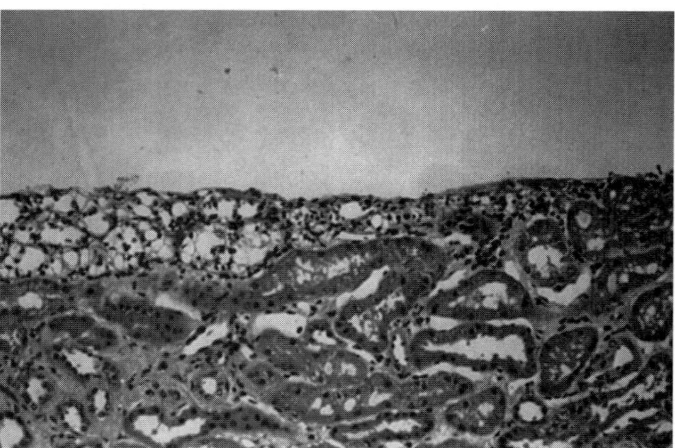

B

Fig. 41-11 Histology of early renal lesions in a VHL patient. Lubensky et al. detected *VHL* gene LOH in microdissected material from 25 of 26 renal lesions, including lesions such as renal cell carcinoma (*A*) and atypical cysts lined by two to three layers of clear epithelial cells (*B*). (*From Lubensky et al.*[67] *Used with permission.*)

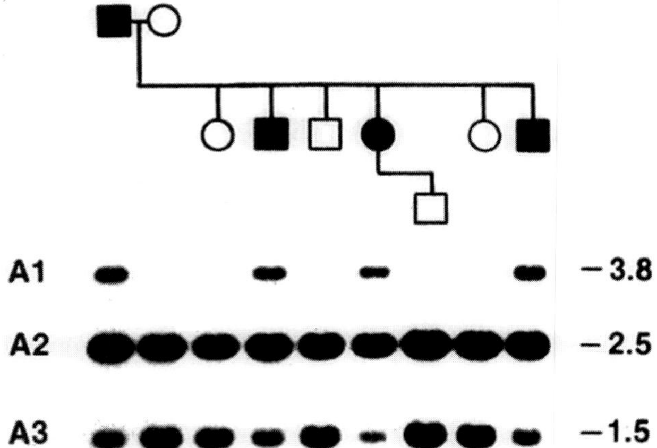

Fig. 41-12 Linkage analysis demonstrating cosegregation of the *A1* allele of the chromosome 3p marker *D3S18* with VHL. The darkened boxes represent individuals affected with VHL. (*From Hosoe et al.*[70] *Used with permission.*)

THE *VHL* GENE IS LOCALIZED TO CHROMOSOME 3

In 1988, Seizinger et al.[68] localized the *VHL* gene to a locus in the telomeric region of the short arm of chromosome 3, in the region of the *cRAF1* oncogene at 3p25. To further characterize the *VHL* gene locus, Lerman et al.[69] isolated a collection of 2000 lambda phage carrying single-copy DNA fragments that were ordered as RFLP markers for construction of a fine linkage map spanning the distal portion of chromosome 3p encompassing the *VHL* locus. These markers made localization and subsequent identification of the *VHL* gene possible. When Hosoe et al.[70] and Richards et al.[71] performed multipoint linkage analysis (Fig. 41-12) with chromosome 3p markers in VHL families, the gene locus was determined to be in a 4-cM interval between *cRAF1* and *D3S18*, an anonymous marker at 3p25.5.

PRESYMPTOMATIC DIAGNOSIS OF VHL BY DNA POLYMORPHISM ANALYSIS

With flanking DNA markers available, Glenn et al.[72] compared the results of DNA linkage analysis with a comprehensive clinical screening examination. Forty-three individuals at risk for developing VHL were informative with polymorphic markers. In 42 of 43 at-risk individuals, polymorphism analysis accurately identified individuals carrying the *VHL* gene among asymptomatic family members.[72] All nine of the at-risk individuals predicted to carry the *VHL* gene were found on clinical examination to have evidence of occult manifestations; no clinical evidence of VHL was detected in 32 of 33 of the at-risk individuals predicted to carry the wild-type allele of the *VHL* gene.[72] The single patient who was classified clinically as having VHL and who was not predicted by linkage analysis to carry the *VHL* gene was a 42-year-old at-risk female who was found to have a solid renal mass. When the mass was removed surgically, a small focus of clear cell renal cell carcinoma was found. When the *VHL* gene was later identified and the mutation in this kindred was determined, this patient was found not to carry a germ-line *VHL* mutation. A somatic *VHL* gene mutation, however, was found subsequently in her tumor,[73] which, as would be predicted, was different from that identified in her affected siblings. She was an example of a *phenocopy*, i.e., an

Table 41-3 Classification of VHL

Type I	VHL without pheochromocytoma
Type II	VHL with pheochromocytoma
Type IIA	Pheochromocytoma, CNS hemangioblastomas, and retinal angiomas
Type IIB	VHL IIA plus pancreatic involvement and renal manifestations (tumors, cysts)

individual who is found to have a tumor in a target organ in a hereditary cancer syndrome who does not carry the *VHL* gene.[72]

VHL: GENOTYPIC HOMOGENEITY/PHENOTYPIC HETEROGENEITY

To further localize the *VHL* gene, over 100 VHL families from North America were evaluated. Different patterns of VHL manifestation appeared among the VHL families. In the initial genetic studies, one large family was identified whose VHL phenotype was markedly distinct from typical VHL. Whereas pheochromocytoma is normally identified in 18 percent of affected VHL individuals, in this kindred, 57 percent (27 of 47) of affected family members were found to have pheochromocytoma. Four of 47 affected family members had spinal or cerebellar hemangioblastomas; none of the affected family members had renal cell carcinoma (0 of 47) or pancreatic cysts (0 of 24).[72,74]

The clinical findings were confirmed by genetic analysis. The family linked to *RAF1* and *D3S18*, markers shown to be linked to typical VHL. Subsequently, a number of families have been characterized with this pattern of VHL, i.e., with pheochromocytomas. These findings formed the initial basis for the classification of VHL kindreds (Table 41-3) as VHL type I (VHL without pheochromocytomas) or VHL type II (with pheochromocytoma).

IDENTIFICATION OF THE *VHL* GENE

Once the *VHL* gene was localized to the 3p25 locus, the area was covered with overlapping yeast artificial chromosomes (YACs) and cosmid-phage contigs.[75] A critical step in the identification of the gene occurred when Yao et al. identified overlapping germ-line deletions in three unrelated VHL patients during the construction of a long-range (2.5-Mb) restriction map of the regions surrounding the *VHL* gene. A cosmid (cosmid 11) was identified that mapped to the smallest nested deletion. Two candidate cDNAs, denoted g7 and g6, were isolated from a (GT11 teratocarcinoma library screened by conserved sequences in cosmid 11. Since previous studies had determined that there was genotypic homogeneity in VHL, the *VHL* gene was considered to be at a single locus. g6 was found to be an unlikely candidate because no mutations were detected in 120 unrelated VHL patients. When inactivating mutations were searched for in constitutional DNA derived from 221 unrelated VHL patients by Southern blot analysis, aberrant bands ranging in size from 4 to 25 kb were detected in 28 of the 221 VHL kindreds. SSCP analysis revealing inactivating mutations that segregated with VHL were identified in three families. These findings (Fig. 41-13) indicated that g7 is the *VHL* tumor-suppressor gene.[75] *VHL* gene expression has been detected in all human tissues tested; the 6- and 6.5-kb transcripts likely represent alternatively spliced forms of g7 mRNA. The human *VHL* gene, which has three exons, encodes a protein of 213 amino acids.

GENETIC DIAGNOSIS OF VHL

The "gold standard" for diagnosis of VHL disease is the identification of germ-line mutations in patients suspected of having the illness. Previously, the best available diagnostic test in at-risk asymptomatic VHL family members was the use of linkage analysis.[72] Now that the *VHL* gene has been identified, germ-line mutation detection can be used to establish the diagnosis of VHL in individuals with clinical pictures suggestive of VHL disease, to identify mutation carriers in at-risk members of VHL families, and to identify the germ-line mutation that characterizes each family. The detection of germ-line mutation initially varied from 39 to 75 percent. Now, with improved methodology, it should be possible to identify germ-line mutations in virtually all families with VHL[76] (Fig. 41-14).

Groups at the National Cancer Institute and the University of Pennsylvania reported detection of germ-line mutations in 100 percent (93 of 93) of VHL families. Improved mutation detection in VHL required the use of panel mutation-detection methods to detect all the types of mutations that produce VHL disease (Fig. 41-15). The methods included quantitative Southern blotting to detect deletions of the entire *VHL* gene, Southern blotting to detect gene rearrangements, fluorescence in situ hybridization to confirm deletions, and complete sequencing of the gene.

GENOTYPE/PHENOTYPE CORRELATIONS

Clinical heterogeneity is a feature of VHL. In order to determine the relationship between *VHL* gene mutations and the clinical

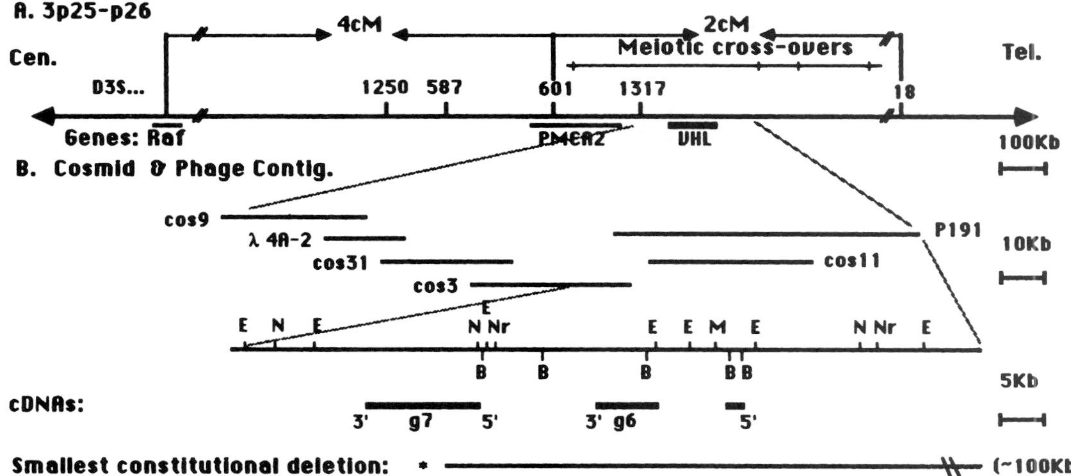

Fig. 41-13 Physical and genetic map encompassing the *VHL* gene locus on chromosome 3p. The *VHL* locus was determined by meiotic mapping and multipoint linkage analysis. The nested deletions identified in the germ-line DNA of the three unrelated VHL patients[153] are shown under the map. (*From Latif et al.*[75] *Used with permission.*)

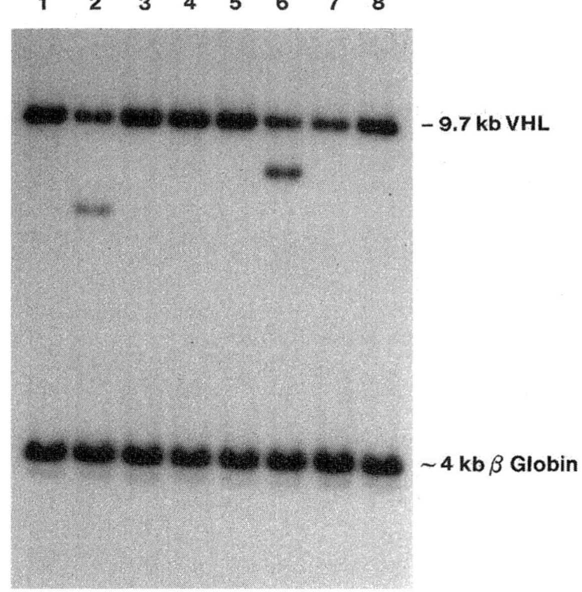

Fig. 41-14 Stolle et al. analyzed in detail the characteristics of the germ-line *VHL* gene in 93 families seen at the NCI. A new method for detection of deletion (or partial deletion) of the *VHL* gene was developed. In normal individuals, a single 22-kb *EcoRI* or 9.7-kb *EcoRI/AseI* fragment was detected by hybridization with the g7 cDNA probe. In individuals with partial deletions of the *VHL* gene, a slower or faster migrating fragment was detected in addition to the normal-sized fragment. A germ-line deletion of the entire *VHL* gene was suspected when there was a reduction of signal intensity of the fragment hybridized to the g7 cDNA. Lane 7 VHL is deleted; lanes 2 and 6 represent partial deletion (*From Stolle et al.*[76] *Used with permission.*)

manifestation of the VHL, Chen et al.[77] searched for *VHL* gene mutations in 114 families (Fig. 41-16). Mutations, including microdeletions/insertions, nonsense mutations, deletions, or missense mutations, were detected in 85 of 114 (75 percent) families. Mutations were detected in each of the three exons, clustering in the 3′ end of exon 1 and the 5′ end of exon 3. There were a small number of mutations in exon 2. While 56 percent of the mutations associated with VHL type I were deletions, nonsense mutations, or microdeletions/insertions, 96 percent of mutations in VHL type II

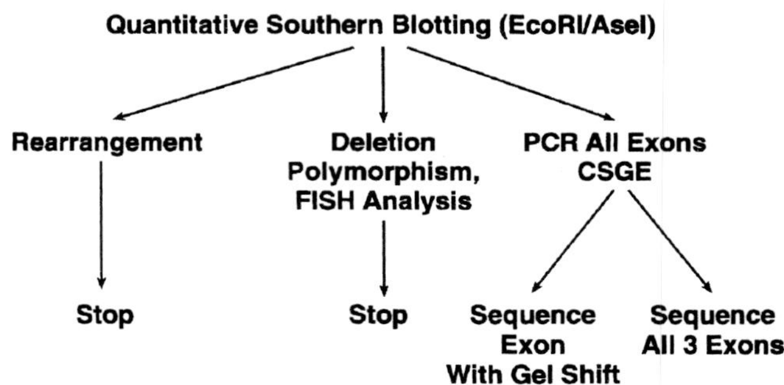

Fig. 41-15 Flowchart of methods used sequentially by Cathy Stolle at the University of Pennsylvania to detect germ-line *VHL* mutations in 100 percent (93 of 93) of VHL families.

(VHL with pheochromocytoma) kindreds were found to be missense mutations. There also was a clustering of VHL type II mutations in a small region in the 5′ end of exon 3 of the *VHL* gene; mutation in codon 238 accounted for 43 percent of the VHL type II mutations.[77] Subsequent studies have confirmed the association of missense mutations with VHL type II families. Brauch et al.[78] identified a missense mutation at nucleotide 505 (T to C) in 14 VHL type II families from the Black Forest region of Germany. This mutation had been identified previously in two VHL type II families living in Pennsylvania (the kindred previously described in the phenotypic heterogeneity section). Haplotype analysis among the 100 patients with the 505 mutation indicated a founder effect.[78] A nucleotide 547 missense mutation also has been described in a large VHL family with pheochromocytoma, with no members affected with renal cell carcinoma.[79] Similar mutation patterns have been detected in families from Europe[80,81] and Japan.[82–84]

Hereditary forms of pheochromocytoma can be found associated with VHL, multiple endocrine neoplasia type 2 (MEN2), or neurofibromatosis type 1. Families with multiple pheochromocytomas in which there is uncertainty about the diagnosis are candidates for *VHL* gene mutation analysis.[78,80,81,83–86] For example, the abdominal imaging studies in Fig. 41-17 are from an 11-year-old boy with pheochromocytoma whose mother had

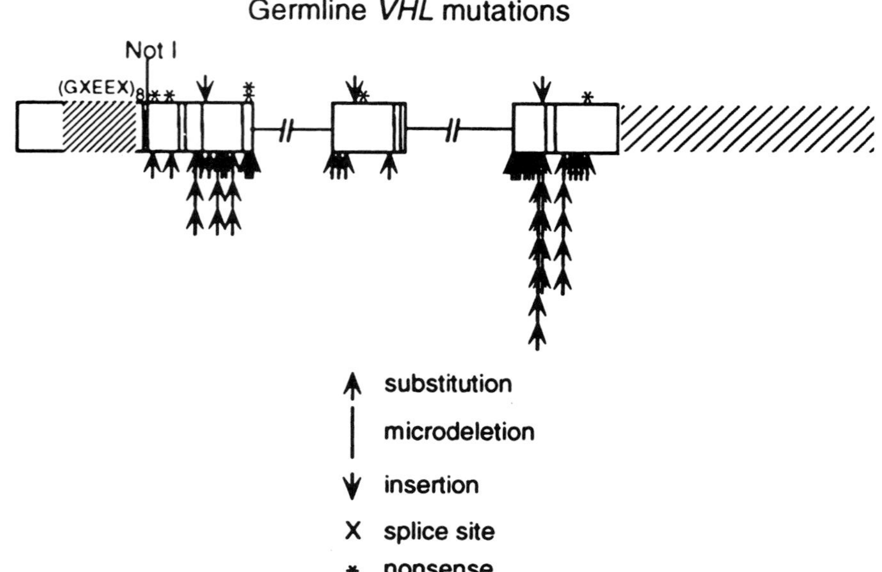

Fig. 41-16 *VHL* gene germ-line mutation distribution in VHL kindreds. The boxes indicate cloned exons. The 3′ UTR and the exon 1 pentameric acidic repeat are indicated by cross-hatching. (*From Chen et al.*[77] *Used with permission.*)

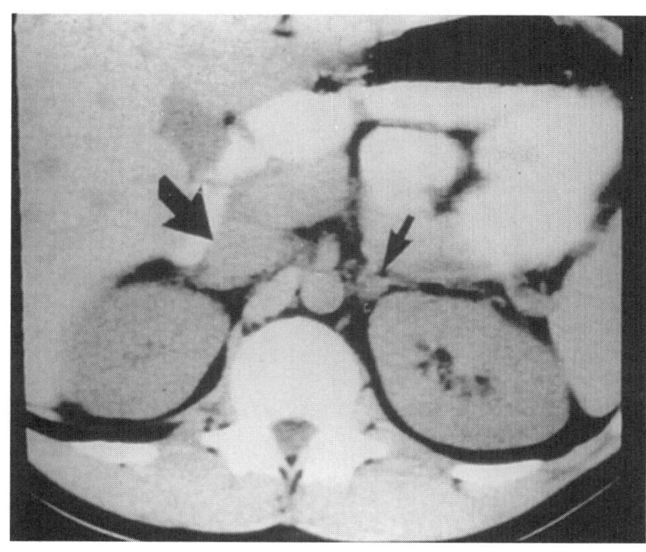

A

B

Fig. 41-17 Abdominal CT scan (*A*) and abdominal MRI examination (*B*) reveal the presence of pheochromocytoma in an 11-year-old child found to have a mutation of the *VHL* gene. (*From Linehan et al.*[152] *Used with permission.*)

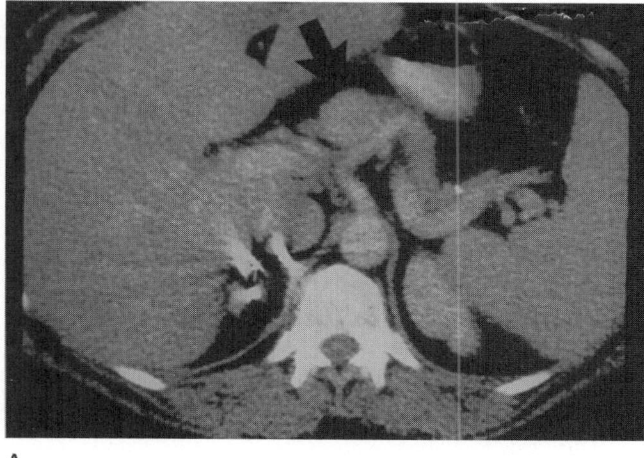

A

B

Fig. 41-18 Abdominal CT scan (*A*) reveals a pancreatic lesion in a woman whose 11-year-old child was found to have a pheochromocytoma. Abdominal ultrasound (*B*) confirmed that the pancreatic lesion is solid. The mass was removed surgically and found to be an islet cell tumor. (*From Linehan et al.*[152] *Used with permission.*)

had a pheochromocytoma removed when she was 11 years of age and whose uncle had died at age 9 with severe hypertension. The clinical impression previously had been that this family was affected with either MEN2 or "familial pheochromocytoma."

When the child's mother underwent abdominal imaging (Fig. 41-18), she was found to have a pancreatic mass that was removed surgically and found to be an islet cell tumor. Germ-line *VHL* gene mutation analysis was performed, and a nucleotide 595 (leucine-phenylalanine) missense mutation was detected, confirming the diagnosis of VHL type II.

When a 25-year-old woman from a pheochromocytoma family (six other members have been diagnosed with pheochromocytoma) was evaluated, a retroperitoneal mass was detected (Fig. 41-19). She was found to have malignant pheochromocytoma with pulmonary metastases. Germ-line *VHL* mutation analysis revealing a missense mutation in exon 2 confirmed the diagnosis of VHL type II.

Penetrance of Different Mutations

There is evidence that the penetrance of the *VHL* gene depends on the particular germ-line mutation. About 60 percent of people with the 505 mutation will develop clinical or radiologic evidence of VHL during their lifetimes (Neumann, unpublished work).

Modifier Genes and VHL

Individuals with identical germ-line *VHL* mutations differ in the degree of disease severity. To search for evidence of genes modifying the expression of *VHL* mutant genes, Webster et al.[87] examined 183 individuals with germ-line *VHL* mutations for the presence and number of retinal angiomas. The number of ocular tumors was significantly correlated in closely related individuals but not in more distantly related individuals. The findings suggested that the development of ocular tumors was determined at an early age and was influenced by genetic or environmental modifier effects that act at multiple sites.

MUTATIONS OF THE *VHL* TUMOR-SUPPRESSOR GENE IN RENAL CARCINOMA

To evaluate the role of VHL in the origin of sporadic, nonhereditary renal cell carcinoma, Gnarra et al.[73] searched for *VHL* gene mutation in tumors from 108 patients with both

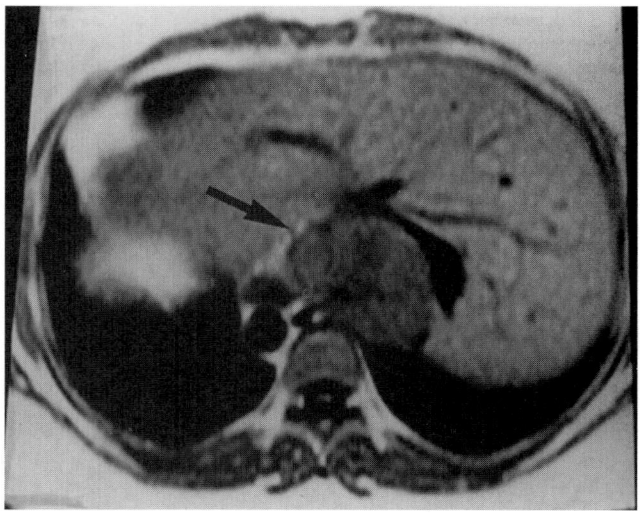

A

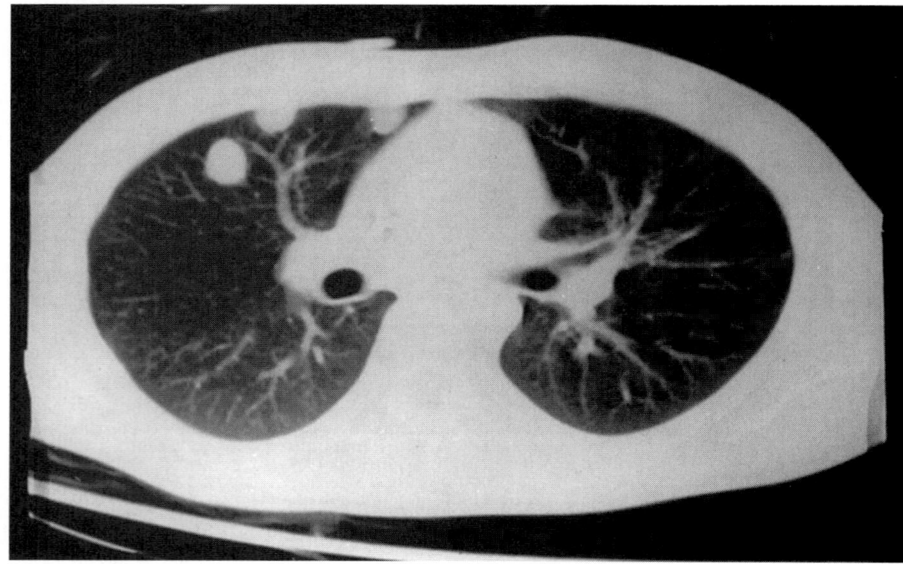

B

Fig. 41-19 Abdominal CT scan (*A*) reveals a retroperitoneal mass in a 25-year-old woman who had had two previous surgical resections of pheochromocytoma. Lung CT scan (*B*) revealed the presence of metastatic foci in the chest. *VHL* gene analysis revealed a mutation in exon 2 of the *VHL* gene, confirming the diagnosis of VHL. (*From Linehan, et al.*[152] *Used with permission.*)

Sporadic renal carcinoma *VHL* mutations

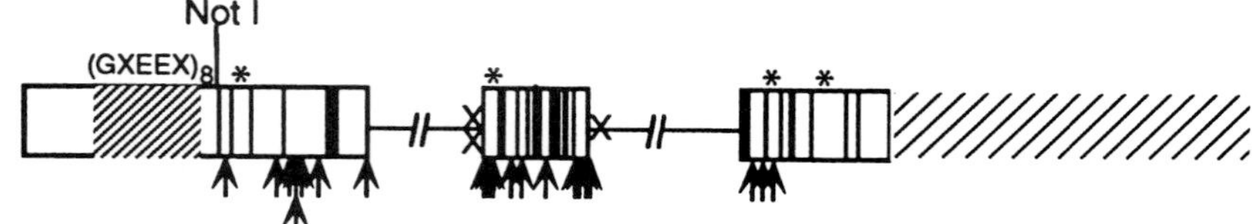

substitution
microdeletion
insertion
X splice site
* nonsense

Fig. 41-20 *VHL* gene mutation distribution in sporadic clear cell renal carcinoma. The boxes indicate cloned exons. The 3′ UTR and the exon 1 pentameric acidic repeat are indicated by cross-hatching. (*From Gnarra et al.*[73] *Used with permission.*)

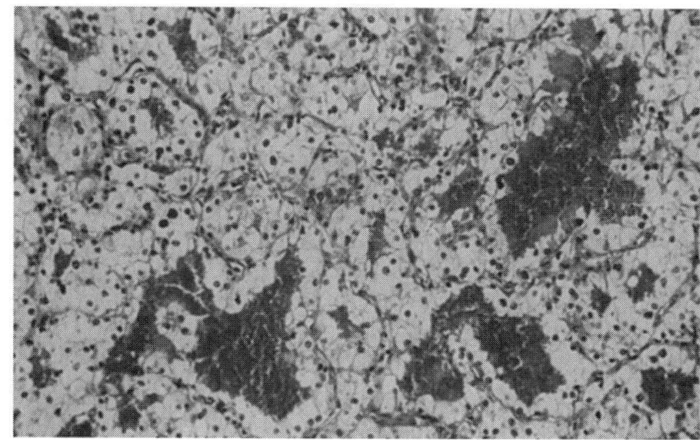

A

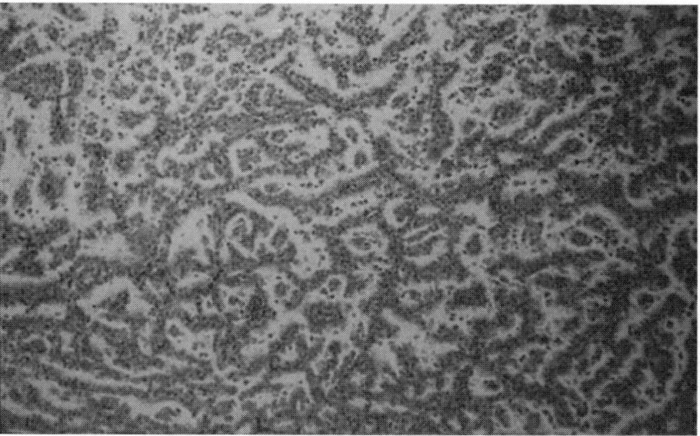

B

Fig. 41-21 Somatic *VHL* gene mutations and LOH are characteristic of clear cell renal carcinoma (*A*) but are not found in papillary renal carcinoma (*B*). (*From Linehan et al.*[152] *Used with permission.*)

localized and advanced renal cell carcinoma (Fig. 41-20). LOH of the *VHL* gene was detected in 98 percent of clear cell renal carcinomas; *VHL* mutations were identified in 57 percent of the samples (Fig. 41-21*A*). Mutations including nucleotide deletions, substitutions, insertions, and nonsense mutations were found in each of the three exons. The presence of splice-site mutations that would eliminate the translation of exon 2 and the high percentage of mutations (45 percent) involving exon 2 indicated that exon 2 may have an important function in the protein.[3,73] The detection of somatic *VHL* mutations in small, clinically localized renal cell carcinomas (< 2 cm) suggests that inactivation of this gene is an early event in renal carcinogenesis.[88] When 119 tumors from 11 different tissues were evaluated, no additional somatic *VHL* gene mutations were detected. Neither chromosome 3 LOH nor *VHL* gene mutations were detected in tumor tissue from patients with papillary renal carcinoma (Fig. 41-21*B*). *VHL* gene mutations have been identified in clear cell renal carcinomas in Japan,[89] Europe,[90–92] and North America.[85]

When tumor tissues from patients with hereditary renal carcinoma characterized by 3;8 translocation[13] were analyzed for *VHL* mutations,[73,93] two of four tumors were found to have mutations of the wild-type *VHL* gene. In this kindred, it is the inherited derivative chromosome 8 carrying the portion of chromosome 3 distal to the breakpoint that is deleted in the kidney tumors and the normal chromosome 3 that is retained.[14] The wild-type *VHL* allele was found to be mutated in the tumors, demonstrating a mechanism of clear cell renal carcinoma tumorigenesis in the chromosome (3;8) translocation family that involves the loss of both copies of the *VHL* gene.[73,93] The association of *VHL* gene mutation and clear cell renal carcinoma in three independent clinical entities [(1) sporadic clear cell renal carcinoma, (2) clear cell renal carcinoma associated with VHL, and (3) clear cell renal carcinoma associated with the 3;8 translocation hereditary clear cell renal carcinoma] demonstrates that inactivation of the *VHL* gene is a critical event in clear cell renal carcinoma. Detection of *VHL* gene inactivation in clear cell renal carcinoma and not in papillary renal carcinoma supports the proposal of a molecular genetic classification of renal carcinoma, papillary versus clear cell renal carcinoma, with clear cell renal carcinoma being characterized by inactivation of the *VHL* gene.

The microdissection techniques for archival DNA[94] provide a method for detection of *VHL* gene mutations in paraffin-embedded material[95] that may furnish clinicians with improved strategies for both diagnosis[96] and classification of renal tumors. Similar methods applied to aspirate cytology may enable improved clarification of whether or not an indeterminate mass in a kidney or another organ is a clear cell renal carcinoma. *VHL* gene mutations were detected when the sporadic forms of other tumors that appear in VHL patients were analyzed. Kanno et al.[97] detected abnormal *VHL* gene SSCP patterns in 7 of 13 sporadic hemangioblastomas, 3 of which were characterized by direct sequencing. Somatic mutations in the three tumors included two missense mutations and one microdeletion, one in exon 1 and two in exon 2. Gilcrease et al.[98] detected a somatic *VHL* gene mutation in 1 of 2 sporadic cystadenomas of the epididymis. *VHL* gene mutations appear to play a role in tumorigenesis in a subset of sporadic epididymal cystadenomas and CNS hemangioblastomas.

SILENCING THE *VHL* GENE BY DNA METHYLATION

Herman et al.[99] demonstrated another potential mechanism for inactivation of the *VHL* gene in clear cell renal carcinoma by showing hypermethylation of the normally unmethylated CpG island in the 5′ region of the gene. The hypermethylation was observed in 5 of 26 (19 percent) clear cell renal carcinomas evaluated. In four of the tumors, one copy of the *VHL* gene was lost; the fifth retained two heavily methylated *VHL* alleles. One of the five tumors had a missense mutation in addition to hypermethylation of the single remaining allele. The other four tumors with *VHL* hypermethylation had no detectable mutations. None of the five tumors expressed the *VHL* gene. When one of the renal cell carcinoma cell lines with a hypermethylated (and silent) *VHL* gene was treated with 5-aza-2′-deoxycytidine, the *VHL* gene was re-expressed. While the extent of hypermethylation of the *VHL* gene in a larger series of tumors and the potential role of agents such as 5-aza-2′-deoxycytidine remain to be determined, this study provides an additional mechanism for inactivation of the *VHL* gene in clear cell renal carcinoma.[99]

CHARACTERIZATION OF THE *VHL* TUMOR-SUPPRESSOR GENE PRODUCT

When the *VHL* gene was identified, the deduced amino acid sequence predicted no significant homology to other proteins. No functional or structural motifs that could provide insight into function of the VHL protein were found. In order to characterize the *VHL* gene product, Duan et al.[100] identified the homologous rat gene that encodes a 185-amino-acid protein with 88 percent sequence identify to the 213-amino-acid human *VHL* gene product. When epitope-tagged human and rat proteins were introduced into cell lines and examined by immunofluorescence microscopy, a number of patterns were observed. The VHL protein was found to be localized to the nucleus and the cytosol but not to the cell surface. Both the human and the rat proteins co-immunoprecipitated a similar set of other protein bands. These included bands at 16 and 9 kDa and a group of bands migrating between 50 and 70 kDa.

A large percentage of both sporadic and hereditary *VHL* gene mutations include missense mutations in the protein. When cDNA constructs containing naturally occurring *VHL* point mutations were tested for co-immunoprecipitation, a number of the mutants appeared to assemble poorly, if at all, with the 16- and 9-kDa proteins.[100] Notable among those which failed to associate with p16 and p9 were proteins with the arginine-to-glutamine or arginine-to-tryptophan mutations at amino acid 167. These correspond to a VHL type II germ-line mutation "hot spot."[77,101] The Trp-117 mutant had diminished but detectable association with the p16 and p9 proteins. However, the Tyr-98 mutants, from a VHL type II kindred, formed complexes that were identical to the wild type. The loss of binding to specific proteins by naturally occurring inactivating mutants suggests functional importance of these complexes and indicates that mutations in different domains of the VHL protein may have a role in determining organ-specific tumorigenesis.[77,101]

VHL Is a Part of a Multiprotein Complex

The finding that the heterotrimer consisting of VHL and the two proteins of 9 and 16 kDa did not form when the VHL protein contained certain naturally occurring missense mutations led to studies to identify these proteins. When the p9 band was sequenced,[102] it was found to match to a sequence in elongin C, a 112-amino-acid protein that had been found to be a subunit of the heterotrimeric transcription elongation factor elongin (SIII).[103] When p16 underwent sequence analysis, a peptide from p16 showed identity to a sequence in elongin B.[102,104] Elongin (SIII) is a heterotrimeric complex consisting of two regulatory subunits (B and C) and a transcriptionally active subunit (A) (Fig. 41-22). The elongin (SIII) complex has been shown to activate transcriptional elongation by mammalian RNA polymerase II by suppressing the transient pausing of the polymerase at sites within the transcription units.[105] The VHL protein, which does not bind with the transcriptionally active subunit of the elongin (SIII) complex, elongin A, tightly and specifically binds to elongin B and C and can prevent their assembly to the transcriptionally active subunit of the elongin (SIII) complex, elongin A.[102] The finding that the cellular transcription factor, elongin (SIII), is a functional target of the VHL protein and that point-mutant derivatives corresponding to naturally occurring *VHL* missense mutations inhibit this interaction initially suggested that the tumor-suppression function

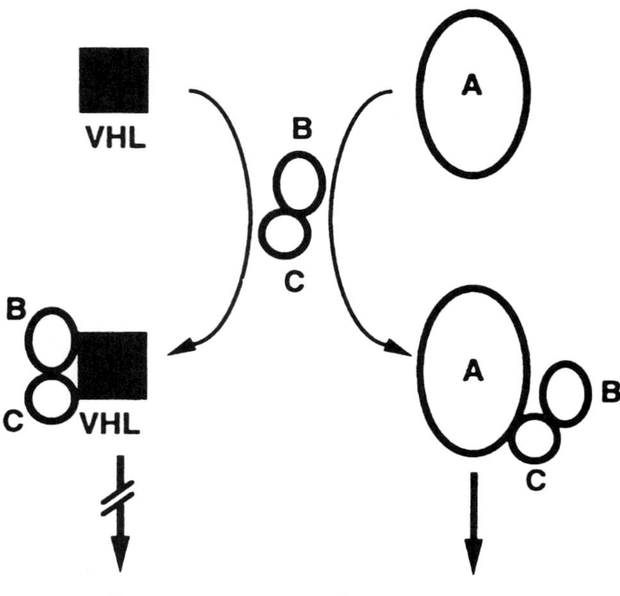

Fig. 41-22 A model for the interaction between elongin (SIII) and VHL. Elongin A forms a heterotrimeric complex with elongin B and C and activates transcription elongation by RNA pol II. VHL binds elongin B and C and inhibits the elongin ABC complex activation of transcriptional elongation. (*From Duan et al.*[102] *Used with permission.*)

of the VHL protein may be related to its ability to inhibit transcriptional elongation.[102,106]

A potential locus for VHL elongin B/C binding has been described by Kibel et al.[106] Aso et al.[107] detected significant sequence homology between residues 547 to 560 of elongin A and VHL residues 155 to 167.[107] Kibel et al.[106] determined that peptides in the VHL residues 157 to 172 fail to inhibit VHL-elongin B and C binding, whereas wild-type residues block the interaction.[107] This region is frequently mutated in sporadic clear cell renal carcinoma and in the germ line of VHL patients. It is the region of the amino acid 167 hot spot.[101]

Identification of Cul-2 as a Component of the VHL Complex

In addition to elongins B and C, labeled immunoprecipitates from cells expressing epitope- tagged VHL revealed a 70-kDa band that was purified for peptide microsequencing. The sequencing revealed a perfect match of the protein to one in the database that had recently been called Cul-2.[108] Cul-2 is one of a family of proteins called *cullins* that are all highly homologous to the *Saccharomyces cerevisiae* protein Cdc53p.[109] The human protein most similar in sequence (30 percent identical) was referred to as Cul-1. In *Caenorhabditid elegans,* Cul-1 mutants cause hyperplasia of certain tissues because of failure of these cells to apoptose. There are currently six human cullins available as sequences in the public database. Cul-2 is the one most closely related to Cul-1. Isolation of the full-length Cul-2 cDNA allowed in vitro assembly studies with VHL.[108] No interaction between VHL and Cul-2 could be detected in the absence of elongins B and C. Consistent with this, mutants of VHL that could not bind elongins B and C did not interact with Cul-2. Only Cul-2 and not Cul-1, Cul-3, or Cul-4 formed stable complexes with VBC. Although binding of Cul-2 to either elongin B or elongin B + C complexes has not been detected, Lonergan et al.[110] have detected complexes containing elongin C and Cul-2 in the absence of VHL. Mutagenesis of Cul-2 revealed a broad region (between amino acids 1 and 90) necessary and sufficient for binding to VBC complexes. This amino terminal region of Cul-2 showed the least homology with other cullins and presumably explains why only Cul-2 is able to interact with VBC complexes.

Recently, significant progress has been made in attempting to understand the structure and function of Cdc53p complexes in *S. cerevisiae.*[109,111] In that organism, these complexes function to target specific proteins for ubiquitin-mediated degradation. Cdc53p is a component of the SCF complex that functions as an E3 ubiquitin ligase that controls several different cell cycle transitions. The most studied transition regulated by this complex is the G1 $\rightarrow$ S transition. The SCF complex is composed of three subunits, Dkp1p, Cdc34p, and Cdc53p. Cdc53p serves as a protein bridge between Skp1p and Cdc34p having nonoverlapping binding sites for each protein. Cdc34p is the enzymatically active ubiquitin ligase subunit, whereas Dkp1p interacts with a variety of F-box proteins such as Cdc4p, Grr1p, and Met30p. While a biochemical function for the VHL complexes has not been directly identified, it is intriguing to extend the homology with the SCF complexes. Analysis of the sequence of elongin C revealed that it has significant homology to Skp1p. Elongin B is a ubiquitin homology domain protein. Elongin A is an F-box protein like *S. cerevisiae* Cdc34p, Grr1p, and Met30p. Despite the observations concerning the biochemistry, cell biology, and phenotypic characterization of the VHL-expressing renal cell carcinoma cells, the biochemical and biologic functions of the VHL protein remain to be determined. Its association with Cul-2 and elongin C, homologues of two components of the yeast SCF complex, suggests that the VHL complex may function by analogy via the targeting of specific proteins for ubiquitin-mediated degradation.

The VHL Protein and Regulation of Cell Cycle Arrest

Renal cell carcinoma cell lines (with inactivating *VHL* gene mutation) grown in cell culture fail to exit the cell cycle when serum is reduced or removed. In marked contrast, kidney cancer cells that express wild-type VHL respond to the removal of serum by withdrawing from the cell cycle.[112] Biochemical analysis of the serum-deprived renal cell carcinoma cells showed marked accumulation of the cyclin-dependent kinase inhibitor p27. The effect on p27 levels can be explained by stabilization of the p27 protein. Whether the rise in p27 levels in VHL-containing renal cell carcinoma cells is a cause or an effect of cell cycle arrest is not yet known.[112]

Posttranscriptional Regulation of Vascular Endothelial Growth Factor mRNA by the *VHL* Product

Sporadic clear cell renal carcinomas are characterized by a high degree of neoangiogenesis. Angiogenesis is also a striking feature in the clinical manifestations of VHL. VHL renal tumors, spinal and cerebellar hemangioblastomas, retinal angiomas, islet cell tumors, and epididymal cystadenomas are markedly hypervascular. A number of polypeptide growth factors have been implicated in the migration, proliferation, and differentiation of vascular endothelial cells, including vascular endothelial growth factor (VEGF). VEGF, which is normally expressed in the brain, kidney, and other tissues, is markedly elevated in renal carcinomas as well as in sporadic and VHL-associated CNS hemangioblastomas.[113–118] When the effect of VHL on VEGF was evaluated, introduction of the wild-type *VHL* gene into renal carcinoma cells with VHL mutations resulted in decreased VEGF mRNA expression.[113,119] Renal cell carcinoma cell lines express high levels of VEGF mRNA and protein. In normal cells, VEGF expression is regulated by multiple factors, including hypoxia, which is an inducer of VEGF mRNA levels. Renal cell carcinoma cell lines show constitutively high levels of VEGF mRNA in both normoxic and hypoxic cells. Introduction of a wild-type, but not a mutant, *VHL* gene into these renal cell carcinoma cells reconstitutes the hypoxia-regulated expression of VEGF mRNA and inhibits VEGF expression under normoxic conditions. An analogous effect is seen in these cells in response to serum deprivation. Only in cells expressing wild-type VHL is VEGF expression suppressed in 10% serum and induced with serum deprivation. Surprisingly, VHL over-expression affected neither VEGF transcription initiation nor elongation, suggesting that VHL regulates VEGF at a post-transcriptional level. Determination of the mechanism of VHL-mediated regulation of VEGF and related genes should lead to significant advances in understanding of the mechanism of tumorigenesis in VHL and sporadic renal cell carcinoma. Interestingly, wild-type VHL repressed the normoxic expression of other hypoxia-induced genes such as the glucose transporter GLUT1 and the platelet-derived growth factor β chain (PDGF-β).[119]

Carbonic Anhydrases and VHL

Recently, Ivanov et al.[120] reported that carbonic anhydrases 9 and 12 are down-regulated by the *VHL* gene.[120] The authors used RNA differential display to compare genes expressed in a VHL-null renal carcinoma cell line or the same cell line expressing wild-type VHL. Increased expression of CA9 and CA12 was found in two VHL-null renal carcinoma cell lines. CA9 and CA12 are single-pass cell membrane-spanning proteins that catalyze the reversal hydration of CO_2. Of particular interest, CA9 is identical to the MN antigen and is the target of the G250 antibody.[121,122] The MN antigen is reported to be characteristic of clear cell renal carcinomas; one antigen that is characteristic of clear cell renal carcinomas is a protein under the control of the *VHL* gene.

DETERMINANTS OF NUCLEAR/CYTOPLASMIC LOCALIZATION OF THE *VHL* GENE PRODUCT

Critical to understanding the function of the *VHL* gene is determination of its location in the cell and the factors that regulate its transport. The VHL protein was shown by Duan et al.[100] to be present in both the nucleus and the cytoplasm. In order to define the determinants of VHL localization, Lee et al.[123] showed that there is a tightly regulated cell density-dependent transport of VHL into and/or out of the nucleus.[123] When cells expressing an epitope-tagged (FLAG) VHL protein were plated in sparse conditions, most of the protein was detected in the nucleus. In densely grown cells, the VHL protein is found in the cytoplasm. Immunofluorescence studies of mutant VHL protein revealed that the C-terminal region of the VHL protein is required for localization to, or retention in, the cytosol. When a frameshift mutant that removes all of exon 3 was examined, VHL was present only in the nucleus in most of the cells grown in both sparse as well as confluent conditions. In contrast, when the entire exon 1 was deleted, the protein remained predominantly in the cytosol under both sparse and confluent conditions[123] (Fig. 41-23). The factors associated with sparse and confluent conditions that determine localization of the VHL protein have not yet been determined. Understanding these factors as well as the genetic determinants of VHL localization should provide significant insights into the function of the *VHL* gene and how inactivation of this gene results in the manifestations that appear in VHL and in sporadic clear cell renal carcinoma.

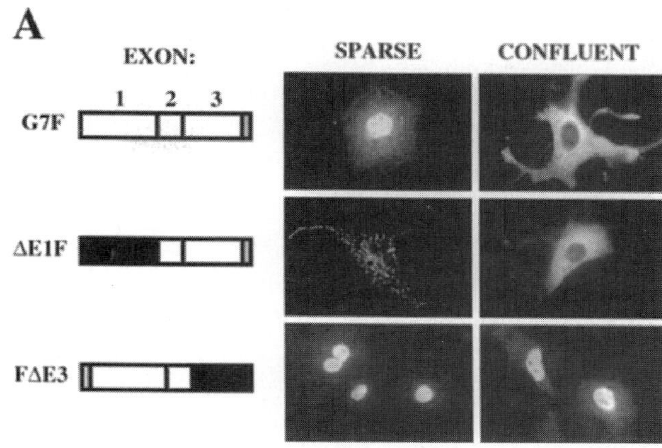

Fig. 41-23 Localization of the *VHL* gene. The wild-type VHL protein is found predominantly in the cytoplasm when transiently transfected COS-7 cells are grown under confluent conditions and in the nucleus under sparse conditions (top panel). When an exon 1 deletion mutant is analyzed, immunofluorescence localizes the protein to the cytoplasm in both sparse and confluent cells. When an exon 3 deletion mutant is introduced into the COS-7 cells, there is striking localization predominantly to the nucleus in both the sparse and confluent conditions. (*From Lee et al.*[123] *Used with permission.*)

Constitutional Translocation of Chromosome 3p and Clear Cell Renal Carcinoma

Several families have been described with an inherited predisposition to develop clear cell renal carcinoma associated with a constitutional balanced translocations involving chromosome 3p and either chromosomes 2, 6, or 8.[13,19,124] Studies of the renal tumors from these families have provided insight into mechanisms of formation of clear cell renal carcinomas. Clear cell renal carcinomas from members of the t(3;8) family and from members of the t(3;2) family showed a loss of the derivative chromosome (the chromosome to which the distal portion of chromosome 3p had been translocated).[124,125] Clear cell renal carcinomas from members of these families also showed somatic mutation of the remaining *VHL* gene in 2 of 4 tumors studied in the t(3,8) family and in 4 of 5 tumors studied in the t(3;2) family.[93,124] The *VHL* mutation found in each renal tumor was different.

These results suggest that clear cell renal carcinomas develop in members of chromosome t(3;8) and t(3;2) translocation families by a series of steps: (1) inheritance of the balanced chromosome 3p translocation, (2) loss of the derivative chromosome bearing the distal portion of chromosome 3p (a somatic event leading to the

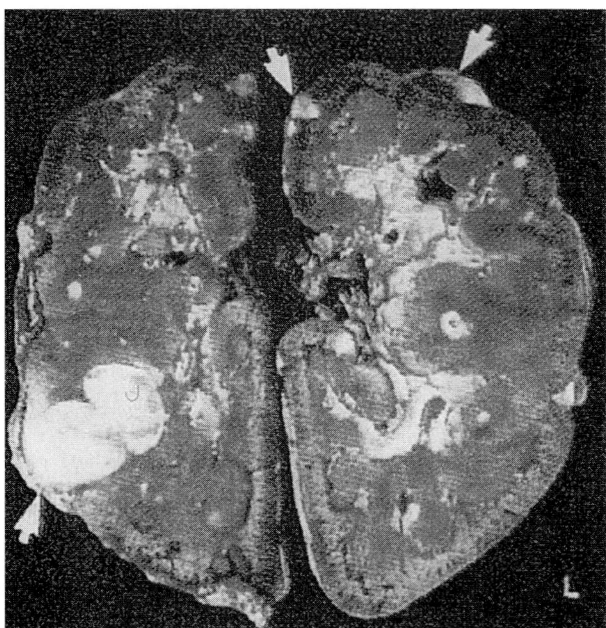

A

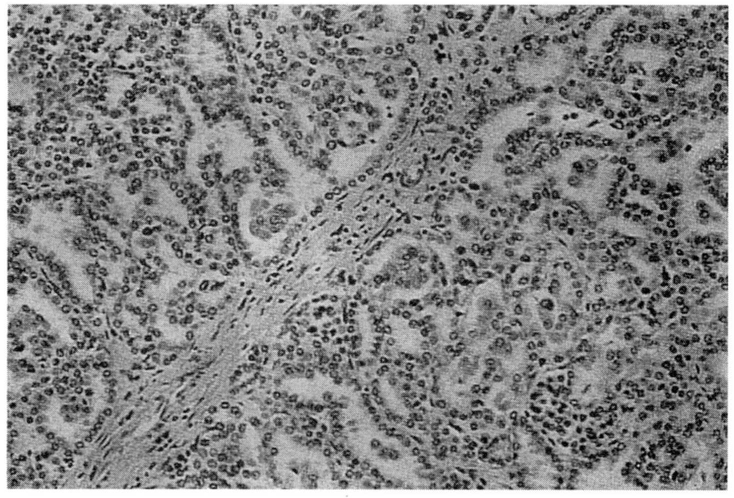

B

Fig. 41-24 ***A.*** **Photograph of renal tumor from patient IV-8 (family 160) with HPRC, a 35-year-old woman treated by bilateral nephrectomy. Arrows point to renal tumors.** ***B.*** **Photomicrograph of renal tumor from patient IV-8. Note papillary histology. (*From Schmidt et al.*[145] *Used with permission.*)**

loss of one copy of the *VHL* gene), and (3) somatic mutation of the *VHL* gene located on the normal chromosome 3. These three events occur within a single renal epithelial cell and initiate malignant transformation. The process of formation of clear cell renal carcinomas in individuals with the chromosome t(3;8) and t(3:2) translocations appears to be a variation of the events leading to sporadic clear cell renal carcinomas.[88] The initiating event in both situations appears to be a loss or inactivation of both copies of the *VHL* gene.

PAPILLARY RENAL CARCINOMA

Five to 10 percent of sporadic renal carcinoma is the papillary histologic type.[3,11,73] Papillary renal carcinoma is significantly less hypervascular and tends to be of lower grade than clear cell renal carcinoma. The clinical course of papillary renal carcinoma may be more indolent than that of clear cell renal carcinoma.[126,127] Sporadic papillary renal carcinoma frequently appears as bilateral, multifocal disease; multiple tumor nodules and areas of atypical hyperplastic growth may appear throughout the kidney.[128,129] Whether the presence of multifocal, bilateral papillary renal carcinoma is due primarily to genetic events, is secondary to an agent such as a renotrophic virus, or is the result of exposure to environmental factors is not known.

Most common among the cytogenetic changes that have been described in tumor tissue from patients with papillary renal carcinoma are those involving trisomy of chromosomes 7, 10, and 17.[33,128,130] More recently, a consistent t(X;1)(p11.2;q21) translocation in papillary renal cell carcinoma has been described as a feature of at least some papillary renal carcinomas.[131–133] Whether or not the t(X;1) translocation represents a distinct subtype of papillary renal cell carcinoma is currently under study.

HEREDITARY PAPILLARY RENAL CELL CARCINOMA (HPRC)

Multigenerational kindreds in which members develop papillary renal cell carcinoma have been described by Zbar et al.[16,17,134] (Fig. 41-24). Affected family members develop multiple tumors of varying size in both kidneys (Fig. 41-25). In this disorder, which has an autosomal dominant inheritance pattern, the renal tumors are the uniformly papillary histologic type.[16]

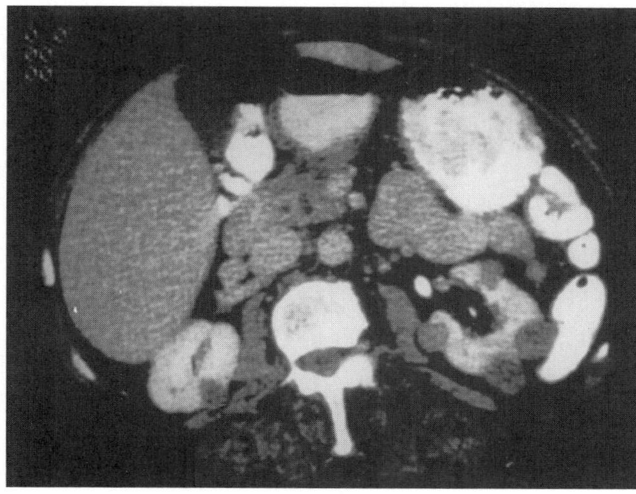

A

B

Fig. 41-25 A CT scan (*A*) and gross anatomy (*B*) of a kidney from an affected individual in an HPRC kindred showing multifocal papillary renal carcinomas. (*From Zbar et al.*[16] *Used with permission.*)

Germ-Line and Somatic Mutations in the Tyrosine Kinase Domain of the *MET* Proto-Oncogene in Papillary Renal Carcinomas

Malignant papillary renal carcinomas are characterized by trisomy of chromosomes 7, 16, and 17 and, in men, by loss of the Y chromosome. The HPRC was localized to chromosome 7q31.1-34 in a 24-cM interval between *D7S496* and *D7S1837*. Among the genes located in the nonrecombinant interval was the *MET* proto-oncogene. Emphasis was placed on the *MET* proto-oncogene because cytogenetic and FISH studies showed chromosome 7 duplication rather than loss, suggesting that the gene responsible for HPRC was a proto-oncogene rather than a tumor-suppressor gene. Also, the *MET* gene was in the same supergene family (receptor tyrosine kinase) as *RET*, a proto-oncogene mutated in another inherited cancer syndrome (MEN2).

Genome Structure of the *MET* Proto-Oncogene

Although the *MET* proto-oncogene was discovered in 1984, its genomic structure had not been determined. As a first step toward mutation analysis, the genomic structure of the *MET* gene was determined.[135] The *MET* gene was found to contain 21 exons. These exons encoded a receptor tyrosine kinase that contains extracellular, transmembrane, juxta membrane and tyrosine kinase domains. Primers were designed for the polymerase chain reaction to test for mutations in *MET* in affected members of HPRC families. Germ-line missense mutations located in the tyrosine kinase domain of the *MET* proto-oncogene were detected in the germ line of affected members of HPRC families and in a subset of sporadic papillary renal carcinomas.

Two large North American families with HPRC were identified with identical mutations in the *MET* proto-oncogene.[136] Affected members of the two families shared the same haplotype within and immediately distal to the *MET* gene, suggesting a founder effect. That is, both families had a common ancestor. The age-dependent penetrance of the *H1112R* mutation was determined (Fig 41-26). The *H1112R* mutation produced a late-onset malignancy of low penetrance. The estimated risk at 40 years of age among carriers was 19 percent (95 percent confidence interval, 5–34 percent).

Duplication of the Chromosome Carrying the Mutant *MET* Allele in HPRC Tumors

Although trisomy of chromosome 7 has been demonstrated in HPRC renal tumors, it was not known whether the process of chromosome duplication in HPRC tumors was random or nonrandom. Sixteen renal tumors from two patients with the *MET H1112R* mutation were studied by FISH and by quantitative PCR to identify which chromosome 7 was duplicated in the tumors.[137] FISH showed trisomy 7 in all renal tumors. In all 16 tumors, there was an increased signal intensity of the microsatellite allele from the chromosome bearing the mutant *MET* allele compared with the chromosome bearing the wild-type *MET*.[137] Similar work was performed independently by the Kovacs laboratory with identical results.[138] The study demonstrates nonrandom duplication of the chromosome bearing the mutated *MET* in hereditary papillary renal carcinomas.

Mutations in the *MET* Proto-Oncogene Produce a Gain of Function

The MET receptor tyrosine kinase transduces motility, proliferation, and morphogenic signals of hepatocyte growth factor/scatter factor in epithelial cells.[139–141] During embryogenesis, the MET receptor HGF/SF pathway is required for normal muscle and liver development. The effect of each MET mutation was examined in biological and biochemical assays.[142]

MET mutants exhibited increased levels of tyrosine phosphorylation and enhanced kinase activity toward an exogenous substrate when compared with wild-type MET. NIH 3T3 cells expressing mutant MET molecules formed foci in vitro and were tumorigenic in nude mice versus wild-type MET. A strong correlation was observed between the enzymatic and biological activity of the MET mutants, indicating that the tumorigenesis is quantitatively related to its level of activation.

Similarities Between Mutations in *MET, RET*, c-*KIT*, and c-*erbB* Proto-Oncogene

There are striking homologies in the location of the mutations observed in the *MET, RET*, c-*KIT*, and c-*erbB* proto-oncogenes.[136,143] c-*KIT* is a receptor tyrosine kinase that is expressed on stem cells in the bone marrow. Activating c-*KIT* mutations have been detected in mastocytosis and can be associated with malignant hematologic disorders.[144] RET, also a receptor tyrosine kinase expressed in thyroid cells, is the receptor for glial-derived growth factor. Germ-line mutations in *RET* are found in the hereditary cancer syndrome MEN2. The c-*erbB* proto-oncogene is an avian proto-oncogene.[145]

All four transmembrane tyrosine kinase receptors have mutations in the tyrosine kinase domains. In four instances, the mutations in *MET* were located in codons homologous to mutation in *RET*, c-*KIT*, or c-*erbB*. The results indicate that there are hot spots for mutation within the tyrosine kinase domain that are common to several receptor tyrosine kinases[145] (Fig. 41-27).

FAMILIAL RENAL ONCOCYTOMAS

At the National Cancer Institute five families were seen in which individuals were affected with bilateral, multiple renal oncocytomas.[146] One identical twin pair was affected with bilateral multiple

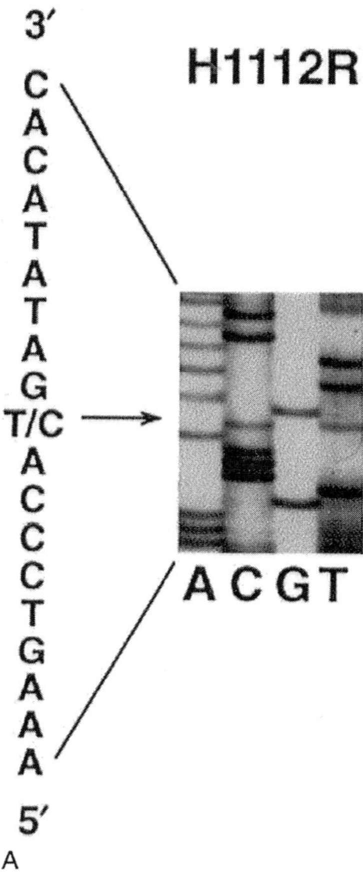

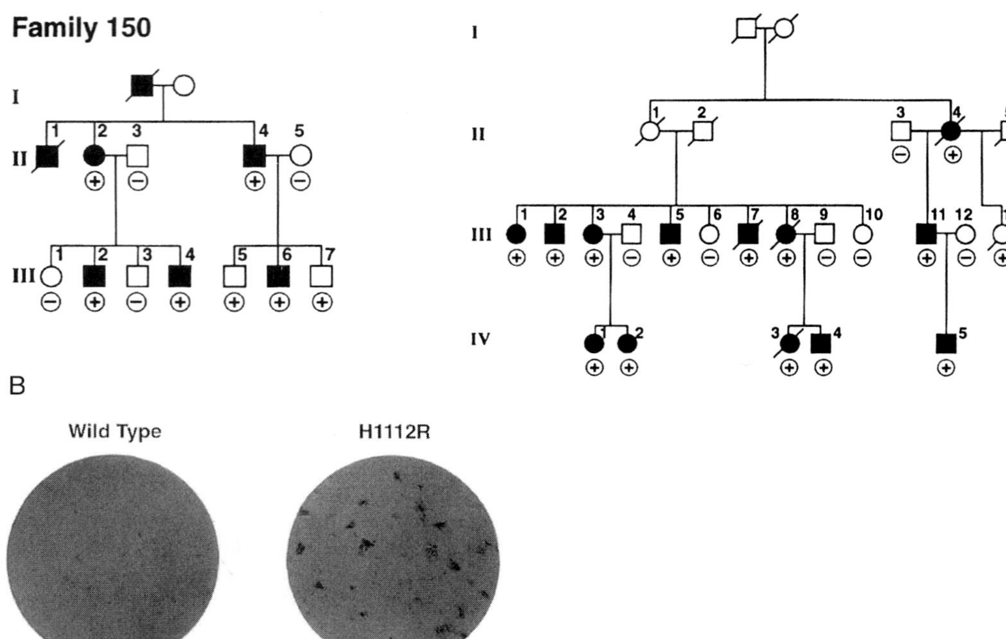

Fig. 41-26 The *H1112R MET* germ-line HPRC mutation identification. ***A.*** The DNA sequence of the region demonstrating the mutation. ***B.*** Segregation of the germ-line mutation with the phenotype (***B***) in pedigrees of two HPRC families, 150 and 160. Individuals predicted not to be carriers of the HPRC gene, −; individuals predicted to be carriers of the HPRC gene, +. The solid symbols represent those found to be affected. ***C.*** The NIH3T3 growth focus induced by wild-type and mutant *MET*. (*From Schmidt et al.*[145] *Used with permission.*)

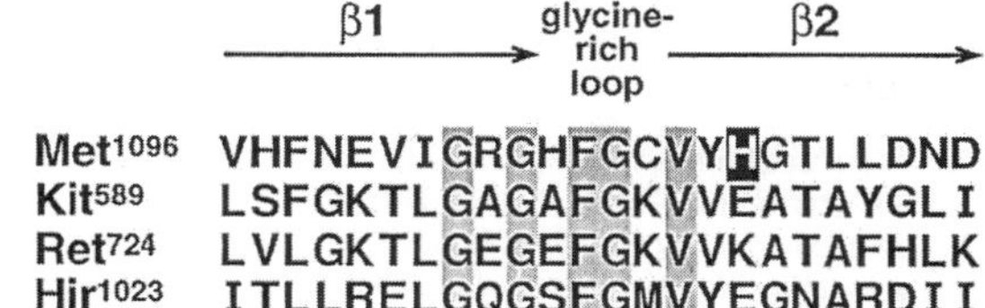

Fig. 41-27 The amino acid sequence of the homologous regions of *HIR, RET,* and *KIT* shown in comparison with *MET* in the region of the *H1112R* mutation. The site of the *H1112R* mutation is outlined in black. The codons conserved in the four proteins are outlined in gray (*From Schmidt et al.*[145] *Used with permission.*)

renal oncocytomas. Because renal oncocytomas were in most cases asymptomatic, occurred at a late age, and required imaging studies for detection, it was initially difficult to detect the hereditary pattern of this disorder. Further studies are in progress to identify the genetic factor that predisposes individuals to the development of renal oncocytomas.

GENETICS OF HEREDITARY RENAL CARCINOMA

There are three forms of hereditary renal carcinoma: VHL, HCRC, and HPRC. VHL is characterized by mutation of the *VHL* gene. Currently, *VHL* gene mutation can be detected in 75 to 99 percent of VHL families. As advanced mutation-detection methods are used (FISH-based deletion analysis, analysis of the 3′UTR, promoter, etc.), the mutation-detection percentage increases. VHL has been categorized as type I and type II, with type II families being characterized by the presence of pheochromocytoma. Nearly all the type II families carry a missense mutation, and there is a VHL type II hot spot in exon 3 of the *VHL* gene. Further studies in progress will determine if there are genotype/phenotype correlations with other VHL-associated tumors, such as CNS hemangioblastoma, pancreatic tumors, and ELST.

The role of genetic and clinical screening programs in the management of individuals at risk for a multisystem hereditary cancer syndrome such as VHL is complex. Unlike some syndromes where testing is not performed routinely in at-risk individuals under the age of 18 because medical intervention is not required, in individuals at risk for VHL germ-line mutations, testing is recommended by most clinicians at an early age. Early intervention may be of significant benefit to affected VHL patients, particularly those with retinal, adrenal, and CNS lesions. Retinal angiomas, which can occur in very young children, are bilateral and multifocal and can cause early loss of vision that eventually may lead to blindness. Treatment with laser therapy is performed with the goal of preservation of vision and with the intent of decreasing the morbidity of VHL-associated retinal angiomas. Pheochromocytoma and CNS hemangioblastomas can appear before the age of 10. Occult pheochromocytoma can be lethal, and early detection of functioning pheochromocytomas is critical. While the benefit of detection of an occult functioning pheochromocytoma is clear, the benefit of detection and treatment of occult, nonfunctioning pheochromocytomas is not yet determined. In some patients, occult CNS hemangioblastomas also can have significant morbidity, including stroke, paralysis, and death. However, longitudinal studies will be needed to determine whether aggressive screening for CNS lesions as well as other manifestations of VHL will enhance quality of life or increase survival.

The role of early diagnosis of VHL-associated renal, pancreatic, and endolymphatic sac tumors is less well defined. Greater understanding of the natural history of these VHL manifestations will be required for determining the most appropriate management of patients with these malignancies. At present, there is no consensus for which patients with VHL-associated renal carcinomas are best treated with surgical resection. Renal cell carcinoma can spread in asymptomatic individuals, and advanced renal carcinoma has been reported as the direct cause of death in one-third of VHL patients.[15,147] As such, physicians managing these patients often recommend removal of the tumors when they have reached a certain size, such as 2.5 to 3 cm. The clinical rationale is that removal of tumors of this size may reduce the incidence of metastasis while preserving quality of life. VHL-associated pancreatic islet cell tumors are malignant lesions that can become metastatic. Surgical resection is often recommended with the intent to prevent metastasis, but prospective trials will be required to define the role of surgery in the management of these tumors. The endolymphatic sac tumors represent a similar clinical challenge. These tumors can have profound manifestations in VHL patients. Patients with ELST may lose total hearing in an ear within a matter of 3 to 4 days. Trials are in progress to determine whether or not early surgical intervention will preserve hearing in VHL patients with ELST.

When tumors that had formed in other organs affected by VHL (such as sporadic cerebellar hemangioblastoma and epididymal cystadenoma) were analyzed, mutations were found. Further studies of these tumors as well as in other sporadic tumors from organs affected in VHL (such as pancreatic tumors, ELST, retinal angiomas, and pheochromocytoma) will be required to determine the role of *VHL* gene inactivation in these neoplasms.

Papillary Renal Carcinoma. Much remains to be learned about the genetics and the subtypes of papillary renal carcinoma. Little is known about the factors associated with the development of multifocal, bilateral sporadic papillary renal carcinoma. The genetic or environmental features that characterize individuals with bilateral, multifocal papillary renal carcinoma with no apparent hereditary feature (no parents, siblings, or offspring involved) remain to be determined.

A number of kindreds have been evaluated in which multiple members (two to six) have clear cell renal carcinoma. Whether or not these findings are coincidental, the result of an undetermined combination of genetic and environmental factors or an example of complex genetics is not yet known.

VHL gene mutation analysis is now an integral aspect in the diagnosis of VHL and of screening of at-risk asymptomatic individuals. Predictions about which types of tumors will appear are possible in some instances, particularly in VHL type II kindreds. Germ-line *VHL* gene mutation analysis is likely to be useful in kindreds with "familial pheochromocytoma" or those with clinical manifestations of MEN2 in whom the diagnosis is in doubt. *VHL* gene mutation analysis may be useful for assisting in the diagnosis of an indeterminate renal mass or in an extra-renal mass in a patient with clear cell kidney cancer.

Patients who present with advanced renal carcinoma have an 8 to 15 percent 2-year survival. Those who are diagnosed with stage I renal carcinoma have a 95 percent 5-year survival. It is possible that detection of an inactivated *VHL* gene will aid in the early diagnosis of clear cell renal carcinoma. Cancer cells, including renal carcinoma cells, may circulate years in advance of the clinical detection of metastasis.[148–151] It is possible that detection of a mutated *VHL* gene in the urine or in circulating cells may provide a method for early diagnosis of this disease.

Ultimately, it is hoped that knowledge of the mechanism of the *VHL* gene and other genes involved in renal carcinoma will lead to the development of targeted methods for early diagnosis, prevention, and treatment of diseases such as sporadic and hereditary renal carcinoma.

ACKNOWLEDGMENTS

We greatly acknowledge the work of our many collaborators and colleagues whose studies are discussed here.

REFERENCES

1. Boring CC, Squires TS, Tong T: Cancer statistics. *CA Cancer J Clin* **44**:7, 1994.
2. Linehan WM, Shipley W, Parkinson D: Cancer of the kidney and ureter, in DeVita VT, Hellman S, Rosenberg SA (eds): *Cancer: Principles and Practice of Oncology*, Philadelphia, Lippincott, 1996, pp 19-46.
3. Linehan WM, Lerman MI, Zbar B: Identification of the VHL gene: Its role in renal carcinoma. *JAMA* **273**:564, 1995.
4. Malker HR, Malker BK, McLaughlin JK, Blot WJ: Kidney cancer among leather workers. *Lancet* **1**:56, 1984.
5. Maclure M: Asbestos and renal adenocarcinoma: A case-control study. *Environ Res* **42**:353, 1987.
6. Maclure M, Willett W: A case-control study of diet and risk of renal adenocarcinoma. *Epidemiology* **1**:430, 1990.
7. Yu MC, Mack TM, Hanisch R, Cicioni C, Henderson BE: Cigarette smoking, obesity, diuretic use, and coffee consumption as risk factors for renal cell carcinoma. *J Natl Cancer Inst* **77**:351, 1986.
8. Chung-Park M, Parveen T, Lam M: Acquired cystic disease of the kidneys and renal cell carcinoma in chronic renal insufficiency without dialysis treatment. *Nephron* **53**:157, 1989.
9. Matson MA, Cohen EP: Acquired cystic kidney disease: Occurrence, prevalence, and renal cancers. *Medicine* **69**:217, 1990.
10. Brennan JF, Stilmant MM, Babayan RK, Siroky MB: Acquired renal cystic disease: implications for the urologist. *Br J Urol* **67**:342, 1991.
11. Kovacs G, Ishikawa I: High incidence of papillary renal cell tumours in patients on chronic haemodialysis. *Histopathology* **22**:135, 1993.
12. Bard RH, Lord B, Fromowitz F: Papillary adenocarcinoma of kidney. *Urology* **19**:16, 1982.
13. Cohen AJ, Li FP, Berg S, Marchetto DJ, Tsai S, Jacobs SC, Brown RS: Hereditary renal-cell carcinoma associated with a chromosomal translocation. *New Engl J Med* **301**:592, 1979.
14. Li FP, Decker H-JH, Zbar B, Stanton VP, Kovacs G, Seizinger BR, Aburantani H, Sandberg AA, Berg S, Hosoe S, Brown RS: Clinical and genetic studies of renal cell carcinomas in a family with a constitutional chromosome 3;8 translocation:genetics of familial renal carcinoma. *Ann Intern Med* **118**:106, 1993.
15. Glenn GM, Choyke PL, Zbar B, Linehan WM: Von Hippel-Lindau disease: Clinical review and molecular genetics, in Anderson EE (ed): *Problems in Urologic Surgery: Benign and Malignant Tumors of the Kidney*. Philadelphia, Lippincott, 1990, pp 312-330.
16. Zbar B, Tory K, Merino M, Schmidt L, Glenn G, Choyke P, Walther MM, Lerman M, Linehan WM: Hereditary papillary renal cell carcinoma. *J Urol* **151**:561, 1994.
17. Zbar B, Glenn G, Lubensky IA, Choyke P, Magnusson G, Bergerheim U, Pettersson S, Amin M, Hurley K, Linehan WM, Walther MM: Hereditary papillary renal cell carcinoma: Clinical studies in 10 families. *J Urol* **153**:907, 1995.
18. Pathak S, Strong LC, Ferrell RE, Trindade A: Familial renal cell carcinoma with a 3:11 chromosome translocation limited to tumor cells. *Science* **217**:939, 1982.
19. Kovacs G, Brusa P, de Riese W: Tissue-specific expression of a constitutional 3;6 translocation: Development of multiple bilateral renal-cell carcinomas. *Int J Cancer* **43**:422, 1989.
20. Zbar B, Brauch H, Talmadge C, Linehan WM: Loss of alleles of loci on the short arm of chromosome 3 in renal cell carcinoma. *Nature* **327**:721, 1987.
21. Anglard P, Brauch TH, Weiss GH, Latif F, Merino MJ, Lerman MI, Zbar B, Linehan WM: Molecular analysis of genetic changes in the origin and development of renal cell carcinoma. *Cancer Res* **51**:1071, 1991.
22. Szucs S, Muller-Brechlin R, DeRiese W, Kovacs G: Deletion 3p: The only chromosome loss in a primary renal cell carcinoma. *Cancer Genet Cytogenet* **26**:369, 1987.
23. Kovacs G, Erlandsson R, Boldog F, Ingvarsson S, Muller-Brechlin R, Klein G, Sumegi J: Consistent chromosome 3p deletion and loss of heterozygosity in renal cell carcinoma. *Proc Natl Acad Sci USA* **85**:1571, 1988.
24. Linehan WM, Miller E, Anglard P, Merino M, Zbar B: Improved detection of allele loss in renal cell carcinomas after removal of leukocytes by immunologic selection. *J Natl Cancer Inst* **81**:287, 1989.
25. Boldog F, Arheden K, Imreh S, Strombeck B, Szekely L, Erlandsson R, Marcsek Z, Sumegi J, Mitelman F, Klein G: Involvement of 3p deletions in sporadic and hereditary forms of renal cell carcinoma. *Genes Chromosom Cancer* **3**:403, 1991.
26. Morita R, Ishikawa J, Tsutsumi M, Hikiji K, Tsukada Y, Kamidono S, Maeda S, Nakamura Y: Allelotype of renal cell carcinoma. *Cancer Res* **51**:820, 1991.
27. Ogawa O, Kakehi Y, Ogawa K, Koshiba M, Sugiyama T, Yoshida O: Allelic loss at chromosome 3p characterizes clear cell phenotype of renal cell carcinoma. *Cancer Res* **51**:949, 1991.
28. Presti JC, Rao PH, Chen Q, Reuter VE, Li FP, Fair WR, Jhanwar SC: Histopathological, cytogenetic, and molecular characterization of renal cortical tumors. *Cancer Res* **51**:1544, 1991.
29. Yoshida HA, Ohyashiki K, Ochi H, Gibas Z, Pontes JE, Prout GR, Huben R, Sandberg AA: Cytogenetic studies of tumor tissue from patients with nonfamilial renal cell carcinoma. *Cancer Res* **46**:2139, 1986.
30. Carroll PR, Murty VVS, Reuter V, Jhanwar S, Fair WR, Whitemore WF, Chaganti RSK: Abnormalities of chromosome region 3p12-14 characterize clear cell renal carcinoma. *Cancer Genet Cytogenet* **26**:253, 1987.
31. Kovacs G, Wilkens L, Papp T, de Riese W: Differentiation between papillary and nonpapillary renal cell carcinomas by DNA analysis. *J Natl Cancer Inst* **81**:527, 1989.
32. Kovacs G: Papillary renal cell carcinoma: A morphologic and cytogenetic study of 11 cases. *Am J Pathol* **134**:27, 1989.
33. Kovacs G, Fuzesi L, Emanual A, Kung HF: Cytogenetics of papillary renal cell tumors. *Genes Chromosom Cancer* **3**:249, 1991.
34. Anglard P, Trahan E, Liu S, Latif F, Merino M, Lerman M, Zbar B, Linehan WM: Molecular and cellular characterization of human renal cell carcinoma cell lines. *Cancer Res* **52**:348, 1992.
35. Choyke PL, Glenn GM, Walther MM, Patronas NJ, Linehan WM, Zbar BZ: Von Hippel Lindau disease: Genetic, clinical and imaging features. *Radiology* **194**:629, 1995.
36. Collins ET: Two cases, brother and sister, with peculiar vascular new growth, probably primarily retinal, affecting both eyes. *Trans Ophthalmol Soc UK* **14**:141, 1894.
37. von Hippel E: Uber eine sehr seltene erkrankrung der netzhaut. *Klin Boebachtungen Arch Ophthalmol* **59**:83, 1904.
38. Lindau A: Studien uber kleinhirncysten bau:pathogenese und beziehungen zur angiomatous retinae. *Acta Pathol Microbiol Scand Suppl* **1**:1, 1926.
39. Melmon KL, Rosen SW: Lindau's disease: Review of the literature and study of a large kindred. *Am J Med* **36**:595, 1964.
40. Poston CD, Jaffe GS, Lubensky IA, Solomon D, Zbar B, Linehan WM, Walther MM: Characterization of the renal pathology of a familial form of renal cell carcinoma associated with von Hippel-Lindau disease: Clinical and molecular genetic implications. *J Urol* **153**:22, 1995.
41. Walther MM, Lubensky IA, Venzon D, Zbar B, Linehan WM: Prevalence of microscopic lesions in grossly normal renal parenchyma from patients with von Hippel-Lindau disease, sporadic renal cell carcinoma and no renal disease: Clinical implications. *J Urol* **154**:2010, 1995.
42. Choyke PL, Filling-Katz MR, Shawker TH, Gorin MB, Travis WD, Chang R, Seizinger BR, Dwyer AJ, Linehan WM: Von Hippel-Lindau disease: Radiologic screening for visceral manifestations. *Radiology* **174**:815, 1990.
43. Jamis-Dow CA, Choyke PL, Jennings SB, Linehan WM, Thakore KN, Walther MM: Small (< 3-cm) renal masses: Detection with CT versus US and pathologic correlation. *Radiology* **198**:785, 1996.
44. Pearson JC, Weiss J, Tanagho EA: A plea for conservation of kidney in renal adenocarcinoma associated with von Hippel-Lindau disease. *J Urol* **124**:910, 1980.
45. Palmer JM, Swanson DA: Conservative surgery in solitary and bilateral renal carcinoma: Indications and technical considerations. *J Urol* **120**:113, 1987.
46. Frydenberg M, Malek RS, Zincke H: Conservative renal surgery for renal cell carcinoma in von Hippel-Lindau's disease. *J Urol* **194**:461, 1993.
47. Walther MM, Choyke PL, Weiss G, Manolatos C, Long J, Reiter R, Alexander RB, Linehan WM: Parenchymal sparing surgery in patients with hereditary renal cell carcinoma. *J Urol* **153**:913, 1995.
48. Walther MM, Thompson N, Linehan WM: Enucleation procedures in patients with multiple hereditary renal tumors. *World J Urol* **13**:248, 1995.
49. Walther MM, Choyke PL, Hayes W, Shawker TH, Thakore K, Alexander RB, Linehan WM: Evaluation of color Doppler intraoperative ultrasound in parenchymal sparing renal surgery. *J Urol* **152**:1984, 1995.

50. Marshall FF, Holdford SS, Hamper UM: Intraoperative sonography of renal tumors. *J Urol* **148**:1393, 1992.
51. Choyke PL, Glenn G, Walther MM, Zbar B, Weiss GH, Alexander RB, Hayes WS, Long JP, Thakore KN, Linehan WM: The natural history of renal lesions in von Hippel-Lindau disease: A serial CT study in 28 patients. *AJR* **159**:1229, 1992.
52. Filling-Katz MR, Choyke PL, Oldfield E, Charnas L, Patronas NJ, Glenn GM, Gorin MB, Morgan JK, Linehan WM, Seizinger BR, Zbar B: Central nervous system involvement in von Hippel-Lindau disease. *Neurology* **41**:41, 1991.
53. Lee J, Dong S, Park WS, Yoo N, Kim S, Kim C, Jang J, Zbar B, Lubensky IA, Linehan WM, Vortmeyer AO, Zhuang Z: Loss of heterozygosity and somatic mutations of the VHL tumor suppressor gene in sporadic cerebellar hemangioblastomas. *Cancer Res* **58**:504, 1998.
54. Vortmeyer AO, Gnarra JR, Emmert-Buck MR, Katz D, Linehan WM, Oldfield EH, Zhuang Z: von Hippel-Lindau gene deletion detected in the stromal cell component of a cerebellar hemangioblastoma associated with von Hippel-Lindau disease. *Hum Pathol* **28**:540, 1997.
55. Robb L, Elefanty AG: The hemangioblast: An elusive cell captured in culture (in process citation). *Bioessays* **20**:611, 1998.
56. Choi K, Kennedy M, Kazarov A, Papadimitriou JC, Keller G: A common precursor for hematopoietic and endothelial cells. *Development* **125**:725, 1998.
57. Maurea S, Cuocolo A, Reynolds JC, Tumeh SS, Begley MG, Linehan WM, Norton JA, Walther MM, Keiser HR, Neumann RD: Iodine-313-metaiodobenzylguanidine scientigraphy in preoperative and post-operative evaluation of paragangliomas: Comparison with CT and MRI. *J Nucl Med* **34**:173, 1993.
58. Keiser HR, Doppman JL, Robertson CN, Linehan WM, Averbuch SD: Diagnosis, localization and management of pheochromocytoma, in Lack EE (ed): *Pathology of the Adrenal Gland*. New York, Churchill-Livingstone, 1990, pp 2372–255.
59. Bouck NP, Polverini PJ: Identification of a new inhibitor of neovascularization controlled by a tumor suppressor gene. *J Northwest Univ Cancer Ctr* **1**:4, 1990.
60. Perry RR, Keiser HJ, Norton JA, Wall RT, Robertson CN, Travis W, Pass HI, Walther MM, Linehan WM: Surgical management of pheochromocytoma with the use of metyrosine. *Ann Surg* **212**:621, 1990.
61. Green JS, Bowmer MI, Johnson GJ: Von Hippel-Lindau disease in a Newfoundland kindred. *Can Med Assoc J* **134**:133, 1986.
62. Seizinger BR: Von Hippel-Lindau disease: A model system for the isolation of tumor suppressor genes associated with the primary genetic mechanisms of cancer. *Adv Nephrol Necker Hosp* **23**:29, 1994.
63. Neumann HPH: Basic criteria for clinical diagnosis and genetic counselling in von Hippel-Lindau syndrome. *Vasa* **16**:220, 1987.
64. Karsdorp N, Elderson A, Wittebol-Post D: Von Hippel-Lindau diseae: New strategies in early detetion and treatment. *Am J Med* **97**:158, 1994.
65. Vortmeyer AO, Choo D, Pack SD, Oldfield E, Zhuang Z: von Hippel-Lindau disease gene alterations associated with endolymphatic sac tumor. *J Natl Cancer Inst* **89**:970, 1997.
66. Tory K, Brauch H, Linehan WM, Barba D, Oldfield E, Filling-Katz M, Seizinger B, Nakamura Y, White R, Marshall FF, Lerman MI, Zbar B: Specific genetic change in tumors associated with von Hippel-Lindau disease. *J Natl Cancer Inst* **81**:1097, 1989.
67. Lubensky IA, Gnarra JR, Bertheau P, Walther MM, Linehan WM, Zhuang Z: Allelic deletions of the VHL gene detected in multiple microscopic clear cell renal lesions in von Hippel-Lindau disease patients. *Am J Pathol* **149**:2089, 1996.
68. Seizinger BR, Rouleau GA, Ozelius LJ, Lane AH, Farmer GE, Lamiell JM, Haines J, Yuen JW, Collins D, Majoor-Krakauer D, et al: Von Hippel-Lindau disease maps to the region of chromosome 3 associated with renal cell carcinoma. *Nature* **332**:268, 1988.
69. Lerman MI, Latif F, Glenn GM, Daniel LN, Brauch H, Hosoe S, Hampsch K, Delisio J, Orcutt M-L, McBride OW, Grzeschik K-H, Takahashi T, Minna J, Anglard P, Linehan WM, Zbar B: Isolation and regional localization of a large collection (2000) of single copy DNA fragments on human chromosome 3 for mapping and cloning tumor suppressor genes. *Hum Genet* **86**:567, 1991.
70. Hosoe S, Brauch H, Latif F, Glenn G, Daniel L, Bale S, Choyke P, Gorin M, Oldfield E, Berman A, Goodman J, Orcutt ML, Hampsch K, Delisio J, Modi W, McBride W, Anglard P, Weiss G, Walther MM, Linehan WM, Lerman MI, Zbar B: Localization of the von Hippel-Lindau disease gene to a small region of chromosome 3. *Genomics* **8**:634, 1990.
71. Richards FM, Maher ER, Latif F, Phipps ME, Tory K, Lush M, Croseey PA, Oostra B, Gustavson KH, Green J, Turner G, Yates JRW, Linehan WM, Affara NA, Lerman M, Zbar B, Ferguson-Smith MA: Detailed genetic mapping of the von Hippel-Lindau disease tumour suppressor gene. *J Med Genet* **30**:104, 1993.
72. Glenn GM, Linehan WM, Hosoe S, Latif F, Yao M, Choyke P, Gorin MB, Chew E, Oldfield E, Manolatos C, Orcutt ML, Walther MM, Weiss GH, Tory K, Jensson O, Lerman MI, Zbar B: Screening for von Hippel-Lindau disease by DNA-polymorphism analysis. *JAMA* **267**:1226, 1992.
73. Gnarra JR, Tory K, Weng Y, Schmidt L, Wei MH, Li H, Latif F, Liu S, Chen F, Duh F-M, Lubensky IA, Duan R, Florence C, Pozzatti R, Walther MM, Bander NH, Grossman HB, Brauch H, Pomer S, Brooks JD, Issacs WB, Lerman MI, Zbar B, Linehan WM: Mutation of the *VHL* tumour suppressor gene in renal carcinoma. *Nature Genet* **7**:85, 1994.
74. Glenn GM, Daniel LN, Choyke P, Linehan WM, Oldfield E, Gorin M, Hosoe S, Latif F, Weiss G, Walther MM, Lerman MI, Zbar B: Von Hippel-Lindau disease:distinct phenotypes suggest more than one mutant allele at the *VHL* locus. *Hum Genet* **87**:207, 1991.
75. Latif F, Tory K, Gnarra J, Yao M, Duh F-M, Orcutt ML, Stackhouse T, Kuzmin I, Modi W, Geil L, Schmidt L, Zhou F, Li H, Wei MH, Glenn G, Richards FM, Crossey PA, Ferguson-Smith MA, Le Paslier D, Chumakov I, Cohen D, Chinault CA, Maher ER, Linehan WM, Zbar B, Lerman MI: Identification of the von Hippel-Lindau disease tumor suppressor gene. *Science* **260**:1317, 1993.
76. Stolle CA, Glenn G, Zbar B, Humphrey JS, Choyke P, Walther MM, Pack S, Hurley K, Ondrey C, Klausner RD, Linehan WM: Improved detection of germline mutations in the von Hippel-Lindau disease tumor suppressor gene. *Hum Mutat* **12**:417, 1998.
77. Chen F, Kishida T, Yao M, Hustad T, Glavac D, Dean M, Gnarra JR, Orcutt ML, Duh FM, Glenn G, Green J, Hsia YE, Lamiell J, Li H, Wei MH, Schmidt L, Tory K, Kuzmin I, Stackhouse T, Latif F, Linehan WM, Lerman M, Zbar B: Germline mutations in the von Hippel-Lindau disease tumor suppressor gene:correlation with phenotype. *Hum Mutat* **5**:66, 1995.
78. Brauch H, Kishida T, Glavac D, Chen F, Pausch F, Hofler H, Latif F, Lerman MI, Zbar B, Neumann HPH: Von Hippel-Lindau (VHL) disease with pheochromocytoma in the Black forest region of Germany: Evidence for a founder effect. *Hum Genet* **95**:551, 1995.
79. Tisherman SE, Tisherman BG, Tisherman SA, Dunmire S, Levey GS, Mulvihill JJ: Three-decade investigation of familial pheochromocytoma. *Arch Intern Med* **153**:2550, 1993.
80. Crossey PA, Eng C, Ginalska-Malinowska M, Lennard TW, Wheeler DC, Ponder BA, Maher ER: Molecular genetic diagnosis of von Hippel-Lindau disease in familial phaeochromocytoma. *J Med Genet* **32**:885, 1995.
81. Neumann HP, Eng C, Mulligan LM, Glavac D, Zauner I, Ponder BA, Crossey PA, Maher ER, Brauch H: Consequences of direct genetic testing for germline mutations in the clinical management of families with multiple endocrine neoplasia, type II (see comments). *JAMA* **274**:1149, 1995.
82. Kanno H, Shuin T, Kondo K, Ito S, Hosaka M, Torigoe S, Fujii S, Tanaka Y, Yamamoto I, Kim I, Yao M: Molecular genetic diagnosis of von Hippel-Lindau disease:analysis of five Japanese families. *Jpn J Cancer Res* **87**:423, 1996.
83. Shuin T, Kondo K, Kaneko S, Sakai N, Yao M, Hosaka M, Kanno H, Ito S, Yamamoto I: Results of mutation analyses of von Hippel-Lindau disease gene in Japanese patients: Comparison with results in United States and United Kingdom (in Japanese). *Hinyokika Kiyo* **41**:703, 1995.
84. Clinical Research Group for VHL in Japan: Germline mutations in the von Hippel-Lindau disease (*VHL*) gene in Japanese VHL. *Hum Mol Genet* **4**:2233, 1995.
85. Whaley JM, Naglich J, Gelbert L, Hsia YE, Lamiell JM, Green JS, Collins D, Neumann PH, Laidlaw J, Li FP, Klein-Szanto AJP, Seizinger BR, Kley N: Germ-line mutations in the von Hipel-Lindau tumor-suppressor gene are similar to von Hippel-Lindau aberrations in sporadic renal cell carcinoma. *Am J Hum Genet* **55**:1092, 1994.
86. Gross DJ, Avishai N, Meiner V, Filon D, Zbar B, Abeliovich D: Familial pheochromocytoma associated with a novel mutation in the von Hippel-Lindau gene. *J Clin Endocrinol Metab* **81**:147, 1996.
87. Webster AR, Richards FM, MacRonald FE, Moore AT, Maher ER: An analysis of phenotypic variation in the familial cancer syndrome von Hippel-Lindau disease: Evidence for modifier effects. *Am J Hum Genet* **63**:1025, 1998.

88. Knudson AG: VHL gene mutation and clear-cell renal carcinomas. *Cancer J* **1**:180, 1995.
89. Shuin T, Kondo K, Torigoe S, Kishida T, Kubota Y, Hosaka M, Nagashima Y, Kitamura H, Latif F, Zbar B, Lerman MI, Yao M: Frequent somatic mutations and loss of heterozygosity of the von Hippel-Lindau tumor suppressor gene in primary human renal cell carcinomas. *Cancer Res* **54**:2852, 1994.
90. Crossey PA, Richards FM, Foster K, Green JS, Prowse A, Latif F, Lerman MI, Zbar B, Affara NA, Ferguson-Smith MA, Maher ER: Identification of intragenic mutations in the von Hippel-Lindau disease tumor suppressor gene and correlation with disease phenotype. *Hum Mol Genet* **3**:1303, 1994.
91. Foster K, Prowse A, van den Berg A, Fleming S, Hulsbeek MMF, Crossey PA, Richards FM, Cairns P, Affara NA, Ferguson-Smith MA, Buys CHCM, Maher ER: Somatic mutations of the von Hippel-Lindau disease tumour suppressor gene in nonfamilial clear cell renal carcinoma. *Hum Mol Genet* **3**:2169, 1994.
92. Bailly M, Bain C, Favrot MC, Ozturk M: Somatic mutations of von Hippel-Lindau (VHL) tumor-suppressor gene in European kidney cancers. *Int J Cancer* **63**:660, 1995.
93. Schmidt L, Li F, Brown RS, Berg S, Chen F, Wei MH, Tory K, Lerman MI, Zbar B: Mechanism of tumorigenesis of renal carcinomas associated with the constitutional chromosome 3;8 translocation. *Cancer J* **1**:191, 1995.
94. Zhuang Z, Bertheau P, Emmert-Buck MR, Liotta LA, Gnarra J, Linehan WM, Lubensky IA: A microdissection technique for archival DNA analysis of specific cell populations in lesions < 1 mm in size. *Am J Pathol* **146**:620, 1995.
95. Zhuang Z, Gnarra JR, Dudley CF, Zbar B, Linehan WM, Lubensky IA: Detection of von Hippel-Lindau disease gene mutations in paraffin-embedded sporadic renal cell carcinoma specimens. *Mod Pathol* **9**:838, 1996.
96. Long JP, Anglard P, Gnarra JR, Walther MM, Merino MJ, Liu S, Lerman MI, Zbar B, Linehan WM: The use of molecular genetic analysis in the diagnosis of renal cell carcinoma. *World J Urol* **12**:69, 1994.
97. Kanno H, Kondo K, Ito S, Yamamoto I, Fujii S, Torigoe S, Sakai N, Masahiko H, Shuin T, Yao M: Somatic mutations of the von Hippel-Lindau tumor suppressor gene in sporadic central nervous system hemangioblastomas. *Cancer Res* **54**:4845, 1994.
98. Gilcrease MZ, Schmidt L, Zbar B, Truong L, Rutledge M, Wheeler TM: Somatic von Hippel-Lindau mutation in clear cell papillary cystadenoma of the epididymis. *Hum Pathol* **26**:1341, 1995.
99. Herman JG, Latif F, Weng Y, Lerman MI, Zbar B, Liu S, Samid D, Duan D-SR, Gnarra JR, Linehan WM, Baylin SB: Silencing of the *VHL* tumor suppressor gene by DNA methylation in renal carcinoma. *Proc Natl Acad Sci USA* **91**:9700, 1994.
100. Duan DR, Humphrey JS, Chen DYT, Weng Y, Sukegawa J, Lee S, Gnarra JR, Linehan WM, Klausner RD: Characterization of the *VHL* tumor suppressor gene product: Localization, complex formation, and the effect of natural inactivating mutations. *Proc Natl Acad Sci USA* **92**:6459, 1995.
101. Gnarra JR, Duan DR, Weng Y, Humphrey JS, Chen DYT, Lee S, Pause A, Dudley CF, Latif F, Kuzmin I, Schmidt L, Duh FM, Stackhouse T, Chen F, Kishida T, Wei MH, Lerman MI, Zbar B, Klausner RD, Linehan WM: Molecular cloning of the von Hippel-Lindau tumor suppressor gene and its role in renal carcinoma. *Biochim Biophys Acta* **1242**:201, 1996.
102. Duan DR, Pause A, Burgess WH, Aso T, Chen DYT, Garret KP, Conaway RC, Conaway JW, Linehan WM, Klausner RD: Inhibition of transcription elongation by the VHL tumor suppressor protein. *Science* **269**:1402, 1995.
103. Garrett KP, Tan S, Bradsher JN, Lane WS, Conaway JW, Conaway RC: Molecular cloning of an essential subunit of RNA polymerase II elongation factor SIII. *Proc Natl Acad Sci USA* **91**:5237, 1994.
104. Garrett KP, Aso T, Bradsher JN, Foundling SI, Lane WS, Conaway RC, Conaway JW: Positive regulation of general transcription factor SIII by a tailed ubiquitin homolog. *Proc Natl Acad Sci USA* **92**:7172, 1995.
105. Aso T, Lane WS, Conaway JW, Conaway RC: Elongin (SIII): A multisubunit regulator of elongation by RNA polymerase II. *Science* **269**:1439, 1995.
106. Kibel A, Iliopoulos O, DeCaprio JA, Kaelin WG Jr: Binding of the von Hippel-Lindau tumor suppressor protein to elongin B and C (see comments). *Science* **269**:1444, 1995.
107. Aso T, Lane WS, Conaway JW, Conaway RC: Elongin (SIII): A multisubunit regulator of elongation by RNA polymerase II (see comments). *Science* **269**:1439, 1995.
108. Pause A, Lee S, Worrell RA, Chen DYT, Burgess WH, Linehan WM, Klausner RD: The von Hippel-Lindau tumor-suppressor gene product forms a stable complex with human CUL-2, a member of the Cdc53 family of proteins. *Proc Natl Acad Sci USA* **94**:2156, 1997.
109. Elledge SJ, Harper JW: The role of protein stability in the cell cycle and cancer. *Biochim Biophys Acta* **1377**:M61, 1998.
110. Lonergan KM, Iliopoulos O, Ohh M, Kamura T, Conaway RC, Conaway JW, Kaelin WGJ: Regulation of hypoxia-inducible mRNAs by the von Hippel-Lindau tumor suppressor protein requires binding to complexes containing elongins B/C and Cul2. *Mol Cell Biol* **18**:732, 1998.
111. Patton EE, Willems AR, Tyers M: Combinatorial control in ubiquitin-dependent proteolysis: Don't Skp the F-box hypothesis. *Trends Genet* **14**:236, 1998.
112. Pause A, Lee S, Lonergan KM, Klausner RD: The von Hippel-Lindau tumor suppressor gene is required for cell cycle exit upon serum withdrawal. *Proc Natl Acad Sci USA* **95**:993, 1998.
113. Gnarra JR, Zhou S, Merrill MJ, Wagner JR, Krumm A, Papavassiliou E, Oldfield EH, Klausner RD, Linehan WM: Post-transcriptional regulation of vascular endothelial growth factor mRNA by the product of the *VHL* tumor suppressor gene. *Proc Natl Acad Sci USA* **93**:10589, 1996.
114. Siemeister G, Weindel K, Mohrs K, Barleon B, Martiny-Baron G, Marme D: Reversion of deregulated expression of vascular endothelial growth factor in human renal carcinoma cells by von Hippel-Lindau tumor suppressor protein. *Cancer Res* **56**:2299, 1996.
115. Berger DP, Herbstritt L, Dengler WA, Marme D, Mertelsmann R, Fiebig HH: Vascular endothelial growth factor (VEGF) mRNA expression in human tumor models of different histologies. *Ann Oncol* **6**:817, 1995.
116. Takahashi A, Sasaki H, Kim SJ, Tobisu K, Kakizoe T, Tsukamoto T, Kumamoto Y, Sugimura T, Terada M: Markedly increased amounts of messenger RNAs for vascular endothelial growth factor and placenta growth factor in renal cell carcinoma associated with angiogenesis. *Cancer Res* **54**:4233, 1994.
117. Sato K, Terada K, Sugiyama T, Takahashi S, Saito M, Moriyama M, Kakinuma H, Suzuki Y, Kato M, Kato T: Frequent overexpression of vascular endothelial growth factor gene in human renal cell carcinoma. *Tohoku J Exp Med* **173**:355, 1994.
118. Wizigmann-Voos S, Breier G, Risau W, Plate KH: Up-regulation of vascular endothelial growth factor and its receptors in von Hippel-Lindau disease-associated and sporadic hemangioblastomas. *Cancer Res* **55**:1358, 1995.
119. Iliopoulos O, Jiang C, Levy AP, Kaelin WG, Goldberg MA: Negative regulation of hypoxia-inducible genes by the von Hippel-Lindau protein. *Proc Natl Acad Sci USA* **93**:10595, 1996.
120. Ivanov SV, Kuzmin I, Wei MH, Pack S, Geil L, Johnson BE, Stanbridge EJ, Lerman MI: Down-regulation of transmembrane carbonic anhydrases in renal cell carcinoma cell lines by wild-type von Hippel-Lindau transgenes (in process citation). *Proc Natl Acad Sci USA* **95**:12596, 1998.
121. Oosterwijk E, Ruiter DJ, Hoedemaeker PJ, Pauwels EK, Jonas U, Zwartendijk J, Warnaar SO: Monoclonal antibody G 250 recognizes a determinant present in renal-cell carcinoma and absent from normal kidney. *Int J Cancer* **38**:489, 1986.
122. McKiernan JM, Buttyan R, Bander NH, Stifelman MD, Katz AE, Chen MW, Olsson CA, Sawczuk IS: Expression of the tumor-associated gene *MN:* A potential biomarker for human renal cell carcinoma. *Cancer Res* **57**:2362, 1997.
123. Lee S, Chen DYT, Humphrey JS, Gnarra JR, Linehan WM, Klausner RD: Nuclear/cytoplasmic localization of the *VHL* tumor suppressor gene product is determined by cell density. *Proc Natl Acad Sci USA* **93**:1770, 1996.
124. Koolen MI, van der Meyden AP, Bodmer D, Eleveld M, van der Looij E, Brunner H, Smits A, van den Berg E, Smeets D, Geurts vK: A familial case of renal cell carcinoma and a t(2;3) chromosome translocation. *Kidney Int* **53**:273, 1998.
125. Li FP, Decker HJH, Zbar B, Stanton VP, Kovacs G, Seizinger BR, Aburatani H, Sandberg AA, Berg S, Hosoe S, Brown RS: Clinical and genetic studies of renal cell carcinomas in a family with a constitutional chromosome 3;8 translocation. *Ann Intern Med* **118**:106, 1993.
126. Mydlo JH, Bard RH: Analysis of papillary renal adenocarcinoma. *Urology* **30**:529, 1987.
127. Boczko S, Fromowitz FB, Bard RH: Papillary adenocarcinoma of kidney. *Urology* **14**:491, 1979.

128. Kovacs G: Papillary renal cell carcinoma: A morphologic and cytogenetic study of 11 cases. *Am J Pathol* **134**:27, 1989.
129. Kovacs G, Hoene E: Multifocal renal cell carcinoma: A cytogenetic study. *Virchows Arch [A]* **412**:79, 1987.
130. Hughson MD, Johnson LD, Silva FG, Kovacs G: Nonpapillary and papillary renal cell carcinoma: A cytogenetic and phenotypic study. *Mod Pathol* **6**:449, 1993.
131. Shipley JM, Birdsall S, Clark J, Crew J, Gill S, Linehan WM, Gnarra J, Fisher S, Craig IW, Cooper CS: Mapping the X chromosome breakpoint in two papillary renal cell carcinoma cell lines with a t(X;1)(p11.2;q21.2) and the first report of a female case. *Cytogenet Cell Genet* **71**:280, 1995.
132. Suijkerbuijk RF, Meloni AM, Sinke RJ, de Leeuw B, Wilbrink M, Janssen HA, Geraghty MT, Monaco AP, Sandberg AA, Geurts van Kessel A: Identification of a yeast artificial chromosome that spans the human papillary renal cell carcinoma-associated t(X;1) breakpoint in Xp11.2. *Cancer Genet Cytogenet* **71**:164, 1993.
133. Meloni AM, Dobbs RM, Pontes JE, Sandberg AA: Translocation (X;1) in papillary renal cell carcinoma: A new cytogenetic subtype. *Cancer Genet Cytogenet* **65**:1, 1993.
134. Zbar B, Lerman M: Inherited carcinomas of the kidney, in *Advances in Cancer Research*. 1998, pp 163-201.
135. Duh FM, Scherer SW, Tsui LC, Lerman MI, Zbar B: Gene structure of the human *MET* proto-oncogene. *Oncogene* **15**:1583, 1997.
136. Schmidt L, Duh F-M, Chen F, Kishida T, Glenn G, Choyke P, Scherer SW, Zhuang Z, Lubensky IA, Dean M, Allikmets R, Chidambaram A, Bergerheim UR, Feltis TJ, Casadevall C, Zamarron A, Bernues M, Richard S, Lips CJM, Walther MM, Tsui L, Geil L, Orcutt ML, Stackhouse T, Lipan J, Slife L, Brauch H, Decker J, Niehans G, Hughson MD, Moch H, Storkel S, Lerman MI, Linehan WM, Zbar B: Germline and somatic mutations in the tyrosine kinase domain of the *MET* proto-oncogene in papillary renal carcinomas. *Nature Genet* **16**:68, 1997.
137. Zhuang Z, Park WS, Pack S, Schmidt L, Pak E, Pham T, Weil RJ, Candidus S, Lubensky IA, Linehan WM, Zbar B, Weirich G: Trisomy 7-harboring non-random duplication of the mutant MET allele in hereditary papillary renal carcinomas. *Nature Genet* **20**:66, 1998.
138. Fischer J, Palmedo G, von Knobloch R, Bugert P, Prayer-Galetti T, Pagano F, Kovacs G: Duplication and overexpression of the mutant allele of the *MET* proto-oncogene in multiple hereditary papillary renal cell tumours. *Oncogene* **17**:733, 1998.
139. Park M, Dean M, Kaul K, Braun MJ, Gonda MA, Vande WG: Sequence of *MET* protooncogene cDNA has features characteristic of the tyrosine kinase family of growth-factor receptors. *Proc Natl Acad Sci USA* **84**:6379, 1987.
140. Weidner KM, Sachs M, Birchmeier W: The Met receptor tyrosine kinase transduces motility, proliferation, and morphogenic signals of scatter factor/hepatocyte growth factor in epithelial cells. *J Cell Biol* **121**:145, 1993.
141. Bladt F, Riethmacher D, Isenmann S, Aguzzi A, Birchmeier C: Essential role for the c-met receptor in the migration of myogenic precursor cells into the limb bud (see comments). *Nature* **376**:768, 1995.
142. Jeffers M, Schmidt L, Nakaigawa N, Webb C, Weirich G, Kishida T, Zbar B, Woude GV: Activating mutations for the Met tyrosine kinase receptor in human cancer. *Proc Natl Acad Sci USA* **94**:11445, 1997.
143. Schmidt L, Junker K, Weirich G, Glenn G, Choyke P, Lubensky IA, Zhuang Z, Jeffers M, Woude GV, Neumann H, Walther MM, Linehan WM, Zbar B: Two North American families with hereditary papillary renal carcinoma and identical novel mutations in the *MET* proto-oncogene. *Cancer Res* **58**:1719, 1998.
144. Buttner C, Henz BM, Welker P, Sepp NT, Grabbe J: Identification of activating c-kit mutations in adult- but not in childhood-onset indolent mastocytosis: A possible explanation for divergent clinical behavior. *J Invest Dermatol* **111**:1227, 1998.
145. Schmidt L, Junker K, Nakaigawa N, Kinjerski T, Weirich G, Miller M, Lubensky I, et al.: Novel mutations of the *MET* proto-oncogene in papillary renal carcinomas. *Oncogene* **18**:2343, 1999.
146. Weirich G, Glenn G, Junker K, Merino M, Storkel S, Lubensky IA, Choyke P, Pack S, Amin M, Walther MM, Linehan WM, Zbar B: Familial renal oncocytoma: Clinicopathologic study of 5 families. *J Urol* **160**:335, 1998.
147. Horton WA, Wong V, Eldridge R: Von Hippel-Lindau disease: Clinical and pathological manifestations in nine families with 50 affected members. *Arch Intern Med* **136**:769, 1976.
148. Pontes JE, Pescatori E, Connelly R, Hashimura T, Tubbs R: Circulating cancer cells in renal-cell carcinoma. *Prog Clin Biol Res* **348**:1, 1990.
149. Liotta LA, Kleinerman J, Seidel GM: Quantitative relationships of intravascular tumor cells, tumor vessels and pulmonary metastasis following tumor implantation. *Cancer Res* **34**:997, 1974.
150. Buttler TP, Gullino PM: Quantitation of cell shedding into efferent blood of mammary adenocarcinoma. *Cancer Res* **35**:512, 1975.
151. Moreno JG, Croce CM, Fischer R, Monne M, Vihko P, Mulholland SG, Gomella LG: Detection of hematogenous micrometastasis in patients with prostate cancer. *Cancer Res* **52**:6110, 1992.
152. Linehan WM, Klausner RD: Renal carcinoma, in Vogelstein B, Kinzler K (eds): *The Genetic Basis of Human Cancer*. New York: McGraw-Hill, 1998, pp 455–473.
153. Yao M, Latif F, Kuzmin I, Stackhouse T, Zhou FW, Tory K, Orcutt ML, Duh FM, Richards F, Maher E, La Forgia S, Huebner K, Le Pasilier D, Linehan WM, Lerman M, Zbar B: Von Hippel-Lindau disease: Identification of deletion mutations by pulsed field gel electrophoresis. *Hum Genet* **92**:605, 1993.

CHAPTER 42

Multiple Endocrine Neoplasia Type 2

B. A. J. Ponder

1. **Multiple endocrine neoplasia type 2 (MEN 2) is an uncommon autosomal disorder of tumor formation and developmental abnormalities which affects about 1 in 30,000 individuals. It is characterized by the occurrence of C-cell tumors of the thyroid (medullary thyroid carcinoma), often in association with tumors of the adrenal medulla (pheochromocytoma) and parathyroid hyperplasia or adenoma. Developmental abnormalities, which occur in a minority of cases, principally affect the autonomic nerve plexuses of the intestine. The thyroid C cells, adrenal medulla, and intestinal autonomic plexuses but not the parathyroid glands are derived from neural ectoderm.**
2. **Distinct clinical subtypes of MEN 2 are defined by the combination of tissues affected and the presence or absence of developmental abnormalities. In MEN 2A, thyroid C cells, adrenal medulla, and parathyroids may all be involved, but developmental abnormalities are rare. In familial MTC (FMTC), only thyroid C-cell tumors are seen; there are no developmental abnormalities. In MEN 2B, thyroid C cells and adrenal medullary tumors are common, but parathyroid abnormality is uncommon; there are constant developmental abnormalities involving hyperplasia of the intestinal autonomic nerve plexuses and disorganized growth of peripheral nerve axons in the lips, oral mucosa, and conjunctiva, giving rise to a characteristic facies. The onset of thyroid and adrenal tumors in MEN 2B tends to occur early, and their behavior may be more aggressive.**
3. **The gene for MEN 2 was identified by positional cloning. It lies on chromosome 10q11.2. This gene, *ret,* is a previously known receptor tyrosine kinase. Mutations in *ret* in MEN 2A and FMTC result in constitutive activation of the receptor; in MEN 2B, the extent of activation is unclear, but the substrate specificity of the tyrosine kinase may be altered. There are clear correlations between specific mutations in *ret* and the phenotypes that result. Loss-of-activity mutations in *ret* result in Hirschsprung disease of the colon and rectum (HSCR), in which there is an absence of intestinal autonomic nerve plexuses, in distinction to the hyperplasia in MEN 2B. In a few families, MEN 2A and HSCR coexist, apparently as a result of the same *ret* mutation; the mechanism for this is not understood. *ret* is unusual among tumor-predisposing genes in that MEN 2 mutations result in gain of function; it is not a tumor-suppressor gene.**
4. **The tumors characteristic of MEN 2 also occur in a nonhereditary form. Somatic mutations of *ret* are found in these tumors, but almost all are of the same type as the germ-line mutations characteristic of MEN 2B, which alter the substrate specificity of the tyrosine kinase. This may imply that *ret* mutations of the type seen in MEN 2A and FMTC, which result in activation of a normal tyrosine kinase domain, are for the most part effective in tumorigenesis only during a restricted period in development.**
5. **MEN 2 is a good example of an inherited cancer syndrome in which screening of family members leads to early diagnosis and effective treatment by thyroidectomy and adrenalectomy. Since each of the tissues involved in tumor formation secretes a characteristic product (calcitonin, epinephrine, parathyroid hormone), biochemical monitoring of family members at risk provides a sensitive means of early detection. This can now be refined by predictive genetic testing for the characteristic *ret* mutations.**

Multiple endocrine neoplasia (MEN) is characterized by the occurrence of tumors that involve two or more endocrine glands in a single patient or in close relatives. There are two types of MEN syndrome,[1] with distinct patterns of tissue involvement (Table 42-1). Multiple endocrine neoplasia type 1 (MEN 1), sometimes called *Wermer syndrome,*[1–3] includes tumors of parathyroid, pituitary, and pancreatic islet cells and less frequently adrenocortical, carcinoid, and multiple lipomatous tumors.[4–6] MEN 1 is dominantly inherited; the predisposing locus has been mapped by linkage to chromosome 11q13,[7] and the gene has been identified recently.[7a] There is no evidence to suggest genetic heterogeneity. Multiple endocrine neoplasia type 2 (MEN 2), sometimes called *Sipple syndrome* and previously called *MEA II* or *MEN II,* although MEN 2 is now preferred, includes tumors of the thyroid C cells and adrenal medulla and hyperplasia or adenoma of the parathyroids.[8–10] There also may be various developmental abnormalities, which are described below. The predisposing gene for MEN 2 is *ret,* a receptor tyrosine kinase that maps to chromosome 10q11.2. The great majority of MEN 2 families have detectable mutations in *ret,* but a few are unaccounted for,[11] and genetic heterogeneity remains a possibility.[12]

Patients occasionally have been described as having tumors that are a combination of those associated with MEN 1 and MEN 2, e.g., pituitary tumors and pheochromocytoma. It is unclear whether these are more than chance occurrences[13] and whether there is an additional MEN "overlap" syndrome. A spectrum of endocrine tumors that overlaps that of MEN 1 and MEN 2 is seen in some inbred strains of rats[14,15] and in transgenic mice homozygous for loss of activity of the retinoblastoma gene, which have been reported to develop thyroid C-cell and pituitary tumors. The human MEN 1 and MEN 2 syndromes are genetically and almost always clinically distinct. Familial pheochromocytomas occur in two other human inherited cancer syndromes: von

A list of standard abbreviations is located immediately preceding the index in each volume. Nonstandard abbreviations used in this chapter include: MEN 1 = multiple endocrine neoplasia type 1; MEN 2 = multiple endocrine neoplasia type 2; FMTC = familial medullary thyroid carcinoma; MTC = medullary thyroid carcinoma; HSCR = Hirschsprung disease of the colon and rectum.

Table 42-1 Endocrine Involvement in the MEN Syndromes

MEN 1	MEN 2
Parathyroid	Thyroid C cells
Anterior pituitary	Adrenal medulla
Pancreatic islets	Parathyroid
Adrenal cortex	

Hippel-Lindau (VHL) syndrome (see Chap. 41) and neurofibromatosis type 1 (see Chap. 39).

CLINICAL ASPECTS OF MEN 2

Three clinical types of MEN 2 [MEN 2A, MEN 2B, and familial medullary thyroid carcinoma (FMTC)] are distinguished by the combination of tissues involved[16–18] (Table 42-2).

The Component Tumors of MEN 2

As in the other inherited cancer syndromes, each of the component tumors of MEN 2 also has a nonhereditary counterpart.

Medullary Thyroid Carcinoma. The characteristic tumor of MEN 2 is the medullary thyroid carcinoma (MTC), which is derived from the C cells of the thyroid. These are malignant tumors, metastasizing usually at a stage when the primary tumor is 5 to 10 mm in diameter, at first locally within the neck and then to distant sites.[19,20] The C cells and the tumors derived from them secrete the hormone calcitonin. This provides a valuable marker for early diagnosis and for following the later course of disease.[21] There is no obvious syndrome of calcitonin overproduction.

Pheochromocytoma. The tumor derived from the adrenal medulla is the pheochromocytoma. Generally these tumors are nonmalignant, at least until they are of large size.[22] They commonly secrete epinephrine and norepinephrine, which, if undetected, can lead to fatal hypertensive episodes, especially in situations such as general anesthesia and childbirth.

Parathyroid. The parathyroid abnormalities in MEN 2 are benign, either hyperplasia or the formation of true benign adenomas.[23] Parathyroid involvement is often clinically silent but may present with symptomatic hypercalcemia or renal stones.

THE CLINICAL TYPES OF MEN 2 SYNDROMES

MEN 2A

Clinical Features. MEN 2A is the most common type, accounting for about 65 percent of families that could be classified in a recent international survey of *ret* mutations in MEN 2 families.[11] The penetrance of *ret* mutations in MEN 2A is incomplete.[24] About 70 percent of gene carriers develop symptomatic disease within their lifetimes, with MTC as the usual first manifestation. Almost all gene carriers can, however, be detected by biochemical screening for MTC by age 40 (Fig. 42-1; see below). On average, about 50 percent of gene carriers will develop pheochromocytoma, and perhaps 5 to 10 percent will develop symptomatic parathyroid disease, but the pattern varies considerably both between and within families.[24] Some of the variation between families can be attributed to different mutant *ret* alleles (see below); the contribution of genetic background, environment, and chance to within-family variation has not been elucidated.

Table 42-2 Patterns of Tissue Involvement in the MEN 2 Syndromes

	MEN 2A	MEN 2B	FMTC
Thyroid C cells	Tumor	Tumor	Tumor
Adrenal medulla	Tumor	Tumor	Not involved
Parathyroid	Hyperplasia/ benign tumor	Not involved	Not involved
Enteric ganglia	Normal*	Hyperplasia	Normal
Other developmental abnormalities	None	Various†	None

*Usually there is no abnormality of enteric ganglia in MEN 2A, but a few families have been described in which there is absence of ganglia from a variable length of the intestine in some individuals.

†Includes musculoskeletal abnormalities and others; see text.

Incidence. The incidence of MEN 2A has not been documented accurately. An attempt to identify all new cases of MTC (hereditary and nonhereditary) in a 2-year period in the United Kingdom, using ascertainment from cancer registries and requests for calcitonin estimations from regional assay laboratories, suggested an overall incidence of about 1 per 1 million per year.[25] Wide variations in the number of registrations between different registries suggested, however, that the data may not be very accurate. It generally is assumed that 20 to 25 percent of MTCs are heritable. This figure is not based on a systematic population-based study but derives largely from two observations: In early clinical studies, about 15 percent of consecutive cases of MTC had an evident family history[19,20,26]; in later series in which families of apparently isolated cases were investigated further by more careful history taking or by genetic or biochemical screening, up to 10 percent showed familial involvement.[27,28] Together, these figures add up to about 20 to 25 new cases of MEN 2 (all types) per year in the United Kingdom (population 55 million).

New Mutations. Some apparently sporadic cases of MTC are new mutations to the hereditary disease. The frequency is not known precisely. There are a few documented cases,[29] and MEN 2 mutations occur on many different haplotypes, indicating separate origins.[30] However, many MEN 2A families have been traced back through several generations, suggesting that founder mutations are not uncommon. This contrasts with MEN 2B, where new mutations are more usual.[31]

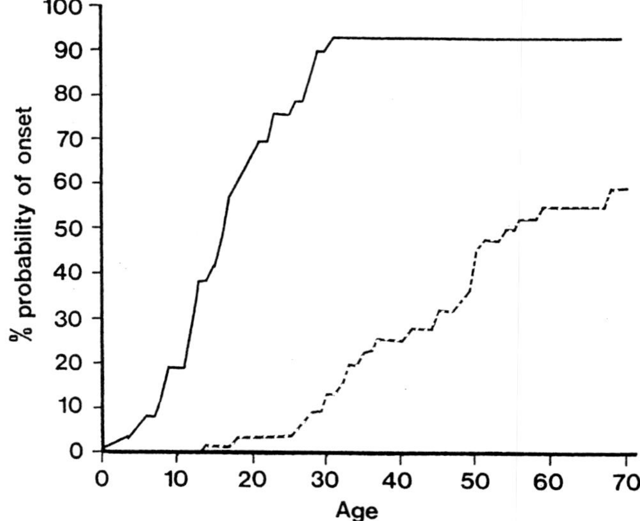

Fig. 42-1 Age-related probability of detection of disease in MEN 2A. Shown is the probability that an individual with the gene for MEN 2A will have presented to medical attention (dotted line) or be detectable by a pentagastrin stimulation test (solid line) by a given age. (*Reproduced with permission from Easton et al: Am J Hum Genet 44:208, 1989. Published by University of Chicago Press.*)

Clinical Variants. No developmental abnormalities are known to be consistently associated with MEN 2A. There are, however, two clinical variants. A small number of families have been described in which several individuals have an itchy skin lesion in the interscapular area with histologic features of lichen amyloidosis.[32,33] A dermatomal distribution in one family[33] suggested a neurologic basis for the lesion, but this remains unsubstantiated. Several families have been described in which there is cosegregation of MEN 2A (or FMTC) and Hirschsprung disease of the colon and rectum (HSCR), with individuals having both phenotypes.[34–37] This is a surprising and intriguing observation, because the *ret* mutations in MEN 2 are thought to result in activation of the gene, whereas those typical of HSCR are associated with loss of activity. It is almost certainly significant that each of the MEN 2/HSCR families described to date has one of two specific *ret* mutations (see below).

Familial MTC

Clinical Features and Definition. The term *familial MTC* denotes families in which MTC is the only abnormality. The original evidence for a separate category of site-specific MTC came from two large kindreds in the United States in which there were multiple cases of MTC but no evidence, either clinically or on biochemical screening, of adrenal or parathyroid involvement.[18] A particular feature of these families was the late onset and low mortality of the tumors. There were no developmental abnormalities. The categorization of FMTC as a distinct variety of MEN 2 was justifiable in these extensive kindreds and subsequently has received support from mutational analysis of the *ret* gene that indicates that the spectrum of mutations in families designated as having FMTC is indeed different from (although overlapping) that described in MEN 2A.[11] Nevertheless, the inconstant occurrence of adrenal or parathyroid involvement in MEN 2A families clearly leads to a difficulty in the classification of small families in which MTC is the only feature: Is the family truly FMTC or a MEN 2A family in which by chance the adrenal or parathyroid components have not yet manifested? As more data are collected, it may be possible to classify families with respect to risks of different tumors on the basis of the *ret* mutation that is present (see below). For the present, however, an arbitrary definition has been generally adopted: To qualify as FMTC, a family should have at least four individuals with proven MTC and no clinical or biochemical evidence of an adrenal or parathyroid abnormality either in the affected members or in available first-degree relatives.[38] Families that fail to meet these criteria either because there are fewer affected cases or because clinical or biochemical data are not available are assigned to an "MEN 2—other" or "undefined" category. Clinical impressions as well as the results of *ret* mutation analysis indicate that FMTC is less common than MEN 2A.

MEN 2B

Clinical Features. MEN 2B is probably the least common variety of MEN 2 but is the most clearly distinct. MTC and pheochromocytoma are common, as in MEN 2A, but tend to present at a younger age (18 and 24 years for MTC and pheochromocytoma in MEN 2B compared with 38 years for MTC in MEN 2A (EuroMEN collaboration, unpublished data).[39] Parathyroid involvement in MEN 2B is rare or absent.[22] The main distinguishing features of MEN 2B are the consistent developmental abnormalities.[17,40–46] A characteristic facies (Fig. 42-2) with thick blubbery lips, nodules on the anterior tongue and the conjunctivae, and thickening of the corneal nerves visible on ophthalmologic examination results from disorganized growth of axons, leading to thickening and irregularity of peripheral nerves.[40,41] (Note, however, that the corneal nerve thickening may be difficult to score.[42]) Hyperplasia of the intrinsic autonomic ganglia in the wall of the intestine leads to disordered gut motility,[43] which commonly presents in infancy or childhood as failure to thrive or alternating episodes of constipation and diarrhea. These abnormalities can be recognized on rectal biopsy. A generalized hypotonia ("floppy baby") has been described in newborn infants.[44] There may be a variety of skeletal abnormalities, including pes cavus, slipped femoral epiphyses, pectus excavatum, and bifid ribs,[45] and a general abnormality of body shape with features resembling those of Marfan syndrome but without the aortic, palatal, or lens abnormalities. Delayed puberty has been noted in a few girls with MEN 2B; the mechanism is unclear. Impotence in men is neurologic in origin.

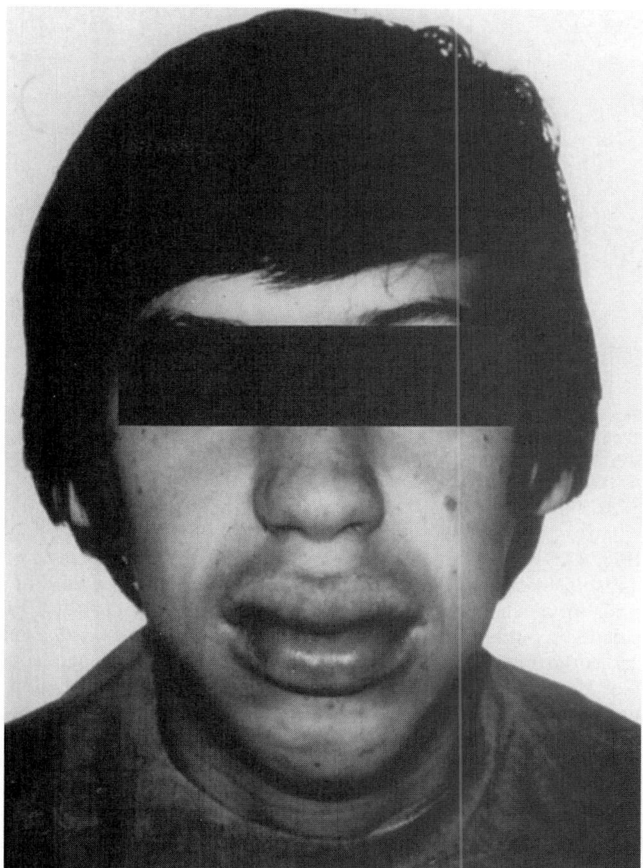

Fig. 42-2 Typical facies of MEN 2B showing the prominent "blubbery" lips caused by neuroma tissue.

New Mutations. The earlier onset of tumors and the developmental abnormalities presumably confer a reproductive disadvantage. As a result, perhaps one-half of all MEN 2B cases result from new mutations.[31] As in retinoblastoma and neurofibromatosis type 1, new mutations occur predominantly on the chromosome from the male parent.[46] It has been suggested that the sex of the transmitting parent also may affect the probability that the disease will manifest in a male or a female child, with an excess of affected female children among the offspring of transmitting males.[46] An interesting commentary on these findings was written by Sapienza.[47]

Differences Between Hereditary and Nonhereditary Tumors: Multifocal Hyperplasia

The histologic appearances of the fully developed MTC, pheochromocytoma, or parathyroid adenomas of MEN 2 patients are indistinguishable from those of nonhereditary cases. However, just as familial cancers at any site are commonly multiple and associated with multiple preneoplastic changes in the target tissue, in the MEN 2 syndromes there are multiple foci of hyperplasia in the target tissues before the development of overt tumors[48,49]

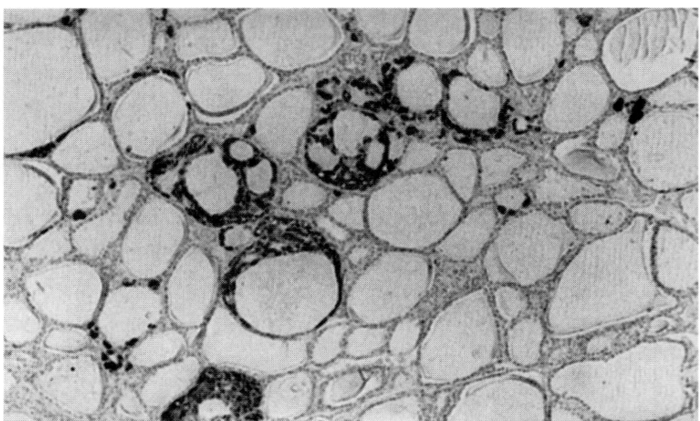

Fig. 42-3 C-cell hyperplasia in MEN 2A thyroid. Prominent groups of C cells are demonstrated by immunochemistry for calcitonin among the thyroid follicles which are unstained. (*Photograph courtesy of Dr. G. Thomas.*)

(Fig. 42-3). This may provide a histologic basis for recognition of an isolated case as being of the hereditary type and provides the basis for biochemical screening to detect the increased amounts of calcitonin or catecholamines produced by the hyperplastic C cells and adrenal medulla.[21] The biochemical test for C-cell hyperplasia (see "Biochemical Screening" below) is made more sensitive by the use of a stimulus (usually intravenous pentagastrin or calcium) that causes the C cells to release stored calcitonin into the circulation. Measurement of calcitonin levels before and after the stimulus provides an indication of C-cell mass. The test is sufficiently sensitive to detect C-cell hyperplasia before the stage of progression to invasive tumor, and surgery based on presymptomatic calcitonin screening is likely to be curative.[21]

Other Causes of C-Cell Hyperplasia. It is important to note that although it is a useful indication of hereditary disease, C-cell hyperplasia may not be completely specific for MEN 2. Increased C-cell numbers (although possibly in a different histologic pattern) have been described in autopsy samples from the general population,[50–52] and there are several well-documented instances in which members of MEN 2 families have had thyroidectomy on the basis of increased calcitonin levels on screening and the thyroid histology has been reported as C-cell hyperplasia but subsequent genetic testing has shown them not to have inherited the familial MEN 2 mutation.[53,54] There may be genetic or nongenetic influences on C-cell mass independent of the MEN 2 mutation that complicate the assessment of C-cell hyperplasia.

Diagnostic Criteria for MEN 2

Failure to Recognize Hereditary Disease. A recent survey for the Royal College of Physicians in the United Kingdom[25] showed that the diagnosis of MEN 2 often is missed. The possibility of hereditary disease in an apparently isolated case of MTC is discounted or not pursued with sufficient vigor.

Part of the problem may stem from terminology. An isolated case of MTC is often referred to as *sporadic*. *Sporadic* in turn is often incorrectly used to signify *nonhereditary*, and so clinicians may come to regard any isolated case as nonhereditary. In fact, of course, a sporadic case may be hereditary, lacking a family history because the phenotype was not manifest in immediate relatives (MEN 2 is incompletely penetrant; see Fig. 42-1), because the history has been poorly taken, or because the case is a new mutation (particularly common in MEN 2B, and in such cases, the diagnosis should be signaled by the associated phenotype) (see Fig. 42-2).

Evaluation of an Apparently Sporadic Case. Guidelines for estimating the probability that an apparently isolated patient presenting with MTC at a given age is in fact hereditary are given by Ponder et al.[55] An apparently sporadic case of MTC, pheochromocytoma, or parathyroid disease should be evaluated carefully for the possibility of MEN 2 first by taking a detailed family history (with special attention to possible indications of the MEN 2 syndrome—goiter, possible hypertensive sudden death, renal stones) and second by evaluation of the surgical specimen for evidence of multifocal hyperplasia.

GENETIC LOCI

Genetic Loci Involved in Germ-Line Mutations in MEN 2

The great majority of MEN 2 families show linkage to chromosome 10q11.2 and have demonstrable mutations in *ret*[11] (Table 42-3). Most published reports suggest that around 10 to 15 percent of FMTC families and families with fewer than four cases of MTC (in the "MEN 2—other" category) have not been found to have *ret* mutations,[11] even though in some of these families the known coding region of *ret* has been examined carefully. Probably some mutations are missed, even on careful analysis. Evidence in support of this comes from the report of a German group who describe a previously undetected "hot spot" for mutations in codons 790 and 791 of *ret* (exon 13) in families with FMTC and a single family with MEN 2A. This group claims to be able to detect *ret* mutation in 100 percent of their MEN 2 families.[55a] A further possibility, not completely excluded, is that another locus also predisposes primarily to MTC, possibly with low penetrance.[12] There have been occasional reports of "MTC-only" families in which there is evidence against linkage on chromosome 10q, but the linkage results have relied on C-cell hyperplasia as the MEN 2 phenotype. Because C-cell hyperplasia can be a difficult phenotype to define,[50–54] it is uncertain how these results should be interpreted.

Genetic Loci Involved in Somatic Mutations

Loss of heterozygosity (LOH) studies show a low level of chromosomal instability in MTC and pheochromocytomas. Mulligan et al.,[56] in a systematic search, identified six chromosomal regions that showed a frequency of LOH of 10 percent or more in a combined series of MTC and pheochromocytoma: 1p, 3p, 3q, 11p, 13, and 22. There were no clear differences between sporadic and familial tumors. Losses are rarely seen at the *ret* locus on chromosome 10q. Chromosome 1p is the most frequently involved in both MTC and pheochromocytoma.[56,57] In almost all cases, the entire chromosome arm is lost. This is not associated with isochromosome 1q formation.[56] A localized region of loss at 1p32 was reported[57] but appears not to be a consistent finding in

Table 42-3 Percentages of MEN 2 Families with Different Phenotypes in Which *ret* Mutations Have Been Detected

Phenotype	No. of Families	Mutation +ve(%)	Mutation −ve (%)
MEN 2A			
MTC, pheochromocytoma, PTH	94	91 (97)	3 (3)
MTC, pheochromocytoma, no PTH	96	95 (99)	1 (1)
MTC, PTH, no pheochromocytoma	13	13 (100)	0 (0)
MEN 2B	79	75 (95)	4 (5)
FMTC*	34	30 (88)	4 (12)
Other MTC*	161	136 (85)	25 (15)
Total	477	440 (92)	37 (8)

*See text.

SOURCE: Data from the International Mutation Consortium.[11]

other studies. No mutations have been identified in candidate genes lying within the regions of LOH.

SPECIFIC GENES

ret is the only gene known to be involved in the inherited predisposition to MEN 2 and the only gene known to cause a predisposition to MTC. Germ-line mutations in other genes may predispose to pheochromocytoma in VHL syndrome (see Chap. 41) and neurofibromatosis type 1 (see Chap. 22). It is not clear whether there is an additional syndrome of site-specific pheochromocytoma or whether all these families will fall within VHL. Germ-line mutations in the Menin gene in MEN 1 predispose to parathyroid tumors.[4–6]

Mutations of *ret* in MEN 2

Identification of *ret* as a Proto-Oncogene. The *ret* proto-oncogene is a cell-surface glycoprotein that is a member of the receptor tyrosine kinase (RTK) family.[58] The name *ret* is an acronym for "*re*arranged during *t*ransfection," reflecting the original identification of *ret* as a chimeric oncogene formed by rearrangement during transfection assays using DNA from human lymphomas and gastric tumors.[59] Three different rearranged versions of *ret* have since been described *in vivo*, specifically in papillary thyroid carcinomas (which arise from thyroid follicular epithelial cells and are therefore distinct from the C-cell-derived MTC).[60–62] These rearranged versions are termed *ret PTC-1, -2,* and *-3*. In each case, the effect of the rearrangement, which occurs as a somatic event, is to fuse the tyrosine kinase region of *ret* with different activating sequences that are expressed in thyroid epithelial cells. The fused activating genes contribute a new N-terminal portion to the ret protein that is capable of dimerization, leading to activation of the tyrosine kinase domain independent of any ligand. Mutations of the *ret-PTC* type are not seen in MEN 2-related tumors.

Identification of *ret* in MEN 2. *ret* lies in the region of the MEN 2 locus defined by linkage analysis and was therefore a candidate gene.[63,64] At that time, *ret* was known as a proto-oncogene, whereas all the tumor-predisposing genes identified to that point acted as suppressor genes. The plausibility of *ret* as a candidate was, however, strengthened by the first reports that the *ret* knockout mouse had a phenotype that resembled HSCR[65] and the known association of MEN 2 and HSCR in some families. Mutation analysis of *ret* in MEN 2 families revealed mutations in the extracellular domain of the gene in MEN 2A and FMTC[66–68] and subsequently in the tyrosine kinase domain in MEN 2B.[69–71]

***ret* Structure.** The coding sequence consists of 21 exons in a genomic sequence of approximately 55 kb.[72,73] The protein exists in three main 39 alternatively spliced forms of 1072 to 1114 amino acids.[74] There is a cleavable signal sequence of 28 amino acids; an extracellular domain, which is glycosylated and has a conserved[75,76] cysteine-rich region close to the cell membrane and a region of cadherin homology further out[77]; a transmembrane domain; and a tyrosine kinase domain with a short interkinase region of 27 amino acids (Fig. 42-4). Further details of the structure are given in references 72–74 and 78–80.

Ligands for the *ret* Receptor. Three ligands have so far been identified: glial cell line-derived neurotrophic factor (GDNF),[81] neurturin,[81a] and persephin.[81b] These are structurally related secreted proteins that are widely expressed in the nervous system and in other tissues and promote the survival of neurons during development.[81c,81d] Each signals through a multicomponent receptor consisting of *ret* and one of the GFRα family of glycosylphosphatidylinositol (GP1)-linked proteins.[81e,81f,81g,81h,84,85] GFRα1 is the preferred ligand-binding protein for GDNF; GFRα2, for neurturin; and GFRα4, for persephin.[81e,81f,81h] Mouse knockouts of the *GDNF* gene have a phenotype similar to that of *ret* knockouts.[82,83] The distinct and overlapping roles of the different *ret*-ligand combinations in development are currently under study.

Germ-Line *ret* Mutations in MEN 2. A summary of the mutations is given in Table 42-3 and Fig. 42-4. With one

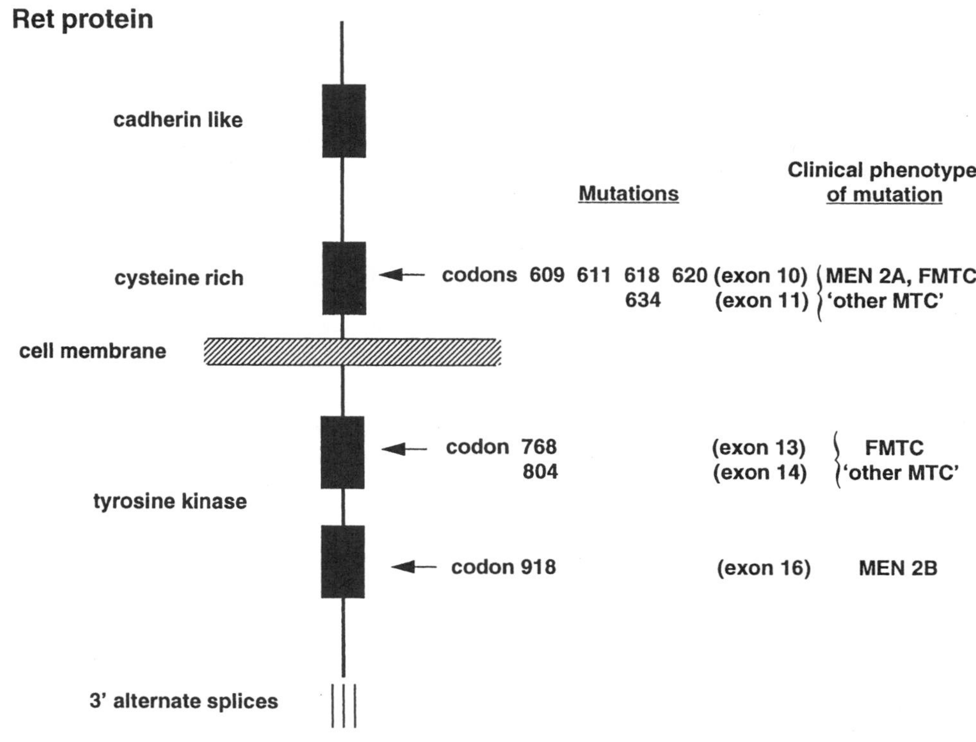

Fig. 42-4 The main features of the protein encoded by the *ret* proto-oncogene and the sites of the mutations in the different clinical varieties of MEN 2.

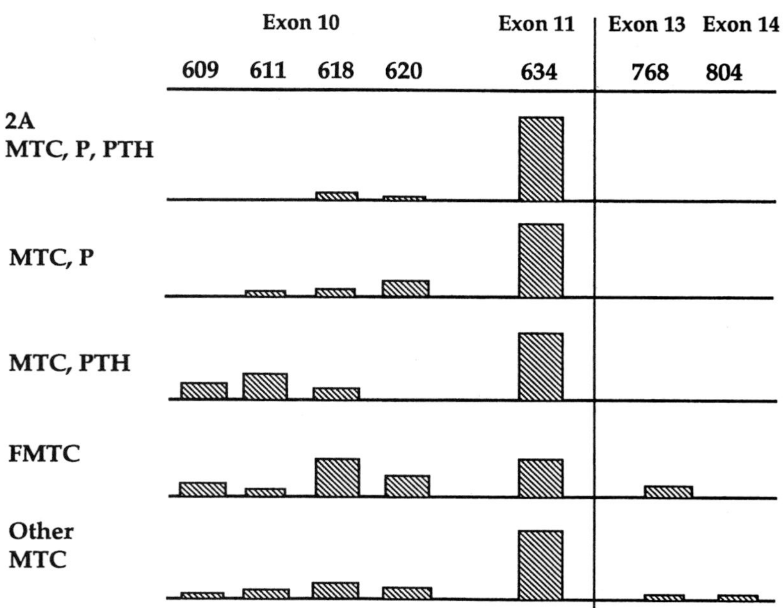

Fig. 42-5 Proportion of mutations in different codons of *ret* in different phenotypic subtypes of MEN 2A, FMTC, and other MTC families. Based on data from the International *ret* Mutation Consortium summarized in Table 42-3.

exception, an in-frame insertion,[85a] all MEN 2 germ-line mutations so far identified are point mutations that lead to amino acid substitution.

Mutations in MEN 2A and FMTC. The majority of mutations in MEN 2A and FMTC lie in one of five cysteine codons in the cysteine-rich region of the extracellular domain[11,38] and result in substitution of the cysteine by another amino acid. A few mutations in families with MTC have been found in exons 13, 14, and 15 of the intracellular domain,[86,87] and a single MEN 2A family has been reported with mutation in codon 790 (exon 13)[55a] (see Figs. 42-4 and 42-5). Figure 42-5 shows clearly that there is a correlation between the codon involved in the mutation and the MEN 2 phenotype.[11] In families with MEN 2A with both pheochromocytoma and parathyroid involvement, almost all the mutations are in codon 634; in MEN 2A families lacking pheochromocytoma and in FMTC, codons 609, 611, 618, and 620 are more frequently involved. This correlation is highly significant; 160 of 186 families with at least one proven case of pheochromocytoma have mutations in codon 634, compared with 18 of 43 families with no evidence of pheochromocytoma ($p < 0.0001$).[11,11a] There also may be an effect not only of the position of the cysteine codon but of the particular amino acid substitution involved. Mutations at codon 634 seen in MEN 2 include all the possible amino acid substitutions allowed by the coding sequence. The most common changes are cysteine to arginine (C634R; TGC → CGC) and cysteine to tyrosine (C634Y; TGC → TAC), which may reflect the known frequency of T → C and G → A changes rather than the particular biologic significance of these substitutions. Nevertheless, it is intriguing that while C634R was present in 88 of 169 MEN 2A families with a codon 634 mutation, none of 9 FMTC families with a codon 634 mutation had this change.[11] Furthermore, Mulligan et al.[38] found a highly significant association between the C634R mutation, compared with all other 634 mutations, and the presence in the family of parathyroid disease. This, however, has not so far been replicated in an independent study.[11a] Four families (three meeting the criteria for FMTC and one "other") have been identified with a glu → asp mutation in codon 768 (exon 13),[86,87] and two families with MTC have been placed in the "other" category with a leu → val mutation in codon 804 (exon 14).[86] Mutations in codons 790 and 791 have been reported in several small families with MTC and one with MEN 2A.[55a] Thus mutations in this region of the intracellular domain seem mostly to be specifically associated with MTC rather than with pheochromocytoma or parathyroid disease, although the MEN 2A family with codon 790 mutation indicates that this correlation may not be absolute.

Mutations in MEN 2B. Some 95 percent of MEN 2B families reported to date have an identical mutation: methionine → threonine in codon 918 of exon 16.[11,69–71,88] Each of four families lacking this mutation had typical and well-documented phenotypic features.[89] In four families without M918T mutation, a mutation of A883F recently has been reported.[89a,89b]

Mutations in Families with MEN 2 and HSCR. Each of the 17 or so families reported has a mutation in either cys 609, cys 618, or cys 620.[33,37,90,90a,90b,90c] No other mutation has been found after careful examination of the remainder of the gene in these families, and so the conclusion must be that the same mutation can result in apparently contrasting phenotypes in the same individual. Families with HSCR alone with no evidence of MEN 2 also have been reported to have missense mutations in cysteine codons 609 and 620.[35,36]

Expression of *ret* in Development. Three of the tissues principally involved in MEN 2 — thyroid C cells, adrenal medulla, and intestinal autonomic ganglia — are derived from neural ectoderm.[91] The parathyroids are derived from the endoderm of the third and fourth pharyngeal pouches. The lineage relationships between C cells and other cells of neuroectodermal origin are still unclear, but the origin of C cells from vagal neural crest and the biochemical similarities with enteric neurons[92] suggest that they share a common precursor with enteric neurons and ultimately with the sympathoadrenal progenitor that is the precursor of chromaffin cells and sympathetic neurons.[93]

In situ hybridization studies during mouse and rat development show that *ret* is expressed in the neural crest-derived cells that migrate from the region of the hindbrain into the posterior pharyngeal arches and from there to form the thyroid C cells and the vagal neural crest that gives rise to the intestinal autonomic nerves.[94,95] *ret* is also expressed in migrating cells derived from the trunk neural crest as they coalesce alongside the aorta to form the sympathetic ganglia and the chromaffin cells that will form the adrenal medulla and in the endoderm of the pharyngeal pouches that give rise to the parathyroids.[94,96] The expression of *ret* is therefore consistent with a role in the development and differentiation of the tissues that are involved in MEN 2. It is perhaps surprising that *ret* homozygous knockout mice appear at birth to have absent intestinal autonomic ganglia but normal C cells and adrenal medulla.[65] The mice die at this stage, probably of respiratory or kidney failure resulting from other developmental defects, and so the possible role of *ret* expression in postnatal development cannot be assessed. However, the tentative conclusion must be that while disordered *ret* expression can lead to tumor formation, normal *ret* expression is not necessary for C-cell or adrenal medullary development up to the time of birth. A caveat is that while the C cells and adrenal medulla may appear grossly normal, the development of the cells may have been perturbed in some way that is not readily apparent. There is a further possibility, with some evidence to support it, that the C-cell population is heterogeneous, with only some C cells expressing *ret*.[95,97] It may be, therefore, that the C cells that are seen in the knockout mice are only one component of the population, with the other component being absent.

In the later stages of embryogenesis in the mouse and in rodent and human thyroid and adrenal medullas after birth, there appears to be only weak and patchy expression of *ret* by the criteria of *in situ* hybridization and immunohistochemistry.[95,97] In most MTCs and pheochromocytomas, by contrast, *ret* is expressed at high levels.[98,99] At present, nothing is known about the role of *ret* in C-cell or adrenal medullary development or in the adult glands. The mechanism and significance of the apparent increase in the expression in tumors are uncertain but may in part have a trivial explanation in terms of stabilization of the *ret* mRNA or protein as a result of the mutation.[100]

Function of *ret* at the Cellular Level. *ret* is a receptor tyrosine kinase (RTK). Binding of ligand results in dimerization of the receptor, activation of the tyrosine kinase, and initiation of onward signaling pathways.[101] Evidence is slowly accumulating,[102–106,106a,106b] but there is no coherent picture of the signaling events that follow *ret* activation. Analysis is complicated by the three 39 alternative splice forms of *ret,* which might be predicted from the sequence context of their tyrosines to differ in the affinity with which they bind different signaling molecules and may therefore signal through different pathways, and by the likelihood (supported by some evidence[106]) that the pathways of signaling are specific for different cell types, which implies that studies should be done in cells that resemble as closely as possible those involved in MEN 2.

Consequences of *ret* Mutations. Transfection experiments[101,104] have shown that both the MEN 2A (cys 634 arg) and the MEN 2B (met 918 thr) mutations lead to activation of *ret* tyrosine kinase. The evidence is of two types: (1) biologic, in which transfection of mutant but not wild-type *ret* induces transformation of NIH 3T3 cells and differentiation of rat PC12 (pheochromocytoma) cells, and (2) biochemical, in which the *ret* protein becomes phosphorylated on tyrosine and acquires tyrosine kinase activity against added substrates.

Extracellular Domain Cysteine Mutations. The cysteine mutations activate *ret* by inducing covalent dimerization[101,104,107,108] (Fig. 42-6). The genotype-phenotype correlation observed with different cysteine mutations is probably explained by quantitative differences in signaling. The different cysteine mutants have been shown to differ both in their efficiency of dimerization and in their maturation to the fully glycosylated form, which is necessary for insertion into the plasma membrane. Either or both of these differences may be responsible for differences in the level of *ret* activation.[108a,108b]

The Met 918 Thr MEN 2B Mutation. This mutation has proved to be of considerable interest because one effect of the mutation is to convert the substrate specificity of the *ret* tyrosine kinase from that typical of a receptor tyrosine kinase (RTK) to that typical of a cytoplasmic tyrosine kinase. It also confers some activity on the receptor, independent of dimerization (see below).

Residue 918 is predicted from modeling studies to lie at the base of a pocket in the protein that is involved in substrate

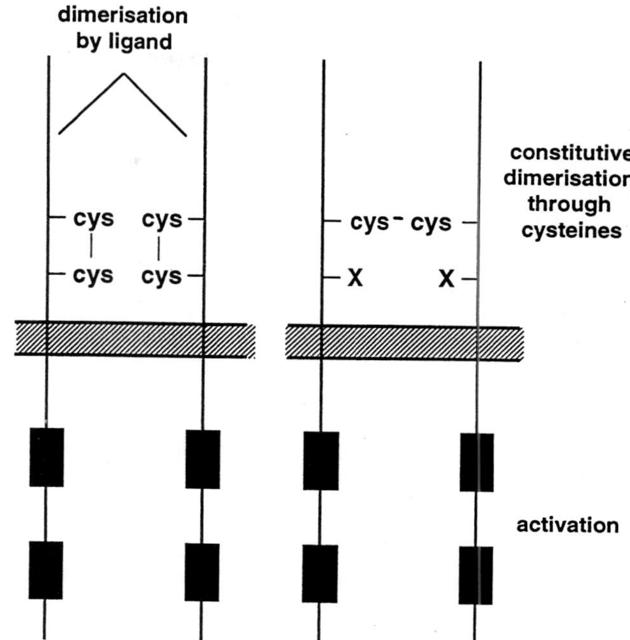

Fig. 42-6 Constitutive activation of *ret* as a result of mutation of a cysteine in the extracellular domain.

binding.[58,69] The substitution of threonine for methionine is predicted to alter the dimensions of the pocket and thus the substrate specificity. Tyrosine kinases fall into two classes: RTKs and cytoplasmic tyrosine kinases. Almost all RTKs have methionine at the equivalent position to codon 918, whereas almost all cytoplasmic tyrosine kinases have threonine (Fig. 42-7).[58] Songyang et al.[109] used degenerate peptide libraries to demonstrate that whereas RTKs prefer hydrophobic amino acids at positions 11 and 13 downstream of the target tyrosine in their substrate, cytoplasmic tyrosine kinases prefer a hydrophilic residue at 11 and a hydrophobic residue at 13. These different amino acid contexts flanking the tyrosine provide different preferred substrates for different groups of SH2 domains on signaling molecules and hence the possibility of different pathways of downstream signaling.

When wild-type (equivalent to MEN 2A) and MEN 2B *ret* tyrosine kinases were compared for their ability to phosphorylate model substrates, a clear shift toward the specificity characteristic of a cytoplasmic tyrosine kinase was seen with the MEN 2B mutation.[109] The inference that the MEN 2B mutation has altered the pathway of downstream signaling is supported by the observation that activated MEN 2B *ret* differs from activated wild-type *ret* both in the pattern of tyrosine phosphorylation of the *ret* protein itself[110] and in the patterns of tyrosine phosphorylations seen in cell extracts.[104]

The MEN 2B mutation does not lead to covalent dimerization of *ret*.[104] However, there is *in vitro* evidence that it does lead to activation of the receptor through an intramolecular mechanism.[101,104,105] Activation by this mechanism may be further

Cytoplasmic - Q G A K F P I/V K W T A P E A A/L-

Receptor - S Q G R I P I/V K/R W M A I/P E S L-

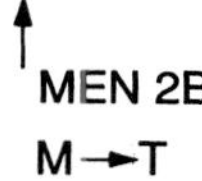

Fig. 42-7 Amino acid sequence of consensus receptor and cytoplasmic tyrosine kinases in the substrate binding region of Hanks domain VIII, showing the mutation characteristic of MEN 2B.

enhanced by ligand binding, and the combined result may be a higher activity than is conferred by the cysteine MEN 2A mutations. It is unclear whether this increased activity, or the altered substrate specificity, is responsible for the characteristic features of the MEN 2B phenotype.

The 768 and 804 Mutations. The glu 768 asp mutation[86,87] involves a residue that is highly conserved in different receptor tyrosine kinases (RTKs). Modeling suggests a possible effect both on ATP binding and on substrate specificity, each of which is being tested experimentally. The val 804 leu mutation[86] also affects a conserved residue, but no modeling studies have been reported.

Genes Involved in Somatic Mutations

The genetic events in the progression of MEN 2 tumors and in the initiation and progression of the related nonhereditary tumors are largely unknown. Baylin et al.[111] showed that the tumors are clonal. Several candidate oncogenes have been screened for mutations or altered expression (N-*ras,* Ha-*ras,* N-*myc,* c-*myc,* 1-*myc,* c-*mos,* β nerve growth factor, and the low-affinity nerve growth factor receptor).[112,113] Apart from one report of overexpression of N-*myc* in 6 of 21 MTCs analyzed by *in situ* hybridization,[114] all the studies were negative.

The role of mutations of *ret* in sporadic tumors is of some interest. In the inherited cancer syndromes, nonhereditary tumors often have mutations in the same gene that shows germ-line mutations in hereditary cases. In MEN 2 this is partly true, with an interesting twist. Among 157 apparently sporadic MTCs in the literature, 39 percent are reported to have a somatic mutation in *ret* codon 918 (the MEN 2B mutation), but mutations of the cysteine codons characteristic of MEN 2A and FMTC are uncommon, probably on the order of 1 to 3 percent.[28,67,115,115a,115b] Somatic mutations in the intracellular domain are seen a little more frequently, e.g., codon 768 in 4 of 72 sporadic MTCs[87,87a,116] and codons 790 and 791 in 11 tumors[55] and codon 883 in exon 15 in 4 of 111 MTCs[116,117] (Eng et al., unpublished data). In pheochromocytomas, the picture is slightly different. Six of 112 (5 percent) sporadic pheochromocytomas had a mutation in the *ret* codon 918,[118,119] 2 of 112 had proven somatic mutations of codon 634,[119,120] and a further 3 tumors have been reported with novel somatic mutations affecting the 39 splice acceptor site of exon 9, codons 632 through 633, and codon 925.[118,121] None of 32 non-MEN 2–associated parathyroid lesions was found to have *ret* mutations.[122] No *ret* mutations have been found in sporadic or hereditary neuroblastoma.[122a]

Detailed study of codon 918 mutations in sporadic MTCs by PCR analysis of microdissected portions of primary tumors and metastases has shown that the tumors are most often mosaic for the mutation; i.e., there are mutant and nonmutant clones, implying that the 918 mutation is not the initiating event in formation of sporadic MTC.[123] One tumor was found to have different areas with codon 918 and codon 883 mutations. Mosaicism for codon 918 mutation also was found in two of three MEN 2A tumors studied, in which a germ-line codon 634 also was present.

Synthesis: Speculation on How *ret* Mutations Result in Tumor Formation

Carlson et al.[124] showed that induction of raf-1 signaling in TT cells (an MTC cell line bearing a codon 634 mutation)[125] results in both differentiation and silencing of *ret* expression. Possibly, during development, C cells move from a "predetermined" to a terminally differentiated state in which *ret* expression is reduced and the potential for proliferation is lost.[124] Inappropriate continued activation of *ret* by a cysteine mutation may override the differentiation program, allowing continued proliferation and the hyperplasias seen in MEN 2. In this scheme, the effects of mutations in the different cysteine codons may depend on the degree of activation that resulted. The combined HSCR/MEN 2 phenotype occasionally seen with mutations of cys 609, cys 618, and cys 620 may (speculatively) be a result of these mutations causing inappropriate activation of *ret* sufficient to result in tumor formation but insufficient to sustain the development of enteric neurons. If these mutations also impaired ligand binding, any reinforcement of *ret* activation by that means would be reduced. The lack of developmental abnormalities in MEN 2A and FMTC compared with MEN 2B may be the case because although the timing of *ret* signaling is inappropriate, the pathways of signaling are normal and the degree of activation of *ret* signaling is probably less. Similarly, the preponderance of MEN 2B-type somatic mutations in tumors could occur because once they are past a certain stage of differentiation and development, thyroid C cells and adrenal medullary cells are no longer susceptible to transformation by increased *ret* activity alone but are susceptible to the altered pathways of signaling induced by the MEN 2B mutation, or because MEN 2B mutations are associated with a higher level of activation. The lack of parathyroid involvement in MEN 2B may be the case either because the MEN 2B-specific signaling pathways are not present in parathyroid cells or because the MEN 2B mutations, unlike MEN 2A, still retain partial dependence on ligand binding for activity and the ligand may not be present in parathyroid tissue. Evidence is not currently available to distinguish any of these alternatives but may become available through studies of transgenic models in which the design of both mutant *ret* and ligand can be modulated.

Implications for Diagnosis

Biochemical Screening. Regular screening by biochemical testing and imaging, followed by surgery where necessary, has been shown to be effective in preventing mortality and morbidity in MEN 2 families.[21,126–128]

In families with MEN 2A or FMTC, it is generally recommended that screening be started at about 4 to 5 years of age, continued annually until about age 20, and then possibly (this is controversial) continued at rather wider intervals until age 35. Screening should consist of measurement of plasma calcitonin after stimulation with intravenous pentagastrin, calcium, or both combined[21,127,128]; blood pressure measurement; urinary or plasma catecholamines; possibly imaging of the adrenals; and serum calcium levels. Thyroid surgery should consist of total thyroidectomy and central node dissection with conservation of normal parathyroid *in situ* or autotransplantation to the forearm.[129] It is controversial whether after the detection of a unilateral adrenal abnormality one or both adrenals should be removed.[130] The risks of serious problems from pheochromocytoma developing subsequently in the remaining adrenal must be balanced against the inconvenience and possible dangers of life after adrenalectomy and hormone replacement. Current opinion generally favors bilateral adrenalectomy. There is no consensus about screening for MEN 2B. Because of the sometimes early development and aggressive nature of the thyroid tumor, screening for MTC in a *ret* mutation-positive child of a known MEN 2B patient probably should start by age 1 year.[131,132] Normal calcitonin levels may be high in infants, and screening results may be difficult to interpret. In this situation, some clinicians have advocated thyroidectomy on the basis of the MEN 2B phenotype alone. Greater certainty can now be provided by DNA testing for the MEN 2B mutation.

Although generally effective, biochemical screening has several problems. The stimulated calcitonin tests are somewhat unpleasant, and compliance is not always good. Occasional false-positive results have been obtained, and results on successive tests that fluctuate at and just above the normal level are common and a frequent cause of anxiety to physicians and family members. Finally, there is the problem of whether to initiate a program of screening for the families of apparently sporadic cases of one of the MEN 2 component tumors. Although many physicians are reluctant to burden a family with these tests, not following such a screening program will inevitably lead to missing some opportunities for early diagnosis.

DNA Testing. The number of distinct *ret* mutations that occur in MEN 2 is small. One of these mutations can be detected in over 90 percent of patients. DNA testing is therefore relatively simple and is now in routine clinical use.[53]

In a family known to have MEN 2 in which the causative mutation can be identified, DNA testing of unaffected family members at risk will eliminate those who do not have the mutation from the need for biochemical screening and simplify the decision to have surgery in those whose screening results are equivocal. Increasingly, opinion is moving toward a recommendation for thyroidectomy in childhood on the basis of DNA testing alone, without waiting for biochemical testing to show abnormalities indicative of C-cell hyperplasia. This may seem surprising given that the chances of presentation with symptomatic disease in MEN 2A are only on the order of 50 percent by age 50[24] and that a good biochemical screen for early disease is available. It probably reflects a mixture of concern about continued compliance with the biochemical screening and the possibility that equivocation over borderline results may lead to surgery being carried out too late; there is also the view that thyroidectomy even in young children has low morbidity and that the best thing for the child and family is to deal with the problem and put it behind them. Because of the lower probability of adrenal disease and the much greater morbidity of adrenalectomy, prophylactic removal of the adrenals is not advised except when there is evidence of abnormality.

The genotype-phenotype correlations outlined above[11] may provide some indication of the probability of adrenal or parathyroid involvement, but at present the data are too few and the overlaps too great to recommend that mutation data be used to exclude families from adrenal or parathyroid screening.

DNA Testing in an Apparently Sporadic Case. DNA testing plays an important role in determining which apparently sporadic cases have heritable disease. All apparently sporadic cases of MTC should be offered DNA testing. If the patient is dead, normal or tumor tissues from pathology specimens may be tested. The limited range of mutations makes this technically feasible in most cases, and since MEN 2A-type mutations are uncommon as somatic events, they can be interpreted as probably germ line in origin even if they are found in tumor (the same does not, of course, apply to MEN 2B mutations). If there is no family history on careful review and no evidence of C-cell hyperplasia on the thyroidectomy specimen, the probability of hereditary disease will vary according to the age at diagnosis of the index case but is almost certainly well below 10 percent.[27,55] In this case, failure to find a mutation in exons 10, 11, 13, 14, and 16 of *ret* excludes MEN 2A with 99 percent probability[11] and, if there is no abnormal phenotype, MEN 2B as well. The residual probability of FMTC or "MTC only" familial disease is a little higher, since up to 10 percent of such families have no detectable *ret* mutation, but it is still probably below 2 percent. It remains a matter of clinical judgment, according to the circumstances and perceptions of each family, whether to pursue biochemical screening of family members at these levels of risk. On the one hand, one does not wish to lose any possibility of early diagnosis and treatment of a potentially lethal and unpleasant cancer (but possibly the FMTC, which is most likely to be missed, could be treated satisfactorily at clinical presentation); on the other hand, one does not want to run the risk of unnecessarily "medicalizing" a family over a period of many years.

Direct mutation testing of unselected cases of apparently sporadic pheochromocytomas suggests that roughly 5 percent may carry a *ret* mutation and that another 5 percent will have a VHL mutation[119] (see Chap. 41). Mutation screening of apparently sporadic cases of pheochromocytoma for MEN 2A and VHL mutations is probably worthwhile. The incidence of occult MEN 2 among apparently sporadic cases of parathyroid hyperplasia and adenoma appears to be low,[122] and unless there are other suggestive features, DNA screening probably is not justified. Children presenting with Hirschsprung disease should be tested for *ret* mutation and, if a mutation is found in exons 10 or 11, for thyroid C-cell tumor.

ACKNOWLEDGMENTS

B. A. J. Ponder is a Gibb Fellow of The Cancer Research Campaign [CRC].

REFERENCES

1. Thakker RV, Ponder BAJ: Multiple endocrine neoplasia. *Clin Endocrinol Metab* **2**:1031, 1988.
2. Thakker RV: Multiple endocrine neoplasia type 1, in Grossman A (ed): *Clinical Endocrinology.* Oxford, Blackwell, 1992, p 597.
3. Wermer P: Multiple endocrine adenomatosis: Multiple hormone producing tumours: A familial syndrome. *Clin Gastroenterol* **3**:671, 1974.
4. Marx SJ, Vinik AI, Santen RJ, Floyd JC, Mills JL, Green J: Multiple endocrine neoplasia type 1: Assessment of laboratory tests to screen for the gene in a large kindred. *Medicine* **65**:226, 1986.
5. Vasen HFA, Lamers CBHW, Lips CJM: Screening for multiple endocrine neoplasia syndrome type 1: A study of 11 kindreds in the Netherlands. *Arch Intern Med* **149**:2717, 1989.
6. Trump D, Farren B, Wooding C, Pang JT, Besser GM, Buchanan KD, Edwards CR, et al: Clinical studies of multiple endocrine neoplasia type 1 (MEN 1). *Q J Med* **89**:653, 1996.
7. Larsson C, Skogseld B, Oberg K. Nakamura Y, Nordenskjold M: Multiple endocrine neoplasia type 1 gene maps to chromosome 11 and is lost in insulinoma. *Nature* **332**:85, 1988.

7a. Chandrasekharappa SC, et al: Positional cloning of the gene for multiple endocrine neoplasia type 1. *Science* **276**:404, 1997.

8. Smith DP, Ponder BAJ: The MEN 2 syndromes and the role of the *ret* protooncogene. *Adv Cancer Res* **70**:199, 1996.
9. Schimke RN: Genetic aspects of multiple endocrine neoplasia. *Annu Rev Med* **35**:25, 1984.
10. Cancer WG, Wells SA: Multiple endocrine neoplasia type 2A. *Curr Probl Surg* **22**:7, 1985.
11. Eng C, Clayton D, Schuffenecker I, et al: The relationship between specific *ret* protooncogene mutations and disease phenotype in multiple endocrine neoplasia type 2: International RET Mutation Consortium. *JAMA* **276**:1575, 1996.

11a. Schuffenecker I, Virally Monod M, Brohet R, Goldgar D, Conte Devolx C, Leclerc L, Chabre O, et al: Risk and penetrance of primary hyperparathyroidism in multiple endocrine neoplasia type 2A families with mutations at codon 634 of the *ret* protooncogene. *J Clin Endocrinol Metab* **83**:487, 1998.

12. Nelkin BD, De Bustros AC, Mabrey M, Baylin SB: The molecular biology of medullary thyroid carcinoma. *JAMA* **261**:3130, 1989.
13. Schimke RN: Multiple endocrine neoplasia: How many syndromes? *Am J Med Genet* **37**:375, 1990.
14. DeLellis RA, Nunnemacher G, Bitman WR, Gagel RF, Tashjian AH, Blount M, Wolfe HJ: C-cell hyperplasia and medullary thyroid carcinoma in the rat. *Lab Invest* **40**:140, 1979.
15. Sass B, Rabstein LS, Madison R, Nims AM, Peters RL, Kelloff GJ: Evidence of spontaneous neoplasms in F344 rats throughout the natural life-span. *J Natl Cancer Inst* **54**:1449, 1975.
16. Schimke KN, Hartmann WH, Prout TE, Rimoin DL: Syndrome of bilateral pheochromocytoma, medullary thyroid carcinoma and multiple neuromas. *N Engl J Med* **279**:1, 1968.
17. Khairi MRA, Dexter RN, Burzynoki NJ, Johnson CC Jr: Mucosal neuroma, pheochromocytoma and medullary thyroid carcinoma: Multiple endocrine neoplasia type 3. *Medicine* **54:89, 1975.**
18. Farndon JR, Leight GS, Dilley WG, Baylin SB, Smallridge RC, Harrison TC, Wells SA Jr: Familial medullary thyroid carcinoma without associated endocrinopathies: A distinct clinical entity. *Br J Surg* **73**:278, 1986.
19. Chong GC, Beaths OH, Sizemore GW, Woolmer LH: Medullary carcinoma of the thyroid gland. *Cancer* **35**:695, 1975.
20. Saad MF, Ordonez NG, Rashid RK, Guido JJ, Hill CS Jr, Hickey RC, Samaan NA: Medullary carcinoma of the thyroid: A study of the clinical features and prognostic factors in 161 patients. *Medicine* **63**:319, 1984.
21. Gagel RF, Tashjian AH, Cummings T, Papathanasopoulos N, Kaplan MM, Delellis RA, Wolfe HJ, et al: The clinical outcome of prospective screening for multiple endocrine neoplasia type 2A. *N Engl J Med* **318**:478, 1988.

22. Dralle H, Schurmeyer TH, Kotzerke TH, Kemnitz J, Crosse H, von zur Muhlen A: Surgical aspects of familial phaeochromocytoma. *Hormone Metab Res Suppl Series* **21**:34, 1989.
23. Van Heerden JA, Kent RB, Sizeman GW, Grant CS, ReMine WH: Primary hyperparathyroidism in patients with multiple endocrine neoplasia syndromes. *Arch Surg* **118**:533, 1983.
24. Easton DF, Ponder MA, Cummings T, Gagel RF, Hansen HH, Reichlin S, Tashjian AH Jr, et al: The clinical and age-at-onset distribution for the MEN 2 syndrome. *Am J Hum Genet* **44**:208, 1989.
25. Harris R, Williamson P: Confidential enquiry into counselling for genetic disorders. *J R Coll Phys Lond* **30**:316, 1991.
26. Sizemore GW, Carney JA, Hunter H II: Epidemiology of medullary carcinoma of the thyroid gland: A 5-year experience (1971–1976). *Surg Clin North Am* **57**:633, 1977.
27. Ponder BAJ, Finer M, Coffey R, Harmer CL, Maisey M, Ormerod MG, Pembrey ME, et al: Family screening in medullary thyroid carcinoma presenting without a family history. *Q J Med* **252**:299, 1986.
28. Eng C, Mulligan LM, Smith DP, Healey CS, Frilling A, Raue F, Neumann HPH, et al: Mutation of the *RET* pro-oncogene in sporadic medullary thyroid carcinoma. *Genes Chromosom Cancer* **12**:209, 1995.
29. Mulligan LM, Eng C, Healey CS, Ponder MA, Feldman CL, Li P, Jackson CE, et al: A *de novo* mutation of the *RET* proto-oncogene in a patient with MEN 2A. *Hum Mol Genet* **3**:1007, 1994.
30. Narod SA, Lavone MF, Morgan K, Calmettes C, Solbol H, Goodfellow PJ, Lenoir GM: Genetic analysis of 24 French families with multiple endocrine neoplasia type 2A. *Am J Hum Genet* **51**:469, 1992.
31. Norum RA, Lafreniere RC, O'Neal LW, Nikolai TF, Delaney JP, Sisson JC, Sobol H: Linkage of the multiple endocrine neoplasia type 2B gene (MEN 2B) to chromosome 10 markers linked to MEN 2A. *Genomics* **8**:313, 1990.
32. Gagel RF, Levy ML, Donovan DT, Alford BR, Wheeler T, Tschen JA: Multiple endocrine neoplasia type 2A associated with cutaneous lichen amyloidosis. *Ann Intern Med* **111**:802, 1989.
33. Chabre O, Labat F, Berthod F, Jarel V, Bachelot Y: Cutaneous lesions associated with multiple endocrine neoplasia type 2A: Lichen amyloidosis or notalgia paresthetica? *Henry Ford Hosp Med J* **40**:245, 1992.
34. Verdy M, Weber AM, Roy CC, Morin CL, Cadotte M, Brochu P: Hirschsprung's disease in a family with multiple endocrine neoplasia type 2. *J Paediatr Gastroenterol Nutr* **1**:603, 1982.
35. Mulligan LM, Eng C, Attie T, Lyonnet S, Marsh DJ, Hyland VJ, Robinson BG, et al: Diverse phenotypes associated with exon 10 mutations of the *RET* proto-oncogene. *Hum Mol Genet* **3**:2163, 1994.
36. Angrist M, Bolk S, Thiel B, Puffenberger EG, Hofstra RM, Buys CHCM, Cass DT, et al: Mutation analysis of the *RET* receptor tyrosine kinase in Hirschsprung's disease. *Hum Mol Genet* **4**:821, 1995.
37. Borst MJ, van Camp JM, Peacock ML, Decker RA: Mutation analysis of multiple endocrine neoplasia type 2A associated with Hirschsprung disease. *Surgery* **117**:386, 1995.
38. Mulligan LM, Eng C, Healey CS, Clayton D, Kwok JBJ, Gardner E, Ponder MA, et al: Specific mutations of the *RET* proto-oncogene are related to disease phenotype in MEN 2A and FMTC. *Nature Genet* **6**:70, 1994.
39. Vasen HFA, Kruseman ACN, Berkel H: Multiple endocrine neoplasia syndrome type 2: the value of screening and central registration: A study of 15 kindreds in the Netherlands. *Am J Med* **83**:487, 1987.
40. Dyck PJ, Carney A, Sizemore GW: Multiple endocrine neoplasia type 2B: Phenotype recognition. *Ann Neurol* **6**:302, 1979.
41. Khalil MK, Lorenzetti DWC: Eye manifestations in medullary carcinoma of the thyroid. *Br J Ophthalmol* **64**:789, 1980.
42. Kinoshita S, Tanaki F, Ohasi Y, Ikeda M, Takai S: Incidence of prominent corneal nerves in multiple endocrine neoplasia type 2A. *Am J Ophthalmol* **111**:307, 1991.
43. Carney JA, Go VLW, Sizemore GW, Hayles AB: Alimentary-tract ganglioneuromatosis: A major component of the syndrome of multiple endocrine neoplasia, type 2B. *N Engl J Med* **295**:1287, 1976.
44. Fryns JP, Chrzanowska K: Mucosal neuromata syndrome [MEN type IIb (III)]. *J Med Genet* **25**:703, 1988.
45. Carney JA, Bianco AJ, Sizeman GW, Hayles AB: Multiple endocrine neoplasia with skeletal manifestations. *J Bone Joint Surg* **63A**:405, 1981.
46. Carlson KM, Bracamontes J, Jackson CE, Clark R, Lacroix A, Wells SA Jr, Goodfellow PJ: Parent of origin effects in multiple endocrine neoplasia type 2B. *Am J Hum Genet* **55**:1076, 1994.
47. Sapienza C: Parental origin effects, genomic imprinting and sex-ratio distortion: Double or nothing? *Am J Hum Genet* **55**:1073, 1994.
48. Wolfe HJ, Melvin KEW, Cervi-Skinner SJ: C cell hyperplasia preceding medullary thyroid carcinoma. *New Engl J Med* **289**:437, 1973.
49. Block MA, Jackson CE, Greenawald KA, Yott JB, Tashjian AH: Clinical characteristics distinguishing hereditary from medullary thyroid carcinoma. *Arch Surg* **115**:142, 1980.
50. O'Toole K, Genoglio-Prieser C, Pushparag N: Endocrine changes associated with the aging process: III. Effect of age on the number of calcitonin immunoreactive cells in the thyroid gland. *Hum Pathol* **16**:991, 1985.
51. Gibson WGH, Peng TC, Croker BP: C cell nodules in adult human thyroid: A common autopsy finding. *Am J Clin Pathol* **75**:347, 1981.
52. Gibson WGH, Peng TC, Croker BP: Age-associated C-cell hyperplasia in the human thyroid. *Am J Pathol* **106**:388, 1982.
53. Lips CJM, Landsvater RM, Hoppener JWM, Geerdink RA, Blijham G, Jansen-Schillhorn van Veen JM, van Gils APG, et al: Clinical screening as compared with DNA analysis in families with multiple endocrine neoplasia type 2A. *N Engl J Med* **331**:828, 1994.
54. Wolfe HJ, Kaplan M, Cummings T, Ponder BAJ, Ponder M, Gardner G, Papi L, et al: Re-evaluation of histologic ceriteria for C cell hyperplasia in MEN 2A using genetic recombinant markers. *Henry Ford Hosp J Med* **40**:312, 1992.
55. Ponder BAJ, Ponder MA, Coffey R, Pembrey ME, Gagel RP, Telenius-Berg M, Semple P, et al: Risk estimation and screening in families of patients with medullary thyroid carcinoma. *Lancet* **1**:397, 1988.
55a. Berndt I, Reuter M, Saller B, Frank-Raue K, Groth P, Grussendorf M, Raue F, et al: A new hot spot for mutations in the *ret* protooncogene causing familial medullary thyroid carcinoma and multiple endocrine neoplasia. *J Clin Endocrinol Metab* **83**:770, 1998.
56. Mulligan LM, Gardner E, Smith BA, Mathew CGP, Ponder BAJ: Genetic events in tumor initiation and progression in multiple endocrine neoplasia. *Genes Chrom Cancer* **6**:166, 1993.
57. Moley JF, Brother MB, Fong CT, White PS, Baylin SB, Nelkin B, Wells SA, et al: Consistent association of 1p loss of heterozygosity with phaeochromocytomas from patients with multiple endocrine neoplasia type 2 syndromes. *Cancer Res* **52**:770, 1992.
58. Hanks SK, Quinn AM, Hunter T: The protein kinase family: Conserved features and deduced phylogeny of the catalytic domain. *Science* **241**:42, 1988.
59. Takahashi M, Cooper GM: *RET* fusion protein encodes a fusion protein homologous to tyrosine kinases. *Mol Cell Biol* **7**:1378, 1987.
60. Grieco M, Santoro M, Berlingieri MT, Melillo RM, Donghi R, Bonzgarzone I, Pierotti MA, et al: PTC is a novel rearranged form of the *RET* proto-oncogene and is frequently expressed in vivo in human papillary thyroid carcinomas. *Cell* **60**:557, 1990.
61. Bongarzone I, Monzini N, Borrello MG, Carcano C, Ferraresi G, Arighi E, Mondellini P, et al: Molecular characterisation of a thyroid fusion-sapecific transforming sequence formed by the fusion of *ret* tyrosine kinase and the regulatory subunit R1 of cyclic AMP-dependent protein kinase A. *Mol Cell Biol* **13**:358, 1993.
62. Santoro M, Dathan NA, Berlingieri MT, Bongarzone I, Paulin C, Grieco M, Pierotti MA, Vecchio G, Fusco A: Molecular characterisation of RET/PTC3, a novel rearranged version of the *RET* protooncogene in a human papillary thyroid carcinoma. *Oncogene* **9**:509, 1994.
63. Gardner E, Mullian LM, Eng C, Healey CS, Kwok JAJ, Ponder MA, Ponder BAJ: Haplotype analysis of MEN 2 mutations. *Hum Mol Genet* **3**:1771, 1994.
64. Mole SE, Mulligan LM, Healey CS, Ponder BAJ, Tunnacliffe A: Localisation of the gene for multiple endocrine neoplasia type 2A to a 480 kb region in chromosome band 10q11.2. *Hum Mol Genet* **2**:247, 1993.
65. Schuchardt A, D'Agati V, Larrson-Blomberg L, Constantini F, Pachnis V: The c-*ret* receptor tyrosine kinase gene is required for the development of the kidney and the enteric nervous systrem. *Nature* **367**:380, 1994.
66. Mulligan LM, Kwok JBJ, Healey CS, Elsdon M, Eng C, Gardner E, Love DR, et al: Germ-line mutations of the *RET* proto-oncogene in multiple endocrine neoplasia type 2A. *Nature* **363**:458, 1993.
67. Donis-Keller H, Dou S, Chi D, Carlson KM, Toshima K, Lairmore TC, Howe JR, et al: Mutations in the *RET* proto-oncogene are associated with MEN 2A and FMTC. *Hum Mol Genet* **2**:851, 1993.
68. Schuffenecker I, Billaud M, Calender A, Chambe B, Ginet N, Calmettes C, Modigliani E, et al: *RET* proto-oncogene mutations in French MEN 2A and FMTC families. *Hum Mol Genet* **3**:1939, 1994.

69. Carlson KM, Dou S, Chi D, Scavarda N, Toshima K, Jackson CE, Wells SA, et al: Single missense mutation in the tyrosine kinase catalytic domain of the *RET* protoncogene is associated with multiple endocrine neoplasia type 2B. *Proc Natl Acad Sci USA* **91**:1579, 1994.
70. Eng C, Smith DP, Mulligan LM, Nagai MA, Healey CS, Ponder MA, Gardner E, et al: Point mutation within the tyrosine kinase domain of the *RET* proto-oncogene in multiple endocrine neoplasia type 2B and related sporadic tumours. *Hum Mol Genet* **3**:237, 1994.
71. Hofstra RMW, Landsvater RM, Ceccherini I, Stulp RP, Stelwagen T, Luo Y, Pasini B, et al: A mutation in the *RET* proto-oncogene associated with multiple endocrine neoplasia type 2B and sporadic medullary thyroid carcinoma. *Nature* **367**:375, 1994.
72. Ceccherini I, Hofstra RMW, Luo Y, Stulp RP, Barone V, Stelwagen T, Bocciardi R, et al: DNA polymorphisms and conditions for SSCP analysis of the 20 exons of the *ret* proto-oncogene. *Oncogene* **9**:3025, 1994.
73. Kwok JBJ, Gardner E, Warner JP, Ponder BAJ, Mulligan LM: Structural analysis of the human *ret* proto-oncogene using exon trapping. *Oncogene* **8**:2575, 1993.
74. Myers SM, Eng C, Ponder BAJ, Mulligan LM: Characterisation of *ret* protooncogene 39 splicing variants and polyadenylation sites: A novel C terminus for *ret*. *Oncogene* **11**:2039, 1995.
75. Iwamoto I, Taniguchi M, Asai N, Ohkusu K, Nakashima I, Takahashi M: cDNA cloning of mouse *ret* proto-oncogene and its sequence similarity to the cadherin superfamily. *Oncogene* **8**:1087, 1993.
76. Sugaya R, Ishimaru S, Hosoya T, Saigo K, Emori Y: A *Drosophila* homology of human protooncogene *ret* transiently expressed in embryonic neuronal precursor cells including neuroblast and CNS cells. *Mech Dev* **45**:139, 1994.
77. Schneider R: The human protooncogene *ret:* A communicative cadherin? *Trends Biochem Sci* **17**:468, 1992.
78. Lorenzo MJ, Eng C, Mulligan LM, Stonehouse TJ, Healey CS, Ponder BAJ, Smith DP: Multiple mRNA isoforms of the human ret protooncogene generated by alternate splicing. *Oncogene* **10**:1377, 1995.
79. Takahashi M, Buma Y, Iwamoto T, Iwaguma Y, Ikeda H, Hiai H: Cloning and expression of the *ret* protooncogene encoding a tyrosine kinase with two potential transmembrane domains. *Oncogene* **3**:571, 1988.
80. Asai N, Iwashita T, Matsumama M, Takahashi M: Mechanism of activation of the *ret* protooncogene by multiple endocrine neoplasia type 2A mutations. *Mol Cell Biol* **15**:1613, 1995.
81. Liu LF-H, Doherty DH, Uke JD, Behtash S, Collins F: GDNF: A glial cell line-derived neurotrophic factor for mid-brain dopaminergic neurons. *Science* **260**:1130, 1993.
81a. Kotzbauer PT, Lampe PA, Heuckeroth RO, Golden JP, Creedon DJ, Johnson EMJ, et al: Neurturin, a relative of glial-cell-line-derived neurotrophic factor. *Nature* **384**:467, 1996.
81b. Milbrandt J, de Sauvage FJ, Fahrner TJ, Baloh RH, Leitner ML, Tansey MG: Persephin, a novel neurotrophic factor related to GDNF and neurturin. *Neuron* **20**:245, 1998.
81c. Buj-Bello A, Buchman VL, Horton A, Rosenthal A, Davies AM: GDNF is an age-specific survival factor for sensory and autonomic neurons. *Neuron* **15**:821, 1995.
81d. Trupp M, Ryden M, Jornvall H, Funakoshi H, Timmusk T, Arenas E, Ibanez CF: Peripheral expression and biological activities of GDNF, a new neurotrophic factor for avian and mammalian peripheral neurons. *J Cell Biol* **130**:137, 1995.
81e. Klein RD, Sherman D, Ho WH, Stone D, Bennett GL, Moffat B, Vandlen R, et al: A GPI-linked protein that interacts with *Ret* to form a candidate neurturin receptor. *Nature* **387**:717, 1997.
81f. Buj-Bello A, Adu J, Pinon LGP, Horton A, Thompson J, Rosenthal A, Chinchetru M, et al: Neurturin responsiveness requires a GPI-linked receptor plus the *Ret* receptor tyrosine kinase. *Nature* **387**:721, 1997.
81g. Trupp M, Raynoschek C, Belluardo N, Ibanez CF: Multiple GPI-anchored receptors control GDNF-dependent and independent activation of the c-*ret* receptor tyrosine kinase. *Mol Cell Neurosci* **11**:47, 1998.
81h. Enokido Y, de Sauvage F, Hongo J-A, Ninkina N, Rosenthal A, Buchman VL, Davies AM: GFRa-4 and the tyrosine kinase *Ret* form a functional receptor complex for persephin. *Curr Biol* **8**:1019, 1998.
82. Sanchez MP, Silos-Santiago I, Frisen J, He B, Lira SA, Barbacid M: Renal agenesis and the absence of enteric neurons in mice lacking GDNF. *Nature* **382**:70, 1996.
83. Pichel JG, Shen L, Sheng HZ, Granholm A-C, Drago J, Grinberg A, Lee EJ, et al: Defects in enteric innervation and kidney development in mice lacking GDNF. *Nature* **382**:73, 1996.
84. Treanor JS, Goodman L, de Sauvage F, Stone DM, Poulsen KT, Beck CD, Gray C, et al: Characterisation of a multicomponent receptor for GDNF. *Nature* **382**:80, 1996.
85. Jing S, Wen D, Yu Y, Holst PL, Luo Y, Fang M, Tamir R, et al: GDNF-induced activation of the *ret* protein tyrosine kinase is mediated by GDNF-α, a novel receptor for GDNF. *Cell* **85**:1113, 1996.
85a. Hoppner W, Ritter MM: A duplication of 12bp in the critical cysteine rich domain of the *ret* protooncogene results in a distinct phenotype of multiple endocrine neoplasia type 2A. *Hum Mol Genet* **6**:587, 1997.
86. Bolino A, Schuffenecker I, Luo Y, Seri M, Silengo M, Tocco T, Chabrier G, et al: RET mutations in exons 13 and 14 of FMTC patients. *Oncogene* **10**:2415, 1995.
87. Eng C, Smith DP, Mulligan LM, Healey CS, Zvelebil MJ, Stonehouse TJ, Ponder MA, et al: A novel point mutation in the tyrosine kinase domain of the *RET* proto-oncogene in sporadic medullary thyroid carcinoma and in a family with FMTC. *Oncogene* **10**:509, 1995.
87a. Eng C, Mulligan LM, Smith DP, Healey CS, Frilling A, Raue F, Neumann HPH, et al: Low frequency of germline mutations in the *ret* protooncogene in patients with apparently sporadic medullary thyroid carcinoma. *Clin Endocrinol* **43**:123, 1995.
88. Rossel M, Schuffenecker I, Schlumberger M, Bonnardel C, Modigliani E, Gardet P, Navarro J, et al: Detection of a germ line mutation at codon-918 of the *ret* protooncogene in French MEN 2B families. *Hum Genet* **95**:403, 1995.
89. Toogood AA, Eng C, Smith DP, Ponder BAJ, Shalet SM: No mutation at codon 918 of the *ret* gene in a family with multiple endocrine neoplasia type 2B. *Clin Endocrinol* **43**:759, 1995.
89a. Smith DP, Houghton C, Ponder BAJ: Germline mutation of RET codon 883 in two cases of *de novo* MEN 2B. *Oncogene* **15**:1213, 1997.
89b. Gimm O, Marsh DJ, Andrew SD, Frilling A, Dahia PLM, Mulligan LM, Zajac JD, et al: Germline dinucleotide mutation in codon 883 of the *RET* protoncogene in multiple endocrine neoplasia type 2B without codon 918 mutation. *J Clin Endocrinol Metab* **82**:3902, 1997.
90. Landsvater RM, Jansen RPM, Hofstra RMW, Buys CHCM, Lips CJM, Ploos van Amstel HK: Mutation analysis of the *ret* protooncogene in Dutch families with MEN 2 and FMTC. *Hum Genet* **97**:11, 1996.
90a. Decker RA, Peacock ML, Watson P: Hirschsprung disease in MEN 2A: Increased spectrum of *RET* exon genotypes and strong genotype-phenotype correlation. *Hum Mol Genet* **7**:129, 1998.
90b. Peretz H, Luboshitsky R, Baron E, Biton A, Gershoni R, Usher S, Grynberg E, et al: Cys 618 Arg mutation in the *RET* protooncogene associated with familial medullary thyroid carcinoma and maternally transmitted Hirschsprung disease suggesting a role for imprinting. *Hum Mutat* **10**:155, 1997.
90c. Romeo G, Ceccherini I, Celli J, Priolo M, Betsos N, Bonardi G, Seri M, Yin L, et al: Association of multiple endocrine neoplasia type 2A and Hirschsprung disease. *J Intern Med* **243**:515, 1998.
91. Le Douarin N: *The Neural Crest*. Cambridge, UK, Cambridge University Press, 1982.
92. Tamir H, Liu K-P, Playette RF, Hsuing S-C, Adlersberg M, Nurez EA, Gershon MD: *J Neurosci* **9**:1199, 1989.
93. Anderson DJ: Molecular control of cell fate in the neural crest: The sympathoadrenal lineage. *Annu Rev Neurosci* **16**:129, 1993.
94. Pachnis V, Maukoo B, Constantini F: Expression of the c-*ret* proto-oncogene during mouse embryogenesis. *Development* **119**:1005, 1993.
95. Tsuzuki T, Takahashi M, Asai N, Iwashita T, Matsuyene M, Asai J: Spatial and temporal expressio of the *ret* proto-oncogene product in embryonic, infant and adult rat tissues. *Oncogene* **10**:191, 1995.
96. Van der Geer P, Wiley S, Lai VK-M, Olivier JP, Gish GD, Stephens R, Kaplan D, et al: A conserved amino terminal shc domain binds to glycophosphotyrosine motifs in activated receptors and phosphopep-tides. *Curr Biol* **5**:404, 1995.
97. Durbec PL, Larsson-Blomberg WB, Schuchardt A, Constantini P, Pachnis V: Common origin and developmental dependence on c-*ret* of subsets of enteric and sympathetic neuroblasts. *Development* **122**:349, 1996.
98. Fabien N, Paulin C, Santoro M, Berger B, Grieco M: The *ret* protooncogene is expressed in normal human parafollicular thyroid cells. *Int J Oncol* **4**:623, 1994.
99. Santoro M, Rosati R, Grieco M, Berlinger M, D'Amato GLC, de Franciscis V, Fusco A: The *ret* proto-oncogene is consistently expressed in human pheochromocytoma and thyroid medullary carcinomas. *Oncogene* **5**:1595, 1990.

100. Miya A, Yamamoto M, Morimoto H, Tanaka N, Shin E, Karakawa K, Toyoshima K, et al: Expression of the *ret* proto-oncogene in human medullary thyroid carcinomas and pheochromocytomas of MEN 2A. *Henry Ford Hosp Med J* **40**:215, 1992.
101. Pawson T, Schlessinger J: SH2 and SH3 domains. *Curr Biol* **3**:434, 1993.
102. Borrello MG, Pelicci G, Arighi E, De Filippis L, Greco A, Bongarzone I, Rizzetti MG, et al: The oncogenic versions of the *Ret* and *Trk* tyrosine kinases bind Shc and Grb2 adaptor proteins. *Oncogene* **9**:1661, 1994.
103. Santoro M, Wong WT, Aroca P, Santos E, Matoskova B, Grieco M, Fusco A, Di Fiore PP: An epidermal growth factor receptor/ret chimera generates mitogenic and transforming signals: Evidence for a *ret*-specific signalling pathway. *Mol Cell Biol* **14**:663, 1994.
104. Pandey A, Duan H, Di Fiore PP, Dixit VM: The *ret* receptor protein tyrosine kinase associates with the SH2-containing adapter protein Grb10. *J Biol Chem* **270**:21461, 1995.
105. Santoro M, Carlomagno F, Romanova A, Bottaro DP, Dathan NA, Grieco M, Fusco A, et al: Activation of *RET* as a dominant transforming gene by germ line mutations of MEN 2A and MEN 2B. *Science* **267**:381, 1995.
106. Iwashita T, Asai N, Murakami H, Matsuyama M, Takahashi M: Identification of tyrosine residues that are essential for transforming activity of the *ret* proto-oncogene with MEN 2A or MEN 2B mutation. *Oncogene* **12**:481, 1996.
106a. Xing S, Furminger TL, Tong Q, Jhiang SM: Signal transduction pathways activated by *ret* oncoproteins in phaeochromocytoma cells. *J Biol Chem* **273**:4909, 1997.
106b. Durick K, Gill GN, Taylor S: Shc and Enigma are both required for mitogenic signalling by *ret/ptc2*. *Mol Cell Biol* **18**:2298,1998.
107. Van Weering DHJ, Medema JP, van Puijenbroek A, Burgering BMT, Baas PD, Bos JL: Ret receptor tyrosine kinase activates extracellular signal regulated kinase Z in SK-N-Mc cells. *Oncogene* **11**:2207, 1995.
108. Wada M, Asai N, Tsuzuki T, Maruyama S, Ohiwa M, Imai T, Funahashi H, et al: Detection of *ret* homodimers in MEN 2A associated phaeochromocytomas. *Biochem Biophys Res Commun* **218**:606, 1996.
108a. Carlomagno F, Salvatore G, Cirafici AM, DeVita G, Mellillo RM, de Franciscus V, Billaud M, et al: The different *ret* activating capability of mutations of cysteine 620 or cysteine 634 correlates with multiple endocrine neoplasia type 2 phenotype. *Cancer Res* **57**:391, 1997.
108b. Ito S, Iwashita T, Asai N, Mutakami H, Iwata Y, Sobue G, Takahashi M: Biological properties of *ret* with cysteine mutations correlate with multiple endocrine neoplasia type 2A, familial medullary thyroid carcinoma and Hirschsprungs disease phenotype. *Cancer Res* **57**:2870, 1997.
109. Songyang Z, Carraway KL III, Eck MJ, Harrison SC, Feldman RA, Mohammadi M, Schlessinger J, et al: Catalytic specificity of protein-tyrosine kinases is critical for selective signalling. *Nature* **373**:539, 1995.
110. Liu X, Vega QC, Decker RA, Plandey A, Worby CA, Dixon JE: Oncogenic *RET* receptors display different autophosphorylation sites and substrate binding specificities. *J Biol Chem* **271**:5309, 1996.
111. Baylin SB, Gann DS, Hsu SH: Clonal origin of inherited medullary thyroid carcinoma and phaeochromocytoma. *Science* **193**:321, 1976.
112. Moley JF, Brother MB, Wells SA, Spengler BA, Bredler JL, Brodeur GM: Low frequency of ras gene mutations in neuroblastomas, phaeochromocytomas and medullary thyroid cancers. *Cancer Res* **51**:1596, 1991.
113. Moley JF, Wallin GK, Brother MB, Kim M, Wells SA Jr, Brodeur GM: Oncogene and growth factor expression in MEN 2 and related tumours. *Henry Ford Hosp Med J* **40**:284, 1992.
114. Boultwood J, Wyllie FS, Williams GD, Wynford Thomas D: N-*myc* expression in neoplasia of human thyroid C cells. *Cancer Res* **48**:4073, 1988.
115. Zedenius J, Wallin G, Hamberger B, Nordenskjold M, Weber G, Larsson C: Somatic and MEN2A *de novo* mutations identified in the *ret* protooncogene by screening of sporadic MTCs. *Hum Mol Genet* **3**:1259, 1994.
115a. Shirahama S, Ogura K, Takami H, Itoh K, Tohsen T, Miyauchi A, Nakamura Y: Mutational analysis of the *RET* protooncogene in 71 Japanese patients with medullary thyroid carcinoma. *J Hum Genet* **43**:101, 1998.
115b. Jhiang SM, Fithian L, Weghorst CM, Clark OH, Falko JM, Odorisio TM, Mazzaferri EL: *Ret* mutation screening in MEN 2 patients and discovery of a novel mutation in a sporadic medullary thyroid carcinoma. *Thyroid* **6**:115, 1996.
115c. Ixalinin V, Frilling A: 27bp deletion in the ret protooncogene as a somatic mutation associated with medullary thyroid carcinoma. *J Mol Med* **76**:365, 1998.
115d. Romei C, Elisei R, Pinchera A, Ceccherini I, Molinari E, Mancusi F, Martino E, et al: Somatic mutations of the *ret* protooncogene in sporadic medullary thyroid carcinoma are not restricted to exon 16 and are associated with tumour recurrence. *J Clin Endocrinol Metab* **81**:1619, 1996.
116. Marsh DJ, Andrew SD, Learoyd DL, Pojer R, Eng C, Robinson BG: Deletion-insertion mutation encompassing *RET* codon 634 is associated with medullary thyroid carcinoma. *Hum Mutat* Suppl **1**:3, 1998.
117. Dou S, Chi D, Carlson KM, Moley JA, Wells SA Jr, Donis-Keller H: *RET* proto-oncogene mutations associated with sporadic cases of medullary thyroid carcinoma. *Fifth International Workshop on Multiple Endocrine Neoplasia, Karolinska Inst*, Stockholm, Sweden, 1994, p 3.
118. Beldjord C, Desclaux-Arramond F, Raffin-Sanson M, Corvol J-C, De Keyzer Y, Luton J-P, Plouin P-F, et al: The *ret* proto-oncogene in sporadic phaeochromocytomas: Frequent MEN 2-like mutations and new molecular defects. *J Clin Endocrinol Metab* **80**:2063, 1995.
119. Eng C, Crossey PA, Mulligan LM, Healey CS, Houghton C, Prowse A, Chew SL, et al: Mutations of the *ret* protooncogene and the Von Hippel-Lindau disease tumour suppressor gene in sporadic and syndromic phaeochromocytoma. *J Med Genet* **32:934, 1995.**
120. Komminoth P, Kunz EK, Matias-Guiu X, Hiort O, Christensen G, Colomer A, Rother J, et al: Analysis of *ret* protooncogene point mutations distinguishes heritable from non-heritable thyroid carcinomas. *Cancer* **76**:479, 1995.
121. Lindor NM, Honchel R, Khosla S, Thibodeau SN: Mutations in the *ret* plrotooncogene in sporadic phaeochromocytomas. *J Clin Endocrinol Metab* **80**:627, 1995.
122. Padberg BC, Schroder S, Jochum W, Kastendieck H, Roth J, Heitz PU, Komminoth P: Absence of *ret* protooncogene point mutations in sporadic hyperplastic and neoplastic lesions of the parathyroid gland. *Am J Pathol* **147**:1600, 1995.
122a. Hofstra RMW, Cheng NC, Hausen C, Stulp RP, Stelwagen T, Clausen N, Tommerup N, et al: No mutations found by *ret* screening in sporadic and hereditary neuroblastoma. *Hum Genet* **97**:362, 1996.
123. Eng C, Mulligan LM, Healey CS, Houghton C, Frilling A, Raue F, Thomas GA, et al: Heterogeneous mutation of the *RET* proto-oncogene in subpopulations of medullary thyroid carcinoma. *Cancer Res* **56**:2167, 1996.
124. Carson EB, McMahon M, Baylin SB, Nelkin BD: *Ret* gene silencing is associated with Raf-1-induced medullary thyroid carcinoma cell differentiation. *Cancer Res* **55**:2048, 1995.
125. Carlomagno F, Salvatore D, Santoro M, de Franciscis V, Quadro L, Panariello L, Colantuoni V, et al: Point mutation of the *RET* proto-oncogene in the TT human medullary thyroid carcinoma cell line. *Biochem Biophys Res Commun* **207**:1022, 1995.
126. Ponder BAJ: Medullary carcinoma of the thyroid, in Peckham M, Pinedo, Veronesi U (eds): *Oxford Textbook of Oncology*, vol 2. Oxford, UK, Oxford Medical Publications, 1996, p 2110.
127. Telenius-Berg M, Berg B, Hamberger B: Impact of screening on prognosis in the multiple endocrine neoplasia type 2 syndromes: Natural history and treatment results in 105 patients. *Henry Ford Hosp Med J* **32**:225, 1984.
128. Wells SA, Baylin SB, Leight GS, Dale JK, Dilley WG, Farndon JR: The importance of early diagnosis in patients with hereditary medullary thyroid carcinoma. *Ann Surg* **195**:595, 1982.
129. Malletta LE, Blewins T, Jordan PM, Noon GP: Autogenous parathyroid grafts for generalized primary parathyroid hyperplasia: Contrasting outcome in sporadic hyperplasia versus multiple endocrine neoplasia type 1. *Surgery* **101**:738, 1987.
130. Jansson S, Tisell LE, Fjalling M, Lindberg S, Jacobson L, Zacharison BF: Early diagnosis of and surgical strategy for adrenal medullary disease in MEN II gene carriers. *Surgery* **103**:11, 1988.
131. Vasen HFA, van der Feltz M, Raue F, Kruseman AN, Koppeschaar HPF, Pieters G, Seif FJ, et al: The natural course of multiple endocrine neoplasia type IIb. *Arch Intern Med* **251**:1250, 1992.
132. Samaan NA, Draznin MB, Halpin RE, Bloss RS, Hawkins E, Lewis RA: Multiple endocrine syndrome type IIb in early childhood. *Cancer* **68**:1832, 1991.

CHAPTER 43

Multiple Endocrine Neoplasia Type 1

Stephen J. Marx

1. **Multiple endocrine neoplasia type 1 (MEN1) is an autosomal dominant disorder with endocrine tumors of the parathyroids, the enteropancreatic neuroendocrine tissues, the anterior pituitary, and foregut carcinoid. Associated nonendocrine tumors include facial angiofibromas, skin collagenomas, and lipomas.**
2. **Most of the tumors are benign and produce symptoms and signs by oversecreting hormones (parathyroid hormone, gastrin, prolactin, etc.). Associated gastrinomas and foregut carcinoid tumors have a substantial malignant potential.**
3. **The most common endocrinopathy is primary hyperparathyroidism with several features different from features in sporadic parathyroid adenoma. Hyperparathyroidism in MEN1 is expressed earlier than in sporadic adenoma; 50 percent of gene carriers express it by ages 18 to 30. Most MEN1 patients have multiple parathyroid tumors and, after successful subtotal parathyroidectomy, have a high likelihood of late recurrence. Hyperparathyroidism can exacerbate the simultaneous Zollinger-Ellison syndrome in MEN1.**
4. **The *MEN1* gene was identified by positional cloning in 1997. Its sequence predicted a novel protein termed *menin*.**
5. ***MEN1* germ-line mutations have been found in over 80 percent of MEN1 families and in a similar fraction of patients with sporadic MEN1. Clinical use of germ-line *MEN1* mutation testing can give valuable information. It does not have the urgency of germ-line *RET* mutation testing for MEN2a or MEN2b.**
6. **Certain sporadic endocrine and nonendocrine tumors often show somatic *MEN1* mutation. In fact, *MEN1* is the known gene most commonly mutated in sporadic parathyroid adenoma, gastrinoma, insulinoma, and bronchial carcinoid tumor.**
7. ***MEN1* is likely a tumor-suppressor gene, since most MEN1 tumors and many sporadic endocrine tumors with *MEN1* mutation show inactivation (recognized as loss of heterozygosity) of the normal allele at 11q13, the *MEN1* locus.**
8. **The *MEN1*-encoded protein, menin, is mainly located in the nucleus. It binds to and inhibits junD, an AP1 transcription factor. It shows no protein homologies. Most germ-line or somatic *MEN1* mutations predict truncation of the menin protein and are thus likely to cause inactivation of menin function. Inactivation-type mutation further supports menin's predicted role as a tumor suppressor.**

A list of standard abbreviations is located immediately preceding the index in each volume. Nonstandard abbreviations used in this chapter include: MEN1 = multiple endocrine neoplasia type 1; MEN2 = multiple endocrine neoplasia type 2; Z-E = Zollinger-Ellison; BAO = basal acid output; MAO = maximal acid output; LOH = loss of heterozygosity.

DEFINITIONS AND HISTORY

Multiple endocrine neoplasia is a broad term that encompasses many distinct disorders. Literally interpreted, it includes all patients and families with endocrine neoplasia in more than one tissue type. Thus it includes patients with two coincidental endocrine neoplasms such as parathyroid adenoma and pituitary microadenoma, and it can include patients with a neoplasm that stimulates another tumor, such as pancreatic islet tumor secreting growth hormone-releasing hormone, which causes pituitary hyperplasia.

Within this broad definition, multiple endocrine neoplasia type 1 (MEN1) and multiple endocrine neoplasia type 2 (MEN2) stand out as occurring repeatedly in sporadic cases and also within families. The main endocrine expressions of MEN1 are parathyroid tumor, enteropancreatic neuroendocrine tumor, anterior pituitary tumor, and foregut carcinoid tumor. Nonendocrine expressions include lipoma, facial angiofibroma, and skin collagenoma (Table 43-1).

The first description of a patient with MEN1 is generally attributed to Erdheim.[1] He reported in 1903 the autopsy of a patient with acromegaly, pituitary adenoma, and four enlarged parathyroids. Familial transmission of MEN1 was established in 1953-1954 by Moldawar[2,3] and Wermer.[4] Subsequently, *Wermer's syndrome* has been an eponym for MEN1. With delineation of sporadic gastrinoma[5–7] and prolactinoma[8,9] as clinical entities in 1955 and 1971, respectively, they were almost simultaneously recognized as possible components of MEN1. In the 1970s and 1980s, knowledge about MEN1 advanced with the development of new and improved radioimmunoassays for hormones and other peptides. During this time, the clinical spectrum of MEN1 also changed with advances in pharmacology, such as acid secretion-blocking drugs for Zollinger-Ellison syndrome[10–13] and dopamine agonists for prolactinoma.[14] Important surgical advances also were made, beginning with total gastrectomy for Zollinger-Ellison syndrome through improved pituitary microsurgery and use of new pre- and intraoperative tumor imaging methods.[15–17,17b,17c]

The genetic etiology of MEN1 has been clarified only recently. Larsson *et al.*[18] showed in 1988 that the *MEN1* gene was likely a tumor-suppressor gene, based on MEN1 tumors showing loss of the normal allele from chromosome 11. At the same time, these authors reported tight genetic linkage of MEN1 to the *PYGM* locus at 11q13. The *MEN1* gene was identified in 1997.[19]

CLINICAL ASPECTS

Prevalence

There are no population-based studies of the prevalence of MEN1. Autopsy series have estimated a prevalence of 2.5 per 1000.[20,21] However, biochemical tests have suggested a prevalence of 0.01 to 0.175 per 1000.[22–25]

Table 43-1 Summary Features of Multiple Endocrine Neoplasia Type 1 with Estimated Average Penetrance (in Parentheses) among Patients Expressing the *MEN1* Gene

Endocrine Features	Nonendocrine Features
Parathyroid adenomas (90%)	Facial angiofibromas (85%)
Enteropancreatic tumor	Lipomas (30%)
Gastrinoma (40%)	Collagenomas (70%)
Insulinoma (10%)	Ependymoma (< 1%)
Pancreatic polypeptide or nonfunctioning (20%)*	
Other—glucagonoma, VIPoma, somatostatinoma, etc. (2%)	
Anterior pituitary tumor	
Prolactinoma (25%)	
Other—growth hormone/prolactin, growth hormone, ACTH, etc. (5%)	
Nonsecreting (10%)	
Foregut carcinoid tumor	
Thymic carcinoid (2%)	
Bronchial carcinoid (4%)	
Gastric enterochromaffin-like tumor (10%)	
Other tumor: adrenal cortex (5%), pheochromocytoma (< 1%)	

* Does not include near 100% prevalence of nonfunctioning and clinically silent tumors, which are detected incidental to pancreaticoduodenal surgery in MEN1.

An alternate estimate can be derived from the fraction of MEN1 among patients with evaluation for single-tissue endocrine tumor. Primary hyperparathyroidism is likely to be one main source of MEN1 case ascertainment; the fraction of MEN1 among patients with primary hyperparathyroidism has been estimated at 1 to 18 percent.[26] The cause for this variable fraction is not known, but selection bias is likely. The true fraction is probably 2 to 3 percent; this, combined with a population annual incidence of 0.5 per 1000 for primary hyperparathyroidism,[27] gives an estimate of MEN1 annual incidence of 0.015 per 1000.

Among patients with Zollinger-Ellison syndrome, the prevalence of MEN1 has been 16 to 38 percent, much higher than that of MEN1 among sporadic primary hyperparathyroidism.[25,28,29] Among patients with pituitary tumor, the prevalence of MEN1 has been 2.7 to 5 percent[30–32] but as high as 14 percent among prolactinoma patients.[32]

Familial versus Sporadic Cases

The majority of cases of MEN1 are familial. In a British series, there were 36 sporadic cases versus 220 familial cases among 62 families.[33] In our series (Marx et al., unpublished), there are 40 sporadic cases versus approximately 450 familial cases in 65 families. Sporadic cases, of course, may have unrecognized familial MEN1.

Diagnostic Criteria

Similar broad diagnostic criteria have been used informally by most groups.[19,33] MEN1 is usually defined as a patient with an endocrine tumor in two (not necessarily simultaneously) of the three major tissue systems (parathyroid, enteropancreatic neuroendocrine, and anterior pituitary). This is to say, carcinoid tumor, lipoma, facial angiofibroma, and certain other features (see Table 43-1) have not been used traditionally for ascertainment. *Familial* MEN1 is defined as a family that includes at least one patient with MEN1 and at least one first-degree relative with an endocrine tumor in one of the three principal MEN1-associated tissues. It is understood that these operational criteria will encompass, occasionally, several disorders that are not caused by *MEN1* mutation. Similarly, some, presumably small, kindreds with MEN1 will not meet these criteria.

Expressions of MEN1 by Tissue System

Benign and Malignant Neoplasia. An important feature of MEN1 is that most of its main expressions are determined by the hormone(s) that are oversecreted. Thus MEN1 is expressed mainly as hyperparathyroidism, Zollinger-Ellison (Z-E) syndrome, and hyperprolactinemia. The neoplasms in general are small and benign. Only the pituitary tumor, and much less commonly a pancreatic islet tumor, can produce clinical signs through a local mass effect. At the same time, MEN1 is a genuine familial cancer syndrome. Gastrinomas, thymic carcinoid, and bronchial carcinoid all are common expressions of MEN1 with a substantial malignant potential. Some less common expressions (see below) also have substantial malignant potential. Malignant enteropancreatic neuroendocrine tumor and malignant carcinoid account for one-third of deaths among MEN1 patients.[34]

Parathyroid Gland

Primary Hyperparathyroidism as the Most Common Endocrinopathy in MEN1. Primary hyperparathyroidism is the most common endocrine expression of MEN1,[35–41] with 87 to 100 percent prevalence among carriers expressing any endocrinopathy (see Table 43-1). Among obligate carriers of the *MEN1* gene, approximately 50 percent will express hyperparathyroidism by ages 18 to 25 and 90 percent by age 50.[33,39–41] Rare carriers do not express the trait at any age.[42] The prevalences for other endocrinopathies vary widely, depending largely on the methods to test the tissue.

Primary Hyperparathyroidism in MEN1 Differs from Sporadic Occurrences. Most features of primary hyperparathyroidism in MEN1 are similar to those in sporadic primary hyperparathyroidism.[24,33,43,44] These include a long early asymptomatic stage, generally low morbidity, and rapid amelioration after parathyroidectomy. Typical symptoms and signs include weakness, kidney stones, and back pain. Hypercalcemic crisis[45] or parathyroid cancer[46,47] is extremely rare, and one of two reported cancer cases[46] has been reinterpreted as not parathyroid cancer (JJ Shepherd, personal communication).

However, the hyperparathyroidism in MEN1 also has important differences from that in sporadic cases (Table 43-2). Primary hyperparathyroidism begins earlier in MEN1, with 50 percent of carriers expressing this by ages 18 to 25,[33,39–41] with recognition as early as age 8.[33] Clinically important primary hyperparathyroidism in MEN1 is rare before age 15. The female-to-male ratio is 1.0 in MEN1 versus 3.0 in sporadic hyperparathyroidism. It can cause osteopenia in young adults.[47b] Primary hyperparathyroidism can exacerbate Z-E syndrome (see below) in MEN1 (Fig. 43-1). This can influence a decision toward parathyroid surgery for this criterion, which is not relevant in sporadic hyperparathyroidism. On the other hand, because of excellent stomach acid control by antisecretory drugs, concommitant Z-E syndrome is usually not a sole indication for parathyroid surgery in MEN1.

Parathyroid gland clinical biology differs in MEN1 and sporadic cases. In sporadic cases there is usually a single benign parathyroid tumor (adenoma). In MEN1, multiple parathyroid glands are usually enlarged, and the enlargement is highly asymmetric.[48,49] These are multiple adenomas, not diffuse hyperplasia. Surgical outcomes differ in MEN1 from outcomes in sporadic cases. Because of the multiplicity of tumors and the associated occurrence of occasional tumor in unusual locations, postoperative persistence of hyperparathyroidism in MEN1 can be 40 to 60 percent with inexperienced surgeons[50] and as high as 10 percent with experienced surgeons.[49–52] The desire, in MEN1, to identify all four parathyroid glands and to remove all but part of one results in an increased rate of postoperative hypoparathyroidism, as high as 30 percent.[49,52,53] While rare in sporadic cases,[54] in MEN1, postoperative late recurrent primary hyperparathyroidism

Table 43-2 Distinguishing Features Among Three Categories of Primary Hyperparathyroidism

Feature	Sporadic Adenoma(s)	Multiple Endocrine Neoplasia Type 1	Familial Hypocalciuric Hypercalcemia
Percent of all hyperparathyroids	94	2	2
Heredity	Sporadic	Autos. dom.	Autos. dom.
Hypercalcemia onset age (year)	50–60	15–25	0 (at birth)
Sex ratio (F:M)	3:1	1:1	1:1
Calcium in urine	High	High	Normal to low
PTH in serum	High	High	Normal (15% high)
Endocrine tumors outside parathyroid	No	Often	No
Parathyroid gland pathology	Adenoma, often one	Adenoma, multiple	Hyperplasia, mild
Surgical result*			
Immediate cure (%)	95%	92%	Below 5%
Persistence (%)	5%	10%	Above 95%
Hypoparathyroidism (%)	2%	5%	2%
Late recurrence (%)	2%	Above 50%	NA†

*Surgical results are for patients with appropriate preoperative evaluation and with an experienced parathyroid surgeon. Hypoparathyroidism is not considered a "cure."

†NA = Not applicable, since virtually no operations lead to stable normocalcemia in familial hypocalciuric hypercalcemia.

reaches very high rates with time, 50 percent after 8 to 12 years.[50,51]

Enteropancreatic Neuroendocrine Tissues

Overview. As with parathyroid tumors, enteropancreatic neuroendocrine tumors develop at younger ages and in more sites (multiplicity) in MEN1 than in sporadic cases.[33,41] The enteropancreatic neuroendocrine tumors in MEN1 are virtually always multiple at the time of surgery.[55] Although primary hyperparathyroidism is usually present when the enteropancreatic neuroendocrine tumor expresses itself, in a small fraction of cases, Z-E syndrome or insulinoma can be expressed first.[56b]

The enteropancreatic neuroendocrine tumors in MEN1 usually present with symptoms of hormone release rather than symptoms of tumor expansion or metastasis.[56,57] In fact, such hormone-oversecreting tumors may be too small to be imaged.[57]

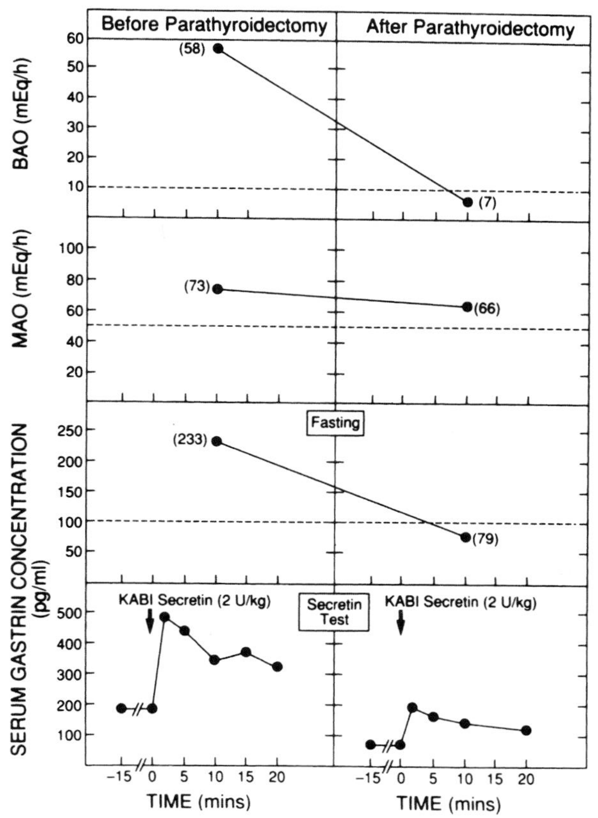

Fig. 43-1 The gastrin-gastric acid axis in a patient with MEN1 with Zollinger-Ellison syndrome, before and after normalization of serum calcium through parathyroidectomy. Successful parathyroidectomy caused remission in typical expressions of gastrinoma. Panels show BAO, MAO, and gastrin fasting or after intravenous secretin. Dashed lines are upper limits of normal, (*From Metz et al.*[60] Used with permission.)

Hormone Oversecretion and Storage in Tumors. Among the enteropancreatic neuroendocrine tumors in MEN1, gastrinoma is expressed most commonly at up to 54 percent.[45,57–59] Insulinoma is expressed second most commonly in MEN1, as often as 21 percent.[45,57] Glucagonoma, VIPoma, growth hormone-releasing factor-secreting tumor, intestinal carcinoid, and somatostatinoma each have been much less frequent (see Table 43-1). Furthermore, MEN1 patients can express more than one enteropancreatic neuroendocrine tumor. Conversely, MEN1 occurs in approximately 20 percent of patients with Z-E syndrome, 4 percent with insulinoma, and 33 percent with GRFoma.[60]

Nonfunctional endocrine tumors are a major component of MEN1. Although only one tumor may hypersecrete a hormone and cause symptoms and signs, typically there are many associated pancreatic islet tumors. While these may synthesize hormonal peptides, they do not oversecrete them. Still they have the potential to cause subsequent oversecretion and/or cancer.[61]

Histologic evaluations of the MEN1 pancreas from surgical specimens have shown multiple tumors in about 50 percent,[55,62,63] but diffuse micronodules (diameter 0.5 cm) have been found in all.[62] The rates of positivity of immunostaining in 201 macro- or micronodules were pancreatic polypeptide (26 percent), glucagon (24 percent), insulin (23 percent), gastrin (4 percent), and no hormone (18 percent)[48]; this study was done before recognition of the frequent extrapancreatic locations of gastrinomas in MEN1.[57,62] There do not appear to be important components of diffuse islet hyperplasia or nesidioblastosis (islets budding from ducts) in the MEN1 pancreas.

Gastrinoma. Z-E syndrome is a symptom complex resulting from gastrinomas. Gastrinomas originate in the pancreatic islets or proximal duodenum.[6,64–66] The initial syndrome was the triad of (1) non-beta islet cell tumor of the pancreas, (2) gastric acid hypersecretion, and (3) severe peptic ulcers of the stomach and small intestine. With increasing awareness of the disease, and with ready availability of acid-blocking drugs, the disease is now seen in milder and different forms (see below).[58,59,67] All the usual features of Z-E syndrome result from gastrin's ability to stimulate secretion of acid from the stomach.

Gastrinomas in sporadic and familial MEN1 are mostly in the "gastrinoma triangle," the duodenum or pacreatic head.[57–59,64,68–71] The specific distribution (concentrated in the duodenum) of MEN1 gastrinomas within this zone may differ from that of sporadic gastrinomas, of which 40 to 80 percent occur in the pancreas.[59,65,69,70,72] Furthermore, while most sporadic gastrinomas are solitary and large, those in MEN1 are often multiple, small, and submucosal.[64] Gastrinoma in MEN1 versus sporadic has been suggested to have lesser[59,65,73] or similar malignant propensity.[59,65,74,75] "Milder" malignancy can be an artefact from earlier ascertainment age; however, it is clear that metastases can occur,[58,64,75] and they can dominate the clinical picture.[76–78]

Many gastrinomas in MEN1 occur after age 40.[33,57,59,65] Abdominal pain is the most common symptom, and symptoms of gastrointestinal (GI) reflux occur in up to two-thirds of patients. Some patients do not show these symptoms despite high acid output.[60] Diarrhea can be associated; in 10 to 30 percent of patients it is the sole symptom or sign. The diarrhea is a direct consequence of acid oversecretion with associated (1) high fluid secretion into bowel, (2) inactivation of pancreatic enzymes, and (3) mucosal ulceration.[58,59,76,79,80] Whereas atypical ulcer location was once common in Z-E syndrome, current practices recognize most ulcers in locations similar to locations with idiopathic peptic disease.[58,59]

Gastrinoma should be evaluated in any MEN1 patient with the symptoms listed above. Furthermore, fasting gastrin should be measured periodically in asymptomatic MEN1 patients older than age 20. The most useful tests for diagnosis are acid output, fasting gastrin, and stimulated gastrin. Endoscopy, because of widespread availability, is often used as a substitute for acid measurements. This is not optimal.

The upper limit for basal acid output (BAO) in the absence of acid-reducing surgery is 15 meq/h for both genders.[58,59,81] This criterion alone is insufficient for diagnosis of Z-E syndrome. There are many false positives (such as some cases of idiopathic peptic disease, a much more common disorder)[58,59] and some false negatives (exemplified by the postparathyroidectomy state)[82] (see Fig. 43-1). Maximal acid output (MAO) after subcutaneous pentagastrin (6 mg/kg) correlates with parietal cell mass.[57,58,68] However, the variability of this response and of the BAO/MAO ratio give them little diagnostic use.[58,59,76,79] Documentation of fasting gastric pH above 3.0 in a patient not taking acid-blocking medications can exclude Z-E syndrome. In a patient with hypergastrinemia, this can establish hypo- or achlorhydria (Table 43-3).

The clinical diagnosis of gastrinoma depends on documentation of dysregulated hypersecretion of gastrin. Virtually all cases have high fasting gastrin levels.[76,77] With the widespread use of acid-blocking drugs, drug-induced hypergastrinemia has become the most common condition to exclude[85] (see Table 43-3). Another consideration is hypochlorhydria, which is very common among patients with sporadic primary hyperparathyroidism (both states are concentrated among women beyond age 50). Another consideration specific to MEN1 is the interaction of gastrinoma and hyperparathyroidism. Z-E syndrome can diminish or even enter remission after successful parathyroidectomy[85] (see Fig. 43-1). It is not known if parathyroidectomy slows the growth of the gastrinomas.

Two separate gastrin measurements should be made because values can fluctuate. Most cases of Z-E syndrome show a gastrin level above 1000 pg/ml, more than 10-fold above the upper limit of normal. With gastric acid below 3.0, the diagnosis is established. When the diagnosis is uncertain, provocative testing for hypergastrinemia should be done. Stimulants have included secretin, calcium infusion, and a standardized meal. The most effective stimulus is secretin. The criterion for an abnormal response is a positive change of serum gastrin greater than 200 pg/ml.[58,59,86]

Once the diagnosis has been established, management must combine acid control, which may be accomplished pharmacologically, and tumor evaluation. The mainstay of tumor evaluation is imaging with radioactive octreotide. This agent is usually effective in distinguishing local from metastatic gastrinoma.[87–89]

Insulinoma. Insulinoma is expressed in 10 to 20 percent of patients with familial MEN1.[37,90] Onset has been as early as age 6 years. Mean age of onset is younger in MEN1 than in sporadic cases (age 30 versus 45 years).[33,41] Although they are associated with multiple islet tumors, their high surgical cure rate suggests that (1) the insulinoma syndrome in MEN1 usually results from one hypersecreting adenoma, and (2) the adenoma is usually large and often the largest islet tumor in that patient.[91–93]

The most common expression of insulinoma is neuroglycopenia, often worst on fasting and relieved by eating sweets. Once suspected, hypoglycemia should be documented during symptoms and during fasting. Other possible etiologies should be excluded, including prescribed medications, surreptitious use of hypoglycemic agents, wasting, hypoadrenalism, and growth hormone deficiency (in children). The most reliable test is a supervised fast. Most patients show hypoglycemia (sugar 40 mg/dl) and neuroglycopenic symptoms by 48 h, but apparently negative tests should be carried to 72 h. Glucose, insulin, C-peptide, and proinsulin fraction should be measured at the time of hypoglycemia.[94] The single most useful indicator is an insulin concentration above 6 mU/ml at the time of hypoglycemia. This establishes insulin mediation of hypoglycemia; however, it does not exclude surreptitious use of insulin or sulfonylureas or hypoglycemia caused by antibodies against the insulin receptor.

Treatment of insulinoma in MEN1 is surgery. Insulinoma in MEN1 is usually benign. Failed initial operation was common in the past.[95] Because of the frequent association with multiple nonfunctioning islet tumors, it is desirable to identify the approximate location of insulin hypersecretion before resection. This can be done most effectively by selective arteriography with calcium infusion.[96] Transhepatic venous sampling has high yield, but it is not widely available, and it has substantial potential for morbidity.[97] Individual tumors are often small and are best localized with intraoperative ultrasound.[15,98] Noninvasive imaging methods, including octreotide radionuclide scanning, have low sensitivity for insulinoma, based on experience with sporadic insulinoma.[97] Approximately 15 percent of MEN1 insulinomas recur late after surgery; this could reflect insulinoma malignancy,

Table 43-3 Causes of Fasting Hypergastrinemia

With Deficient Gastric Acid Production	With Gastric Acid Production
Medications	Retained gastric antrum syndrome
Histamine H_2-receptor antagonists	Small bowel resection
Blockers of stomach acid pump	Chronic gastric outlet obstruction
Atrophic gastritis (includes pernicious anemia)	Antral G-cell hyperplasia or hyperfunction
Chronic renal failure	Gastrinoma
Postvagotomy/gastric resection	Laboratory error

benign insulinoma resected incompletely, or an independently arising insulinoma.

Glucagonoma. Glucagonomas are islet tumors causing a syndrome of a specific dermatitis, weight loss, glucose intolerance, and anemia.[99–101] The specific skin rash is termed *migratory necrolytic erythema.*[102,103] Glucagonoma is rare in MEN1 (3 percent), and glucagonoma patients rarely have MEN1. Most tumours occur after age 40. They are usually in the pancreatic body or tail and large at presentation,[98,103] with 50 to 80 percent showing metastases at presentation.[100,101] Glucose intolerance characteristically predates recognition of glucagonoma by 5 years.[101] Glucose intolerance in MEN1 is more often idiopathic or secondary to Cushing syndrome.

VIPoma. VIPomas are enteropancreatic neuroendocrine tumors that oversecrete vasoactive intestinal protein (VIP). They cause severe watery diarrhea ("pancreatic cholera," a misnomer), hypokalemia, and hypochlorhydria.[105–109] This is sometimes called *Verner-Morrison syndrome* and sometimes called *WDHA syndrome,* for watery diarrhea, hypokalemia, and achlorhydria. Over 80 percent are in the pancreas,[110,111] but several occur in intestinal carcinoid or pheochromocytoma.[112] In children (age 2–4 years), the tumor is usually an extrapancreatic ganglioneuroma or ganglioneuroblastoma[111] and is not associated with MEN1. Just as glucagonomas, VIPomas in adults present usually after age 40 and are usually large and metastatic. Associated hypercalcemia in up to 50 percent of patients may be caused by tumor secretion of parathyroid hormone-related peptide, but in MEN1 this must be distinguished from associated primary hyperparathyroidism.

GRFoma. Growth hormone-releasing factor (GRF or GHRH) can be oversecreted by a tumor, a GRFoma. This is a rare tumor that stimulates the pituitary to release excessive growth hormone.[113,114] Approximately one-third of GRFomas are associated with MEN1.[115–117] GRFomas occur in the lung (53 percent), pancreas (30 percent), or small intestine (10 percent). They are often large and metastatic at presentation.[115,118] GRF is a 44-amino-acid peptide. Its oversecretion results in somatotroph hyperplasia and growth hormone excess. Most cases of growth hormone excess (with or without MEN1) are caused by primary tumor of the pituitary. GRFoma is diagnosed by finding growth hormone excess and high blood levels of GRF.

Somatostatinoma. Somatostatin-secreting tumor causes a syndrome of mild diabetes mellitus, gall bladder disease, weight loss, and anemia.[119,120] There is a frequent association of this rare tumor with MEN1 or with MEN2, but its prevalence in an MEN1 population seems very low. Most somatostatinomas are in the pancreatic head.[121,122] Fewer are in the proximal duodenum or ampulla of Vater. At presentation, most are large and metastatic. Commonly, somatostatin is the "second" hormone secreted by the tumor.[122] Somatostatin is a 14-amino-acid peptide with multiple inhibitory effects on the GI tract. It inhibits release of many hormones, including insulin, gastrin, and growth hormone. It decreases stomach acid secretion; decreases bile flow and gall bladder contractility; decreases pancreatic enzyme and fluid secretion; and decreases absorption of lipid, D-xylose, vitamin B_{12}, and folate.[123] All these actions contribute to its presentations.

PPomas and Nonfunctional Pancreatic Endocrine Tumors. PPomas are pancreatic tumors that oversecrete pancreatic polypeptide but do not cause a recognizable syndrome.[55,124–128] Nonfunctional tumors may or may not produce a hormonal peptide, but they do not secrete enough to cause a recognizable syndrome.[57,121,126] Nonfunctional tumors or PPomas, if they cause symptoms, do so by local or metastatic growth. They are among the most common tumors in MEN1,[45,55,61,127] but because they do not cause endocrine symptoms, they have received limited attention.[61] The finding of multiple pancreatic islet tumors is a strong predictor of MEN1.[61–63] If these tumors cause symptoms through growth, they are usually in the pancreatic head, large, and malignant.

Carcinoid Tumor of Bronchus or Thymus. Carcinoid tumors occur in derivatives of foregut, midgut, or hindgut. Carcinoid tumor in MEN1 is in foregut derivatives (bronchi, thymus, stomach, pancreas, duodenum).[129] This contrasts with sporadic carcinoid, which is predominantly hindgut in origin.[130] Unlike the equal sex distribution of sporadic bronchial carcinoid, female sex predominates by 4:1 in MEN1. Thymic carcinoids are 90 percent male in sporadic cases as well as in MEN1.[129]

Common presentations of mediastinal carcinoid in MEN1 are through mass effect, incidental to chest imaging, or incidental to prophylactic thymectomy (for primary hyperparathyroidism in MEN1). Carcinoid tumors of the bronchus or thymus in MEN1 rarely cause the carcinoid syndrome or secrete serotonin. They occasionally oversecrete histamine, which is converted to 5-hydroxyindoleacetic acid and measurable in urine. Occasionally, they cause an atypical carcinoid syndrome with facial flushing, lacrimation, headache, and bronchoconstriction; the biochemical cause is not known. Bronchial and thymic carcinoid can oversecrete endocrine peptides including ACTH,[132,133] GHRH,[134] calcitonin, and others. Sporadic carcinoid tumors are often malignant, and this also has been found in thymic carcinoid in MEN1.[131]

Gastric ECLomas. Histamine-secreting enterochromaffin-like cells (ECL cells) are prominent among the endocrine cells of the human gastric oxyntic mucosa. In sporadic cases they produce tumors unrelated to hypergastrinemia. In MEN1, these ECLomas (also termed *gastric carcinoids*) are associated with hypergastrinemia.[135–137] It is thought that hypergastrinemia is associated with ECL cell stimulation. This has been seen in animal models and in pernicious anemia. However, ECLomas are uncommon in association with sporadic gastrinoma.[65,135,136] Gastric ECLomas have no associated hormonal syndrome, and their natural history is unknown. They have been recognized in up to 15 percent of MEN1 patients incidental to endoscopies for gastrinoma.[138] Their malignant potential in MEN1 may be substantial.[139]

GI Tract Carcinoid Tumor. Carcinoid tumors are structurally indistinguishable from other enteropancreatic neuroendocrine tumors; thus the term *carcinoid tumor* has sometimes been applied to all these tumors.[57,65] Carcinoid of the midgut or hindgut is somewhat common in the general population, but there seems to be no real association of these latter carcinoids with MEN1. The non-MEN1 carcinoid of the terminal ileum often metastasizes to the liver, secretes serotonin, and can cause the carcinoid syndrome.[58,130,140]

Carcinoid Tumor Syndrome. Carcinoid tumors can secrete a variety of bioactive peptides and small molecules.[58,130,140] Carcinoid tumor syndrome is a complex thought to result from these products. It includes episodes of flushing, diarrhea, abdominal cramping, wheezing, dyspnea, and palpitations. Blood pressure falls rather than rises. It usually arises when a midgut carcinoid tumor metastasizes to the liver. It can arise from bronchial carcinoid without metastases. Most foregut carcinoids in MEN1 do not produce this syndrome.

Anterior Pituitary Tumor

Symptoms and signs of pituitary tumor are evident in 10 to 30 percent of symptomatic MEN1 patients. The symptoms and signs of pituitary tumor have age, sex, and hormone distributions (MEN1 shows some enrichment for prolactin[32]) similar to those in tumors not associated with MEN1.[33,38,41] The sex ratio favors women because the majority of tumors are prolactinomas (40–75 percent), with approximately 10 percent secreting prolactin and growth hormone, 10 percent growth hormone only, and 5 percent

ACTH.[140] Oversecretion of luteinizing hormone/follicle-stimulating hormone (LH/FSH) or thyroid-stimulating hormone (TSH) are even less common. Five percent are hormone nonsecreting and important because they present by mass effect (hypopituitarism, pituitary apoplexy, visual compromise).

Aside from mass effect, prolactinoma is recognized as galactorrhea, amenorrhea, and/or infertility in women. Hypogonadism may occur in men. Biochemical diagnosis depends mainly on a fasting prolactin level above 300 ng/ml (upper normal about 12 ng/ml). Milder elevations occur too but are hard to distinguish from loss of inhibition through stalk compression. Imaging is a useful supplement for diagnosis and management. Excellent images can be obtained with gadolinium-enhanced magnetic resonance imaging (MRI). As for prolactinoma, the features of other hormone-secreting pituitary tumors are similar in MEN1 and sporadic cases.

Other Tissue Features of MEN1

Thyroid Neoplasms. Thyroid follicular adenoma has long been recognized as an occasional association in MEN1,[36] but no detailed analysis has established a significant connection.

Primary Adrenocortical Neoplasms. Rare patients with MEN1 have shown hypercortisolism or hyperaldosteronism.[36,95,142] Analyses of adrenal cortical enlargement in MEN1 indicated frequent silent enlargement in 30 to 40 percent.[142] Adrenocortical cancer has been reported.[143]

Pheochromocytoma. Unilateral pheochromocytoma has been encountered in 7 cases of familial MEN1.[144b] However, tumor documentation has so far been incomplete in each. All the same, it seems likely that this is a true but uncommon feature of MEN1.

Lipoma. While a common neoplasm, lipoma is especially common in MEN1, at 20 to 30 percent of patients.[36,145] Lipomas may occur anywhere, single or multiple. Large visceral lipomas can be noted by imaging or at laparotomy.

Skin Lesions. One survey of 32 MEN1 patients showed multiple facial angiofibromas in 88 percent.[145] These were clinically and histologically identical to the lesions in tuberous sclerosis. Another highly specific finding was collagenomas in 72 percent. Confetti-like hypopigmented macules (6 percent) and multiple gingival papules (6 percent) were other findings that previously had been associated with tuberous sclerosis.

Intrafamilial Homogeneity of MEN1

Prolactinoma Variant. One or two unusual expressions of MEN1 sometimes occur in a small kindred, such as a kindred with hyperparathyoridism, two cases of Cushing's disease, and no enteropancreatic tumor.[146] Such associations may be rare and random events. Ideally, large kindreds are preferred for efforts to recognize an unusual phenotype. Three large MEN1 kindreds (9–83 affected members) have shown a high frequency of prolactinoma (35–65 percent) but a low frequency of gastrinoma (2.5–11 percent).[147–151] The largest family also showed 14 percent carcinoid tumors.[151] The trait in these families has been termed the *prolactinoma variant* of MEN1, with $MEN1_{Burin}$ applied to the similar subfamilies about the Burin peninsula of Newfoundland.

In an extraordinarily large MEN1 pedigree from Tasmania, prolactinoma was found commonly (50 percent) in two branches but uncommonly in others. Although gastrinoma was not included in the analysis, the observations were used to suggest that the "prolactinoma phenotype" required a second mutation other than that causing MEN1.[152]

Other Possible Variants of MEN1

Hyperparathyroidism Variant. Several kindreds, reported initially as isolated familial hyperparathyroidism, subsequently expressed features of MEN1.[37] One large kindred showed only minimal features of MEN1 on follow-up.[37,153] Another large kindred showed likely linkage to 11q13 with a LOD (Logarithm of the odds) score of 2.1 and no other features of MEN1.[154] There are types of familial primary hyperparathyroidism not caused by the *MEN1* gene (see below). It is not yet known if *MEN1* mutation can cause a stable phenotype of isolated hyperparathyroidism.

Insulinoma Variant. Several MEN1 kindreds showed disproportional prevalence of insulinoma with little gastrinoma.[37,39]

Cancer Variant. Most gastrinomas are multiple in MEN1.[64] A high, though undetermined, fraction have metastasized by the time they cause symptoms. In some kindreds, gastrinomas have seemed particularly aggressive.[39] In one large kindred, there was clustering of enteropancreatic malignancy cases, suggesting that modifiers determined penetrance of this *MEN1* expression.[155] This question requires additional study.

Earliest Penetrance by Organ

In general, expression of MEN1 begins with slowly developing hyperparathyroidism between the ages of 15 and 30 years. In planning biochemical and genetic screening programs, it is helpful to know about frequency and severity of very early expressions. There is little information on these points. The earliest reported expressions in MEN1 have been as follows: primary hyperparathyroidism at age 8,[33] prolactinoma at age 5,[156] and insulinoma at age 6.[56b]

TREATMENT OF MEN1

Treatment of the multiple expressions of MEN1 is not covered here. Suffice it to say that treatment can be complex and expensive. In general, each hormone-oversecreting tumor must be handled as an independent disorder requiring pharmacologic or surgical management.[158] Mild expressions (such as mild hyperparathyroidism) may only require periodic monitoring, whereas malignant expressions may prove refractory to most measures.

DIFFERENTIAL DIAGNOSIS

As pleiomorphic as it is, MEN1 has a potentially long list of conditions from which it must be distinguished. Conditions to be covered here are those which are the most relevant clinically and also those which may have special relevance with regard to understanding the metabolic pathway disturbed in MEN1.

Sporadic Multiple Endocrine Neoplasia

Any combination of endocrine neoplasia in more than one tissue is multiple endocrine neoplasia. Some such cases may be expressions of *MEN1* germ-line mutation. Some others could be termed *MEN1 phenocopies*.

Pancreatic islet tumors can cause secondary endocrine tumors when the primary pancreatic tumor secretes "ectopically" ACTH[159,160] or growth hormone-releasing hormone.[161]

Some reports, based on single cases, are probably random coincidences.[162] There has been an association between primary hyperparathyroidism and nonmedullary thyroid cancer,[163,164] perhaps independent of the association attributable to radiation (see below). There have been other endocrine tumors with prolactinoma[165–168] or with acromegaly.[169,170] Some of the more intriguing cases have combined components of MEN1 and MEN2 within a single patient.[170–182]

A relation between radiation and thyroid neoplasia has been long recognized.[183,184] More recently, a relation between radiation and parathyroid neoplasia also has been recognized. Parathyroid and thyroid neoplasia, when they coexist, are often a consequence of prior radiation exposure.[184–193] The thyroid neoplasms may be uni- or multifocal and benign or malignant; the parathyroid tumors are almost always benign and sometimes multiple.

Table 43-4 Syndromes of Hereditary Endocrine Neoplasia with Proven or Presumed Clonal Basis for Tumors*

Multiple Endocrine Neoplasia	Single Endocrine Neoplasia in Syndrome of Multiple Neoplasia	Isolated Endocrine Neoplasia
Multiple endocrine neoplasia type1	Hyperparathyroidism–jaw tumor syndrome	Hyperparathyroidism
Multiple endocrine neoplasia type 2a and type 2b	Cowden syndrome	Pituitary tumor
Von Hippel-Lindau syndrome	Neurofibromatosis type 1	Insulinoma
Carney complex	Li-Fraumeni syndrome	Carcinoid
McCune-Albright syndrome*	Tuberous sclerosis	Thyroid oxyphil

* Fibrous dysplasia in McCune-Albright syndrome is likely a mosaic proliferation that includes the clonal mutation.[197] This may not be neoplastic and has not been tested in other pathologic tissues in this syndrome.

Hereditary Endocrine Neoplasia

There is a spectrum of hereditary endocrine neoplasias (Table 43-4). However, MEN1 is the only one for which endocrine/metabolic hyperfunctions are the principal manifestation.

Disorders Affecting Multiple Endocrine Organs

McCune-Albright Syndrome. The McCune-Albright syndrome combines features of sporadic and hereditary neoplasia. The McCune-Albright syndrome is a complex of polyostotic fibrous dysplasia, café-au-lait skin pigmentation, and any among the following endocrine disorders: sexual precocity, hyperthyroidism, growth hormone oversecretion, and adrenal hyperfunction.[194] This is usually caused by an activating mutation in Gs-α, a subunit of the stimulatory G-protein involved in signal transduction.[195] The mutation is apparently lethal in the germ line, but it can occur early in ontogeny so that the carrier is a mosaic. The mutation appears to cause tumor in tissues where overproduction of cyclic AMP leads to cell proliferation.[196] Fibrous dysplasia of bone, which is not clearly neoplastic, is composed of a mixture of cells with mutated *Gsα* and cells without mutated *Gsα* in this syndrome.[197]

Multiple Endocrine Neoplasia Type 2. MEN2[198] consists of neoplasms of thyroid C-cells, adrenal medulla, and parathyroid. A distinct, more morbid variant, MEN2b, has low penetrance for parathyroid tumors but has ganglioneuromas, submucosal neuromas, and a marfanoid habitus. MEN2 is caused usually or always by mutation of the *RET* gene on chromosome 10. It encodes the catalytic subunit of a membrane-bound tyrosine kinase whose normal ligands include glial cell-derived growth factor and nurturin. The mutations in MEN2 are in focused regions of the *RET* gene, and all are believed to be activating mutations. Because MEN2 rarely presents as hyperparathyroidism alone,[199] MEN2 is not difficult to distinguish from MEN1.

Carney Complex. Carney complex is a rare autosomal dominant complex of myxomas (cardiac, cutaneous, and breast), pigmented skin lesions, and endocrine tumors.[200,201] The endocrinopathies include pigmented bilateral adrenal lesions (often cortisol hypersecreting), acromegaly, Sertoli or Leydig cell tumor of testis, and thyroid neoplasms.[202] The disorder is usually but not linked to chromosome 2p or to 17q.[203,204]

Von Hippel-Lindau Syndrome. This disorder is characterized by hemangioblastoma of the central nervous system (CNS), retinal angiomatosis, renal clear cell carcinoma, visceral cysts, and pheochromocytoma.[205] Pancreatic cysts and pancreatic islet cell tumors are associated. The islet cell tumors occur in 10 percent, are usually nonfunctional, and can be benign or malignant.[206] Patients with this disease also rarely show other endocrine tumor such as carcinoid, prolactinoma, and medullary thyroid cancer.[207] The *VHL* gene functions by a tumor-suppressor mechanism, is at chromosome 3p, and has been cloned.[208] It encodes a protein that may interact with several other proteins important in the cell cycle.[209]

Hereditary Disorders Affecting One Endocrine Organ (Likely Clonal)

Cloned Tumor-Suppressor Genes with Endocrine Tumor as a Minor Feature. Li-Fraumeni syndrome (*p53* inactivating mutations) can be expressed as many types of cancer. Adrenal cancer occurs in about 1 percent of patients with the Li-Fraumeni syndrome.[210]

Cowden syndrome (*PTEN* inactivating mutations) is expressed most often as breast cancer and hamartomas. Thyroid neoplasia is seen in some 50 percent of patients with Cowden syndrome (about 20 percent of the thyroid neoplasms are malignant).[211]

Neurofibromatosis type 1 causes neural disturbances including café-au-lait spots, neurofibromas, benign and malignant tumors of the nervous system, Lisch nodules of the iris, and mental retardation.[212] Pheochromocytoma occurs in about 1 percent. Hyperparathyroidism, usually a single adenoma, has been associated at least 11 times.[213] It is unclear if this is a random association; 17q loss of heterozygosity (LOH) analysis in parathyroid tumors could clarify this question. Rare associations include duodenal somatostatinoma[214] and adrenocortical adenoma.[215,216] The *NF1* gene is on 17q, functions as a tumor suppressor, and has been cloned.[217] It encodes a protein, neurofibromin, with a GTPase activating protein-like domain that down-regulates GTP-bound ras.

Familial Hyperparathyroidism and Jaw Tumors. About 20 families have been described with parathyroid tumors and fibroosseus jaw tumors.[218] The parathyroid tumors sometimes have a micro- or macrocystic appearance.[219] Parathyroid cancer also has occurred in 10% of these cases. Other features clearly associated in one large family are Kidney cysts, Wilms tumor, and nephroblastoma.[220] The trait in most of these families has been linked to chromosome 1q21-32, and there was LOH about this locus in renal hamartomas and in parathyroid tumors, suggesting cause by a tumor-suppressor gene at this locus.[220–222] Two large families with autosomal dominant hyperparathyroidism plus parathyroid cancer[223,224] may express this disorder but were not originally tested for linkage to chromosome 1q.

Isolated Hyperparathyroidism. Isolated familial hyperparathyroidism has been described in many, mostly small kindreds. Some undoubtedly have MEN1,[37] others have familial hypocalciuric hypercalcemia (see below), few likely have the hyperparathyroidism–jaw tumor syndrome, while others probably have still different disorders. Most transmission patterns have been consistent with autosomal dominant transmission, with one suggesting a recessive mode.[225] Unusual features in some families have been early age of onset, severe hypercalcemia, and occasionally tumor of one parathyroid gland.[226,227] In one report, three or four tumors representing different kindreds showed LOH at chromosome 13q, raising the possibility of germ-line mutation in a tumor-suppressor gene in that region.[228]

Isolated Pancreatic Islet Tumors. There are two reports of familial insulinoma without other endocrinopathy.[229,230] In each kindred, this was seen in a father and a daughter.

Isolated Pituitary Tumors. Acromegaly alone has been seen in several families.[231,232] Haplotype and tumor LOH studies in one family suggested that the tumor might be an expression of *MEN1* germ-line mutation.[237] Four small families have had prolactinomas in first-degree relatives.[238]

Isolated Carcinoid Tumors. Occasionally, carcinoid tumors show familial clustering independent of MEN1.[239–243] The tumors have been in the terminal ileum or appendix (five families) or in the duodenum (one family).

Hereditary Disorders Affecting One Endocrine Tissue (Likely Polyclonal or Hyperplastic)

Hypocalciuric Hypercalcemia and Neonatal Severe Primary Hyperparathyroidism. The hereditary disorder most often requiring differentiation from MEN1 is familial hypocalciuric hypercalcemia (FHH), also termed *familial benign hypercalcemia.*[244] This is an autosomal dominant form of hypercalcemia with a prevalence similar to that of MEN1. Features that distinguish it from MEN1 are highlighted (see Table 43-2). In FHH, serum calcium level (if tested) is high near birth, and its degree of elevation remains stable throughout life. In FHH, urine calcium level is usually in the normal range; as a result, there is no increased incidence of calcium urolithiasis. A useful diagnostic index in hypercalcemic patients is the ratio of calcium clearance over creatinine clearance. Values in FHH are usually below 0.01, whereas those in typical primary hyperparathyroidism are usually above. Parathyroid hormone (PTH) levels are typically normal in FHH.[245] The parathyroid glands are normal to minimally enlarged,[246] and subtotal parathyroidectomy is followed by persistent hypercalcemia in FHH. FHH is usually or always a disturbance in calcium recognition by the parathyroid cells and perhaps by the renal tubular cells.[247] Most familial cases are linked to chromosome 3q and can be attributed to mutations in a parathyroid cell surface calcium-sensing receptor (*CaS-R*).[248] Cases in rare kindreds are linked to chromosome 19p, 19q, or other loci.[249,250]

FHH patients with homozygous inactivating mutation of the *CaS-R* express extremely severe neonatal primary hyperparathyroidism with impressive enlargement of all parathyroid glands and with serum total calcium generally above 4 mM.[251,252]

Hyperplasia in Endocrine Tissue Other than Parathyroid. Mutation in one of several genes has been identified as a cause of endocrine polyclonal hyperfunction limited to one, presumed hyperplastic tissue and not associated with a multiple neoplasia syndrome (Table 43-5). The resulting syndromes all begin in the neonatal period and vary from hyperparathyroidism,[248] to hyperthyroidism,[253] to testotoxicosis (isosexual male precocious puberty),[254] or to hyperinsulinism.[255–258,258b]

These genes generally show a relatively organ-specific expression pattern. Their encoded proteins include three serpentine G-protein-coupled membrane receptors (the calcium ion-sensing receptor of the parathyroid gland, the TSH receptor of the thyroid follicular cell, and the LH/HCG receptor of Leydig cells) and four proteins involved in glucose recognition by the pancreatic beta cell (two nonhomologous membrane subunits of the ATP-sensitive potassium channel and two cytoplasmic enzymes that determine ATP concentration). Each functions in recognition by a hormone-secreting cell of a major extracellular factor that regulates hormone secretion by that cell (see Table 43-5). The neonatal onset or lack of postnatal latency interval seems to reflect this disturbance in hormone secretory regulation, independent of a period for clonal cell accumulation.

The underlying endocrine gland histology often suggests a diffuse or polyclonal process[246,259,260,260a]; endocrine malignancy is not an expression of these hereditary syndromes. However, mutation of the *TSH-R* or of the *LH/CG-R* also has been implicated in sporadic, clonal neoplasm of the thyrocyte and Leydig cell,

Table 43-5 Cloned Genes Whose Mutation Can Cause Hereditary Hyperfunction of One (Presumably Hyperplastic or Polyclonal) Endocrine Tissue

Syndrome	Oversecreted Hormone	Gene Mutation(s)*	Extracellular Sensor Pathway Disturbed
Hypocalciuric hypercalcemia	PTH	$CaS\text{-}R^-$ †	Parathyroid cell response to serum ionized calcium
Neonatal severe primary hyperparathyroidism	PTH	$CaS\text{-}R^- \times CaS\text{-}R^-$	Parathyroid cell response to serum ionized calcium
Juvenile thyrotoxicosis	T_3/T_4	$TSH\text{-}R^+$	Thyrocyte response to serum TSH
Testotoxicosis	Testosterone	$LH/CG\text{-}R^+$	Leydig cell response to serum LH
Persistent hyperinsulinemic hypoglycemia of infancy	Insulin	$SUR^- \times SUR1^-$	Pancreatic islet beta cell response to blood glucose
Persistent hyperinsulinemic hypoglycemia of infancy	Insulin	$Kir6.2^- \times Kir6.2^-$	Pancreatic islet beta cell response to blood glucose
Persistent hyperinsulinemic hypoglycemia of infancy	Insulin	GK^+	Pancreatic islet beta cell response to blood glucose
Persistent hyperinsulinemic hypoglycemia of infancy	Insulin	$GLUD1^+$	Pancreatic islet beta cell response to blood glucose

* Gene abbreviations: *Ca-SR* = calcium ion-sensing receptor (mainly on plasma membrane of parathyroid cell); *TSH-R* = receptor for thyroid stimulating hormone (mainly on plasma membrane of thyrocyte); *LH/CG-R* = receptor for luteinizing hormone or chorionic gonadotropin (in males, mainly on plasma membrane of Leydig cells); *SUR1* = sulfonylurea receptor (part of ATP-sensitive K^+ channel of pancreatic beta cells); *Kir6.2* = inward rectifying K^+ channel subunit (part of ATP-sensitive K^+ channel of pancreatic beta cells); *GK* = glucokinase; *GLUD1*=glutamate dehydrogenase.

† Mutation momenclature: − = inactivating mutation; + = activating mutation; × = accompanied by a second, in these cases mutated, allele (i.e., homozygous mutation).

respectively, and thus could even contribute to malignancy in these tissues.[261,262] Most of the preceding features (excepting involvement in sporadic neoplasia) and mechanisms contrast in important ways with features of the genes for MEN1 and other multiple neoplasia syndromes.[258b]

CELLULAR EXPRESSIONS OF MEN1

MEN1 Growth Factor

A growth factor was detected in MEN1 plasma when incubated with cultured parathyroid cells.[263–266] High levels were independent of age among adults.[267] Preliminary data pointed to high levels even in young, asymptomatic *MEN1* gene carriers.[268] This growth factor shared many features with FGF-2 or basic fibroblast growth factor, including size, immunologic epitopes, and reactivity toward endothelium.[269,270] The FGF family is small, but all members are potent mitogens.[271] The growth activity in MEN1 plasma could be tumor-derived. However, parathyroid tumors apparently have been excluded as the source.[266] Pituitary tumor is a possible source because the circulating growth activity fell after treatment of pituitary tumors by surgery or medication.[272]

Any role for a circulating growth factor in MEN1 remains unknown. It could be an unimportant by-product of the neoplastic process. It could be an autocrine or paracrine factor that escapes into the circulation. It could be a circulating factor that acts on one or more target tissues to help initiate the neoplastic process. Since the *MEN1* gene is a tumor suppressor, the MEN1 growth factor is not likely to be a product of the *MEN1* gene. However, it remains possible that overexpression of the MEN1 growth factor is an early, albeit downstream, consequence of inactivation of one or both copies of the *MEN1* gene. An early phase in MEN1 angiofibroma may be clonal proliferation of perivascular cells.[272b]

Chromosomal Instability

Several studies have suggested increased frequency of chromosomal breakage in MEN1. Cultured lymphocytes in familial MEN1 showed increased frequency of gaps and chromatid-type abnormalities.[273] Lymphocytes also showed increased chromosomal breakage.[274] Lastly, cultured lymphocytes and cultured fibroblasts from MEN1 patients showed increased chromosomal instability.[275]

GENETIC LOCI

Hereditary Patterns

Genetic Linkage

Near Homogeneity. In 1988, Larsson first reported, in three Swedish kindreds, genetic linkage of MEN1 tract to *PYGM* (muscle phosphorylase locus) at chromosome 11q13.[18] This was confirmed in a single large American kindred, with MEN1 linked to *INT-2* at 11q13.[276] Subsequently, many MEN1 kindreds showed similar linkage to several probes at 11q13. The kindreds have been in Japan,[277] Asia,[278] Finland,[279] and North America,[280] plus England, France, Tasmania, and Sweden.[281] A workshop-based survey of 87 families (including many of those cited above) suggested that the trait was linked to 11q13 in all kindreds evaluated to that point.[282]

Prolactinoma Variant. The largest kindreds with the prolactinoma variant of MEN1 are located almost solely in Newfoundland, Canada. This variant has been termed $MEN1_{\text{Burin}}$, after the Burin Peninsula where most patients live.[148] Linkage of MEN1 to 11q13 was demonstrated in those kindreds.[283] Furthermore, a common founder for the four apparently separate families with $\text{MEN1}_{\text{Burin}}$ was suggested by finding linkage to the same allele of *PYGM* in each Newfoundland family[283] and strongly supported by a detailed demonstration of a shared 11q13 haplotype and a shared *MEN1* mutation.[284]

Locus Heterogeneity. Subsequently, one large kindred almost meeting the criteria of MEN1 (but no member showed two major MEN1 features) raised the possibility of locus heterogeneity, since their MEN1 trait was not linked to 11q13.[285] This kindred had several features that would be unusual for MEN1. In generation 1 there was a patient with primary hyperparathyroidism. In generation 2 there were (1) a patient with acromegaly, (2) a patient with acromegaly and possible hyperparathyroidism, and (3) an asymptomatic carrier. In generation 3 there was a patient with prolactinoma. Screening suggested that other members may express the trait in mild forms. Linkage analysis of affected patients excluded 11q13. This kindred could be categorized, alternately, as showing familial pituitary tumors (see also above and below).

Rare Situations

Twins. MEN1 was described in a pair of identical twins. Their disease expressions differed, though not strikingly.[286] At age 25, both had hyperparathyroidism and prolactinoma. One also had gastrinoma and Cushing disease. Few other twin pairs have been reported in the accumulated experience.[286a] The stochastic nature of the tumors makes interindividual variability likely.

Possible Homozygotes. A sibship was reported in which apparently unrelated parents each were likely heterozygotes for MEN1.[287] Linkage analysis suggested that two of three siblings were homozygotes (double heterozygotes) for MEN1. Their features of MEN1 were not unusually severe or early in onset, although both (a male and a female) had unexplained infertility. Another sibship includes two remotely related parents with $\text{MEN1}_{\text{Burin}}$, the prolactinoma variant of MEN1.[148,284] They had two children. One seemed unaffected, and a daughter expressed galactorrhea at age 23 (presumed prolactinoma) and died at age 30 of an invasive thymic carcinoid without expressing hyperparathyroidism. Her *MEN1* allele status or *MEN1* mutation status was not known.

Sporadic MEN1

There have been many reports of sporadic MEN1 cases.[36] These cases have two, three, or more features of MEN1. Some such cases represent coincidental occurrence of common plus uncommon diseases. Many others, however, are likely expressions of the *MEN1* gene (see below, *MEN1* germ-line mutations among sporadic cases).

Endocrine tumor in a single tissue system is also a predictable expression of the *MEN1* gene. This had not been possible to test rigorously until the *MEN1* gene was isolated.[288] In the near future, *MEN1* germ-line mutation will be explored in sporadic primary hyperparathyroidism (particularly that caused by multiple parathyroid tumors and that in younger patients), sporadic Z-E syndrome, and sporadic pituitary tumor.

11q13 LOSS OF HETEROZYGOSITY

MEN1 Tumors and Tissues

Endocrine Tumors. Larsson reported in 1988 that two MEN1 insulinomas had loss of alleles from the chromosome 11 copy, inherited from the unaffected parent.[18] This led to their prediction that the *MEN1* gene would be a tumor-suppressor gene; i.e., it would cause tumors by a sequential gene inactivation mechanism in the tumor precursor cell(s) ("two hit" hypothesis).[289,290] Subsequently, depending on the probes and on variable normal DNA contamination of tumor DNA, 11q13 LOH has been shown to be frequent in MEN1 tumors of the parathyroids[292–296] and pituitary,[297] approaching 100 percent of tumors following microdissection.[297–301] 11q13 LOH also has been found in 85 percent of nongastrinoma pancreatic islet tumors,[302] in 40 percent of gastrinomas,[302] and in 75 percent of gastric carcinoids.[303] Fewer MEN1 carcinoids and lipomas have been tested, but approximately 50 percent of each type show 11q13 LOH.[304] It is likely that the 11q13 LOH rate in MEN1 tumors would be near 100 percent if near-in probes were used with noncontaminated tumor DNA specimens. Adrenal cortex shows generally silent bilateral enlargement in about a third of MEN1 patients; 11q13 LOH was not found.[142]

Studies of MEN1 tumors have suggested involvement of other tumor-suppressor genes in addition to *MEN1*. In particular there was 1p LOH in 21 percent of MEN1 parathyroids.[305] And comparative genomic hybridization studies of multiple tumors from one patient showed losses from large regions of seven chromosomes, including chromosome 11.[306] There has been no extensive survey in MEN1 to determine the full extent of other genes that may cooperate in development of these neoplasms.

Nonendocrine Tumors. Three MEN1 angiofibromas did not show 11q13 LOH.[304] It is notable that two angiofibromas in tuberous sclerosis also did not show LOH at either of the two tuberous sclerosis disease loci.[307] Both diseases are associated with other tumors that show LOH at the locus of the germ-line mutation; however, it was uncertain if the syndrome-associated angiofibromas were neoplasms or other dysplasias. If they were neoplasms, they might have a large stromal/fibrous component, and the neoplastic component may not have been sufficiently cleared from normal tissue admixture to allow LOH to be recognized. Single-cell analysis (FISH or fluorescent *in situ* hybridization) of angiofibroma, collagenoma, and lipoma in MEN1 subsequently showed loss of one *MEN1* allele, establishing that these are neoplasms and "two hit" in development.[309]

Sporadic Tumors

Endocrine Tumors. In general, sporadic tumors have shown about half the frequency of 11q13 LOH as compared with the tumors of the same organs in MEN1, suggesting that mutation of the *MEN1* gene often may contribute to these sporadic tumors and also that other oncogenes and tumor-suppressor genes play an even more important role in these sporadic tumors than in MEN1.[309] Twenty to 60 percent of sporadic parathyroid tumors show 11q13 LOH.[228,291,293,295] 11q13 LOH has been found in 19 percent of sporadic insulinomas[302] and in 45 percent of sporadic gastrinomas, this latter being a similar incidence to that in MEN1 gastrinoma in the same study.[302] Analyses on smaller numbers of sporadic islet tumors have found similar frequencies of 11q13 LOH.[293,311] Sporadic pituitary tumors have shown variable 11q13 LOH, perhaps relating to contamination by normal tissue and to variable informativeness of the probes used: 3 percent (selectively high LOH for prolactinoma?),[293] 33 percent in somatotropinomas,[311] and 15 to 30 percent similarly distributed among 88 nonfunctioning growth hormone-secreting, prolactin-secreting, and ACTH-secreting.[312] One large analysis found approximately 30 percent 11q13 LOH in invasive pituitary tumors versus 3 percent in noninvasive.[313] The highest rate of 11q13 LOH among sporadic tumors has been reported at 78 percent among carcinoids.[314] In this series, 11q13 LOH had similar frequency in carcinoids of the foregut, midgut, and hindgut. However, a more recent report did not find 11q13 LOH in intestinal or rectal carcinoids.[303] One report found 15 percent 11q13 LOH in benign follicular tumors of the thyroid but not in papillary tumors or malignant follicular tumors of the thyroid.[315] Thirty-five percent of aldosteronomas showed 11q13 LOH.[316] A separate analysis found 11q13 LOH in most adrenocortical cancers but in few adrenocortical benign tumors.[317] Not surprisingly, 11q13 LOH also has been found in some endocrine tumors in familial settings different from MEN1: familial hyperparathyroidism[318] and familial acromegaly.[237,319]

Uremic Parathyroids. Renal failure causes a multifactorial enlargement of the parathyroid glands (secondary hyperparathyroidism). Occasionally, the process becomes sufficiently dysregulated as to resist suppression and occasionally to cause PTH-mediated hypercalcemia (tertiary hyperparathyroidism). In either secondary or tertiary hyperparathyroidism, occasionally surgical removal of portions of the parathyroids is the best treatment. Four studies of these abnormal tissues have found that they usually contain monoclonal components.[228,320–322] 11q13 LOH was found in 0 to 16 percent.

Nonendocrine tumors. 11q13 LOH has been found in several tumors without known relation to MEN1. This includes *in situ* and invasive breast cancer[323,324] and cervical cancer.[325,326]

MEN1 GENE

Methods of Discovery

Positional Candidates. The search for the *MEN1* gene was accelerated by findings in 1988 that it was linked to 11q13 and that, since MEN1 tumors showed LOH about this locus, it was likely to be a tumor-suppressor gene.[18] In the ensuing years, the candidate interval was gradually narrowed by identifying kindred members with important meiotic recombinations between *MEN1* and nearby loci.[280,281,327] In addition, several "positional candidate" genes,[328] which had been mapped to this interval, did not show mutation in MEN1 and thus seemed unlikely to be the *MEN1* gene, including *FAU*,[329] *phospholipase C beta*,[330] and *REL A*.[331] In retrospect, it is evident that testing of the few available positional candidates could not have uncovered the *MEN1* gene at that time.

Positional Cloning. Identification of the *MEN1* gene was achieved by positional cloning, a strategy that used a combination of methods.[19] In short, these methods were (1) assemble a large set of overlapping cloned DNA including development of new polymorphic markers therein, (2) narrow the candidate interval using recombinant cases in kindreds and using 11q13 LOH in tumors, (3) identify candidate genes, mainly from genomic sequence in the narrowest candidate interval, and (4) search for mutations in candidate genes by dideoxy fingerprinting and sequencing analysis of MEN1 probands (Fig. 43-2).

A contig (overlapping DNA, cloned in YACs, bacterial artificial clones (BACs), PACs, P1s, and cosmids) was assembled to ensure uninterrupted coverage of 2.8 million bases encompassing the *MEN1* gene.[332] Thirty-three candidate genes were identified in this interval.[333] New polymorphic probes were developed[334] to help narrow the interval through linkage and 11q13 LOH analyses.[301,327]

The candidate interval was narrowed with analysis of recombinants in families (genetic linkage) and with 11q13 LOH in tumors using the newly developed polymorphic probes. Almost 200 tumors were analyzed, mostly from familial MEN1 but some from sporadic cases.[298,301,302] Because PCR reactions with tumor DNA sometimes gave confusing results (unexpected retention of two alleles within a larger zone of allelic loss) attributable to admixture with nontumor DNA, most tumors were microdissected with customized pipettes or with laser capture.[299,300]

The minimal candidate interval from meiotic recombinations was between *D11S1883* and *D11S449*[281,302] (see Fig. 43-2). However 11q13 LOH in four tumors allowed an inward shift of the centromeric border to *PYGM*, and one tumor moved the telomeric border centromerically to *DS11S4936*. Thus the size of the candidate interval had been narrowed from 3000 kb, based on meiotic recombination, down to only 300 kb based on 11q13 LOH.[301]

Genomic sequence for most of the 300-kb interval in the final steps of the search was obtained by "shotgun" sequencing of two BACs and by obtaining additional cosmid sequences available publicly. This sequence was used to identify eight genes in the minimal interval. Segments of seven genes were matched initially

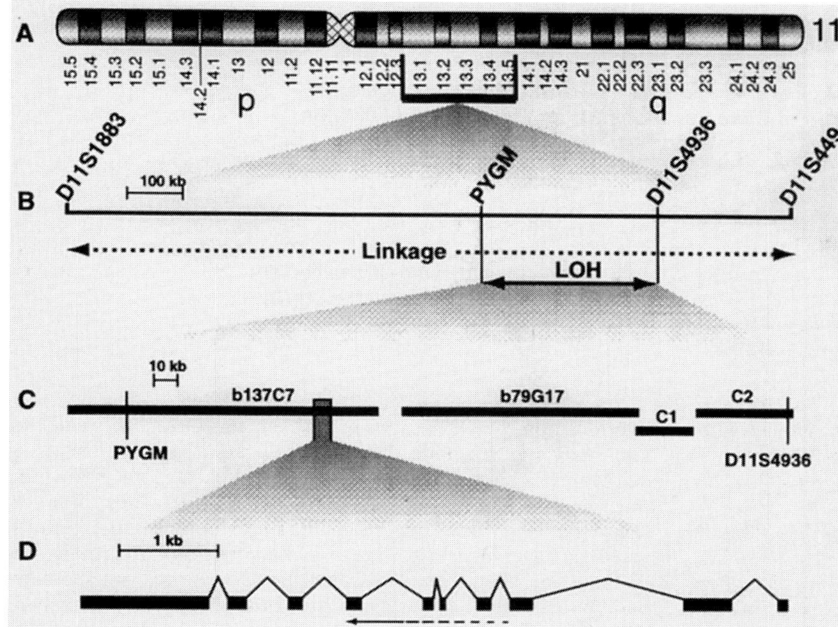

Fig. 43-2 Steps in positional cloning of the *MEN1* gene. Initial genetic linkage to chromosome 11q13 (*A*) was followed by finer mapping by meiotic recombination (an extension of genetic linkage) (*B*) and yet finer mapping by loss of heterozygosity (LOH) analyses in tumors (*C*). Nearly complete bacterial clone coverage was achieved across the most likely interval. Shotgun DNA sequencing revealed eight new candidate genes (*D*). One of these candidates had 10 exons, revealing mutations in 14 MEN1 probands among a testing panel of 15 probands. (*From Chandrasekharappa et al.*[19] *Used with permission.*)

through computer software to publicly available ESTs (expressed sequence tags), and one gene was identified from a computer software prediction of introns and exons.

Mutation Testing of Candidate Genes with a DNA Panel from MEN1 Probands. Full-length cDNA of a candidate transcript was isolated and sequenced. The intron/exon boundaries were determined from comparing the cDNAs and genomic sequences. Candidate genes were tested for mutations, using a DNA panel from probands representing 15 MEN1 kindreds. Mutations were screened by dideoxy fingerprinting, a method that combines features of dideoxy chain termination sequencing and single-strand conformation polymorphism.[335]

Most genes showed occasional polymorphisms (present in normal individuals and MEN1 probands). Only one anonymous gene (*Mu*) showed mutations in many MEN1 probands. Mutations of this anonymous gene were identified in 14 of the 15 probands. The mutations were present in other MEN1-affected family members and not in 142 normal chromosomes. Most mutations were nonsense/stop codons or frameshifts; a few were missense mutations or inframe deletions. These mutations, thereby specific for MEN1, established the identification of the *MEN1* gene.

Germ-Line *MEN1* Mutations

In MEN1 Families. Germ-line mutations in the open reading frame of the *MEN1* gene were found initially in members of 47 of 50 MEN1 kindreds from North America.[336] Germ-line mutation was not evaluated in most of the noncoding 5′, 3′, or intronic portions of the *MEN1* gene. Thus it is apparent that all or most families with typical MEN1 do have germ-line mutations in the open reading frame of this gene. Similar mutation rates also were found in other centers.[319,337–340]

Among Sporadic Cases. Sporadic MEN1, defined as endocrine tumor in two or more of the main MEN1-related tissues, has shown high *MEN1* mutation prevalence, similar to that in familial cases.[42,336,340] Several of these cases were proven to have new mutations, with 10 percent of all mutations being new in an extensive survey.[340]

Repeating *MEN1* Germ-Line Mutations. Eight mutations occurred more than one time among 50 North American MEN1 kindreds.[336] The six mutations occurring twice each did not reflect founder effects but rather mini-hot spots of mutation.[341] The most frequent mutations occurred six (512delC) and five (416delC) times. Haplotype analysis indicated that, like the Newfoundland cluster with R460X and with the prolactinoma variant of MEN1,[283,284] all kindreds in the two large clusters must share a common ancestor.[341] A similar conclusion was possible for a cluster of six Finnish families with 1466del12.[342] The Newfoundland and Finland MEN1 clusters in particular are typical of the founder effects that characterize hereditary diseases in geographically or socially constrained populations.

Genotype/Phenotype Correlations. Three kindreds with the prolactinoma variant of MEN1 were tested to explore possible genotype/phenotype correlations.[147–151,283,284] Two kindreds had germ-line *MEN1* mutations (R460X and Y312X). The third did not have a mutation identified but showed *MEN1* linkage to 11q13 (LOD score 3.25), suggesting that it has an unrecognized *MEN1* mutation. The three presumed different *MEN1* mutations showed no recognizable difference from other *MEN1* mutations.[336] Thus no explanation for the prolactinoma variant could be recognized from the type of *MEN1* mutation. Other explanations for such a phenotype could include other associated polymorphisms in *MEN1,* linked feature in a neighboring gene, *MEN1* mutation occurring in a modifying background, and unrecognized ascertainment bias. MEN1 mutation has been found in six families with isolated hyperparathyroidism, with no specific genotype.[342b]

Possible *MEN1* Phenocopies

Familial Hyperparathyroidism. Familial hyperparathyroidism is sometimes an expression of MEN1.[37] An analysis of five families uncovered *MEN1* mutation in none.[336] The feature in these kindreds making MEN1 less likely was advanced age in most affected members; features against familial hypocalciuric hypercalcemia were that each proband had multiple parathyroid tumors and hypercalciuria. *MEN1* mutation is found in a minority of families with isolated hyperparathyroidism.[342b]

Familial Pituitary Tumors. None among 13 small families with hereditary pituitary tumor, mainly acromegaly, have shown germ-line *MEN1* mutation.[319,342,342c] One of these families (see above)

Table 43-6 Genes Contributing by Mutation to Hereditary and/or Sporadic Parathyroid Tumor, Including Parathyroid Cancer*

	Parathyroid Tumorigenesis from Gain of Gene Function	Parathyroid Tumorigenesis from Loss of Gene Function
Cloned genes	*Cyclin D1 (S)* *RET(H)*	*MEN1 (S & H)* *CaS-R(H)* *RB1(S)* *P53(S)*
Loci of noncloned genes		1q21-32 (hyperpara–jaw tumor) (H) LOH evidence (1p, 6q, 15q, X) (S)

*Abbreviations: *S* = sporadic; *H* = hereditary.

with three members with pituitary tumor also had a member with hyperparathyroidism; the MEN1-like trait in this family was not linked to 11q13.[285,342]

Sporadic Endocrine Tumor as a Possible *MEN1* Phenocopy. As part of evaluations of tumors for somatic *MEN1* mutation (see below), tumor-bearing patients also were evaluated for germ-line *MEN1* mutation. As a result, *MEN1* germ-line mutation was excluded in the following 119 cases of sporadic endocrine tumor: 31 with hyperparathyroidism,[318] 38 with pituitary tumor,[156] 27 with gastrinoma,[345] 12 with insulinoma[345] and 11 with bronchial carcinoid.[347]

Somatic *MEN1* Mutations

A somatic *MEN1* mutation, by definition, arises in a somatic tissue and is not in the germ line of the patient. In fact, germ-line mosaicism is sometimes impossible to exclude. Somatic mutation of the *MEN1* gene has been found in 12 to 21 percent of sporadic parathyroid adenomas,[318,343,344] 33 percent of sporadic gastrinomas,[345,346] 17 percent of sporadic insulinomas,[345] and 36 percent of sporadic bronchial carcinoids.[347] For each of those four tumors, *MEN1* is the gene most frequently known to be mutated. *MEN1* mutation did not correlate with any clinical feature, such as invasivness in a large series of gastrinomas.[347b] The *MEN1* mutation rate has been lower (0–5 percent) in sporadic pituitary tumors, in parathyroid cancer, or in uremic hyperparathyroidism.[156,348,349,349b,349c] In the prior analyses, *MEN1* mutation was associated with 11q13 LOH if this was evaluated. Furthermore, for all but bronchial carcinoid, 11q13 LOH also was found in a similar fraction of tumors without *MEN1* mutation. Most likely, this excess of 11q13 LOH without *MEN1* mutation reflects other mechanisms (such as promoter methylation)[350] for inactivation of the first *MEN1* allele. Additional possibilities include undiscovered *MEN1* mutations and inactivation of other, unknown 11q13 tumor-suppressor gene(s).[351] Despite frequent LOH at 11q13, thyroid tumors have not had somatic *MEN1* mutation.[351b]

Somatic *MEN1* mutation also has been implicated in certain nonendocrine tumors: angiofibroma (2 of 19)[352] and lipoma (1 of 6).[353]

***MEN1* as One of Many Genes Implicated in Parathyroid Tumors.** The *MEN1* gene is frequently mutated in certain endocrine tumors, but it is just one of many genes that can contribute by mutation to endocrine tumorigenesis. By way of illustration, parathyroid tumor is notable for its importance in MEN1 and for the number of genes that have already been implicated in tumor development (Table 43-6). Activating mutation in either of two genes, *RET* or *Cyclin D1,* contributes to parathyroid tumorigenesis.[198,199,354,355] However, *RET* activation has not been found in sporadic parathyroid tumor,[356] and *Cyclin D1* activating mutation has been found in only 4 percent of sporadic parathyroid tumors.[354,355] Other loci of possible gene amplification have been suggested with comparative genome hybridization, but there was insufficient agreement between the two studies to conclude that any one locus was important (see below). Gene inactivation has been recognized more frequently than gene activation in parathyroid tumors. Heterozygous or homozygous mutation of the calcium-sensing receptor is implicated in hereditary variants of hyperparathyroidism (see Table 43-5), but these have not been identified in sporadic parathyroid tumor.[357–359] Inactivation of *RB1* or *p53* is common in sporadic parathyroid cancer but rare in common-variety parathyroid adenoma.[360–364] As yet unidentified genes are also likely to be implicated. The gene for hyperparathyroidism–jaw tumor is probably a tumor suppressor[219] but LOH at this 1q24 locus has not been implicated in sporadic parathyroid tumors. LOH has been identified in several loci in parathyroid tumors[309]; in particular, 1p34 LOH seems about as frequent as 11q13 LOH. Additional loci have been implicated by recognizing chromosomal or subchromosomal DNA loss with comparative genome hybridization.[364,365]

Functions of the *MENI* Gene

The function of the *MEN1* gene is not known.[19] The gene is approximately 9000 bases long with a message of 2800 bases. Across 9 of its 10 exons, it encodes a predicted protein, named *menin,* that is 610 amino acids long. The protein is highly homologous to mouse menin,[365b] but it does not have other known homologies in humans or other species. The encoded menin protein resides all or mainly in the nucleus, and it has two nuclear localization domains near its C-terminus.[366] Menin binds to junD, a jun/fos transcription factor, and it inhibits transcription stimulated by junD. Tumor suppression might arise from a cooperative role of menin and junD.[366b]

Limited information can be derived from the identified mutations (Fig. 43-3). Tumors in different organs show similar *MEN1* mutations. The somatic mutations in tumors are similar to germ-line mutations. Two-thirds of germ-line and somatic mutations predict protein truncation. Thus they are likely inactivating mutations. This is made more likely because each truncating mutation would remove one or both of the C-terminal nuclear localization signals.[366] The inactivating mutations, together with loss of the remaining normal allele in tumors, thus indicate that both alleles had been inactivated in the tumor clone precursor(s). Most genes that cause tumors through inactivation of both alleles are classified as tumor-suppressor genes. This is supported further by overexpression of menin in ras-transformed cells, causing partial suppression of the the tumor phenotype.[366c] The predicted normal function of menin still could be in a pathway of cell birth, cell death, or DNA repair, thus not narrowing the types of function.

The missense *MEN1* mutations are not clustered and thus do not highlight a particularly critical menin region. The related interpretation is that missense mutation at various loci can compromise the molecule.

Only one large deletion, likely eliminating the entire *MEN1* open reading frame, has been reported to date.[367] A large deletion

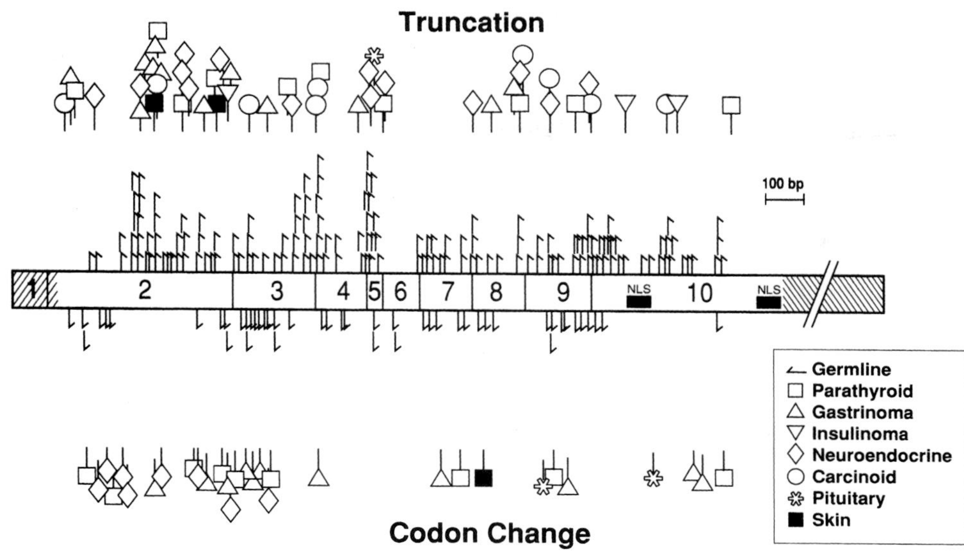

Fig. 43-3 Unique germ-line *MEN1* mutations in families and in sporadic cases. Somatic *MEN1* mutations in diverse tumors are shown separately along the top and bottom of the figure. *MEN1* message is diagrammed with exons numbered; untranslated regions are cross-hatched. Truncating mutations [frameshift mutations, splice error, and nonsense (stop codons) mutations] are shown above the mRNA diagram. Codon shift mutations (missense mutations or in-frame deletions) are shown below. Repeating mutations within germline or somatic category are shown only once. NLS = nuclear localization sequence. One large deletion, likely of the entire *MEN1* gene, is not shown.[367]

excludes menin function as a dominant negative. No unusual phenotype was commented on in this kindred.[367]

IMPLICATIONS FOR DIAGNOSIS

Periodic Biochemical Testing

For Diagnosis of MEN1. The standard of care has been that members of MEN1 kindreds undergo periodic biochemical testing. Recent recommendations have been to begin this testing at age 15[40] or as early as age 8.[33] The latter is based on the projected age when important signs may begin. Parameters for testing such as chromogranin A[367b] must be dictated by clinical importance, cost, and local availability. A cost-effective panel could consist of ionized calcium, parathyroid hormone, and prolactin. Such a panel should be repeated approximately every 2 years. Any patient who does not convert to a positive test by age 30 has far reduced (about 10 percent) likelihood of being a gene carrier. But testing should be continued at longer intervals indefinitely, since no maximal age for conversion to a positive test has been determined.[42]

For Monitoring of MEN1. Patients with established MEN1 should undergo periodic testing for expression of new endocrinopathies and for recurrence of treated endocrinopathies. Monitoring and treatment of recognized hormone excess states are beyond this chapter. Even more so than for diagnostic testing, testing of known carriers must depend on cost and availability (Table 43-7). Sometimes symptoms, such as ulcer or hypoglycemia, will present before an abnormality is found by biochemical testing.

Table 43-7 A Typical Panel of Tests for Periodic Monitoring of a Patient with MEN1 or with *MEN1* Mutation

Parathyroids	Enteropancreatic Neuroendocrine
Ionized calcium (annually) PTH (annually)	Fasting sugar and gastrin (annually) CT scan and Octreoscan (every 5 years; needs more evaluation)
Pituitary	**Carcinoid**
Prolactin (annually) Sella MRI (every 5 years)	CT scan (every 5 years)

Genetic Linkage Testing

Until the isolation of the *MEN1* gene, genetic linkage was the only method to establish that the trait in a family was linked to 11q13 and similarly to make a confident genetic diagnosis in an asymptomatic member of an MEN1 family.[282] After *MEN1* gene discovery, genetic linkage analysis has had less frequent applications. The main use is in the MEN1 family with no *MEN1* mutation identified. There, linkage analysis may establish if the disease is linked to 11q13 or not. Of course, when positive, it also can be used for ascertainment within a family. Where 11q13 linkage testing has been possible in "mutation negative" MEN1 families, it has confirmed linkage to 11q13 in 3 of 4 families.[42,336]

Detection Rates with Mutation Testing

By dideoxy fingerprinting and cycle sequencing, germ-line mutation was recognizable in 47 of 50 families. This implies that virtually every MEN1 family has a mutation in the open reading frame of the *MEN1* gene. The implication is that robust *MEN1* germ-line mutation testing is possible, and this can be applied to families and sporadic cases. Detection rates in academic centers, reporting more than 30 tested MEN1 families and using various detection methods, range from 51 to 94 percent.[56b,144b,336,340,342,342c,367c]

Difficulty of *MEN1* Germ-Line Mutation Testing

Approximately 200 different germ-line *MEN1* mutations are spread over nine coding exons (see Fig. 43-3). Many familial and sporadic MEN1 patients reveal a previously undescribed mutation. There is only limited clustering of mutations in the 3′ two-thirds of exon 2. Thus there is little prospect for test shortcuts directed at several bases or several exons. Furthermore, the relatively high fraction with missense mutations predicts that even if most truncated messages are expressed, a protein truncation type assay would fail to recognize at least one-third of mutations. Of course, within a family or in a population with a founder effect,[19,284,342] simplified tests directed at the known mutation should be used.

Currently available methods (cycle sequencing alone or with dideoxy fingerprinting, with single-strand conformer polymorphism or with heteroduplex analysis) are likely to have similarly high diagnostic yield under carefully controlled conditions. It is likely that these will be developed by academic centers. It is not

Table 43-8 Major Differences Between MEN1 and MEN2a/MEN2b. Some Can Affect Decisions About Gene Testing

The Concerns	MEN1	MEN2a/MEN2b
Gene and locus	*MEN1*, 11q13	*RET*, 10 cen
Encoded protein location and action	Nucleus, unknown action Binds junD	Plasma membrane, tyrosine kinase
How mutation promotes tumor	Gene inactivation	Gene activation
Mutation distribution	Throughout open reading frame	Few exons, few codons
Main clinical expressions	Hormone excess effects	Cancer of C-cells
Gene-testing benefits	Information to MD and patient	Information to MD and patient Cancer prevention or cure
Age to offer mutation test	Rarely before 18 yrs (in U.S.)	5 years in MEN2a; 1 year in MEN2b
False negative rate	10–20%	1–2%

clear if there will be sufficient demand to lead soon to commercial development as well.

Cases for Possible *MEN1* Germ-Line Mutation Testing

Several categories of clinical presentation have rather clear justification for *MEN1* germ-line mutation testing at presentation or after a delay (see 5):

1. An affected member in an MEN1 or MEN1 phenocopy family that has not previously had a member tested. Testing can confirm the diagnosis and also assist in possible development of an inexpensive mutation test for other members, such as based on a specific restriction digest or based on hybridization to allele specific oligonucleotides.
2. A likely affected member of an MEN1 or MEN1 phenocopy family with known familial mutation, concerned for confirmation of mutational status.
3. An unaffected adult in an MEN1 family. Any without mutation would be freed from the recommendation to undergo regular biochemical screening (Table 43-8). Any with mutation would be given opposite recommendations with more confidence.
4. A sporadic case with MEN1 or an MEN1 phenocopy. Certain phenocopies (such as combined hyperparathyroidism and bronchial carcinoid) will have a high likelihood of mutation, while others (such as sporadic hyperparathyroidism) will have low likelihood.
5. Rarely an unaffected child in an MEN1 family. The consensus of the U.S. genetics community is that children in the United States generally should not be offered genetic testing that will not have a major effect on their immediate care.[368] Early testing deprives them of their right to decide as an adult whether to undergo such testing.

Issues for Genetic Counseling

The issues to consider for counseling are, in general, covered in detail in the body of this chapter. Several additional points can be made. The similarity in names leads to confusion among some patients and among some physicians between MEN1 and MEN2, but the differences are more important than their similarities (see Table 43-8). Above all, *RET* gene testing in MEN2a or MEN2b carries major therapeutic implications (possible prevention or cure of cancer)[198]; major therapeutic implications are uncommon from *MEN1* gene testing in MEN1. A patient education manual, which has been updated regularly, is available on the international communications Web at *http://www.niddk.nih.gov/health/endo/pubs/fmen1/fmen1.htm*.[369]

MEN1 generally does not have major effects on fertility. Primary hyperparathyroidism in a mother is considered a risk factor for pregnancy complications.[370] However, the mild hyperparathyroidism that is common in MEN1 rarely leads to complications for mother or child. MEN1 in a fetus is not a pregnancy risk factor for fetus or mother. Prolactinoma can clearly impair fertility in women or men, and it should be monitored during pregnancy. Most women (and men) with prolactinoma are able to conceive when treated with a dopamine agonist.[371]

ACKNOWLEDGMENTS

I wish to thank many collaborators who contributed to our work on MEN1, particularly those in the NIH intramural programs, including Sunita K. Agarwal, MaryBeth Kester, Christina Heppner, Young S. Kim, Paul K. Goldsmith, Monica C. Skarulis, Allen M. Spiegel, and A. Lee Burns (All National Institute of Diabetes and Digestive and Kidney Diseases), Sirandanahalli C. Guru, Judith S. Crabtree, Pachiapan Manickam, Francis S. Collins, and Settara C. Chandrasekharappa (All National Human Genome Research Institute), Michael R. Emmert-Buck, Larissa V. Debelenko, Zhengping Zhuang, Irina A. Lubensky, and Lance A. Liotta (National Cancer Institute). I am also indebeted for many contributions from John L. Doppman, H. Richard Alexander, Mark S. Boguski, Thomas L. Darling, Lee S. Weinstein, William F. Simonds, and many members of the NIH Interinstitute Endocrine Program. Many persons outside NIH also made important contributions, particularly Bruce A. Roe, Jane S. Green, Joseph E. Green III, and also many patients and their families.

REFERENCES

1. Erdheim J: Zur normalen und pathologischen histologie der glandula throidea, parathyroidea, und hypophysis. *Beitr Z Pathol Anat* **33**:158, 1903.
2. Moldawer MP: Case records of the Massachusetts General Hospital, case 39501. *N Engl J Med* **249**:990, 1953.
3. Moldawer MP, Nardi GL, Raker JW: Concomitance of multiple adenomas of the parathyroids and pancreatic islet cells with tumor of the pituitary a syndrome with familial incidence. *Am J Med Sci* **228**:190, 1954.
4. Wermer P: Genetic aspects of adenomatosis of endocrine glands. *Am J Med* **16**:363, 1954.
5. Schmid JR, Labhart A, Rossier PH: Relationship of multiple endocrine adenomas to the syndrome of ulcerogenic islet cell adenomas (Zollinger-Ellison): Occurrence of both syndromes in one family. *Am J Med* **31**:343, 1961.
6. Zollinger RM, Ellison EH: Primary peptic ulceration of the jejunum associated with islet cell tumors of the pancreas. *Ann Surg* **142**:709, 1955.
7. Gregory RH, Tracy HJ, French JM, Sircus W: Extraction of a gastrin-like substance from a pancreatic tumor in a case of Zollinger-Ellison syndrome. *Lancet* **1**:1040, 1960.
8. Lewis UJ, Singh RN, Seavey BK: Human prolactin: Isolation and some properties. *Biochem Biophys Res Commun* **44**:1169, 1971.
9. Malarkey WB: Prolactin and the diagnosis of pituitary tumors. *Annu Rev Med* **30**:249, 1979.

10. Howard JM, Chremos AN, Collen MJ: Famotidine, a new potent long acting histamine H_2-receptor antagonist: comparison with cimetidine and ranitidine in the treatment of Zollinger-Ellison syndrome. *Gastroenterology* **188**:1026, 1985.
11. Metz DC, Pisegna JR, Fishbeyn VA, Benya RV, Jensen RT: Control of gastric acid hypersecretion in the management of patients with Zollinger-Ellison syndrome. *World J Surg* **17**:468, 1993.
12. Frucht H, Maton PN, Jensen RT: Use of omeprazole in patients with Zollinger-Ellison syndrome. *Dig Dis Sci* **36**:394, 1991.
13. Maton PN, Vinayek R, Frucht H: Long term efficacy and safety of omeprazole in patients with Zollinger-Ellison syndrome. *Gastroenterology* **97**:827, 1989.
14. Bevan JS, Webster J, Burke CW, Scanlon MF: Dopamine agonists and pituitary tumor shrinkage. *Endocr Rev* **13**:220, 1992.
15. Norton JA, Cromack DT, Shawker TH: Intraoperative ultrasonographic localization of islet cell tumors: A prospective comparison to palpation. *Ann Surg* **207**:160, 1988.
16. Norton JA, Shawker TH, Jones BL, Spiegel AM, Marx SJ, Fitzpatrick L, Aurbach GD, Doppman JL: Intraoperative ultrasound and reoperative parathyroid surgery: an initial evaluation. *World J Surg* **10**:631, 1986.
17. Doppman JL: Tumor localization in multiple endocrine neoplasia type 1. *Ann Intern Med* **129**:484, 1998.
17b. Norton JA: Intraoperative methods to stage and localize pancreeatic and duodenal tumors. *Ann Oncol* **10**(Suppl 4):182, 1999.
17c. Tonelli F, Spini S, Tommasi M et al: Intraoperative PTH measurement in patients with MEN1 syndrome and hyperparathyroidism. *World J Surg* In press.
18. Larsson C, Skogseid B, Oberg K, Nakamura Y, Nordenskjold M: Multiple endocrine neoplasia type 1 gene maps to chromosome 11 and is lost in insulinoma. *Nature* **332**:85, 1988.
19. Chandrasekharappa SC, Guru SC, Manickam P, Olufemi S-E, Collins FS, Emmert-Buck MR, Debelenko LV, Zhuang Z, Lubensky IA, Liotta LA, Crabtree JS, Wang Y, Roe BA, Weiseman J, Bogusky MS, Agarwal SK, Kester MB, Kim YS, Heppner C, Dong Q, Spiegel AM, Burns AL, Marx SJ: Positional cloning of the gene for multiple endocrine neoplasia type 1. *Science* **276**:404, 1997.
20. Lips CJM, Vasen HFA, Lamers CBHW, Berdjis CC: Polyglandular syndrome: II. Multiple endocrine adenomas in man: A report of 5 cases and a review of the literature. *Oncologia* **15**:288, 1962.
21. Lips CJM, Vasen HFA, Lamers CBHW: Multiple endocrine neoplasia syndromes. *CRC Crit Rev* **2**:117, 1984.
22. Eberle F, Grun R: Multiple endocrine neoplasia, type I (MEN1). *Ergeb Inn Med* **46**:76, 1981.
23. Oberg K, Skogseid B, Eriksson B: Multiple endocrine neoplasia type 1 (MEN-1): Clinical, biochemical and genetical investigations. *Acta Oncologia* **28**:383, 1989.
24. Betts JB, O'Malley BP, Rosenthal FD: Hyperparathyroidism: A prerequisite for Zollinger-Ellison syndrome in multiple endocrine adenomatosis type 1. *Q J Med* **193**:69, 1980.
25. Watson RGP, Johnston CF, O'Hare MMT, Anderson JR, Wilson BG, Collins JS, Sloan JM, Buchanan KD: The frequency of gastrointestinal endocrine tumors in a well defined population — Northern Ireland. *Q J Med* **72**:647, 1985.
26. Brandi ML, Marx SJ, Aurbach GD, Fitzpatrick LA: Familial multiple endocrine neoplasia type I: A new look at pathophysiology. *Endocr Rev* **8**:391, 1987.
27. Heath H III, Hodgson S, Kennedy MA: Primary hyperparathyroidism: Incidence, morbidity, and potential economic impact in a community. *N Engl J Med* **302**:189, 1980.
28. Bardram L, Stage JG: Frequency of endocrine disorders in patients with the Zollinger-Ellison syndrome: A collective surgical experience. *Scand J Gastroenterol* **20**:233, 1985.
29. Farley DR, van Heerden JA, Grant CS, Miller LJ, Ilstrup DM: The Zollinger-Ellison syndrome: A collective surgical experience. *Ann Surg* **215**:561, 1992.
30. Schaaf L, Gerschner M, Geissler W, Eckert B, Seif FJ, Usadel KH: The importance of multiple endocrine neoplasia syndromes in differential diagnosis. *Klin Wochenschr* **68**:669, 1990.
31. Scheithauer BW, Laws ER Jr, Kovacs K, Horvath E, Randall RV, Carney JA: Pituitary adenomas of the multiple endocrine neoplasia type I syndrome. *Semin Diagn Pathol* **4**:205, 1987.
32. Corbetta S, Pizzocaro A, Peracchi M, Beck-Peccoz P, Faglia G, Spada A: Multiple endocrine neoplasia type 1 in patients with recognized pituitary tumors of different types. *Clin Endocrinol* **47**:507, 1997.
33. Trump D, Farren B, Wooding C, Pang JT, Besser GM, Buchanan KD, Edwards CR, Heath DA, Jackson CE, Jansen S, Lips K, Monson JP, O'Halloran D, Sampson J, Shalet SM, Wheeler MH, Zink A, Thakker RV: Clinical studies of multiple endocrine neoplasia type 1 (MEN1). *Q J Med* **89**:563, 1996.
34. Doherty GM, Olson JA, Frisella MM, Lairmore TC, Wells SA Jr, Norton JA: Lethality of multiple endocrine neoplasia type 1. *World J Surg* **22**:581, 1998.
35. Majewski JT, Wilson SD: The MEA-I syndrome: An all or none phenomenon? *Surgery* **86**:475, 1979.
36. Ballard HS, Frame B, Hartsock RJ: Familial multiple endocrine adenoma-peptic ulcer complex. *Medicine* **43**:481, 1964.
37. Marx SJ, Spiegel AM, Levine MA, Rizzoli RE, Lasker RD, Santora AC II, Downs RW, Aurbach GD: Familial hypocalciuric hypercalcemia: The relation to primary parathyroid hyperplasia. *N Engl J Med* **307**:416, 1982.
38. Vasen HFA, Lamers CBHW, Lips CJM: Screening for multiple endocrine neoplasia syndrome type I. *Arch Intern Med* **149**:2717, 1989.
39. Skogseid B, Eriksson B, Lundqvist G: Multiple endocrine neoplasia type 1: A 10-year prospective screening study in four kindreds. *J Clin Endocrinol Metab* **73**:281, 1991.
40. Marx SJ, Vinik AI, Santen RJ, Floyd JC Jr, Mills JL, Green JE III: Multiple endocrine neoplasia type I: Assessment of laboratory tests to screen for the gene in a large kindred. *Medicine* **65**:226, 1986.
41. Skarulis MC: Clinical expressions of MEN1 at NIH. *Ann Intern Med* **129**:484, 1998.
42. Giraud S, Choplin H, Teh B, Lespinasse J, Jouvet A, Labat-Moleur F, Lenoir G, Hamon B, Hamon P, Calender A: A large multiple endocrine neoplasia type 1 family with clinical expression suggestive of anticipation. *J Clin Endocrinol Metab* **82**:3487, 1997.
43. Samaan NA, Ovais S, Ordonez NG, Choksi UA, Selvin RV, Hickey RC: Multiple endocrine syndrome type 1: Clinical laboratory findings, and management in five families. *Cancer* **64**:741, 1989.
44. Lamers CBHW, Froeling PGAM: Clinical significance of hyperparathyroidism in familial multiple endocrine adenomatosis type I (MEA I). *Am J Med* **66**:422, 1979.
45. Eberle F, Grun R: Multiple endocrine neoplasia, type I (MEN I), in Frick P, Harnack G-A, Kochsiek K, Martini GA, Prade A (eds): *Advances in Internal Medicine and Pediatrics*. Berlin, Springer-Verlag, 1981, p 77.
46. Shepherd JJ: Latent familial multiple endocrine neoplasia in Tasmania. *Med J Aust* **142**:395, 1985.
47. Wu CW, Huang CI, Tsai ST, Chiang H, Liu W-Y, P'eng F-K: Parathyroid carcinoma in a patient with non-secretory pituitary tumor: A variant of multiple endocrine neoplasia type-I? *Eur J Surg Oncol* **18**:517, 1992.
47b. Burgess JR, David R, Greenaway TM, Parameswaran V, Shepherd JJ: Osteoporosis in multiple endocrineoplasia type 1. *Arch Surg* **134**:1119, 1999.
48. Marx SJ, Menczel J, Campbell G, Aurbach GD, Spiegel AM, Norton JA: Heterogeneous size of the parathyroid glands in familial multiple endocrine neoplasia type 1. *Clin Endocrinol* **35**:521, 1991.
49. Hellman P, Skogseid B, Juhlin C, Akerstrom G, Rastad J: Findings and long-term result of parathyroid surgery in multiple endocrine neoplasia type 1. *World J Surg* **16**:718, 1992.
50. Rizzoli R, Green J III, Marx SJ: Primary hyperparathyroidism in familial multiple endocrine neoplasia type I. *Am J Med* **78**:468, 1985.
51. Burgess JR, David R, Parameswaran V, Greenaway TM, Shepherd JJ: The outcome of subtotal parathyroidectomy for the treatment of hyperparathyroidism in multiple endocrine neoplasia type 1. *Arch Surg* **133**:126, 1998.
52. Prinz RA, Gamvros OI, Sellu D, Lynn JA: Subtotal parathyroidectomy for primary chief cell hyperplasia of the multiple endocrine neoplasia type I syndrome. *Ann Surg* **193**:26, 1981.
53. van Heerden JA, Kent RB III, Sizemore GW, Grant CS, ReMine WH: Primary hyperparathyroidism in patients with multiple endocrine neoplasia syndromes. *Arch Surg* **118**:533, 1983.
54. Rudberg C, Akerstrom G, Palmer M, Ljunghall S, Adami HO, Johansson H, Grimelius L, Thoren L, Bergstrom R: Later results of operation for primary hyperparathyroidism in 441 patients. *Surgery* **99**:643, 1986.
55. Le Bodic M-F, Heymann M-F, Lecompte M, Berger N, Berger F, Louvel A, De Micco C, Patey M, De Mascarel A, Burtin F, Saint-Andre J-P: Immunohistochemical study of 100 pancreatic tumors in 28 patients with multiple endocrine neoplasia, type 1. *Am J Surg Pathol* **20**:1378, 1996.
56. Benya RV, Metz DC, Venzon DJ, Fishbeyn VA, Strader DB, Orbuch M, Jensen RT: Zollinger-Ellison syndrome can be the initial

endocrine manifestation in patients with multiple endocrine neoplasia-type I. *Am J Med* **5**:436, 1994.

56b. Giraud S, Zhang CX, Serova-Sinilnikova O, Wautot V, Salandre J, Buisson N, Waterlot C, Bauters C, Porchet N, Aubert J-P, Emy P, Cadiot G, Delemer B, Chabre O, and 27 additional coauthors: Germline mutation analysis in patients with multiple endocrine neoplasia type 1 and related disorders. *Am J Hum Genet* **63**:455, 1998.

57. Norton JA, Levin B, Jensen RT: Cancer of the endocrine system, in DeVita VT Jr, Hellman S, Rosenberg SA (eds): *Cancer: Principles and Practice of Oncology*. Philadelphia, Lippincott, 1993, p 1335.

58. Metz DC, Jensen RT: Endocrine tumors of the pancreas, in Haubrich WB, Berk JE, Schaffner F (eds): *Bockus Gastroenterology*. Philadelphia, Saunders, 1994, p 3002.

59. Jensen RT, Gardner JD: Gastrinoma, in Go VLW, Brooks FP, DiMagno EP (eds): *The Exocrine Pancreas*. New York, Raven Press, 1993.

60. Metz DC, Jensen RT, Bale A, Skarulis MC, Eastman RC, Nieman L, Norton JA, Friedman E, Larsson C, Amorosi A, Brandi ML, Marx SJ: Multiple endocrine neoplasia type 1: Clinical features and management, in Bilezekian JP, Levine MA, Marcus R (eds): *The Parathyroids*. New York, Raven Press, 1994, p 591.

61. Skogseid B, Oberg K, Eriksson B, Juhlin C, Grandberg D, Akerstrom G, Rastad J: Surgery for asymptomatic pancreatic lesion in multiple endocrine neoplasia type I. *World J Surg* **7**:872, 1996.

62. Kloppel G, Sillemar S, Stamm B, Hacki WH, Heitz PN: Pancreatic lesions and hormonal profile in pancreatic tumors in multiple endocrine neoplasia type I. *Cancer* **57**:1824, 1986.

63. Thompson NW, Lloyd RU, Nishiyama RH: MEN-1 pancreas: A histological and immunohistochemical study. *World J Surg* **8**:561, 1984.

64. Pipeleers-Marichial M, Somers G, Willems G: Gastrinomas in the duodenum of patients with multiple endocrine neoplasia type 1 and the Zollinger-Ellison syndrome. *N Engl J Med* **322**:723, 1990.

65. Jensen RT, Gardner JD: Zollinger-Ellison syndrome: Clinical presentation, pathology, diagnosis and treatment, in Dannenberg A, Zakim D (eds): *Peptic Ulcer and Other Acid-Related Diseases*. New York, Academic Research Association, 1991, p 117.

66. Norton JA, Doppman JL, Jensen RT: Curative resection in Zollinger-Ellison syndrome: Results of a 10 year prospective study. *Ann Surg* **215**:8, 1992.

67. Ruszniewski P, Podevin P, Cadiot G, Marmuse JP, Mignon M, Vissuzaine C, Bonfils S, Lehy T: Clinical anatomical, and evolutive features of patients with the Zollinger-Ellison syndrome combined with type I multiple endocrine neoplasia. *Pancreas* **8**:295, 1993.

68. Neuburger P, Lewin M, Bonfils S: Parietal and chief cell population in four cases of the Zollinger-Ellison syndrome. *Gastroenterology* **63**:937, 1972.

69. Norton JA, Doppman JL, Collen MJ: Prospective study of gastrinoma localization and resection in patients with Zollinger-Ellison syndrome. *Ann Surg* **204**:468, 1986.

70. Stabile BE, Morrow DJ, Passaro E Jr: The gastrinoma triangle: Operative implications. *Am J Surg* **147**:25, 1984.

71. Norton JA, Jensen RT: Unresolved issues in the management of patients with Zollinger-Ellison syndrome. *World J Surg* **15**:151, 1991.

72. Zollinger RM, Ellison EH, Fabri PJ, Johnson J, Sparks J, Carey LC: Primary peptic ulceration of the jejunum associated with islet cell tumors: Twenty-five year appraisal. *Ann Surg* **192**:422, 1980.

73. Oberg K, Skogseid B, Eriksson B: Multiple endocrine neoplasia type 1 (MEN-1). *Acta Oncol* **28**:383, 1989.

74. Zollinger RM: Gastrinoma factors influencing prognosis. *Surgery* **97**:49, 1985.

75. Podevin P, Ruszniewski P, Mignon M: Management of multiple endocrine neoplasia type 1 (MEN1) in Zollinger-Ellison syndrome. *Gastrenterology* **98**:A230, 1990.

76. Jensen RT, Gardner JD, Raufman J-P: Zollinger-Ellison syndrome: Current concepts and management. *Ann Intern Med* **98**:59, 1983.

77. Weber HC, Venzon DJ, Lin JT, Fishbein VA, Orbuch M, Strader DB, Gibril F, Metz DC, Fraker DL, Norton JA, Jensen RT: Determinants of metastatic rate and survival in patients with Zollinger-Ellison syndrome: A prospective long-term study. *Gastroenterology* **108**:1637, 1995.

78. Jensen RT: Management of the Zollinger-Ellison syndrome in patients with multiple endocrine neoplasia type 1. *Ann Intern Med* **243**:477, 1998.

79. Isenberg JI, Walsh JH, Grossman MI: Zollinger-Ellison syndrome. *Gastroenterology* **65**:140, 1973.

80. Shimoda SS, Saunders DR, Rubin C: The Zollinger-Ellison syndrome with steatorrhea: Mechanisms of fat and vitamin B_{12} malabsorption. *Gastroenterology* **55**:705, 1968.

81. Feldman M: Gastric secretion, in Sleisenger MH, Fordtran JS (eds): *Gastrointestinal Disease*. Philadelphia, Saunders, 1983, p 541.

82. Norton JA, Cornelius MJ, Doppman JL: Effect of parathyroidectomy in patients with hyperparathyroidism and multiple endocrine neoplasia type I. *Surgery* **102**:958, 1987.

83. Yonda RJ, Ostroff JW, Ashbaugh CD, Guis MS, Goldberg HI: Zollinger-Ellison syndrome with a normal screening gastrin level. *Dig Dis Sci* **34**:1929, 1989.

84. Wolfe MM, Jensen RT: Zollinger-Ellison syndrome. *N Engl J Med* **317**:1200, 1987.

85. Metz DC, Pisegna JR, Fishbeyn VA, Benya RV, Jensen RT: Current maintenance doses of omeprazole in Zollinger-Ellison syndrome are too high. *Gastroenterology* **103**:1498, 1992.

86. Frucht H, Howard JM, Slaff JE: Secretin and calcium provocative tests in patients with Zollinger-Ellison syndrome: A prospective study. *Ann Intern Med* **111**:713, 1989.

87. Krenning EP, Kwekkeboom DJ, Oei HY, de Jong RJB, Dop FJ, Reubi JC, Lambers SWJ: Somatostatin-receptor scintigraphy in gastroenteropancreatic tumors. *Ann NY Acad Sci* **733**:416, 1994.

88. Gibril F, Reynolds JC, Doppman JL, Chen CC, Venzon DJ, Termanini B, Weber HC, Stewart CA, Jensen RT: Somatostatin receptor scientigraphy: A prospective study of its sensitivity compared to other imaging modalities in detecting primary and metastatic gastrinomas. *Ann Intern Med* **125**:26, 1996.

89. Termanini B, Gibril F, Reynolds JC, Doppman JL, Chen CC, Sutliffe VE, Jensen RT: Value of somatostatin receptor scintigraphy: A prospective study in gastrinoma of its effect on clinical management. *Gastroenterology* **112**:335, 1997.

90. Galbut DL, Markowitz AM: Insulinoma: Diagnosis, surgical management and long term followup. Review of 41 cases. *Am J Surg* **139**:682, 1980.

91. Rasbach DA, van Heerden JA, Telander RL, Grant CS, Carney A: Surgical management of hyperinsulinism in the multiple endocrine neoplasia type 1 syndrome. *Arch Surg* **123**:584, 1985.

92. Pasieka JL, McLoed MK, Thompson NW, Burney RE: Surgical approach to insulinomas. Assessing the need for preoperative localization. *Arch Surg* **127**:442, 1992.

93. van Heerden JA, Edis AJ, Service FJ: Surgical aspects of insulinomas. *Ann Surg* **189**:677, 1992.

94. Eastman RC, Kahn CR: Hypoglycemia, in Moore WT, Eastman EC (eds): *Diagnostic Endrocrinology*. Toronto, BC Decker, 1990, p 183.

95. Boukhman MP, Karam JH, Shaver J, Siperstein AE, Duh Q-Y, Clark OH: Insulinoma: Experience from 1950 to 1995. *West J Med* **169**:98, 1998.

96. Doppman JL, Miller DL, Chang R: Insulinomas: Localization with selective intrarateral injection of calcium. *Radiology* **178**:237, 1991.

97. Doherty GM, Doppman JL, Shawker TH, Miller DL, Eastman RC, Gorden P, Norton JA: Results of a propective strategy to diagnose, localize and resect insulinomas. *Surgery* **110**:989, 1991.

98. Grant CS, van Heerden JA, Charboneau JW, James EM, Reading CC: Insulinoma: The value of intraoperative ultrasonography. *Arch Surg* **123**:843, 1988.

99. Boden G: Glucagonomas and insulinomas. *Gastroenterol Clin North Am* **18**:831, 1989.

100. Leichter SB: Clinical and metabolic aspects of glucagonoma. *Medicine* **59**:100, 1980.

101. Guillausseau PJ, Guillausseau C, Villet R: Les glucagonomas. Aspect Cliniques biologiques, Anatomo-pathologiques et therapeutiques (Revue général de 130 cas). *Gastroenterol Clin Biol* **6**:1029, 1982.

102. Wilkinson DS: Necrolytic migratory erythema with carcinoma of the pancreas. *Trans St Johns Hosp Dermatol Soc* **59**:244, 1973.

103. Mallison CN, Bloom SR, Warin AP: A glucagonoma syndrome. *Lancet* **2**:1, 1974.

104. Holst JJ: Hormone producing tumors of the gastrointestinal tract, in Cohen S, Soloway RD (eds): *Glucagon-Producing Tumors*. New York, Churchill-Livingstone, 1985, p 57.

105. Verner JV, Morrison AB: Endocrine pancreatic ilset disease with diarrhea: Report of a case due to diffuse hyperplasia of non beta islet tissue with a review of 54 additional cases. *Arch Intern Med* **133**:492, 1974.

106. Matsumoto KK, Peter JB, Schultze RG: Watery diarrhea and hypokalemia associated with pancreatic islet cell adenoma. *Gastroenterology* **50**:231, 1966.

107. Mekhjian H, O'Dorisio TM: VIPoma syndrome. *Semin Oncol* **14**:282, 1987.
108. Kane MG, D'Dorisio TM, Krejs GJ: Production of secretory diarrhea by intravenous infusion of vasoactive intestinal peptide. *N Engl J Med* **309**:1482, 1983.
109. Namihara Y, Achord JL, Subramony C: Multiple endocrine neoplasia, type 1, with pancreatic cholera. *Am J Gastroenterol* **82**:794, 1987.
110. Welbourn RB, Wood SM, Polak JM, Bloom SR: Pancreatic endocrine tumors, in Bloom SR, Polak JM (eds): *Gut Hormones*. New York, Churchill-Livingstone, 1981, p 547.
111. Long RG, Bryant MG, Mitchell SJ, Adrian TE, Polak JM, Bloom SR: Clinicopathological study of pancreatic and ganglioneuroblastoma tumors secreting vasoactive intestinal polyeptide (Vipomas). *Br Med J* **282**:1767, 1981.
112. Capella C, Polak JM, Butta R: Morphologic patterns and diagnostic criteria of VIP-producing endocrine tumors: A histologic, histochemical, ultrastructural and biochemical study of 32 cases. *Cancer* **52**:1860, 1983.
113. Rivier J, Spress J, Thorner M, Vale W: Characterization of a growth-hormone releasing factor from a human pancreatic islet cell tumor. *Nature* **300**:276, 1982.
114. Thorner M, Perryman RI, Cronin MJ: Somatotroph hyperplasia. *J Clin Invest* **70**:965, 1982.
115. Sano T, Asa SL, Kovacs K: Growth hormone releasing-producing tumors: Clinical, biochemical and morphological manifestations. *Endocr Rev* **9**:357, 1988.
116. Asa SL, Singer W, Kovacs K, Horvath E, Murray D, Colapinto N, Thorner MO: Pancreatic endocrine tumour producing growth hormone-releasing hormone associated with multiple endocrine neoplasia type I syndrome. *Acta Endocrinol* **115**:331, 1987.
117. Barkan AL, Shenker Y, Grekin RJ: Acromeglay from ectopic GHRH secretion by malignant carcinoid tumor: Successful treatment with long-acting somatostain analogue SMS. *Cancer* **61**:221, 1986.
118. Sano T, Yamasaki R, Saito H: Growth hormone releasing hormone (GHRH)-secreting pancreatic tumor in a patient with multiple endocrine neoplasia type 1. *Am J Surg Pathol* **11**:810, 1987.
119. Larsson LI, Hirsch MA, Holst JJ: Pancreatic somatostatinoma: Clinical features and physiologic implications. *Lancet* **1**:666, 1977.
120. Ganda OP, Weir GC, Soeldner JS: Somatostatinoma: A somatostatin-containing tumor of the endocrine pancreas. *N Engl J Med* **296**:963, 1977.
121. Vinik AI, Strodel WE, Eckhauser FE, Moattari AR, Lloyd R: Somatostatinomas, Ppomas and neurotensinomas. *Semin Oncol* **14**:263, 1987.
122. Boden G, Shimoyama R: Hormone-producing tumors of the gastrointestinal tract, in Cohen S, Soloway RD (eds): *Somatostatinoma*. New York, Churchill-Livingstone, 1985, p 85.
123. Yamada T, Chiha T: The gastrointestinal system, in Makhlouf GM (ed): *Handbook of Physiology*, sec 6: *Somatostatin*. Bethesda, MD, American Physiological Society, 1979, p 431.
124. Eckhauser FE, Cheung PS, Vinik A, Strodel WE, Lloyd R, Thompson NW: Nonfunctioning malignant neuroendocrine tumors of the pancreas. *Surgery* **100**:978, 1986.
125. Kent RB, van Heerden JA, Weiland LH: Nonfunctioning islet cell tumors. *Ann Surg* **193**:185, 1981.
126. O'Dorisio TM, Vinik AI: Pancreatic polypeptide and mixed peptide-producing tumors of the gastrointestinal tract, in Cohen S, Soloway RD (eds): *Contemporary Issues in Gastroenterology*. Edinburgh, Churchill-Livingstone, 1984, p 117.
127. Takahashi H, Nakano K, Adachi Y: Multiple nonfunctional pancreatic islet cell tumor in multiple endocrine neoplasia type 1: A case report. *Acta Pathol Jpn* **38**:667, 1988.
128. Heitz PU, Kasper M, Polak JM, Kloppel G: Pancreatic endocrine tumors: immunocytochemical analysis of 125 tumors. *Hum Pathol* **13**:163, 1982.
129. Duh Q-Y: Carcinoids associated with multiple endocrine neoplasia syndromes. *Am J Surg* **154**:142, 1987.
130. Godwin JD: Carcinoid tumors. An analysis of 2837 cases. *Cancer* **36**:560, 1975.
131. Teh BT, McArdle J, Chan SP, Menon J, Hartley L, Pullan P, Ho J, Khir A, Wilkinson S, Larsson C, Cameron D, Shepherd J: Clinicopathologic studies of thymic carcinoids in multiple endocrine neoplasia type 1. *Medicine* **76**:21, 1997.
132. Pass HI, Doppman JL, Nieman L: Management of the ectopic ACTH syndrome due to thoracic carcinoids. *Ann Thorac Surg* **50**:52, 1990.
133. Doppman JL, Pass HI, Nieman LK: Detection of ACTH-producing bronchial carcinoid tumors: MR imaging vs CT. *AJR* **156**:39, 1991.
134. Glikson M, Gil-Ad I, Calun E, Dresner R: Acromegaly due to ectopic growth hormone-releasing hormone secretion by a bronchial carcinoid tumour: Dynamic hormonal responses to various stimuli. *Acta Endocrinol (Copenh)* **125**:366, 1991.
135. Maton PN, Dayal Y: Clinical implication of hypergastrinemia, in Dannenberg A, Zakim D (eds): *Peptic Ulcer and Other Acid-Related Diseases*. New York, Academic Research Association, 1993, p 213.
136. Frucht H, Maton PN, Jensen RT: Use of omeprazole in patients with Zollinger-Ellison syndrome. *N Engl J Med* **322**:723, 1990.
137. Jensen RT: Gastrinoma as a model for prolonged hypergastrinemia, in Walsh JH (ed): *Gastrin*. New York, Raven Press, 1993.
138. Benya RV, Metz DC, Hijazi YM, Fishbeyn VA, Pisegna JR, Jensen RT: Fine needle aspiration cytology for the evaluation of submucosal nodules in patients with Zollinger-Ellison sndrome. *Am J Gastroenterol* **88**:258, 1993.
139. Bordi C, Falchetti A, Azzoni C, D'Adda T, Canavese G, Guariglia A, Santini D, Tomasetti P, Brandi ML: Aggressive forms of gastric neuroendocrine tumors in multiple endocrine neoplasia type 1. *Am J Surg Pathol* **21**:1075, 1997.
140. Thompson GB, van Heerden JA, Martin JK, Scutt AJ, Ilstrup DM, Carney JA: Carcinoma of the gastrointestinal tract: Presentation, management, and prognosis. *Surgery* **98**:1054, 1985.
141. Scheithauer BW, Laws ER Jr, Kovacs K, Horvath E, Randall RV, Carney JA: Pituitary adenomas of the multiple endocrine neoplasia type I syndrome. *Semin Diagn Pathol* **4**:205, 1987.
142. Skogseid B, Larsson C, Lindgren PG, Kvanta E, Rastad J, Theodorsson E, Wide L, Wilander E, Oberg K: Clinical and genetic features of adrenocortical lesions in multiple endocrine neoplasia type 1. *J Clin Endorcrinol Metab* **75**:76, 1992.
143. Houdelette P, Chagnon A, Dumotier J, Marthan E: Corticosurrenalome malin dans le cadre d'un syndrome de Wermer. *J Chir (Paris)* **126**:385, 1989.
144. Marx SJ, Agarwal SK, Kester MB, Heppner C, Kim YS, Skarulis MC, James LA, Goldsmith PK, Saggar SK, Park SY, Spiegel AM, Burns AL, Debelenko LV, Zhuang Z, Lubensky IA, Liotta LA, Emmert-Buck MR, Guru SC, Manickam P, Crabtree J, Erdos MR, Collins FS, Chandrasekharappa SC: Multiple endocrine neoplasia type 1: Clinical and genetic features of the hereditary endocrine neoplasias. *Rec Prog Horm Res* **54**:397, 1999.
144b. Dackiw APB, Cote GJ, Fleming JB, Schultz PN, Stanford P, Vassilopoulous-Sellin R, Evans DB, Gagel RF, Lee JE: Screening for MEN1 mutations in patients with atypical endocrine neoplasia.. *Surgery* **126**:1097, 104 1999.
145. Darling TN, Skarulis MC, Steinberg SM, Marx SJ, Spiegel AM, Turner M: Multiple facial angiofibromas and collagenomas in patients with multiple endocrine neoplasia type 1. *Arch Dermatol* **133**:853, 1997.
146. Gaitan D, Loosen PT, Orth DN: Two patients with Cushing's disease in a kindred with multiple endocrine neoplasia type 1. *J Clin Endocrinol Metab* **76**:1580, 1993.
147. Hershon KS, Kelly WA, Shaw CM, Schwartz R, Bierman EL: Prolactinomas as part of the multiple endocrine neoplastic syndrome type 1. *Am J Med* **74**:713, 1983.
148. Farid NR, Buehler S, Russell NA, Maroun FB, Allerdice P, Smyth HS: Prolactinomas in familial multiple endocrine neoplasia syndrome type 1. *Am J Med* **69**:874, 1980.
149. Bear JC, Urbina RB, Fahey JF, Farid NR: Variant multiple endocrine neoplasia I (MEN I-Burin): Further studies and non-linkage to HLA-1. *Hum Hered* **35**:15, 1985.
150. Marx SJ, Powell D, Shimkin PM, Wells SA, Ketcham AS, McGuigan JE, Bilezikian JP, Aurbach GD: Familial hyperparathyroidism: Mild hypercalcemia in at least nine members of a kindred. *Ann Intern Med* **78**:371, 1973.
151. Green JS: Development implementation and evaluation of clinical and genetic screening programs for hereditary tumor syndromes. Ph.D. thesis, Memorial University, Newfoundland, Canada, 1995.
152. Burgess JR, Shepherd JJ, Parameswaran V, Hoffman L, Greenaway TM: Prolactinomas in a large kindred with multiple endocrine neoplasia type 1: Clinical features and inheritance pattern. *J Clin Endocrinol Metab* **81**:1841, 1996.
153. Goldsmith RE, Sizemore GW, Chen I, Zalme E, Altemeier WA: Familial hyperparathyroidism description of a large kindred with physiologic observations and a review of the literature. *Ann Intern Med* **842**:36, 1976.
154. Kassem M, Zhang X, Brask S, Ericksen EF, Mosekilde L, Kruse TA: Familial isolated primary hyperparathyroidism. *Clin Endocrinol* **41**:415, 1994.

155. Burgess JR, Greenaway TM, Parameswaran V, Challis DR, David R, Shepherd JJ: Enteropancreatic malignancy associated with multiple endocrine neoplasia type 1: Risk factors and pathogenesis. *Cancer* **83**:428, 1998.
156. Zhuang Z, Ezzat SZ, Vortmeyer AS, Weil R, Oldfield EH, Park WS, Pack S, Huang S, Agarwal SK, Guru SC, Manickam P, Debelenko LV, Kester MB, Olufemi SE, Heppner C, Burns AL, Spiegel AM, Marx SJ, Chandrasekharappa SC, Collins FS, Emmert-Buck MR, Liotta L, Asa SL, Lubensky IA: Mutations of the MEN1 tumor suppressor gene in pituitary tumors. *Cancer Res* **57**:5446, 1997.
158. Arnold A (ed): *Endocrine Neoplasms*. Boston, Kluwer Academic Publishers, 1997.
159. Maton PN, Gardner JD, Jensen RT: Cushing's syndrome in patients with Zollinger-Ellison syndrome. *N Engl J Med* **315**:1, 1986.
160. Kloppel G, Heitz PU: Pancreatic endocrine tumors. *Pathol Res Pract* **183**:155, 1988.
161. Melmed S, Ezrin C, Kovacs K, Goodman RS, Frohman LA: Acromegaly due to secretion of growth hormone by an ectopic pancreatic islet-cell tumor. *N Engl J Med* **312**:9, 1986.
162. Schimke RN: Multiple endocrine adenomatosis syndrome. *Adv Intern Med* **21**:249, 1976.
163. Calcatera TC, Paglia D: The coexistence of parathyroid adenoma and thyroid carcinoma. *Laryngoscope* **89**:1166, 1979.
164. Simpson RJ, Moss J Jr: Parathyroid adenoma and nonmedullary thyroid carcinoma association. *Otolaryngol Head Neck Surg* **101**:584, 1989.
165. Doumith R, Gennes JL, Cabane JP, Zygelman N: Pituitary prolactinoma, adrenal aldosterone producing adenoma, gastric schwannoma and clonic polyadenomas: A possible variant of multiple endocrine neoplasia (MEN) type 1. *Acta Endocrinol* **100**:189, 1982.
166. Holland OB, Gomez-Sanchez CE, Kem DC, Weiberger MH, Kramer NJ, Higgins JR: Evidence against prolactin stimulation of aldosterone in normal subjects and in patients with primary hyperaldosteronism, including a patient with primary hyperaldosteronismn and prolactin producing pituitary macroadenoma. *J Clin Endocrinol Metab* **45**:1064, 1977.
167. Blumenkopf B, Boekelheide K: Neck paraganglinoma with a pituitary adenoma: Case report. *J Neurosurg* **57**:426, 1982.
168. Nelson DR, Stachura ME, Dunlap DB: Case report: Ileal carcinoid tumor complicated by retroperitoneal fibrosis and prolactinoma. *Am J Med Sci* **296**:129, 1988.
169. Barzilay J, Heatley GJ, Cushing GW: Benign and malignant tumors in patients with acromegaly. *Arch Intern Med* **151**:1629, 1991.
170. Anderson RJ, Lufkin EG, Sizemore GW, Carney JA, Sheps SG, Silliman YE: Acromegaly and pituitary adenoma with pheochromocytoma: A variant of multiple endocrine neoplasia. *Clin Endocrinol* **14**:605, 1981.
171. Morris JA, Tymms DJ: Oat cell carcinoma, pheochromocytoma and carcinoid tumors — Multiple APUD neoplasia. A case report. *J Pathol* **131**:107, 1980.
172. Farhi F, Dikman SH, Lawson W, Cobin RH, Zak FG: Paragangliomatosis associated with multiple endocrine adenomas. *Arch Pathol Lab Med* **100**:495, 1976.
173. Hansen OP, Hansen M, Hansen HH, Rose B: Multiple endocrine adenomatosis of the mixed type. *Acta Med Scand* **200**:327, 1976.
174. Cameron D, Spiro HM, Lansberg L: Zollinger-Ellison syndrome with multiple endocrine adenomatosis type II. *N Engl J Med* **299**:152, 1978.
175. Janson KL, Roberts JA, Varela M: Multiple endocrine adenomatosis: In support of the common origin theories. *J Urol* **119**:161, 1978.
176. Alberts MW, Mcmeekin JO, George JM: Mixed multiple endocrine neoplasia syndromes. *JAMA* **244**:1236, 1980.
177. Cusick JF, Ho KC, Hagen TC, Kun LE: Granular-cell pituicytoma associated with multiple endocrine neoplasia type 2. *J Neurosurg* **56**:594, 1982.
178. Manning GS, Stevens KA, Stock JL: Multiple endocrine neoplasia type 1: Association with marfanoid habitus, optic atrophy, and other abnormalities. *Arch Intern Med* **143**:2315, 1983.
179. Bertnard JH, Ritz P, Reznik Y, Grollier G, Potier JC, Evrad C, Mahoudeau JA: Sipple's syndrome associated with a large prolactinoma. *Clin Endocrinol* **27**:607, 1987.
180. Jerkins TW, Sacks HS, O'Dorisio TM, Tuttle S, Solomon SS: Medullary carcinoma of the thyroid, pancreatic nesidioblastosis and microadenosis, and pancreatic polypeptide hypersecretion: A new association and clinical and hormonal response to a long-acting somatostatin analog. *J Clin Endocrinol Metab* **64**:1313, 1987.
181. Maton PN, Norton JA, Nieman LK, Doppman JL, Jensen RT: Multiple endocrine neoplasia type II with Zollinger-Ellison syndrome caused by a solitary pancreatic gastinoma. *JAMA* **262**:535, 1989.
182. Reschini E, Catania A, Airaghi L, Manfredi MG, Crosignani PG: Scintigraphic study of extra-adrenal ganglioneuroma in a patient with overlap between multiple endocrine neoplasia types 1 and 2. *Clin Nucl Med* **17**:573, 1992.
183. Modan B, Baidatz D, Mart H, Steinitz R, Levin SG: Radiation-induced head and neck tumors. *Lancet* I 277, 1975.
184. Schneider AB, Shore-Freedman E, Weinstein RA: Radiation-induced thyroid and other head and neck tumors: Occurrence of multiple tumors and analysis of risk factors. *J Clin Endocrinol Metab* **63**:107, 1986.
185. Rosen IB, Strawbridge HG, Bain J: A case hyperparathyroidism associated with radiation of the head and neck area. *Cancer* **36**:1111, 1975.
186. Tisell LE, Carlsson S, Lindberg S, Ragnhult I: Autonomous hyperparathyroidism: A possible late complication of neck radiotherapy. *Acta Chir Scand* **142**:889, 1976.
187. Hedman I, Hansson G, Lundberg LM, Tisell LE: A clinical evaluation of radiation-induced hyperparathyroidism based on 148 surgically treated patients. *World J Surg* **8**:96, 1984.
188. Christmas TJ, Chapple CR, Noble JG, Milroy EJG, Cowie AGA: Hyperparathyroidism after neck irradiation. *Br J Surg* **75**:873, 1988.
189. Fujiwara S, Spoto R, Ezaki HAB, Akiba S, Neriishi K, Kodama K, Hosada Y, Shimaoka K: Hyperparathyroidism among atomic bomb survivors in Hiroshima. *Radiat Res* **130**:372, 1992.
190. Printz RA, Paloyan E, Lawrence AM, Pickleman JR, Braithwaite S, Brooks MH: Radiation-associated hyperparathyroidism: A new syndrome? *Surgery* **822**:276, 1977.
191. Tisell LE, Hansson G, Lindberg S, Ragnhult I: Hyperparathyroidism in persons treated with X-rays for tuberculous cervical adenitis. *Cancer* **40**:846, 1977.
192. Cohen J, Gierlowski TC, Schneider AB: A prospective study of hyperparathyroidism in individuals exposed to radiation in childhood. *JAMA* **264**:581, 1990.
193. Katz A, Braunstein GD: Clinical, biochemical and pathologic features of radiation-associated hyperparathyroidism. *Arch Intern Med* **143**:79, 1983.
194. Weinstein LS: Other skeletal diseases of G proteins — McCune-Albright syndrome, in Bilezikian J, Raisz L, Rodan G (eds): *Principles of Bone Biology*. New York, Academic Press, 1996, p 877.
195. Weinstein LS, Shenker A, Gejman PV, Merino MJ, Friedman E, Spiegel AM: Activating mutations of the stimulatory G protein in the McCune-Albright syndrome. *N Engl J Med* **325**:1688, 1991.
196. Landis CA, Masters SB, Spada A, Pace AM, Bourne HR, Vallar L: GTPase inhibiting mutations activate the subunit of Gs and stimulate adenylyl cyclase in human pituitary tumors. *Nature* **340**:692, 1989.
197. Bianco P, Kuznetsov SA, Riminucci M, Fisher LW, Spiegel AM, Robey PG: Reproduction of human fibrous dysplasia of bone in immunocompromised mice by transplanted mosaics of normal and Gsalpha-mutated skeletal progenitor cells. *J Clin Invest* **101**:1737, 1998.
198. Ponder B: Multiple endocrine neoplasia type 2, in Scriver CR, Beaudet A, Sly WS, Valle D, Vogelstein B (eds): *Metabolic and Molecular Bases of Inherited Disease*, 8th ed. New York, McGraw-Hill, 2000.
199. Schuffenecker I, Virally-Monod M, Brohet R, Goldgar D, Conte-Devolx B, Leclerc L, Chabre O, Boneu A, Caron J, Houdent C and the Groupe D'Etude des Tumeurs a Calcitonine: Risk and penetrance of primary hyperparathyroidism in multiple endocrine neoplasia type 2A families with mutations at codon 634 of the RET proto-oncogene. *J Clin Endocrinol Metab* **83**:487, 1998.
200. Schweitzer-Cagianut M, Froesch ER, Hedinger C: Familial Cushing's syndrome with primary adrenocortical microadenomatosis (primary adrenocortical nodular dysplasia). *Acta Endocrinol (Copenh)* **94**:529, 1980.
201. Carney JA, Gordon H, Carpenter PC, Shenoy BV, Go VLW: The complex of myxomas, spotty pigmentation and endocrine overactivity. *Medicine* **64**:270, 1985.
202. Stratakis CA, Courcoutsakis NA, Abati A, Filie A, Doppman JL, Carney JA, Shawker T: Thyroid gland abnormalities in patients with the syndrome of spotty skin pigmentation, myxomas, endocrine overactivity, and schwannomas (Carney complex). *J Clin Endocrinol Metab* **82**:2037, 1997.
203. Stratakis CA, Carney JA, Lin JP, Papaniccolaou DA, Karl M, Kastner DL, Pras E, Chrousos GP: Carney complex, a familial multiple

neoplasia and lentiginosis syndrome: Analysis of 11 kindreds and linkage to the short arm of chromosome 2. *J Clin Invest* **97**:699, 1996.

204. Basson CT, MacRae CA, Korf B, Merliss A: Genetic heterogeneity of familial atrial myxoma syndromes (Carney complex). *Am J Cardiol* **79**:994, 1997.
205. Linehan WM, Klausner R: Renal carcinoma, in Scriver CR, Beaudet A, Sly WS, Valle D, Vogelstein B (eds): *Metabolic and Molecular Bases of Inherited Disease*, 8th ed. New York, McGraw-Hill, 2000.
206. Lubensky IA, Pack S, Ault D, Vortmeyer AO, Libutti SK, Choyke PL, Walther MM, Linehan WM, Zhuang ZP: Multiple neuroendocrine tumors of the pancreas in von Hipple-Lindau disease patients. *Am J Pathol* **153**:1, 1998.
207. Neumann HPH: Basic criteria for clinical diagnosis and genetic counseling in von Hippel-Lindau syndrome. *J Vasc Dis* **16**:220, 1987.
208. Latif F, Tory K, Gnara J, Yao M, Duh FM, Orcutt ML, Stackhouse T, Kuzmin I, Modi W, Geil L: Identification of the von Hipple-Lindau disease tumor suppressor gene. *Science* **260**:1317, 1993.
209. Pause A, Lee S, Worrell RA, Chen DY, Burgess WH, Linehan WM, Klausner RD: The von Hippel-Landau tumor-suppressor gene product forms a stable complex with human CUL-2, a member of the Cdc53 family of proteins. *Proc Natl Acad Sci USA* **94**:2156, 1997.
210. Malkin D: Li-Fraumeni syndrome, in Scriver CR, Beaudet A, Sly WS, Valle D, Vogelstein B (eds): *Metabolic and Molecular Bases of Inherited Disease*, 8th ed. New York, McGraw-Hill, 2000.
211. Eng C, Parsons R: Cowden syndrome, in Scriver CR, Beaudet A, Sly WS, Valle D, Vogelstein B (eds): *Metabolic and Molecular Bases of Inherited Disease*, 8th ed. New York, McGraw-Hill, 2000.
212. Guttman GH, Collins FS: Neurofibromatosis, in Scriver CR, Beaudet A, Sly WS, Valle D, Vogelstein B (eds): *Metabolic and Molecular Bases of Inherited Disease*, 8th ed. New York: McGraw-Hill, 2000.
213. Weinstein RS, Harris RL: Hypercalcemic hyperparathyroidism and hypophosphatemic osteomalacia complicating neurofibromatosis. *Calcif Tissue Int* **46**:261, 1990.
214. Swinburn BA, Yeong ML, Lane MR, Nicholson GI, Holdaway IM: Neurofibromatosis associated with somatostatinoma: A report of two patients. *Clin Endocrinol* **28**:353, 1988.
215. Sartori P, Symons JC, Taylor NF, Grant OB: Adrenal cortical adenoma in a 13 year old girl with neurofibromatosis. *Acta Paediatr Scand* **78**:476, 1989.
216. DeAngelis LM, Kelleher MB, Kalmon DP, Fetell MR: Multiple paragangliomatosis in neurofibromatosis: A new neuroendocrine neoplasia. *Neurology* **37**:129, 1987.
217. Cawthon RM, Weiss R, Xu C, Viskochill D, Culver M, Stevens J, Robertson M, Dunn D, Gesteland R, O'Connel P, White R: A major segment of the neurofibromatosis type 1 gene: cDNA sequence, genomic structure, and point mutations. *Cell* **62**:193, 1990.
218. Jackson CE, Norum RA, Boyd SB, Talpos GB, Wilson SD, Taggart T, Mallette LE: Hereditary hyperparathyroidism and multiple ossifying jaw fibromas: A clinically and genetically distinct syndrome. *Surgery* **108**:1006, 1990.
219. Mallette LE, Malini S, Rappaport MP, Kirkland JL: Familial cystic parathyroid adenomatosis. *Ann Intern Med* **107**:54, 1987.
220. Teh BT, Farnebo F, Kristoffersson U, Sundelin B, Cardinal J, Axelson R, Yap A, Epstein M, Heath H III, Cameron D, Larsson C: Autosomal dominant primary hyperparathyroidism and jaw tumor syndrome associated with renal hamartomas and cystic kidney disease: Linkage to 1q21-q32 and loss of the wild type allele in renal hamartomas. *J Clin Endocrinol Metab* **81**:4204, 1996.
221. Szabo J, Heath B, Hill VM, Jackson CE, Zarbo RJ, Mallette LE, Chew SL, Besser GM, Thakker RV, Huff V, Leppert MF, Heath H III: Hereditary hyperparathyroidism–jaw tumor syndrome: The endocrine tumor gene HRPT2 maps to chromosome 1q21-q31. *Am J Hum Genet* **56**:944, 1995.
222. Teh BT, Farnebo F, Twigg S, Kristoffersson U, Sundelin B, Cardinal J, Axelson R, Yap A, Epstein M, Heath H III, Camerson D, Larsson C: Familial isolated hyperparathyroidism maps to the hyperparathyroidism–jaw tumor locus in 1q21-q32 in a subset of families. *J Clin Endocrinol Metab* **83**: 2114, 1998.
223. Wassif WS, Moniz CF, Friedman E, Wong S, Weber G, Nordenskjold M, Peters TJ, Larsson C: Familial isolated hyperparathyroidism: A distinct genetic entity with an increased risk of parathyroid cancer. *J Clin Endocrinol Metab* **77**:1485, 1993.
224. Streeten E, Weinstein LS, Norton JA, Mulvihill JJ, White B, Friedman E, Jaffe G, Brandi ML, Stewart K, Zimering MB, Spiegel AM, Aurbach GD, Marx SJ: Studies in a kindred with parathyroid carcinoma. *J Clin Endocrinol Metab* **75**:362, 1992.
225. Law WM Jr, Hodgson S, Heath H III: Autosomal recessive inheritance of familial hyperparathyroidism. *N Engl J Med* **309**:650, 1983.
226. Allo M, Thompson NW: Familial hyperparathyroidism caused by solitary adenomas. *Surgery* **92**:486, 1982.
227. Huang SM, Duh O-Y, Shaver J, Siperstein AE, Kraimp JL, Clark OH: Familial hyperparathyroidism without multiple endocrine neoplasia. *World J Surg* **21**:22, 1997.
228. Farnebo F, Teh B, Dotzenrath C, Wassif WS, Svensson A, White I, Betz R, Goretzki P, Sandelin K, Farnebo LO, Larsson C: Differential loss of heterozygosity in familial, sporadic, and uremic hyperparathyroidism. *Hum Genet* **99**:342, 1997.
229. Tragl KH, Mayr WR: Familial islet cell adenomatosis. *Lancet* **1**:426, 1977.
230. Maioli M, Cicarese M, Pacifico A, Tonolo G, Ganau A, Cossu S, Tanda F, Realdi G: Familial insulinoma: Description of two cases. *Acta Diabetol* **29**:38, 1992.
231. Kinnamon JEC: Heredity and symptoms in acromegaly. *Acta Otolaryngol* **82**:230, 1976.
232. Kurisaka M, Takei Y, Tsubokawa T, Motiyasu N: Growth hormone-secreting pituitary adenoma in uniovular twin brothers: Case report. *Neurosurgery* **8**:226, 1981.
233. Jones MK, Evans PJ, Jopnes IR, Thomas JP: Familial acromegaly. *Clin Endocrinol (Oxf)* **20**:355, 1984.
234. Abbassioun K, Fatourechi V, Amirjamshidi A, Meibodi NA: Familial acromegaly with pituitary adenoma: Report of three affected siblings. *J Neurosurg* **64**:510, 1986.
235. Pestell RG, Alford FP, Best JD: Familial acromegaly. *Acta Endocrinol (Copenh)* **121**:286, 1989.
236. Benlian P, Giraud S, Lahlou N, Roger M, Blin C, Holler C, Lenoir G, Sallandre J, Calender A, Turpin G: Familial acromegaly: A specific clinical entity. Further evidence from the genetic study of a three-generation family. *Eur J Endocrinol* **133**:451, 1995.
237. Yamada S, Yoshimoto K, Sano T, Takada K, Itakura M, Usui M, Teramoto A: Inactivation of the tumor suppressor gene on 11q13 in brothers with familial acrogigantism without multiple endocrine neoplasia type 1. *Clin Endocrinol Metab* **82**:239, 1997.
238. Berezin M, Karasik A: Familial prolactinoma. *Clin Endocrinol* **42**:483, 1995.
239. Eschbach JW, Rinaldo JA: Metastatic carcinoid: A familial occurrence. *Ann Intern Med* **57**:647, 1962.
240. Anderson RE: A familial instance of appendiceal carcinoid tumors. *Am J Surg* **111**:738, 1966.
241. Wale RJ, William JA, Veeley AH: Familial occurrence in carcinoid tumors. *Aust NZ J Surg* **53**:325, 1983.
242. Moertel CG, Dockerty MB: Familial occurrence of metastasizing carcinoid tumors. *Ann Intern Med* **78**:389, 1973.
243. Yeatman TJ, Sharp JV, Kimura AK: Can susceptibility to carcinoid tumors be inherited? *Cancer* **63**:390, 1989.
244. Marx SJ, Attie M, Levine MA, Spiegel AM, Downs RW Jr, Lasker RD: The hypocalciuric or benign variant of familial hypercalcemia: Clinical and biochemical features in fifteen kindreds. *Medicine* **60**:397, 1981.
245. Firek AF, Kao PC, Heath H III: Plasma intact parathyroid hormone (PTH) and PTH-related peptide in familial benign hypercalcemia: Greater responsiveness to endogenous PTH than in primary hyperparathyroidism. *J Clin Endocrinol Metab* **72**:541, 1991.
246. Thorgeirsson U, Costa J, Marx SJ: The parathyroid glands in familial hypocalciuric hypercalcemia. *Hum Pathol* **12**:229, 1981.
247. Attie MF, Gill JR Jr, Stock JL, Spiegel AM, Downs RW Jr, Levine MA, Marx SJ: Urinary calcium excretion in familial hypocalciuric hypercalcemia: Persistence of relative hypocalciuria after induction of hypoparathyroidism. *J Clin Invest* **72**:667, 1983.
248. Brown EM, Pollak M, Seidman CE, Seidman JG, Chou YHW, Riccardi D, Herbert SC: Calcium-ion-sensing cell-surface receptors. *N Engl J Med* **333**:234, 1995.
249. Heath H III, Jackson CE, Otterud B, Leppert MF: Genetic linkage analysis in familial benign (hypocalciuric) hypercalcemia: Evidence for locus heterogeneity. *Am J Hum Genet* **53**:193, 1993.
250. Trump D, Whyte MP, Wooding C, Pang JT, Pearce SHS, Kocher DV, Thakker RV: Linkage studies in a kindred from Oklahoma, with familial benign (hypocalciuric) hypercalcaemia (FBH) and developmental elevations in serum parathyroid hormone levels, indicate a third locus for FBH. *Hum Genet* **96**:183, 1995.
251. Pollack MR, Chou YHW, Marx SJ, Steinman B, Cole DEC, Brandi ML, Papopoulos SE, Menko F, Hendy GN, Brown EM, Seidman CE, Seidman JG: Familial hypocalciuric hypercalcemia and neonatal

severe hyperparathyroidism: Effects of mutant gene dosage on phenotype. *J Clin Invest* **93**:1108, 1994.

252. Pearse SHR, Trump D, Wooding C, Besser GM, Hew SL, Grant DB, Heath DA, Hughes IA, Paterson CR, Whyte MP, Thakker RV: Calcium-sensing receptor mutations in familial benign hypercalcemia and neonatal hyperparathyroidism. *J Clin Invest* **96**:2683, 1995.
253. Tonacchera M, Van Sande J, Cetani F, Swillens S, Schvartz C, Winiszewski L, Portmann L, Dumont JE, Vassart G, Parma J: Functional characteristics of three new germline mutations of the thyrotropin receptor gene causing autosomal dominant toxic thyroid hyperplasia. *J Clin Endocrinol Metab* **81**:547, 1996.
254. Shenker A, Laue L, Kosugi S, Merendino JJ, Menegishi T, Cutler GB Jr: A constitutively activating mutation of the luteinizing-hormone receptor in familial male precocious puberty. *Nature* **365**:652, 1993.
255. Thomas PM, Cote GJ, Wohlik N, Haddad B, Mathew PM, Rabel W, Aguilar-Bryan L, Gagel RF, Bryan J: Mutations in the sulfonylurea receptor gene in familial persistent hyperinsulinemic hypoglycemia of infancy. *Science* **268**:426, 1995.
256. Thomas PM, Ye Y, Lightner E: Mutation of the pancreatic islet inward rectifier Kir6.2 also leads to familial persistent hyperinsulinemic hypoglycemia of infancy. *Hum Mol Genet* **11**:1809, 1996.
257. Glaser B, Kesavan P, Heyman M, Davis E, Cuesta A, Buchs A, Stanley CA, Thornton PS, Permutt MA, Matschinsky FM, Herold KC: Familial hyperinsulinism caused by an activating glucokinase mutation. *N Engl J Med* **338**:226, 1998.
258. Stanley CA, Lieu YK, Hsu BY, Burlina AB, Greenberg CR, Hopwood NJ, Perlman K, Rich BH, Zammarchi E, Poncz M: Hyperinsulinism and hyperammonemia in infants with regulatory mutations of the glutamate dehydrogenase gene. *N Engl J Med* **338**:1352, 1998.

258b. Marx SJ: Contrasting paradigms for hereditary hyperfunction of endocrine cells. *J Clin Endocrinol Metab* **84**:3001, 1999.

259. Ho C, Conner DA, Pollak MR, Ladd DJ, Kifor O, Warren HB, Brown EM, Seidman JG, Seidman CE: A mouse model of human familial hypocalciuric hypercalcemia and neonatal severe hyperparathyroidism. *Nature Genet* **11**:389, 1995.
260. Vassart G: New pathophysiological mechanisms in hyperthyroidism. *Horm Res* **48(suppl 4)**:47, 1997.

260a. Verkarre V, Fournet J-C, de Lonlay P, Gross-Morand M-S, Devillers M, Rahier J, Brunelle F, Robert J-J, Nihoul-Fekete C, Saudubray J-M, Junien C: Paternal mutation of the sulfonylurea receptor (SUR1) gene and maternal loss of 11p15 imprinted genes lead to persistent hyperinsulinism in focal adenomatous hyperplasia. *J Clin Invest* **102: 1286, 1998.**

261. Parma J, Duprez L, Van Sande J, Hermans J, Roomans P, Van Vliet G, Costagliola S, Rodien P, Dumont JE, Vassart G: Diversity and prevalence of somatic mutations in the thyrotrophin receptor and Gs alpha genes as a cause of toxic thyroid adenomas. *J Clin Endocrinol Metab* **82**:2695, 1997.
262. Liu G, Duranteau L, Monroe J, Doyle DA, Carel J-C, Shenker A: A novel somatic mutation of the lutrophic receptor (LHR) gene in leydig cell adenoma, in *Program and Abstracts of the 80th Annual Meeting of the Endocrine Society*, 1998 (abstract), p 62.
263. Brandi ML, Fitzpatrick LA, Coon HG, Aurbach GD: Bovine parathyroid cells: Cultures maintained for more than 140 population doublings. *Proc Natl Acad Sci USA* **83**:1709, 1986.
264. Sakaguchi K, Santora A, Zimering M, Curcio F, Aurbach GD, Brandi ML: Functional epithelial cell line cloned from rat parathyroid glands. *Proc Natl Acad Sci USA* **84**:3269, 1987.
265. Brandi ML, Ornberg R, Sakaguchi K, Curcio F, Fattorossi A, Lelkes P, Matsui T, Zimering M, Aurbach GD: Establishment and characterization of a clonal line of parathyroid endothelial cells. *FASEB J* **4**:3152, 1990.
266. Brandi ML, Aurbach GD, Fitzpatrick LA: Parathyroid mitogenic activity in plasma from patients with familial multiple endocrine neoplasia type 1. *N Engl J Med* **314**:1287, 1985.
267. Marx SJ, Sakagucki K, Green JE III, Aurbach GD, Brandi ML: Mitogenic activity on parathyroid cells in plasma from members of a large kindred with multiple endocrine neoplasia type 1. *J Clin Endocrinol Metab* **67**:149, 1988.
268. Friedman E, Larsson C, Amorosi A, Brandi ML, Bale A, Metz D, Jensen RT, Skarulis M, Eastman RC, Nieman L, Norton JA, Marx SJ: Multiple endocrine neoplasia type 1: Pathology pathophysiology, and differential diagnosis, in Bilezekian JP, Levine MA, Marcus R (eds): *The Parathyroids*. New York, Raven Press, 1994, p 647.
269. Zimering MB, Brandi ML, DeGrange DA, Marx SJ, Streeten E, Katsumata N, Murphy PR, Sato Y, Friesen HG, Arubach GD: Circulating fibroblast growth factor-like substance in familial multiple endocrine neoplasia type 1. *J Clin Endocrinol Metab* **70**:149, 1990.
270. Bikealvi A, Klein S, Pintucci G, Rifkin DB: Biological roles of fibroblast growth factor-2. *Endocr Rev* **18**:26, 1997.
271. Brem H, Klagsbrun M: The role of fibroblast growth factors and related oncogenes in tumor growth. *Cancer Treat Res* **63**:211, 1992.
272. Zimering MB, Katsumata N, Sato Y, Brandi ML, Aurbach GD, Marx SJ, Friesen HG: Increeased basic fibroblast growth factor in plasma from multiple endocrine neoplasia type 1: Relation to pituitary tumor. *J Clin Endocrinol Metab* **76**:1182, 1993.

272b. Vortmeyer AO, Boni R, Pack SD, Darling TN, Zhuang Z: Perivascular cells harboring multiple endocrine neoplasia type 1 alteration are neoplastic cells in angiofibromas. *Cancer Res* **59**:274, 1999.

273. Gustavsson KH, Jansson R, Oberg K: Chromosomal breakage in multiple endocrine adenomatosis (type 1 and II). *Clin Genet* **23**:143, 1983.
274. Benson L, Gustavson KH, Rastad J, Akerstrom G, Oberg K, Ljunghall S: Cytogenetical investigations in patient with primary hyperparathyroidism and multiple endocrine neoplasia type 1. *Hereditas* **108**:227, 1988.
275. Scappaticci S, Maraschio P, Del Ciotto N, Fossati GS, Zonta A, Fraccarp M: Chromosome abnormalities in lymphocytes and fibroblasts of subjects with multiple endocrine neoplasia type 1. *Cancer Genet Cytogenet* **52**:85, 1991.
276. Bale SJ, Bale AE, Stewart K, Dachowski L, McBride OW, Glaser T, Green JE III, Mulvihill JJ, Brandi ML, Sakaguchi K, Aurbach GD, Marx SJ: Linkage analysis of multiple endocrine neoplasia type 1 with int-2 and other markers on chromosome 11. *Genomics* **4**:320, 1989.
277. Sakurai A, Katai M, Itakura Y, Nakajima K, Baba K, Hashizume K: Genetic screening in hereditary multiple endocrine neoplasia type 1: Absence of a founder effect among Japanese families. *Jpn J Cancer Res* **87**:985, 1996.
278. Teh BT, Hii SI, David R, Parameswaran V, Grimmond S, Walters MK, Tan TT, Nancarrow DJ, Chan SP, Mennon J, Larsson C, Zaini A, Khalid AK, Shepherd JJ, Cameron DP, Hayward NK: Multiple endocrine neoplasia type (MEN1) in two Asian families. *Hum Genet* **94**:468, 1994.
279. Kytola S, Leisti J, Winqvist R, Salmela P: Improved carrier testing for multiple endocrine neoplasia, type 1, using new microsatellite-type DNA markers. *Hum Genet* **96**:449, 1995.
280. Smith CM, Wells SA, Gerhard DS: Mapping eight new polymorphisms in 11q13 in the vicinity of multiple endocrine neoplasia type 1: Identification of a new distal recombinant. *Hum Genet* **96**:377, 1995.
281. Courseaux A, Grosgeorge J, Gaudray P, Pannett AAJ, Forbes SA, Williamson C, Bassett D, Thakker RV, Teh BT, Farnebo F, Shepherd J, Skogseid B, Larsson C, Giraud S, Zhang CX, Salandre J, Calender A: The European Consortium on MEN1: Definition of the minimal MEN1 candidate area based on a 5-Mb integrated map of proximal 11q13. *Genomics* **37**:354, 1996.
282. Larsson C, Calender A, Grimmond S, Giraud S, Hayward NK, Teh BT, Farnebo F: Molecular tools for presymptomatic testing in multiple endocrine neoplasia type 1. *J Intern Med* **2328**:239, 1995.
283. Petty EM, Green JS, Marx SJ, Taggart RT, Farid N, Bale AE: Mapping the gene for hereditary hyperparathyroidism and prolactinoma (MEN1-Burin) to chromosome 11q: Evidence for a founder effect in patients from Newfoundland. *Am J Hum Genet* **54**:1060, 1994.
284. Olufemi SE, Green JS, Manickam P, Guru SC, Agarwal SK, Kester MB, Dong Q, Burns AL, Spiegel AM, Marx SJ, Coillins FS, Chandrasekharappa SC: A common ancestral mutation in the MEN1 gene is likely responsible for the prolactinoma variant (MEN1-Burin) in four kindreds from Newfoundland. *Hum Mutat* **11**:264, 1998.
285. Stock JL, Warth MR, Teh BT, Coderre JA, Overdorf JH, Baumann G, Hintz RL, Hartman ML, Seizinger BR, Larsson C, Aronin N: A kindred with a variant of multiple endocrine neoplasia type 1 demonstrating frequent expression of pituitary tumors but not linked to the multiple endocrine neoplasia type 1 locus at chromosome region 11q13. *J Clin Endocrinol Metab* **82**:486, 1997.
286. Bahn RS, Scheithauer BW, van Heerden JA, Laws ER Jr, Horvath E, Gharib H: Nonidentical expressions of multiple endocrine neoplasia type 1 in identical twins. *Mayo Clin Proc* **61**:689, 1986.

286a. Flanagan DE, Armitage M, Clein GP, Thakker RV: Prolactinoma presenting in identical twins with multiple endocrine neoplasia type 1. *Clin Endocrinol* **45**:117, 1996.

287. Brandi ML, Weber G, Svensson A, Falchetti A, Tonelli F, Castello R, Furlani L, Scappaticci S, Fraccaro M, Larsson C: Homozygotes for the autosomal dominant neoplasia syndrome (MEN1). *Am J Hum Genet* **53**:1167, 1993.
288. Muhr C, Ljunghall S, Akerstrom G, Palmer M, Bergstrom K, Enoksson P, Lundqvist G, Wide L: Screening for multiple endocrine neoplasia syndrome (type 1) in patients with primary hyperparathyroidism. *Clin Endocrinol* **20**:153, 1984.
289. de Mars R: Published discussion, *23rd Annual Symposium of Fundamental Cancer Research.* Baltimore, Williams & Wilkins, 1969, p 105 (abstract).
290. Knudson AG: Mutation and cancer: Statistical study of retinoblastoma. *Proc Natl Acad Sci USA* **68**:820, 1971.
291. Friedman E, Sakaguchi K, Bale AE, Falchetti A, Streeten A, Zimering MB, Weinstein LS, McBride WO, Nakamura Y, Brandi ML, Norton JA, Aurbach GD, Spiegel AM, Marx SJ: Clonality of parathyroid tumors in familial multiple endocrine neoplasia type 1. *N Engl J Med* **321**:213, 1989.
292. Thakker RV, Bouloux P, Wooding C, Chotai K, Broad PM, Spurr NK, Besser GM, O'Riordan JLH: Association of parathyroid tumors in multiple endocrine neoplasia type 1 with loss of alleles on chromosome 11. *N Engl J Med* **321**:218, 1989.
293. Bystrom C, Larsson C, Blomberg C, Sandelin K, Falkermern U, Skogseid B, Oberg K, Werner S, Nordenskhold M: Localization of the MEN 1 gene to a small region within chromosome 11q13 by deletion mapping in tumors. *Proc Natl Acad Sci USA* **87**:1968, 1990.
294. Radford DM, Ashley SM, Wells SA, Gerhard DS: Loss of hetrozygosity of markers on chromosome 11 in tumors from patients with multiple endocrine neoplasia syndrome type 1. *Cancer Res* **50**:6529, 1990.
295. Friedman E, DeMarco L, Gejman PV, Norton JS, Bale AE, Aurbach GD, Spiegel AM, Marx SJ: Allelic loss from chromosome 11 in parathyroid tumors. *Cancer Res* **525**:6804, 1992.
296. Morelli A, Falchetti A, Amorosi A, Tonelli F, Bearzi I, Ranaldi R, Tomassetti P, Brandi ML: Clonal analysis by chromsome 11 microsatellite-PCR of microdissected parathyroid tumors from MEN1 patients. *Biochem Biophys Res Commun* **227**:736, 1996.
297. Weil RJ, Vortmeyer AO, Huang S, Huang S, Boni R, Lubensky IA, Pack S, Marx SJ, Zhuang Z, Oldfield EH: 11q13 Allelic loss in pituitary tumors in patients with multiple endocrine neoplasia type 1. *Clin Cancer Res* **4**:1673, 1998.
298. Lubensky IA, Debelenko LV, Zhuang Z, Emmert-Buck MR, Dong Q, Chandrasekharappa SC, Guru SC, Manickam P, Olufemi SE, Marx SJ, Spiegel AM, Collins FS, Liotta LA: Allelic deletions in chromosome 11q13 in multiple tumors from individual MEN1 patients. *Cancer Res* **56**:5272, 1996.
299. Zhuang Z, Bertheau P, Emmert-Buck MR, Liotta LA, Gnarra J, Linehan WM, Lubensky IA: A microdissection technique for archival DNA analysis of specific cell populations in lesions, 1 mm in size. *Am J Pathol* **146**:620, 1995.
300. Emmert-Buck MR, Bonner RF, Smith PD, Chuaqui RF, Zhuang Z, Goldstein SR, Weiss RA, Liotta LA: Laser capture microdissection. *Science* **274**:998, 1996.
301. Emmert-Buck MR, Lubensky IA, Dong Q, Manickam P, Guru SC, Kester MB, Olufemi S-E, Agarwal SK, Burns AL, Spiegel AM, Collins FS, Marx SJ, Zhuang Z, Liotta LA, Chandrasekharappa SC, Debelenko LV: Localization of the MEN1 gene based on tumor LOH analysis. *Cancer Res* **57**:1855, 1997.
302. Debelenko LV, Zhuang Z, Emmert-Buck MR, Chandrasekharappa SC, Manickam P, Guru SC, Marx SJ, Spiegel AM, Collins FS, Jensen RT, Liotta LA, Lubensky IA: Allelic deletions on chromosome 11q13 in MEN1-associated and sporadic duodenal gastrinomas and pancreatic endocrine tumors. *Cancer Res* **157**:2238, 1997.
303. Debelenko LV, Emmert-Buck MR, Zhuang Z, Epshteyn E, Moskaluk CA, Jensen RT, Liotta LA, Lubensky IA: The multiple endocrine neoplasia type 1 gene locus is involved in the pathogenesis of type II gastric carcinoids. *Gastroenterology* **113**:773, 1997.
304. Dong Q, Debelenko L, Chandrasekharappa S, Emmert-Buck MR, Zhuang Z, Guru SC, Manickam P, Skarulis M, Lubensky IA, Liotta LA, Collins FS, Marx SJ, Spiegel AM: Loss of heterozygosity at 11q13: Analysis of pituitary tumors, lung carcinoids, lipomas, and other uncommon tumors in familial multiple endocrine neoplasia type 1. *J Clin Endocrinol Metab* **82**:1416, 1997.
305. Williamson C, Pannett A, Pang JT, McCarthy M, Sherppard MN, Monson JP, Clayton RN, Thakker RV: Localisation of a tumour suppressor gene causing endocrine tumours to a four centimorgan region on chromosome 1, in *Program and Abstracts of the Endocrinology Society*, 1996, p 961 (abstract).
306. Kytola S, Makinen MJ, Kahkonen M, Teh BT, Leisti J, Salmela P: Comparative genomic hybridization studies in tumors from a patient with multiple endocrine neoplasia type 1. *Eur J Endocrinol* **139**:202, 1998.
307. Henske EP, Scheithauer BW, Short MP, Wollmann R, Nahmias J, Hornigold N, Slegtenhorst M, Welsh CT, Kwiatkowski DJ: Allelic loss is frequent in tuberous sclerosis kidney lesions but rare in brain lesions. *Am J Hum Genet* **59**:400, 1996.
308. Pack S, Turner ML, Zhuang Z, Vortmeyer AO, Boni R, Skarulis M, Marx SJ, Darling TN: Cutaneous tumors in patients with multiple endocrine neoplasia type 1 show allelic deletions of the MEN1 gene. *J Invest Dermatol* **11**:438, 1998.
309. Tahara H, Smith AP, Gaz RD, Cryns VL, Arnold A: Genomic localization of novel candidate tumor suppressor gene loci in human parathyroid adenomas. *Cancer Res* **56**:599, 1996.
310. Eubanks PJ, Sawicki MP, Samara GJ, Gratti R, Nakamura Y, Tsao D, Johnson C, Hurwitz M, Wan YJ, Passaro E: Putative tumor-suppressor gene on chromosome 11 is important in sporadic endocrine tumor formation. *Am J Surg* **167**:180, 1994.
311. Thakker RV, Pook MA, Wooding C, Boscaro M, Scanarini M, Clayton RN: Association of somatotrophinomas with loss of alleles on chromsome 11 and with gsp mutations. *J Clin Invest* **91**:2815, 1993.
312. Boggild MD, Jenkinson S, Pistorello M, Boscaro M, Scanarini M, McTernan P, Perrett CW, Thakker RV, Clayton RN: Molecular genetic studies of sporadic pituitary tumors. *J Clin Endocrinol Metab* **78**:387, 1994.
313. Bates AS, Farrell WE, Bicknell EJ, McNicol AM, Talbots AJ, Broome JC, Perrett CW, Thakker RV, Clayton RN: Allelic deletion in pituitary adenomas reflects aggressive biological activity and has potential value as a prognostic marker. *J Clin Endocrinol Metab* **82**:818, 1997.
314. Jakobovitz O, Devora N, DeMarco L, Barbosa AJA, Simoni FB, Rechavi G, Friedman E: Carcinoid tumors frequently display genetic abnormalities involving chromosome 11. *J Clin Endocrinol Metab* **81**:3164, 1996.
315. Matsuo K, Tang SH, Fagin JA: Allelotype of human thyroid tumors: Loss of chromosome 11q13 sequences in follicular neoplasms. *Mol Endocrinol* **5**:1873, 1991.
316. Iida A, Blake K, Tunny T, Klemm S, Stowasser M, Hayward N, Gordon R, Nakamura Y, Imai TK: Allelic losses on chromosome band 11q13 in aldosterone-producing adrenal tumors. *Genes Chromosom Cancer* **12**:73, 1995.
317. Heppner C, Reincke M, Agarwal SK, Mora P, Allolio B, Burns AL, Spiegel AM, Marx SJ: MEN1 gene analysis in sporadic adrenocortical neoplasms. *J Clin Endocrinol Metab* **84**:216, 1999.
318. Heppner C, Kester MB, Agarwal SK, Debelenko LV, Emmert-Buck MR, Guru SC, Manickam P, Olufemi SE, Skarulis MC, Doppman JL, Alexander RH, Kim YS, Saggar SK, Lubensky IA, Zhuang Z, Liotta LA, Chandrasekharappa SC, Collins FS, Spiegel AM, Burns AL, Marx SJ: Somatic mutation of the MEN1 gene in parathyroid tumors. *Nature Genet* **16**:375, 1997.
319. Tanaka C, Yoshimoto K, Yamada S, Lnishioka H, Moritani M, Yamaoka T, Itakura M: Absence of germ-line mutations of the multiple endocrine neoplasia type 1 (MEN1) gene in familial pituitary adenoma in contrast to MEN1 in Japanese. *J Clin Endocrinol Metab* **83**:960, 1998.
320. Falchetti A, Bale AE, Amorosi A, Bordi C, Cicci P, Bandini S, Marx SJ, Brandi ML: Progression of uremic hyperparathyroidism involves allelic loss on chromosome 11. *J Clin Endocrinol Metab* **76**:139, 1993.
321. Arnold A, Brown MF, Urena P, Gaz RD, Sarfati E, Drueke TB: Monoclonality of parathyroid tumors in chronic renal failure and in primary parathyroid hyperplasia. *J Clin Invest* **95**:2047, 1995.
322. Farnebo F, Farnebo L-O, Nordenstrom J, Larsson C: Allelic loss on chromosome 11 is uncommon in parathyroid glands of patients with hypercalcemic secondary hyperparathyroidism. *Eur J Surg* **163**:331, 1997.
323. Zhuang Z, Merino MJ, Chuaqui R, Liotta LA, Emmert-Buck MR: Identical allelic loss on chromosome 11q13 in microdissected *in situ* and invasive human breast cancer. *Cancer Res* **55**:467, 1995.
324. Chuaqui RF, Zhuang Z, Emmert-Buck MR, Liotta LA, Merino MJ: Analysis of loss of heterozygosity on chromosome 11q13 in atypical ductal hyperplasia and *in situ* carcinoma of the breast. *Am J Pathol* **150**:297, 1997.

325. Srivatsan ES, Misra BC, Venugopalan M, Wilczynski SP: Loss of heterozygosity for alleles on chromosome 11 in cervical carcinoma. *Am J Hum Genet* **49**:868, 1991.
326. Popescu NC, Zimonjic DB: Alterations of chromosome 11q13 in cervical carcinoma cell lines. *Am J Hum Genet* **58**:422, 1996.
327. Debelenko LV, Emmert-Buck MR, Manickam P, Kester MB, Guru SC, DiFranco EM, Olufemi SE, Agarwal SK, Lubensky IA, Zhuang Z, Burns AL, Spiegel AM, Liotta LA, Collins FS, Marx SJ, Chandrasekharappa SC: Haplotype analysis defines a minimal interval for the multiple endocrine neoplasia type 1 (MEN1) gene. *Cancer Res* **57**:1039, 1997.
328. Collins FS: Positional cloning moves from perditional to traditional. *Nature Genet* **9**:347, 1995.
329. Kas K, Weber G, Merregaert J, Michiels L. Sandelin K, Skogseid B, Thompson N, Nordenskjold M, Larsson C, Friedman E: Exclusion of FAU as the multiple endocrine neoplasia type 1 (MEN1) gene. *Hum Mol Genet* **2**:349, 1993.
330. DeWit MJ, Landsvater RM, Sinke RJ, van Kessel A, Lips CJ, Hoppener JW: Exclusion of the phosphatidylinositol-specific phospholipase C beta 3 (PLC beta 3) gene as candidate for the multiple endocrine neoplasia type 1 (MEN1) gene. *Hum Genet* **99**:133, 1997.
331. Landsvater RM, DeWit MJ, Peterson LF, Sinke RJ, van Kessel AD, Lips CJM, Hoppener JWM: Exclusion of the nuclear factor-kB3 (REL A) gene as candidate for the multiple endocrine neoplasia type (MEN1) gene. *Biochem Mol Med* **60**:76, 1997.
332. Guru SC, Olufemi S-E, Manickam P, Cummings C, Gieser LM, Pike BM, Bittner ML, Jiang Y, Chinnault AC, Nowack NJ, Brzozowska A, Crabtree JS, Wang Y, Roe BA, Weisemann J, Boguski MS, Agarwal SK, Burns AL, Spiegel AM, Marx SJ, Flejter WL, de Jong PJ, Collins FS, Chandrasekharappa SC: A 2.8 Mb clone contig of the multiple endocrine neoplasia type 1 (MEN1) region at 11q13. *Genomics* **42**:436, 1997.
333. Guru SC, Agarwal SK, Manickam P, Olufemi S-E, Crabtree JS, Weisemann J, Kester MB, Kim YS, Wang Y, Emmert-Buck MR, Liotta LA, Spiegel AM, Boguski MS, Roe BA, Collins FS, Marx SJ, Burns AL, Chandrasekharappa SC: A transcript map for the 2.8 Mb region containing the multiple endocrine neoplasia type 1 (MEN1) locus. *Genome Res* **7**:725, 1997.
334. Manickam P, Guru SC, Debelenko LV, Agarwal SK, Olufemi S-E, Weisemann JM, Boguski M, Crabtree JS, Wang Y, Roe BA, Lubensky IA, Zhuang Z, Kester MB, Burns AL, Spiegel AM, Marx SJ, Liotta LA, Emmert-Buck MR, Collins FS, Chandrasekharappa SC: Eighteen new polymorphic markers in the multiple endocrine neoplasia type 1 (MEN1) region. *Hum Genet* **101**:102, 1997.
335. Sarkar G, Yoon HS, Sommer SS: Dideoxy fingerprinting (ddF): A rapid and efficient screen for the presence of mutations. *Genomics* **13**:441, 1992.
336. Agarwal SK, Kester MB, Debelenko LV, Heppner C, Emmert-Buck MR, Skarulis MC, Doppman JL, Kim YS, Lubensky IA, Zhuang Z, Green JS, Guru SC, Manickam P, Olufemi SE, Liotta LA, Chandrasekharappa SC, Collins FS, Spiegel AM, Burns AL, Marx SJ: Germline mutations of the MEN1 gene in familial multiple endocrine neoplasia type 1 and related states. *Hum Mol Genet* **7**:1177, 1997.
337. Lemmens I, Van de Ven WJM, Kas K, Zhang CX, Giraud S, Wautot V, Buisson N, De Witte K, Salandre J, Lenoir G, Pugeat M, Calender A, Parente F, Quincey D, Gaudray P, De Wit MJ, Lips CJM, Hoppener JWM, Khodaei S, Grant AL, Weber G, Kytola S, Teh BT, Farnebo F, Phelan C, Hayward N, Larsson C, Pannett AJ, Forbes SA, Bassett JHD, Thakker RV: The European Consortium on MEN1: Identification of the multiple endocrine neoplasia type 1 (MEN1) gene. *Hum Mol Genet* **6**:1177, 1997.
338. Mayr B, Apenberg S, Rothamel T, von zur Muhlen A, Brabant G.: Menin mutations in patients with multiple endocrine neoplasia type 1. *Eur J Endocrinol* **137**:684, 1997.
339. Shimizu S, Tsukada T, Futami H, Ui K, Kameya T, Kawanaka M, Uchiyama S, Aoki A, Yasuda H, Kawano S, Ito Y, Kanbe M, Obara T, Yamaguchi K: Germline mutations of the MEN1 gene in Japanese kindred with multiple endocrine neoplasia type 1. *Jpn J Cancer Res* **88**:1029, 1997.
340. Bassett JHD, Forbes SA, Pannett AAJ, Lloyd SE, Christie PT, Wooding C, Harding B, Besser GM, Edwards CR, Monson JP, Sampson J, Wass JAH, Wheeler MH, Thakker RV: Characterization of the mutations in patients with multiple endocrine neoplasia type 1. *Am J Hum Genet* **62**:232, 1998.
341. Agarwal SK, Debelenko LV, Kester MB, Guru SC, Manickam P, Olufemi SE, Skarulis MC, Heppner C, Crabtree JS, Lubensky IA, Zhuang Z, Kim YS, Chandrasekharappa SC, Collins FS, Liotta LA, Spiegel AM, Burns AL, Emmert-Buck MR, Marx SJ: Analysis of recurrent germline mutations in the MEN1 gene encountered in apparently unrelated families. *Hum Mutat* **12**:75, 1998.
342. Teh BT, Kytola S, Farnebo F, Bergman L, Wong FK, Weberf G, Hayward N, Larsson C, and a Clinical Diagnosis Group: Mutation analysis of the MEN1 gene in multiple endocrine neoplasia type 1, familial acromegaly and familial isolated hyperparathyroidism. *J Clin Endocrinol Metab* **83**:2621, 1998.
342b. Kassem M, Kruse TA, Wong FK, Larsson C, Teh BT: Familial isolated hyperparathyroidism as a variant of multiple endocrine neoplasia type 1 in a large Danish pedigree. *J Clin Endocrinol Metab* **85**:165, 2000.
342c. Poncin J, Abs R, Velkeniers B, Bonduelle M, Abramawicz M, Legros JJ, et al: Mutation analysis of the *MEN1* gene in Belgian patients with multiple endocrine neoplasia type 1 and related diseases. *Hum Mut* **13**:54, 1999.
343. Farnebo F, Teh BT, Kytola S, Svensson A, Phelan C, Sandelinm K, Thompson NW, Hoog A, Weber G, Farnebo L-O, Larsson C: Alterations of the MEN1 gene in sporadic parathyroid tumors. *J Clin Endocrinol Metab* **83**:2627, 1998.
344. Carling T, Correa P, Hessman O, Hedberg J, Skogseid B, Lindberg D, Rastad J, Westin G, Akerstrom G: Parathyroid MEN1 gene mutations in relation to clinical characteristics of nonfamilial primary hyperparathyroidism. *J Clin Endocrinol Metab* **83**:2960, 1998.
345. Zhuang Z, Vortmeyer AO, Pack S, Huang S, Pham TA, Wang C, Park WS, Agarwal SK, Debelenko LV, Kester MB, Guru SC, Manickam P, Olufemi SE, Yu F, Heppner C, Skarulis MC, Venzon DJ, Emmert-Buck MR, Spiegel AM, Chandrasekharappa SC, Collins FS, Burns AL, Marx SJ, Jensen RT, Liotta LA, Lubensky IA: Somatic mutations of the MEN1 tumor suppressor gene in sporadic gastrinomas and insulinomas. *Cancer Res* **57**:4682, 1997.
346. Wang EH, Ebrahimi SA, Wu AY, Kashefi C, Passaro E Jr, Sawicki MP: Mutation of the menin gene in sporadic pancreatic endocrine tumors. *Cancer Res* **58**:4417, 1998.
347. Debelenko LV, Brambilla E, Agarwal SK, Swalwell JI, Kester MB, Lubensky IA, Zhuang Z, Guru SC, Manickam P, Olufemi S-E, Chandrasekharappa SC, Crabtree JS, Kim YS, Heppner C, Burns AL, Spiegel AM, Marx SJ, Collins FS, Travis WB, Emmert-Buck MR: Identification of MEN1 gene mutations in sporadic carcinoid tumors of the lung. *Hum Mol Genet* **6**:2285, 1997.
347b. Goebel SU, Heppner C, Burns AL, Marx SJ, Spiegel AM, Zhuang Z, et al: Genotype/phenotype correlation of *MEN1* gene mutations in sporadic gastrinomas. *J Clin Endocrinol Metab* **85**:116–123, 2000.
348. Prezant TR, Levine J, Melmed S: Molecular characterization of the MEN1 tumor suppressor gene in sporadic pituitary tumors. *J Clin Endocrinol Metab* **83**:1388, 1998.
349. Tanaka C, Kimura T, Yang P, Moritani M, Yamaoka T, Yamada S, Sano T, Yoshimoto K, Itakura M: Analysis of loss of heterozygosity on chromosome 11 and infrequent inactivation of the MEN1 gene in sporadic pituitary adenomas. *J Clin Endocrinol Metab* **83**:2631, 1998.
349b. Imanishi Y, Palanisamy N, Tahara H, Vickery A, Cryns VL, Gaz RD, et al: Molecular pathogenetic analysis of parathyroid carcinoma. *J Bone Min Res* **14**(Suppl 1):S421 (abstract), 1999.
349c. Imanishi Y, Tahara H, Salusky I, Goodman W, Brandi ML, Drucke TB, et al: *MEN1* gene mutations in refractory hyperparathyroidism of uremia. *J Bone Min Res* **14**(Suppl 1):S446 (abstract), 1999.
350. Herman, JG, Latif F, Weng Y, Lerman MI, Zbar B, Liu S, Samid D, Duan DS, Gnarra JR, Linehan WM: Silencing of the VHL tumor-suppressor gene by DNA methylation in renal carcinoma. *Proc Natl Acad Sci USA* **91**:9700, 1994.
351. Chakrabarti R, Srivatsan ES, Wood TF, Eubanks PJ, Ebrahimi SA, Gatti RA, Passaro E, Sawicki MP: Deletion mapping of endocrine tumors localizes a second tumor supressor gene on chromosome band 11q13. *Genes Chromosom Cancer* **22**:130, 1998.
351b. Nord B, Larsson C, Wong FK, Wallin G, Teh BT, Zedenius J: Sporadic follicular thyroid tumors of a 200-kb region in 11q13 without evidence for mutations in the *MEN1* gene. *Genes Chromosomes* **35**, 1999.
352. Boni R, Vortmeyer AO, Pack S, Park WS, Burg G, Hofbauer G, Darling T, Liotta L, Zhuang Z: Somatic mutations of the MEN1 tumor suppressor gene detected in sporadic angiofibromas (abstract). *Mod Pathol* **11**:47A, 1998.
353. Vortmeyer AO, Boni R, Pak E, Pack S, Zhuang Z: Multiple endocrine neoplasia 1 gene alterations in MEN1-associated and sporadic lipomas. *J Natl Cancer Inst* **90**:398, 1998.

354. Motokura T, Bloom T, Kim HG, Juppner H, Ruderman JV, Kronenberg HM, Arnold A: A novel cyclin encoded by a bcl-1 linked candidate oncogene. *Nature* **350**:512, 1991.

355. Hsi ED, Zukerberg LF, Yang WI, Arnold A: Cyclin D1/PRAD1 expression in parathyroid adenomas: An immunohistochemical study. *J Clin Endocrinol Metab* **81**:1736, 1996.

356. Pausova Z, Soliman E, Amizuka N, Janicic N, Konrad EM, Arnold A, Goltzman D, Hendy GN: Role of the RET proto-oncogene in sporadic hyperparathyroidism and in hyperparathyroidism of multiple endocrine neoplasia type 2. *J Clin Endocrinol Metab* **81**:2711, 1996.

357. Hosokawa Y, Pollak MR, Brown EM, Arnold A: Mutational analysis of the extracellular Ca(2+)-sensing receptor gene in human parathyroid tumors. *J Clin Endocrinol Metab* **80**:3107, 1995.

358. Thompson DB, Samowitz WS, Odelberg S, Davis RK, Szabo J, Heath H III: Genetic abnormalities in sporadic parathyroid adenomas: Loss of heterozygosity for chromosome 3q markers flanking the calcium receptor locus. *J Clin Endocrinol Metab* **80**:3377, 1995.

359. Kifor O, Moore FD Jr, Wang P, Goldstein M, Vassilev P, Kifor I, Hebert SC, Brown EM: Reduced immunostaining for the extracellular Ca^{2+}-sensing receptor in primary and uremic secondary hyperparathyroidism. *J Clin Endocrinol Metab* **81**:1598, 1996.

360. Cryns VL, Rubio MP, Thor AD, Louis DL, Arnold A: P53 abnormalities in human parathyroid carcinoma. *J Clin Endocrinol Metab* **78**:1320, 1994.

361. Cryns VL, Thor AD, Xu HJ, Hu SH, Wierman ME, Vickery AL Jr, Benedict WF, Arnold A: Loss of the retinoblastoma tumor-suppressor gene in parathyroid carcinoma. *N Engl J Med* **330**:757, 1994.

362. Dotzenrath C, Teh BT, Farnebo T, Cupisti K, Svensson A, Toell A, Goretzki P, Larsson C: Allelic loss of the retinoblastoma tumor suppressor gene: A marker for aggressive parathyroid tumors? *J Clin Endocrinol Metab* **81**:3194, 1996.

363. Pearce SH, Trump D, Woodling C, Sheppard MN, Clayton RN, Thakker RV: Loss of heterozygosity studies at the retinoblastoma and breast cancer susceptibility (BRCA2) loci in pituitary, parathyroid, pancreatic and carcinoid tumors. *Clin Endocrinol* **45**:195. 1996.

364. Palanisamy N, Imanishy Y, Rao PH, Tahara H, Chaganti RSK, Arnold A: Novel chromosomal abnormalities identified by comparative genomic hybridization in parathyroid adenomas. *J Clin Endocrinol Metab* **83**:1766, 1998.

365. Agarwal SK, Schrock E, Kester MB, Burns AL, Heffess CS, Reid T, Marx SJ: Comparative genome hybridization analysis of human parathyroid tumors. *Cancer Genet Cytogenet* **106**:30, 1998.

365b. Guru SC, Crabtree JS, Brown KD, Dunn KJ, Manickam P, Prasad BN, Wangsa D, Burns AL, Spiegel AM, Marx SJ, Pavan WJ, Collins FS, Chandrasekharappa SC: Isolation, genomic organization and expression analysis of *Men*1, the murine homolog of the MEN1 gene. *Mammalian Genome* **10**:592–596, 1999.

366. Guru SC, Goldsmith PK, Burns AL, Marx SJ, Spiegel AM, Collins FS, Chandrasekharappa SC: Menin, the product of the MEN1 gene, is a nuclear protein. *Proc Natl Acad Sci USA* **95**:1630, 1998.

366b. Agarwal SK, Guru SC, Heppner C, Erdos MR, Collins M, Park SY, Saggar S, Chandrasekharappa SC, Collins FS, Spiegel AM, Marx SJ, Burns AL: Menin interacts with the AP1 transcrition factor JunD and represses JunD activated transcription. *Cell* **96**:143, 1999.

366c. Kim YS, Burns AL, Goldsmith PK, Heppner C, Park SY, Chandrasekharappa SC, Collins FS, Spiegel AM, Marx SJ: Stable overexpression of *MEN1* suppresses tumorigenictiy of *RAS*. *Oncogene* **18**:5936, 1999.

367. Kishi M, Tsukada T, Shimizu S, Futami H, Ito Y, Kanbe M, Obara T, Yamaguchi K: A large germline deletion of the MEN1 gene in a family with multiple endocrine neoplasia type 1. *Jpn J Cancer Res* **81**:1, 1998.

367b. Granberg D, Stridsberg M, Seensalu R, Eriksson B, Lundqvist G, Oberg K, Skogseid B: Plasma chromogranin A in patients with multiple endocrin neoplasia type 1. *J Clin Endocrinol Metab* **84**:2712, 1999.

367c. Mutch MG, Dilley WG, Sanjurjo F, DeBenedetti MK, Doherty G, Wells SA Jr, et al: Germline mutations in the multiple endocrine neoplasia type 1 gene: Evidence for frequent splicing defects. *Hum Mutat* **13**:175, 1999.

368. American Society of Human Genetics Board of Directors and the American College of Medical Genetics Board of Directors: Points to consider: Ethical, legal, and psychosocial implications of genetic testing in children and adolescents. *Am J Hum Genet* **57**:1233, 1995.

369. Marx SJ: Familial multiple endocrine neoplasia type 1. NIH publication no 96-3048, 1997.

370. Kohlmeier L, Marcus R: Calcium disorders of pregnancy. *Endocrinol Metab Clin North Am* **1**:15, 1995.

371. Ciccarelli E, Camanni F: Diagnosis and drug therapy of prolactinoma. *Drugs* **51**:954, 1996.

CHAPTER 44

Malignant Melanoma

Alexander Kamb ▪ Meenhard Herlyn

1. **Melanoma is one of the more common cancers in the United States and is increasing rapidly in occurrence. Environmental factors, particularly sun exposure, have been strongly implicated in melanoma risk.**
2. **An accumulation of evidence points to a set of genetic changes that underlie the evolution from melanocyte to metastatic melanoma. In addition, a significant fraction of the disease is familial, suggesting that specific genes regulate susceptibility. Study of familial melanoma provides one route to identification of genes that contribute to all melanomas, including the more common sporadic form.**
3. **The investigation of somatic lesions in melanoma tumors and cell lines has permitted clinicians and molecular geneticists to focus on defined regions in the genome. Several chromosomal areas have been delineated based on various types of analyses. These regions exhibit loss of heterozygosity (LOH) and, in some cases, homozygous deletions. The most commonly observed abnormality in melanoma is LOH and homozygous deletion at 9p21. Chromosomal aberrations at 9p21 may occur early in tumor development, although certain results suggest that their ultimate effect may be manifested later.**
4. **Linkage analysis of melanoma-prone kindreds also identified 9p21 as the site of a potential tumor-suppressor gene involved in melanoma susceptibility. Interestingly, initial linkage studies were hindered by use of dysplastic nevi as the phenotypic trait rather than melanoma itself, emphasizing the importance of phenotype definition in linkage analysis. The melanoma susceptibility locus discovered at 9p21, called *MLM,* is inherited as a dominant allele with penetrance that ranges upward from 50 percent. Its expressivity is highly variable.**
5. **The identity of *MLM* has been determined largely through deletion mapping in melanoma cell lines. It encodes a negative growth regulator called p16, the expression of which causes cell cycle arrest. p16 is part of a growth-control pathway that involves cyclin-dependent kinases, cyclins, and the retinoblastoma gene product Rb. An impressive list of experiments supports a role for p16 not only in melanoma formation but also in the genesis of many other tumors. p16 inactivation may occur in nearly half of all advanced human cancers.**
6. **Genes other than *p16* also play a part in melanoma formation. One of these is cyclin-dependent kinase 4 (cdk4), a target of *p16's* biochemical inhibitory activity. *CDK4* is mutated in some tumors and in the germ line of rare familial melanoma cases. It is only the second germ-line oncogene to be described. Through cdk4 and Rb, *p16* is tied into the basic cell cycle control apparatus.**
7. **The identification of genes involved in familial and sporadic melanoma raises the possibility of gene-based tests for cancer predisposition and for the classification of tumors. *p16,* as the primary genetic element in familial melanoma, is an interesting case study for genetic testing. Technical and economic issues are especially important in this realm. With respect to somatic gene testing, technical concerns are superseded by the pressing need to demonstrate clinical utility of information about *p16* status in tumors. Therapeutic implications of genetic discoveries are not insignificant but remain largely speculative and long term.**

Melanoma is a malignancy that originates from melanocytes, the pigment-producing cells in skin. Melanocytes generate a light-absorbing shield of melanin that protects the skin from damage caused by ultraviolet (UV) radiation. They transfer much of this pigment to keratinocytes in the suprabasal skin layers via dendritic connections. It is ironic that melanocytes themselves are among the targets of UV, spurred into malignant growth by the agent they are intended to counter. Melanocytes arise from neural crest-derived progenitors that migrate from the developing central nervous system into the skin and are homogeneously distributed at the junction between the epidermal and dermal layers. Born of colonists themselves, it is perhaps not surprising that melanocytes, when fully transformed, are as aggressive and migratory as any tumor cells. Melanocytes are present in the skin at roughly equal densities in all the races.[1] Dark-skinned people do not have more melanocytes; rather, each melanocyte produces, on average, more melanin pigment than melanocytes from light-skinned people. Consequently, individuals differ little in the numbers of precursor cells that can give rise to melanomas.

Several factors have contributed recently to a heightened awareness of melanoma. People are more conscious of the dangers imposed by sun exposure. Melanoma, like lung cancer, is gaining a reputation as a neoplasm on the rise, a cancer whose incidence is profoundly affected by controllable environmental influences. In addition, genetic principles that underlie the disease are beginning to emerge.[2]

Melanoma responds poorly to chemical and radiation therapy, and the most effective treatment is surgical excision before the tumor is well advanced.[3] Early detection thus is of paramount importance. Because the skin lesions are relatively easy to spot, frequent examination and prompt treatment are highly successful medical strategies. On the other hand, clinical and histologic diagnosis of early lesions remains difficult and controversial. For individuals who have hundreds of moles, diagnosis is especially problematic. Partly because of the efficacy of early detection, genetic analysis of melanoma offers hope in a comprehensive plan to limit the morbidity of the disease. Genetic tests may provide the means to assess risk and recognize individuals who require more intensive observation. Although genetic studies in melanoma have lagged somewhat behind other neoplasias such as colon cancer, the future appears bright in the effort to understand the biology of melanoma, predict its clinical behavior, and eventually discern how to defeat it.[4]

INCIDENCE OF MELANOMA

The overall melanoma incidence in the United States currently is nearly 40,000 cases per year, placing it significantly below only prostate, breast, lung, and colon cancers in occurrence.[5] The

A list of standard abbreviations is located immediately preceding the index in each volume. Nonstandard abbreviations used in this chapter include: LOH = loss of heterozygosity; DNS = dysplastic nevus syndrome.

population-averaged lifetime risk of developing melanoma can be as high as 1 in 60 in particular groups; more typically, it is 1 in 90.[6,7] This rate of occurrence is increasing rapidly, more so than for any other cancer site except lung. Since the 1930s, the incidence of melanoma has jumped nearly 20-fold.[7] The reason is likely related to the fashion for tanning and outdoor activities. The development of melanoma is strongly influenced by genetic as well as environmental factors—especially exposure to UV.[8] This is dramatically illustrated by epidemiologic studies that relate melanoma incidence to ethnographic and geographic factors. Melanoma is nearly three times more common in southern latitudes of the United States than in the northern United States.[3] The highest incidence of melanoma occurs in Queensland, Australia, whereas one of the lowest occurs in South India. Both these regions have a high degree of sun exposure. The difference is that Australians are largely light-skinned, whereas South Indians are dark-skinned. Thus, the genetics of skin color interact with sunlight exposure to determine the overall rate of melanoma.

DEVELOPMENT OF MELANOMA

Clinical Features

Melanoma presents in a variety of clinically distinct forms: superficial spreading melanoma, lentigo maligna melanoma, acral lentigious melanoma, and nodular melanoma.[3] At least two of these types, lentigo maligna melanoma and superficial spreading melanoma, may exist for several years in a preinvasive state, providing a long window of opportunity for removal. Once the lesion thickens and begins to invade, the prognosis worsens considerably. The survival of melanoma patients correlates strongly with the thickness of the primary lesion and its degree of invasion into the dermis. If the lesion is clinically localized, the 5-year survival rate is 85 percent.[3]

Specific genetic components are presumed to account for the morphologic features that distinguish the various clinical forms of melanoma. One important goal of melanoma research is to identify genes that influence the phenotype of the tumor. Thus it is helpful to develop a tractable experimental system in which to study tumor progression. Fortunately, some of the features of melanoma *in situ* can be reproduced in tissue culture.[9]

Often it is useful to classify cells in culture based not on the clinical criteria described earlier but on a scheme with a more chronologic emphasis. The transition from normal melanocyte to metastatic melanoma occurs in a series of defined stages. Each stage is characterized broadly by changes in morphology and growth properties (Fig. 44-1). The first abnormal state that is recognizably different from the melanocyte is the nevus cell. This cell type differs little in microscopic appearance from a normal melanocyte, yet it can contain random chromosomal abnormalities. The next stage is the premalignant melanoma, discernible often as a raised mole that has acquired atypical architectural and cytologic features. This premalignant lesion can evolve further into a primary melanoma that is capable of breaking through the dermal layer into the underlying blood vessels. Finally, the most insidious form, metastatic melanoma, arises from the primary lesion. This end stage is invasive, migratory, and ultimately, if unchecked, kills the patient. The secondary sites of metastasis include brain, bone, lung, and liver.

Models of Melanoma in Tissue Culture

Much has been learned about the properties of the different melanoma stages by study of cells in culture. The overall pattern of melanoma, as of other cancer types, involves progressive loss of dependence on exogenous growth signals as melanocytes evolve toward malignancy (Table 44-1). For example, normal melanocytes placed in culture require phorbol ester, basic fibroblast

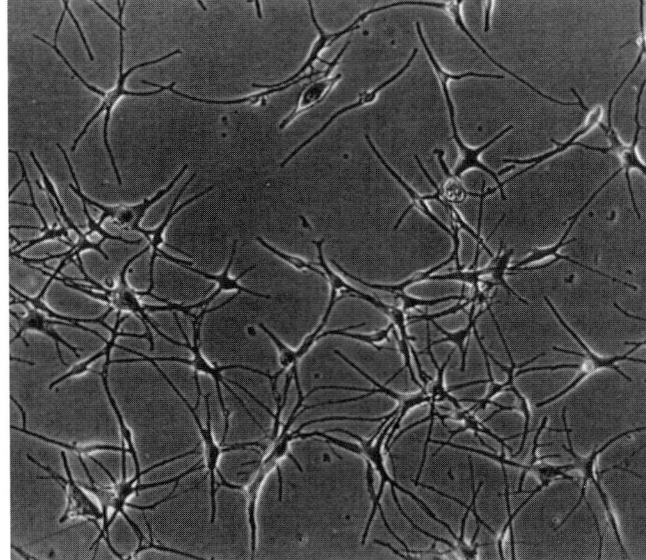

A

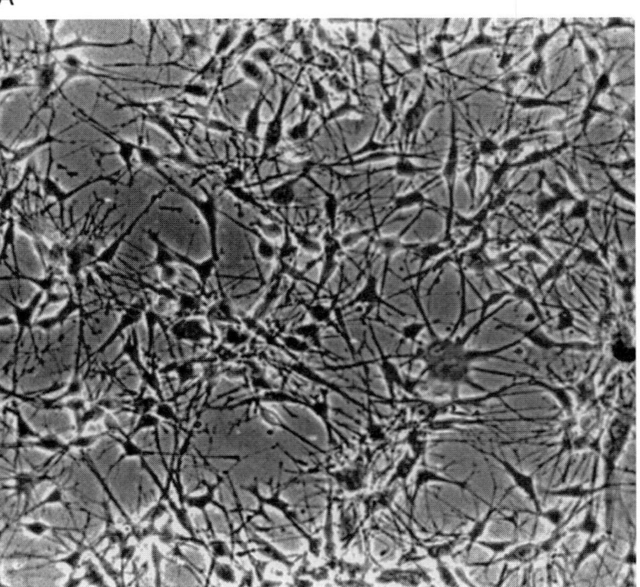

B

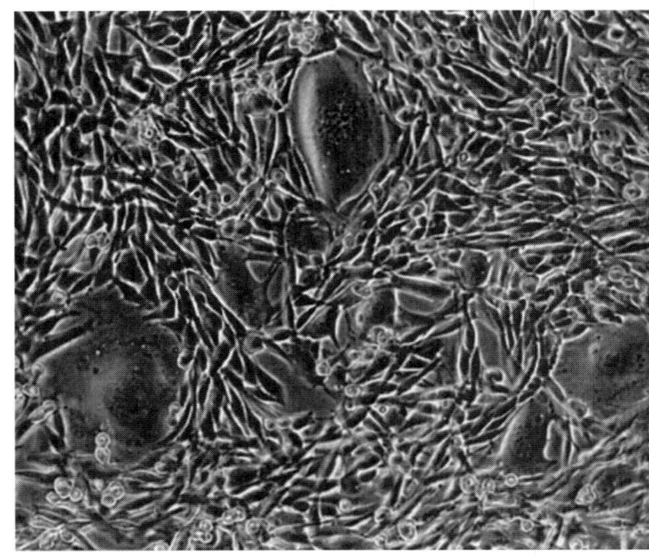

C

Fig. 44-1 Cells in culture. *A.* Normal melanocytes. *B.* Nevus cells. *C.* Metastatic melanoma cells.

Table 44-1 Culture Characteristics of Normal Melanocytes and Cells from Nonmalignant Primary and Metastatic Melanocytic Lesions

Parameter	Melanocytes	Nevus	Primary Melanoma		Metastatic Melanoma
			Early	Late	
Chromosomal abnormalities	None	None (few random)	(#1, 6, 7, 9) Nonrandom	(#1, 6, 7, 9) Nonrandom	(#1, 6, 7, 9, 11) Nonrandom
Life span (doublings)	Finite (< 60)	Finite (< 50)	Infinite (> 100)	Infinite (> 100)	Infinite (> 100)
Response to phorbol ester	Stimulation	Stimulation	Inhibition	Inhibition	Inhibition
Growth factor requirements	I, FGF, aMSH, TPA*	Same as melanocytes†	I only	None	None
Growth in soft agar (percent)	< 0.001	0.001–3 (average 0.9)	5–10 (average 8)	5–20	5–70 (average 25)
Growth in nude mice (percent)	None	None	80	100	100

*I = insulin; FGF = basic fibroblast growth factor; αMSH = α-melanocyte stimulating hormone. †Cultures are often independent of FGF and/or TPA.

growth factor, α-melanocyte-stimulating factor, and insulin-like growth factor 1. However, most lines derived from early melanomas no longer require phorbol ester. By the time metastases appear, the cells have lost their dependence on any of these factors. They grow rapidly in culture dishes without special serum factors. Behavior of cells in culture that have been established from clinically defined stages of melanoma is presumed relevant to the transitions that occur as melanocytes evolve in the body toward metastatic melanoma. Thus thorough characterization of such cell lines is likely to be of great value in understanding the biology of melanoma.

GENETICS OF MELANOMA

Genetic analysis of melanoma has two aspects: the study of predisposition in melanoma-prone kindreds and the study of somatic genetic alterations that occur as tumors evolve in the body. Both approaches have considerable appeal and, as described in the following, may converge on the same set of genes important in melanoma development.

Somatic Genetics of Melanoma Tumors

Melanomas, like practically all tumors, progressively accumulate abnormalities in their DNA as they evolve more malignant traits.[10,11] These abnormalites include chromosomal losses, duplications, translocations, and deletions. In addition to cytogenetically detectable aberrations, melanomas incorporate more subtle somatic changes such as microsatellite variability and point mutations.[12–15] Which of these changes are causal in tumorigenesis and which are merely the effect of the transformed state are difficult questions to answer in many cases.

9p21 Loss of Heterozygosity

One of the most consistent somatic changes in melanomas is the loss of chromosomal material from the short arm of chromosome 9 (9p).[11,16,17] This cytogenetic abnormality is observed in over half of malignant melanomas. Some studies suggest that the initial change involving loss of heterozygosity (LOH) on 9p is a relatively early event in melanoma development, occurring before the primary lesion matures.[11] More recent work has demonstrated that a large fraction of the 9p abnormalities ultimately are detected as homozygous deletions of 9p21 in advanced malignancies.[18] Whether or not the homozygous deletions are present at an earlier stage in tumor development remains an open question, although some studies suggest that they may be a later phenomenon.[19] If so, the role of the early LOH lesions in melanoma is unclear. In a subsequent section, the molecular identity of the 9p21 tumor suppressor is discussed.

Other LOH Sites

Chromosomal abnormalities other than 9p LOH also have been observed as common features in primary melanoma tumors[11] (Table 44-2). These include LOH regions on 3p, 6q, 10q, 11q, and 17p. 3p and 10q losses are detected in tumors less than 1.5 mm in thickness, suggesting that hypothetical tumor-suppressor loci located on these chromosomal arms may be important at earlier stages of melanoma formation. 6q, 11q, and 17p LOH is detected only in more invasive tumors. Homozygous deletions at a specific site on 3p have been described recently.[20] These deletions frequently remove a gene termed *FHIT*, suggesting that it may be the relevant tumor-suppressor locus in the region. However, the *FHIT* location on 3p is a fragile site, prone to rearrangement, and further studies are necessary to establish a causal relationship between *FHIT* inactivation and tumor growth. 17p contains the *p53* tumor-suppressor gene, and although point mutations in *p53* are relatively uncommon in melanomas, *p53* may account for a fraction of 17p LOH.[21,22] Additional regions of abnormality on 1p, 3q, and 17q have been described in melanoma cell lines and metastases.[23–27] 17q contains the metastasis-suppressor gene *NM23* and the *NF1* tumor-suppressor gene, a gene found to be mutated in some melanoma cell lines.[27–29] The *PTEN* tumor-suppressor gene located on 10q is likely the underlying cause of 10q LOH because the gene is altered in a significant percentage of melanoma tumors and cells lines.[30]

Kindred Analysis

Apart from skin tone, predisposition to melanoma may be strongly influenced by heredity. As early as 1952, the familial nature of nonocular melanoma was described, and current estimates indicate that 5 to 10 percent of all melanoma cases may have a genetic basis.[30,31] This heritable component is inferred from melanoma cases that cluster in specific families. The definition of familiality varies, but typically, melanoma patients who have at least one

Table 44-2 Loss of Heterozygosity in Primary Melanoma Specimens

Chromosome Arm	Percent LOH
1p	5
3p	19
3q	14
6q	31
9p	47
9q	19
10q	31
11q	17
13q	9
17p	16
17q	4
22q	6

SOURCE: Data are taken from Ref. 11. Experiments on each chromosome arm involved 21 to 41 informative samples.

first-degree relative with melanoma are classified as familial cases. For first-degree relatives of melanoma patients, the increased risk is calculated to be 2.0; with a relative under age 50 affected, the risk is 6.5.[32,33]

Based on the commonly accepted figures, over 90 percent of melanomas are predicted to be of a nongenetic, or sporadic, origin, percentages similar to those reported for other cancer sites such as breast and colon the Sporadic melanoma truly may be independent of heredity, arising solely from random wear and tear that occur during a lifetime. Alternatively, it may be caused by multiple genes or weakly penetrant alleles that modify an individual's risk modestly but, in aggregate, strongly affect the overall incidence of disease in a population.

Dysplastic Nevus Syndrome

During the past few decades, numerous families with multiple cases of melanoma have been identified.[34–36] Individuals in many of these kindreds were reported to have unusual numbers of large nevi, and the nevus count on the skin was shown to be a risk factor for melanoma.[37] A variety of pathologic studies suggested that certain nevi could be classified as dysplastic and, therefore, more likely to produce melanomas.[38,39] These nevi resemble the clinically miniature early superficial spreading melanomas.[3] Such observations gave rise to the notion of a disease, dysplastic nevus syndrome (DNS), characterized by frequent occurrence of atypical moles and increased risk of melanoma.

MLM

Some DNS/melanoma kindreds served as the basis for genetic linkage analysis in which molecular genetic markers positioned at various places throughout the genome were tested for linkage to DNS and to melanoma. Because dysplastic nevi are believed to be precursors to melanomas, initial attempts to determine a genetic basis for melanoma focused on DNS. However, these attempts were hindered by the difficulties of diagnosis and classification of moles. A reported linkage assignment on 1p36 was not reproduced in other families.[40–46] When the phenotype was restricted to melanoma itself, definitive linkage was obtained with markers in 9p21[47] (Fig. 44-2). This linkage study produced a cumulative Lod score (base 10 logarithm of the odds of linkage) of nearly 13, suggesting a probability of linkage in excess of 1 trillion to 1; one large kindred had a Lod score of nearly 6. The genetic locus identified by linkage analysis was designated *MLM*.

The history of the discovery of *MLM* is an ideal example of the importance of phenotypic definition to linkage analysis.[48] DNS proved to be an unreliable phenotype, difficult to diagnose objectively. The use of melanoma itself as the primary phenotypic trait reduced the number of affecteds in the analysis but placed the phenotypic definition on a firm, objective foundation. This definition provided the key to identification of *MLM*.

MLM is inherited in a dominant Mendelian fashion; a single defective germ-line copy of the gene predisposes to melanoma. The penetrance of the disease gene, the likelihood that an individual carrier will develop melanoma by age 80, has been estimated at 53 percent using three 9p21-linked kindreds.[49] More recent studies suggest that the penetrance may vary depending on the particular allele and/or the kindreds under consideration. In some kindreds, the penetrance appears to approach 100 percent.[50] However, in general, as with many other cancer-predisposition genes, inheritance of a defective *MLM* allele increases the *probability* of melanoma; it does not guarantee illness. For melanoma, the increased lifetime risk caused by inheritance of predisposing *MLM* alleles is roughly 50-fold. This risk depends on the level of sun exposure.[49]

MLM behaves as a classic tumor-suppressor locus. Although the increased risk is dominantly inherited, the mutant locus acts in cells as a recessive. Tumors that arise in *MLM* gene carriers invariably lose the wild-type chromosome by deletion or nondisjunction.[51] This feature accords with the proposal of Knudson based originally on studies of the retinoblastoma (*RB1*) tumor-suppressor gene.[52] In the general case of a tumor-suppressor gene, two "hits" are required to inactivate the locus, one for the maternal copy and one for the paternal copy. In familial cancers, one hit occurs through inheritance of a defective allele. Thus a single somatic event is necessary to complete the functional inactivation of the locus.

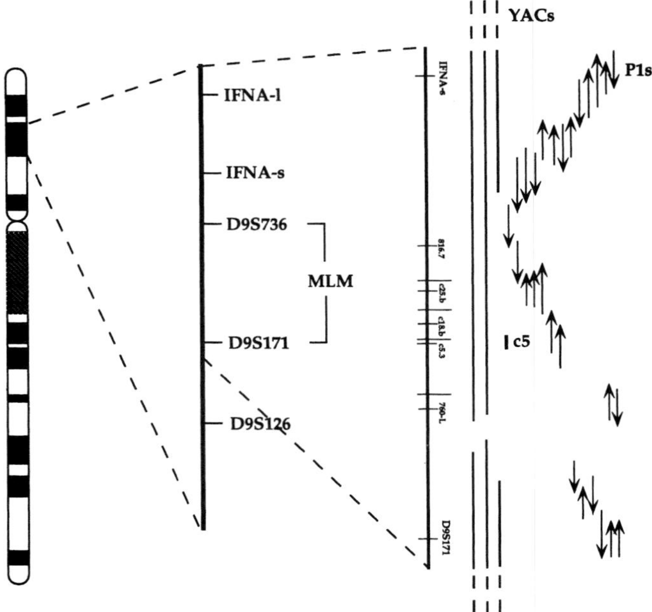

Fig. 44-2 Genetic and physical maps of 9p21 region containing *MLM*. A cartoon of human chromosome 9 is shown with the 9p21 region expanded. Shown are 5 microsatellite markers; *MLM* maps between *D9S736* and *D9S171* by recombinant analysis. This region was aligned to a physical map of P1, yeast artificial chromosome (YAC), and cosmid clones. Several new markers were generated, some of which are shown (e.g., c5.3). In addition, the location of cosmid c5 is shown. This cosmid contains sequences from *p15* and *p16*.

The relationship between nevi and melanoma remains unclear. The role of nevi as melanoma precursors has not been disputed, but the genetic underpinnings of mole incidence and size are unresolved. No simple genetic basis for nevi has been discovered. Nevertheless, *MLM* may influence mole size and number. A comparison of *MLM* carriers and noncarriers revealed that carriers had roughly 50 percent more nevi.[49] If real, the phenotypic effect is dominant or codominant, involving inheritance of a single defective *MLM* copy. This deduction has implications for the role of *MLM* in melanocyte biology.

GENES THAT INFLUENCE MELANOMA

p16

Following the establishment of melanoma linkage to 9p21 markers, an effort to isolate *MLM* was undertaken. However, isolation of the gene proceeded largely without recourse to the 9p21-linked kindreds (see Fig. 44-2). Instead, cell lines were used as the primary tools for gene localization. Previous work had revealed the presence of melanoma cell lines with large homozygous deletions in 9p21.[16,17] This implied that the genetic locus *MLM* and a tumor-suppressor locus presumed to underlie the 9p21 deletions might be one and the same. Under this assumption, standard positional cloning methods of recombinant chromosome analysis were bypassed in favor of the simpler strategy of deletion breakpoint localization in cell lines.

In one study, a collection of nearly 100 melanoma cell lines was assembled to identify and map deletion breakpoints in 9p21.[18] Roughly 60 percent of these lines proved to have detectable

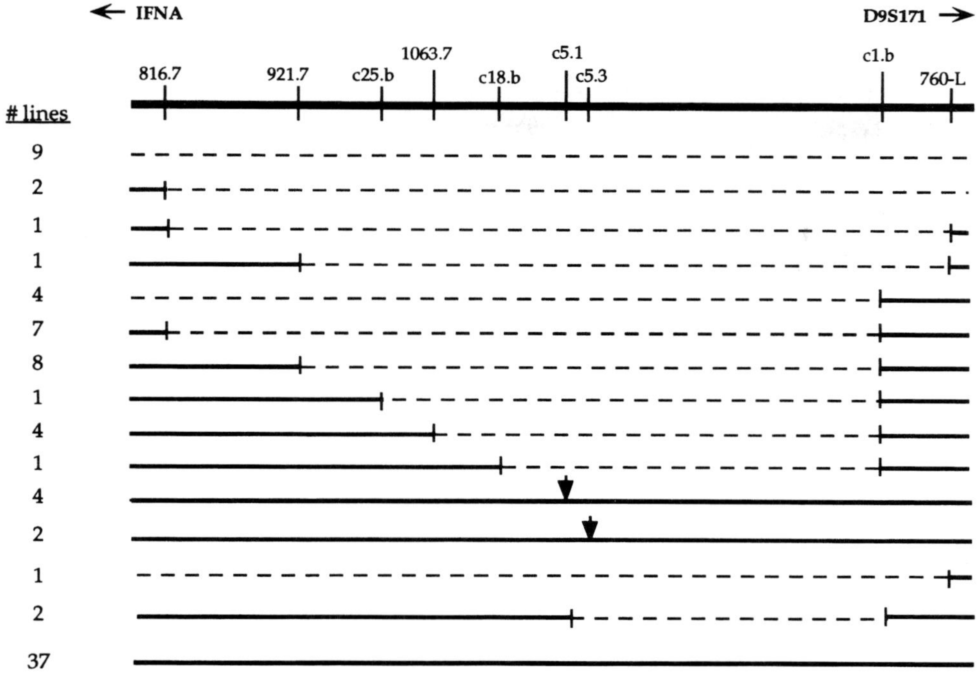

Fig. 44-3 Homozygous deletions in melanoma cell lines. Markers used to detect homozygous deletions are shown above. Melanoma cell lines are grouped into families based on which markers are missing, indicated by dashed lines. The two arrows show homozygous deletions that remove a single marker. The number of cell lines per family is listed on the left.

homozygous deletions, and the deletions clustered around a single site in 9p21 (Fig. 44-3). This site contained two genes, one that encoded the previously identified cyclin-dependent kinase (CDK) inhibitor p16, and the second subsequently shown to encode the related CDK inhibitor p15.[53–57] A variety of deletional and DNA sequence-based studies soon pointed to *p16* (also designated *P16INK4A, MTS1, CDKN2*) as the relevant locus. Inactivating point mutations were found in the *p16* coding sequence but not in *p15* in cell lines and tumors.[54,58,59] In addition, no homozygous deletions were found that removed *p15* but left *p16* intact.[60] In contrast, there were several examples of deletions that left *p15* intact but selectively removed *p16.*

Clinching evidence for the role of *p16* in tumorigenesis was obtained through study of the gene in 9p21-linked families. Linked *p16* sequence variants were found in many, although not all, of these kindreds[61–66] (Table 44-3). Several of the sequence variants obviously were disruptive to the protein causing truncation of the predicted product, and several other missense changes subse-

Table 44-3 Parameters Associated with Melanoma-Prone Kindreds and Mutations

Kindred	Lod Score	Cases	Cases with Haplotype or Mutation	Mutation	Effect
3346	5.97	21	21	—	—
1771	3.57	12	12	Val126Asp	Missense
3137	1.90	17	16	—	—
1764	1.04	4	4	—	—
3012	0.64	4	4	Gly101Trp	Missense
3006	0.19	6	3	—	—
D4	1.22	6	6	Del(218-237)	Frameshift
2482	1.65	—	—	—	—
377	1.64	—	—	—	—
1016	1.41	6	6	Val126Asp	Missense
1017	1.24	4	4	Gly101Trp	Missense
567	1.08	4	4	Arg58Ter	Stop
479	1.03	5	5	Val126Asp	Missense
2884	0.52	2	2	IVS2+1	Splice
909	0.47	—	—	—	—
2209	0.24	—	—	—	—
928	0.12	4	6	Gly101Trp	Missense
481	0.00	3	3	Gly101Trp	Missense
873	−0.03	2	3	Arg87Pro	Missense
373	−0.34	3	3	Asn71Ser	Missense

NOTE: Lod scores for the first five kindreds were calculated for markers between IFNA and D9S171.[63] The Lod score for D4 was computed using D9S171.[66] Note that this mutation was misreported in the original work. Lod scores for the last 12 kindreds were calculated for IFNA.[62] A number of other studies have reported germ-line p16 mutations that are not listed here.[51,64,67]

quently were shown to encode defective p16 molecules.[67–69] *p16* germ-line mutations are found rarely in sporadic cases and in familial cases that do not manifest strong signs of 9p21 linkage. For instance, in 38 patients who meet the typical definition of familiality but who were not part of extended 9p21-linked kindreds, no *p16* mutations were detected.[62] Based on such studies, it is likely that *p16* accounts for a fraction of the total melanoma incidence that is generally considered to be familial. To date, there are no firm estimates for the population frequency of predisposing *MLM* alleles. Extrapolation from some of the work previously cited suggests a frequency in the U.S. population of no more than 1 in a few thousand.[60,64]

Through remarkable serendipity, two individuals homozygous for a predisposing *MLM* allele have been identified.[65] Both homozygous persons carried two copies of the same mutant *p16* allele that contains a deletion of 19 base pairs, an allele that is prevalent especially in melanoma-prone families in Holland. The chance intermarriage of two gene carriers from relatively isolated Dutch villages produced the homozygous individuals. Interestingly, the homozygous gene carriers were normal, except that one of them developed two primary melanomas by age 15. The other individual, however, lived to the age of 55 with no melanomas, although she died of an internal adenocarcinoma. It is worth noting that the melanoma patient had numerous nevi, whereas the other carrier was relatively mole-free. The latter individual, however, had offspring, some of whom were classified as DNS cases. These facts demonstrate two important aspects of *p16* function. First, *p16* is not essential for normal development or viability, a conclusion confirmed by the recent demonstration of viable *p16* knockout mice.[70] Second, *p16* mutations have variable expressivity; phenotypic effects may depend on unknown genetic factors as well as environmental factors, including but perhaps not restricted to sun exposure.

The weight of the evidence strongly supports the view that *p16* is *MLM*. As is the case with many familial tumor suppressors, *p16* germ-line mutations increase cancer risk, whereas *p16* somatic mutations also occur in sporadic tumors during the transition toward malignancy.

p15

A continuing mystery is the existence of kindreds that are definitely 9p21-linked but for whom mutations cannot be found in *p16*[60,61] (see Table 44-3). These kindreds served as the initial impetus to explore *p15* as a candidate for a second melanoma-susceptibility gene on 9p21. *p15* has considerable sequence similarity to *p16* (77 percent at the protein level in humans) and encodes a protein with biochemical behavior nearly identical to p16.[56,57] It is located within 20 kb of *p16* on chromosome 9 and likely was derived from *p16* by gene duplication, divergence, and in the human lineage, a gene conversion event.[71] Both proteins cause growth arrest when overexpressed in certain cell lines and in normal cells.[59,67,72,73] *p15* regulation, however, is markedly different from *p16*. *p15* is induced by transforming growth factor beta (TGF-β); *p16* is not.[56] This adds further interest to the possible role of p15 in cancer, since TGF-β is an important regulator of cell growth. Despite the obvious appeal of *p15* as an alternative *MLM*-like gene, no germ-line mutations have been reported so far in *p15*.[59]

*E1β/p19^ARF^*

Another potential tumor suppressor is encoded at the *p16* locus, although its role in cancer is obscure (Fig. 44-4). The gene, termed $p19^{ARF}$ or $p16^{E1\beta}$, actually overlaps the *p16* coding sequence.[74–76] The $p16^{E1\beta}$ transcript originates from a promotor distinct from the normal *p16* promotor. This second upstream promotor produces a transcript that contains the second and third coding exons of *p16* (*E2* and *E3*) but incorporates an alternative first exon (*E1β*) in place of the normal first exon of *p16* (see Fig. 44-3). The reading frame used to encode *p16* is closed immediately upstream of the *E1β-E2* junction, suggesting that if this frame were used for

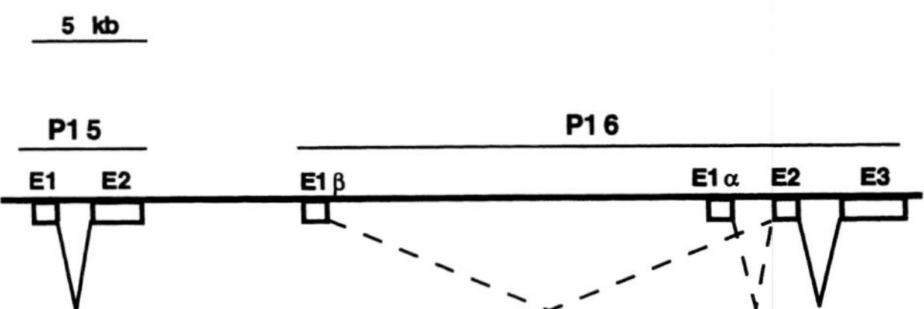

Fig. 44-4 The *p16* locus is complex. The relative position of *p16* coding exons (1 and 2) and *p16* exons are shown. Dashed lines indicate an alternative splice that distinguishes the *E1β* transcript from the *p16* transcript.

translation, a truncated *p16* molecule missing the first third of the protein would result. No such protein has been detected *in vivo*. An alternative reading frame (*ORF2*), however, potentially encodes a protein of 19 kDa; hence the name $p19^{ARF}$. This protein bears no homology to any known protein sequence. However, it is conserved between mouse and human.[71,77]

The *E1β* exon is deleted selectively in several melanoma cell lines, leaving the *p16* transcript and protein intact. This implies an important role for $p16^{E1\beta}$ in the tumor-suppressor function of the *p16* locus. No *E1β* mutations have been observed in the germ lines of familial cases. Moreover, no *E1β*-specific point mutations have been detected in cell lines or tumors.[74]

Antibodies raised against $p19^{ARF}$ detect a 19-kDa protein *in vivo*, and overexpression of $p19^{ARF}$ causes cessation of cell growth.[77] However, unlike p16 and other CDK inhibitors, $p19^{ARF}$ does not inhibit cdk4 *in vitro*. Paradoxically, the level of the *E1β* transcript increases as quiescent T cells enter the cell cycle.[74] In addition, comparison of human and mouse sequences reveals that the reading frame predicted to encode $p19^{ARF}$ is no more conserved than the other alternative to the *p16* reading frame (*ORF3*).[71,74] Thus there is little evidence for evolutionary selective pressure on the $p19^{ARF}$ protein. The $p19^{ARF}$ protein binds to mdm2, which in turn interacts with p53, thus potentially tying the p53 and p16 pathways together.[79–81] $E1\beta/p19^{ARF}$ may represent one of the more bizarre genes in the mammalian genome: a member of a complex locus; transcribed from a separate, independently regulated promotor; overlapping a gene that is translated in a different reading frame; and both genes participating in the cell cycle regulatory apparatus.

CDK4

On the heels of the discovery that *p16* germ-line mutations predispose to melanoma, a second melanoma-predisposition gene was uncovered. A fraction of melanoma-prone families that are not linked to 9p21 segregate mutations in a gene that encodes one of the targets of p16's inhibitory activity, cdk4.[79] These mutations affect a single site in the *CDK4* coding sequence that renders the molecule resistant to p16 binding and inhibition. The identical lesion also has been observed as a somatic mutation in a sporadic melanoma.[80] Thus *CDK4* behaves as a proto-oncogene; the mutant form is converted into an overactive growth promotor, an oncogene. This is only the second example of germ-line mutations in a proto-oncogene. The other example is the *RET* proto-oncogene, germ-line mutations in which predispose to the cancer-susceptibility syndrome multiple endocrine neoplasia 2A.[81] Based on the observed frequency of mutations, kindreds that segregate *CDK4* mutations may be tenfold less frequent than *p16* kindreds.

A Growth-Control Pathway in Melanocytes

The identification of *CDK4* germ-line mutations in melanoma-prone kindreds is exciting for another reason. cdk4, p16, Rb, and D cyclins comprise part of a growth-control pathway that operates in a variety, perhaps all, tissues[82] (Fig. 44-5). Several lines of evidence suggest that p16 inhibits cdk4, which has the consequence of preventing phosphorylation of Rb protein. Hypophos-

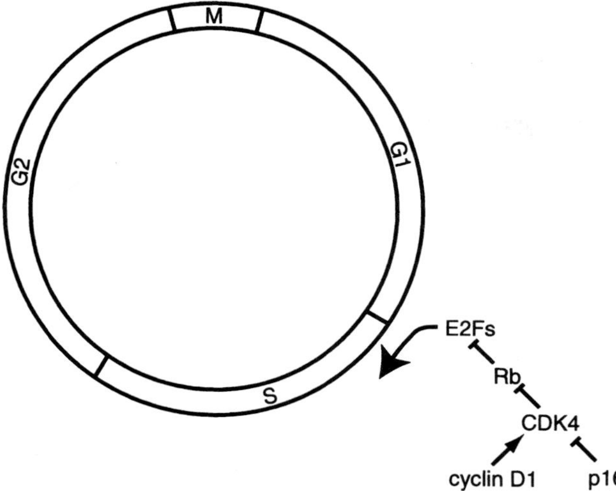

Fig. 44-5 The cell cycle and the p16 growth-control pathway. Eukaryotic cell division is broken up into four phases: G1, during which the cell prepares to synthesize DNA; S, the phase of DNA replication; G2 during which the cell prepares for mitosis; and M, the mitotic period. The transition between G1 and S is monitored carefully by the cell. p16, acting through cdk4 and Rb, exercises its control over cell division at this point. Arrows indicate a positive effect; blunt-ended lines an inhibitory effect.

phorylated Rb binds transcription factors such as members of the *E2F* family, interfering with their ability to activate transcription of genes involved in DNA synthesis.[83] Sporadic tumors seldom contain mutations in more than one component of this pathway, an observation that supports the mutually dependent function of the genes.[84–87] In contrast, mutations in *p53,* although rare in melanoma, occur as frequently in *p16*-positive tumors as in *p16*-negative tumors, an indication that p53 and p16 function in separate pathways of growth control.[13] It should be emphasized, however, that p19^{ARF} may link the two pathways in some functional sense. p16, cdk4, and Rb thus play a central part in the regulation of the cell cycle. They may comprise a primary circuit that integrates information relevant in the decision to proceed through the first stage of cell division and DNA replication.

To date, three of the four known components of the pathway have been implicated in hereditary cancer syndromes: *CDK4, p16,* and *RB1.* Curiously, *RB1* mutant gene carriers do not suffer from excessive melanoma but rather from a specific childhood tumor of the eye.[88] Why the phenotype of *CDK4* and *p16* mutations differs from the *RB1* mutant phenotype is unclear, but it emphasizes the complexity of the growth-control pathways that operate in cells.

The evidence that *p16* is an important cancer gene is compelling. Germ-line mutations in *p16* increase melanoma risk. Deletions in *p16,* as well as a smaller number of point mutations, are found in a large percentage of melanomas and many other cancer types.[89] In melanoma tumors and cell lines, the large majority of point mutations that are detected have the hallmarks of UV-induced changes, signs of the link between UV and *p16* inactivation in tumors.[58,90,91] Loss of *p16* expression owing to methylation has been reported in a variety of cell lines.[92–94] Overexpression of p16 in a range of cell types causes arrest at the G1/S checkpoint in the cell cycle.[67,70,73] Mice in which the *p16* gene has been inactivated by homologous recombination are cancer-prone.[70] p16 functions *in vitro* as a biochemical inhibitor of cdk4, a protein known to promote passage through the G1/S checkpoint. Taken together, this body of data leaves little doubt that *p16* plays a key role in a variety of human cancers but does not delineate the precise nature of the role.

p16 and Other CDK Inhibitors

Many other CDK inhibitors have been identified including p15, p18, p21, p27, and p57.[56,95–102] All, including p16, are expressed in a wide variety of tissues.[74] The biochemical behavior of p16 protein differs little from, for example, p15.[56] All CDK inhibitors, when overexpressed in particular cell types, induce cell cycle arrest. Yet *p16* appears to be a special case. None of the other genes is mutated at appreciable frequencies in tumors or cell lines.[59,103–105] The physiologic function of p16 that may distinguish it from other CDK inhibitors, rendering it more vulnerable to mutational inactivation, is not obvious.

Attempts to define the physiologic function of p16 *in vivo* have focused on two general areas: its role in programmed cell death, or apoptosis, and its role in cellular senescence. In one model system, p16 expression correlated with protection from apoptosis, a finding that does not explain why tumor cells would dispense with *p16.*[106] More germane, perhaps, *p16*-deficient mouse cells are highly sensitive to oncogenic transformation and readily form colonies in culture.[70] This result suggests that loss of p16 expression may contribute to immortalization. Other studies have reported an increase in p16 levels as cells approach senescence, followed by a fall as cells become immortalized.[107–109] Based on this correlation, it seems reasonable to propose a role for p16 in suppressing immortalization. To achieve this effect, p16 must work through Rb. Consequently, Rb and the other components of the p16 pathway are implicated as accessory molecules in the control of cellular life span. This proposed role for p16 leaves unexplained the early 9p LOH events in melanoma development.

p16 Mutations and Predisposition to Nonmelanoma Cancers

It is perplexing given the widespread involvement of *p16* in sporadic cancer that *p16* mutant gene carriers are predisposed only to melanoma. Some studies have suggested an association between pancreatic cancer and melanoma in certain families, but a clear role for *MLM* in cancers besides melanoma has been difficult to prove.[51,110] A simple explanation may lie in considerations about rate-limiting steps in tumorigenesis. If, as the data begin to suggest, p16 inactivation is a relatively late step in tumor development, its removal may not be rate-limiting in most tumor types. For reasons that are obscure, p16 inactivation may be important at an earlier stage in melanoma formation, or it may be the final brake that is released in cells that suffer an environmental insult in the form of UV exposure and consequent high rates of mutation. It is more complicated, although not impossible, to hypothesize a role for *p16* mutations both early during melanoma formation in nevi and later in the escape from senescence.

GENETICS AND MELANOMA DIAGNOSIS

Germ-Line Testing for Melanoma Susceptibility

With identification of the major genetic factors underlying hereditary melanoma, *p16* and, to a lesser extent, *CDK4,* the possibility of germ-line testing for melanoma risk has arrived. Contrary to many other types of genetic testing, a melanoma-predisposition screen has certain clear advantages. First, in principle, the results of such a test provide valuable information to guide behavior. If an individual tests positive (i.e., carries a high-risk allele), steps can be taken to avoid sun exposure and to maintain vigilance for abnormal growths on the skin. Such behavior not only would diminish the chance of melanoma but also would facilitate early detection and removal of the lesion, by far the most successful approach to combating the disease. Second, although many independent sequence changes have been described, the *p16* gene is small, consisting of only 158 codons. By contrast, coding sequences of the breast cancer-susceptibility genes *BRCA1* and *BRCA2* are huge, roughly 12 and 25 times the size of *p16*, respectively.[111,112] The relatively small size of *p16* should reduce dramatically the technical difficulties and cost associated with a genetic screen. In the case of *CDK4*, a screen that targets a single codon may be sufficient.[79]

Excitement about the value of a melanoma-susceptibility screen is blunted somewhat by other considerations, especially the economic realities of such a test. The combined gene frequency of *p16* and *CDK4* predisposing alleles is low. Thus, for random, population-based screening, the *a priori* probability of getting a positive result is very small, a disincentive to pay for such a test. In addition, the possibility of missing *MLM* mutations that fall outside the coding sequence must be considered. Several kindreds that show a strong indication of 9p21 linkage appear to have wild-type *p16* coding regions.[61,62] This suggests that a percentage of *p16* mutations fall outside the coding sequences or that a second *MLM* gene resides in 9p21. Either a test must be devised to detect such mutations, or the test may have limited informativeness.

The greatest value of a melanoma-susceptibility test may apply to individuals at higher risk of melanoma than the majority of the population. These include people with many moles and people with affected relatives. With roughly 40,000 melanoma cases per year in the United States, such a test might be relevant to over 100,000 people every year. If the criterion of numerous nevi also is used, the number of higher-risk individuals may exceed 1 million. This is a potential market size that may drive development of a commercial test, but whether a specialized melanoma genetic test could be economically self-sustaining in the short term remains debatable. It may make more sense to provide an *MLM* test when the costs of such gene-based diagnostic screens are lower or when it becomes part of a larger panel of susceptibility gene tests.

Somatic Gene Testing

An alternative to germ-line *p16* and *CDK4* testing is afforded by the potential for somatic gene testing in tumors. *p16* is one of the most frequently altered genes in human cancer, inactivated in perhaps half of all advanced tumors.[54] Here, economic considerations contribute a strong impulse for test development, providing certain criteria can be met. First, there is a slew of technical issues that involve detection of *p16* alterations in cancer cells: homozygous deletions, the most common form of *p16* inactivation, methylated DNA, and other somatic changes. Detection of such disparate lesions is a particularly significant problem in tumors that are invariably adulterated by normal somatic cells.[60] Second, the clinical relevance of such a somatic *p16* gene test must be demonstrated firmly. The test must prove useful in the diagnosis or prognosis of cancer. Most desirable would be test results that aid in customization of cancer therapy. Clinical studies that address these issues are critically important. At least one report so far details the significance of *p16* gene status as a prognostic indicator in childhood acute lymphocytic leukemia.[113] Thus there is the exciting possibility that *p16* gene tests, as well as tests for multiple other cancer genes, ultimately may supplement or replace traditional modes of subjective histologic analysis in the classification and treatment of tumors.

GENETICS AND MELANOMA THERAPY

Advances in understanding the genetics of melanoma so far have had little impact on treatment, nor are they likely to have a rapid effect in the future. The difficulties of translating genetic knowledge into practical therapeutic advances are immense. Here, as in the traditional approach to cancer therapy, the challenge is to achieve specificity. An effective therapeutic agent must target cancer cells and leave normal cells relatively unharmed. With some of the molecules that regulate melanoma development now in hand, it is at least possible to formulate potential strategies.

Targeting cdk4

Immunotherapy tailored to abnormal cdk4 molecules offers a route to novel melanoma therapy. Indeed, T cells have been identified that recognize tumor cells that harbor mutant cdk4 proteins.[80] One of the weaknesses of this approach, however, is the small number of tumors likely to have sustained cdk4 alterations. Thus a treatment that targets mutant cdk4 is unlikely to have general success in combating the vast majority of melanomas.

Complementation of Defective *p16* Genes in Tumors

An alternative approach is to devise treatments that rely on *p16*. Because *p16* mutations occur in many tumors besides melanoma, the investment in such a treatment likely would have benefits that extend well beyond melanoma. Once again, however, specificity and delivery are key factors. Simple reintroduction of functional *p16* sequences into tumor cells causes growth arrest.[114,115] However, the sequences also arrest normal cells.[73] Therefore, a strategy that depends on restored expression of p16 in tumor cells must include either a means for selective delivery of *p16* into tumor cells or a mechanism for regulated expression that permits normal cell growth.

Manipulating the Cell Cycle

Small-molecule drugs that mimic p16 may find some use in cancer treatment and are currently under development by certain pharmaceutical companies. However, the issue of selectivity remains problematic here as with gene therapy.

Finally, it may be possible to use cell cycle regulators such as p16 to protect normal cells from the ravages of conventional chemo- or radiotherapy. If a method for specific induction of growth arrest in normal cells could be found, a state of temporary arrest could be induced in normal cells that would endow them with resistance to subsequent cytotoxic treatments. This general concept has been explored in the past.[116–119] *p16* provides a new molecular tool to study the value of such an approach. At least in one model system, p16 expression causes reversible cell cycle arrest that protects cells from chemotherapeutics.[120] The challenge in this approach is to achieve a general protection of normal tissues by reversible induction of p16 or other regulators. The strategy is attractive because the induction does not need to be selective. Many tumors have lost the function of the p16 growth-control pathway, either by mutation of *p16* itself or by alteration of downstream components such as cdk4 or Rb. Thus most tumors would not respond to an agent that induces p16 expression by entering a state of arrest. Only normal cells, which maintain the integrity of the p16 pathway, would arrest and be rendered resistant to cytotoxic treatments.

REFERENCES

1. Clark WH: The skin, in Rubin E, Farber JL (eds): *Pathology*. Philadelphia, Lippincott, 1988.
2. Kamb A: Human melanoma genetics. *J Invest Dermatol Symp Proc* **1**:177, 1996.
3. Fitzpatrick TB, Sober AJ, Mihm MC Jr: Malignant melanoma of the skin, in Braunwald E, Isselbacher KJ, Petersdorf RG, Wilson JD, Martin JB, Fauci AS (eds): *Principles of Internal Medicine*. New York, McGraw-Hill, 1987.
4. Fearon ER, Vogelstein B: A genetic model for colorectal tumorigenesis. *Cell* **61**:759, 1990.
5. National Cancer Institute: *1987 Annual Cancer Statistics Review*. NIH publication no 88-2789, 1988.
6. Sober AJ, Lew RA, Koh HK, Barnhill RL: Epidemiology of cutaneous melanoma. *Dermatol Clin* **9**:617, 1991.
7. Nigel DS, Fridman RJ, Kopf AW: The incidence of malignant melanoma in the United States: Issues as we approach the 21st century. *J Am Acad Dermatol* **34**:839, 1996.
8. Green A, Swerdlow AJ: Epidemiology of melanocytic nevi. *Epidemiol Rev* **11**:204, 1989.

9. Herlyn M: *Molecular and Cellular Biology of Melanoma*. Austin, TX, RG Landes, 1993.
10. Fountain JW, Bale SJ, Housman DE, Dracopoli NC: Genetics of melanoma. *Cancer Surv* **9**:645, 1990.
11. Healy E, Rehman I, Angus B, Rees JL: Loss of heterozygosity in sporadic primary cutaneous melanoma. *Genes Chromosom Cancer* **12**:152, 1995.
12. Walker GJ, Palmer JM, Walters MK, Nancarrow DJ, Hayward NK: Microsatellite instability in melanoma. *Melanoma Res* **4**:267, 1994.
13. Gruis NA, Weaver-Feldhaus J, Liu Q, Frye C, Ecles R, Orlow I, Lacombe L, Ponce-Castoneda V, Lianes E, et al: Genetic evidence in melanoma and bladder cancers that p16 and p53 function in separate pathways of tumor suppression. *Am J Pathol* **146**:1199, 1995.
14. Peris K, Keller G, Chimenti S, Amantea A, Derl H, Hofler H: Microsatellite instability and loss of heterozygosity in melanoma. *J Invest Dermatol* **105**:625, 1995.
15. Quinn AG, Healy E, Rehman I, Sikkink S, Rees JL: Microsatellite instability in human non-melanoma and melanoma skin cancer. *J Invest Dermatol* **104**:309, 1995.
16. Olopade OI, Jenkins R, Linnenbach AJ, et al: Molecular analysis of chromosome 9p deletion in human solid tumors. *Proc Am Assoc Cancer Res* **21**:318, 1990.
17. Fountain JW, Karayiorgou M, Ernstoff MS, Kirkwood JM, Vlock DR, Titus-Ernstoff L, Bouchard B, Vijayasaradhi S, Houghton AN, Lahti J, et al: Homozygous deletions within human chromosome band 9p21 in melanoma. *Proc Natl Acad Sci USA* **89**:10557, 1992.
18. Weaver-Feldhaus J, Gruis NA, Neuhausen S, Le Paslier D, Stockert E, Skolnick MH, Kamb A: Localization of a putative tumor suppressor gene by using homozygous deletions in melanomas. *Proc Natl Acad Sci USA* **91**:7563, 1994.
19. Reed JA, Loganzo F Jr, Shea CR, Walker GJ, Flores JF, Glending JM, Bogdany JK, Shiel MJ, Haluska FG, Fountain JW, Albino AP: Loss of expression of the p16/cyclin-dependent kinase inhibitor 2 tumor suppresser gene in melanocytic lesions correlates with invasive stage of tumor progression. *Cancer Res* **55**:2713, 1995.
20. Sozzi G, Veronese ML, Negrini M, Baffa R, Cotticelli MG, Inoue H, Tornielli S, Pilotti S, De Gregorio L, Pastorino U, Pierotti MA, Ohta M, Huebner K, Croce CM: The *FHIT* gene 3p14.2 is abnormal in lung cancer. *Cell* **85**:17, 1996.
21. Volkenandt M, Schlegel U, Nanus DM, Albino AP: Mutational analysis of the human *p53* gene in malignant melanoma cell lines. *Pigment Cell Res* **4**:35, 1991.
22. Levin DB, Wilson K, Valadares de Amorim G, Webber J, Kenny P, Kusser W: Detection of *p53* mutations in benign and dysplastic nevi. *Cancer Res* **55**:4278, 1995.
23. Balaban GB, Herlyn M, Clark WH Jr, Nowell PC: Karyotypic evolution in human malignant melanoma. *Cancer Genet Cytogenet* **19**:113, 1986.
24. Dracopoli ND, Alhadeff B, Houghton AN, Old LJ: Loss of heterozygosity at autosomal and X-linked loci during tumor progression in a patient with melanoma. *Cancer Res* **47**:3995, 1987.
25. Cowan JM, Halaban R, Francke U: Cytogenetic analysis of melanocytes from premalignant nevi and melanomas. *J Natl Cancer Inst* **80**:1159, 1988.
26. Horsman DE, White VA: Cytogenetic analysis of uveal melanoma: Consistent occurrence of monosomy 3 and trisomy 8q. *Cancer* **71**:811, 1993.
27. Andersen LB, Fountain JW, Gutmann DH, Tarle SA, Glover TW, Dracopoli NC, Housman DE, Collins FS: Mutations in the neurofibromatosis 1 gene in sporadic melanoma cell lines. *Nature Genet* **3**:118, 1993.
28. Johnson MR, Look AT, DeClue JE, Valentine MB, Lowy DR: Inactivation of the *NF1* gene in human melanoma and neuroblastoma cell lines without impaired regulation of *GRP.ras. Proc Natl Acad Sci USA* **90**:5539, 1993.
29. Welch DR, Chen P, Miele ME, McGary CT, Bower JM, Stanbridge EJ, Weissman BE: Microcell-mediated transfer of chromosome 6 into metastatic human C8161 melanoma cells suppresses metastasis but does not inhibit tumorigenicity. *Oncogene* **9**:255, 1994.
30. Teng DH, Hu R, Lin H, Davis T, Iliev D, Frye C, Swedlund B, Hansen KL, Vinson VL, Gumpper KL, Ellis L, El-Nagger A, Frazier M, Jasser S, Langford LA, Lee J, Mills GB, Pershouse MA, Pollack RE, Tornos C, Troncoso P, Yung WK, Fujii G, Berson A, Steck PA, et al: MMAC1/PTEN mutations in primary tumor specimens and tu cell lines *Cancer Res* **57**:5221, 1997.
31. Cawley EP: Genetic aspects of malignant melanoma. *Arch Dermatol* **65**:440, 1952.
32. Greene MH, Fraumeni JF Jr: The hereditary variant of malignant melanoma, in Clark WH Jr, Goldman LI, Mastrangelo MJ (eds): *Human Malignant Melanoma*. New York, Grune and Stratton, 1979.
33. Wallace DC, Exton LA, McLeod GR: Genetic factor in malignant melanoma. *Cancer* **27**:1262, 1971.
34. Goldgar DE, Easton DF, Cannon-Albright LA, Skolnick MH: A systematic population-based assessment of cancer risk in first degree relatives of cancer probands. *J Natl Cancer Inst* **86**:1600, 1994.
35. Turkington RW: Familial factors in malignant melanoma. *JAMA* **192**:77, 1965.
36. Smith EE, Henley WS, Knox JM, Lane M: Familial melanoma. *Arch Intern Med* **117**:820, 1966.
37. Anderson DE, Smith JL Jr, McBride CM: Hereditary aspects of malignant melanoma. *JAMA* **200**:741, 1967.
38. Swerdlow AJ, English J, Mackie RM, O'Doherty CJ, Hunter JAA, Clark J: Benign nevi associated with high risk of melanoma. *Lancet* **2**:168, 1984.
39. Clark WH, Reimer RR, Greene M, Ainsworth AM, Mastrangelo M: Origin of familial malignant melanomas from heritable melanocyte lesions. *Arch Dermatol* **114**:732, 1978.
40. Lynch HT, Frichot BC, Lynch J: Familial atypical multiple mole melanoma syndrome. *J Med Genet* **15**:352, 1978.
41. Greene MH, Goldin LR, Clark WH, et al: Familial malignant melanoma: Autosomal dominant trait possibly linked to the Rhesus locus. *Proc Natl Acad Sci USA* **80**:6071, 1983.
42. Bale SJ, Dracopoli NC, Tucker, MA, Clark WH Jr, Fraser MC, Stanger BZ, Green P, Donis-Keller H, Housman DE, Green MH: Mapping the gene for hereditary cutaneous malignant melanoma-dysplastic nevus to chromosome 1p. *N Engl J Med* **320**:1367, 1986.
43. van Haeringen A, Bergman W, Nolen MR, van der Kooij-Meijs E, Hendrikse I, Wijnen JT, Khan PM, Klasen EC, Frants RR: Exclusion of the dysplastic nevus syndrome (DNS) locus from the short arm of chromsome 1 by linkage studies in Dutch families. *Genomics* **5**:61, 1989.
44. Cannon-Albright LA, Goldgar DE, Wright EC, et al: Evidence against the reported linkage to the cutaneous melanoma-dysplastic nevus syndrome locus to chromosome 1p36. *Am J Human Genet* **46**:912, 1990.
45. Kefford RF, Salmon J, Shaw HM, Donald JA, McCarthy WH: Hereditary melanoma in Australia: Variable association with dysplastic nevi and absence of genetic linkage to chromosome 1p. *Cancer Genet Cytogenet* **51**:45, 1991.
46. Nancarrow DJ, Palmer JM, Walters MK, Kerr BM, Hofner GJ, Garske L, McLeod GR, Hayward NK: Exclusion of the familial melanoma locus (*MLM*) from the *PND/DIS47* and *MYCL1* regions of chromosome arm 1p in 7 Australian pedigrees. *Genomics* **12**:18, 1992.
47. Goldstein AM, Dracopoli NC, Engelstein M, Fraser MC, Clark WH Jr, Tucker MA: Linkage of cutaneous malignant melanoma/dysplastic nevi to chromosome 9p, and evidence for genetic heterogeneity. *Am J Hum Genet* **54**:489, 1994.
48. Cannon-Albright LA, Goldgar DE, Meyer LJ, Lewis CM, Anderson DE, Fountain JW, Hegi ME, Wiseman RW, Petty EM, Bale AE, Olopade OI, Diaz MO, Kwiatkowski DJ, Piepkorn MW, Zone JJ, Skolnick MH: Assignment of a locus for familial melanoma, *MLM,* to chromosome 9p 13-p22. *Science* **258**:1148, 1992.
49. Skolnick MH, Cannon-Albright LA, Kamb A: Genetic predisposition to melanoma. *Eur J Cancer* **30**:1991, 1994.
50. Cannon-Albright LA, Meyer LJ, Goldgar DE, Lewis CM, McWhorter WP, Jost M, Harrison D, Anderson DE, Zone JJ, Skolnick MH: Penetrance and expressivity of the chromosome 9p melanoma susceptibility locus (*MLM*). *Cancer Res* **54**:6041, 1994.
51. Walker GJ, Hussussian CJ, Flores JF, Glendening JM, Haluska FG, Drocopoli NC, Hayward NK, Fountain JW: Mutations of the *CDKN2/p16INK4* gene in Australian melanoma kindreds. *Hum Mol Genet* **4**:1845, 1995.
52. Gruis NA, Sandkuijl LA, van der Velden PA, Bergman W, Frants RR: CDKN2 explains part of the clinical phenotype in Dutch familial atypical multiple-mole melanoma (FAMMM) syndrome families. *Melanoma Res* **5**:169, 1995b.
53. Knudson AG: Mutation and cancer: Statistical study of retinoblastoma. *Proc Natl Acad Sci USA* **68**:820, 1971.
54. Serrano M, Hannon GJ, Beach D: A new regulatory motif in cell-cycle control causing specific inhibition of cyclin D/CDK4. *Nature* **366**:704, 1993.
55. Kamb A, Gruis NA, Weaver-Feldhaus J, Liu Q, Harshman K, Tavtigian SV, Stockert E, Day RS, Johnson BE, Skolnick MH: A cell cycle regulator potentially involved in genesis of many tumor types. *Science* **264**:436, 1994.

56. Nobori T, Miura K, Wu DJ, Lois A, Takabayashi K, Carson DA: Deletions of the cyclin-dependent kinase-4 inhibitor gene in multiple human cancers. *Nature* **368**:753, 1994.
57. Hannon GJ, Beach D: p15INK4B is a potential effector of TFG-β–induced cell cycle arrest. *Nature* **371**:257, 1994.
58. Jen J, Harper JW, Bigner SH, Bigner DD, Papadopoulos N, Markowitz S, Wilson JKV, Kinzler KW, Vogelstein B: Deletion of *p16* and *p15* genes in brain tumors. *Cancer Res* **54**:6353, 1994.
59. Liu Q, Neuhausen S, McClure M, Frye C, Weaver-Feldhaus J, Gruis NA, Eddington K, Allalunis-Turner MJ, Skolnick MH, Fujimura FK, Kamb A: *CDKN2* (*MTS1*) tumor suppressor gene mutations in human tumor cell lines. *Oncogene* **10**:1061, 1995.
60. Stone S, Dayananth P, Jiang P, Weaver-Feldhaus JM, Tavtigian SV, Skolnick MH, Kamb A: Genomic structure, expression, and mutational analysis of the *P15* (*MTS2*) gene. *Oncogene* **11**:987, 1995.
61. Kamb A, Liu Q, Harshman K, Tavtigian SV: Response to rate of *p16* (*MTS1*) mutations in primary tumors with 9p loss. *Science* **265**:416, 1994.
62. Hussussian CJ, Struewing JP, Goldstein AM, Higgins PAT, Ally DS, Sheahan MD, Clark WHJ, Tucker MA, Dracopoli NC: Germline *p16* mutations in familial melanoma. *Nature Genet* **8**:15, 1994.
63. Kamb A, Shattuck-Eidens D, Eeles R, Liu Q, Gruis NA, Ding W, Hussey C, Tran T, Miki Y, Weaver-Feldhaus J, McClure M, Aitken JF, Anderson DE, Bergman W, Frants R, Goldgar DE, Green A, MacLennan R, Martin NG, Meyer LJ, Youl P, Zone JJ, Skolnick MH, Cannon-Albright LA: Analysis of the *p16* gene (*CDKN2*) as a candidate for the chromosome 9p melanoma susceptibility locus. *Nature Genet* **8**:22, 1994.
64. Borg A, Johannsson U, Johannsson O, Hakansson S, Westerdahl J, Masback A, Olsson H, Ingvar C: Novel germline *p16* mutation in familial malignant melanoma in southern Sweden. *Cancer Res* **56**:2497, 1996.
65. Holland EA, Beaton SC, Becker TM, Grulet OM, Peters BA, Rizos H, Kefford RF, Mann GJ: Analysis of the *p16* gene, *CDKN2,* in 17 Australian melanoma kindreds. *Oncogene* **11**:2289, 1995.
66. Gruis NA, van der Velden PA, Sandkuijl LA, Prins DE, Weaver-Feldhaus J, Kamb A, Bergman W, Frants RR: Homozygotes for *CDKN2* (*p16*) germline mutation in Dutch familial melanoma kindreds. *Nature Genet* **10**:351, 1995.
67. Liu L, Lassam NJ, Slingerland JM, Bailey D, Cole D, Jenkins R, Hogg D: Germline *p16INK4A* mutation and protein dysfunction in a family with inherited melanoma. *Oncogene* **11**:405, 1995.
68. Koh J, Enders GH, Cynlacht BD, Harlow E: Tumor-derived p16 alleles encoding proteins defective in cell-cycle inhibition. *Nature* **375**:506, 1995.
69. Ranade K, Hussussian CJ, Sikorski RS, Varmus HE, Goldstein AM, Tucker MA, Serrano M, Hannon GJ, Beach D, Dracopoli NC: Mutations associated with familial melanoma impair *p16INK4* function. *Nature Genet* **10**:114, 1995.
70. Yang R, Gombart AF, Serrano M, Koeffler P: Mutational effects on the *p16INK4a*. *Cancer Res* **55**:2503, 1995.
71. Serrano M, Lee H, Chin L, Cordon-Cardo C, Beach D, DePinho RA: Role of the *INK4a* locus in tumor suppression and cell mortality. *Cell* **85**:27, 1996.
72. Jiang P, Stone S, Wagner R, Wang S, Dayananth P, Kozak CA, Wold B, Kamb A: Comparative analysis of *Homo sapiens* and *Mus musculus* cyclin-dependent kinase (CDK) inhibitor genes *p16* (*MTS1*) and *p15* (*MTS2*). *J Mol Evol* **41**:795, 1995.
73. Serrano M, Gomez-Lahoz E, DePinho RA, Beach D, Bar-Sagi D: Inhibition of ras-induced proliferation and cellular transformation by *p16INK4*. *Science* **267**:249, 1995.
74. Lukas J, Parry D, Aagaard L, Mann DJ, Bartkova J, Strauss M, Peters G, Bartek J: Retino-blastoma-protein-dependent cell-cycle inhibition by the tumor suppressor *p16*. *Nature* **375**:503, 1995.
75. Stone S, Jiang P, Dayannanth P, Tavtigian SV, Katcher H, Parry D, Peters G, Kamb A: Complex structure and regulation of the *P16* (*MTS1*) locus. *Cancer Res* **55**:2988, 1995.
76. Mao L, Merlo A, Bedi G, Shapiro GI, Edwards CD, Rollins BJ, Sidransky DA: A novel *p16INK4A* transcript. *Cancer Res* **55**:2995, 1995.
77. Duro D, Bernard O, Della Valle V, Berger R, Larsen CJ: A new type of p161INK4/MTS1 gene transcript expressed in B-cell malignancies. *Oncogene* **11**:212, 1995.
78. Quelle D, Zindy F, Ashmun RA, Sherr CJ: Alternative reading frames of the *INKa* tumor suppressor gene encode two unrelated proteins capable of inducing cell cycle arrest. *Cell* **83**:993, 1995.
79. Pomerantz J, Schreiber-Agus N, Liegeois NJ, et al: The Ink4a tumor suppressor gene product, p19Arf, interacts with MDM2 and neutralizes MDM2's inhibition of p53. *Cell* **92**:713, 1998.
80. Zhang Y, Xiong Y, Yarbrough WG: ARF promotes MDM2 degradation and stabilizes p53: ARF-INK4a locus deletion impairs both the Rb and p53 tumor suppression pathways. *Cell* **92**:725, 1998.
81. Kamijo T, Weber JD, Zambetti G, et al: Functional and physical interactions of the ARF tumor suppressor with p53 and Mdm2. *Proc Natl Acad Sci USA* **95**:8292, 1998
82. Glendening JM, Flores JF, Wlaker GJ, Stone S, Albino AP, Fountain JW: Homozygous loss of the *p15INK4B* gene (and not the *p16INK4* gene) during tumor progression in a sporadic melanoma patient. *Cancer Res* **55**:5531, 1995.
83. Zuo L, Weger J, Yang Q, Goldstein AM, Tucker MA, Walker GJ, Hayward N, Dracopoli NC: Germline mutations in the *p16INK4a* binding domain of CDK4 in familial melanoma. *Nature Genet* **12**:97, 1996.
84. Wolfel T, Hauer M, Schneider J, Serrano M, Wolfel C, Klehmann-Hieb E, De Plaen E, Hankeln T, Meyer zum Buschenfelde KH, Beach D: A *p16INK4a*-insensitive CDK4 mutant targeted by cytolytic T lymphocytes in human melanoma. *Science* **269**:1281, 1995.
85. Mulligan LM, Kwok JBJ, Healey CS, Elsdon MJ, Gardner E, Love DR, Moore JK, Papi L, Ponder MA, Telenius H, Tunnacliffe A, Ponder BAJ: Germ-line mutations of the *RET* proto-oncogene in multiple endocrine neoplasia type 2A. *Nature* **363**:774, 1993.
86. Sherr CJ: G1 phase progression: Cycling on cue. *Cell* **79**:551, 1994.
87. Lukas J, Petersen BO, Holm K, Bartek J, Helin K: Deregulated expression of E2F family members induces S-phase entry and overcomes *p16INK4A*-mediated growth suppression. *Mol Cell Biol* **16**:1047, 1996.
88. He J, Allen JR, Collins VP, Allalunis-Turner MJ, Godbout R, Day RS 3d, James CD: CDK4 amplification is an alternative mechanism to *p16* gene homozygous deletion in glioma cell lines. *Cancer Res* **54**:5804, 1994.
89. Okamoto A, Demetrick DJ, Spillare EA, Hagiwara K, Hussain SP, Bennett WP, Forrester K, Gerwin B, Serrano M, Beach DH, et al: Mutations and altered expression of *P16INK4* in human cancer. *Proc Natl Acad Sci USA* **91**:11045, 1994.
90. Otterson GA, Dkatzke RA, Coxon A, Kin YW, Kaye FJ: Absence of p16INK4 protein is restricted to the subset of lung cancer lines that retains wildtype RB. *Oncogene* **9**:3375, 1994.
91. Aagaard L, Lukas J, Bartkova J, Kjerulff AA, Strauss M, Bartek J: Aberrations of p16Ink4 and retinoblastoma tumor-suppressor genes occur in distinct sub-sets of human cancer cell lines. *Int J Cancer* **61**:115, 1995.
92. DeVita VT, Hellman S, Rosenberg SA: *Cancer: Principles and Practice of Oncology*. Philadelphia, Lippincott, 1989.
93. Kamb A: Cell-cycle regulators and cancer. *Trends Genet* **11**:136, 1995.
94. Maestro R, Boiocchi M: Sunlight and melanoma: An answer from MTS1 (p16). *Science* **267**:15, 1995.
95. Pollock PM, Yu F, Qiu L, Parsons PG, Hayward NK: Evidence for UV induction of *CDKN2* mutations in melanoma cell lines. *Oncogene* **11**:663, 1995.
96. Herman JG, Merlo A, Mao L, Issa JJ-P, Davidson NE, Sidransky D, Baylin SB: Inactivation of the *CDKN2/p16/MTS1* gene is frequently associated with aberrant DNA methylation in all common human cancers. *Cancer Res* **55**:4525, 1995.
97. Merlo A, Herman JG, Mao L, Lee DJ, Gabrielson E, Burger PC, Baylin SB, Sidransky D: 5′ CpG island methylation is associated with transcriptional silencing of the tumour suppressor *p16/CDKN2/MTS1* in human cancers. *Nature Med* **1**:686, 1995.
98. Gonzalez-Zulueta M, Bender CM, Yang AS, Nguyen T, Beart RW, Van Tornout JM, Jones PA: Methylation of the 5′ CpG island of the *p16/CDKN2* tumor suppressor gene in normal and transformed human tissues correlates with gene silencing. *Cancer Res* **55**:4531, 1995.
99. El-Deiry WF, Tokino T, Velculescu VE, Levy DB, Parsons R, Trent JM, Lin D, Mercer WE, Kinzler KW, Vogelstein B: WAF1, a potential mediator of p53 tumor suppression. *Cell* **75**:817, 1993.
100. Gu W, Turck CW, Morgan DO: Inhibition of CDK2 activity *in vivo* by an associated 20K regulatory subunit. *Nature* **366**:707, 1993.
101. Harper JW, Adami GR, Wei N, Keyomarsi K, Elledge KK: The p21 Cdk-interacting protein Cip1 is a potent inhibitor of G1 cyclin-dependent kinases. *Cell* **75**:805, 1993.
102. Xiong Y, Hannon GJ, Zhang H, Casso D, Kobayashi R, Beach D: p21 is a universal inhibitor of cyclin kinases. *Nature* **366**:701, 1993.
103. Polyak K, Lee M-H, Bromage HE, Koff A, Roberts JM, Tempst P, Massague J: Cloning of p27Kip1, a cyclin-dependent kinase inhibitor

and a potential mediator of extracellular antimitogenic signals. *Cell* **78**:59, 1994.
104. Toyoshima H, Hunter T: p27, a novel inhibitor of G1 cyclin-Cdk protein kinase activity, is related to p21. *Cell* **78**:67, 1994.
105. Guan K-L, Jenkins CW, Li Y, Nichols MA, Wu X, O'Keefe CL, Matera AG, Xiong Y: Growth suppression by p18, a p16INK4/MTS1 and p14INK4B/MTS2-related CDK6 inhibitor, correlates with wild-type pRb function. *Genes Dev* **8**:2939, 1994.
106. Lee MH, Reynisdottir I, Massague J: Cloning of p57KIP2, a cyclin-dependent kinase inhibitor with unique domain structure and tissue distribution. *Genes Dev* **9**:639, 1995.
107. Kawamata N, Seriu T, Koeffler HP, Bartram CR: Molecular analysis of the cyclin-dependent kinase inhibitor family: *p16(CDKN2/MTS1/INK4A)*, *p18(INK4C)* and *p27(Kip1)* genes in neuroblastomas. *Cancer* **77**:570, 1996.
108. Orlow I, Iavorone A, Crider-Miller SJ, Bonilla F, Latres E, Lee MH, Gerald WL, Massague J, Weissman BE, Cordon-Cardo C: Cyclin-dependent kinase inhibitor p57/KIP2 in soft tissue sarcomas and Wilms tumors. *Cancer Res* **56**:1219, 1996.
109. Rusin MR, Okamoto A, Chorazy M, Czyzewski K, Harasim J, Spillare EA, Hagiwara K, Hussain SP, Xiong Y, Demetrick DJ, Harris CC: Intragenic mutation of the *p16(INK4)*, *p15(INK4B)* and *p18* genes in primary non-small-cell lung cancers. *Int J Cancer* **65**:734, 1996.
110. Wang J, Walsh K: Resistance to apoptosis conferred by Cdk inhibitors during myocyte differentiation. *Science* **273**:359, 1996.
111. Reznikoff CA, Yeager TR, Belair CD, Savelieva E, Puthenveettil JA, Stadler WM: Elevated p16 at senescence and loss of p16 at immortalization in human papillomavirus 16 E6, but not E7, transformed human uroepithelial cells. *Cancer Res* **56**:2886, 1996.
112. Hara E, Smith R, Parry D, Tahara H, Stone S, Peters G: Regulation of p16/CDKN2 expression and its implications for cell immortalization and senescence. *Mol Cell Biol* **16**:859 1986.
113. Rogan EM, Bryan TM, Hukku B, Maclean K, Chang AC, Moy EL, Englezou A, Warneford SG, Dalla-Pozza L, Reddel RR: Alterations in p53 and p16INK4 expression and telomere length during spontaneous immortalization of Li-Fraumeni syndrome fibroblasts. *Mol Cell Biol* **15**:475, 1986.
114. Bergman W, Watson P, de Jong J, Lunch HT, Fusaro RM: Systemic cancer and the FAMMM syndrome. *Br J Cancer* **61**:932, 1990.
115. Miki Y, Swensen J, Shattuck-Eidens D, et al: A strong candidate for the breast and ovarian cancer susceptibility gene *BRCA1*. *Science* **266**:66, 1994.
116. Tavtigian SV, Simard J, Rommens J: The complete *BRCA2* gene and mutations in chromosome 13Q-linked kindreds. *Nature Genet* **12**:1, 1996.
117. Heyman M, Rasool O, Borgonovo Brandter L, et al: Prognostic importance of *p15INK4B* and *p16INK4* gene inactivation in childhood acute lymphocytic leukemia. *J Clin Oncol* **14**:1512, 1996.
118. Jin X, Nguyen D, Zhang WW, Kyritsis AP, Roth JA: Cell cycle arrest and inhibition of tumor cell proliferation by the *p16INK4* gene mediated by an adenovirus vector. *Cancer Res* **55**:3250, 1995.
119. Fueyo J, Gomez-Manzano C, Yung WK, Clayman GL, Liu TJ, Bruner J, Levin VA, Kyritsis AP: Adenovirus-mediated *p16/CDKN2* gene transfer induces growth arrest and modifies the transformed phenotype of glioma cells. *Oncogene* **12**:103, 1996.
120. Pardee AB, James LJ: Selective killing of transformed baby hamster kidney (BHK) cells. *Cell Biol* **72**:4994, 1975.
121. Hartwell LH, Kastan MB: Cell cycle control and cancer. *Science* **266**:1821, 1994.
122. Kohn KW, Jackman J, O'Connor PM: Cell cycle control and cancer chemotherapy. *J Cell Biochem* **54**:440, 1994.
123. Darzynkiewicz Z: Apoptosis in anticancer strategies: Modulation of cell cycle or differen-tiation. *J Cell Biochem* **58**:151, 1995.
124. Stone S, Dayananth P, Kamb A: Reversible, p16-mediated cell cycle arrest as protection from chemotherapy. *Cancer Res* **56**:3199, 1996.

CHAPTER 45

Cowden Syndrome

Charis Eng ■ Ramon Parsons

1. **Cowden syndrome (CS) is an autosomal dominant disorder characterized by multiple hamartomas and a risk of breast and thyroid cancers.**
2. **The great majority of tumors, including those of the thyroid and breast, are benign. Up to 10 percent of affected individuals develop nonmedullary thyroid carcinoma, and up to 50 percent of affected females develop breast cancer.**
3. **The pathognomonic hamartoma is the trichilemmoma, a benign tumor of the infundibulum of the hair follicle.**
4. **The susceptibility gene for CS is a tumor-suppressor gene as evidenced by loss of heterozygosity in the *PTEN* region of 10q23 in various tumors and by transfection.**
5. **The CS gene *PTEN* was isolated by a combination of genetic mapping analyses, somatic genetics, and a candidate gene approach. *PTEN*, located on 10q23.3, encodes a 403-amino acid protein, which contains a phosphatase signature motif and has sequences homologous to tensin.**
6. **PTEN is a dual-specificity lipid phosphatase. PTEN is the 3-phosphatase for phosphotidylinositol-3,4,5-triphosphate and, hence, coordinately regulates the cell survival factor PKB/Akt via the PI3 kinase signaling pathway.**
7. **Germ line mutations in *PTEN* have been found in CS families as well as in the related but distinct hamartoma disorder Bannayan-Ruvalcaba-Riley syndrome. These mutations result in predicted protein truncation or likely loss of function, hence supporting its predicted function as a tumor suppressor.**
8. **Somatic mutations of *PTEN* occur in a broad spectrum of sporadic tumors, which is almost always biallelic. However, alternate mechanisms of PTEN inactivation do occur.**

INTRODUCTION

Cowden syndrome (CS) [MIM 158350], named after Rachel Cowden, is an autosomal dominant inherited cancer syndrome characterized by multiple hamartomas, which are benign hyperplastic disorganized growths, involving organ systems derived from all three germ cell layers and a risk of breast and thyroid cancers.[1] Females with CS have been reported to have as high as a 67 percent risk of fibrocystic disease of the breasts and a 25 to 50 percent lifetime risk of developing adenocarcinoma of the breast.[2,3] This maximum lifetime risk exceeds that of the general population in the United States (11 percent). Furthermore, affected individuals are said to have a 3 to 10 percent lifetime risk of developing epithelial thyroid carcinoma:[3–5] this, too, exceeds that of the general population (1 percent).

The CS susceptibility gene, *PTEN*, is located on chromosome sub-band 10q23.3.[6,7]

CLINICAL ASPECTS

Incidence

CS has not been well recognized; as of 1993, there were approximately 160 reported cases in the world literature.[8] From an informal population-based study, the estimated gene frequency is one in one million.[6] Because of frequencies such as this, CS is often listed as rare, but exponents of the field suspect that it is much more common than believed. Because of the variable, protean and often subtle external manifestations of CS, many cases remain undiagnosed[9,10] (Eng, unpublished). Indeed, between two centers in the United States dedicated to the study of Cowden syndrome, over 80 cases have been ascertained (Eng & Peacocke, unpublished). These cases are not included in those reported prior to 1993. Further, each of the features of CS could occur in the general population as well, thus confounding recognition of this disease. Despite the apparent rarity of CS, the syndrome is worthy of note from both scientific and clinical viewpoints.

Because CS is likely underdiagnosed, a true count of the fraction of isolated cases (defined as no obvious family history) and familial cases (defined as two or more related affected individuals) cannot be performed. From the literature and the experience of both major U.S. CS centers, the majority of CS cases are isolated. As a broad estimate, perhaps 10 to 50 percent of CS cases are familial.

Diagnostic Criteria

Cowden syndrome usually presents by the late 20s. It has variable expression and, probably, an age-related penetrance, although the exact penetrance is unknown. By the third decade, 99 percent of affected individuals would have developed the mucocutaneous stigmata although any of the features could be present already (see Tables 45-1 and 45-2; Fig. 45-1). Because the clinical literature on CS consists mostly of reports of the most florid and unusual families, or case reports by subspecialists interested in their respective organ systems, the spectrum of component signs is unknown. Despite this, the most commonly reported manifestations are mucocutaneous lesions; thyroid abnormalities; fibrocystic disease and carcinoma of the breast; gastrointestinal hamartomas; multiple, early-onset uterine leiomyoma; macrocephaly (specifically, megalencephaly); and mental retardation (Table 45-1).[3–5,11] Pathognomonic mucocutaneous lesions are trichilemmomas and papillomatous papules (Table 45-2; Fig. 45-1). Because of the lack of uniform diagnostic criteria for CS prior to 1995, a group of individuals, the International Cowden Consortium, interested in systematically studying this syndrome, arrived at a set of consensus operational diagnostic criteria (Table 45-2).

The two most commonly recognized cancers in CS are carcinoma of the breast and thyroid.[3] By contrast, in the general population, lifetime risks for breast and thyroid cancers are approximately 11 percent (in women) and 1 percent, respectively. Breast cancer has yet to be observed in men with CS. In women with CS, lifetime risk estimates for the development of breast cancer range from 25 to 50 percent.[3–5,12] The mean age at diagnosis is likely 10 years earlier than breast cancer occurring in the general population.[3,5] Although Rachel Cowden died of breast cancer at the age of 31[1,2] and the earliest recorded age at diagnosis of breast cancer is 14,[3] the great majority of breast cancers are diagnosed after the age of 30 to 35 (range 14 to 65).[5]

The lifetime risk for thyroid cancer can be as high as 10 percent in males and females with CS. Because of small numbers, it is unclear if the age of onset is truly earlier than that of the general population. Histologically, thyroid cancer is predominantly

Table 45-1 Common Manifestations of Cowden Syndrome

Mucocutaneous lesions (90–100%)
Trichilemmomas
Acral keratoses
Verucoid or papillomatous papules
Thyroid abnormalities (50–67%)
Goiter
Adenoma
Cancer (3–10%)
Breast lesions
Fibroadenomas/Fibrocystic disease (76% of affected females)
Adenocarcinoma (25–50% of affected females)
Gastrointestinal lesions (40%)
Hamartomatous polyps
Macrocephaly (38%)
Gentiourinary abnormalities (44% of females)
Uterine leiomyoma (multiple, early onset)

follicular carcinoma, although papillary histology has also been obseved, albeit rarely[3,4,11] (Eng, unpublished observations). Medullary thyroid carcinoma has yet to be observed in patients with CS.

Benign tumors are also common in CS. Apart from those of the skin, benign tumors or disorders of breast and thyroid are the most frequently noted and likely represent true component features of this syndrome (Table 45-1). Fibroadenomas and fibrocystic disease of the breast are common signs in CS, as are follicular adenomas and multinodular goiter of the thyroid. An unusual central nervous system tumor, cerebellar dysplastic gangliocytoma or Lhermitte-Duclos disease, has only recently been associated with CS.[13,14]

Other malignancies and benign tumors have been reported in patients or families with CS (Tables 45-3 and 45-4). Exponents of this field believe that endometrial carcinoma could be a component tumor of CS as well. Whether each of these tumors is a true component of CS, or whether some are coincidental findings, is as yet unknown.

Differential Diagnosis

With the variable expression of Cowden syndrome, this disorder can be considered a great imitator of many syndromes. A few differential diagnoses to consider include neurofibromatosis type 1 (NF1), basal cell nevus syndrome (Gorlin syndrome), Proteus syndrome, Darier-White disease, and Bannayan-Ruvalcaba-Riley syndrome (BRR). NF-1 is an autosomal-dominant inherited cancer syndrome with many features. The only two consistent features are café-au-lait macules and fibromatous tumors of the skin. The plexiform neuroma is highly suggestive of NF1. The susceptibility gene for this syndrome has been isolated.[15,16] Because of the large size of the gene, direct mutation analysis is still not practical. In informative families, linkage analysis is feasible for predictive testing purposes and is 98 percent accurate.[17] Basal cell nevus

Table 45-2 International Cowden Syndrome Consortium Operational Criteria for the Diagnosis of Cowden Syndrome (Ver. 1996)*

Pathognomonic Criteria
Mucocutanous lesions:
Trichilemmomas, facial
Acral keratoses
Papillomatous papules
Mucosal lesions
Major Criteria
Breast CA
Thyroid CA. esp. follicular thyroid carcinoma
Macrocephaly (Megalencephaly) (say, $<$ 97%ile)
Lhermitte-Duclos disease (LDD)
Minor Criteria
Other thyroid lesions (e.g., adenoma or multinodular goiter)
Mental retardation (say, IQ $\leq$ 75)
GI hamartomas
Fibrocystic disease of the breast
Lipomas
Fibromas
GU tumors (e.g., uterine fibroids) or malformation
Operational Diagnosis in an Individual:
1. Mucocutanous lesions alone if:
a) there are 6 or more facial papules, of which 3 or more must be trichilemmoma, or
b) cutaneous facial papules and oral mucosal papillomatosis, or
c) oral mucosal papillomatosis and acral keratoses, or
d) palmo plantar keratoses, 6 or more
2. 2 major criteria but one must include macrocephaly or LDD
3. 1 major and 3 minor criteria
4. 4 minor criteria
Operational Diagnosis in a Family Where One Individual Is Diagnostic for Cowden
1. The pathognomonic criterion/ia
2. Any one major criterion with or without minor criteria
3. Two minor criteria

*Operational diagnostic criteria are reviewed and revised on a continuous basis as new clinical information becomes available.

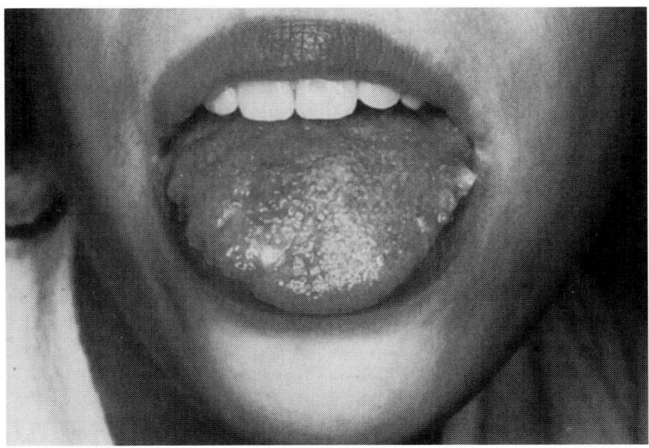

A

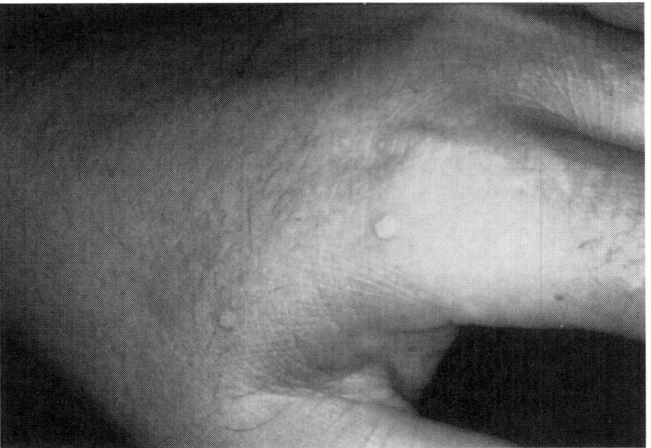

B

Fig. 45-1 Characteristic mucocutaneous features of Cowden syndrome. *A*, Scrotal tongue comprising papillomatous papules. *B*, Papillomatous papules of the skin. (*Reprinted from Eng and Parsons*[101] *with permission from the publisher and authors.*)

Table 45-3 Reported Malignancies in Patients with Cowden Syndrome

Central nervous system
Glioblastoma multiforme
Mucocutaneous
Squamous cell carcinoma
Basal cell carcinoma
Malignant melanoma
Merkel cell carcinoma
Breast
Adenocarcinoma
Endocrine
Nonmedullary thyroid carcinoma
Pulmonary
Non–small cell carcinoma
Gastrointestinal
Colorectal carcinoma
Hepatocellular carcinoma
Pancreatic carcinoma
Genitourinary
Uterine carcinoma
Ovarian carcinoma
Transitional cell carcinoma of the bladder
Renal cell carcinoma
Other
Liposarcoma

syndrome is an autosomal dominant condition characterized by basal cell nevi, basal cell carcinoma, and diverse developmental abnormalities. In addition, affected individuals can develop other tumors and cancers, such as fibromas, hamartomatous gastric polyps, and medulloblastomas. However, the dermatologic findings and developmental features in Cowden syndrome and basal cell nevus syndrome are markedly different. For instance, the palmer pits together with the characteristic facies of the latter are never seen in CS. The susceptibility gene for basal cell nevus syndrome has recently been isolated and is the human homolog of the Drosophila *patched* gene, *PTC* on 9q22-31.[18] Linkage analysis and mutation analysis are (technically) possible. However, because it is not known what proportion of patients with this syndrome will actually have mutations in *PTC*, predictive testing based on mutation analysis alone should be deferred until more data become available. Proteus syndrome could be considered in the differential diagnosis of CS because of the common theme of overgrowth.[19] However, many of the rest of the features of Proteus syndrome, such as the skeletal abnormalities, hemihypertrophy, hypertrophy of the skins of the soles and macrodactyly, are rarely, if ever seen, in CS. BRR is probably a group of autosomal dominant disorders characterized by macrocephaly, hamartomas, and telangiectasias.[20,21] This may sound quite similar to CS but the dermatologic findings in CS are quite distinct. Further genetic delineation for BRR is discussed below. Finally, Darier-White disease is an autosomal dominant disorder characterized by keratotic, often oozing, papules in the "seborrheic areas" of the skin, and sometimes can be confused with CS. Nonetheless, the dermatologic findings of these two syndromes, especially at the microscopic level, are distinct. The susceptibility locus for Darier-White disease has been mapped to 12q23-24.1.[22,23]

Although Peutz-Jeghers syndrome (PJS) might be initially considered in the differential diagnosis, it can be quickly discarded. The pigmentation of the peroral region in this autosomal dominant hamartoma syndrome is pathognomonic.[24,25] Further, the histology of the hamartomas in Peutz-Jeghers patients is unique. They are unlike the hamartomatous polyps seen in CS and in juvenile polyposis. Clinically, while Peutz-Jeghers polyps are often symptomatic (intussusception, rectal bleeding), CS polyps are rarely so. At a molecular genetic level, PJS is distinct

Table 45-4 Noncutaneous Benign Lesions Reported in Cowden Syndrome

Nervous system
Lhermitte-Duclos disease
Megencephaly
Glioma
Meningioma
Neuroma
Neurofibroma
Bridged sella turcica
Mental retardation
Breast
Fibrocystic disease
Fibroadenoma
Hamartoma
Gynecomastia of male breast
Thyroid
Goiter
Adenoma
Thyroiditis
Thyroglossal duct cyst
Hyperthyroidism
Hypothyroidism
Gastrointestinal
Hamartomatous polyposis of entire tract
Diverticuli of colon and sigmoid
Ganglioneuroma
Leiomyoma
Hepatic hamartoma
Genitourinary
Female
Leiomyomas
Ovarian cysts
Vaginal and vulvar cysts
Various developmental anomalies (e.g., duplicated collecting system)
Male
Hydrocele
Varicocele
Hypoplastic testes
Skeletal
Craniomegaly
Adenoid facies
High arched palate
Hypoplastic zygoma
Kyphoscoliosis
Pectus excavatum
Bone cysts
Rudimentary sixth digit
Other
Hypoplastic vulva
Atrial septal defect
Arteriovenous malformations
Eye cataracts
Retinal angioid streaks

from CS.[26–28] There is a small but finite subset of juvenile polyposis cases that are noted to have "congenital anomalies."[29] Syndromologists have wondered whether these should truly be considered under the rubric of juvenile polyposis or whether they are really misclassified CS or BRR cases (see below).

Histology

Like other inherited cancer syndromes, multifocality and bilateral involvement is the rule. Hamartomas are the hallmark of CS. These are classic hamartomas in general, and are benign tumors that comprise all the elements of a particular organ, but in a

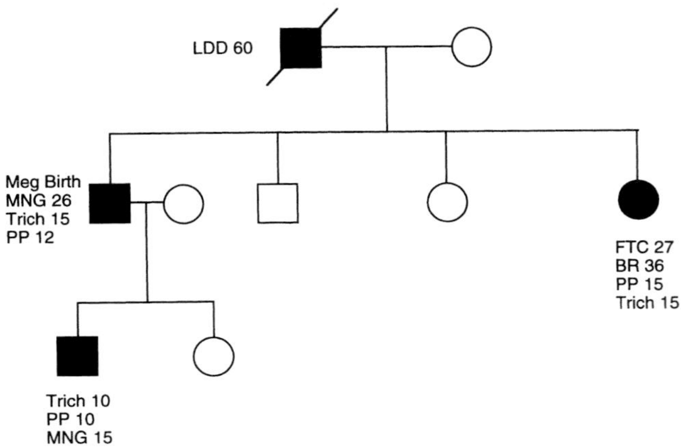

Fig. 45-2 Hypothetical CS family pedigree. *LDD*, Lhermitte-Duclos disease; *Meg* megencephaly; *MNG*, multinodular goiter; *Trich*, trichilemmoma; *PP*, papillomatous papules; *FTC*, follicular thyroid carcinoma; *BR*, breast adenocarcinoma. (*Reprinted from Eng and Parsons*[101] *with permission from the publisher and authors.*)

disorganized fashion. Of note, the hamartomatous polyps found in this syndrome are different in histomorphology from Peutz-Jeghers polyps, which have a distinct appearance. A preliminary report examining the gastrointestinal manifestations of nine patients from six unrelated CS kindreds found that all patients examined had colonic nonadenomatous hamartomatous polyps.[30] Additionally, a majority had acanthosis of the esophagus.[30]

With regard to the individual cancers, even of the breast and thyroid, there has yet to be a systematic study published. Recently, however, one study attempted to look at benign and malignant breast pathology in CS patients. Although these are preliminary studies, without true matched controls, it is, to date, the only study that examines breast pathology in a series of CS cases. Breast histopathology from 59 cases belonging to 19 CS women was systematically analyzed.[10] Thirty-five specimens had some form of malignant pathology. Of these, 31 (90 percent) had ductal adenocarcinoma, 1 had tubular carcinoma, and 1 had lobular carcinoma-in-situ. Sixteen of the 31 had both invasive and in situ (DCIS) components of ductal carcinoma, while 12 had DCIS only, and 2 had only invasive adenocarcinoma. Interestingly, it was noted that 19 of these carcinomas appeared to have arisen in the midst of densely fibrotic hamartomatous tissue.

Benign thyroid pathology is more common in CS than malignant pathology. Multinodular goiter and thyroid adenomas are often noted. Follicular thyroid carcinomas are much more common than papillary histology.[3,11,12] No systematic study of thyroid pathology in CS has been performed.

GENETICS

Inheritance patterns in families with CS implicate an autosomal dominant pattern.[3,14] Figure 45-2 is a pedigree of an hypothetical CS family. Expression is variable and true penetrance is unknown, although it is likely to be high and age-related. It is believed by some that the penetrance is 90 percent by the age of 20.[6] The precise penetrance will be clarified after further study of the susceptibility gene within families and affected individuals.

Cytogenetic and nonsystematic genetic analyses reported prior to 1996 were uninformative with regard to the localization of the CS-susceptibility gene and to the nature of the gene.[14,31–33]

Linkage Analysis Localizes *CS* to 10q22-23

A total autosomal genome scan, using dinucleotide repeat markers at 10 to 20-cM intervals, was performed in 12 classic CS families, comprising 40 affected individuals, in a collaborative study performed by the International Cowden Syndrome Consortium.[6] Regions containing candidate genes such as *BRCA1*, *BRCA2*, *APC*, *hMSH2*, *hMLH1*, *hPMS1/2*, *RB1*, *p53*, *p16/MTS1*, *RET*, and *ATM* were excluded. Markers in the region of chromosome sub-band 10q22-23 revealed significant evidence for linkage to CS, with Zmax of 8.92 ($\theta = 0.02$) for the marker D10S573. Despite the clinical variability and diverse ethnic origin of the studied families, no genetic heterogeneity was observed among the 12 families who originated from the U.S., U.K., France, and the Netherlands. Further genetic analysis revealed a new recombinant placing the consensus critical interval centromeric of D10S541.[7] Taken together with previous recombinant[6] and somatic genetic[34–36] data, this recombinant helped place the putative gene between the markers D10S215 and D10S541, a region of < 1 cM.

PTEN AS COWDEN SYNDROME SUSCEPTIBILITY GENE

A novel candidate tumor-suppressor gene *PTEN* was located precisely in the CS critical interval.

Two groups searching for putative tumor-suppressor genes on chromosome sub-band 10q23, and a third searching for novel products with tyrosine phosphatase homologies, independently isolated a novel gene, *PTEN/MMAC1/TEP1*.[37–39] The gene comprises 9 exons and likely spans a genomic distance of over 120 kb.[37,38] The 1209-bp coding sequence is predicted to encode a 403-amino acid protein. Sequence analysis of the open reading frame demonstrated a protein tyrosine phosphatase domain and homology to tensin and auxilin.[37,38] Hence, this new gene was dubbed *PTEN* for *P*hosphatase and *T*ensin homolog deleted on chromosome *Ten*. Further examination of the regions of homology revealed that the phosphatase domain of PTEN contained the consensus (I/V)-H-C-X-A-G-X-X-R-(S/T) motif found in all tyrosine phosphatases.[40] The PTEN phosphatase domain shares the closest homologies with that of CDC-14, PRL-1 (phosphatase of regenerating liver) and BVP (baculovirus phosphatase).[37] These phosphatases belong to a sub-class of tyrosine phosphatases called dual-specificity phosphatases, which remove phosphate groups from tyrosine, as well as from serine and threonine. *In vitro*, PTEN has been shown to act as a dual specificity phosphatase[41] and as a lipid 3-phosphatase, converting phosphatidyl inositol-3,4,5-triphosphate (PIP3) to phosphatidyl inositol-4,5-diphosphate.[42] Subsequently, in an *in vivo* murine model, PTEN has been proven to be a lipid phosphatase whose substrate is PIP3.[43] PIP3 mediates growth factor-induced activation of intracellular signaling, in particular through the serine-threonine kinase Akt/PKB, a known cell survival-promoting factor.[44,45] Phosphorylation of Akt, in particular at Thr308 and Ser473 residues, has been proposed to be essential for its activation. And, indeed, it has been shown that when PTEN levels are low, P-Akt levels are high, which in theory, should represent an antiapoptotic signal. This coordinate control of PTEN/P-Akt has been shown to be true in a murine knockout model,[43] as well as in human brain and hematologic malignancies[46,47] (see below).

The PTEN homology to the amino terminus of tensin and auxilin is approximately 35 percent over 160 amino acids[37] (Salgia & Eng, unpublished). The phosphatase signature motif lies within this region. In fact, the homologous domains of tensin and auxilin share many amino acid residues with the phosphatase consensus site.[48] Because the signature motifs of tensin and auxilin lack the full complement of residues, it is believed that these two molecules cannot hydrolyze phosphopeptides. However, these proteins may form a pocket capable of binding phosphoprotein substrates. Although the real function of the phosphatase-like domains is unknown, given the current state of knowledge, some believe that these domains can bind phosphopeptides in a manner distinct from PTB and SH2 domains.[48–50]

To determine if *PTEN* is involved in the pathogenesis of sporadic breast, brain, kidney, and prostate cancers, cell lines and a few primary tumors were examined for mutations in this gene. Homozygous deletions, insertions, frameshift, and nonsense *PTEN* mutations were indeed found in 19 of 80 glioblastoma, 4 of 4

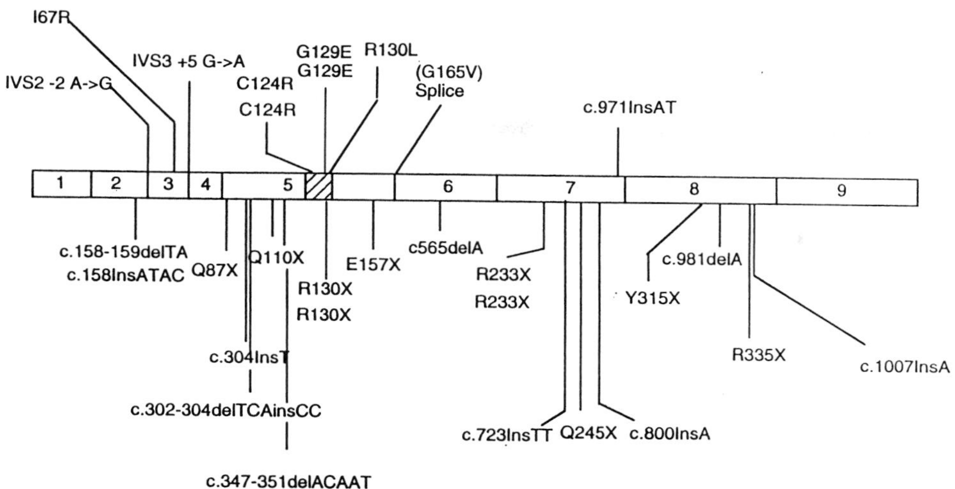

Fig. 45-3 Diagram of *PTEN* showing position and nature of germ line mutations in a single series of CS families. Hatched box within exon 5 represents the phosphatase signature motif. (See text for details.)

prostate cancer, 1 of 4 kidney cancer, and 6 of 74 breast cancer cell lines, xenografts, and primary tumors combined. Somatic mutation of *PTEN* is nearly always accompanied by loss of the wild-type allele. From these data, it would appear that mutations in *PTEN* are etiologic for some sporadic breast, prostate, kidney, and brain cancers. From these genetic analyses, it may be concluded that PTEN seems to behave like a classic tumor suppressor.

To determine if germ line *PTEN* mutations could be etiologic for CS, the groups led by Eng and Parsons chose 5 CS families (utilizing 12 affected and 8 unaffected individuals) for analysis.[7] All five met the International Cowden Consortium operational diagnostic criteria for CS as outlined above (Table 45-2). Four of these families were described before and were linked to 10q22-23.[6] The fifth family was comprised of two brothers who showed 10q22-23 haplotype sharing, but no further family members are available to us. In addition, hamartomas from one of these two brothers and from one member of one of the four 10q-linked families demonstrated LOH in the region between D10S579/S215 and D10S541.[35]

Initial mutation analysis demonstrated that four of these five classic CS families harbored germ line *PTEN* mutations.[7] Three of the five CS families were shown to have germ line heterozygous mutations in this exon (Fig. 45-3). A three-generation CS family was found to have a G to T substitution at codon 157, which resulted in a nonsense mutation within the putative phosphatase domain and immediately after the phosphatase signature motif. Two families shared an identical missense mutation, G129E, which is a nonconservative amino acid alteration occurring in one of the conserved Glycines of the phosphatase signature motif (see above). The identical mutations did not arise on a similar haplotype, arguing against a founder effect in this instance. *PTEN* mutations segregated with CS within each family. No unaffected family member carried these mutations. The fourth family had a truncating mutation in exon 7, R233X. In each family, the family-specific germ line *PTEN* mutation segregated with disease but not in unaffected family members or normal controls. No germ line mutations were detected in the fifth family despite sequencing of all 9 exons using a PCR-based approach.

Given these data, *PTEN* was most likely the susceptibility gene for CS. Further support that *PTEN* is indeed the susceptibility gene came when several other groups confirmed that germ line mutations in *PTEN* are associated with CS.[51–55]

PTEN Mutation Spectrum and Preliminary Genotype-Phenotype Correlations in Cowden Syndrome

In the single largest series of CS cases ascertained under the strict operational diagnostic criteria of the International Cowden Consortium,[12] 37 unrelated families were examined for frequency and spectrum of germ line *PTEN* mutations.[56] Of these 37, 30 (81 percent) had germ line mutations (Fig. 45-3). The 30 mutations were scattered along the length of the gene except for exons 1, 4, and 9. Exons 5, 7, and 8 together contain 77 percent of all mutations; 43 percent of all mutations were found in exon 5, which encodes the phosphatase core motif, although exon 5 only represents 20 percent of the entire coding sequence. Each mutation was unique except for four, C124R, G129E, R130X, and R233X, each of which occurred twice. These were likely not due to founder effects as 10q22-24 haplotypes were not shared. The G129E mutation has been shown to abrogate lipid phosphatase activity.[57]

An exploratory genotype-phenotype association analysis was performed in these 37 CS families. Two potential associations were noted. The first is the association between the presence of detectable germ line mutation in *PTEN* and the presence of malignant breast disease. The second is the association between the presence of missense mutation and/or position of mutation within the phosphatase core motif or 5′ of it and the development of multiorgan disease. Because most missense mutations occur within the core motif, it is unclear whether the nature and/or position of the mutation are significant. One could imagine that while missense mutations could disrupt phosphatase activity, the ability to bind substrate is maintained. In this scenario, substrates are sequestered but not dephosphorylated. Conceivably, this could lead to multiorgan involvement. Obviously, given the relatively small numbers, a second larger independent cohort needs to be accrued for genotype-phenotype analyses. If proven true, these preliminary associations might be helpful in tailoring medical management with regard to surveillance. It is also suspected that with a larger series, other associations might be found as well.

Germ line *PTEN* Mutations in Bannayan-Ruvalcaba-Riley Syndrome: *CS* and *BRR* are Allelic

Bannayan-Ruvalcaba-Riley syndrome (MIM 153450) comprises three related, overlapping autosomal dominant syndromes, Bannayan-Zonana syndrome, Ruvalcaba-Myhre-Smith syndrome, and Riley-Smith syndrome. BRR is characterized by onset at birth, or shortly thereafter, macrocephaly, hamartomas, hemangiomas, lipomatosis, and pigmented macules of the glans penis.[58–60] Some believe that benign thyroid disease may be a part of BRR, but malignancy has never been rigorously demonstrated to be a component of this syndrome.[60]

Germ line mutations in *PTEN* have been found in BRR,[61] thus demonstrating that CS and BRR are allelic. *PTEN* mutations occur in slightly over half of all BRR cases, whether familial or isolated.[56] While the great majority of *PTEN* mutations in CS occur within exon 5, which encodes the phosphatase domain, thus far, none of the BRR mutations occur in that exon, although numbers are small. Interestingly, CS and BRR families share at least one mutation, R233X in exon 7. At least one missense mutation S170P in exon 6, well distal of the phosphatase motif, has been shown to abrogate phosphatase activity.[41]

IMPLICATIONS FOR DIAGNOSIS AND PREDICTIVE TESTING

With the identification of *PTEN* as the susceptibility gene for CS and the original linkage studies indicating no genetic heterogeneity, it is theoretically possible to perform direct mutation analysis of *PTEN* for molecular diagnosis of CS. Direct mutation analysis has advantages over linkage analysis because it can be performed even if only one individual is available. If a germ line *PTEN* mutation was detected in a previously undiagnosed individual, or in an individual with an unclear clinical presentation, then the diagnosis is obvious. If, however, no germ line *PTEN* mutation was found in such an individual, then the result should be considered nondiagnostic. Until the mutation frequency and mutation spectrum of *PTEN* in CS is comprehensively determined, exclusion of a CS diagnosis in a "new" case based on mutation analysis alone should not be done.

If a family specific mutation is already known, then screening for that particular mutation in as yet unaffected family members yields results that are 100 percent accurate, barring administrative error. If a family specific mutation cannot be identified in a family that clearly fits the International Cowden Consortium operational diagnostic criteria for CS, then predictive testing based on direct mutation analysis is not possible. However, in the rare instances where the family is large and many affected members are available, then linkage analysis using makers within and closely flanking *PTEN* (D10S1765, D10S579 or D10S215, D10S2491/S2492, and D10S541) might be considered.

Interestingly, families or individuals with only breast and thyroid cancers, or a CS-like phenotype that does not fulfill the diagnostic criteria of the International Cowden Consortium, have a low frequency of germ line *PTEN* mutation of approximately 2 percent.[62]

Because approximately half of BRR cases have germ line *PTEN* mutations,[56] in theory, it is possible to use this as a molecular diagnostic test. The presence of a germ line *PTEN* mutation in an individual with some or all stigmata of BRR (as above) is diagnostic of the syndrome. The absence of a mutation in this case is nondiagnostic. As with CS, in the presence of a family specific *PTEN* germ line mutation, predictive testing may be offered to as yet unaffected individuals (but see below).

Although initially believed to be a locus for juvenile polyposis syndrome (JPS; MIM 174900),[63] *PTEN* has likely been excluded.[64–67] Further, the first susceptibility gene for JPS has been identified as *SMAD4/DPC4* on 18q21.1.[66,68,69] It seemed plausible, therefore, that other susceptibility genes for the remainder of JPS could be members of the *SMAD* family as well as other members in the broader SMAD/TGFβ pathway.[67,70] However, mutation scanning of *SMAD1*, *SMAD2*, *SMAD3*, and *SMAD5* in 30 unrelated *SMAD4* mutation negative JPS cases did not reveal any germ line mutations in these genes.[71]

GENETIC COUNSELING AND MEDICAL MANAGEMENT

The key to proper genetic counseling in CS is recognition of the syndrome. Families with CS should be counseled as for any autosomal dominant trait with high penetrance. What is unclear, however, is the variability of expression between and within families. We suspect that there are CS families who have nothing but trichilemmomas and, therefore, never come to medical attention.

The two most serious and established component tumors in CS are breast cancer and nonmedullary thyroid cancer. Patients with CS, or those who are at risk for CS, should undergo surveillance for these two cancers. Beginning in their teens, these individuals should undergo annual physical examinations paying particular attention to the thyroid examination. Beginning in their mid-20s, women with CS, or those at risk for it, should be encouraged to perform monthly breast self-examinations and to have careful breast examinations during their annual physicals. The value of annual imaging studies is unclear because there are no objective data available. Nonetheless, we usually recommend annual mammography and/or breast ultrasounds performed by skilled individuals in at-risk women-beginning at age 30 or 5 years earlier than the earliest breast cancer case in the family, whichever is younger. Some women with CS develop severe, sometimes disfiguring, fibroadenomas of the breasts well before age 30. This situation should be treated individually. For example, if the fibroadenomas cause pain, or if they make breast cancer surveillance impossible, then some have advocated prophylactic mastectomy.[2]

Whether other tumors are true components of CS is unknown. It is believed, however, that endometrial carcinomas and, possibly, skin cancers, might be true features of CS as well. For now, surveillance for other organs should follow the American Cancer Society guidelines, although proponents of CS will advise routine skin and uterine surveillance as well.

No formal studies have shown that BRR is associated with an increased risk of malignancy. However, one wonders if those BRR cases with germ line *PTEN* mutations carry a similar risk of malignancy as CS. In the instance where a BRR family has an identical mutation as several CS families, R233X,[35,61] it would be prudent to treat that family as if it were a CS family. Further, until additional data become available, it might be conservative to manage all BRR families with germ line *PTEN* mutations like CS families with respect to cancer formation and surveillance.

The key to successful management of CS and likely BRR patients and their families is a multi-disciplinary team. There should always be a primary care provider, usually a general internist, who orchestrates the care of such patients, some of whom will need the care of surgeons, gynecologists, dermatologists, oncologists, and geneticists at some point.

Somatic *PTEN* Mutations in Sporadic Tumors

It is not uncommon to find somatic mutations in Gene-X in a proportion of sporadic counterpart tumors of an inherited cancer syndrome whose susceptibility gene is Gene-X. Both at the cytogenetic and molecular levels, deletions along chromosome 10 have been observed in sporadic tumors of the thyroid, breast, brain, endometrium, and melanoma, all sporadic counterpart tumors of CS.

Deletions, represented by LOH of anonymous polymorphic markers residing on chromosome 10 have been prominent among both benign and malignant epithelial thyroid tumors.[72] However, prior to 1996, the CS critical region, defined by the markers D10S215 and D10S564 on 10q22-24, had not been examined in thyroid tumors. Subsequently, LOH of markers within this critical interval is demonstrated in nonmedullary thyroid tumors.[34] Surprisingly, however, the frequency of deletion within this interval is higher in the benign tumors when compared to malignant ones of European origin. When *PTEN* was identified as the CS susceptibility gene, direct mutation analysis revealed that *PTEN* is mutated (either intragenic mutation or whole-gene deletion) in 23.3 percent of benign adenomas as compared to 6.1 percent of malignant epithelial carcinomas.[73] However, the only intragenic point mutation was a somatic frameshift mutation in a single papillary thyroid carcinoma. This observation suggests that the pathogenesis of adenomas and carcinomas may proceed along two different pathways, and that the adenoma-carcinoma sequence is not the rule in epithelial thyroid neoplasia. The data are surprising in that epithelial thyroid malignancies does occur in 3 to 10 percent of CS patients[3,12], creating the expectation that a larger proportion of sporadic thyroid carcinomas are associated with somatic *PTEN* alteration. However, one must recall that benign thyroid disease occurs in 50 to 67 percent of CS individuals, far outnumbering the frequency of thyroid carcinoma. In this manner, the situation in sporadic thyroid tumors almost mirrors that in CS.

In contrast to thyroid tumors, at least of European origin, somatic *PTEN* mutations appear to occur in 20 to 44 percent of glioblastoma multiforme, the highest grade glial tumor, but rarely in lower grade tumors of glial differentiation, confirming initial predictions.[38,74–77] The broad range in somatic *PTEN* mutation frequency seems to depend on the sample selection, sample size, mutation detection technology employed, and the extent of mutation and deletion analysis performed. The 20 percent mutation prevalence occurred in a large series of 331 unselected glioneural tumors, 142 of which were glioblastoma multiforme.[76] The 44 percent mutation prevalence occurred in a small series of 25 glioblastomas selected for the presence of LOH of 10q markers after extensive mutation analysis by direct sequence analysis and deletion analysis using microsatellite markers.[75] In at least one study, it appears that somatic *PTEN* mutations occurred in high-grade brain tumors that were diagnosed in older individuals.[74] Although the numbers are small, the presence of somatic *PTEN* mutation was not associated with prognosis.[74] Similarly, in a study with the 142 glioblastomas, presence or absence of somatic *PTEN* alteration did not correlate with overall survival.[76] In this same study, age at diagnosis was similar in patients, regardless of mutation status. Nonetheless, while *PTEN* seems to be shown to play a role in progression to advanced disease, another as yet unidentified gene(s) telomeric to this region, on 10q25-26, might be implicated in initiation of glial tumors of all grades.[77] In contrast to tumors of the glioneural line, only 1 anaplastic meningioma of 75 meningiomas of various grades was found to have somatic *PTEN* mutation,[78] and no deletions were noted. To date, three series report somatic *PTEN* mutation in 34 to 50 percent of apparently sporadic endometrial carcinoma.[79–81] Interestingly, the frequency is much higher (86 percent) in those of endometrioid histology with microsatellite instability.[79] Corroborating this link between endometrioid histology and *PTEN* mutation, a single study has shown that ovarian carcinomas of endometrioid, but not other, histology is associated with a high frequency of deletion (43 percent) and somatic intragenic mutations (21 percent).[82] In the latter instance, all tumors with intragenic *PTEN* mutations also had loss of the other allele. Further, somatic mutations have been observed in 20 percent of endometrial hyperplasias unrelated to coexisting atypia.[83] In two studies examining melanoma cell lines, either homozygous deletions or somatic intragenic mutations were noted in 20 to 26 percent and 8 to 17 percent of cell lines, respectively.[84,85] Among 17 uncultured primary melanomas, one tumor had a homozygous deletion and the other a somatic 17-bp duplication in exon 7 (10 percent mutation frequency), predicted to result in a truncated protein.[85]

While cell line work on breast cancer shows a high frequency of mutation,[37,38] examination of *PTEN* in primary carcinomas has not borne out this high mutation frequency.[36,86–88] In one study of 54 unselected primary breast carcinomas, only 1 true somatic mutation was noted.[86] Even when selected for 10q23 hemizygous deletion, only 1 of 14 samples had a somatic intragenic mutation.[88] However, the 10q region has not previously shown prominent LOH. Yet, deletions in the region of *PTEN* occur in almost half of primary breast carcinomas.[36,87,88] Intragenic point mutation is, however, rare. In one study, hemizygous deletion of *PTEN* and the 10q23 region occurred with any frequency only in invasive carcinomas of the breast, but not in in situ cancers, and appeared to be associated with loss of estrogen receptor.[88] A similar situation seems to exist in prostate cancer. Initial analyses reveal a high frequency of deletion and intragenic mutations.[37,38] One study, which examined 80 prostate carcinomas, found 23 tumors (28.7 percent) with deletion of 10q23 and presumably *PTEN*.[89] Of the 23 tumors with deletions, 10 (43 percent) harbored *PTEN* intragenic mutations as well. Note should be made that the majority of mutations were found in metastatic tumors. Other analyses using unselected primary prostate carcinomas did not show such a high frequency of "second hit" intragenic *PTEN* mutation.[90,91] In the first study, while 49 percent of these tumors harbor somatic hemizygous whole-gene deletion, only one tumor has a somatic *PTEN* missense mutation. In a subsequent study, only 8 homozygous deletions were found among 60 samples of localized prostate carcinoma; no intragenic mutations were noted.[91] These data, of course, may be easily reconciled by invoking the "mutated in multiple advanced cancers" hypothesis. The primary breast and prostate carcinomas are derived from archival material, mainly surgical specimens from early stage disease. It may be argued that the frequency of somatic intragenic mutations increases with increasing stage, similar to that observed in tumors of the glioneural line. Alternatively, instead of being altered at the genomic level, it is altogether possible that total *PTEN* expression is actually decreased or lost, as demonstrated in advanced prostate cancer.[92]

The status of PTEN is interesting in hematologic malignancies. Three reports concur that the minority (4 to 30 percent) of hematologic malignancies carries intragenic *PTEN* mutation or hemizygous deletion.[46,93,94] Such cell lines had a *PTEN* mutation frequency of 22 to 30 percent.[46,93] However, when these cell lines were examined at the protein level, over 70 percent had either no PTEN or markedly reduced PTEN.[46] More interestingly, lack of PTEN protein did not always reflect decreased transcript levels, which in turn did not always reflect structural DNA haplo insufficiency.[46] Therefore, in human malignancies, there are several mechanisms of PTEN inactivation, not only DNA-level mutations. Further, in human hematologic malignancies, Akt does appear to be coordinately controlled by PTEN, although other pathways are almost certainly involved as well.[46]

Mutation Spectrum in Cowden Syndrome vs. Sporadic Primary Glioneural Tumors

When mutations in a cancer-susceptibility gene can occur in the germ line as well as somatically, the spectrum of mutations may either be similar or quite distinct. Although the *PTEN* mutation spectrum in the germ line and in tumors is still preliminary, there appears to be a difference. The spectrum in primary glioneural tumors was chosen as an example of somatic mutation spectra because the most data has accrued on these tumors.[74–76] As noted above, the majority of *CS PTEN* mutations occur in exons 5, 7, and 8, with 43 percent of a single series occurring in exon 5, encoding the phosphatase motif. In contrast, the spectrum in primary glioblastomas is broader, with mutations occurring in all exons, with only 23 percent of all somatic mutations in exon 5 (which represents 20 percent of the coding sequence). As in CS, missense mutations in sporadic glioblastomas seem to occur in the 5′ exons. However, while 20 percent are missense mutations in CS, almost twice that (38 percent) are missense mutations in glioblastomas. It is unclear as yet whether somatic missense mutations and/or somatic mutations in the 5′ exons is correlated with poorer prognosis, as might be extrapolated from the germline work in CS.

PTEN Acts as a Tumor Suppressor

While the genetic evidence which points to PTEN as a tumor suppressor — broad spectrum of mutations scattered throughout the gene, truncating mutations, and location of the gene in a region of LOH — is strong and agrees with the original Knudson two-hit definition,[95] it is genetically based. Functional demonstration that a protein suppresses tumor development is still required. When functional wild-type PTEN was transfected into a series of glioma cell lines that carry *PTEN* mutations, growth suppression was observed.[96,97] Introduction of wild-type PTEN into glioma cell lines without obvious endogenous *PTEN* mutation did not cause growth suppression. This is *in vitro* functional evidence that PTEN does act as a tumor suppressor, at least in glioma cell lines. When PTEN was overexpressed in NIH 3T3 cells, it appeared that cell migration was inhibited while antisense PTEN enhanced migration.[98] Evidence for PTEN interaction with focal adhesions kinases (FAK) was given when integrin-mediated cell spreading and focal adhesion formation were down-regulated by wild-type but not mutant PTEN; PTEN must interact with FAK to reduce its tyrosine phosphorylation.[98] This leads to the hypothesis that PTEN functions as a phosphatase by negatively regulating cell interactions with the extracellular matrix, with implications for cell migration and metastatic potential.

Recently, PTEN has been shown to have 3-phosphatase activity against phosphatidyl inositol-3,4,5-triphosphate[42,43,57] (see above). In a glioma cell-line model, Furnari and colleagues demonstrated that growth suppression was dependent on the lipid phosphatase activity of PTEN.[99] Interestingly, under stressful conditions, such as serum starvation, PTEN-mediated growth suppression was secondary to G1 cell-cycle block and not apoptosis, as would be predicted by PTEN's key relationship in the PI3 kinase/Akt pathway.[99]

Murine Models of *Pten*

Several murine models of *Pten* have been developed.[43,100] In one model, *Pten* was disrupted by homologous recombination such that exons 4 and 5 were removed. In this case, *Pten* inactivation resulted in embryonic lethality: the *Pten* −/− embryonic stem (ES) cells formed primitive, abnormal embryoid bodies, and failed to differentiate into the three embryonal germ layers, thus indicating that Pten is significant in embryonic development,[100] a fact that was predicted from clinical studies of both CS and BRR (see above). *Pten*+/− and ES cell chimera-derived mice resulted in hyperplastic-dysplastic changes in the skin, prostate, and colon. Further, these mice developed germ cell, gonadostromal, thyroid, and colon tumors. Although the manifestations of the skin and colon are reminiscent of, but not similar to, features of CS and BRR, the remainder of the murine phenotype is completely different from human CS and BRR. In CS patients, germ cell, gonadostromal, and colon tumors are not considered part of the spectrum.[3,5] Interestingly, the thyroid tumor in a single chimera was a papillary adenocarcinoma.[100] Although papillary thyroid carcinomas have been described in CS,[12] they are in the rare minority; the vast majority of thyroid malignancies in CS are of follicular histology. Further, in a single series of approximately 40 unrelated CS families, the two otherwise classic CS families with papillary thyroid carcinoma were shown not to have germ line *PTEN* mutations[56] (Eng, unpublished results). In the second murine hemizygous knockout model, *Pten* was generated by targeted disruption of exons 3 to 5. These mice succumbed to thymic lymphomas, which showed LOH of the wild-type allele. In general, lymphomas are not components of CS or BRR. While neither murine model mimics CS, these models are useful in delineating the function of PTEN and the response of PTEN-deficient cells.

ACKNOWLEDGMENTS

We gratefully acknowledge the CS and BRR patients and their families for the continuous inspiration for our work, the members of our laboratories, and our collaborators.

REFERENCES

1. Lloyd KM, Denis M: Cowden's disease: A possible new symptom complex with multiple system involvement. *Ann Intern Med* **58**:136, 1963.
2. Brownstein MH, Wolf M, Bilowski JB: Cowden's disease. *Cancer* **41**:2393, 1978.
3. Starink TM, van der Veen JPW, Arwert F, de Waal LP, de Lange GG, Gille JJP, et al: The Cowden syndrome: A clinical and genetic study in 21 patients. *Clin Genet* **29**:222, 1986.
4. Hanssen AMN, Fryns JP: Cowden syndrome. *J Med Genet* **32**:117, 1995.
5. Longy M, Lacombe D: Cowden disease. Report of a family and review. *Ann Genet* **39**:35, 1996.
6. Nelen MR, Padberg GW, Peeters EAJ, Lin AY, van den Helm B, Frants RR, et al: Localization of the gene for Cowden disease to 10q22-23. *Nat Genet* **13**:114. 1996.
7. Liaw D, Marsh DJ, Li J, Dahia PLM, Wang SI, Zheng Z, et al: Germline mutations of the *PTEN* gene in Cowden disease, an inherited breast and thyroid cancer syndrome. *Nat Genet*; **16**:64, 1997.
8. Lyons CJ, Wilson CR, Horton JC: Association between meningioma and Cowden's disease. *Neurology* **43**:1436, 1993.
9. Haibach H, Burns TW, Carlson HE, Burman KD, Deftos LJ: Multiple hamartoma syndrome (Cowden's disease) associated with renal cell carcinoma and primary neuroendocrine carcinoma of the skin (Merkel cell carcinoma). *Am J Clin Pathol* **97**:705, 1992.
10. Schrager CA, Schneider D, Gruener AC, Tsou HC, Peacocke M: Clinical and pathological features of breast disease in Cowden's syndrome: An underrecognised syndrome with an increased risk of breast cancer. *Hum Pathol* **29**:47, 1997.
11. Mallory SB: Cowden syndrome (multiple hamartoma syndrome). *Dermatol Clin* **13**:27, 1995.
12. Eng C: Cowden syndrome. *J Genet Counsel* **6**:181, 1997.
13. Padberg GW, Schot JDL, Vielvoye GJ, Bots GTAM, de Beer FC: Lhermitte-Duclos disease and Cowden syndrome: A single phakomatosis. *Ann Neurol* **29**:517, 1991.
14. Eng C, Murday V, Seal S, Mohammed S, Hodgson SV, Chaudary MA, et al: Cowden syndrome and Lhermitte-Duclos disease in a family: A single genetic syndrome with pleiotropy? *J Med Genet* **31**:458, 1994.
15. Viskochil D, Buchberg AM, Xu G, Cawthon RM, Stevens J, Wolff RK, et al: Deletions and translocation interrupt a cloned gene at the neurofibromatosis type 1 locus. *Cell* **62**:187, 1990.
16. Wallace MR, Marchuk DA, Anderson LB, Letcher R, Oden HM, Saulino AM, et al: Type 1 neurofibromatosis gene: Identification of a large transcript disrupted in three NF1 patients. *Science* **249**:181, 1990.
17. Ward K, O'Connell P, Carey J, Leppert M, Jolley S, Plaetke R, et al: Diagnosis of neurofibromatosis 1 by using tightly linked, flanking DNA markers. *Am J Hum Genet* **46**:943, 1990.
18. Johnson RL, Rothman AL, Xie J, Goodrich LV, Bare JW, Bonifas JM, et al: Human homolog of *patched*, a candidate gene for the basal cell nevus syndrome. *Science* **272**:1668, 1996.
19. Gorlin RJ: Proteus syndrome. *J Dysmorphol* **2**:8, 1984.
20. Higginbottom MC, Schultz P: The Bannayan syndrome: An autosomal dominant disorder consisting of macrocephaly, lipomas and hemangiomas, and risk for intracranial tumours. *Pediatrics* **69**:632, 1982.
21. Halal F, Silver K: Slowly progressive macrocephaly with hamartomas: A new syndrome? *Am J Med Genet* **33**:182, 1989.
22. Bashir R, Munro CS, Mason S, Stephenson A, Rees JL, Strachan T: Localisation of a gene for Darier's disease. *Hum Mol Genet* **2**:1937, 1993.
23. Craddock N, Dawson E, Burge S, Parfitt L, Mant B, Roberts Q, et al: The gene for Darier's disease maps to chromosome 12q23-24.1. *Hum Mol Genet* **2**:1941, 1993.
24. Eng C, Blackstone MO. Peutz-Jeghers syndrome. *Med Rounds* **1**:165, 1988.
25. Rustgi AK. Medical progress — Hereditary gastrointestinal polyposis and nonpolyposis syndromes. *N Engl J Med* **331**:1694, 1994.
26. Hemminki A, Tomlinson I, Markie D, Järvinen H, Sistonen P, Bjrkqvist A-M, et al: Localisation of a susceptibility locus for Peutz-Jeghers syndrome to 19p using comparative genomic hybridization and targeted linkage analysis. *Nat Genet* **15**:87, 1997.
27. Hemminki A, Markie D, Tomlinson I, Avizienyte E, Roth S, Loukola A, et al: A serine/threonine kinase gene defective in Peutz-Jeghers syndrome. *Nature* **391**:184, 1998.
28. Jenne DE, Reimann H, Nezu J-I, Friedel W, Loff S, Jeschke R, et al: Peutz-Jeghers syndrome is caused by mutations in a novel serine threonine kinase. *Nat Genet* **18**:38, 1998.
29. Coburn MC, Pricolo VE, DeLuca FG, Bland KI: Malignant potential in intestinal juvenile polyposis syndromes. *Ann Surg Oncol* **2**:386, 1995.
30. Weber HC, Marsh D, Lubensky I, Lin A, Eng C: Germline *PTEN/MMAC1/TEP1* mutations and association with gastrointestinal manifestations in Cowden disease. *Gastroenterology* **114S**:G2902, 1998.
31. Carlson HE, Burns TW, Davenport SL, Luger AM, Spence MA, Sparkes RS, et al: Cowden disease: Gene marker studies and measurements of epidermal growth factor. *Am J Hum Genet* **38**:908, 1986.
32. Starink TM, van der Veen JP, Goldschmeding R: Decreased natural killer cell activity in Cowden's syndrome [letter]. *J Am Acad Dermatol* **15**:294, 1986.
33. Willard W, Borgen P, Bol R, Tiwari R, Osbourne M: Cowden's disease. A case report with analysis at the molecular level. *Cancer* **69**:2969, 1992.

34. Marsh DJ, Zheng Z, Zedenius J, Kremer H, Padberg GW, Larsson C, et al: Differential loss of heterozygosity in the region of the Cowden locus within 10q22-23 in follicular thyroid adenomas and carcinomas. *Cancer Res* **57**:500, 1997.
35. Marsh DJ, Dahia PLM, Coulon V, Zheng Z, Dorion-Bonnet F, Call KM, et al: Allelic imbalance, including deletion of *PTEN/MMAC1*, at the Cowden disease locus on 10q22-23, in hamartomas from patients with Cowden syndrome and germline *PTEN* mutation. *Genes Chromosomes Cancer* **21**:61, 1998.
36. Feilotter HE, Coulon V, McVeigh JL, Boag AH, Dorion-Bonnet F, Duboué B, et al: Analysis of the 10q23 chromosomal region and the *PTEN* gene in human sporadic breast carcinoma. *Br J Cancer* **79**:718, 1999.
37. Li J, Yen C, Liaw D, Podsypanina K, Bose S, Wang S, et al: *PTEN*, a putative protein tyrosine phosphatase gene mutated in human brain, breast and prostate cancer. *Science* **275**:1943, 1997.
38. Steck PA, Pershouse MA, Jasser SA, Yung WKA, Lin H, Ligon AH, et al: Identification of a candidate tumour suppressor gene, *MMAC1*, at chromosome 10q23.3 that is mutated in multiple advanced cancers. *Nat Genet* **15**:356, 1997.
39. Li D-M, Sun H: TEP1, encoded by a candidate tumor suppressor locus, is a novel protein tyrosine phosphatase regulated by transforming growth factor B. *Cancer Res* **57**:2124, 1997.
40. Tonks NK, Neel BG: From form to function: signaling by protein tyrosine phosphatases. *Cell* **87**:365, 1996.
41. Myers MP, Stolarov J, Eng C, Li J, Wang SI, Wigler MH, et al: PTEN, the tumor suppressor from human chromosome 10q23, is a dual specificity phosphatase. *Proc Natl Acad Sci USA* **94**:9052, 1997.
42. Maehama T, Dixon JE: The tumor suppressor, PTEN/MMAC1, dephosphorylates the lipid second messenger phosphoinositol 3,4,5-triphosphate. *J Biol Chem* **273**:13375, 1998.
43. Stambolic V, Suzuki A, de la Pompa JL, Brothers GM, Mirtsos C, Sasaki T, et al: Negative regulation of PKB/Akt-dependent cell survival by the tumor suppressor PTEN. *Cell* **95**:1, 1998.
44. Burgering BM, Coffer PJ: Protein kinase B (c-Akt) in phosphotidylinositol-3-OH kinase signal transduction. *Nature* **376**:599, 1995.
45. Kulik G, Klippel A, Weber MJ: Anti-apoptotic signalling by the insulin-like growth factor I receptor, phosphatidylinositol 3-kinase and Akt. *Mol Cell Biol* **17**:1595, 1997.
46. Dahia PLM, Aguiar RCT, Alberta J, Kum J, Caron S, Sills H, et al: PTEN is inversely correlated with the cell survival factor PKB/Akt and is inactivated by diverse mechanisms in haematologic malignancies. *Hum Mol Genet* **8**:185, 1999.
47. Haas-Kogan D, Shalev N, Wong M, Mills G, Yount G, Stokoe D: Protein kinase B (PKB/Akt) activity is elevated in glioblastoma cells due to mutation of the tumor suppressor *PTEN/MMAC1*. *Curr Biol* **8**:1195, 1998.
48. Haynie DT, Ponting CP: The N-terminal domains of tensin and auxilin are phosphatase homologues. *Protein Sci* **5**:2643, 1996.
49. Jungbluth A, Eckerskorn C, Gerisch G, Lottspeich F, Stocker S, Schweiger A: Stress-induced tyrosine phosphorylation of actin in *Dictyostelium* cells and localization of the phosphorylation site to tyrosine-53 adjacent to the *DNase*I binding loop. *FEBS Lett* **375**:87, 1995.
50. Lo SH, Janmey PA, Hartwig JH, Chen LB: Interactions of tensin with actin and identification of its three distinct actin-binding domains. *J Cell Biol* **125**:1067, 1994.
51. Tsou HC, Teng D, Ping XL, Broncolini V, Davis T, Hu R, et al: Role of *MMAC1* mutations in early onset breast cancer: causative in association with Cowden's syndrome and excluded in *BRCA1*-negative cases. *Am J Hum Genet* **61**:1036, 1997.
52. Nelen MR, van Staveren CG, Peeters EAJ, Ben Hassel M, Gorlin RJ, Hamm H, et al: Germline mutations in the *PTEN/MMAC1* gene in patients with Cowden disease. *Hum Mol Genet* **6**:1383, 1997.
53. Lynch ED, Ostermeyer EA, Lee MK, Arena JF, Ji H, Dann J, et al: Inherited mutations in *PTEN* that are associated with breast cancer, Cowden syndrome and juvenile polyposis. *Am J Hum Genet* **61**:1254, 1997.
54. Tsou HC, Ping XL, Xie XX, Gruener AC, Zhang H, Nini R, et al: The genetic basis of Cowden's syndrome: Three novel mutations in PTEN/MMAC1/TEP1. *Hum Genet* **102**:467, 1998.
55. Kohno T, Takahashi M, Fukutomi T, Ushio K, Yokota J: Germline mutations of the *PTEN/MMAC1* gene in Japanese patients with Cowden disease. *Jpn J Cancer Res* **89**:471, 1998.
56. Marsh DJ, Coulon V, Lunetta KL, Rocca-Serra P, Dahia PLM, Zheng Z, et al: Mutation spectrum and genotype-phenotype analyses in Cowden disease and Bannayan-Zonana syndrome, two hamartoma syndromes with germline *PTEN* mutation. *Hum Mol Genet* **7**:507, 1998.
57. Myers MP, Pass I, Batty IH, van der Kaay J, Storalov JP, Hemmings BA, et al: The lipid phosphatase activity of PTEN is critical for its tumor suppressor function. *Proc Natl Acad Sci USA* **95**:13513, 1998.
58. Bannayan GA: Lipomatosis, angiomatosis, and macrencephalia: A previously undescribed congenital syndrome. *Arch Pathol* **92**:1, 1971.
59. Zonana J, Rimoin DL, Davis DC: Macrocephaly with multiple lipomas and hemangiomas. *J Pediatr* **89**:600, 1976.
60. Gorlin RJ, Cohen MM, Condon LM, Burke BA: Bannayan-Riley-Ruvalcaba syndrome. *Am J Med Genet* **44**:307, 1992.
61. Marsh DJ, Dahia PLM, Zheng Z, Liaw D, Parsons R, Gorlin RJ, et al: Germline mutations in *PTEN* are present in Bannayan-Zonana syndrome. *Nat Genet* **16**:333, 1997.
62. Marsh DJ, Caron S, Dahia PLM, Kum JB, Frayling IM, Tomlinson IPM, et al: Germline *PTEN* mutations in Cowden syndrome-like families. *J Med Genet* **35**:881, 1998.
63. Olschwang S, Serova-Sinilnikova OM, Lenoir GM, Thomas G: *PTEN* germline mutations in juvenile polyposis coli. *Nat Genet* **18**:12, 1998.
64. Marsh DJ, Roth S, Lunetta K, Hemminki A, Dahia PLM, Sistonen P, et al: Exclusion of *PTEN* and 10q22-24 as the susceptibility locus for juvenile polyposis syndrome (JPS). *Cancer Res* **57**:5017, 1997.
65. Riggins GJ, Hamilton SR, Kinzler KW, Vogelstein B: Normal *PTEN* gene in juvenile polyposis. *J Neg Obs Genet Oncol* **1**:1, 1998. http://128.220.85.41:5002/MCGI/SEND1^WEBUTLTY(1378,1)/1674326758.
66. Howe JR, Ringold JC, Summers RW, Mitros FA, Nishimura DY, Stone EM: A gene for familial juvenile polyposis maps to chromosome 18q21.1. *Am J Hum Genet* **62**:1129, 1998.
67. Eng C, Peacocke M: *PTEN* and inherited hamartoma-cancer syndromes. *Nat Genet* **19**:223, 1998.
68. Howe JR, Roth S, Ringold JC, Summers RW, Jarvinen HJ, Sistonen P, et al: Mutations in the *SMAD4/DPC4* gene in juvenile polyposis. *Science* **280**:1086, 1998.
69. Houlston R, Bevan S, Williams A, Young J, Dunlop M, Rozen P, et al: Mutations in *DPC4* (*SMAD4*) cause juvenile polyposis syndrome, but only account for a minority of cases. *Hum Mol Genet* **7**:1907, 1998.
70. Eng C, Ji H: Molecular classification of the inherited hamartoma polyposis syndromes: Clearing the muddied waters. *Am J Hum Genet* **62**:1020, 1998.
71. Bevan S, Woodford-Richens K, Rozen P, Eng C, Young J, Dunlop M, et al: Screening SMAD1, SMAD2, SMAD3 and SMAD5 for germline mutations in juvenile polyposis syndrome. *Gut* **45**:406, 1999.
72. Zedenius J, Wallin G, Svensson A, Grimelius L, Hoog A, Lundell G, et al: Allelotyping of follicular thyroid tumors. *Hum Genet* **96**:27, 1995.
73. Dahia PLM, Marsh DJ, Zheng Z, Zedenius J, Komminoth P, Frisk T, et al: Somatic deletions and mutations in the Cowden disease gene, *PTEN*, in sporadic thyroid tumors. *Cancer Res* **57**:4710, 1997.
74. Rasheed BKA, Stenzel TT, McLendon RE, Parsons R, Friedman AH, Friedman HS, et al: *PTEN* gene mutations are seen in high-grade but not in low-grade gliomas. *Cancer Res* **37**:4187, 1997.
75. Wang SI, Puc J, Li J, Bruce JN, Cairns P, Sidransky D, et al: Somatic mutations of *PTEN* in glioblastoma multiforme. *Cancer Res* **57**:4183, 1997.
76. Dürr E-M, Rollbrocker B, Hayashi Y, Peters N, Meyer-Puttlitz B, Louis DN, et al: *PTEN* mutations in gliomas and glioneuronal tumours. *Oncogene* **16**:2259, 1998.
77. Maier D, Zhang ZW, Taylor E, Hamou MF, Gratzl O, van Meir EG, et al: Somatic deletion mapping on chromosome 10 and sequence analysis of *PTEN/MMAC1* point to the 10q25-26 region as the primary target in low-grade and high-grade gliomas. *Oncogene* **16**:3331, 1998.
78. Peters N, Wellenreuther R, Rollbrocker B, Hayashi Y, Meyer-Puttlitz B, Dürr E-M, et al: Analysis of the *PTEN* gene in human meningiomas. *Neuropathol Appl Neurobiol* **24**:3, 1998.
79. Tashiro H, Blazes MS, Wu R, Cho KR, Bose S, Wang SI, et al: Mutations in *PTEN* are frequent in endometrial carcinoma but rare in other common gynecological malignancies. *Cancer Res* **57**:3935, 1997.
80. Kong D, Suzuki A, Zou T-T, Sakurada A, Kemp LW, Wakatsuki S, et al: *PTEN1* is frequently mutated in primary endometrial carcinomas. *Nat Genet* **17**:143, 1997.
81. Risinger JI, Hayes AK, Berchuck A, Barrett JC: *PTEN/MMAC1* mutations in endometrial cancers. *Cancer Res* **57**:4736, 1997.
82. Obata K, Morland SJ, Watson RH, Hitchcock A, Chnevix-Trench G, Thomas EJ, et al: Frequent PTEN/MMAC mutations in endometrioid but not serous or mucinous epithelial ovarian tumors. *Cancer Res* **58**:2095, 1998.

83. Maxwell GL, Risinger JL, Gumbs C, Shaw H, Bentley RC, Barrett JC, et al: Mutation of the *PTEN* tumor suppressor gene in endometrial hyperplasias. *Cancer Res* **58**:2500, 1998.
84. Guldberg P, Thor Straten P, Birck A, Ahrenkiel V, Kirkin AF, Boyd J: Mutation analysis of the putative tumor suppressor gene *PTEN/MMAC1* in primary breast carcinomas. *Cancer Res* **57**:3657, 1997.
85. Tsao HS, Zhang X, Benoit E, Haluska FG: Identification of *PTEN/MMAC1* alterations in uncultured melanomas and melanoma cell lines. *Oncogene* **16**:3397, 1998.
86. Rhei E, Kang L, Bogomoliniy F, Federici MG, Borgen PI, Boyd J: Mutation analysis of the putative tumor suppressor gene *PTEN/MMAC1* in primary breast carcinomas. *Cancer Res* **57**:3657, 1997.
87. Singh B, Ittman MM, Krolewski JJ: Sporadic breast cancers exhibit loss of heterozygosity on chromosome segment 10q23 close to the Cowden disease locus. *Genes Chromosomes Cancer* **21**:166, 1998.
88. Bose S, Wang SI, Terry MB, Hibshoosh H, Parsons R. Allelic loss of chromosome 10q23 is associated with tumor progression in breast carcinomas. *Oncogene* **17**:123, 1998.
89. Cairns P, Okami K, Halachmi S, Halachmi N, Esteller M, Herman JG, et al: Frequent inactivation of *PTEN/MMAC1* in primary prostate cancer. *Cancer Res* **57**:4997, 1997.
90. Feilotter HE, Nagai MA, Boag AH, Eng C, Mulligan LM: Analysis of PTEN and the 10q23 region in primary prostate carcinomas. *Oncogene* **16**:1743, 1998.
91. Wang SI, Parsons R, Ittman M: Homozygous deletion of the PTEN tumor suppressor gene in a subset of prostate adenocarcinomas. *Clin Cancer Res* **4**:811, 1998.
92. Whang YE, Wu X, Suzuki H, Reiter RE, Tran C, Vessella RL, et al: Inactivation of the tumor suppressor PTEN/MMAC1 in advanced human prostate cancer through loss of expression. *Proc Natl Acad Sci USA* **95**:5246, 1998
93. Sakai A, Thieblemont C, Wellmann A, Jaffe ES, Raffeld M: *PTEN* gene alterations in lymphoid neoplasms. *Blood* **92**:3410, 1998.
94. Gronbaek K, Zeuthen J, Guldberg P, Ralfkiaer E, Houjensen K: Alterations of the *MMAC1/PTEN* gene in lymphoid malignancies. *Blood* **91**:4388, 1998.
95. Knudson AG: Mutation and cancer: Statistical study of retinoblastoma. *Proc Natl Acad Sci USA* **68**:820, 1971.
96. Furnari FB, Lin H, Huang H-JS, Cavanee WK: Growth suppression of glioma cells by PTEN requires a functional catalytic domain. *Proc Natl Acad Sci USA* **94**:12479, 1997.
97. Cheney IW, Johnson DE, Vaillancourt M-T, Avanzini J, Morimoto A, Demers GW, et al: Suppression of tumorigenicity of glioblastoma cells by adenovirus-mediated *MMAC1/PTEN* gene transfer. *Cancer Res* **58**:2331, 1998.
98. Tamura M, Gu J, Matsumoto K, Aota S-I, Parsons R, Yamada KM: Inhibition of cell migration, spreading and focal adhesions by tumor suppressor PTEN. *Science* **280**:1614, 1998.
99. Furnari FB, SuHuang H-J, Cavanee WK: The phosphoinositol phosphatase activity of *PTEN* mediates a serum-sensitive G1 growth arrest in glioma cells. *Cancer Res* **58**:5002, 1998.
100. Di Cristofano A, Pesce B, Cordon-Cardo C, Pandolfi PP: *Pten* is essential for embryonic development and tumour suppression. *Nat Genet* **19**:348, 1998.
101. Eng C, Parsons R. Cowden syndrome, in Vogelstein B, Kinzler KW (eds): *The Genetic Basis of Human Cancer*. New York, McGraw-Hill, 1998, p. 519.

CHAPTER 46

Skin Cancer (Including Nevoid Basal Cell Carcinoma Syndrome)

Jonathan L. Rees

1. **Nonmelanoma skin cancer is the most common malignancy in many Caucasian populations. Approximately 80 percent of the tumors are basal cell carcinomas (BCCs), the majority of the remaining 20 percent being squamous cell carcinomas (SCCs). Putative precursor lesions, such as actinic keratoses, are even more common. Basal cell carcinomas and squamous cell carcinomas are readily diagnosed on the basis of clinical and histopathologic appearance. Basal cell carcinomas rarely metastasize, and although squamous cell carcinomas have a low rate of metastasis, overall case fatality is low. Surgical therapy or radiotherapy is highly effective.**
2. **The main environmental cause is ultraviolet radiation, and the major genetic influence is through the major physiologic adaptation to ultraviolet radiation, namely, pigmentation. Studies of coat color in the mouse suggest that over 100 loci are involved in determining pigmentation, and to date, the loci important in accounting for differences in pigmentary characteristics between different human populations are largely unknown. Recently, mutations in the melanocortin 1 receptor (MC1R), a receptor for melanocyte-stimulating hormone, have been shown to be strongly associated with red hair and fair skin.**
3. **Familial disorders characterized by a simple Mendelian inheritance pattern probably account for fewer than 1 percent of all cases of skin cancer. The most common disorder is the nevoid basal cell carcinoma syndrome (NBCCS, Gorlin syndrome), an autosomal dominant disorder with an estimated minimum prevalence of 1 in 56,000 in a U.K. population. Nevoid basal cell carcinoma syndrome is characterized by multiple BCCS, a high incidence of other neoplasms including medulloblastomas, ocular abnormalities, and a variety of developmental abnormalities including odontogenic keratocysts. The gene for nevoid basal cell carcinoma syndrome was mapped by several groups to 9q22-31 and has been identified as the human homologue (*PTC*) of the *Drosophila* gene *patched* (*ptc*). Mutations of *PTC* have been found in NBCCS probands and in sporadic BCC as well as in a range of central nervous system (CNS) tumors including medulloblastomas, which are a feature of the NBCCS syndrome. Loss of heterozygosity data is compatible with its role as a tumor suppressor, and some developmental anomalies, such as the odontogenic keratocysts, also may fit the two-hit model. The other developmental anomalies suggest a dosage effect. The pattern of expression in the mouse is compatible with its putative role in developmental abnormalities in the human. *PTC* acts in the Hedgehog signaling pathway so as to inhibit the action of *smoothened* (*SMO*); mutations of *patched* therefore may exert similar effects to activating mutations of *smoothened,* a model supported by the recent identification of activating mutations of *SMO* in sporadic BCCs.**
4. **There is no inherited syndrome principally characterized by an elevated risk of squamous cell carcinoma (increased rates of SCC and BCC are seen in xeroderma pigmentosum). The Ferguson Smith syndrome (self-healing epitheliomata of Ferguson Smith) is characterized by lesions that clinically and pathologically resemble squamous cell carcinomas but are distinct because they involute spontaneously. On a worldwide basis, the syndrome is extremely rare. The Ferguson Smith syndrome maps to the same locus as the nevoid basal cell carcinoma syndrome. It is not known at present whether the two conditions are allelic or caused by separate genes.**
5. ***p53* mutations are common in both BCC and SCC. Nonmelanoma skin cancers, however, are not a feature of the Li-Fraumeni syndrome. The mutational spectrum in nonmelanoma skin cancer with frequent C → T and CC → TT transitions strongly supports ultraviolet radiation as the relevant mutagen.**
6. **Although BCCs and SCCs show frequent *p53* mutations and *ras* mutations have been described in both tumor types, loss of heterozygosity studies show clear differences between the two tumor types. In BCCs, which usually are diploid, allelic loss is uncommon and is almost entirely confined to the Gorlin locus on 9q. By contrast, in SCC, the fractional allelic loss is 25 to 30 percent, with loss of heterozygosity being common on chromosomes 3, 9, 13, and 17. Loss of heterozygosity studies clearly distinguish SCC from BCC, keratoacanthoma (a regressing form of nonmelanoma skin cancer), and other rarer tumor types, including appendageal tumors.**

Based on their underlying biology and clinical behavior, skin cancers are usefully classified according to their cell of origin: melanoma from melanocytes or melanocyte precursors (melanoma skin cancer) and nonmelanoma skin cancer (NMSC), the majority of which are derived from the major cell type of the epidermis, the keratinocyte. There are two common types of NMSC, basal cell

A list of standard abbreviations is located immediately preceding the index in each volume. Nonstandard abbreviations used in this chapter include: NMSC = nonmelanoma skin cancer; BCC = basal cell carcinoma; SCC = squamous cell carcinoma; NBCCS = nevoid basal cell carcinoma syndrome; LOH = loss of heterozygosity; KA = keratoacanthoma.

carcinoma (BCC) and (cutaneous) squamous cell carcinoma (SCC). A small number of tumors arise from other cell types of the epidermis or dermis including Merkel cells and endothelial cells, and although they are technically nonmelanoma skin cancers, they have little in common with the keratinocyte-derived tumors and will not be discussed further. Melanoma skin cancer is discussed in Chap. 44. Xeroderma pigmentosum is associated with dramatically increased rates of both NMSC and melanoma skin cancer and is dealt with in Chap. 28.

Because NMSC has a low case-fatality rate and often is treated outside the hospital setting, and because some lesions may be treated without histologic confirmation, incidence data for NMSC are notoriously unreliable.[1] Nevertheless, for predominantly Caucasian populations in many parts of the world, NMSC is the most common human malignancy.[2–5] It is estimated that in the United States over three-quarters of a million individuals present with NMSC every year, accounting for over one-third of all incident cancers. Approximately 80 percent of NMSCs are BCCs, with most of the remaining 20 percent being SCCs. In areas with high ambient ultraviolet radiation and a predominantly Caucasian population, such as Australia, over half the population over the age of 40 have NMSCs or cognate lesions.[1,6–8] The relative neglect of serious study of NMSC probably reflects a number of facts, most notably the relative ease and success of surgical or other destructive therapy.[9–12] Although in part this may be attributed to the ease of their detection, their visibility, is not a complete explanation because melanomas are equally, if not more, visible and yet show a significant mortality. Recent work has shown that even when keratinocytes have accumulated multiple genetic abnormalities and when by conventional histopathologic criteria they show considerable dedifferentiation, their clinical behavior is relatively benign in comparison with other epithelial malignancies.[13,14] Given the frequency of NMSC and that ultraviolet radiation, the main cause of NMSC, is the most ubiquitous human carcinogen, it is tempting to speculate that evolutionary constraints on keratinocytes make them relatively resistant to the adoption of an aggressive malignant phenotype.

ETIOLOGY

The population contribution of single-gene disorders to NMSC is dwarfed by the influence of ultraviolet radiation. Clinically characterized single-gene disorders such as the nevoid basal cell carcinoma syndrome (Gorlin syndrome) and the Ferguson Smith syndrome (self-healing epitheliomata of Ferguson Smith) and other rarer syndromes account for fewer than 1 percent of incident cases of NMSC. Even in these disorders, expressivity is influenced by the biology of the response to ambient ultraviolet radiation. In black skin BCC may be entirely absent in the nevoid BCC syndrome (highlighting the inadequacy of the syndrome name), whereas in countries with high ambient ultraviolet radiation such as Australia, the age of presentation is markedly younger than in countries in more temperate latitudes.[15–18] Despite the small contribution from these characterized Mendelian syndromes, the genetic contribution to NMSC is considerable, as can be appreciated by considering the relation between pigmentary status, cancer risk, and ultraviolet exposure.[19,20]

Proof of the importance of ultraviolet radiation in the causation of NMSC comes from several sources.[1,19–21] First, both SCC and BCC are most common on sun-exposed body sites (although there are differences in body-site distribution between the two tumors, suggesting that other factors may be important or that the quantitative relation with ultraviolet radiation differs between BCC and SCC). Second, the results of forced or voluntary population migrations, most notably of individuals of Anglo-Saxon origin to Australia, support a role for sun exposure.[1,20] Within genetically homogeneous populations, tumor rates are inversely proportional to distance from the equator, with rates, for instance, being higher in Brisbane than in Melbourne. Third, the mutational spectra of target genes such as *p53* directly implicate a role for ultraviolet radiation mutagenesis in NMSC.[22,23] Fourth, NMSC rates are orders of magnitude different between human populations with different pigmentary characteristics.[24–26] Finally, some, but possibly not all, forms of iatrogenically administered ultraviolet radiation cause NMSC.[27,28] It is salutary to remember that the color of one's skin and the ability to tan in response to ultraviolet radiation are largely the result of an evolutionary tradeoff between the need to protect against solar damage in areas of high ambient ultraviolet radiation and the need to ensure that adequate ultraviolet B radiation reaches the spinous and basal layers of skin to ensure adequate vitamin D synthesis to avoid metabolic bone disease.[20,29–31] The genetic basis of these pigmentary differences is likely to be complex. In the mouse, over a hundred loci are known to be important in determining coat color, although recent candidate approaches based on the melanocortin 1 receptor (MC1R) may explain the predisposition of those with red hair and/or pale skin to NMSC.[32–35] Although ultraviolet radiation is the major cause of NMSC, other etiologic factors with smaller attributable risks include ionizing radiation, chemical carcinogens, and some forms of iatrogenic immunosuppression.[10,11,36]

BASAL CELL CARCINOMA

Basal cell carcinomas are characteristically indolent, small, pearly edged lesions with accompanying telangiectasia and an ulcerated center occurring most commonly on the face or less commonly on the upper trunk or elsewhere.[11,12,37–39] They are the most common tumor in the United States, with over 750,000 incident cases per year.[40] Histologically, the tumors show downgrowths of keratinocytes from the epidermis lined by palisades of cells resembling basal cells. There are a number of clinicopathologic variants with differences in clinical behavior, although the molecular basis for these differences is unknown, and different tumor subtypes may be seen in the same individual. Differentiation with features of eccrine or hair epithelia may occur. Although BCCs are invasive and can track down nerves or invade underlying tissues such as bone, metastasis is extremely uncommon (<1 in 4000) and calls into question the diagnosis.[11,12,41] Destruction of the tumor using a variety of modalities including surgical excision, curetting, and cautery, cryotherapy, or radiotherapy is usually curative. BCCs are a central feature of the nevoid basal cell carcinoma syndrome and the Bazex-Dupre-Christol syndrome.

Nevoid Basal Cell Carcinoma Syndrome (Gorlin Syndrome) (OMIM 109400)

Nevoid basal cell carcinoma syndrome (NBCCS) is inherited as an autosomal dominant fashion with a high rate (40 percent) of new mutations and an estimated minimum incidence in a U.K. population of 1 in 56,000.[42] Fewer than 0.5 percent of patients presenting with a BBC will have NBCCS, although the proportion will be higher in patients presenting with a BCC at an early age or with multiple tumors. Patients show a characteristic facial appearance, an increased frequency of a number of neoplasms, most notably BCCs, odontogenic keratocysts, and a variety of other developmental abnormalities.[42–44] Gorlin recently has reviewed the clinical features.[18] Cutaneous signs include the development of multiple (up to several hundred or more) BCCs and palmar-plantar pits. BCCs occur most commonly on the face, neck, or upper trunk and histologically are identical to sporadic BCCs. Tumors commonly appear at or after puberty, but presentation appears to be influenced by the amount of ambient ultraviolet radiation and other cutaneous characteristics. In blacks, BCCs may be uncommon or not seen at all, whereas among whites in Australia, the average age of BCC presentation is relatively young.[15,16] Tumors have been reported as early as 2 years of age. BCCs do not occur in about 10 percent of documented cases of NBCCS. The clinical appearance of the lesions is said to be distinctive and may resemble benign cutaneous lesions, including skin tags or seborrhoeic warts or melanocytic nevi.[18] Gorlin reports that before puberty these lesions are harmless and that only a minority change and become aggressive.[18] Palmar or plantar pits occur in over half the cases, more commonly on the hands than feet, and are more common in adults than in children. Typically, they are several millimeters across, have a telangiectatic base, and are clinically distinct from the pits seen in Darier disease. BCC may develop in the bases of the pits.

Patients with NBCCS are at increased risk of a number of other neoplasms, benign or malignant, including medulloblastoma (approximately 5 percent), meningioma, cardiac fibromas, and ovarian sarcomas and fibromas (15 percent). Patients also show a variety of other developmental defects: multiple odontogenic keratocysts that are often asymptomatic and peak during the second or third decade and occur in up to 85 percent of subjects; a characteristic facial appearance with frontal and biparietal bulging, prominent supraorbital ridges, and a low occiput and a long mandible (such patients are often tall, with some showing a marfanoid build); and a variety of skeletal manifestations including bifid ribs, short fourth metacarpals, and cortical defects of the long bones. Ophthalmic abnormalities such as squint or cataract are also seen in 25 percent of patients.[17] Patients with unilateral cutaneous signs have been described.[45] It seems likely that some of the many patients who present with multiple BCCs may be forme frustes of the NBCCS syndrome.

Genetic Loci Involved in BCC

Mapping of NBCCS by several groups to 9q22-31 and the finding of loss of heterozygosity (LOH) in up to 70 percent of sporadic BCCs suggests an underlying tumor-suppressor gene important in both familial and sporadic BCC.[46,47] Loss of the same wild-type allele in multiple BCCs from the same individual with NBCCS is in keeping with this.[48] There is no evidence of genetic heterogeneity.

The gene underlying NBCCS was identified recently using positional cloning strategies by two groups and has been found to be the human homologue (*PTC*) of the *Drosophila* gene *ptc*.[49,50] *PTC* is a 23-exon gene spanning 34 kb and consists of an open reading frame of 4242 nucleotides encoding a putative protein of 1296 amino acids, which shows 39 percent identity and 60 percent similarity to its *Drosophila* counterpart.[49–51] Over 15 different mutations of *PTC* have been identified in approximately one-third of individuals with NBCCS, as well as in variable numbers (20–50 percent) of sporadic BCCs and in other tumors, including medulloblastomas characteristic of the NBCCS syndrome, and sporadic medulloblastomas.[52–57] Why a higher proportion of *PTC* mutations has not been found in sporadic or familial cases is not yet clear. There is no evidence of locus heterogeneity, but because *PTC* is a large gene, mutations may have been missed for technical reasons, or alternatively, other mechanisms of inactivation may occur. Whereas some of the abnormalities such as the odontogenic keratocysts may, like BCC, be explained by a two-hit mechanism, the widespread developmental abnormalities suggest a dosage effect and, of course, fall outside the strict Knudson paradigm for the recessive nature at the cellular level of tumor-suppressor genes.[58] Little genotype-phenotype correlation between the various mutations and clinical phenotype has been reported so far.[59] Most mutations of *PTC* in BCC are truncations leading to presumed loss of function, and about 40 percent have the hallmark of ultraviolet radiation-induced damage.[49,50,57]

Work in *Drosophila* and other model organisms has facilitated understanding the oncogenic role of the patched signaling pathway. *PTC* encodes a transmembrane receptor for the secreted ligand Sonic Hedgehog (SHH). In the absence of SHH, *PTC* inhibits Smoothened (SMO), an adjacent transmembrane receptor. SMO in humans is believed to activate a family of genes including *Gli1* and, through this pathway, activates transcription of a number of genes, including *PTC* itself, *TGFβ*, and the *Wnt* class of genes. From this model it would be predicted that activating mutations of SMO may produce similar effects to loss of function of *PTC* and that *Gli* expression would increase with either loss of *PTC* function or activation of *Smoothened*. Recent experiments have provided support for this model. First, activation mutations of *Smoothened* have been described recently in sporadic BCCs, and transgenic mice with mutated *Smoothened* under a basal keratin promoter develop changes consistent with those seen in human BCC.[60,61] Second, transgenic mice for SHH under the control of the K14 promoter developed many of the cutaneous features of NBCCS with multiple BCCs like epidermal proliferations.[62,63] Interestingly, transplantation of the skin from these mice to SCID mice resulted in a normalization of the phenotype, suggesting the importance of mesenchymal interaction in these tumours (as is believed to be the case in humans). Third, following the transgenic SHH experiments, mutations of SHH have been found in sporadic BCC.[64] Finally, as would be expected, *PTC* and *Gli1* are overexpressed in human BCC and, in keeping with the presumed hair follicle origin of BCC, are normally expressed in the developing follicle.[63,65] It seems likely that mutations of other components of these pathways may be involved in sporadic BCC.

Other Genetic Targets in BCC

Unusually for an epithelial malignancy LOH studies on sporadic BCC show a low frequency of allele loss (at loci other than the NBCCS locus that is lost in up to 70 percent of BCCs), a result in keeping with the usual diploid nature of these tumors.[47,66,67] LOH of 14 to 33 percent for chromosome arm 1q has been reported, but otherwise, LOH appears uncommon, unless it is confined to small areas that have not been examined. Interestingly, despite the presence of *p53* mutation, LOH of 17p is uncommon, but a second inactivating *p53* mutation on the remaining allele is relatively common.[47,68,69]

Mutations of *p53*, *ras*, and a GTPase-activating protein have been described in BCC. Abnormal expression of *p53* is common in BCC and, depending on the antibody and exact immunocytochemical method employed, is increased compared with normal skin in upward of 50 percent of tumors.[69–74] In many instances this increased expression represents overexpression of wild-type sequence.[69] Various studies have reported the presence of *p53* mutations in BCC. As with SCC, the mutation spectrum reflects in large part the particular characteristics of ultraviolet radiation mutagenesis with frequent C → T transitions at (dipyrimidine sites) and double CC → TT transitions, with the result that the mutation "hot spots" differ from those seen in many internal malignancies.[22,23,75,76] The absolute rate of *p53* mutation in BCC varies considerably between different studies, ranging from 20 to 60 percent.[68,69,77,78] These differences may be accounted for by small statistical sample sizes and technical factors, particularly relating to the difficulties in separating stromal or inflammatory elements in small tumors, but also could conceivably represent genuine differences in molecular epidemiology. The presence of more than one *p53* point mutation, one on each allele, perhaps reflects the high ultraviolet radiation mutagenic load skin is exposed to.[68,69]

Ras mutations are common in the murine chemical carcinogenesis model of skin cancer, and investigators early on examined human NMCS including BCC for the presence of such changes.[79,80] Activating mutations of *ras* could be expected based on the known properties and base specificity of ultraviolet radiation-induced mutations. As for *p53*, and possibly for similar reasons, *ras* mutation rates show a wide scatter between 0 and 30 percent.[77,80–82] There is one report of mutations of the GTPase-activating protein (which is involved in down-regulating ras proteins and in signal transduction) in 3 of 21 BCCs.[83] To date, there are no studies showing a relation between the presence of specific genetic change and clinical behavior or histologic subtype of BCC, nor has a definite precursor lesion been identified, although some authors have identified *p53* immunopositive clones harboring *p53* mutations close to clinically obvious BCC.[78,81,84] It remains possible, perhaps likely, that these lesions are precursors of other types of NMSCs.[72]

Bazex-Dupre-Christol Syndrome (OMIM 301845)

This is an extremely uncommon X-linked dominant condition characterized by multiple BCCs developing in the second and third decades and follicular atrophoderma present from birth or early childhood.[85–88] Hypotrichosis and other abnormalities may be present. The BCCs may resemble those seen in the NBCCS. It has been mapped to Xq24-27.[89]

Rombo Syndrome (MIM 180730)

There is one report of this syndrome that was transmitted through four generations consistent with an autosomal dominant trait. BCCs were described together with vermiculate atrophoderma, abnormal eyelashes and eyebrows, and in one case, trichoepitheliomas.

SQUAMOUS CELL CARCINOMA

SCCs are invasive tumors with the ability to metastasize that have a histologic resemblance to differentiated suprabasal keratinocytes.[4,10,39,90,91] They usually arise on sun-exposed skin, grow quicker than BCCs, and produce a more indurated, untidy keratotic lesion with ulceration. There may be associated signs of ultraviolet radiation damage to skin, including actinic keratoses. Histology shows aberrant differentiation, frequent mitoses, and variable degrees of dysplasia. Metastasis rates are between 0.1 and 4 percent, but the overall mortality is low.[4,10,91,92] Cutaneous SCCs are less aggressive in their biologic behavior than other keratinocyte-derived tumors such as those of the oral cavity or cervix and SCC of the lip, which are also caused by ultraviolet radiation exposure.[10,91] There is some evidence that SCC arising in the sites of thermal burns or in sites of chronic inflammation may behave more aggressively.[10] Most cutaneous SCCs are readily amenable to surgery or radiotherapy.

Whereas there are no clinically identified precursor lesions for BCC, some SCCs are thought to arise from actinic keratoses or areas of Bowen disease (*in situ* carcinoma).[10,93] Actinic keratoses are focal areas of cutaneous dysplasia characterized clinically by redness and scaling that are usually only minimally indurated or show no induration.[93,94] They are usually multiple, and their body-site distribution mirrors cumulative ultraviolet radiation exposure, being high on the scalps of balding men, face, and backs of hands and lower arms.[94] Epidemiologic studies in Australia report a prevalence for actinic keratoses of around 50 percent over age 40 and that the risk of progression from a single actinic keratosis to a SCC is less than 1:1000 per year.[1,95] One-quarter of actinic keratoses may resolve spontaneously over a 1-year period, whereas approximately half of SCCs arise in a preexisting actinic keratosis, with the other half apparently arising *de novo*.[95,96] Actinic keratoses are at least 15 times more common than SCC.[1] Sporadic SCCs, unlike keratoacathomas or the epitheliomata of Ferguson Smith, show no significant propensity to clinical regression.[10] There are no single-gene disorders that specifically feature SCCs. (Ferguson Smith tumors, although showing certain similarities, are distinct.)

Genetic Change in SCC

Aneuploidy is common in SCC (unlike BCC), occurring in between 20 and 80 percent of patients. SCCs show distinct patterns of LOH compared with other noncutaneous squamous cell cancers and other skin tumors such as BCCs or keratoacanthomas.[67,97,98] LOH in SCC is especially common on chromosomes 3 (25 percent), 9 (40 percent), and 17 (40 percent), with an overall fractional allelic loss of 30 percent.[14,47] With the exception of chromosome 17 and *p53*, the identity of the underlying putative tumor-suppressor genes for cutaneous SCC are unknown. Loss of 3p is common in other keratinocyte squamous malignancies including oral carcinoma, but the target gene is at present unknown: *FHIT* mutations were not found in one study of cutaneous SCC.[99,100] The target gene(s) underlying LOH on chromosome 9 also is unknown. Current data suggest that the NBCCS or the Ferguson Smith locus is not a primary target in SCC; rather, deletion mapping studies suggest an area of 9p that includes *p16* and *p15*.[101,102] Studies examining these genes for mutation have not been reported, nor have other areas of 9p been excluded.[103]

Brash first showed that *p53* mutations were common in SCC but, perhaps more important, showed that the pattern of mutation involving frequent C→T and CC→TT transitions bore the molecular footprint of ultraviolet radiation-induced mutagenesis.[22] Ultraviolet radiation can influence the carcinogenic process in a number of ways.[20] Ultraviolet radiation is mutagenic, in animal systems can act as a tumor promoter, and there is evidence in animals, if not in humans, that local and systemic immunosuppression induced by ultraviolet radiation may be important in skin carcinogenesis. The finding of ultraviolet radiation-induced mutations was therefore important direct proof of the mutagenic role of ultraviolet radiation in human skin cancer (the increased incidence of SCC in patients with xeroderma pigmentosum could, although perhaps not very convincingly, be attributed to the ultraviolet radiation-induced abnormalities of immune function or to effects on tumor promotion). Subsequent studies have in large part confirmed the earlier findings, although not unfamiliarly for studies of genetic change in NMSC, the absolute rates of *p53* mutation in SCC vary considerably from 10 to over 60 percent.[22,76,77,82,104,105] These differences may reflect genuine epidemiologic differences, technical factors, or statistical sampling errors, since most studies were relatively small. There is a suggestion that the type of mutations may vary in different studies. Studies of premalignant lesions such as Bowen disease and actinic keratoses also show a high rate of *p53* mutation.[106,107] It is not known whether preinvasive lesions harboring *p53* mutations are more likely to progress to SCC than those without mutation, although given the frequency of nonprogression, even with *p53* mutations, the majority of actinic keratoses would be expected to regress or at least not progress. In contrast with BCC, where allelic loss is uncommon, as with many other malignancies, loss of the remaining wild-type allele is common in SCC. It remains possible that there are targets other than *p53* on chromosome 17.[14]

The timing of *p53* mutation during SCC development and the role *p53* plays in keratinocyte physiology also have been examined.[23,107] Wild-type p53 protein expression is increased in human skin following exposure to doses of ultraviolet radiation too small to induce erythema.[108–110] Increased expression is seen with ultraviolet A, B, and C, although when normalized so that equal amounts of erythema are produced, the largest increase is seen for ultraviolet B.[108] The pattern of induction throughout the epidermis is not easily explained on the basis of the known penetration characteristics of the various wavebands of ultraviolet radiation.[108] It is widely assumed that the up-regulation of *p53* expression in response to ultraviolet radiation is a direct result of DNA damage, although more modest increases are seen following a range of stimuli that are not known to cause DNA damage.[109] The functional significance of the increased expression is not clear. For instance, individuals with the Li-Fraumeni syndrome harboring *p53* mutations do not show an excess of NMSC, nor has photosensitivity been reported in this group of patients (although I have seen one such patient). In an attempt to assess the function of *p53*, Brash and colleagues irradiated mice null for *p53* and showed that the number of sunburn cells formed in response to ultraviolet radiation was diminished.[107] (Sunburn cells are defined morphologically and are thought to represent apoptotic—probably basal—keratinocytes.[111,112]) They argued that wild-type *p53* plays an important role in facilitating apoptosis in response to DNA damage and that loss of this function would allow clonal expansion of mutated clones, thus implicating a role for ultraviolet radiation in mutagenesis and tumor promotion.[107,113] It remains unclear why the increase in *p53* expression following ultraviolet B radiation is seen throughout both the proliferative and terminally differentiated compartment.[108] No increase in sunburn cell formation following irradiation was reported in mice carrying a mutant *p53* transgene.[114]

The timing of *p53* mutations in the development of SCC also has been studied. Sensitive techniques such as the ligase-mediated PCR that do not rely on the presence of a clonally expanded group of cells have shown that *p53* mutations can be identified in normal sun-exposed skin and in irradiated cultured keratinocytes.[115] Clusters of *p53* immunopositive cells harboring *p53* mutation also have been described close to BCC and in sun-exposed skin in the absence of any clinical tumor, and although these could represent BCC precursors, perhaps it is more likely that they are related to SCC development.[72,81,113,116,117] It has been suggested that because dissection of different regions of actinic keratoses shows no heterogeneity for *p53* mutation, then *p53* mutation may be the initiating event in SCC development.[107] Given the high proliferative rate of many actinic keratoses, this argument is not decisive, since other changes may have occurred already. In keeping with this, recent work has shown that in many actinic keratoses, increased proliferation, elevated wild-type *p53* expression, changes in p21$^{waf/cip1}$ expression, and chromosomal loss all occur without or before *p53* mutation.[14] There may be many pathways to SCC development, and within certain limits, the order of genetic change may not be critical. The high rate of regression and the low rate of progression to SCC raise the possibility that actinic keratoses and SCC are cognate phenomena, both responses to ultraviolet radiation-induced genetic damage, and that the rare apparent progression from an actinic keratosis to an SCC is the result of misdiagnosis of early *in situ* SCC as actinic keratosis.[118,119] The finding of higher rates of genetic change in actinic keratosis than in SCC, although compatible with this, does not prove it, and the hypothesis remains speculative.[14,120]

As with BCC, a number of studies have looked for *ras* mutations in SCC. Although some early studies reported a high frequency of *ras* mutations (principally of H-*ras* at codon 12), as has been found in studies of other human cancers, later results have qualified earlier work, with lower mutation rates being reported. Rates therefore vary from 0 to 46 percent in different studies.[77,80,121–123] There is some evidence that *ras* mutation rates are higher in some risk groups such as patients with xeroderma pigmentosum than in control tumors.[124–126] Definitive studies conducted simultaneously on samples from different populations are required. In addition to studies of point mutations of *ras,* there are reports of alteration in *ras* expression, gene amplification, or gene deletion that appear particularly common in tumors occurring on the basis of xeroderma pigmentosum.[124,125]

Keratoacanthoma

Keratoacanthomas (KAs) are interesting tumors that, although sharing histologic and clinical overlap with SCC, are defined by their history of spontaneous regression.[39,127,128] Characteristically, KAs develop over the course of a few months and show rapid growth resulting in lesions a few centimeters across, with a keratin plug and a cellular shoulder, before regressing leaving a scar. KAs show many similarities to SCCs, and because the defining feature of a KA is natural regression, in clinical practice where lesions are excised or biopsied, differentiation from SCC is often problematic. KAs are distinct from the self-healing epitheliomata of Ferguson Smith.[129]

Even in the face of their interesting natural history, KAs have received little serious attention. Various theories have been proposed to account for their regressing course: that they have a viral pathogenesis, that they are follicular tumors and that their growth pattern mimics the hair follicle's anagen and telogen, and that they are SCCs that are immunologically rejected by the host.[127,128,130] There are particular diagnostic problems with any analysis of these tumors because the "gold standard" of distinction between a KA and an SCC relies on natural history, which is compromised by removal or biopsy.

Studies conflict as to the frequency of aneuploidy in KA and whether it is possible to clearly distinguish KA from SCC on the basis of ploidy[67,97,131] (although subsequent allelotyping of KA and SCC suggest that differences are likely[98]). Increases in *p53* expression have been described, although definitive studies of mutation rates have not been reported.[77,80,121–123] *Ras* mutations have been described in a small number of tumors, and an attempt has been made to link the presence of mutation with regression rather than progression.[136,137] A recent study of LOH in KAs showed a low fractional allelic loss based on examination of 26 autosomes of only 1.3 percent, with only sporadic loss seen.[98] This suggests clear differences from SCC (score of 30 percent) and makes it likely that KAs and SCCs are different *de novo* rather than KAs being the result of a successful immunologic attack on an SCC.[14,47,130] LOH at the Ferguson Smith locus was uncommon.[98]

Ferguson Smith Syndrome (OMIM 132800)

This syndrome was described originally in a single individual, and the familial nature of the disorder was recognized only later.[129,132,133] It is inherited as an autosomal dominant fashion, has been reported to skip generations, and the largest series all originate from Scotland, with the possibility that they all derive from a single mutation in the late eighteenth century.[132] The incidence is unknown, but worldwide the tumors appear exceptionally rare. Clinically, the condition is characterized by the presence of recurrent lesions identical to SCCs that develop over a few months and then resolve spontaneously, leaving a depressed scar. More than one lesion may be present at the same time. Histologically, the lesions are well-differentiated SCCs rather than KAs[127] (although many workers still refer to them as KAs or argue that they are indeed a form of familial KA). Tumors may present in the second decade but occur more commonly later in life. Tumors on the face and scalp are common, and although most tumors occur on sun-exposed areas, tumors have been reported on the anus and the perineum.[134] There are no associated extracutaneous features, and while disabling and destructive with tumors capable of underlying infiltration, they do not usually affect mortality. There are reports of genuine SCC with metastases developing in individuals with the Ferguson Smith syndrome.[129] The disorder may be unilateral.[134]

In studies of 13 British families, linkage has been shown to 9q22-31, the same locus as for the NBCCS.[135] Whether the two disorders are allelic or reflect mutations of two different genes is not known.[136] Studies of LOH in Ferguson Smith tumors have not been published, and it remains possible that the target gene is not a tumor suppressor.

Muir Torre Syndrome (OMIM 158320)

This is best considered part of the Lynch type 2 family cancer syndrome secondary to an underlying defect in mismatch repair.[137–139] The cutaneous manifestations are characterised by sebaceous gland tumors, including sebaceous adenomas, sebaceous epitheliomas, and sebaceous carcinomas, and less commonly KAs.[140] The syndrome is inherited as an autosomal dominant trait, but expressivity is variable.[141] The true incidence is unknown, but I suspect that the cutaneous aspects are widely underdiagnosed or misdiagnosed. Replication errors have been demonstrated in the cutaneous tumors, including tumors such as actinic keratoses not considered part of the syndrome (replication errors are otherwise uncommon in NMSC).[142,143]

Epidermodysplasia Verruciformis (OMIM 226400)

This disorder is characterized by the onset in childhood of a combination of plane wart, red plaque, and pityriasis versicolor-like lesions in which a range of human papillomavirus types may be identified, with the development of SCCs on sun-exposed areas later, and depressed cell-mediated immunity.[144,145] The mode of inheritance is unclear, although the majority of reports favor an autosomal recessive inheritance.[144] The condition is extremely rare, and apart from identification of new papillomaviruses, it has received little genetic attention.[145]

Dyskeratosis Congenita (OMIM 305000)

SCCs of the skin and other epithelia have been reported in this condition, which is characterized by leukoplakia, nail dystrophy, and cutaneous atrophy and pigmentation.[146,147] It is usually an X-linked recessive syndrome, although other patterns of inheritance have been described.[146,152] The X-linked form has been mapped to Xq28 and is the result of mutations in the gene coding for dyskerin (*DKC1*).[148,149]

APPENDAGEAL TUMORS

BCC and SCC aside, there are a large number of different types of epidermal tumors of varying degrees of aggressiveness that on a clinicopathologic basis are believed to relate to the pilosebaceous unit or eccrine or apocrine sweat glands.[150,151] They are uncommon in comparison with BCC or SCC and often are only correctly diagnosed after histologic examination. The vast majority of tumors are solitary and occur without any family history. Examination of a range of appendageal tumors for LOH showed a low frequency of LOH at selected loci and failed to find any consistent pattern, a finding perhaps not surprising given their pathologic heterogeneity and relatively benign clinical course.[84] Particular familial syndromes that usually are characterized by multiple tumors include Cowden syndrome (multiple hamartoma syndrome, OMIM 158350), an autosomal dominant trait comprising multiple hair follicle tumors, oral papillomas, and breast cancer, which maps to 10q22-23 and is due to mutations in the *PTEN* gene; familial trichoepithelioma (OMIM 132700), which recently has been mapped tentatively to 9p (see below); and familial cyclindromatosis (turban tumors, OMIM 132700), which maps to 16q12-q13 and that shows LOH for this locus in the tumors.[129,152–154] Mutations of *PTC* also have been described in sporadic trichoepitheliomas, a benign hair follicle-related tumor with many similarities to BCCs, although no *PTC* mutations were seen in two familial cases.[155] Clinical and pathologic diagnosis in appendageal tumors is often difficult, and some individuals suffer from more than one type of tumor. It is likely that genetic strategies may assist in understanding the nosology and relation of the different tumors.

COMPLEX TRAITS AND SKIN CANCER SUSCEPTIBILITY

In numerical terms, the contribution of the highly penetrant single-gene disorders described earlier to NMSC is small, accounting for perhaps fewer than 1 percent of cases. Nevertheless, the genetic influence on skin cancer development is considerable. Although ultraviolet radiation is viewed as the major environmental cause of NMSC, this is true in large part only because populations adapted to areas of low ambient ultraviolet radiation have in the relatively recent evolutionary past migrated to areas of high exposure.[20,156] The major genetic determinant of NMSC worldwide therefore is pigmentation (and any other genetic determinants of the cutaneous response to ultraviolet radiation). Blacks have rates of NMSC greater than 50-fold lower than whites, and Japanese who have migrated to areas of higher ultraviolet radiation still show rates 4 to 12 times lower than those seen in Caucasians (although differences in sun-exposure habits cannot be excluded entirely).[24,157–159] Even within Caucasian populations, rates vary perhaps fivefold between those with red hair or who tend to burn rather than tan (and who are often red-haired or of Irish, or Welsh, or Scottish — so-called Celtic — ancestry) and those who tan rather than burn from southern Europe.[160,161] Although the genetics of pigmentation appear complex with, in the mouse, upward of a 100 loci involved in determining coat color, there are in humans single loci effecting pigmentation that exert considerable effects on skin cancer rates.[33,162] For instance, oculocutaneous albinos living in areas of high ambient ultraviolet radiation show dramatically increased risks of NMSC, and without appropriate care and sun avoidance, they may die from complications of their tumors in early adult life.[157,163–165]

Recently, associations between variants of the melanocortin 1 receptor and the inability to tan and red hair have been described.[34,166,167] The melanocortin 1 receptor is a receptor for melanocyte-stimulating hormone and is present on a range of cells including melanocytes and keratinocytes. Genetic analyses in the mouse (and other mammals) have shown that melanocyte-stimulating hormone controls the switch from the production of pheomelanin (red/yellow melanin) to eumelanin (black/brown melanin), an action antagonized by agouti.[32,168] Although eumelanin is photoprotective, pheomelanin has poor sunscreen activities and actually may generate free radicals in response to ultraviolet radiation.[169–171] Over 75 percent of the population of the United Kingdom has been shown to harbor coding region variants of the MC1R, with three alleles in particular (Arg151Cys, Arg160Trp, and Asp294His) looking as though they are functionally important. Evidence for loss of function in transient transfection assays for the Arg151Cys variant has been published recently.[172] The majority of individuals with bright red hair are compound heterozygotes for these alleles, and family studies suggest that as operationally defined, the trait often approximates to a recessive model. That other loci are important in determining the red hair phenotype, however, came from twin studies in which different (hair color) phenotypes in discordant twins concordant for the MC1R locus were seen.[167] An overrepresentation of particular MC1R putative mutant alleles has been reported in melanoma and non-melanoma skin cancer.[166,173] It is likely that there are a number of other genetic influences on NMSC development of unknown magnitude, including the relation between immunologic aspects of cutaneous function and tumor risk.[174,175] Associations have been reported between NMSC and glutathione *S*-transferase GSTM1 polymorphisms, between HLA haplotypes and NMSC, and between NMSC and genetic determinants of susceptibility to the immunosuppressive actions of ultraviolet radiation.[176–179] The influence of differences in DNA repair rates on NMSC is discussed in Chap. 28 and references 180 and 181.

REFERENCES

1. Marks R: An overview of skin cancers: Incidence and causation. *Cancer* **75**(suppl):607, 1995.
2. Gallagher RP, Ma B, McLean DI, Yang CP, Ho V, Carruthers JA, Warshawski LM: Trends in basal cell carcinoma, squamous cell carcinoma, and melanoma of the skin from 1973 through 1987. *J Am Acad Dermatol* **23**:413, 1990.
3. Glass AG, Hoover RN: The emerging epidemic of melanoma and squamous cell skin cancer. *JAMA* **262**:2097, 1989.
4. Preston DS, Stern RS: Nonmelanoma cancers of the skin. *N Engl J Med* **327**:1649, 1992.
5. Green A: Changing patterns in incidence of non-melanoma skin cancer (review). *Epithel Cell Biol* **1**(1):47, 1992.
6. Marks R, Jolley D, Dorevitch AP, Selwood TS: The incidence of non-melanocytic skin cancers in an Australian population: Results of a five-year prospective study. *Med J Aust* **150**(9):475, 1989.
7. Kricker A, English DR, Randell PL, Heenan PJ, Clay CD, Delaney TA, Armstrong BK: Skin cancer in Geraldton, Western Australia: A survey of incidence and prevalence. *Med J Aust* **152**:399, 1990.
8. Marks R, Staples M, Giles GG: Trends in non-melanocytic skin cancer treated in Australia: The second national survey. *Int J Cancer* **53**(4):585, 1993.
9. Fleming ID, Amonette R, Monaghan T, Fleming MD: Principles of management of basal and squamous cell carcinoma of the skin. *Cancer* **75**(suppl):699, 1995.
10. Kwa RE, Campana K, Moy RL: Biology of cutaneous squamous cell carcinoma. *J Am Acad Dermatol* **26**:1, 1992.
11. Miller SJ: Biology of basal cell carcinoma, part 1. *J Am Acad Dermatol* **24**:1, 1991.
12. Miller SJ: Biology of basal cell carcinoma, part 2. *J Am Acad Dermatol* **24**:161, 1991.

13. Rehman I, Quinn AG, Healy E, Rees JL: High frequency of loss of heterozygosity in actinic keratoses, a usually benign disease. *Lancet* **344**:788, 1994.
14. Rehman I, Takata M, Wu YY, Rees JL: Genetic change in actinic keratoses. *Oncogene* **122**:483, 1996.
15. Goldstein AM, Pastakia B, DiGiovanna JJ, Poliak S, Santucci S, Kase R, Bale AE, Bale SJ: Clinical findings in two African-American families with the nevoid basal cell carcinoma syndrome (NBCC) (review). *Am J Med Genet* **50**(3):272, 1994.
16. Shanley S, Ratcliffe J, Hockey A, Haan E, Oley C, Ravine D, Martin N, Wicking C, Chenevix-Trench G: Nevoid basal cell carcinoma syndrome: Review of 118 affected individuals (review). *Am J Med Genet* **50**(3):282, 1994.
17. Evans DG, Ladusans EJ, Rimmer S, Burnell LD, Thakker N, Farndon PA: Complications of the naevoid basal cell carcinoma syndrome: Results of a population based study. *J Med Genet* **30**(6):460, 1993.
18. Gorlin RJ: Nevoid basal-cell carcinoma syndrome. *Medicine* **66**(2):98, 1987.
19. IARC: IARC *Monographs on the Evaluation of Carcinogenic Risks to Humans: Solar and Ultraviolet Radiation*. Lyon, France: IARC, World Health Organization, 1992, p 55.
20. Report of an advisory group on non-ionising radiation: Board statement on effects of ultraviolet radiation on human health and health effects from ultraviolet radiation.Chilton, Didcot, Oxon: National Radiation Protection Board, 1995, p 6(2). Documents of the NRPB.
21. Urbach F, Rose DB, Bonnem RDH, Urbach F, Rose DB, Bonnem RDH, Bonnem M, eds: *Genetic and Environmental Carcinogenesis*. Baltimore: Williams & Wilkins; 1972, pp 355–371.
22. Brash DE, Rudolph JA, Simon JA, Lin A, McKenna GJ, Baden HP, Halperin AJ, Ponten J: A role for sunlight in skin cancer: UV-induced *p53* mutations in squamous cell carcinoma. *Proc Natl Acad Sci* USA **88**:10124, 1991.
23. Brash DE, Ziegler A, Jonason AS, Simon JA, Kunula S, Leffel DJ: Sunlight and sunburn in human skin cancer: *p53,* apoptosis, and tumour promotion. *J Invest Dermatol Symp* **1**(suppl):136S, 1996.
24. Scotto J, Fears TR, Fraumeni JF: *Incidence of Non-Melanoma Skin Cancer in the United States*. Washington, National Institutes of Health, 1983.
25. Fleming ID, Barnawell JR, Burlison PE, Rankin JS: Skin cancer in black patients. *Cancer* **35**(3):600, 1975.
26. Weinstock MA: Epidemiology of nonmelanoma skin cancer: Clinical issues, definitions, and classification. *J Invest Dermatol* **102**(suppl):4S, 1994.
27. Stern RS: Risks of cancer associated with long-term exposure to PUVA in humans: Current status — 1991. *Blood Cells* **18**:91, 1992.
28. Bhate SM, Sharpe GR, Marks JM, Shuster S, Ross WM: Prevalence of skin and other cancers in patients with psoriasis. *Clin Exp Dermatol* **18**(5):401, 1993.
29. Bodmer WF, Cavalli-Sforza LL: *Genetics, Evolution and Man*. San Fransisco, WH Freeman, 1976.
30. Freemon FR, Loomis WF: Vitamin D and skin pigments. *Science* **158**(801):579, 1967.
31. Loomis WF: Skin-pigment regulation of vitamin-D biosynthesis in man. *Science* **157**(788):501, 1967.
32. Jackson IJ: Molecular and developmental genetics of mouse coat color. *Annu Rev Genet* **28**:189, 1994.
33. Jackson IJ: Mouse coat colour mutations: A molecular genetic resource which spans the centuries. *Bioessays* **13**(9):439, 1991.
34. Valverde P, Healy E, Jackson I, Rees JL, Thody AJ: Variants of the mealnocyte-stimulating hormone receptor gene are associated with red hair and fair skin in humans. *Nature Genet* **11**:328, 1995.
35. Smith R, Healy E, Siddiqui S, Flanagan N, Steijlen PM, Rosdahl I, Jacques JP, Rogers R, Turner R, Jackson IJ, Birch-Machi MA, Rees JL: Melanocortin 1 receptor variants in an Irish population. *J Invest Dermatol* **111**(1):119, 1998.
36. Bouwes Bavinck JM, Vermeer BJ, Claas FHJ, Schegget JT, Van Der Woude FJ: Skin cancer and renal transplantation. *J Nephrol* **7**(5):261, 1994.
37. Lang PJJ, Maize JC, Friedman RJ, Rigel DS, Kopf AW, Harris MN, Baker D, eds: *Cancer of the Skin*. Philadelphia, Saunders, 1991, pp 35–73.
38. Mackie RM: *Skin Cancer*, 2d ed. London, Martin Dunitz, Ltd, 1996, pp 112–132.
39. Mackie RM, Champion RH, Burton JL, Ebling FJG, eds: *Textbook of Dermatology*, 5th ed. London, Blackwell Scientific, 1992, pp 1505–1524.
40. Miller DL, Weinstock MA: Nonmelanoma skin cancer in the United States: Incidence. *J Am Acad Dermatol* **30**:774, 1994.
41. Lo JS, Snow SN, Reizner GT, Mohs FE, Larson PO, Hruza GJ: Metastatic basal cell carcinoma: Report of twelve cases with a review of the literature (see comments) (review). *J Am Acad Dermatol* **24**(5:pt 1):715, 1991.
42. Evans DG, Ladusans EJ, Rimmer S, Burnell LD, Thakker N, Farndon PA: Complications of the naevoid basal cell carcinoma syndrome: Results of a population based study. *J Med Genet* **30**(6):460, 1993.
43. Gorlin RJ, Goltz RW: Multiple nevoid basal-cell epithelioma, jaw cysts and bifid rib. *N Engl J Med* **262**(18):908, 1960.
44. Bale AE, Gailani MR, Leffell DJ: Nevoid basal cell carcinoma syndrome. *J Invest Dermatol* **103**(suppl):126S, 1994.
45. Sharpe GR, Cox NH: Unilateral naevoid basal cell carcinoma syndrome: An individually controlled study of fibroblast sensitivity to radiation. *Clin Exp Dermatol* **15**:352, 1990.
46. Farndon PA, Mastro RGD, Evans DGR, Kilpatrick MW: Location of gene for Gorlin syndrome. *Lancet* **339**:581, 1992.
47. Quinn AG, Sikkink S, Rees JL: Basal cell carcinomas and squamous cell carcinomas of human skin show distinct patterns of chromosome loss. *Cancer Res* **54**(17):4756, 1994.
48. Bonifas JM, Bare JW, Kerschmann RL, Epstein EH: Parental origin of chromosome 9q22.3-q31 lost in basal cell carcinomas from basal cell nevus syndrome patients. *Hum Mol Genet* **3**:447, 1994.
49. Hahn H, Wicking C, Zaphiropoulos PG, Gailani MR, Shanley S, Chidambaram A, Vorechovsky I, Holmberg E, Unden AB, Gillies S, Negus K, Smyth I, Pressman C, Leffell DJ, Gerrard B, Goldstein AM, Dean M, Toftgard R, Chenevix-Trench G, Wainwright B, Bale AE: Mutations of the human homologue of *Drosophila patched* in the nevoid basal cell carcinoma syndrome. *Cell* **85**(6):841, 1996.
50. Johnson RL, Rothman AL, Xie JW, Goodrich LV, Bare JW, Bonifas JM, Quinn AG, Myers RM, Cox DR, Epstein EH Jr, Scott MP: Human homologue of *patched*, a candidate gene for the basal cell nevus syndrome. *Science* **272**(5268):1668, 1996.
51. Hahn H, Christiansen J, Wicking C, Zaphiropoulos PG, Chidambaram A, Gerrard B, Vorechovsky I, Bale AE, Toftgard R, Dean M, Wainwright B: A mammalian *patched* homolog is expressed in target tissues of *sonic hedgehog* and maps to a region associated with developmental abnormalities. *J Biol Chem* **271**(21):12125, 1996.
52. Chidambaram A, Goldstein AM, Gailani MR, Gerrard B, Bale SJ, DiGiovanna JJ, Bale AE, Dean M: Mutations in the human homologue of the *Drosophila patched* gene in Caucasian and African-American nevoid basal cell carcinoma syndrome patients. *Cancer Res* **56**(20):4599, 1996.
53. Lench NJ, Telford EA, High AS, Markham AF, Wicking C, Wainwright BJ: Characterisation of human patched germ line mutations in naevoid basal cell carcinoma syndrome. *Hum Genet* **100**(5-6):497, 1997.
54. Raffel C, Jenkins RB, Frederick L, Hebrink D, Alderete B, Fults DW, James CD: Sporadic medulloblastomas contain *PTCH* mutations. *Cancer Res* **57**(5):842, 1997.
55. Wolter M, Reifenberger J, Sommer C, Ruzicka T, Reifenberger G: Mutations in the human homologue of the *Drosophila* segment polarity gene patched (*PTCH*) in sporadic basal cell carcinomas of the skin and primitive neuroectodermal tumors of the central nervous system. *Cancer Res* **57**(13):2581, 1997.
56. Xie J, Johnson RL, Zhang X, Bare JW, Waldman FM, Cogen PH, Menon AG, Warren RS, Chen LC, Scott MP, Epstein EH Jr: Mutations of the *patched* gene in several types of sporadic extracutaneous tumors. *Cancer Res* **57**(12):2369, 1997.
57. Aszterbaum M, Rothman A, Johnson RL, Fisher M, Xie JW, Bonifas JM, Zhang XL, Scott MP, Epstein EH Jr: Identification of mutations in the human *patched* gene in sporadic basal cell carcinomas and in patients with the basal cell nevus syndrome. *J Invest Dermatol* **110**(6):885, 1998.
58. Levanat S, Gorlin RJ, Fallet S, Johnson DR, Fantasia JE, Bale AE: A two-hit model for developmental defects in Gorlin syndrome. *Nature Genet* **12**(1):85, 1996.
59. Wicking C, Shanley S, Smyth I, Gillies S, Negus K, Graham S, Suthers, Haites N, Edwards M, Wainwright B, Chenevix-Trench G: Most germ-line mutations in the nevoid basal cell carcinoma syndrome lead to a premature termination of the *patched* protein, and no genotype-phenotype correlations are evident. *Am J Hum Genet* **60**(1):21, 1997.
60. Xie J, Murone M, Luoh SM, Ryan A, Gu Q, Zhang C, Bonifas JM, Lam CW, Hynes M, Goddard A, Rosenthal A, Epstein EHJ,

de Sanvage FJ: Activating Smoothened mutations in sporadic basal-cell carcinoma. *Nature* **391**(6662):90, 1998.
61. Reifenberger J, Wolter M, Weber RG, Megahed M, Ruzicka T, Lichter P, Reifenberger G: Missense mutations in *SMOH* in sporadic basal cell carcinomas of the skin and primitive neuroectodermal tumors of the central nervous system. *Cancer Res* **58**(9):1798, 1998.
62. Fan H, Oro AE, Scott MP, Khavari PA: Induction of basal cell carcinoma features in transgenic human skin expressing sonic hedgehog. *Nature Med* **3**(7):788, 1997.
63. Dahmane N, Lee J, Robins P, Heller P, Ruiz: Activation of the transcription factor Gli1 and the sonic hedgehog signalling pathway in skin tumours. *Nature* **389**(6653):876, 1997.
64. Oro AE, Higgins KM, Hu Z, Bonifas JM, Epstein EHJ, Scott MP: Basal cell carcinomas in mice overexpressing sonic hedgehog. *Science* **276**(5313):817, 1997.
65. Unden AB, Zaphiropoulos PG, Bruce K, Toftgard R, Stahle-Backdahl M: Human patched (PTCH) mRNA is overexpressed consistently in tumor cells of both familial and sporadic basal cell carcinoma. *Cancer Res* **57**(12):2336, 1997.
66. Bare JW, Lelbo RV, Epstein EH: Loss of heterozygosity at chromosome 1q22 in basal cell carcinomas and exclusion of the basal cell nevus syndrome gene from this site. *Cancer Res* **52**:1494, 1992.
67. Newton JA, Camplejohn RS, McGibbon DH: A flow cytometric study of the significance of DNA aneuploidy in cutaneous lesions. *Br J Dermatol* **117**:169, 1987.
68. Ziegler A, Leffell DJ, Kunala S, Sharma HW, Gailani M, Simon JA, Halperin AJ, Baden HP, Shapiro PE, Bale AE, et al: Mutation hotspots due to sunlight in the *p53* gene of nonmelanoma skin cancers. *Proc Natl Acad Sci USA* **90**(9):4216, 1993.
69. Campbell C, Quinn AG, Angus B, Rees JL: The relation between *p53* mutation and p53 immunostaining in non-melanoma skin cancer. *Br J Dermatol* **129**:235, 1993.
70. McGregor JM, Yu CC, Dublin EA, Levison DA, Macdonald DM: Aberrant expression of p53 tumour-suppressor protein in non-melanoma skin cancer. *Br J Dermatol* **127**:463, 1992.
71. McNutt NS, Saenz-Santamaria C, Volkenandt M, Shea CR, Albino AP: Abnormalities of p53 protein expression in cutaneous disorders (editorial, review). *Arch Dermatol* **130**:225, 1994.
72. Rees JL: *p53* and the origins of skin cancer (editorial, comment). *J Invest Dermatol* **104**(6):883, 1995.
73. Ro YS, Cooper PN, Lee JA, Quinn AG, Harrison D, Lane D, Horne CH, Rees JL, Angus B: p53 protein expression in benign and malignant skin tumours. *Br J Dermatol* **128**:237, 1993.
74. Rees J: Genetic alterations in non-melanoma skin cancer (review). *J Invest Dermatol* **103**(6):747, 1994.
75. Hollstein M, Sidransky D, Vogelstein B, Harris CC: *p53* mutations in human cancers. *Science* **253**:49, 1991.
76. Dumaz N, Stary A, Soussi T, Daya-Grosjean L, Sarasin A: Can we predict solar ultraviolet radiation as the causal event in human tumours by analysing the mutation spectra of the *p53* gene? (review). *Mutat Res* **307**(1):375, 1994.
77. Moles JP, Moyret C, Guillot B, Jeanteur P, Guihou J, Theillet C, Basset-Seguin N: *p53* gene mutations in human epithelial skin cancers. *Oncogene* **8**:583, 1993.
78. Gailani MR, Leffell DJ, Ziegler A, Gross EG, Brash DE, Bale AE: Relationship between sunlight exposure and a key genetic alteration in basal cell carcinoma. *J Natl Cancer Inst* **88**(6):349, 1996.
79. Burns PA, Bremner R, Balmain A: Genetic changes during mouse skin tumorigenesis (review). *Environ Health Perspect* **93**:41, 1991.
80. Campbell C, Rees JL: The role of ras gene mutations in murine and human skin carcinogenesis. *Skin Cancer* **8**:245, 1993.
81. Urano Y, Asano T, Yoshimoto K, Iwahana H, Kubo Y, Kato S, Sasaki S, et al: Frequent p53 accumulation in the chronically sun-exposed epidermis and clonal expansion of p53 mutant cells in the epidermis adjacent to basal cell carcinoma. *J Invest Dermatol* **104**:928, 1995.
82. Kubo Y, Urano Y, Yoshimoto K, Iwahana H, Fukuhara K, Arase S, Itakura M: *p53* gene mutations in human skin cancers and precancerous lesions: comparison with immunohistochemical analysis. *J Invest Dermatol* **102**(4):440, 1994.
83. Friedman E, Gejman PV, Martin GA, McCormick F: Nonsense mutations in the C-terminal SH2 region of the GTPase activating protein (*GAP*) gene in human tumours. *Nature Genet* **5**:242, 1993.
84. Takata M, Quinn AG, Hashimoto K, Rees JL: Low frequency of loss of heterozygosity at the nevoid basal cell carcinoma locus and other selected loci in appendageal tumors. *J Invest Dermatol* **106**(5):1141, 1996.
85. Bazex A, Dupre A, Christol B: Atrophodermaie folliculaire, proliferations basocellulaires et hypothichose. *Ann Dermatol Syphiol* **93**:241, 1966.
86. Viksnins P, Berlin A: Follicular atrophoderma and basal cell carcinomas: The Bazex syndrome. *Arch Dermatol* **113**(7):948, 1977.
87. Goeteyn M, Geerts ML, Kint A, De Weert J: The Bazex-Dupre-Christol syndrome. *Arch Dermatol* **130**:337, 1994.
88. Kidd A, Carson L, Gregory DW, De Silva D, Holmes J, Dean JCS, Haites N: A Scottish family with Bazex-Dupre-Christol syndrome: Follicular atrophoderma, congenital hypotrichosis, and basal cell carcinoma. *J Med Genet* **33**(6):493, 1996.
89. Vabres P, Lacombe D, Rabinowitz LG, Aubert G, Anderson CE, Taieb A, Bonafe JL, Hors-Cayla MC: The gene for Bazex-Dupre-Christol syndrome maps to chromosome Xq. *J Invest Dermatol* **105**(1):87, 1995.
90. Mackie RM: *Skin Cancer*, 2d ed. London, Martin Dunitz, Ltd, 1996, pp 133–156.
91. Rowe DE, Carroll RJ, Day CL: Prognostic factors for local recurrence, metastasis, and survival rates in squamous cell carcinoma of the skin, ear, and lip. *J Am Acad Dermatol* **26**:976, 1992.
92. Lund HZ: How often does squamous cell carcinoma of the skin metastasize. *Arch Dermatol* **92**:635, 1965.
93. Callen JP, Friedman RJ, Rigel DS, Kopf AW, Harris MN, Baker D, eds: *Cancer of the Skin*. Philadelphia, Saunders, 1991, pp 27–34.
94. Sober AJ, Burstein JM: Precursors to skin cancer. *Cancer* **75**(suppl):645, 1995.
95. Marks R, Rennie G, Selwood TS: Malignant transformation of solar keratoses to squamous cell carcinoma. *Lancet* **1**:795, 1988.
96. Marks R, Foley P, Goodman G, Hage BH, Selwood TS: Spontaneous remission of solar keratoses: the case for conservative management. *Br J Dermatol* **115**:649, 1986.
97. Stephenson TJ, Cotton DW: Flow cytometric comparison of keratoacanthoma and squamous cell carcinoma (letter). *Br J Dermatol* **118**(4):582, 1988.
98. Waring AJ, Takata M, Rehman I, Rees JL: Loss of heterozygosity analysis of keratoacanthoma reveals multiple differences from cutaneous squamous cell carcinoma. *Br J Cancer* **73**(5):649, 1996.
99. Roz L, Wu CL, Porter S, Scully C, Speight P, Read A, Sloan P, et al: Allelic imbalance on chromosome 3p in oral dysplastic lesions: An early event in oral carcinogenesis. *Cancer Res* **56**(6):1228, 1996.
100. Sikkink SK, Rehman I, Rees JL: Deletion mapping of chromosome 3p and 13q and preliminary analysis of the *FHIT* gene in human nonmelanoma skin cancer. *J Invest Dermatol* **109**(6):801, 1997.
101. Quinn AG, Sikkink S, Rees JL: Delineation of two distinct deleted regions on chromosome 9 in human non-melanoma skin cancers. *Genes Chromosome Cancer* **11**:222, 1994.
102. Quinn AG, Campbell C, Healy E, Rees JL: Chromosome 9 allele loss occurs in both basal and squamous cell carcinomas of the skin. *J Invest Dermatol* **102**:300, 1994.
103. Puig S, Ruiz A, Lázaro C, Castel T, Lynch M, Palou J, Vilalta A, Weissenbach J, Mascaro J-M, Estivill X: Chromosome 9p deletions in cutaneous malignant melanoma tumors: The minimal deleted region involves markers outside the *p16 (CDKN2)* gene. *Am J Hum Genet* **57**(2):395, 1995.
104. Sato M, Nishigori C, Zghal M, Yagi T, Takebe H: Ultraviolet-specific mutations in *p53* gene in skin tumors in xeroderma pigmentosumpatients. *Cancer Res* **53**:2944, 1993.
105. Pierceall WE, Mukhopadhyay T, Goldberg LH, Ananthaswamy HN: Mutations in the *p53* tumor suppressor gene in human cutaneous squamous cell carcinomas. *Mol Carcinog* **4**(6):445, 1991.
106. Campbell C, Quinn AG, Ro YS, Angus B, Rees JL: *p53* mutations are common and early events that precede tumor invasion in squamous cell neoplasia of the skin. *J Invest Dermatol* **100**:746, 1993.
107. Ziegler A, Jonason AS, Leffell DJ, Simon JA, Sharma HW, Kimmelman J, Remington L, Jacks T, Brash DE: Sunburn and *p53* in the onset of skin cancer. *Nature* **372**:773, 1994.
108. Campbell C, Quinn AG, Angus B, Farr PM, Rees JL: Wavelength specific patterns of *p53* induction in human skin following exposure to UV radiation. *Cancer Res* **53**:2697, 1993.
109. Healy E, Reynolds NJ, Smith M, Campbell C, Farr PM, Rees JL: Dissociation between erythema and *p53* expression in human skin: Effects of UVB irradiation and skin irritants. *J Invest Dermatol* **103**:493, 1994.
110. Hall PA, McKee PH, Menage HD, Dover R, Lane DP: High levels of *p53* protein in UV-irradiated normal human skin. *Oncogene* **8**:203, 1993.
111. Young AR: The sunburn cell. *Photodermatology* **4**:127, 1987.

112. Danno K, Horio T: Sunburn cell: Factors involved in its formation. *Photochem Photobiol* **45**:683, 1987.
113. Jonason AS, Kunala S, Price GJ, Restifo RJ, Spinelli HM, Persing JA, Leffell DJ, Tarone RE, Brash DE: Frequent clones of *p53*-mutated keratinocytes in normal human skin. *Proc Natl Acad Sci USA* **93**(24):14025, 1996.
114. Li G, Mitchell DL, Ho VC, Reed JC, Tron VA: Decreased DNA repair but normal apoptosis in ultraviolet-irradiated skin of *p53*-transgenic mice. *Am J Pathol* **148**(4):1113, 1996.
115. Nakazawa H, English D, Randell PL, Nakazawa K, Martel N, Armstrong BK, Yamasaki H: UV and skin cancer: Specific *p53* gene mutation in normal skin as a biologically relevant exposure measurement. *Proc Natl Acad Sci USA* **91**:360, 1994.
116. Ren ZP, Hedrum A, Ponten F, Nister M, Ahmadian A, Lundeberg J, Uhlen M, Ponten J: Human epidermal cancer and accompanying precursors have identical *p53* mutations different from *p53* mutations in adjacent areas of clonally expanded non-neoplastic keratinocytes. *Oncogene* **12**(4):765, 1996.
117. Ren ZP, Ahmadian A, Ponten F, Nister M, Berg C, Lundeberg J, Uhlen M, Ponten J: Benign clonal keratinocyte patches with *p53* mutations show no genetic link to synchronous squamous cell precancer or cancer in human skin. *Am J Pathol* **150**(5):1791, 1997.
118. Marks R: Premalignant disease of the epidermis: The Parkes Weber lecture 1985. *J R Coll Phys Lond* **20**(2):116, 1986.
119. Harvey I, Shalom D, Marks RM, Frankel SJ: Non-melanoma skin cancer (review). *Br Med J* **299**(6708):1118, 1989.
120. Rees JL, Altmeyer P, Hoffman K, Stücker M, eds: *Skin Cancer and UV Radiation*. Berlin, Spriner-Verlag, 1997, pp 700–708.
121. Anathaswamy HN, Pierceall WE: Molecular alterations in human skin tumors. Klein-Szanto AJP, Anderson MW, Barrett JC, Slaga TJ, eds *Comparative Molecular Carcinogenesis* New York, Wiley, 1992, pp 61–84.
122. Van der Schroeff J, Evers LM, Boot AJM, Bos JL: *ras* oncogene mutations in basal cell carcinomas and squamous cell carcinomas of human skin. *J Invest Dermatol* **94**:423, 1990.
123. Spencer JM, Kakhn SM, Jiang W, DeLeo VA, Weinstein IB: Activated *ras* genes occur in human actinic keratoses, premalignant precursors to squamous cell carcinomas. *Arch Dermatol* **131**:796, 1995.
124. Suarez HG, Daya-Grosjean L, Schlaifer D, Nardeux P, Renault G, Bos JL, Sarasin A: Activated oncogenes in human skin tumors from a repair-deficient syndrome, xeroderma pigmentosum. *Cancer Res* **49**(5):1223, 1989.
125. Daya-Grosjean L, Robert C, Drougard C, Suarez H, Sarasin A: High mutation frequency in *ras* genes of skin tumors isolated from DNA repair deficient xeroderma pigmentosum patients. *Cancer Res* **53**:1625, 1993.
126. Ishizaki K, Tsujimura T, Nakai M, Nishigori C, Sato K, Katayama S, Kurimura O, Yoshikawa K, Imamura S, Ikenaga M: Infrequent mutation of the *ras* genes in skin tumors of xeroderma pigmentosum patients in Japan. *Int J Cancer* **50**:382, 1992.
127. Straka BF, Grant-Kels JM, Friedman RJ, Rigel DS, Kopf AW, Harris MN, Baker D, eds: *Cancer of the Skin*. Philadelphia, Saunders, 1991, pp 390–407.
128. Schwartz RA: Keratoacanthoma (review). *J Am Acad Dermatol* **30**(1):1, 1994.
129. Mackie RM: *Skin Cancer*, 2d ed. London, Martin Dunitz, Ltd, 1996, pp 30–51.
130. Patel A, Halliday GM, Cooke BE, Barneston RS: Evidence that regression in keratoacanthoma is immunologically mediated: A comparison with squamous cell carcinoma. *Br J Dermatol* **131**:789, 1994.
131. Herzberg AJ, Kerns BJ, Pollack V, Kinney RB: DNA image cytometry of keratoacanthoma and squamous cell carcinoma. *J Invest Dermatol* **97**:495, 1991.
132. Ferguson-Smith MA, Wallace DC, James ZH, Renwick JH: Multiple self-healing squamous epithelioma. *Birth Defects* **7**(8):157, 1971.
133. Ferguson-Smith J: Multiple primary, self-healing epitheliomata of the skin. *Br J Dermatol* **60**:315, 1948.
134. Rook A, Moffatt JL: Multiple self-healing epitheliomata of Ferguson Smith type: Report of a case of ulilateral distribution. *Arch Dermatol* **74**:525, 1956.
135. Goudie DR, Yuille MAR, Leversha MA, Furlong RA, Carter NP, Lush MJ, Affara NA, Ferguson-Smith MA: Multiple self healing squamous epitheliomata (*ESS1*) mapped to chromosome 9q22-q31 in families with common ancestry. *Nature Genet* **3**:165, 1993.
136. Richards FM, Goudie DR, Cooper WN, Jene Q, Barroso I, Wicking C, Wainwright BJ, Ferguson-Smith MA: Mapping the multiple self-healing squamous epithelioma (*MSSE*) gene and investigation of xeroderma pigmentosum group A (*XPA*) and *PATCHED* (*PTCH*) as candidate genes. *Hum Genet* **101**(3):317, 1997.
137. Lynch HT, Fusaro RM, Roberts L, Voorhees GJ, Lynch JF: Muir-Torre syndrome in several members of a family with a variant of the cancer family syndrome. *Br J Dermatol* **113**:295, 1985.
138. Papadopoulos N, Nicolaides NC, Wei Y-F, Ruben SM, Carter KC, Rosen CA, Haseltine WA, Fleischmann RD, Fraser CM, Adams MD, Venter JC, Hamilton SR, Petersen GM, Watson P, Lynch HT, Peltomakl P, Mecklin J-P, de la Chapelle A, Kinzler KW, Vogelstein B: Mutation of a *mut*L homolog in hereditary colon cancer. *Science* **263**:1625, 1994.
139. Nyström-Lahti M, Parsons R, Sistonen P, Pylkkänen L, Aaltonen LA, Leach FS, Hamilton SR, Watson P, Bronson E, Fusaro R, Cavalieri J, Lynch J, Lanspa S, Smyrk T, Lynch P, Drouhard T, Kinzler KW, Vogelstein B, Lync HT, de la Chapelle A, Peltomäkl P: Mismatch repair genes on chromosomes 2p and 3p account for a major share of hereditary nonpolyposis colorectal cancer families evaluable by linkage. *Am J Hum Genet* **55**:659, 1994.
140. Schwartz RA, Torre DP: The Muir-Torre syndrome: A 25-year retrospect. *J Am Acad Dermatol* **33**(1):90, 1995.
141. Hall NR, Murday VA, Chapman P, Williams MA, Burn J, Finan PJ, Bishop DT: Genetic linkage in Muir-Torre syndrome to the same chromosomal region as cancer family syndrome. *Eur J Cancer* **30A**(2):180, 1994.
142. Honchel R, Halling KC, Schaid DJ, Pittelkow M, Thibodeau SN: Microsatellite instability in Muir-Torre syndrome. *Cancer Res* **54**:1159, 1994.
143. Quinn AG, Healy E, Rehman I, Sikkink S, Rees JL: Microsatellite instability in human non-melanoma and melanoma skin cancer. *J Invest Dermatol* **104**:309, 1995.
144. Jablonska S, Friedman RJ, Rigel DS, Kopf AW, Harris MN, Baker D, eds: *Cancer of the Skin*. Philadelphia, Saunders, 1991, pp 101–116.
145. Majewski S, Jablonska S: Epidermodysplasia verruciformis as a model of human papillomavirus-induced genetic cancer of the skin. *Arch Dermatol* **131**(11):1312, 1995.
146. Davidson HR, Connor JM: Dyskeratosis congenita. *J Med Genet* **25**(12):843, 1988.
147. Connor JM, Teague RH: Dyskeratosis congenita: Report of a large kindred. *Br J Dermatol* **105**(3):321, 1981.
148. Arngrimsson R, Dokal I, Luzzatto L, Connor JM: Dyskeratosis congenita: Three additional families show linkage to a locus in Xq28. *J Med Genet* **30**(7):618, 1993.
149. Heiss NS, Knight SW, Vullimany TJ, Klauck SM, Wiemann S, Mason PJ, Poustk A, Dokal I: X-linked dyskeratosis congenita is caused by mutations in a highly conserved gene with putative nucleolar functions. *Nature Genet* **19**:32, 1998.
150. Hashimoto K, Friedman RJ, Rigel DS, Kopf AW, Harris MN, Baker D, eds: *Cancer of the Skin*. Philadelphia, Saunders, 1991, pp 209–218.
151. Mackie RM: *Skin Cancer*, 2d ed. London, Martin Dunitz, Ltd, 1996, pp 242–277.
152. Nelen MR, van Staveren WC, Peeters EA, Hassel MB, Gorlin RJ, Hamm H, Lindboe CF, Fryns JP, Sijmons RH, Woods DG, Mariman EC, Padberg GW, Kremer H: Germline mutations in the PTEN/MMAC1 gene in patients with Cowden disease. *Hum Mol Genet* **6**:1383, 1997.
153. Biggs PJ, Wooster R, Ford D, Chapman P, Mangion J, Quirk Y, Easton DF, Burn J, Atratton MR: Familial cylindromatosis (turban tumour syndrome) gene localised to chromosome 16q12-q13: Evidence for its role as a tumour suppressor gene. *Nature Genet* **11**(4):441, 1995.
154. Harada H, Hashimoto K, Ko MSH: The gene for multiple familial trichoepithelioma maps to chromosome 9p21. *J Invest Dermatol* **107**(1):41, 1996.
155. Vorechovsky I, Unden AB, Sandstedt B, Toftgard R, Stahle-Backdahl M: Trichoepitheliomas contain somatic mutations in the overexpressed *PTCH* gene: Support for a gatekeeper mechanism in skin tumorigenesis. *Cancer Res* **57**(21):4677, 1997.
156. Kricker A, Armstrong BK, English DR: Sun exposure and non-melanocytic skin cancer (review). *Cancer Causes Control* **5**(4):367, 1994.
157. Halder RM, Bridgeman-Shah S: Skin cancer in African Americans (review). *Cancer* **75**(suppl 2):667, 1995.
158. Chuang TY, Reizner GT, Elpern DJ, Stone JL, Farmer ER: Nonmelanoma skin cancer in Japanese ethnic Hawaiians in Kauai, Hawaii: An incidence report. *J Am Acad Dermatol* **33**(3):422, 1995.
159. Weinstock MA, Grob JJ, Stern RS, MacKie RM, Weinstock MA, eds: *Epidemiology, Causes and Prevention of Skin Diseases*. London, Blackwell Scientific, 1998, pp 121–128.

160. Kricker A, Armstrong BK, English DR, Heenan PJ: Pigmentary and cutaneous risk factors for non-melanocytic skin cancer: A case-control study. *Int J Cancer* **48**:650, 1991.
161. Urbach F, Rose DB, Bonnem RDH, Urbach F, Rose DB, Bonnem RDH, Bonnem M, eds: *Genetic and Environmental Carcinogenesis*. Baltimore, Williams & Wilkins, 1971, pp 355–371.
162. Barsh GS: The genetics of pigmentation: From fancy genes to complex traits. *Trends Genet* **12**(8):299, 1996.
163. Spritz RA: Molecular genetics of oculocutaneous albinism (review). *Hum Mol Genet* **3**(spec no):1469, 1994.
164. Lookingbill DP, Lookingbill GL, Leppard B: Actinic damage and skin cancer in albinos in northern Tanzania: Findings in 164 patients enrolled in an outreach skin care program. *J Am Acad Dermatol* **32**(4):653, 1995.
165. Luande J, Henschke CI, Mohammed N: The Tanzanian human albino skin: Natural history. *Cancer* **55**(8):1823, 1985.
166. Valverde P, Healy E, Sikkink S, Haldane F, Thody AJ, Carothers A, Jackson IJ, Rees JL: The ASP84GLU variant of the melanocortin 1 receptor (*MC1R*) is associated with melanoma. *Hum Mol Genet* **5**:1663, 1996.
167. Box NF, Wyeth JR, O'Gorman LE, Martin NG, Sturm RA: Characterization of melanocyte stimulating hormone receptor variant alleles in twins with red hair. *Hum Mol Genet* **6**(11):1891, 1997.
168. Cone RD, Lu D, Koppula S, Vage DI, Klungland H, Boston B, Chen W, Orth DN, Pouton C, Kesterson RA: The melanocortin receptors: Agonists, antagonists, and the hormonal control of pigmentation (review). *Recent Prog Horm Res* **51**:287, 1996.
169. Hill HZ: The function of melanin or six blind people examine an elephant. *Bioessays* **14**(1):49, 1992.
170. Thody AJ, Priestly GC, eds: *Molecular Aspects of Dermatology*. New York, Wiley, 1993, pp 55–73.
171. Persad S, Menon IA, Haberman HF: Comparison of the effects of UV-visible irradiation of melanins and melanin-hematoporphyrin complexes from human black and red hair. *Photochem Photobiol* **37**(1):63, 1983.
172. Frändberg PA, Doufexis M, Kapas S, Chhajlani V: Human pigmentation phenotype: A point mutation generates nonfunctional MSH receptor. *Biochem Biophys Res Commun* **245**(2):490, 1998.
173. Rees JL, Birch-Machin M, Flanagan N, Healy E, Philipp S, Todd C: Melanocortin 1 receptor (MCR1). *Ann NY Acad Sci* 1999, in press.
174. Streilein JW, Taylor JR, Vincek V, Kurimoto I, Shimizu T, Tie C, Golomb C: Immune surveillance and sunlight-induced skin cancer. *Immunol Today* **15**(4):174, 1994.
175. de Berker D, Ibbotson S, Simpson NB, Matthew JNS, Idle JR, Rees JL: Reduced experimental contact sensitivity in squamous cell but not basal cell carcinomas of the skin. *Lancet* **345**:425, 1995.
176. Heagerty AH, Fitzgerald D, Smith A, Bowers B, Jones P, Fryer AA, Zhao L, Alldersea J, Strange RC: Glutathione *S*-transferase GSTM1 phenotypes and protection against cutaneous tumours. *Lancet* **343**:266, 1994.
177. Bouwes Bavinck JN, Claas FHJ: The role of HLA molecules in the development of skin cancer. *Hum Immunol* **41**:173, 1994.
178. Czarnecki D, Tait B, Nicholson I, Lewis A: Multiple non-melanoma skin cancer: Evidence that different *MHC* genes are associated with different cancers. *Dermatology* **188**:88, 1994.
179. Streilein JW, Taylor JR, Vincek V, Kurimoto I, Richardson J, Tie C, Medema J-P, Golomb C: Relationship between ultraviolet radiation-induced immunosuppression and carcinogenesis. *J Invest Dermatol* **103**(suppl):107S, 1994.
180. Wei Q, Matanoski GM, Farmer ER, Hedayati MA, Grossman L: DNA repair and aging in basal cell carcinoma: A molecular epidemiology study. *Proc Natl Acad Sci USA* **90**:1614, 1993.
181. Hall J, English DR, Artuso M, Armstrong BK, Winter M: DNA repair capacity as a risk factor for non-melanocytic skin cancer: A molecular epidemiological study. *Int J Cancer* **58**:179, 1994.

CHAPTER 47

Breast Cancer

Fergus J. Couch ▪ Barbara L. Weber

1. **Breast cancer is the most frequently diagnosed cancer in Western women and the leading cause of death in U.S. women aged 40 to 55. Breast cancer is heterogeneous in its clinical, genetic, and biochemical profile. The large majority of affected women present with a breast mass or mammographic abnormality as the only clinically detectable manifestation of disease, yet approximately 30 percent of women diagnosed with breast cancer go on to develop metastatic disease that ultimately is fatal.**
2. **Numerous risk factors for the development of breast cancer have been identified. Family history suggesting an inherited component in the development of some breast cancers is one of the strongest known risk factors. It is estimated that 15 to 20 percent of women with breast cancer have a family history of the disease, with approximately 5 percent of all breast cancers attributable to dominant susceptibility alleles. Two major breast cancer susceptibility genes (*BRCA1* and *BRCA2*) have been identified; others are being actively sought.**
3. **Breast cancer may present in a preinvasive form or an invasive form. Treatment depends on the stage at diagnosis, patient age at the time of diagnosis, and the presence or absence of the estrogen receptor in tumor cells. The prognosis is largely dependent on the stage at diagnosis.**
4. ***BRCA1* is a highly penetrant breast cancer susceptibility gene on chromosome 17q21 that is thought to account for 20 to 30 percent of inherited breast cancers. Families with germ-line mutations in *BRCA1* have an autosomal dominant inheritance pattern of breast cancer as well as an increased incidence of ovarian cancer. The mutation spectrum of *BRCA1* is well defined, and functional links to transcription regulation, cellular response to DNA damage, and development are becoming evident.**
5. ***BRCA2* is a highly penetrant breast cancer susceptibility gene on chromosome 13q12-13 that is thought to account for 10 to 20 percent of inherited breast cancers. Families with germ-line mutations in *BRCA2* also have an autosomal dominant inheritance pattern of breast cancer, an increased incidence of ovarian cancer that is less striking that that with *BRCA1,* and an increased incidence of male breast cancer. The mutation spectrum of *BRCA2* is well defined, and functional links also have been made to transcription regulation, cellular response to DNA damage, and development.**
6. **Sporadic breast cancers have been studied extensively for molecular changes that may provide clues to etiology, prognosis, and improved treatment approaches. Growth factors and their receptors, intracellular signaling molecules, regulators of cell cycling, adhesion molecules, and proteases have all been shown to be altered in sporadic breast cancer.**

Breast cancer is among the most common human cancers, representing 32 percent of all incident cancers in the United States. Currently, more than 180,000 women in the United States and almost 1 million women worldwide are diagnosed with breast cancer every year.[1] Because of the magnitude of the public health problem, the desire to reduce the impact of this disease on American women, and the suitability of breast cancer as a model for the study of the molecular basis of cancer, an increasing number of investigators have focused on this disease in recent years. As a result, tremendous strides have been made in identifying susceptibility genes for breast cancer, defining regions of the human genome that harbor unidentified breast cancer-related genes, and characterizing a number of genes that are somatically altered in sporadic breast cancers. In turn, advances in these areas provide the reagents necessary to translate scientific discoveries into clinical practice as a means of improving the detection, treatment, and ultimately, prevention of breast cancer. In an effort to catalogue this large body of knowledge, this chapter provides (1) an overview of the clinical aspects of breast cancer, (2) a detailed description of the two recently isolated breast cancer susceptibility genes, *BRCA1* and *BRCA2*, (3) information on genes that contribute to less common inherited breast cancer susceptibility syndromes, (4) a summary of the genomic regions thought to harbor unidentified breast cancer-related genes, (5) a synopsis of genes that have been implicated in the development and progression of sporadic breast cancer, and (6) a review of the clinical uses of these genes for predisposition testing, disease detection, prognostication, and therapy selection.

CLINICAL ASPECTS OF BREAST CANCER

Incidence and Mortality

Breast cancer is the leading cause of death for American women between the ages of 50 and 55.[2] The most recent data suggest that 12 percent of all American women (1 in 8) will be diagnosed with breast cancer, and approximately 30 percent of the women diagnosed with breast cancer will die of the disease. Overall, there are more than 50,000 deaths from breast cancer every year in the United States alone. Adding to this concern is the fact that breast cancer incidence in the United States has been rising steadily since 1930, with an average increase of 1.2 percent per year, as reported by the Connecticut Tumor Registry.[3] The incidence in all age groups has increased, with the greatest increase occurring in older women.[4] Many investigators have attempted to explain these data, and while it appears that the advent of screening mammography and the aging of the population play a role in the increasing incidence of breast cancer, the increase reflects a real trend, suggesting that environmental or lifestyle changes may be effecting an increase in the number of breast cancers that develop. However, it is important to evaluate the age-adjusted risk for breast cancer because breast cancer risk rises steeply with age. Data from the National Cancer Institute Surveillance Program indicate that a 35-year-old woman has a risk

A list of standard abbreviations is located immediately preceding the index in each volume. Nonstandard abbreviations used in this chapter include: DCIS = ductal carcinoma *in situ*; LCIS = lobular carcinoma *in situ*; LFS = Li-Fraumeni syndrome; PJS = Peutz-Jeghers syndrome; LOH = loss of heterozygosity.

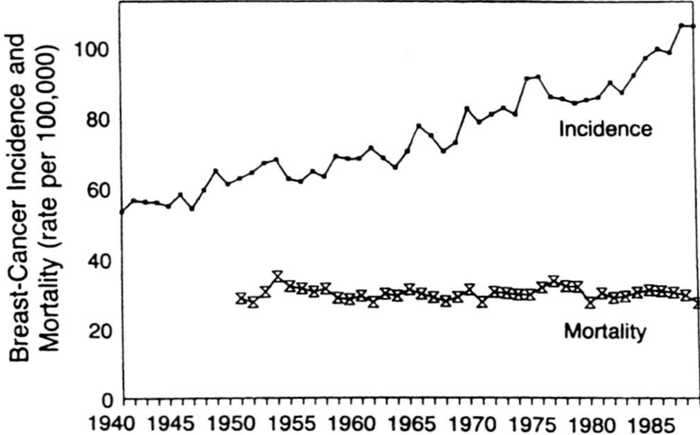

Fig. 47-1 Breast cancer incidence and mortality trends. Incidence of breast cancer in the United States from 1940 to 1985 is indicated by closed circles. Mortality rates, indicated by Xs, have remained fairly constant despite the rising incidence. (*Used with permission from Holford et al.*[5])

of 1 in 2500, a 50-year-old woman has a risk of 1 in 50, and it is not until age 85 that risk reaches 1 in 8. Interestingly, while incidence rates have been increasing steadily, mortality rates have remained relatively constant[5] (Fig. 47-1). This constancy in the face of increasing incidence may be explained by better reporting, increases in less aggressive forms of the disease, improved detection strategies, and/or improvements in treatment.

Risk Factors

The search for breast cancer risk factors is based on a desire to explain the rising incidence of breast cancer and an obvious interest in identifying modifiable lifestyle or environmental factors that will reduce the likelihood of developing breast cancer in individual women. The best-studied and most significant risk factor is a family history of breast cancer. While shared exposure to another risk factor cannot be excluded, this most commonly represents heritable factors that increase the likelihood of developing breast cancer. The breast cancer susceptibility genes *BRCA1* and *BRCA2* represent the most dramatic examples, but since they probably account for only 15 to 20 percent of the breast cancer that clusters in families,[6] it is clear that other, less penetrant, but more common heritable factors remain to be identified. Relative risk for breast cancer with respect to family history ranges from 1.4 for a woman whose mother was diagnosed with breast cancer after age 60[7,8] to 150 for a 40-year-old woman with an inherited *BRCA1* alteration.[9] Weaker risk factors for breast cancer include early age at menarche (relative risk 1.2),[10] nulliparity (relative risk 2.0),[11] and late age at menopause (relative risk 2.0).[12] Pike and colleagues postulated that these factors all reflect an increased number of menstrual cycles compared with multiparous women and that this is the underlying risk factor; work on this hypothesis is ongoing.[13] Additionally, terminal differentiation of breast epithelial cells does not occur until the onset of lactation after the completion of a full-term pregnancy. This final stage of differentiation may confer increased resistance to carcinogens. Radiation exposure is clearly a risk factor, with significant increases in breast cancer observed among atomic bomb survivors (maximum relative risk 13),[14,15] and in women who received mantle radiation for Hodgkin disease as children (incidence ratio 75.3).[16] Additional factors that have appeared as risk factors in some but not all studies include bottle feeding as opposed to breast feeding, alcohol intake greater than two drinks per day, a high-fat diet, prolonged oral contraceptive use, and estrogen replacement therapy.[17,18] Risk factor data are summarized in Table 47-1.

Histology of Breast Cancer

Breast carcinoma arises from the epithelium of the mammary gland, which includes the milk-producing lobules and the ducts that carry milk to the nipple (Fig. 47-2). Malignant transformation of the stromal, vascular, or fatty components of the breast is not included in this definition and is extremely rare. These facts may largely explain why breast size is not a risk factor for breast cancer, since all women have a similar amount of breast epithelium, whereas breast size is determined largely by the amount of stromal and fatty tissue. The transition from normal to malignant breast epithelium has not been as well studied as the parallel changes in colonic epithelium; however, there is increasing evidence that the breast epithelium undergoes a transformation from normal to hyperplasic, followed by the appearance of atypia in association with the hyperplasia, ultimately becoming malignant. Malignant cells continue to evolve from noninvasive carcinoma, typified by ductal carcinoma *in situ* (DCIS), to invasive carcinoma, and ultimately, to cells with metastatic potential.

Lobular Carcinoma *in Situ*. Lending confusion to the progression from normal to malignant epithelium is the entity of lobular carcinoma *in situ* (LCIS), which is not a preinvasive lesion but appears to be a marker of increased risk for the development of invasive cancer. LCIS was not identified as a clinical entity until 1941 and originally was believed to be the precursor lesion of invasive lobular carcinoma. Since its original description, LCIS has been recognized as a purely histologic diagnosis. Clinical diagnosis is not possible because LCIS does not form a palpable lesion and therefore cannot be identified on physical examination, and because it is not visible on mammography. Thus the diagnosis of LCIS always is made as an incidental finding on a breast biopsy obtained for diagnosis of an adjacent lesion. In addition, the incidence of LCIS in the general population is unknown because the nature of the diagnosis precludes studies based on mammographic screening. Evidence that LCIS is a marker lesion and not a

Table 47-1 Risk Factors for Breast Cancer

Risk Factor	Risk Category	Relative Risk	References
Family history	Mother $>$ 60	1.4	7
	Two first-degree relatives	4–6	8
BRCA1/BRCA2 mutations	Carriers	150 (at age 40)	9
Age at menarche	$<$14	1.3	10
Age at menopause	$>$55	1.5	12
Parity	No full-term birth	1.9	11
Benign breast disease	Atypical hyperplasia	4.0	18
Radiation	Atomic bomb survivors	13	14,15
	Mantle radiation for Hodgkin disease	75	16

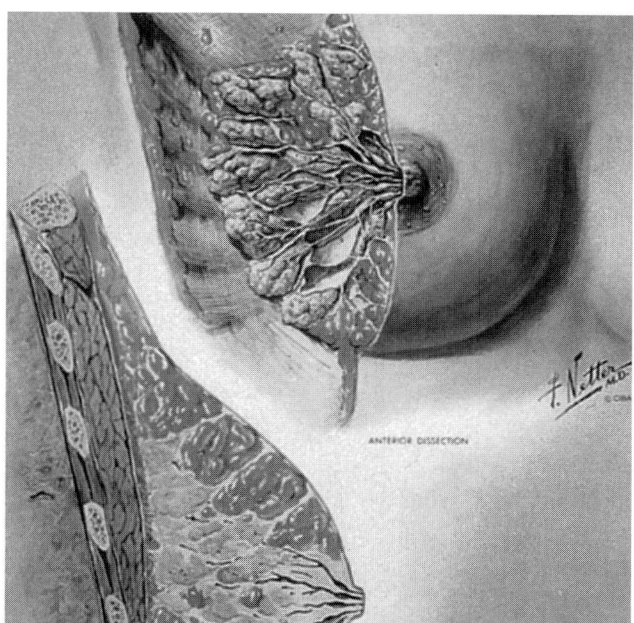

Fig. 47-2 Normal breast architecture. The breast is shown partially dissected from an anterior view (above) and in a sagittal section. Mammary ducts are seen radiating out from the nipple and terminating in milk-producing lobules. Fat and stoma surround and interdigitate with the ductal and lobular structure.

true malignant lesion comes from studies demonstrating that it is frequently multicentric and/or bilateral and that the invasive cancer that may develop subsequently is likely to occur distant from the known focus of LCIS and is more often of ductal rather than lobular histology.[19] The risk of invasive breast cancer after a diagnosis of LCIS has been the subject of many studies; the series with the longest follow-up was reported by Rosen and colleagues at the Memorial Sloan-Kettering Cancer Institute.[20] In this cohort, followed for a mean of 24 years, 37 percent of the women with LCIS who were not lost to follow-up developed invasive breast cancer; more than half these women developed an invasive lesion within at least 15 years following the initial diagnosis of LCIS. When the data were analyzed with the assumption that all the women lost to follow-up remained cancer-free, the percentage of patients developing invasive disease dropped to 31 percent.[20] Because of the substantial risk of invasive carcinoma and the inability to predict where it will occur in the breasts of a woman with LCIS, the treatment of LCIS presents a conundrum. Currently, patients are offered a choice between frequent mammographic surveillance and bilateral mastectomies. This widely discrepant choice is, for obvious reasons, a difficult one and seems particularly harsh when considering the emphasis on breast conservation for the treatment of invasive disease.

Although there has been considerable speculation that LCIS represents a histologic marker of genetic predisposition to breast cancer, recent work suggests that this may not be the case. In a study of 436 women with familial breast cancer and an equal number of age-matched controls selected randomly from a general hospital, Lakhani and colleagues provided evidence that LCIS was underrepresented in the familial cohort, including the subset of known *BRCA1* and *BRCA2* mutation carriers, compared with the controls (3 versus 6 percent, $p < 0.013$).[21] Data suggest that women with LCIS and a family history of breast cancer may be more likely to develop invasive cancer than those with LCIS alone[22]; however, no studies that compare invasive cancer risk in women with a family history of LCIS with that of women with no family history have been reported. Thus the question of whether family history and LCIS represent compounding risk factors remains unanswered.

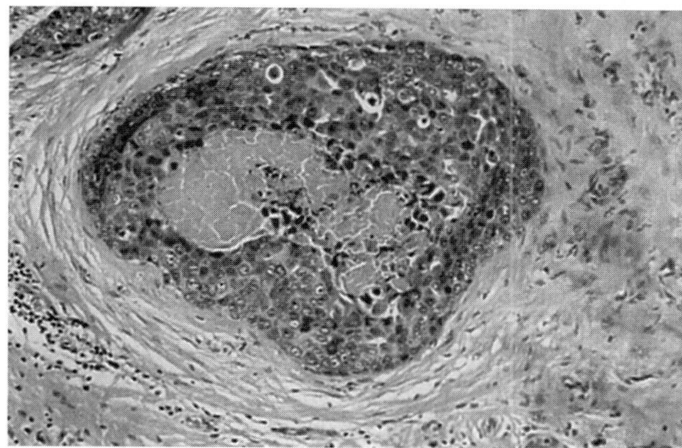

Fig. 47-3 Ductal carcinoma *in situ*. A focus of comedo-type DCIS is shown stained with hematoxylin and eosin. The malignant cells are wholly contained within the duct and do not invade the surrounding stroma. The central region is filled with necrotic cellular debris.

Ductal Carcinoma *in Situ*. Unlike LCIS, DCIS is considered a true precursor lesion of invasive ductal carcinoma (Fig. 47-3). Historically, patients presented with a palpable breast mass, a nipple discharge, or both. Before the use of mammography, pure DCIS lesions without an invasive component were uncommon, constituting only 1 to 5 percent of all breast cancer cases.[23] Patients were treated with total mastectomy. However, after the widespread dissemination of screening mammography, the clinical picture of DCIS changed radically, with 50 to 60 percent of DCIS being diagnosed solely as a mammographic abnormality and pure DCIS representing more than 30 percent of breast cancers diagnosed by screening mammography.[24] The most common mammographic manifestation of DCIS is clustered microcalcifications. Information on the risk of progression from DCIS to invasive cancer is limited because until recently patients were treated with total mastectomy. While this is essentially 100 percent effective in preventing disease progression and death, the natural history of the lesion was obscured by the procedure. Estimates from small series of patients inadvertently treated with biopsy alone suggest that 30 to 50 percent of DCIS lesions evolve into invasive cancer within 6 to 10 years of diagnosis.[25,26] In nearly all these patients, the invasive cancer occurred at or near the original biopsy site and was of ductal histology.

As noted earlier, historically treatment of DCIS consisted of mastectomy, and in women with multifocal lesions, this is still the treatment of choice. However, recent data suggest that when the lesion is localized, lumpectomy followed by radiation does not compromise survival, allowing breast conservation for women who choose this approach.[27] A large, randomized clinical trial designed to confirm this observation and validate this treatment is being conducted by the National Surgical Adjuvant Breast and Bowel Project (NSABP).

It is clear that DCIS alone or in association with an invasive lesion may be found in women with breast cancer caused by germline mutations in the breast cancer susceptibility genes *BRCA1* or *BRCA2*. However, recent data suggest that the frequency of DCIS may be lower in inherited breast cancers than in age-matched unselected controls.[21] The biologic meaning of this finding is unclear but could reflect an early transition from noninvasive to invasive breast cancer and/or an invasive tumor with a rapid growth rate. This would result in a lesion where the noninvasive component may be too small to be clinically recognizable or where the ratio of invasive to noninvasive cancer in a given lesion makes the detection of the noninvasive component difficult.

Invasive Breast Cancer. Invasive breast cancer may be ductal or lobular in histologic type, and while there are a few distinguishing clinical features, the natural history and treatment of the two

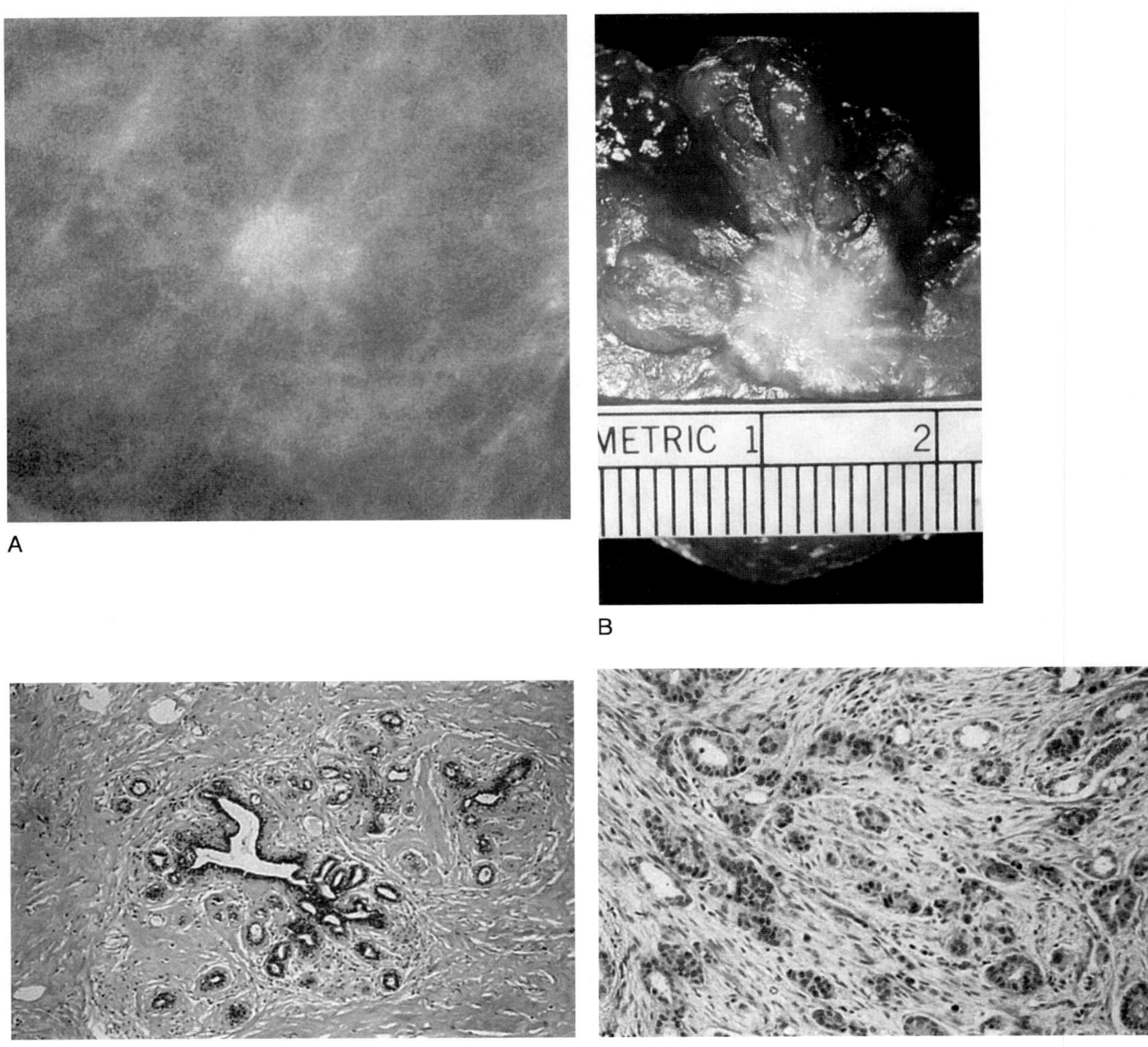

Fig. 47-4 Invasive breast cancer. *A.* Mammogram showing a spiculated mass with poorly defined borders that is characteristic of an invasive breast cancer. *B.* Invasive ductal carcinoma gross pathology. An unfixed biopsy specimen illustrates the gross pathologic correlates of the mammogram. The hard white invasive cancer extends into the breast in all directions with no defined border and numerous stellate extensions. *C.* Normal breast histopathology. The ducts are shown cut in cross section lined with a single layer of ductal epithelium. The surrounding stroma stains pink in this preparation (hematoxylin and eosin). *D.* Invasive ductal carcinoma histopathology. Malignant epithelial cells are characterized by large pleomorphic nuclei invading the breast stroma individually and in clusters and forming ductlike structures in some cases.

lesions are virtually identical. About 80 percent of invasive breast cancers are ductal carcinomas. Infiltrating lobular carcinoma is less common, representing only 5 to 10 percent of breast cancers. The remainder of invasive breast cancer consists of a variety of "special types," including tubular cancer, characterized by prominent tubule formation; medullary carcinoma, a lesion that appears poorly differentiated under the microscope but is thought to have a more favorable prognosis than other breast cancers[28]; and mucinous (or colloid) carcinoma, characterized by the abundant accumulation of extracellular mucin, bulky tumors, and a good prognosis.[17] Of particular note is the fact that approximately 15 percent of invasive carcinomas are not detectable mammographically, particularly invasive lobular carcinomas. The clinical implication of this false-negative rate is that mammography alone is not sufficient for the evaluation of a breast mass. In the presence of a palpable breast mass, a negative mammogram should be followed by ultrasound and/or biopsy. A cystic lesion on ultrasound may be presumed benign and aspirated or followed. A solid or complex lesion should be subjected to excisional biopsy. The mammographic and histopathologic appearance of invasive breast cancer is illustrated in Fig. 47-4.

The treatment and prognosis of a woman with breast cancer are strongly influenced by the stage at the time of diagnosis. Multiple staging systems have been proposed, but the most commonly used system is the one adopted by both the American Joint Committee (AJC) and the International Union against Cancer (UICC).[29] This staging system is a detailed TNM (tumor, nodes, metastasis) system but can be summarized as in Table 47-2. Data compiled from several studies with extensive follow-up suggest that 10-year disease-free survival rates for women with invasive breast cancer

Table 47-2 AJC and IUCC Staging System for Breast Cancer

State 0	Carcinoma *in situ*
Stage I	Tumor ≤ 2 cm, negative axillary nodes
State II	Tumor from 2–5 cm and/or mobile positive axillary nodes
Stage III	Tumor > 5 cm and/or fixed axillary nodes; inflammatory breast cancer
Stage IV	Distant metastases beyond ipsilateral axillary nodes

are approximately 80 percent for women diagnosed with stage I disease, decreasing to 55 percent (stage II), 40 percent (stage III), and 10 percent (stage IV) as the stage at diagnosis increases[30,31] (Fig. 47-5).

Since breast cancer is considered a systemic disease at the time of detection, treatment is designed to achieve two distinct goals: (1) local control of the tumor in the breast and the ipsilateral axillary lymph nodes and (2) eradication of clinically occult systemic micrometastases. Local control may be obtained in most cases by mastectomy alone or by lumpectomy (removal of the tumor with histologically negative margins) followed by radiation therapy to the affected breast. Lumpectomy without radiation is associated with a 35 percent local recurrence rate and thus is considered unacceptable[32] and is rarely used. Since multiple randomized studies have shown that the breast-conserving approach of lumpectomy and radiation does not compromise survival compared with mastectomy, this therapeutic choice is often left to the individual patient. Relative contraindications to the use of breast conservation are related to the presence of a multicentric or multifocal tumor, extensive DCIS in association with an invasive tumor, or a large tumor (> 5 cm). Large tumors are particularly problematic in a small breast, where the cosmetic result associated with a complete excision may be compromised by the relative amount of tissue that must be removed to obtain clear margins around the tumor. However, the choice of procedure generally is dictated only by personal preference (some patients feel more comfortable with removal of the entire breast despite data supporting the safety of lumpectomy) and convenience (some patients choose mastectomy to avoid 6 to 7 weeks of daily radiotherapy treatments).

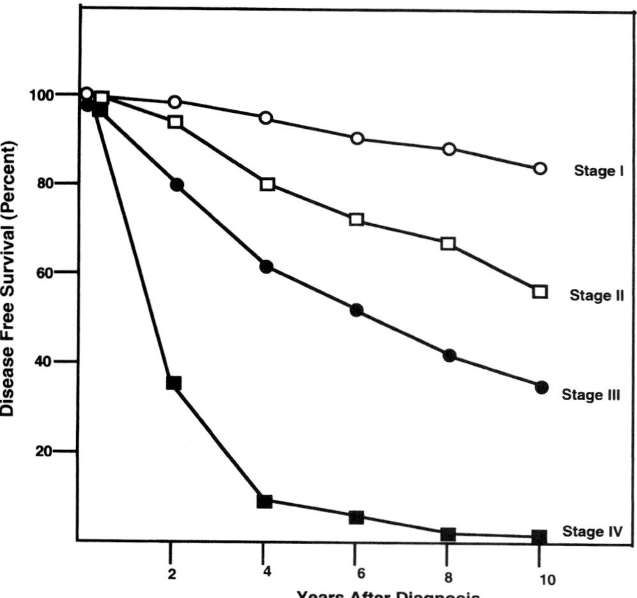

Fig. 47-5 Stage-specific survival for breast cancer. Survival at 2-year intervals is indicated by stage (IUCC). Stage I: open circles; stage II: open squares; stage III: shaded circles; stage IV: shaded squares.

Table 47-3 Adjuvant Treatment Options for Women with Breast Cancer

Patient Characteristics	Standard Treatment
Premenopausal	
Tumor < 1 cm, node negative	None
Tumor ≥1 cm, node negative	Chemotherapy with tamoxifen if ER+
Tumor ≥1 cm, node positive	Chemotherapy with tamoxifen if ER+
Postmenopausal	
Tumor < 1 cm, node negative	None
Tumor ≥1 cm, node negative, ER+	Tamoxifen or observation
Tumor ≥1 cm, node negative, ER –	Chemotherapy or observation
Tumor ≥1 cm, node negative, ER+	Tamoxifen ± chemotherapy
Tumor ≥1 cm, node negative, ER –	Chemotherapy

Once local control has been achieved by one of the two surgical options just discussed, adjuvant therapy may be used to reduce the likelihood of a systemic recurrence. Often confusing to patients, the decision to use adjuvant chemotherapy is not dictated by the choice of local therapy but by the stage of disease and the menopausal status of the patient. The adjuvant regimens most commonly used include a 3- to 6-month course of chemotherapy and/or a prolonged course of the partial estrogen antagonist tamoxifen. Surgical oophorectomy (removal of both ovaries) performed after local therapy also has been shown to reduce the risk of systemic recurrence in premenopausal patients. While the needs of each patient must be addressed individually, generalizations can be made about the choice of therapy (Table 47-3). First, there is increasing evidence that women with tumors less than 1 cm in diameter without involved axillary nodes do not require adjuvant therapy. The 10-year survival rates for women in this category exceed 90 percent, and the relative benefit derived from adjuvant treatment adds little to this excellent prognosis. In contrast, numerous studies support the use of adjuvant therapy in premenopausal women with tumors greater than 1 cm in diameter regardless of nodal status. In this setting, chemotherapy is associated with the greatest increase in overall survival, with tamoxifen generally being added for women with tumors that appear to be hormonally responsive by virtue of expressing the estrogen receptor (ER). More controversial is the treatment of postmenopausal women because tamoxifen alone may be of benefit equivalent to that of chemotherapy, obviating the need for chemotherapy in postmenopausal women with ER-positive tumors. Postmenopausal women with ER-negative tumors without involved axillary nodes may receive no adjuvant therapy or be given a course of chemotherapy depending on a number of variables, including the size and grade of the tumor as well as the general health status of the patient. Postmenopausal women with involved axillary nodes may receive chemotherapy and/or tamoxifen depending on their ER status. Chemotherapy may be administered for 3 to 6 months, is given in the outpatient setting, and generally is well tolerated. The most commonly employed regimens include cyclophosphamide and doxorubicin or cyclophosphamide, methotrexate, and 5-fluorouracil. A taxane increasingly is becoming an important part of this regimen. Tamoxifen is self-administered orally and is taken daily for a minimum of 5 years after the diagnosis.

Finally, autologous bone marrow transplantation is an experimental adjuvant therapy approach that may be an option for women with a high risk of systemic relapse. These women generally are defined by the presence of 10 or more involved axillary lymph nodes or by the presence of inflammatory breast cancer, a particularly aggressive form of invasive carcinoma that presents clinically with diffuse breast pain, swelling, and redness.

Ten-year survival rates for patients with both these clinical entities are only 15 to 20 percent in the absence of systemic therapy. Conventional-dose chemotherapy, which may improve survival by 10 to 15 percent, is still associated with 10-year recurrence rates of 60 to 65 percent.[33]

Autologous bone marrow transplantation for breast cancer was designed as a means of delivering very high doses of chemotherapy that would be fatal in the absence of a method for protecting bone marrow stem cells from the toxic effects of treatment. In this setting, bone marrow cells may be harvested directly from the iliac crest or by pheresis of stem cells from peripheral blood. Stem cells are stored (by freezing) during intensive chemotherapy and reinfused into the patient when the drugs have been cleared. While this approach is promising, the long-term results are not available.

The interventions just described are of clear benefit in reducing the risk of recurrence; nonetheless, overall, at least 30 percent of patients with breast cancer will relapse and die of the disease. Metastatic disease (stage IV) may be extremely variable in course. Ten-year survival rates are dismal at 5 to 10 percent,[33] with the median survival for patients with metastatic disease being approximately 18 months. However, while some patients with metastatic breast cancer may succumb within months of a recurrence, others, particularly those with metastases to bone as the only site of disease, may do well with minimally progressive disease for years. Time to recurrence is also extremely variable, since some patients will relapse with aggressive drug-resistant tumors within weeks of the completion of adjuvant therapy and some patients will have disease-free intervals of up to 30 years before ultimate disease recurrence.

Treatment for metastatic disease must be individualized but may include chemotherapy, hormonal therapy, and palliative radiation therapy. Surgical resection of chest wall recurrences after mastectomy may be indicated in some patients. Unfortunately, treatment of metastatic breast cancer is uniformly considered palliative. The only exception at present may be a subset of patients who achieve complete remission of all clinically detectable tumors with standard chemotherapy and then undergo autologous bone marrow transplantation. While early studies suggested that 10 to 15 percent of these patients may attain durable complete remissions[34], recent studies have failed to show a benefit of this approach.[34b]

THE GENETICS OF BREAST CANCER

Breast cancer is a complex and heterogeneous disease caused by interactions of both genetic and nongenetic factors; however, a family history of breast cancer has long been recognized as a significant risk factor, as evidenced by the fact that familial clustering of breast cancer was first described by physicians in ancient Rome.[35] The first modern documentation of familial clustering of breast cancer was published in 1866 by a French surgeon who reported 10 cases of breast cancer in four generations of his wife's family; four other women in this family died as a result of hepatic tumors that may well have been metastatic breast cancer.[36] In 1984, Williams and Anderson were the first to provide statistical evidence for an autosomal dominant breast cancer susceptibility gene with age-related penetrance, using segregation analysis to compare various models that might explain the pattern of aggregation of breast cancer in families.[37] This model was supported in 1988 by Newman and colleagues,[38] and the hypothesis was proven correct in 1994 with isolation of the susceptibility gene *BRCA1*.[39]

Two high-penetrance breast cancer susceptibility genes have been identified (*BRCA1* and *BRCA2*),[39–41] and others are being actively sought. Breast cancer in families with germ-line mutations in these genes appears as an autosomal dominant trait, as predicted by previous work. In addition, mutations in several other genes such as *TP53, MSH2,* and *PTEN* have been identified as rare causes of hereditary breast cancer. Finally, it is very likely that other lower-penetrance genes are responsible for inherited susceptibility to breast cancer in families in which the incidence of breast cancer is higher than that in the general population, but the susceptibility inheritance pattern does not fit the classic model of Mendelian inheritance.

Given the strong influence of molecular genetics in medicine in recent years, there is a tendency to assume that familial clustering of disease results from a genetically inherited predisposition. However, other explanations for familial clustering of breast cancer are possible, including (1) geographically limited environmental exposure to carcinogens that might affect an extended family living in close proximity, (2) culturally motivated behavior that alters the risk factor profile such as age at first live birth and contraceptive choice, and (3) socioeconomic influences that, for example, may result in differing dietary exposures. In addition, multiple, complex inherited genetic factors are likely to influence the extent to which a risk factor for breast cancer plays a role in any single individual; such modifying effects are likely to be shared among genetically similar members of an extended family. Nonetheless, while noninherited factors certainly play a role in familial clustering of breast cancer, recent advances have provided unequivocal evidence for the presence of breast cancer susceptibility genes that are directly responsible for 5 to 10 percent of all breast cancers.

Breast cancer due to inherited susceptibility has several distinctive clinical features: Age at diagnosis is considerably lower than in sporadic cases, the prevalence of bilateral breast cancer is higher, and the presence of associated tumors in affected individuals is noted in some families. Associated tumors may include ovarian, colon, prostate, and endometrial cancers and sarcomas.[42] However, breast cancer due to inherited susceptibility does not appear to be distinguished by histologic type, metastatic pattern, or survival characteristics. The study of *BRCA1* and *BRCA2*[39,40] has greatly expanded our knowledge of inherited susceptibility breast cancer, and the study of these and other genes continues at a rapid pace.

BRCA1

Clinical Features of Affected Families. In 1990, chromosome 17q21 was identified as the location of a susceptibility gene for early-onset breast cancer now termed *BRCA1*.[39] Linkage between the genetic marker D17S74 on 17q21 and the appearance of ovarian cancer in several large kindreds was subsequently demonstrated.[43] A collaborative study of more than 200 families suggested that breast/ovarian cancer was linked to markers in this region in more than 90 percent of families with apparent autosomal dominant transmission of breast cancer and at least one case of ovarian cancer. Linkage between breast cancer and genetic markers on 17q12-q21 was observed in just 45 percent of families with breast cancer only. However, the percentage of site-specific breast cancer families in this study attributed to *BRCA1* mutations rose to almost 70 percent when the median age of onset of breast cancer in the families was less than 45 years.[9] As greater numbers of breast cancer families have been screened for mutations in *BRCA1,* it has become apparent that the role of *BRCA1* in familial breast and/or ovarian cancer may have been overestimated. These data were collected from the largest, most severely affected families that were suitable for linkage analysis, thereby introducing substantial ascertainment bias. Recent studies of the complete spectrum of families (from 3 to 12 affected members) that present at high-risk breast cancer clinics suggest that *BRCA1* mutations are responsible for 20 to 30 percent of familial breast cancer and 10 to 20 percent of familial ovarian cancer.[44–47] While the families used in these studies most likely include cancer clusters not associated with a dominant susceptibility gene, it is clear that *BRCA1* is responsible for far less familial breast cancer than the widely quoted estimate of 45 percent.[9]

As described earlier, breast cancer in highly penetrant families appears as a classic Mendelian trait of autosomal dominant

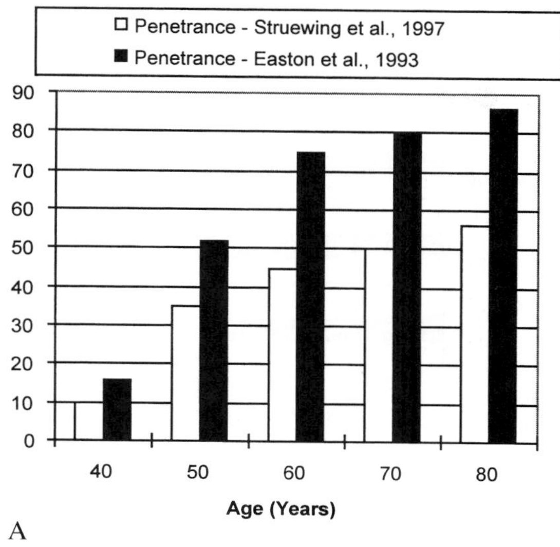

Fig. 47-6 Breast and ovarian cancer risks associated with *BRCA1* and *BRCA2* mutations. *A.* Age-adjusted penetrance for breast cancer in *BRCA1* and *BRCA2* mutation carriers comparing data from Easton et al.[48] and Struewing et al.[49] *B.* Age-adjusted penetrance for ovarian cancer in *BRCA1* and *BRCA2* mutation carriers comparing data from Easton et al.[48] and Struewing et al.[49]

transmission with high penetrance, with almost 50 percent of the children of carriers developing breast and/or ovarian cancer by age 85. Female mutation carriers are estimated to have an 87 percent lifetime risk of developing breast cancer[9] and a 40 to 60 percent lifetime risk of developing ovarian cancer[48] (Fig. 47-6). Approximately 20 percent of female *BRCA1* mutation carriers will develop breast cancer by age 40 years, 51 percent by age 50 years, and 87 percent by age 70. *BRCA1* mutation carriers also have an increased incidence of bilateral breast cancer. In a study of 33 families with evidence of germ-line mutations in *BRCA1* conducted by the Breast Cancer Linkage Consortium, the cumulative risk of developing a second breast cancer was estimated to be 65 percent for mutations carriers who live to age 70.[48] However, ascertainment bias again affects these risk estimates.

However, studies of families segregating *BRCA1* mutations have shown that in many cases the mutations are nonpenetrant. By focusing on founder mutations in the Ashkenazi population, Struewing and colleagues estimated the penetrance of *BRCA1* and *BRCA2* mutations in this population at 56 and 16 percent, respectively[49] (Fig. 47-6). Results from three additional population-based studies using estimates of *BRCA1* and *BRCA2* prevalence suggest that the risk for breast and ovarian cancer by age 80 years in mutation carriers is 73.5 and 27.8 percent, respectively.[50] Thus it is likely that different mutations, variable genetic background, and differential exposure to certain risk factors result in a great variation in penetrance. Currently, penetrance for breast cancer is thought to range between 56 and 86 percent.[51]

Risk for other cancers also may be increased in the presence of an inherited *BRCA1* mutation. Data published in 1993 from a study of a large Icelandic breast/ovarian cancer family suggested that prostate cancer may be a component of the *BRCA1* syndrome.[52] Subsequently, the Breast Cancer Linkage Consortium estimated a relative risk of 3.33 for prostate cancer in males thought to carry *BRCA1* germ-line mutations and a relative risk of 4.11 for colon cancer.[53] It is important to note that the excess colon cancer risk reflects the experience of only a few families, suggesting either very low penetrance with regard to colon cancer or a limited number of specific mutations that increase colon cancer risk. No significant excesses were observed for cancers originating from other anatomic sites.[53] Male breast cancer is only rarely associated with *BRCA1* germ-line mutations.

To determine whether tumors that arise as a result of *BRCA1* mutations have clinical and pathologic characteristics that differ from those of sporadic tumors, Lynch and colleagues analyzed 180 tumors from hereditary breast/ovarian or site-specific breast cancer families.[54] Ninety-eight of the 180 tumors were considered as a subset more likely than the remainder to result from *BRCA1* mutations on the basis of linkage analysis or the presence of ovarian cancer in the family. Patients in both subgroups were significantly younger than the population average for women with breast cancer. In addition, the "*BRCA1* group" was found to have more aneuploid and more high S-phase tumors, but surprisingly, disease-free survival was longer in this group than in the group thought less likely to have *BRCA1* mutations. Tubular and lobular cancers were less common in the group where the presence of *BRCA1* mutations was suspected. These investigators suggested that *BRCA1* mutations may result in tumors with adverse pathologic indicators but a paradoxically better survival than expected. Unfortunately, this study was performed before it was possible to determine which tumors were actually attributable to *BRCA1* mutations. Subsequent studies of the pathobiology of breast tumors associated with *BRCA1* verified that these tumors are often high grade and tend to be estrogen and progesterone receptor negative[20,55–59] (Fig. 47-7). One further study suggested a correlation between the absence of *BRCA1* in the nucleus of cells from *BRCA1* tumors and high proliferative rate.[60] However, the possibility that these tumors are associated with a paradoxically better survival has not been substantiated.

Several more recent studies have shown that survival for carriers of *BRCA1* mutations may be similar to that of sporadic breast cancer patients when controlling for stage of diagnosis,[61,62] and a study of Ashkenazi Jewish *BRCA1* mutation carriers suggested that *BRCA1* mutation is an adverse prognostic factor.[63] Genetic studies of *BRCA1*-related breast and ovarian tumors by comparative genome hybridization indicate that these tumors have high levels of amplification and deletion, suggesting that the tumors are genetically unstable and highly proliferative.[64,65] Several regions of amplification and deletion were identified in familial breast tumors, but not in sporadic breast tumors, whereas amplification of 2q24-q32 accounted for the only apparent difference between familial and sporadic ovarian tumors.[65]

Several environmental factors have been identified that modify the risk of breast and ovarian cancer in *BRCA1* mutation carriers.

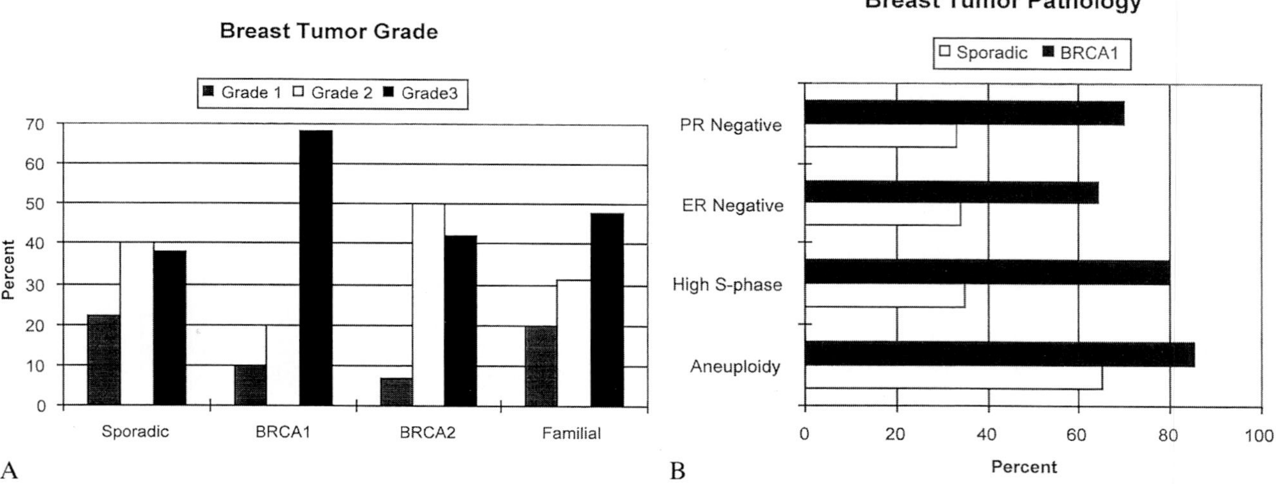

Fig. 47-7 Pathologic features of *BRCA1* and *BRCA2* breast cancers. *A.* Grade distribution of sporadic *BRCA1, BRCA2,* and combined familial breast tumors. (*Used with permission from MR Stratton.*[21]) *B.* Frequency of pathobiologic characteristics of sporadic and *BRCA1*-related breast tumors. PR refers to the progesterone receptor, and ER refers to the estrogen receptor. (Data from refs. 21,30,56, and 62.)

A recent study reported that women who smoke and have *BRCA1* or *BRCA2* mutations have a lower risk of breast cancer.[66] Subjects who smoked more than 4 pack-years had a lower breast cancer risk (odds ratio of 0.46, 95% CI = 0.27–0.80) than nonsmokers. One explanation for this observation is based on the relationship of estrogen to breast cancer and on the fact that women smokers are found to have lower levels of estrogen on average. This study is preliminary and needs to be repeated, taking into account the clustering of cases within specific families and adjusting for other effectors of circulating estrogen levels in the subjects.

Another recent study also reported that oral contraceptives may reduce the risk of ovarian cancer in *BRCA1* or *BRCA2* mutation carriers.[67] The odds ratio for ovarian cancer associated with any use of oral contraceptives was 0.5 (95% CI = 0.3–0.8). Oral contraceptive use for greater than 6 years was associated with a 60 percent risk reduction. While this result supports previous observations that oral contraceptives are protective for ovarian cancer, no consideration was given to the possible increased risk of breast cancer in this study. The study also contained a possible source of bias in the control group. First, many of the controls did not have a defined *BRCA1* or *BRCA2* mutation. Second, many of the controls who were assessed for ovarian cancer development had previously undergone prophylactic oophorectomy. And third, the controls contained a significantly lower proportion of Ashkenazi Jewish individuals than the study population. These findings await further confirmation.

It also is becoming clear that modifying genes affect the penetrance of *BRCA1* mutations.[68] In the first study to assess the role of potential modifiers of *BRCA1* penetrance, rare alleles at the *HRAS1* (*Harvey ras* proto-oncogene) VNTR were associated with an increased risk of ovarian cancer in individuals with a *BRCA1* mutation.[69] Recently, it has been reported that the common *APC I1307K* variant that occurs in 6 percent of the Ashkenazi Jewish population and has been associated with colorectal neoplasia is also associated with an increased risk of developing breast cancer in the Ashkenazi population.[70] In this study, 10.4 percent of individuals with breast cancer (unselected for family history of breast cancer) carried the variant in comparison with 6.8 percent of unaffected Ashkenazi controls. The frequency of the variant in carriers of *BRCA1* and *BRCA2* mutations was significantly greater than in controls (OR = 1.9, 95% CI = 1.2–3.0), suggesting an association between *BRCA1/2* mutations and the *APC* variant. However, no association between breast cancer risk and the *APC* variant was seen in patients without *BRCA1* or *BRCA2* mutations (OR = 1.4, 95% CI = 1.0–1.8),[70] nor was age at onset of breast cancer afffected by the presence of *I1307K* mutation.

Isolation of *BRCA1*. No information was available on the structure and function of the *BRCA1* gene before its identification in 1994; thus positional cloning was used by several groups in an attempt to isolate the gene. These efforts began in 1990 with identification of chromosome 17q21 as the location of *BRCA1*. Initial linkage analysis was performed on seven families and yielded a maximum cumulative Lod score of 5.98.[71] Several groups adopted linkage analysis and positional cloning strategies in an attempt to locate the *BRCA1* gene. In late 1994, this effort culminated in identification of the *BRCA1* gene by Miki and colleagues.[39]

BRCA1 is a novel gene composed of 24 exons, with an mRNA that is 7.8 kb in length, and 22 coding exons translating into a protein of 1863 amino acids (Fig. 47-8). The entire gene covers approximately 80 kb of genomic sequence. The structure of *BRCA1* is unusual, with most exons in the expected 100- to 500-bp size, but with exon 11 (approximately 3500 bp) constituting approximately 60 percent of the coding region of the gene (see Fig. 47-8). The functional or evolutionary significance of this unusual structure is unknown. Exon 4 is thought to be an artifact of the isolation method and is omitted from the gene sequence. The BRCA1 protein contains a zinc-binding RING finger motif near the N-terminus and two BRCT (*BRCA1* C-terminal) domains in tandem (motif 1: amino acids 1653–1736; motif 2: amino acids 1760–1855). The RING finger motif has been identified in numerous transcription factors and cofactors involved in both DNA and protein binding, suggesting a role for *BRCA1* in transcription regulation, while the BRCT motifs have been found in a number of proteins involved in cell cycle control and DNA repair.[72]

The murine homologue of *BRCA1* has been characterized by several groups.[73–75] The mouse cDNA sequence predicts a protein of 1812 amino acids, 51 residues shorter than the human cDNA. The human and mouse proteins display 58 percent identity and 73 percent similarity, with perfect conservation in the RING finger domain near the N-terminus and high homology in a putative acidic transactivation domain at the C-terminus.[73] The canine form of *BRCA1* also has been identified and sequenced and, similar to the murine form, displays greater than 80 percent identity in both the RING domain and in 80 amino acids at the C-terminus containing the acidic transactivation domain.[76] Finally, a fragment of the rat *BRCA1* gene containing the RING domain has been

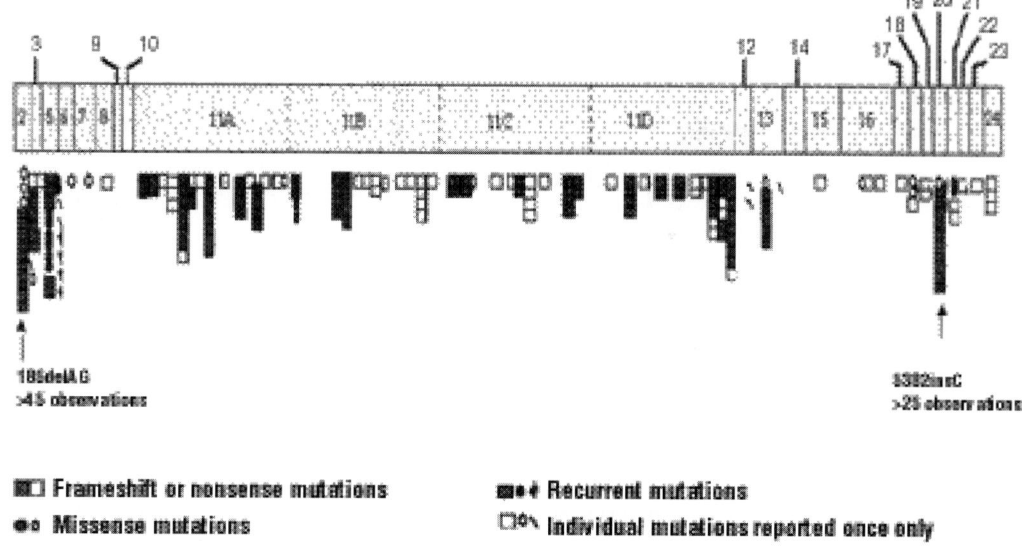

Fig. 47-8 Structure and mutation spectrum of *BRCA1.* Diagram demonstrating even distribution of mutations across the *BRCA1* coding sequence. The 24 exons of *BRCA1* are represented by vertical lines within the gene. Mutations are depicted beneath the *BRCA1* exon where the mutation occurrs. Mutations are categorized according to recurrance and mutation type, as shown in the accompanying key. The idiogram was copied from the Breast Cancer Information Core (BIC) Web site and was generated by Simon Gayther, Cambridge, U.K.

sequenced and shown to have high homology with the human form.[77]

Mutational Spectrum. Since the identification of *BRCA1,* more than 500 sequence variations have been detected (see Fig. 47-8). Initial reports described eight disease-associated mutations within the gene,[39,78] followed shortly afterward by an increasing number of novel mutations.[79–81] Surprisingly, almost all described mutations are germ-line mutations, with *BRCA1* mutations being extremely rare in sporadic breast and ovarian tumors,[82–85] suggesting that *BRCA1* coding-region mutations play a limited role in the development of sporadic breast cancer. A single individual has been reported to be homozygous for a *BRCA1* mutation, inheriting the same mutation from each parent.[86] This homozygous individual is developmentally normal but was diagnosed with breast cancer at age 32.

A variety of mutation-detection techniques have been used to identify *BRCA1* mutations, including SSCP,[79,80,87] protein truncation assays,[88,89] multiplex heteroduplex analysis,[90] conformation-sensitive gel electrophoresis,[44,91] and most commonly, direct sequencing. Details of these techniques are available on the Breast Cancer Information Core (BIC) Web site: *http://www.nchgr.nih.gov/dir/Intramural_Res/Lab_transfer/Bic/.* A report from 1996 describing the first 254 sequence variants in the *BRCA1* gene showed that 55 percent of the mutations were located in exon 11 (which contains 62 percent of the gene-coding sequence), suggesting that sequence alterations are scattered evenly throughout *BRCA1.*[92] In this early summary, the great majority of mutations resulted in truncation or absence of the protein product. This number included frameshift and nonsense mutations, splice variants that also create frameshifts and stop codons in the gene, and ill-defined noncoding region mutations. The remaining sequence variants were nontruncating missense mutations within the *BRCA1* coding sequence. The four noncoding region mutations were inferred from inactivation of transcription of one allele of *BRCA1.*[39,93,94] The specific DNA alterations that result in inactivation of transcription in these samples have not been determined. Serova and colleagues also identified various regions of the *BRCA1* cDNA that when mutated led to complete loss of the allele-specific transcript, presumably as a result of destabilization and degradation of mRNA.[94]

Analysis of more than 500 *BRCA1* mutations in the BIC database suggests that the data for the earlier study were biased toward truncating mutations. It is now believed that approximately 30 percent of all *BRCA1* mutations are missense alterations. This group of sequence alterations includes defined disease-associated mutations, polymorphisms, and unclassified variants. Several *BRCA1* missense mutations are thought to inactivate *BRCA1* function. The C61G variant is thought to alter the structure of the RING finger domain,[95] which is known to bind both the BARD[96] and BAP[97] proteins. The C64G variant originally was reported as a RING finger missense mutation; however, this variant could also result in altered splicing and a frameshift within *BRCA1* due to the formation of a cryptic slice site. In addition, a G $\rightarrow$ C transversion at nucleotide 117 in the Kozak site of the *BRCA1* gene recently has been postulated to alter translation of the BRCA1 protein.[98] Several missense mutations from the exon 17–21 region of *BRCA1,* which is now known to encode a transcription activation domain, also have been shown to ablate *BRCA1* function by a yeast growth assay.[99] The assay also was successful in identifying several nonfunctional polymorphisms. In the absence of functional assays, frequency data currently are being used to predict the role of missense mutation in disease. However, conclusive evidence awaits the establishment of a robust *BRCA1* functional assay.

Two studies have determined that large genomic deletions form part of the constellation of *BRCA1* mutations. Mazoyer and colleagues identified a 1.7-kb deletion within *BRCA1* that was postulated to result from inter-Alu recombination.[100] Three genomic deletions within the *BRCA1* gene have been shown to account for 30 percent of *BRCA1* mutations in the Dutch-Belgian high-risk breast cancer population.[101] The high frequency of Alu-related repetitive sequences in the intronic regions of *BRCA1* is thought to facilitate the formation of these deletions by homologous recombination.

Two studies have identified a genotype-phenotype correlation,[93,102] suggesting that mutations in the 5′ half of *BRCA1* predispose to both breast and ovarian cancer, whereas mutations closer to the 3′ portion of the gene are predominantly associated with site-specific breast cancer. This correlation is rarely seen in the *BRCA1* populations from the United States but holds up well in the majority of European studies. Mutations occurring in two terminal regions of *BRCA1* may be associated with a more severe phenotype, as defined by high tumor grade,[103] suggesting that these two regions may be important in the control of mammary cell growth.

The two most common mutations in *BRCA1* are 185delAG and 5382insC.[92] These mutations have been shown to occur at a frequency of 8 and 1.2 per 1000 individuals in the Ashkenazi Jewish population,[49,104] as compared with the overall frequency of *BRCA1* mutations in an unselected Caucasian population of about 1 in 1500, suggesting the presence of a founder effect in the Ashkenazi Jewish population. This observation has been expanded to include the Moroccan Iraqi and Yemenite Jewish populations.[105] Analysis of germ-line *BRCA1* mutations in Jewish and non-Jewish women with early onset breast cancer indicated that approximately 21 percent of Jewish women who develop breast cancer before age 40 may carry the 185delAG mutation.[106,107] Preliminary screening of unselected Ashkenazi Jewish patients showed that 20 to 60 percent with ovarian cancer and 30 percent with early onset breast cancer carried either the 185delAG *BRCA1* mutation or the 6174delT *BRCA2* mutation.[108–110]

Haplotype analysis of 185delAG *BRCA1* mutation carriers has identified two common haplotypes within the Ashkenazi Jewish population.[111] These studies suggest that although these are ancestral mutations, several founder populations may have arisen independently. The location of the mutation in a tandem AG repeat suggests that this may be a hypermutable region. Other haplotype studies have identified three common haplotypes in a large series of breast and ovarian cancer cases using four common polymorphisms.[112] No association was found between the presence of the common haplotypes and breast or ovarian cancer, suggesting that common polymorphisms in *BRCA1* do not make a significant contribution to development of breast or ovarian cancer. However, the same study suggested that the Gln356Arg polymorphism may be associated with a protective effect against breast cancer and thus actually may be a gain-of-function mutation.

A number of studies have investigated the frequency of *BRCA1* mutations in subpopulations. Founder mutations identified thus far include the G5193A mutation in three Icelandic families,[113] the 3745delT and IVS1-2A → G mutations in the Finnish population,[114] and the185delAG and 5382insC mutations in the Ashkenazi Jewish,[49] Hungarian,[115] and Russian[116] populations. Common genomic deletions have been found in the Dutch-Belgian population,[101] along with the 1675delA mutation in the Norwegian population.[117] King and Szabo recently presented a comprehensive review of many of these studies.[118]

A number of large mutation screening studies of women with breast and/or ovarian cancer with and without a family history of breast and/or ovarian cancer also have been completed in an effort to define the prevalence of *BRCA1* mutations in certain subsets of the population and to determine risk estimates for women conforming to the selection criteria. Studies of *BRCA1* mutations in women with early onset breast cancer have shown that approximately 10 percent of unselected breast cancer patients under 40 years of age carry *BRCA1* mutations. Similarly, only 7 percent of site-specific breast cancer families carry mutations. In comparison, 17 to 20 percent of all breast cancer families including those with breast and ovarian cancer possess *BRCA1* mutations. This indicates that ovarian cancer within a family is a strong predictor of the presence of a *BRCA1* mutation.[44] The data also suggest that other, as yet unidentified genes exist that predispose to early onset breast cancer and site-specific breast cancer. A number of other studies have validated these results and have extended the studies to show that only 7 percent of breast cancer patients under 45 years of age with an affected first-degree relative carried *BRCA1* mutations.[119] In a similar study and the first to consider *BRCA1* mutation prevalence in the African-American population, it was reported that 3 percent of Caucasians and less than 1 percent of African-Americans with breast cancer unselected for family history possessed *BRCA1* mutations.[120] Cumulatively, these data suggest that *BRCA1* mutations are rare in those individuals who do not have a significant family history of breast and/or ovarian cancer. Similar studies have not yet been reported for Hispanics, Asians, Native Americans, and other ethnic populations. A summary of these studies is presented in Table 47-4.[44,45,47,49,92,94,108,110,119–123]

Table 47-4 Germ-line BRACA1 and BRCA2 Mutations in Select Populations

Population	No. of Cases	Percent with Germ-line Mutations
BRCA1		
High-risk families*		
Britain	339	21%
France	160	24%
Sweden	106	23%
USA	238	26.5%
High-risk Ashkenazi Jewish		
Israel	42	38%
Early onset breast cancer, non-Ashkenazi Jewish		
USA, < 40 y	94	13%
USA, < 32 y	73	12.3%
Japan, < 35, bilateral	103	4%
Early onset breast cancer, Ashkenazi		
USA, < 40 y	39	21%
Population based		
USA, Jewish	5318	1.15%
US Breast cancer cases (North Carolina)		
White	120	3.3%
Black	88	8%
US breast cancer cases (Seattle)		
< 35 y	193	6.2%
< 45 y, 1st degree affected	208	7.2%
BRCA2		
High-risk families		
Finland	100	11%
Sweden	106	11.3%
Europe	22	27%
USA	238	13%
High-risk Ashkenazi Jewish		
Israel	42	21%
Early onset breast cancer, non-Ashkenazi Jewish		
USA, < 32	73	2.7%
Early onset breast cancer, Ashkenazi Jewish		
Israel, < 40 y	43	7%
Population based		
Washington, D.C., Jewish	5318	1.11%
Male breast cancer (USA)		
Family history	50	14%
Unselected	54	3.7%

*High-risk families have three or more cases of female breast and/or any cases of ovarian cancer.

NOTE: All cases represent individuals affected with breast cancer.[118] Visit the BIC Web site at for a comprehensive listing at: http://ruly70.medfac.leidenuniv.nl/~devilee/screen.htm.

Clinical Utility of Mutation Testing. Testing for *BRCA1* and *BRCA2* mutations is now widely available both commercially and in research studies. One problem associated with mutation screening is the identification of missense mutations that cannot be classified as either benign variants or disease-associated mutations. Approximately 20 percent of all identified variants reported in the BIC database excluding common polymorphisms are missense mutations. Improvement in the identification of disease-associated variants awaits the development of functional assays for the *BRCA1* and *BRCA2* genes. A second difficulty is the recent realization that current mutation screening technology may fail to identify as many as 20 to 30 percent of mutations in families linked to the *BRCA1* and *BRCA2* genes. A third problem associated with testing is the observation that perhaps only 40 percent of high-risk breast cancer families are associated with *BRCA1* and *BRCA2* mutations. Thus a high percentage of mutation tests will produce negative results.

In an attempt to improve the selection of patients for mutation testing, several laboratories have generated frequency tables and models based on screening of high-risk women that predict the presence of a *BRCA1* mutation. The first study of this kind identified *BRCA1* mutations in 169 women with breast cancer from high-risk families containing from 1 to 11 cases of breast cancer. A probability model was developed that predicts the presence of a *BRCA1* mutation by considering family characteristics, including (1) average age of onset of breast cancer in the family, (2) Ashkenazi Jewish ancestry, (3) presence of ovarian cancer, and (4) presence of breast and ovarian cancer in a single individual.[44] A second *BRCA1* predictive model used frequency data from mutation studies of several hundred individuals to provide probabilities for the presence of a *BRCA1* mutation. Probability tables were provided for (1) number of breast cancers, (2) number of ovarian cancers, and (3) age of onset of the individual.[46] A third group generated a mathematical model for predicting the presence of *BRCA1* or *BRCA2* mutations. Estimates of *BRCA1* and *BRCA2* mutation frequencies and age-specific incidence rates for breast and ovarian cancer were used to predict the presence of a mutation. The model is based on the cancer status of all first- and second-degree relatives and the age of onset of affected individuals.[124] Thus the probability that an individual from a high-risk family has a *BRCA1* or *BRCA2* mutation can be estimated using one or more of the models described earlier.

Molecular Biology of *BRCA1*. *BRCA1* does not appear to be a member of a known gene family on the basis of sequence analysis, other than as a member of a widespread group of cell cycle control and DNA repair genes that contain BRCT domains. Southern blotting of human genomic DNA detects a single band, suggesting that only one copy is present in the human genome. Northern blotting of human and mouse tissue with a *BRCA1* probe has been performed by a number of laboratories. Initial reports using a *BRCA1* fragment as a probe described a 7.8-kb RNA and several splice variants formed as a result of alternate splicing at the 5′ end of the transcript.[39,125,126] Subsequent work with a probe representing the complete coding region of *BRCA1* identified several additional transcripts. Three of these variants have been identified as (1) an in-frame deletion of exon 11, (2) a deletion of exon 11 117 bp from the 5′ splice acceptor, and (3) an in-frame deletion of exon 10.[127,128] Of greatest significance is the observation that deletion of exon 11 results in removal of the nuclear localization signal of *BRCA1*. Thus the proteins encoded by the exon 11-deleted forms of *BRCA1* may be localized in the cytoplasm of the cell. The functional significance of these isoforms is under investigation.

The two regions of near 100 percent homology between human and murine *BRCA1* have been studied in detail by several groups. The N-terminal RING finger domain has been screened extensively for a DNA-binding function with no success reported. Studies of protein-protein interaction by yeast twin-hybrid analysis has resulted in the identification of a BRCA1-binding protein termed *BRCA1 activator protein-1* (BAP1)[97] that is thought to function as a ubiquitin hydrolase that enhances BRCA1-mediated

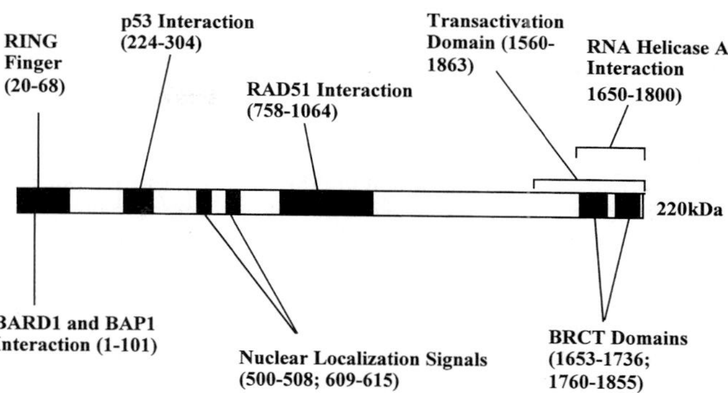

Fig. 47-9 Functional domains of *BRCA1*. Idiogram of the 220-kDa BRCA1 protein depicting known functional domains. Domains are shown as filled areas within the diagram.

cell growth suppression. BAP and BRCA1 co-localize in the cell nucleus. A second protein shown to bind the RING finger of BRCA1 has been termed *BARD1*.[129] This protein contains a zinc finger domain and two BRCT domains that are commonly found in proteins involved in DNA repair. BARD1 colocalizes with BRCA1 in the cell nucleus during S phase but not G phase of the cell cycle.[130] BRCA1 also complexes with Rad51[131] and BRCA2.[132] Since both these proteins have been associated with cellular response to double-strand DNA breaks, this further suggests a role for BRCA1 in DNA damage repair.

Studies of the C-terminal acidic activation domain by yeast two-hybrid and mammalian two-hybrid assays have shown that this region of BRCA1, as well as the complete BRCA1 protein, can function as a coactivator of transcription, as detailed below[133–135] (Fig. 47-9). BRCA1 also has been shown to bind to the oligomerization domain of p53.[136] The interaction between BRCA1 and p53 has been associated with activation of p21 expression, leading to a cell cycle pause.[137] These data suggest that BRCA1 functions as a coactivator of p53-regulated transcription. Finally, BRCA1 has been shown to bind to the RNA polymerase II holoenzyme through RNA helicase A[138,139] and to the transcription coactivator and histone acetylase CREB-binding protein (CBP).[140] The association of BRCA1 with these proteins also suggests that BRCA1 functions as a transcriptional coactivator and forms a key component of the bridge between DNA-binding transcription factors and RNA polymerase II.

In addition, a novel kinase activity has been copurified with amino acids 329–435 of BRCA1.[141] This activity does not involve protein kinase A (PKA), protein kinase C (PKC), or casein kinase II (CKII). However, the purification of a kinase activity supports the observation that BRCA1 is a phosphoprotein and suggests that this kinase may play a role in regulation of BRCA1 function.

***BRCA1* Gene Regulation.** Shortly after identification of *BRCA1*, the sequence of 1345 bp of genomic DNA proximal to the putative transcription start site was identified.[125] This 1345-bp region was notable for the inclusion of the putative promoters of both the *BRCA1* gene and the *1A1.3B* gene, a homologue of CA-125 encoding a protein of unknown function that is overexpressed in some ovarian tumors. These genes are located head to head with transcription start sites located 295 bp apart, raising the possibility that sharing of promoters between the two genes acts as a regulatory mechanism. Physical mapping of the *BRCA1* region identified a large duplicated region containing the 5′ end of the *BRCA1* gene; a partial pseudogene of *BRCA1* containing exons 1A, 1B, and 2; the functional *1A1.3B* gene; and a *1A1.3B* pseudogene containing exons 1A, 1B, and 3.[125] A second transcription start site for *BRCA1* also was identified that initiates transcription in an alternative exon 1 located in intron 1. Thus two promoters for *BRCA1* have been located separated by approximately 2 kb of genomic DNA. These *BRCA1* promoters contain consensus binding elements for multiple transcription factors including p53 and AP2, although no data are available concerning the functionality of these sites. Studies of the *BRCA1* promoter detected CpG methylation of a CREB (cAMP-responsive element-binding) site in breast tumors but not in normal tissues, suggesting that methylation of regulatory sequences in the *BRCA1* promoter may be a method of inactivation of *BRCA1* in breast tumors.[142] A further report of hypermethylation of two of seven sporadic breast carcinomas with no methylation of normal tissues supports this hypothesis.[143]

***BRCA1* and Estrogen Response.** Little is known about the transcriptional regulation of the *BRCA1* gene, although BRCA1 mRNA and protein levels have been shown to be altered by some steroid hormones in an indirect manner.[144–147] In these studies, estrogen, as well as a mixture of estrogen and progesterone, has been shown to increase BRCA1 mRNA and protein levels in human cell line[144,145] and mRNA levels in animal models; however, protein levels were not analyzed in this system.[147] This induction appears to result indirectly in association with the increased cellular proliferation and DNA synthesis following estrogen exposure and not from direct activity of the estrogen receptor on the *BRCA1* promoter.[148,149] This is evidenced by the fact that putative estrogen response elements in the *BRCA1* promoter fails to respond to 17-β-estradiol,[148] and application of cyclohexamide to block protein synthesis inhibits the induction of *BRCA1* expression.[150]

Subcellular Localization of BRCA1. The subcellular localization of BRCA1 was studied initially by cell fractionation and immunofluorescence of breast cancer cell lines, "normal" breast epithelial cell lines, and breast tumor tissue. BRCA1 was detected in the nucleus of the normal cells and in the cytoplasm or in both the cytoplasm and the nucleus of almost all breast cancer cell lines through the use of three polyclonal BRCA1 antibodies.[151] Staining of primary cells from pleural effusions and cells in tissue sections also provided evidence that BRCA1 was located predominantly in the cytoplasm of malignant cells, suggesting that subcellular mislocalization of BRCA1 may be a mechanism by which BRCA1 plays a role in the pathogenesis of sporadic breast tumors. However, a similar study performed by Scully and colleagues using fixed tissue sections and BRCA1 monoclonal antibodies demonstrated localization of BRCA1 to the nucleus in every section analyzed. This group also tested a variety of methods of tissue fixation and determined that technical variation may lead to apparent cytoplasmic localization of BRCA1.[152] To add to this confusion, BRCA1 was noted to have homology to a granin consensus sequence. Granins are proteins that are secreted and modified to form bioactive peptides that act on the cell surface. In studies by Jensen and colleagues, polyclonal antibodies against the last 20 C-terminal amino acids identified a 190-kDa protein localized to the cytoplasm, Golgi network, and secretory vesicles.[153] Fractionation studies and confocal imaging supported these results, the latter purportedly identifying the protein they believed to be BRCA1 being released from a secretory body on the extracellular surface. Subsequent experiments indicate that the two polyclonal antibodies used by Jensen and colleagues detect BRCA1 as well as EGF-R and HER-2/*neu* and that it is the latter two proteins that are detected on the extracellular surface and in the Golgi network.[154] Immunofluorescence studies of BRCA1 using a variety of BRCA1 polyclonal and monoclonal antibodies have demonstrated that BRCA1 transfected into cell lines is localized in the nucleus, whereas BRCA1 splice forms or mutants deleted for the consensus nuclear localization signal in exon 11 are located in the cytoplasm.[127] The current consensus is that BRCA1 is localized to the nucleus in normal cells; however, no consensus has been reached concerning the location of BRCA1 in cells from breast cancer lines or tumors. Therefore, it is unknown whether aberrant localization of BRCA1 is a mechanism by which BRCA1 plays a role in the development of sporadic breast cancer. A functional consensus nuclear localization signal in BRCA1 exon 11 has been identified[127] (see Fig. 47-9), multiple laboratories have replicated the initial observation that BRCA1 is a nuclear protein, and the controversy is largely resolved.

***BRCA1* and Tumor Suppression.** Before its isolation, *BRCA1* was predicted to function as a tumor-suppressor gene based on frequent loss of heterozygosity in *BRCA1*-associated tumors, where the deleted region invariantly included the wild-type allele.[155,156] These data suggested that malignant transformation occurs when both functional copies of *BRCA1* are lost, a pattern indicative of a tumor-suppressor gene. After isolation of the gene, Thompson and colleagues demonstrated that the presence of antisense oligonucleotides complementary to BRCA1 RNA significantly increased the growth rate of MCF-7 cells in comparison with untreated cells, indicating that reduction of BRCA1 RNA levels was associated with an increased growth rate in these cells.[157] Analysis of BRCA1 RNA levels in tumors also suggested that *BRCA1* was down-regulated in sporadic tumors compared with normal breast epithelium. Subsequent studies using NIH-3T3 fibroblasts indicated that BRCA1 antisense RNA could reduce native BRCA1 RNA levels and result in a transformed phenotype in these cells. This group also demonstrated that nontumorigenic NIH-3T3 cells formed tumors in nude mice when treated with antisense BRCA1 RNA.[102] The growth-inhibitory properties of BRCA1 were then tested in animal models and cell lines. Retroviral transfer of wild-type BRCA1 inhibited the growth of two breast cancer cell lines and three ovarian cancer cell lines. Finally, it was demonstrated that the development of MCF-7 tumors in nude mice was inhibited in the presence of wild-type BRCA1 and unaffected by the presence of mutant BRCA1, adding further support to the hypothesis that *BRCA1* functions as a tumor suppressor.[102]

Further study of the role of BRCA1 in cell growth control has proved difficult because of consistent problems with the development of cell lines stably transfected with wild-type BRCA1, since transfected cells die rapidly in culture. Shao and colleagues analyzed this phenomenon and determined that constitutive expression of an exon 11-deleted form of BRCA1 results in induction of apoptosis, especially notable in conjunction with serum starvation or calcium ionophore treatment.[158] However, the use of the deleted form of BRCA1 complicates the interpretation of this study and suggests that further evidence is required in order to associate BRCA1 with apoptosis.

Of note, a recent report described the characterization of a novel breast cancer cell line derived from the breast carcinoma of a germ-line *BRCA1* mutation carrier. The patient carried a 5382insC mutation in *BRCA1,* and the tumor demonstrated loss of the wild-type *BRCA1* allele. Thus the cell line only contains a truncated form of the *BRCA1* gene that may or may not retain some level of function. While a number of additional genetic alterations have been identified in this cell line (a *p53* mutation, a *PTEN* deletion, and others), further cellular studies of *BRCA1* function will be greatly enhanced by the availability of this breast epithelial *BRCA1* mutant cell line.[159]

***BRCA1* and the Cell Cycle.** A connection between *BRCA1* and the cell cycle was suggested originally by studies of breast cancer cell lines treated with estrogen, which demonstrated that BRCA1 and cyclin A RNA levels increased in parallel in response to the hormone treatment.[144] It is now known that BRCA1 is a nuclear phosphoprotein that is phosphorylated in a cell cycle-dependent manner.[160] The greatest expression and phosphorylation of BRCA1 are observed in the S and M phases of the cell cycle. Cyclin-dependent kinase 2 and cyclin D- and A-associated kinases bind to and phosphorylate BRCA1, suggesting that BRCA1 function may be regulated by cyclin-dependent kinase phosphorylation. Subsequent studies showed that BRCA1 RNA levels were highest in rapidly growing cells, decreased after growth factor withdrawal, and increased at the G1/S phase boundary in synchronized cells.[145] BRCA1 RNA levels also were reduced in senescent cells and cells treated with transforming growth factor beta (TGFβ), indicating that BRCA1 expression is sensitive to *in vitro* growth conditions and may play a role in G1/S phase checkpoint control or merely be up-regulated at this point in the cell cycle in response to cellular messages. Vaughan and colleagues described similar findings and extended their analysis to include BRCA1 protein levels. In this study, induction of BRCA1 occurred before the initiation of DNA synthesis at the G1/S boundary.[146] Finally, overexpression of the BRCT transactivation domain led to increased growth rate through loss of a colchicine-induced G2/M block.[161] The cumulative data suggest that BRCA1 plays a role in cell cycle checkpoint control and is regulated by kinases and phosphatases that are known to play a role in the regulation of the cell cycle.

BRCA1 and Development. The first studies of the role of BRCA1 in development were performed by *in situ* hybridization of mouse embryos. Whole-mount embryos hybridized with mouse BRCA1 probe indicated that BRCA1 was widely expressed in many developing tissues, suggesting that BRCA1 may play a role in tissue development, possibly as a ubiquitous transcription factor.[147] Northern blots of mouse mammary gland RNAs also were used to demonstrate that BRCA1 was highly expressed in the mouse gland during pregnancy, remaining above pregestational levels at least 4 weeks after postlactational regression of the mammary epithelium. These results suggest that BRCA1 is involved in cell proliferation in breast epithelial cells and is regulated at least secondarily by ovarian hormone changes during pregnancy.

Further studies have supported the observation that BRCA1 is expressed in proliferating cells of embryos in the mammary gland during morphogenesis and in most adult tissues. BRCA1 exhibited a hormone-independent expression pattern in the oocytes, granulosa cells, and thecal cells of developing ovarian follicles and in the mitotic spermatogenia and meiotic spermatocytes of the testes.[162]

Gowen and colleagues produced the first *BRCA1* nullizyous mice. The disrupted allele was generated by the complete deletion of *BRCA1* exon 11 and flanking intron sequences, resulting in embryonic lethality 10 to 13 days after conception.[163] Abnormalities were most evident in the neural tube, with 40 percent of the embryos exhibiting spina bifida and anencephaly. In all homozygous null mice, the neuroepithelium appeared disorganized, with excessive cell growth as well as increased cell death. This report substantiated the work of Marquis and colleagues,[147] suggesting that *BRCA1* plays an important role in early murine development.

Hakem and colleagues also reported on the development of homozygous null *BRCA1* mice. The construct used for the generation of these mice was made by targeted deletion of exons 5 and 6, introducing stop codon in all three reading frames. The early truncation of the protein, coupled with deletion of a portion of the RING finger domain, was expected to yield a severely affected phenotype. These homozygous null mice have a phenotype slightly different from that of mice produced by Koller and colleagues and die before day 7.5 of embryogenesis.[164] The death of mutant embryos before gastrulation was postulated to result from failure of the proliferative burst necessary for the development of early germ layers. No increase in apoptosis was detected in these mice, but cell proliferation was reduced. These results again suggest a role for BRCA1 as a growth activator in early development. Further analysis demonstrated that the absence of BRCA1 was associated with reduced expression of mdm-2 and cyclin E, whereas expression of the cyclin-dependent kinase (cdk) inhibitor p21 was dramatically increased.

Liu and colleagues also generated a mouse with homozygous disruptions in *BRCA1* by replacing 186 bp of exon 11 with a neomycin resistance gene, resulting in protein truncation. These animals die at 4.5 to 8.5 days of embrogenesis.[165] The embryos fail to form egg cylinders and are unable to complete gastrulation. The difference between the Koller mice and the Liu mice may be accounted for by mouse strain differences and by stability differences in the mutant transcripts of *BRCA1*. Finally, Ludwig and colleagues reported that loss of p53 in association with loss of BRCA1 by deletion of exon 2 in a $BRCA1^{-/-}$, $p53^{-/-}$ embryo resulted in a less severe phenotype than that observed in the $BRCA1^{-/-}$ embryo. The *BRCA1/p53* double nullizygous mutants were significantly more advanced developmentally than the $BRCA1^{-/-}$ mice and survived to 9.5 days of embryogenesis.[166] These data support the data described above that suggest that p53 and BRCA1 are functionally associated. The accumulating data increasingly suggest that BRCA1 plays a role in cell cycle regulation, but how this function is associated with tumor suppression and early embryonic development is not yet understood.

***BRCA1* and Transcription.** As noted earlier, *BRCA1* contains a C-terminal transactivation domain,[133,134] as first defined by the yeast two-hybrid system. The transactivation domain was mapped to the region of the protein encoded by exons 21–24 using deletion constructs of *BRCA1* fused to the Gal4 DNA binding domain in both the yeast and mammalian systems. The ability of the transactivation domain to activate a Gal4 promoter was ablated by the addition of specific missense mutations in both hosts.[99,134] It also was shown that expression of human BRCA1 in *Saccharomyces cereviseae* resulted in a small-colony or slow-growth phenotype. Expression of mutant *BRCA1* failed to produce the small-colony effect, leading to the suggestion that the yeast growth assay could be used as a functional assay for C-terminal *BRCA1* mutations.[99] The transactivation domain of *BRCA1* coincides with the position of the second BRCT domain, suggesting that the BRCT domain can, but does not always, function as an activation domain.[167] Thus different proteins may use this domain for diverse functions. As mentioned previously, BRCA1 has been shown to physically interact with the BARD1 protein.[129] The presence of a DNA-binding zinc finger domain and two BRCT domains suggests that BARD1 functions as a member of transcriptional complexes, and the association between the two proteins further implicates BRCA1 in this process of transcription.

The association between BRCA1 and transcription was further strengthened when Somasundaram and colleagues demonstrated that BRCA1 was capable of activating the p21 promoter.[137] This activation was reported initially as p53-independent and resulted in a partial S phase block and a reduction of DNA synthesis in SW480 p53 null cells. Missense mutations in the *BRCA1* transactivation domain resulted in decreases in p21 induction. Subsequent studies determined that the p21, mdm2, and bax promoters could all be activated by BRCA1 in a p53-dependent manner and that amino acids 261–314 of BRCA1 physically interacted with the oligomerization domain of p53[135,136] (see Fig. 47-9). Hanafusa and colleagues were unable to validate the p53-independent transactivating potential of BRCA1[135] but provided supporting data for the role of BRCA1 as a coactivator of p53-dependent transcription.

In support of this role, Scully and colleagues demonstrated that BRCA1 interacts with the RNA polymerase II holoenzyme[168] (see Fig. 47-9). Other investigators have shown that BRCA1 colocalizes with PCNA at DNA replication forks and transcription sites and interacts specifically with RNA helicase A.[138] Finally, it has been suggested that BRCA1 associates with CBP and modulates histone transacetylase activity[140] and complexes with BRCA1 in the S phase of the cell cycle and in response to DNA damage. The amalgamation of these studies strongly suggests that one of the primary roles of BRCA1 in the cell is to function as a coactivator of transcription. No evidence has yet been presented that BRCA1 can directly bind DNA.

BRCA1 and Cellular Response to DNA Damage. A substantial amount of evidence implicating BRCA1 in the response to DNA damage has been generated. BRCA1 nullizygous embryos present with the same phenotype at 6.5 days of embryogenesis as seen in Rad51 nullizygous embryos.[169] BRCA1 also colocalizes with Rad51 and BARD1 to nuclear foci during S phase of the cell cycle in mitotic cells and coimmunoprecipitates.[130,131] Rad51 is a RecA homologue and has been implicated in double-strand DNA break repair and recombination in yeast.[170] In meiotic cells, the BRCA1 and Rad51 proteins colocalize to axial filaments of the synaptonemal complex. The S phase foci disperse in response to hydroxyurea, ultraviolet radiation, mitomycin C, or gamma irradiation[168] and are not associated with altered phosphorylation states of BRCA1. Following dispersal, BRCA1, BARD1, and Rad51 accumulate at PCNA replication structures. A similar study demonstrated that hydrogen peroxide also induces BRCA1 phosphorylation and nuclear focus dispersal and suggests that BRCA1 undergoes cyclic hyperphosphorylation in the cell cycle and in response to DNA damage.[171] These studies implicate BRCA1 in several different DNA damage-associated pathways. Further attempts to identify damaging agents and response pathways involving BRCA1 showed that adriamycin and ultraviolet irradiation was associated with down-regulated BRCA1 expression in a mutant p53 ovarian cancer cell line,[172] suggesting that BRCA1-associated DNA damage response may be dependent on p53 function. However, in a separate study, overexpression of wild-type BRCA1 increased prostate cancer cell line sensitivity to adriamycin and drug-induced apoptosis and reduced efficiency of single-strand DNA break repair.[173] Resistance to *cis*-diamine dichloroplatinum (CDDP) also has been associated with induction of BRCA1 expression, and antisense BRCA1 expression has been associated with CDDP sensitivity.[174]

Finally, *BRCA1* nullizygous mouse embryonic stem cells have been shown to be hypersensitive to ionizing radiation and hydrogen peroxide and are unable to perform preferential transcription-coupled repair of oxidative DNA damage, as measured by thymine glycol removal.[175] Ultraviolet radiation damage of the transcribed strand was unaffected by the absence of BRCA1. Taken together, these data suggest that BRCA associates with Rad51 and plays a role in transcription-coupled double-strand DNA damage repair. However, it is possible that BRCA1 is also involved in other mechanisms of DNA damage repair that are uncoupled from transcription.

A recent commentary introduced the concept of gatekeeper and caretaker genes in cancer initiation and progression. In this model, caretaker genes including *BRCA1* and *BRCA2* do not promote tumor initiation directly but function to regulate genome stability. Elimination of the caretaker function leads to eventual mutation of gatekeeper genes that directly initiate tumorigenesis.[176] The discovery that cells without functional BRCA1 are hypersensitive to DNA damage supports this hypothesis. Further evidence comes from the observation that *p53* mutations are significantly more common in *BRCA1*-associated breast tumors than in sporadic tumor controls.[177] In addition, an increased frequency of *p53* mutations was found in association with loss of heterozygosity at the *BRCA1* and *BRCA2* loci in breast carcinomas.[178] Mutations in *p53* also were found in 80 percent of *BRCA1*-associated ovarian tumors, suggesting that *p53* mutations are important in but perhaps not essential for *BRCA1*-associated tumorigenesis.[179] In this case, mutation of *BRCA1* may lead to increased genome instability, resulting in mutation of the gatekeeper *p53* gene and subsequent tumor formation.

BRCA2

Clinical Features of Affected Families. Initial progress toward the identification of a second breast cancer susceptibility gene came from a linkage analysis of 22 families with multiple cases of early onset female breast cancer and at least one case of male breast cancer. Twelve of these families also had at least one individual diagnosed with ovarian cancer.[180] All 22 families were analyzed for linkage between breast cancer and genetic markers flanking the *BRCA1* candidate region on chromosome 17. A maximum Lod score of −6.63 was obtained, providing strong evidence against linkage to *BRCA1* in these families. This study demonstrated that only a small proportion of breast cancer families with at least one case of male breast cancer were likely to be associated with germ-line mutations in *BRCA1*, arguing strongly for the existence of at least one additional breast cancer susceptibility gene, now known to be *BRCA2*. Shortly after the appearance of this report, a large collaborative group succeeded in identifying linkage in large female and male breast cancer families between polymorphic genetic markers on chromosome 13q12-13 and the disease phenotype.[181] A genomewide linkage search, using 15 large breast cancer families, located a familial early onset breast cancer susceptibility gene (*BRCA2*) in a 6-cM region between the markers D13S289 and D13S267, with a maximum total multipoint Lod score of 9.58, 5 cM proximal to D13S260. *BRCA2*, which was identified in late 1995, has a cancer risk profile similar but not identical to that of *BRCA1*.

A number of studies have been carried out in an attempt to define lifetime risk for breast and ovarian cancer in carriers of *BRCA2* mutations. The first studies of this type focused only on *BRCA1* mutation carriers, and only recently have estimates become available for *BRCA2* carriers. Initial reports from families used for linkage analysis estimated that lifetime breast cancer risk for *BRCA2* mutation carriers is 86 percent, and lifetime ovarian cancer risk is 27 percent.[182] While significantly above the general population risk of 1 percent, the *BRCA2*-associated ovarian cancer risk is lower than the 40 to 60 percent lifetime risk of ovarian cancer associated with *BRCA1* mutations found in the same type of heavily affected families (see Fig. 47-6). Predictably, when using a more population-based ascertainment strategy, more recent analyses of the Ashkenazi Jewish population estimated that a lower lifetime BRCA2-associated risk of breast cancer is 56 percent, whereas the lifetime risk for ovarian cancer is 10 to 20 percent.[49] Thus these risks are often presented as ranging between 56 and 86 percent for breast cancer and between 10 and 27 percent for ovarian cancer.

In contrast to *BRCA1*, *BRCA2* mutations are associated with a 6 percent lifetime risk of male breast cancer. Although in absolute terms this represents significantly less cancer risk to men than to women, the relative risk represents a similar 100-fold increase over the general population risk. Elevated risks for the development of prostate, pancreatic, non-Hodgkin lymphoma, basal cell carcinoma, and other cancers may be associated with *BRCA2* mutations but remain poorly defined.

Like *BRCA1* tumors, *BRCA2* tumors have been reported as highly proliferative and may be of either ductal or lobular origin. A significant increase in tubule formation was identified in these tumors, along with aneuploidy and high S phase fraction.[21] These tumors are often high grade (see Fig. 47-7),[21,56,57] and in a recent study of tumors from Icelandic 999del5 mutation carriers, many were shown to be estrogen and progesterone receptor positive.[183] This is in contrast to *BRCA1*-associated tumors, which are often ER negative.

Isolation of *BRCA2*. After demonstration of the linkage of familial breast cancer to chromosome 13q12-13, several laboratories began evaluating families not linked to *BRCA1* for linkage to this region, particularly those with male breast cancer cases. Icelandic pedigrees with male breast cancer cases were shown to be linked to chromosome 13q12-13, and a common haplotype was identified, suggesting a common founder.[184] An unexpected addition to the fine mapping of the *BRCA2* region was provided by the identification of a homozygous somatic deletion in a single pancreatic cancer[185] that spanned a region estimated at 250 kb.

Sequence data from a 900-kb region thought to contain *BRCA2* were completed by DNA sequencing groups at the Sanger Center and Washington University, and the assembled sequence was released over the Internet, greatly facilitating this effort. The

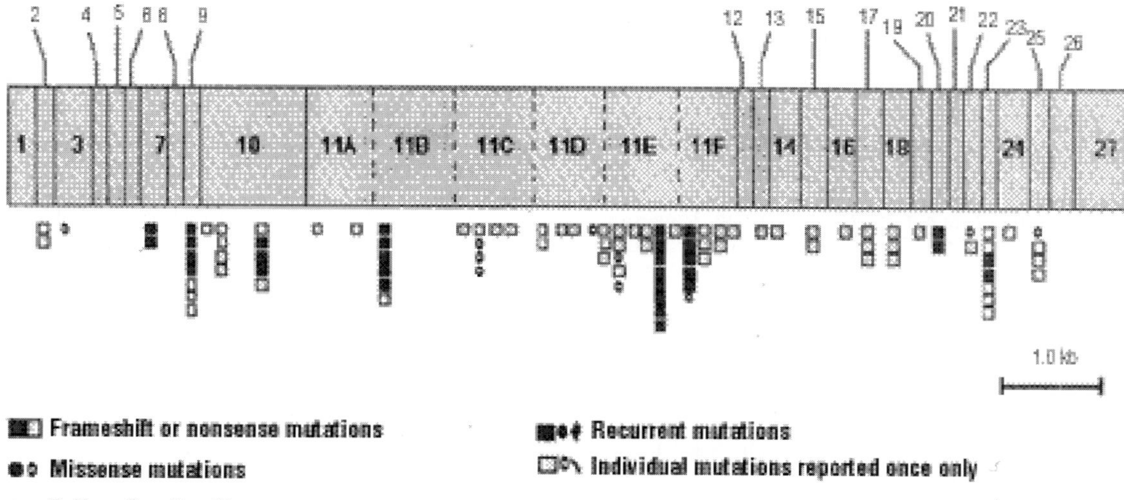

Fig. 47-10 Structure and mutation spectrum of *BRCA2*. The 27 exons of the *BRCA2* cDNA are shown as sections within the *BRCA2* gene structure. Mutations are drawn as boxes beneath the exons of the gene in which they were detected and are categorized by frequency and mutation type. The idiogram was copied from the Breast Cancer Information Core (BIC) Web site and was generated by Simon Gayther, Cambridge, U.K.

culmination of this effort was the identification of a partial sequence of the *BRCA2* gene[40] and six mutations that truncated the putative BRCA2 protein. Shortly afterward, the complete cDNA sequence of *BRCA2* was published by another collaborative group.[41]

The *BRCA2* cDNA is approximately 11.5 kb in length and is contained within 70 kb of genomic DNA. The coding region is 10.4 kb in length and is composed of 26 exons, with exon 1 forming part of the 5′ untranslated region. Like *BRCA1, BRCA2* has a large exon 11 (4.8 kb) and has no significant homology to any previously described gene (Fig. 47-10). *BRCA2* does not appear to be a member of a known gene family on the basis of sequence analysis and Southern blotting of human genomic DNA. Northern blotting using a *BRCA2* fragment as a probe described an 11.4-kb RNA with no predominant splice variants. The BRCA2 protein is composed of 3418 amino acids and has an estimated molecular mass of 384 kDa.[41]

Neither *BRCA2* cDNA nor protein contain previously defined functional domains (Fig. 47-11). However, eight copies of a 30- to 80-amino-acid repeat (BRC repeats) are encoded by exon 11. Comparison of sequences from several species demonstrates that the repeats are conserved but that exon 11 in general is poorly conserved.[186,187] The functional significance of the conserved repeats remains controversial, but at least some of the repeats form the binding site for the interaction between BRCA2 and Rad51 (discussed below).

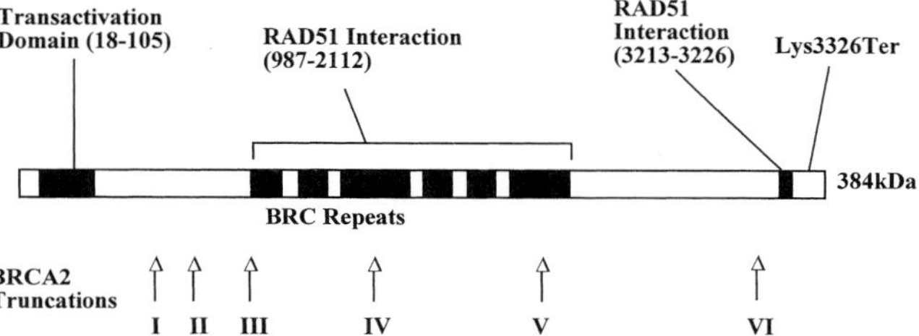

Fig. 47-11 Functional domains of *BRCA2*. The known functional domains of the BRCA2 protein including the N-terminal transactivation domain, the C-terminal Rad51 binding site, and the central Rad51-binding BRC repeats are depicted as black boxes within the diagram. The position of mutations leading to truncations in several *BRCA2* homozygous mutant mice are depicted as arrows beneath the gene.

BRCA2 is expressed in most human tissues at very low levels, with higher expression in testes.[41] The murine *BRCA2* gene has been identified and sequenced, and a similar pattern exists in the mouse.[188,189] The murine cDNA encodes a protein of 3329 amino acids that shares 59 percent identity with human BRCA2. However, identity is higher in certain regions, including the putative transactivation domain encoded by exon 3, the BRC repeats encoded by exon 11, and the C-terminus of the protein between amino acids 2414 and 3092 with 77 percent identity. The complete rat *BRCA2* sequence also is available and displays 58 percent identity with human *BRCA2* over 3343 amino acids. The mouse and rat genes are 73 and 72 percent identical, respectively, to the human gene.

Mutational Spectrum. More than 250 *BRCA2* mutations have been defined to date[40,41,190–196] (see Fig. 47-10), with a tabulated list available on the BIC Web site (*http//www.nchgr.nih.gov/dir/Intramural_research/Lab_transfer/Bic/*). Interestingly, several similarities with *BRCA1* are apparent. First, *BRCA2* mutations span the entire coding region of the gene, adding little information on important functional regions and making mutation screening in this very large gene difficult. No mutation hotspots have been detected. Second, 70 percent of mutations reported to date are truncating mutations created mainly by small insertions and deletions, again adding little in the way of clues for defining functional regions. Missense mutations in the *BRCA2* gene account for approximately 30 percent of all variants detected in this gene (see Fig. 47-10). As with *BRCA1,* a number of these variants have not been classified as either polymorphisms, benign rare variants, or disease-causing mutations. One example, however, is likely to be the G2901N mutation, which recently was detected in three siblings with ovarian cancer. Evidence supporting the disease association of this mutation is that the glycine residue and the surrounding amino acids are conserved in human, mouse, and chicken, and the mutation was not present in 220 controls and was found only in affected members of the family. Definitive evidence awaits a functional assay.

Several mutations have been identified in *BRCA2,* which have helped to delimit specific functional domains. One variant of particular importance is the Lys3326ter alteration, which truncates the BRCA2 protein close to the C-terminus. Analysis of families with this variant showed that the putative mutation did not segregate with breast cancer in the family.[198] Furthermore, families were identified that carried other truncating *BRCA2* mutations along with the Lys3326ter variant. This observation indicates that the discrete C-terminus of *BRCA2* is not important for normal protein function and that Lys3326ter is a nonfunctional polymorphism. Another potentially useful mutation is a 126-bp deletion in exon 23 that does not create a frameshift, suggesting that the protein encoded by exon 23 may be important for BRCA2 function.[190] In addition, a large 5068-bp genomic deletion in *BRCA2* spanning from intron 2 to intron 3 removes the exon 3 transactivation domain and is expected to alter the putative transcription-associated function of BRCA2,[199] whereas two missense mutations, V1283G and T1302N, in the BRC repeats have been shown to ablate the ability of BRCA2 to repair methylmethane sulfonate-induced DNA damage.[200] Thus the analysis of mutations within the gene has partially validated the role of BRCA2 in transcription regulation and DNA repair.

Several founder mutations have been identified in the *BRCA2* gene in specific populations. The 6174delT mutation has been found in the Ashkenazi Jewish population at a prevalence of 1.2 percent, with a total of 2.5 percent of the entire Ashkenazi Jewish population now thought to carry one of three specific *BRCA1* and *BRCA2* mutations.[201] No human homozygotes of any of the three founder mutations have been reported, suggesting that the null phenotype involving any of these three mutations is an embryonic lethal. However, double mutants with one *BRCA1* mutation and one *BRCA2* mutation have been noted by numerous groups. Studies of the *BRCA2* gene in the Icelandic population have determined that a founder effect also exists in that population, with the majority of high-risk breast and ovarian cancer patients sharing a common haplotype flanking *BRCA2,*[184] which is associated with a 999del5 mutation.[202] It also has been shown that 8.5 percent of breast cancer patients, 7.9 percent of ovarian cancer patients, and 2.7 percent of prostate cancer patients under 65 years of age in Iceland carry the 999del5 mutation. Finally, founder mutations have been identified in Finland. These include the IVS23-2A $\rightarrow$ G mutation and the 999del5 mutation, which suggests that individuals from Finland may have introduced this mutation into Iceland.[114] Analysis of haplotypes associated with nine recurrent mutations in *BRCA2* provides evidence of common origins of each founder *BRCA2* mutation.[111]

Mutations in the *BRCA2* gene have been identified in individuals with apparently sporadic ovarian cancer at a prevalence of less than 1 percent, in comparison with a prevalence of 10 percent for *BRCA1*.[203] Mutations also have been detected in 7.3 percent of germ-line pancreatic carcinomas.[204] No mutations have been reported in sporadic meningiomas[205] or in sporadic breast cancer. Few studies have been performed on *BRCA2* because of the difficulty in screening the entire coding sequence for mutations. However, one study has shown that *BRCA2* mutations account for only 2.7 percent of breast cancer in women under 32 years of age,[122] suggesting that *BRCA2* contributes to fewer cases of early onset breast cancer than does *BRCA1*. In a large study of Ashkenazi Jewish breast cancer patients, 7 percent of women with breast cancer diagnosed under age 40 years and 5 percent of those diagnosed over age 50 years carried the 6174delT mutation. In those with breast cancer and no family history, 4.5 percent were accounted for by 6174delT.[110] The same study determined that cumulatively the common *BRCA1* and *BRCA2* mutations failed to account for 79 percent of high-incidence breast cancer families and 35 percent of high-risk breast and ovarian cancer families in the Ashkenazi Jewish population. This suggests that other *BRCA1* and *BRCA2* mutations may have been overlooked because of the focus on the founder mutations and also that other breast cancer predisposition genes remain to be identified. This observation is supported by recent studies suggesting that the prevalence of *BRCA2* mutations in high-risk breast cancer families appears to have been overestimated. These studies found *BRCA2* mutations in 10 to 20 percent of high-risk breast and/or ovarian cancer families (Table 47-4), whereas earlier studies suggested that *BRCA2* mutations accounted for up to 35 percent of familial breast and/or ovarian cancer.[45,47,49,108,110,118,121,122,190,206–208]

Molecular Biology of BRCA2. The regions of high homology between human and murine BRCA2 have been studied by several groups; however, little functional data are available to date. Of note, exon 3 has been shown to encode a transactivation domain,[197] using a mammalian one-hybrid system, and the BRC repeats have been shown to bind the Rad51 a DNA repair protein, as does a C-terminal domain,[188,189] suggesting a role for BRCA2 in DNA repair. Most recently, BRCA2 has been shown to interact with BRCA1 (as discussed earlier), suggesting that the two proteins function in the same pathway.[132] This hypothesis makes sense teleologically, since mutations in each of the two genes produce an almost identical phenotype.

The sequence of the single BRCA2 promoter has been available since the entire *BRCA2* region was sequenced by groups at Washington University in St. Louis and at the Sanger Center. Interestingly, the promoter does not appear to contain either a CCAAT box or a TATA box. The BRCA2 promoter contains consensus binding elements for multiple transcription factors, including the arylhydrocarbon receptor AP2 and SP1; however, no data are available concerning the functionality of these sites. Little is known about the transcriptional regulation of the *BRCA2* gene.

BRCA2 has been detected in the nucleus of MCF7 breast cancer cells. Cells were fractionated into nuclear and cytoplasmic fractions and probed on western blots with TFIIH, p89, and β-tubulin as controls for nuclear and cytoplasmic proteins. BRCA2 was detected predominantly in the nucleus.[208] BRCA2 also has been localized to the nucleus by transfection of cells with a GFP-tagged BRCA2 construct.[132] A series of basic amino acids including the sequence KKRR beginning at amino acid 3382 of the human BRCA2 protein has been suggested as a consensus nuclear binding site.[189]

BRCA2 and the Cell Cycle. Shortly after the identification of *BRCA2,* the gene was shown to be regulated in a cell cycle-dependent manner and in association with cellular proliferation. Levels of BRCA2 are low in G1 but increase as the cell approaches the G1/S boundary. Highest levels of BRCA2 are detected in S phase. Expression of BRCA2 also was shown to be independent of bulk DNA synthesis.[209] A second study reported that BRCA2 RNA levels were maintained through the S and G2/M phases of the cell cycle.[210] The cell cycle kinetics of BRCA2 are similar to the kinetics of BRCA1 and suggest that these proteins are coordinately regulated.

BRCA2 and Development. The first studies of the role of BRCA2 in development were performed by *in situ* hybridization of mouse embryos similarly to BRCA1. BRCA2 hybridization to whole-mount embryos showed widespread expression in many developing tissues, suggesting that BRCA2 may play a role in tissue development, possibly as a ubiquitous transcription factor.[211] Further studies have supported the observation that BRCA2 is expressed in proliferating cells of embryos in the mammary gland during morphogenesis and in most adult tissues. Similar to BRCA1, BRCA2 exhibited a hormone-independent expression pattern in the oocytes, granulosa cells, and thecal cells of developing ovarian follicles and in the mitotic spermatogenia and meiotic spermatocytes of the testes.[162] However, the time course of BRCA2 expression in spermatogonia was delayed relative to BRCA1, possibly suggesting distinct roles for BRCA1 and BRCA2 in meiosis.

Sharan and colleagues produced the first *BRCA2* nullizygous mice. The null allele was generated by the deletion of *BRCA2* exon 11 encoding amino acids 626–1437 and resulted in embryonic lethality at day 8.5 of embryogenesis at the same time that BRCA2 expression levels were detected in the normal animals.[212] However, unlike *BRCA1* nullizygous animals, mesoderm formation had begun prior to developmental arrest. Heterozygous mice were healthy and fertile. Suzuki and colleagues also demonstrated that embryos nullizygous for *BRCA2* due to deletion of exons 10 and 11 die before day 9.5 of development.[213] Cellular proliferation was shown to be inhibited, and p21 levels were increased. The death of the *BRCA2* nullizygous mice during early postimplantation suggests a role for BRCA2 in cellular proliferation and development. Embryos nullizygous for both *BRCA1* and *BRCA2* exhibited a *BRCA1* nullizygous phenotype.[166] In this case, the *BRCA2* mutation involved a large deletion of exon 11. *BRCA2/p53* nullizygous embryos had a partially rescued phenotype, surviving to 11.5 days of embryogenesis. These data suggest that p53 and BRCA2 are functionally associated similar to BRCA1 and p53.

Each of the three nullizygous embryos just described involved mutations that truncated the BRCA2 protein in the region encoded by exon 10 or early exon 11 and eliminated the BRC repeats. However, viable nullizygous *BRCA2* mice also have been generated by two groups.[214,215] In these animals, truncation of BRCA2 occurred in regions encoded by the central and 3′ sections of exon 11 and by exon 27. Each of these alleles removes the C-terminal *Rad51* interaction domain of *BRCA2*. The allele described by Connor and colleagues contains seven of the eight BRC repeats,[215] whereas the Friedman *et al.*[214] mice retain three of the four BRC repeats. These animals are sickly and growth-retarded but survive to adulthood. Levels of p21 and p53 were elevated in mouse embryo fibroblasts derived from these animals. The data suggest that the presence of at least three BRC repeats is essential for regulation of embryonic development and cellular proliferation by BRCA2.

***BRCA2* and Transcription.** BRCA2 contains an N-terminal transactivation domain,[197] as defined by the yeast two-hybrid system and the mammalian one-hybrid system (Fig. 47-11). This BRCA2 transactivation domain was segregated into repression and activation domains. The ability of the domain to transactivate a Gal4 promoter was ablated by the addition of a Y42C missense mutation located in exon 3 of the *BRCA2* gene. BRCA2 has not been shown to interact with the RNA polymerase II holoenzyme; however, studies have demonstrated that BRCA2 complexes with BRCA1 and with RAD51.[132,210] The association with BRCA1 has not been shown to be a direct interaction, but the formation of a protein complex does support the hypothesis that BRCA2 may function as a coactivator or corepressor of transcription similarly to BRCA1. RAD51 has been shown to bind to both p53 and the RNA polymerase II holoenzyme, suggesting a role for this protein in regulation of transcription, perhaps through transcription-coupled double-strand DNA break repair.[169] Evidence that BRCA2 can bind DNA directly has yet to be presented.

BRCA2 and Cellular Response to DNA Damage. Several experiments have supported the hypothesis that BRCA2 plays a role in double-strand break repair. Hasty and colleagues successfully identified a C-terminal portion of mouse BRCA2 as a RAD51-binding protein in a two-hybrid screen in yeast (see Fig. 47-11). Further analysis by this group and others demonstrated that Rad51 binds to a 36-amino-acid domain (residues 3196–3232).[212,216] These amino acids are 95 percent conserved between mouse and human BRCA2, suggesting that the domain is important for BRCA2 function. As mentioned previously, Rad51 is a human homologue of *Escherchia coli* RecA and of yeast ScRad51, a member of the RAD52 epistasis group. ScRad51 is involved in mitotic and meiotic recombination and double-strand DNA break repair in yeast,[170] the human form of which associates with BRCA1 in S phase of the cell cycle.[168] Several other studies expanded on this discovery, showing that RAD51 also binds to the BRC repeats of BRCA2. Wong and colleagues reported that residues 98 to 339 of human RAD51 interact with a 59-amino-acid region within each of the eight BRC repeats[210] (see Fig. 47-11). Katagiri found that RAD51 bound to at least two regions of BRCA2 involving residues 982 to 1066 and 1139 to 1266.[217] More recently, RAD51 was shown to bind directly to the four 5′ BRC repeats and was shown to form complexes in vivo by coimmunoprecipitation. In contrast to previous studies, RAD51 was shown not to bind the four 3′ BRC repeats or at the C-terminus of BRCA2.[200] While it is unclear which BRC repeats bind RAD51, it is now well established that BRCA2 binds RAD51 at several positions and thus likely plays a role in response to double-strand breaks and in both mitotic and meiotic recombination.

Further evidence supporting this role for BRCA2 has been provided by studies of *BRCA2* mutant embryos. The first such evidence was provided by the homozygous mutant embryos generated by Sharan and colleagues that display hypersensitivity to ionizing radiation.[189] Following exposure of these mutant embryos to 400 rads of γ-irradiation at day 3.5 of development, the inner cell mass outgrowth of these embryos was completely ablated, and this effect not seen in heterozygous or normal embryos. The number of trophoblast cells also was greatly reduced in the homozygous mutant embryos. Mouse embryo fibroblasts (MEF) from viable *BRCA2* homozygous mutant animals with mutations 3′ of the BRC repeats are also hypersensitive to agents that create double-strand DNA breaks.[215,218,219] This suggests that the BRC repeats may be necessary for development of the embryo but may not be essential for radiation resistance because even in the presence of these repeats the MEF cells are hypersensitive to radiation damage in comparison with controls. Thus the C-terminal Rad51 interaction domain or other as yet unidentified C-terminal domains may regulate the DNA damage response function of BRCA2.

Studies of a pancreatic cell line (CAPAN-1) expressing truncated BRCA2 have shown these cells to be hypersensitive to methyl methanesulfonate (MMS) treatment.[200] CAPAN-1 cells carry the 6174delT common Ashkenazi Jewish *BRCA2* mutation of one allele and a deletion of the wild-type allele. Introduction of wild-type BRCA2 into these cells conferred resistance to MMS, whereas introduction of BRCA2 with BRC repeat deletions or missense mutations in the BRC repeats had no effect. This suggests that the BRC repeats and the interaction between RAD51 and BRCA2 is essential for repair of MMS-induced DNA damage. Further studies by Abbott and colleagues showed that CAPAN-1 cells are highly sensitive to double-strand DNA break-inducing drugs such as etoposide and to ionizing radiation.[220] Thus it is likely that binding of RAD51 to both the BRC repeats and the C-terminal interaction domain is important for the DNA damage-repair function of BRCA2. Tumors in mice derived from CAPAN-1 injection also demonstrated hypersensitivity to radiation and mitoxantrone, suggesting that irradiation or treatment with DNA-damaging agents may be a useful method for elimination of BRCA2 null cells.[220]

The discovery that cells without functional BRCA2 are sensitive to DNA damage supports the hypothesis that *BRCA2* is a caretaker of the genome. Further evidence comes from the observation that *p53* mutations are significantly more common in *BRCA2*-associated breast tumors[221] and ovarian tumors[179] than in sporadic tumor controls.

Rare Causes of Inherited Breast Cancer Syndromes

Li-Fraumeni Syndrome. Li-Fraumeni syndrome (LFS), now known to be associated with germ-line mutations in *TP53*, was first identified as a syndrome in 1969 in a description of four kindreds in which cousins or sibs had childhood soft tissue sarcomas and other relatives had excessive cancer occurrence.[222] Subsequent epidemiologic efforts resulted in enumeration of the major component neoplasms, including breast cancer, soft tissue sarcomas and ostersarcomas, brain tumors, leukemias, and adrenocortical carcinomas, with several additional tumor types likely to merit inclusion.[223,224] Segregation analysis of families identified through a family member with sarcoma confirmed the autosomal dominant pattern of transmission of cancer susceptibility, with age-specific penetrance functions estimated to reach 90 percent by age 70. Nearly 30 percent of tumors in reported families occur before age 15 years.[224]

The pattern of breast cancer in LFS families is remarkable. Among 24 LFS families currently under study, 44 women have been diagnosed with breast cancer, of whom 77 percent were between the ages of 22 and 45 years.[225] Bilateral disease was documented in 25 percent of these women; 11 percent had additional primary tumors. It has been suggested that males may have later onset tumors in LFS families because they tend not to get breast cancer, which is so dramatic among female LFS family members.

As noted previously, in 1990, germ-line mutations were identified in the *p53* tumor-suppressor gene (*TP53*) in affected members of LFS families.[226,227] Mutations were clustered in the conserved sequences of the gene (exons 5 through 9), an observation that was thought to increase the significance of these findings. Additional families meeting the classic criteria for the clinical syndrome of LFS have been evaluated for the presence of germ-line alterations in *p53*. Approximately 50 percent of such carefully defined families have had alterations identified in the *p53* gene. While mutations are more frequently identified in hotspots within the conserved sequences, they have been seen throughout the gene.[228–232] *p53* genes ostensibly normal by sequencing but abnormal in a functional assay or with regard to expression also have been observed.[233,234] The prevalence of germ-line *TP53* alterations among women diagnosed with breast cancer before age 40 has been estimated at less than 1 percent.[235,236] It is therefore a rare explanation for breast cancer occurrence in the population; nonetheless, *p53* mutation screening formed the basis for the first predisposition testing programs for breast cancer susceptibility. However, the low prevalence of *TP53* mutations in the general population, and the profound psychological impact of such testing have kept this genetic test from widespread application. The role of *TP53* in LFS and breast cancer is discussed further in Chap. 37.

Cowden Disease. Cowden disease, also known as the *multiple hamartoma syndrome,* is a rare autosomal dominant familial cancer syndrome that is characterized by an increased risk of breast cancer, genodermatosis, and multiple, more variable clinical features. The most consistent and characteristic findings are mucocutaneous lesions, including multiple facial trichilemmomas, papillomatosis of the lips and oral mucosa, and acral keratoses. Vitiligo and angiomas also have been reported. The syndrome is inherited in an autosomal dominant mode with variable expressivity and complete penetrance of the dermatologic lesions by age 20.[237]

Benign proliferations in other organ systems are common in patients with Cowden disease, including thyroid goiter, thyroid adenomas, gastrointestinal polyps, uterine leiomyomas, and lipomas. Nonmalignant abnormalities of the breast similarly are noted in these patients and include fibroadenomas, fibrocystic lesions, areolar and nipple malformations, and ductal epithelial hyperplasia.[237–239] Central nervous system involvement was recognized only recently and includes megaencephaly, epilepsy, and gangliocytomas of the cerebellum.[240,241]

A marked increase in breast cancer incidence compared with the general population was observed in a series of recently published cases of Cowden disease.[239] Breast neoplasms occurred in 10 of the 21 female patients; the lesions were bilateral in 4 of these women. Lesions were said to be exclusively intraductal in 2 of the 10 women; however, given the fact that these are true precursor lesions, these intraductal carcinomas are likely to represent a manifestation of the underlying genetic defect. Additional cases of Cowden disease have been published, bringing the number of reported patients to 83, of whom 51 are female.[237] Thus the total number of women with breast cancer and Cowden disease totals 15 (29 percent), with bilateral invasive tumors in 4 women. Since many of the women in these families are still alive and at risk of developing breast cancer, the number of these women with breast cancer is likely to increase, increasing current estimates for the lifetime risk of developing breast cancer in women with this syndrome. However, increased recognition of Cowden disease could continue to disproportionately increase the number of Cowden patients without breast cancer and ultimately reduce estimates of the breast cancer rate. The gene for Cowden disease recently was mapped to chromosome 10q22-23 by linkage analysis of 12 families from four different countries.[242] Haplotype analysis demonstrated that all 12 families were linked to this locus, indicating that Cowden disease is a single-gene disorder.

A candidate tumor-suppressor gene *PTEN/MMAC1/TEP1* (phosphatase and tensin homologue/mutated in multiple advanced cancers 1/TGFβ-regulated and epithelial cell–enriched phophatase 1) was recently identified on chromosome 10q23.[242–245] Somatic mutations in the gene were identified in cancer cell lines and in 70 percent of primary glioblastomas and 60 percent of advanced prostate, breast, and kidney tumors.[244] Subsequently, mutations were identified in the *PTEN* gene in the germ line of Cowden disease patients.[246,247] Several more mutations identified in Cowden disease patients demonstrated that *PTEN* mutations are causative of Cowden disease and associated breast cancer.[248] In the same study, certain Cowden disease families were shown to have no *PTEN* coding-region mutations, suggesting that the mutations in these families are not readily detectable by PCR-based strategies or that other Cowden disease genes remain to be identified. Germ-line and somatic *PTEN* mutations have not been detected in sporadic breast cancers or in early onset breast cancers, suggesting that only breast cancer in association with the Cowden disease phenotype is caused by *PTEN* mutations. A *PTEN* pseudogene also has been identified.[249] The presence of the pseudogene may result in coamplification of pseudogene and functional gene fragments when using PCR-based mutation screening strategies. Thus accumulated variants in the pseudogene may be mistaken for mutations within the functional *PTEN* gene.

The PTEN protein has dual-specificity tyrosine phosphatase activity[245] and can dephosphorylate serine, threonine, or tyrosine residues. PTEN has homology to tensin, an SH2 domain actin-binding cytoskeletal protein localized to focal adhesions.[246] PTEN also contains a PDZ-binding domain at the C-terminus.[247] Thus PTEN also may function as an assembly factor for protein signaling complexes.

Peutz-Jeghers Syndrome. Peutz-Jeghers syndrome (PJS) is a rare autosomal dominant disorder characterized by gastrointestinal hamartomas and macular melanotic pigmentation of the mucosa, lips, fingers, and toes.[250] Pigmented lesions often appear at 1 to 2 years of age and accumulate with age. PJS predisposes to cancers of the gastrointestinal tract,[251] respiratory tract,[252] urinary tract,[253] female genital tract,[254] breast,[255] and ovary.[256] The female genital tract tumors are rare and not well recognized and include Sertoli cell tumors,[257] sex cord tumors with annular tubules (SCTAT),[258] and adenoma malignum of the cervix.[259] A recent follow-up study of 34 PJS patients identified a relative risk for cancer in females of 20 and of 7 in males.[260] A total of 6 cases of breast cancer were reported in the 34 individuals, and 50 percent of women with PJS developed a gynecologic or breast malignancy.

A PJS locus was recently mapped to chromosome 19p13.3 by a combination of comparative genome hybridization and loss of heterozygosity (LOH) studies in tumors, followed by linkage studies of PJS families.[261] Subsequently, the PJS gene, *LKB1* (*STK11*), was identified as a serine-threonine kinase.[262] Mutation screening in 12 patients determined that most mutations result in truncation of the STK11 protein product by creating a premature stop codon or by intragenic deletion.[262] Thus *STK11* is the first kinase gene associated with hereditary cancer that is inactivated by mutations. A series of mutation studies of *STK11* in sporadic breast,[263] colon,[264] and testicular[265] tumors has failed to identify any variants, suggesting that the involvement of *STK11* in these cancers is limited to those associated with an inherited predis-

Table 47-5 Causes of Inherited Breast Cancer Syndromes

	Clinical Manifestations	Mutation	Inheritance
Li-Fraumeni syndrome	Breast cancer, sarcoma, brain tumors, leukemia, adrenocortical carcinoma	*TP53*	Autosomal dominant
Cowden disease	Mucocutaneous lesions, angiomas, hamartomatous polyps of the colon, breast, and thyroid cancer	*PTEN*	Autosomal dominant
Muir-Torre syndrome	Gastrointestinal and genitourinary tumors, skin and breast tumors	*MLH1, MSH2*	Autosomal dominant
Peutz-Jeghers syndrome	Melanin deposits, hamartomatous polyps of the colon, breast, ovary, cervical, uterine, and testicular tumors	*LKB1/STK11*	Autosomal dominant
Ataxia-telangiectasia	Cerebellar ataxia, oculocutaneous telangiectasias, radiation hypersensitivity, lymphoma, leukemia, and breast tumors	*ATM*	Autosomal recessive

position. Further studies have determined that a small number of PJS families are not linked to the *STK11* locus, suggesting the presence of another PJS gene elsewhere in the genome.[266]

Muir-Torre Syndrome. Muir-Torre syndrome, a variant of Lynch syndrome type II, is the eponym given to the association between multiple skin tumors and multiple benign and malignant tumors of the upper and lower gastrointestinal and genitourinary tracts.[267,268] Many of the manifestations are common lesions (basal cell carcinomas, keratoacanthomas, colonic diverticula) that occur at younger ages but in a distribution similar to that in the general population. Inheritance of this syndrome is autosomal dominant with high penetrance.[268] Females with the syndrome reportedly have an increased risk of breast cancer, particularly after menopause, although lifetime risk has not been calculated.[269] Five genes responsible for inherited forms of colon cancer not associated with polyposis recently were described, including *MLH1* and *MSH2, PMS1, PMS2,* and *MSH6.*[270–274] Mutations in these genes are thought to lead to the development of hereditary nonpolyposis colorectal cancer (HNPCC) through loss of the ability to repair damaged DNA, accumulation of replication errors, and genome instability. Since various malignancies in Muir-Torre syndrome display microsatellite instability similar to that seen in colon cancer patients with HNPCC, it was postulated that mutations in one or more HNPCC-related genes may be the underlying defect in Muir-Torre syndrome. This observation was verified recently by linkage and mutation analysis demonstrating that mutations in *MSH2* predispose to Muir-Torre syndrome.[275] A truncating mutation in *MLH1* also has been detected in a Muir-Torre syndrome family.[276] Further discussion of the role of *MLH1* and *MSH2* in carcinogenesis is presented in Chap. 32.

Ataxia-Telangiectasia. Ataxia-telangiectasia (AT) is an autosomal recessive disorder that is characterized by cerebellar ataxia, oculocutaneous telangiectasias, radiation hypersensitivity, and an increased incidence of malignancy. Chromosomal fragility and resulting DNA rearrangements are thought to result from the genetic defect that underlies the clinical syndrome of AT. AT is characterized by an autosomal recessive pattern of inheritance, with the complete clinical syndrome occurring only in homozygous individuals. Of note, AT homozygotes, accounting for 3 to 11 live births per million,[277] are estimated to have a risk of cancer that is 60 to 180 times greater than that of the general population.[278] Cancers observed in association with AT include non-Hodgkin lymphoma (nearly 100 percent lifetime risk) and a significant but lower risk of developing breast cancer, ovarian cancer, lymphocytic leukemia, and malignancies of the oral cavity, stomach, pancreas, and bladder. However, breast cancer risk in AT mutation carriers does not approach the risk observed in women with inherited mutations in *p53, BRCA1,* or *BRCA2.* Initially, reports of increased susceptibility to cancer were limited to homozygous AT mutation carriers, who represent approximately 0.2 to 0.7 percent of the general population in the United States.[278] However, a study published in 1987 suggested that AT heterozygotes who do not display the typical neurologic findings seen in homozygotes have a fivefold increased incidence of breast cancer.[279] This finding was particularly significant given that AT heterozygotes represent up to 7 percent of the general population[277] and that screening mammography, a source of ionizing radiation, could possibly contribute to the increased breast cancer incidence seen in this population. However, this study has been criticized for methodologic flaws, including small sample size, inappropriateness of the control group, and lack of quantitation of radiation exposure. In addition, two groups have analyzed a total of 80 families with evidence for an inherited form of breast cancer for linkage between breast cancer and genetic markers flanking the AT locus on chromosome 11, finding strong evidence against this association.[280,281] Both groups concluded that the contribution of AT mutations to familial breast cancer is likely to be minimal. Nonetheless, since AT results from an alteration in the ability to repair DNA damage, the hypothesis that AT heterozygotes may have a decreased capacity to repair DNA could explain an increased susceptibility to cancer in such individuals. The AT gene (*ATM*) on human chromosome 11q22 has been identified[282] and is described in detail in Chap. 29. On the basis of preliminary work, it appears that heterozygote carriers of *ATM* mutations are not at significantly increased risk of developing breast cancer. A summary of the clinical and genetic characteristics of the rare genetic syndromes associated with increased breast cancer risk is presented in Table 47-5.

Other Breast Cancer Susceptibility Loci

A large number of genes have been implicated in breast cancer tumorigenesis through identification of mutations in tumors, and several of these genes are discussed later in this chapter. Two genes in addition to those described earlier have been implicated in familial breast cancer susceptibility by identification of mutations that segregate with the disease in families or by linkage analysis. First, the estrogen receptor (ER) has been suggested as a candidate locus for familial late onset breast cancer susceptibility.[283] One extended family with eight women with late onset breast cancer was identified with a single haplotype flanking the ER locus that consistently segregated with the disease, yielding a maximum Lod score of 1.85. The frequent expression of the ER in breast cancer is associated with responsiveness to hormonal treatment and a favorable prognosis. Therefore, mutations in the ER may modify the hormonal response in breast epithelium and potentially result in inherited susceptibility to breast cancer. However, no mutations associated with inherited cancer have been identified in the ER, although several somatic mutations have been identified in breast cancer biopsies and established breast cancer cell lines.[284]

Another breast cancer susceptibility locus has been proposed on chromosome 8p12-22[285] based on linkage analysis of several breast cancer families with polymorphic genetic markers on chromosome 8p. This analysis yielded a maximum Lod score of 2.51 using the polymorphic markers NEFL and D8S259. Several groups have attempted to reproduce this result with little success. However, the region is thought to harbor tumor-suppressor genes involved in sporadic prostate cancer[286] and sporadic breast tumors,[285] as defined by LOH studies. Studies of male breast tumors identified 83 percent LOH at one marker on chromosome 8p and two distinct regions of loss on chromosome 8p12-21.3 and 8p22.[287] These data suggest that a tumor-suppressor gene functioning as an inherited susceptibility gene may be involved in breast cancer pathogenesis in a small subset of families, especially those with cases of male breast cancer. As whole-genome linkage studies commence in an effort to identify other familial breast cancer susceptibility genes, the 8p12-22 region will be at the forefront as a strong candidate locus.

Somatic Alterations in Breast Cancer

Another approach to understanding the pathogenesis of breast cancer is the study of noninherited (sporadic) breast cancers. This is an important complementary approach to the study of germ-line alterations for several reasons. First, the large majority of breast cancers do not arise as a result of inherited mutations in single breast cancer susceptibility genes, and sporadic tumors may have fundamental molecular genetic differences. Second, genes that are frequently dysregulated or mutated in sporadic breast cancer are candidate genes for susceptibility loci, as was demonstrated with *p53* and LFS. Third, the study of genetic alterations per se, such as mutations, deletions, and amplifications, provides clues to the mechanisms that result in the genomic instability that is inherent in cancer cells. This section provides a summary of chromosomal regions commonly deleted in breast cancer (resulting in LOH), as well as an overview of genes that are mutated or dysregulated in sporadic breast cancers. Some of these genetic alterations have been identified as markers of particularly aggressive tumor behavior, whereas a few have become potential therapeutic targets. A summary of the genes altered in sporadic breast cancers is given in Table 47-6.

Table 47-6 Somatic Alterations in Breast Cancer

Gene/Region	Modification	Frequency
Growth factors and receptors		
EGFR	Overexpression	20–40%
HER-2/neu	Overexpression	20–40%
FGF1/FGF4	Overexpression	20–30%
TGFα	Overexpression	Not reported
Intracellular signaling molecules		
Ha-ras	Mutation	5–10%
c-src	Overexpression	50–70%
Regulators of cell cycle		
TP53	Mutation/inactivation	30–40%
RB1	Inactivation	20%
Cyclin D	Overexpression	35–45%
TGFβ	Dysregulation	Not reported
Adhesion molecules and proteases		
E-cadherin	Reduced/absent	60–70%
P-cadherin	Reduced/absent	30%
Cathepsin D	Overexpression	20–24%
MMPs	Increased expression	20–80%
Other genes		
bcl-2	Overexpression	30–45%
c-*myc*	Amplification	5–20%
nm23 (*NME1*)	Decreased expression	Not reported

Loss of Heterozygosity. Loss of heterozygosity has long been associated with the presence of tumor-suppressor genes in DNA because the analysis of many tumors has demonstrated that the wild-type allele of a mutated tumor-suppressor gene is often lost during tumorigenesis. In the case of germ-line mutations in tumor-suppressor genes, as suggested by Knudsen's "two hit" hypothesis,[288] individuals from "cancer families" inherit an inactivating mutation in one allele of the implicated tumor-suppressor gene in all cells. Therefore, only one somatic event is required to inactivate the remaining copy, making the development of cancer a much more common event than it is in individuals born without the "first hit." The mechanism by which LOH occurs is not known, but the end result is physical deletion of large regions of chromosomes. LOH has been studied in detail in sporadic and familial breast tumors, resulting in identification of many putative tumor-suppressor loci. A subset of these loci is likely to function as inherited breast cancer susceptibility loci.

The most common regions of LOH in breast cancer are located on chromosomes 17p, 17q, 16q, 13q, 11p, 1p, 3p, 6q, 7q, 18q, and 22q.[289–293] Many other loci have been identified. The 17q LOH region originally was thought to harbor the *BRCA1* gene, but more complete analysis has identified at least three and as many as six independent regions on chromosome 17q, only one of which contains *BRCA1*.[294–297] LOH also has been associated with the *BRCA2* gene on chromosome 13q12-13. These data demonstrate that the known inherited susceptibility genes are associated with LOH in tumors and that other susceptibility genes may be isolated from other LOH regions.

The 17p LOH region can be divided into two separate loci, one containing *TP53* on 17p13.1 and a second, more distal region on 17p13.3.[298] Two candidate tumor-suppressor genes have been isolated from the 17p13.3 region.[299] Studies of chromosome 1 also have identified multiple regions of loss on 1p13, 1p31, and 1p32-p34 and 1p36.2 in the same region as the neuroblastoma gene.[300,301] Three regions of LOH have been identified on chromosome 11 at 11p15.5, 11q13, and 11q22-qter, with 19, 23, and 37 to 43 percent LOH, respectively, demonstrated in a group of breast tumors. More detailed mapping has suggested that as many as five different LOH regions exist on chromosome 11q22-q24.[302] Significant association between LOH on chromosomes 11p15, 17q21, and 3p also has been detected, suggesting that the putative tumor-suppressor genes at these loci may function together in a tumorigenic pathway.[291] LOH has been detected on chromosomes 16q22.1 and 16q22.4-qter in a large number of breast tumors[303]; this is of interest because chromosome 16q is the location of the E-cadherin gene, which has been implicated in metastasis of sporadic breast cancers. Further discussion of the role of E-cadherin in breast cancer can be found below. Finally, an association has been seen between LOH on chromosomes 9p, 3p, and 6q,[304] suggesting the existence of a tumorigenic pathway involving all these loci. Another example of cooperativety between distant loci was reported by Smith and colleagues,[305] who analyzed 133 breast cancers for *TP53* mutations and LOH on 13 chromosome arms. In this series, *TP53* mutations were strongly associated with LOH at two specific loci: 3p24-26 ($p < 0.001$) and 7q31 ($p < 0.05$). Surprisingly, there was no association between *TP53* mutations and LOH at 17p, the site of the *p53* gene, suggesting that breast cancers frequently have only one defective *TP53* allele.

Many sites of LOH correspond with the location of known tumor-suppressor genes. Examples include the *DCC* gene on chromosome 18q, with 52 percent LOH in breast tumors, and the *APC* gene on chromosome 5q21.[306] These genes have been screened for mutations in familial breast cancer samples, and none has been identified, seemingly eliminating these LOH regions as candidate loci for inherited susceptibility genes. However, it is possible that tumor-suppressor genes other than *DCC* and *APC* exist in these locations. The previously described *I1307K* variant may account for the association of LOH with the *APC* gene.

Recently, investigators began analyzing atypical ductal hyperplasia, a precancerous lesion of the breast, for LOH, which has been demonstrated on chromosomes 16q and 17p in these lesions.[307] Analysis of DCIS, a malignant but noninvasive lesion of the breast, resulted in the identification of LOH on chromosomes 8p, 13q, 16q, 17p, and 17q.[308] These results suggest that known genes such as *BRCA1, BRCA2,* and *p53* or unknown tumor-suppressor genes in these chromosomal regions are altered as the first steps in breast tumorigenesis and may provide clues to the location of additional breast cancer susceptibility genes. LOH in breast cancer also has been tracked in stages from primary tumors to the onset of metastasis, demonstrating LOH on chromosome 7q31 at all stages[309] and suggesting that LOH of chromosome 7q31 is another early event in breast tumorigenesis.

Growth Factor Receptors. An important class of genes frequently altered in sporadic breast cancer are members of the epidermal growth factor receptor (EGFR) family of growth factor receptors. The members of this family of proto-oncogenes (*EGFR, erbB*-2 or *HER*-2*/neu, erbB*-3, and *erbB*-4) all share extensive homology and encode transmembrane glycoproteins with tyrosine kinase activity. They become oncogenic through gene amplification or overexpression at the mRNA and protein levels, leading to aberrations in signal transduction pathways and deregulation of cellular proliferation.[310] All the members of this family have been described as overexpressed in breast carcinoma; the most extensively studied receptors, EGFR and erbB-2, are known to be overexpressed in 20 to 40 percent of breast cancers.[311–316]

Recent work has revealed a complex system of interaction between the various members of the EGFR family, as well as cross-regulation between growth factor-activated signal transduction pathways and estrogen-responsive pathways. For example, estrogen receptor-positive breast cancer cell lines that overexpress erbB-2 demonstrate decreased erbB-2 protein expression in response to treatment with estradiol or EGF.[317] The erbB-2 pathway also has been linked to the *ras* oncogene signal transduction pathway and activation of mitogen-activated protein kinase (MAPK),[318,319] suggesting that cooperation between various oncogenes may be important in breast tumorigenesis. Overexpression of erbB-2 has been associated with a less favorable prognosis in patients with breast cancer, particularly in tumors with involvement of axillary lymph nodes.[315,320,321] It also has been reported that overexpression of erbB-2 identifies a subgroup of patients who are more resistant to chemotherapy, and a recent study suggested that higher doses of chemotherapy with regimens containing doxorubicin can in part overcome this effect.[322] In fact, overexpression of p185/c-erbB2 renders cells resistant to tamoxifen.[323] In addition, ER-positive patients who overexpress erbB-2 are less likely to have a clinically significant response to the estrogen antagonist tamoxifen and have overall shorter survival than do patients with ER-positive, erbB-2-negative tumors.[324] Finally, evidence is accumulating that down-regulation of erbB-2 protein levels with monoclonal antibodies or antisense oligonucleotides may be useful therapeutically. p185HER2/neu monoclonal antibodies have antiproliferative effects *in vitro* on cells that overexpress erbB-2 and sensitize human breast cancer cells to tumor necrosis factor.[325] In addition, erbB-2 antisense oligonucleotides[326] can inhibit the proliferation of breast cancer cells. Down-regulation of EGFR using antisense oligonucleotides also has been shown to result in down-regulation of protein kinase A and reduced growth potential in breast cancer cells.[327] Furthermore, neutralizing antibodies against EGFR and HER2/neu result in down-regulation of vascular endothelial growth factor and reduced angiogenesis.[328]

Of note, the well-described growth factor transforming growth factor alpha (TGFα) is a member of the EGF family and is a ligand for EGFR. Elevated expression of TGFα consistently has been associated with neoplastic transformation, with transgenic mouse models providing direct evidence for the role of TGFα in malignant transformation of breast epithelium. In this regard, metallothionein-directed expression of TGFα in transgenic mice and constitutive TGFα expression promote uniform epithelial hyperplasia of several organs and induce postlactational secretory mammary adenocarcinomas.[329]

The fibroblast growth factors (FGFs) and their receptors (FGFRs) also are thought to play a role in breast cancer. However, since specific genetic alterations in FGFs or FGFRs have not been reported in breast tumors, their causal role in breast tumorigenesis is less clear than that of EGFR or HER-2/neu. This large group of proteins may be involved in cell transformation by deregulated activation of a receptor tyrosine kinase through an autocrine mechanism. FGF signaling activates the STAT1 and p21 pathways and inhibits the estrogen response and cell proliferation in breast cancer cells.[330] Acidic FGF (FGF1) and basic FGF (FGF2) initially were identified as heparin-binding growth factors that stimulate the proliferation of vascular endothelium. They are expressed in a number of tumors and have strong angiogenic properties.[331,332] Basic FGF also is known to down-regulate Bcl-2 and induce apoptosis.[333] Acidic FGF plays a role in estrogen-independent cell growth regulation and anti-estrogen-resistant growth of MCF-7 cells.[330] FGF3, initially identified as int-2 because it is activated by the insertion of murine mammary tumor provirus, is associated with the transformation of murine mammary epithelium. At least nine FGFs and four FGFRs have been identified. A recent study of seven of the nine known family members and all four known receptors in a panel of 10 tumor cell lines and 103 breast tumor samples provided evidence for FGF1 and FGF2 expression in almost all samples, as well as limited expression of FGF5, FGF6, FGF7, and FGF9. FGF3 was not expressed in any sample, and FGF4 and FGF8 were not assayed. FGF8 recently has been shown to be expressed at high frequency in breast tissues.[334]

Intracellular Signaling Molecules. While it is clear that overexpression and/or mutation of mediators of intracellular signaling play a key role in malignant transformation, relatively little work has focused on the specific role of these molecules in the development of breast cancer. However, recent work suggests that dysregulation of several signaling pathways intersects directly with many breast cancer-related proteins such as the receptor tyrosine kinases. The proto-oncogene *Ha-ras* is the most extensively studied example of the involvement of signaling pathways in breast cancer development. Additionally, work in the past few years has produced evidence that rare *Ha-ras* alleles are associated with inherited susceptibility to breast cancer.[335] More recent work suggests that these rare alleles may be associated with altered penetrance of the major breast cancer susceptibility gene *BRCA1*.[69] However, the mechanism underlying this association remains unclear. Some investigators have suggested that the presence of the rare alleles is a marker of genomic instability that predisposes to cancer, whereas others have suggested that function may be altered by changes in *ras* regulatory regions or that mutations in genes in close physical proximity to the *Ha-ras* locus that are therefore genetically linked may be the underlying cause of the increase in cancer susceptibility associated with these alleles.

Experimental models have been used to determine whether chemically induced breast neoplasia is associated with *Ha-ras* changes. Using the spontaneously immortalized but nontransformed breast line MCF10A, loss of one *Ha-ras* allele and induction of a mutation in the remaining allele at the first position of codon 12 have been observed after carcinogen exposure.[336] These changes were associated with the ability of these cells to form colonies in soft agar, but not with the emergence of tumorigenesis in animals.

There is evidence that while *ras* coding region mutations occur in less than 10 percent of breast cancers, the pathway *ras* services may be deregulated in breast cancer more frequently. Bland and colleagues examined 85 breast cancer specimens with immunohistochemical staining for the presence of multiple oncogene products, including *Ha-ras,* and correlated the results with the clinical outcome.[337] The oncogenes with the strongest prognostic correlation to survival were *Ha-ras* and c-*fos.* Coexpression of c-*myc* and *Ha-ras* with c-*fos* also correlated with an increased likelihood of recurrence and decreased survival. Other studies also suggested cooperativity between *Ha-ras* and both rat c-erbB-2 and human TGFα in transformation but similarly demonstrated that additional genetic changes are required for a fully tumorigenic phenotype.[338] Finally, a link has been established between the expression of *Ha-ras* and the appearance of the multidrug resistance phenotype. Transfection of the breast cell line MCF-10A with c-*Ha-ras* and c-*erbB*-2 results in up-regulation of the *mdr-1* gene (multidrug resistance-1), appearance of the protein product on the cell surface, and the multidrug resistance phenotype.[339] Transfection with either proto-oncogene alone has no effect, strongly suggesting cooperativity. As noted earlier, the association between c-erbB-2 expression and breast cancer prognosis has been investigated extensively, and recent work suggests that erbB-2 expression may correlate with Ha-ras expression.[340] Interestingly, in this study, if chemotherapy is included in the model, tumors coexpressing Ha-ras and c-erbB-2 are less responsive to both chemotherapy and the partial estrogen antagonist tamoxifen.

The signaling pathway involving the proto-oncogene c-*src* also has been linked to genetic alterations in breast cancer. Specifically, the phosphotyrosine residues of receptor tyrosine kinases serve as binding sites for proteins that contain SRC homology 2 (SH2) domains. Using glutathione-*S*-transferase fusion proteins containing the SH2 region, it has been demonstrated that in human breast carcinoma cell lines the SH2 domain binds to activated EGFR and to p185her2/neu. These investigators also have shown that endogenous pp60c-src is tightly associated with tyrosine-phosphorylated EGFR, raising the possibility that this association may be an integral part of malignant transformation of breast epithelium.[341] In a related study, protein tyrosine kinase activity was assayed in 72 primary breast cancer specimens; increased activity compared with normal breast tissue was identified in all 72 samples. In this study, at least 70 percent of the cytosolic protein tyrosine kinase activity originated from the presence of the c-*src* oncogene product.[342] Since cytosolic protein tyrosine kinase activity parallels malignancy in breast tumors,[343] and since most of this activity is precipitated by anti-src antibodies, it appears likely c-*src* plays a significant role in the manifestation of breast cancer.[342]

Regulators of the Cell Cycle. Accumulating evidence indicates that derangements in the protein machinery that normally regulates passage through the cell cycle are critical contributors to uncontrolled cell growth and cancer.[344,345] *TP53* (encoding p53) initially was regarded as a tumor-suppressor gene that is deleted or mutated in a large number of human tumors from a variety of tissue types. p53 was known to have DNA-binding and transcriptional activation domains, and more recent work has established that p53 plays a central role in regulating progression through the cell cycle. The strongest link between *TP53* mutations and breast cancer comes from the increased incidence of early onset breast cancer seen in LFS, the family cancer syndrome caused by germline alterations in *TP53.*[226] Additional evidence for the involvement of *TP53* in breast cancer comes from studies demonstrating decreased ability to form tumors in nude mice and reduced capacity for growth in soft agar when wild-type *TP53* in a retroviral vector is introduced into breast cancer cell lines with mutated *TP53.* Alterations in *TP53* in breast cancer may be detected by analyzing the coding region for mutations[236,346] or in some cases by using antibody demonstrating aberrant localization or altered levels of p53. *TP53* mutations have been detected in 15 to 45 percent of human breast cancer specimens in several studies.[347–350] Of note, several groups have investigated racial differences in the *TP53* mutations found in breast cancer. While striking differences between Caucasian and African-American patients in the type and/or frequency of *TP53* mutations have not been reported, significantly lower survival rates have been reported in association with *TP53* mutations in black patients compared with white patients (four- to fivefold excess death rate, $p < 0.012$).[351]

Interestingly, *TP53* mutations do not appear to be evenly distributed among the various histologic types of breast cancer. In one series, 148 human breast cancers were surveyed for *TP53* mutations, with mutations identified in 39 percent of medullary cancers and 26 percent of invasive ductal lesions but only 12 percent of invasive lobular cancers. No *TP53* mutations were detected in the 19 mucinous and 8 papillary carcinomas examined.[352] In all studies where survival data were available, *TP53* mutations were associated with a significantly poorer prognosis. Finally, *TP53* mutations have been reported in approximately 15 percent of DCIS lesions.[349]

In addition to mutations, alterations in the subcellular location of p53 have been noted in breast cancer specimens compared with normal breast epithelium. In an analysis of 27 breast cancers, sequestration of p53 in the cytoplasm was demonstrated in 37 percent of the breast cancers analyzed, overexpression of nuclear p53 in another 30 percent of tumors, and complete lack of staining in the remaining 33 percent.[353] While other studies have not found p53 alterations in all samples studied, these data suggest that p53 alterations are among the most common genetic changes found in breast carcinoma.

The relationship between *TP53* mutations and the chemoresistance of breast cancer cells was suggested initially by a report hinting that specific mutations in the DNA-binding domain of p53 lead to primary resistance to doxorubicin, one of the most widely used and most effective chemotherapeutic agents for breast cancer.[354] In this study, 11 of 63 tumors had mutations in this region. Four of these 11 patients progressed on doxorubicin, as opposed to only 2 of 52 patients without p53 DNA-binding region mutations. Among the patients with p53 DNA-binding-domain mutations who did respond to doxorubicin, most relapsed within 3 months of treatment. Similar data were reported in a second study reporting a smaller benefit from chemotherapy, hormonal therapy, and radiation in patients with tumors harboring *TP53* mutations.[355]

The retinoblastoma tumor-suppressor gene (*RB1*) appears to play a role in breast tumorigenesis in at least a proportion of cases; however, *RB1* has not been as well characterized in breast cancer as *TP53.* Like p53, RB regulates cell cycle progression, with dephosphorylated RB acting to halt cell cycle progression in G1. The link between *RB1* and breast cancer was first suggested by studies demonstrating structural rearrangements and inactivation of *RB1* in breast cancer.[356,357] This observation was followed by work demonstrating that estradiol decreases expression of RB, fueling speculation that estogren may act as a tumor promoter by decreasing expression of critical tumor-suppressor genes.[358] Further evidence for the role of RB1 in breast cancer was provided by demonstration that using retroviral-mediated gene transfer, wild-type RB1 introduced into breast cancer cells with a known *RB1* mutation results in decreased tumorgenicity in nude mice and a reduction in anchorage-independent growth.[359]

Current estimates suggest that *RB1* may be inactivated in approximately 20 percent of breast cancers.[360] One group of investigators described the incidence of RB1 alterations in 96 primary breast cancers and related their findings to patient and tumor characteristics, as well as oncogene amplifications and *TP53* mutations.[361] In this series, RB1 alterations were found to occur more frequently in ER-positive tumors and less frequently in tumors with HER2/neu or c-myc amplification. RB1 alterations were associated with small (< 2 cm) tumors without axillary node involvement. In contrast, a study of 197 breast cancer specimens using immunohistochemistry to evaluate the expression of RB1[362] suggested that loss of RB1 expression was correlated with the presence of axillary nodal metastasis; however, neither group of investigators was able to demonstrate a correlation with relapse-free or overall survival.

Various cyclins accumulate at cell cycle checkpoints and complex with cdks. Binding of a cdk to a specific cyclin partner activates the kinase activity of the cdk, which in turn phosphorylates and activates downstream target proteins that are necessary to propel the cell into the next phase of the cell cycle.[363,364] Overproduction of cyclins and cdks or their presence at an inappropriate time would be expected to cause unregulated cell division. Consequently, these molecules are candidate proto-oncogenes. In one of the first studies of the role of cyclins in breast carcinoma, 20 breast cancer cell lines were assayed for expression of cyclin A, B1, C, D1, D2, D3, and E; increased expression of one or more cyclins was demonstrated in 7 of 20 lines (35 percent). Five of the seven displayed increased expression of cyclin D1. This group also noted cyclin D1 overexpression in 45 percent of 124 primary breast cancers.[363] Cyclin D1, which regulates the G1/S transition, recently was identified as the *PRAD1* oncogene located at chromosome 11q13.[364] Cyclin D1 overexpression appears to be a relatively early event in tumor development.[365,366] Evidence for the early involvement of cyclin D in breast cancer was provided by Steeg and colleagues, who demonstrated cyclin D1 overexpression in 18 percent of benign breast lesions but in 76 percent of low-grade DCIS, 87 percent of high-grade DCIS, and 83 percent of infiltrating ductal cancers.[367] Significantly lower frequencies of overexpression were seen in a recent study, where 39 percent of atypical ductal hyperplasia, 43 percent of DCIS, and 48 percent of invasive carcinoma demonstrated overexpression of cyclin D1.[368] Cyclin D1 overexpression also has been identified in up to 80 percent of invasive lobular carcinomas of the breast.[369] Induced expression of cyclin D1 in breast cancer cells leads to an increase in the proportion of cells progressing through G1 and removes the requirement for growth factor stimulation normally necessary for completion of the cell cycle.[370] Overexpression of cyclin D1 in 30 to 50 percent of breast tumors does not correlate with observations of cyclin D1 gene amplification in 15 percent of tumors. Thus a mechanism other than amplification leads to overexpression and oncogenesis. A more recent analysis of cyclin D1-null mice provides an interesting and not unexpected link with mammary development as these mice do not undergo the massive mammary epithelial proliferation associated with pregnancy despite a normal ovarian hormone response.[371] Finally, Cyclin D1 is capable of activating the estrogen receptor in the absence of estrogen and independently of cdk4 activation.[372,373] This suggests that overexpression of cyclin D1 may exhibit some of its oncogenic effect through regulation of ER-responsive genes. However, one group found that this activation can be inhibited by tamoxifen,[373] while the other group states that antiestrogens do not inhibit ER activation.[372]

Tumor-specific mutations are rare in the p27Kip1 and cyclin E cell cycle regulators. However, levels of expression of these genes can be altered by posttranscriptional mechanisms. Thus, by observing protein levels, Porter and colleagues demonstrated that p27 and cyclin E correlate with survival in early onset breast cancer patients.[374]

The growth inhibitory protein of transforming growth factor beta (TGFβ) is thought to exert its effect on cell growth through inhibition of cell cycle progression. Because a number of tumorigenic cell lines have lost responsiveness to TGFβ, it is believed to play a role in tumor suppression, with malignant transformation being partially dependent on the loss of TGFβ expression or function. The growth-inhibitory effects of TGFβ are initiated by binding to cell surface TGFβ receptors. After ligand-receptor binding, multiple molecular targets have been suggested, including down-regulation of c-myc and cyclin expression, accumulation of hypophosphorylated RB, and inactivation of cdk2 and cdk4.[375] Work in this area is ongoing, but any one of these effects potentially could result in G1 arrest. Of particular interest in regard to breast cancer, TGFβ is hormonally regulated. Jeng and colleagues demonstrated that TGFβ isoforms are differentially regulated,[376] with TGFβ_2 and TGFβ_3 levels being suppressed by estrogen with little effect on TGFβ_1 levels. While early work suggested that TGFβ (isoforms not specified) is induced to high levels by the growth inhibitory estrogen antagonist tamoxifen,[377] later work demonstrated that short exposure (6 h) to tamoxifen resulted in a slight decrease in TGFβ_1 protein, whereas longer exposure had no effect. Thus the increase in unfractionated TGFβ in response to tamoxifen probably is due to increases in TGFβ_2 and/or TGFβ_3.[378] Paradoxically, while TGFβ is a strong growth inhibitor of normal mammary tissue, recent evidence suggests that enhanced TGFβ secretion correlates with aggressive malignant behavior. This was first demonstrated with the growth-stimulatory effect of TGFβ_1 on the breast cancer cell lines T47D and MCF-7.[379] In support of these studies, the breast cancer cell line MCF-7, transfected with TGFβ_1 cDNA, formed tumors in ovariectomized mice in the absence of estrogen supplementation, whereas the parental MCF-7 cells did not.[380] Prominent TGFβ_1 expression also has been associated with axillary lymph node metastases ($p < 0.015$), but this association was not found in tumors that expressed both TGFβ_1 and TGFβ_2.[381] In a study of 50 breast cancers, one group reported that 90 percent expressed TGFβ_1, 78 percent expressed TGFβ_2, and 94 percent expressed TGFβ_3, with 74 percent of the tumors expressing all three isoforms. Expression of all three isoforms was more likely to be associated with lymph node metastases than with the expression of one or two isoforms ($p < 0.025$).[382] However, other studies have not confirmed the usefulness of TGFβ expression as a prognostic factor in breast cancer.[383]

Regulators of Apoptosis. Apoptosis, the genetically programmed process of active (energy-requiring) cell death, is clearly important in understanding both neoplastic transformation and resistance to cytotoxic chemotherapy in breast cancer. Apoptosis can be induced by a variety of stimuli, including withdrawal of growth factors, DNA damage, viral infection, and expression of p53.[384] Since emerging evidence suggests that cytotoxic chemotherapy may exert a major effect on cancer cells by inducing apoptosis in response to chemotherapy-induced DNA damage, resistance to chemotherapy in some cases may result from inhibition of the apoptotic response.[385]

The proto-oncogene *bcl*-2, which normally functions to suppress apoptosis in a variety of cell types, has been studied extensively in several human cancers, including breast carcinoma, where it is overexpressed in 30 to 45 percent of cases.[386,387] Bcl-2 expression in human breast tissue varies dramatically throughout the menstrual cycle, suggesting that bcl-2 regulation is hormone-dependent.[388] Consistent with this hypothesis is the finding that bcl-2 expression is increased in ER-positive tumors and further increases after treatment with tamoxifen.[386] Conversely, bcl-2 expression is down-regulated in tumors expressing aberrant p53.[389] However, no genetic alterations that would increase bcl-2 levels have been reported in breast cancers.

c-myc**.** Numerous investigators have examined the role of the c-*myc* proto-oncogene in breast cancer with variable results. c-*myc* amplification was examined in 89 Norwegian breast cancer patients without axillary node involvement; amplification was noted in only one tumor.[390] However, another group used immunohistochemical methods to study 206 breast carcinomas and reported nuclear staining in 12 percent and cytoplasmic staining in 95 percent of these tumors. The presence of cytoplasmic staining was associated with increased disease-free survival compared with patients with tumors where c-myc was detected in the nucleus.[391] Finally, a study of 42 invasive breast cancers and 11 normal breast tissues suggested that while c-myc as detected by immunohistochemistry was present in both normal and malignant tissues, the level of expression in tumors was higher than it was in normal breast tissue.[392]

Cell Adhesion Molecules. Normal mammary epithelial cells are arranged in two layers: (1) a luminal epithelium and (2) a basal layer composed of myoepithelial cells and a small number of basal or stem cells. The basal layer is highly proliferative and is in direct contact with the basement membrane. During mammary carcinogenesis, tumor cells must escape normal adhesion mechanisms and traverse the basement membrane to invade surrounding structures. In this setting, interactions between breast carcinoma cells and their microenvironment are important determinants of the growth, invasion, and metastatic potential of tumor cells. In an effort to elucidate these interactions, researchers have investigated cell adhesion mechanisms, proteolytic enzymes, and the paracrine stimulation of growth factor receptors.[393]

Several factors participate in the maintenance of normal cell-cell and cell-matrix interactions. Cell-cell interactions are mediated via desmosomes and cadherin-containing junctions. In adult breast tissue, E-cadherin is expressed in normal ductal epithelial cells, and a reduction in E-cadherin expression is being investigated as a possible marker of invasive and metastatic potential. P-cadherin normally is expressed only in embryonal cells and in the basal layer of the adult epithelium. In examining cell-cell interactions, one study of 11 cases of invasive breast carcinoma suggested that in histologically normal areas, myoepithelial cells contain higher levels of cell-matrix adhesion molecules than do luminal epithelial cells.[394] In these normal areas, both myoepithelial and luminal cells have cadherin-containing junctions necessary for cell-cell interactions. In regions containing invasive carcinoma, normal E-cadherin staining was maintained in 10 of 11 cases, but β-catenin, the cytoplasmic component of E-cadherin-mediated junctions, was down-regulated or was distributed in an irregular punctate pattern. Similar findings were reported in a study of 26 primary breast carcinomas in which E-cadherin expression was decreased or lost in 63 percent of cases and α-catenin was reduced or absent in 81 percent of cases.[395] In this study, all patients with known metastatic disease at the time of biopsy had abnormal β-catenin staining, suggesting a role for β-catenin in maintaining normal cell-cell interactions. In keeping with other studies, expression of both E- and P-cadherin in 57 invasive breast carcinomas was noted to be altered, with reduced E-cadherin expression in 67 percent of tumors and abnormal P-cadherin in the luminal cells of 30 percent of invasive carcinomas.[396] All specimens with abnormal P-cadherin staining were histologic grade III and also revealed decreased E-cadherin expression. Of note, while an earlier study observed P-cadherin expression in lobular carcinomas of all grades,[397] P-cadherin expression in ductal carcinomas has been limited to high-grade lesions. These findings suggest that in some aggressive breast carcinomas, decreased or absent E-cadherin may be replaced by P-cadherin. This association between reduced E-cadherin staining and an aggressive histologic appearance also was noted in 109 patients with invasive ductal carcinomas, with an association between reduced E-cadherin expression and reduced disease-free survival in univariate analysis (5-year DFS = 70 percent in the E-cadherin positive group; DFS = 38 percent in the reduced E-cadherin group; $p = 0.027$).[398] However, longer follow-up and further validation will be required to determine whether E-cadherin is an independent predictor of disease prognosis.

Matrix Metalloproteinases. Extracellular proteinases are believed to be important in modulating both cell-matrix interactions and the degradation of the basement membrane necessary for invasion and metastasis. The matrix metalloproteinases (MMPs) include the gelatinases MMP-2 (gelatinase A) and MMP-9 (gelatinase B). The gelatinases, which are secreted as zymogens and are activated by cell membrane-associated proteins, have specific activity against type IV collagen, a component of the basement membrane.[399] This collagenase activity, the results of specific inhibition studies, and higher levels of immunostaining in invasive breast cancers (relative to preinvasive cancers) implicate these MMPs in tumor invasiveness.[393,400] Membrane-type metalloproteinase (MT-MMP), another member of the MMP family, has been postulated to be the membrane-associated activator of MMP-2. The inhibitory component of this pathway consists of tissue inhibitors of metalloproteinase (TIMP-1 and -2). TIMPs are believed to exert their inhibitory activity by direct binding with the activated MMPs.

In an analysis of MMP-8, MMP-9, and TIMP-1 expression in breast cancer cells, protein levels were measured in the tumor tissue of 53 breast cancer patients.[401] MMP-8 and MMP-9 appeared to be coordinately regulated, and both were elevated in invasive tumors. However, increased levels of the MMP inhibitor TIMP-1 also were found in association with increased levels of the MMPs. These findings do not support earlier data suggesting that metastatic potential is associated with decreased TIMP-1 expression.

Of great interest is whether these proteases are produced by tumor cells or surrounding "normal" stromal cells, and if they are produced by stromal cells, whether the tumor cells are able to induce the expression of proteases. In an attempt to address this question, *in situ* hybridization was used to demonstrate that MT-MMP mRNA was expressed exclusively in the stromal cells in 83 of 83 human tumor specimens (including breast) analyzed.[402] In contrast, using an antibody directed against MT-MMP, protein was detected on the surface of invasive carcinoma cells.[403] This apparent discrepancy also has been described for MMP-2, with MMP-2 mRNA detected in tumor fibroblasts but MMP-2 protein detected in carcinoma cells.[404] Taken together with earlier studies suggesting that conditioned medium or the membrane fraction from breast carcinoma lines up-regulates the expression of MMP-2 in fibroblasts,[405,406] these findings suggest close interaction between tumor and stromal cells. A unifying hypothesis is that both MT-MMP and MMP-2 are produced in peritumor fibroblasts in response to the paracrine stimulation of carcinoma cells, that MT-MMP may activate MMP-2 on the stromal cell membrane, that the enzymes are secreted into the extracellular matrix, that each binds to the surface of malignant cells, and that one or both enzymes subsequently may be internalized by tumor cells.

Cathepsins. The cathepsins are another class of proteases that may affect the invasive and metastatic potential of malignant cells. These proteins are expressed at low levels in all cells, and once they are auto-activated, they have enzymatic activity against several matrix proteins, including those in the basement membrane. Levels of cathepsin expression in breast cancer have been studied as possible prognostic markers. Cathepsin D expression has been examined by immunostaining of 151 breast carcinomas, with "strong" cathepsin D expression detected in 22 percent of cases correlating with the nonductal histologic type ($p = 0.0243$) and metastases at the time of diagnosis ($p = 0.0068$) but not with tumor size, histologic grade, lymph node metastases, or ER/PR status. On univariate analysis, "strong" cathepsin D staining appeared to predict a significantly worse prognosis (median survival < 40 months in the high-cathepsin D group, median survival not yet reached at 140 months of follow-up in the low-cathepsin D group; $p = 0.047$). In multivariate analysis, however, no significant correlation between "strong" cathepsin D staining and prognosis persisted after adjusting for other known prognostic markers.[407] The relationship between cathepsin D and other pathologic features has been investigated in a large series of 1752 primary breast cancer patients. In this study, cathepsin D was associated with tumor size and grade and the presence or absence of nodal metastasis. On multivariate analysis performed on 489 patients from this series, cathepsin D independently predicted relapse-free survival and overall survival.[408] While the reason for the discrepancy between the findings of these two studies is not clear; it may be that the scoring of the intensity of cathepsin D staining as a continuous variable and the larger sample size of later study allowed detection of the prognostic significance of this marker.

Mediators of Metastasis. In addition to the well-characterized cell adhesion molecules and matrix metalloproteases that are thought to play a role in the development of metastatic breast cancer, *NME1* (encoding nm23) is a gene that is difficult to characterize with regard to its normal function and as result of decreased expression.[409] *NME1* was isolated initially as a gene that is differentially expressed in melanoma cells with discrepant metastatic potential.[410] The highest level of nm23 expression is seen in cells with low metastatic potential. Shortly after the isolation of *NME1,* data were presented suggesting that NME1 is differentially expressed in human breast cancers, with low NME1 mRNA levels found in association with histopathologic indicators of high metastatic potential.[411] These data are supported by studies demonstrating that transfection of NME1 into human MDA-MB-435 breast carcinoma cells reduces the metastatic potential of these cells when injected into the mammary fat pad of mice. Reduction in metastatic potential was associated with decreased ability of cells to form colonies in soft agar and an altered response to TGFβ.[412] Murine developmental studies also demonstrated a role for nm23 in the functional differentiation of the mammary gland. In this study, NME1 expression increased with functional differentiation of the mammary gland in nulliparous and pregnant animals.[413] Howlett and colleagues subsequently demonstrated a link between nm23 and human breast epithelial differentiation by using a culture system designed to mimic breast stroma. In this system, transfected breast cancer cell lines that overexpressed nm23 regained several aspects of the normal phenotype, including acinar formation, basement membrane production, and eventual growth arrest.[414] In investigations of the biologic function of NME1, it became clear that this gene is identical to PUF, a factor known to alter myc transcription *in vitro*.[415] However, data suggesting that nm23 can function as a growth inhibitor[414] led to confusion about how nm23 can be both a tumor suppressor and an activator of the proto-oncogene c-*myc*. It is possible that this is due to a tissue-specific effect, since NME1 expression is increased in aggressive neuroblastomas but is reduced in aggressive breast cancers.[416]

CLINICAL IMPLICATIONS OF BREAST CANCER SUSCEPTIBILITY

As was discussed in this chapter, advances in molecular genetics have provided data that allow risk estimation for women with inherited mutations in dominant cancer susceptibility genes and prognostic determinations for women with sporadic breast cancer. Unfortunately, our ability to make clinically useful interventions on the basis of these data remains limited. Prospective studies that allow an estimation of risk reduction from prophylactic surgical intervention are unavailable, and the science of chemoprevention is in its infancy. There are limited data available to assess the efficacy of enhanced surveillance programs for individuals at high risk of developing breast cancer. Finally, there is little information available about the interaction of multiple risk factors, so recommendations regarding modification of exposure to hormonal agents or dietary changes in the face of increased breast cancer risk caused by family history may be premature. Thus, in counseling women at increased risk of breast cancer, clinicians rely almost entirely on clinical judgment and the wishes of the women being counseled. Women at increased risk of breast cancer are offered the options of increased surveillance and prophylactic surgery and may be eligible for chemoprevention as part of an approved research protocol.

For women diagnosed with breast cancer, whether inherited or sporadic, prognostic information is most useful when coupled with targeted therapeutic approaches, very few of which exist. Identification of highly aggressive tumors is of little benefit if we have only the standard treatment to offer. The challenge for the future is to learn to use data on the molecular characteristics of an individual tumor to benefit patients and, ultimately, to prevent the development of breast cancer.

RECOMMENDATIONS FOR WOMEN WITH INHERITED SUSCEPTIBILITY TO BREAST CANCER

As noted earlier, it is not known whether increased surveillance will reduce breast cancer-related mortality in high-risk women. Furthermore, women from high-risk breast cancer families are well aware that mammography and clinical breast examination may not detect premalignant lesions. In the face of a striking family history and close personal losses, these women may be unconvinced that mammography and clinical breast examination offer the protection they seek. Such women often inquire about prophylactic mastectomy in the absence of other preventive options. There are few prospective data demonstrating the efficacy of prophylactic mastectomy in this setting. Furthermore, there are theoretical considerations that call into question the rationale for prophylactic surgery. Current surgical technique does not allow the complete removal of all breast tissue in a prophylactic total mastectomy. Since a germ-line mutation will be present in all residual breast tissue, individuals may remain at increased risk after surgery. Similarly, prophylactic oophorectomy does not guarantee protection from ovarian carcinoma, since tumors may arise spontaneously in the peritoneal reflection. These uncertainties make it difficult to counsel individuals about the potential benefits of these procedures. Nonetheless, the anxiety faced by women who harbor mutations in a breast cancer susceptibility gene can be overwhelming. Women must be presented with available data and allowed to make decisions that reflect their needs but do not offer a false sense of security.

Current recommendations include breast examination and mammography every 6 to 12 months beginning between the ages of 25 and 35 for women at increased risk of breast cancer resulting from direct or indirect molecular demonstration of a breast cancer-related genetic mutation.[417,418] Although no data exist to determine whether an increased frequency of clinical examination and screening mammography in this population reduces mortality, there are preliminary data that *BRCA1*-related tumors may have a faster growth rate than do sporadic tumors.[419] In addition, patient anxiety may be allayed somewhat by offering the option of two mammograms per year. Prophylactic mastectomy may be an option for interested women, who should be provided with information regarding the limited evidence for or against risk reduction by this procedure.

In women with a documented *BRCA1* or *BRCA2* mutation, pelvic examinations with transvaginal ultrasound every 6 to 12 months for those under age 40 and/or those still interested in childbearing may be of benefit. Prophylactic oophorectomy at the completion of childbearing or at the time of menopause is recommended by the American College of Obstetrics and Gynecology; however, there is a low but measurable incidence of peritoneal malignancies after oophorectomy that may derive from peritoneal cells, which are at similar risk for malignant transformation and are not removed by oophorectomy. It may be prudent for women at increased risk of breast cancer to avoid the use of exogenous estrogens when possible, since no data exist regarding the effect of estrogens on the penetrance of susceptibility genes in breast cancer. However, a dilemma arises in that there may be some benefit to taking oral contraceptives to reduce ovarian cancer risk and in that heart disease and osteoporosis are more prevalent in women who do not use estrogen replacement therapy after menopause.

ACKNOWLEDGMENTS

We are extremely grateful to Stacy Schierts and Colleen Schehl for assistance with the preparation of this chapter.

REFERENCES

1. Kelsey JL, Horn-Ross PL: Breast cancer: Magnitude of the problem and descriptive epidemiology. *Epidemiol Rev* **15**:7, 1993.

2. Miller BA: Causes of breast cancer and high risk groups, incidence and demographics, in Harris JR, Hellman S, Henderson IC, Kinne DW (eds): *Breast Diseases*. Philadelphia, Lippincott, 1991, p 119.
3. Miller BA, Feuer EJ, Hankey BF: The increasing incidence of breast cancer since 1982: Relevance of early detection. *Cancer Causes Control* **2**:67, 1991.
4. Glass A, Hoover RN: Changing incidence of breast cancer (letter). *J Natl Cancer Inst* **80**:1076, 1988.
5. Holford TR, Roush GC, McKay LA: Trends in female breast cancer in Connecticut and the United States. *J Clin Epidemiol* **44**:29, 1991.
6. Slattery ML, Kerber RA: A comprehensive evaluation of family history and breast cancer risk: The Utah Population Database (see comments). *JAMA* **270**:1563, 1993.
7. Colditz GA, et al: Family history, age, and risk of breast cancer: Prospective data from the Nurses' Health Study (see comments) [published erratum appears in *JAMA* **270**:1548, 1993]. *JAMA* **270**:338, 1993.
8. Gail MH, et al: Projecting individualized probabilities of developing breast cancer for white females who are being examined annually (see comments). *J Natl Cancer Inst* **81**:1879, 1989.
9. Easton DF, Bishop DT, Ford D, Crockford GP: Genetic linkage analysis in familial breast and ovarian cancer: Results from 214 families. The Breast Cancer Linkage Consortium. *Am J Hum Genet* **52**:678, 1993.
10. Kampert JB, Whittemore AS, Paffenbarger RS Jr: Combined effect of childbearing, menstrual events, and body size on age-specific breast cancer risk. *Am J Epidemiol* **128**:962, 1988.
11. White E: Projected changes in breast cancer incidence due to the trend toward delayed childbearing. *Am J Public Health* **77**:495, 1987.
12. Trichopoulos D, MacMahon B, Cole P: Menopause and breast cancer risk. *J Natl Cancer Inst* **48**:605, 1972.
13. Pike MC, Spicer DV, Dahmoush L, Press MF: Estrogens, progestogens, normal breast cell proliferation, and breast cancer risk. *Epidemiol Rev* **15**:17, 1993.
14. Tokunaga M, et al: Incidence of female breast cancer among atomic bomb survivors, 1950–1985. *Radiat Res* **138**:209, 1994.
15. McGregor H, et al: Breast cancer incidence among atomic bomb survivors, Hiroshima and Nagasaki, 1950–69. *J Natl Cancer Inst* **59**:799, 1977.
16. Bhatia S, et al: Breast cancer and other second neoplasms after childhood Hodgkin's disease (see comments]. *N Engl J Med* **334**:745, 1996.
17. Harris JR, Lippman ME, Veronesi U, Willett W: Breast cancer (1) (see comments). *N Engl J Med* **327**:319, 1992.
18. Dupont WD, Page DL: Risk factors for breast cancer in women with proliferative breast disease. *N Engl J Med* **312**:146, 1985.
19. Kinne DW: Clinical measurement of lobular carcinoma in situ, in Harris JR, Hellman S, Henderson IC, Kinne DW (eds): *Breast Diseases*. Philadelphia, Lippincott, 1985, pp 239–244.
20. Rosen PP, Kosloff C, Lieberman PH, Adair F, Braun DW Jr: Lobular carcinoma *in situ* of the breast: Detailed analysis of 99 patients with average follow-up of 24 years. *Am J Surg Pathol* **2**:225, 1978.
21. Consortium BCL: Pathology of familial breast cancer: Differences between breast cancers in carriers of *BRCA1* or *BRCA2* mutations and sporadic cases. Breast Cancer Linkage Consortium (see comments). *Lancet* **349**:1505, 1997.
22. Haagensen CD, Bodian C, Haagensen DE Jr: *Breast Carcinoma, Risk and Detection*. Philadelphia, Saunders, 1981, p. 238.
23. Rosner D, Bedwani RN, Vana J, Baker HW, Murphy GP: Noninvasive breast carcinoma: Results of a national survey by the American College of Surgeons. *Ann Surg* **192**:139, 1980.
24. Baker LH: Breast Cancer Detection Demonstration Project: Five-year summary report. *Cancer J Clin* **32**:194, 1982.
25. Page DL, Dupont WD, Rogers LW, Landenberger M: Intraductal carcinoma of the breast: Follow-up after biopsy only. *Cancer* **49**:751, 1982.
26. Rosen PP, Braun DW Jr, Kinne DE: The clinical significance of pre-invasive breast carcinoma. *Cancer* **46**:919, 1980.
27. Solin LJ, et al: Ten-year results of breast-conserving surgery and definitive irradiation for intraductal carcinoma (ductal carcinoma *in situ*) of the breast. *Cancer* **68**:2337, 1991.
28. Fisher ER, et al: Medullary cancer of the breast revisited. *Breast Cancer Res Treat* **16**:215, 1990.
29. American Joint Committee on Cancer: *Manual for Staging for Breast Carcinoma*. Philadelphia, Lippincott, 1989.
30. Harris JR: Staging of breast carcinoma, in Harris JR, Hellman S, Henderson IC, Kinne DW (eds): *Breast Diseases*. Philadelphia, Lippincott, 1991, p 330.
31. Clark GM, Sledge GW Jr, Osborne CK, McGuire WL: Survival from first recurrence: Relative importance of prognostic factors in 1015 breast cancer patients. *J Clin Oncol* **5**:55, 1987.
32. Fisher B, Anderson S, Redmond C: Reanalysis and results after 12 years follow-up in a randomized clinical trial comparing total mastectomy with lumpectomy with or without irradiation in the treatment of breast cancer. *N Engl J Med* **333**:1456, 1995.
33. Valero V, Buzdar AU, Hortobagyi GN: Locally advanced breast cancer. *Oncologist* **1**:8, 1996.
34. Peters WP: High-dose chemotherapy with autologous bone marrow transplantation for the treatment of breast cancer: Yes. *Import Adv Oncol* 215, 1995.
34b. Stadtmauer EA, O'Neill A, Goldstein LJ, Crilley PA, Mangan KF, Ingle JN, Brodsky I, et al: Conventional-does chemotherapy compared with high-dose chemotherapy plus autologous hematopoietic stem-cell transplatation for metastatic breast cancer. *N Engl J Med* **342**:1069, 2000.
35. Lynch HT, et al: Genetic heterogeneity and familial carcinoma of the breast. *Surg Gynecol Obstet* **142**:693, 1976.
36. Broca: *Taite de tumerus*. Asselin, 1866.
37. Williams WR, Anderson DE: Genetic epidemiology of breast cancer: Segregation analysis of 200 Danish pedigrees. *Genet Epidemiol* **1**:7, 1984.
38. Newman B, Austin MA, Lee M, King MC: Inheritance of human breast cancer: Evidence for autosomal dominant transmission in high-risk families. *Proc Natl Acad Sci USA* **85**:3044, 1988.
39. Miki Y, et al: A strong candidate for the breast and ovarian cancer susceptibility gene *BRCA1*. *Science* **266**:66, 1994.
40. Wooster R, et al: Identification of the breast cancer susceptibility gene *BRCA2* (see comments) [published erratum appears in *Nature* **379(6567)**:749, 1996]. *Nature* **378**:789, 1995.
41. Tavtigian SV, et al: The complete *BRCA2* gene and mutations in chromosome 13q-linked kindreds (see comments). *Nature Genet* **12**:333, 1996.
42. Nelson CL, et al: Familial clustering of colon, breast, uterine, and ovarian cancers as assessed by family history. *Genet Epidemiol* **10**:235, 1993.
43. Narod SA, et al: Familial breast-ovarian cancer locus on chromosome 17q12-q23 (see comments). *Lancet* **338**:82, 1991.
44. Couch FJ, et al: *BRCA1* mutations in women attending clinics that evaluate the risk of breast cancer (see comments). *N Engl J Med* **336**:1409, 1997.
45. Stoppa-Lyonnet D, et al: *BRCA1* sequence variations in 160 individuals referred to a breast/ovarian family cancer clinic: Institut Curie Breast Cancer Group (see comments). *Am J Hum Genet* **60**:1021, 1997.
46. Shattuck-Eidens D, et al: *BRCA1* sequence analysis in women at high risk for susceptibility mutations: Risk factor analysis and implications for genetic testing (see comments). *JAMA* **278**:1242, 1997.
47. Frank TS, et al: Sequence analysis of *BRCA1* and *BRCA2:* Correlation of mutations with family history and ovarian cancer risk. *J Clin Oncol* **16**:2417, 1998.
48. Easton DF, Bishop DT, Ford D, Crockford GP, Consortium BCL: Breast and ovarian cancer incidence in *BRCA1* mutation carriers. *Lancet* **343**:962, 1994.
49. Struewing JP, et al: The risk of cancer associated with specific mutations of *BRCA1* and *BRCA2* among Ashkenazi Jews (see comments). *N Engl J Med* **336**:1401, 1997.
50. Whittemore AS, Gong G, Itnyre J: Prevalence and contribution of *BRCA1* mutations in breast cancer and ovarian cancer: Results from three U.S. population-based case-control studies of ovarian cancer. *Am J Hum Genet* **60**:496, 1997.
51. Brody LC, Biesecker BB: Breast cancer susceptibility genes: *BRCA1* and *BRCA2*. *Medicine* **77**:208, 1998.
52. Arason A, Barkardottir RB, Egilsson V: Linkage analysis of chromosome 17q markers and breast-ovarian cancer in Icelandic families and possible relationship to prostatic cancer. *Am J Hum Genet* **52**:711, 1993.
53. Ford D, Easton DF, Bishop DT, Narod SA, Goldgar DE: Risks of cancer in *BRCA1*-mutation carriers: Breast Cancer Linkage Consortium. *Lancet* **343**:692, 1994.
54. Lynch HT, Marcus J, Watson P, Page D: Distinctive clinicopathologic features of *BRCA1*-linked hereditary breast cancer. *Proc ASCO* **13**:56, 1994.
55. Marcus JN, et al: Hereditary breast cancer: Pathobiology prognosis and *BRCA1* and *BRCA2* gene linkage (see comments). *Cancer* **77**:697, 1996.

56. Karp SE, et al: Influence of *BRCA1* mutations on nuclear grade and estrogen receptor status of breast carcinoma in Ashkenazi Jewish women. *Cancer* **80**:435, 1997.
57. Robson M, et al: *BRCA*-associated breast cancer: Absence of a characteristic immunophenotype. *Cancer Res* **58**:1839, 1998.
58. Wagner TM, et al: *BRCA1*-related breast cancer in Austrian breast and ovarian cancer families: Specific *BRCA1* mutations and pathological characteristics. *Int J Cancer* **77**:354, 1998.
59. Eisinger F, et al: Germ line mutation at *BRCA1* affects the histoprognostic grade in hereditary breast cancer. *Cancer Res* **56**:471, 1996.
60. Jarvis EM, Kirk JA, Clarke CL: Loss of nuclear *BRCA1* expression in breast cancers is associated with a highly proliferative tumor phenotype. *Cancer Genet Cytogenet* **101**:109, 1998.
61. Johannsson OT, Ranstam J, Borg A, Olsson H: Survival of *BRCA1* breast and ovarian cancer patients: A population-based study from southern Sweden (see comments). *J Clin Oncol* **16**:397, 1998.
62. Verhoog LC, et al: Survival and tumour characteristics of breast-cancer patients with germline mutations of *BRCA1*. *Lancet* **351**:316, 1998.
63. Foulkes WD, Wong N, Rozen F, Brunet JS, Narod SA: Survival of patients with breast cancer and *BRCA1* mutations (letter). *Lancet* **351**:1359, 1998.
64. Tirkkonen M, et al: Distinct somatic genetic changes associated with tumor progression in carriers of *BRCA1* and *BRCA2* germ-line mutations. *Cancer Res* **57**:1222, 1997.
65. Tapper J, et al: Genetic changes in inherited and sporadic ovarian carcinomas by comparative genomic hybridization: Extensive similarity except for a difference at chromosome 2q24-q32. *Cancer Res* **58**:2715, 1998.
66. Brunet JS, et al: Effect of smoking on breast cancer in carriers of mutant *BRCA1* or *BRCA2* genes (see comments). *J Natl Cancer Inst* **90**:761, 1998.
67. Narod SA, et al: Oral contraceptives and the risk of hereditary ovarian cancer: Hereditary Ovarian Cancer Clinical Study Group (see comments). *N Engl J Med* **339**:424, 1998.
68. Easton D: Breast cancer genes: What are the real risks? (news). *Nature Genet* **16**:210, 1997.
69. Phelan CM, et al: Ovarian cancer risk in *BRCA1* carriers is modified by the HRAS1 variable number of tandem repeat (VNTR) locus. *Nature Genet* **12**:309, 1996.
70. Redston M, Nathanson K, Yuan ZQ: The APC I1307K allele and cancer risk in a community-based study of Ashkenazi Jews. *Nature Genet* **20**:62, 1998.
71. Hall JM, et al: Linkage of early-onset familial breast cancer to chromosome 17q21. *Science* **250**:1684, 1990.
72. Bork P, et al: A superfamily of conserved domains in DNA damage-responsive cell cycle checkpoint proteins. *FASEB J* **11**:68, 1997.
73. Abel KJ, et al: Mouse *Brca1:* Localization sequence analysis and identification of evolutionarily conserved domains. *Hum Mol Genet* **4**:2265, 1995.
74. Bennett LM, et al: Isolation of the mouse homologue of *BRCA1* and genetic mapping to mouse chromosome 11. *Genomics* **29**:576, 1995.
75. Sharan SK, Wims M, Bradley A: Murine *Brca1:* Sequence and significance for human missense mutations. *Hum Mol Genet* **4**:2275, 1995.
76. Szabo CI, et al: Human, canine and murine *BRCA1* genes: Sequence comparison among species. *Hum Mol Genet* **5**:1289, 1996.
77. Chen KS, Shepel LA, Haag JD, Heil GM, Gould MN: Cloning genetic mapping and expression studies of the rat *Brca1* gene. *Carcinogenesis* **17**:1561, 1996.
78. Futreal PA, et al: *BRCA1* mutations in primary breast and ovarian carcinomas. *Science* **266**:120, 1994.
79. Castilla LH, et al: Mutations in the *BRCA1* gene in families with early-onset breast and ovarian cancer. *Nature Genet* **8**:387, 1994.
80. Friedman LS, et al: Confirmation of *BRCA1* by analysis of germline mutations linked to breast and ovarian cancer in ten families. *Nature Genet* **8**:399, 1994.
81. Simard J, et al: Common origins of *BRCA1* mutations in Canadian breast and ovarian cancer families. *Nature Genet* **8**:392, 1994.
82. Merajver SD, et al: Somatic mutations in the *BRCA1* gene in sporadic ovarian tumours. *Nature Genet* **9**:439, 1995.
83. Hosking L, et al: A somatic *BRCA1* mutation in an ovarian tumour (letter). *Nature Genet* **9**:343, 1995.
84. Takahashi H, et al: Mutation analysis of the *BRCA1* gene in ovarian cancers. *Cancer Res* **55**:2998, 1995.
85. Matsushima M, et al: Mutation analysis of the *BRCA1* gene in 76 Japanese ovarian cancer patients: Four germline mutations but no evidence of somatic mutation. *Hum Mol Genet* **4**:1953, 1995.
86. Boyd M, Harris F, McFarlane R, Davidson HR, Black DM: A human *BRCA1* gene knockout (letter). *Nature* **375**:541, 1995.
87. Inoue R, et al: Germline mutation of *BRCA1* in Japanese breast cancer families. *Cancer Res* **55**:3521, 1995.
88. Hogervorst FB, et al: Rapid detection of *BRCA1* mutations by the protein truncation test. *Nature Genet* **10**:208, 1995.
89. Plummer SJ, et al: Detection of *BRCA1* mutations by the protein truncation test. *Hum Mol Genet* **4**:1989, 1995.
90. Gayther SA, et al: Rapid detection of regionally clustered germ-line *BRCA1* mutations by multiplex heteroduplex analysis: UKCCCR Familial Ovarian Cancer Study Group. *Am J Hum Genet* **58**:451, 1996.
91. Ganguly T, Dhulipala R, Godmilow L, Ganguly A: High throughput fluorescence-based conformation-sensitive gel electrophoresis (F-CSGE) identifies six unique *BRCA2* mutations and an overall low incidence of *BRCA2* mutations in high-risk *BRCA1*-negative breast cancer families. *Hum Genet* **102**:549, 1998.
92. Couch FJ, Weber BL: Mutations and polymorphisms in the familial early-onset breast cancer (*BRCA1*) gene: Breast Cancer Information Core. *Hum Mutat* **8**:8, 1996.
93. Gayther SA, et al: Germline mutations of the *BRCA1* gene in breast and ovarian cancer families provide evidence for a genotype-phenotype correlation. *Nature Genet* **11**:428, 1995.
94. Serova O, et al: A high incidence of *BRCA1* mutations in 20 breast-ovarian cancer families. *Am J Hum Genet* **58**:42, 1996.
95. Brzovic PS, Meza J, King MC, Klevit RE: The cancer-predisposing mutation *C61G* disrupts homodimer formation in the NH_2-terminal *BRCA1* RING finger domain. *J Biol Chem* **273**:7795, 1998.
96. Wu GS, et al: KILLER/DR5 is a DNA damage-inducible p53-regulated death receptor gene (letter). *Nature Genet* **17**:141, 1997.
97. Jensen DE, et al: *BAP1:* A novel ubiquitin hydrolase which binds to the *BRCA1* RING finger and enhances *BRCA1*-mediated cell growth suppression. *Oncogene* **16**:1097, 1998.
98. Papa S, et al: Identification of a possible somatic *BRCA1* mutation affecting translation efficiency in an early-onset sporadic breast cancer patient (letter). *J Natl Cancer Inst* **90**:1011, 1998.
99. Humphrey JS, et al: Human *BRCA1* inhibits growth in yeast: Potential use in diagnostic testing. *Proc Natl Acad Sci USA* **94**:5820, 1997.
100. Puget N, et al: A 1-kb Alu-mediated germ-line deletion removing *BRCA1* exon 17. *Cancer Res* **57**:828, 1997.
101. Petrij-Bosch A, et al: *BRCA1* genomic deletions are major founder mutations in Dutch breast cancer patients [published erratum appears in *Nature Genet* **17(4)**:503, 1997]. *Nature Genet* **17**:341, 1997.
102. Holt JT, et al: Growth retardation and tumour inhibition by *BRCA1* (see comments). *Nature Genet* **12**:298, 1996.
103. Sobol H, et al: Truncation at conserved terminal regions of BRCA1 protein is associated with highly proliferating hereditary breast cancers. *Cancer Res* **56**:3216, 1996.
104. Tonin P, et al: *BRCA1* mutations in Ashkenazi Jewish women (letter). *Am J Hum Genet* **57**:189, 1995.
105. Bar-Sade RB, et al: The 185delAG *BRCA1* mutation originated before the dispersion of Jews in the diaspora and is not limited to Ashkenazim. *Hum Mol Genet* **7**:801, 1998.
106. FitzGerald MG, et al: Germ-line *BRCA1* mutations in Jewish and non-Jewish women with early-onset breast cancer (see comments). *N Engl J Med* **334**:143, 1996.
107. Offit K, et al: Germline *BRCA1* 185delAG mutations in Jewish women with breast cancer (see comments). *Lancet* **347**:1643, 1996.
108. Levy-Lahad E, et al: Founder *BRCA1* and *BRCA2* mutations in Ashkenazi Jews in Israel: Frequency and differential penetrance in ovarian cancer and in breast-ovarian cancer families (see comments). *Am J Hum Genet* **60**:1059, 1997.
109. Muto MG, Cramer DW, Tangir J, Berkowitz R, Mok S: Frequency of the *BRCA1* 185delAG mutation among Jewish women with ovarian cancer and matched population controls. *Cancer Res* **56**:1250, 1996.
110. Abeliovich D, et al: The founder mutations 185delAG and 5382insC in *BRCA1* and 6174delT in *BRCA2* appear in 60% of ovarian cancer and 30% of early-onset breast cancer patients among Ashkenazi women. *Am J Hum Genet* **60**:505, 1997.
111. Neuhausen SL, et al: Haplotype and phenotype analysis of nine recurrent *BRCA2* mutations in 111 families: Results of an international study. *Am J Hum Genet* **62**:1381, 1998.
112. Dunning AM, et al: Common *BRCA1* variants and susceptibility to breast and ovarian cancer in the general population. *Hum Mol Genet* **6**:285, 1997.

113. Bergthorsson JT, et al: Chromosome imbalance at the 3p14 region in human breast tumours: High frequency in patients with inherited predisposition due to BRCA2. *Eur J Cancer* **34**:142, 1998.
114. Huusko P, et al: Evidence of founder mutations in Finnish *BRCA1* and *BRCA2* families (letter). *Am J Hum Genet* **62**:1544, 1998.
115. Ramus SJ, et al: Analysis of *BRCA1* and *BRCA2* mutations in Hungarian families with breast or breast-ovarian cancer (letter). *Am J Hum Genet* **60**:1242, 1997.
116. Gayther SA, et al: Variation of risks of breast and ovarian cancer associated with different germline mutations of the *BRCA2* gene. *Nature Genet* **15**:103, 1997.
117. Dorum A, et al: A *BRCA1* founder mutation, identified with haplotype analysis, allowing genotype/phenotype determination and predictive testing. *Eur J Cancer* **33**:2390, 1997.
118. Szabo CI, King MC: Population genetics of *BRCA1* and *BRCA2* (editorial; comment). *Am J Hum Genet* **60**:1013, 1997.
119. Malone KE, et al: *BRCA1* mutations and breast cancer in the general population: Analyses in women before age 35 years and in women before age 45 years with first-degree family history (see comments). *JAMA* **279**:922, 1998.
120. Newman B, et al: Frequency of breast cancer attributable to *BRCA1* in a population-based series of American women (see comments). *JAMA* **279**:915, 1998.
121. Hakansson S, et al: Moderate frequency of *BRCA1* and *BRCA2* germ-line mutations in Scandinavian familial breast cancer (see comments). *Am J Hum Genet* **60**:1068, 1997.
122. Krainer M, et al: Differential contributions of *BRCA1* and *BRCA2* to early-onset breast cancer (see comments). *N Engl J Med* **336**:1416, 1997.
123. Katagiri T, et al: Mutations in the *BRCA1* gene in Japanese breast cancer patients. *Hum Mutat* **7**:334, 1996.
124. Berry DA, Parmigiani G, Sanchez J, Schildkraut J, Winer E: Probability of carrying a mutation of breast-ovarian cancer gene *BRCA1* based on family history (see comments). *J Natl Cancer Inst* **89**:227, 1997.
125. Brown MA, Xu C, Nicolai H: The 59 end of the *BRCA1* gene lies within a duplicated region of human chromosome 17q21. *Cancer Res* **12**:2507, 1996.
126. Fetzer S, Tworek HA, Piver MS, Dicioccio RA: An alternative splice site junction in exon 1a of the *BRCA1* gene (letter). *Cancer Genet Cytogenet* **105**:90, 1998.
127. Thakur S, et al: Localization of *BRCA1* and a splice variant identifies the nuclear localization signal. *Mol Cell Biol* **17**:444, 1997.
128. Wilson CA, et al: Differential subcellular localization expression and biological toxicity of *BRCA1* and the splice variant *BRCA1*-delta11b. *Oncogene* **14**:1, 1997.
129. Wu LC, et al: Identification of a RING protein that can interact in vivo with the *BRCA1* gene product. *Nature Genet* **14**:430, 1996.
130. Jin Y, et al: Cell cycle-dependent colocalization of *BARD1* and *BRCA1* proteins in discrete nuclear domains. *Proc Natl Acad Sci USA* **94**:12075, 1997.
131. Scully R, et al: Association of *BRCA1* with *Rad51* in mitotic and meiotic cells. *Cell* **88**:265, 1997.
132. Chen J, Silver DP, Walpita D, Cantor SB, Gazdar AF, Tomlinson G, Couch FJ, Weber BL, Ashley T, Livingston DM, Scully R: Stable interaction between the products of the BRCA1 and BRCA2 tumor suppressor genes in mitotic and meiotic cells. *Mol Cell* **2**:317, 1998.
133. Chapman MS, Verma IM: Transcriptional activation by *BRCA1* (letter; comment). *Nature* **382**:678, 1996.
134. Monteiro AN, August A, Hanafusa H: Evidence for a transcriptional activation function of *BRCA1* C-terminal region. *Proc Natl Acad Sci USA* **93**:13595, 1996.
135. Ouchi T, Monteiro AN, August A, Aaronson SA, Hanafusa H: *BRCA1* regulates p53-dependent gene expression. *Proc Natl Acad Sci USA* **95**:2302, 1998.
136. Zhang H, et al: *BRCA1* physically associates with *p53* and stimulates its transcriptional activity. *Oncogene* **16**:1713, 1998.
137. Somasundaram K, et al: Arrest of the cell cycle by the tumour-suppressor *BRCA1* requires the CDK-inhibitor p21WAF1/CiP1. *Nature* **389**:187, 1997.
138. Anderson SF, Schlegel BP, Nakajima T, Wolpin ES, Parvin JD: *BRCA1* protein is linked to the RNA polymerase II holoenzyme complex via RNA helicase A. *Nature Genet* **19**:254, 1998.
139. Scully R, et al: *BRCA1* is a component of the RNA polymerase II holoenzyme. *Proc Natl Acad Sci USA* **94**:5605, 1997.
140. Cui JQ, et al: *BRCA1* splice variants *BRCA1a* and *BRCA1b* associate with CBP co-activator. *Oncol Rep* **5**:591, 1998.
141. Burke TF, et al: Identification of a *BRCA1*-associated kinase with potential biological relevance. *Oncogene* **16**:1031, 1998.
142. Mancini DN, et al: CpG methylation within the 5′ regulatory region of the *BRCA1* gene is tumor specific and includes a putative CREB binding site. *Oncogene* **16**:1161, 1998.
143. Dobrovic A, Simpfendorfer D: Methylation of the *BRCA1* gene in sporadic breast cancer. *Cancer Res* **57**:3347, 1997.
144. Gudas JM, Nguyen H, Li T, Cowan KH: Hormone-dependent regulation of *BRCA1* in human breast cancer cells. *Cancer Res* **55**:4561, 1995.
145. Gudas JM, et al: Cell cycle regulation of *BRCA1* messenger RNA in human breast epithelial cells. *Cell Growth Diff* **7**:717, 1996.
146. Vaughn JP, et al: *BRCA1* expression is induced before DNA synthesis in both normal and tumor-derived breast cells. *Cell Growth Diff* **7**:711, 1996.
147. Marquis ST, et al: The developmental pattern of *Brca1* expression implies a role in differentiation of the breast and other tissues. *Nature Genet* **11**:17, 1995.
148. Marks JR, et al: *BRCA1* expression is not directly responsive to estrogen. *Oncogene* **14**:115, 1997.
149. Romagnolo D, et al: Estrogen upregulation of *BRCA1* expression with no effect on localization. *Mol Carcinogen* **22**:102, 1998.
150. Spillman MA, Bowcock AM: *BRCA1* and *BRCA2* mRNA levels are coordinately elevated in human breast cancer cells in response to estrogen. *Oncogene* **13**:1639, 1996.
151. Chen Y, et al: Aberrant subcellular localization of *BRCA1* in breast cancer (see comments) [published erratum appears in *Science* **270**:5241, 1995]. *Science* **270**:789, 1995.
152. Scully R, Ganesan S, Brown M: Localization of *BRCA1* in human breast and ovarian cancer cells. *Science* **272**:122, 1996.
153. Jensen RA, et al: *BRCA1* is secreted and exhibits properties of a granin (see comments). *Nature Genet* **12**:303, 1996.
154. Wilson CA, et al: *BRCA1* protein products: Antibody specificity. *Nature Genet* **13**:264, 1996.
155. Chamberlain JS, et al: *BRCA1* maps proximal to D17S579 on chromosome 17q21 by genetic analysis. *Am J Hum Genet* **52**:792, 1993.
156. Smith SA, Easton DF, Evans DG, Ponder BA: Allele losses in the region 17q12-21 in familial breast and ovarian cancer involve the wild-type chromosome. *Nature Genet* **2**:128, 1992.
157. Thompson ME, Jensen RA, Obermiller PS, Page DL, Holt JT: Decreased expression of *BRCA1* accelerates growth and is often present during sporadic breast cancer progression. *Nature Genet* **9**:444, 1995.
158. Shao N, Chai YL, Shyam E, Reddy P, Rao VN: Induction of apoptosis by the tumor suppressor protein *BRCA1*. *Oncogene* **13**:1, 1996.
159. Tomlinson GE, et al: Characterization of a breast cancer cell line derived from a germ-line *BRCA1* mutation carrier. *Cancer Res* **58**:3237, 1998.
160. Chen Y, et al: *BRCA1* is a 220-kDa nuclear phosphoprotein that is expressed and phosphorylated in a cell cycle-dependent manner [published erratum appears in *Cancer Res* **56**:17, 1996]. *Cancer Res* **56**:3168, 1996.
161. Larson JS, Tonkinson JL, Lai MT: A *BRCA1* mutant alters G2-M cell cycle control in human mammary epithelial cells. *Cancer Res* **57**:3351, 1997.
162. Blackshear PE, et al: *Brca1* and *Brca2* expression patterns in mitotic and meiotic cells of mice. *Oncogene* **16**:61, 1998.
163. Gowen LC, Johnson BL, Latour AM, Sulik KK, Koller BH: *Brca1* deficiency results in early embryonic lethality characterized by neuroepithelial abnormalities. *Nature Genet* **12**:191, 1996.
164. Hakem R, et al: The tumor suppressor gene *Brca1* is required for embryonic cellular proliferation in the mouse. *Cell* **85**:1009, 1996.
165. Liu CY, Flesken-Nikitin A, Li S, Zeng Y, Lee WH: Inactivation of the mouse *Brca1* gene leads to failure in the morphogenesis of the egg cylinder in early postimplantation development. *Genes Dev* **10**:1835, 1996.
166. Ludwig T, Chapman DL, Papaioannou VE, Efstratiadis A: Targeted mutations of breast cancer susceptibility gene homologs in mice: Lethal phenotypes of *Brca1, Brca2, Brca1/Brca2, Brca1/p53,* and *Brca2/p53* nullizygous embryos. *Genes Dev* **11**:1226, 1997.
167. Shore D: *RAP1:* A protean regulator in yeast. *Trends Genet* **10**:408, 1994.
168. Scully R, et al: Dynamic changes of *BRCA1* subnuclear location and phosphorylation state are initiated by DNA damage. *Cell* **90**:425, 1997.

169. Lim DS, Hasty P: A mutation in mouse *rad51* results in an early embryonic lethal that is suppressed by a mutation in *p53*. *Mol Cell Biol* **16**:7133, 1996.
170. Shinohara A, Ogawa H, Ogawa T: Rad51 protein involved in repair and recombination in *S. cerevisiae* is a RecA-like protein [published erratum appears in *Cell* **71**:180, 1992]. *Cell* **69**:457, 1992.
171. Thomas JE, Smith M, Tonkinson JL, Rubinfeld B, Polakis P: Induction of phosphorylation on *BRCA1* during the cell cycle and after DNA damage. *Cell Growth Diff* **8**:801, 1997.
172. Fan S, et al: Down-regulation of *BRCA1* and *BRCA2* in human ovarian cancer cells exposed to adriamycin and ultraviolet radiation. *Int J Cancer* **77**:600, 1998.
173. Fan S, et al: *BRCA1* as a potential human prostate tumor suppressor: Modulation of proliferation damage responses and expression of cell regulatory proteins. *Oncogene* **16**:3069, 1998.
174. Husain A, He G, Venkatraman ES, Spriggs DR: *BRCA1* up-regulation is associated with repair-mediated resistance to cis-diamminedichloroplatinum(II). *Cancer Res* **58**:1120, 1998.
175. Gowen LC, Avrutskaya AV, Latour AM, Koller BH, Leadon SA: *BRCA1* required for transcription-coupled repair of oxidative DNA damage. *Science* **281**:1009, 1998.
176. Kinzler KW, Vogelstein B: Cancer-susceptibility genes: Gatekeepers and caretakers (news; comment). *Nature* **386**:761, 1997.
177. Crook T, Crossland S, Crompton MR, Osin P, Gusterson BA: *p53* mutations in *BRCA1*-associated familial breast cancer (letter). *Lancet* **350**:638, 1997.
178. Tseng SL, et al: Allelic loss at *BRCA1, BRCA2,* and adjacent loci in relation to *TP53* abnormality in breast cancer. *Genes Chromosom Cancer* **20**:377, 1997.
179. Rhei E, et al: Molecular genetic characterization of *BRCA1*- and *BRCA2*-linked hereditary ovarian cancers. *Cancer Res* **58**:3193, 1998.
180. Stratton MR, et al: Familial male breast cancer is not linked to the *BRCA1* locus on chromosome 17q. *Nature Genet* **7**:103, 1994.
181. Wooster R, et al: Localization of a breast cancer susceptibility gene *BRCA2* to chromosome 13q12-13. *Science* **265**:2088, 1994.
182. Ford D, et al: Genetic heterogeneity and penetrance analysis of the *BRCA1* and *BRCA2* genes in breast cancer families: The Breast Cancer Linkage Consortium. *Am J Hum Genet* **62**:676, 1998.
183. Agnarsson BA, et al: Inherited *BRCA2* mutation associated with high grade breast cancer. *Breast Cancer Res Treat* **47**:121, 1998.
184. Gudmundsson J, et al: Frequent occurrence of *BRCA2* linkage in Icelandic breast cancer families and segregation of a common *BRCA2* haplotype. *Am J Hum Genet* **58**:749, 1996.
185. Schutte M, et al: An integrated high-resolution physical map of the DPC/BRCA2 region at chromosome 13q12. *Cancer Res* **55**:4570, 1995.
186. Bignell G, Micklem G, Stratton MR, Ashworth A, Wooster R: The BRC repeats are conserved in mammalian BRCA2 proteins. *Hum Mol Genet* **6**:53, 1997.
187. Bork P, Blomberg N, Nilges M: Internal repeats in the BRCA2 protein sequence (letter). *Nature Genet* **13**:22, 1996.
188. Sharan SK, Bradley A: Murine *Brca2:* Sequence map position and expression pattern. *Genomics* **40**:234, 1997.
189. McAllister KA, et al: Characterization of the rat and mouse homologues of the *BRCA2* breast cancer susceptibility gene. *Cancer Res* **57**:3121, 1997.
190. Couch FJ, et al: *BRCA2* germline mutations in male breast cancer cases and breast cancer families. *Nature Genet* **13**:123, 1996.
191. Neuhausen S, et al: Recurrent *BRCA2* 6174delT mutations in Ashkenazi Jewish women affected by breast cancer. *Nature Genet* **13**:126, 1996.
192. Phelan CM, et al: Mutation analysis of the *BRCA2* gene in 49 site-specific breast cancer families (see comments) [published erratum appears in *Nature Genet* **13(3)**:374, 1996]. *Nature Genet* **13**:120, 1996.
193. Lancaster JM, et al: *BRCA2* mutations in primary breast and ovarian cancers. *Nature Genet* **13**:238, 1996.
194. Miki Y, Katagiri T, Kasumi F, Yoshimoto T, Nakamura Y: Mutation analysis in the *BRCA2* gene in primary breast cancers. *Nature Genet* **13**:245, 1996.
195. Teng DH, et al: Low incidence of *BRCA2* mutations in breast carcinoma and other cancers. *Nature Genet* **13**:241, 1996.
196. Takahashi H, et al: Mutations of the *BRCA2* gene in ovarian carcinomas. *Cancer Res* **56**:2738, 1996.
197. Milner J, Ponder B, Hughes-Davies L, Seltmann M, Kouzarides T: Transcriptional activation functions in *BRCA2* (letter; see comments). *Nature* **386**:772, 1997.
198. Mazoyer S, et al: A polymorphic stop codon in *BRCA2* (letter). *Nature Genet* **14**:253, 1996.
199. Nordling M, et al: A large deletion disrupts the exon 3 transcription activation domain of the *BRCA2* gene in a breast/ovarian cancer family. *Cancer Res* **58**:1372, 1998.
200. Chen PL, et al: The BRC repeats in *BRCA2* are critical for *RAD51* binding and resistance to methyl methanesulfonate treatment. *Proc Natl Acad Sci USA* **95**:5287, 1998.
201. Tonin P, et al: Frequency of recurrent *BRCA1* and *BRCA2* mutations in Ashkenazi Jewish breast cancer families (see comments). *Nature Med* **2**:1179, 1996.
202. Thorlacius S, et al: A single *BRCA2* mutation in male and female breast cancer families from Iceland with varied cancer phenotypes (see comments). *Nature Genet* **13**:117, 1996.
203. Rubin SC, et al: Clinical and pathological features of ovarian cancer in women with germ-line mutations of *BRCA1* (see comments). *N Engl J Med* **335**:1413, 1996.
204. Goggins M, et al: Germline *BRCA2* gene mutations in patients with apparently sporadic pancreatic carcinomas. *Cancer Res* **56**:5360, 1996.
205. Kirsch M, Zhu JJ, Black PM: Analysis of the *BRCA1* and *BRCA2* genes in sporadic meningiomas. *Genes Chromosom Cancer* **20**:53, 1997.
206. Schubert EL, et al: *BRCA2* in American families with four or more cases of breast or ovarian cancer: Recurrent and novel mutations variable expression penetrance and the possibility of families whose cancer is not attributable to *BRCA1* or *BRCA2* (see comments). *Am J Hum Genet* **60**:1031, 1997.
207. Friedman LS, et al: Mutation analysis of *BRCA1* and *BRCA2* in a male breast cancer population. *Am J Hum Genet* **60**:313, 1997.
208. Bertwistle D, et al: Nuclear location and cell cycle regulation of the BRCA2 protein. *Cancer Res* **57**:5485, 1997.
209. Vaughn JP, et al: Cell cycle control of *BRCA2*. *Cancer Res* **56**:4590, 1996.
210. Wong AKC, Pero R, Ormonde PA, Tavtigian SV, Bartel PL: *RAD51* interacts with the evolutionarily conserved BRC motifs in the human breast cancer susceptibility gene brca2. *J Biol Chem* **272**:31941, 1997.
211. Rajan JV, Marquis ST, Gardner HP, Chodosh LA: Developmental expression of *Brca2* colocalizes with *Brca1* and is associated with proliferation and differentiation in multiple tissues. *Dev Biol* **184**:385, 1997.
212. Sharan SK, et al: Embryonic lethality and radiation hypersensitivity mediated by *Rad51* in mice lacking *Brca2* (see comments). *Nature* **386**:804, 1997.
213. Suzuki A, et al: *Brca2* is required for embryonic cellular proliferation in the mouse. *Genes Dev* **11**:1242, 1997.
214. Friedman LS, et al: Thymic lymphomas in mice with a truncating mutation in *Brca2*. *Cancer Res* **58**:1338, 1998.
215. Connor F, et al: Tumorigenesis and a DNA repair defect in mice with a truncating *Brca2* mutation. *Nature Genet* **17**:423, 1997.
216. Mizuta R, et al: RAB22 and RAB163/mouse BRCA2: Proteins that specifically interact with the RAD51 protein. *Proc Natl Acad Sci USA* **94**:6927, 1997.
217. Katagiri T, et al: Multiple possible sites of BRCA2 interacting with DNA repair protein RAD51. *Genes Chromosom Cancer* **21**:217, 1998.
218. Patel KJ, et al: Involvement of *Brca2* in DNA repair. *J Clin Monit Comput* **1**:347, 1998.
219. Morimatsu M, Donoho G, Hasty P: Cells deleted for *Brca2* COOH terminus exhibit hypersensitivity to gamma-radiation and premature senescence. *Cancer Res* **58**:3441, 1998.
220. Abbott DW, Freeman ML, Holt JT: Double-strand break repair deficiency and radiation sensitivity in *BRCA2* mutant cancer cells (see comments). *J Natl Cancer Inst* **90**:978, 1998.
221. Gretarsdottir S, et al: *BRCA2* and *p53* mutations in primary breast cancer in relation to genetic instability. *Cancer Res* **58**:859, 1998.
222. Li FP, Fraumeni JF: Soft-tissue sarcomas breast cancer and other neoplasms: Familial syndrome? *Ann Intern Med* **71**:747, 1969.
223. Li FP, Fraumeni JF, Mulvihill JJ: A cancer family syndrome in 24 kindreds. *Cancer Res* **48**:5358, 1988.
224. Strong LC, Williams WR, Tainsky MA: The Li-Fraumeni syndrome: From clinical epidemiology to molecular genetics. *Am J Epidemiol* **135**:190, 1992.
225. Li FP: Unpublished data, 1997.
226. Malkin D, et al: Germ line *p53* mutations in a familial syndrome of breast cancer sarcomas and other neoplasms (see comments). *Science* **250**:1233, 1990.
227. Srivastava S, Zou ZQ, Pirollo K, Blattner W, Chang EH: Germ-line transmission of a mutated *p53* gene in a cancer-prone family with Li-Fraumeni syndrome (see comments). *Nature* **348**:747, 1990.

228. Law JC, Strong LC, Chidambaram A, Ferrell RE: A germ line mutation in exon 5 of the *p53* gene in an extended cancer family. *Cancer Res* **51**:6385, 1991.
229. Santibanez-Koref MF, et al: *p53* germline mutations in Li-Fraumeni syndrome. *Lancet* **338**:1490, 1991.
230. Srivastava S, et al: Detection of both mutant and wild-type p53 protein in normal skin fibroblasts and demonstration of a shared "second hit" on *p53* in diverse tumors from a cancer-prone family with Li-Fraumeni syndrome. *Oncogene* **7**:987, 1992.
231. Brugieres L, et al: Screening for germ line *p53* mutations in children with malignant tumors and a family history of cancer. *Cancer Res* **53**:452, 1993.
232. Sameshima Y, et al: Detection of novel germ-line *p53* mutations in diverse-cancer-prone families identified by selecting patients with childhood adrenocortical carcinoma. *J Natl Cancer Inst* **84**:703, 1992.
233. Frebourg T, et al: Germ-line mutations of the *p53* tumor suppressor gene in patients with high risk for cancer inactivate the p53 protein. *Proc Natl Acad Sci USA* **89**:6413, 1992.
234. Barnes DM, et al: Abnormal expression of wild type p53 protein in normal cells of a cancer family patient. *Lancet* **340**:259, 1992.
235. Sidransky D, et al: Inherited *p53* gene mutations in breast cancer. *Cancer Res* **52**:2984, 1992.
236. Borresen AL, et al: Screening for germ line *TP53* mutations in breast cancer patients. *Cancer Res* **52**:3234, 1992.
237. Starink TM: Cowden's disease: Analysis of fourteen new cases. *J Am Acad Dermatol* **11**:1127, 1984.
238. Wood DA, Darling HH: A cancer family manifesting multiple occurrences of bilateral carcinoma of the breast. *Cancer Res* **3**:509, 1943.
239. Brownstein MH, Wolf M, Bikowski JB: Cowden's disease: A cutaneous marker of breast cancer. *Cancer* **41**:2393, 1978.
240. Padberg GW, Schot JD, Vielvoye GJ, Bots GT, de Beer FC: Lhermitte-Duclos disease and Cowden disease: A single phakomatosis (see comments). *Ann Neurol* **29**:517, 1991.
241. Eng C, et al: Cowden syndrome and Lhermitte-Duclos disease in a family: A single genetic syndrome with pleiotropy? *J Med Genet* **31**:458, 1994.
242. Nelen MR, et al: Localization of the gene for Cowden disease to chromosome 10q22-23. *Nature Genet* **13**:114, 1996.
243. Steck PA, et al: Identification of a candidate tumour suppressor gene *MMAC1* at chromosome 10q23.3 that is mutated in multiple advanced cancers. *Nature Genet* **15**:356, 1997.
244. Li J, et al: *PTEN:* A putative protein tyrosine phosphatase gene mutated in human brain breast and prostate cancer (see comments). *Science* **275**:1943, 1997.
245. Li DM, Sun H: TEP1, encoded by a candidate tumor suppressor locus, is a novel protein tyrosine phosphatase regulated by transforming growth factor beta. *Cancer Res* **57**:2124, 1997.
246. Liaw D, et al: Germline mutations of the *PTEN* gene in Cowden disease, an inherited breast and thyroid cancer syndrome. *Nature Genet* **16**:64, 1997.
247. Nelen MR, et al: Germline mutations in the *PTEN/MMAC1* gene in patients with Cowden disease. *Hum Mol Genet* **6**:1383, 1997.
248. Tsou HC, et al: The role of *MMAC1* mutations in early-onset breast cancer: Causative in association with Cowden syndrome and excluded in *BRCA1*-negative cases. *Am J Hum Genet* **61**:1036, 1997.
249. Chiariello E, Roz L, Albarosa R, Magnani I, Finocchiaro G: *PTEN/MMAC1* mutations in primary glioblastomas and short-term cultures of malignant gliomas. *Oncogene* **16**:541, 1998.
250. Jeghers H, McKusick VA, Katz KH: Generalized intestinal polyposis and melanin spots of the oral mucosa lips and digits: A syndrome of diagnostic significance. *N Engl J Med* **241**:993, 1949.
251. Utsunomiya J, Gocho H, Miyanaga T: Peutz-Jeghers syndrome: Its natural course and management. *Johns Hopkins Med J* **136**:71, 1975.
252. Jancu J: Peutz-Jeghers syndrome: Involvement of the gastrointestinal and upper respiratory tracts. *Am J Gastroenterol* **56**:545, 1971.
253. Sommerhaug RG, Mason T: Peutz-Jeghers syndrome and ureteral polyposis. *JAMA* **211**:120, 1970.
254. Chen KT: Female genital tract tumors in Peutz-Jeghers syndrome. *Hum Pathol* **17**:858, 1986.
255. Riley E, Swift M: A family with Peutz-Jeghers syndrome and bilateral breast cancer. *Cancer* **46**:815, 1980.
256. Young RH, Scully RE: Mucinous ovarian tumors associated with mucinous adenocarcinomas of the cervix: A clinicopathological analysis of 16 cases. *Int J Gynecol Pathol* **7**:99, 1988.
257. Cantu JM, Rivera H, Ocampo-Campos R: Peutz-Jeghers syndrome with feminizing Sertoli cell tumor. *Cancer* **46**:223, 1980.
258. Scully RE: Sex cord tumor with annular tubules: A distinctive ovarian tumor of the Peutz-Jeghers syndrome. *Cancer* **25**:1107, 1970.
259. Sristava PJ, Keeney GL, Podratz KC: Disseminated cervical adenoma malignum and bilateral ovarian sex cord tumors with annular tubules associated with Peutz-Jeghers syndrome. *Gynecol Oncol* **53**:256, 1994.
260. Boardman LA: Unpublished data, 1998.
261. Hemminki A, Tomlinson I, Markie D: Localization of a susceptibility locus for PJS to 19p using comparative genomic hybridization and targeted linkage analysis. *Nature Genet* **15**:87, 1997.
262. Hemminki A, et al: A serine/threonine kinase gene defective in Peutz-Jeghers syndrome. *Nature* **391**:184, 1998.
263. Bignell GR, et al: Low frequency of somatic mutations in the LKB1/Peutz-Jeghers syndrome gene in sporadic breast cancer. *Cancer Res* **58**:1384, 1998.
264. Wang ZJ, Taylor F, Curchman M: Genetic pathways of colorectal carcinogenesis rarely involve the *PTEN* and *LKB1* genes outside the inherited hamartoma syndromes. *Am J Pathol* **153**:363, 1998.
265. Avizienyte E: Somatic mutations in *LKB1* are rare in sporadic colorectal and testicular tumors. *Cancer Res* **58**:2087, 1998.
266. Olschwang S, Markie D: Peutz-Jeghers disease: Most but not all families are compatible with linkage to 19p13.3. *J Med Genet* **35**:42, 1998.
267. Muir EG, Bell AJ, Barlow KA: Multiple primary carcinomata of the colon duodenum and larynx associated with kerato-acanthomata of the face. *Br J Surg* **54**:191, 1967.
268. Hall NR, Williams MA, Murday VA, Newton JA, Bishop DT: Muir-Torre syndrome: A variant of the cancer family syndrome. *J Med Genet* **31**:627, 1994.
269. Anderson DE: An inherited form of large bowel cancer: Muir's syndrome. *Cancer* **45**:1103, 1980.
270. Papadopoulos N, et al: Mutation of a *mutL* homolog in hereditary colon cancer (see comments). *Science* **263**:1625, 1994.
271. Bronner CE, et al: Mutation in the DNA mismatch repair gene homologue *hMLH1* is associated with hereditary nonpolyposis colon cancer. *Nature* **368**:258, 1994.
272. Fishel R, et al: The human mutator gene homolog *MSH2* and its association with hereditary nonpolyposis colon cancer [published erratum appears in *Cell* **77**:167, 1994]. *Cell* **75**:1027, 1993.
273. Leach FS, et al: Mutations of a *mutS* homolog in hereditary nonpolyposis colorectal cancer. *Cell* **75**:1215, 1993.
274. Nicolaides NC, et al: Genomic organization of the human *PMS2* gene family. *Genomics* **30**:195, 1995.
275. Kolodner RD, et al: Structure of the human *MSH2* locus and analysis of two Muir-Torre kindreds for *msh2* mutations [published erratum appears in *Genomics* **28(3)**:613, 1995]. *Genomics* **24**:516, 1994.
276. Bapat B, et al: The genetic basis of Muir-Torre syndrome includes the *hMLH1* locus (letter). *Am J Hum Genet* **59**:736, 1996.
277. Swift M, et al: The incidence and gene frequency of ataxia-telangiectasia in the United States. *Am J Hum Genet* **39**:573, 1986.
278. Morrell D, Cromartie E, Swift M: Mortality and cancer incidence in 263 patients with ataxia-telangiectasia. *J Natl Cancer Inst* **77**:89, 1986.
279. Swift M, Morrell D, Massey RB, Chase CL: Incidence of cancer in 161 families affected by ataxia-telangiectasia (see comments). *N Engl J Med* **325**:1831, 1991.
280. Cortessis V, et al: Linkage analysis of DRD2, a marker linked to the ataxia-telangiectasia gene in 64 families with premenopausal bilateral breast cancer. *Cancer Res* **53**:5083, 1993.
281. Wooster R, et al: Absence of linkage to the ataxia telangiectasia locus in familial breast cancer. *Hum Genet* **92**:91, 1993.
282. Savitsky K, et al: A single ataxia telangiectasia gene with a product similar to PI-3 kinase (see comments). *Science* **268**:1749, 1995.
283. Zuppan P, Hall JM, Lee MK, Ponglikitmongkol M, King MC: Possible linkage of the estrogen receptor gene to breast cancer in a family with late-onset disease. *Am J Hum Genet* **48**:1065, 1991.
284. Sluyser M: Mutations in the estrogen receptor gene. *Hum Mutat* **6**:97, 1995.
285. Kerangueven F, Essioux L, Dib A: Loss of heterozygosity and linkage analysis in breast carcinoma: Indication for a putative third susceptibility gene on the short arm of chromosome 8. *Oncogene* **10**:1023, 1995.
286. Latil A, et al: Genetic alterations in localized prostate cancer: Identification of a common region of deletion on chromosome arm 18q. *Genes Chromosom Cancer* **11**:119, 1994.
287. Chuaqui RF, et al: Loss of heterozygosity on the short arm of chromosome 8 in male breast carcinomas. *Cancer Res* **55**:4995, 1995.
288. Knudson AG Jr: Mutation and cancer: Statistical study of retinoblastoma. *Proc Natl Acad Sci USA* **68**:820, 1971.

289. Callahan R, et al: Genetic and molecular heterogeneity of breast cancer cells. *Clin Chim Acta* **217**:63, 1993.
290. Cleton-Jansen AM, et al: At least two different regions are involved in allelic imbalance on chromosome arm 16q in breast cancer. *Genes Chromosom Cancer* **9**:101, 1994.
291. Gudmundsson J, et al: Loss of heterozygosity at chromosome 11 in breast cancer: Association of prognostic factors with genetic alterations. *Br J Cancer* **72**:696, 1995.
292. Morelli C, et al: Characterization of a 4-Mb region at chromosome 6q21 harboring a replicative senescence gene. *Cancer Res* **57**:4153, 1997.
293. Huang H, Qian C, Jenkins RB, Smith DI: Fish mapping of YAC clones at human chromosomal band 7q31.2: Identification of YACS spanning FRA7G within the common region of LOH in breast and prostate cancer. *Genes Chromosom Cancer* **21**:152, 1998.
294. Cropp CS, Champeme MH, Lidereau R, Callahan R: Identification of three regions on chromosome 17q in primary human breast carcinomas which are frequently deleted. *Cancer Res* **53**:5617, 1993.
295. Kirchweger R, et al: Patterns of allele losses suggest the existence of five distinct regions of LOH on chromosome 17 in breast cancer. *Int J Cancer* **56**:193, 1994.
296. Nagai MA, et al: Five distinct deleted regions on chromosome 17 defining different subsets of human primary breast tumors. *Oncology* **52**:448, 1995.
297. Phelan CM, et al: Consortium study on 1280 breast carcinomas: Allelic loss on chromosome 17 targets subregions associated with family history and clinical parameters. *Cancer Res* **58**:1004, 1998.
298. Cornelis RS, et al: Evidence for a gene on 17p13.3 distal to *TP53* as a target for allele loss in breast tumors without *p53* mutations. *Cancer Res* **54**:4200, 1994.
299. Schultz DC, et al: Identification of two candidate tumor suppressor genes on chromosome 17p13.3. *Cancer Res* **56**:1997, 1996.
300. Mathew S, Murty VV, Bosl GJ, Chaganti RS: Loss of heterozygosity identifies multiple sites of allelic deletions on chromosome 1 in human male germ cell tumors. *Cancer Res* **54**:6265, 1994.
301. Bieche I, Khodja A, Lidereau R: Deletion mapping in breast tumor cell lines points to two distinct tumor-suppressor genes in the 1p32-pter region, one of deleted regions (1p36.2) being located within the consensus region of LOH in neuroblastoma. *Oncol Rep* **5**:267, 1998.
302. Kerangueven F, et al: Loss of heterozygosity in human breast carcinomas in the ataxia telangiectasia Cowden disease and *BRCA1* gene regions. *Oncogene* **14**:339, 1997.
303. Dorion-Bonnet F, Mautalen S, Hostein I, Longy M: Allelic imbalance study of 16q in human primary breast carcinomas using microsatellite markers. *Genes Chromosom Cancer* **14**:171, 1995.
304. Eiriksdottir G. et al: Loss of heterozygosity on chromosome 9 in human breast cancer: Association with clinical variables and genetic changes at other chromosome regions. *Int J Cancer* **64**:378, 1995.
305. Smith HS, et al: Molecular aspects of early stages of breast cancer progression. *J Cell Biochem Suppl* **17G**:144, 1993.
306. Medeiros AC, Nagai MA, Neto MM, Brentani RR: Loss of heterozygosity affecting the *APC* and *MCC* genetic loci in patients with primary breast carcinomas. *Cancer Epidemiol Biomark Prevent* **3**:331, 1994.
307. Lakhani SR, Collins N, Stratton MR, Sloane JP: Atypical ductal hyperplasia of the breast: Clonal proliferation with loss of heterozygosity on chromosomes 16q and 17p. *J Clin Pathol* **48**:611, 1995.
308. Radford DM, et al: Allelotyping of ductal carcinoma in situ of the breast: deletion of loci on 8p, 13q, 16q, 17p, and 17q. *Cancer Res* **55**:3399, 1995.
309. Champeme MH, Bieche I, Beuzelin M, Lidereau R: Loss of heterozygosity on 7q31 occurs early during breast tumorigenesis. *Genes Chromosom Cancer* **12**:304, 1995.
310. Bacus SS, Zelnick CR, Plowman G, Yarden Y: Expression of the erbB-2 family of growth factor receptors and their ligands in breast cancers: Implication for tumor biology and clinical behavior. *Am J Clin Pathol* **102**:S13, 1994.
311. Slamon DJ, Godolphin W, Jones LA: Studies of the *Her-2/neu* proto-oncogene in human breast and ovarian cancer. *Science* **244**:707, 1989.
312. Kraus MH, Issing W, Miki T, Popescu NC, Aaronson SA: Isolation and characterization of ERBB3, a third member of the ERBB/epidermal growth factor receptor family: Evidence for overexpression in a subset of human mammary tumors. *Proc Natl Acad Sci USA* **86**:9193, 1989.
313. Lewis S, et al: Expression of epidermal growth factor receptor in breast carcinoma. *J Clin Pathol* **43**:385, 1990.
314. Hawkins RA, et al: Epidermal growth factor receptors in intracranial and breast tumours: Their clinical significance. *Br J Cancer* **63**:553, 1991.
315. Paik S, et al: Pathologic findings from the National Surgical Adjuvant Breast and Bowel Project: Prognostic significance of erbB-2 protein overexpression in primary breast cancer. *J Clin Oncol* **8**:103, 1990.
316. Clark GM, McGuire WL: Follow-up study of *HER-2/neu* amplification in primary breast cancer. *Cancer Res* **51**:944, 1991.
317. Antoniotti S, et al: Oestrogen and epidermal growth factor down-regulate erbB-2 oncogene protein expression in breast cancer cells by different mechanisms. *Br J Cancer* **70**:1095, 1994.
318. Janes PW, Daly RJ, deFazio A, Sutherland RL: Activation of the *Ras* signalling pathway in human breast cancer cells overexpressing *erbB*-2. *Oncogene* **9**:3601, 1994.
319. Nowak F, Jacquemin-Sablon A, Pierre J: Expression of the activated p185erbB2 tyrosine kinase in human epithelial cells leads to MAP kinase activation but does not confer oncogenicity. *Exp Cell Res* **231**:251, 1997.
320. Toikkanen S, Helin H, Isola J, Joensuu H: Prognostic significance of *HER*-2 oncoprotein expression in breast cancer: A 30-year follow-up (see comments). *J Clin Oncol* **10**:1044, 1992.
321. Gusterson BA, et al: Prognostic importance of c-*erbB*-2 expression in breast cancer: International (Ludwig) Breast Cancer Study Group (see comments). *J Clin Oncol* **10**:1049, 1992.
322. Thor AD, et al: *erbB*-2, *p53,* and efficacy of adjuvant therapy in lymph node-positive breast cancer (see comments). *J Natl Cancer Inst* **90**:1346, 1998.
323. Yu D, et al: Overexpression of both *p185c-erbB2* and *p170mdr-1* renders breast cancer cells highly resistant to Taxol. *Oncogene* **16**:2087, 1998.
324. Leitzel K, et al: Elevated serum c-erbB-2 antigen levels and decreased response to hormone therapy of breast cancer. *J Clin Oncol* **13**:1129, 1995.
325. Sleijfer S, Asschert JG, Timmer-Bosscha H, Mulder NH: Enhanced sensitivity to tumor necrosis factor-alpha in doxorubicin-resistant tumor cell lines due to down-regulated c-*erbB2*. *Int J Cancer* **77**:101, 1998.
326. Colomer R, Lupu R, Bacus SS, Gelmann EP: erbB-2 antisense oligonucleotides inhibit the proliferation of breast carcinoma cells with *erbB*-2 oncogene amplification. *Br J Cancer* **70**:819, 1994.
327. Ciardiello F, et al: Down-regulation of type I protein kinase A by transfection of human breast cancer cells with an epidermal growth factor receptor antisense expression vector. *Breast Cancer Res Treat* **47**:57, 1998.
328. Petit AM, et al: Neutralizing antibodies against epidermal growth factor and ErbB-2/neu receptor tyrosine kinases down-regulate vascular endothelial growth factor production by tumor cells in vitro and in vivo: Angiogenic implications for signal transduction therapy of solid tumors. *Am J Pathol* **151**:1523, 1997.
329. Sandgren EP, Luetteke NC, Palmiter RD, Brinster RL, Lee DC: Overexpression of TGF alpha in transgenic mice: Induction of epithelial hyperplasia pancreatic metaplasia and carcinoma of the breast. *Cell* **61**:1121, 1990.
330. Johnson MR, Valentine C, Basilico C, Mansukhani A: FGF signaling activates STAT1 and p21 and inhibits the estrogen response and proliferation of MCF-7 cells. *Oncogene* **16**:2647, 1998.
331. Burgess WH, Maciag T: The heparin-binding (fibroblast) growth factor family of proteins. *Annu Rev Biochem* **58**:575, 1989.
332. Penault-Llorca F, et al: Expression of FGF and FGF receptor genes in human breast cancer. *Int J Cancer* **61**:170, 1995.
333. Wang Q, et al: Basic fibroblast growth factor downregulates *Bcl-2* and promotes apoptosis in MCF-7 human breast cancer cells. *Exp Cell Res* **238**:177, 1998.
334. Tanaka A, et al: High frequency of fibroblast growth factor (FGF) 8 expression in clinical prostate cancers and breast tissues immunohistochemically demonstrated by a newly established neutralizing monoclonal antibody against FGF 8. *Cancer Res* **58**:2053, 1998.
335. Conway K, et al: *Ha-ras* rare alleles in breast cancer susceptibility. *Breast Cancer Res Treat* **35**:97, 1995.
336. Zhang PL, Calaf G, Russo J: Allele loss and point mutation in codons 12 and 61 of the c-*Ha-ras* oncogene in carcinogen-transformed human breast epithelial cells. *Mol Carcinogen* **9**:46, 1994.
337. Bland KI, Konstadoulakis MM, Vezeridis MP, Wanebo HJ: Oncogene protein co-expression: Value of *Ha-ras,* c-*myc,* c-*fos,* and *p53* as prognostic discriminants for breast carcinoma (see comments). *Ann Surg* **221**:706, 1995.

338. Ciardiello F, et al: Additive effects of c-*erbB*-2, c-*Ha-ras,* and transforming growth factor-alpha genes on in vitro transformation of human mammary epithelial cells. *Mol Carcinogen* **6**:43, 1992.
339. Sabbatini AR, et al: Induction of multidrug resistance (MDR) by transfection of MCF-10A cell line with c-*Ha-ras* and c-*erbB*-2 oncogenes. *Int J Cancer* **59**:208, 1994.
340. Giai M, Roagna R, Ponzone R: Prognostic and predictive relevance of c-*erB*-2 and *ras* expression in node-positive and negative breast cancer. *Anticancer Res* **14**:1441, 1994.
341. Luttrell DK, et al: Involvement of *pp60c-src* with two major signaling pathways in human breast cancer. *Proc Natl Acad Sci USA* **91**:83, 1994.
342. Ottenhoff-Kalff AE, et al: Characterization of protein tyrosine kinases from human breast cancer: Involvement of the c-*src* oncogene product. *Cancer Res* **52**:4773, 1992.
343. Hennipman A, van Oirschot BA, Smits J, Rijksen G, Staal GE: Tyrosine kinase activity in breast cancer benign breast disease and normal breast tissue. *Cancer Res* **49**:516, 1989.
344. Hunter T, Pines J: Cyclins and cancer. II: Cyclin D and CDK inhibitors come of age (see comments). *Cell* **79**:573, 1994.
345. Marx J: How cells cycle toward cancer (news). *Science* **263**:319, 1994.
346. Hollstein M, Sidransky D, Vogelstein B, Harris CC: *p53* mutations in human cancers. *Science* **253**:49, 1991.
347. Deng G, et al: Loss of heterozygosity and *p53* gene mutations in breast cancer. *Cancer Res* **54**:499, 1994.
348. Andersen TI, et al: Prognostic significance of *TP53* alterations in breast carcinoma. *Br J Cancer* **68**:540, 1993.
349. Elledge RM, Fuqua SA, Clark GM, Pujol P, Allred DC: William L. McGuire Memorial Symposium: The role and prognostic significance of *p53* gene alterations in breast cancer. *Breast Cancer Res Treat* **27**:95, 1993.
350. Saitoh S, et al: *p53* gene mutations in breast cancers in midwestern U.S. women: Null as well as missense-type mutations are associated with poor prognosis. *Oncogene* **9**:2869, 1994.
351. Shiao YH, Chen VW, Scheer WD, Wu XC, Correa P: Racial disparity in the association of *p53* gene alterations with breast cancer survival. *Cancer Res* **55**:1485, 1995.
352. Marchetti A, et al: *p53* mutations and histological type of invasive breast carcinoma. *Cancer Res* **53**:4665, 1993.
353. Moll UM, Riou G, Levine AJ: Two distinct mechanisms alter *p53* in breast cancer: Mutation and nuclear exclusion. *Proc Natl Acad Sci USA* **89**:7262, 1992.
354. Aas T, et al: Specific *p53* mutations are associated with *de novo* resistance to doxorubicin in breast cancer patients. *Nature Med* **2**:811, 1996.
355. Bergh J, Norberg T, Sjogren S, Lindgren A, Holmberg L: Complete sequencing of the *p53* gene provides prognostic information in breast cancer patients, particularly in relation to adjuvant systemic therapy and radiotherapy. *Nature Med* **1**:1029, 1995.
356. T'Ang A, Varley JM, Chakraborty S, Murphree AL, Fung YK: Structural rearrangement of the retinoblastoma gene in human breast carcinoma. *Science* **242**:263, 1988.
357. Lee EY, et al: Inactivation of the retinoblastoma susceptibility gene in human breast cancers. *Science* **241**:218, 1988.
358. Gottardis MM, et al: Regulation of retinoblastoma gene expression in hormone-dependent breast cancer. *Endocrinology* **136**:5659, 1995.
359. Wang NP, To H, Lee WH, Lee EY: Tumor suppressor activity of *RB* and *p53* genes in human breast carcinoma cells. *Oncogene* **8**:279, 1993.
360. Fung YK, T'Ang A: The role of the retinoblastoma gene in breast cancer development. *Cancer Treat Res* **61**:59, 1992.
361. Berns EM, et al: Association between *RB-1* gene alterations and factors of favourable prognosis in human breast cancer without effect on survival. *Int J Cancer* **64**:140, 1995.
362. Sawan A, et al: Retinoblastoma and *p53* gene expression related to relapse and survival in human breast cancer: An immunohistochemical study. *J Pathol* **168**:23, 1992.
363. Buckley MF, et al: Expression and amplification of cyclin genes in human breast cancer. *Oncogene* **8**:2127, 1993.
364. Motokura T, Bloom T, Kim HG: A *BCL1*-linked candidate oncogene, which is rearranged in parathyroid tumors, encodes a novel cyclin. *Nature* **350**:512, 1991.
365. Bartokova J, Lukas J, Muller H: Cyclin D1 protein expression and function in human breast cancer. *Int J Cancer* **57**:353, 1994.
366. Zhang SY, Caamano J, Cooper F, Guo X, Klein-Szanto AJ: Immunohistochemistry of cyclin D1 in human breast cancer. *Am J Clin Pathol* **102**:695, 1994.
367. Weinstat-Saslow D, et al: Overexpression of cyclin D mRNA distinguishes invasive and *in situ* breast carcinomas from non-malignant lesions (see comments). *Nature Med* **1**:1257, 1995.
368. Alle KM, Henshall SM, Field AS, Sutherland RL: Cyclin D1 protein is overexpressed in hyperplasia and intraductal carcinoma of the breast. *Clin Cancer Res* **4**:847, 1998.
369. Oyama T, Kashiwabara K, Yoshimoto K, Arnold A, Koerner F: Frequent overexpression of the cyclin D1 oncogene in invasive lobular carcinoma of the breast. *Cancer Res* **58**:2876, 1998.
370. Musgrove EA, Lee CS, Buckley MF, Sutherland RL: Cyclin D1 induction in breast cancer cells shortens G1 and is sufficient for cells arrested in G1 to complete the cell cycle. *Proc Natl Acad Sci USA* **91**:8022, 1994.
371. Sicinski P, et al: Cyclin D1 provides a link between development and oncogenesis in the retina and breast. *Cell* **82**:621, 1995.
372. Zwijsen RM, et al: CDK-independent activation of estrogen receptor by cyclin D1. *Cell* **88**:405, 1997.
373. Neuman E, et al: Cyclin D1 stimulation of estrogen receptor transcriptional activity independent of cdk4. *Mol Cell Biol* **17**:5338, 1997.
374. Porter PL, et al: Expression of cell-cycle regulators p27Kip1 and cyclin E alone and in combination correlate with survival in young breast cancer patients (see comments). *Nature Med* **3**:222, 1997.
375. Alexandrow MG, Moses HL: Transforming growth factor beta and cell cycle regulation. *Cancer Res* **55**:1452, 1995.
376. Jeng MH, ten Dijke P, Iwata KK, Jordan VC: Regulation of the levels of three transforming growth factor beta mRNAs by estrogen and their effects on the proliferation of human breast cancer cells. *Mol Cell Endocrinol* **97**:115, 1993.
377. Knabbe C, et al: Evidence that transforming growth factor-beta is a hormonally regulated negative growth factor in human breast cancer cells. *Cell* **48**:417, 1987.
378. Perry RR, Kang Y, Greaves BR: Relationship between tamoxifen-induced transforming growth factor beta 1 expression cytostasis and apoptosis in human breast cancer cells (see comments). *Br J Cancer* **72**:1441, 1995.
379. Croxtall JD, Jamil A, Ayub M, Colletta AA, White JO: TGF-beta stimulation of endometrial and breast-cancer cell growth. *Int J Cancer* **50**:822, 1992.
380. Arteaga CL, Dugger TC, Winnier AR, Forbes JT: Evidence for a positive role of transforming growth factor-beta in human breast cancer cell tumorigenesis. *J Cell Biochem Suppl* **17G**:187, 1993.
381. Walker RA, Dearing SJ, Gallacher B: Relationship of transforming growth factor beta 1 to extracellular matrix and stromal infiltrates in invasive breast carcinoma. *Br J Cancer* **69**:1160, 1994.
382. MacCallum J, et al: Expression of transforming growth factor beta mRNA isoforms in human breast cancer (see comments). *Br J Cancer* **69**:1006, 1994.
383. Dublin EA, Barnes DM, Wang DY, King RJ, Levison DA: TGF alpha and TGF beta expression in mammary carcinoma. *J Pathol* **170**:15, 1993.
384. Thompson CB: Apoptosis in the pathogenesis and treatment of disease. *Science* **267**:1456, 1995.
385. Fisher DE: Apoptosis in cancer therapy: Crossing the threshold. *Cell* **78**:539, 1994.
386. Johnston SR, et al: Modulation of *Bcl*-2 and *Ki-67* expression in oestrogen receptor-positive human breast cancer by tamoxifen. *Eur J Cancer* **30A**:1663, 1994.
387. Joensuu H, Pylkkanen L, Toikkanen S: Bcl-2 protein expression and long-term survival in breast cancer. *Am J Pathol* **145**:1191, 1994.
388. Sabourin JC, et al: *bcl-2* expression in normal breast tissue during the menstrual cycle. *Int J Cancer* **59**:1, 1994.
389. Haldar S, Negrini M, Monne M, Sabbioni S, Croce CM: Down-regulation of *bcl-2* by *p53* in breast cancer cells. *Cancer Res* **54**:2095, 1994.
390. Ottestad L, et al: Amplification of c-*erbB*-2, *int-2,* and c-*myc* genes in node-negative breast carcinomas: Relationship to prognosis. *Acta Oncol* **32**:289, 1993.
391. Pietilainen T, et al: Expression of c-myc proteins in breast cancer as related to established prognostic factors and survival. *Anticancer Res* **15**:959, 1995.
392. Pavelic ZP, et al: c-*myc,* c-*erbB*-2, and *Ki-67* expression in normal breast tissue and in invasive and noninvasive breast carcinoma. *Cancer Res* **52**:2597, 1992.
393. Porter-Jordan K, Lippman ME: Overview of the biologic markers of breast cancer. *Hematol Oncol Clin North Am* **8**:73, 1994.

394. Glukhova M, Koteliansky V, Sastre X, Thiery JP: Adhesion systems in normal breast and in invasive breast carcinoma. *Am J Pathol* **146**:706, 1995.
395. Rimm DL, Sinard JH, Morrow JS: Reduced alpha-catenin and E-cadherin expression in breast cancer (see comments). *Lab Invest* **72**:506, 1995.
396. Palacios J, et al: Anomalous expression of P-cadherin in breast carcinoma: Correlation with E-cadherin expression and pathological features. *Am J Pathol* **146**:605, 1995.
397. Rasbridge SA, Gillett CE, Sampson SA, Walsh FS, Millis RR: Epithelial (E-) and placental (P-) cadherin cell adhesion molecule expression in breast carcinoma. *J Pathol* **169**:245, 1993.
398. Siitonen SM, et al: Reduced E-cadherin expression is associated with invasiveness and unfavorable prognosis in breast cancer. *Am J Clin Pathol* **105**:394, 1996.
399. Stetler-Stevenson WG: Type IV collagenases in tumor invasion and metastasis. *Cancer Metastas Rev* **9**:289, 1990.
400. Yu M, Sato H, Seiki M, Thompson EW: Complex regulation of membrane-type matrix metalloproteinase expression and matrix metalloproteinase-2 activation by concanavalin A in MDA-MB-231 human breast cancer cells. *Cancer Res* **55**:3272, 1995.
401. Duffy MJ, et al: Assay of matrix metalloproteases types 8 and 9 by ELISA in human breast cancer. *Br J Cancer* **71**:1025, 1995.
402. Okada A, et al: Membrane-type matrix metalloproteinase (*MT-MMP*) gene is expressed in stromal cells of human colon breast and head and neck carcinomas. *Proc Natl Acad Sci USA* **92**:2730, 1995.
403. Sato H, et al: A matrix metalloproteinase expressed on the surface of invasive tumour cells (see comments). *Nature* **370**:61, 1994.
404. Polette M, et al: Gelatinase A expression and localization in human breast cancers: An *in situ* hybridization study and immunohistochemical detection using confocal microscopy. *Virchows Arch* **424**:641, 1994.
405. Ito A, Nakajima S, Sasaguri Y, Nagase H, Mori Y: Co-culture of human breast adenocarcinoma MCF-7 cells and human dermal fibroblasts enhances the production of matrix metalloproteinases 1, 2, and 3 in fibroblasts. *Br J Cancer* **71**:1039, 1995.
406. Noel AC, et al: Coordinate enhancement of gelatinase A mRNA and activity levels in human fibroblasts in response to breast-adenocarcinoma cells. *Int J Cancer* **56**:331, 1994.
407. Aaltonen M, Lipponen P, Kosma VM, Aaltomaa S, Syrjanen K: Prognostic value of cathepsin-D expression in female breast cancer. *Anticancer Res* **15**:1033, 1995.
408. Gion M, et al: Relationship between cathepsin D and other pathological and biological parameters in 1752 patients with primary breast cancer. *Eur J Cancer* **31A**:671, 1995.
409. Steeg PS, et al: Evidence for a novel gene associated with low tumor metastatic potential. *J Natl Cancer Inst* **80**:200, 1988.
410. Rosengard AM, et al: Reduced Nm23/Awd protein in tumour metastasis and aberrant *Drosophila* development. *Nature* **342**:177, 1989.
411. Bevilacqua G, Sobel ME, Liotta LA, Steeg PS: Association of low nm23 RNA levels in human primary infiltrating ductal breast carcinomas with lymph node involvement and other histopathological indicators of high metastatic potential. *Cancer Res* **49**:5185, 1989.
412. Leone A, Flatow U, VanHoutte K, Steeg PS: Transfection of human *nm23-H1* into the human MDA-MB-435 breast carcinoma cell line: Effects on tumor metastatic potential colonization and enzymatic activity. *Oncogene* **8**:2325, 1993.
413. Steeg PS, et al: *Nm23* and breast cancer metastasis. *Breast Cancer Res Treat* **25**:175, 1993.
414. Howlett AR, Petersen OW, Steeg PS, Bissell MJ: A novel function for the *nm23-H1* gene: Overexpression in human breast carcinoma cells leads to the formation of basement membrane and growth arrest (see comments). *J Natl Cancer Inst* **86**:1838, 1994.
415. Postel EH, Berberich SJ, Flint SJ, Ferrone CA: Human c-*myc* transcription factor PuF identified as nm23-H2 nucleoside diphosphate kinase, a candidate suppressor of tumor metastasis (see comments). *Science* **261**:478, 1993.
416. Chang CL, et al: *Nm23-H1* mutation in neuroblastoma (letter). *Nature* **370**:335, 1994.
417. Hoskins KF, et al: Assessment and counseling for women with a family history of breast cancer: A guide for clinicians. *JAMA* **273**:577, 1995.
418. Burke W, et al: Recommendations for follow-up care of individuals with an inherited predisposition to cancer: II. *BRCA1* and *BRCA2*. Cancer Genetic Studies Consortium (see comments). *JAMA* **277**:997, 1997.
419. Lakhani SR, Sloane JP, Gusterson BA: Pathology of familial breast cancer: Differences between breast cancers in carriers of *BRCA1* or *BRCA2* mutations and sporadic cases. *Lancet* **349**:1505, 1997.

CHAPTER 48

Colorectal Tumors

Kenneth W. Kinzler ■ Bert Vogelstein

1. **Colorectal tumors progress through a series of clinical and histopathologic stages ranging from single crypt lesions (aberrant crypt foci) through small benign tumors (adenomatous polyps) to malignant cancers (carcinomas). This progression is the result of a series of genetic changes that involve activation of oncogenes and inactivation of tumor-suppressor genes.**
2. **There are several inherited predispositions to colorectal cancer. The two best characterized and most pronounced are hereditary nonpolyposis colorectal cancer (HNPCC) and familial adenomatous polyposis (FAP). Patients with HNPCC inherit defective DNA mismatch repair genes (see Chap. 32). Although HNPCC and FAP are both associated with a marked predisposition to colorectal cancer, they only account for a small fraction of colorectal cancers. Most colorectal cancers occur in the absence of a recognized inherited factor and are considered sporadic.**
3. **The majority of mutations contributing to colorectal tumorigenesis are acquired in the tumor cell (i.e., somatic). To date, over a dozen genes have been found to be somatically mutated in colorectal cancer. Four genetic events are particularly common in colorectal cancers and have been described at the molecular level. These include activation of *RAS* oncogenes and inactivation of tumor-suppressor genes on chromosomes 5q, 17p, and 18q.**
4. **Activating mutations of one of the *RAS* oncogenes occur in about 50 percent of colorectal cancers and in a similar percentage of adenomas larger than 1.0 cm in diameter. The majority of these mutations affect the *c-Ki-RAS* gene, with the rest affecting the *N-RAS* gene. The RAS proteins are homologous to G proteins and are believed to play a role in signal transduction.**
5. **The tumor-suppressor gene on chromosome 17p has been identified as the *p53* gene. The *p53* gene is inactivated in at least 85 percent of colorectal cancers but rarely in benign tumors. Inactivation of *p53* is most often due to a missense mutation combined with a loss of the other allele. Biochemical studies of the p53 protein suggest that it functions through transcriptional activation of genes controlling cell birth and cell death, such as the cyclin-dependent kinase inhibitor p21WAF1/CIP1. The p53 protein has been shown to bind to specific recognition elements within the promoters of these genes. Mutant p53 is defective in these activities.**
6. **Three candidate tumor-suppressor genes, *DCC, SAMD4/DPC4,* and *SMAD2,* have been isolated from chromosome 18q. At least one copy of these genes is lost in 70 percent of colorectal cancers and in over 40 percent of large adenomas with foci of carcinomatous transformation. Somatic alterations, including homozygous deletions, point mutations, or insertions, have been detected in all three candidate genes, with mutations of *SMAD4* being most frequent. However, mutations of these genes cannot account for the majority of 18q chromosome loss events, suggesting that additional mechanism of inactivation or other undefined tumor-suppressor genes are playing a role. Additional studies will be necessary to fully understand the role of 18q losses in colorectal tumorigenesis.**
7. **The tumor-suppressor gene on chromosome 5q has been identified as the *APC* gene. In addition to causing FAP through germ-line transmission, mutations of the *APC* gene occur somatically in over 80 percent of sporadic colorectal tumors, whether benign or malignant. Almost all these mutations, like the inherited mutations causing FAP, are predicted to result in truncation of the APC protein. Mutation of the *APC* gene is the earliest genetic event yet identified in colorectal tumorigenesis, with mutations being identified in lesions as small as a few crypts. At the biochemical level, one critical function of APC is inhibition of β-catenin/Tcf–mediated transcription. Mutation of *APC* leads to increased β-catenin/Tcf–mediated transcription of growth-promoting genes including the *c-MYC* oncogene. In rare tumors with wild-type APC, increased β-catenin/Tcf–mediated transcription results from mutations of β-catenin that render it resistant to the inhibitory effects of APC.**
8. **Despite the requirement for multiple somatic mutations to drive the neoplastic process, several inherited predispositions can result from inheritance of a single defective gene, as noted earlier. The genes responsible for cancer predispositions can be grouped broadly into three categories of defects: *caretakers, gatekeepers,* and *landscapers.* Examples of all three defects exist for colon cancer. Caretaker defects are typified by the DNA mismatch repair alterations observed in HNPCC. While these defects do not act directly to affect cellular growth, they act as caretakers, reducing the accumulation of mutations that arise during the normal replication of DNA. Defects in DNA mismatch repair lead to a genetic instability that accelerates the progression of cancer. In contrast, patients with FAP inherit truncating mutations of the *APC* tumor-suppressor gene. *APC* functions as a gatekeeper, directly regulating the growth of colorectal epithelial cells. As a result of inheriting a mutant gatekeeper gene, patients with FAP develop hundreds of benign colorectal tumors, some of which progress to carcinomas. The third category of predispositions results from landscaper defects. Landscaper defects do not directly affect cancer cell growth but contribute to abnormal stromal environment that contributes to the neoplastic transformation of the overlying epithelium. The increased risk of colorectal cancer observed in juvenile polyposis syndrome and Peutz-Jeghers syndrome may be the result of landscaper defects.**
9. **The analysis of mutations in colorectal tumors at various stages of their development allows definition of a model for**

A list of standard abbreviations is located immediately preceding the index in each volume. Nonstandard abbreviations used in this chapter include: ACF = aberrant crypt foci; FAP = familial adenomatous polyposis coli; GS = Gardner syndrome; HNPCC = hereditary nonpolyposis colorectal cancer; JPS = juvenile polyposis syndrome.

colorectal tumor development. Mutations in the *APC* gene appear to initiate this process, resulting in small tumors representing the clonal growth of a single cell. One of the cells in this small tumor may acquire an additional mutation (often in the *K-RAS* gene), allowing it to overgrow surrounding cells and resulting in a larger tumor. Subsequent waves of clonal expansion are driven by sequential mutations in the 18q suppressor and *p53* genes. Along with this expansion comes further cellular disorganization and eventually the ability to invade and metastasize. While this accumulation of multiple genetic changes is driven by growth advantages, it also can be facilitated by an innate genetic instability. In a small but significant fraction of cancers, this genetic instability is due to a defect in DNA mismatch repair. In the majority of cancers, accumulation of genetic changes is facilitated by a chromosomal instability, perhaps associated with defects in mitotic spindle checkpoints.

CLINICAL FEATURES

Incidence and Scope

Colorectal cancer is the second leading cause of cancer death in the United States. In 1998, there were an estimated 131,000 new cases of colorectal cancers and 56,000 deaths from this disease.[1] The cases are roughly equally distributed between the sexes. The average age of incidence of colon cancer in the United States is 67 years,[2] and over 90 percent of colon cancer deaths occur in individuals over the age of 55.[3] Approximately 5 percent of the population develop colorectal cancer, and this figure is expected to rise as life expectancy increases.[3] Furthermore, when nonmalignant colorectal tumors are considered, up to half the population is affected.[4–6]

Histopathology

A single layer of epithelial cells lines the invaginations (crypts) of the colon and rectum (Fig. 48-1). As is true throughout the digestive tract, these crypts substantially increase the surface area occupied by the epithelium. Four to six stem cells at the base of each crypt give rise to the three major epithelial cell types (absorptive cells, mucus-secreting goblet cells, and neuroepithelial cells). The cells multiply in the lower third of the crypt and differentiate in the upper two-thirds. The journey from the base of the crypt to its apex, where the epithelial cells are extruded, takes 3 to 6 days.[7,8]

Normally, the birth rate of the colonic epithelial cells precisely equals the rate of loss from the crypt apex to the lumen of the bowel. If the birth/loss ratio increases, a neoplasm results (a *neoplasm* is here defined as any abnormal accumulation of cells originating from a single progenitor cell). A tumor of the colon is often first observed clinically as a polyp, a mass of cells protruding from the bowel wall (Fig. 48-2). There are predominantly two types of polyps, which can be distinguished histologically but not

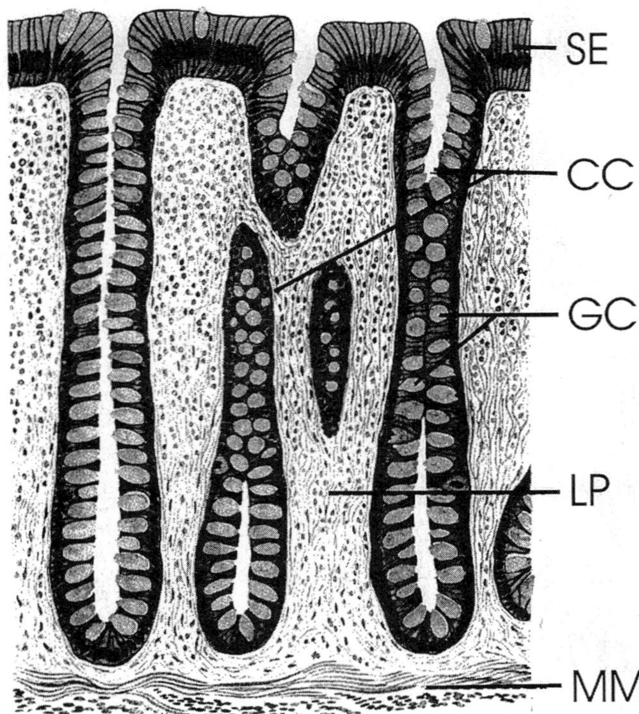

Fig. 48-1 Histology of normal colon. Examples of surface epithelium (SE), colonic crypts (CC), goblet cells (GC), lamina propria (LP), and muscularis mucosa (MM) are marked. (*Used with permission from Clara et al.*[417])

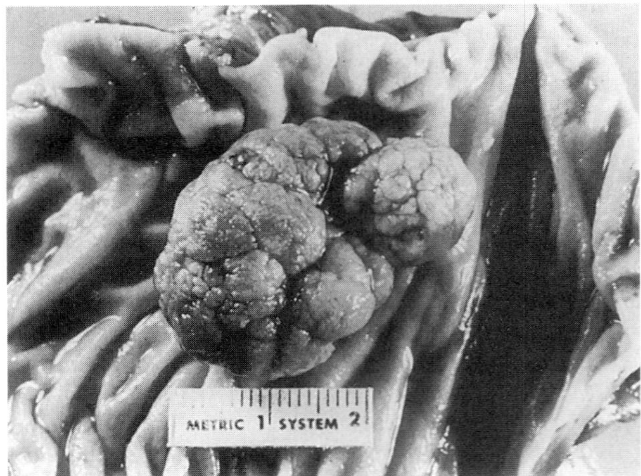

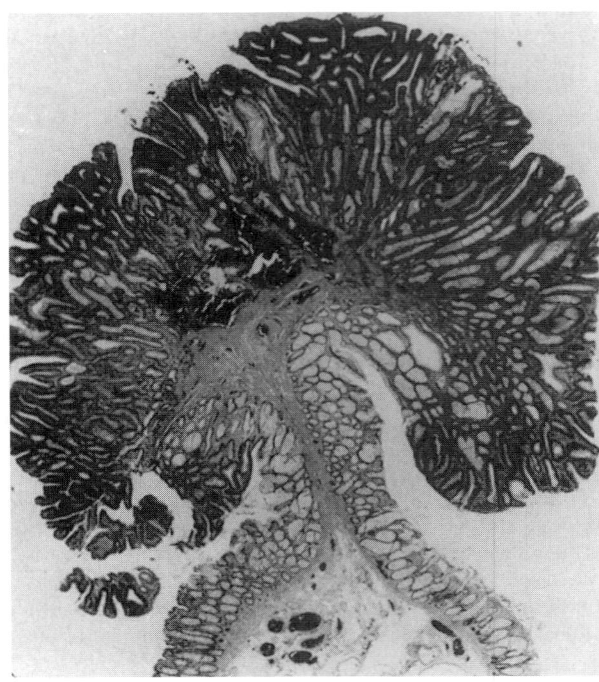

Fig. 48-2 Morphology of a colonic polyp showing its pedunculated nature. (*A*) A macroscopic view of a large tubular adenoma. (*B*) A cross section of a tubular adenoma with a clearly visible stalk. (*Used with permission from Kent and Mitros.*[9])

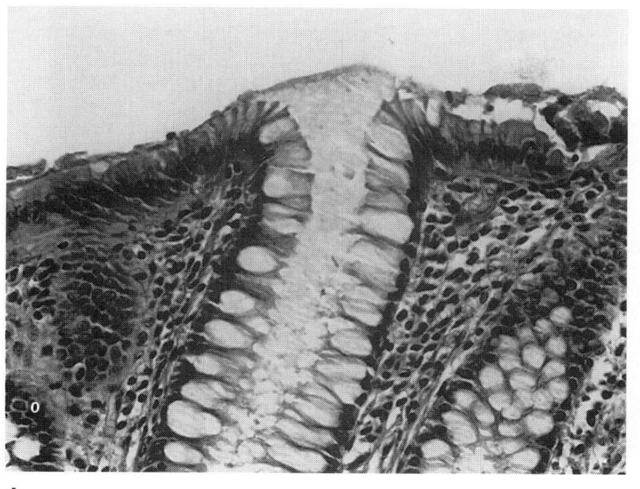

A

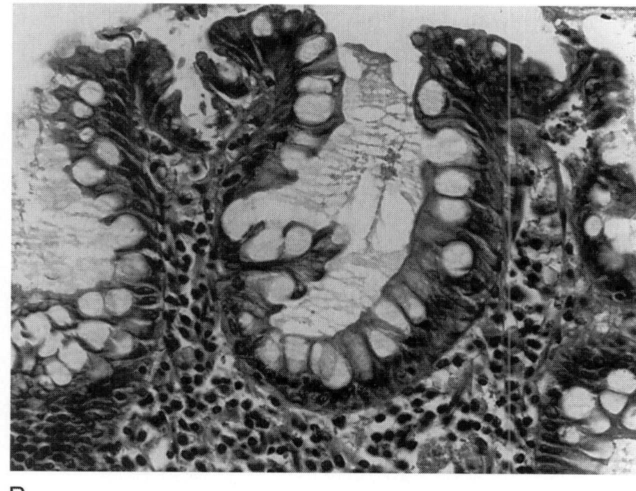

B

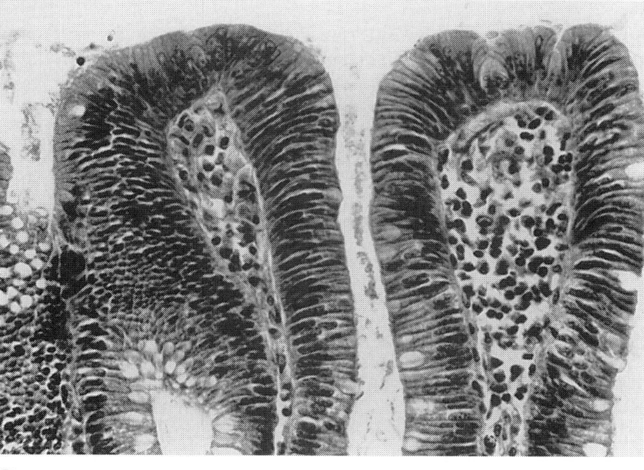

C

Fig. 48-3 Histopathology of colonic polyps. Panels show high-power views of hematoxylin and eosin–stained sections of normal colonic mucosa, (*A*) a hyperplastic polyp (nondysplastic), and an adenomatous polyp (dysplastic) (*B*), respectively. Note (*C*) the increased disruption of normal architecture present in the adenomatous polyp compared with the hyperplastic polyp. (*From Dr. Stanley R. Hamilton, Johns Hopkins University School of Medicine, Baltimore MD.*)

by their external appearance.[9] The nondysplastic or hyperplastic type consists of large numbers of cells that have a normal morphology (Fig. 48-3*B*). The cells are lined up in a single row along the basement membrane, and these polyps apparently have little tendency to become neoplastic. The other polyp type (adenomatous) is dysplastic, i.e., has an abnormal intracellular and intercellular organization (see Fig. 48-3*C*). Several layers of epithelial cells, in addition to the one adjacent to the basement membrane, are evident; the nuclei of the epithelial cells are larger than normal; and their position within the cell is often aberrant. Crypts crowd together in a kaleidoscopic pattern. As adenomas grow in size, they become more dysplastic. They also are more likely to contain "villous" components, i.e., fingerlike projections of dysplastic crypts that can be distinguished from the smooth contour of the less advanced "tubular" adenomas. As adenomas progress, they are more likely to become malignant, defined as the ability to invade surrounding tissues and travel to distant organs through direct spread or transport by blood vessels and lymphatics (metastasis). Malignant tumors are not necessarily larger or more dysplastic than benign tumors; their sole determining feature is invasiveness. Adenocarcinomas are the most common malignant tumor of the colon, although other cancers (e.g., lymphomas, sarcomas) that arise from nonepithelial cells occur occasionally.[10] As noted earlier, polyps are the earliest clinical manifestation of colorectal neoplasia, but methylene blue staining or microscopic examination of the colonic mucosa also can detect lesions affecting one or a small number of crypts (Fig. 48-4). These lesions are termed *aberrant crypt foci* (ACF) and, like their larger counterparts, can be either dysplastic (microadenomas) or nondysplastic.

Colorectal neoplasia is not a rare condition. About 5 percent of individuals 40 to 50 years of age have adenomatous polyps, as do about half of those over 70 years old.[4–6] These figures are even higher when ACF are considered. Adenomas less than 10 mm in diameter have a very low probability of developing a focus of malignancy, whereas tumors larger than 10 mm have a 15 percent chance of becoming malignant over a 10-year period.[11] Benign tumors are easily removed by colonoscopy or surgery. Malignant tumors are usually excisable by surgery, but if they have already metastized, additional therapy is necessary. The most common site of metastasis is the mesenteric lymph nodes.[2] These lymph nodes are usually excised at the time of the initial surgery for the cancer. If distant metastasis has occurred (to the peritoneal surface or liver), surgery will not be curative. Patients with metastatic disease are usually treated with radiation and/or chemotherapeutic agents (adjuvant therapy). Although such treatments can induce remissions of many months, they are usually not curative, as evidenced by the fact that about 40 percent of patients with colorectal cancer die from their disease within 5 years of diagnosis despite adjuvant treatment.[1]

Inherited Predispositions

Familial colorectal cancers can be divided broadly into two groups: those characterized by the presence of multiple benign colorectal polyps (polyposis) and those characterized by the absence of polyposis. Several types of polyposis syndromes have

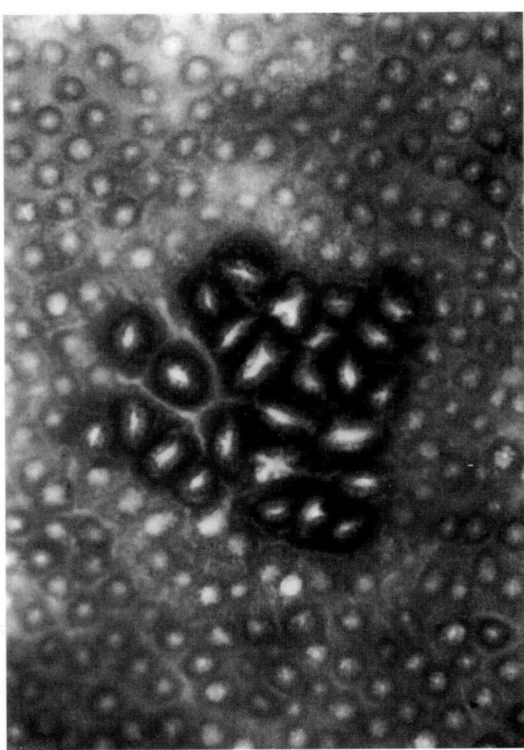

Fig. 48-4 Morphology of an ACF. Macroscopic view of an ACF after staining with methylene blue. (*From Dr. Stanley R. Hamilton, Johns Hopkins University School of Medicine, Baltimore, MD.*)

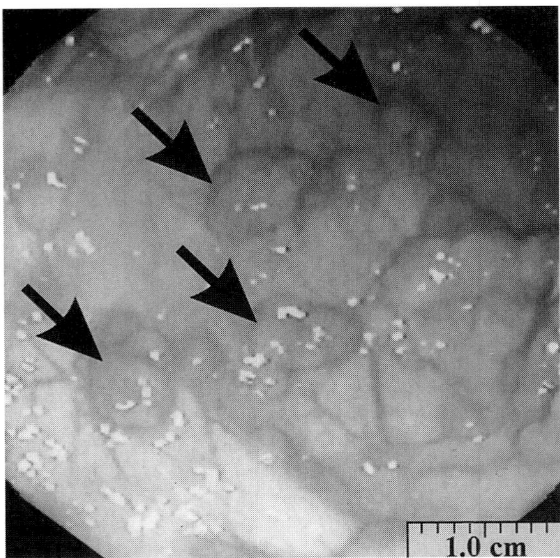

Fig. 48-5 Polyposis in an FAP patient. Colonoscopic view of polyps in a patient with FAP. (*Used with permission from Kinzler and Vogelstein.*[418])

been described, including familial adenomatous polyposis coli (FAP), Peutz-Jegher syndrome (see Chap. 34), familial juvenile polyposis (see Chap. 35), Cowden syndrome (see Chap. 45), Cronkhite-Canada syndrome, and hyperplastic polyposis. We will limit our discussion of the polyposis syndromes to FAP and its variants because its pathogenesis has been proven to be especially relevant to sporadic colorectal tumorigenesis.

FAP is inherited in autosomal dominant fashion, and affected individuals develop hundreds to thousands of adenomatous polyps during their lifetime (Fig. 48-5). The polyps are first observed during the second decade of life and increase in number over the next two decades. The histologic and biologic features of these polyps are indistinguishable from those of sporadic adenomatous polyps that develop in the general population. Although an individual polyp in an FAP patient is no more likely to progress to cancer than a sporadic polyp with the same degree of dysplasia, their large numbers in FAP patients essentially guarantee that some will progress to cancer. Indeed, the median age for colorectal cancer in untreated FAP patients is about 40.[12] Thus prophylactic colectomies are performed routinely on FAP patients to reduce their risk of cancer. Although about 1 in 5000 to 10,000 individuals is affected with FAP in the United States,[13] less than 1 percent of all colon cancers occur in FAP patients. Patients with FAP are also at increased risk for cancers of the thyroid, small intestine, stomach, and brain.[12,14] Variants of FAP have been described that include all the colonic manifestations of FAP plus varied extracolonic manifestations.[15,16] The most common variant is Gardner syndrome (GS), which is characterized by soft tissue tumors, osteomas, dental abnormalities, and congenital hypertrophy of the retinal pigment epithelium (CHRPE).[15] Still other attenuated variants of FAP are characterized by a reduced number of intestinal polyps (10 to 100).[17,18] Finally, many cases of Turcot syndrome, which is characterized by the presence of central nervous system (CNS) tumors in combination with familial predisposition to colorectal cancer, are variants of FAP.[14] As detailed below, FAP and its variants can now be traced to germ-line mutations of the *APC* gene. Molecular, physiologic, and epidemiologic studies all suggest that FAP represents a defect in the control of tumor initiation.

It is estimated that hereditary nonpolyposis colorectal cancer (HNPCC) accounts for about 2 to 4 percent of colorectal cancer in the Western world.[19] Like FAP patients, HNPCC patients develop colorectal cancer at a median age of approximately 42 years (see Chap. 32 for a detailed review).[20] However, unlike FAP patients, HNPCC patients do not have a marked increase in the number of precursor adenomas. Thus, until recently, HNPCC kindred have had to be defined operationally. The standard clinical criterion for HNPCC included the identification of at least three first-degree relatives in at least two different generations with colorectal cancer, with at least one individual affected at less than 50 years of age. The identification of the underlying genetic defect now allows a genetic definition.[21] It is now known that the majority of HNPCC patients inherit a defect in DNA mismatch repair (*MMR*) genes. Tumors arising in these patients are DNA mismatch repair deficient and as a result are genetically unstable and progress rapidly to cancer. Thus, in contrast to FAP, the defect in HNPCC primarily affects tumor progression. In addition to colorectal cancer, HNPCC patients are at increased risk for other cancers, including those of the uterus, ovary, and brain.[21] Indeed, those cases of Turcot syndrome which are not due to germ-line defects in *APC* usually have germ-line defects in an *MMR* gene.[14]

Other Genetic Factors

The majority of patients with colorectal cancer do not have first-degree relatives with colorectal cancer, and therefore, the cancers are considered sporadic. Only about 3 to 5 percent of all colorectal cancers occur in individuals with well-characterized inherited predispositions such as those described earlier. However, several studies suggest a broader role for inheritance.[22–24] For example, the relatives of patients with sporadic colon cancers also have an increased risk for colon cancer; detailed studies of this phenomenon have suggested a dominant inheritance of susceptibility to adenomatous polyps and associated cancers.[23,24] Furthermore, it has been estimated that such inherited susceptibility could account for 15 to more than 50 percent of the total colorectal cancers in the population at large. Although these studies await to be confirmed through identification of the specific genetic factors involved, it is reasonable to assume that hereditary factors, when combined with environmental factors (see below), determine the aggregate risk for colorectal cancer. Whether the hereditary factors turn out to be embodied in a few major genes, rather than in a synergistic combination of multiple genes, remains to be determined.

Environmental Factors

While inherited genetic factors can clearly play an important role in the development of colon cancers, they are by no means the sole determinant.[25] This point is well illustrated by classic studies of Japanese immigrants to the United States. Historically, the incidence of colon cancer has been low in Japan, whereas the incidence of gastric cancer has been high. Japanese populations that moved to the United States show a progressive increase in colorectal cancer.[26] Today, this change in cancer incidence is being repeated on a larger scale in Japan, where the incidence of gastric cancer is declining, while the incidence of colon cancer is increasing.[27] These changes have been hypothesized to be due to the westernization of the Japanese diet. Epidemiologic studies indicate that certain diets[28–32] are associated with increased risk for colorectal cancer. The components of these diets that are responsible for the effects on risk and the mechanisms underlying such effects have not yet been fully elucidated. Presumably, they affect either the incidence of mutations or the ability of mutated cells to expand clonally.

MOLECULAR GENETICS OF COLORECTAL CANCER

Clonal Nature of Colorectal Cancers

The clonal nature of tumors is a critical feature of the somatic mutation/clonal evolution model of carcinogenesis.[33] In this model, a single cell acquires a mutation providing a selective growth advantage that allows its progeny to outnumber those of neighboring cells (Fig. 48-6). From within this clonal population, a single cell may acquire a second mutation, providing an additional growth advantage that allows further clonal expansion. Repeated cycles of mutation followed by clonal expansion eventually lead to a fully developed malignant tumor.

The clonal nature of human colorectal tumors was first demonstrated using techniques based on X chromosome inactivation in females. Only a single X chromosome is active in any somatic cell of a female. This inactivation occurs early during embryogenesis and is random with regard to which copy of the X chromosome (maternal or paternal) is inactivated in any given cell. The pattern of X inactivation is transmitted in a highly stable manner to progeny cells. The inactivation is also accompanied by changes in methylation of cytosine residues on the inactivated X

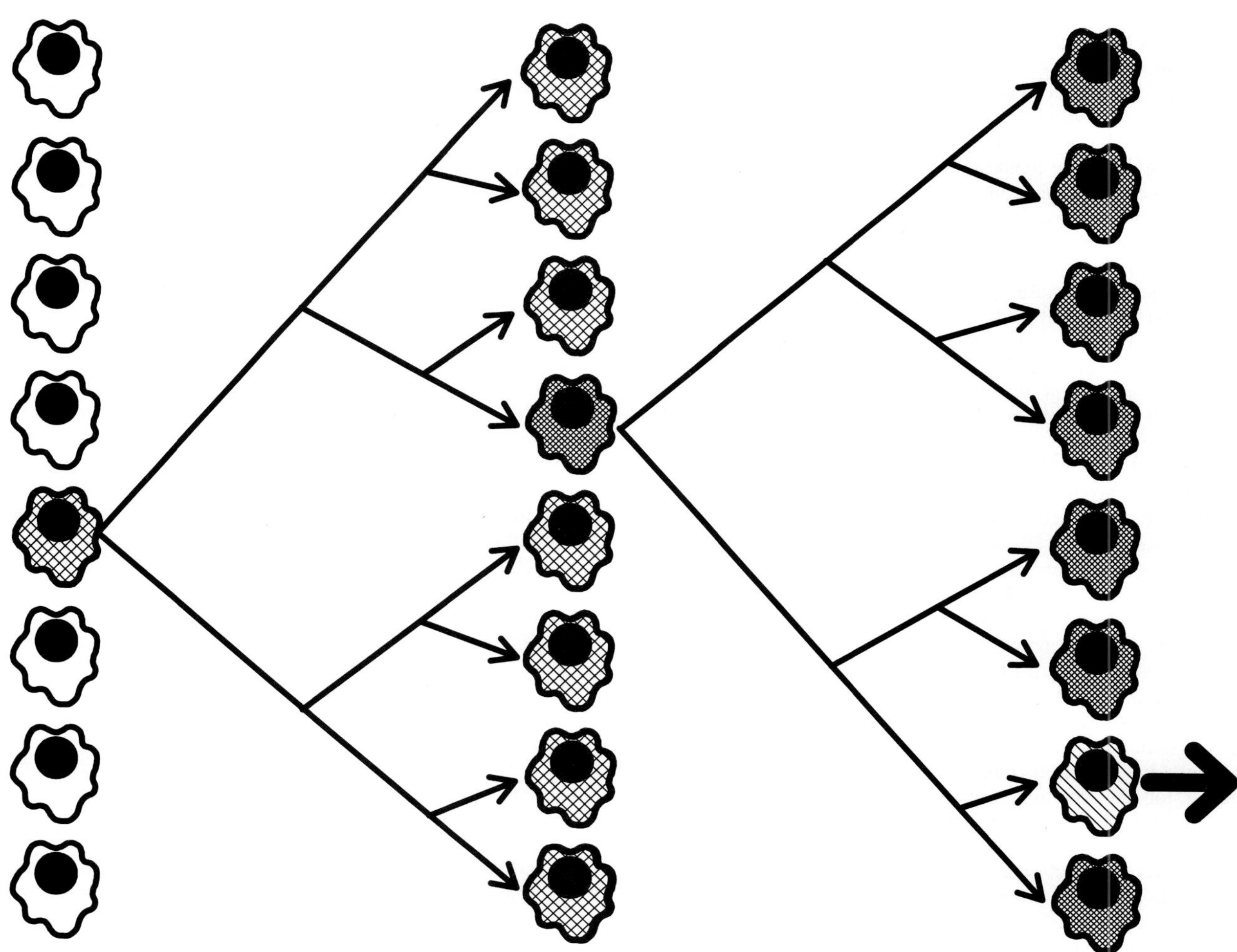

Fig. 48-6 Clonal evolution of tumor cells. A normal cell suffers a mutation that gives it a slight growth advantage. With time, this clone expands, and one of the progeny cell acquires another mutation providing an additional growth advantage. After several rounds of mutation followed by expansion, a malignant tumor results. The expansion phase is important because it provides additional targets for subsequent mutation. Without this expansion, mutations would be so infrequent that multiple genetic changes would be unlikely to occur, and tumors would be very rare.

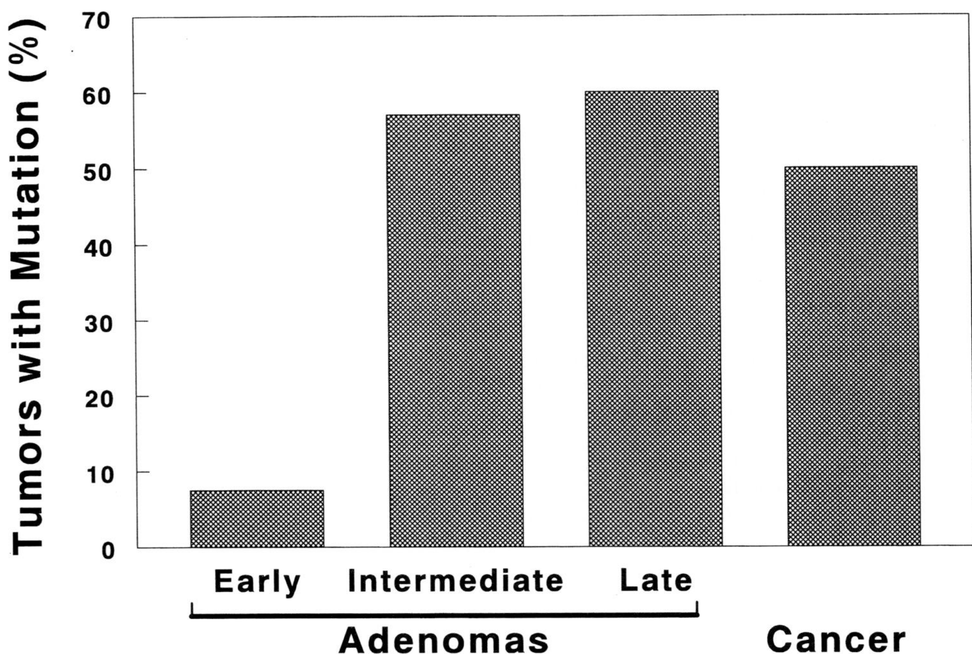

Fig. 48-7 Frequency of *RAS* mutations in colorectal tumors. Early adenomas were defined as less than 1.0 cm; intermediate adenomas were larger than 1.0 cm but without foci of carcinomatous transformation; late adenomas were larger than 1.0 cm and contained at least one focus of carcinomatous transformation; the cancers were adenocarcinomas of the colon. Tumors were assessed for *RAS* mutations as described.[45]

chromosome. Thus methylation-sensitive restriction enzymes in combination with restriction fragment length polymorphism can be used to distinguish which copy of the X chromosome is inactivated.[34] When this type of analysis is performed on small portions of normal colonic mucosa, the inactivation of X is equally distributed between the maternal and paternal copies. In contrast, when benign or malignant colorectal tumors are analyzed, they are found to display a monoclonal pattern of X inactivation.[35,36] The monoclonal nature of these tumors was further demonstrated using autosomal polymorphic markers that demonstrated clonal chromosomal losses.[36] These observations were consistent with cytogenetic studies that had demonstrated clonal chromosomal abnormalities in many carcinomas[37–39] and a major fraction of adenomas.[40–42] Subsequently, the identification of somatic point mutations in specific growth-controlling genes provided conclusive proof of the monoclonal nature of human colorectal tumors.

The *RAS* Oncogenes

The first breakthrough in the molecular genetics of colorectal tumors was the identification of *RAS* gene mutations.[43–45] The first *RAS* genes were identified as the transforming components of the Kirsten and Harvey rat sarcoma virus genomes (see Chap. 25). Three cellular *RAS* genes, *K-RAS, H-RAS,* and *N-RAS,* were later identified and shown to transform cells in tissue culture when mutated.[46,47] Specific point mutations of *K-RAS* or *N-RAS* are found in approximately 50 percent of colorectal adenomas larger than 1.0 cm and in 50 percent of carcinomas; *RAS* mutations are seen rarely in adenomas less than 1.0 cm in size[45] (Fig. 48-7). The lack of mutations in smaller adenomas suggests that *RAS* mutations are acquired during adenoma progression. Direct evidence for this premise comes from microdissection studies demonstrating subpopulations of adenoma cells that have acquired *RAS* mutations.[48] *RAS* mutations are not limited to dysplastic colorectal lesions; 100 percent of nondysplastic ACF and 25 percent of hyperplastic polyps have *RAS* mutations.[49,50] However, these nondysplastic lesions appear to be largely self-limited with respect to their potential for neoplastic progression. Regardless of the lesion's histology, most of the mutations identified (85 percent) are in codons 12 and 13 of *K-RAS,* with the rest affecting codon 61 of *K-RAS* or *N-RAS.* These studies clearly indicate that *RAS* oncogene mutations play a role during the development of a significant fraction of colorectal tumors. However, they also suggest that many tumors can develop in the absence of *RAS* mutations or fail to progress in the presence of one. The importance of *RAS* in colorectal tumorigenesis also has been emphasized by the finding that colorectal tumor cells in which the mutated *RAS* gene has been removed by homologous recombination still grow indefinitely *in vitro* but lose their ability to form tumors in nude mice.[51]

The *RAS* oncogenes encode 21-kDa monomeric proteins with homology to G proteins.[52] Like G proteins, RAS can bind GTP and catalyze its hydrolysis to GDP. RAS is active only when bound to GTP, with the hydrolysis to GDP leading to inactivation. The ratio of GTP-RAS to GDP-RAS is higher in cells containing mutant *RAS* genes than in cells with only wild-type *RAS* gene products. The altered ratio is due to decreased hydrolysis of GTP to GDP. However, the intrinsic GTPase activities of wild-type and mutant RAS do not usually account for this difference. The interaction of RAS with a cellular GTPase-activating protein (GAP) is apparently responsible for the difference. The GTPase activity of wild-type RAS is stimulated by GAP, whereas mutant RAS fails to respond to GAP.[53] Interestingly, the gene responsible for neurofibromatosis type 1 (NF1) has been found to have GAP activity (see Chap. 39).[54–57] This is interesting in light of the fact that many colon cancers do not contain *RAS* gene mutations. Accordingly, a mutation of NF1 has been reported to occur in a colon tumor that did not have a *RAS* mutation.[58]

Tumor-Suppressor Genes in Colorectal Cancers

The first molecular evidence for the role of tumor-suppressor genes in colorectal tumorigenesis came from the study of allelic losses.[36,45,59–63] Tumor-suppressor genes can be inactivated in a variety of ways, including point mutations, rearrangements, and deletions. Many of the deletions include entire chromosomal arms or even whole chromosomes. These large deletions can be detected using polymorphic markers that distinguish the two alleles present in the germ line.[64] Comparison of the alleles present in the tumor tissue with those in normal tissue allows the identification of deletions as loss of heterozygosity (LOH). When colorectal cancers were examined using at least one polymorphic marker for each nonacrocentric autosomal arm, certain arms were found to be frequently lost[63] (Fig. 48-8). Most frequently implicated were chromosomes 5q, 8p, 17p, and 18q, which were lost in 36, 50, 73, and 75 percent of the cases, respectively. This frequent loss of

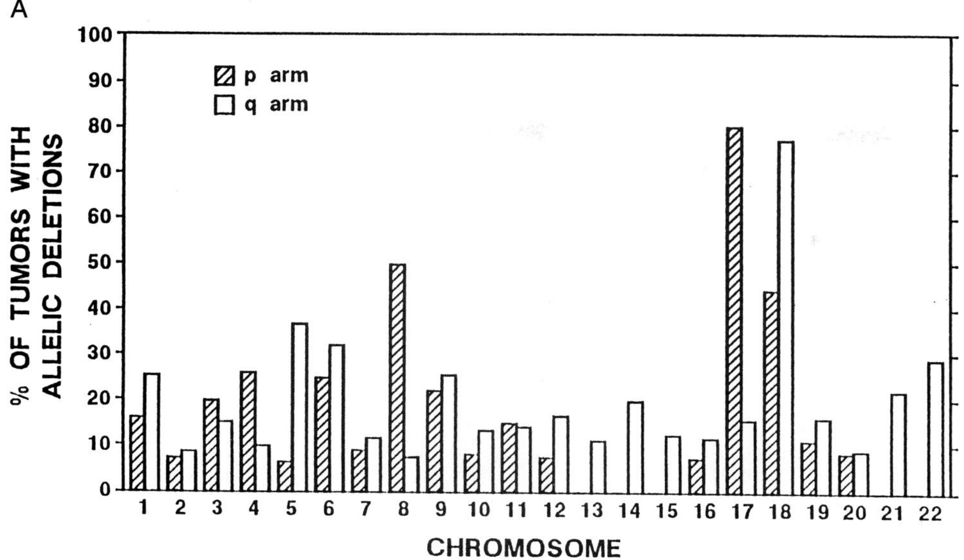

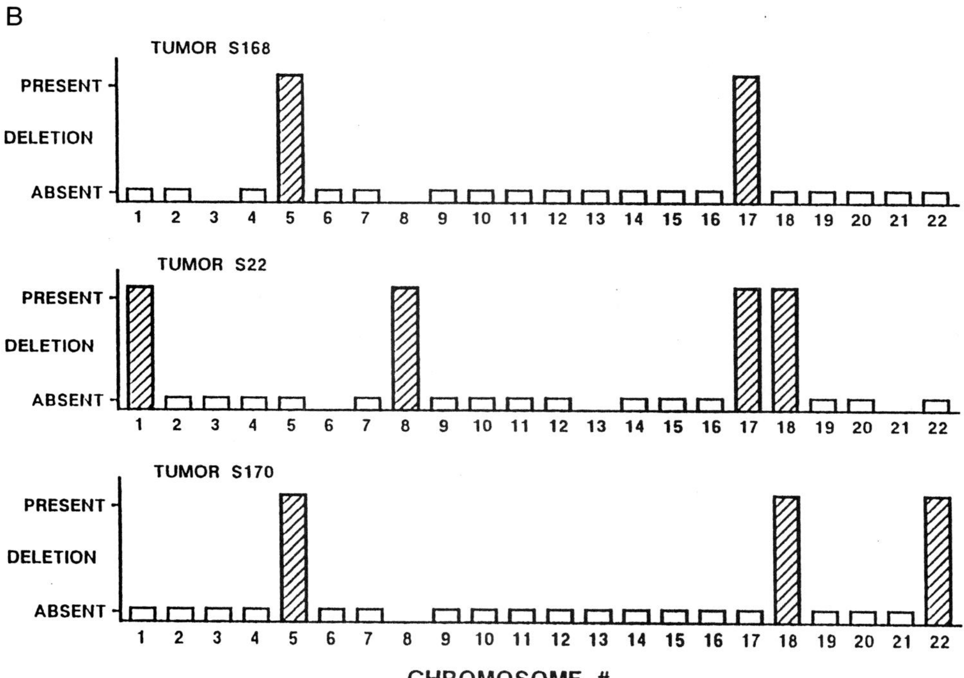

Fig. 48-8 Chromosomal losses in colorectal cancers. (*A*) Frequency of allelic deletions for individual chromosome arms in colorectal carcinomas. Allelic losses were scored in 56 colorectal carcinomas using polymorphic marker for all nonacrocentric autosomal arms.[63] Values for loss are expressed as a percentage of informative cases showing allelic loss. (*Used with permission from Fearon and Vogelstein.*[381]) (B) Allelic losses in three individual tumors (S168, S22, and S170) are shown. Long bars indicate a deletion; short bars indicate no deletion; the lack of an informative marker is indicated by the absence of a bar. Note that although there is a significant trend for loss of chromosomes 5, 8, 17, and 18, the exact pattern in individual tumors varies.

specific chromosomes has been taken to represent one step in the inactivation of a tumor-suppressor gene residing on the lost chromosome. The LOH analyses generally were consistent with karyotypic studies that had shown frequent losses of the same chromosomes.[37–39] To date, presumptive tumor-suppressor genes located on chromosomes 5q, 17p, and 18q have been identified. Chromosome losses, analyzed by LOH or karyotype, obviously underestimate the prevalence of suppressor gene alterations in colorectal tumors because small deletions, rearrangements, or point mutations are not detected in such analyses.

Chromosome 17p: The *p53* Gene

The first tumor-suppressor gene implicated in the development of colorectal tumors was the *p53* gene on chromosome 17p. The existence of a tumor-suppressor gene on 17p was suggested by the aforementioned allelic loss,[36,45,60,62,63] as well as by cytogenetic studies.[38,39] Loss of 17p sequences was detected in 75 percent of cancers, whereas 17p sequences were rarely lost in adenomas, suggesting that inactivation of the 17p tumor-suppressor gene was a relatively late event in colorectal tumorigenesis[45] (Fig. 48-9).

The *p53* gene was identified originally in 1979 by virtue of its expression in cells infected with tumor viruses.[65–67] During the first 10 years of its study, the cellular *p53* gene was considered to be a proto-oncogene. This was in part because of its increased expression in tumors and also because *p53* was apparently able to transform rat embryo fibroblasts in collaboration with *RAS* oncogenes.[68–70] However, subsequent studies have indicated that the wild-type *p53* gene is a tumor-suppressor gene, not a proto-oncogene. Studies on colorectal tumors were critical to this realization.[71] As mentioned earlier, chromosome 17p losses were noted frequently in colorectal tumors. To further localize the position of the putative tumor-suppressor gene on this chromosome, a large panel of polymorphic markers was used to analyze numerous colorectal cancer cases. The common region of deletion (i.e., the chromosomal region consistently lost in tumors containing any loss of chromosome 17p) was mapped to a region centered

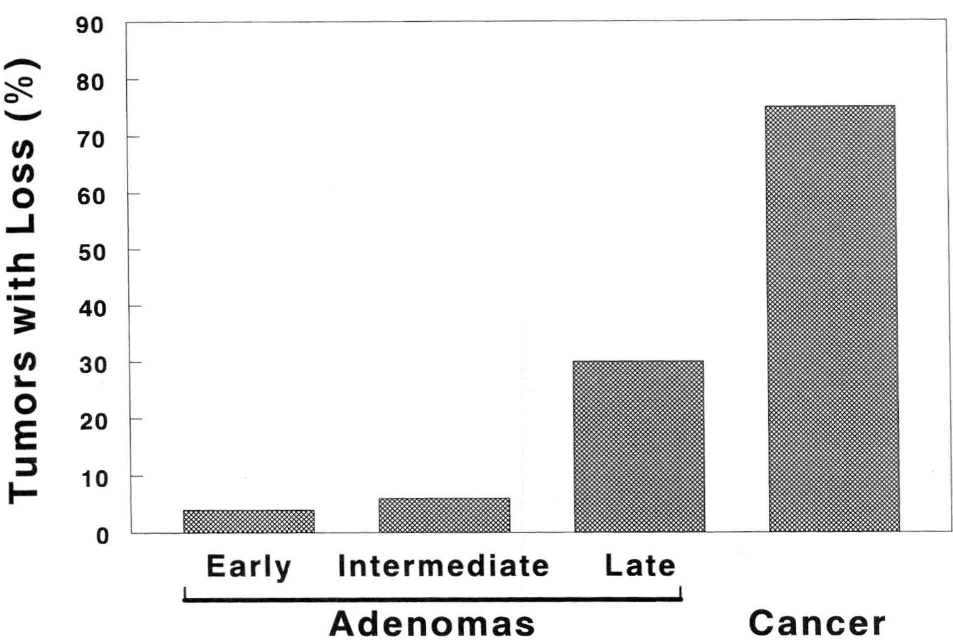

Fig. 48-9 Frequency of 17p losses in colorectal tumors. Tumor classes are defined as in Fig. 48-7. Values for chromosome 17p losses are expressed as a percentage of informative cases showing allelic loss.

at 17p13.1. Based on Knudson's hypothesis,[72] it was hypothesized that the loss of 17p13 removed one copy of a putative suppressor gene from the cell, while the remaining copy was mutant. Because *p53* was known to reside at 17p13 and had been implicated previously in neoplasia (albeit as an oncogene), it was tested to see if it fit Knudson's hypothesis. The remaining *p53* gene from a colorectal tumor that had lost one *p53* allele was sequenced. It was found to harbor a missense mutation at codon 143, changing alanine to valine. The mutation was somatic; i.e., it was not present in the normal colon of the same patient. Further analysis identified somatic mutations in the remaining *p53* gene in 24 of 28 colorectal tumors that had undergone allelic loss of 17p.[73] The majority of these mutations were missense and clustered into four regions that are conserved among mammals, amphibians, birds, and fish (Figs. 48-10 and 48-11).

The frequent allelic loss of 17p, coupled with mutation of the remaining copy of *p53,* strongly suggested that *p53* was a tumor-suppressor gene. Several other observations reinforced this idea. It was found that the wild-type *p53* gene, but not the mutant *p53* gene, could inhibit the growth of transformed cells in culture. This was first demonstrated in rodent cell fibroblasts[74,75] and later in human cancers of the colon[76] and other tissues.[77–79] Conversely, it was found that mutant, but not wild-type, *p53* genes could transform rat embryo fibroblasts in cooperation with *RAS* oncogenes (the presumably normal *p53* genes used for the initial studies on transformation by *p53* turned out to contain a mutation).[80,81] In Friend virus–induced erythroleukemias, the *p53* gene was found to be inactivated by proviral integration.[82–84] The p53 protein appears to be inactivated by viruses in some human cancers as well. In cervical cancers, the human papilloma virus E6 protein binds to the *p53* gene product[85] and inhibits its functional properties.[86] Finally, studies of other human tumor types, including lung, breast, brain, bladder and liver, show that *p53* is frequently mutated, just as in the colon.[87] In fact, the mutations observed in some of these tumors have provided clues as to the responsible mutagen.[88] For example, a specific mutation at codon 249 in liver tumors suggests a role for aflatoxins,[89–91] pyrimidine dimer mutations in skin tumors are consistent with a role for ultraviolet light,[92] and the pattern of mutations in lung cancers suggests mutagens in tobacco smoke as the culprits.[93] It has been estimated that over half the total malignancies in the world involve inactivation of *p53*.

How does *p53* exert its tumor-suppressor effect? The biochemical properties of p53 protein provide some answers to this question. The *p53* gene encodes a 393-amino-acid phosphoprotein (Fig. 48-11). Biophysical studies of the p53 protein indicate that it exists as a tetramer.[94,95] The region responsible for this tetramerization has been mapped to the carboxyl terminus,[96] between amino acids 344 to 393, and this tetramerization appears to be critical for defining the biochemical properties of p53.[97] The most compelling property is the ability of wild-type p53 to bind DNA in a sequence-specific manner.[98] Analysis of numerous human and artificially constructed sequences that bind p53 *in vitro* allowed definition of a consensus binding site composed of two copies of the 10-bp motif 5′-PuPuPuC(A/T)(A/T)GPyPyPy-3′.[99–101] One copy of this binding site is insufficient for binding, but binding is preserved even when the two copies are separated by as much as 13 bp. The complete p53 binding site is thus composed of four copies of the 5-bp half site 5′-PuPuPuC(A/T) (A/T)-3′ arranged in opposing directions. The ability of p53 to form tetramers could account for the fourfold symmetry of the binding site.

The fact that tumor-derived mutant p53 proteins nearly always have a reduced ability to bind DNA in a sequence-specific manner accentuates the importance of this activity.[98–100,102,103] The three-dimensional structure of a p53-DNA complex provides a biochemical understanding of the effects of these mutations.[104] Indeed, the Arg 248 and Arg 273 residues, which are the most frequently targeted residues for somatic mutations, were observed to directly contact DNA (Fig. 48-12).

What does this DNA binding accomplish in the cell? The amino terminus of p53 (codons 20–42) has an acidic domain that is similar to those in other transcription factors[81,105–107] (see Fig. 48-11). When this domain is fused to a DNA-binding protein, it conveys the ability to activate transcription.[81,105,106] Additional evidence for the role of p53 as a transcription factor comes from the studies of artificial genes containing a p53 binding site upstream of a reporter gene.[100,108] Expression of wild-type p53 in the presence of these reporter constructs results in strong transcriptional activation of the reporter molecule. The activation of transcription is proportional to the strength of p53 binding, and no transactivation is seen with constructs containing mutated binding sites that no longer bind p53. Additionally, p53 can mediate transactivation of genes containing p53 binding sites in

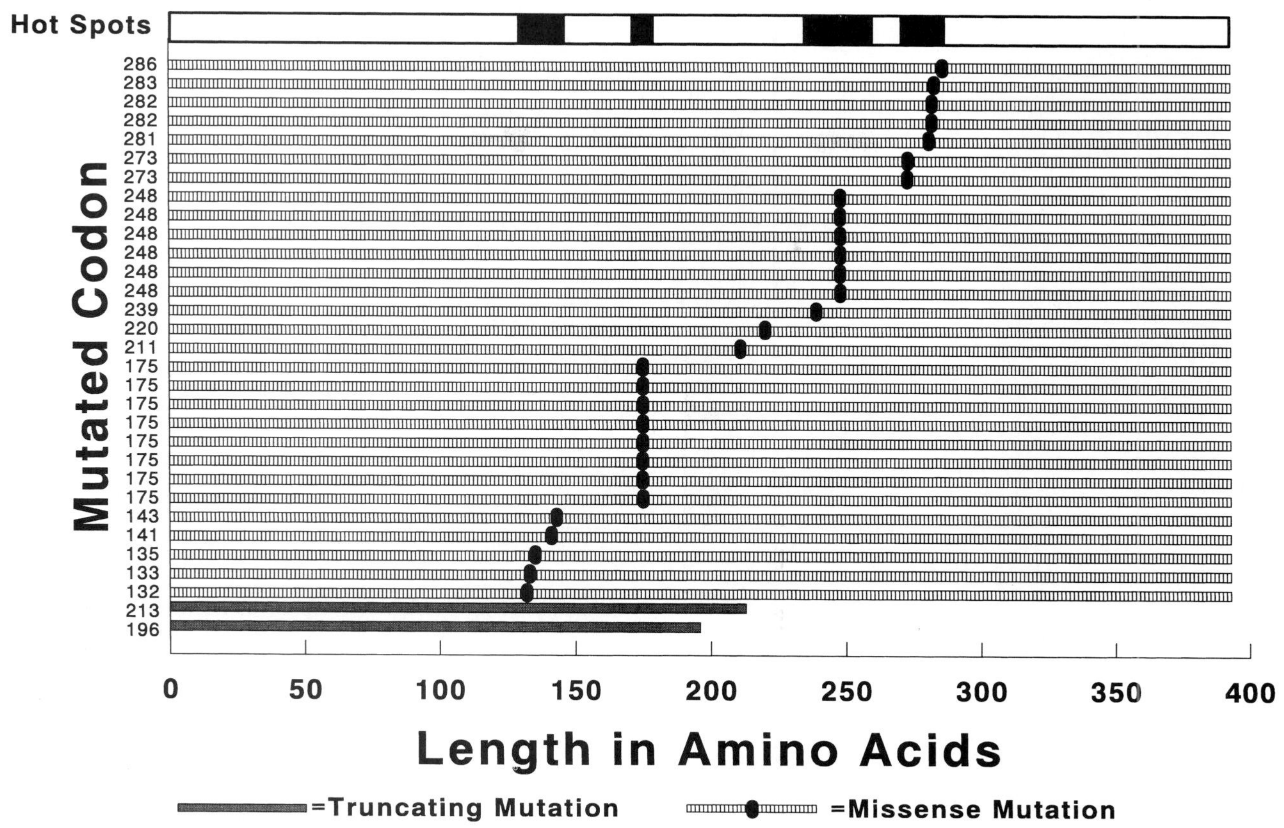

Fig. 48-10 Mutation of *p53* in colorectal tumors. Thirty-one *p53* mutations are illustrated.[73] Length of bar indicates region of *p53* translation terminated normally or by a somatic nonsense mutation. Cross bars indicate the locations of somatic missense mutations.

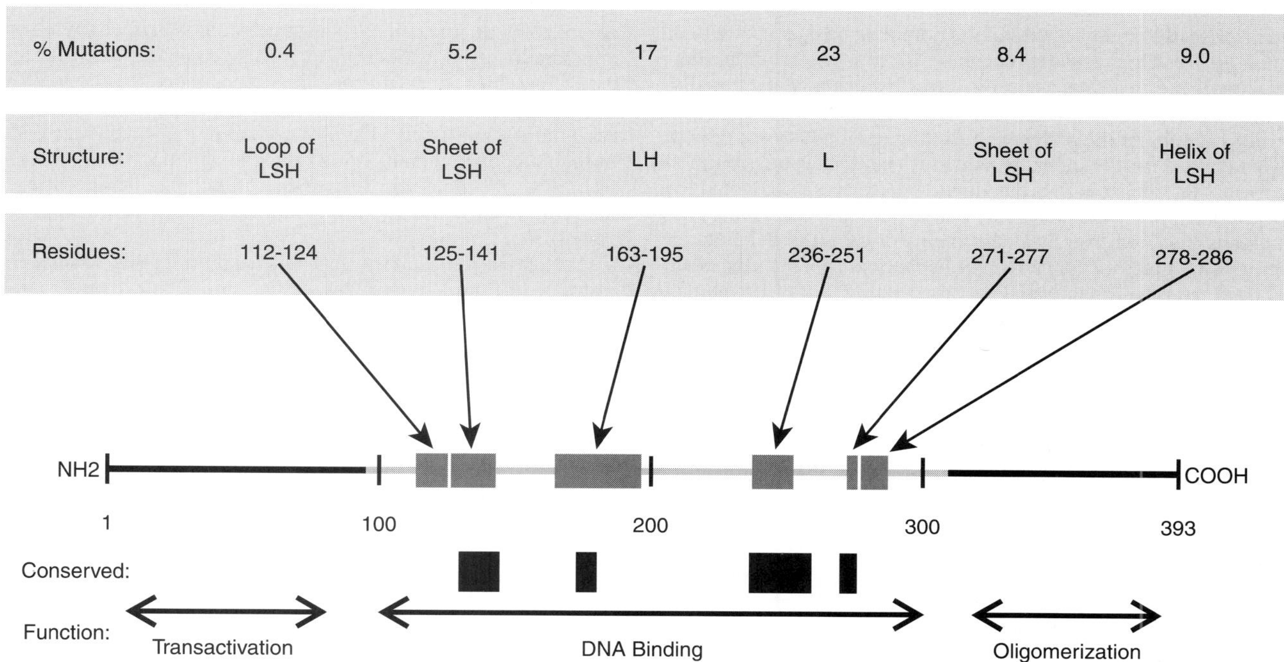

Fig. 48-11 Mutations as they relate to structural domains of p53. Mutations within the indicated region are taken from compiled data (from Greenblatt et al.[419]). Structural domains were determined by x-ray crystallography of the region indicated in yellow.[104] L, LH, and LSH indicate loop, loop-helix, and loop-sheet-helix, respectively. Function domains are indicated and conserved domains are indicated at the bottom. (*Modified with permission from Vogelstein and Kinzler.*[420])

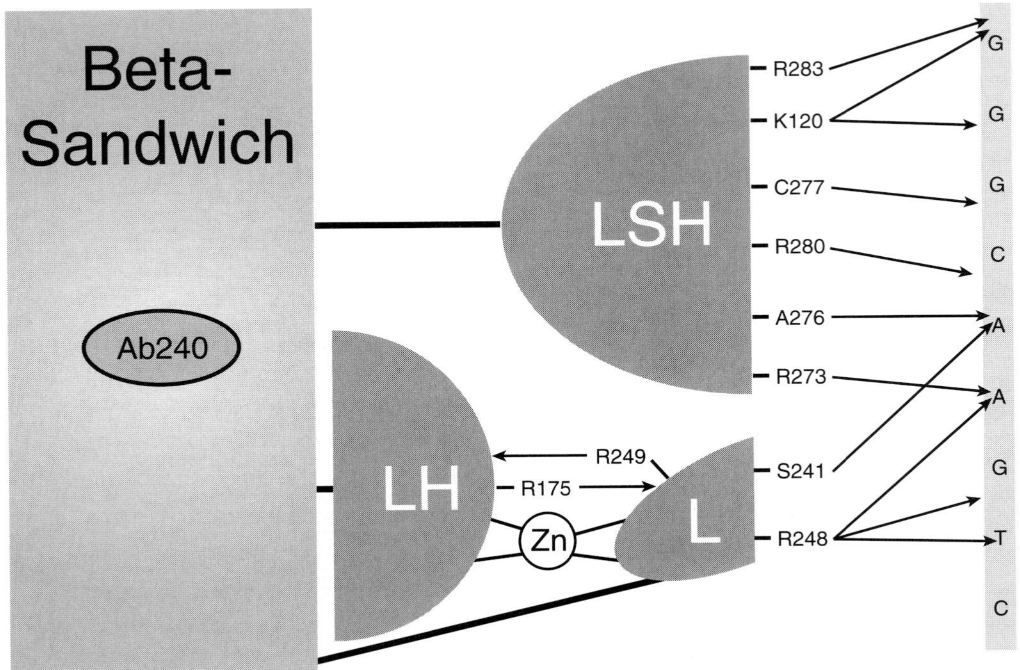

Fig. 48-12 Key structural elements of p53-DNA binding. Based on the crystal structure in Cho et al.[104] L, LH, and LSH indicate loop, loop-helix, and loop-sheet-helix, respectively. Residues are indicated in single-letter code, and DNA contacts are indicated by arrows. For simplicity, only one strand is shown with arrows pointing to bases indicating a base contact and arrows pointing between bases indicating contacts to sugar or phosphate groups. (*Used with permission from Vogelstein and Kinzler.*[420])

yeast.[108,109] As expected due to the lack of specific DNA binding, mutant p53 proteins are devoid of transactivation activity. Moreover, mutant p53 is able to suppress transactivation by wild-type p53 in a dominant negative manner.[108] This suppression was found to be due to the ability of mutant p53 to inhibit wild-type p53 binding to DNA, likely through the formation of inactive hetero-oligomers between wild-type and mutant p53 molecules.

Taken together, these studies suggest the following model for p53 function[110]: Wild-type p53 is hypothesized to bind to specific sequences within the promoters of growth-inhibitory genes and activate their transcription. If a tumor acquires an inactivating missense mutation in one copy of the *p53* gene, p53 activity in the cell is reduced (in part because of the dominant negative activity of mutant p53). The resulting decrease in expression of growth-inhibitory genes leads to a selective growth advantage. Eventually, the residual wild-type activity is completely eliminated by loss of the normal copy of the *p53* gene, resulting in an additional growth advantage and further clonal expansion. This scenario is common in tumors of the colon, brain, lung, breast, skin, and bladder. Occasionally, *p53* is inactivated by nonsense or splice-site mutations that lead to truncated proteins or by gross deletions of one or both copies of the *p53* gene. In cervical cancers, it appears that p53 is often inactivated by association with the human papilloma virus–produced E6 protein.[85,86] Similarly, p53 appears to be inactivated in some tumors by the product of the *MDM2* gene.[111–113] The *MDM2* gene was identified originally by virtue of its amplification in transformed mouse cells[114] and is often amplified in human sarcomas, particularly the malignant fibrous histiocytoma subclass.[112]

Direct evidence for this model has come from the identification of genes transcriptionally regulated by p53. To date, at least 20 genes have been identified that are regulated by p53.[115–133] These genes appear to affect a variety of cellular processes including apoptosis,[117,118,126] cell cycle arrest,[116,127] and negative regulation of the p53 pathway itself.[115] One of the first to be characterized and best understood of these downstream pathways is that containing p21$^{WAF1/CIP1}$.[116,134–136] p53 directly induces the expression of p21$^{WAF1/CIP1}$ via binding to three consensus binding sites located within 2.3 kb of the transcription start site.[116,137] p21$^{WAF1/CIP1}$ in turn inhibits growth by inducing a G1 cell cycle arrest.[116,134] This arrest is due to the ability of p21$^{WAF1/CIP1}$ to bind to and inhibit cyclin-dependent kinases.[135,138] Consistent with this, disruption of the p21$^{WAF1/CIP1}$ genes by homologous recombination eliminates the ability of p53 to induce a G1 arrest in colorectal cancer cells[139,140] and (to a lesser extent) in mouse fibroblasts.[141,142]

As indicated above, p53 induces a variety of genes, and accordingly, the growth-inhibitory effects of p53 on the cell are not limited to a G1 arrest. p53 also can produce a sustained G2 arrest that requires p21$^{WAF1/CIP1}$[143] and the p53-inducible gene *14-3-3σ*.[127,144] In a subset of colon cancers, restoration of p53 function can result in apoptosis rather than cell cycle arrest.[145] Although the specific mechanism for p53-induced apoptosis in colorectal epithelial cells remains unclear, it is likely to involve the transcriptional activation of apoptosis-promoting genes. Candidates for such apoptosis-promoting genes include *BAX*[117,118] and the *PIGs*.[145] The definitive identification of the specific genes essential for p53-induced apoptosis will require their inactivation by homologous recombination; analogously, the essential role of p21 in cell cycle arrest became compelling only after its inactivation by homologous recombination was shown to abrogate this arrest.

In summary, it appears that when p53 is called to duty, it is instructed to stop cell growth at all cost. To achieve this goal, the p53 commando has been granted a large arsenal of growth-inhibitory weapons that allow it to function in diverse cellular environments. If all attempts at growth control fail, p53 induces cellular suicide (the "doomsday" weapon of last resort).

Although p53 function is beginning to be understood at the cellular and biochemical levels, its strategic role at the organism level still remains elusive. Mice with both copies of *p53* inactivated by homologous recombination are viable and develop normally, albeit with a predisposition to lymphomas and, to a lesser extent, other tumors.[146–148] Furthermore, individuals with Li-Fraumeni syndrome inherit a mutated *p53* gene and are normal except for an increased risk of leukemia, breast carcinoma, soft tissue sarcoma, brain tumor, and osteosarcoma.[149,150] These results suggest that p53 function is not essential to the normal cell under most circumstances. However, p53 may be critical to normal cells when stressed. Normal cells arrest their growth in response to x-ray- or drug-induced DNA damage, whereas cells with mutant p53 are only partially blocked and continue to divide.[151–153] This has prompted the suggestion that p53 in part protects the integrity of the genome by preventing propagation of cells with DNA damage.[154] Other forms of stress in addition to DNA damage can induce p53 function. For example, hypoxia, such as that found in poorly vascularized tumors, can induce p53 expression and p53-dependent apoptosis in mouse cells.[155,156] Moreover, cells lacking p53 were shown to have a selective advantage in such an environment.[156] Likewise, excess mitogenic signals from overexpression of Myc,[157,158] E1A,[159] or E2F-1[160–162] can induce p53-mediated apoptosis. This induction is dependent on $p19^{ARF}$ and is distinct from induction by hypoxia and DNA damage.[163–168] In addition to DNA damage, hypoxia, and mitogenic stimulation, changes in adhesion, redox, or rNTP levels status can modulate p53 activity (reviewed in Giaccia and Kastan[169]). Many of these pathways ultimately lead to activation of p53 by post-translational modification of p53 or by interference with the negative regulatory protein Mdm2 (reviewed in Giaccia and Kastan[169]). The physiologic importance of appropriate regulation of p53 has been elegantly illustrated by the ability of deletion of *p53* to rescue the lethality of Mdm2 null mice.[170]

Further information about the regulation and function of p53 is provided in Chap. 37. While a great deal has been learned about the function of p53 and models for its role in tumorigenesis can be proposed (Fig. 48-13), several fundamental questions remain unanswered. For example, it is not understood why patients with Li-Fraumeni syndrome do not have a higher incidence of colon cancer. Nor are the intracellular mediators that determine the expression levels of p53 in normal and tumor cells fully elucidated. Finally, while some insight into the ability of p53 to induce growth arrest have been made, our understanding of its ability to induce apoptosis is less developed. These answers have

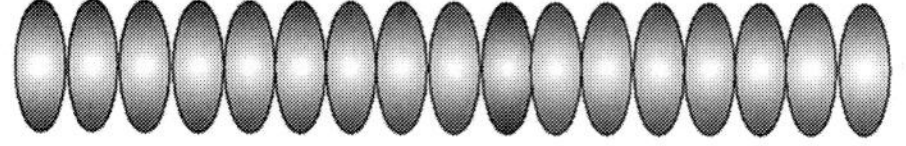

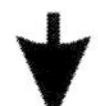
Mutation in Tumor Initiating Gene
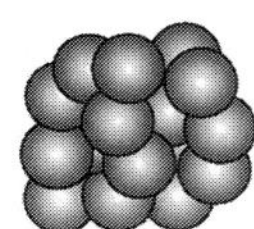

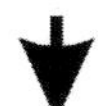
Additional Mutations
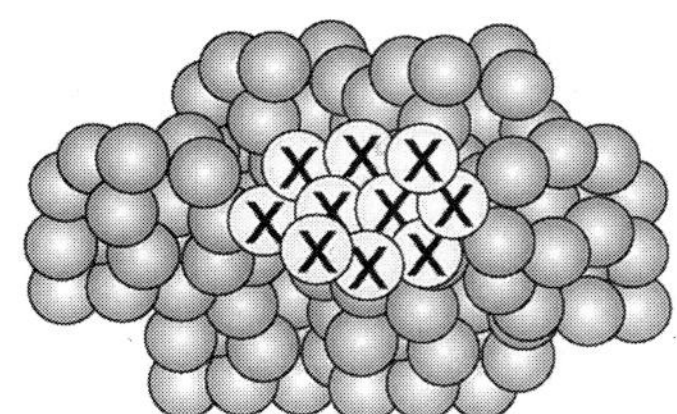

Large Tumor, Central Hypoxia Induces p53, Resulting in Growth Arrest/Apoptosis

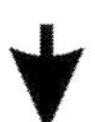
p53 Mutation
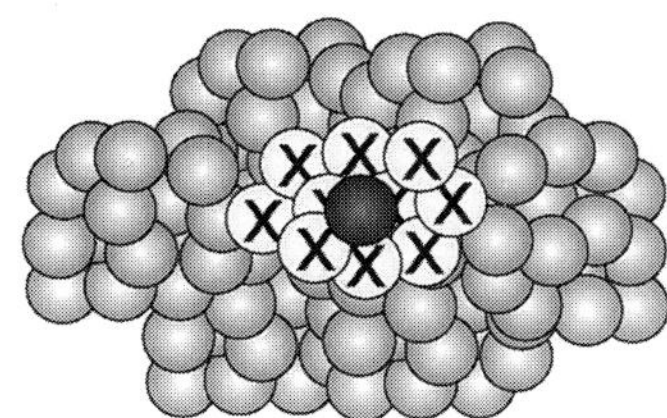

Clonal Expansion
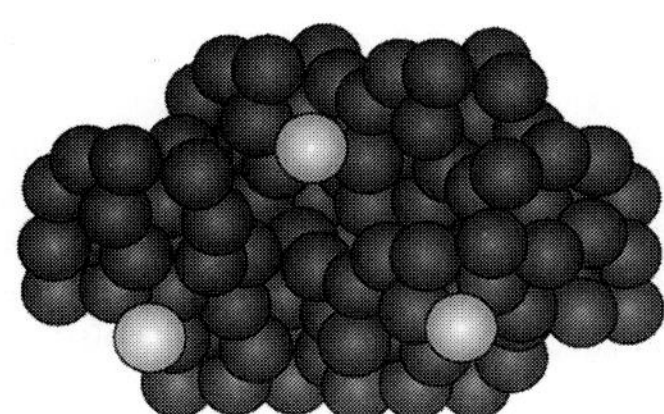

p53 Mutant Cells Become the Predominant Cells in the Tumor

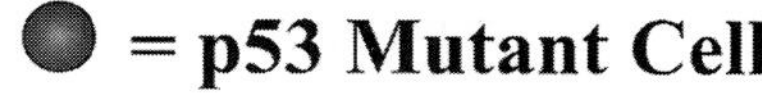
= p53 Mutant Cell

Fig. 48-13 Function of p53 in tumor development. Model of why *p53* mutations occur late in tumorigenesis and lead to selective survival in the adverse environment of a tumor. In this example, hypoxia is the selecting factor, although other adverse conditions also may operate in tumors. (*Used with permission from Kinzler and Vogelstein.*[421])

been amplified recently with identification of structural and functional homologues to *p53* on chromosomes 1p (p73)[171] and 3q (p63, p51, and p40).[172–174] Although products from both loci share p53's ability to inhibit growth, these genes do not appear to play the same central role in human cancers as does *p53*.

Chromosome 18q: The *DCC, SMAD4,* and *SMAD2* Genes

As with *p53,* the first evidence for a tumor-suppressor gene on chromosome 18q came from the study of chromosomal losses in colorectal cancers.[36,45,62,63] One copy of chromosome 18q is lost in 73 percent of sporadic colorectal cancers and in 47 percent of large adenomas with foci of carcinomatous growth, but the loss occurs infrequently in less advanced adenomas[45] (Fig. 48-14). In the clinical arena, three studies have demonstrated that 18q loss is associated with an unfavorable outcome in stage II colorectal cancers,[175–177] although another has not.[178] On the molecular side, several candidate tumor-suppressor genes have been identified in this region, but efforts to positively pinpoint the culprit genes have been complicated by the inability to identify a candidate gene displaying intragenic mutations in the majority of cases.

The first candidate tumor-suppressor gene was isolated during attempts to map the chromosome 18q losses in human colorectal cancer with molecular techniques.[179] Analysis of 60 cancers with a series of polymorphic markers along 18q localized the most common region of deletion to 18q21. One marker from this region identified one carcinoma with a somatic point mutation that could create a novel splice acceptor site and a second with a complete (homozygous) loss of sequences from this region. Thorough analysis of a 370-kb region flanking this marker, using a variety of techniques, revealed a single expressed gene termed *DCC* for *deleted in colorectal cancer.* The *DCC* gene encodes a 10-kb transcript with a 4347-bp open reading frame.[179,180] The coding portion of the transcript is distributed within 29 exons occupying 1350 kb.[181]

The primary structure of DCC provides important clues to how DCC might function. If initiation occurs at the first methionine of the open reading frame, it would encode a 1447-amino-acid protein. DCC protein has several structural features, indicating that it is a membrane protein.[179,180] The amino-terminal end has a 25-amino-acid hydrophobic leader sequence, and an apparent membrane-spanning region divides the protein into an 1100-amino-acid extracellular domain and a 324-amino-acid intracytoplasmic domain. The intracytoplasmic domain shows no obvious homologies to previously sequenced proteins. The extracellular domain shows extensive homology to the cell adhesion molecule N-CAM and to other related cell surface glycoproteins. Specifically, the extracellular domain contains four immunoglobulin-like C2 domains and six fibronectin type III repeats. Some of the suspected properties of DCC derived from the primary sequence have been confirmed by direct analysis of the DCC protein. Cell surface labeling studies documented a cell surface localization for the DCC protein. Immunocytochemical analysis of cells expressing high levels of DCC revealed membrane staining concentrated at points of cell-cell contact.[180] Immunohistochemical studies of human tissues indicate that DCC protein is expressed in differentiating cells, particularly in the intestinal epithelium and brain.[182] Consistent with the preceding observations, the DCC protein was shown to be a receptor for netrin, a laminin-related protein involved in guidance of developing axons.[183–185]

The precise role of *DCC* in colorectal cancer has been difficult to define, in part due to its large size and its lack of expression in colorectal cancers. While the *DCC* transcript is expressed in many tissues, including the colonic mucosa, most colorectal cancers fail to express an intact *DCC* transcript, consistent with its potential role as a tumor suppressor.[179,186] Unfortunately, this lack of expression complicates mutational analysis in that mutations leading to such loss of expression need not be limited to the coding portions of *DCC.* Despite this, a small number of somatic mutations of *DCC,* including small insertions and point mutations, have been identified in human tumors.[179,181] Southern blot analysis of DCC has revealed two intronic point mutations by chance, and detailed analysis of 7 of *DCC*'s 29 coding exons in 30 colorectal cancers identified one somatic missense mutation.[179,181] In addition, three homozygous mutations affecting DCC have been described in colorectal cancer cells.[179,186] Homozygous deletions of *DCC* also were observed in 2 of 91 human germ cell cancers screened by Southern blot analysis.[187] Moreover, the lack of expression of DCC in a subset of tumors with mismatch repair deficiency may be due to an unusually large expansion of a repeat in a DCC intron.[179,181] Loss of DCC protein expression has prognostic value and is associated with an unfavorable outcome in stage II and III colorectal cancers.[188–191] These immunohistochemical studies support the previous observations that

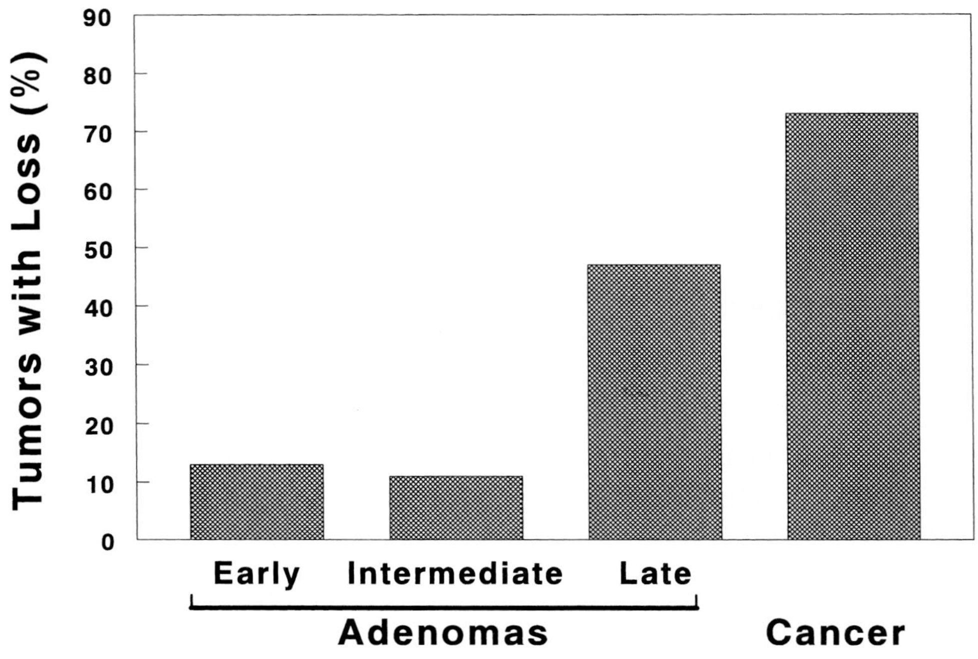

Fig. 48-14 Frequency of 18q losses in colorectal tumors. Tumor classes are defined as in Fig. 48-7. Values for chromosome 18q losses are expressed as a percentage of informative cases showing allelic loss.

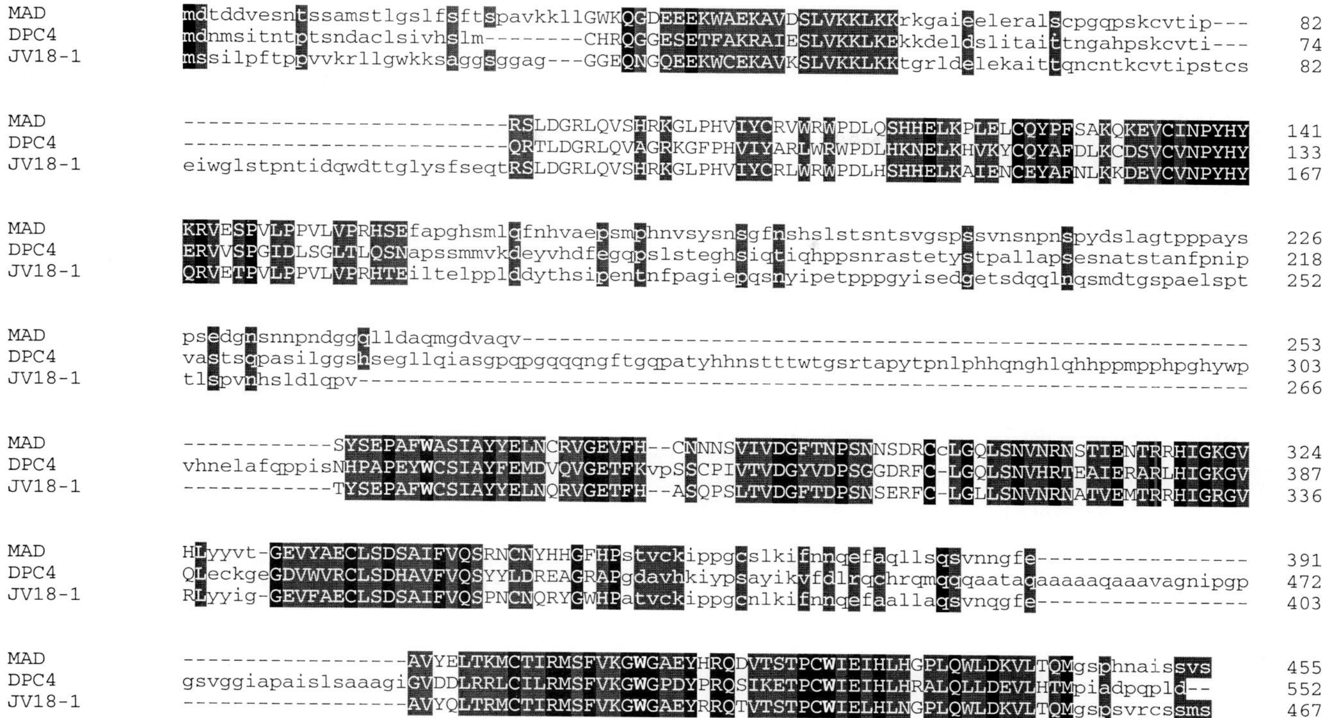

Fig. 48-15 Homology between *SMAD4*, *SMAD2*, and *Drosophila Mad*. The amino acid sequences of *Mad*,[196] *SMAD4* (DPC4),[193] and *SMAD2* (JV18-1)[207] were aligned and shaded by the means of their pairwise score using the MACAW multiple alignment software.[422]

chromosome 18q loss carries an unfavorable prognosis and suggest that the target of such losses is DCC. However, because the mechanisms underlying the loss of DCC expression are not yet known, it is not possible to conclusively implicate DCC as this target from these data. To date, no germ-line mutations of *DCC* have been found. A small fraction of mice with targeted inactivation of one copy of *DCC* showed multiple intestinal tumors or lethal brain tumors that are not observed in normal mice, but the number of mice with these neoplastic phenotypes was not high enough to draw statistically significant conclusions supporting a role for DCC in murine tumorigenesis.[192]

A second tumor-suppressor gene was identified on chromosome 18q21 during the course of investigation of chromosome 18q losses in pancreatic cancers.[193] Chromosome 18q losses occur in nearly 90 percent of pancreatic cancer.[194] Detailed analysis of pancreatic tumors losses identified a marker that revealed homozygous deletions that did not overlap with *DCC*. Characterization of this minimally deleted region identified a single expressed gene, termed *deleted in pancreatic cancer 4 (DPC4)*.[193] Further analysis of *DPC4* revealed that it was homozygously deleted in 25 of 84 pancreatic carcinomas (30 percent). Sequencing analysis of *DPC4* in 27 pancreatic cancers without homozygous mutations identified six intragenic mutations including one splice site, one missense, and four truncating mutations. Together these findings suggest a critical role for *DPC4* inactivation in pancreatic cancers.

DPC4 encodes a 552-residue protein with significant homology to the *Drosophila* mothers against Dpp (Mad) protein as well as *Caenorhabditis elegans* Mad homologues (Fig. 48-15). These proteins have been implicated in the signaling pathway of the transforming growth factor-beta (TGFβ) superfamily of signaling polypeptides.[195–197] This is of particular interest in light of the fact that TGFβ suppresses the growth of most normal cells and many cancer cells are resistant to the growth-suppressing affects of TGFβ (reviewed in Fynan and Reiss[198] and Brattain *et al.*[199]). Indeed, mutations of the TGFβ receptor have been identified in a subset of human colorectal cancers.[200–202] In colorectal cancer cells, DPC4 was shown to be required for TGFβ and activin signaling by specific disruption of the *DPC4* loci through homologous recombination.[203] At the biochemical level, DPC4 functions in this pathway as a sequence-specific transcription activator.[204–206] To date, over a half dozen human Mad homologues (*SMAD*s) have been identified,[193,197,207–211] and *DPC4* has been redesignated *SMAD4*. Interestingly, *SMAD2*[207,208] and *SMAD7*,[210–212] in addition to *DPC4/SMAD4*, also map to chromosome 18q21, providing additional candidate tumor-suppressor genes. In contrast to SMAD2 and DPC4/SMAD4, SMAD7 appears to function antagonistically in TGFβ signaling, making it less appealing as a candidate tumor-suppressor gene.[210,211]

Mutational analysis of *DPC4/SMAD4* in 18 human colorectal cancers with 18q losses identified one homozygous deletion, one nonsense mutation, and three somatic missense mutations.[186] Analysis of *SMAD2* in the same 18 tumors identified one homozygous deletion that did not affect *DPC4/SMAD4* or *DCC* and a 42-bp deletion.[207] Intact *SMAD4/DPC4* and *SMAD2* transcripts were detected in the remaining tumors. In a separate study, analysis of *SMAD2* in 66 colorectal cancers identified four missense mutations.[208] Three of these mutations were shown to be functionally defective, as assessed by their abnormal TGFβ-induced phosphorylation and *Xenopus* mesoderm induction.[208] Other studies have found somatic mutations of *DPC4/SMAD4* or *SMAD2* in colorectal,[213] lung,[214] and stomach[215] cancers. However, in each case, mutations of *DPC4/SMAD4* could only account for the minority of 18q losses, suggesting that mutations remained undetected or that another chromosome 18q gene is the primary target of the 18q losses in these tumors. Germ-line mutations of *DPC4/SMAD4* are observed in a subset of individuals with juvenile polyposis syndrome (JPS). Individuals with JPS develop multiple juvenile polyps (distinct from adenomas) and are at an increased risk for colorectal cancer. The *SMAD4* mutations in JPS may lead to colorectal neoplasia only indirectly, since the mutations appear to initially affect stromal cells rather than the epithelial precursors of cancers (see Chap. 35).[216] In mice, inactivation of one copy of *Dpc4/Smad4* does not lead to increased rate of spontaneous tumors.[217,218]

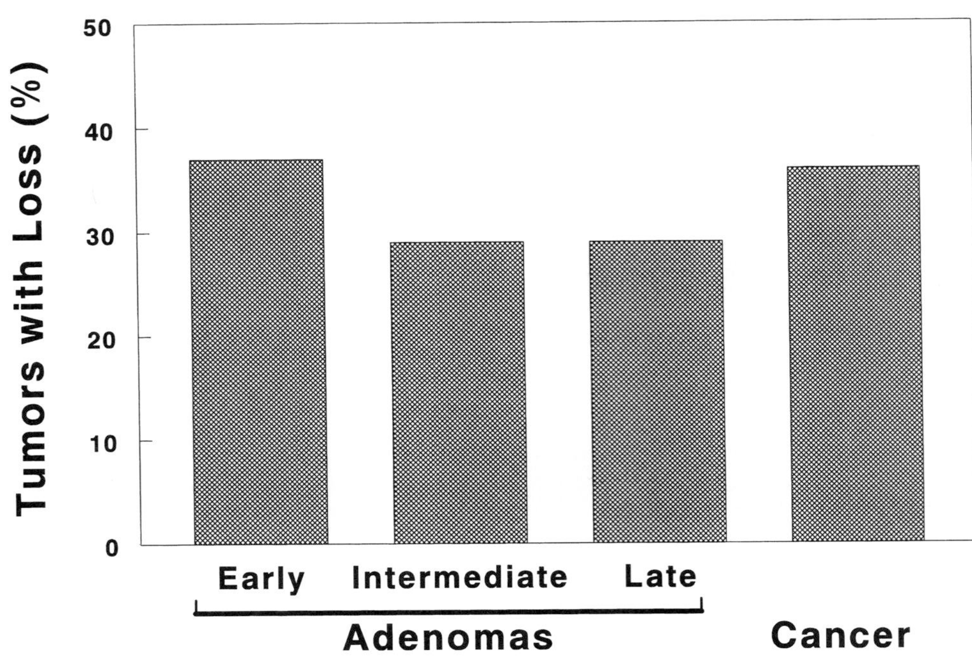

Fig. 48-16 Frequency of 5q losses in colorectal tumors. Tumor classes are defined as in Fig. 48-7. Values for chromosome 5q losses are expressed as a percentage of informative cases showing allelic loss.

However, inactivation of both copies of *Dpc4/Smad4* did accelerate the progression of tumors arising in mice with a concurrent inactivation of *Apc*.[219] Interestingly, whereas homozygous inactivation of *Smad2*[220,221] or *Smad4*[217,218] is embryonically lethal, certain mouse strains with homozygous inactivation of *Smad3* are viable and develop metastatic colorectal cancer.[222]

Studies employing chromosome transfer demonstrated the ability of chromosome 18q to eliminate or reduce the growth of human colon cancer cells in nude mice.[223,224] In both colorectal cancer and squamous carcinoma cell lines, suppression by chromosome 18 is associated with restoration of TGFβ sensitivity.[224,225] In the squamous carcinoma cell lines, loss of this suppression is associated with loss of *DPC4/SMAD4* but not *DCC*.[225] Evidence for the growth-suppressive effect of DCC has come from antisense studies. When DCC expression in rat cells is inhibited by *DCC* antisense sequences, the cells become anchorage-independent *in vitro* and form tumors in nude mice.[226,227] Conversely, when DCC expression vectors are used to express DCC in human keratinocytes lacking DCC expression, tumorigenicity in nude mice is suppressed.[228] A molecular basis for these observations was provided recently when it was found that DCC induces apoptosis through a novel mechanism requiring receptor proteolysis.[229]

A variety of data point to the existence of a tumor-suppressor gene(s) on chromosome 18q in a number of human cancers. In some cancers, the inactivation of *DPC4/SMAD4* is clearly the target of these loss events. However, mutations of *DPC4/SMAD4* do not appear to account for most cases of chromosome 18q loss, so other known or yet-to-be-discovered candidate tumor-suppressor genes are likely to be the culprit(s) in the majority of cases.

Chromosome 5q: The *APC* Gene

Two lines of evidence suggested that a putative tumor-suppressor gene located on chromosome 5q was of particular interest. The first line of evidence came from the study of FAP, an inherited predisposition to colorectal cancer. The seminal clue to the location of the gene causing FAP came from a patient with polyposis and a constitutional interstitial deletion of 5q that was visible on cytogenetic analysis.[230] This observation suggested that a suppressor gene on chromosome 5q was responsible for the patient's condition. This suggestion was confirmed and extended by linkage analysis, which established linkage of FAP to chromosome 5q21 markers in all kindreds analyzed.[231–233]

The second line of evidence came from the study of allelic losses in sporadic colorectal tumors. Chromosome 5q losses were reported to occur in 20 to 50 percent of colorectal cancers, depending on the region of chromosome 5q assessed.[45,59,62,63,234–237] Even more important, the loss of chromosome 5 sequences occurred as frequently in small benign colorectal tumors as in larger malignant tumors[45] (Fig. 48-16). These observations suggested that inactivation of a tumor-suppressor gene on chromosome 5q occurs frequently and early during tumor formation.

These two lines of evidence converged with the identification of a small region of chromosome 5q21 that was altered in the germ line of FAP patients and in sporadic colorectal cancers. Four genes were mapped to this region [*MCC, TB2 (DP1), SRP19,* and *APC*].[238,239] One of these genes (*APC*, for *adenomatous polyposis coli*) was found to be mutated in the germ line of FAP patients[240,241] and in sporadic colorectal tumors.[240] The *APC* gene contains an open reading frame of 8538 bp that would encode a 2843-amino-acid protein if translation initiated at the first methionine. This coding sequence is distributed over 15 exons and is remarkable in that the last exon contains a 6579-bp uninterrupted open reading frame. Several alternatively spliced forms of *APC* are known to exist, including variants that affect the coding region.[239,241–243]

The *APC* gene has been examined in over 500 FAP kindreds.[244,245] The most successful of these analyses have identified intragenic mutations in roughly 80 percent of the kindreds examined.[246] The majority of the remaining kindreds also have mutations of the *APC* gene that result in deletion of large portions of the gene or reduce its expression.[247] These latter mutations are difficult to detect because they can be masked by the normal allele.[248] The nature of the intragenic mutations so far documented is quite striking, with more than 95 percent predicted to result in truncation of the APC protein (based on 176 mutations compiled in Nagase and Su[244]). The truncating mutations are largely the result of nonsense point mutations (33 percent) or small insertions (6 percent) and deletions (55 percent) that lead to frameshifts.[244] The majority of mutations occur in the first half of the last exon (Fig. 48-17). A few missense changes have been identified, but it is currently not known whether these missense changes are functional or merely represent rare variants; at least one has been shown not to segregate with the disease.[249]

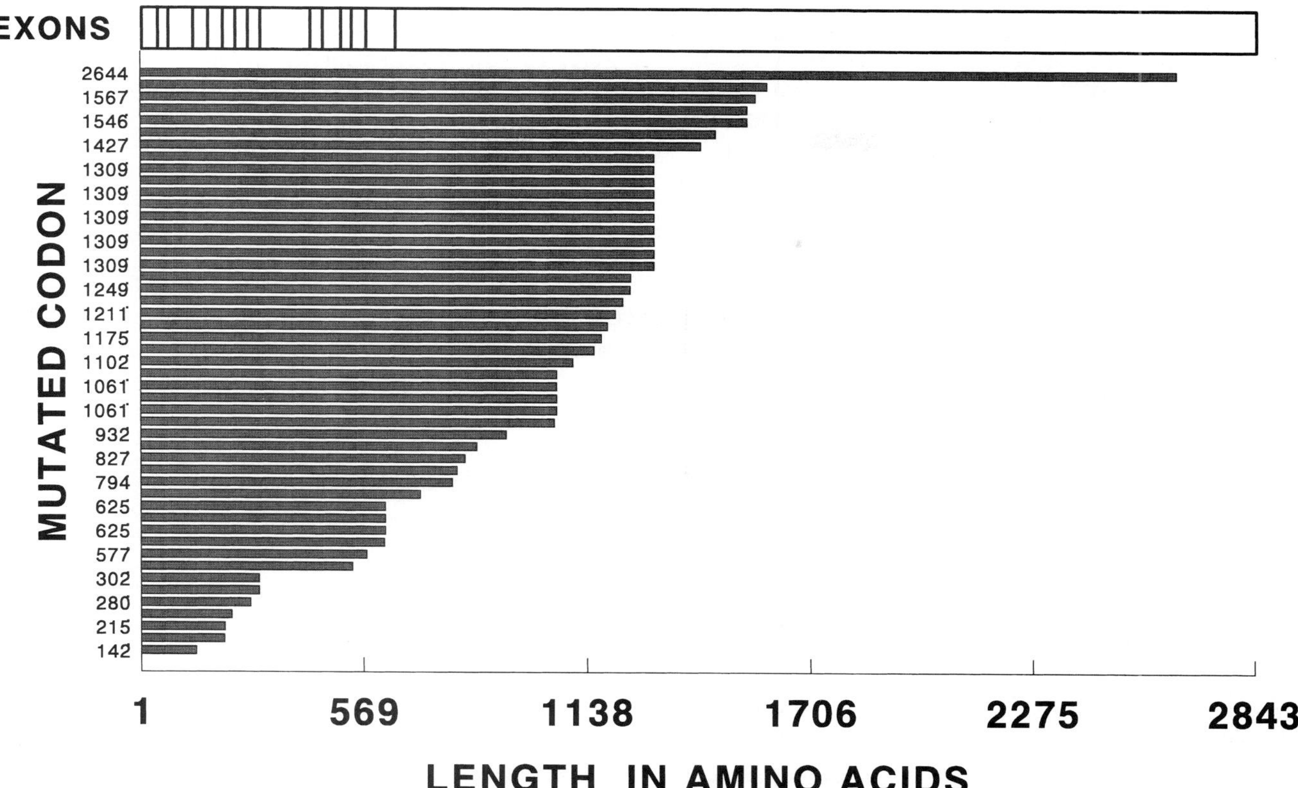

Fig. 48-17 Mutation of the *APC* gene in the germ line of FAP patients. Truncating *APC* mutations from 49 independent FAP kindreds are illustrated (Miyoshi et al.[423]). Four missense changes are not shown because it is not known whether they represent rare variants or true (functional) mutations. Lengths of bars indicate the region of *APC* translated until terminated by either a nonsense or frameshift mutation.

The phenotypic manifestations of FAP vary considerably and in some cases can be correlated with a specific *APC* mutation (Fig. 48-18). For example, congenital hypertrophy of the retinal pigment epithelium (CHRPE) is associated with truncating mutations between codons 463 and 1387.[250–252] Truncating mutations between codon 1403 and 1578 are associated with increased extracolonic disease, particularly desmoid tumors and mandibular lesions, but patients with such mutations do not exhibit CHRPE.[252–254] Similarly, colonic manifestations have been shown to vary with the position of the mutation. Truncating mutations amino-terminal to codon 157[18] or at the extreme carboxyl-terminal end[255–259] are associated with an attenuated form of FAP in which patients develop a relatively small number of polyps (0–100). Some studies have suggested that mutations between codons 1250 and 1464 are associated with an increased number of colorectal tumors.[260,261] In contrast, patients with identical mutations can develop dissimilar clinical features. For example, some patients with identical truncating mutations develop features of GS (mandibular osteomas and desmoid tumors), whereas others do not.[240,262] Likewise, only a small number of patients within any kindred develop brain tumors, hepatoblastomas, or thyroid cancers, even though there is a clear predisposition to these tumors associated with germ-line *APC* mutations.[12,14]

APC's role in colorectal tumorigenesis is not limited to FAP; it also plays a critical role in the development of sporadic colorectal tumors.[263–265] It is estimated that at least 80 percent of colorectal tumors have somatic mutations of the *APC* gene.[263–265] The nature and distribution of somatic mutations identified in sporadic tumors resemble those observed in FAP patients (Fig. 48-19). Over 95 percent of the mutations are predicted to result in truncations of the APC protein, due to either splice-site mutations (7 percent), nonsense mutations (40 percent), or insertions (12 percent) or deletions (41 percent) that lead to frameshifts (based on 75 mutations from Miyoshi et al.[263] and Powell et al.[264]). Two observations suggest that mutation of *APC* is an early, perhaps initiating event in sporadic colorectal tumorigenesis. First, the frequency of *APC* mutations is just as high in small benign tumors as in cancers.[50,263,264] This is in marked contrast to mutations of other genes (such as those in *RAS* or *p53*), which appear only as tumors progress. Second, mutations of *APC* have been found in the earliest sporadic lesions analyzed, including those as small as a few crypts (ACF).[50,266]

In addition to FAP and sporadic colorectal cancers, studies of *APC* in individuals with a modest predisposition to colorectal cancer revealed a novel mechanism for cancer predisposition. Genetic testing of an individual with multiple polyps and a family history of late-onset colorectal cancer revealed a missense substitution in codon 1307 (I1307K).[267] This change was present in approximately 6 percent of Ashkenazi Jews but rarely in the general population.[267–269] Among Ashkenazim, the I1307K allele was found to be more common in colorectal cancer patients and in individuals with a family history of colorectal cancer than in the Ashkenazi population at large.[267] In the families of I1307K colorectal cancer survivors, the I1307K allele was found to be associated with individuals with polyps or cancer in a highly nonrandom manner.[267,270] Together the preceding data suggested an increased risk (1.8-fold) for colorectal cancer for I1307K carriers. However, the mechanistic basis for this increased risk was unclear because previously only truncating mutations of *APC* had been shown to be disease-causing. This mechanism became clear, however, on analysis of the codon 1307 region in tumors. Sequencing of the *APC* gene in tumors from individuals with the I1307K variant revealed the presence of somatic truncating mutations in the immediate vicinity of the codon 1307 change in

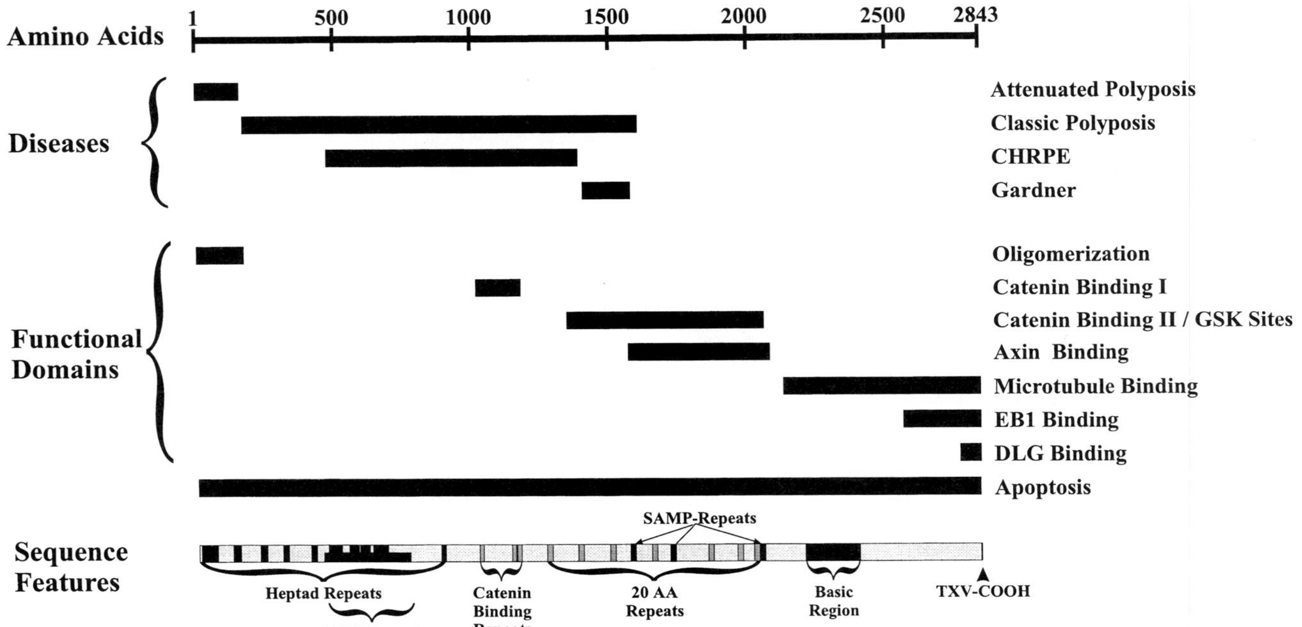

Fig. 48-18 Functional and disease-related domains of *APC*. Disease map: The location of truncating *APC* mutations has been shown to correlate with the extent of colonic and extracolonic manifestations. Truncating mutations prior to codon 157[18] or at the extreme C-terminal end[255–259] are associated with a reduced number of colorectal polyps, whereas the majority of mutations are associated with more pronounced polyposis and occur between codon 169 and 1600.[244] Mutations in codons 463 to 1387 are associated with congenital hypertrophy of the retinal pigment epithelium (CHRPE).[250–252] Mutations in codons 1403 to 1578 have been associated with an increased incidence of extracolonic manifestations.[252–254] Functional domains and sequence features: N-terminal residues 1 to 171 are sufficient for oligomerization.[287,288] This oligomerization is thought to be mediated by the heptad repeats.[238,241,287] APC binds to β-catenin through two motifs, the first comprising three 15-amino-acid repeats located between residues 1020 and 1169.[289,290] A second region, comprising seven 20-amino-acid repeats between residues 1324 and 2075,[241] binds to β-catenin and also acts as substrate for GSK phosphorylation.[293,310] Phosphorylation is thought to occur at SXXXS sites within the 20-amino-acid repeats.[293] Axin homologues bind to three SAMP repeats located between residues 1561 and 2057 of *APC*.[295] When transiently overexpressed, full-length APC decorates the microtubule cytoskeleton. The C-terminus of APC is required for this association, and residues 2130 to 2843 are sufficient.[265,301] Two proteins have been shown to associate with the C-terminus of APC. Residues 2560 to 2843 are sufficient to bind EB-1, a highly conserved 30-kDa protein of unknown function.[300] Residues 2771 to 2843 are sufficient to bind DLG, a human homologue of the *Drosophila* disk large tumor-suppressor gene[303]; the three C-terminal residues of APC (TXV) probably mediate this binding. Expression of full-length APC in colorectal cancer cell lines results in apoptosis, but the regions required for this activity have not been precisely defined.[285] Residues 453 to 767 contain 7 copies of a repeat consensus found in the *Drosophila* segment polarity gene product armadillo,[424] and residues 2200 to 2400 correspond to a basic region.[241] (*Modified with permission from Kinzler and Vogelstein.*[418])

48 percent of the tumors.[267] Each of these somatic changes was found to affect the K allele of *APC* rather than the I allele. Taken together, these data suggest that the I1307K change predisposes to colorectal polyps and cancer by creating a premutation, i.e., a genomic region that is predisposed to subsequent somatic mutation. As expected with a mutation that causes only a 1.8-fold increase in risk, such risk increases are difficult to detect using standard epidemiologic methods in small samples of patients. However, several studies have documented an association with colorectal cancer consistent with a 1.5- to 2-fold increase.[267,268,271,272] Other studies could exclude a markedly increased risk but did not have the power to exclude or implicate a modest increase.[273–275] Given the difficulties associated with population studies, examination of the aforementioned somatic mutations may provide a better estimate of the increased risk associated with I1307K. Two studies of somatic mutations suggest that approximately 43 percent of the colorectal cancers that arise in I1307K carriers are attributed to the I1307 change.[267,276] If it is assumed that I1307K patients with colorectal cancer are representative of all I1307K individuals, this would translate to a relative risk of 1.7, in excellent agreement with the epidemiologic studies. The larger implications of the Ashkenazi work are that classic mutations in tumor-suppressor genes can lead to severe disease (like polyposis), while less obvious mutations in the same genes also can lead to milder predispositions to the same tumor types. Indeed, other missense mutations of *APC* have been suggested to lead to colorectal cancer predisposition in the absence of polyposis.[271]

Evidence for an important role of *APC* in tumorigenesis has been supported by the study of mice with germ-line inactivation of the murine homologue of *APC* (*mAPC*). Three such mouse lineages have been reported, and all three have an increased risk for intestinal tumors.[277–279] The first and best described of these is the multiple intestinal neoplasia (Min) strain of mice.[280] The Min mouse was established from a C57BL/6J male mouse treated with ethylnitrosurea and bred for inherited traits. Min mice exhibit an autosomal dominantly inherited predisposition to multiple intestinal neoplasia and on a susceptible background develop an average of 30 to 50 intestinal tumors by the age of 90 days.[280,281] This phenotype is not exactly like that of FAP patients, since the mouse adenomas are largely found in the small intestine rather than in the colon, whereas the reverse is true in FAP patients. The Min phenotype was traced to a single nonsense mutation resulting in the truncation of mApc protein at codon 850.[277] Similar phenotypes to Min are observed in mouse lineages derived by homologous recombination to specifically inactivate *mAPC*.[278,279] The nature of the mutations in all these mice is similar to those observed in the germ line of FAP patients, making these mice good models of FAP at both the phenotypic and genotypic levels. Furthermore, because these mouse models share at least one important genetic defect with sporadic human colorectal tumors, they may prove to be a good model for colorectal tumorigenesis in general.

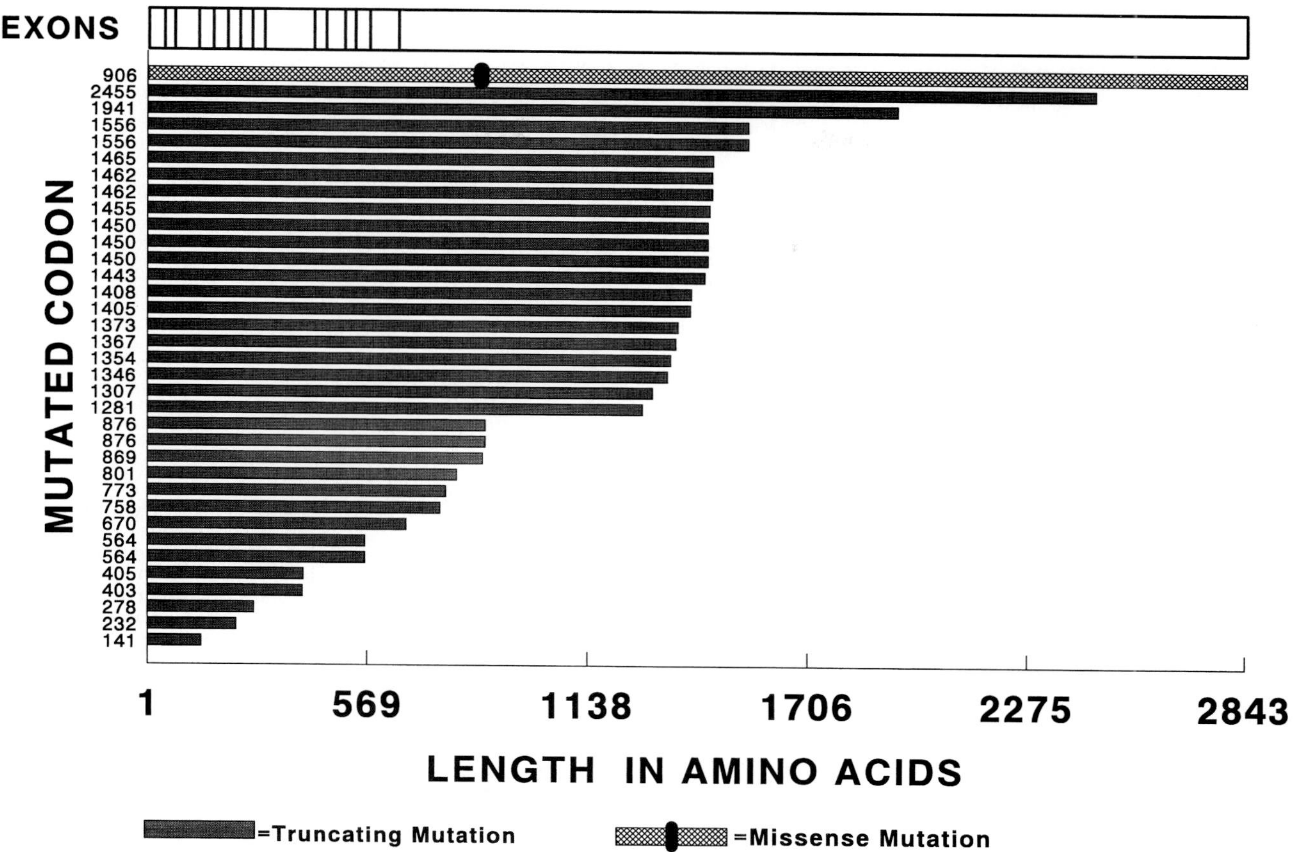

Fig. 48-19 Somatic *APC* mutations in sporadic colorectal tumors. Thirty-five *APC* mutations from 16 adenomas and 26 carcinomas are illustrated (Powell et al.[264]). Lengths of bars indicate the region of *APC* translated until terminated by either a nonsense or frameshift mutation. Cross bar indicates the location of the single somatic missense mutation identified.

Do both copies of the *APC* gene need to be inactivated for it to exert its affect on tumor development, as Knudson's tumor-suppressor gene model would suggest? Studies of *APC* mutations in primary sporadic colorectal tumors suggest that at least a third of both benign and malignant tumors have no normally functioning *APC* gene.[263,264] Studies of primary tumors from FAP patients identify a second inactivating mutation in about 80 percent of the tumors. Both these studies undoubtedly represent underestimates of the true extent of inactivation of both alleles due to the difficulties in analyzing primary human tumors. However, studies of APC protein in colorectal cancer cell lines indicate that most (26 of 32) were totally devoid of full-length APC protein.[265] Similarly, inactivation of both alleles of the *mAPC* gene occurs almost without exception in Min tumors and can be detected in lesions so small that they can only be observed at the microscopic level.[282,283] Together these data strongly suggest that both copies of *APC* must be inactivated during tumorigenesis. This notion is further supported by the rapid development of adenomas after disruption the *Apc* gene in mice with conditional targeting of the *Apc* locus.[284]

What is APC's normal function that is so critical to prevention of intestinal tumor development? Expression of wild-type APC in colorectal epithelial cells with *APC* mutations results in apoptosis, suggesting that APC may control the cell death process.[285] Immunohistochemical analysis indicates that APC protein is apparently located at the basolateral membrane in colorectal epithelial cells, with expression increasing as cells migrate to the top of the crypt.[265,286] Since loss of cells from the top of crypts is an important homeostatic process in the colon, it is easy to imagine how disruption of such a "death signal" could lead to neoplasia.

The primary structure of APC provides few clues as to how it might mediate such functions (see Fig. 48-18). Residues 453 to 767 contain seven copies of repeat consensus found in the *Drosophila* segment polarity gene *armadillo*. The amino-terminal third of *APC* contains several heptad repeats of the type that mediate oligomerization by a coiled-coil structure.[287,288] These regions may mediate homo-oligomerization between mutant and wild-type proteins and could theoretically cause a dominant negative effect, although no such effect has been demonstrated biologically. In addition, seven 20-amino-acid repeats have been identified between residues 1324 and 2075.[241]

Although the preceding sequence features have provided some insights into the function of APC, the identification of proteins that interact with APC has yielded even more tantalizing clues. To date, over a half dozen APC protein interactions have been described, including β-catenin,[289,290] γ-catenin,[291,292] GSK-3β,[293] AXIN family proteins,[294–299] EB-1,[300] microtubules,[301,302] and hDLG.[303] Two of these proteins, EB-1 and hDLG, bind to the C-terminus of APC. *EB-1* encodes a highly conserved 30-kDa protein[300] that is associated with cytoplasmic and spindle microtubules.[304] In yeast, an *EB-1* homologue is required for a cytokinesis checkpoint.[305] The second C-terminal interacting gene product is the human homologue of the *Drosophila* tumor-suppressor gene disks large (*DLG*).[303] Since virtually all *APC* mutations result in loss of the C-terminus of the APC protein (see Figs. 48-17 and 48-19), these data suggest that hDLG and/or EB-1 may be essential for APC's growth-controlling function.

The most penetrating insights into APC function have come from studies of the interaction between β-catenin and APC.[289,290] The central third of APC contains two classes of β-catenin–binding repeats, one of which is modulated by phosphorylation[293]

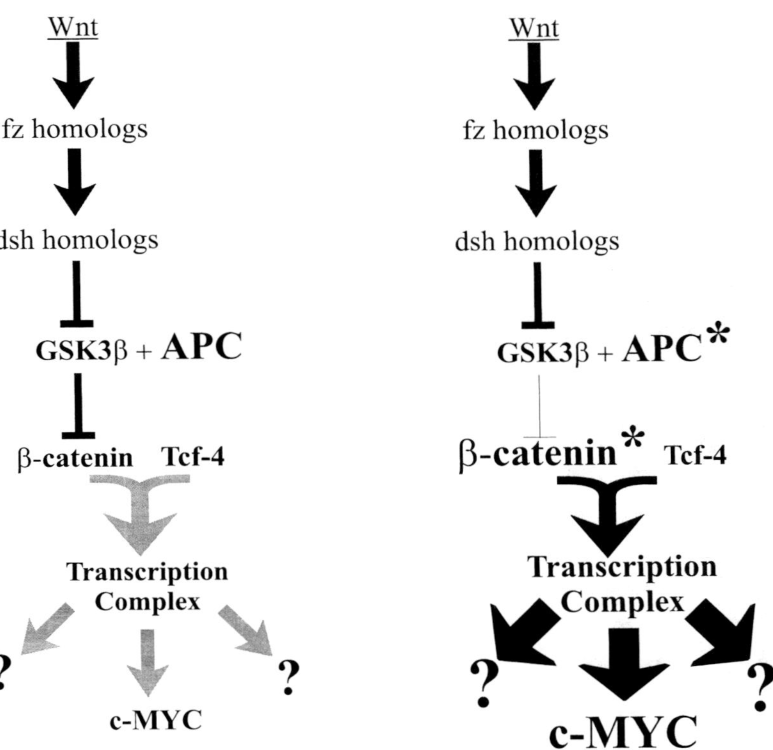

Fig. 48-20 The Wg/Wnt pathway ultimately results in β-catenin/Tcf–mediated transcription. APC cooperates with GSK-3β to degrade β-catenin and inhibit β-catenin/Tcf–mediated transcription. Inactivating mutations of APC or activating mutations of β-catenin can alleviate this inhibition resulting in increased transcription of growth promoting genes. One of these growth-promoting genes is *c-MYC*. See the text for additional detail.

(see Fig. 48-18). Although many mutant APC proteins retain some β-catenin binding, virtually all mutant APC proteins lack at least one type of β-catenin–binding repeat.

The β-catenin association links APC to two apparently diverse cellular processes. The first process is related to cellular adhesion. The catenins originally were identified as cytoplasmic proteins that bind to cadherins, a family of calcium-dependent homophilic cell adhesion molecules. Several studies have indicated that β-catenin is necessary for cadherin-mediated cell adhesion.[306] Given that binding of β-catenin to cadherins or to APC is mutually exclusive, it is possible that APC could modulate such adhesion as part of its tumor-suppressing function. APC additionally could act as a downstream communicator of adhesion status, linking cadherin-catenin complexes to other cellular components.

The second process involving APC has been elucidated by studies of the wingless (Wg) and Wnt signaling pathways in *Drosophila, Xenopus,* and mouse. *β-Catenin* and *armadillo* (the *Drosophila* homologue of *β-catenin*) have been firmly implicated as signal transducers in these pathways.[307–309] This link was fortified by the observation that the APC-β-catenin complex is physically associated with a second member of this pathway, the ZW3/GSK3β protein kinase.[293] Moreover, this kinase was found to promote β-catenin binding to APC, presumably by phosphorylation of APC class II binding sites[293] (see Fig. 48-18). The functional consequence of this binding is the ubiquitin-dependent proteosomal degradation of β-catenin.[310–312] Consistent with this, epistasis evaluations in *Drosophila* suggest that Wg signaling inhibits ZW3 function and that active ZW3 can inhibit β-catenin signaling. Finally, studies in *Xenopus* and mouse suggest that Wnt signaling ultimately results in formation of a heteromeric complex containing β-catenin and members of the Tcf/Lef family of HMG box transcription factors.[313,314] Taken together, these observations suggest that APC works in concert with ZW3/GSK3β to inhibit β-catenin–induced transcription. Given that this pathway had been implicated previously in neoplasia by the ability of truncated β-catenin to transform cells in culture[315] and the involvement of Wnt signaling in breast tumorigenesis in mice,[16] it was plausible that the β-catenin–APC interaction contributed to the tumor-suppressive function of APC. Further analysis of this pathway in colorectal cancers provided strong support for this notion.[317,318] Constitutive activity of this pathway as measured by β-catenin/Tcf–mediated transcription was elevated in colorectal cancer cell lines but not in cancer cell lines from other organs, and wild-type APC could specifically down-regulate this activity when transfected into appropriate reporter cells. Furthermore, APC mutants derived from colon cancers and FAP patients were deficient in this down-regulating activity. Compelling evidence for the importance of β-catenin came from the study of the rare tumors that lacked APC mutations. Approximately half these tumors possessed β-catenin mutations in the N-terminal regulatory domain.[318–321,322] These mutations render β-catenin superactive and relatively resistant to the effects of APC.[318] These findings strongly suggest that excess β-catenin/Tcf signaling contributes to colorectal tumorigenesis (Fig. 48-20). In the majority of cancers, this is achieved by mutations of the *APC* gene that prevent its inhibition of β-catenin. In a significant fraction of the remaining tumors, this is achieved by dominant activating β-catenin mutations that render the protein insensitive to APC/GSK-3β–mediated degradation. Similar oncogenic mutations of β-catenin have been observed in other human[323–328] and rodent[324,329,330] cancers. These observations led to the prediction that the increased β-catenin/Tcf–mediated transcription ultimately results in expression of genes that promote cell growth or inhibit cell death (see Fig. 48-20). This expectation was confirmed recently by identification of the *c-MYC* oncogene as a direct downstream target of β-catenin/Tcf–mediated transcription.[331] Interestingly, this observation is consistent with previous studies that indicated that restoration of chromosome 5 to colorectal cancer cells was associated with a decrease in c-MYC expression.[332] Other β-catenin/Tcf downstream targets have also been identified.[332a,332b,332c,332d,332e] Whether all of APC tumor-suppressive effects are related to inhibition of β-catenin/Tcf–mediated transcription remains to be determined. In this regard, it is interesting to note that mice with transgenic expression of activated β-catenin in their intestinal epithelial cells did not develop intestinal tumors but did show abnormal intestinal cell homeostasis.[333] Likewise, mice with transgenic expression of an activated β-catenin in their keratinocytes underwent *de novo* hair follicle morphogenesis but also developed hair follicle tumors.[334] Mice engineered to lack Tcf-4 by homologous recombination showed depletion of intestinal epithelial stem cell compartment.[335] Thus β-catenin/Tcf signaling plays a critical role in regulation of epithelial cell homeostasis, and loss of regulation of this pathway by APC contributes to neoplastic transformation of several cell types. Why germ-line *APC* mutations lead largely to colorectal neoplasia, rather than to more widespread tumorigenesis, remains a mystery. An APC homologue (APCL) that shares APC's ability to interact with β-catenin has been described recently.[336,337] It will be interesting to determine whether APCL functions like APC in noncolonic tissues, with the resulting redundancy perhaps explaining the cell type specificity of APC tumorigenesis.

Other Genetic Changes

MCC. During the search for the gene responsible for FAP, a second gene from chromosome 5q21 was identified that was somatically mutated in sporadic colorectal cancers.[338] The *MCC* gene, for *mutated in colorectal cancer,* is located less than 250 kb away from the *APC* gene[238,239,339] and was chosen for further study because Southern blot analysis revealed a colon carcinoma with a somatic rearrangement. The *MCC* gene transcript contains a 2511-bp open reading frame that is distributed over 17 exons. Detailed analysis of all 17 coding exons identified specific point mutations in 6 of 90 colorectal carcinomas examined. All 6 mutations were predicted to alter the MCC protein either by amino acid substitution or by altered splicing. However, it is unlikely that mutations of *MCC* play a major role in the development of colorectal cancer.[338,340] Comparison of *MCC* with *APC* reveals some interesting similarities in addition to their proximity in the genome. Although the significance of *MCC* mutations in colorectal tumors is not clear, these similarities raise the possibility that *MCC* and *APC* may function along the same pathway.

Gene Amplification. The specific amplification of a small region of the genome (gene amplification) frequently activates oncogenes in some tumor types. One indication of gene amplification is the cytogenetic observation of double-minute chromosomes. These chromosomes are known to harbor amplified sequences. Although double-minute chromosomes have been reported in a significant fraction of primary colorectal cancers,[341] amplification of specific, well-characterized genes has been described rarely in colon cancers. Isolated cases of *c-MYB,*[342] *c-MYC,*[343–346] *NEU,*[345,347,348] and *cyclin*[349] gene amplification have been reported. It is notable that those few colorectal cancers with demonstrable gene amplification are indistinguishable from other colorectal cancers in histology and behavior. It is likely that amplification of these genes, as well as additional (as yet unidentified) oncogenes, contributes to tumor progression, especially at late stages. More recently, it has been reported that *aurora*[350,351] and *Fas decoy*[352] genes are amplified in a subset of colorectal tumors. Although these reports are certainly intriguing, it is often difficult to distinguish true amplification from chromosome imbalance by the techniques used in these studies. Confirmation of the specific amplification of these genes with other techniques and documentation of the importance of these amplifications in colorectal tumorigenesis are eagerly awaited.

Modifying Loci. The existence of genetic loci that modify the risk for colorectal cancer has long been suspected but has been difficult to prove in humans. However, the Min model provides a clear-cut example of a modifying locus in mice. Depending on the inbred mouse strain harboring this mutation, the number of polyps varies significantly.[281] Linkage analysis has demonstrated that a single locus (*MOM1,* for *modifier of Min*) on mouse chromosome 4 accounts for much of this difference between strains.[353] Recently, the *MOM1* gene has been identified as that encoding secreted phospholipase A2 (sPLA2).[354,355] Unfortunately, studies of sPLA2 in humans suggest that it is not a major modifier of colorectal cancer risk.[356]

Gene Expression

One of the most difficult issues in cancer research involves the evaluation of gene expression. Although the expression of numerous genes is different in tumor cells than in normal cells, the significance of these differences is uncertain. For example, the expression of various oncogenes, particularly *c-MYC,*[346,357] a variety of mucins,[358] growth factors and their receptors,[347,359,360] carcinoembryonic antigens,[361] cell surface glycoproteins,[362,363] and enzymes involved in DNA replication and cell division[364] are increased in neoplastic colon cells. Whether these increases in expression drive the process of tumorigenesis or are simply the *result* of the abnormal growth or microenvironment of cancer is impossible to determine at present. Some of the abnormally expressed gene products are likely to play an important role in mediating the biologic effects of the mutant genes discussed in this chapter. Recent results linking *c-MYC* expression to *APC* mutation provide an excellent example of this principle.[331] Other changes in gene expression are likely to be insignificant with regard to pathogenesis. The advent of several new technologies for the analysis of gene expression hopefully will lead to advances in this important area.[365–368] Indeed, using just one of these new approaches,[367] it was possible to analyze over 300,000 transcripts from human cancer cells and identify hundreds of genes that were differentially expressed between normal and tumor tissue.[369] While a complete understanding of the behavior of a neoplastic cell will require a full knowledge of these differentially expressed genes, their large numbers and inherent complexity illustrate why the study of genetic alterations has been so useful.

Methylation

The only known covalent modification of DNA in normal mammalian cells occurs at the fifth position of cytosine at 5′-CG-3′ dinucleotides. In most somatic cells, 80 percent of these dinucleotides are methylated, and such methylation has been implicated in the control of gene expression and chromosome condensation.[370] In cancer cells, a generalized hypomethylation of the genome occurs relatively early during colorectal tumorigenesis and can be observed even in small adenomas.[371,372] Hypermethylation of specific 5′-CG-3′–rich sites also occurs.[373] The causes and effects of these methylation differences are not understood. Hypomethylation is not likely due to the underexpression of methylase activity, because such activity is not decreased in tumors.[374] Changes in methylation of genes, unlike the mutations of genes noted earlier, are not clonal changes in that any specific 5′-CG-3′dinucleotide is methylated differently in only a fraction of the tumor cell population. Nevertheless, these changes could have significant effects on tumor cell biology. For example, decreased methylation could in part allow expression of genes that normally should be silent, such as those required for cellular invasion (proteinases) or growth at metastatic sites (cell surface receptors for growth factors or extracellular matrices). Additionally, it has been demonstrated experimentally that reduced methylation of DNA can lead to aberrant chromosome condensation and adherence of the decondensed regions to one another.[375] This, in turn, could result in abnormal chromosome segregation, particularly chromosome loss, which, as noted earlier, is one of the most common mechanisms for inactivating tumor-suppressor genes. Conversely, increased methylation could lead to silencing of genes important for growth suppression. Indeed, methylation changes have been implicated in the silencing of the *hMLH1* DNA mismatch repair gene in tumors with mismatch repair deficiency[376] and in silencing of the *p16* tumor-suppressor gene in colorectal cancers in general.[377,378] The evidence implicating methylation in colorectal tumorigenesis is not limited to the methylation changes observed in tumors but also includes direct experimental evidence. For example, the hypermethylation of *hMLH1* can be reversed with the demethylating agent 5-aza-cytidine, leading to expression of *hMLH1* and reconstitution of mismatch repair activity.[376] Treatment of cells with 5-aza-cytidine has been shown to be oncogenic *in vitro* and *in vivo*, suggesting a proneoplastic role of decreased methylation *in vivo*.[379] On the other hand, mice with a genetic deficiency for methyltransferase are resistant to intestinal tumors resulting from *mAPC* mutations, and this resistance is potentiated by 5-aza-cytidine.[380] While the evidence implicating methylation changes in tumorigenesis continues to mount, additional studies will be necessary to clarify the significance of these changes and the mechanisms responsible for the differences between methylation in normal and neoplastic cells.

A Genetic Model for Colorectal Tumorigenesis

In molecular terms, the process of colorectal tumor evolution represents the acquisition of sequential mutations[381,382] (Fig. 48-21). Mutations in *APC* seem to be required to initiate the adenomatous process, resulting in the clonal growth of a single cell. In most cases, it appears that inactivation of both alleles of *APC* is both necessary and sufficient for tumor initiation. In rare cases, mutations of β-catenin can substitute for *APC* mutations.[381,382] A small polyp that results from these initial mutations may remain dormant for decades. Eventually, however, one of the cells of this small tumor acquires an additional mutation (often in the *K-RAS* gene), allowing it to overgrow its sister cells and resulting in a larger tumor. Subsequent waves of clonal expansion are driven by further mutations in other genes [particularly the 18q tumor suppressor(s) and *p53*], and along with this expansion comes further dysplasia. When a cell has acquired sufficient mutations (generally affecting at least four genes), it acquires the ability to invade and metastasize and is observed clinically as a malignancy.

There are several points worth noting about the preceding model. First, not every tumor needs to acquire each of the mutations indicated. For example, only half of all colorectal cancers have *RAS* mutations. It is likely that other yet unidentified mutated genes can substitute for *RAS* mutations. Second, it is likely that other genetic events are required for cancer development. Even so, this model predicts that at least seven genetic events (i.e., one oncogene mutation and six mutations to inactivate three tumor-suppressor genes) typically are required for a cancer to develop. Finally, the order of mutations can have a significant impact on tumorigenic process. For example, as noted earlier, nondysplastic ACF with *RAS* gene mutations are remarkably common.[49,50] However, these cells, unlike their dysplastic *APC* mutant counterparts, appear to have little or no potential to form clinically important tumors. Similarly, patients with germ-line mutations of *p53* do not develop polyposis[383] despite that fact that *p53* mutations occur in over 80 percent of colorectal cancers.[73] Therefore, although it is clear that *p53* can play a role in colorectal tumorigenesis, it is equally clear that it cannot initiate the process in a fashion similar to *APC*. Thus it appears that it is not simply the accumulation of mutations but rather also their order that determines the propensity for neoplasia and that only a subset of the genes that can affect cell growth actually can initiate the neoplastic process. This subset of tumor-suppressor genes has been deemed *gatekeepers*.[384]

It is notable that the genes identified in colorectal tumors affect almost all the cellular compartments (i.e., *RAS* at the inner surface of the cell membrane, *APC* in the cytoplasm, and *p53* in the nucleus). This suggests that human cells have evolved several levels of cellular protection against neoplasia and that many of these protective mechanisms must be disassembled before cancer can fully develop. Even at the malignant stage, however, the tumor continues to evolve, developing subclones with varying degrees of aneuploidy, drug or radiation resistance, and metastatic capability. This whole process, from appearance of a tiny adenomatous tumor to invasion by a carcinoma, takes 20 to 40 years, perhaps reflecting the time required to sequentially mutate the relevant genes and generate clonal expansions.

It has long been suspected that this accumulation of genetic changes may be facilitated by genetic instability.[385–387] In the case of colorectal cancer, tangible proof of this premise came with the identification of defects in DNA mismatch repair in HNPCC patients (see Chap. 32) and in a subset of sporadic colorectal cancers.[388–390] These tumors display an increased rate of small intragenic mutations[391] that can drive the neoplastic process. However, defects in DNA mismatch repair occur in only about 13 percent of all colorectal cancers.[388–390] Recently, there has been growing evidence of a genetic instability that operates in the remaining colorectal cancers. *Aneuploidy*, defined as an abnormal complement of chromosomes, is a classic characteristic of most solid tumors. Until recently, it was not clear whether an abnormal karyotype was the result of a true genetic instability. In this regard, it is interesting to note that cancers with instability due to a defect in DNA mismatch repair generally have a normal karyotype, whereas the remaining cancers are generally aneuploid. Careful measurement of chromosomal losses in colorectal cancer cell lines revealed that aneuploid lines had a persistent and marked increase in chromosomal gains and losses compared with diploid lines.[392] This instability was termed a *chromosomal instability* (CIN) and could be transferred in a dominant manner in cell fusion experiments.[392] Subsequent studies showed that the CIN phenotype was associated with functional defects of mitotic checkpoints.[393] In a small fraction of colorectal cancers, somatic mutations of the mitotic checkpoint gene *BUB1* probably account for the mitotic checkpoint defect and resulting CIN.[393] Thus it appears that most colorectal cancers possess some form of genetic instability that drives the neoplastic process (see Fig. 48-21). In a minority of cancers, this instability is due to a defect in DNA mismatch repair and results in an increased rate of small intragenic mutations. In the majority of cancers, a chromosomal instability exists that manifests as losses and gains of whole chromosomes or

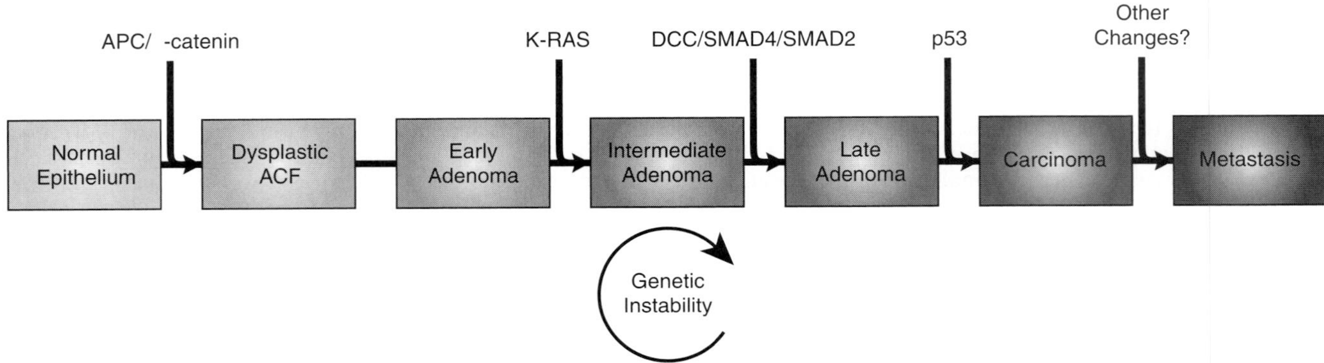

Fig. 48-21 T > A genetic model for colorectal tumorigenesis. See text for explanation. (*Modified with permission from Fearon and Vogelstein.*[381])

large chromosomal regions. The subset of tumor-suppressor genes that prevents such genetic instabilities has been deemed *caretakers*.[384] Although in a few cases CIN can be traced to defects in a specific gene, the genetic basis of CIN is unknown in the great majority of cases, providing a significant challenge for future research.[394]

This chapter has focused on gene alterations that contribute to the neoplastic process in a direct and cell autonomous manner. Mutations of *APC* (gatekeeper) or DNA mismatch repair genes (caretakers) are examples of such alterations that can result in highly penetrant predispositions to colorectal cancer. The third category of predispositions results from *landscaper* defects. Landscaper defects do not directly affect cancer cell growth but contribute to an abnormal stromal environment that contributes to the neoplastic transformation of the overlying epithelium. The cancer predispositions associated with such landscapers would be expected to be weaker than that observed with a gatekeeper such as *APC*. The increased risk of colorectal cancer observed in JPS and perhaps also inPeutz-Jeghers syndrome, characterized by the intestinal hamartomatous polyps, may be the result of landscaper defects. In the lesions associated with these syndromes, the epithelium does not initially show any neoplastic changes, but rather it is the underlying mesenchymal tissue that appears to be affected. This abnormal mesenchymal growth may create a microenvironment that facilitates that neoplastic transformation of the overlying epithelium. However, because both genes (*PTEN*[395,396] and *SMAD4*[193]) that have been implicated in this pathway can directly affect growth of epithelial cells as well, additional studies will be necessary to distinguish a weak gatekeeper effect from a landscaper effect.

PROSPECTUS

Despite the advances made in understanding the genetics of colorectal tumorigenesis, many questions remain unanswered. First, other chromosomes besides 5q, 17p, and 18q are lost in subsets of colorectal cancers. The identification of the culprit genes on these chromosomes has not been accomplished. It is unclear whether these other genes are simply responsible for the evolution of tumor heterogeneity at late stages of the process or play a more fundamental role in tumorigenesis. Second, about one-half of all colorectal tumors develop without a *RAS* mutation, and a small fraction of tumors apparently do not have abnormalities of *p53* or *APC/β-catenin*. The mechanism that allows such alterations to be bypassed could prove to be very important. Perhaps such tumors develop mutations of other genes in the same pathway that have the same physiologic effects. Third, the biochemical and physiologic functions of oncogenes and tumor-suppressor genes have yet to be fully worked out in cells *in vitro*, much less in the complex environment that exists in tissues *in vivo*. Finally, inherited genetic factors affecting colon cancer risk in the general population have yet to be defined.

Diagnosis

One of the first benefits derived from the study of colorectal cancer genetics is improved diagnosis. Already, knowledge of the genetic bases for FAP and HNPCC is allowing presymptomatic diagnosis in affected families (see Chap. 49). Demonstration that an individual member of such a family has not inherited the disease can have significant impact, reducing the discomfort and expense of repeated medial examinations as well as the anxiety associated with disease expectation. Genetic diagnosis also could be performed *in utero*, although substantial ethical questions are inherent in such diagnoses when the relevant disease is not necessarily lethal and when mortality, if it occurs at all, is delayed until adulthood. Presymptomatic testing also will have significant clinical implications with the advent of pharmacologic intervention for the possible prevention of polyposis in FAP patients (see below).

Specific gene mutations also may be used as the basis of a very specific test for presymptomatic diagnosis of colorectal tumors in the general population. Tumor cells shed into the stool can be identified by the presence of their mutant *RAS* genes in DNA isolated from stool samples.[397–401] Mutant genes were detected in stool from patients with benign as well as malignant tumors and could be observed in relatively small tumors as well as large ones. Application of this strategy to other mutations known to occur in colorectal tumors could significantly improve the applicability of this test. Numerous additional studies of course will be required to determine whether such assays will lead to improved detection of colorectal neoplasia in a cost-effective manner.

The analysis of genetic changes in colorectal cancers also has been shown to have prognostic value.[175] While *RAS* oncogene mutations and chromosome 5q losses do not show any prognostic utility, chromosome 17p and 18q losses each provide independent prognostic information. Chromosome 17p and 18q losses are associated with distant metastases and poorer prognosis.[175–177,188–191] This analysis represents the first step in the application of molecular genetics to the management of colorectal cancer patients. In the future, one can imagine that the choice of chemotherapeutic regimen will depend on the specific genetic changes present in the patient's tumor.

PREVENTION AND TREATMENT

One of the most important purposes of studying colorectal tumorigenesis lies in the hope that this will lead to better treatment and/or prevention of the disease. The notion that more effective drugs to treat colorectal tumors can be developed is furthered by the apparent success of some conventional drug treatments. Several studies have indicated that the nonsteroidal anti-inflammatory drug (NSAID) sulindac can cause tumor regression in FAP patients.[402–409] Hope that such treatment may prove useful for the general public comes from epidemiologic studies of colon cancer in aspirin users.[410–412] Many of these studies have shown that the use of aspirin, another NSAID, is associated with a reduced colon cancer death risk. Evaluation of these and other drugs may be greatly facilitated by testing in Min mice. Indeed, several studies have already demonstrated the ability of NSAIDs to reduce the incidence of intestinal tumors in the Min mouse.[413–415] Ultimately, it is hoped that the study of cancer genes and their biologic consequences will lead to the knowledge-based development of much more specific and effective chemopreventive and chemotherapeutic agents. In this regard, the identification of specific genetic alterations that commonly underlie human cancers has yielded considerable excitement because it is clear that such changes provide targets that are unique to the cancer cell. However, most of these mutations result in loss of function of a tumor-suppressor gene. Restoration of such function represents a formidable therapeutic challenge because most commonly used drugs are designed to inhibit an activity rather than replace the function of a protein. Fortunately, detailed studies of the tumor-suppressive pathway often reveal consequences of mutations that are more readily targeted. For example, while it is hard to imagine a small drug replacing the function of the 300-kDa APC protein, it is easy to conceive of a drug that inhibits the elevated *β*-catenin/Tcf–mediated transcription that results from inactivation of APC. Likewise, it is also simple to imagine the development of agents that exploit the checkpoint defects that arise from mutations in *p53* or are associated with the CIN phenotype.[140,394,416] Future and ongoing studies undoubtedly will provide additional targets for therapeutic intervention.

REFERENCES

1. *Cancer Facts & Figures 1998*. Atlanta, American Cancer Society, 1998.
2. Beart RW: Colorectal cancer, in Holleb AI, Fink DJ, Murphy GP (eds): *American Cancer Society Textbook of Clinical Oncology*. Atlanta, American Cancer Society, 1991, pp 213-218.

3. Cohen AM, Shank B, Friedman MA: Colorectal cancer, in De Vita V, Hellman S, Rosenberg S (eds): *Cancer: Principles and Practice of Oncology*. Philadelphia, Lippincott, 1989, p 895.
4. Ransohoff D, Lang C: Screening for colorectal cancer. *N Engl J Med* **325**:37, 1991.
5. Jass JR, Stewart SM: Evolution of hereditary non-polyposis colorectal cancer. *Gut* **33**:783, 1992.
6. Lieberman D: Cost-effectiveness of colon cancer screening. *Am J Gastroenterol* **86**:1789, 1991.
7. Lipkin M, Bell B, Shelrock P: Cell proliferation kinetics in the gastrointestinal tract of man. *J Clin Invest* **42**:767, 1963.
8. Shorter RG, Moertel CG, Titus JL, Reitemeier RJ: Cell kinetics of in the jejenum and rectum of man. *Am J Dig Dis* **9**:760, 1964.
9. Kent TH, Mitros FA: Polyps of the colon and small bowel, polyp syndromes, and the polyp-carcinoma sequence, in Norris HT (eds): *Pathology of the Colon, Small Intestine, and Anus,* Vol 2. New York, Churchill-Livingstone, 1983, p 167.
10. Cooper HS: Carcinoma of the colon and rectum, in Norris HT (eds): *Pathology of the Colon, Small Intestine and Anus,* Vol 2. New York, Churchill-Livingstone, 1983, p 201.
11. Stryker SJ, Wolff BG, Culp CE, Libbe SD, Ilstrup DM, MacCarty RL: Natural history of untreated colonic polyps. *Gastroenterology* **93**:1009, 1987.
12. Giardiello FM: Gastrointestinal polyposis sydromes and hereditary nonpolyposis colorectal cancer, in Rustgi AK (eds): *Gastrointestinal Cancers: Biology, Diagnosis, and Therapy*. Philadelphia, Lippincott-Raven, 1995, pp 367–377.
13. Bussey HJ, Veale AM, Morson BC: Genetics of gastrointestinal polyposis. *Gastroenterology* **74**:1325, 1978.
14. Hamilton SR, Liu B, Parsons RE, et al: The molecular basis of Turcot's syndrome. *N Engl J Med* **332**:839, 1995.
15. Gardner E, Richards R: Multiple cutaneous and subcutaneous lesions occurring simultaneously with hereditary polyposis and osteomatosis. *Am J Hum Genet* **5**:139, 1953.
16. Bulow S: Extracolonic manifestations of familial adenomatous polyposis, in Herrera L (eds): *Familial Adenomatous Polyposis*. New York, Alan R Liss, 1990, p 109.
17. Spirio L, Otterud B, Stauffer D, et al: Linkage of a variant or attenuated form of adenomatous polyposis coli to the adenomatous polyposis coli (*APC*) locus. *Am J Hum Genet* **51**:92, 1992.
18. Spirio L, Olschwang S, Groden J, et al: Alleles of the *APC* gene: An attenuated form of familial polyposis. *Cell* **75**:951, 1993.
19. Ponz de Leon M, Sassatelli R, Benatti P, Roncucci L: Identification of hereditary nonpolyposis colorectal cancer in the general population: The 6-year experience of a population-based registry. *Cancer* **71**:3493, 1993.
20. Lynch HT, Smyrk T, Jass JR: Hereditary nonpolyposis colorectal cancer and colonic adenomas: Aggressive adenomas? *Semin Surg Oncol* **11**:406, 1995.
21. Lynch HT, Smyrk T, Lynch JF: Overview of natural history, pathology, molecular genetics and management of HNPCC (Lynch syndrome). *Int J Cancer* **69**:38, 1996.
22. Burt RW, Bishop DT, Cannon LA, Dowdle MA, Lee RG, Skolnick MH: Dominant inheritance of adenomatous colonic polyps and colorectal cancer. *N Engl J Med* **312**:1540, 1985.
23. Cannon-Albright LA, Skolnick MH, Bishop DT, Lee RG, Burt RW: Common inheritance of susceptibility to colonic adenomatous polyps and associated colorectal cancers. *N Engl J Med* **319**:533, 1988.
24. Houlston RS, Collins A, Slack J, Morton NE: Dominant genes for colorectal cancer are not rare. *Ann Hum Genet* **56**:99, 1992.
25. Willett W: The search for the causes of breast and colon cancer. *Nature* **338**:389, 1989.
26. Haenszel W, Kurihara M: Studies of Japanese migrants: I. Mortality from cancer and other diseases among Japanese in the United States. *J Natl Cancer Inst* **40**:43, 1968.
27. Lee JA: Recent trends of large bowel cancer in Japan compared to United States and England and Wales. *Int J Epidemiol* **5**:187, 1976.
28. Armstrong B, Doll R: Environmental factors and cancer incidence and mortality in different countries, with special reference to dietary practices. *Int J Cancer* **15**:617, 1975.
29. Pickle LW, Greene MH, Ziegler RG, et al: Colorectal cancer in rural Nebraska. *Cancer Res* **44**:363, 1984.
30. Willett WC, Stampfer MJ, Colditz GA, Rosner BA, Speizer FE: Relation of meat, fat, and fiber intake to the risk of colon cancer in a prospective study among women. *N Engl J Med* **323**:1664, 1990.
31. Burkitt DP: Epidemiology of cancer of the colon and rectum. *Cancer* **28**:3, 1971.
32. Bingham S, Williams DR, Cole TJ, James WP: Dietary fibre and regional large-bowel cancer mortality in Britain. *Br J Cancer* **40**:456, 1979.
33. Nowell PC: The clonal evolution of tumor cell populations. *Science* **194**:23, 1976.
34. Vogelstein B, Fearon ER, Hamilton SR, Feinberg AP: Use of restriction fragment length polymorphisms to determine the clonal origin of human tumors. *Science* **227**:642, 1985.
35. Vogelstein B, Fearon ER, Hamilton SR, et al: Clonal analysis using recombinant DNA probes from the X-chromosome. *Cancer Res* **47**:4806, 1987.
36. Fearon ER, Hamilton SR, Vogelstein B: Clonal analysis of human colorectal tumors. *Science* **238**:193, 1987.
37. Martin P, Levin B, Golomb HM, Riddell RH: Chromosome analysis of primary large bowel tumors: A new method for improving the yield of analyzable metaphases. *Cancer* **44**:1656, 1979.
38. Reichmann A, Martin P, Levin B: Chromosomal banding patterns in human large bowel cancer. *Int J Cancer* **28**:431, 1981.
39. Muleris M, Salmon RJ, Zafrani B, Girodet J, Dutrillaux B: Consistent deficiencies of chromosome 18 and of the short arm of chromosome 17 in eleven cases of human large bowel cancer: A possible recessive determinism. *Ann Genet* **28**:206, 1985.
40. Mark J, Mitelman F, Dencker H, Norryd C, Tranberg KG: The specificity of the chromosomal abnormalities in human colonic polyps: A cytogenetic study of multiple polyps in a case of Gardner's syndrome. *Acta Pathol Microbiol Scand [A]* **81**:85, 1973.
41. Mitelman F, Mark J, Nilsson PG, Dencker H, Norryd C, Tranberg KG: Chromosome banding pattern in human colonic polyps. *Hereditas* **78**:63, 1974.
42. Reichmann A, Martin P, Levin B: Chromosomal banding patterns in human large bowel adenomas. *Hum Genet* **70**:28, 1985.
43. Bos JL, Fearon ER, Hamilton SR, et al: Prevalence of ras gene mutations in human colorectal cancers. *Nature* **327**:293, 1987.
44. Forrester K, Almoguera C, Han K, Grizzle WE, Perucho M: Detection of high incidence of *K-ras* oncogenes during human colon tumorigenesis. *Nature* **327**:298, 1987.
45. Vogelstein B, Fearon ER, Hamilton SR, et al: Genetic alterations during colorectal-tumor development. *N Engl J Med* **319**:525, 1988.
46. Bishop JM: Molecular themes in oncogenesis. *Cell* **64**:235, 1991.
47. Weinberg RA: Oncogenes and tumor suppressor genes. *CA Cancer J Clin* **44**:160, 1994.
48. Shibata D, Schaeffer J, Li ZH, Capella G, Perucho M: Genetic heterogeneity of the *c-K-ras* locus in colorectal adenomas but not in adenocarcinomas. *J Natl Cancer Inst* **85**:1058, 1993.
49. Pretlow TP, Brasitus TA, Fulton NC, Cheyer C, Kaplan EL: *K-ras* mutations in putative preneoplastic lesions in human colon. *J Natl Cancer Inst* **85**:2004, 1993.
50. Jen J, Powell SM, Papadopoulos N, et al: Molecular determinants of dysplasia in colorectal lesions. *Cancer Res* **54**:5523, 1994.
51. Shirasawa S, Furuse M, Yokoyama N, Sasazuki T: Altered growth of human colon cancer cell lines disrupted at activated *Ki-ras*. *Science* **260**:85, 1993.
52. Bourne HR, Sanders DA, McCormick F: The GTPase superfamily: Conserved structure and molecular mechanism. *Nature* **349**:117, 1991.
53. Haubruck H, McCormick F: *Ras* p21: Effects and regulation. *Biochim Biophys Acta* **1072**:215, 1991.
54. Xu GF, Lin B, Tanaka K, et al: The catalytic domain of the neurofibromatosis type 1 gene product stimulates *ras* GTPase and complements *ira* mutants of *S. cerevisiae*. *Cell* **63**:835, 1990.
55. Martin GA, Viskochil D, Bollag G, et al: The GAP-related domain of the neurofibromatosis type 1 gene product interacts with *ras* p21. *Cell* **63**:843, 1990.
56. Ballester R, Marchuk D, Boguski M, et al: The *NF1* locus encodes a protein functionally related to mammalian GAP and yeast IRA proteins. *Cell* **63**:851, 1990.
57. Bollag G, McCormick F: Differential regulation of rasGAP and neurofibromatosis gene product activities. *Nature* **351**:576, 1991.
58. Li Y, Bollag G, Clark R, et al: Somatic mutations in the neurofibromatosis 1 gene in human tumors. *Cell* **69**:275, 1992.
59. Solomon E, Voss R, Hall V, et al: Chromosome 5 allele loss in human colorectal carcinomas. *Nature* **328**:616, 1987.
60. Monpezat JP, Delattre O, Bernard A, et al: Loss of alleles on chromosome 18 and on the short arm of chromosome 17 in polyploid colorectal carcinomas. *Int J Cancer* **41**:404, 1988.
61. Okamoto M, Sasaki M, Sugio K, et al: Loss of constitutional heterozygosity in colon carcinoma from patients with familial polyposis coli. *Nature* **331**:273, 1988.

62. Law DJ, Olschwang S, Monpezat JP, et al: Concerted nonsyntenic allelic loss in human colorectal carcinoma. *Science* **241**:961, 1988.
63. Vogelstein B, Fearon ER, Kern SE, et al: Allelotype of colorectal carcinomas. *Science* **244**:207, 1989.
64. Cavenee WK, Dryja TP, Phillips RA, et al: Expression of recessive alleles by chromosomal mechanisms in retinoblastoma. *Nature* **305**:779, 1983.
65. DeLeo AB, Jay G, Appella E, Dubois GC, Law LW, Old LJ: Detection of a transformation-related antigen in chemically induced sarcomas and other transformed cells of the mouse. *Proc Natl Acad Sci USA* **76**:2420, 1979.
66. Linzer DI, Levine AJ: Characterization of a 54-kilodalton cellular SV40 tumor antigen present in SV40-transformed cells and uninfected embryonal carcinoma cells. *Cell* **17**:43, 1979.
67. Lane DP, Crawford LV: T antigen is bound to a host protein in SV40-transformed cells. *Nature* **278**:261, 1979.
68. Eliyahu D, Raz A, Gruss P, Givol D, Oren M: Participation of p53 cellular tumour antigen in transformation of normal embryonic cells. *Nature* **312**:646, 1984.
69. Parada LF, Land H, Weinberg RA, Wolf D, Rotter V: Cooperation between gene encoding p53 tumour antigen and *ras* in cellular transformation. *Nature* **312**:649, 1984.
70. Jenkins JR, Rudge K, Currie GA: Cellular immortalization by a cDNA clone encoding the transformation-associated phosphoprotein p53. *Nature* **312**:651, 1984.
71. Baker SJ, Fearon ER, Nigro JM, et al: Chromosome 17 deletions and *p53* gene mutations in colorectal carcinomas. *Science* **244**:217, 1989.
72. Hethcote HW, Knudson AG Jr: Model for the incidence of embryonal cancers: Application to retinoblastoma. *Proc Natl Acad Sci USA* **75**:2453, 1978.
73. Baker SJ, Preisinger AC, Jessup JM, et al: *p53* gene mutations occur in combination with 17p allelic deletions as late events in colorectal tumorigenesis. *Cancer Res* **50**:7717, 1990.
74. Finlay CA, Hinds PW, Levine AJ: The *p53* proto-oncogene can act as a suppressor of transformation. *Cell* **57**:1083, 1989.
75. Eliyahu D, Michalovitz D, Eliyahu S, Pinhasi-Kimhi O, Oren M: Wild-type p53 can inhibit oncogene-mediated focus formation. *Proc Natl Acad Sci USA* **86**:8763, 1989.
76. Baker SJ, Markowitz S, Fearon ER, Willson JK, Vogelstein B: Suppression of human colorectal carcinoma cell growth by wild-type p53. *Science* **249**:912, 1990.
77. Diller L, Kassel J, Nelson CE, et al: p53 functions as a cell cycle control protein in osteosarcomas. *Mol Cell Biol* **10**:5772, 1990.
78. Mercer WE, Shields MT, Amin M, et al: Negative growth regulation in a glioblastoma tumor cell line that conditionally expresses human wild-type p53. *Proc Natl Acad Sci USA* **87**:6166, 1990.
79. Chen PL, Chen YM, Bookstein R, Lee WH: Genetic mechanisms of tumor suppression by the human *p53* gene. *Science* **250**:1576, 1990.
80. Hinds PW, Finlay CA, Quartin RS, et al: Mutant p53 DNA clones from human colon carcinomas cooperate with ras in transforming primary rat cells: A comparison of the "hot spot" mutant phenotypes. *Cell Growth Diff* **1**:571, 1990.
81. Raycroft L, Wu HY, Lozano G: Transcriptional activation by wild-type but not transforming mutants of the *p53* anti-oncogene. *Science* **249**:1049, 1990.
82. Mowat M, Cheng A, Kimura N, Bernstein A, Benchimol S: Rearrangements of the cellular *p53* gene in erythroleukaemic cells transformed by Friend virus. *Nature* **314**:633, 1985.
83. Hicks GG, Mowat M: Integration of Friend murine leukemia virus into both alleles of the *p53* oncogene in an erythroleukemic cell line. *J Virol* **62**:4752, 1988.
84. Ben David Y, Prideaux VR, Chow V, Benchimol S, Bernstein A: Inactivation of the *p53* oncogene by internal deletion or retroviral integration in erythroleukemic cell lines induced by Friend leukemia virus. *Oncogene* **3**:179, 1988.
85. Werness BA, Levine AJ, Howley PM: Association of human papillomavirus types 16 and 18 E6 proteins with p53. *Science* **248**:76, 1990.
86. Scheffner M, Werness BA, Huibregtse JM, Levine AJ, Howley PM: The E6 oncoprotein encoded by human papillomavirus types 16 and 18 promotes the degradation of p53. *Cell* **63**:1129, 1990.
87. Hollstein M, Shomer B, Greenblatt M, et al: Somatic point mutations in the *p53* gene of human tumors and cell lines: Updated compilation. *Nucl Acids Res* **24**:141, 1996.
88. Vogelstein B, Kinzler KW: Carcinogens leave fingerprints. *Nature* **355**:209, 1992.
89. Hsu IC, Metcalf RA, Sun T, Welsh JA, Wang NJ, Harris CC: Mutational hotspot in the *p53* gene in human hepatocellular carcinomas. *Nature* **350**:427, 1991.
90. Bressac B, Kew M, Wands J, Ozturk M: Selective G to T mutations of *p53* gene in hepatocellular carcinoma from southern Africa. *Nature* **350**:429, 1991.
91. Ozturk M: *p53* mutation in hepatocellular carcinoma after aflatoxin exposure. *Lancet* **338**:1356, 1991.
92. Brash DE, Rudolph JA, Simon JA, et al: A role for sunlight in skin cancer: UV-induced *p53* mutations in squamous cell carcinoma. *Proc Natl Acad Sci USA* **88**:10124, 1991.
93. Hollstein M, Sidransky D, Vogelstein B, Harris CC: *p53* mutations in human cancers. *Science* **253**:49, 1991.
94. Stenger JE, Mayr GA, Mann K, Tegtmeyer P: Formation of stable p53 homotetramers and multiples of tetramers. *Mol Carcinogen* **5**:102, 1992.
95. Jeffrey PD, Gorina S, Pavletich NP: Crystal structure of the tetramerization domain of the *p53* tumor suppressor at 1.7 angstroms. *Science* **267**:1498, 1995.
96. Milner J, Medcalf EA: Cotranslation of activated mutant *p53* with wild type drives the wild-type p53 protein into the mutant conformation. *Cell* **65**:765, 1991.
97. Hupp TR, Meek DW, Midgley CA, Lane DP: Regulation of the specific DNA binding function of p53. *Cell* **71**:875, 1992.
98. Kern SE, Kinzler KW, Bruskin A, et al: Identification of p53 as a sequence-specific DNA-binding protein. *Science* **252**:1708, 1991.
99. El-Deiry WS, Kern SE, Pietenpol JA, Kinzler KW, Vogelstein B: Definition of a consensus binding site for p53. *Nature Genet* **1**:45, 1992.
100. Funk WD, Pak DT, Karas RH, Wright WE, Shay JW: A transcriptionally active DNA-binding site for human p53 protein complexes. *Mol Cell Biol* **12**:2866, 1992.
101. Tokino T, Thiagalingam S, El-Deiry WS, Waldman T, Kinzler KW, Vogelstein B: p53 tagged sites from human genomic DNA. *Hum Mol Genet* **3**:1537, 1994.
102. Bargonetti J, Friedman PN, Kern SE, Vogelstein B, Prives C: Wild-type but not mutant p53 immunopurified proteins bind to sequences adjacent to the SV40 origin of replication. *Cell* **65**:1083, 1991.
103. Kern SE, Kinzler KW, Baker SJ, et al: Mutant p53 proteins bind DNA abnormally in vitro. *Oncogene* **6**:131, 1991.
104. Cho Y, Gorina S, Jeffrey PD, Pavletich NP: Crystal structure of a p53 tumor suppressor-DNA complex: Understanding tumorigenic mutations. *Science* **265**:346, 1994.
105. Fields S, Jang SK: Presence of a potent transcription activating sequence in the p53 protein. *Science* **249**:1046, 1990.
106. O'Rourke RW, Miller CW, Kato GJ, et al: A potential transcriptional activation element in the p53 protein. *Oncogene* **5**:1829, 1990.
107. Unger T, Nau MM, Segal S, Minna JD: *p53:* A transdominant regulator of transcription whose function is ablated by mutations occurring in human cancer. *EMBO J* **11**:1383, 1992.
108. Kern SE, Pietenpol JA, Thiagalingam S, Seymour A, Kinzler KW, Vogelstein B: Oncogenic forms of *p53* inhibit p53-regulated gene expression. *Science* **256**:827, 1992.
109. Scharer E, Iggo R: Mammalian p53 can function as a transcription factor in yeast. *Nucl Acids Res* **20**:1539, 1992.
110. Vogelstein B, Kinzler KW: p53 function and dysfunction. *Cell* **70**:523, 1992.
111. Momand J, Zambetti GP, Olson DC, George D, Levine AJ: The *mdm-2* oncogene product forms a complex with the p53 protein and inhibits p53-mediated transactivation. *Cell* **69**:1237, 1992.
112. Oliner JD, Kinzler KW, Meltzer PS, George DL, Vogelstein B: Amplification of a gene encoding a p53-associated protein in human sarcomas. *Nature* **358**:80, 1992.
113. Oliner JD, Pietenpol JA, Thiagalingam S, Gyuris J, Kinzler KW, Vogelstein B: Oncoprotein MDM2 conceals the activation domain of tumour suppressor *p53*. *Nature* **362**:857, 1993.
114. Fakharzadeh SS, Trusko SP, George DL: Tumorigenic potential associated with enhanced expression of a gene that is amplified in a mouse tumor cell line. *EMBO J* **10**:1565, 1991.
115. Wu X, Bayle JH, Olson D, Levine AJ: The *p53-mdm-2* autoregulatory feedback loop. *Genes Dev* **7**:1126, 1993.
116. El-Deiry WS, Tokino T, Velculescu VE, et al: *WAF1,* a potential mediator of *p53* tumor suppression. *Cell* **75**:817, 1993.
117. Miyashita T, Krajewski S, Krajewska M, et al: Tumor suppressor *p53* is a regulator of *bcl-2* and *bax* gene expression in vitro and in vivo. *Oncogene* **9**:1799, 1994.

118. Miyashita T, Reed JC: Tumor suppressor *p53* is a direct transcriptional activator of the human *bax* gene. *Cell* **80**:293, 1995.
119. Madden SL, Galella EA, Riley D, Bertelsen AH, Beaudry GA: Induction of cell growth regulatory genes by p53. *Cancer Res* **56**:5384, 1996.
120. Lehar SM, Nacht M, Jacks T, Vater CA, Chittenden T, Guild BC: Identification and cloning of *EI24,* a gene induced by p53 in etoposide-treated cells. *Oncogene* **12**:1181, 1996.
121. Amson RB, Nemani M, Roperch JP, et al: Isolation of 10 differentially expressed cDNAs in p53-induced apoptosis: Activation of the vertebrate homologue of the *Drosophila* seven in absentia gene. *Proc Natl Acad Sci USA* **93**:3953, 1996.
122. Rouault JP, Falette N, Guehenneux F, et al: Identification of BTG2, an antiproliferative p53-dependent component of the DNA damage cellular response pathway. *Nature Genet* **14**:482, 1996.
123. Fiscella M, Zhang H, Fan S, et al: Wip1, a novel human protein phosphatase that is induced in response to ionizing radiation in a p53-dependent manner. *Proc Natl Acad Sci USA* **94**:6048, 1997.
124. Nishimori H, Shiratsuchi T, Urano T, et al: A novel brain-specific p53-target gene, *BAI1,* containing thrombospondin type 1 repeats inhibits experimental angiogenesis. *Oncogene* **15**:2145, 1997.
125. Varmeh-Ziaie S, Okan I, Wang Y, et al: *Wig-1,* a new p53-induced gene encoding a zinc finger protein. *Oncogene* **15**:2699, 1997.
126. Polyak K, Xia Y, Zweier JL, Kinzler KW, Vogelstein B: A model for p53 induced apoptosis. *Nature* **389**:300, 1997.
127. Hermeking H, Lengauer C, Polyak K, et al: 14-3-3s is a p53-regulated inhibitor of G2/M progression. *Mol Cell* **1**:3, 1997.
128. Urano T, Nishimori H, Han H, et al: Cloning of *P2XM,* a novel human P2X receptor gene regulated by p53. *Cancer Res* **57**:3281, 1997.
129. Kimura Y, Furuhata T, Urano T, Hirata K, Nakamura Y, Tokino T: Genomic structure and chromosomal localization of *GML* (GPI-anchored molecule-like protein), a gene induced by p53. *Genomics* **41**:477, 1997.
130. Sheikh MS, Burns TF, Huang Y, et al: p53-dependent and -independent regulation of the death receptor *KILLER/DR5* gene expression in response to genotoxic stress and tumor necrosis factor alpha. *Cancer Res* **58**:1593, 1998.
131. Takei Y, Ishikawa S, Tokino T, Muto T, Nakamura Y: Isolation of a novel *TP53* target gene from a colon cancer cell line carrying a highly regulated wild-type *TP53* expression system. *Genes Chromosom Cancer* **23**:1, 1998.
132. Mashimo T, Watabe M, Hirota S, et al: The expression of the *KAI1* gene, a tumor metastasis suppressor, is directly activated by p53. *Proc Natl Acad Sci USA* **95**:11307, 1998.
133. Utrera R, Collavin L, Lazarevic D, Delia D, Schneider C: A novel p53-inducible gene coding for a microtubule-localized protein with G2-phase-specific expression. *EMBO J* **17**:5015, 1998.
134. Harper JW, Adami GR, Wei N, Keyomarsi K, Elledge SJ: The p21 Cdk-interacting protein Cip1 is a potent inhibitor of G1 cyclin-dependent kinases. *Cell* **75**:805, 1993.
135. Xiong Y, Hannon GJ, Zhang H, Casso D, Kobayashi R, Beach D: p21 is a universal inhibitor of cyclin kinases. *Nature* **366**:701, 1993.
136. Noda A, Ning Y, Venable SF, Pereira-Smith OM, Smith JR: Cloning of senescent cell-derived inhibitors of DNA synthesis using an expression screen. *Exp Cell Res* **211**:90, 1994.
137. El-Deiry WS, Tokino T, Waldman T, et al: Topological control of p21(Waf1/Cip1) expression in normal and neoplastic tissues. *Cancer Res* **55**:2910, 1995.
138. Elledge SJ, Harper JW: Cdk inhibitors: On the threshold of checkpoints and development. *Curr Opin Cell Biol* **6**:847, 1994.
139. Waldman T, Kinzler KW, Vogelstein B: P21 is necessary for the p53-mediated G(1) arrest in human cancer cells. *Cancer Res* **55**:5187, 1995.
140. Waldman T, Lengauer C, Kinzler KW, Vogelstein B: Uncoupling of S phase and mitosis induced by anticancer agents in cells lacking p21. *Nature* **381**:713, 1996.
141. Deng C, Zhang P, Harper JW, Elledge SJ, Leder P: Mice lacking p21CIP1/WAF1 undergo normal development, but are defective in G1 checkpoint control. *Cell* **82**:675, 1995.
142. Brugarolas J, Chandrasekaran C, Gordon JI, Beach D, Jacks T, Hannon GJ: Radiation-induced cell cycle arrest compromised by p21 deficiency. *Nature* **377**:552, 1995.
143. Bunz F, Dutriaux A, Lengauer C, et al: Requirement for p53 and p21 to sustain G2 arrest after DNA damage. *Science* **282**:1497, 1998.
144. Chan T, Hermeking H, Kinzler K, Vogelstein B: Unpublished observation, 1998.
145. Polyak K, Waldman T, He T-C, Kinzler KW, Vogelstein B: Genetic determinants of p53 induced apoptosis and growth arrest. *Genes Dev* **10**:1945, 1996.
146. Lowe SW, Schmitt EM, Smith SW, Osborne BA, Jacks T: p53 is required for radiation-induced apoptosis in mouse thymocytes. *Nature* **362**:847, 1993.
147. Clarke AR, Purdie CA, Harrison DJ, et al: Thymocyte apoptosis induced by p53-dependent and independent pathways. *Nature* **362**:849, 1993.
148. Donehower LA, Harvey M, Slagle BL, et al: Mice deficient for p53 are developmentally normal but susceptible to spontaneous tumours. *Nature* **356**:215, 1992.
149. Malkin D, Li FP, Strong LC, et al: Germ line *p53* mutations in a familial syndrome of breast cancer, sarcomas, and other neoplasms. *Science* **250**:1233, 1990.
150. Srivastava S, Zou ZQ, Pirollo K, Blattner W, Chang EH: Germ-line transmission of a mutated *p53* gene in a cancer-prone family with Li-Fraumeni syndrome. *Nature* **348**:747, 1990.
151. Kastan MB, Onyekwere O, Sidransky D, Vogelstein B, Craig RW: Participation of p53 protein in the cellular response to DNA damage. *Cancer Res* **51**:6304, 1991.
152. Kuerbitz SJ, Plunkett BS, Walsh WV, Kastan MB: Wild-type p53 is a cell cycle checkpoint determinant following irradiation. *Proc Natl Acad Sci USA* **89**:7491, 1992.
153. Kastan MB, Zhan Q, el-Deiry WS, et al: A mammalian cell cycle checkpoint pathway utilizing p53 and GADD45 is defective in ataxia-telangiectasia. *Cell* **71**:587, 1992.
154. Lane DP: Cancer: *p53,* guardian of the genome. *Nature* **358**:15, 1992.
155. Graeber TG, Peterson JF, Tsai M, Monica K, Fornace AJ Jr, Giaccia AJ: Hypoxia induces accumulation of p53 protein, but activation of a G1-phase checkpoint by low-oxygen conditions is independent of p53 status. *Mol Cell Biol* **14**:6264, 1994.
156. Graeber TG, Osmanian C, Jacks T, et al: Hypoxia-mediated selection of cells with diminished apoptotic potential in solid tumours. *Nature* **379**:88, 1996.
157. Hermeking H, Eick D: Mediation of *c-Myc*-induced apoptosis by p53. *Science* **265**:2091, 1994.
158. Wagner AJ, Kokontis JM, Hay N: *Myc*-mediated apoptosis requires wild-type p53 in a manner independent of cell cycle arrest and the ability of p53 to induce p21waf1/cip1. *Genes Dev* **8**:2817, 1994.
159. Lowe SW, Ruley HE: Stabilization of the *p53* tumor suppressor is induced by adenovirus 5 E1A and accompanies apoptosis. *Genes Dev* **7**:535, 1993.
160. Qin XQ, Livingston DM, Kaelin WG Jr, Adams PD: Deregulated transcription factor E2F-1 expression leads to S-phase entry and p53-mediated apoptosis. *Proc Natl Acad Sci USA* **91**:10918, 1994.
161. Shan B, Lee WH: Deregulated expression of E2F-1 induces S-phase entry and leads to apoptosis. *Mol Cell Biol* **14**:8166, 1994.
162. Wu X, Levine AJ: p53 and E2F-1 cooperate to mediate apoptosis. *Proc Natl Acad Sci USA* **91**:3602, 1994.
163. Bates S, Phillips AC, Clark PA, et al: p14ARF links the tumour suppressors *RB* and *p53*. *Nature* **395**:124, 1998.
164. Kamijo T, Weber JD, Zambetti G, Zindy F, Roussel MF, Sherr CJ: Functional and physical interactions of the *ARF* tumor suppressor with *p53* and *Mdm2*. *Proc Natl Acad Sci USA* **95**:8292, 1998.
165. Pomerantz J, Schreiber-Agus N, Liegeois NJ, et al: The *Ink4a* tumor suppressor gene product, p19Arf, interacts with MDM2 and neutralizes MDM2's inhibition of p53. *Cell* **92**:713, 1998.
166. de Stanchina E, McCurrach ME, Zindy F, et al: E1A signaling to p53 involves the p19 (*ARF*) tumor suppressor. *Genes Dev* **12**:2434, 1998.
167. Zhang Y, Xiong Y, Yarbrough WG: *ARF* promotes MDM2 degradation and stabilizes p53: ARF-INK4a locus deletion impairs both the *Rb* and *p53* tumor suppression pathways. *Cell* **92**:725, 1998.
168. Zindy F, Eischen CM, Randle DH, et al: *Myc* signaling via the *ARF* tumor suppressor regulates p53-dependent apoptosis and immortalization. *Genes Dev* **12**:2424, 1998.
169. Giaccia AJ, Kastan MB: The complexity of p53 modulation: Emerging patterns from divergent signals. *Genes Dev* **12**:2973, 1998.
170. Montes de Oca Luna R, Wagner DS, Lozano G: Rescue of early embryonic lethality in *mdm2*-deficient mice by deletion of *p53*. *Nature* **378**:203, 1995.
171. Kaghad M, Bonnet H, Yang A, et al: Monoallelically expressed gene related to p53 at 1p36, a region frequently deleted in neuroblastoma and other human cancers. *Cell* **90**:809, 1997.
172. Osada M, Ohba M, Kawahara C, et al: Cloning and functional analysis of human p51, which structurally and functionally resembles p53. *Nature Med* **4**:839, 1998.

173. Trink B, Okami K, Wu L, Sriuranpong V, Jen J, Sidransky D: A new human *p53* homologue. *Nature Med* **4**:747, 1998.
174. Yang A, Kaghad M, Wang Y, et al: *p63,* a *p53* homolog at 3q27-29, encodes multiple products with transactivating, death-inducing, and dominant-negative activities. *Mol Cell* **2**:305, 1998.
175. Jen J, Kim H, Piantadosi S, et al: Allelic loss of chromosome 18q and prognosis in colorectal cancer. *N Engl J Med* **331**:213, 1994.
176. Martinez-Lopez E, Abad A, Font A, et al: Allelic loss on chromosome 18q as a prognostic marker in stage II colorectal cancer. *Gastroenterology* **114**:1180, 1998.
177. Ogunbiyi OA, Goodfellow PJ, Herfarth K, et al: Confirmation that chromosome 18q allelic loss in colon cancer is a prognostic indicator. *J Clin Oncol* **16**:427, 1998.
178. Carethers JM, Hawn MT, Greenson JK, Hitchcock CL, Boland CR: Prognostic significance of allelic lost at chromosome 18q21 for stage II colorectal cancer. *Gastroenterology* **114**:1188, 1998.
179. Fearon ER, Cho KR, Nigro JM, et al: Identification of a chromosome 18q gene that is altered in colorectal cancers. *Science* **247**:49, 1990.
180. Hedrick L, Cho KR, Fearon ER, Wu TC, Kinzler KW, Vogelstein B: The *DCC* gene product in cellular differentiation and colorectal tumorigenesis. *Genes Dev* **8**:1174, 1994.
181. Cho KR, Oliner JD, Simons JW, et al: The *DCC* gene: Structural analysis and mutations in colorectal carcinomas. *Genomics* **19**:525, 1994.
182. Hedrick L, Cho KR, Boyd J, Risinger J, Vogelstein B: *DCC:* A tumor suppressor gene expressed on the cell surface. *Cold Spring Harb Symp Quant Biol* **57**:345, 1992.
183. Keino-Masu K, Masu M, Hinck L, et al: Deleted in colorectal cancer (*DCC*) encodes a netrin receptor. *Cell* **87**:175, 1996.
184. Chan SS, Zheng H, Su MW, et al: *UNC-40,* a *C. elegans* homologue of *DCC* (deleted in colorectal cancer), is required in motile cells responding to UNC-6 netrin cues. *Cell* **87**:187, 1996.
185. Kolodziej PA, Timpe LC, Mitchell KJ, et al: Frazzled encodes a *Drosophila* member of the DCC immunoglobulin subfamily and is required for CNS and motor axon guidance. *Cell* **87**:197, 1996.
186. Thiagalingam S: Evaluation of chromosome 18q in colorectal cancers. *Nature Genet* **13**:343, 1996.
187. Murty VV, Li RG, Houldsworth J, et al: Frequent allelic deletions and loss of expression characterize the *DCC* gene in male germ cell tumors. *Oncogene* **9**:3227, 1994.
188. Shibata D, Reale MA, Lavin P, et al: The DCC protein and prognosis in colorectal cancer. *N Engl J Med* **335**:1727, 1996.
189. Reymond MA, Dworak O, Remke S, Hohenberger W, Kirchner T, Kockerling F: DCC protein as a predictor of distant metastases after curative surgery for rectal cancer. *Dis Colon Rectum* **41**:755, 1998.
190. Goi T, Yamaguchi A, Nakagawara G, Urano T, Shiku H, Furukawa K: Reduced expression of deleted colorectal carcinoma (DCC) protein in established colon cancers. *Br J Cancer* **77**:466, 1998.
191. Yamamoto H, Itoh F, Kusano M, Yoshida Y, Hinoda Y, Imai K: Infrequent inactivation of *DCC* gene in replication error-positive colorectal cancers. *Biochem Biophys Res Commun* **244**:204, 1998.
192. Fazeli A, Dickinson SL, Hermiston ML, et al: Phenotype of mice lacking functional deleted in colorectal cancer (*DCC*) gene. *Nature* **386**:796, 1997.
193. Hahn SA, Schutte M, Hoque ATMS, et al: *Dpc4,* a candidate tumor suppressor gene at human chromosome 18q21.1. *Science* **271**:350, 1996.
194. Hahn SA, Seymour AB, Hoque AT, et al: Allelotype of pancreatic adenocarcinoma using xenograft enrichment. *Cancer Res* **55**:4670, 1995.
195. Hursh DA, Padgett RW, Gelbart WM: Cross regulation of decapentaplegic and ultrabithorax transcription in the embryonic visceral mesoderm of *Drosophila. Development* **117**:1211, 1993.
196. Sekelsky JJ, Newfeld SJ, Raftery LA, Chartoff EH, Gelbart WM: Genetic characterization and cloning of mothers against *dpp,* a gene required for decapentaplegic function in *Drosophila melanogaster. Genetics* **139**:1347, 1995.
197. Savage C, Das P, Finelli AL, et al: *Caenorhabditis elegans* genes *Sma2, Sma-3,* and *Sma-4* define a conserved family of transforming growth factor beta pathway components. *Proc Natl Acad Sci USA* **93**:790, 1996.
198. Fynan TM, Reiss M: Resistance to inhibition of cell growth by transforming growth factor-beta and its role in oncogenesis. *Crit Rev Oncogen* **4**:493, 1993.
199. Brattain MG, Howell G, Sun LZ, Willson JK: Growth factor balance and tumor progression. *Curr Opin Oncol* **6**:77, 1994.
200. Markowitz S, Wang J, Myeroff L, et al: Inactivation of the type II TGF-beta receptor in colon cancer cells with microsatellite instability. *Science* **268**:1336, 1995.
201. Parsons R, Myeroff LL, Liu B, et al: Microsatellite instability and mutations of the transforming growth factor beta type II receptor gene in colorectal cancer. *Cancer Res* **55**:5548, 1995.
202. Grady WM, Rajput A, Myeroff L, et al: Mutation of the type II transforming growth factor-beta receptor is coincident with the transformation of human colon adenomas to malignant carcinomas. *Cancer Res* **58**:3101, 1998.
203. Zhou S, Buckhaults P, Zawel L, et al: Targeted deletion of *Smad4* shows it is required for TGF-β and activin signalin in colorectal cancer cells. *Proc Natl Acad Sci USA* **95**:2412, 1998.
204. Yingling JM, Datto MB, Wong C, Frederick JP, Liberati NT, Wang XF: Tumor suppressor *Smad4* is a transforming growth factor beta–inducible DNA binding protein. *Mol Cell Biol* **17**:7019, 1997.
205. Zawel L, Dai JL, Buckhaults P, et al: Human *Smad3* and *Smad4* are sequence-specific transcription activators. *Mol Cell* **1**:611, 1998.
206. Dennler S, Itoh S, Vivien D, ten Dijke P, Huet S, Gauthier JM: Direct binding of *Smad3* and *Smad4* to critical TGF beta–inducible elements in the promoter of human plasminogen activator inhibitor-type 1 gene. *EMBO J* **17**:3091, 1998.
207. Riggins GJ, Kinzler KW, Vogelstein B, Thiagalingam S: *Mad*-related genes in the human. *Nature Genet* **13**:347, 1996.
208. Eppert K, Scherer SW, Ozcelik H, et al: *MADR2* maps to 18q21 and encodes a TGF-beta-regulated MAD-related protein that is mutated in colorectal carcinoma. *Cell* **86**:543, 1996.
209. Riggins GJ, Kinzler KW, Vogelstein B, Thiagalingam S: Frequency of *Smad* gene mutations in human cancers. *Cancer Res* **57**:2578, 1997.
210. Hayashi H, Abdollah S, Qiu Y, et al: The MAD-related protein Smad7 associates with the TGF-beta receptor and functions as an antagonist of TGF-beta signaling. *Cell* **89**:1165, 1997.
211. Nakao A, Afrakhte M, Moren A, et al: Identification of *Smad7,* a TGF-beta–inducible antagonist of TGF-beta signalling. *Nature* **389**:631, 1997.
212. Roijer E, Moren A, ten Dijke P, Stenman G: Assignment of the *Smad7* gene (*MADH7*) to human chromosome 18q21.1 by fluorescence in situ hybridization. *Cytogenet Cell Genet* **81**:189, 1998.
213. MacGrogan D, Pegram M, Slamon D, Bookstein R: Comparative mutational analysis of *DPC4* (*Smad4*) in prostatic and colorectal carcinomas. *Oncogene* **15**:1111, 1997.
214. Uchida K, Nagatake M, Osada H, et al: Somatic in vivo alterations of the *JV18-1* gene at 18q21 in human lung cancers. *Cancer Res* **56**:5583, 1996.
215. Powell SM, Harper JC, Hamilton SR, Robinson CR, Cummings OW: Inactivation of *Smad4* in gastric carcinomas. *Cancer Res* **57**:4221, 1997.
216. Howe JR, Roth S, Rigold JC, et al: Mutations in the *SMAD4/DPC4* gene in juvenile polyposis. *Science* **280**:1086, 1998.
217. Yang X, Li C, Xu X, Deng C: The tumor suppressor *SMAD4/DPC4* is essential for epiblast proliferation and mesoderm induction in mice. *Proc Natl Acad Sci USA* **95**:3667, 1998.
218. Sirard C, de la Pompa JL, Elia A, et al: The tumor suppressor gene *Smad4/Dpc4* is required for gastrulation and later for anterior development of the mouse embryo. *Genes Dev* **12**:107, 1998.
219. Takaku K, Oshima M, Miyoshi H, Matsui M, Seldin MF, Taketo MM: Intestinal tumorigenesis in compound mutant mice of both *Dpc4* (*Smad4*) and *Apc* genes. *Cell* **92**:645, 1998.
220. Nomura M, Li E: *Smad2* role in mesoderm formation, left-right patterning and craniofacial development. *Nature* **393**:786, 1998.
221. Waldrip WR, Bikoff EK, Hoodless PA, Wrana JL, Robertson EJ: *Smad2* signaling in extraembryonic tissues determines anterior-posterior polarity of the early mouse embryo. *Cell* **92**:797, 1998.
222. Zhu Y, Richardson JA, Parada LF, Graff JM: *Smad3* mutant mice develop metastatic colorectal cancer. *Cell* **94**:703, 1998.
223. Tanaka K, Oshimura M, Kikuchi R, Seki M, Hayashi T, Miyaki M: Suppression of tumorigenicity in human colon carcinoma cells by introduction of normal chromosome 5 or 18. *Nature* **349**:340, 1991.
224. Goyette MC, Cho K, Fasching CL, et al: Progression of colorectal cancer is associated with multiple tumor suppressor gene defects but inhibition of tumorigenicity is accomplished by correction of any single defect via chromosome transfer. *Mol Cell Biol* **12**:1387, 1992.
225. Reiss M, Santoro V, de Jonge RR, Vellucci VF: Transfer of chromosome 18 into human head and neck squamous carcinoma cells: Evidence for tumor suppression by *Smad4/DPC4*. *Cell Growth Diff* **8**:407, 1997.

226. Narayanan R, Lawlor KG, Schaapveld RQ, et al: Antisense RNA to the putative tumor-suppressor gene *DCC* transforms Rat-1 fibroblasts. *Oncogene* **7**:553, 1992.
227. Lawlor KG, Telang NT, Osborne MP, et al: Antisense RNA to the putative tumor suppressor gene "deleted in colorectal cancer" transforms fibroblasts. *Ann NY Acad Sci* **660**:283, 1992.
228. Klingelhutz AJ, Hedrick L, Cho KR, McDougall JK: The *DCC* gene suppresses the malignant phenotype of transformed human epithelial cells. *Oncogene* **10**:1581, 1995.
229. Mehlen P, Rabizadeh S, Snipas SJ, Assa-Munt N, Salvesen GS, Bredesen DE: The *DCC* gene product induces apoptosis by a mechanism requiring receptor proteolysis. *Nature* **395**:801, 1998.
230. Herrera L, Kakati S, Gibas L, Pietrzak E, Sandberg A: Gardner syndrome in a man with an interstitial deletion of 5q. *Am J Med Genet* **25**:473, 1986.
231. Leppert M, Dobbs M, Scambler P, et al: The gene for familial polyposis coli maps to the long arm of chromosome 5. *Science* **238**:1411, 1987.
232. Bodmer W, Bailey C, Bodmer J, et al: Localization of the gene for familial adenomatous polyposis on chromosome 5. *Nature* **328**:614, 1987.
233. Nakamura Y, Lathrop M, Leppert M, et al: Localization of the genetic defect in familial adenomatous polyposis within a small region of chromosome 5. *Am J Hum Genet* **43**:638, 1988.
234. Ashton Rickardt PG, Dunlop MG, Nakamura Y, et al: High frequency of *APC* loss in sporadic colorectal carcinoma due to breaks clustered in 5q21-22. *Oncogene* **4**:1169, 1989.
235. Delattre O, Olschwang S, Law DJ, et al: Multiple genetic alterations in distal and proximal colorectal cancer. *Lancet* **2**:353, 1989.
236. Sasaki M, Okamoto M, Sato C, et al: Loss of constitutional heterozygosity in colorectal tumors from patients with familial polyposis coli and those with nonpolyposis colorectal carcinoma. *Cancer Res* **49**:4402, 1989.
237. Ashton Rickardt PG, Wyllie AH, Bird CC, et al: *MCC*, a candidate familial polyposis gene in 5q.21, shows frequent allele loss in colorectal and lung cancer. *Oncogene* **6**:1881, 1991.
238. Kinzler KW, Nilbert MC, Su LK, et al: Identification of *FAP* locus genes from chromosome 5q21. *Science* **253**:661, 1991.
239. Joslyn G, Carlson M, Thliveris A, et al: Identification of deletion mutations and three new genes at the familial polyposis locus. *Cell* **66**:601, 1991.
240. Nishisho I, Nakamura Y, Miyoshi Y, et al: Mutations of chromosome 5q21 genes in *FAP* and colorectal cancer patients. *Science* **253**:665, 1991.
241. Groden J, Thliveris A, Samowitz W, et al: Identification and characterization of the familial adenomatous polyposis coli gene. *Cell* **66**:589, 1991.
242. Horii A, Nakatsuru S, Ichii S, Nagase H, Nakamura Y: Multiple forms of the *APC* gene transcripts and their tissue-specific expression. *Hum Mol Genet* **2**:283, 1993.
243. Thliveris A, Samowitz W, Matsunami N, Groden J, White R: Demonstration of promoter activity and alternative splicing in the region 5′ to exon 1 of the *APC* gene. *Cancer Res* **54**:2991, 1994.
244. Nagase H, Su Y: Mutations of the *APC* (adenomatous polyposis coli) gene. *Hum Mutat* **2**:425, 1993.
245. Laurent-Puig P, Beroud C, Soussi T: *APC* gene: Database of germline and somatic mutations in human tumors and cell lines. *Nucl Acids Res* **26**:269, 1998.
246. Powell SM, Petersen GM, Krush AJ, et al: Molecular diagnosis of familial adenomatous polyposis. *N Engl J Med* **329**:1982, 1993.
247. Laken SJ, Papadopoulous N, Petersen GM, et al: Analysis of masked mutations in familial adenomatous polyposis. *Proc Natl Acad Sci USA* **96**:2322, 1999.
248. Papadopoulos N, Leach FS, Kinzler KW, Vogelstein B: Monoallelic mutation analysis (MAMA) for identifying germline mutations. *Nature Genet* **11**:99, 1995.
249. Groden J, Gelbert L, Thliveris A, et al: Mutational analysis of patients with adenomatous polyposis: Identical inactivating mutations in unrelated individuals. *Am J Hum Genet* **52**:263, 1993.
250. Olschwang S, Tiret A, Laurent-Puig P, Muleris M, Parc R, Thomas G: Restriction of ocular fundus lesions to a specific subgroup of *APC* mutations in adenomatous polyposis coli patients. *Cell* **75**:959, 1993.
251. Wallis YL, Macdonald F, Hulten M, et al: Genotype-phenotype correlation between position of constitutional *APC* gene mutation and CHRPE expression in familial adenomatous polyposis. *Hum Genet* **94**:543, 1994.
252. Caspari R, Olschwang S, Friedl W, et al: Familial adenomatous polyposis: Desmoid tumours and lack of ophthalmic lesions (CHRPE) associated with *APC* mutations beyond codon 1444. *Hum Mol Genet* **4**:337, 1995.
253. Davies D, Armstrong J, Thakker N, et al: Severe Gardner syndrome in families with mutations restricted to a specific region of the *APC* gene. *Am J Hum Genet* **57**:1151, 1995.
254. Dobbie Z, Spycher M, Mary J-L, et al: Correlation between the development of extracolonic manifestations in FAP patients and mutations beyond codon 1403 of the *APC* gene. *J Med Genet* **33**:274, 1996.
255. Friedl W, Meuschel S, Caspari R, et al: Attenuated familial adenomatous polyposis due to a mutation in the 3′ part of the *APC* gene: A clue for understanding the function of the APC protein. *Hum Genet* **97**:579, 1996.
256. Walon C, Kartheuser A, Michils G, et al: Novel germline mutations in the *APC* gene and their phenotypic spectrum in familial adenomatous polyposis kindreds. *Hum Genet* **100**:601, 1997.
257. Soravia C, Berk T, Madlensky L, et al: Genotype-phenotype correlations in attenuated adenomatous polyposis coli. *Am J Hum Genet* **62**:1290, 1998.
258. Pedemonte S, Sciallero S, Gismondi V, et al: Novel germline *APC* variants in patients with multiple adenomas. *Genes Chromosom Cancer* **22**:257, 1998.
259. Brensinger JD, Laken SJ, Luce MC, et al: Variable phenotype of familial adenomatous polyposis in pedigrees with 3′mutation in the *APC* gene. *Gut* **43**:548, 1998.
260. Gayther S, Wells D, SenGupta S, et al: Regionally clustered *APC* mutations are associated with a severe phenotype and occur at a high frequency in new mutation cases of adenomatous polyposis coli. *Hum Mol Genet* **3**:53, 1994.
261. Nagase H, Miyoshi Y, Horii A, et al: Correlation between the location of germ-line mutations in the *APC* gene and the number of colorectal polyps in familial adenomatous polyposis patients. *Cancer Res* **52**:4055, 1992.
262. Giardiello FM, Krush AJ, Petersen GM, et al: Phenotypic variability of familial adenomatous polyposis in 11 unrelated families with identical *APC* gene mutation. *Gastroenterology* **106**:1542, 1994.
263. Miyoshi Y, Nagase H, Ando H, et al: Somatic mutations of the *APC* gene in colorectal tumors: Mutation cluster region in the *APC* gene. *Hum Mol Genet* **1**:229, 1992.
264. Powell SM, Zilz N, Beazer-Barclay Y, et al: *APC* mutations occur early during colorectal tumorigenesis. *Nature* **359**:235, 1992.
265. Smith KJ, Johnson KA, Bryan TM, et al: The *APC* gene product in normal and tumor cells. *Proc Natl Acad Sci USA* **90**:2846, 1993.
266. Smith AJ, Stern HS, Penner M, et al: Somatic *APC* and *K-ras* codon 12 mutations in aberrant crypt foci from human colons. *Cancer Res* **54**:5527, 1994.
267. Laken SJ, Petersen GM, Gruber SB, et al: Familial colorectal cancer in Ashkenazim due to a hypermutable tract in *APC*. *Nature Genet* **17**:79, 1997.
268. Woodage T, King SM, Wacholder S, et al: The *APCI1307K* allele and cancer risk in a community-based study of Ashkenazi Jews. *Nature Genet* **20**:62, 1998.
269. Lothe RA, Hektoen M, Johnsen H, et al: The *APC* gene I1307K variant is rare in Norwegian patients with familial and sporadic colorectal or breast cancer. *Cancer Res* **58**:2923, 1998.
270. Petersen GM, Parmigiani G, Thomas D: Missense mutations in disease genes: A Bayesian approach to evaluate causality. *Am J Hum Genet* **62**:1516, 1998.
271. Frayling IM, Beck NE, Ilyas M, et al: The *APC* variants I1307K and E1317Q are associated with colorectal tumors, but not always with a family history. *Proc Natl Acad Sci USA* **95**:10722, 1998.
272. Rozen P, Shomrat R, Strul H, et al: Prevalence of the I1307K *APC* gene variant in Israel Jews of differing ethnic origin and risk for cancer. *Gastroenterology* **16**:54, 1999.
273. Petrukhin L, Dangel J, Vanderveer L, et al: The I1307K *APC* mutation does not predispose to colorectal cancer in Jewish Ashkenazi breast and breast-ovarian cancer kindreds. *Cancer Res* **57**:5480, 1997.
274. Abrahamson J, Moslehi R, Vesprini D, et al: No association of the I1307K *APC* allele with ovarian cancer risk in Ashkenazi Jews. *Cancer Res* **58**:2919, 1998.
275. Yuan ZQ, Kasprzak L, Gordon PH, Pinsky L, Foulkes WD: I1307K *APC* and *hMLH1* mutations in a non-Jewish family with hereditary non-polyposis colorectal cancer. *Clin Genet* **54**:368, 1998.

276. Gryfe R, Di Nicola N, Gallinger S, Redston M: Somatic instability of the *APC* I1307K allele in colorectal neoplasia. *Cancer Res* **58**:4040, 1998.
277. Su LK, Kinzler KW, Vogelstein B, et al: Multiple intestinal neoplasia caused by a mutation in the murine homolog of the *APC* gene. *Science* **256**:668, 1992.
278. Fodde R, Edelmann W, Yang K, et al: A targeted chain-termination mutation in the mouse *Apc* gene results in multiple intestinal tumors. *Proc Natl Acad Sci USA* **91**:8969, 1994.
279. Oshima M, Oshima H, Kitagawa K, Kobayashi M, Itakura C, Taketo M: Loss of *Apc* heterozygosity and abnormal tissue building in nascent intestinal polyps in mice carrying a truncated *Apc* gene. *Proc Natl Acad Sci USA* **92**:4482, 1995.
280. Moser AR, Pitot HC, Dove WF: A dominant mutation that predisposes to multiple intestinal neoplasia in the mouse. *Science* **247**:322, 1990.
281. Moser AR, Dove WF, Roth KA, Gordon JI: The *Min* (multiple intestinal neoplasia) mutation: Its effect on gut epithelial cell differentiation and interaction with a modifier system. *J Cell Biol* **116**:1517, 1992.
282. Luongo C, Moser AR, Gledhill S, Dove WF: Loss of *Apc+* in intestinal adenomas from *Min* mice. *Cancer Res* **54**:5947, 1994.
283. Levy DB, Smith KJ, Beazer-Barclay Y, Hamilton SR, Vogelstein B, Kinzler KW: Inactivation of both *APC* alleles in human and mouse tumors. *Cancer Res* **54**:5953, 1994.
284. Shibata H, Toyama K, Shioya H, et al: Rapid colorectal adenoma formation initiated by conditional targeting of the *Apc* gene. *Science* **278**:120, 1997.
285. Morin PJ, Vogelstein B, Kinzler KW: Apoptosis and *APC* in colorectal tumorigenesis. *Proc Natl Acad Sci USA* **93**:7950, 1996.
286. Miyashiro I, Senda T, Matsumine A, et al: Subcellular localization of the APC protein: Immunoelectron microscopic study of the association of the APC protein with catenin. *Oncogene* **11**:89, 1995.
287. Joslyn G, Richardson DS, White R, Alber T: Dimer formation by an N-terminal coiled coil in the APC protein. *Proc Natl Acad Sci USA* **90**:11109, 1993.
288. Su LK, Johnson KA, Smith KJ, Hill DE, Vogelstein B, Kinzler KW: Association between wild type and mutant *APC* gene products. *Cancer Res* **53**:2728, 1993.
289. Rubinfeld B, Souza B, Albert I, et al: Association of the *APC* gene product with beta-catenin. *Science* **262**:1731, 1993.
290. Su LK, Vogelstein B, Kinzler KW: Association of the APC tumor suppressor protein with catenins. *Science* **262**:1734, 1993.
291. Hulsken J, Birchmeier W, Behrens J: E-cadherin and APC compete for the interaction with beta-catenin and the cytoskeleton. *J Cell Biol* **127**:2061, 1994.
292. Rubinfeld B, Souza B, Albert I, Munemitsu S, Polakis P: The APC protein and E-cadherin form similar but independent complexes with alpha-catenin, beta-catenin, and plakoglobin. *J Biol Chem* **270**:5549, 1995.
293. Rubinfeld B, Albert I, Porfiri E, Fiol C, Munemitsu S, Polakis P: Binding of GSK3-beta to the APC-beta-catenin complex and regulation of complex assembly. *Science* **272**:1023, 1996.
294. Ikeda S, Kishida S, Yamamoto H, Murai H, Koyama S, Kikuchi A: Axin, a negative regulator of the Wnt signaling pathway, forms a complex with GSK-3beta and beta-catenin and promotes GSK-3beta-dependent phosphorylation of beta-catenin. *EMBO J* **17**:1371, 1998.
295. Behrens J, Jerchow BA, Wurtele M, et al: Functional interaction of an axin homolog, conductin, with beta-catenin, APC, and GSK3beta. *Science* **280**:596, 1998.
296. Yamamoto H, Kishida S, Uochi T, et al: Axil, a member of the Axin family, interacts with both glycogen synthase kinase 3beta and beta-catenin and inhibits axis formation of *Xenopus* embryos. *Mol Cell Biol* **18**:2867, 1998.
297. Kishida S, Yamamoto H, Ikeda S, et al: Axin, a negative regulator of the wnt signaling pathway, directly interacts with adenomatous polyposis coli and regulates the stabilization of beta-catenin. *J Biol Chem* **273**:10823, 1998.
298. Hart MJ, de los Santos R, Albert IN, Rubinfeld B, Polakis P: Downregulation of beta-catenin by human Axin and its association with the APC tumor suppressor, beta-catenin and GSK3 beta. *Curr Biol* **8**:573, 1998.
299. Nakamura T, Hamada F, Ishidate T, et al: Axin, an inhibitor of the Wnt signalling pathway, interacts with beta-catenin, GSK-3beta and APC and reduces the beta-catenin level. *Genes Cells* **3**:395, 1998.
300. Su LK, Burrell M, Hill DE, et al: APC binds to the novel protein EB1. *Cancer Res* **55**:2972, 1995.
301. Munemitsu S, Souza B, Muller O, Albert I, Rubinfeld B, Polakis P: The *APC* gene product associates with microtubules in vivo and promotes their assembly in vitro. *Cancer Res* **54**:3676, 1994.
302. Smith KJ, Levy DB, Maupin P, Pollard TD, Vogelstein B, Kinzler KW: Wild-type but not mutant *APC* associates with the microtubule cytoskeleton. *Cancer Res* **54**:3672, 1994.
303. Matsumine A, Ogai A, Senda T, et al: Binding of *APC* to the human homolog of the *Drosophila* discs large tumor suppressor protein. *Science* **272**:1020, 1996.
304. Berrueta L, Kraeft SK, Tirnauer JS, et al: The adenomatous polyposis coli-binding protein EB1 is associated with cytoplasmic and spindle microtubules. *Proc Natl Acad Sci USA* **95**:10596, 1998.
305. Muhua L, Adames NR, Murphy MD, Shields CR, Cooper JA: A cytokinesis checkpoint requiring the yeast homologue of an APC-binding protein. *Nature* **393**:487, 1998.
306. Kemler R: From cadherins to catenins: Cytoplasmic protein interactions and regulation of cell adhesion. *Trends Genet* **9**:317, 1993.
307. Perrimon N: The genetic basis of patterned baldness in *Drosophila*. *Cell* **76**:781, 1994.
308. Gumbiner BM: Signal transduction of beta-catenin. *Curr Opin Cell Biol* **7**:634, 1995.
309. Peifer M: Regulating cell proliferation: As easy as APC. *Science* **272**:974, 1996.
310. Munemitsu S, Albert I, Souza B, Rubinfeld B, Polakis P: Regulation of intracellular beta-catenin levels by the adenomatous polyposis coli (APC) tumor-suppressor protein. *Proc Natl Acad Sci USA* **92**:3046, 1995.
311. Aberle H, Bauer A, Stappert J, Kispert A, Kemler R: Beta-catenin is a target for the ubiquitin-proteasome pathway. *EMBO J* **16**:3797, 1997.
312. Orford K, Crockett C, Jensen JP, Weissman AM, Byers SW: Serine phosphorylation-regulated ubiquitination and degradation of beta-catenin. *J Biol Chem* **272**:24735, 1997.
313. Behrens J, von Kries JP, Kuhl M, et al: Functional interaction of beta-catenin with the transcription factor LEF-1. *Nature* **382**:638, 1996.
314. Molenaar M, van de Wetering M, Oosterwegel M, et al: XTcf-3 transcription factor mediates beta-catenin-induced axis formation in *Xenopus* embryos. *Cell* **86**:391, 1996.
315. Whitehead I, Kirk H, Kay R: Expression cloning of oncogenes by retroviral transfer of cDNA libraries. *Mol Cell Biol* **15**:704, 1995.
316. Nusse R, Varmus HE: *Wnt* genes. *Cell* **69**:1073, 1992.
317. Korinek V, Barker N, Morin PJ, et al: Constitutive transcriptional activation by a beta-catenin-Tcf complex in *APC-/-* colon carcinoma. *Science* **275**:1784, 1997.
318. Morin PJ, Sparks AB, Korinek V, et al: Activation of beta-catenin-Tcf signaling in colon cancer by mutations in beta-catenin or APC. *Science* **275**:1787, 1997.
319. Iwao K, Nakamori S, Kameyama M, et al: Activation of the beta-catenin gene by interstitial deletions involving exon 3 in primary colorectal carcinomas without adenomatous polyposis coli mutations. *Cancer Res* **58**:1021, 1998.
320. Ilyas M, Tomlinson IP, Rowan A, Pignatelli M, Bodmer WF: Beta-catenin mutations in cell lines established from human colorectal cancers. *Proc Natl Acad Sci USA* **94**:10330, 1997.
321. Kitaeva MN, Grogan L, Williams JP, et al: Mutations in beta-catenin are uncommon in colorectal cancer occurring in occasional replication error-positive tumors. *Cancer Res* **57**:4478, 1997.
322. Sparks AB, Morin PJ, Vogelstein B, Kinzler KW: Mutational analysis of the APC/b-catenin/Tcf pathway in colorectal cancer. *Cancer Res* **58**:1130, 1998.
323. Rubinfeld B, Robbins P, El-Gamil M, Albert I, Porfiri E, Polakis P: Stabilization of beta-catenin by genetic defects in melanoma cell lines. *Science* **275**:1790, 1997.
324. de la Coste A, Romagnolo B, Billuart P, et al: Somatic mutations of the beta-catenin gene are frequent in mouse and human hepatocellular carcinomas. *Proc Natl Acad Sci USA* **95**:8847, 1998.
325. Voeller HJ, Truica CI, Gelmann EP: Beta-catenin mutations in human prostate cancer. *Cancer Res* **58**:2520, 1998.
326. Miyoshi Y, Iwao K, Nagasawa Y, et al: Activation of the beta-catenin gene in primary hepatocellular carcinomas by somatic alterations involving exon 3. *Cancer Res* **58**:2524, 1998.
327. Palacios J, Gamallo C: Mutations in the beta-catenin gene (*CTNNB1*) in endometrioid ovarian carcinomas. *Cancer Res* **58**:1344, 1998.
328. Zurawel RH, Chiappa SA, Allen C, Raffel C: Sporadic medulloblastomas contain oncogenic beta-catenin mutations. *Cancer Res* **58**:896, 1998.

329. Dashwood RH, Suzui M, Nakagama H, Sugimura T, Nagao M: High frequency of beta-catenin (*ctnnb1*) mutations in the colon tumors induced by two heterocyclic amines in the F344 rat. *Cancer Res* **58**:1127, 1998.
330. Takahashi M, Fukuda K, Sugimura T, Wakabayashi K: Beta-catenin is frequently mutated and demonstrates altered cellular location in azoxymethane-induced rat colon tumors. *Cancer Res* **58**:42, 1998.
331. He TC, Sparks AB, Rago C, et al: Identification of c-MYC as a target of the APC pathway. *Science* **281**:1509, 1998.
332. Rodriguez-Alfageme C, Stanbridge EJ, Astrin SM: Suppression of deregulated c-MYC expression in human colon carcinoma cells by chromosome 5 transfer. *Proc Natl Acad Sci USA* **89**:1482, 1992.
332a. Tetsu O, McCormick F: Beta-catenin regulates expression of cyclin D1 in colon carcinoma cells. *Nature* **398**:422, 1999.
332b. Shtutman M, Zhurinsky J, Simcha I, Albanese C, D'Amico M, Pestell R, Ben-Ze'ev A: The cyclin D1 gene is a target of the beta-catenin/LEF-1 pathway. *Proc Natl Acad Sci USA* **96**:5522, 1999.
332c. Mann B, Gelos M, Siedow A, Hanski ML, Gratche A, Ilyas M, Bodmer WF, Moyer MP, Riecken EO, Buhr HJ, Hanski C: Target genes of beta-catenin-T cell-factor/lymphoid-enhancer-factor signaling in human colorectal carcinomas. *Proc Natl Acad Sci USA* **96**:1603, 1999.
332d. Roose J, Huls G, van Beest M, Moerer P, van der Horn K, Goldschmeding R, Logtenberg T, Clevers H: Synergy between tumor suppressor APC and the beta-catenin-Tcf4 target Tcf1. *Science* **285**:1923, 1999.
332e. He TC, Chan TA, Vogelstein B, Kinzler KW: PPARdelta is an APC-regulated target of nonsteroidal anti-inflammatory drugs. *Cell* **99**:335, 1999.
333. Wong MH, Rubinfeld B, Gordon JI: Effects of forced expression of an NH2-terminal truncated beta-catenin on mouse intestinal epithelial homeostasis. *J Cell Biol* **141**:765, 1998.
334. Gat U, DasGupta R, Degenstein L, Fuchs E: *De novo* hair follicle morphogenesis and hair tumors in mice expressing a truncated beta-catenin in skin. *Cell* **95**:605, 1998.
335. Korinek V, Barker N, Moerer P, et al: Depletion of epithelial stem-cell compartments in the small intestine of mice lacking Tcf-4. *Nature Genet* **19**:379, 1998.
336. Nakagawa H, Murata Y, Koyama K, et al: Identification of a brain-specific APC homologue, APCL, and its interaction with beta-catenin. *Cancer Res* **58**:5176, 1998.
337. van Es J, Kirkpatrick C, van de Wetering M, et al: A homologue of the adenomatous polyposis coli tumor suppressor gene. *Curr Biol* **9**:105, 1999.
338. Kinzler KW, Nilbert MC, Vogelstein B, et al: Identification of a gene located at chromosome 5q21 that is mutated in colorectal cancers. *Science* **251**:1366, 1991.
339. Hampton GM, Ward JR, Cottrell S, et al: Yeast artificial chromosomes for the molecular analysis of the familial polyposis *APC* gene region. *Proc Natl Acad Sci USA* **89**:8249, 1992.
340. Curtis LJ, Bubb VJ, Gledhill S, Morris RG, Bird CC, Wyllie AH: Loss of heterozygosity of *MCC* is not associated with mutation of the retained allele in sporadic colorectal cancer. *Hum Mol Genet* **3**:443, 1994.
341. Barker PE: Double minutes in human tumor cells. *Cancer Genet Cytogenet* **5**:81, 1982.
342. Alitalo K, Winqvist R, Lin CC, de la Chapelle A, Schwab M, Bishop JM: Aberrant expression of an amplified *c-myb* oncogene in two cell lines from a colon carcinoma. *Proc Natl Acad Sci USA* **81**:4534, 1984.
343. Alitalo K, Schwab M, Lin CC, Varmus HE, Bishop JM: Homogeneously staining chromosomal regions contain amplified copies of an abundantly expressed cellular oncogene (*c-myc*) in malignant neuroendocrine cells from a human colon carcinoma. *Proc Natl Acad Sci USA* **80**:1707, 1983.
344. Alexander RJ, Buxbaum JN, Raicht RF: Oncogene alterations in primary human colon tumors. *Gastroenterology* **91**:1503, 1986.
345. Meltzer SJ, Ahnen DJ, Battifora H, Yokota J, Cline MJ: Protooncogene abnormalities in colon cancers and adenomatous polyps. *Gastroenterology* **92**:1174, 1987.
346. Finley GG, Schulz NT, Hill SA, Geiser JR, Pipas JM, Meisler AI: Expression of the *myc* gene family in different stages of human colorectal cancer. *Oncogene* **4**:963, 1989.
347. Tal M, Wetzler M, Josefberg Z, et al: Sporadic amplification of the *HER2/neu* protooncogene in adenocarcinomas of various tissues. *Cancer Res* **48**:1517, 1988.
348. D'Emilia J, Bulovas K, D'Ercole K, Wolf B, Steele G Jr, Summerhayes IC: Expression of the *c-erbB-2* gene product (p185) at different stages of neoplastic progression in the colon. *Oncogene* **4**:1233, 1989.
349. Leach FS, Elledge SJ, Sherr CJ, et al: Amplification of cyclin genes in colorectal carcinomas. *Cancer Res* **53**:1986, 1993.
350. Zhou H, Kuang J, Zhong L, et al: Tumour amplified kinase STK15/BTAK induces centrosome amplification, aneuploidy and transformation. *Nature Genet* **20**:189, 1998.
351. Bischoff JR, Anderson L, Zhu Y, et al: A homologue of *Drosophila aurora* kinase is oncogenic and amplified in human colorectal cancers. *EMBO J* **17**:3052, 1998.
352. Pitti RM, Marsters SA, Lawrence DA, et al: Genomic amplification of a decoy receptor for Fas ligand in lung and colon cancer. *Nature* **396**:699, 1998.
353. Dietrich WF, Lander ES, Smith JS, et al: Genetic identification of *Mom-1,* a major modifier locus affecting Min-induced intestinal neoplasia in the mouse. *Cell* **75**:631, 1993.
354. MacPhee M, Chepenik K, Liddell R, Nelson K, Siracusa L, Buchberg A: The secretory phospholipase A2 gene is a candidate for the *Mom1* locus, a major modifier of ApcMin-induced intestinal neoplasia. *Cell* **81**:957, 1995.
355. Cormier RT, Hong KH, Halberg RB, et al: Secretory phospholipase Pla2g2a confers resistance to intestinal tumorigenesis. *Nature Genet* **17**:88, 1997.
356. Riggins GJ, Markowitz S, Wilson JK, Vogelstein B, Kinzler KW: Absence of secretory phospholipase a(2) gene alterations in human colorectal cancer. *Cancer Res* **55**:5184, 1995.
357. Melhem MF, Meisler AI, Finley GG, et al: Distribution of cells expressing myc proteins in human colorectal epithelium, polyps, and malignant tumors. *Cancer Res* **52**:5853, 1992.
358. Ogata S, Uehara H, Chen A, Itzkowitz SH: Mucin gene expression in colonic tissues and cell lines. *Cancer Res* **52**:5971, 1992.
359. Ciardiello F, Kim N, Saeki T, et al: Differential expression of epidermal growth factor-related proteins in human colorectal tumors. *Proc Natl Acad Sci USA* **88**:7792, 1991.
360. Koenders PG, Peters WH, Wobbes T, Beex LV, Nagengast FM, Benraad TJ: Epidermal growth factor receptor levels are lower in carcinomatous than in normal colorectal tissue. *Br J Cancer* **65**:189, 1992.
361. Gold P, Freedman SO: Demonstration of tumor-specific antigens in human colonic carcinomata by immunological tolerance and absorption techniques. *J Exp Med* **121**:439, 1965.
362. Ransom JH, Pelle B, Hanna MG Jr: Expression of class II major histocompatibility complex molecules correlates with human colon tumor vaccine efficacy. *Cancer Res* **52**:3460, 1992.
363. Tsioulias G, Godwin TA, Goldstein MF, et al: Loss of colonic HLA antigens in familial adenomatous polyposis. *Cancer Res* **52**:3449, 1992.
364. Calabretta B, Kaczmarek L, Ming PM, Au F, Ming SC: Expression of *c-myc* and other cell cycle-dependent genes in human colon neoplasia. *Cancer Res* **45**:6000, 1985.
365. Adams MD, Kerlavage AR, Fleischmann RD, et al: Initial assessment of human gene diversity and expression patterns based upon 83 million nucleotides of Cdna sequence. *Nature* **377**:3, 1995.
366. Liang P, Pardee AB: Differential display of eukaryotic messenger RNA by means of the polymerase chain reaction. *Science* **257**:967, 1992.
367. Velculescu VE, Zhang L, Vogelstein B, Kinzler KW: Serial analysis of gene expression. *Science* **270**:484, 1995.
368. Schena M, Shalon D, Davis RW, Brown PO: Quantitative monitoring of gene expression patterns with a complementary DNA microarray. *Science* **270**:467, 1995.
369. Zhang L, Zhou W, Velculescu VE, Kern SE, Hruban RH, Hamilton SR, Vogelstein B, Kinzler KW: Gene expression profiles in normal and cancer cells. *Science* **276**:1268 1997.
370. Bird A: The essentials of DNA methylation. *Cell* **70**:5, 1992.
371. Goelz SE, Vogelstein B, Hamilton SR, Feinberg AP: Hypomethylation of DNA from benign and malignant human colon neoplasms. *Science* **228**:187, 1985.
372. Feinberg AP, Gehrke CW, Kuo KC, Ehrlich M: Reduced genomic 5-methylcytosine content in human colonic neoplasia. *Cancer Res* **48**:1159, 1988.
373. Silverman AL, Park JG, Hamilton SR, Gazdar AF, Luk GD, Baylin SB: Abnormal methylation of the calcitonin gene in human colonic neoplasms. *Cancer Res* **49**:3468, 1989.

374. El-Deiry WS, Nelkin BD, Celano P, et al: High expression of the DNA methyltransferase gene characterizes human neoplastic cells and progression stages of colon cancer. *Proc Natl Acad Sci USA* **88**:3470, 1991.
375. Schmid M, Haaf T, Grunert D: 5-Azacytidine-induced undercondensations in human chromosomes. *Hum Genet* **67**:257, 1984.
376. Herman JG, Umar A, Polyak K, et al: Incidence and functional consequences of *hMLH1* promoter hypermethylation in colorectal carcinoma. *Proc Natl Acad Sci USA* **95**:6870, 1998.
377. Baylin SB, Makos M, Wu JJ, et al: Abnormal patterns of DNA methylation in human neoplasia: Potential consequences for tumor progression. *Cancer Cells* **3**:383, 1991.
378. Herman JG, Merlo A, Mao L, et al: Inactivation of the *CDKN2/p16/MTS1* gene is frequently associated with aberrant DNA methylation in all common human cancers. *Cancer Res* **55**:4525, 1995.
379. Landolph JR, Jones PA: Mutagenicity of 5-azacytidine and related nucleosides in C3H/10T 1/2 clone 8 and V79 cells. *Cancer Res* **42**:817, 1982.
380. Laird P, Jackson-Grusby L, Fazeli A, et al: Suppression of intestinal neoplasia by DNA hypomethylation. *Cell* **81**:197, 1995.
381. Fearon ER, Vogelstein B: A genetic model for colorectal tumorigenesis. *Cell* **61**:759, 1990.
382. Vogelstein B, Kinzler KW: The multistep nature of cancer. *Trends Genet* **9**:138, 1993.
383. Garber JE, Goldstein AM, Kantor AF, Dreyfus MG, Fraumeni JF Jr, Li FP: Follow-up study of twenty-four families with Li-Fraumeni syndrome. *Cancer Res* **51**:6094, 1991.
384. Kinzler KW, Vogelstein B: Cancer-susceptibility genes: Gatekeepers and caretakers. *Nature* **386**:761, 1997.
385. Loeb LA: Mutator phenotype may be required for multistage carcinogenesis. *Cancer Res* **51**:3075, 1991.
386. Hartwell L: Defects in a cell cycle checkpoint may be responsible for the genomic instability of cancer cells. *Cell* **71**:543, 1992.
387. Heim S, Mitelman F: Cytogenetic analysis in the diagnosis of acute leukemia. *Cancer* **70**:1701, 1992.
388. Ionov Y, Peinado MA, Malkhosyan S, Shibata D, Perucho M: Ubiquitous somatic mutations in simple repeated sequences reveal a new mechanism for colonic carcinogenesis. *Nature* **363**:558, 1993.
389. Thibodeau SN, Bren G, Schaid D: Microsatellite instability in cancer of the proximal colon. *Science* **260**:816, 1993.
390. Aaltonen LA, Peltomaki P, Leach FS, et al: Clues to the pathogenesis of familial colorectal cancer. *Science* **260**:812, 1993.
391. Eshleman JR, Lang EZ, Bowerfind GK, et al: Increased mutation rate at the hprt locus accompanies microsatellite instability in colon cancer. *Oncogene* **10**:33, 1995.
392. Lengauer C, Kinzler KW, Vogelstein B: Genetic instability in colorectal cancers. *Nature* **386**:623, 1997.
393. Cahill DP, Lengauer C, Yu J, et al: Mutations of mitotic checkpoint genes in human cancers. *Nature* **392**:300, 1998.
394. Lengauer C, Kinzler KW, Vogelstein B: Genetic instabilities in human cancers. *Nature* **396**:643, 1998.
395. Li J, Yen C, Liaw D, et al: *PTEN,* a putative protein tyrosine phosphatase gene mutated in human brain, breast, and prostate cancer. *Science* **275**:1943, 1997.
396. Steck PA, Pershouse MA, Jasser SA, et al: Identification of a candidate tumour suppressor gene, *MMAC1,* at chromosome 10q23.3 that is mutated in multiple advanced cancers. *Nature Genet* **15**:356, 1997.
397. Sidransky D, Tokino T, Hamilton SR, et al: Identification of *ras* oncogene mutations in the stool of patients with curable colorectal tumors. *Science* **256**:102, 1992.
398. Smith-Ravin J, England J, Talbot IC, Bodmer W: Detection of *c-Ki-ras* mutations in faecal samples from sporadic colorectal cancer patients. *Gut* **36**:81, 1995.
399. Hasegawa Y, Takeda S, Ichii S, et al: Detection of *K-ras* mutations in DNAs isolated from feces of patients with colorectal tumors by mutant-allele-specific amplification (MASA). *Oncogene* **10**:1441, 1995.
400. Villa E, Dugani A, Rebecchi AM, et al: Identification of subjects at risk for colorectal carcinoma through a test based on K-ras determination in the stool. *Gastroenterology* **110**:1346, 1996.
401. Nollau P, Moser C, Weinland G, Wagener C: Detection of *K-ras* mutations in stools of patients with colorectal cancer by mutant-enriched PCR. *Int J Cancer* **66**:332, 1996.
402. Waddell WR, Ganser GF, Cerise EJ, Loughry RW: Sulindac for polyposis of the colon. *Am J Surg* **157**:175, 1989.
403. Rigau J, Pique JM, Rubio E, Planas R, Tarrech JM, Bordas JM: Effects of long-term sulindac therapy on colonic polyposis. *Ann Intern Med* **115**:952, 1991.
404. Labayle D, Fischer D, Vielh P, et al: Sulindac causes regression of rectal polyps in familial adenomatous polyposis. *Gastroenterology* **101**:635, 1991.
405. Giardiello FM, Hamilton SR, Krush AJ, et al: Treatment of colonic and rectal adenomas with sulindac in familial adenomatous polyposis. *N Engl J Med* **328**:1313, 1993.
406. Nugent K, Farmer K, Spigelman A, Williams C, Phillips R: Randomized controlled trial of the effect of sulindac on duodenal and rectal polyposis and cell proliferation in patients with familial adenomatous polyposis. *Br J Surg* **80**:1618, 1993.
407. Winde G, Gumbinger HG, Osswald H, Kemper F, Bunte H: The NSAID sulindac reverses rectal adenomas in colectomized patients with familial adenomatous polyposis: Clinical results of a dose-finding study on rectal sulindac administration. *Int J Colorectal Dis* **8**:13, 1993.
408. Debinski H, Trojan J, Nugent K, Spigelman A, Phillips R: Effect of sulindac on small polyps in familial adenomatous polyposis. *Lancet* **345**:855, 1995.
409. Winde G, Schmid K, Schlegel W, Fischer R, Osswald H, Bunte H: Complete reversion and prevention of rectal adenomas in colectomized patients with familial adenomatous polyposis by rectal low-dose sulindac maintenance treatment: Advantages of a low-dose nonsteroidal anti-inflammatory drug regimen in reversing adenomas exceeding 33 months. *Dis Colon Rectum* **38**:813, 1995.
410. Kune GA, Kune S, Watson LF: Colorectal cancer risk, chronic illnesses, operations, and medications: Case control results from the Melbourne Colorectal Cancer Study. *Cancer Res* **48**:4399, 1988.
411. Rosenberg L, Palmer JR, Zauber AG, Warshauer ME, Stolley PD, Shapiro S: A hypothesis: Nonsteroidal anti-inflammatory drugs reduce the incidence of large-bowel cancer. *J Natl Cancer Inst* **83**:355, 1991.
412. Thun MJ, Namboodiri MM, Heath CW Jr: Aspirin use and reduced risk of fatal colon cancer. *N Engl J Med* **325**:1593, 1991.
413. Beazer-Barclay Y, Levy DB, Moser AM, et al: Sulindac suppresses tumorigenesis in the Min mouse. *Carcinogenesis* **17**:1757, 1996.
414. Jacoby RF, Marshall DJ, Newton MA, et al: Chemoprevention of spontaneous intestinal adenomas in the APC-Min mouse by the nonsteroidal anti-inflammatory drug piroxicam. *Cancer Res* **56**:710, 1996.
415. Boolbol SK, Dannenberg AJ, Chadurn A, et al: Cyclooxygenase-2 overexpression and tumor formation are blocked by sulindac in a murine model of familial adenomatous polyposis. *Cancer Res* **56**:2556, 1996.
416. Waldman T, Zhang Y, Dillehay L, et al: Cell-cycle arrest versus cell death in cancer therapy. *Nature Med* **3**:1034, 1997.
417. Clara M, Herschel K, Ferner H: *Atlas of Normal Microscopic Anatomy of Man*. New York, Urban & Schwarzenberg, 1974.
418. Kinzler KW, Vogelstein B: Lessons from hereditary colon cancer. *Cell* **87**:159, 1996.
419. Greenblatt MS, Bennett WP, Hollstein M, Harris CC: Mutations in the *p53* tumor suppressor gene: Clues to cancer etiology and molecular pathogenesis. *Cancer Res* **54**:4855, 1994.
420. Vogelstein B, Kinzler K: Tumour-suppressor genes: X-rays strike p53 again. *Nature* **370**:174, 1994.
421. Kinzler KW, Vogelstein B: Life (and death) in a malignant tumour. *Nature* **379**:19, 1996.
422. Altschul SF, Gish W, Miller W, Myers EW, Lipman DJ: Basic local alignment search tool. *J Mol Biol* **215**:403, 1990.
423. Miyoshi Y, Ando H, Nagase H, et al: Germ-line mutations of the *APC* gene in 53 familial adenomatous polyposis patients. *Proc Natl Acad Sci USA* **89**:4452, 1992.
424. Peifer M, Berg S, Reynolds AB: A repeating amino acid motif shared by proteins with diverse cellular roles. *Cell* **76**:789, 1994.

CHAPTER 49

Genetic Testing for Familial Cancer

Gloria M. Petersen ▪ Ann-Marie Codori

1. **Cancer gene discoveries have led to important changes in the clinical practice of cancer risk assessment. Genetic tests, in conjunction with family history information, can be used to a) clarify the diagnosis of inherited cancer syndromes in patients with tumors and b) provide information about cancer susceptibility to asymptomatic persons in high-risk families. The promise of cancer gene testing is reduced cancer incidence and mortality through directed prevention and screening.**
2. **In addition to the medical and health benefits of cancer gene testing, the power to identify high-risk persons has led to considerable discussion of the implications from consumer, epidemiologic, technologic, ethical, legal, policy, psychological, and genetic counseling perspectives.**
3. **Cancer gene testing can include a variety of modalities, including linkage, direct detection when the mutation is known, and mutation analysis, such as protein truncation test or sequencing. In addition, tests for microsatellite instability in colon tumors and gene expression assays may provide indirect evidence supporting a diagnosis of hereditary nonpolyposis colorectal cancer.**
4. **Commercial availability of germline cancer gene tests (i.e., BRCA1, BRCA2, APC, hMSH2, hMLH1, p16, NF2) has outpaced the awareness among health professionals of the need for careful implementation of testing algorithms and patient education on the issues.**
5. **Surveys of persons at varying risks for cancer show that most persons are interested in having a gene test. The actual uptake of cancer gene testing has been more modest; the decision to undergo gene testing is influenced by psychosocial factors, including perception of cancer risk, perceived ability to cope with gene test results, depression, and fear of insurance discrimination. Among persons who are tested, there appears to be no significant short-term (1–3 months) psychological distress following disclosure of results.**
6. **Cancer genetic risk assessment is a multistep process and incorporates medical, psychological, genetic, and counseling dimensions. Clinical indications and a model algorithm for cancer risk assessment and gene testing are provided. For persons who are at risk for cancer, gene test interpretation will depend upon whether the specific germline cancer gene mutation is known for the family. Careful evaluation of the pedigree for characteristic aggregation of tumor types among affected individuals and availability of affected persons for testing are important issues in implementing genetic testing.**
7. **Health professionals will need to be aware of the variety of issues that contribute to the process of helping patients to understand their risk, make informed decisions, and appreciate the implications for cancer prevention and risks for other family members. Genetic counseling is an essential component of cancer genetic risk assessment services.**

The translation of cancer gene discoveries into the clinical setting by the introduction of genetic testing has undergone a remarkable evolution in a few short years. Cancer genetic testing has become a significant focus from a variety of perspectives because it represents a potentially powerful means to identify high-risk individuals. From a medical and public health perspective, cancer genetic testing provides a more precise way to intervene with measures that may detect cancer at an earlier stage or to prevent cancer altogether. From a patient or consumer perspective, cancer genetic testing offers a new way to learn about individual and family cancer risk but also raises concern about job and insurance discrimination. From an epidemiologic perspective, cancer genetic testing provides a means to better understand the etiology of cancer through the interaction of genetic and environmental factors and to better characterize cancer risk. From the technologic perspective, cancer genetic testing represents an application that mandates development of faster and more cost-effective assays that are clinically valid. From the ethical, legal, and policy perspective, cancer genetic testing reinforces and recasts the basic premise that genetic information is different and requires special protection. Finally, from the psychological and counseling perspective, cancer genetic testing is part of a challenging multidimensional process that involves communication with patients about different types of risk information and requires that patients understand the implications, benefits, and risks.

The confluence of these perspectives and the intensity with which their proponents have addressed genetic testing are due to several factors: the inherent appeal of perceived benefit from cancer genetic knowledge, the potential impact on a broad segment of the population, and the concern that the public and health professional communities are unprepared for this new technology. In this nascent period of gene testing for cancer risk, few of the issues are fully resolved and many continue to arise. This chapter reviews cancer genetic testing from different perspectives and provides an overview of the current status of clinical cancer risk assessment and genetic testing.

PERSPECTIVES ON CANCER GENETIC TESTING

Medical and Public Health Perspective

The identification of genes that are responsible for hereditary forms of cancer has resulted in efforts to apply this knowledge clinically, primarily in the form of gene tests. There is no doubt that information derived from genetic testing will lead in many

Table 49-1 Hereditary syndromes with increased cancer risk and identified susceptibility genes and chromosomal localizations

Syndrome	Predominate Tumor Types	Chromosome	Gene	Reference
Ataxia telangiectasia	Breast cancer, chromosome breakage/rearrangement syndrome	11q22.3	*ATM*	154
Cowden disease	Multiple hamartomas of skin and mucous membranes, breast cancer, thyroid cancer, renal cell adenocarcinoma, dysplastic cerebellar gangliocytoma	10q23	*PTEN*	155, 156
Familial adenomatous polyposis	Multiple colorectal adenomas	5q21	*APC*	157, 158
Familial gastric cancer	Gastric cancer	16q22.1	*CDH1*	159
Familial melanoma	Melanoma, glioblastoma, lung cancer	9p21	*CDKN* [2]*(p16)*	160
Gorlin syndrome	Nevoid basal cell carcinoma of skin	9q	*NBCCS*	161–163
Hereditary breast-ovarian cancer syndrome	Breast, ovarian, prostate carcinoma; increased risk of other tumors	17q21 13q12–q13	*BRCA1* *BRCA2*	150, 151
Hereditary nonpolyposis colorectal cancer	Colon, endometrial, ovarian, stomach, small bowel, ureteral carcinomas	2p16 3p21 2q31–q33 7q11.2 2p16	*hMsh2* *hMLH1* *hPMS1* *hPMS2* *hMSH6*	81, 83 164
Hereditary prostate cancer	Prostate carcinoma	1q24–25 Xq27–28	*HPC1* *HPCX*	165, 166
Li-Fraumeni syndrome	Leukemia, soft-tissue sarcoma, osteosarcoma, brain tumor, breast and adrenal cortical carcinoma	17p13	*TP53*	167
Multiple endocrine neoplasia type 1	Parathyroid, endocrine pancreas, and pituitary tumors	11q	*MEN–1*	168
Multiple endocrine neoplasia type 2a	Medullary thyroid carcinoma, pheochromocytoma	10q11.2	*RET*	169
Multiple endocrine neoplasia type 2b	Familial medullary thyroid carcinoma	10q11.2	*RET*	170, 171
Neurofibromatosis type 1	Multiple peripheral neurofibromas, optic glioma, neurofibrosarcoma	17q11.2	*NF1*	172–176
Neurofibromatosis type 2	Central schwannomas and meningiomas, acoustic neuromas	22q11.2	*NF2*	177
Peutz-Jeghers syndrome	Multiple gastrointestinal tract polyps hamartomatous and adenomatus cancer of intestinal tract, pancreas, ovary, testis, breast, uterus	19p13.3	*STK11*	178, 179
Retinoblastoma	Retinoblastomas, osteosarcomas	13q14	*RB*	180, 181
von Hippel–Lindau syndrome	Renal cell carcinoma, pheochromocytoma, hemangioblastoma	3p25–p26	*VHL*	182

instances to an improvement in cancer risk assessment and clinical management of cancer patients and their families.[1,2] In conjunction with family history information, gene tests can be used to clarify the diagnosis of inherited cancer syndromes in patients with tumors and to provide information about cancer susceptibility to asymptomatic persons in high-risk families. Table 49-1 summarizes some hereditary cancer syndromes, detailed elsewhere in this volume, for which genetic testing can potentially improve cancer risk management of patients and their families.

Genetic testing for cancer holds the promise of reducing cancer mortality through timely screening and early intervention in those with predisposing mutations. The anticipated health benefits of testing rest on the assumption that persons at increased risk for cancer will be given options for preventive screening regimens or other interventions (such as prophylactic surgery or chemoprevention). Several decision analysis studies have evaluated the theoretical health and cost benefits of cancer gene testing for retinoblastoma[3] and familial adenomatous polyposis (FAP),[4,5] and those of management decisions (surveillance and prophylactic surgery) for hereditary breast cancer,[6,7] and hereditary colorectal cancer[8] and have generally found that the use of genetic test information or targeted interventions in cancer gene mutation carriers can be an improvement over conventional methods of cancer prevention. The parameters and construction of these decision analysis models vary, and some may only approximate the actual clinical situation, but they do appear to support the concept that genetic testing has a valid medical rationale.

It is becoming apparent that gene tests can and will change the way in which cancer risk assessment will be performed.[1,2,9–13] Indeed, certain gene tests (APC, RET, RB1, VHL) may now be considered part of the standard management of the respective hereditary cancer syndrome families, while the medical benefit of other gene tests (hMSH2, hMLH1, hPMS1, hPMS2, BRCA1, BRCA2, and p53) is presumed but not established.[14] The gene test outcome for an individual patient or at-risk family member can lead to more informed and directed recommendations for preventive interventions. As a general example, Fig. 49-1 illustrates the way in which colon cancer risk assessment has been conventionally performed. That is, health professionals often evaluate family histories of persons at risk for colon cancer who seek to learn their cancer risk but less often assess family histories of patients with colon cancer. Conventional risk assessment is based almost exclusively on evaluation of the family history, after which cancer screening recommendations can be made, tailored according to whether an inherited syndrome can be diagnosed. Fig. 49-2 illustrates a potential scenario in which colon cancer gene

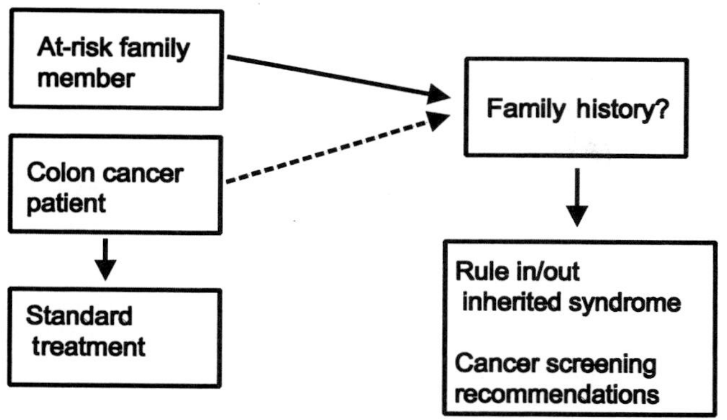

Fig. 49-1 Current view of conventional colon cancer risk assessment.

tests will alter this process. When gene tests are offered in conjunction with family history evaluation, not only will the two sources of information help make a firmer diagnosis, but clinical management of colon cancer patients may be influenced by this diagnosis. Likewise, more refined follow-up recommendations may be given to at-risk persons, whether they test positive or negative for a colon cancer gene. Genetic testing for cancer risk carries psychosocial implications that should be communicated through careful genetic counseling to persons considering cancer gene tests, both patients and family members. On one hand, genetic counseling will entail directive counseling toward cancer prevention where indicated, but on the other, it will entail communication about complex issues related to heredity, genetic test performance, probabilities, and uncertainty of outcome.

From the public health perspective, cancer gene discoveries may potentially be translated into genetic screening programs to identify high-risk groups to whom interventions (lifestyle modification, chemoprevention, or early detection) can be more effectively applied. There is agreement that much research is required prior to implementing any kind of public health program that involves genetic screening for cancer.[15–18] There is a need for more research into the issues surrounding technical and policy implications when applied to large-scale screening.[19] There is also a need to understand the frequency and attributable risks of cancer susceptibility genes and the efficacy and effectiveness of interventions in susceptible individuals, including examination of the premise that health prevention behaviors would be enhanced by knowledge of one's genetic susceptibility status. The difficulties are underscored by a recent study using decision analysis to investigate the role of genetic screening in cancer prevention. Grann and coworkers found that the theoretical cost-benefit ratio and survival rate would make screening all Ashkenazi Jewish women for specific BRCA1 and BRCA2 mutations cost-effective only if prophylactic surgery were performed on mutation carriers.[20]

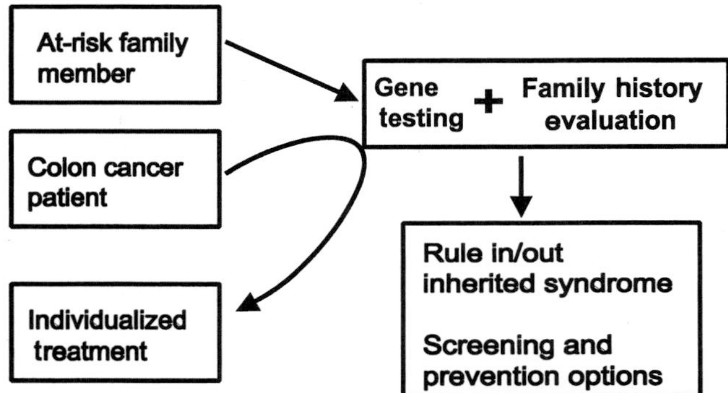

Fig. 49-2 Future view of colon cancer risk assessment.

Patient/Consumer Perspective

A variety of studies have found that there is great interest in cancer genetic testing across all risk groups, whether for breast, ovarian, prostate, or colon cancers.[21–29] Studies among first-degree relatives of cancer patients have found that when presented with the hypothetical possibility of cancer genetic testing, the majority of respondents probably or definitely want genetic testing. Cancer risk perception is increased among those with a positive family history, and these individuals may be more likely to choose genetic testing to learn more about their cancer risk.[25–31] Generally, those with a family history of a given disorder are more likely to engage in disease prevention behaviors for that disorder,[32–34] and most persons tend to overestimate their personal risk of cancer[25] or probability of carrying a cancer gene mutation.[35] Adherence to screening recommendations after genetic testing is likely to be associated with pre-genetic testing screening behavior[32–34,36] and with previous symptoms suggestive of cancer.[37]

In clinical and research experience, the reasons patients give for wanting cancer genetic testing are cancer worry and/or desire to know if more screening tests are needed (personal cancer risk concern), childbearing concerns or need to learn if one's children are at risk (concern for relatives), and wanting to take better care of oneself (general health concern).[30,31,38–41] As will be discussed later, there are a number of psychosocial factors that influence the actual decision to have a cancer gene test. Among those that can damp interest are perceived inability to cope with the gene test result and worry about insurance discrimination.

Epidemiologic Perspective

The epidemiologic challenges offered by genetic testing are threefold. First, it is necessary to understand the frequency, attributable risk, and heterogeneity of cancer-associated gene mutations. In general, the mutations in genes that are known to be associated with hereditary forms of cancer (e.g., breast cancer[42]) are not common, and obtaining estimates is complicated by the logistic difficulties of conducting population-based genetic testing, and by ethnic variation. For example, certain types of BRCA1, BRCA2, and APC mutations are more common in the Ashkenazi Jewish population,[43–45] and certain hMLH1 mutations are more common in the Finnish population, due to a founder effect.[46,47] In addition, it is recognized from a number of studies that not all hereditary forms of cancer are accounted for by the currently known genes.[48,49]

Second, the opportunity to understand genetic and nongenetic contributions to cancer causation is enhanced by the existence of persons, either with or without clinical manifestations of malignancy, who are known to carry cancer gene mutations. The respective roles of genes and environment may be more efficiently addressed in such defined risk groups. While studying more common polymorphisms of genes associated with metabolism of carcinogens has been one strategy to investigate this relationship, it may be increasingly possible to study high-penetrance cancer gene mutations. For example, Brunet and coworkers examined the relationship of smoking to breast cancer risk using only BRCA1 or BRCA2 mutation carriers and found a protective effect of smoking.[50] While this result contradicts our widespread understanding of the more typical harmful effect of smoking, this study design yielded an example of the type of knowledge that can be obtained from samples of gene-tested patients.

Third, the necessity to more carefully characterize and communicate cancer risk has been reinforced by cancer genetic testing.[51,52] In particular, there are two main ways in which risk associated with cancer gene mutations is usually given to patients: (1) *The probability that a person will carry a cancer gene mutation*, given information such as age, gender, ethnicity, and family history. A number of studies have investigated ways to estimate these risks and have obtained varying results, depending upon the subjects studied and the factors employed in computing risks.[53–56] Predictive models have been developed for hereditary breast and ovarian cancer[57–59] and for hereditary nonpolyposis colorectal cancer (HNPCC).[60] (2) *The probability that a mutation carrier is going to develop cancer* (also termed *lifetime risk* or *penetrance* of a gene mutation). These studies are more difficult to perform, but estimates have been made, using both high-risk samples and larger population studies.[44,61–63] As the volume of gene-tested persons increases, the current methods for computing risks will be refined to more accurately inform the risk assessment process.

Technology Perspective

Two of the most consistent patterns to emerge from genetic studies of inherited cancer syndromes are that there are many causal mutations in associated loci and that many families have unique mutations. Thus, testing laboratories will have to develop a variety of different strategies for detecting mutations in patients or diagnosing at-risk individuals in cancer-carrying families.[64–66] These tests range from linkage analysis[67–69] and single-stranded conformational polymorphism analysis[70] to protein truncation tests[71,72] and direct end-to-end DNA sequencing and allele specific oligonucleotide assays.[64] The relative merits and drawbacks of mutation detection approaches have been reviewed elsewhere,[64–66,73,74] and different laboratories vary in their strategies for gene testing. Potential new strategies include DNA chip technology,[64] conversion of diploidy to haploidy,[75] and mass spectrometry,[76] but it is unlikely that there will ever be tests that meet the ideal criteria for DNA-based genetic tests, as set forth by Eng and Vijg:[64] 100% sensitivity, 100% specificity, cost-effectiveness (< $100 per gene or combination of genes), throughput and speed of testing that fit into clinical laboratory routine, and being user friendly.

Because of the relatively high sophistication of current mutation analysis technology, it is not necessarily a simple process for the clinician to understand and interpret the potential implications of gene test results. The Task Force on Genetic Testing of the National Institutes of Health–Department of Energy Working Group on the Ethical, Legal, and Social Implications of Human Genome Research has set forth general principles on gene testing relative to gene test validation and testing laboratory quality control[77] and has proposed revisions to policies regulating laboratories that perform gene tests, which notably mandate the inclusion of clinical validation of tests.[78] This group argues that gene tests are different from other clinical tests because of the complexities in assessment and interpretation and that they require more intake information. In addition, it says health care providers must describe the features of the genetic test, including potential consequences, prior to testing. When a clearcut test result is obtained, either because a disease-predisposing mutation is detected (positive gene test) or because a mutation is not detected in an at-risk person from a family where a known mutation is segregating (true negative gene test), the subsequent counseling and management options are more apparent. Inconclusive or uninformative negative gene tests will occur when no mutation is detected in a cancer family but, because of the limitations of the testing method, a mutation in the tested locus (or elsewhere) cannot be ruled out. At-risk members in these families should not reduce their vigilance in cancer screening.

Tissue sources for clinical gene testing. The most common tissue source for gene testing is leukocyte DNA; a simple blood sample is often all that is required to perform a gene test. DNA obtained from paraffin-embedded tissue blocks obtained at surgery is also an option, if an affected relative is deceased or obtaining a blood sample is not feasible.

Specific tumor DNA studies may also yield information to aid in the diagnosis of inherited susceptibility to cancer. In the case of HNPCC, a special tumor analysis to identify microsatellite instability (MSI, also known as replication error [RER]) can be performed.[79,80] In this analysis, DNA from both normal tissue and tumor tissue is analyzed by highly polymorphic microsatellite DNA markers and their banding patterns compared. Allele alterations (band shifts) seen between tumor and normal DNA suggest that the patient may have an impaired ability to repair DNA, which is an indirect assessment of forms of HNPCC that are due to mutations in mismatch repair genes (hMSH2, hMLH1, hPMS1, and hPMS2).[79–83] Because MSI analysis is less time consuming and expensive than gene tests based on mutation analysis, it offers a useful first screening test for HNPCC.[55]

The utility of gene expression assays in tumors as an adjunct to germline mutation detection in a genetically heterogeneous syndrome has also been evaluated. For example, in the case of a suspected HNPCC mutation carrier whose tumor is MSI-positive, immunohistochemistry expression assays of hMSH2 and hMLH1 may help to identify which gene to sequence.[84,85] RNA expression assays of BRCA1 have been investigated as a means of screening for germline mutations.[86]

Commercial availability of testing. With the discovery of specific genes responsible for inherited cancer syndromes, commercial laboratories have been quick to invest in the development of marketable gene tests. Among the cancers that may affect a larger segment of the population, hereditary breast and ovarian cancer (*BRCA1, BRCA2*), HNPCC (*hMSH2, hMLH1*), FAP and its variants (*APC*), hereditary melanoma (*p16*), and neurofibromatosis type 2 (*NF2*) now have commercially available gene tests.[14,87–89]

The widening commercial availability of germline cancer gene tests has outpaced the awareness among health professionals of the need for careful implementation of testing algorithms and patient education on the issues.[88,89] There have been calls for caution in moving genetic tests out of the research labs and into the commercial labs[87,90–94] until their impact and the effectiveness of cancer prevention strategies can be studied. Specifically, some professional organizations advise that genetic testing and counseling for cancer risk may be safely integrated into clinical practice only after there have been studies of gene frequencies and associated cancer risks, test sensitivity and specificity, the efficacy of interventions for decreasing cancer morbidity and mortality, counseling methods, and genetic discrimination among those found to be at high risk.[92–94]

Ethical, Legal, and Policy Perspective

The ethical, legal, and policy issues in genetic testing have been discussed in numerous reviews and position statements,[92–103] and certain themes are emerging. Perhaps the most important overarching theme is that genetic information is different from other types of information (whether medical, demographic, or social), because of implications for future risk of disease and because of implications for other relatives. As a result, genetic testing that reveals intrinsic genetic status mandates special consideration.

As with all ethical dilemmas, there are no absolute right or wrong answers to many of the questions raised by cancer genetic testing. Inherent in medical and genetic service is the principle of beneficence. Discussions and decisions related to genetic testing can further be guided by the relevant principles of bioethics identified by the Committee on Assessing Genetic Risks of the National Academy of Sciences and Institute of Medicine,[91] including: respect for autonomy, privacy, confidentiality, and equity. These have implications for shaping how clinicians should approach and manage cancer patients and their families. Some common ethical issues for clinicians to consider are the right to know/not to know, sharing of genetic information, coercion by family members to participate in genetic testing, privacy of medical and genetic information, reproductive decision-making, and testing of minors.

The legal and social ramifications of genetic susceptibility testing for cancer are also taking shape. Some issues that may have

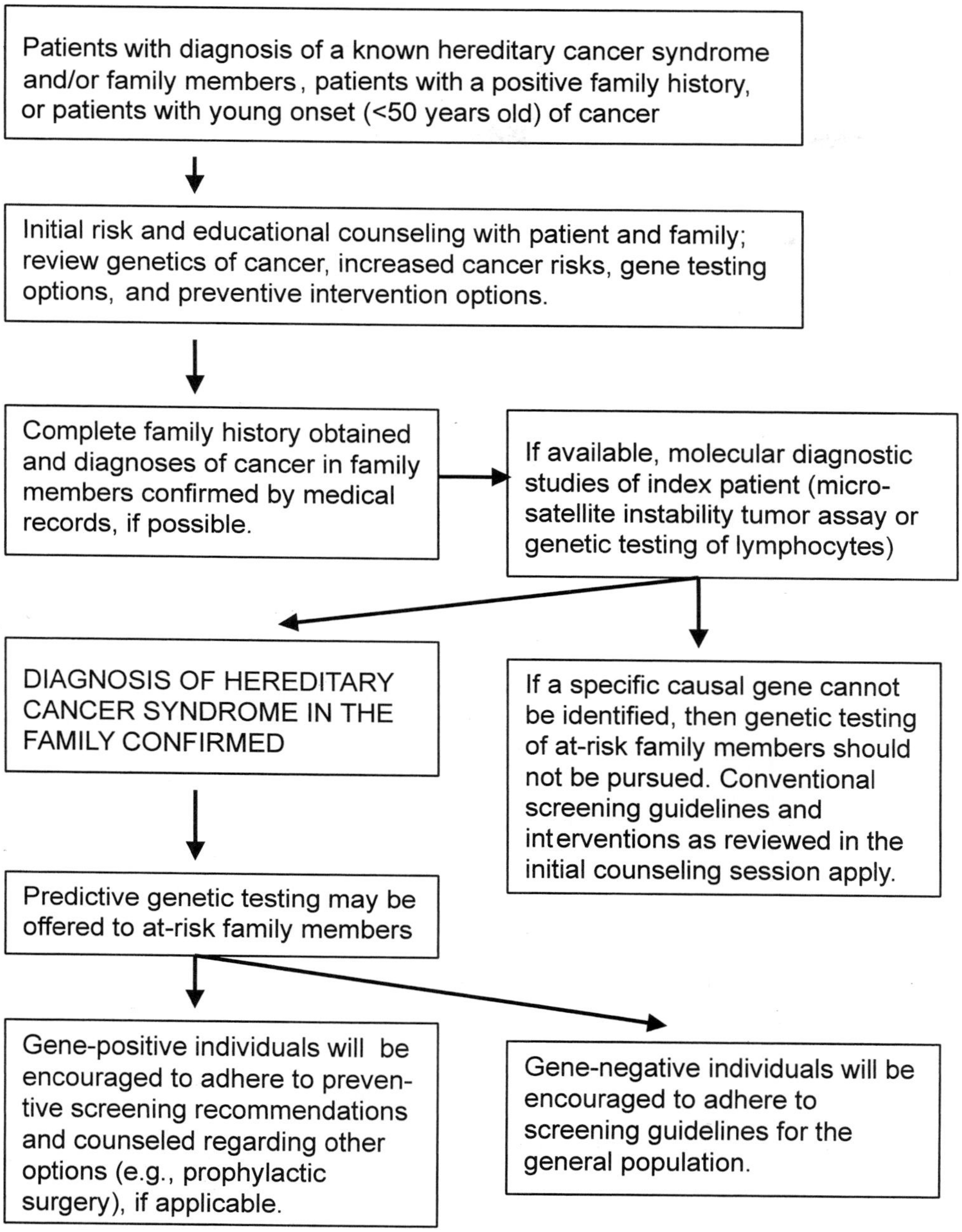

Patients with diagnosis of a known hereditary cancer syndrome and/or family members, patients with a positive family history, or patients with young onset (<50 years old) of cancer

↓

Initial risk and educational counseling with patient and family; review genetics of cancer, increased cancer risks, gene testing options, and preventive intervention options.

↓

Complete family history obtained and diagnoses of cancer in family members confirmed by medical records, if possible.

→ If available, molecular diagnostic studies of index patient (micro-satellite instability tumor assay or genetic testing of lymphocytes)

DIAGNOSIS OF HEREDITARY CANCER SYNDROME IN THE FAMILY CONFIRMED

If a specific causal gene cannot be identified, then genetic testing of at-risk family members should not be pursued. Conventional screening guidelines and interventions as reviewed in the initial counseling session apply.

↓

Predictive genetic testing may be offered to at-risk family members

Gene-positive individuals will be encouraged to adhere to preventive screening recommendations and counseled regarding other options (e.g., prophylactic surgery), if applicable.

Gene-negative individuals will be encouraged to adhere to screening guidelines for the general population.

Fig. 49-3 Basic algorithm for cancer risk assessment that employs gene testing.

legal implications for clinicians are disclosing benefits, risks, and limitations of cancer genetic testing; following up and recontacting patients and family members when new information emerges; maintaining confidentiality of genetic information; and warning of inherited cancer risk ("genetic transferability") to others.

Privacy of genetic information. Genetic information should be considered confidential, and it is incumbent upon health professionals and laboratories to exercise all means of preventing unauthorized disclosure of gene test results to third parties. In practice, it is recommended that results should be released only to those individuals to whom the patient has consented or requested in writing to have them released, and care should be taken to minimize the likelihood that results will become available to unauthorized persons or organizations.[77] Garber and Patenaude point out, however, that physicians may breach confidentiality unintentionally by placing information in medical charts that may be reviewed by insurers or other third parties.[96] The dilemma is that omitting this information compromises the patient's future medical care, yet including the information would compromise the ability of the patient or family members to obtain health, life, or disability insurance (and therefore coverage for preventive screening tests or procedures).

Another crucial issue is the revelation of gene test results to family members. As shown in Fig. 49-3, the optimal algorithm for gene testing of at-risk persons is to first test a family member who is affected with cancer; this patient must be willing to have the resulting genetic information shared with relatives. It is an important principle of gene testing that health care providers have an obligation to the person being tested not to inform other family members without the permission of the person tested.[77,91] There are also circumstances in which certain individuals may not want their test results known, yet by virtue of the pedigree structure this information will become known (e.g., an identical twin of a gene-positive patient); or family members may refuse to have their gene test results shared. The resolution of these issues may not always be easy, but it will call for careful planning and thorough genetic counseling with the family members involved, well before gene test results are made available.[103–105]

Risk of genetic discrimination. Persons at risk for cancer face other risks in the form of genetic discrimination (insurance, employment, educational, or other opportunities). Insurance companies may use genetic information, much as they use any other medical information, to underwrite an insurance policy. In these cases, insurance companies may deny insurance to those whom they consider to be at too great a risk for an illness or to those with pre-existing conditions.[106,107] Such denials are predicted to become more commonplace as new predisposition tests are developed.[108,109] Billings *et al.*[108] and Lapham *et al.*[107] have identified cases in which insurance or employment discrimination has occurred. They found discrimination against the "asymptomatic ill"—those with a genetic predisposition who remain healthy—who usually lost their insurance after undertaking preventive care. Overall, the problems encountered included difficulty obtaining coverage, finding or retaining employment, and being given permission for adoptions. Insurance problems often arose when people tried to alter existing policies because of relocations or job changes. Information provided by physicians often had little or no influence on the adverse outcomes. Many people dealt with this by giving incomplete or dishonest information.[107,108]

With respect to discrimination in the workplace, there may be risk of loss of employability if gene status or genetic risk of cancer is known or required by employers.[110] Recent attempts to remedy this include laws to protect access to health insurance, including the Health Insurance Portability and Accountability Act, which took effect in July 1997; protection of access to employment by an interpretation of the Americans with Disabilities Act of 1990 to include genetic information, and state laws to prevent genetic information from being used in employment considerations.

Psychological and Genetic Counseling Perspective.

The areas of psychological importance in cancer genetic testing include interest in and uptake of testing, impact of both positive and negative gene test results on cancer prevention behaviors and interventions (e.g., prophylactic surgery), and genetic testing of children.[111]

Uptake of cancer genetic testing. It has been observed in a number of studies that while interest in a hypothetical cancer gene test may be high, the actual uptake rates are more modest, even when persons are offered the gene test at no monetary cost. A person's decision to have a gene test is affected by a number of factors, including demographic, psychological, social, and personality.[38–41,112,113] Indeed, research suggests that psychological rather than medical factors appear to predominate in decisions about genetic testing. For example, Codori and coworkers[38] found that strength of cancer family history did not predict a patient's decision to be tested for HNPCC. Instead, tested persons had greater perceived confidence in their ability to cope with a positive test, thought more frequently about cancer, and had greater perceived risk for developing colorectal cancer. Of some concern was the fact that gene test decliners also were less likely to have had a colonoscopy, leading the authors to posit that those who choose not to take cancer gene tests may also be those who are unlikely to undertake the surveillance interventions. Bowen *et al.* suggest that while clinicians may think of the benefit of genetic testing as a medical decision, the predominance of emotion and self-perception of risk may lead to difficulties in patient-provider communication.[114] To overcome this barrier, some at-risk persons may need more psychological support and counseling to increase perceived ability to handle unfavorable medical information. One lesson from the research thus far is that recognition of psychologically vulnerable persons may require different or tailored genetic counseling to prompt appropriate screening behaviors in those persons who might otherwise avoid screening.

Psychological consequences of positive gene tests. A favorable balance of health benefits versus costs depends on determining whether the medical benefits will outweigh any psychological "side effects." For at-risk persons, cancer gene testing is not without potential side effects, as it may pose risks to psychological well-being and to the very cancer prevention practices it is meant to promote. These risks derive from several factors, including the predictable stress reaction that can follow the delivery of unfavorable medical information.

Surveys of persons at risk for cancer have shown that they expect significant distress in the face of a positive cancer gene test. Eighty percent of 121 female first-degree relatives of ovarian cancer patients reported that they would become depressed if they tested positive for a breast cancer mutation; 77 percent reported that they would become anxious.[30] Similarly, 60 percent of male and female first-degree relatives of colon cancer patients reportedly expected to become depressed and 52 percent anxious upon receiving a positive gene test.[31] It is possible that distress caused by a positive gene test may interfere with subsequent preventive health behavior. This has been shown in other situations: Of women notified of an abnormal mammogram, those who experienced high levels of psychological distress after notification were less likely to perform subsequent breast self-exam than those with moderate levels of distress;[115] persons psychologically distressed after having been notified of their risk for hypertension adhered less to their medication regimens;[116] and distressed persons delay seeking medical attention for possible cancer symptoms[117]

There is concern that persons distressed by their cancer risk will make irrevocable decisions to have unproven prophylactic surgeries.[118] This prediction has some support from a study of first-degree relatives of breast cancer patients. Those who subsequently chose prophylactic mastectomy were more anxious and had higher levels of cancer worry than women who later chose continued screening or a chemoprevention trial.[119] The finding suggests that women undertake prophylactic surgery to more fully eliminate their cancer risk. However, prophylactic mastectomy, while effective,[120] does not eliminate breast cancer risk,[121,122] and some of the women studied may never develop cancer. Moreover, basing decisions on probabilistic genetic information means that short-term relief from cancer worry could be followed by regret if later, more definitive information reveals that the surgery was unnecessary.

A positive genetic test can have favorable psychological consequences, including removal of uncertainty and being better able to prepare for future events, as has been seen in Huntington disease[123,124] and FAP.[10] Surveys of persons at risk for cancer suggest that they anticipate benefits from "bad news." For example, 68 percent of first-degree relatives of ovarian cancer patients reported that they would feel more "in control" of their lives even if they tested positive.[125] Several studies that measured psychological parameters at baseline and 1 to 3 months following gene testing have found no adverse reactions in persons who received positive test results: Lerman *et al.* studied 279 male and female members of *BRCA1*-linked hereditary breast and ovarian cancer families and found no short-term increased depression or functional impairment in those who tested gene positive.[112] Croyle and coworkers found that distress declines after gene testing but that women who are mutation positive for *BRCA1* experience more distress than noncarriers in followup.[126] In a study of 42 children at risk for FAP and their parents, Codori *et al.* also did not observe any significant increase in distress or behavioral problems in the gene-positive children.[127] The response to genetic testing is likely complex,[128] and research to examine these observations in the context of longer-term impact are ongoing.

Psychological Consequences of Negative Gene Tests. Those whose receive negative gene tests often experience relief at removal of uncertainty and doubt.[10,112,127] These persons are likely to be spared anxiety-provoking,[10,129] costly, and sometimes invasive screening procedures and to be relieved to know that their children's and their own personal risk for cancer is no greater than in the general population.

It is possible that some proportion of those who learn that they do not carry the cancer gene mutation in their family are at risk for psychological distress. In Huntington disease, "survivor guilt" was reported in 25 percent of people who tested negative,[130] and individual cases of depression and marital disruption have been reported.[130,131] Twenty-five percent of persons at risk for colon cancer predict feeling guilty, and 50 percent expect to continue worrying about cancer even after learning that they are noncarriers.[31] Similar rates were reported by women at risk for breast and ovarian cancer.[125]

Genetic Testing of Children. There has been debate on the appropriateness of genetic testing of minors, particularly for cancers that have their onset later in adulthood or for which there is no intervention to change the outcome. The medical and legal ramifications need to be explored and the interests of the children and their parents weighed.[91,132] Issues to consider include assessment of the significance of the potential benefits and harms of the gene test, determination of the decision-making capacity of the child, and advocacy on behalf of the child.[132,133] Certainly, the medical benefit to the child should be the primary justification for gene testing of children.

Certain hereditary cancer syndromes (e.g., multiple endocrine neoplasia type 2, FAP, retinoblastoma) involve onset of tumors in childhood and warrant genetic testing of children[10,12,134,135] because interventions are feasible.[91] Genetic testing of children requires special counseling adjusted to their age level, taking into consideration their awareness of cancer risk and perceptions of family attitudes toward cancer.[10] While screening and prophylactic surgery for gene-positive persons are currently available modalities, there is potential for chemoprevention or other interventions for which initiation in childhood would be most effective.[136] This would reopen the issue of performing gene tests in childhood for cancer syndromes that have their onset in adulthood.[9]

In summary, the available data suggest that interest in cancer gene testing may be high but that actual uptake may be more modest, being affected by psychological factors. The data also suggest that there may be psychological risks from cancer genetic testing, including emotional distress from positive and negative test results, unintended and inappropriate decreases in cancer screening behavior, irrevocable decisions made in a state of anxiety, false reassurances about cancer risk, distressing and unwanted genetic knowledge, and insurance and employment discrimination. These issues warrant carefully planned implementation of testing protocols. These factors, in large measure, call for sensitive, thorough preparation and follow-up, including education and psychological evaluation and support.

CURRENT STATUS OF CANCER RISK ASSESSMENT AND GENETIC TESTING

Cancer Risk Assessment Clinical Services

Within the last several years, there have been numerous clinical initiatives to provide cancer genetic risk assessment and genetic testing services.[137–140] Many are located in major medical university or comprehensive cancer center settings, but an increasing number of health professionals in health maintenance organization and private practice settings have begun to offer cancer genetic testing. While clinical geneticists and genetic counselors can provide this service, it is more often the case that the medical specialties that are generally associated with treatment of cancer have begun to recognize the importance of providing this component of a comprehensive service to their patients. In particular, professional societies of clinical oncologists, surgeons, and oncology nurses have initiated educational programs to keep their members current.[141–144]

The cancer risk assessment service is interdisciplinary (medicine, genetics, genetic counseling) and at a minimum should include a physician (oncologist or clinical geneticist), and genetic counselor, or nurse/nurse practitioner with cancer genetics experience. The service should have access to resource support personnel, including social workers, psychologists, specialists in cancer treatment and management, and ethicists, and to genetic testing laboratories certified under Clinical Laboratory Improvement Act (CLIA) regulations.

Indications for Cancer Risk Assessment

The increased understanding of the relationship of clinical features, epidemiology, and aggregation of cancers in families has allowed the compilation of guidelines to clues for clinicians that would warrant further evaluation for familial or hereditary cancer:[1,13,137]

- A cancer occurring at an unusually young age compared with the usual presentation of that type of cancer
- Multifocal development of cancer in a single organ or bilateral development of cancer in paired organs
- Development of more than one primary tumor of any type in a single individual
- Family history of cancer of the same type in a close relative(s)
- High rate of cancer within a family
- Occurrence of cancer in an individual or a family exhibiting congenital anomalies or birth defects
- Ashkenazi Jewish heritage
- Family known to segregate a hereditary gene mutation

More recently, resources for clinical cancer genetics have become available, in the form of both textbooks[1,13] and handbooks,[137] Internet-based resources and government-sponsored programs, such as the National Cancer Institute's Cancer Genetics Network, Cancer Information Service, and the Physician Data Query (PDQ) database, are other emerging new resources (Table 49-2).

Indications for Cancer Gene Tests

At this time, cancer gene tests have two primary clinical applications. When affected individuals are tested, gene tests may be used to molecularly diagnose an inherited cancer syndrome. When asymptomatic persons are tested, gene tests may be used to identify whether or not they are at increased risk because they carry a known predisposing mutation. The appropriate use of gene tests, particularly in determining who should be tested, is relatively straightforward in clearcut hereditary cancer syndrome families. However, this distinction is rapidly becoming blurred as further characterization of cancer gene loci appears to indicate that gene tests may be used for familial cancers due to mutations associated with lower penetrance in families that do not fit known criteria for hereditary syndromes, or for screening specific populations in which cancer susceptibility genes occur at high frequency.

Testing Affected Individuals to Clarify the Diagnosis. A patient with cancer might be offered gene testing to rule in or out a suspected inherited syndrome. In this case, there may be indications from family history or from clustering of specific tumors in family members suggestive of a hereditary syndrome (such as leukemia, soft-tissue sarcoma, brain tumors, or breast cancer in Li-Fraumeni syndrome[145]). Table 49-1 lists some of the tumor types that are associated with known cancer syndromes. Gene tests may also be offered to patients with apparently sporadic cancer if the cancer occurs at an unusually young age or if the patient has other stigmata suggestive of a hereditary syndrome. For

Table 49-2 Internet-Based Cancer Genetics Resources

Resource	Internet (Web Page) Address	Description
Alliance of Genetic Support Group	http://www.geneticalliance.org/index.html	Nonprofit organization that addresses the concerns of people with, and at risk for, genetic conditions.
American Cancer Society	http://www.cancer.org/	Nationally recognized non profit organization site contains a variety of information on cancer.
Association of Cancer Online Resources – Breast Cancer Information Clearinghouse	http://www.acor.org/	Established in 1994, this contains a directory of organizations that provide information and support for breast cancer patients and their families and access to online discussion groups.
Avon Breast Cancer Awareness Crusade	http://www.avoncrusade.com/	Avon's Internet crusade to provide more women, particularly low-income, minority, and older women, with access to breast cancer education and early detection screening services.
Cancer and Genetics	http://www.cancergenetics.org/	The Robert H. Lurie Comprehensive Cancer Center of Northwestern University site contains information for the genral public, primary care physician, nurse practitioners, and other health care professionals.
Cancer Genetics Network	http://www.-dccps.ims.nci.nih.gov/CGN/	Newly established network sponsored by the National Cancer Institute.
Cancer Information Network	http://www.cancernetwork.com/	Containing separate sections for professional and patients, this site is a good source of facts and news on various cancers.
Cancer information Service	http://cis.nih.gov/	Sponsored by the National Cancer Institute, this site is the home of the national information and education network, available at 1-800-4-CANCER, that provides the most up-to-date and accurate information on cancer.
CancerNet	http://cancernet.nci.nih.gov/	Sponsored by the National Cancer Institute, this site provides access to several NCI databases, including the PDQ (Physician Data Query) and Cancerlit.
Clinical Genetics: Information for Genetic Professionals	http://www.kumc.edu/gec/geneinfo.html	University of Kansas Medical Center site contains clinical, research, and educational resources for genetics professionals.
Division of Cancer Epidemiology and Genetics	http://www-dceg.ims.nci.nih.gov/index.html	Part of the National Cancer Institute, this site contains information on population-based research on environmental and genetic determinants of cancer.
ELSI	http://www.nhgri.nih.gov/ELSI/	The Ethical, Legal, and Social Implications program is a branch of the National Human Genome Research Institute, established in 1990 to address issues related to human gene mapping research.
Healthfinder	http://www.healthfinder.gov/	Developed by the U.S. Department of Health and Human Services, this site contains links to over 1400 health-related sites.
Human Genome Project	http://www.nhgri.nih.gov/HGP/	Home of the international effort to determine the DNA sequence of the entire human genome.
InteliHealth	http://www.intelihealth.com/IH/ihtlH	Developed by Aetna U.S. Healthcare and the Johns Hopkins University Hospital and Health System, this comprehensive site contains information for both consumers and professional.
International Collaborative Group on Hereditary Non-polyposis Colorectal Cancer	http://www.nfdht.nl/	Mainly for physicians and researchers, this site contains a mutation database and a set of clinical guidelines.
Johns Hopkins Breast Center	http://www.med.jhu.edu/breastcenter/	This site is the Internet link to the Johns Hopkins Oncology Center, a National Cancer institute–designated Comprehensive Cancer Center.
Johns Hopkins Colon Cancer Center	http://www.hopkins-coloncancer.org/	This site is the Internet link to the Johns Hopkins Breast Cancer Center, part of the Johns Hopkins Oncology Center, a National Cancer Institute–designated Comprehensive Cancer Center
Medscape Oncology	http://oncology.medscape.com/Home/Topics//oncology.html	A commercial, comprehensive web service for both clinicians and consumers.
National Cancer Institute	http://www.nci.nih.gov/	The U.S. goverment's primary agency for cancer research and training.
National Institutes of Health	http://www.nih.gov/	One of eight agencies that make up the Public Health Service in the Department of Health and Human Services.
Office of Genetics and Disease Prevention	http://www.cdc.gov/genetics/	Maintained by the Centers for Disease Control and Prevention, this site contains information on the impact of human genetic research and the Human Genome Project on public health and disease prevention, including HuGE Net.

Table 49-2 (Continued).

Resource	Internet (Web page) Address	Description
OncoLink: Genetics and Cancer	http://Oncolink.upenn.edu/causeprevent/genetics/	Part of the University of Pennsylvania Cancer Center OncoLink site.
Principles and Recommendation: Task Force on Genetic Testing	http://www.med.jhu.edu/tfgtelsi/promoting/	Final report of the Task Force on Genetic Testing, a workiong group of the National Institutes of Health and Department of Energy human genome programs.
The Susen G. Komen Foundation	http:/www.komen.org	For both patients and professionals, this site contains information on breast cancer detection and coping as well as grant and funding opportunities.
US TOO International, Inc.	http://www..ustoo.com/	Home to the largest prostate cancer support group in the world, this site provides access to information on prostate cancer and to counseling and educational meetings.

example, FAP might be suspected in a patient who has multiple colonic adenomas, congenital hypertrophy of the retinal pigment epithelium, and desmoid tumor[146] but no family history of colon polyps or cancer. *APC* gene testing is an indicated diagnostic test, as such a patient could have a *de novo* mutation in the *APC* gene.[147] If the *APC* gene test is positive, the patient can be presumed to have FAP and his or her children to be at 50 percent risk for inheriting the mutation.

Because genetic heterogeneity is seen in some hereditary cancer phenotypes, gene tests may be used help to identify the specific locus that is involved. For example, Turcot syndrome, a rare colon polyposis/cancer syndrome associated with central nervous system malignancies, has been shown to be genetically heterogeneous, with at least three loci (*APC, hMLH1,* and *hPMS2*) that independently produce a similar clinical picture.[148] Patients from suspected hereditary breast cancer families may need to be tested for at least two genes, *BRCA1* and *BRCA2*, because both genes may produce similar family histories.[149–151]

Testing At-risk Individuals for Inherited Susceptibility to Cancer. Asymptomatic at-risk persons from known hereditary cancer syndrome families may benefit from gene testing. In particular, when a mutation in a cancer gene is known to be segregating in the family, at-risk persons who test negative for the mutation may be relieved of years of surveillance, while persons who test positive for the mutation may approach the screening regimen with greater willingness to adhere to the recommendations.

When a mutation is not known to segregate in a cancer family, or if the diagnosis of a cancer syndrome is less clearcut, gene testing of at-risk persons in these families is more problematic. Often there is not a living family member with cancer who can undergo gene testing to identify the mutation. In such instances a negative gene test result in an at-risk person is not a "true" negative result that places him or her at the general population's risk for that cancer. Rather, this person has an "inconclusive" or "uninformative" negative test result that does not rule out other cancer gene loci, or even other mutations in the tested locus that the gene test was not able to detect. A person receiving an inconclusive test result should continue to maintain a cancer surveillance regimen as though no gene test was ever done.

Cancer Genetic Risk Assessment Process

The risk assessment process has multiple steps and incorporates multiple dimensions: medicine, psychology, genetics, and counseling. Health professionals trained in cancer genetics will need to have an awareness of the variety of issues that contribute to the process of helping patients to understand their risk, make informed decisions, and appreciate the implications for cancer prevention and risks for other family members.

Algorithm for genetic testing. With due consideration given to the issues surrounding cancer gene testing, a basic algorithm for integrating gene tests in cancer risk assessment can be constructed (Fig. 49-3). In this algorithm, eligible persons might include patients with a diagnosis of a known hereditary cancer syndrome and/or family members, patients with a positive family history, and patients with young onset of cancer (generally before age 50). Such patients should receive initial face-to-face counseling about cancer risk, with an educational component that includes a review of the genetics of the specific cancer(s) relevant to the patient, factors influencing increased cancer risk, and preventive intervention options, all adjusted to each patient's level of understanding. If it has not already been done, a detailed family history should be elicited and follow-up confirmation of cancer diagnoses in family members obtained, if possible.

The novel aspect of cancer risk assessment is genetic testing. The gene test may consist of mutation analysis or of tumor analysis for microsatellite instability (in the case of colorectal cancer). Following initial counseling, a careful explanation of the risks and benefits of the gene test should be given to the patient, with ample opportunity to check understanding and to answer questions or concerns. Genetic testing may not necessarily be the best option for some patients or families and should be entered into voluntarily, after careful deliberation on the implications.

If a specific causal gene mutation cannot be identified, then genetic testing of at-risk family members should not be pursued. Conventional screening guidelines and interventions as reviewed in the initial counseling session apply. If a specific causal gene mutation is identified, then the diagnosis of the corresponding hereditary cancer syndrome can be confirmed. In this instance, genetic counseling and predictive gene testing may be offered to at-risk family members who may wish to have this test done.

If an at-risk person tests positive for the gene, then he or she will be encouraged to adhere to preventive screening recommendations specific to the hereditary syndrome and counseled regarding other options, such as prophylactic surgery or chemoprevention, if applicable. In the case of FAP, hereditary breast and ovarian cancer, and HNPCC, recommendations have been developed, mostly based on expert opinion.[1,122,147,152]

If an at-risk person from a family in which the mutation in the cancer gene is known to segregate tests negative for the mutation, then he or she will be encouraged to adhere to cancer screening guidelines for the general population.

Genetic counseling in cancer gene testing. *Genetic counseling must accompany genetic testing, because of the implications for family members and for reproductive decision-making.* While a conventional, non genetic diagnostic test pertains primarily to the health of the person who has been tested, a genetic test often has implications for the health of other relatives, such as offspring, parents, and siblings. For example, a person who learns that he or she has a gene for an autosomal dominant form of cancer immediately knows that all of his or her offspring have a 50 percent risk of having inherited the mutation and his or her grandchildren a 25 percent risk. When an affected person tests positive, without prior evidence that the cancer was hereditary, the entire family may be suddenly suspected to be at increased risk for cancer. An identical twin cannot be tested without automatically revealing the co-twin's status, whether or not she or he wants the information. Similarly, a person at 25 percent risk for cancer (i.e., with an affected grandparent and healthy at-risk parent) who tests positive for the mutation automatically reveals a genetic diagnosis to the at-risk parent. Thus, genetic information may have serious implications for many persons who were not even tested.

Pre-test Counseling. *Genetic counseling accompanying gene tests for inherited cancer risk should include*:

a) Educating the family about the clinical and management aspects of hereditary cancer, the risks of cancer within the syndrome, and the consequences of receiving gene-positive or gene-negative test results, including the recommended screening guidelines for each possible test outcome.

b) Exploration of the issues related to the family history and experiences with cancer. These experiences can be multigenerational and include quite personal involvement with relatives who have died from cancer and/or who had oncologic or surgical interventions. Family relationships can be profoundly marked by issues such as guilt and blame, and personal and familial identity may be strongly linked with cancer status. Other issues include the denial of disease risk or stigmatization of cancer within the family and the acceptability, convenience, and affordability of screening regimens. Thus, genetic testing is imbued with meaning for certain patients far beyond its function as a simple determiner of genetic status. The at-risk patient may have pre-formed, well-entrenched conceptions of what having cancer entails, and family relationships and identity may be strongly linked with disease or gene status. Understanding of the patient's perspective is crucial so that it can be taken into account in assisting her or him to adjust to genetic test results.

c) Exploration of the perception of risk and its meaning and anticipated meaning of any test results. With parents of at-risk minor children, time should also be devoted to discussing how and when the test results and risk will be communicated to the children. In certain countries, employability or loss of insurability (life or health) is a risk, although the magnitude of this risk is at present unknown.

Informed Consent for Gene Testing. The decision to move forward with the gene test should be freely made by the at-risk person after carefully considering the consequences of genetic testing. It is strongly recommended that a consent form that outlines the meaning of test results and the consequences of the gene test be utilized.[14,77,91,153] If patients are to make fully informed decisions about gene testing, the informed consent process must include discussions of several complex issues, listed below. This is a time-consuming process and can require at least an hour of counseling time. The genetic counseling process that accompanies gene testing should incorporate the basic elements of informed consent, including:[14,153]

- Information on the specific test being performed
- Implications of a positive and a negative result
- Possibility that the test will not be informative
- Options for risk estimation without genetic testing
- Risk of passing a mutation to children
- Technical accuracy of the test
- Fees involved in testing and counseling
- Risks of psychological distress
- Risks of insurance or employer discrimination
- Confidentiality issues
- Options for and limitations of medical surveillance and screening following testing

Disclosure and Post-disclosure Counseling. Disclosure of gene test results, which can occur 2 weeks to 2 months later, depending upon the laboratory, provides another opportunity to meet again with the at-risk family member, explore the meaning of the test, and discuss in a more substantial way the likely follow-up regimen and cancer risks to future offspring.

For persons who test positive for the tested cancer gene, we recommend a third, follow-up session (either by telephone or in person), in which the patient is allowed a second opportunity, free from the initial emotional reaction to the test result, to ask questions about clinical management and the clinician can determine if referral to a mental health professional for additional support is indicated.

SUMMARY

In summary, new research developments in the molecular genetics of cancer have led to the feasibility of cancer genetic testing for many patients and family members. Gene tests have the potential to identify high-risk persons, and gene tests results will have clinical implications for cancer risk management: Conventional preventive recommendations can be modified in light of gene test results such that those at higher risk for cancer (gene positive) will be identified for increased cancer surveillance, while those at lower risk (true gene negative) may be reassured. There is a very real potential for misinterpretation of inconclusive gene test results. The new genetic technology also has psychosocial consequences for patients and families and ethical, legal, and policy implications for health care providers. Genetic counseling is an important added component in cancer risk assessment and management, particularly in helping those at risk to understand the variety of implications gene test results have in the context of their experience with cancer and intervention options.

REFERENCES

1. Offit K: *Clinical Cancer Genetics: Risk Counseling and Management*. New York, Wiley-Liss, 1998.
2. Ponder B: Genetic testing for cancer risk. *Science* **278**:1050, 1997.
3. Noorani HZ, Khan HN, Gallie BL, Detsky AS: Cost comparison of molecular versus conventional screening of relatives at risk for retinoblastoma. *Am J Hum Genet* **59**:301, 1996.
4. Cromwell DM, Moore RD, Brensinger JD, Petersen GM, Bass EB, Giardiello FM: Cost analysis of alternative approaches to colorectal screening in familial adenomatous polyposis. *Gastroenterology* **114**:893, 1998.
5. Bapat B, Noorani H, Cohen Z, Berk T, Mitri A, Gallie B, Pritzker K, et al: Cost comparison of predictive genetic testing versus conventional screening for familial adenomatous polyposis. *Gut* **44**:698, 1999.
6. Schrag D, Kuntz KM, Garber JE, Weeks JC: Decision analysis—effects of prophylactic mastectomy and oophorectomy on life expectancy among women with BRCA1 or BRCA2 mutations. *N Engl J Med* **336**:1465, 1997.
7. Grann VR, Panageas KS, Whang W, Antman KH, Neugut AI: Decision analysis of prophylactic mastectomy and oophorectomy in BRCA1-positive or BRCA2-positive patients. *J Clin Oncol* **16**:979, 1998.
8. Syngal S, Weeks JC, Schrag D, Garber JE, Kuntz KM: Benefits of colonoscopic surveillance and prophylactic colectomy in patients with hereditary nonpolyposis colorectal cancer mutations. *Ann Intern Med* **129**:787, 1998.
9. Knudson AG: Hereditary cancers: from discovery to intervention. *J Natl Inst Cancer Monogr* **17**:5, 1995.
10. Petersen GM, Boyd PA: Gene tests and counseling for colorectal cancer risk: Lessons from familial polyposis. *J Natl Inst Cancer Monogr* **17**:67, 1995.
11. Li FP, Garber JE, Friend SH, Strong LC, Patenaude AF, Juengst ET, Reilly PR, et al: Recommendations on predictive testing for germ line p53 mutations among cancer-prone individuals. *J Natl Cancer Inst* **84**:1156, 1992.
12. Neumann HPH, Eng C, Mulligan LM, Glavac D, Zäuner I, Ponder BAJ, Crossey PA, et al: Consequences of direct genetic testing for

germline mutations in the clinical management of families with multiple endocrine neoplasia, type II. *JAMA* **274**:1149, 1995.

13. Hodgson SV, Maher ER: *A Practical Guide to Human Cancer Genetics*. Cambridge, Cambridge University Press, 1993.
14. Statement of the American Society of Clinical Oncology: Genetic testing for cancer susceptibility. *J Clin Oncol* **14**:1730, 1996.
15. Li FP: Cancer control in susceptible groups: Opportunities and challenges. *J Clin Oncol* **17**:719, 1999.
16. Khoury MJ: Genetic epidemiology and the future of disease prevention and public health. *Epidemiol Rev* **19**:175, 1997.
17. Perera FP: Environment and cancer: Who are susceptible? *Science* **278**:1068, 1997.
18. Kelloff GJ, Boone CW, Crowell JA, Nayfield SG, Hawk E, Malone WF, Steele VE, et al: Risk biomarkers and current strategies for cancer chemoprevention. *J Cell Biochem Suppl* **25**:1, 1996.
19. Holtzman NA: Scale-up technology: Moving predictive tests for inherited breast, ovarian, and colon cancers from the bench to the bedside and beyond. *J Natl Cancer Inst Monogr* **17**:95, 1995.
20. Grann VR, Whang W, Jacobson JS, Heitjan DF, Antman KH, Neugut AI: Benefits and costs of screening Ashkenazi Jewish women for BRCA1 and BRCA2. *J Clin Oncol* **17**:494, 1999.
21. Tambor ES, Rimer BK, Strigo TS: Genetic testing for breast cancer susceptibility: Awareness and interest among women in the general population. *Am J Med Genet* **68**:43, 1997.
22. Andrykowski MA, Munn RK, Studts JL: Interest in learning of personal genetic risk for cancer: A general population survey. *Prev Med* **25**:527, 1996.
23. Lerman C, Seay J, Balshem A, Audrain J: Interest in genetic testing among first-degree relatives of breast cancer patients. *Am J Med Genet* **57**:385, 1995.
24. Graham ID, Logan DM, Hughes-Benzie R, Evans WK, Perras H, McAuley LM, Laupacis A, Stern H: How interested is the public in genetic testing for colon cancer susceptibility? Report of a cross-sectional population survey. *Cancer Prev Control* **2**:167, 1998.
25. Petersen GM, Larkin E, Codori A-M, Wang C-Y, Booker SV, Bacon J, Giardiello FM, Boyd PA: Attitudes toward colon cancer gene testing: Survey of relatives of colon cancer patients. *Cancer Epidemiol Biomark Prev* **8**:337, 1999.
26. Glanz K, Grove J, Lerman C, Gotay C, Le Marchand L: Correlates of intentions to obtain genetic counseling and colorectal cancer gene testing among at-risk relatives from three ethnic groups. *Cancer Epidemiol Biomark Prev* **8**:329, 1999.
27. Smith KR, Croyle RT: Attitudes toward genetic testing for colon cancer risk. *Am J Public Health* **85**:1435, 1995.
28. Struewing JP, Lerman C, Kase RG, Giambarresi TR, Tucker MA: Anticipated uptake and impact of genetic testing in hereditary breast and ovarian cancer families. *Cancer Epidemiol Biomark Prev* **4**:169, 1995.
29. Bratt O, Kristoffersson U, Lundgren R, Olsson H: Sons of men with prostate cancer: Their attitudes regarding possible inheritance of prostate cancer, screening, and genetic testing. *Urology* **50**:360, 1997.
30. Lerman C, Daly M, Masny A, Balshem A: Attitudes about genetic testing for breast-ovarian cancer susceptibility. *J Clin Oncol* **12**:843, 1994.
31. Lerman C, Marshall J, Audrain J, Gómez-Caminero A: Genetic testing for colon cancer susceptibility: Anticipated reactions of patients and challenges to providers. *Int J Cancer* **69**:58, 1996.
32. Rodríguez C, Plasencia A, Schroeder DG: Predictive factors of enrollment and adherence in a breast cancer screening program in Barcelona. *Soc Sci Med* **40**:1155, 1995.
33. Kelly RB, Shank JC: Adherence to screening flexible sigmoidoscopy in asymptomatic patients. *Med Care* **30**:1029, 1992.
34. Kendall C, Hailey BJ: The relative effectiveness of three reminder letters on making and keeping mammogram appointments. *Behav Med* **19**:29, 1993.
35. Bluman LG, Rimer BK, Berry DA, Borstelmann N, Iglehart JD, Regan K, Schildkraut J, Winer EP: Attitudes, knowledge, and risk perceptions of women with breast and ovarian cancer considering testing for BRCA1 and BRCA2. *J Clin Oncol* **17**:1040, 1999.
36. Kash KM, Holland JC, Halper MS, Miller DG: Psychological distress and surveillance behaviors of women with a family history of breast cancer. *J Natl Cancer Inst* **84**:24, 1992.
37. Champion VL: Compliance with guidelines for mammography screening. *Cancer Detect Prev* **16**:253, 1992.
38. Codori A-M, Petersen GM, Miglioretti DL, Larkin EK, Bushey MT, Young C, Brensinger JD, et al: Attitudes toward colon cancer gene testing: Factors predicting test uptake. *Cancer Epidemiol Biomark Prev* **8**:345, 1999.
39. Jacobsen PB, Valdimarsdottir HB, Brown KL, Offit K: Decision-making about genetic testing among women at familial risk for breast cancer. *Psychosomat Med* **59**:459, 1997.
40. Lynch HT, Watson P, Tinley S, Snyder C, Durham C, Lynch J, Kirnarsky Y, et al: An update on DNA-based BRCA1/BRCA2 genetic counseling in hereditary breast cancer. *Cancer Genet Cytogenet* **109**:91, 1999.
41. Evans DG, Maher ER, Macleod R, Davies DR, Craufurd D: Uptake of genetic testing for cancer predisposition. *J Med Genet* **34**:746, 1997.
42. Newman B, Mu H, Butler LM, Millikan RC, Moorman PG, King M-C: Frequency of breast cancer attributable to BRCA1 in a population-based series of American women. *JAMA* **279**:915, 1995.
43. Struewing JP, Beliovich D, Peretz T, Avishai N, Kaback MM, Collins FS, Brody LC: The carrier frequency of the BRCA1 185delAG mutation is approximately 1 percent in Ashkenazi Jewish individuals. *Nature Genet* **11**:198, 1995.
44. Struewing JP, Hartge P, Wacholder S, Baker SM, Berlin M, McAdams M, Timmerman MM, et al: The risk of cancer associated with specific mutations of BRCA1 and BRCA2 among Ashkenazi Jews. *N Engl J Med* **336**:1401, 1997.
45. Laken SJ, Petersen GM, Gruber SB, Oddoux C, Ostrer H, Giardiello FM, Hamilton SR, et al: Familial colorectal cancer in Ashkenazim due to a hypermutable tract in APC. *Nat Genet* **17**:79, 1997.
46. Nyström-Lahti M, Kristo P, Nicolaides NC, Chang SY, Aaltonen LA, Moisio AL, Järvinen HJ, et al: Founding mutations and Alu-mediated recombination in hereditary colon cancer. *Nat Med* **1**:1203, 1995.
47. Moisio AL, Sistonen P, Weissenbach J, de la Chapelle A, Peltomaki P: Age and origin of two common MLH1 mutations predisposing to hereditary colon cancer. *Am J Hum Genet* **59**:1243, 1996.
48. Serova OM, Mazoyer S, Puget N, Dubois V, Tonin P, Shugart YY, Goldgar D, et al: Mutations in BRCA1 and BRCA2 in breast cancer families: Are there more breast cancer-susceptibility genes? *Am J Hum Genet* **60**:486, 1997.
49. Liu B, Parsons R, Papadopoulos N, Nicolaides NC, Lynch HT, Watson P, Jass JR, et al: Analysis of mismatch repair genes in hereditary non-polyposis colorectal cancer patients. *Nature Med* **2**:169, 1996.
50. Brunet JS, Ghadirian P, Rebbeck TR, Lerman C, Garber JE, Tonin PN, Abrahamson J, et al: Effect of smoking on breast cancer in carriers of mutant BRCA1 or BRCA2 genes. *J Natl Cancer Inst* **90**:761, 1998.
51. Bottorff JL, Ratner PA, Johnson JL, Lovato CY, Joab SA: Communicating cancer risk information: The challenges of uncertainty. *Patient Educ Counseling* **33**:67, 1998.
52. Welch HG, Burke W: Uncertainties in genetic testing for chronic disease. *JAMA* **280**:1525, 1998.
53. Cornelis RS, Vasen HFA, Meijers-Heijboer H, Ford D, van Vliet M, van Tilborg AAG, Cleton FJ, et al: Age at diagnosis as an indicator of eligibility for BRCA1 DNA testing in familial breast cancer. *Hum Genet* **95**:539, 1995.
54. Rubin SC, Blackwood MA, Bandera C, Behbakht K, Benjamin I, Rebbeck TR, Boyd J: BRCA1, BRCA2, and hereditary nonpolyposis colorectal cancer gene mutations in an unselected ovarian cancer population—relationship to family history and implications for genetic testing. *Am J Obstet Gynecol* **178**:670, 1998.
55. Aaltonen LA, Salovaara R, Kristo P, Canzian F, Hemminki A, Peltomaki P, Chadwick RB, et al: Incidence of hereditary nonpolyposis colorectal cancer and the feasibility of molecular screening for the disease. *N Engl J Med* **338**:1481, 1998.
56. Shattuck-Eidens D, Oliphant A, McClure M, McBride C, Gupte J, Rubano T, Pruss D, et al: BRCA1 sequence analysis in women at high risk for susceptibility mutations. *JAMA* **278**:1242, 1997.
57. Couch FJ, DeShano ML, Blackwood MA, Calzone K, Stopfer J, Campeau L, Ganguly A, et al: BRCA1 mutations in women attending clinics that evaluate the risk of breast cancer. *N Engl J Med* **336**:1409, 1997.
58. Berry DA, Parmigiani G, Sánchez J, Winder E: Probability of carrying a mutation of breast ovarian cancer gene BRCA1 based on family history. *J Natl Cancer Inst* **89**:227, 1997.
59. Parmigiani G, Berry D, Aguilar O: Determining carrier probabilities for breast cancer-susceptibility genes BRCA1 and BRCA2. *Am J Hum Genet* **62**:145, 1998.
60. Wijnen JT, Vasen HFA, Khan PM, Zwinderman AH, Vanderklift H, Mulder A, Tops C, et al: Clinical findings with implications for genetic

testing in families with clustering of colorectal cancer. *N Engl J Med* **339**:511, 1998.

61. Ford D, Easton DF, Bishop DT, Narod SA, Goldgar DE, Breast Cancer Linkage Consortium: Risks of cancer in BRCA1 mutation carriers. *Lancet* **343**:692, 1994.
62. Aarnio M, Mecklin JP, Aaltonen LA, Nyström-Lahti M, Järvinen HJ: Life-time risk of different cancers in hereditary non-polyposis colorectal cancer (HNPCC) syndrome. *Int J Cancer* **64**:430, 1995.
63. Aarnio M, Sankila R, Pukkala E, Salovaara R, Aaltonen LA, de la Chapelle A, Peltomäki P, et al: Cancer risk in mutation carriers of DNA-mismatch-repair genes. *Int J Cancer* **81**:214, 1999.
64. Hawkins JR: *Finding Mutations*. New York, Oxford University Press, 1997.
65. Cotton RGH: *Mutation Detection*. Oxford, Oxford University Press, 1997.
66. Eng C, Vijg J: Genetic testing: The problems and the promise. *Nature Biotechnol* **15**:422, 1997.
67. Petersen GM, Slack J, Nakamura Y: Screening guidelines and premorbid diagnosis of familial adenomatous polyposis using linkage. *Gastroenterology* **100**:1658, 1991.
68. Maher ER, Bentley E, Payne SJ, Latif F, Richards FM, Chiano M, Hosoe S, et al.: Presymptomatic diagnosis of von Hippel-Lindau disease with flanking DNA markers. *J Med Genet* **29**:902, 1992.
69. Shimotake T, Iwai N, Yanagihara J, Tokiwa K, Tanaka N, Yamamoto M, Takai S: Prediction of affected MEN2A gene carriers by DNA linkage analysis for early total thyroidectomy: A progress in clinical screening program for children with hereditary cancer syndrome. *J Pediatr Surg* **27**:444, 1992.
70. Gayther SA, Sud R, Wells D, Tsioupra K, Delhanty JD: Rapid detection of rare variants and common polymorphisms in the APC gene by PCR-SSCP for presymptomatic diagnosis and showing allele loss. *J Med Genet* **32**:568, 1995.
71. Powell SM, Petersen GM, Krush AJ, Booker S, Jen J, Giardiello FM, Hamilton SR, et al: Molecular diagnosis of familial adenomatous polyposis. *N Engl J Med* **329**:1982, 1993.
72. Luce MC, Marra G, Chauhan DP, Laghi L, Carethers JM, Cherian SP, Hawn M, et al: In vitro transcription/translation assay for the screening of hMLH1 and hMSH2 mutations in familial colon cancer. *Gastroenterology* **109**:1368, 1995.
73. Forrest S, Cotton R, Landegren U, Southern E: How to find all those mutations. *Nature Genet* **10**:375, 1996.
74. Cotton RGH: Detection of unknown mutations in DNA: A catch-22. *Am J Hum Genet* **59**:289, 1996.
75. Papadopoulos N, Leach FS, Kinzler KW, Vogelstein B: Monoallelic mutation analysis (MAMA) for identifying germline mutations. *Nat Genet* **11**:99, 1995.
76. Laken SJ, Jackson PE, Kinzler KW, Vogelstein B, Strickland PT, Groopman JD, Friesen MD: Genotyping by mass spectrometric analysis of short DNA fragments. *Nat Biotechnol* **16**:1352, 1998.
77. Holtzman NA, Watson MS (eds): *Promoting Safe and Effective Genetic Testing in the United States. Final Report of the Task Force on Genetic Testing*. Baltimore, Johns Hopkins University Press, 1998.
78. Holtzman NA, Murphy PD, Watson MS, Barr PA: Predictive genetic testing: From basic research to clinical practice. *Science* **278**:602, 1997.
79. Rodríguez-Bigas MA, Boland CR, Hamilton SR, Henson DE, Jass JR, Khan PM, Lynch H, et al: A National Cancer Institute workshop on hereditary nonpolyposis colorectal cancer syndrome: Meeting highlights and Bethesda Guidelines. *J Natl Cancer Inst* **89**:1758, 1997.
80. Boland CR, Thibodeau SN, Hamilton SR, Sidransky D, Eshleman JR, Burt RW, Meltzer SJ, et al: A National Cancer Institute workshop on microsatellite instability for cancer detection and familial predisposition: Development of international criteria for the determination of microsatellite instability in colorectal cancer. *Cancer Res* **58**:5248, 1998.
81. Leach FS, Nicolaides N, Papadopoulos N, Liu B, Jen J, Parsons R, Peltomäki P, et al: Mutations of a MutS homolog in hereditary nonpolyposis colorectal cancer. *Cell* **75**:1215, 1993.
82. Papadopoulos N, Nicolaides NC, Wei Y-F, Ruben SM, Carter KC, Rosen CA, Haseltine WA, et al: Mutation of a mutL homolog in hereditary colon cancer. *Science* **263**:1625, 1994.
83. Nicolaides NC, Papadopoulos N, Liu B, Wei Y-F, Carter KC, Ruben SM, Rosen CA, et al: Mutations of two PMS homologues in hereditary nonpolyposis colon cancer. *Nature* **371**:75, 1994.
84. Thibodeau SN, French AJ, Cunningham JM, Tester D, Burgart LJ, Roche PC, McDonnell SK, et al: Microsatellite instability in colorectal cancer: Different mutator phenotypes and the principal involvement of hMLH1. *Cancer Res* **58**:1713, 1998.
85. Cunningham JM, Kim CY, Tester DJ, Christensen ER, Parc Y, Halling K, Burgart LJ, et al: The frequency and mechanism of defective DNA mismatch repair in unselected colorectal carcinomas. *Am Assn Cancer Res Proc* **40**:243, 1999.
86. Kainu T, Kononen J, Johansson O, Olsson H, Borg A, Isola J: Detection of germline BRCA1 mutations in breast cancer patients by quantitative messenger RNA in situ hybridization. *Cancer Res* **56**:2912, 1996.
87. Hubbard R, Lewontin RC: Pitfalls of genetic testing. *N Engl J Med* **334**:1192, 1996.
88. Giardiello FM, Brensinger JD, Petersen GM, Luce MC, Hylind LM, Bacon JA, Booker SV, et al: The use and interpretation of commercial APC gene testing for familial adenomatous polyposis. *N Engl J Med* 336:823, 1997.
89. Cho MK, Sankar P, Wolpe PR, Godmilow L: Commercialization of BRCA1/2 testing: Practitioner awareness and use of a new genetic test. *Am J Med Genet* **83**:157, 1999.
90. Nelson NJ: Caution guides genetic testing for hereditary cancer genes. *J Natl Cancer Inst* **88**:70, 1996.
91. Andrews LB, Fullarton JE, Holtzman NA (eds): *Assessing Genetic Risks: Implications for Health and Social Policy*. Washington, DC: National Academy Press, 1994.
92. National Advisory Council for Human Genome Research: Statement on use of DNA testing for presymptomatic detection of cancer risk. *JAMA* **271**:785, 1994.
93. Statement of the American Society of Human Genetics on genetic testing for breast and ovarian cancer predisposition. *Am J Hum Genet* **55**:i, 1994.
94. National Action Plan on Breast Cancer: Position paper: Hereditary susceptibility testing for breast cancer. *J Clin Oncol* **14**:1738, 1996.
95. Rothstein MA: Genetic testing: employability, insurability, and health reform. *Monogr Natl Cancer Inst* **17**:87, 1995.
96. Garber JE, Patenaude AF: Ethical, social and counseling issues in hereditary cancer susceptibility. *Cancer Surv* **25**:381, 1995.
97. Kash KM: Psychosocial and ethical implications of defining genetic risk for cancers. *Ann NY Acad Sci* **768**:41, 1995.
98. Patenaude AF: The genetic testing of children for cancer susceptibility: Ethical, legal and social issues. *Behav Sci Law* **14**:393, 1996.
99. Wilfond BS, Rothenberg KH, Thomson EJ, Lerman C: Cancer genetic susceptibility testing—ethical and policy implications for future research and clinical practice. *J Law Med Ethics* **25**:243, 1997.
100. Davis JG: Predictive genetic tests: Problems and pitfalls. *Ann NY Acad Sci* **833**:42, 1997.
101. Grady C: Ethics and genetic testing. *Adv Intern Med* **44**:389, 1999.
102. Ad Hoc Committee on Genetic Testing/Insurance Issues: Genetic testing and insurance. *Am J Hum Genet* **56**:327, 1995.
103. American Society of Human Genetics Social Issues Subcommittee on Familial Disclosure: Professional disclosure of familial genetic information. *Am J Hum Genet* **62**:474, 1998.
104. Lerman C, Peshkin BN, Hughes C, Isaacs C: Family disclosure in genetic testing for cancer susceptibility: Determinants and consequences. *J Health Care Law Policy* **1**:353, 1998.
105. Clayton EW: What should the law say about disclosure of genetic information to relatives? *J Health Care Law Policy* **1**:373, 1998.
106. ASHG Background Statement: Genetic testing and insurance. *Am J Hum Genet* **56**:327, 1995.
107. Lapham EV, Kozma C, Weiss JO: Genetic discrimination: Perspectives of consumers. *Science* **274**:621, 1996.
108. Billings PR, Kohn MA, de Cuevas M, Beckwith J, Alper JS, Natowicz MR: Discrimination as a consequence of genetic testing. *Am J Hum Genet* **50**:476, 1992.
109. Natowicz MR, Alper JK, Alper JS: Genetic discrimination and the law. *Am J Hum Genet* **50**:465, 1992.
110. Billings PR, Beckwith J: Genetic testing in the workplace: A view from the USA. *Trends Genet* **8**:198, 1992.
111. Hopwood P: Psychological issues in cancer genetics: Current research and future priorities. *Patient Educ Counseling* **32**:19, 1997.
112. Lerman C, Narod S, Schulman K, Hughes C, Gómez-Caminero A, Bonney G, Gold K, et al: BRCA1 testing in families with hereditary breast-ovarian cancer. A prospective study of patient decision making and outcomes. *JAMA* **275**:1885, 1996.
113. Lerman C, Hughes C, Trock BJ, Myers RE, Main D, Bonney A, Abbaszadegan MR, et al: Genetic testing in families with hereditary nonpolyposis colon cancer. *JAMA* **281**:1618, 1999.

114. Bowen DJ, Patenaude AF, Vernon SW: Psychosocial issues in cancer genetics: From the laboratory to the public. *Cancer Epidemiol Biomark Prev* **8**:326, 1999.
115. Lerman C, Trock B, Rimer BK, Jepson C, Brody D, Boyce A: Psychological side effects of breast cancer screening. *Health Psychol* **10**:259, 1991.
116. Macdonald LA, Sackett DL, Haynes RB, Taylor DW: Labelling in hypertension: A review of the behavioural and psychological consequences. *J Chron Dis* **37**:933, 1984.
117. Greenwald HP, Becker SW, Nevitt MC: Delay and noncompliance in cancer detection: A behavioral perspective for health planners. *Milbank Mem Fund Quart* **56**:212, 1978.
118. Biesecker BB, Boehnke M, Calzone K, Markel DS, Garber JE, Collins FS, Weber BL: Genetic counseling for families with inherited susceptibility to breast and ovarian cancer. *JAMA* **269**:1970, 1993.
119. Stefanek ME, Helzlsouer KJ, Wilcox PM, Houn F: Predictors of and satisfaction with bilateral prophylactic mastectomy. *Prev Med* **24**:412, 1995.
120. Hartmann LC, Schaid DJ, Woods JE, Crotty TP, Myers JL, Arnold PG, Petty PM, et al: Efficacy of bilateral prophylactic mastectomy in women with a family history of breast cancer. *N Engl J Med* **340**:77, 1999.
121. King M-C, Rowell S, Love SM: Inherited breast and ovarian cancer. What are the risks? What are the choices? *JAMA* **269**:1975, 1993.
122. Burke W, Daly M, Garber J, Botkin J, Kahn MJE, Lynch P, McTiernan A, et al: Recommendations for follow-up care of individuals with an inherited predisposition to cancer. II. *BRCA1* and *BRCA2*. *JAMA* **277**:997, 1997.
123. Codori AM, Brandt J: Psychological costs and benefits of predictive testing for Huntington's disease. *Am J Med Genet* **54**:174, 1994.
124. Wiggins S, Whyte P, Huggins M, Adam S, Theilmann J, Bloch M, Sheps SB, et al: The psychological consequences of predictive testing for Huntington's disease. *N Engl J Med* **327**:1401, 1992.
125. Lerman C, Daly M, Masney A, Balshem A: Attitudes about genetic testing for breast-ovarian cancer susceptibility. *J Clin Oncol* **12**:843, 1994.
126. Croyle RT, Smith KR, Botkin JR, Baty B, Nash J: Psychological responses to BRCA1 mutation testing: Preliminary findings. *Health Psychol* **16**:63, 1997.
127. Codori A-M, Petersen GM, Corazzini K, Bacon J, Loth DM, Boyd PA, Brandt J, et al: Genetic testing for cancer in children: Short-term psychological impact. *Arch Pediatr Adolesc Med* **150**:1131, 1996.
128. Dudok deWit AC, Tibben A, Duivenvoorden HJ, Niermeijer MF, Passchier J: Predicting adaptation to presymptomatic DNA testing for late onset disorders: Who will experience distress? Rotterdam Leiden Genetics Workgroup. *J Med Genet* **35**:745, 1998.
129. Lerman C, Rimer BK: Psychosocial impact of cancer screening. *Oncology* **7**:67, 1993.
130. Codori AM, Brandt J: Psychological costs and benefits of predictive testing for Huntington's disease. *Am J Med Genet* **54**:174, 1994.
131. Huggins M, Bloch M, Wiggins S, Adam S, Suchowersky O, Trew M, Klimek M, et al: Predictive testing for Huntington disease in Canada: Adverse effects and unexpected results in those receiving a decreased risk. *Am J Med Genet* **42**:508, 1992.
132. The American Society of Human Genetics Board of Directors and the American College of Medical Genetics Board of Directors: ASHG/ACMG Report. Points to consider: Ethical, legal, and psychosocial implications of genetic testing in children and adolescents. *Am J Hum Genet* **57**:1233, 1995.
133. Grosfeld FJM, Lips CJM, Beemer FA, van Spijker HG, Brouwers-Smalbraak GJ, ten Kroode HFJ: Psychological risks of genetically testing children for a hereditary cancer syndrome. *Patient Educ Counseling* **32**:63, 1997.
134. Learoyd DL, Marsh DJ, Richardson AL, Twigg SM, Delbridge L, Robinson BG: Genetic testing for familial cancer. Consequences of RET proto-oncogene mutation analysis in mutliple endocrine neoplasia, type 2. *Arch Surg* **132**:1022, 1997.
135. Gallie BL, Dunn JM, Chan HSL, Hamel PA, Phillips RA: The genetics of retinoblastoma: Relevance to the patient. *Pediatr Clin North Am* **38**:299, 1991.
136. Giardiello FM, Hamilton SR, Krush AJ, Piantadosi S, Hylind LM, Celano P, Booker SV, et al: Treatment of colonic and rectal adenomas with Sulindac in familial adenomatous polyposis. *N Engl J Med* **328**:1313, 1993.
137. Lindor NM, Greene MH, Mayo Familial Cancer Program: The concise handbook of family cancer syndromes. *J Natl Canc Inst* **90**:1039, 1998.
138. Lynch HT, Fitzsimmons ML, Lynch J, Watson P: A hereditary cancer consultation clinic. *Nebr Med J* **74**:351, 1989.
139. McKinnon WC, Guttmacher AE, Greenblatt MS, Compas BE, May S, Cutler RE, Yandell DW: The familial cancer program of the Vermont cancer center: Development of a cancer genetics program in a rural area. *J Genet Counseling* **6**:131, 1997.
140. Stadler MP, Mulvihill JJ: Cancer risk assessment and genetic counseling in an academic medical center: Consultands' satisfaction, knowledge, and behavior in the first year. *J Genet Counseling* **7**:279, 1998.
141. American Society of Clinical Oncology: Resource document for curriculum development in cancer genetics education. *J Clin Oncol* **15**:2157, 1997.
142. Niederhuber JE: Genetic testings for cancer: The surgeon's critical role. *J Am Coll Surg* **188**:74, 1999.
143. Webb MJ: Genetic testing and management of the cancer patient and cancer families. *Obstet Gynecol Symposium* **187**:449, 1998.
144. Engelking C: Genetics in cancer care: Confronting a Pandora's box of dilemmas. *Oncol Nurs Forum* **22**:27, 1995.
145. Li FP, Fraumeni JF Jr, Mulvihill JJ, Blattner WA, Dreyfus MG, Tucker MA, Miller RW: A cancer family syndrome in twenty-four kindreds. *Cancer Res* **48**:5358, 1988.
146. Herrera L (ed.): *Familial Adenomatous Polyposis*. New York, Liss, 1990.
147. Petersen GM, Brensinger J: Gene tests and genetic counseling in familial adenomatous polyposis. *Oncology* **10**:89, 1996.
148. Hamilton SR, Liu B, Parsons RE, Papadopoulos N, Jen J, Powell SM, Krush AJ, et al: The molecular basis of Turcot's syndrome. *N Engl J Med* **332**:839, 1995.
149. Ford D, Easton DF: The genetics of breast and ovarian cancer. *Br J Cancer* **72**:805, 1995.
150. Futreal PA, Liu Q, Shattuck-Eidens D, Cochran C, Harshman K, Tavtigian S, Bennett LM, et al: BRCA1 mutations in primary breast and ovarian carcinomas. *Science* **266**:120, 1994.
151. Tavtigian SV, Simard J, Rommens J, Couch F, Shattuck-Eidens D, Neuhausen S, Merajver S, et al: The complete BRCA2 gene and mutations in chromosome 13q-linked kindreds. *Nature Genet* **12**:333, 1996.
152. Burke W, Petersen G, Lynch P, Botkin J, Daly M, Garber J, Kahn MJE, et al: Recommendations for follow-up care of individuals with HNPCC-associated mutations. *JAMA* **277**:915, 1997.
153. Geller G, Botkin JR, Green MJ, Press N, Biesecker BB, Wilfond B, Grana G, et al: Genetic testing for susceptibility to adult-onset cancer. The process and content of informed consent. *JAMA* **277**:1467, 1997.
154. Savitsky K, Bar-Shira A, Gilad S, Rotman G, Ziv Y, Vanagaite L, Tagle DA, et al: A single ataxia telangiectasia gene with a product similar to PI-3 kinase. *Science* **268**:1749, 1995.
155. Li J, Yen C, Liaw D, Podsypanina K, Bose S, Wang SI, Puc J, et al: PTEN, a putative protein tyrosine phosphatase gene mutated in human brain, breast, and prostate cancer. *Science* **275**:1943, 1997.
156. Liaw D, Marsh DJ, Li J, Dahia PL, Wang SI, Zheng Z, Bose S, et al: Germline mutations of the PTEN gene in Cowden disease, an inherited breast and thyroid cancer syndrome. *Nature Genet* **16**:64, 1997.
157. Kinzler KW, Nilbert MC, Su L-K, Vogelstein B, Bryan TM, Levy DB, Smith KJ, et al: Identification of FAP locus genes from chromosome 5q21. *Science* **253**:661, 1991.
158. Groden J, Thliveris A, Samowitz W, Carlson M, Gelbert L, Albertsen H, Joslyn G, et al: Identification and characterization of the familial adenomatous polyposis coli gene. *Cell* **66**:589, 1991.
159. Guilford P, Hopkins J, Harraway J, McLeod M, McLeod N, Harawira P, Taite H, et al: E-cadherin germline mutations in familial gastric cancer. *Nature* **392**:402, 1998.
160. Kamb A, Shattuck-Eidens D, Eeles R, Liu Q, Gruis NA, Ding W, Hussey C, et al: Analysis of the p16 gene (CDKN2) as a candidate for the chromosome 9p melanoma susceptibility locus. *Nat Genet* **8**:23, 1994.
161. Farndon PA, Del Mastro RG, Evans DGR, Kilpatrick MW: Location of the gene for Gorlin syndrome. *Lancet* **339**:581, 1992.
162. Reis A, Kuster W, Linss G, Gebel E, Fuhrmann W, Groth W, Kuklik M, et al: Localisation of gene for the nevoid basal cell carcinoma syndrome. *Lancet* **339**:617, 1992.
163. Gailani MR, Bale SJ, Leffell DJ, DiGiovanna JJ, Peck GL, Poliak S, Drum MA, et al: Developmental defects in Gorlin syndrome related to a putative tumor suppressor gene on chromosome 9. *Cell* **69**:111, 1992.
164. Miyaki M, Konishi M, Tanaka K, Kikuchi-Yanoshita R, Muraoka M, Yasuno M, et al: Germline mutation of MSH6 as the cause of

hereditary nonpolyposis colorectal cancer. *Nat Genet* **17**:271, 1997.
165. Smith JR, Freije D, Carpten JD, Grönberg H, Xu J, Isaacs SD, Brownstein MJ, et al: Major susceptibility locus for prostate cancer on chromosome 1 suggested by a genome-wide search. *Science* **274**:1301, 1996.
166. Xu J, Meyers D, Freije D, Isaacs S, Wiley K, Nusskern D, Ewing C, et al: Evidence for a prostate cancer susceptibility locus on the X chromosome. *Nature Genet* **20**:175, 1998.
167. Malkin D, Li FP, Strong LC, Fraumeni JF Jr., Nelson CE, Kim DH, Kassel J, et al: Germ line p53 mutations in a familial syndrome of breast cancer, sarcomas, and other neoplasms. *Science* **250**:1233, 1990.
168. Larsson C, Skogseid B, Oberg K, Nakamura Y, Nordenskjold M: Multiple endocrine neoplasia type 1 gene maps to chromosome 11 and is lost in insulinoma. *Nature* **332**:85, 1988.
169. Mulligan LM, Kwok JBJ, Healey CS, Elsdon MJ, Eng C, Gardner E, Love DR, et al: Germ-line mutations of the RET proto-oncogene in multiple endocrine neoplasia type 2A. *Nature* **363**:458, 1993.
170. Hofstra RM, Landsvater RM, Ceccherini I, Stulp RP, Stelwagen T, Luo Y, Pasini B, et al: A mutation in the RET proto-oncogene associated with multiple endocrine neoplasia type 2B and sporadic medullary thyroid carcinoma. *Nature* **367**:375, 1994.
171. Carlson KM, Dou S, Chi D, Scavarda N, Toshima K, Jackson CE, Wells SA Jr., et al: Single missense mutation in the tyrosine kinase catalytic domain of the RET protooncogene is associated with multiple endocrine neoplasia type 2B. *Proc Natl Acad Sci USA* **91**:1579, 1994.
172. Rouleau GA, Wertelecki W, Haines JL, Hobbs WJ, Trofatter JA, Seizinger BR, Martuza RL, et al: Genetic linkage of bilateral acoustic neurofibromatosis to a DNA marker on chromosome 22. *Nature* **329**:246, 1987.
173. Barker D, Wright E, Nguyen K, Cannon L, Fain P, Goldgar D, Bishop DT, et al: Gene for von Recklinghausen neurofibromatosis is in the pericentromeric region of chromosome 17. *Science* **236**:1100, 1987.
174. Seizinger BR, Rouleau GA, Ozelius LJ, Lane AH, Faryniarz AG, Chao MV, Huson S, et al: Genetic linkage of von Recklinghausen neurofibromatosis to the nerve growth factor receptor gene. *Cell* **49**:589, 1987.
175. Wallace MR, Marchuk DA, Andersen LB, Letcher R, Odeh HM, Saulino AM, Fountain JW, et al: Type 1 neurofibromatosis gene: Identification of a large transcript disrupted in three NF1 patients. *Science* **249**:181, 1990.
176. Cawthon RM, Weiss R, Xu GF, Viskochil D, Culver M, Stevens J, Robertson M, et al: A major segment of the neurofibromatosis type 1 gene: cDNA sequence, genomic structure, and point mutations. *Cell* **62**:193, 1990.
177. Trofatter JA, MacCollin MM, Rutter JL, Murrell JR, Duyao MP, Parry DM, et al.: A novel moesin-, ezrin-, radixin-like gene is a candidate for the neurofibromatosis 2 tumor suppressor. *Cell* **75**:826, 1993.
178. Hemminki A, Markie D, Tomlinson I, Avizienyte E, Roth S, Loukola A, Bignell G, et al: A serine/threonine kinase gene defective in Peutz-Jeghers syndrome. *Nature* **391**:184, 1998.
179. Jenne DE, Reimann H, Nezu J-I, Friedel W, Loff S, Jeschke R, Müller O, et al: Peutz-Jeghers syndrome is caused by mutations in a novel serine threonine kinase. *Nature Genet* **18**:38, 1998.
180. Cavenee WK, Hansen MF, Nordenskjold M, Kock E, Maumenee I, Squire JA, Phillips RA, et al: Genetic origin of mutations predisposing to retinoblastoma. *Science* **228**:501, 1985.
181. Lee W-H, Bookstein R, Hong F, Young L-J, Shew J-Y, Lee EYP: Human retinoblastoma susceptibility gene: Cloning, identification, and sequence. *Science* **235**:1394, 1987.
182. Latif F, Tory K, Gnarra J, Yao M, Duh F-M, Orcutt ML, Stackhous T, et al: Identification of the von Hippel-Lindau disease tumor suppressor gene. *Science* **260**:1317, 1993.

CHAPTER 50

Pancreatic Cancer

Ralph H. Hruban ▪ Charles J. Yeo ▪ Scott E. Kern

1. Pancreatic ductal adenocarcinoma is the fifth leading cause of cancer death in the United States. It is estimated that approximately 27,600 Americans were diagnosed with pancreatic cancer in 1997. It is a nearly uniformly fatal disease, and the mortality rate closely follows that of the incidence. Pancreatic cancer presents clinically with pain, with symptoms related to obstruction of the biliary or pancreatic ducts, or with protean symptoms such as weight loss and cachexia.

2. Although most carcinomas of the pancreas appear to be sporadic, a number of anecdotal case reports and case-control studies suggest that as many as 10 percent of all cases of pancreatic carcinoma are hereditary. The gene or genes responsible for the familial aggregation of pancreatic cancer largely are unknown, but germ-line mutations in the *BRCA2* gene and, less commonly, in the *p16* gene, have been shown to predispose to pancreatic cancer, although with incomplete penetrance.

3. The profile of genetic mutations in pancreatic cancer is distinct from other neoplasms. The K-*ras* oncogene is commonly activated by somatic mutations in pancreatic cancer, whereas three tumor-suppressor genes are commonly inactivated. Ninety percent or more of pancreatic cancers harbor activating point mutations in codon 12 of K-*ras*. The *p16* tumor-suppressor gene is inactivated in 90 to 100 percent of pancreatic cancers, *p53* in 50 to 75 percent, and *DPC4* in 50 percent. In addition, occasional somatic mutations of the *RB1*, *MKK4*, *LKB1*, and *TGFβ* receptor genes also have been reported. Various gene amplifications affect a minority of carcinomas.

4. Inactivation of the *DPC4* gene may be rather specific for pancreatic neoplasia. *DPC4* is inactivated in as few as 15 percent of colorectal cancers and in less than 10 percent of other major cancer types. Dpc4 belongs to a class of proteins that mediate signals of the TGFβ superfamily.

5. Microsatellite instability (RER+) is seen in a small minority (~4 percent) of pancreatic cancers. These RER+ cancers have a characteristic histologic appearance and frequently have wild-type K-*ras* genes.

6. Pancreatic cancer is likely to harbor changes in additional yet uncharacterized genes. Chromosome arms with unexplained losses of heterozygosity at frequencies of greater than 40 percent in pancreatic cancer include 1p, 6p, 8p, 12q, 13q, 21q, and 22q.

7. A large number of pancreatic cancers have been karyotyped. Double minute chromosomes, possibly representing gene amplification, were identified in 8 percent of pancreatic cancers in one study. These karyotyping studies also provide an understanding of the structural basis for genetic losses identified at the molecular level. Sites having loss of heterozygosity tend to correspond to sites of karyotypic abnormalities in individual tumors.

8. The diagnosis of pancreatic cancer is suspected based on clinical findings and often can be confirmed with radiologic and endoscopic techniques. Effective screening tests are not available yet.

A list of standard abbreviations is located immediately preceding the index in each volume. Nonstandard abbreviations used in this chapter include: HNPCC = hereditary nonpolyposis colorectal carcinoma; FAMM = familial atypical mole-multiple melanoma; LOH = loss of heterozygosity; RDA = representational difference analysis.

Adenocarcinoma of the pancreas is one of the most aggressive of human malignancies. It typically presents late in the course of the disease, with nonspecific symptoms. As a result, patients with pancreatic cancer have an extremely poor prognosis, with an overall 5-year survival rate of less than 5 percent.[1] However, those patients with early, surgically resectable carcinomas have a substantially improved prognosis. Clearly, early detection of the carcinoma, before it has spread beyond the pancreas, is the key to the successful treatment of patients with pancreatic carcinoma. A better understanding of the molecular genetic alterations in pancreatic cancer may lead to the development of new tests to detect this cancer earlier.

Until recently, our understanding of the genetics of pancreatic cancer was very incomplete. In large part, this was because of difficulties presented by the carcinomas themselves. Pancreatic cancers induce a prominent nonneoplastic reaction. As a result, the neoplastic cells constitute only a small minority of the cells in the tumor. This problem of low neoplastic cellularity has hampered the molecular analyses of pancreatic cancer. Recent efforts, however, have overcome this obstacle by selectively enriching for neoplastic cells by propagating the cancers in tissue culture or in immunodeficient mice. Once a mutation is identified in these enriched populations, it can be confirmed by a sensitive assay of the original primary tumor. Indeed, these techniques are a major advance in our ability to analyze pancreatic cancers, and pancreatic cancer now boasts an extensive molecular description.[2] Whereas much of what is known about pancreatic cancer has been learned by the study of sporadic pancreatic cancers, some genes that have been identified in sporadic carcinomas also have been found to play a role in the development of inherited forms of pancreatic cancer.

In this chapter we will focus on the advances in our understanding of the molecular genetic alterations in human ductal adenocarcinoma of the pancreas, since this tumor type accounts for the majority of pancreatic neoplasms.

CLINICAL ASPECTS OF ADENOCARCINOMA OF THE PANCREAS

Incidence

Adenocarcinoma of the pancreas is the fifth leading cause of cancer death in the United States.[1] In 1998, approximately 28,000 new cases of pancreas cancer were diagnosed in the United States, and nearly the same number died from it.[1] These patients are mostly elderly.[3] The incidence of pancreatic cancer increases steadily with age, and approximately 80 percent of the cancers occur in the seventh and eight decades of life.[4] Pancreatic cancer is extremely uncommon before the age of 40, although cases have been reported in children.[5] Pancreatic cancer appears to occur slightly more commonly in men than in women and, in the United States, in African-Americans more frequently than in whites.[3,4] The incidence of pancreatic cancer is higher among Jews than among non-Jews, and it is higher in Western industrialized countries than it is in the third world.[6,7] Among white males, the incidence and mortality rates from pancreatic cancer have been decreasing slowly since the 1970s, but during this same period of time, the mortality rates among African-American women have increased slightly.[1]

A number of environmental factors have been studied as possible etiologic agents in the development of pancreatic cancer, and cigarette smoking has the highest association with pancreatic cancer.[3,8–11] For example, smoking during college has been associated with a 2.6-fold risk of developing pancreatic cancer.[12] In addition, the risk of developing pancreatic cancer increases in relation to the duration of smoking and the number of cigarettes smoked.[4,13]

Diets high in meat and fat and low in fiber also may predispose to the development of pancreatic cancer, but the role of alcohol consumption is less clear.[4,13–17] Based on an early well-publicized study, coffee was once thought to be a possible risk factor for the development of pancreatic cancer. This study, however, had serious methodologic flaws, and coffee is now not felt to be a significant risk factor.[15,16] Thus age and cigarette smoking remain the greatest risk factors for developing pancreatic cancer.

Familial Patterns of Pancreatic Cancer

Almost all cancers show a tendency to aggregate in families, but the fraction of cancer that is hereditary varies substantially among different cancer types.[18] There have been a number of case reports in the literature that suggest that there is a familial form of pancreatic cancer.[19–34] For example, Lynch et al. described 47 individuals with pancreatic cancer in 18 families in which multiple family members had pancreatic cancer.[20] The age of onset (median 70 years), histologic types, and survival times of these 47 patients were comparable with published data on unselected patients with pancreatic cancer, and there appeared to be an autosomal dominant mode of transmission in several of the families.[20,34] Based on these family studies, it has been suggested that as many as 10 percent of the cases of pancreatic cancer are hereditary.[24] Similarly, Ghadirian et al. interviewed 179 patients with pancreatic cancer and 179 controls matched for gender and age, and they reported that 7.8 percent of the patients with pancreatic cancer had a family history of pancreatic cancer, compared with only 0.6 percent of control patients without pancreatic cancer ($p < 0.01$).[35] Fernandez et al. also studied the relationship of family history to the development of pancreatic cancer.[36] They conducted a case-control study in northern Italy of 362 patients with histologically confirmed pancreatic cancer and 1408 controls admitted to the hospital for acute, nonneoplastic, non-digestive tract disorders.[36] Significantly more of the patients with pancreatic cancer had a family history of pancreatic cancer than did the controls (RR = 3.0). From their data they estimated that 3 percent of newly diagnosed pancreatic cancers were familial.[36] Similarly, we recently analyzed 212 kindreds enrolled in the National Familial Pancreas Tumor Registry (NFPTR).* *Familial* pancreatic kindreds were defined as those families in which there had been at least two first-degree relatives diagnosed with pancreatic cancer, and we found that second-degree relatives of patients with familial pancreatic cancer are at increased risk for developing pancreatic cancer .[37]

*The National Familial Pancreas Tumor Registry, The Johns Hopkins Hospital, Department of Pathology, Meyer 7-181, 600 N. Wolfe Street, Baltimore, MD 21287. (410) 955-9132; (410) 955-0115 (fax); e-mail: *rhuban@welchlink.welch.jhu.edu.*

Thus anecdotal reports and several case-control studies suggest that between 3 and 10 percent of pancreatic cancers are caused by inherited factors, and even second-degree relatives of patients with pancreatic cancer are at increased risk for developing the disease.

Diagnosing Pancreatic Cancer

Although the pancreas is located deep in the retroperitoneal space, it can be visualized with sophisticated imaging techniques.[38] Spiral (or helical) computed tomography (CT) is the best of these techniques, and other commonly used techniques include real-time ultrasonography, magnetic resonance imaging (MRI), angiography, endoscopic retrograde cholangiopancreatography, and endoscopic ultrasonography. Despite the introduction of these new techniques, the death rate for pancreatic carcinoma has not changed significantly. This is not surprising, since the biggest determinant of patient outcome is stage at diagnosis, and these tools do not currently influence the timing of patient presentation.[38] The survival rate for pancreatic cancer will not improve significantly until new tests are developed to screen for the disease before patients become symptomatic.

Although all the imaging techniques may reveal a suspicious mass in the pancreas, the "gold standard" for diagnosing pancreatic cancer remains histopathology. Tissue for microscopic examination can be obtained either by fine-needle aspiration, by tissue needle core biopsy, or by excisional biopsy at the time of laparotomy.[38,39] Again, as was true for imaging, the need for biopsy is likely to be apparent only after the disease has advanced.[40]

Pathology of Pancreatic Cancer

The most common type of exocrine pancreatic cancer is the duct cell adenocarcinoma.[41–43] The majority of these cancers arise in the head of the pancreas (60 percent) and the remainder in the body (13 percent), tail (5 percent) or infiltrate diffusely throughout the gland (21 percent).[42] By light microscopy, adenocarcinomas of the pancreas are composed of neoplastic glands infiltrating a dense nonneoplastic stroma (Fig. 50-1). Numerous inflammatory cells, including lymphocytes, also are frequently admixed with the tumor cells. This nonneoplastic host response is characteristic of pancreatic cancers, and it must be considered when conducting molecular analyses of allelic loss, since DNA isolated from most pancreatic cancers contains predominantly normal DNA. Perineural (Fig. 50-2) and vascular invasion is seen frequently in pancreatic cancers, as is infiltration of adjacent structures and metastases to regional lymph nodes (Fig 50-3).

Infiltrating adenocarcinoma of the pancreas frequently is associated with dramatic histologic changes in the pancreatic ducts and ductules. The normal pancreatic ducts and ductules are lined by a single layer of cuboidal to columnar epithelial cells, but in most pancreata with cancer this epithelium is regionally replaced by a proliferative epithelium with varying degrees of cytologic and architectural atypia.[44] There is no uniform nomenclature for these duct lesions, but the term *flat hyperplasia* refers to a uniform increase in the mucin content of the epithelial cells. The term *papillary hyperplasia without atypia* refers to the presence of papillae lined by columnar cells. The term *atypical papillary hyperplasia* designates papillary lesions with nuclear enlargement, increased nuclear-to-cytoplasmic ratio, loss of cellular polarity, and nuclear pleomorphism.[43,45,46] The histology of selected duct lesions is illustrated in Fig. 50-4.

These various duct lesions are more common in pancreata with cancer than they are in pancreata without cancer.[45–48] For example, Cubilla and Fitzgerald compared the duct changes in 227 pancreata with pancreatic cancer with the duct changes in 100 age- and sex-matched controls without pancreatic cancer.[45] They found that papillary lesions were three times more common in the pancreata obtained from patients with pancreatic cancer than they

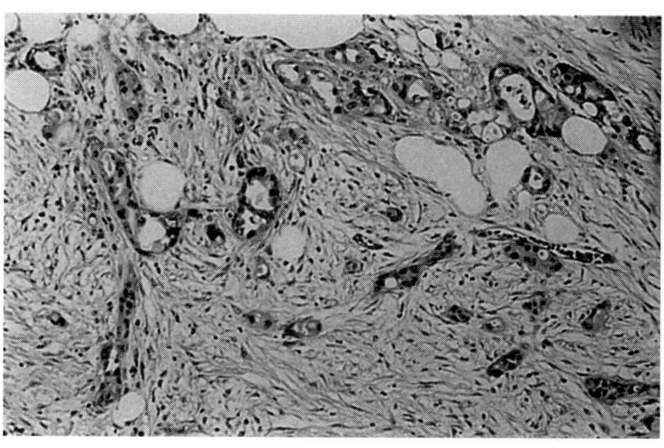
A

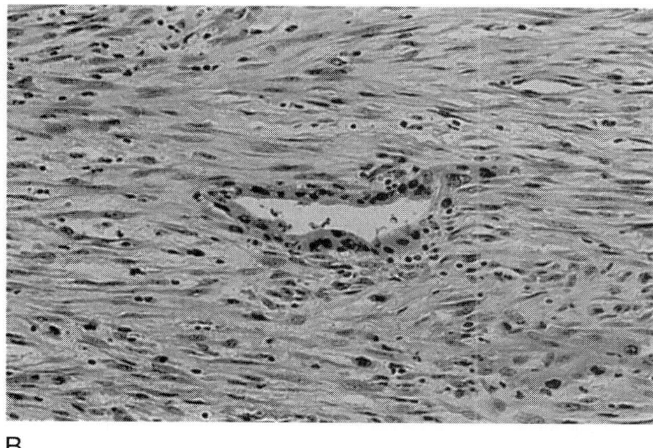
B

Fig. 50-1 Infiltrating adenocarcinoma of the pancreas. Note the haphazard arrangement of markedly atypical glands (*A*) and the intense nonneoplastic inflammatory and fibroblastic response elicited by the carcinoma (*B*). (*A,B* both hematoxylin and eosin).

were in pancreata obtained from patients without pancreatic cancer and that atypical papillary lesions were seen only in pancreata with pancreas cancer.[45] These findings have been confirmed by Kozuka et al. and Pour et al.[47,48] More recently Furukawa et al., using three-dimensional mapping techniques, have demonstrated a stepwise progression from mild dysplasia to severe dysplasia in pancreatic duct lesions.[46] These results suggest that infiltrating cancers of the pancreas arise from precursors in the pancreatic ducts—that there is a progression in the pancreas from flat mucinous lesions (Fig. 50-4*A*), to papillary lesions without atypia (Figs. 50-4*A–C*), to papillary lesions with atypia (Fig. 50-4*D*), to *in situ* carcinoma, to infiltrating adenocarcinoma[41,43,49] (see Figs. 50-1 and 50-2). This hypothesis, however, is based on observations of fixed static specimens. Serial samples taken over time would be needed to demonstrate that, in fact, these lesions in pancreatic ducts can progress to infiltrating cancer.[49] Brat et al. have recently done just that, in a series of patients followed after partial pancreatectomy. Brat et al. reported three patients in whom papillary duct lesions with atypia were documented 17 months, 9 years, and 10 years before the development of an infiltrating cancer of the pancreas.[43,49] These morphologic observations therefore strongly suggest that just as there is a progression from adenoma to infiltrating cancer in the colorectum, so too is there a progression from intraductal papillary lesions to infiltrating cancer in the pancreas.[49] Furthermore, these results suggest that these lesions in the pancreatic ducts are not in actuality hyperplasias but instead represent part of the neoplastic process.

GENETIC LOCI

Genetic Loci Involved in Hereditary Pancreatic Cancer

It has proven difficult to perform classic linkage studies in families with pancreatic cancer because of the small size of most kindreds and the short life expectancy of patients with carcinoma of the pancreas. Nonetheless, analyses of families in which there is an aggregation of pancreatic cancer may provide clues as to which genes are involved in hereditary pancreatic cancer.

Families with an aggregation of pancreatic cancer can be divided into three general groups: (1) those associated with known syndromes, (2) those in which there is an aggregation of pancreatic cancers but not part of a known syndrome, and (3) those in which there is an association of pancreatic with nonpancreatic cancers.

Syndromes Associated with Pancreatic Cancer. Several well-characterized genetic syndromes have been shown to predispose affected family members to the development of pancreatic cancer.[33,37] These include hereditary pancreatitis, hereditary nonpolyposis colorectal carcinoma (HNPCC, Lynch syndrome), a subset of the familial atypical mole-multiple melanoma

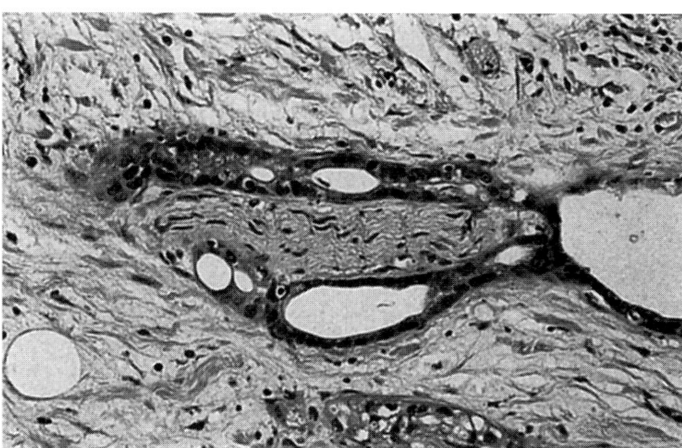

Fig. 50-2 Infiltrating adenocarcinoma of the pancreas growing along a nerve. Pain is a common symptom of pancreatic cancer (hematoxylin and eosin).

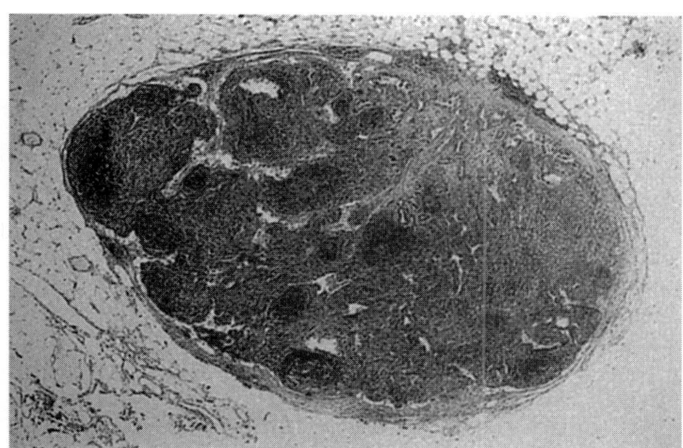

Fig. 50-3 Metastatic adenocarcinoma of the pancreas in a lymph node. The carcinoma has metastasized to the upper right-hand corner of this node (hematolylin and eosin).

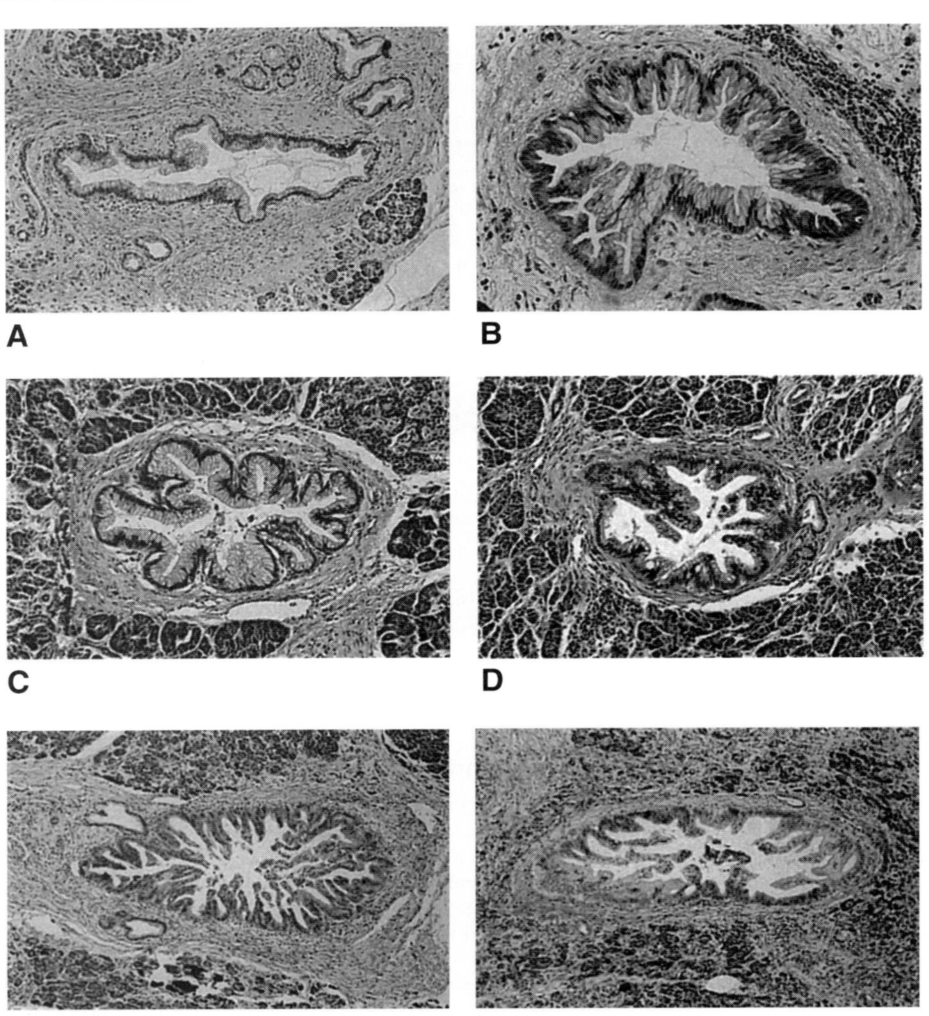

Fig. 50-4 Duct lesions, also called *hyperplasias,* from pancreata with cancer. Note the progression from (top row, *A-C*) flat lesions (*A*), to papillary lesions without atypia (*B, C*), to (bottom row, *D-F*) papillary lesion with atypia (*D*), to papillary lesions with marked atypia (*E, F,* carcinoma *in situ*) (all hematoxylin and eosin).

(FAMMM) syndrome, the Peutz-Jeghers syndrome, familial breast cancer (*BRCA2*), and ataxia telangiectasia[33,34] (Table 50-1).

Hereditary Pancreatitis. Hereditary pancreatitis is an autosomal dominant disorder with incomplete penetrance characterized by recurrent episodes of severe pancreatitis in blood-related family members over two generations.[50–53] There is often an early age of onset of the pancreatitis, and the patients frequently develop chronic pancreatitis. Men are affected at the same rate as women.[34] Familial pancreatitis recently has been shown by Whitcomb et al. to be caused by mutations in the *cationic trypsinogen* gene on 7q35.[53,54] These authors constructed a 500-member pedigree from a U.S. kindred centered in eastern Kentucky and Western Virginia, and using microsatellite markers

Table 50-1 Hereditary Syndromes Associated with Pancreatic Cancer

Syndrome	Mode of Inheritance	Gene	Chromosome Locus	Manifestation
Hereditary pancreatitis	AD	*cationic trypsinogen*	7q35	Recurrent episodes of severe pancreatitis occurring at an early age
HNPCC	AD	*MSH2*	2p	Cononic, endometrial, and stomach cancers; mutator penotype
		MLH1	3p	
		PMS2	7p	
		PMS1	2q	
FAMMM	AD	*p16*	9p	Multiple nevi, atypical nevi, melanomas
Peutz-Jeghers	AD	*LKB1*	19p	Hamartomatous polyps of the gastrointestinal tract, mucocutaneous melanin macules
Familial breast cancer 2	AD	*BRCA2*	13q	Breast, ovarian, and pancreatic cancer
Ataxia telangiectasia	AR	*ATM*	11q22–23	Cerebellar ataxia, oculocutaneous telangiectasia, thymic hypoplasia

NOTE: HNPCC = hereditary nonpolyposis colorectal cancer; FAMMM = familial atypical mole–multiple melanoma; AD = autosomal dominant; AR = autosomal recessive.

and linkage analysis, they were able to establish cosegregation between the familial pancreatitis phenotype and the 7q35 locus.[53] The *cationic trypsinogen* gene resides at 7q35, and Whitcomb et al. demonstrated that an Arg-His substitution at residue 117 of this gene segregates with the hereditary pancreatitis in some families.[54] Mutations at this site block the inactivation of trypsin, resulting in autodigestion of the pancreas. The mechanism by which pancreatitis leads to the development of pancreatic cancer is not clear; however, some have suggested that the increased risk of pancreatic cancer observed in patients with chronic pancreatitis is secondary to chronic injury and regeneration from the pancreatitis itself.[33,55,56]

HNPCC. Hereditary nonpolyposis colorectal cancer is another syndrome that predisposes affected individuals to pancreatic cancers.[19,34] This syndrome is characterized by the autosomal dominant transmission of a predisposition to colonic cancer in association with other cancers, including endometrial, stomach, and pancreatic cancer.[23,57–59] HNPCC is caused by germ-line mutations in one of the DNA mismatch repair genes.[60–65] These genes include *hMSH2, hMSH1, hPMS2, hPMS1, hMSH6/GTBP,* and *hMSH3*, and they code for proteins that repair single-base-pair changes and small insertions/deletions that occur during DNA replication.[61,62,66–69] When one of these genes is inactivated in a neoplasm, the neoplastic cells accumulate mutations in small noncoding regions of the genome called *microsatellite repeats,* resulting in changes in length of these repeats, a phenotype called *microsatellite instability.* Of note, replication errors, such as those found in HNPCC, are found in approximately 4 percent of pancreatic cancers,[67,70,71] and as noted previously, pancreatic cancer has been reported in some HNPCC kindreds.[23,57–59]

Peutz-Jeghers. The Peutz-Jeghers syndrome is a hereditary disease with an autosomal dominant pattern of inheritance characterized by hamartomatous polyps of the gastrointestinal tract and mucocutaneous melanocytic macules.[72] Forty-eight percent of 31 patients with Peutz-Jeghers syndrome followed by Giardiello et al. developed cancer, and 4 of these cancers were pancreatic cancer.[73] This represents a 100-fold excess of pancreatic cancer compared with that expected. The Peutz-Jeghers syndrome recently has been shown to be caused by germ-line mutations in the *LKB1/STK11* gene on 19p.[74,75] *LKB1* has strong homology to a cytoplasmic *Xenopus* serine threonine protein kinase, *XEEK1*. Peutz-Jeghers is therefore the first cancer-susceptibility syndrome to be identified that is attributable to inactivating mutations in a protein kinase.[74,75] Su et al. recently have demonstrated loss of the wild-type *LKB1* allele in a pancreatic cancer from a patient with a germ-line *LKB1* mutation and the Peutz-Jeghers syndrome.[76]

FAMMM. A subset of patients with the FAMMM syndrome appear to be at increased risk for developing pancreatic cancer.[21,33,34] The FAMMM syndrome is inherited in an autosomal dominant fashion and is characterized by multiple nevi, multiple atypical nevi, and multiple cutaneous malignant melanomas.[21,77,78] Germ-line mutations in *p16* have been shown to segregate with the increased risks of pancreatic cancer in some kindreds with the FAMMM syndrome.[77,78] Of interest, although the risk of pancreatic cancer is increased in these kindreds, it is not a highly penetrant trait. In these families there may be a tendency for mutations at the C-terminal end of the *p16* gene to be associated with a higher penetrance for pancreatic cancer.[79]

Ataxia Telangectasia. Patients with ataxia telangiectasia also may be at increased risk for developing pancreatic cancer.[33,34] Ataxia telangiectasia is characterized by progressive cerebellar ataxia with degeneration of Purkinje cells, telangiectasias (primarily conjuctival), thymic hypoplasia with cellular and humoral immunodeficiencies, and oculomotor apraxia. Ataxia telangiectasia is inherited in an autosomal recessive pattern, and the gene responsible for this syndrome has been cloned recently. The *ATM* gene resides on chromosome 11q22-23, and it encodes for a protein that is similar to several yeast and mammalian phosphatidylinositol 3′ kinases involved in mitogenic signal transduction, meiotic recombination, and cell cycle control.[80] Patients with ataxia telangiectasia are at increased risk for developing a number of neoplasms, including ovarian cancer, biliary cancer, gastric cancer, leukemia, lymphoma, and possibly pancreatic cancer.[33,34,80]

Families with an Aggregation of Pancreatic Cancer. Although a number of well-characterized syndromes have been associated with an increased risk of pancreatic cancer, the majority of pancreatic cancers cannot be explained in this way. In many families, pancreatic cancer occurs independent of a known syndrome. For example, Henry Lynch at Creighton University has reported over 30 extended families with multiple cases of pancreatic carcinoma.[19–25,34] He identified a suspected autosomal dominant mode of transmission in some of his pedigrees and estimated that between 5 and 10 percent of all pancreatic cancers have a hereditary origin.[24,34] Lynch notes, however, that the clustering of a cancer in a family does not necessarily mean that the cancer is hereditary. Environmental exposures need to be considered. For example, it is possible that several members of a family developed cancer because they each had smoked cigarettes.[33] Nonetheless, these families provide a unique opportunity to study efficiently the clinical patterns and genetics of pancreatic cancer.

We therefore established the National Familial Pancreas Tumor Registry (NFPTR) at Johns Hopkins in 1994 . This is now one of the largest registries of families in which more than one family member is affected with pancreatic cancer.* One hundred and forty-nine families with two or more first-degree relatives having cancer of the pancreas have enrolled in this registry as of July 29, 1998. The average age at diagnosis for patients with pancreatic cancer in these families (65.5 years) does not appear to differ from the age of onset of pancreatic carcinomas that are apparently sporadic.[37] Ninety-nine of the kindreds involved two family members: 68 parent-child pairs and 31 sibling-sibling pairs. Fifty of the 149 kindreds had three to five affected family members (Table 50-2). Approximately 20 percent of the patients with pancreatic cancer enrolled in this registry developed a second cancer.[37] These cancers included breast cancer, colon cancer, melanoma, bladder cancer, lung cancer, and prostate cancer. [37] As discussed previously, analyses of the kindred enrolled in this registry have demonstrated that second-degree relatives of patients from kindreds with familial pancreatic cancer are at increased risk for developing pancreatic cancer compared with second-degree relatives of patients from families in which only one first-degree relative developed pancreatic cancer (3.7 percent versus 0.6 percent, $p < 0.0001$).[37] Nonpancreatic cancers also were increased in second-degree relatives of the familial pancreatic cancer cases (27.2 percent versus 12.1 percent, $p < 0.0001$). The other types of cancer that developed in these patients included breast cancer, lung cancer, and colon cancer.[37]

Members of these registries, as well as those of registries created for other cancer types, are an important resource that can be used to determine the contribution of environmental risk factors, the patterns of inheritance of pancreatic cancer, and the types and prevalence of other tumor types (such as melanoma, breast cancer, and ovarian cancer) in familial pancreatic cancer.[81,82] The results of these analyses should provide a basis for counseling families with a familial aggregation of pancreatic cancer.

Families in Which There Is an Association of Pancreatic with Nonpancreatic Cancers. Several other cancers, including those

*The National Familial Pancreas Tumor Registry, The Johns Hopkins Hospital, Department of Pathology, Meyer 7-181, 600 N. Wolfe Street, Baltimore, MD 21287. (410) 955-9132; (410) 955-0115 (fax); e-mail: *rhuban@welchlink.welch.jhu.edu.*

Table 50-2 **Kindred Enrolled in the National Familial Pancreas Tumor Registry as of 7/29/98 in Which Two or More First-Degree Relatives Have Pancreatic Cancer**

Description of Kindred	Number of Kindreds	Total No. of Pancreas Cancer Cases
One generation		
2 siblings	31	62
3 siblings	10	30
4 siblings	2	8
5 siblings	1	5
2 siblings and 1 third-degree relative	4	9
2 siblings and 2 third-degree relatives	1	3
Two generations		
Parent, 1 offspring	68	136
Parent, 2 offspring	6	18
Parent, 3 offspring	3	12
Parent, 1 offspring, 1 sibling	7	21
Parent, 1 offspring, 3 siblings	1	5
Parent, 2 offspring, 1 sibling	1	4
Parent, offspring, sibling, 1 second-degree relative	1	4
Parent, offspring, sibling, 1 third-degree relative	1	4
Parent, offspring, 1 second-degree relative	2	6
Parent, 1 offspring, 1 third-degree relative	3	9
Three generations		
Grandparent, parent, grandchild	3	9
Grandparent, parent, grandchild, 1 first-degree relative	2	8
Grandparent, parent, grandchild, 2 first-degree relatives	1	5
Grandparent, parent, grandchild, 1 third-degree relative	1	4
TOTAL	149	362

of the breast and ovary, have been associated with pancreatic cancer in some families.[34] Tulinius et al. analyzed the cancer risk for family members of 947 randomly selected female breast cancer patients in the Icelandic Cancer Registry.[83] They found more cases of pancreatic cancer than expected in male first-degree relatives of the breast cancer patients ($RR = 1.66$).[83] Kerber and Slattery, in a case-control study of the Utah Population Database, found that a family history of pancreatic cancer is significantly associated with an increased risk of ovarian cancer.[84] From this Kerber and Slattery estimate that a family history of pancreatic cancer accounted for 4.8 percent of the cases of ovarian cancer.[84] Similarly, genetically defined subsets of families with familial melanoma and with familial breast cancer have been found to have an increased incidence of pancreatic cancer.[77,78,85–88]

Currently, a minority of the cases in which there is an aggregation of pancreatic cancer can be accounted for by known syndromes or by an association of nonpancreatic with pancreatic cancers. Each form of familial pancreatic cancer has, however, provided insights and fresh opportunities to study the genetics of pancreatic cancer. In turn, the results of these analyses will provide insight into the etiology of pancreatic cancers that are apparently sporadic.

Genetic Loci Involved in Sporadic Pancreatic Cancer

Three general approaches have been taken in the search for the genetic loci involved in the development of pancreatic cancer. The identity of specific chromosomes lost or gained by the pancreatic cancer can be determined by the karyotypes of metaphase spreads obtained from fresh cancers. These cytogenetic studies provide structural information about the mechanisms responsible for the loss or gain of genetic material, but the resolution of this technique is limited. More detailed information can be obtained by looking for loss of heterozygosity (LOH) using a panel of molecular probes specific for each chromosome arm. Such allelotypes were used in the identification of the novel *DPC4* tumor-suppressor gene in a panel of pancreatic cancers and in defining the roles of the *p16* and *p53* genes. Finally, the relatively new technique of representational difference analysis (RDA) has been applied to pancreatic cancer. RDA is a method for isolating DNA fragments that are present in only one of two nearly identical complex genomes. It uses subtraction hybridization methods and has been shown to enrich for difference products over 1 million-fold. RDA is a particularly attractive technique for isolating new tumor-suppressor genes because it can strongly favor the enrichment of homozygously deleted regions. Homozygous deletions are smaller than most heterozygous losses, and so this technique promises to focus attention on smaller regions of the genome to serve as candidate loci for new tumor-suppressor genes.

Karyotype of Sporadic Pancreatic Cancer. A number of recurrent chromosome abnormalities have been identified in sporadic pancreatic cancers, providing clues to the specific genes involved in the pathogenesis of pancreatic cancer.[89–92] Griffin et al. have karyotyped 62 primary pancreatic cancers resected at The Johns Hopkins Hospital and found clonally abnormal karyotypes in 44 of the cancers.[91,92] The karyotypes generally were complex and included both numerical and structural changes. Losses were more frequent than gains and included a high prevalence of losses of chromosomes 18, 13, 12, 17, and 6. The losses of chromosome 6q were confirmed by fluorescent *in situ* hybridization using a biotin-labeled microdissection probe from 6q24-ter. The most frequent whole-chromosome gains were of chromosomes 20 and 7. Recurrent structural abnormalities most frequently involved 1p, 3p, 11p, 17p, 1q, 6q, and 19q.[91,92] In addition, double-minute chromatin bodies suggestive of gene amplification were identified in six of the cancers. These karyotype studies, when combined with smaller reports by Johansson et al., suggest that chromosomes 1p, 3p, 6q, and 11p may harbor yet unidentified tumor-suppressor genes.[89,91,92] More recently Höglund et al. have combined karyotyping with fluorescence *in situ* hybridization to demonstrate that chromosome 19 aberrations are common in pancreatic cancer.[93]

Allelotype of Sporadic Pancreatic Cancer. Hahn et al. and Seymour et al. have allelotyped two series of pancreatic cancers.[70,94] High frequencies (60 percent) of allelic loss were found at 1p, 9p, 17p, and 18q, whereas moderate frequencies (40–60 percent) of allelic loss were seen at 3p, 6p, 8p, 10q, 12q, 13q, 18p, 21q, and 22q.[70,94] These patterns of allelic loss suggest regions of the genome as harboring candidate tumor-suppressor loci. For example, the *p53* gene is located on 17p, and 17p was lost in 100 percent of the cancers allelotyped by Hahn et al.[70] Similarly, the *DPC4* gene on 18q and the *p16* gene on 9p each suffered LOH in nearly 90 percent of the tumors.[70] In these studies, chromosome 1p had the highest frequency of allelic loss (67 percent) not accounted for by a known tumor-suppressor gene.

Allelotype and karyotype studies produce different kinds of information, and a comparison of these results provides new insight into the structural basis of the molecular genetic alterations. Brat et al. recently compared the chromosomal abnormalities of primary pancreatic adenocarcinomas, as determined by classic cytogenetics, with the molecular changes, as determined by the studies of LOH, in the same cancers.[95] In the 14 cancers with abnormal karyotypes, 65 percent (123 of 188) of the chromosomal arms with molecular LOH were associated with karyotypic structural abnormalities. Karyotypic changes accounting for these losses included 83 whole-chromosomal losses, 18 partial deletions, 9 isochromosomes, 8 additions, and 5 translocations. The greatest degree of correlation between the cytogenetic and molecular studies was found at sites of known tumor-suppressor genes such as *p53*, *DPC4*, *p16*, and *BRCA2*. These results generally validate both techniques and indicate that, in pancreatic cancer, large structural abnormalities can account for two-thirds of the LOH. Of note, there were 13 chromosomes that had extensive regions of LOH yet appeared normal on karyotypic analysis. This finding suggests that chromosome loss with reduplication of the remaining chromosome occurs in pancreatic cancer.[95] Finally, homozygous deletions tended to be small and were not detected in the karyotype analyses.

RDA Applied to Sporadic Pancreas Cancer. As discussed previously, RDA is a powerful technique that can be used to isolate small regions of homozygous deletion in a cancer. Schutte et al. applied RDA to a sporadic pancreatic cancer and identified a homozygous deletion that mapped to a 180-kb region on chromosome 13q.[96] This deletion mapped to the area of the *BRCA2* locus, and the map of this deletion provided the first published partial sequences of the *BRCA2* gene, including exon 2 and intron 24.[96] The mapping of this deletion, a critical advance aiding in the discovery of the *BRCA2* gene by Stratton et al. and by Myriad Genetics, provided the first clue that the *BRCA2* was a tumor-suppressor gene as opposed to a proto-oncogene and showed that *BRCA2* served such a role in the pancreas.[97,98]

SPECIFIC GENES

Specific Genes Involved in Hereditary Pancreatic Cancer

The short life expectancy of patients with pancreatic carcinoma has made it difficult to perform classic linkage studies on families with pancreatic cancer. Simply put, it is extremely unusual to find more than one patient alive with disease at a time in any family. Because of these difficulties, most studies of familial pancreatic cancer have relied on the candidate gene approach. In this approach, a tumor-suppressor gene that is known to be inactivated in sporadic pancreatic cancers is selected as the candidate gene, and then germ-line tissues from affected individuals from families in which there is an aggregation of pancreatic cancer can be tested for mutations in this candidate gene. This approach is possible because, at the molecular level, familial and sporadic forms of cancer often involve the same genes.[99] For example, familial adenomatous polyposis (FAP) has been shown to be caused by inherited mutations in the *APC* gene, and inactivation of *APC* is a common and early event in sporadic adenocarcinomas of the colon.[100,101] Similarly, missense germ-line mutations in the *RET* proto-oncogene are responsible for the multiple endocrine neoplasia type 2 (MEN2) syndrome, and these same mutations have been identified in sporadic medullary carcinomas.[102,103]

The candidate gene approach has been applied to familial pancreatic cancer, and in a few of the families, the pancreatic cancers appear to be caused by germ-line mutations in the *p16*, *LKB1*, or *BRCA2* gene.[104,105] In contrast, a number of these families have been examined for germ-line mutations in *DPC4*, but to date, none have been found.[79]

Germ-Line *p16* Mutations in Pancreatic Cancer Families. The *p16* (*MTS1/p16/CDKN2*) gene is genetically inactivated in approximately 80 percent of sporadic adenocarcinomas of the pancreas.[71] In 40 percent of these cancers, these inactivations are caused by homozygous deletions of the gene and in another 40 percent by intragenic mutations in one allele coupled with loss of the second allele. *p16* therefore would appear to be a good candidate to examine in patients with familial pancreatic cancers. Moskaluk et al. analyzed 21 kindreds with familial pancreatic carcinoma for germ-line mutations in *p16* and in the related *CDK4* gene.[104] Kindreds known to have the FAMMM syndrome were excluded. Germ-line *CDK4* mutations were not seen, and germ-line *p16* mutation were identified in only one family. The mutation was found in two individuals affected with pancreatic cancer in this family, and the alteration destroyed the donor splice site of intron 2, causing premature termination after the addition of two new codons at the 3′ end of exon 2.[104] Of interest, one of the two carriers in this kindred also had a melanoma, suggesting that this kindred, in fact, had the FAMMM syndrome. All other patients in this series were found to be wild type for both *p16* and for *CDK4*.[104] Thus germ-line *p16* mutations could account for the pancreatic cancers in only 1 (5 percent) of the 21 kindreds studied with familial pancreatic cancer, and they were seen in a patient who also had melanoma. Germ-line mutations in *p16* therefore should be suspected when there is an aggregation of both melanoma and pancreatic cancer in a family.[77,78]

Germ-Line *BRCA2* Mutations in Pancreatic Cancer Families. The *BRCA2* gene was another logical choice for the candidate gene approach. *BRCA2* may play a role in the development of sporadic pancreatic cancer. Twenty-five to 35 percent of sporadic pancreatic cancers show LOH at the *BRCA2* locus on 13q, and karyotypic losses of chromosome 13 are common in pancreatic cancer.[70,89,91,92,94] Furthermore, a critical advance in the discovery of *BRCA2* was the identification of a homozygous deletion of the *BRCA2* locus in a pancreatic cancer.[96,97] Finally, as noted previously, there have been some reports suggesting that the risk of pancreatic cancer is increased in families of breast cancer patients and in carriers of *BRCA2* mutations.[83,85–88] Goggins et al. therefore screened a panel of 41 adenocarcinomas of the pancreas for *BRCA2* mutations.[105] Four of the 41 cancers had both a loss of one allele of *BRCA2* and a mutation in the second allele. Three of these four mutations were present in the germ-line. The three germ-line mutations identified included two germ-line 6174 delT at codon 1982 and a germ-line 2481 insT mutation.[105] Because of these findings, the utility of a cross-sectional population screen was evaluated. Normal tissues from 245 consecutive surgical patients with adenocarcinoma of the pancreas were screened near the 6174 nucleotide. Sequence analysis of this limited region of the *BRCA2* gene revealed two additional germ-line mutations, a 6174 delT mutation and a second nearby 6158 insT mutation. Thus a total of 5 germ-line mutations in *BRCA2* were identified. Remarkably, only 1 of the 5 patients with germ-line mutations had

Table 50-3 Genetic Alterations in Apparently Sporadic Pancreatic Carcinomas

Genes	Chromosome Locus	Mechanism of Inactivation	Frequency (%)
Oncogenes			
K-*ras*	12	Point mutations codons 12, 13	80–100
Tumor-suppressor genes			
p16	9p	Homozygous deletion, LOH and IM, hypermethylation	95
p53	17p	LOH and IM	50–75
DPC4	18q	Homozygous deletion, LOH and IM	50
BRCA2	13q	Germ-line IM and acquired LOH	4–7
MKK4	17p	Homozygous deletion, LOH and IM	4
LKB1	19p	Homozygous deletion, LOH and IM	5
RB	13q	Mutation/small deletion	0–7
Genome maintenance genes			
hMSH2, hMLH1, hPMS1, hPMS2, hMSHG/GTBP, hMSH3	Multiple	Often undetermined; gives phenotype of microsatellite instability	4

NOTE: LOH = loss of heterozygosity; IM = intragenic mutation; AD = autosomal dominant; AR = autosomal recessive.

a relative with breast cancer, and 1 had a relative with prostate cancer. None had a family history of pancreatic cancer.[105] Ozcelik et al. confirmed these findings by Goggins and estimated that 10 percent of pancreatic cancers in Ashkenazi Jews are caused by germ-line *BRCA2* 6174 delT mutations and suggested that carriers of the 6174 delT mutation have a 10-fold increased risk of developing pancreatic cancer.[106]

Germ-line mutations in *BRCA2* therefore represent the most common inherited predisposition to pancreatic carcinoma identified to date, and the results of screening for *BRCA2* mutations suggest that the classic definition of a familial case of pancreatic cancer is too stringent. Clearly, some cases of pancreatic cancer that appear sporadic are, in fact, caused by inherited mutations in *BRCA2*.

***LKB1*.** As noted previously, the Peutz-Jeghers syndrome is associated with an increased risk of pancreatic cancer,[73] and Su et al. have demonstrated recently loss of the wild-type *LKB1* allele in a pancreatic cancer obtained from a patient with the Peutz-Jeghers syndrome and a germ-line *LKB1* mutation.[76]

Absence of Germ-Line *DPC4*, K-*ras* and *p53* Mutations in Pancreatic Cancer Families. The recently discovered *DPC4* gene was an attractive candidate gene to study in families with pancreatic cancer.[107] *DPC4* was identified in a locus of consensus homozygous deletions in sporadic pancreatic carcinomas. It is biallelically inactivated in almost 50 percent of pancreatic carcinomas.[107] Moskaluk et al. therefore sequenced the complete *DPC4* coding sequence of 25 individuals from 11 separate kindreds with a familial aggregation of pancreatic carcinoma, but no mutations were found.[79] Similarly, the K-*ras* oncogene frequently is activated and the *p53* tumor suppressor frequently is inactivated in pancreatic carcinomas, but to date, germ-line mutations have not been identified in either of these two genes in patients with familial or sporadic cancer.[107,108]

In summary, the gene or genes responsible for the majority of cases of familial pancreatic cancer have not yet been identified. A small minority of these cases may be caused by germ-line mutations in *p16*, particularly in patients in whom there is a family history of melanoma. Germ-line mutations in *BRCA2* also predispose to the development of pancreatic cancer, and because of their low penetrance, these mutations appear responsible for some cases of pancreatic cancer that appear to be sporadic.

Specific Genes Involved in Sporadic Pancreatic Cancer (Table 50-3)

The development of an adenocarcinoma of the pancreas is complex and involves the accumulation of mutations in the K-*ras* oncogene and in numerous tumor-suppressor genes. K-*ras* appears to be activated in the vast majority of pancreatic cancers, whereas the tumor-suppressor genes *p53*, *p16*, *DPC4*, and *BRCA2* frequently are inactivated.[108] These mutations dysregulate the cell cycle and lead to inappropriate cell proliferation. Of interest, a high concordance of *DPC4* and *p16* inactivation ($p < 0.007$) has been reported in pancreatic cancer, suggesting that inactivation of the *p16/RB* pathway might increase the selective pressure for subsequent mutations of *DPC4* in this tumor type.[2] This section will begin with a discussion of K-*ras*, the most frequently altered gene in pancreatic cancer, and it will then be followed by a discussion of the tumor-suppressor genes that are most frequently inactivated in pancreatic cancer. It will conclude with a discussion of microsatellite instability in pancreatic cancer.

Activation of K-*ras*. Oncogenes encode for proteins that, when overexpressed or activated by a mutation, possess transforming properties. In normal cells, K-*ras* is a proto-oncogene that encodes for a G protein involved in signal transduction.[109] Point mutations in codons 12, 13, or 61 of K-*ras* activate the gene product.[110] These mutations impair the intrinsic GTPase activity of this protein and cause it to be constitutively active in signal transduction.[109] K-*ras* is the most frequently mutated gene in pancreatic cancer, with reported mutation rates ranging 71 to 100 percent.[108,111–124] This is the highest reported prevalence of K-*ras* mutations in any tumor type. The vast majority of these mutations occur in codon 12 of K-*ras*.[108] These mutations appear to be early events in the development of pancreatic neoplasia. This has been demonstrated by studies of the noninvasive duct lesions that are found in the pancreata with and without cancer.[125] In humans and in the Syrian golden hamster animal model of pancreatic neoplasia, these duct lesions have been shown to harbor activating point mutations in K-*ras*.[125–133] For example, several investigators have microdissected the pancreatic duct lesions from pancreata obtained from patients without cancer, and they have shown that these noninvasive duct lesions can harbor activating clonal mutations in K-*ras*.[125,128,129] Thus activation of the K-*ras* oncogene appears to be a fairly early event in the development of adenocarcinoma of the pancreas. Furthermore, as will be discussed later, the high prevalence of K-*ras* mutations in invasive cancers, their presence early in the neoplastic process, and the limitation of these mutations largely to a pair of codons all make K-*ras* a promising marker for a molecular-based test to detect early pancreatic carcinomas.

Amplification of Oncogenes

The most common amplicon in pancreatic cancer (10 percent of the cases) also was the first to be identified. Originally found as the amplification of the *PD-1* gene, the leading current candidate to explain the amplification on chromosome 19q is the *AKT2* gene.[134,135] Other sites of amplification exist, however, at much lower frequencies.[136]

Tumor-Suppressor Genes. Tumor-suppressor genes differ from oncogenes in that tumor-suppressor genes normally function to restrict the expansion of cell populations. Their loss, by deletion or mutation, leads to dysregulated cell growth.

p53 Inactivation. The *p53* tumor-suppressor gene is inactivated in more than half of all pancreatic carcinomas.[2,117,137–143] In almost all these cancers this inactivation occurs by loss of one allele coupled with an intragenic mutation of the other. Evidence for the loss of one allele comes from allelotyping and karyotyping studies that have identified 17p as a site of frequent loss in pancreatic cancers.[70,91,92,94] When sequenced, the second allele of *p53* is mutated in about 50 to 75 percent of the cancers.[2,121,140] The majority of mutations reported have been transitions (pyrimidine-to-pyrimidine or purine-to-purine) in the conserved regions of the gene. Redston et al. and Rozenblum et al. also noted a high prevalence of small frameshift mutations in the *p53* gene in pancreatic cancers.[2,140] p53 is a nuclear DNA-binding protein that acts as a G1/S checkpoint, and it also plays a role in the induction of apoptosis.[144–148] Inactivation of *p53* in pancreatic cancers therefore results in the loss of two important controls of cell number, the initiation of replication and the induction of cell death.

p16 Inactivation. *p16* is a tumor-suppressor gene that is inactivated in a variety of tumors.[149] *p16* resides on chromosome 9p, and as noted earlier, 9p was found to be a frequent site of allelic loss in allelotypes of pancreatic cancer.[70,94] Caldas et al. demonstrated loss of one allele of *p16* accompanied by sequence changes in *p16* in the second allele in 38 percent of tumors.[70,71,94,150–154] Furthermore, Caldas et al. demonstrated homozygous deletions of *p16* in nearly 40 percent of the tumors. Therefore, *p16* is genetically inactivated in nearly 80 percent of pancreatic cancers. In addition, Schutte et al. demonstrated that *p16* is inactivated by hypermethylation of its promoter in most of the remaining cancers.[155,156] *p16* inhibits the promotion of the cell cycle by competing with cyclin D in binding to CDK4, preventing CDK4 from phosphorylating the RB protein. Hypophosphorylated RB protein binds and may sequester transcription factors that otherwise promote the G1/S transition, whereas hyperphosphorylation of RB releases these factors.[157] Therefore, the inactivation of *p16* in approximately 95 percent of pancreatic cancers dysregulates another important cell cycle checkpoint.

DPC4. One of the most frequently lost chromosome arms in both the allelotypes and karyotypes of pancreatic cancer is 18q.[91,92,94,158] Based on this observation, Hahn et al. performed detailed genome scanning of 18q on a panel of pancreatic carcinomas.[107] These analyses not only confirmed the high frequency of LOH on 18q but also revealed a consensus locus of homozygous deletions. These homozygous deletions did not include the *DCC* locus. Further positional cloning of the locus lead to the discovery of the *DPC4* gene. This tumor-suppressor gene, also known as *SMAD4*, is biallelically inactivated in almost 50 percent of pancreatic carcinomas.[107] In 30 percent, this inactivation is by homozygous deletion, and in 20 percent, by loss of one allele coupled with an intragenic mutation of the other.[107] Remarkably, although *DPC4* appears to be a common target of inactivation in pancreatic cancer, it is only infrequently inactivated in other neoplasms.[159] The specificity of *DPC4* inactivation for pancreatic cancer suggests that the *DPC4* status may be useful in determining if a particular metastatic carcinoma in a patient had arisen in the pancreas.

DPC4 has homology to the Smad family of proteins, and the Smad proteins play a role in signal transduction from transforming growth factor beta (TGFβ) superfamily cell surface receptors.[160–163] Normally, TGFβ provides a growth-inhibitory signal to epithelial cells.[164] When TGFβ binds to the TGFβ receptor, it promotes the dimerization of the TGFβ receptors type I and type II, which in turn activate the kinase activity of the TGFβ type I receptor.[164] The signal is transferred to Smad proteins by phosphorylation. These proteins then complex with *DPC4,* and relocalization to the nucleus occurs.[165]

The importance of *DPC4* in TGFβ signaling was proven conclusively by Zhou et al.[166] They homozygously deleted the *DPC4* gene of cultured human colonic cancer cells using homologous recombination and demonstrated that this deletion abrogated signaling from TGFβ, as well as from the TGFβ family member activin.[166] Takaku et al. demonstrated the importance of *DPC4* (*Smad4*) inactivation in tumorigenesis.[167] They made mice that were compound heterozygotes to mutant *APC* and *DPC4* alleles. Because these genes lie close on the same chromosome in mice, an LOH event results in a tumor lacking functional copies of both genes.[167] The intestinal neoplasms that developed in these mice were unusually invasive and had a greater stromal response than did neoplasms that developed in simple *APC* mutant mice.[167] Therefore, by extension, the inactivation of *DPC4* in pancreatic cancer may lead to the loss of an important pathway in TGFβ-related signaling, and it may play a significant role in the malignant progression of these tumors.

Mutations in Multiple Genes in Pancreatic Cancer. Rozenblum et al. have determined the status of K-*ras*, *p53*, *p16*, *DPC4,* and *BRCA2* in a series of 42 pancreatic carcinomas.[2] This extensive molecular analysis of a series of cancers provides a unique opportunity to determine if there are any relationships among the mutations in these various genes. All 42 carcinomas harbored a mutation in codon 12 of K-*ras,* and inactivation of all three tumor-suppressor genes occurred in 37 percent of the cancers.[2] A high concordance was found between *DPC4* and *p16* inactivation ($p < 0.007$), suggesting that inactivation of the p16/RB pathway increased the selective pressure for subsequent mutations of *DPC4.* Of note, one carcinoma carried a germ-line mutation in *BRCA2* and eight additional selected genetic events, highlighting the complexity of the molecular genetic events responsible for the development of pancreatic cancer. Furthermore, small homozygous deletions appear to be a common mechanism for inactivating tumor-suppressor genes in pancreatic cancer. One or more homozygous deletions were found in 64 percent of the cancers.[71,107,159,168]

Other Tumor-Suppressor Genes. A number of other tumor-suppressor genes appear to be inactivated in only a small minority of pancreatic carcinomas. For example, the *MKK4* gene on 17p encodes for the mitogen-activated protein kinase 4 (MKK4) protein. MKK4 is an important component of a stress- and cytokine-induced signal transduction pathway involving the mitogen-activated protein kinase (MAPK) proteins.[169] Su et al. recently have confirmed the findings of Teng et al. that *MKK4* is inactivated in about 4 percent of pancreatic carcinomas.[169] Two percent of the carcinomas harbored an intragenic mutation coupled with LOH, and in 2 percent *MKK4* was inactivated by homozygous deletion.[169] Some of the allelic loss patterns did not extend to the *p53* locus on 17p, and inactivation of *MKK4* may therefore explain some of the LOH seen on 17p in pancreatic adenocarcinomas.

Chromosome 19p is also frequently lost in pancreatic cancer, and as discussed earlier, the gene responsible for the Peutz-Jeghers syndrome, *LKB1*, has been identified recently at 19p13.3.[74,75,93] Höglund et al. karyotyped a series of pancreatic cancers and reported that structural arrangements of chromosome 19 resulting in loss of 19p were common.[93] Su et al. extended these studies and demonstrated, at the molecular level, that *LKB1* is indeed inactivated in 5 percent of apparently sporadic pancreatic carcinomas.[76] In 1 to 2 percent of the cancers this was by homozygous deletion and in 3 to 4 percent by LOH coupled with an intragenic mutation. The inactivation of *LKB1* in both familial (Peutz-Jeghers syndrome) and sporadic pancreatic cancers confirms the hypothesis that the same genes are frequently responsible for the development of both sporadic and familial forms of cancer.[99]

Although one report suggested that *APC* might be inactivated in pancreatic cancers, more detailed studies, which examined large numbers of pancreatic cancers, demonstrated that inactivation of *APC* or its pathway partner *β-catenin* is rare to absent in pancreatic cancers.[94,170–172] These genes are almost universally mutated in colorectal neoplasia, and the absence of *APC* pathway alterations in pancreatic cancer demonstrates further that the mutation spectrum of pancreatic carcinoma is distinct from that seen in other gastrointestinal neoplasms.

There have been conflicting reports on the expression levels of the *DCC* gene product in pancreatic carcinomas, but no genetic alterations, including homozygous deletions, have been reported to date for *DCC* in pancreatic cancer.[70,107,173]

Mutations of *RB* are reported in pancreatic cancer, but at a very low rate. Huang et al. found that immunohistologic staining for RB expression was lost in 3 of 30 pancreatic cancers. In one of these three cases a truncating mutation was found, and in a second a missense mutation was verified by DNA sequencing.[94,173–175]

Microsatellite Instability. Goggins et al. screened 82 xenografted sporadic adenocarcinomas of the pancreas for DNA replication errors (RER+) using polymerase chain reaction amplification of microsatellite markers.[67] Three (3.7 percent) of the 82 carcinomas were RER+ and contained associated mutations in the *TGFBRII* gene. In contrast to typical gland-forming adenocarcinomas of the pancreas, all these RER+ carcinomas were poorly differentiated and had expanding borders and a prominent syncytial growth pattern[67] (Fig. 50-5). Furthermore, all the RER+ carcinomas were K-*ras* wild type, and the one case that was karyotyped showed a near diploid pattern. These data by Goggins et al. suggest that DNA replication errors occur in approximately 4 percent of pancreatic carcinomas and that wild-type K-*ras* gene status coupled with the histologic findings of poor differentiation, a syncytial growth pattern, and pushing borders should suggest the possibility of DNA replication errors in carcinomas of the pancreas.

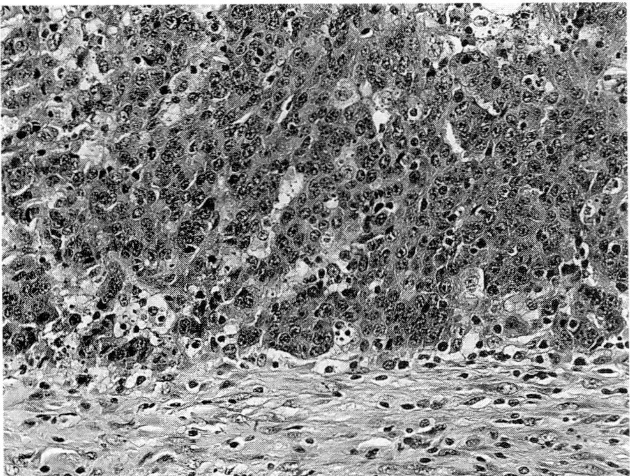

Fig. 50-5 Pancreatic carcinoma with DNA replication errors (RER+). RER+ carcinomas of the pancreas are associated with wild-type K-*ras* and poor differentiation, a syncytial growth pattern, and pushing borders.

IMPLICATIONS FOR DIAGNOSIS

There are no molecular tests currently being used to screen for pancreatic carcinomas. However, the recent advances in our understanding of how molecular biology can be used to screen for cancer, coupled with an improved understanding of the molecular genetics of this tumor, provide several avenues for developing such a test.[176] Probably the best example is the K-*ras* oncogene. K-*ras* is a particularly attractive target for a molecular screening test for pancreatic cancer for three reasons. First, the vast majority of pancreatic carcinomas harbor mutations in K-*ras*, suggesting that K-*ras* will be a sensitive genetic marker.[108,111–124] Second, mutations in this oncogene essentially are limited to two codons, and so a limited number of probes can be employed to detect these mutations, greatly simplifying the analyses.[108] Finally, as discussed earlier, these mutations appear to be early events in the development of pancreatic neoplasia, suggesting that K-*ras* could be used to detect early and therefore curable cancers.[125–129,137] Indeed, K-*ras* mutations have been used to identify cells shed from pancreatic cancers in pancreatic juice samples, in cytologic preparations, and in stool and blood specimens.[122,129,130,177–183] For example, Caldas et al. screened stool specimens obtained from patients with chronic pancreatitis, cholangiocarcinoma, and pancreatic cancer.[129] They found K-*ras* mutations in stool specimens from nine patients. Six of these nine patients had pancreatic cancer, and in five of the six cases the mutation found in the patients' invasive pancreatic cancer was the same as the one identified in the stool. In the remaining four patients, mutations identified in the stool were identical to those present in duct lesions (duct hyperplasias) found in the patients' resected pancreatic specimens.[129] This study established that screening for genetic alterations can be used to detect rare cells shed from pancreatic cancers. It also demonstrated that an improved understanding of the genetic alterations in duct lesions and in early invasive pancreatic cancers will be essential for the development of genetic-based screening tests. A significant investigative effort has therefore been focused on defining the genetic alterations in duct lesions in the pancreas. The majority of duct lesions examined to date have been found to harbor activating point mutations with codon 12 of the K-*ras* oncogene,[125,126,128–133,177,184] and some duct lesions with cytologic and architectural atypia have been shown to accumulate the *p53* gene product to immunohistologically detectable levels, suggesting that those duct lesions harbor *p53* mutations.[137,185] More recently, Moskaluk et al. examined duct lesions adjacent to infiltrating pancreatic cancers known to harbor inactivating *p16* mutations, and one-third of these duct lesions harbored *p16* alterations.[132] Wilentz et al. have confirmed that *p16* is inactivated in duct lesions using immunohistochemical stains.[186] Importantly, these genetic alterations in K-*ras*, *p53*, and *p16* occur while the neoplasm is still *in situ*, before it has spread beyond the pancreatic duct system.

In addition to leading to the development of new screening tests for early pancreatic neoplasms, an improved understanding of the genetics of pancreatic cancer will lead to the discovery of additional germ-line mutations in cancer-causing genes that predispose to pancreatic cancer, and geneticists will be able to screen at-risk individuals for these germ-line mutations. Carriers of germ-line mutations can then be clinically screened more thoroughly and may even choose prophylactic surgery, while those found not to carry germ-line mutations will have their anxiety relieved and can be spared unnecessary screening tests.

Clearly, we need to advance our understanding of the molecular genetics of pancreatic cancer so that new tests can be developed that are both sensitive and specific for early stages of this disease.

ACKNOWLEDGMENTS

We would like to thank Michele Heffler for her assistance, energy, and enthusiasm in preparing this manuscript and Flo Falatko for her tireless dedication to the National Familial Pancreas Tumor Registry. For the latest on pancreatic cancer, visit our Web site (*http://pathology.jhu.edu/pancreas*).

REFERENCES

1. Parker SL, Tong T, Bolden S, Wingo PA: Cancer statistics, 1997. *CA Cancer J Clin* **47**:5, 1997.
2. Rozenblum E, Schutte M, Goggins M, et al: Tumor-suppressive pathways in pancreatic carcinoma. *Cancer Res* **57**:1731, 1997.
3. Gold EB, Goldin SB: Epidemiology of and risk factors for pancreatic cancer. *Surg Oncol Clin North Am* **7**:67, 1998.
4. Gold EB: Epidemiology of and risk factors for pancreatic cancer. *Surg Clin North Am* **75**:819, 1995.
5. Taxy JB: Adenocarcinoma of the pancreas in childhood: Report of a case and a review of the English language literature. *Cancer* **37**:1508, 1976.
6. Newill VA: Distribution of cancer mortality among ethnic subgroups of the white population in New York City, 1953-1958. *J Natl Cancer Inst* **26**:405, 1961.
7. Seidman H: Cancer death rates by site and sex for religions and socioeconomic groups in New York City. *Environ Res* **3**:234, 1970.
8. Durbec JP, Chevillotte C, Bidart JM, Berthezene P, Sarles H: Diet, alcohol, tobacco, and risk of cancer of the pancreas: A case-control study. *Br J Cancer* **47**:463, 1983.
9. Ghadirian P, Simard A, Baillargeon J: Tobacco, alcohol, and coffee and cancer of the pancreas: A population-based, case-control study in Quebec, Canada. *Cancer* **67**:2664, 1991.
10. Doll R, Peto R: Mortality in relation to smoking: Twenty years observation on male British doctors. *Br Med J* **2**:1525, 1976.
11. Kahn HA: The Dorn study of smoking and mortality among U.S. Veterans: Report on eight and one-half years of observation. *Natl Cancer Inst Monogr* **19**:1, 1966.
12. Whittemore AS, Paffenbarger RS Jr, Anderson D, Lee JE: Early precursors of pancreatic cancer in college men. *J Chron Dis* **36**:251, 1983.
13. Howe GR, Ghadirian P, DeMesquita HB, et al: A collaborative case-control study of nutrient intake and pancreatic cancer within the search programme. *Int J Cancer* **51**:365, 1992.
14. Hirayama T: Epidemiology of pancreatic cancer in Japan. *Jpn J Clin Oncol* **19**:208, 1989.
15. Gold EB, Gordis L, Diener MD, Seltser R, Boitnott JK, Bynum TE, Hutcheon DF: Diet and other risk factors for cancer of the pancreas. *Cancer* **55**:460, 1985.
16. LaVecchia C, Liati P, Decarlie A, Negri E, Franceschi S: Coffee consumption and risk of pancreatic cancer. *Int J Cancer* **40**:309, 1987.
17. Velema JP, Walker AM, Gold EB: Alcohol and pancreatic cancer: Insufficient epidemiiologic evidence for a causal relationship. *Epidemiol Rev* **8**:28, 1986.
18. Li FP: Molecular epidemiology studies of cancer in families. *Br J Cancer* **68**:217, 1993.
19. Lynch HT, Voorhees GJ, Lanspa S, McGreevy PS, Lynch J: Pancreatic carcinoma and hereditary nonpolyposis colorectal cancer: A family study. *Br J Cancer* **52**:271, 1985.
20. Lynch HT, Fitzsimmons ML, Smyrk TC, Lanspa SJ, Watson P, McClellan J, Lynch JF: Familial pancreatic cancer: Clinicopathologic study of 18 nuclear families. *Am J Gastroenterol* **85**:54, 1990.
21. Lynch HT, Fusaro RM: Pancreatic cancer and the familial atypical multiple mole melanoma (FAMMM) syndrome. *Pancreas* **6**:127, 1991.
22. Lynch HT, Fusaro L, Lynch JF: Familial pancreatic cancer: A family study. *Pancreas* **7**:511, 1992.
23. Lynch HT, Smyrk TC, Watson P, et al: Genetics, natural history, tumor spectrum, and pathology of hereditary nonpolyposis colorectal cancer: An updated review. *Gastroenterology* **104**:1535, 1993.
24. Lynch HT: Genetics and pancreatic cancer. *Arch Surg* **129**:266,1994.
25. Lynch HT, Fusaro L, Smyrk T, Watson P, Lanspa S, Lynch J: Medical genetic study of eight pancreatic cancer-prone families. *Cancer Invest* **13**:141, 1995.
26. Bergman W, Watson P, de Jong J, Lynch HT, Fusaro RM: Systemic cancer and the FAMMM syndrome. *Br J Cancer* **61**:932, 1990.
27. Dat N, Sontag S: Pancreatic carcinoma in brothers. *Ann Intern Med* **97**:282, 1982.
28. Ehrenthal D, Haeger L, Griffin T, Compton C: Familial pancreatic adenocarcinoma in three generations. *Cancer* **59**:1661, 1987.
29. Grajower MM: Familial pancreatic cancer. *Ann Intern Med* **98**:111, 1983.
30. Katkhouda N, Mouiel J: Pancreatic cancer in mother and daughter. *Lancet* **2**:747, 1986.
31. MacDermott RP, Kramer P: Adencarcinoma of the pancreas in four siblings. *Gastroenterology* **65**:137, 1973.
32. Reimer R, Fraumeni JF Jr, Ozols R, Bender R: Pancreatic cancer in father and son. *Lancet* **1**:911, 1977.
33. Lumadue JA, Griffin CA, Osman M, Hruban RH: Familial pancreatic cancer and the genetics of pancreatic cancer. *Surg Clin North Am* **75**:845, 1995.
34. Lynch HT, Smyrk T, Kern SE, et al: Familial pancreatic cancer: a review. *Semin Oncol* **23**:251, 1996.
35. Ghadirian P, Boyle P, Simard A, Baillargeon J, Maisonneuve P, Perret C: Reported family aggregation of pancreatic cancer within a population-based case-control study in the Francophone community in Montreal, Canada. *Int J Pancreatol* **10**:183, 1991.
36. Fernandez E, La Vecchia C, D'Avanzo B, Negri E, Franceschi S: Family history and the risk of liver, gallbladder, and pancreatic cancer. *Cancer Epidemiol Biomark Prev* **3**:209, 1994.
37. Hruban RH, Petersen GM, Ha PK, Kern SE: Genetics of pancreatic cancer: From genes to families. *Surg Oncol Clin North Am* **7**:1, 1998.
38. Moossa AR, Gamagami RA: Diagnosis and staging of pancreatic neoplams. *Surg Clin North Am* **75**:871, 1995.
39. Christoffersen P, Poll P: Preoperative pancreas aspiration biopsies. *Acta Pathol Microbiol Immunol Scand (Suppl)* **212**:28, 1970.
40. American Cancer Society: *Cancer Facts and Figures 1996*. New York, 1996 (abstract).
41. DiGiuseppe JA, Yeo CJ, Hruban RH: Molecular biology and the diagnosis and treatment of adenocarcinoma of the pancreas. *Adv Anat Pathol* **3**:139, 1996.
42. Solcia E, Capella C, Klöppel G: *Tumors of the Pancreas*. 3rd Series, Armed Forces Institute of Pathology, Washington, DC, 1997.
43. Wilentz RE, Hruban RH: Pathology of cancer of the pancreas. *Surg Oncol Clin North Am* **7**:43, 1998.
44. Wilentz RE, Slebos RJC, Hruban RH: Screening for pancreatic cancer using techniques to detect altered gene products, in Reber HA (ed): *Advances in Pancreatic Cancer*. 1997.
45. Cubilla AL, Fitzgerald PJ: Morphological lesions associated with human primary invasive nonendocrine pancreas cancer. *Cancer Res* **36**:2690, 1976.
46. Furukawa T, Chiba R, Kobari M, Matsuno S, Nagura H, Takahashi T: Varying grades of epithelial atypia in the pancreatic ducts of humans: Classification based on morphometry and multilvariate analysis and correlated with positive reactions of carcinoembryonic antigen. *Arch Pathol Lab Med* **118**:227, 1994.
47. Kozuka S, Sassa R, Taki T, et al: Relation of pancreatic duct hyperplasia to carcinoma. *Cancer* **43**:1418, 1979.
48. Pour PM, Sayed S, Sayed G: Hyperplastic, preneoplastic and neoplastic lesions found in 83 human pancreases. *Am J Clin Pathol* **77**:137, 1982.
49. Brat DJ, Lillemoe KD, Yeo CJ, Warfield PB, Hruban RH: Progression of pancreatic intraductal neoplasias to infiltrating adenocarcinoma of the pancreas. *Am J Surg Pathol* **22**:163, 1998.
50. de la Garza M, Hill ID, Lebenthal E: Hereditary pancreatitis, in Go VLW, DiMango EP, Gardner JD, et al (eds): *The Pancreas: Biology, Pathobiology, and Disease*, vol 2. New York, Raven Press, 1993, p 1095.
51. Davidson P, Costanza D, Swieconek JA, Harris JB: Hereditary pancreatitis: A kindred without gross aminoaciduria. *Ann Intern Med* **68**:88, 1968.
52. Comfort MW, Steinberg AG: Pedigree of a family with hereditary chronic relapsing pancreatitis. *Gastroenterology* **21**:54, 1952.

53. Whitcomb DC, Preston RA, Aston CE, et al: A gene for hereditary pancreatitis maps to chromosome 7q35. *Gastroenterology* **110**:1975, 1996.
54. Whitcomb DC, Gorry MC, Preston RA, et al: Hereditary pancreatitis is caused by a mutation in the cationic trypsinogen gene. *Nature Genet* **14**:141, 1996.
55. Ekbom A, McLaughlin JK, Karlsson B-M, Nyren O, Gridley G, Adami H-O, Fraumeni JF J: Pancreatitis and pancreatic cancer: A population-based study. *J Natl Cancer Inst* **86**:625, 1994.
56. Lowenfels AB, Maisonneuve P, Cavallini G, et al: Pancreatitis and the risk of pancreatic cancer. *New Engl J Med* **328**:1433, 1993.
57. Lynch HT, Krush AJ: Heredity and adenocarcinoma of the colon. *Gastroenterology* **53**:517, 1967.
58. Lynch HT, Krush AJ, Guirgis H: Genetic factors in families with combined gastrointestinal and breast cancer. *Am J Gastroenterol* **59**:31, 1973.
59. Lynch HT, Schuelke GS, Kimberling WJ, et al: Hereditary non-polyposis colorectal cancer (Lynch syndromes I and II): II. Biomarker studies. *Cancer* **56**:939, 1985.
60. Liu B, Parsons R, Papadopoulos N, et al: Analysis of mismatch repair genes in hereditary non-polyposis colorectal cancer patients. *Nature Med* **2**:169, 1996.
61. Leach FS, Nicolaides NC, Papadopoulos N, et al: Mutations of a *mutS* homolog in hereditary nonpolyposis colorectal cancer. *Cell* **75**:1215, 1993.
62. Fishel R, Lescoe MK, Rao MRS, et al: The human mutator gene homolog *MSH2* and its association with hereditary nonpolyposis colon cancer. *Cell* **75**:1027, 1993.
63. Aaltonen LA, Peltomaki P, Mecklin J-P, et al: Replication errors in benign and malignant tumors from hereditary nonpolyposis colorectal cancer patients. *Cancer Res* **54**:1645, 1994.
64. Thibodeau SN, Bren G, Schaid D: Microsatellite instability in cancer of the proximal colon. *Science* **260**:816, 1993.
65. Ionov Y, Peinado MA, Malkhosyan S, Shibata D, Perucho M: Ubiquitous somatic mutations in simple repeated sequences reveal a new mecanism for colonic carcinogenesis. *Nature* **363**:558, 1993.
66. Strand M, Prolla TA, Liskay RM, Petes TD: Destabilization of tracts of simple repetitive DNA in yeast by mutations affecting DNA mismatch repair. *Nature* **365**:274, 1993.
67. Goggins M, Offerhaus GJA, Hilgers W, et al: Pancreatic adenocarcinomas with DNA replication errors (RER+) are associated with wild-type k-*ras* and characteristic histopathology: poor differentiation, a syncytial growth pattern, and pushing borders suggest RER+. *Am J Pathol* **152**:1501, 1998.
68. Parsons R, Li G-M, Longley MJ, et al: Hypermutability and mismatch repair deficiency in RER+ tumor cells. *Cell* **75**:1227, 1993.
69. Kunkel TA: Slippery DNA and diseases. *Nature* **365**:207, 1993.
70. Hahn SA, Seymour AB, Hoque ATMS, et al: Allelotype of pancreatic adenocarcinoma using xenograft enrichment. *Cancer Res* **55**:4670, 1995.
71. Caldas C, Hahn SA, da Costa LT, et al: Frequent somatic mutations and homozygous deletions of the *p16* (*MTS1*) gene in pancreatic adenocarcinoma. *Nature Genet* **8**:27, 1994.
72. Bowlby LS: Pancreatic adenocarcinoma in an adolescent male with Peutz-Jeghers syndrome. *Hum Pathol* **17**:97, 1986.
73. Giardiello FM, Welsh SB, Hamilton SR, et al: Increased risk of cancer in the peutz-jeghers syndrome. *New Engl J Med* **316**:1511, 1987.
74. Jenne DE, Reimann H, Nezu J, et al: Peutz-Jeghers syndrome is caused by mutations in a novel serine threonine kinase. *Nature Genet* **18**:38, 1998.
75. Hemminki A, Markie D, Tomlinson I, et al: A serine/threonine kinase gene defective in Peutz Jeghers syndrome. *Nature* **391**:184, 1998.
76. Su GH, Hruban RH, Bansal RK, et al: Germline and somatic mutations of the *STK11/LKB1* Peutz-Jeghers gene in pancreatic and biliary cancers. *Am J Pathol* **154**:1835, 1999.
77. Whelan AJ, Bartsch D, Goodfellow PJ: Brief report: a familial syndrome of pancreatic cancer and melanoma with a mutation in the *CDKN2* tumor-suppressor gene. *New Engl J Med* **333**:975, 1995.
78. Goldstein AM, Fraser MC, Struewing JP, et al: Increased risk of pancreatic cancer in melanoma-prone kindreds with p16 *INK4* mutations. *New Engl J Med* **333**:970, 1995.
79. Moskaluk CA, Hruban RH, Schutte M, et al: Polymerase chain reaction and cycle sequencing of DPC4 in the analysis of familial pancreatic carcinoma. *Diagn Mol Pathol* **6**:85, 1997.
80. Savitsky K, Bar-Shira A, Gilad S, et al: A single ataxia telangiectasia gene with a product similar to P1-3 kinase. *Science* **268**:1749, 1995.
81. Aston CE, Banke MG, McNamara PJ, et al: Segregation analysis of pancreatic cancer (abstract). *Am J Hum Genet* **61:A194, 1997.**
82. Crowley KE, Aston CE, MacNamara PJ, et al: Familial aggregation of other cancers in families with pancreatic cancer (abstract). *Am J Hum Genet* **61:A196, 1997.**
83. Tulinius H, Olafsdottir GH, Sigvaldason H, Tryggvadottir L, Bjarnadottir K: Neoplastic diseases in families of breat cancer patients. *J Med Genet* **31**:618, 1994.
84. Kerber RA, Slattery ML: The impact of family history on ovarian cancer risk. *Arch Intern Med* **155**:905, 1995.
85. Thorlacius S, Olafsdottir G, Tryggvadottir L, et al: A single BRCA2 mutation in male and female breast cancer families from Iceland with varied cancer phenotypes. *Nature Genet* **13**:117, 1996.
86. Phelan CM, Lancaster J, Tonin P, et al: Mutation analysis of the *BRCA2* gene in 49 site-specific breast cancer families. *Nature Genet* **13**:120, 1996.
87. Couch FJ, Farid LM, DeShano ML, et al: *BRCA2* germline mutations in male breast cancer cases and breast cancer families. *Nature Genet* **13**:123, 1996.
88. Berman DB, Costalas J, Schultz DC, Grana G, Daly M, Godwin AK: A common mutation in BRCA2 that predisposes to a variety of cancers is found in both Jewish Ashkenazi and non-Jewish individuals. *Cancer Res* **56**:3409, 1996.
89. Johansson B, Bardi G, Heim S, et al: Nonrandom chromosomal rearrangements in pancreatic carcinomas. *Cancer* **69**:1674, 1992.
90. Johansson B, Mandahl N, Heim S, Mertens F, Andrén-Sandberg Å, Mitelman F: Chromosome abnormalities in a pancreatic adenocarcinoma. *Cancer Genet Cytogenet* **37**:209, 1989.
91. Griffin CA, Hruban RH, Long PP, Morsberger LA, Douna-Issa F, Yeo CJ: Chromosome abnormalities in pancreatic adenocarcinoma. *Genes Chromosom Cancer* **9**:93, 1994.
92. Griffin CA, Hruban RH, Morsberger L, et al: Consistent chromosome abnormalities in adenocarcinoma of the pancreas. *Cancer Res* **55**:2394, 1995.
93. Höglund M, Gorunova L, Andrén-Sandberg Å, Dawiskiba S, Mitelman F, Johansson B: Cytogenetic and fluorescence in situ hybridization analyses of chromosome 19 aberrations in pancreatic carcinomas: Frequent loss of 19p13.3 and gain of 19q13.1-13.2. *Genes Chromosom Cancer* **21**:8, 1998.
94. Seymour A, Hruban RH, Redston MS, et al: Allelotype of pancreatic adenocarcinoma. *Cancer Res* **54**:2761, 1994.
95. Brat DJ, Hahn SA, Griffin CA, Yeo CJ, Kern SE, Hruban RH: The structural basis of molecular genetic deletions: An integration of classical cytogenetic and molecular analyses in pancreatic adenocarcinoma. *Am J Pathol* **150**:383, 1997.
96. Schutte M, daCosta LT, Hahn SA, et al: Identification by representational difference analysis of a homozygous deletion in pancreatic carcinoma that lies within the *BRCA2* region. *Proc Natl Acad Sci USA* **92**:5950, 1995.
97. Wooster R, Bignell G, Lancaster J, et al: Identification of the breast cancer susceptibility gene *BRCA2*. *Nature* **378**:789, 1995.
98. Tavtigian SV, Simard J, Rommens J, et al: The complete *BRCA2* gene and mutations in chromosome 13q linked kindreds. *Nature Genet* **12**:335, 1996.
99. Knudson AG: Mutation and cancer: Statistical study of retinoblastoma. *Proc Natl Acad Sci USA* **68**:820, 1971.
100. Powell SM, Petersen GM, Krush AJ, et al: Molecular diagnosis of familial adenomatous polyposis. *New Engl J Med* **329**:1982, 1993.
101. Powell SM, Zilz N, Beazer-Barclay Y, et al: *APC* mutations occur early during colorectal tumorigenesis. *Nature* **359**:235, 1992.
102. Mulligan L, Kwok JBJ, Healey CS, et al: Germ-line mutations of the *RET* proto-oncogene in multiple endocrine neoplasia type 2A. *Nature* **363**:458, 1993.
103. Blaugrund JE, Johns MM Jr, Eby YJ, Ball DW, Baylin SB, Hruban RH, Sidransky D: *RET* proto-oncogene mutations in inherited and sporadic medullary thyroid cancer. *Hum Mol Genet* **3**:1895, 1994.
104. Moskaluk CA, Hruban RH, Lietman A, et al: Low prevalence of $p16^{INK4a}$ and CDK4 mutations in familial pancreatic carcinoma. *Hum Mutat* **12**:70, 1998.
105. Goggins M, Schutte M, Lu J, et al: Germline *BRCA2* gene mutations in patients with apparently sporadic pancreatic carcinomas. *Cancer Res* **56**:5360, 1996.
106. Ozcelik H, Schmocker B, DiNicola N, et al: Germline BRCA2 6174delT mutations in Ashkenazi Jewish pancreatic cancer patients. *Nature Genet* **16**:17, 1997.

107. Hahn SA, Schutte M, Hoque ATMS, et al: *DPC4*, a candidate tumor suppressor gene at human chromosome 18q21.1. *Science* **271**:350, 1996.
108. Hruban RH, van Mansfeld ADM, Offerhaus GJA, et al: K-*ras* oncogene activation in adenocarcinoma of the human pancreas: A study of 82 carcinomas using a combination of mutant-enriched polymerase chain reaction analysis and allele-specific oligonucleotide hybridization. *Am J Pathol* **143**:545, 1993.
109. Barbacid M: *Ras* genes. *Annu Rev Biochem* **56**:779, 1987.
110. Scheffzek K, Ahmadian MR, Kabsch W, Wiesmuller L, Lautwein A, Schmitz F, Wittinghofer A: The Ras-RasGAP complex: Structural basis for GTPase activation and its loss in oncogenic *ras* mutants. *Science* **277**:333, 1997.
111. Almoguera C, Shibata D, Forrester K, Martin J, Arnheim N, Perucho M: Most human carcinomas of the exocrine pancreas contain mutant c-K-*ras* genes. *Cell* **53**:549, 1988.
112. Smit VTHBM, Boot AJM, Smits AMM, Fleuren GJ, Cornelisse CJ, Bos JL: K-*ras* codon 12 mutations occur very frequently in pancreatic adenocarcinomas. *Nucleic Acids Res* **16**:7773, 1988.
113. Mariyama M, Kishi K, Nakamura K, Obata H, Nishimura S: Frequency and types of point mutation at the 12th codon of the c-Ki-*ras* gene found in pancreatic cancers from Japanese patients. *Jpn J Cancer Res* **80**:622, 1989.
114. Grünewald K, Lyons J, Frolich A, et al: High frequency of Ki-*ras* codon 12 mutations in pancreatic adenocarcinomas. *Int J Cancer* **43**:1037, 1989.
115. Nagata Y, Abe M, Motoshima K, Nakayama E, Shiku H: Frequent glycine-to-aspartic acid mutations at codon 12 of c-Ki-*ras* gene in human pancreatic cancer in Japanese. *Jpn J Cancer Res* **81**:135, 1990.
116. Tada M, Yokosuka O, Omata M, Ohto M, Isono K: Analysis of ras gene mutations in biliary and pancreatic tumors by polymerase chain reaction and direct sequencing. *Cancer* **66**:930, 1990.
117. Berrozpe G, Schaeffer J, Peinado MA, Real FX, Perucho M: Comparative analysis of mutations in the *p53* and K-*ras* genes in pancreatic cancer. *Int J Cancer* **58**:185, 1994.
118. Motojima K, Urano T, Nagata Y, Shiku H, Tsunoda T, Kanematsu T: Mutations in the Kirsten-*ras* oncogene are common but lack correlation with prognosis and tumor stage inhuman pancreatic carcinoma. *Am J Gastroenterol* **86**:1784, 1991.
119. Motojima K, Urano T, Nagata Y, Shiku H, Tsurifune T, Kanematsu T: Detection of point mutations in the Kirsten-*ras* oncogene provides evidence for the multicentricity of pancreatic carcinoma. *Ann Surg* **217**:138, 1993.
120. Pellegata NS, Losekoot M, Fodde R, et al: Detection of K-*ras* mutations by denaturing gradient gel electrophoresis (DGGE): A study on pancreatic cancer. *Anticancer Res* **12**:1731, 1992.
121. Pellegata NS, Sessa F, Renault B, Bonato MS, Leone BE, Solcia E, Ranzani GN: K-*ras* and *p53* gene mutations in pancreatic cancer: ductal and nonductal tumors progress through different genetic lesions. *Cancer Res* **54**:1556, 1994.
122. Suzuki H, Yoshida S, Ichikawa Y, et al: Ki-ras mutations in pancreatic secretions and aspirates from two patients without pancreatic cancer. *J Natl Cancer Inst* **86**:1547, 1994.
123. Tabata T, Fujimori T, Maeda S, Yamamoto M, Saitoh Y: The role of *ras* mutation in pancreatic cancer, precancerous lesions, and chronic pancreatitis. *Int J Pancreatol* **14**:237, 1993.
124. Yashiro T, Fulton N, Hara H, et al: Comparison of mutations of ras oncogen in human pancreatic exocrine and endocrine tumors. *Surgery* **114**:758, 1993.
125. DiGiuseppe JA, Hruban RH, Offerhaus GJA, Clement MJ, van den Berg FM, Cameron JL, van Mansfeld ADM: Detection of K-*ras* mutations in mucinous pancreatic duct hyperplasia from a patient with a family history of pancreatic carcinoma. *Am J Pathol* **144**:889, 1994.
126. Cerny WL, Mangold KA, Scarpelli DG: K-*ras* mutation is an early event in pancreatic duct carcinogenesis in the syrian golden hamster. *Cancer Res* **52**:4507, 1992.
127. Tada M, Omata M, Ohto M: *Ras* gene mutations in intraductal papillary neoplasms of the pancreas: Analysis in five cases. *Cancer* **67**:634, 1991.
128. Yanagisawa A, Ohtake K, Ohashi K, Hori M, Kitagawa T, Sugano H, Kato Y: Frequent c-Ki-*ras* oncogene activation in mucous cell hyperplasias of pancreas suffering from chronic inflammation. *Cancer Res* **53**:953, 1993.
129. Caldas C, Hahn SA, Hruban RH, Redston MS, Yeo CJ, Kern SE: Detection of K-*ras* mutations in the stool of patients with pancreatic adenocarcinoma and pancreatic ductal hyperplasia. *Cancer Res* **54**:3568, 1994.
130. Berthélemy P, Bouisson M, Escourrou J, Vaysse N, Rumeau JL, Pradayrol L: Identification of K-*ras* mutations in pancreatic juice in the early diagnosis of pancreatic cancer. *Ann Intern Med* **123**:188, 1995.
131. Sugio K, Molberg K, Albores-Saavedra J, Virmani AK, Koshimoto Y, Gazdar AF: K-*ras* mutations and allelic loss at 5q and 18q in the development of human pancreatic cancers. *Int J Pancreatol* **21**:205, 1997.
132. Moskaluk CA, Hruban RH, Kern SE: *p16* and K-*ras* gene mutations in the intraductal precursors of human pancreatic adenocarcinoma. *Cancer Res* **57**:2140, 1997.
133. Tada M, Ohashi M, Shiratori Y, et al: Analysis of K-*ras* gene mutation in hyperplastic duct cells of the pancreas without pancreatic disease. *Gastroenterology* **110**:227, 1996.
134. Cheng JQ, Ruggeri B, Klein WM, Sonoda G, Altomare DA, Watson DK, Testa JR: Amplification of *AKT2* in human pancreatic cells and inhibition of *AKT2* expression and tumorgenicity by antisense RNA. *Proc Natl Acad Sci* **93**:3636, 1996.
135. Batra SK, Metzgar RS, Hollingsworth MA: Isolation and characterization of a complementary DNA (PD-1) differentially expressed by human pancreatic ductal cell tumors. *Cell Growth Differ* **2**:385, 1991.
136. Wallrapp C, Müeller-Pillasch F, Solinas-Toldo S, et al: Characterization of a high copy number amplification at 6q24 in pancreatic cancer identifies *c-myb* as a candidate oncogene. *Cancer Res* **57**:3135, 1997.
137. DiGiuseppe JA, Hruban RH, Goodman SN, et al: Overexpression of p53 protein in adenocarcinoma of the pancreas. *Am J Clin Pathol* **101**:684, 1994.
138. Casey G, Yamanaka Y, Friess H, et al: *p53* mutations are common in pancreatic cancer and are absent in chronic pancreatitis. *Cancer Lett* **69**:151, 1993.
139. Nakamori S, Yashima K, Murakami Y, et al: Association of *p53* gene mutations with short survival in pancreatic adenocarcinoma. *Jpn J Cancer Res* **86**:174, 1998.
140. Redston MS, Caldas C, Seymour AB, Hruban RH, da Costa L, Yeo CJ, Kern SE: *p53* mutations in pancreatic carcinoma and evidence of common involvement of homocopolymer tracts in DNA microdeletions. *Cancer Res* **54**:3025, 1994.
141. Scarpa A, Capelli P, Mukai K, Zamboni G, Oda T, Iacono C, Hirohashi S: Pancreatic adenocarcinomas frequently show *p53* gene mutations. *Am J Pathol* **142**:1534, 1993.
142. Suwa H, Yoshimura T, Yamaguchi N, et al: K-*ras* and *p53* alterations in genomic DNA and transcripts of human pancreatic adenocarcinoma cell lines. *Jpn J Cancer Res* **85**:1005, 1994.
143. Weyrer K, Feichtinger H, Haun M, et al: *p53,* Ki-*ras,* and DNA ploidy in human pancreatic ductal adenocarcinomas. *Lab Invest* **74**:279, 1996.
144. Yonish-Rouach E, Resnitzky D, Lotem J, Sach L, Kimchi A, Oren M: Wildtype p53 induces apoptosis of myeloid leukemic cells that is inhibited by interleukin-6. *Nature* **352**:345, 1991.
145. Bates S, Vousden KH: p53 in signaling checkpoint arrest or apoptosis. *Curr Opin Genet Dev* **6**:12, 1996.
146. Kern SE, Pietenpol JA, Thiagalingam S, Seymour A, Kinzler KW, Vogelstein B: Oncogenic forms of p53 inhibit p53-regulated gene expression. *Science* **256**:827, 1992.
147. Kern SE, Kinzler KW, Bruskin A, Jarosz D, Friedman P, Prives C, Vogelstein B: Identification of p53 as a sequence-specific DNA-binding protein. *Science* **252**:1708, 1991.
148. Yin Y, Tainsky MA, Bischoff FZ, Strong LC, Wahl GM: Wild-type p53 restores cell cycle control and inhibits gene amplification in cells with mutant *p53* alleles. *Cell* **70**:937, 1992.
149. Kamb A, Gruis NA, Weaver-Feldhaus J, et al: A cell cycle regulator potentially involved in genesis of many tumor types. *Science* **264**:436, 1994.
150. Hu YX, Watanabe H, Ohtsubo K, Yamaguchi Y, Ha A, Okai T, Sawabu N: Frequent loss of p16 expression and its correlation with clinicopathological parameters in pancreatic carcinoma. *Clin Cancer Res* **3**:1473, 1997.
151. Huang L, Goodrow TL, Zhang S, Klein-Szanto AJP, Chang H, Ruggeri BA: Deletion and mutation analyses of the *P16/MTS-1* tumor-suppressor gene in human ductal pancreatic cancer reveals a higher frequency of abnormalities in tumor-derived cell lines than in primary ductal adenocarcinomas. *Cancer Res* **56**:1137, 1996.
152. Bartsch D, Shevlin DW, Callery MP, Norton JA, Wells SA, Goodfellow PJ: Reduced survival in patients with ductal pancreatic adenocarcinoma associated with *CDKN2* mutation. *J Natl Cancer Inst* **88**:680, 1996.
153. Naumann M, Savitskaia N, Eilert C, Schramm A, Kalthoff H, Schmiegel W: Frequent codeletion of *p16/MTS1* and *p15/MTS2* and genetic alterations in *p16/MTS1* in pancreatic tumors. *Gastroenterology* **110**:1215, 1996.

154. Bartsch D, Shevlin DW, Tung WS, Kisker O, Wells SA, Goodfellow PJ: Frequent mutations of *CDKN2* in primary pancreatic adenocarcinomas. *Genes Chromosom Cancer* **14**:189, 1995.
155. Herman JG, Merlo A, Mao L, et al: Inactivation of the *CDKN2/p16/MTS1* gene is frequently associated with aberrant DNA methylation in all common human cancer. *Cancer Res* **55**:4525, 1995.
156. Schutte M, Hruban RH, Geradts J, et al: Abrogation of the *Rb/p16* tumor-suppressive pathway in virtually all pancreatic carcinomas. *Cancer Res* **57**:3126, 1997.
157. Whyte P: The retinoblastoma protein and its relatives. *Semin Cancer Biol* **6**:83, 1995.
158. Longnecker DS: The quest for preneoplastic lesions in the pancreas. *Arch Pathol Lab Med* **118**:226, 1994.
159. Schutte M, Hruban RH, Hedrick L, et al: *DPC4* gene in various tumor types. *Cancer Res* **56**:2527, 1996.
160. Niehrs C: Mad connection to the nucleus. *Nature* **381**:561, 1996.
161. Derynck R, Gelbart WM, Harland RM, et al: Nomenclature: Vertebrate mediators of TGFβ family signals. *Cell* **87**:173, 1996.
162. Riggins GJ, Thiagalingam S, Rozenblum E, et al: Mad-related genes in the human. *Nature Genet* **13(3)**:347, 1996.
163. Grau AM, Zhang L, Wang W, et al: Induction of p21^{waf1} expression and growth inhibition by transforming growth factor β involve the tumor suppressor gene *DPC4* in human pancreatic adenocarcinoma cells. *Cancer Res* **57**:3929, 1997.
164. Polyak K: Negative regulation of cell growth by TGFβ. *Biochim Biophys Acta* **1242**:185, 1996.
165. White RL: Tumor suppressing pathways. *Cell* **92**:591, 1998.
166. Zhou S, Buckhaults P, Zawel L, et al: Targeted deletion of Smad4 shows it is required for transforming growth factor β and activin signaling in colorectal cancer cells. *Proc Natl Acad Sci USA* **95**:2412, 1998.
167. Takaku K, Oshima M, Miyoshi H, Matsui M, Seldin MF, Taketo MM: Intestinal tumorigenesis in compound mutant mice of both *Dpc4(Smad4)* and *Apc* genes. *Cell* **92**:645, 1998.
168. Hahn SA, Hoque ATMS, Moskaluk CA, et al: Homozygous deletion map at 18q21.1 in pancreatic cancer. *Cancer Res* **56**:490, 1996.
169. Su GH, Hilgers W, Shekher M, Tang D, Yeo CJ, Hruban RH, Kern SE: Alterations in pancreatic, biliary, and breast carcinomas support *MKK4* as a genetically targeted tumor-suppressor gene. *Cancer Res* 58:2339, 1998.
170. Horii A, Nakatsuru S, Miyoshi Y, et al: Frequent somatic mutations of the *APC* gene in human pancreatic cancer. *Cancer Res* **52**:6696, 1992.
171. Yashima K, Nakamori S, Murakami Y, et al: Mutations of the adenomatous polyposis coli gene in the mutation cluster region: Comparison of human pancreatic and colorectal cancers. *Int J Cancer* **59**:43, 1994.
172. McKie AB, Filipe MI, Lemoine NR: Abnormalities affecting the *APC* and *MCC* tumour suppressor gene loci on chromosome 5q occur frequently in gastric cancer but not in pancreatic cancer. *Int J Cancer* **55**:598, 1993.
173. Barton CM, McKie AB, Hogg A, et al: Abnormalities of the *RB1* and *DCC* tumor suppressor genes: uncommon in human pancreatic adenocarcinoma. *Mol Carcinog* **13**:61, 1995.
174. Ruggeri B, Zhang S-Y, Caamano J, DiRado M, Flynn SD, Klein-Szanto AJP: Human pancreatic carcinomas and cell lines reveal frequent and multiple alterations in the *p53* and *Rb-1* tumor-suppressor genes. *Oncogene* **7**:1503, 1992.
175. Huang L, Lang D, Geradts J, Obara T, Klein-Szanto AJP, Lynch HT, Ruggeri BA: Molecular and immunochemical analyses of RB1 and cyclin D1 in human ductal pancreatic carcinomas and cell lines. *Mol Carcinog* **15**:85, 1996.
176. Hruban RH, van der Riet P, Erozan Y, Sidransky D: Molecular biology and the early detection of carcinoma of the bladder: The case of Hubert H. Humphrey. *New Engl J Med* **330**:1276, 1994.
177. Tada M, Omata M, Kawai S, Saisho H, Ohto M, Saiki RK, Sninsky JJ: Detection of *ras* gene mutations in pancreatic juice and peripheral blood of patients with pancreatic adenocarcinoma. *Cancer Res* **53**:2472, 1993.
178. Apple SK, Hecht JR, Novak JM, Nieberg RK, Rosenthal DL, Grody WW: Polymerase chain reaction-based K-*ras* mutation detection of pancreatic adenocarcinoma in routine cytology smears. *Am J Clin Pathol* **105**:321, 1996.
179. Brentnall TA, Chen R, Kimmey MB, et al: *Ras* mutations and microsatellite instability detected in ERCP-derived pancreatic juice from patients with pancreatic cancer (abstract). *Gastroenterology* **108:A452, 1995.**
180. Iguchi H, Sugano K, Fukayama N, et al: Analysis of Ki-*ras* codon 12 mutations in the duodenal juice of patients with pancreatic cancer. *Gastroenterology* **110**:221, 1996.
181. Kondo H, Sugano K, Fukayama N, et al: Detection of point mutations in the K-*ras* oncogene at codon 12 in pure pancreatic juice for diagnosis of pancreatic carcinoma. *Cancer* **73**:1589, 1994.
182. Uehara H, Nakaizumi A, Baba M, et al: Diagnosis of pancreatic cancer by K-*ras* point mutation and cytology of pancreatic juice. *Am J Gastroenterol* **91**:1616, 1996.
183. Wilentz RE, Chung CH, Sturm PDJ, et al: Detection of K-*ras* mutations in duodenal fluid-derived DNA from patients with pancreatic cancer. *Cancer* **82**:96, 1998.
184. Hruban RH, Yeo CJ, Kern SE: Screening for pancreatic cancer, in Kramer B, Provok P, Gohagan J (eds): *Screening Theory and Practice*. New York, Marcel Dekker 1998.
185. Hameed M, Marrero AM, Conlon KC, et al: Expression of p53 nucleophosphoprotein in *in situ* pancreatic ductal adenocarcinoma: An immunohistochemical analysis of 100 cases (abstract). *Lab Invest* **70**:132A, 1994.
186. Wilentz RE, Geradts J, Maynard R, et al: Inactivation of the *p16 (INK4A)* tumor-suppressor gene in pancreatic duct lesions: loss of intranuclear expression. *Cancer Res.* **58**:4740, 1998.

CHAPTER 51

Ovarian Cancer

Louis Dubeau

1. **Ovarian carcinomas are the fifth leading cause of death from cancer among women. These tumors are morphologically similar to those arising from Müllerian-derived gynecologic organs despite the ovary itself not being embryologically derived from Müllerian ducts.**
2. **That ovarian carcinomas rarely spread outside the pelvic and abdominal cavities should facilitate usage of molecular genetic tests to document the presence or absence of residual tumor cells in treated patients.**
3. **Ovarian carcinomas are thought to arise from the mesothelial layer lining the ovarian surface. This theory does not account for the Müllerian-like appearance of these tumors and remains unproven.**
4. **The development of a suitable animal model for ovarian carcinomas is complicated by the low frequencies of these tumors in lower mammals. That such tumors are associated with frequent ovulation in birds supports theories linking incessant ovulation to risk of ovarian cancer in humans.**
5. ***In vitro* cultures of cells regarded as possible candidates for the origin of ovarian carcinomas, as well as of benign ovarian tumors, are available. Such cultures provide experimental systems to clarify the association between these different cell types and ovarian tumorigenesis.**
6. **Ovarian epithelial tumors are a good model to study tumor development because they are subdivided into benign, low malignant potential, and different grades of malignant subgroups which can each be regarded as representing varying degress of neoplastic transformation.**
7. **Although most ovarian carcinomas occur sporadically, a significant proportion arise in individuals with familial predisposition to this disease. The best-characterized genetic determinants of such predisposition are inherited mutations in either the *BRCA1* gene (familial breast/ovarian cancer syndrome) or in genes coding for mismatch repair enzymes (Lynch II syndrome).**
8. **Molecular genetic changes distinguishing ovarian cystadenomas, LMP tumors, and different grades of carcinomas from each other have been described. A gene that possibly escapes X chromosome inactivation may control the development of tumors of low malignant potential. Abnormalities in the same gene may be associated with increased biological aggressiveness in carcinomas.**
9. **Molecular genetic studies suggest that benign and malignant ovarian epithelial tumors are usually not part of a disease continuum. Benign tumors that progress to malignancy are probably those that are predisposed to such progression from their onset because of the presence of molecular genetic abnormalities associated with malignancy.**
10. **A genetic model for ovarian epithelial tumor development can be formulated based on known molecular genetic differences between benign, low malignant potential, and malignant tumors.**

A list of standard abbreviations is located immediately preceding the index in each volume. Additional abbreviations used in this chapter include: LMP = low maligant potential

CLINICOPATHOLOGIC FEATURES OF OVARIAN CARCINOMAS

Ovarian carcinoma is the fifth leading cause of death from cancer among women in the United States. This heterogeneous group of tumors includes several histopathologic subtypes, such as serous, mucinous, endometrioid, clear cell, as well as other less common forms.[1] One of the most intriguing features of these different subtypes is their striking resemblance to carcinomas arising from other organs of the female genital tract. For example, serous ovarian carcinomas are morphologically similar to epithelial tumors arising in the fallopian tubes. Mucinous carcinomas resemble those arising in endocervix. Endometrioid ovarian carcinomas are similar to carcinomas of the endometrium. Clear-cell tumors are likewise similar to a variant of endometrial carcinomas. These morphologic similarities are difficult to reconcile with there being no fallopian, endocervical, or endometrial-like epithelia present in normal ovaries. In addition, whereas the above organs are derived embryologically from the Müllerian ducts, the ovary is thought to be of mesonephric origin. The histogenesis of ovarian epithelial tumors is, therefore, still unclear, greatly complicating the development screening protocols for precursor lesions or early disease.

Ovarian carcinomas usually remain confined to the pelvic and abdominal cavities even at advanced disease stages. Thus, these tumors should be suitable for molecular genetic tests aimed at documenting the presence of residual disease following completion of adjuvant chemotherapy protocols. Recent studies[2] suggest that the presence of measurable levels of the enzyme telomerase in abdominal washings of patients may be a useful indicator of active disease for that purpose.

CURRENT THEORIES ABOUT THE CELL OF ORIGIN OF OVARIAN EPITHELIAL TUMORS

According to the currently favored theory, ovarian epithelial tumors arise in the mesothelial layer lining the ovarian surface (surface epithelium).[1] This cell layer may invaginate to create small cysts, which eventually lose their connection to the ovarian surface and may give rise to ovarian tumors. That ovarian epithelial tumors resemble tumors of Müllerian origin is often explained by the suggestion that the ovarian surface epithelium is not the direct precursor of ovarian epithelial neoplasms; instead, it must first undergo metaplasia to become Müllerian-like. If this hypothesis is correct, knowledge of the factors responsible for such metaplastic changes could lead to effective approaches for the prevention of ovarian cancer. Indeed, if metaplasia of the ovarian surface epithelium is a necessary step preceding tumor development, controlling this step would put us one step ahead of the cancer. However, the above theory is largely based on morphologic observations and remains unproved.[3] Recently, an argument was made that the components of the secondary Müllerian system, which include rete ovarii, paraovarian Müllerian rests, and endosalpingiosis, as well as pathologic conditions such as endometriosis, may be the site of origin of ovarian carcinomas.[3]

ANIMAL MODELS

Development of a suitable animal model for spontaneous ovarian carcinoma is complicated by these tumors being rare in most animals, including lower mammals. Knowledge of the reasons for the relatively low incidence of spontaneous ovarian epithelial tumors in lower mammals as compared to humans could provide important clues about the origin and risk factors of the human tumors. That tumors resembling human ovarian carcinomas are frequently present in the domestic hen[2] may prove particularly relevant. The high frequency of ovarian tumors in those animals has been linked to the activity of incessant egg production.[4] Wild hens or other wild birds, in which continuous egg production is not artificially induced, do not develop ovarian tumors. These observations are intriguing in light of the extensive epidemiologic data suggesting an association between incessant ovulation and risk of ovarian cancer in humans.[5] Such studies indicate that interruption of chronic menstrual cycling by either pregnancy or anovulatory drugs has an important protective effect against this disease.[5] Recent findings that the *BRCA1* gene, which is important for familial predisposition to breast and ovarian cancer, is strongly expressed in cells responding to pituitary gonadotropin hormones,[6] and that ovaries from patients with familial predisposition to the above cancers show various changes related to ovulatory activity,[7] provide additional support for a link between ovulatory activity and ovarian cancer development. These observations raise the possibility that ovarian carcinomas result from an artifact of civilization, that of incessant ovulation, as chronic menstrual cycling was unlikely in early humans due to more frequent pregnancies and longer lactation periods.

In Vitro MODELS

Several authors succeeded in culturing mesothelial cells lining the surface of ovaries of either adult humans or experimental animals, and were able to keep the cells in culture over several passages.[8–10] Cultures of epithelial cells derived from rete ovarii were also reported.[11] Godwin *et al.*[12] reported a high transformation rate in cultured ovarian surface mesothelial cells, suggesting that they may indeed be prone to malignant development. Support for the hypothesis that such cells may be prone to undergo metaplastic changes comes from the demonstration that steroid hormone responsiveness, a characteristic of Müllerian-derived epithelia, was induced by v-*ras* transformation in cultured ovarian surface epithelial cells.[13]

Several strains of ovarian cystadenomas, which are benign tumors of the same cell lineage as carcinomas, were recently developed and characterized.[14] Given the divergent differentiation pathways of ovarian epithelial tumors and ovarian surface mesothelium, and because definitive evidence that the former originates in the latter is still missing, these strains may constitute attractive models to investigate the molecular mechanisms of ovarian tumor progression in *in vitro* environments.

OVARIAN EPITHELIAL TUMORS AS A MODEL FOR TUMOR DEVELOPMENT

In addition to being an important clinical entity, ovarian epithelial tumors are attractive for studying tumor development because they can be subdivided into well-defined and phenotypically stable categories that may be regarded as representing varying degrees of neoplastic transformation (Fig. 51-1). Cystadenomas are made up of the same cell type as carcinomas, but are readily distinguished from the latter based on their total absence of invasive or metastatic abilities. Ovarian tumors of low malignant potential (LMP) are histologically more complex than cystadenomas and show some histopathologic features that are normally associated

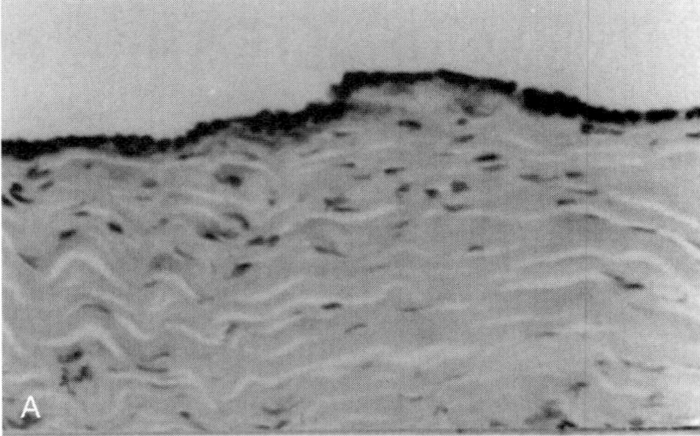

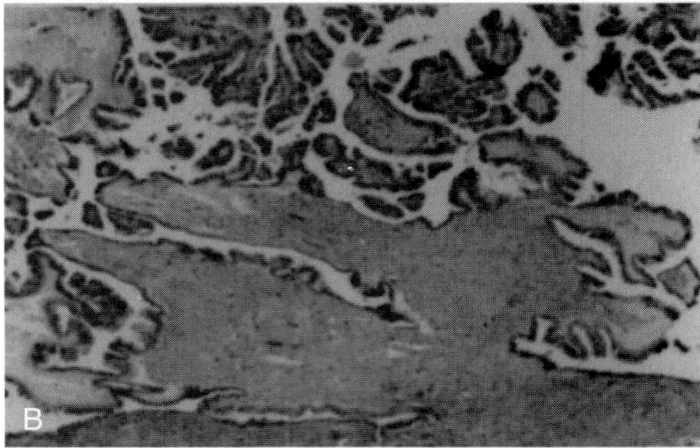

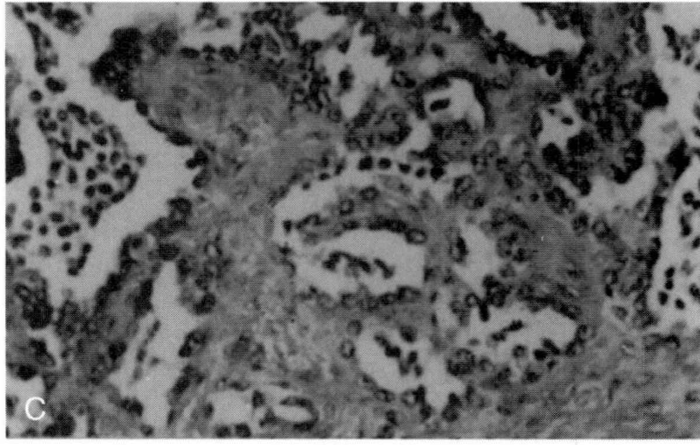

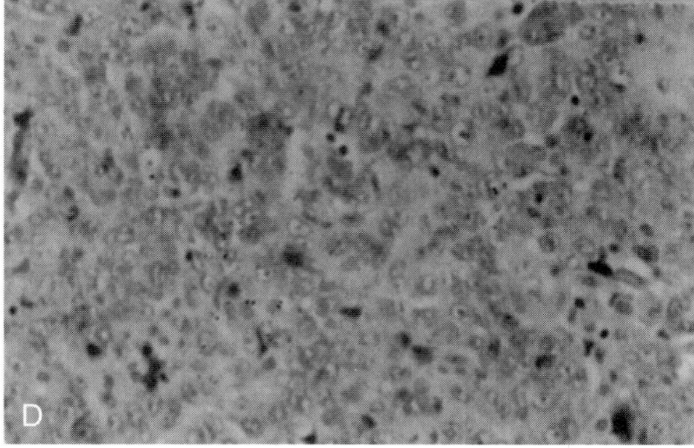

Fig. 51-1 Components of the ovarian epithelial tumor model. *A* Cystadenoma: Incessant but ordered cell proliferation. *B.* Low malignant potential: Disorganized cell proliferation resulting in complex histologic architectures. *C.* Low grade carcinoma: Invasive and metastatic; incessant but ordered cell proliferation allowing maintenance of glandular or other specialized structures. *D.* High grade carcinoma: Invasive and metastatic; disorganized cell proliferation resulting in solid and amorphous tumor blocks.

with carcinomas, but have absent (or greatly reduced) invasive abilities.[1,15] The further subdivision of ovarian carcinomas into low and high histologic grades allows further dissection of their phenotypic features. Low-grade carcinomas form organized structures, such as glandular acini, whereas high-grade lesions form solid, poorly organized cell masses according to the criteria used in Fig. 51-1, which were adopted in the author's laboratory because of their simplicity and reproducibility.

FAMILIAL PREDISPOSITION TO OVARIAN CARCINOMA

Although this review focuses primarily on sporadic ovarian epithelial tumors, it is estimated that up to 10 percent of ovarian carcinomas occur in individuals with familial predisposition to this disease. Most familial ovarian cancers appear to fall into one of two major syndromes. The first syndrome is the familial breast and ovarian cancer syndrome that is associated with inherited mutations in the *BRCA1* and *BRCA2* genes. Tumors belonging to this group may show different clinicopathologic characteristics than sporadic ovarian tumors show,[16] and it has been suggested that their spectrum of somatic molecular genetic abnormalities may also be different.[17] Some features, however, are similar to those seen in sporadic ovarian cancers. For example, incessant ovulatory activity, which is an important risk factor for sporadic cancers, also increases disease risk in patients with germ-line mutations in either of these two genes. The second group of familial ovarian cancers is that associated with Lynch II syndrome, which is characterized by predisposition to cancers of the colon, endometrium, and ovary, and which is associated with inherited abnormalities in genes coding for mismatch repair enzymes. Both syndromes are described more fully in other chapters and are not discussed further here.

MOLECULAR CHANGES DISTINGUISHING DIFFERENT SUBTYPES OF OVARIAN EPITHELIAL TUMORS

A number of abnormalities involving cellular proto-oncogenes, including HER-2/*neu*,[18] AKT2,[19] c-*fms*,[20] Bcl-2,[21] FGF-3,[22] and *met*,[23] were described in ovarian carcinomas. Abnormalities involving tumor-suppressor genes such as *p53*,[24–27] *SPARC*,[28] and *nm23*,[29] were also reported. Novel genes were isolated based on their down-regulation in ovarian tumors, and may function as tumor suppressors,[30–32] although their exact roles in ovarian tumorigenesis are still unclear. Data on frequencies of losses of heterozygosity on various chromosomes are extensive, including several complete allelotypes.[33–35] In addition, comprehensive cytogenetic analyses of ovarian tumors have been reported.[36–39] Specific molecular abnormalities were shown to be associated with disease prognosis[21,22,40,41] and specific genes, such as *HER-2/neu*[42–44] and *p53*,[45] have been evaluated as potential targets for gene therapy. A comprehensive review of these data are beyond the scope of this chapter, which focuses on molecular genetic studies presented in the context of the ovarian epithelial tumor model described in Fig. 51-2. The intent of this chapter is to provide insights into the molecular genetic changes controlling the different tumor subtypes shown in Fig. 51-1, in order to develop a molecular genetic model for ovarian tumorigenesis similar to what was first achieved with colorectal cancer.[46]

The complexity of molecular genetic changes present in ovarian carcinomas clearly increases with increasing tumor histologic grades.[35,37,47,48] This observation is in agreement with classical tumor progression theories.[49] Grades of ovarian carcinomas, however, are not only a function of the mere number of molecular genetic abnormalities present in a given tumor genome as specific molecular abnormalities appear strongly associated with high histologic grades.[35,37,47,48,50,51] Thus, whereas losses of heterozygosity affecting certain chromosomes, such as 6q, 17p, and 17q, appear frequently in ovarian tumors of all histologic grades,[35] losses in chromosome 13 are frequent only in those of high histologic grades.[50,51] It may be that the gene(s) targeted by losses of heterozygosity in chromosome 13 control(s) a different cellular pathway associated perhaps with differentiation or other determinants of tumor grade, but not with cell-cycle regulation. Proof of this hypothesis awaits identification and characterization of the gene(s) targeted by these losses of heterozygosity.

Recent data[35,37] also provide insights into the molecular genetic differences distinguishing ovarian carcinomas from the noninvasive and nonmetastatic ovarian epithelial tumors (Fig. 51-2). Examination of the distribution and frequencies of losses of heterozygosity in these various tumor subtypes showed that such losses, which are frequent in ovarian carcinomas, are rare in the biologically less aggressive ovarian epithelial tumors (with the exception of losses affecting the X chromosome in LMP tumors discussed below).[35] Thus, the underlying defects responsible for loss of heterozygosity usually result in malignancy, implying that tumor-suppressor gene inactivation, which is an important consequence of such losses, is not a feature of cystadenoma or LMP tumor development.[35] Other published molecular genetic differences between the different subtypes of ovarian tumors mentioned in Fig. 51-2 include the presence of p53 mutations,[27,52] which is strongly associated with malignant tumors, and changes in DNA methylation,[53] which are associated with both LMP tumors and carcinomas, but not with cystadenomas. Telomerase, an enzyme necessary for unlimited cell growth, is usually not detected in cystadenomas, whereas it is expressed in most LMP tumors and carcinomas.[54]

The only exception to the rarity of losses of heterozygosity in LMP tumors are losses affecting the X chromosome, which are present in about 50 percent of cases.[35] The target(s) of the allelic losses involving this chromosome in LMP tumors is not known, although the candidate chromosomal region was recently narrowed down considerably.[55] That the reduced allele invariably affects the inactive copy of this chromosome suggests that the targeted gene(s) escapes X inactivation. This suggestion is attractive because individuals born with a single X chromosome (Turner syndrome)[56] show abnormal ovarian development (gonadal dysgenesis). Thus, the presence of the inactive X chromosome is necessary for normal ovarian development and it is conceivable that abnormalities in the same gene during adult life may lead to tumorigenesis. The X chromosome is also thought to be important for the establishment of *in vitro* immortality,[57,58] and was recently implicated in the development of prostate cancer.[59]

ARE OVARIAN CYSTADENOMAS, LMP TUMORS, AND CARCINOMAS PART OF A DISEASE CONTINUUM?

Whether ovarian cystadenomas, LMP tumors, and carcinomas represent distinct disease processes or are part of a disease continuum is important to our understanding of ovarian tumor development and is relevant to the clinical management of cystadenomas and LMP tumors. Arguments in favor of a disease continuum come from morphologic observations that areas that are histologically indistinguishable from typical ovarian cystadenomas are sometimes found contiguous to carcinomas.[60] The most straightforward interpretation for these lesions, which are sometimes called cystadenocarcinomas, is that the histologically malignant areas arose from the preexisting morphologically benign areas. This interpretation implies that any molecular genetic change associated with carcinomas, but that are normally not present in solitary cystadenomas, should be confined to the histologically malignant portions of cystadenocarcinomas. However, losses of heterozygosity and *p53* mutations, which are frequent in carcinomas and absent, or at least very rare, in solitary cystadenomas, are usually concordant in all portions of ovarian cystadenocarcinomas, including the morphologically benign areas.[27,61] Concordance for aneuploidy was likewise shown in different regions of cystadenocarcinomas using interphase

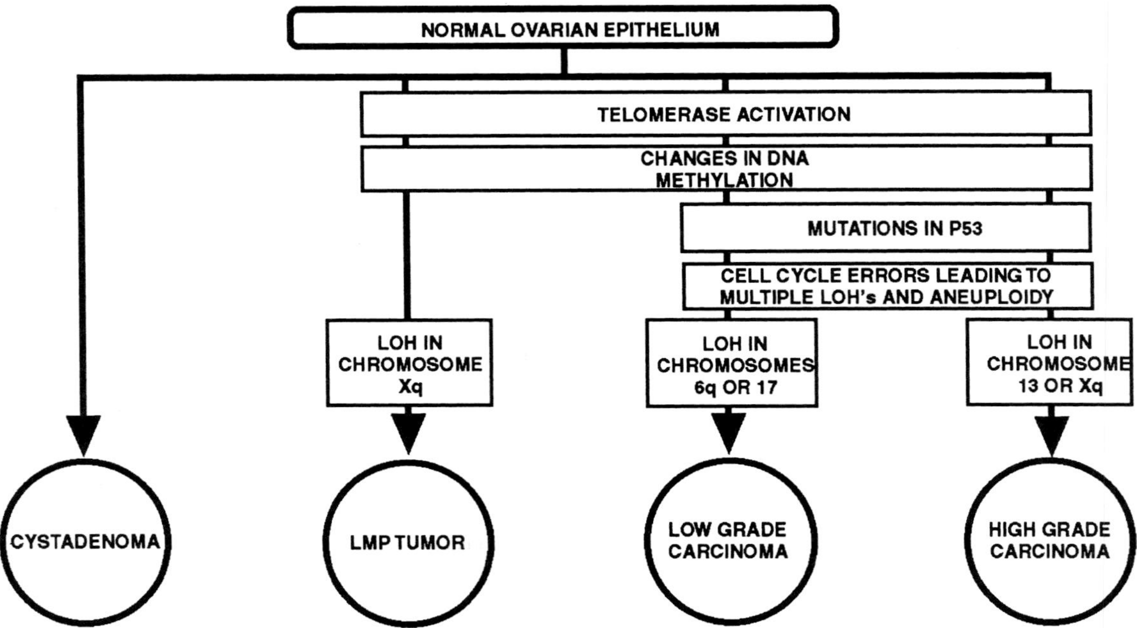

Fig. 51-2 A genetic model for sporadic (nonfamilial) ovarian epithelial tumor development.

cytogenetic approaches.[62] It seems clear based on these observations that histologically benign portions of cystadenocarcinomas are genetically different from typical (solitary) cystadenomas.[27,61] This conclusion supports the idea that cystadenomas do not generally progress to malignancy unless they carry a genetic predisposition to such progression, such as a mutation in the *p53* gene.[27]

A GENETIC MODEL FOR NONFAMILIAL OVARIAN EPITHELIAL TUMOR DEVELOPMENT

The genetic model in Fig. 51-2 is a working hypothesis based on information reviewed in the last section. Little is known about the genetic determinants of ovarian cystadenomas. These tumors appear to share few features with their malignant counterparts and may arise from a different mechanism. In contrast, some molecular changes, such as telomerase expression[54] and global changes in DNA methylation,[53] appear to be shared both by LMP tumors and carcinomas. These observations emphasize the merit of subdividing the biologically less aggressive ovarian tumors into cystadenomas and LMP tumors, in spite of the apparent clinically benign nature of the latter.[63] LMP tumors also show frequent losses of heterozygosity targeting a specific region of the inactive copy of the X chromosome. These changes, by themselves, are not sufficient to induce invasive and metastatic behavior because they occur in LMP tumors. However, if losses affecting the X chromosome occur in tumors where the malignant phenotype is already present, these may result in increased biological aggressiveness. This last conclusion accounts for the observation that losses affecting the X chromosome, although rare in low-grade carcinomas, are frequent in high-grade tumors.[35] Mutations in *p53*, as well as multiple losses of heterozygosity, the latter presumably resulting from cell-cycle errors that may be facilitated by the former, lead to the development of carcinomas. Specific losses of heterozygosity (such as in chromosome 13 or Xq) may be associated with specific features of the malignant phenotype, such as cellular differentiation, and may lead to higher tumor histologic grades. In contrast, losses in chromosomes 6q or 17 may be more directly associated with the malignant phenotype *per se* and are compatible with all histologic grades.

The nature of the specific genes targeted by the allelic deletions mentioned in the above model, as well as the exact consequences of other molecular genetic changes, such as in DNA methylation, are still largely unknown. These questions are the focus of current research efforts and significant progress is likely in the near future. These advances will result in a more comprehensive understanding of the mechanisms of ovarian epithelial tumors at the molecular level, and should also provide a basis for novel screening, diagnostic, and therapeutic approaches that are likely to improve the clinical management of these important tumors of women.

REFERENCES

1. Scully RE: Ovarian tumors. *Am J Pathol* **87:**686, 1977.
2. Duggan B, Wan M, Yu M, Roman L, Muderspach L, Delgadillo E, Li W-Z, Martin S, Dubeau L: Detection of ovarian cancer cells: Comparison of a telomerase assay and cytologic examination. *J Natl Cancer Inst* **90:**238, 1998.
3. Dubeau L: The cell of origin of ovarian epithelial tumors and the ovarian surface epithelium dogma: Does the emperor have no clothes? *Gynecol Oncol* **72:**437, 1999.
4. Fredrickson TN: Ovarian tumors of the hen. *Environ Health Perspect* **73:**35, 1987.
5. Whittemore AS, Harris R, Intyre J, Group CC: Characteristics relating to ovarian cancer risk: Collaborative analysis of 12 U.S. case-control studies. *Am J Epidemiol* **136:**1184, 1992.
6. Wan M, Sangiorgi F, Felix JC, Dubeau L: Association of BRCA1 with gonadotropin-responsive cells. *Lancet* **348:**192, 1996.
7. Salazar H, Godwin AK, Daly MB, Laub PB, Hogan WM, Rosenblum N, Boente MP, Lynch HT, Hamilton TC: Microscopic benign and invasive neoplasms and a cancer-prone phenotype in prophylactic oophorectomies. *J Natl Cancer Inst* **88:**1810, 1996.
8. Nicosia SV, Johnson JH, Streibel EJ: Growth characteristics of rabbit ovarian mesothelial (surface epithelial) cells. *Int J Gynecol Pathol* **4:**58, 1985.
9. Siemens CH, Auersperg N: Serial propagation of human ovarian surface epithelium in tissue culture. *J Cell Physiol* **134:**347, 1988.
10. Tsao SW, Mok SC, Fey EG, Fletcher JA, Wan TS, Chew EC, Muto MG, Knapp RC, Berkowitz RS: Characterization of human ovarian surface epithelial cells immortalized by human papilloma viral oncogenes (HPV-E6E7 ORFs). *Exp Cell Res* **218:**499, 1995.
11. Dubeau L, Velicescu M, Sherrod AE, Schreiber G, Holt G: Culture of human fetal ovarian epithelium in a chemically defined, serum-free medium: A model for ovarian carcinogenesis. *Anticancer Res* **10:**1233, 1990.
12. Godwin AK, Testa JR, Handel LM, Liu Z, Vanderveer LA, Tracey PA, Hamilton TC: Spontaneous transformation of rat ovarian surface

epithelial cells: Association with cytogenetic changes and implications of repeated ovulation in the etiology of ovarian cancer. *J Natl Cancer Inst* **84:**592, 1992.

13. Pan J, Roskelley CD, Luu The V, Rojiani M, Auersperg N: Reversal of divergent differentiation by ras oncogene-mediated transformation. *Cancer Res* **52:**4269, 1992.
14. Luo MP, Gomperts B, Imren S, DeClerck YA, Ito M, Velicescu M, Felix JC, Dubeau L: Establishment of long-term *in vitro* cultures of human ovarian cystadenomas and LMP tumors and examination of their spectrum of expression of matrix-degrading proteinases. *Gynecol Oncol* **67:**277, 1997.
15. Bell DA: Ovarian surface epithelial-stromal tumors. *Hum Pathol* **22:**750, 1991.
16. Johannsson OT, Idvall I, Anderson C, Borg A, Barkardottir RB, Egilsson V, Olsson H: Tumour biological features of BRCA1-induced breast and ovarian cancer. *Eur J Cancer* **33:**362, 1997.
17. Rhei E, Bogomolniy F, Federici MG, Maresco DL, Offit K, Robson ME, Saigo PE, Boyd J: Molecular genetic characterization of BRCA1- and BRCA2-linked hereditary ovarian cancers. *Cancer Res* **58:**3193, 1998.
18. Press MF, Jones LA, Godolphin W, Edwards CL, Slamon DJ: HER-2/neu oncogene amplification and expression in breast and ovarian cancers. *Prog Clin Biol Res* **354A:**209, 1990.
19. Bellacosa A, DeFeo D, Godwin AK, Bell DW, Cheng JQ, Altomare DA, Wan M, Dubeau L, Scambia G, Masciullo V, Ferrandina G, Panici PB, Mancuso S, Neri G, Testa JR: Molecular alterations of the AKT2 oncogene in ovarian and breast carcinomas. *Int J Cancer* **64:**280, 1995.
20. Chambers SK, Wang Y, Gertz RE, Kacinski BM: Macrophage colony-stimulating factor mediates invasion of ovarian cancer cells through urokinase. *Cancer Res* **55:**1578, 1995.
21. Herod JJ, Eliopoulos AG, Warwick J, Niedobitek G, Young LS, Kerr DG: The prognostic significance of Bcl-2 and p53 expression in ovarian carcinoma. *Cancer Res* **56:**2178, 1996.
22. Rosen A, Sevelda P, Klein M, Dobianer K, Hruza C, Czerwenka K, Hanak H, Vavra N, Salzer H, Leodolter S, Medl M, Spona J: First experience with FGF-3 (INT-2) amplification in women with epithelial ovarian cancer. *Br J Cancer* **67:**1122, 1993.
23. Di-Renzo MF, Olivero M, Katsaros D, Crepaldi T, Gaglia P, Zola P, Sismondi P, Comoglio PM: Overexpression of the Met/HGF receptor in ovarian cancer. *Int J Cancer* **58:**658, 1994.
24. Teneriello MG, Ebina M, Linnoila RI, Henry M, Nash JD, Park RC, Birrer MJ: p53 and Ki-ras gene mutations in epithelial ovarian neoplasms. *Cancer Res* **53:**3103, 1993.
25. Mazars R, Pujol P, Maudelonde T, Jeanteur P, Theillet C: p53 mutations in ovarian cancer: A late event? *Oncogene* **6:**1685, 1991.
26. Kohler MF, Marks JR, Wiseman RW, Jacobs IJ, Davidoff AM, Clarke-Pearson DL, Soper JT, Bast RC, Berchuck A: Spectrum of mutation and frequency of allelic deletion of the p53 gene in ovarian cancer. *J Natl Cancer Inst* **85:**1513, 1993.
27. Zheng J, Benedict WF, Xu H-J, Hu S-X, Kim TM, Velicescu M, Wan M, Cofer KF, Dubeau L: Genetic disparity between morphologically benign cysts contiguous to ovarian carcinomas and solitary cystadenomas. *J Natl Cancer Inst* **87:**1146, 1995.
28. Mok SC, Chan WY, Wong KK, Muto MG, Berkowitz RS: SPARC, an extracellular matrix protein with tumor-suppressing activity in human ovarian epithelial cells. *Oncogene* **12:**1895, 1996.
29. Mandai M, Konishi I, Koshiyama M, Mori T, Arao S, Tashiro H, Okamura H, Nomura H, Hiai H, Fukumoto M: Expression of metastasis-related nm23-H1 and nm23-H2 genes in ovarian carcinomas: Correlation with clinicopathology, EGFR, c-erbB-2, and c-erbB-3 genes, and sex steroid receptor expression. *Cancer Res* **54:**1825, 1994.
30. Mok SC, Chan WY, Wong KK, Cheung KK, Lau CC, Ng SW, Baldini A, Colitti CV, Rock CO, Berkowitz RS: DOC-2, a candidate tumor suppressor gene in human epithelial ovarian cancer. *Oncogene* **16:**2381, 1998.
31. Schultz DC, Vanderveer L, Berman BD, Hamilton TC, Wong AJ, Godwin AK: Identification of 2 candidate tumor suppressor genes on chromosome 17.p13.3. *Cancer Res* **56:**1997, 1996.
32. Abdollahi A, Godwin AK, Miller PD, Getts LA, Schultz DC, Taguchi T, Testa JR, Hamilton TC: Identification of a gene containing zinc-finger motifs based on lost expression in malignantly transformed rat ovarian surface epithelial cells. *Cancer Res* **57:**2029, 1997.
33. Sato T, Saito H, Morita R, Koi S, Lee JH, Nakamura Y: Allelotype of human ovarian cancer. *Cancer Res* **51:**5118, 1991.
34. Cliby W, Ritland S, Hartmann L, Dodson M, Halling KC, Keeney G, Podratz KC, Jenkins RB: Human epithelial ovarian cancer allelotype. *Cancer Res* **53:**2393, 1993.
35. Cheng PC, Gosewehr JA, Kim TM, Velicescu M, Wan M, Zheng J, Felix JC, Cofer KF, Luo P, Biela BH, Godorov G, Dubeau L: Potential role of the inactivated X chromosome in ovarian epithelial tumor development. *J Natl Cancer Inst* **88:**510, 1996.
36. Pejovic T: Genetic changes in ovarian cancer. *Ann Med* **27:**73, 1995.
37. Iwabuchi H, Sakamoto M, Sakunaga H, Ma YY, Carcangiu ML, Pinkel D, Yang Feng TL, Gray JW: Genetic analysis of benign, low-grade, and high-grade ovarian tumors. *Cancer Res* **55:**6172, 1995.
38. Thompson FH, Emerson J, Alberts D, Liu Y, Guan XY, Burgess A, Fox S, Taetle R, Weinstein R, Makar R, Powell D, Trent J: Clonal chromosome abnormalities in 54 cases of ovarian carcinoma. *Cancer Genet Cytogenet* **73:**33, 1994.
39. Persons DL, Hartmann LC, Herath JF, Borell TJ, Cliby WA, Keeney GL, Jenkins RB: Interphase molecular cytogenetic analysis of epithelial ovarian carcinomas. *Am J Pathol* **142:**733, 1993.
40. Henriksen R, Wilander E, Oberg K: Expression and prognostic significance of Bcl-2 in ovarian tumors. *Br J Cancer* **72:**1324, 1995.
41. Berchuck A, Kamel A, Whitaker R, Kerns B, Olt G, Kinney R, Soper JT, Dodge R, Clarke Pearson DL, Marks P, McKenzie S, Yin S, Bast RC: Overexpression of HER-2/neu is associated with poor survival in advanced epithelial ovarian cancer. *Cancer Res* **50:**4087, 1990.
42. Yu D, Matin A, Xia W, Sorgi F, Huang L, Hung MC: Liposome-mediated in vivo E1A gene transfer suppressed dissemination of ovarian cancer cells that overexpress HER-2/neu. *Oncogene* **11:**1383, 1995.
43. Hung MC, Matin A, Zhang Y, Xing X, Sorgi F, Huang L, Yu D: HER-2/neu-targeting gene therapy — a review. *Gene* **159:**65, 1995.
44. Pietras RJ, Fendly BM, Chazin VR, Pegram MD, Howell SB, Slamon DJ: Antibody to HER-2/neu receptor blocks DNA repair after cisplatin in human breast and ovarian cancer cells. *Oncogene* **9:**1829, 1994.
45. Mujoo K, Maneval DC, Anderson SC, Gutterman JU: Adenoviral-mediated p53 tumor suppressor gene therapy of human ovarian carcinoma. *Oncogene* **12:**1617, 1996.
46. Fearon ER, Vogelstein B: A genetic model for colorectal tumorigenesis. *Cell* **61:**759, 1990.
47. Zheng JP, Robinson WR, Ehlen T, Yu MC, Dubeau L: Distinction of low grade from high grade human ovarian carcinomas on the basis of losses of heterozygosity on chromosomes 3, 6, and 11 and HER-2/neu gene amplification. *Cancer Res* **51:**4045, 1991.
48. Dodson MK, Hartmann LC, Cliby WA, DeLacey KA, Keeney GL, Ritland SR, Su JQ, Podratz KC, Jenkins RB: Comparison of loss of heterozygosity patterns in invasive low-grade and high-grade epithelial ovarian carcinomas. *Cancer Res* **53:**4456, 1993.
49. Nowell PC: The clonal evolution of tumor cell populations. *Science* **194:**23, 1976.
50. Kim TM, Benedict WF, Xu H-J, Hu S-X, Gosewehr J, Velicescu M, Yin E, Zheng J, D'Ablaing G, Dubeau L: Loss of heterozygosity on chromosome 13 is common only in the biologically more aggressive subtypes of ovarian epithelial tumors and is associated with normal retinoblastoma gene expression. *Cancer Res* **54:**605, 1994.
51. Dodson MK, Cliby WA, Xu H-J, DeLacey KA, Hu S-X, Keeney GL, Li J, Podratz KC, Jenkins RB, Benedict WF: Evidence of functional RB protein in epithelial ovarian carcinomas despite loss of heterozygosity at the RB locus. *Cancer Res* **54:**610, 1994.
52. Wertheim I, Muto MG, Welch WR, Bell DA, Berkowitz RS, Mok SC: P53 gene mutation in human borderline epithelial ovarian tumors. *J Natl Cancer Inst* **86:**1549, 1994.
53. Cheng PC, Schmutte C, Cofer KF, Felix JC, Yu MC, Dubeau L: Alterations in DNA methylation are early, but not initial events in ovarian tumorigenesis. *Br J Cancer* **75:**396, 1997.
54. Wan M, Li W-Z, Duggan B, Felix J, Zhao Y, Dubeau L: Telomerase activity in benign and malignant epithelial ovarian tumors. *J Natl Cancer Inst* **89:**437, 1997.
55. Edelson MI, Lau CC, Colitti CV, Welch WR, Bell DA: A one-centimorgan deletion unit on chromosome Xq12 is commonly lost in borderline and invasive epithelial ovarian tumors. *Oncogene* **16:**197, 1998.
56. Turner HH: A syndrome of infantilism, congenital webbed neck, and cubitus valgus. *Endocrinol* **23:**566, 1938.
57. Klein CB, Conway K, Wang XW, Bhamra RK, Lin XH, Cohen MD, Annab L, Barrett JC, Costa M: Senescence of nickel-transformed cells by an X chromosome: Possible epigenetic control. *Science* **251:**796, 1991.
58. Wang XW, Lin X, Klein CB, Bhamra RK, Lee YW, Costa M: A conserved region in human and Chinese hamster X chromosomes can induce cellular senescence of nickel-transformed Chinese hamster cell lines. *Carcinogenesis* **13:**555, 1992.

59. Monroe KA, Yu MC, Kolonel LN, Coetzee GA, Wilkens LR, Ross RK, Henderson BE: Evidence of an X-linked or recessive genetic component to prostate cancer risk. *Nat Med* **1**:827, 1995.
60. Puls LE, Powell DE, DePriest PD, Gallion HH, Hunter JE, Kryscio RJ, van Nagell JR: Transition from benign to malignant epithelium in mucinous and serous ovarian cystadenocarcinoma. *Gynecol Oncol* **47**:53, 1992.
61. Zheng J, Wan M, Zweizig S, Velicescu M, Yu MC, Dubeau L: Histologically benign or low-grade malignant tumors adjacent to high-grade ovarian carcinomas contain molecular characteristics of high-grade carcinomas. *Cancer Res* **53**:4138, 1993.
62. Wolf NG, Abdul-Karim FW, Schork NJ, Schwartz S: Origins of heterogeneous ovarian carcinomas. A molecular cytogenetic analysis of histologically benign, low malignant potential, and fully malignant components. *Am J Pathol* **149**:511, 1996.
63. Kurman RJ, Trimble CL: The behavior of serous tumors of low malignant potential: Are they ever malignant? *Int J Gynecol Pathol* **12**:120, 1993.

CHAPTER 52

Endometrial Cancer

Lora Hedrick Ellenson

1. **Endometrial carcinoma is the most common malignancy of the female genital tract in the United States. In 1998 there were approximately 36,100 newly diagnosed cases of endometrial carcinoma and 6,300 deaths occurred as a result of this cancer.**
2. **Endometrial carcinoma is the most common noncolorectal carcinoma in women belonging to hereditary nonpolyposis colorectal carcinoma (HNPCC) families. Thus, mutations in the DNA mismatch repair genes (*hMSH2, hMLH1, hPMS1,* and *hPMS2*) that cause HNPCC are also thought to cause endometrial carcinoma in this setting.**
3. **Endometrial carcinoma encompasses two broad categories of malignant epithelial tumors that arise from endometrial epithelium. Epidemiologic and clinical features can distinguish them. Recently, it has been recognized that there are distinct histologic features of endometrial carcinomas that correlate, for the most part, with the two categories. The histologic types are called endometrioid carcinoma and uterine serous carcinoma. Recent molecular studies suggest that there may be differences in the molecular profiles of the two categories of endometrial carcinoma. Furthermore, it is suggested that these molecular differences may contribute to the differences in the clinical behavior of the tumor types.**
4. **Approximately 20 percent of sporadic endometrial carcinomas demonstrate microsatellite instability, yet only a fraction of these tumors have mutations in one of the four known DNA mismatch repair genes that cause HNPCC. Microsatellite instability has not been identified in uterine serous carcinomas, and may represent a molecular phenotype confined to endometrioid carcinomas.**
5. **The most common molecular abnormalities identified, to date, in endometrial carcinoma are *PTEN* mutations, microsatellite instability, K-*ras* mutations, and p53 gene mutations. *PTEN* is a recently identified tumor-suppressor gene on chromosome 10q23. Mutations in *PTEN* are the most common molecular alteration yet identified in endometrial cancer with 40–50 percent harboring such mutations. It appears that mutations in *PTEN* may be important early in the development of endometrioid carcinoma, as they are found in 20 percent of hyperplastic precursor lesions. K-*ras* mutations are thought to occur in 10–30 percent of endometrial carcinomas, and may also represent a relatively early alteration in endometrioid carcinoma, as mutations are present in atypical hyperplastic lesions.**
6. **p53 mutations are found in 10–30 percent of endometrial carcinomas. Recent data suggest that the majority occur in uterine serous carcinoma and in high-grade and high-stage endometrioid carcinomas. p53 mutations are very common in endometrial intraepithelial carcinoma, the precursor of uterine serous carcinoma, and may, therefore, occur early in the pathogenesis of this aggressive type of endometrial carcinoma. Statistical analyses of p53 overexpression by immunohistochemistry have found that it is an independent indicator of poor prognosis.**
7. **The molecular genetics of endometrial carcinoma are just beginning to be elucidated. To date, only p53 overexpression offers promise as a useful molecular diagnostic tool.**

CLINICAL ASPECTS

Incidence

Endometrial cancer is the fifth leading cause of cancer in women worldwide, with approximately 150,000 cases diagnosed each year. In the United States, it is the most common malignancy of the female genital tract, with 36,100 newly diagnosed cases and roughly 6,300 deaths estimated in 1998.[1] It should be noted that the term *endometrial cancer* encompasses both malignant epithelial tumors (carcinomas) and malignant mesenchymal tumors (sarcomas). Because more than 95 percent of endometrial cancers are carcinomas, the terms *endometrial cancer* and *endometrial carcinoma* are often used synonymously in the literature.

Most cases of endometrial carcinoma are thought to be sporadic; however, some clearly have a hereditary basis. Mothers and sisters of women with endometrial carcinoma have 2.7 times the risk of developing endometrial carcinoma when compared to controls.[2] The vast majority of endometrial carcinomas recognized as inherited occur in affected women belonging to hereditary nonpolyposis colorectal cancer (HNPCC) families. HNPCC is an autosomal dominantly inherited disease, and members of HNPCC families have an increased risk of developing a number of different types of cancer, especially colorectal cancer.[3] Notably, endometrial carcinoma is the most common extracolonic cancer in HNPCC families.[4] Women who are gene carriers of HNPCC have a tenfold increased risk, compared to the general population, of developing endometrial carcinoma; however, the percentage of endometrial cancers due to HNPCC is not well defined.[5] A small amount of literature has suggested the possibility of a site-specific form of inherited endometrial carcinoma, but there are insufficient data to conclusively prove its existence as a clinical genetic entity.[6]

Clinical Behavior and Histology

The endometrium forms the lining of the uterine cavity and is a complex tissue composed of both glandular epithelial and stromal components. Endometrial carcinoma arises from the epithelial component, with most tumors displaying glandular differentiation. It most commonly arises in perimenopausal and postmenopausal women. In most cases, women with endometrial carcinoma seek medical attention for abnormal vaginal bleeding, and endometrial tissue is obtained by biopsy or curettage for a definitive microscopic diagnosis.

Although endometrial carcinoma is classically thought of as a single disease, there is substantial evidence to support that it consists of two broad categories of malignant epithelial tumors.

A list of standard abbreviations is located immediately preceding the index in each volume. Nonstandard abbreviations used in this chapter include: HNPCC = hereditary nonpolyposis colorectal carcinoma; LOH = loss of heterozygosity.

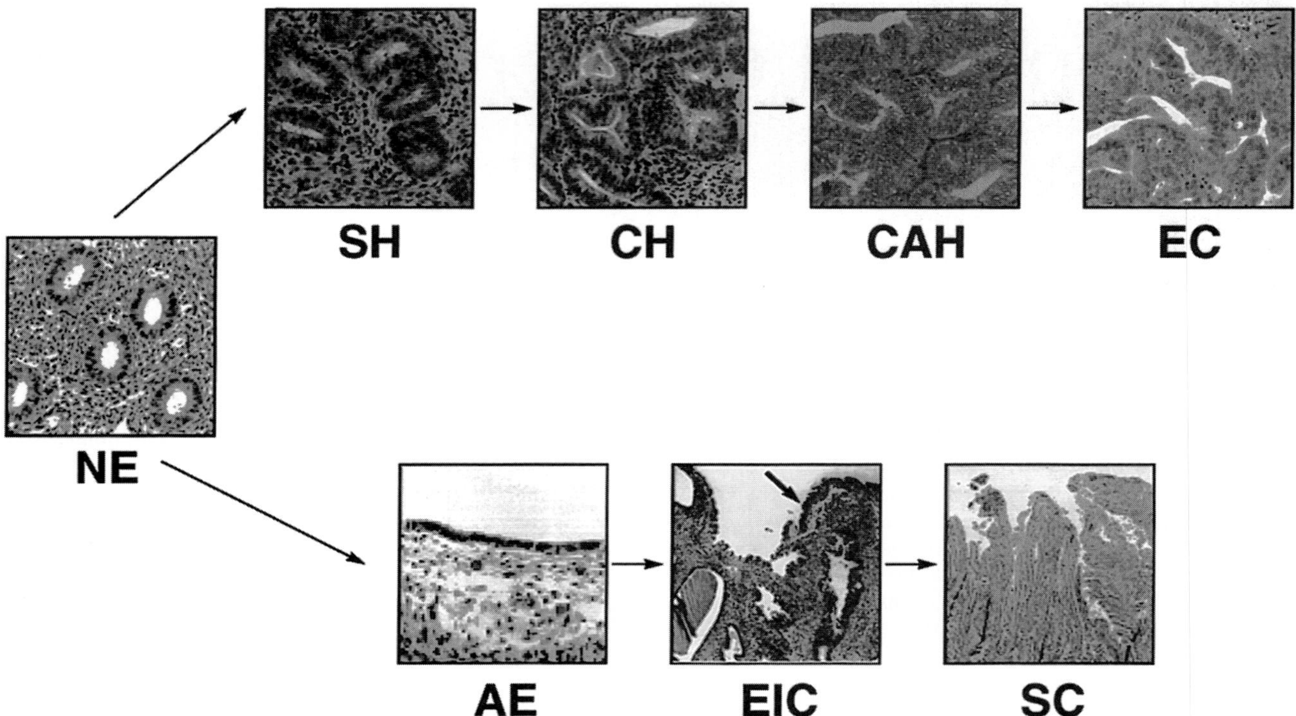

Fig. 52-1 Progression model of the two types of endometrial carcinoma. The development of endometrioid carcinoma (EC) from normal epithelium (NE) arises over time through a series of hyperplastic lesions that increase in both architectural complexity and cytologic atypia from simple hyperplasia (SH) to complex hyperplasia (CH) and finally complex atypical hyperplasia (CAH). Uterine serous carcinoma (SC) develops in the setting of atrophic endometrium (AE) from a precursor lesion called endometrial intraepithelial carcinoma (EIC).

The initial data suggesting the existence of two distinct types of endometrial carcinoma came from epidemiologic and clinical studies.[7] Recently it became apparent that these clinically defined categories of tumors correlate, for the most part, with specific light microscopic features.

Briefly, the initial clinical studies recognized that one group of women with endometrial carcinoma often have a history of exposure to estrogen, are slightly younger (mean age of 59) than the overall mean for the disease, and have tumors that usually behave in a relatively indolent manner. This group has been designated Type I endometrial carcinoma, and is often referred to as "estrogen-related."[8] Histologically, the majority of Type I tumors tend to have architectural features that resemble the appearance of normal endometrial glands, and are called endometrioid carcinomas to denote this resemblance. They are generally low-grade (i.e., well differentiated), low-stage (confined to the uterus), and have a good prognosis. Both epidemiologic and light microscopic studies have suggested that this type of carcinoma develops from normal epithelium, under the influence of estrogen stimulation, through a continuum of histopathologically recognizable lesions called hyperplasias (Fig. 52-1). Hyperplasia is defined as a proliferation of abnormal shaped and sized endometrial glands that leads to an imbalance in the normal glandular/stromal ratio of the endometrium. This proliferative process can, over time, undergo an increase in architectural complexity and cytologic atypia until it is difficult to distinguish from carcinoma, with the notable exception that there is a lack of detectable stromal invasion.[9] Hyperplasia, at any stage, can cause abnormal vaginal bleeding. As a result, many cases come to clinical attention and are treated prior to the development of frankly invasive carcinoma.

Type II carcinoma, in contrast to Type I, is unrelated to estrogenic stimulation (non-estrogen-related), occurs in older women (mean age of 68), and demonstrates aggressive behavior. Virtually all Type II carcinomas are composed of cuboidal cells showing marked cytologic atypia and nuclear pleomorphism that grow in either a glandular or papillary architecture.[10] These features are strikingly similar to those of the more common serous carcinoma of the ovary, giving rise to the name uterine serous carcinoma to distinguish them from primary serous ovarian tumors. By definition, serous carcinomas of the endometrium are all high-grade, frequently have extrauterine spread by the time of diagnosis, and carry a poor prognosis, behaving much like ovarian serous carcinomas.[11] Serous tumors of the endometrium generally arise in the setting of an atrophic, not a hyperplastic, endometrium. Recently, a putative precursor of uterine serous carcinoma has been described and termed endometrial intraepithelial carcinoma (Fig. 52-1).[12] It is characterized by a replacement of the preexisting endometrial epithelium with markedly atypical cells that are virtually indistinguishable from the cells found in invasive uterine serous carcinoma. Endometrial intraepithelial carcinoma, even in the absence of definitive invasion in the uterus, can be associated with intra-abdominal carcinoma illustrating the aggressive nature of this neoplastic endometrial process.

It is important to recognize that the histology of endometrial carcinoma is more complicated than presented above. For example, there are several other minor histologic variants of endometrial carcinoma (e.g., mucinous, villoglandular, and clear cell). The appropriate category in which these histologic variants belong is not well established. These histologic variants are rare and poorly understood, and are not considered further in this chapter.

That the two major types of endometrial carcinoma are distinct has been further supported by recent molecular studies, as is discussed in detail below. Until recently, many of the molecular genetic studies of endometrial carcinoma have failed to adequately recognize and separately study the two major types of tumors, creating a body of literature that is often difficult to interpret, as becomes evident later in this chapter.

HEREDITARY ENDOMETRIAL CARCINOMA

The only well-established form of inherited endometrial carcinoma is associated with HNPCC. Over the past several years, the genes responsible for the majority of families that meet the clinical criteria for HNPCC have been identified and cloned. Furthermore, the HNPCC families in which linkage studies have been informative demonstrate linkage to loci subsequently found to harbor one of the known genes. For these reasons, the discussion of the genetic loci and the specific genes involved in inherited endometrial carcinoma are combined.

HNPCC is discussed in great detail in Chap. 32. Therefore, it is presented only briefly here, with an emphasis on endometrial carcinoma. HNPCC is the most common hereditary family cancer syndrome and is transmitted as an autosomal dominant trait. It is clinically defined by these criteria: (a) at least three relatives with colorectal cancer with one a first-degree relative of the other two; (b) the presence of tumors in at least two successive generations; and (c) one family member affected by colorectal cancer before the age of 50.[13] Endometrial carcinoma is not a required criterion for the clinical definition of HNPCC. However, the International Collaborative Group on HNPCC has recognized that if these criteria are strictly followed, families with a high incidence of endometrial carcinoma, as well as colorectal carcinoma, would be excluded. Although the actual percentage of all endometrial carcinoma due to HNPCC is not known, it has been shown that the cumulative incidence of endometrial carcinoma in women belonging to HNPCC kindreds is 20 percent by age 70, in contrast to 3 percent in the general population.[5]

Genetic Loci and Specific Genes

As previously stated, endometrial carcinoma is the most common extracolonic tumor that occurs in HNPCC families. Linkage analysis of several large HNPCC kindreds identified susceptibility loci on the short arms of chromosomes 2 and 3.[14,15] Informative linkage studies have determined linkage to either of these two chromosomal arms in the majority of HNPCC families. However, in a small number of families linkage to either of these regions is lacking.

Over the past several years four genes have been identified that cause HNPCC in most of the kindreds meeting the clinical criteria of this inherited family cancer syndrome. The cloning of these genes resulted from the propitious coincidence of several different lines of scientific investigation, including studies aimed at identifying genes that play a role in human tumors, and others aimed at understanding fundamental molecular processes in microbial organisms.

Investigators were analyzing microsatellites (small repetitive sequences) in DNA isolated from tumors arising in HNPCC family members and found alterations in the length of microsatellite DNA sequences when compared to germ-line DNA from the same patients.[16] Other investigators reported a similar molecular phenotype in approximately 20 percent of sporadic colorectal tumors.[17,18] This molecular phenotype was referred to as microsatellite instability or replication errors. Microsatellite instability and its role, if any, in the neoplastic process was unclear. Shortly after the discovery of microsatellite instability in both sporadic and HNPCC-associated colorectal carcinomas, a study was published demonstrating that mutations in DNA mismatch repair genes led to a 100- to 700-fold increase in the instability of simple dinucleotide repeat sequences in the simple eukaryote *S. cerevisiae*.[19] This observation, along with previous work in both *E. coli* and *S. cerevisiae*, provided a crucial connection between microsatellite instability and mutations in DNA mismatch repair genes. This connection led to the ultimate identification of human DNA mismatch repair genes and opened a new avenue of cancer research.

In a very short time, four human homologues of microbial DNA mismatch repair genes were cloned. At a somewhat later date a fifth gene involved in DNA mismatch repair, *GTPB*, was cloned, but it will not be discussed here.[20,21] The four human DNA mismatch repair genes known to cause HNPCC are named *hMSH2, hMLH1, hPMS1*, and *hPMS2*, in keeping with their microbial homologues, and are located on chromosomes 2p, 3p, 2q, and 7q, respectively.[22–26] The physical maps of *hMSH2* and *hMLH1* have shown that their locations correlate with chromosomal loci determined to have genetic linkage to HNPCC. The linkage and physical mapping data provided additional information suggesting that DNA mismatch repair genes play a role in the pathogenesis of neoplasms arising in HNPCC kindreds. Subsequent studies documented germ-line mutations in one of these four human mismatch repair genes in affected members of most HNPCC kindreds, with the *hMSH2* and *hMLH1* genes accounting for the vast majority. At present, there is not a reported difference in the frequency of endometrial carcinoma among the HNPCC kindreds that carry mutations in the different genes.

The contribution of how microsatellite instability and defects in the DNA mismatch repair system contributed to tumorigenesis remained unproved. In microorganisms, the DNA mismatch repair system was known to detect and repair mispaired bases introduced during replication of the cellular genome. Furthermore, microbial organisms lacking a functional DNA mismatch repair system have a marked increase in the rate at which mutations accumulate. In mammalian cells, the DNA mismatch repair system has been much less well characterized, but it is thought to have a similar function to its microbial counterpart. Microsatellite DNA sequences in both humans and microorganisms are prone to undergo alterations in their length (explaining their highly polymorphic nature) during DNA replication. Therefore, it follows that microsatellite DNA sequences might demonstrate numerous alterations in the absence of an intact DNA mismatch repair system. This suggests that microsatellite instability may simply serve as a marker of an increased rate of mutation caused by an underlying defect in the DNA mismatch repair system. This led directly to the notion that lack of a functional mismatch repair system would result in an increased rate of mutations in oncogenes and tumor-suppressor genes, thus predisposing cells to the accumulation of mutations now thought to be a cornerstone of the neoplastic process. In support of this idea, studies have demonstrated an increase in the rate of point mutations in an expressed gene (HPRT) in a mismatch repair-deficient mammalian cell line. The identification of mutations in DNA mismatch repair genes in human tumors created a new class of cancer-causing genes called mutator genes.

The high frequency of endometrial carcinoma in HNPCC families indicates that the genes responsible for HNPCC are involved in the pathogenesis of endometrial carcinoma in this setting. A review of the literature does not provide a straightforward analysis of mutations in women with endometrial carcinoma belonging to HNPCC families. Clearly, further studies of HNPCC-associated endometrial carcinomas are needed.

Sporadic Endometrial Carcinoma

As alluded to earlier, the identification and characterization of the genetic loci and specific genes involved in endometrial tumorigenesis have been hampered by the inadequate recognition of the distinct types of endometrial carcinomas. Much of the problem is related to the classification scheme, described earlier, being initially described in 1983 and only recently gaining widespread acceptance. In addition, uterine serous (Type II) carcinomas are relatively rare, comprising approximately 10 percent of all sporadic endometrial carcinomas. Consequently, and understandably, many of the studies have not clearly stated the type (or types) of endometrial carcinomas that were included. Additionally, many studies that have classified the tumors lack significant numbers to enable the results of the different tumor types to be assessed independently. When possible, this chapter discusses the molecular genetics of sporadic endometrial carcinoma in the context of these two tumor types.

Genetic Loci

Over the past several years a number of loss of heterozygosity (LOH) studies have attempted to locate regions of the genome that may harbor tumor-suppressor genes that play a role in endometrial tumorigenesis. In combining the results of the major studies, LOH has been detected on these chromosomes: 1, 3, 6, 8p, 9p, 9q, 10q, 11, 13, 14q, 15, 16q, 17p, 18p, 18q, 20, 21, and 22q.[28–32] A review of the literature reveals substantial variation in the regions that have been found to undergo LOH in endometrial carcinoma, and there are only several regions from this long list that have shown significant LOH in more than one study. These include loci on chromosomes 3p, 10q, 17p, and 18q. The 3p LOH is striking, as several candidate tumor-suppressor genes and the *hMLH1* gene map to this chromosome. The target(s) of 3p LOH have not yet been determined in endometrial carcinoma. Two separate groups of investigators have reported between 35 and 40 percent LOH of a region of 10q, and one group has suggested that there may be two discrete regions of 10q that undergo LOH.[29,31] A range of 9 to 35 percent of endometrial carcinomas has been reported to show 17p LOH. A recent study of uterine serous carcinoma detected LOH of 17p, specifically 17p13.1, in 100 percent of informative cases.[33] Because most of the LOH studies did not specify the tumor type, it will be of interest in the future to determine the percentage of each type that have 17p LOH. LOH of chromosome 18q has been found in three studies, all of which included tumors from Japanese women, with the highest reported frequency of 33 percent.[28,30,32] Other studies have failed to detect 18q LOH, including two studies confined to the analysis of tumors from American women, as well as one exclusively of Japanese women. Although 14q LOH has been identified in only one study, the association of 14q LOH with a poor prognosis led the authors to suggest that 14q LOH may indicate aggressive tumor behavior.[30] Interestingly, the authors note that several of the tumors with 14q LOH were uterine serous carcinomas. Further studies are necessary to confirm the possible association of 14q LOH and aggressive behavior of endometrial carcinoma.

As is easily imaginable, the variability among the LOH studies has hindered the identification of novel regions of the genome that may be important in the development of endometrial carcinoma. The reason(s) for the variability between studies are uncertain, but there are many possible explanations. For example, the polymorphic markers used in the various studies are not identical, and if relatively small deletions are responsible for LOH in endometrial carcinoma, the critical regions may only be detected with very specific markers. Furthermore, many of the studies have failed to carefully report the histologic types of the tumors analyzed. If the histologic types, which reflect the distinct categories of endometrial carcinoma, have different underlying molecular genetic alterations, the results of such studies may depend heavily on the types of tumors studied. This point is of further interest, as many studies have included tumors from Japanese and American patients and there is some evidence suggesting differences in the molecular basis of endometrial carcinomas in these two populations.

Specific Genes

The discussion of the specific genes is divided into three sections according to the general classification of genes currently recognized as cancer-causing genes: (a) mutator genes, (b) oncogenes, and (c) tumor-suppressor genes.

Mutator Genes. Due to the association of endometrial carcinoma and HNPCC, presumably sporadic cases of endometrial carcinoma were analyzed for instability of microsatellite DNA sequences. In several studies, microsatellite instability was detected in approximately 20 percent of endometrial tumors.[34–36] Given the association of microsatellite instability and mutations in human DNA mismatch repair genes, it seemed likely that mutations in these genes may be involved in the development of sporadic endometrial carcinomas that displayed microsatellite instability. A mutational analysis of four of the known DNA mismatch repair genes (*hMSH2, hMLH1, hPMS1*, and *hPMS2*) found that only a small number of sporadic endometrial carcinomas with microsatellite instability had mutations in one of these four genes.[37] In addition, mutations of *hMSH2* and *hMLH1* have been found in two endometrial carcinoma cell lines (HEC59 and AN_{3CA}) that demonstrate microsatellite instability.[38] These findings are similar to those seen in cases of microsatellite instability-positive sporadic colorectal cancers. The recent literature has found that the vast majority of microsatellite instability-positive sporadic endometrial carcinomas demonstrate hypermethylation of the hMLH1 promoter. This, in turn, is thought to be related to lack of expression of hMLH1 and the disruption of DNA mismatch repair.[38a,38b]

Finally, a recent study found that 34 cases of uterine serous carcinoma failed to demonstrate microsatellite instability.[39] The observed difference in the frequency between endometrial and uterine serous carcinoma is statistically significant and provides support for differences in the molecular pathogenesis of the two most common types of endometrial carcinoma.

Oncogenes. A number of oncogenes have been studied over the years, yet there are very few that have been found to be altered in a substantial number of endometrial carcinomas. The proto-oncogene recognized as mutated most commonly in endometrial carcinoma is K-*ras*. It has been shown, in a number of independent studies, to be mutated in 10 to 30 percent of endometrial carcinomas.[40–45] K-*ras* is a member of the *ras* gene family that consists of three closely related genes (H-*ras*, K-*ras*, and N-*ras*). The H-*ras* gene was discovered due to its ability to transform an immortalized rodent cell line, and its identification led to the cloning of the two other family members. Each of the *ras* genes encodes a 21-kDa guanine nucleotide-binding protein (p21) that transduces signals from activated transmembrane receptors to protein kinases that regulate cell growth and differentiation. The oncogenic mutations occur most commonly at codons 12, 13, and 61 and result in a gain-of-function. The mutant *ras* proteins have a decreased ability to interact with the GTPase-activating protein called *ras*-GAP, reducing their ability to interact with the GTPase-activating protein *ras*-GAP, and reducing their ability to hydrolyze guanosine triphosphate (GTP) to guanosine diphosphate (GDP). Hence, the mutant *ras* protein remains in the GTP-bound or activated state. In endometrial carcinoma, most mutations are found in codon 12. A recent study of American patients, that separated the two types of endometrial carcinoma, found that 11.6 percent of endometrioid carcinomas contained codon 12 mutations, whereas uterine serous carcinomas were all negative for codon 12 mutations.[46] The numbers were not statistically significant; however, it suggests that K-*ras* mutations may be differentially mutated in the different types of endometrial carcinoma. K-*ras* mutations have also been found in complex atypical hyperplasia (the precursor of endometrioid carcinoma) leading investigators to suggest that K-*ras* mutations may be a relatively early event in endometrial tumorigenesis.[43–45] Investigators have analyzed the association of K-*ras* mutations with prognosis, but the results have been conflicting.

There are a small number of studies showing alterations in the expression and/or amplification of the *HER-2/neu* gene in endometrial carcinoma. *HER-2/neu* is a member of the epidermal growth factor receptor gene family. It encodes a transmembrane tyrosine kinase receptor and is overexpressed in a subset of breast and ovarian cancers. The data on this gene in endometrial carcinoma are limited, but several studies have shown that it is overexpressed in 11 to 59 percent of tumors, and amplified in 14 to 21 percent of tumors.[47,48] One study revealed that overexpression and amplification of *HER-2/neu* were associated with a poor prognosis, and a multivariate analysis indicated that overexpres-

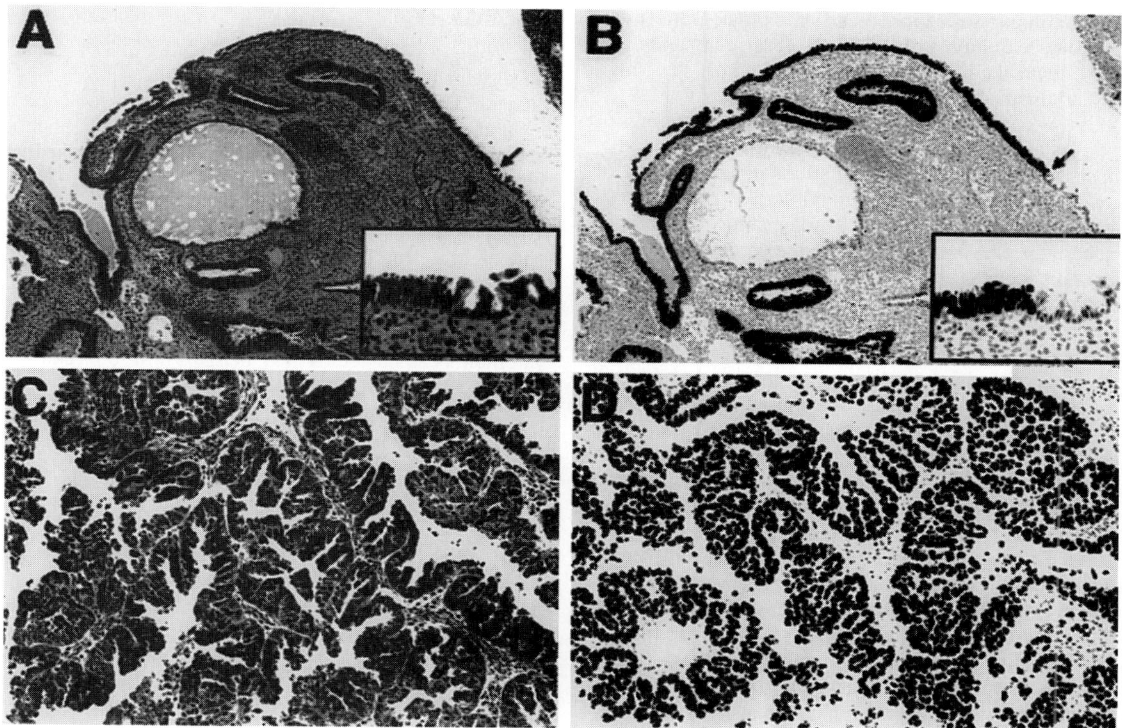

Fig. 52-2 Immunohistochemistry of p53 in uterine serous carcinoma and its precursor endometrial intraepithelial carcinoma. Endometrial intraepithelial carcinoma (EIC) arises abruptly from atrophic endometrium (*A*) and shows intense positive staining (*B*). A typical uterine serous carcinoma (*C*) also shows intense, diffuse staining for p53 protein (*D*). (Reprinted with permission from Tashiro H, et al.[33])

sion was an independent prognostic factor.[49,50] Independent studies have suggested that overexpression may be more common in uterine serous carcinomas.[51]

Recently, there have been several studies looking at expression of the *bcl-2* gene in endometrial carcinoma and hyperplasia. The *bcl-2* gene product prevents cells from undergoing apoptosis and is overexpressed in a number of different types of human tumors. The results of the studies in endometrial carcinoma are contradictory, with some demonstrating increased expression in endometrial carcinomas and others finding it decreased.[52,53] However, the results of several studies have found expression in normal proliferative endometrium and an absence of expression in normal secretory endometrium. These results suggest that *bcl-2* may play a role in the normal endometrial cycle. Hence, further studies on endometrial carcinoma seem needed to determine if *bcl-2* has a role in endometrial tumorigenesis.

Tumor-Suppressor Genes. As is true in many tumors, the *p53* gene has been the most extensively studied gene in endometrial carcinoma. *p53* is the prototype tumor-suppressor gene and it is the most frequently mutated gene in human cancers. It encodes a nuclear phosphoprotein with an apparent molecular weight of 53 kDa. For obvious reasons, this gene has been under intensive investigation for many years. Recent studies have begun to elucidate the mechanisms by which *p53* controls cell growth (reviewed in reference 54). Briefly, it has been found that p53 expression increases, posttranscriptionally, in response to DNA damage, resulting in a G1/S cell-cycle arrest. It is thought that this arrest gives cells the opportunity to repair the damaged DNA such that mutations are not fixed in the genomic template and, in turn, passed to daughter cells after cell division is complete. It has also been found that elevations in *p53* gene expression can lead to apoptosis. Recent data suggest that transcriptional activation of $p21^{WAF1}$ by p53 is important in the G1/S arrest, but is not essential for apoptosis. Evidently, given its ubiquitous involvement in human tumorigenesis, mutations that inactivate the *p53* gene provide a significant growth-promoting affect on many cell types.

Evaluation of p53 in endometrial carcinoma has largely been by immunohistochemistry, and overexpression of the protein has been reported in anywhere from 11 to 45 percent of endometrial carcinomas.[55–57] Evaluation of the data is troublesome due to a lack of description of the staining patterns (intensity and percent of cells staining) and the types of tumors analyzed. The staining pattern may be of utmost importance, as it is thought that detection of p53 by immunohistochemistry reflects the presence of mutations in the gene. Many studies have shown that there is considerable variability in staining and that only intense, diffuse staining may accurately predict the presence of mutations. One large study demonstrated that positive staining was more common in high-grade (41.7 percent) than in low-grade (12 percent) tumors, and another study revealed it more frequently in high-stage (41 percent) than in low-stage (9 percent) tumors.[56,58] Furthermore, when the tumor types have been separated, a higher frequency of staining is noted in uterine serous carcinomas (66 to 86 percent) as compared to the endometrioid type (Fig. 52-2).[33,59] Several studies have shown that overexpression of p53 by immunohistochemistry is an independent prognostic variable, predicting a poor prognosis.[57,60]

Analyses have also shown a wide range (9.5 to 23 percent) in the frequency of p53 mutations in endometrial carcinoma.[59,61] Again, these differences may be due to the types, grades, and stages of tumors analyzed. Many of the mutational studies have consistently shown that mutations are more common in high-grade tumors, and a recent study analyzing only uterine serous carcinomas detected mutations in 90 percent of tumors.[33] The strong association of p53 mutations and uterine serous carcinoma may offer an explanation for the prognostic significance of p53 overexpression and its association with a poor outcome.

Many of the p53 studies have focused on the clinical utility of the results. Recent studies suggest that they may also provide meaningful information about the molecular pathogenesis of endometrial carcinoma. As mentioned earlier, a putative precursor of uterine serous carcinoma has been described and p53 immunohistochemical studies revealed positivity in a very high percentage of endometrial intraepithelial carcinoma (Fig. 52-2).[62] This finding is in contrast to the very infrequent staining of atypical hyperplasia, the precursor of endometrioid carcinoma. Mutational analyses have shown that mutations in exons 5 to 8 of the *p53* gene are present in a majority of endometrial intraepithelial carcinomas (78 percent), suggesting, along with the high frequency of p53 mutations in uterine serous carcinoma, that *p53* mutations occur early in the pathogenesis of this tumor type.[33] It is reasonable to speculate that early mutation of the *p53* gene may be an important determinant of the aggressive biological behavior of uterine serous carcinoma, resulting in the poor outcome of patients with this tumor type.

Several recent studies have shown that mutations in *PTEN*, a tumor-suppressor gene located on chromosome 10q23.3, are common in endometrial carcinoma.[63,64,65] Approximately 40 to 50 percent of endometrioid carcinomas contain *PTEN* mutations, making it the most frequently mutated gene yet identified in this tumor type. The small number of uterine serous carcinomas analyzed for *PTEN* mutations are negative; however, before mutations in this tumor type are excluded more cases of serous carcinoma should be analyzed. Interestingly, *PTEN* mutations are more frequent in microsatellite instability-positive tumors than in those that lack instability.[63,64] Although the biological basis of this association is not yet understood it may represent an important finding with regards to the molecular pathogenesis of endometrioid carcinoma. Furthermore, *PTEN* mutations have been identified in approximately 20 percent of complex hyperplasias, with and without atypia, suggesting that *PTEN* mutations occur early in the pathogenesis of at least some endometrial carcinomas.[66,67] The predicted amino acid sequence of *PTEN* reveals significant homology to both tensin, a protein located in focal cell adhesions, and tyrosine phosphatases.[68] Biochemical studies have since shown that *PTEN* encodes a dual-specificity phosphatase, and substrates of PTEN are currently under investigation.[69] In addition, several studies have implicated a role for PTEN in signal transduction pathways.[70,71] In sum, the high frequency of *PTEN* mutations in endometrial carcinoma and their presence in hyperplastic lesions imply that inactivation of *PTEN* plays a significant role in its development. Clearly, the role of *PTEN* in endometrial tumorigenesis will be actively pursued in the near future.

Finally, a recent study found mutations in the β-catenin gene in 13 percent of endometrial carcinomas, and an accumulation of β-catenin protein in 38 percent of endometrial carcinomas.[53a] This finding is of considerable interest as it suggests a role for the *Wnt* signaling pathway, a pathway commonly involved in colorectal tumorigenesis, in the development of endometrial carcinoma. Additional studies are needed to determine the significance of this pathway in endometrial tumorigenesis.

IMPLICATIONS FOR DIAGNOSIS

As endometrial carcinoma remains poorly understood at the molecular level, there are very few molecular markers that are currently helpful in its diagnosis. The only gene, at present, with potential usefulness as a diagnostic tool is *p53*. It is very possible that *p53* immunohistochemistry may aid in the recognition of uterine serous carcinoma and its precursor lesion, endometrial intraepithelial carcinoma. The ability to consistently recognize this tumor, particularly in its early stages, may lead to better treatment approaches for this very aggressive tumor type. However, future studies are needed to better define the quality and quantity of *p53* immunostaining that accurately identify this type of tumor in the endometrium. In addition, *p53* staining may help identify the more aggressive subset of endometrioid tumors that should perhaps be treated more rigorously than those subsets that lack positive staining.

SUMMARY

The role of steroid hormones and their receptors in the development of endometrial carcinoma is excluded from this chapter. This is not an oversight, but little is known at the genetic level about how they contribute to the neoplastic phenotype in the endometrium. It is an area that deserves attention in the future. Finally, there is much to be learned about the molecular basis of endometrial carcinoma. Hopefully, future investigations will more vigilantly include a record of the distinct histologic types of endometrial carcinoma and their specific molecular genetic alterations so that we can come to understand the distinct genetic differences, and similarities, of the two major types of endometrial carcinoma. If the molecular underpinnings of these two types of carcinoma can be determined, perhaps new tools can be developed for more effective diagnosis and treatment of this common malignancy of women.

REFERENCES

1. Lardis SH, Murray T, Bolden S, Wingo PA: Cancer Statistics. *Cancer J Clin* **48**:6, 1998.
2. Schildkraut JM, Risch N, Thompson WD: Evaluating genetic association among ovarian, breast, and endometrial cancer: Evidence for a breast/ovarian cancer relationship. *Am J Hum Genet* **45**:521, 1989.
3. Watson P, Lynch HT: The tumor spectrum in HNPCC. *Anticancer Res* **14**:1635, 1994.
4. Watson P, Lynch HT: Extracolonic cancer in hereditary nonpolyposis colorectal cancer. *Cancer* **71**:679, 1993.
5. Watson P, Vasen HFA, Mecklin JP, Jarvinen H, Lynch HT: The risk of endometrial cancer in hereditary nonpolyposis colorectal cancer. *Am J Med* **96**:516, 1994.
6. Sandles LG, Shulman LP, Elias S, Photopulos GJ, Smiley LM, Posten WM, Simpson JL: Endometrial adenocarcinoma: Genetic analysis suggesting heritable site-specific uterine cancer. *Gynecol Oncol* **47**:167, 1992.
7. Bokhman JV: Two pathogenetic types of endometrial carcinoma. *Gynecol Oncol* **15**:10, 1983.
8. Kurman RJ: *Blaustein's Pathology of the Female Genital Tract*. New York: Springer-Verlag, 1994.
9. Kurman RJ, Kaminski PF, Norris HJ: The behavior of endometrial hyperplasia: A long-term study of "untreated" hyperplasia in 170 patients. *Cancer* **56**:403, 1985.
10. Sherman ME, Bitterman P, Rosenheim NB, Delgado G, Kurman RJ: Uterine serous carcinoma. A morphologically diverse neoplasm with unifying clinicopathologic features. *Am J Surg Pathol* **16**:600, 1992.
11. Hendrickson M, Ross J, Eifel P, Martinez A, Kempson R: Uterine papillary serous carcinoma a highly malignant form of endometrial adenocarcinoma. *Am J Surg Pathol* **6**:93, 1982.
12. Ambros RA, Sherman ME, Zahn CM, Bitterman P, Kurman RJ: Endometrial intraepithelial carcinoma: A distinctive lesion specifically associated with tumors displaying serous differentiation. *Hum Pathol* **26**:1260, 1995.
13. Vasen HFA, Mecklin JP, Meera Khan P, Lynch HT: Hereditary non-polyposis colorectal cancer. *Lancet* **338**:877, 1991.
14. Lindblom A, Tannergard P, Werelius B, Nordenskjold M: Genetic mapping of a second locus predisposing to hereditary non-polyposis colon cancer. *Nat Genet* **5**:279, 1993.
15. Peltomäki P, Aaltonen LA, Sistonen P, Pylkkänen L, Mecklin J-P, Jarvinen H, Green JS, JR, J, Weber JL, Leach FS, Petersen GM, Hamilton SR, de la Chapelle A, Vogelstein B: Genetic mapping of a locus predisposing to human colorectal cancer. *Science* **260**:810, 1993.
16. Aaltonen LA, Peltomäki P, Leach FS, Sistonen P, Pylkkänen L, Mecklin JP, Jarvinen H, Powell SM, Jen J, Hamilton SR, Petersen GM, Kinzler KW, Vogelstein B, de la Chapelle A: Clues to the pathogenesis of familial colorectal cancer. *Science* **260**:812, 1993.
17. Thibodeau SN, Bren G, Schaid D: Microsatellite instability in cancer of the proximal colon [see comments]. *Science* **260**:816, 1993.
18. Ionov Y, Peinado MA, Malkhosyan S, Shibata D, Perucho M: Ubiquitous somatic mutations in simple repeated sequences reveal a new mechanism for colonic carcinogenesis. *Nature* **363**:558, 1993.
19. Strand M, Prolla TA, Liskay RM, Petes TD: Destabilization of tracts of simple repetitive DNA in yeast by mutations affecting DNA mismatch repair. *Nature* **365**:274, 1993.

20. Palombo F, Gallinari P, Iaccarino I, Lettieri T, Hughes M, D'Arrigo A, Truong O, Hsuan JJ, Jiricny J: GTBP, a 160-kilodalton protein essential for mismatch-binding activity in human cells. *Science* **268**:1912, 1995.
21. Papadopoulos N, Nicolaides NC, Liu B, Parsons R, Lengauer C, Palombo F, D'Arrigo A, Markowitz S, Willson JK, Kinzler KW, Jirichy J, Vogelstein B: Mutations of GTBP in genetically unstable cells [see comments]. *Science* **268**:1915, 1995.
22. Papadopoulos N, Nicolaides NC, Wei YF, Ruben SM, Carter KC, Rosen CA, Haseltine WA, Fleischmann RD, Fraser CM, Adams MD, Venter JC, Hamilton SR, Peterson GM, Watson P, Lynch HT, Peltomaki P, Mecklin J, de la Chapelle A, Kinzler KW, Vogelstein B: Mutation of a mutL homolog in hereditary colon cancer [see comments]. *Science* **263**:1625, 1994.
23. Nicolaides NC, Papadopoulos N, Liu B, Wei YF, Carter KC, Ruben SM, Rosen CA, Haseltine WA, Fleischmann RD, Fraser CM, Adams MD, Venter JC, Dunlop MG, Hamilton SR, Petersen GM, de la Chapelle A, Vogelstein B, Kinzler KW: Mutations of two PMS homologues in hereditary nonpolyposis colon cancer. *Nature* **371**:75, 1994.
24. Bronner CE, Baker SM, Morrison PT, Warren G, Smith LG, Lescoe MK, Kane M, Earabino C, Lipford J, Lindblom A, Tannergard P, Bollag RJ, Godwin AR, Ward DC, Nordenskjold M, Fishel R, Kolodner R, Liskay RM: Mutation in the DNA mismatch repair gene homologue hMLH1 is associated with hereditary non-polyposis colon cancer. *Nature* **368**:258, 1994.
25. Fishel R, Lescoe MK, Rao MR, Copeland NG, Jenkins NA, Garber J, Kane M, Kolodner R: The human mutator gene homolog MSH2 its association with hereditary nonpolyposis colon cancer. *Cell* **75**:1027, 1993.
26. Leach FS, Nicolaides NC, Papadopoulos N, Liu B, Jen J, Parsons R, Peltomaki P, Sistonen P, Aaltonen LA, Nystrom LM, Guan JZ, Meltzer PS, Yu J, Kao F, Chen DJ, Cerosaletti KM, Fournier REK, Todd S, Lewis T, Leach RJ, Naylor SL, Weissenbach J, Mecklin J, Jarvinen H, Petersen GM, Hamilton SR, Green J, Jass J, Watson P, Lynch HT, Trent JM, de la Chapelle A, Kinzler KW, Vogelstein B: Mutations of a mutS homolog in hereditary nonpolyposis colorectal cancer. *Cell* **75**:1215, 1993.
27. Eshleman JR, Markowitz SD, Donover S, Lang EZ, Lutterbaugh JD, Li G, Longley M, Modrich P, Veigl ML, Sedwick WD: Diverse hypermutability of multiple expressed sequence motifs present in a cancer with microsatellite instability. *Oncogene* **12**:1425, 1996.
28. Imamura T, Arima T, Kato H, Miyamoto S, Sasazuki T, Wake N: Chromosomal deletions and K-ras gene mutations in human endometrial carcinomas. *Int J Cancer* **51**:47, 1992.
29. Jones MH, Koi S, Fujimoto I, Hasumi K, Kato K, Nakamura Y: Allelotype of uterine cancer by analysis of RFLP and microsatellite polymorphisms: Frequent loss of heterozygosity on chromosome arms 3p, 9q, 10q, 17p. *Genes Chromosomes Cancer* **9**:119, 1994.
30. Fujino T, Risinger JI, Collins NK, Liu F-S, Nishii H, Takahashi H, Westphal E- M, Barrett JC, Sasaki H, Kohler MF, Berchuck A, Boyd J: Allelotype of endometrial carcinoma. *Cancer Res* **54**:4294, 1994.
31. Peiffer SL, Herzog TJ, Tribune DJ, Mutch DG, Gersell DJ, Goodfellow PJ: Allelic loss of sequences from the long arm of chromosome 10 and replication errors in endometrial cancers. *Cancer Res* **55**:1922, 1995.
32. Okamoto A, Sameshima Y, Yamada Y, Teshima S-I, Terashima Y, Terada M, Yokota J: Allelic loss on chromosome 17p and p53 mutations in human endometrial carcinoma of the uterus. *Cancer Res* **51**:5632, 1991.
33. Tashiro H, Isacson C, Levine R, Kurman RJ, Cho KR, Hedrick L: p53 gene mutations are common in uterine serous carcinoma and occur early in their pathogenesis. *Am J Pathol* **150**:177, 1997.
34. Burks RT, Kessis TD, Cho KR, Hedrick L: Microsatellite instability in endometrial carcinoma. *Oncogene* **9**:1163, 1994.
35. Duggan BD, Felix JC, Muderspach LI, Tourgeman D, Zheng J, Shibata D: Microsatellite instability in sporadic endometrial carcinoma. *J Natl Cancer Inst* **86**:1216, 1994.
36. Risinger JI, Berchuck A, Kohler MF, Watson P, Lynch HT, Boyd J: Genetic instability of microsatellites in endometrial carcinoma. *Cancer Res* **53**:5100, 1993.
37. Katabuchi H, van Rees B, Lambers AR, Ronnett BM, Blazes MS, Leach FS, Cho KR, Hedrick L: Mutations in DNA mismatch repair genes are not responsible for microsatellite instability in most sporadic endometrial carcinomas. *Cancer Res* **55**:5556, 1995.
38. Boyer JC, Umar A, Risinger JI, Lipford JR, Kane M, Yin S, Barrett JC, Kolodner RD, Kunkel TA: Microsatellite instability, mismatch repair deficiency, and genetic defects in human cancer cell lines. *Cancer Res* **55**:6063, 1995.
38a. Esteller M, Levine R, Baylin SB, Ellenson LH, Herman JG: MLH1 promoter hypermethylation is associated with the microsatellite instability phenotype in sporadic endometrial carcinomas. *Oncogene* **17**:2413, 1998.
38b. Simpkins SB, Bocker T, Swisher EM, Mutch DG, Gersell DJ, Kovatich AJ, Palazzo JP, Fishel R, Goodfellow PJ: MLH1 promoter methylation and gene silencing is the primary cause of microsatellite instability in sporadic endometrial cancers. *Hum Mol Genet* **8**:661, 1999.
39. Tashiro H, Lax SF, Gaudin PB, Isacson C, Cho KR, Hedrick L: Microsatellite instability is uncommon in uterine serous carcinoma. *Am J Pathol* **150**:75, 1997.
40. Mizuuchi H, Nasim S, Kudo R, Silverberg SG, Greenhouse S, Garrett CT: Clinical implications of k-ras mutations in malignant epithelial tumors of the endometrium. *Cancer Res* **52**:2777, 1992.
41. Ignar-Trowbridge D, Risinger JI, Dent GA, Kohler M, Berchuck A, McLachlan JA, Boyd J: Mutations of the Ki-ras oncogene in endometrial carcinoma. *Am J Obstet Gynecol* **167**:227, 1992.
42. Fujimoto I, Shimizu Y, Hirai Y, Chen J-I, Teshima H, Hasumi K, Masubuchi K, Takahashi M: Studies on ras oncogene activation in endometrial carcinoma. *Gynecol Oncol* **48**:196, 1993.
43. Duggan BD, Felix JC, Muderspach LI, Tsao J-L, Shibata DK: Early mutational activation of the c-Ki-ras oncogene in endometrial carcinoma. *Cancer Res* **54**:1604, 1994.
44. Enomoto T, Fujita M, Inoue M, Rice JM, Nakajima R, Tanizawa O, Nomura T: Alterations of the p53 tumor suppressor gene and its association with activation of the c-K-ras-2 proto-oncogene in premalignant and malignant lesions of the human uterine endometrium. *Cancer Res* **53**:1883, 1993.
45. Sasaki H, Nishii, Takahashi H, Tada A, Furusato M, Terashima Y, Siegal GP, Parker SL, Kohler MF, Berchuck A, Boyd J: Mutations of the ki-ras proto-oncogene in human endometrial hyperplasia and carcinoma. *Cancer Res* **53**:1906, 1993.
46. Caduff RF, Johnston CM, Frank TS: Mutations of the Ki-ras oncogene in carcinoma of the endometrium. *Am J Pathol* **146**:182, 1995.
47. Esteller M, Garcia A, Martinez i Palones JM, Cabero A, Reventos J: Detection of c-erbB-2/neu and fibroblast growth factor-3/INT-2 but not epidermal growth factor receptor gene amplification in endometrial cancer by differential polymerase chain reaction. *Cancer* **75**:2139, 1995.
48. Czerwenka K, Lu Y, Heuss F: Amplification and expression of the c-erbB-2 oncogene in normal, hyperplastic, and malignant endometria. *Int J Gynecol Pathol* **14**:98, 1995.
49. Pisani AL, Barbuto DA, Chen D, Ramos L, Lagasse LD, Karlan BY: Her-2/neu, p53, and DNA analyses as prognosticators for survival in endometrial carcinoma. *Obstet Gynecol* **85**:729, 1995.
50. Saffari Jones LA, El-Naggar A, Felix JC, George J, Press MF: Amplification and overexpression of HER2/neu (c-erbB2) in endometrial cancers: Correlation with overall survival. *Cancer Res* **55**:5693, 1995.
51. Khalifa MA, Mannel RS, Haraway SD, Walker J, Min K-W: Expression of EGFR, HER-2/neu, p53, and PCNA in endometrioid, serous papillary, and clear cell endometrial adenocarcinomas. *Gynecol Oncol* **53**:84, 1994.
52. Yamauchi N, Sakamoto A, Uozaki H, Iihara K, Machinami R: Immunohistochemical analysis of endometrial adenocarcinoma for bcl-2 and p53 in relation to expression of sex steroid receptor and proliferative activity. *Int J Gynecol Pathol* **15**:202, 1996.
53. Henderson GS, Brown KA, Perkins SL, Abbott TM, Clayton F: bcl-2 is down-regulated in atypical endometrial hyperplasia and adenocarcinoma. *Mod Pathol* **9**:430, 1996.
53a. Fukuchi T, Sakamoto M, Tsuda H, Maruyama K, Nozawa S, Hirohashi S. β-Catenin mutation in carcinoma of the uterine endometrium. *Cancer Res* **58**:3526, 1998.
54. Kastan MB, Canman CE, Leonard CJ: p53, cell cycle control and apoptosis: Implications for cancer. *Cancer Metastasis Rev* **14**:3, 1995.
55. Inoue M, Okayama A, Fujita M, Enomoto T, Sakata M, Tanizawa O, Ueshima H: Clinicopathological characteristics of p53 overexpression in endometrial cancers. *Int J Cancer* **58**:14, 1994.
56. Kohler MF, Berchuck A, Davidoff AM, Humphrey PA, Dodge RK, Iglehart JD, Soper JT, Clarke-Pearson DL, Bast RC, Marks JR: Overexpression and mutation of p53 in endometrial carcinoma. *Cancer Res* **52**:1622, 1992.
57. Ito K, Watanabe K, Nasim S, Sasano H, Sato S, Yajima A, Silverberg SG, Garrett CT: Prognostic significance of p53 overexpression in endometrial cancer. *Cancer Res* **54**:4667, 1994.
58. Jiko K, Sasano H, Ito K, Ozawa N, Sato S, Yajima A: Immunohistochemical and in situ hybridization analysis of p53 in human endometrial carcinoma of the uterus. *Anticancer Res* **13**:305, 1993.

59. Kihana T, Hamada K, Inoue Y, Yano N, Iketani H, Murao S-I, Ukita M, Matsuura S: Mutation and allelic loss of the p53 gene in endometrial carcinoma. *Cancer* **76**:72, 1995.
60. Geisler JP, Wiemann MC, Zhou Z, Miller GA, Geisler HE: p53 as a prognostic indicator in endometrial cancer. *Gynecol Oncol* **61**:245, 1996.
61. Honda T, Kato H, Imamura T, Gima T, Nishida J, Sasaki M, Hosi K, Sato A, Wake N: Involvement of p53 gene mutations in human endometrial carcinomas. *Int J Cancer* **53**:963, 1993.
62. Sherman ME, Bur ME, Kurman RJ: p53 in endometrial cancer and its putative precursors: Evidence for diverse pathways of tumorigenesis. *Hum Pathol* **26**:1268, 1995.
63. Tashiro H, Blazes MS, Wu R, Cho KR, Bose S, Wang SI, Li J, Parsons R, Hedrick Ellenson L: Mutations in PTEN are frequent in endometrial carcinoma but rare in other common gynecologic malignancies. *Cancer Res* **57**:3935, 1997.
64. Kong D, Suzuki A, Zou T, Sakurada A, Kemp LW, Wakatsuki S, Yokoyama T, Yamakawa H, Furukawa T, Sato M, Ohuchi N, Sato S, Yin J, Wang S, Abraham JM, Souza RF, Smolinski KM, Meltzer SJ, Horii A: PTEN is frequently mutated in primary endometrial carcinomas. *Nat Genet* **17**:143, 1997.
65. Risinger JI, Hayes K, Berchuck A, Barrett JC: PTEN/MMAC1 mutations in endometrial cancers. *Cancer Res* **57**:4736, 1997.
66. Levine RL, Cargile CB, Blazes MS, van Rees B, Kurman RJ, Hedrick Ellenson L: PTEN mutations and microsatellite instability in complex atypical hyperplasia, a precursor lesion to uterine endometrioid carcinoma. *Cancer Res* **58**:3254, 1998.
67. Maxwell GL, Risinger JI, Gumbs C, Shaw H, Bentley RC, Barrett JC, Berchuck A, Futreal PA: Mutation of the PTEN tumor suppressor gene in endometrial hyperplasia. *Cancer Res* **58**:2500, 1998.
68. Li J, Yen C, Liaw D, Podsypanina K, Bose S, Wang SI, Puc J, Miliaresis C, Rodgers L, McCombie R, Bigner SH, Giovanella BC, Ittmann M, Tycko B, Hibshoosh H, Wigler MH, Parsons R: PTEN, a putative protein tyrosine phosphatase gene mutated in human brain, breast, and prostate cancer. *Science* **275**:1943, 1997.
69. Meyers MP, Stolarov JP, Eng C, Li J, Wang S, Wigler MH, Parsons R, Tonks NK: P-TEN, the tumor suppressor from human chromosome 10q23, is a dual-specificity phosphatase. *Proc Natl Acad Sci U S A* **94**:9052, 1997.
70. Maehama T, Dixon JE: The tumor suppressor, PTEN/MMAC1, dephosphorylates the lipid second messenger, phosphatidylinositol 3,4,5-triphosphate. *J Biol Chem* **273**:13375, 1998.
71. Tamura M, Gu J, Matsumoto K, Aota S, Parsons R, Yamada KM: Inhibition of cell migration, spreading, and focal adhesions by tumor suppressor PTEN. *Science* **280**:1614, 1998.

CHAPTER 53

Cervical Cancer

Kathleen R. Cho

1. **Based on available worldwide statistics, cervical cancer is the second most common cause of cancer-related mortality in women. Cervical cancers are curable when detected early, and the implementation of effective screening programs has reduced the incidence of and mortality from cervical cancer in industrialized countries substantially.**
2. **Neoplastic processes are undoubtedly complex, and cervical tumorigenesis is no exception. Like other adult solid tumors, cervical cancer appears to develop and progress largely as a consequence of activating mutation of oncogenes coupled with inactivation of tumor-suppressor genes. Alterations of such genes have profound effects on the exquisite control of cell growth and differentiation present in normal cells. Based on currently available information, it appears that inherited factors do not play a major role in cervical tumorigenesis.**
3. **Cervical cancer is different from most other common malignancies in that it is strongly associated with an infectious agent (human papillomavirus, HPV). This strong association has been used to great advantage in the research laboratory because the HPVs provide powerful tools with which to examine the molecular mechanisms underlying cervical tumor development and progression.**
4. **Most studies have focused on the E6 and E7 transforming proteins of the oncogenic HPV types. E6 and E7 interfere with function of the cellular tumor-suppressor proteins p53 and pRB via protein-protein interactions. By interfering with cell cycle control and DNA repair mechanisms, oncogenic HPVs appear to contribute indirectly to cervical tumorigenesis by promoting genetic instability and the accumulation of mutations in HPV-infected cells.**
5. **Relatively few specific genes have been identified that are often altered in cervical carcinomas, although frequent amplification of *c-myc* and *HER2-neu* has been reported. However, other cytogenetic and molecular genetic studies suggest that genes on chromosomes 1, 3, 5, 11, and others are likely to play important roles in cervical tumorigenesis. Intensive efforts are currently underway to identify specific genes targeted by alterations of these chromosomes.**
6. **Animal models of papillomavirus-associated tumorigenesis have been developed, including several species-specific systems. More recently, production of transgenic animals expressing HPV transforming proteins have provided new insights into the mechanisms by which HPVs contribute to cervical cancer.**
7. **Cervical cancers are particularly attractive targets for preventive and antitumor vaccines because they virtually always contain tumor-specific antigens (HPV proteins).**

A list of standard abbreviations is located immediately preceding the index in each volume. Nonstandard abbreviations used in this chapter include: SILs = squamous intraepithelial lesions; LSILs = low-grade squamous intraepithelial lesions; HSILs = high-grade squamous intraepithelial lesions; HPV = human papillomavirus.

CLINICAL ASPECTS

Incidence

Of cancers affecting women worldwide, cervical cancer is second only to breast cancer in both incidence and mortality.[1] Nearly 500,000 women are diagnosed with cervical cancer each year, and many die of the disease. The majority of cervical cancer patients are socioeconomically disadvantaged and thus without access to routine gynecologic care and screening for precancerous lesions. As a result, cervical cancer is particularly prevalent in many developing nations.

Notably, carcinomas of the cervix usually are curable if detected early. In the United States, the incidence and death rate from cervical cancer have decreased markedly over the last few decades, largely because of early detection and effective treatment of noninvasive precursor lesions and minimally invasive carcinomas. In the United States during 1997, there were approximately 14,500 new cervical cancer cases and 4800 cervical cancer deaths.[2] Estimates of the prevalence of precursor lesions, collectively referred to as *squamous intraepithelial lesions* (SILs), range from 0.5 to 6.5 percent of the American female population and include at least 50,000 new cases of carcinoma *in situ* each year.

Histopathology

The cervix includes both vaginal (ectocervical) and internal (endocervical) portions. The ectocervix is covered by stratified squamous epithelium, whereas the endocervix is lined by mucin-producing columnar epithelium that invaginates into the underlying stroma to form gland-like structures. Most cervical cancers are of squamous-type differentiation and arise within a specific region of the cervix referred to as the *transformation zone.* The transformation zone is an area in which, via a process called *squamous metaplasia,* the columnar epithelium located at the junction between the ectocervix and endocervix is replaced by squamous epithelium. Less commonly, cervical carcinomas arise from the endocervical columnar/glandular epithelium (adenocarcinomas).

During the development of squamous carcinomas, metaplastic squamous cells within the transformation zone undergo distinctive morphologic changes reflecting a progression from normal epithelium to carcinoma (Fig. 53-1). Lesions confined to the epithelium can be categorized as low-grade squamous intraepithelial lesions (LSILs) or high-grade squamous intraepithelial lesions (HSILs) depending on their specific morphologic features. Histopathologically, the intraepithelial lesions are characterized by changes reflecting abnormal cellular proliferation and differentiation. LSILs (previously called *mild* or *low-grade dysplasias*) show mild expansion of the proliferative zone in the basal and parabasal portions of the epithelium. Cells toward the surface are arranged haphazardly and often contain enlarged, pleomorphic, and hyperchromatic nuclei surrounded by clear halos. Collectively, these changes are referred to as *koilocytotic atypia.* The HSILs show even greater expansion of the proliferative zone, with mitotic figures often identified in the middle and upper portions of the epithelium. Koilocytotic atypia usually is less prominent than in LSILs, but the cells are more crowded and disorganized, have

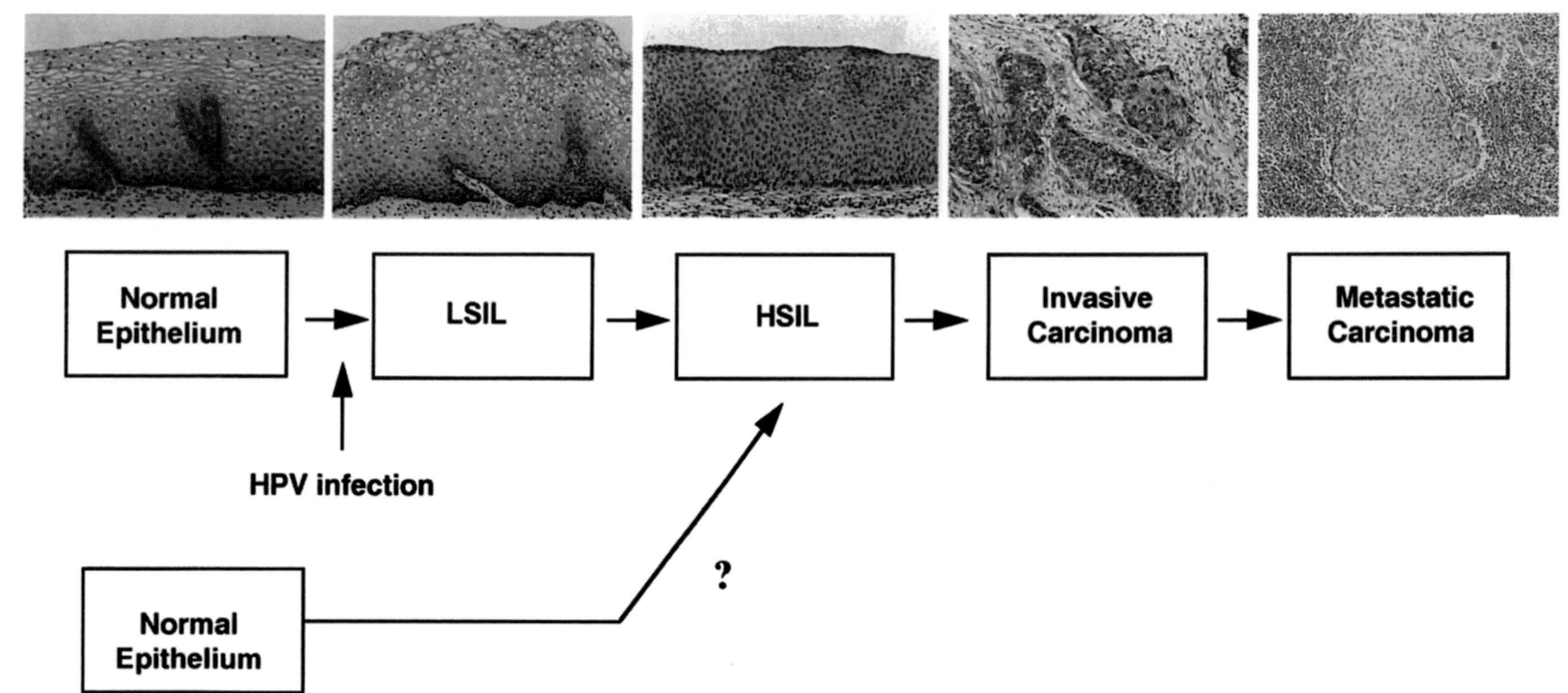

Fig. 53-1 Cervical tumorigenesis is associated with distinctive morphologic changes that reflect a progression from normal epithelium to carcinoma. HPV infection is an early, if not initiating, event in this process. Although all high-grade squamous intraepithelial lesions (HSILs) may not arise from low-grade lesions (LSILs), invasive carcinomas are almost always found in association with their HSIL precursors.

higher nuclear to cytoplasmic ratios, and show loss of polarity. The HSIL category includes lesions previously characterized as moderate and high-grade dysplasias as well as *in situ* carcinomas. Although HSILs may not always arise from preexisting LSILs, virtually all invasive squamous carcinomas arise from untreated HSILs.[3]

Biologic Behavior

If left untreated, SILs can either regress spontaneously, persist, or progress to a more advanced lesion. Based on several previous studies, it appears that the likelihood an LSIL will regress is about 60 percent, whereas the likelihood of progression to invasive carcinoma is only 1 percent.[4] In contrast, the highest grade of intraepithelial lesions regress only 33 percent of the time, and progression to invasive carcinoma occurs in greater than 12 percent of patients. Clearly, high-grade lesions are much more likely to progress to frank malignancy than those of low grade, but not all HSILs will progress to carcinoma, even if left untreated. Presently, lesions that will progress cannot be distinguished from those which will regress based on morphologic features alone.

Women with preinvasive and even early invasive cervical lesions usually are asymptomatic. Hence, without a strategy for early detection, those who develop cervical cancer would be more likely to be diagnosed with late-stage and often incurable disease. Fortunately, exfoliated cervical cells can be collected easily and examined microscopically, following staining, with the method originally described by Papanicolau. Detection of abnormal cells on these "Pap smears" is followed by diagnostic biopsy. Although some clinicians elect to closely follow patients with LSILs, some low-grade and virtually all high-grade lesions are treated by excisional biopsy or other ablative modalities such as laser therapy, cryotherapy, or electrocautery.

Even invasive cancers, when detected early, usually are cured by surgery alone. The 5-year survival of patients with tumors showing less than 3.0 mm of stromal invasion and maximum width of less than 7.0 mm (FIGO stage IA1) is nearly 100 percent.[5] Unfortunately, a substantial number of women in the United States fail to obtain even routine gynecologic care. As a consequence, nearly 50 percent of U.S. women with cervical cancer are diagnosed when the disease is stage II or higher.[6] Women with clinically visible cancers almost always report abnormal vaginal bleeding. Patients with high-stage disease usually are treated with surgery or radiation.

Cervical Cancer as an Infectious Disease

Essentially all human tumors are thought to arise because of mutations in oncogenes, tumor-suppressor genes, and genes encoding proteins involved in DNA damage recognition and repair. These mutations may be acquired somatically or inherited in the germ line. Based on the information available to date, it appears that inherited factors do not play a major role in cervical tumorigenesis, although some investigators have noted an association between the incidence of cervical cancer and particular major histocompatibility complex (MHC) alleles (HLA-DQ3 and, to a lesser extent, HLA-DR6).[7,8] Recently, Banks and colleagues reported a sevenfold increased risk of cervical cancer in individuals homozygous for the Arg allele at the polymorphic codon 72 of the *p53* tumor-suppressor gene.[9] Interestingly, the Arg allele was found to be more susceptible to human papillomavirus (HPV) E6-mediated degradation than the Pro allele (see discussion of E6 function below). Thus increased cervical cancer risk associated with the Arg/Arg genotype is plausible based on what is known about the mechanisms by which HPVs contribute to cervical tumorigenesis. Unfortunately, several larger case-control studies in a variety of populations could not find evidence to support this association.[9a–9e]

Although the contribution of inherited factors to cervical cancer risk remains uncertain, there is no doubt that cervical cancer is strongly associated with an infectious agent. The past few years have seen a remarkable convergence of several lines of investigation convincingly implicating involvement of certain types of HPVs in the development of cervical carcinoma. More recent molecular studies also have provided insight into probable mechanisms by which oncogenic HPVs contribute to cervical neoplasia.

Despite the fact that cervical cancer may, in many respects, be thought of as an infectious disease, it is important to recognize that of the millions of women infected by HPVs, only a small subset actually develops cervical cancer. This observation suggests that in the majority of patients, host immune surveillance may play an important role in limiting the growth and/or promoting regression of HPV-induced lesions. Humoral immunity does not appear to be a critical factor in controlling viral infection, particularly once the virus has entered the cell. Rather, HPV infection is more likely limited in most patients by the cell-mediated immune response.[10]

THE ROLE OF HPV INFECTION IN CERVICAL TUMORIGENESIS

Over 90 percent of invasive cervical carcinomas have been shown to contain DNA sequences from particular HPV types.[11] Papillomaviruses are small DNA viruses composed of an approximately 8-kb double-stranded circular genome enclosed by a 55-nm viral capsid. Over 100 different HPV types have been characterized on the basis of differences in DNA sequence, and a single host may be infected by multiple different HPVs. Based on extensive examination of the association of different HPV types with exophytic condylomas (genital warts), SILs, and cervical cancers, genital HPVs can be broadly classified into two groups: those associated with benign lesions (primarily HPVs 6 and 11) and those associated with invasive carcinomas (primarily HPVs 16 and 18). This classification into low-risk (non-cancer-associated) and high-risk (cancer-associated) types is reflected by *in vitro* evidence that cloned DNA of high-risk, but not low-risk, HPVs can efficiently immortalize primary human keratinocytes.[12–14] Moreover, only the E6 and E7 open reading frames of the high-risk HPV genome are required for this immortalization function.[15]

Nearly all invasive cervical cancers contain high-risk HPV sequences, providing compelling evidence for HPV infection as a causative factor. However, several lines of evidence suggest that HPV infection alone is insufficient to generate the fully malignant phenotype. First, while the HPV *E6* and *E7* genes from high-risk viruses can cooperate to efficiently immortalize primary cells in culture, a fully transformed phenotype is only seen after many *in vitro* cell doublings. Second, although infection with high-risk HPV types is very common, only a small percentage of infected women develop invasive cervical cancer. Third, those who develop cancer generally do so long after initial infection with HPV (many years in most cases). These observations suggest that in addition to infection with a high-risk HPV type, other events are required for the development of cervical cancer. Presumably, these events include alterations of oncogenes and tumor-suppressor genes in cervical cells harboring the HPV genome.

Functional Consequences of HPV Oncoprotein Expression

Given that infection with high-risk HPVs contributes to the pathogenesis of cervical cancer, studies over the past decade have sought to investigate the molecular mechanisms underlying HPV-associated tumor development. The HPV E6 and E7 oncoproteins have been shown to interact directly with tumor-suppressor gene products. Specifically, the E6 oncoprotein of high-risk HPV types 16 and 18 binds the tumor-suppressor protein p53 with much higher affinity than E6 of low-risk HPV types 6 and 11, and this binding appears to promote p53 degradation via the ubiquitin pathway.[16,17] The interaction between high-risk HPV E6 and p53 is mediated by a third protein, called *E6-AP,* that functions as a ubiquitin ligase in the ubiquitination of p53.[18–20] The HPV16 E7 protein has been shown to bind the retinoblastoma tumor-suppressor protein p105-RB (and other members of the RB family) with much greater affinity than its low-risk counterpart, presumably inactivating pRB's tumor-suppressor function.[21–23] Comparable to the p53-E6 interaction, studies by Boyer *et al.* provide evidence for E7-induced enhanced degradation of Rb protein via the ubiquitin-proteasome pathway.[23a]

Since high-risk HPV infection provides a means with which to inactivate these tumor suppressors through protein-protein interactions, it is not surprising that most HPV-positive cervical carcinomas and carcinoma-derived cell lines lack *p53* and *pRB* mutations.[24,25] However, a few HPV-positive tumors have been shown to contain *p53* gene mutations, suggesting that in at least some cases the gene mutation confers an additional growth advantage to the HPV-infected cell.[26–28] Other studies support the notion that *p53* gene mutation may play a role in the progression of at least some cervical tumors, since *p53* point mutations have been identified more frequently in metastases arising from HPV-positive cervical carcinomas than in primary tumors.[29]

The functional consequences of *p53* and *pRB* inactivation by HPV oncoproteins have been addressed by several studies. Cells damaged by irradiation or DNA strand-breaking drugs arrest in the late G1 portion of the cell cycle, presumably allowing the cells to repair DNA damage and avoid accumulation of genetic lesions.[30–32] This cell cycle arrest is temporally associated with accumulation of wild-type p53 protein and is not seen in cells lacking p53 or in those expressing mutant *p53* genes. When the HPV16 E6 protein is expressed in cells exhibiting a normal DNA damage response, baseline p53 protein levels are reduced dramatically, and the cell cycle arrest following DNA damage is abolished.[33,34] Hence high-risk HPVs may indirectly contribute to cervical tumorigenesis by promoting genomic instability and the accumulation of mutations in HPV-infected cells. HPV16 E7 also has been shown to effectively abrogate the p53-dependent growth arrest in response to DNA damage.[35–37] Several studies suggest that this may be explained by a role for pRB downstream of p53 in the growth-arrest pathway (Fig. 53-2). Abrogation of this important cellular response by the HPV transforming proteins suggests a plausible mechanism for the accelerated accumulation of genetic alterations necessary for cervical tumor progression that occurs in the setting of high-risk HPV infection.

There are several types of genetic alterations that may arise as a consequence of *p53* and *pRB* inactivation and the resulting abrogation of the growth arrest in response to DNA damage. When high-risk (HPV16) E6 is introduced into human fibroblasts, the cells show a marked increase in their ability to amplify drug-resistance genes in response to drug treatment.[38] In contrast, low-risk (HPV6) E6 has no effect. The idea that high-risk HPV infection may enhance gene amplification is particularly interesting because frequent amplification of *c-myc, HER2-neu,* and as yet unidentified gene(s) on the long arm of chromosome 3 (3q) has been reported in cervical cancers.[39–42] At least one study suggests that *c-myc* amplification may be a useful marker of poor prognosis, since patients whose tumors had *c-myc* amplification suffered early relapse more frequently than those whose tumors lacked the alteration.[40] The gains of chromosome 3q sequences also are particularly interesting because they appear to occur at the transition from severe dysplasia (HSIL) to invasive squamous carcinoma.[42] Specifically, over-representation of chromosome 3q sequences was observed in 90 percent of carcinomas but in less than 10 percent of HSILs, suggesting that the 3q gains may confer the potential for stromal invasion to affected cells.

Another genetic alteration that occurs frequently at the transition from HSIL to invasive carcinoma is integration of the viral genome into the host DNA. In condylomas and most SILs, the HPV genome is maintained as an episome (a free circular molecule replicating independently of the cellular genome). Regardless of HPV type, the production of progeny virions in these lesions is tightly linked to squamous epithelial differentiation.[43] In contrast, the majority of invasive carcinomas contain high-risk HPV DNA integrated into human chromosomal DNA as one or multiple tandem copies.[44,45] During the process of integration, substantial portions of the HPV genome may be deleted, but the *E6* and *E7* open reading frames virtually always are retained. Although several studies have failed to find a common site in the host genome where the virus integrates, viral integration almost invariably disrupts elements of the HPV genome (i.e., *E1* and/or *E2*) that regulate expression of the *E6* and *E7* transforming genes.[46] Not surprisingly, integration of HPV16 DNA into the genome of cervical epithelial cells was found to correlate with a selective growth advantage *in vitro*, providing further support for the notion that viral integration is an important step for *in vivo* tumor progression.[47] High-risk HPVs may themselves contribute to integration of HPV DNA into the host genome. Indeed, studies have shown that the frequency of foreign DNA integration is enhanced in cells expressing high-risk but not low-risk HPV E6 and E7.[48]

In other studies, inactivation of *p53* by the HPV16 E6 protein was found to increase the rate of spontaneous mutagenesis (particularly point mutations and small insertions or deletions) in human cells.[49] Interestingly, HPV16 E7 expression had no effect on the rate of mutagenesis, suggesting that the type of genetic alteration detected by this assay is enhanced by *p53* but not by *pRB* inactivation. A plausible explanation for this finding may be provided by the observation that p53's role in suppressing tumorigenesis is not likely to be restricted to its participation in

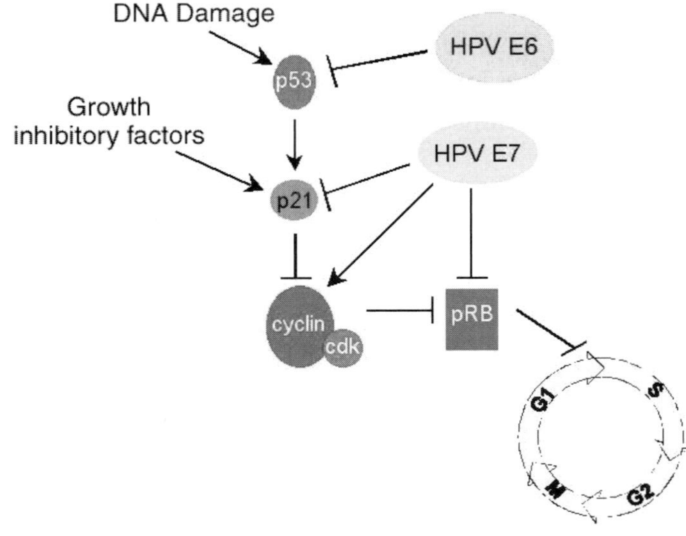

Fig. 53-2 A representation of the DNA damage-induced cell cycle checkpoint pathway in mammalian cells. DNA damage results in accumulation of the p53 protein. Accumulation of wtp53 increases levels of p21$^{waf1/cip1}$, which in turn inhibits activation of cyclin-cdk complexes. pRB therefore remains in the unphosphorylated (active) state, and pRB-associated E2F transcription factors are unable to activate transcription of genes required for progression from G1 into S phase. Consequently, cells arrest in late G1. High-risk HPVs can disrupt the pathway at multiple points: through interaction of E6 with p53 and, further downstream, through the effects of E7 on pRB, p21, and the G1 cyclins. (*Modified with permission from Alani and Münger K: Human papillomaviruses and associated malignancies. J Clin Oncol 16:330-337, 1998.*)

the DNA damage-response pathway. p53 is thought to play a more direct role in DNA repair also, because it has been found to be associated with other proteins involved in DNA repair such as the DNA helicases ERCC3/XPB and RPA.[49]

Clearly, we are beginning to develop an understanding of the molecular mechanisms underlying the difference in oncogenic potential between the high- and low-risk HPVs. The E6 and E7 proteins encoded by the low-risk HPVs appear to have substantially less impact on p53 and pRB function than their high-risk counterparts. However, it remains possible, if not likely, that the oncogenic potential of the various HPV types is owing to additional factors beyond their ability to directly interfere with p53 and pRB function. For example, in addition to its interaction with E6-AP, HPV E6 has been shown to bind to a putative calcium-binding protein called *ERC-55,* and the transforming ability of *E6* mutants was found to correlate with ERC-55 binding activity.[50] E6 proteins encoded by high-risk HPVs are also able to bind to the PDZ domain of HDLG, the mammalian homologue of the *Drosophila* disks large tumor-suppressor protein, which in turn has been shown to interact with the *APC* (adenomatous polyposis coli) tumor-suppressor gene product.[51,52] These findings raise the intriguing possibility that the interaction of HPV E6 with hDLG may represent a mechanism with which to inactivate APC function that bypasses the need for *APC* gene mutation. Additional studies are needed to further explore this possibility. The E6 transforming protein of bovine papillomavirus 1 (BPV1) has been shown to interact with the focal adhesion protein paxillin.[53,54] Paxillin is thought to participate in the transduction of signals from the plasma membrane to focal adhesions and the actin cytoskeleton. Hence E6-mediated disruption of the actin fiber network could alter important signal transduction pathways that regulate cell cycle control and cellular differentiation programs. HPV E7 has been shown to interact with a number of nuclear and cytoplasmic proteins, suggesting that the interaction of E7 with pRB is one of several protein-protein interactions relevant for cellular transformation.[54a] For example, E7 can bind and inactivate the cyclin-dependent kinase inhibitors p21 and p27, and expression of E7 leads to increased expression of the G1 cyclins A and E.[55–58] G1 cyclin-cdk complexes are important in regulating the phosphorylation status of pRB, which in turn regulates cell growth mediated by the E2F family of transcription factors.[59–61] In other studies, expression of HPV16 E6/E7 was shown to lead to increased cellular levels of cyclin B and $p34^{cdc2}$, suggesting that the HPV oncoproteins may affect other portions of the cell cycle in addition to the G1S checkpoint.[62]

The role of other HPV proteins in cellular transformation is also being actively investigated. E5 has been shown to act as a mitogen, presumably through growth factor receptor signal transduction pathways, and to induce anchorage-independent growth of immortalized fibroblasts in an epidermal growth factor (EGF)-dependent fashion.[63]

OTHER GENETIC LOCI IMPLICATED IN CERVICAL TUMORIGENESIS

Both cytogenetic and molecular genetic analyses have been used in an attempt to identify additional loci frequently altered during cervical tumorigenesis. In general, cytogenetic studies have failed to identify consistent specific chromosomal rearrangements or other karyotypic abnormalities in cervical cancer cells. Structural and numerical abnormalities of chromosome 1 have been reported most frequently.[64,65]

Other investigators have performed allelotype analyses of cervical carcinomas in an attempt to localize tumor-suppressor loci. In one study of 35 uterine cancers (including both endometrial and cervical carcinomas), high frequencies of allelic loss (i.e., >35 percent) were found at loci on chromosomes 3p, 9q, 10q, and 17p.[66] In another study of 53 primary cervical carcinomas, more than 25 percent of informative tumors had allelic losses involving chromosomes 1q, 3p, 3q, 4q, 5p, 5q, 6p, 10q, 11p, 18p, and Xq.[67] Frequent deletions on 3p and 11p have been confirmed by other studies.[68–70] Deletion mapping of chromosome 3p has localized common regions of deletion to 3p13-14.3 and 3p13-p21.1.[68,69] The 3p losses are particularly interesting in part because deletions of this region are common not only in cervical carcinomas but also in several other tumor types, including clear cell renal carcinomas, lung carcinomas, and nasopharyngeal carcinomas. Recently, a candidate tumor-suppressor gene, *FHIT* at 3p14.2, was cloned.[71] Aberrant *FHIT* transcripts have been identified in several different tumor types, including esophageal, stomach, breast, and colon carcinomas.[71,72] The gene spans a fragile site called *FRA3B* that was found independently to contain a spontaneous HPV16 integration site.[73] Altered *FHIT* transcripts and markedly reduced or absent Fhit protein expression have been demonstrated in roughly 70 percent of primary cervical carcinomas but not in normal cervix, suggesting that *FHIT* inactivation may be important in cervical cancer pathogenesis.[74]

Functional studies have provided yet additional evidence suggesting involvement of tumor-suppressor genes in the development and/or progression of cervical cancer. For example, transfer of chromosome 11 into HeLa cells (derived from an HPV18-positive cervical carcinoma) and SiHa cells (derived from an HPV16-positive cervical carcinoma) resulted in complete suppression of tumorigenicity.[75,76] Similarly, expression of the *DCC* gene in keratinocytes transformed by HPV18 and nitrosomethylurea resulted in suppression of tumorigenicity, and tumorigenic reversion was associated with loss or rearrangement of transfected *DCC* sequences.[77]

ANIMAL MODELS

A better understanding of the role of HPV infection in the pathogenesis of cervical cancer undoubtedly will enhance our ability to effectively manage patients with this disease. Although *in vitro* systems are very powerful, they are often limited in their ability to provide insights into the processes driving neoplastic progression. Thus a long-standing goal of HPV and cervical cancer researchers has been to develop effective animal models of HPV-induced tumors. Such models, in addition to leading to improved preventive, diagnostic, and therapeutic strategies, also may facilitate identification of genetic and environmental cofactors that may profoundly influence both tumor development and progression.

The strong association of HPV infection with cervical tumorigenesis led to great optimism that useful animal models of cervical cancer could be developed easily. In general, animal models of viral diseases require a source of infectious virus and a susceptible host. Unfortunately, both have been problematic with respect to HPVs. These viruses are notoriously difficult to culture, largely because HPV virions are only produced in highly differentiated keratinocytes. Successful culture of HPV was not achieved until 1992.[78] To further complicate matters, infection with the various types of papillomaviruses is species-specific, and HPVs do not infect nonhuman species. Thus several models of papillomavirus-associated oncogenesis have been developed in species-specific systems, including those in rabbits, rodents, cattle, dogs, and non-human primates.[79,80] Fortunately, many researchers have successfully circumvented the species specificity of papillomaviruses by expressing viral genes in transgenic animals. Several groups have produced transgenic mice expressing high-risk HPV transforming genes.[79,80] Increased propensity to develop tumors has been observed in all transgenic lineages, with the specific location and type of tumor determined largely by the nature of the promoter used to express the transgenes. Transgenic mice expressing the *E6* and *E7* oncogenes of HPV16 under control of the β-actin promoter or α-A-crystallin promoter develop neuroepithelial carcinomas and lens tumors, respectively.[81,82] In one study, mice expressing the same genes under the control of the mouse mammary tumor virus promoter developed large testicular seminomas, whereas another group reported the development of salivary gland carcinomas, lymphomas, and cutaneous histiocytomas.[83,84] In the latter study, 77 percent of the female transgenic mice also developed dysplastic and/or hyperplastic changes in the cervix and vagina, although no anogenital tumors were observed. Probably the most illustrative transgenic model system is that recently described by Arbeit and colleagues.[85] These investigators generated transgenic mice expressing the early region of the HPV16 genome under the control of the human keratin-14 promoter. The mice developed squamous carcinomas exclusively in the vagina and cervix when treated chronically with 17β-estradiol. Although the mechanisms for the synergism between chronic estrogen exposure and expression of HPV oncoproteins in squamous carcinogenesis remain to be determined, this animal model system is likely to prove invaluable in future studies.

IMPLICATIONS FOR DIAGNOSIS AND TREATMENT

HPV proteins provide tumor-specific antigens in the great majority of cervical carcinomas, and hence it should be feasible to develop prophylactic or antitumor vaccines to effectively prevent or treat cervical cancer.[86] The development of such vaccines has been hindered, at least in part, by the difficulty in propagating HPVs in culture and by only relatively recent availability of good animal model systems. Nonetheless, substantial progress has been made in the last few years. For example, several investigators are working to develop prophylactic vaccines based on the use of genetically engineered papillomavirus-like particles to elicit neutralizing anti-HPV antibodies or cell-mediated immune response.[87,88] Preliminary studies in animals have been encouraging. Alternative approaches also have been employed. Noncapsid papillomavirus antigens (those consistently present in cervical cancer cells) are preferentially routed for MHC class I presentation, which typically is deficient in cervical cancer cells.[10] Thus a reasonable approach for an antitumor vaccine is one that attempts to route such antigens into the MHC class II processing and presentation pathway via the endosomal and lysosomal cellular compartments. In a recent study, Wu and colleagues fused a target tumor antigen (HPV16 E7) to a sequence of the lysosomal protein LAMP-1 in order to direct the antigen into the endosomal and lysosomal compartments and enhance MHC class II presentation of E7 peptides.[89] Expression of the fusion protein in appropriate recipient cells resulted in enhanced presentation to CD4+ cells in vitro. Moreover, *in vivo* immunization experiments using recombinant vaccinia viruses in mice demonstrated that immunization with the chimeric protein resulted in increased E7-specific lymphoproliferative activity, antibody titers, and cytotoxic T-lymphocyte activity compared with immunization with wild-type E7. In more recent studies, these investigators were able to use the same recombinant viral vaccines to cure mice with small established tumors.[90] Clinical trials of this type of vaccine in cervical cancer patients are likely to follow in the near future.

Certainly, another major goal of cervical cancer researchers in the future will be to identify specific genes involved in the progression of premalignant lesions. The identification of such genes is critical for developing potential screening protocols to augment those currently based on cytopathologic screening of Papanicolau smears alone. The knowledge gained also may prove useful for designing novel and more sensible therapeutic strategies as well as more reliable methods that can be used to predict which intraepithelial lesions may be more likely to progress to invasive disease.

REFERENCES

1. Beral V, Hermon C, Muñoz N, Devesa SS: Cervical cancer. *Cancer Surv* **19-20**:265, 1994.
2. Parker SL, Tong T, Bolden S, Wingo PA: Cancer statistics, 1997. *CA* **47**:5, 1997.
3. Kiviat NB, Critchlow CW, Kurman RJ: Reassessment of the morphological continuum of cervical intraepithelial lesions: Does it reflect different stages in the progression to cervical carcinoma? in Muñoz N, Bosch FX, Shah KV, Meheus A (eds): *The Epidemiology of Cervical Cancer and Human Papillomavirus*. Lyon: International Agency for Research on Cancer, 1992, pp 59-66.
4. Östör AG: Natural history of cervical intraepithelial neoplasia: A critical review. *Int J Gynecol Pathol* **12**:186, 1993.
5. Benedet JL, Anderson GH: Stage IA carcinoma of the cervix revisited. *Obstet Gynecol* **87**:1052, 1996.
6. Jessup JM, McGinnis LS, Winchester DP, Eyre H, Fremgen A, Murphy GP, Menck HR: Clinical highlights from the National Cancer Data Base: 1996. *CA* **46**:185, 1996.
7. Wank R, Thomssen C: High risk of squamous cell carcinoma of the cervix for women with HLA-DQw3. *Nature* **352**:723, 1991.
8. Helland A, Borresen AL, Kaern J, Ronningen KS, Thorsby E: HLA antigens and cervical carcinoma (letter, comment). *Nature* **356**:23, 1992.
9. Storey A, Thomas M, Kalita A, Harwood C, Gardiol D, Mantovani F, Breuer J, [JKM4]et al: Role of a p53 polymorphism in the development of human papillomavirus-associated cancer. *Nature* 393:229, 1998.

9a. Helland A, Langerod A, Johnsen H, Olsen AO, Skovlund E, Borresen-Dale AL: p53 polymorphism and risk of cervical cancer. *Nature* **396**: 530, 1998.

9b. Hildesheim A, Schiffman M, Brinton LA, Fraumeni JF Jr, Herrero R, Bratti MC, Schwartz P, Mortel R, Barnes W, Greenberg M, McGowan L, Scott DR, Martin M, Herrera JE, Carrington M: p53 polymorphism and risk of cervical cancer. *Nature* **396**: 531, 1998.

9c. Josefsson AM, Magnusson PK, Ylitalo N, Quarforth-Tubbin P, Ponten J, Adami HO, Gyllensten UB: p53 polymorphism and risk of cervical cancer. *Nature* **396**: 531, 1998.

9d. Klaes R, Ridder R, Schaefer U, Benner A, von Knebel Doeberitz M: No evidence of p53 allele-specific predisposition in human papillomavirus-associated cervical cancer. *J Mol Med* **77**: 299, 1999.

9e. Minaguchi T, Kanamori Y, Matsushima M, Yoshikawa H, Taketani Y, Nakamura Y: No evidence of correlation between polymorphism at codon 72 of p53 and risk of cervical cancer in Japanese patients with human papillomavirus 16/18 infection. *Cancer Res* **58**: 4584, 1998.

10. Altmann A, Jochmus I, Rösl F: Intra- and extracellular control mechanisms of human papillomavirus infection. *Intervirology* **37**:180, 1994.
11. Bosch FX, Manos MM, Muñoz N, Sherman ME, Jansen AM, Peto J, Schiffman MH, Moreno V, Kurman R, Shah KV: Prevalence of human papillomavirus in cervical cancer: A worldwide perspective. International Biological Study on Cervical Cancer (IBSCC) study Group. *J Natl Cancer Inst* **87**:796, 1995.
12. Pirisi L, Yasumoto S, Feller M, Doniger J, DiPaolo JA: Transformation of human fibroblasts and keratinocytes with human papillomavirus type 16 DNA. *J Virol* **61**:1061, 1987.
13. Pecoraro G, Morgan D, Defendi V: Differential effects of human papillomavirus type 6, 16, and 18 DNAs on immortalization and transformation of human cervical epithelial cells. *Proc Natl Acad Sci USA* **86**:563, 1989.
14. Woodworth CD, Doniger J, DiPaolo JA: Immortalization of human foreskin keratinocytes by various human papillomavirus DNAs corresponds to their association with cervical carcinoma. *J Virol* **63**:159, 1989.
15. Hawley-Nelson P, Vousden KH, Hubbert NL, Lowy DR, Schiller JT: HPV16 E6 and E7 proteins cooperate to immortalize human foreskin keratinocytes. *EMBO J* **8**:3905, 1989.
16. Werness BA, Levine AJ, Howley PM: Association of human papillomavirus types 16 and 18 E6 proteins with p53. *Science* **248**:76, 1990.
17. Scheffner M, Werness BA, Huibregtse JM, Levine AJ, Howley PM: The E6 oncoprotein encoded by human papillomavirus types 16 and 18 promotes the degradation of p53. *Cell* **63**:1129, 1990.
18. Huibregtse JM, Scheffner M, Howley PM: A cellular protein mediates association of p53 with the E6 oncoprotein of human papillomavirus types 16 or 18. *EMBO J* **10**:4129, 1991.
19. Huibregtse JM, Scheffner M, Howley PM: Cloning and expression of the cDNA for E6-AP, a protein that mediates the interaction of the human papillomavirus E6 oncoprotein with p53. *Mol Cell Biol* **13**:775, 1993.
20. Scheffner M, Huibregtse JM, Vierstra RD, Howley PM: The HPV-16 E6 and E6-AP complex functions as a ubiquitin-protein ligase in the ubiquitination of p53. *Cell* **75**:495, 1993.
21. Dyson N, Howley PM, Münger K, Harlow E: The human papillomavirus 16 E7 oncoprotein is able to bind to the retinoblastoma gene product. *Science* **243**:934, 1989.

22. Dyson N, Guida P, Münger K, Harlow E: Homologous sequences in adenovirus E1A and human papillomavirus E7 proteins mediate interaction with the same set of cellular proteins. *J Virol* **66**:6893, 1992.
23. Davies RC, Hicks R, Crook T, Morris JDH, Vousden K: Human papillomavirus type 16 E7 associates with a histone H1 kinase and with p107 through sequences necessary for transformation. *J Virol* **67**:2521, 1993.
23a. Boyer SN, Wazer DE, Band V: E7 protein of human papilloma virus-16 induces degradation of retinoblastoma protein through the ubiquitin-proteasome pathway. *Cancer Res* **56**:4620, 1996.
24. Scheffner M, Münger K, Byrne JC, Howley PM: The state of the *p53* and *retinoblastoma* genes in human cervical carcinoma cell lines. *Proc Natl Acad Sci USA* **88**:5523, 1991.
25. Crook T, Wrede D, Vousden KH: *p53* point mutation in HPV negative human cervical carcinoma cell lines. *Oncogene* **6**:873, 1991.
26. Helland A, Holm R, Kristensen G, Kaern J, Karlsen F, Trope C, Nesland JM, Borresen AL: Genetic alterations of the *tp53* gene, p53 protein expression, and HPV infection in primary cervical cancers. *J Pathol* **171**:105, 1993.
27. Fujita M, Inoue M, Tanizawa O, Iwamoto S, Enomoto T: Alterations of the *p53* gene in human primary cervical carcinoma with and without human papillomavirus infection. *Cancer Res* **52**:5323, 1992.
28. Kessis TD, Slebos RJC, Han S, Shah KV, Bosch FX, Muñoz N, Hedrick L, Cho KR: *p53* gene mutations and *mdm2* amplification are uncommon in primary carcinomas of the uterine cervix. *Am J Pathol* **143**:1398, 1993.
29. Crook T, Vousden KH: Properties of *p53* mutations detected in primary and secondary cervical cancers suggest mechanisms of metastasis and involvement of environmental carcinogens. *EMBO J* **11**:3935, 1992.
30. Kastan MB, Onyekwere O, Sidransky D, Vogelstein B, Craig RW: Participation of p53 protein in the cellular response to DNA damage. *Cancer Res* **51**:6304, 1991.
31. Kuerbitz SJ, Plunkett BS, Walsh WV, Kastan MB: Wild-type p53 is a cell cycle checkpoint determinant following irradiation. *Proc Natl Acad Sci USA* **89**:7491, 1992.
32. Kastan MB, Zhan Q, El-Deiry WS, Carrier F, Jacks T, Walsh W, Plunkett B, Vogelstein B, Fornace AJ Jr: A mammalian cell cycle checkpoint pathway utilizing p53 and GADD45 is defective in ataxia-telangiectasia. *Cell* **71**:587, 1992.
33. Kessis TD, Slebos RJC, Nelson WG, Kastan MB, Plunkett BS, Han SM, Lorincz AT, Hedrick L, Cho KR: Human papillomavirus 16 E6 expression disrupts the p53-mediated cellular response to DNA damage. *Proc Natl Acad Sci USA* **90**:3988, 1993.
34. Foster SA, Demers GW, Etscheid BG, Galloway DA: The ability of human papillomavirus E6 proteins to target p53 for degradation in vivo correlates with their ability to abrogate actinomycin D-induced growth arrest. *J Virol* **68**:5698, 1994.
35. Hickman ES, Picksley SM, Vousden KH: Cells expressing HPV16 E7 continue cell cycle progression following DNA damage induced p53 activation. *Oncogene* **9**:2177, 1994.
36. Demers GW, Foster SA, Halbert CL, Galloway DA: Growth arrest by induction of p53 in DNA damaged keratinocytes is bypassed by human papillomavirus 16 E7. *Proc Natl Acad Sci USA* **91**:4382, 1994.
37. Slebos RJ, Lee MH, Plunkett BS, Kessis TD, Williams BO, Jacks T, Hedrick L, Kastan MB, Cho KR: p53-dependent G1 arrest involves pRB-related proteins and is disrupted by the human papillomavirus 16 E7 oncoprotein. *Proc Natl Acad Sci USA* **91**:5320, 1994.
38. White AE, Livanos EM, Tlsty TD: Differential disruption of genomic integrity and cell cycle regulation in normal human fibroblasts by the HPV oncoproteins. *Genes Dev* **8**:666, 1994.
39. Baker VV, Hatch KD, Shingleton HM: Amplification of the *c-myc* proto-oncogene in cervical carcinoma. *J Surg Oncol* **39**:225, 1988.
40. Ocadiz R, Sauceda R, Cruz M, Graef AM, Gariglio P: High correlation between molecular alterations of the *c-myc* oncogene and carcinoma of the uterine cervix. *Cancer Res* **47**:4173, 1987.
41. Mitra AB, Murty VVVS, Pratap M, Sodhani P, Chaganti RSK: *ERBB2* (*HER2/neu*) oncogene is frequently amplified in squamous cell carcinoma of the uterine cervix. *Cancer Res* **54**:637, 1994.
42. Heselmeyer K, Schrock E, du Manoir S, Blegen H, Shah K, Steinbeck R, Auer G, Ried T: Gain of chromosome 3q defines the transition from severe dysplasia to invasive carcinoma of the uterine cervix. *Proc Natl Acad Sci USA* **93**:479, 1996.
43. Chow LT, Broker TR: Papillomavirus DNA replication. *Intervirology* **37**:150, 1994.
44. Dürst M, Kleinheinz A, Hotz M, Gissman L: The physical state of human papillomavirus type 16 DNA in benign and malignant genital tumours. *J Gen Virol* **66**:1515, 1985.
45. Cullen AP, Reid R, Champion M, Lorincz AT: Analysis of the physical state of different human papillomavirus DNAs in intraepithelial and invasive cervical neoplasia. *J Virol* **65**:606, 1991.
46. Choo KB, Pan CC, Han SH: Integration of human papillomavirus type 16 into cellular DNA of cervical carcinoma: Preferential deletion of the *E2* gene and invariable retention of the long control region and the *E6/E7* open reading frames. *Virology* **161**:259, 1987.
47. Jeon S, Allen-Hoffmann BL, Lambert PF: Integration of human papillomavirus type 16 into the human genome correlates with a selective growth advantage of cells. *J Virol* **69**:2989, 1995.
48. Kessis TD, Connolly DC, Hedrick L, Cho KR: Expression of HPV16 E6 or E7 increases integration of foreign DNA. *Oncogene* **13**:427, 1996.
49. Havre PA, Yuan JL, Hedrick L, Cho KR, Glazer PM: *p53* inactivation by HPV16 E6 results in increased mutagenesis in human cells. *Cancer Res* **55**:4420, 1995.
50. Chen JJ, Reid CE, Band V, Androphy EJ: Interaction of papillomavirus E6 oncoproteins with a putative calcium-binding protein. *Science* **269**:529, 1995.
51. Kiyono T, Hiraiwa A, Fujita M, Hayashi Y, Akiyama T, Ishibashi M: Binding of high-risk human papillomavirus E6 oncoproteins to the human homologue of the *Drosophila* discs large tumor suppressor protein. *Proc Natl Acad Sci USA* **94**:11612, 1997.
52. Matsumine A, Ogai A, Senda T, Okumura N, Satoh K, Baeg GH, Kawahara T, [JKM13]et al: Binding of *APC* to the human homologue of the *Drosophila* discs large tumor suppressor protein. *Science* 272:1020, 1996.
53. Tong X, Howley PM: The bovine papillomavirus E6 oncoprotein interacts with paxillin and disrupts the actin cytoskeleton. *Proc Natl Acad Sci USA* **94**:4412, 1997.
54. Tong X, Salgia R, Li JL, Griffin JD, Howley PM: The bovine papillomavirus E6 protein binds to the LD motif repeats of paxillin and blocks its interaction with vinculin and the focal adhesion kinase. *J Biol Chem* **272**:33373, 1997.
54a. Zwerschke W, Jansen-Durr P: Cell transformation by the E7 oncoprotein of human papillomavirus type 16: Interactions with nuclear and cytoplasmic target proteins. *Adv Cancer Res* **78**:1, 2000.
55. Zerfass-Thome K, Zwerschke W, Mannhardt B, Tindle R, Botz JW, Jansen-Durr P: Inactivation of the cdk inhibitor p27 (kip1) by the human papillomavirus type 16 E7 oncoprotein. *Oncogene* **13**:2323, 1996.
56. Jones DL, Alani RM, Münger K: The human papillomavirus E7 oncoprotein can uncouple cellular differentiation and proliferation in human keratinocytes by abrogating $p21^{Cip1}$-mediated inhibition of cdk2. *Genes Dev* **11**:2101, 1998.
57. Funk JO, Waga S, Harry JB, Espling E, Stillman B, Galloway DA: Inhibition of CDK activity and PCNA-dependent DNA replication by p21 is blocked by interaction with the HPV-16 E7 oncoprotein. *Genes Dev* **11**:2090, 1997.
58. Zerfass K, Schulze A, Spitkovsky D, Friedman V, Henglein B, Jansen-Durr P: Sequential activation of cyclin E and cyclin A gene expression by human papillomavirus type 16 E7 through sequences necessary for transformation. *J Virol* **69**:6389, 1995.
59. Ewen ME, Sluss HK, Sherr CJ, Matsushime H, Kato J, Livingston DM: Functional interactions of the retinoblastoma protein with mammalian D-type cyclins. *Cell* **73**:487, 1993.
60. Kato J, Matsushime H, Hiebert SW, Ewen ME, Sherr CJ: Direct binding of cyclin D to the retinoblastoma gene product (pRb) and pRb phosphorylation by the cyclin D-dependent kinase CDK4. *Genes Dev* **7**:331, 1993.
61. Hinds PW, Mittnacht S, Dulic V, Arnold A, Reed SI, Weinberg RA: Regulation of retinoblastoma protein functions by ectopic expression of human cyclins. *Cell* **70**:993, 1992.
62. Steinmann KE, Pei XF, Stoppler H, Schlegel R: Elevated expression and activity of mitotic regulatory proteins in human papillomavirus-immortalized keratinocytes. *Oncogene* **9**:387, 1994.
63. Straight SW, Hinkle PM, Jewers RJ, McCance DJ: The E5 oncoprotein of human papillomavirus type 16 transforms fibroblasts and effects the downregulation of the epidermal growth factor receptor in keratinocytes. *J Virol* **67**:4521, 1993.
64. Atkin NB, Baker MC: Chromosome 1 in 26 carcinomas of the cervix uteri: Structural and numerical changes. *Cancer* **44**:604, 1979.
65. Sreekantaiah C, De Braekeleer M, Haas O: Cytogenetic findings in cervical carcinoma: A statistical approach. *Cancer Genet Cytogenet* **53**:75, 1991.
66. Jones MH, Koi S, Fujimoto I, Hasumi K, Kato K, Nakamura Y: Allelotype of uterine cancer by analysis of RFLP and microsatellite

polymorphisms: Frequent loss of heterozygosity on chromosome arms 3p, 9q, 10q, and 17p. *Genes Chromosom Cancer* **9**:119, 1994.
67. Mitra AB, Murty VVVS, Li RG, Pratap M, Luthra UK, Chaganti RSK: Allelotype analysis of cervical carcinoma. *Cancer Res* **54**:4481, 1994.
68. Jones MH, Nakamura Y: Deletion mapping of chromosome 3p in female genital tract malignancies using microsatellite polymorphisms. *Oncogene* **7**:1631, 1992.
69. Kohno T, Takayama H, Hamaguchi M, Takano H, Yamaguchi N, Tsuda H, Hirohashi S, [JKM14]et al: Deletion mapping of chromosome-3p in human uterine cervical cancer. *Oncogene* **8**:1825, 1993.
70. Srivatsan ES, Misra BC, Venugopalan M, Wilczynski SP: Loss of heterozygosity for alleles on chromosome 11 in cervical carcinoma. *Am J Hum Genet* **49**:868, 1991.
71. Ohta M, Inoue H, Cotticelli MG, Kastury K, Baffa R, Palazzo J, Siprashvili Z, [JKM15]et al: The *FHIT* gene, spanning the chromosome 3p14.2 fragile site acid renal carcinoma-associated t(3-8) breakpoint, is abnormal in digestive tract cancers. *Cell* **84**:587, 1996.
72. Negrini M, Monaco C, Vorechovsky I, Ohta M, Druck T, Baffa R, Huebner K, Croce CM: The *FHIT* gene at 3p14.2 is abnormal in breast carcinomas. *Cancer Res* **56**:3173, 1996.
73. Wilke CM, Hall BK, Hoge A, Paradee W, Smith DI, Glover TW: FRA3B extends over a broad region and contains a spontaneous HPV16 integration site: Direct evidence for the coincidence of viral integration sites and fragile sites. *Hum Genet* **5**:187, 1996.
74. Greenspan DL, Connolly DC, Wu R, Lei RY, Vogelstein JTC, Kim Y, Mok JE, [JKM17]et al: Loss of *FHIT* expression in cervical carcinoma cell lines and primary tumors. *Cancer Res* **57**:4692, 1997.
75. Oshimura M, Kugoh H, Koi M, Shimizu M, Yamada H, Satoh H, Barrett JC: Transfer of a normal human chromosome 11 suppresses tumorigenicity of some but not all tumor cell lines. *J Cell Biochem* **42**:135, 1990.
76. Saxon PJ, Srivatsan ES, Stanbridge EJ: Introduction of human chromosome 11 via microcell transfer controls tumorigenic expression of HeLa cells. *EMBO J* **5**:3461, 1986.
77. Klingelhutz AJ, Hedrick L, Cho KR, McDougall JK: The *DCC* gene suppresses the malignant phenotype of transformed human epithelial cells. *Oncogene* **10**:1581, 1995.
78. Meyers C, Frattini MG, Hudson JB, Laimins LA: Biosynthesis of human papillomvirus from a continuous cell line upon epithelial differentiation. *Science* **257**:971, 1992.
79. Brandsma JL: Animal models of human-papillomavirus-associated oncogenesis. *Intervirology* **37**:189, 1994.
80. Griep AE, Lambert PF: Role of papillomavirus oncogenes in human cervical cancer: Transgenic animal studies. *Proc Soc Exp Biol Med* **206**:24, 1994.
81. Arbeit JM, Münger K, Howley PM, Hanahan D: Neuroepithelial carcinomas in mice transgenic with human papillomavirus type 16 E6/E7 ORFs. *Am J Pathol* **142**:1187, 1993.
82. Griep AE, Herber R, Jeon S, Lohse JK, Dubielzig RR, Lambert PF: Tumorigenicity by human papillomavirus type 16 E6 and E7 in transgenic mice correlates with alterations in epithelial cell growth and differentiation. *J Virol* **67**:1373, 1993.
83. Kondoh G, Murata Y, Aozasa K, Yutsudo M, Hakura A: Very high incidence of germ cell tumorigenesis (seminomagenesis) in human papillomavirus type 16 transgenic mice. *J Virol* **65**:3335, 1991.
84. Sasagawa T, Kondoh G, Inoue M, Yutsudo M, Hakura A: Cervical/vaginal dysplasias of transgenic mice harbouring human papillomavirus type 16 *E6-E7* genes. *J Gen Virol* **75**:3057, 1994.
85. Arbeit JM, Howley PM, Hanahan D: Chronic estrogen-induced cervical and vaginal squamous carcinogenesis in human papillomavirus type 16 transgenic mice. *Proc Natl Acad Sci USA* **93**:2930, 1996.
86. Galloway DA: Human papillomavirus vaccines: A warty problem. *Infect Agents Dis* **3**:187, 1994.
87. Greenstone HL, Nieland JD, de Visser KE, De Bruijn ML, Kirnbauer R, Roden RB, Lowy DR, Kast WM, Schiller JT: Chimeric papillomavirus virus-like particles elicit antitumor immunity against the E7 oncoprotein in an HPV16 tumor model. *Proc Natl Acad Sci USA* **95**:1800, 1998.
88. Balmelli C, Roden R, Potts A, Schiller J, De Grandi P, Nardelli-Haefliger D: Nasal immunization of mice with human papillomavirus type 16 virus-like particles elicits neutralizing antibodies in mucosal secretions. *J Virol* **72**:8220, 1998.
89. Wu TC, Guarnieri FG, Stavely-O'Carroll KF, Viscidi RP, Levitsky HI, Hedrick L, Cho KR, August JT, Pardoll DM: Engineering an intracellular pathway for major histocompatibility complex class II presentation of antigens. *Proc Natl Acad Sci USA* **92**:11671, 1995.
90. Lin KY, Guarnieri FG, Staveley-O'Carroll KF, Levitsky HI, August JT, Pardoll DM, Wu T-C: Treatment of established tumors with a novel vaccine that enhances major histocompatibility class II presentation of tumor antigen. *Cancer Res* **56**:21, 1996.

CHAPTER 54

Bladder Cancer

Paul Cairns ▪ David Sidransky

1. **Bladder cancer is the fifth most common male cancer among Americans. Almost all bladder cancer in the United States is composed of transitional cell carcinoma. Familial cases are rare and usually part of the Lynch syndrome. Smoking is perhaps the greatest risk factor for sporadic disease.**
2. **Cytogenetic studies have identified a number of chromosomal changes in bladder cancer. Low-grade noninvasive tumors are usually diploid, whereas high-grade invasive tumors often contain gross aneuploidy. Monosomy of chromosome 9 is the most common abnormality seen in this disease.**
3. **Few proto-oncogene mutations or amplifications have been described in bladder cancer. However, chromosomal deletions are very common on chromosomes 9p, 17p, and 13q. Candidate genes inactivated at these loci include *p16, p53,* and *Rb,* respectively. Moreover, *p53* and *Rb* mutations usually are seen in flat (carcinoma *in situ*) or invasive lesions and are correlated with a poor prognosis.**
4. **Many bladder cancers appear as multifocal disease at presentation. Molecular studies have shown that multiple tumors in the same patient arise from the uncontrolled spread of a single progenitor cell. These tumors then proceed through variable genetic events during progression. A preliminary molecular progression model for bladder cancer suggests that chromosome 9p is an early loss event in most tumors. Conversely, loss of chromosomes 17p and 14q is more often associated with flat lesions and invasive tumors.**
5. **Genetic alterations can be detected in the urine sediment of patients with bladder cancer. Microsatellite analysis allows detection of loss of heterozygosity (LOH) or genomic instability in primary tumor and urine DNA. Pilot studies suggest that most bladder tumors can be detected by DNA analysis. Moreover, these approaches are amenable to automated techniques suitable for the clinical setting.**

CLINICAL ASPECTS

Bladder cancer is the fifth most common male cancer among Americans.[1] There are over 50,000 new cases diagnosed yearly, with a male/female ratio of almost 3:1. There is no pathognomonic sign or symptom for bladder cancer, but most patients present with microscopic hematuria. Occasionally, gross hematuria and pain also can lead to the diagnosis. This year alone over 11,000 patients will die from advanced and/or metastatic disease.[1]

There are few reports of familial bladder cancer.[2] Clinical cases of bladder cancer owing to hereditary predisposition probably represent 1 percent or less of all tumors. The estimated relative risk of developing the disease, even with an affected family member under the age of 45, is only 1.45 per person.[3] The greatest risk for inherited urothelial cancer probably occurs as part of the Lynch syndrome (hereditary nonpolyposis colorectal cancer, HNPCC).[4] In this syndrome, there is a high risk of bladder cancer, but it is often overshadowed by the high risk of other neoplasms, including colon cancer and uterine cancer.

Almost all bladder cancers in the United States are composed of transitional cell carcinoma (TCC). Bladder irritation or infections such as schistosomiasis can predispose to specific types of bladder cancer. In areas such as Egypt where these infection rates are high, squamous carcinoma is very common.[5] Exposure to certain chemical compounds including analgesics also may predispose to an increased risk of urothelial cancer.[6,7]

In the United States, cigarette smoking is perhaps the single greatest risk factor for bladder cancer. Compared with nonsmokers, smokers have been estimated to have a twofold increased risk of developing the disease. It is also clear that this risk may be dose-related, and in a similar fashion to lung cancer, patients who stop smoking develop an intermediate risk that begins to subside with increasing age.[8–10]

PATHOLOGY

The vast majority of bladder cancer originates in the urothelium, the characteristic transitional cell urothelial lining in the urinary tract.[11] Moreover, many tumors are already multifocal at presentation. A major and overwhelming distinction between superficial and invasive disease involves penetration into the lamina propria. The prognosis for invasive disease is much worse and depends on grade and stage. Although 85 to 95 percent of bladder cancers are TCCs, mixed tumors occasionally with squamous cell or adenocarcinoma elements are also found. Despite its low frequency in the United States, squamous cell carcinoma, for the reasons mentioned earlier, may be the most common malignancy in Egypt. Adenocarcinoma, thought to arise from the trigone of the bladder, occurs in less than 2 percent of all bladder cancers. A particular subset of adenocarcinomas also may arise from the urachus remnant located over the dome of the bladder.

There are two separate and clearly defined entities of superficial bladder cancer presentation.[12,13] The treatment for these two distinct clinical entities of bladder cancer is quite unique, since the outcome and prognosis of each are quite different.

Primary flat lesions with carcinoma *in situ* are notorious for their high likelihood of recurrence and progression.[14,15] A large retrospective study demonstrated that 40 percent of the patients with carcinoma *in situ* developed invasive disease within 5 years.[13] Papillary tumors have a strong propensity to recur, and over 70 percent of patients have a second primary lesion, usually within 2 years.[16,17] However, these lesions have no more than a 20 percent lifetime risk of progression to invasive tumors. Molecular studies have already shed some light as to the different genetic changes that may determine the morphologic appearance and progression of these two very different clinical and pathologic presentations of superficial bladder cancer.[18–20]

CHROMOSOMAL ABNORMALITIES

Neoplastic cells of the transitional cell epithelium contain many structural and numerical chromosomal changes that appear with some consistency.[21,22] These chromosomal changes in tumor cells

A list of standard abbreviations is located immediately preceding the index in each volume. Nonstandard abbreviations used in this chapter include: CGH = comparative genomic hybridization; ECFR = epidermal growth factor receptors; HNPCC = hereditary nonpolyposis colorectal cancer; LOH = loss of heterozygosity; TCC = transitional cell carcinoma.

include the underrepresentation or abnormally high numbers of chromosomes (aneuploidy) and the presence of easily identifiable structurally abnormal chromosomes that are stably inherited from one cell to another (markers). In general, it has been found that low-grade noninvasive tumors are associated with a normal (diploid) number of 46 chromosomes or with numerical deviations of only a few chromosomes. High-grade invasive tumors, on the other hand, are usually associated with gross aneuploidy and often contain marker chromosomes. The presence of marker chromosomes in low-grade noninvasive tumors has been associated with a strong tendency for recurrence and progression.[22]

Cytogenetic reports on bladder cancer have demonstrated the consistent gain or loss of specific chromosomes or chromosomal regions in most tumors.[22] Cytogenetic studies have identified loss of chromosome 9 as a very frequent change in bladder tumors.[23–25] These studies often described monosomy of chromosome 9 as the most common karyotypic change.[23] Loss of chromosome 10 or deletions of only a portion of 10q also have been described as the only karyotypic abnormality.[24,25] Another specific chromosomal abnormality in bladder cancer was first reported as an isochromosome of chromosome 5p. This appears cytogenetically as a symmetric duplication of the short arm of chromosome 5, specific for a subset of bladder cancers. Deletions and translocations of chromosome 5 are also frequently reported.[24,26]

In addition to traditional cytogenetics, novel methods now allow easier identification of genomic amplifications. A method called *comparative genomic hybridization* (CGH) allows fluorescent identification of amplified genomic regions in human cancers.[27,28] Recent CGH analysis of bladder cancer identified several areas of amplification and confirmed other areas of deletions.[29] Amplifications not previously seen by cytogenetics or molecular studies were identified on chromosomes 3p, 10p, 12q, 17q, 18p, and 22q. Thus, in many ways, CGH has become complementary to traditional cytogenetic and molecular studies.

GENETIC LOCI

As mentioned previously, there have been very few reported cases of inherited bladder cancer. Families have been described without any evidence of cytogenetic abnormalities.[2] Recently, a family was identified with a translocation of 20q and 5p.[30] In addition to bladder cancer, this family also demonstrated metastatic melanoma. In this family, however, a putative oncogene or tumor-suppressor gene has not been identified.

Sporadic Loci

Proto-oncogenes. Despite the initial discovery of a *ras* mutation in a bladder carcinoma cell line, very few *ras* gene mutations have been detected in primary TCC of the bladder.[31] It now appears that less than 10 percent of primary bladder tumors contain *ras* gene mutations.[32,33] Some investigators have observed increased expression of ras protein, but this result remains unproven because of questions about the specificity of the antibodies used.[34]

Growth factors are a class of proteins that bind to specific cell surface receptors, inducing a variety of responses including mitoses in susceptible target cells. Several laboratories have independently studied the expression of urothelial epidermal growth factor receptors (EGFR) using either immunohistochemistry to detect message with antibodies to various portions of the EGFR or autoradiography with isotope-labeled ligand.[18] Most groups have found a higher density of receptors on malignant cells compared with normal epithelium.[18,35] Moreover, epidermal growth factors are excreted in high concentrations in human urine, allowing incubation continually with normal premalignant and malignant urothelial cells. EGFRs are normally found only on the basal cell layer of the bladder epithelium. They also can be richly expressed on the superficial layers of malignant tissue. This abnormal distribution of receptors presumably allows greater access of malignant transitional cells to urinary epidermal growth factor (EGF) and has led investigators to suspect that EGF plays a role in the development and growth of bladder cancer.[18] Others have reported that the *EGFR* gene is expressed mostly in high-grade invasive tumors, and increased staining has been correlated with increased stage and death from disease in patients with Ta or T1 lesions.[36,37] However, other investigators have found no gross abnormalities at the DNA level; thus overexpression may be owing to an increase in mRNA transcription alone.[38] The *c-erbB1* proto-oncogene that maps to chromosome 7 encodes the *EGFR* gene. Interestingly, trisomy of chromosome 7 is a frequent genetic observation in bladder tumors and could lead to an increase in EGFR expression in tumor cells.[21,22] Another gene on chromosome 7, *MET*, is a candidate proto-oncogene in bladder cancer because mutations of *MET* have been found in hereditary and sporadic papillary renal tumors with trisomy 7.[39] We have sequenced 48 primary bladder tumors and found no mutation of the critical exons of the tyrosine kinase domain.

DNA amplification and increased levels of expression of *c-erbB2* have been reported as well as alterations of *c-myc* and *c-src*.[40–43] However, gross alterations or amplifications of these genes have been described rarely in primary bladder tumors. Although many proto-oncogenes have been identified in human tumors, very few have been found to be consistently altered in bladder cancer. In contrast, chromosomal loss and inactivation of tumor-suppressor genes have been found to play a significant role in progression of bladder tumors.

Chromosomal Deletions and Tumor-Suppressor Genes. Southern analysis with RFLP markers followed by the recent availability of highly polymorphic small repeat sequences known as *microsatellites* has allowed genome-wide assessment of chromosomal loss in bladder cancer.[44–48] The most common loss is the genetic event identified as loss of chromosome 9.[49] Deletion of chromosome 9 appears to be just as common in superficial tumors and invasive tumors. Inactivation of a putative tumor-suppressor gene on chromosome 9 is therefore a key candidate for the initiating event in bladder carcinoma. Careful mapping of chromosome 9 with microsatellite markers has revealed that there are at least two distinct regions of loss: one on chromosome 9p21 and the second on chromosome 9q.[50–52] Southern blot analysis, comparative multiplex PCR, and FISH analysis have revealed the presence of small homozygous deletions of 9p21 in primary bladder tumors.[53,54] These deletions also have been seen in cell lines and have been implicated in the genesis of a variety of tumor types.[55,56]

Another common area of allelic loss is on chromosome 17p. Losses of 17p have correlated with mutations of *p53* and occur predominantly in invasive bladder tumors.[57,58] However, a subset of superficial tumors, especially flat lesions, has been found to contain a higher rate of 17p loss.[19,59]

Southern blot analysis of primary bladder tumors with polymorphic markers has revealed frequent loss of chromosome 13q at the *Rb* locus.[45] Loss of 13q also has been associated with tumors of high stage, and immunohistochemical studies recently have confirmed that *Rb* is the major target of 13q deletions in bladder tumors.[60]

A number of other areas of allelic loss have been identified in bladder cancer. Chromosome 11p loss originally was described by Southern blot analysis and has been confirmed by microsatellite analysis.[44,47,48] Although both Wilms' tumor loci are candidate targets for the deletion of 11p observed in bladder cancer, bladder tumors are not seen in the spectrum of urogenital abnormalities or as second primary malignancies in Wilms' tumors.[61]

Losses of 3p, 4, 5q, 8, 14q, and 18q also have been reported.[19,47,48,62] Two distinct regions of loss have been identified on chromosome 4, one on 4p and one on 4q.[63,64] There also has been a report of two distinct regions of loss on chromosome 14, one on proximal and one on distal 14q. These losses of chromosome 14q correlated closely with increasing grade and stage.[65]

The Clonal Origin of Bladder Cancer

Many bladder tumors present as multifocal disease at diagnosis. The concept of field cancerization was described originally by Slaughter to explain the occurrence of multiple skip lesions and second primary tumors in patients with aerodigestive tract tumors.[66] This hypothesis also was extended to bladder tumorigenesis to describe the possible presence of a field defect secondary to continued exposure of exogenous and endogenous compounds excreted in urine.[11]

We have examined the hypothesis of field cancerization in bladder cancer using molecular genetic techniques.[67] We tested tumors from four female patients with a method that analyzes X chromosome inactivation, which can determine whether tumors were derived from the same precursor cell. This technique was complimented by analysis of allelic loss on various chromosomes, as described previously. In each patient examined, all tumors had the same X chromosome inactivation, whereas normal bladder retained the same polyclonal X chromosome inactivation pattern as expected. Moreover, each of the evaluable tumors from a given patient had lost the same chromosome 9 allele, commonly found early in progression. Later events in progression, such as 17p and 18q loss, were not shared by different tumors from the same patient, implying that multiple tumors in the same patient arose from the uncontrolled early spread of a single transformed cell. These tumors then proceeded through independent and variable genetic events during progression. If a field defect existed, one would expect multiple independent transforming events in each tumor, implying a multiclonal origin for these lesions.

Since this study, other investigators have confirmed the hypothesis that most multiple tumors in the bladder arise from a single progenitor cell. In another study, multiple tumors from 28 of 30 patients were found to contain the same X chromosome inactivation pattern, implying evolution from the same progenitor cell.[68] This understanding about bladder cancer genesis has implications for our understanding of tumor progression and may be useful for cancer diagnosis (see below). It also has allowed the designation of a preliminary progression model for bladder cancer.

Molecular Progression Model

As mentioned previously, careful characterization of genetic alterations within histopathologic lesions at various stages of progression allows the delineation of a molecular progression model. We have previously defined a simple progression model for bladder cancer.[18] In this model, critical allelic losses have been placed in various steps of progression, but oncogenes are not demonstrated because they are involved, so far, in only a minority of primary bladder tumors at the genetic level. Critical steps in this model include initiation of bladder cancer owing to the inactivation of a putative tumor-suppressor gene on chromosome 9, loss of *p53* function from the preinvasive to invasive state, and a variety of other genetic alterations associated with invasion and metastasis.

One interesting aspect of this progression model is the distinct differences between the progression of flat and papillary superficial lesions. Both these lesions share a high frequency of chromosome 9 loss that remains almost unchanged during the progression to invasive tumors. However, loss of chromosome 17p is far more frequent in flat lesions and has been associated with inactivation of the *p53* gene.[19,59,69] This is intriguing because inactivation of *p53* may lead to accumulation of further genetic changes and the propensity of these lesions to acquire a more invasive phenotype. Another distinct change is loss of chromosome 14q. 14q deletion is almost exclusively seen in flat lesions or invasive tumors and virtually absent in papillary lesions.[69] Interestingly, the frequency of 14q loss is even higher in flat lesions than in invasive tumors, suggesting that not all invasive tumors arise from flat lesions. 14q loss thus may lead to the initiation of flat lesions, from which only a fraction may continue to progress to invasive tumors. In this way, invasive tumors may be the final progression pathway for some papillary lesions and many flat lesions. Further characterization of the critical gene on chromosome 14q may lead to a better understanding of the events that lead to the development of flat lesions and their propensity for invasion.[65]

Specific Genes

Germ-Line Mutations. Although there is no common or defined syndrome for familial bladder cancer, familial uroepithelial tumors have been reported. Often these cases appear as a manifestation of the cancer family syndrome, known as *Lynch syndrome* (HNPCC).[4] Of the many neoplasms that occur in these families, TCC is the fourth most common, affecting individuals who manifest TCC alone, TCC and colon cancer, or TCC and other carcinomas.[70,71] Interestingly, in Lynch syndrome, TCC is predominant in the upper tract in contrast to sporadic TCC.

Mutations of mismatch repair genes, including *MSH2, MLH1, PMS1,* and *PMS2,* have been found to be responsible for the majority of cases.[72–75] These genes are involved in DNA mismatch repair and belong to a highly conserved group of repair proteins. As in other sporadic tumors from this syndrome, bladder tumors display characteristic genetic instability manifested by shifts or changes in the repeat size of microsatellite markers.[76] These shifts are actually expansions and contractions of small DNA repeat elements. Approximately 2 percent of all sporadic bladder tumors display characteristic microsatellite instability associated with Lynch syndrome and mismatch repair.[76]

Somatic Mutations. A candidate gene on chromosome 9p21, *p16* (*CDKN2/MTS-1*), is the most common inactivated gene in bladder cancer.[56,77] This gene has been found to be mutated in familial melanoma and pancreatic cancer.[78,79] Although a few point mutations are observed in bladder cancer cell lines, the vast majority of primary tumors with loss of heterozygosity (LOH) of 9p21 do not contain obvious mutations of *p16*.[80,81] This finding pointed to alternative mechanisms for gene inactivation or, potentially, that a second tumor-suppressor gene resided nearby. Recently, we have shown that homozygous deletions of chromosome 9p21 stretching into the *p16* locus are quite common in primary bladder tumors.[54] Much of the controversy surrounding this locus stems from difficulty in identifying homozygous deletions in primary tumors because of contaminating nonneoplastic cells. However, using the strategy of fine microsatellite mapping, homozygous deletions can be identified by the apparent retention of one or two closely spaced markers among a large region demonstrating LOH.[54] These results were confirmed in a number of cases by Southern blot and FISH analyses demonstrating the specificity of the technique. It is now clear that at least 50 percent of all bladder tumors contain a homozygous deletion that includes *p16*. Moreover, we have demonstrated other alternative mechanisms of inactivation including methylation of the *p16* promoter leading to transcriptional block and inactivation of *p16*.[82] Although methylation is common in many other tumor types, inactivation of *p16* by methylation is still uncommon in bladder cancer. The *p16* locus is quite complex and codes for a second transcript called *ARF*. This distinct protein appears to be involved in a separate p53 pathway. Although its exact role in tumor progression is not clear, deletion of the *p16* locus may inactivate genes involved in two critical tumor-suppressor gene pathways, *Rb* and *p53*.[83] Further analysis of a putative second tumor-suppressor locus on chromosome 9 is hampered in bladder cancer by the wide occurrence of monosomy, perhaps indicating inactivation of a gene on chromosome 9q. Although the *patched* gene, inactivated in Gorlin's syndrome and sporadic basal cell carcinoma, has been found on chromosome 9q, an important role in bladder cancer has not been defined.[84,85,85a,85b] Mutations of *p53* are ubiquitous in human cancer, and bladder cancer is no exception.[86] Losses of 17p have correlated well with sequence analysis of *p53* mutations and occur predominantly in invasive bladder tumors.[57] However, a subset of superficial tumors, especially flat lesions, has been found to contain these mutations. Importantly, a large study based on immunohistochemical analysis of *p53* demonstrated a significant decrease in overall survival for *p53* positive patients versus those with tumors that were *p53* negative.[87] It was implied that mutation of *p53* was an independently poor prognostic factor regardless of stage or therapy. Inactivation of *p53* is critical in many tumor types.[86] It has been postulated that *p53* is a critical regulator of response to DNA damage.[88] The appropriate presence of wild-type *p53* leads to growth arrest in the presence of damage and perhaps to apoptosis with excessive damage. Cells that lack p53 protein are unable to undergo a normal G1/S arrest and perhaps propagate further accumulated genetic damage.

A number of lines of evidence also point to a role for the *Rb* gene in bladder carcinogenesis. Immunohistochemical studies have confirmed that *Rb* is the target of 13q deletions in most bladder cancers.[60] A substantially worse prognosis for those tumors with negative standing also has been reported.[89,90] Moreover, reintroduction of the *Rb* gene leads to slowing of cell growth and tumorigenicity in bladder carcinoma cells.[91] The regulatory function of the Rb protein appears to be controlled by phosphorylation during the G1S phase of the cell cycle.[92] p16, one of a number of CDK inhibitors, is also critical for this pathway. In many ways, inactivation of both *p16* and *Rb* may be redundant, and in fact, tumors have demonstrated inactivation of one or the other of these genes but generally not both.[88] Analysis of *Rb* and *p16* status directly in bladder cancer has not been done on the same tumors. It is tempting to speculate, however, that the cyclin D1/p16/Rb pathway is vital in bladder cancer as in many other tumor types.

Bladder tumors are occasionally seen in patients with Cowden syndrome,[93] which arises from mutation of the *PTEN/MMAC1* tumor-suppressor gene located at chromosome 10q23.[94] Point mutations and homozygous deletions of *PTEN/MMAC1* have been found in a subset of bladder tumors with chromosome 10q LOH and are associated with advanced disease.[95]

IN VITRO SYSTEMS

In vitro models have been essential for much of the molecular work done on bladder cancers. Transformation of bladder epithelial cell lines that harbor allelic losses similar to those seen in primary human tumors have helped in the cloning of critical tumor-suppressor genes.[96,97] Transfection of human cell lines followed by reintroduction into animal bladders or renal capsules also have been important models.[98] Transfection of indolent transitional cell carcinoma with proto-oncogenes will not only increase expression of epidermal growth factor receptors but also can increase proliferate responses to epidermal growth factor as well.[99] Moreover, transfection of tumor-suppressor genes leads to diminished growth in these models. Furthermore, these models may be useful to test therapeutic efficacy before clinical trials.[100]

IMPLICATIONS FOR DIAGNOSIS

Microsatellite DNA markers are not only used for mapping primary tumors but also can be used for tumor detection. Microsatellite markers allow detection of LOH or genomic instability in primary tumors.[101] In a blinded study, urine samples from 25 patients with suspicious bladder lesions were analyzed by microsatellite analysis and compared with normal DNA from the same patients. Microsatellite changes matching those in the tumor were detected in the urine sediment in 19 of the 20 patients (95 percent) who were diagnosed with bladder cancer. Urine cytology detected cancer cells in only 50 percent of these same samples.[101]

The most common microsatellite abnormality detected in urine was LOH at critical chromosomal loci.[101] As mentioned earlier in the molecular progression model, early changes including loss of chromosome 9p and 14q were instrumental in the diagnosis of these patients. Moreover, although widespread microsatellite instability is only associated with Lynch syndrome, occasional microsatellite alterations are not uncommon. These microsatellite expansions or deletions are rare in small repeats but are more common in larger repeats, including tri- and tetranucleotides repeat sequences.[102] It appears that certain repeats are more susceptible to alterations and can be found with a relatively high frequency in many sporadic tumors including bladder cancers. At least 15 percent of the patients in this study were diagnosed by microsatellite alterations that would not have been diagnosed by LOH.[101]

In the study, tumors of all grades and stages were detected, including the difficult to diagnose low-grade papillary tumors.[101] In many cases that were considered atypical but not diagnostic for cancer by cytology, the correct diagnosis was established by molecular analysis. Importantly, control patients without cancer did not demonstrate any of the abnormalities. In a second pilot study where patients were monitored for bladder cancer recurrence, molecular analysis was sensitive, identifying 10 of 11 recurrences. Moreover, at least 2 patients had a positive molecular analysis several months before a recurrence was definitively identified by cystoscopy.[103] The ability to automate this technique with fluorescent labeling and microcapillary electrophoresis may make this a rapidly useful clinical test.[104] The final implementation awaits the completion of large prospective clinical trials to assess overall efficacy.

The recent explosion in our understanding of the genetic events that underlie the progression of human cancer has allowed us to consider novel approaches for diagnosis and treatment. For bladder cancer, a preliminary progression model already suggests specific genetic differences between papillary and flat lesions that may be critical for the treatment of these patients. These models also have led to the development of molecular markers that promise exquisite specificity and sensitivity for the early detection of cancer and for diagnosis of recurrent cases. The fact that most recurrent disease is owing to the expansion of a single progenitor cell may allow us to develop rational therapeutic targets. Critical changes such as *p53* that may lead to a poor outcome also may yield novel, specific therapeutic strategies. It is certain that the future promises to bring exciting new discoveries that will bring molecular biology closer to the forefront of clinical medicine.

REFERENCES

1. Parker SL, Tong T, Bolden S, Wingo PA: Cancer statistics, 1996. *CA* **5**:27, 1996.
2. Schulte PA: The role of genetic factors in bladder cancer. *Cancer Detect Prev* **11**(3-6):379, 1988.
3. Kantor AF, Hartge P, Hoover RN, Fraumeni JF Jr: et al: Familial and environmental interaction in bladder cancer. *Int J Cancer* **35**:703, 1985.
4. Lynch HT: Genetics, natural history, tumor spectrum, and pathology of hereditary nonpolyposis colorectal cancer: An updated review. *Gastroenterology* **104**(5):1535, 1993.
5. Tawfik HN: Carcinoma of the urinary bladder associated with schistosomaisis in Egypt: The possible causal relationship. *Int Symp Princes Takamatsu Cancer Res Fund* **18**:197, 1987.
6. McCredie M, Stewart JH, Ford JM, MacLennan RA, et al: Phenacetin analgesics and cancer of the bladder or renal pelvis in women. *Br J Urol* **55**:220, 1983.
7. Piper JM, Tonocia J, Matanoski GM: Heavy phenacetin use and bladder cancer in women aged 20 to 49 years. *N Engl J Med* **313**:292, 1985.
8. Silverman DT, Hartge P, Morrison AS, Devesa SS, et al: Epidemiology of bladder cancer. *Hematol Oncol Clin North Am* **6**:1, 1992.
9. Augustine A, Hebert JR, Kabat GC, Wynder EL, et al: Bladder cancer in relation to cigarette smoking. *Cancer Res* **48**:4405, 1988.
10. Burch JD, Rohan TE, Howe GR, Risch HA, Hill GB, Steele R, Miller AB, et al: Risk of bladder cancer by source and type of tobacco exposure: A case study. *Int J Cancer* **44**:622, 1989.
11. Fair WR, Fuks ZY, Scher HI: Cancer of the bladder, in Devita VT, Hellman S, Rosenberg SA (eds): *Cancer: Principles and Practices of Oncology*. Philadelphia, Lippincott, 1993, pp 1052–1072.
12. Friedell GH, Soloway MS, Hilgar AG, Farrow GM, et al: Summary of workshop on carcinoma in situ of the bladder. *J Urol* **136**:1047, 1986.

13. Tannenbaum M, Romas NA, Droller MJ: The pathobiology of early urothelial cancer, in Skinner DG, Leiskovsky G (eds): *Genitourinary Cancer.* Philadelphia, Saunders, 1988.
14. Althausen AF, Prout GR Jr, Daly JJ: Noninvasive papillary carcinoma of the bladder associated with carcinoma *in situ*. *J Urol* **116**:575, 1976.
15. Farrow GM, Utz DC, Rife CC, Greene LF, et al: Clinical observation of sixty cases of *in situ* carcinoma of the urinary bladder. *Cancer Res* **37**:2794, 1977.
16. Heney NM, Ahmed S, Flanagan MJ: Superficial bladder cancer: Progression and recurrence. *J Urol* **130**:1083, 1983.
17. Fitzpatrick JM, West AB, Butler MR: Superficial bladder tumors (stage pTa, grade 1 and 2): The importance of recurrence pattern following initial resection *J Urol* **135**:920, 1986.
18. Sidransky D, Messing E: Molecular genetics and biochemical mechanisms in bladder cancer: Oncogenes, tumor suppressor genes, and growth factors. *Urol Clin North Am* **19**(4):629, 1992.
19. Dalbagni S, Presti JC, Reuter VE, Fair WR, Cordon-Cardo C: Genetic alterations in bladder cancer. *Lancet* **342**:469, 1993.
20. Spruck CH, Ohneseit PF, Gonzalez M, Esrig D, Miyao N, Tsai YC, Lerner SP, Schmütte C, Yang AS, Cote R, Dubeau L, Nichlos PW, Hermann GG, Steven K, Horn T, Skinner DG, Jones PA: Two molecular pathways to transition cell carcinoma of the bladder. *Cancer Res* **54**:784, 1994.
21. Sandberg AA: *The Chromosomes in Human Cancer and Leukemia*, 2d ed. New York, Elsevier Science, 1990.
22. Sandberg AA: Chromosome changes in bladder cancer: Clinical and other correlations. *Cancer Genet Cytogenet* **19**(1-2):163, 1986.
23. Smeets W, Pauwels R, Laarakkers L, Debruyne F, Geraedts J: Chromosomal analysis of bladder cancer: III. Nonrandom alterations. *Cancer Genet Cytogenet* **29**(1):29, 1987.
24. Berger CS, Sandberg AA, Todd IAD, Pennington RD, Haddad FS, Hecht BK, Hecht F: Chromosomes in kidney, ureter, and bladder cancer. *Cancer Genet Cytogenet* **23**:1, 1986.
25. Gibas Z, Prout GJ, Connolly JG, Prontes JE, Sandberg AA: Nonrandom chromosomal changes in transitional cell carcinoma of the bladder. *Cancer Res* **44**(3):1257, 1984.
26. Gibas Z, Prout GR, Pontes JE, Connolly JG, Sandberg AA: A possible specific chromosome change in transitional cell carcinoma of the bladder. *Cancer Genet Cytogenet* **19**(3):229, 1986.
27. Kallioniemi A, Kallioniemi OP, Sudar D, Rutovitz D, Gray JW, Waldman F, Pinkel D: Comparative genomic hybridization for molecular cytogenetic analysis of solid tumors. *Science* **258**(5083):818, 1992.
28. du Manoir S, Speicher MR, Joos S, Schrock E, Popp S, Dohner H, Kovacs G, Robert M, Lichter P, Cremer T: Detection of complete and partial chromosome gains and losses by comparative genomic *in situ* hybridization. *Hum Genet* **90**(6):590, 1993.
29. Voorter C, Joos S, Vallinga M, Poddighe P, Schalken J, du Manoir S, Ramaekers Lichter P, Hopman A: Detection of chromosomal imbalances in transitional cell carcinoma of the bladder by comparative genomic hybridization. *Am J Pathol* **146**(6):1341, 1995.
30. Schoenberg M, Kiemeney L, Walsh PC, Griffin CA, Sidransky D: Germline translocation t(5)(p15) and familial transitional cell carcinoma. *J Urol* **155**(3):1035, 1996.
31. Reddy EP, Reynolds RK, Santos E, Barbacid M: A point mutation is responsible for the acquisition of transforming properties by the T24 human bladder carcinoma oncogene. *Nature* **300**(5888):149, 1982.
32. Knowles MA, Williamson M: Mutation of Hras is infrequent in bladder cancer: Confirmation by single conformation polymorphism analysis, designed restriction fragment length polymorphisms, and direct sequencing. *Cancer Res* **53**:133, 1993.
33. Fujita J, Srivastava SK, Kraus MH, Rhim JS, Tronick SR, Aaronson SA: Frequency of molecular alterations affecting *ras* proto-oncogenes in human urinary tract tumors. *Proc Natl Acad Sci USA* **82**(11):3849, 1985.
34. Viola MV, Fromowitz F, Oravez S, Deb S, Schlom J: *ras* oncogene p21 expression is increased in premalignant lesions and high grade bladder carcinoma. *J Exp Med* **161**:1213, 1985.
35. Messing EM, Reznikoff CA: Normal and malignant urothelium: In effects of epidermal growth factor. *Cancer Res* **47**:2230, 1987.
36. Neal DE, Marsh C, Bennett MK, Abel PD, Hall RR, Sainsbury JR, Harris AL: Epidermal receptors in human bladder cancer: Comparison of invasive and superficial tumours. *Lancet* **1**(8425):366, 1985.
37. Neal DE, Sharples L, Smith K, Fennelly J, Hall RR, Harris AL: The epidermal growth factor receptor and the prognosis of bladder cancer. *Cancer* **65**:1619, 1990.
38. Berger MS, Greenfield C, Gullick WJ, Haley J, Downward J, Neal DE, Harris AL, Waterfieldm MD: Evaluation of epidermal growth factor receptors in bladder tumours. *Br J Cancer* **56**:533, 1987.
39. Schmidt L, Duh F-M, Chen F, Kishida T, Glenn G, Choyke P, Scherer SW, Zhuang Z, Lubensky Dean M, Allikmets R, Chidambaram, Bergerheim UR, Feltis JR, Casadevall C, Zamarron A, Bernues M, Richard S, Lips C, Walther MM, Tsui LC, Geil L, Orcutt ML, Stackhouse T, Lipan J, Slife L, Brauch H, Decker J, Niehans G, Hughson M, Moch H, Storkel S, Lerman MI, Linehan WM, Zbar B: Germline and somatic mutations in the tyrosine kinase domain of the *MET* proto-oncogene in papillary renal carcinomas. *Nature Genet* **16**:68, 1997.
40. Wright C, Mellon K, Neal DE, Johnston P, Corbett IP, Horne CH: Expression of c-erbB2 protein product in bladder cancer. *Br J Cancer* **62**:764, 1990.
41. Masters JR, Vesey SG, Munn CF, Evan GI, Watson JV: c-myc oncoprotein levels in bladder cancer. *Urol Res* **16**(5):341, 1988.
42. Del-Senno L, Maestri I, Piva R, Hanau S, Reggiani A, Romano A, Russo G: Differential hypomethylation of the *c-myc* proto in bladder cancers at different stages and grades. *J Urol* **142**:146, 1989.
43. Fanning P, Bulovas K, Saini KS: Elevated expression of $pp60^{c\text{-}src}$ in low grade bladder carcinomas. *Cancer Res* **52**:1457, 1992.
44. Fearon ER, Feinberg AP, Hamilton SH, Vogelstein B: Loss of genes on the short arm of chromosome 11 in bladder cancer. *Nature* **318**(6044):377, 1985.
45. Cairns P, Proctor AJ, Knowles MA: Loss of heterozygosity at the *Rb* locus is frequent and correlates with muscle invasion in bladder carcinoma. *Oncogene* **6**:2305, 1991.
46. Tsai YC, Nichols PW, Hiti AL, Williams Z, Skinner DG, Jones PA: Allelic losses of chromosomes 9, 11, and 17 in human bladder cancer. *Cancer Res* **50**:44, 1990.
47. Presti JC, Reuter VW, Galan T, Fair WR, Cordon C: Molecular genetic alterations in superficial and locally advanced human bladder cancer. *Cancer Res* **51**:5405, 1991.
48. Knowles MA, Elder PA, Williamson M, Cairns JP, Shaw ME, Law MG: Allelotype of human bladder cancer. *Cancer Res* **54**:531, 1994.
49. Cairns P, Shaw ME, Knowles MA: Initiation of bladder cancer may involve deletion of a tumor suppressor gene on chromosome 9. *Oncogene* **8**:1083, 1993.
50. Ruppert JM, Tokino K, Sidransky D: Evidence for two bladder cancer suppressor loci on human chromosome 9. *Cancer Res* **53**:5093-5095, 1993.
51. Cairns P, Shaw ME, Knowles MA: Preliminary mapping of the deleted region of chromosome 9 in bladder cancer. *Cancer Res* **53**:1230, 1993.
52. Linnenbach AJ, Pressler LB, Seng BA, Kimmel BS, Tomaszewski JE, Malkowicz SB: Characterization of chromosome 9 deletions in transitional cell carcinoma by microsatellite assay. *Hum Mol Genet* **2**(9):1407, 1993.
53. Cairns P, Tokino K, Eby Y, Sidransky D: Homozygous deletions of 9p21 in primary human bladder tumors detected by comparative multiplex PCR. *Cancer Res* **54**(6):1422, 1994.
54. Cairns P, Polascik TJ, Eby Y, Tokino K, Califano J, Merlo A, Mao L, Herath J, Jenkins R, Westra W, Rutter JL, Buckler A, Gabrielson E, Tockman M, Cho KR, Hedrick L, Bova GS, Isaacs W, Koch W, Schwab D, Sidransky D: Frequency of homozygous deletion at p16/CDKN2 in primary human tumors. *Nature Genet* **11**(2):210, 1995.
55. Olopade OI, Buchhagen DL, Malik K, Sherman J, Nobori T, Bader S, Nau MM, Gazdar AF, Minna J, Diaz MO: Homozygous loss of the interferon genes defines the critical region on 9p that is deleted in lung cancers. *Cancer Res* **53**:2410, 1993.
56. Kamb A, Gruis NA, Weaver-Feldhaus J, Liu Q, Harshmann K, Tavtigian SI, Stockert E, Day IIIRD, Johnson BE, Skolnick MH: A cell cycle regulator potentially involved in genesis of many tumor types. *Science* **264**:436, 1994.
57. Sidransky D, von Eschenbach A, Tsai YC, Jones P, Summerhayes I, Marshall F, Meera P, Green P, Hamilton SR, Frost P, Vogelstein E: Identification of *p53* gene mutations in bladder cancers and urine samples. *Science* **252**:706, 1991.
58. Habuchi T, Ogawa O, Kaheki Y, Sugiyama T, Yoshida O: Allelic loss of chromosome 17p in urothelial cancer: Strong association with invasive phenotype. *J Urol* **148**:1595, 1992.
59. Fujimoto K, Yamada Y, Okajima E: Frequent association of *p53* mutation in invasive bladder cancer. *Cancer Res* **52**:1393, 1992.
60. Xu HJ, Cairns P, Hu SX, Knowles MA, Benedict WF: Loss of Rb protein expression in primary bladder cancer correlates with loss of heterozygosity at the *Rb* locus and tumor progression. *Int J Cancer* **53**(5):781, 1993.
61. Hawkins MM, Draper GJ, Smith RA: Cancer among 1348 offspring of survivors of childhood cancer. *Int J Cancer* **43**(6):975, 1989.

62. Wu S, Storer BE, Bookland EA, Klingelhutz AJ, Gilchrsit KW, Meisner LF, Oyasu R, Reznikoff CA: Nonrandom chromosome losses in stepwise neoplastic transformation in vitro of human uroepithelial cells. *Cancer Res* **51**:3323, 1991.
63. Elder PA, Bell SM, Knowles MA: Deletion of two regions on chromosome 4 in bladder carcinoma: Definition of a critical 750-kb region at 4p16.3. *Oncogene* **9**(12):3433, 1994.
64. Polascik TJ, Cairns P, Chang WY, Schoenberg MP, Sidransky D: Distinct regions of allelic loss on human chromosome 4 in primary bladder carcinoma. *Cancer Res* **55**(22):5396, 1995.
65. Chang WY, Cairns P, Schoenberg MP, Polasick TJ, Sidransky D: Novel suppressor loci on chromosome 14q in primary bladder cancer. *Cancer Res* **55**(15):3246, 1995.
66. Slaughter DL, Southwick HW, Smejkal W: Field cancerization in oral stratified squamous epithelium: Clinical implications of multicentric origin. *Cancer* **6**:963, 1953.
67. Sidransky D, Frost P, Von Eschenbach A, Oyasu R, Preisinger AC, Vogelstein B: Clonal origin of bladder cancer. *N Engl J Med* **326**:737, 1992.
68. Miyao N, Tsai YC, Lerner SP, Olami AF, Spruck CH, Gonzalez-Zuleta M, Nichols PW, Skinner DG, Jones PA: Role of chromosome 9 in human bladder cancer. *Cancer Res* **53**(17):4066, 1993.
69. Rosin MP, Cairns P, Epstein JI, Schoenberg MP, Sidransky D: An allelotype of carcinoma *in situ* of the human bladder. *Cancer Res* **55**:5213, 1995.
70. Vasen HF, Offerhaus GJ, den Hartog Jager FC, Menko FH, Nagengast FM, Griffioen G, van Hogezand RB, Heintz : The tumour spectrum in hereditary non-polyposis colorectal cancer: A study of 24 kindreds in the netherlands. *Int J Cancer* **46**(1):31, 1990.
71. Lynch HT, Ens JA, Lynch JF: The Lynch syndrome II and urological malignancies. *J Urol* **143**:24, 1990.
72. Cleaver JE: It was a very good year for DNA repair. *Cell* **76**:1, 1994.
73. Bronner CE, Baker SM, Morrison PT, Warren G, Smith LG, Lescoe MK, Kane M, Earabino C, Lipford J, Lindbla Tannergard P, Bollag RJ, Godwin AR, Ward DC, Nordenskjold M, Fishel R, Kolodner R, Liskay RM: Mutation in the DNA mismatch repair gene homologue *hMLH1* is associated with hereditary non-polyposis colon cancer. *Nature* **368**:258, 1994.
74. Nicolaides NC, Popadopoulos N, Liu B, Wei YF, Carter KC, Ruben SM, Rosen CA, Haseltine WA, Fleischmann RD, Fraser CM, Adams MD, Venter JC, Dunlop M, Hamilton SR, Petersen GM, de la Chapelle A, Vogelstein B, Kinzler KW: Mutations of two PMS homologues in hereditary nonpolyposis colon cancer. *Nature* **371**:75, 1994.
75. Liu B, Parsons R, Papadopoulos N, Nicolaides NC, Lynch HT, Watson P, Jass JR, Dunlop M, Wyllie A, Peltomaki P, de la Chapelle Hamilton SR, Vogelstein B, Kinzler H: Analysis of mismatch repair genes in hereditary non-polyposis colorectal cancer patients. *Nature Med* **2**(2):169, 1996.
76. Gonzalez M, Ruppert JM, Tokino K, Tsai YC, Spruck CH III, Miyao N, Nichols PW, Hermann GG, Horn T, Steven K, Summerhayes IC, Sidransky D, Jones PA: Microsatellite instability in bladder cancer. *Cancer Res* **53**:5620, 1993.
77. Serrano M, Hannon GJ, Beach D: A new regulatory motif in cell control causing specific inhibition of cyclin D^{CDK4}. *Nature* **366**:704, 1993.
78. Hussussian CJ, Struewing JP, Goldstein AM, Higgins PAT, Ally DS, Sheahan M, Clark WH Jr, Tucker MA, Dracopoli NC: Germline *p16* mutations in familial melanoma. *Nature Genet* **8**:15, 1994.
79. Caldas C, Hahn SA, da Costa LT, Redston MS, Schutte M, Seymour AB, Weinstein CL, Hruban R, Yeo CJ, Kern SE: Frequent somatic mutations and homozygous deletions of the *p16* (*MTS1*) gene in pancreatic adenocarcinoma. *Nature Genet* **8**:27, 1994.
80. Cairns P, Mao L, Merlo A, Lee DJ, Schwab D, Eby Y, Tokino K, van der Riet P, Blaugrand JE, Sidransky D: Rates of *p16* (*MTS1*) mutations in primary tumors with 9p loss. *Science* **256**:415, 1994.
81. Spruck CH, Gonzalez-Zuleta M, Shibata A, Simoneau AR, Lin M-F, Gonzales F, Tsai Y, Jones PA: *p16* gene in uncultured tumors. *Nature* **370**:183, 1994.
82. Merlo A, Herman JG, Mao L, Lee DJ, Schwab D, Burger PC, Baylin SB, Sidransky D: 59 CpG island methylation is associated with transcriptional silencing of the tumour suppressor *p16/CDKN2/MTS1* in human cancers. *Nature Med* **7**(1):686, 1995.
83. Zhang Y, Xiong Y, Yarbrough WG: ARF promotes MDM2 degradation and stabilizes p53: ARF-INK4a locus deletion impairs both the *RB* and *p53* tumor suppression pathways. *Cell* **92**:725, 1998.
84. Johnson RL, Rothman AL, Xie J, Godrich LV, Bare JW, Bonifas JM, Quinn AG, Myers RM, Cox DR, Epstein EH, Scott MP: Human homologue of *patched,* a candidate gene for the basal cell nevus syndrome. *Science* **272**:1668, 1996.
85. Hahn H, Wicking C, Zaphiropoulos PG, Gailani MR, Shanley S, Chidambaram, Vorechovsky I, Holmberg E, Unden A, Gillies S, Negus K, Smyth I, Pressman C, Leffell DJ, Gerrard B, Goldstein AM, Dean M, Toftgard R, Chenevix-Trench G, Wainwright B, Bale AE: Mutations of the human homologue of *Drosophila patched* in the nevoid basel cell carcinoma syndrome. *Cell* **85**:841, 1996.
85a. McGarvey TW, Maruta Y, Tomaszewski JE, Linnenbach AJ, Malkowicz SB: PTCH gene mutations in invasive transitional cell carcinoma of the bladder. *Oncogene* **17**:1167, 1998.
85b. Simoneau AR, Spruck CH 3rd, Gonzalez-Zulueta M, Gonzalgo ML, Chan MF, Tasi YC, Dean M, Steven K, Horn T, Jones PA: Evidence for two tumor suppressor loci accosicated with proximal chromosome 9p to q and distal chromosome 9q in bladder cancer and the initial screening for GASI and PTC mutations. *Cancer Res* **56**:5039, 1996.
86. Hollstein M, Sidransky D, Vogelstein B, Harris C: *p53* mutations in human cancer. *Science* **253**:49, 1991.
87. Esrig D, Elmajian D, Groshen S, Freeman JA, Stein JP, Chen SC, Nicholls Skinner DG, Jones PA, Cote RJ: Accumulation of nuclear p53 and tumor progression in bladder cancer. *New Engl J Med* **331**(19):1259, 1994.
88. Hartwell LH, Kastan MB: Cell cycle control and cancer. *Science* **266**(5192):1821, 1994.
89. Cordon-Cardo C, Wartinger D, Petrylak D, Dalbagni G, Fair WR, Fuks Z, Renter VE: Altered expression of retinoblastoma gene product: Prognostic indicator in bladder cancer. *J Natl Cancer Inst* **84**:1251, 1992.
90. Logothetis CJ, Xu HJ, Ro JY, Hu SX, Sahin A, Ordonez N, Benedict WF: Altered expression of retinoblastoma protein and known prognostic variables in locally advanced bladder cancer. *J Natl Cancer Inst* **84**:1256, 1992.
91. Takahashi R, Hashimoto T, Hu HJ, Hu SX, Matsui T, Miki T, Bigo-Marshall H, Aaronson SA, Benedict WF: The retinoblastoma gene functions as a growth and tumor suppressor in human bladder carcinoma cells. *Proc Natl Acad Sci USA* **88**:5257, 1991.
92. Mihara K, Cao XR, Yen A, Chandler S, Driscoll B, Murphree AL, T'Ang A, Fung Y: Cell cycle regulation of phosphorylation of human *Rb* gene product. *Science* **246**:1300, 1989.
93. Starink TM, Van Der Veen JPW, Arwert F, De Waal LP, De Lange GG, Gille JJP, Eriksson AW: The Cowden syndrome: A clinical and genetic study in 21 patients. *Clin Genet* **29**:222, 1986.
94. Liaw D, Marsh DJ, Li J, Dahia PLM, Wang SI, Zheng Z, Bose S, Call KM, Tsou HC, Peacocke M, Eng C, Persons R: Germline mutations of the *PTEN* gene in Cowden disease, an inherited breast and thyroid cancer syndrome. *Nature Genet* **16**:64, 1997.
95. Cairns P, Evron E, Okami K, Halachmi N, Esteller M, Herman JG, Bose S, Wang SI, Persons R, Sidransky D: Point mutation and homozygous deletion of *PTEN/MMAC1* in primary bladder cancers. *Oncogene* **16**:3215, 1998.
96. Reznikoff CA, Kao C, Messing EM, Newton M, Swaminathan S: A molecular genetic model of human bladder carcinogenesis. *Semin Cancer Biol* **4**(3):143, 1993.
97. Kao C, Wu SQ, Bhatthacharya M, Meisner LF, Reznikoff CA: Losses of 3p, 11p, and 13q in EJ/ras simian virus 40 human uroepithelial cells. *Genes Chromosom Cancer* **4**(2):158, 1992.
98. Theodorescu D, Cornil I, Fernandez BJ, Kerbel RS: Over-expression of normal and mutated forms of *HRAS* induces orthotopic bladder invasion in a human transitional cell carcinoma. *Proc Natl Acad Sci USA* **87**(22):9047, 1990.
99. Theodorescu D, Cornil I, Sheehan C, Man MS, Kerbel RS: *Ha-ras* induction of the invasive phenotype results in up of epidermal growth factor receptors and altered responsiveness to epidermal growth factor in human papillary transitional cell carcinoma cells. *Cancer Res* **51**(16):4486, 1991.
100. Theodorescu D, Connors KM, Groce A, Hoffman RM, Kerbel RS: Lack of influence of c-ras expression on the drug sensitivity of human bladder cancer histocultured in three. *Anticancer Res* **13**(4):941, 1993.
101. Mao L, Schoenberg MP, Scicchitano M, Erozan YS, Merlo A, Schwab D, Sidransky D: Molecular detection of primary bladder cancer by microsatellite analysis. *Science* **271**:659, 1996.
102. Mao L, Lee DJ, Tockman MS, Erozan YS, Askin F, Sidransky D: Microsatellite alterations as clonal markers in the detection of human cancer. *Proc Natl Acad Sci USA* **91**:9871, 1994.
103. Steiner G, Schoenberg MP, Linn JF, Mao L, Sidransky D: Detection of bladder cancer recurrence by microsatellite analysis of urine. *Nature Med* **3**(6): 621, 1997.
104. Wang Y, Ju J, Carpenter BA, Atherton JM, Sensabaugh GF, Mathies RA: Rapid sizing of short tandem repeat alleles using capillary array electrophoresis and energy fluorescent primers. *Anal Chem* **67**(1):1197, 1995.

CHAPTER 55

Stomach Cancer

Steven M. Powell

1. **Adenocarcinoma comprises the vast majority of malignant tumors arising from the stomach. Gastric carcinoma is a significant worldwide health burden, second only to lung tumors as a leading cause of cancer deaths. Significant geographic and temporal variances are observed in this cancer's incidence, predominantly of the intestinal type. Epidemiologic studies indicate a strong environmental component in the acquisition of this cancer. Developing countries that are noted to have a high prevalence of *Helicobacter pylori* infection early in life are distinctly prone to having high rates of gastric adenocarcinomas. Most gastric cancers are identified in advanced stages that present in the later decades of adult life, commonly resulting in a lethal outcome shortly thereafter.**
2. **Gastric cancers exhibit heterogeneity in clinical, biologic, and genetic aspects. Multiple pathologic classifications of gastric adenocarcinomas exist, including those with morphologic and histologic criteria. The TNM staging system is generally used as the basis for prognostication in this cancer, with depth of infiltration being an important parameter. Most cases of stomach cancer are sporadic in nature, with rare reports of inherited gastric cancer predisposition traits that can involve germ-line E-cadherin alterations or in conjunction with the hereditary nonpolyposis colon cancer disease entity.**
3. **Cytogenetic studies have been unsuccessful in identifying an obvious significant chromosomal aberration in gastric cancers. Loss of heterozygosity studies and comparative genomic hybridization analyses have identified several loci with significant allelic loss, thus indicating the possibility of harboring a tumor-suppressor gene important in gastric tumorigenesis. The exact target(s) of loss or gain in most of these chromosomal regions, including 4q, 5q, 9p, 17p, 18q, and 20q, remains to be clarified. Additionally, evidence of Epstein-Barr virus infection can be found in a minority of gastric cancer patients.**
4. **Multiple somatic alterations have been described in gastric carcinomas at the molecular level. The significance of these changes in gastric tumorigenesis remains to be established in most instances. The *p53* gene is consistently altered in a majority of gastric cancer cases. Microsatellite instability and associated alterations of the transforming growth factor βII receptor, *IGFRII, BAX, E2F-4, MSH3,* and *MSH6* genes are found in a subset of gastric carcinomas. Cell adhesion abnormalities such as E-cadherin or associated molecule alterations may play an important role in diffuse-type gastric cancer development. A detailed, clear working model of gastric tumorigenesis has yet to be formulated. Thus improved diagnostic, prognostic, therapeutic, and preventive strategies are eagerly awaited for gastric carcinomas. Critical molecular alterations that are prevalent in these cancers, once fully characterized, ultimately may provide new avenues to combat this lethal disease.**

A list of standard abbreviations is located immediately preceding the index in each volume. Nonstandard abbreviations used in this chapter include: HNPCC = hereditary nonpolyposis colon cancer; LOH = loss of heterozygosity.

CLINICAL ASPECTS

Gastric adenocarcinoma is the predominant cancer of the stomach, accounting for over 95 percent of cases. Lymphomas, leiomyosarcomas, and carcinoid lesions represent only a minority of stomach tumors. Once the leading cause of cancer deaths in the United States, the incidence of gastric cancer in developed countries has declined dramatically.[1] Adenocarcinomas of the gastroesophageal junction that commonly arise from Barrett's esophagus, on the other hand, appear to be on the rise most recently in several populations for unclear reasons.[2,3] Adenocarcinoma of the stomach remains a leading cause of cancer death worldwide and continues to be responsible for the majority of cancer deaths in developing countries.[4,5]

Most cases of gastric cancer appear to occur sporadically without an obvious inherited component. It is estimated that up to 10 percent of gastric cancer cases are related to a familial component. Familial clustering has been observed in 12 to 25 percent of cases.[6] Case-control studies suggest a small but consistent increased risk of gastric cancer in first-degree relatives of patients with gastric adenocarcinoma.[7–9]

A well-characterized inherited predisposition syndrome potentially involving gastric cancer development is hereditary nonpolyposis colon cancer (HNPCC), which includes potential tumor development in a variety of tissue types.[10] Germ-line genetic abnormalities of mismatch repair genes underlying this disease entity have been unveiled recently, as discussed in Chap. 32. The isolation of these genes should allow better definition of the fraction of gastric cancers that result from this inherited cancer predisposition trait. Interestingly, fewer gastric cancers have been noted to be associated with HNPCC, correlating with the recent general decline in incidence of gastric cancer in developed countries.

Rare kindreds exhibiting site-specific gastric cancer predilection have been reported, occasionally associated with other inherited abnormalities.[11–13] Notably, Napoleon Bonaparte's family was afflicted with this cancer. A few kindreds manifesting a diffuse, poorly differentiated gastric cancer predisposition trait have been shown recently to harbor E-cadherin alterations in their germ line that cosegregate with these cancers.[14] There has even been a report of gastric carcinoma in an extended Li-Fraumeni kindred.[15]

Epidemiology

Significant geographic variability in incidence both internationally and intranationally is observed. In the early 1990s, incidence rates varied from 60.1 per 100,000 in Costa Rica to 7.3 per 100,000 in the United States.[16] Epidemiologic studies that include migration and temporal analyses indicate that environmental factors, especially in the first decades of life, are important in the etiology of gastric cancers.[17,18] Notably, a consistent predominance of gastric cancers in males (approximately 2:1 ratio) is seen across worldwide populations.

Helicobacter pylori infection has been implicated recently as an etiologic factor in gastric cancer development, both adenocarcinoma and primary non-Hodgkin lymphoma.[19–21] Evidence continues to accumulate that this infection, especially when contracted early in life, as commonly occurs in developing countries, leads to chronic gastric inflammation with subsequent fivefold to sixfold risk of gastric cancer development.[22] This risk of cancer development in infected persons depends on as yet unidentified cofactors, and its pathophysiological mechanism remains to be elucidated. Similarly, chronic gastritis and resulting atrophy from pernicious anemia appear to be associated with an increased risk, albeit small, of gastric cancer development.[23]

Evidence of Epstein-Barr virus (EBV) infection has been demonstrated in a small proportion (approximately 10 percent) of gastric carcinomas by *in situ* hybridization with specific RNA probes.[24–27] The monoclonal nature of EBV genomes in virtually all neoplastic cells of these tumors along with significant prior antibody levels suggests that infection by this virus may not be so latent. The classic proteins associated with cell transformation of EBV infection, LMP1 and EBNA2, do not appear to be expressed in these gastric cancers; however, EBNA1 was shown to be expressed in most virus-associated tumor cells.[27,28] A significant lymphoid infiltration and tendency toward prolonged survival have been observed in gastric cancers harboring detectable EBV. Further studies are needed to determine the role of this infection in human gastric tumorgenesis.

Dietary irritants (i.e., salts or preservatives) and potential carcinogens (i.e., nitrates) have been suggested as etiologic factors of gastric cancer,[29] yet no specific agent has been indicted definitively. Additionally, several protective factors such as fruits, vegetables, ascorbic acid, α-tocopherol, onions, and gastric acidity have been indicated, yet the precise agents responsible for a specific action remain elusive. Molecular studies may help clarify these issues.

Pathology

Gastric adenocarcinomas display several distinct morphologic, histologic, and biologic characteristics. Thus multiple tumor classification systems have been created to characterize these lesions pathologically in attempts to confer their natural history. Lauren described histopathologic subtypes of gastric adenocarcinomas as intestinal type (expansive or gland-forming) or diffuse type (infiltrative or scattered neoplastic cells), and this classification is widely applied.[30] Evidence continues to accumulate suggesting that these two subtypes of gastric cancer arise in different settings and have distinctive biologic behavior.[31] Intestinal-type gastric adenocarcinomas tend to predominante in high-risk geographic regions, arise in association with precursor lesions (i.e., chronic atrophic gastritis or intestinal metaplasia), and occur more distally and later in life (usually after the sixth decade of life), whereas diffuse-type gastric cancers appear to have a relatively constant incidence, arise without identifiable precursor lesions, and present earlier in life and more diffusely in the stomach. Additionally, intestinal-type gastric cancers tend to spread hematogenously to the liver, whereas diffuse-type gastric cancers tend to spread more contiguously into the peritoneum. Moreover, although some molecular alterations are shared, distinct genetic abnormalities appear to occur with specific biologic phenotypes (see below).

Additional histologic classifications for gastric carcinoma have been developed (i.e., World Health Organization[32] and Ming[33]) that involve tissue architecture and differentiation criteria. The traditional classification of Borman is based on morphologic criteria.[34] Goeski has even developed criteria that examine mucin content and degree of cellular atypia as potentially distinctive prognostic features of gastric tumors.[35,36]

The TMN staging classification[37] is used primarily in staging cancers at diagnosis to assess resectability and prognoses. The primary tumor's depth is one of the most important parameters in this determination. The concept of early gastric adenocarcinomas[35] (tumors confined to the mucosa or submucosa) originated in Japan,[38] and patients are observed to have much better 5-year survival rates (over 90 percent) versus more advanced lesions (less than 20 percent for stage III or IV). Unfortunately, most cases of gastric cancer are diagnosed in more advanced stages, for which effective systemic therapy is limited and surgery reserved for palliation. Mass screening programs in high-risk regions such as Japan have helped in diagnosing some of these cancers at earlier stages, but significant improvements in diagnosis, prognostication, and therapy are eagerly awaited to make a substantial impact on this cancer's mortality.

ALTERED GENETIC LOCI

Large kindreds with an obvious highly penetrant inherited predisposition for the development of gastric cancer, having the potential power to link disease markers, are rare. Three Maroi kindreds with significant occurrence of diffuse gastric carcinomas were identified and found to have underlying germ-line E-cadherin mutations that cosegregated with disease.[14] HNPCC with underlying mismatch repair gene alterations is the only other well-defined inherited trait with germ-line mutations known to predispose to gastric cancer development. Of note, the blood group A phenotype was reported to be associated with gastric cancers[39,40] and the blood group O phenotype with gastric ulcers.[41] Interestingly, *H. pylori* was shown to adhere to the Lewis^b blood group antigen and may be an important host factor that facilitates this chronic infection and subsequent risk of gastric cancer development.[42] Further studies are awaited to clarify this or any other host factor with genetic determinants that might predispose toward the development of gastric cancer.

Most molecular analyses of this cancer have involved studies of sporadic tumors for critical, acquired alterations. Cytogenetic studies of gastric adenocarcinomas are few in number and have failed to identify any consistent or noteworthy chromosomal abnormalities. A variable number of numerical or structural aberrations have been reported in gastric cancer cells, including those involving chromosomes 3 (rearrangements), 6 (deletion distal to 6q21), 8 (trisomy), 11 (11p13-p15 aberrations), and 13 (monosomy and translocations).[43–46] Alone, these findings are not compelling for a specific role in gastric tumorigenesis and may represent only nonspecific changes accompanying transformation.

Comparative genomic hybridization (CGH) analyses of xenografted and primary gastric and gastroesophageal junctional adenocarcinomas have revealed several regions of consensus change in DNA copy number.[47,48] Chromosomal arms 4q, 5q, 9p, 17p, and 18q showed frequent decreases in DNA copy number. On the other hand, chromosomes 7, 8, and 20q showed frequent increases in DNA copy number of cases analyzed in this fashion.

Loss of heterozygosity (LOH) analyses have identified several arms and regions of chromosomes that may contain tumor-suppressor genes important in gastric tumorigenesis. Genetic loci observed to be significantly lost in gastric tumors include those located on the following chromosomal arms: 17p (over 60 percent at the *p53* locus),[49] 18q (over 60 percent at the *DCC* locus),[50] and 5q (30 to 40 percent at or near the *APC* locus).[49,51,52] Less frequent but significant allelic losses have been reported on chromosome arms 1p, 1q, 7q, and 13q.[53] A 13-cM region between D1S201 and D1S197 on chromosome 1p commonly lost in gastric cancers has been delineated, but the critical target remains to be identified.[54] Moreover, a locus on 7q (D7S95) has been associated with peritoneal metastasis when lost.[55] Known, as well as candidate, tumor-suppressor genes have been isolated in some of these frequently lost regions, as described below, but the actual targets of genetic loss that provide gastric neoplastic cells with additional survival or growth advantages for clonal expansion remain to be clarified for many of these loci.

SPECIFIC MOLECULAR ALTERATIONS

The *p53* gene has been demonstrated consistently to be significantly altered in gastric adenocarcinomas. Allelic loss occurs in over 60 percent of patients, and mutations are identified in approximately 30 to 50 percent of patients depending on the mutational screening method employed [i.e., single-stranded conformational polymorphism (SSCP) assay or degenerative gradient gel electrophoresis assay] and sample sizes.[56] Some mutations of *p53* have even been identified in early dysplastic and apparent intestinal metaplasia gastric lesions. In general, however, alterations of this gene occur more frequently in the advanced stages of dysplasia in both histopathologic subtypes. The spectrum of mutations in this gene within gastric tumors appears similar to that which occurs in other cancers with a predominance of base transitions, especially at CpG dinucleotides. Inactivation of this important cell cycle regulator appears to confer a growth advantage and allow clonal expansion of transformed cells. Many studies have used immunohistochemical analysis of tumors in an effort to detect excessive expression of p53 as an indirect means to identify mutations of this gene, but this assay does not appear to have consistent prognostic value in patients with gastric cancers.[57,58]

Microsatellite instability has been found in a significant portion of sporadic gastric carcinomas.[59–61] Variability in classification of instability or histopathologic subtype and number of loci examined in studies account for some variation of this phenotype's frequency, with a trend toward more frequent occurrence in intestinal-type cancers at more advanced stages observed, although noted in early lesions as well (i.e., adenomas). The degree of genome-wide instability also varies, with more severe instability (e.g., >2 abnormal loci) associated with subcardial intestinal or atypical types. A negative association with p53 alterations also has been suggested, indicating different paths of alterations accumulating in individual gastric tumors. Studies have indicated less frequent lymph node or vessel invasion, prominant lymphoid infiltration, and better prognosis in those gastric cancers which displayed significant microsatellite instability.[59,62,63] However, it remains to be proven if this phenotype is a prognostic marker for improved survival, as suggested in colon cancers. The alterations responsible for producing this phenotype in a subset of sporadic gastric cancers remain to be elucidated.

At least one important target of the instability in those cancers displaying abnormally sized microsatellites appears to be the transforming growth factor beta (TGF-β) type II receptor. A study of gastric cancers displaying the microsatellite instability phenotype revealed that a majority (5 of 7) contained mutated TGF-β type II receptors at a polyadenine tract within its gene.[64] Moreover, altered TGF-β type II receptor genes could be found in gastric cancers not displaying microsatellite instability. Several gastric cancer cell lines resistant to the growth inhibitory and apoptotic effects of TGF-β were shown to have altered TGF-β type II genes (deletions and amplifications) and transcripts (truncated or absent).[65] Thus TGF-β type II receptor mutation appears to be a critical event in the development of at least a subset of gastric cancers, allowing escape from the growth control of TGF-β. Additional genes with simple tandom repeat sequences within their coding regions found to be altered in gastric cancers displaying microsatellite instability include *BAX, IGFRII, hMSH3, hMSH6,* and *E2F-4*.[66–68]

As mentioned earlier, E-cadherin germ-line mutations have been found in several large kindreds exhibiting a strong predisposition to diffuse gastric cancer development. Several sporadic gastric cancers also have displayed altered E-cadherin, mainly in diffuse cases. Reduced E-cadherin expression determined by immunohistochemical analysis was noted often (92 percent of 60 patients) in gastric carcinomas and observed to be significantly associated with diffuse-type cancers and more undifferentiated neoplastic cells (i.e., signet ring cells).[69] Genetic abnormalities of the E-cadherin gene (located on chromosome 16q22.1) and transcripts also have been demonstrated in diffuse gastric cancers.[70] Half of 26 diffuse gastric carcinomas had abnormal E-cadherin transcripts detected by reverse transcription PCR (RT-PCR) analysis that were not seen in noncancerous tissue from the same patients. Moreover, a study of 10 gastric cancer cell lines displaying loose intercellular adhesion found absent E-cadherin transcripts in four lines and insertions or deletions in two other lines.[71] Splice-site alterations producing exon deletion and skipping, large deletions including allelic loss, and point mutations of the E-cadherin gene were all demonstrated in these diffuse-type cancers, some even exhibiting alterations in both alleles. In comparison of RT-PCR products from normal tissue and tumor tissue from patients, allelic expression imbalance of E-cadherin also has been shown in a porportion (42 percent of 35 informative cases) of gastric carcinomas.[72] E-cadherin is a transmembrane, calcium-ion-dependent adhesion molecule (important in epithelial cell homotypic interactions) that, when decreased in expression, is associated with invasive properties.[73] Additionally, α-catenin, which binds to the intracellular domain of E-cadherin and links it to actin-based cytoskeletal elements, was noted to have reduced immunohistochemical expression in 70 percent of 60 gastric carcinomas and correlated with infiltrated growth and poor differentiation.[74]

LOH studies suggest that chromosome 5q harbors at least one tumor-suppressor gene important in the development of gastric cancers.[49,51,52,75,76] The exact target(s), however, of this loss in gastric tumors is not fully clarified. Several somatic *APC* mutations, mostly missense in nature and of relatively low frequency, have been reported in Japanese patients with gastric adenocarcinomas and adenomas using ribonuclease protection or SSCP assays for partial screening.[77] On the other hand, several other reports including Japanese patients have not identified significant *APC* mutations in gastric carcinomas on similar partial screening analysis of the commonly mutated region and include direct nucleotide sequencing and the sensitive in vitro synthesis protein assay.[76,78–80] Interestingly, an increased risk of gastric cancer associated with familial adenomatous polyposis (patients with germ-line *APC* mutations) has been reported in high-risk regions such as Asia,[81,82] whereas no increased risk was exhibited in other populations.[83,84] Significant allelic loss (30 percent) at the *APC* locus suggests the existence of a tumor-suppressor gene important in gastric tumorigenesis nearby. Indeed, alternative loci have been mapped to commonly deleted regions in gastric cancers (the interferon regulatory factor 1 loci and D5S428)[75] and esophageal cancers (5q31.1).[85] Thus future studies should help define the important gene(s) on chromosome 5q, which is critically involved in gastric tumorigenesis.

The targets of loss on other chromosomes implicated to harbor important tumor-suppressor gene(s) in gastric cancer also remain to be defined. Significant allelic loss (60 percent) has been noted at the *DCC* locus on chromosome 18q in gastric cancers.[50] Only one of 35 gastric cancers contained an intragenic mutation of *Smad4* along with allelic loss, suggesting that this *MADD* homologue gene is infrequently altered in gastric tumorigenesis.[86]

Evidence of a tumor-suppressor loci on chromosome 3p has accumulated from a variety of studies, including allelic loss in primary gastric tumors (46 percent) and homozygous deletion in a gastric cancer cell line (KATO III).[87] A candidate tumor-suppressor gene, *FHIT,* recently isolated from the FRA3B site at 3p14.2, was reported to have abnormal transcripts of deleted exons in 5 of 9 gastric cancers in addition to transcript abnormalities noted in esophagus, colon, lung, and head and neck cancers as well.[88–90] One somatic missense mutation was identified in exon 6 of the *FHIT* gene during a coding region analysis of 40 gastric carcinomas.[91] Significant abnormalities of the *FHIT* gene were not observed in a study of 31 colorectal cancer patients.[92] Addtional studies should help clarify the role *FHIT* plays in gastric tumorigenesis.

The *c-met* gene encodes a tyrosine kinase receptor for the hepatocyte growth factor. Amplification of the *c-met* gene was reported to be associated with scirrhous-type gastric cancers.[93] Northern blot analyses of gastric cancer cell lines and resected primary carcinomas compared with paired nonneoplastic tissue showed overexpression of a 7.0-kb transcript of the *c-met* gene in 48 percent of 31 cancers, predominantly of the well-differentiated type.[94] Moreover, a 6.0-kb *c-met* transcript appeared to be preferentially expressed in scirrhous gastric tumor cells and correlated with latter stages of tumor development. Tumor and stromal cell interactions have been implicated with this growth factor and receptor signal system as well as involvement of multiple others, including epidermal growth factor (which is expressed in approximately one-quarter of gastric cancers), transforming growth factor alpha (TGF-α), interleukin-1a, criptor, amphiregulin, platelet-derived growth factor, K-sam, and others.[53,95] Telomerase activity has been detected by a PCR-based assay frequently in the late stages of gastric tumors (85 percent of 66 patients) and is associated with a poor prognosis.[96] The expression of telomerase, a ribonucleoprotein DNA polymerase, and stabilization of telomeres have been noted to be concomitant with immortalization in tumor cells.[97] Specific alterations and the true prevalence of significant changes in these genes or gene products in gastric tumors remain to be characterized.

Another potential marker of poor prognosis is overexpression of *c-erbB-2,* a transmembrane tyrosine kinase receptor proto-oncogene. Amplification of *c-erbB-2* has been demonstrated in a small subset of gastric cancers, approximately 10 percent.[98] Several reports have shown amplification or increased expression of erbB-2 immunohistochemically in gastric tumors to be associated with a worse prognosis.[99] Furthermore, enhanced expression of erbB-2 recently has been demonstrated to occur more frequently in gastric cancers displaying microsatellite instability.[100] The specific genetic or epigenetic alterations underlying these immunohistochemical findings remain to be characterized.

A number of other alterations have been reported in gastric carcinomas that remain to be defined, as well as the role they play in gastric tumorigenesis. Several splice variants of a transmembrane glycoprotein, CD44, seem to be preferentially expressed in gastric tumors cells.[101] Membrane-type matrix metalloproteinase was expressed preferentially in some gastric cancer cells with colocalization and activation of the zymogen proMMP-2.[102] Both loss and overexpression of Bc1-2 and nm23 have been reported in several gastric cancers, making their role unclear. Amplification of cyclin E and increased plasminogen activation have been reported as well in several gastric tumors.[103] A somatic mitochondrial deletion of 50 bp was even demonstrated in four gastric adenocarcinomas.[104]

Activation of the oncogene *K-ras* appears to be rare in gastric tumorigenesis.[79,105,106] Although allelic loss was noted in 18 percent of gastric tumors at the locus for p16 on chromosome 9p, no inactivating somatic mutations were detected in over 70 patients screened by PCR-SSCP analysis.[107] No methylation abnormalities or genetic alterations of cycle regulators such as p16, p21, or p27 have as yet been reported.

IMPLICATIONS

Identification of important genetic alterations in gastric tumorigenesis has important practical as well as biologic implications. As evident from molecular genetic characterization of colorectal tumor development, genetic markers with potential clinical utility in diagnosis, prognosis, and therapeutic guidance can be discovered. A clear molecular working model of gastric tumorigenesis has yet to be delineated, but as genetic alterations are better characterized in these cancers, critical changes may emerge to provide new opportunities of earlier diagnosis, improved prognostication, and more rational design of therapeutic agents and preventive strategies. Since most gastric cancers are diagnosed in late stages of development with concomitant poor prognosis and little chance of cure, genetic changes occurring early and frequently may enable identification of truly premalignant gastric lesions that would be beneficial to remove or warrant intervention in some manner. Directed screening efforts for this cancer are a pressing issue, and molecular markers may help address this important matter.

Characterization of somatic changes in these gastric tumors also may expose specific environmental factors (e.g., fingerprints[108]) and strongly indict agents for further mechanistic studies. Additionally, identification of a genetic predisposition marker for the development of gastric cancer may facilitate more effective preventive and screening programs. Identifying critical molecular alterations and defining the role played in gastric tumorigenesis also may provide unique opportunities for improved chemopreventive or chemotherapeutic agents to be developed and given at more opportune times.

Finally, since gastric cancer appears to be a rather heterogeneous disease biologically and genetically, characterization of the various pathways and events along the way should afford multiple opportunities to design more specific and therefore more effective therapies in the treatment of this tumor. For example, antibodies to the oncoprotein erbB-2 and epidermal growth factor receptor have shown promise in inhibiting growth of gastric cancer cell lines and xenografts.[95,109] Moreover, current systemic therapies are generally ineffective in controlling gastric cancer growth. Opportunities to explore whether a genetic marker's status such as p53 in these tumors will guide more effective therapy are welcomed. Improved prognostic markers are also eagerly awaited to help guide more aggressive surgical or systemic therapies (i.e., chemotherapy and/or radiotherapy) and ultimately may be derived from the molecular alterations indicated earlier or from as yet unidentified critical change in gastric cancer cells.

ACKNOWLEDGMENTS

This work was supported in part by NIH Grant CA67900-01 and a Foundation AGA Research Scholarship award.

REFERENCES

1. Correa P, Chen V: Gastric cancer. *Cancer Surv* **19/20**:55, 1994.
2. Blot WJ, Devesa SS, Kneller RW: Rising incidence of adenocarcinoma of the esophagus and gastric cardia. *JAMA* **265**:1287, 1991.
3. Locke RG, Talley NJ, Carpenter HA, Harmsen WS, Zinsmeister AR, Melton LJ: Changes in the site- and histology-specific incidence of gastric cancer during a 50-year period. *Gastroenterology* **109**:1750, 1995.
4. Parkin DM, Pisani P, Ferlay J: Estimates of the worldwide incidence of eighteen major cancers in 1985. *Int J Cancer* **54**:594, 1993.
5. Boffetta P, Parkin DM: Cancer in developing countries. *CA* **44**:81, 1994.
6. Goldgar DE, Easton DF, Cannon-Albright LA, Skolnock MH: Systematic population-based assessment of cancer risk in first-degree relatives of cancer probands. *J Natl Cancer Inst* **86**:1600, 1994.
7. La Vecchia C, Negri E, Franceschi S, Gentile A: Family history and the risk of stomach and colorectal cancer. *Cancer* **70**:50, 1992.
8. Zangheiri G, Di Gregorio C, Sacchetti R, et al: Familial occurrence of gastric cancer in the 2-year experience of a population-based registry. *Cancer* **66**:2047, 1990.
9. Graham S, Lilienfeld AM: Genetic studies of gastric cancer in humans: An appraisal. *Cancer* **11**:957, 1958.
10. Lynch HT, Smyrk TC, Watson P, Lanspa SJ, Lynch JF, Lynch PM, Cavalieri RJ, Boland CR: Genetics, natural history, tumor spectrum, and pathology of hereditary nonpolyposis colorectal cancer. *Gastroenterology* **104**:1535, 1993.
11. Maimon SN, Zinninger MM: An analysis of 5 stomach cancer families in the state of Utah. *Cancer* **14**:1005, 1953.
12. Woolf CM, Isaacson EA: An analysis of 5 stomach cancer families in the state of Utah. *Cancer* **1961**:1005, 1961.
13. Triantafillidis JK, Kosmidis P, Kottardis S: Genetic studies of gastric cancer in humans: An appraisal. *Cancer* **11**:957, 1958.
14. Guilford P, Hopkins J, Harraway J, McLeod M, McLeod N, Harawira P, Taite H: E-cadherin germline mutations in familial gastric cancer. *Nature* **392**:402–405, 1998.

15. Varley JM: An extended Li-Fraumeni kindred with gastric carcinoma and a codon 175 mutation of *TP53*. *J Med Genet* **32**:942–945, 1995.
16. Parker SL, Tong T, Bolden S, Wingo PA: Cancer statistics. *CA* **46(1)**:5, 1996.
17. Haenszel W, Kurihara M, Segi M, Lee RK: Stomach cancer among Japanese in Hawaii. *J Natl Cancer Inst* **49**:969, 1972.
18. Correa P, Haenszel W: Epidemiology of gastric cancer, in Correa P, Haenszel W (eds): *Epidemiology of Cancer of the Digestive Tract*. The Hague, The Netherlands: Martinus Hijhoff, 1972, p 58.
19. Parsonnet J, Hansen S, Rodriguez L, Gelb AB, Warnke RA, Jellum E, Orentreich N, Vogelman JH, Friedman GD: *Helicobacter pylori* infection and gastric lymphoma. *New Engl J Med* **330**:1267, 1994.
20. Parsonnet J, Friedman GD, Vandersteen DP, Chang Y, Vogelman JH, Orenreich N, Sibley RK: *Helicobacter pylori* infection and the risk of gastric carcinoma. *N Engl J Med* **325**:1127, 1991.
21. Nomura A, Stemmerman GN, P-HC, Kato I, Perez-Perez GI, Blaser MJ: *Helicobacter pylori* infection and gastric carcinoma among Japanese Americans in Hawaii. *N Engl J Med* **325**:1132, 1991.
22. Blaser MJ, Chyou PH, Nomura A: Age at establishment of *Helicobacter pylori* infection and gastric carcinoma, gastric ulcer, and duodenal ulcer risk. *Cancer Res* **55**:562, 1995.
23. Elsborg L, Mosbech J: Pernicious anaemia as a risk factor in gastric cancer. *Acta Med Scand* **206**:315, 1979.
24. Rowlands DC, Ito M, Mangham DC, Reynolds G, Herlost H, Fielding JWL, Newbold KM, Jones EL, Young LS, Niedobitek G: Epstein-Barr virus and carcinomas: Rare association of the virus with gastric adenocarcinomas. *Br J Cancer* **68**:1014, 1993.
25. Shibata D, Weiss LM: Epstein-Barr virus-associated gastric adenocarcinoma. *Am J Pathol* **140**:769, 1992.
26. Imai S, Koizumi S, Sugiura M, Toyunaga M, Uemura Y, Yanamoto N, Tanaka S, Sato E, Osato T: Gastric carcinoma: Monoclonal epithelial malignant cells expressing Epstein-Barr virus latent infection protein. *Proc Natl Acad Sci USA* **91**:9131, 1994.
27. Gulley ML, Pulitzer DR, Eagan PA, Schneider BG: Epstein-barr virus infection is an early event in gastric carcinogenesis and is independent of bcl-2 expression and p53 accumulation. *Hum Pathol* **27(1)**:19, 1996.
28. Murray PG, Nieddobitek G, Kremmer E, Grasser F, Reynolds GM, Cruchley A, Williams DM, Muller-Lantzsh N, Young LS: *In situ* detection of the Epstein-Barr virus-encoded nuclear antigen 1 in oral hairy leukoplakia and virus-associated carcinomas. *J Pathol* **178**:44, 1996.
29. Fuchs CS, Mayer RJ: Gastric carcinoma. *N Engl J Med* **333(1)**:32, 1995.
30. Lauren P: The two histological main types of gastric carcinoma: Diffuse and so-called intestinal-type carcinoma. *Acta Pathol Microbiol Scand* **64**:31, 1965.
31. Correa P, Shiao YH: Phenotypic and genotypic events in gastric carcinogenesis. *Cancer Res* **54**:1941, 1994.
32. Oota K, Sobin LH: Histological typing: Gastric and esophageal carcinogenesis, in *International Histological Classification of Tumors*. Geneva, World Health Organization, 1977.
33. Ming S-C: Gastric carcinoma: A pathobiological classification. *Cancer* **39**:2475, 1977.
34. Borrmann R: Gushwulste de magens and duodenums, in Henke F, Lubarsh O (eds): *Handbuch der Speziellen Pathologischen Anatomie und Histologie*. Berlin, Springer, 1926, p 865.
35. Dixon MF, Martin JG, Sue-Ling HM, Wyatt JI, Quirke P, Johnston D: Goseki grading in gastric cancer: Comparison with existing systems of grading and its reproducibility. *Histopathology* **25**:309, 1994.
36. Goseki N, Takizawa T, Koike M: Differences in the mode of extension of gastric cancer classified by histological type: New histological classification of gastric carcinoma. *Gut* **33**:606, 1992.
37. Sobin LH, Wittekind Ch (eds): *International Union Against Cancer (UICC): TNM Classification of Malignant Tumors* 5th ed. New York: John Wiley, 1997
38. Hirota T, Ming S-C, Itabashi M: *Pathology of early gastric cancer*, in *Gastric Cancer*, in Nishi M, Ichikawa, H, Nakajima T, Maruyama K, Tahara E (eds): Tokyo, New York, Springer-Verlag p. 66–86.
39. Aird I, Bentall H: A relationship between cancer of stomach and ABO groups. *Br J Med* **1**:799, 1953.
40. Haenszel W, Kurihara M, Locke F, Shimuzu K, Segi M: Stomach cancer in Japan. *J Natl Cancer Inst* **56**:265, 1976.
41. Clarke CA, Cowan WK, Edwards JW, Howel-Evans AW, McConnell RB, Woodrow JC, Sheppard PM: The relation of ABO bloodgroups to duodenal and gastric ulceration. *Br Med J* **4940**:643, 1955.
42. Boren T, Per F, Roth KA, Larson G, Normark S: Attachment of *Helicobacter pylori* to human gastric epithelium mediated by blood group antigens. *Science* **262**:1892, 1993.
43. Seruca R, Castedo S, Correia C, Gomes P, Carneiro F: Cytogenetic findings in eleven gastric carcinomas. *Cancer Genet Cytogenet* **68**:42–48, 1993.
44. Rodriguez E, Ladanyi M, Altorki N, Albino AP, Kelsen DP: 11p13-15 is a specific region of chromosomal rearrangement in gastric esophageal adenocarcinomas. *Cancer Res* **50**:6410–6416, 1990.
45. Ochi H, Douglass H, Sandberg AA: Cytogenetic studies in primary gastric cancer. *Cancer Genet Cytogenet* **22**:295, 1986.
46. Panani AD, Ferti A, Malliaros S, Raptis S: Cytogenetic study of 11 gastric adenocarcinomas. *Cancer Genet Cytogenet* **81**:169, 1995.
47. El-Rifai W, Harper JC, Cummings OW, Hyytinen E, Frierson HF, Knuutila S, Powell SM: Consistent genetic alterations in xenografts of proximal stomach and gastroesophageal junction adenocarcinomas. *Cancer Res* **58**:34, 1998.
48. Moskaluk CA, Hu J, Perlman EJ: Comparative genomic hybridization of esophageal and gastroesophageal adenocarcinomas reveals consensus areas of DNA gain and loss. *Genes Chromosom Cancer* **22**:305, 1998.
49. Sano T, Tsujino T, Yoshida K, Nakyama H, Haruma K, Ito H, Nakamura Y, Kajiyama G, Tahara E: Frequent loss of heterozygosity on chromosomes 1q, 5q and 17q in human gastric carcinomas. *Cancer Res* **51**:2926, 1991.
50. Uchino S, Hitoshi T, Masayuki N, Jun Y, Terada M, Saito T, Kobayashi M, Sugimura T, Hirohashi S: Frequent loss of heterozygosity at the *DCC* locus in gastric cancer. *Cancer Res* **52**:3099, 1992.
51. McKie AB, Filipe I, Lemoine NR: Abnormalities affecting the *APC* and *MCC* tumour suppressor gene loci on chromosome 5q occur frequently in gastric cancer but not in pancreatic cancer. *Int J Cancer* **55**:598, 1993.
52. Rhyu MG, Park WS, Jung YJ, Choi SW, Meltzer SJ: Allelic deletions of *MCC, APC* and *p53* are frequent late events in human gastric carcinogenesis. *Gastroenterology* **106**:1584, 1994.
53. Tahara E, Semba S, Tahara H: Molecular biological observations in gastric cancer. *Semin Oncol* **23(3)**:307, 1996.
54. Ezaki T, Yanagisawa A, Ohta K, Aiso S, Watanabe M, Hibi T, Kato Y, Nakajima T, Ariyama T, Inzawa J, Nakamura Y, Horii A: Deletion mapping chromosome 1p in well-differentiated gastric cancer. *Br J Cancer* **73**:424, 1996.
55. Kuniyasu H, Yasui W, Yokosaki H: Frequent loss of heterozygosity of the long arm of chromosome 7 is often associated with progression of human gastric carcinoma. *Cancer* **59**:597, 1994.
56. Beroud C, Soussi T: *p53* and *APC* gene mutations: Software and databases. *Nucl Acids Res* **25(1)**:138, 1997.
57. Gabber HE, Muller W, Schneiders A, Meier S, Hommel G: The relationship of p53 expression to the prognosis of 418 patients with gastric carcinoma. *Cancer* **76(5)**:720, 1995.
58. Hurlimann J, Saraga EP: Expression of p53 protein in gastric carcinomas. *Am J Surg Pathol* **18(12)**:1247, 1994.
59. Seruca R, Santos NR, David L, Constancia M, Barroca H, Carneiro F, Seixas M, Peltomaki R, Lothe R, Sobrinho-Simoes M: Sporadic gastric carcinomas with microsatellite instability display a particular clinicopathologic profile. *Int J Cancer* **64**(1):32–6, 1995.
60. Strickler JG, Zheng J, Shu Q, Burgart LJ, Alberts SR, Shibata D: *p53* mutations and microsatellite instability in sporadic gastric cancer: When guardians fail. *Cancer Res* **54**:4750, 1994.
61. Chong J-M, Fukayama M, Hayashi Y, Takizawa T, Koike M, Konishi M, Kikuchi-Yanoshita R, Miyaki M: Microsatellite instability in the progression of gastric carcinoma. *Cancer Res* **54**:4595, 1994.
62. Nakashima H, Hiroshi I, Mori M, Ueo H, Ikeda M, Akiyoshi T: Microsatellite instability in Japanese gastric cancer. *Cancer Suppl* **75(6)**:1503, 1995.
63. Dos Santos NR, Seruca R, Constancia M, Seixas M, Sobrinho-Simoes M: Microsatellite instability at multiple loci in gastric carcinoma: Clinicopathologic implications and prognosis. *Gastroenterology* **110**:38, 1996.
64. Myeroff LL, Ramon P, Kim S-J, Hedrick L, Cho KR, Orth K, Mathis M, Kinzler K, Lutterbaugh J, Park K, Bang Y-J, Lee HY, Park J-G, Lynch H, Roberts AB, Vogelstein B, Markowitz SD: A transforming growth factor β receptor type II gene mutation common in colon and gastric but rare in endometrial cancers. *Cancer Res* **55**:5545, 1995.
65. Park K, Kim S-J, Bang Y-J, Park J-G, Kim NK, Roberts AB, Sporn MB: Genetic changes in the transforming growth fact beta (TGF-β) type II receptor gene in human gastric cancer cells: Correlation with sensitivity to growth inhibition by TGF-β. *Proc Natl Acad Sci USA* **91**:8772, 1994.
66. Yamamoto H, Sawai H, Perucho M: Frameshift somatic mutations in gastrointestinal cancer of the microsatellite mutator phenotype. *Cancer Res* **57**:4420, 1997.

67. Souza RF, Appel R, Jing Y, Wang S, Smolinski KN, Abraham JM, Zou T, Shi Y, Lei J, Cottrell J, Cymes K, Biden K, Simms L, Leggett B, Lynch PM, Frazier M, Powell SM, Harpaz N, Sugimura H, Young J, Meltzer SJ: Microsatellite instability in the insulin-like growth factor II receptor gene in gastrointestinal tumours. *Nature Genet* **14**:255, 1996.
68. Souza RF, Yin J, Smolinski KN, Zou TT, Wang S, Shi YQ, Ryu MG, Cottrell J, Abraham JM, Biden K, Simms L, Leggett B, Bova GS, Frank T, Powell SM, Sugimura H, Young J, Harpaz N, Shimizu K, Matsuvara N, Melzer SJ: Frequent mutations of the E2F-4 cell cycle gene in primary human gastrointestinal tumors. *Cancer Res* **57**:2350, 1997.
69. Mayer B, Johnson JP, Leitl F, Jauch KW, Heiss MM, Schildberg FW, Birchmeier W, Funke I: E-cadherin expression in primary and metastatic gastric cancer: Down-regulation correlates with cellular dedifferentiation and glandular disintegration. *Cancer Res* **53**:1690, 1993.
70. Becker KF, Atkinson MJ, Reich U, Becker I, Nekarda H, Siewart JR, Hofler H: E-cadherin gene mutations provide clues to diffuse type gastric carcinomas. *Cancer Res* **54**:3845, 1994.
71. Oda T, Kanai Y, Oyama T, Yoshiura K, Shimoyama Y, Birchmeier W, Sugimura T: E-cadherin gene mutations in human gastric carcinoma cell lines. *Proc Natl Acad Sci USA* **91**:1858, 1994.
72. Becker KF, Hofler H: Frequent somatic allelic inactivation of the E-cadherin gene in gastric carcinomas. *J Natl Cancer Inst* **87**(14):1082, 1995.
73. Birchmeier W, Behrens J: Cadherin expression in carcinomas: Role in the formation of cell junctions and the prevention of invasiveness. *Biochem Biophys Acta* **1198**:11, 1994.
74. Matsui S, Shiozaki H, Masatoshi I, Shigeyuke T, Doki Y, Kadowaki T, Iwazawa T, Shimaya K, Nagafuchi A, Tsukita S, Mori T: Immunohistochemical evaluation of α-catenin expression in human gastric cancer. *Virchows Archov* **424**:375–381, 1997.
75. Tamura G, Ogaswara S, Nishizuka S, Sakata K, Maesawa C, Suzuki Y, Tershima M, Saito K, Satodate R: Two distinct regions of deletion on the long arm of chromosome 5 in differentiated adenocarcinomas of the stomach. *Cancer Res* **56**:612, 1996.
76. Powell SM, Cummings OW, Mullen JA, Asghar A, Fuga G, Piva P, Minacci C, Megha T, Piero T, Jackson CE: Characterization of the *APC* gene in sporadic gastric adenocarcinomas. *Oncogene* **12**:1953, 1996.
77. Nagase H, Nakamura Y: Mutation of the *APC* (adenomatous polyposis coli) gene. *Hum Mutat* **2**:425, 1993.
78. Ogaswara S, Maesawa C, Tamura G, Satodate R: Lack of mutations of the adenomatous polyposis coli gene in oesophageal and gastric carcinomas. *Virchows Arch* **424**(6):607, 1994.
79. Maesawa C, Tamura G, Suzuki Y, Ogasawara S, Sakata K, Kashiwaba M, Satodate R: The sequential accumulation of genetic alterations characteristic of the colorectal adenoma-carcinoma sequence does not occur between gastric adenoma and adenocarcinoma. *J Pathol* **176**:249, 1995.
80. Sud R, Talbot IC, Delhanty JD: Infrequent alterations of the *APC* and *MCC* genes in gastric cancers from British patients. *Oncogene* **21**:1104, 1996.
81. Utsunomiya J: The concept of hereditary colorectal cancer and the implications of its study, in Utsunomiya J, Lynch HT (eds): *Hereditary Colorectal Cancer.* Tokyo, Springer-Verlag, 1990, p 3.
82. Park JG, Park KJ, Ahn YO, Song IS, Choi KW, Moon HY, Choo SY, Kim JP: Risk of gastric cancer among Korean familial adenomatous polyposis patients. *Dis Colon Rectum* **53**:996, 1992.
83. Offerhaus GJA, Giardello FM, Krush AJ, Booker SV, Tersmette AC, Kelley NC, Hamilton SR: The risk of upper gastrointestinal cancer in familial adenomatous polyposis. *Gastroenterology* **102**:1980, 1992.
84. Burt RW: Polyposis syndromes, in Yamada T, Alpers TH (eds): *Textbook of Gastroenterology.* New York, Lippincott, 1991.
85. Ogaswara S, Tamura G, Maesawa C, Suzuki Y, Iishida K, Satoh N, Uesugi N, Saito K, Satodate R: Common deleted region of the long arm of chromosome 5 in esophageal carcinoma. *Gastroenterology* **110**:52, 1996.
86. Powell SM, Harper J, Hamilton S, Robinson C, Cummings OW: Inactivation of *Smad4* in gastric carcinomas. *Cancer Res* **57**:4221, 1997.
87. Kastury K, Baffa R, Druck T, Cotticelli MG, Inoue H, Massimo N, Rugge M, Huang D, Croce CM, Palazzo J, Huebner K: Potential gastrointestinal tumor suppressor locus at the 3p14.2FRA3b site identified by homozygous deletions in tumor cell lines. *Cancer Res* **56**:978, 1996.
88. Ohta M, Hiroshi I, Citticelli MG, Kastury K: The *FHIT* gene, spanning the chromosome 3p14.2 fragile site and renal carcinoma-associated t(3;8) breakpoint, is abnormal in digestive tract cancers. *Cell* **84**:587, 1996.
89. Sozzi G, Verosnese ML, Negrini M, Baffa R, Cotticelli MG, Enoue H, Tornielli S, Pilotti S, De Gregorio L, Pastorino U, Pierotti MA, Ohta M, Huebner K, Croce CM: The *FHIT* gene at 3p14.2 is abnormal in lung cancer. *Cell* **85**:17, 1996.
90. Virgilio L, Shuster M, Gollin SM, Veronese ML, Ohta M, Huebner K, Croce CM: *FHIT* gene alterations in head and neck squamous cell carcinomas. *Proc Natl Acad Sci USA* **93**:9770, 1996.
91. Gemma A, Hagiwara K, Ke Y, Burke LM, Khan MA, Nagashima M, Bennett WP, Harris CC: *FHIT* mutations in human primary gastric cancer. *Cancer Res* **57**:1435, 1997.
92. Thiagalingam S, Lisitsyn NA, Hamaguchi M, Wigler MH, Willson JKV, Markowitz SD, Leach FS, Kinzler KW, Vogelstein B: Evaluation of *FHIT* gene in colorectal cancers. *Cancer Res* **56**:2936, 1996.
93. Kuniyasu H, Yasui W, Kitadai Y, Yokosaki H, Ito H, Tahara E: Frequent amplification of the *c-met* gene in scirrhous type stomach cancer. *Biochem Biophys Res Commun* **189**:227, 1992.
94. Kuniyasu H, Yasui W, Kitadai Y, Tahar E: Aberrant expression of *c-met* mRNA in human gastric carcinomas. *Int J Cancer* **55**:72, 1993.
95. Tokunaga A, Onda M, Okuda T, Teramoto T, Fijita I, Mizutani T, Kiyama T, Yoshiyuki T, Nishi K, Matsukura N: Clinical significance of epidermal growth factor (EGF), EGF receptor, and *c-erbB-2* in human gastric cancer. *Cancer* **75**:1418, 1995.
96. Hiyama E, Yokoyama T, Tatsumato N, Hiyama K, Imamura Y, Murakami Y: Telomerase activity in gastric cancer. *Cancer Res* **55**:3258–3262, 1995.
97. Kim JW, Piatyszek MA, Prowse MA, Harley KR, West CB, Peter LC, Ho GMC, Woodring EN, Weinrich SL, Shay JW: Specific association of human telomerase activity with immortal cells and cancer. *Science* **266**:2011, 1994.
98. Ooi A, Kobayashi M, Mai M, Nakanishi I: Amplification of *c-erbB2* in gastric cancer: Detection in formalin-fixed, paraffin-embedded tissue by fluorescence *in situ* hybridization. *Lab Invest* **78**(3):345, 1997.
99. Mizutani T, Onda M, Tokunaga A, Yamanaka N, Sugisaka Y: Relationship of c-erbB-2 protein expression and gene amplification to invasion and metastasis in human gastric cancer. *Cancer* **72**:2083, 1993.
100. Lin J-T, Wu MS, Shun C-T, Lee W-J, Wang T-H: Occurrence of microsatellite instability in gastric carcinoma is associated with enhanced expression of erbB-2 oncoprotein. *Cancer Res* **55**:1428, 1995.
101. Dammrich J, Vollmers HP, Heider K-H, Muller-Hermelink H-K: Importance of different CD44v6 expression in human gastric intestinal and diffuse type cancers for metastatic lymphogenic spreading. *J Mol Med* **73**:395, 1995.
102. Nomura H, Hiroshi S, Motoharu S, Masyoshi M, Yasunori O: Expression of membrane-type matrix metalloproteinase in human gastric carcinomas. *Cancer Res* **55**:3263, 1995.
103. Tahara E: Molecular mechanism of stomach carcinogenesis. *J Cancer Res Clin Oncol* **119**:265, 1993.
104. Burgart LJ, Zheng J, Shu Q, Strickler JG, Shibata D: A somatic mitochondrial mutation in gastric cancer. *Am J Pathol* **147**(4):1105, 1995.
105. Kihana T, Tsuda H, Teruyuki H, Shimosato Y, Hiromi S, Terada M, Hirohashi S: Point mutation of *c-Ki-ras* oncogene in gastric adenoma and adenocarcinoma with tubular differentiation. *Jpn J Cancer Res* **82**:308, 1991.
106. Koshiba M, Ogawaa O, Habuchi T, Hamazaki S, Thoshihide S: Infrequent *ras* mutation in human stomach cancers. *Jpn J Cancer Res* **84**:163–167, 1993.
107. Igaki H, Sasaki H, Tachimori Y, Watanabe H, Kimura T, Harada Y, Sugimura T, Tarada M: Mutation frequency of the *p16/CDKN2* gene in primary cancers in the upper digestive tract. *Cancer Res* **55**:3421, 1995.
108. Vogelstein B, Kinzler KW: Carcinogens leave finger prints. *Nature* **355**:209, 1992.
109. Kasprzyk PG, Song SU, Di Fiore PP, King CR: Therapy of an animal model of human gastric cancer using a combination of Anti-erbB-2 monoclonal antibodies. *Cancer Res* **52**:2771, 1992.

CHAPTER 56

Prostate Cancer

William B. Isaacs ▪ G. Steven Bova

1. **Prostate cancer is the most commonly diagnosed cancer in men. The incidence of this disease shows strong age, race, and geographic dependence, with African Americans and Asians being examples of high- and low-risk populations, respectively.**
2. **Although no hereditary prostate cancer genes have been cloned, familial clustering data and segregation analyses are consistent with the existence of dominant high-risk alleles for prostate cancer. Genome-wide scans for linkage in prostate cancer families have implicated loci on 1q and Xq as harboring prostate cancer-susceptibility genes.**
3. **Deletion of sequences from the short arm of chromosome 8 is perhaps the most frequent chromosomal alteration in prostate cancer, occurring at high frequency even in precursor lesions. Gain of sequences on chromosome 8q and loss of sequences on 13q are only slightly less common than 8p loss of heterozygosity (LOH). Gain and deletion of chromosome 7 sequences, along with deletions of chromosomes 5q, 6q, 10q, and 16q, are also frequent events in the prostate cancer cell genome. The genes driving the apparent selection of these abnormalities are largely unknown.**
4. **Methylation of a CpG island in the promoter of the *GSTP1* gene is the most common genomic alteration yet identified in prostate cancer, occurring in virtually every case. The common inactivation of this carcinogen-defense pathway suggests a potentially important role of environmental carcinogens during prostatic carcinogenesis.**
5. **Although mutations of *p53, PTEN, Rb, ras, CDKN2,* and other tumor-suppressors and oncogenes have been detected at varying frequencies in prostate cancer, no single gene has been identified as being mutated in the majority of prostate cancers.**
6. **The androgen receptor gene, when either mutated or amplified, may play a critical role in prostate tumorigenesis both at the early stages and during progression to androgen-insensitive disease. Polymorphic variants of the androgen receptor and other genes involved in androgen metabolism that differ in their biologic activity may modulate risk for prostate cancer or for the tendency to develop more aggressive forms of this disease.**
7. **Prostate cancers vary tremendously in their biologic aggressiveness. The ability of various genetic alterations to serve as much-needed molecular diagnostic and prognostic indicators is being evaluated.**

CLINICAL ASPECTS

Incidence

In 1990, prostate cancer became the most common form of cancer (other than skin cancer) diagnosed in the U.S. male. In 1997, over 200,000 new prostate cancer cases were diagnosed, accounting for over 35 percent of all cancers affecting men, and over 40,000 deaths resulted from this disease.[1] The number of prostate cancers diagnosed in the United States has been increasing since 1972 and in particularly dramatic fashion since 1988. This increase is due primarily to changes in methods used to detect the disease [e.g., the use of serum prostate-specific antigen (PSA)] as well as interest in detecting this disease (increased awareness and screening), coupled with what appears to be an actual but slight increase in the true incidence rate.[2]

The incidence of prostate cancer shows strong age, race, and geographic dependence. It is primarily a disease of older men, with the incidence rate for men over age 65 being 20-fold greater than that for men between 50 and 54 years of age. Less than 1 percent of cases are diagnosed under the age of 40, reaching a peak frequency of approximately 1 in 7 in the eighth and ninth decades of life.[3] This disease is uncommon in Asian populations and common in Scandinavian countries, and the highest incidence (and mortality) rates known are in African-American males, with the latter being twofold higher than for American white males.[4]

The *initiation* of prostate cancer, i.e., the formation of a histologically identifiable lesion, is a very frequent event, occurring in the nearly one-third of men over age 45.[5] Fortunately, the majority of such lesions do not progress to clinically detectable tumors. Interestingly, the rate of histologic cancer incidence is roughly the same worldwide,[6,7] suggesting an important role for environmental factors as potential promoting agents to explain the large regional differences observed in the incidence of clinically detectable disease.[8] In addition to environmental factors, studies of familial aggregation of this disease have suggested that between 5 and 10 percent of prostate cancers may be directly attributable to the inheritance of prostate cancer-susceptibility alleles (see below) that may act as genetic factors driving this progression independent of environmental exposure. Thus, as with numerous other cancers, there is evidence for both genetic and environmental factors in the etiology of prostate cancer, with the majority of disease most likely being a result of interaction of the two.[9]

Prostate cancer develops in two different regions of the gland, with most lesions (~80 percent) being found in the periphery, where more often than not the disease is multifocal. The remainder of cancers are found in a periurethral region, termed the *transition zone.*[10] Curiously, it is the latter region of the prostate in which the virtually ubiquitous process of benign prostatic hyperplasia (BPH) occurs.[11] Based primarily on this regional difference in the incidence of benign and malignant growth and on the fact that stromal cell proliferation is typically a major component of BPH, these benign lesions are not thought to be the precursors of invasive adenocarcinoma in the prostate. Instead, *prostatic intraepithelial neoplasia* (PIN) is the term given to characteristic foci of dysplastic ductal and acinar cells thought to be the precursor lesions of this disease.[12]

Diagnostic Criteria

Previously, the development of symptoms, either due to local disease resulting primarily in voiding dysfunction or due to disseminated disease commonly resulting in bone pain, has been the initial sign of prostatic malignancy, resulting in many men being diagnosed with advanced disease. This situation has changed

A list of standard abbreviations is located immediately preceding the index in each volume. Nonstandard abbreviations used in this chapter include: PSA = prostate-specific antigen; PIN = prostatic intraepithelial neoplasia; LOH = loss of heterozygosity.

dramatically with the use of PSA as a screening tool, which, when combined with digital rectal examination and transrectal ultrasound, results in a much greater ability to detect prostate cancer while it is still confined to the gland. The use of these latter methods is primarily responsible for the approximately threefold increase in incidence rates observed since 1988,[2] as well as the tremendous decline in the percentage of patients diagnosed annually with disseminated disease.

PSA is a serine protease with a chymotrpysin-like substrate specificity. It is normally secreted by the prostate in large amounts into the seminal plasma.[13] The PSA level in the bloodstream of men is normally below 4 ng/ml, although this varies with age.[14] With prostate pathology, this level can increase, in particularly dramatic fashion in the case of carcinoma. A current focus of intense research effort is on the ability to accurately interpret slightly elevated PSA levels that can be indicative of either benign or malignant disease.[15–17] Serum PSA detection after prostatectomy or other treatment for prostate cancer is a very reliable indication of disease progression.[18]

The histology of normal, cancerous, and benign hyperplastic prostate is illustrated in Fig. 56-1. Prostate cancer is graded based on tissue architectural patterns according to the system proposed by the Gleason.[19] Because of the common morphologic heterogeneity, two different grades are given for the first and second most prevalent patterns, and the sum of these two grades is added to give the Gleason score. Staging is categorized using the TNM (tumor, node, metastasis) classification.[20]

Unique Features of Prostate Carcinoma

Several features tend to distinguish adenocarcinoma of the prostate from other common cancers. The following list is not exhaustive but serves to highlight important questions in prostate cancer biology for which there is little understanding at the molecular level: (1) extreme age dependence of incidence—although the most common malignancy in men, this disease does not appear (at least in a clinically detectable form) at significant rates until the sixth decade of life (incidence of 1 in 2 million below the age of 40[3]); (2) slow growth rate-doubling times measured in years are not uncommon[21] (Does this slow growth rate simply explain the age-dependent incidence of prostate cancer?); (3) sensitivity to androgens—most prostate cancers respond to androgen ablation therapy, although virtually all become insensitive to this treatment; (4) multifocality—the prostate of a man diagnosed with prostate cancer contains an average of five apparently independent lesions[22] (these lesions are genetically heterogeneous, both inter- and intratumorally,[23–25] and this multifocality is independent of family history of prostate cancer[22]); and (5) lack of ability to establish cell lines in vitro from clinical specimens of prostate cancer (after hundreds of attempts by numerous investigators, only a handful of cell lines exist). Recent establishment of a series of useful human prostate cancer xenografts[26–30] has provided an important research alternative.

GENETIC LOCI

Hereditary Prostate Cancer

Although no prostate cancer-susceptibility genes have been cloned, there is substantial evidence that a hereditary form of this disease exists. A positive family history of prostate cancer is one of the strongest risk factors identified for this disease.[31–35] Segregation analyses of familial aggregation patterns suggest that these observations are most consistent with the existence of one or more hereditary prostate cancer genes that act in an autosomal dominant fashion to confer greatly increased risk of disease.[35–37] It is estimated that approximately 9 percent of all prostate cancer is attributable to such gene(s), although in the case of early-onset disease (i.e., diagnosis before age 55), a greater proportion (40 percent) may be due to an inherited susceptibility.[35,38]

Studies supporting the existence of hereditary forms of prostate cancer have led to the initiation of genome-wide searches for loci contributing to hereditary prostate cancer. The first such scan for linkage, reported by Smith et al.,[39] resulted in suggestive evidence for prostate cancer-susceptibility loci on several chromosomes, including 1q, 4q, 5p, 7p, 13q, and Xq. Statistically significant evidence was achieved for the locus 1q24-25 (*HPC1*). Families linked to *HPC1* tended to have an early mean age of diagnosis (under 65 years) and large number of affected members (> 4).[40] While three subsequent studies have corroborated linkage to *HPC1*,[40–42] three additional studies found no clear evidence for *HPC1*-predisposed disease within their study populations,[43–45] although evidence of linkage to a novel locus at 1q42.2-43 was observed in one report.[45] The disparity in these studies emphasizes the common set of obstacles for linkage detection in hereditary prostate cancer, most prominently, a high phenocopy rate and genetic locus heterogeneity.

A further confounding issue in prostate cancer linkage studies is the lack of a clear delineation of the mode(s) of inheritance. Although segregation analyses of familial prostate cancer have supported autosomal dominant inheritance, several population-based studies have reported a statistically significant excess risk of prostate cancer in men with affected brothers compared with those with affected fathers, consistent with the hypothesis of an X-linked, or recessive, model of inheritance.[46–50] Interestingly, in a follow-up study to the initial genome-wide search for prostate cancer linkage, Xu et al.[51] reported linkage to the X chromosome (q27-28) in a large collection of multiplex prostate cancers from North America and Europe. More precise information on inherited prostate cancer and its molecular mechanisms will have to await the cloning of the responsible genes.

As a result of various epidemiologic studies over the past four decades, a link between prostate and breast cancer etiology has been suspected.[52–56] More recent studies have demonstrated an association between *BRCA1* and *BRCA2* mutations and the incidence of prostate cancer in carriers.[57–60] The most direct evidence for a role of these genes in prostate cancer susceptibility comes from the study by Struewing et al.[60] of Ashkenazi men known to harbor *BRCA1* or *BRCA2* gene mutations. In this cohort, the rate of prostate cancer diagnosis by age 70 was 16 percent, compared with 3.8 percent for nonmutation carriers. Other studies examining a role for these genes in prostate cancer have been less supportive of a prominent effect. Lehrer et al.[61] reported an absence of *BRCA1* and *BRCA2* founder mutations in Ashkenazi prostate cancer cases, although only a limited number of these men reported a positive family history of the disease. Langston et al.[62] found a *BRCA1* 185delAG mutation in an affected member of a Jewish prostate cancer family, although no other family members were tested. A study of multiplex Ashkenazi Jewish prostate cancer families did not find elevated rates of common mutations in either *BRCA1* or *BRCA2*.[63] Overall, germ-line mutations in these genes are likely to account for only a small proportion of familial prostate cancer.

Sporadic Disease

Chromosomal Alterations in Sporadic Disease. Initial loss of heterozygosity (LOH) studies indicated that chromosomes 8p, 10q, and 16q may harbor prostate tumor-suppressor genes. These studies have been confirmed and extended to include chromosomes 7q and 13q as regions of frequent allelic loss.[64]

Chromosome 8. Of the regions analyzed, the short arm of chromosome 8 has received the most attention because it appears to be the most frequent site of LOH in prostate cancers, occurring in the majority of patients examined. Two or possibly three distinct region of LOH occur on this chromosomal arm, with the region 8p21-12 being deleted in the majority of prostate cancer precursor lesions (PIN), and more distally, 8p22 is deleted in most adenocarcinomas.[65–70] In this latter region, a homozygous deletion of approximately 1 megabase has been observed.[71]

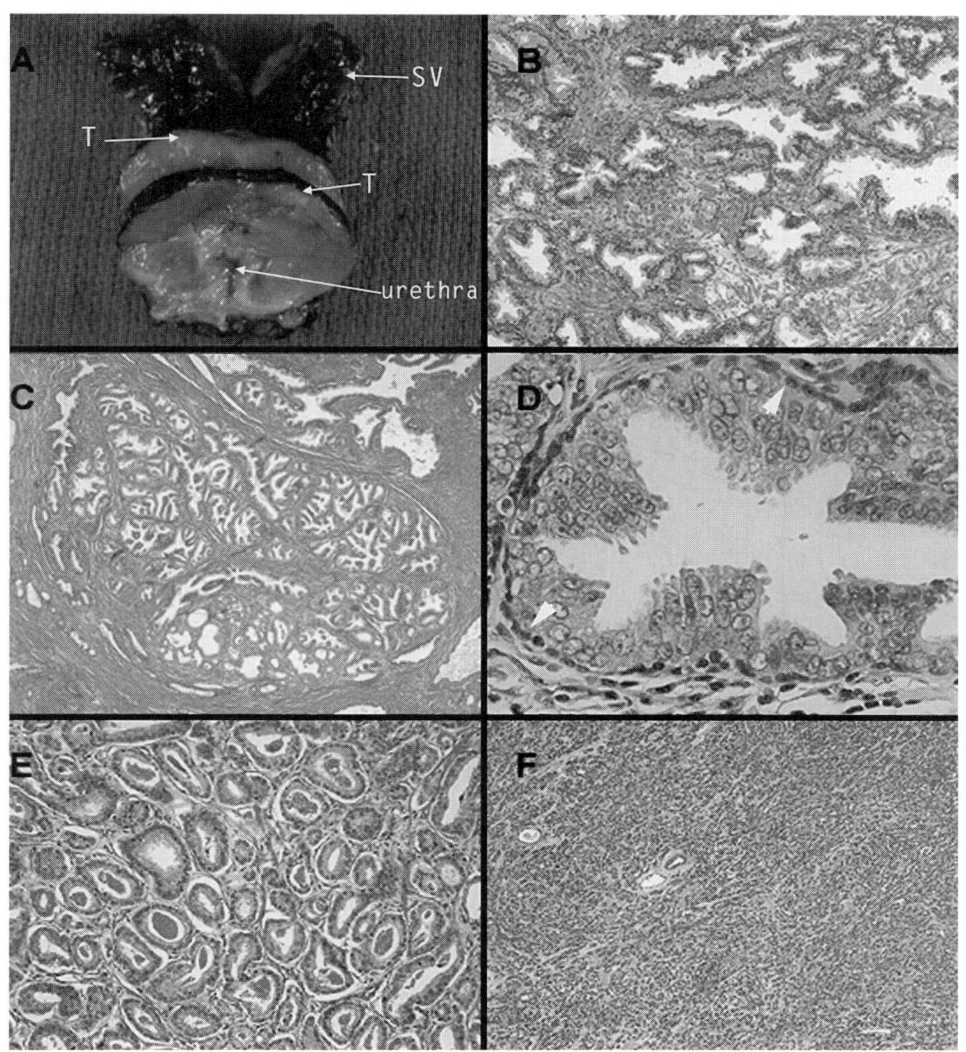

Fig. 56-1 Representative prostate histology. (*A*) Gross radical prostatectomy specimen. Serial section of the gland from apex to base. Bilateral tumor occurrence in the posterior portion (marked T). The position of the urethra is labeled. SV, seminal vesicles. (*B*) Normal. Histology of normal prostate. Open glands varying in size and form are separated by abundant stromal tissue (×20). (*C*) Benign prostatic hyperplasia (BPH). Well-defined nodule of crowded but non infiltrative, benign glands (×20). (*D*) Prostatic intraepithelial neoplasia (PIN). Cytologically malignant cells within a single architecturally benign gland. Note the presence of basal epithelial cell layer (*arrowheads*) (×400). (*E*) Prostate adenocarcinoma. Low-grade (Gleason 2 + 2 = 4). Closely packed single, round glands, separated by scant stroma (×20). (*F*) Prostate adenocarcinoma. High grade (Gleason 5 + 5 = 10). Glandular differentiation is absent; sheets of anaplastic cells occasionally intermixed with smooth muscle fibers (×20). (*Photographs kindly provided by Joseph D. Kronz, M.D., and Jurgita Sauvageot.*)

The first reports of chromosome 8p abnormalities in prostate cancer were cytogenetic studies that suggested that loss of chromosome 8p material was correlated with loss of androgen responsiveness.[72] The finding of chromosome 8p LOH was first described by Bergerheim et al.[73] in a study of primary and metastatic deposits of prostate cancer. Since then, subregional deletion analysis of chromosome 8p in prostate cancer has been performed using a variety of molecular methods, all of which have confirmed a high frequency of loss in this region, especially but not exclusively within chromosome band 8p22.[24,65–68,73–80] The rate of 8p22 loss reported in these regions varies from 32 to 65 percent in primary tumors and 65 to 100 percent in DNA derived from metastases.

Separate discrete regions of loss in more proximal regions including 8p21[67,70] and 8p12[68,70] have been described. Frequent loss (63 percent) of portions of 8p21-p12 have been identified in PIN lesions,[69] suggesting that a gene in this area may become frequently inactivated at a relatively early stage in prostate tumorigenesis. Evidence of heterogeneity of 8p LOH among different PIN lesions within the same gland was observed.[69] A combined CGH, Southern, and microsatellite study has shown loss of chromosome 8p22-p12 in 80 percent of prostate cancer lymph node metastases,[81] and microcell transfer of human chromosome 8 into a rat prostate cancer cell line has been reported to suppress metastatic ability.[82] An association of chromosome 8p loss and higher stage has been reported.[68]

A candidate tumor-suppressor gene, termed *N33,* located in a homozygously deleted region of chromosome 8p22 has been identified that is expressed in many normal tissues but not in some cancers, most notably those of the colon.[83] The contribution of this gene to prostatic carcinogenesis awaits further clarification.

The frequent loss of sequences on chromosome 8p provides a marker to determine the similarity or difference between primary prostate cancers and their metastases. This approach has been used to determine the concordance rates for 8p loss in a series of PIN, primary, and metastatic lesions obtained from the same patient.[24] Cases were observed in which there was a complete concordance in that all samples of cancer had retained or lost the same 8p marker, but there also were cases in which the PIN sample would show loss but not the primary tumor or the lymph node tumor samples. In addition, there were cases that showed differences among the multiple primary lesions within the prostate. These data and similar findings[23] demonstrate the complex genetic relationship that exists between primary and metastatic lesions and suggest that the primary prostate cancer that gives rise to a given metastatic deposit is not easily predicted on the basis of morphologic characteristics.

Concomitant with deletion of sequences from the short arm, chromosome 8 is frequently affected by gain of sequences on the long arm. First observed by Southern analysis,[65] a CGH study of lymph node metastases indicated that 85 percent of such tumors showed evidence of 8q gain, making this the most common numerical alteration observed in this study.[81] Van den Berg et al.[84] reported that gain of 8q sequences in prostate cancer was highly correlated with disease progression, and similarly, in the CGH study of Visakorpi et al.,[79] gain of 8q sequences was seen in 89 percent of tumor recurrences after hormonal therapy, whereas only 6 percent of primary tumors showed this alteration. An obvious candidate gene that may be the target of these amplification events in prostate cancer is the oncogene *c-myc* located at 8q24, although most of the amplification events on 8q are large, suggesting that many genes are affected. At present, the overall contribution of the *c-myc* gene to progression of prostate cancer is undefined.

Chromosome 7. Similar to chromosome 8, chromosome 7 also frequently undergoes both gain and loss events in prostate cancer. Trisomy 7 is common in both PIN[23] and cancer lesions,[85–89] and gain of chromosome 7 has been observed in 30 to 56 percent of cases in CGH studies.[70,80] The association of chromosome 7 aneusomy with advanced stage[88,90] and poor prognosis[89] indicates that gain of chromosome 7 material may play an important role in progression of some prostate cancers. Likewise, loss of discrete portions of chromosome 7q in prostate cancer,[91–94] with the most frequent region of deletion appearing at 7q31.1, suggests that this region also may harbor a gene important in tumor progression, since tumors deleting this region are usually of high grade and stage.

Chromosome 10. Cytogenetic analyses of prostate cancer have not revealed consistent chromosomal deletions (see refs. 87 and 95–97), which might provide information regarding the location of tumor-suppressor genes. However, an early study[98] employing direct preparations of prostate cancer cells, showed that four of four patients with late-stage prostate carcinomas exhibited chromosome 10q deletions and three of four exhibited chromosome 7q deletions. Since that time, alterations of the long arm of chromosome 10, while by no means ubiquitous, have been the most consistently observed karyotypic abnormality in prostate cancer. Initial studies examining chromosome 10 by RFLP analysis found losses solely on 10q[99] or on both arms of chromosome 10.[73] A number of reports since then using both RFLP and microsatellite analysis have found loss of chromosome 10 in 29 to 48 percent of informative cases, with a complex pattern of loss being observed, including monosomy and loss of 10p alone, loss of portions of 10p and 10q, and loss of sequences on 10q alone.[100–103] The most common region of deletion on the short and long arms has been mapped to 10p11.2 and 10q23.1, respectively (see *PTEN* below).

Chromosome 16q. Carter et al.[99] observed LOH of markers on chromosome 16q in approximately 30 percent of clinically localized tumors, whereas Bergerheim et al.[73] found a higher rate (56 percent) in a series of metastatic and localized tumors. Deletion mapping data presented in this latter study suggested that the critical region was located between D16S4 and 16qter. Employing a series of cosmid contigs in a FISH analysis, Cher et al.[104] suggested that the common region of loss was more distally located between 16q23.1 and 16qter.

Chromosome 17. Studies of loss of chromosome 17 sequences have focused primarily on two regions, one being in the vicinity of the *p53* gene at 17p13.1 and the other being in the area of the *BRCA1* gene on the proximal long arm. Allelic of loss the *p53* gene and distal markers is generally low in early-stage primary prostate cancer (< 20 percent), a finding consistent with the low frequency of *p53* gene mutations found in these tumors (see below). A study by Brooks et al.[105] demonstrates that there is a higher rate of 17p loss in higher-grade and later-stage prostate cancers but that this loss is not correlated with an increasing frequency of *p53* mutations, suggesting the presence of perhaps another tumor-suppressor gene that may contribute to the LOH events on this chromosomal arm.

Brothman et al.[106] and Williams et al.[107] used a variety of approaches to implicate a region on the proximal long arm of chromosome 17 in the vicinity of the *BRCA1* gene at 17q21 as harboring a gene important in prostate carcinogenesis. By using a series of P1 clones in a FISH analysis, these workers were able to demonstrate that the common region of loss did not include *BRCA1* but was more distal, implicating a different gene in this region. These results are critical because it has been suggested repeatedly that the *BRCA1* gene may play an important role in prostate carcinogenesis, although little direct evidence of this has been reported.

Chromosome 18. Initial studies implicating chromosome 18 as harboring a prostate tumor-suppressor gene found LOH of markers in the vicinity of the *DCC* gene at band 21.2 on the long arm of this chromosome at rates of between 20 and 40 percent.[73,78,99] Latil et al.[74] found that one-third of clinically localized prostate cancers show loss of markers on 18q and suggest that the common region of deletion lies between the centromere and D18S19, located at 18q22.1, although a subsequent study narrowed this region, excluding *DCC*. Examinations of the *DPC4* gene at 18q21.1 in prostate cancer revealed an absence of inactivating mutations of this pancreatic tumor-suppressor gene.[108,109]

CGH Studies of Prostate Cancer. Visakorpi et al.[79] used comparative genomic hybridization (CGH) to survey the genome of a series of both untreated, localized prostate cancers and tumors from patients failing hormonal therapy. This study found chromosome 8p to be the most frequently deleted, followed by 13q, 6q, 16q, 18q, and 9p. In a series of nine advanced prostate cancers, there was a significant increase in deletions of chromosome 5q and gains of chromosomes 7p, 8q, and X when compared with untreated primary tumor samples. Similarly, Cher et al.[81] used CGH combined with Southern and microsatellite analyses to study a series of over 31 advanced prostate cancers (primarily lymph node deposits of prostate cancer). As expected, a high frequency of chromosome 8p loss was seen (71 percent). This study also revealed that portions of chromosome 13 were just as commonly deleted (65 percent), followed by chromosomes 17p (52 percent), 10q22.1-qter (42 percent), 2cen-q31 (42 percent), 16q (42 percent), 5cen-q23.3 (39 percent), and 6q14-q23.2 (39 percent). Increases in copy number of sequences on chromosome 8q were observed in 81 percent of samples, with gains of chromosomes 1q, 2p, 3p and q, 7p and q, and 11p being observed in over 40 percent of the samples. Although the CGH analysis was not able to detect a case containing a homozygous deletion on chromosome 8p22, in general, the concordance between the CGH data and that obtained by either Southern or microsatellite analysis was excellent, with agreement observed at 215 to 233 (92 percent) of informative loci. Thus these studies confirm previous studies of allelic loss in prostate cancer and at the same time greatly expand the chromosomal regions implicated as harboring "prostate cancer genes."

SPECIFIC GENES

Sporadic Disease

A number of genes have been found to be mutated in prostate cancer, including *p53, PTEN, Rb, RAS, CDKN2,* androgen receptor (*AR*), *MXI1,* and *POLB,* although the latter two, located on chromosomes 10q25 and 8p11.2, respectively, remain to be confirmed. *RAS* mutations are uncommon (< 5 percent of cases),[110–112] as are point mutations of *Rb,*[113] although loss of one copy of *Rb* readily occurs. To date, the most consistently observed site of point mutations is the *p53* gene, and these mutations are common only in advanced disease. Microsatellite instability is uncommon but detectable in prostate cancer,[114–117] and the *hPMS2* gene has been shown to be mutated in a prostate cancer cell line that exhibits this phenotype.[118]

p53. *p53* mutations are uncommon in localized disease but become quite frequent in deposits of metastatic prostate cancer, particularly those to bone.[119–125] Observed heterogeneity of *p53* mutations within different tumors in the same gland and within different regions of the same gland appears to be a unique feature of prostate cancer.[25] Furthermore, LOH and point mutation of *p53* do not appear to be tightly coupled in this disease.[105]

PTEN. A series of studies has examined prostate cancer specimens for alterations in the dual-function phosphatase gene *PTEN* and found that this gene is inactivated by a combination of mechanisms including hemi- and homozygous deletion,[126–129] point mutation,[126–128] and promoter methylation.[129] These changes are observed most commonly in advanced disease and may play a role in the acquisition of metastatic potential.

Rb. The importance of *Rb* gene inactivation in prostate cancer was suggested initially by the studies of Bookstein et al.,[130,131] who demonstrated the presence of inactivating mutations in the *Rb* gene in clinical specimens of prostate cancer, as well as the ability of reintroduction of a cloned copy of *Rb* to suppress the tumorigenicity of DU145 prostate cancer cells, which had been shown to produce a nonfunctional truncated Rb protein. Combined CGH and LOH studies reveal that one copy of *Rb* is lost in advanced prostate cancer at rates approaching 80 percent,[81] although limited sequencing studies suggest that point mutations are present in less than 20 percent of clinical samples.[113] Immunohistochemical studies of *Rb* expression demonstrate lack of expression in 10 to 22 percent of tumors, with a questionable correlation between tumor LOH of *Rb* and lack of expression.[132,133] These data, together with LOH events on 13q that do not include *Rb,* suggest the presence of an additional or alternative prostate tumor-suppressor gene near the *Rb* locus.[133]

CDKN2. Much attention has been focused on the *p16/CDKN2* gene, a negative regulator of cell cycle progression located at chromosome 9p21, since the finding of frequent homozygous deletions in a wide variety of cancer cell lines.[134] A relatively high frequency of homozygous (~20 percent)[135] and hemizygous losses of *CDKN2* have been observed in clinical specimens of prostate cancer.[136] In the latter case, loss events in the vicinity of the *CDKN2* gene are more common in metastatic deposits of prostate cancer (43 versus 20 percent in primary tumors), and in a small but detectable fraction of tumors (~15 percent), the *CDKN2* gene shows evidence of inactivation by promoter methylation.[136] Whether all the allelic loss events at 9p21 in prostate cancer are associated with *CDKN2* inactivation or whether they reflect inactivation of a neighboring gene, e.g., *p15,* has not been determined.

Androgen Receptor. The role of androgen in normal prostate physiology is unquestioned, since these hormones are strictly required for normal development and maintenance of prostate growth and function. However, the role of androgens and androgen receptors in prostate cancer is much less clear, and recent studies have generated a great deal of renewed interest in this pathway[137] and its role in the critical progression of prostate cancer to androgen independence. An initial hypothesis that loss of *AR* gene expression may be important in androgen-independent disease was not supported by several studies that showed continued or even elevated *AR* gene expression in androgen-independent tumors.[138,139] Newmark et al.[140] were the first to report a mutated androgen receptor in a clinical specimen of prostate cancer, found curiously in a localized cancer prior to any hormonal therapy. This and other findings of mutations prior to hormonal therapy[141] would suggest that mutant *AR* may provide a growth advantage even in the presence of normal androgen levels. Kelly et al.[142] and Sartor et al.[143] described a number of patients who underwent a paradoxical response to withdrawal of the antiandrogen flutamide in that a number of clinical parameters (e.g., PSA levels, bone pain) improved on cessation of drug treatment. One explanation proposed for this response is that such patients harbor *AR* gene mutations similar to that found in the prostate cancer cell line LNCaP (Thr to Ala change at codon 868) that alters the ligand specificity of the receptor such that both estrogens and antiandrogens, as well as androgens, can now act as agonists.[144,145] The frequency of such mutations in prostate cancer patients is unknown, but a study by Taplin et al.[146] found that 5 of 10 samples of hormone-refractory prostate cancer metastatic to bone had *AR* mutations and at least two of these mutations resulted in a shift in hormone specificity of the androgen receptor. Finally, Visakorpi et al.[147] demonstrated that up to 30 percent of prostate cancer specimens from men failing hormonal therapy are characterized by increases in copy number of X chromosomal region (q11-q13) containing the androgen receptor. These results suggest that instead of being insensitive to androgen, such tumors may become supersensitive to androgen by an as yet undetermined mechanism or perhaps sensitive to a different nonandrogen steroid hormone. Thus, whereas the precise role of androgen and the androgen receptor in this disease is not known, these studies imply a potential role of this pathway at a critical step in prostate cancer progression.

p27 (CDKN1B). A number of studies report that reduced levels of the cyclin kinase inhibitor p27 are associated with a more aggressive prostate cancer phenotype,[148–151] although the mechanism of this down-regulation is not clear. Interestingly, Kibel et al.[152] described a homozygous deletion of the *p27* gene in a lethal case of prostate cancer and a high frequency of LOH of *p27* in advanced prostate cancers in general. Thus it is possible that, in addition to increased ubiquitin-mediated p27 protein degradation that has been demonstrated in colon and other cancers, in prostate cancer, at least a subset of lesions may inactivate this gene via deletion.

***Bcl-2:* An Inhibitor of Apoptosis.** The *bcl-2* gene, located on chromosome 18q21, is unique among oncogenes in that its expression does not enhance the rate of cell proliferation but instead decreases the rate of cell death.[153,154] The role of *bcl-2* in the development and progression of carcinoma of the prostate has been examined by McDonnell et al.[155] Using immunohistochemical techniques, *bcl-2* is not usually expressed in androgen-dependent prostatic cancer cells, whereas it was expressed in androgen-independent prostatic cancer cells.[155] This observation has been confirmed by Colombel et al.[156] These findings suggest that enhanced expression of bcl-2 protein in carcinomas of the prostate is associated with the transition to androgen independence, although Furuya et al.[157] demonstrated that there are bcl-2 independent pathways to this state as well.

***E-cadherin* and *KAI-1*.** Genes whose down-regulation has been implicated in prostate cancer progression include the cell adhesion molecule genes *E-cadherin* and *KAI-1* located at chromosomes 16q22.1 (a frequent site of LOH) and 11p11.2, respectively.[158] E-cadherin protein levels are frequently reduced in high-grade prostate cancers, and this finding has prognostic significance.[159–161] *KAI-1* was identified by its ability to suppress metastasis in experimental animal studies.[162,163] Although the predominate mechanism for down-regulation of these genes has not been determined, in the case of *E-cadherin,* gene inactivation via promoter methylation has been found commonly in prostate cancer cell lines and at a low but detectable rate in clinical specimens of prostate cancer.

GSTπ. Similarly, the gene for the phase II detoxification enzyme glutathione *S*-transferase π also has been found to be extensively methylated in the promoter region, in a completely cancer-specific fashion, with concomitant absence of expression.[164–166] In fact, this methylation event, being found in over 90 percent of all prostate cancers, as well as in PIN lesions, is the most common genomic alteration yet observed in prostate cancer. The mechanism by which this region becomes specifically methylated in prostate cancer and the basis for its apparent selection in the carcinogenic pathway are unclear at present. Since this enzyme is a key part of an important cellular pathway to prevent damage from a wide range of carcinogens, its inactivation may result in increased susceptibility of prostate tissue to both tumor initiation and progression resulting from an increased rate of accumulated DNA damage. Indeed, reactivation of this or a similar cellular defense pathway, perhaps by dietary intervention, has been proposed as a treatment strategy aimed at blocking the progression of initiated prostate cancer foci.

Hereditary Cases

***AR* Gene.** To date, no germ-line mutations have been identified that confer increased risk for prostate cancer, although multiple efforts are underway to identify such changes in prostate cancer families. Polymorphic variations in a variety of genes, however, have been suggested to modulate an individual's risk of prostate cancer development. A prime example of this is the *AR* gene, which has been implicated as a potentially important gene in modifying prostate cancer risk due to polymorphisms within the gene that result in variable androgen receptor activity. Specifically, there are two polymorphic triplet repeats in exon 1 that code for polyglutamine and polyglycine repeats of varying lengths of between 11 and 31 and 10 and 22 residues, respectively.[167–170] Although variations in the polyglycine repeat length are of unknown biologic consequence, it has been demonstrated that the polyglutamine repeat length is inversely related to the ability of the androgen receptor to stimulate androgen-specific transcriptional activity.[171–173] This is of particular interest because the population with the shortest average glutamine repeat length observed is the African-American population, which has the highest incidence and mortality rates reported for prostate cancer, whereas Asian individuals, who have low risk for prostate cancer, tend to have longer repeat lengths.[167,168] Hakimi et al.[137] have suggested that *AR* genes with shorter repeat lengths may increase the risk of developing more aggressive prostate cancer by virtue of conferring greater sensitivity to androgenic stimulation. Polymorphisms in other genes involved in androgen metabolism also have been implicated in determining one's risk for prostate cancer development (e.g., 5α-reductase, 3β-hydroxysteroid dehydrogenase).[174–177] Further study will be necessary to determine the overall role of these polymorphisms in determining or modifying prostate cancer risk.

Implications for Diagnosis

Whereas localized prostate cancer is readily curable by prostatectomy, there is presently no effective curative therapy for disseminated disease. Thus early detection is a critical aspect in prostate cancer diagnosis, although it is confounded by the presence of neoplastic lesions of limited clinical relevance in most aging men. Once the disease is detected, the ability to accurately determine the biologic aggressiveness of a given prostate cancer is a prime research goal. As mentioned earlier, certain molecular alterations such as gain and loss of sequences on chromosomes 7 and 8 have been shown to have prognostic significance, and loss of expression of the cell adhesion molecules, E-cadherin and possibly KAI-1, is strongly associated with more aggressive disease. In terms of diagnosis, PCR-based detection of methylation of the *GSTP1* promoter offers great potential as a highly sensitive and specific prostate cancer detection tool.[165,166]

New therapeutic approaches based on genetic alterations in prostate cancer cells have been limited, primarily due to lack of progress in the identification of genes that are mutated at high frequency in this disease. However, *p53* gene replacement and PSA (and other prostate-specific) promoter-based targeting of toxic gene expression to the prostate are examples of novel strategies that are under development.[178,179]

REFERENCES

1. Landis SH, Murray T, Bolden S, Wingo PA: Cancer statistics, 1998. *CA* **48**:6, 1998.
2. Brawley OW, Kramer BS: Epidemiology of prostate cancer, in Vogelsang NJ, Scardino PT, Shipley WU, Coffey DS (eds): *Comprehensive Textbook of Genitourinary Oncology*. Baltimore, Williams & Wilkins, 1996, pp 565-572.
3. National Cancer Institute: SEER Program, 1996.
4. Boring CC, Squires TS, Tong T: Cancer statistics, 1992 [published erratum appears in *CA* **42**(2):127,1992]. *CA* **42**:19, 1992.
5. Dhom G: Epidemiologic aspects of latent and clinically manifest carcinoma of the prostate. *J Cancer Res Clin Oncol* **106**:210, 1983.
6. Breslow N, Chan CW, Dhom G, Drury RA, Franks LM, Gellei B, Lee YS, Lundberg S, Sparke B, Sternby NH, Tulinius H: Latent carcinoma of prostate of autopsy in seven areas. *Int J Cancer* **20**:680, 1977.
7. Yatani R, Chigusa I, Akazaki K, Stemmermann GN, Welsh RA, Correa P: Geographic pathology of latent prostatic carcinoma. *Int J Cancer* **29**:611, 1982.
8. Carter BS, Carter HB, Isaacs JT: Epidemiologic evidence regarding predisposing factors to prostate cancer (review). *Prostate* **16**:187, 1990.
9. Taylor JA: Epidemiologic evidence of genetic susceptibility to cancer (review). *Birth Defects* **26**:113, 1990.
10. McNeal JE, Redwine EA, Freiha FS, Stamey TA: Zonal distribution of prostatic adenocarcinoma: Correlation with histologic pattern and direction of spread. *Am J Surg Pathol* **12**:897, 1988.
11. McNeal JE: Origin and evolution of benign prostatic enlargement. *Invest Urol* **15**:340, 1978.
12. Bostwick DG: Prostatic intraepithelial neoplasia (PIN). *Urology* **34**:16, 1989.
13. Lilja H, Abrahamsson PA: Three predominant proteins secreted by the human prostate gland. *Prostate* **12**:29, 1988.
14. Dalkin BL, Ahmann FR, Kopp JB: Prostate specific antigen levels in men older than 50 years without clinical evidence of prostatic carcinoma. *J Urol* **150**:1837, 1993.
15. Oesterling JE: Prostate specific antigen: A critical assessment of the most useful tumor marker for adenocarcinoma of the prostate (review). *J Urol* **145**:907, 1991.
16. Pannek J, Partin AW: The role of PSA and percent free PSA for staging and prognosis prediction in clinically localized prostate cancer. *Semin Urol Oncol* **16**(3):100, 1998.
17. Carter HB, Pearson JD: Prostate-specific antigen velocity and repeated measures of prostate-specific antigen. *Urol Clin North Am* **24**(2):333, 1997.
18. Oesterling JE, Chan DW, Epstein JI, Kimball AW Jr, Bruzek DJ, Rock RC, Brendler CB, Walsh PC: Prostate specific antigen in the preoperative and postoperative evaluation of localized prostatic cancer treated with radical prostatectomy. *J Urol* **139**:766, 1988.
19. Gleason DF: Histologic grading of prostate cancer: A perspective (review). *Hum Pathol* **23**:273, 1992.
20. Montie JE: 1992 staging system for prostate cancer (review). *Semin Urol* **11**:10, 1993.
21. Berges RR, Vukanovic J, Epstein JI, CarMichel M, Cisek L, Johnson DE, et al: Implication of cell kinetic changes during the progression of human prostatic cancer. *Clin Cancer Res* **1**:473, 1995.
22. Bastacky SI, Wojno KJ, Walsh PC, CarMichael MJ, Epstein JI: Pathologocal features of hereditary prostate cancer. *J Urol* **153**:987, 1995.
23. Qian JQ, Bostwick DG, Takahashi S, Borell TJ, Herath JF, Lieber MM, Jenkins RB: Chromosomal anomalies in prostatic intraepithelial neoplasia and carcinoma detected by fluorescence in situ hybridization. *Cancer Res* **55**:5408, 1995.
24. Sakr WA, Macoska JA, Benson P, Grignon DJ, Wolman SR, Pontes JE, Crissman JD: Allelic loss in locally metastatic, multisampled prostate cancer. *Cancer Res* **54**:3273, 1994.
25. Mirchandani D, Zheng J, Miller GJ, Ghosh AK, Shibata DK, Cote RJ, Roy-Burman P: Heterogeneity in intratumor distribution of *p53* mutations in human prostate cancer. *Am J Pathol* **147**:92, 1995.
26. Ellis WJ, Vessella RL, Buhler KR, Bladou F, True LD, Bigler SA, et al: Characterization of a novel androgen-sensitive, prostate-specific antigen-producing prostatic carcinoma xenograft: LuCaP 23. *Clin Cancer Res* **2**:1039, 1996.
27. Klein KA, Reiter RE, Redula J, Moradi H, Zhu XL, Brothman AR, et al: Progression of metastatic human prostate cancer to androgen independence in immunodeficient SCID mice. *Nature Med* **3**:402, 1997.
28. Nagabhushan M, Miller CM, Pretlow TP, Giaconia JM, Edgehouse NL, Schwartz S, et al: CWR22: The first human prostate cancer xenograft with strongly androgen-dependent and relapsed strains both in vivo and in soft agar. *Cancer Res* **56**:3042, 1996.

29. van Weerden WM, de Ridder CM, Verdaasdonk CL, Romijn JC, van der Kwast TH, Schroder FH, et al: Development of seven new human prostate tumor xenograft models and their histopathological characterization. *Am J Pathol* **149**:1055, 1996.
30. Stearns ME, Ware JL, Agus DB, Chang CJ, Fidler IJ, Fife RS, et al: Workgroup 2: Human xenograft models of prostate cancer. *Prostate* **36**:56, 1998.
31. Cannon L, Bishop DT, Skolnick M, Hunt S, Lyon JL, Smart CR: Genetic epidemiology of prostate cancer in the Utah Mormon genealogy. *Cancer Surv* **1**:47, 1982.
32. Meikle AW, Smith JA, West DW: Familial factors affecting prostatic cancer risk and plasma sex-steroid levels. *Prostate* **6**:121, 1985.
33. Spitz MR, Currier RD, Fueger JJ, Babaian RJ, Newell GR: Familial patterns of prostate cancer: a case-control analysis. *J Urol* **146**:1305, 1991.
34. Steinberg GD, Carter BS, Beaty TH, Childs B, Walsh PC: Family history and the risk of prostate cancer. *Prostate* **17**:337, 1990.
35. Carter BS, Beaty TH, Steinberg GD, Childs B, Walsh PC: Mendelian inheritance of familial prostate cancer. *Proc Natl Acad Sci USA* **89**:3367, 1992.
36. Gronberg H, Damber L, Damber JE, Iselius L: Segregation analysis of prostate cancer in Sweden: Support for dominant inheritance. *Am J Epidemiol* **146**:552, 1997.
37. Schaid DJ, McDonnell SK, Blute ML, Thibodeau SN: Evidence for autosomal dominant inheritance of prostate cancer. *Am J Hum Genet* **62**:1425, 1998.
38. Carter BS, Bova GS, Beaty TH, Steinberg GD, Childs B, Isaacs WB, Walsh PC: Hereditary prostate cancer: Epidemiologic and clinical features (review). *J Urol* **150**(3):797, 1993.
39. Smith JR, Freije D, Carpten JD, Gronberg H, Xu J, Isaacs SD,et al: Major susceptibility locus for prostate cancer on chromosome 1 suggested by a genome-wide search (see comments). *Science* **274**:1371, 1996.
40. Gronberg H, Xu J, Smith JR, Carpten JD, Isaacs SD, Freije D, et al: Early age at diagnosis in families providing evidence of linkage to the hereditary prostate cancer locus (*HPC1*) on chromosome 1 [published erratum appears in *Cancer Res* **15**:58(14):3191, 1998]. *Cancer Res* **57**:4707, 1997.
41. Cooney KA, McCarthy JD, Lange E, Huang L, Miesfeldt S, Montie JE, et al: Prostate cancer susceptibility locus on chromosome 1q: a confirmatory study (see comments). *J Natl Cancer Inst* **89**:955, 1997.
42. Guo Y, Sklar GN, Borkowski A, Kyprianou N: Loss of the cyclin-dependent kinase inhibitor p27(Kip1) protein in human prostate cancer correlates with tumor grade. *Clin Cancer Res* **3**:2269, 1997.
43. McIndoe RA, Stanford JL, Gibbs M, Jarvik GP, Brandzel S, Neal CL, et al: Linkage analysis of 49 high-risk families does not support a common familial prostate cancer-susceptibility gene at 1q24-25. *Am J Hum Genet* **61**:347, 1997.
44. Eeles RA, Durocher F, Edwards S, Teare D, Badzioch M, Hamoudi R, et al: Linkage analysis of chromosome 1q markers in 136 prostate cancer families. The Cancer Research Campaign/British Prostate Group U.K. Familial Prostate Cancer Study Collaborators. *Am J Hum Genet* **62**:653, 1998.
45. Berthon P, Valeri A, Cohen-Akenine A, Drelon E, Paiss T, Wohr G, et al: Predisposing gene for early-onset prostate cancer, localized on chromosome 1q42.2-43. *Am J Hum Genet* **62**:1416, 1998.
46. Woolf CM: An investigation of the fammilial aspects of carcinoma of the prostate. *Cancer* **13**:361, 1960.
47. Narod SA, Dupont A, Cusan L, Diamond P, Gomez JL, Suburu R, et al: The impact of family history on early detection of prostate cancer (letter). *Nature Med* **1**:99, 1995.
48. Monroe KR, Yu MC, Kolonel LN, Coetzee GA, Wilkens LR, Ross RK, et al: Evidence of an X-linked or recessive genetic component to prostate cancer risk (see comments). *Nature Med* **1**:827, 1995.
49. Whittemore AS, et al: Family history and prostate cancer risk in black, white, and Asian men in the United States and Canada. *Am J Epidemiol* **141**:732, 1997.
50. Hayes RB, Liff JM, Pottern LM, Greenberg RS, Schoenberg JB, Schwartz AG, et al: Prostate cancer risk in U.S. blacks and whites with a family history of cancer. *Int J Cancer* **60**:361, 1995.
51. Xu J, Meyers D, Freije D, Isaacs S, Wiley K, Nusskern D, et al: Evidence for a prostatecancer susceptibility locus on the X chromosome. *Nature Genet* **20**:175, 1998.
52. Macklin TM: The genetic basis of human mammary cancer, in *Proceedings of the Second National Cancer Conference,* vol 2. New York, 1954, pp 1074-1087.
53. Wynder EL, Hyams L, Shigematsu T: Correlations of international cancer death rates. An epidemiological exercise. *Cancer* **20**:113, 1967.
54. Thiessen EU: Concerning a familial association between breast cancer and both prostatic and uterine malignancies. *Cancer* **34**:1102, 1974.
55. McCahy PJ, Harris CA, Neal DE: Breast and prostate cancer in the relatives of men with prostate cancer. *Br J Urol* **78**:552, 1996.
56. Ekman P, Pan Y, Li C, Dich J: Environmental and genetic factors: A possible link with prostate cancer. *Br J Urol* **79**:35, 1997.
57. Ford D, Easton DF, Bishop DT, Narod SA, Goldgar DE: Risks of cancer in *BRCA1*-mutation carriers. Breast Cancer Linkage Consortium. *Lancet* **343**:692, 1994.
58. Easton DF, Steele L, Fields P, Ormiston W, Averill D, Daly PA, McManus R, Neuhausen SL, Ford D, Wooster R, Cannon-Albright LA, Stratton MR, Goldgar DE: Cancer risks in two large breast cancer families linked to *BRCA2* on chromosome 13q12-13. *Am J Hum Genet* **61**:120, 1997.
59. Sigurdsson S, Thorlacius S, Tomasson J, Tryggvadottir L, Benediktsdottir K, Eyfjord JE, Jonsson E: *BRCA2* mutation in Icelandic prostate cancer patients. *J Mol Med* **75**:758, 1997.
60. Struewing JP, Hartge P, Wacholder S, Baker SM, Berlin M, McAdams M, et al: The risk of cancer associated with specific mutations of *BRCA1* and *BRCA2* among Ashkenazi Jews. *New Engl J Med* **336**:1401, 1997.
61. Lehrer S, Fodor F, Stock RG, Stone NN, Eng C, Song HK, McGovern M: Absence of 185delAG mutation of the *BRCA1* gene and 6174delT mutation of the *BRCA2* gene in Ashkenazi Jewish men with prostate cancer. *Br J Cancer* **78**:771, 1998.
62. Langston AA, Stanford JL, Wicklund KG, Thompson JD, Blazej RG, Ostrander EA: Germ-line *BRCA1* mutations in selected men with prostate cancer (letter). *Am J Hum Genet* **58**:881, 1996.
63. Wilkens EP, Freije D, Xu J, Nusskern D, Suzuki H, Isaacs SD, Wiley K, Bujnovszky P, Walsh PC, Isaacs WB: No evidence for a role of *BRCA1* or *BRCA2* mutations in Ashkenazi Jewish families with hereditary prostate cancer. *Prostate* **39**:280, 1999.
64. Isaacs WB: Molecular genetics of prostate cancer, in Ponder BA, Cavenee WK, Solomon E (eds): *Genetics and Cancer: A Second Look.* Plainview, NY, Cold Spring Harbor Laboratory Press, 1995, pp 357–380.
65. Bova GS, Carter BS, Bussemakers MJ, Emi M, Fujiwara Y, Kyprianou N, Jacobs SC, Robinson JC, Epstein JI, Walsh PC, et al: Homozygous deletion and frequent allelic loss of chromosome 8p22 loci in human prostate cancer. *Cancer Res* **53**:3869, 1993.
66. MacGrogan D, Levy A, Bostwick D, Wagner M, Wells D, Bookstein R: Loss of chromosome arm 8p loci in prostate cancer: Mapping by quantitative allelic imbalance. *Genes Chromosom Cancer* **10**:151, 1994.
67. Trapman J, Sleddens HF, van der Weiden MM, Dinjens WN, Konig JJ, Schroder FH, Faber PW, Bosman FT: Loss of heterozygosity of chromosome 8 microsatellite loci implicates a candidate tumor suppressor gene between the loci D8S87 and D8S133 in human prostate cancer. *Cancer Res* **54**:6061, 1994.
68. Suzuki H, Emi M, Komiya A, Fujiwara Y, Yatani R, Nakamura Y, Shimazaki J: Localization of a tumor suppressor gene associated with progression of human prostate cancer within a 1.2 Mb region of 8p22-p21.3. *Genes Chromosom Cancer* **13**:168, 1995.
69. Emmert-Buck MR, Vocke CD, Pozzatti RO, Duray PH, Jennings SB, Florence CD, Zhuang Z, Bostwick DG, Liotta LA, Linehan WM: Allelic loss on chromosome 8p12-21 in microdissected prostatic intraepithelial neoplasia. *Cancer Res* **55**:2959, 1995.
70. Macoska JA, Trybus TM, Benson PD, Sakr WA, Grignon DJ, Wojno KD, Pietruk T, Powell IJ: Evidence for three tumor suppressor gene loci on chromosome 8p in human prostate cancer. *Cancer Res* **55**:5390, 1995.
71. Bova GS, MacGrogan D, Levy A, Pin SS, Bookstein R, Isaacs WB: Physical mapping of chromosome 8p22 markers and their homozygous deletion in a metastatic prostate cancer. *Genomics* **35**:46, 1996.
72. Konig JJ, Kamst E, Hagemeijer A, Romijn JC, Horoszewicz J, Schroder FH: Cytogenetic characterization of several androgen responsive and unresponsive sublines of the human prostatic carcinoma cell line LNCaP. *Urol Res* **17**:79, 1989.
73. Bergerheim US, Kunimi K, Collins VP, Ekman P: Deletion mapping of chromosomes 8, 10, and 16 in human prostatic carcinoma. *Genes Chromosom Cancer* **3**:215, 1991.
74. Latil A, Baron JC, Cussenot O, Fournier G, Soussi T, Boccon-Gibod L, Le Duc A, Rouesse J, Lidereau R: Genetic alterations in localized prostate cancer: Identification of a common region of deletion on chromosome arm 18q. *Genes Chromosom Cancer* **11**:119, 1994.

75. Macoska JA, Trybus TM, Sakr WA, Wolf MC, Benson PD, Powell IJ, Pontes JE: Fluorescence in situ hybridization analysis of 8p allelic loss and chromosome 8 instability in human prostate cancer. *Cancer Res* **54**:3824, 1994.
76. Cher ML, MacGrogan D, Bookstein R, Brown JA, Jenkins RB, Jensen RH: Comparative genomic hybridization, allelic imbalance, and fluorescence *in situ* hybridization on chromosome 8 in prostate cancer. *Genes Chromosom Cancer* **11**:153, 1994.
77. Matsuyama H, Pan Y, Skoog L, Tribukait B, Naito K, Ekman P, Lichter P, Bergerheim US: Deletion mapping of chromosome 8p in prostate cancer by fluorescence in situ hybridization. *Oncogene* **9**:3071, 1994.
78. Massenkeil G, Oberhuber H, Hailemariam S, Sulser T, Diener PA, Bannwart F, Schafer R, Schwarte-Waldhoff I: *P53* mutations and loss of heterozygosity on chromosomes 8p, 16q, 17p, and 18q are confined to advanced prostate cancer. *Anticancer Res* **14**:2785, 1994.
79. Visakorpi T, Kallioniemi A, Syvanen AC, Hyytinen ER, Karhu R, Tammela T, Isola JJ, Kallioniemi OP: Genetic changes in primary and recurrent prostate cancer by comparative genomic hybridization. *Cancer Res* **55**:342, 1995.
80. Joos S, Bergerheim USR, Pan Y, Matsuyama H, Bentz M, Dumanoir S, Lichter P: Mapping of chromosomal gains and losses in prostate cancer by comparative genomic hybridization. *Genes Chromosom Cancer* **14**:267, 1995.
81. Cher ML, Bova GS, Moore DH, Small EJ, Carroll PR, Pin SS, Epstein JI, Isaacs WB, Jensen RH: Genetic alterations in untreated prostate cancer metastases and androgen independent prostate cancer detected by comparative genomic hybridization and allelotyping. *Cancer Res* **56**:3091, 1996.
82. Ichikawa T, Nihei N, Suzuki H, Oshimura M, Emi M, Nakamura Y, Hayata I, Isaacs JT, Shimazaki J: Suppression of metastasis of rat prostatic cancer by introducing human chromosome 8. *Cancer Res* **54**:2299, 1994.
83. MacGrogan D, Levy A, Bova GS, Isaacs WB, Bookstein R: Structure and methylation-associated silencing of a gene within a homozygously deleted region of human chromosome band 8p22. *Genomics* **35**:55, 1996.
84. Van Den Berg C, Guan XY, Von Hoff D, Jenkins R, Bittner M, Griffin C, Kallioniemi O, Visakorpi T, McGill J, Herath J, Epstein J, Sarosdy M, Meltzer P, Trent J: DNA sequence amplification in human prostate cancer identified by chromosome microdissection: Potential prognostic implications. *Clin Cancer Res* **1**:11, 1995.
85. Macoska JA, Micale MA, Sakr WA, Benson PD, Wolman SR: Extensive genetic alterations in prostate cancer revealed by dual PCR and FISH analysis. *Genes Chromosom Cancer* **8**:88, 1993.
86. Micale MA, Sanford JS, Powell IJ, Sakr WA, Wolman SR: Defining the extent and nature of cytogenetic events in prostatic adenocarcinoma: Paraffin FISH vs metaphase analysis. *Cancer Genet Cytogenet* **69(1)**:7, 1993.
87. Arps S, Rodewald A, Schmalenberger B, Carl P, Bressel M, Kastendieck H: Cytogenetic survey of 32 cancers of the prostate. *Cancer Genet Cytogenet* **66(2)**:93, 1993.
88. Bandyk MG, Zhao L, Troncoso P, Pisters LL, Palmer JL, von Eschenbach AC, Chung LWK, Liang JC, Chung LW: Trisomy 7: A potential cytogenetic marker of human prostate cancer progression. *Genes Chromosom Cancer* **9**:19, 1994.
89. Alcaraz A, Takahashi S, Brown JA, Herath JF, Bergstralh EJ, Larson-Keller JJ, Lieber MM, Jenkins RB: Aneuploidy and aneusomy of chromosome 7 detected by fluorescence *in situ* hybridization are markers of poor prognosis in prostate cancer. *Cancer Res* **54**:3998, 1994.
90. Zitzelsberger H, Szucs S, Weier HU, Lehmann L, Braselmann H, Enders S, Schilling A, Breul J, Hofler H, Bauchinger M: Numerical abnormalities of chromosome 7 in human prostate cancer detected by fluorescence *in situ* hybridization (FISH) on paraffin-embedded tissue sections with centromere-specific DNA probes. *J Pathol* **172**:325, 1994.
91. Zenklusen JC, Thompson JC, Troncoso P, Kagan J, Conti CJ: Loss of heterozygosity in human primary prostate carcinomas: A possible tumor suppressor gene at 7q31.1. *Cancer Res* **54(24)**:6370, 1994.
92. Takahashi S, Shan AL, Ritland SR, Delacey KA, Bostwick DG, Lieber MM, Thibodeau SN, Jenkins RB: Frequent loss of heterozygosity at 7q31.1 in primary prostate cancer is associated with tumor aggressiveness and progression. *Cancer Res* **55(18)**:4114, 1995.
93. Watson DL, Mashal R, Krithivas K, Corless C, Kantoff P, Richie JP, Sklar J: Loss of heterozygosity at chromosomal locus 7q21-q31 in metastatic prostate cancer. *J Urol* **153**:271A, 1995.
94. Takahashi S, Qian J, Brown JA, Alcaraz A, Bostwick DG, Lieber MM, Jenkins RB: Potential markers of prostate cancer aggressiveness detected by fluorescence *in situ* hybridization in needle biopsies. *Cancer Res* **54**:3574, 1994.
95. Brothman AR, Peehl DM, Patel AM, McNeal JE: Frequency and pattern of karyotypic abnormalities in human prostate cancer. *Cancer Res* **50**:3795, 1990.
96. Lundgren R, Mandahl N, Heim S, Limon J, Henrikson H, Mitelman F: Cytogenetic analysis of 57 primary prostatic adenocarcinomas. *Genes Chromosom Cancer* **4**:16, 1992.
97. Micale MA, Mohamed A, Sakr W, Powell IJ, Wolman SR: Cytogenetics of primary prostatic adenocarcinoma: Clonality and chromosome instability. *Cancer Genet Cytogenet* **61**:165, 1992.
98. Atkin NB, Baker MC: Chromosome study of five cancers of the prostate. *Hum Genet* **70**:359, 1985.
99. Carter BS, Ewing CM, Ward WS, Treiger BF, Aalders TW, Schalken JA, Epstein JI, Isaacs WB: Allelic loss of chromosomes 16q and 10q in human prostate cancer. *Proc Natl Acad Sci USA* **87**:8751, 1990.
100. Ittmann M: Allelic loss on chromosome 10 in prostate adenocarcinoma. *Cancer Res* **56**:2143, 1996.
101. Gray IC, Phillips SMA, Lee SJ, Neoptolemos JP, Weissenbach J, Spurr NK: Loss of the chromosomal region 10q23-25 in prostate cancer. *Cancer Res* **55**:4800, 1995.
102. Eagle LR, Yin X, Brothman AR, Williams BJ, Atkin NB, Prochownik EV: Mutation of the *MXI1* gene in prostate cancer. *Nature Genet* **9**:249, 1995.
103. Trybus TM, Burgess AC, Wojno KJ, Glover TW, Macoska JA: Distinct areas of allelic loss on chromosomal regions 10p and 10q in human prostate cancer. *Cancer Res* **56**:2263, 1996.
104. Cher ML, Ito T, Weidner N, Carroll PR, Jensen RH: Mapping of regions of physical deletion on chromosome 16q in prostate cancer cells by fluorescence *in situ* hybridization (FISH). *J Urol* **153(1)**:249, 1995.
105. Brooks JD, Bova GS, Ewing CM, Epstein JI, Carter BS, Piantadosi S, Robinson JC, Isaacs WB: An uncertain role for *p53* alterations in human prostate cancers. *Cancer Res* **56**:3814, 1996.
106. Brothman AR, Steele MR, Williams BJ, Jones E, Odelberg S, Albertsen HM, Jorde LB, Rohr LR, Stephenson RA: Loss of chromosome 17 loci in prostate cancer detected by polymerase chain reaction quantitation of allelic markers. *Genes Chromosom Cancer* **13**:278, 1995.
107. Williams BJ, Jones E, Zhu XL, Steele MR, Stephenson RA, Rohr LR, Brothman AR: Prostatic neoplasm, genes, tumor, *in situ* hybridization, chromosome deletion: Evidence for a tumor suppressor gene distal to *brca1* in prostate cancer. *J Urol* **155**:720, 1996.
108. Schutte M, Hruban RH, Hedrick L, Cho KR, Nadasdy GM, Weinstein CL, et al: *DPC4* gene in various tumor types. *Cancer Res* **56**:2527, 1996.
109. MacGrogan D, Pegram M, Slamon D, Bookstein R: Comparative mutational analysis of *DPC4* (*Smad4*) in prostatic and colorectal carcinomas. *Oncogene* **15**:1111, 1997.
110. Carter BS, Epstein JI, Isaacs WB: *ras* gene mutations in human prostate cancer. *Cancer Res* **50**:6830, 1990.
111. Gumerlock PH, Poonamallee UR, Meyers FJ, deVere White RW: Activated *ras* alleles in human carcinoma of the prostate are rare. *Cancer Res* **51**:1632, 1991.
112. Moul JW, Friedrichs PA, Lance RS, Theune SM, Chang EH: Infrequent *RAS* oncogene mutations in human prostate cancer. *Prostate* **20**:327, 1992.
113. Kubota Y, Fujinami K, Uemura H, Dobashi Y, Miyamoto H, Iwasaki Y, Kitamura H, Shuin T: Retinoblastoma gene mutations in primary human prostate cancer. *Prostate* **27**:314, 1995.
114. Egawa S, Uchida T, Suyama K, Wang C, Ohori M, Irie S, et al: Genomic instability of microsatellite repeats in prostate cancer: Relationship to clinicopathological variables. *Cancer Res* **55**:2418, 1995.
115. Watanabe M, Imai H, Shiraishi T, Shimazaki J, Kotake T, Yatani R: Microsatellite instability in human prostate cancer. *Br J Cancer* **72**:562, 1995.
116. Terrell RB, Wille AH, Cheville JC, Nystuen AM, Cohen MB, Sheffield VC: Microsatellite instability in adenocarcinoma of the prostate. *Am J Pathol* **147**:799, 1995.
117. Cunningham JM, Shan A, Wick MJ, McDonnell SK, Schaid DJ, Tester DJ, et al: Allelic imbalance and microsatellite instability in prostatic adenocarcinoma. *Cancer Res* **56**:4475, 1996.
118. Boyer JC, Umar A, Risinger JI, Lipford JR, Kane M, Yin S, Barrett JC, Kolodner RD, Kunkel TA: Microsatellite instability, mismatch repair

deficiency, and genetic defects in human cancer cell lines. *Cancer Res* **55**:6063, 1995.

119. Visakorpi T, Kallioniemi OP, Heikkinen A, Koivula T, Isola J: Small subgroup of aggressive, highly proliferative prostatic carcinomas defined by p53 accumulation. *J Natl Cancer Inst* **84**:883, 1992.
120. Bookstein R, MacGrogan D, Hilsenbeck SG, Sharkey F, Allred DC: *p53* is mutated in a subset of advanced-stage prostate cancers. *Cancer Res* **53**:3369, 1993.
121. Navone NM, Troncoso P, Pisters LL, Goodrow TL, Palmer JL, Nichols WW, von Eschenbach AC, Conti CJ: p53 protein accumulation and gene mutation in the progression of human prostate carcinoma. *J Natl Cancer Inst* **85**:1657, 1993.
122. Aprikian AG, Sarkis AS, Fair WR, Zhang ZF, Fuks Z, Cordon-Cardo C: Immunohistochemical determination of p53 protein nuclear accumulation in prostatic adenocarcinoma. *J Urol* **151**:1276, 1994.
123. Dinjens WN, van der Weiden MM, Schroeder FH, Bosman FT, Trapman J: Frequency and characterization of *p53* mutations in primary and metastatic human prostate cancer. *Int J Cancer* **56**:630, 1994.
124. Voeller HJ, Sugars LY, Pretlow T, Gelmann EP: *p53* oncogene mutations in human prostate cancer specimens. *J Urol* **151**:492, 1994.
125. Chi SG, deVere White RW, Meyers FJ, Siders DB, Lee F, Gumerlock PH: *p53* in prostate cancer: Frequently expressed transition mutations. *J Natl Cancer Inst* **86**:926, 1994.
126. Cairns P, Okami K, Halachmi S, Halachmi N, Esteller M, Herman JG, Jen J, Isaacs WB, Bova GS, Sidransky D: Frequent inactivation of *PTEN/MMAC1* in primary prostate cancer. *Cancer Res* 15; **57**(22):4997, 1997.
127. Suzuki H, Freije D, Nusskern DR, Okami K, Cairns P, Sidransky D, Isaacs WB, Bova GS: Interfocal heterogeneity of *PTEN/MMAC1* gene alterations in multiple metastatic prostate cancer tissues. *Cancer Res* 15; **58**(2):204, 1998.
128. Vlietstra RJ, van Alewijk DC, Hermans KG, van Steenbrugge GJ, Trapman J: Frequent inactivation of *PTEN* in prostate cancer cell lines and xenografts. *Cancer Res* **58**:2720, 1998.
129. Whang YE, Wu X, Suzuki H, Reiter RE, Tran C, Vessella RL, et al: Inactivation of the tumor suppressor *PTEN/MMAC1* in advanced human prostate cancer through loss of expression. *Proc Natl Acad Sci USA* **95**:5246, 1998.
130. Bookstein R, Shew JY, Chen PL, Scully P, Lee WH: Suppression of tumorigenicity of human prostate carcinoma cells by replacing a mutated *RB* gene. *Science* **247**:712, 1990.
131. Bookstein R, Rio P, Madreperla SA, Hong F, Allred C, Grizzle WE, Lee WH: Promoter deletion and loss of retinoblastoma gene expression in human prostate carcinoma. *Proc Natl Acad Sci USA* **87**:7762, 1990.
132. Ittmann MM, Wieczorek R: Alterations of the retinoblastoma gene in clinically localized, stage B prostate adenocarcinomas. *Hum Pathol* **27**:28, 1996.
133. Cooney KA, Wetzel JC, Merajver SD, Macoska JA, Singleton TP, Wojno KJ: Distinct regions of loss of 13q in prostate cancer. *Cancer Res* **56**:1142, 1996.
134. Kamb A, Gruis NA, Weaver-Feldhaus J, Liu Q, Harshman K, Tavtigian SV, Stockert E, Day RS, Johnson BE, Skolnick MH: A cell cycle regulator potentially involved in genesis of many tumor types (see comments). *Science* **264**:436, 1994.
135. Cairns P, Polascik TJ, Eby Y, Tokino K, Califano J, Merlo A, Mao L, Herath J, Jenkins R, Westra W, Bova GS, et al: Frequency of homozygous deletion at *p16/CDKN2* in primary human tumours. *Nature Genet* **11**:210, 1995.
136. Jarrard D, Bova GS, Ewing CM, Pin SS, Nguyen SH, Baylin SB, Cairns P, Sidransky D, Herman JG, Isaacs WB: Deletional, mutational, and methylation analyses of *CDKN2(p16/MTS1)* in primary and metastatic prostate cancer. *Genes Chromosom Cancer* **19**:90, 1997.
137. Hakimi JM, Rondinelli RH, Schoenberg MP, Barrack ER: Androgen-receptor gene structure and function in prostate cancer. *World J Urol* **14**:329, 1996.
138. Hobisch A, Culig Z, Radmayr C, Bartsch G, Klocker H, Hittmair A: Distant metastases from prostatic carcinoma express androgen receptor protein. *Cancer Res* **55**:3068, 1995.
139. Ruizeveld de Winter JA, Janssen PJ, Sleddens HM, Verleun-Mooijman MC, Trapman J, Brinkmann AO, Santerse AB, Schroder FH, van der Kwast TH: Androgen receptor status in localized and locally progressive hormone refractory human prostate cancer. *Am J Pathol* **144**:735, 1994.
140. Newmark JR, Hardy DO, Tonb DC, Carter BS, Epstein JI, Isaacs WB, Brown TR, Barrack ER: Androgen receptor gene mutations in human prostate cancer. *Proc Natl Acad Sci USA* **89**:6319, 1992.
141. Tilley WD, Buchanan G, Hickey TE, Bentel JM: Mutations in the androgen receptor gene are associated with progression of human prostate cancer to androgen independence. *Clin Cancer Res* **2**:277, 1996.
142. Kelly WK, Scher HI: Prostate specific antigen decline after antiandrogen withdrawal: The flutamide withdrawal syndrome. *J Urol* **149**:607, 1993.
143. Sartor O, Cooper M, Weinberger M, Headlee D, Thibault A, Tompkins A, Steinberg S, Figg WD, Linehan WM, Myers CE: Surprising activity of flutamide withdrawal, when combined with aminoglutethimide, in treatment of "hormone-refractory" prostate cancer [published erratum appears in *J Natl Cancer Inst* 16; **86**(6):463, 1994]. *J Natl Cancer Inst* **86**:222, 1994.
144. Harris SE, Rong Z, Harris MA, Lubahn DD: Androgen receptor in human prostate adenocarcinoma LNCaP/ADEP cells contains a mutation which alters the specificity of the steroid-dependent transcriptional activation region. *Endocrinology* **126**:93, 1990.
145. Veldscholte J, Berrevoets CA, Ris-Stalpers C, Kuiper GG, Jenster G, Trapman J, Brinkmann AO, Mulder E: The androgen receptor in LNCaP cells contains a mutation in the ligand binding domain which affects steroid binding characteristics and response to antiandrogens (review). *J Steroid Biochem Mol Biol* **41**:665, 1992.
146. Taplin ME, Bubley GJ, Shuster TD, Frantz ME, Spooner AE, Ogata GK, Keer HN, Balk SP: Mutation of the androgen-receptor gene in metastatic androgen-independent prostate cancer (see comments). *New Engl J Med* **332**:1393, 1995.
147. Visakorpi T, Hyytinen E, Koivisto P, Tanner M, Keinanen R, Palmberg C, Palotie A, Tammela T, Isola J, Kallioniemi OP: In vivo amplification of the androgen receptor gene and progression of human prostate cancer. *Nature Genet* **9**(4):401, 1995.
148. Guo Y, Sklar GN, Borkowski A, Kyprianou N: Loss of the cyclin-dependent kinase inhibitor p27(Kip1) protein in human prostate cancer correlates with tumor grade. *Clin Cancer Res* **3**:2269, 1997.
149. Yang RM, Naitoh J, Murphy M, Wang HJ, Phillipson J, deKernion JB, et al: Low p27 expression predicts poor disease-free survival in patients with prostate cancer. *J Urol* **159**:941, 1998.
150. Cote RJ, Shi Y, Groshen S, Feng AC, Cordon-Cardo C, Skinner D, et al: Association of p27Kip1 levels with recurrence and survival in patients with stage C prostate carcinoma. *J Natl Cancer Inst* **90**:916, 1998.
151. Cheville JC, Lloyd RV, Sebo TJ, Cheng L, Erickson L, Bostwick DG, et al: Expression of p27kip1 in prostatic adenocarcinoma. *Mod Pathol* **11**:324, 1998.
152. Kibel AS, Schutte M, Kern SE, Isaacs WB, Bova GS: Identification of 12p as a region of frequent deletion in advanced prostate cancer. *Cancer Res* **58**:5652, 1998.
153. Reed JC, Cuddy M, Slabiak T, Croce CM, Nowell PC: Oncogenic potential of *bcl-2* demonstrated by gene transfer. *Nature* **336**:259, 1988.
154. Hockenbery DM: The *bcl-2* oncogene and apoptosis (review). *Semin Immunol* **4**:413, 1992.
155. McDonnell TJ, Troncoso P, Brisbay SM, Logothetis C, Chung LW, Hsieh JT, Tu SM, Campbell ML: Expression of the protooncogene *bcl-2* in the prostate and its association with emergence of androgen-independent prostate cancer. *Cancer Res* **52**:6940, 1992.
156. Colombel M, Symmans F, Gil S, O'Toole KM, Chopin D, Benson M, Olsson CA, Korsmeyer S, Buttyan R: Detection of the apoptosis-suppressing oncoprotein *bcl-2* in hormone-refractory human prostate cancers. *Am J Pathol* **143**:390, 1993.
157. Furuya Y, Krajewski S, Epstein JI, Reed JC, Isaacs JT: Expression of *bcl2* in the progression of human and rodent prostatic cancers. *Clin Cancer Res* **2**:398, 1996.
158. Dong J-T, Suzuki H, Pin SS, Bova GS, Schalken JA, Isaacs WB, Barrett JC, Isaacs JT: Down-regulation of the *KAI1* metastasis suppressor gene during the progression of human prostatic cancer infrequently involves gene mutation and allelic loss. *Cancer Res* **56**: 3091, 1996.
159. Umbas R, Isaacs WB, Bringuier PP, Schaafsma HE, Karthaus HF, Oosterhof GO, Debruyne FM, Schalken JA: Decreased E-cadherin expression is associated with poor prognosis in patients with prostate cancer. *Cancer Res* **54**:3929, 1994.
160. Umbas R, Schalken JA, Aalders TW, Carter BS, Karthaus HF, Schaafsma HE, Debruyne FM, Isaacs WB: Expression of the cellular adhesion molecule E-cadherin is reduced or absent in high-grade prostate cancer. *Cancer Res* **52**:5104, 1992.
161. Morton RA, Ewing CM, Nagafuchi A, Tsukita S, Isaacs WB: Reduction of E-cadherin levels and deletion of the alpha-catenin gene in human prostate cancer cells. *Cancer Res* **53**:3585, 1993.

162. Ichikawa T, Ichikawa Y, Dong J, Hawkins AL, Griffin CA, Isaacs WB, Oshimura M, Barrett JC, Isaacs JT: Localization of metastasis suppressor gene(s) for prostatic cancer to the short arm of human chromosome 11. *Cancer Res* **52**:3486, 1992.
163. Dong J-T, Lamb PW, Rinker-Schaeffer CW, Vukanovic J, Isaacs JT, Barrett JC. KAI-1*:* A metastasis suppressor gene for prostate cancer on human chromosome 11p11.2. *Science* **268**:884, 1995.
164. Lee WH, Morton RA, Epstein JI, Brooks JD, Campbell PA, Bova GS, Hsieh WS, Isaacs WB, Nelson WG: Cytidine methylation of regulatory sequences near the pi-class glutathione *S*-transferase gene accompanies human prostatic carcinogenesis. *Proc Natl Acad Sci USA* **91(24)**:11733, 1994.
165. Lee WH, Isaacs WB, Bova GS, Nelson WG: CG island methylation changes near the *GSTP1* gene in prostatic carcinoma cells detected using the polymerase chain reaction: A new prostate cancer biomarker. *Cancer Epidemiol Biomark Prev* **6**:443, 1997.
166. Brooks JD, Weinstein M, Lin X, Sun Y, Pin SS, Bova GS, et al: CG island methylation changes near the *GSTP1* gene in prostatic intraepithelial neoplasia. *Cancer Epidemiol Biomark Prev* **7**:531, 1998.
167. Edwards A, Hammond HA, Jin L, Caskey CT, Chakraborty R: Genetic variation at five trimeric and tetrameric tandem repeat loci in four human population groups. *Genomics* **12**:241, 1992.
168. Irvine RA, Yu MC, Ross RK, Coetzee GA: The CAG and GGC microsatellites of the androgen receptor gene are in linkage disequilibrium in men with prostate cancer. *Cancer Res* **55**:1937, 1995.
169. Macke JP, Hu N, Hu S, Bailey M, King VL, Brown T, Hamer D, Nathans J: Sequence variation in the androgen receptor gene is not a common determinant of male sexual orientation. *Am J Hum Genet* **53**:844, 1993.
170. Sleddens HF, Oostra BA, Brinkmann AO, Trapman J: Trinucleotide (GGN) repeat polymorphism in the human androgen receptor (*AR*) gene. *Hum Mol Genet* **2**:493, 1993.
171. Chamberlain NL, Driver ED, Miesfeld RL: The length and location of CAG trinucleotide repeats in the androgen receptor N-terminal domain affect transactivation function. *Nucleic Acids Res* **22**:3181, 1994.
172. Kazemi-Esfarjani P, Trifiro MA, Pinsky L: Evidence for a repressive function of the long polyglutamine tract in the human androgen receptor: Possible pathogenetic relevance for the (CAG)n-expanded neuronopathies. *Hum Mol Genet* **4**:523, 1995.
173. Sobue G, Doyu M, Morishima T, Mukai E, Yasuda T, Kachi T, Mitsuma T: Aberrant androgen action and increased size of tandem CAG repeat in androgen receptor gene in X-linked recessive bulbospinal neuronopathy. *J Neurol Sci* **121**:167, 1994.
174. Reichardt JK, Makridakis N, Henderson BE, Yu MC, Pike MC, Ross RK: Genetic variability of the human *SRD5A2* gene: Implications for prostate cancer risk. *Cancer Res* **55**:3973, 1995.
175. Makridakis N, Ross RK, Pike MC, Chang L, Stanczyk FZ, Kolonel LN, et al: A prevalent missense substitution that modulates activity of prostatic steroid 5α-reductase. *Cancer Res* **57**:1020, 1997.
176. Devgan SA, Henderson BE, Yu MC, Shi CY, Pike MC, Ross RK, et al: Genetic variation of 3 beta-hydroxysteroid dehydrogenase type II in three racial/ethnic groups: Implications for prostate cancer risk. *Prostate* **33**:9, 1997.
177. Ross RK, Pike MC, Coetzee GA, Reichardt JK, Yu MC, Feigelson H, et al: Androgen metabolism and prostate cancer: Establishing a model of genetic susceptibility. *Cancer Res* **58**:4497, 1998.
178. Rodriguez R, Schuur ER, Lim HY, Henderson GA, Simons JW, Henderson DR: Prostate attenuated replication competent adenovirus (ARCA) CN706: A selective cytotoxic for prostate-specific antigen-positive prostate cancer cells. *Cancer Res* **57**:2559, 1997.
179. Simons JW, Marshall FF: The future of gene therapy in the treatment of urologic malignancies. *Urol Clin North Am* **25**:23, 1998.

CHAPTER 57

Brain Tumors

Sandra H. Bigner ▪ Roger E. McLendon
Naji Al-dosari ▪ Ahmed Rasheed

1. **Glioblastoma multiforme, the most common malignant primary brain tumor of adults, is characterized by gains of chromosome 7 and losses of chromosome 10, which are seen in up to 80 to 90 percent of patients. Approximately 25 to 30 percent of patients with loss of chromosome 10 have mutations of the *PTEN/MMAC1* gene. More than half of these tumors also contain abnormalities of genes involved in cell cycle control. Specifically, about a third of patients have homozygous deletions of the *CDKN2A* gene, while some tumors with intact *CDKN2A* have loss of expression of the retinoblastoma gene or have amplification of the *CDK4* gene. In addition, approximately one-half of patients have amplification, often with rearrangement, of the epidermal growth factor receptor (*EGFR*) gene.**
2. **Low-grade astrocytomas, particularly anaplastic astrocytomas, as well as low-grade tumors that progress to glioblastomas, contain mutations of the *TP53* gene in up to 50 percent of patients in some series.**
3. **Oligodendrogliomas are frequently characterized by losses of 1p and 19q. The target genes for loss of these regions remain unknown.**
4. **A subset of ependymomas has loss of 22q. Mutation of the neurofibromatosis type 2 (*NF2*) gene has been described in a single patient with an ependymoma. Therefore, whether or not this gene is the target of the 22q loss in these tumors remains speculative.**
5. **The most consistent finding in medulloblastomas, the most common primary malignant brain tumor of children, is loss of 17p. Mapping of the deleted region to distal 17p and a low incidence of *TP53* gene mutations suggest that *TP53* is not the target of 17p loss in these tumors. Approximately 15 percent of patients have mutations of the *PTCH* gene, in association with loss of 9q. The incidence of gene amplification has variously been reported to be from less than 5 to 22 percent in medulloblastomas. The amplified gene is usually *c-myc,* with a few examples of *N-myc* gene amplification.**
6. **Approximately 60 percent of meningiomas and schwannomas have loss of 22q, which is usually associated with *NF2* gene mutations.**

ASTROCYTOMAS

The astrocyte, one form of glial cell that comprises much of the background substance of the brain and spinal cord, is believed to give rise to a large category of primary brain tumors, the astrocytomas. These neoplasms can occur in all areas of the brain and spinal cord in children and adults. Although the vast majority of astrocytic neoplasms occur sporadically, they can be seen in patients with the familial adenomatous polyposis syndrome, the Li-Fraumeni syndrome, and central neurofibromatosis (see Chaps. 37, 40 and 48). The incidence of astrocytomas is approximately 7.0 per 100,000,[1] which means that nearly 20,000 Americans will have an astrocytoma diagnosed each year. The World Health Organization (WHO) classification[2] recognizes four grades of astrocytoma (Fig. 57-1). Grade I astrocytomas are slow-growing, noninfiltrative neoplasms, occurring mainly in children and young adults, and include juvenile pilocytic astrocytomas and gangliogliomas. Grade II astrocytomas are mainly well-differentiated fibrillary astrocytomas, whereas grade III astrocytomas are a more aggressive neoplasm, the anaplastic astrocytoma.[3] The most malignant form of astrocytoma, the grade IV tumor, is the glioblastoma multiforme, which is the most common primary malignant brain tumor of adults. Although these tumors most commonly occur in the cerebral hemispheres of older individuals, they can be seen throughout the brain and spinal cord in patients of all ages.

Chromosomal Abnormalities in Astrocytomas (Table 57-1)

The most consistent chromosomal changes in glioblastomas are gains of chromosome 7, seen in about 80 percent of tumors with abnormal stem lines, losses of chromosome 10 in 60 percent of tumors, losses of 9p in about a third of tumors, and the presence of double minute chromosomes (Dmins) in up to 50 percent of tumors[4–9] (Figs. 57-2 and 57-3).

Genetic Alterations in Astrocytomas

Loss of heterozygosity (LOH) analyses have confirmed losses of all or part of chromosome 10 in more than 90 percent of tumors (Fig. 57-4) in some series and have narrowed the smallest region of overlapping deletion to 10q25.[10,11] Most series also have identified a second region on 10p, and a third site on proximal 10q also has been targeted by some observers.[12–14] Li *et al.*[15] and Steck *et al.*[16] have identified a gene located at 10q23 that was mutated or deleted in a subset of gliomas. This gene, called *PTEN* for phosphatase and tensin homologue deleted on chromosome 10 or *MMAC1* for mutated in multiple advanced cancers, is mutated in 24 to 60 percent of glioblastomas with LOH for 10q[17–21] and in approximately 40 percent of prostatic and endometrial cancers.[22,23] Germline mutations of the *PTEN/MMAC1* gene are seen in Cowden disease and the Bannayan-Zonana syndrome.[24,25] The product of this gene is a protein tyrosine phosphatase, transforming growth factor beta (TGF-β)-regulated and epithelial cell-enriched phosphatase, or TEP1.[26] Although mutations of the *PTEN/MMAC1* gene are common in high-grade astrocytomas (glioblastomas and anaplastic astrocytomas), they are rarely seen in low-grade astrocytomas.[27,28] In addition, among glioblastomas, mutations of this gene are seen more frequently in *de novo* rather than secondary tumors.[29]

Although the *PTEN/MMAC1* gene is clearly implicated in a subset of gliomas, the location of this gene is at 10q23, whereas the most frequent region of overlapping deletions in these tumors is at 10q25-6, and the observation that many astrocytomas with

A list of standard abbreviations is located immediately preceding the index in each volume. Nonstandard abbreviations used in this chapter include: LOH = loss of heterozygosity.

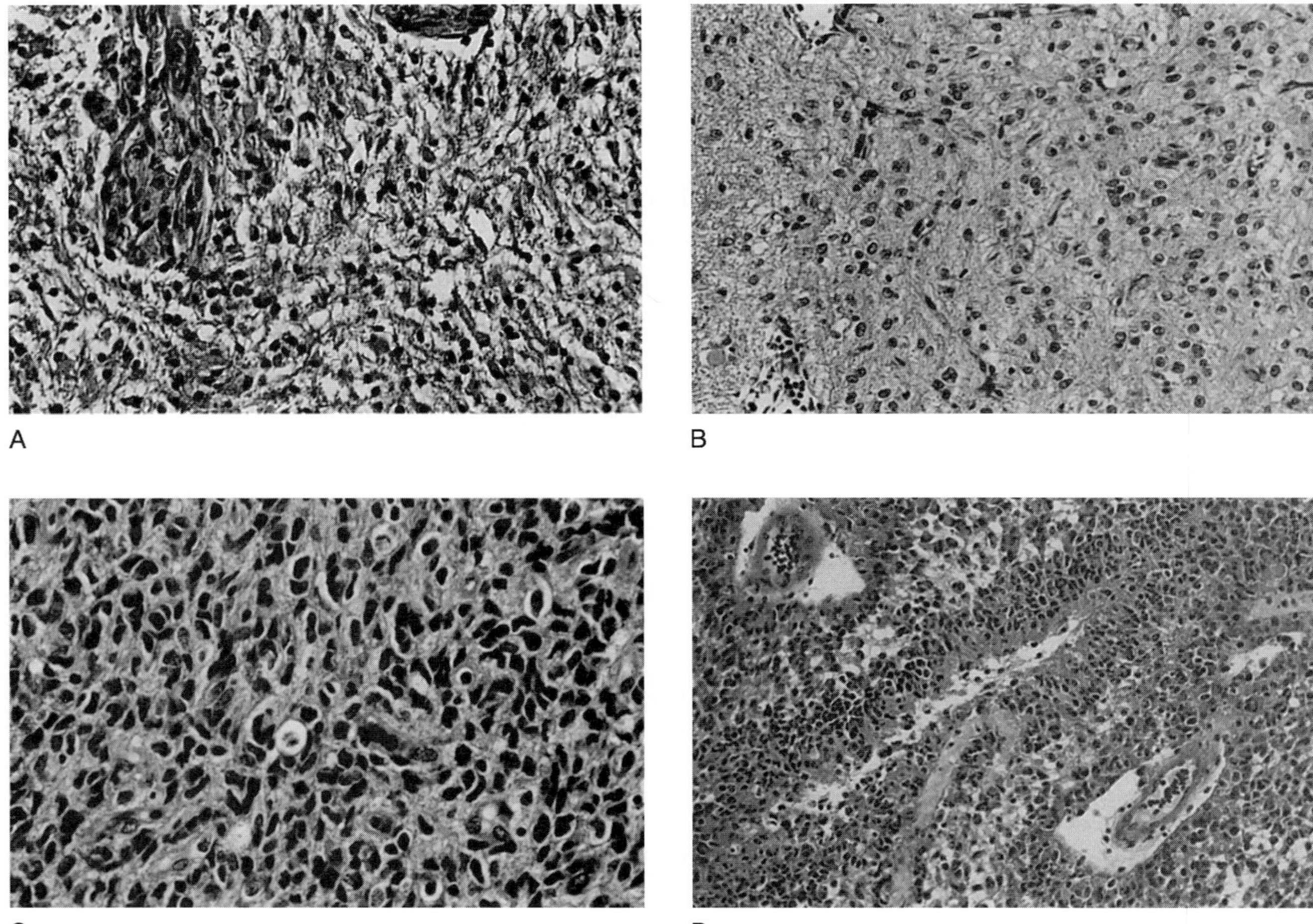

Fig. 57-1 Histology of astrocytomas. (*A*) WHO grade I astrocytomas are largely represented by pilocytic astrocytomas, which are moderately cellular neoplasms formed of bipolar astrocytes that occasionally produce Rosenthal fibers. (*B*) WHO grade II astrocytomas, also known as well-differentiated fibrillary astrocytomas, are composed of unipolar and stellate astrocytes with simplified processes that exhibit mild nuclear pleomorphism and a proliferation index of 1 percent or less. (*C*) Grade III astrocytomas, or anaplastic astrocytomas, are highly cellular neoplasms composed largely of unipolar astrocytes exhibiting nuclear pleomorphism and a brisk proliferation index but lacking in tumor necrosis and vascular proliferation. (*D*) Grade IV astrocytomas, or glioblastomas, form the most malignant end of the spectrum and are characterized by astrocytic neoplasms exhibiting nuclear pleomorphism, brisk proliferation index, vascular proliferation, and/or necrosis with pseudopalisading.

Table 57-1 Chromosomal and Genetic Alterations Characteristic of Specific Types of Brain Tumors

Tumor Type	Chromosomal or LOH Abnormality	Genetic Alteration
Glioblastoma	+7	Unknown
	−9p	*CDKN2A, CDKN2B*
	−10	*PTEN/MMAC1* gene mutation, *DMBT1* deletion?
	−17p	*p53* gene mutation
	Dmins	*EGFR* gene amplification and rearrangement
Oligodendroglioma	−1p, −19q	Unknown
Ependymoma	−22	*NF2* gene mutation?
Medulloblastoma	−17p	Unknonwn
	−9q	*PTCH* gene mutation
	Dmins	*c-myc, N-myc* gene amplification
Meningioma	−22	*NF2* gene mutation
Schwannoma	−22	*NF2* gene mutation

LOH for 10q lack mutations of this gene has raised the possibility that another chromosome 10 gene or genes may be involved in gliomas. Candidate genes in the 10q25 region include *MXI1* and *PAX-2*.[30–32] *DMBT1,* for deleted in malignant brain tumors, is located at 10q25.3-26.1. This gene, which shows homology to the scavenger receptor cysteine-rich superfamily, was shown to be homozygously deleted in 9 of 39 glioblastomas and 2 of 20 medulloblastomas by Mollenhauer et al.[33] Although this gene was not expressed in 4 of 5 brain tumor cell lines, the lack of demonstration of point mutations in these tumors raises the possibility that this gene may not be the target of the deletions.

LOH analyses of astrocytomas revealed that approximately one-third of these tumors have loss of all or part of 17p.[34–45] Unlike the chromosomal deviations described earlier, which are seen mainly in glioblastomas, LOH for 17p occurs in astrocytomas of all grades. Point mutations of the *p53* gene can be demonstrated in the majority of astrocytomas with 17p loss. The mutations are clustered in the same hot spots as are seen in colon, breast, and lung carcinomas. The incidence of *TP53* mutations, confirmed by sequence data, is about 25 percent (73 of 295) in glioblastomas, 34 percent (49 of 144) in anaplastic astrocytomas, and 30 percent (33 of 111) in astrocytomas.[38–40,45–54] Most of the *TP53* studies have concentrated on the conserved exons 5 through 8, but studies that included the entire coding sequence (exons 2–11) have uncovered

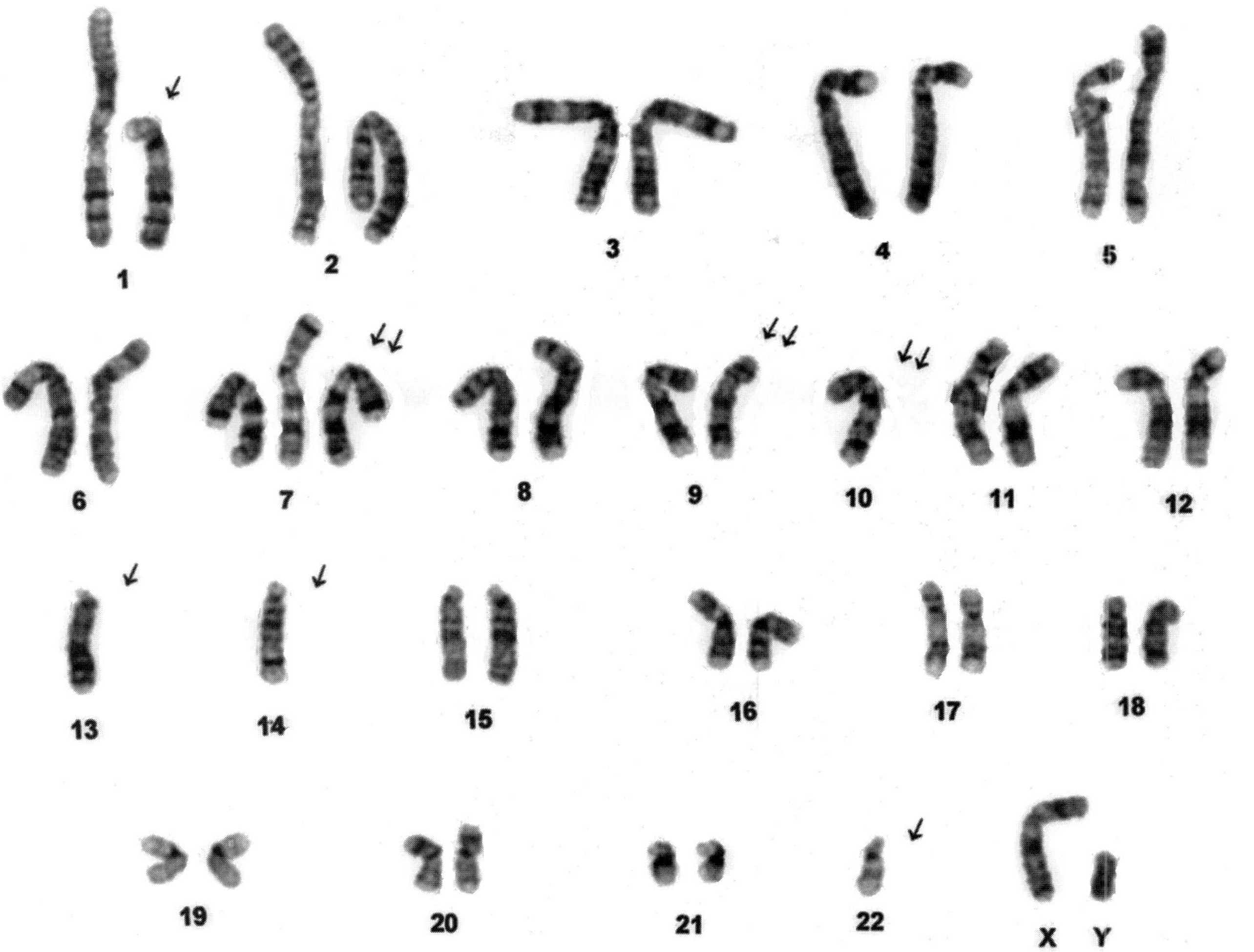

Fig. 57-2 Karyotype of glioblastoma. This Giemsa-trypsin–banded karyotype of glioblasoma xenograft D-643 MG shows gain of chromosome 7, a deletion of 9p, and loss of a chromosome 10 (double arrows). Additional, nonspecific changes are marked with single arrows.

only a handful of mutations outside of exons 5 through 8.[38,40,46,47,50] Similar to colon cancer, codons 175, 248, and 273 are frequently mutated in brain tumors, but the codon that is most frequently mutated in brain is codon 273, whereas in colon it is codon 175.[52] *TP53* mutations are associated with age of the patient. These alterations are rare among pediatric patients[43,45,50,52,55,56] but occur in nearly 50 percent of tumors in young adults, with a much lower incidence (<20 percent) in patients over 50 years of age. Most of the *TP53* mutations identified in astrocytomas are G-to-C > A-to-T transitions located at CpG sites and resemble the pattern of mutations found in colon cancer, sarcomas, and lymphomas.

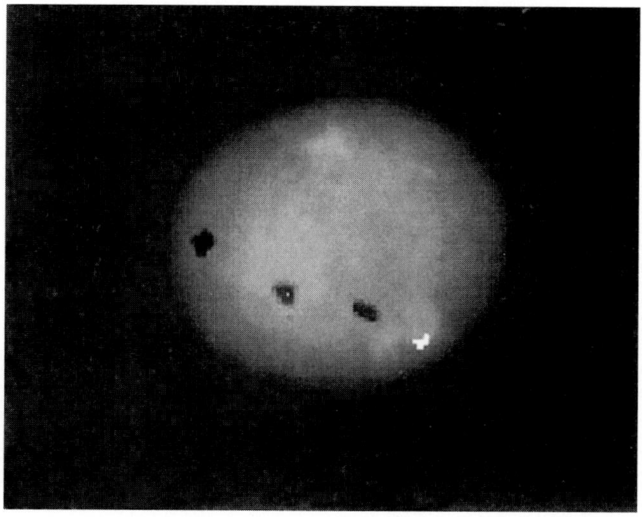

Fig. 57-3 FISH of glioblastoma. This interphase nucleus from a glioblastoma contains three chromosome 7 centromere signals (dark) and one centromere 10 signal (light).

The cytogenetic observation of 9p loss in gliomas prompted evaluation of the α and β interferon genes, which are located at 9p22. Hemizygous or homozygous deletion of interferon genes

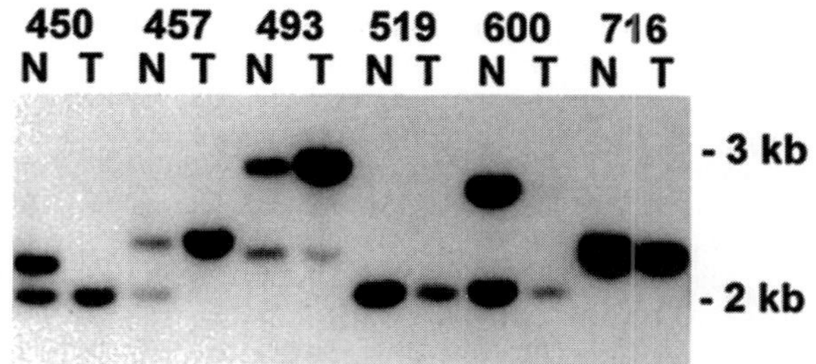

Fig. 57-4 LOH of glioblastoma chromosome 10. A Southern blot of Taq I-digested DNA (5 μg) from blood (N) and glioblastoma tumor (T) was hybridized to the 10q marker D10S25. This marker showed LOH in tumors 450, 457, 493, and 600 and was uninformative in tumors 519 and 716. The size of the alleles ranged from 1.9 to 3 kb.

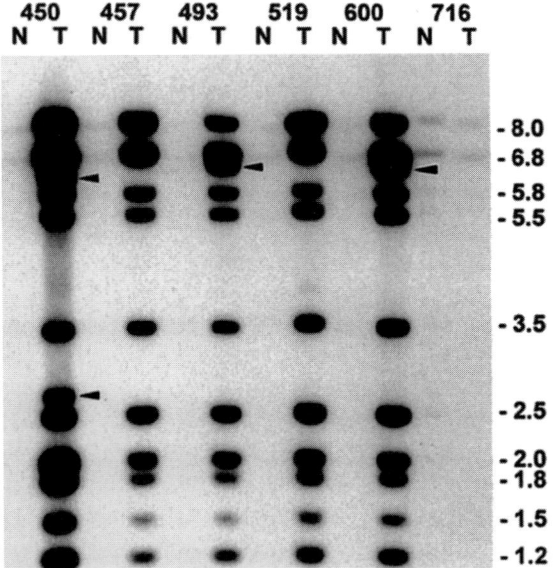

Fig. 57-5 Southern blot gene amplification, glioblastoma. A Southern blot of EcoRI-digested DNA (5 μg) from blood (N) and glioblastoma tumor (T) was hybridized with *EGFR* gene probe pE7. The hybridizing fragments, in samples with normal copy number of the gene (all blood and tumor 716), appear as faint bands, and their sizes (in kb) are indicated on the right. In tumors 457 and 519 the gene was amplified, and in 450, 493, and 600 the gene was amplified and rearranged. Arrows indicate variant bands resulting from gene rearrangement.

was reported in glioma cell lines and in biopsies of high-grade astrocytomas,[57,58] but it was not clear in these early studies whether the interferon genes were the target of 9p deletions in gliomas or were simply located near the region of the target gene. In 1994, the *CDKN2A* and *CDKN2B* genes, which are located at 9p21, were found to be homozygously deleted in various types of tumors including gliomas.[59] By combining data collected on tumor biopsies in several laboratories, the overall incidence of homozygous deletions is 33 percent (98 of 300) in glioblastomas and 24 percent in anaplastic astrocytomas (19 of 79) and for hemizygous deletion or LOH for 9p loci is 24 percent of glioblastomas and 18 percent of anaplastic astrocytomas. The incidence of homozygous deletions of both *CDKN2A* and *CDKN2B* is higher in xenografts, approaching 80 percent in some studies.[60] Among the 23 low-grade astrocytoma biopsies analyzed, none exhibited homozygous deletion, although 5 showed LOH, altogether there have been only 3 cases of mutations, all in glioblastomas.[61–70] The high frequency of homozygous deletions on chromosome 9 and the inclusion of *CDKN2A* and *CDKN2B* gene sequences in the deleted region in most cases has led observers to believe that *CDKN2A* and *CDKN2B* are the target suppressor genes for 9p loss in gliomas. Unlike the *p53* gene, which usually undergoes point mutation, the most common mechanism for *CDKN2A* gene inactivation in gliomas is homozygous deletion. However, alternative mechanisms such as transcriptional silencing by hypermethylation of CpG islands may be responsible for reduced expression in some gliomas with intact *CDKN2A/CDKN2B* genes.[71]

The majority of glioblastomas that possess Dmins contain amplification of the *EGFR* gene.[72] The *EGFR* gene has been shown to be amplified in one-third to one-half of glioblastomas but only in isolated cases of anaplastic astrocytomas and rarely in other lower-grade tumors. In many glioblastomas, the amplified *EGFR* gene is also rearranged[73,74] (Fig. 57-5). The most common class of mutants bears deletion of exons 2 through 7 of the gene, resulting in an in-frame deletion of 801 bp of coding sequence and generation of a glycine residue at the fusion point. This variant receptor, designated EGFRvIII, has been reported in 17 to 62 percent of glioblastomas.[75–80] The tumor cell membrane fractions containing the mutant 140-kDa receptor show a significant elevation in tyrosine kinase activity without its ligand.[81] The mutant is still capable of binding with its ligand but at a significantly reduced affinity.[82]

Relationship Between Cell Cycle Regulators in Astrocytomas

In addition to deletions of the *CDKN2A* and *CDKN2B* genes as discussed earlier, alterations of other genes involved in cell cycle regulation have been described in subsets of astrocytomas. LOH for 13q or loss of expression of the retinoblastoma (*Rb*) gene product has been described in 20 to 40 percent of glioblastomas,[12,37,70,83–86] and amplification of the *CDK4* gene has been described in up to 15 percent of glioblastomas.[64,87] Furthermore, He *et al.*,[86] Biernat,[88] and Ueki *et al.*[70] have shown that most glioblastomas contain only one of these three alterations: (1) *CDKN2A/CDKN2B* deletion, (2) LOH for 13q or loss of *Rb* expression, or (3) *CDK4* gene amplification or increased expression.

Genetic Alterations in the Progression of Gliomas

It has long been recognized that there are two patterns for the development of glioblastomas. The majority of these tumors occur in patients over 50 years of age, in individuals with no previous indication of a brain tumor. A second group of patients involves younger people whose glioblastomas evolve out of lower-grade astrocytomas. Recent studies have provided molecular markers that in many cases distinguish between these two clinical patterns. The *de novo* pathway, occurring in older patients, includes tumors over 50 percent of which contain *EGFR* gene amplification and the majority of which lack *TP53* gene mutations.[42–44,88] Glioblastomas evolving through progression, in contrast, seldom have *EGFR* gene amplification, and more than 50 percent contain *TP53* gene mutations.[41,88–93]

Other molecular markers, including LOH for chromosome 10, *CDKN2A* and *CDKN2B* deletions, *Rb* and *CDK4* abnormalities, and amplification of other oncogenes do not appear to differ in tumors arising through these two pathways.

OLIGODENDROGLIOMAS

Oligodendrogliomas are a type of glioma that occur mainly in the cerebral hemispheres of adults and are derived from the oligodendrocyte. Well-differentiated oligodendrogliomas exhibiting benign cytologic features are considered grade II according to the WHO classification (Fig. 57-6), whereas anaplastic oligoden-

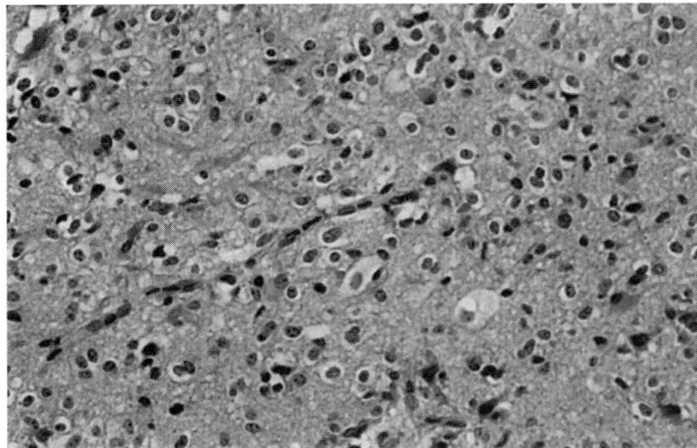

Fig. 57-6 Oligodendrogliomas are characterized by cells with round to oval nuclei surrounded by perinuclear cytoplasmic haloes and usually associated with a fine arcuating network of tubular vessels.

drogliomas exhibiting abundant mitotic activity, necrosis without pseudopalisading, and glomeruloid vascular proliferation are considered grade III tumors. According to data collected by the Surveillance, Epidemiology, and End Results (SEER) Project, the age-adjusted incidence of oligodendroglioma is 0.33 per 100,000.[1]

Chromosomal Abnormalities in Oligodendrogliomas

Although most cytogenetic analyses of oligodendrogliomas have failed to demonstrate consistent findings, LOH studies have shown that loss of 1p and 19q occurs in a substantial proportion of these tumors. Bello *et al.*[94] reported LOH for loci on 1p in up to 100 percent (6 of 6) oligodendrogliomas and in most (5 of 6) anaplastic oligodendrogliomas. Among other types of gliomas, only 2 of 11 glioblastomas exhibited 1p LOH, suggesting that 1p LOH is characteristic of tumors of oligodendroglial origin. A high incidence of 1p loss in tumors of oligodendroglial origin has been confirmed by Reifenberger *et al.*[95] using LOH techniques, and by *in situ* hybridization, Hashimoto *et al.*[96] found deletion of a 1p locus in 9 of 9 oligodendrogliomas.

Analysis with restriction fragment length polymorphism and microsatellite markers showed loss of markers on chromosome 19 in about 63 percent (17 of 27) of grade II oligodendrogliomas, 75 percent (18 of 24) of grade III or anaplastic oligodendrogliomas, and 48 percent (21 of 43) of mixed oligoastrocytomas.[95,97,98] This abnormality also has been reported in about 16 percent (4 of 25) of astrocytomas, 38 percent (13 of 34) of anaplastic astrocytomas, and 28 percent (37 of 130) of glioblastomas tested.[97,98] Loss of loci on 19q was more frequent among oligodendroglial tumors, whereas astrocytic tumors mostly lost 19p alleles.[98] The 19q minimal deletion region has been mapped to a 425-kb region on 19q13.3.[99,100]

EPENDYMOMAS

Ependymomas are a category of glioma derived from the ventricular lining that can occur at many locations within the brain and spinal cord of adults and children predominantly associated with the ventricular system. Favored sites include the posterior fossa (IVth ventricle) in children, the lateral ventricles in adults, and the cauda equina in patients of all ages. Most lesions are classified histologically as grade II (Fig. 57-7), whereas tumors with anaplastic features (anaplastic ependymomas, grade III) are sometimes seen. Central neurofibromatosis (NF type 2) is associated with ependymoma, most commonly of the spinal cord. SEER data indicate an age-adjusted incidence of 0.18 per 100,000.[1]

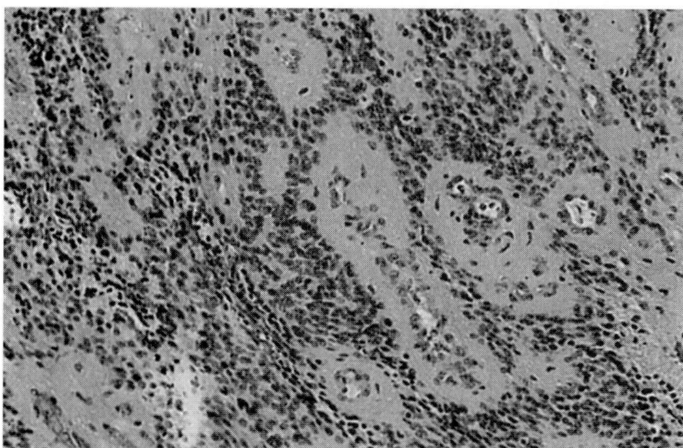

Fig. 57-7 Ependymomas often form perivascular pseudorosettes in which the tumor cells project slender fibrillar processes toward vessels while the nuclei appear excluded to a certain distance.

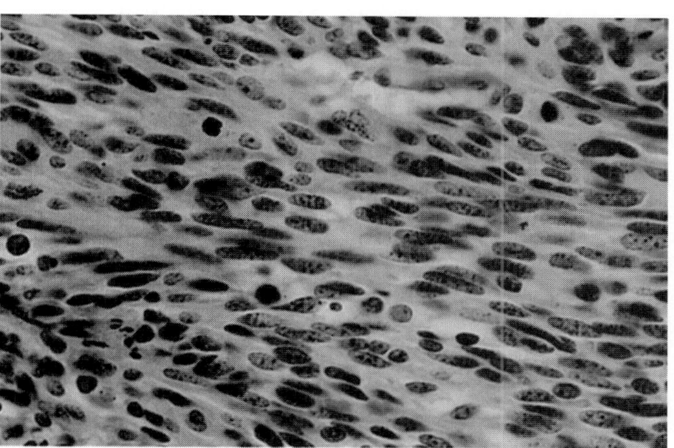

Fig. 57-8 Medulloblastomas are embryonal neoplasms that are markedly cellular, with tumor cells generally exhibiting minimal amounts of cytoplasm. Although the classic growth pattern is that of diffuse sheets of tumor cells, up to a third of cases will show a nodular growth pattern, of uncertain significance.

Chromosomal Abnormalities in Ependymomas

The most common cytogenetic abnormality in ependymomas is loss or structural alteration of chromosome 22, seen as an isolated finding in some patients and as part of a more complex picture in others. This alteration characterizes approximately 10 to 20 percent of patients with abnormal stem lines in most cytogenetic studies, and a similar incidence of chromosome 22 loss has been described in LOH studies.[101–112] Some observers, however, have noted this abnormality in a high proportion of patients by karyotype[103,106,110] or by LOH analysis.[113,114] Since the *NF2* gene is located on 22q, it has been considered as a possible target for loss of this chromosomal region in ependymomas. However, since only one somatic mutation of this gene has been reported among 25 ependymomas that were studied, the role of *NF2* mutations in ependymomas remains speculative.[115]

MEDULLOBLASTOMAS

Medulloblastoma, the most common malignant primary brain tumor of childhood, is a small cell neoplasm that arises in the cerebellum. Owing to the primitive morphology of the cells with lack of differentiation and their resemblance to some poorly differentiated supratentorial neoplasms, these tumors have been called "primitive neuroectodermal tumors (PNET)" by some observers. They are characterized by sheets of small cells with scant cytoplasm and a high mitotic rate (Fig. 57-8). Medulloblastomas are usually a sporadic tumor but can be seen in association with familial adenomatous polyposis (see Chap. 48). In the United Kingdom, the incidence of medulloblastoma has been estimated at 0.5 per 100,000 children less than 15 years old age,[116] with an overall age-adjusted incidence reported by the Central Brain Tumor Registry of the United States (CBTRUS) of 0.2 per 100,000.[117]

Chromosomal Abnormalities in Medulloblastomas

The most common specific chromosomal abnormality in medulloblastomas is loss of 17p, through formation of isochromosome 17q [i(17q)] or by unbalanced translocations[103,104,111,118–123] (Fig. 57-9). By karyotype as well as LOH studies, the incidence of this feature is approximately 30 to 40 percent.[113,124–129] Despite the location of the *TP53* gene on 17p, *TP53* gene mutations are uncommon in these tumors, seen in about 5 percent of cases.[126,128,130–135] This observation, along with mapping of the deleted region to 17p13.1-13.3, which is distal to the *p53* gene, suggests that another as yet undescribed gene is likely to be the target of 17p loss in these tumors.

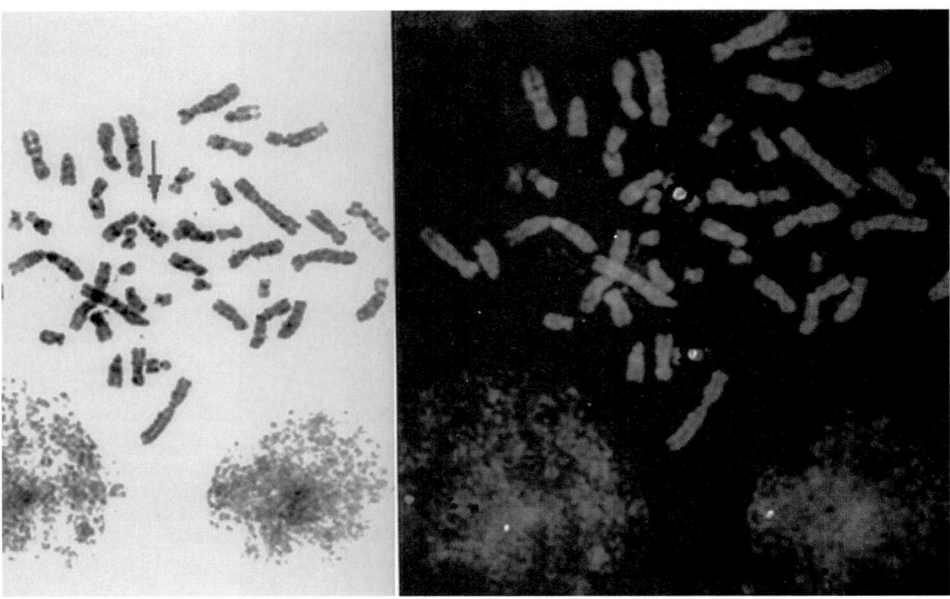

Fig. 57-9 Medulloblastoma with i(17q). The dark label that corresponds to a 17q probe stains the normal q arm of one chromosome 17 and both q arms of the i(17q). The light label marks the 17 centromere in both the normal chromosome 17 and i(17q).

Genetic Alterations in Medulloblastomas

Dmins are seen in about 5 percent of medulloblastoma biopsies but can be identified in almost all permanent cultured cell lines and xenografts derived from these.[118,136] In most samples with Dmins, amplification of the *c-myc* or, less often, the *N-myc* gene can be demonstrated[128,136–142] (Fig. 57-10). The true incidence of *myc* gene amplification is difficult to determine in these tumors because the observed incidence differs according to the method of analysis. However, a recent analysis by comparative genomic hybridization suggested that it may be as high as 18 percent.[143]

The gene for the nevoid basal cell carcinoma (Gorlin) syndrome was mapped to 9q22.3-q31 by linkage analysis. Since patients with this genetic defect are susceptible to developing medulloblastoma, this region was investigated by LOH studies in 3 medulloblastomas from patients with this syndrome and 17 sporadic medulloblastomas by Schofield *et al.*[144] They found loss of this region in both informative cases from Gorlin syndrome patients and in 3 of 17 (18 percent) sporadic tumors. All 3 sporadic tumors with loss were of the desmoplastic type. The Gorlin syndrome gene was identified as *PTCH,* the human homologue of the *Drosophila patched* gene, by Johnson *et al.*[145] and Hahn *et al.*[146] Raffel *et al.*[147] demonstrated mutations of *PTCH* in 3 of 5 sporadic medulloblastomas with 9q LOH. Reports from other laboratories have confirmed *PTCH* mutations in about 15 percent of sporadic medulloblastomas.[148–151] The majority of tumors containing the deletions have desmoplastic histology and exhibit LOH for 9q22. The *PTCH* gene product is a transmembrane receptor for the Sonic hedgehog protein. This observation has prompted investigators to evaluate other members of the *PTCH* gene pathway for alterations in medulloblastoma. Reifenberger *et al.*[152] have described one sporadic medulloblastoma with a mutation of the *SMOH* gene, the product of which is known to complex with *PTCH*.

Medulloblastomas are often seen in Turcot syndrome patients who carry germ-line mutations of the *APC* gene.[153] Although mutations of the *APC* gene have not been demonstrated in sporadic medulloblastomas, the β-catenin gene, the product of which

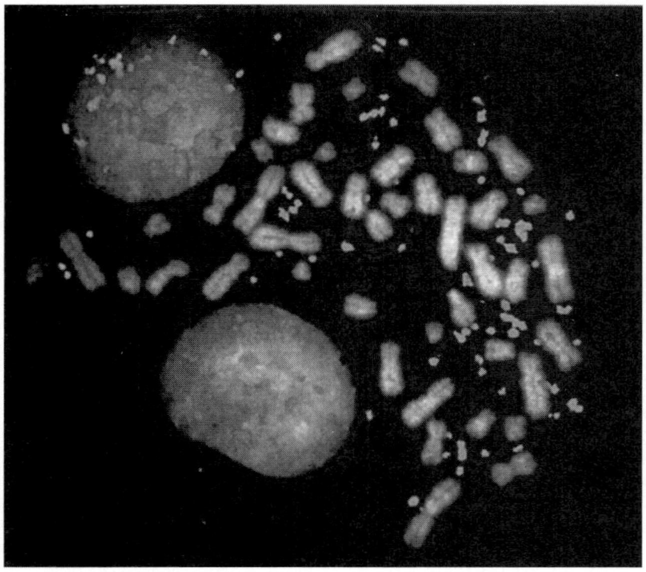

Fig. 57-10 Medulloblastoma with *c-myc* gene amplification. The *c-myc* probe, labeled darkly, is duplicated numerous times, as seen in the interphase nuclei and in the Dmins of a chromosomal spread.

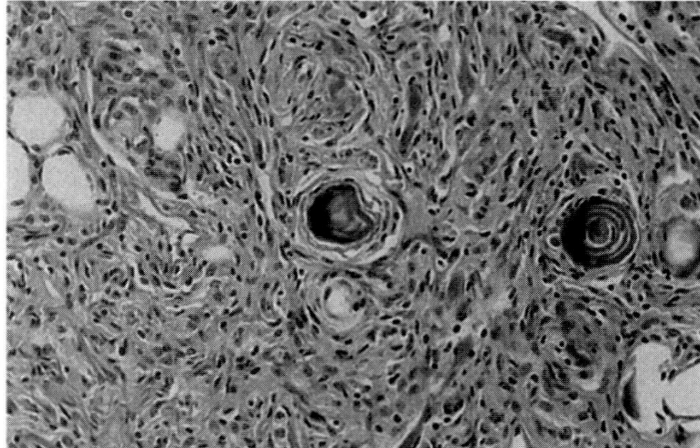

Fig. 57-11 Meningiomas are dural-based neoplasms that grow as noninfiltrating masses, pushing brain away. These spindle cell tumors are often arranged in whorls and cords separated by collagen and occasionally are associated with eosinophilic psammoma bodies.

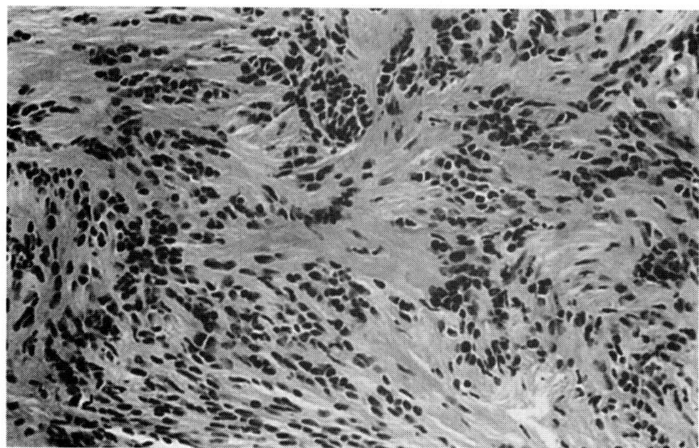

Fig. 57-12 Schwannomas also grow as solid, noninfiltrating tumors but are found along peripheral, and some cranial, nerves. The histologic hallmark of the schwannoma is the Verocay body, which is an anuclear zone formed by palisading tumor cell nuclei.

interacts with the *APC* gene product, has been shown to be mutated in 3 of 67 sporadic medulloblastomas.[154]

MENINGIOMA AND SCHWANNOMA

Meningiomas are slow-growing neoplasms derived from the meningothelial cell that forms the arachnoid membrane. These tumors are composed of swirling sheets of cells with oval nuclei, often forming whorls and psammoma bodies (Fig. 57-11). They are generally considered to be benign, because they often can be excised completely surgically, but occasional cases recur and can show aggressive clinical characteristics. SEER data indicate an age-adjusted incidence of 0.13 per 100,000, although data reported by CBTRUS support a much higher incidence of 2.5 per 100,000.[116,117]

Schwannomas are benign neoplasms, derived from the schwann cell that forms myelin in the peripheral nervous system. They are found attached to cranial or peripheral nerves, with favored sites being the acoustic and other sensory nerves. CBTRUS data report an overall incidence of nerve sheath tumors of 0.7 per 100,000.[117] Histologically, they form masses of spindle-shaped cells and are usually benign (Fig. 57-12). Both schwannomas, particularly bilateral lesions involving the acoustic nerves, and meningiomas are components of central neurofibromatosis type 2, and peripheral schwannomas occur in peripheral neurofibromatosis or NF type 1 (see Chaps. 39 and 40).

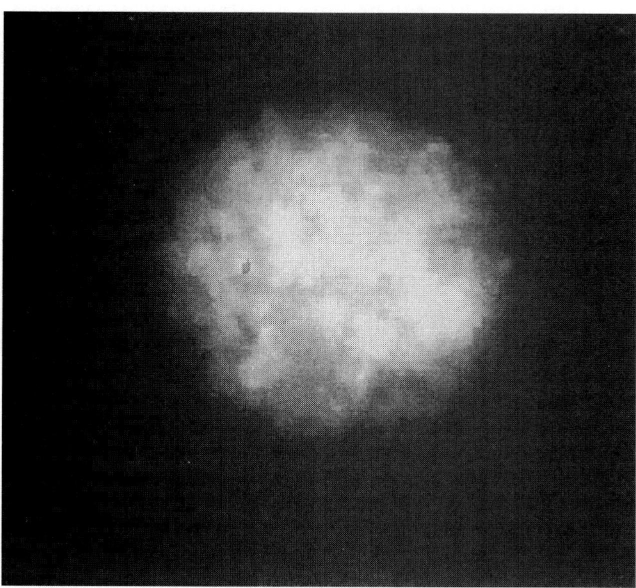

Fig. 57-13 FISH using a chromosome 22 probe in a meningioma. This interphase nucleus from a meningioma contains only one chromosome 22 signal.

Genetic Alterations in Meningiomas and Schwannomas

One of the first chromosomal abnormalities described in a solid human tumor was monosomy for a G-group chromosome.[155] With the implementation of banding techniques, the missing chromosome was identified as number 22 in the early 1970s.[156,157] Loss or deletion of chromosome 22 is the most consistent karyotypic abnormality seen in this tumor type, occurring in about 60 percent of cases[158] (Fig. 57-13). LOH studies confirmed loss of 22q in 40 to 60 percent of both meningiomas and schwannomas.[159–165] This observation, taken together with the occurrence of these tumors in NF2 and linkage studies that localized the NF2 locus to 22q, raised the possibility that the *NF2* gene was the target of chromosome 22 loss in these two tumor types. Isolation of the *NF2* gene and sequencing of this gene in these tumors confirmed that 40 to 60 percent of sporadic meningiomas and schwannomas contain *NF2* gene mutations.[166–172]

REFERENCES

1. Velema JP, Percy CL: Age curves of central nervous system tumor incidence in adults: Variation of shape by histologic type. *J Natl Cancer Inst* **79**:623, 1987.
2. Kleihues P, Burger PC, Scheithauer BW: *Histological Typing of Tumours of the Central Nervous System*, 2nd ed. New York, Springer-Verlag, 1993.
3. Burger PC, Scheithauer BW, Vogel FS: *Surgical Pathology of the Nervous System and Its Coverings*. New York, Churchill-Livingstone, 1991.
4. Rey JA, Bellow J, deCampos JM, Kusak EM, Ramos C, Benitez J: Chromosomal patterns in human malignant astrocytomas. *Cancer Genet Cytogenet* **29**:201, 1987.
5. Bigner SH, Mark J, Burger P, Mahaley MS Jr, Bullard DE, Muhlbaier LH, Bigner DD: Specific chromosomal abnormalities in malignant human gliomas. *Cancer Res* **48**:405, 1988.
6. Jenkins RJ, Kimmel DW, Moertel CA, Schultz CG, Schiethauer BW, Kelly PJ, Dewald GW: A cytogenetic study of 53 human gliomas. *Cancer Genet Cytogenet* **39**:253, 1989.
7. Thiel G, Losanowa T, Kintzel D, Nisch G, Martin H, Vorpahl K, Witkowski R: Karyotypes in 90 human gliomas. *Cancer Genet Cytogenet* **58**:109, 1992.
8. Hecht BK, Turc-Carel C, Chatel M, Grellier P, Gioanni J, Attias R, Gaudray P, Hecht F: Cytogenetics of malignant gliomas: 1. The autosomes with reference to rearrangements. *Cancer Genet Cytogenet* **84**:1, 1995.
9. Debiec-Rychter M, Alwasiak J, Liberski PP, Nedoszytko B, Babinska M, Mrózek K, Imielinski B, Borowska-Lehman J, Limon J: Accumulation of chromosomal changes in human glioma progression: A cytogenetic study of 50 cases. *Cancer Genet Cytogenet* **85**:61, 1995.
10. Fults D, Pedone C: Deletion mapping of the long arm of chromosome 10 in glioblastoma multiforme. *Genes Chromosom Cancer* **7**:173, 1993.
11. Rasheed BK, McLendon RE, Friedman HS, Friedman AH, Fuchs HE, Bigner DD, Bigner SH: Chromosome 10 deletion mapping in human gliomas: A common deletion region in 10q25. *Oncogene* **10**:2243, 1995.
12. Ransom DT, Ritland SR, Moertel CA, Dahl RJ, O'Fallon JR, Scheithauer BW, Kimmel DW, Kelly PJ, Olopade OI, Diaz MO, Jenkins RB: Correlation of cytogenetic analysis and loss of heterozygosity studies in human diffuse astrocytomas and mixed oligo-astrocytomas. *Genes Chromosom Cancer* **5**:357, 1992.
13. Karlbom AE, James CD, Boethius J, Cavenee WK, Collins VP, Nordenskjold M, Larsson C: Loss of heterozygosity in malignant gliomas involves at least three distinct regions on chromosome 10. *Hum Genet* **92**:169, 1993.
14. Kimmelman AC, Ross DA, Liang BC: Loss of heterozygosity of chromosome 10p in human gliomas. *Genomics* **34**:250, 1996.

15. Li J, Yen C, Liaw D, Podsypanina K, Bose S, Wang WI, Puc J, Millaresis C, Rodgers L, McCombie R, Bigner SH, Giovanelia BC, Ittmann M, Tycko B, Hibshoosh H, Wigler MH, Parsons R: *PTEN,* a putative protein tyrosine phosphatase gene mutated in human brain, breast, and prostate cancer. *Science* **273**:1943, 1997.
16. Steck PA, Pershouse MA, Jasser SA, Yung WKA, Lin H, Ligon AH, Langford LA, Baumgard ML, Hattier T, Davis T, Frye C, Hu R, Swedland B, Teng DHF, Tavtigian SV: Identification of a candidate tumour suppressor gene, *MMAC1,* a chromosome 10q23.3 that is mutated in multiple advanced cancers. *Nature Genet* **15**:356, 1997.
17. Wang SI, Pac J, Li J, Brace JN, Cairns P, Sidramsky D, Parsons R: Somatic mutations of *PTEN* in glioblastoma multiforme. *Cancer Res* **57**:4183, 1997.
18. Liu W, James CD, Frederick L, Alderete BE, Jenkins RB: *PTEN/MAC1* mutations and *EGFR* amplification in glioblastomas. *Cancer Res* **57**:5254, 1997.
19. Teng DHJ, Hu R, Lin H, Davis T, Ilev D, Frye C, Swedlund B, Hansen KL, Vinson VL, Gumpper KL, Ellis L, El-Naggar A, Frazier M, Jasser S, Langford LA, Lee J, Mills GB, Perhouse MA, Pollack RE, Tornos C, Troncoso P, Yung WKA, Fujii G, Berson A, Bookstein R, Boten JB, Tavtigian SV, Steck PA: *MMAC1/PTEN* mutations in primary tumor specimens and tumor cell lines. *Cancer Res* **57**:5231, 1997.
20. Fults D, Pedone CA, Thompson GE, Uchiyama CM, Gumpper KL, Iliev D, Vinson VL, Tavtigian SV, Perry WL III: Microsatellite deletion mapping on chromosome 10q and mutation analysis of *MMAC1, FAS,* and *MX11* in human glioblastoma multiforme. *Int J Oncol* **12**:905, 1998.
21. Boström J, Cobbers JMJL, Wolter M, Tabatabai G, Weber RG, Lichter P, Collins VP, Reifenberger G: Mutation of the *PTEN* (*MMAC1*) tumor suppressor gene in a subset of glioblastomas but not in meningiomas with loss of chromosome arm 10q. *Cancer Res* **51**:29, 1998.
22. Cairns P, Okami K, Hatachmi S, Hatachmi N, Esteller M, Herman JG, Jen J, Isaacs WB, Bova GS, Sidransky D: Frequent inactivation of *PTEN/MMAC1* in primary prostate cancer. *Cancer Res* **57**:4997, 1997.
23. Maxwell GL, Risinger JI, Gumbs C, Shaw H, Bentley RC, Barrett JC, Berchuck A, Futreal PA: Mutation of the *PTEN* tumor suppressor gene in endometrial hyperplasias. *Cancer Res* **58**:2500, 1998.
24. Marsh DJ, Dahia PLM, Zheng Z, Liaw D, Parsons R, Gorlin RJ, Eng C: Germline mutations in *PTEN* are present in Bannayan-Zonana syndrome. *Nature Genet* **16**:333, 1997.
25. Marsh DJ, Dahia PLM, Coulon V, Zheng Z, Dorion-Bonnet F, Call KM, Little R, Lin AY, Eles RA, Goldstein AM, Hodgson SV, Richardson A-L, Robinson BG, Weber HC Longy M, Eng C: Allelic imbalance, including deletion of *PTEN/MMAC1,* at the Cowden disease locus on 10q22-23, in hamartomas from patients with Cowden syndrome and germline *PTEN* mutation. *Genes Chromosom Cancer* **21**:61, 1998.
26. Li DM, Sum H: *TEP1,* encoded by a candidate tumor suppressor locus is a novel protein tyrosine phosphatase regulated by transforming growth factor β1. *Cancer Res* **57**:2124, 1997.
27. Rasheed BKA, Stenzel TT, McLendon RE, Parsons R, Friedman AH, Friedman HS, Bigner DD, Bigner SH: *PTEN* gene mutations are seen in high-grade but not in low-grade gliomas. *Cancer Res* **57**:4187, 1997.
28. Duerr EM, Rollbrocker B, Hayashi Y, Peters N, Meyer-Puttlitz B, Louis DN, Schramm J, Wiestler OD, Parsons R, Eng C, von Deimling A: *PTEN* mutations in gliomas and glioneuronal tumors. *Oncogene* **16**:2259, 1998.
29. Tohma Y, Gratas C, Biernat W, Peraud A, Foxuda M, Yonekawa Y, Kleihues P, Ohgaki H: *PTEN* (*MMAC1*) mutations are frequent in primary glioblastomas (*de novo*) but not in secondary glioblastomas. *J Neuropathol Exp Neurol* **57**:684, 1998.
30. Eagle LR, Yin X, Brothman AR, Williams BJ, Atkin NB, Prochownik EV: Mutation of the *MXI1* gene in prostate cancer. *Nature Genet* **9**:249, 1995.
31. Stapleton P, Weith A, Urbanek P, Kozmik Z, Busslinger M: Chromosomal localization of seven *PAX* genes and cloning of a novel family member, *PAX-9*. *Nature Genet* **3**:292, 1993.
32. Wechsler DS, Shelly CA, Petroff CA, Dang CV: *MX11,* a putative tumor suppressor gene, suppresses growth of human glioblastoma cells. *Cancer Res* **57**:4905, 1997.
33. Mollenhauer J, Wiemann S, Scheurlen W, Korn B, Hayashi Y, Wilgenbus KK, von Diemling A, Poustka A: *DMBT1,* a new member of the SRCR superfamily, on chromosome 10q25.3-26.1 is deleted in malignant brain tumours. *Nature Genet* **17**:32, 1997.
34. Eel-Azouzi M, Chung RY, Farmer GE, Martuza RL, Black PM, Rouleau GA, Hettlich C, Hedley-Whyte ET, Zervas NT, Panagopoulos K, Nakamura Y, Gusella JF, Seizinger BR: Loss of distinct regions on the short arm of chromosome 17 associated with tumorigenesis of human astrocytomas. *Proc Natl Acad Sci USA* **86**:7186, 1989.
35. Fults D, Tippets RH, Thomas RJ, Nakamura Y, White R: Loss of heterozygosity for loci on chromosome 17p in human malignant astrocytoma. *Cancer Res* **49**:6572, 1989.
36. James CD, Carlbom E, Nordenskjold M, Collins VP, Cavenee WK: Mitotic recombination of chromosome 17 in astrocytomas. *Proc Natl Acad Sci USA* **86**:2858, 1989.
37. Venter DJ, Bevan KL, Ludwig RL, Riley TEW, Jat PS, Thomas DGT, Noble MD: Retinoblastoma gene deletions in human glioblastomas. *Oncogene* **6**:445, 1991.
38. Fults D, Brockmeyer D, Tullous MW, Pedone CA, Cawthon RM: *P53* mutation and loss of heterozygosity on chromosomes 17 and 10 during human astrocytoma progression. *Cancer Res* **52**:674, 1992.
39. von Deimling A, Eibl RH, Ohgaki H, Louis DN, von Ammon K, Petersen I, Kleihues P, Chung RY, Wiestler OD, Seizinger BR: *p53* mutations are associated with 17p allelic loss in grade II and grade III astrocytoma. *Cancer Res* **52**:2987, 1992.
40. Frankel RH, Bayona W, Koslow M, Newcomb EW: *p53* mutations in human malignant gliomas: Comparison of loss of heterozygosity with mutation frequency. *Cancer Res* **52**:1427, 1992.
41. Lang FF, Miller DC, Koslow M, Newcomb EW: Pathways leading to glioblastoma multiforme: A molecular analysis of genetic alterations in 65 astrocytic tumors. *J Neurosurg* **81**:427, 1994.
42. Leenstra S, Bijlsma EK, Troost D, Oosting J, Westerveld A, Bosch D, Huslebos TJM: Allele loss on chromosomes 10 and 17p and epidermal growth factor receptor amplification in human malignant astrocytoma related to prognosis. *Br J Cancer* **70**:684, 1994.
43. Rasheed BK, McLendon RE, Herndon JE, Friedman HS, Friedman AH, Bigner DD, Bigner SH: Alterations of the *TP53* gene in human gliomas. *Cancer Res* **54**:1324, 1994.
44. Tenan M, Colombo BM, Pollo B, Cajola L, Broggi G, Finocchiaro G: *P53* mutations and microsatellite analysis of loss of heterozygosity in malignant gliomas. *Cancer Genet Cytogenet* **74**:139, 1994.
45. Hermanson M, Funa K, Koopmann J, Maintz D, Waha A, Westermark B, Heldin CH, Wiestler OD, Louis DN, von Deimling A, Nister M: Association of loss of heterozygosity on chromosome 17p with high platelet-derived growth factor alpha receptor expression in human malignant gliomas. *Cancer Res* **56**:164, 1996.
46. Chung R, Whaley J, Kley N, Anderson K, Louis D, Menon A, Hettlich C, Freiman R, Hedley-Whyte ET, Martuza R, Jenkins R, Yandell D, Seizinger BR: *TP53* gene mutations and 17p deletions in human astrocytomas. *Genes Chromosom Cancer* **3**:323, 1991.
47. Mashiyama S, Murakami Y, Yoshimoto T, Sekiya T, Hayashi K: Detection of *p53* gene mutations in human brain tumors by single-strand conformation polymorphism analysis of polymerase chain reaction products. *Oncogene* **6**:1313, 1991.
48. Louis DN: The *p53* gene and protein in human brain tumors. *J Neuropathol Exp Neurol* **53**:11, 1994.
49. Kraus JA, Bolln C, Wolf HK, Neumann J, Kindermann D, Fimmers R, Forster F, Baumann A, Schlegel U: *TP53* alterations and clinical outcome in low grade astrocytomas. *Genes Chromosom Cancer* **10**:143, 1994.
50. Lang FF, Miller DC, Pisharody S, Koslow M, Newcomb E: High frequency of p53 protein accumulation without *p53* gene mutation in human juvenile pilocytic, low grade and anaplastic astrocytomas. *Oncogene* **9**:949, 1994.
51. Alderson LM, Castleberg RL, Harsh GR, Louis DN, Henson JW: Human gliomas with wild-type p53 express bcl-2. *Cancer Res* **55**:999, 1995.
52. Chen P, Iavarone A, Fick J, Edwards M, Prados M, Israel MA: Constitutional *p53* mutations associated with brain tumors in young adults. *Cancer Genet Cytogenet* **82**:106, 1995.
53. Kyritsis AP, Xu R, Bondy ML, Levin V, Bruner JM: Correlation of p53 immunoreactivity and sequencing in patients with glioma. *Mol Carcinogen* **15**:1, 1996.
54. Bogler O, Huang H-JS, Kleihues P, Cavenee WK: The *p53* gene and its role in human brain tumors. *Glia* **15**:308, 1995.
55. Litofsky NS, Hinton D, Raffel C: The lack of a role for p53 in astrocytomas in pediatric patients. *Neurosurgery* **34**:967, 1994.
56. Willert JR, Daneshvar L, Sheffield VC, Cogen PH: Deletion of chromosome arm 17p DNA sequences in pediatric high-grade and juvenile pilocytic astrocytomas. *Genes Chromosom Cancer* **12**:165, 1995.
57. Miyakoshi J, Dobler KD, Allalunis-Turner J, McKean JD, Petruk K, Allen PBR, Aronyk KN, Weir B, Huyser-Wierenga D, Fulton D, Urtsun RC, Day RS III: Absence of *IFNA* and *IFNB* genes from human

malignant glioma cell lines and lack of correlation with cellular sensitivity to interferons. *Cancer Res* **50**:278, 1990.

58. Olopade OI, Jenkins RB, Ransom DT, Malik K, Pomykala H, Nobori T, Cowan JM, Rowley JD, Diaz MO: Molecular analysis of deletions of the short arm of chromosome 9 in human gliomas. *Cancer Res* **52**:2523, 1992.
59. Kamb A, Grui NA, Weaver-Feldhaus J, Liu Q, Harshman K, Tavtigian SV, Stockert E, Day RS, Johnson BE, Skolnick MH: A cell cycle regulator potentially involved in genes of many tumor types. *Science* **264**:436, 1994.
60. Jen J, Harper JW, Bigner SH, Bigner DD, Papadopoulos N, Markowitz S, Wilson JKV, Kinzler KW, Vogelstein B: Deletion of *p16* and *p15* genes in brain tumors. *Cancer Res* **54**:6353, 1994.
61. Ueki K, Rubio MP, Ramesh V, Correa KM, Rutter JL, von Deimling A, Buckler AJ, Gusella JF, Louis DN: *MTS1/CDKN2* gene mutations are rare in primary human astrocytomas with allelic loss of chromosome 9p. *Hum Mol Genet* **3**:1841, 1994.
62. Giani C, Finocchiaro G: Mutation rate of the *CDKN2* gene in malignant gliomas. *Cancer Res* **54**:6338, 1994.
63. He J, Allen JR, Collins VP, Allalunis-Turner MJ, Godbout R, Day RS, James CD: CDK4 amplifications is an alternative mechanism to *p16* gene homozygous deletion in glioma cell lines. *Cancer Res* **54**:5804, 1994.
64. Schmidt EE, Ichimura K, Reifenberger G, Collins VP: *CDKN2* (*p16/MTS1*) gene deletion or CDK4 amplification occurs in the majority of glioblastomas. *Cancer Res* **54**:6321, 1994.
65. Moulton T, Samara G, Chung WY, Yuan L, Desai R, Sist, Bruce J, Tycko B: *MTS1/p16/CDKN2* lesions in primary glioblastoma multiforme. *Am J Pathol* **146**:613, 1995.
66. Nishikawa R, Furnari FB, Lin H, Arap W, Berger MS, Cavenee WK, Su Huang HJ: Loss of P16^{INK4} expression is frequent in high grade gliomas. *Cancer Res* **55**:1941, 1995.
67. Walker DG, Duan W, Popovic EA, Kaye AH, Tomlinson FH, Lavin M: Homozygous deletions of the multiple tumor suppressor gene 1 in the progression of human astrocytomas. *Cancer Res* **55**:20, 1995.
68. Sonoda Y, Yoshimoto T, Sekiya T: Homozygous deletion of the *MTS1/p16* and *MTS2/p15* genes and amplification of the *CDK4* gene in glioma. *Oncogene* **11**:2145, 1995.
69. Li YJ, Hoang-Xuan K, Delattre JY, Poisson M, Thomas G, Hamelin R: Frequent loss of heterozygosity on chromosome 9, and low incidence of mutations of cyclin-dependent kinase inhibitors *p15* (*MTS2*) and *p16* (*MTS1*) genes in gliomas. *Oncogene* **11**:597, 1995.
70. Ueki K, Ono Y, Henson JW, Efird JT, von Deimling A, Louis DN: *CDKN2/p16* or *RB* alterations occur in the majority of glioblastomas and are inversely correlated. *Cancer Res* **56**:150, 1996.
71. Herman JG, Merlo A, Mao L, Lapidus RG, Issa JPJ, Davidson NE, Sidransky D, Baylin SB: Inactivation of the *CDKN2/p16/MTS1* gene is frequently associated with aberrant DNA methylation in all common human cancers. *Cancer Res* **55**:4525, 1995.
72. Bigner SH, Wong AJ, Mark J, Muhlbaier LH, Kinzler KW, Vogelstein B, Bigner DD: Relationship between gene amplification and chromosomal deviations in malignant human gliomas. *Cancer Genet Cytogenet* **29**:165, 1987.
73. Wong AJ, Bigner SH, Bigner DD, Kinzler KW, Hamilton SR, Vogelstein B: Increased expression of the epidermal growth factor receptor gene in malignant gliomas is invariably associated with gene amplification. *Proc Natl Acad Sci USA* **84**:6899, 1993.
74. Bigner SH, Humphrey PA, Wong AJ, Vogelstein B, Mark J, Friedman HS, Bigner DD: Characterization of the epidermal growth factor receptor in human glioma cell lines and xenografts. *Cancer Res* **50**:8017, 1990.
75. Humphrey PA, Wong AJ, Vogelstein B, Zalutsky MR, Fuller GN, Archer GE, Friedman HS, Kwatra MM, Bigner SH, Bigner DD: Anti-synthetic peptide antibody reacting at the fusion junction of deletion-mutant epidermal growth factor receptors in human glioblastoma. *Proc Natl Acad Sci USA* **87**:4207, 1990.
76. Sugawa N, Ekstrand A, James CD, Collins VP: Identical splicing of aberrant epidermal growth factor receptor transcripts from amplified rearranged genes in human glioblastomas. *Proc Natl Acad Sci USA* **87**:8602, 1990.
77. Ekstrand AJ, James CD, Cavenee WK, Seliger B, Pettersson RF, Collins VP: Genes for epidermal growth factor receptor, transforming growth factor alpha, and epidermal growth factor and their expression in human gliomas in vivo. *Cancer Res* **51**:2164, 1991.
78. Ekstrand AJ, Sugawa N, James CD, Collins VP: Amplified and rearranged epidermal growth factor receptor genes in human glioblastomas reveal deletions of sequences encoding portions of the N- and/or C-terminal tails. *Proc Natl Acad Sci USA* **89**:4309, 1992.
79. Moscatello DK, Holgado-Madruga M, Godwin AK, Ramirez G, Gunn G, Zoltick PW, Biegel J, Hayes RL, Wong AJ: Frequent expression of a mutant epidermal growth factor receptor in multiple human tumors. *Cancer Res* **55**:5536, 1995.
80. Wikstrand CJ, Hale LP, Batra SK, Hill ML, Humphrey PA, Kurpad SN, McLendon RE, Moscatello D, Pegram CN, Reist CJ, Traweek T, Wong AJ, Zalutsky MR, Bigner DD: Monoclonal antibodies against EGFRvIII are tumor specific and react with breast and lung carcinomas and malignant gliomas. *Cancer Res* **55**:3140, 1995.
81. Yamazaki H, Fukui Y, Ueyama Y, Tamaoki N, Kawamoto T, Taniguchi S, Shibuya M: Amplification of the structurally and functionally altered epidermal growth factor receptor gene (*c-erbB*) in human brain tumors. *Mol Cell Biol* **8**:1816, 1988.
82. Batra SK, Castelino-Prabhu S, Wikstrand CJ, Zhu X, Humphrey PA, Friedman HS, Bigner DD: Epidermal growth factor ligand-independent, unregulated, cell-transforming potential of a naturally occurring human mutant *EGFRvIII* gene. *Cell Growth Diff* **6**:1251, 1995.
83. James CD, He J, Carlbom E, Dumanski JP, Hansen M, Nordenskjld M, Collins VP, Cavenee WK: Clonal genomic alterations in glioma malignancy stages. *Cancer Res* **48**:5546, 1988.
84. Fults D, Pedone CA, Thomas GA, White R: Allelotype of human malignant astrocytoma. *Cancer Res* **50**:5784, 1990.
85. Henson JW, Schnitker BL, Correa KM, von Deimling A, Fassbender F, Xu HJ, Benedict WF, Yandell DW, Louis DN: The retinoblastoma gene is involved in malignant progression of astrocytomas. *Ann Neurol* **3**:714, 1994.
86. He J, Olson JJ, James CD: Lack of p16^{INK4} or retinoblastoma protein (pRb), or amplification-associated overexpression of cdk4 is observed in distinct subsets of malignant glial tumors and cell lines. *Cancer Res* **55**:4833, 1995.
87. Reifenberger G, Reifenberger J, Ichimura K, Meltzer PS, Collins VP: Amplification of multiple genes from chromosomal region 12q13-14 in human malignant gliomas: Preliminary mapping of the amplicons shows preferential involvement of *CDK4, SAS,* and *MDM2*. *Cancer Res* **54**:4299, 1994.
88. Biernat W, Yohma Y, Yonekawa Y, Kleihues P, Oligaki H: Alterations of cell cycle regulatory genes in primary (*de novo*) and secondary glioblastomas. *Acta Neuropathol* **94**:303, 1997.
89. von Deimling A, von Ammon K, Schoenfeld D, Wiestler OD, Seizinger BR, Louis DN: Subsets of glioblastoma multiforme defined by molecular genetic analysis. *Brain Pathol* **3**:19, 1993.
90. Ohgaki H, Schauble B, zur Hausen A, von Ammon K, Kleihues P: Genetic alterations associated with the evolution and progression of astrocytic brain tumours. *Virchows Arch* **427**:113, 1995.
91. Watanabe K, Tachibana O, Sato K, Yonekawa Y, Kleihues P, Ohgaki H: Overexpression of the EGF receptor and *p53* mutations are mutually exclusive in the evolution of primary and secondary glioblastomas. *Brain Pathol* **6**:217, 1996.
92. Louis DN: Clinicopathogenetic subsets of glioblastoma multiform: From both sides now. *Brain Pathol* **6**:223, 1996.
93. Kleihues P, Ohgaki H: Genetics of glioma progression and the definition of primary and secondary glioblastoma. *Brain Pathol* **7**:1131, 1997.
94. Bello MJ, Vaquero J, de Campos JM, Kusak ME, Sarasa JL, Szez-Castresana J, Pestana A, Rey JA: Molecular analysis of chromosome 1 abnormalities in human gliomas reveals frequent loss of 1p in oligodendroglial tumors. *Int J Cancer* **57**:172, 1994.
95. Reifenberger J, Reifenberger G, Liu L, James CD, Wechsler W, Collins VP: Molecular genetic analysis of oligodendroglial tumors shows preferential allelic deletions on 19q and 1p. *Am J Pathol* **145**:1175, 1994.
96. Hashimoto N, Ichikawa D, Arakawa Y, Date K, Ueda S, Nakagawa Y, Horil A, Nakamura Y, Abe T, Inazawa J: Frequent deletions of material from chromosome arm 1p in oligodendroglial tumors revealed by double-target fluorescence in situ hybridization and microsatellite analysis. *Genes Chromosom Cancer* **14**:295, 1995.
97. von Deimling A, Nagel J, Bender B, Lenartz D, Schramm J, Louis DN, Wiestler OD: Deletion mapping of chromosome 19 in human gliomas. *Int J Cancer* **57**:676, 1994.
98. Ritland SR, Ganju V, Jenkins RB: Region-specific loss of heterozygosity on chromosome 19 is related to the morphologic type of human glioma. *Genes Chromosom Cancer* **12**:277, 1995.
99. Rubio MP, Correa KM, Ueki K, Mohrenweiser HW, Gusella JF, von Deimling A, Louis DN: The putative glioma tumor suppressor gene on

chromosome 19q maps between *APOC2* and *HRC*. *Cancer Res* **54**:4760, 1994.
100. Yong WH, Chou D, Ueki K, Harsh GR IV, von Deimling A, Gusella JF, Mohrenweiser HW, Louis DN: Chromosome 19q deletions in human gliomas overlap telomeric to D19S219 and may target a 425 kb region centromeric to D19S112. *J Neuropathol Exp Neurol* **54**:622, 1995
101. Brown NP, Pearson ADJ, Davison EV, Gardner-Medwin D, Crawford P, Perry RK: Multiple chromosome rearrangements in a childhood ependymoma. *Cancer Genet Cytogenet* **36**:25, 1988.
102. Stratton MR, Darling J, Lantos PL, Cooper CS, Reeves BR: Cytogenetic abnormalities in human ependymomas. *Int J Cancer* **44**:579, 1989.
103. Chadduck WM, Boop FA, Sawyer JR: Cytogenetic studies of pediatric brain and spinal cord tumors. *Pediatr Neurosurg* **17**:57, 1991.
104. Vagner-Capodano AM, Gentet JC, Gambarelli D, Pellissier JF, Gouzien M, Lena G, Genitori L, Choux M, Raybaud C: Cytogenetic studies in 45 pediatric brain tumors. *Pediatr Hematol Oncol* **9**:223, 1992.
105. Weremowicz S, Kupsky WJ, Morton CC, Fletcher JA: Cytogenetic evidence for a chromosome 22 tumor suppressor gene in ependymoma. *Cancer Genet Cytogenet* **61**:193, 1992.
106. Rogatto SR, Casartelli C, Rainho CA, Barbieri-Neto J: Chromosomes in the genes and progression of ependymomas. *Cancer Genet Cytogenet* **69**:146, 1993.
107. Neumann E, Kalousek DK, Norman MG, Stienbok P, Cochrane DD, Goddard K: Cytogenetic analysis of 109 pediatric central nervous system tumors. *Cancer Genet Cytogenet* **71**:40, 1993.
108. Sawyer JR, Sammartino G, Husain M, Boop FA, Chadduck WM: Chromosome aberrations in four ependymomas. *Cancer Genet Cytogenet* **74**:132, 1994.
109. Bijlsma EK, Voesten AMJ, Bijleveld EH, Troost D, Westerveld A, Mérel P, Thomas G, Huslebos TJM: Molecular analysis of genetic changes in ependymomas. *Genes Chromosom Cancer* **13**:272, 1995.
110. Wernicke C, Thiel G, Lozanova T, Vogel S, Kintzel D, Jünisch W, Lehmann K, Witkowski R: Involvement of chromosome 22 in ependymomas. *Cancer Genet Cytogenet* **79**:173, 1995.
111. Agamanolis DP, Malone JM: Chromosomal abnormalities in 47 pediatric brain tumors. *Cancer Genet Cytogenet* **81**:125, 1995.
112. Blaeker H, Rasheed BKA, McLendon RE, Friedman H, Batra SK, Fuchs HE, Bigner SH: Microsatellite analysis of childhood brain tumors. *Genes Chromosom Cancer* **15**:54, 1996.
113. James CD, He J, Carlbom E, Mikkelsen T, Ridderheim PA, Cavenee WK, Collins VP: Loss of genetic information in central nervous system tumors common to children and young adults. *Genes Chromosom Cancer* **2**:94, 1990.
114. Ransom DT, Ritland SR, Kimmel DW, Moertel CA, Dahl RJ, Scheithauer BW, Kelly PJ, Jenkins RB: Cytogenetic and loss of heterozygosity studies in ependymomas, pilocytic astrocytomas, and oligodendrogliomas. *Genes Chromosom Cancer* **5**:348, 1992.
115. Rubio M, Correa KM, Ramesh V, MacCollin MM, Jacoby .B, von Deimling A, Gusella JF, Louis DN: Analysis of the neurofibromatosis 2 gene in human ependymomas and astrocytomas. *Cancer Res* **54**:45, 1994.
116. Stevens MCG, Cameron AH, Muir KR, Parkes SE, Reid H, Whitwell H: Descriptive epidemiology of primary central nervous system tumours in children: A population-based study. *Clin Oncol* **3**:323, 1991.
117. Central Brain Tumor Registry of the United States: Annual Report. Chicago, 1995.
118. Bigner SH, Mark J, Friedman HS, Biegel JA, Bigner DD: Structural chromosomal abnormalities in human medulloblastomas. *Cancer Genet Cytogenet* **30**:91, 1988.
119. Griffin CA, Hawkins AL, Packer RJ, Rorke LB, Emanuel BS: Chromosome abnormalities in pediatric brain tumors. *Cancer Res* **48**:175, 1988.
120. Biegel JA, Rorke LB, Packer RJ, Sutton LN, Schut L, Bonner L, Emanuel S: Isochromosome 17q in primitive neuroectodermal tumors of the central nervous system. *Genes Chromosom Cancer* **1**:139, 1989.
121. Karnes PS, Tran TN, Cui MY, Raffel C, Gilles FH, Barranger JA, Ying KL: Cytogenetic analysis of 39 pediatric central nervous system tumors. *Cancer Genet Cytogenet* **59**:12, 1992.
122. Neumann E, Kalousek DK, Norman MG, Stienbok P, Cochrane DD, Goddard K: Cytogenetic analysis of 109 pediatric central nervous system tumors. *Cancer Genet Cytogenet* **71**:40, 1993.
123. Fuji Y, Hongo T, Hayashi Y: Chromosome analysis of brain tumors in childhood. *Genes Chromosom Cancer* **11**:205, 1994.
124. Thomas GA, Raffel C: Loss of heterozygosity on 6q, 16q and 17p in human central nervous system primitive neuroectodermal tumors. *Cancer Res* **51**:639, 1991.
125. Cogen P, Daneshvar L, Metzger AK, Edwards MSB: Deletion mapping of the medulloblastoma locus on chromosome 17p. *Genomics* **8**:279, 1990.
126. Biegel JA, Burk CD, Barr FG, Emanuel BS: Evidence for a 17p tumor related locus distinct from p53 in pediatric primitive neuroectodermal tumors. *Cancer Res* **52**:3391, 1992.
127. Albrecht S, von Deimling A, Pietsch T, Giangaspero F, Brandnert S, Kleiheust P, Wiestler OD: Microsatellite analysis of loss of heterozygosity on chromosomes 9q, 11p, and 17p in medulloblastoma. *Neuropathol Appl Neurobiol* **20**:74, 1994.
128. Batra SK, McLendon RE, Koo JS, Castelino-Prabhu S, Fuchs E, Krischer JP, Friedman HS, Bigner DD, Bigner SH: Prognostic implications of chromosome 17q deletions in human medulloblastomas. *J Neurooncol* **24**:39, 1995.
129. Scheurlen WG, Senf L: Analysis of the GAP-related domain of the neurofibromatosis type 1 (*NF1*) gene in childhood brain tumors. *Int J Cancer* **64**:234, 1995.
130. Ohgaki H, Eibl RH, Wiestler OD, Yasargil MG, Newcomb EW, Kleihues P: *P53* mutations in nonastrocytic human brain tumors. *Cancer Res* **51**:6202, 1991.
131. Saylors R, Sidransky D, Friedman HS, Bigner SH, Bigner DD, Vogelstein B, Brodeur GM: Infrequent *p53* gene mutations in medulloblastomas. *Cancer Res* **51**:4721, 1991.
132. Cogen PH, Daneshvar L, Metzgar AK, Geoffrey D, Edwards MSB, Sheffield VC: Involvement of multiple chromosome 17p loci in medulloblastoma tumorigenesis. *Am J Hum Genet* **50**:584, 1992.
133. Badiali M, Iolascon A, Loda M, Scheithauer B, Basso G, Trentini G, Giangaspero F: *p53* gene mutations in medulloblastoma, immunohistochemistry, gel shift analysis and sequencing. *Diagn Mol Pathol* **2**:23, 1993.
134. Raffel C, Thomas GA, Tishler DM, Lassof S, Allen JC: Absence of *p53* mutations in childhood central nervous system primitive neuroectodermal tumors. *Neurosurgery* **33**:301, 1993.
135. Adesina AM, Nalbantoglu J, Cavenee WK: *p53* gene mutation and *mdm2* gene amplification are uncommon in medulloblastoma. *Cancer Res* **54**:5649, 1994.
136. Bigner SH, Friedman HS, Vogelstein B, Oakes WJ, Bigner DD: Amplification of the *c-myc* gene in human medulloblastoma cell lines and xenografts. *Cancer Res* **50**:2347, 1990.
137. Raffel C, Gilles FE, Weinberg KI: Reduction to homozygosity and gene amplification in central nervous system primitive neuroectodermal tumors of childhood. *Cancer Res* **50**:587, 1990.
138. Badiali M, Pession A, Basso G, Andreini L, Rigobello L, Galassi E, Giangaspero F: *N-myc* and *c-myc* oncogenes amplification in medulloblastomas: Evidence of particularly aggressive behavior of a tumor with *c-myc* amplification. *Tumori* **77**:118, 1991.
139. Friedman HS, Burger PC, Bigner SH, Trojanowski JQ, Brodeur GM, He X, Wikstrand CJ, Kurtzberg J, Berens ME, Halperin EC, Bigner DD: Phenotypic and genotypic analysis of a human medulloblastoma cell line and transplantable xenograft (D341 Med) demonstrating amplification of *c-myc*. *Am J Pathol* **130**:472, 1988.
140. Wasson JC, Saylors RL, Zelter P, Friedman HS, Bigner SH, Burger PC, Bigner DD, Look AT, Douglass EC, Brodeur GM: Oncogene amplification in pediatric brain tumors. *Cancer Res* **50**:2987, 1990.
141. Batra SK, Rasheed A, Bigner SH, Bigner DD: Oncogenes and antioncogenes in human central nervous system tumors. *Lab Invest* **71**:621, 1994.
142. Pietsch T, Scharman T, Fonatsch CF, Schmidt D, Ockler R, Freihoff D, Albrecht S, Wiestler OW, Zeltzer P, Riehm H: Characterization of five new cell lines derived from human primitive neuroectodermal tumors of the central nervous system. *Cancer Res* **54**:3278, 1994.
143. Schütz BR, Scheurlen W, Krauss J, du Manoir S, Joos S, Bentz M, Lichter P: Mapping of chromosomal gains and losses in primitive neuroectodermal tumors by comparative genomic hybridization. *Genes Chromosom Cancer* **16**:196, 1996.
144. Schofield D, West DC, Anthony DC, Marshal R, Sklar J: Correlation of loss of heterozygosity at chromosome 9q with histological subtype in medulloblastomas. *Am J Pathol* **146**:472, 1995.
145. Johnson RL, Rothamn AL, Xie J, Goodrich LV, Bate JW, Bonifas JM, Quinn AC, Myers RM, Cox DR, Epstein EH Jr, Scott MP: Human homolog of patched, a candidate gene for the basal cell nevus syndrome. *Science* **272**:1668, 1996.
146. Hahn H, Wicking C, Zaphiropoulos C, Gailani MR, Stanley S, Chidanharam A, Vorechovsky J, Holmberg E, Unden AB, Giles S,

Negus K, Smyth I, Pressman C, Leffell DJ, Gerrard B, Goldstein AM, Dean M, Toftgard R, Chenevia-Trench G, Wainwright B, Bale AE: Mutations of the human homologue of *Drosophilia* patched in the nevoid basal cell carcinoma syndrome. *Cell* **85**:841, 1996.

147. Raffel C, Jenkins RB, Frederick L, Hebrink D, Alderete B, Fults DW, James CD: Sporadic medulloblastomas contain *PTCH* mutations. *Cancer Res* **57**:842, 1997.
148. Vorechovsky I, Tingby O, Hartman M, Strmberg B, Nister M, Collins VP, Toftgard R: Somatic mutations in the human homologue of *Drosophilia* patched in primitive neuroectodermal tumours. *Oncogene* **15**:361, 1997.
149. Pietsch T, Waha A, Koch A, Kraus J, Albrecht S, Tonn J, Srensen N, Berthold F, Henk B, Schmandt N, Wolf HK, von Diemling A, Wainwright B, Chenevix-Trench G, Wiestler OD, Wicking C: Medulloblastomas of the desmoplastic variant carry mutations of the human homologue of *Drosophilia* patched. *Cancer Res* **57**:2085, 1997.
150. Wolter M, Reifenberger J, Sommer C, Ruzicka T, Reifenberger G: Mutations in the human homologue of the *Drosophilia* segment polarity gene patched (*PTCH*) in sporadic basal cell carcinomas of the skin and primitive neuroectodermal tumors of the central nervous system. *Cancer Res* **57**:2581, 1997.
151. Xie J, Johnson RL, Zhang X, Bare JW, Waldman FM, Cogen PH, Menon AG, Warren RS, Chen L-C, Scott MP, Epstein EH Jr: Mutations of the *PATCHED* gene in several types of sporadic extracutaneous tumors. *Cancer Res* **57**:2369, 1997.
152. Reifenberger J, Wolter M, Weber RG, Megahed M, Ruzicka T, Lichter P, Reifenberger G: Missense mutations in *SMOH* in sporadic basal cell carcinomas of the skin and primitive neuroectodermal tumors of the central nervous system. *Cancer Res* **58**:1798, 1998.
153. Hamilton SR, Liu B, Parsons RE, Papdopoulos N, Jen J, Powell SM, Krush AJ, Berk T, Cohen Z, Titu B, Burger PC, Wood PA, Taqi F, Booker SV, Petersen GM, Offerhaus GJA, Tersmette AC, Giardiello FM, Vogelstein B, Kinzler KW: The molecular basis of Turcot's syndrome. *N Engl J Med* **392**:839, 1995.
154. Zurawell RH, Chiappa SA, Allen C, Raffel C: Sporadic medulloblastomas contain oncogenic β-catenin mutations. *Cancer Res* **58**:896, 1996.
155. Zang KD, Singer H: Chromosomal constitution of meningiomas. *Nature* **216**:84, 1967.
156. Mark J, Levan G, Mitelman F: Identification by fluorescence of the G chromosome lost in human meningiomas. *Hereditas* **71**:163, 1972.
157. Zankl H, Zang KD: Cytological and cytogenetical studies on brain tumors: IV. Identification of the missing G chromosome in human meningiomas as no. 22 by fluorescence technique. *Hum Genet* **14**:167, 1972.
158. Zang KD: Cytological and cytogenetical studies on human meningioma. *Cancer Genet Cytogenet* **6**:249, 1982.
159. Seizinger BR, De la Monte S, Atkins L, Gusella JF, Martuza RL: Molecular genetic approach to human meningioma: loss of genes on chromosome 22. *Proc Natl Acad Sci USA* **84**:5419, 1987.
160. Dumanski JP, Carlbom E, Collins VP, Nordenskjld M: Deletion mapping of a locus on human chromosome 22 involved in the oncogenesis of meningioma. *Proc Natl Acad Sci USA* **84**:9275, 1987.
161. Seizinger BR, Rouleau G, Ozelius LJ, Lane AH, St George-Hyslop P, Huson S, Gusella JF, Martuza RL: Common pathogenetic mechanism for three tumor types in bilateral acoustic neurofibromatosis. *Science* **236**:317, 1987.
162. Rouleau GA, Wertlecki W, Haines JL, Hobbs WJ, Trofatter JA, Seizinger BR, Martuza RL, Superneau DW, Conneally PM, Gusella JF: Genetic linkage of bilateral acoustic neurofibromatosis to a DNA marker on chromosome 22. *Nature* **329**:246, 1987.
163. Wertelecki W, Rouleau GA, Superneau DW, Forehand LW, Williams JP, Haines JL, Gusella JF: Neurofibromatosis 2: Clinical and DNA linkage studies of a large kindred. *N Engl J Med* **319**:278, 1988.
164. Dumanski JP, Rouleau GA, Nordenskjld M, Collin VP: Molecular genetic analysis of chromosome 22 in 81 cases of meningioma. *Cancer Res* **50**:5863, 1990.
165. Cogen PH, Daneshvar L, Bowcock AM, Metzger AK, Cavalli-Sforza LL: Loss of heterozygosity for chromosome 22 DNA sequences in human meningioma. *Cancer Genet Cytogenet* **53**:271, 1991.
166. Rouleau GA, Merel P, Lutchman M, Sanson M, Zucman J, Marineau C, Hoang-Xuan K, Demczuk S, Desmaze C, Plougastel B, Pulst SM, Lenoir G, Bijlsma E, Fashold R, Dumanski J, deJong P, Parry D, Eldrige R, Aurias A, Delattre O, Thomas G: Alteration in a new gene encoding a putative membrane-organizing protein causes neurofibromatosis type 2. *Nature* **363**:495, 1993.
167. Deprez RHL, Bianchi AB, Groen NA, Seizinger BR, Hagemeijer A, vanDrunen E, Bootsma D, Koper JW, Avezaat CJJ, Kley N, Zwarthoff EC: Frequent *NF2* gene transcript mutations in sporadic meningiomas and vestibular schwannomas. *Am J Hum Genet* **54**:1022, 1994.
168. Ruttledge MH, Xie Y-G, Han F-Y, Peyrard M, Collins V, Nordenskjld M, Dumanski JP: Deletions on chromosome 22 in sporadic meningioma. *Genes Chromosom Cancer* **10**:122, 1994.
169. Ruttledge MH, Sarrazin J, Rangaratnam S, Phelan CM, Twist E, Merel P, Delattre O, Thomas G, Nordenskjld M, Collins VP, Dumanski JP, Rouleau GA: Evidence of the complete inactivation of the *NF2* gene in the majority of sporadic meningiomas. *Nature Genet* **6**:180, 1994.
170. Jacoby LB, MacCollin M, Louis DN, Mohney T, Rubio M-P, Pulaski K, Trofatter JA, Kley N, Seizinger B, Ramesh V, Gusella JF: Exon scanning for mutations of the *NF2* gene in schwannomas. *Hum Mol Genet* **3**:413, 1994.
171. Irving RM, Moffat DA, Hardy DG, Barton DE, Xuereb JH, Raher ER: Somatic *NF2* gene mutations in familial and non-familial vestibular schwannoma. *Hum Mol Genet* **3**:347, 1994.
172. Bijlsma EK, Mérel P, Bosch DA, Westerveld A, Delattre O, Thomas G, Hulsebos TJM: Analysis of mutations in the *SCH* gene in schwannomas. *Genes Chromosom Cancer* **11**:7, 1994.

CHAPTER 58

Lung Cancer

Barry D. Nelkin ▪ Mack Mabry ▪ Stephen B. Baylin

1. **Lung cancer is the leading cause of cancer-related death for both men and women in the United States and the solid tumor with the most defined relationship to a known environmental cause, cigarette smoking. The clinical and biologic aspects of this disease are complex in that four major histologic cancer types, all related to smoking, can arise from the bronchial epithelium, including large cell undifferentiated, squamous cell, adeno-, and small cell lung carcinomas. The first three types, collectively known as non-small cell lung cancer (NSCLC), metastasize later than the small cell tumors (SCLC) and can be cured by early surgery. SCLC is one of the most highly metastatic tumors in humans and has less than a 5 percent 5-year survival rate.**
2. **Hereditary aspects of lung cancer are probably less well understood than for any of the other common forms of solid tumors. There are no well-defined syndromes for inherited lung cancer. However, a growing body of evidence suggests that a complex Mendelian dominant inheritance pattern for genetic predisposition may play a significant role in determining which smokers eventually will get lung tumors. Animal models for carcinogen-induced lung cancers, particularly in mice, suggest a major locus for genetic predisposition to lung adenocarcinoma and may prove useful for defining a gene(s) important to the human disease. The specific gene(s) involved have not been defined, nor have the genetic loci involved been delineated.**
3. **In part because of the poorly defined hereditary aspects of lung cancer, little is known about the precise gene alterations that underly the earliest steps for lung carcinogenesis. However, multiple genetic alterations, in candidate gene regions (loss of heterozygosity at chromosomes 3p, 9p, 13q, and 17p) or in specific candidate genes (*p16, p53,* K-*ras, cyclin D1* genes), have been elucidated for established lung cancers. The most frequent of these changes, and those which occur earliest in disease progression, provide clues for genes involved in both the initial steps and the hereditary aspects of lung neoplasia.**
4. **Further definition of the genes mediating the evolution of lung cancers is essential to establish critically needed markers to facilitate risk assessment for and design of novel tests for early diagnosis of these neoplasms.**

CLINICAL AND BIOLOGIC ASPECTS

In 1996, 177,000 people in the United States were diagnosed with lung cancer, and over 158,000 deaths resulted. Thus, lung cancer is the leading cause of cancer-related death in this country.[1] Ironically, considering the tremendous impact of this disease, lung cancer is arguably the most preventable solid tumor, since 90 percent of all patients with these malignancies develop their disease because of exposure to tobacco products and in virtually all instances through cigarette smoking.[2,3]

One of the difficulties in defining genetic predisposition for lung cancer, for making the diagnosis of this disease, and for treatment is that four major histologies of lung tumors evolve from the bronchial epithelium of smokers, and the precise cellular relationships between these tumor types still are not elucidated. From a clinical perspective, lung cancer can be divided into two treatment groups of four histologic types.[4] Squamous cell, adeno-, and large cell carcinomas are collectively referred to as non-small cell lung cancers (NSCLCs) and comprise approximately 75 percent of all lung tumors. These are different in their treatment approaches and responses from a fourth type, small cell lung cancer (SCLC), which constitutes the remaining 25 percent of lung neoplasms. Each of these major forms of lung cancer is intimately related to cigarette smoking. Of great interest for consideration of genetic predisposition to lung cancer and for studies of the genetic changes in these diseases is that only 10 percent of all smokers at risk develop lung carcinoma.[3] This is so despite the fact that virtually all these individuals have a degree of preneoplastic histologic change in their bronchial epithelium.[5] Also, the average age for diagnosis of lung cancer is approximately 60 years. All these data suggest that the evolution of lung cancer occurs over a protracted period of time and involves multiple genetic changes.

For all the lung cancer types, current therapeutic approaches are less than optimal, as reflected in the high death rate from these malignancies. The initial diagnosis for each tumor type almost always stems from clinical evaluation of a chronic cough, weight loss, dyspnea, hemoptysis, hoarseness, or chest pain in patients with a long history of smoking.[6] For the NSCLC group, successful therapies center on early surgery, since metastases occur later than for SCLC. For patients with the most limited stage of NSCLC at the time of initial diagnosis and surgery, 5-year cure rates are approximately 50 percent.[7,8] For patients with nonresectable initial NSCLC and those with recurrent disease, chemotherapy and irradiation are employed, but long-term response rates are only 35 percent, with a median survival time of only 25 weeks.[9,10]

The clinical course for SCLC is very different than that for NSCLC, as is the mode of and response pattern to treatment. This cancer is one of the most metastatic of all solid tumors and is extremely lethal.[11] Tumor spread occurs so early in the course of the disease that surgery is seldom used as a primary approach even for patients with no objective signs of metastasis at the time of initial diagnosis.[12,13] Treatment approaches rely primarily on combination chemotherapy, with thoracic irradiation added in patients with nonmetastatic disease.[14,15] Ironically, this highly lethal cancer has among the highest initial sensitivity among solid tumors to these approaches.[16] However, recurrent and resistant disease virtually always ensues, and the 5-year survival rate is only 5 percent, with an average survival time of 13 months, even for extensively treated patients presenting with detectable disease limited to the chest.[16]

The division of NSCLC and SCLC into two separate categories is useful for consideration of clinical behavior but is simplistic from a biologic standpoint and for considerations of inherited predisposition for these neoplasms. The heterogeneous histologic types of lung cancers may reflect different cells of origin for each

A list of standard abbreviations is located immediately preceding the index in each volume. Nonstandard abbreviations used in this chapter include: NSCLC = non-small cell lung cancer; SCLC = small cell lung cancer; LOH = loss of heterozygosity.

tumor type within the bronchial epithelium.[17] For example, as discussed in a section that follows on animal models of lung carcinogenesis, the parent cell for bronchoalveolar carcinomas, a subtype of adenocarcinomas, appears to be the type II pneumocyte within the bronchial epithelium. The cellular origins of SCLC are less certain, although they have been of particular interest because this tumor is characterized by having a neuroendocrine phenotype that most closely resembles that of a sparse population of normal neuroendocrine cells found throughout the bronchial epithelium.[18] The complex biology underlying lung cancer evolution is illustrated by the fact that it is not uncommon for individual lung cancers to manifest biochemical features of both SCLC and NSCLC, such as sharing of neuroendocrine features.[19,20] This fact suggests that lung cancers are capable of a transdifferentiation that reflects a common differentiation lineage in which they may arise.[20] This biology, as well as the discussed clinical aspects, must be taken into account in all studies to define the gene defects responsible for evolution of sporadic and inherited forms of these diseases. As will be discussed later, there are some patterns of genetic loci abnormalities and of altered function of tumor-suppressor genes and oncogenes that suggest segregation of specific genetic changes to NSCLC and SCLC.

GENETIC LOCI

Hereditary Cases: Linkage Analyses

The contribution of hereditary factors to the development of lung cancer is probably less well understood than for any of the common forms of solid tumors in humans. Unlike for breast, colon, renal, and other cancers, no distinct familial forms of the common types of lung cancer have been defined. Therefore, specific genetic loci responsible for predisposition to lung tumor development have not been elucidated. However, a building body of evidence indicates that there may be an exceedingly important role for genetic predisposition in determining risk of lung cancer development among smokers. This section briefly reviews the progress in this area and the prospects for defining the specific genetic loci responsible.

Proof that the familial occurrence of lung cancer has a genetic basis is complicated by the central role of cigarette smoking in causing these neoplasms. Smoking rates increased dramatically after World War I in American men, and this trend was followed by a later increase in the incidence of women who smoke.[21] Since there is a lag period of at least 20 years from the initiation of smoking until the development of lung cancer, smoking habits must be taken into account in analyzing multiple family generations.[22] This is especially important for the occurrence of lung cancer in women, since their incidence of smoking has increased dramatically over the past 40 years.[23,24] Finally, there is evidence that the likelihood of an individual choosing to smoke can be highly influenced on a familial basis, and this must be taken into account in all studies of familial lung cancer.[25]

Despite the problems, a growing number of studies over the past 30 years, using increasingly sophisticated statistical methods to factor in influence of smoking and other environmental factors, have demonstrated a twofold or more risk of lung cancer in relatives of patients with this disease.[25] However, the firm link to actual Mendelian inheritance of lung cancer itself still was difficult to establish. The most significant step in documenting this probability has come from the detailed investigations of Sellers and colleagues of a large number of families in southern Louisiana. Using sophisticated epidemiologic approaches that factor in pre- and post-World War I smoking histories of families and the effects of age, sex, and environment, these authors found validation for a Mendelian codominant inheritance pattern for lung cancer among smokers.[25–27] In fact, their data predict, in the population studied, that all smokers eventually develop lung cancer because they inherit a gene(s) that may have a high incidence in the general population.[25–27] As the authors are careful to point out, these results must be verified through studies of other families in other regions. However, the implications are enormous for considering approaches to the control of lung cancer and for identifying specific genetic loci involved in predisposition to these neoplasms.

The cited evidence for the role of true inheritance in the development of lung cancer must be translated into formal searches for the involved genetic loci. The job will not be an easy one for multiple reasons. First, as discussed, the inheritance patterns for lung cancer even within a given family appear complex, and multiple loci may be involved. Second, although an earlier age of onset may be a result of inheriting lung cancer risk genes, particularly in women, disease onset still occurs primarily in older individuals.[25–27] These factors make standard linkage analysis of large kindreds with multiple generations very difficult. Early-age-onset lung cancer certainly occurs.[28–30] However, it remains to be determined whether patients with this phenotype develop their disease via the same mechanisms as do patients with typical late-age-onset lung cancer and whether familial patterns for this phenotype can be delineated to facilitate the search for lung cancer predisposition genes.

In addition, the complex array of lung cancer histologies dictates the need to decipher whether hereditary factors contribute to the occurrence of each major subtype. Recent studies indicate that adenocarcinoma of the lung may be the histologic type most linked to definite familial occurrence.[31,32] Interestingly, this is also the type that has been most associated with the few instances of early-age onset.[28–30,33,34]

Therefore, for all the reasons articulated, definition of the actual genetic loci involved for inherited forms of lung cancer will require acquisition of large numbers of families to facilitate non-classical linkage analyses, such as segregation analyses and sib-pair linkage approaches. Consortium arrangements to conduct such studies are now being established and hopefully will yield at least chromosome assignment for lung cancer predisposition genes within the next several years.

Genetic Loci for Sporadic Forms of Lung Cancer

Cytogenetic Changes. The karyotypes of both SCLC and NSCLC exhibit extensive abnormalities. Whang-Peng et al. showed the first consistent cytogenetic abnormality in lung cancer, deletions on the short arm of chromosome 3, in virtually all SCLC cell lines examined.[35] As discussed in the following section, this observation has been confirmed and extended at the molecular level using polymorphic probes. Testa et al. have shown that in NSCLC primary tumors, an average of 31 clonal karyotypic abnormalities were evident.[36] Among the most common abnormalities were loss of chromosomes 9 and 13 (65 and 71 percent, respectively).

Loss of Heterozygosity. As suggested by the extensive cytogenetic abnormalities, loss of heterozygosity (LOH) is common in lung cancers, as in other solid tumors, and has been studied extensively. Although some LOH loci occur in all lung cancer types, several have distinct incidence differences between subtypes.

LOH areas commonly found in lung cancer are listed in Table 58-1, and those studied most extensively are discussed below. For SCLC, there is a very high incidence (90–100 percent of specimens) of LOH on chromosome 3p in the previously discussed area of frequent cytogenetic loss.[37,38] This last change also often occurs but is less frequent (50–80 percent) in NSCLC. The individual regions of chromosome 3p that are lost differ somewhat among the histologic lung cancer subtypes. Chromosome areas within 3p21 are lost in NSCLC, whereas more distal regions, at 3p25-p26, and more proximal regions, at 3p12-p14, are more often lost in SCLC.[37,38] Studies of SCLC cell lines also have demonstrated areas of homozygous deletion within 3p21 and 3p12-14.[39,40] Importantly, this region is the site for the most common fragile site in the genome, Fra3B. Delineation of these distinct and frequent chromosome 3 LOH areas in lung tumors has

Table 58-1 Commonly Altered Chromosomal Loci in Lung Cancer

Locus	Histologic Subtype	Gene	Frequency
A. Loci with defined tumor suppressor gene			
9p21-p22	SCLC, NSCLC	*p15, p16*	60–70%
13q14	SCLC. NSCLC	*Rb*	75–80%*
17p13.1	SCLC. NSCLC	*p53*	50†–95*
B. Loci without defined tumor suppressor gene			
3p12-p14	SCLC. NSCLC		80†–100%,‡
3p21	NSCLC. SCLC		80†–100*,‡
3p25	SCLC. NSCLC		80†–100*,‡
5q21	SCLC, NSCLC		50%
11q12-q24	NSCLC		65%†
22q	SCLC, NSCLC		55%
C. Other loci commonly (30–50%) altered in lung cancer			
1p, 1q, 2q, 3q, 6q, 7q, 8p, 9p, 11p, 12p, 17q, 18q, 19p, 21q			

*SCLC.
†NSCLC.
‡Combined frequency for LOH on 3p.

prompted intense efforts to identify associated tumor-suppressor genes. As discussed in a section that follows, the search has been difficult, and few, if any, real candidate genes have been delineated to date.

LOH for chromosome region 17p also is extremely frequent in all types of lung cancer and especially in DNA from SCLC (90 percent).[41] The tumor-suppressor gene p53 is located at region 17p13.1 and, as discussed in a later section, is clearly a gene involved in the pathogenesis of established lung cancer.

13q also has a high frequency (75 percent) of LOH in SCLC but a low frequency (15 percent) in NSCLC.[41] As noted in a later section and in Table 58-1, this locus includes the site of the retinoblastoma susceptibility gene (Rb), which is almost always aberrantly expressed or mutated in SCLC.

As discussed previously, 9p is an area of frequent cytogenetic abnormality in NSCLC but not in SCLC. This site is the locus of two separate cyclin-dependent kinase inhibitors (CDKIs), *p15* and *p16*. These genes are described in more detail in a section that follows. Also, there is some evidence that a third tumor-suppressor gene may be located at 9p22-23, and a number of laboratories are attempting to identify genes in this region.[42]

LOH for chromosome 5q is observed in approximately half the SCLC cases studied and is most commonly localized to 5q13-21.[43] The region of loss has been intriguing because the tumor-suppressor gene *APC*, which plays a major role in colon cancer, is located within this region. However, analyses of lung cancers for inactivating mutations of *APC* using an RNAse protection screen have not identified any lesions despite the frequent LOH for this locus.[44]

Listed in Table 58-1 are additional, less well-characterized LOH loci that occur with significant frequency (30–50 percent) in lung cancer. These lesions presumably include loci for tumor-suppressor genes that may be of biologic importance, but more work is required to validate this assumption and to document the importance of these changes within the full spectrum of genetic alterations in lung tumors.

Timing of LOH during Lung Cancer Progression. Several studies have attempted to examine the stages in NSCLC tumor progression at which various genetic lesions accrue. Two groups have shown that 3p loss occurs early in NSCLC and is detectable in hyperplastic, precancerous bronchial lesions.[45,46] Similarly, 9p and 17p loss could be detected in preneoplastic hyperplasia.[47] In one study, K-*ras* mutations were found to occur later in NSCLC development than the preceding LOH changes and were not detectable until the later carcinoma *in situ* stage; another study suggested that the *ras* mutations may occur earlier.[48,49] Allelic loss on chromosomes 2q, 18q, and 22q were relatively uncommon (20–33 percent) in primary NSCLC but were found often (63–83 percent) in brain metastases.[50] These results suggest that these latter genetic lesions provide growth advantages to NSCLC cells late in tumor development. The timing of genetic events in lung carcinogenesis needs much further study and will help to define genes for tumor initiation and clues to those involved in genetic predisposition.

Microsatellite Instability. In hereditary nonpolyposis colon cancer, defects in the mismatch repair pathway, which lead to instability changes in microsatellite repeat sequences, recently have been delineated (see Chap. 32). Instability in microsatellite markers also has been studied by several groups in lung cancers with diverse and occasionally conflicting results. Initial reports indicated that microsatellite markers were more likely to be altered in SCLC compared with NSCLC.[51–53] However, other investigators have found no significant differences. Most recently, it has been reported that microsatellite instability is not observed in SCLC but frequently observed in NSCLC and that the replication error phenotype was more likely in NSCLC metastases and in clinically advanced lung cancers.[52] Whether these conflicting results depend on the microsatellite markers selected for analyses, differences in the selection of cases for study, or technical factors in the assays remains to be determined.

SPECIFIC GENES

Genes Involved in Hereditary Lung Cancer

As mentioned previously, there are no distinct genetic syndromes for lung cancer to help identify gene mutations that specify absolute genetic predisposition to these malignancies. However, there are a few clues to genes for which inherited mutations or patterns of inherited polymorphisms could play a role.

Germ-Line Mutations in Genes Involved in Sporadic Lung Cancer. As noted in a section that follows, mutations in the Ha-*ras* gene occur with frequency in sporadic forms of NSCLC. A rare polymorphism in this gene, which involves differences in numbers of a tandemly arranged reiterated sequence, has been reported to occur with increased frequency in patients with lung cancer.[54] However, subsequent studies have provided conflicting results for the actual linkage of this *ras* polymorphism to lung cancer.[55] The majority of the most recent studies have failed to reveal a predictive relationship, and more work will be required to resolve this issue.

Genetic Syndromes for Other Types of Cancer and the Occurrence of Lung Cancer

There are at least three genetic syndromes that predominantly predispose to other forms of cancer in which lung cancer also may occur. Since these syndromes are so rare, it is not yet clear whether a specific histologic type of lung cancer is favored; moreover, the few reported cases have not yet reached the statistical significance to prove that there is increased incidence of lung cancer associated with these genetic disorders.

Lung cancer may occur with increased frequency in the Li-Fraumeni syndrome (LFS), caused by a germ-line mutation in the *p53* tumor-suppressor gene on chromosome 17p.[56] A substantial fraction of the lung cancers in LFS appear in nonsmokers and young (<45 years) patients, suggesting a biologic effect of LFS on lung cancer development. Similarly, transgenic mice expressing a mutant *p53* gene or lacking *p53* genes can develop lung adenocarcinomas.[57,58]

Patients harboring an inactiving mutation in the *Rb* tumor-suppressor gene on chromosome 13q commonly develop retinoblastoma and osteosarcoma.[59] Primary relatives of bilateral retinoblastoma patients, many of whom are carriers of the mutation, have been reported to develop a variety of secondary cancers, including lung cancer.[60,61] In these studies, several of the lung cancers developed in relatively young (< 55 years) patients.

Bloom syndrome is an exceedingly rare recessive genetic disorder (165 patients reported) that is associated with defects in DNA repair (see Chap. 30). Leukemias and other cancers are quite common in this syndrome. One case of squamous cell carcinoma of the lung has been reported in a 38-year-old Bloom syndrome patient.[62]

Genetic Differences in Capacity to Metabolize Tobacco Carcinogens

Since cigarette smoking is so intimately involved in the development of lung cancer, it has been logical to search for specific lung cancer predisposition genes by investigating genetic differences between individuals in their capacity to metabolize the major carcinogens present in tobacco and in cigarette smoke. Clues to a role for such differences in determining lung cancer risk have emerged. Several enzymes associated with the cytochrome P450 system (CYP) are responsible for metabolizing tobacco carcinogens to forms that can be excreted readily from the body.[63] In so doing, however, functional groups can be altered on the parent molecules that result in enhancement of carcinogenenicity through increased propensity to form bulky DNA adducts. Certain polymorphisms in the discussed enzymes are being associated with differing degrees of metabolic capacity between individuals and increased risk of developing lung cancer. For example, the ability to induce activity of the enzyme CYP2D6 by the antihypertensive drug debrisoquine has been associated with lung cancer risk.[63] The major tobacco carcinogen 4-(methyl-nitrosoamino)-1-(3-pyridyl)-1-butanone (NNK) is a substrate for CYP2D6.[64] High ability for induction of this enzyme now has been correlated with increased incidence of lung cancer (odds ratio of about 7.5 in one study) in several studies.[65,66] Poor ability to induce CYP2D6 was associated with mutations and polymorphisms in the gene.[67] Several studies have challenged the association between CYP2D6 activity and lung cancer risk.[68–70] Work to match allelotypes for these gene changes, using sensitive PCR based assays, with lung cancer incidence in larger populations should resolve these issues over the next several years.

Another cytochrome system enzyme, CYP1A1 (aromatic hydrocarbon hydroxylase, AHH), also demonstrates genetically determined differences between individuals for basal activity and inducibility by tobacco smoke.[63] This enzyme metabolically activates polyaromatic hydrocarbons (PAHs), and levels have been reported to be higher in patients with lung cancer than in control individuals without cancer.[71] Differences in activity of and association of polymorphisms for other CYP enzymes to lung cancer risk alone have been reported.[63] However, for all these enzymes, subsequent studies have yielded conflicting results with regard to tightness of linkage to predisposition and occurrence of lung cancer, and future investigations will be required to resolve these issues.[63]

In addition to the described enzymes that may form carcinogenic metabolites from tobacco-related compounds, other enzymes can influence lung cancer risk by catalyzing detoxication reactions that enhance elimination of the described toxic products. Low or absent activity of one such enzyme, the M1 isoform of glutathione-*S*-transferase (GSTM1), which arises through autosomal recessive inheritance for homozygous deletion of the gene, has been linked to high lung cancer risk.[72] Again, this relationship has been challenged by some studies.[73] However, a recent report of PCR-detected deletion of the *GSTM1* gene showed an odds ratio of approximately 1.5 for linkage of the null phenotype with SCLC and adenocarcinoma of the lung.[72] Similarly, lung cancer patients have been reported to have a higher incidence of a specific *GSTP1* polymorphism associated with increased lung DNA adduct levels.[74] Future studies again will be necessary to establish the precise relationships between GSTM1 or *GSTP1* status and lung cancer risk.

In summary, there is a growing body of data for linking genetic differences in capacity to metabolize tobacco carcinogens with risk for developing lung cancer. The odds ratios being reported indicate that no one of the factors being studied has an overwhelming role in predisposition for an individual smoker to be at the highest risk for lung cancer susceptibility. However, a profile of each of the genetic differences in a given smoker might well define a truly significant indicator of risk status. It is clear, from the studies to date, that existing PCR assays for detecting genetic status of each important metabolizing enzyme require much additional refinement. As these improve, monitoring of inherited capacity for carcinogen metabolism may provide a significant way to assess predisposition to lung cancer in large populations.

Genes Involved in Sporadic Lung Cancer

Despite the large body of data for altered genetic loci in sporadic lung cancer, discussed earlier, few specific genes in these regions have been shown to have a role in lung tumorigenesis. However, as outlined below, alterations in both dominantly acting oncogenes and tumor-suppressor genes do occur in established lung tumors and provide clues to the progression steps for these cancers.

Oncogenes Involved in Sporadic Lung Cancer

***Ras* Family Genes.** As for other solid tumors discussed in this book, mutations in *ras* family genes (see Chap. 25) occur frequently in lung cancer. In NSCLC tumors, *ras* mutations, primarily of K-*ras,* are observed at frequencies that may approach 50 percent of cases, as detected by sensitive PCR-based methods.[75] H-*ras* mutations are observed in NSCLC at a very low frequency, and mutations in N-*ras* are rare.[76–78] K-*ras* mutations are common in adenocarcinomas, less common in squamous cell lung cancers, extremely rare in bronchoalveolar carcinomas, and have not been described in SCLC.[79–84] In NSCLC, the presence of *ras* mutations has been reported to be a negative prognostic factor, especially in patients with adenocarcinomas.[75,82,86]

***myc* Family Genes.** Members of the *myc* family of oncogenes, c-*myc,* N-*myc,* and L-*myc* (see Chap. 25), represent another dominant oncogene family that can be activated in lung cancer, usually by gene amplification. c-*myc* amplification in SCLC appears to be a negative prognostic factor; c-*myc* amplification is three times more common in cancers obtained from treated patients than in tumor specimens from untreated patients.[86–88] Amplification of c-*myc* also correlated with a twofold reduction in median patient survival.[88] A number of investigators have suggested that this poor prognosis occurs because increased c-*myc* protein modifies intrinsic drug resistance to certain treatment modalities.[89,90] Amplification or overexpression of L-*myc* and N-*myc* are also found in SCLC and SCLC cell lines, but the prognostic implications of this overexpression are not certain.[91–93]

Cyclin D. Cyclin D is involved in traversing the G1 cell cycle checkpoint for entry into S phase, at least in part by inactivating the Rb tumor-suppressor protein (see Chap. 23). Thus cyclin D can act as an oncogene. Cyclin D1 is overexpressed in most cases of NSCLC[94,95]; in one recent study,[95] many of these instances of cyclin D1 overexpression were shown to be due to gene amplification. In NSCLC cases with cyclin D1 overexpression, normal Rb expression was seen. Cyclin D1 expression was not commonly seen in SCLC; presumably because the *Rb* gene is consistently altered in SCLC, a second abnormality in the same signal transduction pathway does not confer a further growth advantage.

Tumor-Suppressor Genes Involved in Sporadic Lung Cancer

As discussed in a previous section, there are many common sites of LOH, suggestive of alterations in tumor-suppressor loci in the major forms of lung cancer. However, the specific genes that may have altered function in these chromosome regions have, in the main, not been characterized. Several well-described tumor-suppressor genes are altered in established lung cancers and almost certainly play a role in the evolution of these tumors, especially for progression stages of these cancers. These genes, summarized in Table 58-1, are as follows.

***p53* Gene.** Perhaps the best defined tumor-suppressor gene change in lung cancer is mutation of the *p53* gene. This loss of gene function appears to be the major correlate to the previously discussed very frequent LOH that occurs for chromosome region 17p13.1 in all lung cancer types.[41] *p53* mutations are obviously one of the most common genetic changes in all types of human cancer, and these have been found in 50 percent of NSCLC and 90 percent of SCLC tumors.[96,97] The most frequently observed mutations in these tumors are G > T transversions, and these may reflect bulky DNA adducts resulting from carcinogens found in cigarette smoke.[96] Recently, it has been reported that the tobacco carcinogen benzo[a]pyrenediolepoxide (BPDE) binds directly to the hot spots for the mutations in the *p53* gene found in lung carcinomas.[98] Some studies suggest that lung cancers with *p53* mutations have a worse clinical prognosis, but this relationship remains to be clarified.[99,100]

***p16* Gene.** Alterations in the cyclin-dependent kinase inhibitor encoding gene *p16* occur frequently in lung cancers, as they do in most common forms of human cancer.[101–104] This gene is a strong tumor-suppressor candidate to account for the previously discussed frequent LOH and homozygous deletions that occur at chromosome region 9p21 in lung and other tumor types. As in many tumor types, point mutations in the *p16* gene are rare, and the homozygous deletions are most common in cell culture lines.[104–106] However, this latter change now has been documented in primary lung cancers as well.[105–107] In both cultures and primary tumors, loss of *p16* gene function also occurs frequently via transcriptional silencing associated with abnormal DNA methylation of the transcription start site region.[108] The methylation change occurs in the absence of *p16* gene coding region mutations.[108,109] Both the homozygous deletions of *p16* and the methylation changes occur almost always in NSCLC rather than in SCLC tumors.[108] This is thought to reflect the fact that the *p16* gene functions in the *cyclin D-Rb* gene pathway for control of cell proliferation. Tumor cells appear to require inactivation of only one gene in this pathway.[110–112] Since *Rb* gene mutations are very frequent, as noted below, in SCLC but are much less frequent in NSCLC, inactivation of the *cyclin D-Rb* pathway by loss of *p16* function may be advantageous primarily for NSCLC cells.[110–112]

The precise role for *p16* gene changes in the progression of NSCLC tumors has not been delineated yet. However, this loss of gene function may play a very early role, since, as discussed earlier, LOH and homozygous deletions of chromosome 9p21 have been found in early lung cancer lesions. Further investigations of the role of the *p16* gene in lung carcinogenesis are critical and could be important for understanding of genetic susceptibility for lung cancer.

***Rb* Gene.** The tumor-suppressor gene *Rb,* which plays a critical role in the cyclin D pathway for cell cycle control and is located in chromosome region 13q14, is altered in nearly all SCLC tumors and in 30 to 40 percent of NSCLC.[113–115] In NSCLC, aberrant *Rb* was more common in tumors of higher clinical stage.[115]

***FHIT-1* Gene.** The intense search for altered genes on chromosome 3p, which, as discussed in an earlier section, undergoes frequent LOH changes in both NSCLC and SCLC tumors, has resulted to date in a strong proposal for only one candidate gene. Altered transcription splice products for the *FHIT-1* gene, located in a frequent region of homozygous deletion at 3p14 and in the fragile site region Fra3B, which is disrupted in some familial renal tumors, recently have been described as a frequent characteristic of lung cancers.[116] However, it remains to be determined whether mutations in tumor DNA actually underlie the majority of these different transcripts, and future studies are required to document the importance of *FHIT-1* in pulmonary carcinogenesis.

***PTEN/MMAC1* Gene.** Two recent reports[117,118] document alterations in the *PTEN/MAC1* gene in several SCLC cell lines and in primary SCLC tumors and, less commonly, in NSCLC. PTEN/MMAC1 is a dual specificity phosphatase that is mutated in Cowden disease, which predisposes to several types of cancer, and in Bannayan-Zonana syndrome. However, several earlier reports[119–121] suggested that alterations of the *PTEN/MMAC1* gene in lung cancer are uncommon, and lung cancer is not associated with Cowden disease or Bannayan-Zonana syndrome. Further study, including larger numbers of lung cancers, will be necessary to resolve the role of *PTEN/MMAC1* in lung cancer.

Animal Models for Defining Genetic Aspects of Lung Cancer

Animal models can prove invaluable for clarifying genetic determinants of human cancers, especially for tumors such as lung cancer where little is known about the initial molecular steps underlying tumorigenesis. Multiple animal types, including dogs, mice, and rats, are susceptible to development of either spontaneous lung cancers or lung neoplasms induced by exposure to carcinogens. The carcinogen models may be particularly valuable for determining genetic changes that contribute to predisposition to lung neoplasia and have been especially well studied in the mouse.[122] The most important features of the murine lung cancer models with regard to potential contribution to our understanding of human lung neoplasia will be discussed briefly below.

Controlled exposure of mice to tobacco-related carcinogens, such as NNK, and to various forms of irradiation consistently induce lung tumors. In the main, the lesions have a histology similar to human lung adenocarcinoma and appear to constitute an excellent model for this common form of tumor.[122–124] A particularly important feature of the tumor is that the lesions have been hypothesized to arise in a defined parent cell, the type II pneumocyte.[122,123] This postulation has been further strengthened by the finding that a distinct change, increase in DNA-methyltransferase activity, occurs only in this cell type in the lung immediately after exposure of mice to NNK.[124] Also, following carcinogen exposure, the murine tumors evolve over a distinct course of progression from hyperplasia, to benign appearing adenomas, to frank carcinoma.[122–124] This cellular origin and the ability to examine defined stages of tumor progression offer an excellent opportunity to outline molecular steps responsible for multiple stages of lung tumor progression.

Importantly, susceptibility of mice to the described tumor induction is very strain-dependent, and this genetically determined response relates specifically to lung cancer.[122] This situation provides an opportunity to outline molecular events for predisposition to multiple stages of lung cancer evolution that may have great ramifications for defining genetic steps for human lung cancer. Several approaches to detecting genes responsible for strain susceptibility have been used already. For example, standard linkage analyses have been applied to study generations of mice bred from an initial cross between the A/J mouse, which is very sensitive to tumor induction with NNK exposure, and a resistant strain, the C3H mouse. A major susceptibility locus on distal chromosome 6, termed *Pas1,* has been identified and confirmed in subsequent studies including crosses between the sensitive strain and noninbred mice that are resistant to tumor induction.[122–125]

The gene(s) responsible for the contribution of the described Pas1 locus has not yet been identified but obviously will be of great interest for human lung cancer as well. One interesting candidate, the *Kras2* gene, is near the locus and has been studied in detail. As noted in a previous section, this gene is mutated in a significant percentage of human lung adenocarcinomas and is mutated in an even higher proportion (70 to over 90 percent) of spontaneous and carcinogen-induced murine lung adenocarcinomas as well.[122,123] Furthermore, the alterations in the murine tumors occur very early in the hyperplasia and adenoma stages.[122,123] Intriguingly, in tumors induced in susceptible offspring from crosses between carcinogen-sensitive and -resistant mice, the *Kras2* gene mutations are always in the allele inherited from the sensitive strain.[122] However, the *Kras2* gene does not appear to fall within the tightest area of chromosome linkage on chromosome 6, and the presence of mutations in this gene is as high in tumors from the more resistant strains of mice as in those from sensitive strains.[122] Thus it is felt, at this time, that either the *Kras2* gene mutations are an important step for early progression of the murine tumors but not for the initial steps influenced by inherited susceptibility, or the gene mutations are influenced in some way by a control locus that is contained within the nearby area of tight linkage on chromosome 6.[122]

Subsequent linkage studies to map quantitative trait loci (QTLs) that affect lung cancer incidence or development in mice have detected linkage on chromosomes 4, 6, 9, 10, 11, 12, 17, 18, and 19 (reviewed in ref. 126). Interestingly, the locus on chromosome 4 is near the $p16^{INK4a}$ gene. This locus may be of special importance because in a genome-wide search for LOH in murine lung tumors, the *p16* region was the only region lost consistently, suggesting the presence of a tumor-suppressor gene.[122] Similarly, the frequency of *p16* gene alterations in rat lung tumors is extremely high and consists of homozygous deletions and aberrant promoter region hypermethylation.[127] The relatively weak linkage for the chromosome 4 region to the strain differences in tumor susceptibility suggests that the *p16* gene, or other genes in the LOH area, may, as for *Kras2* mutations, play more of a role in progression than in tumor initiation. Direct studies of alterations in murine homologues of key tumor-suppressor genes for human neoplasia also have been used to search for molecular clues to strain differences in lung tumor susceptibility. No significant incidence for *Rb* or *p53* gene mutations have been found in the murine tumors.[122]

In summary, animal models for lung carcinoma, especially those defined in mice, offer an important opportunity to help define genes that may be central to the development of and genetic predisposition to particularly human lung adenocarcinoma. The difficulty in acquiring large numbers of families with inherited human lung cancer that are suitable for standard linkage analyses emphasizes the importance of using animal models as adjuncts to the study of genetic predisposition to lung cancer in humans. The defined progression stages for the murine carcinogenesis-induced tumors and the differences in strain susceptibility both contribute to the inherent value of using these models to define genes for which human homologues can readily be identified. It will not be surprising if some of the genes discovered will have key roles for lung cancer evolution in both the murine and human settings.

IMPLICATIONS OF GENETIC CHANGES FOR THE DIAGNOSIS AND TREATMENT OF LUNG CANCER

The tremendous impact that lung cancer has on society and the distinct relationship to a known environmental cause for these tumors make this malignancy a prime target for defining genetic markers of risk and for use in early diagnosis. Hopefully, the evidence for an important role for genetic predisposition in determining which smokers develop lung cancer will be followed in the coming years by elucidation of the molecular events involved. In turn, these genetic changes may serve as the best markers for defining risk and marking the earliest stages of lung cancer.

As the best markers emerge, they can be incorporated into diagnostic strategies that are already providing proof of principle for use of genetic changes to provide for early diagnosis of lung cancer, such as the detection of *p53* and *ras* gene mutations in sputum DNA months to years before clinical signs of tumor have been reported.[122] These are retrospective studies in which the precise mutations that appeared in the eventual tumors were known, and prospective investigations will be needed to validate such approaches. However, the ability to use tissue samples obtained by such noninvasive procedures is most encouraging. In fact, other body fluids, including blood and urine, have now been used to detect genetic changes, such as microsatellite instability, that are present in established lung tumors of the patients studied.[128,129] Hopefully, germ-line DNA changes that reflect increased risk for the development of lung cancer also will come to play a role in population screening, since the rate of cigarette smoking remains high and is increasing, especially among young people and women, in many regions of the world.

Some of the genetic changes that already have been defined as frequent events in established lung cancers are being investigated as potential therapeutic targets for lung cancer. Recently, in an initial gene therapy study of patients with lung cancer, regression of tumors injected with a retrovirus for expression of the wild-type *p53* gene, has been reported.[120] Inhibitors of *ras* gene function hold promise for treatment of the many patients with lung cancers that harbor mutations in this family of genes.[131,132] Surely, as other gene alterations important for the various stages of lung cancer progression are discovered, these will present more potential molecular targets for new and novel therapeutic strategies for the current most lethal form of human neoplasia.

REFERENCES

1. Parker SL, Tong T, Bolden S, Wingo PA: Cancer statistics, 1996. *CA* **46**:5, 1996.
2. Ferguson MK, Skosey C, Hoffman PL, Golomb HM: Sex differences in presentation and survival in patients with lung cancer. *J Clin Oncol* **8**:1402, 1990.
3. Mattson ME, Pollack ES, Cullen JW: What are the odds that smoking will kill you. *Am J Public Health* **77**:425, 1987.
4. Pass HI, Mitchell JB, Johnson DH, Turrisi AT: *Lung Cancer: Principles and Practice*. Philadelphia, Lippincott, 1996.
5. Fontana RS, Sanderson DR, Taylor WF: Early lung cancer detection: Results of the initial (prevalence) radiologic and cytologic screening in the Mayo Clinic study. *Am Rev Respir Dis* **130**:561, 1984.
6. Midthun DE, Jett JR: Clinical presentation of lung cancer, in Pass HI, Mitchell JB, Johnson DH, Turrisi AT (eds): *Lung Cancer: Principles and Practice*. Philadelphia, Lippincott, 1996, p 421.
7. Williams DE, Pairolero PC, Davis C, Bernatz PE, Payne WS, Taylor WF, Uhenhopp MA, Fontana RS: Survival of patients surgically treated for stage I lung cancer. *J Thorac Cardiovasc Surg* **82**:70, 1981.
8. Shimizu N, Ando A, Teramoto S, Moritani Y, Nishii K: Outcome of patients with lung cancer detected via mass screening as compared to those presenting with symptoms. *J Surg Oncol* **50**:7, 1992.
9. Einhorn LH, Loehrer PJ, Williams SD, Meyers S, Gabrys T, Nattan SR, Woodburn R, Drasga R, Songer J, Fisher W: Random prospective study of vindesine versus vindesine plus high cisplatin versus vindesine plus cisplatin plus mitomycin C in advanced non lung cancer. *J Clin Oncol* **4**:1037, 1986.
10. Bonomi P: Non small cell lung cancer chemotherapy, in Pass HI, Mitchell JB, Johnson DH, Turrisi AT (eds): *Lung Cancer: Principles and Practice*. Philadelphia, Lippincott, 1996, p 811.
11. Johnson DH, Greco FA: Small cell carcinoma of the lung. *Crit Rev Oncol Hematol* **4**:303, 1986.
12. Miller AB, Fox W, Tall R: Five year follow-up of the Medical Research Council comparative trial of surgery and radiotherapy for the primary treatment of small-celled or oat-celled carcinoma of the bronchus. *Lancet* **2**:501, 1969.
13. Johnson DH: Chemotherapy of small cell lung cancer, in Pass HI, Mitchell JB, Johnson DH, Turrisi AT (eds): *Lung Cancer: Principles and Practice*. Philadelphia, Lippincott, 1996, p 825.
14. Ihde DC: Chemotherapy of lung cancer. *N Engl J Med* **327**:1434, 1992.
15. Murray N, Coy P, Pater J, Hodson I, Arnold Z, Zee BC, Payne D, Kostashuk EC, Evans WK, Dixon P: Importance of timing for thoracic irradiation in the combined modality treatment of limited stage small cell lung cancer. *J Clin Oncol* **11**:336, 1993.

16. Arrigada R, Le Chevalier T, Pignon JP, Riviere A, Monnet I, Chomy P, Tuchais C, Tarayre M, Ruffie P: Initial chemotherapeutic doses and survival in patients with limited small cell lung cancer. *N Engl J Med* **329**:1848, 1993.
17. Gazdar AF, Carney DN, Guccion JG, Baylin SB: Small cell carcinoma of the lung: Cellular origin and relationship to other pulmonary tumors, in Greco FA, Oldham RK, Bunn PA (eds): *Small Cell Lung Cancer.* New York, Grune & Stratton, 1981, p 145.
18. Linnoila RI: in Kaliner MA, Barnes PJ, Kunkel GHH, Baraniuk JN (eds): *Neuropeptides in Respiratory Medicine.* N York, Marcel Dekker, 1994, p 197.
19. Linnoila RI, Mulshine JL, Steinberg SM, Funa K, Matthews MJ, Cotelingam JD, Gazdar AF: Neuroendocrine differentiation in endocrine and non lung carcinomas. *Am J Clin Pathol* **90**:641, 1988.
20. Mabry M, Nelkin BD, Falco JP, Barr LF, Baylin SB: Transitions between lung cancer phenotypes: implications for tumor progression. *Cancer Cell* **3**:53, 1991.
21. Giovino GA, Schooley MW, Zhu BP, Chrismon JH, Tomar SL, Peddicord JP, Merritt RK, Husten CG, Eriksen MP: Surveillance for selected tobacco behaviors: United States, 1900-1994. *MMWR CDC Surveill Summ* **43**:1, 1994.
22. Schottenfeld D: Epidemiology of lung cancer, in Pass HJ, Mitchell JB, Johnson DH, Turrisi AT (eds): *Lung Cancer: Principles and Practice.* Philadelphia, Lippincott, 1996, p 305.
23. Ernster VL: The epidemiology of lung cancer in women. *Ann Epidemiol* **4**:102, 1994.
24. Harris RE, Zang EA, Anderson JI, Wynder EL: Race and sex differences in lung cancer risk associated with cigarette smoking. *Int J Epidemiol* **22**:592, 1993.
25. Sellers TA: Familial predisposition to lung cancer, in Roth JA, Cox JP, Hong WK (eds): *Lung Cancer.* Boston, Blackwell, 1993, p 20.
26. Sellers TA, Bailey JE, Elston RC, Wilson AF, Elston GZ, Ooi WL, Rothschild H: Evidence for mendelian inheritance in the pathogenesis of lung cancer. *J Natl Cancer Inst* **82**:1272, 1990.
27. Sellers TA, Potter JD, Bailey JE, Rich SS, Rothschild H, Elston RC: Lung cancer detection and prevention for an interaction between smoking and predisposition. *Cancer Res* **52**:2694s, 1992.
28. Makimoto T, Tsuchiya S, Nakano H, Watanabe S, Takei Y, Nomoto T, Ishihara S, Saitoh R: Primary lung cancer in young patients. *Nippon Kyobu Shikkan Gakkai Zasshi* **33**:241, 1995.
29. Rocha MP, Fraire AE, Guntupalli KK, Greenberg SD: Lung cancer in the young. *Cancer Detect Prev* **18**:349, 1994.
30. Bourke W, Milstein D, Giura R, Donghi M, Luisetti M, Rubin AH, Smith LJ: Lung cancer in young adults. *Chest* **102**:1723, 1992.
31. Tsuji H, Hara S, Tagawa Y, Kawahara K, Ayabe H, Tomita M: Bilateral bronchiolalveolar carcinoma, showing familial aggregation of lung cancer. *Nippon Kyobu Geka Gakkai Zasshi* **42**:1061, 1994.
32. Ogawa H: Interaction between family history and smoking in lung cancer. *Gan No Rinsho* **33**:575, 1987.
33. Capewell S, Wathen CG, Sankaran R, Sudlow MF: Lung cancer in young patients. *Respir Med* **86**:499, 1992.
34. Larrieu AJ, Jamieson WR, Nelems JM, Fowler R, Yamamoto B, Leriche J, Murray N: Carcinoma of the lung in patients under 40 years of age. *Am J Surg* **149**:602, 1985.
35. Whang-Peng J, Knutsen T, Gazdar A, Steinberg SM, Oie H, Linnoila I, Mulshine J, Nau M, Minna JD: Nonrandom structural and numerical chromosome changes in non-small-cell lung cancer. *Genes Chromosom Cancer* **3**:168, 1991.
36. Testa JR, Siegfried JM, Liu Z, Hunt JD, Feder MM, Litwin S, Zhou J, Taguchi T, Keller SM: Cytogenetic analysis of 63 non cell lung carcinomas: Recurrent chromosome alterations amid frequent and widespread genomic upheaval. *Genes Chromosom Cancer* **11**:178, 1994.
37. Hibi K, Takahashi T, Yamakawa K, Ueda R, Sekido Y, Ariyoshi Y, Suyama M, Takagi H, Nakamura Y: Three distinct regions involved in 3p deletion in human lung cancer. *Oncogene* **7**:445, 1992.
38. Brauch H, Tory K, Kotler F, Gazdar AF, Pettengill OS, Johnson B, Graziano S, Winton T, Buys CH, Sorenson GD: Molecular mapping of deletion sites in the short arm of chromosome 3 in human lung cancer. *Genes Chromosom Cancer* **1**:240, 1990.
39. Rabbitts P, Bergh J, Douglas J, Collins F, Waters J: A submicroscopic homozygous deletion at the D3S3 locus in a cell line isolated from a small cell lung carcinoma. *Genes Chromosom Cancer* **2**:231, 1990.
40. Daly MC, Xiang RH, Buchhagen D, Hensel CH, Garcia DK, Killary AM, Minna JD, Naylor SL: A homozygous deletion on chromosome 3 in a small cell lung cancer cell line correlates with a region of tumor suppressor activity. *Oncogene* **8**:1721, 1993.
41. Yokota J, Wada M, Shimosato Y, Terada M, Sugimura T: Loss of heterozygosity of chromosomes 3, 13, and 17 in small cell carcinoma and on chromosome 3 in adenocarcinoma of the lung. *Proc Natl Acad Sci USA* **84**:9252, 1987.
42. Neville EM, Stewart M, Myskow M, Donnelly RJ, Field JK: Loss of heterozygosity at 9p23 defines a novel locus in non-small cell lung cancer. *Oncogene* **11**:581, 1995.
43. Hosoe S, Ueno K, Shigedo Y, Tachibana I, Osaki T, Kumagai T, Tanio Y, Kawase I, Nakamura Y, Kishimoto T: A frequent deletion of chromosome 5q21 in advanced small cell and non-small cell carcinoma of the lung. *Cancer Res* **54**:1787, 1994.
44. Horii A, Nakatsuru S, Miyoshi Y, Ichii S, Nagase H, Ando H, Yanagisawa A, Tsuchiya E, Kato Y, Nakamura Y: Frequent somatic mutations of *APC* gene in human pancreatic cancer. *Cancer Res* **52**:6696, 1992.
45. Sundaresan V, Ganly P, Haselton P, Rudd R, Sinha G, Bleehen NM, Rabbitts P: *p53* and chromosome 3 abnormalities, characteristic of malignant lung tumours, are detectable in preinvasive lesions of the bronchus. *Oncogene* **7**:1989, 1992.
46. Hung J, Kishimoto Y, Sugio K, Virmani A, McIntire DD, Minna JD, Gazdar AF: Allele-specific chromosome 3p deletions occur at an early stage in the pathogenesis of lung carcinoma. *JAMA* **273**:558, 1995.
47. Kishimoto Y, Sugio K, Hung JY, Virmani AK, McIntire DD, Minna JD, Gazdar AF: Allele loss in chromosome 9p loci in preneoplastic lesions accompanying non-small-cell lung cancers. *J Natl Cancer Inst* **87**:1224, 1995.
48. Sugio K, Kishimoto Y, Virmani AK, Hung JY, Gazdar AF: *K-ras* mutations are a relatively late event in the pathogenesis of lung carcinomas. *Cancer Res* **54**:5811, 1994.
49. Westra WH, Slebos RJ, Offerhaus GJ, Goodman SN, Evers SG, Kensler TW, Askin FB, Rodenhuis S, Hruban RH: *K-ras* oncogene activation in lung adenocarcinomas from former smokers: Evidence that *K-ras* mutations are an early and irreversible event in the development of adenocarcinoma of the lung. *Cancer* **72**:432, 1993.
50. Shiseki M, Kohno T, Nishikawa R, Sameshima Y, Mizoguchi H, Yokota J: Frequent allelic losses on chromosome 2q, 18q, and 22q in advanced non-small cell lung carcinoma. *Cancer Res* **54**:5643, 1994.
51. Merlo A, Mabry M, Gabrielson E, Vollmer R, Baylin SB, Sidransky D: Frequent microsatellite instability in primary small cell lung cancer. *Cancer Res* **54**:2098, 1994.
52. Adachi J, Shiseki M, Okazaki T, Ishimaru G, Noguchi M, Hirohashi S, Yokota J: Microsatellite instability in primary and metastatic lung carcinomas. *Genes Chromosom Cancer* **14**:301, 1995.
53. Shridhar V, Siegfried J, Hunt J, del Mar Alonso M, Smith DI: Genetic instability of microsatellite sequences in many non-small cell lung carcinomas. *Cancer Res* **54**:2084, 1994.
54. Sugimura H, Caporaso NE, Modali RV, Hoover RN, Resau JH, Trump BF, Longeran JA, Krontiris TG, Mann DL, Weston A: Association of rare alleles of the Harvey *ras* protooncogene with lung cancer. *Cancer Res* **50**:1857, 1990.
55. Vineis P, Caporaso N: The analysis of restriction fragment length polymorphism in human cancer: A review from an epidemiologic perspective. *Int J Cancer* **47**:26, 1991.
56. Li FP, Fraumeni JF, Mulvihill JJ, Blattner WA, Dreyfus MG, Tucker MA, Miller RW: A cancer family syndrome in twenty kindreds. *Cancer Res* **48**:5358, 1988.
57. Lavigueur A, Bernstein A: *p53* transgenic mice: Accelerated erythroleukemia induction by Friend virus. *Oncogene* **6**:2197, 1991.
58. Donehower LA, Harvey M, Slagle BL, McArthur MJ, Montgomery CA, Butel JS, Bradley A: Mice deficient for p53 are developmentally normal but susceptible to spontaneous tumours. *Nature* **356**:215, 1992.
59. Goodrich DW, Lee W: The molecular genetics of retinoblastoma. *Cancer Surv* **9**:529, 1990.
60. Strong LC, Herson J, Haas C, Elder K, Chakraborty R, Weiss KM, Majumder P: Cancer mortality in relatives of retinoblastoma patients. *J Natl Cancer Inst* **73**:303, 1984.
61. Sanders BM, Jay M, Draper GJ, Roberts EM: Non-ocular cancer in relatives of retinoblastoma patients. *Br J Cancer* **60**:358, 1989.
62. German J: Bloom syndrome: A Mendelian prototype of somatic mutational disease. *Medicine* **72**:393, 1993.
63. Shields PG, Harris CC: Genetic predisposition to cancer, in Roth JA, Cox JD, Hong WK (eds): *Lung Cancer.* Boston, Blackwell, 1993, p 3.
64. Crespi CL, Penman BW, Gelboin HV, Gonzalez FJ: A tobacco smoke nitrosamine, 4(methylnitrosamino)(3) is activated by multiple cytochrome P450s including the polymorphic human cytchrome P450 2D6. *Carcinogenesis* **12**:1197, 1991.

65. Caporaso NE, Shields PG, Landi MT, Shaw GL, Tucker MA, Hoover R, Sugimura H, Weston A, Harris CC: The debrisoquine metabolic phenotype and DNA assays: Implications of misclassification for the association of lung cancer and the debrisoquine metabolic phenotype. *Environ Health Perspect* **98**:101, 1992.
66. Caporaso NE, Hayes RB, Dosemeci M, Hoover R, Ayesh R, Hetzel M, Idle J: Lung cancer risk, occupational exposure, and the debrisoquine metabolic phenotype. *Cancer Res* **49**:3675, 1989.
67. Gough AC, Miles JS, Spurr NK, Moss JE, Gaedigk A, Eichelbaum M, Wolf CR: Identification of the primary gene defect at the cytochrome P450 CYP2D locus. *Nature* **347**:773, 1990.
68. Shaw GL, Falk RT, Deslauriers J, Frame JN, Nesbitt JC, Pass HI, Issaq HJ, Hoover RN, Tucker MA: Debrisoquine metabolism and lung cancer risk. *Cancer Epidemiol Biomark Prev* **4**:41, 1995.
69. Shaw GL, Falk RT, Frame JN, Weiffenbach B, Nesbitt JC, Pass HI, Caporaso NE, Moir DT, Tucker MA: Genetic polymorphism of CYP2D6 and lung cancer risk. *Cancer Epidemiol Biomark Prev* **7**:215, 1998.
70. Legrand-Andreoletti M, Stucker I, Marez D, Galais P, Cosme J, Sabbagh N, Spire C, Cenee S, Lafitte JJ, Beaune P, Broly F: Cytochrome P450 CYP2D6 gene polymorphism and lung cancer susceptibility in Caucasians. *Pharmacogenetics* **8**:7, 1998.
71. Rudiger HW, Nowak D, Hartmann K, Cerutti PA: Enhanced formation of benzo(a) pyrene: DNA adducts in monocytes of patients with a presumed predisposition to lung cancer. *Cancer Res* **45**:5890, 1985.
72. To-Figueras J, Gene M, Gomez-Catalan J, Galan C, Firvida J, Fuentes M, Rodamilans M, Huguet E, Estape J, Corbella J: Glutathione *S*-transferase M1 and codon 72 p53 polymorphisms in a northwestern Mediterranean population and their relation to lung cancer susceptibility. *Cancer Epidemiol Biomark Prev* **5**:337, 1996.
73. London SJ, Daly AK, Cooper J, Navidi WC, Carpenter CL, Idle JR: Polymorphism of glutathione *S*-transferase M1 and lung cancer risk among African-Americans and Caucasians in Los Angeles County, California. *J Natl Cancer Inst* **87**:1246, 1995.
74. Ryberg D, Skaug V, Hewer A, Phillips DH, Harries LW, Wolf CR, Ogreid D, Ulvik A, Vu P, Haugen A: Genotypes of glutathione *S*-transferase M1 and P1 and their significance for lung DNA adduct levels and cancer risk. *Carcinogenesis* **18**:1285, 1997.
75. Clements NC, Nelson MA, Wymer JA, Savage C, Aquirre M, Garewal H: Analysis of *K-ras* gene mutations in malignant and nonmalignant endobronchial tissue obtained by fiberoptic bronchoscopy. *Am J Respir Crit Care Med* **152**:1374, 1995.
76. Rodenhuis S, Slebos R, Boot AJ, Evers SG, Mooi WJ, Wagenaar SS, van Bodegom PC, Bos JL: Incidence and possible clinical significance of *K-ras* oncogene activation in adenocarcinoma of the human lung. *Cancer Res* **48**:5738, 1988.
77. Mills NE, Fishman CL, Scholes J, Anderson SE, Rom WN, Jacobson DR: Detection of *K-ras* oncogene mutations in bronchoalveolar lavage fluid for lung cancer diagnosis. *J Natl Cancer Inst* **87**:1056, 1995.
78. Suzuki Y, Orita M, Shiraishi M, Hayashi K, Sekiya T: Detection of *ras* gene mutations in human lung cancers by single strand conformation polymorphism analysis of polymerase chain reaction products. *Oncogene* **5**:1037, 1990.
79. Slebos RJC, Evers SG, Wagenaar SS, Rodenhuis S: Cellular protooncogenes are infrequently amplified in untreated non-small cell lung cancer (NSCLC). *Br J Cancer* **59**:76, 1988.
80. Reynolds S, Anna CK, Brown KC, Wiest JS, Beattie EJ, Pero RW, Iglehart JD, Anderson MW: Activated oncogenes in human lung tumors from smokers. *Proc Natl Acad Sci USA* **88**:1085, 1991.
81. Li S, Rosell R, Urban A, Font A, Ariza A, Armengol P, Abad A, Navas JJ, Monzo M: *K-ras* gene point mutation: A stable tumor marker in non-small cell lung carcinoma. *Lung Cancer* **11**:19, 1994.
82. Rosell R, Li S, Skacel Z, Mate JL, Maestre J, Canela M, Tolosa E, Armengol P, Barnadas A, Ariza A: Prognostic impact of mutated *K-ras* gene in surgically resected non cell lung cancer patients. *Oncogene* **8**:2407, 1993.
83. Ohshima S, Shimizu Y, Takahama M: Detection of *c-Ki-ras* gene mutation in paraffin sections of adenocarcinoma and atypical bronchioloalveolar cell hyperplasia of human lung. *Virchows Arch* **424**:129, 1994.
84. Wagner SN, Muller R, Boehm J, Putz B, Wunsch PH, Hofler H: Neuroendocrine neoplasms of the lung are not associated with point mutations at codon 12 of the *Ki-ras* gene. *Virchows Arch [B]* **63**:325, 1993.
85. Rodenhuis S, Slebos RJ: Clinical significance of *ras* oncogene activation in human lung cancer. *Cancer Res* **52**:2665s, 1992.
86. Little CD, Nau MM, Carney DN, Gazdar AF, Minna JD: Amplification and expression of the *c-myc* oncogene in human lung cancer cell lines. *Nature* **306**:194, 1983.
87. Brennan J, O'Connor T, Makuch RW, Simmons AM, Russell E, Linnoila RI, Phelps RM, Gazdar AF, Ihde DC, Johnson BE: *Myc* family DNA amplification in 107 tumors and tumor cell lines from patients with small cell lung cancer treated with different combination chemotherapy regimens. *Cancer Res* **51**:1708, 1991.
88. Johnson BE, Ihde DC, Makuch RW, Gazdar AF, Carney DN, Oie H, Russell E, Nau MM, Minna JD: *c-myc* family oncogene amplification in tumor cell lines established from small cell lung cancer patients and its relationship to clinical status and course. *J Clin Invest* **79**:1629, 1987.
89. Sklar MD, Prochownik EV: Modulation of cis resistance in Friend erythroleukemia cells by *c-myc*. *Cancer Res* **51**:2118, 1991.
90. Niimi S, Nakagawa K, Yokota J, Tsunokawa Y, Nishio K, Terashima Y, Shibuya M, Terada M, Saijo N: Resistance to anticancer drugs in NIH3T3 cells transfected with *c-myc* and/or *c-H-ras* genes. *Br J Cancer* **63**:237, 1991.
91. Nau MM, Brooks BJ, Battey J, Sausville E, Gazdar AF, Kirsch IR, McBride OW, Bertness V, Hollis GF, Minna JD: *L-myc,* a new myc gene amplified and expressed in human small cell lung cancer. *Nature* **318**:69, 1985.
92. Nau MM, Brooks BJ, Carney DN, Gazdar AF, Battey JF, Sausville EA, Minna JD: Human small lung cancers show amplification and expression of the *N-myc* gene. *Proc Natl Acad Sci USA* **83**:1092, 1986.
93. Johnson BE: The role of MYC, JUN, and FOS oncogenes in human lung cancer, in Pass HI, Mitchell JB, Johnson DH, Turisi AT (eds): *Lung Cancer: Principles and Practice*. Philadelphia, Lippincott, 1996, p 83.
94. Schauer IE, Siriwardana S, Langan TA, Sclafani RA: Cyclin D1 overexpression vs retinoblastoma inactivation: Implications for growth control evasion in non-small cell and small cell lung cancer. *Proc Natl Acad Sci USA* **91**:7827, 1994.
95. Marchetti A, Doglioni C, Barbareschi M, Buttitta F, Pellegrini S, Gaeta P, La Rocca R, Merlo G, Chella A, Angeletti CA, Dalla Palma P, Bevilacqua G: Cyclin D1 and retinoblastoma susceptibility gene alterations in non-small cell lung cancer. *Int J Cancer* **75**:187, 1998.
96. Chiba I, Takashi T, Nau MM, D'Amico D, Curiel DT, Misudomi T, Buchhagen DL, Carbone D, Piantadosi S, Koga H: Mutations in the *p53* gene are frequent in primary, resected non-small cell lung cancer. *Oncogene* **5**:1603, 1990.
97. D'Amico D, Carbone D, Mitsudomi T, Nau M, Fedorko J, Russell E, Johnson B, Buchhagen D, Bodner S, Phelps R: High frequency of somatically acquired *p53* mutations in small cell lung cancer cell lines and tumors. *Oncogene* **7**:339, 1992.
98. Denissenko MF, Pao A, Tang M, Pfeifer GP: Preferential formation of benzo[a]pyrene adducts at lung cancer mutational hot spots in p53. *Science* **274**:430, 1996.
99. Quinlan DC, Davidson AG, Summers CL, Warden HE, Doshi HM: Accumulation of p53 protein correlates with a poor prognosis in human lung cancer. *Cancer Res* **52**:4828, 1992.
100. McLaren R, Kuzu I, Dunnill M, Harris A, Lane D, Gatter K: The relationship of p53 immunostaining to survival in carcinoma of the lung. *Br J Cancer* **66**:735, 1992.
101. Serrano M, Hannon GJ, Beach D: A new regulatory motif in cell control causing specific inhibition of cyclin D/CDK4. *Nature* **366**:704, 1993.
102. Sherr CJ: G1 phase progression: Cycling on cue. *Cell* **79**:551, 1994.
103. Larsen C: $p16^{INK4}$: A gene with a dual capacity to encode unrelated proteins that inhibit cell cycle progression. *Oncogene* **12**:2041, 1996.
104. Kamb A, Gruis NA, Weaver J, Liu Q, Harshman K, Tavtigian SV, Stockert E, Day RS, Johnson BE, Skolnick MH: A cell cycle regulator potentially involved in genesis of many tumor types. *Science* **264**:436, 1994.
105. Cairns P, Mao L, Merlo A, Lee DJ, Schwab D, Eby Y, Tokino K, van der Riet P, Blaugrund JE, Sidransky D: Rates of *p16* (*MTS1*) mutations in primary tumors with 9p loss. *Science* **265**:415, 1994.
106. Okamoto A, Hussain SP, Hagiwara K, Spillare EA, Rusin MR, Demetrick DJ, Serrano M, Hannon GJ, Shiseki M, Zariwala M, Xiong Y, Beach DH, Yokota J, Harris CC: Mutations in the $p16^{INK4}/MTS1/CDKN2$, $p15^{INK4}$/MTS2, and *p18* genes in primary and metastatic lung cancer. *Cancer Res* **55**:1448, 1995.
107. Packenham JP, Taylor JA, White CM, Anna CH, Barrett JC, Devereux TR: Homozygous deletions at chromosome 9p21 and mutation analysis of p16 and p15 in microdissected primary non cell lung cancers. *Clin Cancer Res* **1**:687, 1995.

108. Merlo A, Herman JG, Mao L, Lee DJ, Gabrielson E, Burger PC, Baylin SB, Sidransky D: 59 CpG island methylation is associated with transcriptional silencing of the tumour suppressor *p16/CDKN2/MTS1* in human cancers. *Nature Med* **1**:686, 1995.
109. Herman JG, Merlo A, Mao L, Lapidus RG, Issa J, Davidson NE, Sidransky D, Baylin SB: Inactivation of the *CDKN2/p16/MTS1* gene is frequently associated with aberrant DNA methylation in all common human cancers. *Cancer Res* **55**:4525, 1995.
110. Shapiro GI, Edwards CD, Kobzik L, Godleski J, Richards W, Sugarbaker DJ, Rollins BJ: Reciprocal *Rb* inactivation and $p16^{INK4}$ expression in primary lung cancers and cell lines. *Cancer Res* **55**:505, 1995.
111. Otterson GA, Khleif SN, Chen W, Coxon AB, Kaye FJ: *CDKN2* gene silencing in lung cancer by DNA hypermethylation and kinetics of $p16^{INK4}$ protein induction by 5-aza 29deoxycytidine. *Oncogene* **11**:1211, 1995.
112. Otterson GA, Kratzke RA, Coxon A, Kim YW, Kaye FJ: Absence of $p16^{INK4}$ protein is restricted to the subset of lung cancer lines that retains wildtype RB. *Oncogene* **9**:3375, 1994.
113. Sherr CJ: Mammalian G1 cyclins. *Cell* **73**:1059, 1993.
114. Hensel CH, Hsieh CL, Gazdar AF, Johnson BE, Sakaguchi AY, Naylor SL, Lee WH, Lee EY: Altered structure and expression of the retinoblastoma susceptibility gene in small cell lung cancer. *Cancer Res* **50**:3067, 1990.
115. Xu HJ, Hu SX, Cagle PT, Moore GE, Benedict WF: Absence of retinoblastoma protein expression in primary non-small cell lung carcinomas. *Cancer Res* **51**:2735, 1991.
116. Sozzi G, Veronese ML, Negrini M, Baffa R, Cotticelli MG, Inoue H, Tornielli S, Pilotti S, De Gregorio L, Pastorino U, Pierotti MA, Ohta M, Huebner K, Croce CM: The *FHIT* gene at 3p14.2 is abnormal in lung cancer. *Cell* **85**:17, 1996.
117. Kohno T, Takahashi M, Manda R, Yokota J: Inactivation of the *PTEN/MMAC1/TEP1* gene in human lung cancers. *Genes Chromosom Cancer* **22**:152, 1998.
118. Yokomizo A, Tindall DJ, Drabkin H, Gemmill R, Franklin W, Yang P, Sugio K, Smith DI, Liu W: *PTEN/MMAC1* mutations identified in small cell, but not in non-small cell lung cancers. *Oncogene* **17**:475, 1998.
119. Sakurada A, Suzuki A, Sato M, Yamakawa H, Orikasa K, Uyeno S, Ono T, Ohuchi N, Fujimura S, Horii A: Infrequent genetic alterations of the *PTEN/MMAC1* gene in Japanese patients with primary cancers of the breast, lung, pancreas, kidney, and ovary. *Jpn J Cancer Res* **88**:1025, 1997.
120. Kim SK, Su LK, Oh Y, Kemp BL, Hong WK, Mao L: Alterations of *PTEN/MMAC1,* a candidate tumor suppressor gene, and its homologue, *PTH2,* in small cell lung cancer cell lines. *Oncogene* **16**:89, 1998.
121. Okami K, Wu L, Riggins G, Cairns P, Goggins M, Evron E, Halachmi N, Ahrendt SA, Reed AL, Hilgers W, Kern SE, Koch WM, Sidransky D, Jen J: Analysis of *PTEN/MMAC1* alterations in aerodigestive tract tumors. *Cancer Res* **58**:509, 1998.
122. Dragani TA, Manenti G, Pierotti MA: Genetics of murine lung tumors. *Adv Cancer Res* **67**:83, 1995.
123. Belinsky SA, Devereux TR, Maronpot RR, Stoner GD, Anderson MW: Relationship between the formation of promutagenic adducts and the activation of *K-ras* protoncogene in lung tumors from A/J mice treated with nitrosamines. *Cancer Res* **49**:5305, 1989.
124. Belinsky SA, Nikula KJ, Baylin SB, Issa J: Increased cytosine DNA activity is target-cell-specific and an early event in lung cancer. *Proc Natl Acad Sci USA* **93**:4045, 1996.
125. Gariboldi M, Manenti G, Canzian F, Falvella FS, Radice MT, Pierotti MA, Della Porta G, Binelli G, Dragani TA: A major susceptibility locus to murine lung carcinogenesis maps on chromosome 6. *Nature Genet* **3**:132, 1993.
126. Herzog CR, Lubet RA, You M: Genetic alterations in mouse lung tumors: Implications for cancer chemoprevention. *J Cell Biochem Suppl* **28-29**:49, 1997.
127. Swafford DS, Middleton SK, Palmisano WA, Nikula KJ, Tesfaigzi J, Baylin SB, Herman JG, Belinsky SA: Frequent aberrant methylation of $p16^{INK4}$ in primary rat lung tumors. *Mol Cell Biol* **17**:1366, 1997.
128. Mao L, Hruban RH, Boyle JO, Tockman M, Sidransky D: Detection of oncogene mutations in sputum precedes diagnosis of lung cancer. *Cancer Res* **54**:1634, 1994.
129. Chen XQ, Stroun M, Magnenat J, Nicod LP, Kurt A, Lyautey J, Lederrey C, Anker P: Microsatellite alterations in plasma DNA of small cell lung cancer patients. *Nature Med* **2**:1033, 1996.
130. Roth JA, Nguyen D, Lawrence DD, Kemp BL, Carrasco CH, Ferson DZ, Hong WK, Komaki R, Lee JJ, Nesbitt JC, Pisters KMW, Putnam JB, Schea R, Shin DM, Walsh GL, Dolormente MM, Han C, Martin FD, Yen N, Xu K: Retrovirus wild *p53* gene transfer to tumors of patients with lung cancer. *Nature Med* **2**:985, 1996.
131. Sun J, Qian Y, Hamilton AD, Sebti SM: *Ras* CAAX peptidomimetic FTI276 selectivity blocks tumor growth in nude mice of a human lung carcinoma with *K-ras* mutation and *p53* deletion. *Cancer Res* **55**:4243, 1995.
132. James GL, Goldstein JL, Brown MR, Rawson TE, Somers TC, McDowell RS, Crowley CW, Lucas BK, Levinson AD, Marsters JC: Benzodiazepine peptidomimetics: Potent inhibitors of *ras* farnesylation in animal cells. *Science* **260**:1937, 1993.

CHAPTER 59

Hepatocellular Carcinoma

Lynne W. Elmore ▪ Curtis C. Harris

1. **Hepatocellular carcinoma (HCC) is an aggressive malignancy with a poor prognosis. The multifactorial and multistage pathogenesis of HCC has fascinated a wide spectrum of cancer researchers for decades. While a number of etiologic factors have been identified, the elucidation of their mechanistic roles in hepatocarcinogenesis has recently just begun. Clearly, in sub-Saharan Africa and Eastern Asia, viral and chemical carcinogenic components are involved, with the subsequent inactivation of the p53 tumor suppressor gene playing a central role. A better understanding of the molecular pathogenesis of HCC will provide clues for more effective preventive and therapeutic strategies.**
2. **HCC is the predominant cause of cancer mortality in Southern China and sub-Saharan Africa. Infection with hepatitis B virus (HBV) and food contamination with aflatoxin B_1 (AFB_1) are major and possible synergistic risk factors. A number of conditions associated with chronic hepatic inflammation and cirrhosis have also been identified as important etiologic factors worldwide.**
3. **HBV sequences randomly integrate into host chromosomal DNA, resulting in frequent rearrangements. HBV-induced chromosomal aberrations may in part explain the loss of heterozygosity reported on many chromosomes in HCCs. Allelic loss of the short arm of chromosome 17, which includes the p53 tumor suppressor gene, has commonly been found in human HCCs.**
4. **In specific geographic regions of Asia, Africa, and North America with high HCC risk, e.g., Qidong and Tongon, China, southern Africa, and Mexico, a G to T transversion at the third position of codon 249 of p53 has provided a molecular link between dietary AFB_1 exposure and liver cancer development. Data from laboratory studies indicate that this region of p53 is highly sensitive to AFB_1-induced DNA damage and that the resulting mutated protein provides a selective growth advantage in liver cells. Inactivation of p53 gene function may also result from its association with the HBV X protein (HBx). p53 and HBx physically associate, resulting in the inability of p53 to bind specific DNA sequences, transcriptionally transactivate p53-effector genes, associate with critical DNA repair proteins, and induce apoptosis. Abnormalities of the retinoblastoma tumor suppressor gene, typically in advanced lesions and associated with loss of p53, have also been reported in HCCs.**
5. **While mutation and amplification of protooncogenes, e.g., the ras family, are rarely detected in human HCCs, their overexpression is a common finding. *c-myc* and *c-fos* overexpression may result in part from HBV-encoded transcriptional transactivators, which are often expressed and functionally active in HCCs.**
6. **Insulin-like growth factor II (IGF-II) and insulin receptor substrate 1 (IRS-1) are frequently expressed at high levels in HCCs. The insulin growth factor signal transduction pathways may contribute to hepatocarcinogenesis by providing a strong proliferative stimulus, promoting tumor angiogenesis and/or preventing transforming growth factor-β_1(TGF-β_1)-induced apoptosis. Overexpression of transforming growth factor-α also is observed in many HCCs, particularly in those tumors associated with HBV infection.**
7. **A better understanding of the complex pathobiological process of hepatocarcinogenesis has resulted in more effective preventive measures, including the implementation of HBV vaccination programs. The possibility of *p53* as a target for HCC therapy is discussed.**

Hepatocellular carcinoma is one of the most common malignancies worldwide, affecting 250,000 to 1,000,000 individuals annually (reviewed in[1,2]). HCC causes at least 200,000 deaths per year, and in some regions such as Qidong, China, this disease causes 10 percent of all deaths. Both epidemiologists and laboratory researchers have greatly contributed to the understanding of the multifactorial etiology and multistage pathogenesis of HCC[3,4] (Fig. 59-1).

EPIDEMIOLOGY AND ETIOLOGY

The geographic distribution of HCC is highly variable, with Eastern Asia and sub-Saharan Africa being the most prevalent regions (reviewed in[2,5]). Substantial epidemiologic evidence indicates that HBV is a major risk factor for the development of HCC (reviewed in[6]). HBV carriers with chronic active hepatitis have up to a 200-fold greater risk of developing HCC than age-matched noninfected controls.[7–12] Moreover, an estimated 80 percent of HCCs worldwide are in HBV-infected individuals. Aflatoxin B_1 (AFB_1) also is considered to be a significant etiologic agent in certain geographic areas (e.g., Asia, southern Africa, and Mexico) where food contaminated by this mycotoxin is consumed.[13–15] In the high-HCC incidence geographic area of China, exposure to dietary AFB_1 and chronic HBV infection are synergistic risk factors.[15–19] Other etiologic factors for hepatocarcinogenesis include conditions associated with chronic necroinflammatory liver disease and cirrhosis, such as hepatitis C virus (HCV) infection, chronic alcohol-induced liver disease, hemochromatosis, primary biliary cirrhosis, and alpha-1 antitrypsin deficiency.[2,6,20–25] Data from recent case series and case control studies indicate that synergistic interactions may also exist between HBV and HCV in the development of HCC.[26–29]

CHROMOSOMAL AND GENETIC ABNORMALITIES

Little is known regarding the specific alterations responsible for the development or progression of human HCC. Loss of heterozygosity (LOH) has been associated with inactivation of tumor suppressor genes.[30–36] In human HCCs, LOH has been reported on several chromosome arms, including 1p[37–39], 1q[39,40], 2q[39], 4q[38–42], 5q[43,44], 6q[39,45], 8p[39,40,46,47], 8q[38,40,44], 9p[44,48], 9q[39], 10q[40,49], 11p[44,50,51], 11q[44], 13q[39,40,44,51,52] and 17p[38,40,44,52,53] with some occurring irrespective of the presence of HBV infection.[49,54] It is noteworthy that four cases have been reported in which

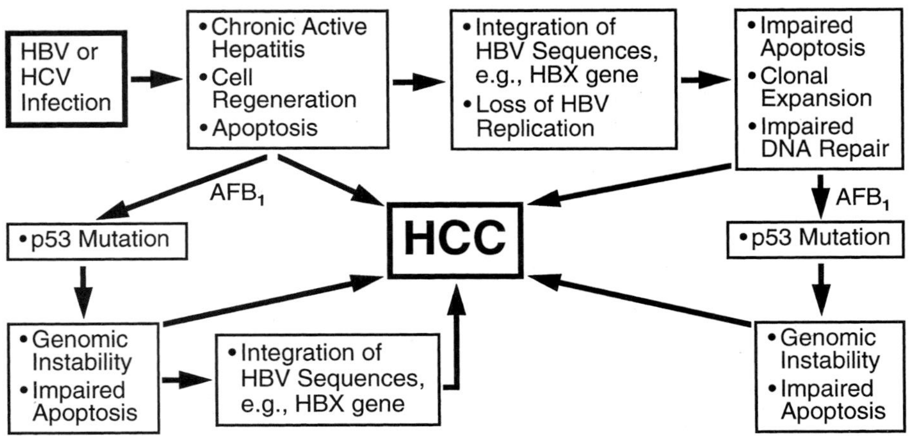

Fig. 59-1 Model of viral-chemical interactions in multistage hepatocellular carcinogenesis.

HBV-associated rearrangements have affected chromosome 17.[35,36,55,56] In two of these[35,36] the rearrangement mapped in the vicinity of the tumor suppressor gene p53, which is located on chromosome 17p13.1.[57] As described below ("Tumor Suppressor Genes"), p53 is the most common LOH site described in human HCCs,[58–62] and data are accumulating to strongly suggest that inactivation of this gene/protein may significantly contribute to the molecular pathogenesis of human HCC. A frequent LOH on 6q at the mannose-6-phosphate/insulin-like growth factor II receptor (M6P/IGF2r) locus in human hepatocellular carcinomas and adenomas has also been reported.[45,63,64] Since this receptor is necessary for both the activation of a growth inhibitor (transforming growth factor β_1 [TGF-β_1])[65] and the degradation of a potent mitogen (insulin growth factor II [IGF-II]),[66] its loss could facilitate liver cell growth.

Most HCCs in HBV carriers contain HBV DNA sequences integrated into the host chromosomal DNA.[6,67] Unlike woodchuck hepatitis virus DNA, which frequently integrates into the c-*myc* or N-*myc* protooncogenes, resulting in either their rearrangement or overexpression,[68,69] the sites of HBV integration in human HCC are highly variable and random.[70,71] Findings of amplification or a single base mutation of some oncogenes have been reported in human HCCs associated with HBV integration, but their incidence is very rare.[72,73] Instead, the sites of cellular DNA at which HBV integrates frequently undergo rearrangements,[74,75] resulting in translocations,[35,55] inverted duplications,[76] deletions,[50,55,77] and possibly recombinatorial events.[2,78] These HBV-induced chromosomal alterations may result in the loss of relevant cellular genes, such as tumor suppressor genes, important in cell cycle control and differentiation.

Tumor Suppressor Genes

The p53 tumor suppressor protein is involved in multiple cellular processes, including cell cycle control, senescence, DNA repair, genomic stability, and apoptosis (reviewed in[79,80]). p53 is functionally inactivated by structural mutations, viral proteins, and endogenous cellular mechanisms in the majority of human cancers.[79,81–83] Certain domains of the p53 gene have been highly conserved, reflecting the functional importance and selection of this protein.[84] The majority of base substitutions fall within the highly conserved central portion of the gene,[85,86] which mediates sequence-specific DNA binding and transcriptional activation[81] (Fig. 59-2). An extensive analysis of p53 gene mutations indicates that the sites and features of DNA base changes differ among the various human tumor types.[82,85] In the case of HCC, a unique mutational spectrum has provided a strong molecular link between carcinogen exposure and cancer development. When primary HCCs in Qidong, China, were examined, we found that 8 of 16 had point mutations at the third position of codon 249, resulting in a G:C to T:A transversion.[88] This finding has been confirmed by others[89,90] and extended to HCCs from southern Africa and North America and Tongon, China.[58,91–93] A dose-dependent relationship between dietary AFB_1 and codon 249^{ser} p53 mutations is observed in these geographic areas (Fig. 59-3). HCCs from geographic areas of low AFB_1 exposure have a different mutational spectrum,[58,94,95] further establishing a positive association between high dietary AFB_1 exposure and 249^{ser} mutations. An analysis of p53 mutations in several human HCC and hepatoblastoma cell lines indicates that this mutational hotspot is specific for liver tumors of hepatocellular origin and does not require the genomic integration of HBV.[96]

Using a highly sensitive genotypic mutation assay, Aguilar et al.[97] have demonstrated the relative abundance of the p53 249^{ser} mutant liver cells of nonmalignant specimens from Qidong when compared to specimens from Thailand and the United States. The biological basis for this frequently observed, early mutational event may be due to the high mutability of the third base at codon 249, as suggested by in vitro studies using human liver cells[98–100]. An alternate, but not mutually exclusive, explanation is that this mutation provides liver cells with a selective growth advantage. Supporting this hypothesis are the following observations: (1) p53-null human liver cancer cells exhibit an enhanced growth rate following transfection with the p53 249^{ser} mutant;[101] (2) introduction of a murine p53 mutation corresponding to human codon 249 into a murine hepatocyte cell line resulted in a selective growth advantage;[102] (3) the 249^{ser} mutant inhibits wild-type p53-mediated apoptosis, resulting in increased cell survival;[103] and (4) the 249^{ser} mutant is more effective than other p53 mutants in inhibiting wild-type p53 transactivation activity in human liver cells[103] (Fig. 59-4). One model concerning the generation of liver cancers with 249^{ser} mutation is that AFB_1 is metabolically activated to form the promutagenic N7dG adduct.[104,105] Enhanced cell proliferation due to chronic active hepatitis then allows both fixation of the G:C → T:A transversion in codon 249 of the p53 gene and selective clonal expansion of cells containing this mutated gene.

While the p53 249^{ser} mutant in HCCs correlates with high risk exposure to AFB_1, the absence of mutations in exons 5–8 of the p53 gene in 50 to 80 percent of HCCs[87,88,91,106,107] suggests that p53 inactivation may be achieved by another mechanism. The finding that p53 protein and HBx interact[108–110] prompted us to evaluate the functional consequences of this association. HBx strongly inhibits p53 sequence-specific binding[109] which is in contrast to the enhanced DNA binding specificity of the transcription factors CREB and AFT-2 when complexed to HBx, a non-DNA binding cotransactivator[111,112]. HBx also blocks p53-mediated transcriptional transactivation in vivo, as well as the in vitro association of p53 with either XPB (ERCC3)[109] or XPD,[113] transcriptional factors involved in nucleotide excision repair.[114–115] Moreover, HBx efficiently abrogates p53-mediataed apoptosis[103] (Fig. 59-5). Recent data indicate that the same carboxyl-terminal domain of HBx (amino acids 111–154)

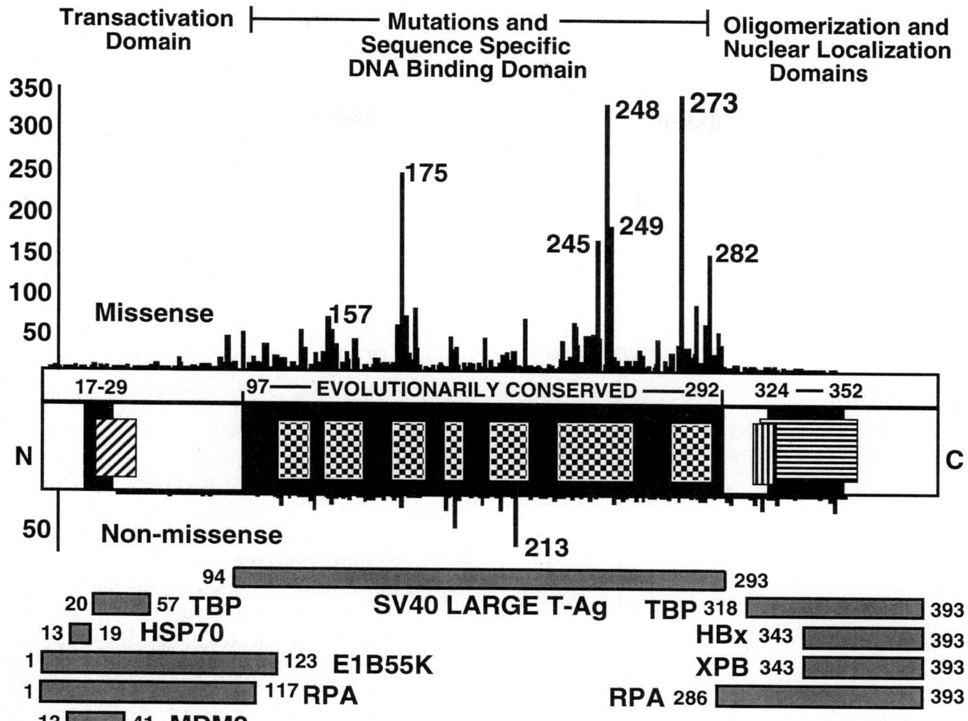

Fig. 59-2 Schematic representation of p53 molecule. The p53 protein consists of 393 amino acids with functional domains, evolutionarily conserved domains, and regions designated as mutational hotspots. Functional domains include the transactivation region (amino acids 20–42; diagonal striped block), sequence-specific DNA-binding region (amino acids 100–293), nuclear localization sequence (amino acids 316–325; vertical striped block), and oligomerization region (amino acids 319–360; horizontal striped block). Cellular or oncoviral proteins bind to specific areas of the p53 protein. Evolutionarily conserved domains (amino acids 17–29, 97–292, and 324–352; black areas) were determined using the MACAW program. Seven mutational hotspot regions within the large conserved domain are identified: amino acids 130–142, 151–164, 171–181, 193–200, 213–223, 234–258, and 270–286; checkered blocks). Functional domains and protein binding sites (gray bars underneath) were compiled from references. Vertical lines above the schematic, missense mutations; lines below schematic, nonmissense mutations.

necessary for binding to p53 (Fig. 59-6) is necessary for sequestering p53 in the cytoplasm and inhibiting p53-mediated apoptosis[116] (Fig. 59-7). The binding of HBx to the extreme carboxyl-terminal domain of p53 appears to inhibit the association of p53 with two putative downstream effectors of p53-mediated apoptosis, namely XPB and XPD[117]. Based on the above data we speculate that inactivation of p53-mediated transcriptional transactivation and apoptosis by HBx could lead to a disruption of normal cellular surveillance mechanisms for repairing and removing damaged cells, thus contributing to genomic instability.

In some cases of HCC, mutation of p53[106,118–121] or possibly inactivation of p53 by MDM-2[122] may be a late event in tumor progression. Tanaka et al.[123] have reported that p53 mutations are closely related to the progression of HCC and that in some cases, malignant cells which acquire the p53 mutations might develop into dedifferentiated subpopulations within a single HCC. Further suggesting an involvement of mutant p53 in the progression of liver cancer is the observation that some nodules consist of both p53 LOH and non-LOH, with the former being associated with cells of more severe cellular atypia.[118] It is noteworthy that abnormalities of the retinoblastoma tumor suppressor gene (Rb) have also been reported in advanced HCCs.[54,124,125,126] In one study, LOH at the Rb gene was detected in 6 of 7 (86 percent) HCCs with a p53 mutation, compared to none of 17 HCCs lacking mutation of p53.[124]

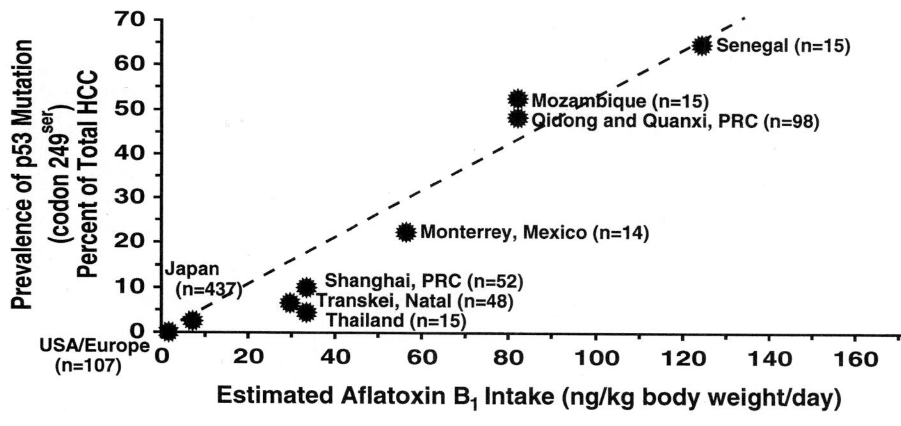

Fig. 59-3 Correlation of estimated aflatoxin B1 dietary exposure and frequency of codon 249^{ser} p53 mutations in hepatocellular carcinoma.

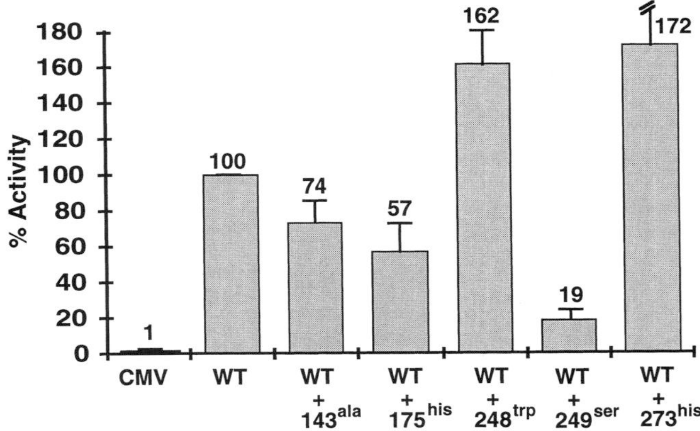

Fig. 59-4 Dominant negative effects of p53 mutants on the transcription of wild-type p53 in a p53-null human liver cancer cell line (Hep-3B).

ONCOGENES

Although activated protooncogenes are found in many spontaneous and experimentally induced HCCs in animal models,[127] no single oncogene has been shown to be preferentially activated in human HCCs.[128–130] By DNA transfection assay in NIH-3T3 cells, activated N-*ras* has been isolated from human HCC tissue; however, the gene was mutated in only a small fraction of the tumor cells.[103] Overexpression of N-*ras*, usually in the absence of a mutation, is often observed in human HCCs,[128,130] while mutations or overexpression of H- and K-*ras* are rare.[132] New oncogenes have been cloned from human HCC tissue,[5,133,134] but their role in hepatocarcinogenesis is unclear.

Mutations and amplification of c-*myc* are rarely detected in human HCCs, but overexpression of this protooncogene is a common finding.[125,130,135] Small studies have also demonstrated frequent overexpression of c-*fos* with an absence of mutations.[125,135,136] The HBV genome contains four open reading frames, two of which are potential transcriptional transactivators (reviewed in[137]). It is well established that HBx is a potent co-transactivator of many viral[138,139] and cellular[138,140–142] promoters including c-*myc*.[143,144] and c-*fos*.[144] The preS/S region of the HBV genome following 3′-truncation[145] also is able to co-transactivate these two protooncogenes.[146] In most cases of HCC, either or both transactivators are expressed and functionally active,[70,146–153] while the other HBV gene products are infrequently detected.[67,148,154] These data indicate that the transcriptional co-transactivation function of HBx and/or preS/S may significantly contribute to the development of HCC. However, considering the multiple functions of HBx, its role in hepatocarcinogenesis may not be limited to its ability to either inactivate p53 functions or transactivate cellular genes. In this regard, HBx can deregulate cell cycle checkpoints,[155] activate the ras-raf-mitogen-activated protein (MAP) kinase[156,157] and protein kinase C signaling cascades,[158,159] stimulate DNA synthesis[155] and cell cycle progression,[160] induce apoptosis,[161] bind to the DNA repair gene XAP-1/UV-DDB,[162,163] complexes with cellular transcrip-

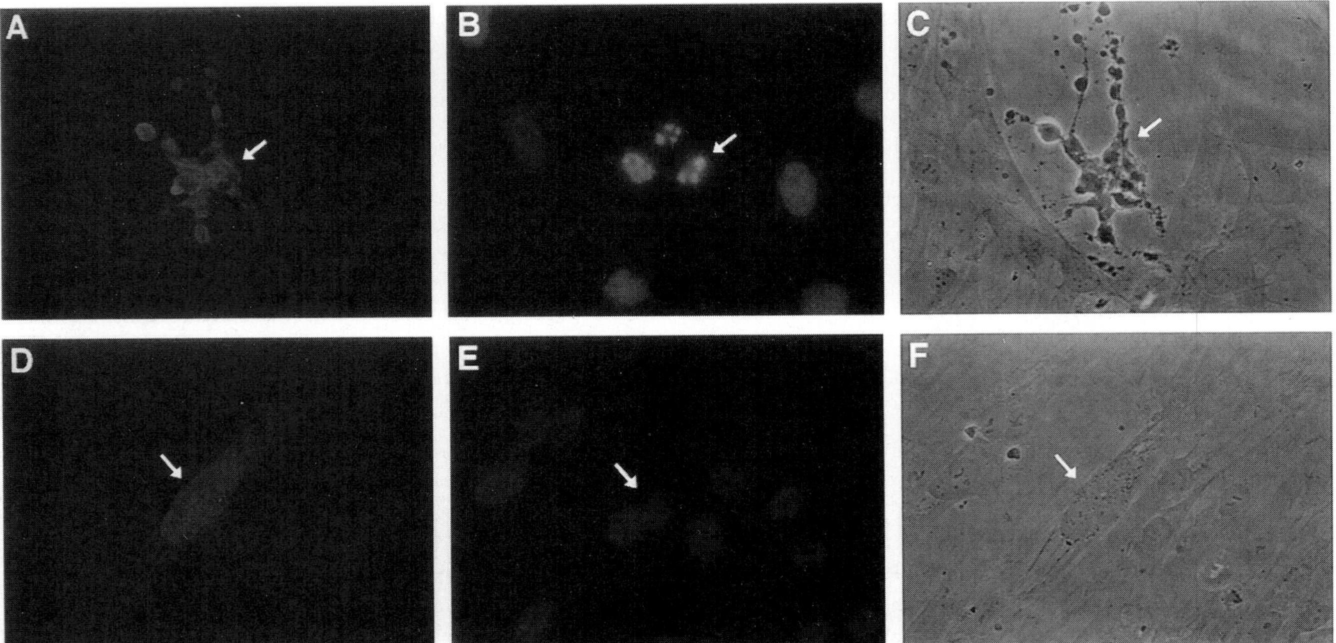

Fig. 59-5 Inhibition of p53-mediated apoptosis by the hepatitis B viral X gene. Induction of apoptosis in normal primary human fibroblasts was achieved by microinjection of a wild-type p53 expression vector. Cells were injected with the wild-type expression vector alone (A–C) or coinjected with wild-type p53 and the HBx gene (D–F). Cells were processed and analyzed as described in ref. 103.

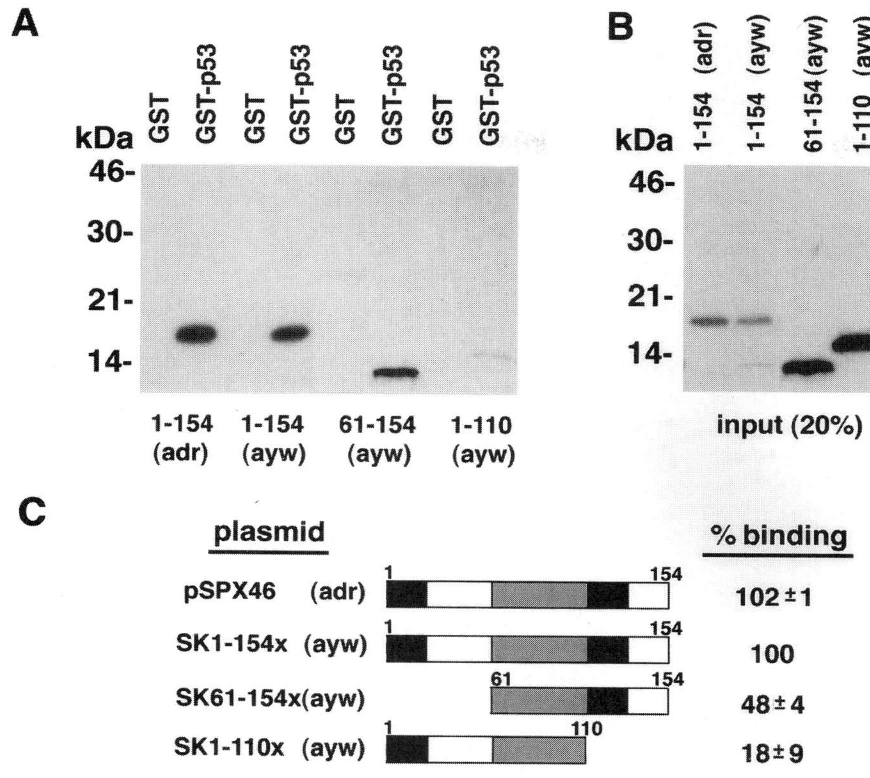

Fig. 59-6 The C-terminal domain of HBx is critical for in vitro association with GST-p53. (*A*) In vitro translated full-length HBx protein (lanes 1–4) and HBx deletion mutants (lanes 5–8) were incubated with glutathione-Sepharose beads loaded with either GST-p53 (lanes 2, 4, 6, 8) or GST (lanes 1, 3, 5, 7); (*B*) To reference input for binding, 20% of the volume of the various in vitro translated HBx proteins used for binding were immunoprecipitated by anti-HBx antibody;[116] (*C*) Schematic representation of full-length and truncated HBx as described in reference,[116] along with a summary of their binding to p53. Percent binding represents the mean ± SD from at least three independent binding assays with values made relative to SK1-154x.

tion factors,[112,164,165] inhibit hepatic serine proteases,[166–168] neoplastically transform rodent cells in vitro,[169,170] and, as a transgene, induce HCCs in mice.[171]

Growth Factors

The insulin growth factors, which include insulin and insulin-like growth factors I and II (IGF-I and -II, respectively), are potent hepatocellular mitogens.[172] IGF-II is overexpressed[66,172–177] and exhibits an allelic-expression imbalance[178–180] in many human HCCs. In some cases of HBV-associated HCCs, HBx may modulate the expression of IGF-II at the transcriptional level.[165,181] Insulin receptor substrate 1 (IRS-1), a main substrate for insulin and insulin-like growth factors I and II, is also highly expressed in many human HCC tumor tissues and cell lines.[178,182] IRS-1 exhibits transforming potential in NIH-3T3 cells, which is dependent in part on the presence of IGF-I.[183] As a transgene, IRS-1 over expression leads to increased hepatocyte DNA synthesis.[182] Collectively, these data indicate that the insulin

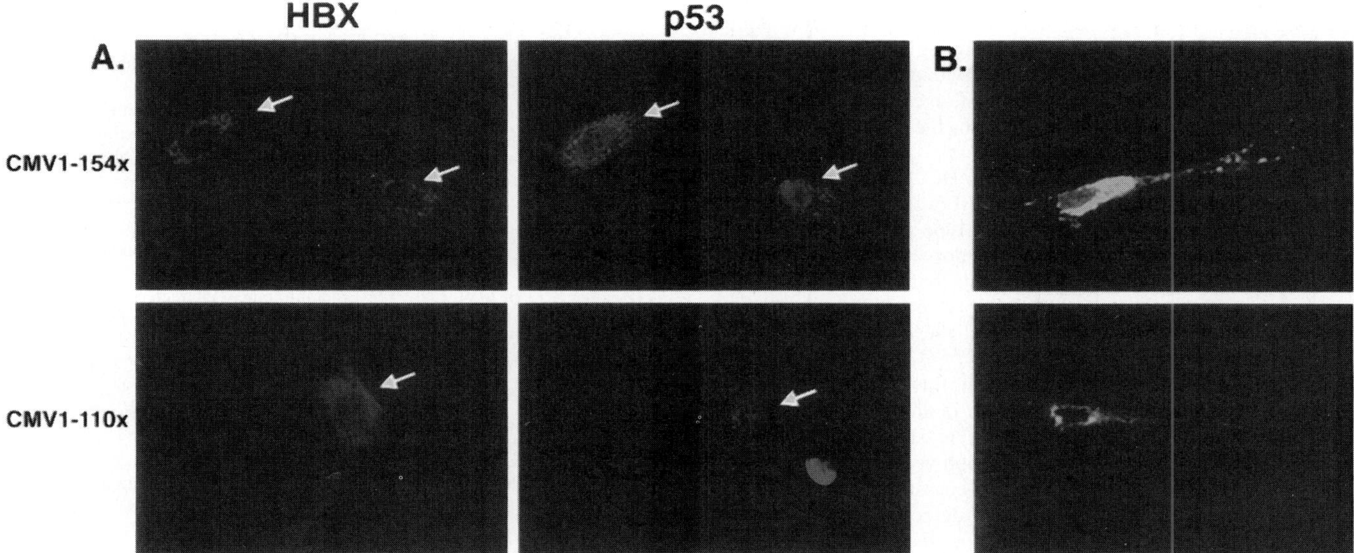

Fig. 59-7 HBx via its carboxyl terminal region sequesters p53 to the cytoplasm. (*A*) Normal human fibroblasts were microinjected with a p53 expression vector and either full-length HBx (CMV-1-154x) or a deletion mutant missing the last 44 amino acids (CMV-1-110x) followed by incubation for 24 hours. Immunostaining was performed as described in reference 116; (*B*) Confocal microscopic analysis of normal human fibroblasts coinjected with p53 and full-length HBx expression vectors. (*Upper*) Representative example of the degree of cytoplasmic sequestration typically observed in fibroblasts over-expressing p53 and HBx. (*Lower*) Fibroblast with all detectable p53 co-localizing with HBx in the cytoplasm.

growth factor signal transduction pathway may provide a critical proliferative stimulus during hepatocarcinogenesis. In addition, IGF-II may promote angiogenesis by upregulating the expression of vascular endothelial growth factor[184,185], a protein which may also play an importnt role in the invasion and metastasis of HCC[186]. Moreover, overexpression of at least one component of this pathway (i.e., IRS-1) may contribute to the development of HCC by preventing TGF-β1-induced apoptosis[187].

Transforming growth factor-α (TGF-α), another potent hepatocellular mitogen, is present at elevated levels in human HCCs, with its detection often being closely linked to HBV infection.[175,188,189] Specifically, TGF-α was detected more frequently in patients whose adjacent nontumorous liver had detectable HBV surface antigen and/or HBV core antigen (91 percent) than in those whose liver lacked these viral protein products (61 percent).[189] It remains unclear, however, whether increased expression of this growth factor is mechanistically related to hepatocarcinogenesis or whether it results from liver regeneration in response to chronic HBV infection. The latter possibility is supported by the finding that elevated TGF-α expression is typically observed in the livers of patients with chronic hepatitis and without HCC.[175] As with IGF-II, TGF-α may promote tumor augiogenesis by upregulating vascular endothelial growth factor.[190]

IMPLICATIONS FOR TREATMENT AND PREVENTION

HCC is regarded as an aggressive malignancy with a poor prognosis.[1,191] Of the more than 250,000 cases diagnosed worldwide annually, less than 3 percent will survive 5 or more years. For some patients, surgical resection or orthotopic liver transplantation offers disease-free survival; however, most must rely on other modes of treatment, which are currently only palliative.[1,192]

Our better understanding of the complex pathobiologic processes during hepatocarcinogenesis has already resulted in more effective preventive measures. Vaccines for HBV are well developed, and vaccination programs are currently being implemented in 85 countries.[193]. The Universal immunization program in Taiwan has resulted in a 10-fold reduction in the hepatitis B carrier rate and has significantly reduced the incidence of hepatocellular carcinoma in children.[194–196] Knowing that AFB_1 is a significant risk factor in the development of HCC, limiting the exposure to this mycotoxin by improving the storage of food grains would be another feasible strategy to decrease the incidence of HCC. The efficiency of this intervention could be monitored by measuring aflatoxin-albumin adducts in the blood of individuals consuming food grains.[197]

The frequent inactivation of p53 in HCCs makes this gene an attractive target for cancer therapy (reviewed in[79]). The development of drugs that would inhibit wild-type p53-HBx interactions may provide a means to rescue p53 tumor suppressor function. In those cases where p53 is mutated, agents that mimic wild-type p53 may be effective. Another possibility is p53 gene therapy. Laboratory studies have demonstrated the efficacy of p53 gene therapy in human cancer cells in vitro[198,199] and as a xenograph in athymic nude mice.[200–202] Based on this success, a phase I protocol for non-small cell lung cancer in humans is underway.[203] While the success of this approach is still speculative, it is encouraging that a p53 cDNA expression vector under the control of an α-fetoprotein promoter was successfully transferred into Hep-3B liver cells using a replication-defective retroviral vector, resulting in decreased cell growth and increased sensitivity to chemotherapy-induced apoptosis in vitro.[204] Vogelstein and coworkers[205] have devised a novel strategy of gene therapy, which may also be a future option for HCCs containing mutant p53. This approach relies on the ability of mutant p53 in tumor cells to selectively bind to exogenously introduced gene products resulting in the transcriptional activation of a toxic gene. As we continue to better understand the molecular pathogenesis of human HCC, clues for additional, rational intervention and therapeutic strategies will likely follow.

ACKNOWLEDGMENTS

The editorial and graphic assistance of Dorothea Dudek and Amy Hancock is greatly appreciated.

REFERENCES

1. Haydon GH, Hayes PC: Hepatocellular carcinoma. *Br J Hosp Med* **53**:74–80, 1995.
2. Sherman M: Hepatocellular carcinoma. *Gastroenterologist* **3**:55–66, 1995.
3. Harris CC: Solving the viral-chemical puzzle of human liver carcinogenesis. *Cancer Epidemiol Biomarkers Prev* **3**:1–2, 1994.
4. Harris CC: The 1995 Walter Hubert Lecture: Molecular epidemiology of human cancer: insights from the mutational analysis of the p53 tumor suppressor gene. *Br J Cancer* **73**:261–269, 1996.
5. Okuda K: Hepatocellular carcinoma: recent progress. *Hepatology* **15**:948–963, 1992.
6. Robinson WS: Molecular events in the pathogenesis of hepadnavirus associated hepatocellular carcinoma. *Annu Rev Med* **45**:297–323, 1994.
7. Beasley RP, Hwang LY, Lin CC, Chien CS: Hepatocellular carcinoma and hepatitis B virus. A prospective study of 22707 men in Taiwan. *Lancet* **2**:1129–1133, 1981.
8. Yeh FS, Yu MC, Mo CC, Luo S, Tong MJ, Henderson BE: Hepatitis B virus, aflatoxins, and hepatocellular carcinoma in southern Guangxi, China. *Cancer Res* **49**:2506–2509, 1989.
9. Beasley RP: Hepatitis B virus. The major etiology of hepatocellular carcinoma. *Cancer* **61**:1942–1956, 1988.
10. McMahon BJ, Lanier AP, Wainwright RB, Kilkenny SJ: Hepatocellular carcinoma in Alaska Eskimos: epidemiology, clinical features, and early detection. *Prog Liver Dis* **9**:643–655, 1990.
11. Iijma T, Saitoh N, Nobutomo K, Nambu M, Sakuma K: A prospective cohort study of hepatitis B surface antigen carriers in a working population. *Gann* **75**:571–573, 1984.
12. Obata H, Hayashi N, Motoike Y, Hisamitsu T, Okuda H, Kobayashi S, Nishioka K: A prospective study on the development of hepatocellular carcinoma from liver cirrhosis with persistent hepatitis B virus infection. *Int J Cancer* **25**:741–747, 1980.
13. Wogan GN: Aflatoxins as risk factors for hepatocellular carcinoma in humans. *Cancer Res* **52**:2114s–2118s, 1992.
14. Harris CC: Hepatocellular carcinogenesis: recent advances and speculations. *Cancer Cells* **2**:146–148, 1990.
15. Ross RK, Yuan JM, Yu MC, Wogan GN, Qian GS, Tu JT, Groopman JD: Urinary aflatoxin biomarkers and risk of hepatocellular carcinoma. *Lancet* **339**:943–946, 1992.
16. Qian GS, Ross RK, Yu MC, Yuan JM, Gao YT, Henderson BE, Wogan GN, et al: A follow-up study of urinary markers of aflatoxin exposure and liver cancer risk in Shanghai, People's Republic of China. *Cancer Epidemiol Biomarkers Prev* **3**:3–10, 1994.
17. Hsia CC, Kleiner DE Jr, Axiotis CA, Di Bisceglie A, Nomura AM, Stemmermann GN, Tabor E: Mutations of p53 gene in hepatocellular carcinoma: role of hepatitis B virus and aflatoxin contamination in the diet. *J Natl Cancer Inst* **84**:1638–1641, 1992.
18. Chen CJ, Yu MW, Liaw YF: Epidemiological characteristics and risk factors of hepatocellular carcinoma. *J Gastroenterol Hepatol* **12**: S294–308, 1997.
19. Lunn RM, Zhang YJ, Wang LY, Chen CJ, Lee PH, Lee CS, Tsai WY et al: p53 mutations, chronic hepatitis B virus infection, and aflatoxin exposure in hepatocellular carcinoma in Taiwan. *Cancer Res* **57**:3471–3477, 1997.
20. Tsukuma H, Hiyama T, Tanaka S, Nakao M, Yabuuchi T, Kitamura T, Nakanishi K et al: Risk factors for hepatocellular carcinoma among patients with chronic liver disease. *N Engl J Med* **328**:1797–1801, 1993.
21. Robinson WS: The role of hepatitis B virus in development of primary hepatocellular carcinoma: Part II. *J Gastroenterol Hepatol* **8**:95–106, 1993.
22. Thompson SC, Lin A, Warren R, Giles G, Crofts N: Risk factors associaated with hepatocellular carcinoma notified to the Anti-Cancer Council of Victoria in 1991-1992. *Aust N Z J Public Health* **21**: 626–630, 1997.

23. Caselmann WH, Alt M: Hepatitis C virus infection as a major risk factor for hepatocellular carcinoma. *J Hepatol* **24**: 61–66, 1996.
24. Izzo F, Cremona F, Ruffolo F, Palaia R, Parisi V, Curley SA: Outcome of 67 patients with hepatocellular cancer detected during screening of 1125 patients with chronic hepatitis. *Ann Surg* **227**:513–518, 1998.
25. Di Bisceglie AM: Hepatitis C and hepatocellular carcinoma. *Hepatology* **26**: 34S–38S, 1997.
26. Yu MW, Chen CJ: Hepatitis B and C viruses in the development of hepatocellular carcinoma. *Crit Rev Oncol Hematol* **17**:71–91, 1994.
27. Kubo S, Nishiguchi S, Tamori A, Hirohashi K, Kinoshita H, Kuroki T: Development of hepatoecellular carcinoma in patients with HCV infection, with or without past HBV infection, and relationship to age at the time of transfusion. *Vox sang* **74**: 129, 1998.
28. Donato F, Boffetta P, Puoti M: A meta-analysis of epidemiological studies on the combined effect of hepatitis B and C virus infections in causing hepatocellular carcinoma. *Int J Cancer* **75**: 347–354, 1998.
29. Tsai JF, Jeng, JE, Ho MS, Chang WY, Hsieh MY, Lin ZY, Tsai JH: Effect of hepatitis C and B virus infection on risk of hepatocellular carcinoma: a prospective study. *Br J Cancer* **76**: 968–974, 1997.
30. Shiraishi M, Morinaga S, Noguchi M, Shimosato Y, Sekiya T: Loss of genes on the short arm of chromosome 11 in human lung carcinomas. *Jpn J Cancer Res* **78**:1302–1308, 1987.
31. Kovacs G, Erlandsson R, Boldog F, Ingvarsson S, Muller R, Klein G, Sumegi J: Consistent chromosome 3p deletion and loss of heterozygosity in renal cell carcinoma. *Proc Natl Acad Sci USA* **85**:1571–1575, 1988.
32. Bodmer WF, Bailey CJ, Bodmer J, Bussey HJ, Ellis A, Gorman P, Lucibello FC et al: Localization of the gene for familial adenomatous polyposis on chromosome 5. *Nature* **328**:614–616, 1987.
33. Solomon E, Voss R, Hall V, Bodmer WF, Jass JR, Jeffreys AJ, Lucibello FC et al: Chromosome 5 allele loss in human colorectal carcinomas. *Nature* **328**:616–619, 1987.
34. Johnson BE, Sakaguchi AY, Gazdar AF, Minna JD, Burch D, Marshall A, Naylor SL: Restriction fragment length polymorphism studies show consistent loss of chromosome 3p alleles in small cell lung cancer patients' tumors. *J Clin Invest* **82**:502–507, 1988.
35. Meyer M, Wiedorn KH, Hofschneider PH, Koshy R, Caselmann WH: A chromosome 17:7 translocation is associated with a hepatitis B virus DNA integration in human hepatocellular carcinoma DNA. *Hepatology* **15**:665–671, 1992.
36. Zhou YZ, Slagle BL, Donehower LA, vanTuinen P, Ledbetter DH, Butel JS: Structural analysis of a hepatitis B virus genome integrated into chromosome 17p of a human hepatocellular carcinoma. *J Virol* **62**:4224–4231, 1988.
37. Zhang W, Hirohashi S, Tsuda H, Shimosato Y, Yokota J, Terada M, Sugimura T: Frequent loss of heterozygosity on chromosomes 16 and 4 in human hepatocellular carcinoma. *Jpn J Cancer Res* **81**:108–111, 1990.
38. Kuroki T, Fujiwara Y, Tsuchiya E, Nakamori S, Imaoka S, Kanematsu T, Nakamura Y: Accumulation of genetic changes during development and progression of hepatocellular carcinoma: loss of heterozygosity of chromosome arm 1p occurs at an early stage of hepatocarcinogenesis. *Genes Chrom Cancer* **13**:163–166, 1995.
39. Nagai H, Pineau P, Tiollais P, Buendia MA, Dejean A: Comprehensive allelotyping of human hepatocellular carcinoma. *Oncogene* **14**: 2927–2933, 1997.
40. Piao Z, Park C, Park JH, Kim H: Allelotype analysis of hepatocellular carcinoma. *Int J Cancer* **75**: 29–33, 1998.
41. Sheu JC: Molecular mechanism of hepatocarcinogenesis. *J Gastroenterol Hepatol* **12**: S309–13, 1997.
42. Chou YH, Chung KC, Jeng LB, Chen TC, Liaw YF: Frequent allelic loss on chromosomes 4q and 16q associated with human hepatocellular carcinoma in Taiwan. *Cancer Lett* **123**:1–6, 1998.
43. Ding SF, Habib NA, Dooley J, Wood C, Bowles L, Delhanty JD: Loss of constitutional heterozygosity on chromosome 5q in hepatocellular carcinoma without cirrhosis. *Br J Cancer* **64**:1083–1087, 1991.
44. Hubbard AL, Harrison DJ, Moyes C, Wyllie AH, Cunningham C, Mannion E, Smith CA: N-acetyltransferase 2 genotype in colorectal cancer and selective gene retention in cancers with chromosome 8p deletions. *Gut* **41**:229–234, 1997.
45. De Souza AT, Hankins GR, Washington MK, Fine RL, Orton TC, Jirtle RL: Frequent loss of heterozygosity on 6q at the mannose 6-phosphate/insulin-like growth factor II receptor locus in human hepatocellular tumors. *Oncogene* **10**:1725–1729, 1995.
46. Emi M, Fujiwara Y, Nakajima T, Tsuchiya E, Tsuda H, Hirohashi S, Maeda Y et al: Frequent loss of heterozygosity for loci on chromosome 8p in hepatocellular carcinoma, colorectal cancer, and lung cancer. *Cancer Res* **52**:5368–5372, 1992.
47. Yuan BZ, Miller MJ, Keck CL, Zimonjic DB, Thorgerison SS, Popescu NC: Cloning, characterization, and chromosomal localizaation of a gene frequently deleted in human liver cancer (DLC-1) homologous to rat RhoGAP. *cancer Res* **58**:2196–2199, 1998.
48. Piao Z, Park C, Lee JS, Yang CH, Choi KY, Kim H: Homozygous delections of the CDKN2 gene and loss of heterozygosity of 9p in primary hepatocellular carcinoma. *Cancer Lett* **122**: 201-207, 1998.
49. Fujimori M, Tokino T, Hino O, Kitagawa T, Imamura T, Okamoto E, Mitsunobu M et al: Allelotype study of primary hepatocellular carcinoma. *Cancer Res* **51**:89–93, 1991.
50. Rogler CE, Sherman M, Su CY, Shafritz DA, Summers J, Shows TB, Henderson A et al: Deletion in chromosome 11p associated with a hepatitis B integration site in hepatocellular carcinoma. *Science* **230**:319–322, 1985.
51. Wang HP, Rogler CE: Deletions in human chromosome arms 11p and 13q in primary hepatocellular carcinomas. *Cytogenet Cell Genet* **48**: 72–78, 1988.
52. Nishida N, Fukuda Y, Kokuryu H, Sadamoto T, Isowa G, Honda K, Yamaoka Y et al: Accumulation of allelic loss on arms of chromosomes 13q, 16q and 17p in the advanced stages of human hepatocellular carcinoma. *Int J Cancer* **51**:862–868, 1992.
53. Nishida N, Fukuda Y, Kokuryu H, Toguchida J, Yandell DW, Ikenega M, Imura H et al: Role and mutational heterogeneity of the p53 gene in hepatocellular carcinoma. *Cancer Res* **53**:368–372, 1993.
54. Fujimoto Y, Hampton LL, Wirth PJ, Wang NJ, Xie JP, Thorgeirsson SS: Alterations of tumor suppressor genes and allelic losses in human hepatocellular carcinomas in China. *Cancer Res* **54**:281–285, 1994.
55. Hino O, Shows TB, Rogler CE: Hepatitis B virus integration site in hepatocellular carcinoma at chromosome 17;18 translocation. *Proc Natl Acad Sci USA* **83**:8338–8342, 1986.
56. Tokino T, Fukushige S, Nakamura T, Nagaya T, Murotsu T, Shiga K, Aoki N et al: Chromosomal translocation and inverted duplication associated with integrated hepatitis B virus in hepatocellular carcinomas. *J Virol* **61**:3848–3854, 1987.
57. McBride OW, Merry D, Givol D: The gene for human p53 cellular tumor antigen is located on chromosome 17 short arm (17p13). *Proc Natl Acad Sci USA* **83**:130–134, 1986.
58. Ozturk M: p53 mutation in hepatocellular carcinoma after aflatoxin exposure. *Lancet* **338**:1356–1359, 1991.
59. Oda T, Tsuda H, Scarpa A, Sakamoto M, Hirohashi S: Mutation pattern of the p53 gene as a diagnostic marker for multiple hepatocellular carcinoma. *Cancer Res* **52**:3674–3678, 1992.
60. Bressac B, Galvin KM, Liang TJ, Isselbacher KJ, Wands JR, Ozturk M: Abnormal structure and expression of p53 gene in human hepatocellular carcinoma. *Proc Natl Acad Sci USA* **87**:1973–1977, 1990.
61. Piao Z, Kim H, Jeon BK, Lee WJ, Park C: Relationship between loss of heterozygosity of tumor suppressor genes and histologic differentiation in hepatocellular carcinoma. *Cancer* **80**: 865–872, 1997.
62. Kishimoto Y, Shiota G, Kamisaki Y, Wada K, Nakamoto K, Yamawaki M, Kotani M, et al: Loss of the tumor suppressor p53 gene at the liver cirrhosis stage in Japanese patients with hepatocellular carcinoma. *Oncology* **54**: 304–310, 1997.
63. Yamada T, De Souza AT, Finkelstein S, Jirtle RL: Loss of the gene encoding mannose 6-phosphate/insulin-like growth factor II receptor is an early event in liver carcinogenesis. *Proc Natl Acad Sci U S A* **94**: 10351–10355, 1997.
64. Piao Z, Choi Y, Park C, Lee WJ, Park JH, Kim H: Deletion of the M6P/IGF2r gene in primary hepatocellular carcinoma. *Cancer Lett* **120**: 39–43, 1997.
65. Takiya S, Tagaya T, Takahashi K, Kawashima H, Kamiya M, Fukuzawa Y, Kobayashi S et al: Role of transforming growth factor beta 1 on hepatic regeneration and apoptosis in liver diseases. *J Clin Pathol* **48**:1093–1097, 1995.
66. Seo JH, Park BC: Expression of insulin-like growth factor II in chronic hepatitis B, liver cirrhosis, and hepatocellular carcinoma. *Gan To Kagaku Ryoho* 22(**Suppl 3**):292–307, 1995.
67. Diamantis ID, McGandy CE, Chen TJ, Liaw YF, Gudat F, Bianchi L: Hepatitis B X-gene expression in hepatocellular carcinoma. *J Hepatol* **15**:400–403, 1992.
68. Fourel G, Trepo C, Bougueleret L, Henglein B, Ponzetto A, Tiollais P, Buendía MA: Frequent activation of N-myc genes by hepadnavirus insertion in woodchuck liver tumours. *Nature* **347**:294–298, 1990.
69. Hsu T, Moroy T, Etiemble J, Louise A, Trepo C, Tiollais P, Buendia MA: Activation of c-myc by woodchuck hepatitis virus insertion in hepatocellular carcinoma. *Cell* **55**:627–635, 1988.

70. Matsubara K, Tokino T: Integration of hepatitis B virus DNA and its implications to hepatocarcinogenesis. *Mol Biol Med* **7**:243–260, 1990.
71. Rogler CE, Chisari FV: Cellular and molecular mechanisms of hepatocarcinogenesis. *Semin Liver Dis* **12**:265–278, 1992.
72. de The H, Marchio A, Tiollais P, Dejean A: A novel steroid thyroid hormone receptor related gene inappropriately expressed in human hepatocellular carcinoma. *Nature* **330**:667–670, 1987.
73. Wang J, Chenivesse X, Henglein B, Brechot C: Hepatitis B virus integration in a cyclin A gene in a hepatocellular carcinoma. *Nature* **343**:555–557, 1990.
74. Ogata N, Tokino T, Kamimura T, Asakura H: A comparison of the molecular structure of integrated hepatitis B virus genomes in hepatocellular carcinoma cells and hepatocytes derived from the same patient. *Hepatology* **11**:1017–1023, 1990.
75. Hino O, Kajino K: Hepatitis virus related hepatocarcinogenesis. *Intervirology* **37**:133–135, 1994.
76. Hino O, Nomura K, Ohtake K, Kawaguchi T, Sugano H, Kitagawa T: Instability of integrated hepatitis B virus DNA with inverted repeat structure in a transgenic mouse. *Cancer Genet Cytogenet* **37**:273–278, 1989.
77. Nakamura T, Tokino T, Nagaya T, Matsubara K: Microdeletion associated with the integration process of hepatitis B virus DNA. *Nucleic Acids Res* **16**:4865–4873, 1988.
78. Hino O, Tabata S, Hotta Y: Evidence for increased in vitro recombination with insertion of human hepatitis B virus DNA. *Proc Natl Acad Sci USA* **88**:9248–9252, 1991.
79. Harris CC: Structure and function of the p53 tumor suppressor gene: clues for rational cancer therapeutic strategies. *J Natl Cancer Inst* **88**:1442–1455, 1996.
80. Ko LJ, Prives C: p53: puzzle and paradigm. *Genes Devel* **10**:1054–1072, 1996.
81. Levine AJ, Momand J, Finlay CA: The p53 tumour suppressor gene. *Nature* **351**:453–456, 1991.
82. Hollstein M, Sidransky D, Vogelstein B, Harris CC: p53 mutations in human cancers. *Science* **253**:49–53, 1991.
83. Greenblatt MS, Bennett WP, Hollstein M, Harris CC: Mutations in the p53 tumor suppressor gene: clues to cancer etiology and molecular pathogenesis. *Cancer Res* **54**:4855–4878, 1994.
84. Soussi T, Caron de Fromentel C, May P: Structural aspects of the p53 protein in relation to gene evolution. *Oncogene* **5**:945–952, 1990.
85. Hollstein M, Rice K, Greenblatt MS, Soussi T, Fuchs R, Sorlie T, Hovig E et al: Database of p53 gene somatic mutations in human tumors and cell lines. *Nucleic Acids Res* **22**:3547–3551, 1994.
86. Hollstein M, Shomer B, Greenblatt M, Soussi T, Hovig E, Montesano R, Harris CC: Somatic point mutations in the p53 gene of human tumors and cell lines: updated compilation. *Nucleic Acids Res* **24**:141–146, 1996.
87. Murakami Y, Hayashi K, Sekiya T: Detection of aberrations of the p53 alleles and the gene transcript in human tumor cell lines by single conformation polymorphism analysis. *Cancer Res* **51**:3356–3391, 1991.
88. Hsu IC, Metcalf RA, Sun T, Welsh JA, Wang NJ, Harris CC: Mutational hotspot in the p53 gene in human hepatocellular carcinomas. *Nature* **350**:427–428, 1991.
89. Scorsone KA, Zhou YZ, Butel JS, Slagle BL: p53 mutations cluster at codon 249 in hepatitis B virus-positive hepatocellular carcinomas from China. *Cancer Res* **52**:1635–1638, 1992.
90. Li D, Cao Y, He L, Wang NJ, Gu J: Aberrations of p53 gene in human hepatocellular carcinoma from China. *Carcinogenesis* **14**:169–173, 1993.
91. Bressac B, Kew M, Wands J, Ozturk M: Selective G to T mutations of p53 gene in hepatocellular carcinoma from southern Africa. *Nature* **350**:429–431, 1991.
92. Soini Y, Chia SC, Bennett WP, Groopman JD, Wang JS, DeBenedetti VM, Cawley H et al: An aflatoxin-associated mutational hotspot at codon 249 in the p53 tumor suppressor gene occurs in hepatocellular carcinomas from Mexico. *Carcinogenesis* **17**:1007–1012, 1996.
93. Yang M, Zhou H, Kong RY, Fong WF, Ren LQ, Liao XH, Wang Y et al: Mutations at codon 249 of p53 gene in human hepatocellular carcinomas from Tongan, China. *Mutat Res* **381**: 25–29, 1997.
94. Oda T, Tsuda H, Scarpa A, Sakamoto M, Hirohashi S: p53 gene mutation spectrum in hepatocellular carcinoma. *Cancer Res* **52**:6358–6364, 1992.
95. Kress S, Jahn UR, Buchmann A, Bannasch P, Schwarz M: p53 mutations in human hepatocellular carcinomas from Germany. *Cancer Res* **52**:3220–3223, 1992.
96. Hsu IC, Tokiwa T, Bennett W, Metcalf RA, Welsh JA, Sun T, Harris CC: p53 gene mutation and integrated hepatitis B viral DNA sequences in human liver cancer cell lines. *Carcinogenesis* **14**:987–992, 1993.
97. Aguilar F, Harris CC, Sun T, Hollstein M, Cerutti P: Geographic variation of p53 mutational profile in nonmalignant human liver. *Science* **264**:1317–1319, 1994.
98. Aguilar F, Hussain SP, Cerutti P: Aflatoxin B1 induces the transversion of G→T in codon 249 of the p53 tumor suppressor gene in human hepatocytes. *Proc Natl Acad Sci USA* **90**:8586–8590, 1993.
99. Cerutti P, Hussain P, Pourzand C, Aguilar F: Mutagenesis of the H-ras protooncogene and the p53 tumor suppressor gene. *Cancer Res* **54**:1934s–1938s, 1994.
100. Mace K, Aguilar F, wang JS, Vautravers P, Gomez-Lechon M, Gonzealea FJ, Groopman J et al: Aflatoxin B1 induced DNA adduct formation and p53 mutations in CYP450-expressing human liver cell lines. *Carcinogenesis* **18**: 1291–1297, 1997.
101. Ponchel F, Puisieux A, Tabone E, Michot JP, Froschl G, Morel AP, Frebourg T et al: Hepatocarcinoma mutant p53 induces mitotic activity but has no effect on transforming growth factor beta 1-mediated apoptosis. *Cancer Res* **54**:2064–2068, 1994.
102. Dumenco L, Oguey D, Wu J, Messier N, Fausto N: Introduction of a murine p53 mutation corresponding to human codon 249 into a murine hepatocyte cell line results in growth advantage, but not in transformation. *Hepatology* **22**:1279–1288, 1995.
103. Wang XW, Gibson MK, Vermeulen W, Yeh H, Forrester K, Sturzbecher HW, Hoeijmakers JHJ, et al: Abrogation of p53-induced apoptosis by the hepatitis B virus X gene. *Cancer Res* **55**:6012–6016, 1995.
104. Guengerich FP, Johnson WW, Ueng Y-F, Yamazaki H, Shimada T: Involvement of cytochrome P450, glutathione S-transferase, and epoxide hydrolase in the metabolism of aflatoxin B1 and relevance to risk of human liver cancer. *Environ Health Perspect* **104**:557–562, 1996.
105. Buss P, Caviezel M, Lutz WK: Linear dose-response relationship for DNA adducts in rat liver from chronic exposure to aflatoxin B1. *Carcinogenesis* **11**:2133–2135, 1990.
106. Hosono S, Chou MJ, Lee CS, Shih C: Infrequent mutation of p53 gene in hepatitis B virus positive primary hepatocellular carcinomas. *Oncogene* **8**:491–496, 1993.
107. Kung YK, Kim CJ, Kim WH, Kim HO, Kang GH, Kim YI: p53 mutation and overexpression in hepatocellular carcinoma and dysplastic nodules in the liver. *Virchows Arch* **432**: 27-32, 1998.
108. Feitelson MA, Zhu M, Duan LX, London WT: Hepatitis B x antigen and p53 are associated in vitro and in liver tissues from patients with primary hepatocellular carcinoma. *Oncogene* **8**:1109–1117, 1993.
109. Wang XW, Forrester K, Yeh H, Feitelson MA, Gu JR, Harris CC: Hepatitis B virus X protein inhibits p53 sequence-specific DNA binding, transcriptional activity, and association with transcription factor ERCC3. *Proc Natl Acad Sci USA* **91**:2230–2234, 1994.
110. Ueda H, Ullrich SJ, Gangemi JD, Kappel CA, Ngo L, Feitelson MA, Jay G: Functional inactivation but not structural mutation of p53 causes liver cancer. *Nat Genet* **9**:41–47, 1995.
111. Maguire HF, Hoeffler JP, Siddiqui A: HBV X protein alters the DNA binding specificity of CREB and ATF-2 by protein-protein interactions. *Science* **252**:842–844, 1991.
112. Williams JS, Andrisani OM: The hepatitis B virus X protein targets the basic region evcine zipper domain of CREB. *Proc Natl Acad Sci USA* **92**:3819–3823, 1995.
113. Jia L, Wang XW, Sun Z, Harris CC: Interactive effects of p53 tumor suppressor gene and hepatitis B virus in hepatocellular carcinogenesis. Tahara E (ed) *In Molecular Pathology of Gastroeuterological Cancer: Application to Clinical Practice*, Tahara E (ed), Tokyo, Springer-Verlag, 1997, pp. 209–218.
114. Schaeffer L, Roy R, Humbert S, Moncollin V, Vermeulen W, Hoeijmakers JH, Cambon P, et al.: DNA repair helicase: a component of BTF2 (TFIIH) basic transcription factor. *Science* **260**:58–63, 1993.
115. Weeda G, van Ham RC, Vermeulen W, Bootsma D, Van der Eb AJ, Hoeijmakers JH: A presumed DNA helicase encoded by ERCC3 is involved in the human repair disorders xeroderma pigmentosum and Cockayne's syndrome. *Cell* **62**:777–791, 1990.
116. Elmore LW, Hancock AR, Chang SF, Wang XW, Chang S, Callahan CP, Geller DA. et al.: Hepatitis B virus X protein and p53 tumor suppressor interactions in the modulation of apoptosis. *Proc Natl Acad Sci USA* **94**:14707–14712, 1997.
117. Wang XW, Yeh H, Schaeffer L, Roy R, Moncollin V, Egly JM, Wang Z, et al.: p53 modulation of TFIIH-associated nucleotide excision repair activity. *Nature Genet* **10**:188–195, 1995.

118. Teramoto T, Satonaka K, Kitazawa S, Fujimori T, Hayashi K, Maeda S: p53 gene abnormalities are closely related to hepatoviral infections and occur at a late stage of hepatocarcinogenesis. *Cancer Res* **54**:231–235, 1994.
119. Jaskiewicz K, Banach L, Izycka E: Hepatocellular carcinoma in young patients: histology, cellular differentiation, HBV infection and oncoprotein p53. *Anticancer Res* **15**:2723–2725, 1995.
120. Mise K, Tashiro S, Yogita S, Wada D, Harda M, Fukuda Y, Mikaye H. et al.: Assessment of the biological malignancy of hepatocellular carcinoma: relationship of clinicopathological facotrs and prognosis. *Clin Cancer Res* **4**:1475–1482, 1998.
121. Qin G, Su J, Ning Y, Duan X, Luo D, Lotlikar PD: p53 protein expression in patients with hepatocellular carcinoma from the high incidence area of Guangxi, Southern China. *Cancer Lett* **121**:203–210, 1997.
122. Qiu SJ, Ye SL, Wu ZQ, TangZY, Liu YK: The expression of the mdm2 gene may be related to the aberration of the p53 gene in human hepatocellular carcinoma. *J Cancer Res Clin Oncol* **124**:253–258, 1998.
123. Tanaka S, Toh Y, Adachi E, Matsumata T, Mori R, Sugimachi K: Tumor progression in hepatocellular carcinoma may be mediated by p53 mutation. *Cancer Res* **53**:2884–2887, 1993.
124. Murakami Y, Hayashi K, Hirohashi S, Sekiya T: Aberrations of the tumor suppressor p53 and retinoblastoma genes in human hepatocellular carcinomas. *Cancer Res* **51**:5520–5525, 1991.
125. Tabor E: Tumor suppressor genes, growth factor genes, and oncogenes in hepatitis B virus-associated hepatocellular carcinoma. *J Med Virol* **42**:357–365, 1994.
126. Ashida K, Kishimoto Y, Nakamoto K, Wada K, Shiota G, Hirooka Y, Kamisaki Y. et al.: Loss of heterozygosity of the retinoblastoma gene in liver cirrhosis accompanying hepatocellular carcinoma. *J Cancer Res Clin Oncol* **123**:489–495, 1997.
127. Pascale RM, Simile MM, Feo F: Genomic abnormalities in hepatocarcinogenesis. Implications for a chemopreventive strategy. *Anticancer Res* **13**:1341–1356, 1993.
128. Gu JR: Molecular aspects of human hepatic carcinogenesis. *Carcinogenesis* **9**:697–703, 1988.
129. Zhang XK, Huang DP, Chiu DK, Chiu JF: The expression of oncogenes in human developing liver and hepatomas. *Biochem Biophys Res Commun* **142**:932–938, 1987.
130. Gu JR, Hu LF, Cheng YC, Wan DF: Oncogenes in human primary hepatic cancer. *J Cell Physiol Suppl* **4**:13–20, 1986.
131. Takada S, Koike K: Activated N-ras gene was found in human hepatoma tissue but only in a small fraction of the tumor cells. *Oncogene* **4**:189–193, 1989.
132. Ogata N, Kamimura T, Asakura H: Point mutation, allelic loss and increased methylation of c-Ha-ras gene in human hepatocellular carcinoma. *Hepatology* **13**:31–37, 1991.
133. Yang SS, Modali R, Parks JB, Taub JV: Transforming DNA sequences of human hepatocellular carcinomas, their distribution and relationship with hepatitis B virus sequence in human hepatomas. *Leukemia* **2**:102S–113S, 1988.
134. Yuasa Y, Sudo K: Transforming genes in human hepatomas detected by a tumorigenicity assay. *Jpn J Cancer Res* **78**:1036–1040, 1987.
135. Arbuthnot P, Kew M, Fitschen W: c-fos and c-myc oncoprotein expression in human hepatocellular carcinomas. *Anticancer Res* **11**:921–924, 1991.
136. Farshid M, Tabor E: Expression of oncogenes and tumor suppressor genes in human hepatocellular carcinoma and hepatoblastoma cell lines. *J Med Virol* **38**:235–239, 1992.
137. Feitelson MA: Biology of hepatitis B virus variants. *Lab Invest* **71**:324–349, 1994.
138. Twu JS, Schloemer RH: Transcriptional trans-activating function of hepatitis B virus. *J Virol* **61**:3448–3453, 1987.
139. Spandau DF, Lee CH: Trans-activation of viral enhancers by the hepatitis B virus X protein. *J Virol* **62**:427–434, 1988.
140. Twu JS, Lai MY, Chen DS, Robinson WS: Activation of protooncogene c-jun by the X protein of hepatitis B virus. *Virology* **192**:346–350, 1993.
141. Aufiero B, Schneider RJ: The hepatitis B virus X-gene product transactivates both RNA polymerase II and III promoters. *EMBO J* **9**:497–504, 1990.
142. Natoli G, Avantaggiati ML, Chirillo P, Costanzo A, Artini M, Balsano C, Levrero M: Induction of the DNA-binding activity of c-jun/c-fos heterodimers by the hepatitis B virus transactivator pX. *Mol Cell Biol* **14**:989–998, 1994.
143. Balsano C, Avantaggiati ML, Natoli G, De Marzio E, Will H, Perricaudet M, Levrero M: Full-length and truncated versions of the hepatitis B virus (HBV) X protein (pX) transactivate the c-myc protooncogene at the transcriptional level. *Biochem Biophys Res Commun* **176**:985–992, 1991.
144. Levrero M, Balsano C, Avantaggiati ML, Natoli G, De Marzio E, Will H: Hepatitis B virus and hepatocellular carcinoma: a possible role for the viral transactivators. *Ital J Gastroenterol* **23**:576–583, 1991.
145. Caselmann WH, Meyer M, Kekulî AS, Lauer U, Hofschneider PH, Koshy R: A trans-activator function is generated by integration of hepatitis B virus preS2/S sequences in human hepatocellular carcinoma DNA. *Proc Natl Acad Sci USA* **87**:2970–2974, 1990.
146. Kekulî AS, Lauer U, Meyer M, Caselmann WH, Hofschneider PH, Koshy R: The preS2/S region of integrated hepatitis B virus DNA encodes a transcriptional transactivator. *Nature* **343**:457–461, 1990.
147. Unsal H, Yakicier C, Marcais C, Kew M, Volkmann M, Zentgraf H, Isselbacher KJ, et al.: Genetic heterogeneity of hepatocellular carcinoma. *Proc Natl Acad Sci USA* **91**:822–826, 1994.
148. Paterlini P, Poussin K, Kew M, Franco D, Brechot C: Selective accumulation of the X transcript of hepatitis B virus in patients negative for hepatitis B surface antigen with hepatocellular carcinoma. *Hepatology* **21**:313–321, 1995.
149. Caselmann WH: Transactivation of cellular gene expression by hepatitis B viral proteins: a possible molecular mechanism of hepatocarcinogenesis. *J Hepatol* **22**:34–37, 1995.
150. Wei Y, Etiemble J, Fourel G, Vitvitski-Trepo L, Buendía MA: Hepadnavirus integration generates virus-cell cotranscripts carrying 3′ truncated X genes in human and woodchuck liver tumors. *J Med Virol* **45**:82–90, 1995.
151. Su Q, Schroder CH, Hofmann WJ, Otto G, Pichlmayr R, Bannash P: Expression of hepatitis B virus X protein in HBV-infected human livers and hepatocellular carcinomas. *Hepatology* **27**:1109–1120, 1998.
152. Su TS, Hwang WL, Yauk YK: Characterization of hepatitis B virus integrant that results in chromosomal rearrangement. *DNA Cell Biol* **17**:415–425, 1998.
153. Kobayashi S, Saigoh Ki, Urashima T, Asano T, Isono K: Detection of hepatitis B virus x transcripts in human hepatocellular carcinoma tissues. *J Surg Res* **73**:97–100, 1997.
154. Laskus T, Radkowski M, Nowicki M, Wang LF, Vargas H, Rakela J: Association between hepatitis B virus core promoter rearrangements and hepatocellular carcinoma. *Biochem Biophys Res Commun* **244**:812–814, 1998.
155. Benn J, Schneider RJ: Hepatitis B virus HBx protein deregulates cell cycle checkpoint controls. *Proc Natl Acad Sci USA* **92**:11215–11219, 1995.
156. Benn J, Schneider RJ: Hepatitis B virus HBx protein activates Ras-GTP complex formation and establishes a Ras, Raf, MAP kinase signaling cascade. *Proc Natl Acad Sci USA* **91**:10350–10354, 1994.
157. Doria M, Klein N, Lucito R, Schneider RJ: The hepatitis B virus HBx protein is a dual specificity cytoplasmic activator of Ras and nuclear activator of transcription factors. *EMBO J* **14**:4747–4757, 1995.
158. Kekulî AS, Lauer U, Weiss L, Luber B, Hofschneider PH: Hepatitis B virus transactivator HBx uses a tumor promoter signalling pathway. *Nature* **361**:742–745, 1993.
159. Luber B, Lauer U, Weiss L, Hohne M, Hofschneider PH, Kekul AS: The hepatitis B virus transactivator HBx causes elevation of diacylglycerol and activation of protein kinase C. *Res Virol* **144**:311–321, 1993.
160. Koike K, Moriya K, Yotsuyanagi H, Iino S, Kurokawa K: Induction of cell cycle progression by hepatitis B virus HBx gene expression in quiescent mouse fibroblasts. *J Clin Invest* **94**:44–49, 1994.
161. Kim H, Lee H, Yum Y: X-gene product of hepatitis B virus induces apoptosis in liver cells. *J Biol Chem* **273**: 381-385, 1998.
162. Lee TH, Elledge SJ, Butel JS: Hepatitis B virus X protein interacts with a probable cellular DNA repair protein. *J Virol* **69**:1107–1114, 1995.
163. Becker SA, Lee TH, Butel JS, Slagle BL: Hepatitis B virus X protein interferes with cellular DNA repair. *J Virol* **72**: 266-272, 1998.
164. Lucito R, Schneider RJ: Hepatitis B virus X protein activates transcription factor NF-kappa B without a requirement for protein kinase C. *J Virol* **66**:983–991, 1992.
165. Lee YI, Lee Y, Bong YS, Hyun SW, Yoo YD, Kim SJ. et al.: The human hepatitis B virus transactivator X gene product regulates Sp1 mediated transcription of an insulin-like growth factor II promoter 4. *Oncogene* **16**: 2367-2380, 1998.
166. Fischer M, Runkel L, Schaller H: HBx protein of hepatitis B virus interacts with the C-terminal portion of a novel human proteasome alpha-subunit. *Virus Genes* **10**:99–102, 1995.

167. Takada S, Kido H, Fukutomi A, Mori T, Koike K: Interaction of hepatitis B virus X protein with a serine protease, tryptase TL2 as an inhibitor. *Oncogene* **9**:341–348, 1994.
168. Takada S, Tsuchida N, Kobayashi M, Koike K: Disruption of the function of tumor-suppressor gene p53 by the hepatitis B virus X protein and hepatocarcinogenesis. *J Cancer Res Clin Oncol* **121**:593–601, 1995.
169. Höhne M, Schaefer S, Seifer M, Feitelson MA, Paul D, Gerlich WH: Malignant transformation of immortalized transgenic hepatocytes after transfection with hepatitis B virus DNA. *EMBO J* **9**:1137–1145, 1990.
170. Shirakata Y, Kawada M, Fujiki Y, Sano H, Oda M, Yaginuma K, Kobayashi M, et al.: The X gene of hepatitis B virus induced growth stimulation and tumorigenic transformation of mouse NIH3T3 cells. *Jpn J Cancer Res* **80**:617–621, 1989.
171. Kim CM, Koike K, Saito I, Miyamura T, Jay G: HBx gene of hepatitis B virus induces liver cancer in transgenic mice. *Nature* **351**:317–320, 1991.
172. Macaulay VM: Insulin-like growth factors and cancer. *Br J Cancer* **65**:311–320, 1992.
173. Su Q, Liu YF, Zhang JF, Zhang SX, Li DF, Yang JJ: Expression of insulin-like growth factor II in hepatitis B, cirrhosis and hepatocellular carcinoma: its relationship with hepatitis B virus antigen expression. *Hepatology* **20**:788–799, 1994.
174. Cariani E, Lasserre C, Seurin D, Hamelin B, Kemeny F, Franco D, Czech MP, et al.: Differential expression of insulin-like growth factor II mRNA in human primary liver cancers, benign liver tumors, and liver cirrhosis. *Cancer Res* **48**:6844–6849, 1988.
175. Park BC, Huh MH, Seo JH: Differential expression of transforming growth factor alpha and insulin-like growth factor II in chronic active hepatitis B, cirrhosis and hepatocellular carcinoma. *J Hepatol* **22**:286–294, 1995.
176. Sohda T, Iwata K, Soejima H, Kamimura S, Shijo H, Yun K: In situ detection of insuline-like growth factor II (IGF2) and H19 gene expression in hepatocellular carcinoma. *J Hum Genet* **43**:49–53, 1998.
177. Sohda T, Kamimura S, Iwata K, Shijo H, Okumura M: Immunohistochemical evidence of insulin-like growth factor II in human small hepatocellular carcinoma with hepatitis C virus infection: relationship to fatty change in carcinoma cells. *J Gastroenterol Hepatol* **12**:224–228, 1997.
178. Takeda S, Kondo M, Kumada T, Koshikawa T, Ueda R, Nishio M, Osada H, et al.: Allelic-expression imbalance of the insulin-like growth factor 2 gene in hepatocellular carcinoma and underlying disease. *Oncogene* **12**:1589–1592, 1996.
179. Aihara T, Noguchi S, Miyoshi Y, Nakano H, Sasaki Y, Nakamura Y, Monden M. et al.: Allelic imbalance of insulin-like growth factor II gene expression in cancerous and precancerous lesions of the liver. *Hepatology* **28**:86–89, 1998.
180. Uchida K, Kondo M, Takeda S, Osada H, Takahashi T, Nakao A: Altered transcriptional regulation of the insulin-like growth factor 2 gene in human hepatocellular carcinoma. *Mol Carcinog* **18**:193–198, 1997.
181. Seo JH, Kim KW, Murakami S, Park BC: Lack of colocalization of HBx Ag and insulin like growth factor II in the livers of patients with chronic hepatitis B, cirrhosis and hepatocelular carcinoma. *J Korean Med Sci* **12**:523–531, 1997.
182. Tanaka S, Mohr L, Schmidt EV, Sugimachi K, Wands JR: Biological effects of human insulin receptor substrate-1 overexpression in hepatocytes. *Hepatology* **26**:598–604, 1997.
183. Ito T, Sasaki Y, Wands JR: Overexpression of human insulin receptor substrate 1 induces cellular transformation with activation of mitogen activated protein kinases. *Mol Cell Biol* **16**:943–951, 1996.
184. Kim KW, Bae SK, Lee OH, Bae MH, Lee MJ, Park BC: Insulin-like growth factor II induced by hypoxia may contribute to angiogenesis of human hepatocellular carcinoma. *Cancer Res* **58**:384–351, 1998.
185. Bae MH, Lee MJ, Bae SK, Lee YM, Park BC, Kim KW: Insulin-like growth factor II (IGF-II) secreted from HepG2 human hepatocellular carcinoma cells shows angiogenic activity. *Cancer Lett* **128**:41–46, 1998.
186. Li XM, Tang ZY, Zhou G, Lui YK, Ye SL: Significance of vascular endothelial growth factor mRNA expression in invasion and metastasis of helpatocellular carcinoma. *J Exp Clin Cancer Res* **17**:13–17, 1998.
187. Tanaka S, Wands JR: Insulin receptor substrate 1 overexpression in human hepatocellular carcinoma cells prevents transforming growth factor beta 1 apoptosis. *Cancer Res* **56**:3391–3394, 1996.
188. Nalesnik MA, Lee RG, Carr BI: Transforming growth factor alpha (TGFalpha) in hepatocellular carcinomas and adjacent hepatic parenchyma. *Hum Pathol* **29**:228–234, 1998.
189. Hsia CC, Axiotis CA, Di Bisceglie AM, Tabor E: Transforming growth factor-alpha in human hepatocellular carcinoma and coexpression with hepatitis B surface antigen in adjacent liver. *Cancer* **70**:1049–1056, 1992.
190. Yamaguchi R, Yano H, Iemura A, Ogasawara S, Haramaki M, Kojiro M: Expression of vascular endothelial growth factor in human hepatocellular carcinoma. *Hepatology* **28**: 68-77, 1998.
191. Di Bisceglie AM, Rustgi VK, Hoofnagle JH, Dusheiko GM, Lotze MT: NIH conference: Hepatocellular carcinoma. *Ann Intern Med* **108**:390–401, 1988.
192. Lin DY, Lin SM, Liaw YF: Non-surgical treatment of hepatocellular carcinoma. *J Gastroenterol Hepatol* **12**:S319–28, 1997.
193. Zuckerman AJ: Prevention of primary liver cancer by immunization. *N Engl J Med* **336**:1906–1907, 1997.
194. Lee CL, Ko YC: Hepatitis B vaccination and hepatocellular carcinoma in Taiwan. *Pediatrics* **99**:351–353, 1997.
195. Chang MH: Hepatitis B: long-term outcome and benefits from mass vaccination in children. *Acta Gastroenterol Belg* **61**:210–213, 1998.
196. Chang MH, Chen CJ, Lai MS, Hsu HM, Wu TC, Kong MS, Liang DC. et al.: Universal hepatitis B vaccination in Taiwan and the incidence of hepatocellular carcinoma in children. Taiwan Childhood Hepatoma Study Group. *N Engl J med* **336**:1855–1859, 1997.
197. Kew MC: Increasing evidence that hepatitis B virus X gene protein and p53 protein may interact in the pathogenesis of hepatocellular carcinoma. *Hepatology* **25**:1037–1038, 1997.
198. Harris CC: p53 Tumor suppressor gene: from the basic research laboratory to the clinic: An abridged historical perspective. *Carcinogenesis* **17**: 1181–1198.
199. Lee JM, Bernstein A: Apoptosis, cancer and the p53 tumor suppressor gene. *Cancer Metastasis Rev* **14**:149–161, 1995.
200. Mullen CA, Blaese RM: Gene therapy of cancer. *Cancer Chemother Biol Response Modif* **15**:176–189, 1994.
201. Clayman GL, el-Naggar AK, Roth JA, Zhang WW, Goepfert H, Taylor DL, Liu TJ: In vivo molecular therapy with p53 adenovirus for microscopic residual head and neck squamous carcinoma. *Cancer Res* **55**:1–6, 1995.
202. Liu TJ, el-Naggar AK, McDonnell TJ, Steck KD, Wang M, Taylor DL, Clayman GL: Apoptosis induction mediated by wild-type p53 adenoviral gene transfer in squamous cell carcinoma of the head and neck. *Cancer Res* **55**:3117–3122, 1995.
203. Roth JA, Nguyen D, Lawrence DD, Kemp BL, Carrasco CH, Ferson DZ, Hong WK. et al.: Retrovirus-mediated wild-type p53 gene transfer to tumors of patients with lung cancer. *Nat Med* **2**:985–991, 1996.
204. Xu GW, Sun ZT, Forrester K, Wang XW, Coursen J, Harris CC: Tissue-specific growth suppression and chemosensitivity promotion in human hepatocellular carcinoma cells by retroviral-mediated transfer of the wild-type p53 gene. *Hepatology* **24**:1264–1268 1996.
205. da Costa LT, Jen J, He TC, Chan TA, Kinzler KW, Vogelstein B: Converting cancer genes into killer genes. *Proc Natl Acad Sci USA* **93**:4192–4196, 1996.

CHAPTER 60

Clinical and Biological Aspects of Neuroblastoma

Garrett M. Brodeur

- **Neuroblastoma, a tumor of the postganglionic sympathetic nervous system, is the most common extracranial solid tumor of childhood.**
- **No environmental exposures or agents have been associated with an increased risk of neuroblastoma. However, a subset has a genetic predisposition that follows an autosomal dominant pattern of inheritance.**
- **Primary tumors generally arise in the adrenal medulla (50 percent) or elsewhere in the abdomen or pelvis (30 percent). Only 20 percent arise in the chest.**
- **Metastases usually are found in the regional lymph nodes, bone, bone marrow, skin, or liver. Paraneoplastic syndromes characteristic of neuroblastomas are seen in a small percentage of patients.**
- **Tissue biopsy or characterization of cells in the bone marrow diagnoses neuroblastomas. Catecholamine metabolites are elevated in the urine in over 90 percent of cases.**
- **There is an international neuroblastoma staging system for categorizing the extent and resectability of the primary tumor and the presence or absence of metastases.**
- **A number of prognostic variables have been identified that allow better prediction of clinical behavior: MYCN amplification, allelic loss of 1p36, gain of 17q, expression of TrkA, tumor cell ploidy, and tumor pathology.**
- **Histologically, neuroblastic tumors can be immature (neuroblastoma), partially mature (ganglioneuroblastoma), or completely mature (ganglioneuroma). However, other features, such as the presence or absence of Schwannian stroma, mitoses, or karyorrhectic cells, may have more prognostic importance.**
- **Localized, resectable tumors can be cured by surgery alone. Unresectable tumors or metastatic disease in infants require mild to moderately intensive chemotherapy. Metastatic disease in older patients, and regional tumors with unfavorable biological features in any age, require intensive chemotherapy, frequently with bone marrow or stem cell rescue.**
- **Screening of infants for neuroblastoma by measuring urinary catecholamine metabolites has resulted in a doubling of the apparent incidence rate in infants with no decrease in advanced disease in older children.**
- **Future therapeutic approaches may be aimed at the induction of differentiation or programmed cell death through retinoid or neurotrophin receptor pathways. Alternate approaches may focus on the product of the MYCN gene, the 1p36 suppressor gene, other specific genetic changes, or antiangiogenesis.**

Few tumors have engendered as much fascination and frustration for clinical and laboratory investigators as neuroblastoma. This tumor of the postganglionic sympathetic nervous system is the most common solid tumor in childhood. Interestingly, some infants with metastatic disease can experience complete regression of their disease without therapy, and some older patients have complete maturation of their tumor into a benign ganglioneuroma. Unfortunately, the majority of patients have metastatic disease that grows relentlessly despite even the most intensive multimodality therapy. Indeed, despite dramatic improvements in the cure rate for other common pediatric neoplasms, such as acute lymphoblastic leukemia or Wilms tumor, the improvement in the overall survival rate of patients with neuroblastoma has been relatively modest.

Recent advances in understanding the biology of neuroblastoma, however, have provided considerable insight into the genetic and biochemical mechanisms underlying these seemingly disparate behaviors. Near triploidy with whole chromosome gains is a characteristic feature of favorable neuroblastoma in infants. High expression of the nerve growth factor receptor (called *TrkA*) is found in the majority of these tumors, and this may mediate either apoptosis or differentiation in these tumors. On the other hand, amplification of the *MYCN* oncogene is found in a substantial number of patients with advanced stages of disease and a poor prognosis. Finally, evidence for allelic loss at 1p, 11q, 14q, or other sites suggests the location of tumor-suppressor genes that may be important in the molecular pathogenesis of more aggressive neuroblastomas. These and other biological observations have given us tremendous insight into mechanisms of malignant transformation and progression, as well as spontaneous differentiation and regression.

The specific genetic changes that have been identified allow tumors to be classified into subsets with distinct biological features and clinical behavior. Indeed, certain genetic abnormalities are very powerful predictors of response to therapy and outcome, and as such, they have become essential components of tumor characterization at diagnosis. Thus, neuroblastoma serves as a model solid tumor in which the genetic and biological analysis of the tumor cells have become conventional determinants of optimal patient management. The challenge of the next decade is to translate this information into more effective and less toxic therapy for these patients.

In this chapter, the epidemiologic, genetic, and pathologic features of neuroblastomas are reviewed. In addition, the essential clinical features of tumor presentation and management are discussed, including several paraneoplastic syndromes that are associated with neuroblastomas. The cytogenetic and molecular

A list of standard abbreviations is located immediately preceding the index in each volume. Nonstandard abbreviations used in this chapter include: BMT = bone marrow transplantation; CCG = Children's Cancer Group; CGH = comparative genomic hybridization; DI = DNA index; Dmins = double-minute chromatin bodies; HSR = homogeneously staining region; HVA = homovanillic acid; INSS = International Neuroblastoma Staging System; LNTR = low-affinity neurotrophin receptor; LOH = loss of heterozygosity; MIBG = meta-iodobenzylguanidine; NGF = nerve growth factor; NSE = neuron-specific enolase; POG = Pediatric Oncology Group; VIP = vasoactive intestinal peptide; VMA = vanillylmandelic acid

genetic features of the tumor cells and their implications are reviewed. Current clinical management is discussed briefly. Finally, the current results of mass screening for neuroblastoma, and the implications for understanding the genetic heterogeneity of this disease, are presented.

EPIDEMIOLOGY

Incidence

Neuroblastomas account for 7 to 10 percent of all childhood cancers. The prevalence is about 1 case per 7500 live births, and there are about 600 new cases of neuroblastoma per year in the United States.[7] This corresponds to an incidence of 10.5 per million per year in Caucasian children and 8.8 per million per year in African-American children less than 15 years of age.[7,8] Evidence indicates that this incidence is fairly uniform throughout the world, at least for industrialized nations. The tumor is slightly more common in boys than in girls, with a male/female sex ratio of 1.2:1 in most large studies.

The median age at diagnosis of 1001 consecutive children with neuroblastoma seen at Pediatric Oncology Group (POG) institutions from 1981 to 1989 is 22 months.[1] Thus, 37 percent of patients are less than 1 year of age, 81 percent are less than 4 years of age, and 97 percent are diagnosed by 10 years of age (Fig. 60-1). Some studies have shown a bimodal age distribution, with an initial peak before 1 year of age and a second peak around 3 years of age.[8,9] This observation suggests that there may be at least two subpopulations of neuroblastoma, the first of which may represent a genetically predisposed subset, as seen in retinoblastoma. Alternatively, there may be two genetically distinct types of neuroblastoma with different ages of onset (see below). However, a bimodal age distribution is not always seen.

Embryology

In 1963, Beckwith and Perrin reported that microscopic neuroblastic nodules, resembling neuroblastoma *in situ*, were found frequently in infants less than 3 months of age who died of other causes.[10] This finding was interpreted initially to indicate that neuroblastomas develop up to 40 times more often than they are detected clinically, but that the tumor regresses spontaneously in the vast majority of cases. However, others subsequently demonstrated that these neuroblastic nodules occurred uniformly in all fetuses studied, peaked between 17 and 20 weeks of gestation, and gradually regressed by the time of birth or shortly after.[11,12] Thus, the microscopic neuroblastic nodules seen in the earlier study were likely remnants of fetal adrenal development. Nevertheless, these neuroblastic cell rests may be the cells from which neuroblastomas develop, at least in the adrenal medulla.

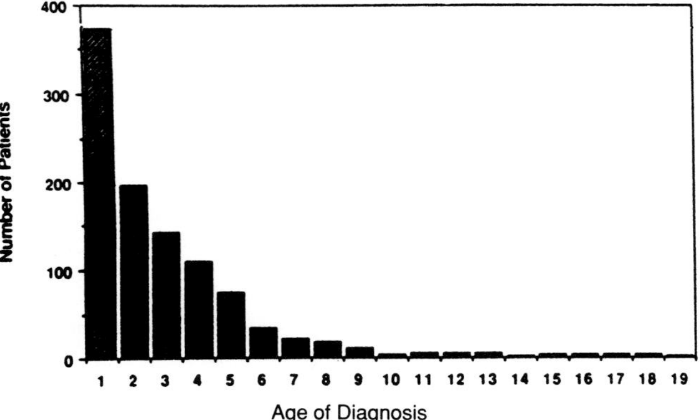

Fig. 60-1 Age at diagnosis in 1001 consecutive patients diagnosed with neuroblastoma in the Pediatric Oncology Group (POG) between 1981 and 1989. (*Reprinted from Brodeur[1] with permission of CV Mosby Year Book.*)

Although some controversy still exists concerning the initial observation of *in situ* neuroblastoma, the latter interpretation is generally accepted.

Microscopic neuroblastic nodules, as described above, would never be detected clinically, nor would they be detected by screening infants for neuroblastoma by measuring urinary catecholamine metabolites (see below). However, the concept of *in situ* neuroblastoma has been used to support the argument that many neuroblastomas arise and regress spontaneously. Indeed, there are a number of well-documented cases in infants with neuroblastoma that have had complete regression of their tumor.[13] The actual frequency of neuroblastomas that are detected clinically and subsequently regress without treatment more likely represents 5 to 10 percent of all neuroblastoma patients.[14–16] However, based on estimates from the mass screening studies, the frequency of true asymptomatic neuroblastomas that regress spontaneously is probably much higher, and may be equal to the number detected clinically (see below).

Environmental Studies

The etiology of neuroblastoma is unknown in most cases, but, based on current information, it appears unlikely that environmental exposures play a major role. There have been a few reports of neuroblastoma associated with the fetal hydantoin, phenobarbital, or alcohol syndromes,[17–19] suggesting that prenatal exposure to these substances may increase the risk of neuroblastoma. However, this association has not been confirmed with certainty. Two studies have reported a weak association between neuroblastoma and paternal occupational exposure to electromagnetic fields, but this was not confirmed in another study.[20–22] The latter group previously had shown an association between maternal use of hair-coloring products, but this also has not been confirmed.[23] Moreover, no prenatal or postnatal exposure to drugs, chemicals, or radiation has been either strongly or consistently associated with an increased incidence of neuroblastoma.

CONSTITUTIONAL GENETICS

Genetic Predisposition

A subset of patients with neuroblastoma exhibits a predisposition to develop this disease, and this predisposition follows an autosomal dominant pattern of inheritance. Knudson and Strong have estimated that as much as 22 percent of all neuroblastomas could be the result of a germinal mutation.[24] Regression analysis of these data from neuroblastoma fits the two-mutation hypothesis proposed by Knudson for the origin of childhood cancer.[25] According to this hypothesis, the nonhereditary form of neuroblastoma would result from two postzygotic (somatic) mutations in a single cell, causing malignant transformation of the cell that then develops into a single tumor. Hereditary tumors would arise in individuals in whom the first mutation is acquired as a prezygotic (germinal) event, so it is present in all cells. Only one additional mutation in any cell of the target tissue would be needed to induce malignant transformation, so these individuals would have a higher incidence of neuroblastoma with a peak incidence at an earlier age. In addition, they may develop tumors at multiple primary sites, either simultaneously or sequentially. If such persons survive, half of their offspring would be carriers of the germinal mutation, with an estimated 63 percent chance of developing neuroblastoma.[24,26]

There have been a number of reports of familial neuroblastoma, as well as bilateral or multifocal disease, consistent with hereditary predisposition, which were reviewed by Kushner and colleagues.[27] The median age at diagnosis of patients with familial neuroblastoma is 9 months, which contrasts with a median age of 22 months for neuroblastoma in the general population. At least 20 percent of patients with familial neuroblastoma have bilateral adrenal or multifocal primary tumors. The concordance for neuroblastoma in monozygotic siblings during infancy suggests that hereditary

Table 60-1 Constitutional Chromosome Abnormalities in Patients with Neuroblastoma

Chromosome Abnormality	Comments	Reference
del(21)(p11); inv(11)(q21q23)	One from each parent	31–33
t(4;7)(p?;q?)	Balanced; normal phenotype	34
t(11;16)(q?;q?)	Balanced; normal phenotype	34
Partial trisomy 2p and monosomy 16p	Congential anomalies	35
Partial trisomy 3q and monosomy 8p	Congenital anomalies	35
Partial trisomy 15q and monosomy 13q	Congenital anomalies	36
Trisomy 18	Congenital anomalies	37
fra(1)(p13.1)	Hereditary fragile site	38
t(1;?)(p36;?)	Mosaic?	39
t(1;17)(p36;q12–21)	Balanced	40, 41
t(1;13)(q22;q12)	Balanced	42
t(8;11)(q22.1;q21)	Balanced	43
t(2;11)(p23;q22)	Balanced	43
t(2;6)(q32.2;q25.3)	Balanced	43
del(1)(p36.2–p36.3)	Dysmorphic, retarded	44
t(1;10)(p22;q21)	Balanced	45, 46

factors may be predominant, whereas the discordance in older twins suggests that random mutations or other factors may play a role.[28] A recent report examined the genetic linkage of neuroblastoma predisposition to several candidate loci in families segregating the disease, but linkage was not found.[29] Nevertheless, an international registry has been developed to identify familial neuroblastoma throughout the world.[29,30]

Constitutional Chromosome Abnormalities

A constitutional predisposition syndrome or associated congenital anomalies have not yet been identified in human neuroblastoma.[5] Several cases of constitutional chromosome abnormalities detected by banding have been reported in individuals with neuroblastoma, but no consistent pattern has emerged as yet (Table 60-1).[31–46] There have been three reports of constitutional abnormalities involving the short arm of chromosome 1, which frequently is deleted or rearranged in neuroblastoma cells. Laureys and colleagues described a patient with neuroblastoma who had a constitutional translocation between chromosomes 1 and 17, with the breakpoint on chromosome 1 in 1p36, the region frequently deleted in neuroblastoma cells.[40,41] A second interesting case, reported by Biegel, had a constitutional deletion of 1p36 and neuroblastoma, confirmed by both cytogenetic and molecular analysis.[44] A third case with a similar deletion was reported by White and colleagues.[47] Together with the frequent deletion of 1p36 in sporadic neuroblastomas, these cases suggested that constitutional deletions or rearrangements involving a gene on 1p36 may play a role in malignant transformation or predisposition to neuroblastoma in some cases. However, a recent report that familial neuroblastoma is not linked to 1p36 suggests that the predominant predisposition locus lies elsewhere.[29]

Two series reporting the routine constitutional karyotype analysis of a series of neuroblastoma patients have identified several cases with balanced translocations, suggesting that balanced translocations per se may be more common than in the general population (Table 60-1).[34,43] No consistent breakpoint has been identified, however, so routine karyotypic analysis is unlikely to be rewarding. Individuals with neuroblastoma who also have mental retardation, dysmorphic features, or other evidence of gross genetic abnormalities should be examined cytogenetically, because this may help identify the neuroblastoma predisposition locus (or loci).[44]

Other Genetic Syndromes

Neuroblastoma has been associated with neurofibromatosis type 1 (von Recklinghausen disease) suggesting that it might be part of a spectrum of syndromes involving maldevelopment of the neural crest.[48–50] However, an analysis of reported instances of the simultaneous occurrence of neuroblastoma and neurofibromatosis in the same patient suggests that these cases probably can be accounted for by chance alone.[51] Aganglionosis of the colon (Hirschsprung disease) is also a disorder of neural crest origin that has been associated with neuroblastoma, but linkage to genes associated with this disorder also has not been seen.[29] A variety of other congenital anomalies and genetic syndromes have been reported in association with neuroblastoma, but no specific abnormality has been identified with increased frequency.[52–54] Interestingly, there may be an increased prevalence of neuroblastoma in patients with Turner syndrome, and a decreased prevalence in patients with Down syndrome, but the reasons for this are unclear.[55–57]

GENETICS OF TUMOR CELLS

Oncogene Activation and Allelic Gain

Amplification of *MYCN* and Other Loci. Some neuroblastomas are characterized cytogenetically by double-minute chromatin bodies (dmins) and homogeneously staining regions (HSRs), which are cytogenetic manifestations of gene amplification (Fig. 60-2).[58–61] However, the gene or genetic region amplified was not known initially. Schwab and others identified a novel *c-myc*-related oncogene that was amplified in a series of neuroblastoma cell lines.[62,63] The amplified sequence, known as *MYCN,* is normally located on the distal short arm of chromosome 2, but maps to the dmins or HSRs in tumors with *MYCN* amplification.[63,64] Apparently a large region from 2p24 (including the *MYCN* locus) becomes amplified initially as extrachromosomal dmins, but may become linearly integrated into a chromosome as one or more HSR, particularly in established cell lines.[65,66]

Brodeur and colleagues have demonstrated that *MYCN* amplification occurs in about 25 percent of primary neuroblastomas from untreated patients (Figs. 60-3 and 60-4).[5,65,67,68] Amplification of *MYCN* is associated predominantly with advanced stages of disease and a poor outcome, but it is also associated with rapid tumor progression and a poor prognosis, even in infants and patients with lower stages of disease.[60,68–71] These studies have been extended to 3000 patients participating in cooperative group protocols in the United States. (Table 60-2).[3–5] *MYCN* amplification can be detected by Southern blot, fluorescence *in situ* hybridization, quantitative PCR, comparative genomic amplification, or other techniques.[66,72]

Interestingly, a consistent pattern was found of *MYCN* copy number (either amplified or unamplified) in different tumor

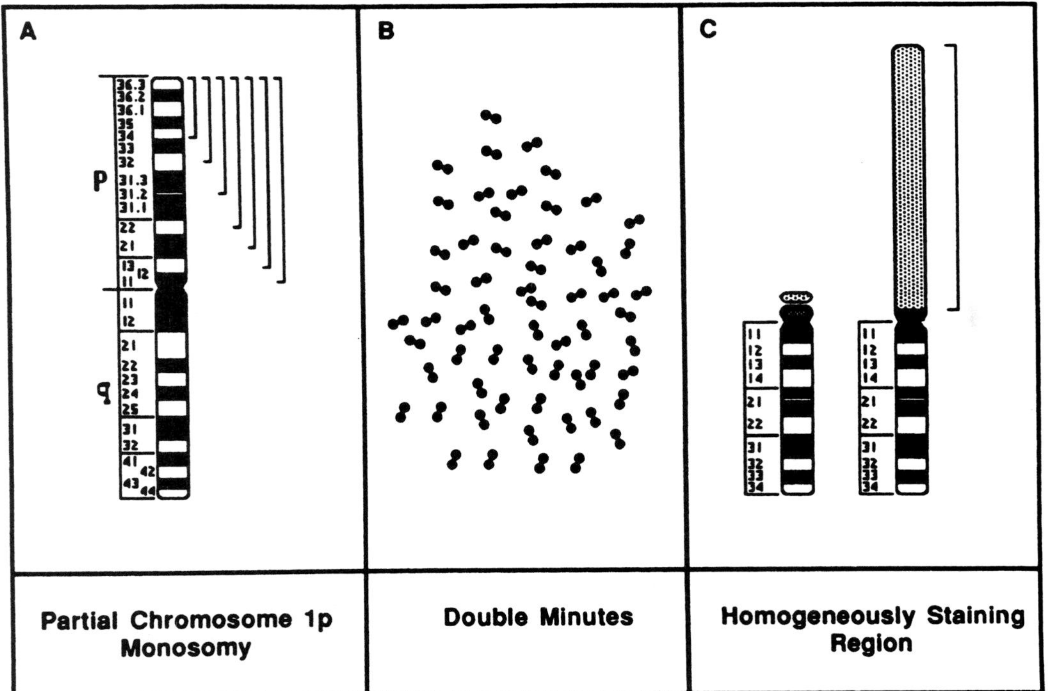

Fig. 60-2 Common cytogenetic abnormalities in human neuroblastomas. Shown are representations of three common cytogenetic abnormalities seen in human neuroblastomas. *A*, Deletions of the short arm of chromosome 1. The brackets indicate that the region deleted in different tumors is variable in terms of its proximal breakpoint, but the distal short arm appears to be deleted in all cases, resulting in partial 1p monosomy. *B*, Extrachromosomal double-minute chromatin bodies (dmins). Dmins are seen in about 30 percent of primary neuroblastomas and are a cytogenetic manifestation of gene amplification. *C*, Homogeneously staining region (HSR). A representative HSR on the short arm of chromosome 13 is shown in this example. HSRs are a cytogenetic manifestation of gene amplification in which the amplified sequences are chromosomally integrated. (*Reprinted from Brodeur*[68] *with permission of Brain Pathology.*)

samples taken from an individual patient, either simultaneously or consecutively.[73] These results suggest that *MYCN* amplification is an intrinsic biological property of a subset of aggressive neuroblastomas, and tumors without amplification at diagnosis rarely, if ever, develop this abnormality subsequently. Currently, neuroblastomas from patients on clinical trials in the United States, Europe, and Japan are routinely assessed for the presence of *MYCN* amplification, because it is a powerful predictor of a poor prognosis.

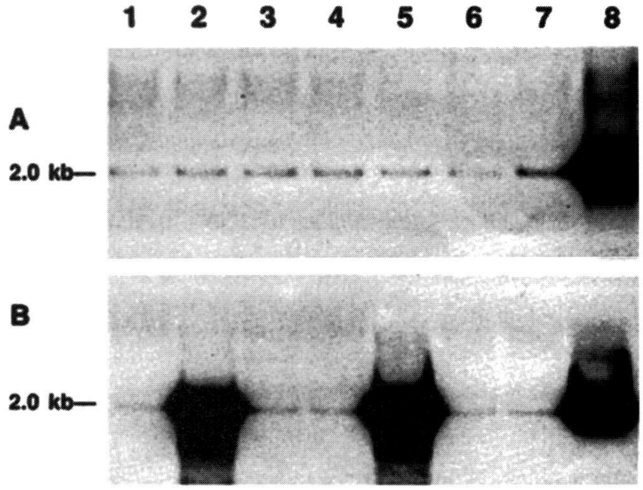

Our studies have also shown a strong correlation between *MYCN* amplification and 1p loss of heterozygosity (LOH).[74–76] Both *MYCN* amplification and deletion of 1p are strongly correlated with a poor outcome and with each other, but it is not yet clear if they are independent prognostic variables.[77–81] Nevertheless, they appear to characterize a genetically distinct subset of very aggressive neuroblastomas. Most cases with *MYCN* amplification also have 1p LOH, but not all cases with 1p LOH have amplification. This suggests that 1p deletion may precede the development of amplification. Indeed, it may be necessary to delete a gene that regulates *MYCN* expression, or one that mediates programmed cell death in the presence of high *MYCN* gene expression, for amplification to occur. Alternatively, there may be an underlying genetic abnormality that leads to genomic instability that predisposes to both 1p LOH and *MYCN* amplification.

About 25 percent of neuroblastomas have *MYCN* amplification, and virtually all of these cases have very high *MYCN* expression at the RNA and protein levels.[70] Indeed, there is heterogeneity in the level of expression of *MYCN* in single-copy tumors, but higher expression in nonamplified tumors does not consistently correlate with a worse outcome.[82–85] It is possible that the level of expression in nonamplified tumors seldom, if ever, exceeds a certain threshold level necessary to confer an unfavorable outcome, whereas almost all tumors with *MYCN* amplification exceed this threshold.[86] Furthermore, activation of *MYCN* by mechanisms other than amplification or overexpression may play an important role.[87] Finally, *DDX1*, a member of the DEAD box family of RNA helicases, is coamplified with *MYCN* in about half the cases.[88–91] However, the clinical significance of this finding is unclear.

Fig. 60-3 Southern blots showing *MYCN* amplification. In both rows, lane 1 represents DNA from a normal lymphoblastoid cell line as a single-copy control, and lane 8 represents DNA from the NGP cell line, with 150 copies of *MYCN* per haploid genome. (Row A). Lanes 2-7 represent 6 neuroblastomas with a single copy of *MYCN* per haploid genome. (Row B). Lanes 2 and 5 show examples of tumors with *MYCN* amplification, whereas the other tumors have the normal single-copy signal. (*Reprinted from Brodeur*[68] *with permission of Brain Pathology.*)

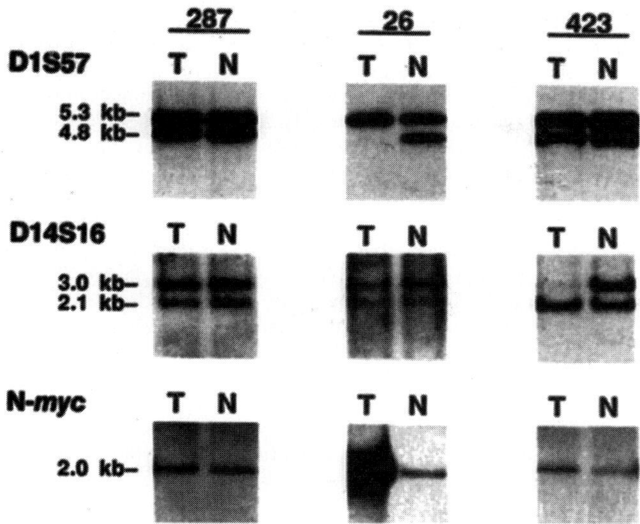

Fig. 60-4 Patterns of genetic change in neuroblastomas. The first row shows assessment of LOH for the short arm of chromosome 1 (1p34) using the hypervariable probe D1S57 and the enzyme *TaqI*. The second row shows assessment of LOH for the long arm of chromosome 14 (14p32) using the probe D14S16 and the enzyme *TaqI*. The third row shows assessment of *MYCN* amplification using the pNB-1probe and *EcoRI* digestion of the DNAs. The first column (patient no. 287) shows no LOH for 1p or 14q, and normal *MYCN* copy number. The second column (patient no. 26) shows LOH for 1p and *MYCN* amplification, without allelic loss for 14q. The third column (patient no. 423) shows LOH for 14q, without LOH for 1p or *MYCN* amplification, which was the second most common pattern of genetic change. (T = tumor DNA; N = normal DNA from the same patient). (*Reprinted from Fong and colleagues*[75] *with permission of Cancer Research.*)

Amplification of Other Loci. We sought evidence for amplification of other oncogenes in a large series of neuroblastomas and tumor-derived cell lines, but none was found.[61] However, there are at least six examples of neuroblastoma cell lines or primary tumors that amplify regions that are remote from the *MYCN* locus at 2p24. These examples include amplification of genes from 2p22 and 2p13 in the IMR-32 cell line, as well as coamplification of *MYCN* and *MDM2* (from 12q13) in the NGP, TR-14, and LS cell lines.[92–95] Finally, there is one report of coamplification of *MYCN* and *MYCL* in a neuroblastoma cell line, which has been seen in at least one primary tumor as well.[4,5,66,96] These findings indicate that more than one locus can be amplified, but no neuroblastoma has been shown to amplify another gene that did not also amplify *MYCN*. Allelic gain of several other loci, such as 2p, 4q, 6p, 7q, 11q, and 18q, has been identified using comparative genomic hybridization (CGH) approaches.[97–102] However, the true prevalence, as well as the biological and clinical significance of these findings, is unclear at present.

Trisomy for 17q. To date, the only other specific karyotypic abnormality that has been detected with increased frequency is trisomy for the long arm of chromosome 17 (17q).[58,77,103] This finding was first noted by conventional cytogenetic studies and by FISH analysis, but its real frequency was not appreciated until recently. Allelotyping and CGH studies have suggested that gain of the long arm of chromosome 17 may occur in over half of all neuroblastomas.[97–101,104] Even accounting for near-triploid cases with gain of the entire chromosome, 17q trisomy may be the most prevalent genetic abnormality identified to date in neuroblastomas. Although gain of 17q can occur independently, it frequently occurs as part of an unbalanced translocation between chromosomes 1 and 17.[101,105–107] The 17q breakpoints vary, but a region has been defined from 17q22-qter that suggests a dosage effect rather than interruption of a gene.[108] Gain of 17q appears to be associated with a more aggressive subset of neuroblastomas, although its significance relative to other genetic and biological markers awaits a large prospective trial and multivariate analysis.

Table 60-2 Correlation between MYCN Amplification and Stage in 3000 Neuroblastomas[2–6]

Stage at Diagnosis	*MYCN* Amplification	3-yr. Survival
Benign ganglioneuromas	0/64 (0%)	100%
Low stages (1, 2)	31/772 (4%)	90%
Stage 4-S	15/190 (8%)	80%
Advanced States (3, 4)	612/1974 (31%)	30%
TOTAL	658/3000 (22%)	50%

Tumor DNA Content: Near-Diploidy vs. Hyperdiploidy. Although the majority of tumors that have been karyotyped are in the diploid range, a substantial number of tumors from patients with lower stages of disease are hyperdiploid or near triploid. The modal karyotype number has been shown to have prognostic value.[109–111] Karyotypic analysis of tumor cells, however, is a tedious process that is generally successful in less than 25 percent of the cases attempted. Flow cytometric analysis of DNA content is a simple and semiautomated way of measuring total cell DNA, which correlates well with modal chromosome number. Recent studies by Look and others demonstrate that determination of the DNA index (DI) of neuroblastomas from infants provides important information that can be predictive of response to particular chemotherapeutic regimens as well as outcome.[112–115] Although this analysis cannot detect specific chromosome rearrangements, such as deletions, translocations, or gene amplification, it is a relatively simple test that correlates with biological behavior, at least in subsets of patients. Unfortunately, the DNA index loses its prognostic significance for patients over 2 years of age.[113] This is probably because hyperdiploid tumors from infants generally have whole chromosome gains without structural rearrangements, whereas hyperdiploid tumors in older patients usually have a number of structural rearrangements as well.

Tumor-Suppressor Genes and Allelic Loss

Chromosome Deletion or Allelic Loss at 1p. Deletion of the short arm of chromosome 1(1p) is a common abnormality that has been identified in 70 to 80 percent of the near-diploid tumors that have been karyotyped (Fig. 60-2).[59,61,103,116,117] However, using DNA polymorphism approaches that do not require tumor cells in mitosis, the actual prevalence is probably closer to 35 percent (Fig. 60-4).[74,76,78–80,118–121] Deletions of chromosome 1 are found more commonly in patients with advanced stages of disease, but the independent prognostic significance of 1p LOH is controversial.[77–81] Distal 1p36 appears to be deleted in almost all cases, including 1p36.2–.3, although the breakpoints are quite variable (Fig. 60-5). Indeed, another area of controversy is whether there is a single site of consistent deletion on distal 1p or two independent sites.[76,119–122] Finally, there is disagreement about whether distal 1p undergoes genomic imprinting, based on preferential parental allelic loss.[123,124] The resolution of these controversies must await additional studies, but it appears clear that at least one (and possibly more) tumor-suppressor gene resides at this locus.[4,5]

Unfortunately, no good candidate for the neuroblastoma tumor-suppressor gene on 1p36 has been identified, but several have been proposed (Fig. 60-5), including the tumor necrosis factor receptor 2 gene,[125] a zinc finger gene called *HKR3*,[126] a cell-cycle control gene called *CDC2L1*,[127] a tumor-suppressor gene in mice called *DAN*,[128] and a *TP53* homolog called *TP73*.[129] Indeed, *TP73* is particularly interesting because of its homology to the prevalent tumor-suppressor gene *TP53*, but mutations have not been identified in neuroblastomas lacking one copy of the gene.[130]

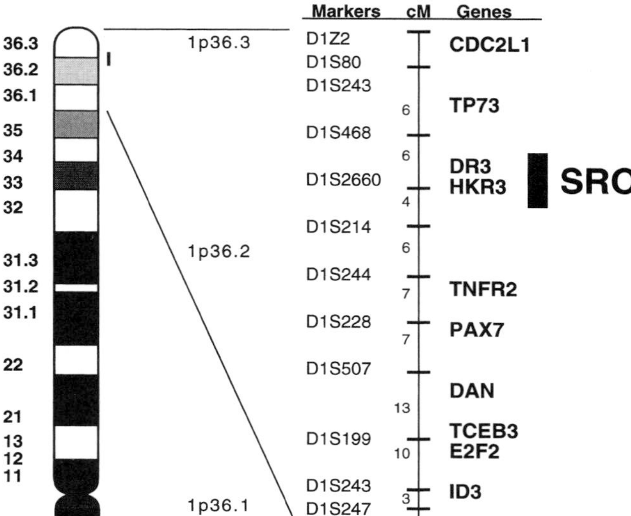

Fig. 60-5 Consistent region of 1p LOH in neuroblastomas. Diagrammatic representation of the short arm of chromosome 1 (1p), as well as the expanded genetic map of 1p36 and the approximate location of several candidates for the neuroblastoma tumor-suppressor gene (shown in bold). Also shown (SRO) is the region of consistent deletion of 1p36 in neuroblastomas (6 cM, 1 to 2 Mb), based on PCR-based polymorphisms. This map is described in more detail by White and colleagues.[47,76] *(Modified from Brodeur[5] with permission of Lippincott-Raven Press.)*

Moreover, with the exception of *HKR3*, these other candidate genes have been excluded from the region of consistent deletion, and careful analysis of *HKR3* has failed to identify any mutations.[47,76,126] Thus, further narrowing of the region of consistent deletion and analysis of candidate genes is required.

Chromosome Deletion or Allelic Loss at 11q, 14q, and Other Sites

Allelic Loss at 11q. Allelic loss of 11q has been detected by analysis of DNA polymorphisms and by CGH techniques.[75,98–101,131,132] In a recent study, 11q allelic loss occurs in 114 of 267 cases (43 percent), making it the most common deletion detected to date in neuroblastomas.[132] 11q deletion was associated with 14q deletion, but it was inversely correlated with 1p deletion and *MYCN* amplification. Interestingly, 11q LOH was associated with decreased event-free survival, but only in patients lacking *MYCN* amplification. Loss of 11q was not associated with other clinical or biological variables.

Allelic Loss at 14q. There is evidence that LOH for the long arm of chromosome 14 also occurs with increased frequency in neuroblastomas (Fig. 60-4).[75,131,133,134] The frequency of 14q allelic loss varies in different studies from 25 percent to 50 percent in several smaller studies, but it appears to be a consistent finding that probably represents loss of another suppressor gene. A more recent study found allelic loss in 64 of 280 cases (23 percent).[135] A consensus region of deletion was found in 14q23–32. There was a strong correlation with 11q allelic loss and an inverse relationship with 1p deletion and *MYCN* amplification. However, no correlation was found with other biological or clinical features or outcome.

Allelic Loss at Other Sites. Deletion or allelic loss has been demonstrated at a variety of other sites by genome-wide allelotyping or by CGH. The most consistent sites, in addition to those mentioned above, include 3p, 4p, 6q, 9p, 13q, and 18q.[98–102,104] However, none of these other sites have been studied in as much detail as the above sites, so their biological or clinical significance is unclear.

Other Tumor-Suppressor Genes

Involvement of TP53. The *TP53* gene, encoding the p53 protein, is one of the most commonly involved genes in human neoplasia. Several studies have examined neuroblastomas for mutation in the *TP53* gene, but mutations are rarely found.[136–140] Nevertheless, there is still controversy about the involvement of this gene in human neuroblastomas. Some reports have shown cytoplasmic sequestration in undifferentiated neuroblastomas, and this impairs the normal G1 checkpoint after DNA damage.[141,142] However, others have demonstrated that, although p53 is primarily located in the cytoplasm, ionizing radiation induces normal translocation to the nucleus of p53 that is capable of inducing G1 arrest.[143] At present this apparent discrepancy remains unresolved.

Involvement of CDK Inhibitors and the Neurofibromatosis 1 Gene. The *CDKN2A* (*INK4A*/p16) gene is deleted or mutated in many types of adult cancer, especially in established cell lines. Nevertheless, three studies have found no evidence of inactivation in neuroblastomas.[144–146] Indeed, two of these studies also examined the related genes *CDKN2B* (*KIP1*/p27) and *CDKN2C* (*INK4C*/p18) genes, but no deletions or rearrangements were found in these genes either.[145,146] One report, however, found frequent loss of 9p in neuroblastomas, and although only one tumor had a missense mutation, a number of others had absence of expression, suggesting inactivation in these cases.[147] Finally, two studies have found evidence of deletions or mutations in the neurofibromatosis 1 (*NF1*) gene in neuroblastoma cell lines, but it is unclear if this occurs commonly in primary tumors.[148,149]

ABNORMAL PATTERNS OF GENE EXPRESSION

Expression of Neurotrophin Receptors

Neuroblastoma cells are derived from sympathetic neuroblasts, and they frequently exhibit features of neuronal differentiation. Indeed, because neuroblastomas may show spontaneous or induced differentiation to ganglioneuroblastoma or ganglioneuroma, the malignant transformation of these cells may result in part from a failure to respond fully to the normal signals to undergo this maturation process. The factors responsible for regulating normal differentiation are not well understood at present, but they probably involve one or several neurotrophin-receptor pathways that signal the cell to differentiate. Recently, three tyrosine kinase receptors for a homologous family of neurotrophin factors were cloned. The main ligand for the *TrkA*, *TrkB,* and *TrkC* receptors is nerve growth factor (NGF), brain-derived neurotrophic factor (BDNF), and neurotrophin-3 (NT-3), respectively; neurotrophin-4/5 (NT-4) appears to function through *TrkB*.[150–159] Another transmembrane receptor binds all the neurotrophins with low affinity (LNTR), but its role in mediating responses to the presence or absence of these homologous ligands is controversial.[150,160,161]

To evaluate the clinical significance of *TrkA* expression in neuroblastomas, we studied the relationship between *TrkA* mRNA expression and patient survival in frozen tumors from 77 children with neuroblastomas and 5 children with ganglioneuromas.[162] High levels of *TrkA* expression (>100 density units) were detected in 63 of the 77 neuroblastomas (82 percent). All tumors that had low-stage and no *MYCN* amplification showed a high level of *TrkA* expression. All but one tumor with *MYCN* amplification, however, had an extremely low or undetectable level of *TrkA* expression. The expression of *TrkA* correlated strongly with survival: the 5-year cumulative-survival rate of the group with a high level of *TrkA* expression was 86 percent, whereas that of the group with a low level of *TrkA* expression was 14 percent ($p < 0.001$). Indeed, the combination of *TrkA* expression and *MYCN* amplification had a strong influence on overall survival (see below). The group with high levels of *TrkA* expression and no *MYCN* amplification showed a cumulative 5-year survival of 87 percent. The patients whose tumors had a

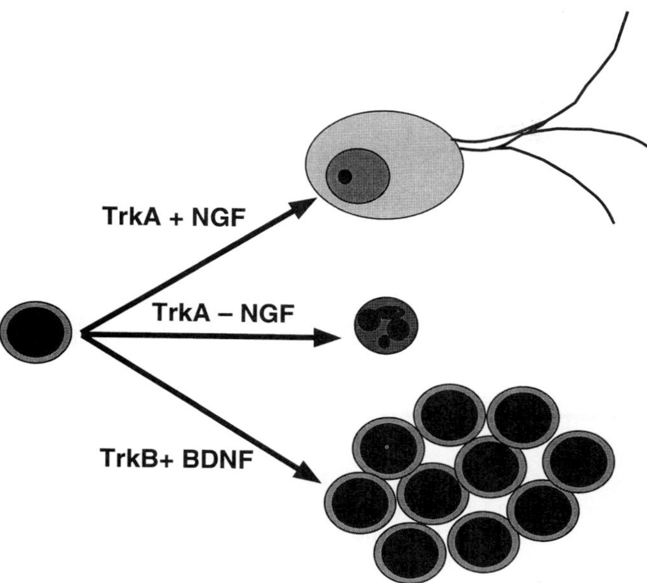

Fig. 60-6 Diagrammatic representation of the potential fates of neuroblastoma cells, depending on the pattern of expression of neurotrophin receptors and the availability of neurotrophins in their microenvironment. Favorable neuroblastoma cells expressing TrkA (with or without TrkC), if deprived of NGF, frequently undergo programmed cell death *in vitro*. These same cells will survive and differentiate if provided with adequate amounts of neurotrophins. In contrast, unfavorable neuroblastomas frequently express TrkB as well as its ligand BDNF. This autocrine loop apparently favors survival of these cells independent of exogenous neurotrophins. Furthermore, these cells generally do not express TrkA (or TrkC), and they do not respond to NGF by undergoing differentiation. (*Modified from Brodeur*[5] *with permission of Lippincott-Raven Press.*)

normal *MYCN* copy number and a low level of expression of *TrkA* had a 50 percent survival ($p = 0.03$), and all patients with *MYCN* amplification died within 2 years. Similar results have been obtained independently by others, supporting the strong correlation between high *TrkA* expression and a favorable outcome.[163–166]

The NGF/*TrkA* pathway may play an important role in the propensity of some neuroblastomas to regress or differentiate in selected patients. The association of *Trk* expression with tumors that have a favorable outcome suggests that it may play some role in the behavior of the tumors. Indeed, the expression of *TrkA* is required for biological responsiveness to NGF. In the presence of ligand, neuronal differentiation is induced and survival is promoted.[167] However, neurotrophic-factor deprivation may lead to programmed cell death (apoptosis) at this stage (Fig. 60-6).[168,169] Thus, the *in vivo* differentiation or regression that is seen either spontaneously or in response to treatment may be mediated by the NGF/*TrkA* pathway.[162]

Recently, we examined the expression and function of *TrkB* and *TrkC* in neuroblastomas. Both of these neurotrophin receptors can be expressed in a truncated form (lacking the tyrosine kinase) and a full-length form. Interestingly, expression of full-length *TrkB* was strongly associated with *MYCN*-amplified tumors.[170] Because these tumors also express the *TrkB* ligand (BDNF), this may represent an autocrine or paracrine loop providing some survival or growth advantage (Fig. 60-6).[171–173] Maturing tumors were more likely to express the truncated *TrkB*, whereas most immature, nonamplified tumors expressed neither.[170] In contrast, the expression of *TrkC* was found predominantly in lower stage tumors, and, like *TrkA*, was not expressed in *MYCN* amplified tumors.[174,175] This suggests that favorable tumors are characterized by the expression of *TrkA* with or without *TrkC*, but unfavorable tumors express full-length *TrkB* plus its ligand *BDNF*.

Expression of *HRAS* and Other Oncogenes

Although *NRAS* was first identified as the transforming gene of a human neuroblastoma cell line, subsequent studies of primary neuroblastomas by ourselves and others indicate that *RAS* activation by mutation of codons 12, 13, 59, or 61 is rare.[176–178] On the contrary, there is evidence that high expression of *HRAS* in neuroblastomas is associated with lower stage and better outcome.[179–181] The pattern of oncogene expression may be used to distinguish neuroblastomas from other histologically similar tumors, such as neuroepithelioma.[182] However, the ultimate clinical utility of the analysis of oncogene expression in neuroblastomas remains to be determined. Thus, in the subset of the patients lacking *MYCN* amplification, there is no consistent evidence to date for amplification or activation of any other oncogene.

Expression of the Multidrug Resistance Genes

Some tumor cells become resistant to a large number of chemotherapeutic agents simultaneously by overexpressing genes that confer this resistance, probably by enhanced efflux of the agents. The genes associated with this phenomenon are the multidrug resistance gene *MDR1* and the gene for multidrug resistance-related protein *MRP*. Most of the investigation of these genes and their encoded proteins has been performed *in vitro*, but their expression and potential clinical significance in neuroblastomas was addressed recently.[183–186] The data concerning the clinical significance of expression of *MDR1* in neuroblastomas are controversial, but the one study examining *MRP* expression shows a strong correlation with advanced clinical stages and a poor prognosis.[183–186] If this is confirmed by a larger independent study, analysis of *MRP* expression could become an important variable to examine to determine a patient's prognosis and to, in turn, influence the choice of agents or the intensity of treatment.

Telomerase Expression and Activity

Hiyama and colleagues[187] have studied 79 neuroblastomas from untreated patients for telomerase activity. They found that 16 had high telomerase activity, 60 had low activity, and 3 had no detectable activity. Interestingly, the three with no activity were among eight with stage 4S, a stage with a special pattern of limited dissemination found in infants whose tumors sometimes undergo spontaneous regression. None of these children died. In fact, only 2 of 60 patients with low activity died, whereas 12 of 16 with high activity died. Interestingly, all 11 with *MYCN* amplification had high activity, including the one patient with stage 4-S who died. These results show a correlation between telomerase activity and outcome of neuroblastoma patients, with a very good outcome seen in the few with no activity and a poor outcome in those with high activity (most with *MYCN* amplification). Thus, the extremes of telomerase activity (high or absent) may provide some useful information, but telomerase activity per se is correlated more with malignancy in general and not with specific types or behavior.[188] In further support of the potential clinical importance of telomerase expression, Reynolds and coworkers have shown a correlation of high expression of the RNA component with stage 4 disease and a poor outcome.[189]

Expression of Apoptosis Genes

Neuroblastoma has the highest rate of spontaneous regression observed in human cancers, and delayed activation of normal apoptotic pathways may play a role in this phenomenon.[190] Activation of programmed cell death can originate from a variety of stimuli, such as the presence or absence of exogenous ligand or from DNA damage. Indeed, NGF withdrawal is an important signal for apoptosis in the developing nervous system, and mediates the elimination of redundant cells. However, other cell surface proteins may be involved with initiation of apoptosis in neuronal cells and neuroblastomas (reviewed by Brodeur and Castle[191]). Members of the tumor necrosis factor receptor (TNFR) family, such as p75 (binds NGF with low affinity) and CD95/FasL (binds Fas ligand), as well as members of the retinoic acid receptor family, can mediate the induction of apoptosis in some neuroblastoma cell lines.[192,193] In addition, increased CD95 expression appears to be an essential component of chemotherapy induced apoptosis in neuroblastomas.[193]

Intracellular molecules responsible for relaying the apoptotic signal include the Bcl-2 family of proteins. *BCL-2* is highly expressed in most neuroblastoma cell lines and primary tumors and the level of expression is inversely related to the proportion of cells undergoing apoptosis and the degree of cellular differentiation.[190,194–198] There have been conflicting reports regarding the correlation between the level of expression of Bcl-2 in primary tumors and prognostic variables,[194,196,197,199,200] but taken together the evidence suggests that there is no significant correlation. However, the Bcl-2 family of proteins may play an important role in acquired resistance to chemotherapy.[201,202] Finally, caspases are the proteolytic enzymes responsible for the execution of the apoptotic signal, and there is evidence that increased expression of interleukin-1β-converting enzyme (ICE, caspase-1) and other caspases in primary neuroblastoma is associated with favorable biological features and improved disease outcome.[203] These observations are consistent with the hypothesis that neuroblastomas prone to undergoing apoptosis are more likely to spontaneously regress and/or respond well to cytotoxic agents.

GENETIC MODEL OF NEUROBLASTOMA DEVELOPMENT

In summary, there is increasing evidence for at least two genetic subsets of neuroblastomas that are highly predictive of clinical behavior. One recently proposed classification takes into account abnormalities of 1p, *MYCN* copy number, and assessment of DNA content, and distinct genetic subsets of neuroblastomas can be identified (Fig. 60-7; Table 60-3).[2–6] The first is characterized by mitotic dysfunction leading to a hyperdiploid or near-triploid modal karyotype, with few if any cytogenetic rearrangements. These tumors lack specific genetic changes like *MYCN* amplification or 1p LOH. These patients are generally less than 1 year of age with localized disease and a very good prognosis. The second is characterized by gross chromosomal aberrations and they generally have a near-diploid karyotype. No consistent abnormality has been identified to date, but 17q gain is common. Within this type, two subsets can be distinguished. One subset is characterized by 11q deletion, 14q deletion, or other changes, but patients in this subset lack *MYCN* amplification and generally lack 1p LOH. Patients with these tumors are generally older with more advanced stages of disease that is slowly progressive and often fatal. The second subset has amplification of *MYCN*, usually with 1p36 LOH. These patients are generally between 1 and 5 years of age with advanced stages of disease that is rapidly progressive and frequently fatal. It is unknown if a tumor from one type ever converts to a less favorable type, but current evidence suggests that they are genetically distinct.[73,113]

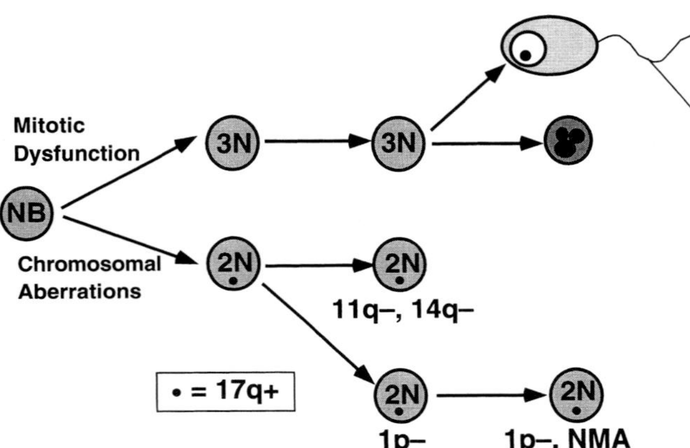

Fig. 60-7 Genetic model of neuroblastoma development. According to this model, all neuroblastomas have a common precursor (NB) and may have a common mutation (the one responsible for familial neuroblastoma). However, a commitment is made to develop into one of two major types. The first type is characterized by mitotic dysfunction leading to a hyperdiploid or near-triploid modal karyotype (3N) with whole chromosome gains, but few if any structural cytogenetic rearrangements. These tumors usually express high levels of TrkA, so they are prone to either differentiation or apoptosis, depending on the presence or absence of NGF in their microenvironment. The second type generally has a near-diploid (2N) or near-tetraploid karyotype but is characterized by gross chromosomal aberrations. No consistent abnormality has been identified to date, but 17q gain is very common. Within this type, two subsets can be distinguished. 11q deletion and/or 14q deletion characterize one subset, whereas the second subset is characterized by 1p LOH, with or without MYCN amplification (NMA). The latter tumors frequently express TrkB plus BDNF, probably representing an autocrine survival pathway. Thus, neuroblastoma represents fundamentally two major types and three subtypes, but they may all arise from a common precursor cell. (*Reprinted from Ambros and Brodeur*[347] *with permission from Lippincott-Raven Press.*)

Table 60-3 Biological/Clinical Types of Neuroblastoma[3–5,347]

Feature	Type 1	Type 2A	Type 2B
MYCN	Normal	Normal	Amplified
DNA Ploidy	Hyperdiploid Near triploid	Near diploid Near tetraploid	Near diploid Near tetraploid
17q gain	Rare	Common	Common
11q, 14q LOH	Rare	Common	Rare
1p LOH	Rare	Rare	Common
TrkA exp.	High	Low or absent	Low or absent
TrkB exp.	Truncated	Low or absent	High (full length)
TrkC exp.	High	Low or absent	Low or absent
Age	Usually <1 yr.	Usually >1 yr.	Usually 1–5 yr.
Stage	Usually 1, 2, 4S	Usually 3, 4	Usually 3, 4
3-yr. Survival	95%	25–50%	20%

Indeed, it is possible that all neuroblastomas have a single mutation in common. This is because one can see the spectrum from ganglioneuroma to metastatic neuroblastoma in a single family.[29,30] However, a commitment is made shortly after to develop into one of two major types: (a) a favorable type characterized by mitotic dysfunction and whole chromosome gains, leading to hyperdiploidy or near triploidy, or (b) an unfavorable type characterized by structural chromosomal rearrangements. The first type of tumors generally expresses high levels of *TrkA*, and these tumors are prone to differentiation or programmed cell death, depending on the presence or absence of NGF. The second type frequently has gain of 17q and expresses little, if any, *TrkA*. However, subsets can be distinguished by different patterns of genetic change (Fig. 60-7). A less aggressive subtype is characterized by deletion of 11q, 14q, or other rearrangements. The most aggressive subtype is characterized by *MYCN* amplification, frequently with 1p LOH, and these tumors frequently express *TrkB* plus *BDNF*, representing an autocrine survival pathway. Thus, neuroblastoma represents fundamentally two different types, but it can be seen as one or three diseases as well, depending on the perspective.

CLINICAL MANIFESTATIONS AND PATTERN OF SPREAD

Primary Tumors

About half of all neuroblastomas originate in the adrenal medulla; 30 percent occur in nonadrenal abdominal sites in the paravertebral ganglia, pelvic ganglia, or the organ of Zuckerkandl; and 20 percent occur in the paravertebral ganglia of the thorax.[1,2] Most primary tumors cause symptoms of abdominal mass or pain. However, because of the paraspinal location of many tumors, they may invade the spinal canal through neural foramina and cause compression of the spinal cord. In the thoracic or upper lumbar region, this usually leads to paraplegia, whereas lower lumbar invasion leads to a cauda equina syndrome with loss of bowel or bladder function. Midline tumors can displace or compress other structures such as the trachea or esophagus, and lead to obstructive symptoms. Finally, involvement of the superior cervical ganglion can produce Horner syndrome, which consists of unilateral ptosis, myosis, and anhydrosis.

Metastatic Disease

Most neuroblastomas are metastatic at the time of diagnosis. Frequent sites of metastasis are: regional or distant lymph nodes, cortical bone, bone marrow, liver, and skin. In infants (<1 year old), a characteristic pattern of small primary tumors with dissemination limited to liver and skin (with or without minimal marrow involvement) is associated with a favorable outcome. This special pattern is referred to as stage 4-S.[204–207] However, in older patients (>1 year old), the dissemination most frequently involves bone marrow and bone, particularly the bones of the skull and orbits. Rarely, disease may spread to lung and brain parenchyma, usually as a manifestation of relapsing or end-stage disease. The outlook for these older patients is very poor, even with intensive multimodality therapy. However, there has been recent progress in elucidating the genetic and biochemical basis of these very different patterns of behavior.

Paraneoplastic Syndromes

Several paraneoplastic syndromes have been associated with neuroblastoma, although each is seen in only 1 to 3 percent of patients. Intractable secretory diarrhea and abdominal distension, sometimes associated with hypokalemia and dehydration (Kerner-Morrison syndrome), is a manifestation of tumor secretion of vasoactive intestinal peptide (VIP).[208,209] VIP is a 28 amino acid polypeptide hormone that is related in structure to glucagon, secretin, and several other polypeptide hormones.[210] It is encoded by the third exon of a large, 6-exon gene that also encodes a closely related polypeptide hormone, PHM-27, in exon 4.[211] However, these two proteins are expressed differentially in some cells.[212] The biological functions of VIP are relaxation of smooth muscle, stimulation of intestinal water and electrolyte secretion, and stimulation of release of other polypeptide hormones.[210] The VIP syndrome usually is associated with ganglioneuroblastoma or ganglioneuroma, and these symptoms resolve after eradication of the tumor.[208,209]

Opsomyoclonus, sometimes called myoclonic encephalopathy, is a syndrome that consists of myoclonic jerking and random eye movement, sometimes associated with cerebellar ataxia. This syndrome has been observed in up to 4 percent of patients.[213–217] Other neuromuscular disorders have been seen in association with neuroblastoma as well, but they are less common. These symptoms may diminish or even disappear with eradication of the tumor, and these patients usually have a favorable outcome from the oncologic perspective.[215] It is, however, becoming increasingly apparent that many patients have residual neurologic abnormalities.[218–220] The symptoms may vary in severity, especially worsening in association with intercurrent illnesses. Recent evidence suggests that the opsoclonus syndrome may be caused by antineuronal autoantibodies.[221–223]

The third paraneoplastic syndrome is due to increased secretion of catecholamines, but this appears to occur in less than 1 percent of patients. The syndrome consists of episodes of tachycardia, palpitations, profuse sweating, and flushing, which is produced by secretion of norepinephrine.[224] Indeed, symptoms attributed to excess catecholamine secretion reportedly were seen in a mother who had a fetus with a neuroblastoma.[225] This syndrome is more common in patients with pheochromocytomas, because these tumors secrete epinephrine, which is a more potent inducer of these symptoms than norepinephrine.

METHODS OF DIAGNOSIS

Diagnostic Criteria

To confirm a diagnosis of neuroblastoma, some histologic evidence that demonstrates neural origin or differentiation by light microscopy, electron microscopy, or immunohistology is usually required. Alternatively, because the bone marrow is frequently involved, some patients are considered to have neuroblastoma based on the presence of "compatible" tumor cells involving the bone marrow, accompanied by increased urinary catecholamine metabolites. Differences in diagnostic criteria used by different groups or countries have led to some difficulties in comparing studies. However, proposals have been made to develop international criteria to confirm a diagnosis of neuroblastoma.[206,207]

Catecholamine Metabolism

When sensitive techniques are used, usually 90 to 95 percent of tumors produce sufficient catecholamines to result in increased urinary metabolites. This provides a great diagnostic advantage in confirming the diagnosis of neuroblastoma, as well as in following disease activity in those patients whose tumors are secretors.[226–228] Fig. 60-8 depicts catecholamine synthesis and metabolism. Although the major pathways and products of catecholamine catabolism are shown, the actual pathways of intracellular and extracellular catecholamine breakdown are more complex.

The precursor amino acids for catecholamine synthesis are phenylalanine and tyrosine. Phenylalanine is converted by phenylalanine hydroxylase to tyrosine (Fig. 60-8). Tyrosine is then converted by tyrosine hydroxylase to 3,4-dihydroxy-phenylalanine (DOPA), which is a catecholamine precursor. DOPA is converted by DOPA decarboxylase to the first catecholamine in the pathway, dopamine. Dopamine is converted by dopamine-β-hydroxylase to norepinephrine, which is then converted by phenylethanolamine-N-methyltransferase to epinephrine. Neuroblastoma cells lack this last enzyme, which is present in adrenal chromaffin cells and pheochromocytomas. The two enzymes primarily responsible for the catabolism of catecholamines are catechol-O-methyl transferase and monoamine oxidase. DOPA and dopamine are converted primarily to homovanillic acid (HVA), whereas norepinephrine and epinephrine are converted primarily to vanillylmandelic acid (VMA). Most laboratories involved in neuroblastoma diagnosis measure both urinary VMA and HVA.

Differential Diagnosis

Because of the many potential clinical presentations, neuroblastoma may be confused with a variety of other neoplasms as well as nonneoplastic conditions. This is particularly a problem in the 5 to 10 percent of tumors that do not produce catecholamines, as well as in the 1 percent or so of patients who do not have an obvious primary tumor.[213–217] Patients with the VIP syndrome can be confused with infectious or inflammatory bowel disease, and those with the opsoclonus-myoclonus and ataxia syndromes can resemble primary neurologic disease. Histologically, neuroblastoma tissue from primary or metastatic sites may be quite undifferentiated, and may be confused with other embryonal pediatric cancers such as rhabdomyosarcoma, Ewing sarcoma, neuroepithelioma, lymphoma, or leukemia (especially megakaryoblastic leukemia). Fortunately, a battery of monoclonal antibodies are being developed that should allow these various disease entities to be made with greater objectivity and confidence.[229–233]

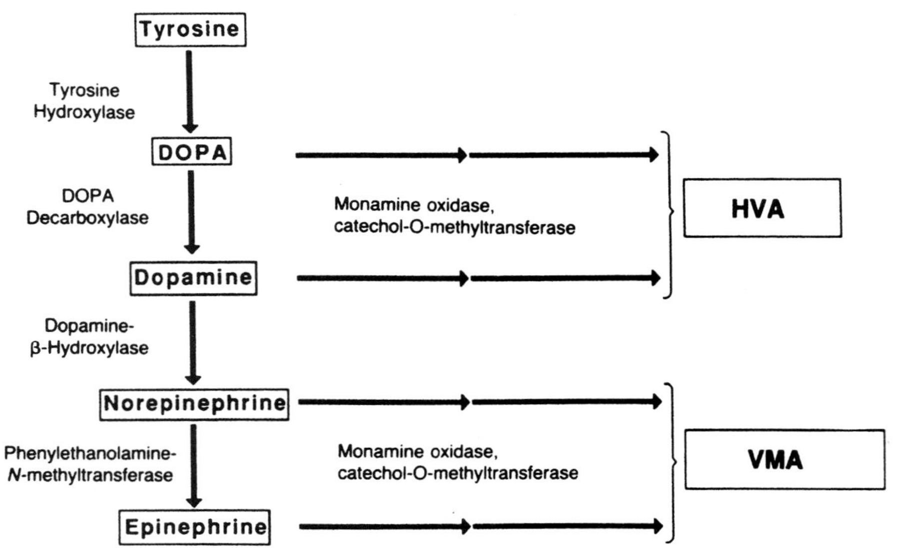

Fig. 60-8 Pathway of catecholamine metabolism. Shown is a simplified diagram of catecholamine synthesis and metabolism. HVA and VMA are the urinary catecholamine metabolites usually measured. (*Repinted from Brodeur*[1] *with permission of Mosby–Year Book.*)

CLINICAL EVALUATION AND STAGING

Diagnostic Testing

A standard set of recommended tests to define the clinical stage or extent of disease has been established.[206,207] Certainly, the more tests that are done, the greater the likelihood of finding disseminated disease. This applies particularly to the number of bone marrow aspirates and biopsies that are done, and the manner in which marrow disease is detected.[234–236] For this purpose, a standard set of immunologic reagents to detect occult neuroblastoma are being developed.[207] This immunocytologic approach may obviate the need for multiple aspirates and biopsies in the future. Uniformity with respect to minimum testing should improve the comparability of studies, but the tests recommended should be available in most medical centers.

The conventional diagnostic imaging modalities include plain radiographs, bone scintigraphy,[237–239] ultrasound,[240] computerized tomography (CT scan),[241,242] and magnetic resonance imaging (MRI scan).[243,244] In addition, the potential specificity and sensitivity of meta-iodobenzylguanidine (MIBG) scintigraphy for evaluation of bone and soft tissue involvement by neuroblastoma is attractive.[245,246] MIBG is taken up by catecholaminergic cells, which includes most neuroblastomas. Radiolabeled MIBG scintigraphy thus has the potential to be a very specific and sensitive method of assessment of the primary tumor and focal metastatic disease. Unfortunately, MIBG scintigraphy is not readily available throughout the industrialized countries of the world.

Tumor Pathology

Neuroblastomas arise from primitive, pluripotential sympathetic nerve cells (sympathogonia), which are derived from the neural crest. These cells differentiate into the different normal tissues of the sympathetic nervous system, such as the spinal sympathetic ganglia, the supporting Schwannian cells, and adrenal chromaffin cells. The three classic histopathologic patterns of neuroblastoma, ganglioneuroblastoma, and ganglioneuroma reflect a spectrum of morphologic and biochemical differentiation. The typical neuroblastoma is composed of small, but uniformly sized, cells containing dense, hyperchromatic nuclei and scant cytoplasm. The presence of neuritic processes, or neuropil, is a pathognomonic feature of all but the most primitive neuroblastoma. The fully differentiated, and benign, counterpart of neuroblastoma is the ganglioneuroma. It is composed of mature ganglion cells, surrounded by a matrix of Schwannian cells and neuropil. Ganglioneuroblastomas are a heterogeneous group of tumors with histopathologic features spanning the extremes of maturation represented by neuroblastoma and ganglioneuroma. Ganglioneuroblastomas may be either focal or diffuse, depending on the pattern seen, but diffuse ganglioneuroblastoma is associated with less aggressive behavior.[247]

Several pathologic classification systems of neuroblastoma have been proposed that have some value in predicting the behavior of the tumor. Some utilize features of neuronal differentiation, whereas others consider the amount of Schwannian stroma, mitotic figures, karyorrhexis, or tumor calcification.[247–249] At the current time the "Shimada" classification is the most popular and has the most clinical utility in predicting outcome.[247] However, in the future, an international neuroblastoma pathology classification based on the Shimada classification will be used.[250] The Schwannian stroma was presumed to arise from the clonal proliferation of malignant cells, because both Schwann cells and neuroblasts are of neural crest origin. Also, neuroblastoma cells in culture could have either a neuronal or a substrate-adherent phenotype.[251] Recent evidence from Ambros and colleagues has shown, however, that the Schwann cells appear to be normal diploid cells that are reactive and infiltrate the tumor.[252] In contrast, the neuroblasts and ganglion cells in such differentiating tumors are near triploid. Thus, the tumors with Schwannian stroma probably make a tropic factor that results in the infiltration and proliferation of these cells.

Staging

The distribution of patients by stage or extent of disease differs depending on the age at diagnosis. For instance, in a consecutive series of 1001 patients enrolled on POG protocols from 1981 to 1989 and staged by the POG staging system, only about 40 percent of patients less than 1 year of age had unresectable or metastatic disease, whereas almost 80 percent of older patients had advanced stages of disease.[1,2,206,207] These findings explain, in part, the generally better outcome of infants with neuroblastoma compared to their older counterparts, but biological differences of the tumors in the two age groups appear to be very important also.

Until recently there were several different staging systems used for neuroblastoma throughout the world.[204,253–257] In general, the various staging systems give comparable results in distinguishing low-stage, good-prognosis patients from high-stage, poor-prognosis patients. However, some of the differences between the staging systems are substantial, particularly as applied to patients with intermediate stages. Therefore, a group of individuals met in 1986 and again in 1991 to formulate an International Neuro-

Table 60-4 International Neuroblastoma Staging System[206,207]

STAGE 1	Localized tumor with complete gross excision, with or without microscopic residual disease; representative ipsilateral lymph nodes negative for tumor microscopically (nodes attached to and removed with the primary tumor may be positive).
STAGE 2A	Localized tumor with incomplete gross excision; representative ipsilateral nonadherent lymp nodes negative for tumor microscopically.
STAGE 2B	Localized tumor with or without complete gross excision, with ipsilateral nonadherent lymph nodes positive for tumor. Enlarged contralateral lymph nodes must be negative microscopically.
STAGE 3	Unresectable unilateral tumor infiltrating across the midline,* with or without regional lymph node involvement; *or* localized unilateral tumor with contralateral regional lymph node involvement; *or* midline tumor with bilateral extension by infiltration (unresectable); *or* by lymph node involvement.
STAGE 4	Any primary tumor with dissemination to distant lymph nodes, bone, bone marrow, liver, skin, and/or other organs (except as defined for Stage 4S).
STAGE 4S	Localized primary tumor (as defined for Stage 1, 2A, or 2B), with dissemination limited to skin, liver, and/or bone marrow† (limited to infants < 1 year of age)

Multifocal primary tumors (e.g., bilateral adrenal primary tumors) should be staged according to the greatest extent of disease, as defined above, followed by a subscript "M" (e.g., 3_M).

*The midline is defined as the vertebral column. Tumors originating on one side and "crossing the midline" must infiltrate to or beyond the opposite side of the vertebral column.

†Marrow involvement in stage 4S should be minimal, i.e., less than 10% of total nucleated cells identified as malignant on bone marrow biopsy or on marrow aspirate. More extensive marrow involvement would be considered to be Stage 4. The MIBG scan (if done) should be negative in the marrow.

blastoma Staging System that would lead to uniformity in staging of patients with neuroblastoma for clinical trials and biological studies around the world.

The International Neuroblastoma Staging System (INSS) is based on clinical, radiographic, and surgical evaluation of children with neuroblastoma.[206,207] This staging system (Table 60-4) utilizes the most important components of previous systems. To distinguish the INSS from previous systems, Arabic numbers are used rather than Roman numerals or letters of the alphabet. Recently, modifications have been proposed in this system to clarify definitions of stages, as well as criteria for diagnosis and response to treatment.[206,207] In addition, suggestions were made to develop biological risk groups that incorporate clinical and laboratory variables in determining prognosis.[207]

PROGNOSTIC CONSIDERATIONS — CLINICAL AND BIOLOGICAL FEATURES

Clinical Features

The most important clinical variables are the stage of disease, the age of the patient at diagnosis, and the site of the primary tumor.[114,258–266] The overall prognosis of patients with stages 1, 2, and 4-S is between 75 and 90 percent, whereas those with stages 3 and 4 have a two-year disease-free survival range of 30 to 40 percent. The outcome of infants less than 1 year of age is substantially better than older patients with the same stage of disease, particularly those with more advanced stages of disease. Patients with primary tumors in the adrenal gland appear to do worse than patients with tumors originating at other sites, particularly the thorax, but this does not appear to add substantially to the prognosis once the variables of age and stage are considered.

Biological Features

A variety of biological variables (pathology, serum markers, genetic features) have been studied that appear to have predictive value as independent prognostic markers in patients with neuroblastoma. The serum markers include ferritin, neuron-specific enolase (NSE), a cell membrane ganglioside (G_{D2}), and lactate dehydrogenase (LDH). The genetic features of the tumor that have been proposed as prognostic markers include tumor-cell DNA index, *MYCN* oncogene copy number, deletion or LOH involving 1p, and unbalanced gain of 17q. Additional markers have been proposed, such as expression of the H-*ras* oncogene, the multidrug resistance gene, or the multidrug resistance-related protein, but the value of these markers is still unclear.[179,180,184–186,267–269] Moreover, no study to date has examined all variables in a large set of patients, so it is somewhat difficult to say which single variable or combination of variables are the most powerful predictors of outcome, in addition to the more conventional clinical features of patient age and stage.

Tumor Pathology

Differentiated histology, such as ganglioneuroblastoma, generally is associated with localized tumors,[248] but this type of histologic classification does not have prognostic value that adds substantially to age and stage. More detailed analysis of histology, such as the classifications by Shimada or Joshi, considers the amount of Schwannian stroma, mitotic figures, karyorrhexis, and calcification.[247,249] These classifications appear to be more powerful predictors of outcome. Soon there will be an international neuroblastoma pathology classification (INPC) that will supersede the abovementioned systems and become the international standard for histopathologic classification, particularly as a prognostic variable.[207,250] Expression of the cell surface glycoprotein CD44 has also been shown to have prognostic significance, with high expression associated with more differentiated tumors and a better outcome.[270–273]

Serum Markers

Ferritin. Analysis of serum from patients with neuroblastoma has determined that ferritin levels are increased in some patients with actively growing tumors.[274–277] Ferritin levels are rarely elevated in patients with low stages of disease, whereas up to half of patients with advanced stages have significant elevations and a much worse outcome. *In vitro* evidence suggests that the tumor cells may produce this ferritin. Increased ferritin levels may be simply a marker of rapid tumor growth and/or large tumor burden. On the other hand, ferritin or iron may be particularly important for growth of neuroblastoma cells. In this regard, it is interesting that some therapeutic approaches are targeting the increased levels of ferritin and iron in patients with advanced disease.

NSE. NSE is a cytoplasmic protein with enolase activity that is associated with neural cells. Analysis of serum NSE from patients with neuroblastoma has indicated that survival is substantially worse in advanced patients with high serum NSE levels.[278–281] Although marked increases in serum NSE were associated with neuroblastomas, mild to moderate elevations were seen with other pediatric tumors, also. Thus, NSE is not as specific as was once thought, but it may have prognostic value, and perhaps it may be useful to follow disease activity and response to treatment in individual patients.

Ganglioside G_{D2}. Several independently derived monoclonal antibodies against neuroblastoma cells recognize gangliosides, which are sialic acid-containing glycosphingolipids. The most characteristic ganglioside on human neuroblastoma cell membranes is called G_{D2}. Not only is the presence of this ganglioside useful for identifying neuroblastoma cells, but also increased levels have been found in the plasma of patients with neuroblastoma. Measurement of circulating G_{D2} may serve as another useful marker of disease activity or response to treatment.[282–285] Indeed, gangliosides shed by tumor cells may play a role in accelerating tumor progression, and antibodies against G_{D2} may be useful for therapy of neuroblastoma as well.[283,286]

LDH. Although it is not specific to neuroblastoma, serum LDH level has been proposed as a prognostic marker for neuroblastoma. Increased LDH levels may be a reflection of rapid cellular turnover or of large tumor burden. Increased levels are more common in patients with extensive or progressive disease, and levels of greater than 1500 μm/ml have been associated with a poor prognosis in infants with neuroblastoma.[287–289]

Genetic Markers

Tumor Cell DNA Index. Tumor cells with an increased DNA content (or "hyperdiploid" karyotype) have been associated with a favorable outcome in infants with neuroblastoma.[109–115,290–293] In addition, hyperdiploid tumors are more likely to have lower stages of disease and require little, if any, therapy, whereas those with a "diploid" DNA content are more likely to have advanced stages of disease and require more intensive therapy. However, this variable appears to be useful primarily for patients less than 1 year of age with advanced stages of disease.[113]

***MYCN* amplification.** The presence of *MYCN* amplification in tumor cells is found predominantly in patients with advanced stages of disease.[67] However, *MYCN* amplification is associated with rapid tumor progression and a poor prognosis, regardless of the age of the patient or the stage of the disease.[60,67–71,113,290] Although not all patients with a poor outcome have *MYCN* amplification, most patients with amplification treated with conventional therapy have rapid progression and die (Fig. 60-9).[1,2]

Allelic Loss for 1p, 11q, or 14q. Finally, there appears to be a strong correlation between 1p deletion and poor event-free survival.[74,76–81,117,273] Because there is an association between *MYCN* amplification and 1p deletion, it remains controversial as to whether this finding has independent prognostic significance.[77–81] Although 11q LOH occurs with substantial frequency and correlates with event-free survival in some series, its overall clinical significance is unclear.[75,98–101,131,132] Finally, 14q LOH does not appear to have prognostic significance other than its association with advanced stages of disease in some studies.[75,131,133–135]

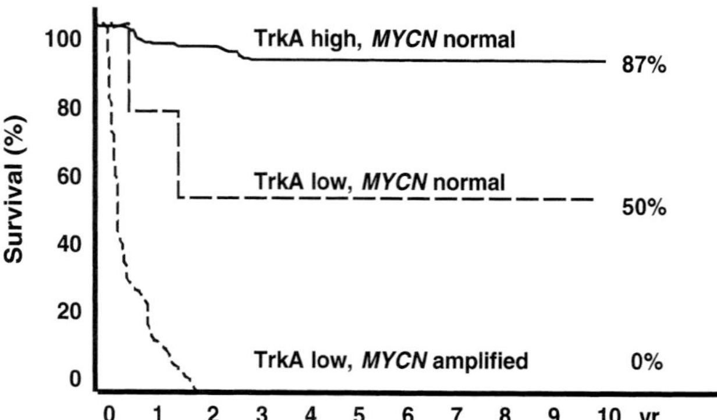

Fig. 60-9 MYCN Amplification, *TrkA* expression and survival in children with neuroblastoma. Survival according to *MYCN* copy number (amplified or not) and *TrkA* expression (high versus low or absent) in 82 children with neuroblastoma. (*Reprinted from Nakagawara*[162] *with permission from the New England Journal of Medicine.*)

Trk Gene Expression. Recent studies suggest that high levels of expression of the *TrkA* gene are associated with a favorable outcome in neuroblastoma patients.[86,162–166] Although prospective studies need to be done to confirm these observations, current evidence suggests that high *TrkA* gene expression may be a very powerful prognostic marker (Fig. 60-9). Indeed, it may predict the propensity of selected tumors to undergo either programmed cell death, leading to regression, or neuronal differentiation, leading to a benign ganglioneuroma. Similar results have been obtained by analysis of *TrkC*, which is also associated with a biologically favorable outcome, but they appear to be a subset of the *TrkA*-positive tumors, so *TrkC* expression does not have independent prognostic significance.[174,175] In contrast, *TrkB* expression is associated with advanced stage tumors with *MYCN* amplification.[170] Tumors expressing *TrkB*, along with its ligand *BDNF*, may have an autocrine survival pathway that provides them with a survival advantage.[170–173]

Biological/Clinical Subsets of Neuroblastoma. As described above, neuroblastomas can be separated into genetically distinct subsets, with characteristic clinical behavior and prognosis (Table 60-4; Fig. 60-7). They represent two fundamentally different types that are either biologically favorable or unfavorable. However, the latter type can be divided into subtypes, based on the pattern of genetic abnormalities, with distinct clinical behavior. This concept has been validated by several recent studies.[113,273,294] Thus, genetic analysis of neuroblastoma cells provides prognostic information that can direct more appropriate choice of treatment.

THERAPEUTIC APPROACHES

The treatment modalities traditionally employed in the management of neuroblastoma are surgery, chemotherapy, and radiotherapy. The role of each is determined by the natural history of individual cases considering stage, age, and biological features. With few exceptions (e.g., patients with localized primary tumors and many infants with 4-S disease), chemotherapy remains the backbone of the multimodality treatment plan. For this discussion, stage is defined by the INSS criteria (Table 60-3).[206,207]

Surgery

Surgery plays a pivotal role in the management of neuroblastoma. Depending on the timing, operative procedures can have diagnostic as well as therapeutic functions.[253,295–298] The goals of primary surgical procedures, performed prior to any other therapy, are to establish the diagnosis, to provide tissue for biological studies, to excise the tumor if feasible, and to stage the tumor surgically. In delayed primary or second-look surgery, the surgeon determines response to therapy and removes residual disease when possible. Surgery can also have palliative benefit for recurrent or progressive disease.

Chemotherapy

Chemotherapy is the predominant modality of management in neuroblastoma. Single-agent phase II trials conducted in patients with recurrent or advanced neuroblastoma have identified a number of effective drugs.[2] Cyclophosphamide, ifosfamide, cisplatin, carboplatin doxorubicin (Adriamycin), and the epipodophyllotoxins (teniposide, VM-26; and etoposide, VP-16) yield complete and partial response rates of 25 to 50 percent, and have become the cornerstone of multiagent regimens. Drug combinations have been developed that take advantage of drug synergism, mechanisms of cytotoxicity, and differences in side effects.[299,300] Treatment of children with advanced stage neuroblastoma using these combinations has resulted in improved response rates with minimal increase in toxicity.[2,301–305]

Radiation Therapy

Neuroblastoma is considered a radiosensitive tumor, and radiotherapy is very effective in achieving local control or palliation.

However, long-term control of neuroblastoma is seldom achieved with radiation therapy alone because of the propensity of this tumor to widespread metastases.[306,307] Historically, radiation has been used in the multimodality management of residual neuroblastoma, bulky unresectable tumors, and disseminated disease. More recently, the role of radiotherapy in neuroblastoma continues to be refined with the improvement in multiagent chemotherapy and the increasing trend toward developing risk-related treatment groups based upon age, stage, and biological features.

Bone Marrow and Stem Cell Transplantation

Attempts have been made to improve on the modest gains of intensive, combined-modality therapy to increase intensity of therapy. Dose-limiting marrow toxicity can be ameliorated to some extent by the use of colony-stimulating factors for the granulocyte or granulocyte-macrophage lineages, which increase the rate of marrow recovery. However, therapy that is more intensive can be administered if accompanied by bone marrow transplantation (BMT). Although allogeneic BMT is practiced by some centers, the most popular approach is autologous BMT, frequently with a purged marrow.[308–318] Marrow purging usually is accomplished by covalently attaching a cocktail of antineuroblastoma antibodies to magnetic beads and mixing beads with the marrow, followed by passing the marrow over powerful magnets.[309,310,319–322] A variation on this approach that is undergoing clinical trials currently is the use of peripheral blood-stem cells (with or without CD34-positive selection) as the source of cells for marrow rescue.[323,324] Although these approaches may increase the median survival of older patients with advanced stages of neuroblastoma, it is not clear that the long-term, disease-free survival has been affected appreciably.

Biologically Based Risk Groups

Most current studies for the treatment of neuroblastoma patients are based on risk groups that consider various biological features (*MYCN* copy number, histopathology, and tumor ploidy in infants) in addition to patient age and INSS stage. Preliminary data, adjusted for age and stage, indicate that analysis of DNA content in infants and *MYCN* copy number in all patients, allow more precise determination of risk.[68,112,113,325] Tumor histopathology by the Shimada classification also appears to be an important independent prognostic marker, at least for certain subsets of patients. It is likely that tumor histopathology as determined by the INPC classification will replace the Shimada classification in these risk assessments.[247] Judging the prognostic impact of other biological variables, such as 1p LOH, 11q LOH, unbalanced 17q gain, *TrkA* expression, or others, must await prospective therapeutic and biological studies.

Second Malignant Neoplasms

Other malignant diseases have been observed in individuals with neuroblastoma, such as pheochromocytoma, brain tumors, acute leukemia, and renal cell carcinoma.[326–330] However, none of these second cancers have occurred with sufficient frequency to indicate a specific relationship between neuroblastoma and any other neoplasm.[331] Furthermore, it is not clear if second malignant neoplasms are more common in survivors who had hereditary predisposition to develop neuroblastoma. Analysis of this question requires more precise methods to detect predisposed individuals, as well as improved patient survival. Thus, it currently appears that most second malignant neoplasms are either coincidental or related to the therapy, so future modifications of treatment aimed at eliminating potentially carcinogenic agents are warranted.

Future Treatment Strategies

The use of dose-intensified chemotherapy combinations, with or without autologous bone marrow transplantation, has produced better immediate disease control in neuroblastoma. Unfortunately, this has not translated into durable remissions in children with high-risk tumors. Future treatment strategies will address: (a) the identification of new drugs and drug combinations; (b) the use of biological agents targeted at killing neuroblastoma cells, such as radiolabeled MIBG or antineuroblastoma antibodies; (c) agents that might induce differentiation, such as retinoic acid or NGF; and (d) antiangiogenesis therapy or other approaches.[332–337]

NEUROBLASTOMA SCREENING STUDIES

Another approach to improve the long-term outcome of patients with neuroblastoma is to identify patients with this disease earlier in the course of their disease. Because neuroblastomas frequently produce increased levels of catecholamines whose metabolites are detectable in the urine, mass urinary screening of infants for neuroblastoma has been undertaken in Japan for over 20 years.[338–341] The rationale of such a mass screening program assumes that patients with aggressive, biologically unfavorable disease and low likelihood of survival evolve over time from more localized, biologically favorable tumors. Alternatively, early detection of patients with biologically unfavorable disease may lead to an improved outcome. Similar efforts have been recently undertaken in North America (especially Quebec, Canada) and in Europe to answer questions concerning the feasibility and utility of screening for neuroblastoma.[342–346]

Studies of the clinical and cytogenetic features of tumors identified as a result of mass screening of infants for neuroblastomas in Japan suggest that the majority of patients identified have lower stages of disease, and virtually all of the tumors are in the hyperdiploid or near-triploid range.[109,291] Previous studies demonstrated that such findings generally are associated with a very favorable outcome.[109–115] Therefore, the results of the screening study have suggested at least two possibilities: either (a) all neuroblastomas begin as tumors with a more favorable genotype and phenotype, and some evolve into more aggressive tumors with adverse genetic features; or (b) there are at least two different subsets of neuroblastoma, and the more favorable group presents earlier, and therefore is the predominant group detected by screening. The accumulating body of genetic information, as discussed above (Table 60-4, Fig. 60-7), is more consistent with the latter explanation.[5,73,113,293,347–351]

In addition to the genetic data discussed above, the accumulating evidence suggests that the prevalence of neuroblastoma in screened populations is increased by 50 to 100 percent over that seen in unscreened populations, and the prevalence of neuroblastoma in patients over 1 year of age has not changed appreciably.[293,343,344,348,351] Taken together with the biological information, this suggests that screening is detecting tumors in a substantial number of patients who likely would never develop symptomatic disease because their tumors would have regressed or matured without therapy. Many of the tumors detected by screening at 6 months of age have favorable biological features and could be cured easily with relatively mild therapy. A few patients with unfavorable biological features have presented clinically during the first 6 to 12 months of age in the screened population, and some have had an unfavorable outcome. It remains to be determined if screening at a later time will permit early detection of tumors with intermediate or unfavorable biological features and thereby improve their prognosis.

FUTURE CONSIDERATIONS

In addition to the improvements and prospects for future therapy discussed herein, there are a variety of areas in which improvement in the management of patients with neuroblastoma may come, including: (a) the identification of individuals with a genetic predisposition to develop this disease; (b) general population screening approaches for early detection and treatment; (c) additional markers besides urinary catecholamine metabolites to follow tumor response to treatment; and (d) better biological characterization of tumors for classification and prognostication.

As improvements occur in the long-term outcome of patients with neuroblastoma, it becomes increasingly important to identify individuals who are predisposed to develop this tumor. Not only will this be useful for the siblings of neuroblastoma patients, but it will also provide useful information for genetic counseling of patients and their offspring. No predisposition locus has been identified as yet, although several loci have been excluded recently, including 1p36.[29] Thus, it appears that the familial neuroblastoma predisposition gene resides elsewhere, although there is the formal possibility that more than one predisposition locus exists. In any case, a genome-wide search is underway to identify the familial neuroblastoma predisposition gene.

The urinary VMA/HVA screening programs in Japan, North America, and Europe initially were very promising, leading to cautious optimism. However, characterization of the tumors identified by screening indicates that the majority of these tumors have favorable biological features, more like those seen in infants with lower stages of disease. Indeed, the screening may just be increasing the prevalence of neuroblastoma by detection of tumors that might regress spontaneously, without lowering the prevalence of more advanced stages of disease in patients over 1 year of age. Indeed, despite this "overdetection," there has been no decrease in the prevalence of neuroblastoma in older patients. Thus, it is not clear if mass screening at an older age will lead to detection of genetically unfavorable, aggressive tumors, or if this early detection will ultimately improve their outcome.

Following the levels of catecholamine metabolites in the urine of patients with neuroblastoma does not appear to be as sensitive as α-fetoprotein or β-human chorionic gonadotropin for following germ-cell tumors. Additional markers have been proposed, including serum ferritin, NSE, G_{D2}, chromogranin A, and others, but none has yet emerged as superior. As more is understood about the biology of neuroblastomas, additional candidates might emerge that could be used to follow response to treatment and to predict early relapse. Such markers might obviate the need for multiple diagnostic imaging studies and marrow sampling in patients in remission.

The biological characterization of neuroblastomas by such features as DNA index, *MYCN* amplification, 1p LOH, *TrkA* expression, and others, has provided powerful prognostic variables. It remains to be determined which will emerge as the most clinically useful prognostic variable when subjected to multivariate analysis. It is possible that these biological features will become more important than clinical distinctions such as age, stage, primary site, and tumor histology. The mandate for the future is to translate promising biological studies into clinical applications, and to continue to look for new insights into mechanisms of neuroblastoma transformation and progression that can be used to clinical advantage.

ACKNOWLEDGMENTS

Some of this material has been published previously.[1–6]

REFERENCES

1. Brodeur GM: Neuroblastoma and other peripheral neuroectodermal tumors, in Fernbach DJ, Vietti TJ (eds): *Clinical Pediatric Oncology.* St. Louis, Mosby–Year Book, 1991, p. 337.
2. Brodeur GM, Castleberry RP: Neuroblastoma, in Pizzo PA, Poplack DG (eds): *Principles and Practice of Pediatric Oncology.* Philadelphia, JB Lippincott, 1997, p. 761.
3. Brodeur GM, Nakagawara A: Molecular basis of clinical heterogeneity in neuroblastoma. *Am J Pediatr Hematol Oncol* **14**:111, 1992.
4. Brodeur GM: Molecular basis for heterogeneity in human neuroblastomas. *Eur J Cancer* **31A**:505, 1995.
5. Brodeur GM, Maris JM, Yamashiro DJ, Hogarty MD, White PS: Biology and genetics of human neuroblastomas. *J Pediatr Hematol Oncol* **19**:93, 1997.
6. Brodeur GM: Clinical and biological aspects of neuroblastomas, in Scriver CR, Beaudet AL, Sly WS, Valle D, Stanbury JB, Wyngaarden JB, Fredrickson DS, Vogelstein B (eds): *The Molecular and Metabolic Basis of Inherited Disease.* New York, McGraw-Hill, 1997, p. 691.
7. Miller RW, Young JLJ, Novakovic B: Childhood cancer. *Cancer* **75**:395, 1995.
8. Voute PA: Neuroblastoma, in Sutow WW, Fernbach DJ, Vietti TJ (eds): *Clinical Pediatric Oncology.* St. Louis, CV Mosby, 1984, p. 559.
9. Sawada T, Sugimoto T, Tanaka T, Kawakatsu H, Ishii T, Matsumura T, Horii Y: Number and cure rate of neuroblastoma cases detected by the mass screening program in Japan: Future aspects. *Med Pediatr Oncol* **15**:14, 1987.
10. Beckwith J, Perrin E: In situ neuroblastomas: A contribution to the natural history of neural crest tumors. *Am J Pathol* **43**:1089, 1963.
11. Turkel SB, Itabashi HH: The natural history of neuroblastic cells in the fetal adrenal gland. *Am J Pathol* **76**:225, 1975.
12. Ikeda Y, Lister J, Bouton JM, Buyukpamukcu M: Congenital neuroblastoma, neuroblastoma in situ, and the normal fetal development of the adrenal. *J Pediatr Surg* **16**:636, 1981.
13. Haas D, Ablin AR, Miller C, Zoger S, Matthay KK: Complete pathologic maturation and regression of stage IVS neuroblastoma without treatment. *Cancer* **62**:818, 1988.
14. Evans AE, Baum E, Chard R: Do infants with stage IV-S neuroblastoma need treatment? *Arch Dis Child* **56**:271, 1981.
15. McWilliams NB: Stage IV-S neuroblastoma: Treatment controversy revisited. *Med Pediatr Oncol* **14**:41, 1986.
16. Carlsen NLT: How frequent is spontaneous remission of neuroblastomas? Implications for screening. *Br J Cancer* **61**:441, 1990.
17. Allen RW, Ogden B, Bentley FL, Jung AL: Fetal hydantoin syndrome, neuroblastoma, and hemorrhagic disease in a neonate. *JAMA* **244**:1464, 1980.
18. Kinney H, Faix R, Brazy J: The fetal alcohol syndrome and neuroblastoma. *Pediatrics* **66**:130, 1980.
19. Seeler RA, Israel JN, Royal JE, Kaye CI, Rao S, Abulaban M: Ganglioneuroblastoma and fetal hydantoin-alcohol syndromes. *Pediatrics* **63**:524, 1979.
20. Spitz MR, Johnson CC: Neuroblastoma and paternal occupation. A case-control analysis. *Am J Epidemiol* **121**:924, 1985.
21. Wilkins JRI, Hundley VD: Paternal occupational exposure to electromagnetic fields and neuroblastoma in offspring. *Am J Epidemiol* **131**:995, 1990.
22. Bunin GR, Ward E, Kramer S, Rhee CA, Meadows AT: Neuroblastoma and parental occupation. *Am J Epidemiol* **131**:776, 1990.
23. Kramer S, Ward E, Meadows AT, Malone KE: Medical and drug risk factors associated with neuroblastoma: A case-control study. *J Natl Cancer Inst* **78**:797, 1987.
24. Knudson AGJ, Strong LC: Mutation and cancer: Neuroblastoma and pheochromocytoma. *Am J Hum Genet* **24**:514, 1972.
25. Knudson AG: Mutation and cancer: Statistical study of retinoblastoma. *Proc Natl Acad Sci U S A* **68**:8820, 1971.
26. Knudson AGJ, Meadows AT: Developmental genetics of neuroblastoma. *J Natl Cancer Inst* **57**:675, 1976.
27. Kushner BH, Gilbert F, Helson L: Familial neuroblastoma: Case reports, literature review, and etiologic considerations. *Cancer* **57**:1887, 1986.
28. Kushner BH, Helson L: Monozygotic siblings discordant for neuroblastoma: Etiologic implications. *J Pediatr* **107**:405, 1985.
29. Maris JM, Kyemba SM, Rebbeck TR, White PS, Sulman EP, Jensen SJ, Allen C, Biegel JA, Yanofsky RA, Feldman GL, Brodeur GM: Familial predisposition to neuroblastoma does not map to chromosome band 1p36. *Cancer Res* **56**:3421, 1996.
30. Maris JM, Chatten J, Meadows AT, Biegel J, Brodeur GM: Familial neuroblastoma: New affected members and a further association with Hirschsprung disease. *Med Pediatr Oncol* **28**:1, 1997.
31. Pegelow CH, Ebbin AJ, Powars D, Towner JW: Familial neuroblastoma. *J Pediatr* **87**:763, 1975.
32. Hecht F, Kaiser-McCaw B: Chromosomes in familial neuroblastoma [letter]. *J Pediatr* **98**:334, 1981.
33. Hecht F, Hecht BK, Northrup JC, Trachtenberg N, Wood ST, Cohen JT: Genetics of familial neuroblastoma: Long-range studies. *Cancer Genet Cytogenet* **7**:227, 1982.
34. Moorhead PS, Evans AE: Chromosomal findings in patients with neuroblastoma. *Prog Cancer Res Ther* **12**:109, 1980.
35. Nagano H, Kano Y, Kobuchi S, Kajitani T: A case of partial 2p trisomy with neuroblastoma. *Jpn J Hum Genet* **25**:39, 1980.
36. Sanger WG, Howe J, Fordyce R, Purtilo DT: Inherited partial trisomy #15 complicated by neuroblastoma. *Cancer Genet Cytogenet* **11**:153, 1984.

37. Robinson MG, McCorquodale MM: Trisomy 18 and neurogenic neoplasia. *J Pediatr* **99**:428, 1981.
38. Rudolph B, Harbott J, Lampert F: Fragile sites and neuroblastoma: Fragile site at 1p13.1 and other points on lymphocyte chromosomes from patients and family members. *Cancer Genet Cytogenet* **31**:83, 1988.
39. Lampert F, Rudolph B, Christiansen H, Franke F: Identical chromosome 1p breakpoint abnormality in both the tumor and the constitutional karyotype of a patient with neuroblastoma. *Cancer Genet Cytogenet* **34**:235, 1988.
40. Laureys G, Speleman F, Opdenakker G, Leroy J: Constitutional translocation t(1;17)(p36;q12-21) in a patient with neuroblastoma. *Genes Chromosomes Cancer* **2**:252, 1990.
41. Laureys G, Speleman F, Versteeg R, van der Drift P, Chan A, Leroy J, Francke U, Opdenakker G, van Roy N: Constitutional translocation t(1;17)(p36.31-p36.13;q11.2-q12.1) in a neuroblastoma patient. Establishment of somatic cell hybrids and identification of PND?A12M2 on chromosome 1 and NF1/SCYA7 on chromosome 17 as breakpoint flanking single copy markers. *Oncogene* **10**:1087, 1995.
42. Michalski AJ, Cotter FE, Cowell JK: Isolation of chromosome-specific DNA sequences from an Alu polymerase chain reaction library to define the breakpoint in a patient with a constitutional translocation t(1;13)(q22;q12) and ganglioneuroblastoma. *Oncogene* **7**:1595, 1992.
43. Bown NP, Pearson ADJ, Reid MM: High incidence of constitutional balanced translocations in neuroblastoma. *Cancer Genet Cytogenet* **69**:166, 1993.
44. Biegel JA, White PS, Marshall HN, Fujimori M, Zackai EH, Scher CD, Brodeur GM, Emanuel BS: Constitutional 1p36 deletion in a child with neuroblastoma. *Am J Hum Genet* **52**:176, 1993.
45. Mead RS, Cowell JK: Molecular characterization of a (1;10)(p22;q21) constitutional translocation from a patient with neuroblastoma. *Cancer Genet Cytogenet* **81**:151, 1995.
46. Roberts T, Chernova O, Cowell JK: Molecular characterization of the 1p22 breakpoint region spanning the constitutional translocation breakpoint in a neuroblastoma patient with a t(1;10)(p22;q21). *Cancer Genet Cytogenet* **100**:10, 1998.
47. White PS, Thompson PM, Jensen SJ, Sulman EP, Sulman EP, Guo C, Maris JM, Hogarty MD, Allen C, Biegel JA, Matise TC, Gregory SG, Reynolds CP, Brodeur GM: Detailed molecular analysis of 1p36 in neuroblastoma. *Eur J Cancer* (in press), 2000.
48. Knudson AGJ, Amromin GD: Neuroblastoma and ganglioneuroma in a child with multiple neurofibromatosis. Implications for the mutational origin of neuroblastoma. *Cancer* **19**:1032, 1966.
49. Bolande R, Towler WF: A possible relationship of neuroblastoma to von Recklinghausen's disease. *Cancer* **26**:162, 1970.
50. Bolande RP: The neurocristopathies: A unifying concept of disease arising in neural crest maldevelopment. *Hum Pathol* **5**:409, 1974.
51. Kushner BH, Hajdu SI, Helson L: Synchronous neuroblastoma and von Recklinghausen's disease: A review of the literature. *J Clin Oncol* **3**:117, 1985.
52. Miller RW, Fraumeni JFJ: Neuroblastoma: Epidemiologic approach to its origin. *Am J Dis Child* **115**:253, 1968.
53. Sy WM, Edmonson JH: The developmental defects associated with neuroblastoma—Etiologic implications. *Cancer* **22**:234, 1968.
54. Nakissa N, Constine LS, Rubin P, Strohl R: Birth defects in three common pediatric malignancies: Wilms' tumor, neuroblastoma and Ewing's sarcoma. *Oncology* **42**:358, 1985.
55. Blatt J, Olshan AF, Lee PA, Ross JL: Neuroblastoma and related tumors in Turner's syndrome. *J Pediatr* **131**:666, 1997.
56. Maris JM, Brodeur GM: Are certain children more likely to develop neuroblastoma? *J Pediatr* **131**:656, 1997.
57. Satge D, Sasco AJ, Carlsen NL, Stiller CA, Rubie H, Hero B, de Bernardi B, de Kraker J, Coze C, Kogner P, Langmark F, Hakvoort-Cammel FG, Beck D, von der Weid N, Parkes S, Hartmann O, Lippens RJ, Kamps WA, Sommelet D: A lack of neuroblastoma in Down syndrome: A study from 11 European countries. *Cancer Res* **58**:448, 1998.
58. Biedler JL, Ross RA, Shanske S, Spengler BA: Human neuroblastoma cytogenetics: Search for significance of homogeneously staining regions and double minute chromosomes. *Prog Cancer Res Ther* **12**:81, 1980.
59. Brodeur GM, Green AA, Hayes FA, Williams KJ, Williams DL, Tsiatis AA: Cytogenetic features of human neuroblastomas and cell lines. *Cancer Res* **41**:4678, 1981.
60. Brodeur GM, Seeger RC, Sather H, Dalton A, Siegel SE, Wong KY, Hammond D: Clinical implications of oncogene activation in human neuroblastomas. *Cancer* **58**:541, 1986.
61. Brodeur GM, Fong CT: Molecular biology and genetics of human neuroblastoma. *Cancer Genet Cytogenet* **41**:153, 1989.
62. Schwab M, Alitalo K, Klempnauer KH, Varmus HE, Bishop JM, Gilbert F, Brodeur G, Goldstein M, Trent JM: Amplified DNA with limited homology to myc cellular oncogene is shared by human neuroblastoma cell lines and a neuroblastoma tumour. *Nature* **305**:245, 1983.
63. Kohl NE, Kanda N, Schreck RR, Bruns G, Latt SA, Gilbert F, Alt FW: Transposition and amplification of oncogene-related sequences in human neuroblastomas. *Cell* **35**:359, 1983.
64. Schwab M, Ellison J, Busch M, Rosenau W, Varmus HE, Bishop JM: Enhanced expression of the human gene N-myc consequent to amplification of DNA may contribute to malignant progression of neuroblastoma. *Proc Natl Acad Sci U S A* **81**:4940, 1984.
65. Brodeur GM, Seeger RC: Gene amplification in human neuroblastomas: Basic mechanisms and clinical implications. *Cancer Genet Cytogenet* **19**:101, 1986.
66. Hogarty MH, Brodeur GM: Oncogene amplification, in Vogelstein B, Kinzler K (eds): *Genetic Basis of Human Cancer.* New York, McGraw Hill, 1998, p. 161–172
67. Brodeur GM, Seeger RC, Schwab M, Varmus HE, Bishop JM: Amplification of N-myc in untreated human neuroblastomas correlates with advanced disease stage. *Science* **224**:1121, 1984.
68. Brodeur GM: Neuroblastoma—Clinical applications of molecular parameters. *Brain Pathol* **1**:47, 1990.
69. Seeger RC, Brodeur GM, Sather H, Dalton A, Siegel SE, Wong KY, Hammond D: Association of multiple copies of the N-myc oncogene with rapid progression of neuroblastomas. *N Engl J Med* **313**:1111, 1985.
70. Seeger RC, Wada R, Brodeur GM, Moss TJ, Bjork RL, Sousa L, Slamon DJ: Expression of N-myc by neuroblastomas with one or multiple copies of the oncogene. *Prog Clin Biol Res* **271**:41, 1988.
71. Brodeur GM, Fong CT, Morita M, Griffith RC, Hayes FA, Seeger RC: Molecular analysis and clinical significance of N-myc amplification and chromosome 1 abnormalities in human neuroblastomas. *Prog Clin Biol Res* **271**:3, 1988.
72. Wasson JC, Brodeur GM: Molecular analysis of gene amplification in tumors, in Dracopoli NC, Haines JL, Korf BR, Moir DT, Morton CC, Seidman CE, Seidman JG, Smith DR (eds): *Current Protocols in Human Genetics.* New York, Greene Publishing and John Wiley & Sons, 1994, p. 10.5.1.
73. Brodeur GM, Hayes FA, Green AA, Casper JT, Wasson J, Wallach S, Seeger RC: Consistent N-myc copy number in simultaneous or consecutive neuroblastoma samples from sixty individual patients. *Cancer Res* **47**:4248, 1987.
74. Fong CT, Dracopoli NC, White PS, Merrill PT, Griffith RC, Housman DE, Brodeur GM: Loss of heterozygosity for the short arm of chromosome 1 in human neuroblastomas: Correlation with N-myc amplification. *Proc Natl Acad Sci U S A* **86**:3753, 1989.
75. Fong CT, White PS, Peterson K, Sapienza C, Cavenee WK, Kern S, Vogelstein B, Cantor AB, Look AT, Brodeur GM: Loss of heterozygosity for chromosome 1 or 14 defines subsets of advanced neuroblastomas. *Cancer Res* **52**:1780, 1992.
76. White PS, Maris JM, Beltinger C, Sulman E, Marshall HN, Fujimori M, Kaufman BA, Biegel JA, Allen C, Hilliard C, Valentine MB, Look AT, Enomoto H, Sakiyama S, Brodeur GM: A region of consistent deletion in neuroblastoma maps within 1p36.2-.3. *Proc Natl Acad Sci U S A* **92**:5520, 1995.
77. Caron H: Allelic loss of chromosome 1 and additional chromosome 17 material are both unfavourable prognostic markers in neuroblastoma. *Med Pediatr Oncol* **24**:215, 1995.
78. Maris JM, White PS, Beltinger CP, Sulman EP, Castleberry RP, Shuster JJ, Look AT, Brodeur GM: Significance of chromosome 1p loss of heterozygosity in neuroblastoma. *Cancer Res* **55**:4664, 1995.
79. Gehring M, Berthold F, Edler L, Schwab M, Amler LC: The 1p deletion is not a reliable marker for the prognosis of patients with neuroblastoma. *Cancer Res* **55**:5366, 1995.
80. Martinsson T, Shoberg P-M, Hedborg F, Kogner P: Deletion of chromosome 1p loci and microsatellite instability in neuroblastomas analyzed with short-tandem repeat polymorphisms. *Cancer Res* **55**:5681, 1995.
81. Caron H, van Sluis P, de Kraker J, Bokkerink J, Egeler M, Laureys G, Slater R, Westerveld A, Voute PA, Versteeg R: Allelic loss of chromosome 1p as a predictor of unfavorable outcome in patients with neuroblastoma. *N Engl J Med* **334**:225, 1996.
82. Nisen PD, Waber PG, Rich MA, Pierce S, Garvin JRJ, Gilbert F, Lanzkowsky P: N-myc oncogene RNA expression in neuroblastoma. *J Natl Cancer Inst* **80**:1633, 1988.

83. Slavc I, Ellenbogen R, Jung W-H, Vawter GF, Kretschmar C, Grier H, Korf BR: myc gene amplification and expression in primary human neuroblastoma. *Cancer Res* **50**:1459, 1990.
84. Chan HSL, Gallie BL, DeBoer G, Haddad G, Ikegaki N, Dimitroulakos J, Yeger H, Ling V: MYCN protein expression as a predictor of neuroblastoma prognosis. *Clin Cancer Res* **3**:1699, 1997.
85. Bordow SB, Norris MD, Haber PS, Marshall GM, Haber M: Prognostic significance of MYCN oncogene expression in childhood neuroblastoma. *J Clin Oncol* **16**:3286, 1998.
86. Nakagawara A, Arima M, Azar CG, Scavarda NJ, Brodeur GM: Inverse relationship between trk expression and N-myc amplification in human neuroblastomas. *Cancer Res* **52**:1364, 1992.
87. Cohn SL, Salwen H, Quasney MW, Ikegaki N, Cowan JM, Herst CV, Kennett RH, Rosen ST, DiGiuseppe JA, Brodeur GM: Prolonged N-myc protein half-life in a neuroblastoma cell line lacking N-myc amplification. *Oncogene* **5**:1821, 1990.
88. Squire JA, Thorner PS, Weitzman S, Maggi JD, Dirks P, Doyle J, Hale M, Godbout R: Co-amplification of *MYCN* and a DEAD box gene (*DDX1*) in primary neuroblastoma. *Oncogene* **10**:1417, 1995.
89. Manohar CF, Salwen HR, Brodeur GM, Cohn SL: Co-amplification and concomitant high levels of expression of a DEAD box gene with MYCN in human neuroblastoma. *Genes Chromosomes Cancer* **14**:196, 1995.
90. George RE, Kenyon RM, McGuckin AG, Malcolm AJ, Pearson ADJ, Lunec J: Investigation of the coamplification of the candidate genes ornithine decarboxylase, ribonucleotide reductase, syndecan-1 and a DEAD box gene, DDX1, with N-myc in neuroblastoma. *Oncogene* **12**:1583, 1996.
91. Amler LC, Shurmann J, Schwab M: The DDX1 gene maps within 400 kbp 5′ to MYCN and is frequently coamplified in human neuroblastoma. *Genes Chromosomes Cancer* **15**:134, 1996.
92. Shiloh Y, Shipley J, Brodeur GM, Bruns G, Korf B, Donlon T, Schreck RR, Seeger R, Sakai K, Latt SA: Differential amplification, assembly and relocation of multiple DNA sequences in human neuroblastomas and neuroblastoma cell lines. *Proc Natl Acad Sci U S A* **82**:3761, 1985.
93. Corvi R, Savelyeva L, Amler L, Handgetinger R, Schwab M: Cytogenetic evolution of MYCN and MDM2 amplification in the neuroblastoma LS tumor and its cell line. *Eur J Cancer* **31A**:520, 1995.
94. Corvi R, Savelyeva L, Breit S, Wenzel A, Handgretinger R, Barak J, Oren M, Amler L, Schwab M: Non-syntenic amplification of MDM2 and MYCN in human neuroblastoma. *Oncogene* **10**:1081, 1995.
95. Van Roy N, Forus A, Myklebost O, Cheng NC, Versteeg R, Speleman F: Identification of two distinct chromosome 12-derived amplification units in neuroblastoma cell line NGP. *Cancer Genet Cytogenet* **82**:151, 1995.
96. Jinbo T, Iwamura Y, Kaneko M, Sawaguchi S: Coamplification of the L-myc and N-myc oncogenes in a neuroblastoma cell line. *Jpn J Cancer Res* **80**:299, 1989.
97. Meddeb M, Danglot G, Chudoba I, Venuat AM, Benard J, Avet-Loiseau H, Vasseur B, Le Paslier D, Terrier-Lacombe MJ, Hartmann O, Bernheim A: Additional copies of a 25 Mb chromosomal region originating from 17q23.1-17qter are present in 90% of high-grade neuroblastomas. *Genes Chromosomes Cancer* **17**:156, 1996.
98. Brinkschmidt C, Christiansen H, Terpe HJ, Simon R, Boecker W, Lambert F, Stoerkel S: Comparative genomic hybridization (CGH) analysis of neuroblastomas—An important methodological approach in paediatric tumour pathology. *J Pathol* **181**:394, 1997.
99. Plantaz D, Mohapatra G, Matthay KK, Pellarin M, Seeger RC, Feuerstein BG: Gain of chromosome 17 is the most frequent abnormality detected in neuroblastoma by comparative genomic hybridization. *Am J Pathol* **150**:81, 1997.
100. Vandesompele J, Van Roy N, Van Gele M, Laureys G, Ambros P, Heimann P, Devalck C, Schuuring E, Brock P, Otten J, Gyselinck J, De Paepe A, Speleman F: Genetic heterogeneity of neuroblastoma studied by comparative genomic hybridization. *Genes Chromosomes Cancer* **23**:141, 1998.
101. Lastowska M, Nacheva E, McGuckin A, Curtis A, Grace C, Pearson A, Bown N: Comparative genomic hybridization study of primary neuroblastoma tumors. United Kingdom Children's Cancer Study Group. *Genes Chromosomes Cancer* **18**:162, 1997.
102. Altura RA, Maris JM, Li H, Boyett JM, Brodeur GM, Look AT: Novel regions of chromosomal loss in familial neuroblastoma by comparative genomic hybridization. *Genes Chromosomes Cancer* **19**:176, 1997.
103. Gilbert F, Feder M, Balaban G, Brangman D, Lurie DK, Podolsky R, Rinaldt V, Vinikoor N, Weisband J: Human neuroblastomas and abnormalities of chromosome 1 and 17. *Cancer Res* **44**:5444, 1984.
104. Takita J, Hayashi Y, Kohno T, Shiseki M, Yamaguchi N, Hanada R, Yamamoto K, Yokota J: Allelotype of neuroblastoma. *Oncogene* **11**:1829, 1995.
105. Van Roy N, Laureys G, Cheng NC, Willem P, Opdenakker G, Versteeg R, Speleman F: 1;17 translocations and other chromosome 17 rearrangements in human primary neuroblastoma tumors and cell lines. *Genes Chromosomes Cancer* **10**:103, 1994.
106. Savelyeva L, Corvi R, Schwab M: Translocation involving 1p and 17q is a recurrent genetic alteration of human neuroblastoma cells. *Am J Hum Genet* **55**:334, 1994.
107. Caron H, van Sluis P, van Roy N, de Kraker J, Speleman F, Voute PA, Westerveld A, Slater R, Versteeg R: Recurrent 1;17 translocations in human neuroblastoma reveal nonhomologous mitotic recombination during the S/G2 phase as a novel mechanism for loss of heterozygosity. *Am J Hum Genet* **55**:341, 1994.
108. Lastowska M, Van Roy N, Bown N, Speleman F, Lunec J, Strachan T, Pearson ADJ, Jackson MS: Molecular cytogenetic delineation of 17q translocation breakpoints in neuroblastoma cell lines. *Genes Chromosomes Cancer* **23**:116, 1998.
109. Hayashi Y, Hanada R, Yamamoto K, Bessho F: Chromosome findings and prognosis in neuroblastoma. *Cancer Genet Cytogenet* **29**:175, 1986.
110. Kaneko Y, Kanda N, Maseki N, Sakurai M, Tsuchida Y, Takeda T, Okabe I, Sakurai M: Different karyotypic patterns in early and advanced stage neuroblastomas. *Cancer Res* **47**:311, 1987.
111. Christiansen H, Lampert F: Tumour karyotype discriminates between good and bad prognostic outcome in neuroblastoma. *Br J Cancer* **57**:121, 1988.
112. Look AT, Hayes FA, Nitschke R, McWilliams NB, Green AA: Cellular DNA content as a predictor of response to chemotherapy in infants with unresectable neuroblastoma. *N Engl J Med* **311**:231, 1984.
113. Look AT, Hayes FA, Shuster JJ, Douglass EC, Castleberry RP, Brodeur GM: Clinical relevance of tumor cell ploidy and N-myc gene amplification in childhood neuroblastoma. A Pediatric Oncology Group Study. *J Clin Oncol* **9**:581, 1991.
114. Oppedal BR, Storm-Mathisen I, Lie SO, Brandtzaeg P: Prognostic factors in neuroblastoma. Clinical, histopathologic, immunohistochemical features, and DNA ploidy in relation to prognosis. *Cancer* **72**:772, 1988.
115. Taylor SR, Blatt J, Constantino JP, Roederer M, Murphy RF: Flow cytometric DNA analysis of neuroblastoma and ganglioneuroma. A 10-year retrospective study. *Cancer* **62**:749, 1988.
116. Brodeur GM, Sekhon GS, Goldstein MN: Chromosomal aberrations in human neuroblastomas. *Cancer* **40**:2256, 1977.
117. Hayashi Y, Kanda N, Inaba T, Hanada R, Nagahara N, Muchi H, Yamamoto K: Cytogenetic findings and prognosis in neuroblastoma with emphasis on marker chromosome 1. *Cancer* **63**:126, 1989.
118. Weith A, Martinsson T, Cziepluch C, Bruderlein S, Amler LC, Berthold F: Neuroblastoma consensus deletion maps to 1p36.1-2. *Genes Chromosomes Cancer* **1**:159, 1989.
119. Takeda O, Homma C, Maseki N, Sakurai M, Kanda N, Schwab M, Nakamura Y, Kaneko Y: There may be two tumor suppressor genes on chromosome arm 1p closely associated with biologically distinct subtypes of neuroblastoma. *Genes Chromosomes Cancer* **10**:30, 1994.
120. Schleiermacher G, Peter M, Michon J, Hugot J-P, Viehl P, Zucker J-M, Magdelénat H, Thomas G, Delattre O: Two distinct deleted regions on the short arm of chromosome 1 in neuroblastoma. *Genes Chromosomes Cancer* **10**:275, 1994.
121. Caron H, Peter M, van Sluis P, Speleman F, de Kraker J, Laureys G, Michon J, Brugieres L, Voute PA, Westerveld A, Slater R, Delattre O, Versteeg R: Evidence for two tumour suppressor loci on chromosomal bands 1p35-36 involved in neuroblastoma: One probably imprinted, another associated with N-myc amplification. *Hum Mol Genet* **4**:535, 1995.
122. Cheng NC, Van Roy N, Chan A, Beitsma M, Westerveld A, Speleman F, Versteeg R: Deletion mapping in neuroblastoma cell lines suggests two distinct tumor suppressor genes in the 1p35-35 region, only one of which is associated with N-myc amplification. *Oncogene* **10**:291, 1995.
123. Caron H, van Sluis P, van Hoeve M, de Kraker J, Bras J, Slater R, Mannens M, Voute PA, Westerveld A, Versteeg R: Allelic loss of chromosome 1p36 in neuroblastoma is of preferential maternal origin and correlates with N-myc amplification. *Nat Genet* **4**:187, 1993.
124. Cheng JM, Hiemstra JL, Schneider SS, Naumova A, Cheung N-KV, Cohn SL, Diller L, Sapienza C, Brodeur GM: Preferential amplification of the paternal allele of the N-myc gene in human neuroblastomas. *Nat Genet* **4**:191, 1993.

125. Beltinger CP, White PS, Maris JM, Sulman EP, Jensen SJ, LePaslier D, Stallard BJ, Goeddel DV, deSauvage FJ, Brodeur GM: Physical mapping and genomic structure of the human TNFR2 gene. *Genomics* **35**:94, 1996.
126. Maris JM, Jensen SJ, Sulman EP, Beltinger CP, Gates K, Allen C, Biegel JA, Brodeur GM, White PS: Cloning, chromosomal localization, and physical mapping and genomic characterization of HKR3. *Genomics* **35**:289, 1996.
127. Lahti JM, Valentine M, Xiang J, Jones B, Amann J, Grenet J, Richmond G, Look AT, Kidd VJ: Alterations in the PITSLRE protein kinase gene complex on chromosome 1p36 in childhood neuroblastoma. *Nat Genet* **7**:370, 1994.
128. Enomoto H, Ozaki T, Takahashi E-i, Nomura N, Tabata S, Takahashi H, Ohnuma N, Tanabe M, Iwai J, Yoshida H, Matsunaga T, Sakiyama S: Identification of human *DAN* gene, mapping to the putative neuroblastoma tumor suppressor locus. *Oncogene* **9**:2785, 1994.
129. Kaghad M, Bonnet H, Yang A, Creancier L, Biscan J, Valent A, Minty A, Chalon P, Lelias J, Dumont X, Ferrara P, McKeon F, Caput D: Monoallelically expressed gene related to p53 at 1p36, a region frequently deleted in neuroblastoma and other human cancers. *Cell* **90**:809, 1997.
130. Ichimiya S, Nimura Y, Sunahara M, Shishikura T, Kageyama H, Nakamura Y, Sakiyama S, Seki N, Ohira M, Kaneko Y, McKeon F, Caput D, Nakagawara A: Genetic analysis of p73 localized at chromosome 1p36.3 in primary neuroblastomas. *Eur J Cancer* (in press), 2000.
131. Srivatsan ES, Ying KL, Seeger RC: Deletion of chromosome 11 and of 14q sequences in neuroblastoma. *Genes Chromosomes Cancer* **7**:32, 1993.
132. Maris JM, Guo C, White PS, Hogarty MD, Thompson PM, Stram DO, Matthay K, K., Seeger RS, Brodeur GM: Chromosome 11q22 allelic deletion is common in neuroblastomas. *Eur J Cancer* (in press), 2000.
133. Suzuki T, Yokota J, Mugishima H, Okabe I, Ookuni M, Sugimura T, Terada M: Frequent loss of heterozygosity on chromosome 14q in neuroblastoma. *Cancer Res* **49**:1095, 1989.
134. Takayama H, Suzuki T, Mugishima H, Fujisawa T, Ookuni M, Schwab M, Gehring M, Nakamura Y, Sugimura T, Terada M, Yokota J: Deletion mapping of chromosomes 14q and 1p in human neuroblastoma. *Oncogene* **7**:1185, 1992.
135. Thompson PM, Kyemba SK, Jensen SJ, Guo C, Maris JM, Brodeur GM, Stram DO, Matthay KK, Seeger RC, White PS: Loss of heterozygosity (LOH) for chromosome 14q in neuroblastoma. *Eur J Cancer* (in press), 2000.
136. Imamura J, Bartram CR, Berthold F, Harms D, Nakamura H, Koeffler HP: Mutation of the p53 gene in neuroblastoma and its relationship with N-myc amplification. *Cancer Res* **53**:4053, 1993.
137. Vogan K, Bernstein M, Brisson L, Leclerc J-M, Brossard J, Brodeur GM, Pelletier J, Gros P: Absence of p53 gene mutations in primary neuroblastomas. *Cancer Res* **53**:5269, 1993.
138. Komuro H, Hayashi Y, Kawamura M, Hayashi K, Kaneko Y, Kamoshita S, Hanada R, Yamamoto K, Hongo T, Yamada M, Tsuchida Y: Mutations of the p53 gene are involved in Ewing's sarcomas but not in neuroblastomas. *Cancer Res* **53**:5284, 1993.
139. Hosoi G, Hara J, Okamura T, Osugi Y, Ishihara S, Fukuzawa M, Okada A, Okada S, Tawa A: Low frequency of the p53 gene mutations in neuroblastoma. *Cancer* **73**:3087, 1994.
140. Castresana JS, Bello MJ, Rey JA, Nebreda P, Queizan A, Garcia-Miguel P, Pestana A: No TP53 mutations in neuroblastomas detected by PCR-SSCP analysis. *Genes Chromosomes Cancer* **10**:136, 1994.
141. Moll UM, LaQuaglia M, Benard J, Riou G: Wild-type p53 protein undergoes cytoplasmic sequestration in undifferentiated neuroblastomas but not in differentiated tumors. *Proc Ntnl Acad Sci U S A* **92**:4407, 1995.
142. Moll UM, Ostermeyer AG, Haladay R, Winkfield B, Frazier M, Zambetti G: Cytoplasmic sequestration of wild-type p53 protein impairs the G1 checkpoint after DNA damage. *Mol Cell Biol* **16**:1126, 1996.
143. Goldman SC, Chen CY, Lansing TJ, Gilmer TM, Kastan MB: The p53 signal transduction pathway is intact in human neuroblastoma despite cytoplasmic localization. *Am J Pathol* **148**:1381, 1996.
144. Beltinger CP, White PS, Sulman EP, Maris JM, Brodeur GM: No CDKN2 mutations in neuroblastomas. *Cancer Res* **55**:2053, 1995.
145. Kawamata N, Seriu T, Koeffler HP, Bartram CR: Molecular analysis of the cyclin-dependent kinase inhibitor family: p16(CDKN2/MTS1/INK4A), p18 (INK4C) and p27 (Kip1) genes in neuroblastomas. *Cancer* **77**:570, 1996.
146. Iolascon A, Giordani L, Moretti A, Tonini GP, Lo Cunsolo C, Mastropietro S, Borriello A, Ragione FD: Structural and functional analysis of cyclin-dependent kinase inhibitor genes (CDKN2A, CDKN2B, and CDKN2C) in neuroblastoma. *Pediatr Res* **43**:139, 1998.
147. Takita J, Hayashi Y, Kohno T, Yamaguchi N, Hanada R, Yamamoto K, Yokota J: Deletion map of chromosome 9 and p16 (CDKN2A) gene alterations in neuroblastoma. *Cancer Res* **57**:907, 1997.
148. The I, Murthy AE, Hannigan GE, Jacoby LB, Menon AG, Gusella JF, Bernards A: Neurofibromatosis type 1 gene mutations in neuroblastoma. *Nat Genet* **3**:62, 1993.
149. Johnson MR, Look AT, DeClue JE, Valentine MB, Lowy DR: Inactivation of the NF1 gene in human melanoma and neuroblastoma cell lines without impaired regulation of GTP-ras. *Proc Ntnl Acad Sci U S A* **90**:5539, 1993.
150. Hempstead BL, Martin-Zanca D, Kaplan DR, Parada LF, Chao MV: High-affinity NGF binding requires coexpression of the trk proto-oncogene and the low-affinity NGF receptor. *Nature* **350**:678, 1991.
151. Kaplan DR, Martin-Zanca D, Parada LF: Tyrosine phosphorylation and tyrosine kinase activity of the trk proto-oncogene product induced by NGF. *Nature* **350**:158, 1991.
152. Kaplan DR, Hempstead BL, Martin-Zanca D, Chao MV, Parada LF: The trk proto-oncogene product: A signal transducing receptor for nerve growth factor. *Science* **252**:554, 1991.
153. Klein R, Jing S, Nanduri V, O'Rourke E, Barbacid M: The trk proto-oncogene encodes a receptor for nerve growth factor. *Cell* **65**:189, 1991.
154. Klein R, Nanduri V, Jing S, Lamballe F, Tapley P, Bryant S, Cordon-Cardo C, Jones KR, Reichardt LF, Barbacid M: The trkB tyrosine protein kinase is a receptor for brain-derived neurotrophic factor and neurotrophin-3. *Cell* **66**:395, 1991.
155. Lamballe F, Klein R, Barbacid M: trkC, a new member of the trk family of tyrosine protein kinases, is a receptor for neurotrophin-3. *Cell* **66**:967, 1991.
156. Squinto SP, Stitt TN, Aldrich TH, Davis S, Bianco SM, Radziejewski C, Glass DJ, Masiakowski P, Furth ME, Valenzuela DM, DiStefano PS, Yancopoulos GD: trkB encodes a functional receptor for brain-derived neurotrophic factor and neurotrophin-3 but not nerve growth factor. *Cell* **65**:885, 1991.
157. Ip NY, Ibanez CF, Nye SH, McClain J, Jones PF, Gies DR, Belluscio L, Le Beau MM, Espinsosa III R, Squinto SP, Persson H, Yancopoulos GD: Mammalian neurotrophin-4: Structure, chromosomal localization, tissue distribution, and receptor specificity. *Proc Natl Acad Sci U S A* **89**:3060, 1992.
158. Berkemeier LR, Winslow JW, Kaplan DR, Nikolics K, Goeddel DV, Rosenthal A: Neurotrophin-5: A novel neurotrophic factor that activates trk and trkB. *Neuron* **7**:857, 1991.
159. Soppet D, Escandon E, Maragos J, Middlemas DS, Reid SW, Blair J, Burton LE, Stanton BR, Kaplan DR, Hunter T, Nikolics K, Parada LF: The neurotrophic factors brain-derived neurotrophic factor and neurotrophin-3 are ligands for the trkB tyrosine kinase receptor. *Cell* **65**:895, 1991.
160. Chao MV, Bothwell MA, Ross AH, Koprowski H, Lanahan AA, Buch CR, Sehgal A: Gene transfer and molecular cloning of the human NGF receptor. *Science* **232**:518, 1986.
161. Hempstead BL, Patil N, Olson K, Chao MV: Molecular analysis of the nerve growth factor receptor. *Cold Spring Harb Symp Quant Biol* **53**:477, 1988.
162. Nakagawara A, Arima-Nakagawara M, Scavarda NJ, Azar CG, Cantor AB, Brodeur GM: Association between high levels of expression of the TRK gene and favorable outcome in human neuroblastoma. *N Engl J Med* **328**:847, 1993.
163. Suzuki T, Bogenmann E, Shimada H, Stram D, Seeger RC: Lack of high-affinity nerve growth factor receptors in aggressive neuroblastomas. *J Natl Cancer Inst* **85**:377, 1993.
164. Kogner P, Barbany G, Dominici C, Castello MA, Raschella G, Persson H: Coexpression of messenger RNA for TRK protooncogene and low affinity nerve growth factor receptor in neuroblastoma with favorable prognosis. *Cancer Res* **53**:2044, 1993.
165. Borrello MG, Bongarzone I, Pierotti MA, Luksch R, Gasparini M, Collini P, Pilotti S, Rizzetti MG, Mondellini P, DeBernardi B, DiMartino D, Garaventa A, Brisgotti M, Tonini GP: TRK and RET protooncogene expression in human neuroblastoma specimens: High-frequency of trk expression in non-advanced stages. *Int J Cancer* **54**:540, 1993.
166. Tanaka T, Hiyama E, Sugimoto T, Sawada T, Tanabe M, Ida N: trkA gene expression in neuroblastoma. *Cancer* **76**:1086, 1995.

167. Levi-Montalcini R: The nerve growth factor 35 years later. *Science* **237**:1154, 1987.
168. Martin DP, Schmidt RE, DiStefano PS, Lowry OH, Carter JG, Johnson EMJ: Inhibitors of protein synthesis and RNA synthesis prevent neuronal death caused by nerve growth factor deprivation. *J Cell Biol* **106**:829, 1988.
169. Koike T, Tanaka S: Evidence that nerve growth factor dependence of sympathetic neurons for survival in vitro may be determined by levels of cytoplasmic free Ca^{2+}. *Proc Natl Acad Sci U S A* **88**:3892, 1991.
170. Nakagawara A, Azar CG, Scavarda NJ, Brodeur GM: Expression and function of TRK-B and BDNF in human neuroblastomas. *Mol Cell Biol* **14**:759, 1994.
171. Kaplan DR, Matsumoto K, Lucarelli E, Thiele CJ: Induction of TrkB by retinoic acid mediates biologic responsiveness to BDNF and differentiation of human neuroblastoma cells. *Neuron* **11**:321, 1993.
172. Acheson A, Conover JC, Fandi JP, DeChiara TM, Russell M, Thadani A, Squinto SP, Yancopoulos GD, Lindsay RM: A BDNF autocrine loop in adult sensory neurons prevents cell death. *Nature* **374**:450, 1995.
173. Matsumoto K, Wada RK, Yamashiro JM, Kaplan DR, Thiele CJ: Expression of brain-derived neurotrophic factor and $p145^{TrkB}$ affects survival, differentiation, and invasiveness of human neuroblastoma cells. *Cancer Res* **55**:1798, 1995.
174. Yamashiro DJ, Nakagawara A, Ikegaki N, Liu X-G, Brodeur GM: Expression of TrkC in favorable human neuroblastomas. *Oncogene* **12**:37, 1996.
175. Ryden M, Sehgal R, Dominici C, Schilling FH, Ibanez CF, Kogner P: Expression of mRNA for the neurotrophin receptor trkC in neuroblastomas with favourable tumour stage and good prognosis. *Br J Cancer* **74**:773, 1996.
176. Ballas K, Lyons J, Jannsen JWG, Bartram CR: Incidence of ras gene mutations in neuroblastoma. *Eur J Pediatr* **147**:313, 1988.
177. Ireland CM: Activated N-ras oncogenes in human neuroblastoma. *Cancer Res* **49**:5530, 1989.
178. Moley JF, Brother MB, Wells SA, Spengler BA, Biedler JL, Brodeur GM: Low frequency of ras gene mutations in neuroblastomas, pheochromocytomas and medullary thyroid cancers. *Cancer Res* **51**:1596, 1991.
179. Tanaka T, Slamon DJ, Shimoda H, Waki C, Kawaguchi Y, Tanaka Y, Ida N: Expression of Ha-ras oncogene products in human neuroblastomas and the significant correlation with a patient's prognosis. *Cancer Res* **48**:1030, 1988.
180. Tanaka T, Slamon DJ, Shimada H, Shimoda H, Fujisawa T, Ida N, Seeger RC: A significant association of Ha-ras p21 in neuroblastoma cells with patient prognosis. *Cancer* **68**:1296, 1991.
181. Tanaka T, Sugimoto T, Sawada T: Prognostic discrimination among neuroblastomas according to Ha-ras/Trk A gene expression. *Cancer* **83**:1626, 1998.
182. Thiele CJ, McKeon C, Triche TJ, Ross RA, Reynolds CP, Israel MA: Differential protooncogene expression characterizes histopathologically indistinguishable tumors of the peripheral nervous system. *J Clin Invest* **80**:804, 1987.
183. Goldstein LJ, Galski H, Fojo A, Willingham M, Lai SL, Gazdar A, Pirker R, Green A, Crist W, Brodeur GM, Grant C, Lieger M, Cossman J, Gottesman MM, Pastan I: Expression of a multidrug resistance gene in human tumors. *J Natl Cancer Inst* **81**:116, 1989.
184. Goldstein LJ, Fojo AT, Ueda K, Crist W, Green A, Brodeur G, Pastan I, Gottesman MM: Expression of the multidrug resistance, MDR1, gene in neuroblastomas. *J Clin Oncol* **8**:128, 1990.
185. Chan HSL, Haddad G, Thorner PS, DeBoer G, Lin YP, Ondrusek N, Yeger H, Ling V: P-glycoprotein expression as a predictor of the outcome of therapy for neuroblastoma. *N Engl J Med* **325**:1608, 1991.
186. Norris MD, Bordow SB, Marshall GM, Haber PS, Haber M: Association between high levels of expression of the multidrug resistance-associated protein (MRP) gene and poor outcome in primary human neuroblastoma. *N Engl J Med* **334**:231, 1996.
187. Hiyama E, Hiyama K, Yokoyama T, Matsuura Y, Piatyszek MA, Shay JW: Correlating telomerase activity levels with human neuroblastoma outcomes. *Nat Med* **1**:249, 1995.
188. Brodeur GM: Do the ends justify the means? *Nat Med* **1**:203, 1995.
189. Reynolds CP, Zuo JJ, Kim NW, Wang H, Lukens JN, Matthay KK, Seeger RC: Telomerase expression in primary neuroblastomas. *Eur J Cancer* **33**:1929, 1997.
190. Oue T, Fukuzawa M, Kusafuka T, Kohmoto Y, Imura K, Nagahara S, Okada A: In situ detection of DNA fragmentation and expression of bcl-2 in human neuroblastoma: Relation to apoptosis and spontaneous regression. *J Pediatr Surg* **31**:251, 1996.
191. Brodeur GM, Castle VP: The role of apoptosis in human neuroblastomas, in Hideman JA, Oive C (eds): *Apoptosis in Cancer Chemotherapy.* Totowa, NJ, Human Press Inc, p. 305.
192. Bunone G, Mariotti A, Compagni A, Morandi E, Della Valle G: Induction of apoptosis by p75 neurotrophin receptor in human neuroblastoma cells. *Oncogene* **14**:1463, 1997.
193. Fulda S, Sieverts H, Friesen C, Herr I, Debatin KM: The CD95 (APO-1/Fas) system mediates drug-induced apoptosis in neuroblastoma cells. *Cancer Res* **57**:3823, 1997.
194. Castle VP, Heidelberger KP, Bromberg J, Ou X, Dole M, Nunez G: Expression of the apoptosis-suppressing protein bcl-2, in neuroblastoma is associated with unfavorable histology and N-myc amplification. *Am J Pathol* **143**:1543, 1993.
195. Hanada M, Krajewski S, Tanaka S, Cazals-Hatem D, Spengler BA, Ross RA, Biedler JL, Reed JC: Regulation of Bcl-2 oncoprotein levels with differentiation of human neuroblastoma cells. *Cancer Res* **53**:4978, 1993.
196. Ramani P, Lu QL: Expression of bcl-2 gene product in neuroblastoma. *J Pathol* **172**:273, 1994.
197. Ikegaki N, Katsumata M, Tsujimoto Y, Nakagawara A, Brodeur GM: Relationship between bcl-2 and myc gene expression in human neuroblastoma. *Cancer Lett* **91**:161, 1995.
198. Hoehner JC, Gestblom C, Olsen L, Pahlman S: Spatial association of apoptosis-related gene expression and cellular death in clinical neuroblastoma. *Br J Cancer* **75**:1185, 1997.
199. Mejia MC, Navarro S, Pellin A, Castel V, Llombart-Bosch A: Study of bcl-2 protein expression and the apoptosis phenomenon in neuroblastoma. *Anticancer Res* **18**:801, 1998.
200. Tonini GP, Mazzocco K, di Vinci A, Geido E, de Bernardi B, Giaretti W: Evidence of apoptosis in neuroblastoma at onset and relapse. An analysis of a large series of tumors. *J Neurooncol* **31**:209, 1997.
201. Dole M, Nunez G, Merchant AK, Maybaum J, Rode CK, Bloch CA, Castle VP: Bcl-2 inhibits chemotherapy-induced apoptosis in neuroblastoma. *Cancer Res* **54**:3253, 1994.
202. Dole MG, Jasty R, Cooper MJ, Thompson CB, Nunez G, Castle VP: Bcl-xL is expressed in neuroblastoma cells and modulates chemotherapy-induced apoptosis. *Cancer Res* **55**:2576, 1995.
203. Nakagawara A, Nakamura Y, Ikeda H, Hiwasa T, Kuida K, Su MS, Zhao H, Cnaan A, Sakiyama S: High levels of expression and nuclear localization of interleukin-1-beta-converting enzyme (ICE) and CPP-32 in human neuroblastomas. *Cancer Res* **57**:4578, 1997.
204. Evans AE, D'Angio GJ, Randolph JA: A proposed staging for children with neuroblastoma. Children's Cancer Study Group A. *Cancer* **27**:374, 1971.
205. D'Angio GJ, Evans AE, Koop CE: Special pattern of widespread neuroblastoma with a favorable prognosis. *Lancet* **1**:1046, 1971.
206. Brodeur GM, Seeger RC: International criteria for diagnosis, staging and response to treatment in patients with neuroblastoma. *J Clin Oncol* **6**:1874, 1988.
207. Brodeur GM, Pritchard J, Berthold F, Carlsen NLT, Castel V, Castleberry RP, De Bernardi B, Evans AE, Favrot M, Hedborg F, Kaneko M, Kemshead J, Lampert F, Lee REJ, Look AT, Pearson ADJ, Philip T, Roald B, Sawada T, Seeger RC, Tsuchida Y, Voute PA: Revisions of the international criteria for neuroblastoma diagnosis, staging and response to treatment. *J Clin Oncol* **11**:1466, 1993.
208. Kaplan S, Holbrook C, McDaniel H, Buntain W, Crist W: Vasoactive intestinal peptide secreting tumors of childhood. *Am J Dis Child* **134**:21, 1980.
209. El Shafie M, Samuel D, Klippel CH, Robinson MG, Cullen BJ: Intractable diarrhea in children with VIP-secreting ganglioneuroblastomas. *J Pediatr Surg* **18**:34, 1983.
210. Said SI: Vasoactive intestinal peptide (VIP): Current status. *Peptides* **5**:143, 1984.
211. Bodmer M, Fridkin M, Gozes I: Coding sequences for vasoactive intestinal peptide and PHM-27 peptide are located on two adjacent exons in the human genome. *Proc Natl Acad Sci U S A* **82**:3548, 1985.
212. Beinfeld MC, Brick PL, Howlett AC, Holt IL, Pruss RM, Moskal JR, Eiden LE: The regulation of vasoactive intestinal peptide synthesis in neuroblastoma and chromaffin cells. *Ann N Y Acad Sci* **527**:68, 1988.
213. Robinson MJ, Howard RN: Neuroblastoma, presenting as myasthenia gravis in a child aged 3 years. *Pediatrics* **43**:111, 1969.
214. Roberts KB, Freeman JM: Cerebellar ataxia and "occult neuroblastoma" without opsoclonus. *Pediatrics* **56**:464, 1975.
215. Altman AJ, Baehner RL: Favorable prognosis for survival in children with coincident opsomyoclonus and neuroblastoma. *Cancer* **37**:846, 1976.

216. Nickerson BG, Hutter JJ: Opsoclonus and neuroblastoma. Response to ACTH. *Clin Pediatr* **18**:446, 1979.
217. Kinast M, Levin HS, Rothner AD, Erenberg G, Wacksman J, Judge J: Cerebellar ataxia, opsoclonus, and occult neural crest tumor. Abdominal computerized tomography in diagnosis. *Am J Dis Child* **134**:1057, 1980.
218. Telander RL, Smithson WA, Groover RV: Clinical outcome in children with acute cerebellar encephalopathy and neuroblastoma. *J Pediatr Surg* **24**:11, 1989.
219. Mitchell WG, Snodgrass SR: Opsoclonus-ataxia due to childhood neural crest tumors: A chronic neurologic syndrome. *J Child Neurol* **5**:153, 1990.
220. Koh PS, Raffensperger JG, Berry S, Larsen MB, Johnstone HS, Chou P, Luck SR, Hammer M, Cohn SL: Long-term outcome in children with opsoclonus-myoclonus and ataxia and coincident neuroblastoma. *J Pediatr* **125**:712, 1994.
221. Noetzel MJ, Cawley LP, James VL, Minard BJ, Agrawal HC: Anti-neurofilament protein antibodies in opsoclonus-myoclonus. *J Neuroimmunol* **15**:137, 1987.
222. Budde-Steffen C, Anderson NE, Rosenblum MK, Graus F, Ford D, Synek BJ, Wray SH, Posner JB: An antineuronal autoantibody in paraneoplastic opsoclonus. *Ann Neurol* **23**:528, 1988.
223. Pranzatelli MR: The neurobiology of the opsoclonus-myoclonus syndrome. *Clin Neuropharmacol* **3**:186, 1992.
224. Kedar A, Glassman M, Voorhess ML, Fisher J, Allen J, Jenis E, Freeman AI: Severe hypertension in a child with ganglioneuroblastoma. *Cancer* **47**:2077, 1981.
225. Mason GA, Hart-Mercer J, Miller EJ, Strang LB, Wynne NA: Adrenaline-secreting neuroblastoma in an infant. *Lancet* **2**:322, 1957.
226. Laug WE, Siegel SE, Shaw KNF, Landing B, Baptista J, Gutenstein M: Initial urinary catecholamine metabolite concentrations and prognosis in neuroblastoma. *Pediatrics* **62**:77, 1978.
227. LaBrosse EH, Com-Nougue C, Zucker JM, Comoy E, Bohuon C, Lemerle J, Schweisguth O: Urinary excretion of 3-methoxy-4-hydroxymandelic acid and 3-methoxy-4-hydroxyphenylacetic acid by 288 patients with neuroblastoma and related neural crest tumors. *Cancer Res* **40**:1995, 1980.
228. Graham-Pole J, Salmi T, Anton AH, Abramowsky C, Gross S: Tumor and urine catecholamines (CATS) in neurogenic tumors. Correlations with other prognostic factors and survival. *Cancer* **51**:834, 1983.
229. Triche TJ, Askin FB, Kissane JM: Neuroblastoma, Ewing's sarcoma, and the differential diagnosis of small-, round-, blue-cell tumors, in Finegold M (eds): *Pathology of Neoplasia in Children and Adolescents*. Philadelphia, WB Saunders, 1986, p. 145.
230. Kemshead JT, Goldman A, Fritschy J, Malpas JS, Pritchard J: Use of panels of monoclonal antibodies in the differential diagnosis of neuroblastoma and lymphoblastic disorders. *Lancet* **1**:12, 1983.
231. Donner K, Triche TJ, Israel MA, Seeger RC, Reynolds CP: A panel of monoclonal antibodies which discriminate neuroblastoma from Ewing's sarcoma, rhabdomyosarcoma, neuroepithelioma, and hematopoietic malignancies. *Prog Clin Biol Res* **175**:367, 1985.
232. Sugimoto T, Sawada T, Arakawa S, Matsumura T, Dakamoto I, Takeuchi Y, Reynolds CP, Kemshead JT, Helson L: Possible differential diagnosis of neuroblastoma from rhabdomyosarcoma and Ewing's sarcoma by using a panel of monoclonal antibodies. *Jpn J Cancer Res* **76**:301, 1985.
233. Moss TJ, Seeger RC, Kindler-Rohrborn A, Marangos PJ, Rajewsky MF, Reynolds CP: Immunohistologic detection and phenotyping of neuroblastoma cells in bone marrow using cytoplasmic neuron specific enolase and cell surface antigens. *Prog Clin Biol Res* **175**:367, 1985.
234. Bostrom B, Nesbit ME, Brunning RD: The value of bone marrow trephine biopsy in the diagnosis of metastatic neuroblastoma. *Am J Pediatr Hematol Oncol* **7**:303, 1985.
235. Franklin IM, Pritchard J: Detection of bone marrow invasion by neuroblastoma is improved by sampling at two sites with both aspirates and trephine biopsies. *J Clin Pathol* **36**:1215, 1983.
236. Moss TJ, Reynolds CP, Sather HN, Romansky SG, Hammond GD, Seeger RC: Prognostic value of immunocytologic detection of bone marrow metastases in neuroblastoma. *N Engl J Med* **324**:219, 1991.
237. Daubenton JD, Fisher RM, Karabus CD, Mann MD: The relationship between prognosis and scintigraphic evidence of bone metastases in neuroblastoma. *Cancer* **59**:1586, 1987.
238. Heisel MA, Miller JH, Reid BS, Siegel SE: Radionuclide bone scan in neuroblastoma. *Pediatrics* **71**:206, 1983.
239. Podrasky AE, Stark DD, Hattner RS, Gooding CA, Moss AA: Radionuclide bone scanning in neuroblastoma: Skeletal metastases and primary tumor localization of 99mTc-MDP. *AJR Am J Roentgenol* **141**:469, 1983.
240. White SJ, Stuck KJ, Blane CE, Silver TM: Sonography of neuroblastoma. *AJR Am J Roentgenol* **141**:465, 1983.
241. Couanet D, Hartmann O, Piekarski JD, Vanel D, Masselot J: The use of computed tomography in the staging of neuroblastomas in childhood. *Arch Pediatr* **38**:315, 1981.
242. Golding SJ, McElwain TJ, Husband JE: The role of computed tomography in the management of children with advanced neuroblastoma. *Br J Radiol* **57**:661, 1984.
243. Fletcher BD, Kopiwoda SY, Strandjord SE, Nelson AD, Pickering SP: Abdominal neuroblastoma: Magnetic resonance imaging and tissue characterization. *Radiology* **155**:699, 1985.
244. Smith FW, Cherryman GR, Redpath TW, Crosher G: The nuclear magnetic resonance appearances of neuroblastoma. *Pediatr Radiol* **15**:329, 1985.
245. Geatti O, Shapiro B, Sisson JC, Hutchinson RJ, Mallette S, Eyre P, Beierwaltes WH: Iodine-131 metaiodobenzylguanidine (131-I-MIBG) scintigraphy for the location of neuroblastoma: Preliminary experience in ten cases. *J Nucl Med* **26**:736, 1985.
246. Voute PA, Hoefnagel CA, Marcuse HR, de Kraker J: Detection of neuroblastoma with ^{131}I-meta-iodobenzylguanidine. *Prog Clin Biol Res* **175**:389, 1985.
247. Shimada H, Chatten J, Newton WA, Jr., Sachs N, Hamoudi AB, Chiba T, Marsden HB, Misugi K: Histopathologic prognostic factors in neuroblastic tumors: Definition of subtypes of ganglioneuroblastoma and an age-linked classification of neuroblastomas. *J Natl Cancer Inst* **73**:405, 1984.
248. Hughes M, Marsden HB, Palmer MK: Histologic patterns of neuroblastoma related to prognosis and clinical staging. *Cancer* **34**:1706, 1974.
249. Joshi V, Cantor A, Altshuler G, Larkin E, Neill J, Shuster J, Holbrook T, Hayes A, Castleberry R: Prognostic significance of histopathologic features of neuroblastoma: A grading system based on the review of 211 cases from the Pediatric Oncology Group [Abstract]. *Proc Am Soc Clin Oncol* **10**:311, 1991.
250. Castleberry RP, Pritchard J, Ambros P, Berthold F, Brodeur GM, Castel V, Cohn SL, De Bernardi B, Dicks-Mireaux C, Frappaz D, Haase GM, Haber M, Jones DR, Joshi VV, Kaneko M, Kemshead JT, Kogner P, Lee REJ, Matthay KK, Michon JM, Monclair R, Roald BR, Seeger RC, Shaw PJ, Shimada H, Shuster JJ: The International Neuroblastoma Risk Groups (INRG): A preliminary report. *Eur J Cancer* **33**:2113, 1997.
251. Ciccarone V, Spengler BA, Meyers MB, Biedler JL, Ross RA: Phenotypic diversification in human neuroblastoma cells: Expression of distinct neural crest lineages. *Cancer Res* **49**:219, 1989.
252. Ambros IM, Zellner A, Roald B, Amann G, Ladenstein R, Printz D, Gadner H, Ambros PF: Role of chromosome 1p and Schwann cells in the maturation of neuroblastoma. *N Engl J Med* **334**:1505, 1996.
253. Nitschke R, Smith EI, Shochat S, Altshuler G, Travers H, Shuster JJ, Hayes FA, Patterson R, McWilliams N: Localized neuroblastoma treated by surgery — A Pediatric Oncology Group Study. *J Clin Oncol* **6**:1271, 1988.
254. Hayes FA, Green AA, Hustu HO, Kumar M: Surgicopathologic staging of neuroblastoma: Prognostic significance of regional lymph node metastases. *J Pediatr* **102**:59, 1983.
255. De Bernardi B, Rogers D, Carli M, Madon E, de Laurentis T, Bagnulo S, di Tullio MT, Paolucci G, Pastore G: Localized neuroblastoma. Surgical and pathological staging. *Cancer* **60**:1066, 1987.
256. Nagahara N, Ohkawa H, Suzuki H, Tsuchida Y, Nakajou T: Staging of neuroblastoma. *J Clin Oncol* **8**:179, 1990.
257. Nakagawara A, Morita K, Okabe I, Uchino J, Ohi R, Iwafuchi M, Matsuyama S, Nagashima K, Takahashi H, Nakajo T, Hirai Y, Tshchida Y, Saeki M, Yokoyama J, Nishi T, Okamoto E, Suita S: Proposal and assessment of Japanese Tumor Node Metastasis postsurgical histopathological staging system for neuroblastoma based on an analysis of 495 cases. Jpn *J Clin Oncol* **21**:1, 1990.
258. Altman AJ, Schwartz AD: Tumors of the sympathetic nervous system, in Altman AJ, Schwartz AD (eds): *Malignant Diseases of Infancy, Childhood and Adolescence*. Philadelphia, WB Saunders, 1983, p. 368.
259. Carlsen NLT, Christensen IJ, Schroeder H, Bro PV, Erichsen G, Hambort-Pedersen B, Jensen KB, Nielsen OH: Prognostic factors in neuroblastomas treated in Denmark from 1943 to 1980. A statistical estimate of prognosis based on 253 cases. *Cancer* **58**:2726, 1986.
260. Coldman AJ, Fryer CJH, Elwood JM, Sonley MJ: Neuroblastoma: Influence of age at diagnosis, stage, tumor site, and sex on prognosis. *Cancer* **46**:1896, 1980.

261. Evans AE, D'Angio GJ, Propert K, Anderson J, Hann H-WL: Prognostic factors in neuroblastoma. *Cancer* **59**:1853, 1987.
262. Grosfeld JL, Schatzlein M, Ballantine TVN, Weetman RM, Baehner RL: Metastatic neuroblastoma: Factors influencing survival. *J Pediatr Surg* **13**:59, 1978.
263. Grosfeld JL: Neuroblastoma in infancy and childhood, in Hays DM (ed): *Pediatric Surgical Oncology*. New York, Grune & Stratton, 1986, p. 63.
264. Jaffe N: Neuroblastoma: Review of the literature and an examination of factors contributing to its enigmatic character. *Cancer Treat Rev* **3**:61, 1976.
265. Jereb B, Bretsky SS, Vogel R, Helson L: Age and prognosis in neuroblastoma. Review of 112 patients younger than 2 years. *Am J Pediatr Hem Oncol* **6**:233, 1984.
266. Kinnier-Wilson LM, Draper GJ: Neuroblastoma, its natural history and prognosis: A study of 487 cases. *BMJ* **3**:301, 1974.
267. Bourhis J, Benard J, Hartmann O, Boccon-Gibod L, Lemerle J, Riou G: Correlation of MDR1 gene expression with chemotherapy in neuroblastoma. *J Natl Cancer Inst* **81**:1401, 1989.
268. Nakagawara A, Kadomatsu K, Sato S-I, Kohno K, Takano H, Akazawa K, Nose Y, Kuwano M: Inverse correlation between expression of multidrug resistance gene and N-myc oncogene in human neuroblastomas. *Cancer Res* **50**:3043, 1990.
269. Corrias MV, Cornaglia-Ferraris P, Di Martino D, Stenger AM, Lanino E, Boni L, Tonini GP: Expression of multidrug resistance gene, MDR1, and N-myc oncogene in an Italian population of human neuroblastoma patients. *Anticancer Res* **10**:897, 1990.
270. Gross N, Beck D, Beretta C, Jackson D, Perruisseau G: CD44 expression and modulation on human neuroblastoma tumours and cell lines. *Eur J Cancer* **31A**:471, 1995.
271. Combaret V, Gross N, Lasset C, Frappaz D, Beretta-Brognara C, Philip T, Beck D, Favrot MC: Clinical relevance of CD44 cell surface expression and MYCN gene amplification in neuroblastoma. *Eur J Cancer* **33**:2101, 1997.
272. Kramer K, Cheung NK, Gerald WL, LaQuaglia M, Kushner BH, LeClerc JM, LeSauter L, Saragovi HU: Correlation of MYCN amplification, Trk-A and CD44 expression with clinical stage in 250 patients with neuroblastoma. *Eur J Cancer* **33**:2098, 1997.
273. Christiansen H, Sahin K, Berthold F, Hero B, Terpe H-J, Lampert F: Comparison of DNA aneuploidy, chromosome 1 abnormalities, MYCN amplification and CD44 expression as prognostic factors in neuroblastoma. *Eur J Cancer* **31A**:541, 1995.
274. Hann HW, Evans AE, Cohen IJ, Leitmeyer JE: Biologic differences between neuroblastoma stage IV-S and IV. Measurement of serum ferritin and E-rosette inhibition in 30 children. *N Engl J Med* **305**:425, 1981.
275. Hann HWL, Evans AE, Siegel SE, Wong KY, Sather H, Dalton A, Hammond D, Seeger RC: Prognostic importance of serum ferritin in patients with stages III and IV neuroblastoma. The Children's Cancer Study Group Experience. *Cancer Res* **45**:2843, 1985.
276. Hann HWL, Stahlhut MW, Evans AE: Basic and acidic isoferritins in the sera of patients with neuroblastoma. *Cancer* **62**:1179, 1988.
277. Silber JH, Evans AE, Fridman M: Models to predict outcome from childhood neuroblastoma: The role of serum ferritin and tumor histology. *Cancer Res* **51**:1426, 1991.
278. Marangos P: Clinical studies with neuron specific enolase. *Prog Clin Biol Res* **175**:285, 1985.
279. Tsuchida Y, Honna T, Iwanaka T, Saeki M, Taguchi N, Kaneko T, Koide R, Tsunematsu Y, Shimizu KI, Makino SI, Hashizume K, Nakajo T: Serial determination of serum neuron-specific enolase in patients with neuroblastoma and other pediatric tumors. *J Pediatr Surg* **22**:419, 1987.
280. Zeltzer PM, Parma AM, Dalton A, Siegel SE, Marangos PJ, Sather H, Hammond D, Seeger RC: Raised neuron-specific enolase in serum of children with metastatic neuroblastoma. *Lancet* **2**:361, 1983.
281. Zeltzer PM, Marangos PJ, Evans AE, Schneider SL: Serum neuron-specific enolase in children with neuroblastoma. Relationship to stage and disease course. *Cancer* **57**:1230, 1986.
282. Ladisch S, Wu ZL: Detection of a tumour-associated ganglioside in plasma of patients with neuroblastoma. *Lancet* **1**:136, 1985.
283. Ladisch S, Kitada S, Hays EF: Gangliosides shed by tumor cells enhance tumor formation in mice. *J Clin Invest* **79**:1879, 1987.
284. Schulz G, Cheresh DA, Varki NM, Yu A, Staffileno LK, Reisfeld RA: Detection of ganglioside GD2 in tumor tissues and sera of neuroblastoma patients. *Cancer Res* **44**:5914, 1984.
285. Schengrund CL, Repman MA, Shochat SJ: Ganglioside composition of human neuroblastomas—Correlation with prognosis. A Pediatric Oncology Group Study. *Cancer* **56**:2640, 1985.
286. Valentino L, Moss T, Olson E, Wang H-J, Elshoff R, Ladisch S: Shed tumor gangliosides and progression of human neuroblastoma. *Blood* **75**:1564, 1990.
287. Quinn JJ, Altman AJ, Frantz CN: Serum lactic dehydrogenase, an indicator of tumor activity in neuroblastoma. *J Pediatr* **97**:89, 1980.
288. Woods WG: The use and significance of biologic markers in the evaluation and staging of a child with cancer. *Cancer* **58**:442, 1986.
289. McWilliams NB, Hayes FA, Shuster JJ, Smith EI, Green A, Castleberry R: Prognostic indicators in babies less than 1 with stage D neuroblastoma [Abstract]. *Pediatr Res* **23**:344A, 1988.
290. Cohn SL, Rademaker AW, Salwen HR, Franklin WA, Gonzales-Crussi F, Rosen ST, Bauer KD: Analysis of DNA ploidy and proliferative activity in relation to histology and N-myc amplification in neuroblastoma. *Am J Pathol* **136**:1043, 1990.
291. Hayashi Y, Habu Y, Fujii Y, Hanada R, Yamamoto K: Chromosome abnormalities in neuroblastomas found by VMA mass screening. *Cancer Genet Cytogenet* **22**:363, 1986.
292. Hayashi Y, Inabada T, Hanada R, Yamamoto K: Chromosome findings and prognosis in 15 patients with neuroblastoma found by VMA mass screening. *J Pediatr* **112**:67, 1988.
293. Kaneko Y, Kanda N, Maseki N, Nakachi K, Okabe I, Sakuri M: Current urinary mass screening or catecholamine metabolites at 6 months of age may be detecting only a small portion of high-risk neuroblastomas: A chromosome and N-myc amplification study. *J Clin Oncol* **8**:2005, 1990.
294. Bourhis J, De Vathaire F, Wilson GD, Hartmann O, Terrier-Lascombe MJ, Boccon-Gibod L, McNally NJ, Lemerle J, Riou G, Bernard J: Combined analysis of DNA ploidy index and N-myc genomic content in neuroblastoma. *Cancer Res* **51**:33, 1991.
295. Kiely EM: The surgical challenge of neuroblastoma. *J Pediatr Surg* **29**:128, 1994.
296. La Quaglia MP, Kushner BH, Heller G, Bonilla MA, Lindsley KL, Cheung NK: Stage 4 neuroblastoma diagnosed at more than 1 year of age: Gross total resection and clinical outcome. *J Pediatr Surg* **29**:1162, 1994.
297. Morris JA, Shochat SJ, Smith EI, Look AT, Brodeur GM, Cantor AB, Castleberry RP: Biological variables in thoracic neuroblastoma: A Pediatric Oncology Group Study. *J Pediatr Surg* **30**:296, 1995.
298. Smith EI, Castleberry RP: Neuroblastoma, in Wells SA Jr. (ed): *Current Problems in Pediatric Surgery*. St. Louis, CV Mosby, 1990, p. 577.
299. Green AA, Hustu HO, Kumar M: Sequential cyclophosphamide and doxorubicin for induction of complete remission in children with disseminated neuroblastoma. *Cancer* **48**:2310, 1981.
300. Hayes FA, Green AA, Casper J, Cornet J, Evans WE: Clinical evaluation of sequentially scheduled cisplatin and VM26 in neuroblastoma; response and toxicity. *Cancer* **48**:1715, 1981.
301. Castleberry RP: Biology and treatment of neuroblastoma. *Pediatr Clin North Am* **44**:919, 1997.
302. Cheung NKV, Heller G: Chemotherapy dose intensity correlates strongly with response, median survival and median progression-free survival in metastatic neuroblastoma. *J Clin Oncol* **9**:1050, 1991.
303. Kushner BH, LaQuaglia MP, Bonilla MA, Lindsley K, Rosenfield N, Yeh S, Eddy J, Gerald WL, Heller G, Cheung NKV: Highly effective induction therapy for stage 4 neuroblastoma in children over 1 year of age. *J Clin Oncol* **12**:2607, 1994.
304. Matthay KK: Neuroblastoma: Biology and therapy. *Oncology* **11**:1857, 1997.
305. Matthay KK, Perez C, Seeger RC, Brodeur GM, Shimada H, Atkinson JB, Black CT, Gerbing R, Haase GM, Stram DO, Swift P, Lukens JN: Successful treatment of stage III neuroblastoma based on prospective biologic staging: A Children's Cancer Group study. *J Clin Oncol* **16**:1256, 1998.
306. Halperin E: Neuroblastoma, in Halperin E, Kun L, Constine L, Tarbell N (eds): *Pediatric Radiation Oncology*. New York, Raven Press, 1989, p. 134.
307. Castleberry RP, Kun L, Shuster JJ, Altshuler G, Smith EI, Nitschke R, Wharam M, McWilliams N, Joshi V, Hayes FA: Radiotherapy improves the outlook for children older than one year with POG stage C neuroblastoma. *J Clin Oncol* **9**:789, 1991.
308. August CS, Serota FT, Koch PA, Burkey E, Schlesinger H, Elkins WL, Evans AE, D'Angio GJ: Treatment of advanced neuroblastoma with supralethal chemotherapy, radiation and allogeneic or autologous marrow reconstitution. *J Clin Oncol* **2**:609, 1984.
309. Gee AP, Graham Pole J: Use of bone marrow purging and bone marrow transplantation for neuroblastoma, in Pochedly C (ed): *Neuroblastoma: Tumor Biology and Therapy*. Boca Raton, FL, CRC Press, 1990, p. 317.

310. Graham-Pole J, Casper J, Elfenbein G, Gee A, Gross S, Janssen W, Koch P, Marcus R, Pick T, Shuster J, Spruce W, Thomas P, Yeager A: High-dose chemoradiotherapy supported by marrow infusions for advanced neuroblastoma: A Pediatric Oncology Group study. *J Clin Oncol* **9**:152, 1991.
311. Hartmann O, Kalifa C, Benhamou E, Patte C, Flamank F, Jullien C, Beaujean F, Lemerle J: Treatment of advanced neuroblastoma with high-dose melphalan and autologous bone marrow transplantation. *Cancer Chemother Pharmacol* **16**:165, 1986.
312. Hartmann O, Benhamou E, Beaujean F, Kalifa C, Lejars O, Patte C, Behard C, Flamant F, Thyss A, Deville A, Vannier JP, Pautard-Muchemble B, Lemerle J: Repeated high-dose chemotherapy followed by purged autologous bone marrow transplantation as consolidation therapy in metastatic neuroblastoma. *J Clin Oncol* **5**:1205, 1987.
313. Philip T, Bernard JL, Zucker JM, Pinkerton R, Lutz P, Bordigoni P, Plouvier E, Robert A, Carton R, Philippe N, Philip I, Chauvin F, Favrot M: High-dose chemoradiotherapy with bone marrow transplantation as consolidation treatment in neuroblastoma: An unselected group of stage IV patients over 1 year of age. *J Clin Oncol* **5**:266, 1987.
314. Philip T, Zucker JM, Bernard JL, et al: Bone marrow transplantation in an unselected group of 65 patients with stage IV neuroblastoma, in Dicke KA, Spitzer G, Jagannath S (eds): *Autologous Bone Marrow Transplantation III*. Houston, TX, University of Texas, 1987, p. 407.
315. Pinkerton CR, Philip T, Biron P, Frapaz D, Philippe N, Zucker JM, Bernard JL, Philip I, Kemshead J, Favrot M: High-dose melphalan, vincristine and total-body irradiation with autologous bone marrow transplantation in children with relapsed neuroblastoma: A phase II study. *Med Pediatr Oncol* **15**:236, 1987.
316. Pritchard J, McElwain TJ, Graham-Pole J: High dose melphalan with autologous marrow for treatment of advanced neuroblastoma. *Br J Cancer* **45**:86, 1982.
317. Seeger R, Moss TJ, Feig SA, Lenarsky C, Selch M, Ramsay N, Harris R, Wells J, Sather W, Reynolds CP: Bone marrow transplantation for poor prognosis neuroblastoma. *Prog Clin Biol Res* **271**:203, 1988.
318. Treleaven JG, Gibson FM, Ugelstad J, Rembaum A, Philip T, Caine GD, Kemshead JT: Monoclonal antibodies and magnetic microspheres for the removal of tumor cells from bone marrow. *Lancet* **1**:70, 1984.
319. Matthay KK, Seeger RC, Reynolds CP, al e: Allogeneic versus autologous purged bone marrow transplantation for neuroblastoma: A report from the Childrens' Cancer Group. *J Clin Oncol* **12**:2382, 1994.
320. Seeger RC, Matthay KK, Villablanca JG, Harris R, Feig SA, Selch M, Stram D, Reynolds CP: Intensive chemoradiotherapy and autologous bone marrow transplantation (ABMT) for high risk neuroblastoma [abstract]. *Proc Am Soc Clin Oncol* **10**:310, 1991.
321. Stram DO, Matthay KK, O'Leary M, Reynolds CP, Haase GM, Atkinson JB, Brodeur GM, Seeger RC: Consolidation chemoradiotherapy and autologous bone marrow transplantation versus continued chemotherapy for metastatic neuroblastoma: A report of two concurrent Children's Cancer Group studies. *J Clin Oncol* **14**:2417, 1996.
322. Zucker JM, Bernard JL, Philip T, Gentet JC, Michon J, Bouffet E: High dose chemotherapy with BMT as consolidation treatment in neuroblastoma—The LMCE 1 unselected group of patients revisited with a median follow up of 55 months after BMT [abstract]. *Proc Am Soc Clin Oncol* **9**:294, 1990.
323. Philip T, Ladenstein R, Lasset C, Hartmann O, Zucker JM, Pinkerton R, Pearson AD, Klingebiel T, Garaventa A, Kremens B, Bernard JL, Rosti G, Chauvin F: 1070 myeloablative megatherapy procedures followed by stem cell rescue for neuroblastoma: 17 years of European experience and conclusions. European Group for Blood and Marrow Transplant Registry Solid Tumour Working Party. *Eur J Cancer* **33**:2130, 1997.
324. Ladenstein R, Philip T, Lasset C, Hartmann O, Garaventa A, Pinkerton R, Michon J, Pritchard J, Klingebiel T, Kremens B, Pearson A, Coze C, Paolucci P, Frappaz D, Gadner H, Chauvin F: Multivariate analysis of risk factors in stage 4 neuroblastoma patients over the age of one year treated with megatherapy and stem-cell transplantation: A report from the European Bone Marrow Transplantation Solid Tumor Registry. *J Clin Oncol* **16**:953, 1997.
325. Bowman LC, Castleberry RP, Altshuler G, Smith EI, Cantor A, Shuster J, Yu A, Look AT, Hayes FA: Therapy based on DNA index (DI) for infants with unresectable and disseminated neuroblastoma (NB): Preliminary results of the Pediatric Oncology Group "Better Risk" study [abstract]. *Med Pediatr Oncol* **18**:364, 1990.
326. Fairchild RS, Kyner JL, Hermreck A, Schimke RN: Neuroblastoma, pheochromocytoma and renal cell carcinoma. Occurrence in a single patient. *JAMA* **242**:2210, 1979.
327. Secker-Walker LM, Stewart EL, Todd A: Acute lymphoblastic leukaemia with t(4;11) follows neuroblastoma: A late effect of treatment? *Med Pediatr Oncol* **13**:48, 1985.
328. Shah NR, Miller DR, Steinherz PG, Garbes A, Farber P: Acute monoblastic leukemia as a second malignant neoplasm in metastatic neuroblastoma. *Am J Pediatr Hem Oncol* **7**:309, 1983.
329. Weh HJ, Kabisch H, Landbeck G, Hossfeld DK: Translocation (9;11)(p21;q23) in a child with acute monoblastic leukemia following 21/2 years after successful chemotherapy for neuroblastoma. *J Clin Oncol* **4**:1518, 1986.
330. Ben-Arush MW, Doron Y, Braun J, Mendelson E, Dar H, Robinson E: Brain tumor as a second malignant neoplasm following neuroblastoma stage IV-S. *Med Pediatr Oncol* **18**:240, 1990.
331. Meadows AT, Baum E, Fossati-Bellani F, Green D, Jenkin RDT, Marsden B, Nesbit M, Newton W, Oberlin O, Sallan SG, Siegel S, Strong LC, Voute PA: Second malignant neoplasms in children: An update from the Late Effects Study Group. *J Clin Oncol* **3**:532, 1985.
332. Cheung NK, Kushner BH, Yeh SDJ, Larson SM: 3F8 monoclonal antibody treatment of patients with stage 4 neuroblastoma: A phase II study. *Int J Cancer* **12**:1299, 1998.
333. Frost JD, Hank JA, Reaman GH, Frierdich S, Seeger RC, Gan J, Anderson PM, Ettinger LJ, Cairo MS, Blazar BR, Krailo MD, Matthay KK, Reisfeld RA, Sondel PM: A phase I/IB trial of murine monoclonal anti-GD2 antibody 14.G2a plus interleukin-2 in children with refractory neuroblastoma: A report of the Children's Cancer Group. *Cancer* **80**:317, 1997.
334. Matthay KK, DeSantes K, Hasegawa B, Huberty J, Hattner RS, Ablin A, Reynolds CP, Seeger RC, Weinberg VK, Price D: Phase I dose escalation of 131I-metaiodobenzylguanidine with autologous bone marrow support in refractory neuroblastoma. *J Clin Oncol* **16**:229, 1998.
335. Meitar D, Crawford SE, Rademaker AW, Cohn SL: Tumor angiogenesis correlates with metastatic disease, N-myc amplification, and poor outcome in human neuroblastoma. *J Clin Oncol* **14**:405, 1996.
336. Villablanca JG, Khan AA, Avramis VI, Seeger RC, Matthay KK, Ramsay NK, Reynolds CP: Phase I trial of 13-cis-retinoic acid in children with neuroblastoma following bone marrow transplantation. *J Clin Oncol* **13**:894, 1995.
337. Wassberg E, Christofferson R: Angiostatic treatment of neuroblastoma. *Eur J Cancer* **33**:2020, 1997.
338. Sawada T, Hirayama M, Nakata T, Takeda T, Takasugi N, Mori T, Maeda K, Koide R, Hanawa Y, Tsunoda A, Shimizu K, Nagahara N, Yamamoto K: Mass screening for neuroblastoma in infants in Japan. *Lancet* **2**:271, 1984.
339. Nishi M, Miyake H, Takeda T, Shimada M, Takasugi N, Sato Y, Hanai J: Effects of the mass screening of neuroblastoma in Sapporo City. *Cancer* **60**:433, 1987.
340. Sawada T, Kidowaki T, Sakamoto I, Hashida T, Matsumura T, Nakagawara M, Kusunoki T: Neuroblastoma. Mass screening for early detection and its prognosis. *Cancer* **53**:2731, 1984.
341. Takeda T, Hatae Y, Nakadate H, Nishi M, Hanai J, Sato Y, Takasugi N: Japanese experience of screening. *Med Pediatr Oncol* **17**:368, 1989.
342. Woods WG, Tuchman M, Bernstein ML, Leclerc J-M, Brisson L, Look T, Brodeur GM, Shimada H, Hann HL, Robison LL, Shuster JJ, Lemieux B: Screening for neuroblastoma in North America. Two-year results from the Quebec project. *Am J Pediatr Hem Oncol* **14**:312, 1992.
343. Woods WG, Lemieux B, Leclerc JM, Bernstein ML, Brisson L, Broussard J, Brodeur GM, Look AT, Robison LL, Schuster JJ, Weitzman S, Tuchman M: Screening for neuroblastoma (NB) in North America: The Quebec Project, in Evans AE, Brodeur GM, Biedler JL, D'Angio GJ, Nakagawara N (eds): *Advances in Neuroblastoma Research*. New York, Wiley Liss, 1994, p. 377.
344. Woods WG, Tuchman M, Robison LL, Bernstein M, Leclerc J-M, Brisson LC, Brossard J, Hill G, Shuster J, Luepker R, Weitzman S, Bunin G, Lemieux B: A population-based study of the usefulness of screening for neuroblastoma. *Lancet* **348**:1682, 1996.
345. Schilling FH, Erttmann R, Ambros PF, Strehl S, Christiansen H, Kovar H, Kabisch H, Treuner J: Screening for neuroblastoma. *Lancet* **344**:1157, 1994.
346. Kerbl R, Urban CHE, Ladenstein R, Ambros IM, Spuller E, Mutz I, Amann G, Kovar H, Gadner H, Ambros PF: Neuroblastoma screening

in infants postponed after the sixth month of age: A trial to reduce "overdiagnosis" and to detect cases with "unfavorable" biologic features. *Med Pediatr Oncol* **29**:1, 1997.

347. Ambross PF, Brodeur GM: The concept of tumorigenesis in neuroblastoma, in Brodeur GM, Sawada T, Tsuchida Y, Voute PA (eds): *Neuroblastoma*. Amsterdam: Elsevier Science, 2000(in press).
348. Bessho F, Hashizume K, Nakajo T, Kamoshita S: Mass screening in Japan increased the detection of infants with neuroblastoma without a decrease in cases in older children. *J Pediatr* **119**:237, 1991.
349. Hachitanda Y, Ishimoto K, Hata J-i, Shimada H: One hundred neuroblastomas detected through a mass screening system in Japan. *Cancer* **74**:3223, 1994.
350. Hayashi Y, Hanada R, Yamamoto K: Biology of neuroblastomas in Japan found by screening. *Am J Pediatr Hem Oncol* **14**:342, 1992.
351. Hayashi Y, Ohi R, Yaoita S, Nakamura M, Kikuchi Y, Konno T, Tsuchiya S, Shiraishi H: Problems of neuroblastoma screen for 6 month olds, and results of second screening for 18 month olds. *J Pediatr Surg* **30**:467, 1995.

PART
5

CHROMOSOMES

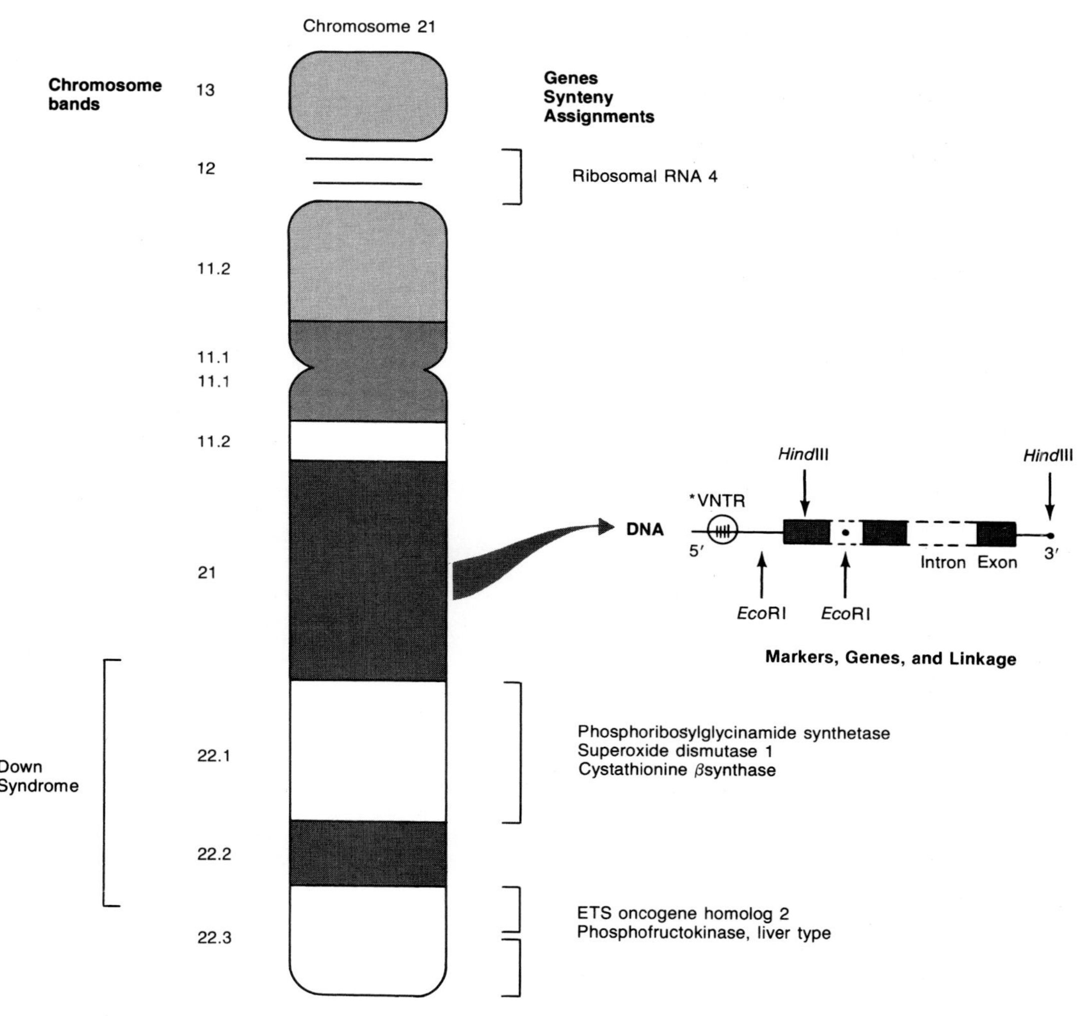
Chromosome 21
Chromosome bands
13
12
11.2
11.1
11.1
11.2
21
22.1
22.2
22.3
Genes Synteny Assignments
Ribosomal RNA 4
Down Syndrome
Phosphoribosylglycinamide synthetase
Superoxide dismutase 1
Cystathionine βsynthase
ETS oncogene homolog 2
Phosphofructokinase, liver type
DNA
*VNTR
HindIII
HindIII
5′
3′
EcoRI
EcoRI
Intron
Exon
Markers, Genes, and Linkage
*VNTR = Variable number tandem repeats

CHAPTER 61

The Sex Chromosomes and X Chromosome Inactivation

Huntington F. Willard

1. **The sex chromosome constitution differs between males and females. The Y chromosome is normally found only in males and is responsible for primary sex determination, but has relatively few other functions. The X chromosome is present in normal males in one copy and in normal females in two copies. X chromosome inactivation acts as a means of dosage compensation by inactivating one of the two X chromosomes in female somatic cells early in development.**
2. **The active and inactive X chromosomes are distinguished by a number of features. In addition to being largely transcriptionally repressed, the inactive X becomes late replicating, heterochromatic (forming the Barr body in interphase nuclei), and extensively methylated at gene control regions. All these features can be used in clinical cytogenetic settings to determine whether an X chromosome is active or inactive. X chromosome inactivation is believed to be random at the blastocyst stage of development. Accordingly, females heterozygous for X-linked traits are mosaic for two cell types that express one or the other X chromosome. Considerable variation occurs in the proportion of the two expected cell types in different individuals. At least 5 to 10 percent of normal females demonstrate extreme skewing of X inactivation, in which a cell type expressing one X predominates over the other cell type. In heterozygotes for an X-linked disorder, this skewing of X inactivation correlates with the degree to which females demonstrate symptoms of the X-linked disease. X inactivation is, therefore, a key determinant of the clinical phenotype in female carriers of X-linked diseases. In several disorders, such as X-linked immunodeficiencies, post-inactivation cell selection is typically observed in affected tissues, and nonrandom X inactivation of the X carrying the mutant allele is observed.**
3. **Not all X-linked genes are subject to X chromosome inactivation. Of the few hundred X-linked genes examined for X inactivation status, several dozen genes have been described that "escape" X inactivation and continue to be expressed from both active and otherwise inactive X chromosomes. These genes are located in several regions of the X chromosome and can be clustered together or interspersed with genes known to be subject to X inactivation. Extrapolating from current studies, it is possible that many hundreds of the expected total of several thousand X-linked genes will escape X inactivation. These genes are candidates to explain the clinical symptoms found in patients with X chromosome aneuploidy in whom additional X chromosomes are invariably inactive.**
4. **X inactivation requires a locus—the X inactivation center—on the long arm of the chromosome in band Xq13.2. In most instances, structurally abnormal X chromosomes found in patients contain the X inactivation center and are nonrandomly inactivated. The *XIST* gene maps within the X inactivation center region and plays a critical role in X inactivation. *XIST* is only expressed from inactive X chromosomes and produces an RNA molecule that remains associated with the inactive X. Although its mechanism(s) of action is not understood completely, *XIST* is useful as a marker for X inactivation, as its expression in patients is, in virtually all instances, correlated with X inactivation.**
5. **Cytogenetic abnormalities of the X and Y chromosomes occur at a frequency of approximately 1 in 500 live births. X chromosome aneuploidy conditions are among the most common chromosome defects. X monosomy (Turner syndrome) occurs in an estimated 1 to 2 percent of all clinically recognized pregnancies, although fewer than 1 percent of these survive to birth. Nondisjunction of the X chromosome is associated with advanced maternal age in both 47,XXX and 47,XXY (Klinefelter syndrome) cases. XY nondisjunction in Klinefelter syndrome is associated with a failure of the two X chromosomes to recombine normally during male meiosis; there is a suggestion that this may be associated with advanced paternal age. Structurally abnormal X chromosomes are detected less frequently and, in the unbalanced state, are almost always late replicating and inactive. The only exceptions to this involve small centric marker or ring chromosomes that do not contain the X inactivation center. Patients with these small abnormal X chromosomes are often mentally retarded, with various phenotypic anomalies, and may represent the clinical consequence of functional disomy of X-linked genes that fail to undergo X inactivation normally. Molecular assays of X inactivation are appropriate for any karyotype involving a structurally abnormal X chromosome.**

THE X AND Y CHROMOSOMES

The X and Y chromosomes are distinguished from the autosomes because they differ between the sexes and because they have their own specific patterns of inheritance. The chromosomes are structurally quite different, but they pair in male meiosis. Unlike other chromosomes, the Y chromosome is thought to be largely

A list of standard abbreviations is located immediately preceding the index in each volume. Nonstandard abbreviations used in this chapter include: *AR* = gene for androgen receptor; *G6PD* = gene for glucose-6-phosphate dehydrogenase; *HPRT* = gene for hypoxanthine phosphoribosyltransferase; Mb = million base pairs of DNA; PDH = pyruvate dehydrogenase; *RPS4X* = gene for ribosomal protein S4; *SHOX*= short stature, homeobox-containing gene; *STS* = gene for steroid sulfatase; *TDF* = gene for testis-determining factor; *XIC* = X inactivation center; *XIST* = gene for inactive X (Xi)-specific transcripts; *ZFX* = gene for X-linked zinc finger protein.

inert, but it has particular significance because of its role in primary sex determination, while the X chromosome uniquely participates in X chromosome inactivation, the process whereby one of the two X chromosomes in female somatic cells becomes inactivated early in development. Abnormalities of X or Y chromosome structure and number are the most common of all chromosomal defects. In addition, X chromosome inactivation plays a significant role in the clinical presentation of metabolic and other inherited diseases in females heterozygous for an X-linked defect. Thus, discussion of the sex chromosomes is highly relevant to considering the molecular and genetic basis of inherited disease and the role of specific X- or Y-linked genes and their expression in determining the phenotype associated with mutant genes or abnormal karyotypes. In this chapter, the structure of the X and Y chromosomes, the general principles of X chromosome inactivation and its consequences, and specific clinical and genetic features of the major sex chromosome aneuploidy conditions, are reviewed.

It has been known for over 70 years that human male and female cells differ in their sex chromosomes[1] and that the difference is visible in interphase, as well as in mitosis.[2] The discovery of sex chromatin masses (also called Barr bodies) in interphase cells of females but not of males revolutionized the early practice of clinical cytogenetics. As a result, abnormalities of sex chromosome constitution were among the first clinical conditions to be recognized as chromosome disorders. The finding that patients with Klinefelter syndrome had two X chromosomes as well as a Y chromosome (karyotype 47,XXY), whereas most Turner syndrome patients had only a single X chromosome (karyotype 45,X), promptly established the crucial role of the Y chromosome in normal male development and demonstrated that abnormal sex chromosome constitutions were associated with an abnormal phenotype.[3,4]

Structure of the Y Chromosome

The structure of the Y chromosome and its role in sexual development have been analyzed at the molecular level and have been reviewed in detail.[5–7] While the basis of sex determination is considered in depth in Chap. 62, the structure of the Y chromosome, particularly how it relates to the X chromosome, is reviewed here.

The Y chromosome consists of two genetically distinct parts. The most distal portion of the short arm (Yp) is shared with the most distal portion of the X chromosome short arm (Xp) and normally recombines with its X chromosome counterpart during male meiosis. Loci in this region, called the pseudoautosomal region, exchange between the two sex chromosomes and are variably linked to gender (i.e., maleness, determined by *TDF*), depending on their distance from the boundary of the pseudoautosomal region (see Chap. 62). The remainder of the Y chromosome (the Y-specific region) does not recombine genetically with the X chromosome and is composed of strictly Y-linked DNA, with the exception of a second pseudoautosomal region involving sequences on the distal long arms of the sex chromosomes.[8] The pseudoautosomal region(s) reflects the role of the Y chromosome as an essential pairing homologue of the X chromosome during male meiosis, while the Y-specific region, including the testis-determining factor gene *TDF*, provides the chromosomal basis of sex determination (see Chap. 62).

The Y chromosome is one of the smallest human chromosomes, with an estimated average size of 60 million base pairs (Mb), less than half the size of the X chromosome. Cytologically, much of the long arm (Yq) is heterochromatic and variable in size, consisting largely of several families of repetitive DNA. The euchromatic portion of the chromosome consists of the Yp pseudoautosomal region (2.6 Mb), the centromere region (approximately 0.5 Mb, but variable among different males), and the DNA of the remainder of Yp and proximal Yq (totaling approximately 30 to 40 Mb).[9,10] A significant proportion of the Y-specific sequences on both Yp and Yq are homologous (but not identical) to sequences on the X chromosome. Although this invites confusion, a distinction can be made. Pseudoautosomal sequences are identical on the X and Y chromosomes, reflecting their frequent meiotic exchange, whereas the Y- and X-homologous sequences on Yp and Yq are only partially related to each other, reflecting their ancient origin from a common ancestral chromosome. While there are relatively few genes encoded on the Y chromosome, they appear to fall into two distinct classes.[6,11] The first class consists of genes that are homologous to X-linked genes and play a role in determining the phenotype associated with some sex chromosome abnormalities. The presence of homologous loci on the two chromosomes is believed to contribute to some of the peculiarities of X chromosome inactivation (see below). The second class of Y-linked gene consists of Y-specific genes that are expressed in the testis and that may be involved in male fertility.[11]

Different deletions of the pseudoautosomal region and Y-specific region of the Y chromosome have been used in an effort to map the precise location of the primary testis-determining region on the short arm of the Y chromosome, as well as other Y-linked phenotypic determinants involving, for example, stature, male infertility, or some of the clinical findings in Turner syndrome.[12–14] The principle of such analyses and their results, especially with regard to the *TDF* gene, are described in depth in Chap. 62.

Structure of the X Chromosome

The X chromosome consists of approximately 160 Mb of DNA and encodes an estimated 2000 to 3000 genes.[15] As of 1999, nearly 1000 X-linked expressed sequences had been characterized in some detail,[15] while several hundred genes (5 to 10 percent of the expected total) had been implicated in X-linked diseases by family studies.[16] By the nature of X-linked patterns of inheritance, females can be either homozygous or heterozygous for X-linked traits, whereas males, because they have only a single X chromosome, are hemizygous (see Chap. 1). Of those X-linked genes known to date, most are X-specific; only pseudoautosomal genes and a few genes mapping outside the pseudoautosomal region have been demonstrated to have functionally equivalent Y chromosome homologues,[11,17] although some genes have related Y-linked sequences that are as yet incompletely understood.[18,19] Thus, for the vast majority of X-linked genes, it is anticipated that mutations will lead to X-linked disorders in males (or to male-lethal events early in development). However, a single pseudoautosomal disorder has been described, involving the short stature, homeobox-containing gene, *SHOX*, with both X- and Y-linked transmission in the same pedigree.[20,21]

Given the relative preponderance of X-linked diseases, the mapping of known genes to the X chromosome and the isolation of their DNA in the context of the Human Genome Project has enormously impacted our understanding of the molecular basis of these disorders and, in some cases, their pathophysiology, while providing molecular tools of significant practical value in medical genetics. The principles behind these advances are, of course, not unique to the X chromosome. However, as many more clinical diseases are known to be determined by genes on the X chromosome (as compared, for example, to any particular autosome or the Y chromosome), the effect of these advances in gene mapping and isolation is more evident. Cytogenetic analysis of the X chromosome has yielded a particularly rich collection of structural abnormalities that have been useful for precisely locating specific X-linked gene defects. For example, DNA from patients with a variety of X chromosome anomalies and clinical syndromes has been used to develop a high-density deletion map covering nearly half of Xp, allowing refined localization of X-linked genes for short stature, ichthyosis, mental retardation, chondrodysplasia punctata, Kallmann syndrome, ocular albinism, and microphthalmia with linear skin defects.[22,23] These studies (and other similar ones focusing on other regions of the chromosome) illustrate nicely the value of collections of patient material for gene mapping and positional cloning.

X CHROMOSOME INACTIVATION

In somatic cells of mammalian females, one of the two X chromosomes in each cell is inactivated at the blastocyst stage, compensating for the dosage difference between females and males who have only one X chromosome. X chromosome inactivation is a unique developmental regulatory event that results in the *cis*-limited inactivation of most of the entire chromosome. Lyon first hypothesized X inactivation in 1961, based on the observation that female mice heterozygous for X-linked traits showed mosaic expression.[24] Beutler also proposed that females were mosaic on the basis of his studies of the X-linked enzyme glucose-6-phosphate dehydrogenase (G6PD) in males and females.[25] The tenets of what is commonly referred to as the Lyon hypothesis are: (a) in normal females, only one of the two X chromosomes present is genetically active, the other being inactivated; (b) X inactivation occurs early in development; (c) the inactive X can be either maternal or paternal in origin and the choice of the X to become inactive is random with respect to parental origin and independent of the choice in other cells in the embryo; and (d) X inactivation is irreversible in somatic cells such that the inactive X in a particular cell remains inactive in all descendants of that cell.[24]

A number of reviews thoroughly summarize much of the original data on X inactivation, both in humans and in other mammals, and extensively discuss many of the theories proposed to explain various aspects of the inactivation process.[26–30] This chapter focuses on the human X chromosome, concentrating on recent developments and advances in the molecular and genetic analysis and understanding of X inactivation, particularly as they relate to medical genetics.

Features of the Inactive X Chromosome

While the inactive X chromosome was first identified cytologically by its heterochromatic nature, there are many features distinguishing the active and inactive X chromosomes. Many of the characteristics appear to be interrelated, and it is as yet unclear which (if any) are causal of inactivation or are, instead, general features of inactive genes and chromatin.[30] As well as yielding insight into the process of inactivation, these features are useful for identification of the inactive X. Even before Lyon correlated the heterochromatic sex chromatin body with the inactive X chromosome, Taylor had identified a late-replicating X chromosome in female cells and suggested that it might be heterochromatic.[31] Studies of replication timing, originally by tritiated thymidine incorporation[32–34] and later by 5-bromodeoxyuridine incorporation followed by fluorescence staining,[35,36] showed that the inactive X chromosome starts and finishes replication later in the cell cycle than the active X in the same cell. Molecular studies of replicating timing based on isolation of newly replicated DNA from different stages of the cell cycle have largely supported earlier cytologic analyses, but importantly have provided substantially greater resolution, at the level of individual genes.[37] The basis for chromosome-wide differences in replication between active and inactive X chromosomes remains unknown, but suggests an intimate relationship between the regulation of gene expression and the temporal and spatial control of chromosomal DNA replication.[38,39]

DNA methylation at the 5′ carbon of cytosine residues in cytosine-guanine dinucleotides (CpG) has long been considered an attractive means of maintaining X chromosome inactivation.[40–42] DNA from the active X chromosome is more efficient in transforming cultured cells than is DNA from the inactive X,[43] indicating that there is some characteristic difference in the DNA between the active and inactive X. Rodent/human somatic cell hybrid lines retaining the human inactive X chromosome can be treated with 5-azacytidine, an inhibitor of DNA methylation, to reactivate genes on the inactive X[44] and restore the transforming competence,[45] establishing that DNA methylation is responsible for the epigenetic change. Methylation-sensitive restriction enzymes, or, more recently, genomic sequencing, can analyze DNA methylation at specific sites on the X chromosome.[46] These data indicated that CpG islands, regions of mammalian DNA unusually high in C + G content with a high frequency of the CpG doublet and found associated with the 5′ end of constitutively expressed genes,[47] are methylated on the inactive, but not the active, X chromosome.[30] These data are consistent with a role for DNA methylation in at least some aspect of the X chromosome inactivation process (see "Mechanisms of X Chromosome Inactivation" below).

The inactive X chromosome is generally more resistant to the action of DNA nucleases than is the active X chromosome,[48,49] and specific sites hypersensitive to nucleases have been identified at the CpG islands of a number of X-linked genes on the active, but not the inactive, X chromosome.[50,51] The binding of proteins that specifically bind methylated DNA[52,53] and inhibit transcription[54] may also contribute to the differential accessibility of the active and inactive X chromosomes to nucleases.[55] As an additional correlate of its genetically repressed state, the chromatin of the inactive X chromosome was found to be complexed with histone molecules (histones H3 and H4) that are significantly less acetylated than the histone found on the active X chromosome in the same cell.[56–58] Histone hypoacetylation is also a feature of X inactivation in marsupials.[59] DNA methylation and histone hypoacetylation are intimately related phenomena and are likely to be partially redundant forms of chromatin modification and gene silencing. The chromatin of the inactive X is also characterized by a novel core histone that is related to histone H2A1, but which has a unique C-terminal sequence.[60] This protein, termed macroH2A1, appears to be preferentially associated with the inactive X in female cells, and thus is the first protein component of the inactive X chromosome to be identified.[60]

The sex chromatin body, or Barr body, is often seen flattened against the inner surface of the nuclear membrane,[2] and *in situ* hybridization with X chromosome "paint" probes shows that sequences from the inactive X tend to be peripheral, with a smoother and rounder shape than those of the active X in the same nucleus.[61] The telomeres of the inactive X chromosome are reported to be much more closely associated with each other than are those of the active X chromosome, suggesting that the inactive X chromosome may be a loop formed by telomere association and attachment to the nuclear membrane.[62] Recent work, however, has concluded that this formation reflects the free motion of the two arms relative to each other in interphase, rather than a looped structure.[63]

Although all these features reinforce the long-range and chromosomal nature of X chromosome inactivation, the causal nature of any of these characteristics in X chromosome inactivation remains unproven.

Activity of X-Linked Genes

While it is generally assumed that most X-linked genes are subject to inactivation and that this inactivation occurs at the transcriptional level, evidence for specific genes being subject to X inactivation is limited. Direct evidence for the transcriptional basis of X inactivation has been presented for only a limited number of genes.[29,64,65] In addition, there are a growing number of genes that have been demonstrated to "escape" X inactivation and to be expressed from both active and (otherwise) inactive X chromosomes (see "The X Inactivation Profile of the X Chromosome" below). The existence of genes that are not subject to X inactivation was first hypothesized by Lyon for genes in common between the X and Y chromosomes in the pseudoautosomal pairing region to explain the phenotypic effect of X chromosome aneuploidies.[66] Cytologic studies have reinforced this concept, as relatively early replicating regions on the inactive X chromosome

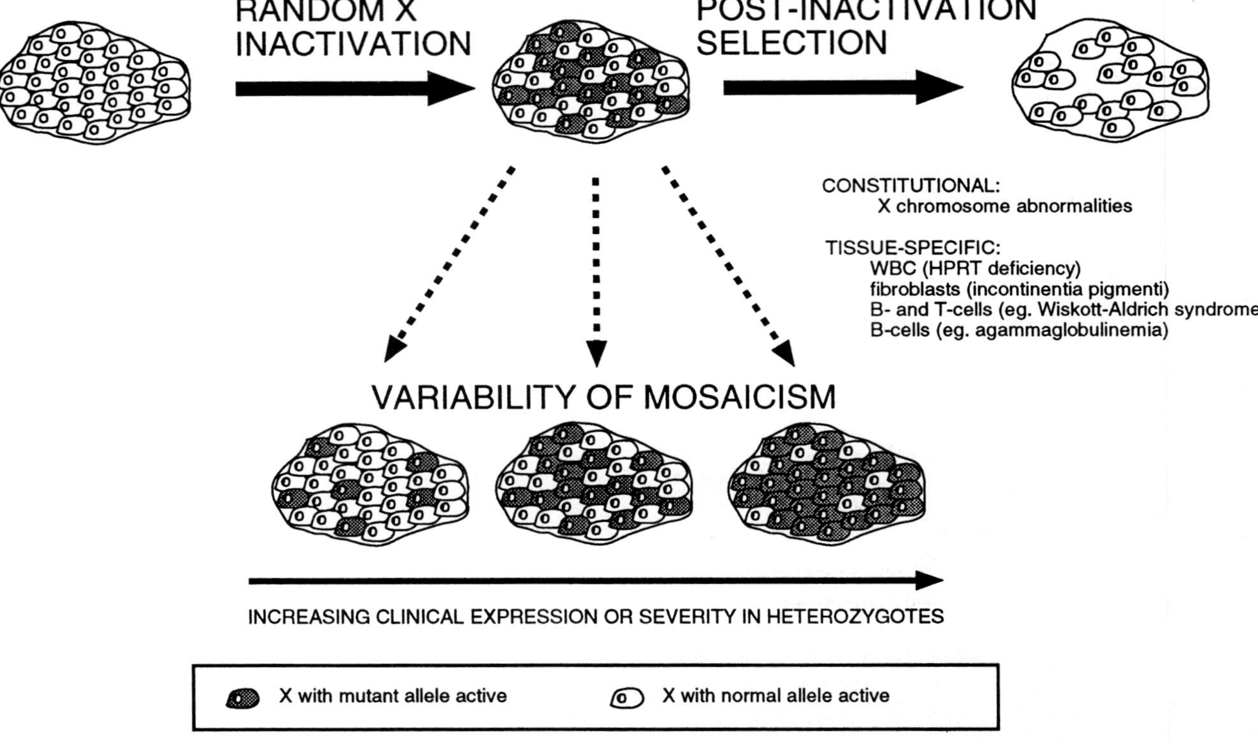

Fig. 61-1 Representation of X chromosome inactivation in female somatic cells. Inactivation early in development is random, with an equal probability a priori that the maternal or paternal X will be active or inactive. However, the distribution of cells expressing alleles from one or the other X chromosome can vary widely, owing either to postinactivation selection against one of the cell types (usually the one expressing a mutant X-linked allele) or to stochastic effects of the choice or subsequent cell proliferation. The phenotype observed in females heterozygous for X-linked traits can also vary widely, with increasing clinical expression or severity correlating with the proportion of cells expressing a mutant allele from the active X chromosome.

have been hypothesized to contain genes being expressed from the inactive X.[67,68]

The original hypothesis of X inactivation was based on the observation of "patchy expression" of X-linked genes,[24] and mosaic expression remains one of the most reliable cellular identifiers of genes that are subject to X inactivation. However, there are a number of different criteria (some stronger than others) that have been used as evidence for X-linked genes being subject to X inactivation. The criteria encompass both the direct assay of expression (of either RNA or protein) and the indirect monitoring of phenotype.

Mosaic Expression of Gene Product. As originally hypothesized, X inactivation is a stable event that is clonally heritable, such that all progeny of a given cell will have the same X chromosomes active and inactive as in the progenitor cell. Therefore, females are a mosaic of two populations of cells in which different X chromosomes are active (Fig. 61-1). By culturing cells in vitro it is possible to isolate homogeneous clonal lineages in which one X is always active and the other X is always inactive. Definitive proof that a gene is subject to inactivation results from identifying clonal populations with different X chromosomes active and showing that one allele (but not both) of the gene in question is being expressed in each population. To unequivocally demonstrate that a clonal population has a specific X chromosome active or inactive requires the presence of a heterozygous genetic marker whose expression is known to be subject to X inactivation. The original characterizable alleles were null alleles or electrophoretic variants, as in the A and B alleles of *G6PD;*[69] however, more recent studies have revealed expressed DNA sequence variants as well.[70–73] Different clonal populations of cells were isolated from females heterozygous for steroid sulfatase (STS) deficiency (X-linked ichthyosis) and also heterozygous for a *G6PD* polymorphism. Both G6PD positive and negative clones (that is, clones with one or the other X chromosome active) were found to express STS activity, despite the fact that the mutant *STS* allele was nonfunctional.[74] These data demonstrated that the normal *STS* gene was expressed even when present on the inactive X chromosome and thus "escapes" X inactivation.

It is not always possible to identify doubly heterozygous disease carriers. In such cases, tissues or cultured cells from females heterozygous for an X-linked disease have been shown to be mosaic for the gene product,[69,75–94] providing evidence that the gene is subject to X inactivation[29] (Table 61-1).

Dosage of Gene Product. In the absence of X inactivation, females would be expected to have twice as much product from X-linked genes as males. Early studies demonstrating that the products of X-linked genes such as factor IX and G6PD were not twice as abundant in females as males were used to support hypotheses of X chromosome inactivation.[25] Recently, dosage at the RNA level was used to argue that the X-linked zinc finger (*ZFX*) and ribosomal protein S4 (*RPS4X*) genes escape X inactivation.[95,96] Such studies must be rigidly controlled for the quantity and quality of RNA being analyzed and are complicated by the fact that expression of "active" genes from the inactive X may be incomplete.[97–99]

Gene Expression in Somatic Cell Hybrids. The isolation of rodent/human somatic cell hybrids that retain the human inactive X without the active X permits the assessment of inactivation for any gene expressed in the hybrid system. By using similar hybrids that retain the active X chromosome, the normal level of expression for the hybrid system can be identified. This method does not require allelic variants of the gene to be studied, but is

Table 61-1 Selected X-Linked Disorders Demonstrating X Chromosome Inactivation*

Disorder	Gene	Map Location
X-linked lactic acidosis	Pyruvate dehydrogenase, E1α subunit	Xp22.1
Duchenne muscular dystrophy	Dystrophin	Xp21.2
Androgen insensitivity syndrome	Androgen receptor	Xq12
Fabry disease	α-Galactosidase	Xq21.3
Gout, excessive purine production	PP-ribose-P synthetase 1	Xq21-q26
Lesch-Nyhan syndrome	HPRT	Xq26
G-6-PD deficiency	G6PD	Xq28
Hunter syndrome	Iduronate sulfatase	Xq28
Chronic granulomatous disease	Cytochrome b-245, β polypeptide	Xp21.1
Ornithine transcarbamylase deficiency	Ornithine transcarbamylase	Xp21.1
Hemolytic anemia	Phosphoglycerate kinase 1	Xq13.3
Glycogen storage disease	Phosphorylase kinase, α2 subunit	Xp22
Fragile X mental retardation	FMR1	Xq27.3
Adrenoleukodystrophy	ATP-binding transporter	Xq28

* Disorders are listed only if there is direct evidence of X inactivation by cloning studies, cell mosaicism in vitro, or somatic cell hybrid expression analysis.

limited to those genes that are expressed in the hybrids (which are generally of fibroblastoid origin).[65,100] Expression of an increasing number of X-linked genes has been analyzed in such systems, providing direct experimental evidence for or against a gene being subject to X inactivation (see "The X Inactivation Profile of the X Chromosome" below).

Mosaic Clinical Expression. There are many disease genes on the X chromosome that have been identified because of their distinctive X-linked inheritance pattern but that have not been cloned, and whose protein product is not known. There is indirect evidence that many of these genes are subject to X inactivation, although definitive proof requires better knowledge of each gene and its product.

If expression of a gene subject to inactivation is localized, then "patches" of expressing and nonexpressing tissue may be observed (Fig. 61-1). Macroscopically visible patches are identifiable in some heterozygous female carriers for a few X-linked diseases[101–106] (Table 61-2). In other diseases, two populations of cells have been identified. These areas of expressing and nonexpressing tissue are assumed to be the result of expression and nonexpression of the disease allele (Fig. 61-1), implying that the gene is subject to X inactivation. However, in none of the cases listed in Table 61-2 (and many others not listed) has it been demonstrated that the patches are, in fact, related to presence or absence of the X-linked gene product.[107–112] It is possible that, in some cases, such patterns reflect phenomena unrelated to X chromosome inactivation, and interpretations based on an assumption of X inactivation must be made with caution.

Because of the long-assumed generality of the initial X chromosome inactivation hypothesis, there is a tendency to interpret all tissue or cell mosaicism for X-linked disease phenotypes in terms of X inactivation. The increasing number of other genes now known to escape X inactivation (see "Genes that

Table 61-2 Selected X-Linked Disorders Demonstrating Mosaicism in Vivo in Heterozygotes, Possibly Reflecting X Chromosome Inactivation

Disorder	Gene (if known)	Mosaicism in Heterozygotes
Chondrodysplasia punctata	Arylsulfatase E*	Pigmentary changes
Amelogenesis imperfecta	Amelogenin	Mottled tooth enamel
Ocular albinism	*OA1*	Irregular fundus pigmentation
Retinitis pigmentosum	Several X-linked forms	Patchy retina, tapetal reflex
Hypohidrotic ectodermal dysplasia	*EDA*	Patchy sweat gland distribution
Lowe syndrome	Inositol polyphosphate-5-phosphatase related	"Snowflake" lenticular opacities
Incontinentia pigmenti	—	Swirling melanin, incomplete dentition
Hypertrichosis	—	Patchy, asymmetric hirsutism
Choroideremia	Rab geranylgeranyl transferase*	Irregular fundus pigmentation
Sideroblastic anemia	*ALAS2*; delta-aminolevulinic synthetase	Two populations of RBC
Alport syndrome	Collagen type IV, α5	Heterogeneous staining with antiglomerular basement membrane antibody

* Gene escapes X inactivation in at least some families, making interpretation of phenotype in carriers uncertain.

Escape X Chromosome Inactivation" below) renders such assumptions unreliable in the absence of direct experimental evidence (as for those disorders listed in Table 61-1).

Clonal Selection in Vivo. In females heterozygous for some X-linked diseases, in tissues where the gene product is required, cells that have the normal allele inactivated can be at a proliferative disadvantage against cells with the normal allele on the active X.[113,114] This results in selection for a population that has only one X chromosome active (Fig. 61-1) and suggests indirectly that the gene is not expressed (or is very poorly expressed) from the inactive X chromosome. For such selection to occur, the defect must be severe and expressed while the affected tissue is still dividing. Such characteristic nonrandom or "skewed" X chromosome inactivation has been observed for a number of disorders, including several X-linked immunodeficiencies,[115] Lesch-Nyhan disease,[82,83] incontinentia pigmenti,[116,117] dyskeratosis congenita,[118–120] several disorders of X-linked mental retardation,[121–125] and severe cases of G6PD deficiency.[126] Importantly, such in vivo selection or differential growth advantage almost invariably results in a clonal population of cells in which the mutant allele is on the inactive X; thus, carrier females for such disorders are characteristically unaffected.[114] For some of these disorders, the presence of nonrandom X inactivation has been used in the past for carrier detection.[120,124,127,128] However, with the increasing availability of the cloned genes, and with the precise molecular defects in individual families being defined, direct DNA diagnosis is appropriate whenever possible.

Table 61-3 Selected X-Linked Disorders Typically Demonstrating Partial Expression of Clinical Phenotype in Heterozygotes

Disorder	Phenotype in Heterozygotes
Adrenoleukodystrophy	Approximately 15% of heterozygotes are symptomatic
Alport syndrome	Hematuria less severe than in males
Charcot-Marie-Tooth disease	Less severe than in males
Ornithine transcarbamylase deficiency	Hyperammonemia; wide range of severity
Fragile X mental retardation	Approximately one-third affected; wide range of severity
Ichthyosis*	Skin abnormalities in some carriers
Kallmann syndrome*	Partial anosmia
Choroideremia*	Abnormal visual field
Lactic acidosis	Progressive neurodegenerative disease; wide range of severity
Coffin-Lowry syndrome	Abnormal digits, mild mental retardation, less severe than in males
Duchenne muscular dystrophy	Mild myopathy in up to 5% of carriers

* Gene escapes X inactivation in at least some families.

Variable Phenotype in Heterozygotes. With the usual exception of those disorders discussed in the previous section, in which nonrandom inactivation is a characteristic of the carrier state, carriers of any X-linked disease allele may show variable or partial expression resulting from different proportions of the affected tissue having the mutant allele inactivated (Fig. 61-1). Because the initial choice of inactivating the maternal or paternal X chromosome is random early in development, variable mosaicism is expected and would occasionally result in a symptomatic carrier female, a finding often termed "unfortunate lyonization." For a wide variety of X-linked diseases, this has been observed[129–138] and can be used as an indirect indication of X inactivation. However, the demonstration of a variable or intermediate phenotype in heterozygotes is unreliable by itself as a criterion for assessing X inactivation, as expression can be variable due to other genetic and/or nongenetic factors; this is particularly true for X-linked disorders in which the phenotype of affected hemizygous males is variable as well. Many well-established X-linked disorders demonstrate partial expression or occasional complete expression in heterozygous females[16] (Table 61-3). Whether these genes are subject to X chromosome inactivation must await confirmation from direct biochemical or molecular studies following firm identification of the gene in question.

For those disorders in which careful analyses were carried out, the data suggest that extreme phenotypic variability in heterozygotes does correlate with clonal variability in X inactivation (e.g., fragile X mental retardation,[139] ornithine transcarbamylase deficiency,[92,140,141] pyruvate dehydrogenase deficiency,[142,143] and Alport syndrome[144]). For example, pyruvate dehydrogenase (PDH) E1a subunit deficiency presents with a relatively broad spectrum of clinical phenotypes in females, ranging from severe lactic acidosis during the newborn period to a progressive neurodegenerative disease with prolonged survival (see Chap. 100). The severity of clinical presentation and the level of residual PDH activity correlates well, but not perfectly, with the proportion of cells in which the mutant allele is on the active X.[142–143] In this and other conditions, however, interpretation is complicated by uncertainty about whether the cells under study are relevant to the disease progression (e.g., leukocytes in fragile X mental retardation[139]) or representative of the tissue being sampled (e.g., liver biopsies in ornithine transcarbamylase deficiency[91]). It may be that different tissues in a given individual are marked by different proportions of one or the other X being active.

At least four of the conditions listed in Tables 61-2 and 61-3 involve X-linked genes that have been shown to escape X chromosome inactivation. Approximately one-fourth of carriers of X-linked ichthyosis are reported to show mild skin defects[145] despite clear evidence that the *STS* gene at least partially escapes inactivation.[74,97] Heterozygotes for X-linked Kallmann syndrome are reported to have mild anosmia and, in some cases,[146] abnormal sexual development.[16] Yet, studies in somatic cell hybrids have clearly demonstrated that the Kallmann syndrome gene escapes X inactivation.[147,148] The third example of a gene escaping X chromosome inactivation is X-linked choroideremia, due to a deficiency of Rab geranylgeranyltransferase, one of a family of GTP-binding proteins regulating vesicular traffic.[149] Carrier females often have patchy pigmentation and show uneven degeneration of the retinal pigment epithelium and choroid,[110] generally interpreted in terms of random X chromosome inactivation.[16] Recent studies, however, have demonstrated that this gene is expressed from both active and inactive X chromosomes and, therefore, escapes X inactivation, at least in a proportion of females.[71] The fourth example is X-linked chondrodysplasia punctata (Table 61-2), which can be caused by mutations in one of a family of sulfatase genes localized to Xp22.3, each of which escapes inactivation.[23] Thus, in both choroideremia and chondrodysplasia punctata, the clinical results obtained with heterozygotes are misleading, and the patchy pigmentation observed in such X-linked disease carriers must have a different underlying basis representing the degenerative nature of the diseases.

In all these cases, the partial expression of the defect in heterozygotes may reflect incomplete dominance, rather than direct effects of X chromosome inactivation. It may be that clinical expression in each of these disorders has a fairly high threshold, in contrast to typical recessive defects in which the threshold for phenotypic expression is thought to be quite low. On the other hand, it is presently impossible to rule out the possibility that X inactivation contributes, because even partial repression of gene expression from the inactive X (as demonstrated, for example, for STS activity[97] and for the choroideremia gene[71]) may be sufficient to create a functionally significant difference between cells

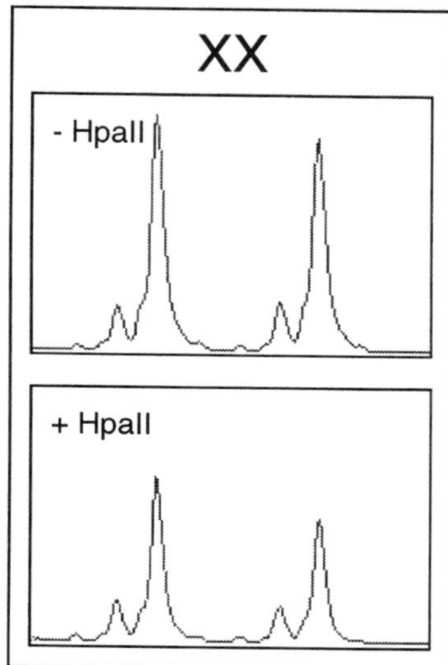

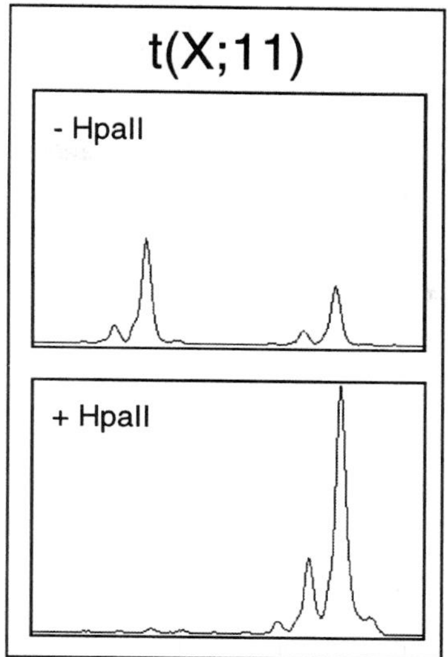

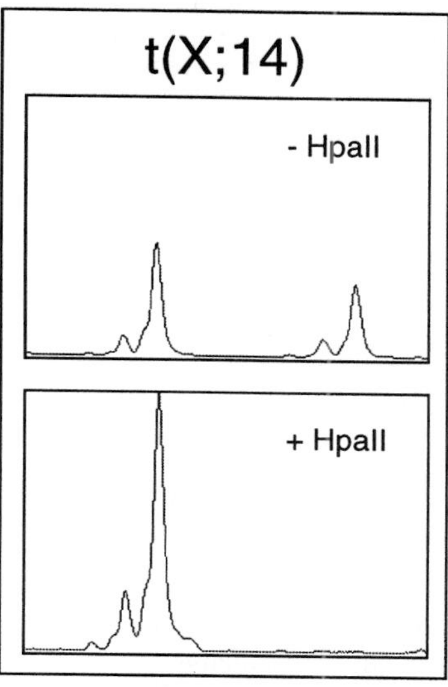

Fig. 61-2 Assay of X inactivation ratio based on androgen receptor (*AR*) DNA methylation differences between the active and inactive X chromosomes, and using the assay of Belmont and colleagues.[159] Heights of major peaks on the electropherograms correspond to relative proportion of DNA with one or the other allele at the AR locus. Top panels correspond to total DNA (both active and inactive X chromosomes). Bottom panels correspond to the inactive X chromosome only. DNA has been digested with *Hpa*II, which cleaves unmethylated DNA on the active X, leaving only methylated DNA on the inactive X chromosome. *Left*: Normal 46,XX female with approximately 60:40 X inactivation ratio. *Center*: Balanced carrier of X;11 translocation, showing preferential inactivation of the normal X and a 0:100 X inactivation ratio. *Right*: Female with unbalanced X;14 translocation, showing preferential inactivation of the abnormal der(X) chromosome and a 100:0 X inactivation ratio.

expressing the normal allele from the active X and cells expressing the normal allele from the inactive X.

Nonrandom (Skewed) X Chromosome Inactivation

There are many instances in chromosomally normal females in which X chromosome inactivation appears to be nonrandom rather than random; that is, tissues of an individual consist predominately (if not exclusively) of cells expressing the same X chromosome, rather than being a mosaic of cells expressing the two different X chromosomes. While in some extreme cases this situation is believed to reflect postinactivation selection (see "Clonal Selection in Vivo" above), in many situations this skewed distribution of the two cell types presumably reflects the stochastic variation expected for a random event operating on a relatively small number of progenitor cells.[113,114]

X chromosome inactivation occurs in the late blastocyst stage of embryogenesis, at about the 32- to 64-cell stage.[26] The number of progenitor cells for individual tissues at this time is presumed to be less, as estimated by clonality studies. For example, the number of hematopoietic stem cells has been estimated to be less than 20.[150–153] Given these relatively small numbers, one predicts on the basis of the binomial distribution that a significant number of females would show distinctly skewed X inactivation purely by chance. Skewed X inactivation can also arise from a number of cryptic selective events early in embryogenesis. For example, confined placental mosaicism may reflect selection against trisomic cells in the embryo itself; in female embryos, this may result in a reduction in the number of embryonic precursor cells at the time of X inactivation and a concomitant increase in the proportion of embryos that show skewing. Indeed, an increased frequency of skewed X inactivation has been detected in cases of confined placental mosaicism relative to controls, suggesting that skewing secondary to confined placental mosaicism may be a contributor to the few percent of newborns that show extreme skewing.[154]

A useful assay to measure patterns of X inactivation is a DNA methylation polymorphism assay to distinguish active from inactive X chromosomes.[155] In such assays, the two X chromosomes in a sample are distinguished by a DNA polymorphism, while the active and inactive X chromosomes are distinguished by characteristic DNA methylation differences (see "Features of the Inactive X Chromosome" above). Samples in which the two X chromosomes are equally methylated at a particular DNA locus demonstrate random X inactivation, whereas those in which only one of the polymorphic bands is methylated demonstrate skewed inactivation. A number of such assays have been developed at different X-linked loci.[155–159] The most informative and widely used assay is based on the androgen receptor (*AR*) locus,[159] and this highly quantitative assay has found widespread usage in both research and clinical settings (Fig. 61-2).

Using such assays, significantly skewed patterns of X chromosome inactivation were demonstrated in fibroblasts or leukocytes in 10 to 20 percent of normal control females.[120,122,152,153,159–166] These studies, which in total surveyed nearly 1000 females, are in general agreement with other estimates of skewed X inactivation based on cell cloning[151,167] or G6PD polymorphisms.[168] These data support nicely the predictions of a binomial distribution, but contradict the often-quoted statement that normal females "should" show 50:50 random X chromosome inactivation. While this may be true on average, there is no such expectation for a given individual or in a given cell lineage. In fact, ratios of 60:40 or 70:30 are common (30 to 40 percent of females in most studies) and more extreme ratios (80:20 or greater) are not rare (at least 10 percent of normal females). Importantly, the proportion of females showing a highly skewed pattern of inactivation (e.g., more extreme than 90:10) increases markedly with age;[152,153,163,164] thus, studies of X inactivation patterns need to be carefully controlled for this variable to establish population norms.

Given that a significant proportion of females in the general population show skewed X inactivation, it can be predicted that an equivalent proportion of females heterozygous for X-linked defects should also demonstrate skewed X inactivation. In some cases, therefore, heterozygous females with the mutant allele present on the active X chromosome in a high proportion of cells in a relevant cell lineage are predicted to show symptoms equivalent to those of affected hemizygous males. Indeed, as described earlier, such affected females are occasionally detected for many X-linked conditions.[129–138,144,169–172]

Recognition of the frequency of skewed X inactivation has significant implications for carrier-detection assays that rely on measurements of X-linked enzyme activities, because samples from females with skewed X inactivation may appear to have normal or near normal activity, despite carrying a mutant allele on the X that is predominantly inactive. Such diagnostic assays are also prone to selective effects in vitro that can result in significant clonality in tissue culture. Studies with both transformed lymphoblasts[173] and chorionic villus samples[142] have demonstrated a high proportion of samples with extreme skewing of X inactivation, suggestive of clonal outgrowths in culture; thus these samples are likely to be unreliable for diagnostic studies that require an accurate reflection of an individual's X inactivation pattern.

Familial Skewed X Chromosome Inactivation. In most of the examples cited above, skewed X inactivation is likely to be attributable to stochastic factors. However, in a few instances, for disorders not typically characterized by nonrandom inactivation, such skewing appears to be familial, suggesting the possibility of inherited factors determining the randomness of X chromosome inactivation.[113,114] Multiple affected females have been described in families with Duchenne muscular dystrophy,[130,174] hemophilia B,[175] Lesch-Nyhan disease,[176] hemophilia A,[177] Fabry disease,[178] and Wiskott-Aldrich syndrome.[179] While such families are rare and while the basis for familial skewed X inactivation has not been determined definitively in any of the reported families to date, they are important for considering the genetic control of X chromosome inactivation.

Preferential X chromosome inactivation is under control of an X-linked locus in the mouse,[30,113,114,180] and thus it might be expected that a similar, perhaps homologous, locus would control X inactivation in humans. Evidence of statistically significant correlations of X inactivation patterns in first-degree female relatives has been presented,[181,182] consistent with such a genetically determined trait. In sufficiently large families, it should be possible to genetically map such a locus.[123,160,161,166] The X inactivation center itself (see "The X Inactivation Center and the *XIST* Gene" below) is an attractive candidate for a gene altered in families demonstrating skewed X chromosome inactivation. In the largest study reported to date, Sapienza and colleagues examined X inactivation in 264 females from 38 families and reported a highly significant sister-sister correlation in lymphocytes, consistent with a *cis*-acting or an imprinting effect.[182] Five families had at least two sisters with skewed X inactivation patterns more extreme than 80:20. The effect could be mapped to genetic markers near the X inactivation center and in Xq25-26.[182]

Skewed X Chromosome Inactivation in Twins. An oddity of twinning is the apparently common occurrence of discordant phenotypes in monozygotic twin females heterozygous for X-linked disorders. At least six sets of twins discordant for Duchenne muscular dystrophy[183,184] and sets of twins discordant for other X-linked conditions, such as Hunter disease[185] and red-green color blindness,[186] have been described. Nonrandom inactivation of the X chromosome carrying the normal allele in one but not both twins has been suggested as the likely basis, and evidence favoring this mechanism has been obtained in several discordant twin pairs using the DNA methylation assays described earlier. In most instances studied, X inactivation in the phenotypically normal co-twin was skewed in the opposite direction; that is, the X chromosome carrying the mutant allele was inactive in most cells.[183,185,186] A different result was reported for monochorionic monozygotic twins, however; the monozygotic twins showed highly correlated X inactivation patterns, indicating that extreme asymmetric splitting of the embryo is not a common mechanism of twin formation, at least not when ascertained because of an affected twin.[187] The available data indicate that commitment to X inactivation precedes the twinning event by at least several cell divisions.[187–189]

Structurally Abnormal X Chromosomes. In all of the above instances, the X chromosomes were structurally normal, and X inactivation was considered in the context of 46,XX karyotypes. Skewed X chromosome inactivation is nearly always observed in individuals with abnormal karyotypes involving structural abnormalities of an X chromosome, such as interstitial or terminal deletions, isochromosomes, or ring chromosomes. In almost all such patients, the structurally abnormal chromosome is inactive in the vast majority of, if not all, cells, presumably reflecting postinactivation selection against those cells in which the normal X was inactive and the abnormal X active[113,114] (Figs. 61-1 and 61-2). As such cells are missing any expressed copy of genes located in the deleted portion of the X, they are presumably at a selective disadvantage. Skewed X inactivation thus has the effect of minimizing the potential genetic imbalance of such abnormalities.[190,191] Because of this preferential inactivation of the abnormal X, X chromosome anomalies are tolerated better than similar abnormalities of autosomes and consequently are more frequently observed. In many instances, the phenotype of females with abnormal X chromosomes is that of Turner syndrome, although more severe phenotypes involving mental retardation and multiple congenital anomalies can be observed (see "Cytogenetic Disorders of the X Chromosome" below).

While completely skewed inactivation of the abnormal X is typical of such karyotypes, it is not invariant. Random X inactivation has been documented in several cases of deleted, duplicated, or insertion X chromosomes.[192–196] As the clinical consequences can be severe when the unbalanced X chromosome is the active X in a significant proportion of cells, this potential outcome should be considered in counseling and molecular assays of X inactivation performed as appropriate.

Nonrandom X inactivation is also observed in the case of X;autosome translocations.[113,114,190,191] If such a translocation is balanced, the normal X chromosome is usually preferentially inactivated (Fig. 61-2), and the two parts of the translocation chromosome remain active, probably as a result of selection against cells in which autosomal genes located adjacent to inactivated X chromosomal material are similarly inactivated.[190,191,197] As expected for a genetically balanced condition, carriers of most balanced translocations are usually clinically unaffected and are ascertained either prenatally or because of clinical defects in their unbalanced offspring. Balanced rearrangements (translocations or inversions) involving a region in the middle of the long arm, however, are often accompanied by ovarian failure or amenorrhea,[198,199] suggesting that normal ovarian development and maintenance requires one or more genes in this region. In rare instances, usually (but not always) involving X chromosome breakpoints near the ends of the two arms in bands Xp22 or Xq28, the normal X can be active in a proportion of cells, with one of the translocation products (but not both) being inactive. These cells appear to be functionally disomic for the portion of the X chromosome that is active in two copies (one on the normal X and one on the active, translocated X), and such findings are associated with mental retardation and other clinical anomalies.[197,200–204] Again, this potential outcome must be recognized in counseling and molecular studies of X inactivation considered for any karyotype with an abnormal X.

In the unbalanced offspring of a balanced carrier, the translocation product is invariably inactivated, while the normal X is active.[190,191] These skewed patterns of inactivation have the general effect of minimizing, but not eliminating, the clinical consequences of the particular chromosomal defect. Depending on the extent to which inactivation spreads from the X chromosome to adjacent autosomal material, the clinical phenotype usually depends on the amount and nature of extra autosomal material present. Spreading of inactivation is a well-recognized, but poorly understood phenomenon. Spreading can partially or even completely ameliorate the expected phenotype due to partial autosomal trisomy;[190,191,205] failure of spreading, however, can result in severe clinical symptoms.[58,206]

In rare instances, an unbalanced translocation chromosome is one that lacks the X inactivation center in Xq13 (see "The X Inactivation Center and the *XIST* Gene" below). In such cases, the translocation product cannot undergo X inactivation and the result is functional disomy. A portion of the X is expressed from two copies, one on the normal active X and one on the translocated portion of the X separated from the X inactivation center.[202,207] The existence of such patients and the clinical abnormalities associated with functional disomy reinforce the significance of and requirement for X chromosome inactivation in normal female development.

One consequence sometimes observed in balanced carriers of X;autosome translocations is that the break itself may cause a mutation by disrupting a gene on the X chromosome at the site of the translocation. Such patients present with a severe form of the relevant X-linked disorder, typical of the phenotype seen in hemizygous males, because the only normal copy of the particular gene (on the normal X) is inactivated in most or all cells as a result of skewed X inactivation. Several X-linked genes were mapped to specific regions of the X chromosome when a typical X-linked phenotype was found in a female who then proved to have an X;autosome translocation. Although expression of an X-linked disease gene can occasionally be seen in chromosomally normal females due to skewed X inactivation (see discussion above), high-resolution chromosome analysis is indicated if a female patient manifests an X-linked phenotype normally seen only in males. The finding of a balanced translocation can often explain the phenotypic expression and show the gene's probable map position on the X chromosome.[208]

Genes that Escape X Chromosome Inactivation

Not all genes on the X chromosome are subject to X chromosome inactivation. Approximately 40 genes on the X chromosome are reported to escape X inactivation, and this number is certain to grow as more genes are identified and studied.[64,65,71,74,100,209] Extrapolating the data to date on genes escaping X inactivation suggests that there may be hundreds of genes that are expressed from both active and inactive X chromosomes. The operational definition of a gene escaping X inactivation is that there is significant expression from the inactive X, although there may not be as much expression as from the active X.[71,97–99] Expression from the inactive X may result either from the gene being refractory to the X inactivation event early in development, or from the inactivation of the gene being unstable (see "Mechanisms of X Chromosome Inactivation" below).

Many, but not all, of the genes that escape X inactivation have a homologous Y-linked locus,[11,17,19,64,65,95,96] consistent with the proposed origin of the sex chromosomes from an original set of autosomes.[8,210–212] Comparison of the evolutionary history of different XY-homologous genes indicates that the determination of whether an X-linked gene escapes inactivation or is subject to inactivation is independent for each gene, possibly as an adaptation to the decay of the homologous Y-linked gene.[19,210,213] If the Y chromosome homologue is expressed, then dosage equivalence between males and females can be maintained without X inactivation.[66] However, for those genes whose Y homologue is not expressed, or when there is not a Y homologue, there must either be an alternative mechanism of dosage compensation or the dosage imbalance between the sexes must be tolerated. A novel variant of dosage compensation has been reported for a synaptobrevin-like gene in the Xq28 pseudoautosomal region. The X-linked homologue is subject to inactivation, while the Y-linked homologue (derived from the inactivated X by meiotic exchange during spermatogenesis) is inactive;[214] thus, dosage equivalence is still maintained between XX and XY individuals.

In most cases, the clinical significance of genes that escape X inactivation is unknown. Of the identified noninactivated genes, only four are associated with known X-linked clinical disorders (X-linked ichthyosis, choroideremia, chondrodysplasia punctata, and Kallmann syndrome) (Tables 61-2 and 61-3). The other genes, however, are candidates to explain clinical symptoms in cases of X chromosome aneuploidy, because in such cases their gene products may be either underexpressed or overexpressed relative to karyotypically normal females.

The X Inactivation Profile of the X Chromosome. As of early 1999, approximately 200 genes had been analyzed for their X inactivation status using the somatic cell hybrid approach described earlier (see "Gene Expression in Somatic Cell Hybrids" above)[209] (Fig. 61-3). This number corresponds to about 10 percent of the total expected number of genes on the chromosome.[15] In total, nearly 40 genes have been described that escape inactivation. While the genes currently $ known to escape X inactivation are distributed widely along the X chromosome,[64,65,95,96,100,209] the distribution appears decidedly nonrandom. First, the pseudoautosomal regions on Xp and Xq contain a number of genes that escape inactivation, and, remarkably, the most distal 10 to 15 Mb of DNA on Xp (consisting of both pseudoautosomal and X-specific regions) contain only genes that escape inactivation (Fig. 61-3). This may reflect the evolutionary origins of this part of the X and suggests that the entire region may have been pseudoautosomal at one point during evolution.[8,212] Second, there are clearly many more genes on Xp that escape inactivation than on Xq. Even excluding the pseudoautosomal region, nearly one-third of all Xp genes tested escape inactivation, as compared to only 2 percent of Xq genes tested.[209]

Many of the regions containing genes escaping X inactivation have been described as being early replicating[36,67,68] and underacetylated[56] on the inactive X chromosome, suggesting that there may be large, cytologically visible domains of genes that escape X inactivation. Consistent with this prediction, a contiguous cluster of at least six genes that all escape inactivation has been described in Xp11.2, one of the regions suspected on cytologic grounds to escape inactivation.[215]

The nonrandom distribution of genes that escape inactivation suggests that different regions of the chromosome may be organized differently. Lyon has suggested that the density of members of the L1 family of long, interspersed repeated DNA elements on the X chromosome may facilitate the spread of X inactivation along this chromosome,[216] a hypothesis that can be examined in more detail as the Human Genome Project progresses. Speculation that the X may have a unique organization is supported by comparative mapping studies that have demonstrated the independent and more recent evolutionary addition of much of the short arm of the X to the modern-day X chromosome, while the long arm ("the ancestral X") has been X-linked for at least 80 to 130 million years.[211,212] This model suggests that sequences on the ancestral X may share properties that render them more likely to be subject to X inactivation than either the more recent Xp sequences or autosomal sequences. Indeed, study of X inactivation in one X;autosome translocation has demonstrated that the frequency of autosomal genes that escape spreading of inactivation is equal to the frequency of Xp genes that escape X inactivation and is, therefore, at least an order of magnitude greater than the frequency of Xq genes that escape inactivation.[205] Whether this is a property of all autosomes requires similar investigation of additional translocations.

The clinical consequences of the X inactivation profile shown in Fig. 61-3 are likely to be substantial. First, the existence of a significant proportion of all X-linked genes that escape inactivation provides a potential explanation for the abnormal phenotypes associated with cases of X aneuploidy and for the well-recognized observation that the phenotype worsens as the number of X chromosomes increases (i.e., 46,XX vs. 47,XXX vs. 48,XXXX vs. 49,XXXXX). This latter finding cannot be explained easily if all X-linked genes undergo inactivation. Second, the profile predicts that imbalance of Xp will be much more poorly tolerated than imbalance of Xq, a prediction that should be accounted for in genetic counseling. Third, it may be that specific phenotypic features of X abnormalities can be associated with overexpression

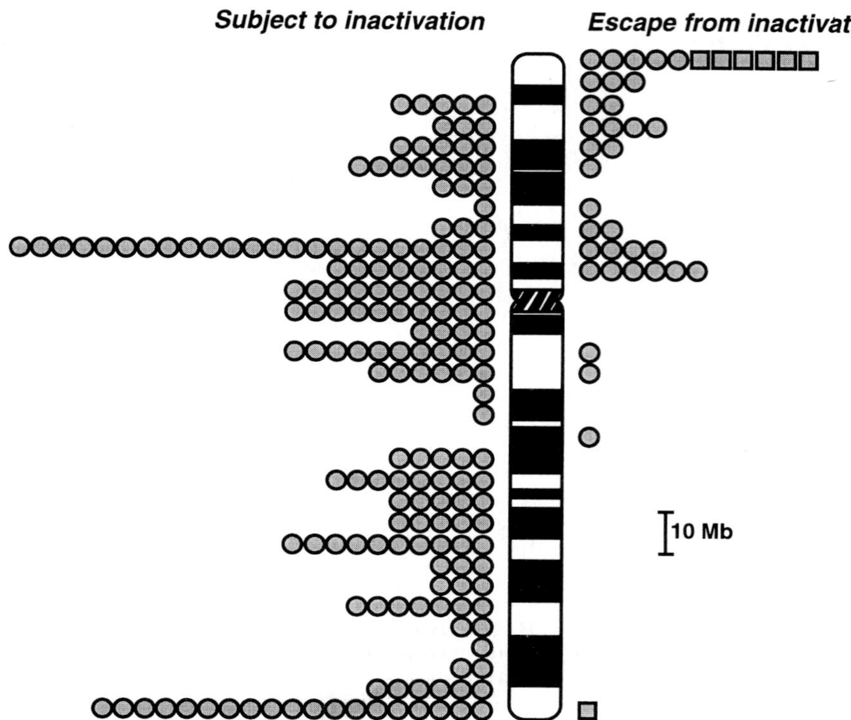

Fig. 61-3 X inactivation profile of the human X chromosome. Each symbol corresponds to a different X-linked gene, assayed by somatic cell hybrid system.[65,100,209] Squares indicate pseudoautosomal loci. A much higher proportion of X-linked genes on Xp escape X inactivation than do genes on Xq.[209] This first-generation profile corresponds to an estimated 10 percent of all X-linked genes.

of particular genes. While this concept is not unique to the X chromosome by any means (see Chap. 63), the fact that relatively few X-linked genes escape inactivation reduces the number of potential candidates whose abnormal gene dosage may underlie a particular constellation of clinical findings. In this respect, karyotype-phenotype correlations may be more direct for partial X aneuploidy than for autosomal defects.

The X Inactivation Center and the *XIST* Gene

Both original and more recent investigations of X chromosome inactivation have emphasized the role of an X-linked locus required in *cis* for inactivation to occur.[191,217–220] The principal evidence for such a locus derives from the observation that when an X chromosome is involved in a balanced translocation to another chromosome, only one of the two products can undergo inactivation, even if inactivation of the other product would have maintained genetic balance.[28–30] The simplest interpretation of such data is that the X inactivation signal requires the presence in *cis* of a critical locus, generally called the X inactivation center (*XIC*). X inactivation requires the presence of at least two copies of the *XIC* on different X chromosomes, because males with a duplication of the portion of the X containing the *XIC* do not demonstrate X inactivation of the duplicated region.[221–223] This, together with the observation that altering the relative dosage of autosomes and X chromosomes (as observed in triploid individuals, for example) can influence the number of active or inactive X chromosomes,[224] argues strongly that the *XIC* is involved as part of a mechanism that "counts" or responds to the number of X chromosomes to ensure the appropriate activity state of X-linked genes, normally one active X per two sets of autosomes.[225,226]

Mapping the X Inactivation Center. The region on the X chromosome that contains the *XIC* has been defined cytogenetically and molecularly by analyzing X chromosome rearrangements that are subject to inactivation.[191,219,220,227,228] There is no convincing or substantiated evidence for more than a single *XIC*, and no chromosome without the *XIC* has been shown definitively to undergo X inactivation. The *XIC* has been mapped to a small region of <1 Mb within band Xq13.2.[220,228] This candidate region is defined by two X chromosome rearrangements, one extending proximally and one distally to the interval. Because genetic imbalance and abnormal phenotypes result from the failure to inactivate structurally abnormal X chromosomes that do *not* contain this locus, other regions of the X chromosome are apparently not sufficient, in the absence of the *XIC*, to sustain X inactivation.[197,201,202,207] However, such examples of functional X disomy are relatively rare and do not account for the entire remainder of the X chromosome. Nonetheless, the series of abnormal inactive X chromosomes that have been used to map the *XIC* are sufficient to rule out any *unique* locus required for X inactivation other than the *XIC* itself.

Alternatively, this region may be absolutely required for survival, rather than having a direct role in X inactivation per se. Indeed, it is intriguing that deletion of this region has never been reported, either on active or inactive X chromosomes, suggesting a possible function in chromosome integrity or an essential role in early development in both males and females, independent of (or in addition to) any role in X inactivation.

Attempts to map the *XIC* using patient material have been complemented by ectopic induction of X inactivation by introducing copies of the mouse *Xic* (including the mouse *Xist* gene, see below) to murine embryonic stem cells and allowing differentiation and X inactivation to occur in vitro. Detailed deletion analysis of a 450-kb region within the *Xic* has shown that X inactivation can be recapitulated in this system by a fragment of the *Xic* as small as 35 to 80 kb.[229–231]

The *XIST* Gene and Its Role in X Chromosome Inactivation. A search for candidate genes mapping to the *XIC* region led to identification of the *XIST* gene.[232] The *XIST* gene gets its acronym from the observation that the gene is expressed only from the inactive X chromosome and not from the active X chromosome [thus, inactive X (Xi)-specific transcripts]. In somatic tissues from karyotypically normal individuals, expression is female-specific. However, males with an inactive X chromosome (e.g., 47,XXY individuals) do express *XIST*, and all normal males express *XIST* during spermatogenesis when inactivation of the single X chromosome is observed.[233–235] *XIST* expression in females is

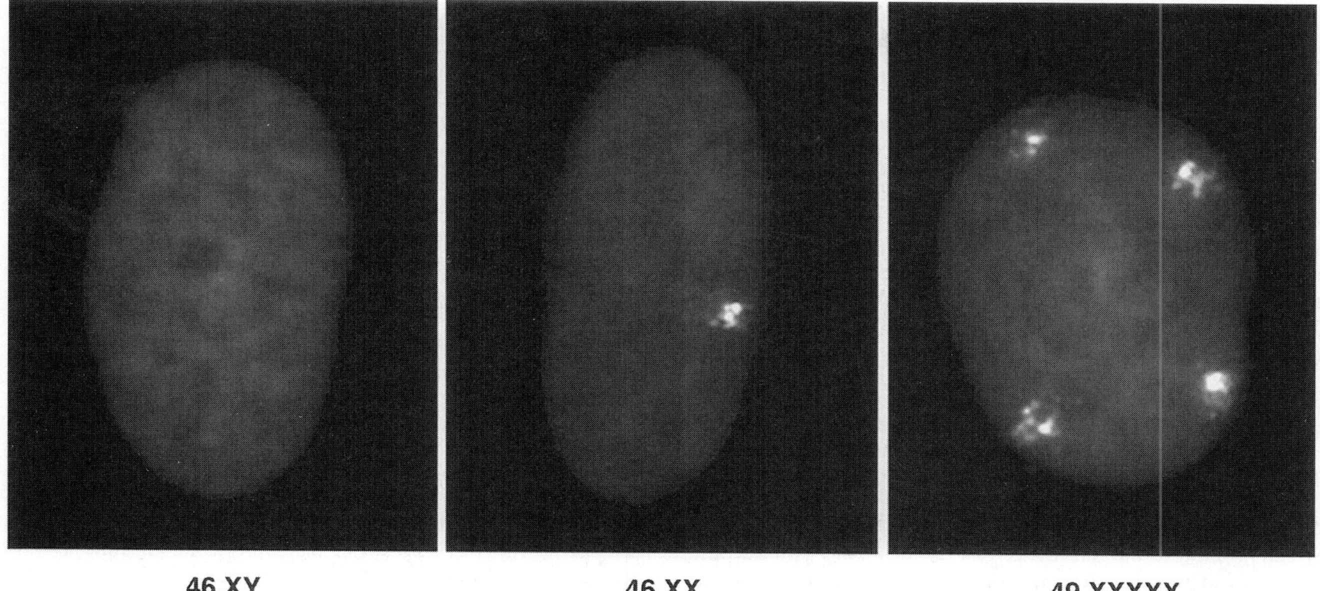

Fig. 61-4 Detection of *XIST* RNA in interphase cells from a normal male, a normal female, and a 49,XXXXX female by RNA fluorescence *in situ* hybridization. Male cells do not express *XIST* RNA. Female cells express *XIST* from the inactive X chromosome, and *XIST* transcripts remain associated with the Barr body complex. Cells from the 49,XXXXX female have four inactive X chromosomes; each expresses *XIST* and forms a distinct *XIST* RNA/Barr body complex.

turned off at about the time of reactivation of the inactive X chromosome during oogenesis.[234] The map location and unique expression pattern of *XIST* strongly suggest that it is either involved in or directly affected by the process of X chromosome inactivation.[220,232]

Similar data have been reported for the homologous mouse gene, *Xist*. *Xist* maps to the corresponding mouse *Xic* interval and is expressed essentially specifically from the inactive X chromosome.[236,237] Both in humans and in mice, the inactive X-specific pattern of expression correlates with methylation of CpG dinucleotides at the 5′ end of the gene only on the active X (i.e., only on the X chromosome that does not express the gene),[238–241] consistent with methylation studies of other X-linked genes showing differential methylation between expressed and nonexpressed copies of the gene (see "Features of the Inactive X Chromosome" above). In the mouse (where such studies can be performed), the accumulation of *Xist* RNA transcripts precedes X chromosome inactivation early in development[242] and is likely, therefore, to be a cause, rather than a consequence, of X inactivation. As mentioned earlier, transgenic experiments have demonstrated that the region of the *Xic* including the *Xist* gene is sufficient for X inactivation to occur in early development, although the exact extent of the regulatory determinants of *Xist* function is unknown.[229–231,243] The promoters of the human and mouse *XIST/Xist* genes appear to be unremarkable,[238,239,244] suggesting that *XIST* is under negative, rather than positive, control.[244] Thus, the effector sequences responsible for *XIST* action presumably lie outside the promoter itself, a conclusion that is supported by the finding that ectopic copies of *Xist* introduced as part of transgenic experiments appear to function only when introduced in multiple copies.[229,230,242,243,245] This result may indicate that the fully functional endogenous *XIC* must have as yet unidentified properties or sequences that are not fully recapitulated by a single copy of the *Xist* gene itself.[245]

RNA transcripts from the *XIST* gene appear to be noncoding, because multiple stop codons were encountered in all potential reading frames, both in the human and mouse genes.[231,246,247] *XIST* transcripts are largely confined to the nucleus, the human *XIST* RNA being associated with the Barr body, the heterochromatic manifestation of the inactive X chromosome in female interphase nuclei[58,247,248] (Fig. 61-4). Similar data have been reported for *Xist* transcripts on the murine X chromosome, with the additional striking finding that the transcripts remain associated with the inactive X during early metaphase.[226,243] *Xist* RNA is excluded from autosomal material in at least some X;autosome rearrangements[249] and shows a banded pattern on the murine inactive X, indicating a nonrandom association of the transcripts with the underlying DNA of the inactive X chromosome.[249] While the mechanism of action of the *XIST/Xist* RNA is open to speculation (see following section), the available sequence data and evolutionary conservation support the hypothesis that at least part of the sequence and/or structure of the RNA itself is important.

Mechanisms of X Chromosome Inactivation. While the precise mechanism(s) of X chromosome inactivation remain to be revealed, the process is generally described in four stages: *recognition* of the number of X chromosomes (sometimes called "counting"); *initiation* early in development; *promulgation* whereby the initial signal is spread to the rest of the chromosome; and *maintenance* of the inactivating signal through successive cell divisions.[28–30] Although this is a theoretically convenient way to visualize events, it may not be accurate in detail, because the hypothesized steps are not generally separable.

The data from studies of X chromosome aneuploidies show that all X chromosomes in excess of one are inactivated (the "n-1 rule") (Fig. 61-4). This finding suggests that the onset of the inactivation process entails two events, the first to "mark" one X chromosome as the active one, and the second to then inactivate all "unmarked" X chromosomes. The presence of two active X chromosomes in triploid and tetraploid individuals suggests that the marking of the active X involves some effect of the autosomal complement.[208] This marking could involve either physical changes in the DNA or epigenetic changes, such as protein binding, membrane attachment, histone deacetylation, or DNA methylation.[27] Evidence that *Xist* itself is involved in the recognition or counting process has come from gene-targeting experiments in mouse that demonstrated that an internally deleted copy of the *Xist* gene cannot be recognized or chosen.[250] Once the single X to remain active has been marked, another factor or inactivation signal could act on any unmarked X chromosomes—none in the case of normal males, one in the case of normal females, and four in the case of an abnormal 49,XXXXX karyotype (Fig. 61-4).

A number of gene-targeting experiments in mouse have demonstrated directly that *Xist* is necessary for X inactivation to occur. A mutation that eliminates *Xist* transcription prevents X inactivation on that chromosome,[251] while two different deletions of portions of the *Xist* transcript itself result in primary nonrandom X inactivation.[250,252] In combination with the ectopic *Xist* transgene experiments summarized in the previous section, these mutations clearly demonstrate that *Xist*, along with adjacent sequences, is both necessary and sufficient for X inactivation to occur and implicate different regions of the *Xist* gene in both recognition/counting and in initiation of inactivation.[226,253] These data are generally consistent with more limited data in humans, including a novel mutation in the promoter of the *XIST* gene that compromises promoter activity and has been detected in two families with skewed X inactivation.[160]

Studies of the initiation of X inactivation in murine embryonic stem cells indicate that commitment to inactivation is accompanied by stabilization of the *Xist* transcripts on the X that will become inactive, followed by transcriptional inactivation (and extensive methylation) of the *Xist* gene on the X that will remain active.[254,255] The factors responsible for converting unstable *Xist* transcripts from both male and female X chromosomes prior to initiation to the more stable transcripts that associate only with the inactive X have not been identified. However, at least in the mouse, this may be determined in part by a switch from a novel upstream promoter whose transcripts are unstable[256] to the constitutive somatic promoter identified earlier in both human and mouse.[240,244]

One of the most intriguing features of X chromosome inactivation is the ability of the inactivation signal to be promulgated along a single X chromosome in *cis*, without affecting the active X chromosome present in the same nucleus. The promulgation signal must distinguish those genes that escape X inactivation[209,215,257] (see "Genes that Escape X Chromosome Inactivation" above), although formally it isn't known whether these genes are never inactivated or whether they are unable to maintain inactivation. In translocations between the X and autosomes, X chromosome inactivation can spread to the translocated material,[205] suggesting that there are not unique X-linked factors associated with each gene subject to inactivation. Promulgation of inactivation could proceed by a locus-by-locus mechanism, although the more commonly proposed mechanisms for a *cis*-limited spread of inactivation are chromosomal in nature,[28,30] presumably involving *XIST* RNA.[249] It is estimated that there are only several hundred to several thousand copies of the RNA per nucleus.[258] As this corresponds to less than one copy of the *XIST* transcript per inactivated gene,[249] the RNA presumably acts by modifying higher-order chromatin structure on the inactive X, in the context of a Barr body-*XIST* RNA complex.[248,249]

All the properties of the inactive X chromosome described earlier could aid in the maintenance of the inactive state, either singly or cooperatively. DNA methylation is most commonly proposed as a secondary mechanism being used to "lock in" the inactive state.[30,39] Extensive methylation of CpG dinucleotides throughout X-linked gene regulatory sequences is well documented[46,50] and may interfere with the binding of transcription factors required for gene expression.[54,55,259,260]

While it is clear that *XIST* is necessary for the initiation of X inactivation early in development, it is less clear what role *XIST* or its RNA plays in maintenance of the inactive state. Deletion of the *XIST* gene from the inactive X either in mouse/human somatic cell hybrids[261] or in leukemic cells[262] does not result in reactivation of the inactive X, indicating that neither the gene nor its transcripts are required for maintenance. Further, reactivation of the transcriptionally silent *XIST* gene on an active X in somatic cell hybrids does not induce inactivation of the X;[263–265] thus, the association of *XIST* RNA with the X chromosome, as well as the initiation of inactivation, must require developmentally regulated steps or factors that are absent from somatic cells.

CYTOGENETIC DISORDERS OF THE X CHROMOSOME

Sex chromosome abnormalities, like abnormalities of the autosomes, can be either numerical or structural. Their incidence in liveborn children is summarized in Table 61-4. X and/or Y chromosome aneuploidy is quite common and, in total, sex chromosome abnormalities are among the most common of all human genetic disorders, with an overall frequency of about 1 in 500 births.[266] The phenotypes associated with these chromosomal defects are generally less severe than those associated with comparable autosomal disorders, because X chromosome inactivation and the apparent low gene content of the Y chromosome minimize the clinical consequences of sex chromosome imbalance. By far the most common sex chromosome defects in live births and fetuses are the trisomic types (47,XXY, 47,XXX, and 47,XYY karyotypes), but all three are rare in spontaneous abortions.[267] In contrast, monosomy for the X (Turner syndrome) is relatively rare in liveborns but is the most common chromosome anomaly reported in abortions.[268]

Structural abnormalities of the sex chromosomes are less common; the most frequently observed defect is an isochromosome of the long arm of the X detected in about 10 to 15 percent of females with Turner syndrome.[269] Mosaicism is more common for sex chromosome abnormalities than for autosomal abnormalities, and in some patients is associated with relatively mild expression of the associated phenotype. Disorders of the sex chromosomes tend to occur as isolated events without apparent predisposing factors, except for an effect of late maternal age in the cases that originate as errors of maternal meiosis I[270] (similar to the effect seen in trisomy 21; see Chap. 63).

The three well-defined syndromes associated with X chromosome aneuploidy are important as causes of infertility, abnormal development, or both. They became of paramount interest to cytogeneticists and medical genetics because their existence and characterization defined the role of the Y chromosome in sex determination (see Chap. 62) and clarified the behavior of supernumerary X chromosomes with respect to X chromosome inactivation.

The first step in the understanding of sex chromosome abnormalities was an explanation of sex chromatin in terms of X chromosome inactivation. Soon after the karyotypic description of the first cases of sex chromosome aneuploidy,[3,4] cytogenetic studies showed that the number of Barr bodies seen in interphase cells was always one less than the total number of X chromosomes per cell. Subsequent studies established that all X chromosomes in excess of one were late replicating and inactivated. Thus, all diploid somatic cells in both males and females have a single active X chromosome, regardless of the total number of Xs or Ys present.[190]

While this observation is central to models describing the initiation of X inactivation, it creates a paradox. If all X chromosomes in excess of one are inactivated, why are abnormal sex chromosome constitutions associated with phenotypic abnormalities? While there is no satisfactory explanation for this as yet, several nonexclusive possibilities are usually invoked. One, the phenotype may reflect a requirement for two active X chromosomes early in development before the initiation of X chromosome inactivation. Second, the increasing number of X-linked genes shown to escape X inactivation may contribute to clinical abnormalities, because the level of their expression is inappropriate in individuals with an abnormal number of X chromosomes.

Klinefelter Syndrome (47,XXY)

Patients with Klinefelter syndrome are tall and thin, with relatively long legs.[271,272] They appear physically normal until puberty, when signs of hypogonadism become obvious. The testes remain small and the secondary sexual characteristics remain underdeveloped. Klinefelter patients are almost always infertile. There is wide variability in clinical presentation.[272] Testosterone replacement therapy can be used to correct androgen deficiency and provide appropriate virilization. Based on a study of 93 unselected male breast cancer patients in Sweden, Klinefelter males have a substantially increased risk of breast cancer.[273]

The incidence of Klinefelter syndrome is about 1 in 500 to 1000 male live births and 1 in 300 spontaneous abortions. Even though the phenotype seems benign compared with autosomal trisomies, half of all 47,XXY conceptions are lost prenatally.[267,268] Less than 10 percent of cases are diagnosed prenatally.[274] About 80 percent of the patients with Klinefelter syndrome have a 47,XXY karyotype.[3] As predicted by the finding that 47,XXY Klinefelter patients are Barr body–positive, one of the two X chromosomes is inactivated and expresses *XIST*.[231] Limited phenotype-karyotype correlations in Klinefelter patients with structurally abnormal X chromosomes suggest that the Klinefelter phenotype is associated with genes mapping to the long arm of the X chromosome.[275]

A 14-year longitudinal study of intelligence and achievement in 47 children with aneuploidy involving an extra X chromosome (principally 47,XXY or 47,XXX karyotypes) suggested milder impairment than generally thought.[276] While verbal comprehension was below that of normal controls, performance IQ did not differ significantly. Relative risk for reading and arithmetic impairment was 2.6 for males. Nonetheless, significant phenotypic variability was stressed in a similar, but independent, study of 42 adolescents with sex chromosome abnormalities.[277]

Combined cytogenetic and molecular investigations of the parental origin and meiotic stage of the nondisjunctional error responsible for the syndrome have found that the extra X chromosome is of paternal origin in half of cases and of maternal origin in half.[278–280] There are no obvious phenotypic differences between patients arising from one parental source or the other. Most (about three quarters) of the cases of maternal origin arise from errors in maternal meiosis I, and maternal age is increased in the cases associated with maternal meiosis I errors, but not in the other cases. In addition to advanced maternal age, maternal meiosis I nondisjunction may be correlated with an increased frequency of meiotic recombination in the vicinity of the X chromosome centromere,[281] suggesting an association between recombination and chromosome nondisjunction (see also Chap. 63). However, another study was unable to confirm this finding.[280]

Nondisjunction can also be associated with a reduction or failure of recombination. Hassold et al.[282] examined recombination in the Xp/Yp pseudoautosomal region in patients with Klinefelter syndrome of paternal origin. They found that most such cases of 47,XXY result from paternal meioses in which the X and Y chromosomes did not recombine, whereas in normal meioses (in which the X and Y chromosomes disjoin properly), recombination was observed. Paternal nondisjunction of the X and Y chromosomes has been reported to be associated with an advanced paternal-age effect.[280]

There are several variants of Klinefelter syndrome with karyotypes other than 47,XXY, including 48,XXYY, 48,XXXY, 49,XXXXY, and others. Phenotypically, the additional X chromosomes cause a correspondingly more severe phenotype (even though the extra X chromosomes are all inactive). Over 100 cases of 49,XXXXY have been reviewed.[283] Radioulnar synostosis, hypogonadism, and mental retardation, as well as congenital heart defects, were prevalent and make this syndrome distinct from typical Klinefelter syndrome. Where analyzed, the extra X chromosomes in cases of 49,XXXXY are of maternal origin,[284,285] suggesting that they originate from sequential nondisjunction in both maternal meiosis I and II.

Trisomy X (47,XXX)

Trisomy X females, though usually above average in stature, are not generally phenotypically abnormal. Some are first identified in infertility clinics, others in institutions for the mentally retarded, but probably many remain undiagnosed. Follow-up studies have shown that 47,XXX girls develop pubertal changes at an appropriate age. Some are capable of reproduction, and virtually all offspring of 47,XXX females are chromosomally normal. About 70 percent of the patients are reported to have learning difficulties,[286] but these may be less severe[276] than originally thought. Severe psychopathology and antisocial behavior appears to be rare; abnormal behavior, while minor, is measurable, particularly during the transition from adolescence to early adulthood.[287]

In 47,XXX cells, two of the X chromosomes are inactivated and late replicating, as suggested originally by the finding of two Barr bodies. Almost all cases result from errors in maternal meiosis and, of these, the majority of the errors are in meiosis I. There is an effect of late maternal age, which is restricted to those patients in whom the error was in maternal meiosis I.[288,289] As in Klinefelter syndrome, maternal meiosis I nondisjunction may be associated with an increase in recombination near the X chromosome centromere.[281]

The tetrasomy X syndrome (48,XXXX) is associated with more serious retardation in both physical and mental development, and the pentasomy X syndrome (49,XXXXX) usually leads to severe developmental retardation with multiple physical defects. The extra X chromosomes are of maternal origin.[284]

Turner Syndrome (45,X)

Unlike patients with other sex chromosome aneuploidies, girls with Turner syndrome can often be identified at birth or before puberty by their distinctive phenotypic features. In liveborn individuals, the phenotype of Turner syndrome includes short stature, ovarian failure, and a number of specific anatomic abnormalities, such as webbed neck, swelling of hands and feet, and coarctation of the aorta.[290,291] The phenotype is presumably due to deficiency for one or more X-linked or Y-linked genes.[13,292] Turner syndrome females are particularly at risk for cardiovascular abnormalities; cardiac screening for both structural and functional defects is recommended.[293] Turner syndrome females account for a significant proportion (estimated to be 6 percent) of all female patients with short stature.[294] The average height is 3 standard deviations below the age-adjusted mean.[295] Growth hormone treatment can lead to an average gain of >6 cm in growth and final adult height, although there is substantial individual variability in this response.[295] A study of morbidity in adult Turner syndrome indicated an increased risk of osteoporotic fractures, diabetes, hypertension, and stroke; average life span was decreased, although risk of cancer was in general not elevated.[296]

The incidence of the Turner syndrome phenotype is approximately 1 in 5000 live female births, much less common than other sex chromosome aneuploidies (Table 61-4). However, at the time of conception, sex chromosome monosomy is much more common, occurring in an estimated 1 to 2 percent of all clinically recognized pregnancies; survival to term is a rare outcome, and over 99 percent of such fetuses abort spontaneously.[269]

The most frequent chromosome constitution in Turner syndrome is 45,X with no second sex chromosome — neither X nor Y.[4] However, about 50 percent of cases have other karyotypes.[269,297,298] About a quarter of Turner syndrome patients have mosaic karyotypes, with only a proportion of cells being 45,X. Other karyotypes include structurally abnormal X chromosomes, such as deletions of the long or short arm, small centric fragments, isochromosomes for the long arm, or X;Y translocations.[269,297] The chromosome constitution is clinically significant.[13] For example, patients with an Xq isochromosome are phenotypically similar to 45,X patients, whereas patients with a deletion of Xp have short stature and congenital malformations, and those with a deletion of Xq often have only gonadal dysfunction. At least 15 percent of females with Turner syndrome contain an isochromosome for Xq, i(Xq). Although these are commonly described as being caused by "misdivision" of the

Table 61-4 Incidence of Sex Chromosome Abnormalities

Sex	Disorder	Karyotype	Incidence
Male	Klinefelter syndrome	47,XXY	1:1,000 males
		48,XXXY	1:25,000 males
		Others	1:10,000 males
	XYY syndrome	47,XYY	1:1,000 males
	Other X or Y chromosome abnormalities		1:1,500 males
	Overall incidence		1:400 males
Female	Turner syndrome	45,X	1:10,000 females
		46,X,i(Xq)	1:50,000 females
		Others	1:15,000 females
	Trisomy X	47,XXX	1:1,000 females
	Other X chromosome abnormalities		1:3,000 females
	Overall incidence		1:650 females

SOURCE: Adapted from Thompson et al.[266]

centromere, the vast majority of i(Xq)'s are dicentric and contain varying amounts of Xp material.[299–301] Thus, aberrant exchange involving sequences in the proximal short arm appears to be the most common mechanism of i(Xq) formation, while misdivision within the centromere proper appears to be quite rare.

In both liveborn and abortus surveys, the single X chromosome in Turner syndrome is maternal in origin in approximately 80 percent of cases;[298,302,303] in other words, the meiotic error is usually paternal. The basis for the unusually high frequency of X or Y chromosome loss in paternal meiosis is unknown. Further, it is not clear why the 45,X karyotype is usually lethal *in utero*, when it is apparently fully compatible with postnatal survival. The parental origin of the single X chromosome has no apparent effect on survival.[304] One suggestion is that survival of a female fetus in early pregnancy depends on the presence of two sex chromosomes, a possibility that derives some support from the high frequency of mosaic karyotypes detected, especially in postnatal surveys.[302,305]

If the Turner syndrome phenotype is due to deficiency of one or more genes, then such genes must reside on both the X and Y chromosomes, because both the X (in the case of normal females) and the Y (in the case of normal males) are capable of "preventing" the lethality *in utero* and the clinical findings associated with Turner syndrome.[290,292] Moreover, because normal females have only one X chromosome active, it must be the inactive X chromosome that protects the fetus from early demise. Such reasoning led Ferguson-Smith to argue that Turner syndrome genes would be among those X-linked genes with Y-linked homologues that escape X chromosome inactivation, even well before the existence of such genes had been demonstrated.[306]

Precise clinical description of patients with and without certain features of Turner syndrome and correlation with molecular description of structural abnormalities of the X chromosome has contributed to the identification of at least some genes thought to be responsible for certain phenotypic effects. In principle, information from such studies may provide information useful for genetic counseling of subjects with partial monosomy X. For example, a novel homeobox gene in the Xp/Yp pseudoautosomal region was implicated in the short stature characteristic of Turner syndrome and other distal Xp chromosome defects.[307–309] Haploinsufficiency for a gene in proximal Xp is associated with ovarian dysfunction, while haploinsufficiency for a pericentromeric gene is tentatively implicated in neck webbing.[309] Based on analysis of 28 apparently nonmosaic cases with partial Xp deletions, one or more Turner syndrome traits (including short stature, ovarian failure, high-arched palate, and autoimmune thyroid disease) could be mapped to the Xp11.2-p22.1 region.[310]

Turner syndrome females have an elevated risk of impaired social adjustment,[286] including significantly low math achievement before age 10.[311] A comparison of Turner syndrome girls with a maternally derived X and those with a paternally derived X provided evidence of significantly worse social cognition skills in those with a maternally derived X.[312] Females with a paternally derived X were better adjusted, with superior verbal and executive function skills that mediate social interactions. Based on this comparison, Skuse et al. suggested the possibility of an X-linked imprinted gene that increases visuospatial memory.[312,313]

Small Ring or Marker X Chromosomes

In additional to those structural abnormalities of the X chromosome discussed earlier [see "Nonrandom (Skewed) X Chromosome Inactivation" and "The X Inactivation Center and the *XIST* Gene" above], several other classes of abnormality are relevant to our current understanding of X chromosome inactivation.

Small ring X chromosomes or centric-marker chromosomes derived from the X are occasionally observed in patients with mental retardation.[314,315] Because mental retardation is not a typical finding of Turner syndrome and the 45,X karyotype, the existence of mental retardation with or without associated physical abnormalities in individuals with 46,X,+marker or 46,X,+ring karyotypes requires explanation. Cohen et al.[316] originally suggested that these small abnormal chromosomes might represent portions of the X chromosome that failed to inactivate because they didn't contain a copy of the X inactivation center. Where analyzed, this hypothesis appears to be supported by molecular and/or cytogenetic studies to examine the presence and/or expression of the *XIST* gene,[317–325] although there are some apparent exceptions.[320,326,327] Some of the uncertainty stems from interpretation of Barr body or late-replication studies. Because small abnormal X chromosomes, if inactivated, may be associated with smaller than normal Barr bodies, and because replication studies of small, centric fragments are difficult, complicated by the typical late replication of centric heterochromatin, it would be valuable to reanalyze as many cases as possible with direct assays for the X inactivation center, using DNA probes from the region (including the *XIST* gene). There are several clearly documented cases that retain the entire *XIST* gene on the marker or ring X, but that fail to express it.[327,328] Migeon et al.[328] have demonstrated directly that several genes normally subject to X inactivation are expressed from ring X chromosomes, thus supporting the functional disomy hypothesis. These findings indicate that studies of *XIST* expression should be performed routinely in cases of 46,X,r(X) karyotypes; normal female levels of *XIST* RNA would be compatible with a typical Turner syndrome phenotype, while absence of *XIST* expression (or absence of the *XIST* gene entirely from the abnormal X) would indicate a more severe phenotype, the severity of which may correlate with the amount of X DNA retained on the ring X.

If the hypothesized association between mental retardation and other abnormalities with ring or marker X chromosomes that fail to undergo X chromosome inactivation is confirmed, then such cases would represent a second class of abnormality due to functional disomy for X-linked genes. Several cases of unbalanced X;autosome translocation have been described in which a portion of the X chromosome is apparently expressed from two copies of the X — a normal X chromosome and the translocated portion of the X separated from the X inactivation center.[165–167] The existence of such patients reinforces the significance of and requirement for X chromosome inactivation in normal female development. Such patients also offer an opportunity to explore phenotype-karyotype correlations for regions of the X chromosome inappropriately expressed as a consequence of failure of X chromosome inactivation.[321,323]

ACKNOWLEDGMENTS

The author thanks Drs. Laura Carrel and Robert Plenge for helpful discussions and Dr. Laura Carrel for numerous contributions to this chapter.

REFERENCES

1. Painter TS: The Y chromosome in mammals. *Science* **53**:503, 1921.
2. Barr ML, Bertram EG: A morphological distinction between neurones of the male and female, and the behaviour of the nucleolar satellite during accelerated nucleoprotein synthesis. *Nature* **163**:676, 1949.
3. Jacobs PA, Strong JA: A case of human sexuality having a possible XXY sex determining mechanism. *Nature* **183**:302, 1959.
4. Ford CE, Jones K, Polani P, de Almeida JC, Briggs JH: A sex chromosome anomaly in a case of gonadal dysgenesis (Turner syndrome). *Lancet* **1**:711, 1959.
5. Burgoyne PS: The role of Y-encoded genes in mammalian spermatogenesis. *Semin Cell Dev Biol* **9**:423, 1998.
6. Burgoyne PS: The mammalian Y chromosome, a new perspective. *Bioessays* **20**:363, 1998.
7. Ramkisoon Y, Goodfellow P: Early steps in mammalian sex determination. *Curr Opin Genet Dev* **6**:316, 1996.
8. Graves JAM, Wakefield MJ, Toder R: The origin and evolution of the pseudoautosomal regions of the human sex chromosomes. *Hum Mol Genet* **7**:1991, 1998.
9. Foote S, Vollrath D, Hilton A, Page DC: The human Y chromosome: overlapping DNA clones spanning the euchromatic region. *Science* **258**:60, 1992.
10. Vogt PH, Affara N, Davey P, Hammer M, Jobling MA, Lau YF, Mitchell M, et al.: Report of the Third International Workshop on Y Chromosome Mapping 1997. *Cytogenet Cell Genet* **79**:1, 1997.
11. Lahn BT, Page DC: Functional coherence of the human Y chromosome. *Science* **278**:675, 1997.
12. Vollrath D, Foote S, Hilton A, Brown LG, Beer-Romano P, Bogan JS, Page DC: The human Y chromosome: A 43-interval map based on naturally occurring deletions. *Science* **258**:52,1992.
13. Ferguson-Smith MA: Genotype-phenotype correlations in individuals with disorders of sex determination and development including Turner syndrome. *Semin Dev Biol* **2**:265, 1991.
14. Cooke HJ, Elliott DJ: RNA-binding proteins and human male infertility. *Trends Genet* **13**:87, 1997.
15. DeLoukas P, Schuler DB, Gyapay G, Beasley EM, Soderlund C, Rodriquez-Tome P, Hui L, et al.: A physical map of 30,000 human genes. *Science* **282**:744, 1998.
16. McKusick VA: *Mendelian Inheritance in Man. Catalogs of Human Genes and Genetic Disorders*, 12th ed. Baltimore, Johns Hopkins University Press, 1998.
17. Watanabe M, Zinn AR, Page DC, Nishimoto T: Functional equivalence of human X- and Y-encoded isoforms of ribosomal protein S4 consistent with a role in Turner syndrome. *Nat Genet* **4**:268, 1993.
18. Schwartz A, Chan DC, Brown LG, Alagappan R, Pettay D, Disteche C, McGillivray B, et al.: Reconstructing hominid Y evolution: X-homologous block, created by XY transposition, was disrupted by Yp inversion through LINE-LINE recombination. *Hum Mol Genet* **7**:1, 1998.
19. Mitchell MJ, Wilcox SA, Watson JM, Lerner JL, Woods DR, Scheffler J, Hearn FP, et al.: The origin and loss of the ubiquitin activating enzyme gene on the mammalian Y chromosome. *Hum Mol Genet* **7**:429, 1998.
20. Belin V, Cusin V, Viot G, Girlich D, Toutain A, Moncla A, Vekemans M, et al.: SHOX mutations in dyschondrosteosis (Leri-Weill syndrome). *Nat Genet* **19**:67, 1998.
21. Shears DJ, Vassal HJ, Goodman FR, Palmer RW, Reardon W, Superti-Furga A, Scambler PJ, et al.: Mutation and deletion of the pseudoautosomal gene SHOX cause Leri-Weill dyschondrosteosis. *Nat Genet* **19**:70, 1998.
22. Wapenaar MC, Bassi MT, Schaefer L, Grillo A, Gerrero GB, Chinault AC, Ballabio A, et al.: The genes for X-linked ocular albinism and microphthalmia with linear skin defects: Cloning and characterization of the critical regions. *Hum Mol Genet* **2**:947, 1993.
23. Franco B, Meroni G, Parenti G, Levilliers J, Bernard L, Gebbia M, Cox L, et al.: A cluster of sulfatase genes on Xp22.3: Mutations in chondrodysplasia punctata (CDPX) and implications for warfarin embryopathy. *Cell* **81**:15, 1995.
24. Lyon MF: Gene action in the X-chromosome of the mouse (Mus musculus L.). *Nature* **190**:372, 1961.
25. Beutler E, Yeh M, Fairbanks VF: The normal human female as a mosaic of X-chromosome activity: Studies using the gene for G-6-PD-deficiency as a marker. *Proc Natl Acad Sci U S A* **48**:9, 1962.
26. Lyon MF: X chromosome inactivation and developmental patterns in mammals. *Biol Rev* **47**:1, 1972.
27. Gartler SM, Riggs AD: Mammalian X-chromosome inactivation. *Ann Rev Genet* **17**:155, 1983.
28. Riggs AD, Pfeifer GP: X chromosome inactivation and cell memory. *Trends Genet* **8**:169, 1992.
29. Brown CJ, Willard HF: Molecular and genetic studies of human X chromosome inactivation. *Adv Dev Biol* **2**:37, 1993.
30. Heard E, Clerc P, Avner P: X chromosome inactivation in mammals. *Ann Rev Genet* **31**:571, 1997.
31. Taylor JH: Asynchronous duplication of chromosomes in cultured cells of Chinese hamster. *Biophys Biochem Cytol* **7**:455, 1960.
32. Gilbert CW, Muldal S, Lajthal LG, Rowley J: Time-sequence of human chromosome duplication. *Nature* **195**:869, 1962.
33. Morishma A, Grumbach MM, Taylor JH: Asynchronous duplication of human chromosomes and the origin of sex chromatin. *Proc Natl Acad Sci U S A* **48**:756, 1962.
34. German J: The pattern of DNA synthesis in the chromosomes of human blood cells. *J Cell Biol* **20**:37, 1964.
35. Latt SA: Microfluorometric detection of deoxyribonucleic acid replication in human metaphase chromosomes. *Proc Natl Acad Sci U S A* **70**:3395, 1973.
36. Willard HF, Latt SA: Analysis of deoxyribonucleic acid replication in human X chromosomes by fluorescence microscopy. *Am J Hum Genet* **28**:213, 1976.
37. Hansen RS, Canfield TK, Fjeld AD, Gartler SM: Role of late replication timing in the silencing of X-linked genes. *Hum Mol Genet* **5**:1345, 1996.
38. Holmquist GP: Role of replication time in the control of tissue-specific gene expression. *Am J Hum Genet* **40**:151, 1987.
39. Riggs AD: DNA methylation and late replication probably aid cell memory, and type I DNA reeling could aid chromosome folding and enhancer function. *Philos Trans R Soc Lond B Biol Sci* **326**:285, 1990.
40. Holliday R, Pugh JE: DNA modification mechanisms and gene activity during development. *Science* **187**:226, 1975.
41. Riggs AD: X inactivation, differentiation, and DNA methylation. *Cytogenet Cell Genet* **14**:9, 1975.
42. Sager R, Kichen R: Selective silencing of eukaryotic DNA. *Science* **189**:426, 1975.
43. Chapman VM, Kratzer PG, Siracusa LD, Quarantillo BA, Evans R, Liskay RM: Evidence for DNA modification in the maintenance of X-chromosome inactivation of adult mouse tissues. *Proc Natl Acad Sci U S A* **79**:5357, 1982.
44. Mohandas T, Sparkes RS, Shapiro LJ: Reactivation of an inactive human X chromosome: Evidence for X inactivation by DNA methylation. *Science* **211**:393, 1981.
45. Venolia L, Gartler SM, Wassman ER, Yen P, Mohandas T, Shapiro LJ: Transformation with DNA from 5-azacytidine-reactivated X chromosomes. *Proc Natl Acad Sci U S A* **79**:2352, 1982.
46. Pfeifer GP, Steigerwald SD, Hansen RS, Gartler SM, Riggs AD: Polymerase chain reaction-aided genomic sequencing of an X chromosome-linked CpG island: Methylation patterns suggest clonal inheritance, CpG site autonomy, and an explanation of activity state stability. *Proc Natl Acad Sci U S A* **87**:8252, 1990.
47. Antequera F, Bird AP: CpG islands, in Jost, JP, Saluz HP (eds): *DNA Methylation: Molecular Biology and Biological Significance*. Basel, Birkhauser Verlag, 1993, p 169.
48. Kerem B-S, Goten R, Richler C, Marcus M, Cedar H: In situ nick-translation distinguishes between active and inactive X chromosomes. *Nature* **304**:88, 1983.
49. Sperling K, Kerem B-S, Goiten R, Kottusch V, Cedar H, Marcus M: DNase I sensitivity in facultative and constitutive heterochromatin. *Chromosoma* **93**:38, 1985.
50. Wolf SF, Migeon BR: Cluster of CpG dinucleotides implicated by nuclease hypersensitivity as control elements of housekeeping genes. *Nature* **314**:467, 1985.
51. Yang TP, Caskey T: Nuclease sensitivity of the mouse HPRT gene promoter region: Differential sensitivity on the active and inactive X chromosomes. *Mol Cell Biol* **7**:2994, 1987.
52. Zhang X-Y, Ehrlich KC, Wang RY-H, Ehrlich M: Effect of site-specific DNA methylation and mutagenesis on recognition by methylated DNA-binding protein from human placenta. *Nucleic Acids Res* **14**:8387, 1986.

53. Meehan RR, Lewis JD, McKay S, Kleiner EL, Bird AP: Identification of a mammalian protein that binds specifically to DNA containing methylated CpGs. *Cell* **58**:499, 1989.
54. Boyes J, Bird A: DNA methylation inhibits transcription indirectly via a methyl-CpG binding protein. *Cell* **64**:1123, 1991.
55. Antequera F, Macloeod D, Bird AP: Specific protection of methylated CpGs in mammalian nuclei. *Cell* **58**:509, 1989.
56. Jeppesen P, Turner BM: The inactive X chromosome in female mammals is distinguished by a lack of H4 acetylation, a cytogenetic marker for gene expression. *Cell* **74**:281, 1993.
57. Boggs BA, Connors B, Sobel RE, Chinault AC, Allis CD: Reduced levels of histone H3 acetylation on the inactive X chromosome in human females. *Chromosoma* **105**:303, 1996.
58. Keohane AM, Barlow AL, Waters J, Bourn D, Turner BM: H4 acetylation, XIST RNA and replication timing are coincident and define X;autosome boundaries in two abnormal X chromosomes. *Hum Mol Genet* **8**:377, 1999.
59. Wakefield MJ, Keohane AM, Turner BM, Graves JAM: Histone underacetylation is an ancient component of mammalian X chromosome inactivation. *Proc Natl Acad Sci U S A* **94**:9665, 1997.
60. Costanzi C, Pehrson JR: Histone macroH2A1 is concentrated in the inactive X chromosome of female mammals. *Nature* **393**:599, 1998.
61. Eils R, Dietzel S, Bertin E, Schrock E, Speicher MR, Ried T, Robert-Nicoud M, et al.: Three-dimensional reconstruction of painted human interphase chromosomes: Active and inactive X chromosome territories have similar volumes but differ in shape and surface structure. *J Cell Biol* **135**:1427, 1996.
62. Walker CL, Cargile CB, Floy KM, Delannoy M, Migeon BR: The Barr body is a looped X chromosome formed by telomere association. *Proc Natl Acad Sci U S A* **88**:6191, 1991.
63. Dietzel S, Eils R, Satzler K, Bornfleth H, Jauch A, Cremer C, Cremer T: Evidence against a looped structure of the inactive human X chromosome territory. *Exp Cell Res* **240**:187, 1998.
64. Disteche CM: Escape from X inactivation in human and mouse. *Trends Genet* **11**:17, 1995.
65. Brown CJ, Carrel L, Willard HF: Expression of genes from the human active and inactive X chromosomes. *Am J Hum Genet* **60**:1333, 1997.
66. Lyon MF: Sex chromatin and gene action in the mammalian X-chromosome. *Am J Hum Genet* **14**:135, 1962.
67. Schempp W, Meer B: Cytologic evidence for three human X chromosomal segments escaping inactivation. *Hum Genet* **63**:171, 1983.
68. Therman E, Sarto GE, Disteche C, Denniston C: A possible active segment on the inactive human X chromosome. *Chromosoma* **59**:137, 1976.
69. Davidson RG, Nitowsky HM, Childs B: Demonstration of two populations of cells in the human female heterozygous for glucose-6-phosphate dehydrogenase variants. *Proc Natl Acad Sci U S A* **50**:481, 1963.
70. Curnutte JT, Hopkins PJ, Kuhl W, Beutler E: Studying X inactivation. *Lancet* **339**:749, 1992.
71. Carrel L, Willard HF: Heterogeneous gene expression from the inactive X chromosome: An X-linked gene that escapes X inactivation in some cell lines but is inactivated in others. *Proc Natl Acad Sci U S A* **96**:7364, 1999.
72. Rupert JL, Brown CJ, Willard HF: Direct detection of nonrandom X chromosome inactivation by use of a transcribed polymorphism in the XIST gene. *Eur J Hum Genet* **3**:333, 1995.
73. Harrison CN, Gale RE, Linch DC: Quantification of X chromosome inactivation patterns using RT-PCR of the polymorphic iduronate-2-sulfatase gene and correlation of the results obtained with DNA-based techniques. *Leukemia* **12**:1834, 1998.
74. Shapiro LJ, Mohandas T, Weiss R, Romeo G: Non-inactivation of an X-linked chromosome locus in man. *Science* **204**:1224, 1979.
75. Brown RM, Dahl HHM, Brown GK: X-chromosome localization of the functional gene for the E1α subunit of the human pyruvate dehydrogenase complex. *Genomics* **4**:174, 1989.
76. Arahata K, Ishihara T, Kamakura K, Tsukahara T, Ishiura S, Baba C, Matsumoto T, Nonaka I, Sugita H: Mosaic expression of dystrophin in symptomatic carriers of Duchenne muscular dystrophy. *N Engl J Med* **320**:138, 1989.
77. Hurko O, Hoffman EP, McKee L, Johns DR, Kunkel LM: Dystrophin analysis in clonal myoblasts derived from a Duchenne muscular dystrophy carrier. *Am J Hum Genet* **44**:820, 1989.
78. Baader SL, Schilling ML, Rosengarten B, Pretsch W, Teutsch FH, Oberdick J, Schilling K: Purkinje cell lineage and the topographic organization of the cerebellar cortex: A view from X inactivation mosaics. *Dev Biol* **174**:393, 1996.
79. Meyer WJI, Migeon BR, Migeon CJ: Locus on human X chromosome for dihydrotestosterone receptor and androgen insensitivity. *Proc Natl Acad Sci U S A* **72**:1469, 1975.
80. Romeo G, Migeon BR: Genetic inactivation of the alpha-galactosidase locus in carriers of Fabry's disease. *Science* **170**:180, 1970.
81. Yen RCK, Adams WB, Lazar C, Becker MA: Evidence for X-linkage of human phosphoribosylpyrophosphate synthetase. *Proc Natl Acad Sci U S A* **75**:482, 1978.
82. Nyhan WL, Bakay B, Connor JD, Markes JF, Keele DK: Hemizygous expression of glucose-6-phosphate dehydrogenase in erythrocytes of heterozygotes for the Lesch-Nyhan syndrome. *Proc Natl Acad Sci U S A* **65**:214, 1970.
83. Rosenbloom FM, Kelley WN, Henderson JF, Seegmiller JE: Lyon hypothesis and X-linked disease. *Lancet* **ii**:305, 1967.
84. Salzmann J, DeMars R, Benke P: Single-allele expression at an X-linked hyperuricemia locus in heterozygous human cells. *Proc Natl Acad Sci U S A* **60**:545, 1968.
85. Linder D, Gartler SM: Glucose-6-phosphate dehydrogenase mosaicism: Utilization as a cell marker in the study of leiomyomas. *Science* **150**:67, 1965.
86. Danes BS, Bearn AG: Hurler's syndrome: A genetic study of clones in cell culture with particular reference to the Lyon hypothesis. *J Exp Med* **126**:509, 1967.
87. Capobianchi MR, Romeo G: Mosaicism for sulfoiduronate sulfatase deficiency in carriers of Hunter's syndrome. *Experentia* **32**:459, 1976.
88. Migeon BR, Sprenkle JA, Liebaers I, Scott JF, Neufeld EF: X-linked Hunter syndrome: The heterozygous phenotype in cell culture. *Am J Hum Genet* **29**:448, 1977.
89. Windhorst DB, Holmes B, Good RA: A newly defined X-linked trait in man with demonstration of the Lyon effect in carrier females. *Lancet* **i**:723, 1967.
90. Beuscher ES, Allings DW, Gallin JI: Use of an X-linked human neutrophil marker to estimate timing of lyonization and size of the dividing stem cell pool. *J Clin Invest* **76**:1581, 1985.
91. Ricciuti FC, Gelehrter TD, Rosenberg LE: X-chromosome inactivation in human liver: Confirmation of X-linkage of ornithine transcarbamylase. *Am J Hum Genet* **28**:332, 1976.
92. Gartler SM, Chen S-H, Fialkow PJ, Giblett ER: X chromosome inactivation in cells from an individual heterozygous for two X-linked genes. *Nat New Biol* **236**:149, 1972.
93. Migeon BR, Huijing F: Glycogen-storage disease associated with phosphorylase kinase deficiency: Evidence for X inactivation. *Am J Hum Genet* **26**:360, 1974.
94. Kirchgessner CU, Warren ST, Willard HF: X inactivation of the FMR1 fragile X mental retardation gene. *J Med Genet* **32**:925, 1995.
95. Schneider-Gadicke A, Beer-Romero P, Brown LG, Nussbaum R, Page DC: The ZFX gene on the human X chromosome escapes X inactivation and is closely related to ZFY, the putative sex determinant on the Y chromosome. *Cell* **57**:1247, 1989.
96. Fisher EMC, Beer-Romero P, Brown LG, Ridley A, McNeil JA, Lawrence JB, Willard HF, Bieber FR, Page DC: Homologous ribosomal protein genes on the human X and Y chromosomes: Escape from X inactivation and implications for Turner syndrome. *Cell* **63**:1205, 1990.
97. Migeon BR, Shapiro LJ, Norum RA, Mohandas T, Axelman J, Dabora RL: Differential expression of steroid sulphatase locus on active and inactive human X chromosome. *Nature* **299**:838, 1982.
98. Carrel L, Hunt PA, Willard HF: Tissue- and lineage-specific variation in inactive X chromosome expression of the murine Smcx gene. *Hum Mol Genet* **5**:1361, 1996.
99. Sheardown S, Norris D, Fisher A, Brockdorf N: The mouse Smcx gene exhibits developmental and tissue specific variation in degree of escape from X inactivation. *Hum Mol Genet* **5**:1355, 1996.
100. Esposito T, Gianfrancesco F, Diccodicola A, D'Esposito M, Nagaraja R, Mazzarella R, D'Urso M, et al.: Escape from X inactivation of two new genes associated with DXS6974E and DXS7020E. *Genomics* **43**:183, 1997.
101. Happle R: Skin markers of X-linked dominant chondrodysplasia punctata. *Arch Dermatol* **115**:931, 1979.
102. Witkop CJ: Partial expression of sex-linked recessive amelogenesis imperfecta in females compatible with the Lyon hypothesis. *Oral Surg* **23**:174, 1967.
103. Maguire AM , Maumenee IH: Iris pigment mosaicism in carriers of X-linked ocular albinism cum pigmento. *Am J Ophthal* **107**:298, 1989.

104. Falls HF, Cotterman CW: Choroidoretinal degeneration: A sex-linked form in which heterozygous women exhibit a tapetal-like reflex. *Arch Ophthal* **40**:685, 1984.
105. Jay B: X-linked retinal disorders and the Lyon hypothesis. *Trans Ophthalmol Soc UK* **104**:836, 1985.
106. Passerge E, Fries E: X chromosome inactivation in X-linked hypohidrotic ectodermal dysplasia. *Nat New Biol* **245**:58, 1973.
107. Gardner RJM, Brown N: Lowe's syndrome: Identification of carriers by lens examination. *J Med Genet* **13**:449, 1976.
108. Wieacker P, Zimmer J, Ropers HH: X inactivation patterns in two syndromes with probable X-linked dominant, male lethal inheritance. *Clin Genet* **28**:238, 1985.
109. Macias-Flores MA, Garcia-Cruz, Rivera H, Escobar-Lujan M, Melendrez-Vega A, Rivas-Campos D, Rodriguez-Collaco F, Morenao-Arellano I, Cantu JM: A new form of hypertrichosis inherited as an X-linked dominant trait. *Hum Genet* **66**:66, 1984.
110. Karna J: Choroideremia, a clinical and genetic study of 84 Finnish patients and 126 female carriers. *Acta Ophthalmol* **176**:1, 1986.
111. Pinkerton PH: X-linked hypochromic anaemia. *Lancet* **i**:1106, 1967.
112. Kashtan C, Fish AJ, Kleppel M, Yoshioka K, Michael AF: Nephritogenic antigen determinants in epidermal and renal basement membranes of kindreds with Alport-type familial nephritis. *J Clin Invest* **78**:1035, 1986.
113. Belmont JW: Genetic control of X inactivation and processes leading to X inactivation skewing. *Am J Hum Genet* **58**:1101, 1996.
114. Puck JM, Willard HF: X inactivation in females with X-linked disease. *N Engl J Med* **338**:325, 1998.
115. Belmont JW: Insights into lymphocyte development from X-linked immune deficiencies. *Trends Genet* **11**:112, 1995.
116. Migeon BR, Axelman J, de Beur SJ, Valle D, Mitchell GA, Rosenbaum KN: Selection against lethal alleles in females heterozygous for incontinentia pigmenti. *Am J Hum Genet* **44**:100, 1989.
117. Parrish JE, Scheuerle AE, Lewis RA, Levy ML, Nelson DL: Selection against mutant alleles in blood leukocytes is a consistent feature in incontinentia pigmenti type 2. *Hum Mol Genet* **5**:1777, 1996.
118. Vulliamy TJ, Knight SW, Dokal I, Mason PJ: Skewed X inactivation in carriers of X-linked dyskeratosis congenita. *Blood* **90**:2213, 1997.
119. Devriendt K, Matthijs G, Legius E, Schollen E, Blockmans D, van Geet C, Degreef H, et al.: Skewed X chromosome inactivation in female carriers of dyskeratosis congenita. *Am J Hum Genet* **60**:581, 1997.
120. Ferraris AM, Forni GL, Mangerini R, Gaetani GF: Nonrandom X chromosome inactivation in hemopoietic cells from carriers of dyskeratosis congenita. *Am J Hum Genet* **61**:458, 1997.
121. Orstavik KH, Orstavik RE, Naumova AK, D'Adamo P, Gedeon A, Bolhuis PA, Barth PG, Toniolo D: X chromosome inactivation in carriers of Barth syndrome. *Am J Hum Genet* **63**:1457, 1998.
122. Orstavik KH, Orstavik RE, Eiklid K, Transbjaerg L: Inheritance of skewed X chromosome inactivation in a large family with an X-linked recessive deafness syndrome. *Am J Med Genet* **64**:31, 1996.
123. Plenge RM, Tranebjaerg L, Jensen PKA, Schwartz C, Willard HF: Evidence that mutations in the X-linked DDP gene cause incompletely penetrant and variable skewed X inactivation. *Am J Hum Genet* **64**:759, 1999.
124. Gibbons RJ, Suthers GK, Wilkie OM, Buckle VJ, Higgs DR: X-linked alpha thalassemia/mental retardation syndrome: Localization to Xq12-q21.31 by X inactivation and linkage analysis. *Am J Hum Genet* **51**:1136, 1992.
125. Ploos van Amstel JK, Terhal PA, VandenBoogaard M, Hennekam R, Beemer F, Pearson PL, Sinke RJ: Skewed X inactivation in a large family with Wilson-Turner syndrome [Abstract]. *Am J Hum Genet* **63**:A380, 1998.
126. Filosa S, Giacometti N, Wangwei C, De Mattia D, Pagnini D, Alfinito F, Schettini F, et al.: Somatic cell selection is a major determinant of the blood cell phenotype in heterozygotes for glucose-6-phosphate dehydrogenase mutations causing severe enzyme deficiency. *Am J Hum Genet* **59**:887, 1996.
127. Winkelstein JA, Fearon E: Carrier detection of the X-linked primary immunodeficiency diseases using X chromosome inactivation analysis. *J Allergy Clin Immunol* **85**:1090, 1990.
128. Puck JM: The role of molecular genetics in carrier detection and prenatal diagnosis of immunodeficiencies. *Curr Opin Pediatr* **3**:855, 1993.
129. Revesz R, Schuler D, Goldschmidt B, Elodi S: Extreme bias in X inactivation in a female with hemophilia B. *J Med Genet* **9**:396, 1972.
130. Moser H, Emery A: The manifesting carrier in Duchenne muscular dystrophy. *Clin Genet* **5**:271, 1974.
131. Dusi S, Poli G, Berton G, Catalano P, Fornasa C, Peserico A: Chronic granulomatous disease in an adult female with granulomatous cheilitis: Evidence for an X-linked pattern of inheritance with extreme lyonization. *Acta Haematol* **84**:49, 1990.
132. Matthews PM, Benjamin D, Van Bakel I, Squier MV, Nicholson LV, Sewry C, Barnes PR, Hopkin J, Brown R, Hilton-Jones D, et al.: Muscle X inactivation patterns and dystrophin expression in Duchenne muscular dystrophy carriers. *Neuromuscul Disord* **5**:209, 1995.
133. Bottomley SS, Wise PD, Wasson EG, Carpenter NJ: X-linked sideroblastic anemia in ten female probands due to ALAS2 mutations and skewed X chromosome inactivation [Abstract]. *Am J Hum Genet* **63**:A352, 1998.
134. Yoshioka M, Yorifuji T, Mituyoshi I: Skewed X inactivation in manifesting carriers of Duchenne muscular dystrophy. *Clin Genet* **53**:102, 1998.
135. Chan V, Chan VW, Yip B, Chim CS, Chan TK: Hemophilia B in a female carrier due to skewed inactivation of the normal X chromosome. *Am J Hematol* **58**:72, 1998.
136. Guo C, Van Damme B, Vanrenterghem Y, Devriendt K, Cassiman JJ, Marynen P: Severe Alport phenotype in a woman with two missense mutations in the same COL4A5 gene and preponderant inactivation of the X chromosome carrying the normal allele. *J Clin Invest* **95**:1832, 1995.
137. Nomura Y, Onigata K, Nagashima T, Yutani S, Mochizuki H, Nagashima K, Morikawa A: Detection of skewed X inactivation in two female carriers of vasopressin type 2 receptor gene mutation. *J Clin Endocrinol Metab* **82**:3434, 1997.
138. Aral B, de Saint Basile G, Al-Garawi S, Kamoun P, Ceballos-Picot I: Novel nonsense mutation in the HPRT gene and nonrandom X inactivation causing Lesch-Nyhan syndrome in a female patient. *Hum Mutat* **7**:52, 1996.
139. Rousseau F, Heitz D, Oberle I, Mandel J-L: Selection in blood cells from female carriers of the fragile X syndrome: Inverse correlation between age and proportion of active X chromosomes carrying the full mutation. *J Med Genet* **28**:830, 1991.
140. Rowe PC, Newman SL, Brusilow SW: Natural history of symptomatic partial ornithine transcarbamylase deficiency. *N Engl J Med* **314**:541, 1986.
141. Batshaw ML, Msall M, Beaudet AL, Trojak J: Risk of serious illness in heterozygotes for ornithine transcarbamylase deficiency. *J Pediatr* **108**:236, 1986.
142. Brown RM, Fraser NJ, Brown GK: Differential methylation of the hypervariable locus DXS255 on active and inactive X chromosomes correlates with the expression of a human X-linked gene. *Genomics* **7**:215, 1990.
143. Brown RM, Brown GK: X chromosome inactivation and the diagnosis of X-linked disease in females. *J Med Genet* **30**:177, 1993.
144. Nakanishi K, Iijima K, Kuroda N, Inoue Y, Sado Y, Nakamura H, Yoshikawa N: Comparison of alpha5(IV) collagen chain expression in skin with disease severity in women with X-linked Alport syndrome. *J Am Soc Nephrol* **9**:1433, 1998.
145. Went LN, DeGroot WP, Sanger R, Tippett P, Gavin J: X-linked ichthyosis: Linkage relationship with the Xg blood groups and other studies in a large Dutch kindred. *Ann Hum Genet* **32**:333, 1969.
146. Sparkes RS, Simpson RW, Paulsen CA: Familial hypogonadotropic hypogonadism with anosmia. *Arch Intern Med* **121**:534, 1968.
147. Franco B, Guioli S, Pragliolоa A, Incerti B, Bardoni B, Tonlorenzi R, Carrozzo R, et al.: A gene deleted in Kallmann's syndrome shares homology with neural cell adhesion and axonal path-finding molecules. *Nature* **353**:529, 1991.
148. Legouis R, Haardelin JP, Levillers J, Claverie JM, Compain S, Wunderle V, Millasseau P, et al.: The candidate gene for the X-linked Kallmann syndrome encodes a protein related to adhesion molecules. *Cell* **67**:423, 1991.
149. Seabra MC, Borwn MS, Goldstein JL: Retinal degeneration in choroideremia: Deficiency of Rab geranylgeranyltransferase. *Science* **259**:377, 1993.
150. Fialkow PJ: Primordial cell pool size and lineage relationships of five human cell types. *Ann Hum Genet* **37**:39, 1973.
151. Puck JM, Stewart CC, Nussbaum RL: Maximum likelihood analysis of human T-cell X chromosome inactivation patterns: Normal women versus carriers of X-linked severe combined immunodeficiency. *Am J Hum Genet* **50**:742, 1992.
152. Tonon L, Bergamaschi G, Dellavecchia C, Rosti V, Lucotti C, Malabarba L, Novella A, et al.: Unbalanced X chromosome inactivation in haemopoietic cells from normal women. *Br J Haematol* **102**:996, 1998.

153. Gale RE, Wheaden H, Boulos P, Linch DC: Tissue specificity of X chromosome inactivation patterns. *Blood* **83**:2899, 1994.
154. Lau AW, Brown CJ, Penaherrera M, Langlois S, Kalousek DK, Robinson WP: Skewed X chromosome inactivation is common in fetuses or newborns associated with confined placental mosaicism. *Am J Hum Genet* **61**:1353, 1997.
155. Vogelstein B, Fearon ER, Hamilton SR, Feinberg AP: Use of restriction fragment length polymorphisms to determine the clonal origin of human tumors. *Science* **227**:642, 1985.
156. Maestrini E, Rivella S. Tribioli C, Rocchi M, Camerino G, Santachiara-Benerecetti S, Parolini O, et al.: Identification of novel RFLPs in the vicinity of CpG islands in Xq28: Application to the analysis of the pattern of X chromosome inactivation. *Am J Hum Genet* **50**:156, 1992.
157. Hendriks RW, Chen ZY, Hinds H, Schuurman RKB, Craig IW: An X chromosome inactivation assay based on differential methylation of a CpG island coupled to a VNTR polymorphism at the 5′ end of the monoamine oxidase A gene. *Hum Mol Genet* **1**:187, 1992.
158. Carrel L, Willard HF: An assay for X inactivation based on differential methylation at the fragile X locus, FMR1. *Am J Med Genet* **64**:27, 1996.
159. Allen RC, Zoghbi HY, Moseley AB, Rosenblatt HM, Belmont JW: Methylation of HpaII and HhaI sites near the polymorphic CAG repeat in the human androgen-receptor gene correlates with X chromosome inactivation. *Am J Hum Genet* **51**:1229, 1992.
160. Plenge RM, Hendrich BD, Schwartz C, Arena JF, Naumova A, Sapienza C, Winter RM, Willard HF: A promoter mutation in the XIST gene in two unrelated families with skewed X chromosome inactivation. *Nat Genet* **17**:353, 1997.
161. Naumova AK, Plenge RM, Bird LM, Leppert M, Morgan K, Willard HF, Sapienza C: Heritability of X chromosome inactivation phenotype in a large family. *Am J Hum Genet* **58**:1111, 1996.
162. Lanasa MC, Hogge WA, Kubik CJ, Ness RJ, Hoffman EP: A subset of recurrent spontaneous abortion is caused by X-linked lethal traits [Abstract]. *Am J Hum Genet* **63**:A6, 1998.
163. El Kassar N, Hetet G, Briere J, Grandchamp B: X chromosome inactivation in healthy females: Incidence of excessive lyonization with age and comparison of assays involving DNA methylation and transcript polymorphisms. *Clin Chem* **44**:61, 1998.
164. Busque L, Mio R, Mattioli J, Brais E, Blais N, Lalonde Y, Maragh M, Gilliland DG: Nonrandom X inactivation patterns in normal females: Lyonization ratios vary with age. *Blood* **88**:59, 1996.
165. Gale RE, Mein CA, Linch DC: Quantification of X chromosome inactivation patterns in haematological samples using the DNA PCR-based HUMARA assay. *Leukemia* **10**:362, 1996.
166. Pegoraro E, Whitaker J, Mowery-Rushton P, Surti U, Lanasa M, Hoffman EP: Familial skewed X inactivation: A molecular trait associated with high spontaneous abortion rate maps to Xq28. *Am J Hum Genet* **61**:160, 1997.
167. Migeon BR: Studies of skin fibroblasts from 10 families with HGPRT deficiency, with reference to X chromosomal inactivation. *Am J Hum Genet* **23**:199, 1971.
168. Nance WE: Genetic tests with a sex-linked marker, glucose-6-phosphate dehydrogenase. *Cold Spring Harb Symp Quant Biol* **29**:415, 1964.
169. Coleman R, Genet SA, Harper JI, Wilkie AOM: Interaction of incontinentia pigmenti and factor VIII mutations in a female with biased X inactivation, resulting in haemophilia. *J Med Genet* **30**:497, 1993.
170. Nisen PD, Waber PG: Nonrandom X chromosome DNA methylation patterns in hemophiliac females. *J Clin Invest* **83**:1400, 1989.
171. Kling S, Coffey AJ, Ljung R, Sjorin E, Nilsson IM, Holberg L, Giannelli F: Moderate haemophilia B in a female carrier caused by preferential inactivation of the paternal X chromosome. *Eur J Haematol* **47**:257, 1991.
172. Ruttum MS, Lewandowski MF, Bateman JB: Affected females in X-linked congenital stationary night blindness. *Ophthalmol* **99**:747, 1992.
173. Migeon BR, Axelman J, Stetten G: Clonal evolution in human lymphoblast cultures. *Am J Hum Genet* **42**:742, 1988.
174. Reddy BK, Anandavalli TE, Reddi OS: X-linked Duchenne muscular dystrophy in an unusual family with manifesting carriers. *Hum Genet* **67**:460, 1984.
175. Taylor SAM, Deugau KV, Lillicrap DP: Somatic mosaicism and female-to-female transmission in a kindred with hemophilia B (factor IX deficiency). *Proc Natl Acad Sci U S A* **88**:39, 1991.
176. Marcus S, Steen AM, Andersson B, Lambert B, Kristoffersson U, Francke U: Mutation analysis and prenatal diagnosis in a Lesch-Nyhan family showing nonrandom X inactivation interfering with carrier detection tests. *Hum Genet* **89**:395, 1992.
177. Ingerslev J, Schwartz M, Lamm LU, Kruse TA, Bukh A, Stenbjerg S: Female hemophilia A in a family with seeming extreme bidirectional lyonization tendency: Abnormal premature X chromosome inactivation? *Clin Genet* **35**:41, 1989.
178. Ropers HH, Wienker TF, Grimm T, Schroetter K, Bender K: Evidence for preferential X chromosome inactivation in a family with Fabry disease. *Am J Hum Genet* **29**:361, 1977.
179. Parolini O, Ressmann G, Haas OA, Pawlowsky J, Gadner H, Knapp W, Holter W: X-linked Wiskott-Aldrich syndrome in a girl. *N Engl J Med* **338**:291, 1998.
180. Cattanach BM, Pollard CE, Perez JN: Controlling elements in the mouse X-chromosome 1. Interaction with X-linked genes. *Genet Res* **14**:223, 1969.
181. Azofeifa J, Voit T, Hubner C, Cremer M: X chromosome methylation in manifesting and healthy carriers of dystrophinopathies: Concordance of activation ratios among first-degree female relatives and skewed inactivation as cause of their affected phenotypes. *Hum Genet* **96**:167, 1995.
182. Naumova AK, Olien L, Bird LM, Smith M, Verner AE, Leppert M, Morgan K, Sapienza C: Genetic mapping of X-linked loci involved in skewing of X chromosome inactivation in the human. *Eur J Hum Genet* **6**:552, 1999.
183. Richards CS, Watkins SC, Hoffman EP, Schneider NR, Milsark W, Katz KS, Cook JD, Kunkel LM, Cortada JM: Skewed X inactivation in a female MZ twin results in Duchenne muscular dystrophy. *Am J Hum Genet* **46**:672, 1990.
184. Lupski JR, Garcia CA, Zoghbi HY, Hoffman EP, Fenwick RG: Discordance of muscular dystrophy in monozygotic twins: Evidence supporting symmetric splitting of the inner cell mass in a manifesting carrier of Duchenne dystrophy. *Am J Med Genet* **40**:354, 1991.
185. Winchester B, Young E, Geddes S, Genet S, Hurst J, Middelton-Price H, Williams N, Webb M, Habel A, Malcolm S: Female twin with Hunter disease due to nonrandom inactivation of the X chromosome: A consequence of twinning. *Am J Med Genet* **44**:834, 1992.
186. Jorgensen AL, Philip J, Raskind WH, Matsushita M, Christensen B, Dreyer V, Motulsky AG: Different patterns of X inactivation in MZ twins discordant for red-green color vision deficiency. *Am J Hum Genet* **51**:291, 1992.
187. Monteiro J, Derom C, Vlietinck R, Kohn N, Lesser M, Gergersen PK: Commitment to X inactivation precedes the twinning event in monochorionic MZ twins. *Am J Hum Genet* **63**:339, 1998.
188. Puck JM: The timing of twinning: more insights from X inactivation. *Am J Hum Genet* **63**:327, 1998.
189. Goodship J, Carter J, Burn J: X inactivation patterns in monozygotic and dizygotic female twins. *Am J Med Genet* **61**:205, 1996.
190. Therman E, Patau K: Abnormal X chromosomes in man: Origin, behavior and effects. *Humangenetik* **25**:1, 1974.
191. Mattei MG, Mattei JF, Ayme S, Giraud F: X-autosome translocations: Cytogenetic characteristics and their consequences. *Hum Genet* **61**:295, 1982.
192. Carrozzo R, Arrigo G, Rossi E, Bardoni B, Cammarata M, Gandulia P, Gatti R, Zuffardi O: Multiple congenital anomalies, brain hypomyelination, and ocular albinism in a female with dup(X) (pter → q24::q21.32 → qter) and random inactivation. *Am J Med Genet* **72**:329, 1997.
193. Migeon BR, Stetten G, Tuck-Muller C, Axelman J, Jani M, Dungy D: Molecular characterization of a deleted X chromosome (Xq13.3-q21.31) exhibiting random inactivation. *Somat Cell Mol Genet* **21**:113, 1995.
194. Vasquez AI, Rivera H, Bobadilla L, Crolla JA: A familial Xp + chromosome, dup (Xq26.3-qter). *J Med Genet* **32**:891, 1995.
195. Wolff DJ, Gustashaw KM, Zurcher V, Ko L, White W, Weiss L, VanDyke DL, Schwartz S, Willard HF: Deletions in Xq26.3-q27.3 including FMR1 result in a severe phenotype in a male and variable phenotypes in females depending on the X inactivation pattern. *Hum Genet* **100**:256, 1997.
196. Vust A, Riordan D, Wickstrom D, Chudley AE, Dawson AJ: Functional mosaic trisomy of 1q12-1q21 resulting from X-autosome insertion translocation with random inactivation. *Clin Genet* **54**:70, 1998.
197. Schmidt M, DuSart D: Functional disomies of the X chromosome influence the cell selection and hence the X inactivation pattern in

females with balanced X-autosome translocations: A review of 122 cases. *Am J Med Genet* **42**:161, 1992.

198. Therman E, Laxova R, Susman B: The critical region on the human Xq. *Hum Genet* **85**:455, 1990.
199. Simpson JL: Reproductive technologies and genetic advances in obstetrics and gynecology. *Int J Gynecol Obstet* **38**:261, 1992.
200. Ballabio A, Andria G: Deletions and translocations involving the distal short arm of the human X chromosome: Review and hypotheses. *Hum Mol Genet* **1**:221, 1992.
201. DuSart D, Kalitsis P, Schmidt M: Noninactivation of a portion of Xq28 in a balanced X-autosome translocation. *Am J Med Genet* **42**:156, 1992.
202. Ishikiriyama S, Iai M, Tanabe Y: Lack of X inactivation: Loss of one X inactivation center in a case with mos45,X,-21+der(21)t(X;21)(p21.3;p11.2)/46,X,t(X;21)(p21.3;p11.2). *Am J Med Genet* **47**:41, 1993.
203. Wolff DJ, Schwartz S, Montgomery T, Zackowski JL: Random X inactivation in a girl with a balanced t(X;9) and an abnormal phenotype. *Am J Med Genet* **77**:401, 1998.
204. Correa-Cerro LS, Rivera H, Vasquez AI: Functional Xp disomy and de novo t(X;13)(q10;q10) in a girl with hypomelanosis of Ito. *J Med Genet* **34**:161, 1997.
205. White WM, Willard HF, VanDyke DL, Wolff DJ: The spreading of X inactivation into autosomal material of an X;autosome translocation: Evidence for a difference between autosomal and X chromosomal DNA. *Am J Hum Genet* **63**:20, 1998.
206. Preis W, Barbi G, Liptay S, Kennerknecht I, Schwemmle S, Pohlandt F: X;autosome translocation in three generations ascertained through an infant with trisomy 16p due to failure of spreading of X-inactivation. *Am J Med Genet* **61**:117, 1996.
207. Gustashaw KM, Zurcher V, Dickerman LH, Stallard R, Willard HF: Partial X chromosome trisomy with functional disomy of Xp due to failure of X inactivation. *Am J Med Genet* **53**:39-45, 1994.
208. Jacobs PA, Hunt PA, Mayer M, Bart RD: Duchenne muscular dystrophy in a female with an X;autosome translocation: Further evidence that the DMD locus is at Xp21. *Am J Hum Genet* **33**:513, 1981.
209. Carrel L, Cottle A, Goglin KC, Willard HF: A first-generation X inactivation profile of the human X chromosome. *Proc Natl Acad Sci* **96**:14440, 1999.
210. Charlesworth B: Sex chromosomes: Evolving dosage compensation. *Curr Biol* **8**:R931, 1998.
211. Graves JAM, Disteche CM, Toder R: Gene dosage in the evolution and function of mammalian sex chromosomes. *Cytogenet Cell Genet* **80**:94, 1998.
212. Ellis NA: Human sex chromosome evolution, in Jackson M, Strachan T, Dover G (eds): *Human Genome Evolution*. Oxford, BIOS Scientific Publishers, 1996, p 229.
213. Jegalian K, Page DC: A proposed path by which genes common to mammalian X and Y chromosomes evolve to become X inactivated. *Nature* **394**:776, 1998.
214. D'Esposito M, Ciccodicola A, Gianfrancesco F, Esposito T, Flagiello L, Mazzarella R, Schlessinger D, D'Urso M: A synaptobrevin-like gene in the Xq28 pseudoautosomal region undergoes X inactivation. *Nat Genet* **13**:227, 1996.
215. Miller AP, Willard HF: Chromosomal basis of X chromosome inactivation: Identification of a multigene domain in Xp11.21-p11.22 that escapes X inactivation. *Proc Natl Acad Sci U S A* **95**:8709, 1998.
216. Lyon MF: X chromosome inactivation, a repeat hypothesis. *Cytogenet Cell Genet* **80**:133, 1998.
217. Russell LB: Mammalian X-chromosome action: Inactivation limited in spread and in region of origin. *Science* **140**:976, 1963.
218. Lyon MF: Cytogenetics [Discussion], in *Second International Conference on Congenital Malformations*. New York, International Medical Congress, 1963, p 67.
219. Therman E, Sarto GE, Patau K: Center for Barr body condensation on the proximal part of the human Xq: A hypothesis. *Chromosoma* **44**:361, 1974.
220. Brown CJ, Lafreniere RG, Powers VE, Sebastio G, Ballabio A, Pettigrew AL, Ledbetter DH, et al.: Localization of the X inactivation center on the human X chromosome in Xq13. *Nature* **349**:82, 1991.
221. Muscatelli F, Lena D, Mattei MG, Fontes M: A male with two contiguous inactivation centers on a single X chromosome: Study of X inactivation and XIST expression. *Hum Mol Genet* **1**:115, 1992.
222. Schmidt M, DuSart D, Kalitsis P, Leversha M, Dale S, Sheffield L, Toniolo D: Duplications of the X chromosome in males: Evidence that most parts of the X chromosome can be active in two copies. *Hum Genet* **86**:519, 1991.
223. Apacik C, Cohen M, Jakobeit M, Schmucker B, Schuffenhauer S, Thurn und Taxis E, Genzel-Boroviczeny O, Stengel-Rutkowski S: Two brothers with multiple congenital anomalies and mental retardation due to disomy (X)(q12 → q13.3) inherited from the mother. *Clin Genet* **50**:63, 1996.
224. Jacobs PA, Matsuyama AM, Buchanan IM, Wilson C: Late replicating X chromosomes in human triploidy. *Am J Hum Genet* **31**:446, 1979.
225. Willard HF: X chromosome inactivation, XIST, and pursuit of the X inactivation center. *Cell* **86**:5, 1996.
226. Panning B, Jaenisch R: RNA and the epigenetic regulation of X chromosome inactivation. *Cell* **93**:305, 1998.
227. Mattei MG, Mattei JF, Vidal I, Giraud F: Structural anomalies of the X chromosome and inactivation center. *Hum Genet* **56**:401, 1981.
228. Leppig KA, Brown CJ, Bressler SL, Gustashaw K, Pagon RA, Willard HF, Disteche CM: Mapping of the distal boundary of the X inactivation center in a rearranged X chromosome from a female expressing XIST. *Hum Mol Genet* **2**:883, 1993.
229. Lee JT, Strauss WM, Dausman JA, Jaenisch R: A 450-kb transgene displays properties of the mammalian X inactivation center. *Cell* **86**:83, 1996.
230. Lee JT, Lu N, Han Y: Genetic analysis of the mouse X inactivation center defines an 80-kb multifunction domain. *Proc Natl Acad Sci U S A* **96**:3836, 1999.
231. Herzing L, Romer JT, Horn JM, Ashworth A: Xist has properties of the X chromosome inactivation centre. *Nature* **386**:272, 1997.
232. Brown CJ, Ballabio A, Rupert JL, Lafreniere RG, Grompe M, Tonlorenzi R, Willard HF: A gene from the region of the human X inactivation centre is expressed exclusively from the inactive X chromosome. *Nature* **349**:38, 1991.
233. McCarrey JR, Dilworth DD: Expression of Xist in mouse germ cells correlates with X chromosome inactivation. *Nat Genet* **2**:200, 1992.
234. Richler C, Soreq H, Wahrman J: X inactivation in mammalian testis is correlated with inactive X-specific transcription. *Nat Genet* **2**:192, 1992.
235. Salido EC, Yen PH, Mohandas TK, Shapiro LJ: Expression of the X inactivation-associated gene XIST during spermatogenesis. *Nat Genet* **2**:196, 1992.
236. Borsani G, Tonlorenzi R, Simmler MC, Dandalo L, Arnaud D, Capra V, Grompe M, Pizzati A, Muzay D, Lawrence C, Willard HF, Avner P, Ballabio A: Characterisation of a murine gene expressed from the inactive X chromosome. *Nature* **351**:325, 1991.
237. Brockdorff N, Ashworth A, Kay GF, Cooper P, Smith S, McCabe VM, Norris DP, Penny GD, Patel D, Rastan S: Conservation of position and exclusive expression of mouse Xist from the inactive X chromosome. *Nature* **351**:329, 1991.
238. Hendrich B, Brown CJ, Willard HF: Evolutionary conservation of possible functional domains of the human and mouse XIST genes. *Hum Mol Genet* **2**:663, 1993.
239. Allaman-Pillet N, Djemai A, Bonny C, Schorderet DF: Methylation status of CpG sites and methyl-CpG binding proteins are involved in the promoter regulation of the mouse Xist gene. *Gene Expr* **7**:61, 1998.
240. Komura J, Sheardown SA, Brockdorff N, Singer-Sam J, Riggs AD: In vivo ultraviolet and dimethyl sulfate footprinting of the 5′ region of expressed and silent Xist alleles. *J Biol Chem* **272**:10975, 1997.
241. McDonald LE, Paterson CA, Kay GF: Bisulfite genomic sequencing-derived methylation profile of the Xist gene throughout early mouse development. *Genomics* **54**:379, 1998.
242. Kay GF, Penny GD, Patel D, Ashworth A, Brockdorff N, Rastan S: Expression of Xist during mouse development suggests a role in the initiation of X chromosome inactivation. *Cell* **72**:171, 1993.
243. Lee JT, Jaenisch R: Long-range cis effects of ectopic X inactivation centres on a mouse autosome. *Nature* **386**:275, 1997.
244. Hendrich BD, Willard HF: Identification and characterization of the human XIST gene promoter: Implications for models of X chromosome inactivation. *Nucleic Acids Res* **25**:2661, 1997.
245. Heard E, Mongelard F, Arnaud D, Avner P: Xist yeast artificial chromosome transgenes function as X-inactivation centers only in multicopy arrays and not as single copies. *Mol Cell Biol* **19**:3156, 1999.
246. Brockdorff N, Ashworth A, Kay GF, McCabe VM, Norris DP, Cooper PJ, Swift S, Rastan S: The product of the mouse Xist gene is a 15-kb inactive X-specific transcript containing no conserved ORF and located in the nucleus. *Cell* **71**:515, 1992.
247. Brown CJ, Hendrich BD, Rupert JL, Lafreniere RG, Xing Y, Lawrence J, Willard HF: The human XIST gene: Analysis of a 17-kb inactive

X-specific RNA that contains conserved repeats and is highly localized within the nucleus. *Cell* **71**:527, 1992.
248. Clemson CM, McNeil JA, Willard HF, Lawrence JB: XIST RNA paints the inactive X chromosome at interphase: Evidence for a novel RNA involved in nuclear/chromosome structure. *J Cell Biol* **132**:259, 1996.
249. Duthie SM, Nesterova TB, Formstone EJ, Keohane AM, Turner BM, Zakian SM, Brockdorff N: Xist RNA exhibits a banded localization on the inactive X chromosome and is excluded from autosomal material in cis. *Hum Mol Genet* **8**:195, 1999.
250. Marahrens Y, Loring J, Jaenisch R: Role of the Xist gene in X chromosome counting. *Cell* **92**:657, 1998.
251. Penny GD, Kay GF, Sheardown SA, Rastan S, Brockdorff N: Requirement for Xist in X chromosome inactivation. *Nature* **379**:131, 1996.
252. Clerc P, Avner P: Role of the region 3′ to Xist exon 6 in the counting process of X chromosome inactivation. *Nat Genet* **19**:249, 1998.
253. Carrel L, Willard HF: Counting on Xist. *Nat Genet* **19**:211, 1998.
254. Panning B, Dausman J, Jaenisch R: X chromosome inactivation is mediated by Xist RNA stabilization. *Cell* **90**:907, 1997.
255. Sheardown SA, Duthie SM, Johnston CM, Newall AET, Formstone EJ, Arkell RM, Nesterova TB, et al.: Stabilization of Xist RNA mediates initiation of X chromosome inactivation. *Cell* **91**:99, 1997.
256. Johnston CM, Nesterova TB, Formstone EJ, Newall AET, Duthie SM, Sheardown SA, Brockdorff N: Developmentally regulated Xist promoter switch mediates initiation of X inactivation. *Cell* **94**:809, 1998.
257. Mohandas T, Geller RL, Yen PH, Rosendorff J, Bernstein R, Yoshida A, Shapiro LJ: Cytogenetic and molecular studies on a recombinant human X chromosome: Implications for the spreading of X chromosome inactivation. *Proc Natl Acad Sci U S A* **84**:4954, 1987.
258. Buzin CH, Mann JR, Singer-Sam J: Quantitative RT-PCR assays show Xist RNA levels are low in mouse female adult tissue, embryos and embryoid bodies. *Development* **120**:3529, 1994.
259. Hornstra IK, Yang TP: Multiple in vivo footprints are specific to the active X allele of the X-linked HPRT gene 5′ region: Implications for X chromosome inactivation. *Mol Cell Biol* **12**:5345, 1992.
260. Boyes J, Bird A: Repression of genes by DNA methylation depend on CpG density and promoter strength: Evidence for involvement of a methyl-CpG binding protein. *EMBO J* **11**:327, 1992.
261. Brown CJ, Willard HF: The human X inactivation centre is not required for maintenance of X chromosome inactivation. *Nature* **368**:154, 1994.
262. Rack KA, Chelly J, Gibbons RJ, Rider S, Benjamin D, Lafreniere RG, Oscier D, et al.: Absence of the XIST gene from late-replicating isodicentric X chromosomes in leukaemia. *Hum Mol Genet* **3**:1053, 1994.
263. Clemson CM, Chow JC, Brown CJ, Lawrence JB: Stabilization and location of Xist RNA are controlled by separate mechanisms and are not sufficient for X inactivation. *J Cell Biol* **142**:13, 1998.
264. Hansen RS, Canfield TK, Stanek AM, Keitges EA, Gartler SM: Reactivation of XIST in normal fibroblasts and a somatic cell hybrid: Abnormal localization of XIST RNA in hybrid cells. *Proc Natl Acad Sci U S A* **95**:5133, 1998.
265. Tinker AV, Brown CJ: Induction of XIST expression from the human active X chromosome in mouse/human somatic cell hybrids by DNA demethylation. *Nucleic Acids Res* **26**:2935, 1998.
266. Thompson MW, McInnes RR, Willard HF: *Genetics in Medicine*, 5th ed. Philadelphia, WB Saunders, 1991.
267. Boue A, Boue J, Gropp A: Cytogenetics of pregnancy wastage. *Ann Rev Genet* **14**:1, 1985.
268. Burgoyne PS, Holland K, Stephens R: Incidence of numerical chromosome anomalies in human pregnancy: Estimation from induced and spontaneous abortion data. *Hum Reprod* **6**:555, 1991.
269. Hook EB, Warburton D: The distribution of chromosomal genotypes associated with Turner syndrome: Livebirth prevalence rates and evidence for diminished fetal mortality and severity in genotypes associated with structural X abnormalities or mosaicism. *Hum Genet* **64**:24, 1983.
270. Lamb NE, Freeman SB, Savage-Austin A, Pettay D, Taft L, Hersey J, Gu Y, et al.: Susceptible chiasmate configurations of chromosome 21 predispose to non-disjunction in both maternal meiosis I and meiosis II. *Nat Genet* **14**:400, 1996.
271. Klinefelter HF, Reifenstein EC, Albright F: Syndrome characterized by gynecomastia, aspermatogenesis, without aleydigism and increased excretion of follicle stimulating hormone. *J Clin Endocrinol* **2**:615, 1942.
272. Smyth CM, Bremner WJ: Klinefelter syndrome. *Arch Intern Med* **158**:1309, 1998.
273. Hultborn R, Hanson C, Kopf I, Verbience I, Warnhammar E, Weimarck A: Prevalence of Klinefelter syndrome in male breast cancer patients. *Anticancer Res* **17**:4293, 1997.
274. Abramsky L, Chapple J: 47,XXY and 47,XYY: estimated rates of and indication for postnatal diagnosis with implications for prenatal counseling. *Prenat Diagn* **17**:363, 1997.
275. Patil S, Bartley JA, Hanson JW: Association of the X chromosomal region q11-q22 and Klinefelter syndrome. *Clin Genet* **19**:343, 1981.
276. Rovet J, Netley C, Bailey J, Keenan M, Stewart D: Intelligence and achievement in children with extra X aneuploidy: A longitudinal perspective. *Am J Med Genet* **60**:356, 1995.
277. Bender GB, Linden MG, Robinson A: Neuropsychological impairment in 42 adolescents with sex chromosome abnormalities. *Am J Med Genet* **48**:169, 1993.
278. Jacobs PA, Hassold T, Whittington E, Butler G, Collyer S, Keston M, Lee M: Klinefelter's syndrome: An analysis of the origin of the additional chromosome using molecular probes. *Ann Hum Genet* **52**:93, 1988.
279. Harvey J, Jacobs PA, Hassold T, Pettay D: The parental origin of 47,XXY males. *Birth Defects Orig Artic Ser* **26**:289, 1991.
280. Lorda-Sanchez I, Binkert F, Maechler M, Robinson WP, Schinzel AA: Reduced recombination and paternal age effect in Klinefelter syndrome. *Hum Genet* **89**:524, 1992.
281. Morton NE, Keats BJ, Jacobs PA, Hassold T, Pettay D, Harvey J, Andrews V: A centromere map of the X chromosome from trisomies of maternal origin. *Ann Hum Genet* **54**:39, 1990.
282. Hassold TJ, Sherman SL, Pettay D, Page DC, Jacobs PA: XY chromosome nondisjunction in man is associated with diminished recombination in the pseudoautosomal region. *Am J Hum Genet* **49**:253, 1991.
283. Peet J, Weaver DD, Vance GH: 49,XXXXY, a distinct phenotype. Three new cases and review. *J Med Genet* **35**:420, 1998.
284. Hassold T, Pettay D, May K, Robinson A: Analysis of nondisjunction in sex chromosome tetrasomy and pentasomy. *Hum Genet* **85**:648, 1990.
285. David D, Marques RA, Garreiro MH, Moreira I, Boavida MG: Parental origin of extra chromosomes in persons with X chromosome tetrasomy. *J Med Genet* **29**:595, 1992.
286. Ratcliffe SG, Paul N (eds): Prospective studies on children with sex chromosome aneuploidy. *Birth Defects Orig Artic Ser* **22**:1, 1986.
287. Harmon RJ, Bender BG, Linden MG, Robinson A: Transition from adolescence to early adulthood: Adaptation and psychiatric status of women with 47,XXX. *J Am Acad Child Adolesc Psychiatry* **37**:286, 1998.
288. May KM, Jacobs PA, Lee M, Ratcliffe S, Robinson A, Nielsen J, Hassold TJ: The parental origin of the extra X chromosome in 47,XXX females. *Am J Hum Genet* **46**:754, 1990.
289. Hassold T, Arnovitz K, Jacobs PA, May K, Robinson D: The parental origin of the missing or additional chromosome in 45,X and 47,XXX females. *Birth Defects Orig Artic Ser* **26**:297, 1990.
290. Zinn AR, Page DC, Fisher EMC: Turner syndrome: The case of the missing sex chromosome. *Trends Genet* **9**:90, 1993.
291. Saenger P: Turner's syndrome. *N Engl J Med* **335**:1749, 1996.
292. Zinn AR, Ross JL: Turner syndrome and haploinsufficiency. *Curr Opin Genet Dev* **8**:322, 1998.
293. Sybert VP: Cardiovascular malformations and complications in Turner syndrome. *Pediatrics* **101**:E11, 1998.
294. Gicquel C, Gaston V, Cabrol S, LeBouc Y: Assessment of Turner syndrome by molecular analysis of the X chromosome in growth-retarded girls. *J Clin Endocrin Metab* **83**:1472, 1998.
295. Plotnick L, Attie KM, Blethen SL, Sy JP: Growth hormone treatment of girls with Turner syndrome: The National Cooperative Growth Study experience. *Pediatrics* **102**:479, 1998.
296. Gravolt CH, Juul S, Naeraa RW, Hansen J: Morbidity in Turner syndrome. *J Clin Epidemiol* **51**:147, 1998.
297. Jacobs PA, Betts PR, Cockwell AE, Crolla JA, Mackenzie MJ, Robinson DO, Youings SA: A cytogenetic and molecular reappraisal of a series of patients with Turner's syndrome. *Ann Hum Genet* **54**:209, 1990.
298. Jacobs P, Dalton P, James R, Mosse K, Power M, Robinson D, Skuse D: Turner syndrome, a cytogenetic and molecular study. *Ann Hum Genet* **61**:471, 1997.
299. Wolff DJ, Miller AP, Van Dyke DL, Schwartz S, Willard HF: Molecular definition of breakpoints associated with human Xq isochromosomes: Implications for mechanisms of formation. *Am J Hum Genet* **58**:154, 1993.

300. James RS, Dalton P, Gustashaw K, Wolff DJ, Willard HF, Mitchell C, Jacobs PA: Molecular characterization of isochromosomes of Xq. *Ann Hum Genet* **61**:485, 1997.
301. Sullivan BA, Willard HF: Stable dicentric X chromosomes with two active centromeres. *Nat Genet* **20**:227, 1998.
302. Hassold T, Pettay D, Robinson A, Uchida I: Molecular studies of parental origin and mosaicism in 45,X conceptuses. *Hum Genet* **89**:647, 1992.
303. Lorda-Sanchez I, Binkert F, Maechler M, Schinzel A: Molecular study of 45,X conceptuses: Correlation with clinical findings. *Am J Med Genet* **42**:487, 1992.
304. Mathur A, Stekol L, Schatz D, Maclaren NK, Scott ML, Lippe B: The parental origin of the single X chromosome in Turner syndrome: Lack of correlation with parental age or clinical phenotype. *Am J Hum Genet* **48**:682, 1991.
305. Held KR, Kerber S, Kaminsky E, Singh S, Goetz P, Seemanova E, Goedde HW: Mosaicism in 45,X Turner syndrome: Does survival in early pregnancy depend on the presence of two sex chromosomes? *Hum Genet* **88**:288, 1992.
306. Ferguson-Smith MA: Karyotype-phenotype correlations in gonadal dysgenesis and their bearing on the pathogenesis of malformations. *J Med Genet* **2**:142, 1965.
307. Rao E, Weiss B, Fukami M, Rump A, Niesler B, Mertz A, Muroya K, et al.: Pseudoautosomal deletions encompassing a novel homeobox gene cause growth failure in idiopathic short stature and Turner syndrome. *Nat Genet* **16**:54, 1997.
308. Ellison JW, Wardak Z, Young MF, Gehron Robey P, Laig-Webster M, Chiong W: PHOG, a candidate gene for involvement in the short stature of Turner syndrome. *Hum Mol Genet* **6**:1341, 1997.
309. James RS, Coppin B, Dalton P, Dennis NR, Mitchell C, Sharp AJ, Skuse DH, et al.: A study of females with deletions of the short arm of the X chromosome. *Hum Genet* **102**:507, 1998.
310. Zinn AR, Tonk VS, Chen Z, Flejter WL, Gardner HA, Guerra R, Kushner H, et al.: Evidence for a Turner syndrome locus or loci at Xp11.2-p22.1. *Am J Hum Genet* **63**:1757, 1998.
311. Mazzocco MM: A process approach to describing mathematics difficulties in girls with Turner syndrome. *Pediatrics* **102**:492, 1998.
312. Skuse DH, James RS, Bishop DVM, Coppin B, Dalton P, Aamodt-Leeper G, Bacarese-Hamilton M, et al.: Evidence from Turner syndrome of an imprinted X-linked locus affecting cognitive function. *Nature* **387**:705, 1997.
313. Skuse DH: Genomic imprinting of the X chromosome: A novel mechanism for the evolution of sexual dimorphism. *J Lab Clin Med* **133**:23, 1999.
314. Kushnick T, Irons TG, Wiley JE, Gettig EA, Rao KW, Bowyer S: 45X/46X,r(X) with syndactyly and severe mental retardation. *Am J Med Genet* **28**:567, 1987.
315. VanDyke DL, Wiktor A, Roberson JR, Weiss L: Mental retardation in Turner syndrome. *J Pediatr* **118**:415, 1991.
316. Cohen MM, Sandberg AA, Takagi N, MacGillivray MH: Autoradiographic investigations of centric fragments and rings in patients with stigmata of gonadal dysgenesis. *Cytogenet* **6**:254, 1967.
317. VanDyke DL, Wiktor A, Palmer CG, Miller DA, Witt M, Babu VR, Worsham MJ, Roberson JR, Weiss L: Ullrich-Turner syndrome with a small ring X chromosome and presence of mental retardation. *Am J Med Genet* **43**:996, 1992.
318. Grompe M, Rao N, Elder F, Caskey CT, Greenberg F: 45,X/46,X,+r(X) can have a distinct phenotype different from Ullrich-Turner syndrome. *Am J Med Genet* **42**:39, 1992.
319. Lindgren V, Chen C, Bryke CR, Lichter P, Page DC, Yang-Feng TL: Cytogenetic and molecular characterization of marker chromosomes in patients with mosaic 45,X karyotypes. *Hum Genet* **88**:393, 1992.
320. Dennis NR, Collins AL, Crolla JA, Cockwell AE, Fisher AM, Jacobs PA: Three patients with ring (X) chromosomes and a severe phenotype. *J Med Genet* **30**:482, 1993.
321. Wolff DJ, Brown CJ, Schwartz S, Duncan AMV, Surti U, Willard HF: Small marker X chromosomes lack the X inactivation center: Implications for karyotype/phenotype correlations. *Am J Hum Genet* **55**:87, 1994.
322. Collins AL, Cockwell AE, Jacobs PA, Dennis NR: A comparison of the clinical and cytogenetic findings in nine patients with a ring (X) cell line and 16 45,X patients. *J Med Genet* **31**:528, 1994.
323. Cole H, Huang B, Salbert BA, Brown J, Howard-Peebles PN, Black SH, Dorfmann A, Febles OR, Stevens CA, Jackson-Cook C: Mental retardation and Ullrich-Turner syndrome in cases with 45,X/46,X,+mar: Additional support for the loss of the X-inactivation center hypothesis. *Am J Med Genet* **52**:136, 1994.
324. Guillen DR, Lowichik A, Schneider NR, Cohen DS, Garcia S, Zinn AR: Prune-belly syndrome and other anomalies in a stillborn fetus with a ring X chromosome lacking XIST. *Am J Med Genet* **70**:32, 1997.
325. Tumer Z, Wolff D, Silahtaroglu AN, Orum A, Brondum-Nielsen K: Characterization of a supernumerary small marker X chromosome in two females with similar phenotypes. *Am J Med Genet* **76**:45, 1998.
326. Yorifuji T, Muroi J, Kawai M, Uematsu A, Sasaki H, Momoi T, Kaji M, Yamanaka C, Furusho K: Uniparental and functional X disomy in Turner syndrome patients with unexplained mental retardation and X-derived marker chromosomes. *J Med Genet* **35**:539, 1998.
327. Jani MM, Torshia BS, Pai GS, Migeon BR: Molecular characterization of tiny ring X chromosomes from females with functional X chromosome disomy and lack of cis X inactivation. *Genomics* **27**:182, 1995.
328. Migeon BR, Luo S, Jani M, Jeppesen P: The severe phenotype of females with tiny ring X chromosomes is associated with inability of these chromosomes to undergo X inactivation. *Am J Hum Genet* **55**:497, 1994.

CHAPTER 62

SRY and Primary Sex-Reversal Syndromes

Peter N. Goodfellow ▪ Malcolm A. Ferguson-Smith
J. Ross Hawkins ▪ Giovanna Camerino

1. **Male differentiation in humans is determined by the testis-determining gene, *SRY*, which is located on the short arm of the Y chromosome adjacent to the pseudoautosomal region.**
2. **Cytogenetic studies of infertile males have revealed rare individuals with an apparently normal 46,XX karyotype. The majority of these sex-reversed XX males have inherited a small fragment of the Y chromosome, which includes *SRY*, transferred to the short arm of one of their X chromosomes.**
3. ***SRY* mutations are found in 15 percent of XY females with pure gonadal dysgenesis.**
4. **SRY induces the differentiation of Sertoli cells in the developing gonad. Sertoli cells produce anti-Mullerian hormone, which causes regression of the female internal genitalia; they also induce Leydig cells to secrete the androgens necessary for the development of male internal and external genitalia. Any genetic or environmental factor that prevents testis differentiation in 46,XY embryos leads to the development of a sex-reversed XY female.**
5. **This chapter reviews the role of *SRY* in primary sex-reversal syndromes.**

In all mammals, sexual differentiation in the early embryo is a consequence of the development of the gonadal ridge into either a testis or an ovary. A central role for the testis in sex determination was established in the 1940s by the embryonic castration experiments of Jost, who showed that removal of the undifferentiated gonads before a critical stage in male rabbit embryos led to female differentiation of the internal and external genitalia.[1] Unilateral castration of male embryos led to ipsilateral female differentiation of the genital ducts and male differentiation of the ducts contralaterally. This indicated the local action of androgenic hormones secreted by each testis.

The first signs of testicular differentiation occur in the supporting cell lineage of the embryonic gonad, which surrounds the incoming germ cells.[2] These cells enlarge into Sertoli cells, which organize to form tubular structures within the gonad. In addition to providing sustenance to the maturing germ cells, the Sertoli cells secrete anti-Mullerian hormone (AMH, also known as Mullerian-inhibiting hormone), which causes regression of the Mullerian ducts (the anlage of the uterus, fallopian tubes, and upper vagina).[3] Sertoli cells also may induce the embryonic interstitial (Leydig) cells to secrete the androgens that stimulate the mesonephric (Wolffian) ducts to differentiate into seminal vesicles, vasa deferentia, and epididymes. The production of androgens also masculinizes the external genitalia. Another function of Sertoli cells is to inhibit meiosis in spermatogonia until puberty, when a further wave of differentiation in both cell types is initiated by the hypothalamus through the anterior pituitary. Testis differentiation occurs in the absence of germ cells, emphasizing the critical role of the Sertoli cell in male differentiation.[4]

Jost's studies revealed that the ovaries develop later than the testes. In the absence of Sertoli-cell differentiation, the supporting cell lineage of the undifferentiated gonad become follicular cells that surround the incoming oogonia to form primordial follicles. The oogonia enter the prophase of first meiosis, where they remain in meiotic arrest until ovulation. Because no AMH is produced, the Mullerian ducts develop into the uterus, fallopian tubes, and upper vagina. The Wolffian ducts atrophy. It is important to emphasize that failure of early development of the undifferentiated gonad in a male embryo, through either a genetic defect or environmental agent, will lead to female differentiation, that is, sex reversal. Partial failure in gonadal development may lead to sexual ambiguity.

An important conclusion of these experiments is the distinction between sex determination, the process of choosing to make a testis, and sexual differentiation, the consequent differentiation of the male and female phenotypes. Errors in sex determination cause *primary sex reversal*; errors in sex differentiation cause *secondary sex reversal*.

The XX:XY chromosomal basis of sex determination in humans was first described by Painter in 1923.[5] However, for half a century, it was not clear whether the primary sex-determining signal was due to the Y chromosome or, as in *Drosophila melanogaster*, dependent on the X chromosome:autosome ratio. This was resolved in 1959 with the discovery that, in both mice and humans, individuals with a single X chromosome are female, whereas those with two X chromosomes and a Y are male.[6–8] Thus, the Y chromosome must carry a dominant determinant for testis development. Because the nature of this determinant (whether the product of a single gene, multiple genes, or repetitive DNA) was unknown, it was referred to as the testis determining factor (*TDF*). The same determinant in the mouse was named *Tdy* (testis determinant on the Y).

Cytogenetic analysis of patients with chromosome rearrangements eventually led to the conclusion that the sex-determining gene must be located on the short arm of the Y chromosome.[9] For many years, the interpretation of cytogenetic studies had been confounded by the difficulties of interpreting chromosomal rearrangements in the era before chromosomal banding became routine.[10] Another difficulty in interpretation was caused by the frequent occurrence of mosaicism for a 45X cell line that had lost the rearranged Y chromosome. If this cell line is dominant in the gonad, female differentiation will occur. These patients either have features of Turner syndrome without masculinization or features of Turner syndrome with genital ambiguity resulting from asymmetrical or mixed gonadal dysgenesis (unilateral streak gonad and unilateral rudimentary testis). All patients are sterile and have one

A list of standard abbreviations is located immediately preceding the index in each volume. Nonsandard abbreviations used in this chapter include: AMH = anti-Mullerian hormone; TDF = testis determining factor; Tdy = testis determinant on the Y; *ZFY* = zinc finger Y gene.

or more of a series of characteristic stigmata that include short stature, webbed neck, peripheral lymphedema, hypoplastic nails, short fourth metacarpals, multiple pigmented nevi, shield chest, congenital heart disease, and sexual infantilism.[11]

The precise location of the sex-determining gene and its identification by positional cloning was achieved by the molecular analysis of the genomes of XX males and XY females.

XX males appeared to be examples of sex reversal in which male differentiation has occurred despite the presence of an apparently normal 46,XX female karyotype.[12] Clinically, those affected are infertile males with small testes and the endocrinologic features of the Klinefelter syndrome, namely gynecomastia, elevated gonadotropins, and characteristic testicular histopathology, including prepubertal atrophy of the seminiferous tubules, absent germ cells, and clumping of abnormal Leydig cells.[13] Unlike the classical 47,XXY Klinefelter patient, intelligence is normal and the average height is at the normal average for females. Extensive search for sex chromosomal mosaicism involving 46,XY or 47,XXY cells, for example, has been unsuccessful in these cases, and there was wide speculation about the origin of the apparent sex reversal. A particularly attractive hypothesis was proposed by Ferguson-Smith who suggested that exchange between the X and Y chromosome might result in the cryptic transfer of the sex-determining region from the Y to the X chromosome.[14] This hypothesis was based on the ideas of Koller and Darlington[15] and is supported by the unusual inheritance patterns of two serologic antigens: occasionally the Xg blood group was not inherited by XX males, suggesting X chromosome deletions,[14,16] and in one XX male, the presence of the Y-linked regulator of the 12E7 antigen implied inheritance of Y chromosome sequences.[17] Additional support for the X-Y exchange model came from high-resolution prometaphase banding in XX males; in a few cases, additional chromosomal material could be seen at the end of one X chromosome.[18–20]

The cloning of sequences from the Y chromosome provided the tools for confirming the X-Y interchange model for the origin of XX males.[21] The cloned probes were used for analyzing the structure of the Y chromosome and the genomes of XX males.[22] In agreement with the suggestions of Koller and Darlington for rat sex chromosomes, the human Y chromosome was shown to be composed of two parts: a region shared by the X and Y chromosome and a differential region specific to each sex chromosome. In the shared region, recombination occurs in male meiosis, and genetic markers in this region segregate independent of sexual phenotype or are partially sex linked.[23,24] Burgoyne introduced the term *pseudoautosomal* to describe this inheritance pattern, and the shared region is often called the *pseudoautosomal region*.[25] Recombination in the pseudoautosomal region has several unusual features:

- Fifty percent recombination occurs between the telomere and the boundary of the shared region in male meiosis; in female meiosis only a few percent recombination is found in the same region.[26–28] This unusually large sex bias is due to elevation of the rate of recombination in males, because the pseudoautosomal region is only 2.6 Mb in size.[29,30]
- Despite the high rate of genetic exchange within the shared region, only a single, obligate recombination occurs in each meiotic event.[27]
- The boundary between the shared and sex-specific regions is an abrupt loss of sequence homology.[31]

The abrupt sequence barrier to recombination does not exert a position effect, and the rate of exchange between the sex chromosomes is constant between the telomere and the boundary.[27,28,32] Circumstantial evidence is consistent with the shared region being essential for pairing, segregation, and fertility in males.[33,34] The Y-specific region includes the sex-determining region and, by definition, cannot normally participate in recombination between the sex chromosomes.

The X-Y interchange model makes several predictions about XX males:

- Y sequences, including the sex-determining gene, should be present due to a terminal exchange between the sex chromosomes.
- The Y sequences should be on the paternal X chromosome.
- The amount of Y material present should be variable, depending on the position of the breakpoint on the Y chromosome.
- The breakpoint on the X chromosome also should vary.

All of these predictions have been confirmed at the molecular level:

- The majority of XX males (>80 percent) have inherited Y-derived sequences.[21,35–37]
- By *in situ* hybridization with Y-specific probes, these sequences are located on the end of the short arm of the X chromosome.[38–40]
- Different XX males have inherited varying portions of the Y chromosome short arm, and this has been used to construct deletion (or fragment) maps of the Y chromosome.[22,41–43]
- The fragments are terminal because the pseudoautosomal region of the Y chromosome is inherited intact along with the Y-specific sequences. The point of the abnormal exchange also varies on the X chromosome.[44–48]

The mechanism that generates the abnormal exchange is only partially defined. A plausible hypothesis is that misalignment during association of the sex chromosomes is followed by recombination within partially homologous sequences. This hypothesis is supported by the discovery of breakpoint cluster regions or "hot spots" for ectopic recombination.[49,50] Detailed analysis of one hot spot in XX males (and in XY females, as explained below) has shown that recombination frequently occurs between two homologous genes, *PPKY* and *PPKX,* which are oriented in the same direction on the Y chromosome and X chromosome, respectively.[51]

The X-Y interchange model also provides an explanation for XY females, which has been confirmed by molecular analysis. Surprisingly, XY females with terminal deletions of the Y chromosome are much rarer than exchange XX males. The phenotype of exchange XY females is similar to patients with Turner syndrome but without short stature.[52–56] This similarity suggests that prenatal lethality, which is also found in Turner syndrome, may be the explanation for the comparative rarity of these patients.

The deletion maps of the Y chromosome, constructed in different laboratories using different Y probes and different patient samples, all placed the sex-determining region in a distal position in the Y-specific region adjacent to the pseudoautosomal region.[22,42,43] Within this region, a novel gene, *ZFY* (zinc finger Y gene), was subsequently identified.[41] However, five XX individuals, with testicular development, were found to have inherited the Y chromosome pseudoautosomal boundary and 35 kb of Y-specific sequence. This region does not include *ZFY.*[35] A careful search of the 35 kb of Y-specific sequence revealed the presence of a gene that was conserved and present on the Y chromosome in all eutherian mammals.[57,58] This gene was named *SRY* in humans and *Sry* in mice (sex-determining region Y gene). *SRY* has the predicted properties of *TDF*:

- *SRY* and *Sry* map to the smallest portion of the human and murine Y chromosomes that are known to be sex determining.[35,57,58]
- *Sry* is expressed in the somatic cells of the mouse gonadal ridge immediately prior to testicular development.[59,60]
- Some XY females with gonadal dysgenesis have suffered mutations in *SRY*; the majority of these mutations are *de novo* [61,62] (Table 62-1). In the mouse, a *de novo* deletion of *Sry* is associated with XY sex reversal.[57]
- A 14-kb fragment of the mouse Y chromosome, which includes *Sry,* can cause female-to-male sex reversal in transgenic mice.[63]

Table 62-1 List of *SRY* Mutations in XY Females

Codon Change	Amino Acid Number	Change	Phenotype	DNA Binding	Inheritance	References
CAA → TAA	2	Q → X	POF		*De novo*	87
TAT → TAA	3	Y → X			*De novo*	80
AGT → AAT	18	S → N	PGD		Familial, father not mosaic	86
TCT AGG (Ins T) → TCT TAG	43	K → X			*De novo*	143
GTG → CTG	60	V → L			Familial, father not mosaic	62
GTG → GCG	60	V → A	TH		ND	144
CGA → GGA	62	R → G			*De novo*	145
ATG → ATA	64	M → I		Weak	*De novo*	62
ATG → AGG	64	M → R			*De novo*	143
TTC → GTC	67	F → V			Familial, father mosaic	92
TTC → GTC	67	F → V			*De novo*	143
ATC → AAC	68	I → T			*De novo*	82
TGG → TAG	70	W → X			*De novo*	146
CAG → TAG	74	Q → X			ND	145
AGG → AAT	75	R → N			(Likely) *de novo*	147
ATG → ACG	78	M → T			*De novo*	145
CGA → TGA	86	R → X			ND	148
ATC → ATG	90	I → M		Near normal	Familial, father not mosaic	90
ATC → ATG	90	I → M			ND	149
AGC → GGC	91	S → G			Familial, father mosaic	93
AAG → TAG	92	K → X			ND	150
CAG → TAG	93	Q → X			*De novo*	151
GGA → CGA	95	G → R		No binding	*De novo*	146
CAG → TAG	97	Q → X			Familial, father mosaic	152
CTT → CAT	101	L → H	TH		*De novo*	88
AAA → ATA	106	K → I		Very weak	ND	90
TGG → TAG	107	W → X			ND	153
TGG → TAG	107	W → X			ND	154
CCA → CGA	108	P → R			ND	155
CCA (ΔA)	109	Frameshift			*De novo*	90
TTC → TCC	109	F → S		Normal	Familial, father not mosaic	156
GCA → ACA	113	A → T			*De novo*	157
AGA GAG (ΔAGAG)	121/122	Frameshift			*De novo*	61
CCG → CTG	125	P → L			Familial, father mosaic	93
TAT → TAA	127	Y → X			*De novo*	82
TAT → TAA	127	Y → X			*De novo*	158
TAT → TGT	127	Y → C		No binding	ND	159
CCT → CGT	131	P → R			(Likely) *de novo*	160
CGG → TGG	133	R → W			ND	145
CGG → TGG	133	R → W			*De novo*	80
TTG → TAG	163	L → X			Familial, father not tested	81
Extragenic variants						
−2027	A to G (5′ to ORF)				Familial—in father, but not controls	83
−75	G to A (5′ to ORF)				Father not tested, absent from controls	84
1097	C to T (3′ to ORF)				Familial—in father, but not controls	80
Deletion beginning 1.7 kb 5′ to ORF					*De novo*	82
Deletion beginning 2–3 kb 3′ to ORF			PGD		*De novo*	85

DNA and amino acid numbers are based on the position of the "A" base of the initiator methionine codon (ATG) being position "1." The *SRY* HMG box runs from codons 58 to 137. All phenotypes are complete gonadal dysgenesis, unless stated. DNA binding studies were only performed in some cases.

Δ = deletion; X = termination codon; ND = not determined; POF = premature ovarian failure; TH = 46, XY true hermaphrodite; PGD = partial gonadal dysgenesis; ORF = open reading frame; kb = kilobases.

Taken together, these results demonstrate a role for *SRY* in sex determination and equate *SRY* with *TDF*.

SRY encodes a protein of 240 amino acids which is capable of sequence-specific binding to DNA using a motif known as the *HMG box*.[64,65] This motif is found in several classes of DNA binding proteins, including several that are known to be transcription factors.[66] Unlike other transcription factors, the SRY protein does not contain any other recognizable motifs, and this has led to the hypothesis that it functions partly as scaffold protein in chromatin.[67] Further discussions of the properties of the *SRY* gene and protein can be found in recent reviews.[68–71]

Obviously, *SRY* cannot be the only gene that is needed to make a testis, but genetic analysis has proved that it is the only gene on the Y chromosome that is needed for sex determination. This unique property makes *SRY* central to the sex determination process. Other genes have been identified that are needed for correct sex determination and differentiation in mammals, but all of these genes have additional roles not related to their functions in sex determination.[72]

It is a consistent theme that clinical material has been exploited to study the complexities of sex determination. Obviously this relationship is reciprocal, and in this review we will consider how knowledge of the genetics and biology of *SRY* has been used to understand and classify sex-reversal syndromes in humans.

XY FEMALES

Because female sex differentiation occurs if testis determination is blocked,[1] errors in male sex determination lead to ovarian development in 46,XY embryos. In the absence of two X chromosomes, the ovaries degenerate (gonadal dysgenesis) to form streak gonads. Secondary sexual characteristics are absent or poorly developed (sexual infantilism), but the external and internal genitalia are female. The postpubertal gonad is composed of a thin streak of ovarian stroma lying in the broad ligament close to the distal end of the fallopian tube (oviduct). There are no primordial follicles. Occasionally, small aggregates of several hundred cells, believed to be abnormal XY germ cells, are seen in characteristic "cell nests" within the ovarian stroma. These usually degenerate and form calcified bodies in the older patient. The cell nests are prone to neoplastic transformation and may form gonadoblastomas, an embryonic cell tumor capable of differentiation into a variety of types of neoplasms, including typical dysgerminoma and choriocarcinoma.[73] The tumors often grow to a large size, sometimes occupying the whole pelvis. After surgical removal, the prognosis is good. Breast development occurs only in patients with greater than usual amounts of ovarian stroma, and this is often associated with gonadoblastoma.[74] It is recommended that dysgenic gonads in XY females always be removed once skeletal growth is complete. Patients who are of normal stature and show none of the features of Turner syndrome are commonly described in the literature as having "pure gonadal dysgenesis" or "complete gonadal dysgenesis";[75] occasionally the term *Swyer syndrome* has been used.[76]

Incomplete development of the testis can be due to an error in either testis determination or differentiation. The sex-reversed phenotype results from reduced testosterone and AMH production with corresponding failure of regression of the Mullerian ducts, failure of induction of the Wolffian ducts, and failure of masculinization of the external genitalia. The phenotype is highly variable and depends on the amount of testosterone production. Unilateral inhibition of testis development causes female differentiation of the internal ducts unilaterally, usually associated with ambiguity of the external genitalia. These sex-reversed patients have been described as suffering from *mixed gonadal dysgenesis* or *partial gonadal dysgenesis*.

Some XY females have normal testicular development but have suffered defects in the hormonal cascade needed for masculinization of the habitus. This group includes patients with defects in androgen production and patients with target organ insensitivity to androgens. A detailed discussion of these individuals is outside the scope of this review.

SRY-Negative XY Females

This condition is uncommon and is invariably associated with gonadal dysgenesis.[52–56] Patients are usually taller than the average for normal women due to the effect of Y-specific[77] or pseudoautosomal[78] genes for stature. Features of Turner syndrome are present in cases in which loss of *SRY* is associated with an extensive contiguous, chromosomal deletion of the short arm of the Y chromosome. In most cases the Y pseudoautosomal boundary is lost, and the Y chromosome deletion is due to an X-Y interchange. Rarely, Y-autosome translocations can also cause *SRY* loss.[79]

XY Females with *SRY* Mutations

Mutations in the *SRY* gene have been found in 10 to 20 percent of reported XY patients with complete gonadal dysgenesis (Table 62-1). The majority of mutations are located in the region of the gene that encodes the HMG-box domain of the *SRY* protein. This clustering may be due in part to ascertainment bias (some groups have only tested this region of the gene) and is unexpected given the viability of individuals with deletions of the *SRY* gene. The biochemical consequences of the mutations in the HMG-box region have been studied in only a few cases; however, most mutations either abolish or severely affect DNA binding of the mutated protein (Table 62-1), a result consistent with structural analyses of the *SRY* protein.[70] Outside of the region that encodes the HMG box, two nonsense mutations have been reported in the third and forty-third codons of the gene,[80] and there is a single report of nonsense mutation in the 3′ coding region.[81] The paucity of mutations and the absence of missense mutations may be a consequence of the lack of functional importance of these regions. A similar paucity of mutations has been found outside of the coding region. A large deletion beginning 1.7 kb from the *SRY* start codon has been found in one sex-reversed patient.[82] Kwok et al. searched for mutations in the 2 kb immediately 5′ to the open reading frame in 49 patients and found only one possible mutation in a patient with complete gonadal dysgenesis. Because the patient's father appeared to share the same mutation, the relationship of the mutation to the phenotype could not be proven.[83] A similar mutation in the region 5′ to the open reading frame has been described by Poulat et al.[84]

In 46XY individuals with partial gonadal dysgenesis and 46XY true hermaphrodites, mutations in *SRY* are rare. In two publications, mutations have been described in partial gonadal dysgenesis: in one case, a *de novo* interstitial deletion was found 3′ to the *SRY* open reading frame;[85] more recently, a familial case was found with a missense mutation at codon 18.[86] In the absence of biochemical data, it is unclear how these mutations are related to the phenotypes observed. Brown et al. have reported a nonsense mutation in the second codon of *SRY* in a 46XY patient with sex reversal and partial ovarian function.[87] Mutations also have been found in a true hermaphrodite. In one case, the patient had both wild-type and mutant *SRY* sequences; the lymphocytes had the wild-type sequence and the ovotestis had both wild type and mutant sequences. Surprisingly, two different *SRY* mutations were observed.[88] One of these mutations was described as a *de novo* missense mutation in the HMG-box region of the gene.[88]

Familial XY Gonadal Dysgenesis

There are a number of accounts in the literature of siblings with XY gonadal dysgenesis. In a few families, inherited sequence variants in the *SRY* gene have been found.[64,89–93] For two of the families, the SRY proteins corresponding to the variants have been tested and shown to have reduced in vitro DNA-binding activity. These results strongly implicate *SRY* mutations as the cause of the disorder but pose the paradox of why the sex reversal occurs only in some individuals. Two plausible explanations are either the segregation of a polymorphic locus that interacts with *SRY* or a stochastic variation dependent on the reduced, but not negligible, activity of the *SRY* protein. Another explanation for the familial cases is paternal mosaicism for wild-type and mutant *SRY* genes, as has been shown by Hines et al. in a family with two 46XY sex-reversed siblings.[92]

Not all familial cases are due to mutations in *SRY*; some appear to have a pattern of inheritance consistent with an X-linked trait. In others, sex-limited autosomal-dominant inheritance is possible.[94–96] A similar phenotype of familial pure gonadal dysgenesis, but without gonadoblastoma, is described in 46,XX females.

XY Females with Testicular Regression (Vanishing Testis, Congenital Anorchia, and Testicular Agenesis)

The term *testicular regression* has been coined to describe individuals with a 46,XY karyotype who show variable masculinization of the internal and external genitalia without evidence of testicular or ovarian differentiation.[97–99] Obviously, phenotypic overlap with gonadal dysgenesis patients is likely. Molecular studies have failed to uncover mutations in *SRY*.[85] In one consanguineous family, both 46XX and 46XY agonadal sisters were found.[100]

46XY patients with gonadal dysgenesis without associated phenotypes and without detected mutations in *SRY* may have suffered mutations in regions of the *SRY* gene and its flanking sequence not subjected to mutational analysis. Alternatively, mutations may have occurred in other genes in the sex determination pathway that have not yet been defined.

XY Sex Reversal Associated with Multiple Congenital Abnormalities

Several genes with multiple roles in development also have been implicated in the sex-determination process; alterations of these genes often have multiple phenotypic consequences in addition to gonadal dysgenesis. In some cases, such as *DAX1*[101] and *SOX9*,[102] there are data for sex-specific gene expression in the genital ridge of embryonic mice that strongly suggest a direct role in sex determination. In other cases, such as *WT1*, the gene is needed for gonad formation.

- Campomelic dysplasia and *SOX9*. Sex reversal can occur in XY individuals with campomelic dysplasia, a severe form of skeletal dysplasia associated with dysmorphic features, including cardiac defects.[103] This autosomal-dominant syndrome is caused by haploinsufficiency for the *SOX9* gene.[104–106] *SOX9* is a member of the *SOX* gene family that is defined by sharing sequence homology to *SRY* in the HMG-box region.[57,107] Campomelic dysplasia and *SOX9* are reviewed in this volume by Schafer (see Chap. 253).
- XY sex reversal and *DAX1*. Duplications of a 160-kb region of the short arm of the X chromosome (within Xp21.3) cause sex reversal and multiple congenital anomalies in 46XY patients.[108,109] Within this region is the gene *DAX1*.[110] Mutations in *DAX1* cause X-linked adrenal hypoplasia congenita but do not affect male development. Elegant experiments in transgenic mice have shown that *DAX1* acts antagonistically to *SRY*.[110]
- XY sex reversal and autosomal rearrangements. Several unbalanced translocations and deletions involving loss of part of the short arm of chromosome 9 have been associated with failure of masculinization of the external genitalia and persistence of Mullerian ducts.[111–114] Recently, Raymond et al. have mapped a human homologue of *dsx2* to the critical region of the short arm of chromosome 9.[115] The *Drosophila melanogaster* sex-determining gene *dsx2* is the first gene to be implicated in sex determination in both the fruit fly and the nematode *Caenorhabditis elegans*; it would be remarkable if the same gene is involved in mammalian sex determination. Sex reversal also has been associated with chromosomal rearrangements of the long arm of chromosome 10[116,117] and the short arm of chromosome 1.[118]
- X-linked α-thalassemia mental retardation syndrome. X-linked α-thalassemia associated with severe mental retardation and multiple congenital abnormalities is caused by mutations in *ATRX*, a DNA helicase gene.[119,120] Some mutations in the C-terminal region of this gene are associated with 46XY gonadal dysgenesis.
- Wilms tumor, Denys-Drash syndrome, and Frasier syndrome. Mutations in the Wilms tumor gene, *WT1*, can cause abnormalities in development of both kidneys and gonads (Denys-Drash syndrome) as well as predisposing to Wilms tumor.[121,122] In Frasier syndrome, splice site mutations in *WT1* have been reported to result in complete gonadal dysgenesis and late-onset kidney failure.[123–125]

Errors in Secondary Sexual Differentiation

These conditions, which result from a number of metabolic defects, are outside the scope of this review, but they are described elsewhere in this volume:

- Androgen insensitivity syndrome (testicular feminization) caused by mutations in the androgen receptor (see Chap. 160)
- 5-α-reductase deficiency resulting in pseudohermaphroditism (see Chap. 160)
- Errors in steroid enzyme biosynthesis, including deficiencies in 20,22-desmolase, 3-β-ol-dehydrogenase, 17-ketosteroid reductase and 17-α-hydroxylase (see Chap. 159)
- Persistent Mullerian duct syndrome caused by mutations in the gene encoding either AMH or the AMH receptor (see Chap. 160)

XX MALES

XX males have a phenotype similar to that found in Klinefelter syndrome.[77] The habitus is male, but with small testes and stature reduced to within the normal female range. Patients are infertile because of breakdown of the germinal epithelium caused by the presence of two X chromosomes in spermatogenesis. The absence of germ cells is associated with elevated serum levels of gonadotropins. Androgen production may be compromised, and gynecomastia is found in many patients in adolescence. Intelligence is usually within the normal range. The majority of XX males have inherited *SRY*.

SRY-Positive XX Males

X-Y interchange can be demonstrated in about 80 percent of XX males by testing their DNA for the presence of the Y-specific pseudoautosomal boundary.[35,126] All these patients have so far also tested positive for *SRY*. Although clustering of breakpoints on the X and Y chromosomes has been described,[49–51] there is variation in the size of the fragment of the Y short arm that has been inherited in different XX males.[58,127] The amount of the short arm of the X chromosome lost in the X-Y interchange varies from a small part of the pseudoautosomal region to a substantial region, which includes the Xg and STS loci.[127] The size of both the deletion of the X chromosome and the transferred fragment of the Y chromosome could affect the phenotype of sex-reversed patients. Several genes have been recently mapped to the pseudoautosomal region and the proximal part of the X chromosome.[128–131] A detailed phenotype-genotype study considering the inclusion or exclusion of these genes might provide an explanation for the occasional differences in phenotype noted in XX males.[121,132]

In a few Y sequence–positive XX males, the X-Y interchange has been very small, including *SRY* but without the immediately proximal *ZFY* and *RPS4Y* loci.[35,133] In one study three such patients were described; two had hypospadias and one had bilateral cryptorchidism.[35] One of the hypospadic XX males had a sibling with true hermaphroditism and genital ambiguity due to bilateral ovotestes. The incomplete development of the external genitalia in these cases suggests a position effect that either alters *SRY* expression because of proximity to an X-linked locus or spreading of X-inactivation.

SRY-Negative XX Males

There are a substantial number of XX males (about 20 percent) in whom no Y sequences can be identified by probing for either the Y-specific pseudoautosomal boundary or *SRY*.[35,126] The majority of these Y-negative cases have ambiguity of the external genitalia as described in the paragraphs above. The cause of the sex reversal in these cases is unknown. One possibility is the constitutive activation or inactivation of a gene, normally regulated by *SRY*. The advantage of this hypothesis is that it could account for familial cases.

SRY in XX True Hermaphrodites

True hermaphroditism is a term used to describe individuals who have both testicular and ovarian development. The most common finding is a testis on one side and an ovary on the other (lateral hermaphroditism), with Mullerian ducts suppressed on the side of the testis. Bilateral ovotestes are usually associated with bilateral tubes and a uterus. Unilateral ovary and ovotestis is almost as common as lateral hermaphroditism. The least frequent variety is a unilateral testes and ovotestis; in all such cases the testis has suppressed Mullerian ducts on the ipsilateral side only.[134] The phenotype is characteristic. All adult patients have stature within the normal female range and are of normal intelligence. They invariably present for investigation of ambiguous external genitalia. This usually consists of perineal hypospadias, a vaginal pouch, and variable development of the uterus and fallopian tubes, depending on the exact nature of the ipsilateral gonad. The majority of true hermaphrodites are assigned the male gender and have extensive operations for repair of the phallus and construction of a penile urethra. Virilization occurs at puberty and is usually followed by breast development in which the mammary gland is involved as well as the mammary duct and periductal tissue.

The causes of true hermaphroditism include mosaicism and chimerism.[135] XX/XY chimerism is usually due to double fertilization of an ovum and its polar body.[136] Such individuals are composed of a mixture of the cells of two embryos — one group destined to be testis determining and the other ovary determining. The exact form of gonadal differentiation depends on the proportion of each cell line in the undifferentiated gonad. True hermaphroditism also may occur in 46XX/47XXY somatic-cell mosaics produced by postzygotic nondisjunction in an XXY zygote. Once again, the presence of an active Y chromosome in only a proportion of cells can lead to both testicular and ovarian development in the same individual.

In most true hermaphrodites there is no evidence of either mosaicism or chimerism, and the karyotype is that of an apparently normal female. The Y-specific pseudoautosomal boundary is absent, and there is no other evidence of X-Y interchange.[35,133,137,138]

Although the majority of XX true hermaphrodites are Y sequence–negative, a few exceptions have Y-specific sequences including *SRY.* In one case, a large part of Yp had been exchanged, including *SRY.*[137] The exchange had deleted a substantial part of the X chromosome short arm. If the deleted X chromosome was preferentially inactivated, the partial sex reversal could have been due to variable spread of inactivation into the Y segment.

In three other cases, only a small fragment of the Y chromosome, including *SRY,* had been transferred.[35,133] In these cases, random X-inactivation affecting the *SRY* locus may have been responsible for the presence of both testicular and ovarian development in a manner analogous to that occurring in the XX/XY chimeras.

Familial XX Males and True Hermaphrodites

As noted above, the Y sequence–positive true hermaphrodite described by Palmer et al.[35] had a hypospadic XX male sibling with the same 35-kb Y-specific sequence and a normal XY brother. In this family, it is possible that the father carries a duplication of the sex-determining region of the Y chromosome.

A number of other families are known in which XX true hermaphroditism or XX males, or both, have occurred in the same sibship.[138–140] Those that have been tested are apparently Y sequence–negative cases.[141,142]

SEX DETERMINATION CASCADE AND IMPORTANCE OF STUDYING SEX-REVERSED PHENOTYPES

The identification and cloning of the genes involved in sex determination and the demonstration of their role in sex determination have depended crucially on the analysis of sex-reversed patients. Future progress will require the continued close collaboration between clinicians, molecular biologists, and our colleagues who study model organisms.

REFERENCES

1. Jost A: Recherches sur la differenciation sexuelle de l'embryon de lapin. III. Role des gonades foetales dans la differentiation sexuelle somatique. *Arch Anat Micr Morphol Exp* **36**:271, 1947.
2. McLaren A: Sex determination in mammals. *Trends Genet* **4**:53, 1988.
3. Jost A, Vigier B, Prepin J, Perchellet JP: Studies on sex differentiation in mammals. *Recent Prog Horm Res* **29**:1, 1973.
4. McLaren A: Relation of germ cell sex to gonadal development, in Halvorson HO, Monroy A (eds): *The Origin and Evolution of Sex*. New York, Liss, 1985, p 289.
5. Painter TS: Studies in mammalian spermatogenesis. II. The spermatogenesis in man. *J Exp Zool* **37**:291, 1923.
6. Ford CE, Jones KW, Polani PE, De Almeida JC, Briggs JH: A sex chromosome anomaly in a case of gonadal dysgenesis (Turner's syndrome). *Lancet* **1**:711, 1959.
7. Jacobs PA, Strong JA: A case of human intersexuality having a possible XXY sex determining mechanism. *Nature* **183**:302, 1959.
8. Welshons WJ, Russell LB: The Y chromosome as the bearer of male determining factors in the mouse. *Proc Natl Acad Sci U S A* **45**:560, 1959.
9. Jacobs PA, Ross A: Structural abnormalities of the Y chromosome in man. *Nature* **210**:352, 1966.
10. Davis RM: Localisation of male determining factors in man: A thorough review of structural anomalies of the Y chromosome. *J Med Genet* **18**:161, 1981.
11. Ferguson-Smith MA: Karyotype-phenotype correlations in gonadal dysgenesis and their bearing on the pathogenesis of malformations. *J Med Genet* **2**:142, 1965.
12. de la Chapelle A, Hortling H, Niemi H, Wennstrom J: XX chromosomes in a human male: First case. *Acta Med Scand Suppl* **412**:25, 1964.
13. Ferguson-Smith MA: Sex chromatin, Klinefelter's syndrome and mental deficiency, in Moore KL (ed): *The Sex Chromatin.* Philadelphia, Saunders, 1965, p 277.
14. Ferguson-Smith MA: X-Y chromosomal interchange in the aetiology of true hermaphroditism and of XX Klinefelter's syndrome. *Lancet* **2**:475, 1966.
15. Koller PC, Darlington CD: The genetical and mechanical properties of the sex chromosomes. 1. Rattus norvegicus. *J Genet* **29**:159, 1934.
16. Race RR, Sanger R: *Blood Groups in Man*. London, Blackwell, 1975.
17. de la Chapelle A, Tippett PA, Wetterstrand G, Page D: Genetic evidence of X-Y interchange in a human XX male. *Nature* **307**:170, 1984.
18. Evans HJ, Buckton KE, Spowart G, Carothers AD: Heteromorphic X chromosomes in 46,XX males: Evidence for the involvement of X-Y interchange. *Hum Genet* **49**:11, 1979.
19. Madan K: Chromosome measurements on an XXp+ male. *Hum Genet* **32**:141, 1976.
20. Magenis RE, Webb MJ, McKean RS, Tomar D, Allen LJ, Kammer H, Van Dyke DL, et al.: Translocation(X;Y)(p22.33;p11.2) in XX males: Etiology of male phenotype. *Hum Genet* **62**:271, 1982.
21. Guellaen G, Casanova M, Bishop C, Geldwerth D, Andre G, Fellous M, Weissenbach J: Human XX males with Y single-copy DNA fragments. *Nature* **307**:172, 1984.
22. Page DC: Sex reversal: deletion mapping the male-determining function of the human Y chromosome. *Cold Spring Harb Symp Quant Biol* **51**:1:229, 1986.
23. Simmler MC, Rouyer F, Vergnaud G, Nystrom-Lahti M, Ngo KY, de la Chapelle A, Weissenbach J: Pseudoautosomal DNA sequences in the pairing region of the human sex chromosomes. *Nature* **317**:692, 1985.
24. Cooke HJ, Brown WR, Rappold GA: Hypervariable telomeric sequences from the human sex chromosomes are pseudoautosomal. *Nature* **317**:687, 1985.
25. Burgoyne PS: Genetic homology and crossing over in the X and Y chromosomes of mammals. *Hum Genet* **61**:85, 1982.
26. Goodfellow PJ, Darling SM, Thomas NS, Goodfellow PN: A pseudoautosomal gene in man. *Science* **234**:740, 1986.
27. Weissenbach J, Levilliers J, Petit C, Rouyer F, Simmler MC: Normal and abnormal interchanges between the human X and Y chromosomes. *Development* **101**(Suppl):67, 1987.

28. Rouyer F, Simmler MC, Johnsson C, Vergnaud G, Cooke HJ, Weissenbach J: A gradient of sex linkage in the pseudoautosomal region of the human sex chromosomes. *Nature* **319**:291, 1986.
29. Brown WR: A physical map of the human pseudoautosomal region. *EMBO J* **7**:2377, 1988.
30. Petit C, Levilliers J, Weissenbach J: Physical mapping of the human pseudo-autosomal region; comparison with genetic linkage map. *EMBO J* **7**:2369, 1988.
31. Ellis NA, Goodfellow PJ, Pym B, Smith M, Palmer M, Frischauf AM, Goodfellow PN: The pseudoautosomal boundary in man is defined by an Alu repeat sequence inserted on the Y chromosome. *Nature* **337**:81, 1989.
32. Ellis N, Yen P, Neiswanger K, Shapiro LJ, Goodfellow PN: Evolution of the pseudoautosomal boundary in Old World monkeys and great apes. *Cell* **63**:977, 1990.
33. Gabriel Robez O, Rumpler Y, Ratomponirina C, Petit C, Levilliers J, Croquette MF, Couturier J: Deletion of the pseudoautosomal region and lack of sex-chromosome pairing at pachytene in two infertile men carrying an X;Y translocation. *Cytogenet Cell Genet* **54**:38, 1990.
34. Shapiro LJ, Mohandas T, Yen P, Speed R, Chandley A: The pseudoautosomal region of the X chromosome is necessary for sex chromosome pairing. *Am J Hum Genet* **45(Suppl. 4)**:107, 1989.
35. Palmer MS, Sinclair AH, Berta P, Ellis NA, Goodfellow PN, Abbas NE, Fellous M: Genetic evidence that ZFY is not the testis-determining factor. *Nature* **342**:937, 1989.
36. Affara NA, Ferguson-Smith MA, Tolmie J, Kwok K, Mitchell M, Jamieson D, Cooke A, et al.: Variable transfer of Y-specific sequences in XX males. *Nucleic Acids Res* **14**:5375, 1986.
37. Muller U, Lalande M, Donlon T, Latt SA: Moderately repeated DNA sequences specific for the short arm of the human Y chromosome are present in XX males and reduced in copy number in an XY female. *Nucleic Acids Res* **14**:1325, 1986.
38. Ferguson-Smith MA: Progress in the molecular cytogenetics of man. *Philos Trans R Soc Lond B Biol Sci* **319**:239, 1988.
39. Andersson M, Page DC, de la Chapelle A: Chromosome Y-specific DNA is transferred to the short arm of X chromosome in human XX males. *Science* **233**:786, 1986.
40. Buckle VJ, Boyd Y, Fraser N, Goodfellow PN, Goodfellow PJ, Wolfe J, Craig IW: Localisation of Y chromosome sequences in normal and "XX" males. *J Med Genet* **24**:197, 1987.
41. Page DC, Mosher R, Simpson EM, Fisher EM, Mardon G, Pollack J, McGillivray B, et al.: The sex-determining region of the human Y chromosome encodes a finger protein. *Cell* **51**:1091, 1987.
42. Ferguson-Smith MA, Affara NA, Magenis RE: Ordering of Y-specific sequences by deletion mapping and analysis of X-Y interchange males and females. *Development* **101** (suppl):41, 1987.
43. Vergnaud G, Page DC, Simmler MC, Brown L, Rouyer F, Noel B, Botstein D, et al.: A deletion map of the human Y chromosome based on DNA hybridization. *Am J Hum Genet* **38**:109, 1986.
44. Petit C, de la Chapelle A, Levilliers J, Castillo S, Noel B, Weissenbach J: An abnormal terminal X-Y interchange accounts for most but not all cases of human XX maleness. *Cell* **49**:595, 1987.
45. Rouyer F, Simmler MC, Page DC, Weissenbach J: A sex chromosome rearrangement in a human XX male caused by Alu-Alu recombination. *Cell* **51**:417, 1987.
46. Page DC, Brown LG, de la Chapelle A: Exchange of terminal portions of X- and Y-chromosomal short arms in human XX males. *Nature* **328**:437, 1987.
47. Page DC, de la Chapelle A: The parental origin of X chromosomes in XX males determined using restriction fragment length polymorphisms. *Am J Hum Genet* **36**:565, 1984.
48. Muller U, Lalande M, Donlon TA, Heartlein MW: Breakage of the human Y-chromosome short arm between two blocks of tandemly repeated DNA sequences. *Genomics* **5**:153, 1989.
49. Wang I, Weil D, Levilliers J, Affara NA, de la Chapelle A, Petit C: Prevalence and molecular analysis of two hot spots for ectopic recombination leading to XX maleness. *Genomics* **28**:52, 1995.
50. Weil D, Wang I, Dietrich A, Poustka A, Weissenbach J, Petit C: Highly homologous loci on the X and Y chromosomes are hot-spots for ectopic recombinations leading to XX maleness. *Nat Genet* **7**:414, 1994.
51. Schiebel K, Winkelmann M, Mertz A, Xu X, Page DC, Weil D, Petit C, et al.: Abnormal XY interchange between a novel isolated protein kinase gene, PRKY, and its homologue, PRKX, accounts for one third of all (Y+)XX males and (Y-)XY females. *Hum Mol Genet* **6**:1985, 1997.
52. Blagowidow N, Page DC, Huff D, Mennuti MT: Ullrich-Turner syndrome in an XY female fetus with deletion of the sex-determining portion of the Y chromosome. *Am J Hum Genet* **34**:159, 1989.
53. Levilliers J, Quack B, Weissenbach J, Petit C: Exchange of terminal portions of X- and Y-chromosomal short arms in human XY females. *Proc Natl Acad Sci U S A* **86**:2296, 1989.
54. Disteche CM, Casanova M, Saal H, Friedman C, Sybert V, Graham J, Thuline H, et al.: Small deletions of the short arm of the Y chromosome in 46,XY females. *Proc Natl Acad Sci U S A* **83**:7841, 1986.
55. Magenis RE, Tochen ML, Holahan KP, Carey T, Allen L, Brown MG: Turner syndrome resulting from partial deletion of Y chromosome short arm: Localization of male determinants. *J Pediatr* **105**:916, 1984.
56. Affara NA, Ferguson-Smith MA, Magenis RE, Tolmie JL, Boyd E, Cooke A, Jamieson D, et al.: Mapping the testis determinants by an analysis of Y-specific sequences in males with apparent XX and XO karyotypes and females with XY karyotypes. *Nucleic Acids Res* **15**:7325, 1987.
57. Gubbay J, Collignon J, Koopman P, Capel B, Economou A, Munsterberg A, Vivian N, et al.: A gene mapping to the sex-determining region of the mouse Y chromosome is a member of a novel family of embryonically expressed genes. *Nature* **346**:245, 1990.
58. Sinclair AH, Berta P, Palmer MS, Hawkins JR, Griffiths BL, Smith MJ, Foster JW, et al.: A gene from the human sex-determining region encodes a protein with homology to a conserved DNA-binding motif. *Nature* **346**:240, 1990.
59. Koopman P, Munsterberg A, Capel B, Vivian N, Lovell-Badge R: Expression of a candidate sex-determining gene during mouse testis differentiation. *Nature* **348**:450, 1990.
60. Jeske YW, Mishina Y, Cohen DR, Behringer RR, Koopman P: Analysis of the role of Amh and Fra1 in the Sry regulatory pathway. *Mol Reprod Dev* **44**:153, 1996.
61. Jager RJ, Anvret M, Hall K, Scherer G: A human XY female with a frameshift mutation in the candidate testis-determining gene *SRY. Nature* **348**:452, 1990.
62. Berta P, Hawkins JR, Sinclair AH, Taylor A, Griffiths BL, Goodfellow PN, Fellous M: Genetic evidence equating *SRY* and the testis-determining factor. *Nature* **348**:448, 1990.
63. Koopman P, Gubbay J, Vivian N, Goodfellow P, Lovell-Badge R: Male development of chromosomally female mice transgenic for *Sry. Nature* **351**:117, 1991.
64. Harley VR, Jackson DI, Hextall PJ, Hawkins JR, Berkovitz GD, Sockanathan S, Lovell-Badge R, et al.: DNA binding activity of recombinant *SRY* from normal males and XY females. *Science* **255**:453, 1992.
65. Nasrin N, Buggs C, Kong XF, Carnazza J, Goebl M, Alexander Bridges M: DNA-binding properties of the product of the testis-determining gene and a related protein. *Nature* **354**:317, 1991.
66. Ner SS: HMGs everywhere. *Curr Biol* **2**:208, 1992.
67. Pontiggia A, Rimini R, Harley VR, Goodfellow PN, Lovell-Badge R, Bianchi ME: Sex-reversing mutations affect the architecture of *SRY*-DNA complexes. *EMBO J* **13**:6115, 1994.
68. Goodfellow PN, Lovell-Badge R: SRY and sex determination in mammals. *Annu Rev Genet* **27**:71, 1993.
69. Greenfield A, Koopman P: SRY and mammalian sex determination. *Curr Top Dev Biol* **34**:1, 1996.
70. Werner MH, Huth JR, Gronenborn AM, Clore GM: Molecular determinants of mammalian sex. *Trends Biochem Sci* **21**:302, 1996.
71. Schafer AJ, Goodfellow PN: Sex determination in humans. *Bioessays* **18**:955, 1996.
72. McElreavey K, Fellous M: Sex determining genes. *Trends Endocrinol Metab* **8**:342, 1997.
73. Scully RE: Gonadoblastoma. A review of 74 cases. *Cancer* **25**:1340, 1970.
74. Warner BA, Monsaert RP, Stumpf PG, Kulin HE, Wachtel SS: 46,XY gonadal dysgenesis: Is oncogenesis related to H-Y phenotype or breast development? *Hum Genet* **69**:79, 1985.
75. Harnden DG, Stewart JSS: The chromosomes in a case of pure gonadal dysgenesis. *Br Med J* **5162**:1285, 1959.
76. Swyer GIM: Male pseudohermaphroditism: A hitherto undescribed form. *BMJ* **2**:709, 1955.
77. Ferguson-Smith MA: Genotype-phenotype correlations in individuals with disorders of sex determination and development including Turner's syndrome. *Semin Dev Biol* **2**:265, 1991.

78. Rao E, Weiss B, Fukami M, Rump A, Niesler B, Mertz A, Muroya K, et al.: Pseudoautosomal deletions encompassing a novel homeobox gene cause growth failure in idiopathic short stature and Turner syndrome. *Nat Genet* **16**:54, 1997.
79. Page DC, Fisher EM, McGillivray B, Brown LG: Additional deletion in sex-determining region of human Y chromosome resolves paradox of X,t(Y;22) female. *Nature* **346**:279, 1990.
80. Veitia R, Ion A, Barbaux S, Jobling MA, Souleyreau N, Ennis K, Ostrer H, et al.: Mutations and sequence variants in the testis-determining region of the Y chromosome in individuals with a 46,XY female phenotype. *Hum Genet* **99**:648, 1997.
81. Tajima T, Nakae J, Shinohara N, Fujieda K: A novel mutation localized in the 3′ non-HMG box region of the SRY gene in 46,XY gonadal dysgenesis. *Hum Mol Genet* **3**:1187, 1994.
82. McElreavy K, Vilain E, Abbas N, Costa JM, Souleyreau N, Kucheria K, Boucekkine C, et al.: XY sex reversal associated with a deletion 5′ to the SRY "HMG box" in the testis-determining region. *Proc Natl Acad Sci U S A* **89**:11016, 1992.
83. Kwok C, Tyler Smith C, Mendonca BB, Hughes I, Berkovitz GD, Goodfellow PN, Hawkins JR: Mutation analysis of the 2 kb 5′ to SRY in XY females and XY intersex subjects. *J Med Genet* **33**:465, 1996.
84. Poulat F, Desclozeaux M, Tuffery S, Jay P, Boizet B, Berta P: A mutation in the 5′ non-coding region of the SRY gene in an XY sex reversed patient. *Hum Mutat* (suppl 1):192, 1998.
85. McElreavey K, Vilain E, Barbaux S, Fuqua JS, Fechner PY, Souleyreau N, Doco Fenzy M, et al.: Loss of sequences 3′ to the testis-determining gene, *SRY,* including the Y pseudoautosomal boundary associated with partial testicular determination. *Proc Natl Acad Sci U S A* **93**:8590, 1996.
86. Domenice S, Yumie Nishi M, Correia Billerbeck AE, Latronico AC, Aparecida Medeiros M, Russell AJ, Vass K, et al.: A novel missense mutation (S18N) in the 5′ non-HMG box region of the SRY gene in a patient with partial gonadal dysgenesis and his normal male relatives. *Hum Genet* **102**:213, 1998.
87. Brown S, Yu C, Lanzano P, Heller D, Thomas L, Warburton D, Kitajewski J, et al.: A *de novo* mutation (Gln2Stop) at the 5′ end of the SRY gene leads to sex reversal with partial ovarian function. *Am J Hum Genet* **62**:189, 1998.
88. Braun A, Kammerer S, Cleve H, Lohrs U, Schwarz HP, Kuhnle U: True hermaphroditism in a 46,XY individual, caused by a postzygotic somatic point mutation in the male gonadal sex-determining locus (SRY): molecular genetics and histological findings in a sporadic case. *Am J Hum Genet* **52**:578, 1993.
89. Jager RJ, Pfeiffer RA, Scherer G: A familial amino-acid substitution in SRY can lead to conditional XY sex inversion. *Am J Hum Genet* **49**(suppl):219, 1991.
90. Hawkins JR, Taylor A, Goodfellow PN, Migeon CJ, Smith KD, Berkovitz GD: Evidence for increased prevalence of *SRY* mutations in XY females with complete rather than partial gonadal dysgenesis. *Am J Hum Genet* **51**:979, 1992.
91. Vilain E, McElreavey K, Jaubert F, Raymond JP, Richaud F, Fellous M: Familial case with sequence variant in the testis-determining region associated with two sex phenotypes. *Am J Hum Genet* **50**:1008, 1992.
92. Hines RS, Tho SP, Zhang YY, Plouffe L Jr, Hansen KA, Khan I, McDonough PG: Paternal somatic and germ-line mosaicism for a sex-determining region on Y (*SRY*) missense mutation leading to recurrent 46,XY sex reversal. *Fertil Steril* **67**:675, 1997.
93. Schmitt Ney M, Thiele H, Kaltwasser P, Bardoni B, Cisternino M, Scherer G: Two novel *SRY* missense mutations reducing DNA binding identified in XY females and their mosaic fathers. *Am J Hum Genet* **56**:862, 1995.
94. Simpson JL: *Disorders of Sexual Differentiation.* New York, Academic, 1976.
95. Simpson JL, Blagowidow N, Martin AO: XY gonadal dysgenesis: genetic heterogeneity based upon clinical observations, H-Y antigen status and segregation analysis. *Hum Genet* **58**:91, 1981.
96. Chemke J, Carmichael R, Stewart JM, Geer RH, Robinson A: Familial XY gonadal dysgenesis. *J Med Genet* **7**:105, 1970.
97. Coulam CB: Testicular regression syndrome. *Obstet Gynecol* **53**:44, 1979.
98. Edman CD, Winters AJ, Porter JC, Wilson J, MacDonald PC: Embryonic testicular regression. A clinical spectrum of XY agonadal individuals. *Obstet Gynecol* **49**:208, 1977.
99. Sarto GE, Opitz JM: The XY gonadal agenesis syndrome. *J Med Genet* **10**:288, 1973.
100. Mendonca BB, Barbosa AS, Arnhold IJ, McElreavey K, Fellous M, Moreira Filho CA: Gonadal agenesis in XX and XY sisters: Evidence for the involvement of an autosomal gene. *Am J Hum Genet* **52**:39, 1994.
101. Swain A, Zanaria E, Hacker A, Lovell-Badge R, Camerino G: Mouse Dax1 expression is consistent with a role in sex determination as well as in adrenal and hypothalamus function. *Nat Genet* **12**:404, 1996.
102. Morais da Silva S, Hacker A, Harley V, Goodfellow P, Swain A, Lovell Badge R: Sox9 expression during gonadal development implies a conserved role for the gene in testis differentiation in mammals and birds. *Nat Genet* **14**:62, 1996.
103. Hoefnagel D, Wuster Hill DH, Dupree WB, Benirschke K, Fuld GL: Camptomelic dwarfism associated with XY-gonadal dysgenesis and chromosome anomalies. *Clin Genet* **13**:489, 1978.
104. Cameron FJ, Sinclair AH: Mutations in SRY and SOX9: testis-determining genes. *Hum Mutat* **9**:388, 1997.
105. Wagner T, Wirth J, Meyer J, Zabel B, Held M, Zimmer J, Pasantes J, et al.: Autosomal sex reversal and campomelic dysplasia are caused by mutations in and around the SRY-related gene *SOX9. Cell* **79**:1111, 1994.
106. Foster JW, Dominguez Steglich MA, Guioli S, Kowk G, Weller PA, Stevanovic M, Weissenbach J, et al.: Campomelic dysplasia and autosomal sex reversal caused by mutations in an *SRY*-related gene. *Nature* **372**:525, 1994.
107. Pevny LH, Lovell-Badge R: Sox genes find their feet. *Curr Opin Genet Dev* **7**:338, 1997.
108. Bernstein R, Jenkins T, Dawson B, Wagner J, Dewald G, Koo GC, Wachtel SS: Female phenotype and multiple abnormalities in sibs with a Y chromosome and partial X chromosome duplication: H-Y antigen and Xg blood group findings. *J Med Genet* **17**:291, 1980.
109. Bardoni B, Zanaria E, Guioli S, Floridia G, Worley KC, Tonini G, Ferrante E, et al.: A dosage sensitive locus at chromosome Xp21 is involved in male to female sex reversal. *Nat Genet* **7**:497, 1994.
110. Zanaria E, Muscatelli F, Bardoni B, Strom TM, Guioli S, Guo W, Lalli E, et al.: An unusual member of the nuclear hormone receptor superfamily responsible for X-linked adrenal hypoplasia congenita. *Nature* **372**:635, 1994.
111. Bennett CP, Docherty Z, Robb SA, Ramani P, Hawkins JR, Grant D: Deletion 9p and sex reversal. *J Med Genet* **30**:518, 1993.
112. Crocker M, Coghill SB, Cortinho R: An unbalanced autosomal translocation (7;9) associated with feminization. *Clin Genet* **34**:70, 1988.
113. McDonald MT, Flejter W, Sheldon S, Putzi MJ, Gorski JL: XY sex reversal and gonadal dysgenesis due to 9p24 monosomy. *Am J Hum Genet* **73**:321, 1997.
114. Veitia R, Nunes M, Brauner R, Doco-Fenzy M, Joanny Flinois O, Jaubert F, Lortat-Jacob S, et al.: Deletions of distal 9p associated with 46,XY male to female sex reversal: Definition of the breakpoints at 9p23.3-p24.1. *Genomics* **41**:271, 1997.
115. Raymond CS, Shamu CE, Shen MM, Seifert KJ, Hirsch B, Hodgkin J, Zarkower D: Evidence for evolutionary conservation of sex-determining genes. *Nature* **391**:691, 1998.
116. Wilkie AO, Campbell FM, Daubeney P, Grant DB, Daniels RJ, Mullarkey M, Affara NA, et al.: Complete and partial XY sex reversal associated with terminal deletion of 10q: report of 2 cases and literature review. *Am J Hum Genet* **46**:597, 1993.
117. Chung YP, Hwa HL, Tseng LH, Shyu MK, Lee CN, Shih JC, Hsieh FJ: Prenatal diagnosis of monosomy 10q25 associated with single umbilical artery and sex reversal: Report of a case. *Prenat Diagn* **18**:73, 1998.
118. Wieacker P, Missbach D, Jakubiczka S, Borgmann S, Albers N: Sex reversal in a child with the karyotype 46,XY, dup (1) (p22.3p32.3). *Clin Genet* **49**:271, 1996.
119. Gibbons RJ, Picketts DJ, Villard L, Higgs DR: Mutations in a putative global transcriptional regulator cause X-linked mental retardation with α-thalassemia (ATR-X syndrome). *Cell* **80**:837, 1995.
120. Ion A, Telvi L, Chaussain JL, Galacteros F, Valayer J, Fellous M, McElreavey K: A novel mutation in the putative DNA helicase XH2 is responsible for male-to-female sex reversal associated with an atypical form of the ATR-X syndrome. *Am J Hum Genet* **58**:1185, 1996.
121. Pelletier J, Bruening W, Li FP, Haber DA, Glaser T, Housman DE: WT1 mutations contribute to abnormal genital system development and hereditary Wilms' tumour. *Nature* **353**:431, 1991.
122. Pelletier J, Bruening W, Kashtan CE, Mauer SM, Manivel JC, Striegel JE, Houghton DC, et al.: Germline mutations in the Wilms' tumor suppressor gene are associated with abnormal urogenital development in Denys-Drash syndrome. *Cell* **67**:437, 1991.
123. Kikuchi H, Takata A, Akasaka Y, Fukuzawa R, Yoneyama H, Kurosawa Y, Honda M, et al.: Do intronic mutations affecting splicing of WT1 exon 9 cause Frasier syndrome? *J Med Genet* **35**:45, 1998.

124. Barbaux S, Niaudet P, Gubler MC, Grunfeld JP, Jaubert F, Kuttenn F, Fekete CN, et al.: Donor splice-site mutations in WT1 are responsible for Frasier syndrome. *Nat Genet* **17**:467, 1997.
125. Klamt B, Koziell A, Poulat F, Wieacker P, Scambler P, Berta P, Gessler M: Frasier syndrome is caused by defective alternative splicing of WT1 leading to an altered ratio of WT1 ± KTS splice isoforms. *Hum Mol Genet* **7**:709, 1998.
126. Ferguson-Smith MA, North MA, Affara NA, Briggs H: The secret of sex. *Lancet* **336**:809, 1990.
127. Ferguson-Smith MA, Affara NA: Accidental X-Y recombination and the aetiology of XX males and true hermaphrodites. *Philos Trans R Soc Lond B Biol Sci* **322**:133, 1988.
128. Ogata T, Goodfellow P, Petit C, Aya M, Matsuo N: Short stature in a girl with a terminal Xp deletion distal to DXYS15: Localisation of a growth gene(s) in the pseudoautosomal region. *J Med Genet* **29**:455, 1992.
129. Gianfrancesco F, Esposito T, Montanini L, Ciccodicola A, Mumm S, Mazzarella R, Rao E, et al.: A novel pseudoautosomal gene encoding a putative GTP-binding protein resides in the vicinity of the Xp/Yp telomere. *Hum Mol Genet* **7**:407, 1998.
130. Perry J, Feather S, Smith A, Palmer S, Ashworth A: The human FXY gene is located within Xp22.3: implications for evolution of the mammalian X chromosome. *Hum Mol Genet* **7**:299, 1998.
131. Quaderi NA, Schweiger S, Gaudenz K, Franco B, Rugarli EI, Berger W, Feldman GJ, et al.: Opitz G/BBB syndrome, a defect of midline development, is due to mutations in a new RING finger gene on Xp22. *Nat Genet* **17**:285, 1997.
132. Ballabio A, Bardoni B, Carrozzo R, Andria G, Bick D, Campbell L, Hamel B, et al.: Contiguous gene syndromes due to deletions in the distal short arm of the human X chromosome. *Proc Natl Acad Sci U S A* **86**:10001, 1989.
133. Jager RJ, Ebensperger C, Fraccaro M, Scherer G: A ZFY-negative 46,XX true hermaphrodite is positive for the Y pseudoautosomal boundary. *Hum Genet* **85**:666, 1990.
134. Jones HW, Ferguson-Smith MA, Heller RH: Pathologic and cytogenetic findings in true hermaphroditism: Report of six cases and review of 23 cases from the literature. *Obstet Gynecol* **25**:435, 1965.
135. van Niekerk WA, Retief AE: The gonads of human true hermaphrodites. *Hum Genet* **58**:117, 1981.
136. Gartler SM, Waxman SH, Gilbert E: An XX/XY human hermaphrodite resulting from double fertilisation. *Proc Natl Acad Sci U S A* **48**:332, 1962.
137. Berkovitz GD, Fechner PY, Marcantonio SM, Bland G, Stetten G, Goodfellow PN, Smith KD, et al.: The role of the sex-determining region of the Y chromosome (*SRY*) in the etiology of 46,XX true hermaphroditism. *Hum Genet* **88**:411, 1992.
138. Ramsay M, Bernstein R, Zwane E, Page DC, Jenkins T: XX true hermaphroditism in southern African blacks: An enigma of primary sexual differentiation. *Am J Hum Genet* **43**:4, 1988.
139. Fraccaro M, Tiepolo L, Zuffardi O, Chiumello G, Di Natale B, Gargantini L, Wolf U: Familial XX true hermaphroditism and the H-Y antigen. *Hum Genet* **48**:45, 1979.
140. Kasdan R, Nankin HR, Troen P, Wald N, Pan S, Yanaihara T: Paternal transmission of maleness in XX human beings. *New Engl J Med* **288**:539, 1973.
141. Ramos ES, Moreira Filho CA, Vicente YA, Llorach Velludo MA, Tucci S Jr, Duarte MH, Araujo AG, et al.: SRY-negative true hermaphrodites and an XX male in two generations of the same family. *Hum Genet* **97**:596, 1996.
142. Zenteno JC, Lopez M, Vera C, Mendez JP, Kofman Alfaro S: Two SRY-negative XX male brothers without genital ambiguity. *Hum Genet* **100**:606, 1997.
143. Scherer G, Held M, Erdel M, Meschede D, Horst J, Lesniewicz R, Midro AT: Three novel *sry* mutations in XY gonadal dysgenesis and the enigma of XY gonadal dysgenesis cases without *sry* mutations. *Cytogenet Cell Genet* **80**:188, 1998.
144. Hiort O, Gramss B, Klauber GT: True hermaphroditism with 46,XY karyotype and a point mutation in the SRY gene [Letter; Comment]. *J Pediatr* **126**:1022, 1995.
145. Affara NA, Chalmers IJ, Ferguson-Smith MA: Analysis of the *SRY* gene in 22 sex-reversed XY females identifies four new point mutations in the conserved DNA binding domain. *Hum Mol Genet* **2**:785, 1993.
146. Hawkins JR, Taylor A, Berta P, Levilliers J, Van der Auwera B, Goodfellow PN: Mutational analysis of *SRY*: nonsense and missense mutations in XY sex reversal. *Hum Genet* **88**:471, 1992.
147. Battiloro E, Angeletti B, Tozzi MC, Bruni L, Tondini S, Vignetti P, Verna R, et al.: A novel double nucleotide substitution in the HMG box of the *SRY* gene associated with Swyer syndrome. *Hum Genet* **100**:585, 1997.
148. Cameron FJ, Smith MJ, Warne GL, Sinclair AH: Novel mutation in the *SRY* gene results in 46,XY gonadal dysgenesis. *Hum Mutat* (Suppl)110, 1998.
149. Dork T, Stuhrmann M, Miller K, Schmidtke J: Independent observation of *SRY* mutation I90M in a patient with complete gonadal dysgenesis. *Hum Mutat* **11**:90, 1998.
150. Muller J, Schwartz M, Skakkebaek NE: Analysis of the sex-determining region of the Y chromosome (*SRY*) in sex reversed patients: point-mutation in SRY causing sex-reversion in a 46,XY female. *J Clin Endocrinol Metab* **75**:331, 1992.
151. McElreavey KD, Vilain E, Boucekkine C, Vidaud M, Jaubert F, Richaud F, Fellous M: XY sex reversal associated with a nonsense mutation in SRY. *Genomics* **13**:838, 1992.
152. Bilbao JR, Loridan L, Castano L: A novel postzygotic nonsense mutation in SRY in familial XY gonadal dysgenesis. *Hum Genet* **97**:537, 1996.
153. Iida T, Nakahori Y, Komaki R, Mori E, Hayashi N, Tsutsumi O, Taketani Y, et al.: A novel nonsense mutation in the HMG box of the *SRY* gene in a patient with XY sex reversal. *Hum Mol Genet* **3**:1437, 1994.
154. Tsutsumi O, Iida T, Nakahori Y, Taketani Y: Analysis of the testis-determining gene *SRY* in patients with XY gonadal dysgenesis. *Horm Res* **46** (Suppl 1):6, 1996.
155. Jakubiczka S, Bettecken T, Stumm M, Neulen J, Wieacker P: Another mutation within the HMG-box of the *SRY* gene associated with Swyer syndrome. *Hum Mutat* **13**:85, 1999.
156. Jager RJ, Harley VR, Pfeiffer RA, Goodfellow PN, Scherer G: A familial mutation in the testis-determining gene *SRY* shared by both sexes. *Hum Genet* **90**:350, 1992.
157. Zeng YT, Ren ZR, Zhang ML, Huang Y, Zeng FY, Huang SZ: A new *de novo* mutation (A113T) in HMG box of the *SRY* gene leads to XY gonadal dysgenesis. *J Med Genet* **30**:655, 1993.
158. Kucheria K, Mohapatra I, Ammini AC, Bhargava VL, McElreavey K: Clinical and DNA studies on 46, XY females with gonadal dysgenesis. A report of six cases. *J Reprod Med* **41**:263, 1996.
159. Poulat F, Soullier S, Goze C, Heitz F, Calas B, Berta P: Description and functional implications of a novel mutation in the sex-determining gene *SRY*. *Hum Mutat* **3**:200, 1994.
160. Lundberg Y, Ritzen M, Harlin J, Wedell A: Novel missense mutation (P131R) in the HMG box of *SRY* in XY sex reversal. *Hum Mutat* Suppl 1:328, 1998.

CHAPTER 63

Down Syndrome (Trisomy 21)

Charles J. Epstein

1. The salient clinical features of Down syndrome include several minor malformations or dysmorphic features, which, while not all are invariably present, together constitute the distinctive physical phenotype of the syndrome. Mental retardation and hypotonia are virtually always present, and congenital heart disease (particularly endocardial cushion defects) occurs in about 40 percent of affected individuals. Gastrointestinal anomalies (especially duodenal atresia and Hirschsprung disease) are found in about 5 percent.
2. There is a wide range of ultimate intellectual attainment and rate of psychomotor development, which, to some extent, may be influenced by both environmental and genetic factors. No pharmacologic therapy as yet has been shown to have a beneficial effect. The specific causes of mental retardation have not been elucidated, although decreased nerve cell densities, changes in phospholipid composition, and alterations in certain electrophysiologic properties of the brain and isolated neurons have been demonstrated. The pathologic, metabolic, and neurochemical changes of Alzheimer disease are present after the third decade in the brains of all individuals with Down syndrome, who also have a progressive loss in cognitive functions. Many develop a frank dementia.
3. There is a fifteen- to twentyfold increase in the incidence of leukemia in children with Down syndrome, with acute megakaryoblastic leukemia being particularly frequent among cases of acute nonlymphocytic leukemia. Leukemoid reactions or transient leukemia occurs in infants, as does macrocytosis and increased hematocrit. The activities of several erythrocyte and granulocyte enzymes not coded for by genes on chromosome 21 are increased, and hyperuricemia may be present.
4. Males with Down syndrome are almost invariably infertile, whereas females, while decreased in fertility, are often capable of reproduction. Longitudinal growth is impaired, and there is an increased frequency of thyroid dysfunction in newborns and of thyroid autoantibodies throughout life. A variety of cellular abnormalities are present, including enhanced responses to interferon and β-adrenergic agonists, and possibly small increases in sensitivity to radiation, mutagenic and carcinogenic chemicals, and viruses.
5. The principal causes of death in Down syndrome are infection, congenital heart disease, and malignancy. Longevity has been steadily increasing in recent years, and the life expectancy for individuals without congenital heart disease may be greater than 60 years. The increased susceptibility to infection appears to be the result of abnormalities of the immune system, particularly in the maturation and function of T lymphocytes.
6. In most instances, Down syndrome results from trisomy 21, the presence of an extra chromosome 21 either free or as part of a robertsonian fusion chromosome or isochromosome. Occasional cases result from triplication of just the distal part of the long arm of chromosome 21, or from the presence of trisomy 21/diploid mosaicism. Depending on the frequency and distribution of trisomic cells, mosaic individuals may range from being normal to having the typical phenotypic features of Down syndrome. There is a very strong effect of maternal age, but not of paternal age, on the incidence of trisomy 21. The nondisjunction event leading to the trisomy occurs in the mother about 86 percent of the time, with the maternal error being predominantly (75 percent) in meiosis I. Meiosis I errors are associated with a decreased rate of chromosome 21 recombination; meiosis II errors are associated with an increased rate. No environmental factor has been found to correlate with the occurrence of nondisjunction.
7. The risk for recurrence of nondisjunction is increased in younger mothers ($\leq$30 to 35 years) of children with Down syndrome, and the risk of aneuploid offspring is much higher in mothers who are carriers of balanced robertsonian translocations than in carrier fathers. Prenatal diagnosis by amniocentesis or chorionic villus sampling is capable of detecting fetuses with Down syndrome, and maternal serum triple-marker screening and fetal ultrasonography can each identify a proportion of pregnancies in which a fetus with Down syndrome is present. Fetal cells in maternal blood can be used for the detection of known mutations.
8. Aneuploid phenotypes, while often variable in their expression, are differentiable from one another and are, in terms of overall pattern, specific. Nonspecific effects, while they may occur, are not major determinants of aneuploid phenotypes. Phenotypic variability may result from a combination of genetic, stochastic, and environmental factors. Individual features of aneuploid phenotypes can often be assigned to specific regions of the genome. The existence of a trisomic state results in the production of 50 percent more of the products of genes present on the unbalanced chromosome segment, and these gene dosage effects are, in turn, responsible for the abnormalities of development and function that constitute the aneuploid phenotype.
9. Chromosome 21 is the smallest of the human autosomes, and comprises about 1–1.5 percent of the haploid genome.

A list of standard abbreviations is located immediately preceding the index in each volume. Additional abbreviations used in this chapter include: AD = Alzheimer disease; ALL = acute lymphoblastic leukemia; ANLL = acute nonlymphoblastic leukemia; APP = amyloid precursor protein; CuZnSOD = CuZn-superoxide dismutase; CVS = chorionic villus sampling; DQ = developmental quotient; DS = Down syndrome; ERP = evoked response potential; IQ = intelligence quotient; MI = meiosis I; MII = meiosis II; MoM = multiple(s) of median; MS-AFP = maternal serum α-fetoprotein; SQ = social quotient; Ts16 = trisomy 16.

The long arm is 33.7 megabase pairs in length and contains 225 known and predicted genes. Loss of the short arm, which contains ribosomal RNA genes and other highly repeated DNA sequences, does not impair normal function or development. The physical phenotype of Down syndrome is thought to be produced principally by imbalance of the region which comprises bands distal q22.1 to proximal q22.3, but imbalance of other regions may also contribute to the phenotype.

10. **Gene dosage effects have been demonstrated for several loci on chromosome 21, and work is presently underway to determine whether the increases in gene product activity or concentration have secondary effects on the functions of these gene products. In particular, studies are being done to assess the roles of increased CuZn-superoxide dismutase activity and of increased, and possibly dysregulated, synthesis of the amyloid precursor protein in the pathogenesis of Alzheimer disease.**
11. **Several mouse models have been developed to facilitate studies of the mechanisms of the pathogenesis of Down syndrome. These include several strains of mice segmentally trisomic for chromosome 16, in which the mouse genome homologous to most of human chromosome 21q is triplicated, the trisomy 16/diploid mouse chimera, which is homologous to human trisomy 21/diploid mosaicism, single gene transgenic mice producing increased quantities of individual chromosome 21 gene products, and YAC transgenic mice with segments of human DNA. Abnormalities of learning and behavior have been demonstrated in the segmentally trisomic and YAC-transgenic mice.**

Down syndrome (DS) is the first chromosomal disorder to have been clinically defined,[1] the first (by a week) to be proven actually to be chromosomal in origin—the result of trisomy 21[2–4]—and the most commonly recognized genetic cause of mental retardation. As such, it has been the prototype of human autosomal aneuploidy and the subject of intense clinical, cytogenetic, epidemiologic, and molecular investigation (for recent reviews see references 5 to 16). With the rapid advances in molecular genetics, it is now possible to envision that the genetic structure of human chromosome 21 will be completely defined and that the pathogenic relationship between the presence of an extra set of chromosome 21 genes and the many features of Down syndrome phenotype will be understood.

Although an aneuploid condition such as DS might not ordinarily be considered to be a metabolic disease, it is, in fact, a collection of many metabolic disorders which stem from the presence of extra genes and, as a result, of extra amounts of the products of these genes. Because these gene products must exert their effects largely by their biochemical actions, aneuploidy is no less metabolic than are conditions such as thalassemia or porphyria.[7] Trisomy 21, the cause of DS, can, therefore, be placed on a conceptual continuum, which ranges from the complete absence of one or several genes to a high degree of gene amplification, as occurs in certain malignant states.[17] What is different in aneuploidy from the more conventional metabolic diseases is the number of loci involved, not necessarily how their functions are perturbed by the change in gene number.

CLINICAL ASPECTS OF DOWN SYNDROME

Dysmorphic Features

The most immediately apparent, if not the most serious, manifestations of Down syndrome are the minor dysmorphic features, which collectively constitute its distinctive physical phenotype (Fig. 63-1). A list of these features is presented in Table 63-1. Detailed descriptions of the minor anomalies are contained in Smith and Berg[5] and Pueschel *et al.*[18] Quantitative cephalometric analyses have been used to describe the craniofacial anomalies in persons with DS.[19,20] Not mentioned in Table 63-1, but worthy of note, are two abnormalities of the eye which appear later in life, cataracts and keratoconus.[21]

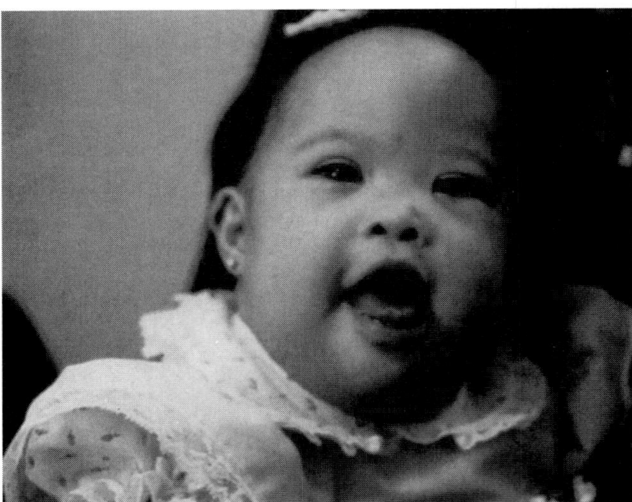

Fig. 63-1 Eight-month-old child with Down syndrome.

Although any single individual will have many of the characteristic features and be easily recognized as having DS, none of these features is present in all persons with DS. Conversely, it is very rare for any single individual with DS to have all the features contained in the list. It should also be remembered that none of the features in the list is unique either to DS or to chromosome abnormalities in general. Accordingly, the presence of one or a few minor dysmorphic features in an otherwise normal individual does not, in itself, signify the existence of a chromosomal abnormality.

In addition to the features listed in Table 63-1, there is a series of dermatoglyphic features that are quite characteristic of DS.[22] These used to play a much greater role in clinical diagnosis than they now do, but they represent, nevertheless, distinctive aspects of the phenotype of DS. Particularly characteristic are the arch tibial

Table 63-1 Physical Characteristics of Down Syndrome

Feature	Frequency, %*
Oblique (upslanting) palpebral fissures	82
Loose skin on nape of neck	81
Narrow palate	76
Brachycephaly	75
Hyperflexibility	73
Flat nasal bridge	68
Gap between first and second toes	68
Short, broad hands	64
Short neck	61
Abnormal teeth	61
Epicanthic folds	59
Short fifth finger	58
Open mouth	58
Incurved fifth finger	57
Brushfield spots	56
Furrowed tongue	55
Transverse palmar crease	53
Folded or dysplastic ear	50
Protruding tongue	47

*Means of frequencies in Table 5-1 of Pueschel et al.[18]

SOURCE: Reprinted by permission from Epstein.[7]

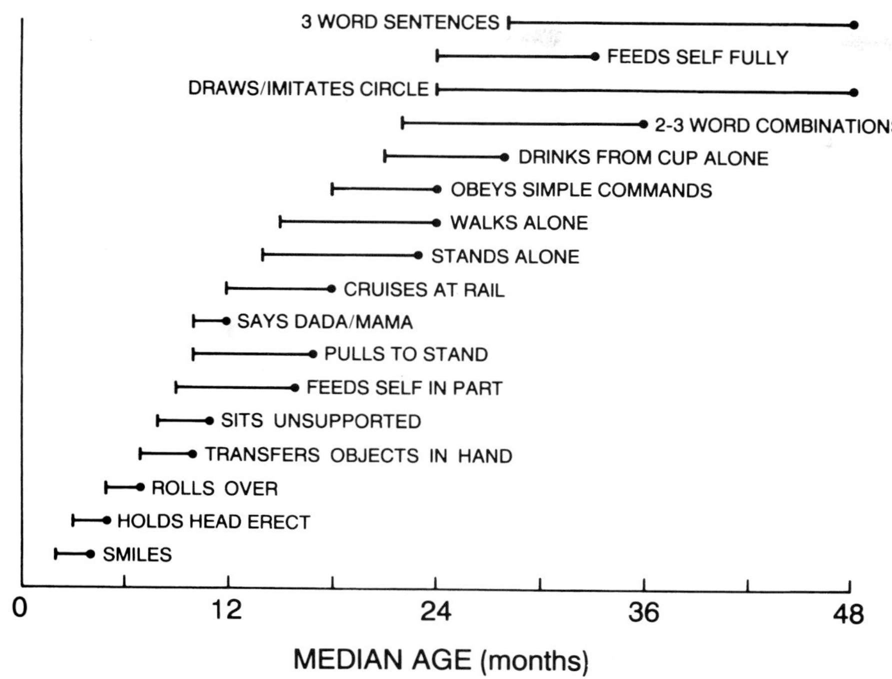

Fig. 63-2 Median time of appearance of developmental landmarks in children with Down syndrome (*) as compared with a normal population (|). *(Data from Share and Veale.*[24]*)*

pattern on the hallucal area of the foot, ulnar loops on the second fingers, and a distal axial palmar triradius. These features, along with ear length (short), the distance between the first and second toes (wide), the internipple distance (< -1 standard deviation [SD]), the presence of Brushfield spots of the iris, and the excessive skinfolds or a fat pad on the neck, can be used to construct an index capable of permitting the diagnosis of 95 percent of patients suspected of having DS with an accuracy of 99.9 percent.[23] In this regard, it is of interest that about 75 to 85 percent of infants clinically suspected of having DS actually have trisomy 21.[23]

Mental Retardation and Neurologic Abnormalities

While the dysmorphic features just discussed are of clinical significance, the condition of overriding clinical importance in DS is, of course, mental retardation. The brain, insofar as it is involved in cognition and other highly integrated mental functions, seems to be the organ most vulnerable to the deleterious effects of autosomal aneuploidy, whichever chromosome is involved. Although structural anomalies of the brain often occur in aneuploid states other than DS, they do not, in themselves, provide a complete explanation for the very severe functional abnormalities that are almost invariably present.

In addition to the effects on intelligence and control of muscle tone early and throughout life, trisomy 21 is also associated with a process of neuronal degeneration during the adult years. This process, which is pathologically identical to Alzheimer disease (AD) (presenile and/or senile dementia), results in significant pathologic changes in the brain and may further compromise the already impaired mental functioning.

Mental Retardation. Although newborns with DS may, with the exception of the profound hypotonia (see "Muscle Tone" below), appear reasonably normal behaviorally, developmental retardation generally becomes obvious during the first several months of life. The attainment of developmental landmarks becomes, on the mean, increasingly more delayed as time goes on. Thus, whereas the average delay may be on the order of 2 months for the very early landmarks (e.g., rolling over, transferring objects), it gradually lengthens and reaches 1 to 2 years for functions that normally appear at about 2 years of age (Fig. 63-2).[24] However, because of the great variability in attainment of landmarks (Fig. 63-3),[25] this delay may or may not be obvious for any single child with DS. For institutionalized individuals, progress continues during the first decade of life, following which there is usually a plateau in mental age.[26] Some individuals may continue to progress mentally for another 5 years or so. There is then a second plateau and ultimately a decline (see "Alzheimer Disease" below).[26]

The conclusions just cited concerning intellectual development in DS were developed based on studies carried out during the 1960s and 1970s. They may be somewhat different now because of changes in social attitudes and education. Nevertheless, many studies of development during the first decade of life indicate that even with DS children reared at home, there is a progressive, virtually linear decline in developmental quotient (DQ) or intelligence quotient (IQ) starting within the first year[25,27] (Fig. 63-4). The same appears to be true of social quotients (SQ).[27] Once again, the wide range of IQs and SQs should be noted. In contrast to these results are the results from a prospective study of infants with DS over the first 3 years of life.[28] In this group, mean DQs, based on the mental scale of the Bayley Scales of Infant Development, remained constant at 55 to 58, although the mean on the motor scale dropped from 67 at 6 months to 53 at 3 years. Cardiac status did not significantly influence mental development, but it did influence motor development.[28] Both mental and motor development appeared to correlate with muscle tone.[28,29]

Genetic and Environmental Effects. In rare instances, children with DS without known mosaicism have attained IQs above 80 and have performed in the low average range.[30] Young men with DS have even written books,[31,32] and another, a well-known television actor, has coauthored one.[33] Although these instances must be considered unusual, they do point out the variability of the syndrome and raise the question of what factors do or could influence mental development. One possible factor is, of course, the intrinsic genetic differences among individuals. An approach to looking at this has been to examine the relationship between parental education levels or IQs and the IQs of their children with DS. Despite evidence against the existence of such correlations,[34] two studies have affirmed the association. In one group of children reared at home and followed longitudinally, the mean DQ or IQ at

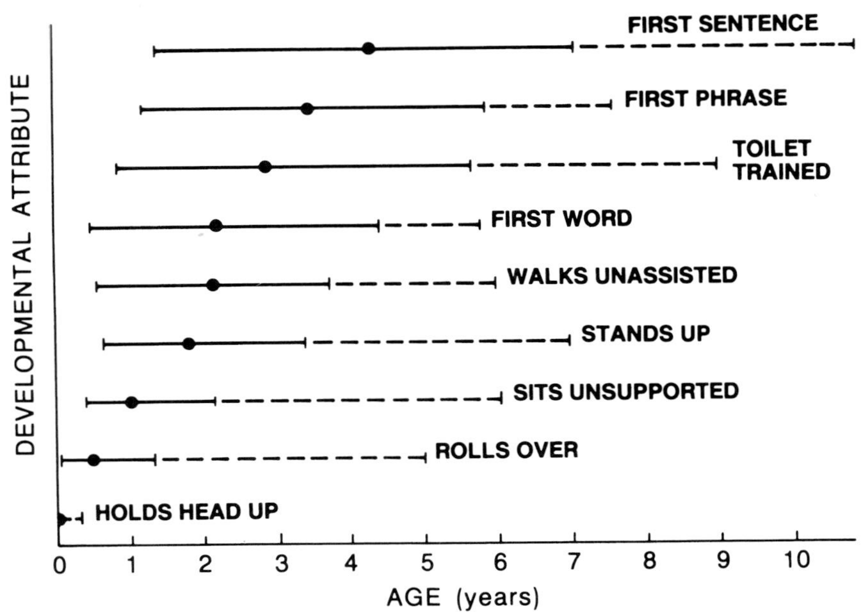

Fig. 63-3 Mean and range of time of appearance of developmental landmarks in children with Down syndrome. The vertical marks to the left of the dashed lines indicate the upper limits for 95 percent of the Down syndrome group. For sitting, standing, walking, and speaking the first word, the figures given are for boys. (*Data from Melyn and White.*[25])

a mean age of about 6 years was 74.6±12 for children of mothers with ≥ 16 years of schooling and 58.8±12 for children of mothers with < 12 years of schooling.[35] In another group with a mean age of 5.2 years, the IQs were 70.3 and 28.8, respectively, when the fathers' schooling was similarly scored.[36]

The results just cited are consistent with a genetic basis for the differences in the IQs of persons with DS, and there is no reason to believe that such genetic influences should not be operating.

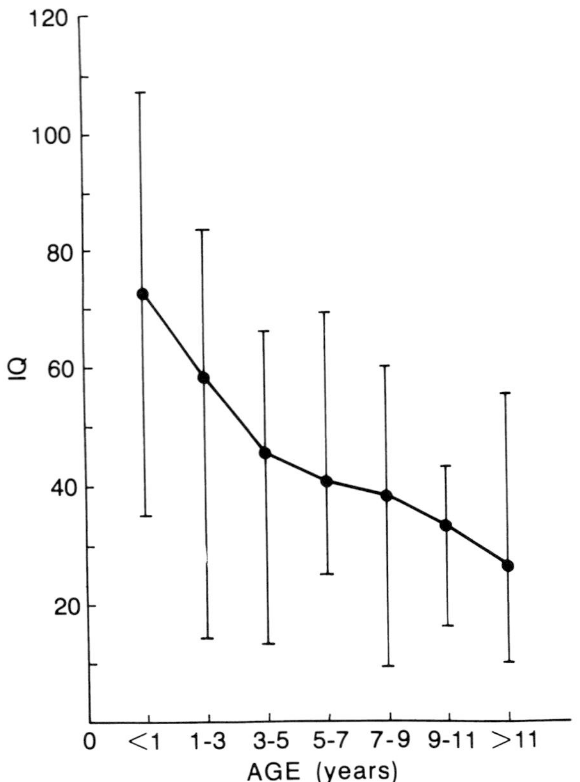

Fig. 63-4 Mean and observed range of intelligence quotient (IQ) of children with Down syndrome as a function of age. (*Data from Morgan.*[27])

However, some authors have argued to the contrary,[26] and it is also possible, of course, that social and educational practices relating to the child are influenced by parental IQ and/or education, and that these environmental factors also play a role. Evidence for the potential impact of environmental factors on intellectual development stems principally from two sources: studies of the outcomes of home-reared versus institutionalized persons with DS, and the results of early intervention programs.

A study of children reared at home showed a positive benefit, with an increase in IQ of ≥ 17 points at 9 to 10 years of age.[37] Similarly, early intervention with intellectual and motor stimulation starting in infancy has also been described as having a positive effect on development.[34,37,38] Both short-term[39] and long-term[37,38] gains have been claimed, although these conclusions are not always based on carefully controlled investigations and the performance of such controlled studies poses problems of its own.[40] In one study in which a control group was used, early intervention and preschool stimulation resulted in a mean increase in IQ of 6.3 points above control levels at 9 to 10 years of age; but the early intervention and preschool stimulation did not significantly alter the gradual decline in IQ when the subjects were followed longitudinally over a 10-year period.[37] The long-term effects of early intervention programs remain to be proven. While it does appear that evidence exists that early intervention can have a positive effect on early development,[41,42] particularly in the domains of fine coordination, self-help skills, and DQ/IQ scores,[43] research in this area is difficult for a variety of reasons,[40] and definitive conclusions are difficult to obtain. However, one evaluation of 21 early intervention demonstration studies indicated that IQ gains receded over time to the levels of the control group or comparison database and that, although primary school performance is critically lacking in many subjects, social acceptance in school is relatively good.[43]

Cognitive Impairment. A considerable literature on the nature of the cognitive impairment in DS has developed and is critically reviewed in detail by Gibson.[26] Unfortunately, much of this literature has been criticized as being characterized by "the relatively poor quality of research design and data management.... It has been possible to reach conclusions, on a tentative basis, by assuming that consensus has power and methodological error is randomly distributed. Both arguments are subject to dispute."[26] Personality stereotypes attributed to individuals with DS have also been seriously questioned and probably have little validity.[24,44] Nevertheless, it was recently asserted that adults with DS show less maladaptive behaviors than do other adults with similar chronological ages and DQs.[45]

Despite the questions about stereotypes, the present state of affairs seems to be well summarized as follows:[46]

> *Although delays appear already in young DS infants in all areas, it seems that, given the appropriate stimulating environment, it is not really until the DS child reaches school age that the delays start to cause problems serious enough to require very intensive and specialized training. The major problem seems to be the lack of ability to handle more advanced cognitive strategies and processes. Thus, in whichever area of development one may look at, the inability to comprehend instructions, to plan alternative approaches to the problem, to attend to several variables at one time, or to express oneself clearly to another to be able to receive help, for example, are all deficiencies which are serious enough to be a major hindrance in pursuing a "normal" life.*

Relative to other mentally retarded individuals, persons with Down syndrome are reported to have greater difficulty in recalling sequences of verbal information presented aurally, particularly when there is no supporting extralinguistic context.[47] Specific deficits in linguistic structure, both syntax and phonology, are also present,[48] and these are impaired relative to other verbal abilities such as communicative function and vocabulary knowledge.[49,50] Anomalous dominance (lateralization) of language has been observed in young adults with DS,[51] and altered interregional correlations of rates of glucose utilization are believed to reflect the abnormalities of language function.[52]

Nadel[53] characterizes the situation with Down syndrome as follows: "Cognitive development in Down syndrome individuals appears slower than normal, with some qualitative quirks that suggest rather selective deficits in rule-based systems, such as number and grammar." The identification of these selective deficits is of considerable importance in understanding the nature of the cognitive impairment produced by trisomy 21. With new methods of psychological investigation being applied to DS, an understanding of the specific nature of the intellectual deficits in DS and their neurologic and biochemical bases should ultimately be obtained.

Muscle Tone. Perhaps the single most characteristic feature of DS in newborns and infants is hypotonia, and several investigators regard it as a universal finding.[54] In a longitudinal study, the muscle tone of DS newborns was rated as 1.6 ± 0.84 (SD) and 1.5 ± 0.70 for males and females, respectively, increasing to 2.8 ± 0.28 and 2.7 ± 0.33, respectively, at 2 years of age (with 0 = extremely, 1 = moderately, and 2 = mildly hypotonic; 3 = normal).[55] During the first year of life, tone was significantly less in infants with moderate to severe congenital heart disease.[55] Tone was also rated as decreased in older children, aged 4 to 17 years, with a mean of 2.74 versus a control mean of 3.14.[56] Patellar reflexes, a stretch reflex response considered to be related to the involuntary reflex responses that are the genesis of muscle tone, were also less smooth and less brisk (2.32 cm versus 6.06 cm in controls) in the DS group.[56] Grip strength was also decreased at all ages between 4 and 17 years, and there was a positive and significant correlation between strength and tone ($r = 0.65$, $p < 0.01$).[56]

The basis for the decreased muscle tone is unknown. It is not the result of a decrease in the concentration of 5-hydroxytryptamine (serotonin) in the peripheral blood;[57] 5-hydroxytryptophan was found to induce infantile spasms in 14 percent of infants receiving the drug.[58] Similarly, vitamin B_6 administration, which also elevates blood serotonin, had no beneficial effects on tone or development.[57,59] It has been reported, however, that dietary manipulations intended to increase central serotonin levels did reduce self-injurious behavior in an adult with DS.[60]

Other Neurologic Abnormalities. In infancy, there is, in addition to the hypotonia, delayed dissolution of early reflexes and automatisms — grasp reflexes, the Moro response, and automatic stepping.[54] Abnormal or deficient responses have been noted in the traction response, position in ventral suspension, and the patellar jerk. In later years, atlantoaxial/atlanto-occipital instability presents a risk to about 15 to 20 percent of children with DS, although symptomatic manifestations appear to be rare.[61,62]

Seizures have been reported in 1 to 17 percent of persons with Down syndrome.[63–65] In one study,[64] with 8.1 percent of a cohort of 405 persons with DS having seizures, 40 percent of these, usually infantile spasms and tonic-clonic seizures with myoclonus, began during the first year of life. Seizures in another 40 percent, usually tonic-clonic, partial simple, or partial complex, began in the third decade. Seizures beginning after 35 years of age are considered indicative of the development of AD, as is the loss of the ability to identify odors.[66] In this study, febrile seizures were very rare. However, another study reported febrile seizures in 5.3 percent of persons with DS and afebrile seizures in 7.9 percent.[67]

Attempts at Therapy. In addition to the unsuccessful trials with 5-hydroxytryptophan, numerous other agents have been used in an attempt to improve the development of children with DS.[68] Prominent among these are the so-called orthomolecular approaches based on the administration of mixtures of vitamins, minerals, thyroid hormone, and other substances.[69–70] Despite claims for remarkable successes — with IQ reported to increase between 10 and 25 points over a 4- to 8-month period[69] – these results have not been duplicated in carefully controlled trials.[71,72] Another approach has been sicca-cell therapy in which lyophilized embryonic animal cells are injected at frequent intervals. Again, contrary to the claims of its proponents,[73] controlled trials have not shown this form of therapy to have any efficacy.[74] There is, in fact, considerable concern that it may be dangerous.

It was recently suggested that the administration of piracetam, a nootropic agent,[75,76] might be of benefit, but, at present, no form of pharmacologic therapy is known to have a reproducibly beneficial effect on the signs or symptoms of DS.

Neuropathology. Like so many aspects of DS, there has been considerable disagreement about the frequency and nature of anatomic abnormalities of the brain. However, the present consensus is that in the majority of patients with Down syndrome the results of neuropathologic study are normal.[77,78] Although histologic findings have been inconsistent, brain weight is in the low-normal range, and the size of the cerebellum and brainstem may be reduced to an even greater extent.[79] The relative volume of the cerebellum does not decrease significantly with age.[80] Frontal-occipital length is shortened, secondary to reduced frontal lobe growth, and there is narrowing of the superior temporal gyri in about a third of cases.[81] Among the semispecific findings in DS are nerve cell heterotopias in the white layers of the cerebellum and vermis, which are found in 16 percent of infantile and fetal DS brains.[77] These heterotopias are attributed to a disturbance or retardation of embryonal cell migration. The anterior commissure in adults with Down syndrome is reduced in cross-sectional area.[82]

Detailed neuronal architecture, studied with Golgi-type preparations, has been analyzed in a handful of cases. Because of the limitations in numbers, all reports must be viewed with caution. There appears to be a diminution and/or abnormality of dendritic spines in infants and children with DS, including atrophy rather than expansion of the dendritic tree of the visual cortex.[83] This dendritic atrophy continues into adulthood, and becomes even more pronounced when AD develops.[84,85] These abnormalities of spine morphology and number are probably nonspecific, and can probably be interpreted as representing secondary changes in neurons that are metabolically or otherwise affected by the trisomic state.

Other evidence for defects in brain histogenesis has also been reported. This includes a poverty of granular cells, possibly the aspinous stellate cells, throughout the cortex and, in individuals ranging in age from newborn to 14 years, of decreased neuronal densities in layers II and IV of the occipital cortex (area 17).[86] This decrease averaged 30 percent during the first year and 20 to 25 percent thereafter. In young infants, the cell layers of the visual cortex are poorly defined,[83] and diminution in the number of hypothalamic neurons has also been observed.[87] Synaptic density in the neocortex has been reported as normal, although presynaptic and postsynaptic width and length may be reduced.[83] Similarly, the surface area of synaptic contact may be lower than normal in the occipital cortex.[86] A reduction in the number of inferior olivary neurons has been reported.[88]

In fetal DS cortex, the activity of choline acetyltransferase and concentration of N-CAM were normal.[89] Although cholinergic muscarinic receptors were found reduced in the superior colliculus and substantia nigra of two stillborns with DS,[90] the activities of cholinergic markers were found to be normal in several regions of brains from infants with DS.[91] However, there appears to be a doubling of the number of S100 protein immunoreactive cells, presumably astroglia, in the hippocampus.[83]

From the above, it is obvious that a clear picture of the state of the "wiring" of the brain in DS does not emerge. Although there is accumulating evidence for abnormalities of neuronal differentiation and migration in fetal and infant brains, it is not certain, if the developmental plasticity of the young brain is taken into account, how many of the changes are permanent or functionally significant.

Neurochemistry. It has been reported that all the phospholipids of myelin contain reduced amounts of monounsaturated fatty acids but do not have unequivocally abnormal amounts of polyunsaturated fatty acids (PUFA).[92] The opposite, however, seems to be true of synaptosomal phospholipids, with reduced proportions of PUFA and normal amounts of monounsaturated fatty acids being found. Monounsaturated fatty acids are reduced in sphingomyelin. The basis for these abnormalities, which are also found in phenylketonuria, is unknown, and it is unclear whether they result in[92] or from[93] other developmental and functional abnormalities of the nervous system. Abnormal ratios of phosphoglycerides were also noted in fetal DS brains, and it was speculated that these alterations could result in membrane abnormalities, and consequently in functional disturbances.[94]

Neurophysiology. Biochemical analyses, while providing valuable information about the chemical structure of elements of the nervous system, do not directly speak to the question of alterations in function. Unfortunately, there are few data that really bear on this issue, and they principally involve electrophysiological studies of one type or another. There are no specific EEG patterns associated with DS, and the observed abnormalities are not well correlated with specific behavioral or neurologic signs and symptoms.[95] It has been suggested, however, that there is an incomplete postnatal development of neuronal interconnections or an immaturity of cerebral development.[96,97] These conclusions were considered to be consistent with the independently described histologic findings of dendritic abnormalities mentioned earlier. Although some of the physiological observations that underlie them are in question,[98] some supportive evidence has come from work on the spectral analysis of EEG, which showed that the most important deviation from normal was a reduction in relative α power.[99]

Somewhat closer to the issue of neuronal function in DS are the studies of visual- and auditory-evoked potentials. Significant differences in patterns are found between DS and other retarded and nonretarded subjects, which differences have been interpreted as indicating that there is abnormal neural activity in numerous neural systems ranging from sensory to cognitive in DS.[100] As summarized by Courchesne,[100] the evoked-response potential (ERP) evidence relating to DS indicates reduced inhibitory control, reduced selectivity and specificity of responsiveness, increased neural responsiveness, abnormalities in the timing of neural responses, and abnormal mechanisms involved in temporal integration and information storage. ERP and reaction time results from children with DS have indicated slower processing of certain types of auditory information and an altered scalp distribution of amplitudes of some ERP components in comparison to both chronological and mental age controls.[101] In young adults with DS, auditory brain stem response detection levels were elevated, response amplitude was reduced, and latency intensity functions were significantly steeper than in a matched nonretarded control group.[102] The meaning of these differences remains to be established, but they do not appear to be attributable to the presence of hearing deficits, even though mild to moderate high-frequency loss or abnormal impedance are found in as many as 73 percent of adults with DS.[102,103] The abnormal responses have been attributed to both structural and neurochemical alterations.[104] Following median-nerve stimulation, interpeak latencies were significantly prolonged in DS, and impaired impulse conduction in the proximal part of the brachial plexus, posterior roots and/or posterior column-medial lemniscal pathway was inferred.[105] Sensory conduction from the upper cervical cord to the sensory cortex appeared normal.

In addition to the *in vivo* studies of neuronal function, functional studies of DS neurons have been done on fetal and infant dorsal root ganglia neurons cultured *in vitro*, and it was found that several physiological parameters were altered. It was postulated that the greater rate of depolarization of trisomic neurons observed at resting potentials was the result of activation of residual fast-sodium channels that also have a faster course of activation.[106] Although there is no evidence to prove it, it has been speculated that similar abnormalities may also occur in central nervous system neurons and could be the neurologic basis of the mental retardation in DS.[107] These inferences are, of course, speculative.

Fetal DS cortical neurons cultured *in vitro* were found to degenerate spontaneously and to undergo apoptosis under conditions in which diploid control neurons did not.[108] Free radical scavengers or catalase could prevent this degeneration, which was associated with increased lipid peroxidation and intracellular reactive oxygen species, but SOD or an NO synthase inhibitor could not prevent it.

Neuropharmacology. Considerable interest has focused on peripheral neurotransmitter function in DS. Hypersensitivity to the mydriatic effect of atropine has been repeatedly confirmed.[109] There is still debate, however, about its cardioacceleratory effect, and both increased[110] and normal[111] sensitivity have been reported. The activity of the enzyme dopamine-β-hydroxylase, which converts dopamine to norepinephrine, is significantly decreased in the plasma of individuals with DS.[112] Nevertheless, the plasma concentration of norepinephrine is normal or increased.[112] Studies of cerebrospinal fluid (CSF) monoamine metabolism in young adults with DS that showed increased concentrations of CSF 5-hydroxyindoleacetic acid (5-HIAA) and norepinephrine were interpreted as indicating an increased turnover of monoamines. However, this alteration was not believed to be related to cognitive decline with age.[113,114]

Platelet Serotonin. A considerable literature has accumulated on abnormalities of tryptophan metabolism and platelet serotonin (5-hydroxytryptamine) in DS, with the latter being of particular interest because of its possible relevance to understanding central nervous system neurotransmitter function. The principal observation is that the concentration of serotonin is decreased in whole blood to about 65 percent of normal, a decrease that is attributable to a reduction in the level of platelet serotonin to levels as low as 35 to 40 percent of normal.[115] Studies of serotonin uptake by platelets demonstrate a reduced rate of influx,[115] which has been attributed to a reduction in Na^+/K^+-ATPase activity with concomitant abnormalities of sodium, potassium, and/or calcium fluxes.[116] On the basis of observations made on transgenic mice with elevated activities of CuZn-superoxide dismutase (CuZn-SOD), in which similar decreases in platelet uptake were found, the DS platelet abnormality has been attributed to the 50 percent increase in CuZnSOD activity found in all DS cells.[117]

It has been suggested that the platelet, with its uptake and storage of amines, can serve as a model for synaptosomes in the central nervous system.[118] However, although direct studies of serotonin concentration and uptake in central nervous system neurons have not been conducted, the CSF concentration of 5-HIAA, the principal catabolite of serotonin, is not significantly reduced in DS.[119] Furthermore, the content of serotonin in the striatum of CuZnSOD transgenic mice with threefold elevated CuZnSOD activity is normal.[120] Therefore, it remains to be shown whether the platelet abnormalities have any relevance for central nervous system function.

Response to β-Adrenergic Agonists and Other Fibroblast Abnormalities. When skin fibroblasts obtained from a variety of sources were treated with 1 μM isoproterenol, the cyclic adenosine monophosphate (cAMP) content of trisomy 21 cells increased to 29 times the initial level in 10 min, in comparison with the 2.5 to 3.2 times increase observed in diploid cells and in cells trisomic for chromosomes other than 21—a ninefold difference.[121] Epinephrine had a similar although less pronounced effect, and epinephrine-induced platelet aggregation (supposedly an α-adrenergic function in platelets) was produced at a considerably lower concentration with trisomy 21 than with control platelets.[122] These alterations in response could not be attributed to increased adenylate cyclase or decreased phosphodiesterase activity, nor to a gene dosage effect at the receptor level. These observations suggest the existence of some type of alteration in the function of a membrane receptor-controlled system, which could have important implications for a variety of physiological and developmental processes in which catecholamines and cAMP are involved. Unfortunately, related work has not yet been done in cells other than fibroblasts, so it is difficult to know how generalizable the results are.

The uptake and incorporation into lipid of inositol by trisomy 21 fibroblasts is increased to about three times normal.[123] By contrast, trisomic fibroblasts are deficient (by 50 percent) in the release of prostaglandin E_2 (PGE_2).[124] As was postulated to explain the decreased uptake of serotonin by trisomic platelets, the defect in PGE_2 release has been attributed to the elevated level of CuZnSOD in the cells which is presumed to affect arachidonic acid metabolism.

Alzheimer Disease. The possibility of a relationship between DS and dementia has been recognized for over 100 years[125] and between DS and AD (as defined pathologically) for over 50 years.[126] This relationship is now well-established.[127–130] The consensus of a large number of reports is that the brains of adults with DS possess all the pathological and neurochemical hallmarks of AD. Detailed morphometric analyses suggest that the pathological changes found in adult DS brains may differ quantitatively in some areas from those found in AD,[129,131] but the order of progression of involved areas appears to be the same in DS as in AD.[132] It has also been reported that the astrocytic reaction is more marked in DS than AD.[133]

The time of appearance and the frequency of the lesions of AD in DS have been matter of particular concern, because the interest in the relationship between the two conditions has been as much a function of the early and generalized appearance of the lesions as of the nature of the lesions themselves. In an extensive autopsy series, which included 347 cases of DS, 5 of 312 (1.6 percent) brains from individuals dying under the age of 40 (20 to 38 years) and 35 of 35 (100 percent) from individuals over the age of 40 (42 to 69 years) had the gross pathologic changes of AD.[134] Of the latter, 60 percent were described as severe and comparable to the most advanced cases of AD, and 40 percent were mild to moderate. In a study of 100 brains of institutionalized individuals with DS, senile plaques and tangles were found in all cases over 30 years of age, and brain weights were generally below the mean −2 SD from the second decade on.[135] It is, therefore, generally believed that the neuropathologic changes of AD are almost universal over the age of 35 years.[136] Based on immunocytochemical analyses, it is claimed that the deposition of the β/A4 amyloid protein in the brains of persons with DS begins 50 years earlier than it does in normal brains, possibly as the result of overexpression of the amyloid precursor protein (APP) gene.[137] However, ubiquitin-immunoreactive dystrophic neurites have been observed in the gray matter of brains of persons with DS as young as 6 years of age, prior to the time of amyloid deposition, as compared with 29 years of age in control brains.[138]

Clinical Manifestations. Although the pathology may be virtually invariant in its occurrence, a significant proportion of adults with DS do not appear to have dementia by any criteria. Furthermore, some persons with DS who are thought to be demented are instead suffering from major depression.[139] It has been estimated that only about 25 percent of adults with DS are demented;[140] however, frequencies ranging from 45 percent to 100 percent (after age 60 years), depending on age, have also been reported.[141–144] In one prospective study involving both institutionalized and noninstitutionalized adults with DS, 84 percent of demented individuals had seizures, 20 percent had parkinsonian features, and all showed loss of brain tissue by computerized tomography (CT), especially in the temporal lobes.[144] In two institutionalized populations, the mean age of onset of dementia was between 51 and 54 years, and the mean duration of dementia in the patients who died was about 5 years.[145,146]

The relationship between numbers of tangles and plaques and the degree of dementia in DS is not known. However, it has been proposed that the number of these abnormalities must exceed a threshold value before symptoms and signs appear—a threshold which for some reason is higher in DS than in non-DS individuals.[146] Alternatively, as suggested by Mann *et al.*,[147] although senile plaques and neurofibrillary tangles are reliable semiquantitative markers for the presence of AD, "there is no compelling evidence that they, by themselves, actually cause dementia, though they obviously make a contribution to it through the damaging effect they inflict. . . ."

CT has demonstrated increased CSF volume and accelerated rates of lateral ventricle and suprasellar cistern dilatation in demented adults with DS.[148–150] Likewise, dementia is associated with reductions of glucose metabolic rates, as measured by positron emission tomography, in the parietal and temporal motor areas, which are not seen in nondemented adults with DS[151] and with an increase in the latency of the auditory P300 event-related potential.[152] On routine magnetic resonance imaging, persons with DS had a higher prevalence and severity of atrophy and white matter lesions, both of which increased with age, and of T2 hypointensity of the basal ganglia, which did not.[153]

Irrespective of whether frank dementia occurs, there appears to be a progressive loss of a variety of intellectual functions and receptive language not attributable simply to mental retardation in many, if not all, older individuals with DS.[141,154–156] Furthermore, nondemented older adults with DS appear to manifest a selective pattern of neuropsychologic reductions as compared with young adults with DS.[157] These reductions include a diminished ability to form long-term memories and impaired visuospatial construction. Intermediate memory span and language seem to be spared, although language function was already significantly impaired. The consistent impairment of visuospatial construction with sparing of language is thought to distinguish the findings in the nondemented adults with DS from those characteristic of early to intermediate Alzheimer-type dementia.[157]

The belief that intellectual decline is inevitable in adults with DS has been challenged.[158] Based both on cross-sectional and relatively short-term longitudinal studies, it is claimed that only a third of persons with DS over 35 years of age show intellectual deterioration. Another study has claimed that only 4 of 91 persons with mild and moderate mental retardation between 31 and 63 years of age could be considered as being demented.[159]

Predisposing Factors. A study of over 100 adults with DS has shown that males are three times more likely than females to develop clinical AD.[160] However, another study indicated that females are affected earlier and have higher densities of neurofibrillary tangles. Because of the discovery that the presence of the apolipoprotein E allele $\varepsilon 4$ is a risk factor for the development of both sporadic and familial AD unrelated to DS, numerous studies have been done to determine whether the same is true in DS. Presence of the $\varepsilon 4$ allele has been reported to be associated with a higher frequency of clinical AD,[160] a tendency to an earlier age of onset of dementia,[161] poorer language ability,[162] more rapid cognitive decline,[163] and earlier age of death.[164] A meta-analysis that reviewed several studies indicated that there was little evidence for reduced survival to adulthood of persons with the homozygous $\varepsilon 4 \varepsilon 4$ genotype.[165]

For a discussion of the pathogenesis of AD in DS, see "Pathogenesis of Specific Features of Down Syndrome" below.

Major Congenital Malformations

Despite the presence of many dysmorphic features in DS, relatively few major malformations are produced by trisomy 21. Those that do occur are quite specific and principally involve two systems — the heart and the gastrointestinal tract.

Congenital Heart Disease. The most frequent major congenital abnormality in DS is congenital heart disease, and 16 to 62 percent of children have been reported as being affected.[166] The most unbiased estimates for living children range from 29 to 39 percent.[167,168] In unselected DS abortuses, 45 percent were found to have forms of congenital heart disease that would not be expected to close after birth,[77] and an overall estimate of 40 percent appears to be reasonable. A variety of estimates also exist for the frequencies of specific cardiac lesions in affected children: atrioventricular canal, 18 to 54 percent (mean: 39 percent); ventricular septal defect, 27 to 43 percent (mean: 31 percent); atrial septal defect, 2 to 17 percent (mean: 9 percent); tetralogy of Fallot, 1 to 15 percent (mean: 6 percent); patent ductus arteriosus, 2 to 24 percent (mean: 9 percent).[190] In the fetal cases, 73 percent of those with cardiac anomalies were judged to have an atrioventricular canal.[168] Despite the variety of lesions described, it is believed that most represent variations of a common problem in the formation of the venous inflow tract of the heart, although other lesions, such as aortic arch anomalies, can also occur.[77] In a survey of institutionalized adults with mental retardation, unsuspected aortic regurgitation or mitral valve prolapse was detected in 20 percent of DS persons as compared to 6 percent of controls.[169]

Survival of children with congenital heart disease is better than was formerly believed, and 80 percent survival to 15 years of age with atrioventricular canal defects has been reported.[170] Development of pulmonary hypertension is generally considered to occur earlier and more severely in children with DS with congenital heart disease,[171] although this conclusion has been disputed.[172] Abnormal development of the lung parenchyma and of the pulmonary vasculature, which could contribute to the development of pulmonary hypertension, may also be present. Pulmonary hypoplasia characterized by a diminished number (<50 percent of normal) of alveoli in relation to acini and a reduction in total alveolar surface area has been reported to be independent of the presence of heart disease.[173] Reduction of airway branching and a thinning of the medial layer of the small pulmonary arteries have also been described.[174,175]

Gastrointestinal Tract Abnormalities. Although much less common than congenital heart disease, there is nevertheless an increased frequency of specific intestinal anomalies in DS. In an aggregate of five series, the most characteristic lesion was duodenal stenosis or atresia, sometimes with annular pancreas, with a frequency of 2.5 percent, followed by imperforate anus (1 percent), Hirschsprung disease (0.56 percent), and tracheoesophageal fistula or esophageal atresia (0.43 percent).[176] Conversely, 5.9 percent of infants with Hirschsprung disease had DS,[177] as did 28 percent of patients with duodenal atresia or stenosis[176] and 20 percent with annular pancreas.[178]

Leukemia and Leukemoid Reactions

Incidence. An increased incidence of leukemia has long been recognized in DS. Estimates of the relative risk have ranged from 10 to 18 times normal in children up to 16 years of age,[179,180] and adults over 20 years also have an excessive rate of mortality from leukemia.[181] The distribution of leukemia by type is shown in Table 63-2. Congenital and newborn cases (<1 year of age) are predominantly acute nonlymphoblastic leukemia (ANLL), but from age 3 years and up, the distribution of types is the same for both DS and non-DS subjects.[182,183] The age of onset of ANLL is younger in DS than in diploid patients, but the ages are the same for acute lymphoblastic leukemia (ALL).[184] The length of survival of DS individuals after diagnosis of ALL is shorter than that of diploid individuals.

Acute Megakaryoblastic Leukemia. Although major emphasis has been placed on ALL and ANLL, it should be noted that the latter may include other forms of leukemia, such as acute megakaryoblastic leukemia, in addition to acute myelocytic leukemia.[185] It has been suggested that acute megakaryoblastic leukemia may be much more common in DS than previously suspected. Of 24 cases of leukemia in DS seen over a 10-year period at a single hospital, 4 (17 percent) originally diagnosed as having ALL were believed to have this form of leukemia. It has

Table 63-2 Types of Leukemia in Down Syndrome

			Proportion of Types (%)		
Sources of Cases	**Age**	**Total Cases**	**ALL**	**ANLL**	**AUL**
Acute leukemia group B[182]	< 1 month	5	20.0	80.0	—
	1 month–19 years	41	69.8	30.2	—
Rosner and Lee[182]	< 1 month	47	42.1	57.9	—
	1 month–19 years	229	69.1	30.9	—
Oxford study of childhood cancer[183]	< 1 year	10	10.0	80.0	10.0
	1–2 years	25	44.4 (82.2)*	52.0 (13.7)	4.0 (4.1)
	3–14	35	80.0 (79.2)	17.1 (18.2)	2.9 (2.6)

ALL = acute lymphoblastic leukemia; ANLL = acute nonlymphoblastic leukemia; AUL = acute undifferentiated or unspecified leukemia.
Proportions in non-Down syndrome population in parentheses.

SOURCE: Reprinted by permission from Epstein.[7]

been estimated that 20 to 40 percent of all cases of acute leukemia and leukemoid reactions or transient leukemia are of this type.[186] Conversely, most cases of acute megakaryoblastic leukemia in young children are thought to occur in individuals with trisomy 21 or trisomy 21/2n mosaicism, and the overall incidence of this form of leukemia may be 200 to 400 times greater in the DS than in the chromosomally normal population.[186]

Response to Therapy. The response of children with DS to therapy differs from that of chromosomally normal patients.[187] For so-called ALL, which could include misdiagnosed, and hence inappropriately treated, acute megakaryoblastic leukemia,[186] remission induction is reduced (80 percent vs 94 percent in non-DS cases) and mortality is higher (14 percent vs 3 percent), with death resulting principally from infection.[187] The 5-year survival is also decreased (50 percent vs 65 percent), but this is mainly attributable to the initial failure to induce a remission. In contrast, children with DS with acute myelogenous leukemia have a very high rate of event-free survival after chemotherapy. Their myeloblasts have a greatly enhanced sensitivity to 1-β-D-arabinofuranosylcytosine, which has been attributed to enhanced metabolism of this drug.[188] Severe methotrexate toxicity at standard therapeutic doses has also been demonstrated.[189] This toxicity was postulated to result from increased tetrahydrofolic acid demand, and hence greater sensitivity to an antifolate agent, because of a presumed increased rate of purine synthesis. It has also been suggested that a decreased rate of methotrexate clearance may be responsible.[190]

Leukemoid Reactions. A high frequency of "transient" acute leukemia, transient myeloproliferative syndrome, or leukemoid reaction has been reported to be present in newborns with DS.[182] In these cases, there is apparently a complete remission, and it is believed by most investigators that the affected individuals never had true leukemia at all. Rather, they appear to have had what has been termed ineffective regulation of granulopoiesis masquerading as congenital leukemia.[191] Unlike true acute leukemia, there are normal numbers of granulocytes and macrophage stem cells (CFU-GM) in the bone marrow,[192–194] there are ultrastructural differences between leukemoid and true leukemic blast cells,[195] and the mean maternal age is lower.[196] However, as in true leukemia, the abnormal cellular proliferation appears to be clonal in nature.[197,198] That the presence of an extra chromosome 21 is of importance in this condition is borne out by several cases of such leukemoid reactions described in phenotypically normal trisomy 21/2n mosaics, in which the abnormally proliferating cell population was always trisomic for chromosome 21.[192,199] It has been proposed that disomic homozygosity for a locus on the long arm of chromosome 21 proximal to the centromere, arising from meiosis II nondisjunction, may be involved in the genesis of leukemoid reactions.[196,200]

The relationship between leukemoid reactions and true leukemia still remains to be defined. While it is, of course, possible that they are unrelated, it is tempting to try to visualize some significant relationship between two such infrequent aberrations affecting leukocyte proliferation. Furthermore, the finding of other hematologic abnormalities in trisomic newborns, especially an increased hematocrit, but also including either thrombocytosis or thrombocytopenia,[201,202] is compatible with the notion of a generalized abnormality in stem-cell regulation. It has been suggested, although not shown, that there is an extensive congenital defect of bone marrow function in DS newborns, possibly due to the presence of a marrow-stimulating humoral substance.[203]

A view dissenting from the prevailing one — that the leukemoid reactions and true leukemia are distinct entities — has been published.[186,204] This dissenting view holds that leukemoid reactions are transient but true leukemia, which most often is acute megakaryoblastic leukemia. In most cases, this leukemia regresses spontaneously, but in about 25 percent it recurs during the first 3 years of life, again as acute megakaryoblastic leukemia.

Immunologic Defects

The immunologic status of individuals with DS has been the subject of intensive investigation for many years, primarily because of clinical observations suggesting that they are more susceptible to a variety of infectious diseases[205] and, as was just discussed, to the development of leukemia. Infection still constitutes the leading cause of death of trisomic individuals (see "Life Expectancy and Causes of Death" below). In general, the literature (summarized in references 5, 7, and 206) has been characterized by considerable disagreement and contradiction stemming, in large part, from differences in subject selection (age, institutionalized vs noninstitutionalized), choice of control subjects, and the methods used. Nevertheless, a picture of immunologic impairment associated with DS still emerges.

Antibodies. The consensus is that serum IgG is elevated, particularly in older subjects. However, there are reports of normal IgG levels and, in newborns, of decreased concentrations.[7,206] The situation with regard to IgM and IgA is less clear. Serum concentrations of IgM have been reported as decreased, normal, and even increased, and the differences do not appear to be age-related. Similarly, IgA has been reported to be decreased, normal, and increased. A transition from normal levels in children to elevated levels in adults may explain some of the discrepancy.[206]

T Lymphocytes. Quantitative studies of peripheral blood T lymphocytes reveal a reduction, often quite small, in the proportion or absolute number of T lymphocytes,[206] although normal proportions or numbers of T and B lymphocytes in DS children have also been seen.[207] The proportion of T-helper cells (CD4+) is decreased, resulting in a decreased, perhaps reversed (<1.0) ratio of helper to suppressor (CD8+) cells,[208] Furthermore, peripheral blood T cells have a decreased number of cells expressing the T-cell receptor-α,β (TCRα,β) complex, elevated numbers expressing TCRγ,δ, and a decreased proportion of CD4+, CD45RA+ naive T cells, suggesting that the DS thymus is inefficient in the release of functionally mature T cells.[209] There appears to be an age dependence in the proliferative response to phytohemagglutinin (PHA) of DS lymphocytes, but not of normal lymphocytes.[206] Allogeneic mixed lymphocyte proliferative responses are decreased, as are PHA-induced interleukin-2 production and cytotoxic T-lymphocyte activity.[206,210]

Response to Antigens. Studies of the *in vitro* response of DS T lymphocytes to specific antigens demonstrate normal responses to purified protein derivative (PPD) and to staphylococcal, streptococcal, and Sendai virus antigens.[211,212] In contrast, significantly reduced responses, as measured by proliferation, interleukin-2 production, and *in vitro* antibody production, to tetanus toxoid and to influenza virus antigens have been found.[208,213] Further dissection of this system has shown that the depressed proliferative response to influenza virus antigen results from a diminished responsiveness of T-helper cells rather than from an increased T-suppressor activity.[213] An intrinsic defect in B-cell antibody production has also been noted, as has a defect in the enhancement of B-cell antibody production by T-helper cells. The *in vitro* observations on tetanus toxoid and influenza antigens are compatible with reports of diminished *in vivo* responses to tetanus toxoid and typhoid vaccine[214] (although normal responses were found by other investigators),[215] influenza vaccine,[216] bacteriophage ΦX174,[217] pneumococcal polysaccharide,[218] recombinant hepatitis B vaccine,[219] and exposure to hepatitis infection.[220] Decreased natural antibody titers have also been found.[221]

Thymus. Further evidence implicating abnormalities of the T-lymphocyte system in the immunologic defects of DS derives from anatomic and functional abnormalities of the thymus.[206] In comparison to age-matched controls, thymuses from infants with DS from 1 day to 15 months of age have marked lymphoid depletion, with a thin cortex and poor corticomedullary demarcation.[222] The Hassall corpuscles are increased in size and frequently cystic.[222] The presence of lower proportions of cells bearing high levels of the TCRα,β complex and of CD3, a signal-transducing complex for the T-cell receptor, in thymuses of children with DS and the increase in the proportions of cells with these markers with age are indicative of delayed maturation of T cells within the thymus.[223] In addition, DS thymuses contain elevated levels of IFN-γ and TNF-α mRNA expressing cells, and there is mast cell hyperplasia and overexpression of class I MHC, CD18, and ICAM-1.[224] DS thymocytes also have a greater than normal sensitivity to inhibition of IL-4-induced proliferation by IFN-γ and TNF-α.[225] Taken together, these findings are indicative of abnormal thymocyte maturation and cytokine dysregulation in the DS thymus, possibly initiated by gene dose-related increased sensitivity to IFN-γ and to overexpression of CD18 (LFA-1β).[224]

Hematologic Alterations

Red Cells. In addition to the neonatal hematologic abnormalities just cited, several other erythrocyte and leukocyte alterations are found in DS. Macrocytosis is commonly observed, with the mean corpuscular volume increased 11 to 14 percent above control values.[225] The enzymes, glutamic oxalacetic transaminase (AST), glucose-6-phosphate dehydrogenase (G-6-PD), 6-phosphogluconate dehydrogenase, adenosine deaminase, and catechol-O-methyltransferase, are increased 15 to 60 percent,[226–228] but membrane ATPase activity (total, Mg^{2+}, and Na^+, K^+) is decreased by 60 to 70 percent.[229] The red cell adenine nucleotides have been variously reported as increased, decreased, or unchanged,[227,230,231] and it is not clear why there has been such variability in the results obtained.

Leukocytes. Several enzymes are increased in activity in leukocytes, including alkaline phosphatase, acid phosphatase, galactose-1-phosphate uridyltransferase, and G-6-PD.[226] The increases in acid and alkaline phosphatases, and in G-6-PD, are found in both granulocytes and lymphocytes. A variety of abnormalities in leukocyte function, of unknown physiological significance, have been reported.[232–234] No satisfactory explanation has been provided for the numerous alterations in the activities of enzymes, none of which are coded for by chromosome 21, in DS erythrocytes and leukocytes, or for the increased size of the DS erythrocytes. However, these observations do highlight the difficulty in attempting to infer the locations of genes for enzymes based on putative dosage effects on their activities in erythrocytes and leukocytes. The same nongene dosage-related increases in enzyme activity are not observed in cultured fibroblasts or other nucleated cells.[235]

Hyperuricemia

Increases in serum uric acid levels have been reported by several investigators,[236] with the increases ranging from 16 to 44 percent. A particularly thorough study found a mean increase of 44 percent in trisomic individuals, with significant differences from normal being found in all age groups.[237] Because urinary uric acid excretion was, if anything, increased, it was inferred that the hyperuricemia was the result of purine overproduction. Other suggestions regarding the etiology of the hyperuricemia have been made, including increased degradation of purines resulting from enhanced leukocyte turnover[238] or associated with an increased adenosine deaminase activity.[227,239] The increased enzyme activity could also be an effect of increased synthesis, rather than a cause of increased degradation. Furthermore, the issue of overproduction (or increased purine degradation) versus diminished excretion has still not been fully resolved, and the role of increased purine biosynthetic enzyme activity (see "Secondary Effects" below) remains to be determined. At issue with regard to the latter is whether the cellular concentrations of these enzymes control the flux of metabolites through the purine biosynthetic pathway.

Endocrine Abnormalities

Thyroid Dysfunction and Autoimmunity. Both hypothyroidism and hyperthyroidism have been reported in individuals with DS. In newborn infants studied in a statewide newborn screening program, 1.1 percent with DS had congenital hypothyroidism. This was persistent in 8, an incidence 28 times that of the general population.[240] An increase in thyroid antibodies was not detected. In children aged 4 months to 3 years studied retrospectively, 3 of 49 (6.1 percent) had congenital hypothyroidism, 1 had acquired hypothyroidism, and 1 had acquired hyperthyroidism; 13 had mildly elevated thyroid-stimulating hormone (TSH) but normal thyroxine levels.[241] Only the two patients with acquired disease had thyroid antibodies. Mean TSH levels were increased and mean reverse triiodothyronine (T_3) levels were decreased in children with DS.[242] In institutionalized adults with DS, hypothyroidism was found in 17 percent, hyperthyroidism in 2.5 percent, and goiter in 18 percent.[243] Although these results would suggest a progressive age-dependent increase in thyroid antibodies and disease in DS, contradictory results were obtained in a study that demonstrated a high frequency of antibodies against thyroglobulin in DS subjects of all ages from 1 to 50 years.[244] T_3 levels were reported to be lower in DS persons with AD than in those without.[245] However, an age-dependent increase in hepatitis B surface antigen (HBsAg) was observed, and the frequency of HBsAg carriers was higher in individuals with thyroid antibodies (mean = 41.8 percent vs control mean = 19.7 percent) than in those without.[244] The etiology of the thyroid abnormalities is not known, but it has been speculated that they are related in part to the abnormalities of the immune function described above. Although it is often stated that persons with DS have a propensity to developing autoimmune disorders, this is not well documented except for thyroid autoantibodies.

Diabetes. The prevalence of type 1 diabetes mellitus appears to be greater than in the non-DS population, but glycemic control was as good as was observed in the control population.[246]

Growth and Stature. Newborns with DS are slightly smaller, on the mean, than chromosomally normal infants, with length being reduced by about 0.5 SD of the mean.[247] The mean head circumference at birth is reduced about 1 SD from the normal, but the growth velocity of the head parallels the normal until age 5 to 6 months, after which it levels off just below 2 SD below the normal mean.[248] After correcting for potential confounding influences, the mean reduction of weight, in comparison with the birthweight of sibs, was found to be 0.24 kg, about 7 percent.[249] In a Swedish group, mean length was reduced at birth by 1.5 SD in females and 0.5 SD in males, and mean height was reduced by 3 SD at age 3 years.[250] This reduction in stature persists throughout life, with the difference from normal individuals becoming greater with increasing age. Similarly, in a longitudinally studied home-reared Japanese group, mean stature was reduced >1 SD up to 24 months of age and ≥ 3 SD after 30 months.[251] The lower limbs were disproportionately short, and incremental growth rates for both total stature and lower limb length were significantly decreased at all ages up to 4 years. A similar decrease in growth velocity was also observed in home-reared American children with DS, and mean bone age was reduced and had greater variance than normal at 24 and 30 months.[247]

In a longitudinal 12-year study of institutionalized children and adolescents with DS, standing and sitting mean heights were both reduced >2 SD in comparison with a normal noninstitutionalized control population.[252] Because bone age was retarded in the DS subjects, these differences were less in the prepubertal years. The stability of the growth pattern between 10 and 18 years of age was the same in both the DS and control groups, and final adult heights were considered to be equally predictable from the heights at 10 years of age in both groups. It was concluded, therefore, that the biologic mechanisms that regulate growth in this age range are not appreciably altered in DS.[252]

Growth charts for children with DS have been developed.[252] A diminished growth rate is most apparent in infancy and in adolescence, and children with congenital heart disease are smaller in stature and weight than those without. In addition to shortness of stature, children and adults with DS tend to be overweight.[253,254] In the latter, an increase in the proportion of body fat on the order of 50 percent or more has been noted in both males and females, and it has been suggested that both environmental (poor diet, lack of activity) and genetic factors may be involved.[254]

Growth Factors. In an attempt to define a specific mechanism for the reduction in growth, measurements of growth hormone and somatomedins have been carried out. Plasma growth hormone levels do not appear to be reduced in children with DS,[255] and serum insulin-like growth factor 1 (IGF-1) is increased during the first 2 years of life.[250] However, rather than undergoing the normal twofold increase in concentration between early childhood and adult life, IGF-1 remains constant throughout life. In contrast, the serum concentration of IGF-2 is normal, as are the levels of insulin and somatomedin receptors in the brains of fetuses with DS.[256,257] Treatment of DS children between 3.5 and 6.5 years of age with growth hormone resulted in increases in the levels of both immunoreactive IGF-1 and IGF-2, the former to normal range, and 50 to 200 percent increases in growth velocity.[255] Similarly, treatment of 13 children with recombinant human growth hormone increased mean growth velocity to 2.25 times pretreatment values.[258] The significance of these findings is presently unclear, but they do suggest that the growth impairment in DS may result from specific growth regulatory defects rather than being a general or nonspecific effect of the aneuploid condition.

Reproduction

Sterility in Males. There is only one documented case of reproduction by a male with trisomy 21,[259] although males with mosaic trisomy 21 have fathered both normal and trisomic offspring.[260] The principal defect in reproduction appears to be in spermatogenesis, with all degrees of impairment—from mild reduction to total arrest—having been reported for males with DS between 16 and 52 years of age.[261] In a few cases, the impairment was so mild as to be compatible with fertility, at least as judged histologically.[262] Sperm counts in nine cases were reported as greatly reduced in five and as zero in four.[263] Penile and testicular size have been described as normal in adolescents,[264] although diminished testicular size approaching that found in Klinefelter syndrome was reported for 17 individuals with a mean age of 30.7 years.[265] In the latter group, significantly elevated levels of FSH (about 3 times control levels) were observed in both young and old individuals and of LH (increased about 1.5 times) only in individuals over 30 years of age.[265] Although a control group was not studied, apparently normal levels of FSH, LH, and testosterone were reported in adolescents reared at home;[264] normal plasma testosterone levels were found in other studies as well.[266]

The cause of the spermatogenic arrest in males with DS is unknown. It has been suggested that it is the result of a direct interference by the extra autosome with meiosis, possibly because the extra chromosome 21 associates with the sex vesicle.[261] A similar impairment of spermatogenesis has been observed in mice heterozygous for robertsonian fusion translocations, albeit in a balanced state.[267] It is also possible, although untested, that the trisomic state is itself, by a dosage effect, deleterious to spermatogenesis. While failure of spermatogenesis may be a sufficient explanation of fertility in males, other factors probably also play a role. These may include a decrease in libido and a diminished opportunity for sexual intercourse.

Fertility in Females. In contrast to the apparent total sterility of males, reproduction has been documented in females. At least 24 women with DS have had children, including a stillborn pair of twins, of which 10 of 25 had trisomy 21.[260] Although equal numbers of disomic and euploid gametes might be expected, a proportion of less than 0.5 for trisomic offspring at term is consistent with the high fetal mortality of trisomy 21. Histologic examination of the ovaries of females with DS between birth and 14.5 years of age revealed an absence or retardation of follicle growth, with a reduced number of antral follicles,[268] and there was no evidence for ovulation in 4 of 13 (31 percent) institutionalized women with DS.[269]

Life Expectancy and Causes of Death

Longevity. With the changing patterns of institutionalization and of the utilization and methods of medical and surgical therapy provided to persons with DS, it is difficult to obtain accurate current figures for life expectancy. Comprehensive reviews of earlier studies[270,271] indicate that mean life expectancy has improved dramatically in the last half-century since the estimate of 9 years in 1929.[272] This increase in life expectancy is presumed to be the result of improved medical and social care of persons with DS at all ages. This conclusion is supported by the finding that, within a single country, survival rates during the first 5 years of life were reduced from 0.80 in the region with good pediatric care to 0.59 in the region with inferior care.[273]

The major determinant of survival during the first decade of life, and especially the first 4 to 5 years, is the presence or absence of congenital heart disease. Recent results from Japanese,[274] Danish,[275] and Canadian[276,277] studies are presented in Table 63-3. Long-term survival rates and life expectancy are not calculated with regard to the presence of congenital heart disease, but its impact is, in part, revealed by comparison of the survival rates of the total DS population with those alive at age 10 and by the increase in total life expectancy during the first 5 years of life (Table 63-3).[276] When compared with the background (whole) population, the life expectancy of an individual with DS at any point in time is 10 to 20 years less, with the difference being greater for females than for males.[276] Furthermore, the absolute fractional survival rates for institutionalized individuals are 0.10 to 0.15 lower than for persons with DS living outside of institutions.[270] When compared with other mentally retarded persons, whether institutionalized or not, one study reported that the survival rates of individuals with DS were not significantly different until age 30, but then became lower thereafter.[277] In another study, however, the DS survival rates were lower at all ages than in a control mentally retarded population.[277]

Mortality. Earlier studies recorded the major causes of death in DS as respiratory disease, including pneumonia (23 to 41 percent), congenital heart disease (30 to 35 percent), other infectious diseases (2 to 15 percent), malignancy (2 to 9 percent), and "senility" and stroke (0 to 9 percent).[270,278–280] In an analysis of the causes of death of persons with DS who died in 1976, it was found that age-corrected rates for deaths from pneumonia were increased 5.6 times and constituted 16 percent of the total deaths observed.[278] For congenital anomalies (83 percent of which were congenital heart disease), the increase was 4.7 times with 38 percent of the total; for leukemia and lymphatic neoplasms, 1.7 and 1.30 times and 3.0 percent and 1.1 percent, respectively. Increased rates for other types of infectious diseases, including kidney infections, influenza, enteritis, and meningitis, were also found. Congenital defects (mainly heart disease) were the leading cause of death up to age 35 years. The increased mortality from pneumonia and congenital anomalies (heart disease) was found over all age groups, while that for leukemia was increased at ages 1 to 4 and 20 to 34 years and for lymphatic neoplasms for 20 to 34 years. Mortality rates for cancers at other sites were greatly diminished (to 0.32, or less than expected), as were the rates for ischemic heart disease (0.57) and cirrhosis of the liver (0.44).

Table 63-3 Survival Rates and Life Expectancy in Down Syndrome

<table>
<tr><th rowspan="3">Age</th><th colspan="4">Rate of Survival in Japanese Study</th><th colspan="3">Rate of Survival in Danish Study</th><th colspan="2" rowspan="2">Rate of Survival in Canadian Study</th></tr>
<tr><th colspan="2">Without CHD</th><th colspan="2">With CHD</th><th rowspan="2">Total Population</th><th rowspan="2">Population Alive at Age 10 Years</th><th rowspan="2">Estimated Life Expectancy, Years</th></tr>
<tr><th>Male</th><th>Female</th><th>Male</th><th>Female</th><th>Without CHD</th><th>With CHD</th></tr>
<tr><td>0</td><td></td><td></td><td></td><td></td><td></td><td></td><td>46.5</td><td></td><td></td></tr>
<tr><td>1</td><td>0.98</td><td>1.00</td><td>0.85</td><td>0.89</td><td>0.92</td><td></td><td>49.5</td><td>0.91</td><td>0.67</td></tr>
<tr><td>5</td><td>0.96</td><td>0.97</td><td>0.72</td><td>0.77</td><td>0.84</td><td></td><td>50.0</td><td>0.87</td><td>0.62</td></tr>
<tr><td>10</td><td>0.96</td><td>0.95</td><td>0.70</td><td>0.77</td><td>0.83</td><td></td><td>45.9</td><td>0.85</td><td>0.57</td></tr>
<tr><td>20</td><td></td><td></td><td></td><td></td><td>0.80</td><td>0.97</td><td>37.1</td><td></td><td></td></tr>
<tr><td>30</td><td></td><td></td><td></td><td></td><td>0.75</td><td>0.92</td><td>29.2</td><td>0.79</td><td>0.50</td></tr>
<tr><td>40</td><td></td><td></td><td></td><td></td><td>0.71</td><td>0.86</td><td>20.8</td><td colspan="2">0.70</td></tr>
<tr><td>50</td><td></td><td></td><td></td><td></td><td>0.64</td><td>0.77</td><td>12.4</td><td colspan="2">0.61</td></tr>
<tr><td>60</td><td></td><td></td><td></td><td></td><td>0.40</td><td>0.49</td><td>6.3</td><td colspan="2">0.44</td></tr>
<tr><td>68</td><td></td><td></td><td></td><td></td><td></td><td></td><td></td><td colspan="2">0.14</td></tr>
<tr><td>70</td><td></td><td></td><td></td><td></td><td>0.10</td><td>0.12</td><td>5.1</td><td></td><td></td></tr>
</table>

CHD = congenital heart disease.

SOURCE: Data from Masaki et al.,[274] Dupont et al.,[275] and Baird and Sadovnick.[276,277]

Alterations in Cultured Cells

Several aspects of the DS phenotype have been defined in cultured cells which represent an enhanced responsiveness to external stimuli. Although in many instances the differences between trisomic and diploid cells are relatively small, in some cases they are quite marked. One such difference, in the responsiveness of cultured fibroblasts to β-adrenergic agonists, is discussed in "Neuropharmacology" above.

Response to Interferon. Because of the location of the gene for the interferon-α/β receptor (IFNAR1) on chromosome 21, the responsiveness of DS cells to interferon has been examined in detail. The results indicate that trisomic cells have an enhanced sensitivity to several biologic actions of IFN-α.[281–285] Subsequently, it was determined that a second component of this receptor, coded for by IFNAR2, is also located on chromosome 21. The enhanced functional and biochemical responses to IFN-α have, therefore, been attributed to the presence of an increased copy of each of these IFN-α receptor genes (see below). Although the IFN-γ receptor gene is not located on chromosome 21, enhanced responses of DS cells to IFN-γ have also been observed,[282,283] and these appear to be due to the fact that a component of the IFN-γ receptor, referred to as a transducer or accessory factor, is coded for by the gene IFNGR2 on chromosome 21. DS cells may also be more responsive in general to a variety of external stimuli acting through cell-surface receptors.

Cell Proliferation. In continuous cell culture, the rate of cell population doubling of matched pairs of fibroblasts decreased linearly with time, with the DS cells always having a slightly lower rate (about 10 to 15 percent).[286] Furthermore, the cumulative number of population cell doublings was reduced by 20 percent (from a mean of 51.5 to 40) in the cultured DS cells. In contrast to these results, which suggest some degree of impairment of cell proliferation *in vitro*, other workers also using matched fibroblasts found that the mean number of cumulative population doublings was not reduced and that doubling times were not significantly increased.[287,288] However, each of these means had a substantial standard deviation. At present, therefore, the data favoring or denying a difference in proliferative rates and cumulative population doublings seem to be about equally persuasive.

Sensitivity to Radiation and Chemicals. Because of the increased susceptibility of children with DS to the development of leukemia, considerable interest is focused on the sensitivity of trisomic cells to mutagenic and carcinogenic agents, including radiation, chemicals, and viruses. The objective of these studies is to determine whether there is an intrinsic defect in DS cells that might make them more susceptible to oncogenic transformation. All of these studies are summarized in detail in reference 7.

Radiation. There are numerous reports describing an increased radiosensitivity of trisomic lymphocytes as measured by a variety of techniques and at different stages of the cell cycle. When data from several of these reports were summarized,[7] the most striking conclusion was that an effect, when one is present, is relatively small — the increased production of aberrations by trisomic cells being on the order of 1.1 to 2.1 times. In some experiments, when the dose of irradiation or the stage of the cell cycle at which radiation occurred was changed, the effect was no longer detectable. Based on experiments demonstrating a decreased survival of irradiated DS lymphoblastoid lines, it has been proposed that there is defective repair rather than an increased amount of x-ray-induced damage.[289] Experiments on irradiated peripheral blood lymphocytes have also been interpreted as indicating enhanced chromosomal radiosensitivity resulting from a developmentally regulated repair deficiency.[290]

Mutagenic and Carcinogenic Chemicals. Data on the effects of mutagenic and carcinogenic chemicals, generally alkylating agents, on the induction of chromosome aberrations in trisomic cells are more limited than for radiation. For the present, the published data are insufficient to support a conclusion that trisomic cells are inherently more sensitive to mutagenic or carcinogenic chemicals.[7]

Effects of Viruses. Another probe of the sensitivity of DS lymphocytes to chromosomal damage is viral infection, either spontaneous or induced by vaccination. Measles infection is reported to increase the number of chromosome breaks per cell 4.8 times in individuals with DS, whereas the increase in normal subjects was only 1.2 times.[291] Similarly, the number of chromosome breaks per cell immediately after chickenpox infection increased 2.8 times in DS but only 1.8 times in normal individuals.[292] These data are insufficient to know what significance to attach to them.

The situation with the SV40 transformation of DS fibroblasts is similar to that described earlier for cell proliferation and sensitivity to radiation. There seems to be something different between DS and diploid cells, albeit a difference that is generally small in magnitude. But, the results are not always consistent, their interpretation is unclear, and their significance is uncertain.[7] Despite the great amount of effort devoted to them, the outcome of these investigations must be considered as disappointing.

THE CHROMOSOMAL BASIS AND EPIDEMIOLOGY OF DOWN SYNDROME

Types of Chromosome Abnormalities

Down syndrome is the phenotypic manifestation of trisomy 21. As such, it occurs when an extra copy of chromosome 21 is present in the genome, whether as a free chromosome (Fig. 63-5), part of a robertsonian (rob) fusion chromosomes, or, in rare instances, as part of a reciprocal translocation (Fig. 63-6). All cells of the body are trisomic, except for the 2 to 4 percent of cases in which mosaicism exists. In cases in which mosaicism exists, two populations of cells, one diploid and one trisomic, are present, with the number and distribution of trisomic cells being sufficient to cause the DS phenotype to manifest itself (see "Mosaicism" below). The proportions of the various cytogenetic forms of trisomy 21 are shown in Table 63-4. As can be seen in these data, the vast majority of cases are 47,+21, with the other categories constituting ≤5 percent each.

The data in Table 63-4 represent means for all cases of DS, independent of maternal age. Since the frequency of 47,+21 is a function of maternal age, whereas the other forms of aneuploidy-producing DS do not appear to be, its proportion and that of 47,+21/46 mosaicism rise progressively with maternal age while that of the robertsonian translocations decreases (Table 63-5). Of the cases associated with robertsonian translocations between chromosome 21 and one of the D-group chromosomes (i.e., chromosomes 13 to 15), approximately 40 to 45 percent are familial, in that they are inherited from a cytogenetically balanced parent of genotype 45,-D,-21,+rob(D;21).[295] For the G-group robertsonian translocations, only about 4 percent are familial.[295] When considered together with the age dependence of nontrans-

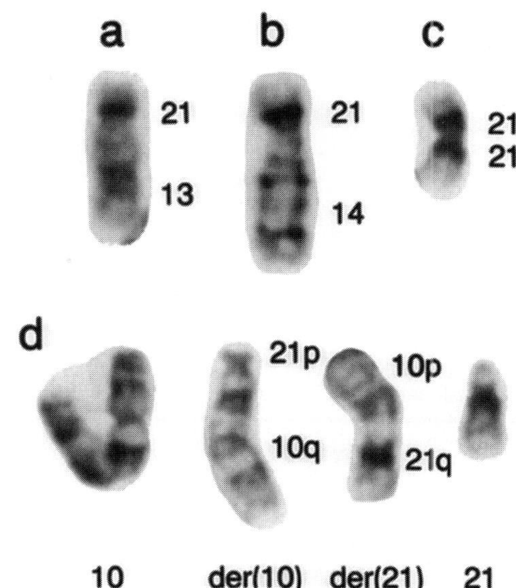

Fig. 63-6 Translocations predisposing to the occurrence of Down syndrome. G-banded chromosomes. *A-C*, Robertsonian translocations. *A*, rob(13;21). *B*, rob(14;21), the most common translocation predisposing to Down syndrome. *C*, rob(21;21). All children of a balanced carrier of the latter translocation have Down syndrome since the complementary product, monosomy 21, is not viable. *D*, rcp(10;21)(p11;p12). This is a reciprocal translocation in which the end of the short arm of a chromosome 21 is translocated to the short arm of a chromosome 10 near the centromere, and most of the short arm of the chromosome 10 is translocated to the short arm of the chromosome 21 near the centromere. The resulting chromosomes appear to have the short arm (p) of 21 on the long arm (q) of 10 [der(10)] and the short arm of 10 on the long arm of 21 [der(21)] (der = derivative). Down syndrome occurs by 3:1 nondisjunction in which chromosomes der(10), der(21), and 21 all migrate to the same pole at the first meiotic division. Robertsonian translocation rob(21;22) and other reciprocal translocations involving chromosome 21 can also give rise to Down syndrome. (*Courtesy of Dr. Steven A. Schonberg, University of California, San Francisco.*)

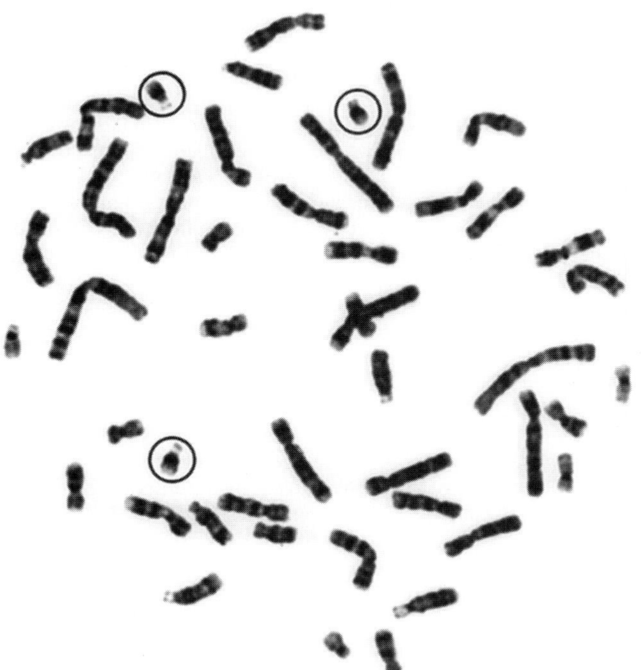

Fig. 63-5 Metaphase spread of G-banded chromosomes from person with trisomy 21. The three chromosomes 21 are circled. (*Courtesy of Dr. Steven A. Schonberg, University of California, San Francisco.*)

location trisomy 21, the likelihood that a child with DS has an unbalanced translocation of familial origin falls from 2.2 percent at a maternal age of 20 years to 1.0 percent at age 30, 0.4 percent at age 35, and 0.1 percent at age 40.[296]

The cytogenetic abnormalities just described involve most or all of chromosome 21, whether free or as part of a robertsonian fusion chromosome (in which case only the long arm, 21q, is present in an extra copy). However, there are, as has been noted, rare cases in which only part of the long arm of the chromosome is triplicated, and such cases have been used to define the region of chromosome 21 responsible for the DS phenotype. This type of analysis is discussed in "Down Syndrome Region" below. Even rarer are reports of cases of phenotypic DS in which the chromosomes appeared normal, but modern molecular and cytogenetic approaches now permit very small triplicated regions to be detected. However, two sibs with "clinically typical" DS and no cytogenetic or molecular evidence of increased numbers of any of 10 chromosome 21 sequences and genes have been born to consanguineous parents, suggesting the existence of an autosomal recessive phenocopy of DS.[297]

Mosaicism

Trisomy 21 mosaicism (47,+21/46) may result from either meiotic or mitotic nondisjunction. In meiotic nondisjunction, the extra chromosome 21 is lost from a cell soon after fertilization occurs. In mitotic nondisjunction, nondisjunction occurs during early embryogenesis to generate both 47,+21 and 45,−21 cell populations, with the monosomic cells presumably being lost during embryonic and fetal life. Based on analysis of maternal

Table 63-4 Types of Chromosome Abnormalities in Individuals with Down Syndrome

	Proportion (%)	
Cytogenetic Abnormality	By Direct Observation	Corrected for Ascertainment Bias
47,+21	89.3–93.9	93–96
47,+21/46 mosaicism	1.0–3.7	2–4
Robertsonian translocations		2–5
46, − 14,+rob(14;21)	1.5–3.4	—
46, − 13,+rob(13;21)	0.1–0.6	—
46, − 15,+rob(15;21)	0.2–0.6	—
46, − 21,+rob(21;21)	1.6–2.1	—
46, − 22,+rob(21;22)	0.1–0.3	—
Reciprocal translocations	0.2–0.3	<1

Source: From Thuline and Pueschel[293] and Hook.[294]

ages at time of birth, it has been estimated that about 20 percent of phenotypically recognized mosaics may be of mitotic origin.[298] It has also been suggested that there is an increased loss of chromosome 21 with age, leading to an increased prevalence of low level mosaicism.[299] Mosaicism for the other types of chromosome abnormalities leading to the presence of an extra chromosome 21q can also exist.

Detection of Mosaicism. Trisomy 21 mosaicism is generally recognized in one of three ways: during the cytogenetic investigation of typical cases of DS; during the evaluation of so-called mild or possible cases of DS or of mildly retarded and/or dysmorphic children without any obvious diagnosis; and in the course of studies on parents who have had more than one child with trisomy 21. In the latter instances, particularly when the proportion of trisomic cells may be quite low, there are serious methodological problems involved in the detection and quantitation of a mosaic state — including in defining whether mosaicism is actually present or, conversely, whether mosaicism can be considered as being reasonably well excluded.[294] One such problem occurs because the proportions of trisomic cells in peripheral blood lymphocytes are generally lower than in skin fibroblasts cultured from the same individual.[298,300] Furthermore, the detected proportion of mosaicism can change with time.[301–303] Some of the difficulties in detection should be alleviated by cytogenetic analysis based on the use of chromosome-specific probes *in situ* in interphase cells,[204] a procedure which would permit a large number of cells to be analyzed. For these reasons, estimates of both the frequency of trisomy 21 mosaicism and the proportions of trisomic and diploid cells in mosaic individuals must be considered as only approximate. Nevertheless, it has been estimated that parental mosaicism, as defined by the detection of at least two trisomic cells, is present in about 3 percent of females (i.e., 1.5 percent of parents) having one child with trisomy 21;[305,306] if only one trisomic cell is accepted as evidence of mosaicism, the frequency rises to 4.3 percent of families.[305] The mosaic individuals in these families, while phenotypically normal, may have proportions of trisomic cells as high as 20 to 25 percent in lymphocytes and fibroblasts,[298] although ≤6 percent[306] or even ≤3 percent[305] for lymphocytes is more usual.

Table 63-5 Types of Chromosome Abnormalities in Individuals with Down Syndrome as a Function of Maternal Age

	Cytogenetic Abnormality (%)		
Maternal Age (Years)	47,+21	47,+21/46 Mosaicism	46,rob(−;21)
15–19	84.9	5.0	10.1
20–24	89.8	1.2	9.0
25–29	91.1	2.1	6.9
30–34	92.7	2.7	4.5
35–39	97.2	1.4	1.5
40–44	97.1	2.0	1.7
≥44	96.6	2.3	1.1

Source: From Hook.[294]

Phenotypes of Mosaics. If mosaic cases ascertained from cytogenetic evaluation because of presumed or suspected DS, or because of mental retardation, are considered, there does not appear to be any correlation between mental development and the proportion of trisomic cells present in either peripheral blood lymphocytes[307,308] or fibroblasts,[308] although such a correlation had been claimed for the latter.[309] No data are available that would permit an assessment of the degree of mosaicism in other tissues of the body, particularly the brain, as is now possible in animal model systems (see "Chimeric Mice" and "Transgenic Mice" below). Nevertheless, when considered as a group, the mean intelligence (IQ) and developmental quotients (DQ) for the mosaic cases do appear to be somewhat higher, perhaps 10 to 20 points, than in matched individuals with nonmosaic trisomy 21.[307] But because of the wide variability, the existence of mosaicism *per se* is not of great prognostic value.[307,310] The physical phenotype can be quite variable, ranging from "typical" DS to only mental retardation and very subtle dysmorphic features. Congenital heart disease appears to occur very infrequently, if at all.[308] Although mosaicism associated with clinical abnormality and parental mosaicism have been discussed as though they were separate entities, they really ought to be considered as different points on a continuum ranging from no clinically detectable abnormalities to the full DS phenotype. There are undoubtedly many mosaic individuals who are not recognized because there is no reason to carry out the extensive chromosome studies that would be required to detect the existence of chromosomal mosaicism.

A case of dementia without mental retardation was reported in a 45-year-old woman with mosaicism for what cytogenetically appeared to be a trisomic cell line containing an isochromosome 21q.[311] The affected person had a few of the minor dysmorphic features of DS, and the degree of mosaicism was low in the blood (≤5 percent), but varied from 0 to 100 percent in skin fibroblast cultures. Another case of dementia was reported in a 41-year-old woman with 5 percent mosaicism (presumably in blood) who had a child with trisomy 21.[312] These cases are of interest in light of the suggestions that sporadic AD dementia may be the result of somatic trisomy 21 in the brain[313] and that toxic products released by trisomic cells, such as amyloid precursor protein (APP), might lead to the degeneration of normal diploid neurons (see "Pathogenesis of Specific Features of Down Syndrome" below). A case of trisomy 21 *without* the phenotype of DS has been attributed to mosaicism in tissues other than blood lymphocytes and fibroblasts (the placenta had 27 percent diploid cells).[314]

Parental Origin of Extra Chromosome 21

A population-based analysis using DNA markers has shown that maternal nondisjunction accounts for 86 percent of all cases of trisomy 21, with 75 percent of cases occurring at meiosis I (MI) and 25 percent at meiosis II (MII).[315] The maternal age effect was greater for MII than MI errors. Nine percent of cases were paternally derived (50 percent MI, 50 percent MII), and 5 percent were somatic in origin. In another study, all of eight *de novo* (nonfamilial) robertsonian (14q;21q) translocations were maternal in origin.[316] By contrast, 21q;21q chromosomes, originally also thought to be robertsonian fusion chromosomes, have been shown to be 21q isochromosomes in most, but not all, instances.[317,318] Of 22 isochromosomes studied, 12 were paternal and 8 were maternal in origin.

Maternal Age and the Incidence of Down Syndrome

It has long been recognized that the risk of having a child with DS increases with maternal age and that the distribution of maternal age in the population of women having children is the primary determinant of the overall incidence of DS.[319] From 1960 to 1978, the proportion of women in the United States giving birth who were ≥ 35 years of age declined from 10.9 to 4.5 percent, and the estimated crude incidence of DS fell from 1.33 to 0.99 per 1000 births.[319] Because of changes over the years in the proportions of cases actually ascertained, it is difficult to determine with certainty whether there have been any changes in age-specific incidence rates. These rates appear to have remained constant.[294]

Effect of Maternal Age on Incidence. A variety of estimates of the incidence of DS in the newborn population have been made, and most figures are in the vicinity of 1 per 1000 live births.[294] The figures can be broken down to provide maternal age-specific rates, which appear to be constant over time,[320] and these rates are shown in Table 63-6. Although it has been suggested otherwise, there is no evidence that the rate levels off at the upper extreme of maternal age (≥ 46 years).[322] On the other hand, there is a suggestion that the rate is slightly higher for mothers under 20 years of age.[294] Overall, the rate of DS increases quite gradually in a linear fashion, about 0.04 to 0.05 per 1000 per year until about age 30 to 31 years. There is then an apparently abrupt shift to more of an exponential pattern of increase. It is not clear whether this represents a true change in the mechanism(s) responsible for nondisjunction or actually derives from two processes, one constant, and one exponential, which coexist throughout the childbearing years.[294]

Table 63-6 Maternal Age Dependence of Down Syndrome Fetuses and Liveborns

	Rate per 1000		
Maternal Age, Years	Liveborn Infants	Amniocentesis	Chorionic Villus Sampling
20	0.58	—	—
25	0.80	—	—
30	1.04	—	—
33	1.57	—	—
35	2.59	3.9	4.2
37	4.28	6.4	7.5
38	5.50	8.1	10.0
39	7.07	10.4	13.4
40	9.09	13.3	17.9
42	15.04	21.7	31.7
44	24.89	35.5	56.4
46	41.22	58.0	(100.2)

SOURCE: From Hook[294] and Hook et al.[321]

Rates in Fetuses. The estimates for the incidence of DS in the newborn population are corrected for underreporting, a quite serious problem in the compilation of accurate statistics. Even so, the rates observed at birth are still only two-thirds the rates observed in fetuses monitored by midgestational amniocentesis (Table 63-6).[294,321] These differences are attributable in whole or in part to fetal death leading to spontaneous abortion between the time the amniocentesis is performed and term. In a survey of pregnancies in which 47,+21 was detected at the 16th to 18th week of gestation and therapeutic abortion was not carried out, over 20 percent of the DS fetuses died *in utero*.[323] When frequencies observed at amniocentesis were compared with those found at chorionic villus sampling at about 10 weeks of gestation, it appeared that about 21 percent of affected fetuses died between these two time points.[321] Overall, it is estimated that ≈30 percent of DS fetuses survive to term.[294,324]

Causes of the Maternal Age Effect. Despite decades of investigation, it is fair to say that we do not understand the basis of the very strong effect of maternal age on incidence. This effect is so strong that it has been estimated that the majority of oocytes, or at least of recognizable pregnancies of women ≥ 40 years of age, may be aneuploid.[325] Several types of hypotheses have been advanced, and, in considering these possibilities, it should be remembered that both age-dependent and age-independent factors may be operating simultaneously.[326]

Aging of Ova. Hypotheses in this category hold that cumulative events, either intrinsic or extrinsic (environmental) in origin, lead to a breakdown in meiosis, and, in turn, to nondisjunction. Such events could be either an age-dependent decay in spindle fibers or their components, or a failure in nucleolar breakdown on the one hand, or an accumulation of the effects of radiation, hormonal imbalances, infection, or the like. Few data are available to support the latter possibilities (see "Environmental and Other Factors" below), and the former are still quite inferential and based primarily on work in animals.[327] Hypotheses of this type would be compatible with the predominantly MI origin of nondisjunction.

Delayed Fertilization. Because of a declining rate of coitus in older couples, and also a probably low rate in very young mothers, it was postulated that delayed fertilization, with "aging" of the ovum after ovulation, could be responsible for the age-dependence of nondisjunction.[328] Experimental evidence from animals supports this notion, but many objections have been raised.[326] In particular, a mechanism involving postovulatory events would have to work at the level of MII, not MI, as is most frequent in human aneuploidy. The finding of an increased frequency of DS, as well as of dizygous twins and males, among the offspring of Orthodox Jewish women is thought to be consistent with this proposal (although aging of sperm could also be a factor).[329]

Aging of Sperm. A hypothesis has been advanced that aging of sperm in the male reproductive tract, associated with infrequent coitus, is responsible for the maternal age effect in cases of DS in which the extra chromosome 21 is derived from the father,[330] an assumption that must be reconfirmed using paternally derived cases proven by molecular means. In addition, it is suggested that such aging of sperm explains the excess frequency of DS in unwed teenage mothers and that it may possibly play a role at all maternal ages.

The Production-Line Hypothesis. Based on studies in the mouse, a "production-line" hypothesis was proposed which states that oocytes with greater numbers of chiasmata are formed earlier during embryogenesis and are ovulated earlier in adult life than are

Table 63-7 Environmental and Other Factors Considered in the Etiology of Down Syndrome

Factor	Consensus
Seasonality	No consistent effect
Infectious disease	No consistent effect
Socioeconomic status	No effect
Ethnic and racial differences	No effect except for high incidence in non-Ashkenazi Jews in Israel
Birth order (independent of maternal age)	No significant effect
Consanguinity (paternal) and inbreeding	Possibly an increase in incidence: fourfold increase in risk in Kuwait
Exogenous agents	
Sex hormones (contraceptive use)	No consistent effect
Spermicides	No effect
Fluoride in water	No effect
Tobacco	Perhaps a slight decrease in incidence
Caffeine, alcohol, marijuana	Unknown
Radiation	Mixed reports; probably no consistent effect
Thyroid autoantibodies	Inconsistent reports

SOURCE: From Hook,[294] Crowley et al.,[335] Kline and Stein,[347] Warburton,[348] Janerich and Bracken,[349] and references in text.

oocytes with fewer chiasmata.[331] A decrease in chiasmata would result in an increased frequency of univalents during MI and, it is believed, in nondisjunction. At present, the evidence favoring such a production line or a relationship between MI univalents and nondisjunction appears to be weak.[326]

***Relaxation of Selection* In Utero.** In contrast to all the foregoing hypotheses, which operate at the level of prezygotic events associated with meiosis, the fifth major hypothesis is that there is a decrease in the rate of abortion of aneuploid embryos and fetuses, rather than in their rate of production. However, failure to find a maternal age effect for DS resulting from robertsonian translocations of the rob(D;21) type[332] would not be compatible with this proposal, and neither would consideration of cases of trisomy 21/2n mosaicism.[333] Selection, if it occurs, is considered likely to be very early in pregnancy, prior to the time of recognizable spontaneous abortions.[334] Nevertheless, it is believed by one investigator that the "indirect evidence…must be regarded as making a presumptive (but not definitive) case for selection effects."[334] Others, in contrast, believe "that it is some factor in the adult maternal environment which is the real cause of age-related aneuploidy."[326]

It is clear that no consistent explanation can be given for the maternal age effects. In the end, it is likely that a variety of factors will be shown to interact and to be of importance.[335] Furthermore, these age-related factors may or may not ultimately explain the basic mechanisms leading to aneuploidy, the nature of which is a subject of considerable debate.[10,336]

Paternal Age Effects on Incidence. In contrast to the very strong effect of maternal age, the age of the father has only a small, if any, effect on incidence. Claims that a paternal age effect exists[337] have been opposed on methodological grounds,[338] and no paternal age effect was found in trisomic spontaneous abortions.[339] Furthermore, direct examination of the chromosomal constitution of sperm from men of different ages did not reveal a paternal age effect in the frequency of aneuploid sperm.[340]

Causes of Nondisjunction

Reduced Recombination. Analyses of the chromosomes 21 of persons with DS demonstrate altered rates of recombination in the maternal meioses that gave rise to them. Reduced rates of recombination in the proximal region of the chromosome are associated with MI errors and an increased rate, again proximally, with MII errors.[341–344] These very important findings are believed to be consistent with the hypothesis that alterations in chiasma formation initiated during MI may lead to malsegregation at either MI or II, and hence to nondisjunction. The decrease in recombination at MI may be manifested cytologically by the appearance of functional univalent (rather than bivalent) chromosomes at MI, presumably as the result of precocious centromeric division.[345]

Environmental and Other Factors. Many environmental and other factors have been considered with regard to their potential roles in the etiology of nondisjunction and causation of trisomy 21, and the question of the role of paternal exposure to environmental agents, acting either directly on spermatogenesis or indirectly on oogenesis, has also been raised.[346] A list of the factors, most of which have given inconsistent (seasonality, infectious disease, sex hormones, radiation) or negative results, is given in Table 63-7. Three items do, however, require specific discussion. The first is the observed increase in the rate of DS in the offspring of West Jerusalem Jewish women of North African or Asian origin, with incidence rates of 2.1 to 2.4 per 1000 live births.[350] No explanation for this more than twofold increase has been provided. The second factor is inbreeding and consanguinity, on which studies have been done to obtain evidence for the participation of recessive traits in the etiology of nondisjunction. While the data are quite susceptible to different interpretations, depending on the statistical analyses used,[294,351] the finding of a fourfold increase in trisomy 21 within consanguineous matings, after controlling for maternal age and birth order, is compatible with a role for genetic factors[352] operating by undefined mechanisms.

The third factor, maternal thyroid autoimmunity and thyroid disease, had been regarded as the only factor which, aside from advanced maternal age, consistently indicated an increased maternal risk for trisomy 21.[335,353] Other types of autoantibodies were also reported as being increased.[335] However, an association between the presence of thyroid antibodies and the risk of DS was not found in a large case-control study, and prospective testing of pregnant women for such antibodies was not recommended.[354]

Recurrence Risks

Trisomy 21. Does the birth of one child with trisomy 21 predispose to the birth of another? In analyses based on live birth data, the recurrence risk was estimated as 1.4 percent for maternal age <30 years in the pregnancy at risk, and 0.5 percent for women ≥ 30 years.[294] These risks are quite approximate and are based on relatively few cases. Figures based on amniocentesis data are presented in Table 63-8. These data indicate that women under 30 to 35 years of age who have a child with trisomy 21 have a significantly increased risk of having another, while the increased risk is little, if any, over the usual maternal age-dependent incidence if the mother at risk is older.[348] As noted earlier, the risk to liveborn infants is about two-thirds the figures given in Table

Table 63-8 Recurrence Risks at Amniocentesis for Trisomy 21 and for All Trisomies after Birth of a Child with Trisomy 21

Maternal Age at Birth of Index Case (Years)	Maternal Age at Amniocentesis (Years)			
	<30 Trisomy 21	≥30 All Trisomies (%)	<35 Trisomy 21	≥35 All Aneuploidy (%)
<30	0.78 (1.18) [8.1 ×]*	0.68 (1.02) [2.5 ×]	—	—
≥30		0.76 (1.19) [1.0 ×]	—	—
All ages			0.6 (1.3)	1.2 (1.6)

*Increase over expected frequency.

SOURCE: From Warburton[348] for < or ≥ 30 and Stene et al[351] for < or ≥ 35.

63-8, or about 0.8 to 1.1 percent for a major chromosome abnormality in each maternal age group. The dichotomy between the increases in risks to the younger and older mothers of index cases is consistent with the belief that cases occurring in younger mothers result principally from causes that are maternal age-independent.[348] Despite one report to the contrary,[355] second-degree relatives do not appear to be at significantly increased risk.[356]

Translocations. Although *de novo* robertsonian translocations appear unlikely to recur, a recurrence risk as high as 2.6 percent was calculated for DS resulting from rob(21q;21q) because of the finding of mosaicism or a pericentric inversion in one member each of 4 of 112 sets of parents.[357]

When a robertsonian translocation causing DS is inherited, the risks to future offspring depend on parental sex (Table 63-9).[358–360] For translocations inherited from the mother, the risks are in the range of 10 to 15 percent, whereas they are only 1 to 2 percent when the father is the carrier. The reason for this difference is not known. However, for the rare case of balanced parental 45, −21, −21,+rob(21q;21q), the risk of DS from a 46, −21,+rob(21q;21q) chromosome constitution is 100 percent, because the only other possible chromosome arrangement (45, −21) is not compatible with viability.

Prenatal Diagnosis

Several methods are employed to screen pregnancies for DS. The first two, amniocentesis and chorionic villus sampling (CVS), are used for a limited segment of the childbearing population. The third, maternal serum screening, can be carried out on all pregnant women. The fourth and newest approach is based on visualization of the fetus by ultrasonography. The principal indications for amniocentesis and CVS to detect chromosomally abnormal fetuses are the birth of a previous child with trisomy 21 or another chromosome disorder, a carrier state for a robertsonian or other translocation in one of the parents, advanced maternal age, and a calculated elevated risk based on maternal serum screening (see below). Several other nonchromosomal indications also exist. One other potential screening procedure—detection of fetal cells in the maternal circulation—is also under development.

Table 63-9 Risks for Unbalanced Progeny When One Parent Is the Carrier of a Robertsonian or Reciprocal Translocation

Translocation	Parent Carrying	Livebirth, % Abnormal	At Amniocentesis, % Abnormal
rob(Dq;21q)	Mother	10–11	15
	Father	2.4	—
rob(21q;22q)	Mother	14	16
	Father	1–2	—
t(21;)*		—	10

*Ascertained through infants with unbalanced translocations.

SOURCE: From Stene[358] and Hamerton[359] for liveborns. Boué and Gallano[360] for amniocentesis.

Amniocentesis and Chorionic Villus Sampling. In most prenatal diagnosis programs, a maternal age of ≥35 years has been used as a threshold for determining when amniocentesis or chorionic villus sampling is indicated. However, because of the distribution of ages of women having children, only a minority of children with DS are born to mothers ≥35 years of age. Thus, in the period 1968 to 1976, only 4.5 percent of total births occurred in this age group, accounting for only 23.1 percent of all infants with DS.[319] Similar figures were obtained for births about a decade later.[361] In 1983, only 7.2 percent of live births occurred in women ≥35 years of age, about half of whom sought amniocentesis;[362] 18.6 percent of births occurred to women from 30 to 34 years of age. Based on these data, it could be estimated from the maternal-age-dependence of DS that 27 percent of all DS pregnancies could be detected by amniocentesis or CVS if half of pregnant women ≥30 years of age were monitored.[362] This is nearly double the figure detectable by prenatal diagnosis at or after 35 years of age.

Conventional amniocentesis is usually carried out at 14 to 16 weeks of gestation and CVS at 8 to 12 weeks. However, early amniocentesis at 11 to 12 weeks of gestation is also being used. The choice of procedure is a function of several factors, including safety (with midtrimester amniocentesis believed to be somewhat less risky than CVS in terms of fetal mortality), methods available for pregnancy termination, desire of the parents to be tested prior to the time the pregnancy becomes obvious and/or fetal quickening occurs, and the time that prenatal care is first sought. Compared to midtrimester amniocentesis, early amniocentesis has been found to be associated with an increased risk of fetal loss (7.6 percent vs 5.9 percent) and talipes equinovarus (1.3 percent vs 0.1 percent), the latter possibly because of increased amniotic fluid leakage.[363] Despite earlier concerns, CVS carried out between 9 and 12 weeks of gestation is not associated with an increased frequency of limb reduction defects.[364] The detection of chromosomally abnormal fetuses follows the expected maternal age dependence, and the figures for DS detected at amniocentesis and at CVS have already been presented in Table 63-6.

Maternal Serum Screening. As second-trimester maternal serum α-fetoprotein (MS-AFP) screening programs for neural-tube defects were being implemented during the early 1980s, it was noted that pregnancies with DS were associated with lower than normal levels of MS-AFP.[365,366] These findings were soon extended to amniotic fluid AFP values,[367] and in both instances the median value of AFP concentration was 0.64 to 0.72 that found in normal pregnancies.[366,367] Similar results have also been found for MS-AFP values obtained as early as the eighth week of gestation.[368] The lower serum AFP levels in DS pregnancies have been attributed to decreased AFP protein production or content in the fetal DS liver.[369] It has been suggested that the lower AFP levels during pregnancy may be related in mechanism to the somewhat decreased concentrations of serum albumin (a homologous and closely linked protein) in children and adults.[370] However, a relative decrease in MS-AFP occurs even in the presence of neural-tube abnormalities that greatly increase amniotic fluid AFP,[371] suggesting that serum AFP concentrations may not be directly related to amniotic fluid concentrations.

Maternal serum screening has been extended into triple-marker screening, in which levels of human chorionic gonadotropin (hCG) and unconjugated estriol (uE_3) are also measured. hCG, as well as total or free β-hCG subunit and free α-hCG subunit, is elevated in DS, and approximately 56 percent of pregnancies with DS have levels of hCG >2 multiples of the median (MoM).[372] Low serum levels (median values of 0.73 to 0.75 MoM) of unconjugated estriol are also found in DS pregnancies.[373,374] The three values are then mathematically combined, along with age, to determine the risk that the fetus has DS.

In most screening programs, a series of gestation age-dependent cutoffs are established so that the risk of DS in the identified pregnancy is in the range of 1 in 190 to 1 in 380, the latter being close to the risk at age 35 when amniocentesis or CVS is considered indicated. Women whose calculated risks are greater than these values are offered amniocentesis for the purpose of fetal karyotyping. In a meta-analysis of 20 studies involving nearly 200,000 pregnancies, it was found that, in women of all ages, the median detection rate (sensitivity) was 67 percent with a cutoff of 1 in 190 to 200, 71 percent at 1 in 250 to 295, and 73 percent at 1 in 350 to 390.[375] The median false positive rates ranged from 4 to 8 percent. Independently of the cutoff used, both sensitivity and the false positive rate increased with maternal age.

Ultrasonography. Several ultrasonographic signs of DS have been described and proposed as prenatal screening procedures, including shortening of the humerus (expressed as a reduced ratio of humerus length to biparietal diameter) and femur, thickening of the nuchal fold, and renal pyelectasis.[376] These measurements appear to be useful as screening procedures, particularly when combined.[377] When combined with maternal age and with assays of free β-hCG and of pregnancy-associated plasma protein A (PAPP-A, which may be decreased in DS pregnancies), measurement of nuchal translucency thickness between 10 and 15 weeks of gestation, with ≥ 3 mm taken as positive, will detect between 80 and 87 percent of fetuses with trisomy 21 with a false positive rate of 5 percent.[378,379]

Detection of Fetal Cells in the Maternal Circulation. Efforts are being made to develop screening and diagnostic procedures based on the detection and analysis of fetal nucleated erythrocytes, lymphocytes, or trophoblast cells in the maternal circulation,[380] or on the analysis of whole blood.[381] The hope is that this approach will become a noninvasive replacement for invasive procedures such as amniocentesis and CVS. Many technical difficulties need to be overcome before fetal cell analysis will permit the accurate diagnosis of a cytogenetic disorder such as DS. However, it is possible to diagnose sickle cell disease and thalassemia by PCR analysis of nucleated erythroblasts microdissected from microscope slides after being isolated by reaction with anti-CD-71 (transferrin receptor) coupled to magnetic beads and staining for fetal or embryonic hemoglobin.[382]

GENERAL PRINCIPLES OF THE EFFECTS OF ANEUPLOIDY

The problem of defining how an extra copy of all or part of chromosome 21 results in the phenotype of DS is a specialized case of the general problem of explaining how chromosome imbalance involving any part of the genome produces abnormalities of function and development. Accordingly, any principles that can be derived from an examination of the effects of a large number of aneuploid states should assist in solving the specific problem of DS. The conclusions of such an examination[7] are presented in the following sections.

Differentiability of Phenotypes

Aneuploid phenotypes, while frequently overlapping, are differentiable from one another. Thus, while the same dysmorphic features or congenital malformations may be part of the phenotype of two or more different aneuploid states,[383] the patterns of individual aneuploid states are specific enough to permit them to be distinguished from one another clinically. By using quantitative methods of pattern analysis, it is possible to distinguish very closely related aneuploid states that might, at first glance, appear to be very similar, or even identical with one another, and to conclude that "although there are few if any physical features which are exclusive to a particular chromosomal defect, the pattern of defects is distinct."[384]

Specificity and Variability of Phenotypes

Although there may be a significant degree of variability in the expression of the phenotype of a given type of chromosome imbalance, the phenotype, in terms of overall pattern, is nonetheless a specific one. As was already discussed with regard to the phenotype of Down syndrome and as the data in Table 63-1 illustrate, no single phenotypic feature, with the possible exceptions of mental retardation and hypotonia, is present all the time. The same is even true within families in the case of hereditary forms of DS — as for example in the family studied by Korenberg *et al.*[385] In fact, if randomly selected series of cases of duplications in sibs reported in the literature are compared with regard to the concordance for the abnormal features which they exhibit, the mean concordance for all sets of sibs is about 75 percent.[7] Even aneuploid identical twins may not be completely concordant.[386] Nevertheless, as has just been discussed, it is still possible to recognize individual aneuploid states based on the overall pattern of defects.

Sources of Variability. Variability in phenotypic expression stems from three sources — genetic, stochastic, and extrinsic — with extrinsic subsuming all nongenetic influences except for those randomly generated developmental events which are referred to as "stochastic." Genetic factors can be thought of as being of two kinds — differences in the precise genetic constitution of the chromosomes or chromosome segments that are unbalanced, or, conversely, differences in the balanced remainder of the genome. With regard to the latter, a state of chromosome imbalance does not operate in a vacuum but is superimposed on the overall genetic constitution of the person or animal — a genetic constitution that, except in identical twins, necessarily differs from individual to individual. The great differences in development encompassed within the concept of "normal" are such that it is not surprising that the genetic perturbations associated with aneuploidy do not always act in a uniform matter. What is perhaps more surprising is that relatively subtle phenotypic manifestations, such as the facies in DS, can be detected so readily, even when superimposed on vastly different genetic backgrounds. Direct evidence for the operation of genetic factors in the determination of phenotypes has been obtained from work on experimentally produced mouse aneuploids.[7,387]

Another potential source of variability in the phenotype is gametic imprinting, in which there is differential expression of individual loci depending on whether they are on a maternally or paternally derived chromosome[388] (see also Chap.15). However, there are no data available that implicate imprinting as a source of variability in any trisomic state. Furthermore, the overwhelmingly frequent derivation of the extra chromosome 21 from the mother would argue against imprinting as a significant factor.

Stochastic and Environmental Factors. Stochastic factors refer to the inherent variability normally present in any developmental process so that, all else being equal, more than one outcome is possible. The operation of such factors in the genesis of endocardial cushion defects in DS has been postulated (see

"Congenital Heart Disease" below) and a more general treatment has been developed.[389] Perhaps the best evidence for the existence of such factors is the lack of complete concordance for single congenital abnormalities in identical twins.[390] A major implication of the existence of stochastic factors is that relatively weak genetic perturbations, such as might exist in aneuploid states, may not always be sufficient to lead consistently to the appearance of a particular abnormality.

Extrinsic or environmental factors refer to everything else that could affect expression of the aneuploid phenotype. Included are variations in maternal anatomy and metabolism, as well as specific external agents that might act as teratogens. In practice, it may be difficult to distinguish extrinsic from stochastic factors, and there is no experimental evidence actually demonstrating the existence of extrinsic factors.

Genetic Basis of Phenotypic Features

Individual phenotypic features can often be assigned or mapped to specific regions of the genome.

The features of segmental aneuploidies can often be combined to generate the phenotypes of combined aneuploidies.

These two principles are complements of one another. The first states that it is possible to dissect an aneuploid phenotype so as to assign particular features to specific regions of the unbalanced genome. The best examples of this phenotypic mapping, which, it must be admitted, is still relatively crude, are derived from duplications and deletions of chromosome 13[7,391,392] and from the several small deletion or contiguous gene syndromes[393] (see also Chap. 65). The second principle holds that it is possible to construct a complex aneuploid phenotype by combining the individual features attributable to imbalance of particular regions within the entire unbalanced region of the genome.

Statement of these two principles, however, is not intended to negate the fact that the combination of segmental aneuploidies may, through an interaction of the effects produced by each, result either in the expression of new phenotypic features not characteristic of either alone or in the masking of certain features characteristic of one or both. The existence of such interactive effects, especially those involved in the development of new phenotypic features, indicates that particular abnormalities need not—indeed, should not—always be attributed to imbalance of only a single locus. Nevertheless, it is not unlikely that it will often turn out to be the case that only a single locus is involved.

When considering mechanisms that underlie the pathogenesis of the phenotypes of aneuploid states, I consider the implications of these principles to be this: It is legitimate to look for and to expect to find specific mechanisms to explain the relationships between particular phenotypic characteristics and the imbalance of individual loci or sets of loci. Contributions to the phenotype are likely to come from all parts of the unbalanced genome and not from just one or a very few loci. While some loci may have a greater phenotypic effect or representation than others, it is the cumulative effect of imbalance of many loci that determines the overall phenotype. As complicated as the relationships between genetic loci and phenotypic effects may be, and with whatever element of randomness they may be associated, these relationships should nonetheless exist and be discoverable. The generation of aneuploid phenotypes is not, therefore, a game of chance, but is an exercise of the conventional rules of developmental genetics and developmental biology.

Nonspecific Effects of Aneuploidy. In making the statements just presented, I am explicitly rejecting arguments that *the* or even *a* major determinant of aneuploid phenotypes operates by mechanisms that may be considered as nonspecific in nature.[7,394] These nonspecific mechanisms could include alterations in the cell cycle,[395] general retardation of development,[396] disruption of developmental and physiological homeostasis,[397] and generalized regulatory disturbances.[398] While such mechanisms could conceivably operate to affect some aspects of the aneuploid phenotype, any major role for them would have the force of obscuring the relationships expressed in the first three principles above, which clearly do exist.

Mechanisms of the Effects of Aneuploidy

The term *mechanisms* is used in the plural, and this is important. My overall sense of the clinical, theoretical, and experimental considerations applicable to an understanding of the effects of aneuploidy is that no single mechanism can explain how aneuploidy produces its deleterious consequences. There is no simple solution to the problem of aneuploidy—only a series of multifaceted individual solutions, each applicable to a particular aneuploid state.

Gene Dosage Effects. Despite the absence of general validation for all types of loci, I use the existence of proportional gene dosage effects as the starting premise for a detailed exploration of a variety of potential mechanisms.[7] Dosage compensation, such as exists for X-linked loci in mammals and for some autosomal loci in Drosophila,[399] does not appear to occur for autosomal loci in humans, although it has been reported that h2-calponin gene expression in lymphocytes is reduced to a normal level by methylation in the adjacent CpG island.[400] However, as is discussed below with regard to the amyloid precursor protein locus, it is possible that proportional changes in the expression of specific loci can be obscured by some type of dysregulative process that is secondary to the imbalance of the same or of other loci.

Precedents for Mechanisms. For the most part, clinical or experimental precedents for potential mechanisms, if they exist at all, are derived from the study of inherited metabolic diseases and not of aneuploid states *per se*. It is necessary, therefore, to be quite careful to discriminate between the effects of changes in the concentration of gene products as opposed to the effects of either qualitative alterations or the total absence of the products. Keeping this in mind, it is possible to make arguments that changes in the concentrations of enzymes, structural proteins, transport system components, regulatory molecules, receptors, and cell-surface constituents can each produce an effect on the development or functioning of an organism.[7] However, not all types of mechanisms are likely to be of equal importance in all situations.

Unfortunately, from the point of view of trying to understand the pathogenesis of DS, it is, in general, easier to come to grips with monosomies than trisomies, because lack of a product seems, at least in theory, to lead to more severe effects than does an excess in nearly any type of system under consideration. It is, therefore, not difficult to understand why monosomies as a group should do less well than the corresponding trisomies. Nevertheless, it is still necessary to explain the abnormalities associated with the trisomies, and certain systems—in particular, receptors, cell-surface recognition and adhesion molecules, growth factors and morphogens, and specific regulatory molecules—are quite attractive as candidates for playing a major role in the pathogenesis of trisomic phenotypes.[7]

The principal precedents for a significant role for regulatory molecules are derived from the studies of somatic-cell hybrids, which point to the existence of *trans*-acting regulatory molecules that can modulate the expression of differentiated function.[7] Because these effects, which are quite dosage-dependent, are highly specific in nature, it is expected that regulatory disturbances in aneuploid cells are highly specific as well. It is not surprising, therefore, that the considerable experimental evidence now available, while not actually disproving the existence of such specific regulatory effects, does argue against the existence of generalized regulatory abnormalities in aneuploid cells, including those with trisomy 21.[7,401,402]

In making judgments about the likely impact of the various mechanisms on the generation of aneuploid phenotypes, I do not distinguish between effects on morphogenesis and effects on function. Such a distinction would be, to some extent, an arbitrary one, because any perturbation of cellular growth and function during the period of morphogenesis could certainly affect tissue differentiation and morphogenesis.

THE PATHOGENESIS OF DOWN SYNDROME

The Structure of Chromosome 21

Chromosome 21 is the smallest of the human autosomes, constituting approximately 1–1.5 percent of the length of the haploid genome. The genetic length has been estimated to be 46 cM (assuming a total length of 2700 cM for the human genome)[403] but a later estimate based on molecular mapping data is a sex-averaged genetic length of 77.1 cM for 21q.[404]

In physical terms, chromosome 21 is an acrocentric chromosome with the centromere very close to one end and with a very small short arm. The short arm (21p) terminates in a satellite region that may vary in size. Proximal to the satellite is the stalk (secondary constriction), which, as the nucleolar organizer region (NOR), contains multiple copies of the ribosomal RNA genes (*RNR4*) and stains characteristically with silver.[405] The degree of silver staining appears to be a representation of the molecular activity of the ribosomal RNA genes that the chromosome contains.[406] The region of 21p adjacent to the centromere contains highly repeated DNA sequences, none of which are unique to chromosome 21.[407]

The major part of chromosome 21 is the long arm (21q), which has a characteristic banding pattern consisting of three or four bands at low resolution, and as many as 11 dark and light bands resolvable by prometaphase banding (Fig. 63-7).[408] With one possible exception, all genes of known function (other than for ribosomal RNA) are located on this arm of chromosome 21, and only this arm is essential for normal development and function. The centromere proximal half of 21q, with half of the DNA, contains only 10 percent of expressed sequences.[409] The presence of a robertsonian fusion chromosome in which the short arms of two acrocentric chromosomes (sometimes both chromosomes 21) are deleted, does not cause detectable abnormalities if the genome is otherwise balanced.

As one of the first triumphs of the Human Genome Project, the sequence of the long arm of chromosome 21 has been completed with an estimated 99.7% coverage.[410] This arm has a length of 33.7 megabase pairs and is relatively gene-poor, with less than half the number of identified genes found on the similarly sized chromosome 22. It contains 127 known genes, 98 predicted genes (of which 69% have no similarity to known proteins), and 59 pseudogenes. Among the known genes are at least 10 kinases, 5 genes in the ubiquitination pathway, 5 cell adhesion molecules, 7 ion channels, 5 members of the interferon receptor family, and several transcription factors. About 22.4% of the chromosome consists of interspersed Alu sequences and LINE1 elements.

The Down Syndrome Region. Cases in which only part of chromosome 21 is triplicated have been intensively studied to arrive at a phenotypic map, which will permit a correlation of particular phenotypic features of DS with specific regions or loci of the chromosome. Nearly all studies reported so far were carried out before molecular markers became available, and only rough phenotypic maps could be constructed.[411] In these studies, the phenotype was characterized mainly on subjective grounds, and quantitative diagnostic approaches[23,384] have not been used. However, protocols for carrying out such studies are now developed and published.[412] The consensus of the earlier studies is that the full DS phenotype, as manifested by mental retardation, congenital heart disease, characteristic facial appearance, hand anomalies, and dermatoglyphic changes, appears when band 21q22 is duplicated, and of this, sub-band 21q22.1, and probably 21q22.2, is required.[413] It had been estimated that this region carries 50 to 100 genes,[414] although this figure may be revised now that the chromosome has been sequenced.[410]

Several groups have recently used molecular analyses to define the extent of the triplication of regions of chromosome 21 and have then used the results to generate phenotypic maps. Korenberg and collaborators[415,416] and Delabar and collaborators[417] summarized these studies. In the latter study, short stature, joint hyperlaxity, hypotonia, mental retardation, and various minor anomalies were mapped to the region *D21S55*, and six facial and dermatologic abnormalities were mapped to the *D21S55-MX1* interval, which extends into 21q22.3. These authors speculate that one or just a few genes may be responsible for the DS phenotype. In contrast, Korenberg and collaborators,[416,417] who partition the phenotype in terms of penetrance and expressivity (because virtually no component of the phenotype is expressed in all individuals with complete trisomy 21), contend that there is evidence for contributions of genes outside the *D21S55* region, especially in the proximal part of 21q. However, even by this analysis, the region responsible for congenital heart disease is confined to the distal part of 21q, and it is inferred that just one gene or cluster of genes is responsible. One version of a phenotypic map of chromosome 21 based on molecular analysis,

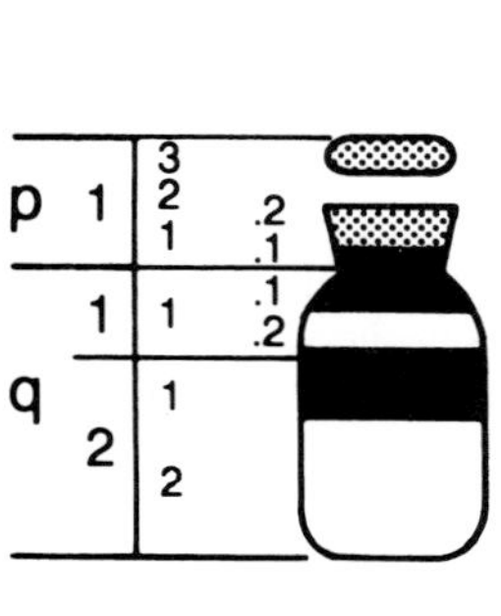

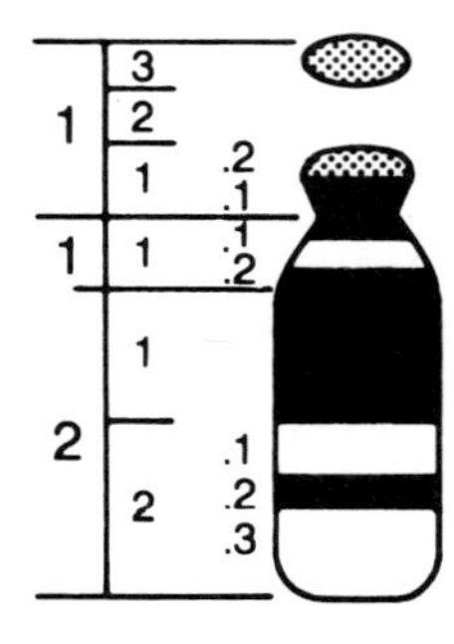

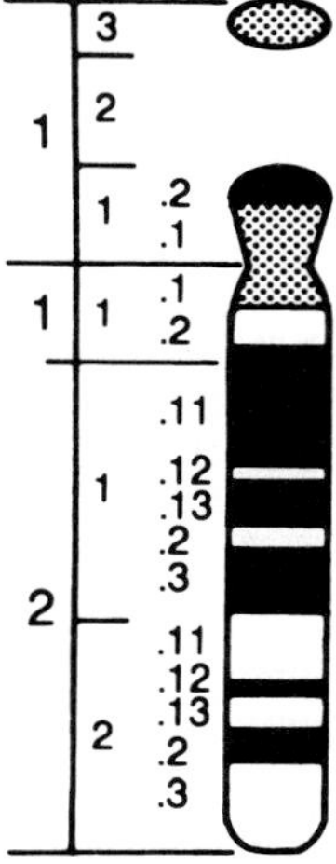

TOTAL BANDS 400 550 850

Fig. 63-7 Giemsa banding patterns of chromosome 21 at increasing degrees of resolution. (*Redrawn from Yunis[408] and reprinted by permission of WB Saunders Company.*)

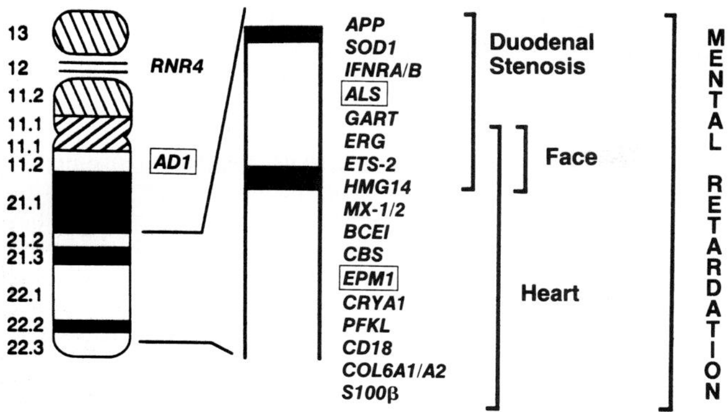

Fig. 63-8 Phenotypic map of human trisomy 21 based on molecular and cytogenetic analysis of cases with triplication of part of chromosome 21. (*Modified by Dr. Julie Korenberg from Korenberg.*[411])

which defines the region responsible for some of the facial features of DS and the limits of the regions involved in the congenital heart disease and the duodenal stenosis is shown in Fig. 63-8.[411]

Effects of Imbalance of Chromosome 21 Loci

Gene Dosage Effects. As noted above, the immediate consequence (or primary effect) of an aneuploid state is a gene dosage effect for each of the loci present on the unbalanced chromosome or chromosome segment. Such gene dosage effects have been reported for nine chromosome 21 loci and are summarized in Table 63-10. With the exception of APP in brain from fetuses and possibly of S100β in cerebellum of young children with DS,[421,423] the measured increases in activities or concentrations in trisomic cells were very close to the theoretically expected values of 1.5. Taken in the aggregate, these results confirm the existence of quite precise gene dosage effects in cells aneuploid for chromosome 21.

Secondary Effects. Although the known chromosome 21 loci and their products represent but a small fraction of the genetically active loci present on chromosome 21, it is still of interest whether imbalance of any of them has detectable phenotypic (secondary) effects as a result of the gene dosage effect. For *IFNAR1*, *IFNAR2*, and *IFNGR2* it is possible to ascribe the secondary effects of enhanced sensitivity to the interferons to the ≈1.5 times increase in receptor component numbers. No measurements of intracellular metabolic flux have been made that would permit any inferences to be drawn about the significance of the increased phosphofructokinase, cystathionine β-synthase, or phosphoribosylglycineamide synthetase (PRGS) activities, although it has been suggested the increased activity of PRGS (and of the other activities, PAIS and PGFT, which are part of the same complex) may result in increased *de novo* purine biosynthesis in trisomic individuals, and consequently in hyperuricemia.[414]

Table 63-10 Gene Dosage Effects in Trisomy 21

Locus	Function Assayed	Ts/2n*
APP	Amyloid precursor protein (APP) concentration in serum	1.48
	APP mRNA concentration in fetal brain	3.8–4.6
CBS	Cystathionine β-synthase activity in stimulated lymphocytes	1.61
CD18	Binding of antibody against LFA-1β to lymphoblastoid lines	1.57†
IFNAR1	Interferon-α binding to fibroblasts	1.57
HMG14	HMG-14 protein and mRNA concentrations in fibroblasts and fetal brain	1.67
PFKL	Phosphofructokinase activity in red cells and fibroblasts	1.46
PRGS	Phosphoribosylglycinamide synthetase activity in fibroblasts	1.56
SOD1	Superoxide dismutase-1 activity in red cells, fibroblasts, platelets, lymphocytes, brain, and granulocytes	1.52
S100b	Protein S-100, beta subunit mRNA, and protein concentrations in cerebellum	1.80

HMG = high mobility group.
*Mean ratio of activity in or binding to trisomic (Ts) and diploid (2n) cells.
†Mean of value for α in geometric model.[420]

SOURCE: References 7, 137, and 418–423.

Superoxide Dismutase. Even though the phenotypic mapping results presented earlier indicate that the visible phenotype of DS, along with mental retardation, can occur in the absence of triplication of *SOD1*, the locus for CuZnSOD, virtually all individuals with DS do have an extra copy of this locus. Therefore, consideration of the possible effects of having an extra copy of this gene is still in order. CuZnSOD catalyzes the dismutation of the superoxide radicals, O_2^-, to H_2O_2, which is then metabolized to water by glutathione peroxidase or catalase. It is generally regarded as a protective enzyme, and numerous examples exist of beneficial effects of exogenously added enzyme.[7,424] However, because the H_2O_2 generated as a result of CuZnSOD action is itself toxic and may, in combination with O_2^-, give rise to the even more dangerous hydroxyl radical (OH·), it has been argued that increased CuZnSOD activity may, under certain circumstances, have a deleterious effect, particularly in the brain.[425] In humans, it remains an open question whether increased CuZnSOD activity has any effect on the balance of oxygen metabolites and, if it does, whether this altered balance causes deleterious effects. Measurements of 8-hydroxy-2′-deoxyguanosine, a marker of DNA oxidation, in brain from adults with DS did not reveal any increase and were interpreted as providing evidence against increased damage resulting from reactive oxygen species.[426] By contrast, the cortex of fetal brain was reported as showing evidence of increased lipid peroxidation and of protein oxidation (carbonyls and glycated products).[427] *In vitro* studies with trisomic fibroblasts have demonstrated a modestly increased resistance to challenge with paraquat, a superoxide generator.[428] Animal models, described below, are now being used to investigate this problem.

Pathogenesis of Specific Features of Down Syndrome

Studies of the pathogenesis of specific components of the DS phenotype have concentrated principally on congenital heart disease, leukemia, and Alzheimer disease, and these are discussed in detail in the following sections. However, many of the other components of the phenotype, such as the craniofacial abnormalities, the gastrointestinal anomalies, and the characteristic dermatoglyphic changes, have also been the subjects of investigation and speculation.[12] With the rapid identification of new genes on chromosome 21, the speculation has increased, but no mechanistic links between increased expression of any gene, or set of genes, and any component of the phenotype have been established.

Congenital Heart Disease. A hypothesis has been developed to explain the high frequency but not invariant occurrence of congenital heart disease in DS, as well as the range of lesions observed.[429] Based on the experimental observation that lung and endocardial cushion fibroblasts derived from fetuses with trisomy 21 are more adhesive *in vitro* than control fetuses,[430] it is proposed that there is a chromosome 21-determined increase, perhaps on the order of 50 percent, in the concentration of an adhesive molecule on the surface of the endocardial cells which give rise to the endocardial cushions. Using a computer simulation of a stochastic model of endocardial cell migration, division, and adhesion, conditions could be defined that would result in complete fusion under normal circumstances and in failure of fusion in the expected 40 percent of instances when the concentration of the adhesion molecule is increased in DS. That fusion fails to occur in some, but not all, cases, results from the stochastic nature of the processes of migration and division, processes that cannot be completely specified genetically. Similar mechanisms may be operative in congenital heart disease of other etiologies, as well as in other types of congenital defects, whether chromosomally, monogenically, or multifactorially determined.

It also has been suggested that abnormal development of the cranial neural crest may play a role in the cardiac malformations, as well as in the short neck and the defects of the face, ear, thymus, and gastrointestinal tract.[431] However, experimental evidence has not shown endocardial cushion defects to be the common consequence of neural crest ablation.

Leukemia. The argument that trisomy 21 should itself be regarded as the predisposing factor in the development of leukemia has been developed at great length.[432] The evidence cited includes the data cited above on the incidence of leukemia and on the relationship of leukemoid reactions to the presence of trisomic cells in trisomy 21/2n mosaics, as well as the fact that trisomy 21, alone or with other types of chromosome imbalance, is the most common acquired change in the leukemic cells in ALL (31 percent in children, 7 percent in adults), and one of the most common in ANLL (7 percent in children, 5 percent in adults), occurring in constitutionally diploid individuals. The equating of such acquired aneuploidy with a constitutional abnormality has raised strong objections, however, as has the idea that constitutional trisomy 21 is directly responsible for acute leukemia in DS. Nevertheless, a relationship clearly exists.

Although the situation in DS has been compared to that which exists with chromosomal deletions that predispose individuals to the development of malignancy,[432] there is at present no real evidence to support such an argument. Furthermore, unlike the malignancies associated with deletions, with frequencies of one-third or higher in chromosomally abnormal individuals, the frequency of leukemia in DS, however high the relative risk, is still one or two orders of magnitude lower, suggesting that another type of mechanism might be operative.

The possibility that factors such as increased susceptibility to radiation, chemical, and/or virus-induced chromosomal genetic damage and transformation are involved in the susceptibility to leukemogenesis provided the rationale for the studies in these areas described earlier. The evidence concerning an increased sensitivity of trisomic cells is still far from persuasive. Therefore, claims for a causal relationship between increased susceptibility to chromosomal damage and increased susceptibility to leukemia must be viewed with caution.

Another possibility is an altered host defense or tumor surveillance system related to abnormalities of lymphocyte function or of the response to interferon. Insofar as the latter is concerned, the result would be a paradoxical one, because it might be expected (although there is no real evidence pro or con) that enhanced sensitivity to interferon should be protective against malignancy rather than increasing susceptibility. With regard to the immune system itself, an analogy has been drawn between the situation in DS and the association of leukemia with a variety of primary immunodeficiency disorders, and it has been speculated that the leukemoid reactions might be the result of a lack of homeostatic control within the lymphoid system, which results, in turn, from a deficiency of suppressor T lymphocytes.[433] Possible roles for increased SOD activity,[434] or for increased expression of the *ETS2* oncogene, have also been suggested. Finally, children with transient leukemia or ANLL subtype 7 have an increase in "atypical" constitutional phenotypes, are almost always male, and may have increased disomic homozygosity in proximal 21q.[435]

We are thus left with many possibilities, but none proven. In the end, the explanation might derive from some still undefined factor or from a combination of factors, both of the type considered here and yet to be discovered. This factor or factors might operate alone or be superimposed on the potentially enhanced proliferative capacity of trisomic hemopoietic stem cells.

Alzheimer Disease. Earlier, numerous anatomic, histologic, biochemical, and functional changes in the nervous systems of young individuals with DS were discussed. It is presumed that some combination of these abnormalities results in the impaired cognitive functioning that we denote as mental retardation. No precise mechanisms have been worked out, and it is still not known to what extent the functional or physiological defects, as opposed to structural abnormalities, actually determine the intellectual outcome.

A number of proposals have been put forward to explain the development of AD in adults with DS[7,13,436] and these can be summarized in two principal categories. The first is that the genetic imbalance present in trisomy 21 indirectly causes AD by enhancing the susceptibility of the brain to exogenous agents that cause AD, either by causing the nervous system to be intrinsically defective from early in life, and therefore predisposed to degenerative changes, or by causing premature aging. With regard to the latter possibility, there is no hard evidence that premature aging is a consequence of trisomy 21[7]—in fact, the major point in favor of such an assumption is the existence of AD itself. The nervous system very likely is intrinsically abnormal from early in life. However, it is not obvious how the observed deficiencies and defects predispose to degenerative changes later in life, particularly because no exogenous agents have yet been shown to cause AD.

The second category of proposals is that the genetic imbalance in trisomy 21 directly causes AD because the increased dosage of one chromosome 21 locus or more results in increased activities or concentrations of one or more gene products, which, in turn, produce injury to the brain. In other words, an AD gene is actually present on chromosome 21. One candidate for the responsible gene product has been CuZnSOD,[415] and the potential deleterious effects of increased SOD activity already have been discussed. A more serious candidate is APP.[437]

Amyloid Precursor Protein. Because the amyloid β/A4 protein is deposited in the neuritic plaques and cerebral blood vessels of the brains of individuals with AD, whether associated with DS or not, it was predicted that this protein might be determined by chromosome 21.[438] This has, in fact, been found to be the case, and several families with familial AD have been discovered to have mutations in the *APP* gene.[439–441]

Of great potential importance, insofar as the development of AD in persons with DS is concerned, is the evidence for overproduction of APP mRNA in the brains of fetuses with DS and (see below) in mouse fetuses with trisomy 16. In three fetal brains, the average abundance of the APP-695 isoform was 4.6-times normal, and of the protease domain-containing isoform(s), 3.8-times normal.[421] In adult DS brains, there is an overexpression of the APP-751 and 770 isoforms in the hippocampal formation and the caudate putamen.[422] It may be postulated that such overproduction, if sustained, could lead to the early accumulation of APP that has been observed in the brains of young persons with DS,[137] and that this accumulation may have toxic effects on neurons which are already impaired. A relevant observation is the absence of any clinical or pathologic evidence of AD in a 78-year-old woman with DS resulting from segmental trisomy 21 with only two copies of *APP*.[443]

One other point relating to AD and DS requires mention, and that is the observation that the frequency of Down syndrome is increased in family members of persons with AD.[444,445] This finding led to the suggestion that there is a "unitary genetic etiology" to both conditions in which a postulated genetic defect of microtubules and microfilaments leads both to the neurofibrillary tangles and other degenerative changes of AD, and to the meiotic abnormalities causing trisomy 21.[444] The validity of this notion is unproved. It has also been speculated that endocrine factors may also be involved in the genesis of both DS and AD.[446]

Animal Models of Down Syndrome

That many of the consequences of aneuploidy in humans arise during the period of morphogenesis places a special obstacle in the way of their investigation. Research on events occurring during gestation, especially early gestation, is both technically impractical and, at present and for the near future, ethically and legally impossible. It is for this reason that interest has turned to the development of models.

In a sense, there are numerous models for studying the effects of aneuploidy.[7] Thus, heterozygosity for an enzyme deficiency is a model for deletion of one enzyme locus; an increased concentration of an adhesive molecule in an *in vitro* aggregation experiment is a model for a duplication of the relevant gene; and a 2s × 1s somatic-cell hybrid can be regarded, depending on the circumstances, as a model for either tetrasomy or monosomy. Models of this type are very helpful, and their usefulness will increase as we begin to identify more loci of interest. However, none of these types of models enables us to deal with complex developmental or functional issues or to appreciate the consequences of aneuploidy at the level of the whole organism. We hope that this is what specific organismic models of aneuploidy will do for us.

Because ultimate concern is with humans and with human disease, we require models that duplicate the human condition—in developmental and functional terms—as closely as possible. No model can be exact because no other organism duplicates the human with respect to all the human biologic and genetic attributes. Nevertheless, models based on other mammals, which share numerous biologic similarities with humans, seem most appropriate. Primates with the genetic and clinical equivalent of trisomy 21 and DS have been observed.[447,448] but do not offer significant advantages over humans for investigational purposes. Therefore, the mouse has been the model animal of choice for several reasons, including ease of manipulation and genetic control, and the similarities to humans in the processes of morphogenesis and (probably) of central nervous system function, in neurobiologic if not psychologic terms. Furthermore, despite considerable rearrangement of the mammalian genome, sizable chromosomal regions carrying many genes remain intact and structurally similar in both humans and mice.[449] However, models based on the mouse are not without problems. It may not always be easy, or even possible, to obtain postnatally viable animals when sizable regions of the genome are unbalanced.[7] Furthermore, even if it were possible, these animals will never be able to duplicate the higher central nervous system functions, such as cognition, which are so vulnerable to the effects of aneuploidy in humans. As difficult as it to define mental retardation in an aneuploid human, it is even more difficult to specify the proper functional homology in an aneuploid mouse.

The modeling of human trisomy 21 in the mouse started at the two ends of the possible spectrum of such models: the trisomic mouse with an extra copy of mouse chromosome 16, the mouse chromosome that most closely resembles human chromosome 21 and, at the other extreme, the mouse with an extra copy or copies of a single human chromosome 21 gene—a transgenic mouse. Recently, however, several intermediate possibilities, with duplications of only parts of mouse chromosome 16 or the insertion of mouse or human yeast artificial chromosome (YAC) transgenes, were developed.[450,451]

Mouse Trisomy 16. To create a mouse model for human trisomy 21, genes and anonymous sequences known to be present on chromosome 21 were mapped on the mouse genome by a variety of genetic techniques. All the loci in 21q, except for those in the distal part of band 21q22.3 beyond MX1, outside the region responsible for the facial features of DS, map to the distal part of mouse chromosome 16[410,452] (see also http://www.informatics.jax.org). The loci not on mouse chromosome 16 were mapped to mouse chromosomes 10 and 17.

Mouse chromosome 16 is certainly not completely homologous to human chromosome 21, because genes present on the former map to other human chromosomes, and, as already indicated, not all human chromosome 21 genes map to mouse chromosome 16.[452] Furthermore, mouse chromosome 16 is about 35 percent larger than that of human chromosome 21 in terms of total genetic length in centimorgans. Therefore, trisomy for all of mouse 16, while reproducing much of genetic imbalance associated with human trisomy 21, results in an overall degree of imbalance that is more extensive than in the human trisomy.

Phenotype of Ts16. Trisomy 16 fetuses are generated by using males doubly heterozygous for two robertsonian chromosomes that share an arm (chromosome 16).[453] These animals usually begin to die at day 14 of gestation, but many survive to, but not beyond, term. The salient phenotypic features of these trisomic mice included massive edema *in utero*, flat snout, short neck, abnormal brain development, hematopoietic and immunologic abnormalities with multiple stem-cell deficiencies, and congenital heart disease with both conotruncal anomalies (in virtually all fetuses) and endocardial cushion defects (in about half).[7,454–456]

Three abnormalities of the Ts16 nervous system are of interest with regard to the investigation of mechanisms involved in the development of AD in persons with DS. One is concerned with the regulation of the expression of APP. Because the gene for APP is carried on mouse chromosome 16, gene dosage considerations would lead to an expectation of a 1.5-fold increase in APP mRNA synthesis and concentration. However, a detailed analysis of APP mRNA expression in Ts16 has revealed a tissue-dependent dysregulation of the synthesis of APP mRNA.[457] At fetal day 15, there is no significant difference between Ts16 and controls in the skin, but Ts16 brain shows a twofold increase, and even greater increases are found in lung, kidney, heart, and placenta. In brains of adult trisomy 16 ↔ 2n chimeras, which are only 40 to 50 percent Ts16 in composition, the APP mRNA concentration appears even more dysregulated and is increased by threefold.[457] Taken together, the Ts16 data point to a dysregulation of APP mRNA synthesis which could be related either to the increased number of copies of this gene, to a more general effect on the expression certain genes in the trisomic cells, or, most likely, to a combination of both.

The second nervous system abnormality of interest in Ts16 mice concerns the behavior of transplanted neurons. When fetal Ts16 basal forebrain cells were transplanted into or abutting the dentate gyrus of the hippocampus of a normal host, neuronal survival and abundant neurite outgrowth were observed.[458] However, 6 months after transplantation, a striking atrophy (by 25 percent in cross-sectional area) of the transplanted Ts16 cholinergic neurons was noted. This atrophy could be prevented by a fimbria-fornix lesion, which causes the release of trophic factors, such as nerve growth factor (NGF), but in this instance, the control neurons also enlarged and the Ts16 neurons were still smaller (by 16 percent) than normal.

Third, when inoculated intracerebrally with the scrapie prion, Ts16 ↔ 2n chimeras had an accelerated incubation period, a more fulminant course, and an earlier time of death than did 2n ↔ 2n chimeric controls.[460]

Segmental Mouse Trisomy 16. Because of the genetic discrepancies between mouse chromosome 16 and human chromosome 21, considerable effort was put into the development of segmentally trisomic mice in which only the human chromosome 21 homologous region was triplicated (Fig. 63-9). Such animals, designated Ts65Dn, were made by Davisson and collaborators.[450,461] The trisomic animals, which are generated as tertiary trisomics from a radiation-induced translocation, T(16;17)65Dn, do not have the major anomalies present in Ts16. Rather, their salient phenotypic abnormalities are confined to the central

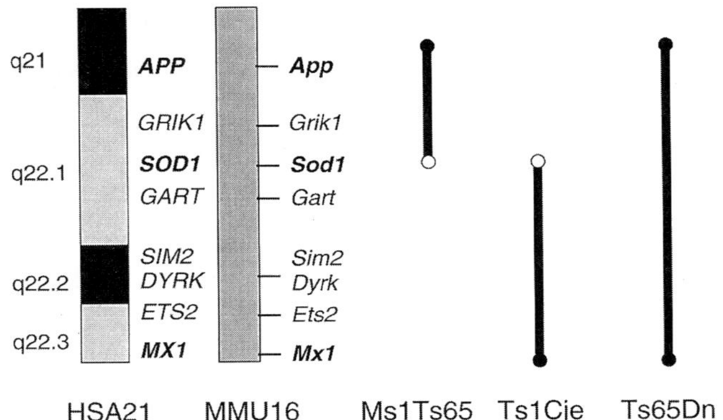

Fig. 63-9 Regions of triplication in segmental trisomies of mouse chromosome 16 (MMU16) showing regions of homology with human chromosome 21 (HSA21). Gene symbols: *APP, App*; amyloid precursor protein; *GRIK1, Grik1*, glutamate receptor, ionotropic, kainate 1; *SOD1, Sod1*, superoxide dismutase 1; *GART, Gart*, glycinamide phosphoribosyltransferase; *SIM2, Sim2*, homolog 2 of Drosophila *single-minded*; *DYRK, Dyrk*, dual-specificity tyrosine phosphorylation-regulated kinase, homolog of Drosophila *minibrain*; *ETS2, Ets2*, avian erythroblastosis virus E26 (V-*ets*) oncogene homolog 2; *MX1*, homolog of murine myxovirus (influenza) resistance 1; *Mx1*, myxovirus (influenza) resistance 1. (*Courtesy of Dr. Haruhiko Sago, University of California, San Francisco.*)

nervous system, although they do exhibit male sterility. They have major deficits in learning and behavior.[461–465] They also show abnormalities in cholinergic neurons in the basal forebrain,[462] in long-term potentiation (LTP) and depression,[466] and in hippocampal cAMP generation.[467] The pattern of behavioral and learning deficits suggests impairment of both hippocampal spatial learning and of prefrontal functions, and the LTP and cAMP abnormalities are also indicative of hippocampal dysfunction. Furthermore, the finding of an age-dependent loss of function and atrophy of cholinergic neurons in the medial septum of the basal forebrain, possibly related to an abnormality of nerve growth factor transport, are also consistent with hippocampal dysfunction.[462]

Ts65Dn mice have rapidly replaced Ts16 as the model of choice for DS. Because none of the major abnormalities present in Ts16 are found in Ts65Dn, with the important exception of the time-dependent atrophy of the basal forebrain cholinergic neurons, the relevance of Ts16 to the understanding of the pathogenesis of the cardiac, immunologic, fetal edema, and other anomalies associated with DS must questioned.

Two additional segmental Ts16 mice have been developed. The first, Ts1Cje, was derived from a balanced 12;16 translocation produced in association with inactivation of *Sod1* by homologous recombination.[468] These animals are functionally trisomic for the region of mouse chromosome 16 distal to *Sod1* (Fig. 63-9), which still includes the region responsible for the major phenotypic abnormalities in DS. They are somewhat less impaired in learning than are the Ts65Dn animals and do not exhibit degeneration of the cholinergic neurons.[468] The second segmental trisomic, designated Ms1CjeTs65Dn, was derived by breeding Ts65Dn females with T(12;16)1Cje males. One of the products obtained is a mouse that is segmentally trisomic for the region that represents the difference between Ts65Dn and Ts1Cje — the region homologous to the proximal part of human 21q down to *SOD1* (Fig. 63-9).[469] These animals have only minimal learning deficits, but they are still not normal, indicating the major genes responsible for the behavioral and learning abnormalities of Ts65Dn are located distal to *Sod1*. The ability to generate these various segmental trisomics and to compare their phenotypes directly provides a precedent for the systematic creation of smaller and smaller segmental trisomics and the dissection of the trisomic phenotype.

Transgenic Mice. In contrast to the formation of trisomic animals, an approach that permits the analysis of the effects of increased dosage of individual human chromosome 21 genes is the construction of transgenic mice. Several strains of such transgenic mice carrying *SOD1*, the gene for human CuZnSOD, have been made and shown to have from 1.6- to 6-fold increased activities of CuZnSOD in the brain and other tissues.[470] Several effects of this increased activity of CuZnSOD have been found. Transgenic mouse platelets, with 1.7- to 2.7-times normal CuZnSOD activities, had diminished levels of serotonin and decreased rates of serotonin accumulation. Dense granules from transgenic platelets also had a decreased rate of serotonin uptake, which was attributed to a diminished pH gradient across the granule membrane such as had been found in PC12 cells transfected with the CuZnSOD gene.[117,471] These findings are, of course, very similar to those described for DS platelets, and it is tempting to ascribe this particular aspect of the DS phenotype to increased activity of CuZnSOD. With regard to whether these observations on platelets might have any implications for the central nervous system, it is worth noting that the content of serotonin in the striatum of transgenic mice, with about three times control CuZnSOD activity, was found to be normal.[120] Also, as in fibroblasts from persons with DS, transgenic mouse cells had a reduction in prostaglandin E_2 and prostaglandin D_2 biosynthesis in primary fetal cells, and in the cerebellum and hippocampus.[124]

The same strains of transgenic mice used for the serotonin and prostaglandin studies were also used for the analysis of neuromuscular junctions, because it has been reported that the neuromuscular junctions of tongue muscles from persons with DS demonstrate terminal axon degeneration, alterations in the end plates, and increased calcium and copper concentrations. Similarly, the neuromuscular junctions of the transgenic tongue muscles were abnormal, with atrophy, degeneration, withdrawal, and destruction of terminal axons, development of multiple small terminals, decreased ratio of terminal axon area to postsynaptic membrane, and hyperplastic secondary folds.[472,473] These changes were considered to be similar to those found in aging animals and, therefore, possibly the result of premature aging.[117] A similar inference was made with regard to changes in the morphology of neuromuscular junctions — as reflected by nerve terminal length, number of nerve terminal branching points, and the incidence of sprouting — in the hind limb muscles of transgenic mice.[474] A decrease in mossy fiber innervation of the hippocampus was also observed.[475]

The abnormalities in transgenic tissues just discussed are presumed mediated by alterations in the metabolism of oxygen free radicals resulting from the increased CuZnSOD activity (this enzyme mediating the first step in the ultimate conversion of superoxide anions to water). In these instances, the outcome was deleterious in that the transgenic tissues were structurally or functionally abnormal. However, there is considerable evidence that increased CuZnSOD activity can have beneficial effects under conditions of acute oxidative stress.[476–478] Also of potential relevance to the DS phenotype are the observations that the CuZnSOD transgenic mice also have anatomic abnormalities of the thymus and premature thymic involution.[479,480]

The significance of the results obtained with transgenic mice with more than a 1.5-fold increase in CuZnSOD activity to the pathogenesis of DS remains to be confirmed by studies on animals with the same degree of increase as is found in the human situation. Nevertheless, the findings do suggest that even relatively small increases in the activity of a single enzyme can have major developmental and functional consequences.

Limited work has been done with other types of transgenic mice carrying individual human chromosome 21 genes or their murine homologues. Although they do not develop the full pathology of AD, mice expressing the human APP-751 isoform gene do have diffuse and amorphous extracellular deposits of β-amyloid which resemble those of early AD.[481] They also manifest deficits in spatial learning.[482] However, transgenic mice with high expression of APP genes that carry mutations associated with familial AD disease, develop a pathology more closely resembling that of AD,[483] especially when a mutant presenilin 1 gene is also present.[484] Transgenic mice overexpressing the Ets2 transcription factor develop craniofacial and other skeletal anomalies, with brachycephaly and short necks, thought to resemble anomalies found in DS and mouse Ts16.[485] However, similar anomalies are not found in any of the segmental trisomics of chromosome 16, even though *Ets2* is present in three copies.[461,468] Overexpression of *HMG14* results in abnormalities of the thymus and epithelial cysts.[486]

The transgenes just described all involve loci present on mouse chromosome 16 as well as human chromosome 21, which makes the absence of similar findings in trisomic mice involving the same regions of concern. The following two loci, however, are represented on mouse chromosome 10, and the trisomic models are, therefore, not relevant. Transgenic mice overexpressing the gene for the protein subunit S100β were reported to be hyperactive, with delays in learning, and to manifest astrocytosis, axonal proliferation, and a significant loss of dendrites in the hippocampus.[487,488] Transgenic mice overexpressing liver-type phosphofructokinase had elevated activity during fetal life but not during adult life.[489] However, perhaps of greater interest is that transgenic PC12 cells showed an alteration in the rate of glycolysis consistent with the change in phosphofructokinase isozyme composition.[490] These results indicate that a change in the proportion of enzyme subunits can have a significant effect on metabolism.

Another approach to the generation of transgenic models for Down syndrome is insertion of genomic segments larger than individual genes in the form of yeast artificial chromosomes. A noteworthy success is the creation of a series of transgenic animals carrying segments of the human 21q22.2 region.[451] Several of the transgenic strains derived had abnormalities of learning and behavior. In one strain, the deficits were similar to, but less severe than, those that were observed with the segmental trisomies Ts1Cje and Ts65Dn.[491] Because the major, and possibly only, gene in the integrated segment of human DNA (designated 152F7tel) was the human *minibrain* gene (*DYRK*), a homologue of a gene expressed in the developing Drosophila brain, it was suggested that imbalance of this locus is responsible for the observed abnormalities.

THE PERSON WITH DOWN SYNDROME

Although this chapter was written principally from the point of view of the relationship between the genetic imbalance present in trisomy 21 and the phenotype that ensues, it must be remembered that DS may create many problems for the individuals who have it, for their families, and for society in general. Because specific forms of therapy are not available, other than surgery for congenital heart disease and major gastrointestinal anomalies, the issue of medical management has not been discussed except to indicate some of the forms of therapy that were found not to be useful. Similarly, only brief mention was made of the educational and psychological aspects of management. However, much has happened in recent years to improve the well-being of individuals with DS and their place in society, and more still needs to be done. For recent discussions of these important aspects of DS, see references 6 and 492 to 494.

REFERENCES

1. Down JLH: Observation on an ethnic classification of idiots. *London Hosp Clin Lect Rep* **3**:259, 1866.
2. Lejeune J, Gauthier M, Turpin R: Les chromosomes humains en culture de tissus. *C R Acad Sci* **248**:602, 1958.
3. Jacobs PA, Baikie AG, Court Brown WM, Strong JA: The somatic chromosomes in mongolism. *Lancet* **1**:710, 1959.
4. Lejeune J, Gauthier M, Turpin R: Etude des chromosomes somatiques de neuf enfants mongoliens. *C R Acad Sci* **248**:1721, 1959.
5. Smith GF, Berg JM: *Down's Anomaly.* Edinburgh, Churchill Livingstone, 1976.
6. Pueschel SM, Rynders JE (eds): *Down Syndrome. Advances in Biomedicine and the Behavioral Sciences.* Cambridge, MA, Ware, 1982.
7. Epstein CJ: *The Consequences of Chromosome Imbalance. Principles, Mechanisms, and Models.* New York, Cambridge University Press, 1986.
8. Epstein CJ (ed): *The Neurobiology of Down Syndrome.* New York, Raven, 1986.
9. McCoy EE, Epstein CJ (eds): *The Oncology and Immunology of Down Syndrome.* New York, Liss, 1987.
10. Hassold TJ, Epstein CJ (eds): *Molecular and Cytogenetic Studies of Non-Disjunction.* New York, Liss, 1989.
11. Patterson D, Epstein CJ (eds): *Molecular Genetics of Chromosome 21 and Down Syndrome.* New York, Wiley-Liss, 1990.
12. Epstein CJ (ed): *The Morphogenesis of Down Syndrome.* New York, Wiley-Liss, 1991.
13. Nadel L, Epstein CJ (eds): *Down Syndrome and Alzheimer Disease.* New York, Wiley-Liss, 1992.
14. Epstein CJ (ed): *The Phenotypic Mapping of Down Syndrome and Other Aneuploid Conditions.* New York, Wiley-Liss, 1993.
15. Epstein CJ, Hassold T, Lott IT, Nadel L, Patterson D (eds): *Etiology and Pathogenesis of Down Syndrome.* New York, Wiley-Liss, 1995.
16. Trisomy 21 (Down syndrome). *Am J Med Genet Suppl* **7**:1990.
17. Epstein CJ: Aneuploidy in mouse and man, in Vogel F, Sperling K (eds): *Human Genetics: Proceedings of the 7th International Congress, Berlin, 1986.* Heidelberg, Springer-Verlag, 1987, p 260.
18. Pueschel SM, Sassaman EA, Scola PS, Thuline HC, Stark AM, Horrobin M: Biomedical aspects in Down syndrome, in Pueschel SM, Rynders JE (eds): *Down Syndrome. Advances in Biomedicine and the Behavioral Sciences.* Cambridge, MA, Ware, 1982, p 169.
19. Fischer-Brandies H: Cephalometric comparison between children with and without Down's syndrome. *Eur J Orthod* **10**:255, 1988.
20. Farkas LG, Posnick JC, Hreczko T: Anthropometry of the head and face in ninety-five Down syndrome patients, in Epstein CJ (ed): *The Morphogenesis of Down Syndrome.* New York, Wiley-Liss, 1991, p 53.
21. Hestnes A, Sand T, Fostad K: Ocular findings in Down's syndrome. *J Ment Defic Res* **35**:194, 1991.
22. Reed T: Dermatoglyphic findings in Down syndrome: A summary of over seven hundred cases, in Epstein CJ (ed): *The Morphogenesis of Down Syndrome.* New York, Wiley-Liss, 1991, p 277.
23. Rex AP, Preus M: A diagnostic index for Down syndrome. *J Pediatr* **100**:903, 1982.
24. Share JB, Veale AM: *Developmental Landmarks for Children with Down's Syndrome.* Dunedin, New Zealand, University of Otago Press, 1974.
25. Melyn MA, White DT: Mental and developmental milestones of noninstitutionalized Down's syndrome children. *Pediatrics* **52**:542, 1973.
26. Gibson D: *Down's Syndrome. The Psychology of Mongolism.* Cambridge, UK, Cambridge University Press, 1978.
27. Morgan SB: Development and distribution of intellectual and adaptive skills in Down syndrome children: Implications for early intervention. *Ment Retard* **17**:247, 1979.
28. Schnell RR: Psychomotor development, in Pueschel SM (ed): *The Young Child with Down Syndrome.* New York, Human Sciences, 1984, p 207.
29. Gath A, Gumley D: Down's syndrome and the family: Follow-up of children first seen in infancy. *Dev Med Child Neurol* **26**:500, 1984.
30. Kouseff BG: Trisomy 21 with average intelligence? *Birth Defects* **14(6C)**:323, 1978.
31. Hunt N: *The World of Nigel Hunt.* New York, Garrett, 1967.
32. Kingsley J, Levitz M: *Count Us In: Growing Up with Down Syndrome.* New York, Harcourt Brace, 1994.
33. Burke C, McDaniel JB: *A Special Kind of Hero.* New York, Doubleday, 1991.
34. Bennett FC, Sells CJ, Brand C: Influences on measured intelligence in Down's syndrome. *Am J Dis Child* **133**:700, 1979.
35. Sharav T, Collins R, Schlomo L: Effect of maternal education of prognosis of development in children with Down syndrome. *Pediatrics* **76**:387, 1985.
36. Libb JW, Myers GJ, Graham E, Bell B: Correlates of intelligence and adaptive behavior in Down's syndrome. *J Ment Defic Res* **27**:205, 1983.

37. Ludlow JR, Allen LM: The effect of early intervention and preschool stimulus on the development of the Down's syndrome child. *J Ment Defic Res* **23**:29, 1979.
38. Sharav T, Shlomo L: Stimulation of infants with Down syndrome: Long-term effects. *Ment Retard* **24**:81, 1986.
39. Sloper P, Glenn SM, Cunningham CC: The effect of intensity of training on sensorimotor development in infants with Down's syndrome. *J Ment Defic Res* **30**:149, 1986.
40. Bricker D: Further notes on early intervention, in Pueschel SM, Tingey C, Rynders JE, Crocker AC, Crutcher DM (eds): *New Perspectives on Down Syndrome*. Baltimore, PH Brookes, 1987, p 171.
41. Spiker D: Early intervention for young children with Down syndrome: New directions in enhancing parent-child synchrony, in Pueschel SM, Rynders JE (eds): *Down Syndrome. Advances in Biomedicine and the Behavioral Sciences*. Cambridge, MA, Ware, 1982, p 331.
42. Hanson MJ: Early intervention for children with Down syndrome, in Pueschel SM, Tingey C, Rynders JE, Crocker AC, Crutcher DM (eds): *New Perspectives on Down Syndrome*. Baltimore, PH Brookes, 1987, p 149.
43. Gibson D, Harris A: Aggregated early intervention effects for Down's syndrome persons: Patterning and longevity of benefits. *J Ment Defic Res* **32**:1, 1988.
44. Bridges FA, Cicchetti D: Mothers' ratings of the temperament characteristics of Down syndrome infants. *Dev Psychol* **18**:238, 1982.
45. Collacott RA, Cooper SA, Branford D, McGrother C: Behaviour phenotype for Down's syndrome. *Br J Psychiatry* **172**:85, 1998.
46. Hartley XY: A summary of recent research into the development of children with Down syndrome. *J Ment Defic Res* **30**:1, 1986.
47. Kernan KT: Comprehension of syntactically indicated sequence by Down's syndrome and other mentally retarded adults. *J Ment Defic Res* **34**:169, 1990.
48. Fowler A: Language abilities in children with Down syndrome: Evidence for a specific syntactic delay, in Cicchetti D, Beeghly M (eds): *Children with Down Syndrome. A Developmental Perspective*. New York, Cambridge University Press, 1990, p 302.
49. Beeghly M, Weiss-Perry B, Cicchetti D: Beyond sensorimotor functioning: Early communicative and play development of children with Down syndrome, in Cicchetti D, Beeghly M (eds): *Children with Down Syndrome: A Developmental Perspective*. New York, Cambridge University Press, 1990, p 339.
50. Miller J: The developmental asynchrony of language development in children with Down syndrome, in Nadel L (ed): *The Psychobiology of Down Syndrome*. Cambridge, MA, MIT Press, 1988, p 167.
51. Giencke S, Lewandowski L: Anomalous dominance in Down syndrome young adults. *Cortex* **25**:93, 1989.
52. Horowitz B, Schapiro MB, Grady CL, Rapoport SI: Cerebral metabolic pattern in young adult Down's syndrome subjects: Altered intercorrelations between regional rates of glucose utilization. *J Ment Defic Res* **34**:237, 1990.
53. Nadel L: Down syndrome in psychobiological profile, in Nadel L (ed): *The Psychobiology of Down Syndrome*. Cambridge, MA, MIT Press, 1988, p 369.
54. Cowie VA: *A Study of the Early Development of Mongols*. London, Pergamon, 1970.
55. Yessayan L, Pueschel SM: Neurological investigations, in Pueschel SM (ed): *The Young Child with Down Syndrome*. New York, Human Sciences, 1984, p 263.
56. Morris AF, Vaughan SE, Vaccaro P: Measurement of neuromuscular tone and strength in Down's syndrome children. *J Ment Defic Res* **26**:41, 1982.
57. Pueschel SM, Reed RB, Cronk CE: Evaluation of the effect of 5-hydroxytryptophan and/or pyridoxine administration in young children with Down syndrome, in Pueschel SM (ed): *The Young Child with Down Syndrome*. New York, Human Sciences, 1984, p 59.
58. Coleman M: Infantile spasms associated with 5-hydroxytryptophan administered in patients with Down's syndrome. *Neurology* **21**:911, 1971.
59. Coleman M, Sobel S, Bhagavan HN, Coursin D, Marquardt A, Guay M, Hunt C: A double-blind study of vitamin B_6 in Down's syndrome infants. Part 1—clinical and biochemical results. *J Ment Defic Res* **29**:233, 1985.
60. Gedye A: Dietary increase in serotonin reduces self-injurious behaviour in a Down's syndrome adult. *J Ment Defic Res* **34**:195, 1990.
61. Pueschel SM, Findley TW, Furia J, Gallagher PL, Scola GH, Pezzulo JC: Atlantoaxial instability in Down syndrome: Roentgenographic, neurologic, and somatosensory-evoked potential studies. *J Pediatr* **110**:515, 1987.
62. Pueschel SM, Scola FH: Atlantoaxial instability in individuals with Down syndrome: Epidemiologic, radiographic, and clinical studies. *Pediatrics* **80**:555, 1987.
63. Trauner DA, Bellugi U, Chase C: Neurologic features of Williams and Down syndromes. *Pediatr Neurol* **5**:166, 1989.
64. Pueschel SM, Louis S, McKnight P: Seizure disorders in Down syndrome. *Arch Neurol* **48**:318, 1991.
65. Johannsen P, Christensen JEJ, Goldstein H, Nielsen VK, Mai J: Epilepsy in Down syndrome—Prevalence in three age groups. *Seizure* **5**:121, 1996.
66. McKeown DA, Doty RL, Pel DP, Frye RE, Simms I, Mester A: Olfactory function in young adolescents with Down's syndrome. *J Neurol Neurosurg Psychiatry* **61**:412, 1996.
67. Romano C, Tine A, Fazio G, Rizzo R, Colognola RM, Sorge G, Bergonzi P, Pavone L: Seizure in patients with trisomy 21. *Am J Med Genet Suppl* **7**:298, 1990.
68. Share JB: Review of drug treatment for Down's syndrome persons. *Am J Ment Defic* **80**:388, 1976.
69. Harrell RF, Capp RH, Davis DR, Peerless J, Ravitz LR: Can nutritional supplements help mentally retarded children? An exploratory study. *Proc Natl Acad Sci USA* **78**:574, 1981.
70. Turkel H, Nusbaum I: *Medical Treatment of Down Syndrome and Genetic Diseases*, 4th ed. Southfield, MI, Ubiotica, 1985.
71. Smith GF, Spiker D, Peterson CP, Cicchetti D, Justice P: Use of megadoses of vitamins and minerals in Down syndrome. *J Pediatr* **105**:228, 1984.
72. Bumbalo TS, Morelewicz HV, Berens DL: Treatment of Down's syndrome with the "U" series of drugs. *JAMA* **187**:361, 1964.
73. Schmid F: Cell therapy: Experimental basis and clinics. *Cytobiol Rev* **2**:65, 1980.
74. Pruess JB, Fewell RR: Cell therapy and the treatment of Down syndrome: A review of research. *Trisomy 21* **1**:3, 1985.
75. Gouliaev AH, Senning A: Piracetam and other structurally related nootropics. *Brain Res Brain Res Rev* **19**:180, 1994.
76. Vernon MW, Sorkin EM: Piracetam: An overview of its pharmacological properties and a review of its therapeutic use in senile cognitive disorders. *Drugs Aging* **1**:17, 1991.
77. Rehder H: Pathology of trisomy 21, in Burgio GR, Fraccaro M, Tiepolo L, Wolf U (eds): *Trisomy 21: An International Symposium*. Berlin, Springer-Verlag, 1981, p 57.
78. Gullotta F, Rehder H, Gropp A: Descriptive neuropathology of chromosomal disorders in man. *Hum Genet* **57**:337, 1981.
79. Crome L, Cowie V, Slater E: A statistical note of cerebellar and brain stem weight in mongolism. *J Ment Defic Res* **10**:69, 1966.
80. Aylward EH, Habbak R, Warren AC, Pulsifer MB, Barta PE, Jerram M, Pearlson GD: Cerebellar volume in adults with Down syndrome. *Arch Neurol* **54**:209, 1997.
81. Schmidt-Sidor B, Wisniewski KE, Shepard TH, Sersen EA: Brain growth in Down syndrome subjects 15–22 weeks of gestational age and birth to 60 months. *Clin Neuropathol* **9**:181, 1990.
82. Sylvester PE: The anterior commissure in Down's syndrome. *J Ment Defic Res* **30**:19, 1986.
83. Becker L, Mito T, Takashima S, Onodera K: Growth and development of the brain in Down syndrome, in Epstein CJ (ed): *The Morphogenesis of Down Syndrome*. New York, Wiley-Liss, 1991, p 133.
84. Takashima S, Ieshima A, Nakamura H, Becker LE: Dendrites, dementia and the Down syndrome. *Brain Dev* **2**:131, 1989.
85. Ferrer I, Gullotta F: Down's syndrome and Alzheimer's disease: Dendritic spine counts in the hippocampus. *Acta Neuropathol* **79**:680, 1990.
86. Wisniewski KE, Laure-Kamionowska M, Connell F, Wen GY: Neuronal density and synaptogenesis in the postnatal stage of brain maturation in Down syndrome, in Epstein CJ (ed): *The Neurobiology of Down Syndrome*. New York, Raven, 1986, p 29.
87. Wisniewski KE, Bobinski M: Hypothalamic abnormalities in Down syndrome, in Epstein CJ (ed): *The Morphogenesis of Down Syndrome*. New York, Wiley-Liss, 1991, p 153.
88. Pine SS, Landing BH, Shankle WR: Reduced inferior olivary neuron number in early Down syndrome. *Pediatr Pathol Lab Med* **17**:537, 1997.
89. Brooksbank BWL, Walker D, Balazs R, Jorgensen OS: Neuronal maturation in the fetal brain in Down's syndrome. *Early Hum Dev* **18**:237, 1989.
90. Florez J, delArco C, Gonzalez A, Pascual J, Pazos A: Autoradiographic studies of neurotransmitter receptors in the brain of newborn infants with Down syndrome. *Am J Med Genet Suppl* **7**:301, 1990.

91. Kish S, Karlinsky H, Becker L, Gilbert J, Rebbetoy M, Chang L-J, DeStefano L, et al: Down's syndrome individuals begin life with normal levels of brain cholinergic markers. *J Neurochem* **52**:1183, 1989.
92. Shah SN: Fatty acid composition of lipids of human brain myelin and synaptosomes: Changes in phenylketonuria and Down's syndrome. *Int J Biochem* **10**:477, 1979.
93. Banik NL, Davison AN, Palo J, Savolainen H: Biochemical studies on myelin isolated from the brains of patients with Down's syndrome. *Brain* **98**:213, 1975.
94. Brooksbank BWL, Martinez M, Balazs R: Altered composition of polyunsaturated fatty acyl groups in phosphoglycerides of Down's syndrome fetal brain. *J Neurochem* **44**:869, 1985.
95. Ellingson RJ, Eisen JD, Otterberg G: Clinical electroencephalographic observation on institutionalized mongoloids confirmed by karyotype. *Electroenceph Clin Neurophysiol* **34**:193, 1973.
96. Elul R, Hanley J, Simmons JQ III: Non-Gaussian behavior of the EEG in Down's syndrome suggests decreased neuronal connections. *Acta Neurol Scand* **51**:21, 1975.
97. Tangye SR: The EEG and incidence of epilepsy in Down's syndrome. *J Ment Defic Res* **23**:17, 1979.
98. Galbraith GC: Unique EEG and evoked response patterns in Down syndrome individuals, in Epstein CJ (ed): *The Neurobiology of Down Syndrome*. New York, Raven, 1986, p 109.
99. Schmid RG, Sadowsky K, Weinman H-M, Tirsch WS, Poppl SJ: Z-transformed EEG power spectra of children with Down syndrome vs a control group. *Neuropediatrics* **16**:218, 1985.
100. Courchesne E: Physioanatomical consideration in Down syndrome, in Nadel L (ed): *The Psychobiology of Down Syndrome*. Cambridge, MA, MIT Press, 1988, p 291.
101. Lincoln AJ, Courchesne E, Kilman BA, Galambos R: Neuropsychological correlates of information-processing by children with Down syndrome. *Am J Ment Defic* **89**:403, 1985.
102. Widen JE, Folsom RC, Thompson G, Wilson WR: Auditory brainstem responses in young adults with Down syndrome. *Am J Ment Defic* **91**:472, 1987.
103. Squires N, Ollo C, Jordan R: Auditory brain stem responses in the mentally retarded: Audiometric correlates. *Ear Hear* **7**:83, 1986.
104. Seidl R, Hauser E, Nernet G, Marx M, Freilinger M, Lubec G: Auditory evoked potentials in young patients with Down syndrome. Event-related potentials (Ps) and histaminergic system. *Brain Res Cogn Brain Res* **5**:301, 1997.
105. Kakigi R: Short-latency somatosensory evoked potentials following median nerve stimulation in Down's syndrome. *Electroencephalogr Clin Neurophysiol* **74**:88, 1989.
106. Caviedes P, Ault B, Rapoport SI: The role of altered sodium currents in action potential abnormalities of cultured dorsal root ganglion neurons from trisomy 21 (Down syndrome) human fetuses. *Brain Res* **510**:229, 1990.
107. Nieminen K, Suarez-Isla BA, Rapoport SI: Electrical properties of cultured dorsal root ganglia neurons from normal human and trisomy 21 human fetal tissue. *Brain Res* **474**:246, 1988.
108. Busciglio J, Yankner BA: Apoptosis and increased generation of reactive oxygen species in Down's syndrome neurons *in vitro*. *Nature* **378**:776, 1995.
109. Sacks B, Smith S: People with Down's syndrome can be distinguished on the basis of cholinergic dysfunction. *J Neurol Neurosurg Psychiatry* **52**:1294, 1989.
110. Harris WS, Goodman RM: Hyper-reactivity to atropine in Down's syndrome. *N Engl J Med* **279**:407, 1968.
111. Wark HJ, Overton JH, Marian P: The safety of atropine premedication in children with Down's syndrome. *Anesthesia* **38**:871, 1983.
112. Lake CR, Ziegler MG, Coleman M, Kopin IJ: Evaluation of the sympathetic nervous system in trisomy-21 (Down's syndrome). *J Psychiatr Res* **15**:1, 1979.
113. Schapiro MB, Kay AD, Max C, Ryker AK, Haxby JV, Kaufman S, Milstien S, Rapoport SI: Cerebrospinal fluid monoamines in Down's syndrome adults at different ages. *J Ment Defic Res* **31**:259, 1987.
114. Schapiro MB, Creasey W, Schwartz M, Haxby JV, White B, Moore A, Rapoport SI: Quantitative CT analysis of brain morphometry in adult Down's syndrome at different ages. *Neurology* **37**:1424, 1987.
115. Bayer SM, McCoy EE: A comparison of the serotonin and ATP content in platelets from subjects with Down's syndrome. *Biochem Med* **9**:225, 1974.
116. McCoy EE, Enns L: Current status of neurotransmitter abnormalities in Down syndrome, in Epstein CJ (ed): *The Neurobiology of Down Syndrome*. New York, Raven, 1986, p 73.
117. Groner Y, Avraham KB, Schickler M, Yarom R, Knobler H: Clinical symptoms of Down syndrome are manifested in transgenic mice overexpressing the human Cu/Zn-superoxide dismutase gene, in Patterson D, Epstein CJ (eds): *Molecular Genetics of Chromosome 21 and Down Syndrome*. New York, Wiley-Liss, 1990, p 233.
118. Paasonen MK: Platelet 5-hydroxytryptamine as a model in pharmacology. *Ann Med Exp Biol Fenn* **46**:416, 1968.
119. Lott IT, Murphy DL, Chase TN: Down's syndrome. Central monoamine turnover in patients with diminished platelet serotonin. *Neurology* **22**:967, 1972.
120. Przedborski S, Kostic V, Jackson-Lewis V, Naini AB, Fahn S, Carlson E, Epstein CJ, et al: Increased CuZn-superoxide dismutase activity confers resistance to MPTP-induced neurotoxicity in transgenic mice. *J Neurosci* **12**:1658, 1992.
121. McSwigan JD, Hanson DR, Lubiniecki A, Heston LL, Sheppard JR: Down syndrome fibroblasts are hyperresponsive to β-adrenergic stimulation. *Proc Natl Acad Sci USA* **78**:7670, 1981.
122. Sheppard JR, McSwigan JD, Wehner JM, White JG, Shows TB, Jakobs KH, Schultz G: The adrenergic responsiveness of Down syndrome cells, in Sheppard JR, Anderson VE, Eaton JW (eds): *Membranes and Genetic Disease*. New York, Liss, 1982, p 307.
123. Fruen BR, Lester BR: Down's syndrome fibroblasts exhibit enhanced inositol uptake. *Biochem J* **270**:119, 1990.
124. Minc-Golomb D, Knobler H, Groner Y: Gene dosage of CuZnSOD and Down's syndrome: Diminished prostaglandin synthesis in human trisomy 21, transfected cells and transgenic mice. *EMBO J* **10**:2219, 1991.
125. Fraser J, Mitchell A: Kalmuc idiocy: Report of a case with autopsy; with notes on sixty-two cases. *J Ment Sci* **22**:169, 1876.
126. Struwe F: Histopathologische Untersuchungen uber Entstehung und Wesen der senilen Plaques. *Z Ges Neurol Psychiatry* **122**:291, 1929.
127. Epstein CJ, Anneren KG, Foster D, Groner Y, Prusiner SB, Smith SA: Pathogenetic relationships between Down syndrome and Alzheimer's disease: Studies with animal models, in Davies P, Finch CE (eds): *Banbury Report 27: Molecular Neuropathology of Aging*. Cold Spring Harbor, NY, Cold Spring Harbor Laboratory, 1987, p 339.
128. Williams RS, Matthyse S: Age-related changes in Down syndrome brain and the cellular pathology of Alzheimer disease. *Prog Brain Res* **70**:49, 1986.
129. Mann DM: The pathological association between Down syndrome and Alzheimer disease. *Mech Ageing Dev* **43**:99, 1988.
130. Hardy J: The Alzheimer family of disease: Many etiologies, one pathogenesis? *Proc Natl Acad Sci U S A* **94**:2025, 1997.
131. Mann DMA, Yates PO, Marcyniuk B, Ravindra CR: Loss of neurons from cortical and subcortical areas in Down's syndrome patients at middle age. Quantitative comparisons with younger Down's patients and patients with Alzheimer's disease. *J Neurol Sci* **80**:79, 1987.
132. Hyman BT: Down syndrome and Alzheimer disease, in Nadel L, Epstein CJ (eds): *Down Syndrome and Alzheimer Disease*. New York, Wiley-Liss, 1992.
133. Jorgensen OS, Brooksbank BWL, Balazs R: Neuronal plasticity and astrocytic reaction in Down syndrome and Alzheimer disease. *J Neurol Sci* **98**:63, 1990.
134. Malamud N: Neuropathology of organic brain syndromes associated with aging, in Gartz CM (ed): *Aging and the Brain*. New York, Raven, 1972, p 63.
135. Wisniewski KE, Wisniewski HM, Wen GY: Occurrence of neuropathological changes and dementia of Alzheimer's disease in Down syndrome. *Ann Neurol* **17**:278, 1985.
136. Whalley LB, Buckton KE: Genetic factors in Alzheimer's disease, in Glen AIM, Whalley LJ (eds): *Alzheimer's Disease. Early Recognition of Potentially Reversible Defects*. Edinburgh, UK, Churchill Livingstone, 1979, p 36.
137. Rumble B, Retallack R, Hilbich C, Simms G, Multhaup G, Martins R, Hockey A, Montgomery P, Beyreuther K, Masters CL: Amyloid A4 protein and its precursor in Down's syndrome and Alzheimer's disease. *N Engl J Med* **320**:1446, 1989.
138. Mattiace LA, Kress Y, Davies P, Ksiezak-Reding H, Yen S-H, Dickson DW: Ubiquitin-immunoreactive dystrophic neurites in Down's syndrome brains. *J Neuropathol Exp Neurol* **50**:547, 1991.
139. Warren AC, Holroyd S, Folstein MF: Major depression in Down's syndrome. *Br J Psychiatry* **155**:202, 1989.
140. Wisniewski KE, Dalton AJ, McLachlan C, Wen GY, Wisniewski HM: Alzheimer's disease in Down's syndrome: Clinicopathologic studies. *Neurology* **35**:957, 1985.
141. Thase ME, Liss L, Smeltzer D, Maloon J: Clinical evaluation of dementia in Down's syndrome. *J Ment Defic Res* **26**:239, 1982.

142. Lai F, Williams RS: A prospective study of Alzheimer disease in Down syndrome. *Arch Neurol* **46**:849, 1989.
143. Franceschi M, Comola F, Piattoni F, Gualandri W, Canal N: Prevalence of dementia in adult patients with trisomy 21. *Am J Med Genet Suppl* **7**:306, 1990.
144. Lai F: Clinicopathologic features of Alzheimer disease in Down syndrome, in Nadel L, Epstein CJ (eds): *Down Syndrome and Alzheimer Disease*. New York, Wiley-Liss, 1992.
145. Evenhuis HM: The natural history of dementia in Down's syndrome. *Arch Neurol* **47**:263, 1990.
146. Wisniewski HM, Rabe A: Discrepancy between Alzheimer-type neuropathology and dementia in people with Down syndrome. *Ann NY Acad Sci* **477**:247, 1986.
147. Mann DMA, Royston MC, Ravindra CR: Some morphometric observations on the brains of patients with Down's syndrome: Their relationship to age and dementia. *J Neurol Sci* **99**:153, 1990.
148. Schapiro MB, Luxenberg JS, Kaye JA, Haxby JV, Friedland RP, Rapoport SI: Serial quantitative CT analysis of brain morphometrics in adult Down's syndrome at different ages. *Neurology* **39**:1349, 1989.
149. LeMay M, Alvarez N: The relationship between enlargement of the temporal horns of the lateral ventricles and dementia in aging patients with Down syndrome. *Neuroradiology* **99**:153, 1990.
150. Pearlson GD, Warren AC, Starkstein SE, Aylward EH, Kumar AJ, Chase GA, Folstein MF: Brain atrophy in 18 patients with Down syndrome: A CT study. *AJNR* **11**:811, 1990.
151. Schapiro MB, Grady CL, Kumar A, Herscovitch P, Haxby JV, Moore AM, White B, Friedland RP, Rapoport SI: Regional cerebral glucose metabolism is normal in young adults with Down syndrome. *J Cereb Blood Flow Metab* **10**:199, 1990.
152. Muir WJ, Squire I, Blackwood DHR, Speight M, St. Clair DM, Oliver C, Dickens P: Auditory P300 response in the assessment of Alzheimer's disease in Down syndrome: A 2-year follow-up study. *J Ment Defic Res* **32**:455, 1988.
153. Roth GM, Sun B, Greensite FS, Lott IT, Dietrich RB: Premature aging in persons with Down syndrome: MR findings. *Am J Neuroradiol* **17**:1283, 1996
154. Schapiro MB, Haxby JV, Grady CL, Rapoport SI: Cerebral glucose utilization, quantitative tomography, and cognitive function in adult Down syndrome, in Epstein CJ (ed): *The Neurobiology of Down Syndrome*. New York, Raven, 1986, p 89.
155. Thase ME, Tigner R, Smeltzer DJ, Liss L: Age-related neuropsychological deficits in Down's syndrome. *Biol Psychiatry* **19**:571, 1984.
156. Young EC, Kramer BM: Characteristics of age-related language decline in adults with Down syndrome. *Ment Retard* **29**:75, 1991.
157. Haxby JV: Neuropsychological evaluation of adults with Down's syndrome: Patterns of selective impairment in non-demented old adults. *J Ment Defic Res* **33**:193, 1989.
158. Fenner ME, Hewitt KE, Torpy DM: Down's syndrome: Intellectual and behavioral functioning during adulthood. *J Ment Defic Res* **31**:241, 1987.
159. Devenny DA, Silverman WP, Hill AL, Jenkins E, Sersen EA, Wisniewski KE: Normal ageing in adults with Down's syndrome: longitudinal study. *J Intellect Disabil Res* **40**:208, 1996.
160. Schipf N, Kapell D, Nightingale B, Rodriguez A, Tycko B, Mayeaux R: Earlier onset of Alzheimer's disease in men with Down syndrome. *Neurology* **50**:991, 1998.
161. Prasher VP, Chowdhury TA, Rowe BR, Bain SC: ApoE genotype and Alzheimer's disease in adults with Down syndrome: Meta-analysis. *Am J Ment Retard* **102**:103, 1997.
162. Alexander GE, Saunders AM, Szczepanik J, Strassburger TL, Pietrini P, Dani A, Furey ML et al: Relation of age and apolipoprotein E to cognitive function in Down syndrome adults. *Neuroreport* **8**:1835, 1997.
163. Del Bo R, Comi GP, Bresolin N, Castelli E, Conti E, Degiuli A, Ausenda CD, Scarlato G: The apolipoprotein E $\varepsilon 4$ allele causes a faster decline of cognitive performances in Down's syndrome subjects. *J Neurol Sci* **145**:87, 1997.
164. Tyrell J, Cosgrave M, Hawi Z, McPherson J, O'Brien C, McCalvert J, McLaughlin M, et al: A protective effect of apolipoprotein E $\varepsilon 2$ allele on dementia in Down's syndrome. *Biol Psychiatry* **43**:397, 1998.
165. Edland SD, Wijsmanm EM, Schoder-Ehri GL, Leverenz JB: Little evidence of reduced survival to adulthood of apoE $\varepsilon 4$ homozygotes in Down's syndrome. *Neuroreport* **8**:3463, 1997.
166. Pueschel SM: Cardiology, in Pueschel SM, Rynders JE (eds): *Down Syndrome. Advances in Biomedicine and the Behavioral Sciences*. Cambridge, MA, Ware, 1982, p 203.
167. Fabia J, Drolette M: Malformations and leukemia in children with Down's syndrome. *Pediatrics* **45**:60, 1970.
168. Buckley LP: Cardiac assessments, in Pueschel SM (ed): *A Study of the Young Child with Down Syndrome*. New York, Human Sciences, 1983, p 351.
169. Goldhaber SZ, Brown WD, Robertson N, Rubin IL, St. John Sutton MG: Aortic regurgitation and mitral valve prolapse with Down's syndrome: A case-control study. *J Ment Defic Res* **32**:333, 1988.
170. Bull C, Rigby ML, Shinebourne EA: Should management of complete atrioventricular canal defect be influenced by coexistent Down syndrome? *Lancet* **1**:1147, 1985.
171. Clapp S, Perry BL, Farooki ZQ, Jackson WL, Karpawich PP, Hakimi M, Arciniegas E, et al: Down's syndrome, complete atrioventricular canal, and pulmonary vascular obstructive disease. *J Thorac Cardiovasc Surg* **100**:115, 1990.
172. Wilson SK, Hutchins GM, Neill CA: Hypertensive pulmonary vascular disease in Down syndrome. *J Pediatr* **95**:722, 1979.
173. Cooney TP, Thurlbeck WM: Pulmonary hypoplasia in Down's syndrome. *N Engl J Med* **307**:1170, 1982.
174. Yamaki S, Horiuchi T, Sekino Y: Quantitative analysis of pulmonary vascular disease in simple cardiac anomalies with the Down syndrome. *Am J Cardiol* **51**:1502, 1983.
175. Schloo BL, Vawter GF, Reid LM: Down syndrome: Patterns of disturbed lung growth. *Hum Pathol* **22**:919, 1991.
176. Levy J: The gastrointestinal tract in Down syndrome, in Epstein CJ (ed): *The Morphogenesis of Down Syndrome*. New York, Wiley-Liss, 1991, p 245.
177. Garver KL, Law JC, Garver B: Hirschsprung disease: A genetic study. *Clin Genet* **28**:503, 1985.
178. Milunsky A, Fisher JH: Annular pancreas in Down's syndrome. *Lancet* **2**:575, 1968.
179. Miller RW: Neoplasia and Down's syndrome. *Ann NY Acad Sci* **171**:637, 1970.
180. Evans DIK, Steward JK: Down's syndrome and leukaemia. *Lancet* **2**:1322, 1972.
181. Scholl T, Stein Z, Hansen H: Leukemia and other cancers, anomalies and infections as causes of death in Down's syndrome in the United States during 1976. *Dev Med Child Neurol* **24**:817, 1982.
182. Rosner F, Lee SL: Down's syndrome and acute leukemia: Myeloblastic or lymphoblastic? *Am J Med* **53**:203, 1972.
183. Stiller CA, Kinnier Wilson LM: Down syndrome and leukaemia. *Lancet* **2**:1343, 1981.
184. Robison LL, Nesbit ME Jr, Sather HN, Level C, Shahidi N, Kennedy MS, Hammond D: Down syndrome and acute leukemia in children: A 10-year retrospective survey from Children's Cancer Study Group. *J Pediatr* **105**:235, 1984.
185. Lewis DS, Thompson M, Hudson E, Liberman MM, Samson D: Down's syndrome and acute megakaryoblastic leukemia. Case report and review of the literature. *Acta Haematol* **70**:236, 1983.
186. Zipursky A, Peeters M, Poon A: Megakaryoblastic leukemia and Down's syndrome — A review, in McCoy EE, Epstein CJ (eds): *The Oncology and Immunology of Down Syndrome*. New York, Liss, 1987, p 33.
187. Robison LL, Neglia JP: Epidemiology of Down syndrome and childhood acute leukemia, in McCoy EE, Epstein CJ (eds): *The Oncology and Immunology of Down Syndrome*. New York, Liss, 1987, p 19.
188. Taub JW, Matherly L, Stout, ML, Buck SA, Gurney JG, Ravindranath Y: Enhanced metabolism of 1-β-D-arabaninofuranosylcytosine in Down syndrome cells: A contributing factor to the superior event-free survival of Down syndrome children with acute myeloid leukemia. *Blood* **87**:3395, 1996.
189. Peeters M, Poon A: Down syndrome and leukemia: Unusual clinical aspects and unexpected methotrexate sensitivity. *Eur J Pediatr* **146**:416, 1987.
190. Garre ML, Relling MV, Kalwinsky D, Dodge R, Crom WR, Abromowitch M, Pui C-H, Evans WE: Pharmacokinetics and toxicity of methotrexate in children with Down syndrome and acute lymphocytic leukemia. *J Pediatr* **111**:606, 1987.
191. Ross JD, Moloney WC, Desforges JF: Ineffective regulation of granulopoiesis masquerading as congenital leukemia in a mongoloid child. *J Pediatr* **63**:1, 1963.
192. Heaton DC, Fitzgerald PH, Fraser GJ, Abbott GD: Transient leukemoid proliferation of the cytogenetically unbalanced +21 cell line of a constitutional mosaic boy. *Blood* **57**:883, 1981.
193. Barak Y, Mogilner BM, Karov Y, Nir E, Schlesinger M, Levin S: Transient acute leukaemia in a newborn with Down's syndrome.

Prediction of its reversibility by bone marrow cultures. *Acta Paediatr Scand* **71**:699, 1982.
194. Rogers PC, Kalousek DK, Denegri JF, Thomas JW, Baker MA: Neonate with Down's syndrome and transient congenital leukemia. In vitro studies. *Am J Pediatr Hematol Oncol* **5**:59, 1983.
195. Eguchi M, Sakakibara H, Suda J, Ozawa T, Hayashi Y, Sato T, Kojima S, Furukawa T: Ultrastructural and ultracytochemical differences between transient myeloproliferative disorder and megakaryoblastic leukaemia in Down's syndrome. *Br J Haematol* **73**:315, 1989.
196. Iselius L, Jacobs P, Morton N: Leukaemia and transient leukaemia in Down syndrome. *Hum Genet* **85**:477, 1990.
197. Miyashita T, Asada M, Fujimoto J, Inaba T, Takihara Y, Sugita K, Bessho F, et al: Clonal analysis of transient myeloproliferative disorder in Down's syndrome. *Leukemia* **5**:56, 1991.
198. Kurahashi H, Hara J, Yumura-Yagi K, Murayama N, Inoue M, Ishihara S, Tawa A, et al: Monoclonal nature of transient abnormal myelopoiesis in Down's syndrome. *Blood* **77**:1161, 1991.
199. Seibel NL, Sommer A, Miser J: Transient neonatal leukemoid reactions in mosaic trisomy 21. *J Pediatr* **104**:251, 1984.
200. Niikawa N, Deng H-X, Abe K, Harada N, Okada T, Tsuchiya H, Akaboshi I, et al: Possible mapping of the gene for transient myeloproliferative syndrome at 21q11.2. *Hum Genet* **87**:561, 1991.
201. Miller JC, Scherrill JG, Hathaway WE: Thrombocythemia in the myeloproliferative disorders of Down's syndrome. *Pediatrics* **40**:847, 1967.
202. Miller M, Cosgriff JM: Hematological abnormalities in newborn infants with Down syndrome. *Am J Med Genet* **16**:173, 1983.
203. Weinberger MM, Oleinick A: Congenital marrow dysfunction in Down's syndrome. *J Pediatr* **77**:273, 1970.
204. Rogers P, Denegri JF, Thomas JW, Kalousek D, Gillen J, Baker MA: Down's syndrome — leukemia vs pseudoleukemia. *Blood* **52**(suppl 1): 273, 1978.
205. Siegel M: Susceptibility of mongoloids to infections. I. Incidence of pneumonia, influenza A and *Shigella dysenteriae*(Sonne). *Am J Hyg* **48**:53, 1948.
206. Ugazio AG, Maccario R, Notarangelo LD, Burgio GR: Immunology of Down syndrome: A review. *Am J Med Genet Suppl* **7**:204, 1990.
207. Epstein CJ, Epstein LB: T-lymphocyte function and sensitivity to interferon in trisomy 21. *Cell Immunol* **51**:303, 1980.
208. Philip R, Berger A, McManus NH, Warner NH, Peacock MA, Epstein LB: Abnormalities of the in vitro cellular and humoral response to bacterial and viral antigens with concomitant numerical alterations in lymphocyte subsets in Down syndrome (trisomy 21). *J Immunol* **136**:1661, 1986.
209. Murphy M, Epstein LB: Down syndrome (DS) peripheral blood contains phenotypically mature CD3+TCRα,β+ cells but abnormal proportions of TCRα,β+, TCRγ,δ+ and CD4+CD45RA+ cells. Evidence for an inefficient release of mature T cells by the DS thymus. *Clin Immunol Immunopathol* **62**:245, 1992.
210. Gerez L, Madar L, Arad G, Sharav T, Reshef A, Ketzinel M, Sayar D, et al: Aberrant regulation of interleukin-2 but not of interferon-γ gene expression in Down syndrome (Trisomy 21). *Clin Immunol Immunopathol* **58**:251, 1991.
211. Fowler I, Hollingsworth DR: Response to stimulation in vitro of lymphocytes from patients with Down's syndrome. *Proc Soc Exp Biol Med* **144**:475, 1973.
212. Funa K, Anneren G, Alm GV, Mjorksten B: Abnormal interferon production and NK cell responses to interferon in children with Down's syndrome. *Clin Exp Immunol* **56**:493, 1984.
213. Epstein LB, Philip R: Abnormalities of the immune response to influenza antigen in Down syndrome (trisomy 21), in McCoy EE, Epstein CJ (eds): *The Oncology and Immunology of Down Syndrome*. New York, Liss, 1987, p 163.
214. Siegel M: Susceptibility of mongoloids to infection. II. Antibody response to tetanus toxoid and typhoid vaccine. *Am J Hyg* **48**:63, 1948.
215. Griffiths AW, Sylvester PE: Mongols and non-mongols compared in their response to active tetanus immunization. *J Ment Defic Res* **11**:263, 1967.
216. Gordon MC, Sinha SK, Carlson SD: Antibody responses to influenza vaccine in patients with Down's syndrome. *Am J Ment Defic* **75**:391, 1971.
217. Lopez V, Ochs HD, Thuline HC, Davis SD, Wedgwood RS: Defective antibody response to bacteriophage ΦX174 in Down syndrome. *J Pediatr* **86**:207, 1975.
218. Nurmi T, Leinonen M, Haiva V-M, Tiilikainen A, Kouvalainen K: Antibody response to pneumococcal vaccine in patients with trisomy-21 (Down's syndrome). *Clin Exp Immunol* **48**:485, 1982.
219. Van Damme P, Vranck R, Meheus A: Immunogenicity of a recombinant DNA hepatitis B vaccine in institutionalized patients with Down's syndrome. *Vaccine* **8**(suppl):S53, 1990.
220. Hollinger FB, Goyal RK, Hersh T, Powell HC, Schulman RJ, Melnick JL: Immune response to hepatitis virus type B in Down's syndrome and other mentally retarded patients. *Am J Epidemiol* **95**:356, 1972.
221. Fekete G, Kulcsar G, Dan P, Nasz I, Schuler D, Dobos M: Immunological and biological investigations in Down's syndrome. *Eur J Pediatr* **138**:59, 1982.
222. Levin S, Schlesinger M, Handzel Z, Hahn T, Altman Y, Czernobilsky B, Boss J: Thymic deficiency in Down's syndrome. *Pediatrics* **63**:80, 1979.
223. Murphy M, Epstein LB: Down syndrome (trisomy 21) thymuses have a decreased proportion of cells expressing high levels of TCRα,β and CD3. *Clin Immunol Immunopathol* **55**:453, 1990.
224. Murphy M, Insoft RM, Pike-Nobile, Epstein LB: A hypothesis to explain the immune defects in Down syndrome, in Epstein CJ, Hassold T, Lott IT, Nadel L, Patterson D (eds): *Etiology and Pathogenesis of Down Syndrome*. New York, Wiley-Liss, 1995, p 147.
225. Eastham RD, Jancar J: Macrocytosis in Down's syndrome and during long-term anticonvulsant therapy. *J Clin Pathol* **23**:296, 1970.
226. Hsia DY-Y, Justice P, Smith GF, Dowben RM: Down's syndrome. A critical review of the biochemical and immunological data. *Am J Dis Child* **121**:153, 1971.
227. Puukka R, Puukka M, Leppilampi M, Linna S-L, Kouvalainen K: Erythrocyte adenosine deaminase, purine nucleoside phosphorylase and phosphoribosyltransferase activity in patients with Down's syndrome. *Clin Chim Acta* **126**:275, 1982.
228. Brahe C, Serra A, Morton NE: Erythrocyte catechol-O-methyltransferase activity: Genetic analysis in nuclear families with one child affected by Down syndrome. *Am J Med Genet* **21**:373, 1985.
229. Xue Q-M, Shen D-G, Dong W: ATPase activity of erythrocyte membrane in patients with trisomy 21 (Down's syndrome). *Clin Genet* **26**:429, 1984.
230. Kedziora J, Hubner H, Kanski M, Jeske J, Keyko W: Efficiency of the glycolytic pathway in erythrocytes of children with Down's syndrome. *Pediatr Res* **6**:10, 1972.
231. Stocchi V, Magnani M, Cucchiarini L, Novelli G, Dallapiccola B: Red blood cell adenine nucleotides. Abnormalities in Down syndrome. *Am J Med Genet* **20**:131, 1985.
232. Barkin RM, Weston WL, Humbert JR, Maire F: Phagocytic function in Down syndrome — I. Chemotaxis. *J Ment Defic Res* **24**:243, 1980.
233. Barkin RM, Weston WL, Humbert JR, Sunada K: Phagocytic function in Down syndrome — II. Bactericidal activity and phagocytosis. *JMent Defic Res* **24**:251, 1980.
234. Barroeta O, Nungaray L, Lopez-Osuna M, Armendares S, Salamanca F, Kretschmer RR: Defective monocyte chemotaxis in children with Down's syndrome. *Pediatr Res* **17**:292, 1983.
235. Hsia DY-Y, Nadler HL, Shih L-Y: Biochemical changes in chromosomal abnormalities. *Ann N Y Acad Sci* **155**:716, 1968.
236. Pueschel SM: Biomedical aspects in Down syndrome: Biochemistry, in Pueschel SM, Rynders JE (eds): *Down Syndrome. Advances in Biomedicine and the Behavioral Sciences*. Cambridge, MA, Ware, 1982, p 249.
237. Pant SS, Moser HW, Krane SM: Hyperuricemia in Down's syndrome. *J Clin Endocrinol Metab* **28**:472, 1968.
238. Mellman WJ, Raab SD, Oski FA, Tedesco TA: Abnormal leukokinetics in 21 trisomy. *Ann N Y Acad Sci* **155**:1020, 1968.
239. Puukka R, Puukka M, Perkkila L, Kouvalainen K: Levels of some purine metabolizing enzymes in lymphocytes from patients with Down syndrome. *Biochem Med Metabol Biol* **36**:45, 1986.
240. Fort P, Lifshitz F, Bellisario R, Davis J, Lanes R, Pugliese M, Richman R, et al: Abnormalities of thyroid function in infants with Down syndrome. *J Pediatr* **104**:545, 1984.
241. Cutler AT, Benezra-Obeiter R, Brink SJ: Thyroid function in young children with Down syndrome. *Am J Dis Child* **140**:479, 1986.
242. Lejeune J, Peeters M, de Blois M-C, Bergere M, Grillot A, Rethore M-O, Vallee G, et al: Fonction thyroidienne et trisomie 21 exces de TSH et deficit en rT. *Ann Genet* **31**:137, 1988.
243. Sare Z, Ruvalcaba RHA, Kelley VC: Prevalence of thyroid disorder in Down syndrome. *Clin Genet* **14**:154, 1978.
244. Ugazio AG, Jayakar S, Marcioni AF, Dose M, Monafo V, Pasquali F, Burgio GR: Immunodeficiency in Down's syndrome: Relationship between presence of human thyroglobulin antibodies and HBsAg carrier status. *Eur J Pediatr* **126**:139, 1977.
245. Percy ME, Dalton AJ, Markovic VD, Crapper McLachlan DR, Gera E, Hummel JT, Rusk ACM, et al: Autoimmune thyroiditis associated with

mild "subclinical" hypothyroidism in adults with Down syndrome: A comparison of patients with and without manifestations of Alzheimer disease. *Am J Med Genet* **36**:148, 1990.
246. Anwar AJ, Walker JD, Frier BM: Type 1 diabetes mellitus and Down's syndrome: Prevalence, management and diabetic complications. *Diabet Med* **15**:160, 1998.
247. Cronk CE, Pueschel SM: Anthropometric studies, in Pueschel SM (ed): *A Study of the Young Child with Down Syndrome*. New York, Human Sciences, 1983, p 105.
248. Palmer CGS, Cronk C, Pueschel SM, Wisniewski KE, Laxova R, Crocker AC, Pauli RM: Head circumference of children with Down syndrome (0–36 months). *Am J Med Genet* **42**:61, 1992.
249. Pueschel SM, Rothman KJ, Ogilby JD: Birth weight of children with Down's syndrome. *Am J Ment Defic* **80**:442, 1976.
250. Sara VR, Gustavson K-H, Anneren G, Hall K, Wetterberg L: Somatomedins in Down's syndrome. *Biol Psychiatry* **18**:803, 1983.
251. Ikeda Y, Higurashi M, Hirayama M, Ishikawa N, Hoshina H: A longitudinal study on the growth of stature, lower limb and upper limb length in Japanese children with Down's syndrome. *J Ment Defic Res* **21**:139, 1977.
252. Rarick GL, Seefeldt V: Observations from longitudinal data on growth in stature and sitting height of children with Down's syndrome. *J Ment Defic Res* **18**:63, 1974.
253. Cronk C, Crocker AC, Pueschel SM, Shea AM, Zackai E, Pickens G, Reed RB: Growth charts for children with Down syndrome: 1 month to 18 years of age. *Pediatrics* **81**:102, 1988.
254. Bronks R, Parker AW: Anthropometric observation of adults with Down syndrome. *Am J Ment Defic* **90**:110, 1985.
255. Anneren G, Sara VR, Hall K, Tuvemo T: Growth and somatomedin responses to growth hormone in Down's syndrome. *Arch Dis Child* **61**:48, 1986.
256. Anneren G, Enberg G, Sara VR: The presence of normal levels of serum immunoreactive insulin-like growth factor 2 (IGF-2) in patients with Down's syndrome. *Ups J Med Sci* **89**:274, 1984.
257. Sara VR, Sjogren B, Anneren G, Gustavson K-H, Forsman A, Hall K, Wahlstrom J, et al: The presence of normal receptors for somatomedin and insulin in fetuses with Down's syndrome. *Biol Psychiatry* **19**:591, 1984.
258. Torrado C, Bastian W, Wisniewski KE, Castells S: Treatment of children with Down syndrome and growth retardation with recombinant human growth hormone. *J Pediatr* **119**:478, 1991.
259. Sheridan R, Llerena J Jr, Matkins S, Debenham P, Cawood A, Bobrow M: Fertility in a male with trisomy 21. *J Med Genet* **26**:294, 1989.
260. Jagiello G: Reproduction in Down syndrome, in de la Cruz FF, Gerald PS (eds): *Trisomy 21 (Down Syndrome). Research Perspectives*. Baltimore, University Park Press, 1981, p 151.
261. Johannisson R, Gropp A, Winking H, Coerdt W, Rehder H, Schwinger E: Down's syndrome in the male. Reproductive pathology and meiotic studies. *Hum Genet* **63**:132, 1983.
262. Shroder J, Lydecken K, de la Chapelle A: Meiosis and spermatogenesis in G-trisomic males. *Humangenetik* **13**:15, 1971.
263. Stearns PE, Droulard KE, Sahhar FH: Studies bearing on fertility of male and female mongoloids. *Am J Ment Defic* **65**:37, 1960.
264. Pueschel S, Orson JM, Boylan JM, Pezzullo JC: Adolescent development in males with Down syndrome. *Am J Dis Child* **139**:236, 1985.
265. Campbell WA, Lowther J, McKenzie I, Price WH: Serum gonadotrophins in Down's syndrome. *J Med Genet* **19**:98, 1982.
266. Hasen J, Boyar RM, Shapiro LR: Gonadal function in trisomy 21. *Horm Res* **12**:345, 1980.
267. Gropp A, Winking H, Redi C: Consequences of robertsonian heterozygosity: Segregational impairment of fertility versus male-limited sterility, in Crosignani PG, Rubin BL (eds): *Serono Clinical Colloquia on Reproduction 3. Genetic Control of Gamete Production and Function*. London, Academic/Grune & Stratton, 1982, p 115.
268. Hojager B, Peters H, Byskov AG, Faber M: Follicular development in ovaries of children with Down syndrome. *Acta Paediatr Scand* **67**:637, 1978.
269. Tricomi V, Valenti C, Hall JE: Ovulatory patterns in Down's syndrome. A pilot study. *Am J Obstet Gynecol* **89**:651, 1964.
270. Thase ME: Longevity and mortality in Down's syndrome. *J Ment Defic Res* **26**:177, 1982.
271. Fryers T: Survival in Down's syndrome. *J Ment Defic Res* **30**:101, 1986.
272. Penrose LS: The incidence of mongolism in the general population. *J Ment Sci* **9**:10, 1949.
273. Mastroiacovo P, Bertollini R, Corchia C: Survival of children with Down syndrome in Italy. *Am J Med Genet* **42**:208, 1992.
274. Masaki M, Higurashi M, Iijima K, Ishikawa N, Tanaka F, Fujii T, Kuroki Y, et al: Mortality and survival for Down syndrome in Japan. *Am J Hum Genet* **33**:629, 1981.
275. Dupont A, Vaeth M, Vedebech P: Mortality and life expectancy of Down's syndrome in Denmark. *J Ment Defic Res* **30**:111, 1986.
276. Baird PA, Sadovnick AD: Life expectancy in Down syndrome. *J Pediatr* **110**:849, 1987.
277. Baird PA, Sadovnick AD: Life tables for Down syndrome. *Hum Genet* **82**:291, 1989.
278. Scholl T, Stein Z, Hansen H: Leukemia and other cancers, anomalies, and infections as causes of death in Down's syndrome in the United States during 1976. *Dev Med Child Neurol* **24**:817, 1982.
279. Oster J, Mikkelsen M, Nielsen A: Mortality and life-table in Down's syndrome. *Acta Paediatr Scand* **64**:243, 1975.
280. Balarjan R, Donnan SPB, Adelstein AM: Mortality and causes of death in Down's syndrome. *J Epidemiol Community Health* **36**:127, 1982.
281. Epstein CJ, Epstein LB: Genetic control of the response to interferon in man and mouse. *Lymphokines* **8**:277, 1983.
282. Epstein CJ, Weil J, Epstein LB: Abnormalities in the interferon response and immune systems in Down syndrome: Studies in human trisomy 21 and mouse trisomy 16, in McCoy EE, Epstein CJ (eds): *The Oncology and Immunology of Down Syndrome*. New York, Liss, 1987, p 191.
283. Weil J, Tucker G, Epstein LB, Epstein CJ: Interferon induction of (2′–5′) oligoisoadenylate synthetase in diploid and trisomy 21 fibroblasts: Relation of dosage of the interferon receptor gene (IFRG). *Hum Genet* **65**:108, 1983.
284. Weil J, Epstein CJ, Epstein LB, Van Blerkom J, Xuong NH: Computer-assisted analysis demonstrates that polypeptides induced by natural and recombinant interferon-α are the same and that several have related primary structures. *Antiviral Res* **3**:303, 1983.
285. Yap WH, Teo TS, Tan YH: An early event in the interferon-induced transmembrane signaling process. *Science* **234**:355, 1986.
286. Schneider EL, Epstein CJ: Replication rate and lifespan of cultured fibroblasts in Down's syndrome. *Proc Soc Exp Biol Med* **141**:1092, 1972.
287. Hoehn H, Simpson M, Bryant EM, Rabinovitch PS, Salk D, Martin GM: Effects of chromosome constitution on growth and longevity of human skin fibroblast cultures. *Am J Med Genet* **7**:141, 1980.
288. Carmeliet G, Hauman R, Dom R, David G, Fryns J-P, Van Den Berghe H, Cassiman J-J: Growth properties and in vitro life span of Alzheimer disease and Down syndrome fibroblasts. A blind study. *Mech Ageing Dev* **53**:17, 1990.
289. Tarone RE, Liao K, Robbins JH: Effects of DNA-damaging agents on Down syndrome cells: Implications for defective DNA-repair mechanisms, in McCoy EE, Epstein CJ (eds): *The Oncology and Immunology of Down Syndrome*. New York: Liss, 1987, p 93.
290. Shafik HM, Au WW, Legator MS: Chromosomal radiosensitivity of Down syndrome lymphocytes at different stages of the cell cycle. *Hum Genet* **78**:71, 1988.
291. Higurashi M, Tamura T, Nakatake T: Cytogenetic observations in cultured lymphocytes from patients with Down's syndrome and measles. *Pediatr Res* **7**:582, 1973.
292. Higurashi M, Tada A, Miyahara S, Hirayama M: Chromosome damage in Down's syndrome induced by chickenpox infection. *Pediatr Res* **10**:189, 1976.
293. Thuline HC, Pueschel SM: Cytogenetics in Down syndrome, in Pueschel SM, Rynders JE (eds): *Down Syndrome. Advances in Biomedicine and the Behavioral Sciences*. Cambridge, MA, Ware, 1982, p 133.
294. Hook EB: Epidemiology of Down syndrome, in Pueschel SM, Rynders JE (eds): *Down Syndrome. Advances in Biomedicine and the Behavioral Sciences*. Cambridge, MA, Ware, 1982, p 11.
295. Giraud F, Mattei JF: Aspects epidemiologues de la trisomy 21. *J Genet Hum* **23**(suppl):1, 1975.
296. Albright SG, Hook EB: Estimates of the likelihood that a Down's syndrome child of unknown genotype is a consequence of familial translocation. *Am J Hum Genet* **30**:107A, 1978.
297. Ahlbom BE, Goetz P, Korenberg JR, Petterson U, Seemanova E, Wadelius C, Zech L, et al: Molecular analysis of chromosome 21 in a patient with a phenotype of Down syndrome and apparently normal karyotype. *Am J Med Genet* **63**:566, 1996.
298. Richards BW: Investigation of 142 mosaic mongols and mosaic parents of mongols; cytogenetic analysis and maternal age at birth. *J Ment Defic Res* **18**:199, 1974.

299. Jenkins EC, Schupf N, Genovese M, Ye LL, Kapell D, Canto B, Harris M, et al: Increased low-level chromosome 21 mosaicism in older individuals with Down syndrome. *Am J Med Genet* **68**:147, 1997.
300. Ford CE: Nondisjunction, in Burgio GR, Fraccaro M, Tiepolo L, Wolf U (eds): *Trisomy 21: An International Symposium*. Berlin, Springer-Verlag, 1981, p 103.
301. Uchida IA, Wheland T: A rare case of mosaic Down syndrome 46,XY/46,XY, −21,+i(21q). *Clin Genet* **17**:271, 1980.
302. Wilson MG, Towner JW, Forsman I: Decreasing mosaicism in Down's syndrome. *Clin Genet* **17**:335, 1980.
303. Taysi K, Kohn G, Mellman WJ: Mosaic mongolism, II. Cytogenetic studies. *J Pediatr* **76**:880, 1970.
304. Kuo W-L, Tenjiu H, Segraves R, Pinkel D, Golbus MS, Gray J: Detection of aneuploidy including chromosomes 13, 18, or 21, by fluorescence in situ hybridization (FISH) to interphase and metaphase amniocytes. *Am J Hum Genet* **49**:112, 1991.
305. Uchida JA, Freeman VCP: Trisomy 21 Down syndrome. Parental mosaicism. *Hum Genet* **70**:246, 1985.
306. Harris DJ, Begleiter ML, Chamberlin J, Hankins L, Magenis RE: Parental trisomy 21 mosaicism. *Am J Hum Genet* **34**:125, 1982.
307. Fishler K, Koch R, Donnell GN: Comparison of mental development in individuals with mosaic and trisomy 21 Down's syndrome. *Pediatrics* **58**:744, 1976.
308. Kohn G, Taysi K, Atkins TE, Mellman WJ: Mosaic mongolism. I. Clinical correlation. *J Pediatr* **76**:874, 1970.
309. Rosencrans CJ: The relationship of normal/21-trisomy mosaicism and intellectual development. *Am J Ment Defic* **72**:562, 1968.
310. Carlin ME, Leon S, Gilbert JD: A comparison between a trisomy 21 child (probably mosaic) with normal intelligence and a mosaic Down syndrome population. *Birth Defects* **14**(6C):327, 1978.
311. Schapiro MB, Kumar A, White B, Fox D, Grady CL, Haxby JV, Friedland RP, et al: Dementia without mental retardation in mosaic translocation in Down syndrome. *Brain Dysfunct* **3**:165, 1990.
312. Rowe IF, Ridler MAC, Gibberd FB: Presenile dementia associated with mosaic trisomy 21 in a patient with a Down syndrome child. *Lancet* **2**:229, 1989.
313. Li J, Xu M, Zhou H, Ma J, Potter H: Alzheimer presenilins in the nuclear membrane, interphase kinetochores, and centrosomes suggest a role in chromosome segregation. *Cell* **90**:917, 1997.
314. Avramopolous D, Kennerknecht I, Barbi G, Eckert D, Dedlabar JM, Maunoury C, Halberg A, et al: A case of apparent trisomy 21 without the Down's syndrome phenotype. *J Med Genet* **34**:597, 1997.
315. Yoon PW, Freeman SB, Sherman SL, Taft LF, Gu Y, Pettay D, Flanders WD, et al: Advanced maternal age and the risk of Down syndrome characterized by the meiotic stage of the chromosome error: A population based study. *Am J Hum Genet* **58**:628, 1996.
316. Petersen MB, Adelsberger PA, Schinzel AA, Binkert F, Hinkel GK, Antonarakis SE: Down syndrome due to de novo robertsonian translocation t(14q;21q): DNA polymorphism analysis suggests that the origin of the extra 21q is maternal. *Am J Hum Genet* **49**:529, 1991.
317. Antonarakis SE, Adelsberger PA, Petersen MB, Binkert F, Schinzel AA: Analysis of DNA polymorphisms suggests that most de novo dup(21q) chromosomes in patients with Down syndrome are isochromosomes and not translocations. *Am J Hum Genet* **47**:968, 1990.
318. Shaffer LG, Jackson-Cook CK, Meyer J, Brown JA, Spence JE: A molecular genetic approach to the identification of isochromosomes of chromosome 21. *Hum Genet* **86**:375, 1991.
319. Adams MM, Erickson JD, Layde PM, Oakley GP: Down's syndrome. Recent trends in the United States. *JAMA* **246**:758, 1981.
320. Baird PA, Sadovnick AD: Maternal age-specific rates for Down syndrome: Changes over time. *Am J Med Genet* **29**:917, 1988.
321. Hook EB, Cross PK, Jackson L, Pergament E, Brambati B: Maternal age-specific rates of 47,+21 and other cytogenetic abnormalities diagnosed in the first trimester of pregnancy in chorionic villus biopsy specimens: Comparison with rates expected from observations at amniocentesis. *Am J Hum Genet* **42**:797, 1988.
322. Hook EB, Cross PK, Regal RR: The frequency of 47,+21, 47,+18 and 47,+13 at the uppermost extremes of maternal ages: Results on 56,094 fetuses studied prenatally and comparisons with data on live-births. *Hum Genet* **68**:211, 1984.
323. Hook EB: Spontaneous deaths of fetuses with chromosomal abnormalities diagnosed prenatally. *N Engl J Med* **299**:1036, 1978.
324. Boue J, Deluchat CC, Nicolas H, Boue A: Prenatal losses of trisomy 21, in Burgio GR, Fraccaro M, Tiepolo L, Wolf U (eds): *Trisomy 21: An International Symposium*. Berlin: Springer-Verlag, 1981, p 183.
325. Hassold T, Chiu D: Maternal age-specific rates of numerical chromosome abnormalities with special reference to trisomy. *Hum Genet* **70**:11, 1985.
326. Bond DJ, Chandley AC: *Aneuploidy*. Oxford, UK, Oxford University Press, 1983.
327. Chandley AC: Maternal aging as the important etiological factor in human aneuploidy, in Dellarco VL, Voytek PE, Hollaender A (eds): *Aneuploidy. Etiology and Mechanisms*. New York, Plenum, 1985, p 409.
328. German J: Mongolism, delayed fertilization and human sexual behavior. *Nature* **217**:516, 1968.
329. Sharav T: Aging gametes in relation to incidence, gender, and twinning in Down syndrome. *Am J Med Genet* **39**:116, 1991.
330. Martin-De Leon PA, Williams MB: Sexual behavior and Down syndrome: The biological mechanism. *Am J Med Genet* **27**:693, 1987.
331. Henderson SA, Edwards RG: Chiasma frequency and maternal age in mammals. *Nature* **218**:22, 1968.
332. Hook EB: Down syndrome rates and relaxed selection of older maternal ages. *Am J Hum Genet* **35**:1307, 1983.
333. Peters GB, Ford JH, Nicholl JK: Trisomy 21 mosaicism and maternal age effect. *Lancet* **1**:1202, 1987.
334. Hook EB: Maternal age, paternal age, and human chromosome abnormality: Nature, magnitude, etiology, and mechanisms of effects, in Dellarco VL, Voytek PE, Hollaender A (eds): *Aneuploidy. Etiology and Mechanisms*. New York, Plenum, 1985, p 117.
335. Crowley PH, Hayden TL, Gulati DK: Etiology of Down syndrome, in Pueschel SM, Rynders JE (eds): *Down Syndrome. Advances in Biomedicine and the Behavioral Sciences*. Cambridge, MA, Ware, 1982, p 89.
336. Dellarco VL, Voytec PE, Hollaender A (eds): *Aneuploidy. Etiology and Mechanisms*. New York, Plenum, 1985.
337. Stene E, Stene J, Stengel-Rutkowski S: A reanalysis of the New York State prenatal diagnosis data on Down's syndrome and paternal age effects. *Hum Genet* **77**:299, 1987.
338. Cross PK, Hook EB: An analysis of paternal age and 47,+21 in 35,000 new prenatal cytogenetic diagnosis data from the New York State Chromosome Registry: No significant effect. *Hum Genet* **77**:307, 1987.
339. Hatch M, Kline J, Levin B, Hutzler M, Warburton D: Paternal age and trisomy among spontaneous abortions. *Hum Genet* **85**:355, 1990.
340. Martin RH, Rademaker A: The effect of age on the frequency of sperm chromosome abnormalities in normal men. *Am J Hum Genet* **39**:123A, 1986.
341. Antonarakis SE, Down Syndrome Collaborative Group: Parental origin of the extra chromosome in trisomy 21 as indicated by analysis of DNA polymorphisms. *N Engl J Med* **324**:872, 1991.
342. Warren AC, Chakravarty A, Wong C, Slaugenhaupt SA, Halloran SL, Watkins PC, Metaxotou C, et al: Evidence for reduced recombination on the nondisjoined chromosomes 21 in Down syndrome. *Science* **237**:652, 1987.
343. Lamb NE, Freeman SB, Savage-Austin A, Pettay D, Taft L, Hersey J, Gu Y, et al: Susceptible chiasmata configurations of chromosome 21 predispose to non-disjunction in both maternal MI and MII. *Nat Genet* **14**:400, 1996.
344. Lamb NE, Feingold E, Savage A, Avramopolous D, Freeman SB, Gu Y, Hallberg A, et al: Characterization of susceptible chiasma configurations that increase the risk for maternal nondisjunction of chromosome 21. *Hum Mol Genet* **6**:1391, 1997.
345. Angell R: Mechanism of chromosome nondisjunction in human oocytes. In Epstein CJ, Hassold T, Lott IT, Nadel L, Patterson D (eds): *Etiology and Pathogenesis of Down Syndrome*. New York, Wiley-Liss, 1995, p 13.
346. Olshan AF, Baird PA, Teschke K: Paternal occupational exposures and the risk of Down syndrome. *Am J Hum Genet* **44**:646, 1989.
347. Kline J, Stein Z: Environmental causes of aneuploidy: Why so elusive? in Dellarco VL, Voytek PE, Hollaender A (eds): *Aneuploidy, Etiology and Mechanisms*. New York, Plenum, 1985, p 149.
348. Warburton D: Genetic factors influencing aneuploidy frequency, in Dellarco VL, Voytek PE, Hollaender A (eds): *Aneuploidy, Etiology and Mechanisms*. New York, Plenum, 1985, p 133.
349. Janerich DT, Bracken MB: Epidemiology of trisomy 21: A review and theoretical analysis. *J Chron Dis* **39**:1079, 1986.
350. Hook EB, Harlap S: Differences in maternal age-specific rates of Down syndrome between Jews of European origin and of North African or Asian origin. *Teratology* **20**:243, 1979.
351. Stene J, Stene E, Mikkelsen M: Risk for chromosome abnormality at amniocentesis following a child with a non-inherited chromosome

aberration. A European collaborative study in prenatal diagnoses 1981. *Prenat Diagn* **4**(Spec Iss):81, 1984.
352. Alfi OS, Chang R, Azen SP: Evidence for genetic control of nondisjunction in man. *Am J Hum Genet* **32**:477, 1980.
353. Fialkow PJ, Thuline HC, Hecht F, Bryant J: Familial predisposition to thyroid disease in Down's syndrome: Controlled immunochemical studies. *Am J Hum Genet* **23**:67, 1971.
354. Torfs CP, van den Berg BJ, Oechsli FW, Christianson RE: Thyroid antibodies as a risk factor for Down syndrome and other trisomies. *Am J Hum Genet* **47**:727, 1990.
355. Tamaren J, Spuhler K, Sujansky E: Risk of Down syndrome among second- and third-degree relatives of a proband with trisomy 21. *Am J Med Genet* **15**:393, 1983.
356. Berr C, Borghi E, Rethore M-O, Lejeune J, Alperovitch A: Risk of Down syndrome in relatives of trisomy 21 children. A case-control study. *Ann Genet* **33**:137, 1990.
357. Steinberg C, Zackai EH, Eunpu DL, Mennuti MT, Emanuel BS: Recurrence rate for de novo 21q21q translocation Down syndrome: A study of 112 families. *Am J Med Genet* **17**:523, 1984.
358. Stene J: Statistical inference on segregation ratios for D/G-translocations, when the families are ascertained in different ways. *Ann Hum Genet* **34**:93, 1970.
359. Hamerton J: *Human Cytogenetics*. New York, Academic, 1971, vol I.
360. Boue A, Gallano P: A collaborative study of the segregation of inherited chromosome structural rearrangements in 1356 prenatal diagnoses. *Prenat Diagn* **4**(Spec Iss):45, 1984.
361. Huether CA: Projection of Down's syndrome births in the United States 1979–2000 and the potential effects of prenatal diagnosis. *Am J Public Health* **73**:1186, 1983.
362. Crandall BF, Lebherz TB, Tarsh K: Maternal age and amniocentesis: Should this be lowered to 30? *Prenat Diagn* **6**:237, 1986.
363. The Canadian Early and Mid-Trimester Amniocentesis Trial (CEMAT) Group: Randomized trial to assess safety and fetal outcome of early and midtrimester amniocentesis. *Lancet* **351**:242, 1998.
364. Kuliev A, Jackson L, Froster U, Brambati B, Simpson JL, Verlinsky Y, Ginsberg N, et al: Chorionic villus sampling safety. *Am J Obstet Gynecol* **174**:807, 1996.
365. Merkatz IR, Nitowsky HN, Macri JN, Johnson WE: An association between low maternal serum α-fetoprotein and fetal chromosomal abnormalities. *Am J Obstet Gynecol* **148**:886, 1984.
366. Cuckle HS, Wald NJ, Lindenbaum RH: Maternal serum alpha-fetoprotein measurement: A screening test for Down syndrome. *Lancet* **1**:926, 1984.
367. Cuckle HS, Wald NJ, Lindenbaum RH, Jonasson J: Amniotic fluid AFP levels and Down syndrome. *Lancet* **1**:290, 1985.
368. Brambati B, Simoni G, Bonacchi I, Piceni L: Fetal chromosomal aneuploidies and maternal serum alpha-fetoprotein levels in first trimester. *Lancet* **2**:165, 1986.
369. Kronquist KE, Draezen E, Keener SL, Nicholas TW, Crandall BF: Reduced fetal hepatic alpha-fetoprotein levels in Down syndrome. *Prenat Diagn* **10**:739, 1990.
370. Voigtlander T, Vogel F: Low alpha-fetoprotein and serum albumin levels in Morbus Down may point to a common regulatory mechanism. *Hum Genet* **71**:276, 1985.
371. Macri JN, Buchanan PD, Gold MP: Low α-fetoprotein and trisomy. *Lancet* **2**:405, 1986.
372. Bogart MH: Current and future modes of prenatal diagnosis, in Lott IT, McCoy EE (eds): *Down Syndrome: Advances in Medical Care*. New York, Wiley-Liss, 1992, p 13.
373. Haddow JE, Palomaki GE, Knight GJ, Canick JA: Maternal serum unconjugated estriol levels are lower in the presence of fetal Down syndrome. *Am J Obstet Gynecol* **163**:1372, 1990.
374. Crandall BF, Golbus MS, Goldberg JD, Matsumoto M: First-trimester maternal serum unconjugated oestriol and alpha-fetoprotein in fetal Down's syndrome. *Prenat Diagn* **11**:377, 1991.
375. Conde-Agudelo A, Kafury-Goeta AC: Triple-marker test as screening for Down syndrome: a meta-analysis. *Obstet Gynecol Surv* **53**:369, 1998.
376. Vintzileos AM, Egan JFX: Adjusting the risk for trisomy 21 on the basis of second-trimester ultrasonography. *Am J Obstet Gynecol* **172**:837, 1995.
377. Nadel AS, Bromley B, Frigoletto FD Jr, Benacerraf BR: Can the presumed risk of autosomal trisomy be decreased in fetuses of older women following a normal sonogram? *J Ultrasound Med* **14**:297, 1995.
378. Snijders RJM, Johnson S, Sebire NJ, Noble PL, Nicolaides KH: First-trimester ultrasound screening for chromosomal defects. *Ultrasound Obstet Gynecol* **7**:216, 1996.
379. Wald NJ, Hackshaw AK: Authors reply. *Prenat Diagn* **18**:521, 1998.
380. Bianchi DW: Progress in the genetic analysis of fetal cells circulating in maternal blood. *Curr Opin Obstet Gynecol* **9**:121, 1997.
381. Bianchi DW, Williams JM, Sullivan LM, Hanson FW, Klinger KW, Shuber AP: PCR quantitation of fetal cells in maternal blood in normal and aneuploid pregnancies. *Am J Hum Genet* **61**:822, 1997.
382. Cheung M-C, Goldberg JD, Kan YW: Prenatal diagnosis of sickle cell anaemia and thalassemia by analysis of fetal cells in maternal blood. *Nat Genet* **14**:264, 1996.
383. Lewandowski RC Jr, Yunis JJ: Phenotypic mapping in man, in Yunis JJ (ed): *New Chromosomal Syndromes*. New York, Academic, 1977, p 369.
384. Preus M, Ayme S: Formal analysis of dysmorphism: Objective methods of syndrome definition. *Clin Genet* **23**:1, 1983.
385. Korenberg JR, Kawashima H, Pulst S-M, Ikeuchi T, Ogasawara N, Yamamoto K, Schonberg S, et al: Molecular definition of a region of chromosome 21 that causes features of the Down syndrome phenotype. *Am J Hum Genet* **47**:236, 1990.
386. Elder FFB, Ferguson JW, Lockhart LH: Identical twins with deletion 16q syndrome: Evidence that 16q12.2-q13 is the critical band region. *Hum Genet* **67**:233, 1984.
387. Epstein CJ: The mouse trisomies: Experimental systems for the study of aneuploidy, in Kalter H (ed): *Issues and Reviews in Teratology*. New York, Plenum, 1985, p 171.
388. Bartolomei MS, Tilghman SM: Genomic imprinting in mammals. *Annu Rev Genet* **31**:493, 1997.
389. Matthysse S, Deutsch C: Convergence and chaos in morphogenesis, in Epstein CJ (ed): *The Morphogenesis of Down Syndrome*. New York, Wiley-Liss, 1991, p 19.
390. Vogel F, Motulsky AG: *Human Genetics. Problems and Approaches*, 3d ed. Berlin, Springer-Verlag, 1996.
391. Wenger SL, Steel MW: Meiotic consequences of pericentric inversions of chromosome 13. *Am J Med Genet* **9**:275, 1981.
392. Yunis JJ, Lewandowski RC: High-resolution cytogenetics. *Birth Defects* **19**(5):11, 1983.
393. Schmickel RD: Contiguous gene syndromes: A component of recognizable syndromes. *J Pediatr* **109**:231, 1986.
394. Epstein CJ: Aneuploidy and morphogenesis, in Epstein CJ (ed): *The Morphogenesis of Down Syndrome*. New York, Wiley-Liss, 1991, p 1.
395. Mittwoch U: Mongolism and sex: A common problem of cell proliferation? *J Med Genet* **9**:92, 1971.
396. Aziz MA: Possible "atavistic" structure in human aneuploids. *Am J Phys Anthropol* **54**:347, 1981.
397. Shapiro BL: Down syndrome — A disruption of homeostasis. *Am J Med Genet* **14**:241, 1983.
398. Krone W, Wolf U: Chromosomes and protein variation, in Brock DJH, Mayo O (eds): *The Biochemical Genetics of Man*. London, Academic, 1978, p 93.
399. Devlin RH, Holm DG, Grigliatti TA: Autosomal dosage compensation in Drosophila melanogaster stains trisomic for the left arm of chromosome 2. *Proc Natl Acad Sci USA* **79**:1200, 1982.
400. Kuromitsu J, Yamashita H, Kataoka H, Takahara T, Muramatsu M, Sekine T, Okamoto N, et al: A unique downregulation of h2-calponin gene expression in Down syndrome: A possible attenuation mechanism for fetal survival by methylation at the CpG island in the trisomic chromosome 21. *Mol Cell Biol* **17**:707, 1997.
401. Weil J, Epstein CJ: The effect of trisomy 21 on the patterns of polypeptide synthesis in human fibroblasts. *Am J Hum Genet* **31**:478, 1979.
402. Klose J, Zeindl E, Sperling K: Analysis of protein patterns in two-dimensional gels of cultured human cells with trisomy 21. *Clin Genet* **28**:987, 1982.
403. Morton NE, Lindsten J, Iselius L, Yee S: Data and theory for a revised chiasma map of man. *Hum Genet* **62**:266, 1982.
404. Shimizu N, Antonarakis SE, Van Broeckhoven C, Patterson D, Gardiner K, Nizetic D, Créau N, et al: Report of the fifth international workshop on human chromosome 21 mapping 1994. *Cytogenet Cell Genet* **70**:148, 1995.
405. Evans HJ, Buckland RA, Pardue ML: Location of the genes coding for 18S and 28S ribosomal RNA in the human genome. *Chromosoma* **48**:405, 1974.
406. Miller DA, Tantravahi R, Dev VG, Miller OJ: Frequency of satellite associations of human chromosomes is correlated with amount of Ag-staining of the nucleolus organizer region. *Am J Hum Genet* **29**:490, 1977.
407. Kurnit DM, Neve RL, Morton CC, Bruns GAP, Ma NSF, Cox DR, Klinger HP: Recent evolution of DNA sequence homology in the

pericentromeric regions of human acrocentric chromosomes. *Cytogenet Cell Genet* **38**:99, 1984.
408. Yunis JJ: Chromosomes and cancer: New nomenclature and future directions. *Hum Pathol* **12**:494, 1981.
409. Gardiner K: Clonability and gene distribution on human chromosome 21: Reflections of junk DNA content? *Gene* **205**:39, 1997.
410. Hattori H, Fujiyama A, Taylor TD, Watanabe H, Yada T, Park H-S, Toyoda A, et al: The DNA sequence of human chromosome 21. *Nature* **405**:311, 2000.
411. Korenberg JR: Down syndrome phenotypic mapping, in Epstein CJ (ed): *The Morphogenesis of Down Syndrome*. New York, Wiley-Liss, 1991, p 43.
412. Epstein CJ, Korenberg JR, Anneren G, Antonarakis SE, Ayme S, Courchesne E, Epstein LB, et al: Protocols to establish genotype-phenotype correlations in Down syndrome. *Am J Hum Genet* **49**:207, 1991.
413. Summitt RL: Chromosome specific segments that cause the phenotype of Down syndrome, in de la Cruz FF, Gerald PS (eds): *Trisomy 21 (Down Syndrome). Research Perspectives*. Baltimore, University Park Press, 1981, p 225.
414. Patterson D, Jones C, Scoggin C, Miller YE, Graw S: Somatic cell genetic approaches to Down's syndrome. *Ann N Y Acad Sci* **396**:69, 1982.
415. Korenberg JR: Mental modelling. *Nat Genet* **11**:109, 1985.
416. Korenberg JR, Chen X-N, Schipper R, Sun Z, Gonsky R, Gerwehr S, Carpenter N, et al: Down syndrome phenotypes: The consequences of chromosome imbalance. *Proc Natl Acad Sci USA* **91**:4997, 1994.
417. Delabar JM, Theophile D, Rahmani Z, Chettouh Z, Blouin JL, Prieur M, Noel B. et al: Molecular mapping of twenty-four features of Down syndrome on chromosome 21. *Eur J Hum Genet* **1**:114, 1993.
418. Anneren KG, Korenberg JR, Epstein CJ: Phosphofructokinase activity in fibroblasts aneuploid for chromosome 21. *Hum Genet* **76**:63, 1987.
419. Arias S, Paradisi I, Rolo M: Cystationine beta-synthase (CBS) location excluded from 21pter → q11, but confirmed to 21q, by gene dosage in trisomy 21. *Cytogenet Cell Genet* **40**:570, 1985.
420. Bardsley WG, McMurray BP, Robson A, D'Souza S, Taylor GM: Analysis of gene-dosage effects on the expression of CD18 by trisomy 21 lymphoblastoid cell-lines using a statistical model to fit flow cytometry profiles. *Hum Genet* **86**:181, 1990.
421. Neve RL, Finch EA, Dawes LR: Expression of the Alzheimer amyloid precursor gene transcript in the human brain. *Neuron* **1**:669, 1988.
422. Pash J, Smithgall T, Bustin M: Chromosomal protein HMG-14 is overexpressed in Down syndrome. *Exp Cell Res* **193**:232, 1991.
423. Marks A, O'Hanlon D, Lei M, Percy ME, Becker LE: Accumulation of S100β mRNA and protein in cerebellum during infancy in Down syndrome and control subjects. *Mol Brain Res* **36**:343, 1996.
424. Halliwell B, Gutteridge JMC: *Free Radicals in Biology and Medicine*. Oxford, UK, Clarendon, 1985.
425. Sinet P-M: Metabolism of oxygen derivatives in Down's syndrome. *Ann N Y Acad Sci* **396**:83, 1982.
426. Seidl R, Greber S, Schuller E, Bernert G, Cairns N, Lubec G: Evidence against increased oxidative DNA-damage in Down brain. *Neurosci Lett* **235**:137, 1997.
427. Odetti P, Angelini G, Dapino D, Zaccheo D, Garibaldi S, Dagna-Bricarelli F, Piombo G, et al: Early glycoxidation damage in brains from Down's syndrome. *Biochem Biophys Res Commun* **243**:849, 1998.
428. Huang T-T, Carlson EJ, Leadon SA, Epstein CJ: Relationship of resistance to oxygen free radicals to CuZn superoxide dismutase activity in transgenic, transfected, and trisomic cells. *FASEB J* **6**:903, 1992.
429. Kurnit DM, Aldridge JF, Matsuoka R, Matthyse S: Increased adhesiveness of trisomy 21 cells and atrioventricular canal malformations in Down's syndrome: A stochastic model. *Am J Med Genet* **20**:385, 1985.
430. Wright TC, Destrempes M, Orkin R, Kurnit DM: Increased adhesiveness of Down syndrome fetal fibroblasts in vitro. *Proc Natl Acad Sci USA* **81**:2426, 1984.
431. Kirby ML: Neural crest and the morphogenesis of Down syndrome with special emphasis on cardiovascular development, in Epstein CJ (ed): *The Morphogenesis of Down Syndrome*. New York, Wiley-Liss, 1991, p 215.
432. Rowley JD: Down syndrome and acute leukemia: Increased risk may be due to trisomy 21. *Lancet* **2**:1020, 1981.
433. Ugazio AG: Down's syndrome: Problems of immunodeficiency, in Burgio GR, Fraccaro M, Tiepolo L, Wolf U (eds): *Trisomy 21: An International Symposium*. Berlin, Springer-Verlag, 1981, p 33.
434. Teyssier JR, Behar C, Bajolle F, Potron G: Selective involvement of cells carrying extra chromosome 21 in a child with acute nonlymphocytic leukaemia. *Lancet* **1**:290, 1984.
435. Shen JJ, Williams BJ, Zipursky A, Doyle J, Sherman SL, Jacobs PA, Shugar AL, et al: Cytogenetic and molecular studies of Down syndrome individuals with leukemia. *Am J Hum Genet* **56**:915, 1995.
436. Epstein CJ: Down's syndrome and Alzheimer's disease: What is the relation? in Glenner GG, Wurtman RI (eds): *Advancing Frontiers in Alzheimer's Disease Research*. Austin, TX, University of Texas Press, 1987, p 155.
437. Yankner BA, Mesulam M-M: β-amyloid and the pathogenesis of Alzheimer's disease. *N Engl J Med* **325**:1849, 1991.
438. Glenner GG: On causative theories in Alzheimer's disease. *Hum Pathol* **16**:435, 1985.
439. Goate AM, Chartier-Harlin MC, Mullan MC, Brown J, Crawford F, Fidani L, Guiffra A, et al: Segregation of a missense mutation in the amyloid precursor protein gene with familial Alzheimer's disease. *Nature* **349**:704, 1991.
440. Chartier-Harlin M-C, Crawford F, Houlden H, Warren A, Hughes D, Fidani L, Goate A, et al: Early-onset Alzheimer's disease caused by mutation at codon 717 of the β-amyloid precursor protein gene. *Nature* **353**:844, 1991.
441. Murrell J, Farlow M, Ghetti B, Benson MD: A mutation in the amyloid precursor protein associated with hereditary Alzheimer's disease. *Science* **254**:97, 1991.
442. Neve RL, Dawes LR, Yankner BA, Benowitz LI, Rodriguez W, Higgins GA: Genetics and biology of the Alzheimer amyloid precursor, in Coleman P, Higgins G, Phelps C (eds): *Progress in Brain Research*. New York, Elsevier Science, 1990, vol 86, p 257.
443. Prasher VP, Farrer MJ, Kessling AM, Fisher EM, West RJ, Barber PC, Butler AC. Molecular mapping of Alzheimer-type dementia in Down's syndrome. *Ann Neurol* **43**:380, 1998.
444. Heston LL, Mastri AR, Anderson VE, White J: Dementia of the Alzheimer type. Clinical genetics, natural history, and associated conditions. *Arch Gen Psychiatry* **38**:1085, 1981.
445. Van Duijn CM, Clayton D, Chandra V, Fratiglioni L, Graves AB, Heyman A, Jorm AF, et al: Familial aggregation of Alzheimer's disease and related disorders: A collaborative re-analysis of case-control studies. *Int J Epidemiol* **20**(suppl 2):S13, 1991.
446. Finch CE: The evolution of ovarian oocyte decline with aging and possible relationships with Down syndrome and Alzheimer disease. *Exp Gerontol* **29**:299, 1994.
447. McClure HM, Belden KJ, Pieper WA, Jacobson CB: Autosomal trisomy in a chimpanzee: Resemblance to Down's syndrome. *Science* **165**:1010, 1969.
448. Andrle M, Fiedler W, Rett A, Ambros P, Schweizer D: A case of trisomy 22 in Pongo pygmaeus. *Cytogenet Cell Genet* **24**:1, 1979.
449. Nadeau JH, Taylor BA: Lengths of chromosomal segments conserved since divergence of man and mouse. *Proc Natl Acad Sci USA* **81**:814, 1984.
450. Davisson M: Segmental trisomy of murine chromosome 16: A new model system for studying Down syndrome, in Patterson D, Epstein CJ (eds): *Molecular Genetics of Chromosome 21 and Down Syndrome*. New York, Wiley-Liss, 1990, p 263.
451. Smith DJ, Zhu Y, Zhang J-L, Cheng J-F, Rubin EM: Construction of a panel of transgenic mice containing a contiguous 2-Mb set of YAC/P1 clones from human chromosome 21q22.2. *Genomics* **17**:425, 1995.
452. Reeves RH, Cabin DE: Mouse chromosome 16. *Mouse Genome Special* **7**:S264, 1997.
453. Gropp A, Kolbus U, Giers D: Systematic approach to the study of trisomy in the mouse. II. *Cytogenet Cell Genet* **14**:42, 1975.
454. Epstein CJ, Cox DR, Epstein LB: Mouse trisomy 16: An animal model of human trisomy 21 (Down syndrome). *Ann N Y Acad Sci* **450**:157, 1985.
455. Oster-Granite ML, Gearhart JD, Reeves RH: Neurobiological consequences of trisomy 16 in mice, in Epstein CJ (ed): *The Neurobiology of Down Syndrome*. New York, Raven, 1986, p 137.
456. Grausz H, Richtsmeier JT, Oster-Granite ML: Morphogenesis of the brain and craniofacial complex in trisomy 16 mice, in Epstein CJ (ed): *The Morphogenesis of Down Syndrome*. New York, Wiley-Liss, 1991, p 169.
457. Holtzman DM, Bayney RM, Li YW, Khosrovi H, Berger CN, Epstein CJ, Mobley WC: Dysregulation of gene expression in mouse trisomy 16, an animal model of Down syndrome. *EMBO J* **11**:619, 1992.
458. Holtzman DM, Li YW, DeArmond SJ, McKinley MP, Gage FH, Epstein CJ, Mobley WC: Mouse model of neurodegeneration: Atrophy

of basal forebrain cholinergic neurons in trisomy 16 transplants. *Proc Natl Acad Sci USA* **89**:1383, 1992.

459. Cox DR, Smith SA, Epstein LB, Epstein CJ: Mouse trisomy 16 as an animal model of human trisomy 21 (Down syndrome): Formation of viable trisomy 16↔diploid mouse chimeras. *Dev Biol* **101**:416, 1984.
460. Epstein CJ, Foster DB, DeArmond SJ, Prusiner SB: Acceleration of scrapie in trisomy 16↔diploid aggregation chimeras. *Ann Neurol* **29**:95, 1991.
461. Reeves RH, Irving NG, Moran TH, Wohn A, Kitt C, Sisodia SS, Schmidt C, et al: A mouse model for Down syndrome exhibits learning and behaviour deficits. *Nat Genet* **11**:177, 1995.
462. Holtzman DM, Santucci D, Kilbridge J, Chua-Couzens J, Fontana DJ, Daniels SE, Johnson RM, et al: Developmental abnormalities and age-related neurodegeneration in a mouse model of Down syndrome. *Proc Natl Acad Sci USA* **93**:13333, 1996.
463. Coussons-Read ME, Crnic LS: Behavioral assessment of the Ts65Dn mouse, a model for Down syndrome: Altered behavior in the elevated plus maze and the open field. *Behav Genet* **26**:7, 1996.
464. Demas GE, Nelson RJ, Krueger BK, Yarowsky PJ: Impaired spatial working and reference memory in segmental trisomy (Ts65Dn) mice. *Behav Brain Res* **90**:199, 1998.
465. Escorihuela RM, Fernandez-Teruel A, Vallina IF, Baamonde C, Lumbreras MA, Dierssen M, Tobena A, et al: A behavioral assessment of Ts65Dn mice: A putative Down syndrome model. *Neurosci Lett* **199**:143, 1995.
466. Siarey RJ, Stoll J, Rapoport SI, Galdzicki Z: Altered long-term potentiation in the young and old Ts65Dn mouse, a model for Down syndrome. *Neuropharmacology* **36**:1549, 1997.
467. Dierssen M, Vallina IF, Baamonde C, Lumbreras MA, Martinez-Cue C, Calatuyud SG, Florez J: Impaired cyclic AMP production in the hippocampus of a Down syndrome murine model. *Brain Res Dev Brain Res* **95**:122, 1996.
468. Sago H, Carlson EJ, Smith DJ, Kilbridge J, Rubin EM, Mobley WC, Epstein CJ, et al: Ts1Cje, a partial trisomy 16 mouse model for Down syndrome. Exhibits learning and behavioral abnormalities. *Proc Natl Acad Sci USA* **95**:6256, 1998.
469. Sago H, Carlson EJ, Smith DJ, Kilbridge J, Rubin EM, Crnic LS, Mobley WC, et al: Genetic dissection of the region associated with behavioral abnormalities in mouse models of Down syndrome. Submitted for Publication.
470. Epstein CJ, Avraham KB, Smith S, Elroy-Stein O, Lovett M, Rotman G, Bry C, Groner Y: Transgenic mice with increased CuZn-superoxide dismutase activity: Animal model of dosage effects in Down syndrome. *Proc Natl Acad Sci USA* **84**:8044, 1987.
471. Elroy-Stein O, Groner Y: Impaired neurotransmitter uptake in PC12 cells overexpressing human Cu-Zn-superoxide dismutase — Implication for gene dosage effects in Down syndrome. *Cell* **52**:259, 1988.
472. Avraham KB, Schickler M, Sapoznikov D, Yarom R, Groner Y: Down's syndrome: Abnormal neuromuscular junction in tongue of transgenic mice with elevated levels of human Cu/Zn-superoxide dismutase. *Cell* **54**:823, 1988.
473. Yarom R, Sapoznikov D, Havivi Y, Avraham KB, Schickler M, Groner Y: Premature aging changes in neuromuscular junction of transgenic mice with an extra human CuZnSOD gene: A model for tongue pathology in Down's syndrome. *J Neurol Sci* **88**:41, 1988.
474. Avraham KB, Sugarman H, Rotshenker S, Groner Y: Down's syndrome: Morphological remodeling and increased complexity in the neuromuscular junction of transgenic CuZn-superoxide dismutase mice. *J Neurocytol* **20**:208, 1991.
475. Barkats M, Bertholet JY, Venault P, Ceballos-Picot I, Nicole A, Phillips J, Moutier R, et al: Hippocampal mossy fiber changes in mice transgenic for the human copper-zinc superoxide dismutase gene. *Neurosci Lett* **160**:24, 1993.
476. Chan PH, Yang GY, Chen SF, Carlson E, Epstein CJ: Cold-induced brain edema and infarction are reduced in transgenic mice overexpressing CuZn superoxide dismutase. *Ann Neurol* **29**:482, 1991.
477. Kinouchi H, Epstein CJ, Mizui T, Carlson E, Chen SF, Chan PH: Attenuation of focal cerebral injury in transgenic mice overexpressing CuZn-superoxide dismutase. *Proc Natl Acad Sci USA* **88**:11158, 1991.
478. Chan PH, Chu L, Chen SF, Carlson EJ, Epstein CJ: Reduced neurotoxicity in transgenic mice overexpressing human CuZn-superoxide dismutase. *Stroke* **21**(suppl III):III-80, 1990.
479. Peled-Kamar M, Lotem J, Okon E, Sachs L, Groner Y: Thymic abnormalities and enhanced apoptosis of thymocytes and bone marrow cells in transgenic mice overexpressing Cu/Zn-superoxide dismutase: implications for Down syndrome. *EMBO J* **14**:4985, 1995.
480. Nabarra B, Casanova M, Paris D, Nicole A, Toyoma K, Sinet PM, Ceballos I, et al: Transgenic mice overexpressing the human Cu/Zn-SOD gene: Ultrastructural studies of a premature thymic involution model of Down's syndrome (trisomy 21). *Lab Invest* **74**:617, 1996.
481. Higgis LS, Holtzman DM, Rabin J, Mobley WC, Cordell B: Transgenic mouse brain histopathology resembles early Alzheimer disease. *Ann Neurol* **35**:598, 1994.
482. D'Hooge R, Nagels G, Westland CE, Mucke L, De Deyn PP: Spatial learning deficit in mice expression human 751-amino acid beta-amyloid precursor protein. *Neuroreport* **4**:2807, 1996.
483. Sturchler-Pierrat C, Abramowski D, Duke, M, Wiederhold KH, Mistl C, Rothacher S, Ledermann B, et al: Two amyloid precursor protein transgenic mouse models with Alzheimer disease-like pathology. *Proc Natl Acad Sci U S A* **94**:13287, 1997.
484. Holcomb L, Gordon MN, McGowan E, Yu X, Benkovic S, Jantzen P, Wright K, et al: Accelerated Alzheimer-type phenotype in transgenic mice carrying both mutant amyloid precursor protein and presenilin 1 transgenes. *Nat Med* **4**:97, 1998.
485. Sumarsono SH, Wilson TJ, Tymms MJ, Venter DJ, Corrick CM, Kola R, Lahoud MH, et al: Down's syndrome-like skeletal abnormalities in Ets2 transgenic mice. *Nature* **379**:534, 1996.
486. Bustin M, Alfonso PJ, Pash JM, Ward JM, Gearhart JD, Reeves RH: Characterization of transgenic mice with an increased content of chromosomal protein HMG-14 in their chromatin. *DNA Cell Biol* **14**:997, 1995.
487. Reeves RH, Yao J, Crowley MR, Buck S, Zhang X, Yarowsky P, Gearhart JD, et al: Astrocytosis and axonal proliferation in the hippocampus of S100β transgenic mice. *Proc Natl Acad Sci U S A* **91**:5359, 1994.
488. Whitaker-Azmita PM, Wingate M, Borella A, Gerlai R, Roder J, Azmita EC: Transgenic mice overexpressing the neurotrophic factor S-100 beta show neuronal cytoskeletal and behavioral signs of altered aging processes: implications for Alzheimer's disease and Down's syndrome. *Brain Res* **776**:51, 1997.
489. Elson A, Levanon D, Weiss Y, Groner Y: Overexpression of liver-type phosphofructokinase (PFKL) in transgenic-PFKL mice: Implication for gene dosage in trisomy 21. *Biochem J* **299**:409, 1994.
490. Groner Y: Transgenic models for chromosome 21 gene dosage effects, in Epstein CJ, Hassold T, Lott IT, Nadel L, Patterson D (eds): *Etiology and Pathogenesis of Down Syndrome*. New York, Wiley-Liss, 1995, p 193.
491. Smith DJ, Stevens ME, Sudanagunta SP, Bronson RT, Makhinson M, Watabe AM, O'Dell TJ, et al: Functional screen of 2 Mb of human 21q22.2 in transgenic mice implicates *minibrain* in the learning defects associated with Down syndrome. *Nat Genet* **16**:28, 1997.
492. Lott IT, McCoy EE (eds): *Down Syndrome. Advances in Medical Care*. New York, Wiley-Liss, 1992.
493. Nadel L, Rosenthal D (eds): *Down Syndrome. Living and Learning in the Community*. New York, Wiley-Liss, 1995.
494. Annerén G, Johansson I, Kristiansson I-L, Lööw L: *Downs Syndrom. En bok for föräldrar och personal*. Stockholm, Liber Utbildning AB, 1996.

CHAPTER 64

The Fragile X Syndrome

Stephen T. Warren ▪ Stephanie L. Sherman

1. **Fragile X syndrome (MIM 309550) is an X-linked dominant disorder with reduced penetrance. Although not as frequent as once believed, the syndrome remains a relatively common form of inherited mental retardation. The syndrome typically presents in males with moderate mental retardation, characteristic, but subtle, facial features of a prominent jaw and large ears, and macroorchidism after puberty. Penetrant females are typically less severely affected.**
2. **Fragile X syndrome derives its name from a characteristic fragile site at Xq27.3 that is found in a proportion of chromosomes in metaphase spreads from appropriately cultured cells of affected males and many penetrant females. Coincident with this fragile site, is a CGG repeat within the 5′-untranslated region (UTR) of the fragile X mental retardation gene 1, designated FMR1 (GenBank L29074). Among normal individuals, the *FMR1* repeat is polymorphic in length and content, often punctuated by AGG interruptions. The most frequent normal allele in Caucasians contains 30 repeats and 2 AGG interruptions at positions 10 and 20. In affected individuals, this repeat is expanded over 230 repeats, with a mean of approximately 780 repeats. Thus, fragile X syndrome is among a unique class of human disorders resulting from unstable repeats, which are referred to as *dynamic mutations*. When the *FMR1* repeat is expanded to this degree, the *FMR1* gene becomes hypermethylated and transcriptionally silent. This is referred to as the *full mutation* to distinguish it from the premutation allele. Premutation alleles are found in nonpenetrant male carriers and many female carriers. The length of these alleles falls between that of the normal repeats and full mutations. Premutation alleles are exquisitely unstable upon transmission and the progression to the full mutation in offspring is dependent upon the length of the maternal premutation. This relationship explains the unusual inheritance patterns and the reduced penetrance of this disorder.**
3. **Fragile X syndrome is found among all ethnic groups studied. The prevalence in the general population is approximately 1/4500 males. Only 50 percent of females carrying the full mutation are penetrant, due to random X-inactivation. Because females only inherit maternal full mutations, the expected female prevalence is 1/9000. Premutation carriers are found in approximately 1/400 females and 1/1000 males.**
4. **Molecular laboratory diagnosis has now superseded cytogenetic testing for the fragile site, although routine karyotype analysis remains indicated in all cases of undiagnosed mental retardation. Molecular diagnostics routinely involve Southern blot studies, which provide information on the repeat length and methylation status. PCR studies can more accurately size normal and premutation alleles and, in some laboratories, can provide an initial screen for full mutations. Antibody detection of the *FMR1*-encoded protein, FMRP, is often a very useful test as the lack of FMRP is the cause of this syndrome. Indeed, a small but significant class of patients owe their disease to more typical mutations, such as deletions, which all predict null alleles. Significantly, missense mutations appear markedly infrequent, with the single exception of severely affected patients with a I304N mutation. Protein studies can be carried out quickly and inexpensively by a histochemical analysis of blood smears or, more accurately, by conventional Western analysis.**
5. **FMRP, the deficient protein in fragile X syndrome, is a selective RNA-binding protein that shuttles between the nucleus and cytoplasm. At steady state, most FMRP is cytoplasmic and associated as a ribonucleoprotein complex to translating polyribosomes or endoplasmic reticulum-associated ribosomes. In neurons, FMRP can also be found at the base of dendritic spines and may participate in the remodeling of the spine following synaptic activity. Thus, the loss of FMRP may directly influence neuronal plasticity resulting in cognitive deficit.**

HISTORY

Johnson[1] noted an excess of males among mentally retarded individuals as early as 1897. In his report, he mentioned a 24 percent excess of retarded males relative to females according to the US census figures, but gave no explanation for this excess. In 1938, Penrose[2] also noted the high male:female ratio in the Colchester survey of institutionalized individuals and suggested that the male majority was due to biases in ascertainment: (a) Males more often were identified as mentally retarded because of the higher expectation for males than for females. (b) Males exhibited aggressive behavior more often than females and therefore were more likely to be institutionalized. No genetic explanation for the excess of males was considered at this time or for many years. In 1969, Lehrke[3] was the first to argue persuasively that the preponderance of mentally retarded males was due to X-linked genes, and that X-linked mental retardation (XLMR) may be responsible for a substantially large proportion of mental retardation (MR). He suggested that the contribution of XLMR had gone largely unnoticed due to the lack of obvious clinical symptoms.[3]

In 1971, Turner et al.[4] suggested that XLMR in individuals with no other clinical signs should be considered as a distinct

A list of standard abbreviations is located immediately preceding the index in each volume. Additional abbreviations used in this chapter include: ATL1 to ATL4 = numbered single nucleotide polymorphisms from the Atlanta Center; FEN1 = flap endonuclease 1; FLAG = a synthetic epitope tag; *FMR1* = fragile X mental retardation gene 1; FMRP = fragile X mental retardation protein; FXR1 = fragile X-related gene 1; *FXR2* = fragile X-related gene 2; KH = ribonucleoprotein K-homology; MR = mental retardation; mRNP = messenger ribonucleoprotein; NES = nuclear export signal; NLS = nuclear localization signal; POF = premature ovarian failure; RGG box = protein sequence of Arg-Gly-Gly; UTR = untranslated region; RNP = ribonucleoprotein; SNP = single nucleotide polymorphism; STR = short-tandem repeats; XLMR = X-linked mental retardation.

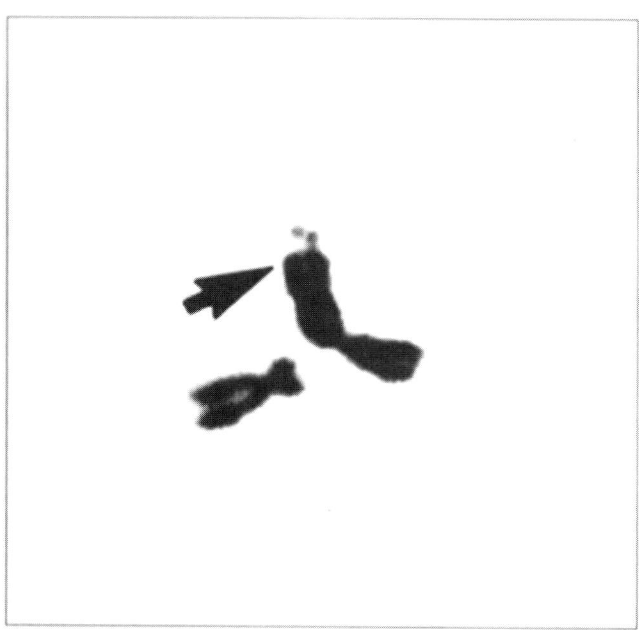

Fig. 64-1 Partial metaphase spread of an affected male with fragile X syndrome showing the fragile site at Xq27.3 (arrow).

diagnostic category. They suggested that one of the earliest XLMR pedigrees published by Martin and Bell,[5] as well as others,[6–8] fit in this category. Thus, by the mid-1970s the importance of nonspecific-XLMR had been recognized, but it was acknowledged that this group was etiologically heterogeneous.

In 1969, Lubs[9] reported a unique cytogenetic marker on the X chromosome observed in four retarded males in a family with XLMR (Fig. 64-1). However, this was thought to be an isolated finding and was not considered relevant to the diagnosis of XLMR. Four years later, a second XLMR family with a cytogenetic marker was reported, but the report was written in Portuguese and published in Brazil,[10] and, unfortunately, went largely unnoticed. However, by the late 1970s it was realized that nonspecific-XLMR associated with a cytogenetic marker located on the end of the long arm of the X chromosome was not uncommon[11,12] and that the cytogenetic marker may be a useful diagnostic tool. Confirmation of the original observation was delayed primarily because expression of the marker depended on culturing cells under particular conditions. In 1977, Sutherland[13] showed that the cell culture medium must be deficient in folic acid or thymidine to stimulate expression. This marker is known as the fragile X site because of its appearance as a gap or break in the chromosome arm.

Macroorchidism was shown to be associated with some forms of XLMR in 1971 by Escalante et al.,[14] and subsequently by others.[15,16] Endocrine and germinal function of the large testes were shown to be normal.[17] In 1975, Turner et al.[16] showed that macroorchidism was also associated with some XLMR families segregating for the cytogenetic marker.

Finally, the pedigree originally published by Martin and Bell[5] was reevaluated by Richards et al.[18] and found to show both macroorchidism and the cytogenetic marker on the X chromosome. In recognition of the first published pedigree, XLMR associated with the X chromosome cytogenetic marker was originally named the Martin-Bell syndrome. Now it is called the fragile X syndrome, referring to the association of the unique cytogenetic marker, the fragile X site. The term *Martin-Bell* is now routinely used to describe the classical facial characteristics associated with the fragile X syndrome.

The importance of the identification of a cytogenetic marker that could distinguish one type of XLMR from the others cannot be overstated. An individual was diagnosed with the fragile X syndrome if he or she had 2 percent or more cells with the fragile X site. This cytogenetic test was thought to be quite accurate for identifying males with the fragile X syndrome and less so for fragile X syndrome females. Based on this test, prevalence estimates of the fragile X syndrome in predominantly Caucasian populations ranged from 1/2500 to 1/1250 in males and from 1/5000 to 1/6666 in females.[19] Once the gene for fragile X syndrome was identified, a more accurate molecular diagnostic test was available. These figures were found to be high, primarily due to nearby fragile sites unrelated to the fragile X syndrome. Irrespective, the fragile X syndrome is one of the most frequent forms of identified inherited MR.

In addition to determining the frequency of the disorder in the population, the unique cytogenetic marker enabled examination of the inheritance pattern in the subset of fragile X-related XLMR pedigrees. Initially, the characterization of the inheritance pattern of the fragile X syndrome was thought to be a simple task: fragile X-related MR was known to be transmitted as an X-linked trait and to cosegregate with the marker on the X chromosome, the fragile X site. However, there were several observations that were exceptions to the simple rules of X-linked inheritance, which were noted even before the fragile X syndrome was fully delineated. Martin and Bell[5] reported two apparently normal brothers who both had affected grandsons. In 1963, Dunn et al.[7] posed several questions based on the inheritance pattern observed in a large XLMR pedigree: (a) Through whom did the defect enter the pedigree? (b) Why was there a deficiency of affected males? (c) Did the males and females of low-normal intelligence have the disease in a mild form? (d) Was this defect inherited by X-linked recessive transmission rather than dominant X-linked transmission?

Using segregation analysis of families with the fragile X syndrome, Sherman et al.[20,21] identified specific characteristics of the inheritance pattern of fragile X-related MR that differentiated it from other X-linked traits. First, no new mutations were predicted; thus, all mothers of affected sons were carriers. Second, 20 percent of males who carried the mutation did not express any clinical or cognitive symptoms. Third, a relatively high proportion of the female carriers expressed MR, although they were usually more mildly affected than males. Fourth, the risk of fragile X syndrome in offspring depended on the sex and phenotype of the carrier parent: (a) Daughters of nonexpressing carrier males were rarely, if ever, mentally impaired, whereas daughters of nonexpressing carrier females had about a 30 percent chance of having daughters with fragile X syndrome. (b) Cognitively impaired female carriers had a higher risk of having offspring with fragile X syndrome than those who were cognitively normal. (c) The risk of having an offspring with fragile X syndrome increased in each succeeding generation, a phenomenon called "anticipation." Once the fragile X syndrome mutation was identified and found to be a "dynamic" trinucleotide repeat mutation, the biological basis for the unusual inheritance pattern of the fragile X-related MR was provided.

THE FMR1 GENE

Identification

The *FMR1* gene was identified through positional cloning efforts in 1991.[22] However, a great deal of earlier work was instrumental in making this discovery possible. The observation of the fragile site at Xq27.3 among individuals in affected pedigrees (see above), the X-linked nature of the disorder, and several linkage studies[23–34] all pointed toward the vicinity of the fragile X site as the most likely location of the causal mutation. Several approaches were taken to refine this localization. Bell et al.[35] and Vincent et al.[36] showed that probes close to the fragile X site were able to discern abnormally methylated pulsed-field-gel electrophoresis fragments, suggesting both an abnormal methylation state

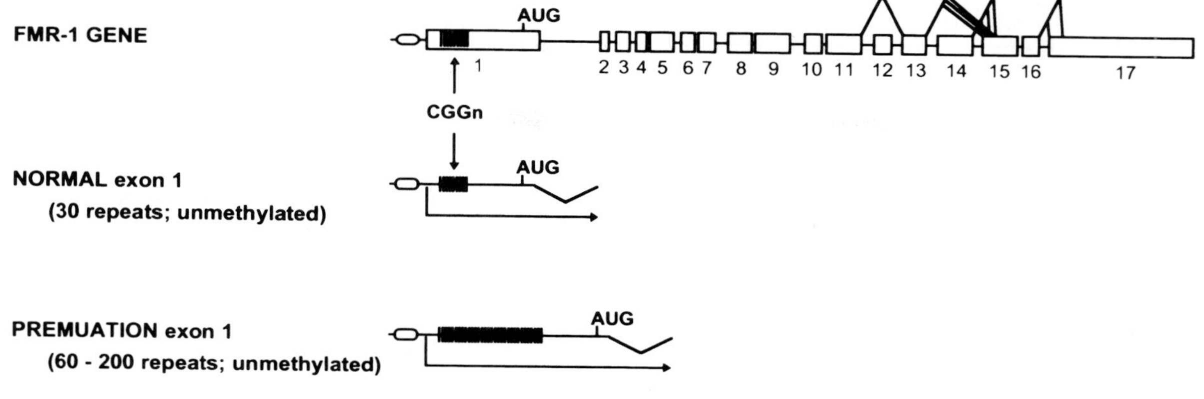

Fig. 64-2 Diagram of the *FMR1* gene showing the promoter (oval) and 17 exons (boxes) as well as the CGG repeat (vertical bars). Note alternative splicing between exons 11 and 12, 13 and 15, 14 and 15, and 16 and 17. Variation in the CGG repeat tract is shown for the three major classes of alleles (normal, premutation, and full mutation). Filled in promoter of the full mutation indicated CpG methylation and transcriptional silencing of FMR1. (*Modified from Warren and Nelson.*[333] *Used by permission.*)

on affected chromosomes and narrowing the critical region to approximately a megabase (Mb). Others used a somatic cell genetic approach[37,38] that proved both insightful and useful. Using somatic cell hybrids, Ledbetter et al.,[39] and later Warren et al.,[40] first found evidence suggesting that a reiterated DNA sequence was involved in fragile X syndrome by studying the behavior of the human fragile X chromosome in somatic cell hybrids. Warren et al. [40,41] exploited somatic cell hybrids to physically define the fragile X site using translocations between the human X chromosome and rodent chromosomes with the breakpoints falling within the smallest critical region defined by multipoint linkage studies. Using these breakpoint-containing hybrids as physical mapping reagents, the fragile X repeat region was cloned,[42–44] including the *FMR1* gene itself.[22] Two cDNA clones were initially identified, and together were found to carry the entire coding sequence of *FMR1*.[22] The mRNA for *FMR1* is 4362 bp, including a long (1.8-kb) 3′ untranslated region (UTR). The open reading frame is 656 amino acids. The CGG trinucleotide repeat responsible for mutations in the majority of fragile X syndrome cases was found to be present at the 5′ end of one of these cDNAs, and was later shown to be located within the 5′-UTR of the *FMR1* transcript.[45]

Allelic Forms of FMR1

In more than 95 percent of cases, the fragile X syndrome is caused by a single type of mutation, the unstable expansion of the CGG trinucleotide of the *FMR1* gene (Fig. 64-2).[22, 43,44, 46,47] There are essentially four allelic forms of the *FMR1* gene, with respect to the repeat length, found in the population, and they are referred to as normal, intermed iate or gray zone, premutation, and full mutation (Table 64-1). The normal form usually contains, on average, 29 to 31 CGG repeats, and is usually interspersed with 1 to 3 single AGG sequences found approximately every 9 to 10 CGG repeats.[42,46,48–53] The region is highly polymorphic with respect to the number of repeats (ranging from 6 to 50 repeats) and the number and position of the interspersed AGG sequences.

Normally, the repeat region is stable when transmitted from parent to child. It has been suggested that loss of the AGG interspersed sequences or an increase in the number of perfect CGG repeats causes the repeat region to become unstable (see

Table 64-1 Charateristics of FMRI CGG Repeat Alleles and Carrier Status

Category	Number of Repeats	Methylation Status	Presence of FMR1 mRNA/protein	Stability: Transmission	Stability: Somatic	Overt Clinical Phenotype
Normal	6–60	unmethylated	+/+	stable	stable	normal
Intermediate	41–60	unmethylated	+/+	stability depends on length of 3′ pure repeat	stable	normal
Premutation	60–200	unmethylated	+/+	unstable	most often stable	normal
Full	>200	methylated	−/−	unstable	unstable	affected
Mosaic	pre- and full-size alleles	pre—unmethylated full—methylated	reduced/reduced (depends on proportion of premutation alleles)	unstable	unstable	affected
Methylation exceptions	>200	a proportion of alleles with no methylation	reduced/reduced (depends on proportion of premutation alleles)	unstable	unstable	affected

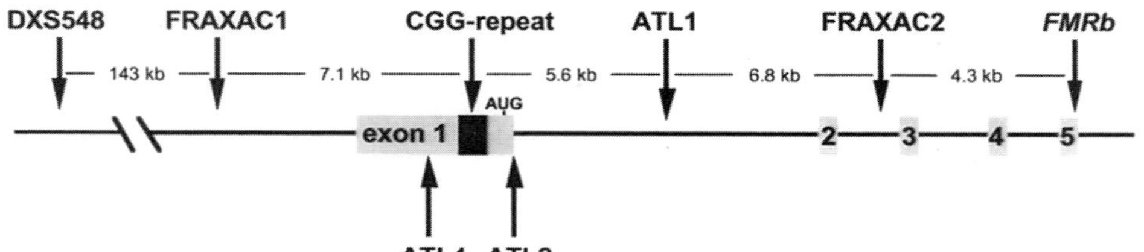

Fig. 64-3 Polymorphic loci surrounding the CGG repeat of *FMR1* used in haplotype analysis.

Mechanism of Expansion below), and to expand in size when transmitted from parent to child.[49,50,52–54] This unstable form of the gene is called a premutation and usually consists of 50 to 200 repeats. Premutation carriers, male and female, usually do not exhibit overt clinical symptoms related to the mutation. The transcription of the *FMR1* gene, the stability of mRNA, and the synthesis of FMRP seem to be unaffected for alleles in the premutation size range, at least in lymphoblastoid cells.[55] However, female premutation carriers are at high risk for having offspring with the fragile X syndrome, as premutation alleles of greater than 60 repeats almost always expand in size during transmission.

There is obvious overlap between the so-called "normal" and "premutation" allele size ranges. Alleles in this overlap, between 40 and 60 repeats, are called intermediate or gray zone alleles. Some proportion of these alleles is unstable and will expand a few repeats during transmission. The instability appears to be related to the length of pure 3′ repeat sequence; unstable alleles have at least 34 to 50 pure 3′ CGG repeats.[54, 56,57] In most populations, the frequency of intermediate alleles is about 2 to 4 percent.[58–60] The frequency of unstable intermediate alleles is thought to be about 1 percent of the general population, although epidemiologic studies have not been done to confirm this figure.

The full mutation form of the *FMR1* gene consists of over 200 repeats and is abnormally hypermethylated. Consequently, no mRNA is produced,[61–63] and the lack of the gene product FMRP, an RNA-binding protein, is responsible for the MR.[64] Because *FMR1* is X-linked, males have more severe expression of the phenotype associated with the syndrome as compared with females.

Full mutations show instability in both the germ line and somatic cell lines. The evidence for somatic instability is based on Southern blotting analyses of DNA extracted from peripheral blood. The full mutation can appear as a single band, discrete multiple bands, or, often, a smear.[65] In addition, some full-mutation carriers have unmethylated premutation-sized bands, which presumably produce FMRP. These are referred to as "mosaics." The frequency of such mosaic carriers depends on the technique used to detect the small proportion of premutation alleles but ranges from 6 to 41 percent in full-mutation males.[66,67] Lastly, another class of full-mutation alleles is comprised of those with over 200 repeats, but which are only partially methylated or completely unmethylated. This class is rare and is usually found in a mosaic state in DNA from peripheral blood. Among individuals with reduced methylation, FMRP levels appeared to be reduced in nonneuronal biopsy tissues in a few cases.[68,69] Feng et al.[68] presented evidence that *FMR1* transcripts containing large expansions are not well translated. Thus, methylation status and the repeat length among the transcribed alleles influence the amount of FMRP produced by mosaic individuals. Moreover, it should be considered that nearly all laboratory evaluation of *FMR1* and its expression is based on nonneuronal tissue. Given the frequent degree of mosaicism involving both methylation and repeat length, clinical correlations with such data may not be accurate in the individual patient.

Gene Structure and Expression

The *FMR1* gene maps precisely within the gap of the fragile X site at Xq27.3.[70,71] The gene is composed of 17 exons spanning approximately 40 kb.[54] The entire gene has been completely sequenced within 185,775 bp of contiguous sequence (GenBank L29074) and is transcribed centromeric to telomeric. No additional genes have been identified in the sequenced region.

A number of polymorphisms, in addition to the CGG repeats, have been described in the vicinity of the *FMR1* gene. Several of these have been utilized in studies to track background chromosomes. Three microsatellites (DXS548,[72] FRAXAC1, and FRAXAC2[73]) have been characterized extensively, as have the single nucleotide polymorphisms (SNPs) FMRa and FMRb,[49] and the more recently described SNPs ATL1 through ATL4.[74] The *FMR1* gene structure and positions of these polymorphisms are shown in Fig. 64-3.

Several of the *FMR1* exons are alternatively spliced, leading to a number of potentially different mRNAs and protein isoforms.[45,75] Numerous distinct isoforms of FMRP, including some with alternative reading frames resulting in shorter C-termini and strikingly altered biochemical properties, have been predicted (see Biochemistry of FMRP below). Western blot analysis demonstrates several protein products ranging from 70 to 80 kDa.[76,77] Widespread expression of *FMR1* is seen in both human and mouse embryos.[78,79] The protein product of the *FMR1* gene has been found present in many adult and fetal tissues, but is most evident in neurons.[80] In 8- and 9-week-old human fetuses, *FMR1* mRNA was observed in the nervous system, retina, and several nonneuronal tissues, and in the 25 week-old human fetal brain, mRNA expression was observed in nearly all differentiated structures, with the highest level in cholinergic neurons of the nucleus basalis magnocellularis, and in pyramidal neurons of hippocampus.[78] Similar concentration of FMRP is found in brain neurons throughout various brain regions, although the apparent high level of expression in certain brain regions was thought to reflect neuron density rather than enhanced expression.[81] High levels of *FMR1* are also found in cells of the testis, primarily spermatogonia.[80,82] In epithelia, a decreasing gradient of *FMR1* expression is observed from the layer of dividing cells to more differentiated cells.[80] For example, in skin, the dermis layer is negative for expression while the epidermis exhibits a decreasing gradient of *FMR1* expression from the basal layer of dividing cells to the keratinized layer. These data also point to the common misstatement in the literature regarding *FMR1* expression as being ubiquitous; it is better stated as being widespread, as some cell types clearly have undetectable expression. Hergersberg et al.[83] produced transgenic mice with the *FMR1* promoter driving the β-galactosidase reporter gene. Five transgenic mouse lines showed lacZ expression in the brain, in particular, in neurons of the hippocampus and the granular layer of the cerebellum. Expression of the reporter gene was also detected in Leydig cells and spermatogonia in the testis, in many epithelia of adult mice, and in the two other steroidogenic cell types, adrenal cortex cells and ovarian follicle cells. Embryonic tissues, which showed strong activity of the reporter gene, included the telencephalon, the genital ridge, and the notochord. The expression of FMRP in the brain and testes is consistent with the major phenotypic aspects of the disorder.

Gene Conservation

The *FMR1* coding sequence is highly conserved in vertebrate evolution; homologues have been characterized from the mouse,[45] the chicken,[84] and *Xenopus laevis*.[85] The level of predicted amino acid identity from human through *Xenopus* is approximately 90 percent, making *FMR1* more highly conserved than most other proteins. In contrast, homologues from nonvertebrates are not as obvious in databases. While a *Drosophila* gene that has some similarity to *FMR1* has been found, its characterization has yet to be published (G. Dreyfuss, personal communication). Query of the yeast database does not reveal a close homologue; a *Saccharomyces cerevisiae* protein involved in the control of ploidy (*Scp160*), however, reveals conservation of many of the domains found in FMRP. Although *Scp160* shares some biochemical attributes with FMRP,[86,87] it more closely matches the protein vigilin.[88]

Amongst mammals, the *FMR1* gene is also highly conserved at the DNA level. The 5′-UTR has been found to carry CGG repeats in approximately the same location in all placental mammals, as well as marsupials, indicating that the repeat has been conserved over 150 million years of mammalian radiation.[89] In the chicken, which diverged from mammals more than 350 million years ago, the 5′ UTR of *FMR1* contains a CCT repeat, instead of a CGG tract.[84] Although such conservation implies a functional significance to the repeat, no function has yet emerged. Indeed, there may be no function, as a normal individual, expressing normal levels of FMRP, has been reported with a 97-bp microdeletion of the entire CGG repeat with the transcriptional and translational start sites unchanged.[90] Despite this, a 20-kDa human protein, which specifically binds to the double-stranded CGG repeat of *FMR1*, has been identified.[91,92] Although the function of this protein is unclear, its mere presence suggests that the CGG repeat, or other similar repeats in the genome, serve some function.

FMR1 MUTATIONS

FMR1 Mutations Other Than Repeat Expansions

The fragile X syndrome is clinically defined as an MR syndrome, with a distinctive phenotypic constellation of signs, in association with the folate-sensitive fragile site at Xq27.3; it is caused by a singular *FMR1* mutation, that being the unstable expansion of a CGG trinucleotide repeat in the 5′-UTR.[22,43,44,46,47] Other mutations of *FMR1* are encountered, but at a much-reduced frequency as compared to the repeat expansion mutation. Aside from a single missense mutation discussed below,[93] these mutations typically predict null outcomes for *FMR1* expression, such as deletions[94–102] and point mutations leading to frameshifts and/or abnormal exon splicing.[103,104] These patients usually present with a more or less typical fragile X syndrome phenotype, but without expression of the cytogenetic fragile site. Thus, these patients provide evidence that expression of the fragile site requires repeat expansion, and that there do not appear to be genes near *FMR1* that contribute to the fragile X phenotype. Indeed, *FMR1* appears to be located in a rather gene-poor region, as very large deletions have also been reported with little change in the clinical presentation. For example, a 3-Mb deletion of *FMR1* was found in a patient with typical fragile X syndrome;[105] a deletion of a portion of *FMR1* and 7 to 10 Mb of proximal sequence was identified in a patient with typical fragile X syndrome;[106] and a 9-Mb distal deletion extending 500 kb proximal to *FMR1* was observed in a typical patient with obesity and anal atresia.[107] A 13-Mb deletion of *FMR1* extending 1 Mb telomeric and approximately 12 Mb centromeric in a patient with profound mental retardation, fragile X facies, and lower limb skeletal defects and contractures has been reported,[108] along with a patient with typical fragile X syndrome and Hunter syndrome, carrying a 5 Mb deletion extending from proximal (centromeric) *FMR1* through the IDS locus.[109] Taken together, these data suggest that there are no clinically evident genes within a Mb flanking either side of *FMR1*.

Some of the smaller deletions of *FMR1* show evidence for preferential sites of breakage. At least four patients have been reported in whom one of the breakpoints is within the CGG repeat itself.[94,110,111] In most of these instances, the deletion was derived from a premutation allele, indicating that the instability of the premutation can lead to deletions as well as expansion, although it remains to be seen if these two outcomes of premutations are mechanistically linked. An intriguing series of patients has been described with common deletion breakpoints between 53 and 75 bp upstream of the CGG repeat.[94,96] Although most of these breakpoints are immediately distal to sequences similar to a chi-like element, the mechanism of these deletions remains unclear.

FMR1 Expansions in Families

Prevalence. As mentioned previously, chromosome analysis was the diagnostic tool used until 1992 to detect the fragile X syndrome-associated fragile site located at Xq27.3. This cytogenetic test was not ideal for several reasons. First, it lacked the sensitivity to detect the mutation in nonexpressing heterozygous females and premutation carrier males. Secondly, the presence of nearby fragile sites, *FRAXE* and *FRAXF* led to false positive results. Finally, chromosome analysis is labor-intensive and expensive, prohibiting large-scale population testing. In terms of the sensitivity of the test with respect to the fragile X syndrome (i.e., the probability of fragile X expression given an individual has the fragile X syndrome), the presence of the fragile X site is a good diagnostic marker for fragile X-related MR in males and a relatively good one for fragile X-related MR in females. Prevalence studies based on the cytogenetic test are reviewed in Sherman et al.[19]

The advent of DNA-based testing enables identification of both expressing and nonexpressing carriers, and is relatively less expensive than cytogenetic testing. The diagnostic test determines the size of the repeat region. Thus, it can be used to identify pre- and full-mutation carriers. This test has close to 100 percent specificity and is approximately 98 percent sensitive, missing only those cases with point mutations or small deletions. It is now the test of choice in a clinical setting (see Molecular Diagnostics below regarding criteria for testing).

The limitation of the cytogenetic test to determine the prevalence of fragile X syndrome was recognized when studies of Turner et al.[112] and Webb et al.[113] were reanalyzed by testing fragile X-positive males, using the DNA diagnostic test for fragile X syndrome.[113a] They found an indication of a high false positive rate (29 to 62 percent) in both studies and attributed most to the expression of other fragile X sites. On final analysis, the prevalence of the fragile X syndrome was estimated to be approximately 1/4000 males.

Subsequent studies using the DNA diagnostic test surveyed target populations (i.e., those with some defined intellectual disability) and extrapolated to the general population using the assumption that individuals with the fragile X syndrome would only be identified in that target population. To date, the fragile X syndrome has been identified in every studied ethnic group.[19] Studies to compare the prevalence among ethnic groups are limited. One study conducted in Israel found that the majority of families diagnosed with fragile X syndrome were Tunisian Jews;[114] thus, the prevalence may vary in isolated populations. However, in larger admixed populations, there is little evidence of prevalence differences.[58] A representative set of studies for males, published since 1996, is summarized in Table 64-2. Comparisons between studies of the prevalence among specific types of target populations cannot be made because of differences in the definitions of MR, and because of the methods of ascertainment (e.g., clinical referral versus surveys). However, the prevalence in the general population ranges from 1/2380 to 1/6045, with most studies finding around 1/4500.

The prevalence of the fragile X syndrome in females has not been estimated empirically but only inferred. First, based on the dynamics of the mutation, the frequency of carriers of full mutations is equal in males and females. This is the result of the absence of paternal transmission. The absence of paternal

Table 64-2 Prevalence of the Fragile X Syndrome in Males in Target Populations and Projected General Population (References from 1996 to 1998).

Reference	Country	Target Population	N. of positive/N. of tested	Estimate Prevalence	
				Target Pop'n*	General (95% CI†)
Faradz et al.[189]	Indonesia (primarily Javanese)	Schools for mild DD, miminum dysmorphology, no cytogenetic abnormality	5/262	Mild MR: 1.9%	
de Vries et al.[390]	South-west Netherlands	Schools and institutes for mentally retarded, no known etiology	Mild MR: 4/333 Mod/sev.: 5/533	Mild MR: 2.0% Mod/sev.: 2.4%	1/6045 (1/9981-1/3851)
Patsalis et al.[60]	Hellenic population of Greece and Cyprus	Referred clinical population of idiopathic mental retardation	8/611	MR: 1.3%	1/4246 (1/16440-1/1333)
Murray et al.[59]	Wessex, U.K.	Special education needs school population of unknown etiology	5/1013	SEN: 0.5%	1/4994 (1/11112-1/2364)
Elbaz et al.[391]	Guadeloupe, French West Indies	Special education needs school population of unknown etiology	11/163	SEN: 6.7%	1/2359 (1/4484-1/1276)
Mazzocco et al.[315]	Baltimore, MD (including Caucasians and African-Americans)	Preschool children referred for language delay	1/379	Language delay: 0.3%	
Goldman et al.[392]	South African Blacks	Institutionalized males with idiopathic mental retardation	9/148	MR: 6.1% Mild: 4.2% Sev.: 7.8%	
Haddad et al.[313]	Brazil	Boys attending schools for the mentally handicaped	5/256	MR: 2.0% Mild: 2.3% Sev.: 1.6%	
Crawford et al.[58]	Atlanta, GA	Special education needs school population	Caucasian: 4/1972 African-Amer: 1/421	SEN: Caucasian: 0.3% African-Amer: 0.2%	Caucasian: 1/3448 (1/7143-1/1742) African-Amer: 1/4000 (1/16260-1/1244)

*MR = mental retardation; SEN = special education needed; DD = developmental disabilities; Mod = moderate MR; SEV = severe MR.
† Confidence intervals (CI) were based on the total number of individuals in the general population, not on the tested population. Thus, these confidence intervals are underestimates (more narrow) and only provide a guide.

transmission of full mutations, due to both reduced male fitness and repeat stability in spermatogenesis, (see Population Dynamics for further explanation of expected carrier frequencies given the trinucleotide inheritance pattern). Assuming only about 50 percent of female carriers show clinical symptoms of the fragile X syndrome, the prevalence of the symptomatic syndrome in females is approximately 1/9000.

Large surveys to establish the prevalence of premutation male and female carriers are summarized in Table 64-3. The largest surveys to date were conducted by Rousseau et al.[115] They surveyed a large, anonymous sample of males and females from a population of over 600,000 individuals in the Québec City metropolitan area. They used blood samples remaining from a consecutive series of routine hemoglobin/hematocrit or complete blood counts from 10,572 males and 10,624 female outpatients who attended a general hospital in Québec. Forty-one females with 55 repeats or more were identified, leading to a heterozygote carrier frequency of 1/259 (95 percent confidence interval: 1/373 to 1/198).[115] Fourteen males with 54 repeats or more were identified leading to a hemizygote frequency of 1/755 (95 percent confidence interval: 1/1327 to 1/138).

Using the definition of 60 repeats or more as a definition of premutations, the frequencies found in the Quebec study are similar to those found in other large admixed populations (Table 64-3). If we estimate that approximately 1/1000 males and 1/400 females carry a premutation, the female-to-male ratio (2.5:1) is higher than the ratio of 2:1 expected for a simple X-linked dominant disorder, but fits models of inheritance of a dynamic repeat sequence as described below.

Inheritance Pattern of FMR1 Repeat Mutation

Although the exact mechanism that causes expansion of the CGG repeats is unknown, it has been observed that the number of repeats most often increases as it is passed from parent to offspring (Fig. 64-4). Although contractions are also observed,[46,116] all full mutations are derived from premutations, which explains why no new mutations have been observed (i.e., the normal form of the *FMR1* gene becoming a premutation gene), as ancestors of several

Table 64-3 Prevalence of Premutation Carriers (95% Confidence Interval)

Reference	Country	Target Population	Definition of Premutation	Males	Females
Ryynanen et al.[393]	Finland	Pregnant women seeking prenatal care	≥60 repeats		1/246(1/605-1/107)
Reiss et al.[394]	U.S.	Families with other genetic disorders	≥60 repeats	0/416	1/561 (1/10747-1/87)
Rousseau et al.[115]	Quebec, Canada	consecutive hemoglobin/hematocrit or complete blood count on outpatients from a public hosital	≥60 repeats		1/354 (1/515-1/248)
Rousseau et al.[395]	Quebec, Canada	consecutive hemoglobin/hematocrit or complete blood count on outpatients from a public hospital	≥54 repeats	1/755 (1/1327-1/438)	
Murray et al.[59]	Wessex, U.K.	Special education needs school boys	≥60 repeats	1/1013 (1/19406-1/157)	
Dawson et al.[396*]	Manitoba, Canada	Consecutive births	≥60 repeats	1/778 (1/14904-1/120)	0/735
Holden et al.[397]	Ontario, Canada	Consecutive births	≥60 repeats	1/1000 (1/19157-1/155)	
Patsalis et al.[60]	Hellenic population of Greece and Cyprus	Mental retardation of unknown etiology	?	1/305 (1/1763-1/76)	
Crawford et al.[58]	Georgia, U.S.	Special education needs school children	≥60 repeats	1/1206(1/3508-1/534)	1/436(1/1268-1/190)

*These are probably underestimates because of technical difficulties

older generations are not available for study. The dynamic mutation process also explains why the risk for the fragile X syndrome increases in each generation: the number of repeats expands through most transmissions, and after it exceeds 200 repeats, the gene is silenced. The magnitude of the increase is greater when transmitted by a female carrier than by a male carrier. A female carrier has a 50 percent chance of passing the unstable *FMR1* gene to her offspring, as is true for any X-linked gene. The risk of expansion from the female carrier's premutation to the full mutation is high and depends on her repeat number.[19,46,51,57,116,117] For example, less than 5 percent of premutation alleles with less than 60 repeats expand to the full mutation, whereas about 50 percent of those with 60 to 80 repeats, and almost all of those with 90 or more repeats, expand to the full mutation (Fig. 64-5). In keeping with X-linked inheritance, a male premutation carrier has a 100 percent chance of passing his premutation to all of his daughters and to none of his sons. In most cases, his *FMR1* repeat region does not change dramatically when transmitted to his daughters; in fact, the repeat size decreases or remains the same in about 30 to 40 percent of transmissions.[57,118] Interestingly, the rate of contraction is correlated with increasing repeat size in the carrier father.[57,119] The risk of expansion to the full mutation is extremely small, if any.

The pattern of instability of premutation alleles explains the unusual inheritance pattern observed in early segregation studies of the fragile X-related MR.[20,21] The decreased risk of having offspring with fragile X syndrome among mothers of transmitting males compared with mothers of affected males can be explained by the fact that mothers of transmitting males will carry, on average, smaller premutation alleles than those who have affected males. Although not understood, the observation that transmitting males do not have fragile X syndrome daughters is accounted for by the fact that the premutation is rather stable in paternal transmissions as compared to maternal transmissions. This may be related to severe instability of the full mutations in sperm leading to contraction as compared to minimal contraction in eggs with full mutations (see Timing of Expansion below). Other factors that influence the expansion of the premutation, in addition to repeat size and sex of the carrier parent, have been examined, including parental age, origin of the grandparental allele, sex of the offspring,[119] and a familial factor.[57] Only an as yet unidentified familial factor was found to significantly influence rates of expansion. That is, offspring of premutation siblings had more similar repeat expansions than had unrelated offspring.[57] Also, there was a trend for increased rates of expansion to the full mutation among premutation carrier females who received their mutation from fathers as compared to those who received their mutation from mothers,[119] although more data are needed to confirm this finding. Observed associations with parental age[120] and sex of the offspring[121,122] could be explained by an apparent bias resulting from somatic selection against full mutations and timing of the diagnostic test, and by an apparent bias of incomplete testing of sibships, respectively.[119]

Timing of Expansion

Two time periods for the expansion of the premutation have been implicated: meiosis and early embryonic development. Expansion must occur in germ cells (either during premeiotic or meiotic division) in order to explain the increased risk of the fragile X syndrome (i.e., the full mutation) in each succeeding generation (i.e., anticipation). Several observations indicate that postzygotic instability also must occur. First, full mutation carriers are found to

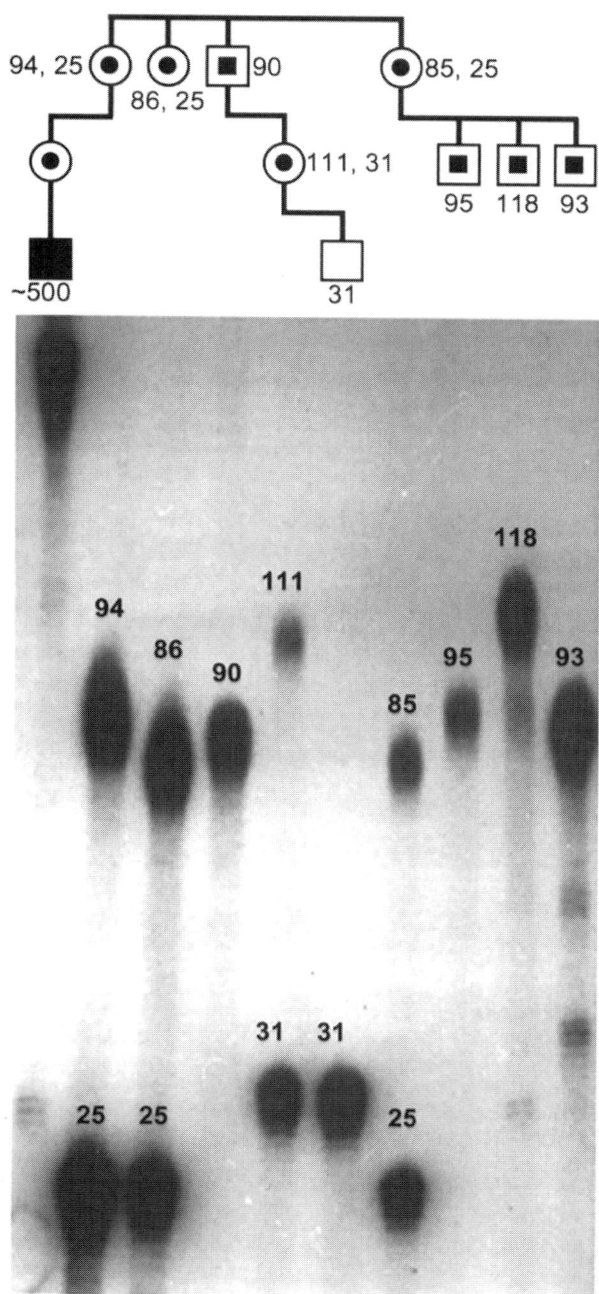

Fig. 64-4 **PCR amplification of the *FMR1* CGG repeat in an affected family. Partially filled symbols indicate premutation allele carriers and the filled symbol is an affected male. Allele repeat numbers are indicated. Note the stability of normal alleles (31 and 25 repeats) when transmitted in contrast to the instability of all larger premutation alleles. (*Modified from Warren and Nelson.*[333] *Used by permission.*)**

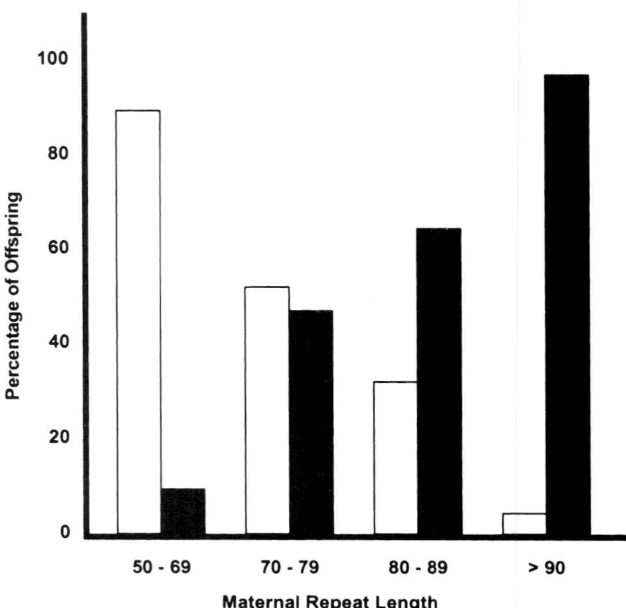

Fig. 64-5 **Probability of either a premutation or a full mutation offspring based upon the maternal premutation repeat length. Percentage of offspring refers to those receiving the mutant allele. *Open bar* premutation; *Fill bar* full mutation. (*Data from Ashley-Koch.*[119])**

be somatic mosaics; that is, repeat sizes vary from tissue to tissue and within a tissue of a full-mutation carrier.[123,124] However, this somatic instability is thought to occur in an early window of postzygotic development because the variability among tissues is not extensive. Reports examining full mutations in fetal tissues[124–126] and in adult postmortem studies[127,128] sometimes show little or no variability among tissues. Furthermore, in vitro studies of cells cultured from different tissues of a full mutation carrier show clonal stability.[126] Data from monozygotic twins also support this idea: some twins show similar patterns, while others show discordant patterns of their *FMR1* alleles in blood,[124,129–131] the inconsistent result indicating instability early in embryogenesis.

The observation that full mutation males have only premutation-size alleles in their sperm[132,133] led Reyniers et al.[132] to propose that expansion from the premutation to the full mutation occurs postzygotically during early embryonic development, but sometime after primordial germ line cells are differentiated. This model also had to include a sex-specific mechanism to explain why expansion to the full mutation occurs only on maternal X-chromosomes. Alternatively, a prezygotic expansion model is possible if selection against full-mutation sperm and contraction to premutations are assumed.

Evidence seems to point to the prezygotic model. Selection against sperm with the full mutation at the protein level does not appear to occur, as the *FMR1* knockout mouse has normal spermatogenesis.[134] However, selection could occur at the level of DNA replication, favoring smaller premutations compared with full mutations. The large number of replication cycles occurring in spermatogenesis may enhance this type of selection[135] and may not require selection but simply the inability of spermatogenesis to maintain lengthy repeats. More directly, Malter et al.[136] showed that the testes of a 13-week full-mutation fetus showed no evidence of premutations, while a 17-week full-mutation fetus exhibited some germ cells with attributes of premutations. These data discount the hypothesis that the germ line is protected from full expansion, and suggest full-mutation contraction in the immature testis. Malter et al.[136] also examined intact ovaries of full mutation fetuses and found only full expansion alleles, but in the unmethylated state. Thus, expansion to the full mutation likely occurs during oogenesis or possibly during very early embryonic development prior to germ line segregation.

The prezygotic expansion model can also explain the characteristics of the observed somatic mosaicism. First, this model predicts that mosaicism results from random contractions of some full mutations, presumably a stochastic process. As predicted, the proportion of full-mutation alleles is almost always higher than premutation alleles in a mosaic individual. Furthermore, if the postzygotic model is true, there should be significant variation in repeat numbers among tissues. Although there is some intertissue variation, it does not seem to be at the level expected for postzygotic expansion. Furthermore, there does seem to be a correlation between the level of mosaicism and the severity of the fragile X syndrome (see Clinical Aspects below). This is not expected if there are large variations among tissues (i.e., peripheral blood versus brain tissue). Also, Moutou et al.[135] predicted from computer simulations of the postzygotic expansion model that the frequency of mosaic offspring would be higher among mothers with smaller premutations. However, there was no such association in a large series of 112 carrier mothers with 212 carrier offspring. Lastly, the ratio of female-to-male carriers of premutations fits the premeiotic model better than the postzygotic model (see Population Dynamics below).

Population Dynamics

Efforts to examine the population dynamics of the fragile X mutation using computer modeling have led to specific predictions that can help elucidate the mechanism of expansion and the factors that influence mutation rates. The cornerstone of all generated models is the underlying estimation of the rates of expansion from one mutant allele to another (transition matrix). All are limited in some way by the lack of empirical data on paternal transmissions and by the small amount of data on maternal transmissions of the premutated allele. Each investigator used a different approach to work with this limitation. For example, Kolehmainen[137] used the empirically derived probabilities from females and extrapolated them to male transmissions. Morris et al.[138] derived probability functions based on the empirical data and used them to determine the transition matrices. Ashley and Sherman[139] assumed an underlying biologic process and fit the parameters of that process to the empirical data to derive transition probabilities. In spite of the different underlying assumptions of each model, several predictions were found to be common to all models.

In a simple two-step model, Winter[140] was the first to show that the predicted frequency of full mutation carrier males at equilibrium is equal to that of full-mutation carrier females. Furthermore, these frequencies only depend on the initial mutation rate from a stable normal allele to a less stable allele still present in the "normal" population (i.e., protomutation) and on the selection against full-mutation carrier males and females. Thus, the number of steps to expand from a premutation allele to the full mutation, the number of premutation alleles, and the rate of transition from one premutation allele to another, have no consequence on the frequency of the fragile X syndrome at equilibrium. This first generalization was found to hold true for all models that assumed a similar pattern of fitness and a lack of expansion of paternal alleles to the full mutation.[137,138,140–143] Thus, assuming complete lack of fitness among males with fragile X syndrome, complete fitness of females with fragile X syndrome (probably an overestimate), and the prevalence among males as 1/4500 (Table 64-2), the mutation rate at equilibrium of the change of a normal allele of less stability (such as an allele with a longer tract of pure CGG repeats) is approximately 7.4×10^{-5}. This estimate is based on a lack of expansion to the full mutation in sperm. If it is assumed that expansion occurs, but that full-mutation sperm are completely selected against, then the mutation rate is estimated to be 11.1×10^{-5} because there would be two levels of complete selection, one against full-mutation sperm of premutation males, and one against males with the fragile X syndrome.[144]

The second generalization is that the frequency of premutation alleles at equilibrium is completely dependent on the probabilities of expansion, as expected.

The third generalization is that the approach to equilibrium is most affected by the transition probabilities and the number of possible steps to proceed from the initial premutation to the full mutation. The approach is (a) inversely proportional to the transition rate of the initial premutation allele to the next, and (b) slowed by the increasing number of steps from the initial premutation to the full mutation. As an example, it takes approximately 180 generations to reach equilibrium assuming a simple 3-step model and an initial transition rate of 0.006[142] or approximately 500 generations assuming an 8-step model and a transition rate of 0.017.[137] The approach to equilibrium does not differ significantly when both meiotic and early embryonic expansion processes are assumed, compared with meiotic expansion only. This observation suggests that the transition probabilities affect the approach to equilibrium much more than pressures of selection. More importantly, predictions concerning magnitude of the mutation rate and the factors that affect the approach to equilibrium (i.e., the expansion mechanism) lead to possible explanations for the association of the fragile X mutation with specific haplotypes (see Haplotype Association Studies below).

Comparison of carrier frequencies predicted at equilibrium for models assuming different time points of expansion is instructive.[144] For models that assume prezygotic expansion and subsequent selection against sperm with full mutations or complete lack of expansion in sperm, the ratio of female to male carrier frequencies of premutation alleles is predicted to be approximately 2.6. In contrast, the model that assumes that prezygotic expansion is similar in egg and sperm, and that subsequent postzygotic expansion is restricted to maternal X-chromosomes, predicts that the female-to-male ratio is approximately 1.2.[139] The observed data from prevalence studies show a 2.5 ratio, which provides indirect evidence for the prezygotic expansion/selection against the full-mutation model.

Ethnic Variation in FMR1 Repeat Alleles

Examination of the variation of the repeat structure, both repeat number and AGG interspersion pattern, in open and closed populations provides information concerning the evolution of the sequence and mutational process. Allele distributions among large admixed racial groups vary significantly, although the overall pattern is similar. For example, the allele distribution among African-Americans is significantly different than that among Caucasians. The difference is primarily due to the lack of intermediate and smaller alleles among African-Americans as compared to Caucasians.[58,145] The allele distributions of a Chinese population also show differences from Caucasians: the most frequent allele is 29 instead of 30 repeats in Caucasians and there is a lack of smaller alleles (20 to 22 repeats).[146] The Japanese allele distribution differs again: the most frequent allele is 28, and there is a higher frequency of alleles with 35 repeats as compared to Caucasians.[147]

With respect to the AGG interspersion pattern, two studies examined closed human populations. Eichler and Nelson[148] studied six closed populations and, despite the extensive genetic isolation and distance among populations (about 200,000 years), found that the structure of the repeat sequence was remarkably conserved. Interestingly, the heterozygosity observed for the *FMR1* alleles among the six closed populations were similar to the average of 30 microsatellite loci in the human genome.[148] Also, the estimated heterozygosity based on the repeat number and AGG pattern was not significantly greater than that based only on repeat number. This suggests that the position of the AGG interruptions has been largely invariant over time. Of course, ethnic differences were observed. For example, Native American alleles were interrupted by more than two AGG repeats,[148,149] compared with open admixed Caucasian alleles that usually have one or two interruptions. Kunst et al.[149] studied nine global populations with origins in Asia, Africa, and Native America, and found that the level of heterozygosity that did exist was correlated with the age and/or genetic history of a particular population. Results from both studies indicated that the ancestral allele structure was $(CGG)_9AGG(CGG)_9AGG(CGG)_9$ (from here on, referred to as 9+9+9, the + indicating the AGG interruption).

Examination of repeat patterns in higher primates shows a somewhat different interspersion pattern than humans.[53,89] Parsimony analysis predicts that expansion of the CGG repeat beyond 20 repeats has occurred in three different primate lineages. In man and gorilla, AGG interruptions occur with higher-order periodicity.[89]

Haplotype-Association Studies

When haplotype studies of tightly linked small-tandem repeat polymorphisms (STRs) surrounding the *FMR1* repeat region were initiated, it was predicted that associations would not be found in large, admixed populations. This expectation was based on basic population genetic principles: a high rate of recurrent mutations should lead to the abnormal allele being found on all haplotype backgrounds at frequencies similar to those found in the sampled population. These expectations were found to be much too simple. The first study to note a haplotype association was that of Richards et al.[150] Using a haplotype based on FRAXAC1 and FRAXAC2 dinucleotide flanking markers (see Fig. 64-3), they found that three haplotypes accounted for only 15 percent of the normal Caucasian population, compared with 58 percent of the fragile X syndrome population. In contrast, one haplotype that was found in 50 percent of the normal population was found in only 18 percent of the fragile X syndrome population. Other investigators saw similar patterns in European populations.[151–158] Using haplotypes based on three flanking STRs (DXS548, FRAXAC1, and FRAXAC2), Macpherson et al.[159] noted that the fragile X mutation was found on a highly diverse set of haplotypes, some of which were in equilibrium with the population, while others were not. Also, the fragile X mutation is found on a few backgrounds observed in the normal population and on backgrounds that have never been seen in the normal population (see review in reference 143). Of course, founder effects were expected, and have been identified in the more genetically isolated populations, such as the Finns[151,160] or the Tunisian Jews.[114] Chiurazzi et al.[161] found that the major fragile X syndrome haplotypes were common to the different European nations and seemed to be distributed along geographical gradients.

Given the confirmed association of specific haplotypes with the fragile X mutation, it would be predicted that the same pattern of associations would be seen among intermediate *FMR1* alleles (40 to 60 repeats). This expectation is based on the assumption that a proportion of intermediate alleles represents the early phase of mutated alleles, those that are already unstable and beginning to expand. Thus, these are assumed to be the pool of susceptible alleles. Surprisingly, only one haplotype was found to be associated with intermediate alleles in both a British[159] and an American population[49] not the expected diversity of haplotypes seen among those associated with the fragile X full mutation. This phenomenon was also seen in a French-Canadian population, although the specific associated haplotype was different than that found in the British and American populations.[115] Results from haplotype studies suggest two alternative hypotheses or a combination of the two models: (a) associations are due to different mutational pathways, each having different rates of mutation and expansion, or (b) associations are due to equilibrium having not been achieved among normal and mutated alleles.

Haplotype studies of normal *FMR1* alleles characterized by repeat number and AGG interspersion patterns are also intriguing, as they, too, reveal significant associations (Fig. 64-6).[48–50,52,53,162] For example, Kunst and Warren[49] examined 172 *FMR1* alleles from a predominantly Caucasian population and based haplotypes primarily on FRAXAC1. These studies revealed that normal alleles with greater than 24 perfect 3′ CGG repeats appeared more frequently on haplotypes overrepresented among fragile X syndrome chromosomes. Similar results were reported by others.[50,52] Both Kunst and Warren[49] and Snow et al.[50] noted that the one haplotype associated with intermediate alleles was less frequent than among fragile X mutations (approximately 50 percent as compared to 25 percent, respectively). One explanation for these results may be that equilibrium between certain predisposed alleles and the fragile X mutation has not yet been attained. Further work on 345 chromosomes from 9 global populations provided support for this hypothesis; the level of heterogeneity of allelic forms correlated with the age and/or genetic history of a particular population.[149] For example, the older African populations showed no haplotype association with the repeat alleles. This contrasts with the strong association observed among Caucasians, and may be due in part to the relatively more recent origin of Europeans as compared to Africans.

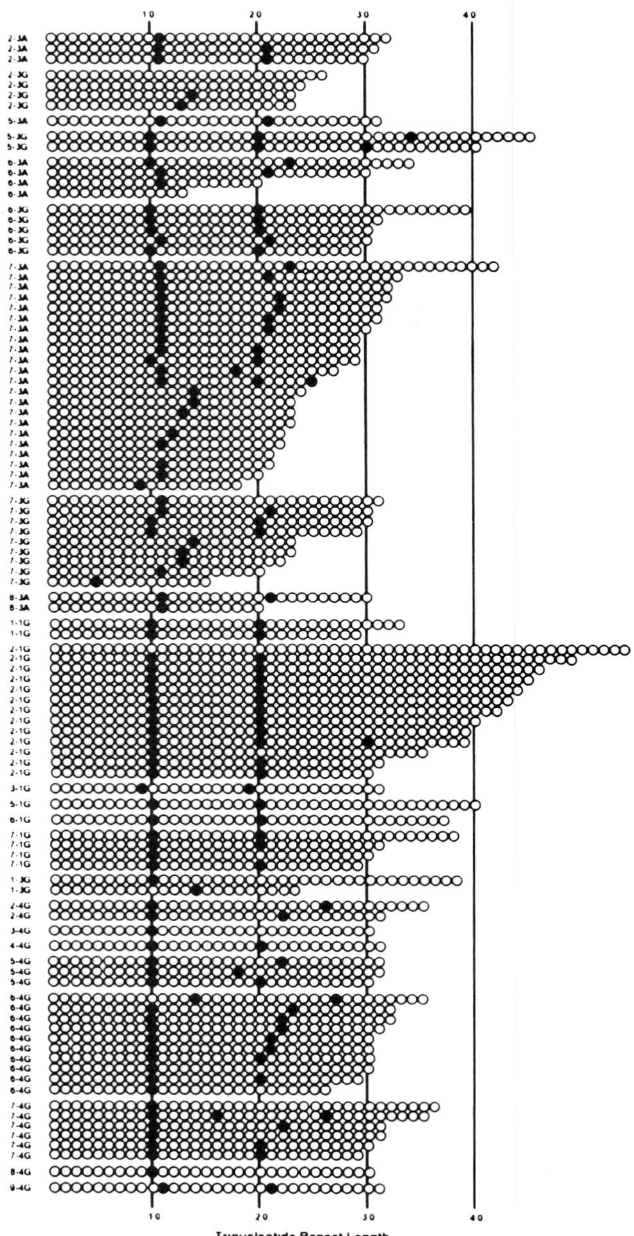

Fig. 64-6 One hundred and one unique normal alleles of *FMR1* based on haplotype and repeat length and complexity. Haplotype is given on the left as alleles for DXS548-AC1, ATL1 as described in Gunter et al.[74] Open circles are CGG repeats and filled circles are AGG interruptions.

Eichler et al.[162] extended the association studies among Caucasians by using haplotypes based on the same three flanking STRs markers (DXS548, FRAXAC1, and FRAXAC2), and defined *FMR1* alleles by repeat number and AGG pattern. Association patterns identified were similar to others,[49,50] but the interpretation differed. Eichler et al.[162] suggested that the observed significant associations in this normal population were due to differential mutational pathways, each having a different rate of the initial mutation and of subsequent expansion. Two general mutational pathways appeared predominant. One was hypothesized to involve the loss of distal AGG interruptions and subsequent large increases in repeat size. It was speculated that asymmetry of the CGG-AGG repeat pattern may influence this mutational process. The other pathway was thought to involve small increases of one or two CGG repeats distal to the most 3′ AGG, indicating some process similar to replication slippage. This pathway was assumed to evolve more slowly toward the hyperexpansion state. The eight-generation family reported by Smits et al.[163] may be an example of this pathway.

Finally, a recent study used single nucleotide polymorphisms (SNPs: ATL1, ATL2, and FMRb) in addition to the three STRs to define the haplotype background of normal and fragile X syndrome chromosomes.[74] The mutation rates of SNPs are usually much lower than those of STRs, and thus may reveal more about the history of various *FMR1* mutations. Use of the more stable SNP markers redefined the relationships between the STR markers and the *FMR1* repeat, which is itself a specialized STR. First, Gunter et al.[74] showed that the variation of the *FMR1* repeat sequence is proportional to the age of the chromosome, as would be expected. For example, there was extensive variation throughout the *FMR1* repeat on the evolutionarily "oldest" chromosomes compared with only 3′ variation on more recent derivative chromosomes. This pattern was also true for the flanking STR markers in that there were more STR haplotypes on the chromosomes of more advanced "age" as defined by the SNP haplotype, compared with the more recent chromosomes. Also, the frequency of fragile X mutations on specific haplotype backgrounds was proportional to the age of the chromosome, as expected.

Interestingly, there were apparent differences in susceptibility to mutational mechanisms leading to instability between what seemed to be similar repeat arrays, 9 + 9 + 9 and 10 + 9 + 9; the 9 + 9 + 9 array appeared more susceptible to instability mechanisms than the 10 + 9 + 9, which appeared to be the more recent mutation.

It is clear that the correct interpretation of the haplotype associations and the repeat structure depends on an understanding of the mutational mechanism responsible for the instability of the repeat and selection pressures, if any, of the repeat structure. There are, clearly, several ways to generate an increased number of 3′ pure CGG repeats, including point mutations, strand slippage, gene conversion, or unequal crossing-over. Although the overall mutation rate of 7.4 to 11.1×10^{-5} is too high to result in founder effects, each specific mutational pathway could occur at much lower rates and, in combination with dynamics of the population, could be expected to be associated with specific haplotype backgrounds.[161] The only way to resolve many of the remaining questions will be direct examination of the repeat unit in model systems.

MECHANISMS OF EXPANSION

The mechanism of trinucleotide repeat expansion remains elusive, and is one of the great mysteries surrounding this entire class of disease. Although unequal exchange has historically led to sequence duplications and deletions, unequal exchange between homologues is not responsible for dynamic mutation. The most obvious data in this regard are the numerous linkage studies carried out of fragile X syndrome families and families segregating other dynamic mutations. An obligatory exchange mechanism of expansion would have been revealed by exchange of flanking markers and/or exaggeration of the genetic distance of a nearby marker. Because none of these events routinely occurred, exchange between homologues does not appear to be necessary. Sister chromatid exchange, however, is possible, but not easily monitored in humans. Similarly, gene conversion events could play a role, but also are more difficult to fully evaluate in humans. However, it should be noted that at least two probable gene conversion events have been reported at *FMR1*.[164,165] Thus, a gene conversion mechanism needs further exploration. Also, reports of very unusual families exhibiting high levels of repeat instability of otherwise normal *FMR1* alleles bring up the issue of *trans*-acting influences on stability, such as familial variation in mismatch repair.[166]

Replication Slippage

A replication-based mechanism based on DNA slippage is favored in the literature, at least for the relatively small increases associated with intermediate or "gray-zone" alleles and smaller premutation alleles. These changes generally involve an increase of 10 repeats or less and are similar in this regard to the other trinucleotide repeat expansion disorders involving CAG repeats. Several reported observations shed some insight into this form of instability. The changes appear polar, chiefly occurring at the 3′ end of the repeat array (relative to the direction of transcription).[48,49] This orientation is evident because of the interspersions of AGG triplets, which themselves appear to stabilize the repeat.[48,49,114,162,167–169] Taken together, a view has emerged that the length of the perfect 3′ repeat tract is critical in determining stability.[48,49] Kunst and Warren[49] showed evidence that alleles with 24 or greater perfect CGG repeats are "predisposed" toward instability, ultimately giving rise to premutations many generations later by occasional small, incremental increases in repeat length. Presumably, with each lengthening of the perfect repeat, the mutation rate of the new "protomutation" allele is greater than the previous allele of the prior generation. Indeed, Eichler et al.[48] demonstrated that when the perfect repeat tract reaches approximately 34 repeats, slippage can be observed in small nuclear families. These alleles, therefore, could change to premutations relatively quickly. However, many of these alleles still harbor one or more 5′ AGG interruptions at positions 10 and 20. Hence, these alleles may have a total repeat length of approximately 54 repeats, clearly within the gray-zone region. Similar total length repeat may, in contrast, contain three AGG interruptions, limiting the length of the perfect repeat, and presumably stabilizing the repeat tract relative to an allele of similar overall length, but with fewer interruptions. Indeed, the mutation rate of the *FMR1* repeat of two males with equivalent overall repeat length was elevated in the male with the longer perfect repeat tract.[169]

Therefore, if one considers that the length of the total *FMR1* repeat is generally an overestimate of the longest perfect repeat tract, the alleles that exhibit attributes of instability are those with approximately 25 to 35 perfect CGG repeats (which typically correspond to alleles with overall repeat lengths of 35 to 55 when considering AGG interruptions)[74] This perfect repeat range is remarkably similar to the length of other trinucleotide repeats, which also exhibit instability and expansion.[170] For example, the CAG repeat responsible for Huntington disease begins exhibiting instability at CAG lengths of greater than 29 repeats.[171] Thus, the relatively modest expansions of less than 20 repeats, seen in the majority of CAG expansions and *FMR1* premutations, may share a similar mechanism because they are dependent on a pure tract of similar-length repeats. Indeed, like *FMR1*, most normal alleles of the ataxin-1 locus (responsible for spinocerebellar ataxia type1) have an interruption of the repeat, while those infrequent alleles without interruptions (and, therefore, longer perfect CAG repeats) comprise the ancestral allelic pool from which expanded, disease-causing alleles are derived.[172] In both situations, such interruptions can also modify structural formations assumed by the repeats.[167]

A mechanism leading to polar variation could be differential fidelity of the leading versus the lagging strands of replication.[49] It has been demonstrated that in prokaryotic systems, the lagging strand is more prone to mutation than the leading strand, and that this mutational asymmetry is influenced by unusual DNA structure.[173] It is believed that if DNA strand slippage occurs within the replicating complex, the lagging strand polymerase elongates off slipped intermediates with a twentyfold higher frequency than the leading strand polymerase.[174] Thus, a single origin of replication near the *FMR1* repeat could result in the striking polarity of variation generated through lagging strand slippage.[49,162] Such a model suggests that the mutation rate leading to variation due to replication asymmetry is directly related to perfect repeat length. As a consequence, the mutation rate becomes extremely high at premutation lengths of 150 to 600 nucleotides (50 to 200 repeats). Such lengths exceed the normal mammalian Okazaki fragment length of 25 to 300 nucleotides.[175] Thus, even those alleles at the threshold of instability with 25 to 35 perfect repeats (75 to 105 nucleotides) could have a substantially increased propensity for slippage.

A model has been proposed in which slippage of perfect repeat Okazaki fragments leads to repeat expansion.[49,162,176] According to this model, for most normal alleles, the repeat region is shorter than most Okazaki fragments and anchored by flanking unique sequence. If longer but interrupted, the interruption could serve to anchor the Okazaki fragment. When the nascent strand contains a long perfect repeat, there is a possibility that the Okazaki fragment is entirely composed of repeats and, without a frame of reference, be prone to slippage. Although such a model may satisfy the observation of modest expansion events, it is not entirely clear how slippage could generate the massive elongation of the repeat when transiting from premutation to full mutation. It is quite possible that two distinct mechanisms may be involved, one involving slippage of modest proportions, and another resulting in massive expansion. However, all possible outcomes of slippage of trinucleotide repeats have not yet been fully explored, and data from simple experimental systems may implicate slippage even in the massive expansion associated with the full mutation.[177,178]

Another model, which is gaining experimental support, was proposed to account for the expansion of trinucleotide repeats. Gordenin et al. proposed that a key player in repeat instability is the RAD 27 endonuclease or, in mammals, the homologue flap endonuclease 1 (FEN1).[179] This endonuclease activity is responsible for the removal of the 5′ ribonucleotide, derived from the RNA primer, from the 5′ end of an Okazaki fragment that is displaced by the growing 3′ end of the preceding Okazaki fragment. The key aspect of FEN1 endonuclease activity is that the substrate (the displaced 5′ end of the Okazaki fragment, or the "flap") must be single-stranded in order to enter the luminal active site.[180] Hence, any intramolecular secondary structure of the flap formed by a trinucleotide repeat tract could result in a FEN1-resistant end. Such an end requires resolution by a recombination or an end-joining mechanism, either of which could lead to expansion of the trinucleotide repeat tract.[179] An appealing aspect of the model is that it accounts for the polar nature of the expansion process observed in actual *FMR1* alleles,[49] and invokes a structural change in the repeat array, which could lead to a threshold for repeat length instability.[181,182] Recent experimental evidence in model systems support this model.[183–186] Freudenreich et al. showed that CTG repeats in *Saccharomyces cerevisiae* were destabilized, and frequently expanded on a RAD27-deficient background.[185] Although the mammalian FEN1 has been cloned,[187] little is understood regarding its developmental and tissue expression patterns, nor has this locus been knocked out in mice. Therefore, evaluation of FEN1 and, by inference, the lagging strand of replication in trinucleotide repeat expansion, is still needed.

Replication Timing

The full mutation, involving both *FMR1* repeat expansion beyond 230 repeats and hypermethylation of the CpG island, has been shown to delay replication of the *FMR1* gene.[188,189] Although *FMR1* is normally rather late-replicating, toward the later stage of S, the full mutation is delayed beyond S into the G2/M boundary.[189] The extent of this effect of the CGG repeat is remarkable, influencing approximately 1.2 Mb surrounding *FMR1*.[190] It has been estimated that the boundaries of delayed replication extend approximately 400 kb centromeric and up to 600 kb telomeric, with the centromeric boundaries similar among different patients' cell lines, while the telomeric boundary varies somewhat.[191] Exposure of full mutation cell lines to the hypomethylation agent, 5-azadeoxycytidine, relieves this replication delay to some degree, suggesting that it is the methylation itself that is influencing replication, rather than just the repeat expansion.[192] Indeed, premutation cell lines, which have rather long repeats relative to any other repeats in the genome, do not significantly reduce replication timing, presumably because they exhibit the normal, hypomethylated state.[190] The mechanism of the delayed replication remains poorly understood. However, chromatin surrounding *FMR1* is less accessible to nucleases,[193,194] and exhibits altered chromatin assembly.[195,196]

Molecular Basis of the Fragile Site

The chromosomal fragile site at Xq27.3 is intertwined with the history of fragile X syndrome. The name of the syndrome, the initial diagnostic tests that led to defining the disorder and its genetics, and, ultimately, the cloning of the *FMR1* gene were based, in part, on the fragile site. Yet, a true understanding of the molecular mechanism of the fragile site remains elusive. It is known that the expanded and methylated CGG repeat is required. This is based on both studies of the fragile X syndrome where repeat length and methylation status is correlated with fragile site expression,[116] as well as those of other rare folate-sensitive fragile sites that also harbor expanded and methylated CGG repeats.[197–201] However, not all expanded trinucleotide repeats lead to fragile sites,[202,203] nor do all fragile sites have expanded trinucleotide repeats,[204–208] although some have expansions of other repetitive units.

The most parsimonious conclusion is that the expansion of the CGG repeat at *FMR1* leads to hypermethylation of the region, with subsequent delayed replication and altered chromatin conformation, as described above. The gap in the metaphase chromosome, identified as the fragile site, appears to be composed of uncondensed DNA,[209,210] and be of a length estimated to be 20 kb coincident with the CGG repeat.[70] It is possible that the fragile site is the CGG repeat region that has slowed replication to the degree that this region has yet to condense with the rest of the metaphase chromosome. Indeed, as discussed above, the full mutation leads to the *FMR1* gene to replicate past S, in the G2/M boundary.[189] Moreover, elongated CGG repeats have been shown in vitro to block replication, perhaps by assuming an unusual structure.[211] Mechanisms that trigger expression of the fragile site (i.e., folate-deficient media, addition of fluorodeoxyuridine, or addition of excess thymidine) may suppress one or more of the deoxynucleotide triphosphate pools to further slow replication, thus potentiating the effect. However, this has yet to be directly tested.

CLINICAL ASPECTS

Males with the Fragile X Syndrome

Somatic. The physical features that are the clinical hallmark of the fragile X syndrome in the typical adult full mutation male are a long narrow face, prominent ears, and large testicles.[212] These features are more prominent in postpubertal males, as compared to prepubertal males (Table 64-4). The long face is sometimes associated with a square chin that becomes more prominent in adulthood (Figs. 64-7 and 64-8). Several investigations discuss unusual growth patterns in fragile X syndrome, including increased birth weights, macrocephaly, increased or decreased height, and an acromegalic appearance in adults.[212] Loesch et al.[213] demonstrated a disturbed growth pattern in males and females with fragile X syndrome, including an increased height throughout childhood, earlier onset of puberty, and a decreased height in adulthood, compared to controls. These findings may be secondary to a proposed hypothalamic dysfunction. Two subtypes

Table 64-4 Percentages of Males with the Full Mutation with Specific Physical Characteristics

	Prepubertal Males (%, n=97)	Pubertal/ Postpubertal Males (%, n=64)
Hallmark features:		
Long face	64	80
Prominent ears	78	66
Macroorchidism (≥3 ml)	54	92
Other common features:		
High arched plate	51	63
Hyperextensible finger joints	81	49
Double jointed thumbs	58	48
Single palmer crease	26	22
Hand calluses	18	52
Flat feet	82	60
Heart murmur or click	16	29

Adapted from Merenstein et al. [269]

of the fragile X syndrome phenotype are also associated with overgrowth: a Soto syndrome-like phenotype with general overgrowth[214] and a Prader Willi-like phenotype associated with extreme obesity with full, round face, small, broad hands/feet, and regional skin hyperpigmentation.[215] Interestingly, these subtypes appear in families with males who have the typical fragile X syndrome phenotype. To date, the cause of the general growth abnormalities in the fragile X syndrome is unknown.

Prominent ears are observed in the majority of affected males who are Caucasian, although prominent ears may not be as evident in other racial groups (Fig. 64-9).[216] This feature is thought to be secondary to an overall connective tissue dysplasia in fragile X syndrome, first noted by Opitz et al.[217] Other features consistent with a connective tissue disorder include hyperextensible finger joints, flat feet, mitral valve prolapse, and velvet-like skin. The etiology of the connective tissue dysplasia is unknown, and no hints are provided by the function of the FMRP.

Macroorchidism, the third clinical feature of the fragile X syndrome triad, occurs in approximately 80 to 95 percent of postpubertal males; the testicular volume is approximately two to three times that of normal males, with a mean volume of about 45 ml.[218] Macroorchidism was noted as early as the fetal stage in one study.[219] The fetal testes showed abnormalities in the ultrastructure, including an increase in glycoprotein granules. Macroorchidism may be secondary to endocrinologic abnormalities associated with fragile X syndrome, as suggested by the dramatic increase in the size of the testes in boys with fragile X syndrome between 10 and 12 years of age.[218] Fryns et al.[220] hypothesized hypothalamic dysfunction in fragile X syndrome males. If true, perhaps such dysfunction may cause an increase in gonadotropins in fragile X syndrome. However, observed levels of gonadotropins in fragile X syndrome are not consistent from one study to another.[212] Thus, current studies are underway to identify the underlying cause of the enlarged testes. It is important to note that men with fragile X syndrome are fertile. Thus, the lack of FMRP does not inhibit spermatogenesis to a significant degree.

There are very few significant medical problems associated with the fragile X syndrome. About 30 percent of infants with fragile X syndrome have recurrent emesis in early childhood, which, in some cases, can lead to failure to thrive.[212] The recurrent emesis seems to be secondary to gastroesophageal reflux. Early studies indicated that approximately 30 percent of children with fragile X syndrome had strabismus; a lower percentage of children had other vision problems.[212]

Other medical problems noted are recurrent otitis media infections (80 percent of children with fragile X syndrome), recurrent sinusitis (20 percent of children with fragile X syndrome), and seizures (20 percent of children with fragile X syndrome).[212] Thus, although children with fragile X syndrome do not have major medical problems, each child should be evaluated for eye and ear problems, as such problems could impede a child's progress toward achieving his or her full potential.

Behavior. The behavioral component of the fragile X syndrome phenotype in males includes hyperarousal, hyperactivity, anxiety, tantrums, and extreme sensitivity to sensations, and sometimes aggression.[212] Some aspects of the behavioral phenotype overlap with autism, including difficulties with social interaction with peers, impaired verbal and nonverbal communication, poor eye contact, tactile defensiveness, hand flapping, hand biting, and other motor stereotypes.[212,221–225] Although the exact cause of these autistic-like features is unknown, some investigators speculate that they may be related to hypersensitivity to sensory stimuli or anxiety.[212,222,224,226] Miller et al.[227] studied individuals with fragile X syndrome and controls using electrodermal activity as a measure of the extent to which an individual responds to stimuli. The measure of skin conductance is an indirect assessment of the sympathetic activity, as the eccrine sweat glands are innervated by the cholinergic fibers of the sympathetic nervous system. They found an enhanced electrodermal response to stimuli, and a lack of normal habituation compared with controls. These findings support a physiologic basis for the enhanced reactions to sensation, and suggest that the sympathetic nervous system is affected in the fragile X syndrome.

Adaptive development (including domains of communication, daily living skills, and socialization) does not seem to differ from

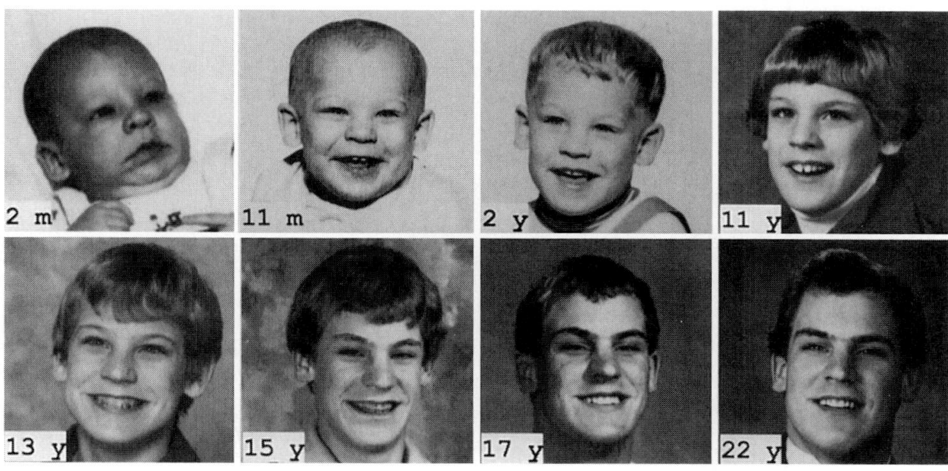

Fig 64-7 Facies of a single full-mutation male from 2 months of age to 22 years.

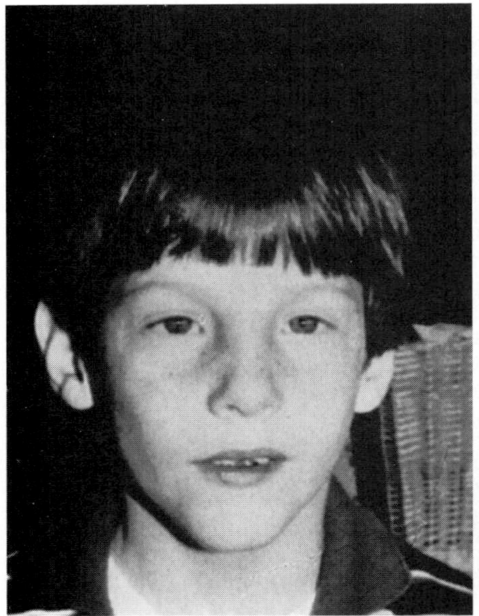

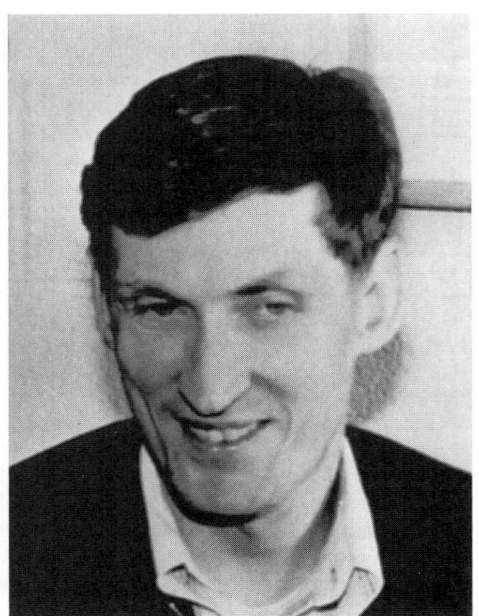

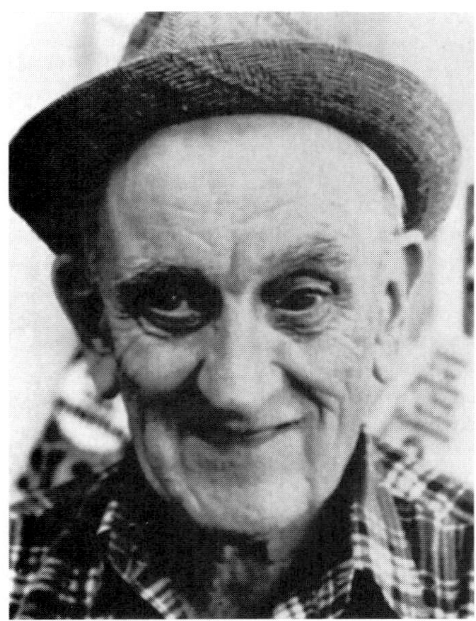

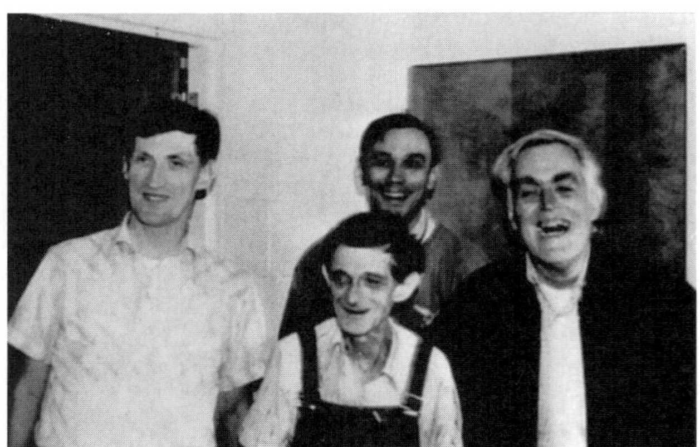

Fig. 64-8 Photographs of institutionalized male patients with the fragile X syndrome. *A* to *C*, Three males, aged 11, 40, and 63. *D*, Individual from panel *B* and his three roommates in a residential home for the mentally retarded. The patients in panel *D* had originally chosen to room with each other because of mutual interests and compatible personalities; during a screening a number of years later, all four men were found to have the fragile X syndrome. (*Courtesy of Brenda Finucane, M.S., and the Elwyn Institute.*)

that expected for mental age.[221,228,229] However fragile X syndrome individuals seem to have relative strengths in daily living skills compared with the adaptive skills in communication and socialization,[221,229,230] but this profile may be true only for adult fragile X syndrome males.[231] Findings from longitudinal and cross-sectional studies suggest that there is significant development of adaptive skills in boys in the 1- to 10-year period. A plateau or stabilization of adaptive development subsequently occurs in late childhood and early adolescence.[231,232] The decline in adaptive development seems to parallel the cognitive trajectory in fragile X syndrome males (see Cognition below).

Cognition. On average, adult males with fragile X syndrome function within the moderately to severely retarded range of

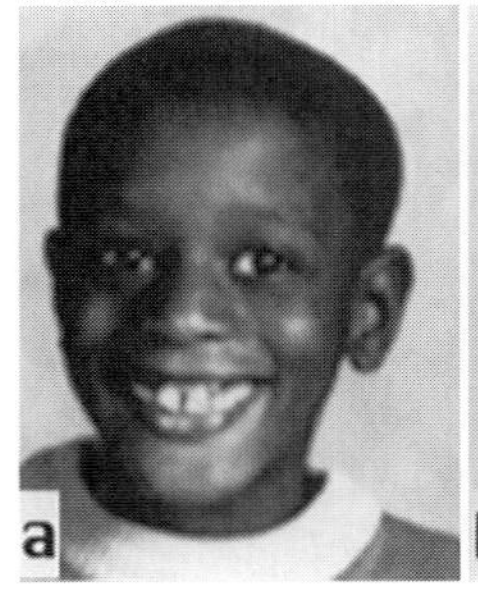

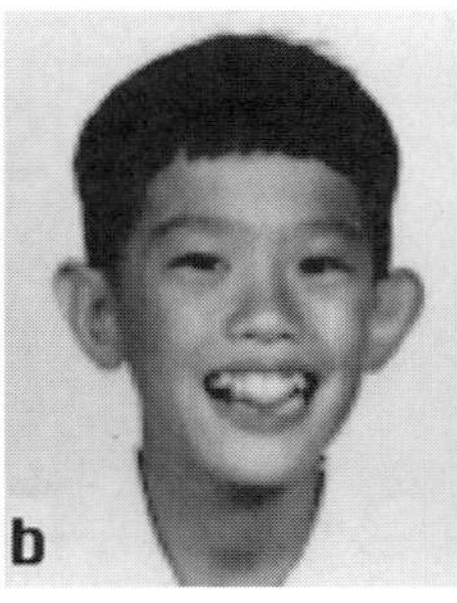

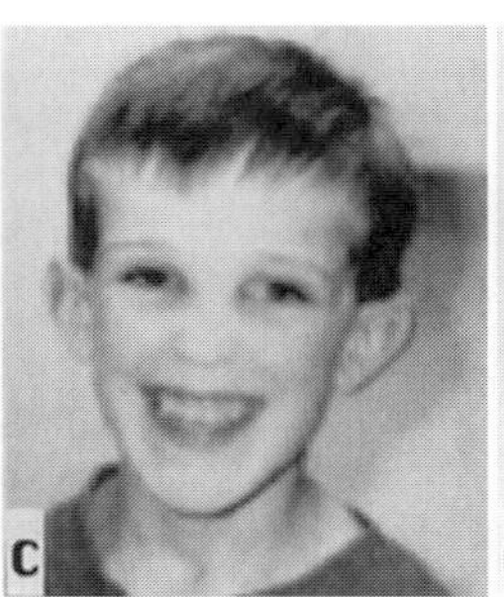

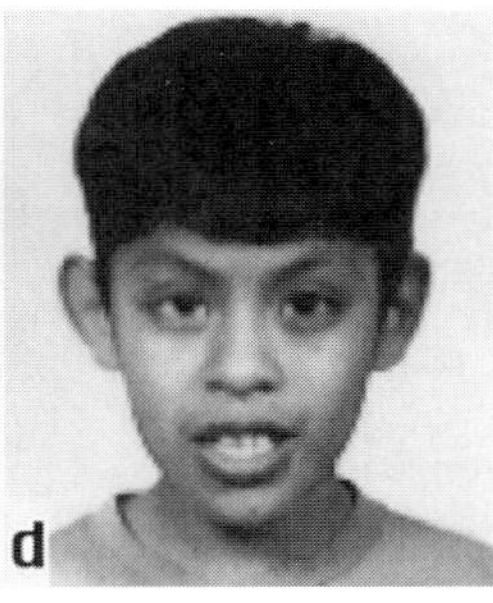

Fig. 64-9 Fragile X syndrome in various ethnic backgrounds. Full mutation males of (*A*) African-American, (*B*) Asian, (*C*) Caucasian, and (*D*) Hispanic background. (*Modified from Jorde et al.*[387] *Used by permission.*)

intelligence, although the spectrum of involvement is quite variable.[233–239] Freund et al.[240] found that 44 percent of a preschool fragile X syndrome group tested in the borderline to average range of IQ. There is now consistent evidence that there is a developmental decline in the IQ of males with fragile X syndrome, although the cause for this decline is unknown. This phenomenon was first shown in cross-sectional studies,[233,236,241] and subsequently confirmed by longitudinal studies.[242–247] It is not clear when or why the decline occurs, some results suggesting that it begins in middle childhood[248] while others suggest around puberty.[242]

Recently, a prospective, longitudinal study has been designed to characterize the early development of males with fragile X syndrome.[249] Based on 46 boys with fragile X syndrome between the ages of 24 and 72 months, preliminary results show: (a) Children varied widely in developmental status with significant differences across individuals in both mean rate and level of performance. (b) The overall development was about half the rate expected for typically developing children. (c) No differences were found in the rates of growth across the five domains including cognition, communication, adaptive, motor, and personal-social. (d) Significant differences were found in the mean levels of performance; thus at every age tested, motor and adaptive domain scores were consistently the highest, and communication and cognition were the lowest. In contrast to the study of Freund et al.,[240] this study found that most children did exhibit significant delays throughout the early childhood years. Differences could be due to small numbers, sample selection, or to the type of measure used. Clearly, more work needs to be done in this area.

Neuropsychology. Most studies indicate consistent areas of weakness for males with fragile X syndrome, including deficits in short-term auditory memory, visual-spatial abilities, visual-motor coordination, and arithmetic skills.[238,250–255] They also show a consistent processing style that indicates that they have problems holding information online as they solve problems (i.e., sequential processing versus simultaneous processing).[234,237,239] In contrast, they seem to have relative strengths in tasks involving long-term memory, perceptual closure, and certain verbal abilities, and thus sometimes appear less affected during preschool years than others with mental retardation.[256]

Abnormalities in both speech production and language competence have been noted consistently for males with the fragile X syndrome. Speech production includes articulation, rate, and prosody. Articulation is consistent with mental age in fragile X syndrome males.[241,257] The rate of speech has been described as rapid and dysrhythmic,[233,241] and has been labeled as "cluttering" to relate a type of verbal clumsiness.[258] Notably, their speech has a harsh or sometimes hoarse vocal quality.[241] Lastly, males with fragile X syndrome have an increase in the repetition of parts of words or whole words.[257]

With respect to language competence, males with fragile X syndrome show varying degrees of impairment of syntatic[257,259] and pragmatic language.[260,261] More recently, two studies showed that specific aspects of the pragmatic competence among males with the fragile X syndrome is unique when compared to individuals with Down syndrome or autism.[262,263] The deviant repetitive language consists of perseveration of words, phrases, and topics, and this aspect of perseveration is greater than would be expected based on mental age, and also differs from the deficits seen in other mental retardation groups. Results from Sudhalter et al.[259,264] suggest that syntactic delays are unrelated to pragmatic deviance.

Memory skills in males show consistent weaknesses. Freund and Reiss[238] showed that males with fragile X syndrome had weaknesses in short-term memory for sentences and a visual memory task, but did relatively well on object memory. Thus, they suggested that memory deficit is not pervasive, but depends on the type of information to be remembered. Males with fragile X syndrome have consistently shown difficulties in remembering sequences or abstract information.[234,237,239] Jakala et al.[265] studied specific aspects of memory in full and premutation males. They found that full-mutation males were impaired, when compared with premutation males, in visual memory, in the learning phase, and delayed recognition of the list-learning task. However, full and premutation males performed similarly in the logical memory task.

Executive functions in males with the fragile X syndrome have not been studied directly, but the preliminary evidence for a deficit comes from the pattern of impairment, as discussed by Bennetto and Pennington.[256] Executive functions can be described as functions that direct behaviors that are goal-directed and future-oriented, and that involve working memory, planning, flexible strategies, and inhibition. Kaufman et al.[266] found that males with fragile X syndrome were able to learn simple tasks, but showed moderate impairments on complex tasks, including delayed alternation and more significant impairments on match-to-sample tasks. These findings are consistent with a deficit in executive functions, as they suggest that tasks requiring the use of working memory or internal representations to guide behavior are difficult for males with fragile X syndrome.

Bennetto and Pennington[256] also suggest that a deficit in executive functions is consistent with some of the behavioral problems observed in males with fragile X syndrome including difficulty with attention control, impulsivity, and difficulty with transitions from one environment to another.

It is now clear that variation in the degree of severity of the fragile X syndrome phenotype in males is related, in part, to characteristics of the *FMR1* mutation that dictate the amount of protein translated.[63,267–270] For example, there was a greater proportion of higher functioning males (IQ >70) who had incomplete or no methylation when compared with more retarded fragile X syndrome males.[271] Using various methods to determine FMRP expression, it has been found that the level of FMRP expression is highly correlated with IQ in pre-/full-mutation mosaic males and partially methylated full-mutation males.[128,272] There is also preliminary evidence to suggest that producing some FMRP (partially methylated full mutation or pre-/full-mutation mosaic) protects an affected male from significant IQ decline.[247]

Full-Mutation Females

Somatic. Overall, females with the full mutation are significantly less affected at all levels, including physical, neuropsychological, and neuroanatomic components, than are males with the full mutation. This is due to X-inactivation of the X-linked *FMR1*,[273] which indicates that some cells of such females are producing FMRP. Because this is a random process, there is a greater range of severity — from essentially no phenotypic expression to profound mental retardation with characteristic physical features of the fragile X syndrome — than is seen among males. The percentage of cells that have the normal X as active, the activation ratio, has been used as a measurement to correlate with various aspects of the phenotype in females. This has been well studied in blood,[268] but not in other tissues, especially not in those target tissues in the central nervous system. There is a correlation between the components of the fragile X syndrome phenotype and severity; thus, females with frank mental retardation usually have typical physical features of the fragile X syndrome, including protruding ears and long face. For example, women with the full mutation more often had a longer face, prominent ears, calluses, and double-jointed thumbs than did either women with the premutation or controls.[274,275] Severity of the phenotype is negatively correlated with the activation ratio, and negatively correlated with the level of FMRP.[128] In one study, the physical symptoms observed among full mutation females were correlated with the number of CGG repeats.[275] The authors speculate that perhaps full mutations with fewer CGG repeat numbers have a tendency to be unmethylated in a proportion of cells in some tissues. These observations were confirmed in an extended study of the same group;[274] however, it remains clear that most symptoms of the fragile X syndrome are not correlated with CGG repeat-size of full mutations.

Behavior. There is considerably less information about the behavior in females with the fragile X syndrome. In general, such females seem to have abnormalities similar in quality to those in males, but which are less severe than those in males.[212,241,276–278] The components that seem to be particularly important are social disability, shyness, anxiety, stereotypic behavior, and hyperactivity.[278–280] These are found among females with the full mutation, irrespective of their level of mental retardation.[278,281–283]

A recent report by Mazzocco et al.[284] examined autistic behaviors among 30 school-age girls with fragile X syndrome and 31 age- and IQ-matched controls. Girls with fragile X syndrome had significantly more autistic behaviors than did the controls. These behaviors were qualitatively similar to those reported for boys with fragile X syndrome, but were not correlated with IQ. Anxiety in girls with fragile X syndrome was positively correlated with abnormal social and communication behaviors. Severity of stereotypic/restricted behaviors was negatively correlated with the activation ratio.

In a study of 29 women with the full mutation, Sobesky et al.[275] found that emotional variables were negatively correlated with neurocognitive variables (i.e., the higher the full scale IQ or more skills related to executive functioning, the lower the *Lie* scale and fewer schizotypal symptoms). The *Lie* scale assesses informant response style and, sometimes, identifies a defensive response set, which is indicated by a tendency to endorse the virtuous behaviors and to deny minor, commonly occurring problems. Thus, the *Lie* scale can suggest unconscious denial of psychological discomfort or a purposeful minimizing of problems. Also, the more physical symptoms present, the higher the *Lie* scale and schizotypal symptoms, and the lower the IQ.

Cognitive. The average mean IQ for all full-mutation carrier females falls in the low-average range of 80 to 90.[256] This figure averages those females with no or only minor learning problems with those with frank mental retardation. Recent studies based on the DNA diagnostic methods show that mental impairment is present in 52 to 82 percent of females with the full mutation.[66,285,286] The variation among studies primarily depends on the selection criteria of females and the method of measuring IQ. There is no consistent evidence of a decline in IQ in females with fragile X syndrome as seen in males.[232,247]

Several studies have examined the association between the size of the full mutation, the activation ratio, and the level of IQ in full-mutation females; results have varied. With respect to size of the full mutation, Abrams et al.[268] and Rousseau et al.[287] found an association with IQ, whereas others did not.[274,286,288,289] As many have suggested, the effect of repeat size is most likely a threshold effect: after 200 repeats, methylation occurs, leading to silencing of the gene. With respect to the activation ratio, the majority of studies have found an association with IQ,[66,128,268,274,275,288,289] although some found no relationship.[286,287] Reiss et al.[288] included the mean parental IQ in their analysis, and found that both the activation ratio and the mean parental IQ contributed about 30 percent to the overall variance of the full-mutation female's IQ. The activation ratio seems to be a better predictor of measures of performance IQ as compared to verbal IQ among fragile X syndrome females.[128,289] It may be a better measure for characteristics in which females with the fragile X syndrome show the greatest impairment.[268,288]

Neuropsychology. There appears to be some specificity in the cognitive profile of females with fragile X syndrome. They tend to show consistent deficits in executive functioning, which is not totally accounted for by their lower IQs.[253,274,275,290–293] Females with fragile X syndrome also show deficits in visual-spatial and nonverbal abilities.[292,294] However, these deficits may not be specific to the fragile X syndrome phenotype, but effects of generally poor cognitive processing.[256] Females with fragile X syndrome also appear to have deficits in verbal memory for rote or abstract information,[238,292,295] and have relative strengths in certain types of verbal memory that impose some external structure.[292,295]

Neuropathology and Neuroanatomy

The relative consistency of the neuropsychologic findings among males and females with the fragile X syndrome suggests that there must be specific central nervous system abnormalities underlying the observed cognitive and behavioral abnormalities. To date, there have been few studies of the anatomic and histologic examination of the brain of an individual with fragile X syndrome.[296,297] These studies showed that there were no gross neuropathologic changes. They did find abnormal dendritic spine morphology (immature, long, and tortuous) with preservation of the neuronal density in the neocortex.

In contrast to neuropathologic studies, there have been relatively more studies on full and premutation carriers that visualize the central nervous system in vivo using MRI. Studies of the structure of the temporal lobe using MRI have shown varying results depending on the age of the study individuals. Reiss et al.[298] found that young males and females with the fragile X syndrome had increased volume of the hippocampus bilaterally and showed an age-related increase in the volume of the hippocampus, and an age-related decrease in volume of the superior temporal gyrus compared with controls. Jakala et al.[265] examined older groups of full- and premutation males and females. They normalized hippocampal volumes by either brain area, or by coronal intracranial area. They found no statistically significant differences in hippocampal volumes normalized for either measure in full-mutation individuals when compared with premutation individuals. Furthermore, the normalized hippocampal volumes of premutation individuals tended to be smaller, not larger, than those of their age- and sex-matched controls. Furthermore, they found age correlated negatively with hippocampal raw volumes and brain areas. Lastly, the study of Jakala et al. did find nonspecific changes indicative of structural abnormalities in temporal lobe structures in greater than 50 percent of full-mutation individuals. These changes included enlargement of ventricular and perivascular spaces, focal hyperintensities in temporal pole white matter, and/or somewhat atypical hippocampal morphology. With respect to age-related changes, both studies were cross-sectional. A need for longitudinal studies is apparent.

With respect to neuropsychologic measures, Reiss et al.[298] did not find any associations between cognitive, behavioral, or developmental measures and the volumes of the four temporal lobe regions studied (right and left hippocampus, right and left superior gyrus) among full-mutation individuals. Interestingly, Jakala et al.[265] found positive correlations between the left normalized hippocampal volumes and performance in many delayed verbal and visual memory tests in only premutation males and females. Thus, performance was better in those with larger left-normalized hippocampal volumes. They speculated that the absence of these correlations in full-mutation males and females could be a reflection of abnormalities in the function of hippocampal circuitries in individuals with the full mutations.

Reiss et al.[277] examined the involvement of the posterior fossa in males and females with fragile X syndrome. Compared with controls, the size of the posterior vermis of the cerebellum was significantly decreased and the fourth ventricle significantly increased in males with the fragile X syndrome. When compared with fragile X syndrome males and controls, the variables describing the posterior vermis and fourth ventricle were intermediate for females with fragile X syndrome. In a study of autistic behaviors among school-age girls with fragile X syndrome and 31 age- and IQ-matched controls, Mazzocco et al.[284] found that the posterior cerebellar vermis area was negatively correlated with measures of communication and stereotypic/restricted behaviors.

Lastly, a study of the neuroanatomy of 51 individuals with fragile X syndrome and matched controls showed that individuals with fragile X syndrome had increased volume of the caudate nucleus and, in males, the lateral ventricle. Both were correlated with IQ. Caudate volume was also correlated with the methylation status of the *FMR1* gene.[131] In addition, these authors studied a pair of monozygous female twins with fragile X syndrome who were discordant for mental retardation. Neuroanatomic differences were localized to the cerebellum, lateral ventricles, and subcortical nuclei.

In summary, when compared to matched controls, males and females appear to have deviations in the size of the cerebellar vermis, fourth ventricle, hippocampus, caudate nucleus, and lateral ventricle. These findings, although not all consistent, suggest that the *FMR1* mutation leads to observable changes in the neuroanatomy that, in turn, may be the cause of the neurodevelopmental disability and behavioral problems associated with the fragile X syndrome. Reiss et al.[131] speculated that the FMRP may be involved in programmed cell death (apoptosis), a process crucial to normal brain development. During normal development, neurons are overproduced and are subsequently pruned back by programmed cell death within the first 2 years of life.[299] It has been suggested that the lack of FMRP may cause a lack of the normal pruning process of neuronal connections early in development. This is consistent with the findings of Comery et al.[300] who showed immature neuronal connections and an increase in dendritic branches in the *FMR1* knockout mouse. Clearly, more studies are necessary to better define anatomic changes, particularly over time, to determine possible interventions or treatment.

Phenotype of Premutation Carriers

Premutation Males. Only one study specifically examined the phenotype of males who carried the premutation. Loesch et al.[301] compared clinical, anthropometric, and psychometric data from a sample of 10 premutation males with those from controls who were primarily married-in relatives of the family. They found that premutation males differed significantly from controls on several cognitive (decreased scores on performance and verbal IQ) and physical measurements (ear length and total facial score). Unfortunately, complete molecular and protein assessments of the premutations were not performed. Clearly, more studies are needed to confirm the phenotype among premutation males.

Jakala et al.[265] studied the hippocampal volumes using MRI in adult males with the full and premutation and normal male controls (n=10 in each group). While the right and left hippocampal volumes, normalized for either brain area or coronal intracranial area, did not differ between full and premutation males, premutation males had smaller left hippocampal normalized volumes than their age- and sex-matched controls. Unfortunately, raw data on controls were not presented and, thus, it is not possible to evaluate the magnitude of this difference.

Premutation Females. The phenotype of premutation females has been studied more intensively than that in premutation males. Intuitively, little or no phenotype is expected due to the presence of an allele with a normal repeat number. However, there is consistent evidence for a somatic phenotype and equivocal evidence for a neuropsychologic phenotype.

Several studies show that carriers with a premutation differ significantly from control individuals in various physical measurements, including overall physical index score and in ear prominence,[274,302] and stature and dermatoglyphics.[301] However, these features are more mild than those observed in full-mutation females.

The most impressive somatic involvement that is consistently found among only premutation carrier females, not full-mutation carriers, is premature ovarian failure (POF). This was first noted in an early study of Cronister et al.,[303] in which they found that premature menopause was present in 8 of 61 normal heterozygotes and in none of the impaired heterozygotes. Later, Schwartz et al.[304] confirmed this observation in a multicenter study in which 24 percent of premutation carriers had POF, whereas only 14 percent of full-mutation carriers and 6 percent of noncarriers had POF. Further studies found this phenomenon,[305,306] and preliminary results from a large international collaboration indicate that among 395 premutation, 128 full-mutation, and 237 noncarrier relatives, 16 percent, 0 percent, and 0.4 percent experienced menopause prior to age 40, respectively.

A possible related phenotype is increased dizygous twinning among premutation carriers only,[307] although increased rates were not confirmed in a prospective study of pregnancy outcomes of carrier females.[19] However, results from a preliminary study found that among 20 pregnancies of premutation carriers with POF, two had produced twins, and that this rate was 10 times higher than that among their noncarrier relatives.[308] As premutation alleles are known to express FMRP,[68] this phenotype is probably caused by a gain-of-function due to increased CGG repeat numbers in the RNA transcripts, rather than by decreased protein levels. Partington et al.[305] suggested that fragile X carriers may produce fewer eggs in utero, leading to premature menopause and an increased rate of dizygous twinning at an earlier age than usual. Alternatively, they suggest that excess dizygous twinning could reflect a programmed excess hypothalamic stimulation of the ovaries resulting in excess follicular usage and earlier menopause.

The neuropsychologic phenotype among premutation females is significantly more subtle, if present at all. We review only studies that used the DNA diagnostic test to classify female carriers as premutation carriers, although there is a wealth of literature on "normal obligate carriers" that includes both pre- and full-mutation carriers (e.g., Mazzocco[292]).

Sobesky et al. examined 92 premutation carriers for measures of emotional problems (Lie scale and schizotypal features), outer ear prominence, physical features, full-scale IQ, and executive functions. Unfortunately, no statistical comparisons were done between this group and the control group, which consisted of 35 noncarrier relatives of fragile X syndrome individuals, although the percentages of females with such problems were intermediate between full-mutation carriers and controls in all but IQ and executive functions. Clearly, the mean IQ and mean executive function variable of premutation women did not differ from controls. No relationships were found between repeat number and these variables. Similar findings related to the Lie scale and schizotypal features among premutation carriers were found in a preliminary study of Steyaert et al.[309] That is, although they found no significant clinical deviation in their population on these scales, low scores on schizotypal features, social introversion, and a so-called faking good profile suggested that individuals may not be aware of some personality characteristics in these areas.

In contrast to these positive findings, Reiss et al.[310] found no phenotype associated with premutation carriers in their study. They examined the neuropsychologic or psychiatric phenotype among 34 adult women with the premutation and 41 matched controls who were mothers of children with nonfragile X-related developmental disabilities. They found no differences related to cognitive abilities or profile, neuropsychologic function, psychiatric diagnoses, or symptoms and self-rated personality profile among the groups. Exploratory analyses showed no significant effect of either the size of repeat or activation ratio on any measure of neurobehavioral function. Both groups had a high lifetime prevalence of major depression, and the authors interpreted this to be related to rearing children with developmental disabilities. Franke et al.[311] found the same trend: premutation carriers and mothers of autistic children had a higher frequency of affective disorders than mothers from the general population. However, they also found that the age-of-onset of psychiatric morbidity in both groups of mothers was earlier than the age when mental retardation was diagnosed in their children. Thus, they concluded that the psychosocial burden of raising a retarded child and/or feelings of guilt could not fully explain the higher frequencies of affective disorders.

Although there is no cognitive deficit among premutation carriers, there may be a specific profile. Allingham-Hawkins et al.[312] studied 14 individuals and found that the mean Verbal and Performance IQs were well within the average range, as was the mean Full-Scale IQ; they observed, however, a trend toward lower Performance IQ compared with Verbal IQ. Interestingly, they also noted that while there was no significant correlation between Full-Scale IQ and CGG repeat size, there was a significant positive correlation between Full-Scale IQ and the proportion of the active X carrying the normal *FMR1* allele in fibroblasts, but not in leukocytes or lymphoblasts. These data need to be confirmed, as the sample size was small.

With respect to neuroanatomic features, similar findings to those in males on normalized hippocampal volumes for full-mutation, premutation, and control females were found by Jakala et al.[265] That is, premutation females had smaller right and left normalized hippocampal volumes than their age- and sex-matched controls. These findings are tantalizing, but need to be confirmed on a large number of individuals.

Phenotype of Intermediate Alleles

Evidence for a phenotypic consequence of alleles with 40 to 60 repeats (referred to as intermediate or gray-zone alleles) is not consistent. Several studies have surveyed populations with special education needs and compared the frequency of intermediate alleles with controls to the population frequency determined by other studies. For example, Murray et al.[59] found a significant excess of intermediate alleles in the schoolboys in classes for intellectual needs in Wessex, England, as compared with the maternal control X chromosome (3.6 percent vs 1.9 percent; $p = 0.039$). The same trend was found for the increased frequency of intermediate alleles among a group of mentally retarded Brazilian males versus a set of controls (6.4 percent vs 2.8 percent; not significant).[313] In contrast, a study of children in special education needs classes in Atlanta, GA, did not find an increased frequency of intermediate alleles relative to maternal X chromosome controls. Other studies have not found the increased rates of the intermediate alleles among clinically referred populations of children with academic difficulties[314] or with language delay[315] as compared with general population frequencies, although no control groups were studied.

Two studies examined the correlation between the full-scale IQ and *FMR1* repeat number.[314,316] Daniels et al.[316] examined the CGG repeat number for three groups: low IQ (mean IQ = 71, n = 35), middle IQ (mean IQ = 103, n = 19), and high IQ (mean IQ = 137, n = 49). They found no difference in the number of *FMR1* CGG repeats for males or females. Mazzocco et al.[314] examined the association between IQ score and the number of repeats in 455 Caucasian and 462 African-American school-aged children referred to developmental pediatrics clinics and found no significant association.

In summary, no obvious cognitive deficit is observed among carriers of intermediate or premutation alleles. However, studies to examine behavioral aspects and cognitive profiles are needed to rule out subtler, but important effects of the CGG repeat.

MOLECULAR DIAGNOSTICS

The laboratory diagnosis of fragile X syndrome has undergone a major advancement since the discovery of the *FMR1* gene. Prior to that time, cytogenetic demonstration of the associated fragile site at Xq27.3 was the major mode of testing.[317–319] However, cytogenetic expression of the fragile site was heavily dependent on the method utilized for fragile site induction, and the skill and experience of the testing laboratory. Although many laboratories became quite proficient at the cytogenetic diagnosis of fragile X syndrome, carrier detection and prenatal diagnosis still posed difficulties.[320–324] DNA testing for the fragile X syndrome has now supplanted the specific cytogenetic test for the fragile X (FRAXA) site and is technically reviewed elsewhere.[51,325–328] It is always important to note, however, that the molecular testing for fragile X syndrome does not eliminate the need for karyotype studies on individuals with undiagnosed mental retardation.

The American College of Medical Genetics[329] made these recommendations regarding whom to test and approaches toward testing:

Individuals for Whom Testing Should Be Considered

- Individuals of either sex with mental retardation, developmental delay, or autism, especially if they have (a) any physical or behavioral characteristics of fragile X syndrome, (b) a family history of fragile X syndrome, or (c) male or female relatives with undiagnosed mental retardation.
- Individuals seeking reproductive counseling who have (a) a family history of fragile X syndrome, or (b) a family history of undiagnosed mental retardation.
- Fetuses of known carrier mothers.
- Patients who have a cytogenetic fragile X test result that is discordant with their phenotype. These include patients who have a strong clinical indication (including risk of being a carrier) and who have had a negative or ambiguous test result, and patients with an atypical phenotype who have had a positive test result.

Approaches to Testing

- DNA analysis is the method of choice if one is testing specifically for fragile X syndrome and associated trinucleotide expansion in the *FMR1* gene.
- If the etiology of mental impairment is unknown, DNA analysis for fragile X syndrome should be performed as part of a comprehensive genetic evaluation, which includes routine cytogenetic analysis. Cytogenetic studies are critical since constitutional chromosome abnormalities have been identified as frequently or more frequently than fragile X mutations in mentally retarded individuals referred for fragile X testing.
- For individuals who are at risk due to an established family history of fragile X syndrome, DNA testing alone is sufficient. If the diagnosis of the affected relative was based on previous cytogenetic testing for fragile X syndrome, then at least one affected relative should be included in DNA testing.
- Prenatal testing of a fetus is indicated following a positive carrier test in the mother. When the mother is a known carrier, DNA testing can be offered to determine whether the fetus inherited the normal or mutant *FMR1* gene. Results from CVS testing must be interpreted with caution because the methylation status of the *FMR1* gene is often not yet established in chorionic villi at the time of sampling. CVS, while a standard technique for prenatal diagnosis, may lead to a situation where follow-up amniocentesis is necessary to resolve an ambiguous result.

Laboratory testing for fragile X syndrome is based upon Southern blot analysis and PCR procedures. Southern blot analysis is designed to either assess repeat length alone, or repeat lengths as well as methylation status of key restriction sites of *FMR1*. The most widely used restriction enzyme for Southern blot assessment of the *FMR1* repeat tract length is *Eco*RI. Digestion of normal genomic DNA with *Eco*RI liberates a 5.2-kb fragment, which includes the *FMR1* promoter region and the first exon containing the CGG repeat. A variety of cloned fragments of this region have been described as probes on Southern analysis (Fig. 64-10).[43,46,65,125,330–333] Although radiolabeling of probes remains common, nonisotopic detection is gaining favor in clinical laboratories.[334] A larger band in premutation and full-mutation males replaces this 5.2-kb band, although the smaller premutations may not be easily discerned. Full-mutation alleles often exhibit a

A

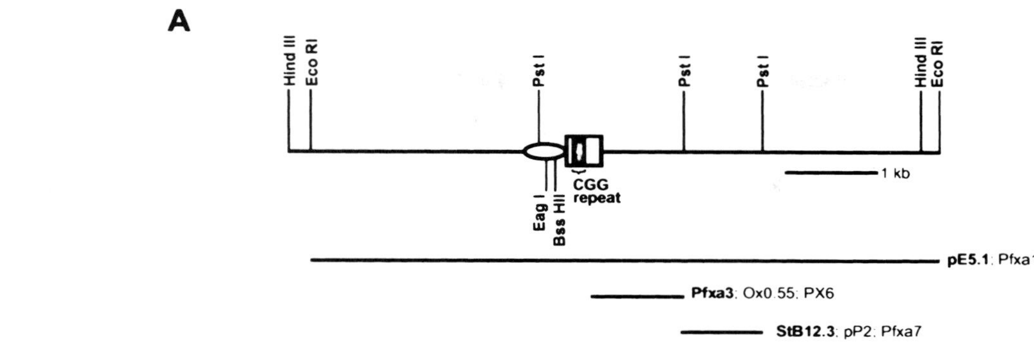

B

DIAGNOSTIC RESTRICTION FRAGMENT LENGTHS BY SOUTHERN ANALYSIS (kb)

	DNA digestion	**Eco RI + [Bss HII *or* Eag I]**		**Hind III + [Bss HII *or* Eag I]**		**Pst I**
	Probe	**pE5.1**	**Pfxa3 *or* StB12.3**	**pE5.1**	**Pfxa3 *or* StB12.3**	**Pfxa3**
Normal 6 - 52 repeats	*Male*	2.4 + 2.8	2.8	2.7 + 2.5	2.5	1.0
	Female	2.4 + 2.8 +5.2*	2.8 + 5.2*	2.7 + 2.5 +5.2*	2.5 + 5.2*	1.0
Premutation 48 - 200 repeats	*Male*	2.4 + **(2.9 - 3.3)**	**2.9 - 3.3**	2.7 + **(2.6 - 3.1)**	**2.6 - 3.1**	**1.1 - 1.6**
	Female	2.4 + 2.8 + **(2.9 - 3.3)** + 5.2**	2.8 + **(2.9 - 3.3)** + 5.2**	2.7 + 2.5 + **(2.6 - 3.1)** + 5.2**	2.5 + **(2.6 - 3.1)** + 5.2**	1.0 + **(1.1 - 1.6)**
Full Mutation >230 repeats	*Male*	**>5.7**	**>5.7**	**>5.7**	**>5.7**	**>1.6**
	Female	2.4 + 2.8 + 5.2* + **>5.7**	2.8 + 5.2* + **> 5.7**	2.7 + 2.5 + 5.2* + **>5.7**	2.8 + 5.2* + **> 5.7**	1.0 + **>1.6**

*Inactive normal X chromosome

**Wider band reflecting inactive normal and premutation X

FIG. 64-10 Diagnostic restriction fragments detected by Southern analysis. *A*, Restriction map surrounding the *FMR1* repeat. Oval, promoter region; Box, exon 1 containing the CGG repeat. Major cloned fragments, used as probes, are shown below. *B*, Table indicating restriction fragment lengths observed using various restriction endonucleases and probes for either sex carrying the three classes of alleles. Sizes are given in kilobases and the bold numbers indicate abnormal fragment lengths. (*Modified from Warren and Nelson.*[333] *Used by permission.*)

smear or a broad band, reflecting the length mosaicism of the repeat in somatic cells. Moreover, some mosaic males may also display a distinctive premutation band in addition to the full mutation bands or smear. More recently, *Hin*dIII was shown to be superior to *Eco*RI because the downstream *Eco*RI site is sometimes refractory to digestion, leading to a partial digest band of 6.4 kb that may be confused with the full mutation or may lead to troublesome shadow bands.[335] In addition, *Bcl*I or *Pst*I digestion results in a smaller normal fragment, which can make identification of premutation length alleles easier to identify by Southern analysis.

In practice, *Eco*RI digestion (or *Hin*dIII digestion) is performed along with a second digestion using a methyl-sensitive restriction enzyme such as *Eag*I or *Bss*HII. Thus, the 5.2-kb *Eco*RI fragment, if unmethylated at these additional sites, is cleaved into a 2.4-kb and a 2.8-kb fragment, with the latter fragment containing the CGG repeat. A typical Southern blot using *Eco*RI and *Bss*HII is shown in Fig. 64-11. The normal male DNA, being unmethylated at two closely adjacent *Bss*HII sites, exhibits these two fragments. Premutation males show the substitution of the 2.8-kb band for a slightly larger band reflecting the size increase due to the premutation. Full-mutation males, however, typically show a banding pattern similar to *Eco*RI alone, with bands larger than 5.2-kb, because the *Bss*HII sites are usually methylated. The determination of methylation status can be particularly useful in evaluation of repeat lengths at the high end of the premutation range where abnormal methylation in a male would be more consistent with the diagnosis of a full mutation rather than a premutation carrier status. In the normal female, the *FMR1* gene is randomly inactivated on one X chromosome in each cell.[273] On the inactive X, the *Bss*HII sites, as well as other nearby methyl-sensitive sites such as *Eag*I, are methylated; the same sites are unmethylated on the active X. Therefore, a 5.2-kb band is observed from the inactive X, while the two smaller bands (2.8 and 2.4 kb), similar to that of the normal male, are observed from the active X of the female.

Females with pre- and full mutations exhibit patterns that are more complex to analyze, because the pattern of bands reflects both normal and abnormal X chromosome alleles. Tables are extremely helpful in interpretation (Fig. 64-10). Remember that it is not possible to accurately render a diagnosis of mental impairment in the absence of clinical information (such as during a prenatal test) when a female carries a full mutation. Empiric data must be relied on. These data indicate that females with full mutations have an approximate 50 to 80 percent risk of having fragile X syndrome (as exhibited by IQ > 85).[285,286,289] Although the ultimate level of performance of individual penetrant females with full mutations cannot be predicted, as a group, they are much less severely affected than males. Females with premutations are sometimes more difficult to detect in this fashion because the 2.8-kb band of the normal X may form a diffuse doublet with a small premutation band; PCR analysis can be extremely useful in this situation.

Prenatal samples, particularly chorionic villus, may not reflect the ultimate methylation state associated with a large repeat length, tending to be less methylated than the fetus itself.[62,336–344] In such cases, diagnosis based on repeat length alone is able to detect the presence of the full mutation. Although this should be sufficient to make the diagnosis, amniocentesis is recommended to confirm the diagnosis by determining hypermethylation in addition

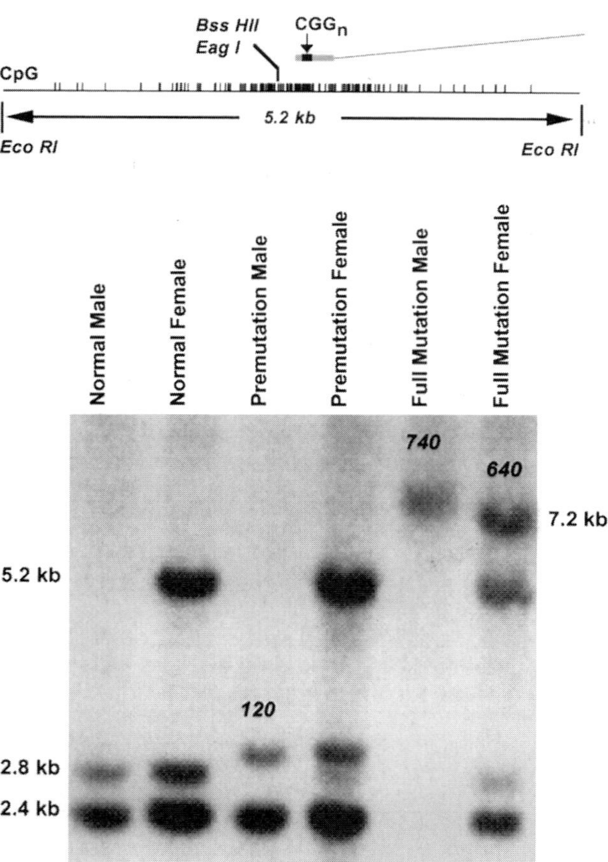

FIG. 64-11 **Southern blot showing normal, premutation and full mutation alleles of either sex.** ***Top,*** **Restriction map showing the first exon of** ***FMR1*** **containing the CGG repeat with CpG dinucleotides indicated by vertical marks.** ***Bottom,*** **Southern blot of DNA from the indicated individuals digested with** ***Eco*****RI and** ***Bss*****hII and probed with pE5.1. Numbers above certain fragments indicate approximate repeat numbers. (*****Modified from Warren and Nelson.***[333] ***Used by permission.*****)**

to the expanded repeat. It is very likely this recommendation will be dropped in the future, because are no reports of full expansions with incomplete methylation in chorionic villus sampling not leading to fully methylated full mutations in amniocytes and/or cord blood samples.

Polymerase chain reaction amplification of the CGG repeat associated with *FMR1* has been greatly improved in recent years, and can accurately determine the repeat size of normal and premutation alleles.[326,336,345–350] Some methods enable observation of full mutations as well, and the use of *Pfu*I polymerase or other proprietary PCR systems has facilitated this assay.[349] However, accurate size determination of the full mutations is generally not possible and usually requires Southern blot confirmation. PCR approaches have also been adapted to assess the methylation status of the *FMR1* gene.[351] Recently, the use of betaine to reduce secondary structure along with *Pfu*I DNA polymerase enabled automated fluorescence sizing of all *FMR1* repeats of less than 100 CGGs.[352]

Antibody Studies

Development of antibodies against FMRP has provided both a critical research tool and a substantial addition to the laboratory diagnosis of fragile X syndrome.[76,353] Western analysis is of most value, as the size of FMRP, as well as abundance, can be validated. This analysis is of particular importance in the analysis of potential *FMR1* deletion/nonsense patients with the clinical picture of fragile X syndrome but without the expansion or methylation of the *FMR1* gene associated with the full mutation.

A more rapid and economical assay has been developed involving immunohistochemistry of blood smears.[354] With this approach, less than 40 percent of the lymphocytes from a full mutation male are labeled and are distinguished from normal male lymphocytes which have a much higher frequency of labeling.[355] This test is quick and economical, working well with both stored blood samples and amniotic fluid cells.[356] While the discrimination of this test appears valid, the background of up to 40 percent positive lymphocytes from affected males who show no FMRP by traditional Western analysis remains to be fully understood. A significant number of the positive cells may be due to mosaicism for smaller, unmethylated repeats. However, not all positive cells are likely to be due to mosaicism because partial expression of FMRP, judged by Western analysis, is not common in full-mutation males. Given the lack of quantitative interpretation of histochemical analysis, the interpretation of percent of positive cells to diagnose mosaic individuals should be viewed with caution. This test is much less specific for females with a full mutation because of the overlap of the proportion of FMRP-positive cells between carriers and controls.[355] Also, because most female carriers are biased for inactivation favoring the expression of the normal *FMR1* gene,[66] most lymphocytes would stain positive and would not accurately reflect inactivation patterns of other tissues. It remains to be seen, however, whether sampling other accessible tissues would avoid this inactivation bias and be a better predictor of brain expression.

BIOCHEMISTRY OF FMRP

The protein product of the *FMR1* gene appears to be the sole determinant, in its absence, for fragile X syndrome. As discussed above, there are no other genes found in the vicinity of *FMR1* that may be influenced by repeat expansion or methylation. Furthermore, and most importantly, a small but significant group of patients has been identified with *FMR1* deletions that are clinically indistinguishable from patients with the more common full-repeat expansion mutation, generating considerable interest regarding the normal function of FMRP and the pathophysiology of its absence.

FMR1 undergoes considerable alternative splicing (Fig. 64-2) with variants of exons 12 and 14 being abundant.[45,75,357] Use of alternative acceptor sites in exon 15 and exon 17 result in downstream frameshifts and unique C-terminal amino acid sequence.[45] Hence, it has been predicted that at least 20 protein isoforms are possible for FMRP.

The molecular masses of the predicted isoforms of FMRP vary between 71.1 kDa and 47.3 kDa. Isoform 7, lacking exon 12, appears to be the most abundant isoform in many cell types.[76,80] Although this isoform has a predicted mass of 68.9 kDa, it migrates through polyacrylamide at an apparent mass of approximately 80 kDa. Besides isoform 7, only three other isoforms are routinely detected in most studied cell types (commonly lymphoblasts), although the precise identity of isoforms has not been rigorously established. As discussed below, certain predicted isoforms have distinctive biochemical attributes that should result in altered function, although none are thought to be commonly expressed.

Protein Domains and Related Genes

Initial homology searches with the *FMR1* cDNA did not reveal any obvious domains that might reveal function. However, in 1993, Ashley et al.[64] and Siomi et al.[353] independently reported that FMRP contains domains commonly found in proteins that interact with RNA. FMRP contains two ribonucleoprotein K homology domains (KH domains), and clusters of arginine and glycine residues (RGG boxes). The KH domains of FMRP are found beginning at residues 222 and 285 of the full-length FMRP (isoform 1; GenBank 457235). The RGG box is generally stated to

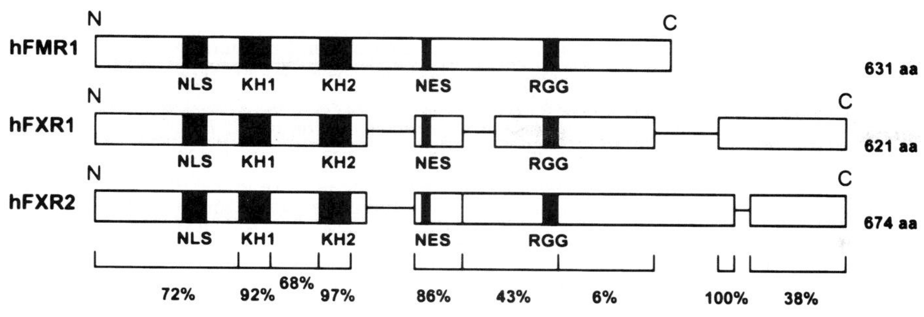

Fig. 64-12 Representation of the protein domains of the human *FMR1* gene family members. Percentages indicate amino acid similarity. (*Modified from Imbert et al.*[388] *Used by permission.*)

begin at residue 530, although several highly similar arginine/glycine-rich regions are found toward the C-terminus.

KH domains individually consist of approximately 40 to 60 amino acids with several invariant hydrophobic domains of isoleucine, leucine, or methionine, as well as a required glycine residue. These domains, as well as nucleocytoplasmic transport signals (see below), are highly conserved among the three *FMR1* gene family members (Fig. 64-12). A wide variety of proteins have been found to contain as few as a single KH-domain, as observed in the yeast alternative splicing factor Mer1p, to 14 copies of the domain in the chicken vigilin protein. Although it remains to be established precisely how KH domains influence RNA binding, it is generally believed that the KH domains bind RNA directly. However, direct RNA binding by KH domains within the context of an intact protein has not been conclusively demonstrated, nor has the three-dimensional crystal structure of a KH domain protein been solved.

RGG boxes are 20- to 25-amino-acid motifs containing repetitions of arginine-glycine-glycine residues often interspersed with aromatic amino acids. RGG boxes are most often observed in conjunction with other RNA-binding domains, as is the case with *FMR1*. Because of this, RGG boxes are generally considered not to be sequence-specific in regard to RNA targets, but are thought to facilitate binding to other domains. Indeed, RGG boxes have been shown to increase specific RNA binding by RNP domains in nucleolin approximately tenfold.

RNA Binding

The presence of two KH domains and RGG boxes allowed the hypothesis to be put forward that *FMR1* is an RNA-binding protein.[358] Two studies demonstrated in vitro RNA-binding activity for *FMR1*.[64,353] Ashley et al.[64] also found that FMRP appears to have a selectivity for a fraction of mRNAs expressed in brain, including its own message. RNA binding has been disrupted by deletions of the C-terminus of the protein, which ablate the RGG sequences.[353] Brown et al.[359] expressed murine Fmrp in baculovirus and affinity-purified FLAG-tagged murine protein. The purified protein was shown to bind directly to both ribonucleotide homopolymers (Fig. 64-13) and human brain mRNA. FLAG-Fmrp exhibited selectivity for binding poly(G) → poly(U) → poly(C) or poly(A). Moreover, purified FLAG-Fmrp bound only to a subset of brain mRNA, including the 3′-UTR of myelin basic protein message and its own message. Recombinant isoform 4, lacking the RGG boxes but maintaining both KH domains, was also purified, and was found to only weakly interact with RNA.

A patient carrying a missense mutation in *FMR1* was identified with unusually severe mental retardation, remarkable macroorchidism, and a violent temperament.[93] The point mutation in this patient alters an isoleucine residue to asparagine at position 304 (I304N) of the common isoform. The Ile in this position is conserved in nearly every protein carrying a KH domain described to date, suggesting a critical role for this residue in the function of the domain. This mutant protein also shows reduced in vitro RNA-binding activity,[360,361] while retaining its ability to form protein-protein interactions with *FXR1* and *FXR2*, the fragile X-related proteins.[362] Recent evidence derived from structural analysis of another member of the KH family, human vigilin, suggests that this mutation destroys the ability of the protein to fold properly.[363] Interestingly, missense mutations within KH domains often cause more severe phenotypes compared to those caused by null mutations. For example, more severe phenotypes have also been reported due to KH domain mutations in the *C. elegans* GLD-1 protein[364] and the *Drosophila* bicaudal -C protein.[365] These more severe phenotypes cannot be explained simply by reduced RNA binding of the corresponding proteins. Because FLAG-purified I304N Fmrp, harboring the I304N mutation, demonstrated RNA binding, it seems that protein-protein interaction may be a more likely cause of the severe phenotype.[359] As discussed below, this

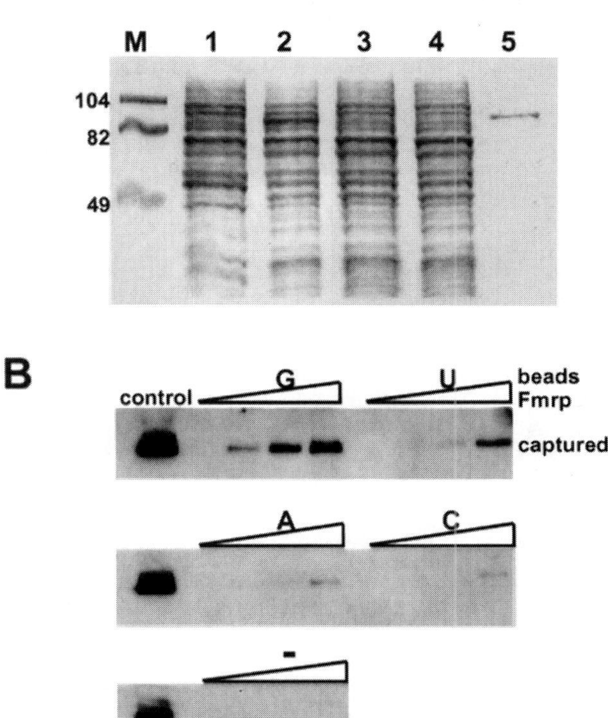

Fig. 64-13 Purified recombinant FMRP shows selective binding to RNA homopolymers. *A,* SDS-PAGE gel of Ponceau S protein staining of *lane 1,* uninfected Sf9 cell lysate; *lane 2,* infected cell lysate load; *lane 3,* anti-FLAG affinity column flow through; *lane 4,* column wash; *lane 5,* eluted FLAG-tagged FMRP. *B,* RNA homopolymer binding. Increasing concentrations (open triangles) of polynucleotide mixed with purified FMRP and agarose conjugated poly(G), poly(U), poly(A), or poly(C), centrifuged, and any bound FMRP captured analyzed by SDS-PAGE and Western blotting. (*Modified from Brown et al.*[359] *Used by permission.*)

appears to be the case by demonstration of the I304N protein associating with a smaller RNP and failing to associate with polyribosomes.[366]

Ribosome Association

Immunolocalization studies with antibodies directed against FMRP revealed that FMRP is predominantly localized in the cytoplasm with a diffuse granular staining pattern.[76,80] Recent reports indicate that FMRP is associated with translating ribosomes.[361,366–368] FMRP-ribosome association is sensitive to low levels of RNase, which removes the mRNAs linking translating polyribosomes without disturbing ribosome assembly.[361,367,369] In addition, EDTA-treatment, which dissociates ribosomes into subunits, releases FMRP into complexes with a similar size range to messenger ribonucleoprotein (mRNP) particles.[366,367] Furthermore, nearly all the cytoplasmic FMRP can be cocaptured with poly-A RNA.[366,369] Taken as a whole, these data suggest that FMRP associates with ribosomes as a component of mRNP particles. Upon translation termination, FMRP seems to dissociate from ribosomes[366] and is ready to be recycled for the next round of translation.

The association of FMRP with translating ribosomes has been observed in many cell and tissue types, including brain neurons. The localization of FMRP in neurons has been analyzed using immunogold electron microscopy with an antibody directed against FMRP.[81] The highest concentration of immunogold particles was seen in the cell body in regions rich in ribosomes. In neuronal processes, immunogold particles were obvious in proximal dendrites. However, no FMRP was detected in axons where ribosomes were absent. In addition, FMRP-immunogold particles were frequently seen in dendritic spines at sites where ribosomes are customarily found. Consistently, neuronal FMRP was also found in synaptosome preparations in association with polyribosomes. The association of FMRP with somatodendritic polyribosomes is certainly consistent with the hypothesis that fragile X mental retardation may be a result of translation abnormality due to the absence of FMRP.

Nucleocytoplasmic Localization

Although FMRP is predominantly localized in the cytoplasm, nuclear staining has been reported.[76,80] It is intriguing to consider that FMRP might enter the nucleus as a part of its normal function. It is known that other RNA-binding proteins shuttle between the nucleus and cytoplasm. Furthermore, FMRP is thought to associate with ribosomes as a component of mRNP particles and most RNP particles are formed in the nucleus. Eberhart et al.[367] utilized FMRP deletion and fusion constructs to delineate a nuclear localization signal (NLS) in the N-terminus of FMRP and a nuclear export signal (NES) encoded by exon 14. The FMRP NES resembles the NES motifs recently described for the HIV-1 Rev protein and protein kinase inhibitor. A 17-amino-acid peptide containing the FMRP NES can direct temperature-dependent nuclear export of a microinjected protein conjugate, whereas a mutant peptide cannot direct export. Immunogold electron microscopy provides further evidence that FMRP is capable of shuttling between the nucleus and the cytoplasm. While FMRP is predominantly in the cytoplasm of neurons, FMRP is detected in the nucleus and in transit through the nuclear pore.[81]

Functional Studies

The subcellular behavior of FMRP, including its selective mRNA binding, nucleocytoplasmic shuttling, and predominant association with cytoplasmic polyribosomes, has led to the hypothesis that FMRP may play a role in nuclear export of its target mRNAs and further present these mRNAs to the translation machinery.[370] The discovery of FMRP polyribosome-association in the neuronal dendritic spine further implies the possible involvement of FMRP in modulating localization and/or translation of its target mRNAs in the appropriate subcellular compartment(s).

Regulation of localized protein synthesis has been demonstrated to be functionally important in cell growth and polarity development. In neurons, the selective localization of translation machinery and a subclass of mRNAs to the postsynaptic sites[371,372] has led to a hypothesis that proteins important for synaptic plasticity may be synthesized near their functional sites. Direct evidence has been found demonstrating that local protein synthesis is required in neurotrophin-induced hippocampal synaptic plasticity.[373] The elevated protein synthesis within the dendritic spine during synaptic development,[374] especially on activation of the metabotropic glutamate receptors,[375] further reinforced the importance of regulated translation in neuronal function. The formation of abnormal dendritic spines due to the lack of FMRP, as found in fragile X patients' brains,[296,297] as well as in the *Fmr1* knockout mice brains,[300] is consistent with the view that fragile X mental retardation may result from protein synthesis abnormality during synapse development.

Until very recently, the functional importance of FMRP-polyribosome association, in relation to translation, was emphasized.[366] The I304N mutation in FMRP, which causes severe fragile X syndrome, abolished FMRP-polyribosome association (Fig. 64-14). The impaired FMRP-polyribosome association does not seem to be a result of failure in RNA binding, as suggested by

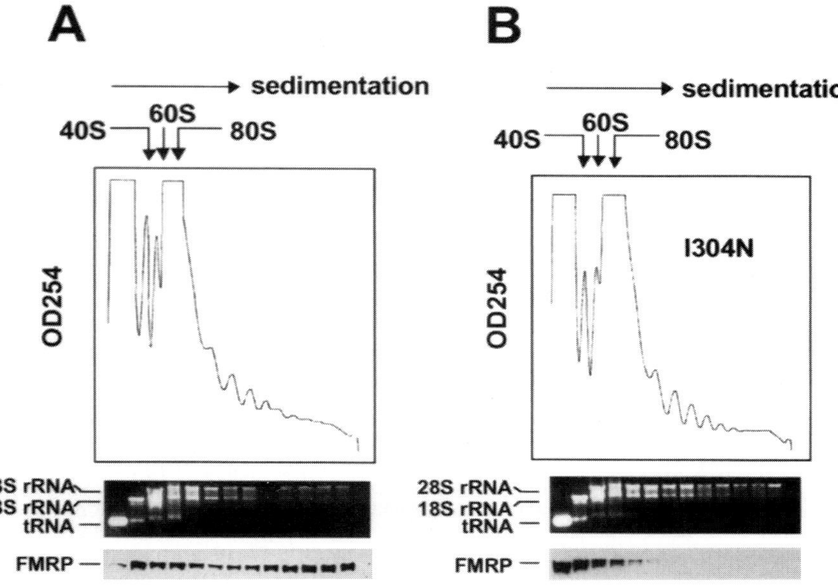

Fig. 64-14 Association of FMRP with polyribosomes is abolished by the I304N mutation. For *A* and *B*, the top panel shows the absorption profile of a 20 percent to 47 percent (w/w) sucrose gradient at 254 nm, with sedimentation and major ribosomal peaks indicated; the middle panel shows the distribution of tRNA and ribosomal RNAs in correlation to the sedimentation profile; and the bottom panel shows the distribution of FMRP in correlation to the sedimentation profile. *A*, Normal FMRP preferentially cosediments with polyribosomes. *B*, Abrogation of FMRP-polyribosome association by the I304N mutation. (*From Feng et al.*[366] *Used by permission.*)

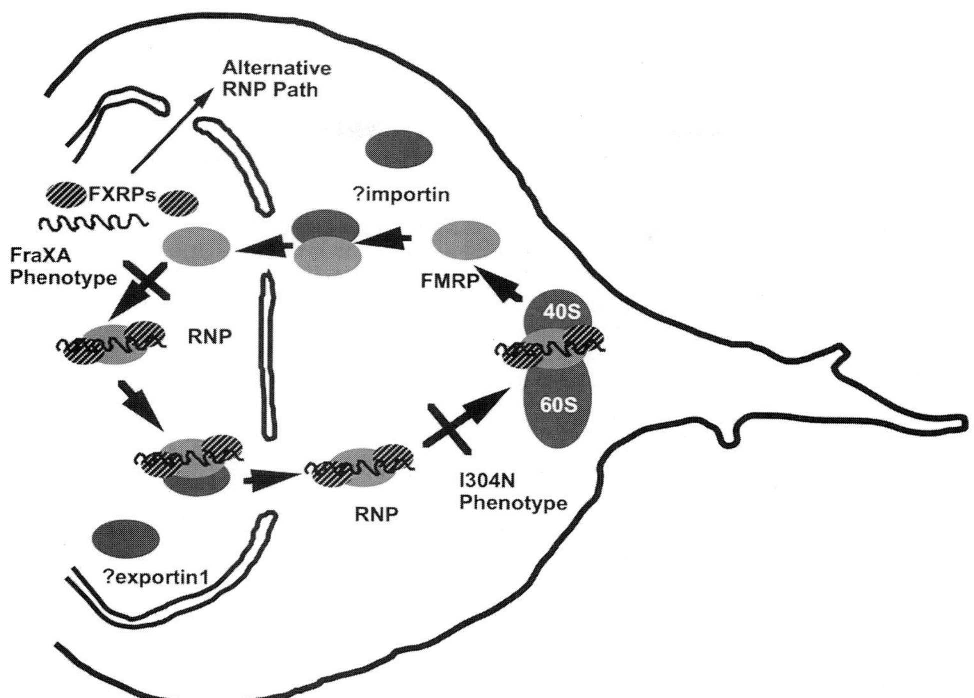

Fig. 64-15 Model depicting known biochemical attributes of FMRP. Cytoplasmic nascent FMRP (black oval) enters the nucleus via its NES possibly interacting with importin. Once in the nucleus, FMRP interacts with several proteins, including the *FXR1* and *FXR2* proteins (striped) and a subset of RNA molecules (black). The RNP is exported out of the nucleus via its NES, possibly by interacting with exportin 1 (hatched). The cytoplasmic RNP then associates with ribosomes (gray) throughout translation. In typical fragile X syndrome lacking FMRP, it is postulated that the RNAs which normally interact with FMRP are exported from the nucleus via alternative RNPs, resulting in translation but perhaps in abnormal quantity, timing, and/or cytoplasmic location. The I304N FMRP binds these RNAs but fails to present them to the ribosome, thus sequestering the RNAs from translation, resulting in a more severe phenotype. (*Modified from Imbert et al.*[388] *Used by permission.*)

previous in vitro study,[360] because the mutant FMRP can be cocaptured with cytoplasmic poly-A RNA similar to normal FMRP.[366] Rather, the inability of the mutant FMRP to associate with polyribosomes most likely results from the formation of abnormally small mRNP particles which fail to be selected for translation. These data suggest that FMRP is important in forming translation-competent mRNP particles, and may further direct their translation in the appropriate subcellular compartment(s). In a typical fragile X patient who lacks FMRP, mRNAs that are normally directed to translation by FMRP may be handled by other mRNPs, possibly including FMRP-related proteins. This scenario may result in partial translation, perhaps abnormally regulated and/or localized in cells such as brain neurons. The dominant formation of abnormal FMRP-mRNP particles that fail to associate with translating polyribosomes by the I304N mutation implies that FMRP-bound mRNAs may be sequestered from translation, thus resulting in the unusually severe fragile X phenotype. A model describing FMRP's involvement in mRNP formation and polyribosome association is postulated in Fig. 64-15.

In addition to modulating mRNA translation and subcellular localization, polyribosmal-mRNPs may also influence mRNA stability; this may occur either by intrinsic endonucleolytic activity as demonstrated by the polysomal messenger ribonuclease,[376] or by increasing the resistance of the bound mRNA to ribonuclease attack. In addition, numerous nuclear RNPs are responsible for mRNA processing. Whether FMRP, especially particular FMRP isoforms that display differential subcellular localization, also is involved in multiple aspects of mRNA metabolism still awaits elucidation. Accumulating evidence points to the possible regulation of mRNP complex formation and mRNA export through phosphorylation and/or methylation of specific mRNA-binding proteins.[377,378] Modification of FMRP and/or its related proteins under the control of growth and neurotransmitter-mediated signals would be conceivable with the predicted function of FMRP in learning and memory. Finally, identification of FMRP's RNA targets should help to define the influence of FMRP in mRNA metabolism, and finally lead to the elucidation of pathogenesis in fragile X syndrome due to the lack of FMRP.

NEUROBIOLOGY OF FMRP

The neurobiologic understanding of FMRP function and the consequence of its absence is critical toward the full appreciation of the pathophysiology of fragile X syndrome. Moreover, it is likely that mechanistic insight into FMRP function should illuminate fundamental processes of learning and cognition. While the advances in neurobiologic function of FMRP have lagged behind the biochemical studies, significant progress has been made, largely due to the use of a knockout mouse model.

Fmr1 Knockout Mouse

A murine model of fragile X syndrome was described by groups led by Oostra and Willems.[134] Using homologous recombination in embryonic stem cells, they interrupted exon 5 of the murine *Fmr1* gene with a neomycin cassette, resulting in the loss of function for this gene. While this mouse model does not recapitulate the actual human expansion mutation, the consequence is the same; thus, this mouse strain should represent an authentic model of the human phenotype. Indeed, testing the knockout animal in various behavioral paradigms revealed a subtle deficit in learning and memory.[379,380] Moreover, the male knockout mice exhibit macroorchidism due to increased Sertoli cell proliferation during testicular development.[381]

The murine model of fragile X syndrome has allowed neurobiologic experiments to be performed in order to gain insight into the human phenotype. Godfraind et al.[382] showed no obvious abnormality in either short-term or long-term potentiation during electrophysiological field recordings in hippocampal slices of the knockout brain. Likewise, Steward et al.[383] did not observe any abnormal dendritic localization for mRNAs coding for microtubule-associated protein 2 (MAP2), calcium/calmodulin-dependent protein kinase II (CAMII kinase), or dendron or activity-regulated cytoskeletal protein (ARC) in knockout brains. These studies, while negative, do serve to rule out obvious possibilities given the current understanding of FMRP function. However, Weiler and coworkers[384] demonstrated that stimulation of the metabotropic glutamate receptor in rat synaptoneurosomes resulted in increased translation of FMRP. This suggests that FMRP translation may be important for normal maturation of synaptic connections. Indeed, the dendritic spines in the knockout mouse appear abnormal, possibly due to impaired spine stabilization and pruning.[300] Thus, an emerging model is that the absence of FMRP, perhaps leading to altered local translation of bound messages, results in a subtle deficit in plasticity of filopodia, resulting in immature spine formation in response to synaptic contact. While much more needs to be understood, combined biochemical and neurobiologic studies of the mouse model should reveal great insight into the pathophysiology of fragile X syndrome and, quite possibly illuminate many aspects of normal human cognition.

TREATMENT

Presently, a treatment or cure related to the primary defect (i.e., lack of FMRP) of the fragile X syndrome does not exist. However, there are a variety of effective interventions that treat the symptoms of the syndrome; these interventions necessitate a multiprofessional approach. An extensive review of treatment is provided by Hagerman and Crontiser.[385] Treatment of the medical problems associated with the fragile X syndrome is obvious and does not differ in approach from that for individuals without the fragile X syndrome. In general, it is essential to maximize vision and hearing to ensure that each individual reaches their potential. The less frequently associated conditions, such as seizures, mitral valve prolapse, or orthopedic problems, need referral to appropriate specialists. Almost all children with the fragile X syndrome benefit greatly from speech and language therapy, and from sensory integration/occupational therapy. Such therapy, particularly sensory integration therapy, provides secondary benefits related to behavior, as it can minimize tantrums, outbursts, or aggression. With respect to learning, children with the fragile X syndrome have significant strengths that can be tapped to affect other areas of learning. For example, special education programs such as the Logo Reading, the Edmark Series, and the Lindamood-Bell can strengthen reading skills.[386] The significant ability to imitate or model is important to recognize in class placement. For example, such children can greatly benefit from inclusion in the regular classroom with the help of an aide, as modeling can help the child learn social skills. Lastly, psychopharmacology can improve behavioral difficulties that sometimes interfere with learning and socialization. For example, stimulant medication has been used to treat the significant hyperactivity and attention-deficit hyperactivity disorder (ADHD) problems of some children with the fragile X syndrome. Other symptoms that have been successfully treated include anxiety, mood lability, and aggression. As with medical problems, application of drugs to help ameliorate behavioral problems is not specific to the child with the fragile X syndrome; however, physicians who work with children with the fragile X syndrome are learning which drugs are most beneficial. Furthermore, as more is learned about the function of the FMRP, specific drugs that can target the altered biochemical conditions resulting from the lack of FMRP will become apparent. With respect to receiving a new diagnosis of the fragile X syndrome, much can be done for the families. Genetic counseling is encouraged to better understand the full spectrum of the syndrome, to determine who is at risk for having children with the fragile X syndrome, and to understand all available options for family planning. It is also beneficial for some families to become involved with parent support groups to discuss their concerns with others who have first-hand experience with issues surrounding the fragile X syndrome. The National Fragile X Foundation (1-800-688-8765) can provide a national and international list of resources and parent groups, as well as educational materials, to families and to health care and educational professionals. (Also see the Web site http://warrenlab.biochem.emory.edu/ for links to various resource and parent groups as well as the Fragile X ListServe, an electronic bulletin board for families.) Although basic research still needs to be done to identify a treatment specific to the cause of the fragile X syndrome, much progress has been made and continues at a rapid pace. Irrespective, interventions specific to the needs of the child with the fragile X syndrome are effective and continue to provide the necessary help to allow such children to reach their full potential.

REFERENCES

1. Johnson GE: Contribution to the psychology and pedagogy of feeble-minded children. *J Psycho-asthenics* **2**:26, 1897.
2. Penrose LS: *A Clinical and Genetic Study of 1280 Cases of Mental Defect*. London, HM Stationery Office, 1938.
3. Lehrke RG: X-linked mental retardation and verbal disability. *Birth Defects Orig Artic Ser* **10**:1, 1974.
4. Turner G, Turner B, Collins E: X-linked mental retardation without physical abnormality: Renpenning's syndrome. *Dev Med Child Neurol* **13**:71, 1971.
5. Martin JP, Bell J: A pedigree of mental defect showing sex-linkage. *J Neurol Psychiatr* **6**:154, 1943.
6. Renpenning H, Gerrard JW, Zaleski WA, Tabata T: Familial sex-linked mental retardation. *Can Med Assoc J* **87**:954, 1962.
7. Dunn HG, Renpenning H, Gerrard JW, Miller JR, Tabata T, Federoff S: Mental retardation as a sex-linked defect. *Am J Ment Defic* **67**:827, 1963.
8. Snyder RD, Robinson A: Recessive sex-linked mental retardation in the absence of other recognizable abnormalities. Report of a family. *Clin Pediatr* **8**:669, 1969.
9. Lubs HA: A marker X chromosome. *Am J Hum Genet* **21**:231, 1969.
10. Escalante JA, Frota-Pessoa O: Retardamento mental, in (ed): *Retardamento Mental*. San Paulo, Sarvier, 1973, p 300.
11. Harvey J, Judge C, Wiener S: Familial X-linked mental retardation with an X chromosome abnormality. *J Med Genet* **14**:46, 1977.
12. Giraud F, Ayme S, Mattei JF, Mattei MG: Constitutional chromosomal breakage. *Hum Genet* **34**:125, 1976.
13. Sutherland GR: Fragile sites on human chromosomes: Demonstration of their dependence on the type of tissue culture medium. *Science* **197**:265, 1977.
14. Escalante JA, Grunspun H, Frota-Pessoa O: Severe sex-linked mental retardation. *J Genet Hum* **19**:137, 1971.
15. Cantu JM, Scaglia HE, Medina M, Gonzalez-Diddi M, Morato T, Moreno ME, Perez-Palacios G: Inherited congenital normofunctional testicular hyperplasia and mental deficiency. *Hum Genet* **33**:23, 1976.
16. Turner G, Eastman C, Casey J, McLeay A, Procopis P, Turner B: X-linked mental retardation associated with macro-orchidism. *J Med Genet* **12**:367, 1975.
17. Ruvalcaba RH, Myhre SA, Roosen-Runge EC, Beckwith JB: X-linked mental deficiency megalotestes syndrome. *JAMA* **238**:1646, 1977.
18. Richards BW, Sylvester PE, Brooker C: Fragile X-linked mental retardation: the Martin-Bell syndrome. *J Ment Defic Res* **25(4)**:253, 1981.
19. Sherman SL, Meadows KL, Ashley AE: Examination of factors that influence the expansion of the fragile X mutation in a sample of conceptuses from known carrier females. *Am J Med Genet* **64**:256, 1996.
20. Sherman SL, Jacobs PA, Morton NE, Froster-Iskenius U, Howard-Peebles PN, Nielsen KB, Partington MW, Sutherland GR, Turner G, Watson M: Further segregation analysis of the fragile X syndrome with special reference to transmitting males. *Hum Genet* **69**:289, 1985.
21. Sherman SL, Morton NE, Jacobs PA, Turner G: The marker (X) syndrome: A cytogenetic and genetic analysis. *Ann Hum Genet* **48**:21, 1984.

22. Verkerk AJ, Pieretti M, Sutcliffe JS, Fu YH, Kuhl DP, Pizzuti A, Reiner O, Richards S, Victoria MF, Zhang FP, et al: Identification of a gene (FMR-1) containing a CGG repeat coincident with a breakpoint cluster region exhibiting length variation in fragile X syndrome. *Cell* **65**:905, 1991.
23. Oostra BA, Hupkes PE, Perdon LF, van Bennekom CA, Bakker E, Halley DJ, Schmidt M, Du Sart D, Smits A, Wieringa B, et al: New polymorphic DNA marker close to the fragile site FRAXA. *Genomics* **6**:129, 1990.
24. Oberle I, Heilig R, Moisan JP, Kloepfer C, Mattei GM, Mattei JF, Boue J, Froster-Iskenius U, Jacobs PA, Lathrop GM, et al: Genetic analysis of the fragile-X mental retardation syndrome with two flanking polymorphic DNA markers. *Proc Natl Acad Sci U S A* **83**:1016, 1986.
25. Mulligan LM, Phillips MA, Forster-Gibson CJ, Beckett J, Partington MW, Simpson NE, Holden JJ, White BN: Genetic mapping of DNA segments relative to the locus for the fragile-X syndrome at Xq27.3. *Am J Hum Genet* **37**:463, 1985.
26. Goonewardena P, Dahl N, Gustavson KH, Holmgren G, Pettersson U: DNA studies of X-linked mental retardation associated with a fragile site at Xq27.3. *Ups J Med Sci Suppl* **44**:155, 1987.
27. Davies KE: DNA studies of X-linked mental retardation associated with a fragile site at Xq27. *Am J Med Genet* **23**:633, 1986.
28. Brown WT, Gross A, Chan C, Jenkins EC, Mandel JL, Oberle I, Arveiler B, Novelli G, Thibodeau S, Hagerman R, et al: Multilocus analysis of the fragile X syndrome. *Hum Genet* **78**:201, 1988.
29. Warren ST, Glover TW, Davidson RL, Jagadeeswaran P: Linkage and recombination between fragile X-linked mental retardation and the factor IX gene. *Hum Genet* **69**:44, 1985.
30. Thibodeau SN, Dorkins HR, Faulk KR, Berry R, Smith AC, Hagerman R, King A, Davies KE: Linkage analysis using multiple DNA polymorphic markers in normal families and in families with fragile X syndrome. *Hum Genet* **79**:219, 1988.
31. Mulley JC, Gedeon AK, Thorn KA, Bates LJ, Sutherland GR: Linkage and genetic counselling for the fragile X using DNA probes 52A, F9, DX13, and ST14. *Am J Med Genet* **27**:435, 1987.
32. Mulley J, Turner G, Bain S, Sutherland GR: Linkage between the fragile X and F9, DXS52 (St14), DXS98 (4D-8) and DXS105 (cX55.7). *Am J Med Genet* **30**:567, 1988.
33. Oberle I, Camerino G, Wrogemann K, Arveiler B, Hanauer A, Raimondi E, Mandel JL: Multipoint genetic mapping of the Xq26-q28 region in families with fragile X mental retardation and in normal families reveals tight linkage of markers in q26-q27. *Hum Genet* **77**:60, 1987.
34. Camerino G, Mattei MG, Mattei JF, Jaye M, Mandel JL: Close linkage of fragile X-mental retardation syndrome to haemophilia B and transmission through a normal male. *Nature* **306**:701, 1983.
35. Bell MV, Hirst MC, Nakahori Y, MacKinnon RN, Roche A, Flint TJ, Jacobs PA, Tommerup N, Tranebjaerg L, Froster-Iskenius U, et al: Physical mapping across the fragile X: Hypermethylation and clinical expression of the fragile X syndrome. *Cell* **64**:861, 1991.
36. Vincent A, Heitz D, Petit C, Kretz C, Oberle I, Mandel JL: Abnormal pattern detected in fragile-X patients by pulsed-field gel electrophoresis. *Nature* **349**:624, 1991.
37. Nussbaum RL, Airhart SD, Ledbetter DH: Expression of the fragile (X) chromosome in an interspecific somatic cell hybrid. *Hum Genet* **64**:148, 1983.
38. Warren ST, Davidson RL: Expression of fragile X chromosome in human-rodent somatic cell hybrids. *Somat Cell Mol Genet* **10**:409, 1984.
39. Ledbetter DH, Ledbetter SA, Nussbaum RL: Implications of fragile X expression in normal males for the nature of the mutation. *Nature* **324**:161, 1986.
40. Warren ST, Zhang F, Licameli GR, Peters JF: The fragile X site in somatic cell hybrids: An approach for molecular cloning of fragile sites. *Science* **237**:420, 1987.
41. Warren ST, Knight SJ, Peters JF, Stayton CL, Consalez GG, Zhang FP: Isolation of the human chromosomal band Xq28 within somatic cell hybrids by fragile X site breakage. *Proc Natl Acad Sci U S A* **87**:3856, 1990.
42. Yu S, Pritchard M, Kremer E, Lynch M, Nancarrow J, Baker E, Holman K, Mulley JC, Warren ST, Schlessinger D, et al: Fragile X genotype characterized by an unstable region of DNA. *Science* **252**:1179, 1991.
43. Oberle I, Rousseau F, Heitz D, Kretz C, Devys D, Hanauer A, Boue J, Bertheas MF, Mandel JL: Instability of a 550-base pair DNA segment and abnormal methylation in fragile X syndrome. *Science* **252**:1097, 1991.
44. Kremer EJ, Pritchard M, Lynch M, Yu S, Holman K, Baker E, Warren ST, Schlessinger D, Sutherland GR, Richards RI: Mapping of DNA instability at the fragile X to a trinucleotide repeat sequence p(CCG)n. *Science* **252**:1711, 1991.
45. Ashley CT, Sutcliffe JS, Kunst CB, Leiner HA, Eichler EE, Nelson DL, Warren ST: Human and murine FMR-1: Alternative splicing and translational initiation downstream of the CGG-repeat. *Nat Genet* **4**:244, 1993.
46. Fu YH, Kuhl DP, Pizzuti A, Pieretti M, Sutcliffe JS, Richards S, Verkerk AJ, Holden JJ, Fenwick RG Jr, Warren ST, et al: Variation of the CGG repeat at the fragile X site results in genetic instability: Resolution of the Sherman paradox. *Cell* **67**:1047, 1991.
47. Kremer EJ, Yu S, Pritchard M, Nagaraja R, Heitz D, Lynch M, Baker E, Hyland VJ, Little RD, Wada M, et al: Isolation of a human DNA sequence which spans the fragile X. *Am J Hum Genet* **49**:656, 1991.
48. Eichler EE, Holden JJ, Popovich BW, Reiss AL, Snow K, Thibodeau SN, Richards CS, Ward PA, Nelson DL: Length of uninterrupted CGG repeats determines instability in the FMR1 gene. *Nat Genet* **8**:88, 1994.
49. Kunst CB, Warren ST: Cryptic and polar variation of the fragile X repeat could result in predisposing normal alleles. *Cell* **77**:853, 1994.
50. Snow K, Tester DJ, Kruckeberg KE, Schaid DJ, Thibodeau SN: Sequence analysis of the fragile X trinucleotide repeat: Implications for the origin of the fragile X mutation. *Hum Mol Genet* **3**:1543, 1994.
51. Snow K, Doud LK, Hagerman R, Pergolizzi RG, Erster SH, Thibodeau SN: Analysis of a CGG sequence at the FMR-1 locus in fragile X families and in the general population. *Am J Hum Genet* **53**:1217, 1993.
52. Hirst MC, Grewal PK, Davies KE: Precursor arrays for triplet repeat expansion at the fragile X locus. *Hum Mol Genet* **3**:1553, 1994.
53. Zhong N, Yang W, Dobkin C, Brown WT: Fragile X gene instability: Anchoring AGGs and linked microsatellites [see comments]. *Am J Hum Genet* **57**:351, 1995.
54. Eichler EE, Richards S, Gibbs RA, Nelson DL: Fine structure of the human FMR1 gene. *Hum Mol Genet* **3**:684, 1994.
55. Feng Y, Lakkis L, Devys D, Warren ST: Quantitative comparison of FMR1 gene expression in normal and premutation alleles. *Am J Hum Genet* **56**:106, 1995.
56. Murray A, Macpherson JN, Pound MC, Sharrock A, Youings SA, Dennis NR, McKechnie N, Linehan P, Morton NE, Jacobs PA: The role of size, sequence and haplotype in the stability of FRAXA and FRAXE alleles during transmission. *Hum Mol Genet* **6**:173, 1997.
57. Nolin SL, Lewis FA, 3rd, Ye LL, Houck GE Jr, Glicksman AE, Limprasert P, Li SY, Zhong N, Ashley AE, Feingold E, Sherman SL, Brown WT: Familial transmission of the FMR1 CGG repeat. *Am J Hum Genet* **59**:1252, 1996.
58. Crawford DC, Meadows KL, Newman JL: Examining the prevalence and phenotype consequence of FRAXA and FRAXE alleles in a large, ethnically diverse special education needs population. *Am J Hum Genet* **64** :495, 1999.
59. Murray A, Youings S, Dennis N, Latsky L, Linehan P, McKechnie N, Macpherson J, Pound M, Jacobs P: Population screening at the FRAXA and FRAXE loci: Molecular analyses of boys with learning difficulties and their mothers. *Hum Mol Genet* **5**:727, 1996.
60. Patsalis PC, Sismani C, Hettinger JA , et al: Molecular screening of fragile X (FRAXA) and FRAXE mental retardation syndromes in the Hellenic population of Greece and Cyprus: Incidence, genetic variation and stability. *Am J Med Gen* **84**:184, 1999.
61. Pieretti M, Zhang FP, Fu YH, Warren ST, Oostra BA, Caskey CT, Nelson DL: Absence of expression of the FMR-1 gene in fragile X syndrome. *Cell* **66**:817, 1991.
62. Sutcliffe JS, Nelson DL, Zhang F, Pieretti M, Caskey CT, Saxe D, Warren ST: DNA methylation represses FMR-1 transcription in fragile X syndrome. *Hum Mol Genet* **1**:397, 1992.
63. McConkie-Rosell A, Lachiewicz AM, Spiridigliozzi GA, Tarleton J, Schoenwald S, Phelan MC, Goonewardena P, Ding X, Brown WT: Evidence that methylation of the FMR-I locus is responsible for variable phenotypic expression of the fragile X syndrome. *Am J Hum Genet* **53**:800, 1993.
64. Ashley CT Jr., Wilkinson KD, Reines D, Warren ST: FMR1 protein: Conserved RNP family domains and selective RNA binding. *Science* **262**:563, 1993.
65. Rousseau F, Heitz D, Biancalana V, Blumenfeld S, Kretz C, Boue J, Tommerup N, Van Der Hagen C, DeLozier-Blanchet C, Croquette MF, et al: Direct diagnosis by DNA analysis of the fragile X syndrome of mental retardation [see comments]. *N Engl J Med* **325**:1673, 1991.

66. Rousseau F, Heitz D, Oberle I, Mandel JL: Selection in blood cells from female carriers of the fragile X syndrome: Inverse correlation between age and proportion of active X chromosomes carrying the full mutation. *J Med Genet* **28**:830, 1991.
67. Nolin SL, Glicksman A, Houck GE Jr, Brown WT, Dobkin CS: Mosaicism in fragile X affected males. *Am J Med Genet* **51**:509, 1994.
68. Feng Y, Zhang F, Lokey LK, Chastain JL, Lakkis L, Eberhart D, Warren ST: Translational suppression by trinucleotide repeat expansion at FMR1. *Science* **268**:731, 1995.
69. Lachiewicz AM, Spiridigliozzi GA, McConkie-Rosell A, Burgess D, Feng Y, Warren ST, Tarleton J: A fragile X male with a broad smear on Southern blot analysis representing 100-500 CGG repeats and no methylation at the *Eag*I site of the FMR-1 gene. *Am J Med Genet* **64**:278, 1996.
70. Verkerk AJ, Eussen BH, Van Hemel JO, Oostra BA: Limited size of the fragile X site shown by fluorescence in situ hybridization. *Am J Med Genet* **43**:187, 1992.
71. Oostra BA, Verkerk AJ: The fragile X syndrome: Isolation of the FMR-1 gene and characterization of the fragile X mutation. *Chromosoma* **101**:381, 1992.
72. Riggins GJ, Sherman SL, Oostra BA, Sutcliffe JS, Feitell D, Nelson DL, van Oost BA, Smits AP, Ramos FJ, Pfendner E, et al: Characterization of a highly polymorphic dinucleotide repeat 150 KB proximal to the fragile X site. *Am J Med Genet* **43**:237, 1992.
73. Richards RI, Holman K, Kozman H, Kremer E, Lynch M, Pritchard M, Yu S, Mulley J, Sutherland GR: Fragile X syndrome: Genetic localisation by linkage mapping of two microsatellite repeats FRAXAC1 and FRAXAC2 which immediately flank the fragile site. *J Med Genet* **28**:818, 1991.
74. Gunter C, Paradee W, Crawford DC, Meadows KA, Newman J, Kunst CB, Nelson DL, Schwartz C, Murray A, Macpherson JN, Sherman SL, Warren ST: Re-examination of factors associated with expansion of CGG repeats using a single nucleotide polymorphism in FMR1. *Hum Mol Genet* **7**:1935, 1998.
75. Verkerk AJ, de Graaff E, De Boulle K, Eichler EE, Konecki DS, Reyniers E, Manca A, Poustka A, Willems PJ, Nelson DL, et al: Alternative splicing in the fragile X gene FMR1. *Hum Mol Genet* **2**:1348, 1993.
76. Verheij C, Bakker CE, de Graaff E, Keulemans J, Willemsen R, Verkerk AJ, Galjaard H, Reuser AJ, Hoogeveen AT, Oostra BA: Characterization and localization of the FMR-1 gene product associated with fragile X syndrome. *Nature* **363**:722, 1993.
77. Verheij C, de Graaff E, Bakker CE, Willemsen R, Willems PJ, Meijer N, Galjaard H, Reuser AJ, Oostra BA, Hoogeveen AT: Characterization of FMR1 proteins isolated from different tissues. *Hum Mol Genet* **4**:895, 1995.
78. Abitbol M, Menini C, Delezoide AL, Rhyner T, Vekemans M, Mallet J: Nucleus basalis magnocellularis and hippocampus are the major sites of FMR-1 expression in the human fetal brain. *Nat Genet* **4**:147, 1993.
79. Hinds HL, Ashley CT, Sutcliffe JS, Nelson DL, Warren ST, Housman DE, Schalling M: Tissue specific expression of FMR-1 provides evidence for a functional role in fragile X syndrome [see comments] [published erratum appears in *Nat Genet* 5(3):312, 1993]. *Nat Genet* **3**:36, 1993.
80. Devys D, Lutz Y, Rouyer N, Bellocq JP, Mandel JL: The FMR-1 protein is cytoplasmic, most abundant in neurons and appears normal in carriers of a fragile X premutation. *Nat Genet* **4**:335, 1993.
81. Feng Y, Gutekunst CA, Eberhart DE, Yi H, Warren ST, Hersch SM: Fragile X mental retardation protein: Nucleocytoplasmic shuttling and association with somatodendritic ribosomes. *J Neurosci* **17**:1539, 1997.
82. Bachner D, Manca A, Steinbach P, Wohrle D, Just W, Vogel W, Hameister H, Poustka A: Enhanced expression of the murine FMR1 gene during germ cell proliferation suggests a special function in both the male and the female gonad. *Hum Mol Genet* **2**:2043, 1993.
83. Hergersberg M, Matsuo K, Gassmann M, Schaffner W, Luscher B, Rulicke T, Aguzzi A: Tissue-specific expression of a FMR1/beta-galactosidase fusion gene in transgenic mice. *Hum Mol Genet* **4**:359, 1995.
84. Price DK, Zhang F, Ashley CT Jr, Warren ST: The chicken FMR1 gene is highly conserved with a CCT 5′-untranslated repeat and encodes an RNA-binding protein. *Genomics* **31**:3, 1996.
85. Siomi MC, Siomi H, Sauer WH, Srinivasan S, Nussbaum RL, Dreyfuss G: FXR1, an autosomal homolog of the fragile X mental retardation gene. *Embo J* **14**:2401, 1995.
86. Wintersberger U, Kuhne C, Karwan A: Scp160p, a new yeast protein associated with the nuclear membrane and the endoplasmic reticulum, is necessary for maintenance of exact ploidy. *Yeast* **11**:929, 1995.
87. Weber V, Wernitznig A, Hager G, Harata M, Frank P, Wintersberger U: Purification and nucleic-acid-binding properties of a Saccharomyces cerevisiae protein involved in the control of ploidy. *Eur J Biochem* **249**:309, 1997.
88. Kugler S, Grunweller A, Probst C, Klinger M, Muller PK, Kruse C: Vigilin contains a functional nuclear localisation sequence and is present in both the cytoplasm and the nucleus. *FEBS Lett* **382**:330, 1996.
89. Eichler EE, Kunst CB, Lugenbeel KA, Ryder OA, Davison D, Warren ST, Nelson DL: Evolution of the cryptic FMR1 CGG repeat. *Nat Genet* **11**:301, 1995.
90. Gronskov K, Hjalgrim H, Bjerager MO, Brondum-Nielsen K: Deletion of all CGG repeats plus flanking sequences in FMR1 does not abolish gene expression. *Am J Hum Genet* **61**:961, 1997.
91. Deissler H, Wilm M, Genc B, Schmitz B, Ternes T, Naumann F, Mann M, Doerfler W: Rapid protein sequencing by tandem mass spectrometry and cDNA cloning of p20-CGGBP. A novel protein that binds to the unstable triplet repeat 5′-d(CGG)n-3′ in the human FMR1 gene. *J Biol Chem* **272**:16761, 1997.
92. Deissler H, Behn-Krappa A, Doerfler W: Purification of nuclear proteins from human HeLa cells that bind specifically to the unstable tandem repeat (CGG)n in the human FMR1 gene. *J Biol Chem* **271**:4327, 1996.
93. De Boulle K, Verkerk AJ, Reyniers E, Vits L, Hendrickx J, Van Roy B, Van den Bos F, de Graaff E, Oostra BA, Willems PJ: A point mutation in the FMR-1 gene associated with fragile X mental retardation. *Nat Genet* **3**:31, 1993.
94. de Graaff E, Rouillard P, Willems PJ, Smits AP, Rousseau F, Oostra BA: Hotspot for deletions in the CGG repeat region of FMR1 in fragile X patients. *Hum Mol Genet* **4**:45, 1995.
95. Wohrle D, Kotzot D, Hirst MC, Manca A, Korn B, Schmidt A, Barbi G, Rott HD, Poustka A, Davies KE, et al: A microdeletion of less than 250 kb, including the proximal part of the FMR-1 gene and the fragile-X site, in a male with the clinical phenotype of fragile-X syndrome. *Am J Hum Genet* **51**:299, 1992.
96. Hammond LS, Macias MM, Tarleton JC, Shashidhar Pai G: Fragile X syndrome and deletions in FMR1: New case and review of the literature. *Am J Med Genet* **72**:430, 1997.
97. Gedeon AK, Baker E, Robinson H, Partington MW, Gross B, Manca A, Korn B, Poustka A, Yu S, Sutherland GR, et al: Fragile X syndrome without CCG amplification has an FMR1 deletion. *Nat Genet* **1**:341, 1992.
98. Tarleton J, Richie R, Schwartz C, Rao K, Aylsworth AS, Lachiewicz A: An extensive de novo deletion removing FMR1 in a patient with mental retardation and the fragile X syndrome phenotype. *Hum Mol Genet* **2**:1973, 1993.
99. Gu Y, Lugenbeel KA, Vockley JG, Grody WW, Nelson DL: A de novo deletion in FMR1 in a patient with developmental delay. *Hum Mol Genet* **3**:1705, 1994.
100. Mannermaa A, Pulkkinen L, Kajanoja E, Ryynanen M, Saarikoski S: Deletion in the FMR1 gene in a fragile-X male. *Am J Med Genet* **64**:293, 1996.
101. Wiegers AM, Curfs LM, Meijer H, Oostra B, Fryns JP: A deletion of 1.6 Kb proximal to the CGG repeat of the FMR1 gene causes fragile X-like psychological features. *Genet Couns* **5**:377, 1994.
102. Hirst M, Grewal P, Flannery A, Slatter R, Maher E, Barton D, Fryns JP, Davies K: Two new cases of FMR1 deletion associated with mental impairment. *Am J Hum Genet* **56**:67, 1995.
103. Lugenbeel KA, Peier AM, Carson NL, Chudley AE, Nelson DL: Intragenic loss of function mutations demonstrate the primary role of FMR1 in fragile X syndrome. *Nat Genet* **10**:483, 1995.
104. Wang YC, Lin ML, Lin SJ, Li YC, Li SY: Novel point mutation within intron 10 of FMR-1 gene causing fragile X syndrome. *Hum Mutat* **10**:393, 1997.
105. Albright SG, Lachiewicz AM, Tarleton JC, Rao KW, Schwartz CE, Richie R, Tennison MB, Aylsworth AS: Fragile X phenotype in a patient with a large de novo deletion in Xq27-q28. *Am J Med Genet* **51**:294, 1994.
106. Trottier Y, Imbert G, Poustka A, Fryns JP, Mandel JL: Male with typical fragile X phenotype is deleted for part of the FMR1 gene and for about 100 kb of upstream region. *Am J Med Genet* **51**:454, 1994.

107. Quan F, Zonana J, Gunter K, Peterson KL, Magenis RE, Popovich BW: An atypical case of fragile X syndrome caused by a deletion that includes the FMR1 gene. *Am J Hum Genet* **56**:1042, 1995.
108. Wolff DJ, Gustashaw KM, Zurcher V, Ko L, White W, Weiss L, Van Dyke DL, Schwartz S, Willard HF: Deletions in Xq26.3-q27.3 including FMR1 result in a severe phenotype in a male and variable phenotypes in females depending upon the X inactivation pattern. *Hum Genet* **100**:256, 1997.
109. Birot AM, Delobel B, Gronnier P, Bonnet V, Maire I, Bozon D: A 5-megabase familial deletion removes the IDS and FMR-1 genes in a male Hunter patient. *Hum Mutat* **7**:266, 1996.
110. van den Ouweland AM, de Vries BB, Bakker PL, Deelen WH, de Graaff E, van Hemel JO, Oostra BA, Niermeijer MF, Halley DJ: DNA diagnosis of the fragile X syndrome in a series of 236 mentally retarded subjects and evidence for a reversal of mutation in the FMR-1 gene. *Am J Med Genet* **51**:482, 1994.
111. Mila M, Castellvi-Bel S, Sanchez A, Lazaro C, Villa M, Estivill X: Mosaicism for the fragile X syndrome full mutation and deletions within the CGG repeat of the FMR1 gene. *J Med Genet* **33**:338, 1996.
112. Turner G, Robinson H, Laing S, Purvis-Smith S: Preventive screening for the fragile X syndrome. *N Engl J Med* **315**:607, 1986.
113. Webb T, Thake A, Todd J: Twelve families with fragile X(q27). *J Med Genet* **23**:400, 1986.
113a. Tumer G, Webb T, Wake S, Robinson H: Prevalence of fragile X syndrome. *Am J Med Genet* **64**:196–197, 1996.
114. Falik-Zaccai TC, Shachak E, Yalon M, Lis Z, Borochowitz Z, Macpherson JN, Nelson DL, Eichler EE: Predisposition to the fragile X syndrome in Jews of Tunisian descent is due to the absence of AGG interruptions on a rare Mediterranean haplotype. *Am J Hum Genet* **60**:103, 1997.
115. Rousseau F, Rouillard P, Morel ML, Khandjian EW, Morgan K: Prevalence of carriers of premutation-size alleles of the FMRI gene and implications for the population genetics of the fragile X syndrome [see comments]. *Am J Hum Genet* **57**:1006, 1995.
116. Yu S, Mulley J, Loesch D, Turner G, Donnelly A, Gedeon A, Hillen D, Kremer E, Lynch M, Pritchard M, et al: Fragile-X syndrome: Unique genetics of the heritable unstable element. *Am J Hum Genet* **50**:968, 1992.
117. Heitz D, Devys D, Imbert G, Kretz C, Mandel JL: Inheritance of the fragile X syndrome: Size of the fragile X premutation is a major determinant of the transition to full mutation. *J Med Genet* **29**:794, 1992.
118. Fisch GS, Snow K, Thibodeau SN, Chalifaux M, Holden JJ, Nelson DL, Howard-Peebles PN, Maddalena A: The fragile X premutation in carriers and its effect on mutation size in offspring. *Am J Hum Genet* **56**:1147, 1995.
119. Ashley-Koch AE, Robinson H, Glicksman AE, Nolin SL, Schwartz CE, Brown WT, Turner G, Sherman SL: Examination of factors associated with instability of the FMR1 CGG repeat. *Am J Hum Genet* **63**:776, 1998.
120. Mornet E, Jokic M, Bogyo A, Tejada I, Deluchat C, Boue J, Boue A: Affected sibs with fragile X syndrome exhibit an age-dependent decrease in the size of the fragile X full mutation. *Clin Genet* **43**:157, 1993.
121. Rousseau F, Heitz D, Tarleton J, MacPherson J, Malmgren H, Dahl N, Barnicoat A, Mathew C, Mornet E, Tejada I, et al: A multicenter study on genotype-phenotype correlations in the fragile X syndrome, using direct diagnosis with probe StB12.3: The first 2,253 cases. *Am J Hum Genet* **55**:225, 1994.
122. Loesch DZ, Huggins R, Petrovic V, Slater H: Expansion of the CGG repeat in fragile X in the FMR1 gene depends on the sex of the offspring. *Am J Hum Genet* **57**:1408, 1995.
123. Wohrle D, Hirst MC, Kennerknecht I, Davies KE, Steinbach P: Genotype mosaicism in fragile X fetal tissues. *Hum Genet* **89**:114, 1992.
124. Devys D, Biancalana V, Rousseau F, Boue J, Mandel JL, Oberle I: Analysis of full fragile X mutations in fetal tissues and monozygotic twins indicate that abnormal methylation and somatic heterogeneity are established early in development. *Am J Med Genet* **43**:208, 1992.
125. Sutherland GR, Gedeon A, Kornman L, Donnelly A, Byard RW, Mulley JC, Kremer E, Lynch M, Pritchard M, Yu S, et al: Prenatal diagnosis of fragile X syndrome by direct detection of the unstable DNA sequence [see comments]. *N Engl J Med* **325**:1720, 1991.
126. Wohrle D, Hennig I, Vogel W, Steinbach P: Mitotic stability of fragile X mutations in differentiated cells indicates early post-conceptional trinucleotide repeat expansion [see comments]. *Nat Genet* **4**:140, 1993.
127. de Graaff E, Willemsen R, Zhong N, de Die-Smulders CE, Brown WT, Freling G, Oostra B: Instability of the CGG repeat and expression of the FMR1 protein in a male fragile X patient with a lung tumor. *Am J Hum Genet* **57**:609, 1995.
128. Tassone F, Hagerman RJ, Ikle DN, et al: FMRP expression as a potential prognostic indicator in fragile X syndrome. *Am J Med Genet* **84**:250, 1999.
129. Malmgren H, Gustavson KH, Wahlstrom J, Arpi-Henriksson I, Bensch J, Pettersson U, Dahl N: Infantile autism—Fragile X: Molecular findings support genetic heterogeneity. *Am J Med Genet* **44**:830, 1992.
130. Kruyer H, Mila M, Glover G, Carbonell P, Ballesta F, Estivill X: Fragile X syndrome and the (CGG)n mutation: Two families with discordant MZ twins. *Am J Hum Genet* **54**:437, 1994.
131. Reiss AL, Abrams MT, Greenlaw R, Freund L, Denckla MB: Neurodevelopmental effects of the FMR-1 full mutation in humans. *Nat Med* **1**:159, 1995.
132. Reyniers E, Vits L, De Boulle K, Van Roy B, Van Velzen D, de Graaff E, Verkerk AJ, Jorens HZ, Darby JK, Oostra B, et al: The full mutation in the FMR-1 gene of male fragile X patients is absent in their sperm. *Nat Genet* **4**:143, 1993.
133. Willems PJ, Van Roy B, De Boulle K, Vits L, Reyniers E, Beck O, Dumon JE, Verkerk A, Oostra B: Segregation of the fragile X mutation from an affected male to his normal daughter. *Hum Mol Genet* **1**:511, 1992.
134. The Dutch-Belgian Fragile X Consortium. Fmr1 knockout mice: A model to study fragile X mental retardation. *Cell* **78**:23, 1994.
135. Moutou C, Vincent MC, Biancalana V, Mandel JL: Transition from premutation to full mutation in fragile X syndrome is likely to be prezygotic. *Hum Mol Genet* **6**:971, 1997.
136. Malter HE, Iber JC, Willemsen R, de Graaff E, Tarleton JC, Leisti J, Warren ST, Oostra BA: Characterization of the full fragile X syndrome mutation in fetal gametes. *Nat Genet* **15**:165, 1997.
137. Kolehmainen K: Population genetics of fragile X: A multiple allele model with variable risk of CGG repeat expansion. *Am J Med Genet* **51**:428, 1994.
138. Morris A, Morton NE, Collins A, Macpherson J, Nelson D, Sherman S: An n-allele model for progressive amplification in the FMR1 locus. *Proc Natl Acad Sci U S A* **92**:4833, 1995.
139. Ashley AE, Sherman SL: Population dynamics of a meiotic/mitotic expansion model for the fragile X syndrome. *Am J Hum Genet* **57**:1414, 1995.
140. Winter RM: Population genetics implications of the premutation hypothesis for the generation of the fragile X mental retardation gene. *Hum Genet* **75**:269, 1987.
141. Sved JA, Laird CD: Population genetic consequences of the fragile-X syndrome, based on the X-inactivation imprinting model. *Am J Hum Genet* **46**:443, 1990.
142. Morton NE, Macpherson JN: Population genetics of the fragile-X syndrome: Multiallelic model for the FMR1 locus. *Proc Natl Acad Sci U S A* **89**:4215, 1992.
143. Morris A, Morton NE, Collins A, Lawrence S, Macpherson JN: Evolutionary dynamics of the FMR1 locus. *Ann Hum Genet* **59**:283, 1995.
144. Sherman SL: The high prevalence of fragile X premutation carrier females: Is this frequency unique to the French Canadian population? [Editorial; Comment]. *Am J Hum Genet* **57**:991, 1995.
145. Meadows KL, Pettay D, Newman J, Hersey J, Ashley AE, Sherman SL: Survey of the fragile X syndrome and the fragile X E syndrome in a special education needs population. *Am J Med Genet* **64**:428, 1996.
146. Zhong N, Liu X, Gou S, Houck GE Jr, Li S, Dobkin C, Brown WT: Distribution of FMR-1 and associated microsatellite alleles in a normal Chinese population. *Am J Med Genet* **51**:417, 1994.
147. Arinami T, Asano M, Kobayashi K, Yanagi H, Hamaguchi H: Data on the CGG repeat at the fragile X site in the non-retarded Japanese population and family suggest the presence of a subgroup of normal alleles predisposing to mutate. *Hum Genet* **92**:431, 1993.
148. Eichler EE, Nelson DL: Genetic variation and evolutionary stability of the FMR1 CGG repeat in six closed human populations. *Am J Med Genet* **64**:220, 1996.
149. Kunst CB, Zerylnick C, Karickhoff L, Eichler E, Bullard J, Chalifoux M, Holden JJ, Torroni A, Nelson DL, Warren ST: FMR1 in global populations. *Am J Hum Genet* **58**:513, 1996.
150. Richards RI, Holman K, Friend K, Kremer E, Hillen D, Staples A, Brown WT, Goonewardena P, Tarleton J, Schwartz C, et al: Evidence of founder chromosomes in fragile X syndrome. *Nat Genet* **1**:257, 1992.

151. Oudet C, von Koskull H, Nordstrom AM, Peippo M, Mandel JL: Striking founder effect for the fragile X syndrome in Finland. *Eur J Hum Genet* **1**:181, 1993.
152. Zhong N, Ye L, Dobkin C, Brown WT: Fragile X founder chromosome effects: Linkage disequilibrium or microsatellite heterogeneity? *Am J Med Genet* **51**:405, 1994.
153. Hirst MC, Knight SJ, Christodoulou Z, Grewal PK, Fryns JP, Davies KE: Origins of the fragile X syndrome mutation. *J Med Genet* **30**:647, 1993.
154. Buyle S, Reyniers E, Vits L, De Boulle K, Handig I, Wuyts FL, Deelen W, Halley DJ, Oostra BA, Willems PJ: Founder effect in a Belgian-Dutch fragile X population. *Hum Genet* **92**:269, 1993.
155. Jacobs PA, Bullman H, Macpherson J, Youings S, Rooney V, Watson A, Dennis NR: Population studies of the fragile X: A molecular approach. *J Med Genet* **30**:454, 1993.
156. Haataja R, Vaisanen ML, Li M, Ryynanen M, Leisti J: The fragile X syndrome in Finland: Demonstration of a founder effect by analysis of microsatellite haplotypes. *Hum Genet* **94**:479, 1994.
157. Malmgren H, Gustavson KH, Oudet C, Holmgren G, Pettersson U, Dahl N: Strong founder effect for the fragile X syndrome in Sweden. *Eur J Hum Genet* **2**:103, 1994.
158. Chiurazzi P, Genuardi M, Kozak L, Giovannucci-Uzielli ML, Bussani C, Dagna-Bricarelli F, Grasso M, Perroni L, Sebastio G, Sperandeo MP, Oostra BA, Neri G: Fragile X founder chromosomes in Italy: A few initial events and possible explanation for their heterogeneity. *Am J Med Genet* **64**:209, 1996.
159. Macpherson JN, Bullman H, Youings SA, Jacobs PA: Insert size and flanking haplotype in fragile X and normal populations: Possible multiple origins for the fragile X mutation. *Hum Mol Genet* **3**:399, 1994.
160. Zhong N, Kajanoja E, Smits B, Pietrofesa J, Curley D, Wang D, Ju W, Nolin S, Dobkin C, Ryynanen M, Brown WT: Fragile X founder effects and new mutations in Finland. *Am J Med Genet* **64**:226, 1996.
161. Chiurazzi P, Destro-Bisol G, Genuardi M, Oostra BA, Spedini G, Neri G: Extended gene diversity at the FMR1 locus and neighboring CA repeats in a sub-Saharan population. *Am J Med Genet* **64**:216, 1996.
162. Eichler EE, Macpherson JN, Murray A, Jacobs PA, Chakravarti A, Nelson DL: Haplotype and interspersion analysis of the FMR1 CGG repeat identifies two different mutational pathways for the origin of the fragile X syndrome. *Hum Mol Genet* **5**:319, 1996.
163. Smits AP, Dreesen JC, Post JG, Smeets DF, de Die-Smulders C, Spaans-van der Bijl T, Govaerts LC, Warren ST, Oostra BA, van Oost BA: The fragile X syndrome: No evidence for any recent mutations. *J Med Genet* **30**:94, 1993.
164. Losekoot M, Hoogendoorn E, Olmer R, Jansen CC, Oosterwijk JC, van den Ouweland AM, Halley DJ, Warren ST, Willemsen R, Oostra BA, Bakker E: Prenatal diagnosis of the fragile X syndrome: Loss of mutation owing to a double recombinant or gene conversion event at the FMR1 locus. *J Med Genet* **34**:924, 1997.
165. van den Ouweland AM, Deelen WH, Kunst CB, Uzielli ML, Nelson DL, Warren ST, Oostra BA, Halley DJ: Loss of mutation at the FMR1 locus through multiple exchanges between maternal X chromosomes. *Hum Mol Genet* **3**:1823, 1994.
166. Mornet E, Chateau C, Taillandier A, Simon-Bouy B, Serre JL: Recurrent and unexpected segregation of the FMR1 CGG repeat in a family with fragile X syndrome. *Hum Genet* **97**:512, 1996.
167. Pearson CE, Eichler EE, Lorenzetti D, Kramer SF, Zoghbi HY, Nelson DL, Sinden RR: Interruptions in the triplet repeats of SCA1 and FRAXA reduce the propensity and complexity of slipped strand DNA (S-DNA) formation. *Biochemistry* **37**:2701, 1998.
168. Eichler EE, Hammond HA, Macpherson JN, Ward PA, Nelson DL: Population survey of the human FMR1 CGG repeat substructure suggests biased polarity for the loss of AGG interruptions. *Hum Mol Genet* **4**:2199, 1995.
169. Kunst CB, Leeflang EP, Iber JC, Arnheim N, Warren ST: The effect of FMR1 CGG repeat interruptions on mutation frequency as measured by sperm typing. *J Med Genet* **34**:627, 1997.
170. Ashley CT Jr, Warren ST: Trinucleotide repeat expansion and human disease. *Annu Rev Genet* **29**:703, 1995.
171. Goldberg YP, Kremer B, Andrew SE, Theilmann J, Graham RK, Squitieri F, Telenius H, Adam S, Sajoo A, Starr E, et al: Molecular analysis of new mutations for Huntington's disease: Intermediate alleles and sex of origin effects [see comments]. *Nat Genet* **5**:174, 1993.
172. Chung MY, Ranum LP, Duvick LA, Servadio A, Zoghbi HY, Orr HT: Evidence for a mechanism predisposing to intergenerational CAG repeat instability in spinocerebellar ataxia type I. *Nat Genet* **5**:254, 1993.
173. Trinh TQ, Sinden RR: Preferential DNA secondary structure mutagenesis in the lagging strand of replication in *E. coli*. *Nature* **352**:544, 1991.
174. Veaute X, Fuchs RP: Greater susceptibility to mutations in lagging strand of DNA replication in *Escherichia coli* than in leading strand. *Science* **261**:598, 1993.
175. Burhans WC, Vassilev LT, Caddle MS, Heintz NH, DePamphilis ML: Identification of an origin of bidirectional DNA replication in mammalian chromosomes. *Cell* **62**:955, 1990.
176. Richards RI, Sutherland GR: Simple repeat DNA is not replicated simply [news]. *Nat Genet* **6**:114, 1994.
177. Ji J, Clegg NJ, Peterson KR, Jackson AL, Laird CD, Loeb LA: In vitro expansion of GGC:GCC repeats: Identification of the preferred strand of expansion. *Nucleic Acids Res* **24**:2835, 1996.
178. Schlotterer C, Tautz D: Slippage synthesis of simple sequence DNA. *Nucleic Acids Res* **20**:211, 1992.
179. Gordenin DA, Kunkel TA, Resnick MA: Repeat expansion — All in a flap? *Nat Genet* **16**:116, 1997.
180. Bambara RA, Murante RS, Henricksen LA: Enzymes and reactions at the eukaryotic DNA replication fork. *J Biol Chem* **272**:4647, 1997.
181. Hirst MC, White PJ: Cloned human FMR1 trinucleotide repeats exhibit a length- and orientation-dependent instability suggestive of in vivo lagging strand secondary structure. *Nucleic Acids Res* **26**:2353, 1998.
182. Chen X, Mariappan SV, Moyzis RK, Bradbury EM, Gupta G: Hairpin induced slippage and hyper-methylation of the fragile X DNA triplets. *J Biomol Struct Dyn* **15**:745, 1998.
183. Kokoska RJ, Stefanovic L, Tran HT, Resnick MA, Gordenin DA, Petes TD: Destabilization of yeast micro- and minisatellite DNA sequences by mutations affecting a nuclease involved in Okazaki fragment processing (rad27) and DNA polymerase delta (pol3-t). *Mol Cell Biol* **18**:2779, 1998.
184. Maurer DJ, O'Callaghan BL, Livingston DM: Mapping the polarity of changes that occur in interrupted CAG repeat tracts in yeast. *Mol Cell Biol* **18**:4597, 1998.
185. Freudenreich CH, Kantrow SM, Zakian VA: Expansion and length-dependent fragility of CTG repeats in yeast. *Science* **279**:853, 1998.
186. Schweitzer JK, Livingston DM: Expansions of CAG repeat tracts are frequent in a yeast mutant defective in Okazaki fragment maturation. *Hum Mol Genet* **7**:69, 1998.
187. Hiraoka LR, Harrington JJ, Gerhard DS, Lieber MR, Hsieh CL: Sequence of human FEN-1, a structure-specific endonuclease, and chromosomal localization of the gene (FEN1) in mouse and human. *Genomics* **25**:220, 1995.
188. Hansen RS, Canfield TK, Lamb MM, Gartler SM, Laird CD: Association of fragile X syndrome with delayed replication of the FMR1 gene. *Cell* **73**:1403, 1993.
189. Torchia BS, Call LM, Migeon BR: DNA replication analysis of FMR1, XIST, and factor 8C loci by FISH shows nontranscribed X-linked genes replicate late. *Am J Hum Genet* **55**:96, 1994.
190. Subramanian PS, Nelson DL, Chinault AC: Large domains of apparent delayed replication timing associated with triplet repeat expansion at FRAXA and FRAXE. *Am J Hum Genet* **59**:407, 1996.
191. Hansen RS, Canfield TK, Fjeld AD, Mumm S, Laird CD, Gartler SM: A variable domain of delayed replication in FRAXA fragile X chromosomes: X inactivation-like spread of late replication. *Proc Natl Acad Sci U S A* **94**:4587, 1997.
192. Yeshaya J, Shalgi R, Shohat M, Avivi L: Replication timing of the various FMR1 alleles detected by FISH: Inferences regarding their transcriptional status. *Hum Genet* **102**:6, 1998.
193. Eberhart DE, Warren ST: Nuclease sensitivity of permeabilized cells confirms altered chromatin formation at the fragile X locus. *Somat Cell Mol Genet* **22**:435, 1996.
194. Luo S, Robinson JC, Reiss AL, Migeon BR: DNA methylation of the fragile X locus in somatic and germ cells during fetal development: Relevance to the fragile X syndrome and X inactivation. *Somat Cell Mol Genet* **19**:393, 1993.
195. Godde JS, Kass SU, Hirst MC, Wolffe AP: Nucleosome assembly on methylated CGG triplet repeats in the fragile X mental retardation gene 1 promoter. *J Biol Chem* **271**:24325, 1996.
196. Wang YH, Gellibolian R, Shimizu M, Wells RD, Griffith J: Long CCG triplet repeat blocks exclude nucleosomes: A possible mechanism for the nature of fragile sites in chromosomes. *J Mol Biol* **263**:511, 1996.

197. Gu Y, Shen Y, Gibbs RA, Nelson DL: Identification of FMR2, a novel gene associated with the FRAXE CCG repeat and CpG island. *Nat Genet* **13**:109, 1996.
198. Gecz J, Gedeon AK, Sutherland GR, Mulley JC: Identification of the gene FMR2, associated with FRAXE mental retardation. *Nat Genet* **13**:105, 1996.
199. Knight SJ, Ritchie RJ, Chakrabarti L, Cross G, Taylor GR, Mueller RF, Hurst J, Paterson J, Yates JR, Dow DJ, Davies KE: A study of FRAXE in mentally retarded individuals referred for fragile X syndrome (FRAXA) testing in the United Kingdom. *Am J Hum Genet* **58**:906, 1996.
200. Ritchie RJ, Knight SJ, Hirst MC, Grewal PK, Bobrow M, Cross GS, Davies KE: The cloning of FRAXF: Trinucleotide repeat expansion and methylation at a third fragile site in distal Xqter. *Hum Mol Genet* **3**:2115, 1994.
201. Nancarrow JK, Kremer E, Holman K, Eyre H, Doggett NA, Le Paslier D, Callen DF, Sutherland GR, Richards RI: Implications of FRA16A structure for the mechanism of chromosomal fragile site genesis. *Science* **264**:1938, 1994.
202. Jalal SM, Lindor NM, Michels VV, Buckley DD, Hoppe DA, Sarkar G, Dewald GW: Absence of chromosome fragility at 19q13.3 in patients with myotonic dystrophy. *Am J Med Genet* **46**:441, 1993.
203. Wenger SL, Giangreco CA, Tarleton J, Wessel HB: Inability to induce fragile sites at CTG repeats in congenital myotonic dystrophy. *Am J Med Genet* **66**:60, 1996.
204. Wilke CM, Hall BK, Hoge A, Paradee W, Smith DI, Glover TW: FRA3B extends over a broad region and contains a spontaneous HPV16 integration site: Direct evidence for the coincidence of viral integration sites and fragile sites. *Hum Mol Genet* **5**:187, 1996.
205. Yu S, Mangelsdorf M, Hewett D, Hobson L, Baker E, Eyre HJ, Lapsys N, Le Paslier D, Doggett NA, Sutherland GR, Richards RI: Human chromosomal fragile site FRA16B is an amplified AT-rich minisatellite repeat. *Cell* **88**:367, 1997.
206. Huang H, Qian J, Proffit J, Wilber K, Jenkins R, Smith DI: FRA7G extends over a broad region: Coincidence of human endogenous retroviral sequences (HERV-H) and small polydispersed circular DNAs (spcDNA) and fragile sites. *Oncogene* **16**:2311, 1998.
207. Hewett DR, Handt O, Hobson L, Mangelsdorf M, Eyre HJ, Baker E, Sutherland GR, Schuffenhauer S, Mao JI, Richards RI: FRA10B structure reveals common elements in repeat expansion and chromosomal fragile site genesis. *Mol Cell* **1**:773, 1998.
208. Mishmar D, Rahat A, Scherer SW, Nyakatura G, Hinzmann B, Kohwi Y, Mandel-Gutfroind Y, Lee JR, Drescher B, Sas DE, Margalit H, Platzer M, Weiss A, Tsui LC, Rosenthal A: Molecular characterization of a common fragile site (FRA7H) on human chromosome 7 by the cloning of a simian virus 40 integration site. *Proc Natl Acad Sci U S A* **95**:8141, 1998.
209. Harrison CJ, Jack EM, Allen TD, Harris R: The fragile X: A scanning electron microscope study. *J Med Genet* **20**:280, 1983.
210. Wen GY, Jenkins EC, Yao XL, Yoon D, Brown WT, Wisniewski HM: Transmission electron microscopy of chromosomes by longitudinal section preparation: Application to fragile X chromosome analysis. *Am J Med Genet* **68**:445, 1997.
211. Usdin K, Woodford KJ: CGG repeats associated with DNA instability and chromosome fragility form structures that block DNA synthesis in vitro. *Nucleic Acids Res* **23**:4202, 1995.
212. Hagerman RJ, Staley LW, O'Conner R, Lugenbeel K, Nelson D, McLean SD, Taylor A: Learning-disabled males with a fragile X CGG expansion in the upper premutation size range. *Pediatrics* **97**:122, 1996.
213. Loesch DZ, Huggins RM, Hoang NH: Growth in stature in fragile X families: A mixed longitudinal study. *Am J Med Genet* **58**:249, 1995.
214. de Vries BB, Robinson H, Stolte-Dijkstra I, Tjon Pian Gi CV, Dijkstra PF, van Doorn J, Halley DJ, Oostra BA, Turner G, Niermeijer MF: General overgrowth in the fragile X syndrome: Variability in the phenotypic expression of the FMR1 gene mutation. *J Med Genet* **32**:764, 1995.
215. de Vries BB, Fryns JP, Butler MG, Canziani F, Wesby-van Swaay E, van Hemel JO, Oostra BA, Halley DJ, Niermeijer MF: Clinical and molecular studies in fragile X patients with a Prader-Willi-like phenotype [see comments]. *J Med Genet* **30**:761, 1993.
216. Schwartz CE, Phelan MC, Pulliam LH, Wilkes G, Vanner LV, Albiez KL, Potts WA, Rogers RC, Schroer RJ, Saul RA, et al: Fragile X syndrome: Incidence, clinical and cytogenetic findings in the black and white populations of South Carolina. *Am J Med Genet* **30**:641, 1988.
217. Opitz JM, Westphal JM, Daniel A: Discovery of a connective tissue dysplasia in the Martin-Bell syndrome. *Am J Med Genet* **17**:101, 1984.
218. Butler MG, Brunschwig A, Miller LK, Hagerman RJ: Standards for selected anthropometric measurements in males with the fragile X syndrome. *Pediatrics* **89**:1059, 1992.
219. Shapiro LR, Wilmot PL: Prenatal diagnosis of the fra(X) syndrome. *Am J Med Genet* **23**:325, 1986.
220. Fryns JP: The female and the fragile X. A study of 144 obligate female carriers. *Am J Med Genet* **23**:157, 1986.
221. Baumgardner TL, Reiss AL, Freund LS, Abrams MT: Specification of the neurobehavioral phenotype in males with fragile X syndrome. *Pediatrics* **95**:744, 1995.
222. Bregman JD, Leckman JF, Ort SI: Fragile X syndrome: Genetic predisposition to psychopathology. *J Autism Dev Disord* **18**:343, 1988.
223. Einfeld S, Molony H, Hall W: Autism is not associated with the fragile X syndrome. *Am J Med Genet* **34**:187, 1989.
224. Cohen IL: Behavioral profiles of autistic and non-autistic fragile X males. *Dev Brain Dysfunct* **8**:252, 1995.
225. Reiss AL, Freund L: Behavioral phenotype of fragile X syndrome: DSM-III-R autistic behavior in male children. *Am J Med Genet* **43**:35, 1992.
226. Belser RC, Sudhalter V: Arousal difficulties in males with fragile X syndrome: A preliminary report. *Dev Brain Dysfunct* **8**:270, 1995.
227. Miller LJ, McIntosh DN, McGrath J, et al: Electrodermal reactivity in patients with fragile X syndrome: A preliminary report. *Am J Med Gen*, **83**:268, 1999.
228. Curfs PM, Schreppers-Tijdink GA, Wiegers AM, van Velzen W, Fryns JP: Adaptive behavior in the fra(X) syndrome: A longitudinal study in eight patients. *Am J Med Genet* **34**:502, 1989.
229. Dykens E, Leckman J, Paul R, Watson M: Cognitive, behavioral, and adaptive functioning in fragile X and non-fragile X retarded men. *J Autism Dev Disord* **18**:41, 1988.
230. Dykens EM, Hodapp RM, Ort SI, Leckman JF: Trajectory of adaptive behavior in males with fragile X syndrome. *J Autism Dev Disord* **23**:135, 1993.
231. Dykens E, Ort S, Cohen I, Finucane B, Spiridigliozzi G, Lachiewicz A, Reiss A, Freund L, Hagerman R, O'Connor R: Trajectories and profiles of adaptive behavior in males with fragile X syndrome: Multicenter studies. *J Autism Dev Disord* **26**:287, 1996.
232. Fisch GS, Simensen R, Arinami T, Borghgraef M, Fryns JP: Longitudinal changes in IQ among fragile X females: A preliminary multicenter analysis. *Am J Med Genet* **51**:353, 1994.
233. Borghgraef M, Fryns JP, Dielkens A, Pyck K, Van den Berghe H: Fragile (X) syndrome: A study of the psychological profile in 23 prepubertal patients. *Clin Genet* **32**:179, 1987.
234. Dykens EM, Hodapp RM, Leckman JF: Strengths and weaknesses in the intellectual functioning of males with fragile X syndrome. *Am J Ment Defic* **92**:234, 1987.
235. Veenema H, Veenema T, Geraedts JP: The fragile X syndrome in a large family. II. Psychological investigations. *J Med Genet* **24**:32, 1987.
236. Chudley AE, Knoll J, Gerrard JW, Shepel L, McGahey E, Anderson J: Fragile (X) X-linked mental retardation I: Relationship between age and intelligence and the frequency of expression of fragil (X)(q28). *Am J Med Genet* **14**:699, 1983.
237. Kemper MB, Hagerman RJ, Altshul-Stark D: Cognitive profiles of boys with the fragile X syndrome. *Am J Med Genet* 30:191, 1988.
238. Freund LS, Reiss AL: Cognitive profiles associated with the fra(X) syndrome in males and females. *Am J Med Genet* **38**:542, 1991.
239. Hodapp RM, Leckman JF, Dykens EM, Sparrow SS, Zelinsky DG, Ort SI: K-ABC profiles in children with fragile X syndrome, Down syndrome, and nonspecific mental retardation. *Am J Ment Retard* **97**:39, 1992.
240. Freund LS, Peebles CD, Aylward E, Reiss AL: Preliminary report on cognitive and adaptive behaviors of preschool aged males with fragile X. *Dev Brain Dysfunct* **8**:245, 1995.
241. Prouty LA, Rogers RC, Stevenson RE, Dean JH, Palmer KK, Simensen RJ, Coston GN, Schwartz CE: Fragile X syndrome: Growth, development, and intellectual function. *Am J Med Genet* **30**:123, 1988.
242. Dykens EM, Hodapp RM, Ort S, Finucane B, Shapiro LR, Leckman JF: The trajectory of cognitive development in males with fragile X syndrome. *J Am Acad Child Adolesc Psychiatry* **28**:422, 1989.
243. Fisch GS, Arinami T, Froster-Iskenius U, Fryns JP, Curfs LM, Borghgraef M, Howard-Peebles PN, Schwartz CE, Simensen RJ,

Shapiro LR: Relationship between age and IQ among fragile X males: A multicenter study. *Am J Med Genet* **38**:481, 1991.
244. Fisch GS, Simensen R, Tarleton J, Chalifoux M, Holden JJ, Carpenter N, Howard-Peebles PN, Maddalena A: Longitudinal study of cognitive abilities and adaptive behavior levels in fragile X males: A prospective multicenter analysis. *Am J Med Genet* **64**:356, 1996.
245. Hodapp RM, Dykens EM, Hagerman RJ, Schreiner R, Lachiewicz AM, Leckman JF: Developmental implications of changing trajectories of IQ in males with fragile X syndrome. *J Am Acad Child Adolesc Psychiatry* **29**:214, 1990.
246. Lachiewicz AM, Gullion CM, Spiridigliozzi GA, Aylsworth AS: Declining IQs of young males with the fragile X syndrome. *Am J Ment Retard* **92**:272, 1987.
247. Wright-Talamante C, Cheema A, Riddle JE, Luckey DW, Taylor AK, Hagerman RJ: A controlled study of longitudinal IQ changes in females and males with fragile X syndrome. *Am J Med Genet* **64**:350, 1996.
248. Hagerman RJ, Schreiner RA, Kemper MB, Wittenberger MD, Zahn B, Habicht K: Longitudinal IQ changes in fragile X males. *Am J Med Genet* **33**:513, 1989.
249. Bailey DB, Hatton DD, Skinner M: Early developmental trajectories of males with fragile X syndrome. *Am J Men Retard* **103** :29, 1998.
250. Theobald TM, Hay DA, Judge C: Individual variation and specific cognitive deficits in the fra(X) syndrome. *Am J Med Genet* **28**:1, 1987.
251. Turk J: The fragile-X syndrome. On the way to a behavioural phenotype. *Br J Psychiatry* **160**:24, 1992.
252. Cianchetti C, Sannio-Fancello G, Fratta AL, Manconi F, Orano A, Pischedda MP, Pruna D, Spinicci G, Archidiacono N, Filippi G: Neuropsychological, psychiatric, and physical manifestations in 149 members from 18 fragile X families. *Am J Med Genet* **40**:234, 1991.
253. Sobesky WE, Pennington BF, Porter D, Hull CE, Hagerman RJ: Emotional and neurocognitive deficits in fragile X. *Am J Med Genet* **51**:378, 1994.
254. Maes B, Fryns JP, Van Walleghem M, Van den Berghe H: Cognitive functioning and information processing of adult mentally retarded men with fragile-X syndrome. *Am J Med Genet* **50**:190, 1994.
255. Crowe SF, Hay DA: Neuropsychological dimensions of the fragile X syndrome: Support for a non-dominant hemisphere dysfunction hypothesis. *Neuropsychologia* **28**:9, 1990.
256. Bennetto L, Pennington BF: The neuropsychology of fragile X syndrome, in Hagerman RJ, Cronister A (eds): *Fragile X syndrome: Diagnosis, Treatment, and Research*. Baltimore, MD, Johns Hopkins University Press, 1996, p 210.
257. Newell K, Sanborn B, Hagerman RJ : Speech and language dysfunction in the fragile X syndrome, in Hagerman RJ, McBogg P (eds): *The Fragile X syndrome: Diagnosis, Biochemistry, and Intervention* . Dillon, CO, Spectra Publishing, 1983, p 175.
258. Hanson DM, Jackson AWD, Hagerman RJ: Speech disturbances (cluttering) in mildly impaired males with the Martin-Bell/fragile X syndrome. *Am J Med Genet* **23**:195, 1986.
259. Sudhalter V, Scarborough HS, Cohen IL: Syntactic delay and pragmatic deviance in the language of fragile X males. *Am J Med Genet* **38**:493, 1991.
260. Madison LS, George C, Moeschler JB: Cognitive functioning in the fragile-X syndrome: A study of intellectual, memory and communication skills. *J Ment Defic Res* **30**:129, 1986.
261. Wolf-Schein EG, Sudhalter V, Cohen IL, Fisch GS, Hanson D, Pfadt AG, Hagerman R, Jenkins E, Brown WT: Speech-language and the fragile X syndrome: Initial findings. *Asha* **29**:35, 1987.
262. Sudhalter V, Cohen IL, Silverman W, Wolf-Schein EG: Conversational analyses of males with fragile X, Down syndrome, and autism: Comparison of the emergence of deviant language. *Am J Ment Retard* **94**:431, 1990.
263. Ferrier LJ, Bashir AS, Meryash DL, Johnston J, Wolff P: Conversational skills of individuals with fragile-X syndrome: A comparison with autism and Down syndrome. *Dev Med Child Neurol* **33**:776, 1991.
264. Sudhalter V, Maranion M, Brooks P: Expressive semantic deficit in the productive language of males with fragile X syndrome. *Am J Med Genet* **43**:65, 1992.
265. Jakala P, Hanninen T, Ryynanen M, Laakso M, Partanen K, Mannermaa A, Soininen H: Fragile-X: Neuropsychological test performance, CGG triplet repeat lengths, and hippocampal volumes. *J Clin Invest* **100**:331, 1997.
266. Kaufmann PM, Leckman JF, Ort SI: Delayed response performance in males with fragile X syndrome. *J Clin Exper Neuropsych* **12**:69, 1990.
267. Loesch DZ, Huggins R, Hay DA, Gedeon AK, Mulley JC, Sutherland GR: Genotype-phenotype relationships in fragile X syndrome: A family study. *Am J Hum Genet* **53**:1064, 1993.
268. Abrams MT, Reiss AL, Freund LS, Baumgardner TL, Chase GA, Denckla MB: Molecular-neurobehavioral associations in females with the fragile X full mutation. *Am J Med Genet* **51**:317, 1994.
269. Merenstein SA, Sobesky WE, Taylor AK, Riddle JE, Tran HX, Hagerman RJ: Molecular-clinical correlations in males with an expanded FMR1 mutation. *Am J Med Genet* **64**:388, 1996.
270. Steyaert J, Borghgraef M, Legius E, Fryns JP: Molecular-intelligence correlations in young fragile X males with a mild CGG repeat expansion in the FMR1 gene. *Am J Med Genet* **64**:274, 1996.
271. Hagerman RJ, Hull CE, Safanda JF, Carpenter I, Staley LW, O'Connor RA, Seydel C, Mazzocco MM, Snow K, Thibodeau SN, et al: High functioning fragile X males: Demonstration of an unmethylated fully expanded FMR-1 mutation associated with protein expression. *Am J Med Genet* **51**:298, 1994.
272. Kaufmann WE, Abrams MT, Chen W, Reiss AL: Genotype, molecular phenotype, and cognitive phenotype: Correlations in fragile X syndrome. *Am J Med Gen* **83**:286, 1999.
273. Kirchgessner CU, Warren ST, Willard HF: X inactivation of the FMR1 fragile X mental retardation gene. *J Med Genet* **32**:925, 1995.
274. Riddle JE, Cheema A, Sobesky WE, Gardner SC, Taylor AK, Pennington BF, Hagerman RJ: Phenotypic involvement in females with the FMR1 gene mutation. *Am J Ment Retard* **102**:590, 1998.
275. Sobesky WE, Taylor AK, Pennington BF, Bennetto L, Porter D, Riddle J, Hagerman RJ: Molecular/clinical correlations in females with fragile X. *Am J Med Genet* **64**:340, 1996.
276. Miezejeski CM, Jenkins EC, Hill AL, Wisniewski K, French JH, Brown WT: A profile of cognitive deficit in females from fragile X families. *Neuropsychologia* **24**:405, 1986.
277. Reiss AL, Aylward E, Freund LS, Joshi PK, Bryan RN: Neuroanatomy of fragile X syndrome: The posterior fossa. *Ann Neurol* **29**:26, 1991.
278. Freund LS, Reiss AL, Abrams MT: Psychiatric disorders associated with fragile X in the young female. *Pediatrics* **91**:321, 1993.
279. Hagerman RJ, Jackson C, Amiri K, Silverman AC, O'Connor R, Sobesky W: Girls with fragile X syndrome: Physical and neurocognitive status and outcome. *Pediatrics* **89**:395, 1992.
280. Lachiewicz AM, Dawson DV: Behavior problems of young girls with fragile X syndrome: Factor scores on the Conners' Parent's Questionnaire. *Am J Med Genet* **51**:364, 1994.
281. Reiss AL, Freund L, Vinogradov S, Hagerman R, Cronister A: Parental inheritance and psychological disability in fragile X females. *Am J Hum Genet* **45**:697, 1989.
282. Reiss AL, Hagerman RJ, Vinogradov S, Abrams M, King RJ: Psychiatric disability in female carriers of the fragile X chromosome. *Arch Gen Psychiatry* **45**:25, 1988.
283. Borghgraef M, Fryns JP, van den Berghe H: The female and the fragile X syndrome: Data on clinical and psychological findings in 7 fra(X) carriers. *Clin Genet* **37**:341, 1990.
284. Mazzocco MM, Kates WR, Baumgardner TL, Freund LS, Reiss AL: Autistic behaviors among girls with fragile X syndrome. *J Autism Dev Disord* **27**:415, 1997.
285. Smits A, Smeets D, Hamel B, Dreesen J, de Haan A, van Oost B: Prediction of mental status in carriers of the fragile X mutation using CGG repeat length. *Am J Med Genet* **51**:497, 1994.
286. Taylor AK, Safanda JF, Fall MZ, Quince C, Lang KA, Hull CE, Carpenter I, Staley LW, Hagerman RJ: Molecular predictors of cognitive involvement in female carriers of fragile X syndrome [see comments]. *JAMA* **271**:507, 1994.
287. Rousseau F, Robb LJ, Rouillard P, Der Kaloustian VM: No mental retardation in a man with 40 percent abnormal methylation at the FMR-1 locus and transmission of sperm cell mutations as premutations. *Hum Mol Genet* **3**:927, 1994.
288. Reiss AL, Freund LS, Baumgardner TL, Abrams MT, Denckla MB: Contribution of the FMR1 gene mutation to human intellectual dysfunction. *Nat Genet* **11**:331, 1995.
289. de Vries BB, Wiegers AM, Smits AP, Mohkamsing S, Duivenvoorden HJ, Fryns JP, Curfs LM, Halley DJ, Oostra BA, van den Ouweland AM, Niermeijer MF: Mental status of females with an FMR1 gene full mutation. *Am J Hum Genet* **58**:1025, 1996.
290. Mazzocco MM, Hagerman RJ, Cronister-Silverman A, Pennington BF: Specific frontal lobe deficits among women with the fragile X gene. *J Am Acad Child Adolesc Psychiatry* **31**:1141, 1992.

291. Mazzocco MM, Hagerman RJ, Pennington BF: Problem solving limitations among cytogenetically expressing fragile X women. *Am J Med Genet* **43**:78, 1992.
292. Mazzocco MM, Pennington BF, Hagerman RJ: The neurocognitive phenotype of female carriers of fragile X: Additional evidence for specificity. *J Dev Behav Pediatr* **14**:328, 1993.
293. Thompson NM, Gulley ML, Rogeness GA, Clayton RJ, Johnson C, Hazelton B, Cho CG, Zellmer VT: Neurobehavioral characteristics of CGG amplification status in fragile X females. *Am J Med Genet* **54**:378, 1994.
294. Borghgraef M, Umans S, Steyaert J, Legius E, Fryns JP: New findings in the behavioral profile of young FraX females. *Am J Med Genet* **64**:346, 1996.
295. Grigsby J, Kemper MB, Hagerman RJ: Verbal learning and memory among heterozygous fragile X females. *Am J Med Genet* **43**:111, 1992.
296. Rudelli RD, Brown WT, Wisniewski K, Jenkins EC, Laure-Kamionowska M, Connell F, Wisniewski HM: Adult fragile X syndrome. Clinico-neuropathologic findings. *Acta Neuropathol* **67**:289, 1985.
297. Hinton VJ, Brown WT, Wisniewski K, Rudelli RD: Analysis of neocortex in three males with the fragile X syndrome. *Am J Med Genet* **41**:289, 1991.
298. Reiss AL, Lee J, Freund L: Neuroanatomy of fragile X syndrome: The temporal lobe. *Neurology* **44**:1317, 1994.
299. Huttenlocher PR: Synaptic density in human frontal cortex: Developmental changes and effects of aging. *Brain Res* **163**:195, 1979.
300. Comery TA, Harris JB, Willems PJ, Oostra BA, Irwin SA, Weiler IJ, Greenough WT: Abnormal dendritic spines in fragile X knockout mice: Maturation and pruning deficits. *Proc Natl Acad Sci U S A* **94**:5401, 1997.
301. Loesch DZ, Hay DA, Mulley J: Transmitting males and carrier females in fragile X — Revisited . *Am J Med Genet* **51**:392, 1994.
302. Hull C, Hagerman RJ: A study of the physical, behavioral, and medical phenotype, including anthropometric measures, of females with fragile X syndrome. *Am J Dis Child* **147**:1236, 1993.
303. Cronister A, Schreiner R, Wittenberger M, Amiri K, Harris K, Hagerman RJ: Heterozygous fragile X female: Historical, physical, cognitive, and cytogenetic features. *Am J Med Genet* **38**:269, 1991.
304. Schwartz CE, Dean J, Howard-Peebles PN, Bugge M, Mikkelsen M, Tommerup N, Hull C, Hagerman R, Holden JJ, Stevenson RE: Obstetrical and gynecological complications in fragile X carriers: A multicenter study. *Am J Med Genet* **51**:400, 1994.
305. Partington MW, Moore DY, Turner GM: Confirmation of early menopause in fragile X carriers. *Am J Med Genet* **64**:370, 1996.
306. Conway GS, Hettiarachchi S, Murray A, Jacobs PA: Fragile X premutations in familial premature ovarian failure. *Lancet* **346**:309, 1995.
307. Turner G, Robinson H, Wake S, Martin N: Dizygous twinning and premature menopause in fragile X syndrome [Letter] [see comments]. *Lancet* **344**:1500, 1994.
308. Vianna-Morgante AM: Twinning and premature ovarian failure in premutation fragile X carriers. *Am J Med Gen* **83**:326, 1999.
309. Steyaert J, Decruyenaere M, Borghgraef M, Fryns JP: Personality profile in adult female fragile X carriers: Assessed with the Minnesota Multiphasic Personality Profile (MMPI). *Am J Med Genet* **51**:370, 1994.
310. Reiss AL, Freund L, Abrams MT, Boehm C, Kazazian H: Neurobehavioral effects of the fragile X premutation in adult women: A controlled study. *Am J Hum Genet* **52**:884, 1993.
311. Franke P, Maier W, Hautzinger M, Weiffenbach O, Gansicke M, Iwers B, Poustka F, Schwab SG, Froster U: Fragile-X carrier females: Evidence for a distinct psychopathological phenotype? *Am J Med Genet* **64**:334, 1996.
312. Allingham-Hawkins DJ, Brown CA, Babul R, Chitayat D, Krekewich K, Humphries T, Ray PN, Teshima IE: Tissue-specific methylation differences and cognitive function in fragile X premutation females. *Am J Med Genet* **64**:329, 1996.
313. Haddad LA, Aguiar MJB, Costa SS, Mingroni-Netto RC, Vianna-Morgante AM, Pena SDJ: Fully mutated and gray-zone FRAXA alleles in Brazilian mentally retarded boys. *Am J Med Genet* **84**:198, 1999.
314. Mazzocco MM, Sonna NL, Teisl JT, Pinit A, Shapiro BK, Shah N, Reiss AL: The FMR1 and FMR2 mutations are not common etiologies of academic difficulty among school-age children. *J Dev Behav Pediatr* **18**:392, 1997.
315. Mazzocco MM, Myers GF, Hamner JL, Panoscha R, Shapiro BK, Reiss AL: The prevalence of the FMR1 and FMR2 mutations among preschool children with language delay. *J Pediatr* **132**:795, 1998.
316. Daniels JK, Owen MJ, McGuffin P, et al: IQ and variation in the number of fragile X CGG repeats: No association in a normal sample. *Intelligence* **19**:45, 1994.
317. Voullaire LE, Webb GC, Leversha M: Fragile X testing in a diagnostic cytogenetics laboratory. *J Med Genet* **26**:439, 1989.
318. de Arce MA, Hecht F, Sutherland GR, Webb GC: Guidelines for the diagnosis of fragile X. *Clin Genet* **29**:95, 1986.
319. Dewald GW, Buckley DD, Spurbeck JL, Jalal SM: Cytogenetic guidelines for fragile X studies tested in routine practice. *Am J Med Genet* **44**:816, 1992.
320. Howard-Peebles PN, Maddalena A: Recent experience in prenatal diagnosis of fragile X. *Am J Med Genet* **43**:162, 1992.
321. Jenkins EC, Brown WT, Wilson MG, Lin MS, Alfi OS, Wassman ER, Brooks J, Duncan CJ, Masia A, Krawczun MS: The prenatal detection of the fragile X chromosome: Review of recent experience. *Am J Med Genet* **23**:297, 1986.
322. Marini T, Pflueger S, Jackson A, Naber S, Karpells S, Naeem R: A five-year experience with fragile X testing. Setting laboratory standards of practice and a cost-effective protocol [published erratum appears in *Diagn Mol Pathol* **6**:304, 1997]. *Diagn Mol Pathol* **6**: 161, 1997.
323. Shapiro LR, Wilmot PL, Fisch GS: Prenatal cytogenetic diagnosis of the fragile X syndrome in amniotic fluid: Calculation of accuracy. *Am J Med Genet* **43**:170, 1992.
324. Tommerup N, Holmgren G, Steinbach P: Fragile X: Carrier detection in pregnancy. *Am J Med Genet* **23**:527, 1986.
325. Murray J, Cuckle H, Taylor G, Hewison J: Screening for fragile X syndrome. *Health Technol Assess* **1**:1, 1997.
326. Rousseau F, Heitz D, Biancalana V, Oberle I, Mandel JL: On some technical aspects of direct DNA diagnosis of the fragile X syndrome. *Am J Med Genet* **43**:197, 1992.
327. Tarleton JC, Saul RA: Molecular genetic advances in fragile X syndrome. *J Pediatr* **122**:169, 1993.
328. Davidow LS, Barberio D, Cao J, McCormick I: An improved fragile X Southern blot probe without the CGGs eliminates background bands. *Mol Cell Probes* **8**:241, 1994.
329. Working Group of the Genetic Screening Subcommittee of the Clinical Practice Committee. American College of Medical Genetics. Fragile X syndrome: Diagnostic and carrier testing. *Am J Med Genet* **53**:380, 1994.
330. Oostra BA, Jacky PB, Brown WT, Rousseau F: Guidelines for the diagnosis of fragile X syndrome. National Fragile X Foundation. *J Med Genet* **30**:410, 1993.
331. Rousseau F, Rehel R, Rouillard P, DeGranpre P, Khandjian EW: High throughput and economical mutation detection and RFLP analysis using a minimethod for DNA preparation from whole blood and acrylamide gel electrophoresis. *Hum Mutat* **4**:51, 1994.
332. Verkerk AJ, deVries BB, Niermeijer MF, Fu YH, Nelson DL, Warren ST, Majoor-Krakauer DF, Halley DJ, Oostra BA: Intragenic probe used for diagnostics in fragile X families. *Am J Med Genet* **43**:192, 1992.
333. Warren ST, Nelson DL: Advances in molecular analysis of fragile X syndrome [see comments]. *JAMA* **271**:536, 1994.
334. el-Aleem AA, Bohm I, Temtamy S, el-Awady M, Awadalla M, Schmidtke J, Stuhrmann M: Direct molecular analysis of the fragile X syndrome in a sample of Egyptian and German patients using non-radioactive PCR and Southern blot followed by chemiluminescent detection. *Hum Genet* **96**:577, 1995.
335. Storm K, Handig I, Reyniers E, Oostra BA, Kooy RF, Willems PJ: Incomplete *Eco*RI digestion may lead to false diagnosis of fragile X syndrome. *Hum Genet* **102**:54, 1998.
336. Brown WT, Nolin S, Houck G Jr, Ding X, Glicksman A, Li SY, Stark-Houck S, Brophy P, Duncan C, Dobkin C, Jenkins E: Prenatal diagnosis and carrier screening for fragile X by PCR. *Am J Med Genet* **64**:191, 1996.
337. Willemsen R, Oosterwijk JC, Los FJ, Galjaard H, Oostra BA: Prenatal diagnosis of fragile X syndrome. *Lancet* **348**:967, 1996.
338. Grasso M, Perroni L, Colella S, Piombo G, Argusti A, Lituania M, Buscaglia M, Giussani U, Grimoldi MG, Bricarelli FD: Prenatal diagnosis of 30 fetuses at risk for fragile X syndrome. *Am J Med Genet* **64**:187, 1996.
339. Brambati B, Tului L, Alberti E: Prenatal diagnosis by chorionic villus sampling. *Eur J Obstet Gynecol Reprod Biol* **65**:11, 1996.

340. Castellvi-Bel S, Mila M, Soler A, Carrio A, Sanchez A, Villa M, Jimenez MD, Estivill X: Prenatal diagnosis of fragile X syndrome: (CGG)n expansion and methylation of chorionic villus samples. *Prenat Diagn* **15**:801, 1995.

341. Iida T, Nakahori Y, Tsutsumi O, Taketani Y, Nakagome Y: The CpG island of the FMR-1 gene is methylated differently among embryonic tissues: Implication for prenatal diagnosis. *Hum Reprod* **9**:1471, 1994.

342. Maddalena A, Hicks BD, Spence WC, Levinson G, Howard-Peebles PN: Prenatal diagnosis in known fragile X carriers. *Am J Med Genet* **51**:490, 1994.

343. Yamauchi M, Nagata S, Seki N, Toyama Y, Harada N, Niikawa N, Masuno I, Kajii T, Hori T: Prenatal diagnosis of fragile X syndrome by direct detection of the dynamic mutation due to an unstable DNA sequence. *Clin Genet* **44**:169, 1993.

344. Suzumori K, Yamauchi M, Seki N, Kondo I, Hori T: Prenatal diagnosis of a hypermethylated full fragile X mutation in chorionic villi of a male fetus. *J Med Genet* **30**:785, 1993.

345. Cao J, Tarleton J, Barberio D, Davidow LS: A simple fragile X PCR assay with 7-deazaguanine-substituted DNA visualized by ethidium bromide. *Mol Cell Probes* **8**:177, 1994.

346. Condorelli DF, Milana G, Dell'Albani P, Roccazzello AM, Insirello E, Pavone L, Mollica F: Routine clinical application of the FRAXA Pfu PCR assay: Limits and utility. *Clin Genet* **50**:366, 1996.

347. Haddad LA, Mingroni-Netto RC, Vianna-Morgante AM, Pena SD: A PCR-based test suitable for screening for fragile X syndrome among mentally retarded males. *Hum Genet* **97**:808, 1996.

348. Hecimovic S, Barisic I, Muller A, Petkovic I, Baric I, Ligutic I, Pavelic K: Expand long PCR for fragile X mutation detection. *Clin Genet* **52**:147, 1997.

349. Chong SS, Eichler EE, Nelson DL, Hughes MR: Robust amplification and ethidium-visible detection of the fragile X syndrome CGG repeat using Pfu polymerase. *Am J Med Genet* **51**:522, 1994.

350. Levinson G, Maddalena A, Palmer FT, Harton GL, Bick DP, Howard-Peebles PN, Black SH, Schulman JD: Improved sizing of fragile X CCG repeats by nested polymerase chain reaction. *Am J Med Genet* **51**:527, 1994.

351. Carrel L, Willard HF: An assay for X inactivation based on differential methylation at the fragile X locus, FMR1. *Am J Med Genet* **64**:27, 1996.

352. Hamdan H, Tynan JA, Fenwick RA, Leon JA: Automated detection of trinucleotide repeats in fragile X syndrome. *Mol Diag* **2**:259, 1997.

353. Siomi H, Siomi MC, Nussbaum RL, Dreyfuss G: The protein product of the fragile X gene, FMR1, has characteristics of an RNA-binding protein. *Cell* **74**:291, 1993.

354. Willemsen R, Mohkamsing S, de Vries B, Devys D, van den Ouweland A, Mandel JL, Galjaard H, Oostra B: Rapid antibody test for fragile X syndrome. *Lancet* **345**:1147, 1995.

355. Willemsen R, Smits A, Mohkamsing S, van Beerendonk H, de Haan A, de Vries B, van den Ouweland A, Sistermans E, Galjaard H, Oostra BA: Rapid antibody test for diagnosing fragile X syndrome: A validation of the technique. *Hum Genet* **99**:308, 1997.

356. Willemsen R, Los F, Mohkamsing S, van den Ouweland A, Deelen W, Galjaard H, Oostra B: Rapid antibody test for prenatal diagnosis of fragile X syndrome on amniotic fluid cells: A new appraisal. *J Med Genet* **34**:250, 1997.

357. Huang T, Li LY, Shen Y, Qin XB, Pang ZL, Wu GY: Alternative splicing of the FMR1 gene in human fetal brain neurons. *Am J Med Genet* **64**:252, 1996.

358. Gibson TJ, Rice PM, Thompson JD, Heringa J: KH domains within the FMR1 sequence suggest that fragile X syndrome stems from a defect in RNA metabolism. *Trends Biochem Sci* **18**:331, 1993.

359. Brown V, Small K, Lakkis L, Feng Y, Gunter C, Wilkinson KD, Warren ST: Purified recombinant Fmrp exhibits selective RNA binding as an intrinsic property of the fragile X mental retardation protein. *J Biol Chem* **273**:15521, 1998.

360. Siomi H, Choi M, Siomi MC, Nussbaum RL, Dreyfuss G: Essential role for KH domains in RNA binding: Impaired RNA binding by a mutation in the KH domain of FMR1 that causes fragile X syndrome. *Cell* **77**:33, 1994.

361. Tamanini F, Meijer N, Verheij C, Willems PJ, Galjaard H, Oostra BA, Hoogeveen AT: FMRP is associated to the ribosomes via RNA. *Hum Mol Genet* **5**:809, 1996.

362. Siomi MC, Zhang Y, Siomi H, Dreyfuss G: Specific sequences in the fragile X syndrome protein FMR1 and the FXR proteins mediate their binding to 60S ribosomal subunits and the interactions among them. *Mol Cell Biol* **16**:3825, 1996.

363. Musco G, Stier G, Joseph C, Castiglione Morelli MA, Nilges M, Gibson TJ, Pastore A: Three-dimensional structure and stability of the KH domain: Molecular insights into the fragile X syndrome. *Cell* **85**:237, 1996.

364. Jones AR, Schedl T: Mutations in gld-1, a female germ cell-specific tumor suppressor gene in *Caenorhabditis elegans*, affect a conserved domain also found in Src-associated protein Sam68. *Genes Dev* **9**:1491, 1995.

365. Mahone M, Saffman EE, Lasko PF: Localized Bicaudal-C RNA encodes a protein containing a KH domain, the RNA binding motif of FMR1 [published erratum appears in *EMBO J* 1;**16**:4152, 1997]. *Embo J* **14**:2043, 1995.

366. Feng Y, Absher D, Eberhart DE, Brown V, Malter HE, Warren ST: FMRP associates with polyribosomes as an mRNP, and the I304N mutation of severe fragile X syndrome abolishes this association. *Mol Cell* **1**:109, 1997.

367. Eberhart DE, Malter HE, Feng Y, Warren ST: The fragile X mental retardation protein is a ribonucleoprotein containing both nuclear localization and nuclear export signals. *Hum Mol Genet* **5**:1083, 1996.

368. Khandjian EW, Corbin F, Woerly S, Rousseau F: The fragile X mental retardation protein is associated with ribosomes. *Nat Genet* **12**:91, 1996.

369. Corbin F, Bouillon M, Fortin A, Morin S, Rousseau F, Khandjian EW: The fragile X mental retardation protein is associated with poly(A)+ mRNA in actively translating polyribosomes. *Hum Mol Genet* **6**:1465, 1997.

370. Eberhart DE, Warren ST: The molecular basis of fragile X syndrome. *Cold Spring Harb Symp Quant Biol* **61**:679, 1996.

371. Steward O, Reeves TM: Protein-synthetic machinery beneath postsynaptic sites on CNS neurons: Association between polyribosomes and other organelles at the synaptic site. *J Neurosci* **8**:176, 1988.

372. Miyashiro K, Dichter M, Eberwine J: On the nature and differential distribution of mRNAs in hippocampal neurites: Implications for neuronal functioning. *Proc Natl Acad Sci U S A* **91**:10800, 1994.

373. Kang H, Schuman EM: A requirement for local protein synthesis in neurotrophin-induced hippocampal synaptic plasticity. *Science* **273**:1402, 1996.

374. Steward O, Falk PM: Protein-synthetic machinery at postsynaptic sites during synaptogenesis: A quantitative study of the association between polyribosomes and developing synapses. *J Neurosci* **6**:412, 1986.

375. Weiler IJ, Greenough WT: Metabotropic glutamate receptors trigger postsynaptic protein synthesis. *Proc Natl Acad Sci U S A* **90**:168, 1993.

376. Chernokalskaya E, Dompenciel R, Schoenberg DR: Cleavage properties of an estrogen-regulated polysomal ribonuclease involved in the destabilization of albumin mRNA. *Nucleic Acids Res* **25**:735, 1997.

377. Chen SH, Schoof JM, Buroker NE, Scott CR: The identification of a (CGG)6AGG insertion within the CGG repeat of the FMR1 gene in Asians. *Hum Genet* **99**:793, 1997.

378. Henry PF, Silver PA: A novel methyltransferase (Hmt1p) modifies poly(A)+-RNA-binding proteins. *Mol Cell Biol* **16**:3688, 1996.

379. D'Hooge R, Nagels G, Franck F, Bakker CE, Reyniers E, Storm K, Kooy RF, Oostra BA, Willems PJ, De Deyn PP: Mildly impaired water maze performance in male Fmr1 knockout mice. *Neuroscience* **76**:367, 1997.

380. Kooy RF, D'Hooge R, Reyniers E, Bakker CE, Nagels G, De Boulle K, Storm K, Clincke G, De Deyn PP, Oostra BA, Willems PJ: Transgenic mouse model for the fragile X syndrome. *Am J Med Genet* **64**:241, 1996.

381. Slegtenhorst-Eegdeman KE, de Rooij DG, Verhoef-Post M, van de Kant HJ, Bakker CE, Oostra BA, Grootegoed JA, Themmen AP: Macroorchidism in FMR1 knockout mice is caused by increased Sertoli cell proliferation during testicular development. *Endocrinology* **139**:156, 1998.

382. Godfraind JM, Reyniers E, De Boulle K, D'Hooge R, De Deyn PP, Bakker CE, Oostra BA, Kooy RF, Willems PJ: Long-term potentiation in the hippocampus of fragile X knockout mice. *Am J Med Genet* **64**:246, 1996.

383. Steward O, Bakker CE, Willems PJ, Oostra BA: No evidence for disruption of normal patterns of mRNA localization in dendrites or dendritic transport of recently synthesized mRNA in FMR1 knockout mice, a model for human fragile-X mental retardation syndrome. *Neuroreport* **9**:477, 1998.

384. Weiler IJ, Irwin SA, Klintsova AY, Spencer CM, Brazelton AD, Miyashiro K, Comery TA, Patel B, Eberwine J, Greenough WT: Fragile X mental retardation protein is translated near synapses in response to neurotransmitter activation. *Proc Natl Acad Sci U S A* **94**:5395, 1997.
385. Hagerman RJ, Cronister A (eds): *Fragile X syndrome: Diagnosis, Treatment and Research.* Baltimore, MD, Johns Hopkins University Press, 1996.
386. Scharfenaker S, O'Connor R, Stackhouse T, Braden M, Hickman L, Gray K: Suggested academic materials for use with fragile X children, in Hagerman RJ, Cronister A (eds): *Fragile X syndrome: Diagnosis, Treatment and Research.* Balitmore, MD, Johns Hopkins University Press, 1996, p 467.
387. Jorde LB, Carey JC, Bamshad MJ, White RL, *Medical Genetics*, 2 ed. 1998, St. Louis, Mosby, p 384.
388. Imbert G, Feng Y, Nelson DL, Warren ST, Mandel J-L : FMR1 and mutations in fragile X syndrome: Molecular biology, biochemistry, and genetics, in Wells RD, Warren ST (eds): *Genetic Instabilities and Hereditary Neurological Diseases.* San Diego, Academic Press, 1998, p 27.
389. Faradz SM, Buckely M, Lam-Po-Tang L, Leigh D, Holden JJ: Molecular screening for fragile-X syndrome among Indonesian children with developmental disability. *Am J Med Gen* **83**:350, 1999.
390. de Vries BB, van den Ouweland AM, Mohkamsing S, Duivenvoorden HJ, Mol E, Gelsema K, van Rijn M, Halley DJ, Sandkuijl LA, Oostra BA, Tibben A, Niermeijer MF: Screening and diagnosis for the fragile X syndrome among the mentally retarded: An epidemiological and psychological survey. Collaborative Fragile X Study Group. *Am J Hum Genet* **61**:660, 1997.
391. Elbaz A, Suedois J, Duquesnoy M, Beldjord C, Berchel C, Merault G: Prevalence of fragile-X syndrome and FRAXE among children with intellectual disability in a Caribbean island, Guadeloupe, French West Indies. *J Intellect Disabil Res* **42**:81, 1998.
392. Goldman A, Krause A, Jenkins T: Fragile X syndrome occurs in the South African black population [Editorial]. *S Afr Med J* 87:418, 1997.
393. Ryynanen M, Heinonen S, Makkonen M, Kajanoja E, Mannermaa A, Pertti K: Feasibility and acceptance of screening for fragile X mutations in low-risk pregnancies. *Eur J Hum Genet* **7**:212, 1999.
394. Reiss AL, Kazazian HH Jr, Krebs CM, McAughan A, Boehm CD, Abrams MT, Nelson DL: Frequency and stability of the fragile X premutation. *Hum Mol Genet* **3**:393, 1994.
395. Rousseau F, Morel ML, Rouillard P, Khandjian EW, Morgan K: Surprisingly low prevalence of FMR1 premutations among males from the general population. *Am J Hum Gen* **59(Suppl)**:A188, 1996.
396. Dawson AJ, Chodirker BN, Chudley AE: Frequency of FMR1 premutations in a consecutive newborn population by PCR screening of Guthrie blood spots. *Biochem Mol Med* **56**:63, 1995.
397. Holden JA, Chalifaux M, Wing M, et al: Distribution and frequency of FMR1 CGG repeat numbers in the general population. *Dev Brain Dysfunct* **8**:405, 1995.

CHAPTER 65

Molecular Cytogenetics of Contiguous Gene Syndromes: Mechanisms and Consequences of Gene Dosage Imbalance

Lisa G. Shaffer ▪ David H. Ledbetter ▪ James R. Lupski

1. **Contiguous gene syndromes (CGS) are disorders caused by chromosomal abnormalities, such as deletions and duplications, which result in an alteration of normal gene dosage. Clinically, each CGS is characterized by a specific and complex phenotype, which was recognized in most cases as a genetic syndrome before knowledge of their cytogenetic etiology. The responsible chromosomal segment is usually small on a cytogenetic scale (<5 Mb), but encompasses multiple genes, some of which are dosage sensitive, and contribute to the phenotype independently.**
2. **CGS may be due to deletions of the X chromosome in males, with resulting structural and functional nullisomy. CGS associated with deletions of Xp22.3 and Xp21 are good examples of regions containing multiple disease genes. Some of the disorders included in these CGS are well-known disease entities due to single gene defects (e.g., Duchenne muscular dystrophy, adrenal hypoplasia congenita, glycerol kinase deficiency).**
3. **For most autosomal loci, deletion causes a reduction of gene dosage to structural and functional monosomy. Haploinsufficiency for specific genes in the critical interval is implicated for del(7)(q11.23q11.23) in Williams syndrome, for del(8)(q24.1q24.1) in Langer-Giedion syndrome, del(17)(p13.3) in Miller-Dieker syndrome, and for del(22)(q11.2q11.2) in DiGeorge syndrome and velocardiofacial syndrome.**
4. **Some human genes show exclusive expression from a single parental homologue and no expression from the other homologue (i.e., genomic imprinting). Imprinting can be tissue-specific, as is the case for the major gene causing Angelman syndrome. Deletion of a chromosome segment containing the active allele of an imprinted gene results in structural monosomy but functional nullisomy (e.g., paternal del(15)(q11.2q13) in Prader-Willi syndrome and maternal del(15)(q11.2q13) in Angelman syndrome). Uniparental disomy for the homologue containing the inactive allele results in structural disomy but functional nullisomy (e.g., maternal disomy 15 in Prader-Willi syndrome and paternal disomy 15 in Angelman syndrome).**
5. **Duplication of chromosomal segments causes increased dosage and gene expression. Beckwith-Wiedemann syndrome can be caused by paternal duplications of 11p15.5 or by paternal uniparental disomy 11. Charcot-Marie-Tooth disease type 1A is caused by duplications within 17p12 including the dosage-sensitive *PMP22* gene. For most cases, Pelizaeus-Merzbacher disease results from duplication of the dosage sensitive *PLP* gene.**
6. **Mechanisms for terminal deletions include telomere healing and telomere capture. Several interstitial deletions and duplications have been shown to result from unequal crossing over between large (>20 kb), low-copy region-specific repeat sequences. The underlying genome architecture likely facilitates large rearrangements of other regions of the genome.**
7. **Molecular technologies, primarily PCR and fluorescence *in situ* hybridization (FISH), have been key to the characterization of CGS and provide powerful and sensitive diagnostic capabilities. For X-linked CGS, multiplex PCR analysis of nullisomic males and FISH analyses of carrier females are efficient strategies for deletion detection. FISH is the method of choice for detection of deletions and translocations in autosomal CGS. Interphase FISH and pulsed-field gel electrophoresis have been used to diagnose chromosomal duplications.**

A list of standard abbreviations is located immediately preceding the index in each volume. Additional abbreviations used in this chapter include: AS = Angelman syndrome; AGS = Alagille syndrome; BWS = Beckwith-Wiedemann syndrome; CGS = contiguous gene syndrome; CDPX = chondrodysplasia punctata; CMT = Charcot-Marie-Tooth disease; DGS = DiGeorge syndrome; DSS = dosage-sensitive sex reversal; HNPP = hereditary neuropathy with liability to pressure palsies; ILS = isolated lissencephaly sequence; LGS = Langer-Giedion syndrome; *LIS1* = gene symbol for lissencephaly 1 gene; MDS = Miller-Dieker syndrome; ME = multiple cartilaginous exostoses; MLS = microphthalmia with linear skin defects; PMD = Pelizaeus-Merzbacher disease; OA1 = X-linked ocular albinism; PSS = Potocki-Shaffer syndrome; PWS = Prader-Willi syndrome; REP = low-copy, region-specific repeat; RSS = Russell-Silver syndrome; SMS = Smith-Magenis syndrome; *SNRPN* = small nuclear ribonucleoprotein-associated peptide N gene; TRPS = trichorhinophalangeal syndrome, including TRPS I and TRPS II syndromes; UPD = uniparental disomy; VCFS = velocardiofacial syndrome; WAGR = syndrome of Wilms tumor, aniridia, genitourinary dysplasia, and mental retardation; and WBS = Williams-Beuren syndrome. See also Table 65-2.

Table 65-1 Features of Contiguous Gene Syndromes

Syndrome described before chromosomal etiology discovered
Cytogenetic abnormalities are sometimes detectable only by high-resolution chromosome analysis
Not all patients have visible cytogenetic abnormalities, but may have submicroscopic deletions or duplications detectable by molecular methods
Specific features of syndrome may occur singly as Mendelian conditions
Multiple, unrelated loci thought to be involved, which are physically contiguous in critical region

Chromosomal abnormalities, such as deletions and duplications, are often characterized by a specific and complex phenotype resulting from an imbalance in the normal dosage of genes located in a particular chromosomal segment. The complex phenotype may have been described as a clinical entity before the discovery of the chromosomal basis of the disease. Schmickel[1] first introduced the term contiguous gene syndrome to describe the involvement of multiple, unrelated genes that were physically close to each other on a chromosome. Different terms have been used to describe these complex disease entities including "microdeletion syndromes" to emphasize the fact that the chromosomal rearrangements are often subtle or submicroscopic, and "segmental aneusomies" to extend the definition to chromosomal duplications and to include imprinting effects.[2–5]

We define contiguous gene syndromes (CGS) as a group of clinically recognizable disorders characterized by a deletion or a duplication of a chromosomal segment spanning multiple disease genes, each potentially contributing to the phenotype independently (Table 65-1). These disease genes may be interspersed among other genes whose dosage imbalance has no effect on the phenotype. In several cases, individual components of the CGS are known Mendelian disorders (e.g., Duchenne muscular dystrophy, glycerol kinase deficiency, and adrenal hypoplasia congenita). In this chapter, we include syndromes for which the involvement of multiple disease genes has been established or is strongly suspected either by genotype/phenotype correlation, or by mapping and cloning of the disease genes contributing to the phenotype. Additionally, we include those deletion syndromes that were classically defined as CGS, but which are now known to be caused by a single gene with pleiotropic effects. We omit reviews of some disorders that have been included as CGS by other authors (e.g., del(13)(q14q14) and retinoblastoma, Chap. 36; del(16)(p13.3) and α-thalassemia; del(17)(q11.2q11.2) and neurofibromatosis, Chap. 39) in which there is no evidence for other specific disease genes except in cases of larger deletions. In addition, syndromes characterized by larger, mostly cytogenetically visible deletions (e.g., del(5)(p15) in the cri-du-chat syndrome or del(4)(p16) in the Wolf-Hirschhorn syndrome), but with little available information on the mapping of disease genes involved, are not included.

CYTOGENETIC AND MOLECULAR METHODS AND RESOLUTION

Chromosome banding techniques, developed in the early 1970s, allow unambiguous identification of each human chromosome and the detection of many large structural abnormalities, including translocations, deletions, and duplications. Banding techniques, particularly G-banding, are routine procedures in all clinical cytogenetics laboratories. A brief overview of the clinical situations that require routine cytogenetic study is given in Chap. 1. The syndromes discussed in this chapter may result from extremely subtle cytogenetic changes that are frequently not detectable by routine banding analysis and require, instead, the application of high-resolution cytogenetic or molecular cytogenetic technologies.

High-Resolution Chromosome Analysis

High-resolution chromosome analysis was introduced in 1976 by Yunis;[6] it involves synchronization of lymphocyte cultures to obtain an enriched population of cells in prophase or prometaphase rather than the middle to late stages of metaphase more characteristic of conventional techniques. A comparative illustration of metaphase and prometaphase chromosomes is shown in Fig. 65-1. Each band seen at metaphase actually represents multiple sub-bands in earlier stages that have "fused together" as the chromosome contracts. Whereas a typical metaphase cell contains on the order of 400 to 500 bands per haploid genome, synchronized chromosome preparations make it possible to visualize up to 2000 bands.[7] For reproducible diagnostic applications, standard ideograms representing human chromosomes at the 400-, 550-, and 850-band stages of resolution have been developed as part of the International System for Human Cytogenetic Nomenclature.[8]

Practically, it is not possible to apply high-resolution chromosome analysis to all clinical cytogenetic studies because of the greatly increased work effort and difficulty of analysis. Therefore, the primary application of high-resolution analysis has come under circumstances in which a particular chromosomal region is to be studied in greater detail.

In fact, despite impressions to the contrary, the microdeletion syndromes were not initially discovered by high-resolution methods. In most cases, a candidate chromosome was identified through routine metaphase chromosome analysis, with high-resolution analysis being subsequently used to characterize the critical region and define the frequency of deletions for a disorder. For example, the first deletions associated with retinoblastoma[9,10] and aniridia-Wilms tumor[11] were described before the development of high-resolution techniques. Likewise, the candidate chromosomes involved in Prader-Willi syndrome[12] and DiGeorge syndrome[13] were initially identified due to gross translocations observed using routine methods and that of Miller-Dieker syndrome by identification of a patient with a ring chromosome[14]

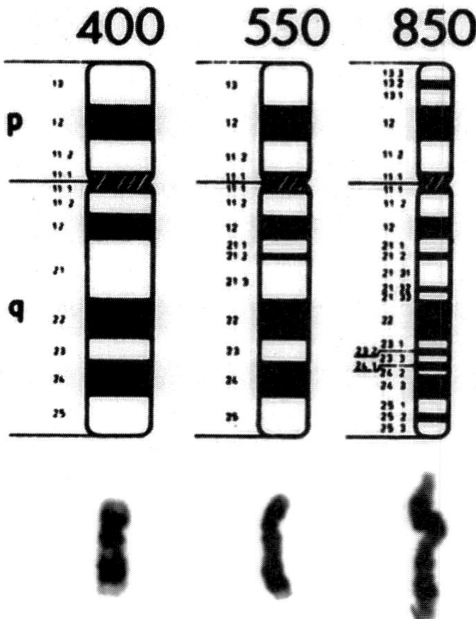

Fig. 65-1 Comparison of routine and high-resolution cytogenetic analysis. An ideogram of human chromosome 17 is shown at the stages of chromosome condensation of approximately 400 (routine), 550, and 850 (high-resolution) bands per haploid genome.[8] Below the ideograms are examples of G-banded chromosomes 17 at approximately the same stages of contraction.

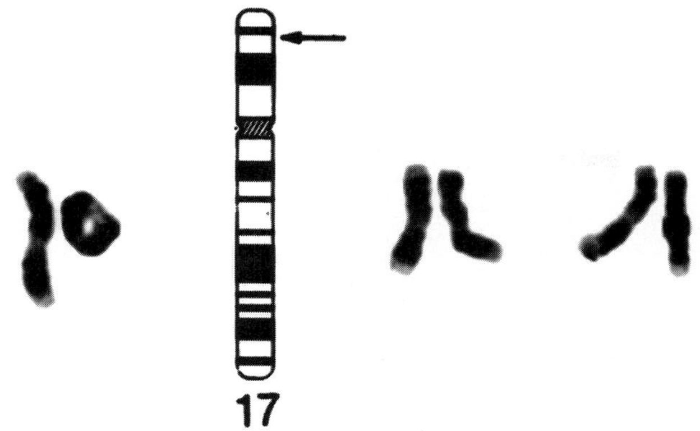

Fig. 65-2 Candidate chromosome for Miller-Dieker syndrome (MDS). On the left is the ring chromosome 17 in an MDS patient, which is easily detectable by routine cytogenetic analysis and which identified chromosome 17 as a candidate chromosome for MDS.[14] In the center, is an ideogram of chromosome 17 at approximately the 850-band stage of resolution,[8] with an arrow indicating the breakpoint of a small, terminal deletion of 17p13 in an MDS patient. To the right are two pairs of chromosomes 17 from this MDS patient showing the small, terminal deletion in the homologue on the right of each pair. This subtle deletion would almost certainly be missed by routine cytogenetic methods and requires the application of high-resolution techniques.

(Fig. 65-2). After the candidate chromosome regions were identified, high-resolution techniques were crucial in the determination of the specific chromosome band or sub-band involved in each disorder (i.e., "critical region"). Many patients previously thought to have normal karyotypes were subsequently found to have deletions too small to be observed using routine cytogenetic methods.

Molecular Cytogenetics

Although important, the gain in resolution due to improved cytogenetic methods has been rather limited. If there are approximately 3×10^9 bp of DNA in the genome, then an average metaphase band (400-band stage) corresponds to about 7.5 Mb. Routine chromosome analysis would thus allow detection of deletions and duplications in the 5- to 10-Mb range. High-resolution chromosome analysis, even at the 1000-band level, only increases the sensitivity of cytogenetic analysis to detection of deletions or duplications in the 3- to 5-Mb range. Those rearrangements smaller than 3 Mb are extremely difficult to detect reliably by current chromosome-banding methods. However, molecular technologies, including PCR, Southern blot analysis, and pulsed-field gel electrophoresis, have been used in the molecular characterization of "submicroscopic" deletions and duplications. Examples of these applications are given below under specific contiguous gene syndromes.

Of particular importance to the study and diagnosis of subtle or submicroscopic chromosome rearrangements has been the development of nonisotopic methods of *in situ* hybridization. The most common methods use fluorescence *in situ* hybridization (FISH).[15,16] It is possible to incorporate fluorescently conjugated nucleotides directly into DNA probes. However, until recently such "direct labeling" strategies have not been as widely used as the alternative methods of "indirect labeling." For these, a DNA probe is labeled with nucleotides conjugated with "reporter" molecules such as biotin or digoxigenin that require detection with an appropriate immunofluorescent reagent to produce the fluorescent signal at the site of probe hybridization. Labeled DNA probes, including unique sequence probes (e.g., cosmids, YAC, or BAC), repetitive sequences (e.g., alpha-satellite repeats), or whole chromosome libraries ("painting probes"), are hybridized to the denatured DNA of metaphase chromosomes or interphase nuclei on glass microscope slides.[15,16] For complex probes, such as cosmids, BAC, and whole-chromosome painting probes, preassociation with an excess of unlabeled DNA is used to "block" the hybridization of *Alu* sequences and other repetitive elements.[17,18]

Examples of FISH analysis are shown in Fig. 65-3. Detection of biotin-labeled DNA can be performed using avidin conjugated to a fluorochrome, such as fluorescein isothiocyanate (FITC). Digoxigenin-labeled DNA can be detected with antidigoxigenin antibodies conjugated to a second fluorochrome such as rhodamine. A variety of other reporter molecules and fluorochromes have been described, allowing the simultaneous hybridization and detection of multiple probes in multicolor FISH analysis.[19] By labeling a probe with either a single fluorochrome or a combination of two or three fluorochromes (i.e., combinatorial labeling), 24 distinct fluorescent patterns can be obtained (Fig. 65-3E).[20,21]

The sensitivity of FISH in detecting submicroscopic (<5 Mb) deletions and translocations has been well documented.[22] Current methods using conventional fluorescence microscopy produce reliable hybridization with single cosmid clones (30 to 40 kb),[23] small contigs of overlapping cosmid clones (80 to 100 kb),[22] or large insert vectors such as BACs. This technology improves sensitivity by almost two orders of magnitude over conventional high-resolution chromosome analysis. This sensitivity can be increased even further, to the detection of probes in the 1-kb range, by the use of high-resolution cooled CCD (charged-coupled device) cameras and digital imaging technology.[16] At present, however, the use of these small probes are beyond the capabilities of most routine diagnostic laboratories.

DIAGNOSIS OF CONTIGUOUS GENE SYNDROMES

Table 65-2 summarizes the location, frequency of visible and submicroscopic rearrangement, and genes known to contribute to the clinical features of the contiguous gene syndromes. Although high-resolution cytogenetic analysis can detect a proportion of deletions in many of the CGS, the relative ease and high sensitivity of FISH analysis has made this the diagnostic method of choice in these disorders (see Fig. 65-3). FISH detection of submicroscopic deletions has been demonstrated for most of these syndromes. Whenever possible, the FISH probe should contain the causative gene and be small enough so that it is completely contained within the common (or minimal) deletion region, yet large enough to be reliably detected and analyzed (see Fig. 65-3A). Patients not demonstrating deletions by FISH for Rubinstein-Taybi syndrome, Alagille syndrome, adrenal hypoplasia congenita, glycerol kinase deficiency, HNPP, trichorhinophalangeal syndrome, and Duchenne muscular dystrophy, are presumed to have a mutation (e.g., point mutations) that is not detectable by this technology in their respective disease genes, or in some cases, potentially another locus. For some syndromes in which a deletion is found in the proband, parental studies should be considered to exclude the presence of a deletion (e.g., DiGeorge syndrome[24]), cryptic translocation (e.g., Miller-Dieker syndrome[22]), inversion (e.g., Miller-Dieker syndrome[22]), or mosaicism (e.g., Smith-Magenis syndrome[25]) that would produce a significant risk of recurrence. This is especially important in the terminal deletion syndromes (e.g., monosomy 1p, Wolf-Hirschhorn syndrome, cri du chat syndrome, and Miller-Dieker syndrome) in which as many as 10 percent of cases are caused by the malsegregation of a parental translocation.[22,26,27]

Additionally, detection of uniparental disomy in Beckwith-Wiedemann syndrome, Russell-Silver syndrome, Prader-Willi syndrome, and Angelman syndrome can be achieved through the use of highly polymorphic markers, such as microsatellite polymorphisms that can be analyzed by PCR, or methylation assays designed to discriminate between maternally inherited and paternally inherited alleles. These studies require parental DNA samples in addition to a proband sample, in order to perform the analysis.

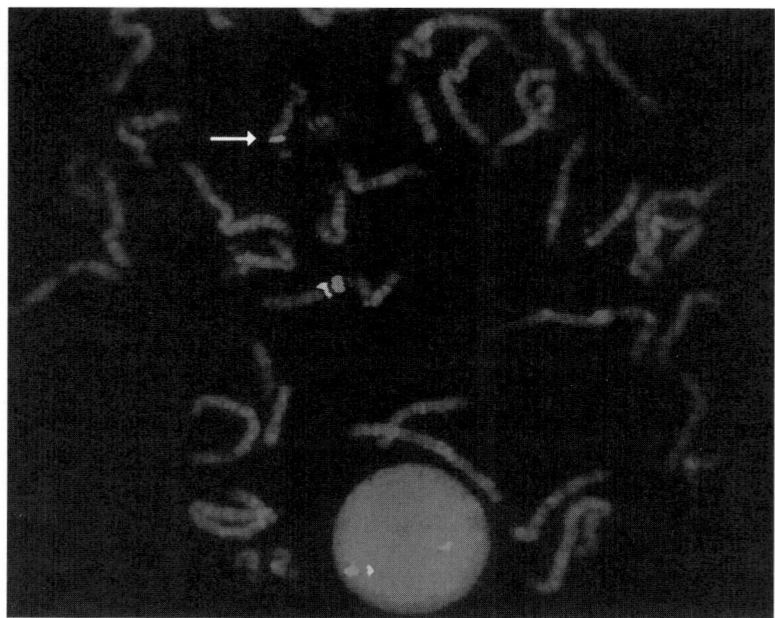

Fig. 65-3 Fluorescence *in situ* hybridization (FISH). Figs. 65-3A, 65-3B, 65-3G, and 65-3J demonstrate the use of unique sequence probes to identify deletions on metaphase chromosomes. Fig. 65-3C demonstrates the use of telomere-region specific probes to identify cryptic deletions and rearrangements. Figs. 65-3D and 65-3E demonstrate the use of multicolored "painting" probes to detect rearrangements of multiple chromosomes simultaneously. Figs. 65-3G, 65-3H, 65-3I, and 65-3K demonstrate the use of unique sequence probes for the identification of a variety of duplications and deletions involving adjacent regions hybridized by the probes. Through the use of this probe set, duplications of 17p11.2 and 17p12, and deletions of the same region can be identified in interphase nuclei. One patient (Fig. 65-3I) showed rearrangements of 17p on each of her homologous chromosomes 17.[427]

Fig. 65-3A FISH using a cosmid containing the ***SNRPN*** gene, mapping to 15q12 on a patient with Prader-Willi syndrome. The control probe hybridizes to the classical satellite DNA on the short arm of chromosome 15. The control probe is labeled with biotin and detected with avidin conjugated to fluorescein (fluoresces green). The test probe is labeled with digoxigenin and detected with antidigoxigenin conjugated to rhodamine (fluoresces red). The normal chromosome 15 shows a control (green) signal and a test (red) signal. The deleted chromosome 15 (arrow) shows only the control (green) signal. This result is seen in Prader-Willi syndrome patients who carry deletions. See Color Plate 2A.

For X-linked deletions, detection of submicroscopic rearrangements and fine characterization of chromosomal breakpoints can be accomplished by molecular analysis. Precise positioning of patients' breakpoints is of fundamental importance for phenotype prediction. Molecular data may lead to the diagnosis of diseases previously overlooked on physical examination.[28,29] In X-linked CGS, male individuals can be directly tested by molecular analysis using Southern blotting or PCR. A deletion of a particular locus will result in absence of a hybridization band, or of a PCR product, respectively. Multiplex PCR tests are available for the detection of deletions involving the Duchenne muscular dystrophy[30] and the steroid sulfatase genes.[31] A PCR test designed for the detection of Xp22.3 CGS is shown in Fig. 65-4. The test allows discrimination between deletions causing isolated X-linked

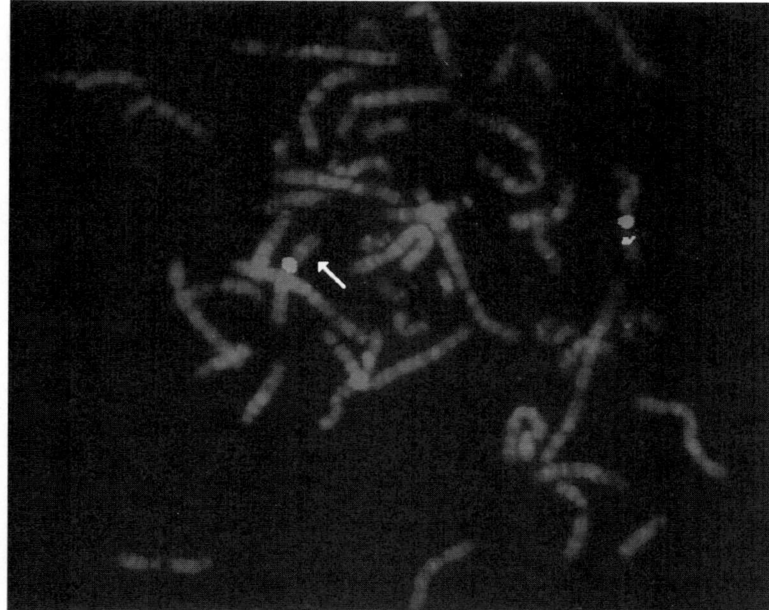

Fig. 65-3B FISH using a cosmid containing exon 51 of the dystrophin encoding DMD gene, mapping to Xp21 on a mother who has an affected son with Duchenne muscular dystrophy. The control probe hybridizes to the alpha-satellite, DNA at the centromere of the X chromosome. The control probe is labeled with biotin and detected with avidin conjugated to fluorescein (fluoresces green). The test probe is labeled with digoxigenin and detected with antidigoxigenin conjugated to rhodamine (fluoresces red). The normal X chromosome shows a control (green) signal and a test (red) signal. The deleted X chromosome (arrow) shows only the control (green) signal. This result is seen in female carriers of DMD deletions.[37a] See Color Plate 2B.

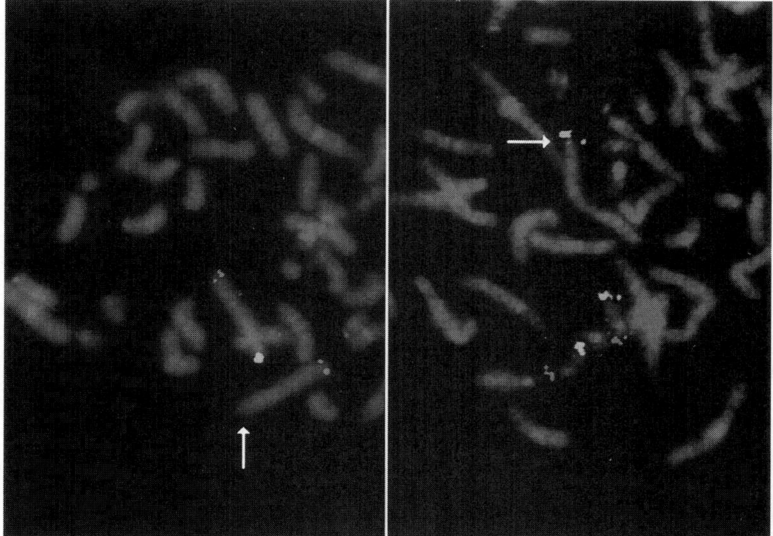

Fig. 65-3C FISH using a cosmids mapping to the telomeres of chromosomes 2 and 17. The short-arm probes are labeled with digoxigenin and detected with antidigoxigenin conjugated to fluorescein (fluoresces green). The long-arm probes are labeled with biotin and detected with antibiotin conjugated to Cy3 (fluoresces red). The left panel shows one normal chromosome 2 with hybridization of the short-arm telomeric probe (fluoresces green) and the long-arm telomeric probe (fluoresces red), and a chromosome 2 that is deleted for the long-arm telomeric probe (arrow). The right panel shows two normal chromosomes 17 with hybridization of the short-arm telomeric probe (fluoresces green) and the long-arm telomeric probe (fluoresces red), and a chromosome 2 that shows hybridization for the chromosome 17 long-arm telomeric probe (arrow). The FISH in this family demonstrated a cryptic translocation between chromosomes 2 and 17 in this child's father. The child's result, shown here, shows monosomy for distal 2q and trisomy for distal 17q using these telomeric probes.[428] See Color Plate 2C.

ichthyosis (Chap. 166) and deletions causing Kallmann syndrome (Chap. 225) and X-linked recessive chondrodysplasia punctata (Chap. 149). Similar tests can be designed for other regions of the X chromosome.

In females (or in XX males), DNA testing can be performed by dosage analysis using Southern blotting. However, this method can lead to erroneous interpretations. FISH analysis is a better method for detection of heterozygous deletions in females. FISH has been used to identify deletions in females for microphthalmia with linear skin defects (MLS; MIM 309801),[32] complex glycerol kinase deficiency,[33] steroid sulfatase deficiency,[34] and intragenic deletions in Duchenne muscular dystrophy (see Fig. 65-3B).[35–37,37a] Once a deletion has been demonstrated using FISH in a family, FISH provides the most reliable, rapid, and direct approach for diagnosing additional family members and for prenatal testing.

Duplications represent a significant diagnostic challenge.[38,39] Detection of dosage differences of heterozygous RFLP and polymorphic STSs can be subject to error. To illustrate, deletion detection of autosomal loci involve detecting a 50 percent reduction in dosage differences (2:1). However, assessment of a duplication requires the detection of a 33 percent increase in dosage (3:2). The use of FISH can greatly enhance the ability to detect duplications (see Figs. 65-3H, 65-3I, and 65-3K). However, because the duplicated segment is often below the resolution obtained in metaphase analysis, FISH must be performed on interphase cells. The proper controls must be used and replication timing must be assessed to distinguish between normal replication of a locus and structural duplication (e.g., CMT1A testing using FISH;[40] Pelizaeus-Merzbacher disease testing[41]). For recurrent duplications, the detection of a novel rearrangement-specific junction fragment using pulsed-field gel electrophoresis of high-molecular-weight DNA is a useful alternative diagnostic approach (see Fig. 65-9) (e.g., Charcot-Marie-Tooth peripheral neuropathy type 1A (CMT1A) testing using PFGE[42] (Chap. 227) or dup(17)(p11.2p11.2);[43] see below).

CONTIGUOUS GENE SYNDROMES RESULT FROM GENE DOSAGE IMBALANCE

CGS result from subtle or submicroscopic deletions or duplications that alter normal gene dosage. Chromosomal rearrangements

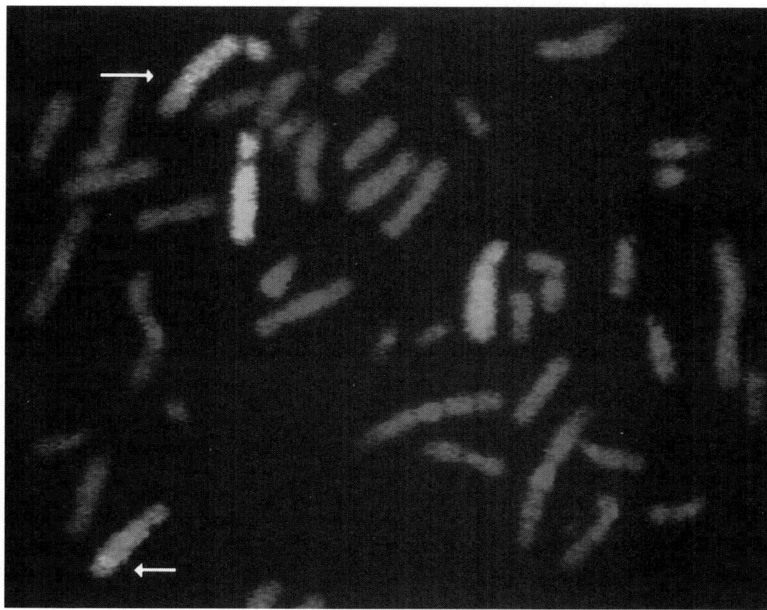

Fig. 65-3D FISH using two painting probes, directly labeled with fluorochromes. Chromosome 4 fluoresces red and chromosome 6 fluoresces green. Arrows indicate the derivative chromosomes of this balanced translocation. See Color Plate 2D.

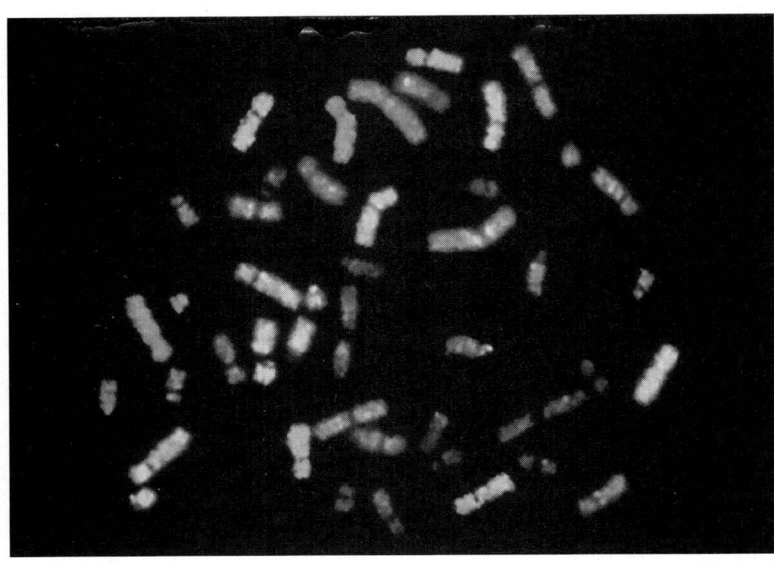

Fig. 65-3E Demonstration of 24-color FISH. Chromosome paints were combinatorially labeled by varying ratios of each fluorochrome to achieve 24 colors simultaneously. Photographed by conventional fluorescence microscopy without pseudocoloring or image processing. (*Used by permission of Thomas Ried, NIH*). See Color Plate 2E.

can cause imbalance of gene dosage in different ways, as shown in Fig. 65-5. Deletions or unbalanced translocations resulting in loss of chromosomal material cause a reduction of gene dosage and, therefore, represent loss-of-function mutations. The simplest example is when the deletion event occurs in a haploid chromosome (X or Y chromosome in males), resulting in structural and functional nullisomy for genes located within the deleted region (Fig. 65-5A). There are several examples of CGS due to interstitial or terminal deletions, or unbalanced translocations, involving the X chromosome (see "X-linked Contiguous Gene Syndromes" below). Typically, these are characterized by full expression of the phenotype in males.

Deletions occurring in autosomes or the X chromosome in females cause structural monosomy (i.e., 50 percent reduction of gene dosage). In some cases, this haploinsufficiency will result in a dominant disease phenotype (Fig. 65-5B). Deletions of 8q24.1 in Langer-Giedion syndrome,[44] deletions of 17p13.3 in Miller-Dieker syndrome,[45] and deletions of 7q11.23 in Williams syndrome[46] are good examples of this mechanism. For X-linked deletions, females typically manifest less severe and more variable phenotypes due to heterozygosity and random X-inactivation.

In some instances, structural monosomy of a particular region of a diploid chromosome may lead to functional nullisomy (Fig. 65-5C). This occurs occasionally when the homologue of a gene contained within the deleted segment has a point mutation on the intact chromosome. Examples include mutations in the *P* gene on the intact homologue in patients with del(15)(q11.2q13) and Prader-Willi syndrome,[47] patients with DiGeorge syndrome and platelet abnormalities,[48] and Smith-Magenis syndrome patients with del(17)(p11.2p11.2) and mutations in the *DFNB3* gene leading to deafness.[49] Alternatively, the locus on the nondeleted homologue can be functionally inactive due to genomic imprinting (e.g., Prader-Willi and Angelman syndromes)[50] or X-chromosome inactivation (e.g., the microphthalmia with linear skin defects syndrome).[51]

Individuals with uniparental disomy may display features of CGS due to functional nullisomy of a particular chromosomal region (Fig. 65-5D). This occurs if a gene (or genes) on a chromosome is subject to imprinting, so that only the paternally derived allele or the maternally derived allele of a gene is actively expressed. Inheritance of both inactive copies would result in functional nullisomy. This mechanism has been described in patients with Prader-Willi and Angelman syndromes.[50]

Constitutional (transmitted in the germ line) rearrangements may be followed by secondary somatic events such as point mutations, deletions, or chromosome losses. This has typically been observed in tumors. In this case, "two hits" (the first being a constitutional rearrangement and the second a somatic event) result in functional nullisomy for genes located in a particular chromosomal region in a specific cell or tissue (Fig. 65-5E). An example of this mechanism is deletion of chromosome 11p13, leading to Wilms tumor.[52] See additional discussions of retinoblastoma and Wilms tumor in Chaps. 36 and 38, respectively.

Both loss-of-function and gain-of-function mutations may cause CGS via gene dosage imbalances. Chromosomal duplications lead to a structural trisomy for genes located within the duplicated region, and may lead to a functional disomy or trisomy depending on the presence or absence of imprinting effects (Fig. 65-5F). This mechanism, characterized by increased gene dosage, has been described for several syndromes. Duplications of 11p15.5, for example, cause Beckwith-Wiedemann syndrome.[53] Functional disomy for specific regions of the X chromosome is another example of increased gene dosage. In this case, a region of the X chromosome, which is normally subject to dosage compensation through X inactivation, is translocated to an autosome and, therefore, can no longer be inactivated. Thus, the functional disomy of genes located in this region may cause a disease phenotype.[54]

Finally, there are instances in which deletions and duplications of the same chromosomal region result in different phenotypes. Patients who carry a duplication of chromosome 17p12 have CMT1A (MIM 118220).[55,56] Conversely, patients with deletions of the same region have hereditary neuropathy with liability to pressure palsies (HNPP; MIM 162500).[57] These diseases, however, cannot be considered a CGS because the phenotypic consequences result from the involvement of a single gene (*PMP22*, Chap. 227). However, these are the most extensively investigated examples to date of disorders definitively caused by a dosage-sensitive gene. In another example, deletion and duplication of the same 5-Mb region on 17p11.2 results in very different phenotypes.[43,58] Deletion of this region results in Smith-Magenis syndrome, while duplication results in a much milder phenotype. Another intriguing example of this mechanism is the Xp21 CGS, in which deletions of a particular region can cause adrenal hypoplasia congenita, while duplications of the same or adjacent region cause sex reversal and abnormalities of gonadal development (Chap. 167).[59–62]

The deletions and duplications involved in CGS may range in size from a few hundred kilobases to several megabases in individual patients. Because there is approximately 1 gene

Color Plates*

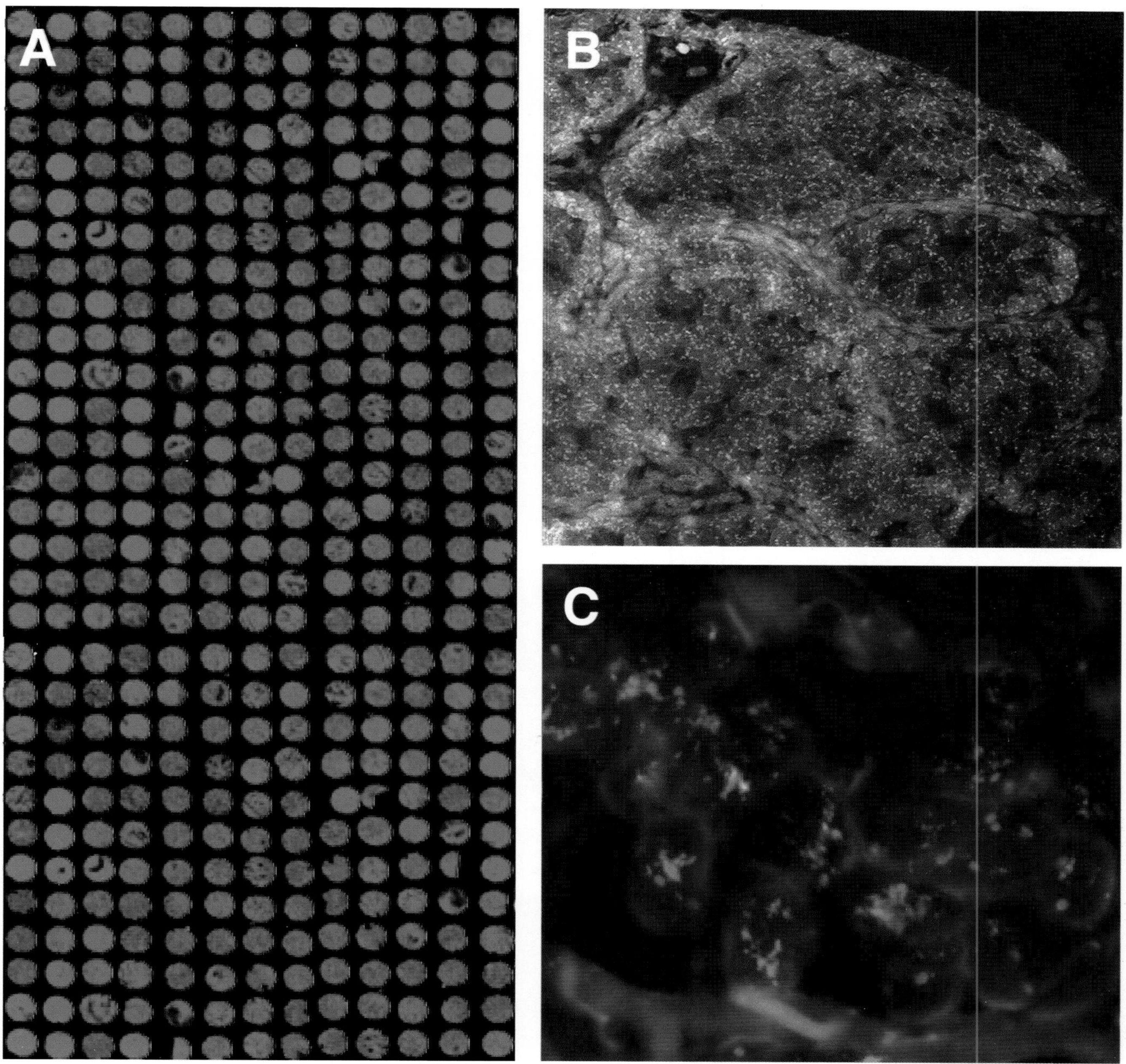

Plate 1 (Fig. 20-10). Detection of androgen receptor (AR) amplification in prostate cancer by FISH on sections of a prostate tissue microarray. *A*, overview of a tissue microarray section containing hundreds of different tumor samples (ϕ 0.6 mm, each). ×3. *B* and *C*, AR amplification with many clustered AR gene signals (red) and a few centromere X signals (green). *B*, ×200; *C*, ×1000.

*The figures in parentheses following the plate numbers have been double-numbered in order to indicate the chapter in which they are discussed and the order of their citation therein.

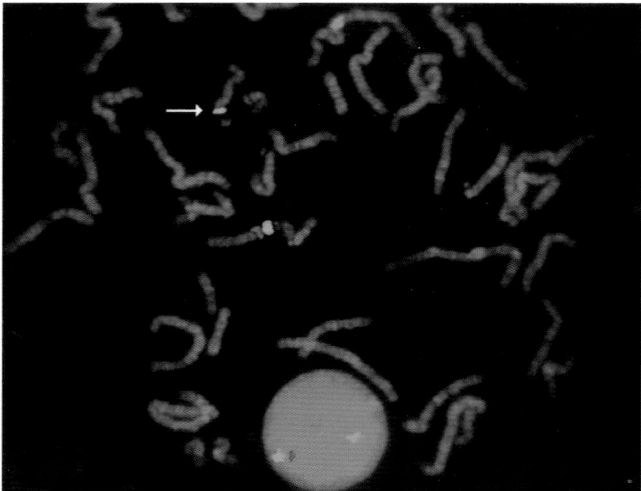

Plate 2A (Fig. 65-3A). FISH using a cosmid containing the SNRPN gene, mapping to 15q12 on a patient with Prader-Willi syndrome. The control probe hybridizes to the classical satellite DNA on the short arm of chromosome 15. The control probe is labeled with biotin and detected with avidin conjugated to fluorescein (fluoresces green). The test probe is labeled with digoxigenin and detected with antidigoxigenin conjugated to rhodamine (fluoresces red). The normal chromosome 15 shows a control (green) signal and a test (red) signal. The deleted chromosome 15 (arrow) shows only the control (green) signal. This result is seen in Prader-Willi syndrome patients who carry deletions.

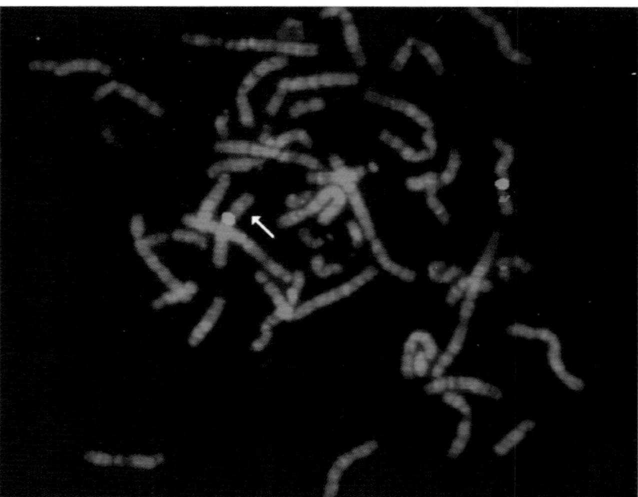

Plate 2B (Fig. 65-3B). FISH using a cosmid containing exon 51 of the dystrophin encoding DMD gene, mapping to Xp21 on a mother who has an affected son with Duchenne muscular dystrophy. The control probe hybridizes to the alpha-satellite DNA at the centromere of the X chromosome. The control probe is labeled with biotin and detected with avidin conjugated to fluorescein (fluoresces green). The test probe is labeled with digoxigenin and detected with antidigoxigenin conjugated to rhodamine (fluoresces red). The normal X chromosome shows a control (green) signal and a test (red) signal. The deleted X chromosome (arrow) shows only the control (green) signal. This result is seen in female carriers of DMD deletions.[37a]

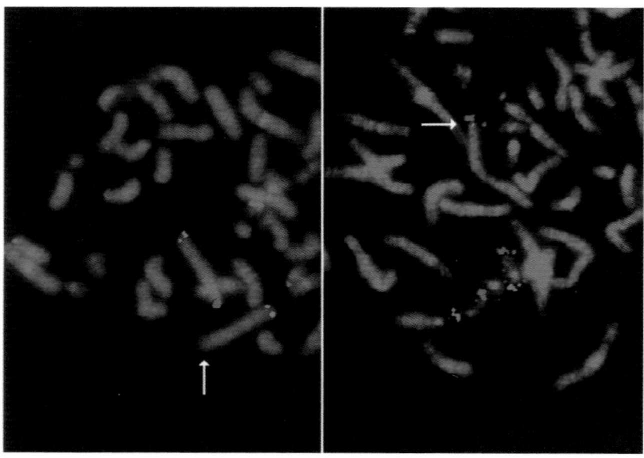

Plate 2C (Fig. 65-3C). FISH using cosmid mapping to the telomeres of chromosomes 2 and 17. The short-arm probes are labeled with digoxigenin and detected with antidigoxigenin conjugated to fluorescein (fluoresces green). The long-arm probes are labeled with biotin and detected with antibiotin conjugated to Cy3 (fluoresces red). The left panel shows one normal chromosome 2 with hybridization of the short-arm telomeric probe (fluoresces green) and the long-arm telomeric probe (fluoresces red), and a chromosome 2 that is deleted for the long-arm telomeric probe (arrow). The right panel shows two normal chromosomes 17 with hybridization of the short-arm telomeric probe (fluoresces green) and the long-arm telomeric probe (fluoresces red), and a chromosome 2 that shows hybridization for the chromosome 17 long-arm telomeric probe (arrow). The FISH in this family demonstrated a cryptic translocation between chromosomes 2 and 17 in this child's father. The child's result, shown here, shows monosomy for distal 2q and trisomy for distal 17q using these telomeric probes.[428]

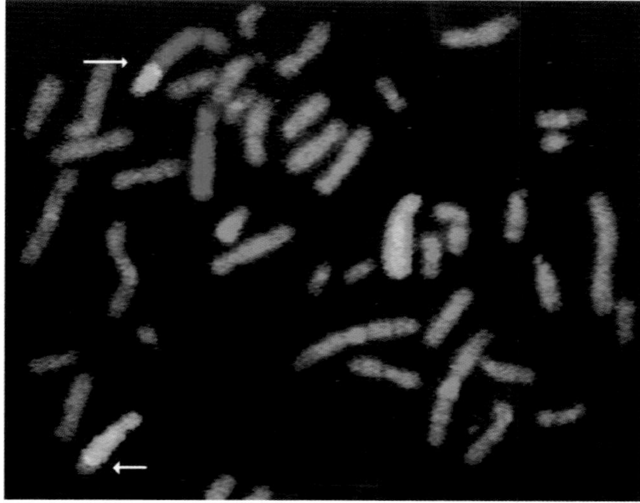

Plate 2D (Fig. 65-3D). FISH using two painting probes, directly labeled with fluorochromes. Chromosome 4 fluoresces red and chromosome 6 fluoresces green. Arrows indicate the derivative chromosomes of this balanced translocation.

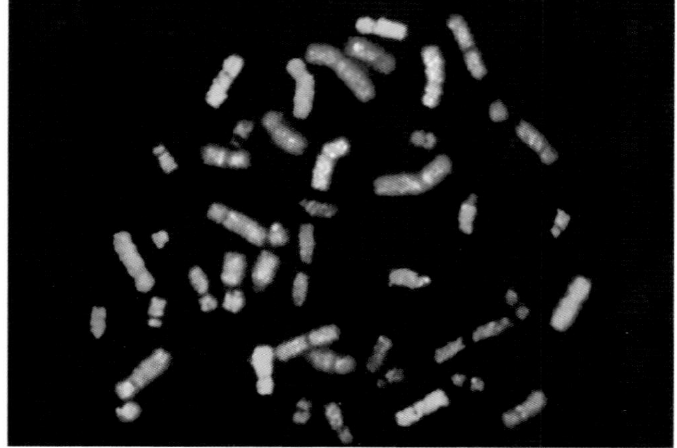

Plate 2E (Fig. 65-3E). Demonstration of 24-color FISH. Chromosome paints were combinatorially labeled by varying ratios of each fluorochrome to achieve 24 colors simultaneously. Photographed by conventional fluorescence microscopy without pseudocoloring or image processing. (Used by permission of Thomas Ried, NIH).

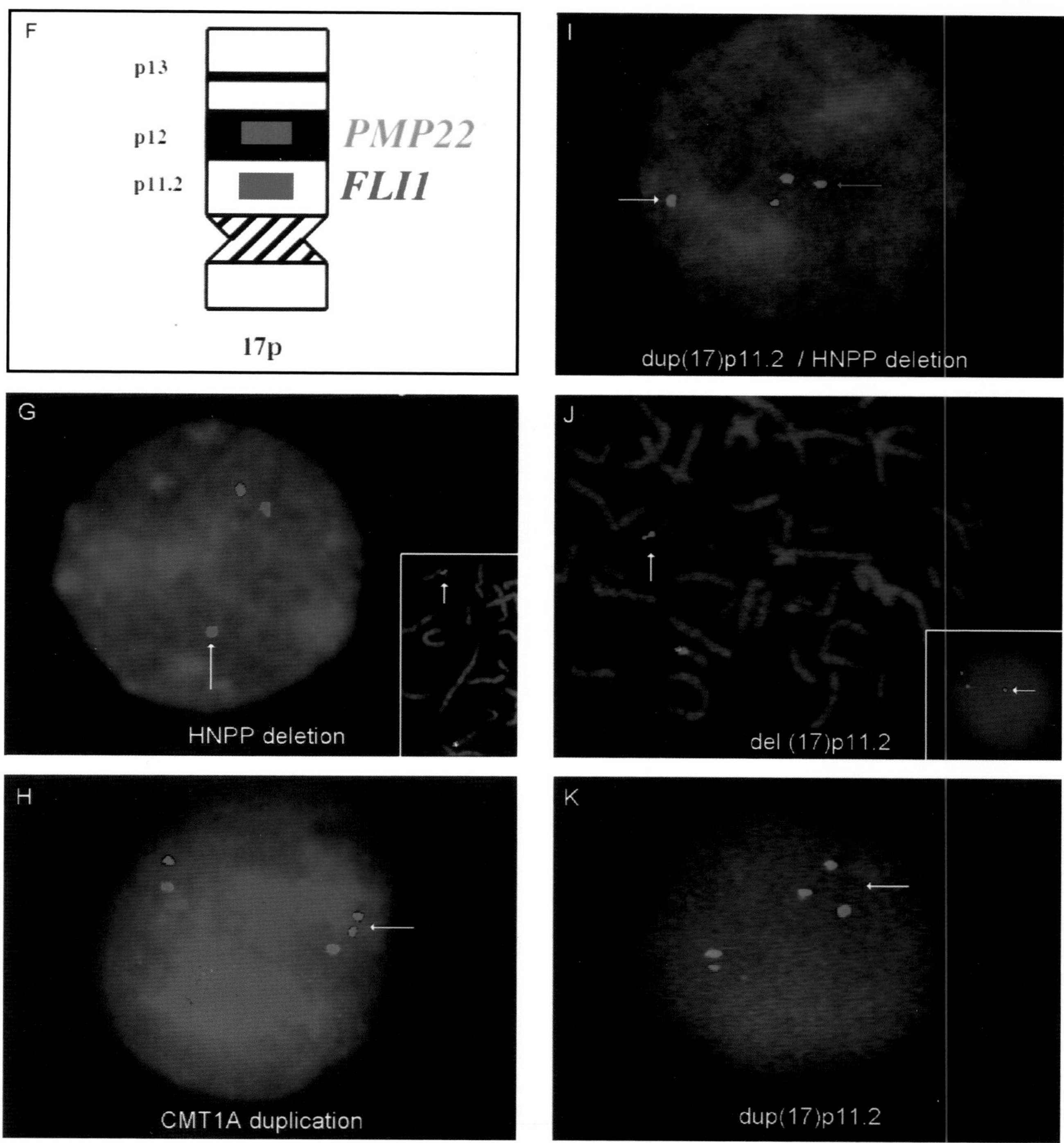

Plate 2F-K (Fig. 65-3F-K). *F*, Ideogram showing 17p and the location of the loci PMP22 and FLI1 to 17p12 and 17p11.2, respectively. The probes are shown in either red (PMP22) or green (FLI1) and this color scheme is used throughout Fig. 65-3G to 65-3K. For each, a cosmid contig containing the FLI1 locus on 17p11.2 is labeled with biotin and detected with avidin conjugated to fluorescein (fluoresces green). A cosmid contig containing the PMP22 gene on 17p12 is labeled with digoxigenin and detected with antidigoxigenin conjugated to rhodamine (fluoresces red). *G*, FISH showing an HNPP deletion in an interphase nucleus and metaphase chromosomes (inset). The normal chromosome 17 shows two signals: a green FLI1 signal and red PMP22 signal. The deleted chromosome 17 (arrow) shows only the green signal, indicating a deletion of the PMP22 locus. This result is seen in HNPP patients who carry deletions. *H*, Interphase FISH showing CMT1A duplication. The normal chromosome 17 shows two signals: a green FLI1 signal and red PMP22 signal. The duplicated chromosome 17 (arrow) shows one green signal and two red signals, indicating a duplication of the PMP22 locus. This result is seen in CMT1A patients who carry duplications. *I*, Interphase FISH showing one chromosome 17 with a deletion for the PMP22 gene on 17p12 (white arrow), while the other homologue shows a duplication for the FLI1 locus on 17p11.2 (red arrow). *J*, FISH using a cosmid contig containing the FLI1 locus, mapping to 17p11.2 on a patient with Smith-Magenis syndrome. The normal chromosome 17 shows two signals: a green FLI1 signal and red PMP22 signal. The deleted chromosome 17 (arrow) shows only the red PMP22 signal, indicating a deletion of the FLI1 locus. This result is seen in Smith-Magenis syndrome patients who carry deletions. *K*, Interphase FISH using a cosmid containing the FLI1 locus, mapping to 17p11.2 on a patient with a dup(17)(p11.2p11.2). The normal chromosome 17 shows two signals: a green FLI1 signal and red PMP22 signal. The duplicated chromosome 17 (arrow) shows one red signal and two green signals, indicating duplication of the region containing the FLI1 locus. This result is consistent with a duplication of 17p11.2.

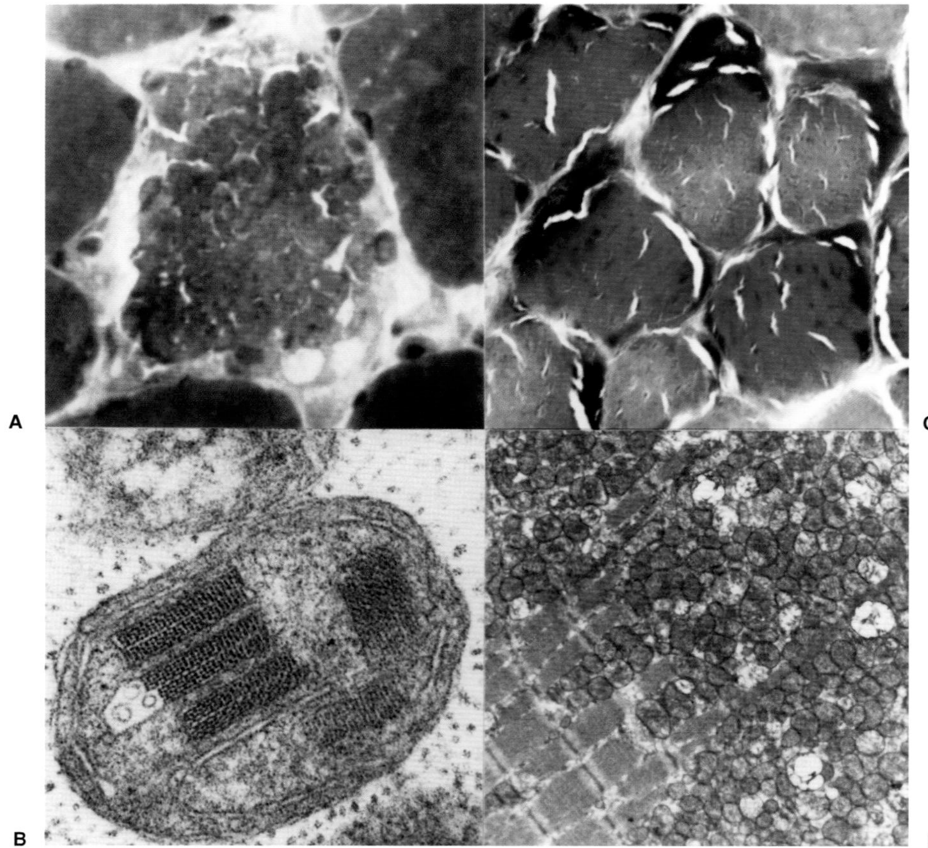

Plate 3 (Fig. 105-16). Mitochondrial myopathy in man and mouse. Panel A and Panel C are skeletal muscle samples from a patient with myoclonic epilepsy and ragged-red fiber disease (MERRF), which is caused by a mutation in the mitochondrially encoded $tRNA^{Lys}$ gene.[279,281] Panel B and Panel D are skeletal muscle samples from a mouse with mitochondrial myopathy and hypertrophic cardiomyopathy resulting from the targeted inactivation of the gene encoding the heart-muscle isoform of the adenine nucleotide translocator (ANT1).[190] Frozen sections showing a single fiber (A) or several fibers (B) were stained with Gomori modified trichrome to show the ragged-red muscle fibers (RRFs). Electron micrographs show (C) an abnormal mitochondrion with paracrystalline arrays in a human RRF, and (D) the abnormal proliferation of mitochondria and degeneration of the contractile elements in a mouse RRF. (Reproduced from Wallace.[825] Used with permission.)

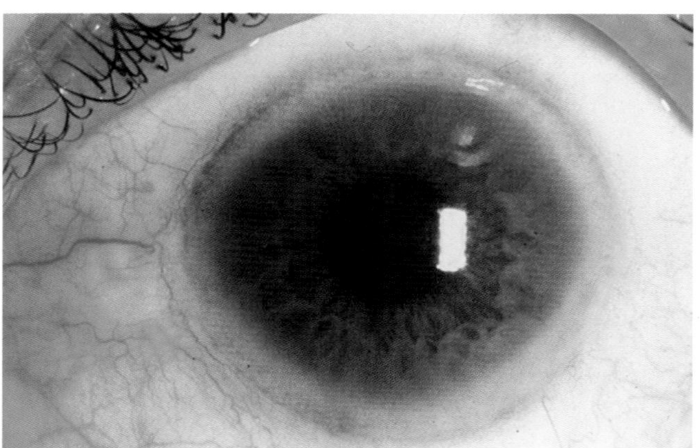

Plate 4 (Fig. 118-5). Corneal opacities in a patient with FLD. Note central stromal haze and prominent peripheral opacification, resembling corneal arcus. The corneal infiltrate composed of numerous minute grayish dots is localized to the parenchyma.

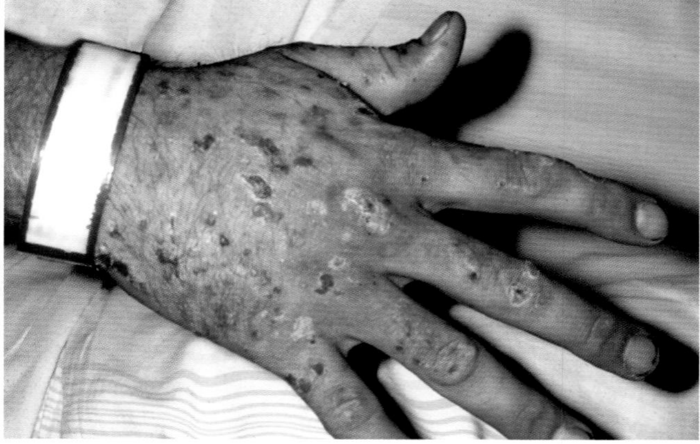

Plate 5 (Fig. 124-20). Chronic, crusted lesions resulting from blistering due to photosensitivity on the dorsum of the hand of a patient with porphyria cutanea tarda (PCT). These occur less commonly on other sun-exposed areas, such as the face, neck, ears, forearms, and feet.

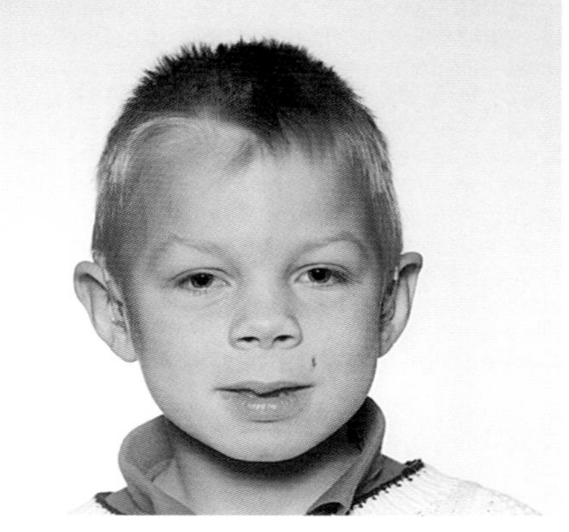

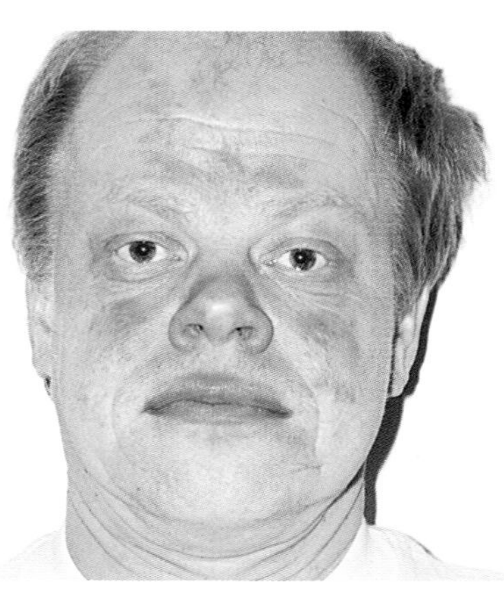

Plate 6 (Fig. 141-2). Facial features of a 9-year-old (left) and 39-year-old patient with aspartylglucosaminuria. The older patient has rosacea-like skin changes with erythema, pustules, and telangiectasias. Facial features associated with AGU are minimal.

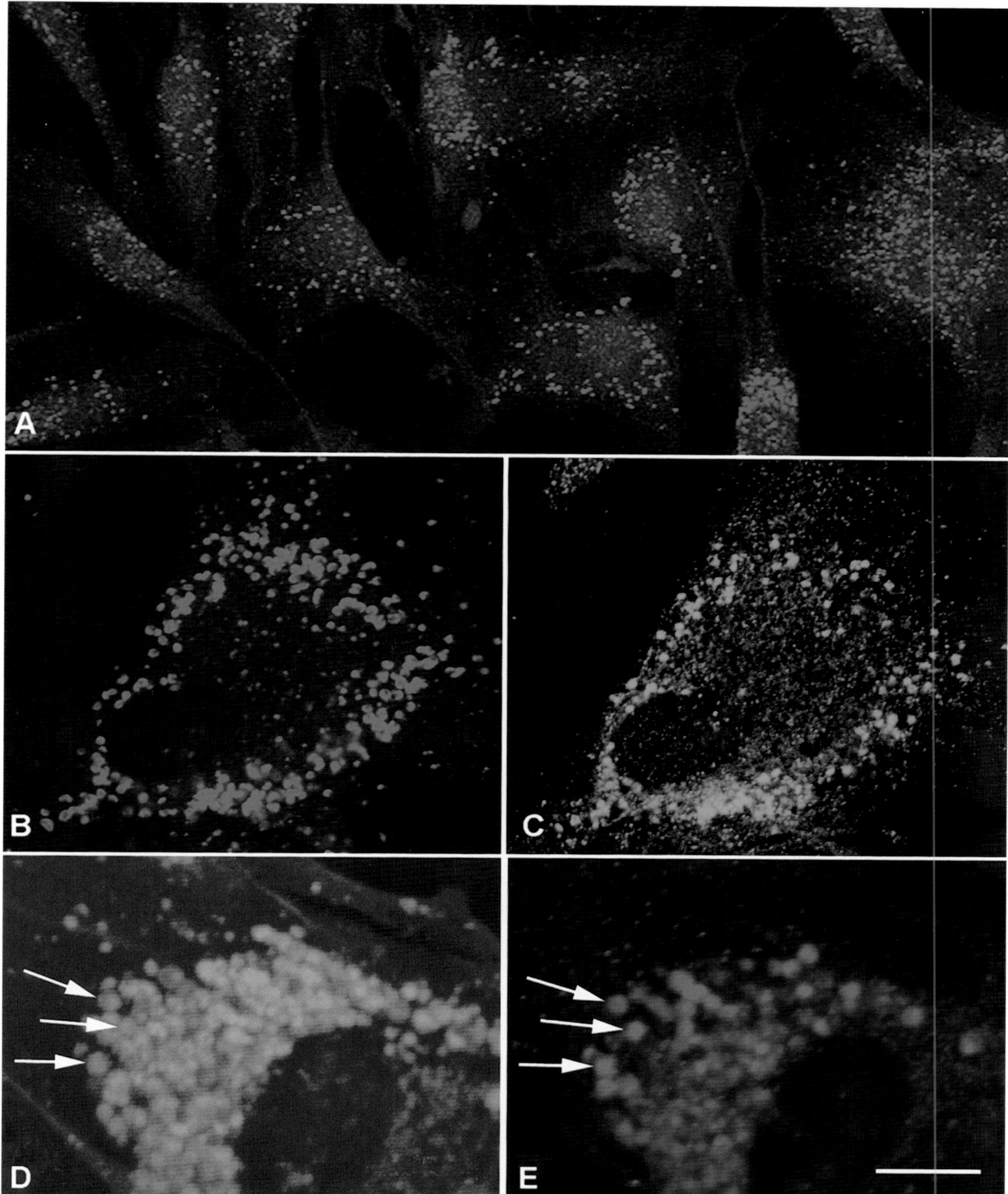

Plate 7 (Fig. 145-10). *A*, Control human fibroblasts incubated with LDL for 24 h, immunostained with antipeptide antibodies to the C-terminus of NPC1 protein, and viewed with confocal fluorescence microscopy. NPC1 immunofluorescence is present in small granules that are distributed throughout the cytoplasm of cells.

B and *C*, Control fibroblast incubated with LDL for 24 h and immunostained with both (B) antibodies to a lysosomal membrane glycoprotein (lamp1) and (C) antipeptide antibodies to the C-terminus of NPC1 protein. The colocalization shows that NPC1 protein (C) is present in lamp1-positive vesicles (B). Note that there are many lamp1-positive lysosomes that do not contain NPC1 protein.

D and *E*, Control fibroblast incubated with LDL and U18666A for 24 h. U18666A causes an accumulation of unesterified cholesterol in lysosomes and Golgi of control cells similar to the cholesterol lipidosis in NP-C cells. Cells were stained with both filipin (D), to visualize unesterified cholesterol, and immunostained with (E) antipeptide antibodies to the C-terminus of NPC1 protein. After drug treatment NPC1 protein (E at arrows) is present in cholesterol-containing lysosomes (D at arrows). Bar = 10 μm.

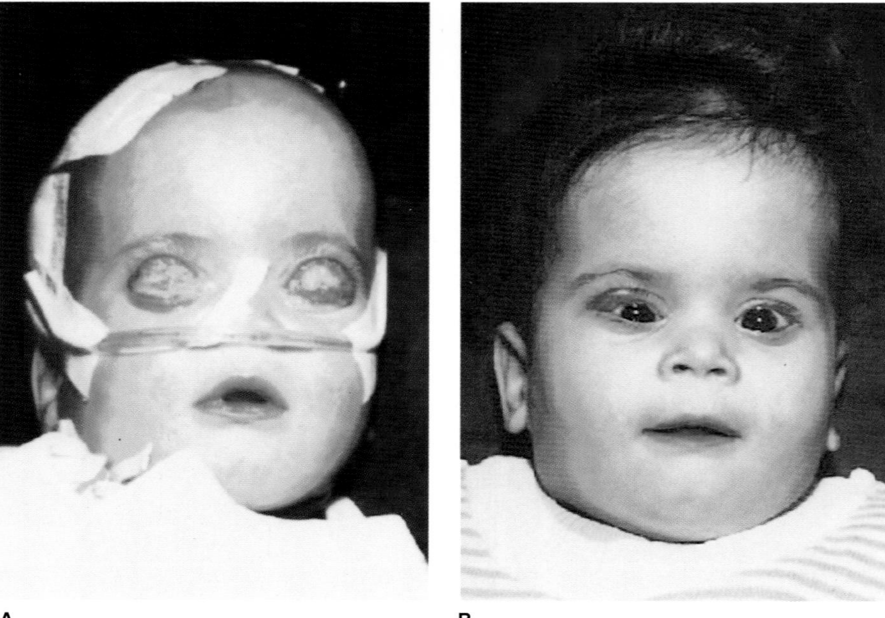

Plate 8 (Fig. 178-7). Panel A is the initial appearance of a child with homozygous plasminogen deficiency resulting in ligneous conjunctivitis. Panel B shows the same child after 7 months of replacement with Lys-plasminogen. (Adapted from Schott et al.[111] Used with permission.)

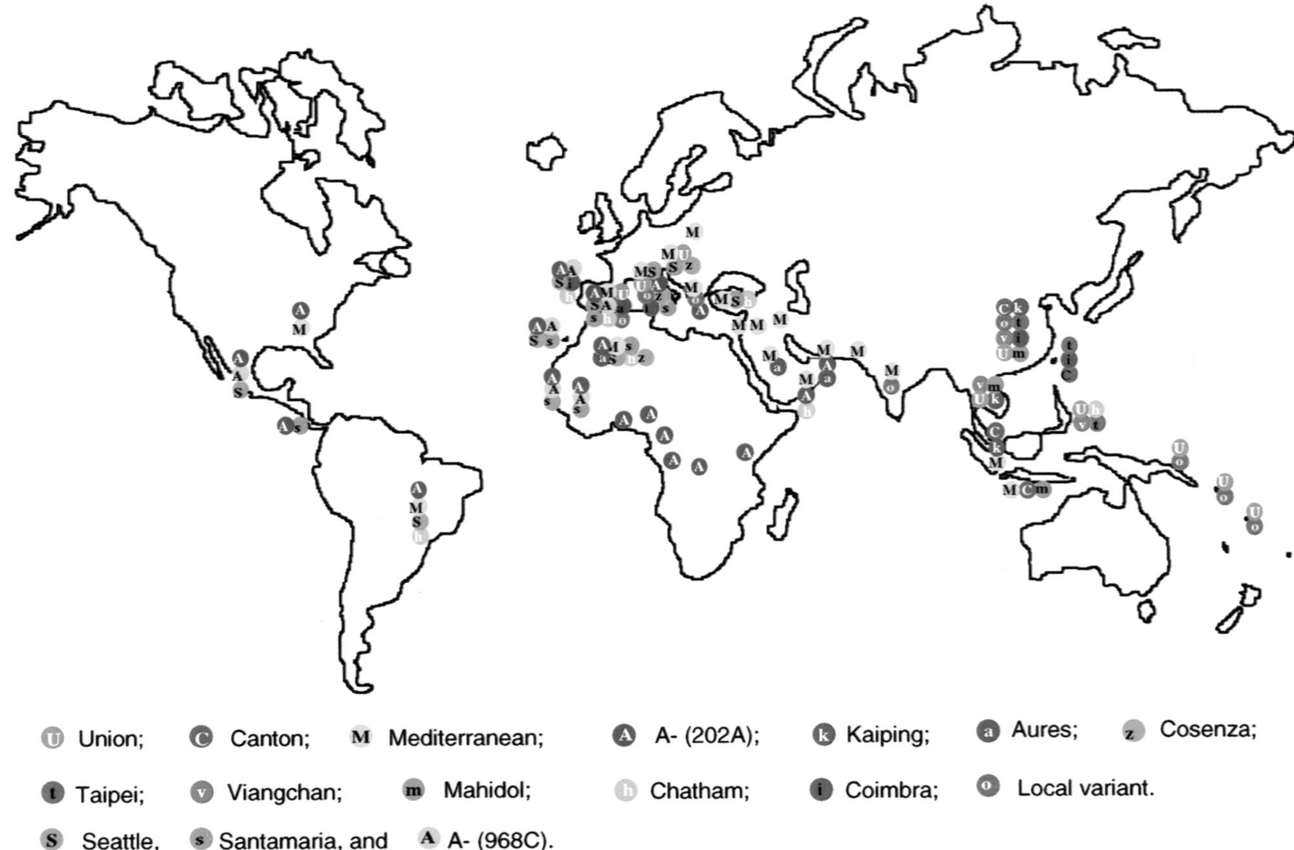

Plate 9 (Fig. 179-8). Worldwide distribution of polymorphic variants of G6PD. The variants in each country are shown in order of prevalence according to these symbols: U = Union; C = Canton; M = Mediterranean; A = A- (202A); k = Kaiping; t = Taipei; v = Viangchan; m = Mahidol; h = Chatham; i = Coimbra; S = Seattle; s = Santamaria; a = Aures; z = Cosenza; A = A- (968C).

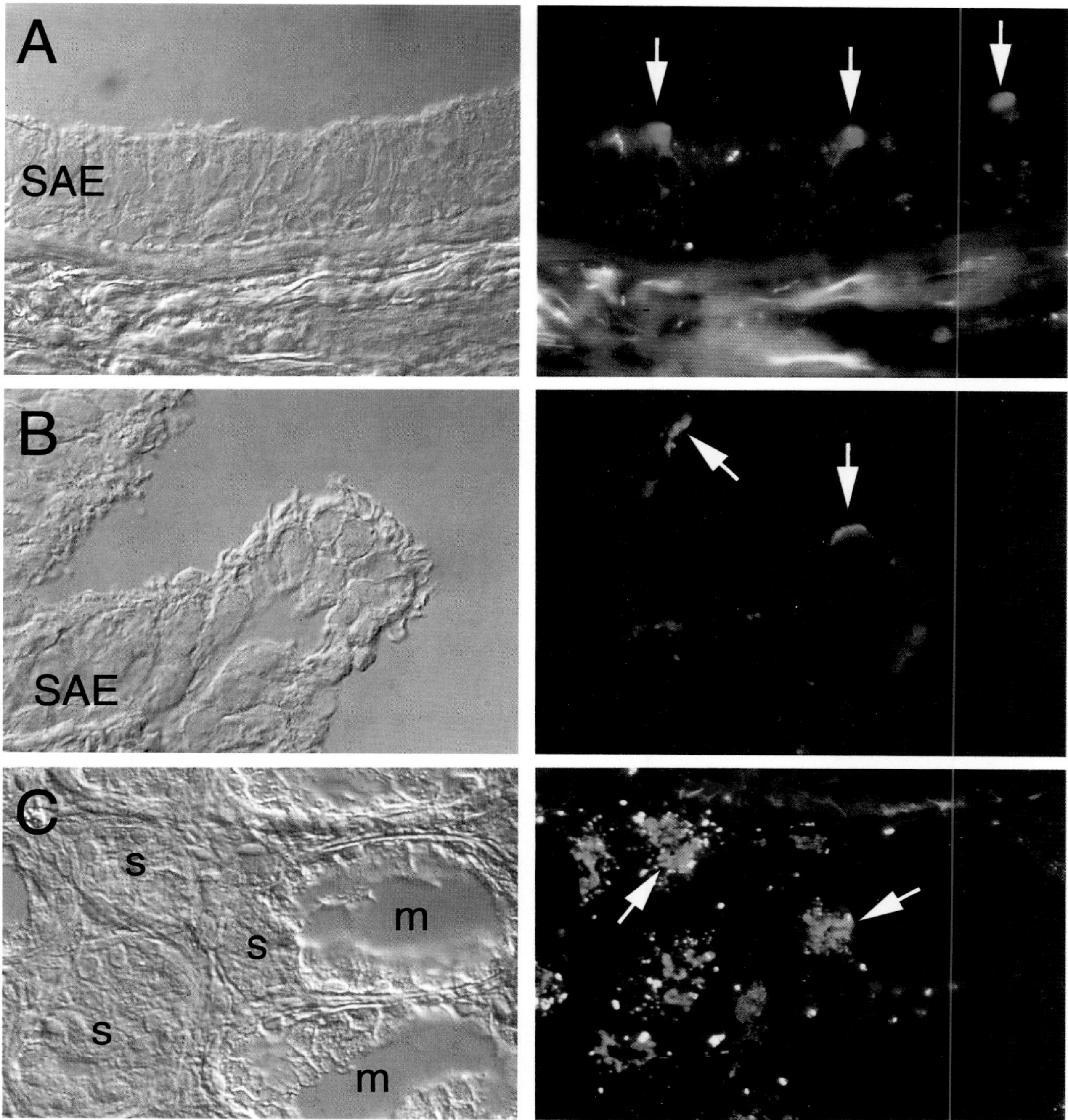

Plate 10 (Fig. 201-23). Immunocytochemical localization of CFTR in the apical membrane of human airway epithelia and in serous cells of submucosal glands. Shown are the surface epithelium of the proximal, *A*, and distal, *B*, airways and submucosal glands, *C*. Panels are Nomarski (left) and fluorescent (right) photomicrographs. SAE indicates surface airway epithelium, s indicates serous cell, and m indicates mucous cell. Bar indicates 35 μm. Arrows point to some areas of CFTR expression. (From Engelhardt.[201,202] Used by permission.)

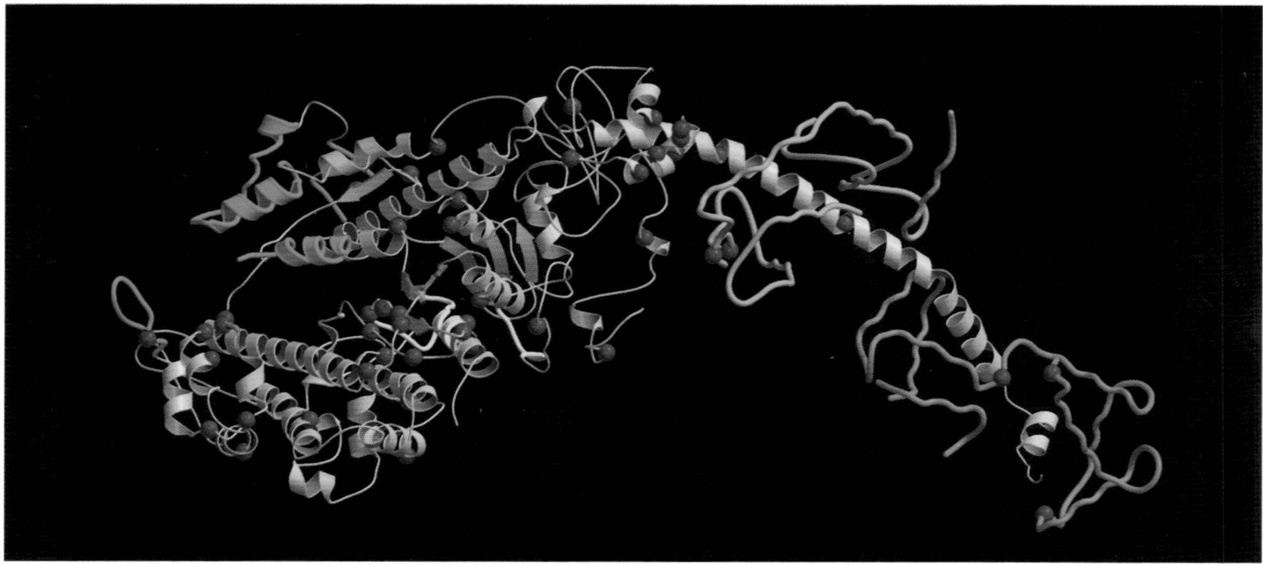

Plate 11 (Fig. 213-13). The location of hypertrophic cardiomyopathy mutations on a computer reconstruction of the 3-dimensional crystal structure of muscle myosin based on coordinates for chicken skeletal muscle myosin. Hypertrophic cardiomyopathy mutations (red spheres) occur throughout the myosin head domain (silver). Myosin residues that interact with actin (green) or ATP (yellow) are indicated. Hypertrophic cardiomyopathy mutations that occur in the essential and regulatory light chains (turquoise and purple, respectively) are also shown.

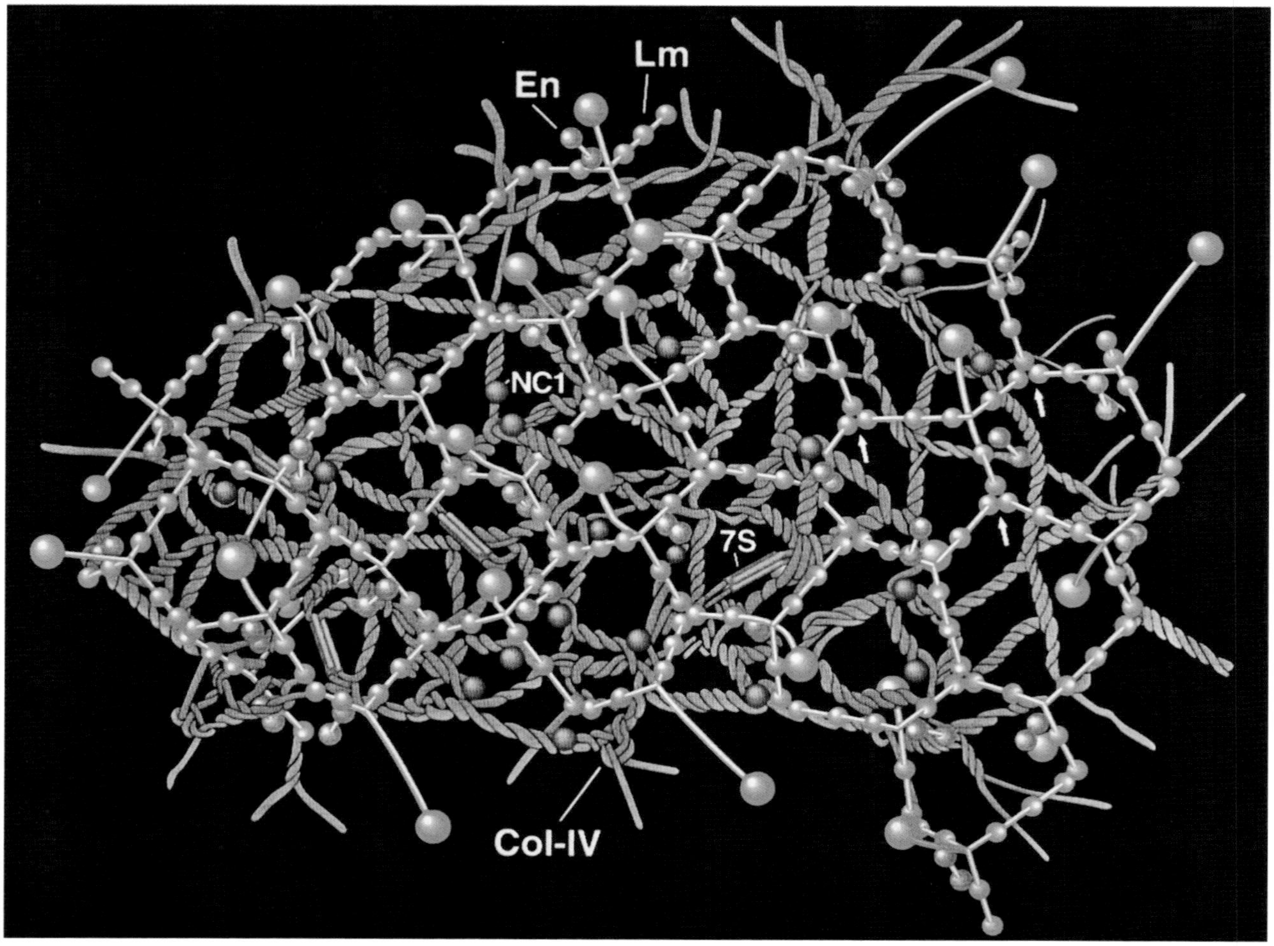

Plate 12 (Fig. 214-3). Hypothetical architecture of the basement membrane. Type IV collagen (Col-IV) and laminin (Lm) form double and interwoven polymer networks. The collagen scaffolding contains lateral, N-terminal tetrameric (7S), and C-terminal globular dimeric (NC1) bonds. The laminin array contains end-to-end interactions of short arms (arrows) and apparently long arms as well. Entactin/nidogen (En) can bridge collagen and laminin. Heparan sulfate proteoglycan (perlecan) complexes are anchored in the network in an unknown where they interact with laminin and collagen through its polyanionic chains in an, as yet unknown. (Courtesy of Dr. Peter Yurchenco, Department of Pathology, Robert-Wood-Johnson Medical School, Piscataway, NJ.)

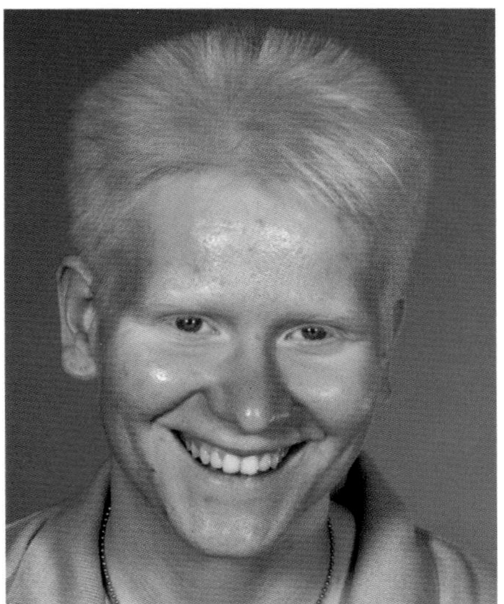

Plate 13 (Fig. 220-8). Young female with OCA1A. No melanin pigment is present. This is the classic tyrosinase-negative OCA phenotype.

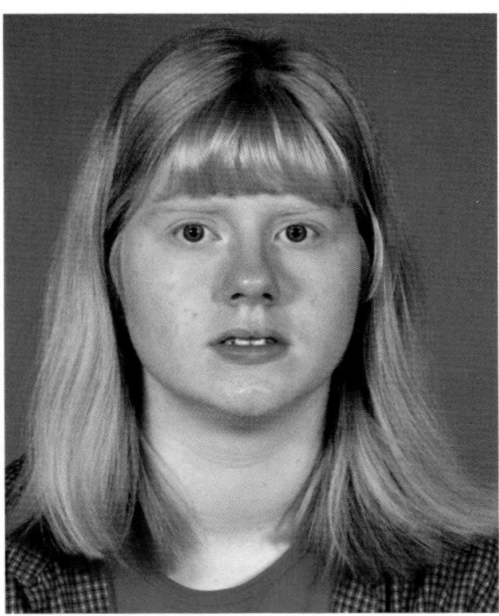

Plate 14 (Fig. 220-10). Young female with OCA1B. The hair was white at birth. This patient now has golden blond hair, dark eyelashes, blue irides, and white skin that tans with sun exposure.

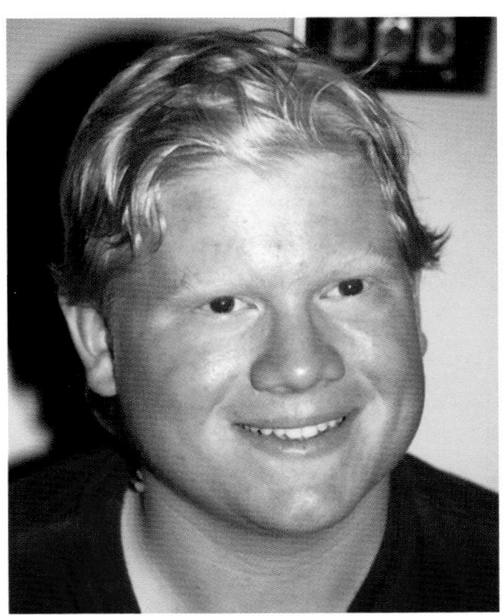

Plate 15 (Fig. 220-12). Young male with OCA2. Hair was light yellow at birth. This individual has yellow/blond scalp and eyelash hair, white skin, and blue irides. The skin does not tan.

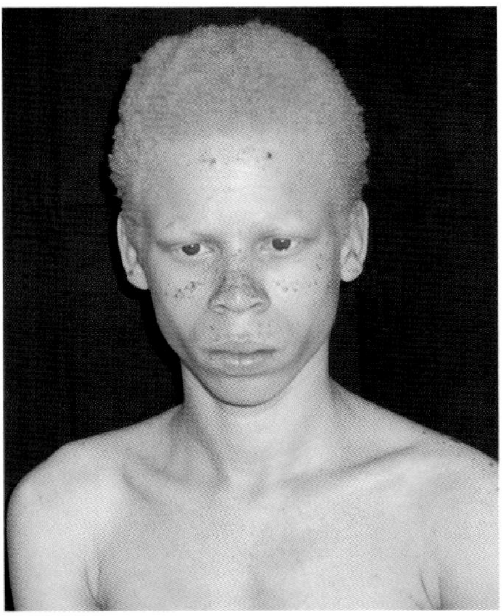

Plate 16 (Fig. 220-13). Young Nigerian male with classic tyrosinase-positive OCA phenotype. Scalp and eyelash hair are yellow. The skin is white and does not tan.

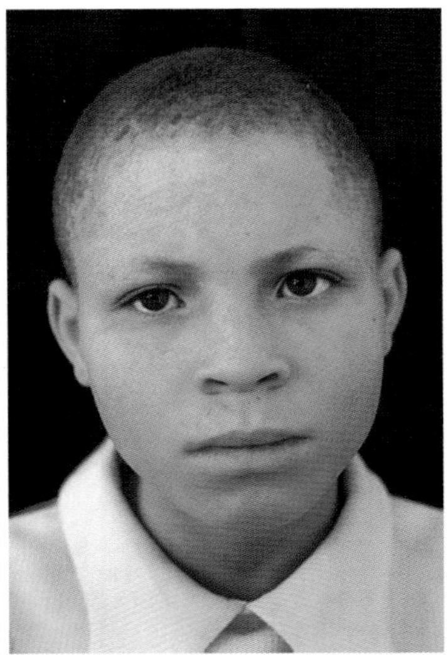

Plate 17 (Fig. 220-14). Young Nigerian female with Brown OCA. Hair, skin, and irides are light brown.

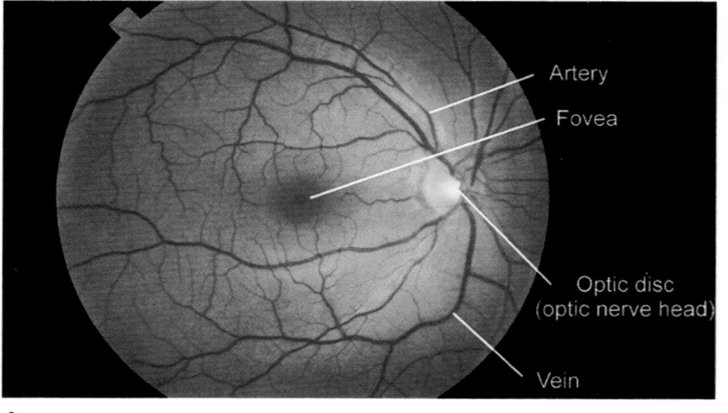

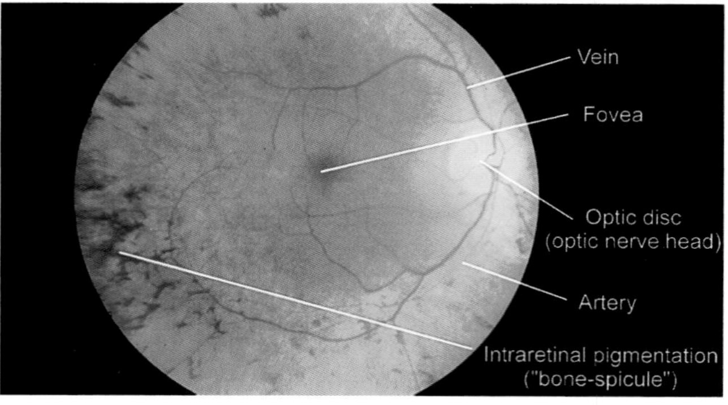

A B

Plate 18 (Fig. 235-1). Normal fundus (A) and a fundus of a patient affected with retinitis pigmentosa (B). The affected fundus has thin retinal blood vessels, a pale optic nerve head, and intraretinal pigment deposits.

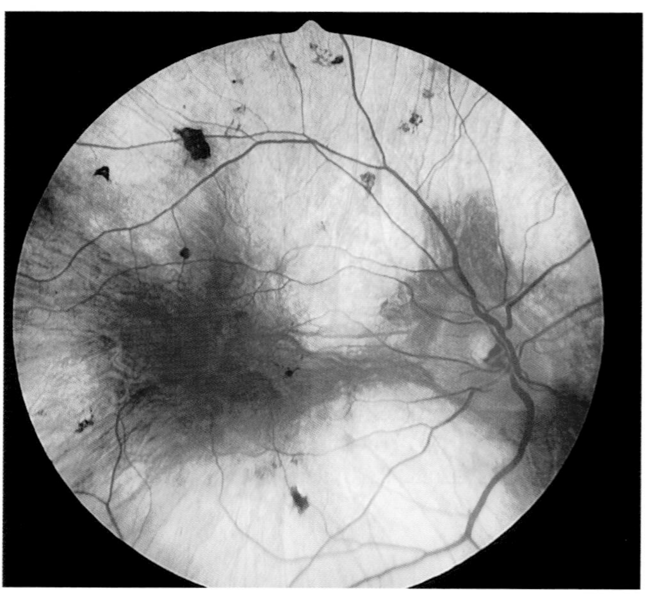

Plate 19 (Fig. 236-1). Fundus of a CHM patient with a deletion of exons 1 and 2 (patient 1167, see Fig. 236-3) at age 30. Note the severe atrophy of the choroid and RPE affecting the entire fundus except for the macular region and the area surrounding the optic disc. At this stage, retinal arteries are still spared.

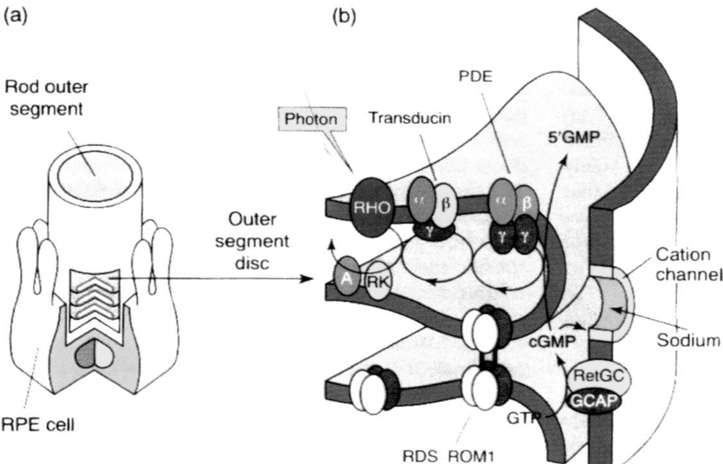

Plate 20 (Fig. 237-2). ***A*****, A rod photoreceptor-retinal pigment epithelial complex and** ***B*****, rod outer-segment discs. The phototransduction pathway: Incident light (photon) photoactivates rhodopsin (RHO), which initiates a cascade reaction involving transducin and phosphodiesterase (PDE). This leads to a relative decrease in intracellular cGMP, closure of sodium channels, and cell hyperpolarization. In the recovery process of photoreceptors, the photoactivated transduction cascade is abolished, and the level of cGMP concentration in photoreceptors is restored to the dark level by the conversion of GTP to 3′,5′-cGMP catalyzed by the guanylate cyclase (RetGC). Regeneration of rhodopsin involves arrestin (A) and rhodopsin kinase (RK). RDS-ROM1 interaction is involved in maintaining rod outer-segment structural integrity. Abbreviations: GCAP, guanylate cyclase activating protein; RDS-ROM1, retinal degeneration slow, rod outer-segment membrane protein. (Used with permission from Gregory-Evans K, Bhattacharya SS: Clinical blindness: Current concepts in the pathogenesis of human outer retinal dystrophies.** ***Trends Genet*** **3:103, 1998.)**

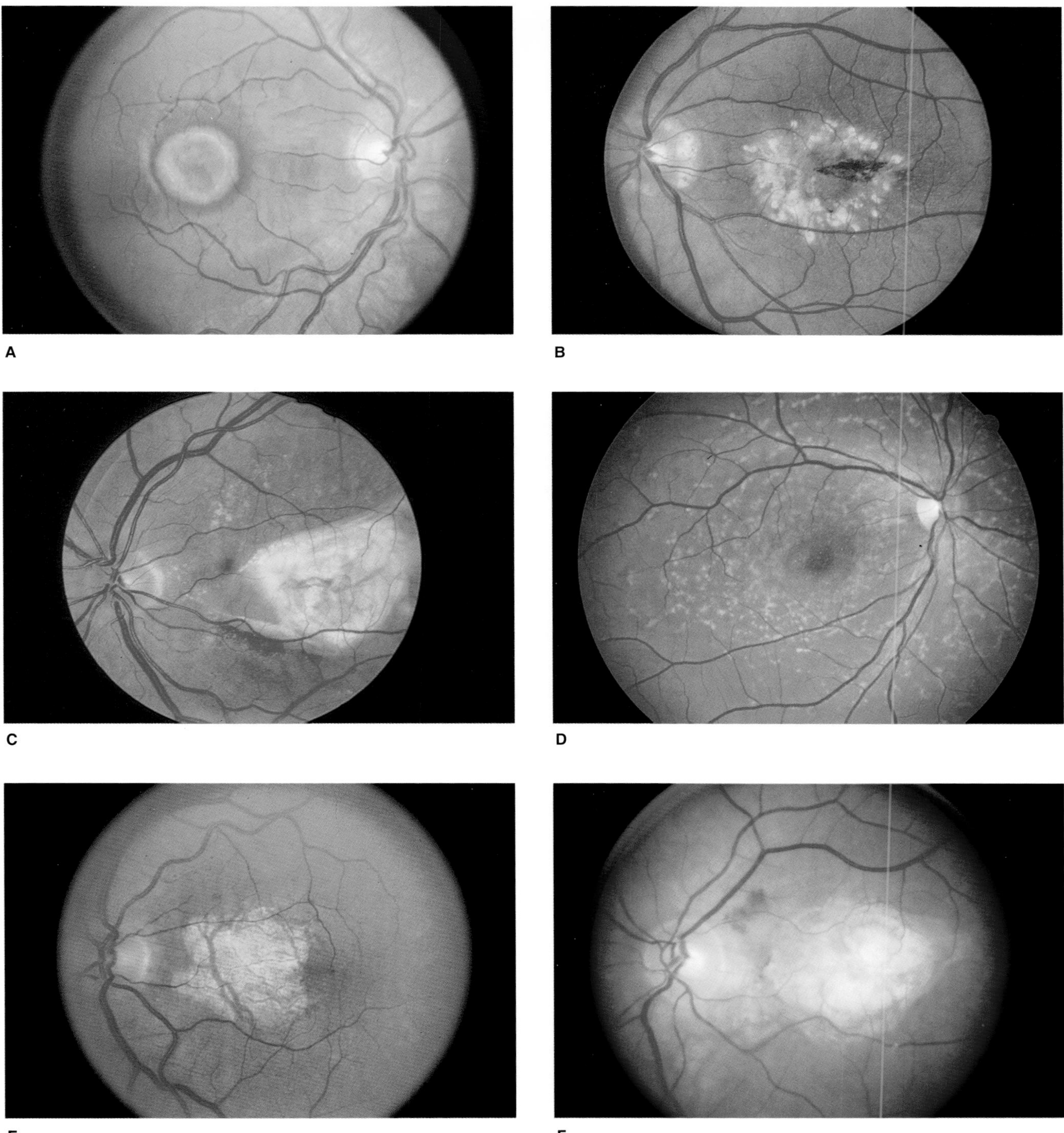

Plate 21 (Fig. 243-1A-F). Clinical manifestations of macular dystrophy and degeneration. *A*, Best disease. The right macula of a 12-year-old boy with a typical "egg yolk" accumulation. Corrected visual acuity is 20/30. Note the normal optic disc, retinal vasculature, and surrounding pigment epithelium. *B*, Doyne honeycomb dystrophy. The left macula of a 45-year-old woman of Swiss-German ancestry who first noted visual distortion at age 27 years. Corrected visual acuity is 20/100. Note the densely packed drusen-like bodies centrally with associated pigment disruption, surrounded by tiny drusen in a radial array. *C*, Sorsby fundus dystrophy. The left macula of a 39-year-old engineer with end-stage disciform macular scarring that began at age 36 years. Two sisters, his mother, and his maternal grandmother each developed disciform macular degeneration before age 40 years. *D*, Stargardt disease/fundus flavimaculatus. The right fundus of a 17-year-old female with slowly progressive loss of central vision over 4 years, now 20/100 in each eye. Note the slight temporal pallor of the optic disc, the fine, sandy atrophy of the pigment epithelium in the fovea, and a myriad of flecks, some circular, some coalescent in short chains inside and just outside the major vascular arcade. *E*, Age-related maculopathy. Geography atrophy: The left macula of a 68-year-old shows a sharply marginated thinning of the retinal pigment epithelium, enhancing visualization of the large choroidal vessels and the deeper sclera. *F*, Age-related maculopathy. Disciform degeneration: The left macula of a 72 year old with a healed white "fibrous" central scar in the shape of a "disc" under the retina.

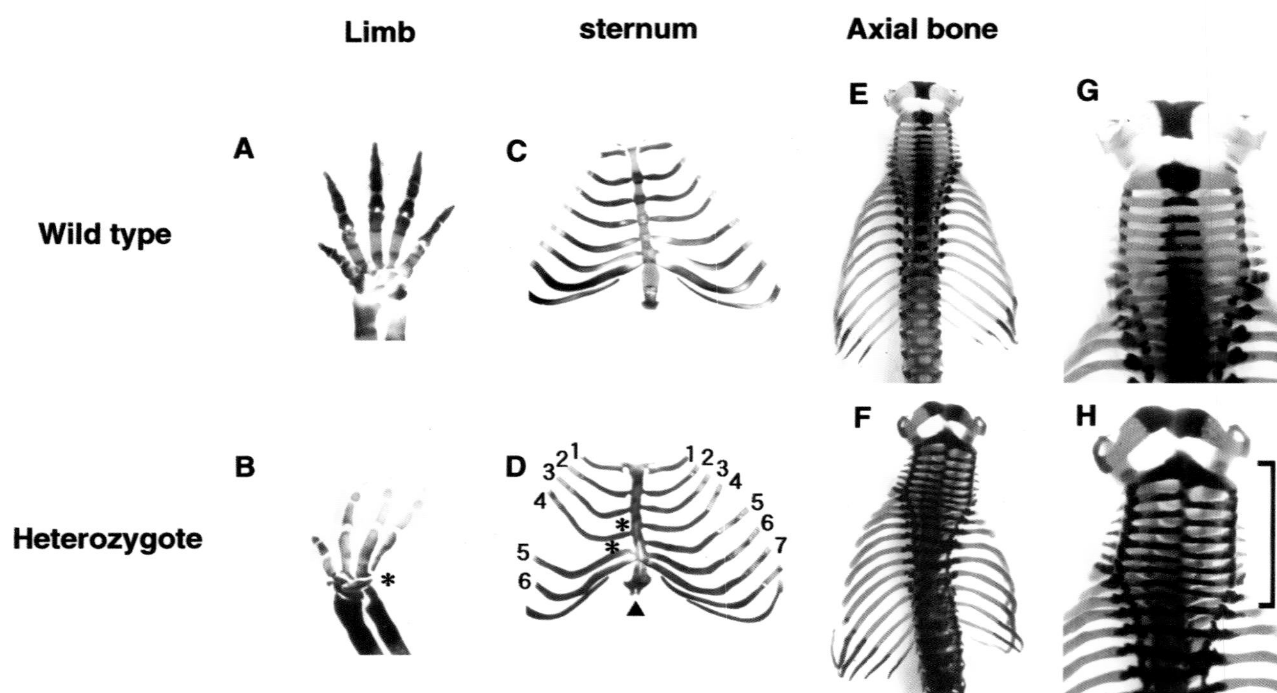

Plate 22 (Fig. 248-11). Severe abnormalities in Cbp heterozygous mice. Bone and cartilage stained specimens of the right forelimbs and sternums of a wild-type (A and C) and a Cbp heterozygote (B and D) mouse. Oligodactyly and misalignment of rib pairs can be observed (*). Only six ribs can be seen on the right side. Dorsal view of the vertebrae of a wild-type (E and G) and a heterozygote (F and H). In the heterozygote, the presence of 10 ribs on the right side, 14 ribs on the left side, asymmetric cervical vertebrae, extra split thoracic vertebrae, and scoliosis were observed. (From Tanaka et al.[143] Copyright 1997; used by permission of National Academy of Sciences U.S.A.)

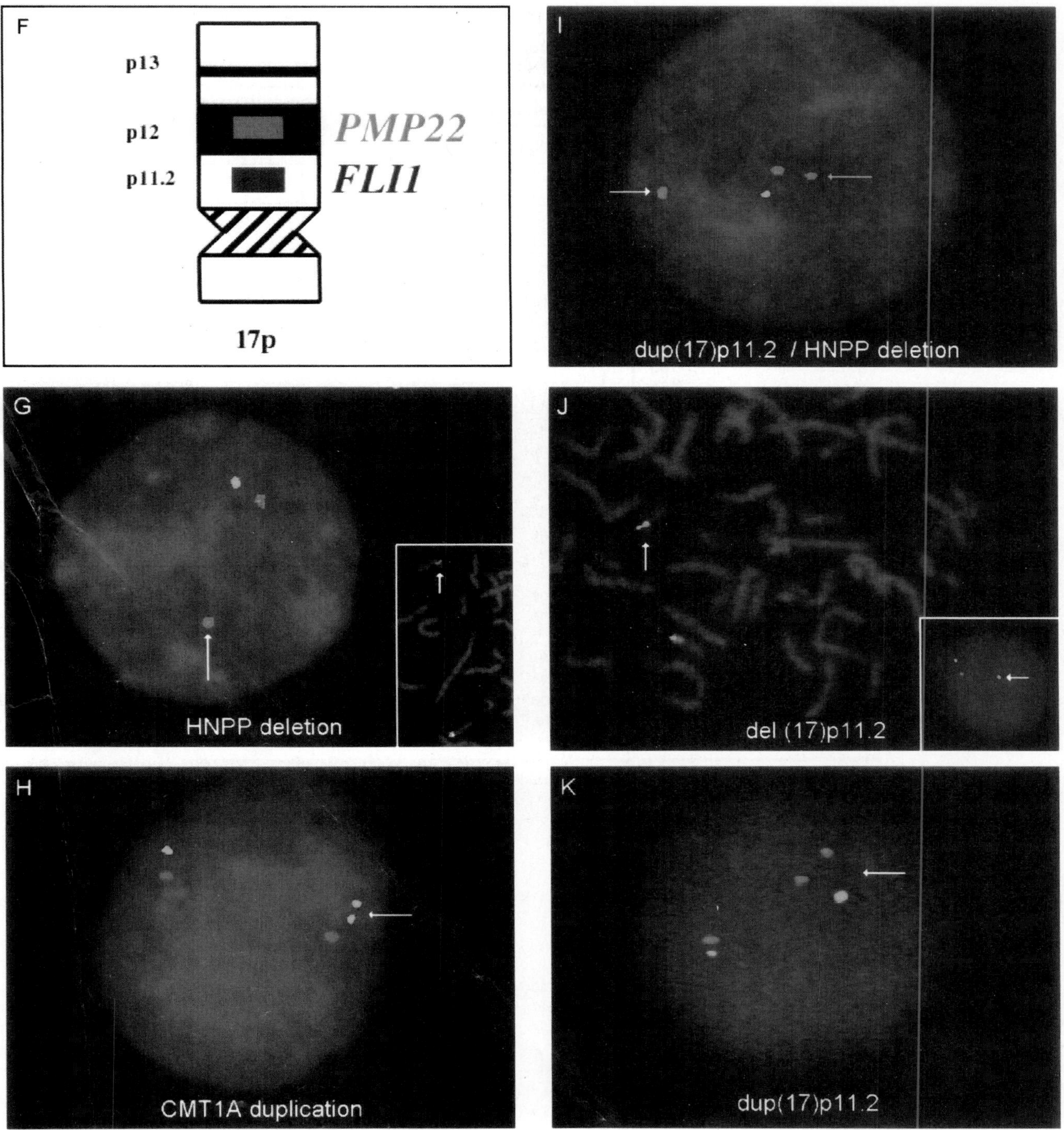

Fig. 65-3F–K *F.* Ideogram showing 17p and the location of the loci *PMP22* and *FLI1* to 17p12 and 17p11.2, respectively. The probes are shown in either red (*PMP22*) or green (*FLI1*) and this color scheme is used throughout Figs. 65-3G to 65-3K. For each, a cosmid contig containing the *FLI1* locus on 17p11.2 is labeled with biotin and detected with avidin conjugated to fluorescein (fluoresces green). A cosmid contig containing the *PMP22* gene on 17p12 is labeled with digoxigenin and detected with antidigoxigenin conjugated to rhodamine (fluoresces red). *G.* FISH showing an HNPP deletion in an interphase nucleus and metaphase chromosomes (inset). The normal chromosome 17 shows two signals: a green *FLI1* signal and red *PMP22* signal. The deleted chromosome 17 (arrow) shows only the green signal, indicating a deletion of the *PMP22* locus. This result is seen in HNPP patients who carry deletions. *H.* Interphase FISH showing CMT1A duplication. The normal chromosome 17 shows two signals: a green *FLI1* signal and red *PMP22* signal. The duplicated chromosome 17 (arrow) shows one green signal and two red signals, indicating a duplication of the *PMP22* locus. This result is seen in CMT1A patients who carry duplications. *I.* Interphase FISH showing a duplication on one chromosome 17 in band p11.2 and a deletion on the other homologue for the *PMP22* gene on 17p12. One chromosome 17 shows a deletion for the *PMP22* gene on 17p12 (white arrow), while the other homologue shows a duplication for the *FLI1* locus on 17p11.2 (red arrow).[427] *J.* FISH using a cosmid contig containing the *FLI1* locus, mapping to 17p11.2 on a patient with Smith-Magenis syndrome. The normal chromosome 17 shows two signals: a green *FLI1* signal and red *PMP22* signal. The deleted chromosome 17 (arrow) shows only the red *PMP22* signal, indicating a deletion of the *FLI1* locus. This result is seen in Smith-Magenis syndrome patients who carry deletions. *K.* Interphase FISH using a cosmid containing the *FLI1* locus, mapping to 17p11.2 on a patient with a dup(17)(p11.2p11.2). The normal chromosome 17 shows two signals: a green *FLI1* signal and red *PMP22* signal. The duplicated chromosome 17 (arrow) shows one red signal and two green signals, indicating duplication of the region containing the *FLI1* locus. This result is consistent with a duplication of 17p11.2. See Color Plates 2F–K.

Table 65-2 Contiguous Gene Syndromes: Chromosomal Localization, Detection of DNA Rearrangements, and Genes Known to Contribute to the Phenotype

Syndrome	Location	Rearrangements		Gene(s)
		Visible	Submicroscopic	
Microdeletions:				
Monosomy 1p	1p36	Most	Unknown	—
Wolf-Hirschhorn	4p16	Most	Few	—
Cri-du-chat	5p15	Most	Few	—
Williams	7q11.23	Few	>90%	*ELN*
TRPS I	8q24.1	Few	~30%	*TRPS1*
Langer-Giedion	8q24.1	75%	Few	*EXT1, TRPS1*
Potocki-Shaffer	11p11.2	Most	One known case	*EXT2*
WAGR	11p13	Most	Unknown	*PAX6, WT1*
Prader-Willi	15q12	~70%	70%	—
Angelman	15q12	~70%	70%	*UBE3A*
Rubinstein-Taybi	16p13.3	None	~10%	*CBP*
Smith-Magenis	17p11.2	Most	Unknown	—
HNPP	17p12	None	85%	*PMP22*
Miller-Dieker	17p13.3	50%	>90%	*LIS1*
Alagille	20p11.23	Rare	6%	*JAG1*
DiGeorge/VCF	22q11.2	~30%	>90%	—
Duchenne MD	Xp21	None	60%	*DMD*
CGKD	Xp21	Few	100%	*DMD, GK, DAX1*
AHC	Xp21	None	13%*	*DAX1*
Steroid Sulfatase	Xp22.3	None	90%	*STS*
Kallmann	Xp22.3	None	10%	*KAL1*
Microduplications:				
BWS	11p15.5	Few	Unknown	*IGF2,* $p57^{KIP2}$
dup 17p11.2	17p11.2	Few	100%	—
CMT1A	17p12	None	>98%	*PMP22*
Sex reversal (DSS)	Xp21	Rare	Unknown	*DAX1*
PMD	Xq22	Rare	70%	*PLP*

*44% of AHC patients have large deletions that include either GK or GK and DMD.

every 30 kb in the human genome, these imbalances may involve 10 to 100 genes. Although it is not known what percentage of genes are dosage sensitive or imprinted in humans, it is likely that these genes represent a minority and that deletion of most genes has no or only minor phenotypic consequence (Fig. 65-6). Thus, molecular characterization of the "critical region" for a CGS will involve identification of all genes within the region, and determination of which genes are primarily responsible for the abnormal phenotype due to dosage or imprinting effects, and whether or not other genes contribute to variability of expression.

IMPLICATIONS FOR PHYSICAL MAPPING AND POSITIONAL CLONING

Panels of cell lines from patients carrying deletions and translocations, most of which have CGS, are available for several chromosomal regions. These panels represent invaluable resources for physical mapping of DNA markers and disease genes. Anonymous DNA probes or cDNA probes can be tested on patients' DNA by Southern blot analysis, PCR, or FISH. Presence or absence of the marker determines the relative positions of loci recognized by DNA markers with respect to patients' chromosomal breakpoints.

Maps of large regions of the genome have been constructed by studying patients with CGS.[63–70] These maps are very helpful for the identification of disease genes involved in CGS. Gene identification is usually achieved by positional cloning, a strategy that allows the isolation of a disease gene based on the knowledge of its physical/genetic location in the genome and with little useful information regarding its function (see Chaps. 1 and 10).[71,72] Syndromes that have varying-sized deletions can be helpful in the identification of disease loci if specific clinical features vary with the size of the deletion.[26,70,73,74] However, if the majority of patients have the same-sized deletion, then the investigator must rely on mutations in patients showing only the partial phenotype, such as supravalvular aortic stenosis in the absence of other features of Williams syndrome,[75,76] or the full phenotype, such as point mutations in *UBE3A* gene in Angelman syndrome patients,[77,78] in order to implicate the candidate gene in the disease phenotype.

X-LINKED CONTIGUOUS GENE SYNDROMES

The three main regions of the X chromosome implicated in CGS (Xp22.3, Xp21, and Xq21) and the disease genes involved in each region are shown in Fig. 65-7. In males, a direct genotype/phenotype correlation can be made, since deletions result in segmental nullisomy. Females carrying X-chromosome rearrangements usually have a normal phenotype. However, females may show an abnormal phenotype if a nonrandom pattern of X-inactivation occurs, causing functional nullisomy, or heterozygotes for loss-of-function alleles may show phenotypic effects, as in ornithine transcarbamylase deficiency, especially under physiological stress (e.g., pregnancy).[4,79,80] Monosomy for the entire X chromosome in females causes Turner syndrome, which is presumed to be the result of functional monosomy for genes located on the X chromosome. It has been hypothesized that the genes involved in the Turner syndrome phenotype must normally be expressed on both the active and inactive X

Map

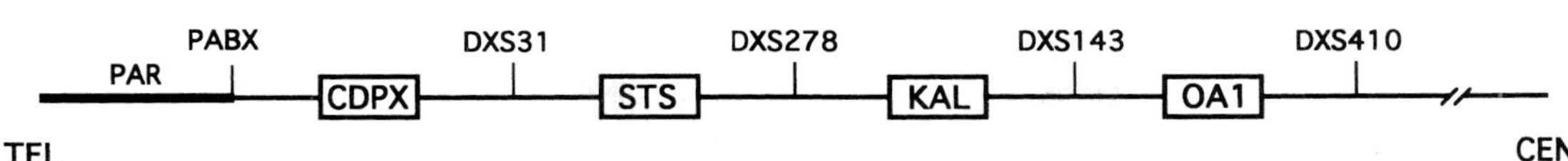

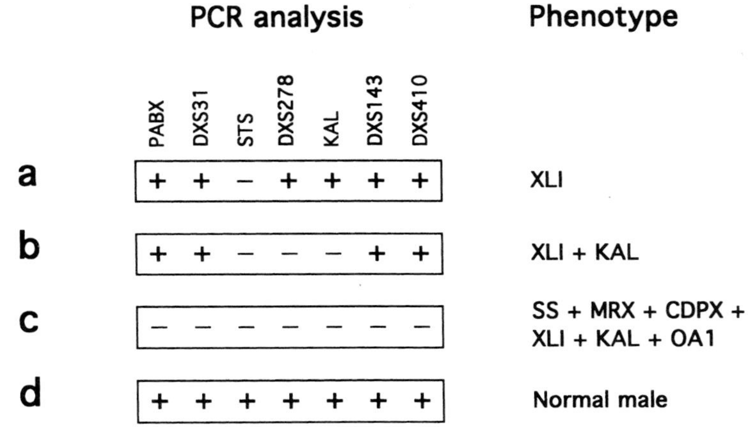

Fig. 65-4 PCR test for Xp22.3 CGS. The order of some of the disease genes and DNA markers in the Xp22.3 region is shown at the top. PABX = pseudoautosomal boundary; PAR = pseudoautosomal region. A seven-loci PCR test has been designed for the detection and partial characterization of Xp22.3 CGS. *A*, Pattern observed in most males with isolated X-linked ichthyosis. *B*, Pattern observed in most males with X-linked ichthyosis associated with Kallmann syndrome. *C*, Pattern observed in males with very complex phenotypes including features of all Xp22.3 diseases. *D*, Normal male pattern.

chromosomes in females and on both the X and Y chromosomes in males.[81]

Xp22.3

The most common recognized chromosomal rearrangements involving the distal short arm of the X chromosome (Xp22.3) are submicroscopic interstitial deletions spanning the steroid sulfatase (*STS*) gene.[82–88] These deletions result in isolated X-linked ichthyosis (XLI; MIM 308100), a dermatologic disorder characterized by dark scaly skin (see Chap. 166). More than 85 percent of patients with X-linked ichthyosis have large molecular deletions (1 to 2 Mb) spanning the entire steroid sulfatase gene.[28,82,83,89]

Kallmann syndrome (KAL; MIM 308700) is characterized by hypogonadotropic hypogonadism and anosmia (see also Chap. 225). The X-linked ichthyosis associated with Kallmann syndrome in males was presumed to be caused by a CGS.[90] Molecular analysis of the deletions in such families was instrumental for both mapping and cloning of the steroid sulfatase gene and Kallmann syndrome gene.[91,92] Many patients with X-linked ichthyosis associated with Kallmann syndrome have been reported (see review[28]). These patients have either interstitial deletions, terminal deletions, or X/Y translocations resulting in loss of terminal Xp.[28] In addition to X-linked ichthyosis and Kallmann syndrome, patients with deletions and translocations involving the Xp22.3 region have other diseases and, therefore, have been included in the spectrum of the Xp22.3 CGS. The genes involved in the Xp22.3 CGS are shown in Fig. 65-7.

Short stature (SS; MIM 312865) was found in all males and females with terminal Xp deletions. The presence of a gene escaping X inactivation located in the human pseudoautosomal region, in which two expressed copies are required for normal height, was postulated[29] and subsequently confirmed.[93,93a] Male patients with terminal Xp deletions frequently have X-linked recessive chondrodysplasia punctata (CDPX; MIM 302950), a bone dysplasia clinically characterized by nasal hypoplasia, focal calcification of cartilage (detectable as radiologic stippling of epiphyses), and distal phalangeal hypoplasia (see review[94]). A patient with isolated X-linked recessive chondrodysplasia punctata carrying an Xp22.3 interstitial deletion has also been reported.[95] The gene causing CDPX is arylsulfatase E.[96] Mutations have been identified in patients with isolated CDPX[96] (see Chap. 149). Patients carrying large terminal deletions involving the steroid sulfatase gene almost invariably have mild mental retardation, unlike patients with smaller terminal deletions or interstitial deletions of only STS. Therefore, a specific locus for mental retardation (MRX; MIM 309530) was assigned to Xp22.3 distal to steroid sulfatase.[29]

X-linked ocular albinism (OA1; MIM 300500) is clinically characterized by impaired visual acuity, nystagmus, strabismus, and photophobia, and by the presence of skin macromelanosomes. X-linked ocular albinism has been described as part of an Xp22.3 CGS in only two cases, one carrying an interstitial deletion[97] and the other a terminal deletion.[51] A patient with isolated X-linked ocular albinism carrying an interstitial, submicroscopic deletion in the Xp22.3 region has been described.[98] The *OA1* gene has been cloned and mutations have been found in patients with isolated ocular albinism (see Chap. 220).[99,100]

Female patients with interstitial deletions, terminal deletions, X/Y translocations, or X/autosomal translocations involving Xp22.3 typically do not show any of the diseases described in affected males, with the exception of short stature (SHOX; MIM 312865). However, very large, male-lethal, Xp22-pter terminal deletions result in a complex developmental defect in heterozygous females. This defect, termed "microphthalmia with linear skin defects syndrome" (MLS; MIM 309801), is characterized by the association of severe microphthalmia with linear skin lesions on the face and neck. It has been hypothesized that in females

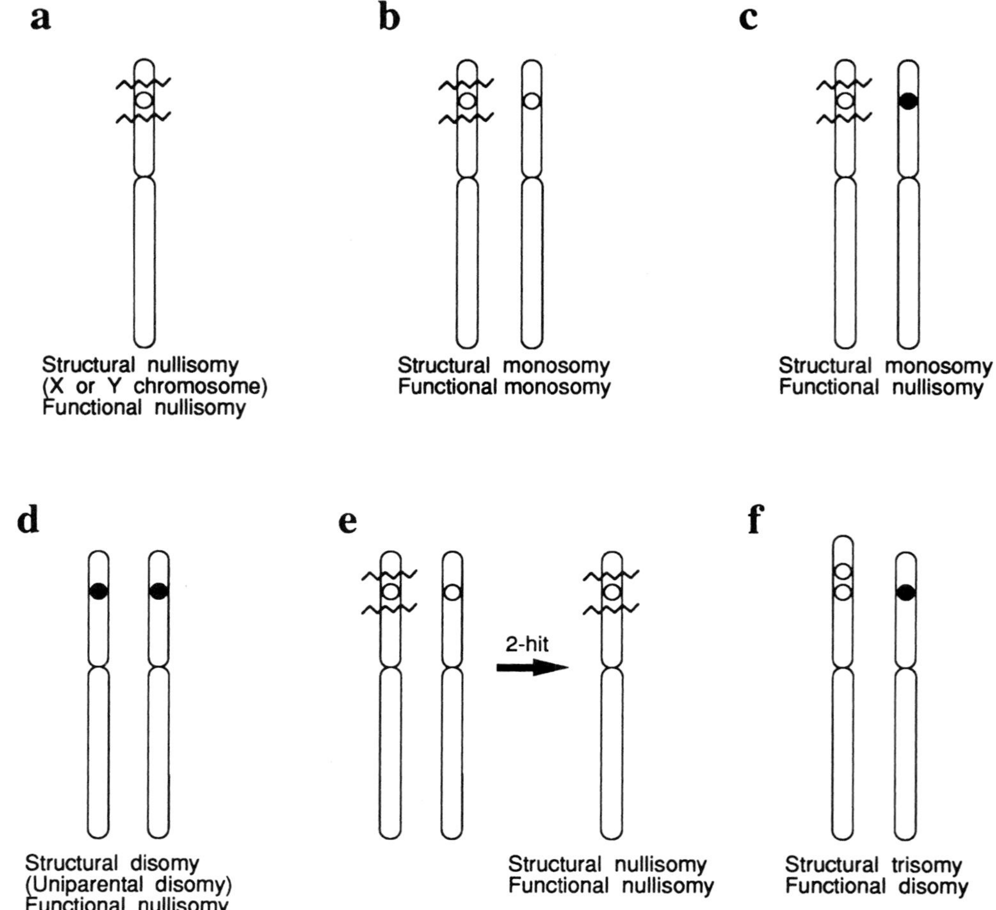

Fig. 65-5 Gene-dosage effects in CGS caused by various chromosomal abnormalities. An open circle indicates an active gene and a black circle indicates an inactive gene. Jagged horizontal lines represent deletion breakpoints. *A*, Deletion of the X or Y chromosome in a hemizygous male produces structural and functional nullisomy for any gene within the deleted interval. *B*, Deletion of one active copy of a gene in an autosomal segment produces structural and functional monosomy. *C*, The gene on the nondeleted homologue (right) is inactive due to imprinting at an autosomal locus or due to X-chromosome inactivation. Deletion of the active copy therefore results in structural monosomy, but functional nullisomy. *D*, Uniparental disomy may produce functional nullisomy even though two structural copies of a gene are present. *E*, In certain tumors, recessive mutations are expressed as a result of structural and functional nullisomy arising from two mutational events. In this example, a constitutional deletion is shown that produces structural and functional monosomy. A second event, loss of the normal homologue, results in structural and functional nullisomy at a cellular level. *F*, A duplication is shown that produces structural trisomy for an autosomal segment. In this example, the duplication involves the active copy of an imprinted gene producing functional disomy.

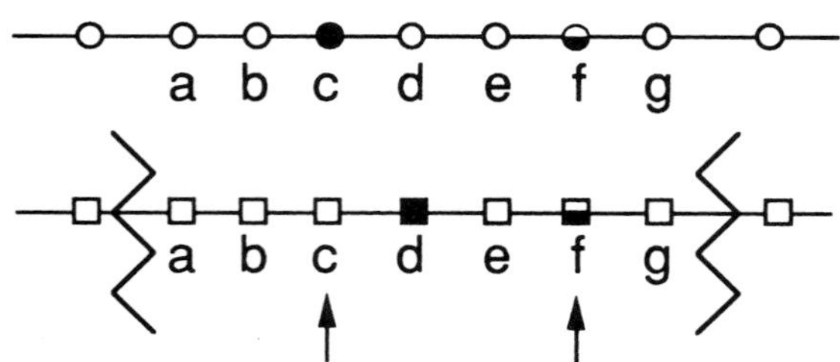

Fig. 65-6 Phenotypic effects of a deletion or duplication result from the dosage imbalance of a subset of genes within the involved segment. Active genes are shown as open circles (maternal homologue) or squares (paternal homologue), and inactive (imprinted) genes are shown as black circles or squares. The jagged vertical lines represent breakpoints of a deleted segment. Most genes are probably not dosage sensitive and not imprinted; therefore, deletion of one copy of the gene results in no phenotypic effects (*a, b, e, g*). Deletion of a dosage sensitive gene (shown as a half-filled circle or square) results in half-normal levels of gene product (*f*). This haploinsufficiency results in an abnormal phenotype. Deletion of the active copy of an imprinted gene (*c*) results in no gene product and produces an abnormal phenotype, while deletion of the inactive copy of an imprinted gene (*d*) does not.

carrying large Xp22-pter terminal deletions, inactivation of the normal X chromosome leads, in some tissues, to functional nullisomy for genes located within the deleted region, causing the MLS phenotype.[28,51]

Several genes have been isolated from the candidate MLS region but whether one or more of these genes cause the MLS phenotype remains to be determined. Two of these genes isolated are a novel rho-GAP (*ARHGAPG*) and a holocytochrome c-synthetase. The third gene is a novel member of the RING finger family midline 1 (*MID1*), and has been isolated near the telomeric boundary of the MLS candidate region. *MID1* is mutated in X-linked Opitz syndrome[101,102] but its role, if any, in MLS has not been established. Because MLS is a deletion syndrome, proving the role of a candidate gene in causing a phenotype will have to await animal studies. Nondeletion MLS patients have been described, but those are rare and it remains to be determined whether they have defects in an Xp22.3-linked gene.[103]

Xp21

The Xp21 CGS has been studied in detail. The first patient diagnosed with an Xp21 CGS had Duchenne muscular dystrophy (DMD; MIM 210200) associated with chronic granulomatous

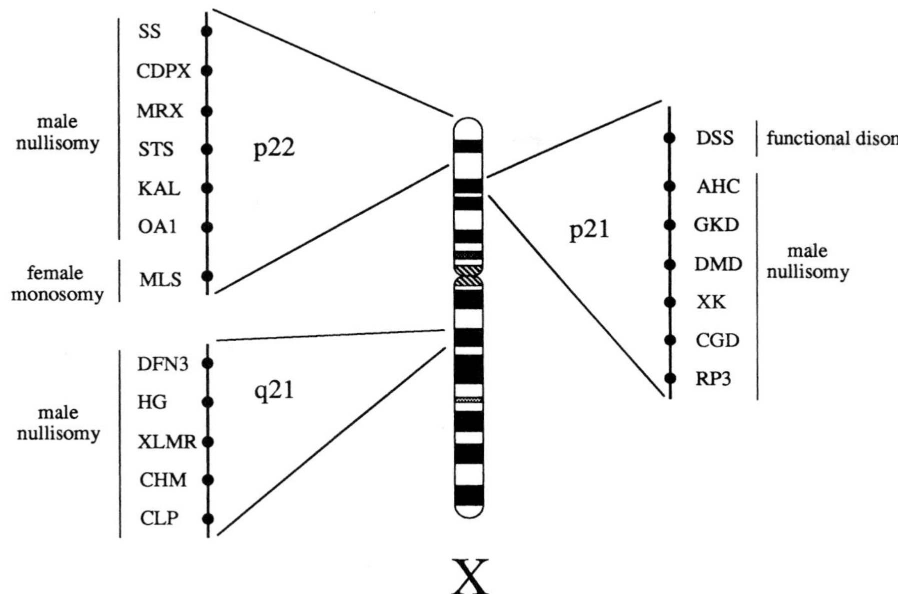

Fig. 65-7 X-linked CGS. Three regions of the X chromosome (Xp22.3, Xp21, and Xq21) implicated in CGS are shown. The position of disease genes within each region is indicated. AHC = adrenal hypoplasia congenita; CDPX = X-linked recessive chondrodysplasia punctata; CGD = chronic granulomatous disease; CHM = choroideremia; CLP = cleft lip and palate; DFN3 = X-linked mixed deafness; DMD = Duchenne muscular dystrophy; DSS = dosage-sensitive sex reversal; GKD = glycerol kinase deficiency; HG = hypergonadotropic hypogonadism; KAL = X-linked Kallmann syndrome; MLS = microphthalmia with linear skin defects; MRX = X-linked mental retardation; OA1 = ocular albinism type 1; OTC = ornithine transcarbamylase deficiency; RP3 = retinitis pigmentosa type 3; SS = short stature; STS = steroid sulfatase; XK = McLeod phenotype; XLMR = X-linked nonspecific mental retardation.

disease (CGD; MIM 306400), retinitis pigmentosa (RP3; MIM 312610), and McLeod phenotype (XK; MIM 314850).[104] Since then, many patients with Xp21 CGS have been identified. The full clinical spectrum of Xp21 CGS can include these diseases: adrenal hypoplasia congenita (AHC; MIM 300200, Chap. 167); glycerol kinase deficiency (GKD; MIM 307030, Chap. 97); Duchenne muscular dystrophy (Chap. 216); McLeod phenotype, chronic granulomatous disease (Chap. 189); retinitis pigmentosa (Chap. 235); and ornithine transcarbamylase deficiency (OTC; MIM 311250, Chap. 85). Some patients with Xp21 deletions have additional clinical features. These include mental retardation, hypogonadotropic hypogonadism, and ophthalmologic features referred to as Oregon eye disease and resembling those of Åland Island eye disease (AIED or OA2; MIM 300600). However, it is not clear whether these additional features represent distinct disease entities or pleiotropic effects of some of the above-mentioned genes.

The disease gene map of the Xp21 region is shown in Fig. 65-7. Molecular studies of patients with Xp21 CGS have been instrumental in the construction of this map by correlating the positions of patients' deletion and translocation breakpoints with their phenotypes. Precise localization of disease genes with respect to deletion breakpoints, and to the position of anonymous DNA markers in the region, has been established (see review[105]). As for the Xp22.3 CGS, study of the Xp21 CGS has been of critical importance for the positional cloning of disease genes in the region. The genes for four disorders have been isolated from Xp21: chronic granulomatous disease,[106] Duchenne muscular dystrophy,[107] glycerol kinase deficiency,[108–110] and adrenal hypoplasia congenita.[111]

Duplications of the distal part of Xp21 in XY individuals can cause sex reversal and abnormal gonadal development.[59–61] Camerino and colleagues characterized the duplicated region and assigned the gene responsible for this phenotype, termed DSS (dosage-sensitive sex reversal), to the adrenal hypoplasia congenita critical region.[62] It is now known to be due to increased dosage of *DAX1*.[112]

Xq21

A few patients carrying Xq21 deletions have been described. Some of these patients had a complex phenotype that could be dissected into these disease entities: choroideremia (CHM; MIM 303100, Chap. 236); mental retardation (XLMR); X-linked mixed deafness (DFN3; MIM 304400); cleft lip and palate (CLP; MIM 303400); and hypergonadotropic hypogonadism (HG; MIM 304350).[113–127]

Choroideremia is a common form of X-linked blindness characterized by progressive dystrophy of the choroid and retina (see Chap. 236). Some of the diseases observed in patients with Xq21 CGS have also been observed as separate genetic entities and have been assigned to the same chromosomal region by linkage studies.[128–131] Patients with submicroscopic deletions showing either isolated choroideremia, or isolated deafness, have been described.[132,133] X/autosomal translocations with breakpoints in Xq21 have been detected in female patients showing features of either choroideremia or mental retardation.[134–137] Positional cloning efforts in Xq21 have led to the isolation of the *REP1* (RAB Escort Protein 1) gene for choroideremia.[138,139]

AUTOSOMAL CONTIGUOUS GENE SYNDROMES

The autosomal CGS discussed in this chapter are presented in order of chromosome number. For each, the chromosomal band that is deleted or duplicated follows the syndrome name. Details of deletion type (terminal or interstitial) are given in each subsection on cytogenetics. Some of these diseases are discussed in separate chapters in this book. Therefore, they will be presented in less detail here and the reader is referred to those chapters.

Monosomy 1p36 (del(1)(p36))

Clinical. The clinical features associated with deletion of the most distal band on the short arm of chromosome 1 were recently delineated.[140,141] Patients show a wide range of features including variable degrees of mental retardation, growth delay, seizures and/or abnormal EEGs, hypotonia, developmental delay, early puberty, orofacial clefting or palatal anomalies, enlarged anterior fontanel, dysmorphic features, deafness, and cardiomyopathy.[140,141] Monosomy 1p36 is one of the most common microdeletion syndromes, with the incidence of the deletion estimated to be about 1 in 10,000 births.[140]

Cytogenetics. The deletion seen in monosomy 1p36 is a terminal deletion of the most distal band on the short arm of chromosome 1. The majority of cases of monosomy 1p36 have been identified through cytogenetic analysis. By molecular analysis and FISH, most deletions are only partial, telomeric deletions of band 1p36 and a few (~15 percent) are interstitial deletions, retaining the original telomere, at the molecular level.[142] For the most part, the size of the deletion and the type of deletion (interstitial or terminal) cannot be distinguished at the light microscope. At the resolution of routine cytogenetic analysis (400 to 550 bands), this deletion is difficult to visualize, accounting for the fact that roughly 50 percent of patients had a "normal" chromosome evaluation prior to the detection of the deletion.[140] Three cases of monosomy 1p36 were identified by using telomeric markers to screen 127 patients with unexplained mental retardation;[143–145] thus, exemplifying the common occurrence of this deletion and the inherent difficulties in visualizing this region by G-banding. Currently, there are 39 reports of "pure" 1p36 deletions and at least 10 other cases of 1p36 deletions due to derivative chromosomes that contain additional segmental aneusomy from other chromosomes.[141] The majority of cases are sporadic. The frequency of parental translocations is about 3 percent.[26] This occurrence is smaller than the frequency of familial translocations in other terminal deletions including cri du chat and Miller-Dieker syndromes, in which about 10 percent of cases are due to the malsegregation of a parental translocation.[22,27]

Molecular Genetics. The deletion sizes have been characterized for 30 patients with monosomy 1p36 using polymorphic microsatellite markers and FISH probes.[26] The deletion sizes were found to be quite variable, with the smallest deletions estimated to be less than 5 Mb and the largest deletions encompassing a genetic distance of up to 32 cM.[26] The occurrence and severity of the clinical findings correlate with the size of the deletions. Patients with the smallest, most telomeric deletions show mild mental retardation, while those with larger deletions show severe mental retardation, seizures, and deafness. The patients with the largest deletions may also have orofacial clefting.[26] The development of this panel of deletion patients and molecular refinement of the deletions will allow for a focused search for genes causing distinct features of the syndrome in specific regions of 1p36. The majority of sporadic deletions (78 percent) occur on the maternally inherited chromosome 1.[26] There are no obvious clinical differences between maternally and paternally derived deletions. This maternal bias may reflect the underlying mechanism of deletion in this region that may be more prone to occur during oogenesis.

Diagnostics. The majority of patients are identified through good quality cytogenetic studies and FISH using very distal 1p probes. Most patients are deleted for loci p1-79 (*D1Z2*), *D1S243*, and *CDC2L1* (*p58*) (MIM 176873). Three patients were identified using telomere screening strategies,[143–145] but about 15 percent of patients have interstitial deletions that are missed using these probes.[142] Parental chromosomes should be investigated to exclude a familial rearrangement that would carry a significant risk for future pregnancies.

Russell-Silver Syndrome (dup(7)(p12p13))

Clinical. The association of prenatal and postnatal growth retardation with relative sparing of the head, triangular facies and other dysmorphic features, and limb and facial asymmetry was first described by Silver[146] and Russell[147] independently. Most cases of Russell-Silver syndrome (RSS; MIM 180860) are sporadic, but a significant number have been reported to be transmitted in an autosomal dominant fashion (see review[148]).

Cytogenetics. A number of chromosomal abnormalities have been associated with the RSS phenotype including deletion of distal 15q,[149] deletion of proximal 8q,[150] and balanced translocations involving 17q.[151,152] No other consistent cytogenetic abnormality was found until recently; two cases of RSS have been described with duplications in the proximal short arm of chromosome 7.[153,154] Although the duplicated regions were slightly different, the common region was from 7p12.1 to 7p13.

Molecular Genetics. In 1988, Spence et al.[155] described a child who had inherited two copies of chromosome 7 from her mother and failed to inherit a chromosome 7 from her father (maternal uniparental disomy 7). In addition to having cystic fibrosis, due to the inheritance of two copies of a mutant CF gene from her mother, she had postnatal growth retardation. Since that time, several reports of maternal UPD 7 with short stature have been published (see reviews[156–158]). Specifically, RSS patients have been investigated for UPD and studies have found that about 10 percent of patients have maternal disomy 7.[159–162] The critical region for an imprinted locus has been narrowed to the short arm of chromosome 7, based on two cases of partial UPD 7 involving just 7p.[163,164] Further refinement, based on the two duplication 7p cases has resulted in a candidate locus.[153,154] The growth factor receptor-binding protein 10 (*GRB10*; MIM 601523) binds both insulin and insulin-like growth-factor receptors. Thus, *GRB10* has a growth suppressing function that would be consistent with the phenotype of growth retardation in RSS patients. *GRB10* has been shown to be imprinted in humans[164a] and mutations have been identified in two RSS patients.[164b] Additionally, the mouse orthologue, *Grb10/Meg1*, shows imprinting.[165] Maternal UPD of this region in mouse produces prenatal growth failure, whereas, paternal UPD of this region produces overgrowth,[166] making this a good candidate for RSS.

Diagnostics. Patients with RSS should be investigated with routine cytogenetic banding methods to exclude a duplication of the short arm of chromosome 7 or other chromosomal abnormalities. Additionally, patients could be investigated for submicroscopic duplications using interphase FISH analysis.[153] For those patients showing a normal karyotype, UPD should be investigated with polymorphic markers for the short arm of chromosome 7. This approach would detect segmental UPD, restricted to 7p, as well as holochromosomic UPD 7. In the future, a methylation-specific assay will likely be developed to detect patients with UPD or imprinting mutations.

Williams Syndrome (del(7)(q11.23q11.23))

Clinical. The clinical features that are now associated with Williams-Beuren syndrome (WBS; MIM 194050) were first independently described by Williams in 1961[167] and Beuren in 1962.[168] Patients have a distinct facial dysmorphism that includes periorbital fullness, stellate pattern of the irides,[169] anteverted nares, long philtrum, and prominent, full lips. Other significant clinical features include infantile hypercalcemia (MIM 143880), mental retardation, gregarious personality, growth deficiency, and considerable cardiac involvement. Cardiovascular anomalies include supravalvular aortic stenosis, peripheral pulmonary artery stenosis, and pulmonic valvular stenosis. Isolated supravalvular aortic stenosis (SVAS; MIM 185500), a congenital narrowing of the ascending aorta, is an autosomal dominant condition that showed linkage to chromosome 7.[170] A family segregating isolated SVAS was shown to have a translocation involving chromosome 7 that disrupted the elastin gene.[171] Additional mutations of the elastin gene in patients with SVAS provided strong evidence for a critical role for elastin in vascular development.[75,76] Given the occurrence of SVAS in WBS, this region was investigated in patients with the disorder. Most cases of WBS are sporadic, although a few families have demonstrated autosomal dominant inheritance.[172] WBS occurs in about 1 in 20,000 to 1 in 50,000 live births.[173]

Cytogenetics. Chromosomal abnormalities in WBS were investigated, with no consistent deletion or rearrangement detected.[174] Given the linkage of SVAS to the long arm of chromosome 7 and the familial t(6;7) associated with SVAS, the elastin gene on chromosome 7 was investigated in patients with WBS and was found to be deleted.[46] Subsequently, deletions of the elastin locus have been found using FISH in greater than 90 percent of WBS patients.[175] Deletions are not reliably detected by routine cytogenetics, but have been localized to 7q11.23 by high-resolution analysis.[176] The deletions are interstitial and occur in a G-negative band, adjacent to the centromere on the long arm of chromosome 7.

Molecular Genetics. Most deletions in patients with WBS are of a consistent size of approximately 2 Mb.[177] The region is flanked by low-copy, region-specific repeats[178] that likely contribute to the deletion process through homologous recombination and unequal crossing over (see "Molecular Mechanisms Leading to Contiguous Gene Syndromes" below).[179,180] The deletion region contains at least 15 known genes.[176] The only gene that has been definitively shown to cause clinical features in WBS is the elastin locus. Functional monosomy for elastin results in the SVAS and is presumed to be responsible for other features in WBS including renal artery stenosis, hypertension, hoarse voice, small genitalia, premature aging of the skin, and perhaps some of the facial characteristics. However, individuals with isolated SVAS due to mutations or small deletions in the elastin gene do not have the facial features, hypercalcemia, or mental retardation. Based on these observations, WBS is considered a true CGS, with other genes likely contributing to the overall phenotype.[175] Although most patients have consistent-sized deletions, a few patients have been described with larger deletions.[181] These patients have more severe mental retardation and many have seizures.[181]

Diagnostics. The deletion in 7q11.23 cannot be reliably detected using routine chromosome analysis. FISH is the only reliable means for detecting the deletions. Greater than 90 percent of patients demonstrate a deletion by FISH using a probe containing the elastin locus.[175]

Langer-Giedion Syndrome (del(8)(q24.1q24.1))

Clinical. The association of sparse hair, a characteristic facial appearance including a pear-shaped nose with bulbous tip and tented alae nasi, and cone-shaped epiphyses was first described by Giedion in 1966,[182] and termed the trichorhinophalangeal syndrome type I (TRPS I; MIM 190350). Affected individuals are usually intellectually normal. In 1969, several groups independently reported patients with features of TRPS I, who, in addition, exhibited multiple cartilaginous exostoses and mental retardation, a combination that has come to be known as the trichorhinophalangeal syndrome type II (TRPS II) or Langer-Giedion syndrome (LGS) (MIM 150230).[183] Other clinical features of LGS may include microcephaly, large, protruding ears, elongated upper lip, micrognathia, lax skin, and short stature.[183,184] Although mental retardation was originally considered a constant feature, intelligence is extremely variable. Approximately 29 percent of patients show normal or borderline intelligence, 17 percent have mild mental retardation, 40 percent are moderately retarded, and 14 percent are profoundly retarded.[184]

TRPS I is inherited as an autosomal dominant disorder. Families with multiple cartilaginous exostoses (ME; MIM 13370) identical with that seen in LGS have been observed with autosomal dominant transmission. LGS is generally a sporadic condition with the notable exception of a set of twins and one case of an affected father and daughter.[184]

Cytogenetics. In 1980, Buhler et al.[185] and Pfeiffer[186] reported cases of LGS with *de novo* interstitial deletions in the long arm of chromosome 8. Subsequently, this was confirmed and the specific location of the deletion determined to be band 8q24.1.[184,187] Approximately 75 percent of LGS patients have cytogenetically detectable deletions in this region by conventional banding or high-resolution chromosome analysis.[44]

These observations led to the hypothesis that LGS was a CGS caused by the deletion of several genes in 8q24.1, including the *TRPS1* gene, the multiple exostoses gene, and a locus or loci causing mental retardation.[1] The finding of a small number of LGS patients with normal intelligence and visible or submicroscopic deletions suggests that the mental retardation locus is not located between the TRPS I and multiple exostoses loci.[44] Mapping of TRPS I to 8q24.1 was initially confirmed by the identification of two patients with visible deletions who had TRPS I but without exostoses or mental retardation.[188,189] A locus for multiple exostoses in 8q24.1 was initially supported by the observation of a patient with a balanced translocation and breakpoint in 8q24.1.[190]

Molecular Genetics. Linkage analysis of families with the autosomal dominant condition hereditary multiple exostoses has demonstrated genetic heterogeneity, with an estimated 70 percent of families showing linkage to 8q24.1.[191] Molecular studies to define the smallest region of overlap among LGS deletions has been reported by two groups,[44,192] and is estimated at less than 2 Mb. In addition to 12 visible deletions, submicroscopic deletions were detected by quantitative Southern blot analysis in two patients with apparently balanced translocations and two patients with apparently normal karyotypes.

The gene for the multiple exostosis I locus has been cloned (EXT1; MIM 133700).[193] Patients with isolated multiple exostoses have shown loss of function mutations in *EXT1*.[194] These patients do not display other features of LGS, lending support to the hypothesis that functional monosomy (haploinsufficiency) causes the multiple exostosis phenotype in LGS and that LGS is a CGS with other genes causing the features associated with TRPS I and the mental retardation. Recently, the gene for the isolated TRPS I phenotype was cloned.[195] The gene contains a putative GATA-binding zinc finger and two potential nuclear localization signals. Some patients were found to have submicroscopic deletions containing this gene, while about 70 percent of patients with the TRPS I phenotype had mutations within the gene. In addition to the identification of the *EXT1* locus in the LGS critical region, the fact that *TRPS1* is deleted in some patients with TRPS I and all patients with LGS; that *TRPS1* is disrupted in two patients with balanced chromosomal abnormalities and TRPS I; and that *TRPS1* contains inactivating mutations in patients with TRPS I, makes LGS a true CGS.

Diagnostics. Many patients with LGS show visible deletions at 8q24.1 using routine cytogenetics. FISH using probes containing the *TRPS1* gene aid in the detection of submicroscopic deletions in TRPS I patients who do not have multiple exostoses,[195] while FISH probes containing the *EXT1* locus are helpful in identifying patients with the full LGS clinical spectrum.[196]

Potocki-Shaffer Syndrome (del(11)(p11.2p12))

Clinical. In 1993, Shaffer et al., reported a family that was segregating an insertional translocation between chromosomes 11 and 13 that resulted in deletion of 11p11.2 in some family members. These individuals had skull defects (wormian bones and biparietal foramina), brachycephaly, developmental delay, mental retardation, and genital anomalies.[197] One family member had multiple exostoses but his sister, who also had the deletion, did not have this trait, so it was concluded that the multiple exostoses were an incidental finding in the brother. Subsequently, additional patients were described with del(11)(p11.2p12) and were all found to have multiple exostoses.[198,199] Radiographic reexamination of the sister from the original family revealed multiple exostoses.[198] The full spectrum of the Potocki-Shaffer syndrome (PSS; MIM 601224) has been delineated to include mental retardation, biparietal foramina, minor facial dysmorphism, multiple cartilaginous exostoses and micropenis in males.[198] In 1990, Lorenz et al. reported a patient with an unusual presentation of acrocephalosyndactyly.[200] Shaffer et al. proposed that although this patient had a normal karyotype, many of the same features were found in the family reported with del(11)(p11.2p12). Upon reexamination of the karyotype, the case reported by Lorenz et al. was found to have a deletion of 11p11.2.[199]

Cytogenetics. The interstitial deletion associated with PSS can be visualized by routine cytogenetic analysis. However, given that the deleted band is the first G-negative band adjacent to the centromere, the deletion may be overlooked.[197–199] In fact, the majority of patients reported to date had at least one "normal" karyotype before the deletion was identified.[197–199] One submicroscopic deletion, detectable by polymorphic microsatellite analysis, has been reported.[199] FISH analysis using a probe containing the multiple exostosis 2 gene (*EXT2*) has been used to confirm a known 11p11.2 deletion.[201]

Molecular Genetics. The extent of the deletion has been delineated and appears relatively large (~20 cM distance).[198,199] Both maternally and paternally derived deletions have been observed.[198,199] The deletion is presumed to include at least three loci contributing to this syndrome; one for multiple exostoses, one for biparietal foramina, and one for mental retardation. This assumption was based on families who segregate autosomal dominant isolated multiple exostoses that are linked to chromosome 11,[202] one family with a smaller deletion in 11p11.2 with multiple exostoses and biparietal foramina but no mental retardation,[199] and large families segregating parietal foramina as an isolated autosomal dominant condition (PFM1; MIM 168500). The multiple exostosis 2 locus was cloned (EXT2; MIM 133701)[203,204] and mutations in isolated multiple exostoses patients have been identified.[204]

Diagnostics. Most patients with PSS will have visible deletions using routine cytogenetic methods. However, given the proximity of this G-negative band to the centromere of chromosome 11 and the fact that the deletion in most patients with PSS was missed initially, FISH using a probe containing the *EXT2* gene should be used in patients with mental retardation and multiple exostoses who do not fit the criteria for Langer-Giedion syndrome.[201]

WAGR Syndrome (del(11)(p12p14))

Clinical. The term WAGR syndrome defines the association of Wilms tumor, aniridia, genitourinary dysplasia, and mental retardation.[205,206] The clinical features, and the genetics of Wilms tumor, or nephroblastoma (MIM 194070), are described in Chap. 38. Aniridia type 2 (AN2; MIM 106210) is a bilateral developmental disorder of the eye, characterized by the complete or partial aplasia or dysplasia of the iris and optic nerve hypoplasia, leading to vision impairment. In some patients, the phenotype can be progressive, owing to cataract, corneal opacification, lens dislocation, and glaucoma.[207] There is genetic evidence that aniridia is the human equivalent of the murine small eye mutation.[208]

Genitourinary abnormalities observed in patients with WAGR syndrome include ambiguous genitalia (pseudohermaphroditism), undescended testes, hypospadias, fused kidneys, urinary tract anomalies, and gonadoblastoma.[11,209–212] The association of these features with a complex nephropathy and with Wilms tumor is also known as the Denys-Drash syndrome.[213] This raises the possibility that the latter clinical entity may be part of the WAGR syndrome.[214] Additional features observed in patients with WAGR syndrome include variable mental retardation, growth retardation, and hemihypertrophy.[11,215,216]

Cytogenetics. The identification of interstitial deletions involving the 11p13 region in patients with WAGR syndrome suggested a common genetic etiology for its various components.[11,217] It was postulated that the complex phenotype observed in patients with WAGR syndrome was the manifestation of a CGS due to a deletion of adjacent genes on 11p13.[11,217] Since then, many patients carrying various types of rearrangements of 11p13, and showing features of the WAGR syndrome, have been identified, lending support to this hypothesis.[216–221]

Molecular Genetics. Molecular characterization of patients carrying 11p13 abnormalities has permitted the assignment of loci involved in specific phenotypic manifestations of the WAGR syndrome.[222–228] Distinction between the Wilms tumor and aniridia loci was possible through the study of patients with familial 11p13 translocations showing isolated aniridia without Wilms tumor.[223,229,230] Furthermore, independent evidence for the presence of an aniridia gene on 11p13 came from linkage studies in families with isolated autosomal dominant aniridia.[228,231]

Several detailed physical maps of 11p13, spanning regions containing deletion and translocation breakpoints from patients with WAGR syndrome, have been constructed.[208,232,233] Overlap cloning of the 11p13 region led to the isolation of the Wilms tumor gene (*WT1*), which encodes a zinc finger-containing transcription factor.[234,235] In Wilms tumor, constitutional heterozygous deletions or mutations involving the Wilms tumor gene are followed by loss of heterozygosity through a somatic-cell event. The genetic mechanism involved in the pathogenesis of Wilms tumor is, therefore, a good example of Knudson's two-hit hypothesis.[236]

There is convincing evidence that the Wilms tumor gene is also involved in the genitourinary abnormalities seen in patients with WAGR syndrome. Point mutations in the Wilms tumor gene were found in patients with Denys-Drash syndrome. These mutations must have a dominant-negative effect based on the evidence that they are present only in one allele of the Wilms tumor gene and that the genitourinary abnormalities found in Denys-Drash patients are far more severe than those observed in WAGR deletions. The molecular mechanisms underlying the dominant-negative nature of these mutations have not yet been identified.[237]

Following the identification of the Wilms tumor gene, "chromosome walking" and "jumping" in 11p13 led to the positional cloning of another disease gene from this region, the aniridia gene.[238] The *PAX6* gene was found to be disrupted in aniridia-associated chromosomal aberrations and to be expressed in all tissues affected in aniridia patients.[238] The identification of point mutations in *PAX6* in patients with sporadic aniridia[239] and of mutations in the murine *Pax6* orthologue in mice with the small-eye phenotype[240] provided definitive evidence for the involvement of this gene in aniridia. However, the possibility still exists that more than one aniridia locus might be present in 11p13.[239] Unlike humans, mice with deletions spanning both the mouse orthologues of the human Wilms tumor and the *PAX6* genes, do not have nephroblastoma.[208]

Diagnostics. Most deletions resulting in WAGR are large, encompassing 11p13 that can be seen using routine banding methods. For those patients showing partial phenotypes, FISH using probes containing *WT1* or *PAX6* may help identify submicroscopic deletions.[241]

Beckwith-Wiedemann Syndrome (dup(11)(p15.5p15.5))

Clinical. Beckwith-Wiedemann syndrome (BWS; MIM 130650) consists of multiple growth abnormalities, including macroglossia, omphalocele, visceromegaly, and gigantism. Importantly, there is an increased predisposition (5 to 20 percent) to several childhood malignancies including Wilms tumor, adrenocortical carcinoma, hepatoblastoma, and rhabdomyosarcoma.[4] Additional discussions of clinical features and the genetics of BWS are found in Chaps. 15, 18, and 38.

Eighty-five percent of BWS cases are sporadic, but a number of familial cases have been reported with or without associated chromosomal aberrations. It is now generally accepted that BWS can be transmitted as a Mendelian trait, influenced by imprinting and that the molecular bases of the disorder is heterogeneous with variable expression (see Chap. 18).

Cytogenetics. Although most BWS patients are cytogenetically normal,[205] a number of cases have been observed with abnormalities involving the most distal band on 11p. At least 15 cases have been reported with unbalanced translocations or other abnormalities that produce partial trisomy for 11p15.5.[53] In all cases in which it has been determined, the origin of the duplicated segment is paternal. In contrast, six cases have been reported with apparently balanced translocations or inversions involving 11p15, and in all cases the abnormality was inherited from the mother.[53]

Molecular Genetics. In familial cases, linkage analysis has confirmed the localization of familial BWS to 11p15.5.[242,243] The most significant finding in sporadic BWS has been the identification of partial paternal uniparental disomy for the distal short arm of chromosome 11 in 20 percent of patients.[244–246] Different from the holochromosomic UPD for chromosome 15 observed in PWS and AS, the UPD in BWS is usually confined to the 11p15 region. All cases analyzed showed isodisomy (homozygosity) for markers in 11p15, but normal biparental inheritance elsewhere on chromosome 11. This indicates that the UPD is a somatic event rather than a meiotic nondisjunction event, resulting in the segmental isodisomy. Evidence for somatic mosaicism for UPD has been observed at the single-cell level,[247] confirming that the UPD arises after fertilization. The molecular genetics of BWS are quite complex, involving genomic imprinting and perhaps several genes. A detailed discussion is presented in Chap. 18.

Diagnostics. Currently the diagnosis of BWS is based on clinical findings. About 20 percent of cases have partial, paternal isodisomy of distal 11p, but the molecular analysis is complicated by the presence of mosaicism. A small percentage of patients demonstrate biallelic expression of *IGF2*, which is normally expressed from only the paternally inherited chromosome 11,[248] and a small number of patients have mutations in the $p57^{KIP2}$ gene.[249] For the majority of the remaining patients, loss of imprinting (LOI) for the gene *LIT1* (long QT intronic transcript 1) appears to be the most common molecular basis causing BWS[250].

Prader-Willi Syndrome (del(15)(q11.2q13))

Clinical. Prader-Willi syndrome (PWS; MIM 176270) was first described in 1956[251] and is a relatively common cause of genetic obesity and mental retardation, with a frequency of approximately 1 in 10,000 to 20,000 births. Severe hypotonia and poor suck during the neonatal period usually requiring gavage feeding characterize this syndrome. Males usually have undescended testes and females may have hypoplastic labia. By 2 to 3 years of age, patients develop hyperphagia leading to obesity unless caloric intake is strictly regulated. A characteristic facial appearance is present including a narrow bitemporal diameter, almond-shaped eyes, upslanting palpebral fissures, and strabismus. Other physical features include short stature, small hands and feet, and fair hair and skin color (hypopigmentation) relative to other family members. The hypopigmentation is a clinical finding suggesting a deletion instead of UPD as the underlying mechanism, because this likely reflects haploinsufficiency of the *P* locus. All individuals with PWS have some degree of cognitive dysfunction, with a wide range of formal IQ scores. Significant behavioral abnormalities are present, including stubbornness, temper tantrums, and poor peer interactions. Excellent reviews of the clinical features and diagnostic criteria for PWS are available.[252–254]

Autosomal recessive and autosomal dominant modes of inheritance had been ascribed to PWS before the finding of a chromosome deletion in most patients.[255] In the great majority of cases, the condition is sporadic. Familial cases of PWS are infrequent, but at least seven cases have been identified with small deletions causing imprinting mutations.[256,257] At least one familial case due to a balanced chromosomal rearrangement is known.[258] Based on the very rare occurrence of familial PWS with normal karyotype, Cassidy[259] estimated the recurrence risk for PWS as less than 1 in 1000 and may reflect gonadal mosaicism for trisomy 15.

Cytogenetics. Hawkey and Smithies[12] first suggested a relationship between chromosome 15 and PWS in 1976. This was based on their patient with a 15;15 Robertsonian translocation and a review of the literature showing several similar abnormalities. Subsequent high-resolution cytogenetic investigation revealed a small, interstitial deletion of proximal 15q in more than half of all PWS patients.[260,261] Using cytogenetic polymorphisms, Butler and coworkers made the interesting observation that the *de novo* interstitial deletions in PWS were paternal in origin.[262,263] It is now recognized that about 70 percent of PWS patients have interstitial deletions in 15q12. The deletion size is about 4 Mb.[264] Given the proximity of this band to the centromere and the variable block of long arm heterochromatin, cytogenetic analysis by G-banding is not always reliable.[265] FISH analysis using a probe contained within the deletion region provides the most reliable means for detecting deletions in the cytogenetics laboratory. Patients with balanced Robertsonian translocations are now recognized to likely have UPD,[156,266] rather than submicroscopic deletions and should be further investigated by DNA polymorphisms or methylation analysis (see "Diagnostics" below).

Molecular Genetics. Several molecular mechanisms can result in PWS: microdeletions of paternal origin in 70 percent of cases; maternal, holochromosomic UPD in about 28 percent of cases; and imprinting mutations in a few (~2 percent) cases. Most patients have consistent-sized deletions of ~4 Mb. The deletion is flanked by ~ 400 kb genomic regions with high sequence identity, which may promote homologous recombination events leading to deletion.[266a,419] Study of PWS patients with atypical deletions or unusual translocations have allowed refinement of the critical region. The PWS region is probably less than 1 Mb and is bounded by D15S13 on the centromeric side,[267] and D15S10 on the telomeric side.[268] This region has been separated from the AS critical region, also mapping to 15q12, by a familial case of AS in which a submicroscopic deletion involving the region from D15S10 to GABRB3 (β_3-subunit of the *GABA* receptor).[269] When the deletion was inherited from a female, children were affected with AS. When the deletion was inherited from a male, there was no phenotypic abnormality. This important case provided strong evidence that PWS and AS were caused by separate loci with AS distal to PWS. The gene causing AS is now known (see "Angelman Syndrome" below).

Patients are considered to have imprinting mutations if they have biparental inheritance of the PWS region, but a maternal methylation pattern on both chromosomes. Methylation is most reliable if analyzed at the CpG island of the 5′ end of *SNRPN*.[270] About half of the patients with imprinting mutations have small deletions very near the major promoter for *SNRPN*.[256,271] These small deletions are consistently of familial origin while patients with imprinting mutations without identifiable deletions are consistently sporadic.[272]

Within the PWS critical region, a number of paternally expressed genes have been identified: *SNRPN* (large and small open reading frame), *IPW* (no open reading frame), *ZNF127*, *NDN* (necdin), and one or two necdin-like genes referred to as *NDNL1* or *MAGEL2*.[256,273,274] In addition, there is evidence for at least 13 paternally expressed transcripts in the PWS region.[275] Any of these transcripts may be causally involved in producing the PWS phenotype. The gene for small nuclear ribonucleoprotein-associated peptide N (*SNRPN*) has been debated to be the PWS gene. As reviewed in Mann and Bartolomei,[273] mice with UPD have been generated that show early postnatal lethality that may be analogous to the hypotonia and poor feeding seen in PWS. Mouse models have also been generated that deleted *Snrpn* and the region containing the imprinting center and these also result in postnatal lethality. Mice that have just an intragenic deletion of *Snrpn* have no lethality or obvious phenotypic features indicating that, at least in mice, mutation involving more than just *Snrpn* is necessary to produce the PWS phenotype. There are conflicting reports as to whether inactivating mutations in mouse necdin cause lethality.[276,277]

Deletion of the *P* gene is likely responsible for the hypopigmentation present in the majority of PWS deletion patients.[278,279] Because paternal and maternal deletions of the *P* gene produce similar phenotypic consequences, this represents a gene dosage effect without imprinting. The *P* locus has also been implicated in type II oculocutaneous albinism (OCA2; MIM 203200) by linkage to this region of chromosome 15,[280] and by identification of recessive mutations.[279] One case of PWS who also had OCA2 was found to have a paternal deletion on one chromosome 15 and a mutation in the *P* locus on the maternal homologue.[47]

Although deletions of chromosome 15 account for the majority of PWS cases, about 30 percent of PWS do not show deletions by cytogenetic or molecular methods. Uniparental disomy (UPD) is now known to account for the majority of nondeletion PWS. UPD, the inheritance of both chromosome homologues from a single parent, was first proposed by Engel in 1980,[281] and first observed in humans by Spence and coworkers in 1988,[155] in a patient with cystic fibrosis and growth retardation who inherited both chromosome 7 homologues from her mother. Since then, UPD has been found for a number of human chromosomes and may be a significant cause of mental retardation and other developmental abnormalities.[282]

Several groups have shown that maternal UPD for chromosome 15 is a common cause of PWS, accounting for approximately 28 percent of cases.[267,283] Maternal UPD leads to paternal deficiency of chromosome 15 and absence of expression of any genes expressed exclusively from the paternal homologue. Interestingly, maternal UPD cases are associated with advanced maternal age, whereas deletion cases of PWS are not.[267,283] Most UPD cases demonstrate maternal heterodisomy (the inheritance of two different maternal homologues) (Fig. 65-8), suggesting a meiosis I nondisjunction event.[267,283,284] Cases of trisomy 15 mosaicism have been observed in chorionic villus cells during prenatal diagnosis for advanced maternal age, but only normal karyotypes were observed at follow-up amniocentesis studies.[285–287] At birth, clinical features of PWS led to molecular investigations and the discovery of maternal UPD. These data suggest a model for the origin of UPD in PWS as shown in Fig. 65-8. Advanced maternal age produces an increased risk for maternal nondisjunction and trisomy 15 conception. Because trisomy 15 is lethal, loss of one chromosome 15 postzygotically would "rescue" this lethal condition. However, if the paternal chromosome 15 is lost (presumed to occur in one-third of cases), maternal UPD 15 results in PWS. Additional discussion on PWS can be found in Chap. 15.

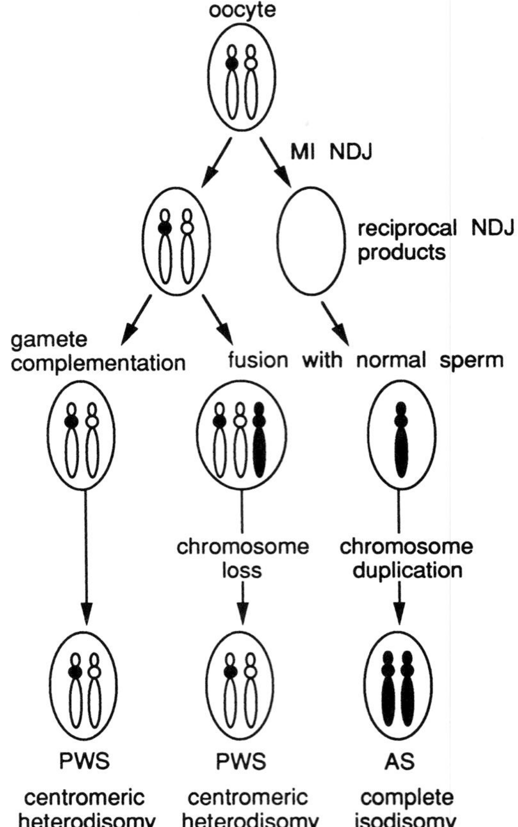

Fig. 65-8 Model for the mechanism of uniparental disomy (UPD) in Prader-Willi and Angelman syndromes. Maternal chromosome 15 homologues are shown in white, with 2 different centromeres white or black, and paternal 15 homologues black. A maternal meiosis I nondisjunction event produces disomic and nullisomic eggs. Fertilization of the disomic egg by a nullisomic sperm (gamete complementation) produces maternal heterodisomy, as does fertilization by a normal sperm with subsequent loss of the paternal homologue. Fertilization of the nullisomic egg by a normal sperm produces monosomy 15, a lethal condition. Subsequent duplication of the single paternal homologue would "rescue" this lethal event and produce AS with complete isodisomy (homozygosity for all markers). (*From Mutirangura et al.*[284] *Used by permission of Human Molecular Genetics.*)

Diagnostics. A joint American Society of Human Genetics/American College of Medical Genetics committee has made diagnostic testing recommendations.[288] The recommendations for patients suspected to have PWS are to perform chromosome analysis to exclude gross structural rearrangements of chromosome 15 or other chromosomal rearrangements and FISH to detect deletions of 15q12 (see Fig. 65-3A). Those patients who have had a prior normal cytogenetic study should be studied by an assay that detects methylation differences within loci of the PWS region. This analysis can detect abnormalities within the region, but cannot distinguish between deletions, UPD, or imprinting mutations. Those patients who show an abnormal methylation pattern should have FISH to confirm a deletion or DNA analysis with polymorphic markers to identify UPD. Abnormal methylation with two methylated copies of the CpG island at *SNRPN* with evidence for biparental inheritance of chromosome 15 defines an imprinting mutation. Analysis can be performed by Southern blotting[270] or with PCR after bisulfite treatment of the DNA.[289,290] Neither the FISH nor the methylation analysis requires parental blood samples to be analyzed. However, analysis of polymorphisms within the PWS region requires a comparison of parental alleles to the child's alleles. The clinical observation of trisomy rescue suggests that it would be prudent to test for UPD in all instances of normal karyotype at amniocentesis following the identification of trisomy 15 in CVS.

Angelman Syndrome (del(15)(q11.2q13))

Clinical. Angelman syndrome (AS; MIM 234400) is associated with severe mental retardation, seizures, and absence of speech development. These patients also have an ataxic gait, inappropriate bouts of laughter, and characteristic facies including a wide mouth, protruding tongue, prominent jaw, and thin upper lip.[291–294] AS patients may also show hypopigmentation, apparently due to deletion and haploinsufficiency of the *P* locus. This feature is the only apparent clinical overlap with PWS other than mental retardation.

AS is sporadic in the majority of cases; however, a number of familial cases have been reported. Because familial cases usually involve affected sibs with normal parents, AS was sometimes erroneously thought to be an autosomal recessive disease.[295] Subsequent to the finding of chromosome 15 abnormalities in the majority of AS cases, linkage analysis in several familial AS cases demonstrated linkage to chromosome 15, consistent with autosomal dominant transmission of an imprinted locus.[296–298] AS occurs in about 1 in 15,000 births.

Cytogenetics. Deletions of chromosome 15 were first described in AS patients in 1987[299] and have subsequently been shown to be present in the majority of patients.[300] Although it was proposed initially that the PWS and AS cytogenetic deletions were of somewhat different size and location in proximal 15q,[301] it has been demonstrated by molecular analysis that the breakpoints of the deletions are the same in the two disorders,[302,303] and the mechanism of deletion involving flanking repeats appears the same.[266a,419] The difference in phenotype is due solely to the differential parental origin of the deletion — exclusively paternal origin of deletions in PWS[262,263,267,304,305] and exclusively maternal origin of deletion in AS.[269,300,306,307] As in PWS, the deletion of 15q12 in AS can be difficult to visualize in some patients due to its proximity to the centromere and pericentromeric heterochromatin.[265] FISH, therefore, provides a more reliable means of detecting these deletions.

Molecular Genetics. Considerable progress has been made in delineating the molecular mechanisms that can result in AS. In AS, paternal disomy has been observed in 3 to 5 percent of cases, but not as frequently as maternal disomy in PWS.[284,308–310] This lack of a maternal homologue is consistent with absence of expression of a gene or genes expressed exclusively from the maternal homologue and has the same effect as maternal deletion of this region. Also different from PWS, paternal disomy in AS more often displays isodisomy (homozygosity) for the entire chromosome (Fig. 65-8).[284,308,309] This is perhaps best explained by a monosomy 15 conception, followed by a postzygotic event that duplicates the single paternal homologue (Fig. 65-8). Because in this case monosomy 15 arises as a result of a maternal nondisjunction event, this is the reciprocal product of the same event producing maternal UPD for chromosome 15. Paternal UPD arising by maternal nondisjunction would be predicted to be associated with advanced maternal age. Too few cases are available for statistical analysis, but in the small number of reported cases, the maternal age is elevated.[284]

Among the remaining patients who do not demonstrate deletions or UPD, 4 to 6 percent have mutations in the *UBE3A* gene, 3 percent have imprinting mutations by methylation analysis, and 10 to 14 percent have no identifiable molecular defect.[311] The *UBE3A* gene encodes the E6-AP ubiquitin-protein ligase. Point mutations, mostly resulting in truncated proteins,[77,78] when inherited on the maternal chromosome, result in functional nullisomy (the paternal copy is silenced in parts of the brain in a tissue-specific manner[312]) and AS.[313,314] More extensive mutation studies of patients without the ~4 Mb deletion, UPD, or imprinting mutation identified loss of function mutations in 75 to 80 percent of families with more than one affected case and in 14 to 23 percent of isolated cases.[315,316] Very large pedigrees with multiple affected individuals can occur with point mutations in *UBE3A*,[297,315] and with imprinting mutations caused by small deletions.[271] As for PWS, imprinting mutations occur usually on an inherited basis involving small deletions in the imprinting center or sporadically with no deletion identified.[272,317] The smallest region of overlap for imprinting center deletions causing AS is found ~5 kb centromeric to the deletions causing PWS and is narrowed to 880 bp.[318,319] The variability of the AS phenotype may be due to genes that modify the basic phenotype caused by maternal deficiency of *UBE3A*. Certainly, this is the case for the light pigmentation seen in AS deletion patients, due to haploinsufficiency of the P protein, but epilepsy may be more severe in deletion patients.[311] Thus, although maternal deficiency for *UBE3A* causes a relatively complete AS phenotype, deletion patients may still be considered as having a CGS.

Diagnostics. Diagnostic testing recommendations were made by a joint American Society of Human Genetics/American College of Medical Genetics committee prior to the identification of the AS gene.[288] The recommendations for patients suspected to have AS are similar to that for PWS. The first step is to perform chromosome analysis to exclude gross structural rearrangements of chromosome 15 or other chromosomes and FISH to detect deletions of 15q12. Those patients who have had a prior normal cytogenetic study should be studied by methylation analysis. Because this assay cannot distinguish between deletions, UPD, or imprinting mutations, those patients who show an abnormal methylation pattern should have FISH to confirm a deletion or DNA analysis with polymorphic markers to identify UPD. Those patients who do not carry a deletion or show an abnormal methylation pattern should be investigated for mutations in the *UBE3A* gene. Unfortunately, a variety of mutations have been identified such that individual mutations must be identified by sequencing *UBE3A*.[315,316]

Rubinstein-Taybi Syndrome (del(16)(p13.3))

Clinical. Rubinstein-Taybi syndrome (RTS; MIM 180849) is a well-defined, complex disorder comprised of facial abnormalities (microcephaly, broad nasal bridge, prominent or beaked nose, downward-slanting palpebral fissures, micrognathia, and ear abnormalities), broad thumbs and toes, and mental retardation. The prevalence at birth has been estimated to be 1 in 125,000.[320] Although autosomal dominant transmission has been occasionally observed, most cases are sporadic. Although Rubinstein-Taybi syndrome was postulated to be a chromosomal syndrome[321] and was listed by Schmickel[1] as an excellent candidate for a CGS, the identification of mutations in a single gene (see below) has redefined the etiology of this disorder.

Cytogenetics. Three unrelated cases of RTS have been identified involving balanced translocations between chromosome 16 and chromosomes 2, 7, or 20.[322] In each case, the breakpoint in chromosome 16 occurred in 16p13.3, suggesting that this was the site of the Rubinstein-Taybi syndrome gene(s). Following this clue, Breuning et al.[322] studied 24 patients with Rubinstein-Taybi syndrome by FISH analysis using cosmid probes in this region of chromosome 16. They identified submicroscopic deletions in 6 of 24 (25 percent) of patients, confirming that 16p13.3 is the location of Rubinstein-Taybi gene(s) and that microdeletions account for a significant percentage of cases. There were no apparent clinical differences between patients with deletions and those without.[323] Subsequent FISH studies have shown that a smaller proportion of patients (~10 percent) have deletions and the remaining patients are likely to have mutations in the *CBP* gene.[324,325]

Molecular Genetics. Using RTS translocation breakpoints and microdeletion patients, the RTS critical region was narrowed to 15 kb.[326] The microdeletions ranged in size from 130 kb to greater than 650 kb. The CREB binding protein (CREBBP or CBP; MIM 600140), a nuclear protein that is a coactivator in cyclic-AMP-regulated gene expression, was shown to be disrupted in RTS patients with translocations.[326] Sequence analysis of *CBP* in nondeletion, nontranslocation patients showed a variety of mutations.[326] Because the clinical findings among deletion RTS patients and patients with *CBP* mutations did not differ, RTS is now considered a condition caused by a single gene with pleiotropic effects. The mutations in *CBP* are all dominant loss-of-function mutations resulting in functional monosomy.

Diagnostics. A minority of RTS patients show gross structural cytogenetic anomalies. Approximately 10 percent of patients will have submicroscopic deletions by FISH.[324,325] Unfortunately, there is not one FISH probe that detects most deletions. Using a panel of 5 cosmid probes spanning the *CBP* gene, Blough et al.[324] found a variety of deletions in RTS patients including deletion of the 5′ end, but not the 3′ end of the gene; deletion extending through both the 5′ and 3′ ends of the gene; deletion of the 3′ end, but not the 5′ end; and an interstitial deletion in the 3′ end of the gene. The majority of patients are presumed to have mutations in the *CBP* gene that are best identified through DNA sequencing or a protein truncation assay.[326]

Smith-Magenis Syndrome (del(17)(p11.2p11.2))

Clinical. In 1986 two groups described a total of 15 patients with an interstitial deletion of 17p11.2 who had very similar phenotypes, including brachycephaly with a broad face and nasal bridge, flat midface, brachydactyly, and mental retardation associated with hyperactivity, and often self-destructive behavior.[327,328] This deletion syndrome has been termed the Smith-Magenis syndrome (SMS; MIM 182290) and is a relatively common recurring cytogenetic deletion. A series of 32 cases confirmed the clinical features described above, and added the common features of speech delay and hoarse, deep voice.[67] In addition, a high percentage of patients have ophthalmologic findings, otolaryngologic abnormalities (including hearing loss), visceral anomalies involving the heart and kidneys, and a significant sleep disturbance.[329] The frequency of Smith-Magenis syndrome has been estimated to be 1 in 25,000,[67] which would make this deletion syndrome more common than cri du chat syndrome (with a frequency of 1 in 50,000),[27] and about as common as Prader-Willi syndrome (at 1 in 10,000 to 20,000).

Cytogenetics. To date, all patients with Smith-Magenis syndrome have visible interstitial deletions of band 17p11.2 detectable by good quality routine cytogenetic analysis.[67] As seen in the Potocki-Shaffer syndrome, the deletion of this very proximal G-negative band on 17p may be overlooked in some cases. A FISH probe was developed containing the human homologue of the *Drosophila melanogaster* Flightless-1 gene (*FLI1*), which was found to map within the SMS critical region.[330] This probe has been deleted in 100 percent of patients tested (L.G. Shaffer and J.R. Lupski, unpublished data). FISH was helpful in reevaluation of two cases suspected to have mosaic deletion who were found to be nonmosaic by FISH, but were shown to have deletions smaller than the common deletion.[331,332]

Molecular Genetics. The deletions in SMS are of consistent size of about 5 Mb.[67–70] The deletion is flanked by low-copy repeat-gene clusters that are likely involved in unequal crossing over events that result in the deletion[58] (see "Molecular Mechanisms Leading to Contiguous Gene Syndromes" below). The reciprocal duplication product has been seen in patients with a milder phenotype that is unrelated to SMS.[43] SMS has been hypothesized to be a CGS[67] and although a number of genes have been directly identified in the deletion region, none have been implicated in the syndrome phenotype.[333]

Diagnostics. The interstitial deletion in 17p11.2 can be visualized using routine banding methods. Currently, FISH can be used to confirm a deletion or exclude a submicroscopic deletion (see Fig. 65-3J). A multiprobe cocktail containing a probe for the PWS/AS region on 15q12, the WBS region on 7q11.23, the DGS/VCFS region on 22q11.2, and the SMS region, identified a 17p11.2 deletion in a patient with developmental delay, referred for cytogenetic analysis.[334] Additionally, interphase FISH has been used to identify duplications of this same genomic region [dup(17)(p11.2p11.2)].[43]

Duplication 17p11.2 (dup(17)(p11.2p11.2))

Clinical. The clinical findings in seven patients with dup(17)(p11.2p11.2) are relatively mild.[43] The patients were ascertained for developmental delay and chromosome analysis revealed an apparently increased band size for the 17p11.2 region. Interphase FISH using the *FLT1* probe from the SMS critical region demonstrated duplications.[43] The phenotype of dup(17)(p11.2p11.2) consists of generally normal-appearing facies for most patients, short stature, mild to borderline mental retardation and behavioral difficulties. Dental abnormalities such as malocclusion and crowded teeth were found in six of seven patients. Notably, no major organ developmental abnormalities were observed, which is in sharp contrast to what is found in patients with SMS who are deleted for the same genomic region.

Cytogenetics. The duplication is difficult to see by routine G-banding and is likely underascertained. By G-banding, the duplication appears as a broader 17p11.2 band. Those patients that have been identified, have been confirmed using FISH on interphase nuclei.[43]

Molecular Genetics. Duplication of 17p11.2 represents the apparent reciprocal recombination of the common deletion found in del(17)(p11.2p11.2) patients with Smith-Magenis syndrome (see "Molecular Mechanisms Leading to Contiguous Gene Syndromes" below). By interphase, multicolor FISH analysis, all duplications were determined to be direct (tandem) in nature.[43]

Diagnostics. The diagnosis of dup(17)(p11.2p11.2) is made by the astute observation of a broader region of the light-staining 17p11.2 band. Confirmation should be made by interphase FISH diagnosis using probes that have been shown to be deleted in the Smith-Magenis syndrome deletion (see Fig. 65-3I and 65-3K).

Miller-Dieker Syndrome (del(17)(p13.3))

Clinical. Miller-Dieker syndrome (MDS) (MIM 247200) is a multiple malformation syndrome characterized by type I lissencephaly and a characteristic facial appearance.[335–337] Lissencephaly is a severe brain malformation whereby the typical convolutions (gyri and sulci) are absent and the brain surface is smooth.[337–339] The specific sequelae of lissencephaly include bitemporal hollowing, a small jaw, and neurologic abnormalities such as severe to profound mental retardation. In addition to the brain abnormalities, a characteristic facial appearance is present in MDS, which includes prominent forehead, bitemporal hollowing, a short nose with upturned nares, protuberant upper lip, thin vermilion border of the upper lip, and small jaw. Lissencephaly can also be observed as an isolated finding with relatively normal facial appearance, which is referred to as isolated lissencephaly sequence (ILS).[337,339,340] The brain malformation may be as severe as in MDS or less severe, with mixed agyria and pachygyria or pachygyria alone. Patients may have subtle facial changes such as bitemporal hollowing and small jaw, but other birth defects are rare. All have profound mental retardation; about half achieve no developmental skills, while the remainder are able to show some social responses, roll over, and make some semipurposeful movements of their hands.

MDS was initially considered an autosomal recessive disorder based on the occurrence of several families with multiple affected sibs.[335] Subsequently, it was shown that most of the known familial cases were due to a parental chromosomal rearrangement.[341] Although most cases of MDS and ILS are now known to be *de novo* deletions or mutations of a chromosome 17 gene, an X-linked form of lissencephaly is well documented and the gene has been identified.[342,343]

Cytogenetics. A chromosomal etiology for MDS was first recognized by the identification of a ring chromosome 17 in a patient with deletion of a small region at distal 17p and distal 17q.[14] Subsequent to this initial report, high-resolution chromosome analysis was performed on a series of MDS patients and identified visible deletions in approximately half.[45] Most abnormalities are *de novo* deletions, but several familial cases have been due to parental balanced translocations and inversions. High-resolution chromosome analysis in 58 ILS patients has been normal with the exception of one *de novo* balanced translocation between chromosome 2 and the X chromosome [46,XX,t(X;2)(q22;p25)] in a female with classic lissencephaly.[337,340,344] This translocation has subsequently been shown to disrupt the doublecortin (DCX; MIM 300121) gene on the X chromosome.[342,343]

Molecular Genetics. A variety of molecular techniques have been used to detect submicroscopic deletions in MDS and ILS patients.[345,346] FISH analysis for detection of submicroscopic deletions in this region has proved to be the most sensitive and efficient method for diagnosis and for mapping the boundaries of patient deletions.[22] With this method, visible or submicroscopic deletions are detected in over 90 percent of MDS patients and in 40 percent of patients with ILS.[22,337,344,347] Importantly, analysis of parents of children in whom a deletion is observed by FISH has revealed the presence of "cryptic" translocations or inversions that were not detectable by high-resolution chromosome analysis.[22] Because a parental rearrangement produces a substantial recurrence risk for unbalanced offspring, it is imperative that parental studies be performed by FISH following the identification of a deletion in a child.

Definition of the smallest region of overlap among a collection of patient deletions revealed a 350-kb "critical region" in MDS and ILS patients,[344] and a gene has been identified in the critical region.[348] Subsequently, it was determined that the 5′ end was chimeric and derived from more distal 17p. The correct 5′ end of the gene was then determined.[349] The *LIS1* gene encodes a subunit of the brain platelet-activating factor acetylhydrolase (*PAFAH*). All truncation mutations and lissencephaly causing point mutations or intragenic deletions result in a reduction in the amount of correctly folded *LIS1* protein.[350] *LIS1* is a microtubule-associated phosphoprotein.[351] Mutations found in ILS patients supports that *LIS1* is responsible for the brain malformation found in MDS and ILS, but that the additional clinical features found in MDS are likely caused by an additional gene(s).[347,349,352] These findings support that MDS is still likely to be a CGS. A knockout for the *LIS1* gene in the mouse has confirmed haploinsufficiency as the underlying molecular mechanism for lissencephaly because heterozygotes have the neuronal migration defects similar to the human brain anomaly.[353]

Diagnostics. Although some patients have visible deletions detectable by routine cytogenetic methods, FISH is the most reliable method for detecting the deletions in MDS and ILS. Probes containing the *LIS1* gene detect deletions in over 90 percent of MDS patients and 40 percent of ILS patients.[347] Parental FISH analyses should be conducted to detect parental translocations. Parents who carry translocations involving 17p13.3 are at substantial risk for having unbalanced offspring.[354] ILS patients not found to have deletions are likely to have point mutations in *LIS1* or *DCX*.[352,355]

Alagille Syndrome (del(20)(p11.23p11.23))

Clinical. Alagille syndrome (AGS; MIM 118450) was first described in 1969,[356] and is characterized by chronic cholestasis due to paucity of intrahepatic bile ducts, typical facial appearance (including broad forehead, deep-set eyes, mild hypertelorism, bulbous tip of the nose, and small pointed chin), peripheral pulmonic stenosis, vertebral anomalies ("butterfly" vertebrae), and posterior embryotoxon of the eye. Many cases are sporadic, but autosomal dominant inheritance with reduced penetrance and variable expressivity is suggested by family studies.[357,358] AGS occurs in about 1 in 70,000 births and is the second most common cause of infantile intrahepatic cholestasis.[359]

Cytogenetics. An interstitial deletion in proximal 20p was first reported in 1986 by Byrne et al.[360] in a patient who was small for gestational age and had features of AGS. At least 15 cases have subsequently been reported with deletions in chromosome 20 involving bands p11.23-p12.2 in association with AGS, confirming this localization and causing its inclusion in the list of CGS disorders.[361,362] However, a prospective study of an additional 14 patients with Alagille syndrome failed to identify any deletions in 20p by high-resolution cytogenetic analysis or limited FISH analysis with a single cosmid probe from this region of chromosome 20.[363] Molecular identification of mutations in the *Jagged 1* (*JAG1*) gene in patients with Alagille syndrome led to the investigation of deletions in patients with AGS. Using a FISH probe containing *JAG1*, 6 percent of AGS patients demonstrated a deletion.[357]

Molecular Genetics. The use of linkage analysis and two AGS families with balanced translocations involving 20p helped narrow the AGS critical region.[364] The region was further narrowed and the candidate gene, *Jagged 1*, was identified.[364,365] *JAG1* encodes a ligand for the transmembrane Notch 1 receptor. Mutations have been identified in 75 percent of patients.[357] A small percentage of patients (6 percent) have microdeletions that include the *JAG1* locus, while the vast majority (69 percent) have a variety of mutations in *JAG1*.[357] The majority of mutations lead to a nonfunctional protein, supporting a gene dosage, haploinsufficiency model in this disease. The finding of *JAG1* mutations in patients with the entire AGS clinical spectrum and in patients with isolated heart defects,[366] is consistent with a single gene defect with variable expressivity and pleiotropic effects.

Diagnostics. Very few AGS patients have visible cytogenetic abnormalities. Even though only 6 percent of patients are deleted by FISH, cytogenetic and FISH analyses rapidly identify abnormalities of 20p. Unfortunately, for the majority of patients not demonstrating a cytogenetic abnormality, more laborious mutation analysis of *JAG1* is needed. To date, only 2 of the 35 mutations identified occurred at the same location in the gene.[357] Therefore, direct sequencing or other methods to detect coding region alterations are the only available options to identify mutations in the majority of AGS patients.

DiGeorge Syndrome/Velocardiofacial Syndrome (del(22)(q11.2q11.2))

Clinical. In 1965, DiGeorge[367] described a patient with hypoparathyroidism and cellular immune deficiency similar to other patients he had seen with absent parathyroids and thymus at autopsy; the condition has become known as DiGeorge syndrome (DGS; MIM 188400). Since then a number of patients have been reported with absent or hypoplastic thymus and absent or hypoplastic parathyroid, frequently in combination with conotruncal-type cardiac malformations (interrupted aortic arch or truncus arteriosus).[368] In fact, congenital heart disease is the most frequent presenting feature in these patients and has been the major contributor to the high morbidity in the first weeks of life. Dysmorphic facial features, including hypertelorism, cleft palate, bifid uvula, and low-set ears, are frequently observed.[368] Most of the patients who survive infancy are mildly to moderately retarded. The incidence of DGS/VCFS has been estimated at 1 in 4000,[369] making it the most common, recognized, microdeletion syndrome.

The velocardiofacial syndrome (VCFS), or Shprintzen syndrome (MIM 192430), was initially described as a separate disorder, unrelated to DiGeorge syndrome. It is characterized by cleft palate, cardiac anomalies, and typical facies, including prominent nose, broad nasal root, narrow palpebral fissures, and retrognathia.[370] It is probably the most common syndrome associated with clefting, with approximately 8 percent of all patients presenting with cleft palate but without cleft lip (see review[370]). Cardiac abnormalities are found in 85 percent of patients, the most common being ventricular septal defect with or without a right aortic arch. Virtually all patients have some degree of learning disability, with microcephaly and mental retardation present in about 40 percent of cases. Other behavioral and psychiatric problems have also been observed. Significant overlap in phenotypic features exists between DGS and VCFS. Stevens et al.[371] first proposed that VCFS represents the inherited form of

DGS. Retrospective review of the literature has led several authors to conclude that many published cases of DGS actually represent VCFS.[370]

The etiology of DGS is heterogeneous, having been associated with several different chromosome abnormalities as well as teratogenic causes including retinoic acid embryopathy and the fetal alcohol syndrome.[372,373] Most cases of DGS are sporadic, but a number of familial cases have been described with apparent autosomal dominant transmission. As discussed above, these familial cases of DiGeorge probably represent the whole clinical spectrum associated with VCFS and deletions of proximal 22q. Additionally, in some families with DGS or VCFS, there are individuals with congenital heart defects but minimal dysmorphism. Because of this, Wilson et al.[24] performed molecular studies on a series of nine cases of familial congenital heart disease. Submicroscopic deletions in 22q11 were identified in five of the nine families. In four cases, the parent who had the deletion had a relatively mild heart anomaly, while in the fifth case, the father had a deletion and was unaffected. Interestingly, the five families with deletions exhibited heterogeneity in the nature of the cardiac anomaly between individuals in the family, while the four families without deletion all had unaffected parents and identical defects in the affected children. These observations provide additional evidence that deletions of 22q11 can have a wide spectrum of clinical expression, even within families.

Cytogenetics. DGS has been reported in association with a number of different chromosome abnormalities, most frequently deletions of proximal 22q and less frequently deletions of 10p13.[374] The specific association with deletion of the proximal portion of the long arm of chromosome 22 was first proposed by de la Chapelle et al. in 1981,[13] based on the observation of an unbalanced translocation producing partial monosomy 22 and a review of previously published monosomy 22 cases. High-resolution cytogenetic studies have identified subtle visible deletions of band 22q11.2 in approximately one-third of cases.[375–377] In VCFS, visible deletions of 22q11.2 have been detected by high-resolution cytogenetic studies in only a small number of cases.[378] Submicroscopic deletions have been identified in the majority of DGS and VCFS patients using Southern blot or FISH analysis.[378–380]

Molecular Genetics. Extensive progress has been made in the molecular characterization of the 22q11.2 CGS. Initial studies used RFLP and dosage analysis of Southern blots to demonstrate the presence of submicroscopic deletions in 22q11 in DGS patients. Combined data from two groups showed that although only about one-third of DGS patients showed cytogenetically detectable deletions, almost 100 percent of patients could be shown to have deletions by molecular methods.[375,376] The smallest region of overlap among these deletions included three common loci that represent a distance of at least 750 kb.[376] There was no apparent correlation between the size of deletion and severity of phenotype, even between patients with visible cytogenetic deletions as compared with those with submicroscopic deletions. FISH analysis with a cosmid probe from the DGS critical region has been demonstrated as an efficient method to detect submicroscopic deletions.[379,380] As described previously for Miller-Dieker syndrome, FISH has become the method of choice for diagnostic studies in DGS.

Molecular studies in VCFS have produced results essentially identical to those in DGS. From two studies, 26 of 27 VCFS patients were demonstrated to have submicroscopic deletions of probes in 22q11 by RFLP or quantitative Southern blot analysis.[378,381,382] With the currently available DNA probes, the deleted region for DGS and VCFS cannot be distinguished.

The deletion in 22q11.2 has been delineated. The common deletion region is 3 Mb in size and is flanked by low-copy repeats.[383] The breakpoints in 22q11.2 deletions associated with the majority of DGS and VCFS patients are identical.[384] Some patients show an alternate breakpoint resulting in smaller (1.5 Mb) deletions.[383,384]

A mouse model has been developed through an engineered heterozygous deletion spanning the region orthologous to human 22q11.2. The mice show defects consistent with DiGeorge syndrome including cardiovascular anomalies.[385] These mutants are important in understanding of the cellular mechanisms leading to developmental abnormalities of the fourth pharyngeal arch arteries.

Diagnostics. The interstitial deletion in proximal 22q cannot be reliably detected by routine G-banding. FISH using probes within the common deletion region have shown that greater than 90 percent of patients are deleted.[378–380] Patients not demonstrating a deletion by FISH for probes in the critical region should have a chromosome analysis to exclude gross structural rearrangements of chromosome 22 or other chromosomes. Some patients with deletions of 10p13-p14 show features of DGS, and FISH with probes from that region has been helpful in identifying these patients.[374] In cases of deletion and given the wide clinical expression, parental chromosomes should be examined using FISH to exclude a familial deletion.

CONTIGUOUS GENE SYNDROMES AND BEHAVIORAL TRAITS

Twin studies, utilizing monozygotic and dizygotic twins separated in infancy and reared apart, provide evidence for strong heritability of many psychologic and behavioral traits.[386] However, genetic linkage analysis and other nonparametric mapping methods have been disappointing in their ability to convincingly demonstrate a specific locus responsible for complex psychologic disorders such as schizophrenia or bipolar disorder. Furthermore, these genetic analysis methods, for the most part, have not been able to identify a single gene responsible for or associated with any psychologic or behavioral trait. One potential exception is the association of a point mutation in the structural gene for monoamine oxidase with an abnormal aggressive behavior in a single Dutch kindred segregating X-linked recessive mental retardation and prominent behavioral disturbances.[387] The only other mammalian study to link a gene alteration to a behavioral trait used mouse knockout technologies and astute observations of the child-rearing behavior of mothers with a *FosB* knockout. These studies showed a defect in nurturing in mice lacking the *FosB* gene.[388]

Many CGS present with specific behavioral or psychologic traits (Table 65-3).[67,389–395] For instance, 67 percent of patients

Table 65-3 Behavioral Phenotypes in Contiguous Gene Syndromes

Syndrome	Deletion	Phenotype
Williams	7q11.23	Gregarious, loquacious, impaired visuospatial recognition
Prader-Willi	15q12 (paternal)	Hyperphagia, obesity, oppositional, mood instability, skin picking, puzzle solving
Angelman	15q12 (maternal)	Paroxysmal laughter, "happy" facies
Smith-Magenis	17p11.2	Self-injurious, aggressive, self-hugging, attention seeking, onychotillomania, polyembolokoilamania
DiGeorge/VCFS	22q11.2	Obsessive behavior and schizophreniform disorders [11/61 (18%) adults had a psychiatric disorder]

with SMS manifest self-destructive behaviors, including onychotillomania (pulling out finger nails and toe nails) and polyembolokoilamania (insertion of foreign objects into bodily orifices).[67] Schizophrenia susceptibility has been associated with the DGS/VCFS interstitial deletion on chromosome 22.[392,393] These behavioral traits can be a useful clinical clue to aid in the diagnosis. Furthermore, evaluation for such behavioral traits is important for management and patient care. However, the existence of such behavioral traits in individuals with specific genomic rearrangements supports the contention that complex behavioral traits may be to some extent genetically determined. Extension of this concept suggests that genes located within the genomic region that is rearranged may be responsible for the behavioral phenotypes. Thus, patients with CGS that present with specific behavioral traits may be important in identifying genes involved in these behaviors.

MOLECULAR MECHANISMS LEADING TO CONTIGUOUS GENE SYNDROMES

In general, there are two genetic levels at which mechanisms for contiguous gene syndromes are operative. The first level involves the mechanisms for generating the chromosomal rearrangement resulting in microdeletion or microduplication. The second genetic level for mechanisms of disease relates to the genes contained within and at the breakpoints of the rearrangement. The gene is still the key in mediating the phenotype, but is altered almost coincidentally by the chromosomal rearrangement. The clinical phenotype may be due to (a) the effects of altered dosage of a single gene (in this sense the term contiguous gene syndrome may be a misnomer) (e.g., RTS and AGS), (b) multiple dosage-sensitive genes independently contributing to the phenotype (the original concept for contiguous gene syndrome as eloquently described by Schmickel[1] (e.g., WBS, PSS, and LGS)), or (c) an imprinted locus within the rearranged genomic region (e.g., PWS, AS, RSS, and BWS).

Mechanisms that explain variability of clinical expression in patients with contiguous gene syndromes may include: (a) variation in the size of the DNA rearrangement in different patients; (b) unmasking of recessive alleles on the remaining chromosome in the case of microdeletions; and (c) stochastic variation of gene expression levels for a subset of genes mapping within the rearrangement.

Mechanisms for Chromosomal Rearrangements

Terminal Deletions. Terminal deletions may vary in size and include those that were initially readily identified using G-banding to those representing cryptic rearrangements, only identified by molecular methods. Molecular analyses have revealed multiple breakpoints for 1p-[26],4p-[396],5p-[397], and 9p-[398] syndromes. However, some evidence for chromosomal breakage hotspots have been detected for the 9p deletion syndrome,[398] in which deletion breakpoints cluster in defined regions. Nevertheless, the nature of the DNA sequence substrates involved in generating the DNA rearrangements for terminal deletions has for the most part not been determined.

A recently proposed mechanism for terminal 11q deletions in Jacobsen syndrome (JBS; MIM 147791) is the expansion of $(CCG)_n$ repeats at the folate-sensitive chromosomal fragile site.[399] A $(CCG)_n$ trinucleotide repeat is located 5′ of *CBL2*, a known proto-oncogene on 11q. Expansion of this trinucleotide repeat causes methylation of the adjacent CpG island; however, the deletion breakpoint is not at the fragile site, but cluster in CCG-repeats.[399a]

By cytogenetic nomenclature convention, terminal deletions are indicated as loss of the chromosomal segment distal to the deletion breakpoint. However, terminal deletions must retain or acquire the repetitive telomeric "cap." Retention of the original telomere is considered an interstitial deletion. Telomere "healing," the *de novo* addition of the repetitive telomeric sequences $(TTAGGG)_n$, has been observed in many species. In humans, molecular analysis of a patient with a terminal deletion of chromosome 16 associated with α-thalassemia demonstrated that the deleted chromosome end was stabilized through telomere healing at a specific recognition site for human telomerase.[400,401] Other terminal deletions have been observed to be stabilized through a mechanism termed "telomere capture." Meltzer et al. studied terminal deletions occurring in human tumors by chromosome microdissection and found that the majority of these apparent terminal deletions represent cryptic subtelomeric translocations involving different partner chromosomes.[402] Recently, chromosome-specific subtelomeric FISH probes that hybridize to unique sequences adjacent to the subtelomeric repeat have been identified.[403,404] These probes have been useful in identifying cryptic translocations and telomeric deletions (see Fig. 65-3C).[405,406] The mechanism for terminal deletion stabilization was investigated in 33 patients with monosomy 1p with the use of these very distal, chromosome-specific, telomere-region probes. Evidence for both telomere healing and telomere capture was observed.[142]

Interstitial Deletions. For some interstitial microdeletions and their corresponding microduplications, a prominent role for unique genome architectural features in recombination leading to rearrangement was recently elucidated. Structural characteristics of the human genome may predispose to DNA rearrangements that can result in human disease traits. Conditions that may result from genome architecture have been referred to as genomic disorders.[407] Low-copy region-specific repeats that flank the genomic region that is rearranged act as substrates for homologous recombination. Nonallelic repeats recombine and this unequal crossing over results in deletion or duplication. These homologous recombination events result in a type of rearrangement that is a function of the orientation of the repeated sequences that act as substrates for homologous recombination.[408] Recombination between direct repeats can lead to deletion and/or duplication of the genetic material between the repeats, while recombination between inverted repeats results in inversion of the intervening genomic sequence. These meiotic recombinations can result in germ cells with a deleted or duplicated chromosomal segment, which may result in an embryo with either a deficiency or an excess of a specific region of the genome.

The CMT1A Duplication/HNPP Deletion Paradigm. CMT1A (MIM 118220) and HNPP (MIM 162500) represent two common inherited disorders of peripheral nerve myelin usually transmitted as autosomal dominant traits (see Chap. 227). CMT1A results from a tandem duplication of a 1.5-Mb region in 17p12, while HNPP results from deletion of the same 1.5-Mb region.[56,57] The 1.5-Mb CMT1A duplication/HNPP deletion genomic region is flanked by a 24,011-bp repeat termed CMT1A-REP.[409,410] The DNA sequences of the flanking CMT1A-REPs are 98.7 percent identical.[410] The duplication and deletion result from reciprocal homologous recombination between flanking proximal and distal CMT1A-REPs.[411,412] Interestingly, two copies of CMT1A-REP are present in humans and chimpanzees, but only one is present in gorillas and other primate species.[413] Thus, a recent evolutionary genomic duplication during speciation resulted in two copies of CMT1A-REP. This provided homologous genomic segments that could be used as substrates for homologous recombination between nonallelic regions resulting in DNA rearrangements.[413,414] Analysis of the products of recombination in multiple patients with either CMT1A duplication or HNPP deletion revealed evidence for a double-stranded break repair model and for potential minimal efficient processing segments (MEPs) required for homologous recombination.[415–417]

The disorders CMT1A and HNPP are clinically distinct (see Table 227-4 in Chap. 227), but both peripheral myelinopathies result from the dosage effects of a single gene, the gene for peripheral myelin protein 22, *PMP22* (GenBank L03203).

Table 65-4 Reciprocal Deletion and Duplication Paradigms for Genetic Disease

Disorder	Unequal (crossing-over)	Common deletion breakpoints	Flanking repeats	Associated duplications
HNPP and CMT1A del/dup 17p12	+	+	+	+
Smith-Magenis Syndrome del 17p11.2 and duplication 17p11.2 syndrome dup 17p11.2	+	+	+	+
Williams syndrome del 7q11.23	+	+	+	N/A
Prader-Willi/Angelman del 15q12	+	+	+	+*
DiGeorge/VCFS del 22q11.2	+	+	+	+*

+Reciprocal recombination demonstrated by molecular analysis.
*Duplication of these regions have been reported but molecular analysis demonstrating that these represent reciprocal recombination products of the common deletion has not yet been achieved.

The *PMP22* gene maps within the 1.5-Mb CMT1A duplication/HNPP deletion region. Both diseases result from a *PMP22* gene dosage effect, with HNPP patients having only one copy of *PMP22*, while CMT1A patients have three copies[414,418] (see Chap. 227).

Homologous Recombination Involving Low-Copy Region-Specific Repeat-Gene Clusters: A Mechanism for Interstitial Microdeletions and Reciprocal Microduplications. SMS is believed to represent a relatively common contiguous gene deletion syndrome that is associated with an approximately 5 Mb deletion in 17p11.2.[70,329] Genetic marker studies revealed a common genomic region deleted in >90 percent of patients.[67–69] This common deletion suggested specific breakpoints that were similar or identical in location in multiple patients. Analysis of the deletion breakpoint region revealed a >200 kb sequence of homology that flanked the common deletion.[58] This large, chromosome 17p11.2 region-specific low-copy repeat was termed SMS-REP.[58] At least four genes have been identified in SMS-REP, but it is not certain (in the absence of complete genome sequence and gene functional studies) whether these genes represent functional copies or pseudogenes. Regardless, these low-copy repeat-gene clusters provide an extensive region of homology. Molecular analysis demonstrated that the deletion breakpoints in most SMS patients occur within the SMS-REP repeat gene clusters.[58] An SMS-REP repeat sequence probe detected a novel junction fragment that is specific to the patients and to their rearranged chromosomes, and of similar size within the limits of resolution of pulsed-field gel electrophoresis (PFGE) (Fig. 65-9). These observations suggest that a precise recombination mechanism involving flanking SMS-REPs mediated the SMS common deletion. The most consistent model to explain the data is one wherein unequal crossing over and homologous recombination occurs between the proximal SMS-REP from one chromosome and the distal SMS-REP from the other.[58] Low-copy region-specific repeat-gene clusters have been identified in the genomic region implicated in and at the breakpoints of DGS/VCFS (del 22q11.2),[383] Williams syndrome (del 7q11.23),[178] and PWS/AS (del 15q12)[266a,419] (Table 65-4).

Duplication 17p11.2 — The Homologous Recombination Reciprocal of the Smith-Magenis Deletion. The hypothesis that homologous recombination and unequal crossing over between SMS-REPs causes duplication of 17p11.2 as the reciprocal event of the SMS deletion was investigated using molecular methods.[43] Seven patients ascertained for mild developmental delay underwent chromosome analysis by G-banding and were found to have an apparently increased band size for 17p11.2. Interphase FISH analysis revealed a direct (tandem) duplication in all patients. Further, these seven patients with *de novo* dup(17)(p11.2p11.2) showed a novel junction fragment that was specific to the patient and their rearranged chromosome, and of similar size within the limits of resolution of PFGE.[43] The same SMS-REP probe that revealed an SMS deletion-specific junction fragment detected the junction fragment in the patients with duplication of 17p11.2. Unequal crossing over of flanking markers was demonstrated by haplotype reconstruction and the genetic markers duplicated in these patients were the same as those deleted in SMS patients with the common deletion. These data are consistent with the hypothesis that homologous recombination and unequal crossing over between SMS-REPs cause the 17p11.2 duplication and the SMS deletion as reciprocal recombination products (Fig. 65-10). Interestingly, the *de novo* dup(17)(p11.2p11.2) may preferentially occur during paternal gametogenesis, similar to what has been observed for *de novo* CMT1A duplication (Chap. 227).

Duplications of segments of the human genome may eventually be shown to be responsible for many human traits.[43,407] The human genome project will delineate genome architectural features, such as low-copy region-specific repeats, that may enable prediction of regions susceptible to rearrangements associated with genomic disorders. Flanking repeat-gene clusters are associated with other genetic loci that undergo recurrent microdeletions.[58,178,264,383] Thus, it remains a distinct possibility that all interstitial chromosomal microdeletion syndromes have corresponding microduplication syndromes that represent the reciprocal recombination products.[43]

Other Potential Mechanisms for Interstitial Chromosomal Duplication

Tandem duplication of chromosomal segments has been recognized as a frequent mutational mechanism in several genetic model systems.[420] The human chromosomal duplications described above for CMT1A and dup(17)(p11.2p11.2) syndromes are mediated by large homologous segments in the human genome and have one discreet size for the duplication that is observed in the overwhelmingly majority of patients. In contrast, the duplications in Pelizaeus-Merzbacher disease (PMD; MIM 312080) differ in size in different patients.[41]

PMD is an X-linked neurodegenerative disorder of the central nervous system myelin (see Chap. 228).[421] It results from a duplication of the dosage sensitive central nervous system myelin gene *PLP* that encodes proteolipid protein.[421–424] The *PLP* duplications are tandem and result from unequal sister chromatid exchanges during male meiosis.[41,425,426] It is presently not known what the nature of the sequences substrates are at the multiple duplication breakpoints. These sequences may share some homology or the multiple rearrangements may result from nonhomologous recombination. The detection of multiple independent breakpoints is reminiscent of what is observed in terminal deletion syndromes at 1p, 4p, 5p, and 9p.

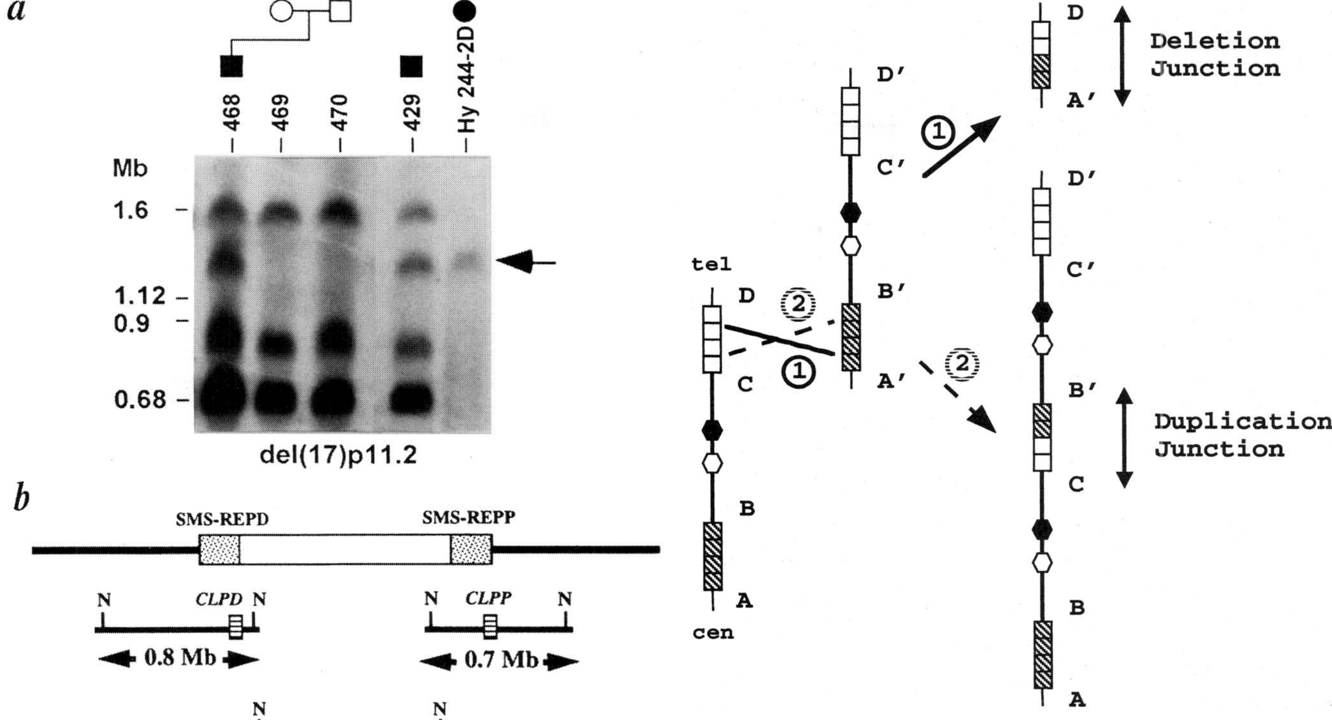

Fig. 65-9 Junction fragment due to recombination of flanking repeat-gene cluster in del(17)(p11.2p11.2). *A*, Southern analysis of PFGE reported high-molecular-weight genomic DNA from two patients with Smith-Magenis syndrome (468 and 429) and unaffected parents (469 and 470) of one patient. In the right lane is genomic DNA of a somatic cell hybrid retaining the del(17)(p11.2p11.2) chromosome from a patient with the SMS common deletion. The Southern blot is probed with a SMS-REP-specific probe, the gene for Coactosin-like protein *CLP*. Molecular size markers on megabases are shown on the left. Note that the junction fragment (jct) is *de novo* (not found in parents). Specific to the rearranged chromosomes (as shown by analysis of the hybrid retaining the del(17)(p11.2p11.2) chromosome) and of similar size in different patients with the common deletion. Also, of note is the disappearance of the cross-hybridizing fragments containing the proximal and distal SMS-REPs on the normal homologue. (*Adapted from Chen et al.*[58] *Used with permission of Nature Genetics*). *B*, Model to interpret the above Southern analysis. Recombination between flanking SMS-REP repeat-gene clusters (proximal SMS-REPP and distal SMS-REPD as stippled boxes). The open rectangle represents the genomic regions of 17p11.2 deleted in SMS patients with the common deletion. The horizontal bold line represents one chromosome 17 homologue, while the diagonally hatched line represents the other homologue. The model for forming the deleted chromosome is unequal crossing over and homologues recombination between flanking repeat gene clusters resulting in a recombinant chromosome with a specific junction fragment.

Fig. 65-10 Molecular mechanisms for microdeletion/microduplication. Misaligned chromosome homologues and the products of unequal crossing over are shown. Vertical rectangles represent low-copy region-specific repeat-gene clusters with proximal or centromeric copies as hatched boxes and distal or telomeric copies as open boxes. The bold vertical centerline represents the region undergoing rearrangement (deletion or duplication) with the filled and open hexagons representing potential dosage sensitive genes. Unique DNA sequence flanking the repeat gene cluster are depicted by the letters A, B, C, and D on one chromosome and A′, B′, C′, and D′ on the other homologue. The model consists of homologous recombination between a distal repeat-gene cluster from one chromosome and a proximal repeat-gene cluster from the other. The unequal crossing over results in recombination products that yield a duplication (dashed arrow labeled 2) or deletion (bold arrow labeled 1). The recombinant chromosomes have novel junction fragments (double-headed vertical arrows) that can now be detected because of the juxtaposition of unique sequences secondary to the recombination (C and B′ for the duplication junction; A and D′ for the deletion junction).

CONCLUSION

Since the last edition of this chapter, tremendous progress has been made in delineation of the critical regions involved in many CGS, identification of the genes contributing to CGS, and in the understanding of the molecular mechanisms which may result in chromosomal deletions and duplications. Some of the syndromes can no longer be considered CGS, based on the identification of mutations in single genes that result in the full phenotypes (AS, AGS, and RTS). For others, many of the causative genes have been identified and will aid in the delineation of all of the adjacent, responsible genes (LGS, PSS, and WBS). Additionally, these syndromes have aided in the understanding of genomic imprinting (AS/PWS, RSS, and BWS). Finally, new syndromes have been elucidated through careful, high quality cytogenetics (1p monosomy and PSS). The molecular mechanisms, mainly involving region-specific low-copy repeats, have been elucidated for a number of interstitial deletions resulting in CGS (DGS, PWS/AS, SMS, and WBS). The mechanism for rearrangement involves homologous recombination and unequal crossing over utilizing the flanking repeats as recombination substrates,[426a] because the deletion sizes are the same among the majority of patients with a given CGS. The delineation of a duplication syndrome, dup(17)(p11.2p11.2), representing the apparent reciprocal recombination product of the SMS deletion suggests that corresponding microduplication syndromes may exist for other genomic regions involved in interstitial microdeletion syndromes. For some of CGS, patient-specific junction fragments have been identified (e.g., SMS and WBS), further supporting a precise homologous recombination mechanism for these interstitial deletions. For other interstitial deletions of varying size and terminal deletions, the molecular mechanisms have yet to be elucidated. However, with the efforts of the human genome project, it is likely that the underlying genome architecture will be uncovered and the mechanisms resulting in these rearrangements will be delineated.

REFERENCES

1. Schmickel RD: Contiguous gene syndromes: A component of recognizable syndromes. *J Pediatr* **109**:231, 1986.
2. Francke U: *Microdeletions and Mendelian Phenotypes.* Berlin, Springer-Verlag, 1987.
3. Emanuel BS: Molecular cytogenetics: Toward dissection of the contiguous gene syndromes. *Am J Hum Genet* **43**:575, 1988.
4. Ledbetter DH, Cavenee WK: Molecular cytogenetics: Interface of cytogenetics and monogenic disorders, in Scriver CR, Beaudet AL, Sly WS, Valle D (eds): *The Metabolic Basis of Inherited Disease*, 6th ed. New York, McGraw-Hill, 1989, p 343.
5. Ballabio A: Contiguous deletion syndromes. *Genes Dev* **1**:25, 1991.
6. Yunis JJ: High resolution of human chromosomes. *Science* **191**:1268, 1976.
7. Yunis JJ: Mid-prophase human chromosomes. The attainment of 2000 bands. *Hum Genet* **56**:293, 1981.
8. ISCN: *An International System for Human Cytogenetic Nomenclature*. Basel, Karger, 1995.
9. Lele KP, Penrose LS, Stallard HB: Chromosome deletion in a case of retinoblastoma. *Ann Hum Genet* **27**:171, 1963.
10. Francke U: Retinoblastoma and chromosome 13. *Cytogenet Cell Genet* **16**:131, 1976.
11. Riccardi VM, Sujansky E, Smith AC, Francke U: Chromosomal imbalance in the aniridia-Wilms tumor association: 11p interstitial deletion. *Pediatrics* **61**:604, 1978.
12. Hawkey CJ, Smithies A: The Prader-Willi syndrome with a 15/15 translocation: Case report and review of the literature. *Med Genet* **13**:152, 1976.
13. de la Chapelle A, Herva R, Koivisto M, Aula P: A deletion in chromosome 22 can cause DiGeorge syndrome. *Hum Genet* **57**:253, 1981.
14. Dobyns WB, Stratton RF, Parke JT, Greenberg F, Nussbaum RL, Ledbetter DH: The Miller-Dieker syndrome: Lissencephaly and monosomy 17p. *J Pediatr* **102**:552, 1983.
15. Trask B: Fluorescence in situ hybridization. *Trends Genet* **7**:149, 1991.
16. Lichter P, Boyle AL, Cremer T, Ward DC: Analysis of genes and chromosomes by nonisotopic in situ hybridization. *Genet Anal* **8**:24, 1991.
17. Lichter P, Cremer T, Tang C-JC, Watkins PC, Manuelidis L, Ward DC: Rapid detection of human chromosome 21 aberrations by in situ hybridization. *Proc Natl Acad Sci U S A* **85**:9664, 1988.
18. Pinkel D, Landegent J, Collins C, Fuscoe J, Segraves R, Lucas J, Gray J: Fluorescence in situ hybridization with human chromosome-specific libraries: Detection of trisomy 21 and translocations of chromosome 4. *Proc Natl Acad Sci U S A* **85**:9138, 1988.
19. Nederlof PM, van der Flier S, Wiegant J, Raap AK, Tanke HJ, Ploem JS, van der Ploeg M: Multiple fluorescence in situ hybridization. *Cytometry* **11**:126, 1990.
20. Schrock E, du Manoir S, Veldman T, Schoell B, Wienberg J, Ferguson-Smith MA, Ning Y, Ledbetter DH, Bar-Am I, Soenksen D, Garini Y, Reid T: Multicolor spectral karyotyping of human chromosomes. *Science* **273**:494, 1996.
21. Speicher MR, Gwyn Ballard S, Ward DC: Karyotyping human chromosomes by combinatorial multi-fluor FISH. *Nat Genet* **12**:368, 1996.
22. Kuwano A, Ledbetter SA, Dobyns WB, Emmanuel BS, Ledbetter DH: Detection of deletions and cryptic translocations in Miller-Dieker syndrome by in situ hybridization. *Am J Hum Genet* **49**:707, 1991.
23. Lichter P, Tang C-JC, Call K, Hermanson G, Evans GA, Housman D, Ward DC: High-resolution mapping of human chromosome 11 by in situ hybridization with cosmid clones. *Science* **247**:64, 1990.
24. Wilson DI, Goodship JA, Burn J, Cross IE, Scambler PJ: Deletions within chromosome 22q11 in familial congenital heart disease. *Lancet* **340**:573, 1992.
25. Zori RT, Lupski JR, Heju Z, Greenberg F, Killian JM, Gray BA, Driscoll DJ, Patel PI, Zackowski JL: Clinical, cytogenetic, and molecular evidence for an infant with Smith-Magenis syndrome born from a mother having a mosaic 17p11.2p12 deletion. *Am J Med Genet* **47**:504, 1993.
26. Wu Y-Q, Heilstedt HA, Bedell JA, May KM, Starkey DE, McPherson JH, Shapira SK, Shaffer LG: Molecular refinement of the 1p36 deletion syndrome reveals size diversity and a preponderance of maternally derived deletions. *Hum Mol Genet* **8**:313, 1999.
27. Niebuhr E: The cri du chat syndrome. *Hum Genet* **44**:227, 1978.
28. Ballabio A, Andria G: Deletions and translocations involving the distal short arm of the human X chromosome: Review and hypotheses. *Hum Mol Genet* **1**:221, 1992.
29. Ballabio A, Bardoni B, Carrozzo R, Andria G, Bick D, Campbell L, Hamel B, Ferguson-Smith MA, Gimelli G, Fraccaro M, Maraschio P, Zuffardi O: Contiguous gene syndromes due to deletions in the distal short arm of the human X chromosome. *Proc Natl Acad Sci U S A* **86**:10001, 1989.
30. Chamberlain JS, Gibbs RA, Ranier JE, Caskey CT: Multiplex PCR for the diagnosis of Duchenne muscular dystrophy, in Innis M, Gelfand D, Sninsky JJ, White T (eds): *PCR Protocols: A Guide to Methods and Applications*. Orlando, FL, Academic Press, 1990, p 272.
31. Ballabio A, Ranier JE, Chamberlain JS, Zollo M, Caskey CT: Screening for steroid sulfatase (STS) gene deletions by multiplex DNA amplification. *Hum Genet* **84**:571, 1990.
32. Lindsay EA, Grillo A, Ferrero GB, Roth EJ, Magenis M, Grompe M, Hulten M, Gould C, Baldini A, Zoghbi HY, Ballabio A: The microphthalmia with linear skin defects (MLS) syndrome: Clinical, cytogenetic and molecular characterization. *Am J Med Genet* **49**:229, 1994.
33. Worley KC, Lindsay EA, Bailey W, Wise J, McCabe ERB, Baldini A: Rapid molecular cytogenetic analysis of X-chromosomal microdeletions: Fluorescence in situ hybridization (FISH) for complex glycerol kinase deficiency. *Am J Med Genet* **57**:615, 1995.
34. Lebo RV, Lynch ED, Golbus MS, Flandermeyer RR, Yen PH, Shapiro LJ: Prenatal in situ hybridization test for deleted steroid sulfatase gene. *Am J Med Genet* **46**:652, 1993.
35. Ried T, Mahler V, Vogt P, Blonden L, van Ommen GJB, Cremer T, Cremer M: Direct carrier detection by in situ suppression hybridization with cosmid clones of the Duchenne/Becker muscular dystrophy locus. *Hum Genet* **85**:581, 1990.
36. Voskova-Goldman A, Peier A, Caskey CT, Richards CS, Shaffer LG: DMD-specific FISH probes are diagnostically useful in the detection of female carriers of DMD gene deletions. *Neurology* **48**:1633, 1997.
37. Rosenberg C, Navajas L, Vagenas DF, Bakker E, Vainzof M, Passos-Bueno MR, Takata RI, van Ommen GJB, Zatz M, den Dunnen JT: Clinical diagnosis of heterozygous dystrophin gene deletions by fluorescence in situ hybridization. *Neuromuscul Disord* **8**:447, 1998.

37a. Ligon AH, Kashork CD, Richards CS, Shaffer LG: Identification of female carriers for Duchenne and Becker muscular dystrophies using a FISH-based approach. *Eur J Hum Genet* **8**:293, 2000.

38. Lupski JR: DNA diagnostics for Charcot-Marie-Tooth disease and related inherited neuropathies. *Clin Chem* **42**:995, 1996.
39. Wise CA, Garcia CA, Davis SN, Heju Z, Pentao L, Patel PI, Lupski JR: Molecular analyses of unrelated Charcot-Marie-Tooth (CMT) disease patients suggest a high frequency of the CMTIA duplication. *Am J Hum Genet* **53**:853, 1993.
40. Shaffer LG, Kennedy GM, Spikes AS, Lupski JR: Diagnosis of CMT1A duplication and HNPP deletions by interphase FISH: Implications for testing in the cytogenetics laboratory. *Am J Med Genet* **69**:325, 1997.
41. Inoue K, Osaka H, Imaizumi K, Nezu A, Takanashi J, Arii J, Murayama K, Ono J, Kikawa Y, Mito T, Shaffer LG, Lupski JR: Proteolipid protein gene duplications causing Pelizaeus-Merzbacher disease: Molecular mechanism and phenotypic manifestations. *Ann Neurol* **45**:624, 1999.
42. Roa BB, Ananth U, Garcia CA, Lupski JR: Molecular diagnosis of Charcot-Marie-Tooth disease type 1A and hereditary neuropathy with liability to pressure palsies. *Lab Medica Int* **12**:22, 1995.
43. Potocki L, Chen K-S, Park S-S, Ostersholm DE, Withers MA, Kimonis V, Summers AM, Meschino WS, Anyane-Yeboa K, Kashork CD, Shaffer LG, Lupski JR: Molecular mechanisms for duplication 17p11.2—The homologous recombination reciprocal of the Smith-Magenis microdeletion. *Nat Genet* **24**:84, 2000.
44. Ludecke HJ, Johnson C, Wagner MJ, Wells DE, Turleau C, Tommerup N, Latos-Bielenska A, Sandig KR, Meinecke P, Zabel B, Horsthemke B: Molecular definition of the shortest region of deletion overlap in the Langer-Giedion syndrome. *Am J Hum Genet* **49**:1197, 1991.

45. Dobyns WB, Curry CJR, Hoyme HE, Turlington L, Ledbetter DH: Clinical and molecular diagnosis of Miller-Dieker syndrome. *Am J Hum Genet* **48**:584, 1991.
46. Ewart AK, Morris CA, Atkinson D, Jin W, Sternes K, Spallone P, Stock AD, Leppert M, Keating MT: Hemizygosity at the elastin locus in a developmental disorder, Williams syndrome. *Nat Genet* **5**:11, 1993.
47. Lee ST, Nicholls RD, Bundey S, Laxova R, Musarella M, Spritz RA: Mutations of the P gene in oculocutaneous albinism, ocular albinism, and Prader-Willi syndrome plus albinism. *N Engl J Med* **330**:529, 1994.
48. Budarf ML, Konkle BA, Ludlow LB, Michaud D, Li M, Yamashiro DJ, McDonald-McGinn D, Zackai EH, Driscoll DA: Identification of a patient with Bernard-Soulier syndrome and a deletion in the DiGeorge/velo-cardio-facial chromosomal region in 22q11.2. *Hum Mol Genet* **4**:763, 1995.
49. Liang Y, Chen KS, Potocki L, Wang A, Fridell RA, Lupski JR, Friedman TB: High frequency hearing loss in an individual with Smith-Magenis syndrome likely due to a missense mutation in MY015 uncovered by del(17)(p11.2p11.2). *Am J Hum Genet* **63**:A333, 1998.
50. Nicholls RD: Genomic imprinting and candidate genes in the Prader-Willi and Angelman syndrome. *Curr Opin Genet Dev* **3**:445, 1993.
51. Wapenaar MC, Bassi MT, Schaefer L, Grillo A, Ferrero GB, Chinault AC, Ballabio A, Zoghbi HY: The genes for X-linked ocular albinism (OA1) and microphthalmia with linear skin defects (MLS): Cloning and characterization of the critical regions. *Hum Mol Genet* **2**:947, 1993.
52. Brown KW, Watson JE, Poirier V, Mott MG, Berry PJ, Maitland NJ: Inactivation of the remaining allele of the WT1 gene in a Wilms' tumor from a WAGR patient. *Oncogene* **7**:763, 1992.
53. Junien C: Beckwith-Wiedemann syndrome, tumourigenesis and imprinting. *Curr Opin Genet Dev* **2**:431, 1992.
54. Schmidt M, du Sart D: Functional disomies of the X chromosome influence the cell selection and hence the X inactivation pattern in females with balanced X-autosome translocations. *Am J Med Genet* **42**:161, 1992.
55. Raeymaekers P, Timmerman V, Nelis E, de Jonghe P, Hoogenduk JE, Baas F, Barker DF, Martin JJ, de Visser M, Bolhuis PA, van Broeckhoven C: Duplication in chromosome 17p11.2 in Charcot-Marie-Tooth neuropathy type 1a (CMT1a). *Neuromuscul Disord* **1**: 93, 1991.
56. Lupski JR, de Oca-Luna RM, Slaugenhaupt S, Pentao L, Guzzetta V, Trask BJ, Saucedo-Cardenas O, Barker DF, Killian JM, Garcia CA, Chakravarti A, Patel PI: DNA duplication associated with Charcot-Marie-Tooth disease type 1A. *Cell* **66**:219, 1991.
57. Chance PF, Alderson MK, Leppig KA, Lensch MW, Matsunami N, Smith B, Swanson PD, Odelberg SJ, Disteche CM, Bird TD: DNA deletion associated with hereditary neuropathy with liability to pressure palsies. *Cell* **72**:143, 1993.
58. Chen KS, Manian P, Koeuth T, Potocki L, Zhao Q, Chinault AC, Lee CC, Lupski JR: Homologous recombination of a flanking repeat gene cluster is a mechanism for a common contiguous gene deletion syndrome. *Nat Genet* **17**:154, 1997.
59. Scherer G, Schempp W, Baccichetti C, Lenzini E, Bricarelli FD, Carbone LDL, Wolf U: Duplication of an Xp segment that includes the ZFX locus causes sex inversion in man. *Hum Genet* **81**:291, 1989.
60. Ogata T, Hawkins JR, Taylor A, Matsuo N, Hata J, Goodfellow PN: Sex reversal in a child with a 46, X, Yp+ karyotype: Support for the existence of a gene(s), located in distal Xp, involved in testis formation. *J Med Genet* **29**:226, 1992.
61. Bardoni B, Floridia G, Guioli S, Peverali G, Anichini C, Cisternino M, Casalone R, Danesino C, Fraccaro M, Zuffardi O, Camerino G: Functional disomy of Xp22-pter in three males carrying a portion of Xp translocation to Yq. *Hum Genet* **91**:333, 1993.
62. Bardoni B, Zanaria E, Guioli S, Floridia G, Worley KC, Tonini G, Ferrante E, Chiumello G, McCabe ERB, Fraccaro M, Zuffardi O, Camerino G: A dosage-sensitive locus at Xp21 is involved in male to female sex reversal. *Nat Genet* **7**:497, 1994.
63. Worley KC, Ellison KA, Zhang YH, Wang D-F, Mason J, Roth EJ, Adams V, Fogt DD, Zhu XM, Towbin JA, Chinault AC, Zoghbi HY, McCabe ERB: Yeast artificial chromosome cloning in the glycerol kinase and adrenal hypoplasia congenita region. *Genomics* **16**:407, 1993.
64. Schaefer L, Ferrero GB, Grillo A, Bassi M-T, Roth EJ, Wapenaar MC, van Ommen GJB, Mohandas TK, Rocchi M, Zoghbi HY, Ballabio A: A high resolution deletion map of human chromosome Xp22. *Nat Genet* **4**:272, 1993.
65. Philippe C, Cremers FPM, Chery M, Bach I, Abbadi N, Ropers HH, Gilgenkrantz S: Physical mapping of DNA markers in the q13-q22 region of the human X chromosome. *Genomics* **17**:147, 1993.
66. Mutirangura A, Jayakumar A, Sutcliffe J, McKenney MJ, Beaudet A, Chinault AC, Ledbetter DH: A complete yeast artificial chromosome (YAC) contig of the Prader-Willi/Angelman syndrome (PWS/AS) region and refined localization of the *SNRPN* gene. *Genomics* **18**:546, 1993.
67. Greenberg F, Guzzetta V, de Oca-Luna M, Magenis RE, Smith ACM, Richter SF, Kondo I, Dobyns WB, Patel PI, Lupski JR: Molecular analysis of the Smith-Magenis syndrome: A possible contiguous-gene syndrome associated with del(17)(p11.2). *Am J Hum Genet* **49**:1207, 1991.
68. Juyal RC, Figuera LE, Hauge X, Elsea SH, Lupski JR, Greenberg F, Baldini A, Patel PI: Molecular analyses of 17p11.2 deletions in 62 Smith-Magenis syndrome patients. *Am J Hum Genet* **58**:998, 1996.
69. Guzzetta V, Franco B, Trask BJ, Zhang H, Saucedo-Cardenas O, De Oca-Luna MR, Greenberg F, Chinault AC, Lupski JR, Patel PI: Somatic cell hybrids, sequence-tagged sites, simple repeat polymorphisms, and yeast artificial chromosomes for physical and genetic mapping of proximal 17p. *Genomics* **13**:551, 1992.
70. Trask BJ, Mefford H, van den Engh G, Massa HF, Juyal RC, Potocki L, Finucane B, Abuelo DN, Witt DR, Magenis E, Baldini A, Greenberg F, Lupski JR, Patel PI: Quantification by flow cytometry of chromosome 17 deletions in Smith-Magenis syndrome patients. *Hum Genet* **98**:710, 1996.
71. Collins FS: Positional cloning: Let's not call it reverse anymore. *Nat Genet* **1**:3, 1992.
72. Ballabio A: The rise and fall of positional cloning? *Nat Genet* **3**:277, 1993.
73. Lupski JR: Charcot-Marie-Tooth disease: Lessons in genetic mechanisms. *Mol Med* **4**:3, 1998.
74. Tassabehji M, Metcalfe K, Karmiloff-Smith A, Carette MJ, Grant J, Dennis N, Reardon W, Splitt M, Read AP, Donnai D: Williams syndrome: Use of chromosomal microdeletions as a tool to dissect cognitive and physical phenotypes. *Am J Hum Genet* **64**:118, 1999.
75. Li DY, Toland AE, Boak BB, Atkinsin DL, Ensing GJ, Morris CA, Keating MT: Elastin point mutations cause an obstructive vascular disease, supravalvular aortic stenosis. *Hum Mol Genet* **6**:1021, 1997.
76. Tassabehji M, Metcalfe K, Donnai D, Hurst J, Reardon W, Burch M, Read AP: Elastin: genomic structure and point mutations in patients with supravalvular aortic stenosis. *Hum Mol Genet* **6**:1029, 1997.
77. Kishino T, Lalande M, Wagstaff J: *UBE3A*/E6-AP mutations cause Angelman syndrome. *Nat Genet* **15**:70, 1997.
78. Matsuura T, Sutcliffe JS, Fang P, Galjaard R-J, Jiang Y-H, Benton CS, Rommens JM, Beaudet AL: De novo truncating mutations in E6-AP ubiquitin-protein ligase gene (*UBE3A*) in Angelman syndrome. *Nat Genet* **15**:74, 1997.
79. Arn PH, Hauser ER, Thomas GH, Herman G, Hess D, Brusilow S: Hyperammonemia in women with a mutation at the ornithine carbamoyltransferase locus. A cause of postpartum coma. *N Engl J Med* **322**:1652, 1990.
80. Ballabio A, Willard HF: Mammalian X-chromosome inactivation and the XIST gene. *Curr Opin Genet Dev* **2**:439, 1992.
81. Fisher EMC, Beer-Romero P, Brown LG, Ridley A, McNeil JA, Lawrence JB, Willard HF, Bieber FR, Page DC: Homologous ribosomal protein genes on the human X and Y chromosomes: Escape from X inactivation and possible implications for Turner syndrome. *Cell* **63**:1205, 1990.
82. Ballabio A, Carrozzo R, Parenti G, Gil A, Zollo M, Persico MG, Gillard E, Affara N, Yates J, Ferguson-Smith AC, Frants RR, Eriksson AW, Andria G: Molecular heterogeneity of steroid sulfatase deficiency: A multicenter study on 57 unrelated patients at DNA and protein levels. *Genomics* **1**:36, 1989.
83. Shapiro LJ, Yen P, Pomerantz D, Martin E, Rolewic L, Mohandas T: Molecular studies of deletions at the human steroid sulfatase locus. *Proc Natl Acad Sci U S A* **86**:8477, 1989.
84. Yen PH, Allen E, Marsh B, Mohandas T, Wang N, Taggart RT, Shapiro LJ: Cloning and expression of steroid sulfatase cDNA and the frequent occurrence of deletions in STS deficiency: Implications for X-Y interchange. *Cell* **49**:443, 1987.
85. Ballabio A, Parenti G, Carrozzo R, Sebastio G, Andria G, Buckle V, Fraser N, Boyd Y, Craig I, Rocchi M, Romeo G, Jobsis AC, Persico MG: Isolation and characterization of a steroid sulphatase cDNA

clone: Genomic deletions in patients with X-linked ichthyosis. *Proc Natl Acad Sci U S A* **84**:4519, 1987.

86. Bonifas JM, Morley BJ, Oakey RE, Kan YW, Epstein EHJ: Cloning of a cDNA for steroid sulfatase: Frequent occurrence of gene deletions in patients with recessive X chromosome-linked ichthyosis. *Proc Natl Acad Sci U S A* **84**:9248, 1987.
87. Conary JT, Lorkowski G, Schmidt B, Pohlmann R, Nagel G, Meyer HE, Krentler C, Cully J, Hasilik A, von Figura K: Genetic heterogeneity of steroid sulfatase deficiency revealed with cDNA for human steroid sulfatase. *Biochem Biophys Res Commun* **144**:1010, 1987.
88. Gillard EF, Affara NA, Yates JRW, Goudie DR, Lambert J, Aitken DA, Ferguson-Smith MA: Deletion of a DNA sequence in eight of nine families with X-linked ichthyosis (steroid sulfatase deficiency). *Nucleic Acids Res* **15**:3977, 1987.
89. Yen PH, Li XM, Tsai SP, Johnson C, Mohandas T, Shapiro LJ: Frequent deletions of the human X chromosome distal short arm result from recombination between low-copy repetitive elements. *Cell* **61**:603, 1990.
90. Ballabio A, Parenti G, Tippett P, Mondello C, di Maio S, Tenore A, Andria G: X-linked ichthyosis due to steroid sulphatase deficiency associated with Kallmann syndrome (hypogonadotropic hypogonadism and anosmia): Linkage relationships with Xg and cloned DNA sequences from the distal short arm of the X chromosome. *Hum Genet* **72**:237, 1986.
91. Franco B, Guioli S, Pragliola A, Incerti B, Bardoni B, Tonlorenzi R, Carrozzo R, Maestrini E, Pieretti M, Taillon-Miller P, Brown CJ, Willard HF, Lawrence C, Persico MG, Camerino G, Ballabio A: A gene deleted in Kallmann's syndrome shares homology with neural cell adhesion and axonal path-finding molecules. *Nature* **353**:529, 1991.
92. Legouis R, Hardelin J-P, Levilliers J, Claverie J-M, Compain S, Wunderle V, Millasseau P, le Paslier D, Cohen D, Caterina D, Bougueleret L, Delemarre-Van de Waal H, Lutfalla G, Weissenbach J, Petit C: The candidate gene for the X-linked Kallmann syndrome encodes a protein related to adhesion molecules. *Cell* **67**:423, 1991.
93. Henke A, Wapenaar MC, van Ommen GJB, Maraschio P, Camerino G, Rappold G: Deletions within the pseudoautosomal region help map three new markers and indicate a possible role of this region in linear growth. *Am J Hum Genet* **49**:811, 1991.
93a. Rao E, Weiss B, Fukami M, Rump A, Niesler B, Mertz A, Muroya K, Binder G, Kirsch S, Winkelmann M, Nordsiek G, Heinrich U, Breuning MH, Ranke MB, Rosenthal A, Ogata T, Rappold GA: Pseudoautosomal deletions encompassing a novel homeobox gene cause growth failure in idiopathic short stature and Turner syndrome. *Nat Genet* **16**:54, 1997.
94. Maroteaux P: Brachytelephalangic chondrodysplasia punctata: A possible X-linked recessive form. *Hum Genet* **82**:167, 1989.
95. Petit C, Melki J, Levilliers J, Serville F, Weissenbach J, Maroteaux P: An interstitial deletion in Xp22.3 in a family with X-linked recessive chondrodysplasia punctata and short stature. *Hum Genet* **85**:247, 1990.
96. Daniele A, Parenti G, d'Addio M, Andria G, Ballabio A, Meroni G: Biochemical characterization of arylsulfatase E and functional analysis of mutations found in patients with X-linked chondrodysplasia punctata. *Am J Hum Genet* **62**:562, 1998.
97. Sunohara N, Sakuragawa N, Satoyoshi E, Tanae A, Shapiro LJ: A new syndrome of anosmia, ichthyosis, hypogonadism and various neurological manifestations with deficiency of steroid sulfatase and arylsulfatase C. *Ann Neurol* **19**:174, 1986.
98. Bassi MT, Bergen AAB, Wapenaar MC, Schiaffino MV, van Schooneveld MJ, Yates JRW, Charles SJ, Meitinger T, Ballabio A: A submicroscopic deletion in a patient with isolated X-linked ocular albinism (OAI). *Hum Mol Genet* **3**:647, 1994.
99. Bassi MT, Schiaffino MV, Renieri A, de Nigris F, Galli L, Bruttini M, Gebbia M, Bergen AA, Lewis RA, Ballabio A: Cloning of the gene for ocular albinism type 1 from the distal short arm of the X chromosome. *Nat Genet* **10**:13, 1995.
100. Schiaffino MV, d'Addio M, Alloni A, Baschirotto C, Valetti C, Cortese K, Puri C, Bassi MT, Colla C, de Luca M, Tacchetti C, Ballabio A: Ocular albinism: Evidence for a defect in an intercellular signal transduction system. *Nat Genet* **23**:108, 1999.
101. Quaderi NA, Schweiger S, Gaudenz K, Franco B, Rugarli EI, Berger W, Feldman GJ, Volta M, Andolfi G, Gilgenkrantz S, Marion RW, Hennekam RC, Opitz JM, Muenke M, Ropers H-H, Ballabio A: Opitz G/BBB syndrome, a defect of midline development, is due to mutations in a new RING finger gene on Xp22. *Nat Genet* **17**:285, 1997.
102. van den Veyver IB, Cormier TA, Jurecic V, Baldini A, Zoghbi HY: Characterization and physical mapping in human and mouse of a novel RING finger gene in Xp22. *Genomics* **51**:251, 1998.
103. Zvulunov A, Kachko L, Manor E, Shinwell E, Carmi R: Reticulolinear aplasia cutis congenita of the face and neck: A distinctive cutaneous manifestation in several syndromes linked to Xp22. *Br J Dermatol* **138**:1046, 1998.
104. Francke U, Ochs HD, de Martinville B: Minor Xp21 chromosome deletion in a male associated with expression of Duchenne muscular dystrophy, chronic granulomatous disease, retinitis pigmentosa, and McLeod syndrome. *Am J Hum Genet* **37**:250, 1985.
105. McCabe ER, Towbin JA, van den Engh G, Trask BJ: Xp21 contiguous gene syndromes: Deletion quantitation with bivariate flow karyotyping allows mapping of patient breakpoints. *Am J Hum Genet* **51**:1277, 1992.
106. Royer-Pokora B, Kunkel LM, Monaco AP: Cloning the gene for an inherited human disorder-chronic granulomatous disease-on the basis of it chromosomal location. *Nature* **322**:32, 1986.
107. Monaco AP, Neve RL, Colletti-Feener C: Isolation of candidate cDNAs for portions of the Duchenne muscular dystrophy gene. *Nature* **323**:646, 1986.
108. Sargent CA, Affara NA, Bentley E, Pelmear A, Bailey DMD, Davey P, Dow D, Leversha M, Aplin H, Besley GTN, Ferguson-Smith MA: Cloning of the X-linked glycerol kinase deficiency gene and its identification by sequence comparison to the Bacillus subtilis homologue. *Hum Mol Genet* **2**:97, 1993.
109. Walker AP, Muscatelli F, Monaco AP: Isolation of the human Xp21 glycerol kinase gene by positional cloning. *Hum Mol Genet* **2**:107, 1993.
110. Guo W, Worley K, Adams V, Mason J, Sylvester-Jackson D, Zhang Y-H, Towbin JA, Fogt DD, Madu S, Wheeler DA, McCabe ERB: Genomic scanning for expressed sequences in Xp21 identifies the glycerol kinase gene. *Nat Genet* **4**:367, 1993.
111. Zanaria E, Muscatelli F, Bardoni B, Strom TM, Guioli S, Guo W, Lalli E, Moser C, Walker AP, McCabe ERB, Meitinger T, Monaco AP, Sassone-Corsi P, Camerino G: An unusual member of the nuclear hormone receptor superfamily responsible for X-linked adrenal hypoplasia congenita. *Nature* **372**:635, 1994.
112. Swain A, Narvaez V, Burgoyne P, Camerino G, Lovell-Badge R: Dax1 antagonizes Sry action in mammalian sex determination. *Nature* **391**:781, 1998.
113. Tabor A, Anderson O, Lundsteen C, Niebuhr E, Sardemann H: Interstitial deletion in the "critical region" of the long arm of the X chromosome in a mentally retarded boy and his normal mother. *Hum Genet* **64**:196, 1983.
114. Rosenberg T, Schwartz M, Niebuhr E, Yang H-M, Sardemann H, Anderson O, Lundsteen C: Choroideremia in interstitial deletion of the X chromosome. *Ophthalmic Paediatr Genet* **7**:205, 1986.
115. Rosenberg T, Niebuhr E, Yang H-M, Parving A, Schwartz M: Choroideremia, congenital deafness and mental retardation in a family with an X chromosomal deletion. *Ophthalmic Paediatr Genet* **8**:139, 1987.
116. Cremers FPM, van de Pol TJR, Wieringa B, Hofker MH, Pearson PL, Pfeiffer RA, Mikkelsen M, Tabor A, Ropers H-H: Molecular analysis of male-viable deletions and duplications allows ordering of 52 DNA probes on proximal Xq. *Am J Hum Genet* **43**:452, 1988.
117. Cremers FPM, van de Pol DJR, Wieringa B, Collins FS, Sankila EM, Siu VM, Flintoff WF, Brunsmann F, Blonden LAJ, Ropers H-H: Chromosomal jumping from the DXS165 locus allows molecular characterization of four microdeletions and a *de novo* chromosome X/13 translocation associated with choroideremia. *Proc Natl Acad Sci U S A* **86**:7510, 1989.
118. Merry DE, Lesko JG, Sosnoski DM, Lewis RA, Lubinsky M, Trask B, van den Engh G, Collins FS, Nussbaum RL: Choroideremia and deafness with stapes fixation: A contiguous gene deletion syndrome in Xq21. *Am J Hum Genet* **45**:530, 1989.
119. Hodgson SV, Robertson ME, Fear CN, Goodship J, Malcolm S, Jay B, Bobrow M, Pembrey ME: Prenatal diagnosis of X-linked choroideremia with mental retardation, associated with a cytologically detectable X-chromosome deletion. *Hum Genet* **75**:286, 1987.
120. Nussbaum RL, Lesko JG, Lewis RA, Ledbetter SA, Ledbetter DH: Isolation of anonymous DNA sequences from within a submicroscopic X chromosomal deletion in a patient with choroideremia, deafness, and mental retardation. *Proc Natl Acad Sci U S A* **84**:6521, 1987.

121. Schwartz M, Rosenberg T, Niebuhr E, Lundsteen C, Sardemann H, Anderson O, Yang H-M, Lamm LU: Choroideremia: Further evidence for assignment of the locus to Xq13-Xq21. *Hum Genet* **74**:449, 1986.
122. Schwartz M, Yang H-M, Niebuhr E, Rosenberg T, Page DC: Regional localization of polymorphic DNA loci on the proximal long arm of the X chromosome using deletions associated with choroideremia. *Hum Genet* **78**:156, 1988.
123. Yang H-M, Lund T, Niebuhr E, Norby S, Schwartz M, Shen L: A deletion panel of the long arm of the X chromosome: Subregional localization of 22 DNA probes. *Hum Genet* **85**:25, 1990.
124. Wells S, Mould S, Robins D, Robinson D, Jacobs P: Molecular and cytogenetic analysis of a familial microdeletion of Xq. *J Med Genet* **28**:163, 1991.
125. Bach I, Robinson D, Thomas N, Ropers H-H, Cremers FPM: Physical fine mapping of genes underlying X-linked deafness and non-fra(X)-X-linked mental retardation of Xq21. *Hum Genet* **89**:620, 1992.
126. Cremers FPM, van de Pol DJR, Diergaarde PJ, Wieringa B, Nussbaum RL, Schwartz M, Ropers H-H: Physical fine mapping of the choroideremia locus using Xq21 deletions associated with complex syndromes. *Genomics* **4**:41, 1989.
127. Cremers FPM, Brunsmann F, Berger W, van Kerkhoff EPM, van de Pol TJR, Wieringa B, Pawlowitzki IH, Ropers HH: Cloning of the breakpoints of a deletion associated with choroideremia. *Hum Genet* **86**:61, 1990.
128. Moore GE, Ivens A, Chambers J, Farrall M, Williamson R, Page DC, Bjornsson A, Arnason A, Jensson O: Linkage of an X chromosome cleft palate gene. *Nature* **326**:91, 1987.
129. Brunner HG, van Bennekom CA, Lambermon EMM, Oei LT, Cremers WR, Wieringa B, Ropers H-H: The gene for X-linked progressive mixed deafness with perilymphatic gusher during stapes surgery (DFN3) is linked to PGK. *Hum Genet* **80**:337, 1988.
130. Wallis C, Ballo R, Wallis G, Beighton P, Goldblatt J: X-linked mixed deafness with stapes fixation in a Mauritian kindred: Linkage to Xq probe pDP34. *Genomics* **3**:299, 1988.
131. Gorski SM, Adams KJ, Birch PH, Friedman JM, Goodfellow PJ: The gene responsible for X-linked cleft palate (CPX) in a British Columbia native kindred is localized between PGK1 and DXYS1. *Am J Hum Genet* **50**:1129, 1992.
132. Bach I, Brunner HG, Beighton P, Ruvalcaba RHA, Reardon W, Pembrey ME, van der Velde-Visser SD, Bruns GA, Cremers CW, Cremers FP, Ropers H-H: Microdeletions in patients with Gusher-associated, X-linked mixed deafness (DFN3). *Am J Hum Genet* **51**:38, 1992.
133. Cremers FP, Sankila EM, Brunsmann F, Jay M, Jay B, Wright A, Pinckers AJ, Schwartz M, van de Pol DJ, Wieringa B, de la Chapelle A, Pawlowitzki IH, Ropers H-H: Deletions in patients with classical choroideremia vary in size from 45 kb to several megabases. *Am J Hum Genet* **47**:622, 1990.
134. Siu VM, Gonder JR, Jung JH, Sergovich FR, Flintoff WF: Choroideremia associated with an X-autosomal translocation. *Hum Genet* **84**:459, 1990.
135. Teboul M, Mujica P, Chery M, Leotard B, Gilgenkrantz S: Balanced X-autosomal translocation and mental retardation. Mapping mental retardation linked to X. *J Genet Hum* **37**:179, 1989.
136. Kaplan J, Gilgenkrantz S, Dufier JL, Frezal J: Choroideremia and ovarian dysgenesis associated with an X;7 *de novo* balanced translocation. Human gene mapping 10: Tenth International Workshop on Human Gene Mapping. *Cytogenet Cell Genet* **51**:1022, 1989.
137. Merry DE, Lesko JG, Siu VM, Flintoff WF, Collins FS, Lewis RA, Nussbaum RL: DXS165 detects a translocation breakpoint in a woman with choroideremia and a *de novo* X;13 translocation. *Genomics* **6**:609, 1990.
138. Cremers FP, van de Pol DJ, van Kerkhoff LP, Wieringa B, Ropers H-H: Cloning of a gene that is rearranged in patients with choroideremia. *Nature* **347**:674, 1990.
139. Merry DE, Janne PA, Landers JE, Lewis RA, Nussbaum RL: Isolation of a candidate gene for choroideremia. *Proc Natl Acad Sci U S A* **89**:2135, 1992.
140. Shapira SK, McCaskill C, Northrup H, Spikes AS, Elder FFB, Sutton VR, Korenberg JR, Greenberg F, Shaffer LG: Chromosome 1p36 deletions: The clinical phenotype and molecular characterization of a common newly delineated syndrome. *Am J Hum Genet* **61**:642, 1997.
141. Slavotinek A, Shaffer LG, Shapira SK: Monosomy 1p36. *J Med Genet* **36**:657, 1999.
142. Kashork CD, Ballif BC, Shapira SK, Shaffer LG: Terminal deletions may not be terminal: FISHing for mechanisms of chromosomal 1p36 deletions using telomere region-specific probes. *Am J Hum Genet* **65**:A385, 1999.
143. Giraudeau F, Aubert D, Young I, Horsley S, Knight S, Kearney L, Vergnaud G, Flint J: Molecular-cytogenetic detection of a deletion of 1p36.3. *J Med Genet* **34**:314, 1997.
144. Slavotinek A, Rosenberg M, Knight S, Gaunt L, Fergusson W, Killoran C, Clayton-Smith J, Kingston H, Campbell RH, Flint J, Donnai D, Biesecker L: Screening for submicroscopic chromosome rearrangements in children with idiopathic mental retardation using microsatellite markers for the chromosome telomeres. *J Med Genet* **36**:405, 1999.
145. Riegel M, Castellan C, Balmer D, Brecevic L, Schinzel A: Terminal deletion, del(1)(p36.3), detected through screening for terminal deletions in patients with unclassified malformation syndromes. *Am J Med Genet* **82**:249, 1999.
146. Silver HD, Kiyasu W, George J, Deamer WC: Syndrome of congenital hemihypertrophy, shortness of stature, and elevated urinary gonadotrophins. *Pediatrics* **12**:368, 1953.
147. Russell A: A syndrome of intrauterine dwarfism recognizable at birth with craniofacial dysostosis, disproportionate short arms and other anomalies. *Proc R Soc Med* **47**:1040, 1954.
148. Patton MA: Russell-Silver syndrome. *J Med Genet* **25**:557, 1988.
149. Rogan PK, Seip JR, Driscoll DJ, Papenhausen PR, Johnson VP, Raskin S, Woodward AL, Butler MG: Distinct 15q genotypes in Russell-Silver and ring 15 syndromes. *Am J Med Genet* **62**:10, 1996.
150. Schinzel AA, Robinson WP, Binkert F, Fanconi A: An interstitial deletion of proximal 8q (q11-q13) in a girl with Silver-Russell syndrome-like features. *Clin Dysmorphol* **3**:63, 1994.
151. Ramirez-Duenas ML, Medina C, Ocampo-Campos R, Rivera H: Severe Silver-Russell syndrome and translocation (17;20) (q25;q13) [see Comments]. *Clin Genet* **41**:51, 1992.
152. Midro AT, Debek K, Sawicka A, Marcinkiewicz D, Rogowska M: Second observation of Silver-Russell syndrome in a carrier of a reciprocal translocation with one breakpoint at site 17q25. *Clin Genet* **44**:53, 1993.
153. Monk D, Wakeling EL, Proud V, Hitchins M, Abu-Amero S, Stanier P, Preece MA, Moore GE: Duplication of 7p11.2-p13, including GRB10, in Silver-Russell syndrome. *Am J Hum Genet* **66**:36, 2000.
154. Joyce CA, Sharp A, Walker JM, Bullman H, Temple IK: Duplication of 7p12.1-p13, including *GRB10* and *IGFBP1*, in a mother and daughter with features of Silver-Russell syndrome. *Hum Genet* **105**:273, 1999.
155. Spence JE, Perciaccante RG, Greig GM, Willard HF, Ledbetter DH, Hejtmancik JF, Pollack MS, O'Brien WE, Beaudet AL: Uniparental disomy as a mechanism for human genetic disease. *Am J Hum Genet* **42**:217, 1988.
156. Shaffer LG, McCaskill C, Adkins K, Hassold TJ: Systematic search for uniparental disomy in early fetal losses: The results and a review of the literature. *Am J Med Genet* **79**:366, 1998.
157. Ledbetter DH, Engel E: Uniparental disomy in humans: Development of an imprinting map and its implications for prenatal diagnosis. *Hum Mol Genet* **4**:1757, 1995.
158. Kotzot D: Abnormal phenotypes in uniparental disomy (UPD): Fundamental aspects and a critical review with bibliography of UPD other than 15. *Am J Med Genet* **82**:265, 1999.
159. Kotzot D, Schmitt S, Bernasconi F, Robinson WP, Lurie IW, Ilyina H, Mehes K, Hamel BC, Otten BJ, Hergersberg M: Uniparental disomy 7 in Silver-Russell syndrome and primordial growth retardation. *Hum Mol Genet* **4**:583, 1995.
160. Preece MA, Price SM, Davies V, Clough L, Stanier P, Trembath RC, Moore GE: Maternal uniparental disomy 7 in Silver-Russell syndrome. *J Med Genet* **34**:6, 1997.
161. Eggermann T, Wollmann HA, Kuner R, Eggermann K, Enders H, Kaiser P, Ranke MB: Molecular studies in 37 Silver-Russell syndrome patients: Frequency and etiology of uniparental disomy. *Hum Genet* **100**:415, 1997.
162. Price SM, Stanhope R, Garrett C, Preece MA, Trembath RC: The spectrum of Silver-Russell syndrome: A clinical and molecular genetic study and new diagnostic criteria. *J Med Genet* **36**:837, 1999.
163. Miyoshi O, Kondoh T, Taneda H, Otsuka K, Matsumoto T, Niikawa N: 47, XX, UPD(7)mat, +r(7)pat/46, XX, UPD(7)mat mosaicism in a girl with Silver-Russell syndrome (SRS): Possible exclusion of the putative SRS gene from a 7p13-q11 region. *J Med Genet* **36**:326, 1999.
164. Eggerding FA, Schonberg SA, Chehab FF, Norton ME, Cox VA, Epstein CJ: Uniparental isodisomy for paternal 7p and maternal 7q in a child with growth retardation. *Am J Hum Genet* **55**:253, 1994.

164a. Blagitko N, Mergenthaler S, Schulz U, Wollmann HA, Craigen W, Eggerman T, Ropers H-H, Kalscheuer VM: Human *GRB10* is imprinted and expressed from the paternal and maternal allele in a highly tissue- and isoform-specific fashion. *Hum Mol Genet* **9**:1587, 2000.

164b. Yoshihashi H, Maeyama K, Kosaki R, Ogata T, Tsukahara M, Goto Y, Hata J, Matsuo N, Smith RJ, Kosaki K: Imprinting of human GRB10 and its mutations in two patients with Russell-Silver syndrome. *Am J Hum Genet* **67**:476, 2000.

165. Miyoshi N, Kuroiwa Y, Kohda T, Shitara H, Yonekawa H, Kawabe T, Hasegawa H, Barton SC, Surani MA, Kaneko-Ishino T, Ishino F: Identification of the Meg1/Grb10 imprinted gene on mouse proximal chromosome 11, a candidate for the Silver-Russell syndrome gene. *Proc Natl Acad Sci U S A* **95**:1102, 1998.

166. Cattanach BM, Kirk M: Differential activity of maternally and paternally derived chromosome regions in mice. *Nature* **315**:496, 1985.

167. Williams JC, Barratt-Boyes BG, Lowe JB: Supravalvular aortic stenosis. *Circulation* **24**:1311, 1961.

168. Beuren AJ: Supravalvular aortic stenosis: A complex syndrome with and without mental retardation. *Orig Art Ser* **8**:45, 1962.

169. Greenberg F, Lewis RA: The Williams syndrome: Spectrum and significance of ocular features. *Ophthalmology* **95**:1608, 1988.

170. Ewart AK, Morris CA, Ensing GJ, Loker J, Moore C, Leppert M, Keating MT: A human vascular disorder, supravalvular aortic stenosis, maps to chromosome 7. *Proc Natl Acad Sci U S A* **90**:3226, 1993.

171. Curran ME, Atkinson DL, Ewart AK, Morris CA, Leppert MF, Keating MT: The elastin gene is disrupted by a translocation associated with supravalvular aortic stenosis. *Cell* **73**:159, 1993.

172. Morris CA, Thomas IT, Greenberg F: Williams syndrome: Autosomal dominant inheritance. *Am J Med Genet* **47**:478, 1993.

173. Greenberg F: Williams syndrome professional symposium. *Am J Med Genet* **6**:85, 1990.

174. Greenberg F, Ledbetter DH: Chromosome abnormalities and Williams syndrome. *Am J Med Genet* **30**:993, 1988.

175. Nickerson E, Greenberg F, Keating MT, McCaskill C, Shaffer LG: Deletions of the elastin gene at 7q11.23 occur in ~90% of patients with Williams syndrome. *Am J Hum Genet* **56**:1156, 1995.

176. Francke U: Williams-Beuren syndrome: genes and mechanisms. *Hum Mol Genet* **8**:1947, 1999.

177. Wu Y-Q, Sutton VR, Nickerson E, Lupski JR, Potocki L, Korenberg JR, Greenberg F, Tassabehji M, Shaffer LG: Delineation of the common critical region in Williams syndrome and clinical correlation of growth, heart defects, ethnicity, and parental origin. *Am J Med Genet* **78**:82, 1998.

178. Peoples R, Franke Y, Wang Y-K, Perez-Jurado L, Paperna T, Cisco M, Francke U: A physical map, including a BAC/PAC clone contig, of the Williams-Beuren syndrome-deletion region at 7q11.23. *Am J Hum Genet* **66**:47, 2000.

179. Urban Z, Helms C, Pekete G, Csiszar K, Bonnet D, Munnich A, Donis-Keller H, Boyd CD: 7q11.23 deletions in Williams syndrome arise as a consequence of unequal meiotic crossover. *Am J Hum Genet* **59**:958, 1996.

180. Dutly F, Schinzel A: Unequal interchromosomal rearrangements may result in elastin gene deletions causing the Williams-Beuren syndrome. *Hum Mol Genet* **5**:1893, 1996.

181. Wu Y-Q, Kepper-Noreuil K, Mullenburg A, Nickerson E, Shaffer LG: A case of Williams syndrome with a large visible cytogenetic deletion. *J Med Genet* **36**:928, 1999.

182. Giedion A: Das Tricho-rhino-phalangeal syndrome. *Helv Paediatr Acta* **21**:475, 1966.

183. Hall BD, Langer LO, Giedion A, Smith DW, Cohen MM, Beals RK, Brandner M: Langer-Giedion syndrome. *Birth Defects* **10**:147, 1974.

184. Langer LO, Krassikoff N, Laxova R, Scheer-Williams M, Lutter LD, Gorlin RJ, Jennings CG, Day DW: The tricho-rhinophalangeal syndrome with exostoses (or Langer-Giedion syndrome): Four additional patients without mental retardation and review of the literature. *Am J Med Genet* **19**:81, 1984.

185. Buhler EM, Buhler UK, Stadler GR, Jani L, Jurik LP: Chromosome deletion and multiple cartilaginous exostoses. *Eur J Pediatr* **133**:163, 1980.

186. Pfeiffer RA: Langer-Giedion syndrome and additional congenital malformations with interstitial deletion of the long arm of chromosome 8:46, XY, del(8)(q13-22). *Clin Genet* **18**:142, 1980.

187. Bowen P, Biederman B, Hoo JJ: The critical segment for the Langer-Giedion syndrome: 8q24.11 → q24.12. *Ann Genet* **28**:224, 1985.

188. Fryns JP, van den Berghe H: 8q24.12 interstitial deletion in trichorhinophalangeal syndrome type 1. *Hum Genet* **74**:188, 1986.

189. Goldblatt J, Smart RD: Tricho-rhino-phalangeal syndrome without exostoses, with an interstitial deletion of 8q23. *Clin Genet* **29**:434, 1986.

190. Ogle RF, Dalzell P, Turner G, Wass D, Yip M-Y: Multiple exostoses in a patient with t(8;11)(q24.11;p15.5). *J Med Genet* **28**:881, 1991.

191. Cook A, Raskind W, Blanton SH, Pauli RM, Gregg RG, Francomano CA, Puffenberger EG, Conrad EU, Schmale G, Schellenberg G, Wijsman E, Hecht JT, Wells D, Wagner MJ: Genetic heterogeneity in families with hereditary multiple exostoses. *Am J Hum Genet* **53**:71, 1993.

192. Parrish JE, Wagner MJ, Hecht JT, Scott CI, Jr, Wells DE: Molecular analysis of overlapping chromosomal deletions in patients with Langer-Giedion syndrome. *Genomics* **11**:54, 1991.

193. Ahn H, Ludecke HJ, Lindow S, Horton WA, Lee B, Wagner MJ, Horsthemke B, Wells DE: Cloning of the putative tumour suppressor gene for hereditary multiple exostoses (EXT1). *Nat Genet* **11**:137, 1995.

194. Wuyts W, van Hul W, De Boulle K, Hendrickx J, Bakker E, Vanhoenacker F, Mollica F, Ludecke HJ, Sayli BS, Pazzaglia UE, Mortier G, Hamel B, Conrad EU, Matsushita M, Raskind WH, Willems PJ: Mutations in the EXT1 and EXT2 genes in hereditary multiple exostoses. *Am J Hum Genet* **62**:346, 1998.

195. Momeni P, Glokner G, Schmidt O, von Holtum D, Albrecht B, Gillessen-Kaesbach G, Hennekam R, Meinecke P, Zabel B, Rosenthal A, Horsthemke B, Ludecke HJ: Mutations in a new gene, encoding a zinc-finger protein, cause tricho-rhino-phalangeal syndrome type 1. *Nat Genet* **24**:71, 2000.

196. Nardmann J, Tranebjaerg L, Horsthemke B, Ludecke HJ: The tricho-rhino-phalangeal syndromes: Frequency and parental origin of 8q deletions. *Hum Genet* **99**:638, 1997.

197. Shaffer LG, Hecht JT, Ledbetter DH, Greenberg F: Familial interstitial deletion 11(p11.12p12) associated with parietal foramina, brachymicrocephaly, and mental retardation. *Am J Med Genet* **45**:581, 1993.

198. Potocki L, Shaffer LG: Interstitial deletion of 11(p11.2p12): A newly described contiguous gene deletion syndrome involving the gene for hereditary multiple exostoses (*EXT2*). *Am J Med Genet* **62**:319, 1996.

199. Bartsch O, Wuyts W, van Hul W, Hecht JT, Meinecke P, Hogue D, Werner W, Zabel B, Hinkel GK, Powell CM, Shaffer LG, Willems PJ: Delineation of a contiguous gene syndrome with multiple exostoses, enlarged parietal foramina, craniofacial dysostosis, and mental retardation, caused by deletions on the short arm of chromosome 11. *Am J Hum Genet* **58**:734, 1996.

200. Lorenz P, Rupprecht E, Tellkamp H: An unusual type of acrocephalosyndactyly with bilateral parietooccipital "encephalocele," micropenis, and severe mental retardation. *Am J Med Genet* **36**:265, 1990.

201. Ligon AH, Potocki L, Shaffer LG, Stickens D, Evans GA: Gene for multiple exostoses (*EXT2*) maps to 11(p11.2p12) and is deleted in patients with a contiguous gene syndrome. *Am J Med Genet* **75**:538, 1998.

202. Wu Y-Q, Heutink P, de Vries BBA, Sandkuijl L, van den Ouweland AMW, Niermeijer MF, Galjaard H, Reyniers E, Willems PJ, Halley DJJ: Assignment of a second locus for multiple exostoses to the pericentromeric region of chromosome 11. *Hum Mol Genet* **3**:167, 1994.

203. Stickens D, Clines G, Burbee D, Ramos P, Thomas S, Hogue D, Hecht JT, Lovett M, Evans GA: The *EXT2* multiple exostoses gene defines a family of putative tumour suppressor genes. *Nat Genet* **14**:25, 1996.

204. Wuyts W, van Hul W, Wauters J, Nemtsova M, Reyniers E, van Hul E, de Boulle K, de Vries BBA, Hendrickx J, Herrygers I, Bossuyt P, Balemans W, Fransen E, Vits L, Coucke P, Nowak NJ, Shows TB, Mallet L, van den Ouweland AMW, McGaughran J, Halley DJJ, Willems PJ: Positional cloning of a gene involved in hereditary multiple exostoses. *Hum Mol Genet* **5**:1547, 1996.

205. Miller RW, Fraumeni JR Jr, Manning MD: Association of Wilms' tumor with aniridia, hemihypertrophy and other congenital malformations. *N Engl J Med* **270**:922, 1964.

206. DiGeorge AM, Harley RDL: The association of aniridia, Wilms tumor and genital abnormalities. *Arch Ophthalmol* **75**:796, 1966.

207. Nelson LB, Spaeth GL, Nowinski TS, Margo CE, Jackson L: Aniridia: A review. *Surv Ophthalmol* **28**:621, 1984.

208. Glaser T, Lane J, Housman D: A mouse model of the Aniridia-Wilms tumor deletion syndrome. *Science* **250**:823, 1990.

209. Pendergrass TW: Congenital anomalies in children with Wilms tumor, a new survey. *Cancer* **37**:403, 1976.
210. Anderson SR, Geertinger P, Larsen H-W, Mikkelsen M, Parving A, Vestermark S, Warburg M: Aniridia, cataract and gonadoblastoma in a mentally retarded girl with deletion of chromosome 11: A clinicopathological case report. *Ophthalmologica* **176**:171, 1978.
211. Junien C, Turleau C, de Grouchy J, Said R, Rethore M-O, Tenconi R, Dufier JL: Regional assignment of catalase (CAT) gene to band 11p13:Association with the aniridia-Wilms' tumor-gonadoblastoma (WAGR) complex. *Ann Genet* **23**:165, 1980.
212. Turleau C, de Grouchy J, Dufier JL, Phuc LH, Schmelck PH, Rappaport R, Nihoul-Fekete C, Diebold N: Aniridia, male pseudohermaphroditism, gonadoblastoma, mental retardation, and del 11p13. *Hum Genet* **57**:300, 1981.
213. Baird PN, Santos A, Groves N, Jadresic L, Cowell JK: Constitutional mutations in the WT1 gene in patients with Denys-Drash syndrome. *Hum Mol Genet* **1**:301, 1992.
214. Jadresic L, Wadey RB, Buckle B, Barratt TM, Mitchell CD, Cowell JK: Molecular analysis of chromosome region 11p13 in patients with Drash syndrome. *Hum Genet* **86**:497, 1991.
215. Fraumeni JF, Geiser CF, Manning MD: Wilms tumor and congenital hemihypertrophy: Report of five new cases and review of literature. *Pediatrics* **40**:886, 1967.
216. Riccardi VM, Hittner HM, Francke U, Yunis JJ, Ledbetter DH, Borges W: The aniridia-Wilms tumor association: The critical role of chromosome band 11p13. *Cancer Genet Cytogenet* **2**:131, 1980.
217. Francke U, Holmes LB, Atkins L, Riccardi VM: Aniridia-Wilms' tumor association: Evidence for specific deletion of 11p13. *Cytogenet Cell Genet* **24**:185, 1979.
218. Slater R, de Kraker J: Chromosome 11 and Wilms tumor. *Cancer Genet Cytogenet* **5**:237, 1982.
219. Nakagome Y, Ise T, Sakurai M, Nakajo T, Okamoto E, Takano T, Nakahori Y, Tsuchida Y, Nagahara N, Takada T, Oshawa Y, Sawaguchi S, Toyosaka A, Kobayashi N, Matsunaga E, Saito S: High-resolution studies in patients with aniridia-Wilms tumor association, Wilms tumor or related congenital abnormalities. *Hum Genet* **67**:245, 1984.
220. Turleau C, de Grouchy J, Tournade M-F, Ganadoux M-F, Junien C: Del 11p/anirida complex. Report of three patients and review of 37 observations from the literature. *Clin Genet* **26**:356, 1984.
221. Yunis JJ, Ramsey NKC: Familial occurrence of the aniridia-Wilms tumor syndrome with deletion 11p13-14.1. *J Pediatr* **96**:1027, 1980.
222. Davis LM, Stallard R, Thomas GH, Couillin P, Junien C, Nowak NJ, Shows TB: Two anonymous DNA segments distinguish the Wilms' tumor and aniridia loci. *Science* **241**:840, 1988.
223. Pettenati MJ, Weaver RG, Burton BK: Translocation t(5;11)(q13.1;p13) associated with familial isolated aniridia. *Am J Med Genet* **34**:230, 1989.
224. Jeanpierre C, Antignac C, Beroud C, Lavedan C, Henry I, Saunders G, Williams B, Glaser T, Junien C: Constitutional and somatic deletions of two different regions of maternal chromosome 11 in Wilms tumor. *Genomics* **7**:434, 1990.
225. Mannens M, Hoovers JMN, Bleeker-Wagemakers E, Redeker E, Bliek J, Overbeeke-Milkert M, Saunders G, Williams B, van Heyningen V, Junien C, Haber D, Speleman F, Heyting C, Slater RM, Leschot NJ, Westerveld A: The distal region of 11p13 and associated genetic diseases. *Genomics* **11**:284, 1991.
226. Hanson IM, Seawright A, van Heyningen V: The human BDNF gene maps between FSHB and HVBS1 at the boundary of 11p13-p14. *Genomics* **13**:1331, 1992.
227. Fantes JA, Bickmore WA, Fletcher JM, Ballesta F, Hanson IM, van Heyningen V: Submicroscopic deletions at the WAGR locus, revealed by a nonradioactive in situ hybridization. *Am J Hum Genet* **51**:1286, 1992.
228. Lyons LA, Martha A, Mintz-Hittner HA, Saunders GF, Ferrell RE: Resolution of the two loci for autosomal dominant aniridia, AN1 and AN2, to a single locus on chromosome 11p13. *Genomics* **13**:925, 1992.
229. Simola K, Knuutila S, Kaitila I, Pirkola A, Pohja P: Familial aniridia and translocation t(4;11)(q22;p13) without Wilms' tumor. *Hum Genet* **63**:158, 1983.
230. Moore J, Hyman S, Antonarakis SE, Mules E, Thomas F: Familial isolated aniridia associated with a translocation involving chromosomes 11 and 22 t(11;22)(p13;q12.20). *Hum Genet* **72**:297, 1986.
231. Mannens M, Bleeker-Wagemakers EM, Bliek J, Hoovers J, Mandjes I, von Tol S, Frants RR, Heyting C, Westerveld A, Slater RM: Autosomal dominant aniridia linked to the chromosome 11p13 markers catalase and D11S141 in a large Dutch family. *Cytogenet Cell Genet* **52**:32, 1989.
232. Bickmore WA, Porteous DJ, Christie S, Seawright A, Fletcher JM, Maule JC, Couillin P, Junien C, Hastie ND, van Heyningen V: CpG islands surround a DNA segment located between translocation breakpoints associated with genitourinary dysplasia and aniridia. *Genomics* **5**:685, 1989.
233. Rose EA, Glaser T, Jones C, Smith CL, Lewis WH, Call KM, Minden M, Champagne E, Bonetta L, Yeter H, Housman DE: Complete physical map of the WAGR region of 11p13 localizes a candidate Wilms' tumor gene. *Cell* **60**:495, 1990.
234. Call KM, Glaser T, Ito CY, Buckler AJ, Pelletier J, Haber DA, Rose EA, Kral A, Yeger H, Lewis WH, Jones C, Housman DE: Isolation and characterization of a zinc finger polypeptide gene at the human chromosome 11 Wilms' tumor locus. *Cell* **60**:509, 1990.
235. Gessler M, Simola KO, Bruns GAP: Cloning of breakpoints of a chromosome translocation identifies the AN2 locus. *Science* **244**:1575, 1989.
236. Knudson AG Jr: Mutation and cancer: statistical study of retinoblastoma. *Proc Natl Acad Sci U S A* **68**:820, 1971.
237. Hastie ND: Dominant negative mutations in the Wilms tumor (WT1) gene cause Denys-Drash syndrome-proof that a tumor-suppressor gene plays a crucial role in normal genitourinary development. *Hum Mol Genet* **1**:293, 1992.
238. Ton CCT, Hirvonen H, Miwa H, Well MM, Monaghan P, Jordan T, van Heyningen V, Hastie ND, Meijers-Heijboer H, Drechsler M, Royer-Pokora B, Collins F, Swaroop A, Strong LC, Saunders GF: Positional cloning and characterization of a paired box- and homeobox-containing gene from the aniridia region. *Cell* **67**:1059, 1991.
239. Jordan T, Hanson I, Zaletayev D, Hodgson S, Prosser J, Seawright A, Hastie N, van Heyningen V: The human PAX6 gene is mutated in two patients with aniridia. *Nat Genet* **1**:328, 1992.
240. Hill RE, Favor J, Hogan BLM, Ton CCT, Saunders GF, Hanson IM, Prosser J, Jordan T, Hastie ND, van Heyningen V: Mouse *small eye* results from mutations in a paired-like homeobox-containing gene. *Nature* **354**:522, 1991.
241. Huff V: Parental origin of WT1 mutations and mental retardation in WAGR syndrome. *Nat Genet* **8**:13, 1994.
242. Ping AJ, Reeve AE, Law DJ, Young MR, Boehnke M, Feinberg AP: Genetic linkage of Beckwith-Wiedemann syndrome to 11p15. *Am J Hum Genet* **44**:720, 1989.
243. Koufos A, Grundy P, Morgan K, Aleck KA, Hadro T, Lampkins BC, Kalbakji A, Cavenee WK: Familial Beckwith-Wiedemann syndrome and a second Wilms tumor locus both map to 11p15.5. *Am J Hum Genet* **44**:711, 1989.
244. Henry I, Bonaiti-Pellie C, Chehensse V, Beldjord C, Schwartz C, Utermann C, Junien C: Uniparental paternal disomy in a genetic cancer-predisposing syndrome. *Nature* **351**:665, 1991.
245. Henry I, Puech A, Riesewijk A, Ahnine L, Mannens M, Beldjord C, Bitoun P, Tournada M-F, Landrieu P, Junien C: Somatic mosaicism for partial paternal isodisomy in Wiedemann-Beckwith syndrome: A post-fertilization event. *Eur J Hum Genet* **1**:19, 1993.
246. Catchpoole D, Lam WW, Valler D, Temple IK, Joyce JA, Reik W, Schofield PN, Maher ER: Epigenetic modification and uniparental inheritance of H19 in Beckwith-Wiedemann syndrome. *J Med Genet* **34**:353, 1997.
247. Bischoff FZ, Feldman GL, McCaskill C, Subramony SH, Hughes MR, Shaffer LG: Single-cell analysis demonstrating somatic mosaicism involving 11p in a patient with paternal isodisomy and Beckwith-Wiedemann syndrome. *Hum Mol Genet* **4**:395, 1995.
248. Weksberg R, Shen DR, Fei Y-L, Song QL, Squire J: Disruption of insulin-like growth factor 2 imprinting in Beckwith-Wiedemann syndrome. *Nat Genet* **5**:143, 1993.
249. Hatada I, Ohashi H, Fukushima Y, Kaneko Y, Inoue M, Komoto Y, Okada A, Ohishi S, Nabetani A, Morisaki H, Nakayama M, Niikawa N, Mukai T: An imprinted gene $p57^{KIP2}$ is mutated in Beckwith-Wiedemann syndrome. *Nat Genet* **14**:171, 1996.
250. Lee MP, DeBaun MR, Mitsuya K, Galonek HL, Brandenburg S, Oshimura M, Feinberg AP: Loss of imprinting of a paternally expressed transcript, with antisense orientation to KVLQT1, occurs frequently in Beckwith-Wiedemann syndrome and is independent of insulin-like growth factor II imprinting. *Proc Natl Acad Sci U S A* **96**:5203, 1999.
251. Prader A, Labhart A, Willi H: Ein syndrom von adipositas, kleinwuchs, kryptorchismus und oligophrenie nach myatonieartigen zustand in neugeborenalter. *Schweiz Med Wochenschr* **86**:1260, 1956.

252. Cassidy SB: Prader-Willi syndrome. *Curr Probl Pediatr* **14**:1, 1984.
253. Holm VJ, Cassidy SB, Butler MG, Hanchett JM, Greenswag LR, Whitman BY, Greenberg F: Prader-Willi syndrome: Consensus diagnostic criteria. *Pediatrics* **912**:398, 1993.
254. Butler MG: Prader-Willi syndrome: Current understanding of cause and diagnosis. *Am J Med Genet* **35**:319, 1990.
255. Hanson JW: A view of the etiology and pathogenesis of Prader-Willi syndrome, in Holm VA, Sulzbacher S, Pipes PL (eds): *Prader-Willi Syndrome*. Baltimore, MD, University Park Press, 1981, p 45.
256. Nicholls RD, Saitoh S, Horsthemke B: Imprinting in Prader-Willi and Angelman syndromes. *Trends Genet* **14**:194, 1998.
257. Horsthemke B, Dittrich B, Buiting K: Imprinting mutations on human chromosome 15. *Hum Mutat* **10**:329, 1997.
258. Hasegawa T, Hara M, Ando M, Osawa M, Fukuyama Y, Takahashi M, Yamada K: Cytogenetic studies of familial Prader-Willi syndrome. *Hum Genet* **65**:325, 1984.
259. Cassidy SB: Recurrence risk in Prader-Willi syndrome. *Am J Med Genet* **28**:59, 1987.
260. Ledbetter DH, Riccardi VM, Airhart SD, Strobel RJ, Keenan BS, Crawford JD: Deletions of chromosome 15 as a cause of the Prader-Willi syndrome. *N Engl J Med* **304**:325, 1981.
261. Ledbetter DH, Mascarello JT, Riccardi VM, Harper VD, Airhart SD, Strobel RJ: Chromosome 15 abnormalities and the Prader-Willi syndrome. A follow-up report of 40 cases. *Am J Hum Genet* **34**:278, 1982.
262. Butler MG, Palmer CG: Parental origin of chromosome 15 deletion in Prader-Willi syndrome. *Lancet* **1**:1285, 1983.
263. Butler MG, Meaney FJ, Palmer CG: Clinical and cytogenetic survey of 39 individuals with Prader-Labhart-Willi syndrome. *Am J Med Genet* **23**:793, 1986.
264. Christian SL, Bhatt NK, Martin SA, Sutcliffe JS, Kubota T, Huang B, Mutirangura A, Chinault AC, Beaudet AL, Ledbetter DH: Integrated YAC contig map of the Prader-Willi/Angelman region on chromosome 15q11-q13 with average STS spacing of 35 kb. *Genome Res* **8**:146, 1998.
265. Delach JA, Rosengren SS, Kaplan L, Greenstein RM, Cassidy SB, Benn PA: Comparison of high-resolution chromosome banding and fluorescence in situ hybridization (FISH) for the laboratory evaluation of Prader-Willi syndrome and Angelman syndrome. *Am J Med Genet* **52**:85, 1994.
266. Nicholls RD, Knoll JHM, Bulter MG, Karam S, Lalande M: Genetic imprinting suggested by maternal heterodisomy in non-deletion Prader-Willi syndrome. *Nature* **342**:281, 1989.
266a. Amos-Landgraf JM, Ji Y, Gottlieb W, Depinet T, Wandstrat AE, Cassidy SB, Driscoll DJ, Rogan PK, Schwartz S, Nicholls RD: Chromosome breakage in the Prader-Willi and Angelman syndromes involves recombination between large, transcribed repeats at proximal and distal breakpoints. *Am J Hum Genet* **65**:370, 1999.
267. Robinson WP, Bottani A, Yagang X, Balakrishman J, Binkert F, Machler M, Prader A, Schinzel A: Molecular, cytogenetic, and clinical investigations of Prader-Willi syndrome patients. *Am J Hum Genet* **49**:1219, 1991.
268. Knoll JHM, Sinnett D, Wagstaff J, Glatt K, Wilcox AS, Whiting PM, Wingrove P, Sikela JM, Lalande M: FISH ordering of reference markers and of the gene for the $\alpha5$ subunit of the γ-aminobutyric acid receptor (GABRA5) within the Angelman and Prader-Willi syndrome chromosomal regions. *Hum Mol Genet* **2**:183, 1993.
269. Hamabe J, Kuroki Y, Imaizumi K, Sugimoto T, Fukushima Y, Yamaguchi A, Izumikawa Y, Niikawa N: DNA deletion and its parental origin in Angelman syndrome patients. *Am J Med Genet* **41**:64, 1991.
270. Kubota T, Sutcliffe JS, Aradhya S, Gillessen-Kaesbach G, Christian SL, Horsthemke B, Beaudet AL, Ledbetter DH: Validation studies of SNRPN methylation as a diagnostic test for Prader-Willi syndrome. *Am J Med Genet* **66**:77, 1996.
271. Ohta T, Buiting K, Kokkonen H, McCandless S, Heeger S, Leisti H, Driscoll DJ, Cassidy SB, Horsthemke B, Nicholls RD: Molecular mechanism of Angelman syndrome in two large families involves an imprinting mutation. *Am J Hum Genet* **64**:385, 1999.
272. Buiting K, Dittrich B, Grob S, Lich C, Buchholz T, Smith E, Reis A, Bürger J, Abeliovich D, Barth-Witte U, Janssen B, Lerer I, van den Ouweland AMW, Halley DJJ, Schrander-Stumpel C, Smeets H, Meineri P, Malcolm S, Gardner A, Lalande M, Nicholls RD, Friend K, Schulze A, Matthijs G, Kokkonen H, Hilbert P, Van Maldergem L, Glover G, Carbonell P, Willems P, Gillessen-Kaesbach G, Horsthemke B: Sporadic imprinting defects in Prader-Willi syndrome and Angelman syndrome: Implications for imprint-switch models, genetic counseling, and prenatal diagnosis. *Am J Hum Genet* **63**:170, 1998.
273. Mann MRW, Bartolomei MS: Towards a molecular understanding of Prader-Willi and Angelman syndromes. *Hum Mol Genet* **8**:1867, 1999.
274. Boccaccio I, Glatt-Deeley H, Watrin F, Roeckel N, Lalande M, Muscatelli F: The human MAGEL2 gene and its mouse homologue are paternally expressed and mapped to the Prader-Willi region. *Hum Mol Genet* **8**:2497, 1999.
275. Lee S, Wevrick R: Identification of novel imprinted transcripts in the Prader-Willi syndrome and Angelman syndrome deletion region: Further evidence for regional imprinting control. *Am J Hum Genet* **66**:848, 2000.
276. Gerard M, Hernandez L, Wevrick R, Stewart CL: Disruption of the mouse necdin gene results in early post-natal lethality. *Nat Genet* **23**:199, 1999.
277. Tsai T-F, Armstrong D, Beaudet AL: Necdin-deficient mice do not show lethality or the obesity and infertility of Prader-Willi syndrome. *Nat Genet* **22**:15, 1999.
278. Gardner JM, Nakatsu Y, Gondo Y, Lee S, Lyon MF, King RA, Brilliant MH: The mouse pink-eyed dilution gene: Association with human Prader-Willi and Angelman syndromes. *Science* **257**:1121, 1992.
279. Rinchik EM, Bultman SJ, Horsthemke B, Lee S-T, Strunk KM, Spritz RA, Avidano KM, Jong MT-C, Nicholls RD: A gene for the mouse pink-eyed dilution locus and for human type II oculocutaneous albinism. *Nature* **361**:72, 1993.
280. Ramsey M, Colman MA, Stevens G, Zwane E, Kromberg J, Farrall M, Jenkins T: The tyrosine-positive oculocutaneous albinism locus maps to chromosome 15q11.2-q12. *Am J Hum Genet* **51**:879, 1992.
281. Engel E: A new genetic concept: Uniparental disomy and its potential effect, isodisomy. *Am J Med Genet* **6**:137, 1980.
282. Engel E: Uniparental disomy revisited: The first twelve years. *Am J Med Genet* **46**:670, 1993.
283. Mascari MJ, Gottlieb W, Rogan PK, Butler MG, Waller DA, Armour JAL, Jeffreys AJ, Ladda RL, Nicholls RD: The frequency of uniparental disomy in Prader-Willi syndrome. Implications for molecular diagnosis. *N Engl J Med* **36**:1599, 1992.
284. Mutirangura A, Greenberg F, Bulter MG, Malcolm S, Nicholls RD, Chakravarti A, Ledbetter DH: Multiplex PCR of three dinucleotide repeats in the Prader-Willi/Angelman critical region (15q11-q13): Molecular diagnosis and mechanism of uniparental disomy. *Hum Mol Genet* **2**:143, 1993.
285. Purvis-Smith SG, Saville T, Manass S, Yip M-Y, Lam-Po-Tang PRL, Duffy B, Johnston H, Leigh D, McDonald B: Uniparental disomy 15 resulting from correction of an initial trisomy 15. *Am J Hum Genet* **50**:1348, 1992.
286. Cassidy SB, Lai L-W, Erickson RP, Magnuson L, Thomas E, Gendron R, Herrmann J: Trisomy 15 with loss of the paternal 15 as a cause of Prader-Willi syndrome due to maternal disomy. *Am J Hum Genet* **51**:701, 1992.
287. Morichon-Delvallez N, Mussat P, Dumez Y, Vekemans M: Trisomy 15 in chorionic villi and Prader-Willi syndrome at birth. *Prenat Diagn* **13**:307, 1993.
288. Cassidy SB, Beaudet AL, Knoll JHM, Ledbetter DH, Nicholls RD, Schwartz S, Butler MG, Watson M: Diagnostic testing for Prader-Willi and Angelman syndromes — Report of the ASHC/ACMC test and technology transfer committee. *Am J Hum Genet* **58**:1085, 1996.
289. Zeschnigk M, Lich C, Buiting K, Doerfler W, Horsthemke B: A single-tube PCR test for the diagnosis of Angelman and Prader-Willi syndrome based on allelic methylation differences at the SNRPN locus. *Eur J Hum Genet* **5**:94, 1997.
290. Kubota T, Das S, Christian SL, Baylin SB, Herman JG, Ledbetter DH: Methylation-specific PCR simplifies imprinting analysis. *Nat Genet* **16**:16, 1997.
291. Robb SA, Pohl KRE, Wilson BJ, Brett EM: The "happy puppet" syndrome of Angelman: Review of the clinical features. *Arch Dis Child* **64**:83, 1989.
292. Clayton-Smith J, Pembrey ME: Angelman syndrome. *J Med Genet* **29**:412, 1992.
293. Clayton-Smith J: Clinical research on Angelman syndrome in the United Kingdom: Observations on 82 affected individuals. *Am J Med Genet* **46**:12, 1993.
294. Laan LA, Haeringen A, Brouwer OF: Angelman syndrome: A review of clinical and genetic aspects. *Clin Neurol Neurosurg* **101**:161, 1999.

295. McKusick VA: *Mendelian Inheritance in Man*. Baltimore, MD, Johns Hopkins University Press, 1992.
296. Wagstaff J, Knoll JHM, Glatt KA, Shugart YY, Sommer A, Lalande M: Maternal but not paternal transmission of 15q11-13-linked nondeletion Angelman syndrome leads to phenotypic expression. *Nat Genet* **1**:291, 1992.
297. Meijers-Heijboer EJ, Sandkuijl L, Brunner HG, Smeets HJM, Hoogeboom AJM, Deelen WH, van Hemel JO, Nelen MR, Smeets DFCM, Niermeijer MF, Halley DJJ: Linkage analysis with chromosome15q11-13 markers shows genomic imprinting in familial Angelman syndrome. *J Med Genet* **29**:853, 1992.
298. Clayton-Smith J, Webb T, Robb SA, Dijkstra I, Willems P, Lam S, Cheng X-J, Pembrey ME, Malcolm S: Further evidence for dominant inheritance at the chromosome 15q11-13 locus in familial Angelman syndrome. *Am J Med Genet* **44**:256, 1992.
299. Magenis RE, Brown MG, Lacy DA, Budden S, LaFranchi S: Is Angelman syndrome an alternate result of del(15)(q11q13)? *Am J Med Genet* **28**:829, 1987.
300. Zackowski JL, Nicholls RD, Gray BA, Bent-Williams A, Gottlieb W, Harris PJ, Waters MF, Driscoll DJ, Zori RT, Williams CA: Cytogenetic and molecular analysis in Angelman syndrome. *Am J Med Genet* **46**:7, 1993.
301. Magenis RE, Toth-Fejel S, Allen LJ, Black M, Brown MG, Budden S, Cohen R, Friedman JM, Kalousek D, Zonana J, Lacy D, LaFranchi S, Lahr M, Macfarlane J, Williams CPS: Comparison of the 15q deletions in Prader-Willi and Angelman syndromes: Specific regions, extent of deletions, parental origin, and clinical consequences. *Am J Med Genet* **35**:333, 1990.
302. Kuwano A, Mutirangura A, Dittrich B, Buiting K, Horsthemke B, Saitoh S, Niikawa N, Ledbetter SA, Greenberg F, Chinault AC, Ledbetter DH: Molecular dissection of the Prader-Willi/Angelman syndrome region (15q11-13) by YAC cloning and FISH analysis. *Hum Mol Genet* **1**:417, 1992.
303. Amos-Landgraf JM, Ji Y, Gottlieb W, Depinet T, Wandstrat AE, Cassidy SB, Driscoll DJ, Rogan PK, Schwartz S, Nicholls RD: Chromosome breakage in the Prader-Willi and Angelman syndromes involves recombination between large, transcribed repeats at proximal and distal breakpoints. *Am J Hum Genet* **65**:370, 1999.
304. Nicholls RD, Knoll JH, Glatt K, Hersh JH, Brewster TD, Graham JM Jr, Wurster-Hill D, Wharton R, Latt SA: Restriction fragment length polymorphisms within proximal 15q and their use in molecular cytogenetics and the Prader-Willi syndrome. *Am J Med Genet* **33**:66, 1989.
305. Hamabe J, Fukushima Y, Harada N, Abe K, Matsuo N, Nagai T, Yoshioka A, Tonoki H, Tsukino R, Niikawa N: Molecular study of the Prader-Willi syndrome: Deletion, RFLP, and phenotype analyses of 50 patients. *Am J Med Genet* **41**:54, 1991.
306. Knoll JHM, Nicholls RD, Magenis RE, Graham JM Jr, Lalande M, Latt SA: Angelman and Prader-Willi syndromes share a common chromosome 15 deletion but differ in parental origin of the deletion. *Am J Med Genet* **32**:285, 1989.
307. Williams CA, Zori RT, Stone JW, Gray BA, Cantú ES, Ostrer H: Maternal origin of 15q11-q13 deletions in Angelman syndrome suggests a role for genomic imprinting. *Am J Med Genet* **35**:350, 1990.
308. Malcolm S, Clayton-Smith J, Nichols M, Robb S, Webb T, Armour JA, Jeffreys AJ, Pembrey ME: Uniparental paternal disomy in Angelman's syndrome. *Lancet* **337**:694, 1991.
309. Nicholls RD, Shashidhar PG, Gottlieb W, Cantú ES: Paternal uniparental disomy of chromosome 15 in a child with Angelman syndrome. *Ann Neurol* **32**:512, 1992.
310. Knoll JHM, Glatt KA, Nicholls RD, Malcolm S, Lalande M: Chromosome 15 uniparental disomy is not frequent in Angelman syndrome. *Am J Hum Genet* **48**:16, 1991.
311. Jiang Y-H, Lev-Lehman E, Bressler J, Tsai T-F, Beaudet AL: Neurogenetics '99: Genetics of Angelman syndrome. *Am J Hum Genet* **65**:1, 1999.
312. Albrecht U, Sutcliffe JS, Cattanach BM, Beechey CV, Armstrong D, Eichele G, Beaudet AL: Imprinted expression of the murine Angelman syndrome gene *Ube3a* in hippocampal and Purkinje neurons. *Nat Genet* **17**:75, 1997.
313. Vu TH, Hoffman AR: Imprinting of the Angelman syndrome gene *UBE3A* is restricted to brain. *Nat Genet* **17**:12, 1997.
314. Rougeulle C, Glatt H, Lalande M: The Angelman syndrome candidate gene *UBE3A*/E6-AP is imprinted in brain. *Nat Genet* **17**:14, 1997.
315. Fang P, Lev-Lehman E, Tsai T-F, Matsuura T, Benton CS, Sutcliffe JS, Christian SL, Kubota T, Halley DJ, Meijers-Heijboer H, Langlois S, Graham JM, Beuten J, Willems P, Ledbetter DH, Beaudet AL: The spectrum of mutations in *UBE3A* causing Angelman syndrome. *Hum Mol Genet* **8**:129, 1999.
316. Malzac P, Webber H, Moncla A, Graham JM, Kukolich M, Williams C, Pagon RA, Ramsdell LA, Kishino T, Wagstaff J: Mutation analysis of *UBE3A* in Angelman syndrome patients. *Am J Hum Genet* **62**:1353, 1998.
317. Burger J, Buiting K, Dittrich B, Gross S, Lich C, Sperling K, Horsthemke B, Reis A: Different mechanisms and recurrence risks of imprinting defects in Angelman syndrome. *Am J Hum Genet* **61**:88, 1997.
318. Farber C, Dittrich B, Buiting K, Horsthemke B: The chromosome 15 imprinting centre (IC) region has undergone multiple duplication events and contains an upstream exon of *SNRPN* that is deleted in all Angelman syndrome patients with an IC microdeletion. *Hum Mol Genet* **8**:337, 1999.
319. Buiting K, Lich C, Cottrell S, Barnicoat A, Horsthemke B: A 5-kb imprinting center deletion in a family with Angelman syndrome reduces the shortest region of deletion overlap to 880 bp. *Hum Genet* **105**:665, 1999.
320. Hennekam RCM, Stevens CA, van de Kamp JJP: Etiology and recurrence risk in Rubinstein-Taybi syndrome. *Am J Med Genet* **6**:56, 1990.
321. Berry AC: Rubinstein-Taybi syndrome. *J Med Genet* **24**:562, 1987.
322. Breuning MH, Dauwerse HG, Fugazza G, Saris JJ, Spruit L, Wijnen H, Tommerup N, van der Hagen CB, Imaizumi K, Kuroki Y, van den Boogaard MJ, de Pater JM, Mariman ECM, Hamel BCJ, Himmelbauer H, Frischauf A-M, Stallings RL, Beverstock GC, van Ommen GJB, Hennekam RCM: Rubinstein-Taybi syndrome caused by submicroscopic deletions within 16p13.3. *Am J Hum Genet* **52**:249, 1993.
323. Hennekam RCM, Tilanus M, Hamel BCJ, Voshart-van Heeren H, Mariman ECM, van Beersum SEC, van den Boogaard MJH, Breuning MH: Deletion at chromosome 16p13.3 as a cause of Rubinstein-Taybi syndrome. Clinical aspects. *Am J Hum Genet* **52**:255, 1993.
324. Blough RI, Petrij F, Dauwerse JG, Milatovich-Cherry A, Weiss L, Saal HM, Rubinstein JH: Variation in microdeletions of the cyclic AMP-responsive element-binding protein gene at chromosome band 16p13.3 in the Rubinstein-Taybi syndrome. *Am J Med Genet* **90**:29, 2000.
325. Wallerstein R, Anderson CE, Hay B, Gupta P, Gibas L, Ansari K, Cowchock FS, Weinblatt V, Reid C, Levitas A, Jackson L: Submicroscopic deletions at 16p13.3 in Rubinstein-Taybi syndrome: Frequency and clinical manifestations in a North American population. *J Med Genet* **34**:203, 1997.
326. Petrij F, Giles RH, Dauwerse HG, Saris JJ, Hennekam RCM, Masuno M, Tommerup N, van Ommen GJB, Goodman RH, Peters DJM, Breuning MH: Rubinstein-Taybi syndrome caused by mutations in the transcriptional co-activator CBP. *Nature* **376**:348, 1995.
327. Smith ACM, McGavran L, Robinson J, Waldstein G, Macfarlane J, Zonona J, Reiss J, Lahr M, Allen L, Magenis E: Interstitial deletion of (17)(p11.2p 11.2) in nine patients. *Am J Med Genet* **24**:393, 1986.
328. Stratton RF, Dobyns WB, Greenberg F, DeSana JB, Moore C, Fidone G, Runge GH, Feldman P, Sekhon GS, Pauli RM, Ledbetter DH: Interstitial deletion of (17)(p11.2p11.2): Report of six additional patients with a new chromosome deletion syndrome. *Am J Med Genet* **24**:321, 1986.
329. Greenberg F, Lewis RA, Potocki L, Glaze D, Parke J, Killian J, Murphy MA, Williamson D, Brown F, Dutton R, McCluggage C, Friedman E, Sulek M, Lupski JR: Multi-disciplinary clinical study of Smith-Magenis syndrome (deletion 17p11.2). *Am J Med Genet* **62**:247, 1996.
330. Chen K-S, Gunaratne PH, Hoheisel JD, Young IG, Gabor Miklos GL, Greenberg F, Shaffer LG, Campbell HD, Lupski JR: The human homologue of the *Drosophila melanogaster* flightless-1 gene (*fli1*) maps within the Smith-Magenis microdeletion critical region in 17p11.2. *Am J Hum Genet* **56**:175, 1995.
331. Juyal RC, Finucane B, Shaffer LG, Lupski JR, Greenberg F, Scott CI, Baldini A, Patel PI: Apparent mosaicism for del(17)(p11.2) ruled out by fluorescence in situ hybridization in a Smith-Magenis syndrome patient. *Am J Med Genet* **59**:406, 1995.
332. Juyal RC, Greenberg F, Mengden GA, Lupski JR, Trask BJ, van den Engh G, Lindsay EA, Christy H, Chen K-S, Baldini A, Shaffer LG, Patel PI: Smith-Magenis syndrome deletion: A case with equivocal cytogenetic findings resolved by fluorescence in situ hybridization. *Am J Med Genet* **58**:286, 1995.

333. Chen K-S, Potocki L, Lupski JR: The Smith-Magenis syndrome (del(17)p11.2): Clinical review and molecular advances. *MRDD Res Rev* **2**:122, 1996.
334. Ligon AH, Beaudet AL, Shaffer LG: Simultaneous, multilocus FISH analysis for detection of microdeletions in the diagnostic evaluation of developmental delay and mental retardation. *Am J Hum Genet* **61**:51, 1997.
335. Jones KL, Gilbert EF, Kaveggia EG, Opitz JM: The Miller-Dieker syndrome. *Pediatrics* **66**:277, 1980.
336. Dobyns WB, Stratton RF, Greenberg F: Syndromes with lissencephaly. I: Miller-Dieker and Norman-Roberts syndromes and isolated lissencephaly. *Am J Med Genet* **18**:509, 1984.
337. Dobyns WB, Reiner O, Carrozzo R, Ledbetter DH: Lissencephaly: A human brain malformation associated with deletion of the L1S1 gene located at chromosome 17p13. *JAMA* **270**:2838, 1993.
338. Barth PG: Disorders of neuronal migration. *Can J Neurol Sci* **14**:1, 1987.
339. Dobyns WB: The neurogenetics of lissencephaly. *Neurol Clin* **7**:89, 1989.
340. Dobyns WB, Elias ER, Newlin AC, Pagon RA, Ledbetter DH: Causal heterogeneity in isolated lissencephaly. *Neurology* **42**:1375, 1992.
341. Stratton RF, Dobyns WB, Airhart SD, Ledbetter DH: New chromosome syndrome: Miller-Dieker syndrome and monosomy 17p13. *Hum Genet* **67**:193, 1984.
342. des Portes V, Pinard JM, Billuart P, Vinet MC, Koulakoff A, Carrie A, Gelot A, Dupuis E, Motte J, Berwald-Netter Y, Catala M, Kahn A, Beldjord C, Chelly J: A novel CNS gene required for neuronal migration and involved in X-linked subcortical laminar heterotopia and lissencephaly syndrome. *Cell* **92**:51, 1998.
343. Gleeson JG, Allen KM, Fox JW, Lamperti ED, Berkovic S, Scheffer I, Cooper EC, Dobyns WB, Minnerath SR, Ross ME, Walsh CA: Doublecortin, a brain-specific gene mutated in human X-linked lissencephaly and double cortex syndrome, encodes a putative signaling protein. *Cell* **92**:63, 1998.
344. Ledbetter SA, Kuwano A, Dobyns WB, Ledbetter DH: Microdeletions of chromosome 17p13 as a cause of isolated lissencephaly. *Am J Hum Genet* **50**:182, 1992.
345. van Tuinen P, Dobyns WB, Rich DC, Summers KM, Robinson TJ, Nakamura Y, Ledbetter DH: Molecular detection of microscopic and submicroscopic deletions associated with Miller-Dieker syndrome. *Am J Hum Genet* **43**:587, 1988.
346. Ledbetter DH, Ledbetter SA, van Tuinen P, Summers KM, Robinson TJ, Nakamura Y, Wolff R, White R, Barker DF, Wallace MR, Collins FS, Dobyns WB: Molecular dissection of a contiguous gene syndrome: Frequent submicroscopic deletions, evolutionarily conserved sequences, and a hypomethylated "island" in the Miller-Dieker chromosome region. *Proc Natl Acad Sci U S A* **86**:136, 1989.
347. Pilz DT, Macha ME, Precht KS, Smith ACM, Dobyns WB, Ledbetter DH: Fluorescence in situ hybridization analysis with *LIS1* specific probes reveals a high deletion mutation rate in isolated lissencephaly sequence. *Genetics* **1**:29, 1998.
348. Reiner O, Carrozzo R, Shen Y, Wehnert M, Faustinella F, Dobyns WB, Caskey CT, Ledbetter DH: Isolation of a Miller-Dieker lissencephaly gene containing G protein β subunit-like repeats. *Nature* **364**:717, 1993.
349. Chong SS, Pack SD, Roschke AV, Tanigami A, Carrozzo R, Smith ACM, Dobyns WB, Ledbetter DH: A revision of the lissencephaly and Miller-Dieker syndrome critical regions in chromosome 17p13.3. *Hum Mol Genet* **6**:147, 1997.
350. Sapir T, Eisenstein M, Burgess HA, Horesh D, Cahana A, Aoki J, Hattori M, Arai H, Inoue K, Reiner O: Analysis of lissencephaly-causing *LIS1* mutations. *Eur J Biochem* **266**:1, 1999.
351. Sapir T, Cahana A, Seger R, Nekhai S, Reiner O: *LIS1* is a microtubule-associated phosphoprotein. *Eur J Biochem* **264**:1, 1999.
352. Pilz DT, Matsumoto N, Minnerath S, Mills P, Gleeson JG, Allen KM, Walsh CA, Barkovich AJ, Dobyns WB, Ledbetter DH, Ross ME: *LIS1* and XLIS (DCX) mutations cause most classical lissencephaly, but different patterns of malformation. *Hum Mol Genet* **7**:2029, 1998.
353. Hirotsune S, Fleck MW, Gambello MJ, Bix GJ, Chen A, Clark GD, Ledbetter DH, McBain CJ, Wynshaw-Boris A: Graded reduction of Pafah1b1 (*Lis1*) activity results in neuronal migration defects and early embryonic lethality. *Nat Genet* **19**:333, 1998.
354. Pollin TI, Dobyns WB, Crowe CA, Ledbetter DH, Bailey-Wilson JE, Smith ACM: Risk of abnormal pregnancy outcome in carriers of balanced reciprocal translocations involving the Miller-Dieker syndrome (MDS) critical region in chromosome 17p13.3. *Am J Med Genet* **85**:369, 1999.
355. Nigro CL, Chong SS, Smith ACM, Dobyns WB, Carrozzo R, Ledbetter DH: Point mutations and an intragenic deletion in *LIS1*, the lissencephaly causative gene in isolated lissencephaly sequence and Miller-Dieker syndrome. *Hum Mol Genet* **6**:157, 1997.
356. Alagille D, Habib EC, Thomassin N: L'atresiedes voies biliaires intrahpatique avec voies biliaires extrahepatiques permeables chez l'enfant. A propos de 25 observations. *Editions Med Flammarion (Paris)* **301**:318, 1969.
357. Krantz ID, Colliton RP, Genin A, Rand EB, Li L, Piccoli DA, Spinner NB: Spectrum and frequency of jagged1 (*JAG1*) mutations in Alagille syndrome patients and their families. *Am J Hum Genet* **62**:1361, 1998.
358. Emerick KM, Rand EB, Goldmuntz E, Krantz ID, Spinner NB, Piccoli DA: Features of Alagille syndrome in 92 patients: Frequency and relation to prognosis. *Hepatology* **29**:822, 1999.
359. Danks DM, Campbell PE, Jack I, Rogers J, Smith AL: Studies of the aetiology of neonatal hepatitis and biliary atresia. *Arch Dis Child* **52**:360, 1977.
360. Byrne JLB, Harrod MJE, Friedman JM, Howard-Peebles PN: del(20p) with manifestations of arteriohepatic dysplasia. *Am J Med Genet* **24**:673, 1986.
361. Anad F, Burn J, Matthews D, Cross I, Davison BCC, Mueller R, Sands M, Lillington DM, Eastham E: Alagille syndrome and deletion of 20p. *J Med Genet* **27**:729, 1990.
362. Schnittger S, Hofers C, Heidemann P, Beermann F, Hansmann I: Molecular and cytogenetic analysis of an interstitial 20p deletion associated with syndromic intrahepatic ductular hypoplasia (Alagille syndrome). *Hum Genet* **83**:239, 1989.
363. Desmaze C, Deleuze JF, Dutrillaux AM, Thomas G, Hadchouel M, Aurias A: Screening of microdeletions of chromosome 20 in patients with Alagille syndrome. *J Med Genet* **29**:233, 1993.
364. Oda T, Elkahloun AG, Pike BL, Okajimi K, Krantz ID, Genin A, Piccoli DA, Meltzer PS, Spinner NB, Collins FS, Chandrasekharappa SC: Mutations in the human *Jagged1* gene are responsible for Alagille syndrome. *Nat Genet* **16**:235, 1997.
365. Li L, Krantz ID, Deng Y, Genin A, Banta AB, Collins CC, Qi M, Trask BJ, Kuo WL, Cochran J, Costa T, Pierpont MEM, Rand EB, Piccoli DA, Hood L, Spinner NB: Alagille syndrome is caused by mutations in human *Jagged1*, which encodes a ligand for Notch1. *Nat Genet* **16**:243, 1997.
366. Krantz ID, Smith R, Colliton RP, Tinkel H, Zackai EH, Piccoli DA, Goldmuntz E, Spinner NB: Jagged 1 mutations in patients ascertained with isolated congenital heart defects. *Am J Med Genet* **84**:56, 1999.
367. DiGeorge AM: Discussions on a new concept of the cellular base of immunology. *J Pediatr* **69**:907, 1965.
368. Conley ME, Beckwith JB, Mancer JFK, Tenckhoff L: The spectrum of the DiGeorge syndrome. *J Pediatr* **94**:883, 1979.
369. Devriendt K, Fryns JP, Mortier G, van Thienen MN, Keymolen K: The annual incidence of DiGeorge/velocardiofacial syndrome. *J Med Genet* **35**:789, 1998.
370. Goldberg R, Motzkin B, Marion R, Scambler PJ, Shprintzen RJ: Velocardiofacial syndrome. A review of 120 patients. *Am J Med Genet* **45**:313, 1993.
371. Stevens CA, Carey JC, Shigeoka AO: DiGeorge anomaly and velocardiofacial syndrome. *Pediatrics* **85**:526, 1990.
372. Greenberg F: What defines DiGeorge anomaly? *J Pediatr* **115**:412, 1989.
373. Scambler PJ: Deletions of human chromosome 22 and associated birth defects. *Curr Opin Genet Dev* **3**:432, 1993.
374. Berend SA, Spikes AS, Kashork CD, Wu JM, Daw SC, Scambler PJ, Shaffer LG: A dual-probe fluorescence in situ hybridization (FISH) assay for detecting deletions associated with VCFS/DiGeorge syndrome I and DiGeorge syndrome II loci. *Am J Med Genet* **91**:313, 2000.
375. Carey AH, Kelly D, Halford S, Wadey R, Wilson D, Goodship J, Burn J, Paul T, Sharkey A, Dumanski J, Nordenskjold M, Williamson R, Scambler PJ: Molecular genetic study of the frequency of monosomy 22q11 in DiGeorge syndrome. *Am J Hum Genet* **51**:964, 1992.
376. Driscoll DA, Budarf ML, Emanuel BS: A genetic etiology for DiGeorge syndrome: Consistent deletions and microdeletions of 22q11. *Am J Hum Genet* **50**:924, 1992.
377. Wilson DI, Cross IE, Goodship JA, Brown J, Scambler PJ, Bain HH, Taylor JFN, Walsh K, Bankier A, Burn J, Wolstenholme J: A prospective cytogenetic study of 36 cases of DiGeorge syndrome. *Am J Hum Genet* **51**:957, 1992.
378. Driscoll DA, Spinner NB, Budarf ML, McDonald-McGinn DM, Zackai EH, Goldberg RB, Shprintzen RJ, Saal HM, Zonana J, Jones

MC, Mascarello JT, Emanuel BS: Deletions and microdeletions of 22q11.2 in velocardiofacial syndrome. *Am J Med Genet* **44**:261, 1992.

379. Lindsay EA, Halford S, Wadey R, Scambler PJ, Baldini A: Molecular cytogenetic characterization of the DiGeorge syndrome region using fluorescence in situ hybridization. *Genomics* **17**:403, 1993.
380. Desmaze C, Scambler P, Prieur M, Halford S, le Deist F, Aurias A: Routine diagnosis of DiGeorge syndrome by fluorescent in situ hybridization. *Hum Genet* **90**:663, 1993.
381. Scambler PJ, Kelly D, Lindsay EA, Williamson R, Goldberg R, Shprintzen RJ, Wilson DI, Goodship JA, Cross IE, Burn J: Velocardiofacial syndrome associated with chromosome 22 deletions encompassing the DiGeorge locus. *Lancet* **339**:1138, 1992.
382. Kelly D, Goldberg R, Wilson D, Lindsay EA, Carey A, Goodship J, Burn J, Cross I, Shprintzen RJ, Scambler PJ: Confirmation that the velocardiofacial syndrome is associated with haploinsufficiency of genes at chromosome 22q11. *Am J Med Genet* **45**:308, 1993.
383. Edelmann L, Pandita RK, Morrow BE: Low-copy repeats mediate the common 3-Mb deletion in patients with velocardiofacial syndrome. *Am J Hum Genet* **64**:1076, 1999.
384. Edelmann L, Pandita RK, Spiteri E, Funke B, Goldberg R, Palanisamy N, Chaganti RS, Magenis E, Shprintzen RJ, Morrow BE: A common molecular basis for rearrangement disorders on chromosome 22q11. *Hum Mol Genet* **8**:1157, 1999.
385. Lindsay EA, Botta A, Jurecic V, Carattini-Rivera S, Cheah Y-C, Rosenblatt HM, Bradley A, Baldini A: Congenital heart disease in mice deficient for the DiGeorge syndrome region. *Nature* **401**:379, 1999.
386. Bouchard TJ, Lykken DT, McGue M, Segal NL, Tellegen A: Source of human psychological differences: The Minnesota study of twins reared apart. *Science* **250**:223, 1990.
387. Brunner HG, Nelen M, Breakefield XO, Ropers H-H, van Oost BA: Abnormal behavior associated with a point mutation in the structural gene for monoamine oxidase A. *Science* **262**:578, 1993.
388. Brown JR, Ye H, Bronson RT, Dikkes P, Greenberg ME: A defect in nurturing in mice lacking the immediate early gene *fosB*. *Cell* **86**:297, 1996.
389. Smith ACM, Dykens E, Greenberg F: Behavioral phenotype of Smith-Magenis syndrome (del 17p11.2). *Am J Hum Genet* **81**:179, 1998.
390. Dykens EM, Smith ACM: Distinctiveness and correlates of maladaptive behavior in children and adolescents with Smith-Magenis syndrome. *J Intellect Disabil Res* **42**:481, 1998.
391. Dykens EM, Finucane BM, Gayley C: Brief report: Cognitive and behavioral profiles in persons with Smith-Magenis syndrome. *J Autism Dev Disord* **27**:203, 1997.
392. Yan W, Jacobsen LK, Krasnewich DM, Guan X-Y, Lenane MC, Paul SP, Dalwadi HN, Zhang H, Long RT, Kumra S, Martin BM, Scambler PJ, Trent JM, Sidransky E, Ginns EI, Rapoport JL: Chromosome 22q11.2 interstitial deletions among childhood-onset schizophrenics and "multidimensionally impaired." *Am J Med Genet* **81**:41, 1998.
393. Karayiorgou M, Morris MA, Morrow B, Shprintzen RJ, Goldberg R, Borrow J, Gos A, Nestadt G, Wolyniec PS, Lasseter VK, Eisen H, Childs B, Kazazian HH, Kucherlapati R, Antonarakis SE, Pulver AE, Housman DE: Schizophrenia susceptibility associated with interstitial deletions of chromosome 22q11. *Proc Natl Acad Sci U S A* **92**:7612, 1995.
394. Greer MK, Brown FR, III, Shashidhar Pai G, Choudry SH, Klein AJ: Cognitive, adaptive, and behavioral characteristics of Williams syndrome. *Am J Med Genet* **74**:521, 1997.
395. Dilts CV, Morris CA, Leonard CO: Hypothesis for development of a behavioral phenotype in Williams syndrome. *Am J Med Genet* **6**:126, 1990.
396. Estabrooks LL, Lamb AN, Aylsworth AS, Callanan NP, Rao KW: Molecular characterisation of chromosome 4p deletions resulting in Wolf-Hirschhorn syndrome. *J Med Genet* **31**:103, 1994.
397. Overhauser J, Huang X, Gersh M, Wilson W, McMahon J, Bengtsson U, Rojas K, Meyer M, Wasmuth JJ: Molecular and phenotypic mapping of the short arm of chromosome 5: Sublocalization of the critical region for the cri du chat syndrome. *Hum Mol Genet* **3**:247, 1994.
398. Christ LA, Crowe CA, Micale MA, Conroy JM, Schwartz S: Chromosome breakage hotspots and delineation of the critical region for the 9p-deletion syndrome. *Am J Hum Genet* **65**:1387, 1999.
399. Jones C, Penny L, Mattina T, Yu S, Baker E, Voullaire L, Langdon WY, Sutherland GR, Richards RI, Tunnacliffe A: Association of a chromosome deletion syndrome with a fragile site within the proto-oncogene *CBL2*. *Nature* **376**:145, 1995.

399a. Jones C, Müllenbach R, Grossfeld P, Auer R, Favier R, Chien K, James M, Tunnacliffe A, Cotter F: Co-localisation of CCG repeats and chromosome deletion breakpoints in Jacobsen syndrome: Evidence for a common mechanism of chromosome breakage. *Hum Mol Genet* **9**:1201, 2000.

400. Wilkie AOM, Lamb J, Harris PC, Finney RD, Higgs DR: A truncated human chromosome 16 associated with α-thalassaemia is stabilized by addition of telomeric repeat $(TTAGGG)_n$. *Nature* **346**:868, 1990.
401. Morin GB: Recognition of a chromosome truncation site associated with α-thalassaemia by human telomerase. *Nature* **353**:454, 1991.
402. Meltzer PS, Guan X-Y, Trent JM: Telomere capture stabilizes chromosome breakage. *Nat Genet* **4**:252, 1993.
403. National Institutes of Health and Institute of Molecular Medicine Collaboration: A complete set of human telomeric probes and their clinical application. *Nat Genet* **14**:86, 1996.
404. Knight SJL, Horsley SW, Regan P, Lawrie NM, Maher EJ, Cardy DLN, Flint J, Kearney L: Development and clinical application of an innovative fluorescence in situ hybridization technique which detects submicroscopic rearrangements involving telomeres. *Eur J Hum Genet* **5**:1, 1997.
405. Precht KS, Lese CM, Spiro RP, Huttenlocher PR, Johnston KM, Baker JC, Christian SL, Kittikamron K, Ledbetter DH: Two 22q telomere deletions serendipitously detected by FISH. *J Med Genet* **35**:939, 1998.
406. Horsley SW, Knight SJL, Nixon J, Huson S, Fitchett M, Boone RA, Hilton-Jones D, Flint J, Kearney L: Del(18p) shown to be a cryptic translocation using a multiprobe FISH assay for subtelomeric chromosome rearrangements. *J Med Genet* **35**:722, 1998.
407. Lupski JR: Genomic disorders: Structural features of the genome can lead to DNA rearrangements and human disease traits. *Trends Genet* **14**:145, 1998.
408. Lupski JR, Weinstock GM: Chromosome rearrangements, in de Bruijn FJ, Lupski JR, Weinstock GM (eds): *Bacterial Genomes; Physical Structure and Analysis*. New York, Chapman and Hall, 1998, p 112.
409. Pentao L, Wise CA, Chinault AC, Patel PI, Lupski JR: Charcot-Marie-Tooth type 1A duplication appears to arise from recombination at repeat sequences flanking the 1.5-Mb monomer unit. *Nat Genet* **2**:292, 1992.
410. Reiter LT, Murakami T, Koeuth T, Gibbs RA, Lupski JR: The human *COX10* gene is disrupted during homologous recombination between the 24-kb proximal and distal CMT1A-REPs. *Hum Mol Genet* **6**:1595, 1997.
411. Chance PF, Abbas N, Lensch MW, Pentao L, Roa BB, Patel PI, Lupski JR: Two autosomal dominant neuropathies result from reciprocal DNA duplication/deletion of a region on chromosome 17. *Hum Mol Genet* **3**:223, 1994.
412. Reiter LT, Murakami T, Koeuth T, Pentao L, Muzny DM, Gibbs RA, Lupski JR: A recombination hotspot responsible for two inherited peripheral neuropathies is located near a *mariner* transposon-like element. *Nat Genet* **12**:288, 1996.
413. Kiyosawa H, Chance PF: Primate origin of the CMT1A-REP repeat and analysis of a putative transposon-associated recombinational hotspot. *Hum Mol Genet* **5**:745, 1996.
414. Boerkoel CF, Inoue K, Reiter LT, Warner LE, Lupski JR: Molecular mechanisms for CMT1A duplication and HNPP deletion. *Ann N Y Acad Sci* **883**:22, 1999.
415. Lopes J, Ravise N, Vandenberghe A, Palau F, Ionasescu V, Mayers M, Levy N, Wood N, Tachi N, Bouche P, Latour P, Ruberg M, Brice A, LeGuern E: Fine mapping of de novo CMT1A and HNPP rearrangements within CMT1A-REPs evidences two distinct sex-dependent mechanisms and candidate sequences involved in recombination. *Hum Mol Genet* **7**:141, 1998.
416. Reiter LT, Hastings PJ, Nelis E, de Jonghe P, van Broeckhoven C, Lupski JR: Human meiotic recombination products revealed by sequencing a hotspot for homologous strand exchange in multiple HNPP deletion patients. *Am J Hum Genet* **62**:1023, 1998.
417. Lopes J, Tardieu S, Silander K, Blair I, Vandenberghe A, Palau F, Ruberg M, Brice A, LeGuern E: Homologous DNA exchanges in humans can be explained by the yeast double-strand break repair model: A study of 17p11.2 rearrangements associated with CMT1A and HNPP. *Hum Mol Genet* **8**:2285, 1999.
418. Lupski JR: Charcot-Marie-Tooth polyneuropathy: Duplication, gene dosage, and genetic heterogeneity. *Pediatr Res* **45**:159, 1999.
419. Christian SL, Fantes JA, Mewborn SK, Huang B, Ledbetter DH: Large genomic duplicons map to sites of instability in the

Prader-Willi/Angelman syndrome chromosome region (15q11-q13). *Hum Mol Genet* **8**:1025, 1999.

420. Lupski JR, Roth JR, Weinstock GM: Chromosomal duplications in bacteria, fruit flies, and humans. *Am J Hum Genet* **58**:21, 1996.
421. Woodward K, Malcolm S: Proteolipid protein gene. Pelizaeus-Merzbacher disease in humans and neurodegeneration in mice. *Trends Genet* **15**:125, 1999.
422. Cremers FPM, Pfeiffer RA, van de Pol TJR, Hofker M, Kruse TA, Wieringa B, Ropers H-H: An interstitial duplication of the X chromosome in a male allows physical fine mapping of probes from the Xq13-q22 region. *Hum Genet* **77**:23, 1987.
423. Ellis D, Malcolm S: Proteolipid protein gene dosage effect in Pelizaeus-Merzbacher disease. *Nat Genet* **6**:333, 1994.
424. Inoue K, Osaka H, Sugiyama N, Kawanishi C, Onishi H, Nezu A, Kimura K, Kimura S, Yamada Y, Kosaki K: A duplicated *PLP* gene causing Pelizaeus-Merzbacher disease detected by comparative multiplex PCR. *Am J Hum Genet* **58**:32, 1996.
425. Woodward K, Kendall E, Vetrie D, Malcolm S: Pelizaeus-Merzbacher disease: Identification of Xq22 proteolipid-protein duplications and characterization of breakpoints by interphase FISH. *Am J Hum Genet* **63**:207, 1998.
426. Mimault C, Giraud G, Courtois V, Cailloux F, Boire JY, Dastugue B, Boespflug-Tanguy O: Proteolipoprotein gene analysis in 82 patients with sporadic Pelizaeus-Merzbacher disease: Duplications, the major cause of the disease, originate more frequently in male germ cells, but point mutations do not. The Clinical European Network on Brain Dysmyelinating Disease. *Am J Hum Genet* **65**:360, 1999.

426a. Shaffer LG, Lupski JR: Molecular mechanisms for constitutional chromosomal rearrangements in humans. *Annu Rev Genet*, **34**:297, 2000.

427. Potocki L, Chen K-S, Koeuth T, Killian J, Iannaccone T, Shapira SK, Kashork CD, Spikes AS, Shaffer LG, Lupski JR: DNA rearrangements on both homologues of chromosome 17 in a mildly delayed individual with a family history of autosomal dominant carpal tunnel syndrome. *Am J Hum Genet* **64**:471, 1999.
428. Bacino CA, Kashork CD, Davino NA, Shaffer LG: Detection of a cryptic translocation in a family with mental retardation using FISH and telomere region-specific probes. *Am J Med Genet* **92**:250, 2000.

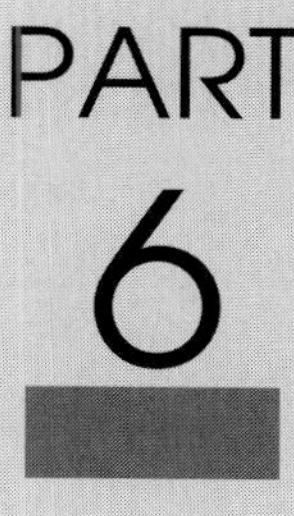

DIAGNOSTIC APPROACHES

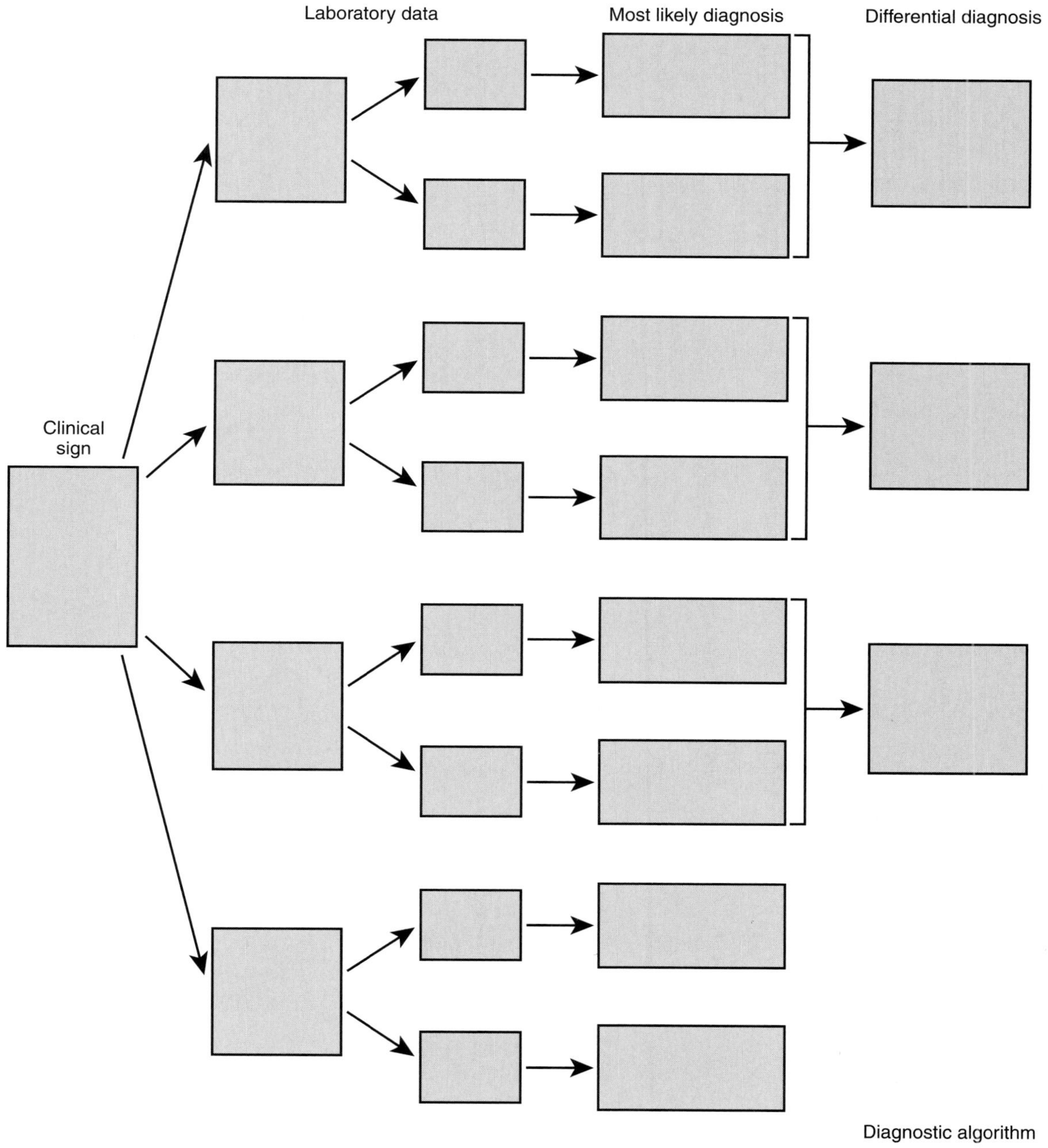

Laboratory data

Most likely diagnosis

Differential diagnosis

Clinical sign

Diagnostic algorithm

CHAPTER 66

Clinical Phenotypes: Diagnosis/Algorithms

Jean-Marie Saudubray ▪ Christiane Charpentier

1. Despite the abundance of new case reports, there is considerable evidence that many inherited metabolic disorders remain undiagnosed or misdiagnosed. There are a number of reasons, the most important of which is the fact that many physicians are not aware of most of the highly specific symptoms or syndromes that are excellent keys to the diagnosis and consequently do not perform comprehensive examinations.
2. From a clinical point of view, all the inborn errors of metabolism can be divided into two large categories:

   Category 1. Diseases that involve only one functional system or affect only one organ or anatomic system. Presenting symptoms are uniform, and diagnosis is usually easy even when the basic biochemical lesion gives rise to systemic consequences.

   Category 2. Diseases in which the basic biochemical lesion either affects a metabolic pathway common to a large number of cells or organs or is restricted to one organ but gives rise to humoral and systemic consequences. Presenting symptoms are very diverse. The central nervous system is frequently involved in advanced disease, and diagnosis may be rendered difficult by the presence of secondary abnormalities. This category includes most inborn errors of intermediary metabolism, diseases of intracellular trafficking, and lysosomal disorders.
3. The second category can be subdivided on the basis of pathophysiology into three groups that are useful for diagnosis.

   Group 1. Diseases that disturb the synthesis or catabolism of complex molecules (lysosomal and peroxisomal disorders; disturbances of intracellular trafficking and secretory protein processing). Clinical symptoms are permanent, progressive, independent of intercurrent events, and unrelated to food intake.

   Group 2. Inborn errors of intermediary metabolism that lead to acute or progressive intoxication caused by accumulation of toxic compounds proximal to the metabolic block. The group includes aminoacidopathies, most organic acidurias, congenital urea cycle defects, and sugar intolerances. In these conditions, a symptom-free interval is followed by clinical signs of acute or chronic intoxication and by recurrent metabolic disturbances. Clinical expression is often late in onset and intermittent. Diagnosis is easy, relying mainly on chromatography of plasma and urine amino acids or organic acids. Treatment involves removing the toxin.

   Group 3. "Energy deficiency" disorders, in which symptoms are caused at least partly by a deficiency in energy production or utilization resulting from an inborn error of intermediary metabolism in liver, myocardium, muscle, or brain. This group includes glycogenosis, gluconeogenesis defects, congenital lactic acidemias, fatty acid oxidation defects, and mitochondrial respiratory chain disorders. These diseases present an overlapping clinical spectrum, and manifestations sometimes result from accumulation of toxic compounds as well as from the deficiency in energy production. Common symptoms include hypoglycemia, hyperlactacidemia, severe generalized hypotonia, myopathy, cardiomyopathy, failure to thrive, cardiac failure, circulatory collapse, sudden infant death syndrome, and congenital malformations, the last suggesting that the abnormal process affected fetal energy pathways.
4. The clinical diagnostic circumstances observed in inborn errors of metabolism are divided in this chapter into eight categories: presentation in the neonatal period, intermittent late-onset acute presentation, progressive neurologic symptoms, ocular symptoms, skin symptoms, hematologic symptoms, visceral symptoms or syndromes, and endocrine symptoms. The following outline expands these categories and constitutes a "table of contents" for the chapter. The approach is developed in the text and tables.

   I. Presentation in the Neonatal Period: "Neonatal Metabolic Distress"
      - A. Identification of children at risk
      - B. Initial approach
      - C. Clinical approach to etiology in metabolic diseases (Table 66-2, 66-3)
      - D. Type I: neurologic deterioration, intoxication type, with ketosis
      - E. Type II: neurologic deterioration, intoxication type, with ketoacidosis: organic acidurias
      - F. Type III: lactic acidosis with neurologic deterioration, "energy-deficiency" type: congenital lactic acidosis
      - G. Type IV
        1. Type IVa: neurologic deterioration, intoxication type, with hyperammonemia and without ketoacidosis: urea cycle defects
        2. Type IVb: neurologic deterioration, energy-deficiency type, without ketoacidosis and without hyperammonemia
      - H. Type V: predominant liver presentation
        1. Type Va: hypoglycemia with hepatomegaly
        2. Type Vb: liver failure with hepatocellular necrosis
        3. Type Vc: cholestatic jaundice
        4. Type Vd: hepatosplenomegaly and storage signs

I. Intrauterine growth retardation
J. Babies born to mothers with acute fatty liver of pregnancy and HELLP syndrome

II. Intermittent Late-Onset Acute Presentation
A. Recurrent attacks of coma, strokes, or vomiting with lethargy, ataxia, or psychiatric symptoms (Table 66-4, 66-5, 66-6)
B. Metabolic acidosis (Table 66-7)
C. Ketosis (Table 66-9)
D. Hyperlactacidemias (Table 66-10)
E. Hypoglycemia: general approach (Table 66-11)
F. Hypoketotic hypoglycemias due to inborn errors of ketogenesis (Fig. 66-1)
G. Reye syndrome (Table 66-12, 66-13)
H. Sudden infant death syndrome (Table 66-14)
I. Recurrent attacks of dehydration (Table 66-15)
J. Exercise intolerance and recurrent myoglobinuria (Table 66-16)
K. Abdominal pain (recurrent attacks) (Table 66-17)
L. Cardiac disorders (acute cardiac failure, heartbeat disorders) (Table 66-18)
M. Bone crisis (Table 66-19)

III. Progressive Neurologic Symptoms
A. Progressive neurologic and mental deterioration
1. Part 1: early in infancy (1 to 12 months) (Tables 66-21, 66-22, 66-23)
2. Part 2: late infancy to early childhood (1 to 5 years) (Tables 66-24, 66-25, 66-26, 66-27)
3. Part 3: late childhood to adolescence (5 to 15 years) (Tables 66-28, 66-29, 66-30, 66-31, 66-32)
4. Part 4: onset in adulthood (15 years to more than 60 years) (Table 66-33)
B. Extrapyramidal signs (dyskinesia, dystonia, choreoathetosis, parkinsonism) (Table 66-34)
C. Deafness (Table 66-35)
D. Hypotonia in the neonatal period and in early infancy (Table 66-36) (see also I. "Acute Symptoms in the Neonatal Period: Neonatal Metabolic Distress")
E. Hyperventilation attacks (Table 66-37)

IV. Ocular Symptoms
A. Cataracts (Table 66-38)
B. Corneal opacity (Table 66-39)
C. Macular cherry red spot (Table 66-40)
D. Retinitis pigmentosa (Table 66-41)
E. Ectopia lentis

V. Skin Symptoms
A. Coarse facies (Table 66-42)
B. Skin lesions (vesicobullous lesions, rashes, photosensitivity, hyperkeratosis, ichthyosis, ulcers, nodules, laxity) (Tables 66-43, 66-44, 66-45, 66-46)
C. Angiokeratoma (Table 66-47)
D. Alopecia (Table 66-48)

VI. Hematologic Symptoms
A. Nonregenerative anemias (macrocytic) (Table 66-49)
B. Nonmacrocytic anemias (due to hemolysis or combined mechanisms) (Table 66-50)
C. Pancytopenia, neutropenia, thrombocytopenia (Table 66-51)
D. Increased neutrophil granulocytes
E. Bleeding tendency (Table 66-52)
F. Acanthocytosis (Table 66-53)

VII. Visceral Symptoms or Syndromes (intestine, liver, heart, lung, kidney)
A. Chronic diarrhea (with failure to thrive, poor feeding, anorexia, hypotonia) (Table 66-54)
B. Hepatomegaly and hepatosplenomegaly (Table 66-55)
C. Liver failure, ascites, edema (Table 66-56)
D. Cardiomyopathy (Table 66-57)
E. Interstitial pulmonary infiltrates (Table 66-58)
F. Tubulopathy (renal Fanconi syndrome and tubular acidosis) (Table 66-59)
G. Renal symptoms (other than tubulopathy) (Table 66-60)

VIII. Endocrine symptoms
A. Diabetes
B. Hypoparathyroidism
C. Primary adrenal insufficiency
D. Growth hormone deficiency
E. Hypogonadism and sterility

EDITORS' NOTE

This chapter is version 2 of an experiment, the first version appeared in the 7th edition of this book. It has been prepared by authors whose clinical experience exceeds that of almost all other persons in the world in their area. As required by its nature, the chapter presents categorical approaches to sick patients for purposes of diagnosis and treatment. However, the patients have disorders in complex, overlapping, noncategorical biologic systems. Accordingly, the authors, the readers, and the editors are currently faced with the classic dilemma of balancing the practicality of categorical thinking against the reality of biologic variation. Compromises were made in seeking that balance. Many of the disorders mentioned in this chapter are topics of extended descriptions in other chapters.

INTRODUCTION

Over 300 human diseases due to inborn errors of metabolism are now recognized, and this number is constantly increasing as new concepts and techniques become available for identifying biochemical phenotypes. However, the incidence of inborn errors may well be underestimated, because diagnostic errors are frequent. Despite the relative abundance of new case reports, there is considerable evidence that many of these disorders remain undetected or misdiagnosed.

A number of factors conspire to make the clinical diagnosis of inborn errors of metabolism difficult. Because individual inborn errors are rare, many physicians do not consider them in acute situations until more common conditions have been ruled out. Moreover, blood and urine samples may be unrevealing unless collected at the right time in relation to an acute episode, because many disorders affecting inborn metabolism produce only intermittent abnormalities.

Neonates have only a limited repertoire of responses to severe overwhelming illness, and the predominant clinical signs and symptoms are nonspecific: poor feeding, lethargy, failure to thrive, and so forth. When infants with undiagnosed inborn errors die, therefore, their deaths are often attributed to sepsis (a common accompaniment of metabolic disorders) or to another common cause. Classic autopsy findings in such cases are also often nonspecific and unrevealing.

Many general practitioners and pediatricians think of inborn errors of metabolism only in relation to certain nonspecific clinical circumstances, such as psychomotor retardation or seizures, and are ignorant of most of the highly specific symptoms that are excellent clues to the diagnosis. Another common mistake is to confuse a "syndrome" — which is a set of symptoms that may have more than one cause — with a specific etiology.

There is still an important gap between clinical description and biologic understanding: Many well-known heritable disorders registered in McKusick catalogues have not been considered from a pathophysiological perspective or subjected to comprehensive biologic evaluation. Examples of well-known syndromes whose biochemical basis has been determined are Zellweger syndrome, in which a generalized peroxisomal dysfunction has been found;[1] Sjögren-Larsson syndrome, now known to be associated with fatty alcohol oxidoreductase deficiency;[2] Canavan disease, now known to involve N-acetylaspartic aciduria;[3,4] and Smith-Lemli-Opitz syndrome, now known to be related to 7,8-dehydrocholesterol dehydrogenase deficiency.[5,5a,5b]

Although most genetic metabolic errors are transmitted as recessive traits, the small size of sibships in developed countries means they are usually encountered as isolated cases. It is important to remember that "hereditary" does not mean "congenital"; many patients have late-onset diseases that do not appear until childhood, adolescence, or even adulthood.

Detection of inborn errors of metabolism relies only in part on screening programs; it depends primarily on a high index of clinical suspicion and coordinated (integrated) access to expert laboratory services. This makes it an absolute necessity to teach primary care physicians a simple method of clinical screening and a protocol for collecting samples to use before initiating sophisticated metabolic investigations.

The growing complexity of such investigations requires close collaboration between physicians, geneticists, and biochemists to gather clinical data and biologic findings. Whenever possible, patients should be referred to specialized centers.

This chapter is an overview of the clinical keys to diagnosis of inherited metabolic disorders. It is largely based on our personal experience over 30 years with more than 1000 patients evaluated at the metabolic and genetic services at Hôpital Necker Enfants-Malades in Paris. Some parts of this chapter have appeared under different guises.[6–8]

CLINICAL CLASSIFICATION OF INBORN ERRORS OF METABOLISM

The vast majority of inborn errors of metabolism involve abnormalities in enzymes and transport proteins. However, all the metabolic disorders can be divided into the following two large categories:

Category 1. Disorders that either involve only one functional system (such as the endocrine system, immune system, coagulation factors, or lipoproteins) or affect only one organ or anatomic system (such as the intestine, renal tubules, erythrocytes, or connective tissue). Presenting symptoms are uniform (e.g., a bleeding tendency in coagulation factor defects or hemolytic anemia in defects of glycolysis), and the correct diagnosis is usually easy to guess even when the basic biochemical lesion gives rise to systemic consequences.

Category 2. Diseases in which the basic biochemical lesion either affects one metabolic pathway common to a large number of cells or organs (e.g., storage diseases due to lysosomal disorders, energy deficiency in mitochondrial disorders) or is restricted to one organ but gives rise to humoral and systemic consequences (e.g., hyperammonemia in urea cycle defects, hypoglycemia in hepatic glycogenosis). The diseases in this category have a great diversity of presenting symptoms. The central nervous system is often involved, and advanced disease can involve many secondary abnormalities that render diagnosis difficult. This category includes most of the inborn errors of intermediary metabolism (defects of carbohydrate, amino acid, or organic acid metabolism, whether primary or secondary to a disturbance of vitamin or metal homeostasis; energy mitochondrial disorders; purine and peroxisomal disorders), diseases of intracellular trafficking (endoplasmic reticulum and Golgi apparatus defects), and lysosomal disorders.

From a pathophysiological perspective, the disorders in this category can be divided into the following three diagnostically useful groups:

Group 1. Diseases that disturb the synthesis or catabolism of complex molecules. Symptoms are permanent, progressive, independent of intercurrent events, and not related to food intake.

All lysosomal disorders belong to this group. These deficiencies (also called storage disorders) lead to the progressive accumulation of undigested substrates, usually complex polymers that cannot be hydrolyzed normally. The polymers accumulate in lysosomes, where they can be seen by light or electron microscopy. The affected tissues are the ones in which the substance is normally catabolized in the largest amounts (circulating lymphocytes, fibroblasts, liver, spleen, conjunctiva, bone marrow, intestinal mucosa).

In peroxisomal biogenesis disorders, many anabolic functions are disturbed, including the biosynthesis of plasmalogens (a major myelin constituent), cholesterol, and bile acids. Generalized peroxisomal β-oxidation deficiency results in a variety of disturbances that are still poorly understood, in part because of an overlap in function between the peroxisomes and other organelles such as the mitochondria and the endoplasmic reticulum (ER). Whatever the exact pathophysiology, these multiple and complex biochemical abnormalities result in a striking disorder of neuronal migration, with malformations and severe neurologic dysfunction. In contrast to the case in lysosomal disorders, there is no intracellular accumulation of undigested polymers. A useful marker for diagnosis is the accumulation of very-long-chain fatty acids and phytanic acid in plasma and low plasmalogen content in membrane erythrocytes. Inborn errors of cholesterol biosynthesis have recently been described[5a,5b,9,10] and are closely related to peroxisome disorders. Their presentation as severe multiple malformations underscores the fact that cholesterol plays a crucial role in specific processes during embryonic development. Their diagnosis relies on the specific determination of low plasma cholesterol and on the plasma profile of cholesterol precursors.

Another group of disorders involves defects of intracellular trafficking and processing of proteins. This group includes alpha-1-antitrypsin deficiency and the congenital defects of glycosylation.[11–14] These disorders are difficult to demonstrate, because they do not resemble simple enzyme-deficiency states. Their diagnosis depends on the measurement of plasma levels of specific proteins, such as α-antitrypsin, glycosylated transferrin, thyroid-binding globulin, or total serum glycoproteins.

Group 2. Inborn errors of intermediary metabolism that lead to an acute or progressive intoxication from accumulation of toxic compounds proximal to the metabolic block. In this group are the aminoacidopathies (phenylketonuria, maple syrup urine disease, homocystinuria, tyrosinemia, etc.), most of the organic acidurias (methylmalonic, propionic, isovaleric, etc.), congenital urea cycle defects, and sugar intolerances (galactosemia, hereditary fructose intolerance). All the conditions in this group present clinical similarities, including a symptom-free interval; clinical signs of "intoxication," which may be either acute (vomiting, lethargy, coma, liver failure, or thromboembolic complications) or chronic (progressive developmental delay or ectopia lentis); and recurrent disturbances (acidosis, ketosis, hyperammonemia). Clinical expression is often late in onset and intermittent. Biologic diagnosis is easy and relies mostly on plasma and urine amino acid or organic acid chromatography. Treatment of these disorders requires removal of the toxin by special diets, exchange transfusion, and peritoneal dialysis or hemodialysis.

Group 3. Inborn errors of intermediary metabolism with symptoms due at least partly to a deficiency in energy production or utilization resulting from a defect in liver, myocardium, muscle, or brain. Included in this group are glycogenosis, gluconeogenesis defects, congenital lactic acidemias (deficiencies of pyruvate carboxylase and pyruvate dehydrogenase), fatty acid oxidation defects, and mitochondrial respiratory chain disorders. These diseases present an overlapping clinical spectrum that sometimes results from both accumulation of toxic compounds and deficient energy production. Symptoms common to this group include hypoglycemia, hyperlactacidemia, severe generalized hypotonia, myopathy, cardiomyopathy, failure to thrive, cardiac failure, circulatory collapse, sudden infant death syndrome (SIDS), and malformations (the last suggesting that the abnormal processes affect the fetal energetic pathways).[15] The recent abundance of reports on inborn errors of the respiratory chain emphasizes the amazing clinical diversity of these disorders and illustrates the ubiquitous role of energy processes at every age and in every organ.[16] Treatment of these disorders, if any, would require adequate energy replacement.

GENERAL CLINICAL CONSIDERATIONS

Age of Onset

Age of onset is a very important concern, not only because each disease has a typical age of onset but also because the mode of expression of a given inborn error of metabolism is closely related to stage of organ development. This is particularly true for inborn errors that involve the nervous system.[17]

Some disorders present at birth, suggesting that the pathologic process interfered with intrauterine development (e.g., peroxisome biogenesis disorders or cholesterol biosynthesis defects), whereas others appear postnatally after a symptom-free interval (e.g., urea cycle defects, maple syrup urine disease [MSUD]) that may extend until childhood or adolescence (e.g., Refsum disease), or even adulthood (e.g., adrenomyeloneuropathy). Variations in age of onset and severity of a given disease sometimes reflect allelic heterogeneity in the mutations, with a resultant wide range of residual enzymatic activity.

Dating the age of onset of a progressive metabolic disease can be difficult. We generally consider the age of onset to be the age at which the first symptom becomes clinically evident. That is easy to determine when the first symptom is acute, such as coma or acute ataxia, but it can be difficult to determine in slowly progressive disorders or when the acute signs are preceded by minor premonitory symptoms that may be missed or misdiagnosed.

Six periods, each corresponding to a specific developmental step, must be considered: birth (congenital), 1 day to 1 month (neonatal period), 1 to 12 months (early infancy), 1 to 5 years (late infancy to early childhood), 5 to 15 years (late childhood to adolescence), and beyond 15 years (adulthood).

Provocative Circumstances

Clinical signs in many inborn errors of intermediary metabolism can transiently or permanently worsen in response to exogenous factors. Table 66-1 lists the most frequent circumstances.

Clinical Diagnostic Circumstances in Inborn Errors of Metabolism

A great diversity of signs and symptoms can lead to diagnosis of inborn errors of metabolism. Besides systematic screening in the general population (as for phenylketonuria) or in at-risk families (in which diagnosis depends on specific biologic tests), there are four basic groups of clinical circumstances in which physicians are faced with metabolic disorders:

1. Acute symptoms in the neonatal period, or so-called metabolic distress (Part I)
2. Late-onset acute and intermittent symptoms (Part II)

Table 66-1 Most Frequent Provocative Circumstances Observed in Inborn Errors of Intermediary Metabolism

Symptoms triggered by	Main disorders
Weaning	Fructose intolerance Fructose diphosphatase deficiency Urea cycle defects Lysinuric protein intolerance Triple H syndrome Maple syrup urine disease Organic acidurias
Fructose	Fructose intolerance Fructose diphosphatase deficiency
Galactose	Galactosemias
Glycerol	Glycerol intolerance
Protein	Urea cycle defects Lysinuric protein intolerance Triple H syndrome Maple syrup urine disease Organic acidurias Hyperinsulinism (with hyperammonemia)
Carbohydrate	Pyruvate dehydrogenase deficiency Respiratory chain disorders Hyperinsulinism
Infection, catabolism, fever, fasting	Aminoacidopathies Organic acidurias Fatty acid oxidation disorders Urea cycle defects Gluconeogenesis defects Glycogenosis defects
Anesthesia, surgery	Thromboembolic accident in homocystinuria All conditions listed above
Drugs	Porphyria Glucose-6-phosphate dehydrogenase deficiency

3. Progressive neurologic symptoms (Part III)
4. Specific symptoms (Part IV to VIII)

Emergencies falling in the first two categories should be approached using a protocol based mainly on the proper application of a few screening tests and on obtaining samples of urine, cerebrospinal fluid (CSF), serum, and tissues at appropriate times.[18,19] In cases of unexpected death, a similar postmortem protocol should be followed (Table 66-2).

Many inborn errors of metabolism are first manifested by specific clinical and biologic signs. Some of these phenotypes are rare and very distinctive (e.g., lens dislocation and thromboembolic accidents in homocystinuria), whereas others are common and rather nonspecific (e.g., hepatomegaly, seizures, mental retardation). We have arbitrarily selected for discussion symptoms about which enough information is available, and we have classified them as neurologic, ocular, skin, hematologic, visceral and endocrine (see corresponding sections below).

Chronic and progressive general symptoms may also occur. Many apparently late-onset acute or "specific" presentations of inherited disorders are often preceded by insidious, nonspecific symptoms such as failure to thrive, vomiting, diarrhea, growth retardation, anorexia, hypotonia, poor muscle mass, or developmental delay. These symptoms are not a priori highly suggestive of an inborn error of metabolism [see "Visceral Symptoms or Syndromes (Intestine, Liver, Heart, Lung, Kidney)" below].

Table 66-2 Initial Investigations

	Basic investigations	Specific investigations
Urine	Smell (special odor) Look (special color) Acetone (Acetest, Ames) Reducing substances (Clinitest, Ames) Keto acids (DNPH) pH (pHstix, Merck) Sulfitest (Merck) Brand reaction Electrolytes (Na^+, K^+) Uric acid (search for hypouricuria)	Urine collection: collect each fresh micturition separately and put it in the refrigerator. Freezing: freeze at −20°C samples collected before treatment and, afterward, an aliquot of 24-h collection on treatment. Do not use for specific investigations without expert metabolic advice.
Blood	Blood cell count Electrolytes (search for anion gap) Glucose, calcium Blood gases (pH, P_{CO_2}, HCO_3H, P_{O_2}) Uric acid Prothrombin time Transaminases (and other liver tests) Ammonemia Lactic and pyruvic acids 3OHbutyrate, acetoacetate Free fatty acids	Plasma, heparinized, 5 ml at −20°C Blood on filter paper (as "Guthrie test") Whole blood 10 to 15 ml collected on EDTA and frozen (for molecular biology studies)
Miscellaneous	Lumbar puncture Chest x-ray Echocardiography, EKG Cerebral ultrasound, EEG	Skin biopsy (fibroblast culture) Cerebrospinal fluid, 1 ml frozen Postmortem: liver, muscle biopsies (macroscopic fragment frozen at −70°C)

I. PRESENTATION IN THE NEONATAL PERIOD: "NEONATAL METABOLIC DISTRESS"

Despite the large number of inborn errors of intermediary metabolism that can be observed in the neonatal period, it is possible to assign most patients to one of five biochemical syndromes. The following method of clinical screening is easy to implement, and we have found it very reliable over the past 30 years. It provides considerable cost-benefit advantages over techniques such as mass screening for acute metabolic errors and is much more rapid, allowing specific treatment to be undertaken within hours in these critically ill neonates. Furthermore, because inherited diseases of intermediary metabolism originate relatively simply in single-gene lesions, our approach is already starting to benefit from the new developments in molecular biology. Despite this sophistication of diagnosis and treatment, the crucial step of early clinical suspicion and diagnosis lies in the hands of the primary care physician.[6,7,8]

Identification of Children at Risk

Clinical diagnosis can be schematized into three steps:

1. At first glance symptoms look apparently nonspecific
2. Apparently nonspecific symptoms included in an evocative clinical context
2. Reappraisal of the child, leading to a clinical diagnosis of an inborn error

These are discussed below.

First Glance. The neonate has a limited repertoire of responses to severe illness and at first glance presents with nonspecific symptoms such as respiratory disorders, hypotonia, poor sucking reflex, vomiting, dehydration, lethargy, or seizures — all of which could easily be attributed to infection or some other common cause. Vomiting associated with abdominal distension sometimes mimics pyloric stenosis or intestinal obstruction. In some cases, the patient will turn out to have had an affected sib who died in infancy and whose death was falsely attributed to sepsis, heart failure, or intraventricular hemorrhage; it is important to review clinical records and autopsy reports critically.

Clinical Context. In the intoxication type of metabolic distress, an extremely suggestive clinical course is seen when a full-term baby born after a normal pregnancy is initially symptom free and normal but then deteriorates relentlessly for no apparent reason and without responding to symptomatic therapy. The interval between birth and onset of clinical symptoms ranges from hours to weeks, depending on the nature of the metabolic block and the environment. In organic acidemias and urea cycle defects, the interval is not necessarily correlated with the protein content of the diet.

Routine investigations in such neonates, including chest radiograph, CSF examination, bacteriologic studies, and cerebral imaging, yield normal results. *The unexpected and "mysterious" deterioration of a child after a normal initial period is the most important signal of the presence of an inherited disease of the intoxication type.* Careful reevaluation of the child's condition is warranted under these circumstances. Signs previously interpreted as nonspecific manifestations of neonatal hypoxia, infection, or other common causes take on a new significance in this context.

Reappraisal of the Child

Neurologic Deterioration. Most inborn errors of both the intoxication or the energy deficiency type are brought to a doctor's attention because of neurologic deterioration. In the intoxication type, the initial symptom-free interval varies in duration depending on the condition.[20] Typically, the first reported sign is poor sucking and feeding, after which the child sinks into an unexplained coma despite supportive measures. At a more advanced state, neurovegetative problems, with respiratory abnormalities, hiccups, apneas, bradycardia, and hypothermia, can appear. In the comatose state, characteristic changes in muscle tone and involuntary movements appear. Generalized hypertonic episodes with opisthotonos are frequent, and boxing or pedaling movements, as well as slow limb elevations, spontaneously or upon stimulation, are observed. Conversely, most nonmetabolic causes of coma are associated with hypotonia, so that the presence of "normal" peripheral muscle tone in a comatose child reflects a relative hypertonia. Another neurologic pattern suggesting metabolic disease is axial hypotonia and limb hypertonia with high-amplitude tremors and myoclonic jerks, which are often mistaken for convulsions. An abnormal urine and body odor is present in some diseases in which volatile metabolites accumulate; the most important examples are the maple syrup odor of MSUD and the sweaty feet odor of isovaleric acidemia (IVA) and type II glutaric acidemia. If one of the preceding symptoms is present, metabolic disorders should be given a high diagnostic priority.

In energy deficiencies, the clinical presentation is less evocative and displays a more variable severity. In many conditions, there is no symptom-free interval. The most frequent symptoms are severe generalized hypotonia, hypertrophic cardiomyopathy, rapidly progressive neurologic deterioration, possible dysmorphism and malformations. However, in contrast to the picture in the intoxication group, lethargy and coma are rarely inaugural signs. Hyperlactacidemia with or without metabolic acidosis is a very frequent symptom.

Few lysosomal disorders with storage symptoms are expressed in the neonatal period. In contrast, most peroxisomal disorders present immediately after birth as dysmorphism and severe neurologic dysfunction.

Seizures. True convulsions occur late and inconsistently in inborn errors of intermediary metabolism, with the exception of pyridoxine-dependent seizures and folinic acid responsive seizures[20a] and some cases of nonketotic hyperglycinemia (NKHG), sulfite oxidase deficiency, and peroxisomal disorders, in which they may be important inaugural elements in the clinical presentation. Convulsions are the only symptom in pyridoxine-dependent convulsions and in folinic acid responsive seizures. These rare disorders should be considered in all cases of refractory seizures in children under 1 year of age. In contrast, newborns with MSUD, organic acidurias, or urea cycle defects rarely experience seizures in the absence of preexisting stupor or coma, or hypoglycemia. The electroencephalogram (EEG) often shows a periodic pattern in which bursts of intense activity alternate with nearly flat segments.

Hypotonia. Hypotonia is a very common symptom in sick neonates. Whereas many nonmetabolic inherited diseases can give rise to severe generalized neonatal hypotonia (mainly all severe fetal neuromuscular disorders), only a few inborn errors of metabolism present as predominant hypotonia in the neonatal period. Discounting disorders in which hypotonia is included in the very evocative clinical context of major bone changes, dysmorphism, malformations, or visceral symptoms, the most severe metabolic hypotonias are observed in hereditary hyperlactacidemias, respiratory chain disorders, urea cycle defects, nonketotic hyperglycinemia, sulfite oxidase deficiency, peroxisomal disorders, and trifunctional enzyme deficiency. In all these circumstances, the diagnosis is mostly based upon occurrence in association with the central hypotonia of lethargy, coma, seizures, and neurologic symptoms in nonketotic hyperglycinemia, sulfite oxidase deficiency, and peroxisomal disorders, and of characteristic metabolic changes in congenital lactic acidosis and urea cycle disorders (hyperammonemia). Severe forms of Pompe disease (α-glucosidase deficiency) can initially mimic respiratory chain disorders or trifunctional enzyme deficiency when generalized hypotonia is associated with cardiomyopathy. However, Pompe disease does not start strictly in the neonatal period. Finally, one of the most frequent diagnoses is Prader-Willi syndrome, in which hypotonia is central and apparently an isolated symptom at birth.

Hepatic Presentation. Three main clinical groups of hepatic symptoms can be identified:

1. Hepatomegaly with hypoglycemia and seizures suggests glycogenosis type I or III, gluconeogenesis defects, or severe hyperinsulinism.
2. Liver failure syndrome (jaundice, hemorrhagic syndrome, hepatocellular necrosis with elevated transaminases, and hypoglycemia with ascites and edema) suggests hereditary fructose intolerance (in the case of a fructose-containing diet), galactosemia, tyrosinemia type I (after 3 weeks), neonatal hemochromatosis, or a respiratory chain disorder.
3. Predominantly cholestatic jaundice with failure to thrive is observed in alpha-1-antitrypsin deficiency, Byler disease, inborn errors of bile acid metabolism, peroxisomal disorders, Niemann-Pick disease type C, congenital defects of glycosylation, cholesterol biosynthesis defect and mevalonic aciduria (the two latter as personal observations).

Hepatic presentations of inherited fatty acid oxidation disorders and urea cycle defects consist of acute steatosis or Reye syndrome with normal bilirubin levels, slightly prolonged prothrombin time, and moderate elevation of transaminases rather than true liver failure, with the exception of 3-hydroxy long-chain acyl-CoA dehydrogenase deficiency (LCHAD), which can present early in life, as cholestatic jaundice and liver failure syndrome. We must emphasize the frequent difficulties in investigating patients with severe hepatic failure. At an advanced stage, many nonspecific symptoms secondary to liver damage can be present. Melituria (galactosuria, glycosuria, fructosuria), hyperammonemia, hyperlactacidemia, short-fasting hypoglycemia, hypertyrosinemia ($>200 \mu M$) and hypermethioninemia (sometimes $>500\ \mu M$) are encountered in advanced hepatocellular insufficiency.

Cardiac Presentation. Sometimes metabolic distress can strike with predominantly cardiac symptoms. Cardiac failure revealing or accompanying a cardiomyopathy (dilated hypertrophy) and most often associated with hypotonia, muscle weakness, and failure to thrive suggests a respiratory chain disorder, Pompe disease, or a fatty acid oxidation disorder. Recent observations suggest that some respiratory chain disorders are tissue specific and are expressed only in the myocardium. The newly discovered multisystemic carbohydrate-deficient glycoprotein syndrome can sometimes present in infancy with cardiac failure due to pericardial effusions and cardiac tamponade. Many defects of long-chain fatty acid oxidation can be revealed by cardiomyopathy and/or heartbeat disorders (atrioventricular block, bundle branch blocks, ventricular tachycardia) resulting in cardiac arrest.[21,21a]

Initial Approach

Once clinical suspicion is aroused, general supportive measures and laboratory investigations must be undertaken immediately (Table 66-2). Abnormal urine odors can best be detected on a drying filter paper or by opening a container of urine that has been closed at room temperature for a few minutes. Although serum ketone body levels reach 0.5 to 1 mM in early neonatal life, acetonuria is an important sign of a metabolic disease and is rarely, if ever, observed in a normal newborn.[22] Its presence is always abnormal in neonates. The dinitrophenylhydrazine (DNPH) test screens for the presence of alpha keto acids, such as are seen in MSUD. The DNPH test can be considered significant only in the absence of glucosuria and acetonuria, which also react with DNPH. Hypocalcemia and elevated or reduced blood glucose are frequently present in metabolic diseases. The physician should be wary of attributing marked neurologic dysfunction merely to these findings.

The metabolic acidosis of organic acidurias is usually accompanied by an elevated anion gap. Urine pH should be below 5; otherwise, renal acidosis is a consideration (see "Metabolic Acidosis" below). Ammonia and lactic acid levels should be determined systematically in newborns at risk. An elevated ammonia level in itself can induce respiratory alkalosis; hyperammonemia with ketoacidosis suggests an underlying organic acidemia. An elevated lactic acid level in the absence of infection or tissue hypoxia is a significant finding. We have often observed moderate hyperlactacidemia (3 to 6 mM) in organic acidemias and in the hyperammonemias; levels greater than 10 mM are frequent in hypoxia. A normal serum pH does not exclude hyperlactacidemia, because neutrality is usually maintained until levels of 5 mM are present. It is important to measure, as often as possible, lactate, pyruvate, 3-hydroxybutyrate (3OHB), and acetoacetate (AA) on a plasma sample deproteinized immediately at the bedside in order to appreciate cytoplasmic and mitochondrial redox states through the measurement of lactate:pyruvate (L:P) and 3OHB:AA ratios, respectively (see "Hyperlactacidemias" below).[23] Some organic acidurias induce granulocytopenia and thrombocytopenia, which may be mistaken for sepsis (see "Pancytopenia, Neutropenia, Thrombocytopenia" below).

It is important to store adequate amounts of plasma, blood spots on filter paper, urine, and CSF; the use of these samples should be carefully planned according to advice from specialists in inborn errors of metabolism. Although not available in most hospital laboratories, some sophisticated analytic procedures (such as amino acid or organic acid chromatography) are available by overnight delivery of frozen plasma to a regional center. It is important to insist, however, that any reference laboratory used for this purpose provide not only prompt test results and reference ranges but also an interpretation of abnormal results.[24]

If the child dies, a diagnosis is still important for genetic counseling. A postmortem protocol for the diagnosis of genetic disease has been proposed that includes taking urine and serum samples, obtaining fibroblasts for culturing (premortem if possible), and performing muscle and liver biopsies (three or more samples of 1 cm^3 each, stored frozen on dry ice or in liquid nitrogen).[18,19]

Once the above clinical and short-term laboratory data have been assembled, specific therapeutic recommendations can be made. The entire process is completed within 2 or 4 h and often makes it unnecessary to wait for sophisticated diagnostic results.

Clinical Approach to Etiologies in Metabolic Diseases

The evaluation procedure just described, in combination with the major clinical presentations (neurologic deterioration, seizures, hypotonia, hepatic and cardiac presentation) can be used to assign most patients to one of five basic syndromes. These are listed in Table 66-3 and described in the following sections. In our experience, type I (MSUD), type II (organic acidurias), type IVa (urea cycle defects), and two diseases in type IVb (nonketotic hyperglycinemia, the most common, and respiratory chain disorders), account for more than 70 percent of the newborn infants with inborn errors of intermediary metabolism. Of course, the experienced clinician will interpret the metabolic data carefully, especially in relation to the time of collection and the treatments that were used. It is important to collect all the biologic data listed in Table 66-2 at the same time. Some very significant symptoms (such as metabolic acidosis and especially ketosis) can be moderate and transient and depend largely on the symptomatic therapy. Conversely, at an advanced state, many nonspecific abnormalities (such as respiratory acidosis, severe hyperlactacidemia, and secondary hyperammonemia) can disturb the primary biologic pattern. This is particularly true in disorders with a rapidly fatal course, such as urea cycle disorders, in which the nearly consistent initial presentation of hyperammonemia with respiratory alkalosis and without ketosis shifts rapidly to a rather nonspecific picture with acidosis and hyperlactacidemia.[6,7,8]

Type I: Neurologic Deterioration, Intoxication Type, with Ketosis

Type I is represented by MSUD (see Chap. 87), one of the commonest acutely toxic aminoacidopathies. After a symptom-free interval of 4 to 5 days, feeding difficulties develop, and the child gradually becomes comatose. Generalized hypertonic episodes with opisthotonos and boxing and pedaling movements, as well as slow limb elevations, are consistently present. A maple syrup odor is present, and the urine DNPH test is strongly positive, whereas urine tests for acetone may be negative. None of our patients with MSUD had an initial blood pH less than 7.30. Sometimes a moderate hyperammonemia can be observed. The diagnosis is confirmed by plasma amino acid chromatography, which displays an elevation of the branched chain amino acids leucine (usually higher than 2 mM), valine, and isoleucine and the presence of alloisoleucine.

Type II: Neurologic Deterioration, Intoxication Type, with Ketoacidosis (Hyperammonemia)

This type includes many of the organic acidurias (see "Organic Acidurias and Multiple Carboxylase Deficiencies," Chapters 93, 94, 156). We have observed more than 70 neonates with such diseases. Feeding difficulties develop by 1 to 4 days of age, and the children then deteriorate into a coma within hours to days. In contrast to infants with MSUD, these patients are acutely ill, dehydrated, and acidotic; they have an increased anion gap and often are hypothermic. The usual approach to such patients is first to exclude adrenogenital syndrome by carefully checking the serum electrolytes for high potassium and low sodium concentrations. Truncal hypotonia and peripheral hypertonia are seen, but high-amplitude limb tremors are the dominant type of abnormal movement. In isovaleric acidemia, a potent sweaty feet odor is present. The urine in the acute phase is positive for ketones, but this highly significant sign can be transient. Neutropenia and thrombocytopenia are also common, sometimes later in the course, and can contribute to confusion with sepsis. Hyperammonemia, sometimes as high as that observed in urea cycle defects, is a nearly constant finding[25] and sometimes predominates. Moderate hypocalcemia is also frequent. In some patients we have observed severe hyperglycemia (higher than 15 mM) with glycosuria before treatment with glucose. These findings, in association with dehydration and ketoacidosis, can suggest neonatal diabetes. The metabolic acidosis and other humoral disturbances observed in organic acidemias may have adverse effects on many different organ systems and may lead to a variety of erroneous diagnoses.[24]

In addition to methylmalonic, propionic, and isovaleric acidurias, modern organic analysis techniques have led to the description of a large number of rare organic acidurias, usually presenting as neurologic deterioration and metabolic acidosis. Of these, glutaric aciduria type II, or multiple acyl CoA dehydrogenase deficiency (MADD),[26] and carnitine acylcarnitine translocase (CAT), type II carnitine palmitoyl transferase (CPT II), very-long-chain acyl CoA dehydrogenase (VLCAD), and hydroxymethylglutaryl CoA lyase[27] deficiencies have many similarities to methylmalonic, propionic, and isovaleric acidurias, except that ketosis is absent and hypoglycemia is frequent. MADD, CAT, CPT II, and VLCAD frequently present as heartbeat disorders, dilated hypertrophic cardiomyopathy, or moderate liver dysfunction, and patients can die unexpectedly, with a clinical picture resembling sudden neonatal death or Reye syndrome.[21,28,29] Sudden infant death and heartbeat disorders occurring in the first week of life are highly suggestive of long-chain mitochondrial fatty acid oxidation disorders (see "Sudden Infant Death Syndrome" and Table 66-18 below). Patients with multiple acyl CoA dehydrogenase deficiency have a sweaty feet odor similar to that in isovaleric aciduria, have severe lactic acidosis, and may have developmental defects.[26] Other very rare conditions in this group are succinyl CoA transferase deficiency[30,31] biotin-dependent multiple carboxylase defects due to holoenzyme synthetase deficiency,[32] short-chain fatty acyl CoA dehydrogenase deficiency,[33,33a] 3-methylglutaconic aciduria,[34] and glycerol kinase deficiency.[35] On the other hand, the literature and our personal experience suggest that organic acidurias such as 3-ketothiolase deficiency,[31] biotin-responsive biotinidase

Table 66-3 Classification of Inborn Errors Presenting in the Neonatal Period

Types	Clinical type	Acidosis/ Ketosis	Other signs	Most usual diagnosis	Elective methods of investigation
I	Neurologic deterioration, intoxication type, abnormal movements, hypertonia	Acidosis 0 DNPH +++ Acetest 0/±	NH_3 N or ↑± Lactate N Blood count N Glucose N Calcium N	MSUD (special odor)	Amino acid chromatography (plasma, urine)
II a)	Neurologic deterioration, intoxication type, dehydration	Acidosis ++ Acetest ++ DNPH 0/±	NH_3 ↑+/++ Lactate N or ↑± Blood count: Leukopenia, thrombocytopenia Glucose N or ↑+ Calcium N or ↓+	Organic acidurias (MMA, PA, IVA, MCD) Ketolysis defects	Organic acid chromatography by GLCMS (urine, plasma) Carnitine (plasma) Carnitine esters (urine, plasma)
b)	Neurologic deterioration, energy deficiency type, with liver or cardiac symptoms	Acidosis ++/± Acetest 0 DNPH 0	NH_3 ↑±/++ Lactate ↑±/++ Blood count N Glucose ↓+/++ Calcium N or ↓+	Fatty acid oxidation and ketogenesis defects (GA II, CPT II, CAT, VLCAD, MCKAT, HMGCoA lyase)	Above, plus: Loading test Fasting test Fatty acid oxidation studies on lymphocytes or fibroblasts
III	Neurologic deterioration, energy deficiency type, polypnea, hypotonia	Acidosis +++/+ Acetest ++/0 Lactate +++/+	NH_3 N or ↑± Blood count: anemia or N Glucose N or ↓± Calcium N	Congenital lactic acidoses (PC, PDH, Krebs cycle, respiratory chain) MCD	Plasma redox states ratios (L:P, 3OHB:AA) Organic acid chromatography (urine) Polarographic studies Enzyme assays (muscle, lymphocytes, fibroblasts)
IV a)	Neurologic deterioration, intoxication type, moderate hepatocellular disturbances, hypotonia, seizures, coma	Acidosis 0 (alkalosis) Acetest 0 DNPH 0	NH_3 ↑+/+++ Lactate N or ↑+ Blood count N Glucose N Calcium N	Urea cycle defects Triple H Fatty acid oxidation defects (GA II, CPT II, VLCAD, LCHAD, CAT)	AAC (plasma, urine) Orotic acid (urine) Liver or intestine enzyme studies (CPS, OTC)
a)	Neurologic deterioration, seizures, myoclonic jerks, severe hypotonia	Acidosis 0 Acetest 0 DNPH 0	NH_3 N Lactate N or ↑+ Blood count N Glucose N	NKH SO ± XO Pyridoxine dependency Peroxisomal disorders Trifunctional enzyme Respiratory chain Neurotransmitter disorders CDG syndrome Cholesterol biosynthesis disorders	AAC (NKH, SO) VLCFA, phytanic acid in plasma (PZO) Acylcarnitine profile (plasma) Lactate (plasma) Neurotransmitters (plasma, urine, CSF) Glycoslated transferrin (plasma) Cholesterol (plasma)
V a)	Hepatomegaly Hypoglycemia	Acidosis ++/+ Acetest +	NH_3 N Lactate ↑+/++ Blood count N Glucose ↓++	Glycogenosis type I (Acetest −) Glycogenosis type III (Acetest ++) Fructose diphosphatase	Fasting test Loading test Enzyme studies (liver, lymphocytes, fibroblasts)
b)	Hepatomegaly Jaundice Liver failure Hepatocellular necrosis	Acidosis +/0 Acetest +/0	NH_3 N or ↑+ Lactate ↑+/++ Glucose N or ↓++	Fructosemia, galactosemia Tyrosinosis type I Neonatal hemochromatosis Respiratory chain disorders	Enzyme studies (fructosemia, galactosemia) Organic acid and enzyme studies (tyrosinosis type I)

Table 66-3 (Continued)

Types	Clinical type	Acidosis/ Ketosis	Other signs	Most usual diagnosis	Elective methods of investigation
c)	Hepatomegaly Cholestatic Jaundice ± Failure to thrive ± Chronic diarrhea	Acidosis 0 Ketosis 0	NH_3 N Lactate N Glucose N	Alpha-1-antitrypsin Inborn errors of bile acid metabolism Peroxisomal disorders CDG syndrome Niemann-Pick type C LCHAD Mevalonate kinase	Protein electrophoresis Organic acid chromatography (plasma, urine, duodenal juice) Acylcarnitine profile VLCFA, phytanic acid, pipecolic acid Glycosylated transferrin Fibroblast studies
d)	Hepatosplenomegaly Storage signs (coarse facies, ascites, hydrops fetalis, macroglossia, bone changes, cherry red spot, vacuolated lymphocytes) ± Failure to thrive ± Chronic diarrhea	Acidosis 0 Acetest 0 Ketosis 0 DNPH 0	NH_3 N Lactate N or ↑ Blood count N Glucose N Hepatic signs ±	G_{M1} gangliosidosis ISSD (sialidosis type II) I-cell disease Niemann-Pick type IA MPS VII Galactosialidosis CDG syndrome	Oligosaccharides, sialic acid Mucopolysaccharides Enzyme studies (lymphocytes, fibroblasts)

3OHB = 3-hydroxybutyrate; AA = acetoacetate; GLCMS = gas liquid chromatography mass spectrometry; L = lactate; P = pyruvate; VLCFA = very-long-chain fatty acids; DNPH = dinitrophenylhydrazine; N = normal (normal values = NH_3 < 80 M; lactate < 1.5 mM; glucose 3.5–5.5 mM); ±, slight; +, moderate; ++, marked; +++, significant/massive; ↑ elevated; ↓ decreased; 0, absent (acidosis) or negative (Acetest, DNPH); AAC = amino acid chromatography; CAT = carnitine acylcarnitine translocase; CPS = carbamyl phosphate synthetase; CPT II = carnitine palmitoyltransferase II; CDG = congenital defects of glycosylation; GA II = glutaric aciduria type II; HMGCoA = 3-hydroxy-3-methylglutaryl coenzyme A; ISSD = infantile sialic acid storage disease; IVA = isovaleric acidemia; LCHAD = 3-hydroxy long-chain acyl CoA dehydrogenase; MCD = multiple carboxylase deficiency; MCKAT = medium-chain 3-ketoacyl coenzyme A thiolase; MMA = methylmalonic acidemia; MPS VII = mucopolysaccharidosis type VII; MSUD = maple syrup urine disease; NKH = nonketotic hyperglycinemia; OTC = ornithine transcarbamylase; PA = propionic acidemia; PC = pyruvate carboxylase; PDH = pyruvate dehydrogenase; PZO = peroxisomal disorders; SO = sulfite oxidase; VLCAD = very-long-chain acyl CoA dehydrogenase; XO = xanthine oxidase

deficiency,[36] and glutaric aciduria type I rarely, if ever, present in the neonatal period. Pyroglutamic aciduria is a rare condition that can start in the first days of life with a severe metabolic acidosis but without either ketosis or abnormalities of blood glucose, lactate, or ammonia. There are no severe neurologic signs, and the clinical picture mimics renal tubular acidosis (see Chap. 121).

Definitive diagnosis of all these organic acidurias is made by identifying a specific acylcarnitine profile by gas chromatography-mass spectrometry (GCMS) and tandem MS-MS of blood and urine. Plasma free carnitine concentrations are always low, with abnormal excretion of specific acylcarnitines. In contrast, plasma and urine amino acid values are often normal, or abnormal in a nonspecific way, with, for example, slight increases in glycine.

Type III: Lactic Acidosis with Neurologic Deterioration, Energy Deficiency Type

The clinical presentation of children with these disorders is diverse. Unlike the previous category, in which moderate acidosis is noted during the evaluation of an acutely ill comatose infant, the main disturbance in type III patients is the acidosis itself, which clinically may be surprisingly well tolerated. The acidosis is sometimes mild. Blood pH is usually normal until lactate concentrations of 5 mM are reached. There is an elevated anion gap, which can be explained in part by the presence of equimolar amounts of lactic acid in the blood. In the absence of adequate treatment, the acidosis often recurs soon after bicarbonate therapy.

If a high lactic acid concentration is found, it is urgent to rule out readily treatable causes, especially hypoxia. Ketosis is present in many of the primary lactic acidemias but is absent in acidosis secondary to tissue hypoxia. Biotin-responsive multiple carboxylase deficiency may present as lactic acidosis, and biotin therapy is indicated in all patients with lactic acidosis of unknown cause after baseline blood and urine samples have been taken.

Primary lactic acidoses form a complex group.[37] A definite diagnosis is often elusive. It is based on specific enzyme assays considered in the light of metabolite levels, redox potential states, and fluxes under fasting and fed conditions (see "Hyperlactacidemias" below); (see also Chapter 100).[23] The defects most frequently demonstrated are pyruvate carboxylase deficiency, pyruvate dehydrogenase deficiency, respiratory chain disorders (complexes I and IV), and multiple carboxylase deficiency (already discussed under type II diseases). Many cases remain unexplained.

In our experience, pyruvate carboxylase deficiencies have a stereotypic biochemical pattern, with an elevated L:P ratio contrasting with a reduced 3-OHB:AA ratio, moderate citrullinemia and hyperammonemia, and hepatic dysfunction. This pattern has been called the "French phenotype" by Robinson.[38] Respiratory chain disorders are frequently observed in the neonatal period. Since the early descriptions,[39] a number of cases have been described.[40] The most frequent symptoms are severe generalized hypotonia (see "Hypotonia in the Neonatal Period and in Early Infancy" below), hypertrophic cardiomyopathy of hypokinetic type (see "Cardiomyopathy" below) with rapid neurologic deterioration, hepatic failure, respiratory failure, and severe lactic acidemia. Some patients have facial dysmorphism and malformations, which have also been observed in infants with a deficiency of the pyruvate dehydrogenase complex and in fumarase deficiency.[15,41,41a]

Type IV

Type IVa: Neurologic Deterioration, Intoxication Type, with Hyperammonemia and Without Ketoacidosis: Urea Cycle

Defects. As mentioned above, this is one of the most important groups of neonatal inborn errors of metabolism. We have investigated more than 70 neonates with these disorders. Primary hyperammonemias due to urea cycle defects have a variable symptom-free interval, sometimes only hours long. A brief hypertonic period and hiccups may occur, after which a profound hypotonic coma rapidly develops, and cardiocirculatory function may be compromised. Coagulation factor depletion, elevated serum aminotransferases, and hepatomegaly, particularly in argininosuccinic acid lyase deficiency, are frequent. The blood ammonia rises precipitously to levels of 400 to 2000 μM or more. Respiratory alkalosis (pH > 7.40) and moderate hyperlactacidemia are frequently observed. An important diagnostic clue to separate urea cycle defects from organic acidurias with hyperammonemia is the universal absence of ketonuria in the former. However, we and others have rarely observed propionic acidemia patients presenting with isolated hyperammonemia without any ketoacidosis, a picture that mimics urea cycle disorders. As already stated, at an advanced stage encephalopathic disorders rapidly give rise to nonspecific findings, including acidosis and hyperlactacidemia.

The two principal urea cycle disorders, which have nondiagnostic amino acid chromatograms, are ornithine transcarbamylase deficiency and carbamylphosphate synthetase deficiency (CPS). The very rare acetyl glutamate synthetase deficiency (AGS) is very similar to CPS but is carbamyl glutamate responsive. The former is the only sex-linked congenital hyperammonemia, the others being autosomal recessive. Plasma citrulline is low in both. Massive orotic acid excretion is present in ornithine transcarbamylase deficiency but absent in CPS and AGS deficiency. Enzyme diagnosis by liver biopsy is the only definitive diagnostic technique for these disorders. Citrullinemia, argininosuccinic aciduria, and argininemia are diagnosed by amino acid chromatography that demonstrates the accumulation of citrulline, argininosuccinate, and arginine, respectively. In the HHH ("triple H") syndrome, hyperammonemia, hyperornithinemia, and homocitrullinemia are present. An especially important diagnostic consideration is transient hyperammonemia of the neonate, in which the patient, often premature and having mild respiratory distress syndrome, falls into a deep coma with severe hyperammonemia, which disappears permanently if initial treatment is successful and does not need any further treatment.[42]

Long-chain fatty acid oxidation disorders (mainly CPT II, carnitine acyltranslocase, and VLCAD deficiencies) can also, though rarely, present in the neonatal period with hyperammonemia mimicking urea cycle disorders. They are associated with hypoglycemia, hepatic dysfunction, muscular and cardiac symptoms, and sudden infant death.[21,28,29]

Type IVb: Neurologic Deterioration Without Ketoacidosis and Without Hyperammonemia. This group has rapidly expanded and encompasses mostly nonketotic hyperglycinemia, sulfite oxidase deficiency, peroxisomal disorders, and neurotransmitter disorders. Nonketotic hyperglycinemia displays a very typical, but not pathognomonic, pattern. It is characterized by coma, hypotonia, and myoclonic jerks appearing at or within a few hours of birth in an infant with no history of perinatal hypoxia. A burst-suppression EEG pattern[43] is always present. The diagnosis rests on the demonstration of elevated plasma glycine levels and especially an elevated cerebrospinal fluid (CSF) plasma glycine ratio. The very rare D-glyceric acidemia shares most of the signs of nonketotic hyperglycinemia, including presence of hyperglycinemia in some patients whereas other patients present with different patterns including metabolic acidosis.

The clinical spectrum of sulfite oxidase and combined sulfite and xanthine oxidase deficiencies[44] includes hypotonia, seizures, myoclonic jerks, microcephaly, and dysmorphic features. Lens dislocation may occasionally be noted as early as the first month of life. This disorder is probably underdiagnosed, because its clinical pattern shares many similarities with common acute fetal distress. In combined sulfite and xanthine oxidase deficiencies due to an abnormal molybdenum cofactor, uric acid concentration is very low in plasma and urine. In both sulfite oxidase deficiencies, sulfites are found in fresh urine in high concentrations (Sulfitest, Merck). Amino acid chromatography performed on immediately deproteinized plasma and on fresh urine shows a specific profile, with high sulfite concentrations in the form of sulfocysteine but a cystine concentration is close to zero.

The common symptoms of peroxisomal disorders presenting in the neonatal period are absence of a symptom-free interval, severe generalized hypotonia, early-onset epileptic seizures, and craniofacial dysmorphism[45] (see Chap. 71); some patients can mimic Werdnig Hoffmann syndrome[45a] diagnosis requires special investigations, including very-long-chain fatty acid, plasmalogen, phytanic acid, bile acid, and pipecolic acid determinations in plasma, urine, and fibroblasts. The most frequent conditions are Zellweger syndrome and neonatal adrenoleukodystrophy. Many other rare variants have recently been described[45b] (see Chaps. 71–75).

Trifunctional enzyme deficiency and VLCAD can present early in the neonatal period as severe generalized hypotonia and lethargy, often associated with cardiac symptoms (myocardiopathy, atrioventricular block), or as sudden death.[21a] The diagnosis relies on plasma acylcarnitine profile determination.

In some patients respiratory chain disorders strike as severe hypotonia without obvious acidosis or hyperlactacidemia.

Aromatic L-amino acid decarboxylase deficiency presents early in the first month as generalized hypotonia, paroxysmal movements of limbs that can mimic those observed in MSUD and organic acidurias, and very suggestive oculogyric crises. The enzyme defect leads to the accumulation of L-dopa and its metabolite 3-methoxytyrosine and of 5-hydroxytryptophan in CSF, plasma, and urine.[46]

Congenital disorders of glycosylation type Ia presents in the neonatal period as axial hypotonia, alternating internal strabismus, and other abnormal eye movements. Many patients present with dysmorphic features, in particular large ears, special face, abnormal adipose tissue distribution (fat pads, tallow), inverted nipples, moderate hepatomegaly, and cerebellar hypoplasia. Some patients have pericardial effusion and cardiomyopathy. The diagnosis is based on plasma glycosylated transferrin determination.

Inborn errors of cholesterol biosynthesis present as congenital disorders with diverse malformations, severe hypotonia, feeding difficulties, and very low plasma cholesterol.[5a,5b,9]

Many other rare inborn errors with nonspecific neurologic dysfunctions and without obvious metabolic disturbances can start in the neonatal period but are most often diagnosed a few months later. Among them 2 methylbutyryl CoA dehydrogenase[46a] and leukotriene C_4 synthesis deficiency[46b,46c] have been recently described. (See also Progressive Neurologic and Mental Deterioration" below; Tables 66-21 and 66-22).

In most diseases of intermediary metabolism, convulsions are a late manifestation. However, they may be important elements in the clinical presentation of most patients with nonketotic hyperglycinemia, sulfite oxidase deficiency, and the peroxisomal disorders described above. They are also the sole symptom in pyridoxine-dependent convulsions and folinic acid responsive seizures. These rare disorders should be considered in all cases of refractory seizures in children under 1 year of age. The clinical response to vitamin B_6 administration is the best way of making the diagnosis in the former. If it can be done without delaying treatment, an EEG should be obtained during the injection of pyridoxine; an immediate improvement in the tracing may be seen.[47] In folinic acid responsive seizures, it is important to collect a CSF sample to search for the characteristic abnormal peak at HPLC, before giving 10 to 20 mg folinic acid. A rapid improvement is observed with the disappearance of the abnormal peak in the CSF.[47a]

Type V: Predominant Hepatic Presentation

The clinical presentation of type V diseases is different from those of the preceding ones.

Type Va. In a first group of disorders, hypoglycemic seizures are often the presenting sign, and hepatomegaly, ketosis, and lactic acidosis are present. The child improves dramatically with IV glucose administration. The main diseases in this group are glucose 6-phosphatase deficiency (type I glycogen storage disease), glycogenosis type III, and fructose 1,6-diphosphatase deficiency. Clinical presentation of phosphoenolpyruvate carboxykinase deficiency in the neonatal period is uncommon and not well defined. Marked hepatocellular dysfunction is uncommon but may occur, especially in fructose 1,6-diphosphatase deficiency.

Type Vb. In a second group of disorders, liver failure syndrome is the predominant manifestation and suggests galactosemia, hereditary fructose intolerance (if the diet contains fructose), tyrosinemia type I (which is always revealed clinically after at least 2 to 3 weeks of life), neonatal hemochromatosis (with normal or disproportionately low serum transaminases), and respiratory chain disorders. Alpha-1-antitrypsin deficiency, Wilson disease, and LCHAD deficiency can rarely present as liver failure early in the first month of life. A new disorder has recently been described in 15 newborns from Finland who all presented with severe fetal growth retardation, lactic acidosis, failure to thrive, hyperaminoaciduria, very high serum ferritin, hemosiderosis of the liver, and early death. The etiology of this syndrome, which appears to be distinct from that of other lactic acidoses and neonatal hemochromatosis, is unknown.[48]

Type Vc. A third group of disorders is revealed by predominant cholestatic jaundice, isolated or associated with failure to thrive and hypotonia. This group encompasses alpha-1-antitrypsin deficiency, Byler disease with intractable pruritus and normal serum gamma-GT, inborn errors of bile acid metabolism, peroxisomal disorders, Niemann-Pick disease type C, carbohydrate-deficient glycoprotein syndrome, and LCHAD deficiency. We have recently observed one patient with Smith-Lemli-Opitz syndrome who presented with a severe cholestatic jaundice associated with the characteristic dysmorphic findings of the syndrome and a patient with mevalonate kinase deficiency who displayed hepatosplenomegaly, jaundice, lymphadenopathy and inflammatory syndrome mimicking a myelodysplastic syndrome.

Type Vd. The last group is composed of disorders presenting as the storage signs listed in Table 66-8. The most important signs are coarse facial features or dysmorphism, macroglossia, hepatosplenomegaly, hydrops fetalis, ascites, edema, stippled epiphyses, periosteal cloaking of long bones and ribs (in sialidosis type II and G_{M1} gangliosidosis), dysostosis multiplex (in most glycoprotein storage diseases), cherry red spot at funduscopy (in G_{M1} gangliosidosis, sialidosis, and galactosialidosis), and vaculoated lymphocytes (in Niemann-Pick disease, I-cell disease, G_{M1} gangliosidosis, sialidosis, mucopolysaccharidosis type VII, and Wolman disease). Interestingly, in some patients, Pearson syndrome[49] or carbohydrate-deficient glycoprotein syndrome can present as hydrops foetalis and simulate storage disorders.[50]

Intrauterine Growth Retardation

Severe intrauterine growth retardation (IUGR) is a frequent finding in a large number of inborn errors that disturb the synthesis or the catabolism of complex molecules, like lysosomal storage disorders, peroxisomal disorders, and cholesterol biosynthesis defects. In most of these cases, many other significant clinical symptoms, like facial dysmorphism, malformations, visceral or neurologic manifestations, lactic acidosis, and liver hemosiderosis, are present. IUGR is also a very frequent finding in a number of nonmetabolic polymalformative syndromes of genetic and nongenetic origin. In rare cases it is a preponderant symptom in respiratory chain disorders. It is the most important presenting sign in babies born to alcoholic or untreated phenylketonuric mothers, in whom it is associated with microcephaly and facial dysmorphism.

Babies Born to Mothers with Acute Fatty Liver of Pregnancy and HELLP Syndrome

Acute fatty liver of pregnancy (AFLP) and hemolysis, elevated liver enzymes, and low platelets (HELPP) syndrome are known to be associated with inborn errors of fatty acid β-oxidation in the fetus, specifically LCHAD deficiency.[51] Recently, CPT I deficiency respiratory chain defects and MCAD deficiency have been found in two unrelated infants born to mothers with AFLP and with HELLP syndrome, respectively, suggesting that an expanding spectrum of metabolic disorders may cause maternal illness in pregnancy.[51,52,52a,52b] An acylcarnitine profile performed on a blood spot collected at birth is mandatory in every neonate born to a mother affected with such a disorder in pregnancy.

II. INTERMITTENT LATE-ONSET ACUTE PRESENTATION

Recurrent Attacks of Coma, Strokes, and Vomiting with Lethargy, Ataxia, and Psychiatric Symptoms

In approximately one-third of patients with inborn errors of intermediary metabolism, disease onset is late; the symptom-free period is often longer than 1 year and may extend into late childhood, adolescence, or even adulthood. Each attack has a rapid course toward either spontaneous improvement or unexplained death despite supportive measures in the intensive care unit. No cause is readily detectable. Recurrent attacks are frequent, and between attacks the person may seem normal. These features make the diagnosis of inborn errors of metabolism in such patients difficult when adequate investigations have not been performed during the acute attack itself. The onset of acute disease may be precipitated by a minor viral infection, fever, or even severe constipation. Excessive protein intake and all conditions that enhance protein catabolism may exacerbate decompensation (see above and Table 66-1). However, sometimes no overt cause is found.

Recurrent attacks of coma, recurrent vomiting with lethargy, and ataxia are the main presentations of these late-onset acute forms. All types of comas in pediatrics can signal inborn errors of metabolism, including those presenting with focal neurologic signs. Neither the age at onset, the accompanying clinical signs (hepatic, digestive, neurologic, psychiatric, etc.), the mode of evolution (improvement, sequelae, death), nor the biologic profile allows an inborn error of metabolism to be ruled out a priori. Tables 66-4, 66-5 and 66-6 summarize the different kinds of comas or acute episodes registered in a series of more than 100 patients investigated at the Clinique de Génétique Médicale, Hôpital Necker Enfants-Malades, Paris, over 30 years. From a clinical point of view, four basic categories can be immediately separated at first glance:

1. Metabolic coma, without focal neurologic signs (Table 66-4)
2. Neurologic coma, with focal signs, seizures, or severe intracranial hypertension (Table 66-5)
3. Hepatic coma, with liver dysfunction or hepatomegaly (Table 66-5)
4. Acute ataxia (Table 66-6)

All the main varieties of metabolic comas may be observed in these late-onset, acute diseases: coma with predominant metabolic acidosis, coma with predominant hyperammonemia, and coma with predominant hypoglycemia (Table 66-4). All combinations of these three major biologic signs are possible: metabolic acidosis with or without ketosis and with or without hyperlactacidemia; hyperammonemia with or without hypoglycemia; and

Table 66-4 Diagnostic Approach to Recurrent Attacks of Coma, Lethargy, and Ataxia Due to Inborn Errors of Metabolism: Metabolic Coma

Predominant Clinical Presentation	Predominant Metabolic Features or Other Important Signs		Most Frequent Diagnosis	Differential Diagnosis
Metabolic coma (without focal neurologic signs) Recurrent vomiting with lethargy	Acidosis (metabolic): pH < 7.20 CO_3H < 10 mmol Pco_2 < 25 mmHg	Ketosis + (Acetest ++) →	Congenital hyperlactacidemias (PC, MCD, respiratory chain) Organic acidurias (MMA, PA, IVA, GA I) MSUD, 3MGA, 3HiBuria Ketolysis defects (OATD, thiolase) Neoglucogenesis defects (FDP, G6P)	→ Diabetes Intoxication Encephalitis
		Ketosis − →	Pyruvate dehydrogenase deficiency Ketogenesis defects (HMG-CoA lyase) Fatty acid oxidation defects Fructose diphosphatase deficiency EPEMA syndrome	
	Hyperammonemia NH_3 > 100 μM Respiratory alkalosis pH > 7.45, Pco_2 < 25 mmHg	Normal glucose →	Urea cycle disorders (OTC, CPS, ASS, AS) HHH, LPI, AGS	→ Reye syndrome Encephalitis Intoxication
		Hypoglycemia →	Fatty acid oxidation disorders HMG-CoA lyase deficiency	
	Hypoglycemia < 2 mM	Acidosis + →	Neoglucogenesis defects MSUD HMG-CoA lyase deficiency	→ Drugs and toxins Recurrent hypoglycemia Fasting hypoglycemia Adrenal insufficiency (and other endocrine etiologies) Hypopituitary coma
		Acidosis →	Fatty acid oxidation disorders (CPT I, CPT II, TL, PSCD, MAD, LCAD, LCHAD, MCAD) HMG-CoA synthetase	
	Hyperlactacidemia > 4 mM	Normal glucose →	"Congenital" hyperlactacidemias PC, MCD, respiratory chain disorders, Krebs (with ketosis), mitochondrial DNA mutations PDH (without ketosis) EPEMA syndrome	
		Hypoglycemia →	Gluconeogenesis defects (FDP, G6P, PC, ketosis variable) Fatty acid oxidation disorders (moderate hyperlactacidemia, no ketosis)	

3HiBuria = 3-hydroxyisobutyric aciduria; 3MGA = 3-methylglutaconic aciduria; AGS =acetylglutamate synthetase; AS = argininosuccinate; ASS = argininosuccinate synthase; CPS = carbamyl phosphate synthetase; CPT = carnitine palmitoyltransferase; EPEMA = encephalopathy, relapsing petechiae, and ethylmalonic aciduria; FDP = fructose diphosphatase; GA I = glutaric acidemia type I; IVA = isovaleric acidemia; LCAD = long-chain acyl CoA dehydrogenase; LCHAD = 3-hydroxy long-chain acyl CoA dehydrogenase; LPI = lysinuric protein intolerance; MAD = multiple acyl CoA dehydrogenase; MCAD = medium-chain acyl CoA dehydrogenase; MCD = multiple carboxylase deficiency; MMA = methylmalonic acidemia; MSUD = maple syrup urine disease; OATD = oxoacid CoA thiolase deficiency; OTC = ornithine transcarbamylase; PA = propionic acidemia; PC = pyruvate carboxylase; PDH = pyruvate dehydrogenase; PSCD = primary systemic carnitine deficiency; TL = carnitine acyl translocase; G6P = glucose 6 phosphatase

Table 66-5 Diagnostic Approach to Recurrent Attacks of Coma, Lethargy, and Ataxia Due to Inborn Errors of Metabolism: Neurologic and Hepatic Comas

Predominant Clinical Presentation	Predominant Clinical Features or Other Important Signs		Most frequent diagnosis	Differential diagnosis
Neurologic coma (with focal signs, seizures, intracranial hypertension)	Cerebral edema Hemiplegia (hemianopsia) Extrapyramidal signs	Biologic signs very variable, can be absent or very moderate if present (see Table 66-7)	MSUD, OTC MSUD, OTC, MMA, PA, PGK MMA, GA I, Wilson disease, homocystinuria (classic)	Cerebral tumor Migraine Encephalitis
	Strokelike episodes Necrosis of the basal ganglia		Urea cycle, MMA, PA, IVA, HMG-CoA Lyase, respiratory chain (MELAS), homocystinuria (classic and variant), CDG, thiamine-responsive megaloblastic anemia, Fabry disease (rarely revealing)	Moyamoya Vascular hemiplegia Cerebral thrombophlebitis Cerebral tumor
	Thromboembolic accidents	Abnormal coagulation Hemolytic anemia	Antithrombin III, protein C or S deficiencies CDG Homocystinuria (classic and variant) Sickle-cell anemia, PGK deficiency	Idem above
Muscular presentation (muscle weakness, recurrent myoglobinuria)	Muscle weakness Muscle pain	Elevated CPK Myoglobinuria	See Table 66-16	
Hepatic coma (hepatomegaly, cytolysis, or liver failure)	Steatosis	Normal bilirubin, slight elevation of transaminases	Fatty acid oxidation defects Urea cycle disorders (OTC, citrullinemia)	Reye syndrome Hepatitis Intoxication
	Liver failure Cirrhosis Chronic hepatic dysfunction	Hyperlactacidemia Hemolytic jaundice	Respiratory chain disorders Wilson disease	

GA I = glutaric acidemia type I; IVA = isovaleric acidemia; MMA = methylmalonic acidemia; MSUD = maple syrup urine disease; OTC = ornithine transcarbamylase; PA = propionic acidemia; PGK = phosphoglycerate kinase; MELAS = mitochondrial encephalopathy with lactic acidosis; CDG = congenital defects of glycosylation

hypoglycemia with or without ketoacidosis. A rather confusing finding in some organic acidurias and ketolytic defects is ketoacidosis with hyperglycemia and glycosuria that mimics diabetic coma. The diagnostic approach to the biologic findings is developed below (see "Metabolic Acidosis," "Ketosis," "Hyperlactacidemias," "Hypoglycemia: General Approach," "Hypoketotic Hypoglycemias Due to Inborn Errors of Ketogenesis" below).

Although most recurrent metabolic comas are not accompanied by neurologic signs other than encephalopathy, we have observed several patients with organic acidemias (methylmalonic, propionic, isovaleric), MSUD, or ornithine transcarbamylase (OTC) deficiency who presented with focal neurologic signs or cerebral edema (Table 66-5). Several of these patients were mistakenly diagnosed as having cerebrovascular accident or cerebral tumor, and two endured neurosurgery. In two patients with classic homocystinuria who were subsequently demonstrated to be vitamin B_6–responsive, the associated disease struck in late childhood with an acute cerebrovascular accident, which was at first mistaken for cerebral thrombophlebitis. A few patients with methylmalonic acidemia have had acute extrapyramidal disease and corticospinal tract involvement after metabolic decompensation. The neurologic findings resulted from bilateral destruction of the globus pallidus with variable involvement of the internal capsule.[53] Cerebellar hemorrhage has also been observed in isovaleric acidemia, propionic acidemia, and methylmalonic acidemia.[54]

Encephalopathy, petechiae, and ethylmalonic acidemia (EPEMA) syndrome is a recently described entity which starts early in infancy and is characterized by the association of progressive encephalopathy with mental retardation, pyramidal signs, and bilateral lesions in the striatum resembling Leigh syndrome; relapsing petechiae; orthostatic acrocyanosis; and recurrent attacks of metabolic decompensation with lactic acidosis and without ketosis, during which there is an increase in ethylmalonic and methylsuccinic excretion. The etiology of this syndrome remains unknown.[55,56] In one patient, a profound defect of cytochrome *c* oxidase activity was found in muscle.[56]

Two patients with 3-hydroxyisobutyric aciduria presenting with recurrent episodes of vomiting and ketoacidotic coma have been described recently.[57] Cyclic vomiting syndrome associated with intermittent lactic acidosis has been described as a revealing sign in mitochondrial DNA mutations.[58,59]

Glutaric aciduria type I can also be revealed by encephalopathic episodes with acute metabolic derangements that occur in connection with gastrointestinal or viral infections and that lead to seizures, coma, paralysis, and loss of all bodily and mental

Table 66-6 Diagnostic Approach to Recurrent Attacks of Coma, Lethargy, and Ataxia Due to Inborn Errors of Metabolism: Ataxia, Psychiatric Symptoms

Predominant Clinical Presentation	Predominant Metabolic Features or Other Important Signs		Most Frequent Diagnosis	Differential Diagnosis
Acute ataxia	Ketoacidosis	Special odor Neutropenia Thrombopenia Hyperglycemia	Late-onset MSUD MMA, PA, IVA (and other organic acidurias)	Diabetes
	Hyperammonemia	Respiratory alkalosis Hepatomegaly	Urea cycle defects (OTC, ASS)	Intoxication
	Hyperlactacidemia	Normal L:P ratio No ketosis Peripheral neuropathy	Pyruvate dehydrogenase deficiency	Encephalitis Migraine
		High L:P ratio Ketosis Cutaneous signs	Multiple carboxylase deficiency Respiratory chain disorders	Cerebellitis (varicella) Polymyoclonia Acetazolamide-responsive ataxia
	No biologic disturbance	Skin rashes, pellagra Sun intolerance	Hartnup disease	Acute exacerbation in chronic ataxias
Psychiatric symptoms (hallucinations, delirium, dizziness, aggressiveness, anxiety, agitation, agony, schizophrenic-like behavior)	Hyperammonemia	Slight liver dysfunction Vomiting Failure to thrive	Urea cycle defects (OTC, ASS, arginase deficiency, LPI)	
	Ketoacidosis	Ataxia Neutropenia	Organic acid disorders, MSUD	
	Portwine urine	Abdominal pain Any kind of neuropathy Vomiting Muscle weakness Cramps Myoglobinuria High CK	Acute intermittent porphyria Hereditary coproporphyria Paroxysmal myoglobinuria (see Table 66-16)	Hysteria
	Positive brand reaction	Stroke Seizures Myelopathy	Methylene tetrahydrofolate reductase	Schizophrenia

ASS = argininosuccinate synthase; IVA = isovaleric acidemia; LPI = lysinuric protein intolerance; MMA = methylmalonic acidemia; OTC = ornithine transcarbamylase; PA = propionic acidemia; MSUD = maple syrup urine disease; CK = creatine kinase

landmarks. Recovery after such episodes is never complete. During these attacks, ketosis, metabolic acidosis, hypoglycemia, and mild hyperammonemia can occur.[60–63]

Mitochondrial myopathy, encephalopathy, lactic acidosis, and stroke (MELAS) syndrome is another important diagnosis to consider in such late-onset and recurrent comas. This syndrome is characterized by onset in childhood with intermittent vomiting, proximal limb weakness, strokelike episodes (hemiparesis, cortical blindness, hemianopsia), lactic acidosis, and ragged red fibers in the muscle or biopsy.[64] Mitochondrial complex I deficiency is the major, if not the only, biochemical cause of this syndrome.[65–69] Complex I deficiency was also found in muscle from a child presenting with MELAS syndrome associated with the angiographic feature of moya moya syndrome.[65]

Early episodic central nervous system problems (stuporous states and/or strokelike attacks) possibly associated with liver insufficiency or cardiac failure (pericardial effusions, cardiac tamponade) have been inaugural symptoms in some cases of congenital defects of glycosylation.[11]

In summary, all the disorders listed should be systematically considered in the expanding differential diagnosis of strokes or strokelike episodes. Probably many other organic acidurias can be potentially revealed by a stroke-like encephalopathy as it is suggested by recent descriptions.[69a,69b] In accordance with this list and to this biologic approach to stroke episodes and recurrent attacks of comas, we emphasize that such vaguely defined and/or undocumented diagnoses as encephalitis, basilar migraine, intoxication, or cerebral thrombophlebitis should be questioned, especially when even moderate ketoacidosis, hyperlactacidemia, or hyperammonemia is present. In fact, these apparent initial acute manifestations are frequently preceded by other premonitory symptoms, which may be unrecognized or misinterpreted. Such symptoms include acute ataxia, persistent anorexia, chronic vomiting, failure to thrive, hypotonia, and progressive developmental delay—all symptoms that are often observed in urea cycle disorders, respiratory chain defects, and organic acidurias.

Certain features or symptoms are characteristic of particular disorders. For example, macrocephaly is a frequent finding in glutaric aciduria type I; unexplained episodes of dehydration may occur in organic acidurias (see "Recurrent Attacks of Dehydration" below); and hepatomegaly at the time of coma is an important although inconsistent finding in fructose diphosphatase deficiency. Severe hematologic manifestations are common in isovaleric acidemia, propionic acidemia, and methylmalonic acidemia; they are usually accompanied by ketoacidosis and coma but are sometimes the presenting problem. Neutropenia is regularly observed in both neonatal and late-onset forms of isovaleric acidemia, propionic acidemia, and methylmalonic acidemia. Thrombocytopenia occurs only in infancy and anemia only in the neonatal period (see "Pancytopenia, Neutropenia, Thrombocytopenia" below). Recurrent infections, particularly with mucocutaneous candidiasis, are common. Relapsing petechiae and orthostatic acrocyanosis are findings evocative of EPEMA syndrome.[55,56]

When coma is associated with hepatic dysfunction, a phenocopy of Reye syndrome involving disorders of fatty acid oxidation and the urea cycle should be considered (see "Reye Syndrome" below). Hepatic coma with liver failure and hyperlactacidemia can be a revealing sign of respiratory chain disorders.[70–72] Finally, hepatic coma with cirrhosis, chronic hepatic dysfunction, hemolytic jaundice, and various neurologic signs (psychiatric, extrapyramidal) is a classic but underdiagnosed manifestation of Wilson disease (see Table 66-5).

Intermittent acute ataxia and abnormal behavior can be the presenting signs of late-onset MSUD and organic acidurias, in which they are associated with ketoacidosis and sometimes with hyperglycemia, which can mimic ketoacidotic diabetes[31] (see "Metabolic Acidosis" below). Late-onset forms of congenital hyperammonemia, mainly partial OTC deficiency, can strike late in childhood or in adolescence with psychiatric symptoms. Because hyperammonemia and liver dysfunction can be mild even at the time of acute attack, these intermittent late-onset forms of urea cycle disorders can easily be misdiagnosed as hysteria, schizophrenia, or intoxication. Acute ataxia associated with peripheral neuropathy is a frequent presenting sign of pyruvate dehydrogenase deficiency; moderate hyperlactacidemia with a normal L:P ratio (see "Hyperlactacidemias" below) supports this diagnosis. Finally, we must remember the patients affected with homocysteine remethylation defects who present with schizophrenia-like, folate-responsive episodes[73] (see "Progressive Neurologic and Mental Deterioration" below).

The initial approach to the late-onset acute forms of inherited metabolic disorders, like the approach to acute "neonatal distresses," is based on the proper use of a few screening tests. As with neonates, the biologic data from these tests (see Table 66-2) must be collected during the acute attack, all at the same time, and both before and after treatment. Some very significant symptoms, such as metabolic acidosis and ketosis, can be moderate and transient and can depend largely on symptomatic therapy. This is also true for hyperammonemia in the late-onset forms of OTC deficiency, in which blood ammonia levels can be only 100 to 150 μM when the child is in deep coma. Similarly, in Reye syndrome, the liver test abnormalities (such as elevated transaminases and lowered prothrombin time) caused by urea cycle disorders and fatty acid oxidation defects are often moderate although significant.[75] Conversely, at an advanced stage, many nonspecific abnormalities (such as acidosis, severe hyperlactacidemia, hyperammonemia, and liver dysfunction) can be secondary consequences of vascular shock.

Metabolic Acidosis

Metabolic acidosis is a very common symptom in pediatrics (see also "Ketosis" below). It can be observed in a large variety of acquired circumstances, including infections, severe catabolic states, tissue anoxia, severe dehydration, and intoxication; All these common causes should be ruled out before considering inborn errors of metabolism. However, it must be stressed that these circumstances can also sometimes trigger acute decompensation for an unrecognized inborn error of metabolism.

Setting aside the effects of specific clinical circumstances, metabolic acidotic states in pediatric patients are understood mainly on the basis of simultaneous determinations of blood gases, electrolytes and anion gap, glucose, lactate, pyruvate, ketone bodies, and ammonia. At the bedside, the physician should check for a special odor and for ketonuria, mellituria, and α-ketoaciduria (DNPH reaction), and should measure urine pH and electrolytes. Urine and plasma samples should be frozen for subsequent metabolic investigations (mostly of amino acids and organic acids). As usual, it is important to collect all laboratory data at the same time and, if possible, before therapy, because therapy can mask some significant symptoms. When disease is advanced, nonspecific abnormalities (such as respiratory acidosis, severe hyperlactacidemia, or secondary hyperammonemia) can mask the primary problem.

The presence or absence of ketonuria associated with metabolic acidosis is the major clinical key to the diagnosis, particularly in the neonatal period, during which significant ketonuria is nearly pathognomonic of an inborn error of metabolism (Table 66-7).

When metabolic acidosis *is not* associated with ketosis, pyruvate dehydrogenase (PDH) deficiency, fatty acid oxidation disorders, and some disorders of gluconeogenesis should be considered, particularly when there is moderate to severe hyperlactacidemia. All these disorders except PDH deficiency have concomitant fasting hypoglycemia. Although fructose diphosphatase and glucose 6-phosphatase deficiencies are classically considered to give rise to ketoacidosis, it has been our experience with several patients that ketosis may be moderate or absent. Interestingly, three patients affected with fructose diphosphatase deficiency were referred to us with the tentative diagnosis of fatty acid oxidation disorders because of low concentrations of ketone bodies during hypoglycemia. When metabolic acidosis occurs with a normal anion gap and without hyperlactacidemia or hypoglycemia, the most frequent diagnosis is renal tubular acidosis (RTA) types I or II, which presents with significant hyperchloremia and alkaline urine (pH >8). In RTA type II, however, urinary pH is below 5 when the patient is profoundly acidotic. A symptomatic hyperammonemia has been recently reported as a secondary consequence in an infant presenting with severe distal renal tubular acidosis.[76] Pyroglutamic aciduria can also present early in life with constant, isolated metabolic acidosis, which can be mistaken for RTA type II. The anion gap is slightly increased, and the urinary pH is below 5.

Metabolic acidoses associated with ketosis (ketoacidotic states) compose the second large group of inherited metabolic disorders. The serum concentration of ketone bodies represents the balance between their production by the liver and their utilization by peripheral tissues. The range of serum ketone body concentration varies with age and nutritional state (Table 66-8). In children, the concentration remains low during the fed state, not exceeding 0.2 mM, except during early neonatal life, when it reaches 0.5 to 1 mM.[77] It increases by amounts related to age and blood glucose during fasting.[78–82] After a 24-h fast, normal children 1 to 7 years of age have ketone body levels of 3 to 6 mM (see Table 66-8).[79] Ketoacidosis is defined as a concentration of ketone bodies greater than 7 mM.[81]

Many metabolic disorders of childhood may lead to ketoacidosis,[31] including:

1. Insulin-dependent diabetes
2. Inborn errors of branched-chain amino acid metabolism, among which the most frequent are the late-onset forms of MSUD and methylmalonic, propionic, and isovaleric acidemias
3. Congenital lactic acidoses, such as multiple carboxylase and pyruvate carboxylase deficiencies
4. Inherited defects in enzymes of gluconeogenesis (glucose 6-phosphatase, fructose 1,6-diphosphatase) and of glycogen synthesis (glycogen synthase)
5. The ketolytic defects represented by the succinyl CoA transferase, 3-ketothiolase, and acetoacetyl CoA thiolase deficiencies

In the first four categories of disorders, hyperketosis is thought to be related mainly to an excess of ketone body production, although this assumption is not always relevant and many mechanisms of ketosis are still to be elucidated. In contrast, ketotic states due to ketolytic defects are mainly caused by decreased peripheral ketone body utilization. When metabolic acidosis is associated with ketosis, the first parameter to be considered is the glucose level, which can be elevated, normal, or low. When ketoacidosis is associated with hyperglycemia, the classic diagnosis is diabetic ketoacidosis. However, organic

Table 66-7 Metabolic Acidosis (pH < 7.30, P_{CO_2} < 30 mm Hg, CO_3H < 15 mmol)

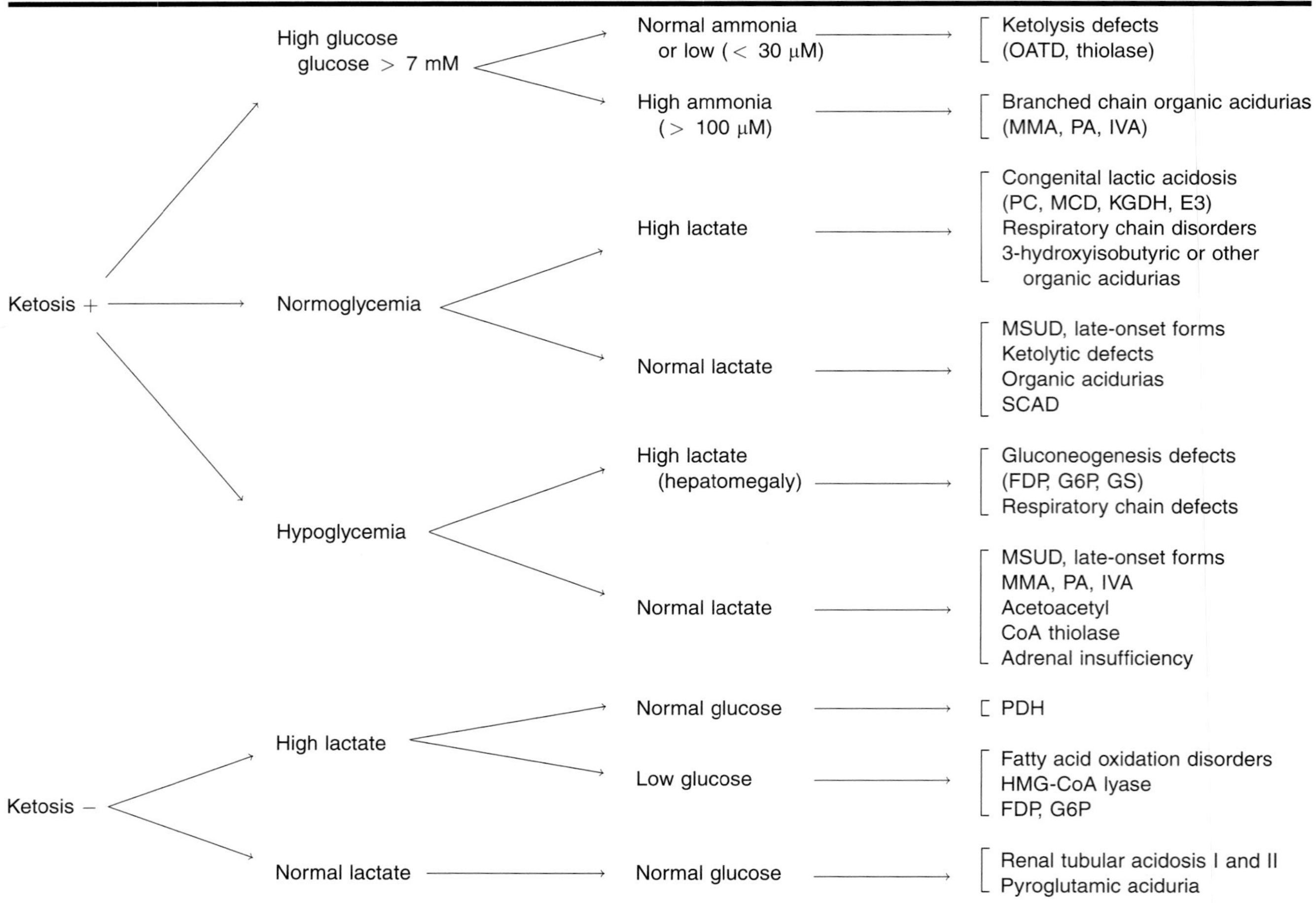

Ketosis	Glucose / lactate	Further finding	Disorders
Ketosis +	High glucose glucose > 7 mM	Normal ammonia or low (< 30 μM)	Ketolysis defects (OATD, thiolase)
Ketosis +	High glucose glucose > 7 mM	High ammonia (> 100 μM)	Branched chain organic acidurias (MMA, PA, IVA)
Ketosis +	Normoglycemia	High lactate	Congenital lactic acidosis (PC, MCD, KGDH, E3) Respiratory chain disorders 3-hydroxyisobutyric or other organic acidurias
Ketosis +	Normoglycemia	Normal lactate	MSUD, late-onset forms Ketolytic defects Organic acidurias SCAD
Ketosis +	Hypoglycemia	High lactate (hepatomegaly)	Gluconeogenesis defects (FDP, G6P, GS) Respiratory chain defects
Ketosis +	Hypoglycemia	Normal lactate	MSUD, late-onset forms MMA, PA, IVA Acetoacetyl CoA thiolase Adrenal insufficiency
Ketosis −	High lactate	Normal glucose	PDH
Ketosis −	High lactate	Low glucose	Fatty acid oxidation disorders HMG-CoA lyase FDP, G6P
Ketosis −	Normal lactate	Normal glucose	Renal tubular acidosis I and II Pyroglutamic aciduria

OATD = oxoacyltransferase; MMA = methylmalonic acid; PA = propionic acid; IVA = isovaleric acid; PC = pyruvate carboxylase; MCD = multiple carboxylase deficiencies; KGDH = ketoglutarate dehydrogenase; E3 = lipoamide oxidoreductase; MSUD = maple syrup urine disease; SCAD = short chain acylCoA dehydrogenase; FDP = fructose biphosphatase; G6P = glucose 6 phosphatase; GS = glycogen synthase; PDH = pyruvate dehydrogenase; HMG-CoA = hydroxymethylglutaryl-CoA.

acidurias such as propionic, methylmalonic, or isovaleric acidemia and ketolytic defects can also be associated with hyperglycemia and glycosuria, mimicking diabetes. The distinction between these conditions is based on ammonia and lactate levels, which are generally increased in organic acidemias and normal or low in ketolytic defects. When ketoacidosis is associated with hypoglycemia, the first classic group of diseases to be considered is the gluconeogenesis and glycogenolysis defects. The main symptoms suggestive of this group of disorders are hepatomegaly and hyperlactacidemia; however, these are not constant findings. When there is no significant hepatomegaly, late-onset forms of MSUD and of organic acidurias must be considered as well. One patient with acetoacetyl CoA thiolase deficiency presented with moderate hypoglycemia.[83] Short-chain acyl CoA dehydrogenase can present as ketoacidosis and normoglycemia, either in the neonatal period or during recurrent attacks in infancy. Affected patients do not consistently excrete characteristic metabolites, which sometimes renders the diagnosis difficult.[84] A classic possibility in the differential diagnosis is adrenal insufficiency, which can strike as a ketoacidotic attack with hypoglycemia.

When blood glucose levels are normal, congenital lactic acidosis must be considered in addition to the disorders discussed above. Metabolic disturbances associated with high or low levels of blood glucose—organic acidurias, congenital lactic acidosis, and ketolytic defects or MSUD—can be differentiated on the basis of blood levels of lactic acid and ammonia, which are elevated in the former group and normal or low in the latter. Among the organic acid disorders, 3-hydroxyisobutyric aciduria can mimic congenital lactic acidosis.[85] According to this schematic approach to inherited ketoacidotic states, a simplistic diagnosis of "fasting ketoacidosis" or "ketotic hypoglycemia" should be questioned when there is concomitant severe metabolic acidosis. Conversely, the rare disorders glycogen synthetase, acetoacetyl CoA thiolase, succinyl CoA transferase, and short chain 3-hydroxy acyl CoA dehydrogenase (SCHAD) deficiencies may be easily missed and mistakenly labeled ketotic hypoglycemia.

Ketosis

While ketonuria should be always considered abnormal in neonates, it is a physiological finding in many circumstances of late infancy, childhood, and even adolescence. Normally, there is an equilibrium between ketone body production by the liver and ketone body consumption by peripheral tissues. However, as a general rule one can assume that hyperketosis at a level that produces metabolic acidosis is not physiological (see "Metabolic Acidosis" above). Conversely, when ketosis is not associated with acidosis, hyperlactacidemia, or hypoglycemia, it is likely to be a normal physiological reflection of the nutritional state (fasting, catabolism, vomiting, medium-chain triglyceride-enriched or other ketotic diets). Of interest are ketolytic defects (succinyl CoA transferase and 3-ketothiolase deficiencies) that can present as permanent moderate ketonuria occurring mainly in the fed state at the end of the day.[31]

Significant fasting ketonuria without acidosis is often observed in glycogenosis type III in childhood, which is always associated with severe hepatomegaly, and in the very rare glycogen synthetase defect in infancy. In both disorders, there is fasting hypoglycemia and postprandial hyperlactacidemia (Table 66-9).

Table 66-8 Normal Levels of Lactate, Ketone Bodies, and Free Fatty Acids in 48 Control Children[56,61]

		1 Month to 1 Year n = 12	1 to 7 Years n = 27	7 to 15 Years n = 9
Lactate, mM (mean ± SD)	Fed state	1.95–3.0 (2.34 ± 0.54)	0.9–1.8 (1.38 ± 0.32)	1.04–1.55 (1.23 ± 0.17)
	Fast 15 h	0.95–2.3 (1.2 ± 0.65)	0.8–1.5 (1.02 ± 0.5)	0.7–0.9 (0.7 ± 0.14)
	Fast 20 h	0.85–1.8 (1.28 ± 0.49)	0.5–1.6 (1.10 ± 0.5)	0.6–0.9 (0.76 ± 0.24)
	Fast 24 h	0.8–1.5 (1.22 ± 0.49)	0.7–1.9 (1.20 ± 0.5)	0.4–1.0 (0.8 ± 0.33)
Lactate:pyruvate (mean ± SD)	Fed state	9–14 (13.4 ± 3.4)	12–18 (15.5 ± 3.7)	8–20 (16.1 ± 6)
	Fast 15 h	10–28 (17.6 ± 8)	11–18 (14.6 ± 4.4)	8–20 (12.6 ± 6)
	Fast 20 h	7–20 (14.5 ± 7)	8–19 (14.3 ± 6.7)	7–22 (12.9 ± 6)
	Fast 24 h	8–19 (14.4 ± 5.5)	10–22 (16 ± 5.5)	7–16 (12 ± 5)
Ketone bodies (KB), mM (3OHB + AA) (mean ± SD)	Fed state	0.10–0.30 (0.18 ± 0.10)	< 0.10	< 0.10 (0.054 ± 0.020)
	Fast 15 h	0.10–0.70 (0.49 ± 0.4)	0.10–2.10 (0.83 ± 0.76)	0.10–0.40 (0.3 ± 0.38)
	Fast 20 h	0.6–3.2 (1.59 ± 1.05)	1.2–3.7 (2.46 ± 1.26)	0.10–1.00 (0.61 ± 0.43)
	Fast 24 h	1.3–3.9 (2.69 ± 1.05)	2.5–5.2 (3.56 ± 1.25)	0.7–1.7 (1.26 ± 1.02)
3OHB:AA (mean ± SD)	Fed state	< 1	< 1	< 1
	Fast 15 h	1.4–2.6 (2.2 ± 0.6)	1.4–3.2 (2.37 ± 0.91)	0.4–2.3 (1.7 ± 1.1)
	Fast 20 h	1.9–3.1 (2.54 ± 0.7)	2.3–3.3 (2.84 ± 0.45)	1.3–2.8 (2.1 ± 0.9)
	Fast 24 h	2.4–2.7 (2.42 ± 0.5)	2.5–3.3 (2.9 ± 0.58)	1.6–3.1 (2.64 ± 0.7)
Free fatty acids (FFA), mM (mean)	Fast 15 h	0.5–1.6 (1.0)	0.6–1.5 (1.1)	0.2–1 (0.7)
	Fast 20 h	0.6–1.3 (0.9)	0.9–2.6 (1.7)	0.6–1.3 (1.0)
	Fast 24 h	1.1–1.6 (1.3)	1.1–2.8 (2.1)	1.0–1.8 (1.4)
FFA:KB (mean)	Fast 15 h	0.6–5.2 (2.3)	0.7–4.0 (2.2)	1.9–10 (5.4)
	Fast 20 h	0.3–1.4 (0.8)	0.4–1.5 (0.8)	0.7–4.6 (2.5)
	Fast 24 h	0.3–0.7 (0.5)	0.4–0.9 (0.6)	0.5–2 (1.5)

3OHB = 3-hydroxybutyrate; AA = acetoacetate.

Finally, ketosis without acidosis is observed in ketotic hypoglycemias of childhood and in association with hypoglycemias due to adrenal insufficiency. SCHAD, short-chain acyl CoA (SCAD) and medium-chain acyl CoA dehydrogenase (MCAD) deficiencies can present as recurrent attacks of ketotic hypoglycemia, since these enzymes are both sufficiently far down the β-oxidation pathway to be able to generate some ketones from long-chain fatty acids.[86] Absence of ketonuria in hypoglycemic states, as well as in fasting and in catabolic circumstances induced by vomiting, anorexia, or intercurrent infections, is an important observation, suggesting an inherited disorder of fatty acid oxidation and ketogenesis (see "Hypoketotic Hypoglycemias Due to Inborn Errors of Ketogenesis" below).

Hyperlactacidemias

Under physiological conditions, blood levels of lactate, pyruvate, acetoacetate, and 3-hydroxybutyrate are determined by carefully regulated pathways for production and utilization, which take place at different sites in the body. The enzymatic defect or defects underlying many inherited diseases are revealed in abnormal blood levels of these compounds. It should be noted that the metabolic profiles for these substrates are very different in the major organs, such as brain, muscle, and liver.

Lactate and pyruvate are normal metabolites. Their plasma levels reflect the equilibrium between their cytoplasmic production from glycolysis and their consumption by the different tissues. Some tissues derive much of their energy from glycolytic activity, and in such circumstances the end product of glycolysis is lactic acid. Lactate is produced mainly in skin (30 percent), erythrocytes (30 percent), brain (16 percent), and muscle (16 percent). Lactate utilization during fasting occurs through gluconeogenesis in liver (60–70 percent) and by mitochondrial oxidation in heart, muscle, and kidney. Blood levels of lactate and pyruvate and the L:P ratio (see Table 66-8) reflect the redox state of the cells. Table 66-8

Table 66-9 Ketosis (see also Metabolic Acidosis)

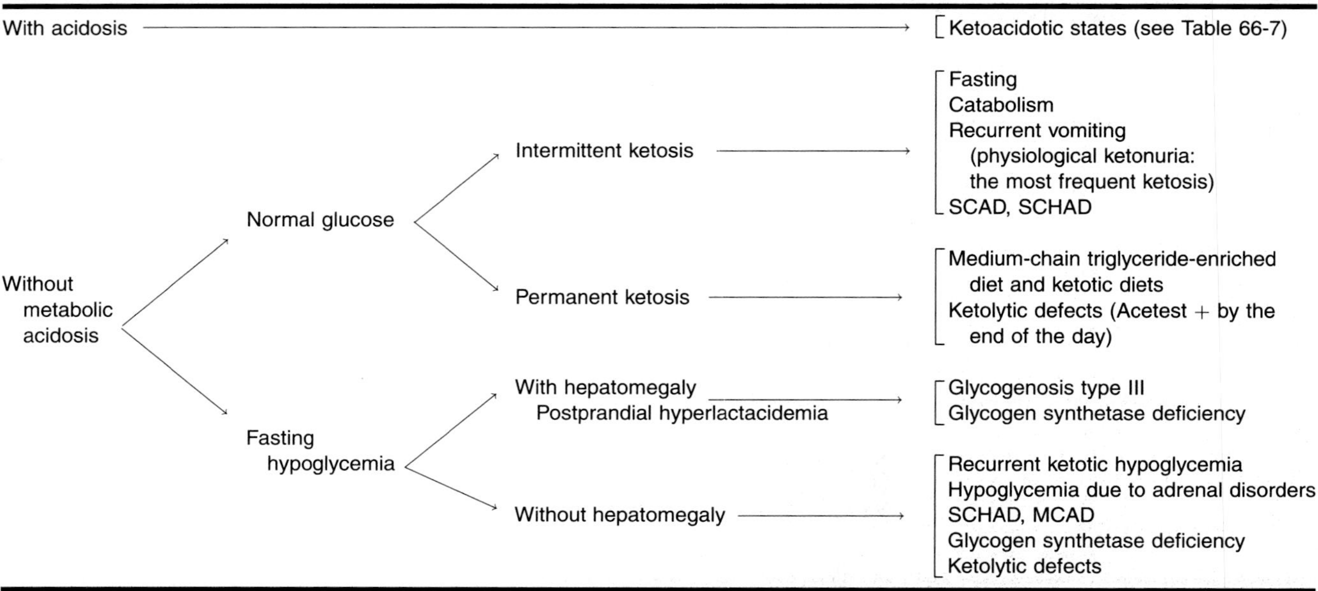

SCAD = short chain acyl CoA dehydrogenase; SCHAD = hydroxy short chain acyl CoA dehydrogenase; MCAD = medium chain acyl CoA dehydrogenase.

gives normal levels of lactate, ketone bodies, and free fatty acids as measured in 48 control children aged 1 month to 15 years[79,87] (see also in ref. 82).

Blood lactate accumulates in circulatory collapse, in hypoxic insult, and in other conditions involving failure of cellular respiration. These conditions must be ruled out before an inborn error of lactate-pyruvate oxidation is sought. Persistent hyperlacticacidemias can result from many acquired conditions, such as chronic diarrheas (as in cow milk intolerance), persistent infections (mainly of the urinary tract), hyperventilation, and hepatic failure. Ketosis is absent in most hyperlactacidemias secondary to tissue hypoxia, while it is a nearly constant finding in most inborn errors of metabolism. On the other hand, the level of lactic acidemia is not discriminating: Some acquired disorders are associated with very high levels, whereas some inborn errors of lactate-pyruvate oxidation cause only moderate hyperlactacidemia. Nutritional state also influences the levels of lactate and pyruvate.

Lactic Acidemias Due to Inborn Errors of Metabolism. Once the organic acidurias, urea cycle defects (mainly citrullinemia), and fatty acid oxidation defects that cause secondary hyperlactacidemia have been excluded as possible diagnoses, four types of disorder remain to be considered:

1. Disorders of liver glycogen metabolism
2. Disorders of liver gluconeogenesis
3. Abnormalities of lactate-pyruvate oxidation, the PDH complex, or the Krebs cycle
4. Deficient activity in one of the components of the respiratory chain

The diagnosis of hyperlactacidemias revolves around certain clinical and metabolic criteria (Table 66-10).[23]

Time of Occurrence of Lactic Acidosis Relative to Feeding. In disorders of gluconeogenesis (fructose diphosphatase and glucose 6-phosphatase deficiencies), hyperlactacidemia (up to 15 mM) reaches its maximum level in the fasted state, when blood glucose is low. Conversely, lactate can drop to normal values in the fed state, when blood glucose is normal. In contrast, in glycogenosis types III and VI and in glycogen synthetase deficiency, hyperlacticacidemia is observed only in the postprandial period in patients on a carbohydrate-rich diet; lactate levels are normal when the patient has been fasting or is hypoglycemic.[88,89] In these disorders, hyperlactacidemia rarely exceeds 6 mM. In pyruvate carboxylase deficiency, hyperlactacidemia is present in both the fed and the fasted state but tends to decrease with a short fast. In disorders of PDH, alpha-ketoglutarate dehydrogenase, and respiratory chain function, maximum lactate levels are observed in the fed state (although all hyperlactacidemias exceeding 7 mM appear more or less permanent). In these disorders, there is a real risk of missing a moderate (although significant) hyperlactacidemia when the level is checked only before breakfast after an overnight fast (as is usual for laboratory determinations).

Use of Ratios: Lactate:Pyruvate, 3-Hydroxybutyrate:Acetoacetate. The second clue to diagnosis is the simultaneous determination of plasma L:P and 3OHB:AA ratios before and after meals. These ratios indirectly reflect cytoplasmic L:P and mitochondrial 3OHB:AA redox potential states. They must be measured in carefully collected blood samples that have been deproteinized immediately; any delay between removal of the blood and deproteinization results in a rapid loss of pyruvate and acetoacetate, resulting in artificial elevation of the L:P and 3OHB:AA ratios. When these cautions are observed, redox ratios provide an excellent tool for classifying congenital hyperlactacidemias.

Three metabolic profiles are nearly pathognomonic for an inborn error of lactate-pyruvate metabolism:[23]

1. When the L:P ratio is normal or low (<10) without hyperketonemia, PDH deficiency is highly probable, regardless of lactate level (which is often only moderately elevated after a meal). If PDH deficiency is suspected, a study of blood lactate after fructose intake can be useful.[90] Loading with dichloroacetate[91] or 2-chloropropionate can also be performed to test *in vivo* PDH activation.
2. When the L:P ratio is very high (>30) in association with paradoxical postprandial hyperketonemia and a normal or low (<1.5) 3OHB:AA ratio, a diagnosis of pyruvate carboxylase deficiency[38,92] or alpha-ketoglutarate dehydrogenase deficiency is virtually certain. The two disorders are differentiated on the basis of glutamate and alpha-ketoglutarate determinations, which are strongly elevated in the latter condition.[93] Biotinidase and holocarboxylase synthetase deficiencies give rise to a

Table 66-10 **Hyperlactacidemias**

Time of occurrence	Main clinical signs	Redox potential states	Diagnosis
Only after feeding (or exacerbated after feeding)	Hepatomegaly Fasting ketotic hypoglycemia	Not diagnostic	Glycogenosis type III Glycogen synthetase
	Neurologic signs Encephalomyopathy	Normal L:P ratio No ketosis	PDH
		L:P high 3OHB:AA low Postprandial hyperketosis	PC (citrullinemia), MCD Alpha-KDH (isolated or multi-ketodecarboxylase)
		L:P high 3OHB:AA high Postprandial ketosis	Respiratory chain (3 methyl glutaconic aciduria, Krebs cycle intermediates) Krebs cycle defects
		L:P high No ketosis	Respiratory chain Krebs cycle defects
Only after fasting (or exacerbated after fasting) or during acute attack	Prominent hepatomegaly Fasting hypoglycemia	Not diagnostic (normal L:P ratio)	Glycogenosis type I Fructose diphosphatase (ketosis inconstant)
	Moderate hepatomegaly Hypoketotic hypoglycemia	Not diagnostic	Fatty acid oxidation disorders (cardiac, muscle symptoms) Fructose diphosphatase
Permanent	Moderate hyperlactacidemia Recurrent attacks of ketoacidosis	Not diagnostic	Organic acidurias (MMA, PA, IVA, and others)
	Predominant hyperammonemia	Not diagnostic	Urea cycle defects (in neonates)
	Predominant fasting hypoglycemia Hepatomegaly	Not diagnostic	Glycogenosis type I Fructose diphosphatase
	Neurologic signs Encephalomyopathy Significant hyperlactacidemia (>7 mM)	Highly diagnostic (see above "after feeding")	Congenital lactic acidemias (see above "after feeding")
	Intrauterine growth retardation Severe hepatic failure Significant hyperlactacidemia in the neonatal period	L:P high	Liver hemosiderosis Respiratory chain disorders Hepatic necrosis (all causes)

AA = acetoacetate; IVA = isovaleric acidemia; KDH = ketoglutarate dehydrogenase; MCD = multiple carboxylase deficiency; MMA = methylmalonic aciduria; PA = propionic acidemia; PC = pyruvate carboxylase; PDH = pyruvate dehydrogenase; L = lactate; P = pyruvate; 3OHB = 3-hydroxybutyrate

metabolic profile similar to that of isolated pyruvate carboxylase deficiency.

3. When both L:P and 3OHB:AA ratios are elevated in association with significant postprandial hyperketonemia, respiratory chain disorders should be suspected.[16,94]

All other situations, especially when the L:P ratio is high without hyperketonemia, are compatible with respiratory chain disorders, but all acquired anoxic conditions should also be ruled out (see above). In such situations, if hyperlactacidemia is moderate (2 to 3 mM), it would be worthwhile to determine the CSF lactate level (in cases with a neurologic presentation) and the L:P ratio after a glucose loading test and/or a physical exercise test (in cases with a muscular or systemic presentation).[82] These tests are not useful when the basal lactate level exceeds 7 mM.

Hypoglycemia: General Approach

Our approach to hypoglycemia is based on four major clinical criteria:[94a]

1. Liver size
2. Characteristic schedule of hypoglycemia (unpredictable or permanent, postprandial or only after fasting)
3. Association with lactic acidosis
4. Association with hyperketosis or hypoketosis

Other clinical signs of interest are neonatal size (head circumference, weight, height); hepatic failure; vascular hypotension; dehydration; short stature later in life; and evidence of encephalopathy, myopathy, or cardiomyopathy. In neonates, glucose infusion rates higher than 10 mg/kg/min to maintain plasma glucose levels within normal limits, and glycemic responses to glucagon infusion are highly characteristic of hyperinsulinism.

Liver size can be used to separate the hypoglycemias into two large groups (Table 66-11), as discussed below.

Hypoglycemia with Permanent Hepatomegaly. Most of the hypoglycemias associated with permanent hepatomegaly are due to inborn errors of metabolism. All conditions, acquired or inherited, that are associated with severe liver failure in the neonatal period or during infancy or childhood can give rise to severe hypoglycemia, which appears after 2 to 3 h of fasting and involves moderate lactic acidosis and no ketosis. When hepatomegaly is the most prominent feature and liver insufficiency is absent, gluconeogenesis defects (involving glucose 6-phosphatase or fructose diphosphatase [FDP]), glycogenosis type III, and glycogen synthetase (GS) deficiency are the most probable diagnoses. However, in some cases of FDP and GS, hepatomegaly can be moderate or absent, even at the time of a hypoglycemia attack. Conversely, moderate hepatomegaly can be present in neonatal forms of hyperinsulinism and is a frequent finding during acute decompensation in fatty acid oxidation disorders. In gluconeogenesis defects, fasting hypoglycemia is classically associated with ketolactic acidosis (see "Metabolic Acidosis" and "Hyperlactacidemias" above). In glycogenosis type III and glycogen synthetase deficiency, the abdomen is prominent and fasting hypoglycemia is associated with hyperketosis, but there is no metabolic acidosis and fasting lactacidemia is low. In contrast,

Table 66-11 Hypoglycemia: General Approach

With permanent hepatomegaly or severe liver dysfunction	Severe liver failure Hepatic necrosis (see Table 66-56)	Permanent short-fast hypoglycemia	Neonatal to early infancy	Galactosemia Fructosemia Tyrosinosis type I Neonatal hemochromatosis Other severe hepatic failure (respiratory chain)
	Cirrhosis	Postprandial hypoglycemia (triggered by fructose) Vomiting	Neonatal to early infancy	Fructose intolerance Glycerol intolerance
		Mental retardation Hypermethioninemia	Early infancy	Glycogenosis type IV SAH hydrolase
	Isolated hepatomegaly	Fasting hypoglycemia and lactic acidosis Ketosis	Infancy	Glycogenosis type I Fructose diphosphatase PEPCK
		Protuberant abdomen Fasting hypoglycemia and ketosis Postprandial hyperlactacidemia	Infancy	Glycogenosis type III Glycogen synthetase
	Hypotonia Failure to thrive Chronic diarrhea	Abnormal glycosylated transferrin	Infancy	CDG syndrome
		Fanconi-like tubulopathy Postprandial hyperglycemia	Infancy	Fanconi-Bickel syndrome (GLUT II mutations)
Without permanent hepatomegaly	With ketoacidosis	Recurrent attacks Hyperlactacidemia	Infancy to childhood	Organic acidurias Late-onset MSUD Ketolysis defects Glycerol kinase Fructose diphosphatase SCHAD, MCAD Respiratory chain disorders
		Dehydration Collapse Hyponatremia	Neonatal to childhood	Adrenal insufficiency
	Acidosis without ketosis	Moderate hyperlactacidemia Reye syndrome (± muscle/cardiac symptoms)	Neonatal to infancy	HMG-CoA lyase (frequent) HMG-CoA synthetase (rare) FAO disorders (frequent) Idiopathic Reye
	Ketosis without acidosis	Fasting hypoglycemia Low lactate levels Small for age Macrocephaly	1–6 years	Recurrent ketotic hypoglycemia Adrenal insufficiency (central or peripheral) SCHAD, MCAD Ketolysis defects
		Unpredictable and postprandial hypoglycemia reactive to glucagon	Neonatal to childhood	Hyperinsulinism: SUR and KIR mutations Glucokinase mutation Glutamate dehydrogenase mutation (with hyperammonemia) Focal hyperplasia (loss of maternal allele on 11p15 chromosome) CDG syndrome Munchausen by proxy
	Without ketosis O2 acidosis	Short stature (inconstant) Short-fast hypoglycemia	Infancy	Growth hormone deficiency and related disorders
		Long-fast hypoglycemia Reye syndrome Acute moderate hepatomegaly Transient cytolysis and slight hepatic insufficiency	Neonatal to infancy	FAO disorders (frequent) HMG-CoA lyase (rare) Fructose diphosphatase (rare) HMG-CoA synthetase (rare)

SAH = S-adenosylhomocysteine; MSUD = maple syrup urine disease; PEPCK = phosphoenolpyruvate carboxykinase; CDG = congenital defects of glycosylation; MCAD = medium chain acyl CoA dehydrogenase; SCHAD = hydroxy short chain acyl CoA dehydrogenase; FAO = fatty acid oxidation; HMG-CoA = hydroxymethylglutaryl CoA.

there is a moderate but significant postprandial hyperlactacidemia that is highly suggestive of these diagnoses. Disorders presenting as hepatic fibrosis and cirrhosis, such as hereditary tyrosinemia type I, can give rise to hypoglycemia. The late-onset form of fructose intolerance is rarely if ever revealed by isolated postprandial hypoglycemic attacks. S-adenosylhomocysteine hydrolase deficiency presents as fasting hypoglycemia and hepatocellular insufficiency, often triggered by high protein or methionine ingestion, and is associated with hepatic fibrosis, mental retardation, and marked hypermethioninemia.[95] A hyperinsulinemic hypoglycemia associated with hepatomegaly can reveal a carbohydrate-deficient glycoprotein (CDG) syndrome.[95a] In Fanconi-Bickel syndrome, fasting hypoglycemia is associated with hepatic glycogenosis and Fanconi's tubulopathy and is due to *GLUT2* mutations.[96]

Hypoglycemia Without Permanent Hepatomegaly. It is important to discover the timing of hypoglycemia and to search for metabolic acidosis and ketosis when the patient is hypoglycemic. Unpredictable postprandial or very short fasting hypoglycemias (2 to 6 h) are mostly due to hyperinsulinism and growth hormone deficiency or related disorders.

When ketoacidosis is present at the time of hypoglycemia, organic acidurias (methylmalonic, propionic, isovaleric, hydroxyisobutyric, methylglutaconic, and methylcrotonic, ketolytic defects (succinyl CoA transferase, 3-ketothiolase), late-onset MSUD, and glycerol kinase deficiencies should be considered. Here, hypoglycemia is very rarely the initial metabolic abnormality. Adrenal insufficiencies (all types) should be systematically considered in the differential diagnosis, especially when vascular hypotension, dehydration, and hyponatremia are present. Severe hypoglycemia with metabolic acidosis and absence of ketosis in the context of Reye syndrome suggests 3-hydroxy-3-methylglutaryl CoA (HMG-CoA) lyase deficiency or fatty acid oxidation disorders (see "Hypoketotic Hypoglycemias Due to Inborn Errors of Ketogenesis" below). Fasting hypoglycemia with ketosis occurring mostly in the morning and in the absence of metabolic acidosis suggests recurrent functional ketotic hypoglycemia, which presents mostly in late infancy or childhood in children who were small for their gestational age or in children with macrocephaly. All types of adrenal insufficiencies (peripheral or central) can share this presentation. Two other disorders, SCHAD and MCAD, can also present as recurrent attacks of ketotic hypoglycemia, as the enzymes involved are both sufficiently far down the β-oxidation pathway to be able to generate some ketones from long-chain fatty acids.[86]

Hypoketotic hypoglycemias encompass several groups of disorders. As already stated, hyperinsulinemic states present as unpredictable or postprandial hypoglycemia, which is dramatically responsive to glucagon (0.5 to 1 mg intramuscularly). In addition to patients with the well-known neonatal "intractable" hypoglycemias due to severe hyperinsulinism, a number of hyperinsulinemic patients present with an unexpected generalized seizure occurring right in the middle of the day at the age of 3 to 12 months or sometimes later. Diagnosis relies mostly on the timing of hypoglycemia and on constant glucagon responsiveness rather than on peripheral plasma insulin measurements, which can be normal even when the patient is hypoglycemic.[97,98] Such patients frequently have neonatal height and weight above the 90th percentile. Absence of ketonuria (a nearly constant finding) with hypoglycemia occurring in the fed state or after a short fast indicates hyperinsulinism. Hyperinsulinisms can be classified into four categories:

1. Criminal hyperinsulinism secondary to insulin injection or to oral administration of antidiabetic drugs (Munchausen by proxy)
2. Pancreatic adenomas, which start most often in late infancy to childhood or even adulthood and are due to monoclonal proliferation of insulin cells
3. Diffuse hyperplasia (nesidioblastosis) secondary to either mutations in *SUR* and *KIR-2* genes, both localized on 11p15 chromosome, which encode for the K-ATP channel,[99–101] or to glucokinase,[102] and glutamate dehydrogenase mutations (the latter two being associated with permanent hyperammonemia)[104]
4. Focal hyperplasia due to a somatic genetic event resulting in loss of a maternal-imprinted region localized on chromosome 11p15 with duplication of the corresponding imprinted paternal chromosome 11p15 region, which also bears a genomic mutation in the *SUR* gene. This loss of heterozygosity is limited to the tumor and is not present in the rest of the pancreas or in systemic DNA[105,106]

From a clinical point of view, once forms associated with hyperammonemia have been recognized, there is no clinical difference between diffuse and focal forms (same age of onset, same neonatal measurements, same severity of hypoglycemia, same usual resistance of hypoglycemia to diazoxide), and classic radiologic investigations (including nuclear magnetic resonance [NMR] echography, and [SCAN]) fail to visualize focal forms.[107] The only way to identify focal hyperplasia preoperatively is by pancreatic venous sampling through portal catheterization[97] and intraoperative histology of three biopsies, performed in the tail, the isthmus, and the head of the pancreas.[108] Pre- and perioperative recognition of focal forms is of major importance, as focal hyperinsulinism can be cured by very limited partial pancreatectomy, while diffuse hyperplasias resistant to medical treatment require nearly total pancreatectomy, which exposes the patient to pancreatic diabetes.[107] Some rare mutations in the proinsulin processing cleavage pathway can give rise to glycemic instability, with alternation of hyper- and hypoglycemia.[109] Very rare autoimmune disorders can lead to the synthesis of autoantibodies directed against insulin receptors, resulting in attacks of hypoglycemia which can mimic hyperinsulinism.[110] In a congenital defect glycosylation. Hypoglycemic hyperinsulinism has also been described as a presenting symptom.[95a]

In hereditary disorders of fatty acid oxidation and in Reye syndrome with hypoketosis, hypoglycemia occurs mostly after fasting.

Growth hormone deficiency and related disorders (Laron dwarfism, insulin growth factor deficiencies, etc.) can present early in infancy as severe hypoketotic hypoglycemia occurring after a 4- to 6-h fast. Hypoglycemia can be a revealing sign before a height abnormality appears.

Hypoketotic hypoglycemia due to inborn errors of ketogenesis and fatty acid oxidation most often presents in a highly suggestive clinical context. It either is integrated in a picture of Reye syndrome or occurs after an overnight fast or a catabolic insult. In this context, the absence of ketonuria in fasting hypoglycemia should always be considered abnormal and very suggestive of a fatty acid oxidation disorder. Hypoketotic hypoglycemia can be the initial symptom or can be associated with other manifestations, either acute (hypotension, heartbeat disorders, cardiac arrest, sudden death) or chronic (tubulopathy, progressive proximal myopathy, cardiomyopathy, peripheral neuropathy). The diagnostic approach to hypoketotic hypoglycemia is presented in Table 66-11.

Hypoketotic Hypoglycemias Due to Inborn Errors of Ketogenesis

About twenty hereditary defects of fatty acid catabolism and ketogenesis have been discovered in patients with manifestations ranging from congenital malformations and SIDS-like deaths to vague malaise in the adult. They include multiple acyl CoA dehydrogenase deficiency caused by defects in electron transport flavoprotein (ETF) or electron transport flavoprotein dehydrogenase (ETFDH), defects of long-chain fatty acid oxidation due to mitochondrial transport disorders (carnitine transporter deficiency, deficiencies of CPT I, CPT II, and translocase), defects of β-oxidation (deficiencies of VLCAD, LCHAD, trifunctional protein [TF], and dienoyl CoA reductase), and deficiencies of medium- and short-chain acyl CoA dehydrogenases (MCAD and

SCAD or SCHAD, respectively), medium-chain 3-ketoacyl CoA thiolase[111] and the two mitochondrial enzymes involved in ketogenesis, HMG-CoA synthetase, and HMG-CoA lyase. The clinical features are diverse. However, hypoketotic hypoglycemia, Reye syndrome–like encephalopathy, sudden infant death, and fasting coma are common features of all these disorders, with or without other manifestations[21] (see also "I. Presentation in the Neonatal Period" above and "Reye Syndrome," "Sudden Infant Death Syndrome," "Exercise Intolerance and Recurrent Myoglobinuria," "Cardiac Disorders," "Progressive Neurologic and Mental Deterioration" [Table 66-25], "Retinitis Pigmentosa," and "Tubulopathy [Renal Fanconi Syndrome and Tubular Acidosis]" below).

Age of onset is an important key to diagnosis. Deficiencies of MCAD and CPT I and primary systemic carnitine deficiency are rarely observed in the neonatal period. Deficiencies of ETF, ETFDH, and CPT II can present in the neonatal period in association with renal cysts and brain dysplasia. Depending on the residual enzyme activity, these disorders have clinical presentations ranging from neonatal coma with severe cardiomyopathy and sudden infant death to late-onset myopathy and recurrent myoglobinuria. The absence of ketonuria during fasting hypoglycemia is always abnormal and is suggestive of a mitochondrial fatty acid oxidation disorder.

In general, long-chain fatty acid disorders involving CPT II, translocase, VLCAD, TF, and LCHAD have more severe clinical signs than MCAD and SCAD deficiencies. These long-chain disorders often begin in infancy and can be revealed by cardiac arrest or shock, which can be easily misdiagnosed as toxic shock, malignant hyperthermia, or heartbeat disorders (see "Cardiac Disorders" below). Massive pericardial effusion has been recently reported in a late-onset type II glutaric acidemia.[112]

All patients who have cardiomyopathy (except those affected with treated carnitine transporter deficiency) are permanently at risk for unexpected death, despite therapy. By contrast, cardiomyopathy and myopathy are not observed in MCAD and CPT I deficiencies.[113] Proximal and distal renal tubulopathy responsive to the addition of medium-chain triglycerides to the diet has been a presenting sign in patients with CPT I deficiency.[114] The occurrence and pathophysiology of neurologic symptoms are unclear. It must be stressed that the depth and duration of coma do not correlate with the degree of hypoglycemia. One condition, LCHAD deficiency, presents as retinitis pigmentosa and progressive peripheral neuropathy, symptoms also commonly observed in peroxisomal disorders.[115,116] Hydroxymethylglutaryl CoA (HMG-CoA) lyase deficiency presents similarly to fatty acid oxidation disorders, with hypoketotic hypoglycemia, Reye syndrome, SIDS, and metabolic acidosis, as HMG-CoA synthetase deficiency, which does not display acidosis.[117] A defect in the transport of long chain fatty acids associated with acute liver failure has been recently identified.[117a] All these conditions can be diagnosed through a protocol based mostly on the plasma and urine carnitine levels, acylcarnitine[118–120] and organic acid profiles at the time of the acute episode, provocative tests between attacks (long-chain/medium-chain triglyceride loading tests, fasting test), and the *in vitro* study of whole fatty acid oxidation on fresh lymphocytes or cultured fibroblasts. It should be emphasized that a normal or nonspecific urinary organic acid pattern and a normal plasma carnitine level, even when measured during acute decompensation, do not necessarily rule out an inherited disorder of fatty acid oxidation.

An algorithm summarizing our current diagnostic approach is proposed in Fig. 66-1.

Reye Syndrome

In 1963, Reye first described a clinical entity in children involving acute encephalopathy and fatty degeneration of the viscera.[121] The Centers for Disease Control and Prevention (CDC) now define Reye syndrome as an acute noninflammatory encephalopathy (alteration in level of consciousness, no CSF pleocytosis, and, if biologic examination is possible, cerebral edema without meningeal or perivascular inflammation) associated with "microvesicular fatty metamorphosis of the liver" (confirmed by biopsy or autopsy) or a significant rise (threefold or greater) of serum transaminases or blood ammonia, having "no more reasonable explanation" for the cerebral and hepatic abnormalities.[122,123] The criteria for diagnosis are not specific and could be more rigorous.[124] Despite strong epidemiologic evidence in the United States and Great Britain that the disorder is associated with salicylate ingestion and influenza B virus infection,[125–127] the exact etiology of the syndrome remains unknown more than 30 years after Reye's description; most believe it is heterogeneous.[75,128,129] The pathophysiology obviously involves a generalized loss of mitochondrial function, which results in a

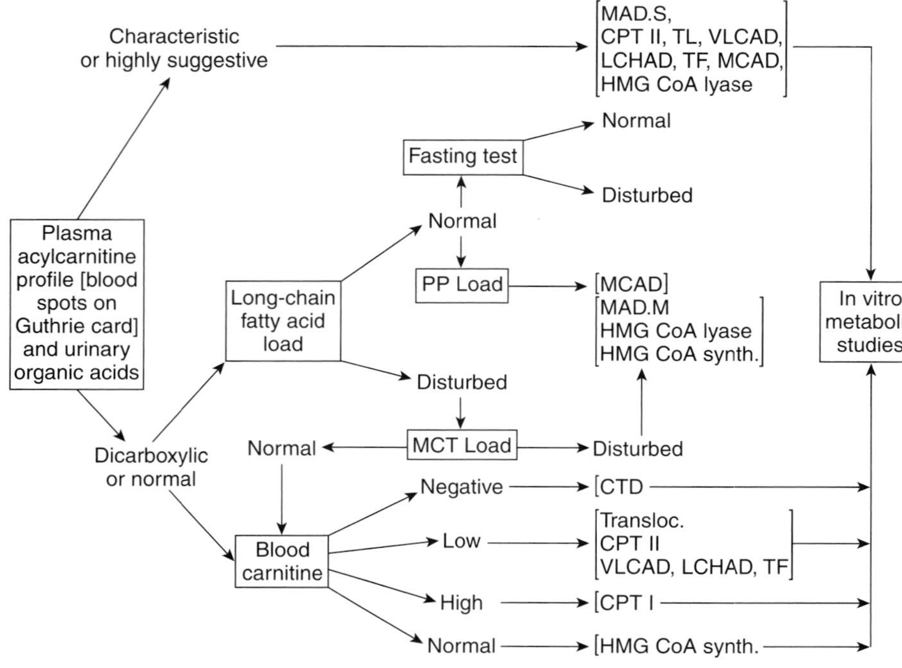

Fig. 66-1 Diagnostic approach to disorders of fatty acid oxidation. MAD(S) = multiple acyl CoA dehydrogenase, severe form; MAD(M) = multiple acyl CoA dehydrogenase, mild form; MCAD = medium-chain acyl CoA dehydrogenase; PP = phenylpropionate; MCT = medium-chain triglyceride; PSCD = primary systemic carnitine deficiency; CPT = carnitine palmitoyl transferase; LCHAD = long-chain acyl CoA dehydrogenase; 3OHLCAD = 3-hydroxyacyl CoA dehydrogenase.

Table 66-12 Inborn Errors of Metabolism Presenting as Reye Syndrome

Disorder	Incidence
Disorders of ureagenesis	Frequent
Partial OTC deficiency	> 100 cases
Partial carbamylphosphate synthase	Rare
Partial argininosuccinic acid synthase	Rare
Lysinuric protein intolerance	Rare
HHH syndrome	Very rare
Disorders of mitochondrial fatty acid oxidation and ketogenesis	Frequent
Carnitine transport defect	< 20
CPT I deficiency	< 20
CPT II deficiency	< 10
Translocase deficiency	Very rare
VLCAD/LCAD	< 20
LCHAD, trifunctional	< 20
MCAD	> 100
Multiple acyl CoA dehydrogenase	< 30
3-HMG-CoA lyase	< 30
Unknown (3-ketoacyl CoA thiolase?)	
Organic acidurias	Frequent
3-methylcrotonyl CoA carboxylase deficiency	< 10
Glutaric aciduria type I	< 30
Respiratory chain disorders	Rare
Others (e.g., MMA, PA, IVA, biotinidase)	Rare
Carbohydrate metabolism	Rare
Fructose intolerance	
Fructose diphosphatase deficiency	
Others (pyruvate carboxylase, etc.)	Very rare
Peroxisomal disorders	Very rare

IVA = isovaleric acidemia; MMA = methylmalonic acidemia; PA = propionic acidemia

Table 66-13 Reye Syndrome: Protocol of Investigation

Urinary organic acid profile
- Basal
- After fasting

Free and total carnitine and acylcarnitine in plasma and urines (acylcarnitine profile can be analyzed from a blood spot collected on filter paper)
- Basal
- After fasting
- After carnitine loading

Long-chain fatty acid loading test (1.5 g/kg by mouth after 8 hour overnight fast). Only when there is no basal disturbance.
- Check plasma glucose, free fatty acids, ketone bodies, acylcarnitine, and urinary organic acids

Phenylpropionate loading test (20 mg/kg by mouth)
- Check urinary organic acid for phenylpropionyl glycine

24-h fasting test (only when there is no basal disturbance)
- Check plasma glucose, free fatty acids, ketone bodies, NH_3, carnitine, lactate, pyruvate, amino acids, urinary organic acids; stop when blood glucose drops to $\leq$ 2.8 mM/liter

Protein load (5 g/kg/day during 1 to 5 days rather than acute load of 1 g/kg)
- Check NH_3, amino acids, orotic acid excretion; get NH_3 levels during emergency
- Perform this loading test only when basal parameters are normal and only under careful medical supervision; stop when NH_3 rises to $\geq$ 100 μM/liter

Enzymatic studies
- Liver: urea cycle enzymes (intestinal biopsy for CPS and OTC)
- Fibroblasts: fatty acid oxidation (palmitate, octanoate, butyrate)
- Lymphocytes: fatty acid oxidation, acyl CoA dehydrogenases, CPT I, CPT II, translocase, ETF, and ETFDH.

CPS = carbamylphosphate synthetase; OTC = ornithine transcarbamylase; CPT = carnitine palmitoyl transferase; ETF = electron transport flavoprotein; ETFDH = electron transfer flavoprotein dehydrogenase

large variety of metabolic disturbances involving especially fatty acyl CoA and fatty acylcarnitine compounds and carnitine metabolism.[130–132]

Within the last decade, an increasing number of inherited metabolic diseases have been described that produce episodes fitting the criteria originally used to define Reye syndrome (Table 66-12). There is now considerable evidence that many of the disorders responsible for Reye syndrome were misdiagnosed in the past because investigations for inborn errors of metabolism were not pursued sufficiently. Another important reason for this underestimation is the necessity of collecting blood and urine specimens for metabolic investigation at an appropriate time in relation to the illness, since most of the disorders affecting the mitochondrial pathways of the urea cycle and fatty acid oxidation (which are the most important group of inborn errors mimicking Reye syndrome) may produce only intermittent abnormalities. Finally, in contrast to the usual belief, a normal or nonspecific urinary organic acid pattern and a normal carnitine plasma level, even at the time of an acute attack, do not rule out an inherited fatty acid oxidation disorder. In a series of 30 patients with a diagnosis of Reye syndrome who were referred to our metabolic unit after recovery, we found specific inborn errors of metabolism in 15 (nine with fatty acid oxidation defects and three with OTC deficiency) and probable but unclassified fatty acid oxidation defects in six others. Our retrospective study of clinical, histologic, and biologic data demonstrated that no symptoms make it possible a priori to distinguish "idiopathic" Reye syndrome from Reye syndrome due to an inborn error of metabolism.[133] The latter all have symptoms and a clinical course compatible with "Reye syndrome." The finding of "no more reasonable explanation" for the encephalitic and hepatic disorders is a vague notion, and the diagnosis may depend on the thoroughness of the investigation. Increased density of the mitochondrial matrix and intracristal widening have been reported in MCAD deficiency,[134] but these data are rarely available in emergency conditions. These considerations emphasize the necessity of performing plasma amino acid chromatography, obtaining urinary organic acid profiles and an acylcarnitine profile (from a blood spot collected on filter paper like a Guthrie card)[118–120] and measuring plasma carnitine levels, ketonuria, and orotic aciduria in the acute phase. When the child survives, "a more reasonable explanation" can be excluded only by performing a complete biologic investigation as described in Table 66-13 (see also "Hypoketotic Hypoglycemias Due to Inborn Errors of Ketogenesis" above) for the diagnostic approach to fatty acid oxidation disorders. When urea cycle defects are suspected (mainly OTC deficiency) and when adequate investigations (amino acid chromatography, orotic acid excretion) have not been performed during the acute phase, we prefer to use long-term protein loading (5 g/kg/day for 1 to 5 days) for testing, rather than the classic short-term protein loading (1 g/kg), which can give a false-negative result. This test should be performed only when basal parameters (amino acids and orotic acid) are not disturbed and only under careful medical supervision.

Sudden Infant Death Syndrome

Strictly speaking, SIDS is the unexpected death of an apparently well infant over 1 month of age for which no explanation can be found despite postmortem examination.[135] It can occur as the result of dramatic cardiac failure, shock, or cardiac arrest in many metabolic situations, particularly respiratory chain disorders and mitochondrial fatty acid oxidation defects (see discussions of these symptoms in this section). Since the reports by Howat *et al.*[136,137] of MCAD deficiency presenting as SIDS, many SIDS cases have been investigated accordingly.

Actually, true SIDS due to an inborn error of metabolism is a rare event despite the large number of publications on the topic and despite the fact that at least 31 metabolic defects are candidates for causes of SIDS[138–154] (see list below). It must be stressed that some of these reports are questionable. For example, a report[146] claiming that glycogen storage disease type I was present in 10 of 38 cases of SIDS had the following flaws: (1) liver size was not reported, even though the children were autopsied and even though hepatomegaly is prominent in glycogen storage disease type I; (2) neither optical nor electron microscopic examination of the liver seems to have been done, although they would have revealed glycogen accumulation if present; (3) glucose 6-phosphatase was assayed after death, although this enzyme is very unstable and postmortem assays are unreliable.

A working party[145] tried to determine the types of metabolic diseases that may present as unexpected infant death. A call was made for a protocol to establish the existence of an inborn error of metabolism in infants who died suddenly. The following inborn errors of metabolism were considered as possible causes of such deaths:

1. Urea cycle defects
2. Organic acidurias (such as methylmalonic, propionic, and isovaleric acidurias)
3. Congenital lactic acidosis (biotinidase, PDH, and respiratory chain defects)[155]
4. Carbohydrate disorders (such as galactosemia, hereditary fructose intolerance, glycogenosis type I, fructose diphosphatase deficiency)
5. Various abnormalities of fatty acid oxidation and ketogenesis

In reality, apart from fatty acid oxidation defects, most of these disorders do not cause true SIDS in previously healthy children but rather result in acute illness with obvious clinical symptoms that precede death by hours or days. In four studies carried out on over 500 unselected SIDS cases in Paris, Lyon, Bristol, and Edinburgh, not one metabolic disorder was detected.[145] In a retrospective evaluation of 844 infants admitted after having survived an apparent life-threatening event, proven or highly suspected inborn errors of metabolism were found in only five patients, four of whom had highly significant clinical symptoms.[156] Conversely, in a more recent series of 103 patients with fatty acid oxidation disorders, we found 20 patients with revealing heartbeat disorders and 5 patients with revealing SIDS during the first week of life.[21,21a]

Table 66-14 shows the protocol for investigating SIDS sibs and near-SIDS cases. It is useful to culture fibroblasts from a skin biopsy sample if biochemical or histologic tests suggest the presence of a fatty acid oxidation defect. Also useful is the measurement of acylcarnitines in plasma or liver tissue, the profile of which is highly characteristic of many fatty acid oxidation disorders (see Chap. 45) In near-SIDS, it is important to collect urine and obtain a blood spot on filter paper during or shortly after the acute attack. Indications for investigating surviving normal sibs are few (Table 66-14); the protocol is the same as that recommended for Reye syndrome (see Table 66-13).

Table 66-14 SIDS: Protocol of Investigation

SIDS
- Gas liquid chromatography-mass spectrometry (GLCMS)
  - Urine
  - CSF
  - Vitreous humor
- *cis*-4-Decenoic acid in plasma
- Carnitine and acylcarnitines in plasma (tandem MS-MS from blood spot)
- Assessment of fatty change
  - Liver
  - Skeletal muscle
  - Heart muscle
- Frozen skin?

Near-SIDS
- During acute attack
  - Urine gas chromatography-mass spectrometry
  - *cis*-4-Decenoic acid in plasma
  - Carnitine and acylcarnitines in plasma (tandem MS-MS from blood spot)
- After acute attack
  - See Table 66-13

SIDS Sibs
- Indications
  - SIDS in sib aged less than 1 month (first week ++)
  - >1 SIDS in siblings
  - Parental consanguinity
  - Diffuse tissue fatty change or suggestive biochemical abnormality in an infant after death
  - Acute unexplained episode triggered by fever, fasting, or immunization in sib
  - Suggestive hepatic, muscular, or cardiac symptoms on clinical examination of sib
- Methods
- See Table 66-13

Recurrent Attacks of Dehydration

In pediatrics, dehydration is a common consequence of diarrhea caused by a variety of enteral or parenteral acute infections. However, it must be kept in mind that these common infectious diseases occasionally trigger acute decompensation for an inborn error of metabolism. Moreover, aside from dehydration due to gastrointestinal losses, some inborn errors of metabolism can present as recurrent attacks of dehydration secondary to polyuria, hyperventilation, or excessive sweating. The main accompanying symptoms (severe diarrhea, salt wasting, ketoacidosis, or failure to thrive) can be used to classify dehydration due to inborn errors of metabolism, as shown in Table 66-15.

Exercise Intolerance and Recurrent Myoglobinuria

Exercise intolerance and recurrent myoglobinuria syndrome[158] is defined as myalgias, cramping, and/or limb weakness associated with elevated serum levels of creatine phosphokinase (CPK) and other sarcoplasmic enzymes (high usually > 100 times upper limit of normal), recurrent pigmenturia, and sometimes acute renal failure. In the last instance, or when the patient is in a comatose state, clinical muscular symptoms can be missed. An important rule is to check serum CPK and for myoglobinuria in such conditions.

In the resting state, muscle is heavily dependent on fatty acid oxidation.[159] During moderate exercise, adenosine triphosphate (ATP) is regenerated using glycolytic precursors and then muscle glycogen for the first 5 to 10 min.[160] After 90 min, the major fuels are free fatty acids and glucose. After 4 h, free fatty acids are used twice as much as carbohydrates. Because of these physiologic requirements, disorders of muscle energy metabolism present in two ways (Table 66-16).

In the glycolytic disorders, exercising muscle is most vulnerable during the initial stages of exercise and during intense exercise when carbohydrates are the main energy source. A "second-wind" phenomenon sometimes develops, probably reflecting a switch from carbohydrate to fatty acid utilization.[161] Clinically, the glycolytic disorders are mostly observed in late childhood, adolescence, or adulthood. Their diagnosis is based largely on an abnormal forearm ischemia test, absence of hyperlactatemia during a physical exercise test, and the muscle

Table 66-15 Attacks of Dehydration

Leading Symptoms	Other signs	Age at onset	Diagnosis
Severe diarrhea: digestive causes	Severe watery acidic diarrhea Glycosuria	Neonatal	Glucose galactose malabsorption Congenital lactase deficiency
	Hydramnios No meconium Severe watery nonacidic diarrhea Metabolic alkalosis Hypokalemia Hypochloremia	Congenital	Congenital chloride diarrhea
	Severe watery diarrhea	After weaning or when sucrose or starch dextrins are added to the diet	Sucrase isomaltase deficiency
	Anorexia Failure to thrive Weight loss (before cutaneous lesions and alopecia)	2–4 weeks or after weaning	Acrodermatitis enteropathica
Ketoacidosis: organic acidurias	Polyuria Polypnea Hyperglycemia Glycosuria	Infancy to early childhood	Diabetic coma Methylmalonic aciduria Propionic acidemia Isovaleric aciduria 3-Ketothiolase deficiency Hydroxyisobutyric aciduria
Failure to thrive, anorexia, poor feeding, polydipsia, polyuria: renal tubular dysfunction	Photophobia Corneal opacities Renal Fanconi Syndrome Rickets Metabolic acidosis	Infancy 3–6 months	Cystinosis
	Hypernatremia Vomiting Psychomotor retardation Spasticity X-linked inheritance	Neonatal to first month	Nephrogenic diabetes insipidus
	Hyperchloremia Metabolic acidosis Alkaline urine pH	Early in infancy	RTA type I (distal): nephrocalcinosis, hypokalemia RTA type II (proximal): Fanconi syndrome, acidic urine pH when profoundly acidotic RTA type IV: hyperkalemia (associated with adrenogenital syndrome or pseudohypoaldosteronism) and obstructive uropathy
	Hypoglycemia Hepatic glycogenosis Fanconi syndrome	Early in infancy	Fanconi-Bickel syndrome (GLUT II mutation)
	Pulmonary infections Chronic diarrhea Salty sweat	Infancy to early childhood	Cystic fibrosis
Salt-losing syndrome: adrenal dysfunction	Severe hyponatremia Ambiguous genitalia	End of first week of life	Congenital adrenal hyperplasias: 21-hydroxylase deficiency (frequent), β-hydroxysteroid dehydrogenase, very severe (rare), desmolase deficiency, very severe (rare)
	Unambiguous genitalia	End of first week	Hypoaldosteronism
	Ambiguous genitalia	Infancy to early childhood	Congenital adrenal hypoplasia Congenital adrenal hyperplasia, late-onset forms
	Unambiguous genitalia		Hypoaldosteronism Pseudohypoaldosteronism
	Hypoketotic hypoglycemia		Fatty acid oxidation disorders (CPT I and II) CDG syndrome

RTA = renal tubular acidosis; GLUT = glucose transporter; CPT = carnitine palmitoyl transferase; CDG = congential disorders of glycosylation.

Table 66-16 Exercise Intolerance and Recurrent Myoglobinuria

Main Clinical Features	Other Important Signs	Age at Onset	Disorders
Stiffness and cramping or weakness typically occurring during initial stages of intense exercise, "second wind" phenomenon	Normal basal glucose and lactate Abnormal forearm ischemic lactate test Absence of hyperlactacidemia after physical exercise test Elevated CK interictally	10–18 years (mean 14)	Glycogenolytic/Glycolytic defects: Phosphorylase (MacArdle syndrome) Phosphofructokinase Phosphoglycerate kinase Phosphoglycerate mutase Lactate dehydrogenase Phosphorylase b kinase
Myalgias, stiffness, and cramping or weakness occurring after mild to moderate prolonged exercise, also triggered by cold, fasting and infections	Normal lactate Fasting hypoketotic hypoglycemia Low ketogenesis after long-chain triglyceride load CK elevation during fasting test	3–18 years (mean 10)	Fatty acid oxidation defects: CPT II deficiency (ubiquitous) VLCAD deficiency (ubiquitous) LCHAD deficiency (ubiquitous) TF deficiency (ubiquitous) SCHAD deficiency (restricted to muscle)
	With hemolytic anemia	30 years	G6PDH deficiency
	No NH_3 elevation after physical exercise test	Variable	Myoadenylate deaminase deficiency
	Hyperlactatemia, high L:P ratio at rest, after meals, or only after physical exercise test Frequent cardiomyopathy or encephalopathy	Childhood to adolescence	Respiratory chain disorders Lipoamide dehydrogenase deficiency
Calf hypertrophy	No significant lactate or glucose abnormality Permanent CK elevation Abnormal dystrophin on muscle biopsy		Duchenne and Becker muscular dystrophy
Clinically Isolated	No significant biologic perturbation Normal muscle biopsy		Normo- and hyperkalemic paralysis Familial recurrent myoglobinuria Repeated attacks in sporadic cases

SCHAD = 3-hydroxy short-chain acyl CoA dehydrogenase; TF = trifunctional enzyme; CK = creatine kinase; G6PDH = glucose 6 phosphate dehydrogenase; CPT II, VLCAD, LCHAD, SCHAD see preceding tables.

magnetic resonance spectroscopy pattern. The CPK level remains elevated in most patients. The most frequent and typical disorder in this group is MacArdle disease due to myophosphorylase deficiency.

In the fatty acid oxidation disorders, attacks of myoglobinuria occur typically after mild to moderate prolonged exercise and are particularly likely when patients are additionally stressed by fasting, cold, or infection. This group is largely dominated by muscle CPT II, VLCAD, LCHAD and trifunctional (TF) deficiencies, which may occur in childhood, in adolescence, or later.[162–165] Recurrent rhabdomyolysis has been recently described in a child with glutaric aciduria type I.[165a] Deficiencies of VLCAD[163] and SCHAD[166] may also present as myopathy.

The diagnosis of all these fatty acid oxidation disorders is based mostly on the plasma acylcarnitine profile and on the demonstration of fasting hypoketotic hypoglycemia, which reflects a fatty acid oxidation defect in the liver but can be absent. An interesting sign is elevation of serum CPK during fasting. Oral loading of long-chain triglycerides provides another test for fatty acid oxidation defects (see "Hypoketotic Hypoglycemia Due to Inborn Errors of Ketogenesis" above). With respect to confirming the diagnosis, it should be stressed that in CPT II, VLCAD, LCHAD, and TF deficiencies, the enzymatic defect is ubiquitous, being expressed especially in circulating lymphocytes or fibroblasts and thus easy to demonstrate without muscle biopsy. Conversely, some fatty acid oxidation enzymes, for example, SCHAD[166] and CPT I,[112] are tissue specific and should be investigated only through muscle biopsy.

In the pathway of purine catabolism, adenylate deaminase deficiency has been suspected to cause exercise intolerance and cramps in a few patients,[167,168] but the relationship between clinical symptoms and the enzyme defect is uncertain. An enzyme defect is to be suspected when there is no significant elevation of blood ammonia during a physical exercise test.

Although respiratory chain disorders are not classically considered to cause recurrent muscle pain and myoglobinuria, the literature and our personal experience[169] provide considerable evidence that these disorders can actually give rise to exercise intolerance and myalgias. In the series of patients (belonging to five families) described by Larsson *et al.*,[170] there was a history of exercise intolerance, dyspnea, palpitation, and recurrent myoglobinuria, in some cases beginning in childhood, with an excessive rise in lactate and pyruvate on exercise. These cases are now thought to be secondary to complex II deficiency of the respiratory chain.[170]

A respiratory chain disorder should be suspected when hyperlactatemia is accompanied by an elevated L:P ratio, either permanently or after meals. Sometimes the lactate abnormality will be found only after an exercise test. In respiratory chain disorders, muscle symptoms are often associated with cardiomyopathy or diverse neurologic signs (encephalomyopathy). A case of lipoamide dehydrogenase deficiency presenting as recurrent myoglobinuria has been described recently in an adult.[171]

Attention has been directed toward myoglobinuria associated with Xp21-linked myopathies. Several patients with Becker muscular dystrophy have had exertional myoglobinuria in adolescence.[158] We have personally observed two such patients who presented with myoglobinuria in childhood (Melki J, Saudubray JM: unpublished observations). This could be a more frequent occurrence, but children with more severe weakness may be protected by their limited capacity for physical exercise. That

Table 66-17 Abdominal Pain (Recurrent Attacks)

Leading Symptoms	Other Signs	Age at Onset	Diagnosis
With meteorism, diarrhea, loose stools	Symptoms appear shortly after drinking milk or sucrose	Adolescence to adulthood	Lactose malabsorption Congenital sucrase maltase deficiency
With vomiting, lethargy	Hyperammonemia		Urea cycle defects (OTC, ASS)
	Ketoacidosis		Organic acidurias (MMA, PA, IVA) Ketolysis defects (succinyl CoA transferase, 3-ketothiolase)
	Hyperlactatemia		Mitochondrial DNA deletion
With neuropathy, paralysis, psychiatric symptoms, respiratory failure	Cutaneous symptoms (skin photosensitivity, abnormal pigmentation, alopecia, hypertrichosis)	Adulthood Adulthood (Infancy)	Porphyria variegata Coproporphyria (homozygous form with hemolytic anemia)
	Black urine	Second decade	Acute intermittent porphyria
	Rickets Liver dysfunction	First decade	Tyrosinemia type I
	Pain in extremities		Aladehydratase deficiency
With predominant hepatomegaly ± splenomegaly	Hypertriglyceridemia	Infancy Second decade	Cholesterol ester storage disease Lipoprotein lipase deficiency
	Neutropenia Failure to thrive Anorexia Lethargy Hyperammonemia	First year	Lysinuric protein intolerance
	Hepatic failure	Infancy	Cholesterol ester storage disease
	Cirrhosis	Adulthood Infancy	Hemochromatosis Cystic fibrosis (rare presentation)
With pain in extremities	Corneal clouding Angiokeratoma	Childhood to adolescence	Fabry disease
	Paralysis Neuropathy	Childhood to adolescence	Aladehydratase deficiency
	Splenomegaly Hemolytic anemia	Childhood	Sickle-cell anemia
With nephrolithiasis		(see this symptom) Table 66-60	
With hemolytic anemia	Neuropathy Paralysis Skin photosensitivity	Infancy	Coproporphyria
	Splenomegaly	Infancy	Hereditary spherocytosis Sickle-cell anemia
With fever, inflammatory syndrome	Rash Arthralgias	Infancy childhood	Mediterranean fever Mevalonic aciduria

ASS = argininosuccinate synthetase; IVA = isovaleric acidemia; MMA = methylmalonic acidemia; PA = propionic acidemia

may be even more true for Duchenne dystrophy, in which weakness is more severe.[158,172]

Finally, despite the various biochemical studies, a number of cases remain undiagnosed. This group will be certainly reduced over the next few years as more extensive biochemical studies, especially on energy metabolism, are developed. It is not yet clear whether normo- and hyperkalemic paralysis due to sodium channel gene mutations may present as exercise intolerance attacks.[173]

Abdominal Pain (Recurrent Attacks)

Table 66-17 contains all pertinent information on recurrent attacks of abdominal pain. Mevalonic aciduria due to mevalonate kinase deficiency can present as recurrent attacks of abdominal pain with fever, skin rashes, arthralgias, and inflammatory syndrome and hyper Ig D.[174,174a]

Cardiac Disorders

Acute cardiac failure and disorders of heart rate can be revealing signs in inborn errors of metabolism (Table 66-18). In most cases, acute cardiac failure is the initial sign. The important metabolic causes of cardiomyopathy are Pompe disease, all long-chain fatty acid oxidation disorders except CPT I deficiency, multiple acyl CoA dehydrogenase deficiency, and respiratory chain disorders. It must be stressed that MCAD deficiency, the most common inborn error of fatty acid mitochondrial catabolism, does not present as cardiomyopathy or cardiac symptoms. Congenital disorders of glycosylation may at times present in infancy as

Table 66-18 Cardiac Failure and Heartbeat Disorders

Cardiac failure revealing or accompanying a cardiomyopathy	Severe hypotonia, short PR interval, high QRS amplitude at EKG, macroglossia	Neonatal to infancy	Pompe disease
	Hypoketotic hypoglycemia attacks, hypotonia	Neonatal to late infancy	Fatty acid oxidation defects (CTD, MAD, TL, CPT II, VLCAD, LCHAD, TF)
	Isolated or with hypotonia and various neurologic signs, hyperlactacidemia	Neonatal to infancy	Respiratory chain disorders (complex I, II, IV, V) Phosphorylase b kinase
With tamponade, pericardial effusions, multiorgan failure	Muscular weakness, strokelike attacks, peculiar fat pads, thick and sticky skin	Neonatal to infancy	Congenital defects of glycosylation
Apparently primitive heartbeat disorders (without evidence of cardiomyopathy)	Hyperkalemia, hyponatremia	Neonatal to infancy	Adrenal dysfunction (see also dehydration, in Table 66-15)
	Hypoparathyroidism, hypocalcemia, prolonged QT interval	Infancy	Congenital hypoparathyroidism Pseudohypoparathyroidism
	Hyperkinetic hemodynamic state, sinus tachycardia	Infancy to childhood	Thiamine-deficient/dependent states
	Arrhythmia, sudden cardiac death, hemolytic anemia, progressive severe neurologic dysfunction	Infancy	Triosephosphate isomerase deficiency
	Collapse, heart rate trouble, hypoketotic hypoglycemia	Neonatal to infancy	Fatty acid oxidation defects (CPT II, VLCAD, LCHAD, TF, MAD)
	Atrioventricular heart block, external ophthalmoplegia, retinal degeneration	Late childhood to adult	Kearns-Sayre syndrome (mitochondrial DNA deletion)

CTD = carnitine transporter defect; LCHAD = 3-hydroxy long-chain acyl CoA dehydrogenase; MAD = multiple acyl CoA dehydrogenase; TF = long-chain trifunctional protein; TL = acylcarnitine translocase.

tamponade with pericardial effusion, multiorgan failure, and characteristic cutaneous and neurologic features.[11,175] Pericardial effusion associated with severe fatty liver has been observed in late onset type II glutaric aciduria.[112] Isolated isobutyryl CoA dehydrogenase deficiency presenting with dilated cardiomyopathy has been recently described.[175a]

Alternatively, heart failure may result from disturbed cardiac rhythm. In congenital hypoparathyroidism and pseudohypoparathyroidism, cardiac failure can be the consequence of severe hypocalcemia with a prolonged QT interval on EKG. In Kearns-Sayre syndrome, atrioventricular block with syncope is a classic sign usually associated with progressive external ophthalmoplegia and retinal degeneration (see "Hyperlactacidemias" above). In the rare disorder triosephosphate isomerase deficiency, which presents early in infancy as hemolytic anemia and progressive neurologic dysfunction, arrhythmia may cause sudden cardiac death. A hyperkinetic hemodynamic state with sinus tachycardia, a classic finding in hyperthyroidism and in thiamine-deficient and dependent states, can be dramatically relieved by thiamine administration. Finally, all long-chain fatty acid oxidation disorders except CPT I deficiency can present in early infancy, even in the neonatal period, with cardiac arrest or hypotension, which is readily misdiagnosed as toxic shock or malignant hyperthermia. Disorders of heart rate (premature ventricular complexes, atrioventricular block, and ventricular tachycardia) are frequent features[21a,28] and could be due to accumulation of long-chain acylcarnitine, which has been shown to promote arrhythmogenesis in the cat heart.[176] In a series of 103 patients with fatty acid oxidation disorders, we found 37 patients with heart rate disorders; in 20 of them, the heart rate disorder was the presenting symptom.[21]

Bone Crisis

Bone pain occurs in the form of osteomalacia or rickets and in three other circumstances (Table 66-19). First, bone pain can occur in sickle-cell anemia and various porphyrias in association with other signs. One particularly important form of painful crisis that occurs early in infancy in sickle-cell anemia is the hand-foot syndrome, which is a dactylitis characterized by sudden onset of painful swelling of the dorsum of the hands and feet. In various porphyrias, bone crisis is associated with abdominal pain, constipation, vomiting, and neuropathy. These crises may also occur in tyrosinemia type I (see also Table 66-17).

Second, bone pain can occur in three progressive neurologic disorders. In the infantile form of Krabbe disease, bone crises are expressed by irritability and incessant crying, which may precede by a few weeks the characteristic psychomotor deterioration with peripheral neuropathy. Similar crises have been observed in defects of biopterin synthesis and in aromatic amino acid decarboxyase deficiency. In late infantile metachromatic leukodystrophy, bone crises are associated with limb hypertonia, muscle weakness, and progressive neurologic deterioration. In Gaucher disease type III, bone crises can precede, accompany, or follow a large variety of neurologic symptoms (myoclonic jerks, ophthalmoplegia, spasticity, abnormal movements, etc.); they appear in late childhood or adolescence and are associated with splenomegaly.

Table 66-19 Bone Crisis (or Pain in Extremities)

Leading Symptoms	Other Signs	Age at Onset	Diagnosis
With bone changes (rickets), osteomalacia, femorotibial bowing	Abdominal distension Alopecia Dental defects Hypotonia Respiratory infection Anemia Hypocalcemia High alkaline phosphatase levels	First year	Calciferol metabolism deficiency (pseudo-vitamin D deficiency, types I and II)
	Short stature Muscle weakness Hypophosphatemia Hypercalciuria	First year	Hereditary hypophosphatemia, rickets with hypercalciuria
	Short stature Hypophosphatemia Hypercalciuria X-linked inheritance	First year	Familial hypophosphatemia, rickets with hypercalciuria
With hemolytic anemia ± abdominal pain	Splenomegaly Failure to thrive Infections Other "crisis"	Infancy to childhood	Sickle-cell anemia (hand-foot syndrome)
	Abdominal pain Vomiting Constipation Muscle weakness Neuropathy	Late childhood to adolescence	Aminolevulinic acid dehydratase deficiency Tyrosinemia type I (hepatic signs) Acute intermittent porphyria Hereditary coproporphyria (cutaneous signs) Porphyria variegata (cutaneous signs)
With progressive neurologic signs	Psychomotor deterioration Irritability Hyperreactivity Dystonia Peripheral neuropathy Hyperproteinorachia	3–6 months	Krabbe disease
	Ataxia Limb hypertonia Peripheral neuropathy Neurologic deterioration Hyperproteinorachia Delay in learning to walk	1–2 years	Metachromatic leukodystrophy, late infantile form Biopterin synthesis defects Aromatic amino acid decarboxylase deficiency
	Hepatosplenomegaly Myoclonic jerks Ophthalmoplegia Osteonecrosis Neurologic deterioration	Late childhood to adolescence	Gaucher disease type III
Apparently isolated (bone crisis as presenting symptom)	With abdominal pain Acroparesthesias Angiokeratoma Corneal opacities X-linked inheritance Rare in female heterozygotes	Childhood to adolescence	Fabry disease
	Bleeding tendency Splenomegaly Moderate pancytopenia Osteonecrosis	Infancy to childhood	Gaucher disease type I

Third, bone pain may occur as an isolated sign. Bone crisis is frequently the presenting symptom in hemizygotic Fabry disease and nonneuronopathic Gaucher disease (type I). The "Fabry crisis" can last from minutes to several days. It consists of agonizing burning pain commencing in the palms and soles and radiating to the proximal extremities. Because it is often associated with fever and elevated erythrocyte sedimentation, it may be confused with rheumatic fever, neurosis, or erythromelalgia. Another item in the differential diagnosis may be metabolic crisis in mevalonic aciduria, which causes arthralgias, morbilliform rash, fever, lymphadenopathy, and hepatosplenomegaly.[174,174a,177] Painful crises are usually triggered by exercise, fatigue, emotional stress, or rapid changes in temperature and humidity. Clinical diagnosis depends on the recognition of specific symptoms (see

"Angiokeratoma" and "Corneal Opacity" below). A "Fabry crisis" is rarely observed in female heterozygotes.

Many patients with Gaucher disease type I (chronic nonneuronopathic) experience episodic pain lasting for days to months in the hips, legs, back, and shoulders. Although osteopenia and osteolysis are common, some patients have neither radiographic, scintigraphic, nor scanographic evidence of bone involvement at the time of the first attack. Rarely, bone crisis precedes hepatosplenomegaly and is the presenting sign of the disease.[178]

III. PROGRESSIVE NEUROLOGIC SYMPTOMS

Progressive Neurologic and Mental Deterioration

A very large number of inborn errors of metabolism can give rise to neurologic symptoms, developmental delay, psychiatric disorders, or mental deterioration. When these symptoms are associated with extraneurologic findings (osseous, cutaneous, visceral, endocrine, sensory, metabolic), the latter are often useful keys to the diagnosis. Indeed, the presence of extraneurologic signs raises a strong probability of finding systemic metabolic disturbances. However, there is still an important gap between clinical descriptions and biologic investigations. Many well-known heritable disorders have not been considered from a pathophysiological viewpoint and have not been subject to comprehensive biochemical evaluation. This problem is illustrated by the story of Canavan disease. N-acetylaspartic aciduria was demonstrated in Canavan disease only in 1988,[3,4] even though the clinical phenotype had been identified in 1949 and the procedure for identifying N-acetylaspartate (urine gas chromatography-mass spectrometry) was available in 1972. Conversely, Schindler's tenacious search for a biochemical defect in two severely handicapped brothers observed in 1985[179] led to the discovery in 1986 by Van Diggelen *et al.*[180] of the new lysosomal defect alpha-N-acetyl galactosaminidase deficiency.

These two examples show how necessary close collaboration among neurochemists, biochemists, molecular biologists, geneticists, specialists in inborn errors of metabolism, and neuropediatricians is for elucidating new genetic defects in neurologic and neuropsychiatric disorders.

Table 66-20 presents a general approach to inborn errors of metabolism involving neurologic and/or mental deterioration. Diseases are classified according to age of onset, presence or absence of associated extraneurologic signs, and the neurologic presentation itself; the last is based largely on the clinical classification of Adams and Lyon.[17] Inborn errors of metabolism with neurologic signs presenting in the neonate (birth to 1 month) and those presenting intermittently as acute attacks of coma, lethargy, ataxia, or acute psychiatric symptoms are presented elsewhere in this chapter (see "Neonate," "Recurrent Attacks of Coma," "Metabolic Acidosis," "Hyperlactacidemias," and "Hypoglycemia" above).

Part 1: Early Infancy (1 to 12 months). We identify three general categories.

Category 1. This category includes disorders associated with extraneurologic symptoms. Visceral signs (e.g., hepatosplenomegaly), coarse facies, dysmorphism, bone changes, and ocular symptoms) appear in lysosomal disorders. A cardiomyopathy, sometimes responsible for cardiac failure, associated with early neurologic dysfunction, failure to thrive, and hypotonia, is suggestive of respiratory chain disorders, sometimes associated with a predominant macrocephaly,[181] D-2-hydroxyglutaric aciduria (with atrioventricular block),[182,183] or congenital disorders of glycosylation.[175] Abnormal hair and cutaneous signs appear in Menkes disease (steely hair), Sjögren-Larsson syndrome (ichthyosis), biotinidase deficiency, and respiratory chain disorders (alopecia, cutaneous rashes).[183a] Peculiar fat pads over the upper outer parts of the buttocks; thick and sticky skin (like "tallow," "peau d'orange"), especially on the legs; and inverted nipples are highly suggestive of congenital defects of glycosylation.[11] A newly recognized glycosylation defect presents early in life with ichthyosis, psychomotor retardation and dwarfism (CDG-If).[183b]

Table 66-20 Progressive Neurologic and Mental Deterioration (see also Coma and Neonatal Deterioration, Tables 66-3, 66-4, and 66-5)

Part 1: Onset Early in Infancy (1 to 12 months)
With extraneurologic symptoms (Table 66-21)
Visceral signs
Hair and cutaneous symptoms
Megaloblastic anemia
Cardiac symptoms
Ocular symptoms
With specific or suggestive neurologic signs (Table 66-22)
Extrapyramidal signs
Macrocephaly, startle response to sound, ocular symptoms
Recurrent attacks of neurologic deterioration
Without suggestive symptoms: nonspecific mental retardation (Table 66-23)
Evidence of developmental arrest
No specific symptoms
Part 2: Onset in Late Infancy to Early Childhood (1 to 5 Years)
With visceral, craniovertebral, or other somatic abnormalities (Table 66-24)
With progressive paraplegia, weakness, hypotonia, or spasticity of the lower limbs due to corticospinal tract involvement or to peripheral neuropathy (Table 66-25)
With unsteady gait and uncoordinated movements due to cerebellar syndrome, sensory defects, or involuntary movements (athetotic choreiform movements)
Without disturbance of organic acid excretion (Table 66-26A)
With disturbance of organic acid excretion (Table 66-26B)
With convulsions, seizures and myoclonus, ataxia, or frequent falling due to intention myoclonus or to cerebellar ataxia (Table 66-27)
Disorders with arrest or regression of psychic and perceptual functions as predominant or only revealing symptom (Table 66-27)
Part 3: Onset in Late Childhood to Adolescence (5 to 15 Years)
With predominant extrapyramidal signs, parkinsonism, dystonia, choreoathetosis (Table 66-28)
With severe neurologic and mental deterioration, diffuse central nervous system disorders, bipyramidal paralysis, incoordination, seizures, visual failure, dementia (Table 66-29)
With visceral signs
Without visceral signs
With polymyoclonia (Table 66-30)
With predominant cerebellar ataxia (Table 66-31)
With significant mental deterioration or dementia
Without mental deterioration or dementia
With predominant polyneuropathy (Table 66-32)
With psychiatric symptoms as the only presenting sign: (Table 66-32).
Part 4: Onset in Adulthood (15 to 70 Years) (Table 66-33)
With predominant ataxia
With predominant psychosis, dementia
With predominant extrapyramidal signs
With predominant hemiparesis, paraparesis, but no mental deterioration
With myoclonic epilepsy

Generalized cyanosis unresponsive to oxygen suggests methemoglobinemia, which is associated with severe hypertonicity in cytochrome b5 reductase deficiency. Kernicterus and athetosis are complications of Crigler-Najjar syndrome. The recently described EPEMA syndrome is characterized by orthostatic acrocyanosis, recurring petechiae, pyramidal signs, mental retardation, and recurrent attacks of lactic acidosis.[55,56] The presence of megaloblastic anemia (see "Nonregenerative Anemias [Macrocytic]" below), sometimes associated with pancytopenia, suggests an inborn error of folate and cobalamin metabolism (Table 66-21).

Ocular symptoms can be highly diagnostic signs, like cherry red spot, optic atrophy, nystagmus, abnormal eye movements, and retinitis pigmentosa (see Table 66-21; see also "Ocular Symptoms" below).

Category 2. This category includes disorders with specific or suggestive neurologic signs. Predominant extrapyramidal symptoms are associated with inborn errors of biopterin and aromatic amino acid metabolism (parkinsonism),[46,184] Lesch-Nyhan syndrome (self-mutilation, choreoathetoid movements), cytochrome b5 reductase deficiency (generalized cyanosis, methemoglobinemia), Crigler-Najjar syndrome ("kernicterus syndrome"), the early-onset form of glutaric aciduria type I (choreoathetosis, severe dystonia), and cerebral creatine deficiency due to guanidinoacetate methyltransferase deficiency.[185,186] Dystonia can also be observed as a subtle but revealing sign in X-linked Pelizaeus-Merzbacher syndrome (laryngeal stridor and nystagmus).

Macrocephaly with startle response to sound, incessant crying, and irritability are frequent early signs in G_{M2} gangliosidosis (Tay-Sachs and Sandhoff diseases), Canavan disease, Alexander disease, infantile Krabbe disease, and glutaric aciduria type I. Macrocephaly can be also a revealing sign in L-2-hydroxyglutaric aciduria[187,188] and in respiratory chain disorders due to complex I deficiency (association with hypertrophic cardiomyopathy).[181]

Recurrent attacks of neurologic crisis associated with progressive neurologic and mental deterioration suggest Leigh disease, which is a poorly defined entity that can present at any age from early in infancy to late childhood with widely varying neurologic symptoms. Leigh disease is not a specific inborn error of metabolism but rather the clinical phenotype of any of several such errors some of which still remain to be identified (Table 66-22). Recurrent strokelike episodes, often associated with anorexia, failure to thrive, and hypotonia, can be revealing symptoms in urea cycle defects (mostly OTC), late-onset MSUD, organic acidurias, glutaric aciduria type I, carbohydrate-deficient glycoprotein syndrome, and respiratory chain disorders. Thromboembolic accidents can be revealing signs of classic homocystinuria and carbohydrate-deficient glycoprotein syndrome.

Angelman syndrome sometimes displays a very suggestive picture, with early-onset encephalopathy, happy puppet appearance, failure to thrive, facial dysmorphism, microcephaly, and epilepsy with a highly suggestive EEG pattern.[189–192] Diagnosis relies on the molecular analysis of chromosome 15, which displays a partial paternal unidisomy.

Category 3. A large number of inborn errors of intermediary metabolism present as nonspecific early progressive developmental delay, poor feeding, hypotonia, some degree of ataxia, seizures, and frequently autistic features. The list has lengthened rapidly as new laboratory techniques have been applied. The relationship between clinical symptoms and biochemical abnormalities is not always firmly established. Many aminoacidopathies that were first described in the late 1950s and 1960s, when plasma and urine amino acid chromatography was systematically used in studying mentally retarded children, must now be questioned as definite causes of neurologic disturbance. This is the case for histidinemia, hyperlysinemia, hyperprolinemia, alpha-aminoadipic aciduria, and Hartnup "disease."

The same story may now be developing with organic acidurias, so that it is more and more important to try to define pathophysiological links between clinical symptoms and metabolic disturbances. Conversely, it is more and more difficult to screen patients on clinical grounds when the clinical symptoms consist only of developmental delay, hypotonia, and convulsions. There is also now considerable evidence that an increasing number of inborn errors of metabolism can masquerade as cerebral palsy, by presenting as permanent impairment of movement or posture. Among the new categories of inborn errors of intermediary metabolism that present as uninformative clinical manifestations are adenylosuccinase deficiency,[193] dihydropyrimidine dehydrogenase deficiency,[194,195] 4-hydroxybutyric aciduria,[196] mevalonic aciduria,[177] fumarase deficiency,[197] trimethylglutaconic aciduria,[198] creatine deficiency syndrome,[186,199,200] the recently described inborn errors of serine biosynthesis,[201,202,202a] 2 methyl, 3-hydroxy butyryl-CoA dehydrogenase deficiency,[202b] methylmalonic semialdehyde dehydrogenase deficiency,[202c] homocystinuria, and Salla disease (sialic acid excretion). Late-onset subacute forms of hyperammonemia (mostly ornithine transcarbamylase deficiency in girls) can also be revealed by an apparently nonspecific early encephalopathy. Inborn errors of neurotransmitter synthesis, especially dopa-responsive dystonia due to cyclohydrolase deficiency,[203] tyrosine hydroxylase deficiency, and aromatic L-amino acid decarboxylase deficiency,[204] in particular can masquerade as cerebral palsy. As a consequence, all patients presenting with unclearly identified cerebral palsy should be investigated with organic acid and neurotransmitter analyses, including the measurement of biogenic amine neurotransmitter metabolites in CSF.[47a,204] These disorders rarely, if ever, give rise to true developmental arrest but rather cause progressive subacute developmental delay (Table 66-23). Recurrent attacks of seizures unresponsive to anticonvulsant drugs occurring in the first year of life secondary to mutations of the blood-brain barrier glucose carrier gene *GLUT1* have been described.[205] The diagnosis relies on the finding of a low glucose level in CSF while a simultaneous blood glucose level is normal.[206]

Part 2: Late Infancy to Early Childhood (1 to 5 years). In this period, diagnosis becomes easier. Five general categories can be defined.

Category 1. When visceral, craniovertebral, ocular, or other somatic abnormalities are present and associated with a slowing or regression of development, diagnosis is usually easy. Mucopolysaccharidosis type I (Hurler syndrome) and II (Hunter syndrome), mucolipidosis type III (pseudo-Hurler polydystrophy), oligosaccharidosis (mannosidosis, fucosidosis, aspartylglucosaminuria), Austin disease, Niemann-Pick disease type C, Gaucher disease type III, and lactosyl ceramidosis are usually easy to recognize. Mucolipidosis type IV, which causes major visual impairment by the end of the first year of life, sometimes associated with dystonia, is detected by finding characteristic cytoplasmic membranous bodies in cells. In SanFilippo syndrome (mucopolysaccharidosis type III), coarse facies and bone changes may be very subtle or absent (see below). Peroxisomal disorders may present in this age group as progressive mental deterioration, retinitis pigmentosa, and deafness, appearing very similar to Usher syndrome type II (Table 66-24).[45,45b] In the recently described pyrroline-5-carboxylate synthetase deficiency, slow progressive neurologic and mental deterioration is associated with severe hypotonia, joint laxity, congenital cataracts, and low plasma citrulline, ornithine, and proline levels with a paradoxical preprandial hyperammonemia.[207,208]

Category 2. Three disorders are revealed by progressive paraplegia and spasticity. Metachromatic leukodystrophy and neuroaxonal dystrophy strike between 12 and 24 months, both present as flaccid paraparesis, hypotonia, and weakness. Cerebrospinal fluid protein content and nerve conduction velocity are disturbed in the former but normal in the latter. Schindler disease is roughly similar to neuroaxonal dystrophy but is often associated with myoclonic

Table 66-21 Progressive Neurologic and Mental Deterioration: Part 1 (1 to 12 months): Category 1: With Obvious Extraneurologic Symptom

Leading Symptom	Other Signs	Age at Onset	Diagnosis
With visceral signs	Hepatosplenomegaly Coarse facies Joint stiffness Cherry red spot Vacuolated lymphocytes Bone changes	0–3 months 6–12 months	Landing disease I-cell disease Sialidosis type II Niemann-Pick disease type A Lactosyl ceramidosis
	Hepatosplenomegaly Opisthotonos Spasticity Vegetative state	1–6 months	Gaucher type II
	Hepatomegaly Digestive signs Retinitis pigmentosa	0–6 months	Peroxisomal disorders Congenital defects of glycosylation
With hair and cutaneous symptoms	Steely, brittle hair Hypopigmentation Hypothermia Osteopenia	3–6 months	Menkes disease (X-linked) Trichothiodystrophy Argininosuccinic aciduria
	Ichthyosis Brittle hair Spastic paraplegia Cataract Retinitis	1–6 months	Sjögren-Larsson syndrome
	Alopecia Cutaneous rashes Ketoacidosis Hyperlactacidemia	3–12 months	Biotinidase deficiency Respiratory chain disorders
	Peculiar fat pads on buttocks Thick, sticky hair Episodic multiorgan failure (liver, cardiac tamponade)	1–3 months	Congenital defects of glycosylation
	Cyanosis (generalized) Methemoglobinemia Hypertonicity	0–6 months	Cytochrome b-5 reductase deficiency
	Kernicterus Athetosis	1–3 months	Crigler-Najjar syndrome
	Acrocyanosis Petechiae Chronic diarrhea Attacks of lactic acidosis	1–3 months	Ethylmalonic aciduria: EPEMA syndrome
With megaloblastic anemia (see Table 66-49)	Failure to thrive Feeding difficulties Pigmentary retinopathy Metabolic acidosis	1–3 months	Inborn errors of folate metabolism Inborn errors of cobalamin metabolism Hereditary orotic aciduria
With cardiac symptoms	Cardiomyopathy Heart failure Heartbeat disorders	Congenital to 6 months	D2-hydroxyglutaric acidemia Respiratory chain disorders Congenital defects of glycosylation
With ocular symptoms	Cherry red spot Hydrops fetalis	0–3 months	Landing disease Galactosialidosis Sialidosis type I
	Myoclonic jerks Macrocephaly	3–12 months	Tay-Sachs disease Sandhoff disease
	Optic atrophy Macrocephaly Nystagmus Epilepsy	1–6 months	Canavan disease
	Nystagmus Macrocephaly Epilepsy	1–6 months	Canavan disease
	Dystonia Stridor	3–12 months	Pelizaeus-Merzbacher disease (X-linked)
	Retinitis pigmentosa		See Table 66-41
	Abnormal eye movements Strabismus Supranuclear paralysis	Neonatal	Aromatic amino acid decarboxylase deficiency Congenital defects of glycosylation Gaucher disease Niemann-Pick disease type C

Table 66-22 Progressive Neurologic and Mental Deterioration: Part 1 (1 to 12 months): Category 2: With Specific or Suggestive Neurologic Signs

Leading Symptom	Other Signs	Age at Onset	Diagnosis
Extrapyramidal signs	Major parkinsonism Hyperphenylalaninemia Abnormal biopterin Abnormal neurotransmitters	0–3 months	Inborn errors of biopterin metabolism Aromatic amino acid decarboxylase deficiency Tyrosine hydroxylase deficiency
	Choreoathetoid movements Self-mutilation Aggressiveness Hyperuricemia	3–6 months	Lesch-Nyhan syndrome (X-linked)
	Bilateral athetosis Hypertonicity Cyanosis Methemoglobinemia	0–6 months	Cytochrome b5 reductase deficiency
	Dystonia Laryngeal stridor Nystagmus	3–12 months	Pelizaeus-Merzbacher disease (X-linked)
	Kernicterus	1–3 months	Crigler-Najjar syndrome
	Acute onset Pseudoencephalitis Choreoathetosis Dystonia	9–12 months	Glutaric aciduria type I
	Low creatinine	6–12 months	Cerebral creatine deficiency (GAMT deficiency)
Macrocephaly	Cherry red spot Myoclonic jerks Startle response to sound Sometimes slight hepatosplenomegaly	6–12 months	Tay-Sachs disease Sandhoff disease
	Megaloencephaly Hyperreactivity Tonic spasms, opisthotonos Optic atrophy Cerebral edema Acetylaspartaturia	3–6 months	Canavan-Van Bogaert-Bertrand (aspartoacylase deficiency) or Alexander disease
	Incessant crying Irritability Dystonia Peripheral neuropathy (abnormal nerve conduction velocity) Hyperproteinorachia	3–6 months	Krabbe disease (infantile)
	Dystonia Choreoathetosis	9–12 months	Glutaric aciduria type I L-2 hydroxyglutaric aciduria
	Developmental delay Progressive irritability Limb hypertonia Cardiomyopathy	1–3 months	Respiratory chain disorders (complex I)
Recurrent attacks of neurologic crisis (see also "Metabolic Coma," Table 66-4)	Mental regression Failure to thrive Hyperventilation attacks Various neurologic signs (optic atrophy, ataxia, peripheral neuropathy, intention tremor)	3–12 months	Leigh disease (pyruvate carboxylase and dehydrogenase, respiratory chain deficiency)
	Strokelike episodes	1–12 months	Urea cycle defects MSUD, organic acidemias, GA I CDG syndrome, respiratory chain disorders
	Thromboembolic accidents	1–12 months	Classic homocystinuria CDG syndrome

CDG = congenital defects of glycosylation; MSUD = maple syrup urine disease; GAI = glutaric acidemia type I.

jerks[179] (Table 66-25). Arginase deficiency is a rare disorder that presents in early infancy to childhood (2 months to 5 years) with progressive spastic diplegia, scissoring or "tiptoe" gait, and developmental arrest. Diagnosis is based on hyperargininemia and high orotic acid excretion[209] (see Chap. 32). A rapidly progressive flaccid paraparesis resembling subacute degeneration of the cord can be the presenting sign of inherited cobalamin synthesis defects, characterized by methylmalonic aciduria associated with homocystinuria (Cbl C) or isolated homocystinuria (Cbl D, G, F).[210,211,211a]

Table 66-23 Progressive Neurologic and Mental Deterioration: Part 1 (1 to 12 months): Category 3: Without Suggestive Neurologic Signs: Nonspecific Mental Retardation

Leading Symptom	Other Signs	Age at Onset	Diagnosis
With evidence of developmental arrest	Infantile spasms Hypsarrhythmia Autistic features	3–12 months	Classic untreated phenylketonuria Inborn errors of biopterin metabolism Peroxisomal disorders Rett syndrome
Without specific symptoms, apparently nonprogressive disorder	Frequent autistic features Poor feeding Failure to thrive Hypotonia Seizures	Variable, congenital to first year	Hyperammonemia (late-onset subacute form) 4-Hydroxybutyric aciduria L-2-Hydroxyglutaric aciduria D-2-Hydroxyglutaric aciduria Mevalonic aciduria
	With diverse neurologic findings simulating cerebral palsy		Adenylosuccinase deficiency Dihydropyrimidine dehydrogenase 3-methylglutaconic aciduria Fumarase deficiency Other organic acidurias Creatine deficiency 3-phosphoglycerate dehydrogenase deficiency 3-phosphoserine phosphatase deficiency Homocystinuria (iridodonesis, lens dislocation) Salla disease (ocular nystagmus) Neurotransmitter disorders Angelman syndrome Blood-brain barrier glucose carrier deficiency

Category 3. When the neurologic picture is dominated by unsteady gait and uncoordinated movements (when standing, walking, sitting, reaching for objects, speaking, or swallowing) several groups of disorders must be considered. Given that an increasing number of inborn errors of intermediary metabolism have been described in the last recent years with such a neurologic presentation, a careful investigation of organic acid metabolism is always mandatory in these clinical circumstances. However, in some well-defined organic acidurias, the metabolic disturbances can be subtle or intermittent, demonstrable only in stressful circumstances. This is particularly emphasized by the recent descriptions of subtle cerebrospinal fluid modification in the so called leukoencephalopathy with vanishing white matter,[211b] and a leukoencephalopathy associated with a disturbance in the metabolism of polyols.[211c]

Disorders in this category without disturbances of urinary organic acid excretion and lactic acid metabolism are the late-onset forms of G_{M1} and G_{M2} gangliosidosis, late infantile Krabbe disease, ataxia-telangiectasia, and carbohydrate-deficient glycoprotein syndrome; each presents with signs suggestive enough to warrant specific investigations (lysosomal leukocyte enzymes in G_{M1}, G_{M2}, and Krabbe disease; plasma glycosylated transferrin in CDG syndrome; immunologic investigations and chromosome analysis in ataxia-telangiectasia) (Table 66-26). A severe early-onset encephalopathy with seizures and myoclonic jerks associated with hepatic symptoms is highly suggestive of Alpers syndrome due to respiratory chain disorders. Creatine deficiency due to guanidinoacetate methyltransferase deficiency can strike in infancy with an extrapyramidal disorder associated with epilepsy, neurologic regression, and failure to thrive. The biologic mark of this defect is the very low plasma and urine creatine levels, but unfortunately, this screening symptom can be lacking.[199,200]

Using a comprehensive organic acid metabolism investigation (including amino acid, urinary organic acid, and plasma acylcarnitine determinations) allows the diagnosis of several intermediary metabolic defects that disturb energy production and give rise to progressive ataxia, intention tremor, and progressive peripheral neuropathy. Pyruvate dehydrogenase deficiency frequently presents as peripheral neuropathy, intermittent ataxia, and slight or moderate hyperlactacidemia (see "Hyperlactacidemias" above). Several respiratory chain disorders first cause ataxia, intention tremor, dysarthria, epilepsy, and myopathy and eventually lead to various multiorgan failures. Lactic acid metabolism should be carefully investigated in all these patients. 3-Hydroxyacyl CoA dehydrogenase deficiency,[115,116,211d] L-2-hydroxyglutaric aciduria,[212] 3-methylglutaconic aciduria, methylmalonic aciduria, and propionic acidemia disturb organic acid excretion significantly, although sometimes only slightly and intermittently. In these disorders, an acylcarnitine profile determined by a tandem MS-MS technique from blood spots collected on dry filter paper, can be very helpful in identifying characteristic acylcarnitine compounds.

Glutaric aciduria type I due to glutaryl CoA dehydrogenase can also present as permanent unsteady gait due to choreoathetosis, with dystonia striking abruptly after an acute episode resembling encephalitis[63] (Table 66-26). The new syndrome biotin-responsive basal ganglia disease can also start before 5 years with such a subacute encephalopathy, dysarthria, dysphagia, external ophthalmoplegia and rapid progress to severe cogwheel rigidity, dystonia and quadriparesis. The only consistent radiological abnormality is central necrosis of the head of the caudates and the involvement of the putamen on brain MRI.[213]

Category 4. Diseases with predominant epilepsy and myoclonus resulting in ataxia and frequent falling include two ceroid lipofuscinoses. Santavuori-Hagberg disease presents as rapidly advancing psychomotor degeneration, myoclonic jerks, blindness, and early flattening of the EEG. Jansky-Bielschowski disease roughly resembles Lennox-Gastaut syndrome (akinetic myoclonic petit mal). There is a typical EEG pattern on slow rate photic stimulation, and vacuolated lymphocytes are present. Late-onset forms of Niemann-Pick disease type C and Gaucher disease are readily suspected because of hepatomegaly and/or splenomegaly. Two other disorders must also be considered: myoclonus epilepsy and ragged fed fibers (MERFF) syndrome, which has been found to be due to mutations in mitochondrial DNA, and Schindler disease, which presents in the second year of life as mental regression, myoclonic seizures, spasticity, optic atrophy, and

Table 66-24 Progressive Neurologic and Mental Deterioration: Part 2 (1 to 5 Years): Category 1: With Visceral, Craniovertebral, Ocular, or Other Somatic Abnormalities

Leading Symptom	Other Signs	Age at Onset	Diagnosis
Coarse facies	Skeletal changes Hepatosplenomegaly Hirsutism Corneal opacities Joint stiffness	2–3 years 1–2 years 3–5 years 2–4 years	Hurler syndrome (mucopolysaccharidosis type I) Hunter syndrome (X-linked) (mucopolysaccharidosis II) Sanfilippo syndrome (mucopolysaccharidosis type III) Pseudo-Hurler polydystrophy (mucolipidosis III)
	Subtle bone changes Hepatosplenomegaly Vacuolated lymphocytes ±Lens/corneal opacities	2–6 years 1–2 years 1–5 years 1–2 years	Mannosidosis (gingival hyperplasia) Fucosidosis (angiokeratoma) Aspartylglucosaminuria (macroglossia, leukopenia, joint laxity) Austin disease (ichthyosis)
Hepatosplenomegaly	Vertical supranuclear ophthalmoplegia Progressive dementia Myoclonic jerks	2–6 years	Niemann-Pick type C and related disorders (late infantile form)
Splenomegaly + hepatomegaly	Osseous lesions Various neurologic signs (ataxia, supranuclear ophthalmoplegia, myoclonus)	1–6 years	Gaucher type III (subacute neuronopathy)
Major visual impairment or ocular signs	Blindness Corneal clouding in first year Cytoplasmic membranous bodies in cells (conjunctiva, fibroblasts, liver, spleen) Dystonia	1–2 years	Mucolipidosis type IV
	Retinitis pigmentosa Deafness	1–5 years	Peroxisomal disorders Usher syndrome type II
	Cataracts Joint laxity Severe hypotonia Low plasma citrulline, ornithine, and proline Preprandial hyperammonemia	1–5 years	Pyrroline-5-carboxylate synthetase deficiency
Joint laxity	Cataracts Severe hypotonia Low plasma citrulline	1–5 years	Pyrroline-5-carboxylate synthetase deficiency

Table 66-25 Progressive Neurologic and Mental Deterioration: Part 2 (1 to 5 Years): Category 2: With Progressive Paraplegia, Weakness, Hypotonia, or Spasticity of the Lower Limbs Due to Corticospinal Tract Involvement or to Peripheral Neuropathy

Leading Symptom	Other Signs	Age at Onset	Diagnosis
Flaccid paraparesis ± pyramidal signs	Abnormal nerve conduction velocity High protein content in CSF fluid Dysarthria Dementia Blindness	12–18 months	Metachromatic leukodystrophy
Flaccid paraparesis	Normal nerve conduction velocity No change in CSF protein Optic atrophy Early mental regression Denervation atrophy on EMG	6–24 months	Neuroaxonal dystrophy (Seitelberger disease) Schindler disease (see also Table 66-27)
	Ataxia resembling subacute degeneration of the cord		Methylmalonic aciduria and homocystinuria (Cbl C) Homocystinuria (Cbl E, F, G)
Progressive spastic diplegia	Scissoring or "tiptoe" gait Irritability Hyperactivity Ataxia Seizures Psychosis Hyperargininemia High orotic acid excretion	2 months to 5 years	Arginase deficiency

Table 66-26 Progressive Neurologic and Mental Deterioration: Part 2 (1 to 5 Years): Category 3: With Unsteady Gait, Uncoordinated Movements Due to Cerebellar Syndrome, Sensory Defects, or Involuntary Movements (Athetotic Choreiform Movements)

Table 66-26a Without Disturbances of Organic Acid Excretion

Main signs	Age at Onset	Diagnosis
Ataxia with choreoathetosis Oculocephalic asynergia Conjunctival telangiectasias Lymphoid tissue node atrophy Sinopulmonary infections Low IgA level	18 months to 3 years	Ataxia-telangiectasia
Ataxia Difficulty in walking Mental deterioration (speech) Spastic quadriparesis Pseudobulbar signs Normal vision, CSF, and nerve conduction velocity	6 months to 4 years	G_{M1} gangliosidosis (Landing disease, late infantile form)
Ataxia Spinocerebellar degeneration Psychotic behavior Spasticity Seizures	2–4 years	G_{M2} gangliosidosis (Tay-Sachs disease, Sandhoff disease) Late infantile form
Ataxia Pyramidal signs (hemiplegia, paraplegia) Vision loss Peripheral neuropathy Normal CSF and nerve conduction velocity in 50% Acute onset common	6 months to 3 years	Krabbe disease (late infantile form)
Ataxia Muscular atrophy in lower extremities Dysequilibrium Dyskinesia Walking tiptoe with support Contractures of the knees Strokelike episodes Abnormal nerve conduction velocity (peripheral neuropathy)	3 months to 6 years	Congenital defects of glycosylation
Seizures and myoclonic jerks Uncoordinated movements Postictal coma Transient hemiplegia Hepatic symptoms (jaundice, high transaminases) Hyperlactatemia	3 months to 3 years	Alpers syndrome (respiratory chain disorders)
Extrapyramidal disorder Dyskinesia Epilepsy Neurologic regression Failure to thrive Low plasma creatinine		Creatine deficiency (GAMT deficiency)
Leukoencephalopathy Ataxia-spasticity Optic atrophy Vanishing white matter	1 to 5 years	Disease of vanishing white matter with hyperglycinorrachia
Ataxia-dysarthria Optic atrophy, nystagmus Mental retardation Leukoencephalopathy	3 months to 5 years	Leukoencephalopathy with disturbance of polyol metabolism

severe osteopenia. This disorder roughly resembles neuroaxonal dystrophy[179] (Table 66-27).

Category 5. Only a few disorders present between 1 and 5 years of age as isolated arrest or regression of psychic and perceptual functions and without significant neurologic or extraneurologic signs. SanFilippo disease is one, although regression of high-level achievements, loss of speech, and agitation usually begin later than 5 years of age. Although not a metabolic disorder, Rett syndrome is another such disease; it should be considered when a girl

Table 66-26 Progressive Neurologic and Mental Deterioration: Part 2 (1 to 5 Years): Category 3: With Unsteady Gait, Uncoordinated Movements Due to Cerebellar Syndrome, Sensory Defects, or Involuntary Movements (Athetotic Choreiform Movements)

Table 66-26b With Disturbances of Organic Acid Excretion

Main signs	Age at Onset	Diagnosis (major excreted compounds shown in parenthesis)
Progressive ataxia Intention tremor Slight extrapyramidal signs Cerebellar atrophy Spongiform encephalopathy L-2-hydroxyglutaric aciduria	2–3 years	L-2-hydroxyglutaric aciduria (L-2-hydroxyglutaric)
Ataxia Peripheral neuropathy Recurrent attacks of lethargy Hyperlactatemia	1–5 years	Pyruvate dehydrogenase deficiency (lactic, pyruvic)
Ataxia Intention tremor Muscular weakness Retinitis pigmentosa Dysarthria Myoclonic epilepsy Associated or not with multiorgan failure	1–5 years	Respiratory chain disorders (lactic acid, Krebs cycle intermediates) MERFF syndrome 3-methylglutaconic aciduria (3-methylglutaconic)
Ataxia Peripheral neuropathy Abnormal nerve conduction velocity Retinitis pigmentosa Progressive cardiomyopathy Recurrent attacks of hypoketotic hypoglycemia and of myoglobinuria	6 months to 4 years	3-hydroxy-acyl CoA dehydrogenase deficiency (3-hydroxydicarboxylic and 3-hydroxy-acylcarnitine esters)
Ataxia Subacute degeneration of the cord Megaloblastic anemia	Infancy to childhood	Methylmalonic aciduria and homocystinuria (CblC) Homocystinuria (CblE, CblF, CblG)
Acute attacks resembling encephalitis, increasingly severe choreoathetosis Macrocephaly Temporal lobe atrophy and bilateral basal ganglia damage	1–3 years	Glutaric aciduria type I (glutaric, methylglutaconic)
Dystonia Athetosis Chronic diarrhea		Methylmalonic acidemia (methylmalonic) Propionic acidemia (methylcitrate, tiglylglycine)

without familial precedent presents between 1 and 2 years of age with autistic behavior, mental regression, special stereotyped movements of the fingers, and microcephaly (Table 66-27).

Part 3: Late Childhood to Adolescence (5 to 15 Years). It is important to separate conditions in which mental functions are primarily affected from "pure" neurologic disorders with normal or subnormal intellectual functioning. According to Adams and Lyon,[17] there are six clinical categories.

Category 1. This category includes disorders that present as predominant extrapyramidal signs (parkinsonian syndrome, dystonia, choreoathetotis) [see "Extrapyramidal Signs (Dyskinesia, Dystonia, Choreoathetosis, Parkinsonism)" below; see also Tables 66-28 and 66-29].

Category 2. This category includes disorders presenting as severe neurologic and mental deterioration and "diffuse" central nervous system disorders. Patients have in common severe neurologic dysfunction with bipyramidal paralysis, incoordination, seizures, visual failure, impaired scholastic performance, and dementia. In association with splenomegaly or hepatomegaly, these signs suggest Niemann-Pick disease type C or Gaucher disease type III. When visceral signs are absent, they may indicate juvenile metachromatic leukodystrophy, X-linked adrenoleukodystrophy, Krabbe disease, juvenile G_{M1} and G_{M2} gangliosidoses, or respiratory chain disorders (Table 66-30). It has been recently described in a patient with peroxisomal biogenesis defect who presented in the second decade of life with peripheral neuropathy, at first mimicking Charcot-Marie-Tooth type II disease, and who shortly thereafter developed a pyramidal syndrome and intellectual deterioration with dementia and neurovegetative state.[45b] The new entity biotinresponsive basal ganglia disease can sometimes also start with such a diffuse central nervous disorder.[213]

Category 3. This category includes disorders presenting as polymyoclonus and epilepsy. The juvenile form of Spielmeyer-Vogt disease (or Batten disease due to *CLN3* gene mutations[214,215]), which presents as loss of sight, retinitis, ataxia, and, at an advanced stage, extrapyramidal signs, should be suspected in this situation.[215] Vacuolated lymphocytes are a nearly constant finding in this disorder. After puberty, Lafora disease is another important diagnostic consideration. Gaucher disease type III, late G_{M2} gangliosidosis, Niemann-Pick disease type C, and

Table 66-27 Progressive Neurologic and Mental Deterioration: Part 2 (1 to 5 Years): Category 4: With Convulsions and With Arrest of Psychic Functions

With Convulsions, Seizures and Myoclonus, Ataxia, Frequent Falling Due to Intention Myoclonus or to Cerebellar Ataxia		
Rapidly advancing psychomotor degeneration Hypotonia Ataxia Myoclonic jerks Early-flattening EEG Blindness	1–2 years	Santavuori-Hagberg disease (infantile ceroid lipofuscinosis)
Akinetic myoclonic petit mal Polymyoclonus Cerebellar ataxia Retinitis pigmentosa Typical EEG on slow rate photic stimulation Vacuolated lymphocytes	2–4 years	Jansky-Bielschowski disease (late infantile ceroid lipofuscinosis) (may be misdiagnosed as Lennox-Gastaut syndrome)
Rapid regression Myoclonic seizures Muscular hypotonia Spasticity Corneal blindness Optic atrophy Severe osteoporosis	6 months to 2 years	Schindler disease (alpha-N-acetyl galactosaminidase deficiency) (roughly similar to neuroaxonal dystrophy)
Myoclonic epilepsy volitional and intentional myoclonias Muscular weakness Cerebellar ataxia Hyperlactacidemia Optic atrophy Deafness	4–15 years	MERFF syndrome (respiratory chain disorders)
With splenomegaly and hepatomegaly Supranuclear ophthalmoplegia Myoclonic epilepsy can be revealing	2–6 years	Niemann-Pick disease type C Gaucher disease type III
Seizures and myoclonic jerks Uncoordinated movements Postictal coma Transient hemiplegia Hepatic symptoms (jaundice, high transaminases) Hyperlactatemia	1–2 years	Alpers syndrome (respiratory chain disorders)
Disorders with Arrest or Regression of Psychic and Perceptual Functions as the Predominant or Only Presenting Symptom*		
Autistic behavior Loss of speech Regression of high-level achievements Stereotyped movements of fingers Acquired microcephaly Secondary epilepsy	1–2 years	Rett syndrome (only in girls; sporadic cases of unknown etiology)
Regression of high-level achievements Loss of speech Agitation Hirsutism without evident bone and facial changes	4–6 years or later	Sanfilippo syndrome

*See also disorders that begin after 5 years of age (Tables 66-29 and 66-32).

respiratory chain disorders can also begin with polymyoclonus as an early important sign (Table 66-30).

Category 4. This category includes diseases presenting as predominant cerebellar ataxia. Friedreich ataxia and other hereditary ataxias must be considered (although previously considered nonmetabolic). They are recognized on clinical and genetic grounds. Abetalipoproteinemia and ataxia-telangiectasia are usually readily suspected because of the associated extraneurologic signs. Peroxisomal disorders,[45b,215a] CDG syndrome, and Refsum disease (which can all present as a peripheral neuropathy and retinitis pigmentosa) can be easily demonstrated by studies of plasma very-long-chain fatty acids, glycosylated transferrin profile, and plasma phytanic acid, respectively. Cerebellar ataxia in the context of progressive mental deterioration, dementia, and epilepsy suggests Lafora disease, cerebrotendinous xanthomatosis, late-onset forms of gangliosidosis, Krabbe disease, Gaucher disease, Niemann-Pick disease type C, or metachromatic leukodystrophy. Respiratory chain disorders can also be revealed by predominant ataxia (Table 66-31).

Table 66-28 Progressive Neurologic and Mental Deterioration Part 3: 5 to 15 Years: Category 1. With Predominant Extrapyramidal Signs, Parkinson Syndrome, Dystonia, Choreoathetosis (See Also Symptom "Extrapyramidal Signs," Table 66-34)

Main signs	Age at Onset	Diagnosis
Torsion Dystonia No mental retardation	6–10 years	Dystonia musculorum deformans
Dystonia of lower extremities Gait difficulties No or minimal axial dystonia Normal intellect Diurnal fluctuation of dystonia Dopa responsive	5–10 years	Segawa disease (GTP cyclohydrolase deficiency)
Lens dislocation Moderate mental retardation Marfanoid morphology	5–15 years	Classic homocystinuria
Progressive disorder of locomotion Dystonic posture Choreoathetosis Severe mental regression Retinitis pigmentosa Acanthocytosis	5–15 years	Hallervorden-Spatz syndrome
Generalized parkinsonian rigidity or gross postural and intention tremor Scholastic failure Psychiatric abnormalities Hepatic signs Kayser-Fleischer ring	10–15 years	Wilson disease
Rigidity Fine tremor abolished by movements Dementia Seizures Dominant inheritance	10–15 years and later	Huntington chorea
Parkinsonism (no tremor) Rigidity Moderate hypokinesia Brisk tendon jerks Difficulties in reading and writing Alacrima Dysphagia due to achalasia Hypoglycemia due to selective cortisol deficiency	10–15 years	Familial glucocorticoid deficiency
Subacute encephalopathy Dysarthria, dysphagia External ophthalmoplegia Cogwheel rigidity Dystonia Central necrosis of basal ganglia	5–10 years	Biotin-responsive basal ganglia disease

Category 5. This category includes diseases presenting as predominant polyneuropathy. Porphyrias and tyrosinemia type I can present in episodes of acute decompensation as polyneuropathy mimicking Guillain-Barré syndrome. Many other disorders can present as late-onset progressive polyneuropathy that can mimic heredataxia, such as Charcot-Marie-Tooth disease or other hereditary ataxias. These disorders include lysosomal diseases (Krabbe disease and metachromatic leukodystrophy), defects of energy metabolism (Leigh disease, respiratory chain disorders, PDH deficiency, LCHAD and trifunctional enzyme deficiencies), abetalipoproteinemia, CDG syndrome, and peroxisomal disorders,[45b,215a] including Refsum disease (see Table 66-32).

Category 6. Finally, some inborn errors of metabolism can appear between five and 15 years of age as psychiatric disorders. Behavioral disturbances (personality and character changes), loss of speech, scholastic failure, mental regression, dementia, psychosis, and a schizophrenia-like syndrome are the most frequent symptoms. Among the disorders listed in Table 66-30, we have personal experience of such a pure psychiatric presentation in SanFilippo disease, X-linked adrenoleukodystrophy, Wilson disease, and classic homocystinuria. In addition to this list of inborn errors that classically present as psychiatric disorders, we and others have observed patients with OTC deficiency who presented with intermittent abnormal behavior and character change until hyperammonemia and coma revealed the true situation (see "Recurrent Attacks of Coma, Strokes, and Vomiting with Lethargy, Ataxia, and Psychiatric Symptoms" above; see also Table 66-6). Homocystinuria due to methylene tetrahydrofolate reductase deficiency has presented as isolated schizophrenia.[73,211,211a]

Part 4: Onset in Adulthood (15 to 70 Years). In adults, neurodegenerative diseases such as psychosis, dementia, ataxia,

Table 66-29 Progressive Neurologic and Mental Deterioration: Part 3: 5 to 15 Years: Category 2. With Severe Neurologic and Mental Deterioration, Diffuse Central Nervous System Disorders, Bipyramidal Paralysis, Incoordination, Seizures, Visual Failure, Dementia

Leading Symptom	Other Signs	Diagnosis
With visceral signs	Hepatosplenomegaly Splenomegaly	Niemann-Pick disease type C Gaucher disease type III
Without visceral signs	Abnormal nerve conduction velocity High CSF protein	Metachromatic leukodystrophy (juvenile form)
	High CSF protein Adrenal dysfunction	Adrenal leukodystrophy (X-linked) (many variants)
	Ophthalmoplegia Peripheral neuropathy Various signs	Leigh disease
	Paraplegia Tremor Ataxia	Krabbe disease (infantile form) G_{M1} and G_{M2} gangliosidoses (juvenile form)
	Multiorgan failure Lactic acidemia	Respiratory chain disorders
	Peripheral neuropathy Pseudo-Charcot-Marie-Tooth disease	Peroxisomal biogenesis defects

epilepsy, dystonia, and peripheral neuropathy can be revealing signs of variant forms of inborn errors. The best known of these are listed in Table 66-33.[210,215a–218] It is highly probable that many other disorders will be discovered in adults in the near future, when neurologists further extend metabolic investigations to late-onset progressive neurologic deterioration, now still considered to be "degenerative," inflammatory, or of vascular origin.

Extrapyramidal Signs (Dyskinesia, Dystonia, Choreoathetosis, Parkinsonism)

Extrapyramidal signs are extremely common in pediatrics. When they are associated with other neurologic symptoms in a severe diffuse central nervous system disorder, it may be difficult to recognize them specifically. When they are predominant, they can be presenting symptoms of a number of inherited metabolic disorders (Table 66-34).

In progressive diseases, the dystonic state can involve all muscles, including the tongue, facio-oropharyngeal, and visceral musculature. Strictly speaking, dystonia is a nonpyramidal disorder in which fluctuating and finally persistent hypertonia is present. However, the term is also often used in neurologic examination to designate a persistent hypertonic state of any kind (even spasticity) that results in a fixed abnormal posture. When muscles are kept continuously in spasm, dystonia eventually results in fixed deformities (pseudocontractures) that contort the body. Athetotic movements in distal parts of the limbs and in the

Table 66-30 Progressive Neurologic and Mental Deterioration: Part 3: 5 to 15 Years: Category 3. With Polymyoclonus

Leading Symptom	Other Signs	Age at Onset	Diagnosis
Generalized epilepsy	Polymyoclonus Dementia Neurologic deterioration Ataxia	14–20 years	Lafora disease
Intellectual deterioration	Loss of sight Retinitis Polymyoclonus Ataxia Extrapyramidal signs Vacuolated lymphocytes	5–12 years	Spielmeyer-Vogt (juvenile neuronal ceroid lipofuscinosis, or Batten disease due to CLN_3 mutations)
Predominant seizures	Myoclonic epilepsy Dementia Splenomegaly Osseous signs	7–10 years	Gaucher disease type III
Cerebellar ataxia	Myoclonic jerks Cherry red spot	4–10 years	Late onset G_{M2} gangliosidosis (Sandhoff disease Tay-Sachs disease)
Hepatomegaly	Splenomegaly Ophthalmoplegia	5–10 years	Niemann-Pick disease type C
Myoclonic epilepsy	Ataxia Lactic acidosis	All ages	Respiratory chain disorders (MERFF, etc.)

Table 66-31 Progressive Neurologic and Mental Deterioration: Part 3: 5 to 15 Years: Category 4. With Predominant Cerebellar Ataxia

Leading Symptom	Other Signs	Age at Onset	Diagnosis
Without significant mental deterioration	Dysarthria Pes cavus Cardiomyopathy	8–15 years	Friedreich ataxia
	Spinocerebellar degeneration		Other hereditary ataxias
	Chronic diarrhea Low cholesterol Retinitis pigmentosa Acanthocytosis Peripheral neuropathy		Abetalipoproteinemia Peroxisomal disorders Congenital defects of glycosylation
	Oculocephalic asynergia Conjunctival telangiectasias		Ataxia-telangiectasia (see age of onset 1–5 years)
	Peripheral neuropathy Retinitis pigmentosa Ichthyosis		Refsum disease
With mental deterioration and dementia			Lafora disease (see above polymyoclonia and later onset in adulthood) Cerebrotendinous xanthomatosis (see later onset in adulthood) G_{M1}, G_{M2} gangliosidoses Gaucher disease Niemann-Pick disease type C Krabbe disease, juvenile form Metachromatic leukodystrophy Respiratory chain disorders

face are frequently associated with dystonia, suggesting that any distinction between athetosis and dystonia is only relative. Resistance to passive movements is variable, tending to be plastic and to vanish suddenly, leaving the limb slack. Parkinsonian syndrome includes rigidity, tremor, and slowness of movement without paralysis.[17] In infants, profound parkinsonism results in hypokinesis, drooling, difficulty swallowing, sweating, pinpoint pupils, oculogyric spasms, truncal hypotonia, increased limb tone, and blank facies with relative preservation of smiling.[184]

In the first year of life, discounting kernicterus secondary to Crigler-Najjar disease type I, only a few inborn errors present as predominant extrapyramidal signs. In patients with inborn errors of tetrahydrobiopterin metabolism (mostly GTP cyclohydrolase deficiency), with the recently described aromatic amino acid decarboxylase deficiency, or with tyrosine hydroxylase deficiency, the neurologic features are highly characteristic whether the disorder involves defective synthesis or recycling of biopterins.[8,46,204] Untreated cases can involve profound parkinsonism accompanied by myoclonic, choreic, or dystonic limb movements and very brisk tendon jerks. Patients with less marked symptoms exhibit different types of movement disorder and/or slow development. Many of the neurologic features can be explained by dopamine and serotonin deficiency.[46,184]

In the rare cytochrome b5 reductase type II deficiency, bilateral athetosis is one of the leading symptoms, with hypertonicity of the limbs, severe mental retardation, and ophthalmoplegia. The presence of cyanosis and methemoglobinemia suggests the diagnosis. Pelizaeus-Merzbacher disease early in life in boys causes laryngeal stridor, nystagmus, and dystonia, the last symptom being easily mistaken for myoclonia.

In late infancy to early childhood (1 to 5 years), glutaric aciduria type I, 3-methylglutaconic aciduria, 4-hydroxybutyric aciduria, a variant form of methylmalonic aciduria and propionic acidemia, and the recently described L-2-hydroxyglutaric aciduria[212] can give rise to extrapyramidal signs. All these disorders can be identified by careful analysis of urinary organic acids. Glutaric aciduria type I should rank high in the differential diagnosis in any child with acute profound dyskinesia or subacute motor delay accompanied by increasingly severe choreoathetosis and dystonia.[63] Most of these patients present acutely with an illness resembling encephalitis. Early macrocephalus is a nearly constant finding in this disorder. In methylmalonic acidemia and propionic acidemia, there can be late-onset extrapyramidal disease and corticospinal tract involvement after metabolic decompensation (see "Recurrent Attacks of Coma, Strokes, or Vomiting with Lethargy, Ataxia, or Psychiatric Symptoms" above). The neurologic findings result from bilateral destruction of the globus pallidus with variable involvement of the internal capsule. This particular presentation is not related to a specific gene defect, as it has been observed irrespective of mutant class type and cobalamin responsivity.[53] Congenital folate malabsorption, which presents early in infancy as severe megaloblastic anemia and failure to thrive, may involve the nervous system in the second year of life, causing athetosis, ataxia, peripheral neuropathy, seizures, mental retardation, and cerebral calcifications.

Lesch-Nyhan syndrome and Pelizaeus-Merzbacher disease, both X-linked, are classic diagnostic considerations in boys who present with predominant extrapyramidal signs in the second year of life. Diagnosis of the latter disorder is based only on clinical and familial findings. Ataxia-telangiectasia may be revealed in the second to third year of life by choreoathetosis. Diagnosis relies on recognition of the characteristic oculocephalic asynergia, ocular telangiectasias, recurrent sinopulmonary infections, lymph node atrophy, and low plasma IgA levels. Dystonic posture can be the (rare) presenting sign of Niemann-Pick disease type C (juvenile dystonic lipidosis) and of Gaucher disease type III, in which it is associated with vertical and lateral supranuclear ophthalmoplegia, respectively. G_{M1} gangliosidosis can present late in adolescence as abnormal movements, dysarthria, and mental regression. In the newly described inborn error of creatine biosynthesis at the level of guanidinoacetate methyltransferase, developmental arrest and severe extrapyramidal disorder can be the presenting signs.

Table 66-32 Progressive Neurologic and Mental Deterioration: Part 3: 5 to 15 Years: Categories 5 and 6

Category 5. With Predominant Polyneuropathy	
Acute attacks	Porphyrias Tyrosinemia type I
Progressive Can mimic heredataxias Charcot-Marie-Tooth disease or other hereditary ataxias	Metachromatic leukodystrophy Krabbe disease Refsum disease Abetalipoproteinemia Leigh disease Respiratory chain disorders PDH deficiency LCHAD deficiency Trifunctional enzyme deficiency CDG syndrome Peroxisomal biogenesis defects α Methyl acyl CoA racemase
Category 6. With Psychiatric Symptoms as the Only Presenting Sign	
Behavior disturbances Personality and character changes Mental regression Dementia Schizophrenia before any significant neurologic or extraneurologic sign	Sanfilippo syndrome Metachromatic leukodystrophy Krabbe disease Niemann-Pick disease type C X-linked adrenoleukodystrophy Leigh disease Spielmeyer-Vogt disease (lipofuscinosis) Hallervorden-Spatz disease Wilson disease Cerebrotendinous xanthomatosis Huntington chorea (juvenile form) OTC deficiency (and other subacute congenital hyperammonemias) Classic homocystinuria Methylene tetrahydrofolate reductase deficiency Cobalamin defects (Cbl C)

PDH = pyruvate dehydrogenase; LCHAD = hydroxyl long chain acyl CoA dehydrogenase; CDG = congenital defects of glycosylation; OTC = ornithine transcarbamylase.

Both are significantly improved by oral supplementation with creatine.[219]

In late childhood (5 to 15 years), dopa-responsive hereditary progressive dystonia (Segawa disease) should be considered when dystonia starts in the lower extremities mostly with gait difficulties and little or no axial dystonia. In most (not all) patients, there is marked diurnal fluctuation of symptoms. Mental development remains normal. Low doses of L-dopa cause marked improvement in a few days or weeks, and symptoms recur immediately after L-dopa is withdrawn.[220,221] Rarely, homocystinuria presents as severe dystonia apparently as the initial symptom, although lens dislocation or iridodonesis is already present.[222]

Hallervorden-Spatz disease is a progressive disorder that may develop at any age between 2 and 15 years or even in adult life, although in most cases it becomes apparent by the age of 15. A progressive disorder of locomotion and movements of the extrapyramidal type are the usual initial manifestations. Rigidity, dystonic postures, and choreoathetosis precede progressive and severe mental deterioration. The diagnosis becomes evident when these very suggestive early manifestations are associated with dementia, retinitis pigmentosa, and acanthocytosis (see also the sections on these symptoms).

In Wilson disease, the neurologic abnormalities do not usually become apparent until the second decade of life or even later. Either of two major, often dissociated, symptoms may be the first manifestation: generalized parkinsonian rigidity involving mainly the facial and oropharyngeal musculature with dysarthria, dysphagia, and facial masking, or gross postural and intention tremor. Psychiatric abnormalities, scholastic failure, loss of emotional control, and subtle impairment of intellectual function are frequently present and can also be presenting signs. Diagnosis relies on hepatic signs (sometimes incipient cirrhosis), presence of a Kayser-Fleischer corneal ring, and copper assay. Familial glucocorticoid deficiency can present late in childhood as parkinsonism, rigidity, and moderate hypokinesia without tremor or dementia.[223]

Finally, early-onset Huntington chorea can present in late childhood or adolescence as rigidity, dementia, seizures, and fine tremor abolished by movements. This autosomal dominant condition can easily be mistaken for schizophrenia.

Deafness

Deafness is difficult to detect in children who have severe mental dysfunction. The cochleopalpebral reflex is of little value in these cases because it is highly influenced by the state of alertness of the infant. Auditory evoked potentials are of great interest here but have not been extensively studied in inborn errors of metabolism. In some inborn errors with symptoms occurring in late childhood and adolescence, peripheral or central types of deafness can be observed, sometimes as the main diagnostic symptom, as in thiamine-responsive megaloblastic anemia, deafness, and diabetes (Table 66-35). In biotin-responsive multicarboxylase defect, deafness occurring in the first years of life is a common complication when the disease has been recognized late or incorrectly treated. In some cases of phosphoribosyl pyrophosphate synthetase superactivity presenting early in infancy as clinical signs of uric acid overproduction, sensorineural deafness associated with hypotonia and autistic features can be helpful for diagnosis.[224,225] In most peroxisomal disorders and in some mucopolysaccharidoses, deafness is a frequent finding. Many

Table 66-33 Progressive Neurologic and Mental Deterioration: Part 4: Onset in Adulthood (15 to 70 Years)

Main Clinical Presentation	Diagnoses
With predominant ataxia	Metachromatic leukodystrophy Hexosaminidase deficiencies Niemann-Pick disease type C Cerebrotendinous xanthomatosis Galactosialidosis 3-methylglutaconic aciduria
With peripheral sensory polyneuropathy	3-hydroxy long-chain acyl CoA dehydrogenase deficiency Trifunctional enzyme deficiency Congenital defects of glycosylation Peroxisomal biogenesis defects α Methyl acyl-CoA racemase
With predominant psychosis, dementia	Metachromatic leukodystrophy Hexosaminidase deficiencies Niemann-Pick disease type C Ceroid lipofuscinosis: Kufs disease Cerebrotendinous xanthomatosis Huntington chorea Wilson disease Lafora disease Ornithine transcarbamylase deficiency Classic homocystinuria Cobalamin defects (Cbl C)
With predominant extrapyramidal signs	G_{M1} gangliosidosis Hexosaminidase deficiencies Niemann-Pick disease type C Ceroid lipofuscinosis: Kufs disease Huntington chorea Wilson disease
With predominant hemiparesis or paraparesis but no mental deterioration	Krabbe disease (late-onset form) Adrenomyeloneuropathy Peroxisomal disorders
With myoclonic epilepsy	Galactosialidosis Sialidosis type I (cherry red spot, myoclonus syndrome) Ceroid lipofuscinosis: Kufs disease Lafora disease

Table 66-34 Extrapyramidal Signs (Dyskinesia, Dystonia, Choreoathetosis, Parkinsonism)

Neonatal to early infancy (birth to 1 year)
- Biopterin synthesis or recycling deficiencies
- Aromatic amino acid decarboxylase deficiency
- Tyrosine hydroxylase deficiency
- 4-Hydroxybutyric aciduria
- Cytochrome b5-reductase deficiency (methemoglobinemia)
- Crigler-Najjar syndrome
- Early onset of Pelizaeus-Merzbacher disease
- Leigh disease

Late infancy to early childhood (1–5 years)
- Glutaric aciduria type I
- 3-Methylglutaconic aciduria
- 2-Hydroxyglutaric aciduria
- 4-Hydroxybutyric aciduria
- Methylmalonic aciduria (variant form)
- Lesch-Nyhan syndrome (X-linked)
- Pelizaeus-Merzbacher disease (X-linked)
- Mucolipidosis type IV
- Congenital folate malabsorption (megaloblastic anemia, failure to thrive)
- Gaucher disease type III (supranuclear ophthalmoplegia)
- Niemann-Pick disease type C (juvenile dystonic lipidosis)
- G_{M1} gangliosidosis ("adult" form)
- Ataxia-telangiectasia
- Leigh disease
- Triosephosphate isomerase deficiency (hemolytic anemia, diffuse weakness)
- Creatine deficiency (guanidinoacetate methyltransferase deficiency)

Late childhood to adulthood (5–15 years)
- Segawa disease (dopa-responsive)
- Classic homocystinuria (lens dislocations)
- Hallervorden-Spatz disease (dementia, retinitis pigmentosa)
- Dystonia musculorum deformans
- Wilson disease (cirrhosis)
- Huntington chorea (dementia, dominant inheritance)
- Spielmeyer-Vogt disease (retinitis pigmentosa, mental deterioration, extrapyramidal signs appearing late in the disease)
- Familial glucocorticoid deficiency
- Leigh disease
- Biotin-responsive basal ganglia disease

well-known genetic syndromes (considered autonomous entities) are similar to or indistinguishable from recently discovered inborn errors of metabolism, for example, Wolfram syndrome and thiamine-responsive megaloblastic anemia,[226–233] Usher syndrome type II and infantile Refsum disease,[234] and various neurologic syndromes (MELAS, MERRF, Kearns-Sayre) that are really inborn errors of the mitochondrial respiratory chain. Deafness is a dominant and frequently revealing sign in the rare β-mannosidosis.[235] An amazing and yet-unexplained association of deafness, nonprogressive encephalopathy, intermittent episodes of coma, and hyperkynureninuria has recently been described.[236]

Hypotonia in the Neonatal Period and in Early Infancy

Hypotonia is a very common nonspecific symptom of sick neonates (see also "Presentation in the Neonatal Period" above). Whereas many nonmetabolic inherited diseases can give rise to severe generalized neonatal hypotonia (mainly all severe fetal neuromuscular disorders), only a few inborn errors of metabolism present in neonates as predominant hypotonia. Aside from disorders in which hypotonia is included in a very suggestive clinical context of major bone changes, dysmorphism, malformations, or visceral symptoms (Table 66-36), the most severe metabolic hypotonias are observed in neonatal distress types III (congenital hyperlactacidemias, respiratory chain disorders), IVa (urea cycle defects), and IVb (nonketotic hyperglycinemia, sulfite oxidase deficiency, peroxisomal disorders, trifunctional enzyme deficiency and congenital disorders of glycosylation). The diagnosis emerges when the associated hypotonia is coupled with lethargy, coma, seizures, and neurologic symptoms in type IVb and with characteristic metabolic changes in type III (lactic acidosis) and type IVa (hyperammonemia). Severe forms of Pompe disease (α-glucosidase deficiency) can mimic respiratory chain disorders when generalized hypotonia is associated with cardiomyopathy. In reality, these two disorders are very different, since Pompe disease is associated with characteristic EKG changes (short PR interval, high-amplitude QRS complex) and vacuolated lymphocytes, whereas respiratory chain disorders present as hypertrophic dilated cardiomyopathy and lactic acidosis (see "Cardiomyopathy" below). Suggestive craniofacial dysmorphism is present only in typical Zellweger syndrome but can be moderate or even absent in variant forms of peroxisomal disorders such as neonatal adrenoleukodystrophy, acyl CoA oxidase deficiency, or peroxisomal biogenesis defects.[45,45a,45b]

Table 66-35 Deafness

Age of Detection	Main Symptoms	Disorders
Neonatal to early infancy	Dysmorphism Severe mental retardation Hypotonia Retinitis pigmentosa Seizures	Zellweger syndrome and variants Rhizomelic chondrodysplasia punctata Acyl CoA oxidase deficiency
	Congenital encephalopathy Episodes of coma	Hyperkynureninuria
	All the above plus intracranial calcifications	Cockayne syndrome Alport syndrome
Late infancy to early childhood	Failure to thrive Hepatomegaly Diarrhea Osteoporosis Retinitis pigmentosa	Infantile Refsum disease
	Gout Arthritis Hyperuricemia Ataxia Hypotonia Psychotic behavior	PRPP synthetase overactivity
	Coarse facies Dysostosis multiplex	Mucopolysaccharidoses types I, II, IV Mannosidosis (alpha and beta) Mucolipidosis type II
	Alopecia Cutaneous rashes Hypotonia, coma Lactic acidosis	Biotinidase deficiency (biotin responsive)
	Megaloblastic anemia Diabetes Responsiveness to thiamine	Megaloblastic anemia, thiamine responsive Wolfram syndrome
	Ichthyosis Hepatomegaly Myopathy Vacuolated lymphocytes	Neutral lipid storage disorder
	Lactic acidosis Short stature Dementia Weakness Ragged red fibers Multiorgan failure Strokes	Mitochondrial encephalomyopathy MELAS, MERRF, and Kearns-Sayre syndromes due to various respiratory chain errors (nuclear mitochondrial gene deletions or insertions)
Late childhood to adolescence and adulthood	Mental retardation Retinitis pigmentosa	Infantile Refsum disease Usher syndrome type II
	Ataxia Peripheral neuropathy Retinitis pigmentosa Ichthyosis Anosmia	Refsum disease (classic form)
	Ptosis Ophthalmoplegia Retinitis pigmentosa Myopathy Atrioventricular dissociation Hyperlactacidemia	Kearns-Sayre syndrome (mitochondrial DNA deletion) and other respiratory chain disorders
	Myoclonic epilepsy Ragged red fibers Ataxia	MERRF syndrome (mitochondrial tRNA Lys mutation)
	Angiokeratoma Mental retardation	β-Mannosidosis

PRPP = phosphoribosylpyrophosphate; MERRF = myoclonic epilepsy with ragged red fibers; MELAS = mitochondrial encephalopathy with lactic acidosis.

Table 66-36 Hypotonia in Neonatal Period and Early Infancy

Leading Symptom	Other Signs	Time When First Seen	Diagnosis
Evocative clinical context (dysmorphism, bone changes, visceral symptoms, malformations)	Main bone changes Hypomineralization Rachitic deformations	Birth to early infancy	Hypophosphatasia (large fontanelle, wide cranial suture) Calciferol metabolism defects Osteogenesis imperfecta (large skull, hyperlaxity, blue sclerae)
	Predominant dysmorphism Psychomotor retardation Malformations	Birth	Peroxisomal disorders (Zellweger syndrome and variants, chondrodysplasia punctata) Smith-Lemli-Opitz syndrome (hexadactyly, swallowing difficulties) Lowe syndrome Chromosomal abnormalities Other multiple-malformation syndromes (mainly those with muscular dystrophy: Walker-Warburg syndrome, Fukuyama muscular dystrophy, etc.)
	Storage disorders Hepatosplenomegaly Ascitic edema Coarse facies	Birth	Lysosomal disorders: Niemann-Pick disease type A G_{M1} gangliosidosis (Landing disease) Galactosialidosis Sialidosis type II I-cell disease
	Hepatomegaly Cholestatic jaundice Failure to thrive	Birth	Peroxisomal disorders Congenital defects of glycosylation
	Cataract Tubulopathy	Birth	Lowe syndrome (X-linked) Respiratory chain disorders
	Severe cardiomyopathy Macroglossia Vacuolated lymphocytes	Neonatal to early infancy	Pompe disease Respiratory chain disorders
Neurologic neonatal distress (see this symptom) Table 66-3	With ketosis and ketoacidosis (type I and II)	Neonatal to first month	MSUD, organic acidurias
	With hyperlactacidemia (type III)	Neonatal to first month	Congenital hyperlactacidemias
	With hyperammonemia (type IVa)	Neonatal to first days	Urea cycle defects, HHH syndrome Lysinuric protein intolerance Transient hyperammonemia
	Without biologic symptoms Seizures Myoclonias	Birth to first days	Nonketotic hyperglycinemia Sulfite oxidase deficiency Peroxisomal disorders Trifunctional enzyme deficiency
Apparently isolated at birth	Massive generalized hypotonia Anemia Fetal distress Hydramnios Arthrogryposis Respiratory failure	Birth	Severe fetal neuromuscular disorders Steinert disease (myotonia in mother) Myasthenia (prostigmin test) Congenital myopathy Hereditary sensorimotor neuropathy (abnormal nerve conduction velocity) Familial dysautonomy Congenital dystrophy (elevated CK) Respiratory chain disorders
	Predominant proximal amyotrophy Paralysis Areflexia	Birth to first weeks	Werdnig-Hoffman disease (SMA type I) Peroxisomal disorders Respiratory chain disorders
	Mental retardation Secondary obesity Minor dysmorphism	Birth	Prader-Willi syndrome (frequent)
	Stridor Dystonia, nystagmus	First months	Pelizaeus-Merzbacher disease (X-linked)

Table 66-37 Hyperventilation Attacks

Leading Symptoms	Other Signs	Age of Onset	Diagnosis
Metabolic acidosis pH < 7.30 P_{CO_2} < 30 mm Hg Base deficit < −10	See "Metabolic Acidosis" Table 66-22 and Table 66-7		
Respiratory alkalosis	Hyperammonemia	Neonatal to childhood	Urea cycle defects (OTC, ASA, ASS) Lysinuric protein intolerance Triple H syndrome Rett syndrome
	Hyperlactacidemia (moderate)	Infancy	Leigh syndrome (PDH, PC, respiratory chain defects, biotinidase deficiency)
	Chronic neurologic dysfunction Mental retardation Vermis atrophy Retinitis pigmentosa	Congenital	Joubert syndrome (with or without associated pipecolic acidemia)
	Mental regression Microcephaly Seizures Abnormal behavior	6 months to 2 years	Rett syndrome

ASA = argininosuccinic aciduria; ASS = argininosuccinate synthetase; PDH = pyruvate dehydrogenase; PC = pyruvate carboxylase; OTC = ornithine transcarbamylase

We have recently observed such a defect that presented in the neonatal period as an isolated generalized hypotonia mimicking Werdnig-Hoffmann syndrome.[45a] A very similar presentation can also be observed in some carbohydrate-deficient glycoprotein syndromes and in a new disorder caused by defective biosynthesis of N-linked oligosaccharides due to glucosidase I deficiency.[236a] Occasionally, the facies of Zellweger syndrome is confused with that of Down syndrome or other chromosomal aberrations. Smith-Lemli-Opitz syndrome types I and II due to 7,8-cholesterol dehydrogenase deficiency present in the neonatal period as severe hypotonia, facial dysmorphism, hexadactyly, and swallowing difficulties.[5,5a,5b,9] Lowe syndrome should be considered in boys who present with congenital cataract, tubulopathy, and minor facial dysmorphism. Prader-Willi syndrome is a significant cause of congenital hypotonia. The syndrome can be confirmed by demonstrating an abnormality of chromosome 15 (see Chap. 7) or in the second year of life when polyphagia and considerable obesity become manifest. As shown in Table 66-36, inborn errors of metabolism rarely appear in neonates as isolated hypotonia.

Hyperventilation Attacks

Central hyperventilation attacks are observed in a limited number of inborn errors, giving rise to hyperammonemia, hyperlactacidemia, and metabolic acidosis. Leigh disease (apparently idiopathic or secondary to inborn errors of metabolism), Joubert syndrome, and Rett syndrome frequently present as hyperventilation attacks (Table 66-37).

IV. OCULAR SYMPTOMS

Cataracts

Although more than 90 percent of congenital cataracts remain unexplained, a number of metabolic disorders give rise to them.[237] Age at onset of cataracts is useful for differential diagnosis (Table 66-38).

At birth, cataracts are a nearly constant sign in X-linked Lowe syndrome. They are also frequently present in peroxisomal biogenesis disorders such as classic Zellweger syndrome, in chondrodysplasia punctata (rhizomelic type), and in Cockayne syndrome. Cataracts can be the only presenting sign in sorbitol dehydrogenase deficiency. Cataracts associated with liver and renal tubular failure in a newborn or during the first month of life may indicate galactose 1-phosphate uridyl transferase or epimerase deficiency. Interestingly, neonatal cataracts have been observed in newborns born to mothers with the so-called marginal galactokinase deficiency and in patients with peripheral epimerase deficiency who were otherwise normal. Cataracts have even been observed in heterozygotes for peripheral epimerase deficiency.[238] These observations support the notion that galactitol accumulation in the lens is a major cause of cataract development.

In infancy, cataracts are the only presenting sign in the different variants of galactokinase deficiencies (total, partial, or marginal maternal) and in diverse galactitol or sorbitol accumulation states of unknown origin. Cataracts can be associated with other typical symptoms in lysosomal disorders (mannosidosis, sialidosis), respiratory chain defects, hypoglycemia of various origins, and the severe form of mevalonic aciduria.

In childhood, cataracts are a sign of hypoparathyroidism and pseudohypoparathyroidism and are observed in up to a quarter of Wilson disease patients. Minute opacities in the anterior fetal Y suture of both lenses, often surrounded by minute satellites, are a frequent finding in lysinuric protein intolerance. The opacities have never been large enough to cause visual impairment and have remained stable in some patients for over 20 years. In Sjögren-Larsson syndrome due to fatty alcohol oxidoreductase deficiency, cataract can accompany the other features of the syndrome (spasticity, mental retardation, ichthyosis, retinitis pigmentosa). In the so-called neutral lipid storage disorder, cataracts, ichthyosis, ataxia, myopathy, hepatomegaly, and vacuolated lymphocytes compose a highly typical syndrome of unknown origin. In the recently described pyrroline 5 carboxylase synthetase deficiency, congenital cataracts are associated with severe hypotonia, joint laxity, slow progressive neurologic and mental deterioration, and low plasma citrulline, ornithine, and proline levels with paradoxical preprandial hyperammonemia.[207,208] Isolated autosomal dominant bilateral cataracts associated with a mutation in the iron-responsive element of L-ferritin mRNA have recently been described.[239,240]

In adults, isolated cataracts can be a sign of heterozygosity for inborn errors of galactose metabolism and possibly for Lowe syndrome. Cataract is a frequent symptom in cerebrotendinous xanthomatosis, which is easily diagnosed from the association of xanthoma, neurodegenerative disorders, ataxia, and mental

Table 66-38 Cataract

Time when first visible	Other important symptoms	Disorders
Congenital (at birth)	Severe hypotonia Facial dysmorphism Tubulopathy	Lowe syndrome (X-linked)
	Dysmorphic features Hypotonia, seizures	Peroxisomal biogenesis defects Zellweger syndrome and variants
	Chondrodysplasia punctata Bone changes (rhizomelic dwarfism)	Chondrodysplasia punctata (rhizomelic type)
	Encephalopathy Retinitis, deafness Intracranial calcifications Facial dysmorphism	Cockayne syndrome
	Isolated	Sorbitol dehydrogenase deficiency
Neonatal (from first week to first month)	Liver failure Jaundice, tubulopathy	Galactosemias (galactose:uridyl transferase and epimerase deficiency)
	Isolated	Peripheral epimerase deficiency (homozygotes and heterozygotes) Marginal maternal galactokinase deficiency
	Possible fortuitous association	3-Phosphoglycerate dehydrogenase deficiency Congenital defects of glycosylation
Infant (from first month to first year)	Isolated	Galactokinase deficiency (total or partial) Galactitol or sorbitol accumulation
	Storage disorders (hepatosplenomegaly, coarse facies, vacuolated lymphocytes)	Sialidosis α-mannosidosis
	Hypoglycemia	Various origins
	Hypotonia Encephalomyopathy, lactic acidosis	Respiratory chain disorders Mevalonic aciduria
Childhood (1 to 15 years)	Isolated High serum ferritin Dominant inheritance	Dominant hyperferritinemia
	Bone changes Hypocalcemia	Hypoparathyroidism Pseudohypoparathyroidism
	Hyperglycemia	Diabetes mellitus
	Hepatic signs Neurologic signs	Wilson disease
	Ichthyosis Spastic paraplegia Retinal degeneration	Sjögren-Larsson syndrome (fatty alcohol oxidoreductase deficiency)
	Osteoporosis Growth retardation Hepatosplenomegaly Hyperammonemia	Lysinuric protein intolerance
	Ichthyosis Ataxia, myopathy Hepatomegaly Vacuolated lymphocytes	Neutral lipid storage disorder (unknown cause)
	Joint laxity Severe hypotonia Neurologic deterioration Low plasma citrulline and proline	Pyrroline-5-carboxylase synthetase deficiency
Adulthood (>15 years)	Isolated	Heterozygosity for galactose uridyltransferase and galactokinase Carrier state for Lowe syndrome Lactose absorbers
	Blindness Retinitis Hyperornithinemia	Ornithine aminotransferase deficiency
	Xanthoma Ataxia Neurodegenerative disorders Psychotic behavior	Cerebrotendinous xanthomatosis
	Hemolytic anemia	Glucose-6-phosphate dehydrogenase deficiency
	Myopathy Myotonia Cardiomyopathy Multiorgan involvement	Steinert disease (cataract can be presenting sign)

Table 66-39 Corneal Opacities

Time when first visible	Major symptoms	Disorders
Early infancy (3–12 months)	Keratitis "Conjunctivitis" Photophobia Hyperkeratosis (sole/plants) Hypertyrosinemia	Tyrosinosis type II (tyrosine aminotransferase)
	Keratoconjunctivitis Photophobia Failure to thrive Renal Fanconi syndrome Rickets	Cystinosis
	"Storage" symptoms Coarse facies Hepatosplenomegaly Bone changes Cardiomyopathy Inguinal hernias	I-cell disease Hurler syndrome (MPS type I, S) Scheie syndrome (MPS type I, M) α-Mannosidosis (infantile form) Maroteaux-Lamy syndrome (MPS type VI)
	Ichthyosis Short stature Mental retardation Hypogonadism X-linked inheritance	Steroid sulfatase
Late infancy to early childhood (1–6 years)	Bone changes Dwarfism Scoliosis Normal intelligence Odontoid hypoplasia	Morquio syndrome (MPS type IV)
	Psychomotor retardation Blindness Retinal degeneration Cytoplasmic inclusions in conjunctiva and fibroblasts	Mucolipidosis type IV (ganglioside sialidase deficiency)
	Cataract Bone changes Hearing loss Mental deterioration	α-Mannosidosis (late-onset form)
	Yellow tonsil Hypocholesterolemia Absence of LDL Polyneuropathy	Tangier disease
	Hemolytic anemia Proteinuria Lipoprotein abnormalities	Lecithin:cholesterol acyltransferase deficiency
Late childhood or adolescence to adulthood	Abdominal pain Pain in extremities Angiokeratoma Rare in heterozygotes	Fabry disease (X-linked)
	Cherry red spot Bone changes Angiokeratoma Neurologic deterioration	Galactosialidosis (juvenile form)
	Kayser-Fleischer ring Hepatic dysfunction Hemolytic crises Extrapyramidal signs Multiorgan involvement	Wilson disease

S = severe; M = mild; MPS = mucopolysaccharidosis

regression. Posterior subcapsular cataracts with onset in the second decade are a nearly constant complication of gyrate atrophy of the choroid and retina, which presents as progressive retinal degeneration, blindness, and hyperornithinemia due to ornithine aminotransferase deficiency (see Chap. 31). Cataracts are the presenting sign in adults (about 10 percent of cases) with Steinert disease.

Corneal Opacity

Corneal opacities are a presenting sign in tyrosinemia type II, cystinosis, mucolipidosis type IV, Tangier disease, lecithin:cholesterol acyltransferase (LCAT) deficiency, and Fabry disease (Table 66-39).

Table 66-40 Macular Cherry Red Spot

Time when first visible	Other important symptoms	Disorders
Neonates	Ascites Edema Coarse facies Hepatosplenomegaly Vacuolated lymphocytes Bone changes	Landing disease (G_{M1} gangliosidosis) Galactosialidosis (early infantile form; neuraminidase deficiency)
	Failure to thrive Hepatosplenomegaly Interstitial pneumonia Neurologic deterioration Vacuolated lymphocytes	Niemann-Pick disease type IA
Infantile (3–12 months)	Bone changes Hepatosplenomegaly	Galactosialidosis (late infantile form)
	Hypotonia Myoclonic jerks Hepatosplenomegaly Macrocephaly Mental regression Startle response to sound	Tay-Sachs disease Sandhoff disease
Late childhood to adulthood	Blindness Myoclonic epilepsy	Sialidosis type I (late-onset form)
	Bone changes Angiokeratoma Corneal opacities Dysmorphism Neurologic deterioration Mental deterioration	Galactosialidosis (juvenile form)

Macular Cherry Red Spot

In some lysosomal disorders, the nerve cells of the retina can be the site of a storage process giving rise to a white ring of lipid-laden neurons that encircles the red, cell-free fovea, resulting in the characteristic macular "cherry red spot" (Table 66-40).

Retinitis Pigmentosa

Retinitis pigmentosa (RP) is the most common form of tapetoretinal degeneration and one of the major causes of hereditary visual impairment.[241] The condition affects approximately 30 percent of patients with visual handicaps seen in specialized practices. RP affects the retinal pigment epithelium and the rods and/or cones (see Chap. 144). The age at onset of RP is variable. Symptoms include indifference to the visual environment, pendular eye movements, and nystagmus. The earliest ophthalmoscopic findings are a dull retinal reflex and threadlike retinal arteries. The electroretinogram is abnormal before there is gross funduscopic evidence of RP.

The pigmentary retinopathies can be divided into two large groups: primary RP, in which the disease process is confined to the eyes, and secondary RP, in which the retinal degeneration is associated with single or multiple organ system disease. Primary RP segregates into autosomal dominant, autosomal recessive, and X-linked traits (see Chap. 144). Secondary RP is most often associated with nervous system involvement, morphologic abnormalities, deafness, myopathy, nephropathy, and skin abnormalities. Some of these conditions are associated with well-defined nonmetabolic genetic syndromes, and others are related to inherited metabolic disorders. An overview of the most frequent inherited metabolic diseases (autosomal and X-linked) associated with RP is presented in Table 66-41.

Although the pathophysiology of retinal degeneration is not known, the occurrence of retinal dysfunction in metabolic disorders suggests that it may be induced by toxic effects of certain metabolites, errors of synthetic pathways, or deficient energy metabolism. In clinical practice, two situations may arise: (1) the patient presents with a known metabolic disorder and retinal dysfunction appears as a manifestation of the disease, or (2) the patient presents with retinal abnormalities and a metabolic disorder is sought. The search will concentrate on

1. Errors of lipid metabolism
2. Errors of peroxisomal function
3. Errors of mitochondrial function, including respiratory chain defects

Important clues to the diagnosis emerge when the disorder is classified according to age of onset and presence of neurologic manifestations, digestive symptoms, or skin problems (Table 66-41).

Ectopia Lentis

Ectopia lentis is a frequent feature of four heritable disorders with systemic manifestations. Numerically, the most important of these is Marfan syndrome, an autosomal dominant inherited disease mainly affecting the connective tissue in the eye, the skeleton, and the cardiovascular system. Symptoms of ectopia lentis usually appear early in life, and the ophthalmologist is often the patient's primary contact in the health care system. With the potentially life-threatening systemic implications of Marfan syndrome and other systemic disorders associated with congenital ectopia lentis, it is of great importance to be aware of the different etiologies of this symptom. Ectopia lentis is the most consistent finding in classic homocystinuria secondary to cystathionine β-synthase deficiency. In this disorder, ectopia lentis, frequently preceded by severe myopia, is a frequent isolated presenting sign. In contrast with the picture in patients with Marfan syndrome, the dislocation is

Table 66-41 Retinitis Pigmentosa

With Neurologic Findings	Age at Onset
Inborn errors of lipid metabolism (nonperoxisomal)	
Abetalipoproteinemia	Infantile
Vitamin E malabsorption	Variable
3-OH-acylCoA dehydrogenase deficiency	Infantile
Sjögren-Larsson syndrome due to fatty alcohol oxidoreductase deficiency	Neonatal
Ceroid lipofuscinosis	
Santavuori-Hagberg disease	Infantile
Jansky-Bieschowsky disease	Late infantile
Spielmeyer-Vogt disease	Juvenile
Peroxisomal disorders	
Zellweger syndrome and variant forms	Neonatal
Neonatal adrenoleukodystrophy	Neonatal
Infantile Refsum disease	Infantile
Isolated β-oxidation defects	Neonatal
Peroxisomal biogenesis defects	Neonatal to infantile
Classic Refsum disease	Late infantile to adulthood
Congenital defects of glycosylation	Infantile
Respiratory chain disorders	Adolescence,
Kearns-Sayre syndrome	adulthood
Others	Variable
Cobalamin (Cbl C) metabolism defect	Neonatal to infantile
Recessive autosomal syndromes without known etiology	
Cockayne (dysmorphism, hypotonia, intracranial calcifications, deafness)	
Hallervorden-Spatz (severe neurologic regression, dystonia, acanthocytosis)	
Laurence-Moon-Biedl (obesity, polydactyly, mental retardation)	
Usher type II (deafness, severe mental retardation)	
Joubert (mental retardation, vermis atrophy, hyperventilation attacks)	
Others (Senior-Loken, Alström, etc.)	
With "Digestive" Symptoms (Failure to Thrive, Osteoporosis, Chronic Diarrhea, Hypolipemia)	
Abetalipoproteinemia	First 6 months
Vitamin E malabsorption	Variable
Infantile Refsum disease	First 6 months
With Cutaneous Symptoms	
Classic Refsum disease	Juvenile
Ichthyosis	
Sjögren-Larsson syndrome	Congenital
Ichthyosis	
Respiratory chain disorders	Juvenile
Cutaneous rashes, sun intolerance	
Isolated	
Gyrate atrophy with ornithine aminotransferase deficiency	Juvenile to adult
Primary retinitis pigmentosa (X-linked or autosomal recessive or dominant)	Variable

usually downward, although it may occur in any direction. Dislocation has only rarely been noted before 2 years of age; it was observed as early as 4 weeks of age in one patient. Plasma and urine amino acid chromatography and plasma total homocysteine determinations are always mandatory, searching for the characteristic hyperhomocysteinemia, before any ophthalmologic surgery.

Ectopia lentis is also frequent and an early manifestation in the very rare disorder sulfite oxidase, whether isolated or associated with xanthine oxidase deficiency (with hypouricuria) secondary to molybdenum cofactor deficiency. In these rare disorders, ectopia lentis is always part of a severe neurologic dysfunction (mental retardation and microcephaly). Ectopia lentis is also part of the Marchesani syndrome.

V. SKIN SYMPTOMS

Coarse Facies

Coarse facies is a highly suggestive sign observed in several lysosomal disorders. In some, it can be a presenting sign; in most it is associated with bone changes (dysostosis multiplex), hepatosplenomegaly, eye changes (corneal clouding, cataract, cherry red spot), various neurologic signs, mental regression, and vacuolated lymphocytes. The diagnosis is aided by urinary screening tests for mucopolysaccharides, oligosaccharides, and determination of bound and free sialic acid in urine,[242–244] but it must be confirmed by enzymatic assays. Patients with a normal enzyme value and with clinical findings or a test result suggestive of a lysosomal disorder will need additional studies to rule out the less common (and less easily diagnosed) disorders such as defects of sphingolipid activator proteins or membrane transport proteins.[244] Given the number of clinical subtypes and variants that have been described for the lysosomal disorders, the clinical picture in a given case is not likely to be typical for any one enzyme defect (Table 66-42). A recent publication suggested that Dubowitz syndrome (an autosomal recessive disorder with growth retardation microcephaly, moderate mental retardation and characteristic facial appearance made of triangular face, bilateral ptosis and small palpebral fissures, flat nasal bridge, and abnormal ears) could be related to a defect in cholesterol biosynthese.[244a]

Skin Lesions (Vesicobullous Lesions, Rashes, Photosensitivity, Hyperkeratosis, Ichthyosis, Ulcers, Nodules, Laxity)

Skin lesions of several types occur in inborn errors of metabolism. Some though not all of these lesions may be grouped into the following four categories:

1. Vesicobullous lesions (Table 66-43)
2. Photosensitivity and skin rashes (Table 66-44)
3. Hyperkeratosis and ichthyosis (Table 66-45)
4. Skin ulceration, skin nodules, and skin laxity (Table 66-46)

Some lesions are highly characteristic and diagnostic and may be presenting signs, such as those in acrodermatitis enteropathica, biotin-responsive multiple carboxylase deficiencies, cutaneous porphyrias, xeroderma pigmentosum,[245] tyrosinemia type II (hyperkeratosis on palms and soles), Sjögren-Larsson syndrome (neonatal ichthyosiform erythroderma), prolidase deficiency (skin ulcers), Farber lipogranulomatosis (subcutaneous nodules), CDG syndrome (peculiar fat pads over the upper outer parts of the buttocks), and the recently described EPEMA syndrome (encephalopathy, petechiae, ethylmalonic aciduria), characterized by orthostatic acrocyanosis and recurring petechiae associated with early-onset encephalopathy and recurrent attacks of lactic acidosis, vasculopathy, and chronic mucoid diarrhea.[55,56,246]

We have observed several patients with methylmalonic and propionic acidurias who presented with generalized pseudostaphylococcal cutaneous epidermolysis accompanying ultimate

Table 66-42 Coarse Facies

Time When First Visible	Other Important Symptoms	Disorders
Neonatal	Hydrops fetalis Ascites Edema	Landing disease Sialidosis type II Galactosialidosis (early infancy) Sly syndrome (MPS type VII) (rare)
	Failure to thrive Hypotonia Joint stiffness Osteoporosis	I-cell disease
Early infancy (3–12 months)	Seizures Myoclonias Spasticity Mental retardation	Fucosidosis type I Sialidosis type II Salla disease
	Inguinal hernias Ear, nose, and throat infections	Hurler syndrome (MPS type I) Sly syndrome (MPS type VII)
1–2 years	Psychomotor retardation Ataxia Seizures	Fucosidosis Mannosidosis
	Quadriplegia Ichthyosis Blindness	Austin disease
	Normal intelligence	Maroteaux-Lamy syndrome
2–6 years	Developmental delay Mental regression	Hunter syndrome (MPS type II) Aspartylglucosaminuria Pseudo-Hurler polydystrophy
	Abnormal behavior	Sanfilippo syndrome (MPS type III) (facies only slightly coarse)

MPS = mucopolysaccharidosis

Table 66-43 Vesicobullous Lesions

Nature and Distribution of Lesions	Other Important Symptoms	Age at Onset	Disorders
Skin rash Symmetric Circumorifice Retroauricular Acral distribution Secondary infection frequent	Watery stools Failure to thrive Mucosal lesions Total alopecia Conjunctivitis Zinc-responsiveness	2–4 weeks or after weaning	Acrodermatitis enteropathica Zinc deficiency
Scaly skin rash Over whole body Prominent on diaper and intertriginous areas Patchy, erythematous exudative circumorifice	Seborrheic dermatitis Keratoconjunctivitis Alopecia Biotin-responsiveness Hypotonia Ketoacidotic coma Hyperlactacidemia Developmental delay	Neonatal to infancy	Holocarboxylase synthetase deficiency (biotin responsive) Biotinidase deficiency (biotin responsive)
Vesicobullous Eczematous eruption Circumorifice Diaper and acral areas, similar to *Staphylococcus epidermolysis* infection Cutaneous detachment Desquamation	Ketoacidosis Failure to thrive Hypotonia Pancytopenia Hyperammonemia Acute decompensation episodes	Infancy	Methylmalonic acidemia Propionic acidemia (may be a presenting sign, or secondary to severe essential amino acid restriction)

Table 66-44 Photosensitivity and Skin Rashes

Nature of Skin Lesions	Other Important Symptoms	Age at Onset	Disorders
Cutaneous fragility Bullous lesions Hypertrichosis Dyspigmentation (alternation of hyperpigmented and hypopigmented areas)	Hemolytic anemia Splenomegaly Pink urine and diaper Major cutaneous signs	Neonatal and late onset form	Congenital erythropoietic porphyria
	Hemolytic anemia Splenomegaly Dark urine Major cutaneous signs	First months	Erythrohepatic porphyria
	Abdominal and neurologic crises	Adulthood	Porphyria variegata
	Abdominal and neurologic crises Hemolytic anemia	Adulthood	Hereditary coproporphyria
	Hepatic siderosis No crisis	Adulthood	Porphyria cutanea tarda
Photosensitivity Pain and edema in extremities	Hepatic failure Gallstones	<5 years	Erythropoietic protoporphyria
Freckling Hypopigmentation and hyperpigmentation of sun-exposed skin Atrophy Telangiectasias Tumors	Tumors Basal carcinomas Malignant melanomas Ocular symptoms One form with progressive neurologic deterioration	1–2 years	Xeroderma pigmentosum (9 varieties)
Skin rashes Sun intolerance Pellagra	Ataxia Recurrent attacks	Infancy to late childhood	Hartnup disease
Skin rashes Sun intolerance Pigmentation dilution	Various neurologic signs Multiorgan failure Hyperlactacidemia	Infancy to childhood	Respiratory chain disorders
Telangiectatic rashes on sun-exposed skin	Growth retardation Thin triangular face Malignancies	Congenital	Bloom syndrome
Recurring petechiae Distal acrocyanosis	Congenital encephalopathy Vasculopathy Mucoid diarrhea Attacks of lactic acidosis	Early in infancy	EPEMA syndrome (ethylmalonic aciduria)

metabolic decompensation leading to death despite supportive measures. Severe skin lesions with vesicobullous and eczematous eruption in the perineal, perioral, and anal areas can occur in methylmalonic and propionic acidemias; the cutaneous involvement can also consist of cheilitis and diffuse erythema with erosions and desquamation resembling the skin lesions of acrodermatitis enteropathica. In some cases, dermatitis may be a presenting sign, while in others, skin lesions have been ascribed to nutitional deficiency due to therapeutic amino acid restrictions.[247,248] In respiratory chain disorders resulting from mitochondrial DNA deletion, mottled pigmentation in photoexposed areas and repeated episodes of cold-triggered erythrocyanosis involving toes and fingers have been described in some patients especially in a syndrome of proximal tubulopathy, diabetes mellitus, and cerebellar ataxia.[183a] Ichthyosis is frequently observed in inborn errors that affect fatty acid metabolism and cholesterol and have been also recently observed in a new disorder of glycosylation (CDG If). The Conradi Hünermann syndrome[183b] has been recently found to be related to sterol $\Delta 8$ isomerase deficiency.[5b,249]

Angiokeratoma

Angiokeratomas are dark (red to blue-black) angiectases that develop slowly in the superficial layers of the skin. The lesions are flat or slightly raised and do not blanch with pressure. Mostly symmetric, their usual distribution is between the umbilicus and knees, mainly on the back, thighs, buttocks, penis, and scrotum. Oral mucosa and conjunctiva are also commonly involved. They may be one of the earliest manifestations in Fabry disease and are also observed in a few other lysosomal disorders (Table 66-47).

Alopecia

Symptoms and signs associated with alopecia are listed in Table 66-48.

VI. HEMATOLOGIC SYMPTOMS

Nonregenerative Anemias (Macrocytic)

Most nonregenerative macrocytic anemias of children are associated with bone marrow megaloblastosis. The vast majority of them are secondary to acquired deficiencies of folate or cobalamin; some are found in the inherited disorders of absorption, transport, or intracellular metabolism of these vitamins. Other inherited metabolic disorders can also give rise to megaloblastic anemia as a presenting symptom—Pearson syndrome due to mitochondrial DNA deletion,[94] thiamine-responsive megaloblastic anemia associated with diabetes and

Table 66-45 Hyperkeratosis and Ichthyosis

Nature of Skin Lesions	Other Important Symptoms	Age at Onset	Disorders
Painful blisters or erosions in palms and soles leading to hyperkeratosis	Keratitis Lacrimation Photophobia "Conjunctivitis" Hypertyrosinemia dramatically responsive to low-tyrosine diet	Infancy to early childhood	Tyrosinemia type II
Neonatal ichthyosiform erythroderma	Spasticity Mental retardation Cataract Retinitis	Neonatal to infancy	Sjögren-Larsson syndrome (fatty alcohol oxidoreductase deficiency)
	Hepatomegaly Slight myopathy Deafness Cataract Ataxia Vacuolated lymphocytes	Neonatal to infancy	Neutral lipid storage disorder
	Corneal opacities Hypogonadism Short stature Mental retardation Chondrodysplasia punctata	<4 months	Steroid sulfatase deficiency (X-linked)
	Psychomotor retardation Feeding problems Growth retardation Partial growth hormone deficiency Scaly, itching skin disease	Early in infancy	Congenital defect of glycosylation (CDG If)
Ichthyosis	Coarse facies Growth retardation Hepatosplenomegaly Bone changes Mental regression Quadriplegia Vacuolated lymphocytes	1–2 years	Austin disease
	Retinitis pigmentosa Ataxia Peripheral neuropathy Deafness	Late childhood to adulthood	Classic Refsum disease (adult form)
Ichthyosis "en bande"	Chondrodysplasia punctata X-linked dominant inheritance Asymmetric body	Childhood to adulthood	Conradi-Hünermann syndrome (Sterol $\Delta 8$ isomerase deficiency) Deletion of terminal short arm of one X chromosome
Ichthyosis Brittle hair	Short stature Mental retardation Dysmorphism	Infancy	Trichothiodystrophy

deafness,[226–232,250] congenital orotic aciduria due to uridine monophosphate (UMP) synthase deficiency, and Lesch-Nyhan syndrome (hypoxanthine phosphoribosyl transferase [HPRT] deficiency) (see Chaps. 50 and 55). With the exception of the last, in most of these disorders—including the inborn errors of folate and vitamin B_{12} metabolism—nonregenerative macrocytic anemia presents early in life and is associated with failure to thrive, anorexia, vomiting, digestive signs, hypotonia, and developmental delay. Aside from folate and vitamin B_{12} measurements, the main clues to diagnosis are to be found by analyzing urine and plasma amino acids and organic acids and measuring the levels of uric acid, glucose, blood gases, and plasma lactate. The presence of homocysteinemia and homocystinuria with low plasma methionine, even when very moderate, is highly suggestive of a remethylation defect of homocysteine to methionine secondary to various inborn errors of vitamin B_{12} metabolism. It is important to deproteinize the sample immediately for measurement of plasma free homocysteine or plasma total homocysteine. The additional presence of methylmalonate in megaloblastic anemia indicates an inborn error of vitamin B_{12} metabolism. Although homocystinuria and methylmalonic aciduria are not classic features of intrinsic factor deficiency and vitamin B_{12} congenital malabsorption defect (Imerslünd-Grasbeck syndrome), we could expect to find such perturbations if they were carefully sought (Table 66-49). Some patients with isolated methylmalonic, propionic, or isovaleric acidemia can present with severe nonregenerative anemia, although this symptom is most often associated with thrombocytopenia and neutropenia (see "Pancytopenia, Neutropenia, Thrombocytopenia" below).

Orotic acid is elevated in urine in congenital orotic aciduria due to UMP synthase deficiency. It is slightly elevated in some cases of congenital folate malabsorption, in which it can coexist with

Table 66-46 Skin Ulceration, Nodules, and Laxity

	Skin Ulceration		
Erythematous dermatitis Ecchymosis Purpuric rash Telangiectasia Skin ulcers on legs resistant to symptomatic treatment Cutaneous infections	Dysmorphic features Cognitive development impairment Ophthalmoplegia Splenomegaly Iminodipeptiduria	Infancy to adulthood (usually 6 years)	Prolidase deficiency
	Skin Nodules		
Nodular subcutaneous swellings near interphalangeal, ankle, wrist, and elbow joints and points of mechanical pressure	Painful, stiff joint Hoarseness Interstitial pneumonia Central nervous system impairment	Neonatal to early infancy	Farber disease (lipogranulomatosis)
Peculiar fat pads over upper outer parts of buttocks Thick, sticky skin Lipoatrophic streaks on lower limbs	Failure to thrive Developmental delay Episodic failure of multiorgan systems	Infancy	Congenital defects of glycosylation
	Skin Laxity, Dysmorphic Scarring, Easy Bruising		
Joint laxity Hypotonia	Inborn errors of collagen synthesis		Ehlers-Danlos syndrome (9 types) (see Chap. 134) Occipital horn syndrome (see Chap. 68) Cutis laxa
			Pyrroline-5-carboxylase synthetase deficiency [208]

Table 66-47 Angiokeratoma

Diagnosis	Major Signs	Age at Onset
Fabry disease	Abdominal pain Acroparesthesias Excruciating pains in extremities Corneal opacities Strokes	Childhood (male hemizygote)
	Isolated angiokeratomas Corneal dystrophy	Adolescence (female heterozygote)
Fucosidosis	Bone changes Coarse facies Hepatosplenomegaly Vacuolated lymphocytes	Infancy
Galactosialidosis	Bone changes Cherry red spot Corneal opacities Neurologic deterioration	Juvenile form (5–20 years)
Aspartylglucosaminuria	Coarse facies Joint laxity Lens opacities Mental regression Vacuolated lymphocytes	1–5 years
β-Mannosidosis	Nerve deafness Mental retardation Aggressive behavior Lymphedema(?)	Adults

Table 66-48 Alopecia and Brittle Hair

Leading Symptoms	Other Signs	Age at Onset	Diagnosis
Neurologic symptoms	Arrested development Sagging cheeks Brittle hair Pili torti Hypothermia Seizures Loss of skills	First 6 months	Menkes syndrome (X-linked)
	Recurrent attacks of coma Hypotonia Ataxia Dermatitis Keratoconjunctivitis Failure to thrive Ketoacidosis Hyperlactacidemia	Neonatal to infancy	Biotin-responsive multiple carboxylase defects Methylmalonic and propionic acidurias
	Myotonia Myopathy Cardiomyopathy	Adulthood	Steinert disease
Bone changes Rickets Osteopenia Dental defects Bone crisis	Hypotonia Muscle weakness Abdominal distension	First year	Calciferol metabolism defects
Cutaneous signs	Skin fragility Easy bruising "Acrogeria" Thin skin on extremities Pneumothorax Gut perforation Arterial bleeding	First year	Ehlers-Danlos syndrome type IV
	Skin photosensitivity Abnormal pigmentation Hemolytic anemia Splenomegaly Black or pink urine	Neonatal and first months	Hepatoerythropoietic porphyria Congenital erythropoietic porphyria
	Hepatic siderosis	Adulthood	Porphyria cutanea tarda
	Periorifice bullous lesions Chronic diarrhea Failure to thrive Hypotonia	First months	Methylmalonic and propionic acidurias Acrodermatitis enteropathica Essential fatty acid deficiency Zinc deficiency
Brittle hair	Mental retardation	Infancy	Menkes syndrome Trichothiodystrophy Argininosuccinic aciduria Citrullinemia

abnormal formiminoglutamic acid (FIGLU) excretion. Nonregenerative anemia with erythroblastophagocytosis can be also the predominant hematologic sign in lysinuric protein intolerance,[251] in which it is frequently associated with failure to thrive, recurrent attacks of hyperammonemic coma, interstitial pneumonia, hepatosplenomegaly, neutropenia, or pancytopenia. The diagnosis relies on plasma amino acid chromatography that displays low lysine, arginine, and ornithine concentrations contrasting with increased excretion of these amino acids in urine (see also "Pancytopenia, Neutropenia, Thrombocytopenia"; see also Table 66-51). Modest elevation of plasma lactic acid (to 5 mM) with mild compensated metabolic acidosis was the almost constant key symptom leading to the elucidation of Pearson syndrome and other respiratory chain disorders. The diagnosis should be entertained when refractory sideroblastic anemia in early infancy is associated with vacuolization of marrow precursors, chronic diarrhea, and modest hyperlactacidemia.[94] Thiamine-responsive megaloblastic anemia is a rare but treatable condition associated with diabetes, deafness, and sometimes neurologic signs (strokes). Clinical diagnosis rests on finding hyperglycemia and deafness (Table 66-49). The gene for this syndrome has been recently localized.[250]

Nonmacrocytic Anemias (Due to Hemolysis or Combined Mechanisms)

Regenerative anemia due to hemolysis or other mechanisms is observed in many inborn errors of metabolism. In addition to erythrocyte glycolytic enzyme deficiencies, microspherocytosis,

Table 66-49 Nonregenerative Anemias (Macrocytic)

Leading Symptoms		Other Important Symptoms	Age at Onset	Diagnosis
Homocystinuria/ homocystinemia (with normal or low plasma methionine)	With methylmalonic aciduria	Proteinuria Low plasma vitamin B_{12} Abnormal Schilling test	First to third year	Congenital vitamin B_{12} malabsorption (Imerslünd-Grasbeck disease)
		Neurologic signs (paresthesia, ataxia) Developmental delay Low plasma vitamin B_{12} Abnormal Schilling test	First to fifth year	Intrinsic factor deficiency
		Pancytopenia Diarrhea, malabsorption Infections Stomatitis Normal plasma vitamin B_{12}	First months	Transcobalamin II deficiency
		Ketoacidosis Thrombocytopenia Hemolytic uremic syndrome Myocardiopathy Interstitial pneumonia Retinitis	First months	Intracellular cobalamin metabolism defect (Cbl C)
	Without methylmalonic aciduria	Infections Seizures Cellular immunodeficiency Normal or high plasma folate Inconstant homocystinuria	First months	Methionine synthase deficiency
		Failure to thrive Pancytopenia Developmental delay	First weeks	Methylcobalamin metabolism defects (Cbl E, G)
Abnormal organic acidurias (MMA, PA, IVA)		Erythroblastopenia Pancytopenia Failure to thrive Ketoacidotic coma	First weeks	Methylmalonic, propionic, and isovaleric acidemias
Orotic aciduria		Severe infections Sparse hair, nail hypoplasia Cellular immunodeficiency Leukopenia Cardiac malformation	First year	Congenital orotic aciduria (UMP synthase deficiency)
		Failure to thrive Mouth ulcers Diarrhea Neurologic signs	First to third month	Congenital folate malabsorption (inconstant orotic aciduria)
		Pancytopenia Erythroblastophagocytosis Interstitial pneumonia Failure to thrive Hyperammonemic coma Splenomegaly Low plasma lysine, arginine, ornithine	Infancy	Lysinuric protein intolerance
Hyperlactacidemia (moderate acidosis)		Pancytopenia Failure to thrive Exocrine pancreas insufficiency Chronic diarrhea, liver failure Vacuolization of marrow precursors Lactic acidemia Diabetes	First month	Bone marrow–pancreas syndrome (Pearson syndrome) Mitochondrial DNA deletion

Table 66-49 (Continued)

Leading Symptoms	Other Important Symptoms	Age at Onset	Diagnosis
Hyperglycemia, glycosuria (diabetes)	Deafness Pancytopenia Strokelike episodes Coarse facies Wolfram syndrome Anemia responsive to thiamine	Infancy to childhood	Thiamine-responsive megaloblastic anemia
Hyperuricemia (>600 μmol/liter) Hyperuricuria (>120 μmol/kg/24h)	Neurologic deterioration Dystonia, athetosis Self-mutilation Nephrolithiasis	Third to sixth month	Lesch-Nyhan syndrome (HGPRT deficiency)
Severe hypofolatemia (plasma and CSF)	Mouth ulcers, fever Diarrhea, failure to thrive Seizures, ataxia Peripheral neuropathy Intracranial calcifications	First to third month	Congenital folate malabsorption
No evident biologic disturbances (sometimes FIGLU excretion or orotic aciduria)	Developmental delay Abnormal behavior Cortical atrophy Neurologic signs	First year to adulthood	Dihydrofolate reductase (?) Glutamate formiminotransferase (FIGLU excretion)

HGPRT = hypoxanthine guanine phosphoribosyl transferase

and hemoglobinopathies, in which chronic hemolytic anemia syndrome is clearly the leading symptom, there are several inborn errors of metabolism that are associated with severe anemia (Table 66-50). In the neonatal period, inborn errors that cause severe hepatic failure can present as anemia. Wilson disease should be considered at any age when an acute hemolytic crisis is associated with liver dysfunction or neurologic signs. Severe anemia is one of the earliest signs in Wolman disease and abetalipoproteinemia (in which it is associated with severe failure to thrive and digestive symptoms). Hemolytic anemia with neurologic deterioration is found in triosephosphate isomerase deficiency[252] and phosphoglycerate kinase deficiency. In the latter, hemolytic crises accompany neurologic crises (hemiplegia and deep coma) (see "Recurrent Attacks of Coma, Strokes, or Vomiting with Lethargy, Ataxia, or Pychiatric Symptoms" above). Two forms of porphyria can present as hemolytic anemia—congenital erythropoietic porphyria, which presents in the neonatal period as severe cutaneous signs and sometimes as severe hepatic dysfunction, and late-onset erythropoietic porphyria. Pseudohemolytic uremic syndrome is observed in cobalamin metabolism defects (Cbl C and methionine synthase deficiency).[253,253a]

In adulthood, hemolytic anemia is a constant finding in lecithin:cholesterol acyltransferase deficiency (in which it is associated with proteinuria and corneal opacities) and in phytosterolemia.

Pancytopenia, Neutropenia, Thrombocytopenia

Pancytopenia, neutropenia, and thrombocytopenia are presenting signs in a small number of inborn errors of metabolism (Table 66-51). Peripheral pancytopenia can exist in Gaucher disease type I or type III (with its characteristic splenomegaly). Pancytopenia in association with nonregenerative macrocytic/megaloblastic anemia, failure to thrive, chronic diarrhea, frequent infections, hypotonia, and developmental delay is found in congenital folate malabsorption, inborn errors of cobalamin metabolism (the Cbl C, Cbl D, Cbl E, and Cbl G defects), organic acidurias (methylmalonic acidemia, propionic acidemia, and isovaleric acidemia), and Pearson syndrome. These conditions are easily mistaken for intestinal malabsorption syndrome, immunodeficiencies, or sepsis. The very rare disorder thiamine-responsive megaloblastic anemia can also present as pancytopenia.

Chronic neutropenia is a constant finding in glycogenosis type Ib (microsomal glucose 6-phosphate carrier defect) and in lysinuric protein intolerance. Diagnosis of glycogenosis type I is based on severe tendency to fasting hypoglycemia and hepatomegaly. Diagnosis of the cause of neutropenia in this clinical context requires a special assay technique for liver glucose 6-phosphate (the liver sample is not frozen to avoid disrupting microsomal membranes). Because of the neutropenia, patients have frequent infections (particularly abscesses) and may present with inflammatory bowel disease. Patients with lysinuric protein intolerance (often misdiagnosed) sometimes present with preponderant hematologic findings that are frequently associated with a great diversity of symptoms, such as malnutrition, failure to thrive, chronic diarrhea, hepatosplenomegaly, interstitial pneumonia, and recurrent metabolic attacks that can lead to psychiatric symptoms. In congenital orotic aciduria due to UMP synthase deficiency, neutropenia is always associated with megaloblastic anemia along with failure to thrive, developmental delay, and frequent infections. Orotic acid excretion is always massive.

Thrombocytopenia is an important sign in at least two situations: (1) in an atypical hemolytic uremic syndrome with ketoacidosis, cardiomyopathy, hypotonia, coma, and interstitial pneumonia, which is highly suggestive of an inborn error of cobalamin metabolism (Cbl C defect),[253] and (2) when severe and persistent thrombocytopenia (<5000/liter) occurs in the context of classic methylmalonic, propionic, or isovaleric acidemia.

Increased Neutrophil Granulocytes

When it is associated with dysmorphia, short arms and legs, failure to thrive and recurrent infections it is mandatory to search for a leukocyte adhesion deficiency II syndrome due to a generalized defect in fucose metabolism.[253b]

Bleeding Tendency

A bleeding tendency can be an alarming symptom in five categories of clinical circumstances, as shown in Table 66-52.

Table 66-50 Nonmacrocytic Anemias (Hemolytic or Due to Combined Mechanisms)

Leading Symptoms	Age at Onset	Diagnosis
Liver failure (jaundice, ascites, edema, low prothrombin time, high transaminases)	Neonatal	Hemochromatosis (neonatal) Any other inborn errors with severe liver failure
	Childhood (<5 years)	Erythropoietic protoporphyria (cutaneous signs, edema, gallstones) Wilson disease
	Adulthood	Wilson disease
Digestive signs (failure to thrive, vomiting, poor feeding, diarrhea, hypotonia)	First weeks	Wolman disease (hepatosplenomegaly, adrenal gland calcifications, vacuolated lymphocytes)
	First months	Abetalipoproteinemia (severe hypocholesterolemia, acanthocytosis) Organic acidemias (pancytopenia) (MMA, PA, IVA, subacute forms) Mevalonic aciduria
Neurologic signs (neurologic deterioration)	1–2 years	Triosephosphate isomerase deficiency (weakness, exercise intolerance, abnormal movements, neurologic deterioration, heartbeat disorders) Phosphoglycerate kinase deficiency (mental retardation, extrapyramidal signs, neurologic crisis: hemiplegia with deep coma; X-linked)
	Childhood (2–5 years)	Abetalipoproteinemia (ataxia, peripheral neuropathy, retinitis, spinocerebellar degeneration) Wilson disease
Metabolic acidosis (pseudotubular acidosis)	Congenital to childhood	Glutathione synthetase deficiency (metabolic acidosis, pyroglutamic aciduria, ataxia, mental retardation)
Cutaneous signs (photosensitivity, dyspigmentation, cutaneous edema, skin ulcers)	Neonatal to first months (late-onset adult form)	Congenital erythropoietic porphyria (splenomegaly, pink urine and diapers)
	Childhood (1–5 years)	Erythropoietic porphyria (hepatic signs, gallstones)
Renal signs (proteinuria, renal failure)	Childhood to adulthood	Lecithin:cholesterol acyltransferase deficiency (corneal opacities, low plasma cholesteryl esters)
Hemolytic uremic syndrome	Neonatal to infancy	Inborn errors of cobalamin (Cblc, methionilne synthase deficiency)
Intravascular hemolytic crisis Nocturnal venous thrombosis Hemoglobinuria		Paroxysmal nocturnal hemoglobinuria (somatic mutation of the *PIGA* gene)
Xanthomas	1–3 years	Phytosterolemia (hypercholesterolemia)
Isolated (chronic hemolytic anemia syndrome: jaundice, gallstones, indirect hyperbilirubinemia), splenomegaly	Neonatal to late infancy	Erythropoietic glycolytic enzyme (PK, PFK, HK, GPI, 2, 3DPM, G6PD, GS, GGS) deficiency Sickle-cell anemias (failure to thrive, painful crisis, chest syndrome, sequestration crisis, aplastic crisis, repeated infections) Congenital Heinz body hemolytic anemia Thalassemia syndromes (bone changes, thalassemic facies) Hereditary microspherocytosis

2,3DPM = 2,3-diphosphoglycerate mutase; GGS = gamma-glutamyl cysteine synthetase; GPI = glucose phosphate isomerase; GS = glutathione synthetase; G6PD = glucose-6-phosphate dehydrogenase; HK = hexokinase; PFK = phosphofructokinase; PIGA = phosphatidylinositol glycosyl ancholin; PK = pyruvate kinase

Acanthocytosis

Acanthocytosis is covered in Table 66-53.

VII. VISCERAL SYMPTOMS OR SYNDROMES (INTESTINE, LIVER, HEART, LUNG, KIDNEY)

Chronic Diarrhea (with Failure to Thrive, Poor Feeding, Anorexia, Hypotonia)

"Digestive" symptoms occur in a wide variety of inborn errors of metabolism (see Table 66-54). Unfortunately, their cause often remains unrecognized, delaying correct diagnosis. Persistent anorexia, feeding difficulties, chronic vomiting, failure to thrive, frequent infections, osteopenia, and generalized hypotonia in the context of chronic diarrhea are the presenting symptoms in a number of inherited and acquired diseases in pediatrics. They are easily misdiagnosed as cow's milk protein intolerance; celiac disease; chronic ear, nose, or throat infections; late-onset chronic pyloric stenosis; fructose intolerance; or diverse intestinal problems. Congenital immunodeficiencies are also frequently considered, although only a few present early in infancy and have such a clinical picture.

From a pathophysiological viewpoint, it is possible to define two groups of inborn errors of metabolism presenting as chronic diarrhea:

Table 66-51 Pancytopenia, Neutropenia, Thrombocytopenia

Leading Symptoms	Major Clinical Findings	Age at Onset	Disorders
Pancytopenia	Major splenomegaly	Variable	Gaucher disease type I and III
		Variable	Other conditions with splenomegaly severe enough to give rise to hypersplenism
	Predominant macrocytic or megaloblastic nonregenerative anemia	Infancy to childhood	Thiamine-responsive megaloblastic anemia (diabetes, deafness, Wolfram syndrome)
		First month	Pearson syndrome due to mitochondrial DNA deletion (failure to thrive, chronic diarrhea, multiorgan failure, lactic acidosis, vacuolization of marrow precursors)
		Early infancy	Transcobalamin II deficiency (diarrhea, malabsorption, infection, stomatitis)
		First weeks	Methylcobalamin metabolism defects: Cbl C, Cbl D, Cbl E, Cbl G (failure to thrive, developmental delay)
	Ketoacidosis, hypotonia, failure to thrive, attacks of coma	Neonatal to infancy	MMA, PA, IVA (frequent infections, hyperammonemia) Mevalonic aciduria Lysinuric protein intolerance
	Chronic diarrhea, failure to thrive	Neonatal to infancy	Folate malabsorption Transcobalamin II deficiency Pearson syndrome Other exocrine pancreas insufficiency (Schwachmann, Johansson-Blizzard syndromes) Mevalonic aciduria Lysinuric protein intolerance
Predominant or isolated neutropenia	Recurrent attacks of hypoglycemia Hepatomegaly Failure to thrive Inflammatory bowel disease Frequent infections	Infancy	Glycogenosis type Ib
	Failure to thrive, chronic diarrhea Recurrent attacks of hyperammonemia Interstitial pneumonia Hepatosplenomegaly Orotic acid excretion (moderate)	Infancy	Lysinuric protein intolerance
	Megaloblastic anemia Failure to thrive Developmental delay Orotic acid excretion (major)	Infancy	Congenital orotic aciduria (UMP synthase deficiency)
	Hyperammonemia Ketoacidotic comas Hypotonia Failure to thrive	Infancy	Organic acidurias (MMA, PA, IVA) Mevalonic aciduria
	Coarse facies, lens opacities, joint laxity, short stature	1–5 years	Aspartylglucosaminuria
Predominant thrombocytopenia	Hemolytic uremic syndrome Ketoacidosis Cardiomyopathy	First weeks to first months	Cobalamin metabolism defect (Cbl C)
	Hyperammonemia Ketoacidosis	Infancy	Organic acidurias (MMA, PA, IVA)

IVA = isovaleric acidemia; LPI = lysinuric protein intolerance; MMA = methylmalonic acidemia; PA = propionic acidemia

1. Disorders of the intestinal membrane or the exocrine function of the pancreas, for example, congenital chloride diarrhea, glucose-galactose malabsorption, lactase and sucrase-isomaltase deficiencies, abetalipoproteinemia type II (Anderson disease), enterokinase deficiency, acrodermatitis enteropathica, or selective intestinal malabsorption of folate and vitamin B_{12}.
2. Disorders that affect several different tissues directly or indirectly and give rise to systemic consequences.

In clinical practice, these groups are sometimes very difficult to distinguish, because a number of specific intestinal disorders can give rise to various systemic clinical consequences. Accordingly, we divide chronic diarrhea due to inborn errors of metabolism into five clinical categories.

Category 1. This category includes severe watery diarrhea resulting in dehydration with onset immediately after birth, after

Table 66-52 Bleeding Tendency

Primitive disorders of homeostasis
von Willebrand disease
Vitamin K-dependent factor deficiency
Afibrinogenemias and dysfibrinogenemias
Factor VIII and XII deficiencies
Bernard-Soulier disease
Glanzmann thrombasthenia
Congenital defects of glycosylation
Severe thrombocytopenias of any origin
Liver failure
α-antitrypsin deficiency
Galactosemias
Fructosemia
Tyrosinemia type I
Wilson disease
Neonatal hemochromatosis
Others
Hepatomegaly or splenomegaly without significant liver dysfunction or thrombocytopenia
Glycogenosis types Ia and Ib
Gaucher disease types I and III
Others
Vasculopathy (recurring petechiae)
EPEMA syndrome (ethylmalonic aciduria)

EPEMA = encephalopathy, petechiae, and ethylmalonic aciduria.

weaning, or after starch dextrins have been added to the diet. It encompasses congenital chloride diarrhea, glucose-galactose malabsorption, lactase and sucrase-isomaltase deficiencies, and acrodermatitis enteropathica (marked by less severe diarrhea).

Category 2. In this category, the clinical picture is dominated by chronic diarrhea associated with malabsorption syndrome, hypocholesterolemia, and osteopenia presenting early in infancy. It includes inborn errors of bile acid metabolism that present as unexplained neonatal cholestatic jaundice,[254] infantile Refsum disease,[45,45b,234,236a,255] and abetalipoproteinemia types I and II. Respiratory chain disorders and Pearson syndrome can also appear early in infancy as severe intestinal malabsorption and exocrine pancreatic insufficiency.[94] The recently described congenital disorder of glycosylation type Ib secondary to phosphomannoisomerase deficiency can strike in the first year of life as protein-losing enteropathy associated with hypotonia, failure to thrive, vomiting, severe hypoglycemia, hepatomegaly, and thrombotic events, as well as life-threatening gastrointestinal bleeding episodes. Daily oral mannose administration is a successful therapy for this new type of the syndrome.[12–14] Congenital liver cirrhosis has been recently described in a patient with highly elevated plasma and urine levels of arabitol, ribitol and erythritol due to transaldolase deficiency.[255a]

Category 3. Disorders in this category are marked by severe failure to thrive, poor feeding, hypotonia, and frequent infections associated with obvious hepatomegaly and splenomegaly. Five inherited disorders can share these clinical features:

1. Glycogenosis type Ib due to defective microsomal glucose 6-phosphate carrier and marked by severe hypoglycemia, neutropenia, recurrent infections, and sometimes inflammatory bowel disease
2. Wolman disease due to lipase deficiency with vacuolated lymphocytes and adrenal gland calcifications
3. X-linked chronic granulomatous disease with dermatitis, recurrent purulent infections, and inflammatory bowel disease
4. Intrinsic factor deficiency resulting in vitamin B_{12} malabsorption with megaloblastic anemia and peripheral neuropathy
5. Lysinuric protein intolerance with neutropenia or pancytopenia, interstitial pneumonia, and recurrent attacks of hyperammonemia

Some patients with lysinuric protein intolerance masquerading as celiac disease have been reported.[256]

Category 4. This category includes disorders with nonregenerative megaloblastic anemia with or without pancytopenia, such as transcobalamin II and intrinsic factor deficiencies, congenital folate malabsorption, and Pearson syndrome.

Table 66-53 Acanthocytosis

Leading Symptoms	Other Signs	Age at Onset	Diagnosis
Gastrointestinal symptoms Failure to thrive Diarrhea Hypotonia	Hepatosplenomegaly Vacuolated lymphocytes Adrenal gland calcifications	First week	Wolman disease
Malabsorption syndrome	Marked hypocholesterolemia Ataxia Peripheral neuropathy Retinitis pigmentosa	First week	Abetalipoproteinemia
Neurologic regression with retinitis pigmentosa	Ataxia Peripheral neuropathy	2–5 years	Abetalipoproteinemia
	Dystonia Choreoathetosis	Second decade	Hallervorden-Spatz syndrome
Acute renal failure Hemolytic anemia Hemolytic uremic syndrome	Failure to thrive Cardiomyopathy Ketoacidosis Leukopenia Thrombocytopenia Interstitial pneumonia Retinitis	1–3 months	Inborn errors of cobalamin (Cbl C)

Table 66-54 **Chronic Diarrhea, Failure to Thrive**

Leading Symptom	Other Signs	Age at Onset	Diagnosis
Severe watery diarrhea, attacks of dehydration	No meconium Nonacidic diarrhea Metabolic alkalosis Hypochloremia and hypochloruria	Birth to infancy	Congenital chloride diarrhea
	Acidic diarrhea sugars Reducing sugars in stools Glucosuria	Neonatal	Glucose galactose malabsorption Lactase deficiency
	Acidic diarrhea Reducing sugars in stools After weaning or after starch dextrins are added to the diet	Neonatal to infancy	Sucrase isomaltase deficiency
Less severe diarrhea (after weaning)	Skin lesions	Neonatal or after weaning	Acrodermatitis enteropathica Alopecia (late onset) Failure to thrive
Fat-soluble vitamin malabsorption, severe hypocholesterolemia Osteopenia Steatorrhea	Unexplained cholestatic jaundice Hepatomegaly Hypotonia Slight mental retardation Retinitis pigmentosa Deafness	Neonatal Infancy	Bile acid synthesis defects Infantile Refsum disease (peroxisomal disorders)
	Protein-losing enteropathy Hepatomegaly Attacks of cholangitis Gastrointestinal bleeding Thromboembolic events Hypoglycemia, hypotonia	Infancy	Congenital defects of glycosylation (Phosphomannoisomerae deficiency)
	Abdominal distension Failure to thrive Anorexia Acanthocytosis Peripheral neuropathy Ataxia Retinitis pigmentosa (all last 3 symptoms after 5 years)	Infancy	Abetalipoproteinemia type I Abetalipoproteinemia type II (no acanthocytes, no neurologic signs)
	Pancreatic insufficiency Neutropenia Pancytopenia	Early in infancy	Pearson syndrome Schwachman syndrome
Severe failure to thrive Anorexia Poor feeding with predominant hepatomegaly (± splenomegaly)	Severe hypoglycemia Inflammatory bowel disease Neutropenia Recurrent infections No splenomegaly	Neonatal to early infancy	Glycogenosis type Ib (glucose-6-phosphate carrier deficiency)
	Hypotonia Vacuolated lymphocytes Adrenal gland calcifications	Neonatal	Wolman disease
	Recurrent infections Inflammatory bowel disease Dermatitis, stomatitis	Infancy	Chronic granulomatosis (X-linked)
	Megaloblastic anemia Stomatitis Muscle weakness Peripheral neuropathy	1–5 years	Intrinsic factor deficiency
	Neutropenia Osteopenia Recurrent attacks of hyperammonemia Interstitial pneumonia	Infancy	Lysinuric protein intolerance
Severe failure to thrive Anorexia Poor feeding with megaloblastic anemia (nonregenerative)	Oral lesion, stomatitis Pancytopenia Peripheral neuropathy Infections, homocystinuria, methylmalonic aciduria	1–2 years	Transcobalamin II deficiency Intrinsic factor deficiency
	Stomatitis, infections Peripheral neuropathy Intracranial calcifications	Infancy	Congenital folate malabsorption

(Continued on next page)

Table 66-54 (Continued)

Leading Symptom	Other Signs	Age at Onset	Diagnosis
	Severe pancytopenia Vacuolization of marrow precursors Exocrine pancreas insufficiency Lactic acidosis	Neonatal	Pearson syndrome
Severe failure to thrive Anorexia Poor feeding Hypotonia No significant hepatosplenomegaly No megaloblastic anemia	Severe hypoproteinemia "Putrefaction" diarrhea	Infancy	Enterokinase deficiency
	Diarrhea after weaning Cutaneous lesion Alopecia Modest diarrhea Low alkaline phosphatase Low plasma zinc	Infancy	Acrodermatitis enteropathica
	Ketoacidosis Metabolic attacks Frequent infections Vomiting	Infancy	Organic acidurias (MMA, PA) Mitochondrial DNA deletions (lactic acidosis)
	Vomiting Lethargy Metabolic attacks Hyperammonemia Frequent infections	Infancy	Urea cycle defects (mainly OTC)
	Lymphopenia Bone changes	Infancy	Adenosine deaminase deficiency
	Developmental delay Recurring petechiae Orthostatic acrocyanosis Recurrent attacks Hyperlactacidemia	Infancy	Ethylmalonic aciduria

OTC = ornithine transcarbamylase; MMA = methylmalonic aciduria; PA = propionic aciduria

Category 5. This category is dominated by failure to thrive, anorexia, hypotonia, and recurrent infections. It can be the first clinical expression in infants who have subacute forms of organic acidurias, urea cycle defects, or adenosine deaminase deficiency. Enterokinase deficiency presents as severe hypoproteinemia and "putrefaction" diarrhea. Acrodermatitis enteropathica presents after weaning and has bullocutaneous perioral lesions and alopecia (see above). A novel clinical phenotype characterized by chronic diarrhea associated with developmental delay, recurring petechiae, orthostatic acrocyanosis, brain MRI abnormalities, recurrent attacks of hyperlactacidemia, and ethylmalonic acid excretion (EPEMA syndrome) has recently been described.[55,56,246]

Hepatomegaly and Hepatosplenomegaly

Hepatomegaly in inborn errors of metabolism occurs in three different circumstances:[257]

1. With manifestations of hepatocellular necrosis
2. With cholestatic jaundice
3. With no prominent hepatic dysfunction

In the first situation, the clinical picture is characterized by some degree of jaundice, edema, ascites, bleeding tendency, and hepatic encephalopathy. In neonates and young infants, several disorders should be considered: galactosemias, hereditary fructose intolerance (if the diet contains fructose), tyrosinemia type I (which always presents clinically after at least 2 to 3 weeks of life), neonatal hemochromatosis (with normal or disproportionately low serum transaminases), and respiratory chain disorders (associated with hypotonia and hyperlactacidemia).[70–72] In late infancy and childhood, Wilson disease and α_1-antitrypsin deficiency are the main concerns. In Wilson disease, the liver disease is usually subacute or chronic (chronic active hepatitis or cirrhosis), but some patients present with fulminant liver failure associated with hemolysis and renal failure. In α_1-antitrypsin deficiency, there may be fulminant liver failure. Absence of an α_1-globulin peak should be sought in all patients with unexplained overwhelming liver disease.[257]

A second group of disorders is revealed by predominant cholestatic jaundice, either isolated or associated with hypotonia. In the neonatal period, this group encompasses α_1-antitrypsin deficiency, neonatal hemochromatosis;[258,259] progressive familial intrahepatic cholestasis (Byler disease with intractable pruritus and normal serum gamma GT), inborn errors of bile acid synthesis,[254] Niemann-Pick disease type C (presenting as giant cell hepatitis), inborn errors of peroxisome metabolism (Zellweger syndrome, infantile Refsum disease, trihydroxycoprostanoyl CoA oxidase deficiency),[45,45b,207] congenital defects of glycosylation,[11–14] and IX[259a] (the latter revealed by a Budd Chiari syndrome), LCHAD deficiency,[21,259b] Smith-Lemli-Opitz syndrome, and mevalonic aciduria (personal unpublished observations).

When hepatomegaly is the main or only presenting symptom of liver disease, a major clinical clue to the diagnosis is the consistency of the liver and the characteristics of its surface. A firm or rock-hard consistency may indicate tyrosinemia type I, galactosemia, glycogenosis type IV, severe neonatal hemochromatosis, α_1-antitrypsin deficiency, Wilson disease, cystic fibrosis (Table 66-55), Niemann-Pick B and C and Gaucher disease.

When the liver consistency is normal or soft and there is associated splenomegaly, the lysosomal disorders should be considered; coarse facies, bone changes, joint stiffness, ocular symptoms, vacuolated lymphocytes, and neurologic deterioration are strongly suggestive of the mucolipidoses and mucopolysaccharidoses. Failure to thrive, anorexia, poor feeding, severe diarrhea, hypotonia, hypothermia, and frequent infections are presenting signs in Niemann-Pick disease type IA, Farber disease, Gaucher disease type II, and Wolman disease, and also in chronic granulomatous disease, glycogenosis type Ib, and lysinuric protein

Table 66-55 Permanent Hepatomegaly or Hepatosplenomegaly

Leading Symptoms			Age at Onset	Diagnosis
With manifestations of hepatocellular necrosis				
Jaundice (mild to severe) Edema, ascites Bleeding tendency Possible neurologic signs Intercurrent sepsis Elevated transaminases Disturbed hepatocellular function (liver failure) Hypoglycemia, hyperammonemia Possible hemolytic anemia			Neonatal to early infancy	Galactosemia (uridyl transferase and epimerase) Fructose intolerance Tyrosinemia type I (after 2 weeks) Neonatal hemochromatosis (low serum transaminases) Respiratory chain disorders 3-Methylglutaconic aciduria 3-hydroxy long-chain acyl CoA dehydrogenase deficiency
			Late infancy to childhood	α_1-antitrypsin deficiency Wilson disease
With cholestatic jaundice				
Yellow brown urine Jaundice Light or acholic stools Pruritus			Neonatal	α_1-antitrypsin deficiency (frequent) Byler disease (progressive familial intrahepatic cholestasis; normal GT) Inborn error of bile acid metabolism (normal GT) Niemann-Pick disease type C Classical Zellweger syndrome and variants Neonatal hemochromatosis Galactosemias, fructosemias (rare) Tyrosinosis type I, cystic fibrosis (rare)
			Infancy	Infantile Refsum disease Trihydroxycoprostanoyl CoA oxidase deficiency Congenital defects of glycosylation 3-hydroxy long-chain acyl CoA dehydrogenase deficiency
With hepatomegaly as only or major presenting symptom of liver disease				
Firm or rock-hard liver consistency with or without splenomegaly and portal hypertension (hepatic fibrosis, cirrhosis)			<1 year	Tyrosinosis type I Galactosemia, fructosemia Glycogenosis type IV Neonatal hemochromatosis
			1–6 years	α_1-antitrypsin deficiency Adenosylhomocysteine hydrolase deficiency (hypermethioninemia, hypoglycemia, mental retardation)
			>6 years	Wilson disease Cystic fibrosis Cholesteryl ester storage disease Glycogenosis type III (rare)
With normal or soft liver consistency	With splenomegaly	Storage disorders Coarse facies, bone changes Joint stiffness Vacuolated lymphocytes Ocular symptoms	Neonatal to early infancy	Landing disease Galactosialidosis (early infantile) Sialidosis type II I-cell disease (mucolipidosis type II)
		Progressive neurologic dysfunction	1–2 years	Austin disease (multiple sulfatase deficiency) Fucosidosis (late infancy to childhood) Galactosialidosis (late infantile) α-Mannosidosis Mucopolysaccharidosis type I (Hurler syndrome)

(Continued on next page)

Table 66-55 (Continued)

With hepatomegaly as only or major presenting symptom of liver disease			
Leading Symptoms		**Age at Onset**	**Diagnosis**
			Mucopolysaccharidosis type VI (Maroteaux-Lamy syndrome)
	Severe failure to thrive Anorexia Poor feeding Neurologic deterioration	Early infancy	Niemann-Pick disease type IA (interstitial pneumonia) Farber disease (interstitial pneumonia, hoarseness, skin nodules, hyperthermia) Gaucher disease type II (acute neuronopathy, spasticity)
	Chronic diarrhea Failure to thrive Anorexia Poor feeding Hypotonia	Early infancy	Wolman disease (adrenal gland calcifications, vacuolated lymphocytes) Lysinuric protein intolerance (neutropenia, recurrent metabolic attacks) Chronic granulomatous disease (recurrent infections, hyperthermia, inflammatory bowel disease) Glycogenosis type Ib (recurrent infections, hypoglycemia, neutropenia)
	Isolated	Late infancy to childhood	Niemann-Pick disease type IB (interstitial pneumonia) Gaucher disease type I (pancytopenia, splenomegaly ++)
	With various neurologic signs Myoclonic jerks Ophthalmoplegia Neurologic deterioration	Late infancy to childhood	Niemann-Pick disease type C Gaucher disease type III (subacute neuronopathic)
Without splenomegaly	Fasting hypoglycemia ± metabolic acidosis Hyperlactacidemia Failure to thrive	Neonatal to late infancy	Glycogenosis types Ia and Ib Glycogenosis type III Fructose diphosphatase deficiency Glycogen synthetase deficiency
	Tubulopathy	Early infancy	Bickel-Fanconi syndrome
	Severe hypotonia Cardiomyopathy Failure to thrive	Early infancy	Pompe disease Respiratory chain disorders Phosphorylase b kinase deficiency Congenital disorders of glycosylation Fatty acid oxidation disorders
	Apparently isolated	Infancy to childhood	Argininosuccinic aciduria (failure to thrive, hyperammonemia) Glycogenosis type VI (phosphorylase and phosphorylase b kinase) (abdominal distension) Cholesteryl ester storage disease (hypercholesterolemia) Neutrallipid storage disorder (ichthyosis, myopathy, vacuolated lymphocytes) Tangier disease (orange tonsils)

intolerance. Hepatosplenomegaly can be the presenting sign in Gaucher disease type I and in Niemann-Pick disease type Ib (with asymptomatic interstitial pneumonia in the latter). In late infancy or childhood, hepatosplenomegaly associated with myoclonic jerks, opthalmoplegia, and neurologic deterioration is a strong argument for the diagnosis of late-onset forms of Niemann-Pick disease type C (without sphingomyelinase deficiency) and subacute neuronopathic Gaucher disease type III.

When hepatomegaly is not associated with splenomegaly, three clinical circumstances should be considered. Situations with fasting hypoglycemia suggest glycogenosis type I or type III (in which the liver can extend down to the iliac crest) or Bickel-Fanconi syndrome (in which glycogenosis is associated with tubulopathy); these patients have a doll-like appearance and short stature. Fructose diphosphatase deficiency is considered when hypoglycemia is associated with recurrent attacks of lactic acidosis triggered by fasting or by intercurrent infections. In argininosuccinic aciduria there can be hepatomegaly and failure to thrive that can mimic hepatic glycogenosis.

Isolated hepatomegaly with protuberant abdomen is a presenting sign of glycogenosis type VI (phosphorylase and phosphorylase b kinase) and is also observed in the rare entities cholesteryl

Table 66-56 **Liver Failure, Ascites, Edema**

Leading Symptoms	Other Signs	Age at Onset	Diagnosis
Hydrops fetalis	Storage disorders (hepatosplenomegaly, coarse facies, dysostosis multiplex)	Congenital	Landing disease Sialidosis type II Galactosialidosis Mucopolysaccharidosis type VII (Sly)
	Hemolytic syndromes (and other congenital anemias)	Congenital	Bart hemoglobinopathy Glycolytic enzymopathies (rare) Pearson syndrome
Isolated liver failure Jaundice Hemorrhagic syndrome Hepatosplenomegaly Hypoglycemia Cytolysis (± hemolytic anemia)	*E. coli* sepsis Cataract Tubulopathy	First days	Galactosemias
	Vomiting Dizziness Tubulopathy	First days	Fructosemias
	Hemolytic anemia	First days	Neonatal hemochromatosis
	Tubulopathy Hemolytic anemia	First weeks to first months	Tyrosinemia type I Respiratory chain disorders
	Yellow-brown urine Jaundice Conjugated bilirubinemia	First months	Cystic fibrosis α_1-antitrypsin LCHAD deficiency
	Recurrent cholangitis	First months	Congenital defects of glycosylation
	Hypoglycemia	After weaning	Fructose intolerance Fructose diphosphatase deficiency
	Hemolytic anemia	Childhood to adolescence	Wilson disease
Liver failure with neurologic symptoms	Hypotonia Failure to thrive Cardiomyopathy Developmental delay Lactic acidosis	Neonatal to infancy	Respiratory chain disorders Glycogenosis type IV (hepatic fibrosis, cirrhosis) Congenital defects of glycosylation
	Mental retardation Hypoglycemia Hypermethioninemia	Infancy to childhood	*s*-Adenosyl-homocysteine hydrolase deficiency
	"Porphyria-like" tubulopathy Acute neurologic crisis	Infancy to childhood	Tyrosinemia type I
Storage disorders Hepatosplenomegaly Cherry red spot Dysotosis multiplex Vacuolated lymphocytes	Coarse facies Failure to thrive "Hepatitis"	Congenital to first weeks	Mucopolysaccharidosis type VII Niemann-Pick disease type A and C (acute forms)
	Coarse facies Decerebration Spasticity Seizures	Congenital to first weeks	Landing disease-sialidosis type II Galactosialidosis
Hepatosplenomegaly Vacuolated lymphocytes	Failure to thrive Vomiting Diarrhea Adrenal calcifications	First week	Wolman disease

LCHAD = hydroxy long chain acyl CoA dehydrogenase.

ester storage disease, Tangier disease, and neutral lipid storage disorders.

Liver Failure, Ascites, Edema

Four clinical groups of metabolic disorders can present as liver failure, ascites, and edema, usually in the neonatal period or infancy (Table 66-56):

1. Lysosomal disorders presenting either as nonimmune hydrops fetalis syndrome or in early infancy with clinical signs of a storage disorder (hepatosplenomegaly, dysostosis multiplex, vacuolated circulating lymphocytes, cherry red spot, and coarse facies).
2. Severe congenital hemolytic anemias giving rise to hydrops fetalis syndrome. The best known is Bart hemoglobinopathy due to absence of functional alpha globin chain. At least one case of Pearson syndrome and congenital defects of glycosylation has presented in the neonatal period as hydrops fetalis.[49,50]
3. The disorders that present most often as liver failure (jaundice, hemorrhagic syndrome, hypoglycemia, hepatosplenomegaly, elevated transaminases) in neonates or young infants are fructosemia, galactosemia, tyrosinemia type I, and, rarely,

Table 66-57 Cardiomyopathy (Primary, Nonobstructive)

Leading Symptoms	Major Clinical Findings	Age at Onset	Disorders
Integrated in an already known or evident clinical picture			
With hepatomegaly Hypoglycemia Abdominal distension Hypotonia		Late infancy to childhood	Glycogenosis type III (amylo-1, 6-glucosidase) Glycogenosis type IV (cirrhosis, hepatic failure)
With storage signs Coarse facies Dysostosis multiplex Hepatomegaly Corneal opacities Inguinal hernias Development delay		Neonatal to infancy	Mucolipidosis type II (I-cell disease), vacuolated lymphocytes
		Infancy 2–6 years	Mucopolysaccharidosis types IH and IS (Hurler syndrome, Scheie syndrome) Mucopolysaccharidosis type II (Hunter syndrome)
		Late infancy	Mucopolysaccharidosis type VI (Maroteaux-Lamy syndrome) Fucosidosis
With obvious neurologic or muscle symptoms		Late infancy to childhood	Freidreich ataxia Steinert disease
Predominant or presenting symptom			
With hypotonia Muscle weakness Failure to thrive	Ketoacidosis Hyperlactacidemia Developmental delay	Early infancy	Respiratory chain disorders (complex I, II, IV) 3-methylglutaconic aciduria (unknown origin) Ketoglutarate dehydrogenase deficiency
	Multiorgan failure Developmental delay Cardiac tamponade Pericardial effusions	Infancy	Congenital defects of glycosylation
	Macroglossia Hepatomegaly Vacuolated lymphocytes EKG changes (short PR interval, high-amplitude QRS complex)	Early infancy	Pompe disease (glycogenosis type II due to α-glucosidase deficiency)
	Myopathy Hypoglycemia Recurrent myoglobinuria	Neonatal to infancy	Fatty acid oxidation disorders (CUD, MAD, VLCAD, LCHAD, TL, LCTP) Phosphorylase b kinase
With hypoketotic hypoglycemia Hepatic signs		Infancy to childhood	Fatty acid oxidation disorders (CUD, MAD, TL, CPT II, VLCAD, LCHAD, LCTP)
With heartbeat disorders Cardiac arrest Cardiovascular collapse		Early in infancy (<1 year)	Fatty acid oxidation disorders (MAD, CPT II, VLCAD, LCHAD, LCTP) Respiratory chain disorders
With macrocytic megaloblastic anemia	Hemolytic uremic syndrome Ketoacidosis Retinopathy	Early infancy	Cobalamin (Cbl C) metabolism defects
	Diabetes Deafness Thiamine responsiveness	Childhood	Thiamine-responsive megaloblastic anemia
Isolated			
		Early infancy to childhood	Respiratory chain disorders (complexes I, II, IV) Phosphorylase b kinase Thiamine-responsive cardiomyopathy

CUD = carnitine uptake defect; MAD = multiple acyl CoA dehydrogenase; VLCAD = very long-chain acyl CoA dehydrogenase; LCHAD = hydroxy long-chain acyl CoA dehydrogenase; TL = translocase; LCTP = long-chain trifunctional; CPT II = carnitine palmitoyl transferase.

fructosebisphosphatase deficiency. Other disorders are α_1-antitrypsin deficiency, cystic fibrosis, neonatal hemochromatosis,[258,259] respiratory chain disorders, and congenital disorders of glycosylation (mostly type Ib).

4. The fourth group presents in early infancy as liver failure and severe neurologic dysfunction. It includes glycogenosis type IV due to a deficiency of branching enzyme and respiratory chain disorders with predominant hepatocellular dysfunction. In both conditions, the liver dysfunction is accompanied by neurologic signs, severe hypotonia, developmental delay, cardiomyopathy, and hyperlactacidemia. Adenosyl-homocysteine hydrolase deficiency with hepatocellular insufficiency, recurrent hypoglycemia, cirrhosis, mental retardation, and hypermethioninemia has been reported.[95]

The hepatic manifestations of inherited fatty acid oxidation disorders and urea cycle defects involve acute steatosis or Reye syndrome. These diseases exhibit normal bilirubin, only slightly prolonged prothrombin time, and moderate elevation of transaminases; true liver failure with ascites and edema is not usual but has been observed in a few cases of LCHAD deficiency.[21,259b]

It can be difficult to study patients with severe hepatic failure, because the liver failure can cause many nonspecific symptoms. Melituria (galactosuria, glycosuria, fructosuria), hyperammonemia, hyperlactacidemia, hypoglycemia, hypertyrosinemia, and hypermethioninemia are all signs of advanced hepatocellular insufficiency. Elevated succinylacetone excretion is specific for tyrosinemia type I due to fumaryl:acetoacetate hydrolase deficiency, but its absence does not rule out this diagnosis. Investigation of parents for evidence of partial enzyme deficiency can be very helpful in diagnosing galactosemia when the patient has undergone transfusion.

Cardiomyopathy

Except for myocardiopathy in an evocative clinical context, as in glycogenoses types III and IV, mucopolysaccharidoses, or mucolipidoses or in well-defined neurodegenerative disorders (Friedreich ataxia, Steinert disease), there are three groups of inborn errors that can be revealed by cardiomyopathy: Pompe disease, respiratory chain disorders, and fatty acid oxidation defects. The car diomyopathy is usually of the hypertrophic and hypokinetic type.(Table 66-57)

In Pompe disease, the cardiomyopathy appears in early infancy and is associated with severe muscle hypotonia, macroglossia, characteristic EKG changes, and vacuolized lymphocytes. The severity of cardiac damage and of gross motor dysfunction contrasts sharply with the normal mental development.

In respiratory chain disorders and in the Krebs cycle disorder α-ketoglutarate dehydrogenase deficiency, cardiomyopathy is associated with hypotonia, myopathy, diverse neurologic signs, and development delay. An important clue is hyperlactacidemia in the fed state with a high L:P ratio and ketosis. A form of 3-methylglutaconic aciduria involves cardiomyopathy and lactic acidemia.

Recent observations suggest that some respiratory chain disorders are tissue-specific and are expressed only in myocardium, as is true for phosphorylase b kinase deficiency.[260–262] This fact highlights the importance of measuring respiratory chain enzyme activity directly in endomyocardial biopsy samples whenever possible.[262] The multisystemic congenital disorders of glycosylalion frequently presents in infancy as cardiac failure due to pericardial effusions and cardiac tamponade,[11,175] or as glutaric aciduria type II.[112]

At least nine of the hereditary defects of fatty acid oxidation involve a cardiomyopathy and/or arrhythmia.[21,21a] Primary systemic carnitine deficiency, caused by a carnitine uptake defect, is the best known. It is dramatically curable by carnitine replacement therapy. In most cases, the cardiomyopathy is associated with hypotonia, hepatic signs, and fasting hypoketotic hypoglycemia. Severe forms of multiple acyl CoA dehydrogenase (glutaric aciduria type II due to electron transport flavoprotein or electron transport flavoprotein dehydrogenase deficiency) and long-chain fatty acid disorders involving CPT II, translocase, VLCAD, LCHAD, and trifunctional enzyme can appear early in infancy, even in the neonatal period, as cardiac arrest or shock (often misdiagnosed as toxic shock or malignant hyperthermia). Except for primary disorders of carnitine metabolism, all patients with fatty acid oxidation disorders who have cardiomyopathy are permanently at risk of unexpected death despite therapy. This susceptibility may result not only from severe energy deprivation,

Table 66-58 Interstitial Pulmonary Infiltrates

Leading Symptoms	Age at Onset	Other Signs	Diagnosis
Hemolytic uremic syndrome	Neonatal to early infancy	Ketoacidosis Hypotonia Cardiomyopathy	Cobalamin (Cbl C) metabolism defect
Storage signs (hepatosplenomegaly)	Neonatal to early infancy (first 3 months)	Hoarseness Joint stiffness Skin nodules Failure to thrive	Farber disease
		Neurologic deterioration Failure to thrive Cherry red spot Vacuolated lymphocytes	Niemann-Pick disease type A
	Infancy to childhood	Abdominal distension No neurologic signs	Niemann-Pick disease type B
		Massive splenomegaly $\pm$neurologic signs Bone crisis	Gaucher disease type I Gaucher disease type III
Isolated or predominant	Infancy to childhood	Failure to thrive Leukopenia Hyperammonemia Osteoporosis	Lysinuric protein intolerance

which can be prevented by medium-chain triglyceride supplementation, but also from accumulation of long-chain acylcarnitine, which has been shown to promote arrhythmia in a feline heart model.[176] In contrast, cardiomyopathy and myopathy are rarely if ever observed in MCAD and CPT I deficiencies. Cardiomyopathy is rare in inborn errors of vitamin B_{12} (Cbl C) and the exceptional case of thiamine-responsive cardiomyopathy that dramatically responds to oral thiamine supplementation.[263]

Interstitial Pulmonary Infiltrates

The radiographic finding of diffuse interstitial pulmonary infiltrates (interstitial pneumonia) is a rare but important sign of several inborn errors (Table 66-58). Affected patients may have no pulmonary symptoms for many years. The radiographic picture often leads to a misdiagnosis of viral pneumonia, particularly when the patient has an intercurrent respiratory illness. Pulmonary infiltrates are a nearly constant finding in the acute form of Farber disease (disseminated lipogranulomatosis) and Niemann-Pick disease type A and are sometimes observed in Gaucher disease types I and III. Interstitial infiltrates, often asymptomatic for years, are found regularly in Niemann-Pick disease type B. Undefined interstitial pneumonia is a potentially lethal complication of lysinuric protein intolerance, which can be also a presenting sign (see Chap. 118). Patients affected with impaired cobalamin metabolism (Cbl C complementation group) may have pneumonia (see also "Renal Symptoms and Thrombocytopenia" above).

Tubulopathy (Renal Fanconi Syndrome and Tubular Acidosis)

Renal Fanconi syndrome accompanies several inborn errors of metabolism (Table 66-59). The syndrome includes polyuria and high free water clearance, normal or low glycemic glycosuria,

Table 66-59 Tubulopathy

Leading Symptom	Other Signs	Age at Onset	Diagnosis
Fanconi syndrome	Acute liver failure	Neonatal to early in infancy	Fructosemia Galactosemia Tyrosinemia type I
	Severe hypotonia Dysmorphia Cataract	Congenital	Lowe syndrome (X-linked)
	Hepatomegaly Glycogenosis Hypoglycemia Failure to thrive Rickets	Infancy	Bickel-Fanconi syndrome (glycogenosis with tubulopathy secondary to GLUT II mutations)
	Anorexia Vomiting Severe failure to thrive Photophobia Corneal deposits	3–12 months	Cystinosis
	Severe myopathy Macroglossia Lactic acidosis	Congenital to first months	Cytochrome c oxidase deficiency and other respiratory chain disorders
	Severe vitamin D: dependent rickets (as presenting sign)	6 months to early childhood	Tyrosinosis type I (subacute or chronic form) Respiratory chain disorders (complex IV or mitochondrial DNA deletion)
Renal tubular acidosis (see also attacks of dehydration, Table 66-15)	Anorexia Failure to thrive Polydipsia, polyuria Nephrocalcinosis Hypokalemia Metabolic acidosis Alkaline urine pH	Early in infancy	RTA type I (distal) (red cell anion exchanges gene mutations)
	Metabolic acidosis Loss of bicarbonate Acidic urine pH in profound acidosis Ketosis Lactic acidosis Neurologic symptoms Hyperuricemia	Early in infancy	RTA type II (proximal) Pyruvate carboxylase deficiency Methylmalonic aciduria
	Metabolic acidosis No ketosis Recurrent attacks of hypoglycemia	6–18 months	Combined distal and proximal RTA CPT I deficiency
Salt loss	See "Dehydration," (Table 66-15)		CPT II deficiency CDG syndrome

RTA = renal tubular acidosis; CPT = carnitine palmitoyl transferase I and II; CDG = congenital defects of glycosylation

generalized aminoaciduria, tubular proteinuria (with massive excretion of β_2-microglobulin and lysozyme), phosphaturia with hypophosphatemia, and excessive renal loss of potassium and sodium bicarbonate leading to hypokalemia, hyponatremia, and acidosis. Hypercalciuria is also massive, and hypouricemia secondary to hyperuricuria is frequently found. In some patients, one or another tubular defect is predominant, resulting in an initial misdiagnosis of Bartter syndrome, diabetes insipidus, or pseudo-hypoaldosteronism.[249,264–266] Rickets due to phosphate loss and impaired vitamin D hormone synthesis can be the initial sign, especially in subacute and chronic forms of tyrosinemia type I and in respiratory chain disorders.[249,266,267] The most frequent inborn errors giving rise to Fanconi syndrome include hereditary fructose intolerance, galactosemia, tyrosinemia type I, X-linked Lowe syndrome, cystinosis, and respiratory chain disorders.

Bickel-Fanconi syndrome is a rare condition that presents within the first year of life as hepatomegaly, abdominal distension due to unclassified glycogen storage disease, hypoglycemia, glycosuria, and galactosuria, failure to thrive, severe tubulopathy, and vitamin D-unresponsive rickets. The pathogenesis of this syndrome has been recently elucidated as being secondary to mutations in the *GLUT2* (glucose-galactose transporter) gene.[96] Many disorders of energy metabolism can give rise to partial or total Fanconi syndrome. They include pyruvate carboxylase deficiency, which most often presents as proximal tubular acidosis with loss of bicarbonate,[268,269] respiratory chain disorders such as cytochrome c oxidase deficiency (complex IV deficiency),[39,267] and mitochondrial DNA deletion.[249,266] Carnitine palmitoyl transferase I deficiency is another cause.[114,270] We have recently observed one patient with carbohydrate-deficient glycoprotein syndrome type I due to phosphomannomutase deficiency and another one with carnitine palmitoyl transferase II deficiency, both of whom presented in the neonatal period with predominant tubulopathy and salt losing (unpublished observations).

Renal Symptoms (Other Than Tubulopathy)

Table 66-60 lists renal symptoms and their corresponding diagnoses. Among them, the methylmalonic aciduria variant with cobalamin Cbl C metabolism defect can present in early infancy as hemolytic uremic syndrome. In subacute forms of methylmalonic aciduria (methylmalonyl CoA mutase deficiency, cobalamin Cbl A and Cbl B mutant complementation groups), renal complications are rare presenting signs. They include reduction in glomerular filtration rates and hyperuricemia.[271,272]

Table 66-60 Renal Symptoms

Symptom	Age at Onset	Diagnosis
Tubulopathy Renal tubular proteinuria	See this symptom, Table 66-59	 Glycogenosis type I
Hemolytic uremic syndrome (see also thrombocytopenia)	Early in infancy	Cobalamin metabolism defect (Cbl C)
Tubulointerstitial nephropathy Glomerulosclerosis	Infancy to early childhood	Methylmalonic aciduria Glycogenosis type I
Acute renal failure with myoglobinuria (see also exercise intolerance)	Childhood to adolescence	Inborn errors of glycolysis, CPT II deficiency and other fatty acid oxidation defects
Nephrolithiasis (major accumulated compound in parentheses)	Infancy to childhood	Cystinuria (cystine) Hyperoxalurias type I and II (oxalic) Xanthine oxidase deficiency (xanthine) Hereditary renal hypouricemia (uric acid) Lesch-Nyhan syndrome (HGPRT) (uric acid) Glycogenosis type I (uric acid) Organic acidurias (uric acid) Molybdenum cofactor metabolism defect (xanthine) Adenine phosphoribosyl transferase deficiency (2-8-hydroxyadenine) PRPP synthase superactivity (uric acid)
Nephrotic syndrome	Congenital to infancy	Respiratory chain disorders Glutaric aciduria type I (isolated observation)
Renal cysts	Congenital (early in embryofetal life)	Zellweger syndrome Multiple acyl CoA dehydrogenase deficiency (glutaric aciduria type II) CPT II deficiency
Abnormal odor (major characteristic in parentheses)	Intermittent, only in acute phases, or depending on food intake	3-methylcrotonyl glycinuria (cat urine) Glutaric aciduria type II (sweaty feet) Isovaleric aciduria (sweaty feet) Trimethylaminuria (fish) Dimethylglycinuria (fish) Maple syrup urine disease (maple syrup, curry) Tyrosinemia type I (boiled cabbage) Phenylketonuria (musty odor) Cystinosis and other hyperaminoacidurias
Abnormal color	Intermittent, only in acute phases, or permanent	Alkaptonuria (black) Myoglobinuria (red) Porphyria (cherry red) Indicanuria (blue)

HGPRT = hypoxanthine guanine phosphoribosyl transferase; PRPP = phosphoribosylpyrophosphate; CPT = carnitine palmitoyl transferase.

Nephrolithiasis is diagnostic of several disorders (Table 66-60). Nephrotic syndrome can be the presenting sign in respiratory chain disorders[266] and has been observed in one case of glutaric aciduria type I.[273] Dimethylglycine dehydrogenase deficiency has been recently found in parents complaining with fish odor and execreting large amounts of dimethylglycine.[273a]

VIII. ENDOCRINE SYMPTOMS

Diabetes

Diabetes can be a presenting sign of respiratory chain disorders; Wolfram syndrome; and diabetes, deafness, and thiamine-responsive megaloblastic anemia. Organic acidurias (methylmalonic, propionic, isovaleric) and 3-ketothiolase deficiency can simulate diabetes.

Hypoparathyroidism

Hypoparathyroidisim has been observed in respiratory chain disorders,[274] in long-chain 3-hydroxyacyl CoA dehydrogenase deficiency,[275] and in mitochondrial trifunctional protein deficiency.[276]

Primary Adrenal Insufficiency

Primary adrenal insufficiency can be observed in respiratory chain disorders,[277] peroxisomal disorders (mostly X-linked adrenoleukodystrophy), and long-chain fatty acid oxidation defects (unpublished observation).

Growth Hormone Deficiency

Growth hormone deficiency has been observed as a presenting sign in respiratory chain disorders, and congenital defects of glycosylation (CDG If).[183b]

Hypogonadism and Sterility

Hypogonadism and sterility are frequent complications of galactosemia in girls.

ACKNOWLEDGMENTS

We thank all our residents, interns, and colleagues who have referred to us almost 25,000 patients in the past 30 years and participated in the investigation of their cases. We are especially grateful to the nurses of the metabolic ward, to Mrs. E. Depondt, dietitian, and to Miss D. Rapoport, psychologist, who were with us at the beginning of our study of inborn errors of metabolism and who are still working in the ward. We also thank Elisabeth Saudubray, who, once more, typed the manuscript efficiently and with an unflagging sense of humor.

REFERENCES

1. Wanders RJA, Kos M, Roest B, Meyer AJ, Schrakamp G, Heymans HSA, Vegelaers WHH, *et al.*: Activity of peroxisomal enzymes and intracellular distribution of catalase in Zellweger syndrome. *Biochem Biophys Res Comm* **123**:1054, 1984.
2. Rizzo WB, Dammann AL, Craft DA: Sjögren-Larsson syndrome: Impaired fatty alcohol oxidation in cultured fibroblasts due to deficient fatty alcohol: Nicotinamide adenine dinucleotide oxidoreductase activity. *J Clin Invest* **81**:738, 1988.
3. Divry P, Vianey-Liaud C, Gay C, Macabeo V, Rapin F, Echenne B: N-acetylaspartic aciduria: Report of three new cases in children with a neurological syndrome associating macrocephaly and leukodystrophy. *J Inherit Metab Dis* **11**:307, 1988.
4. Matalon R, Michels K, Sebesta D, Deanching M, Gashkoff P, Casanova J: Aspartoacylase deficiency and N-acetylaspartic aciduria in patients with Canavan disease. *Am J Hum Genet* **27**:463, 1988.
5. Salen G, Shefer S, Batta AK, Tint GS, Xu G, Honda A, Irons M, *et al.*: Abnormal cholesterol biosynthesis in the Smith-Lemli-Opitz syndrome. *J Lipid Res* **37**:1169, 1996.

5a. Kelley R, Hennekam RCM: The Smith-Lemli-Opitz syndrome. *J Med Genet* **37**:321, 2000.

5b. Moebius FF, Fitzky BU, Glossmann H: Genetic defects in postsqualene cholesterol biosynthesis. *TEM* **11**:106, 2000.

6. Saudubray JM, Ogier de Baulny H, Charpentier C: Clinical approach to inherited metabolic diseases, in Fernandes J, Saudubray JM, Van den Berghe G (eds): *Inborn Metabolic Diseases: Diagnosis and Treatment* 3d ed. Berlin, Springer Verlag, 2000, p 3.
7. Saudubray JM, Ogier H, Bonnefont JP, Munnich A, Lombes A, Hervé F, Mitchell G, *et al.*: Clinical approach to inherited metabolic diseases in the neonatal period: A 20 year survey. *J Inherit Metab Dis* **12**(suppl):25, 1989.
8. Poggi F, Billette de Villemeur T, Munnich A, Saudubray JM: The newborn with suspected metabolic disease: An overview, in Clayton BE, Round JM (eds): *Clinical Biochemistry and the Sick Child* 2d ed. Oxford, Blackwell Scientific Publications, 1994, p 60.
9. Clayton PT: Disorders of cholesterol biosynthesis. *Arch Dis Child* **78**:185, 1998.
10. FitzPatrick D, Keeling JW, Evans MJ, Kan AE, Bell JE, Porteous MEM, Mills K, *et al.*: Clinical phenotype of desmosterolosis. *Am J Med Genet* **75**:145, 1998.
11. Jaeken J, Stibler H, Hagberg B: The carbohydrate-deficient glycoprotein syndrome: A new inherited multisystemic disease with severe nervous system involvement. *Acta Paediatr Scand* **375**(suppl):5, 1991.
12. Niehues R, Hasilik M, Alton G, Körner C, Schiebe-Sukumar M, Koch HG, Zimmer KP, *et al.*: Carbohydrate-deficient glycoprotein syndrome type Ib: Phosphomannose isomerase deficiency and mannose therapy. *J Clin Invest* **101**:1414, 1998.
13. De Koning TJ, Dorland L, Van Diggelen OP, Boonman AMC, de Jong GJ, van Noort WL, de Schryver J, *et al.*: A novel disorder of N-glycosylation due to phosphomannose isomerase deficiency. *Biochem Biophys Res Comm* **245**:38, 1998.
14. Jaeken J, Matthijs G, Saudubray JM, Dionisi-Vici C, Bertini E, De Lonlay P, Henri H, *et al.*: Phosphomannomutase isomerase deficiency: A carbohydrate-deficient glycoprotein syndrome with hepatic-intestinal presentation. *Am J Hum Genet* **62**:1535, 1998.

14a. Grunewald S, Imbach T, Huijben K, Rubio-Gozalbo ME, Verrips A, de Klerk JBC, Stroink H, *et al.*: Clinical and biochemical characteristics of congenital disorder of glycosylation type Ic, the first recognized endoplasmic reticulum defect in N-glycan synthesis. *Ann Neurol* **47**:776, 2000.

15. Clayton PT, Thompson E: Dysmorphic syndromes with demonstrable biochemical abnormalities. *J Med Genet* **25**:463, 1988.
16. Munnich A, Rustin P, Rötig A, Chretien D, Bonnefont JP, Nuttin C, Cormier V, *et al.*: Clinical aspects of mitochondrial disorders. *J Inherit Metab Dis* **15**:448, 1992.
17. Lyon G, Adams RD, Kolodny EH: *Neurology of Hereditary Metabolic Diseases of Children* 2d ed. New York, McGraw-Hill, 1996.
18. Kronick JB, Scriver CR, Goodyer PR, Kaplan PB: A perimortem protocol for suspected genetic disease. *Pediatrics* **71**:960, 1983.
19. Poggi F, Rabier D, Vassault A, Charpentier C, Kamoun P, Saudubray JM: Protocole d'investigations métaboliques dans les maladies héréditaires du métabolisme. *Arch Pédiatr* **1**:667, 1994.
20. Ogier de Baulny H, Saudubray JM: Branched-chain organic acidurias, in Fernandes J, Saudubray JM, Van den Berghe G (eds): *Inborn Metabolic Diseases: Diagnosis and Treatment* 3d ed. Berlin, Springer-Verlag, 2000, p 195.

20a. Hyland K, Buist NRM, Powell BR, Hoffman GF, Rating D, Mc Grath J, Acworth IN: Folinic responsive seizures: a new syndrome? *J Inher Metab Dis* **18**:257, 1995.

21. Saudubray JM, Martin D, de Lonlay P, Touati G, Poggi-Travert F, Bonnet D, Jouvet P, *et al.*: Recognition and management of fatty acid oxidation defects: A series of 107 patients. *J Inher Metab Dis* **22**:488, 1999.

21a. Bonnet D, Martin D, de Lonlay P, Villain E, Jouvet P, Rabier D, Brivet M, *et al.*: Arrhytmias and conduction defects as presenting symptoms of fatty acid oxidation disorders in children. *Circulation* **100**:2248, 1999.

22. Settergren G, Lindblad BS, Persson B: Cerebral blood flow and exchange of oxygen, glucose, ketone bodies, lactate, pyruvate and amino acids in infants. *Acta Paediatr Scand* **65**:343, 1976.
23. Poggi-Travert F, Martin D, Billette de Villemeur T, Bonnefont JP, Vassault A, Rabier D, Charpentier C, *et al.*: Metabolic intermediates in lactic acidosis: Compounds, samples and interpretation. *J Inher Metab Dis* **19**:478, 1996.

24. Burton BK: Inborn errors of metabolism: The clinical diagnosis in early infancy. *Pediatrics* **79**:359, 1987.
25. Cathelineau C, Briand P, Ogier H, Charpentier C, Coudé FX, Saudubray JM: Occurrence of hyperammonemia in the course of 17 cases of methylmalonic acidemia. *J Pediatr* **99**:279, 1981.
26. Goodman SI, Frerman FE, Loehr JP: Recent progress in understanding glutaric acidemias. *Enzyme* **38**:76, 1987.
27. Wysocki SJ, Hahnel R: 3-hydroxy-3-methylglutaryl-coenzyme A lyase deficiency. *J Inherit Metab Dis* **9**:225, 1986.
28. Demaugre F, Bonnefont JP, Colonna M, Cepanec C, Leroux JP, Saudubray JM: Infantile form of carnitine palmitoyltransferase II deficiency with hepatomuscular symptoms and sudden death. *J Clin Invest* **87**:859, 1991.
29. Pande SV, Brivet M, Slama A, Demaugre F, Aufrant C, Saudubray JM: Carnitine-acylcarnitine translocase deficiency with severe hypoglycemia and auriculo ventricular block. *J Clin Invest* **91**:1247, 1993.
30. Tildon JT, Cornblath M: Succinyl-CoA: 3-ketoacidosis in infancy. *J Clin Invest* **51**:493, 1972.
31. Saudubray JM, Specola NB, Middleton B, Lombes A, Bonnefont JP, Jakobs C, Vassault A, *et al.*: Hyperketotic states due to inherited defects of ketolysis. *Enzyme* **38**:80, 1987.
32. Burri BJ, Sweetman L, Nyhan WL: Mutant holocarboxylase synthetase: Evidence for the enzyme defect in early infantile biotin-responsive multiple carboxylase deficiency. *J Clin Invest* **68**:1491, 1981.
33. Amendt BA, Greene C, Sweetman L, Cloherty J, Shih V, Moon A, Teel L, *et al.*: Short chain acyl-CoA dehydrogenase deficiency: Clinical and biochemical studies in two patients. *J Clin Invest* **79**:1303, 1987.
33a. Treacy EP, Lambert DM, Barnes R, Boriack RL, Vockley J, O'Brien LK, Jones PM, *et al.*: Short-chain hydroxyacyl-coenzyme A dehydrogenase deficiency presenting as unexpected infant death: A family study. *J Pediatr* **137**:257, 2000.
34. Divry P, Vianey-Liaud C, Mory O, Ravussin SS: A methylglutaconic aciduria familial neonatal form with fatal onset. *J Inherit Metab Dis* **10**(suppl 2):286, 1987.
35. Francke U, Harper JF, Darras BT, Cowan JM, McCabe ERB, Kohlschutter A, Seltzer WK, *et al.*: Congenital adrenal hypoplasia, myopathy, and glycerol kinase deficiency: Molecular genetic evidence for deletions. *Am J Hum Genet* **40**:212, 1987.
36. Wolf B, Grier RE, Allen RJ, Goodman SI, Kien CL, Parker WD, Howell DM, *et al.*: Phenotypic variation in biotinidase deficiency. *J Pediatr* **103**:233, 1983.
37. Robinson BH, Sherwood WG: Lactic acidaemia. *J Inherit Metab Dis* **7**(suppl 1):69, 1984.
38. Robinson BH, Oei J, Saudubray JM, Marsac C, Bartlett K, Quan F, Gravel RA: The French and North American phenotypes of pyruvate carboxylase deficiency, correlation with biotin containing protein by H3-biotin incorporation, S35-streptavidin labeling and northern blotting with a cloned cDNA probe. *Am J Hum Genet* **40**:50, 1987.
39. Van Biervliet JPGM, Bruinvis L, Ketting D, De Bree PK, Van der Heiden C, Wadman SK, Willems JL, *et al.*: Hereditary mitochondrial myopathy with lactic acidemia, a DeToni-Fanconi-Debré syndrome and a defective respiratory chain in voluntary muscle. *Pediatr Res* **1**:1088, 1977.
40. Di Mauro S, Bonilla E, Zeviani M, Servidei S, DeVivo DC, Schon EA: Mitochondrial myopathies. *J Inherit Metab Dis* **10**(suppl 1):113, 1987.
41. Nyhan WL, Sakati NA: *Diagnostic Recognition of Genetic Diseases*. Philadelphia, Lea-Febiger, 1987.
41a. Kerrigan JF, Aleck KA, Tarby TJ, Bird CR, Heidenreich RA: Fumaric aciduria: Clinical and imaging features. *Ann Neurol* **47**:583, 2000.
42. Ballard RA, Vinocour B, Reynolds JW, Wennburg RP, Merritt A, Sweetman L, Nyhan WL: Transient hyperammonemia of the preterm infant. *N Engl J Med* **299**:920, 1978.
43. Mises J, Moussalli-Salefranque F, Laroque ML, Ogier H, Coudé FX, Charpentier C, Saudubray JM: EEG findings as an aid to the diagnosis of neonatal non ketotic hyperglycinemia. *J Inherit Metab Dis* **5**(suppl 2):117, 1982.
44. Wadman SK, Duran M, Beemer FA, Cats BP, Johnson JL, Rajagopalan KV, Saudubray JM, *et al.*: Absence of hepatic molybdenum cofactor: An inborn error of metabolism leading to a combined deficiency of sulphite oxidase and xanthine dehydrogenase. *J Inherit Metab Dis* **6**:78, 1983.
45. Poggi-Travert F, Fournier B, Poll-The BT, Saudubray JM: Clinical approach to inherited peroxisomal disorders. *J Inherit Metab Dis* **18**(suppl 1):1, 1995.
45a. Baumgartner MR, Verhoeven NM, Jakobs C, Roels F, Espeel M, Martinez M, Rabier D, *et al.*: Defective peroxisome biogenesis with a neuromuscular disorder resembling Werding Hoffmann disease. *Neurology.* **51**:1427, 1998.
45b. Baumgartner MR, Poll The BT, Verhoeven NM, Jakobs C, Espeel M, Roels F, Rabier D, *et al.*: Clinical approach to inherited peroxisomal disorders. Consecutive series of 27 patients *Ann Neurology.* **44**:720, 1998.
46. Hyland K, Surtees RAH, Rodeck C, Clayton PT: Aromatic L-amino acid decarboxylase deficiency: Clinical features, diagnosis and treatment of a new inborn error of neurotransmitter amine synthesis. *Neurology* **42**:1980, 1992.
46a. Gibson KM, Burlingame TG, Hogema B, Jakobs C, Schutgens RBH, Millington D, Roe CR, *et al.*: 2-methylbutyryl-coenzyme A dehydrogenase deficiency: A new inborn error of L-isoleucine metabolism. *Pediat Res* **47**:6, 2000.
46b. Mayatepek E, Flock B: Leukotriene C_4-synthesis deficiency: a new inborn error of metabolism linked to a fatal developmental syndrome. *Lancet* **352**:1514, 1998.
46c. Mayatepek E, Lindner M, Zelezny R, Lindner W, Brandstetter G, Hoffmann GF: A severely affected infant with absence of cysteinyl leukotrienes in cerebrospinal fluid: further evidence that leukotriene C_4-synthesis deficiency is a new neuro-metabolic disorder. *Neuropediatrics* **30**:5, 1999.
47. Bankier A, Turner M, Hopkins IJ: Pyridoxine dependent seizures: A wider clinical spectrum. *Arch Dis Child* **58**:415, 1983.
47a. Hoffmann GF, Surtees RAH, Wevers RA: Cerebrospinal fluid investigations for neurometabolic disorders. *Neuropediatrics* **29**:59, 1998.
48. Fellman V, Rapola J, Pihko H, Varilo T, Raivio KO: Iron-overload disease in infants involving fetal growth retardation, lactic acidosis, liver haemosiderosis, and aminoaciduria. *Lancet* **351**:490, 1998.
49. Kirk J, FitzPatrick D, Lyon A, Thomas A, Smith N, Seller A: Pearson's syndrome presenting as hydrops fetalis. *J Inherit Metab Dis* **19**(suppl 1):75, 1996. (Abstract)
50. Dorland L, De Koning TJ, Toet M, de Vries LS, Van Den Berg IET, Poll-The BT: Recurrent non-immune hydrops fetalis associated with carbohydrate-deficient glycoprotein syndrome. *J Inherit Metab Dis* **20**(suppl 1):88, 1997. (Abstract)
51. Ibdha JA, Bennett MJ, Rinaldo P, Zhao Y, Gibson B, Sims HF, Strauss AW: A fetal fatty-acid oxidation disorder as a cause of liver disease in pregnant women. *N Engl J Med* **340**:1723, 1999.
52. Innes AM, Seargeant LE, Balachandra K, Roe CR, Wanders RJA, Ruiter JPN, Casiro O, *et al.*: Hepatic carnitine palmitoyltransferase I deficiency presenting as maternal illness in pregnancy. *Pediat Res* **47**:1, 2000.
52a. Tein I: Metabolic disease in the fetus predisposes to maternal hepatic complications of pregnancy. *Pediat Res* **47**:6, 2000.
52b. Nelson J, Lewis B, Walters B: The HELLP syndrome associated with fetal medium-chain acyl-CoA dehydrogenase deficiency. *J Inherit Metab Dis* **23**:518, 2000.
53. Heidenriech R, Natowicz M, Hainline BE, Berman P, Kelley RI, Hillman RE, Berry GT: Acute extrapyramidal syndrome in methylmalonic acidemia: "Metabolic stroke" involving the globus pallidus. *J Pediatr* **113**:1022, 1988.
54. Dave P, Curless RG, Steinman L: Cerebellar hemorrhage complicating methylmalonic and propionic acidemia. *Arch Neurol* **41**:1293, 1984.
55. Burlina AB, Dionisi-Vici C, Bennett MJ, Gibson KM, Servidei S, Bertini E, Hale DE, *et al.*: A new syndrome with ethylmalonic aciduria and normal fatty acid oxidation in fibroblasts. *J Pediatr* **124**:79, 1994.
56. Garcia-Silva MT, Ribes A, Campos Y, Garavaglia B, Arenas J: Syndrome of encephalopathy, petechiae, and ethylmalonic aciduria. *Pediatr Neurol* **17**:165, 1997.
57. Sasaki M, Kimura M, Sugai K, Hashimoto T, Yamaguchi S: 3-Hydroxyisobutyric aciduria in two brothers. *Pediatr Neurol* **18**:253, 1998.
58. Boles RG, Chun N, Senadheera D, Wong LJC: Cyclic vomiting syndrome and mitochondrial DNA mutations. *Lancet* **350**:1299, 1997.
59. Chinnery PF, Turnbull DM: Vomiting, anorexia, and mitochondrial DNA disease. *Lancet* **6351**:448, 1997.

60. Goodman SI, Norenberg MD, Shilkes RH, Breslich DJ, Moe PG: Glutaric aciduria: Biochemical and morphologic considerations. *J Pediatr* **90**:746, 1977.
61. Gregersen N, Brandt NJ: Ketotic episodes in glutaryl-CoA dehydrogenase deficiency (glutaric aciduria). *Pediatr Res* **13**:977, 1979.
62. Leibel RL, Shih V, Goodman SI, Bauman ML, McCabe ERB, Zwerdling RG, Bergman I, *et al.*: Glutaric acidemia: A metabolic disorder causing progressive choreoathetosis. *Neurology* **30**:1163, 1980.
63. Superti-Furga A, Hoffmann GF: Glutaric aciduria type 1 (glutaryl-CoA-dehydrogenase deficiency): Advances and unanswered questions. *Eur J Pediatr* **156**:821, 1997.
64. Pavlakis SG, Phillips PC, Di Mauro S: Mitochondrial myopathy, encephalopathy, lactic acidosis and strokelike episodes (MELAS): A distinctive clinical syndrome. *Ann Neurol* **16**:481, 1984.
65. Kotagal S, Peterson PL, Martens ME: Impaired NADH-CoQ reductase activity in a child with Moyamoya syndrome. *Pediatr Neurol* **4**:241, 1988.
66. Ichiki T, Tanaka K, Nishikimi M: Deficiency of subunits of complex I and mitochondrial encephalomyopathy. *Ann Neurol* **23**:287, 1988.
67. Koga Y, Nonaka I, Kobayashi M: Findings in muscle in complex I (NADH coenzyme Q reductase) deficiency. *Ann Neurol* **24**:749, 1988.
68. Kobayashi M, Morishita H, Sugiyama N: Two cases of NADH-coenzyme Q reductase deficiency. Relationship to MELAS syndrome. *J Pediatr* **110**:223, 1987.
69. Nishizawa M, Tanaka K, Shinozawa K: A mitochondrial encephalomyopathy with cardiomyopathy. A case revealing a defect of complex I respiratory chain. *J Neurol Sci* **78**:189, 1987.
69a. Huemer M, Muehl A, Wandl-Vergesslich K, Strobl W, Wanders RJA, Stoeckler-Ipsiroglu S: Stroke-like encephalopathy in an infant with 3-hydroxy-3-methylglutaryl-coenzyme A lyase deficiency. *Eur J Pediatr* **157**:743, 1998.
69b. Steen C, Baumgartner ER, Duran M, Lenhert W, Suormala T, Fingerhut R, Stehn M, *et al.*: Metabolic stroke in isolated 3-methylcrotonyl-Coa carboxylase deficiency. *Eur J Pediatr* **158**:730, 1999.
70. Cormier V, Rustin P, Bonnefont JP, Rambaud C, Vassault A, Rabier D, Parvy P, *et al.*: Hepatic failure in disorders of oxidative phosphorylation with neonatal onset. *J Pediatr* **119**:951, 1991.
71. Vilaseca MA, Briones P, Ribes A, Carreras E, Llacer A, Querol J: Fatal hepatic failure with lactic acidemia, Fanconi syndrome and defective activity of succinate:cytochrome C reductase. *J Inherit Metab Dis* **14**:285, 1991.
72. Parrot-Roulaud F, Carré M, Lamirau T, Letellier T, Malgat M, Mazat JP, Munnich A, *et al.*: Fatal neonatal hepatocellular deficiency with lactic acidosis: A defect of the respiratory chain. *J Inherit Metab Dis* **14**:289, 1991.
73. Freeman JM, Finkelstein JD, Mudd SF: Folate responsive homocystinuria and schizophrenia. *N Engl J Med* **292**:491, 1975.
74. Autret E, Jonville-Béra AP, Llau ME, Bavoux F, Saudubray JM, Laugier J, Devictor D, *et al.*: Reye's syndrome in France: A national register. (unpublished)
75. Hardie RM, Newton LH, Bruce JC, Glasgow JFT, Mowat AP, Stephenson JB, Hall SM: The changing clinical pattern of Reye's syndrome 1982–1990. *Arch Dis Child* **74**:400, 1996.
76. Miller SG, Schwartz GJ: Hyperammonemia with distal renal tubular acidosis. *Arch Dis Child* **77**:441, 1997.
77. Persson B, Gentz J: The pattern of blood lipids, glycero and ketone bodies during the neonatal period, infancy and childhood. *Acta Paediatr Scand* **55**:353, 1966.
78. Saudubray JM, Marsac C, Limal JM, Dumurgier E, Charpentier C, Ogier H, Coudé FX: Variation in plasma ketone bodies during a 24-hour fast in normal and in hypoglycemic children. *J Pediatr* **6**:904, 1981.
79. Bonnefont JP, Specola NB, Vassault A, Lombes A, Ogier H, De Klerk JBC, Munnich A, *et al.*: The fasting test in paediatrics: Application to the diagnosis of pathological hypo- and hyperketotic states. *Eur J Paediatr* **150**:80, 1990.
80. Lamers KJB, Doesburg WH, Gabreels FJM, Romsom AC, Renier WO, Wevers RA, Lemmens WAJG: Reference values of blood components related to fuel metabolism in children after an overnight fast. *Clin Chim Acta* **145**:17, 1985.
81. Robinson AM, Williamson DH: Physiological roles of ketone bodies as substrates and signals in mammalian tissues. *Physiol Rev* **60**:143, 1980.
82. Touati G, Rigal O, Lombès A, Frachon P, Giraud M, Ogier de Baulny H: In vivo functional investigations of lactic acid in patients with respiratory chain disorders. *Arch Dis Child* **76**:16, 1997.
83. Leonard JV, Middleton B, Seakins JW: Acetoacetyl CoA thiolase deficiency presenting as ketotic hypoglycemia. *Pediatr Res* **21**:211, 1987.
84. Bhala A, Willi SM, Rinaldo P, Bennett MJ, Schmidt-Sommerfeld E, Hale DE: Clinical and biochemical characterization of short-chain acyl-coenzyme A dehydrogenase deficiency. *J Pediatr* **126**:910, 1995.
85. Ko FJ, Nyhan WL, Wolff J, Barshop B, Sweetman L: 3-hydroxyisobutyric aciduria: An inborn error of valine metabolism. *Pediatr Res* **30**:322, 1991.
86. Bennett MJ, Weinberger MJ, Kobori JA, Rinaldo P, Burlina AB: Mitochondrial short-chain L-3-hydroxyacyl-coenzyme A dehydrogenase deficiency: A new defect of fatty acid oxidation. *Pediatr Res* **39**:185, 1996.
87. Vassault A, Bonnefont JP, Specola N, Saudubray JM: Lactate, pyruvate, ketone bodies, in Hommes FA (ed): *Techniques in Diagnostic Human Biochemical Genetics*. New York, Wiley-Liss, 1991, p 285.
88. Fernandes J, Koster JF, Grose WFA, Sorgedrager N: Hepatic phosphorylase deficiency: Its differentiation from other hepatic glycogenoses. *Arch Dis Child* **49**:186, 1974.
89. Aynsley-Green A, Williamson DH, Gitzelmann R: The dietary treatment of glycogen synthetase deficiency. *Helv Paediatr Acta* **1**:71, 1977.
90. Stansbie D, Sherriff RJ: Fructose load test — an *in vivo* screening test designed to assess pyruvate dehydrogenase activity and interconversion. *J Inherit Metab Dis* **1**:163, 1978.
91. Coudé FX, Saudubray JM, Demaugre F, Marsac C, Leroux JP: Dichloroacetate as treatment for congenital lactic acidosis. *N Engl J Med* **299**:1365, 1978.
92. Saudubray JM, Marsac C, Charpentier C, Cathelineau L, Besson-Léaud M, Leroux JP: Neonatal congenital lactic acidosis with pyruvate carboxylase deficiency in two siblings. *Acta Paediatr Scand* **65**:717, 1976.
93. Bonnefont JP, Chretien D, Rustin P, Robinson BH, Vassault A, Aupetit J, Charpentier C, *et al.*: Alpha-ketoglutarate dehydrogenase deficiency presenting as congenital lactic acidosis. *J Pediatr* **121**:255, 1992.
94. Rötig A, Cormier V, Blanche S, Bonnefont JP, Ledeist F, Romero N, Schmitz J, *et al.*: Pearson's marrow-pancreas syndrome: A multisystem mitochondrial disorder in infancy. *J Clin Invest* **86**:1601, 1990.
94a. Saudubray JM, de Lonlay P, Touati G, Martin D, Nassogne MC, Castelnau P, Sevin C: Genetic hypoglycaemia in infancy and childhood: Pathophysiology and diagnosis. *J Inherit Metab Dis* **23**:197, 2000.
95. Labrune P, Perignon JL, Rault M, Brunet C, Lutun H, Charpentier C, Saudubray JM, *et al.*: Familial hypermethioninemia partially responsive to dietary restriction. *J Pediatr* **2**:220, 1990.
95a. De Lonlay P, Cuer M, Vuillaumier-Barrot S, Beaune G, Castelnau P, Kretz M, Durand G, *et al.*: Hyperinsulinemic hypoglycemia as a presenting sign in phosphomanno-isomerase deficiency: a new manifestation of carbohydrate deficient glycoprotein treatable with mannose. *J Pediatr* **135**:379, 1999.
96. Santer R, Schneppenheim R, Dombrowski A, Götze H, Steinmann B, Schaub J: Mutations in GLUT2, the gene for the liver-type glucose transporter in patients with Fanconi-Bickel syndrome. *Nature Genet* **17**:324, 1997.
97. Dubois J, Brunelle F, Touati G, Sebag G, Nuttin C, Thach T, Nihoul-Fékété C, *et al.*: Hyperinsulinism in children: Diagnostic value of pancreatic venous sampling correlated with clinical, pathological and surgical outcome in 25 cases. *Pediatr Radiol* **25**:512, 1995.
98. Labrune P, Bonnefont JP, Fékété CN, Nezeloff C, Gepts W, Czernichow P, Rappaport R, *et al.*: Evaluation des méthodes diagnostiques et thérapeutiques de l'hyperinsulinisme du nouveau-né et du nourrisson. *Arch Fr Pediatr* **46**:167, 1989.
99. Thomas PM, Cote GJ, Wohllk N, Haddad B, Mathew PM, Rabl W, Aguilar-Bryan L, *et al.*: Mutations in the sulfonylurea receptor gene in familial persistent hyperinsulinemic hypoglycemia of infancy. *Science* **268**:426, 1995.
100. Nestorowicz A, Wilson BA, Schoor KP, Inagaki N, Gonoi T, Glaser B, Permutt MA: Mutations in the sulfonylurea receptor gene are associated with familial hyperinsulinism in Ashkenazi Jews. *Hum Mol Genet* **5**:1813, 1996.

101. Nestorowicz A, Inagaki N, Gonoi T, Schoor KP, Wilson BA, Glaser B, Landau H, *et al.*: A nonsense mutation in the inward rectifier potassium channel gene, Kir6.2, is associated with familial hyperinsulinism. *Diabetes* **46**:1743, 1997.
102. Glaser B, Kesavan P, Heyman M, Davis E, Cuesta A, Buchs A, Stanley CA, *et al.*: Familial hyperinsulinism caused by an activating glucokinase mutation. *N Engl J Med* **338**:226, 1998.
103. Huijmans JGM, *et al.*: Glutamine synthetase—a new defect of ammonemia disposal, associated with hyperinsulinemic hypoglycemia. *7th International Congress of Inborn Errors of Metabolism*, Vienna, May 21–25, 1997. (Abstract)
104. Stanley CA, Lieu YK, Hsu BYL, Burlina AB, Greenberg CR, Hopwood NJ, Perlman K, *et al.*: Hyperinsulinism and hyperammonemia in infants with regulatory mutations of the glutamate dehydrogenase gene. *N Engl J Med* **338**:1352, 1998.
105. De Lonlay P, Fournet JC, Rahier J, Gross-Morand MS, Poggi-Travert F, Foussier V, Bonnefont JP, *et al.*: Somatic deletion of the imprinted 11p15 region in sporadic persistent hyperinsulinemic hypoglycemia of infancy is specific for focal adenomatous hyperplasia and endorses partial pancreatectomy. *J Clin Invest* **100**:802, 1997.
106. Verkarre V, Fournet JC, De Lonlay P, Gross-Morand MS, Rahier J, Brunelle F, Robert JJ, *et al.*: Paternal mutation of the sulfonylurea receptor (SUR_1) gene and maternal loss of 11p15 imprinted genes lead to persistent hyperinsulinism in focal adenomatous hyperplasia. *J Clin Invest* **102**:1286, 1998.
107. De Lonlay-Debeney P, Poggi-Travert F, Fournet JC, Sempoux C, Dionisi Vici C, Brunelle F, Touati G, *et al.*: Clinical features of 52 neonates with hyperinsulinism. *N Engl J Med* **340**:1169, 1999.
108. Sempoux C, Guiot Y, Lefevre A, Nihoul-Fékété C, Jaubert F, Saudubray JM, Rahier J: Neonatal hyperinsulinemic hypoglycemia: Heterogeneity of the syndrome and keys for differential diagnosis. *J Clin Endocrinol Metab* **83**:1455, 1998.
109. O'Rahilly S, Gray H, Humphreys PJ, Krook A, Polonsky KS, White A, Gibson S, *et al.*: Brief report: Impaired processing of prohormones associated with abnormalities of glucose homeostasis and adrenal function. *N Engl J Med* **23**:1386, 1995.
110. Dozio N, Scavini M, Beretta A, Sarugeri E, Sartori S, Belloni C, Dosio F, *et al.*: Imaging of the buffering effect of insulin antibodies in the autoimmune hypoglycemic syndrome. *J Clin Endocrinol Metab* **83**:643, 1998.
111. Kamijo T, Indo Y, Souri M, Aoyama T, Hara T, Yamamoto S, Ushikubo S, *et al.*: Medium chain 3-ketoacyl-coenzyme A thiolase deficiency: A new disorder of mitochondrial fatty acid β-oxidation. *Pediatr Res* **42**:569, 1997.
112. Hirose S, Hamamoto K, Yoshida I, Inokuchi T, Kogo T, Mitsudome A, *et al.*: Late-onset type II glutaric aciduria with massive pericardial effusion associated with severe fatty liver. *Acta Paediatr* **89**:887, 2000.
113. Tein I, Demaugre F, Bonnefont JP, Saudubray JM: Normal muscle CPT I and CPT II activities in hepatic presentation patients with CPT I deficiency in fibroblasts: Tissue specific isoforms of CPT I? *J Neurol Sci* **93**:229, 1989.
114. Falik-Borenstein ZC, Jordan SC, Saudubray JM, Brivet M, Demaugre F, Edmond J, Cederbaum SD: Renal tubular acidosis in carnitine palmitoyltransferase type 1 deficiency. *N Engl J Med* **327**:24, 1992.
115. Poll-The BT, Bonnefont JP, Ogier H, Charpentier C, Pelet A, Le Fur JM, Jakobs C, *et al.*: Familial hypoketotic hypoglycemia associated with peripheral neuropathy, pigmentary retinopathy and C6-C14 hydroxydicarboxylic aciduria: A new defect in fatty acid oxidation. *J Inherit Metab Dis* **11**(suppl 2):183, 1988.
116. Bertini E, Dionisi-Vici C, Garavaglia B, Burlina AB, Sabatelli M, Rimoldi M, Bartuli A, *et al.*: Peripheral sensory-motor polyneuropathy, pigmentary retinopathy, and fatal cardiomyopathy in long-chain 3-hydroxy-acyl-CoA dehydrogenase deficiency. *Eur J Pediatr* **151**:121, 1992.
117. Thompson GN, Hsu BYL, Pitt JJ, Treacy E, Stanley CA: Fasting hypoketotic coma in a child with deficiency of mitochondrial 3-hydroxy-3-methylglutaryl-CoA synthetase. *N Engl J Med* **337**:1203, 1997.
117a. Al Odaib A, Shneider BL, Bennett MJ, Pober BR, Reyes-Mugica M, Friedman AL, Suchy FJ, *et al.*: A defect in the transport of long-chain fatty acids associated with acute liver failure. *N Engl J Med* **339**:1752, 1998.
118. Millington DS, Kodo N, Norwood DL, Roe CR: Tandem mass spectrometry: A new method for acylcarnitine profiling with potential for neonatal screening for inborn errors of metabolism. *J Inherit Metab Dis* **13**:321, 1990.
119. Millington DS, Terela N, Chace DH, Chen YT, Ding JH, Kodo N, Roe CR: The role of tandem mass spectrometry in the diagnosis of fatty acid oxidation disorders, in Coates P, Tanaka K (eds): *New Developments in Fatty Acid Oxidation*. New York, Wiley-Liss, 1992, p 339.
120. Rashed M, Ozand PT, Bucknall MP, Little D: Diagnosis of inborn errors of metabolism from blood spots by acylcarnitines and amino acids profiling using automated electrospray tandem mass spectrometry. *Pediatr Res* **38**:324, 1995.
121. Reye RDK, Morgan G, Baral J: Encephalopathy and fatty degeneration of the viscera: A disease entity in childhood. *Lancet* **2**:749, 1963.
122. Follow up on Reye's syndrome, United States. *MMWR* **29**:321, 1980.
123. Diagnosis and treatment of Reye syndrome: Consensus conference. *JAMA* **246**:2441, 1981.
124. Reye syndrome, United States. *MMWR* **35**:66, 1986.
125. Corey L, Rubin RJ, Hattwick MAW: A nationwide outbreak of Reye's syndrome: Its epidemiologic relationship to influenza. *Am J Med* **61**:615, 1976.
126. Forsyth BW, Horwitz RI, Acampora D: New epidemiologic evidence confirming that bias does not explain the aspirin/Reye's syndrome association. *JAMA* **17**:2517, 1989.
127. Porter JDH, Robinson PH, Glasgow JFT: Trends in the incidence of Reye's syndrome and use of aspirin. *Arch Dis Child* **65**:826, 1990.
128. DeLong GR, Glick TH: Encephalopathy of Reye's syndrome: A review of pathogenetic hypotheses. *Pediatrics* **69**:53, 1982.
129. Heubi JE, Partin JC, Partin JS, Schubert WK: Reye's syndrome: Current concepts. *Hepatology* **7**:155, 1987.
130. Tracey BM, Cheng KN, Rosankiewickz J, Stacey TE, Chalmers RA: Urinary C6-C12 dicarboxylic acylcarnitines in Reye's syndrome. *Clin Chim Acta* **175**:79, 1988.
131. Tonsgard JH: Serum dicarboxylic acids in patients with Reye's syndrome. *J Pediatr* **109**:440, 1986.
132. Corkey BE, Hale DE, Glennon MC: Relationship between unusual hepatic acylcoenzyme A profile and the pathogenesis of Reye's syndrome. *J Clin Invest* **82**:782, 1988.
133. Billette de Villemeur T, Nuttin C, Poggi F, Carré M, Bonnefont JP, Rabier D, Charpentier C, *et al.*: Metabolic investigations in Reye's syndrome and Reye-like syndrome, in Buts JP, Sokal EM (eds): *Management of Digestive and Liver Disorders in Infants and Children*. Amsterdam, Elsevier, 1993, p 615.
134. Treem WR, Witzleben CA, Piccoli DA: Medium-chain and long-chain acylCoA dehydrogenase deficiency: Clinical, pathologic and ultrastructural differentiation from Reye's syndrome. *Hepatology* **6**:1270, 1986.
135. Valdes-Dapena M: Sudden infant death syndrome: A review of the medical literature 1975–1979. *Pediatrics* **66**:597, 1980.
136. Howat AJ, Bennett MJ, Variend S, Shaw L: Deficiency of medium chain fatty acylcoenzyme A dehydrogenase presenting as the sudden infant death syndrome. *Br Med J* **288**:976, 1984.
137. Howat AJ, Bennett MJ, Variend S, Shaw L, Engel PC: Defects of metabolism of fatty acids in the sudden infant death syndrome. *Br Med J* **290**:1771, 1985.
138. Duran M, Hofkamp M, Rhead WJ, Saudubray JM, Wasman SK: Sudden child death and "healthy" affected family members with medium-chain acyl-Coenzyme A dehydrogenase deficiency. *Pediatrics* **78**:1052, 1986.
139. Roe CR, Millington DS, Maltby DA, Kinnebrew P: Recognition of medium-chain acyl-CoA dehydrogenase deficiency in asymptomatic siblings of children dying of sudden infant death or Reye-like syndromes. *J Pediatr* **108**:13, 1986.
140. Taubman B, Hale DE, Kelley RI: Familial Reye-like syndrome: A presentation of medium-chain acyl-coenzyme A dehydrogenase deficiency. *Pediatrics* **79**:382, 1987.
141. Harpey JP, Charpentier C, Coudé M, Divry P, Paturneau-Jouas M: Sudden infant death syndrome and multiple acyl-coenzyme A dehydrogenase deficiency, ethylmalonic-adipic aciduria, or systemic carnitine deficiency. *J Pediatr* **110**:881, 1987.
142. Johnston K, Newth CJ, Sheu KF, Patel MS, Heldt GP, Schmidt KA, Packman S: Central hypoventilation syndrome in pyruvate dehydrogenase complex deficiency. *Pediatrics* **74**:1034, 1984.
143. Read DTC: The etiology of the sudden infant death syndrome: Current ideas on breathing and sleep and possible links to deranged thiamine neurochemistry. *Aust NZ J Med* **8**:322, 1978.
144. Burton BK, Roach ES, Wolf B, Weissbecker F: Sudden infant death associated with biotinidase deficiency. *Pediatrics* **79**:482, 1987.
145. Emery JL, Mowat AJ, Variend S, Vawter GF: Investigation of inborn errors of metabolism in unexpected infant deaths. *Lancet* **3**:29, 1988.

146. Burchell A: Hepatic microsomal glucose-6-phosphatase system and sudden infant death syndrome. *Lancet* **2**:291, 1989.
147. Lameire N, Mussche M, Baele G, Kint J, Ringoir S: Hereditary fructose intolerance: A difficult diagnosis in the adult. *Am J Med* **65**:416, 1978.
148. Bennett MJ, Powell S: Metabolic disease and sudden, unexpected death in infancy. *Hum Pathol* **25**:742, 1994.
149. Harper RM, Bandler R: Finding the failure mechanism in sudden infant death syndrome. *Nature Med* **4**:157, 1998.
150. Rinaldo P, Stanley CA, Hsu BYL, Sanchez LA, Stern HJ: Sudden neonatal death in carnitine transporter deficiency. *J Pediatr* **131**:304, 1997.
151. Chalmers RA, Stanley CA, English N, Wigglesworth JS: Mitochondrial carnitine-acylcarnitine translocase deficiency presenting as sudden neonatal death. *J Pediatr* **131**:220, 1997.
152. Helweg-Larsen K, Garde E: Sudden natural death in childhood: A review of forensic autopsy protocols in cases of sudden death between the ages of one and five years, 1982–1991, with a special view to sudden unexplained death. *Acta Paediatr* **82**:975, 1993.
153. Cederbaum SD: SIDS and disorders of fatty acid oxidation: where do we go from here? *J Pediatr* **132**:913, 1998.
154. Boles RG, Buck EE, Blitzer MG, Platt MS, Cowan TM, Martin SK, Yoon H, *et al.*: Retrospective biochemical screening of fatty acid oxidation disorders in postmortem livers of 418 cases of sudden death in the first year of life. *J Pediatr* **132**:924, 1998.
155. Santorelli FM, Schlessel JS, Slonim AE, DiMauro S: Novel mutation in the mitochondrial DNA tRNA glycine gene associated with sudden unexpected death. *Pediatr Neurol* **15**:145, 1996.
156. Rebuffat E, Sottiaux M, Goyens P, Blum D, Vamos E, Van Vliet G, Hasaerts D, *et al.*: Sudden infant death syndrome as first expression of metabolic disorder, in Schaub J, Van Hoof F, Vis HL (eds): *Inborn Errors of Metabolism: Nestlé Nutrition Workshop Series* 24th ed. New York, Raven, 1991, p 71.
157. Martin D, Bonnet D, Sevin C, De Lonlay P, Touati G, Poggi-Travert F, Jouvet P, *et al.*: Inborn errors of fatty acid oxidation: A frequent cause of heartbeat disorders in infancy — a series of 37 patients. *Circulation* 1998. (unpublished)
158. Tein I, Di Mauro S, DeVivo DC: Recurrent childhood myoglobinuria. *Adv Pediatr* **37**:77, 1990.
159. Felig P, Wahren J: Fuel homeostasis in exercise. *N Engl J Med* **293**:1078, 1975.
160. Penn AS: Myoglobinuria, in Engel AG, Banker BQ (eds): *Myology*. New York, McGraw-Hill, 1986, p 1785.
161. Rowland LP, Di Mauro S, Layzer RB: Phosphofructokinase deficiency, in Engel AG, Banker BQ (eds): *Myology*. New York, McGraw-Hill, 1986, p 1603.
162. Miyajima H, Orii KE, Shindo Y, Hashimoto T, Shinka T, Kuhara T, Matsumoto I, *et al.*: Mitochondrial trifunctional protein deficiency associated with recurrent myoglobinuria in adolescence. *Neurology* **49**:833, 1997.
163. Vianey-Saban C, Divry P, Brivet M, Nada M, Zabot MT, Mathieu M, Roe CR: Mitochondrial very-long-chain acyl-coenzyme A dehydrogenase deficiency: Clinical characteristics and diagnostic considerations in 30 patients. *Clin Chim Acta* **269**:43, 1998.
164. Smelt AHM, Poorthuis JHM, Onkenhout W, Scholte HR, Andresen BS, van Duinen SG, Gregersen N, *et al.*: Very long chain acyl-coenzyme A dehydrogenase deficiency with adult onset. *Ann Neurol* **43**:540, 1998.
165. Pons R, Roig M, Riudor E, Ribes A, Briones P, Ortigosa L, Baldellou A, *et al.*: The clinical spectrum of long-chain 3-hydroxyacyl-CoA dehydrogenase deficiency. *Pediatr Neurol* **14**:236, 1996.
165a. Wilson CJ, Collins JE, Leonard JV: Recurrent rhabdomyolysis in a child with glutaric aciduria type I. *J Inher Metab Dis* **22**:663, 1999.
166. Tein I, DeVivo DC, Hale DE, Clarke JTR, Zinman H, Laxer R, Shore A, *et al.*: Short-chain L-3-hydroxyacyl-CoA dehydrogenase deficiency in muscle: A new cause for recurrent myoglobinuria and encephalopathy. *Ann Neurol* **30**:415, 1991.
167. Fishbein WN, Armbrustmacher VW, Griffin JL: Myoadenylate deaminase deficiency: A new disease of muscle. *Science* **200**:545, 1978.
168. Keleman J, Rice DR, Bradley WG: Familial myoadenylate deaminase deficiency and exertional myalgia. *Neurology* **32**:857, 1982.
169. Munnich A, Rötig A, Chretien D, Cormier V, Bourgeron T, Bonnefont JP, Saudubray JM, *et al.*: Clinical presentation of mitochondrial disorders in childhood. *J Inherit Metab Dis* **19**:521, 1996.
170. Larsson LE, Linderholm H, Muller R: Hereditary metabolic myopathy with paroxysmal myoglobinuria due to abnormal glycolysis. *J Neurol Neurosurg Psych* **27**:361, 1964.
171. Elpeleg ON, Saada AB, Shaag A, Glustein JZ, Rutenbeek W, Tein I, Halevy J: Lipoamide dehydrogenase deficiency: A new cause for recurrent myoglobinuria. *Muscle Nerve* **20**:238, 1997.
172. Hoffman EP, Kunkel LM, Angelini C: Improved diagnosis of Becker muscular dystrophy by dystrophin testing. *Neurology* **39**:1011, 1989.
173. Plassart E, Elbaz A, Vale-Santos J, Reboul J, Lapie P, Chauveau D, Jurkat-Rott K, *et al.*: Genetic heterogeneity in hypokalemic periodic paralysis (hypoPP). *Hum Genet* **94**:551, 1994.
174. Houten SM, Kuis W, Duran M, de Koning TJ, van Royen-Kerkhof A, Romeijn GJ, Frenkel J, *et al.*: Mutations in MVK, encoding mevalonate kinase, cause hyperimmunoglobulinaemia D and periodic fever syndrome. *Nat Genet* **22**:175, 1999.
174a. Drenth JPH, Cuisset L, Grateau G, Vasseur C, van de Velde-Visser SD, de Jong JGN, Beckmann JS, *et al.*: Mutations in the gene encoding mevalonate kinase cause hyper-IgD and periodic fever syndrome. *Nat Genet* **22**:17, 1999.
175. Kristiansson B, Stibler H, Conradi N, Eriksson BO, Ryd W: The heart and pericardial effusions in CDGS-I (carbohydrate-deficient glycoprotein syndrome type I). *J Inherit Metab Dis* **21**:112, 1998.
175a. Roe CR, Cederbaum SD, Roe DS, Mardach R, Galindo A, Sweetman L: Isolated isobutyryl-Coa dehydrogenase deficiency: an unrecognized defect in human valine metabolism. *Mol Genet Metab* **65**:264, 1998.
176. Corr PB, Creer MH, Yamada KA, Saffitz JE, Sobel BE: Prophylaxis of early ventricular fibrillation by inhibition of acylcarnitine accumulation. *J Clin Invest* **83**:927, 1989.
177. Hoffmann GF, Charpentier C, Mayatepek E, Mancini J, Leichsenring M, Gibson KM, Divry P, *et al.*: Clinical and biochemical phenotype in 11 patients with mevalonic aciduria. *Pediatrics* **91**:915, 1993.
178. Graber D, Flurin-Chollet V, Boulot J, Baunin C, Angosto MJ, Carriere JP: Coxopathie récidivante, manifestation isolée d'une maladie de Gaucher. *Arch Fr Pediatr* **48**:709, 1991.
179. Schindler D, Bishop DF, Wolfe DE, Wang AM, Egge H, Lemieux RU, Desnick RJ: A neuroaxonal dystrophy due to lysosomal alpha-N-acetylgalactosaminidase deficiency. *N Engl J Med* **320**:1735, 1989.
180. Van Diggelen OP, Schindler D, Kleijer WJ, Huijmans JGM, Galjaard H, Linden HU, Peter-Katalinic J, *et al.*: Lysosomal alpha-N-acetylgalactosaminidase deficiency. A new inherited metabolic disease. *Lancet* **2**:804, 1987.
181. Dionisi-Vici C, Ruitenbeek W, Fariello G, Bentlage HA, Wanders RJA, Schägger H, Bosman C, *et al.*: New familial mitochondrial encephalopathy with macrocephaly, cardiomyopathy, and complex I deficiency. *Ann Neurol* **42**:661, 1997.
182. Baker NS, Sarnat HB, Jack RM, Patterson K, Shaw DW, Herndon SP: D-2-Hydroxyglutaric aciduria: Hypotonia, cortical blindness, seizures, cardiomyopathy, and cylindrical spirals in skeletal muscle. *J Child Neurol* **12**:31, 1997.
183. Van der Knaap MS, Jakobs C, Hoffmann GF, Nyhan WL, Hjalmarson O, Herrin JT, Applegarth DA, *et al.*: D-2-Hydroxyglutaric aciduria: Biochemical marker or clinical disease entity? *Ann Neurol* **45**:111, 1999.
183a. Bodemer C, Rotig A, Rustin P, Cormier V, Niaudet P, Saudubray JM, Rabier D, *et al.*: Hair and skin disorders as signs of mitochondrial disease, *Pediatrics* **103**:428, 1999.
183b. Jaeken J, Imbach T, Schenk B, Smeets E, Carchon H, van Schaftingen E, Matthijs G: A newly recognized glycosylation defect with psychomotor retardation, ichthyosis and dwarfism. *J Inherit Metab Dis* **23**(Suppl I):186, 2000.
184. Smith I, Clayton BE, Wolff OH: A new variant of phenylketonuria with progressive neurological illness unresponsive to phenylalanine restriction. *Lancet* **1**:1108, 1975.
185. Stöckler S, Holzbach U, Hanefeld F, Marquardt I, Helms G, Requart M, Hänicke W, *et al.*: Creatine deficiency in the brain: A new treatable inborn error of metabolism. *Pediatr Res* **36**:409, 1994.
186. Ganesan V, Johnson A, Connelly A, Eckhardt S, Surtees RAH: Guanidinoacetate methyltransferase deficiency: New clinical features. *Pediatr Neurol* **17**:155, 1997.
187. Diogo L, Fineza I, Canha J, Borges L, Cardoso ML, Vilarinho L: Macrocephaly as the presenting feature of L-2-hydroxyglutaric aciduria in a 5-month-old boy. *J Inher Metab Dis* **19**:369, 1996.
188. Chen E, Nyhan WL, Jakobs C, Greco CM, Barkovich AJ, Cox VA, Packman S: L-2-Hydroxyglutaric aciduria: Neuropathological corre-

lations and first report of severe neurodegenerative disease and neonatal death. *J Inher Metab Dis* **19**:335, 1996.

189. Vu TH, Hoffman AR: Imprinting of the Angelman syndrome gene, UBE3A, is restricted to brain. *Nat Genet* **17**:12, 1997.
190. Rougeulle C, Glatt H, Lalande M: The Angelman syndrome candidate gene, UBE3A/E6-AP, is imprinted in brain. *Nat Genet* **17**:14, 1997.
191. Clayton-Smith J: Angelman's syndrome. *Arch Dis Child* **67**:889, 1992.
192. Boyd SG, Harden A, Patton MA: The EEG in early diagnosis of the Angelman (happy puppet) syndrome. *Eur J Pediatr* **147**:508, 1988.
193. Jaeken J, Van den Berghe G: An infantile autistic syndrome characterized by the presence of succinylpurines in body fluids. *Lancet* **2**:1058, 1984.
194. Berger R, Stoker-de Vries SA, Wadman SK, Duran M, Breemer FA, De Bree PK, Weits-Binnerts JJ, *et al.*: Dihydropyrimidine dehydrogenase deficiency leading to thymine-uraciluria: An inborn error of pyrimidine metabolism. *Clin Chim Acta* **141**:227, 1984.
195. Wilcken B, Hammond J, Berger R, Wise G, James C: Dihydropyrimidine dehydrogenase deficiency: A further case. *J Inher Metab Dis* **8**(suppl 2):115, 1985.
196. Gibson KM, Christensen E, Jakobs C, Fowler B, Clarke MA, Hammersen G, Raab K, *et al.*: The clinical phenotype of succinic semialdehyde dehydrogenase deficiency (4-hydroxybutyric aciduria): Case reports of 23 new patients. *Pediatrics* **99**:567, 1997.
197. Narayanan V, Diven W, Ahdab-Barmada M: Congenital fumarase deficiency presenting with hypotonia and areflexia. *J Child Neurol* **11**:252, 1996.
198. Straussberg R, Brand N, Gadoth N: 3-Methyl glutaconic aciduria in Iraqi Jewish children may be misdiagnosed as cerebral palsy. *Neuropediatrics* **29**:54, 1998.
199. Schulze A, Hess T, Wevers R, Mayatepek E, Bachert P, Marescau B, Knopp MV, *et al.*: Creatine deficiency syndrome caused by guanidinoacetate methyltransferase deficiency: Diagnostic tools for a new inborn error of metabolism. *J Pediatr* **131**:626, 1997.
200. Stöckler-Ipsiroglu S: Creatine deficiency syndromes: A new perspective on metabolic disorders and a diagnostic challenge. *J Pediatr* **131**:510, 1997.
201. Jaeken J, Detheux M, Van Maldergem L, Foulon M, Carchon H, Van Schaftingen E: 3-Phosphoglycerate dehydrogenase deficiency: An inborn error of serine biosynthesis. *Arch Dis Child* **74**:542, 1996.
202. Jaeken J, Detheux M, Van Maldergem L, Frijns JP, Alliet P, Foulon M, Carchon H, *et al.*: 3-Phosphoglycerate dehydrogenase deficiency and 3-phosphoserine phosphatase deficiency: Inborn errors of serine biosynthesis. *J Inher Metab Dis* **19**:223, 1996.

202a. De Koning TJ, Poll-The BT, Jaeken J: Serine deficiency disorders. *Neuropediatrics* **30**:1, 1999.

202b. Zschocke J, Ijlst L, Brand J, Lindner M, Mayatepek E, Wanders R, Hoffmann GF: 2-methyl-3-hydroxybutyryl-CoA dehydrogenase (MHBD) deficiency — A novel neurodegenerative disorder. *J Inherit Metab Dis* **23**(Suppl 1):199, 2000.

202c. Roe CR, Struys E, Kok RM, Roe DS, Harris RA, Jakobs C: Methylmalonic semialdehyde dehydrogenase deficiency: psychomotor delay and methylmalonic aciduria without metabolic decompensation. *Mol Genet Metab* **65**:35, 1998.

203. Nygaard TG, Warran SP, Levine RA, Naini AB, Chutorian AM: Dopa-responsive dystonia simulating cerebral palsy. *Pediatr Neurol* **11**:236, 1994.
204. Hyland K, Arnold LA, Courtwright KH, Summers JW: Dopa-responsive dystonia, tyrosine hydroxylase deficiency and aromatic L-amino acid decarboxylase deficiency: Multifaceted diseases that can masquerade as cerebral palsy. *Pediatr Res* **43**(suppl):319A, 1998. (Abstract)
205. Siedner G, Garcia Alvarez MB, Yeh JI, O'Driscoll KR, Klepper J, Stump TS, Wang D, *et al.*: GLUT-1 deficiency syndrome caused by haplinsufficiency of the blood-brain barrier hexose carrier. *Nat Genet* **18**:188, 1998.
206. DeVivo DC, Trifiletti RR, Jacobson RI, Ronen GM, Behmand RA, Harik SI: Defective glucose transport across the blood-brain barrier as a cause of persistent hypoglycorrhachia, seizures, and developmental delay. *N Engl J Med* **325**:703, 1991.
207. Kamoun P, Aral B, Saudubray JM: A new inherited metabolic disease: Δ′-pyrroline-5-carboxylate synthetase deficiency. *Bull Acad Nate Med* **182**:131, 1998.
208. Baumgartner M, Hu CA, Almashanu S, Steel G, Obie C, Aral B, Rabier D, *et al.*: Hyperammonemia with reduced ornithine, citrulline, arginine and proline: a new inborn error caused by a mutation in the gene encoding Δ′-pyrroline-5-carboxylate synthase. *Hum Mol Genet*, 2000. In press
209. Prasad AN, Breen JC, Ampola MG, Rosman NP: Argininemia: A treatable genetic cause of progressive spastic diplegia simulating cerebral palsy: Case reports and literature review. *J Child Neurol* **12**:301, 1997.
210. Rosenblatt DS, Aspler AL, Shevell MI, Pletcher BA, Fenton WA, Seashore MR: Clinical heterogeneity and prognosis in combined methylmalonic aciduria and homocystinuria (cblC). *J Inher Metab Dis* **20**:528, 1997.
211. Ogier de Baulny H, Gerard M, Saudubray JM, Zittoun J: Remethylation defects: Guidelines for clinical diagnosis and treatment. *Eur J Pediatr* **157**(suppl2):S77, 1998.

211a. Surtees R: Demyelination and inborn errors of the single carbon transfer pathway. *Eur J Pediatr* **157**(suppl2):S118, 1998.

211b. Van der Knaap MS, Wevers RA, Kure S, Gabreels FJM, Verhoeven NM, van Raaij-Selten B, Jaeken J: Increased cerebrospinal fluid glycine: a biochemical marker for a leukoencephalopathy with vanishing white matter. *J Child Neurol* **14**:728, 1999.

211c. Van der Knaap MS, Wevers RA, Struys EA, Verhoeven NM, Pouwels PJW, Engelke UFH, Feikema W, *et al.*: Leukoencephalopathy associated with a disturbance in the metabolism of polyols. *Ann Neurol* **46**:925, 1999.

211d. Tyni T, Pihko H: Long-chain 3-hydroxyacyl-CoA dehydrogenase deficiency. *Acta Paediatr* **88**:237, 1999.

212. Barth PG, Hoffmann GF, Jaeken J, Lehnert W, Hanefeld F, Van Gennip AH, Duran M, *et al.*: L-2-hydroxyglutaric acidemia: A novel inherited neurometabolic disease. *Ann Neurol* **32**:66, 1992.
213. Ozand PT, Gascon GG, Al Essa M, Joshi S, Al Jishi E, Bakheet S, Al Watban J, *et al.*: Biotin-responsive basal ganglia disease: a novel entity. *Brain* **121**:1267, 1998.
214. Munroe PB, Mitchison HM, O'Rawe AM, Anderson JW, Boustany RM, Lerner TJ, Taschner PEM, *et al.*: Spectrum of mutations in the Batten disease gene, CLN3. *Am J Hum Genet* **61**:310, 1997.
215. Järvelä I, Autti T, Lamminranta S, Aberg L, Raininko R, Santavuori P: Clinical and magnetic resonance imaging findings in Batten disease: Analysis of the major mutation (1.02-kb deletion). *Ann Neurol* **42**:799, 1997.

215a. Ferdinandusse S, Denis S, Clayton PT, Graham A, Rees JE, Allen JT, McLean BN, *et al.*: Mutations in the gene encoding peroxisomal α-methylacyl-Coa racemase cause adult-onset sensory motor neuropathy. *Nature Genet* **24**:188, 2000.

216. Baumann N, Federico A, Suzuki K: Late onset neurometabolic genetic disorders. *Dev Neurosci* **13**:185, 1991.
217. Schaefer J, Jackson S, Dick DJ, Turnbull DM: Trifunctional enzyme deficiency: Adult presentation of a usually fatal β-oxidation defect. *Ann Neurol* **40**:597, 1996.
218. Nievara CC, Biller J, Henderson K, Malkoff M, Sokol D, Wappner R: 3-Methylglutaconic aciduria in young adults. *Neurology* **50**(suppl4):A16, 1998. (Abstract)
219. Stockler S, Hanefeld F, Frahm J: Creatine replacement therapy in guanidinoacetate methyltransferase deficiency, a novel inborn error of metabolism. *Lancet* **348**:789, 1996.
220. Segawa M, Hosaka A, Miyagawa F, Nomura Y, Imai H: Hereditary progressive dystonia with marked diurnal fluctuation. *Adv Neurol* **14**:215, 1976.
221. Deonna T: DOPA-sensitive progressive dystonia of childhood with fluctuations of symptoms—Segawa's syndrome and possible variants. *Neuropediatrics* **17**:81, 1986.
222. Hagberg B, Kyllerman M, Steen G: Dyskinesia and dystonia in neurometabolic disorders. *Neuropediatrics* **10**:305, 1979.
223. Grant DB, Dunger DB, Smith I, Hyland K: Familial glucocorticoid deficiency with achalasia of the cardia associated with mixed neuropathy, long-tract degeneration and mild dementia. *Eur J Pediatr* **151**:85, 1992.
224. Sperling O, Boer P, Persky-Brosh S, Kanarek E, De Vries A: Altered kinetic property of erythrocyte phosphoribosylpyrophosphate synthetase in excessive purine production. *Rev Eur Etud Clin Biol* **27**:703, 1972.
225. Becker MA, Losman MJ, Rosenberg L, Mehlman I, Levinson DJ, Holmes EW: Phosphoribosylpyrophosphate synthetase superactivity: A study of five patients with catalytic defects in the enzyme. *Arthritis Rheum* **29**:880, 1986.
226. Rogers LE, Porter FS, Sidbury JD: Thiamine-responsive megaloblastic anemia. *J Pediatr* **74**:494, 1969.

227. Viana MD, Carvalho RI: Thiamine-responsive megaloblastic anemia and sensorineural deafness associated with deficient alpha-ketoglutarate dehydrogenase activity. *J Pediatr* **83**:235, 1978.
228. Abboud MR, Alexander D, Najjar SS: Diabetes mellitus, thiamine-dependent megaloblastic anemia and sensorineural deafness associated with deficient alpha-ketoglutarate dehydrogenase activity. *J Pediatr* **107**:537, 1985.
229. Mandel H, Berant M, Hazani A, Naveh Y: Thiamine-dependent beriberi in the "thiamine-responsive anemia syndrome." *N Engl J Med* **311**:836, 1984.
230. Rosskamp R: Thiamine-dependent anemia and thrombocytopenia, insulin-dependent diabetes mellitus and sensorineural deafness: Case report and review. *Klin Pädiatr* **197**:315, 1985.
231. Poggi V, Rindi G, Patrini C, De Vizio B, Longo G, Andria G: Studies on thiamine-responsive megaloblastic anemia. *Eur J Paediatr* **148**:307, 1989.
232. Porgna-Pignatti C, Marradi P, Pinelli L, Monetti N, Patrini C: Thiamine-responsive anemia in DIDMOAD syndrome. *J Pediatr* **114**:405, 1989.
233. DIDMOAD (Wolfram) syndrome. *Lancet* **1**:1075, 1986. (Editorial)
234. Poll-The BT, Saudubray JM, Ogier H, Odièvre M, Scotto J, Monnens RJA, Govaerts LCP, *et al.*: Infantile Refsum disease: An inherited peroxisomal disorder: Comparison with Zellweger syndrome and neonatal adrenoleukodystrophy. *Eur J Pediatr* **146**:477, 1987.
235. Cooper A, Hatton CE, Thornley M, Sardharwalla B: Alpha- and beta-mannosidoses. *J Inher Metab Dis* **13**:538, 1990.
236. Cheminal R, Echenne B, Bellet H, Duran M: Congenital non-progressive encephalopathy and deafness with intermittent episodes of coma and hyperkynureninuria. *J Inher Metab Dis* **19**:25, 1996.
236a. Van Coster R, de Praeter C, Gerwig G, Bause E, Nuytinck I, Vliegenthart J, Breuer W, *et al.*: A new disorder caused by defective biosynthesis of N-linked oligosaccharides due to glucosidase I deficiency. *J Inherit Metab Dis* **23**(Suppl 1):186, 2000.
237. Endres W, Shin YS: Cataract and metabolic disease. *J Inher Metab Dis* **13**:509, 1990.
238. Jakobs C, Douwes AC, Brockstedt M, Stellaard F, Endres W, Shin YS: Plasma polyol levels in patients with cataract. *J Inher Metab Dis* **13**:517, 1990.
239. Bonneau D, Winter-Fuseau I, Loiseau MN, Amati P, Berthier M, Oriot D, Beaumont C: Bilateral cataract and high serum ferritin: A new dominant genetic disorder? *J Med Genet* **32**:778, 1995.
240. Beaumont C, Leneuve P, Devaux I, Scoazec JY, Berthier M, Loiseau MN, Grandchamp B, *et al.*: Mutation in the iron responsive element of the L ferritin mRNA in a family with dominant hyperferritinaemia and cataract. *Nat Genet* **11**:444, 1995.
241. Poll-The BT, Billette de Villemeur T, Abitbol M, Dufier JL, Saudubray JM: Metabolic pigmentary retinopathies: Diagnosis and therapeutic attempts. *Eur J Pediatr* **151**:2, 1992.
242. Sewell AC: Urinary oligosaccharides, in Hommes FA (ed): *Techniques in Diagnostic Human Biochemical Genetics*. New York, Wiley-Liss, 1991, p 219.
243. Hommes FA: Determination of bound and free sialic acid in urine, in Hommes FA (ed): *Techniques in Diagnostic Human Biochemical Genetics*. New York, Wiley-Liss, 1991, p 233.
244. Wenger DA, Williams C: Screening for lysosomal disorders, in Hommes FA (ed): *Techniques in Diagnostic Human Biochemical Genetics*. New York, Wiley-Liss, 1991, p 587.
244a. Ahmad A, Amalfitano A, Chen YT, Kishnani PS, Miller C, Kelley R: Dubowitz syndrome: a defect in the cholesterol biosynthetic pathway? *Amer J Med Gen* **86**:503, 1999.
245. Woods CG: DNA repair disorders. *Arch Dis Child* **78**:178, 1998.
246. Ozand PT, Rashed M, Millington DS, Sakati N, Hazzaa S, Rahbeeni Z, Odaib AA, *et al.*: Ethylmalonic aciduria: An organic acidemia with CNS involvement and vasculopathy. *Brain Dev* **16**(suppl):12, 1994.
247. Bodemer C, De Prost Y, Bachollet B, Poggi F, Teillac D, Fraitag S, Saudubray JM: Cutaneous manifestations of methylmalonic and propionic acidaemia: A description based on 38 cases. *Br J Dermatol* **131**:93, 1994.
248. Howard R, Frieden IJ, Crawford D, McCalmont T, Levy ML, Rosenblatt DS, Sweetman L, *et al.*: Methylmalonic acidemia, cobalamin C type, presenting with cutaneous manifestations. *Arch Dermatol* **133**:1563, 1997.
249. Braverman N, Lin P, Obie C, Kelley R, Moebius F, Valle D: Mutations in the gene encoding 3 β-hydroxysteroid $\Delta 8, \Delta 7$-isomerase cause X linked dominant Conradi-Hünermann syndrome. *Nature Genet* **22**:291, 1999.
250. Neufeld EJ, Mandel H, Raz T, Szargel R, Yandava CN, Stagg A, Fauré S, *et al.*: Localization of the gene for thiamine-responsive megaloblastic anemia syndrome, on the long arm of chromosome 1, by homozygosity mapping. *Am J Hum Genet* **61**:1335, 1997.
251. Doireau V, Fenneteau O, Duval M, Perelman S, Vilmer E, Touati G, Schlegel N, *et al.*: Intolérance aux protéines dibasiques avec lysinurie: Aspect caractéristique de l'atteinte médullaire. *Arch Pédiatr* **3**:877, 1996.
252. Poll-The BT, Aicardi J, Girot R, Rosa R: Neurological findings in triose phosphate isomerase deficiency. *Ann Neurol* **17**:439, 1985.
253. Russo PA, Doyon J, Sonsino E, Ogier H, Saudubray JM: Inborn errors of cobalamin metabolism and the hemolytic uremic syndrome, in Kaplan BS, Trompeter RS, Moake JL (eds): *Hemolytic Uremic Syndrome and Thrombotic Thrombocytopenic Purpura*. New York, Marcel Dekker, 1992, p 255.
253a. Labrune P, Zittoun J, Duvaltier I, Trioche P, Marquet J, Niaudet P, Odievre M: Haemolytic uraemic syndrome and pulmonary hypertension in a patient with methionine synthase deficiency. *Eur J Pediatr* **158**:734, 1999.
253b. Marquardt T, Brune T, Luhn K, Zimmer KP, Kornber C, Fabritz L, van der Werft N, *et al.*: Leukocyte adhesion deficiency II syndrome, a generalized defect in fucose metabolism. *J Pediatr* **134**:681, 1999.
254. Clayton PT: Inborn errors of bile acid metabolism. *J Inher Metab Dis* **14**:478, 1991.
255. Mandel H, Meiron D, Schutgens RBH, Wanders RJA, Berant M: Infantile Refsum disease: Gastrointestinal presentation of a peroxisomal disorder. *J Pediatr Gastroenterol Nutr* **14**:83, 1992.
255a. Huck JH, Verhoeven NM, Roos B, Struys EA, Douwes AC, van der Knaap MS, Jakobs C: A new disorder in the pentose phosphate pathway: liver cirrhosis caused by transaldolase deficiency? *J Inherit Metab Dis* **23**(Suppl. 1):172, 2000.
256. Reinoso MA, Whitley C, Jessurun J, Schwarzenberg SJ: Lysinuric protein intolerance masquerading as celiac disease: A case report. *J Pediatr* **132**:153, 1998.
257. Odièvre M: Clinical presentation of metabolic liver disease. *J Inher Metab Dis* **14**:526, 1991.
258. Adams PC, Searle J: Neonatal hemochromatosis: A case and review of the literature. *Am J Gastroenterol* **83**:422, 1998.
259. Barnard JAI, Manci E: Idiopathic neonatal iron-storage disease. *Gastroenterology* **101**:1420, 1991.
259a. Huemer M, Huber WD, Schima W, Moeslingerr D, Holzbach U, Wevers R, Wank H, *et al.*: Budd-Chiari syndrome associated with coagulation abnormalities in a child with carbohydrate deficient glycoprotein syndrome type Ix. *J Pediatr* **136**:691, 2000.
259b. Van Maldergem L, Tuerckx D, Wanders RJ, Vianey-Saban C, van Hoof F, Martin JJ, Fourneau C, *et al.*: Long-chain 3-hydroxyacyl-CoA dehydrogenase deficiency and early-onset liver cirrhosis in two siblings. *Eur J Pediatr* **159**:108, 2000.
260. Mitzuta K, Kashimoto E, Tsutou A, Eishi Y, Takemura T, Narisawa K, Yamamura H: A new type of glycogen storage disease caused by deficiency of cardiac phosphorylase b kinase. *Biochem Biophys Res Comm* **119**:582, 1984.
261. Servidei S, Metlay LA, Chodosh J, Di Mauro S: Fatal infantile cardiopathy caused by phosphorylase b kinase deficiency. *J Pediatr* **113**:82, 1988.
262. Rustin P, Le Bidois J, Chrétien D, Bourgeron T, Piechaud JF, Rötig A, Munnich A, *et al.*: Endomyocardial biopsies for early detection of mitochondrial disorders in hypertrophic myocardiopathies. *J Pediatr* **124**:224, 1994.
263. DiRocco M, Patrini C, Rimini A, Romanengo M, Laforenza U, Borrone C, Rindi G: Infantile thiamine-responsive cardiomyopathy due to defect of thiamine transport. *J Inher Metab Dis* **19**(suppl 1):97, 1996. (Abstract)
264. Broyer M, Guillot M, Gubler MC, Habib R: Infantile cystinosis: Reappraisal of early and late symptoms. *Adv Nephrol* **10**:137, 1981.
265. Lemire J, Kaplan BS: The various renal manifestations of the nephropathic form of cystinosis. *Am J Nephrol* **4**:81, 1984.
266. Niaudet P, Rötig A: The kidney in mitochondrial cytopathies. *Kidney Int* **51**:1000, 1997.
267. Ogier H, Lombes A, Scholte HR, Poll-The BT, Fardeau M, Aicardi J, Vignes B, *et al.*: De Toni-Fanconi-Debré syndrome with Leigh syndrome revealing severe muscle cytochrome C oxidase deficiency. *J Pediatr* **112**:734, 1988.
268. Gruskin AB, Patel MS, Linshaw M, Ettenger R, Huff D, Grover W: Renal function studies and kidney pyruvate carboxylase in subacute necrotizing encephalomyopathy (Leigh's syndrome). *Pediatr Res* **7**:832, 1973.

269. Buist NRM: Is pyruvate carboxylase involved in the renal tubular reabsorption of bicarbonate? *J Inher Metab Dis* **3**:113, 1980.
270. Bergman AJ, Donckerwolcke RA, Duran M, Smeitink JAM, Mousson B, Vianey-Saban C, Poll-The BT: Rate-dependent distal renal tubular acidosis and carnitine palmitoyltransferase I deficiency. *Pediatr Res* **36**:582, 1994.
271. Walter JH, Michalski A, Wilson WM, Leonard JV, Barratt TM, Dillon MJ: Chronic renal failure in methylmalonic acidemia. *Eur J Pediatr* **148**:344, 1989.
272. Broyer M, Guesry P, Burgess EA, Charpentier C, Lemonnier A: Acidémie méthylmalonique avec néphropathie hyperuricémique. *Arch Fr Pediatr* **31**:543, 1974.
272a. Dechaux M, Touati G, Vargas Poussou R, Rabierd D, Saudubray JM: Renal function and followup in children with methylmalonic acidaemia. *J Inherit Metab Dis* **23(Suppl 1)**:97, 2000.
273. Pöge AP, Autschbach F, Korall FK, Mayatepek E: Early clinical manifestation of glutaric aciduria type I and nephrotic syndrome during the first months of life. *Acta Paediatr* **86**:1144, 1997.
273a. Moolenaar SH, Poggi-Bach J, Engelke UFH, Corstiaensen JMB, Heerschap A, de Jong JGN, Binzak BA, *et al.*: Defect in dimethylglycine dehydrogenase, a new inborn error of metabolism: NMR spectroscopy study. *Clinical Chemistry* **45**:459, 1999.
274. Tengan CH, Kiyomoto BH, Rocha MS, Tavares VLS, Gabbai AA, Moraes CT: Mitochondrial encephalomyopathy and hypoparathyroidism associated with a duplication and a deletion of mitochondrial deoxyribonucleic acid. *J Clin Endocrinol Metab* **83**:125, 1997.
275. Tyni T, Rapola J, Palotie A, Pihko H: Hypoparathyroidism in a patient with long-chain-3-hydroxyacyl-coenzyme A dehydrogenase deficiency caused by the G1528C mutation. *J Pediatr* **131**:766, 1997.
276. Dionisi-Vici C, Garavaglia B, Burlina AB, Bertini E, Saponara I, Sabetta G, Taroni F: Hypoparathyroidism in mitochondrial trifunctional protein deficiency. *J Pediatr* **129**:159, 1996.
277. North KN, Korson MS, Krawiecki N, Shoffner JM, Holm IA: Oxidative phosphorylation defect associated with primary adrenal insufficiency. *J Pediatr* **128**:688, 1996.

PART 7

CARBOHYDRATES

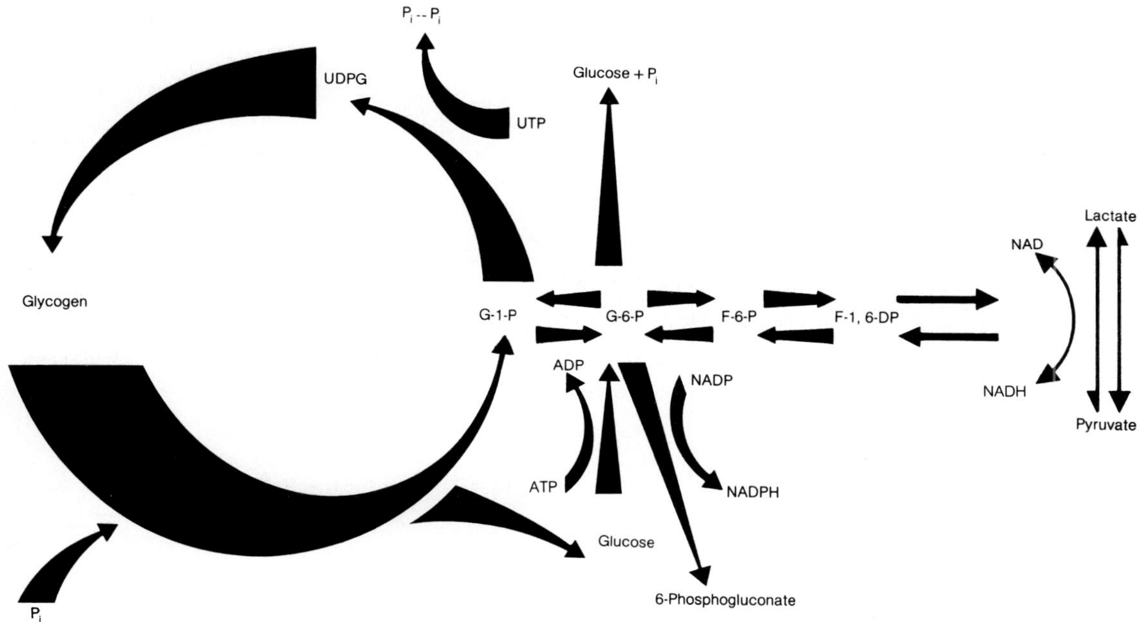

Glycogen metabolism

CHAPTER 67

β-Cell Dysfunction in Type 2 Diabetes: Pathophysiological and Genetic Bases

Steven E. Kahn ▪ Daniel Porte, Jr.

1. **β-Cell dysfunction is an integral component of the pathogenesis of the hyperglycemia of type 2 diabetes mellitus. This dysfunction is associated with decreased insulin secretion as well as a decline in the release of the newly identified β-cell secretory product islet amyloid polypeptide (IAPP or amylin). Production of these hormones by the islet β-cell requires the packaging of their respective propeptides (proinsulin and proIAPP) into secretory granules, where they undergo processing by the proprotein convertases (PC1/3 and PC2) to yield their mature products insulin and IAPP and the inert C-peptide, the latter as a byproduct of proinsulin processing. Proinsulin processing is incomplete, and small amounts of proinsulin are released along with insulin and C-peptide when secretory granule exocytosis is stimulated by glucose and nonglucose secretagogues.**
2. **Glucose-induced exocytosis of the secretory granule requires entry of glucose into the cell via the facilitative glucose transporter Glut-2 followed by its phosphorylation by glucokinase. The subsequent metabolism of glucose results in the production of ATP, which raises the ATP/ADP ratio within the cell and closes the specific ATP-sensitive potassium channel. In the case of the nonglucose secretagogues, these act via the membrane phosphodiesterases or by activation of adenylate cyclase through the guanine-nucleotide binding proteins (G-proteins). All of these mechanisms are dependent on the mobilization of calcium from the extracellular space or from intracellular stores.**
3. **Glucose directly stimulates insulin secretion in a complicated manner involving at least two phases. In addition to stimulating insulin release directly, glucose also potentiates the β-cell response to other secretagogues. The secretory responsiveness of the β-cell is also modulated by other factors including the sensitivity of the peripheral tissues to insulin. The nature of this modulation is compatible with a feedback loop such that β-cell function increases reciprocally as insulin sensitivity declines. Knowledge of the nature of this relationship is important in the interpretation of β-cell-function testing in vivo.**
4. **In type 2 diabetes, β-cell dysfunction is manifest as an absence of the early (first) phase of glucose-induced insulin and IAPP secretion and a reduction in the later (second) phase response. In addition, the ability of glucose to potentiate the β-cell's response to nonglucose secretagogues is diminished. Finally, oscillatory insulin release is also abnormal in subjects with type 2 diabetes. Many of these changes in β-cell function can be demonstrated in subjects at high risk of developing type 2 diabetes at a time when their glucose tolerance is essentially normal. These individuals include women with a history of gestational diabetes or with polycystic ovary syndrome, older subjects, first-degree relatives of individuals with type 2 diabetes, and subjects with impaired glucose tolerance (IGT).**
5. **The etiology of the β-cell dysfunction of type 2 diabetes is incompletely understood. Both genetic and environmental factors are important. Islet mass is reduced by the deposition of islet amyloid which predominantly replaces β-cells. These amyloid deposits are comprised primarily of IAPP. A single amino acid substitution in IAPP has been described in a few Japanese subjects, but this change does not explain the development of islet amyloid in the vast majority of individuals with type 2 diabetes. Thus, the mechanism(s) responsible for islet amyloid deposition do not appear to be related to an abnormality in the IAPP gene but rather to an alteration in IAPP processing and secretion by the β-cell. While β-cell mass is reduced by the deposition of islet amyloid, this is not the sole explanation for its dysfunction, as β-cell mass reduction cannot reproduce the secretory abnormalities observed in the human form of the disease.**

A list of standard abbreviations is located immediately preceding the index in each volume. Additional abbreviations used in this chapter include: AC = adenylate cyclase; ADP = adenosine diphosphate; AIRglucose = acute insulin response to glucose or first-phase insulin response; AIRmax = β-cell secretory capacity or maximal potentiating effect of glucose; ATP = adenosine triphosphate; BMI = body mass index; cAMP = cyclic adenosine monophosphate; CCK = cholecystokinin; CDX = candal-type homeodomain gene; DcoH = DcoH/pterin-4α-carbinolamine dehydratase; DAG = diacylglycerol; GAD = glutamic acid decarboxylase; GDM = gestational diabetes mellitus; GIP = glucose-dependent insulinotropic polypeptide; GIRK-1 = an inward-rectifying potassium channel; GLP = glucagon-like peptide; GLP-1 = glucagon-like peptide 1; GLUT = glucose transporter; GPD = glycerophosphate dehydrogenase; HK = hexokinase; HNF = hepatic nuclear factor; IAPP = islet amyloid polypeptide; IBS = identity by state; IDX-1 = another name for IPF-1; IFG = impaired fasting glucose; IGT = impaired glucose tolerance; IP_3 = inositol 1,4,5-triphosphate; IPF-1 = insulin promoter factor-1; IRI = immunoreactive insulin; ISL-1 = insulin gene transactivator islet; KATP = ATP-sensitive potassium channel; KCNJ-3 = an inward-rectifying potassium channel; KS = Kearns-Sayre; MELAS = mitochondrial encephalopathy, lactic acidosis, and stroke-like episodes; MIDD = maternally inherited diabetes and deafness; MODY = maturity onset diabetes of the young; OGTT = oral glucose tolerance test; PC1/3 = proconvertase 1/3; PC2 = proconvertase 2; PCO = polycystic ovarian disease; PCSK = proprotein convertase; PDX-1 = another name for IPF-1; PHHI = persistent hyperinsulinemic hyperglycemia of infancy; PI/IRI = proportion of immunoreactive insulin comprised of proinsulin; PKA = phosphokinase A; PKC = phosphokinase C; PKN = pyruvate kinase; PLC = phospholipase C; PG50 = β-cell sensitivity to glucose or half-maximal potentiation of the insulin response by glucose; SPECT = single photon emission computed tomography; STF-1 = another name for IPF-1; SU = sulfonylurea; SUR = sulfonylurea receptor; TD = transmission/disequilibrium.

6. Alterations in proinsulin release have also been documented in subjects with type 2 diabetes. Using insulin immunoassays, approximately 15 percent of circulating immunoreactive insulin is comprised of proinsulin in healthy subjects. In patients with type 2 diabetes, this proportion is approximately doubled. Milder alterations have also been demonstrated in subjects who are at high risk of developing type 2 diabetes by virtue of their having had gestational diabetes, or in subjects who subsequently progress to diabetes at a time when they were not hyperglycemic. The explanation for this disproportionate proinsulinemia is debated. It is believed to be either the result of a primary abnormality in β-cell processing or an increase in secretory demand on the β-cell, resulting in the premature release of secretory granules that have not had sufficient time to fully process the proinsulin within them. A few rare genetic alterations in the proinsulin molecule have been documented, but these are not commonly associated with diabetes.
7. Mitochondrial disease-associated syndromes: Muscle and neurologic disorders with maternal inheritance have been identified as mitochondrial gene abnormalities usually due to deletion, duplication, or mutation of specific mitochondrial genes. These are associated with diabetes mellitus and pancreatic β-cell dysfunction. Recent cases have been described with only sensineural hearing loss and diabetes. Clinically the patients present with type 2 diabetes, but progress rather rapidly to insulin dependence. Some cases have GAD and islet cell antibodies, causing confusion with late onset type 1 diabetes. Insulin resistance may occur, but is late in the clinical course. The pancreatic β-cell is assumed to fail because of its high oxidative energy requirement. Clinical heterogeneity is common, presumably because of mitochondrial heteroplasmy and/or modifying genes and environmental effects.
8. Sensorineural hearing loss and diabetes; maternally inherited diabetes and deafness (MIDD): This is the most common mitochondrial syndrome without major neurologic or muscle dysfunction, and is heterogeneous in molecular origin. The most common defect is an A3243G mutation in a tRNA. MIDD is also associated with an A8296G mutation, and occasionally with a T3721C mutation. Identical genetic lesions are clinically heterogeneous.
9. Mitochondrial encephalopathy, lactic acidosis, and stroke-like episodes (MELAS): The A3243 mutation is occasionally associated with a severe neurologic disorder (MELAS). Patients may die young due to severity of the neurologic disorder. If they survive, diabetes is common. Other genetic defects may also present with this phenotype.
10. Kearns-Sayre syndrome (KS): Ophthalmoplegia, pigmentary retinopathy, plus neurologic findings under age 20 are the primary symptoms. Patients usually have a major mitochondrial deletion. Diabetes is frequently present.
11. Maturity onset diabetes of the young (MODY): MODY is a Mendelian genetic syndrome with onset before age 25. Five causative mutations have been identified to date. More kindreds have been recognized, in whom molecular diagnosis is not yet established. To date all cases have impaired β-cell function as the primary defect. Some patients develop insulin resistance and late β-cell failure. Patients are usually lean. The disease occurs worldwide. Prevalence is estimated to be 2 to 5 percent of type 2 diabetes patients. It is characterized by mild to severe insulin deficiency, depending on the specific molecular defect.
12. MODY-1: A mutation of HNF-4α (hepatic nuclear factor-4α). The disease is highly penetrant. One-third of patients require insulin treatment. Interference with glucose metabolism is the postulated defect. Three mutations have been described to date. Most known cases occurred in one large family. Complications may occur.
13. MODY-2: A mutation in glucokinase that usually affects both hepatic and pancreatic isozymes. Hyperglycemia is mild. MODY-2 is usually treated successfully with diet or oral agents. Forty-two mutations have been described to date. Complications were infrequent. Impaired β-cell function is the predominant lesion. Insulin sensitivity is usually normal, but insensitivity may be present late.
14. MODY-3: Mutations affecting HNF-1α (hepatic nuclear factor-1α) are the most common causes of this syndrome to date. Fifty mutations have been described. It is clinically more severe than MODY-2 and progresses relatively rapidly from impaired insulin secretion to insulin deficiency requiring insulin replacement. Complications develop at rates comparable to late onset type 2 diabetes. Patients usually develop hyperglycemia after puberty. It is not associated with obesity, dyslipidemia, or hypertension. Patients may develop insulin resistance with clinical hyperglycemia.
15. Hepatocyte nuclear factor-1β (HNF-1β): Mutations in HNF-1β are rare causes of a MODY-like syndrome. Such mutations may be associated with renal dysfunction.
16. MODY-4: A mutation of insulin promoter factor-1 (IPF-1). Only one family has been identified. Onset of hyperglycemia has been variable (17 to 67 years). The course is mild, and patients respond to diet or oral-agent treatment. One homozygous null mutation resulted in pancreatic agenesis, which was replicated in a targeted deletion in the mouse.
17. Candidate genes for type 2 diabetes mellitus: A large number of candidate genes have been screened. None has been definitely shown as a significant cause of this syndrome. A review of those implicated in β-cell function includes glucokinase; GLUT-2; components of the KATP channel (SUR-1, Kir6.2); the glucagon receptor; IAPP (amylin); GIRK-1; GIRK-2; glucagon; the glucokinase regulatory protein; the glucagon-like protein-1 receptor (GLP-1R); the insulin gene transactivator islet-1 (ISL-1, 1PF-1); the caudal type homeodomain-3 gene (CDX-3); proprotein convertase-2 (PCSK-2); hexokinase-1 (HK-1); mitochondrial FAD-glycerophosphate dehydrogenase (GPD-2); β-cell pyruvate kinase (PKN); and the CCK-β receptor. Many have been associated in some populations, but not others. Some have been associated with impaired β-cell function and/or IGT, but not type 2 diabetes. Some associations are with variants in promoter regions, others with mutations, and still others with nonfunctional polymorphisms. Problems have been related to inadequate sample size, heterogenous populations, ascertainment bias, genetic heterogeneity, inadequate phenotypic characterization, and other methodologic problems. The probable polygenic nature of the syndrome, with factors involving insulin secretion and action, is also a likely contributor to this relative lack of success.
18. Genome-wide scanning: Five groups have published genome-wide scan data in part or in full using the affected sib-pair approach. Only one has reported a potentially significant association in a Mexican-American population identified in Starr County, Texas, as 2Q37 near 2DS125. No other population study has confirmed this finding and, in several studies, linkage was excluded. The locus named NIDDM-1 is under active investigation to identify a mutation. However, no known candidate genes are present in this region.

Type 2 diabetes mellitus is a disease that is now reaching epidemic proportions.[1] It has been well demonstrated that an essential component of the pathogenesis of the hyperglycemia of the syndrome is the presence of β-cell dysfunction, which results in deficient insulin secretion.[2]

It is of interest that until the development of the insulin radioimmunoassay, it was a commonly held belief that type 2 diabetes was associated with a total deficiency of insulin. Thus, it was somewhat of a surprise when the development of this methodology showed that this disorder was not associated with an absolute lack of circulating insulin.[3] The presence of insulin in the circulation was then construed to mean that β-cell dysfunction was not always a component of the disease process. However, with the development of more physiological-based testing, as well as assays for other β-cell peptides related to glucose homeostasis, namely proinsulin, C-peptide, and islet amyloid polypeptide (IAPP or amylin), the importance of alterations in β-cell function to the development of the hyperglycemia of type 2 diabetes is apparent. It is now believed that β-cell function must be deranged for hyperglycemia to develop as part of the type 2 diabetes disease process. In fact, β-cell dysfunction can often be demonstrated in subjects at high risk of subsequently developing type 2 diabetes at a time when they appear otherwise normal.[4] This chapter focuses on studies performed largely in human subjects that have been helpful in delineating the characteristics of β-cell dysfunction and the findings that are associated with the development of type 2 diabetes. Thereafter, the genetic basis for some of these alterations is addressed.

PATHOPHYSIOLOGICAL BASES OF THE β-CELL DYSFUNCTION OF TYPE 2 DIABETES

Normal β-Cell Peptide Biosynthesis and Release

The pancreatic islet comprises a group of cells that are surrounded by the pancreatic exocrine tissue. These islet cells are responsible for synthesizing and releasing a number of different hormones, the classical ones being insulin from the β-cell, glucagon from the A-cell, somatostatin from the D-cell, and the more recently recognized IAPP, also known as amylin, which is a second secretory product of the β-cell. The major secretory product of the β-cell is insulin and this peptide has been most extensively studied as a marker of β-cell function. To understand the basis for normal and abnormal β-cell function, it is important to review briefly the normal biosynthetic and secretory systems operating in the β-cell, using insulin as the prototype.

Insulin mRNA translation in the rough endoplasmic reticulum results in the production of preproinsulin, which is immediately cleaved to proinsulin and then transported from the endoplasmic reticulum to the Golgi apparatus. At the *trans*-Golgi, proinsulin is packaged along with a variety of other products into immature secretory granules. Once formed, these granules mature as they traverse the cell in the regulated secretory pathway to the cell membrane.[5] During this maturation process, each proinsulin molecule is cleaved to produce insulin and C-peptide, thus resulting in the production of equimolar quantities of these two peptides. Insulin condenses in the central portion of the granule, while C-peptide resides in the outer halo, and they remain as such until released on demand by exocytosis. The production of insulin from its precursor proinsulin is an energy-requiring process dependent on ATP and the action of specific processing enzymes (PC1/3 and PC2) that are also located within the secretory granule.[6–8] The activity of these proteases is both pH- and calcium-dependent. The processing of proinsulin to insulin in human islets takes approximately 120 min[9] and generates four conversion intermediates (des 31,32 proinsulin; split 32,33 proinsulin; des 64,65 proinsulin; and split 65,66 proinsulin) before the production of insulin and C-peptide. Insulin production usually exceeds need, so there are unreleased granules that ultimately enter the lysosomal compartment of the β-cell where they undergo crinophagy. Studies in healthy human subjects indicate that proinsulin to insulin processing in the granule is incomplete. Thus, the majority of, but not all, proinsulin is fully processed so that normal subjects release small (1 to 2 percent relative to processed insulin) quantities of proinsulin in response to β-cell stimulation.[10,11]

In addition to the regulated secretory pathway, the β-cell also releases some of its products through the constitutive secretory pathway. This pathway exists in all cell types that typically do not release products in response to secretagogues. For example, the hepatocyte releases albumin through the constitutive secretory pathway and does not exhibit regulated release of this product. The constitutive secretory pathway differs from the regulated pathway in that the rate of release through this pathway is dependent on the rate of new protein synthesis and does not require secretagogue presentation. Further, product entering this pathway is released more rapidly (approximately 20 min in the case of the β-cell) following sorting at the *trans*-Golgi. Finally, the two specific proteases responsible for proinsulin processing in the regulated pathway are not present in the constitutive pathway, so that the entire proinsulin molecule goes essentially unprocessed during its transit in this pathway and little to no insulin and C-peptide are released from it.[5,12]

The process responsible for insulin production appears to apply to the production of IAPP in the β-cell. The larger precursor proIAPP is packaged at the *trans*-Golgi into the same immature secretory granules and is processed by the same processing enzymes responsible for cleaving proinsulin to insulin.[13] These enzymes cleave proIAPP at two dibasic cleavage sites, yielding the mature IAPP peptide and N- and C-terminal flanking peptides.[14] IAPP and insulin exist in the same secretory granules;[15] thus, release of IAPP from the β-cell's regulated pathway usually occurs in parallel with insulin when the cell is acutely stimulated.[16–19] The magnitude of this response is, however, smaller than that of insulin with the molar ratio of processed IAPP to insulin released being on the order of 1 to 2 percent.[17–19] In addition to its release from the regulated pathway, IAPP exits the β-cell via the constitutive secretory pathway. Release of this peptide from the constitutive pathway can occur independently of insulin,[20] and because this default secretory pathway lacks the PC1/3 and PC2, the major secretory product is the larger precursor peptide proIAPP.[12]

Because insulin processing and release have been far more extensively studied, our understanding of β-cell dysfunction as it relates to type 2 diabetes is largely based on studies of this peptide. However, as our knowledge of IAPP production and secretion expands, the importance of this peptide to the β-cell dysfunction of type 2 diabetes is becoming clearer, especially as it relates to the development of the islet amyloid deposits that are so frequently observed in subjects with type 2 diabetes.[21,22] Where appropriate, reference is made to information that is known for both peptides; otherwise, the discussion focuses largely on insulin.

Biochemical Basis of Normal β-Cell Peptide Release

The control of granule exocytosis in the β-cell involves two critical elements: glucose and calcium (Fig. 67-1). Glucose is not only capable of stimulating secretion, but it also modulates the response to a variety of other β-cell stimuli.[2] As is the case for many endocrine cell types, calcium is essential for regulated release of granules from the cell. These effects are mediated by a number of mechanisms that are briefly discussed below.

β-cell regulation of plasma glucose in a narrow range is dependent in large part on the ability of the cell to take up and metabolize glucose. The rate-limiting portion of this process occurs at the early stages when facilitative transport of glucose occurs via the Glut-2 glucose transporter[23] followed by its phosphorylation by glucokinase.[24] The glucokinase found in the islet β-cell is limited in quantity and restricted to very few other cell types. It has a low affinity for glucose, but a high capacity for this substrate. These characteristics separate islet glucokinase from the

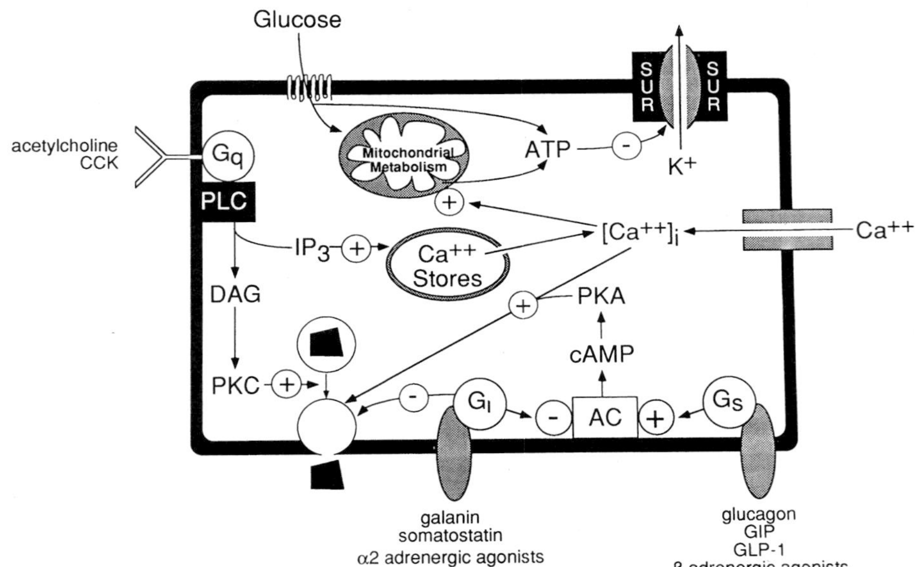

Fig. 67-1 Intracellular signal transduction pathways in the pancreatic β-cell thought to be most important in β-cell secretory granule exocytosis. Glucose is transported into the cell via the GLUT2 glucose transporter and stimulates oxidative metabolism. Other modulators (neurotransmitters and hormones) act via either adenylate cyclase (AC) or phospholipase C (PLC). G_i, G_s, and G_q are heterotrimeric GTPases that couple the action of receptor agonists to AC and PLC. Inhibitors of exocytosis through G_i interfere with cyclic adenosine monophosphate (cAMP) generation, channel activity, and exocytosis itself. Closure of the potassium channel occurs by an increase in the ATP/ADP ratio or following sulfonylurea binding to the sulfonylurea receptor (SUR), which is then followed by calcium influx through the voltage-sensitive L-type calcium channel. CCK = cholecystokinin; DAG = diacylglycerol; GIP = glucose-dependent insulinotropic polypeptide; GLP-1 = glucagon-like peptide 1; IP_3 = inositol 1,4,5-triphosphate; PKA = phosphokinase A; PKC = phosphokinase C. (*Adapted from Wollheim, Lang, and Regazzi.*[260] *Used with permission.*)

high-affinity hexokinase that is also present in the islet but at much lower concentrations. By virtue of the difference in the kinetics of glucokinase, glycolysis by the β-cell is desensitized and thus the threshold for metabolic signaling is higher in the β-cell than in other endocrine cells, which typically contain hexokinase.[25]

Oxidative metabolism of glucose is ultimately required for glucose to stimulate granule exocytosis by closing the ATP-sensitive potassium (KATP) channel.[26,27] The generation of ATP alters the ATP-ADP ratio in the cell. Binding of free ATP to a membrane-associated receptor on the cell results in the depolarization of the cell and closure of the KATP channel. This channel is usually maintained tonically open by the binding of Mg-ADP to a separate receptor on the channel.[28,29] Thus, it can be appreciated that increased glycolysis results in increased ATP generation, reduction of ADP, and closure of the KATP channel, which results in glucose-induced insulin secretion. The KATP channel consists of a specific K-channel protein (Kir 6.2),[30] which is associated with a sulfonylurea receptor protein (SUR-1) that also binds ATP and Mg-ADP.[31] Thus, its closure is also intimately involved in the action of the β-cell secretagogue sulfonylureas. Closure of the KATP channel and membrane depolarization following glucose stimulation or sulfonylurea binding opens voltage-dependent L-type calcium channels, which allows extracellular calcium to enter the intracellular pool of free calcium where it interacts with the exocytotic machinery, resulting in the fusion of the secretory granule with the plasma membrane.

Glucose is also important in regulating pathways that are not dependent on glycolysis. By providing additional phospholipid substrate or by activating membrane phosphodiesterases, glucose increases diacylglycerol (DAG) and inositol triphosphate (IP_3) concentrations. DAG remains as a component of the lipid portion of the cell membrane and, with increases in cytosolic calcium, activates protein kinase C, which, in turn, can phosphorylate β-cell proteins and affect insulin secretion. IP_3 is soluble and is released from the membrane into the cytoplasm where it interacts with the endoplasmic reticulum to release stored calcium.

Activation of adenylate cyclase by various stimuli (for example glucagon, β-adrenergic catecholamines) occurs through the guanine-nucleotide binding proteins (G-proteins). Cyclic-AMP is likely to have various sites of action which involve activation of protein kinase A. One such site may involve exocytosis because elevations of cyclic-AMP can augment β-cell granule exocytosis in the presence of basal cytosolic calcium.

Basal Secretion of the β-Cell Peptides Insulin and IAPP

Insulin and IAPP secretion under basal conditions is phasic, being secreted in a pulsatile manner. The periodicity of insulin release appears to be of two types. Both nonhuman primates[32] and normal human subjects[33,34] release insulin in distinct pulses every 10 to 14 min, superimposed on a longer rhythm of insulin secretion that has a periodicity of 105 to 120 min.[35] IAPP release has similarly been demonstrated to be phasic.[36] While it is not entirely clear whether either or both of these pulsatile rhythms result from an intrinsic β-cell pacemaker or are modulated by other factors, studies performed in vitro using islets[37] and work in vagotomized humans[38] suggest that the shorter oscillations result, at least in part, from an intra-islet pacemaker that, in turn, is influenced by vagal tone. Control of the slower ultradian oscillations may be linked to an oscillating peripheral metabolic signal or an interaction between the insulin response system and insulin's effects on circulating secretagogues, especially glucose.

Glucose Stimulation and Modulation of β-Cell Function

The importance of glucose as a β-cell stimulant following oral ingestion[39] and intravenous administration[40] has been recognized for many years. However, glucose-induced insulin and IAPP secretion is not a linear function of the glucose concentration but a complicated phenomenon comprising at least two phases[41–43] (Fig. 67-2). Both phases commence immediately following glucose administration, but the second phase is only detectable

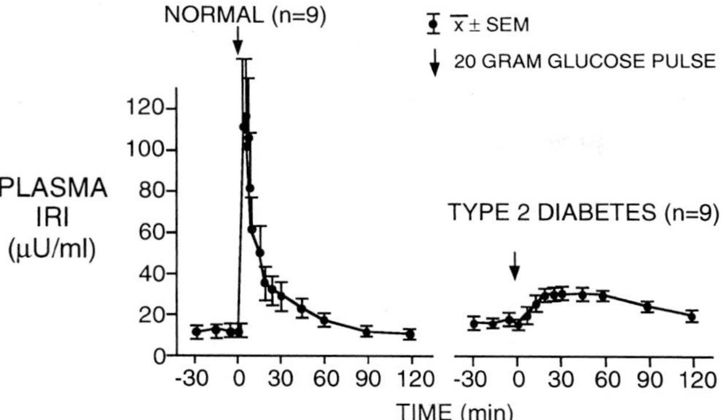

Fig. 67-2 Glucose-induced insulin secretion following an intravenous glucose injection in healthy subjects and individuals with type 2 diabetes. Plasma immunoreactive insulin (IRI) was measured over time. The first-phase response peaks between 3 and 5 min after glucose administration and lasts for approximately 10 min. The second-phase response commences about 2 min after glucose administration but is not evident until about 10 min after glucose administration. It produces a more prolonged pattern of insulin release, which increases continuously or until the stimulus stops. In contrast to first-phase insulin release, the second-phase response is highly dependent on the prestimulus glucose concentration. Because of the dependence of second-phase insulin secretion on the prestimulus plasma glucose level, subjects with type 2 diabetes have a much larger abnormality of the first-phase than second-phase response. (*Reproduced from Pfeifer, Halter, and Porte Jr.*[83] *Used with permission.*)

after the rapid first-phase response has diminished. As detailed subsequently, the glucose-stimulated response is not only related to the magnitude of the glucose stimulus,[44] but also varies based on tissue sensitivity to insulin,[45] with obesity being a major contributor to differences in insulin sensitivity.[40] The importance of insulin sensitivity as a modulator of β-cell function has been underappreciated, and has therefore been partly responsible for erroneous conclusions regarding the role of β-cell dysfunction early in the pathogenesis of type 2 diabetes. Properly interpreting β-cell function in relationship to the prevailing insulin sensitivity may prove important in identifying genes associated with β-cell dysfunction.

A number of other secretagogues, including hormones, gut peptides, and amino acids, are also potent β-cell secretagogues[46] that vary in their capability to provoke an insulin response. Glucose is an important modulator of the magnitude of the β-cell's response to these nonglucose secretagogues, a function that has been called glucose potentiation.[47] The relationship between glucose level and the degree of potentiation follows Michaelis-Menten kinetics, being nonlinear in nature and saturable, reaching a maximum at a glucose level greater than 25 mM (Fig. 67-3).[48] One can analyze this curve and characterize its components into the maximal capacity of glucose to potentiate the β-cell response to a nonglucose stimulus (AIRmax) and the plasma glucose concentration at which half-maximal potentiation of the insulin response occurs (PG50) representing the sensitivity of the system to glucose. Studies examining these two measures under a variety of different natural and experimental conditions demonstrate that they can vary independently.[49–54] Alterations in the ability of glucose to potentiate these responses have been demonstrated in high-risk subjects at a time when they have not yet developed type 2 diabetes.[55]

The ability of elevated glucose levels to enhance insulin release can also be assessed by examining insulin release following sequential clamping of the plasma glucose level at a steady state over a range of glucose concentrations. This clamping can be performed by either infusing glucose at a predetermined rate[47] or by varying the rate of glucose administration to attain a predetermined plasma glucose concentration.[48] The measure obtained in this manner is similar to the potentiation function described above, and is abnormal in subjects with type 2 diabetes or maturity onset diabetes of the young (MODY), as well as in those at high risk for either.[56–59]

Glucose is not only capable of potentiating β-cell function as described above, but it is also capable of modulating the β-cell in its response to a subsequent stimulus shortly after the glucose level has returned to basal. This effect of glucose is called priming.[60] The ability of glucose to prime the human β-cell and thus modulate its response to a subsequent glucose or nonglucose secretagogue has been studied after a glucose infusion lasting 20 h or more.[61–63] This capability of glucose to affect subsequent β-cell responses has been used as a test of β-cell integrity and is abnormal in some subjects with specific genetic β-cell defects, and in others known to have β-cell dysfunction, but in whom no specific genetic abnormality has yet been demonstrated.[56–59,64]

Insulin Sensitivity as a Modulator of β-Cell Function

Regulation of insulin secretion is not limited to glucose and other secretagogues; it is also determined by influences that are more indirect. For instance, it has long been recognized that insulin release is enhanced in obesity,[40,65,66] and this obesity-associated enhancement of insulin secretion affects both the acute responses to glucose and nonglucose secretagogues and the magnitude of oscillatory insulin release.[34,35,67] However, with the development and application of measures of insulin sensitivity, it has become apparent that it is not obesity *per se* that is responsible for the greater insulin responses, but rather that variations in insulin sensitivity are responsible for modulating β-cell function. Thus, in subjects with reduced insulin sensitivity or insulin resistance, as in obesity, pulsatile insulin release and the acute responses to glucose and nonglucose secretagogues are increased.[20] On the other hand, when insulin sensitivity is high, insulin responses are small.

We have examined the nature of the interaction between measures of β-cell function and insulin sensitivity by assessing these two variables in a large cohort of young (<45 years), apparently healthy subjects.[20] The relationship between insulin sensitivity and secretion is nonlinear in nature and best described

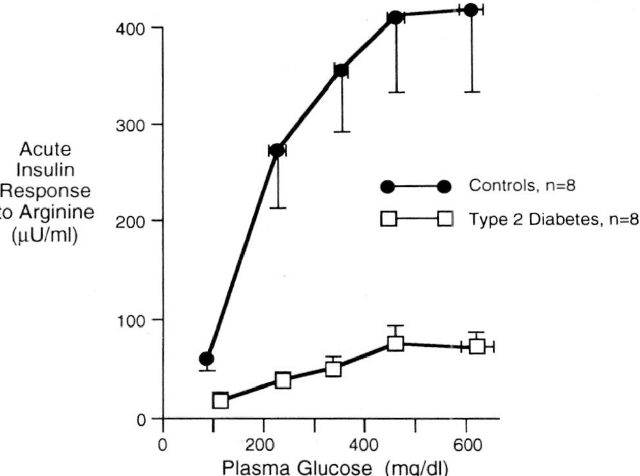

Fig. 67-3 A comparison of acute insulin responses to 5 g i.v. arginine (mean: 2- to 5-min increments) at five matched glucose levels in eight patients with type 2 diabetes mellitus and in eight controls of similar age and body weight. The slope of potentiation is the linear portion of the relation between plasma glucose (100 to 250 mg/dL) and the acute insulin response. It is much flatter in the diabetic group. The maximal insulin response, a measure of β-cell secretory capacity, is the response at a glucose concentration greater than 450 mg/dL. It is also much lower in the diabetic group. The half-maximal glucose level, a measure of β-cell sensitivity to glucose, is between 150 and 200 mg/dL and is unchanged in the diabetic group. (*Reproduced from Ward et al.*[48] *Used with permission.*)

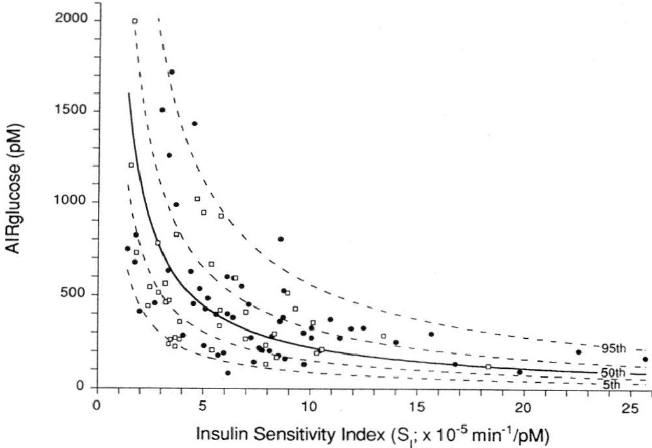

Fig. 67-4 Curvilinear relationship between insulin sensitivity (S_I) and the first-phase insulin response (AIRglucose) in 93 normal subjects (55 males, ● 38 females, ○). The relationship is best described by a hyperbolic function (i.e., insulin sensitivity × β-cell function = constant). Lines depicting the 5th, 25th, 50th, 75th, and 95th percentiles are illustrated. (*Reproduced from Kahn et al.*[45] *Used with permission.*)

by a hyperbolic function. This indicates in general that insulin sensitivity times β-cell function is a constant for a given glucose tolerance. This relationship exists whether β-cell function is examined in response to glucose (Fig. 67-4) or nonglucose stimulation. These variations of insulin release in response to changes in insulin sensitivity are the result of changes in β-cell secretory capacity (AIRmax).[45,49] This hyperbolic relationship also implies that a feedback loop governs the interaction between the β-cell and the peripheral tissues. Thus, for glucose tolerance to remain constant when insulin sensitivity changes, a proportionate reciprocal alteration in insulin output has to occur. If insulin secretion does not change appropriately, glucose tolerance will differ. When insulin secretion is impaired and cannot adapt, the superimposition of insulin resistance is associated with the development of marked hyperglycemia and clinical type 2 diabetes.

The nature of the relationship describing the interaction between insulin sensitivity and insulin secretion also has important implications for the estimation of islet function in humans. As differences in insulin sensitivity must be balanced by reciprocal changes in β-cell function in order to maintain glucose tolerance, it is apparent that, although insulin responses may be identical in two groups of subjects, if insulin sensitivity differs, then glucose tolerance differs between the two groups. Based on the concept that β-cell function should be assessed relative to insulin sensitivity, subjects at risk for developing type 2 diabetes have been shown to have poorer β-cell function than controls.[59,68–70] This is discussed in more detail later.

Islet Amyloid Polypeptide and Pathology of the Islet in Type 2 Diabetes

It has long been recognized that an anatomic abnormality consisting of amorphous deposits in the islet exists in type 2 diabetes.[21] These deposits are amyloid and their presence is associated with a reduction in islet mass.[22,71] Islet amyloid has been demonstrated in up to 90 percent of subjects with the disease in a number of different populations, but much less frequently in individuals with normal glucose tolerance.[72,73] The unique protein component of these deposits is the 37-amino-acid peptide IAPP, which is also known as amylin.[74,75] While the amino acid sequence of human IAPP is inherently amyloidogenic and forms fibrils in vitro, this is not the sole explanation for its propensity to form amyloid in vivo, as healthy subjects and individuals with type 2 diabetes produce and release identical forms of the peptide, yet healthy subjects do not usually develop islet amyloid.[72] In fact, islet amyloid deposits do not appear to result from simple overproduction because simple obesity with high plasma IAPP levels in the absence of type 2 diabetes is not associated with islet amyloid formation.[72]

IAPP is produced in the β-cell and packaged along with insulin into secretory granules so that it is released with insulin when the β-cell is stimulated to release these granules in response to glucose and nonglucose secretagogues administered orally or intravenously.[19,76,77] Because simple overproduction of IAPP is not associated with the development of islet amyloid and type 2 diabetes is associated with abnormalities in IAPP, as well as insulin release (Fig. 67-5), we hypothesize that some secretory change is involved in the pathogenesis of these deposits. However, the mechanism for the initiation of amyloid fibril formation and the ultimate development of the islet deposits is still unclear. It is possible that these changes have genetic, as well as environmental, influences. The recent description of a genetic mutation resulting in an amino acid substitution in the IAPP sequence, which was found to be associated with an earlier age of onset and more severe diabetes in Japanese subjects,[78] supports this hypothesis.

Impaired β-Cell Function in Type 2 Diabetes

Several defects in β-cell function have been demonstrated in type 2 diabetes. This disorder is characterized by the loss of the first-phase insulin response to glucose (Fig. 67-2), a defect that is

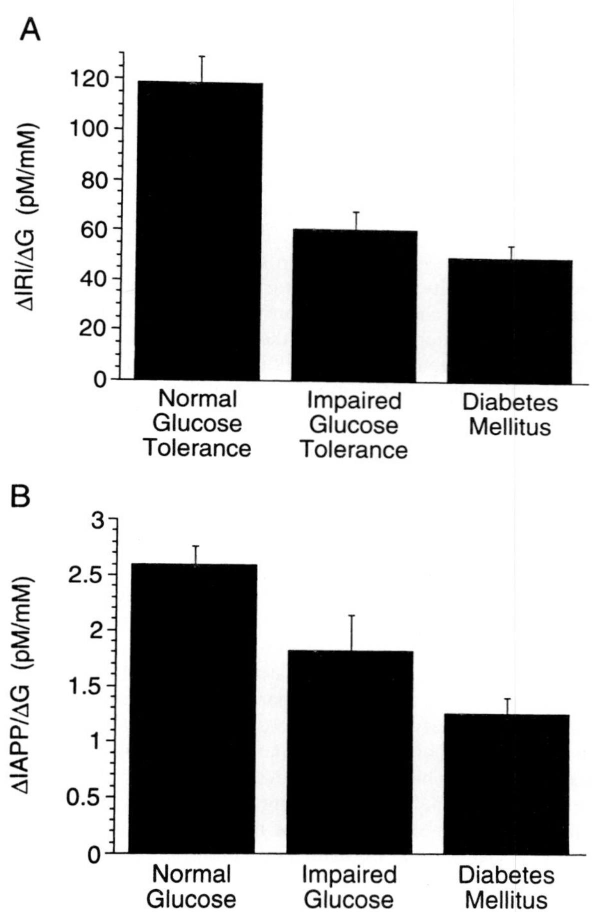

Fig. 67-5 Ratio of the incremental responses of IRI (A) (ΔIRI/ΔG) and IAPP-LI (B) (ΔIAPP/ΔG) to the incremental glucose response over the first 30 minutes following oral glucose ingestion in 94 Japanese-American subjects with varying glucose tolerance. Of the 94 subjects, 56 had normal glucose tolerance, 10 impaired glucose tolerance, and 28 type 2 diabetes. Significant decreases in both the ΔIRI/ΔG ($p < 0.0001$) and ΔIAPP-LI/ΔG ($p < 0.0001$) occurred with decreasing glucose tolerance. (*Reproduced from Kahn et al.*[18] *Used with permission.*)

observed in all individuals with fasting plasma glucose concentrations greater than 7 mM, the diagnostic level for type 2 diabetes.[65,79–81] In fact, this alteration is demonstrable in most individuals whose basal glucose concentration is above 6.4 mM,[81] a level associated with impaired glucose tolerance and impaired fasting glucose. In severely hyperglycemic type 2 diabetes subjects, the first-phase response to glucose may even be paradoxically negative.[82]

While there is an absolute deficiency of first-phase secretion in patients with type 2 diabetes who have fasting hyperglycemia, the presence of higher glucose levels in type 2 diabetes may make the second-phase response appear relatively intact. However, when glucose levels are matched in healthy and type 2 diabetes subjects, it is apparent that a second-phase secretory defect is also characteristic of type 2 diabetes.[48,79,83] Furthermore, the ability of glucose to potentiate the insulin response to nonglucose secretagogues is also reduced in proportion to fasting hyperglycemia.[47,48,84] By examination of the glucose-dose response curve of the relationship between glucose level and insulin response to a nonglucose stimulant, it is apparent that the decrease in glucose potentiation is the result of a reduction in β-cell secretory capacity (reduced AIRmax) without a change in sensitivity of the cell to glucose (unchanged PG50) (Fig. 67-3).[48] Because the reduction in AIRmax is curvilinearly proportionate to the degree of fasting hyperglycemia,[47,48,84] a relatively large decline in AIRmax (approximately 50 to 75 percent) is present at the fasting glucose level diagnostic for type 2 diabetes.

Finally, oscillatory insulin release has also been shown to be defective in type 2 diabetes, involving both the rapid[85] and the more prolonged[86] pulses. These responses are not only reduced in magnitude, but also tend to be haphazard, lacking the typical rapid and slow oscillations present in normal subjects. This early defect in pulsatility may contribute to the pathogenesis of the hyperglycemia because insulin may be more biologically effective when delivered in pulses.[87]

Many of these changes in β-cell function appear to be early events in the pathogenesis of type 2 diabetes. Thus, subjects at high risk exhibit these alterations at a time when they have essentially normal glucose tolerance. It has been argued that some of these alterations may be secondary to the hyperglycemia that occurs in the subjects with type 2 diabetes and even the mild impairments in glucose tolerance that exist in subjects at high risk. However, this does not seem to be the only explanation, as studies in which glucose has been infused for prolonged periods into healthy subjects and thus simulate the change in glucose levels seen in subjects with altered glucose metabolism have failed to reproduce the changes in β-cell function, but rather have demonstrated an effect of glucose to enhance insulin release.[61–63] This adaptation was not observed in a group of type 2 diabetes subjects made similarly hyperglycemic following a period of euglycemia.[64]

While for many years it is has been possible to measure insulin, the discovery of IAPP and the development of assay systems for this peptide were more recent. Thus, the study of its release and alterations in secretion with type 2 diabetes has not been as exhaustive. However, it is apparent from this work that IAPP responses to intravenous and oral glucose are also reduced in subjects with type 2 diabetes and that these reductions parallel those of insulin (Fig. 67-5).[17,18] Furthermore, as with insulin, individuals at high risk of developing type 2 diabetes by virtue of the fact that they have impaired glucose tolerance or are older have IAPP responses that are intermediate between those with normal glucose tolerance and type 2 diabetes (Fig. 67-5).[18,19]

Pathogenesis of the Impaired β-Cell Function of Type 2 Diabetes

Reduced pancreatic β-cell mass is a common anatomic finding in type 2 diabetes at autopsy and appears to be related, in part, to the formation of islet amyloid.[22,71,88,89] However, even a reduction of 50 percent alone does not appear sufficient to explain the observed abnormalities. This conclusion is based in part on studies performed in humans, dogs, and rats that had undergone 50 percent and 65 percent pancreatectomies.[54,90,91] In none of these studies was fasting hyperglycemia observed. Hemipancreatectomy in humans with a first-degree relative with type 1 diabetes mellitus was associated with a reduction in islet secretory responses but not hyperglycemia. The 65 percent reduction in pancreatic mass in the dogs was only associated with mild carbohydrate intolerance in the face of normal fasting glucose, and insulin concentrations and a normal or slightly reduced first-phase insulin response. However, the reduction in the magnitude of the first-phase response was not proportionate to the decrease in β-cell mass as β-cell sensitivity to glucose improved (decreased PG50), thus enhancing the efficiency of insulin release. Persistent hyperglycemia has only been found in two studies. In one study, glucose needed to be infused for weeks in partially pancreatectomized (50 to 65 percent) dogs in order to produce continuous hyperglycemia, while dogs without pancreatic mass reduction did not develop hyperglycemia.[92] In the other study, more than 90 percent of the pancreas had to be removed in rats.[93] Thus, pancreatic resection producing a similar degree of β-cell loss as observed in type 2 diabetes does not produce either the characteristic islet dysfunction seen in type 2 diabetes or persistent hyperglycemia. Therefore it appears that other factor(s) have to be involved in the production of the alterations in islet function that are observed in this disorder. It is possible that many of them have a genetic basis.

Collectively then, experimental observations based on several different approaches suggest that the β-cell dysfunction in type 2 diabetes, which has been characterized as a reduction in β-cell secretory capacity with an apparently "normal" sensitivity of the cell to the potentiating ability of glucose, results from a loss of oscillatory and reduced first-phase insulin secretion followed by progressive loss of β-cell glucose responsiveness. The early abnormalities are most likely due to some defect(s) in the glucose sensing system that precedes a reduction in β-cell mass, but this latter event contributes significantly to the reduction in second-phase insulin secretion that is observed over time.

Defective Insulin Secretion as a Preclinical Feature of Type 2 Diabetes

By studying different groups of subjects at high risk of progression to type 2 diabetes, the potential importance of impaired β-cell function to the pathophysiology of the hyperglycemia of type 2 diabetes has been demonstrated. This work has shown that reduced β-cell function is a predictor of the subsequent development of type 2 diabetes and is present at a time when the fasting plasma glucose concentration is still well within the normal range.[94,95]

Unfortunately, many early studies used the oral glucose tolerance test as a means of evaluating insulin secretion. Difficulty with the interpretation of β-cell function during this test has resulted in a long-standing debate about the importance of β-cell abnormalities in the early stages of the pathogenesis of hyperglycemia.[96] However, recent studies of body adiposity matched subjects with impaired oral glucose tolerance clearly demonstrated the presence of β-cell dysfunction in these individuals,[95,97] thereby confirming data from intravenous testing that demonstrated that defective insulin secretion is present in subjects with impaired glucose tolerance prior to the development of type 2 diabetes.[98,99]

More sophisticated testing using intravenous stimuli has also demonstrated the presence of a subclinical abnormality in β-cell function in individuals at risk of progression at a time when they did not have hyperglycemia. One example is women with a history of gestational diabetes mellitus. This condition is a forerunner for the ultimate development of type 2 diabetes in a large proportion of subjects postpartum.[100] Despite normal fasting plasma glucose levels, these women manifested a reduced first-phase insulin response (Fig. 67-6), although the magnitude of the reduction was not as great as seen in frank type 2 diabetes.[68,70] It is of further interest that this insulin secretory impairment in the women with a

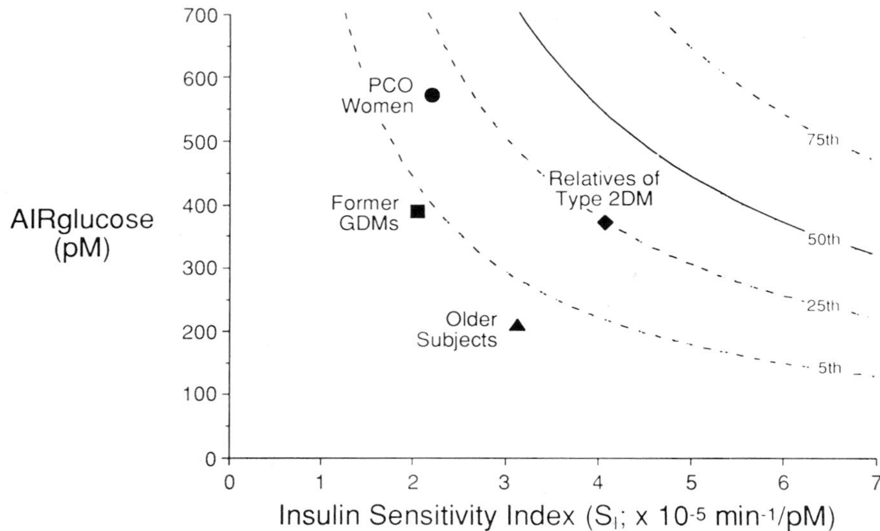

Fig. 67-6 Percentile lines for the relationship between insulin sensitivity (S_I) and the first-phase insulin response (AIRglucose) based on data from 93 normal subjects.[45] Mean data from four other studies are plotted. Thirteen healthy older subjects demonstrate that aging is associated with a reduction in β-cell function.[51] Reduced β-cell function is also manifest in 8 women with a history of gestational diabetes (GDM),[68] 11 women with polycystic ovarian disease (PCO) and a family history of type 2 diabetes,[59] and in 14 subjects with a first-degree relative with type 2 diabetes.[4] The reduction in β-cell function in these groups is compatible with their high risk of subsequently developing type 2 diabetes. (*Reproduced from Kahn.*[4] *Used with permission.*)

history of gestational diabetes was evident despite their being more insulin resistant than their matched controls. The presence of insulin resistance should, if anything, have enhanced insulin release and thus the magnitude of the impairment in β-cell function would have been greater had the relationship between insulin sensitivity and insulin secretion been considered. The importance of insulin sensitivity in the evaluation of the insulin response was also recognized by Johnston et al.[69] in studies in which they examined offspring of a pair of type 2 diabetes parents. They concluded that even though the insulin responses in these high-risk subjects were similar to those in the healthy controls, that these offspring were more insulin resistant meant that they should have been relatively hyperinsulinemic. Thus, the similarity of the responses suggested the presence of a preclinical abnormality in β-cell function characterized by a reduced ability to adapt to insulin resistance. Third, the importance of a family history of type 2 diabetes was highlighted in a recent report of β-cell function in women with polycystic ovary syndrome and a family history of type 2 diabetes.[59] These women, who are at increased risk of developing type 2 diabetes, demonstrated markedly reduced glucose-stimulated first-phase insulin responses, especially when these responses were assessed relative to their degree of insulin sensitivity (Fig. 67-6). Finally, healthy nondiabetic first-degree relatives of individuals with type 2 diabetes demonstrate broad ranges of insulin sensitivity and insulin secretion as shown in Figs. 67-6 and 67-7. However, when these two parameters are assessed in conjunction, it is apparent that many of these subjects have markedly reduced β-cell function relative to their degree of insulin sensitivity, such that their percentile ranking is in the lower range regardless of their absolute β-cell function measurement, perhaps explaining their high risk of subsequently developing type 2 diabetes.

Abnormal oscillatory insulin release is also present before the onset of clinical hyperglycemia. Normoglycemic relatives of subjects with type 2 diabetes manifest a reduction in the pulse frequency and the amplitude of the rapid oscillations.[101] The more prolonged ultradian oscillations are abnormal in individuals with impaired glucose tolerance,[98] as well as in women with polycystic ovary syndrome and a family history of type 2 diabetes.[59] In these subjects who are at high risk of progressing to type 2 diabetes, the periodicity, as well as the amplitude, of these oscillations are altered, as compared to subjects with normal glucose tolerance, with the severity of these alterations being intermediate between normal glucose tolerance and type 2 diabetes.

Studies in subjects with genetic abnormalities associated with MODY highlight the importance of β-cell dysfunction in the absence of insulin resistance to the pathogenesis of hyperglycemia. Many of the individuals that have been studied do not have sufficiently abnormal glucose tolerance to be classified as having diabetes; instead, they have glucose concentrations more commonly observed in impaired glucose tolerance,[102] a condition associated with a high rate of progression to diabetes.[103] In individuals with any one of the five defined genetic abnormalities so far described, reduced β-cell function involving glucose-induced insulin secretion and/or the more prolonged oscillations has been observed and is discussed in greater detail later.

In summary, abnormal β-cell function can be demonstrated to be a characteristic feature in subjects at high risk of subsequent development of type 2 diabetes when sophisticated tests of islet function are employed. The use of these well-characterized tests should provide vital phenotypic information for the further analysis of the genetic basis for type 2 diabetes, as is apparent

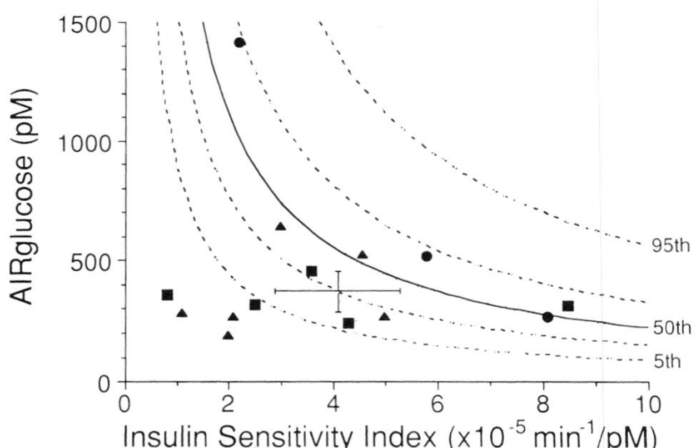

Fig. 67-7 Percentile lines for the relationship between insulin sensitivity (S_I) and the first-phase insulin response (AIRglucose) based on data from 93 normal subjects.[45] Individual data from nondiabetic first-degree relatives of individuals with type 2 diabetes are plotted. These subjects at high risk of developing type 2 diabetes have broad ranges of insulin sensitivity and insulin secretion. However, when these two parameters are assessed in conjunction, it is apparent that many of the subjects have low percentile rankings consistent with their having markedly reduced β-cell function relative to their degree of insulin sensitivity, regardless of their absolute β-cell function measurement. (*Reproduced from Kahn.*[4] *Used with permission.*)

from the examination of many of the recently described genetic abnormalities associated with hyperglycemia.

Alterations in Proinsulin in Type 2 Diabetes

Interpretation of insulin levels in humans is also complicated by the realization that the precursor peptide proinsulin and its related products are present in the circulation and that changes in the quantity of proinsulin and/or closely related precursor products released can occur. Because most insulin assays are incapable of differentiating proinsulin-like molecules from insulin, the reported levels of insulin frequently include a proportion of proinsulin and its conversion intermediates.

In healthy human subjects, approximately 15 percent of the circulating basal insulin immunoreactivity is comprised of proinsulin-like molecules, with the major form being des 31,32 proinsulin.[10,11,104,105] Because the clearance of proinsulin and its intermediates is slower than insulin, when the proportion is examined immediately following release of secretory products by the β-cell, proinsulin-like molecules can be shown to comprise less than 5 percent of total insulin immunoreactivity.[10,11] In subjects with type 2 diabetes, there is a disproportionate increase in the amount of proinsulin-like molecules (increased PI/IRI) circulating in plasma, amounting to, on average, 25 to 30 percent in the basal state.[10,104–111] This observation has been made in many population groups with type 2 diabetes including Caucasians,[10] Pima Indians,[104] Japanese-Americans,[105] and Mexican Americans,[112] and the degree of this alteration is positively related to the magnitude of the elevation in fasting glucose and negatively related to the degree of β-cell secretory capacity.[84] Again, the findings in the basal state in subjects with type 2 diabetes are mirrored following the acute release of granular content. However, the proportion of intact proinsulin and its conversion intermediates does not differ in subjects with normal glucose tolerance and those with hyperglycemia.[11] The implication of these findings is that, in type 2 diabetes, at the time of exocytosis, the granule does not contain a normal complement of fully processed product.

A few studies have examined the relationship between the PI/IRI and type 2 diabetes risk in groups recognized as having a greater chance of progressing to hyperglycemia. Thus, in women with gestational diabetes, an increased PI/IRI has been observed during pregnancy,[113] and this abnormality has also been found to be present when women with a history of gestational diabetes were studied at a time when they were not pregnant.[114] Further support for the concept that an altered PI/IRI may be a forerunner to type 2 diabetes comes from prospective studies in which Japanese-Americans, who subsequently progressed to type 2 diabetes over a 5-year follow-up period, were demonstrated to have an elevated PI/IRI prior to the development of type 2 diabetes, at a time when they had either normal or impaired glucose tolerance.[115] Finally, nondiabetic Mexican-American subjects with a parental history of diabetes have been demonstrated to have an elevated PI/IRI, again suggesting that an increased PI/IRI may be an indicator of β-cell dysfunction in high-risk subjects prior to the development of hyperglycemia.[116]

The explanation for the disproportionate proinsulinemia of type 2 diabetes and its existence in subjects at high risk of developing hyperglycemia has been and continues to be a matter of debate.[117,118] It has been suggested that the increase in proinsulin is a manifestation of an underlying abnormality in β-cell function, is a marker for progressive β-cell failure, and may be genetically determined. Others have argued that this disproportionate increase in proinsulin is simply the result of increased secretory demand on an impaired β-cell that is forced to prematurely release its secretory granules when there has been insufficient time for proinsulin processing to occur. While the etiology of the disproportionate proinsulinemia of type 2 diabetes is not clear, it does appear certain that the answer is not related to mutations of the proinsulin gene; instead, it lies within the inner machinery of the β-cell. To date, only a few, rare familial mutations resulting in amino acid substitutions in the proinsulin molecule have been identified. They are typically not associated with any change in glucose tolerance.[119–121]

GENETIC BASES OF THE β-CELL DYSFUNCTION OF TYPE 2 DIABETES

Mitochondrial Disease and Type 2 Diabetes

Muscle and neurologic disorders that were clinically classified as probable genetic syndromes with maternal inheritance have eventually been shown to be associated with a variety of deletion, duplication, and mutational alterations of specific mitochondrial genes.[122] However, it recently became apparent that some of these neuromuscular mitochondrial syndromes are also associated with type 2 diabetes mellitus, in some cases even without neuromuscular findings.[123]

Mitochondria are critically important for cellular energy production, and their number in individual cells tends to reflect the requirement for oxidative phosphorylation.[122] Thus, some cell types may have up to 1000 per cell, whereas others, such as erythrocytes, have none. Within the mitochondrial matrix there are between 2 and 10 molecules of double-stranded, circular DNA. The entire sequence of the 16,569 base pairs of human mitochondrial DNA is known. Importantly, mitochondrial DNA is largely maternally inherited because essentially all of the cytoplasm and mitochondria are derived from the ovum, and only the spermatozoal head enters to provide nuclear DNA. In addition, mitochondria may replicate independently of the cell cycle. The precise mechanisms for this are not understood. Further, mitochondrial DNA is more susceptible to mutation than nuclear DNA. This is probably because mitochondrial DNA is not protected by histones, and is exposed to a high level of free radicals produced during oxidative phosphorylation. In addition, only one of the five eukaryotic DNA polymerases, gamma, is present in mitochondria, and this polymerase is less efficient in dealing with mismatches than some of the corresponding nuclear enzymes. Because there are a number of mitochondria per cell, when a mutation occurs, the cell will have two populations of mitochondrial DNA: wild-type and mutant. This phenomenon is termed heteroplasmy. Because mitochondrial DNA may segregate unevenly to daughter cells during division, heteroplasmy ratios may vary between daughter cells. If the mutation confers a replication advantage, it may become the dominant form of mitochondrial DNA within a cell, in fact, replacing the original wild-type sequence completely (called homoplasmy). If this occurs in female germ cells, the sequence will be passed on to the offspring. If the novel mitochondrial DNA mutant is highly deleterious, it is likely to be eliminated from the mitochondrial population and homoplasmy of wild-type restored. Presumably, most mutations associated with human disease are relatively benign for replication, leading to persistent heteroplasmy. However, it is generally true that rapidly dividing cells have low levels of heteroplasmy, while slowly dividing cells will have relatively high levels of heteroplasmy, suggesting segregation of mutated mitochondrial DNA in some way. The mitochondrial genome is compact, with no introns and no large noncoding sequences. Thirteen polypeptides, which are all subunits of enzymes of oxidation phosphorylation, are encoded together with 22 transfer RNAs and 2 RNAs required for their intramitochondrial synthesis. Nuclear DNA codes for all of the other subunits of oxidative phosphorylation (the majority). Mitochondria are usually present in excess in cells, and therefore clinical features of phosphorylation deficiency only arise if the levels fall below a threshold. Thus, disordered function may not arise until the level of heteroplasmy is sufficient to interfere with normal function, which may take a considerable period of the patient's life span. Because different tissues have different requirements for oxidative phosphorylation, symptoms will vary greatly depending upon their need for this function.[124]

The first case of mitochondrial disease with diabetes, but not muscle or nerve dysfunction, except for sensorineural hearing loss, was reported in 1992,[123] with an increasing number being reported since that original report. Enough cases of mitochondrial disease with diabetes have been reported that some general comments about the clinical characteristics of these patients and their genetic and clinical heterogeneity can be made.[122,125–128] The general characteristic appears to be an early, selective impairment of insulin secretion. Later, it appears as a global metabolic dysfunction similar to classical type 2 diabetes with insulin resistance and fasting hyperglycemia. The diabetes often progresses to absolute insulin deficiency and the need for insulin treatment. In some cases, an autoantibody to glutamic acid decarboxylase (GAD)[129] or islet cells (ICA)[130] is present. Because these markers are used to assist in the diagnosis of type 1 diabetes, there can be confusion regarding classification. In a detailed analysis of subjects with a known mitochondrial defect from families with associated diabetes, those with normal glucose tolerance or impaired glucose tolerance appear to have either a failure to prime the insulin secretory response by a prolonged glucose infusion or an inability to entrain ultradian insulin secretory oscillations.[128,131] As the disease progresses, clear-cut impaired insulin secretory rates to standard glycemic challenge become obvious, and insulin resistance may develop.[132,133] Because it has been shown that pancreatic islet β-cells are dependent on mitochondrial metabolism for function,[134] and are characterized by high rates of blood flow to the organ and relatively high rates of oxygen consumption, it is assumed that they are a critical tissue, along with nerve and muscle, which depend on mitochondrial oxidative phosphorylation. Despite the general similarities that have been described, there are great differences among individuals in clinical presentation, age of onset, rate of progression, and eventual dependence on insulin. Furthermore, individuals with the same molecularly determined genetic lesion might have different clinical manifestations. Thus, several quite different clinical syndromes may have the same underlying molecular defect. Some of the heterogeneity can be explained by the heteroplasmic nature of the cellular basis for the disease and some by varying genetic backgrounds of the subjects. Thus, reasonable segregation into distinct clinical syndromes is not apparent from the studies that have been performed so far because there is not a good correlation between molecular and clinical findings in many patients.

Specific Mitochondrial Syndromes

Sensorineural Hearing Loss and Diabetes; Maternally Inherited Diabetes and Deafness (MIDD). In 1992, Ballinger et al. reported a single, large pedigree with maternally inherited diabetes and nerve deafness associated with a 10.4-kb deletion of mitochondrial DNA.[123] Further studies of this pedigree have shown the presence of a variety of mitochondrial rearrangements. It is likely that the primary defect is mitochondrial DNA duplication.[125] Shortly afterward, van den Ouweland et al. described a pedigree with maternally inherited diabetes and deafness with a heteroplasmic A to G mutation at 3243 in the $tRNA^{leu(UUR)}$ portion of the mitochondrial genome.[135] This was rather surprising because the same mutation had been previously reported to be associated with the MELAS syndrome (mitochondrial encephalopathy, lactic acidosis, and stroke-like episodes)[136] (see below). In fact, it had been noted for many years that diabetes was sometimes associated with the MELAS syndrome. However, the van den Ouwland case and pedigree, and others reported since, are only affected with diabetes and/or deafness. The clinical diagnosis of diabetes usually, but not always, precedes the detection of clinical sensorineural hearing loss, but the age of presentation in a rather large Japanese population has varied from 11 to 68 years.[137] The diabetes often progressed to sulfonylurea failure (on average, approximately 8 years after the initiation of treatment). Some cases were initially considered to represent the slow onset of type 1 diabetes because of the finding of GAD antibodies, and rather rapid progression to insulin requirement. In this population, approximately 10 percent of such clinically defined slow onset "type 1" patients selected for follow-up were in fact found to be affected by the MIDD syndrome.[137] This syndrome has been estimated to account for approximately 1.3 percent of Japanese patients[137] and 1.5 percent of unselected European cases of type 2 diabetes.[126] However, careful random population screens have not been performed. There are reports of an associated high frequency of abnormal brain MRIs and SPECT imaging studies in such patients, suggesting very subtle neurologic defects in addition to the hearing loss.[129] Occasional cases of cardiomyopathy have been reported with biopsy-proven heteroplasmy for the 3243 A to G mutation.[138] The identical clinical picture has also been associated with several other less-common mitochondrial mutations. The most common of these, the $tRNA^{(lys)}$ 8296 A to G mutation, was estimated to explain 1 percent of Japanese type 2 diabetes cases,[139] and the 3271 T to C $tRNA^{leu(UUR)}$ mutation was estimated to explain one-tenth as many.[140] An explanation for the same molecular lesion in MELAS and MIDD is not clear, nor is there a very good correlation between the degree of heteroplasmy in peripheral tissues and the severity of the diabetes mellitus, suggesting that other genes or environmental factors are important.

Mitochondrial Encephalopathy, Lactic Acidosis, and Stroke-like Episodes (MELAS). This disorder may result in hemiparesis, hemianopia, or cortical blindness. Patients may present with focal seizure. CT scanning reveals low-density areas affecting both the gray and white matter, not necessarily correlating with the clinical features. The neurologic deficit may resolve, or the patient may have recurrent attacks leading to progressive encephalopathy, disability, and death. The 3243 A to G mutation is most common, but others[136,140] have been reported. In those patients who survive long enough, diabetes is a common finding.[122,136]

Kearns-Sayre Syndrome (KS). KS describes patients who present with chronic, progressive, external ophthalmoplegia and pigmentary retinopathy under age 20, together with one or more of the following: ataxia, complete heart block, and cerebral spinal fluid protein concentration of greater than 1 g/liter. The majority of the patients have a mitochondrial DNA deletion on muscle biopsy. Diabetes is frequently associated.[122,141]

Maturity Onset Diabetes of the Young (MODY)

In the great majority of patients with type 2 diabetes, a diagnosis is made in middle age. However, a subclass of this syndrome includes families in whom diabetes can be recognized in children, adolescents, and young adults, which has been termed maturity onset diabetes of the young (MODY).[142] Autosomal dominant inheritance has been established in these families, and specific genetic mutations have been identified. It is the only form of diabetes in which a definite mode of inheritance has been determined. At least five specific mutations have been described, and this does not include all of the families in which a dominant genetic pattern with young family members has been observed. Therefore, more mutations are yet to be discovered. At times, these patients have been confused with type 1 diabetes patients because they are young, some variants lead to relatively severe forms of insulin-deficient diabetes, and by and large most patients with this syndrome are lean. However, most of the patients are ketosis resistant, and even those who need insulin for control of glycemia are not usually ketosis prone. Furthermore, because the more common variety of type 2 diabetes can also be present among these families, it is possible for an individual family member to have both syndromes, and therefore relative insulin deficiency may become more evident in the presence of insulin resistance, obesity, and, during periods of stress, infections or trauma. In some MODY patients, there may be easily diagnosable clinical hyperglycemia, but in other members of the family with the same mutation, much milder degrees of hyperglycemia or glucose intolerance may be present. In the younger members diagnosed by genetic screening, some may have normal glucose tolerance, although when studied carefully, subtle abnormalities of insulin secretion may be detectable. MODY can be suspected and recognized if type 2 diabetes occurs in three or more generations and the pattern of inheritance conforms to autosomal dominant. Families have been diagnosed in Europe, the United States, Japan, and other Asian countries. Progression of hyperglycemia tends to be relatively slow, but this depends somewhat on the specific genetic defect. Glucose tolerance may fluctuate depending on other factors, and variability among family members may be related to other genetic and environmental factors, which can fluctuate over time. In the absence of a specific molecular diagnosis, there may, therefore, be confusion between classical late onset type 2 diabetes, type 1 diabetes of slow onset, and MODY diabetes. The prevalence of MODY is still unknown, and estimates have varied widely from 2–5 percent of patients with type 2 diabetes to 10–20 percent of families with type 2 diabetes. Studies of the insulin secretory defects early in the course of the disease indicate different physiological abnormalities that distinguish among the various genetic mutations.

MODY-1. The R-W pedigree, which includes more than 360 members spanning 6 generations and 74 members with diabetes, including those with MODY, has been studied prospectively since 1958.[57,143] Linkage studies had shown that MODY-1 was linked tightly to markers in chromosome 20, band 20q-13.1, eventually describing a 13-cM interval between markers D20S169 and D20S176.[144] The demonstration in 1996 that mutations in the HNF-1α gene are the cause of MODY-3[145] led the same group to screen the HNF-4α gene for mutations in the R-W pedigree because HNF-4α had been shown to be located between the same critical markers.[146] Furthermore, it had been shown that the HNF-4α protein was a member of the steroid/thyroid hormone receptor superfamily and an upstream regulator of HNF-1α expression.[147] In the R-W pedigree with MODY-1 there was a C → T substitution in codon 130 leading to a threonine to isoleucine substitution and a C → T substitution in codon 268, which generated a nonsense mutation CAG (Gln) → TAG (AM) (Q268X). Both the isoleucine 130 and the amber mutation at codon 268 were present on the same allele.[145]

The clinical data indicate that the nonsense mutation in the HNF-4α gene is highly, but not completely, penetrant. There are some subjects who have normal glucose tolerance and some who have impaired glucose tolerance, but most have clinical hyperglycemia. However, the age of diabetes onset is variable.[145] The family is interesting because one member has type 1 diabetes and one branch has typical type 2 diabetes without the HNF-4α gene mutation. HNF-4α is most highly expressed in liver, kidney, and intestine, but is also present in pancreatic islets and insulinoma cells. It is called a hepatic nuclear factor because it is a key regulator of hepatic gene expression and a major regulator of HNF-1α, which, in turn, activates the expression of a large number of liver-specific genes. Homozygous loss of functional protein in mice leads to embryonic lethality and defects in gastrulation.[148] The phenotype of the heterozygous animals has not been described. It has been hypothesized that the mutation in the R-W family would lead to a protein unable to dimerize or bind to the recognition site and activate transcription, and that impaired function is a result of a deficiency of HNF-4α rather than a dominant negative mechanism.[145] There are no obvious hepatic, renal, or gastrointestinal defects in family members, but detailed investigations of liver glucose metabolism have not been made. Study of marker-positive family members with normal or just impaired fasting glucose shows reduced insulin secretory rates above 7 mM glucose at steady state and an impaired ability to prime β-cell function after a 42-h intravenous glucose infusion[57] (Fig. 67-8). This pattern is different from MODY-2 and MODY-3, despite the relationship between HNF-4α and HNF-1α, the genetic mutation in MODY-3.[56,58] Approximately one-third of affected individuals require insulin treatment, and patients with this form of diabetes may have microvascular complications.

Recently, a second and a third mutation have been associated with MODY-1 or early onset type 2 diabetes. One, a glutamine for glutamic acid substitution in exon 7 (E276Q),[149] was present in all of the diabetic members of the pedigree, plus two unaffected subjects, but was not detected in 75 normal control subjects or 95 U.K. Caucasian subjects with late onset type 2 diabetes. The other is an Arg127/Trp (R127W) mutation located in the T-box region that may play a role in dimerization and DNA binding.[150] None of 53 unrelated nondiabetic Japanese, 53 Chinese, 51 Caucasian, or 57 African-American subjects were positive. The mutation was present in three other members of a family with a dominant pattern of diabetes inheritance, with some members being diagnosed as young as 11 years, consistent with MODY diabetes. However, two family members with early onset disease do not have the mutation and one member with the mutation was only diagnosed at age 90 (Fig. 67-9).

Functional significance of mutations in HNF-4α has been supported by a study of a nonsense mutation (Q268X) in exon 7, the defect in the original family with MODY-1. Mutant and wild-type HNF-4α were expressed, and DNA binding and transcriptional activation studied. The HNF-4α mutant did not bind to the usual HNF-4α binding sites as a homodimer or heterodimer, and exhibited no transcriptional transactivation activity. Furthermore, it does not interact with the wild-type protein in a dominant negative fashion. In embryonic stem cells, the glucose transporter 2 (GLUT-2), the glycolytic enzymes aldolase B and

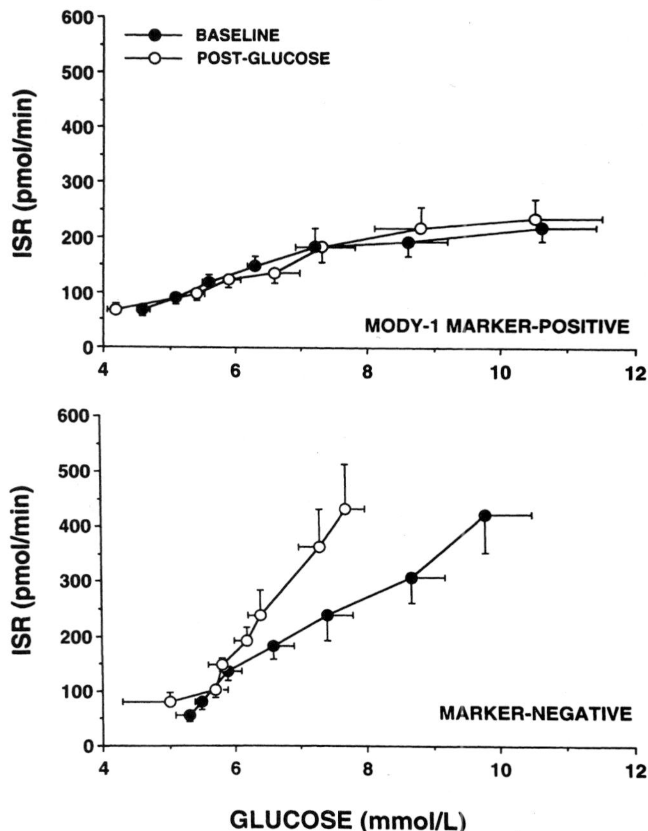

Fig. 67-8 Insulin secretion rates during graded intravenous glucose infusions administered to 6 marker-negative and 10 marker-positive subjects from the R-W MODY-1 family after an overnight fast (baseline) and after a 42-h intravenous infusion of glucose (postglucose) at a rate of 4 to 6 mg · kg^{-1} · min^{-1}. Data expressed as means ± SE. (*Reproduced from Froguel.*[154] *Used with permission.*)

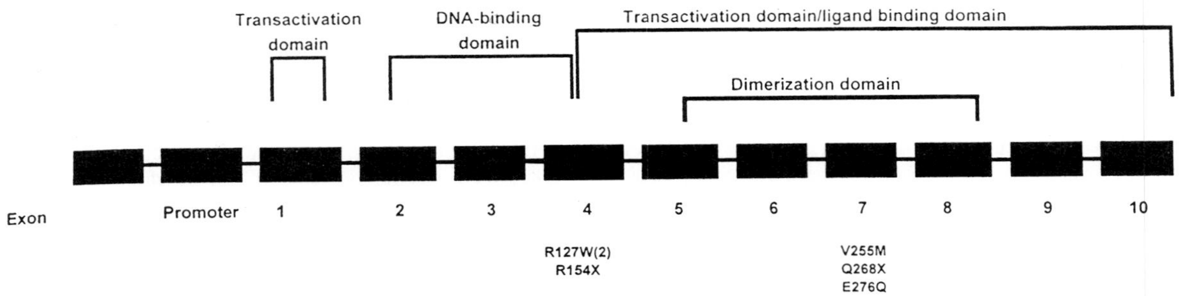

Fig. 67-9 The distribution of HNF-4α gene mutations in MODY-1 families. When there is more than one family with a mutation, the number of families is shown in parentheses. (*Reproduced from Hattersley.*[176] *Used with permission.*)

glyceraldehyde-3-phosphate dehydrogenase, and liver pyruvate kinase were down-regulated, as well as expression of the fatty acid-binding proteins and cellular retinal binding protein, indicating the likely interference with glucose metabolism in the subjects with the HNF-4α mutation to a critical level in the islet.[147]

Linkage between this region has been observed in late onset type 2 diabetes in American Caucasian sib-pairs,[151] and in the same region in French families, diagnosed under age 45, but not in African-American families.[151] Screening the French families found one to contain a mutation of HNF-4α (V391I) which cosegregated with diabetes and deficient insulin secretion.[152] However, this one family does not explain the regional linkage and an additional locus is assumed to be present in type 2 diabetes. A Val/Met 255 mutation was found in HNF-α in 4 of 477 Danish type 2 diabetes patients and in none of 217 glucose-tolerant controls.[153] A Thr/Ile130 variant was present in 4.7 percent of 509 type 2 diabetes patients compared to 1.9 percent in 230 controls. However, in a population of 942 Swedish men, the allele frequency of this variant was similar in IGT, type 2 diabetes, and controls, as it was in a population of 369 young healthy Danes. Furthermore, there is no effect of this mutation on insulin levels in either of these other two populations.[153]

MODY-2. The first candidate gene linkage in the MODY syndrome was described from a study of 16 French families with three or more generations of impaired glucose tolerance or type 2 diabetes, and was found to link to a polymorphic marker adjacent to glucokinase at chromosomal locus 7p.[102] Eventually, a large number of families with 42 different mutations involving all 10 exons in populations distributed worldwide, including all racial types (Caucasian, Black, and Asian) were described[154] (Fig. 67-10). Twenty-eight of these mutations alter the protein sequence by changing one amino acid; six transform the sequence at the site of RNA splicing of an intron-exon or exon-intron junction, resulting in the expression of an abnormal species of messenger RNA; and eight are responsible for the synthesis of a truncated protein by creating a premature termination codon by point mutation or deletion. Most are present in only single families. The enzyme is present at critical levels in the liver and the pancreas, playing an important role in hepatic glucose storage by phosphorylation of glucose after absorption and in the endocrine pancreas by coupling the first step of glucose metabolism to insulin secretion through the generation of ATP and regulation of islet potassium conductance and calcium levels.[155] The missense mutations fall into three main categories: those of conserved active site residues, which generally have a drastic effect on catalytic activity, those predicted to distort enzyme structure, which also tend to show reduced activity, and mutations of surface residues, which may reduce the stability of the structure or affect the conformational change observed on binding of glucose.[156–158] Mutations may also alter the interaction of glucokinase with other proteins such as the glucokinase regulatory protein.[159] Islet glucokinase and hepatic glucokinase are identical from exon 2 through 10, but have a variable exon 1. Most of the mutations are localized in their shared areas. In general, the degree of hyperglycemia is relatively mild, although it can be detected in children. Fewer than 50 percent of subjects present with overt diabetes, but most of the rest demonstrate impaired fasting glucose and/or glucose intolerance. Most of the individuals who carry the mutation are affected before puberty. Long-term complications are relatively unusual with this form of diabetes. Hyperglycemia remains stable, whether treated or not, for many years, and does not progress very fast as in typical type 2 late onset diabetes. Treatment with oral agents is usually satisfactory, and can lead to reasonable

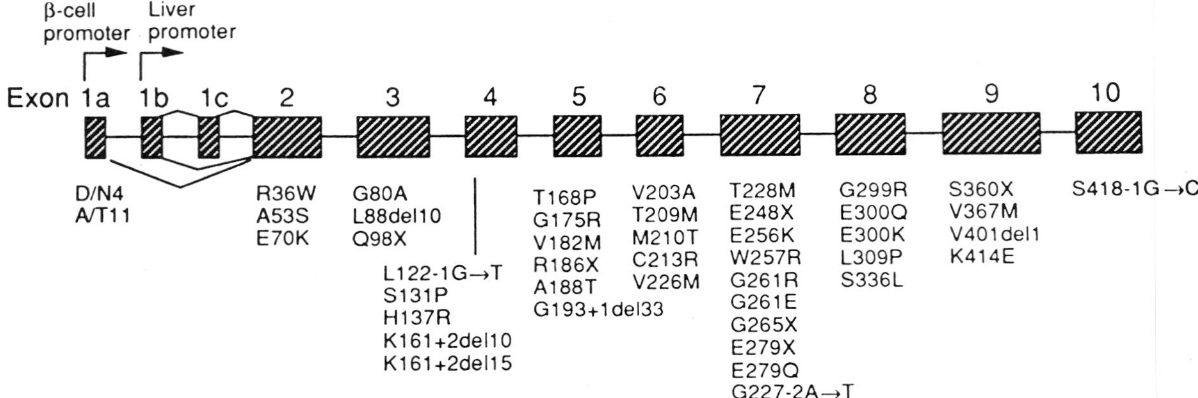

Fig. 67-10 The exon-intron organization of the human glucokinase gene and mutations found in subjects with MODY-2 diabetes. Amino acid residues are numbered as in the β-cell form of human glucokinase. The two amino acid polymorphisms in the unique NH_2-terminal portion of β-cell glucokinase that is encoded by exon 1a are indicated (Asn/Gln-4 [D/N4] and Ala/Thr-11). (*Reproduced from Froguel.*[154] *Used with permission.*)

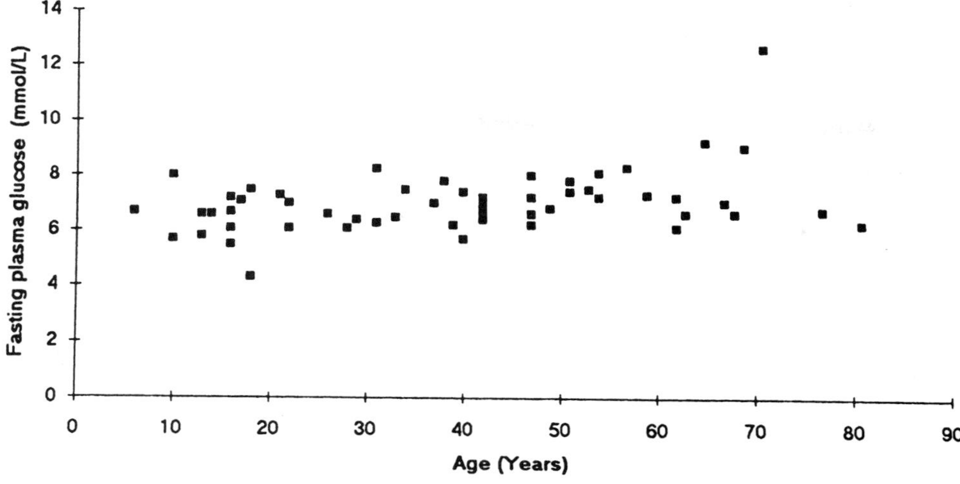

Fig. 67-11 The relationship between age and fasting plasma glucose values in MODY-2 patients with glucokinase mutations. The fasting plasma glucose values increase very gradually with age ($r = 0.41$; $p = 0.002$). (*Reproduced from Tanizawa and Chiu.*[261] *Used with permission.*)

control for many years[142,154,160,161] (Fig. 67-11). Amyloid accumulation in the pancreas was not present in the one case examined with this form of diabetes.[162] It is not known whether this is because of the intrinsic nature of the lesion or the mildness of the hyperglycemia. Obesity is not usually present and hypertension and dyslipidemia are not common. Macrovascular disease is also not common. The major observed functional defect is impaired insulin secretion, but this may not be evident unless sophisticated testing is performed. Twenty-four-hour profiles of affected subjects show persistent, round-the-clock hyperglycemia, but insulin levels are only slightly reduced after meals and are not different at baseline and between meals. However, when glucose levels are matched during continuous infusions, they are reduced by at least 50 percent. At maximal hyperglycemia (i.e., >12 to 15 mM), they are markedly reduced compared to healthy controls[56,161,163] (Fig. 67-12). Islet priming by a 42-h glucose infusion shows a response, but of smaller magnitude than controls, and is quite different than MODY-1 or MODY-3.[57,58,154] After an overnight fast, the entire curve is shifted down and to the right, whereas in MODY-1 the curve is flat throughout, just as it is in MODY-3. In MODY-2, glucose potentiation of arginine-induced insulin secretion is reduced, and glucose suppression of arginine-induced glucagon secretion is impaired.[164] Insulin sensitivity is usually normal, but may be reduced in individuals who are obese or in whom hyperglycemia is severe.[154,165] The average fasting hepatic glycogen content was similar in glucokinase-deficient subjects as compared to control subjects; it increases in both groups after meals, with a continuous pattern throughout the day. However, the net increment in hepatic glycogen content after each meal was 30 to 60 percent lower in glucokinase-deficient subjects than in control subjects. In the 4 h postbreakfast, flux through the gluconeogenesis pathway relative to the direct pathway of glycogen synthesis was higher in the glucokinase-deficient subjects than in control subjects. Thus, glucokinase-deficient subjects have decreased net accumulation of hepatic glycogen, and relatively augmented hepatic gluconeogenesis after meals.[154,166,167] This may implicate mutations in hepatic glucokinase in the pathophysiology of the syndrome. While occasional cases of late onset type 2 diabetes have been reported with mutations in glucokinase,[168] the pattern of inheritance could not be discriminated from that of MODY diabetes, and it is possible that some mutations produce a syndrome so mild that only obesity in middle age or aging-associated insulin resistance will be associated with clinical diagnosis.

MODY-3. In 1995, a genome-wide segregation analysis of highly informative microsatellite markers in 12 French families with MODY diabetes reported the localization of a gene for MODY to the long arm of chromosome 12 in 6 of 12 families.[169] Subsequently, using the identified markers D12S86 and D12S342, four more families from Denmark, the U.S., Germany, and Japan also showed linkage.[170] In 1996, Yamagata et al.

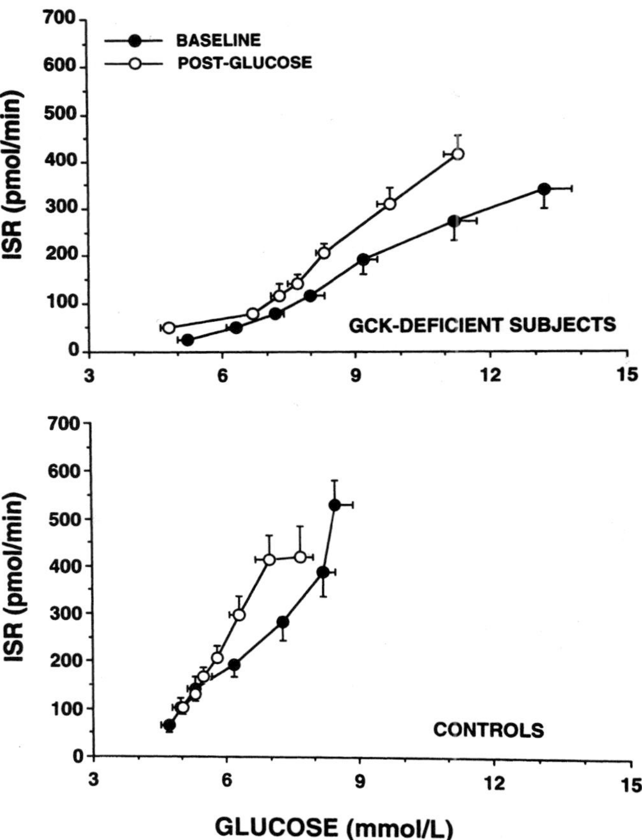

Fig. 67-12 Insulin secretion rates during graded intravenous glucose infusions administered to 6 MODY-2 subjects with glucokinase (GCK) mutations and 6 control subjects after an overnight fast (baseline) and a 42-h intravenous infusion of glucose (postglucose) at a rate of 4 to 6 mg · kg^{-1} · min^{-1}. Administration of the glucose infusion enhanced the insulin secretory response to glucose in both control and glucokinase-deficient subjects. Data are expressed as means ± SE. (*Reproduced from Froguel.*[154] *Used with permission.*)

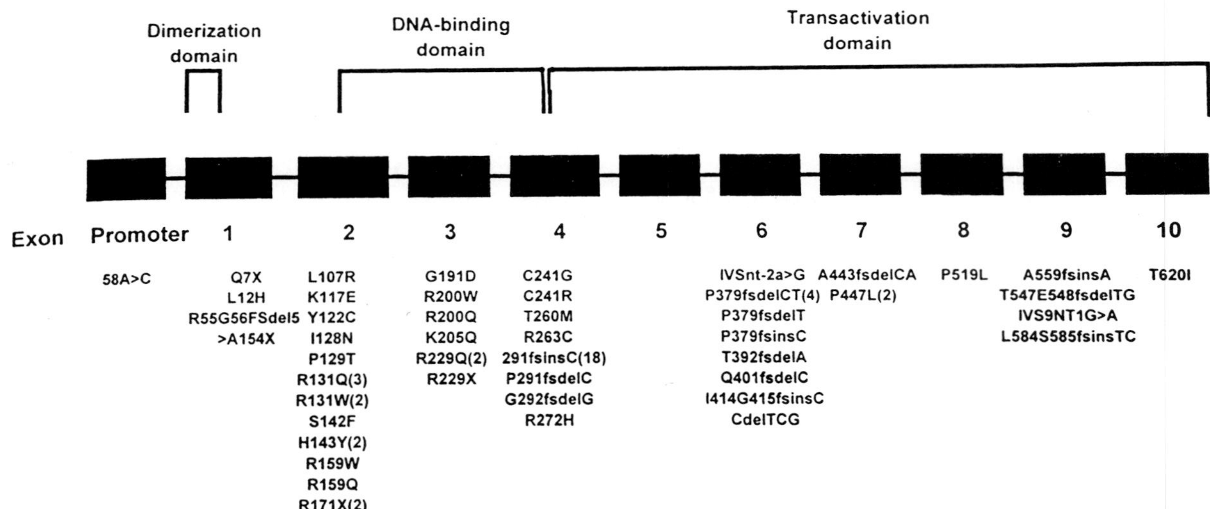

Fig. 67-13 The distribution of HNF-1α gene mutations in MODY-3 diabetes. When there is more than one family with a mutation, the number of families is shown in parentheses. (*Reproduced from Hattersley.*[176] *Used with permission.*)

showed that MODY-3 was the gene encoding the hepatocyte nuclear factor-1α, a transcription factor involved in tissue-specific regulation of liver genes that is also expressed in pancreatic islets and other tissues.[145,171] Seven different mutations in HNF-1α were found to cosegregate with MODY-3 diabetes. More than 50 different mutations have now been identified in MODY-3 families of various populations[172–176] (Fig. 67-13). An insulin secretory defect in the absence of insulin resistance was observed in diabetic and nondiabetic carriers of MODY-3 mutations with a pattern that is distinct from MODY-1 and MODY-2 during sequential glucose infusions.[58,154] In marker-positive NGT subjects, the defect was not observed at glucose levels less than 8 mM, but became evident as glucose rose above this level (Fig. 67-14). Priming was still present in nondiabetic marker-positive subjects, but not in those with clinical hyperglycemia (Fig. 67-15). This is a clinically more severe form of MODY, characterized by a high prevalence of overt diabetes, frequently treated with oral hypoglycemic agents and often requiring insulin.[177] This type of MODY diabetes resembles late onset type 2 diabetes in its natural history with patients

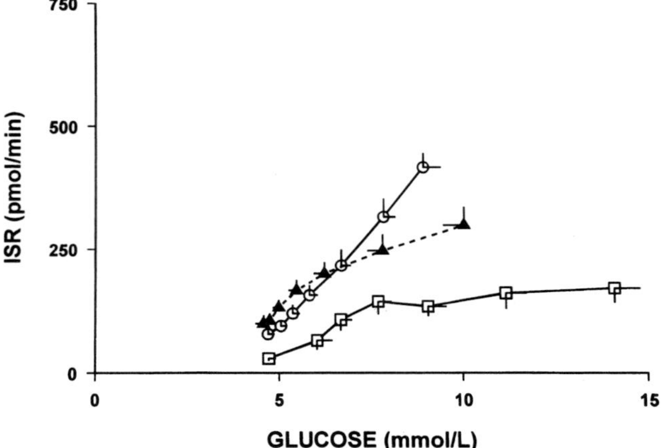

Fig. 67-14 Relationship between average plasma glucose concentrations and insulin secretion rates during the stepped glucose infusion studies in seven diabetic MODY-3 subjects (□), six nondiabetic MODY-3 subjects (▲), and six control subjects (○). The lowest glucose levels and insulin secretion rates were measured under basal conditions, and subsequent levels were obtained during glucose infusion rates of 1, 2, 3, 4, 6, and 8 mg · kg^{-1} · min^{-1}, respectively. (*Reproduced from Byrne et al.*[58] *Used with permission.*)

progressing rapidly from impaired glucose tolerance to overt hyperglycemia with severe deterioration of insulin secretion. Complications, such as proliferative retinopathy, have been observed frequently and at rates comparable to late onset type 2 diabetes. However, there is a low prevalence of obesity, dyslipidemia, and arterial hypertension, and, unlike MODY-2, clinical disease with hyperglycemia usually develops after puberty.[177] HNF-4α is a transcription factor for HNF-1α. There is a mutation in one family with MODY-3 diabetes in the conserved region of the promoter that disrupts the binding site for the transcription factor HNF-4α.[178] This finding suggests that a 50 percent reduction in HNF-1α activity can lead to β-cell dysfunction and hyperglycemia. During screening of 110 Japanese subjects with type 2 diabetes, one patient was found with a mutation at G191D who was diagnosed with hyperglycemia at 64 years of age and who had a sib who was diagnosed with hyperglycemia at 54 years of age. The older sib was known to have to have a normal oral glucose tolerance at age 62.[179] This mutation was not present in 50 unrelated subjects with normal glucose tolerance, and has not been reported in association with MODY diabetes elsewhere. While one group screened early onset Japanese subjects for mutations of this gene and found none,[180] another group reported 7 of 83 such cases (8 percent) so surveyed.[179] Thus, the true frequency of genetic variation in HNF-1α remains to be determined.

Hepatocyte Nuclear Factor-1β (HNF-1β). HNF-1β is a member of a complex transcriptional regulatory network that includes HNF-1α and HNF-4α. It is a homeodomain-containing factor that is structurally related to HNF-1α, and functions as a homodimer or a heterodimer with HNF-1α. They are stabilized by DCoH, which binds to the dimerization domains of HNF-1α and HNF-1β, forming a heterotetrameric complex that enhances transcriptional activity. Both HNF-1β and DCoH are expressed in mouse pancreatic islets. Fifty-seven unrelated Japanese subjects with MODY were screened for mutations in these genes, and one family with a nonsense mutation in codon 177 (R177X) of HNF-1β was found, which, in this family, was associated with diabetes.[181] This family is complex in that the other parent has what appears to be late onset type 2 diabetes with no mutations identified. The truncated protein when expressed does not stimulate transcription of a rat albumin promoter-linked reporter gene or inhibit the activity of wild-type HNF-1β. Further screening has been reported in additional families with early onset type 2 diabetes and a frameshift mutation, with a GG insert in exon 3 of HNF-β for Ala 263, designated A263fsinsGG, found.[182] This MODY family has

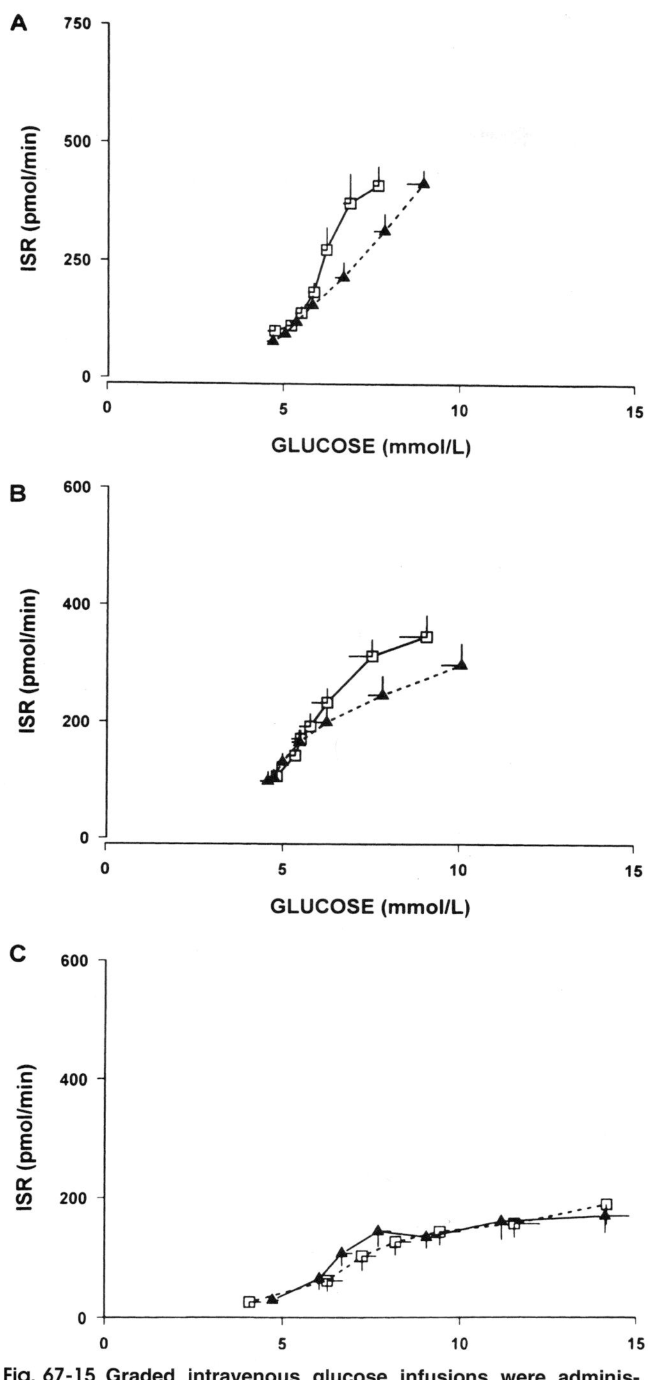

Fig. 67-15 Graded intravenous glucose infusions were administered to six control subjects (*A*), six nondiabetic MODY-3 subjects (*B*), and seven diabetic MODY-3 subjects (*C*) after an overnight fast (baseline, ▲) and after a 42-h intravenous infusion of glucose (postglucose, □) at a rate of 4 to 6 mg · kg^{-1} · min^{-1}. (*Reproduced from Byrne et al.*[58] *Used with permission.*)

diabetes in three generations with renal dysfunction consisting of renal cysts, proteinuria and/or elevated creatinine. The renal lesion may appear first. The other family also had some renal dysfunction and, therefore, this may be a feature of the HNF-1β mutation. Screening of 11 MODY families left from 58 families screened for all known MODY genes in the U.K. was negative for HNF-1β mutations. Four had sufficient numbers to eliminate linkage.[183]

MODY-4. One family with a mutation in the insulin promoter factor-1 (IPF-1) gene was recently reported.[184] IPF-1, also known as IDX-1, STF-1, and PDX-1, regulates both early pancreatic development and the expression of key endocrine β-cell-specific genes, most notably insulin. Targeted homozygous destruction in mice results in pancreatic agenesis.[185] Family studies stimulated by a case with a homozygous inactive mutation in exon 1 of the coding sequence with pancreatic agenesis and neonatal diabetes[186] found a high prevalence of diabetes mellitus with age-dependent autosomal dominant transmission in six generations.[184] Average age of onset of hyperglycemia is 35 years (range: 17 to 67 years). The hyperglycemia is mild, is treated with diet or oral hypoglycemic agents, and clinically resembles MODY diabetes. The association between the mutation and the clinical syndrome was so strong, that the authors suggested the term MODY-4. Screening of 67 Japanese subjects with type 2 diabetes for polymorphisms of exon 2 revealed no mutations.[187]

Genetic Studies of Late Onset Type 2 Diabetes Mellitus

While the pathophysiology of hyperglycemia and type 2 diabetes mellitus is clear, understanding the etiology of the underlying defects at a molecular level and the identification of the genetic defects associated with typical late onset type 2 diabetes have been difficult. This is a complex metabolic disorder with both insulin resistance and impaired β-cell function,[188,189] and both of these defects have primary (i.e., genetic), environmental (e.g., dietary), and secondary (i.e., hyperglycemia-induced) causes. Thus, in the full-blown clinical syndrome, all patients have both findings, and both contribute in varying degrees to the severity of the hyperglycemia. A variety of metabolic studies have demonstrated impaired β-cell function and insulin resistance in family members of subjects with type 2 diabetes,[188,189] and in identical twins of type 2 diabetic patients with normal glucose tolerance, who have a high likelihood of developing the syndrome.[190] It is still not clear in any individual patient, which of these two disorders began first, how much is related to the environment and to genetic dysfunction, and how much of the full-blown syndrome is secondary to the hyperglycemia. There is evidence that both β-cell function[191] and insulin sensitivity[192] are familial traits in certain populations, and abnormalities of insulin secretion and action have been reported to predate the onset of glucose intolerance.[188,189] Nevertheless, there remain many uncertainties regarding progression from normal to impaired glucose tolerance and eventually to fasting hyperglycemia and clinical type 2 diabetes mellitus. For this reason, it has been difficult to identify the genetic defects that are presumed to underlie much of the risk of type 2 diabetes. The most convincing evidence of a genetic factor is derived from twin studies.[193–197] Although there is some variation in reported risk when comparing monozygotic and dizygotic twins, concordance is always higher for monozygotic twins than dizygotic twins. Initial studies reported almost 100 percent concordance in monozygotic twins and roughly 50 percent in dizygotic twins, but ascertainment bias was believed to be a serious problem in the generation of this data. More recent studies suggest that concordance is more likely to be in the 60 to 70 percent range in monozygotic twins and in the 10 to 20 percent range in dizygotic twins. Thus, the relative risk of developing type 2 diabetes in the sib of an identical twin with the disease was increased 2 to 3.4 times compared with nonidentical twins, and this increases with age. Further evidence for genetic factors is the familial aggregation of type 2 diabetes in a variety of ethnic groups and a variation of prevalence among these groups, ranging from as high as 80 percent in subjects such as the Pima Indians whose parents both had early onset diabetes, to the estimates of approximately 5 percent in Caucasian-Americans, 10 percent in African-Americans, 25 percent in Mexican-Americans, and 35 percent in Pima Indians overall.[198] The history of metabolic studies of insulin resistance and insulin secretion in relatives of patients with type 2 diabetes is complex. Suffice it to say that one can quote a 1989 study that found impaired insulin secretion and insulin resistance to be present in impaired glucose tolerance, but that insulin resistance was the only abnormality present in the normal glucose-tolerant first-degree relatives of patients with type 2 diabetes, although this was not universal.[199] Similarly, long-term follow-up of 155 normal glucose-tolerant offspring of two parents with type 2 diabetes, compared with 186 normal control subjects followed for an average of 13 years, demonstrated low glucose clearance and high serum-insulin levels (a marker for insulin resistance) as independent risk factors for the development of diabetes among these offspring.[200] A 1992 study of Mexican-American children of type 2 diabetic parents with normal glucose tolerance demonstrated basal hyperinsulinemia and hyperinsulinemic responses to intravenous glucose challenge during a hyperinsulinemic glucose clamp, consistent with insulin resistance prior to the development of hyperglycemia.[201] However, in 1995, studies of identical Caucasian twin pairs from Denmark who were discordant for type 2 diabetes demonstrated a significant impairment of insulin secretion and insulin action of roughly equal severity in normal glucose-tolerant twins, with both defects more severe in the twins with overt hyperglycemia.[190] And in 1995, a test of 100 subjects of European ancestry with normal glucose tolerance with or without a first-degree type 2 relative, demonstrated a high proportion of first-degree affected relatives with impairment of either first, second, or both phases of insulin secretion, and only rare subjects with impaired insulin action.[202] A similar study of lean first-degree relatives drawn from newspaper advertisements in New Haven, Connecticut, also supported both possibilities with the suggestion that insulin resistance was present in many, but that impaired insulin secretion was present in those with the greatest degrees of insulin resistance.[203] In a subsequent study, glucose-tolerant Caucasian first-degree relatives were compared with normal glucose-tolerant control subjects using a glucose clamp and OGTT.[204] First-phase glucose-induced insulin secretion was not different, but second-phase was reduced. The insulin sensitivity index was not different. However, a different study in Caucasians found hyperinsulinemia independent of obesity in first-degree relatives during a 75 g OGTT.[205] In the same year, another study of offspring of type 2 diabetics was reported.[206] Twenty offspring from parents with low basal C-peptide levels were compared with 18 offspring of high-basal C-peptide parents and 14 controls without a family history. The frequency of IGT was 50 percent in both offspring groups. Acute insulin responses were low in the offspring with low-basal C-peptide (insulin-sensitive) parents and insulin resistance was found-during a euglycemic clamp in the offspring from the high-basal C-peptide (insulin-resistant) parents. The authors conclude that both insulin resistance and impaired β-cell function are independent heritable contributors to type 2 diabetes risk. Thus, the studies continue to show first-degree relatives and monozygotic twins to be at risk and to have abnormalities in insulin secretion and sensitivity, but the type of abnormality and the degree of abnormality appears to vary from study to study, perhaps depending on the population studied, including its age, sex, and racial composition.

For this reason, genetic screening has used diverse phenotypes including clinical diabetes mellitus and specific physiological variables for the testing of candidate genes in both the insulin sensitivity and the insulin secretion pathways as potential contributors to the syndrome. This requires careful and complete phenotyping, which may be difficult and expensive. In addition, positional cloning has been attempted after locating susceptibility genes from either a genome scan using random markers, or discrete regions of a chromosome that are strongly associated with the disease, or one of the physiological markers believed to contribute to the etiology of the disease. The generally disappointing results have now led to the common belief that type 2 diabetes is a polygenic disorder which probably results from several combined gene defects that interact with environmental factors to produce the eventual clinical syndrome. This being the case, it's perhaps not surprising that none of these genetic approaches has been particularly successful in unraveling the important, underlying etiologic factors in late onset type 2 diabetes mellitus. Nevertheless, success using the MODY phenotype has encouraged continuing efforts using more powerful techniques. To date, the study of candidate genes is the most commonly used approach. The reasons for candidacy are numerous. We discuss only those related to insulin secretion. All of the MODY genes discovered so far have been found to result from heterozygous mutations that impair insulin secretion. Two possible approaches are available.[207,208] One relies on sib-pair analysis with the expectation that sharing among sibs is greater than chance for genetic markers associated with diabetes, insulin resistance, or islet dysfunction. As only affected sibs are analyzed, no assumptions are necessary about the mode of inheritance, and defining the nonaffected phenotype is avoided. However, a high degree of heterozygosity is required to optimize sib-pair analysis and identification of those affected is arbitrary, being based on a continuous physiological variable. Identity by descent or identity by state can be utilized. Considering the age of onset of type 2 diabetes, identity by state is the most frequent method, but this requires determination of the frequency of the alleles in an appropriately matched population, and may require a large number of pairs. Until recently, candidate genes have usually been evaluated in populations of unrelated individuals. These studies require careful clinical and metabolic phenotyping in well-matched case and control populations, especially regarding ethnicity and differences in genetic background. Today, many genes have been cloned and sequenced using molecular scanning methods designed to detect changes in nucleotide sequence in fragments of DNA, such as single-strand conformation polymorphism (SSCP) or heteroduplex analysis. An association between a mutation or polymorphism with β-cell dysfunction, impaired glucose tolerance, or diabetes can then be analyzed.

Candidate Genes

Glucokinase. All of the known MODY genes have been considered as possible candidates for gene defects in late onset type 2 diabetes mellitus. Positive associations between type 2 diabetes and particular glucokinase polymorphisms were originally observed in American Blacks and Mauritian Creoles,[209,210] suggesting that the glucokinase locus might be implicated in diabetes in these populations. However, mutations in the coding region were not found. Variants were observed in the liver promoter at -258 and the islet β-cell promoter at -30. A block transversion mutation near this latter region in the rat promoter resulted in a 22 percent reduction in promoter activity in vitro,[211] and the region of the -30 base is known to be completely homologous between rat and human. However, the functional importance of this region in humans is not certain. This variant promoter was associated with an increased frequency of impaired glucose tolerance in a group of middle-aged Japanese men who were surveyed in a population under study in Seattle, and confirmed when this population was resurveyed 5 years later.[212] Further analysis of the population demonstrated an association between this variant and a 30 percent reduction in early insulin responses to oral glucose challenge. This was true whether or not the individual had normal or impaired glucose tolerance. Thus, it was concluded that the -30 promoter variant may be an example of a common genetic variation that increases the risk of impaired glucose tolerance and contributes to the increased frequency of type 2 diabetes in this population, but that the pathophysiology of impaired glucose tolerance is heterogeneous even in this population, and, therefore, multiple factors are probably interacting to produce clinical hyperglycemia. Such subtle changes may be very difficult to detect using standard genetic approaches. It is likely that regulatory regions of genes will have to be scanned, and intermediate phenotypes, such as β-cell function and insulin sensitivity, will be important. For this phenotyping, it is necessary to recognize that insulin sensitivity alters β-cell responses to glucose, and therefore the assessment of β-cell function can be complex. This may explain why populations do not show linkage between the glucokinase locus when clinical diabetes is used as the phenotype,[191,213–216] but may show association with glucose intolerance.[212,217] However, a recent study of β-cell function in Danes showed no association with the promoter variant.[218]

The High-Affinity β-Cell Sulfonylurea Receptor (SUR-1). This molecule couples with an inwardly-rectifying potassium channel (Kir6.2) and acts as a regulatory subunit for coupling glucose metabolism through its nucleotide binding sites for ATP and ADP to regulate the potassium channel and membrane conductance for control of calcium influx and insulin secretion.[219] Its initial cloning in 1995 and localization to 11p15.1[220] suggested the possibility that mutation might be associated with familial persistent hyperinsulinemic hyperglycemia of infancy (PHHI), an autosomal recessive disorder characterized by unregulated insulin secretion and congenital hypoglycemia known to localize to this region. Two separate SUR-1 gene splice-site mutations, which segregated with the disease phenotype, were identified in affected individuals from nine different families.[221] Both mutations resulted in aberrant processing of the RNA sequence and disruption of the putative second nucleotide-binding domain of the SUR protein. A third mutation was subsequently described in another series of families involving a deletion of codon F1388.[222] This particular mutation was expressed and shown to abolish ATP-sensitive potassium channel activity in intact cells. Subsequently, a nonsense mutation in the inward rectifier potassium channel gene was found to be associated with the same phenotype.[223] A nonsense mutation, a tyrosine → stop at codon 12 (Y12X), was also observed in the homozygous state in a single proband.[223] Only one of 78 PHHI probands was positive for this mutation. Subsequently, a series of missense mutations in the SUR-1 molecule was described: H125Q, N188S, F591L, T1139M, R1215Q, G1382S, and R1394H.[224] Most of these generated functional channels in the absence of ATP. However, all but N188S and H125Q had a reduced response to stimulation by MgADP.

Because of the importance of the K channel protein and the β-cell SU binding protein SUR-1 to the K_{ATP} channel, both have been screened for their contribution to type 2 diabetes. In 346 Mexican-American type 2 affected sib-pairs derived from 176 families and an additional 110 ethnically and geographically matched control subjects, no evidence of linkage based on allele sharing for SUR-1 was found.[225] There was no evidence for association based on allele frequencies in patients and control subjects for any microsatellite marker. It was suggested that the SUR gene was not likely to play a major role in this population. One year later, SSCP was used to identify sequence changes in the two nuclear binding site regions of the SUR-1 gene. Eight variants were found and three were evaluated in two northern European Caucasian populations from Utah and the U.K.[226] A silent variation in exon 22, ACC → ACT at nucleotide 761, was more common in patients than in controls with an odds ratio of 3, and an intronic T → C change at position −3 of the exon 24 splice-acceptor site was also more common with an odds ratio of 1.9. The combination occurred in 8.9 percent of patients and in 0.5 percent of control subjects. It was suggested that this locus might be a contributor to type 2 diabetes in northern European Caucasians. A subsequent study partly confirmed an association in type 2 diabetic subjects between morbid obesity and the exon 22 variant at codon 761, although not with the intron 24 variant, except that individuals homozygous for this variant had a more deleterious form of obesity.[227] Sib-pair linkage with type 2 diabetes in French Caucasian families gave no evidence for linkage to the SUR locus, except in one set of obese families. In 1998, 100 Japanese type 2 diabetic patients had the entire coding region examined with the identification of 5 amino acid substitutions and 17 silent mutations.[228] No mutation altered the properties of expressed channels, and it was eventually concluded that SUR-1 mutations did not appear to be major determinants of type 2 susceptibility in Japanese. Finally, 63 type 2 diabetic patients were completely screened from a Danish population.[229] Two missense variants were identified, five silent variants in the coding region, and four intron variants. These variants were examined for association with type 2 diabetes and for a possible influence on insulin and C-peptide secretion after intravenous glucose and tolbutamide in a random sample of unrelated, healthy Danish Caucasians. One variant, a C/T in the silent exon 18 at position 775, and an intron −3c/−3t were found together more frequently in type 2 diabetics than in control subjects. Ten of 300 unrelated, healthy young Danish Caucasians had the combined at-risk genotype associated with a 50 percent reduction in serum C-peptide and a 40 percent reduction in serum insulin responses to tolbutamide, but not glucose injection. In summary, while the sulfonylurea receptor mutants are clearly important to PHHI, so far there is only a possible association with type 2 diabetes mellitus in some populations. Similar screening of the associated potassium channel Kir6.2(Bir) in a small group of 35 Caucasian type 2 subjects detected 5 variants, but subsequent analysis of 306 affected people and 175 controls detected no type 2 diabetes disease association.[230]

GLUT2. GLUT2 is a high K_m (low affinity) glucose transporter expressed in liver, pancreatic islet β-cells, kidney, and intestine. Coupled with glucokinase, GLUT2 has been proposed to act as part of the glucose-sensing mechanism in β-cells.[231] In animal models of type 2 diabetes, GLUT2 is suppressed, and it has therefore been considered a candidate for a type 2 diabetes risk factor. However, in animals the levels of GLUT2 expressed are usually such that glucose transport is not rate limiting, requiring an almost complete absence of GLUT2 in order to impair glucose-induced insulin secretion. Under certain circumstances, where GLUT2 is suppressed in animals or in vitro, there has been retention of glucose-induced insulin secretion.[232,233] In addition, it has been suggested that GLUT2 is not a major β-cell glucose transporter in the human islet as opposed to rodents and many other species.[234] Nevertheless, considerable screening activity has been done. Initial analyses of the GLUT2 locus by population-association studies and linkage analyses (reviewed in Matsubara[235]) failed to show any evidence that it contributes to susceptibility to type 2 diabetes, except for one association study in which molecular scanning of the GLUT2 gene in 48 former gestational diabetic African-American women with overt type 2 diabetes revealed two amino acid substitutions—one in exon 3 and the other in exon 4B.[236] The exon 3 mutation, a C → T Thr 110 Ile, was not more frequent in type 2 patients, but the exon 4 mutation was present in one type 2 diabetic patient, a Val 197 Ile substitution, and was not present in 52 control subjects. Subsequent expression studies demonstrated that the C110T mutation had no effect on glucose transport, but that the G197A mutation abolished transport activity of GLUT2 in *Xenopus* oocytes.[237] No clinical data are available on this patient and no further cases or follow-up have been reported. Subsequently, sib-pair analysis in Pima Indians demonstrated significant linkage between GLUT2 and acute insulin response, but no linkage with type 2 diabetes.[191] Studies in a Japanese group of pedigrees with affected members showed a possible association between a polymorphic marker near the GLUT2 locus, but follow-up in 60 subjects with complete gene scans found three Thr110Ile mutations and one Pro68Leu mutation, which were not associated with disease.[235] In summary, one rare patient has a defective mutant gene, but common association with disease is unlikely.

Glucagon Receptor. In 1995, a screening study of the glucagon receptor gene was reported in a population of Sardinian and French families.[238] Eighty multiplex French type 2 diabetic families were investigated first. The SSCP method revealed six polymorphisms: four in introns, and one silent change in an exon. In exon 2, a single heterozygous missense mutation GGT^{40} → AGT^{40} (Gly40Ser) was identified in 5 of the 80 tested. Subsequently, a further 136 unrelated patients from additional families and 96 unrelated patients from Sardinia were screened. Five of the French subjects were positive, as were 8 of the 96 Sardinian patients. The overall frequency was 4.6 percent in the French and 8.3 percent in Sardinians. Three control groups were tested. Of 159 middle-aged normoglycemic French Caucasians with no family history of diabetes, none was found to carry the mutation; of 183 presumed nondiabetic, nonhypertensive French subjects with no known familial diabetic background, 1 individual was positive; and of 780 randomly chosen individuals, ages 25 to 70, who considered themselves to be nondiabetic upon questioning, 9 (1.2 percent) were carriers. Then, 96 randomly selected individuals from Sardinia were screened. Three were positive. The trend of the two populations was similar. When tested together there was a highly significant association with type 2 diabetes. Linkage was tested using the transmission/disequilibrium (TD) test. The estimated transmission frequency was 0.727, which was significantly higher than the expected value of 0.5. This required subjects with impaired glucose tolerance (IGT), impaired fasting glucose (IFG), or type 2 diabetes to be considered affected, although IGT and IFG combined were also significant. Overt type 2 diabetes assessed alone was not. This receptor variant was expressed in BHK cells and transfected clones tested for binding. Compared to wild-type receptor, labeled glucagon had a threefold lower affinity for the mutant.

Unfortunately, subsequent studies were quite variable and often not confirmatory. Analysis of 383 type 2 diabetic patients in Japan found no one with the Gly40Ser mutation,[239] and similar findings were reported among diabetic patients in the Netherlands.[240] A study of diabetes in the United Kingdom found this mutation to be present in 15 of 1691 patients (2.2 percent), but only in 1 of 425 (0.2 percent) geographically matched controls. However, an increased frequency of the mutation was also found in probands of type 1 diabetes, and it was suggested that the mutation might represent some type of founder effect rather than true association.[241] A further study of 104 German patients found no one with the mutation,[242] and two more Japanese populations were screened with no mutations found in any of the diabetic subjects.[242–244] To further confuse the issue, a separate study in hypertension found an increase in the frequency of this same mutation in a population of individuals with hypertension compared to appropriate controls unrelated to diabetes.[245] Confirming authors postulated that the renal glucagon receptor might be an explanation for this interaction.[246] However, no such relationship was found in hypertensive Sardinian type 2 diabetic subjects, compared to nonhypertensive Sardinian type 2 diabetic subjects.[247] However, a more detailed look at the Sardinian population revealed significant geographic variation within Sardinia in the frequency of this mutation, varying from 1.4 percent in central Sardinia to 7.6 percent in southern Sardinia. Moreover, it was again noticed in a nondiabetic population that there was no relationship between the mutation and hypertension. At this time, 3.6 percent of type 2 diabetic subjects were found to have the mutation, and 4.2 percent of nondiabetic subjects, suggesting that the original report might have been skewed by variable geographic backgrounds in the original study. However, 10 subjects with the mutation were carefully matched for diabetic state, BMI, age, sex, and geographic origin, with 10 patients without the mutation, and a glucagon infusion test was performed to study the ability of glucagon to cause hyperglycemia.[248] Carriers had a significantly lower increment in plasma glucose than wild-type subjects, which was consistent with the reported decreased binding affinity of the mutant in vitro.[249]

Lastly, a Russian group screened its population of 150 unrelated type 2 diabetic patients, and compared it with 109 nondiabetic subjects for the mutation.[250] None of the type 2 diabetics showed the mutation, whereas two of the control subjects were carriers. Thus, it seems unlikely that this mutation is associated with clinical hyperglycemia. It should be remembered, however, that the original report from Sardinia was based largely on the definition of affected as impaired fasting glucose and/or overt diabetes and was not statistically significant when the overt diabetic population was tested alone. Similar association data have been reported with the −30 β-cell glucokinase promoter (see above). This suggests that there may be genetic factors that predispose to impaired glucose tolerance whose impact on blood glucose is modest. Because they are common variants, this effect does not become noticeable when surveying the entire population and comparing overt diabetes while potentially including impaired glucose tolerance and impaired fasting hyperglycemia among the nonaffected populations. Thus, detailed phenotypic characterization may be critical if such variation is a significant contributor to the eventual development of risk for type 2 diabetes in a population.

Other Candidate Genes. A missense mutation of the IAPP or amylin gene (S20G) was reported in 12 of 294 Japanese type 2 diabetes patients screened.[78] None of the 187 controls or 59 type 1 patients was affected. Eight of the 12 were diagnosed under age 35, had severe hyperglycemia requiring insulin treatment, and all had strong family histories of type 2 diabetes. The majority of circulating hormone (84 percent) was mutant by HPLC. The parent who transmitted the mutation was thought to be nondiabetic by history, but had IGT by testing in the three families studied. The authors concluded that the mutation probably only produced IGT unless associated with other unknown susceptibility factors where it led to early onset and increased severity of hyperglycemia or impaired β-cell function. No other studies of this mutation have been reported.

As mentioned in the MODY diabetes section above, several of the MODY genes have been associated with late onset type 2 diabetes, including the mutations usually associated with the MODY syndrome. This includes a Val → Met 255 mutation in HNF-4α[153] and a valine → isoleucine mutation at codon 393.[152] Similarly, an Arg583Gln mutation in the HNF-1α was found in 2 of 245 type 2 diabetic subjects in a Danish population, but in none of the appropriate controls.[251]

A general screen of 19 genes was performed using associated polymorphic markers, including 10 expressed in pancreatic β-cells. Included were two G-coupled inwardly rectifying potassium channels (GIRK-1)(KCNJ-3) and (GIRK-2)(KCNJ-7), plus glucagon; the glucokinase regulatory protein; the glucagon-like protein-1 receptor (GLP-1R); the insulin gene trans-activator islet-1 (ISL-1) and the candal-type homeodomain-3 gene (CDX-3); the proprotein convertase-2 (PCSK-2); hexokinase-1 (HK-1) and the mitochondrial isoenzyme (FAD-glycerophosphate dehydrogenase (GPD-2); as well as the isoform of the pyruvate kinase (PKN), which is expressed in β-cells.[252] The screening was performed in 172 French families selected to have at least two affected sibs. All available sibs, as well as parents, were included. The study population included 751 subjects of whom 573 were considered affected. Individuals were considered affected if they had overt type 2 diabetes mellitus according to the World Health Organization (WHO) criteria, IGT, or impaired fasting glucose with fasting plasma glucose levels greater than 6.1 (110 mg/dL) and a 2-h postload value of >7.8 mM (140 mg/dL). No evidence for linkage was found for any of the genes screened, but suggestive evidence of linkage was observed for the cholecystokinin-B (CCK-B) receptor gene, which is localized at 11p-15.4, in individuals diagnosed with overt hyperglycemia under the age of 45 years. No mutational screening was performed at the time of this publication.

In summary, candidate genes relating to the β-cell have been screened in a variety of populations, but variable results, often conflicting, have been reported, partly attributable to factors including inadequate sample size, heterogeneous populations, ascertainment bias, genetic heterogeneity, inadequate phenotypic characterization, and methodologic problems. Total genome scans have been equally disappointing to date, although not nearly as extensive. This is in marked contrast to MODY diabetes in which this clearly genetically distinct group, which is identified by its clinical genetic characteristics, has begun to reveal its secrets, although even in this much-easier-to-divide-and-segregate subgroup, all of the genes contributing have yet to be discovered, suggesting that there is much work yet to be done.

Genome-Wide Scanning

There are five groups that have assembled the necessary resources, including identification of a suitable population, clinical phenotyping, metabolic studies, and genetic analytic techniques, which are pursuing this approach. However, because the populations vary and the selection criteria are different, it is likely that the outcomes will be different. The first group reported on a population of 217 individuals from 26 families screened from 4000 individuals in a population isolated in western Finland (Botnia), an area of Swedes living in Finland.[253] The total population of the region is 60,000. Over a 5-year period, families with a positive diabetes history at four health centers were recruited to participate in clinical characterization studies with an overall participation rate of 90 percent. In total, 1180 type 2 diabetic patients and 3005 family members were phenotyped. Families containing 3 or more affected individuals, with at least 1 subject having disease onset before age 60 years and another before age 65 years, were selected for analysis. A 10-cM sequence length polymorphic map was made on the 217 individuals and a nonparametric method used for evaluation. This analysis revealed no significant or even suggestive evidence for susceptibility loci predisposing to type 2 diabetes. However, to further phenotype individuals, they selected the early insulin response during the OGTT (30-min insulin level) among affected individuals as an indicator of insulin secretion to rank families. Families were partitioned into four quartiles and the data reanalyzed. In the quartile with the lowest insulin levels, a region near D12S366 on chromosome 12q was highly significant and, with additional markers in this region, evidence for linkage was observed with an approximate LOD score of 3.65. This is the region of the MODY-3 gene, but the lowest quartile families do not fit the usual phenotypic definition of MODY-3 families. Subsequent screening of 86 of these subjects failed to demonstrate a mutation in the HNF-1α gene, suggesting that a nearby gene may be involved.

At about the same time, another sib-pair analysis was performed on a group of Mexican-American families from Starr County, Texas.[254] This group consisted of 408 Mexican-Americans with 330 affected sib-pairs from 170 sibships, located along the Rio Grande River, bordering Mexico. Native-American genes are highly represented among this population. The average distance of the polymorphic markers was 9 cM. Parents were not typed. Allele frequencies were estimated from the family sample. Evidence for linkage was evaluated using two different two-point linkage test statistics. The maximum LOD score was computed using the estimated identity-by-descent probabilities and the possible triangle using an identity-by-state method. One marker at D2S125 showed suggestive evidence for linkage with a LOD score >2.6, $P < 0.0005$. MLS values were increased, but not significantly for other markers in the region. In the identity-by-state tests, this marker had the best evidence for linkage as well. The affected were diagnosed by interview if they were currently taking blood-glucose-lowering medications or had taken such in the past for more than 1 year and were diagnosed over age 30 years. No metabolic measurements were made. Follow-up studies were made in another group of Mexican-Americans consisting of 166 individuals from 76 sibships for a total of 110 affected sib-pairs, and were compared with a group of Japanese affected sib-pairs consisting of 213 individuals from 97 sibships for a total of 140 affected sib-pairs using WHO criteria and an oral glucose tolerance test to determine the affected or current oral hypoglycemic agent or insulin use. Several markers showed some evidence for linkage with type 2 diabetes in this second sample. When combined, only D2S125 met the genome-wide criteria with significant evidence for linkage with IBS chi-square and MLS values in the combined sample of 30.25 ($p < 1 \times 10^{-6}$) and 4.10 ($p < 0.0001$). There was no evidence for linkage in the Japanese population or in a group of heterogeneous non-Hispanic Caucasians who were also screened. All of the known MODY genes, and many of the other candidate genes previously discussed, were also screened, but there was no evidence for linkage in this Mexican-American population. D2S125 is located at 2Q37. No obvious candidate genes are located in this region. A subsequent report of a British affected sib-pair population of 109 type 2 diabetics found no evidence for linkage.[255] A recent genome-scan report in a Finnish population, reported by the FUSION group, excluded linkage with this region.[256] A recent abstract[262] suggests a common single-nucleotide polymorphism UCSNP-43 in the calpain gene (a non-lysosomal cysteine protease) near DS125 showed linkage and association with diabetes. The authors further describe other polymorphisms in the gene which significantly modify risks. None of these polymorphisms were in the coding region of the gene and one haplotype with three polymorphisms (UCSNP-43, -19, and -63) were minimally required to distinguish the high-risk haplotype.

A similar sib-pair analysis of 579 individuals in 32 families of low-income Mexican-American diabetics identified in an epidemiological survey carried out in San Antonio, Texas, eventually yielded 103 sibships containing 349 individuals, 83 of whom were diabetic, yielding 545 sib-pairs. A LOD score >2 was observed for a marker on chromosome 11 and chromosome 6 for 2-h glucose and 1-h glucose, respectively.[257] There was no evidence for linkage at D2S125.

Most recently, an autosomal genome scan for loci linked to prediabetes phenotypes in Pima Indians was reported.[258] Three hundred and sixty-three nondiabetic Pima Indians were genotyped at 516 polymorphic microsatellite markers on all 22 autosomes. Each was chosen because he or she had a full sib who also participated in the studies. A subset of 231 individuals with fasting and 2-h glucose concentrations <7.8 mM during a 75 g oral glucose tolerance test was identified for analyses related to insulin secretion. An intravenous glucose tolerance test and a two-step hyperinsulinemic euglycemic glucose clamp were also performed on all subjects in addition to a large number of other measurements. Seven markers had a positive LOD score of 1.5 or greater for glucose tolerance and four additional markers had LOD scores >2 for fasting and 2-h insulin concentration. There were no LOD scores over 2 for fasting or 2-h glucose concentrations, or for insulin secretion, but there were two LOD scores >2 for insulin action. None of these scores was considered statistically significant for a full genome scan, which has been suggested to require a LOD score of 3.6 for a 5 percent probability. Unfortunately, there was no evidence that any of the physiological markers were linked to D2S125 on distal 2q, which had been identified in Mexican-Americans from Starr County, Texas (a genetically similar group). In addition, they failed to replicate their own data previously reported on linkage of acute insulin response to an area on 1p or linkage to insulin action at 4q. There was no linkage to markers located at the MODY-1, -2, or -3 genes, and there was no linkage to 2-h or fasting glucose concentrations on chromosomes 6 and 11, as reported for Mexican-Americans from San Antonio, Texas. The q-terminal region D22S683-D22S270 mapping to 22q12-13 provided the most significant evidence of linkage to a prediabetic phenotype in the entire genome scan (for fasting plasma glucose concentration). Known genes in this region encode the somatostatin receptor 3 and the structural locus for casein kinase-1 epsilon, neither of which is known to be involved in carbohydrate metabolism directly.

The last major group to propose such work reported its initial research design and metabolic findings in 1998.[259] The FUSION project is a collaborative study between the National Human Genome Research Institute at the NIH and the Department of Epidemiology and Health Promotion at the National Public Health Institute in Helsinki, Finland, in addition to a variety of other academic colleagues in both countries. Based on the genetic isolation of the Finnish population, they have ascertained 495 families with confirmed type 2 diabetes in at least two sibs and no history of type 1 diabetes among first-degree relatives. In a subset, a spouse and offspring were sampled, and participated in an intravenous glucose tolerance test to measure insulin secretion and insulin action. This testing was performed in two nondiabetic offspring in 156 families, with a confirmed nondiabetic spouse. Type 2 diabetes was confirmed by oral glucose tolerance test if no diabetes medication was being given, using WHO criteria. A family was eligible if a proband was diagnosed between age 35 and 60 years and at least one parent was apparently nondiabetic. The study is expected to present data very shortly. A second group for confirming any findings is planned.

In summary, whole genome searches using the affected sib-pair method have been undertaken by a variety of groups to complement the ongoing work on candidate genes. The results to date have been modest, largely because of the difficulties of the effort. It is pointed out by the FUSION group that 400 pairs typed on a 10-cM map will require a 1.8-fold excess risk to siblings of affected individuals at a LOD score of 3.0 with 82 percent power. However, this drops to a LOD score of 1.0 for a 1.4-fold excess risk. It is also pointed out that it would require 800 such pairs to have 70 percent power to detect a locus with an impact estimated by the Starr County investigators for their chromosome 2 finding to produce a LOD score of 3.0, and even this would be reduced to a LOD score of 1.59 if the locus only confers a 1.2-fold excess risk. Thus, it is becoming obvious that detection of genes for type 2 diabetes is going to be extremely complex and difficult if the impact of these genes is relatively modest and their frequencies relatively low or if they interact in some way, which is likely. This probably explains why even the initial efforts have not replicated each other, and no truly significant LOD scores have been observed. This will almost certainly require pooling of data among investigative groups. Fortunately, such efforts have apparently begun.

REFERENCES

1. Harris MI, Flegal KM, Cowie CC, Eberhardt MS, Goldstein DE, Little RR, Wiedmeyer HM, et al.: Prevalence of diabetes, impaired fasting glucose, and impaired glucose tolerance in U.S. adults. The Third National Health and Nutrition Examination Survey, 1988–1994. *Diabetes Care* **21**:518, 1998.
2. Porte D Jr: β-Cells in type II diabetes mellitus. *Diabetes* **40**:166, 1991.
3. Yalow RS, Berson SA: Plasma insulin concentrations in nondiabetic and early diabetic subjects: Determinations by a new sensitive immunoassay technic. *Diabetes* **9**:254, 1960.
4. Kahn SE: Regulation of β-cell function in vivo: From health to disease. *Diabetes Rev* **4**:372, 1996.
5. Halban PA, Irminger JC: Sorting and processing of secretory proteins. *Biochem J* **299**:1, 1994.
6. Davidson HW, Rhodes CJ, Hutton JC: Intraorganellar calcium and pH control proinsulin cleavage in the pancreatic β-cell via two distinct site-specific endopeptidases. *Nature* **333**:93, 1988.
7. Smeekens SP, Steiner DF: Identification of a human insulinoma cDNA encoding a novel mammalian protein structurally related to the yeast dibasic processing protease Kex2. *J Biol Chem* **265**:2997, 1990.
8. Smeekens SP, Avruch AS, LaMendola J, Chan SJ, Steiner DF: Identification of a cDNA encoding a second putative prohormone convertase related to PC2 in AtT20 cells and islets of Langerhans. *Proc Natl Acad Sci U S A* **88**:340, 1991.
9. Sizonenko S, Irminger JC, Buhler L, Deng S, Morel P, Halban PA: Kinetics of proinsulin conversion in human islets. *Diabetes* **42**:933, 1993.
10. Ward WK, LaCava EC, Paquette TL, Beard JC, Wallum BJ, Porte D Jr: Disproportionate elevation of immunoreactive proinsulin in type 2 (non-insulin-dependent) diabetes mellitus and experimental insulin resistance. *Diabetologia* **30**:698, 1987.
11. Kahn SE, Halban PA: Release of incompletely processed proinsulin is the cause of the disproportionate proinsulinemia of NIDDM. *Diabetes* **46**:1725, 1997.
12. Nagamatsu S, Nishi M, Steiner DF: Biosynthesis of islet amyloid polypeptide. Elevated expression in mouse beta TC3 cells. *J Biol Chem* **266**:13737, 1991.
13. Badman MK, Shennan KI, Jermany JL, Docherty K, Clark A: Processing of pro-islet amyloid polypeptide (proIAPP) by the prohormone convertase PC2. *FEBS Lett* **378**:227, 1996.
14. Steiner DF, Ohagi S, Nagamatsu S, Bell GI, Nishi M: Is islet amyloid polypeptide a significant factor in pathogenesis or pathophysiology of diabetes? *Diabetes* **40**:305, 1991.
15. Lukinius A, Wilander E, Westermark GT, Engstrom U, Westermark P: Co-localization of islet amyloid polypeptide and insulin in the B cell secretory granules of the human pancreatic islets. *Diabetologia* **32**:240, 1989.
16. Kahn SE, D'Alessio DA, Schwartz MW, Fujimoto WY, Ensinck JW, Taborsky GJ Jr, Porte D Jr: Evidence of cosecretion of islet amyloid polypeptide and insulin by β-cells. *Diabetes* **39**:634, 1990.
17. Enoki S, Mitsukawa T, Takemura J, Nakazato M, Aburaya J, Toshimori H, Matsukara S: Plasma islet amyloid polypeptide levels in obesity, impaired glucose tolerance and non-insulin-dependent diabetes mellitus. *Diabetes Res Clin Pract* **15**:97, 1992.
18. Kahn SE, Verchere CB, Andrikopoulos S, Asberry PJ, Leonetti DL, Wahl PW, Boyko EJ, et al.: Reduced amylin release is a characteristic of impaired glucose tolerance and type 2 diabetes in Japanese Americans. *Diabetes* **47**:640, 1998.
19. Dechenes CJ, Verchere CB, Andrikopoulos S, Kahn SE: Human aging is associated with parallel reductions in insulin and amylin release. *Am J Physiol* **275**: E785, 1998.
20. Kahn SE, Verchere CB, D'Alessio DA, Cook DL, Fujimoto WY: Evidence for selective release of rodent islet amyloid polypeptide through the constitutive secretory pathway. *Diabetologia* **36**:570, 1993.
21. Opie E: The relation of diabetes mellitus to lesions of the pancreas. Hyaline degeneration of the islets of Langerhans. *J Exp Med* **5**:527, 1901.
22. Westermark P, Wilander E: The influence of amyloid deposits on the islet volume in maturity onset diabetes mellitus. *Diabetologia* **15**:417, 1978.
23. Takeda J, Kayano T, Fukomoto H, Bell GI: Organization of the human GLUT2 (pancreatic beta-cell and hepatocyte) glucose transporter gene. *Diabetes* **42**:773, 1993.
24. Matschinsky F, Liang Y, Kesavan P, Wang L, Froguel P, Velho G, Cohen D, et al.: Glucokinase as pancreatic β-cell glucose sensor and diabetes gene. *J Clin Invest* **92**:2092, 1993.
25. Matschinsky FM: Glucokinase as glucose sensor and metabolic signal generator in pancreatic β-cells and hepatocytes. *Diabetes* **39**:647, 1990.
26. Cook DL, Hales CN: Intracellular ATP directly blocks K+ channels in pancreatic β-cells. *Nature* **311**:271, 1984.
27. Babenko AP, Aguilar-Bryan L, Bryan J: A view of SUR/K_{IR}6.X, K_{ATP} channels. *Annu Rev Physiol* **60**:667, 1998.
28. Ghosh A, Ronner P, Cheong E, Khalid P, Matschinsky FM: The role of ATP and free ADP in metabolic coupling during fuel-stimulated insulin release from islet beta-cells in the isolated perfused rat pancreas. *J Biol Chem* **266**:22887, 1991.
29. Hopkins WF, Fatherazi S, Peter-Riesch B, Corkey BE, Cook DL: Two sites for adenine-nucleotide regulation of ATP-sensitive potassium channels in mouse pancreatic beta-cells and HIT cells. *J Membr Biol* **129**:287, 1992.
30. Inagaki N, Gonoi T, Clement JP, Namba N, Inazawa J, Gonzalez G, Aguilar-Bryan L, et al.: Reconstitution of IKATP: An inward rectifier subunit plus the sulfonylurea receptor. *Science* **270**:1166, 1995.
31. Aguilar-Bryan L, Nichols CG, Wechsler SW, Clement JP 4th, Boyd AE 3rd, Gonzalez G, Herrera-Sosa H, et al.: Cloning of the beta cell high-affinity sulfonylurea receptor: A regulator of insulin secretion [see Comments]. *Science* **268**:423, 1995.
32. Goodner CJ, Walike BC, Koerker DJ, Ensinck JW, Brown AC, Chideckel EW, Palmer J, et al.: Insulin, glucagon, and glucose exhibit synchronous, sustained oscillations in fasting monkeys. *Science* **195**:177, 1977.
33. Lang DA, Matthews DR, Peto J, Turner RC: Cyclic oscillations of basal plasma glucose and insulin concentrations in human beings. *N Engl J Med* **301**:1023, 1979.
34. Hansen BC, Jen KC, Pek SB, Wolfe RA: Rapid oscillations in plasma insulin, glucagon, and glucose in obese and normal weight humans. *J Clin Endocrinol Metab* **54**:785, 1982.
35. Polonsky KS, Given BD, Cauter EV: Twenty-four-hour profiles and patterns of insulin secretion in normal and obese subjects. *J Clin Invest* **81**:442, 1988.
36. Juhl C, Pørksen N, Veldhuis J, Pincus S, Schmitz O: Amylin is secreted in a pulsatile pattern in healthy humans. *Diabetes* **47(Suppl 1)**:A412, 1998.

37. Bergstrom RW, Fujimoto WY, Teller DC, De Haen C: Oscillatory insulin secretion in perifused isolated rat islets. *Am J Physiol* **257**:E479, 1989.
38. Matthews DR, Lang DA, Burnett MA, Turner RC: Control of pulsatile insulin secretion in man. *Diabetologia* **24**:231, 1983.
39. Yalow RS, Berson SA: Immunoassay of endogenous plasma insulin in man. *J Clin Invest* **39**:1157, 1960.
40. Karam JH, Grodsky GM, Forsham PH: Excessive insulin response to glucose in obese subjects as measured by immunochemical assay. *Diabetes* **12**:197, 1963.
41. Porte D Jr, Pupo AA: Insulin responses to glucose: evidence for a two pool system in man. *J Clin Invest* **48**:2309, 1969.
42. Ludvik B, Lell B, Hartter E, Schnack C, Prager R: Decrease of stimulated amylin release precedes impairment of insulin secretion in type II diabetes. *Diabetes* **40**:1615, 1991.
43. Verchere CB, D'Alessio DA, Palmiter RD, Kahn SE: Transgenic mice overproducing human islet amyloid polypeptide have increased insulin storage and secretion. *Diabetologia* **37**:725, 1994.
44. Chen M, Porte D Jr: The effect of rate and dose of glucose infusion on the acute insulin response in man. *J Clin Endocrinol Metab* **42**:1168, 1976.
45. Kahn SE, Prigeon RL, McCulloch DK, Boyko EJ, Bergman RN, Schwartz MW, Neifing JL, et al.: Quantification of the relationship between insulin sensitivity and β-cell function in human subjects. Evidence for a hyperbolic function. *Diabetes* **42**:1663, 1993.
46. Ward WK, Beard JC, Halter JB, Pfeifer MA, Porte D Jr: Pathophysiology of insulin secretion in non-insulin-dependent diabetes mellitus. *Diabetes Care* **7**:491, 1984.
47. Halter JB, Graf RJ, Porte D Jr: Potentiation of insulin secretory responses by plasma glucose levels in man: Evidence that hyperglycemia in diabetes compensates for impaired glucose potentiation. *J Clin Endocrinol Metab* **48**:946, 1979.
48. Ward WK, Bolgiano DC, McKnight B, Halter JB, Porte D Jr: Diminished B-cell secretory capacity in patients with non-insulin-dependent diabetes mellitus. *J Clin Invest* **74**:1318, 1984.
49. Kahn SE, Beard JC, Schwartz MW, Ward WK, Ding HL, Bergman RN, Taborsky GJ Jr, et al.: Increased β-cell secretory capacity as mechanism for islet adaptation to nicotinic acid-induced insulin resistance. *Diabetes* **38**:562, 1989.
50. Kahn SE, Klaff LJ, Schwartz MW, Beard JC, Bergman RN, Taborsky GJ Jr, Porte D Jr: Treatment with a somatostatin analog decreases pancreatic β-cell and whole body sensitivity to glucose. *J Clin Endocrinol Metab* **71**:994, 1990.
51. Kahn SE, Bradbury VL, Beard JC, Cain KC, Fellingham GW, Schwartz RS, Veith RC, et al.: Effect of exercise on insulin action, glucose tolerance and insulin secretion in aging. *Am J Physiol* **258**:E937, 1990.
52. Ortiz-Alonso FJ, Herman WH, Zobel DL, Perry TJ, Smith MJ, Halter JB: Effect of epinephrine on pancreatic β-cell and α-cell function in patients with NIDDM. *Diabetes* **40**:1194, 1991.
53. Kahn SE, Larson VG, Schwartz RS, Beard JC, Cain KC, Fellingham GW, Stratton JR, et al.: Exercise training delineates the importance of B-cell dysfunction to the glucose intolerance of human aging. *J Clin Endocrinol Metab* **74**:1336, 1992.
54. Seaquist ER, Robertson RP: Effects of hemipancreatectomy on pancreatic alpha and beta cell function in healthy human donors. *J Clin Invest* **89**:1761, 1992.
55. Larsson H, Ahren B: Islet dysfunction in obese women with impaired glucose tolerance. *Metabolism* **45**:502, 1996.
56. Byrne MM, Sturis J, Clement K, Vionnet N, Pueyo ME, Stoffel M, Takeda J, et al.: Insulin secretory abnormalities in subjects with hyperglycemia due to glucokinase mutations. *J Clin Invest* **93**:1120, 1994.
57. Byrne MM, Sturis J, Fajans SS, Ortiz FJ, Stoltz A, Stoffel M, Smith MJ, et al.: Altered insulin secretory responses to glucose in subjects with a mutation in the MODY1 gene on chromosome 20. *Diabetes* **44**:699, 1995.
58. Byrne MM, Sturis J, Menzel S, Yamagata K, Fajans SS, Dronsfield MJ, Bain SC, et al.: Altered insulin secretory responses to glucose in diabetic and nondiabetic subjects with mutations in the diabetes susceptibility gene MODY3 on chromosome 12. *Diabetes* **45**:1503, 1996.
59. Ehrmann DA, Sturis J, Byrne MM, Karrison T, Rosenfield RL, Polonsky KS: Insulin secretory defects in polycystic ovary syndrome. Relationship to insulin sensitivity and family history of non-insulin-dependent diabetes mellitus. *J Clin Invest* **96**:520, 1995.
60. Cerasi E: Potentiation of insulin release by glucose in man. I. Quantitative analysis of the enhancement of glucose-induced insulin secretion by pretreatment with glucose in normal subjects. *Acta Endocrinol* **79**:483, 1975.
61. Ward WK, Halter JB, Beard JC, Porte D Jr: Adaptation of β and α cell function during prolonged glucose infusion in human subjects. *Am J Physiol* **246**:E405, 1984.
62. Kahn SE, Bergman RN, Schwartz MW, Taborsky GJ Jr, Porte D Jr: Short-term hyperglycemia and hyperinsulinemia improve insulin action but do not alter glucose action in normal humans. *Am J Physiol* **262**:E518, 1992.
63. Byrne MM, Sturis J, Polonsky JS: Insulin secretion and clearance during low-dose graded glucose infusion. *Am J Physiol* **268**:E21, 1995.
64. Herman WH, Morrow LA, Halter JB: Maladaptation of beta cell function to hyperglycemia in noninsulin-dependent diabetes mellitus. *Diabetes* **37(Suppl 1)**:5A, 1988.
65. Perley MJ, Kipnis DM: Plasma insulin responses to oral and intravenous glucose: Studies in normal and diabetic subjects. *J Clin Invest* **46**:1954, 1967.
66. Bagdade JD, Porte D Jr, Brunzell JD, Bierman EL: Basal and stimulated hyperinsulinism: reversible metabolic sequelae of obesity. *J Lab Clin Med* **83**:563, 1974.
67. Beard JC, Ward WK, Halter JB, Wallum BJ, Porte D Jr: Relationship of islet function to insulin action in human obesity. *J Clin Endocrinol Metab* **65**:59, 1987.
68. Ward WK, Johnston CLW, Beard JC, Benedetti TJ, Halter JB, Porte D Jr: Insulin resistance and impaired insulin secretion in subjects with histories of gestational diabetes mellitus. *Diabetes* **34**:861, 1985.
69. Johnston CLW, Ward WK, Beard JC, McKnight B, Porte D Jr: Islet function and insulin sensitivity in the non-diabetic offspring of conjugal type 2 diabetic patients. *Diabetic Med* **7**:119, 1990.
70. Ryan EA, Imes S, Liu D, McManus R, Finegood DT, Polonsky KS, Sturis J: Defects in insulin secretion and action in women with a history of gestational diabetes. *Diabetes* **44**:506, 1995.
71. Clark A, Wells CA, Buley ID, Cruickshank JK, Vanhegan RI, Matthews DR, Cooper GJS, et al.: Islet amyloid, increased α-cells, reduced β-cells and exocrine fibrosis: Quantitative changes in the pancreas in type 2 diabetes. *Diabetes Res* **9**:151, 1988.
72. Clark A, Saad MF, Nezzer T, Uren C, Knowler WC, Bennett PH, Turner RC: Islet amyloid polypeptide in diabetic and non-diabetic Pima Indians. *Diabetologia* **33**:285, 1990.
73. Bell ET: Hyalinization of the islets of Langerhans in nondiabetic individuals. *Am J Pathol* **35**:801, 1959.
74. Westermark P, Wernstedt C, Wilander E, Hayden DW, O'Brien TD, Johnson KH: Amyloid fibrils in human insulinoma and islets of Langerhans of the diabetic cat are derived from a neuropeptide-like protein also present in normal islets. *Proc Natl Acad Sci U S A* **84**:3881, 1987.
75. Cooper GJS, Willis AC, Clark A, Turner RC, Sim RB, Reid KBM: Purification and characterization of a peptide from amyloid-rich pancreases of type 2 diabetic patients. *Proc Natl Acad Sci U S A* **84**:8628, 1987.
76. Butler PC, Chou J, Carter WB, Wang Y-N, Bu B-H, Chang D, Chang J-K, et al.: Effects of meal ingestion on plasma amylin concentration in NIDDM and nondiabetic humans. *Diabetes* **39**:752, 1990.
77. Ludvik B, Clodi M, Kautzky-Willer A, Capek M, Hartter E, Pacini G, Prager R: Effect of dexamethasone on insulin sensitivity, islet amyloid polypeptide and insulin secretion in humans. *Diabetologia* **36**:84, 1993.
78. Sakagashira S, Sanke T, Hanabusa T, Shirmomura H, Ohagi S, Kumagaye KY, Nakajima K, et al.: Missense mutation of amylin gene (S20G) in Japanese NIDDM patients. *Diabetes* **45**:1279, 1996.
79. Seltzer HS, Allen EW, Herron AL Jr, Brennan MT: Insulin secretion in response to glycemic stimulus: Relation of delayed initial release to carbohydrate intolerance in mild diabetes mellitus. *J Clin Invest* **46**:323, 1967.
80. Cerasi E, Luft R: The plasma insulin response to glucose infusion in healthy subjects and in diabetes mellitus. *Acta Endocrinol* **55**:278, 1967.
81. Brunzell JD, Robertson RP, Lerner RL, Hazzard WR, Ensinck JW, Bierman EL, Porte DJ: Relationships between fasting plasma glucose levels and insulin secretion during intravenous glucose tolerance tests. *J Clin Endocrinol Metab* **42**:222, 1976.
82. Metz SA, Halter JB, Robertson RP: Paradoxical inhibition of insulin secretion by glucose in human diabetes mellitus. *J Clin Endocrinol Metab* **48**:827, 1979.

83. Pfeifer MA, Halter JB, Porte D Jr: Insulin secretion in diabetes mellitus. *Am J Med* **70**:579, 1981.
84. Roder ME, Porte D Jr, Kahn SE: Disproportionately elevated proinsulin levels reflect the degree of impaired B-cell secretory capacity in patients with non-insulin dependent diabetes mellitus. *J Clin Endocrinol Metab* **83**:604, 1998.
85. Lang DA, Matthews DR, Burnett M, Turner RC: Brief, irregular oscillations of basal plasma insulin and glucose concentrations in diabetic man. *Diabetes* **30**:435, 1981.
86. Polonsky KS, Given BD, Hirsch LJ, Tillil H, Shapiro ET, Beebe C, Frank BH, et al.: Abnormal patterns of insulin secretion in non-insulin-dependent diabetes mellitus. *N Engl J Med* **318**:1231, 1988.
87. Matthews DR, Naylor BA, Jones RG, Ward GM, Turner RC: Pulsatile insulin has greater hypoglycemic effect than continuous delivery. *Diabetes* **32**:617, 1983.
88. Saito K, Yaginuma N, Takahashi T: Differential volumetry of A, B, and D cells in the pancreatic islets of diabetic and nondiabetic subjects. *Tohoku J Exp Med* **129**:273, 1979.
89. Kloppel G, Lohr M, Habich K, Oberholzer M, Heitz PU: Islet pathology and the pathogenesis of type 1 and type 2 diabetes mellitus revisited. *Surv Synth Pathol Res* **4**:110, 1985.
90. Ward WK, Wallum BJ, Beard JC, Taborsky GJ Jr, Porte D Jr: Reduction of glycemic potentiation. Sensitive indicator of beta-cell loss in partially pancreatectomized dogs. *Diabetes* **37**:723, 1988.
91. Leahy JL, Bonner-Weir S, Weir GC: Abnormal glucose regulation of insulin secretion in models of reduced B-cell mass. *Diabetes* **33**:667, 1984.
92. Imamura T, Koffler M, Helderman JH, Prince D, Thirlby R, Inman L, Unger RH: Severe diabetes induced in subtotally depancreatized dogs by sustained hyperglycemia. *Diabetes* **37**:600, 1988.
93. Bonner-Weir S, Trent DF, Weir GC: Partial pancreatectomy in the rat and subsequent defect in glucose-induced insulin release. *J Clin Invest* **71**:1544, 1983.
94. Lillioja S, Mott DM, Spraul M, Ferraro R, Foley JE, Ravussin E, Knowler WC, et al.: Insulin resistance and insulin secretory dysfunction as precursors of non-insulin-dependent diabetes mellitus. Prospective studies of Pima Indians. *N Engl J Med* **329**:1988, 1993.
95. Chen K-W, Boyko EJ, Bergstrom RW, Leonetti DL, Newell-Morris L, Wahl PW, Fujimoto WY: Earlier appearance of impaired insulin secretion than of visceral adiposity in the pathogenesis of NIDDM: 5-year follow-up of initially nondiabetic Japanese-American men. *Diabetes Care* **18**:747, 1995.
96. DeFronzo RA, Bonadonna RC, Ferrannini E: Pathogenesis of NIDDM. A balanced overview. *Diabetes Care* **15**:318, 1992.
97. Mitrakou A, Kelley D, Mokan M, Veneman T, Pangburn T, Reilly J, Gerich J: Role of reduced suppression of glucose production and diminished early insulin release in impaired glucose tolerance. *N Engl J Med* **326**:22, 1992.
98. O'Meara NM, Sturis J, Van Cauter E, Polonsky KS: Lack of control by glucose of ultradian insulin secretory oscillations in impaired glucose tolerance and in non-insulin-dependent diabetes mellitus. *J Clin Invest* **92**:262, 1993.
99. Larsson H, Ahren B: Failure to adequately adapt reduced insulin sensitivity with increased insulin secretion in women with impaired glucose tolerance. *Diabetologia* **39**:1099, 1996.
100. O'Sullivan JB: Body weight and subsequent diabetes mellitus. *JAMA* **248**:949, 1982.
101. O'Rahilly S, Turner RC, Matthews DR: Impaired pulsatile secretion of insulin in relatives of patients with non-insulin-dependent diabetes. *N Engl J Med* **318**:1225, 1988.
102. Froguel P, Vaxillaire M, Sun F, Velho G, Zouali H, Butel MO, Lesage S, et al.: Close linkage of glucokinase locus on chromosome 7p to early-onset non-insulin-dependent diabetes mellitus. *Nature* **356**:162, 1992.
103. Saad MF, Knowler WC, Pettitt DJ, Nelson RG, Mott DM, Bennett PH: The natural history of impaired glucose tolerance in the Pima Indians. *N. Eng. J. Med.* **319**:1500, 1988.
104. Saad MF, Kahn SE, Nelson RG, Pettitt DJ, Knowler WC, Schwartz MW, Kowalyk S, et al.: Disproportionately elevated proinsulin in Pima Indians with noninsulin-dependent diabetes mellitus. *J Clin Endocrinol Metab* **70**:1247, 1990.
105. Kahn SE, Leonetti DL, Prigeon RL, Bergstrom RW, Fujimoto WY: Relationship of proinsulin and insulin with noninsulin-dependent diabetes mellitus and coronary heart disease in Japanese American men: Impact of obesity. *J Clin Endocrinol Metab* **80**:1399, 1995.
106. Gorden P, Hendricks CM, Roth J: Circulating proinsulin-like component in man: increased proportion in hypoinsulinemic states. *Diabetologia* **10**:469, 1974.
107. Duckworth WC, Kitabchi AE, Heinemann M: Direct measurement of plasma proinsulin in normal and diabetic subjects. *Am J Med* **53**:418, 1972.
108. Mako ME, Starr JI, Rubenstein AH: Circulating proinsulin in patients with maturity onset diabetes. *Am J Med* **63**:865, 1977.
109. Deacon CF, Schleser-Mohr S, Ballmann M, Willms B, Conlon JM, Creutzfeldt W: Preferential release of proinsulin relative to insulin in non-insulin-dependent diabetes mellitus. *Acta Endocrinol* **119**:549, 1988.
110. Yoshioka N, Kuzuya T, Matsuda A, Taniguchi M, Iwamoto Y: Serum proinsulin levels at fasting and after oral glucose load in patients with type 2 (non-insulin-dependent) diabetes mellitus. *Diabetologia* **31**:355, 1988.
111. Temple RC, Carrington CA, Luzio SD, Owens DR, Schneider AE, Sobey WJ, Hales CN: Insulin deficiency in non-insulin-dependent diabetes. *Lancet* **1**:293, 1989.
112. Haffner SM, Bowsher RR, Mykkanen L, Hazuda HP, Mitchell BD, Valdez RA, Gingerich R, et al.: Proinsulin and specific insulin concentration in high- and low-risk populations for NIDDM. *Diabetes* **43**:1490, 1994.
113. Kautzky-Willer A, Thomaseth K, Ludvik B, Nowotny P, Rabensteiner D, Waldhausl W, Pacini G, et al.: Elevated islet amyloid pancreatic polypeptide and proinsulin in lean gestational diabetes. *Diabetes* **46**:607, 1997.
114. Persson B, Hanson U, Hartling SG, Binder C: Follow-up of women with previous GDM: Insulin, C-peptide, and proinsulin responses to oral glucose load. *Diabetes* **40(Suppl 2)**:136, 1991.
115. Kahn SE, Leonetti DL, Prigeon RL, Bergstrom RW, Fujimoto WY: Proinsulin as a marker for the development of non-insulin dependent diabetes mellitus in Japanese-American men. *Diabetes* **44**:173, 1995.
116. Haffner SM, Stern MP, Miettinen H, Gingerich R, Bowsher RR: Higher proinsulin and specific insulin are both associated with a parental history of diabetes in nondiabetic Mexican-American subjects. *Diabetes* **44**:1156, 1995.
117. Porte D Jr, Kahn SE: Hyperproinsulinemia and amyloid in NIDDM: Clues to etiology of islet β-cell dysfunction? *Diabetes* **38**:1333, 1989.
118. Rhodes CJ, Alarcon C: What beta-cell defect could lead to hyperproinsulinemia in NIDDM? Some clues from recent advances made in understanding the proinsulin-processing mechanism. *Diabetes* **43**:511, 1994.
119. Steiner DF, Tager HS, Chan SJ, Nanjo K, Sanke T, Rubenstein AH: Lessons learned from molecular biology of insulin-gene mutations. *Diabetes Care* **13**:600, 1990.
120. Yano H, Kitano N, Morimoto M, Polonsky KS, Imura H, Seino Y: A novel point mutation in the human insulin gene giving rise to hyperproinsulinemia (proinsulin Kyoto). *J Clin Invest* **89**:1902, 1992.
121. Warren-Perry MG, Manley SE, Ostrega D, Polonsky K, Mussett S, Brown P, Turner RC: A novel point mutation in the insulin gene giving rise to hyperproinsulinemia. *J Clin Endocrinol Metab* **82**:1629, 1997.
122. Sherratt E, Thomas A, Alcolado J: Mitochondrial DNA defects: a widening clinical spectrum of disorders. *Clin Sci* **92**:225, 1997.
123. Ballinger S, Shoffner J, Hedaya E, Trounce I, Polak M, Koontz D, Wallace D: Maternally transmitted diabetes and deafness associated with a 10.4-kb mitochondrial DNA deletion. *Nat Genet* **1**:11, 1992.
124. Gerbitz K, Gempel K, Brdiczka D: Mitochondria and diabetes: Genetic, biochemical, and clinical implications of the cellular energy circuit. *Diabetes* **45**:113, 1996.
125. Ballinger S, Wallace D: Maternally transmitted diabetes and deafness. *Endocrinologist* **5**:104, 1995.
126. Maassen J, Jansen J, Kadowaki T, van den Ouweland J, Hart L, Lemkes H: The molecular basis and clinical characteristics of maternally inherited diabetes and deafness (MIDD), a recently recognized diabetic subtype. *Exp Clin Endocrinol Diabetes* **104**:205, 1996.
127. Maassen J, van den Ouweland M, Hart L, Lemkes H: Maternally inherited diabetes and deafness: a diabetic subtype associated with a mutation in mitochondrial DNA. *Horm Metab Res* **29**:50, 1997.
128. Velho G, Byrne M, Clement K, Sturis J, Pueyo M, Blanche H, Vionnet N, et al.: Clinical phenotypes, insulin secretion, and insulin sensitivity in kindreds with maternally inherited diabetes and deafness due to mitochondrial tRNA Leu(UUR) gene mutation. *Diabetes* **45**:478, 1996.
129. Suzuki Y, Hata T, Miyaoka H, Atsumi Y, Kadowaki H, Taniyama M, Kadowaki T, et al.: Diabetes with the 3243 mitochondrial tRNA Leu(UUR) mutation. *Diabetes Care* **19**:739, 1996.
130. Oka Y, Katagiri H, Yazaki Y, Murase T, Kobayashi T: Mitochondrial gene mutation in islet cell antibody positive patients who were initially non-insulin-dependent diabetics. *Lancet* **342**:527, 1993.

131. Oka Y, Katagiri H, Ishihara H, Asano T, Kikuchi M, Kobayashi T: Mitochondrial diabetes mellitus-glucose-induced signaling defects and beta-cell loss. *Muscle Nerve* **3**:S131, 1995.
132. Gebhart S, Shoffner J, Koontz D, Kaufman A, Wallace D: Insulin resistance associated with maternally inherited diabetes and deafness. *Metabolism* **45**:526, 1996.
133. Kadowaki T, Kadowaki H, Mori Y, Tobe K, Sakuta R, Suzuki Y, Tanabe Y, et al.: A subtype of diabetes mellitus associated with a mutation of mitochondrial DNA. *N Engl J Med* **330**:962, 1994.
134. Kennedy ED, Maechler P, Wollheim CB: Effects of depletion of mitochondrial DNA in metabolism secretion coupling in INS-1 cells. *Diabetes* **47**:374, 1998.
135. van den Ouweland J, Lemkes H, Ruitenbeek W, Sandkuijl L, de Vijlder M, Struyvenberg P, van de Kamp J, et al.: Mutation in mitochondrial tRNA(Leu)(UUR) gene in a large pedigree with maternally transmitted type 2 diabetes mellitus and deafness. *Nat Genet* **1**:368, 1992.
136. Ciafaloni E, Ricci E, Shanske S, Moraes C, Silvestri G, Hirano M, Simonett S, et al.: MELAS: Clinical features, biochemistry, and molecular genetics. *Ann Neurol* **31**:391, 1992.
137. Katagiri H, Asano T, Ishihara H, Inukai K, Anai M, Yamanouchi T, Tsukuda K, et al.: Mitochondrial diabetes mellitus: prevalence and clinical characterization of diabetes due to mitochondrial tRNA Leu(UUR) gene mutation in Japanese patients. *Diabetologia* **37**:504, 1994.
138. Kovalenko S, Tanaka M, Yoneda M, Iakovlev A, Ozawa T: Accumulation of somatic nucleotide substitutions in mitochondrial DNA associated with the 3243 A-to-G tRNA Leu(UUR) mutation in encephalomyopathy and cardiomyopathy. *Biochem Biophys Res Commun* **222**:201, 1996.
139. Kameoka K, Isotani H, Tanaka K, Azukari K, Fujimura Y, Shiota Y, Sasaki E, et al.: Novel mitochondrial DNA mutation in tRNA(Lys) (88296A-G) associated with diabetes. *Biochem Biophys Res Commun* **245**:523, 1998.
140. Tsukuda K, Suzuki Y, Kameoka K, Osawa N, Goto Y, Katagiri H, Asano T, et al.: Screening of patients with maternally transmitted diabetes for mitochondrial gene mutations in the tRNA Leu(UUR) region. *Diabet Med* **14**:1032, 1997.
141. Harvey J, Barnett D: Endocrine dysfunction in Kearns-Sayre syndrome. *Clin Endocrinol* **37**:97, 1992.
142. Tattersall R: Maturity-onset diabetes of the young: a clinical history. *Diabet Med* **15**:11, 1998.
143. Fajans SS: Scope and heterogenous nature of MODY. *Diabetes Care* **13**:49, 1990.
144. Bell GI, Xiang K-S, Newman MV, Wu S-H, Wright LG, Fajans SS, Spielman RS, et al.: Gene for non-insulin-dependent diabetes mellitus (maturity-onset diabetes of the young subtype) is linked to DNA polymorphism on human chromosome 20q. *Proc Natl Acad Sci U S A* **88**:1484, 1991.
145. Yamagata K, Oda N, Kaisaki PJ, Menzel S: Mutations in the hepatocyte nuclear factor-1alpha gene in maturity-onset diabetes of the young (MODY 3). *Nature* **384**:455, 1996.
146. Stoffel M, Le-Beau M, Espinosa R, Bohlander S, Bell CI: A yeast artificial chromosome-based map of the region of the chromosome 20 containing the diabetes-susceptibility gene, MODY1, and a myeloid leukemia-related gene. *Proc Natl Acad Sci U S A* **93**:3937, 1996.
147. Stoffel M, Duncan S: The maturity-onset diabetes of the young (MODY1) transcription factor HNF4α regulates expression of genes required for glucose transport and metabolism. *Proc Natl Acad Sci U S A* **94**:13209, 1997.
148. Chen WS, Manova K, Weinstein C, Duncan SA, Plump AS, Prezioso VR, Bachvarova RF, et al.: Disruption of the HNF-4 gene, expressed in visceral endoderm, leads to cell death in embryonic ectoderm and impaired gastrulation of mouse embryos. *Genes Dev* **8**:2466, 1994.
149. Bulman M, Dronsfield M, Frayling T, Appleton M, Bain S, Ellard S, Hattersley A: A missense mutation in the hepatocyte nuclear factor 4 alpha gene in a UK pedigree with maturity-onset diabetes of the young. *Diabetologia* **40**:859, 1997.
150. Furuta H, Iwasaki N, Oda N, Hinokio Y, Horikawa Y, Yamagata K, Yano N, et al.: Organization and partial sequence of nuclear factor-4α/MODY1 gene and identification of a missense mutation, R127W, in a Japanese family with MODY. *Diabetes* **46**:1653, 1997.
151. Bowden DW, Sale M, Howard TD, Qadri A, Spray BJ, Rothschild CB, Akots G, et al.: Linkage of genetic markers on chromosomes 20 and 12 to NIDDM in Caucasian sib pairs with a history of diabetic nephropathy. *Diabetes* **46**:882, 1997.
152. Hani E, Suaud L, Boutin P, Chevre J, Durand E, Philippi A, Demenais F, et al.: A missense mutation in hepatocyte nuclear factor-4 alpha, resulting in a reduced transactivation activity, in human late-onset non-insulin-dependent diabetes mellitus. *J Clin Invest* **101**:521, 1998.
153. Moller A, Urhammer S, Dalgaard L, Reneland R, Berglund L, Hansen T, Clausen J, et al.: Studies of the genetic variability of the coding region of the hepatocyte nuclear factor-4 alpha in Caucasians with maturity onset NIDDM. *Diabetologia* **40**:980, 1997.
154. Froguel P, Vaxillaire M, Velho G: Genetic and metabolic heterogeneity of maturity-onset diabetes of the young. *Diabetes Rev* **5**:123, 1997.
155. Matchinsky FM: Glucokinase as glucose sensor and metabolic signal generator in pancreatic beta-cells and hepatocytes. *Diabetes* **39**:647, 1990.
156. Gidh-Jain M, Takeda J, et al.: Glucokinase mutations associated with non-insulin-dependent (type 2) diabetes mellitus have decreased activity. *Proc Natl Acad Sci U S A* **90**:1932, 1993.
157. Liang Y, Kevsavan P, Wang LQ, Niswender K, Tanizawa Y, Permutt MA, Magnuson MA, et al.: Variable effects of maturity onset diabetes of youth (MODY)-associated glucokinase mutations on substrate interactions. *Biochem J* **309**:167, 1995.
158. Kesavan P, Wang L, Davis E, Cuesta A, Sweet I, Niswender K, Magnuson M, et al.: Structural instability of mutant beta-cell glucokinase: Implications for the molecular pathogenesis of maturity-onset diabetes of the young (type-2). *Biochem J* **322**:57, 1997.
159. veiga da Cunha M, Courtois S, Michael A, Gosselain E, van Schaftingen E: Amino acid conservation in animal glucokinases: Identification of residues implicated in the interaction with the regulatory protein. *J Biol Chem* **271**:6292, 1996.
160. Velho G, Blanche H, Vaxillaire M, Bellanne-Chantelot C, Pardini V, Timsit J, Passa P, et al.: Identification of 14 new glucokinase mutations and description of the clinical profile of 42 MODY-2 families. *Diabetologia* **40**:217, 1997.
161. Bell G, Pilkis S, Weber I, Polonsky K: Glucokinase mutations, insulin secretion, and diabetes mellitus. *Annu Rev Physiol* **58**:171, 1996.
162. Clark A, de Koning E, Hattersley AT, Hansen BC, Yajnik CS, Poulton J: Pancreatic pathology in non-insulin dependent diabetes (NIDDM). *Diabetes Res Clin Pract* **28(Suppl)**:S39, 1995.
163. Polonsky KS: The β-cell in diabetes: From molecular genetics to clinical research. *Diabetes* **44**:705, 1995.
164. Wajngot A, Alvarsson M, Glaser A, Efendic S, Luthman H, Grill V: Glucose potentiation of arginine-induced insulin secretion in subjects with a glucokinase Glu256Lys. *Diabetes* **43**:1402, 1994.
165. Clement K, Pueyo ME, Vaxillaire M, Rakotoambinina B, Thuiller F, Passa P, Froguel P, et al.: Assessment of insulin sensitivity in glucokinase-deficient subjects. *Diabetologia* **39**:82, 1996.
166. Velho G, Petersen K, Perseghin G, Hwang J, Rothman D, Pueyo M, Cline G, et al.: Impaired hepatic glycogen synthesis in glucokinase-deficient (MODY2) subjects. *J Clin Invest* **98**:1755, 1996.
167. Tappy L, Dussoix P, Iynedjian P, Henry S, Schneiter P, Zahnd G, Jequier E, et al.: Abnormal regulation of hepatic glucose output in maturity-onset diabetes of the young caused by a specific mutation of the glucokinase gene. *Diabetes* **46**:204, 1997.
168. Katagiri H, Asano T, Ishihara H, Inukai K, Anai M, Miyazaki J-I, Tsukuda K, et al.: Nonsense mutation of glucokinase gene in late-onset non-insulin-dependent diabetes mellitus. *Lancet* **340**:1316, 1992.
169. Vaxillaire M, Boccio V, Philippi A, Vigouroux C, Terwilliger J, Passa P, Beckmann J, et al.: A gene for maturity onset diabetes of the young (MODY) maps to chromosome 12q. *Nat Genet* **9**:418, 1995.
170. Menzel S, Yamagata K, Trabb J, Nerup J, Permutt M, Fajans S, Menzel R, et al.: Localization of *MODY3* to a 5-cM region of human chromosome 12. *Diabetes* **44**:1408, 1995.
171. Yamagata K, Furuta H, Oda N, Kaisaki PJ, Menzel S, Cox NJ, Fajans SS, et al.: Mutations in the hepatocyte nuclear factor-4alpha gene in maturity-onset diabetes of the young (MODY1). *Nature* **384**:458, 1996.
172. Vaxillaire M, Rouard M, Yamagata K, Oda N, Kaisaki P, Boriraj V, Chevre J, et al.: Identification of nine novel mutations in the hepatocyte nuclear factor 1 alpha gene associated with maturity-onset diabetes of the young (MODY3). *Hum Mol Genet* **6**:583, 1997.
173. Frayling T, Bulman M, Ellard S, Appleton M, Dronsfield M, Mackie A, Baird J, et al.: Mutations in the hepatocyte nuclear factor-1alpha gene are a common cause of maturity-onset diabetes of the young in the U.K. *Diabetes* **46**:720, 1997.
174. Glucksmann M, Lehto M, Tayber O, Scotti S, Berkemeier L, Pulido J, Wu Y, et al.: Novel mutations and a mutational hotspot in the MODY3 gene. *Diabetes* **46**:1081, 1997.
175. Velho G, Froguel P: Genetic, metabolic and clinical characteristics of maturity onset diabetes of the young. *Eur J Endocrinol* **138**:233, 1998.

176. Hattersley A: Maturity-onset diabetes of the young: clinical heterogeneity explained by genetic heterogeneity. *Diabet Med* **15**:15, 1998.
177. Velho G, Vaxillaire M, Boccio V, Charpentier G, Froguel P: Diabetes complications in NIDDM kindreds linked to the MODY3 locus on chromosome 12q. *Diabetes Care* **19**:915, 1996.
178. Gragnoli C, Lindner T, Cockburn BN, Kaisaki PJ, Gragnoli F, Marozzi G, Bell GI: Maturity-onset diabetes of the young due to a mutation in the hepatocyte nuclear factor-4 α binding site in the promoter of the hepatocyte nuclear factor 1-α gene. *Diabetes* **46**:1648, 1997.
179. Iwasaki N, Oda N, Ogata M, Hara M, Hinokio Y, Oda Y, Yamagata K, et al.: Mutations in the hepatocyte nuclear factor-1alpha/MODY3 gene in Japanese subjects with early- and late-onset NIDDM. *Diabetes* **46**:1504, 1997.
180. Nishigori H, Yamada S, Kohama T, Utsugi T, Shimizu H, Takeuchi T, Tadeda J: Mutations in the hepatocyte nuclear factor-1 alpha gene (MODY3) are not a major cause of early-onset non-insulin-dependent (type 2) diabetes mellitus in Japanese. *J Hum Genet* **43**:107, 1998.
181. Horikawa Y, Iwasaki N, Hara M, Furuta H, Hinokio Y, Cockburn BN: Mutation in hepatocyte nuclear factor-1β gene (TCF2) associated with MODY. *Nat Genet* **17**:384, 1997.
182. Nishigori H, Yamada S, Kohama T, Tomura H, Sho K, Horidawa Y, Bell GI, et al.: Frameshift mutation, A263fsinsGG, in the hepatocyte nuclear factor-1β gene associated with diabetes and renal dysfunction. *Diabetes* **47**:1354, 1998.
183. Beards F, Frayling T, Bulman M, Horikawa Y, Allen L, Appleton M, Bell GI, et al.: Mutations in hepatocyte nuclear factor 1β are not a common cause of maturity-onset diabetes of the young in the U.K. *Diabetes* **47**:1152, 1998.
184. Stoffers DA, Ferrer J, Clarke WL, Habener JF: Early-onset type-II diabetes mellitus (MODY 4) linked to IPF1. *Nat Genet* **17**:138, 1997.
185. Jonsson J, Carlsson L, Edlund T, Edlund H: Insulin-promoter-factor 1 is required for pancreas development in mice. *Nature* **371**:606, 1994.
186. Stoffers DA, Zinkin NT, Stanojevic V, Clarke WL, Habener JF: Pancreatic agenesis attributable to a single nucleotide deletion in the human IPF-1 gene coding sequence. *Nat Genet* **15**:106, 1997.
187. Inoue H, Riggs AC, Tanizawa Y, Ueda K, Kuano A, Liu L, Donis-Keller H, et al.: Isolation, characterization, and chromosomal mapping of the human insulin promoter factor 1 (IPF-1) gene. *Diabetes* **45**:789, 1996.
188. Gerich JE: The genetic basis of type 2 diabetes mellitus: Impaired insulin secretion *versus* impaired insulin sensitivity. *Endocr Rev* **19**:491, 1998.
189. Ferrannini E: Insulin resistance *versus* insulin deficiency in insulin-dependent diabetes mellitus: problems and prospects. *Endocr Rev* **19**:477, 1998.
190. Vaag A, Henriksen J, Madsbad S, Holm N, Beck-Nielsen H: Insulin secretion, insulin action, and hepatic glucose production in identical twins discordant for non-insulin-dependent diabetes mellitus. *J Clin Invest* **95**:690, 1995.
191. Janssen RC, Bogardus C, Takeda J, Knowler WC, Thompson DB: Linkage analysis of acute insulin secretion with GLUT2 and glucokinase in Pima Indians and the identification of a missense mutation in GLUT2. *Diabetes* **43**:558, 1994.
192. Lillioja S, Mott DM, Zawadzki JK, Young AA, Abbott WG, Knowler WC, Bennett PH, et al.: In vivo insulin action is a familial characteristic in nondiabetic Pima Indians. *Diabetes* **36**:1329, 1987.
193. Gottlieb MS, Root HF: Diabetes Mellitus in twins. *Diabetes* **17**:693, 1968.
194. Barnett AH, Eff C, Leslie RDG, Pyke DA: Diabetes in identical twins. A study of 200 pairs. *Diabetologia* **20**:87, 1981.
195. Newman B, Selby JV, King M-C, Slemeda C, Fabsitz R, Friedman GC: Concordance for type 2 (non-insulin-dependent) diabetes mellitus in male twins. *Diabetologia* **30**:763, 1987.
196. Japan Diabetes Society Committee on Diabetic Twins: Diabetes mellitus in twins: A cooperative study in Japan. *Diabetes Res Clin Pract* **5**:271, 1988.
197. Kaprio J, Tuomilehto J, Koshenvuo M, Romanov K, Reunanen A, Eriksson J, Stengard J, et al.: Concordance for type 1 (insulin-dependent) and type 2 (non-insulin-dependent) diabetes mellitus in a population-based cohort of twins in Finland. *Diabetologia* **35**:1060, 1992.
198. Harris MI, Hadden WC, Knowler WC, Bennett PH: Prevalence of diabetes and impaired glucose tolerance and plasma glucose levels in U.S. population aged 20–74 yr. *Diabetes* **36**:523, 1987.
199. Eriksson J, Fransila-Kallunki A, Ekstrand A, Saloranta C, Widen E, Camilla-Schalin MS, Groop L: Early metabolic defects in persons at increased risk for non-insulin dependent diabetes mellitus. *N Engl J Med* **321**:337, 1989.
200. Warram JH, Martin BC, Krolewski AS, Soeldner JS, Kahn CR: Slow glucose removal rate and hyperinsulinemia precede the development of type 2 diabetes in the offspring of diabetic parents. *Ann Int Med* **113**:909, 1990.
201. Gulli G, Ferrannini E, Stern M, Haffner S, DeFronzo R: The metabolic profile of NIDDM is fully established in glucose-tolerant offspring of two Mexican-American NIDDM parents. *Diabetes* **41**:1575, 1992.
202. Pimenta W, Korytkowski M, Mitrakou A, Jenssen T, Yki-Jarvinen H, Evron W, Dailey G, et al.: Pancreatic beta-cell dysfunction as the primary genetic lesion in NIDDM. *JAMA* **273**:1855, 1995.
203. Perseghin G, Ghosh S, Gerow K, Shulman G: Metabolic defects in lean nondiabetic offspring of NIDDM parents. *Diabetes* **46**:1001, 1997.
204. van Haeften T, Dubbeldam S, Zonderland M, Erkelens D: Insulin secretion in normal glucose-tolerant relatives of type 2 diabetic subjects. *Diabetes Care* **21**:278, 1998.
205. Ishikawa M, Pruneda M, Adams-Huet B, Raskin P: Obesity-independent hyperinsulinemia in nondiabetic first-degree relatives of individuals with type 2 diabetes. *Diabetes* **47**:788, 1998.
206. Vauhkonen I, Niskanen L, Vanninen E, Kainulainen S, Uusitupa M, Laakso M: Defects in insulin secretion and insulin action in non-insulin-dependent diabetes mellitus are inherited—Metabolic studies on offspring of diabetic probands. *J Clin Invest* **101**:86, 1998.
207. Ghosh S, Collins F: The geneticist's approach to complex disease. *Annu Rev Med* **47**:333, 1996.
208. Velho G, Froguel P: Genetic determinants of non-insulin-dependent diabetes mellitus: Strategies and recent results. *Diabetes Metab* **23**:7, 1997.
209. Chiu KC, Province MA, Dowse GK, Zimmet PZ, Wagner G, Serjeantson S, Permutt MA: A genetic marker at the GK gene locus for type 2 diabetes mellitus in Mauritian Creoles. *Diabetologia* **35**:632, 1992.
210. Chiu KC, Province MA, Permutt MA: Glucokinase gene is genetic marker for NIDDM in American blacks. *Diabetes* **41**:843, 1992.
211. Shelton KD, Franklin AJ, Khoor A, Beechem J, Magnuson MA: Multiple elements in the upstream glucokinase promoter contribute to transcription in insulinoma cells. *Mol Cell Biol* **12**:4578, 1992.
212. Stone LM, Kahn SE, Fujimoto WY, Deeb SS, Porte D Jr: A variation at position −30 of the B-cell GK gene promoter is associated with reduced B-cell function. *Diabetes* **45**:422, 1996.
213. Elbein SC, Hoffman M, Chiu D, Tanizawa Y, Permutt MA: Linkage analysis of the glucokinase locus in familial type 2 diabetic pedigrees. *Diabetologia* **36**:141, 1993.
214. Zouali H, Vaxillaire M, Lesage S, Sun F, Velho G, Vionnet N, Chiu K, et al.: Linkage analysis and molecular scanning of glucokinase gene in NIDDM families. *Diabetes* **42**:1238, 1993.
215. Cook JTE, Hattersley AT, Christopher P, Bown E, Barrow B, Patel P, Shaw JAG, et al.: Linkage analysis of glucokinase gene with NIDDM in Caucasian pedigrees. *Diabetes* **41**:1496, 1992.
216. McCarthy MI, Hitchins M, Hitman GA, Cassel P, Hawrami K, Morton N, Mohan V, et al.: Absence of linkage suggests a minor role for the glucokinase gene in the pathogenesis of type 2 diabetes in South Indians. *Diabetologia* **36**:633, 1993.
217. McCarthy MI, Hitman GA, Hitchins M, Riikonen A, Stengård J, Nissinen A, Tuomilehto-Wolf E, et al.: Glucokinase gene polymorphisms: A genetic marker for glucose intolerance in a cohort of elderly Finnish men. *Diabet Med* **11**:198, 1994.
218. Urhammer SA, Hansen T, Clausen JO, Eiberg H, Pedersen O: The g/a nucleotide variant at position −30 in the β-cell-specific glucokinase gene promoter has no impact on the β-cell function in Danish Caucasians. *Diabetes* **47**:1359, 1998.
219. Cook DL, Taborsky GJ Jr: B-cell function and insulin secretion, in Porte D Jr, Sherwin RS (eds): *Diabetes Mellitus*, 5th ed. Stamford, CT, Appleton and Lange, 1997, p 49.
220. Aquilar-Bryan L, Nichols CG, Wechsler SW, Clement JP, Boyd AE, Gonzalez G, Herrera-Sosa H, et al.: Cloning of the β-cell high affinity sulfonylurea receptor: a regulator of insulin secretion. *Science* **268**:423, 1995.
221. Thomas P, Cote G, Wohllk N, Haddad B, Mathew P, Rabl W, Aguilar-Bryan L, et al.: Mutations in the sulfonylurea receptor gene in familial persistent hyperinsulinemic hypoglycemia of infancy. *Science* **268**:426, 1995.
222. Nestorowicz A, Wilson B, Schoor K, Inoue H, Glaser B, Landau H, Stanley C, et al.: Mutations in the sulfonylurea receptor gene are associated with familial hyperinsulinism in Ashkenazi Jews. *Hum Mol Genet* **5**:1813, 1996.
223. Nestorowicz A, Inagaki N, Gonoi T, Schoor K, Wilson B, Glaser B, Landau H, et al.: A nonsense mutation in the inward rectifier potassium channel gene, Kir6.2, is associated with familial hyperinsulinism. *Diabetes* **46**:1743, 1997.

224. Shyng S, Ferrigni T, Shepard J, Nestorowicz A, Glaser B, Permutt M, Nichols C: Functional analyses of novel mutations in the sulfonylurea receptor 1 associated with persistent hyperinsulinemic hypoglycemia of infancy. *Diabetes* **47**:1145, 1998.
225. Stirling B, Cox N, Bell G, Hanis C, Spielman R, Concannon P: Linkage studies in NIDDM with markers near the sulphonylurea receptor gene. *Diabetologia* **38**:1479, 1995.
226. Inoue H, Ferrer J, Welling C, Elbein S, Hoffman M, Mayorga R, Warren-Perry M, et al.: Sequence variants in the sulfonylurea receptor (SUR) gene are associated with NIDDM in Caucasians. *Diabetes* **45**:825, 1996.
227. Hani E, Clement K, Velho G, Vionnet N, Hager J, Philippi A, Dina C, et al.: Genetic studies of the sulfonylurea receptor gene locus in NIDDM and in morbid obesity among French Caucasians. *Diabetes* **46**:688, 1997.
228. Ohta Y, Tanizawa Y, Inoue H, Hosaka T, Ueda K, Matsutani A, Repunte V, et al.: Identification and functional analysis of sulfonylurea receptor 1 variants in Japanese patients with NIDDM. *Diabetes* **47**:476, 1998.
229. Hansen T, Echwald S, Hansen L, Moller A, Almind K, Aguilar-Bryan L, Permutt M, et al.: Decreased tolbutamide-stimulated insulin secretion in healthy subjects with sequence variants in the high-affinity sulfonylurea receptor gene. *Diabetes* **47**:598, 1998.
230. Inoue H, Ferrer J, Warren-Perry M, Zhang Y, Millns N, Turner RC, Elbein SC, et al.: Sequence variants in the pancreatic islet beta-cell inwardly rectifying K+ channel Kir6.2 (Bir) gene: Identification and lack of role in Caucasian patients with NIDDM. *Diabetes* **46**:502, 1997.
231. Matschinsky F: A lesson in metabolic regulation inspired by the glucokinase glucose sensor paradigm. *Diabetes* **45**:223, 1996.
232. Liang Y, Cushman SM, Whitesell RR, Natschinsky FM: GLUT1 is adequate for glucose uptake in GLUT2-deficient insulin-releasing beta-cells. *Horm Metab Res* **29**:255, 1997.
233. Chen C, Thorens B, Bonner-Weir S, Weir GC, Leahy JL: Recovery of glucose-induced insulin secretion in a rat model of NIDDM is not accompanied by return of the B-cell GLUT2 glucose transporter. *Diabetes* **41**:1320, 1992.
234. de Vos A, Heimberg H, Quartier E, Huypens P, Bouwens L, Pipeleers D, Schuit F: Human and rat beta cells differ in glucose transporter but not in glucokinase gene expression. *J Clin Invest* **96**:2489, 1995.
235. Matsubara A, Tanizawa Y, Matsutani A, Kaneko T, Kaku K: Sequence variations of the pancreatic islet/liver glucose transporter (GLUT2) gene in Japanese subjects with non-insulin-dependent diabetes mellitus. *J Clin Endocrinol Metab* **80**:3131, 1995.
236. Tanizawa Y, Riggs A, Chiu K, Janssen R, Bell D, Go R, Roseman J, et al.: Variability of the pancreatic islet beta cell/liver (GLUT2) glucose transporter gene in NIDDM patients. *Diabetologia* **37**:420, 1994.
237. Mueckler M, Kruse M, Strube M, Riggs A, Chiu K, Permutt M: A mutation in the Glut2 glucose transporter gene of a diabetic patient abolishes transport activity. *J Biol Chem* **269**:17765, 1994.
238. Hager J, Hansen L, Vaisse C, Vionnet N, Philippi A, Poller W, Velho G, et al.: A missense mutation in the glucagon receptor gene is associated with non-insulin-dependent diabetes mellitus. *Nat Genet* **9**:299, 1995.
239. Fujisawa T, Ikegami H, Yamato E, Takekawa K, Nakagawa Y, Hamada Y, Ueda H, et al.: A mutation in the glucagon receptor gene (Gly40Ser): Heterogeneity in the association with diabetes mellitus. *Diabetologia* **38**:983, 1995.
240. Hart L, Stolk R, Jansen J, Grobbee D: Absence of the Gly40-Ser mutation in the glucagon receptor among diabetic patients in the Netherlands. *Diabetes Care* **18**:1400, 1995.
241. Gough S, Saker P, Pritchard L, Merriman T, Merriman M, Rowe B, Kumar S, et al.: Mutation of the glucagon receptor gene and diabetes mellitus in the UK: Association or founder effect. *Hum Mol Genet* **4**:1609, 1995.
242. Ristow M, Busch K, Schatz H, Pfeiffer A: Restricted geographical extension of the association of a glucagon receptor gene mutation (Gly40Ser) with non-insulin-dependent diabetes mellitus. *Diabetes Res Clin Pract* **32**:183, 1996.
243. Odawara M, Tachi Y, Yamashita K: Absence of association between the Gly(40)Ser mutation in the human glucagon receptor and Japanese patients with non-insulin-dependent diabetes mellitus or impaired glucose tolerance. *Hum Genet* **98**:636, 1996.
244. Ogata M, Iwasaki N, Ohgawara H, Karibe S, Omori Y: Absence of the Gly(40)Ser mutation in the glucagon receptor gene in Japanese subjects with NIDDM. *Diabetes Res Clin Pract* **33**:71, 1996.
245. Fujisawa T, Ikegami H, Babaya N, Ogihara T: Gly40Ser mutation of glucagon receptor gene and essential hypertension in Japanese. *Hypertension* **28**:1100, 1996.
246. Morris B, Chambers S: Hypothesis: Glucagon receptor glycine to serine missense mutation contributes to one in 20 cases of essential hypertension. *Clin Exp Pharmacol Physiol* **23**:1035, 1996.
247. Tonolo G, Melis M, Ciccarese M, Secchi G, Atzeni M, Li L, Luthman H, et al.: Glucagon receptor Gly40Ser amino acid variant in Sardinian hypertensive non-insulin-dependent diabetic patients. *Acta Diabetologica* **34**:75, 1997.
248. Tonolo G, Melis M, Ciccarese M, Secchi G, Atzeni M, Maioli M, Pala G, et al.: Physiological and genetic characterization of the Gly40Ser mutation in the glucagon receptor gene in the Sardinian population. *Diabetologia* **40**:89, 1997.
249. Hansen L, Abrahamsen N, Hager J, Jelinek L, Kindsvogel W, Froguel P, Nishimura E: The Gly40Ser mutation in the human glucagon receptor gene associated with NIDDM results in a receptor with reduced sensitivity to glucagon. *Diabetes* **45**:725, 1996.
250. Babadjanova G, Reincke M, Mora P, Chuchalin A, Allolio B: Polymorphism of the glucagon receptor gene and non-insulin-dependent diabetes mellitus in the Russian population. *Exp Clin Endocrinol Diabetes* **105**:225, 1997.
251. Urhammer S, Rasmussen S, Kaisaki P, Oda N, Yamagata K, Moller A, Fridberg M, et al.: Genetic variation in the hepatocyte nuclear factor-1 alpha gene in Danish Caucasians with late-onset NIDDM. *Diabetologia* **40**:473, 1997.
252. Vionnet N, Hani EH, Lesage S, Philippi A, Hager J, Varret M, Stoffel M, et al.: Genetics of NIDDM in France: Studies with 19 candidate genes in affected sib pairs. *Diabetes* **46**:1062, 1997.
253. Mahtani M, Widen E, Lehto M, Thomas MM Jr, Brayer J, Bryant B, et al.: Mapping of a gene for type 2 diabetes associated with an insulin secretion defect by a genome scan in Finnish families. *Nat Genet* **14**:90, 1996.
254. Hanis C, Boerwinkle E, Chakraborty R, Ellsworth D, Concannon P, Stirling B, Morrison V, et al.: A genome-wide search for human non-insulin-dependent (type 2) diabetes genes reveals a major susceptibility locus on chromosome 2. *Nat Genet* **13**:161, 1996.
255. Thomas A, Sherratt E, Gagg J, Davies S, Majid A, Alcolado J: Genetic linkage study of a major susceptibility locus (D2S125) in a British population of non-insulin dependent diabetic sib-pairs using a simple non-isotopic screening method. *Hum Genet* **101**:212, 1997.
256. Ghosh S, Hauser ER, Magnuson VL, Valle T, Ally DS, Karanjawala ZE, Rayman JB, et al.: A large sample of Finnish diabetic sib-pairs reveals no evidence for a non-insulin-dependent diabetes mellitus susceptibility locus at 2qter. *J Clin Invest* **102**:704, 1998.
257. Stern M, Duggirala R, Mitchell B, Reinhart L, Shivakumar S, Shipman P, Uresandi O, et al.: Evidence for linkage of regions on chromosomes 6 and 11 to plasma glucose concentrations in Mexican Americans. *Genome Res* **6**:724, 1996.
258. Pratley R, Thompson D, Prochazka M, Baier L, Mott D, Ravussin E, Sakul H, et al.: An autosomal genomic scan for loci linked to prediabetic phenotypes in Pima Indians. *J Clin Invest* **101**:1757, 1998.
259. Valle T, Tumomilehto J, Bergman R, Ghosh S, Hauser E, Eriksson J, Nylund S, et al.: Mapping Genes for NIDDM. *Diabetes Care* **21**:949, 1998.
260. Wollheim CB, Lang J, Regazzi R: The exocytotic process of insulin secretion and its regulation by Ca^{2+} and G-proteins. *Diabetes Rev* **4**:276, 1996.
261. Tanizawa Y, Chiu KC: Role of glucokinase in the defective insulin secretion of diabetes, in Flatt PR, Lenzen S (eds): *Frontiers of Insulin Secretion and Pancreatic B-Cell Research.* London, Smith-Gordon, 1994, p 437.
262. Cox NJ, Horikawa Y, Oda N, Hanis CL: Genetic variation in the calpain 10 gene affects susceptibility to type 2 diabetes in Mexican Americans. *Diabetes* **49 (suppl 1)**:A7, 2000.

CHAPTER 68

Insulin Action, Insulin Resistance, and Type 2 Diabetes Mellitus

Simeon I. Taylor

1. **Diabetes mellitus is a syndrome characterized by elevated levels of glucose in the plasma. The American Diabetes Association has recently proposed revised criteria for the diagnosis of diabetes: (a) a fasting plasma glucose level >126 mg/dl, *or* (b) a plasma glucose level >200 mg/dl at 2 h after the ingestion of oral glucose (75 g), *or* (c) random plasma glucose >200 mg/dl.**
2. **Diabetes is a heterogeneous clinical syndrome with multiple etiologies. Type 1 diabetes is caused by destruction of pancreatic beta cells, most often by autoimmune mechanisms. Type 2 diabetes (the most common form of diabetes, accounting for >90 percent of patients) is caused by a combination of two physiological defects: resistance to the action of insulin combined with a deficiency in insulin secretion. Although the molecular basis of the common form of type 2 diabetes has not been elucidated, it is thought to result from genetic defects that cause both insulin resistance and insulin deficiency. Type 2 diabetes generally has onset after the age of 40. Unlike type 1 diabetes, type 2 diabetes is usually associated with relatively mild hyperglycemia, and ketoacidosis seldom develops. Gestational diabetes mellitus is a form of diabetes that has its initial onset during pregnancy, and resolves after the end of the pregnancy.**
3. **Insulin exerts multiple effects upon target cells — especially skeletal muscle, liver, and adipose tissue. In general, insulin promotes storage of fuels (e.g., glycogen and triglyceride), and inhibits the breakdown of stored fuel. To accomplish these general physiological functions, insulin exerts multiple specific actions upon target cells. For example, insulin promotes recruitment of glucose transporters from intracellular vesicles to the plasma membrane, thereby stimulating glucose transport into skeletal muscle and adipocytes. Insulin also regulates many metabolic enzymes, either by increasing or decreasing the level of protein phosphorylation. In addition, insulin regulates the level of intracellular metabolites that regulate enzyme activity by allosteric mechanisms. Finally, insulin regulates the level of gene expression — inducing the expression of some genes (e.g., hepatic glucokinase) and inhibiting expression of other genes (e.g., phosphoenolpyruvate carboxykinase).**
4. **The biologic actions of insulin are mediated by a cell surface receptor. The receptor possesses an extracellular domain that binds insulin, and an intracellular domain that possesses tyrosine-specific protein kinase activity. Insulin binding activates the receptor tyrosine kinase, leading to autophosphorylation of the receptor as well as phosphorylation of several intracellular proteins (e.g., insulin receptor substrates -1, -2, -3, and -4). Insulin-stimulated tyrosine phosphorylation ultimately leads to the activation of multiple downstream signaling pathways. Among these, activation of phosphatidylinositol 3-kinase is the most important in mediating the metabolic actions of insulin. Increasing the cellular content of phosphatidylinositol 3,4,5-trisphosphate activates phosphoinositide-dependent protein kinases (e.g., PDK-1). PDK-1 phosphorylates and activates multiple downstream protein kinases, including protein kinase B, atypical protein kinase C, and p70 S6 kinase. Activation of these protein kinases is responsible for mediating many of the ultimate metabolic actions of insulin, including translocation of GLUT4, activation of glycogen synthesis, and suppressing gluconeogenesis by inhibiting transcription of the gene encoding phosphoenolpyruvate carboxykinase.**
5. **Although the primary causes of insulin resistance have not yet been elucidated in most patients with type 2 diabetes, mutations in the insulin receptor gene have been demonstrated to cause several rare syndromes associated with insulin resistance (e.g., type A insulin resistance, leprechaunism, and the Rabson-Mendenhall syndrome). In general, patients with two mutant alleles are more severely insulin resistant than are patients with one mutant allele. In some cases, the mutation decreases the number of insulin receptors expressed on the cell surface; in other cases, the mutations impair the functions of the insulin receptor (i.e., insulin binding or insulin-stimulated tyrosine kinase activity).**
6. **Recent studies with knockout mice provide animal models for polygenically inherited type 2 diabetes. For example, knockout of the IRS-1 gene leads to insulin resistance, but not diabetes. If this genetic defect in the insulin action pathway is combined with a genetic defect that impairs insulin secretion (e.g., heterozygosity for a null allele of the glucokinase gene), this causes the mice to become diabetic. Furthermore, it is also possible to cause diabetes by heterozygous knockout of two distinct genes in the insulin action pathway (e.g., the genes encoding the insulin receptor and IRS-1). Although knockout mice lacking IRS-1 did not develop diabetes, homozygous knockout of IRS-2 actually caused diabetes. The reason these mice developed diabetes was that knockout of the IRS-2 gene led to two physiological defects: the expected defect in the insulin action pathway plus an unexpected defect in insulin secretion that impaired the ability of the β-cell to compensate for insulin resistance.**
7. **Type 2 diabetes is associated with two physiological defects: insulin resistance and impaired insulin secretion. However,**

the disease evolves over many years, and progresses through multiple stages. Although there is some controversy about the precise sequence of events in the natural history of type 2 diabetes, the following is one formulation of the progressive evolution of type 2 diabetes in a typical patient. Peripheral insulin resistance develops relatively early in the course of the disease. So long as the pancreatic beta cell retains sufficient functional reserve, plasma insulin levels will rise to compensate for the insulin resistance. Nevertheless, the compensation may not be complete, and the patient may develop impaired glucose tolerance and/or impaired fasting glucose. As the disease continues to evolve, there is a progressive impairment in the ability of the beta cell to secrete insulin. This is the time of onset of overt diabetes—that is, at the time when impaired beta cell function prevents the beta cell from compensating for the preexisting insulin resistance. Ultimately, it is hepatic glucose production that determines the magnitude of the elevation in fasting plasma glucose. Thus, in the final stage in the evolution of type 2 diabetes, the liver becomes insulin resistant, and this (combined with impaired insulin secretion plus peripheral insulin resistance) results in severe hyperglycemia and decompensated diabetes.

8. **Although the primary (genetic) causes of insulin resistance are not known, much is known about some factors that contribute to the pathogenesis of insulin resistance. Most patients with type 2 diabetes are obese, and the increase in adiposity is believed to be an important causal factor in the development of insulin resistance. The increase in adipose tissue is associated with an increase in plasma free fatty acid levels, which promotes hepatic glucose production and inhibits peripheral glucose utilization. In addition, the diabetic state leads to a vicious cycle in which insulin deficiency and hyperglycemia both exacerbate insulin resistance and further impair insulin secretion. There is evidence that "glucose toxicity" is not directly caused by hyperglycemia, but rather that the effects are mediated by glucosamine, the levels of which are elevated in response to hyperglycemia.**
9. **Among the therapies for type 2 diabetes, at least two drugs (troglitazone and metformin) are said to function as insulin sensitizers. Troglitazone, a ligand for the peroxisome proliferator-activated receptor-γ, is thought to act directly upon adipose tissue, thereby exerting indirect effects to increase insulin sensitivity in skeletal muscle. Metformin exerts its principal action to suppress hepatic glucose production. In addition, by reducing the mass of adipose tissue, weight loss also increases insulin sensitivity. However, even therapies that work by other mechanisms (e.g., insulin and sulfonylureas) exert indirect effects to increase insulin sensitivity—for example, by alleviating the adverse effects of glucose toxicity.**

INTRODUCTION

Diabetes mellitus is a major public health problem that afflicts ~5 percent of the population, and is a major cause of morbidity due to blindness, renal failure, and amputations. Furthermore, diabetes is among the most common causes of death because it causes premature cardiovascular disease, cerebrovascular disease, and renal failure.[1]

Diabetes is characterized by abnormal elevations in the level of plasma glucose, and is caused by a deficiency of insulin and/or resistance to the action of the hormone. It is not a single disease, but rather a clinical syndrome characterized by an elevated level of plasma glucose, and also a predisposition to develop chronic complications such as retinopathy, neuropathy, nephropathy, and macrovascular disease.[2] There are many types of diabetes, each with a different cause. Diabetes can result from defects in either insulin secretion or insulin action. For example, insulin deficiency due to autoimmune destruction of pancreatic beta cells causes type 1 diabetes mellitus.[3] In contrast, insulin resistance due to mutations in the insulin receptor gene can cause diabetes despite supranormal levels of insulin in plasma.[4–6] Type 2 diabetes mellitus is a polygenic disease that results from combined defects in both insulin secretion and insulin action. This complexity led one author to refer to diabetes as the "geneticist's nightmare."[7] Fortunately, with the advent of the methods of modern molecular genetics, it is possible to begin to elucidate the molecular basis of each specific form of diabetes.

So far, the most dramatic progress has been made in relatively rare variants of diabetes that are characterized by simple patterns of inheritance.[4–6,8–16] With continued improvement in the power of the methods of molecular genetics, it seems likely that the future will bring major breakthroughs in our understanding of the common forms of diabetes mellitus. This chapter focuses upon mechanisms of insulin action and insulin resistance; issues related to insulin secretion are discussed in Chap. 67.

INSULIN ACTION

Physiology

Insulin exerts multiple actions throughout the body to regulate energy metabolism. After a meal, pancreatic β-cells secrete insulin, which directs the body to store fuel (e.g., triglyceride in adipose tissue and glycogen in liver and muscle). Furthermore, insulin inhibits the mobilization of stored fuels.[17,18] Similarly, insulin stimulates protein synthesis while inhibiting protein breakdown.[19,20] To fully understand the effects of insulin, it is necessary to review energy metabolism in more detail (Fig. 68-1).

Carbohydrate Metabolism. Circulating glucose serves as fuel for many tissues. Some tissues (e.g., erythrocytes) are obliged to metabolize glucose because they lack the mitochondrial enzymes required to metabolize alternative substrates such as fatty acids. Tissues such as muscle are capable of metabolizing either glucose or alternative fuels including free fatty acids and ketone bodies. The brain preferentially uses glucose in the fed state.[17,21,22] Because free fatty acids (FFA) bound to albumin in the plasma cannot pass through the blood-brain barrier, the brain cannot metabolize FFA as a source of fuel. Although the brain is capable of metabolizing water-soluble ketone bodies, the levels of ketone bodies are too low in the fed state to provide a significant fraction of the brain's energy needs. However, with prolonged starvation, ketone body levels rise to the point that they can replace glucose as a major source of fuel for the brain.

Glucose has several alternative fates within the cell (Fig. 68-1); the major pathways for glucose metabolism include storage in the form of glycogen, metabolism through the glycolytic pathway, and metabolism through the pentose cycle. Insulin plays a central role in regulating these pathways:

Glycogen synthesis: Glucose is phosphorylated to yield glucose 6-phosphate, and eventually converted into the nucleotide sugar UDP-glucose prior to incorporation into glycogen. In the fed state, the liver stores approximately 70 grams of glycogen; this is adequate to provide sufficient glucose for a fast of approximately 8 h duration.[23] The final step in the synthesis of glycogen is catalyzed by the enzyme glycogen synthase. In the reverse pathway, glucose 1-phosphate is derived from glycogen by phosphorolysis, in a step catalyzed by the enzyme glycogen phosphorylase. The enzyme glucose 6-phosphatase is required to release glucose into the blood. Because glucose 6-phosphatase is present only in liver and kidney, these are the only tissues that can break down glycogen to provide glucose to other cells in the body. In tissues like muscle, glucose (actually, glucose 6-phosphate) derived from glycogen is available only for metabolism within the same cell in which it was produced.

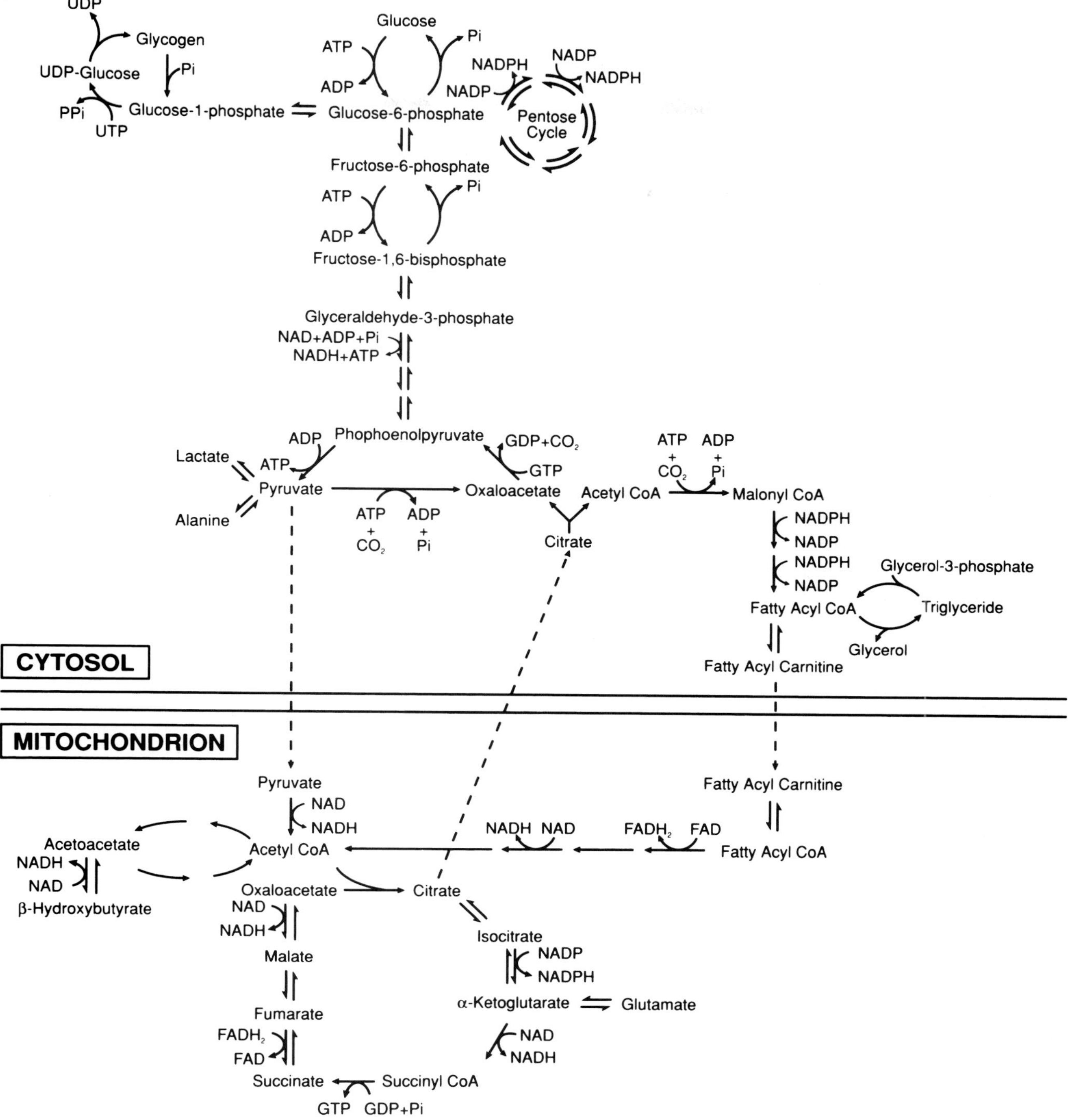

Fig. 68-1 Principal pathways of energy metabolism. The figure summarizes the general outlines of the central pathways of carbohydrate and triglyceride metabolism. Additional details are available in standard biochemistry textbooks.

Insulin activates the enzyme glycogen synthase, thereby accelerating the incorporation of glucose into glycogen.[24–26] In a reciprocal fashion, insulin inhibits glycogen breakdown by inactivating the enzyme glycogen phosphorylase. Counterregulatory enzymes such as epinephrine and glucagon exert effects that are the opposite of insulin upon both pathways.

Glycolytic pathway: In the glycolytic pathway, glucose is metabolized to pyruvate (or lactate). As a by-product of glycolysis, ATP is produced. While this is a minor source of ATP in tissues with active oxidative phosphorylation, anaerobic glycolysis is the major source of ATP in cells that lack mitochondria (e.g., erythrocytes). Even in skeletal muscle, glycolysis may be the major source of ATP under conditions of anaerobic exercise. In addition to ATP, the glycolytic pathway provides precursors for the synthesis of important molecules such as amino acids (e.g., transamination of pyruvate to yield alanine). Most of the enzymes in the glycolytic pathway are present in such high activity that they catalyze equilibrium reactions. Because the reactants and products are at near-equilibrium, the free energy change is approximately zero, and the reaction is said to be "reversible." However, a few reactions are "irreversible" because the enzymes are present in relatively limited activity so that the products of the reaction do not achieve equilibrium levels. In general, metabolic regulation is exerted at these irreversible (nonequilibrium) reactions. There are at least three irreversible reactions within the glycolytic pathway: the phosphorylation reactions catalyzed by hexokinase and phosphofructokinase, and the pyruvate kinase reaction in which ATP is synthesized.[27–29] All three enzymes are the targets for metabolic regulation. Insulin increases the flux through these three steps in insulin-sensitive tissues. The pathway of gluconeogenesis is functionally the reverse of glycolysis. In the case of the reversible reactions, the same enzymes function in both glycolysis and gluconeogenesis. However, different enzymes are required to catalyze the "irreversible" reactions.[28–30] In gluconeogenesis, fructose 1,6-bisphosphatase and glucose 6-phosphatase are the enzymes that remove phosphate from fructose 1,6-bisphosphate and glucose 6-phosphate, respectively. (Note that these are simple phosphatase reactions that are not coupled to the synthesis of ATP.) Synthesis of phosphoenolpyruvate from pyruvate is accomplished by the sequential actions of two enzymes: pyruvate carboxylase and phosphoenolpyruvate carboxykinase.

Pentose cycle: The pentose cycle is a side pathway, leading to the synthesis of NADPH as a consequence of oxidative decarboxylation of glucose 6-phosphate. This pathway has at least two functions: to provide a portion of the NADPH required for biosynthetic pathways (e.g., the synthesis of fatty acids from acetyl CoA), and to provide certain sugars required for synthesis of specialized cellular components (e.g., ribose for synthesis of nucleic acids). The reactions in the pentose cycle are reversible reactions. Thus, the flux through the pathway serves primarily to replenish the intermediates that are utilized in other pathways. Insulin tends to increase the flux through the pentose cycle. For example, inasmuch as insulin stimulates the synthesis of fatty acids from glucose, the utilization of NADPH will be increased by insulin. As NADPH is utilized in biosynthetic pathways, additional NADPH will be synthesized in the pentose cycle to replace that which was utilized.[31–34]

Lipid Metabolism. Triglyceride is the major form in which fuel is stored in the human body. Indeed, because the energy content of adipose tissue (~8 kcal/g) is much higher than lean tissue (~1 kcal/g), triglycerides provide a much more efficient depot in which to store energy than does glycogen.[17,18] Triglycerides consist of one molecule of glycerol esterified with three molecules of fatty acid. Hormone-sensitive lipase is the enzyme responsible for mobilizing stored triglycerides. This enzyme is activated by epinephrine, and inhibited by insulin.[35,36] After the triglyceride is hydrolyzed, the glycerol moiety undergoes further metabolism—for example, conversion to glucose by gluconeogenesis in the liver. The fatty acids can either be metabolized in peripheral tissues such as skeletal muscle, or can be converted to ketone bodies within the liver. However, fatty acids (with the exception of the small fraction of fatty acids with an odd number of carbon atoms) cannot be converted to glucose. Thus, when excess glucose is converted into fatty acids for the purpose of storing energy, this is a truly irreversible reaction. The mitochondrial enzyme pyruvate dehydrogenase converts pyruvate into acetyl CoA. While the substrate pyruvate can be converted into glucose, the reaction product acetyl CoA cannot be converted into glucose because mammalian tissues lack the enzymes required to reverse this biochemical process.

The irreversibility of the pyruvate dehydrogenase reaction suggests that it would be an important target for metabolic regulation. Insulin activates pyruvate dehydrogenase, thereby favoring the synthesis of fatty acids and triglycerides (e.g., in liver and adipose tissue).[37–42] In other tissues (e.g., skeletal muscle), activation of pyruvate dehydrogenase provides acetyl CoA for oxidation in the Krebs cycle.[43,44] In the liver, acetyl CoA has two major alternative fates: conversion to ketone bodies or incorporation into the fatty acid component of triglycerides.[45–48] Under conditions where pyruvate dehydrogenase is activated (e.g., in the presence of insulin), the acetyl CoA will be directed toward fatty acids for storage in the form of triglyceride. In contrast, in the absence of insulin, acetyl CoA is derived primarily from β-oxidation of fatty acids rather than from oxidation of pyruvate. Under these conditions, the acetyl CoA is directed toward synthesis of ketone bodies.

Protein Metabolism. Insulin exerts global effects on total protein metabolism: to promote protein synthesis while inhibiting protein degradation.[19,20] These global effects correlate with importance of proteins in energy metabolism. During prolonged fasting, proteins are degraded to provide substrate for gluconeogenesis. Indeed, the accelerated degradation of protein is among the most important adverse effects of starvation.

In addition to the global effect of insulin to promote protein synthesis, insulin also regulates the expression of many genes. The major physiological roles of proteins relate to their functions as enzymes, structural components, plasma proteins, hormones, and so on. Depending upon the physiological role of a particular protein, insulin may exert either a positive or negative effect upon its level of expression.[49,50] For example, enzymes that are involved in fuel storage (e.g., hepatic glucokinase) tend to be induced in response to insulin.[51] In contrast, insulin tends to inhibit the expression of genes encoding enzymes in catabolic pathways (e.g., hepatic phosphoenolpyruvate carboxykinase).[52]

Biochemistry and Cell Biology

Considerable progress has been made toward elucidating the detailed mechanisms of insulin action at the molecular level.[53,54] The pathways of insulin action can be divided into three phases (Fig. 68-2). The first phase of the pathway is initiated when insulin binds to the extracellular domain of its receptor, and activates the protein tyrosine kinase located in the intracellular domain of the receptor. The third portion of the pathway comprises the end results of insulin action—for example, stimulation of glucose transport, regulation of activities of various enzymes, and regulation of gene expression. The second phase of the pathway is comprised of the multiple steps that couple activation of the tyrosine kinase to the final events in insulin action. Although much has been learned about the first and last portions of the insulin action pathway, many gaps remain in our understanding of the middle portion. The following is a summary of the principal mechanisms whereby insulin regulates metabolism in target cells.

Insulin Receptor. The insulin receptor is a glycoprotein expressed on the surface of classical target cells for insulin action (e.g., hepatocytes, adipocytes, and muscle) as well as other cells (e.g., erythrocytes and monocytes). The receptor is the product of a single gene located on the short arm of human chromosome 19 (bands p13.2 → p13.3).[55] The mature receptor is derived from a 190,000-kilodalton precursor molecule as a result of extensive posttranslational processing, including proteolytic cleavage of the proreceptor into separate α- and β-subunits.[56–58] The subunits assemble into a heterotetrameric $\alpha 2\beta 2$ species, which is held together by disulfide bonds and noncovalent interactions (Fig. 68-3). The α-subunit is entirely extracellular, and contains the insulin-binding domain. The β-subunit has a single transmembrane domain, which allows it to span the plasma membrane. Its extracellular domain anchors the α-subunit to the plasma membrane, while the intracellular portion of the β-subunit possesses enzymatic activity as a tyrosine-specific protein kinase.[59,60] Activation of the receptor tyrosine kinase is a necessary step required to mediate the action of insulin upon target cells.[5,6,53,54,61–65] Insulin binding triggers phosphorylation of at least seven tyrosine residues in the intracellular domain of the β-subunit.[53,66–68] Although this is sometimes referred to as "autophosphorylation," it is thought to occur via transphosphorylation, with one β-subunit in the heterotetrameric $\alpha 2\beta 2$ structure phosphorylating the other β-subunit.

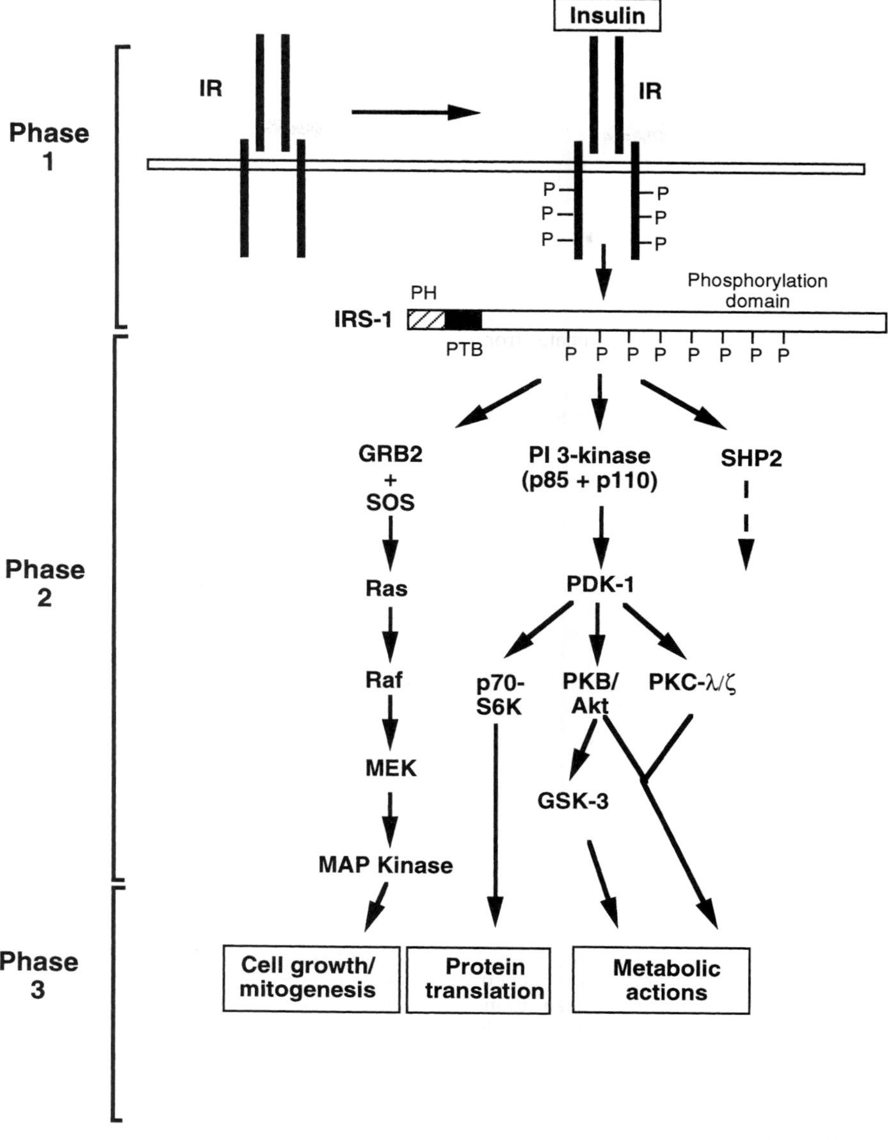

Fig. 68-2 Mechanisms of insulin action. The pathways of insulin action can be divided into three phases. The first phase of the pathway is initiated when insulin binds to the extracellular domain of its receptor, and activates the protein tyrosine kinase to phosphorylate substrates such as IRS-1, -2, -3, and -4. The second phase of the pathway includes several cascades of kinases that mediate the multiple biologic actions of insulin. These include phosphoinositide kinase-1 (PDK-1), protein kinase B (PKB/Akt), protein kinase C-λ/ζ, p70 S6 kinase, as well as the Raf/MEK/MAP kinase pathway downstream from Ras. In addition, phase 2 includes SH2-containing phosphotyrosine phosphatase-2 (SHP2). Phase 3 of the pathway consists of the final biologic effects of insulin—for example, the metabolic actions of insulin: translocation of GLUT4 glucose transporters to the plasma membrane; activation of the synthesis of glycogen, triglycerides, and protein; inhibition of gluconeogenesis, glycogenolysis, lipolysis, and proteolysis; regulation of specific gene expression (e.g., inhibition of transcription of the phosphoenolpyruvate carboxykinase gene). In addition to its metabolic actions, insulin also triggers various other biologic actions—for example, promotion of cell growth (mitogenic action of insulin), stimulating the translation of mRNA into protein, and regulating cell differentiation. The figure presents a somewhat oversimplified view of the coupling of signaling pathways (phase 2) to particular biologic responses (phase 3). Nevertheless, activation of PI 3-kinase appears to be upstream from most (if not all) the metabolic actions of insulin, and the Ras pathway appears to participate primarily in the growth-promoting effects of insulin rather than the metabolic effects. The third portion of the pathway comprises the end results of insulin action—e.g., stimulation of glucose transport, regulation of activities of various enzymes, and regulation of gene expression. The second phase of the pathway is comprised of the multiple steps that couple activation of the tyrosine kinase to the final events in insulin action.

The principal sites of receptor phosphorylation are located in three clusters in the intracellular domain (Fig. 68-3):

1. *Activation loop.* There are three tyrosine phosphorylation sites (Tyr^{1158}, Tyr^{1162}, and Tyr^{1163}) in the "activation loop."[69–71] Determination of the three-dimensional structure of the insulin receptor tyrosine kinase domain explained how phosphorylation of tyrosine residues in the activation loop leads to activation of the insulin receptor tyrosine kinase (Fig. 68-4).[69–71] Tyr^{1162} is located near the active site of the enzyme, and blocks the binding of other protein substrates. In addition, the unphosphorylated enzyme assumes a conformation that does not permit binding of MgATP, the phosphate donor for the reaction. The kinase is inactive because neither ATP nor the protein substrate can bind. When all three Tyr residues in the activation loop become phosphorylated, the

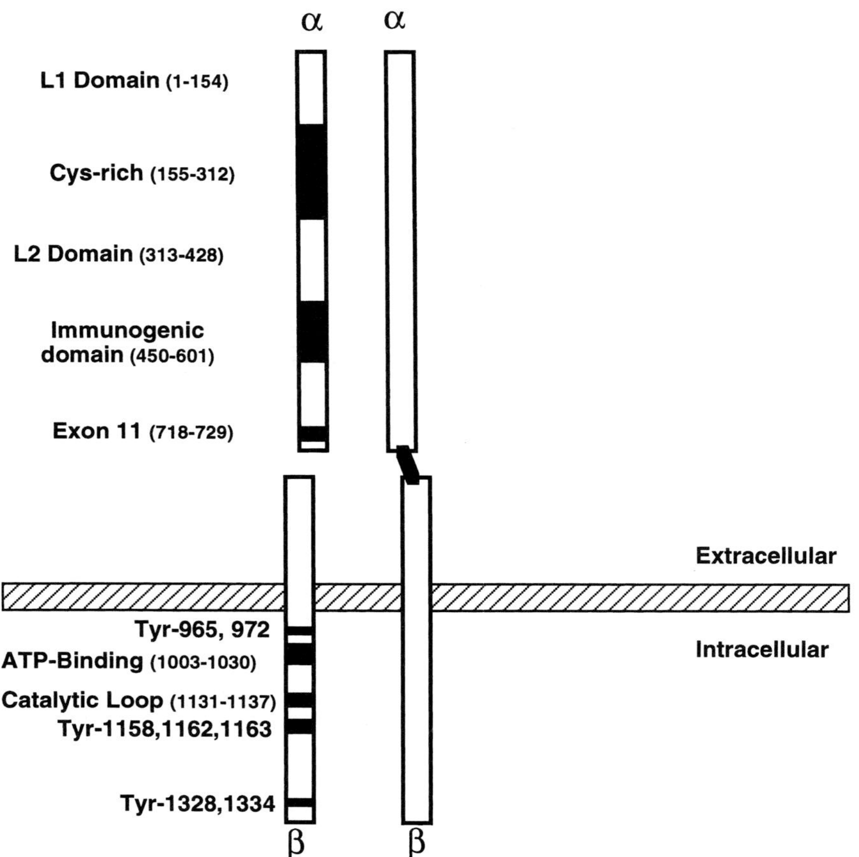

Fig. 68-3 Subunit structure of the insulin receptor. The insulin receptor has a heterotetrameric structure, consisting of two α- and two β-subunits.[5,6,294] The subunits are held together by noncovalent interactions as well as disulfide bonds. In addition to intrasubunit disulfide bonds (especially within the cysteine-rich domain of the α-subunit), there are α-α and α-β intersubunit disulfide bonds. There appear not to be β-β intersubunit disulfide bonds. The two distinct subunits are derived by proteolytic cleavage of a common precursor molecule encoded by a single gene containing 22 exons. The amino acid residues encoded by each exon are indicated on the right side of the figure. Key structural landmarks are indicated on the left side of the figure. The glycine-centered repeats consist of loosely conserved motifs that are homologous to sequences in receptors of the epidermal growth factor receptor family. The best-conserved feature in the motif is a central glycine residue that has been predicted to allow for a "turn" in the polypeptide chain conformation. In addition, there are usually hydrophobic amino acids located at positions 2, 5, and 8 amino acid residues upstream from the glycine residue. There are 4 or 5 of these repeats in each of two domains of the α-subunit (amino acid residues 1 to 154 and 313 to 428). Current evidence suggests that insulin binds primarily to the N-terminal half of the α-subunit. Human autoantibodies to the insulin receptor primarily recognize epitopes in the major immunogenic domain (amino acid residues 450 to 601). The sequence corresponding to exon 11 undergoes variable splicing leading to the existence of two isoforms of the insulin receptor, either containing or lacking amino acid residues 718 to 729. The seven major tyrosine phosphorylation sites are tyrosine residues 960, 972, 1158, 1162, 1163, 1328, and 1334. Tyr^{972} is thought to participate in binding of insulin receptor substrate-1. The Gly-X-Gly-X-X-Gly. . .Lys motif that characterizes ATP binding domains is located at amino acid residues 1003–1030. The seven amino acid residues in the catalytic loop are thought to play a role in catalyzing the phosphotransferase reaction and in determining substrate specificity.

kinase undergoes a conformational change permitting the active site to bind its substrates. This conformational change leads to activation of the receptor, and phosphorylation of multiple intracellular protein substrates.

2. *Juxtamembrane domain.* There are two tyrosine phosphorylation sites (Tyr^{965} and Tyr^{972}) in the juxtamembrane domain. Tyr^{972} is located in an Asn-Pro-Xaa-Tyr motif. Phosphorylation of this motif creates a binding site for the highly conserved phosphotyrosine binding (PTB) domains of several proteins that serve as substrates for phosphorylation by the insulin receptor, including insulin receptor substrates (IRS)-1, IRS-2, IRS-3, IRS-4, and Shc (see "Substrates for Phosphorylation by the Insulin Receptor" below).[54,72–74] When the PTB domain of an IRS protein binds to pTyr^{972} in the juxtamembrane domain of the phosphorylated insulin receptor, this places the IRS protein in a position that favors phosphorylation by the kinase domain of the receptor.
3. *C-terminal domain.* There are two tyrosine phosphorylation sites (Tyr^{1328} and Tyr^{1334}) in the C-terminal domain. Tyr^{1334} is located in a Tyr-Xaa-Xaa-Met motif. Phosphorylation of this motif creates a binding site for Src homology 2 (SH2) domains in the p85 regulatory subunit of phosphatidylinositol (PI) 3-kinase.[75,76] (SH2 domains are a conserved family of structural elements characterized by the ability to bind phosphotyrosine residues. SH2 domains in different proteins differ with respect to their specificity to bind particular phosphotyrosine residues, depending upon the amino acid sequence located downstream from the phosphotyrosine.) Although the SH2 domains of PI 3-kinase can bind to pTyr^{1334} of the insulin receptor, the physiological significance is controversial. While activation of the insulin tyrosine kinase leads to activation of PI 3-kinase, direct binding to the C-terminus of the insulin receptor is not thought to be the major mechanism. Rather, as discussed in "Substrates Containing Phosphotyrosine Binding Domains," PI 3-kinase binds bivalently to pTyr-Xaa-Xaa-Met motifs in IRS proteins, and this is primarily responsible for mediating activation of PI 3-kinase.[54,77]

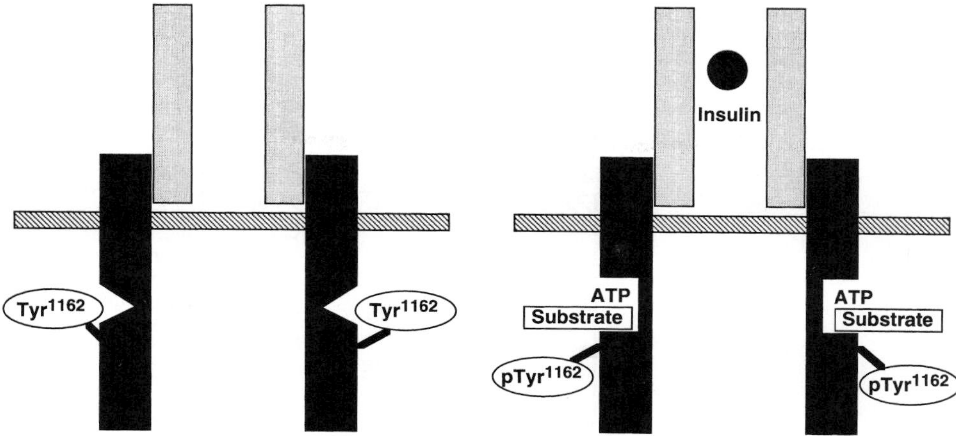

Fig. 68-4 Phosphorylation of tyrosine residues in the "activation loop" leads to activation of the insulin receptor tyrosine kinase. This illustrates a hypothetical mechanism for ligand-stimulated activation of the insulin receptor tyrosine kinase. The model is based upon the three-dimensional structure of the isolated insulin receptor tyrosine kinase as determined by x-ray crystallography.[69–71] In the inactive insulin receptor kinase (shown on the left), Tyr[1162] blocks the active site so that substrates cannot bind. In contrast, when the tyrosine residues in the "activation loop" (including Tyr[1162]) become phosphorylated (shown on the right), Tyr[1162] moves out of the way, and there is a conformational change that allows for binding of ATP and protein substrate so that the kinase reaction can proceed.

Substrates for Phosphorylation by the Insulin Receptor. The activated insulin receptor phosphorylates multiple intracellular proteins, both on the plasma membrane and in the cytoplasm.[77–86] What determines which proteins are phosphorylated by the receptor? To be a substrate, a protein must contain Tyr residues located in sequences that conform to the substrate specificity of the insulin receptor tyrosine kinase. In addition, it is necessary for an enzyme to bind to its substrate in order to catalyze its biochemical reaction. There are at least two different classes of substrates, each of which binds to the insulin receptor by a different mechanism.

Substrates Containing Phosphotyrosine Binding (PTB) Domains. PTB domains are found in IRS proteins (IRS-1, -2, -3, and -4) and also in Shc.[54,72–74] Several lines of evidence suggest that IRS proteins are important mediators of the metabolic actions of insulin action in vivo. Knockout mice lacking either IRS-1 or IRS-2 develop insulin resistance.[54,87–89] In addition, overexpression of IRS proteins mimics insulin action in adipose cells,[90–92] and overexpression of a dominant negative mutant of IRS-3 inhibits insulin action.[92]

All four IRS proteins share the same general architecture (Fig. 68-5). At the N-terminus, there is a highly conserved amino acid sequence (~100 amino acids) called a pleckstrin homology (PH) domain. This is followed by the PTB domain (see the "Insulin Receptor" section), which is also ~100 amino acids in length. The PH domain and the PTB domain have remarkably similar three-dimensional conformations even though their amino acid sequences do not resemble one another closely.[93] Whereas PTB domains bind phosphotyrosine residues, PH domains are believed to bind phosphatidylinositol (PI) derivatives (e.g., PI 3,4,5-trisphosphate; PIP3). The C-terminal domains of the IRS proteins vary in length, and the amino acid sequences are not well conserved. Nevertheless, all four IRS proteins contain multiple tyrosine phosphorylation sites with the potential to bind SH2 domains of downstream signaling molecules. For example, all four IRS proteins contain pTyr-Xaa-Xaa-Met motifs that bind to the tandem SH2 domains in the p85 regulatory subunit of PI 3-kinase, thereby activating the catalytic p110 subunit of the enzyme (Fig. 68-6).[54] Activation of PI 3-kinase is believed to mediate most, if not all, the metabolic actions of insulin.[53,94] In addition, IRS proteins contain binding sites for SH2 domains contained in other signaling molecules. For example, some IRS proteins can bind the SH2 domain-containing protein tyrosine phosphatase-2 (SHP-2) and growth factor receptor binding protein-2 (Grb-2). Binding to SHP-2 leads to activation of the phosphatase, which is believed to be a positive downstream element in a signaling pathway.[95] Grb-2 contains a Src homology-3 (SH3) domain that binds to proline-rich sequences in a protein named Sos (the mammalian homolog of the Drosophila son-of-sevenless protein) (Fig. 68-7).[96,97] Sos is a guanine nucleotide exchange protein that promotes binding of GTP to Ras, in exchange for release of GDP, thereby activating Ras. Shc also contains a binding site for the SH2 domain of Grb-2, and tyrosine phosphorylation of Shc provides another mechanism to mediate insulin-induced activation of Ras.[98]

Activation of Ras activates c-raf,[99–101] a serine/threonine-specific protein kinase that phosphorylates MEK.[101,102] MEK, in turn, is a protein kinase with M_r-50,000 that phosphorylates MAP kinase (mitogen-activated protein kinase).[101,103,104] There are multiple isoforms of MAP kinase, including ERK1 and ERK2 (M_r-44,000 and M_r-42,000, respectively).[105,106] Activation of

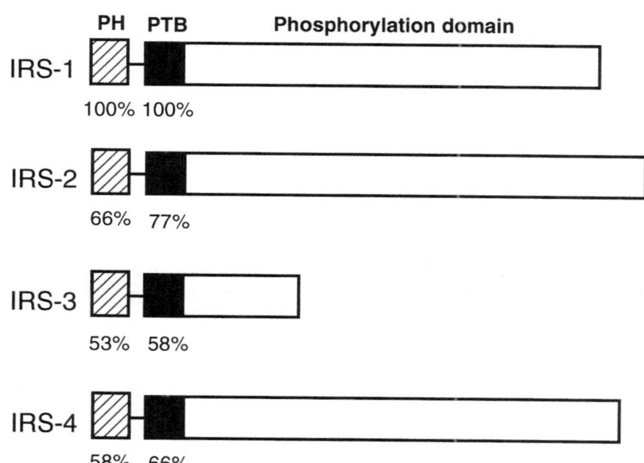

Fig. 68-5 Structure of insulin receptor substrate (IRS) proteins.[77–81] IRS proteins are characterized by several structural domains. There is a high degree of homology in the two domains in the N-terminal region of the proteins: pleckstrin homology (PH) and phosphotyrosine binding (PTB) domains. The PH domain binds polyphosphoinositides (e.g., phosphatidylinositol 3,4,-(bis)phosphate), and the PTB domain binds phosphotyrosine residues in the context of Asn-Pro-Xaa-pTyr sequences. In addition, all four IRS proteins contain C-terminal sequences of varying lengths that contain multiple tyrosine phosphorylation sites that represent binding sites for SH2 domains in various signaling proteins.

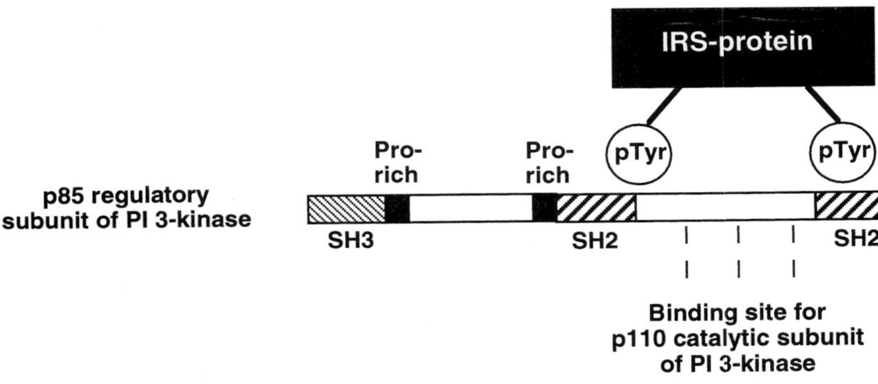

Fig. 68-6 Activation of phosphatidylinositol (PI) 3-kinase. This isoform of PI 3-kinase consists of a catalytic subunit (p110; M_r-110,000) and a regulatory subunit (p85; M_r-85,000). The p85 regulatory subunit contains two SH2 domains with selectivity for pTyr residues in the context of pTyr-(Met/Xaa)-Xaa-Met motifs. When both SH2 domains are simultaneously bound to pTyr residues, this leads to activation of the catalytic activity of p110.

MAP kinases requires phosphorylation on both a tyrosine residue and a threonine residue. Because current evidence suggests that the Ras/Raf/MEK/MAP kinase pathway does not play an important role in mediating the *metabolic* actions of insulin, it will not be emphasized in this chapter.[94,107] Nevertheless, the pathway downstream from Ras is important in mediating some of the mitogenic actions of insulin.

Substrates That Are Integral Membrane Proteins. Because of their location in the plasma membrane, integral membrane proteins are present at a high "local concentration" in the vicinity of the insulin receptor (which is also an integral plasma membrane protein). This physical proximity promotes binding of the substrate to the receptor. The first integral membrane protein identified as a substrate for phosphorylation by the insulin receptor was pp120/HA4.[82–84] Its cytoplasmic domain contains a phosphorylation site that is predicted to bind to the SH2 domain of SHP2.[108] Of course, integral membrane protein substrates such as pp120 may also contain other, as yet unrecognized, binding sites for insulin receptors.

Recently, two other integral membrane proteins have been identified as substrates for phosphorylation by the insulin receptor: SHP substrate-1 (SHPS-1),[85] and signal-regulatory protein (SIRP).[86] All three substrates (pp120/HA4, SHPS-1, and SIRP) are glycoproteins with similar structural features: extracellular domains containing "immunoglobulin-like loops," a single transmembrane domain, and short intracellular domains containing sites for tyrosine phosphorylation. In addition, when SHPS-1 and SIRP become phosphorylated, they bind SHP-1 and SHP-2. Furthermore, SIRP was demonstrated to exert an inhibitory effect upon signaling through receptor tyrosine kinases.

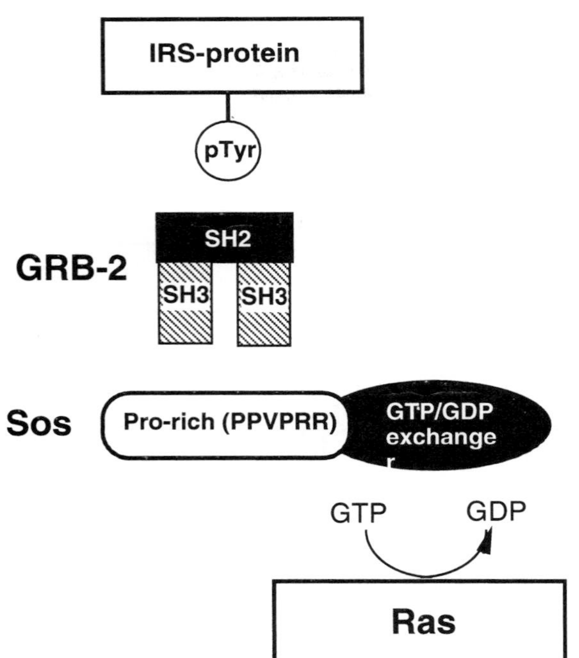

Fig. 68-7 The role of growth factor receptor binding protein-2 (Grb-2) and son-of-sevenless (Sos) in activating Ras. Sos possesses activity as a guanine nucleotide exchange factor for Ras. In addition, Sos contains proline-rich sequences that bind to SH3 domains of Grb-2. When pTyr residues in various signaling molecules (e.g., IRS-1) bind to the SH2 domain of Grb-2, this activates the guanine nucleotide exchange factor of Sos, thereby promoting exchange of GTP for GDP in the guanine nucleotide binding site of Ras and activating Ras.

Downstream from PI 3-kinase. As expected for a hormone that triggers a large number of responses in a wide variety of cell types, insulin action is complex and involves multiple downstream signaling pathways. A complete discussion of all these pathways is beyond the scope of this chapter. Rather, the chapter will focus upon pathways downstream from PI 3-kinase because of the importance in mediating the well-known metabolic actions of insulin.

PI 3-kinase consists of two distinct subunits: an M_r-85,000 regulatory subunit (p85) and an M_r-110,000 catalytic subunit (p110).[53,109] p85 contains two SH2 domains, both of which bind phosphotyrosine residues contained in pTyr-X-X-Met or pTyr-Met-X-Met motifs.[75] When phosphotyrosine-containing proteins bind to the SH2 domains of p85, this leads to activation of the catalytic activity of p110.[110–112] Bivalent binding (i.e., to both SH2 domains in p85) is required to achieve maximal activation of the PI 3-kinase.[113] When target cells are exposed to insulin, this activates the insulin receptor to phosphorylate IRS proteins (i.e., IRS-1, -2, -3, and -4), all four of which contain multiple potential tyrosine phosphorylation sites that activate PI 3-kinase.[77–81] In addition, it has been demonstrated directly that treatment of target cells with insulin leads to the association of activated PI 3-kinase with IRS-1, -2, and -3.[54] Several lines of evidence support the hypothesis that PI 3-kinase mediates the metabolic actions of insulin action. First, inhibitors of PI 3-kinase (e.g., wortmannin) block insulin action.[53] Second, if cells are transfected with inactive mutants of p85, this also inhibits insulin action.[94] Third, expression of constitutively active mutants of PI 3-kinase mimics insulin action.[114] On the other hand, when p85α was knocked out in mice, this did not impair insulin action. Rather knockout mice lacking p85α exhibited increased insulin sensitivity and a tendency to develop hypoglycemia.[115] Although the mechanism of this unexpected observation is not completely understood, it was demonstrated that alternative isoforms of regulatory subunits of PI 3-kinase bind to p110 when p85α is absent.

Phosphoinositide-dependent Kinases. PI 3-kinase phosphorylates PI associated with cell membranes. The products include PIP3, a phospholipid that binds to PH domains in several signaling proteins. Furthermore, production of PIP3 triggers activation of a cascade of serine/threonine protein kinases (Fig. 68-2) including phosphoinositide-dependent kinases (PDK), protein kinase B (PKB, also known as Akt), and atypical isoforms of protein kinase C (PKC), and p70 S6 kinase. An understanding of the biochemistry of these enzymes is beginning to emerge.

PDK-1 is an enzyme that participates in the pathways that activate PKB and atypical PKC. Activation of PKB will be discussed in some detail to illustrate the biochemical mechanisms. (The existence of multiple isoforms for many of these protein kinases will be overlooked in order to simplify the discussion.) Activation of PKB requires phosphorylation of two amino acid residues: Thr^{308} and Ser^{473}.[116–119] PDK-1, the enzyme that phosphorylates Thr^{308} in PKB, has been studied extensively and its cDNA has been cloned.[117] In contrast, PDK-2, the putative enzyme that phosphorylates Ser^{473} in PKB, has not been characterized at the molecular level. In fact, it has been suggested that PDK-2 may not exist as a distinct enzyme, but that PDK-1 might phosphorylate both amino acid residues.[120] Both PDK-1 and PKB contain PH domains that can bind PIP3.[117,121,122] Biochemical studies have suggested that PIP3 promotes phosphorylation of PKB by binding to the PH domain of PKB, thereby making it a better substrate for phosphorylation by PDK-1. However, when a mutant form of PKB lacking a PH domain was expressed in various cell lines, this was capable of being activated in response to insulin.[123] If the PH domain of PKB is not required for activation of PKB, there must be another mechanism whereby PIP3 activated phosphorylation of PKB — for example, for PIP3 to bind directly to the PH domain of PDK-1.

Protein Kinases B and C. Insulin has been shown to activate PKB in adipocytes.[124] If wild type PKB or a constitutively activated mutant of PKB is overexpressed by transfection of cells, this mimics insulin's action to translocate GLUT4 transporters to the plasma membrane.[125–127] These data suggest that PKB has the potential to trigger GLUT 4 translocation. Furthermore, at least in rat adipose cells, expression of a kinase-inactive mutant of PKB partially blocks insulin action.[126] Although this observation is consistent with the hypothesis that PKB participates in the pathway of insulin action, the fact that kinase-inactive PKB does not completely inhibit insulin action raises the possibility that there may be multiple, redundant pathways that mediate insulin action. Indeed, studies in 3T3-L1 cultured adipocytes suggest that PKC-λ may be the major mediator of insulin-induced translocation of GLUT4 in that cell type.[128,129] Insulin action was inhibited by a dominant negative mutant of PKC-λ, but not by a dominant negative mutant of PKB, in 3T3-L1 cells. It is possible that atypical PKC (e.g., PKC-λ or -ζ) may also participate in the insulin action pathway in rat adipocytes — for example, in parallel to the pathway mediated by PKB.[130] Taken together, available evidence suggests that both PKB and atypical PKC mediate insulin action, but that the relative importance of the two pathways may vary depending upon the cell type and/or the species.

The pathway downstream from PKB and/or PKC has not yet been completely elucidated. For example, it is not known how activation of PKB and/or PKC promotes translocation of GLUT4 to the plasma membrane. However, biochemical mechanisms downstream from PKB have been elucidated in other pathways. For example, PKB phosphorylates glycogen synthase kinase-3 (GSK-3), thereby inactivating the enzyme and decreasing the phosphorylation of glycogen synthase (Fig. 68-2). Because phosphorylation of glycogen synthase leads to inactivation of the enzyme, inhibition of GSK-3 favors activation of glycogen synthase. This provides at least a partial explanation of how insulin activates glycogen synthase.[107,131] Furthermore, PKB phosphorylates the forkhead transcription factor, FKHRL1, thereby promoting association with 14-3-3 proteins and retention in the cytoplasm. Because the presence of FKHRL1 in the nucleus promotes apoptosis, PKB-mediated phosphorylation of FKHRL1 provides a mechanism to explain the anti-apoptotic effect of insulin and insulin-like growth factors.[132]

p70 S6 Kinase. Insulin also leads to the activation of p70 S6 kinase, an M_r-70,000 protein kinase that phosphorylates ribosomal protein S6.[101,133] Interestingly, activation of p70 S6 kinase promotes translation of a class of mRNAs that contain an oligopyrimidine tract at their transcriptional start, including mRNAs encoding ribosomal proteins and elongation factors. The p70 S6 kinase undergoes multisite phosphorylations, apparently catalyzed by several protein kinases, including PDK-1, which appears to play a central role in mediating insulin-stimulated activation of p70 S6 kinase.[133,134] In addition, there is evidence that MAP kinases, PKC-1 and PKB, may also lead (either directly or indirectly) to phosphorylation of p70 S6 kinase.[133,135] Furthermore, it is noteworthy that similar mechanisms appear to mediate insulin-stimulated phosphorylation of 4E-BP-I (also known as PHAS-I), another protein that contributes to the regulation of translation. The nonphosphorylated form of 4E-BP-I binds to eukaryotic initiation factor 4E (eIF4E).[136–139] When 4E-BP-I binds to eIF4E, this inhibits translation of mRNAs with 5′-caps. Insulin-stimulated phosphorylation of 4E-BP-I causes the protein to dissociate from eIF4, thereby promoting protein synthesis.

Furthermore, rapamycin inhibits the actions of insulin to activate p70 S6 kinase[140] and to stimulate phosphorylation of 4E-BP-I.[141] These observations suggest that phosphorylation of p70 S6 kinase and 4E-BP-I is also regulated by the mTOR (mammalian target of rapamycin) protein kinase. Although the role of mTOR has not been fully elucidated, it has been suggested that mTOR may inhibit a phosphatase responsible for dephosphorylating p70 S6 kinase and 4E-BP-I. When mTOR is inhibited, this putative phosphatase mediates dephosphorylation of p70 S6 kinase and 4E-BP-I.[141,142]

Cyclic AMP Phosphodiesterase. Under some circumstances, insulin leads to a decrease in the cellular content of cyclic AMP by activating cyclic AMP-phosphodiesterase activity.[143,144] This may contribute to the mechanism whereby insulin decreases the phosphorylation state of metabolic enzymes such as hormone-sensitive lipase and glycogen phosphorylase.

Biologic Responses to Insulin within the Target Cell. As stated in the section on "Biochemistry and Cell Biology," the insulin action pathway is divided into at least three parts. The first part is mediated by the insulin receptor, and consists of insulin binding and tyrosine phosphorylation. There are many branches in the second part of the pathway. Multiple proteins become tyrosine phosphorylated, and multiple downstream signaling pathways become activated (e.g., PI 3-kinase and Ras). Although much progress has been made in elucidating the molecular details of the second part of the pathway, there is much that remains unknown. Nevertheless, a lot is known about the final part of the insulin action pathway — that is, the end effects of insulin upon the target cell. Because insulin exerts such a very large number of effects, it is beyond the scope of this chapter to enumerate all of them. However, this chapter will provide examples of some of the principal mechanisms involved in the final part of the pathway.

Recruitment of Glucose Transporters to the Plasma Membrane. The ability of insulin to stimulate glucose transport into skeletal muscle was among the first recognized biologic actions of insulin.[145] The mechanism of this phenomenon has been defined over the past 50 years. Glucose transport into cells is facilitated by protein molecules in the plasma membrane.[146] There is a family of such glucose transporters (Table 68-1); four of the transporters are particularly well characterized. All the members of this family are similar in size, with M_r ~40,000–50,000 daltons. As shown in Fig. 68-8, glucose transporters are integral membrane proteins with 12 putative transmembrane domains. GLUT1 is responsible for constitutive glucose transport in many cells.[147] Most GLUT1

Table 68-1 Selected Members of Family of Glucose Transport Proteins

Isoform	Chromosome (human)	Tissue distribution
GLUT1	1p35	Most tissues (e.g., brain, erythrocytes, placenta, kidney)
GLUT2	3q26	Hepatocyte, pancreatic β-cell
GLUT3	12p13	Brain
GLUT4	17p13	Skeletal muscle, heart, adipocytes

molecules are localized in the plasma membrane. In contrast, other glucose transporters are expressed in a more tissue-specific fashion. GLUT2 is expressed primarily in hepatocytes and pancreatic islets.[148,149] GLUT3 is expressed in the brain as well as certain other tissues.[150] GLUT4 is particularly expressed in tissues in which glucose transport is subject to regulation by insulin, including skeletal muscle, cardiac muscle, and adipose tissue.[151–155] In the absence of insulin, the majority of GLUT4 molecules are localized in intracellular vesicles. In the presence of insulin, these vesicles are recruited to the plasma membrane where the vesicles fuse with the plasma membrane, thereby inserting their complement of glucose transporters into the membrane (Fig. 68-9).[156,157] Insulin exerts a large effect to stimulate glucose transport in some cell types—for example, a twentyfold increment in the rate of glucose transport in adipocytes. Insulin recruits a comparably large number of GLUT4 molecules in these cell types. While there is also some recruitment of GLUT1 molecules to the cell surface in some cell types, the magnitude of the recruitment of GLUT1 transporters is much smaller than is observed with GLUT4 transporters.[158]

The molecular mechanism whereby insulin stimulates recruitment of vesicles containing glucose transporters is not completely understood. However, current evidence suggests that insulin both stimulates exocytosis and inhibits endocytosis of glucose transporters.[159–161] Recent data have provided insights into the molecular mechanisms that may regulate the ability of GLUT4-containing vesicles to undergo translocation, docking, and fusion with the plasma membrane. Interestingly, the mechanisms resemble the mechanisms involved in exocytosis of synaptic vesicles. Although a detailed discussion of these complex mechanisms is beyond the scope of this chapter, the broad outlines will be summarized. There are multiple proteins that participate in the complex processes of vesicle docking and fusion with target membranes. Vesicle-associated membrane protein 2 (VAMP2) and/or VAMP3 appear to function as the vesicle SNAP receptors on GLUT4-containing vesicles.[162] Syntaxin 4 functions as the target SNAP receptor on the plasma membrane. Binding of syntaxin 4 to VAMP2 and/or VAMP3 appears to be required for translocation of GLUT4 to the plasma membrane. There are multiple additional proteins that participate in and regulate these processes. For example, in the absence of insulin, Munc 18c binds to syntaxin 4, thereby preventing VAMP2 from binding to syntaxin 4.[163] Insulin induces dissociation of the syntaxin 4/Munc 18c complex. The detailed mechanisms of how insulin regulates translocation of GLUT4 continue to be actively investigated.

Inhibition of Protein Phosphorylation. The enzymes of glycogen metabolism were among the first proteins recognized to undergo reversible phosphorylation-dephosphorylation cycles as a mechanism to regulate enzymatic activity.[164,165] Similarly, other enzymes have been demonstrated to be regulated by serine/threonine-specific phosphorylation—for example, the hormone-sensitive triglyceride lipase,[166] pyruvate dehydrogenase,[37–42] and hepatic pyruvate kinase.[28] Insulin decreases the phosphorylation

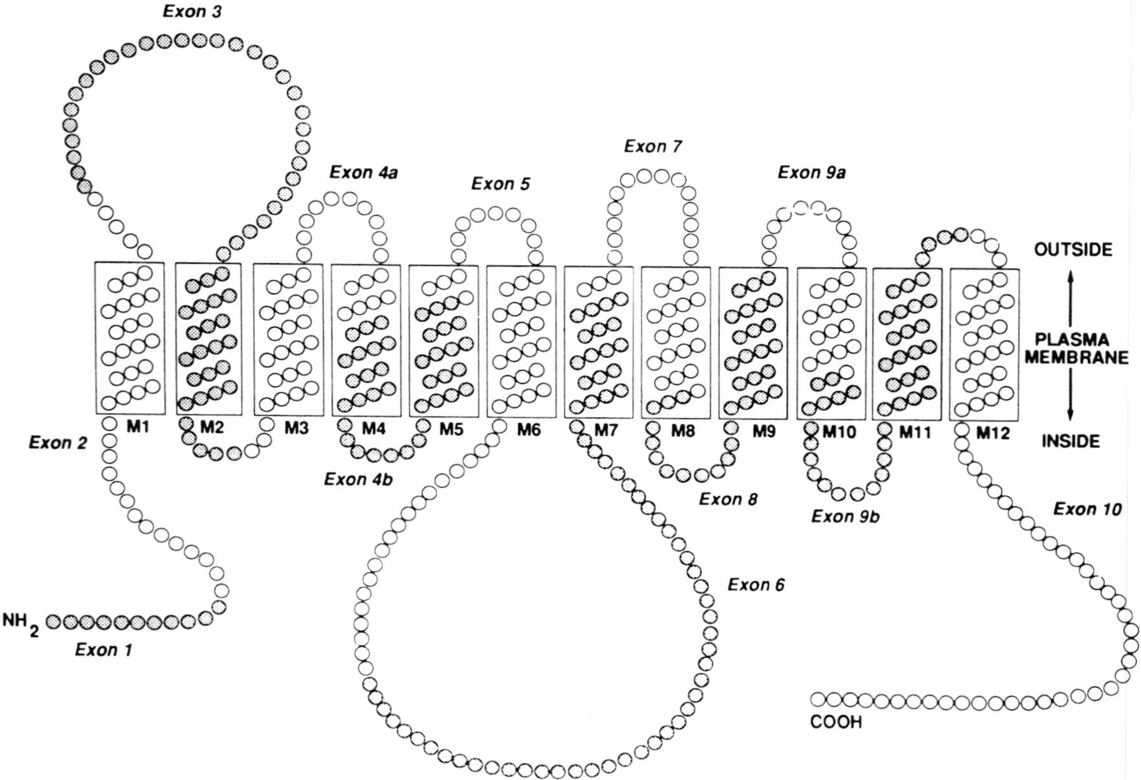

Fig. 68-8 Structure of glucose transporter molecules. This cartoon depicts the proposed structure of glucose transporters with 12 membrane spanning domains (M1 to M12). The circles depict amino acid residues. Amino acids encoded by a given exon are indicated by either open or shaded circles, alternating every other exon. (*Reproduced from Bell et al.*[449] *Used with permission.*)

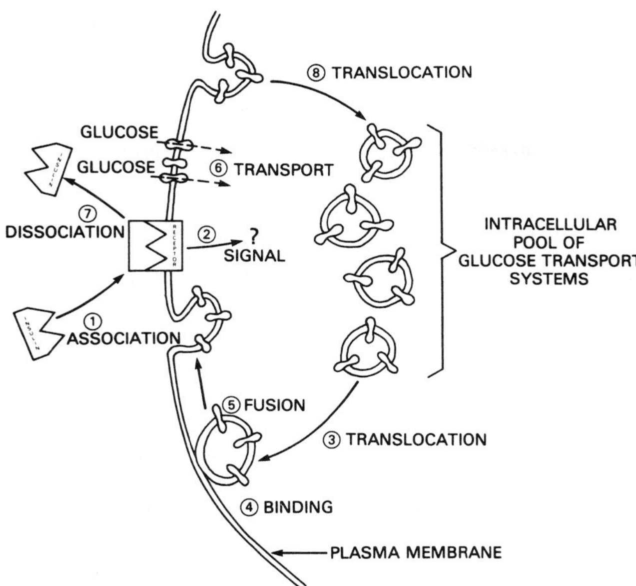

Fig. 68-9 Recruitment of glucose transporters. In the absence of insulin, the majority of GLUT4 glucose transporters are localized in intracellular vesicles, with relatively few GLUT4 glucose transporters being located on the cell surface. Insulin stimulates the recruitment of intracellular glucose transporters to the cell surface. Presumably, intracellular vesicles move to the plasma membrane, and fuse with the plasma membrane thereby increasing the number of glucose transporters on the cell surface. (*Contributed by Drs. Ian Simpson and Samuel Cushman.*)

state of all of these enzymes; in contrast, agents that increase the cellular content of cyclic AMP promote phosphorylation of these enzymes. In the case of enzymes that are active in the fed state (e.g., glycogen synthase, pyruvate kinase, and pyruvate dehydrogenase), phosphorylation leads to inhibition of enzyme activities. However, in the case of enzymes that are active in the fasted state (e.g., glycogen phosphorylase and hormone-sensitive triglyceride lipase), phosphorylation leads to activation of the enzyme.

6-Phosphofructo-2-kinase/fructo-2,6-bisphosphatase is a dual activity enzyme that is regulated by phosphorylation-dephosphorylation (Fig. 68-10).[28] This enzyme is responsible for both synthesis and degradation of fructose-2,6-bisphosphate, a messenger molecule that serves as an allosteric modifier of two key enzymes in the regulation of the balance between glycolysis and glycogenolysis: 6-phosphofructo-1-kinase and fructo-1,6-bisphosphatase (see "Regulation of Enzymatic Activity by Allosteric Modifiers" below). 6-Phosphofructo-2-kinase/fructo-2,6-bisphosphatase can be phosphorylated by cyclic AMP-dependent protein kinase. Phosphorylation leads to activation of fructo-2,6-bisphosphatase and reciprocal inhibition of 6-phosphofructo-2-kinase. Insulin can lead to dephosphorylation of the enzyme. Accordingly, insulin increases the level of fructose-2,6-bisphosphate, while agents that increase cyclic AMP lead to decreased levels of fructose-2,6-bisphosphate.

Regulation of Enzymatic Activity by Allosteric Modifiers. There are multiple examples of allosteric modifiers that participate in the mechanism of insulin action. Several example will be discussed:

1. *Regulation of 6-phosphofructo-1-kinase and fructo-1,6-bisphosphatase:* 6-Phosphofructo-1-kinase is a glycolytic enzyme that converts fructose-6-phosphate into fructose-1,6-bisphosphate. This enzyme is inhibited by ATP and citrate.[28–30] In contrast, AMP and fructose-2,6-bisphosphate are activators of the enzyme. Accordingly, when ATP is plentiful, the ATP/AMP ratio is elevated, and this leads to inhibition of glycolysis. Conversely, when ATP/AMP ratios are low, the rate of glycolysis will be increased leading to generation of ATP. These homeostatic mechanisms create a negative feedback loop that tends to maintain ATP/AMP ratios at a constant value. Similarly, when levels of citrate (an intermediate of the tricarboxylic acid cycle) are high, glycolysis will be inhibited, thereby decreasing the supply of citrate. In contrast to these metabolic intermediates, fructose-2,6-bisphosphate is a messenger molecule that is regulated directly by hormonal regulation of the bifunctional enzyme 6-phosphofructo-2-kinase/fructo-2,6-bisphosphatase. By increasing levels of fructose-2,6-bisphosphate, insulin activates 6-phosphofructo-1-kinase, thereby accelerating the metabolism of glucose through the glycolytic pathway.[28,29] In a reciprocal fashion, increased levels of fructose-2,6-bisphosphate lead to inhibition of the gluconeogenic pathway by inhibiting the enzyme fructo-1,6-bisphosphatase.
2. *Regulation of hepatic pyruvate kinase:* As summarized in "Inhibition of Protein Phosphorylation" above, insulin increases the level of fructose-2,6-bisphosphate (Fig. 68-10), thereby activating 6-phosphofructo-1-kinase and inhibiting fructo-1,6-bisphosphatase. This leads to an increase in the levels of fructose-1,6-bisphosphate.[28,29] In addition to functioning as a metabolic intermediate, fructose-1,6-bisphosphate also serves as a regulator of hepatic pyruvate kinase. Indeed, fructose-1,6-bisphosphate activates pyruvate kinase by two mechanisms.[27,28] First, fructose-1,6-bisphosphate is an allosteric activator of pyruvate kinase. Second, fructose-1,6-bisphosphate inhibits phosphorylation of pyruvate kinase. Since phosphorylation leads to inactivation of pyruvate kinase, inhibition of phosphorylation leads to activation of the enzyme. At least two other molecules contribute importantly as allosteric inhibitors of hepatic pyruvate kinase: ATP and alanine.
3. *Regulation of carnitine palmitoyltransferase I:* Long-chain fatty acids are esterified with coenzyme A in the cytosol. Cytosolic fatty acyl CoA serves as a substrate for synthesis of

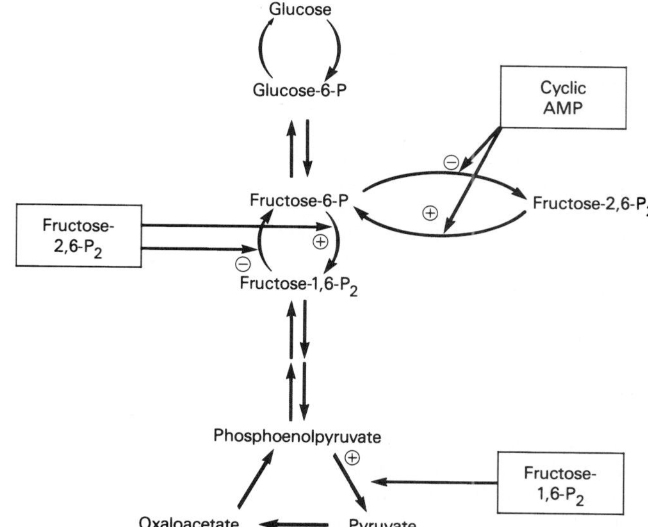

Fig. 68-10 Role of fructose-2,6-bisphosphate in the regulation of glycolysis and gluconeogenesis. Cyclic AMP stimulates phosphorylation of the bifunctional enzymes 6-phosphofructo-2-kinase/fructose-2,6-bisphosphatase, thereby activating the phosphatase and inhibiting the kinase activity. This sets into motion a series of events that inhibits the "forward" flux through the glycolytic pathway and increases the "backward" flux through gluconeogenic pathway. This leads to a reduction of fructose-2,6-bisphosphate levels, thereby increasing the activity of fructose-1,6-bisphosphatase and decreasing the activity of 6-phosphofructo-1-kinase. Consequently, there is a decrease in the levels of fructose-1,6-bisphosphate, and a decrease in the activity of pyruvate kinase.[28]

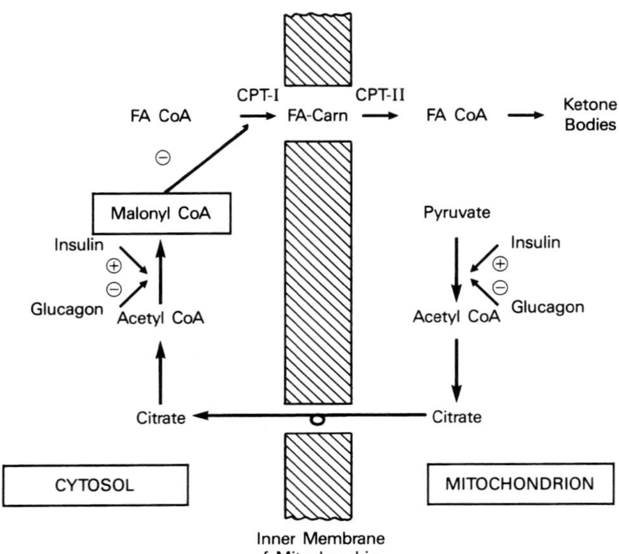

Fig. 68-11 Role of malonyl CoA in regulating ketogenesis. In the presence of insulin, the pathways of lipogenesis are active in the liver. For example, the high activities of pyruvate dehydrogenase and acetyl-CoA carboxylase lead to high levels of malonyl CoA. Because malonyl CoA is an inhibitor of carnitine palmitoyl transferase I (CPT-I), the high levels of malonyl CoA inhibit transport of fatty acids into the mitochondrion for β-oxidation and ketogenesis. When levels of insulin are low and levels of glucagon are high (e.g., in uncontrolled diabetes mellitus), levels of malonyl CoA are low and CPT-I becomes disinhibited. This favors ketogenesis. These reciprocal regulatory mechanisms minimize futile cycling by ensuring that the opposing processes of ketogenesis and fatty acid biosynthesis are not both activated at the same time.

triglycerides and phospholipids. However, oxidation of fatty acyl CoA takes place within mitochondria. Accordingly, the subcellular localization of the fatty acyl CoA determines its metabolic fate — whether to the anabolic pathway of triglyceride synthesis in the cytosol, or to the catabolic pathways of β-oxidation and ketogenesis within mitochondria.[45–48] Because the inner mitochondrial membrane is not permeable to fatty acyl CoA, it contains a transport system that facilitates the transport of fatty acyl CoA. This transport requires at least two distinct enzymes: carnitine palmitoyltransferase I (CPT I) and carnitine palmitoyltransferase II (CPT II) (Fig. 68-11). Both enzymes catalyze a reversible interconversion between fatty acyl CoA and fatty acyl carnitine. CPT I (located on the outer aspect of the inner mitochondrial membrane) synthesizes fatty acyl carnitine using extramitochondrial fatty acyl CoA as substrate. CPT II (located on the inner aspect of the inner mitochondrial membrane) is responsible for reversing the reaction to generate intramitochondrial fatty acyl CoA. The activity of carnitine palmitoyltransferase I (CPT I) is regulated by the levels of an allosteric inhibitor, malonyl CoA. Malonyl CoA is an intermediate in the anabolic pathway of fatty acid biosynthesis. Insulin stimulates pyruvate dehydrogenase and acetyl CoA carboxylase, thereby promoting fatty acid biosynthesis.[37–40,167,168] Activation of acetyl-CoA carboxylase leads to increased production of malonyl CoA, thereby inhibiting carnitine palmitoyltransferase I, which, in turn, leads to inhibition of fatty acid oxidation, and ketogenesis. Thus, there is a reciprocal relationship between fatty acid biosynthesis (a process stimulated by insulin) and fatty acid oxidation/ketogenesis (processes that are inhibited by insulin).

Regulation of Gene Expression. Insulin regulates gene expression.[169] Presently available data suggest that the effects of insulin to regulate gene transcription may result from phosphorylation of transacting factors that bind to specific nucleotide sequences in regulatory domains of individual genes. Some genes are subject to positive regulation by insulin. For example, insulin stimulates transcription of genes encoding glyceraldehyde 3-phosphate dehydrogenase,[170,171] glucokinase,[51] and 6-phosphofructo-2-kinase/fructo-2,6-bisphosphatase.[28] Conversely, insulin inhibits the rate at which the phosphoenolpyruvate carboxykinase (PEP-CK) gene is transcribed.[169,172]

Recent work has begun to shed considerable insight into the detailed molecular mechanisms that mediate insulin's inhibitory effect upon transcription of the genes encoding PEP-CK and insulin-like growth factor binding protein-1 (IGFBP-1). Insulin response elements (IRE) have been identified upstream of the coding sequences of both genes. The core IRE is a 7-base-pair consensus sequence: T(G/A)TTTTG. Interestingly, this IRE is a binding site for transcription factors in a family containing hepatocyte nuclear factor-3 (HNF-3) and forkhead transcription factors.[173,174] Genetic studies in the *C. elegans* model system have provided strong evidence that the daf-16 forkhead transcription factor mediates transcriptional effects downstream from daf-2, the *C. elegans* ortholog of the insulin receptor.[175,176] Furthermore, based upon the *C. elegans* model system, PI 3-kinase and protein kinase B also participate in this signaling pathway. Similar results have been obtained in mammalian systems. FKHRL1[132,177] and AFX,[178] two members of the family of forkhead transcription factors, have been demonstrated to be substrates of PKB. Furthermore, insulin stimulates phosphorylation of both transcription factors. In both cases, the effects of insulin are inhibited (at least partially) by inhibitors of PI 3-kinase. In addition, there appears to be an alternative pathway whereby insulin can trigger phosphorylation of AFX; this PI 3-kinase independent pathway is mediated by Ras.[178] Binding of HNF-3, FKHRL1, or AFX to the IRE can stimulate transcription of the PEP-CK and IGFBP-1 genes.[132,173,174,178] At least in the case of FKHRL1, it has been demonstrated that PKB-mediated phosphorylation promotes binding to 14-3-3 proteins, resulting in retention in the cytosol and inhibition of translocation into the nucleus.[132] Taken together, these data provide a mechanism whereby insulin can inhibit transcription of the genes encoding PEP-CK, IGFBP-1, and probably other genes as well. By promoting phosphorylation of forkhead transcription factors, insulin leads to sequestration of the proteins in the cytosol, thereby inhibiting the positive effects upon gene transcription.

"OFF" SIGNALS

Insulin action is crucial to promote efficient storage of fuels after a meal. However, it is also necessary to have mechanisms that terminate insulin action once the ingested nutrients have been appropriately stored. The understanding of the nature of these "off" signals has lagged behind the understanding of the molecular mechanisms that mediate insulin action. Nevertheless, this section will briefly review the nature of the "off" signals.

Endocytosis

Insulin binding triggers receptor endocytosis. This is a complex multistep process. First, insulin activates the receptor tyrosine kinase. Phosphorylation of tyrosine residues in the receptor leads to the release of receptors from microvillous domain of the plasma membrane, and migration to clathrin-coated pits.[179] The receptor is endocytosed through a clathrin-coated pit mechanism. Multiple structural motifs in the cytoplasmic domain of the receptor are required for endocytosis, presumably to allow for interactions with intracellular proteins that participate in endocytosis.[180–184] As a result of endocytosis, insulin receptors translocate to intracellular vesicles called endosomes, with the ligand binding domain of the receptor located inside the vesicle. Endosomes contain proton pumps that acidify the lumen of the vesicle, and the acidic pH promotes dissociation of insulin.[185,186] In addition, endosomes deliver insulin to lysosomes for degradation. Indeed, receptor-mediated endocytosis is the principal mechanism whereby insulin is cleared from the plasma.[187–190] Two alternative fates are available to intracellular insulin receptors. The receptors can either be recycled to the plasma membrane for reutilization or they can be delivered to lysosomes for degradation. Because insulin accelerates the degradation of insulin receptors, this provides a mechanism whereby hyperinsulinemia can lead to down-regulation of the number of insulin receptors on the cell surface.[191,192]

Protein Tyrosine Phosphatases

Because the insulin receptor tyrosine kinase plays a necessary role in mediating insulin action, logically there must be phosphotyrosine phosphatases that reverse the action of the kinase. Indeed, it has been shown that vanadate, a nonspecific inhibitor of phosphotyrosine phosphatases, can mimic insulin action.[193–195] There are numerous phosphotyrosine phosphatases, several of which are able to dephosphorylate insulin receptors under some experimental conditions.[196–200] Furthermore, there must be phosphotyrosine phosphatases that act upon the various substrates of the insulin receptor (e.g., IRS-1, -2, -3, and -4). In a recent study, a knockout mouse lacking phosphotyrosine phosphatase (PTP)-1B exhibited increased insulin sensitivity.[201] This has focused attention upon the role of PTP-1B as an element in the switch that terminates insulin signaling.

Several mechanisms have been proposed to determine the in vivo specificity of phosphotyrosine phosphatases:

Tissue distribution. Several tissues are particularly important as targets for the metabolic actions of insulin: skeletal muscle, cardiac muscle, adipose tissue, and liver. Thus, the phosphotyrosine phosphatases expressed in those tissues are likely the most relevant candidates to serve as "off" switches for the metabolic actions of insulin.

Intracellular localization. It is necessary for an enzyme to interact directly with its substrate (in this case, a phosphotyrosine-containing protein). Therefore, physiologically relevant phosphotyrosine phosphatases must be located (at least transiently) in proximity to the insulin receptor and/or its substrates.[190]

Enzymatic specificity. Enzymes such as serine/threonine kinases exhibit considerable specificity for the amino acid sequence flanking the phosphorylation site. However, tyrosine kinases and phosphotyrosine phosphatases appear to be considerably less specific with respect to the amino acid sequences flanking the tyrosine residue.[202]

Serine-Threonine Phosphorylation

The insulin receptor possesses intrinsic tyrosine kinase activity, and undergoes phosphorylation on tyrosine residues in response to insulin.[59,60] This process has been studied extensively because of the central role of tyrosine phosphorylation in mediating insulin action. However, insulin also stimulates phosphorylation of serine and threonine residues in the insulin receptor.[59] While the significance of phosphorylation of the receptor on serine/threonine residues is less well understood, there is some evidence suggesting that serine/threonine phosphorylation may lead to inhibition of receptor tyrosine kinase activity.[203–205] Indeed, serine/threonine phosphorylation of insulin receptors has been proposed to be the cause of insulin resistance in some patients with polycystic ovarian syndrome.[206]

Like the insulin receptor itself, insulin receptor substrates undergo phosphorylation on serine/threonine residues, and this phosphorylation appears to antagonize insulin action.[207–213] Several kinases have been proposed to mediate this type of inhibitory phosphorylation of serine/threonine residues in IRS-1, including protein kinase B,[211] protein kinase C,[209,210] and glycogen synthase kinase-3.[214] Interestingly, insulin exerts opposite effects upon these enzymes, activating PKB and PKC, but inhibiting GSK-3. This creates the possibility of complex regulatory mechanisms to regulate the activity of the insulin-signaling pathway. Although incompletely understood, this is the subject of active research interest.

COUNTERREGULATORY HORMONES

Insulin is the predominant hormone promoting glucose utilization and preventing hyperglycemia. However, there are multiple endocrine mechanisms that oppose insulin action.[215] These hormones tend to prevent hypoglycemia, and help to correct hypoglycemia if it occurs. The multiplicity of counterregulatory factors testifies to the importance of providing adequate fuel to the peripheral tissues. Throughout most of evolution, hypoglycemia and nutritional shortages represented great threats.[216] Health problems due to superabundance of nutrition (e.g., obesity and hyperglycemia) have become important very recently in history.

When glucose levels fall, this provides a stimulus for secretion of several counterregulatory hormones: epinephrine, glucagon, growth hormone, and cortisol (Table 68-2).[217] Secretion of epinephrine, glucagon, and growth hormone is elicited when plasma glucose levels fall below 65 to 70 mg/dl. Secretion of cortisol requires plasma glucose to fall below 55 to 60 mg/dl. When plasma glucose levels fall below 50 mg/dl, hypoglycemic symptoms often develop, and plasma norepinephrine levels increase because of release from sympathetic neurons.

Intravenous insulin tolerance tests provide an experimental model for acute development of hypoglycemia. This approach has helped to elucidate the roles of counterregulatory hormones in the recovery from insulin-induced hypoglycemia.[218–220] When secretion of glucagon, growth hormone, and insulin is inhibited by administration of somatostatin, this prolongs the duration and severity of insulin-induced hypoglycemia. Replacement of glucagon (but not growth hormone) prevents this effect of somatostatin, demonstrating that glucagon plays an important role in defending against hypoglycemia. In the presence of normal amounts of glucagon, administration of α- and β-adrenergic blockers has little effect upon recovery from insulin-induced hypoglycemia. However, in glucagon-deficient individuals, α- and β-adrenergic blockade exacerbates the defect in recovery from hypoglycemia. In conclusion, glucagon plays the most important role in the defense against hypoglycemia. Deficiency of epinephrine exacerbates the adverse effects of glucagon deficiency, but epinephrine does not play a major role in the presence of glucagon. Growth hormone and cortisol do not appear to play major roles in preventing the acute development of hypoglycemia, but may play more important roles in chronic situations.

Glucagon and epinephrine act primarily upon the liver to bring about their effects to protect against hypoglycemia. Both hormones increase hepatic glucose production by stimulating glycogenolysis and enhancing gluconeogenesis.[26,218,221] Glucagon acts through receptors on the surface of the hepatocyte. These

Table 68-2 Glycemic Thresholds for Eliciting Secretion of Counterregulatory Hormones or Hypoglycemic Symptoms*

Response	Plasma glucose (mg/dl)
Symptoms	53 ± 2
Secretion of counterregulatory hormones	
Epinephrine	69 ± 2
Glucagon	68 ± 2
Growth hormone	66 ± 2
Cortisol	58 ± 3
Norepinephrine	51 ± 3

*Insulin was infused intravenously in six hourly steps in order to decrease the plasma glucose concentration[217] from 90 to 40 mg/dl in six steps of 10 mg/dl. Hormone levels and symptoms were compared with 10 subjects in whom euglycemia (90 mg/dl) was maintained for 6 h. Arterialized venous plasma glucose concentrations were used to calculate glycemic thresholds.

receptors are coupled through the stimulatory GTP binding protein Gs to activation of adenylate cyclase.[222–224] Elevated levels of cyclic AMP promote glycogenolysis and gluconeogenesis. Epinephrine may exert its effects through two distinct receptors: α_1- and β_2-adrenergic receptors. Like glucagon receptors, β_2-adrenergic receptors are coupled through the stimulatory GTP binding protein G_s to activation of adenylate cyclase.[225] α_1-Adrenergic receptors are coupled through a different GTP binding protein to activation of phospholipase C.[226] This leads to hydrolysis of phosphatidylinositol 4,5-bisphosphate, yielding diacylglycerol and inositol 1,4,5-trisphosphate (IP3). IP3 leads to mobilization of intracellular Ca^{2+}, while diacylglycerol plus Ca^{2+} leads to the activation of protein kinase C.[227]

DEFINITION AND CLASSIFICATION OF DIABETES

Definition

Diabetes mellitus is defined by high levels of glucose in plasma. The criteria to diagnose diabetes are based upon epidemiological data linking hyperglycemia to chronic diabetic complications.[2,228,229] Recently, the American Diabetes Association has recommended a revised set of diagnostic criteria,[2] which will be summarized in this chapter. (Different criteria are used for diagnosis of diabetes in pregnant women — see "Modified Criteria to Diagnose Gestational Diabetes Mellitus.")

The revised criteria provide three ways to diagnose diabetes:

1. *Fasting plasma glucose:* Normal fasting plasma glucose (FPG) is defined to be <110 mg/dl (6.1 mM). Diabetes is diagnosed if the FPG ≥126 mg/dl (7 mM). If FPG is in the range between normal and diabetic (110 mg/dl ≤ FPG < 126 mg/dl), this is called impaired fasting glucose. To apply these diagnostic criteria, the patient must have fasted (i.e., no caloric intake) for at least 8 hr.
2. *Oral glucose tolerance test:* An oral glucose tolerance test (OGTT) consists of administering a solution containing 75 g of glucose. The normal ranges for an OGTT are based upon studies of healthy people eating an adequate diet. Therefore, to obtain an interpretable result from an OGTT, the subject should have eaten a normal diet with a normal amount of carbohydrate for at least three days prior to the test.[230,231] Glucose tolerance is said to be normal if the plasma glucose is <140 mg/dl (7.8 mM) at 2 hr. Diabetes is diagnosed if the plasma glucose ≥200 mg/dl (11.1 mM) at 2 hr. If the 2 hr plasma glucose is intermediate between normal and diabetic (140 mg/dl ≤ 2 hr PG < 200 mg/dl), this is defined as impaired glucose tolerance.
3. *"Casual" hyperglycemia in association with classic symptoms:* If patients have classic symptoms of diabetes (polyuria, polydipsia, or unexplained weight loss), then it is possible to diagnose diabetes if a "casual" determination of plasma glucose ≥ 200 mg/dl (11.1 mM).

Regardless of which criterion is used, the diagnosis must be confirmed on a second day using any of the three criteria. This change in the definition of diabetes was motivated primarily by pragmatic considerations. First, it is simpler and less expensive to base a diagnosis on a determination of the fasting plasma glucose rather than to carry out an oral glucose tolerance test. Second, there is less variability in the measurement of the fasting glucose level than in the data obtained from an oral glucose tolerance test. By choosing a test with less variability, this minimizes the confusion that arises if the diagnosis changes from day to day because of random variation of the laboratory test. Nevertheless, there is evidence that the change in the definition has resulted in a change in diagnosis for some individuals.[232,233] For example, epidemiological data suggest that the new definition results in fewer people being diagnosed with type 2 diabetes. Fortunately, in general, it is the patients with the mildest hyperglycemia (as judged by measurements of hemoglobin A1c) who will be reassigned from the diagnostic category of "diabetes" to "impaired fasting glucose."

Classification

Diabetes mellitus is a heterogeneous syndrome, characterized by hyperglycemia and a predisposition to develop chronic complications such as retinopathy, neuropathy, nephropathy, and atherosclerotic macrovascular disease. The American Diabetes Association has attempted to devise a classification scheme based upon the etiology of disease. However, because the precise cause of diabetes is not yet known in most patients, this effort is only partially successful. Nevertheless, the American Diabetes Association classification scheme provides a useful starting point for discussion of the multiple forms of diabetes.

Type 1 Diabetes Mellitus. Type 1 diabetes is caused by destruction of pancreatic beta cells. In most patients, this results from selective destruction of beta cells by autoimmune mechanisms, although other unknown mechanisms may be responsible in some patients. Type 1 diabetes is characterized by a near-total deficiency of insulin, and a requirement for insulin therapy to prevent diabetic ketoacidosis and sustain life. Indeed, prior to the availability of insulin therapy, this disease was fatal over a relatively short time period.[234] Most commonly, this form of the disease has its onset prior to the age of 20; this was the origin of the obsolete name "juvenile-onset type diabetes mellitus." Type 1 diabetes is discussed in detail in Chap. 69.

Type 2 Diabetes Mellitus. Type 2 diabetes is the most common form of diabetes, accounting for >90 percent of patients with the disease. It is caused by two physiological defects: resistance to the action of insulin combined with a deficiency in insulin secretion. However, the molecular defects causing type 2 diabetes are not known. Even in the absence of therapy, patients with type 2 diabetes mellitus do not ordinarily develop diabetic ketoacidosis, although they may occasionally develop ketoacidosis if stressed by acute illness. Most commonly, this form of the disease has its onset after the age of 40; this was the origin of the obsolete name "adult-onset type diabetes mellitus." The syndrome of maturity-onset type diabetes of youth (MODY) was originally considered to be a form of type 2 diabetes.[10] However, now that specific mutations have been identified as causes of MODY, it is classified under "other specific types of diabetes." Because all five MODY genes cause diabetes by impairing insulin secretion,[9,11–14] they are discussed in Chap. 67. Similarly, mutations in the insulin receptor gene cause syndromes that resemble type 2 diabetes in that the patients are not insulin-dependent. Nevertheless, because the specific disease-causing mutations are known, this form of diabetes is also classified under "other specific types of diabetes" (see below).

The American Diabetes Association Report of the Expert Committee on Diagnosis and Classification states, "There are probably many different causes of this form of diabetes, and it is likely that the proportion of patients in this category [of type 2 diabetes] will decrease in the future as identification of specific pathogenic processes and genetic defects permits better differentiation among them and a more definitive subclassification. Although the specific etiologies of this form of diabetes are not known, autoimmune destruction of beta cells does not occur, and patients do not have any of the other causes of diabetes...."[2] According to this definition, the entity of type 2 diabetes may eventually vanish if research is successful in identifying all of the causes of the syndrome. However, it may be preferable to revise the classification scheme to allow patients with defined defects to retain the diagnosis of type 2 diabetes.

By excluding the presence of autoimmune destruction of beta cells, the American Diabetes Association classification scheme implicitly excludes the syndrome of "latent autoimmune diabetes of adults" (LADA)[235,236] from being classified as a form of type 2 diabetes. In many patients, LADA evolves over time into type 1 diabetes; that is, the patients may eventually become insulin-dependent. However, these patients may have non-insulin-dependent physiology for many years, and their disease may be indistinguishable from type 2 diabetes. Furthermore, it is possible that there are other similarities between LADA and type 2 diabetes. Type 2 diabetes is a polygenic disease, and it is likely that patients have inherited a number of "diabetes genes"—for example, one or more genes causing insulin deficiency and one or more genes causing insulin resistance. Patients with LADA may have inherited typical type 2 "diabetes genes" that cause insulin resistance in combination with typical type 1 diabetes genes that cause autoimmune destruction of pancreatic beta cells. These problems in classifying certain patients are the inevitable result of trying to devise an "etiological" classification scheme at a time when the causes of diabetes are not understood. As our knowledge of the disease grows, it will eventually be possible to resolve these issues.

Obesity is an important factor that predisposes to the development of type 2 diabetes. In previous classification schemes, "non-insulin-dependent diabetes" (type 2 diabetes) was subdivided into two categories: type 2 diabetes associated with obesity, and type 2 diabetes in the absence of obesity, although it is not clear whether these are really distinct entities. In any case, progress has been made in identifying specific genetic causes of obesity—at least in relatively rare forms of obesity. It seems appropriate to classify genetic forms of obesity together with Prader-Willi syndrome under the classification III.H. "Other Genetic Syndromes Sometimes Associated with Diabetes" (see below).

Other Specific Types of Diabetes. Initially, this category was intended to include forms of diabetes that are caused by another disease, but has been expanded to include all forms of diabetes for which the cause is known. There are several unfortunate aspects of this definition:

1. Some conditions are really risk factors that precipitate diabetes in some, but not all patients—for example, therapy with glucocorticoids or thiazide diuretics. It is possible that people with a genetic tendency to develop type 2 diabetes are at increased risk to develop these forms of secondary diabetes, and that the patients may really be part of the same spectrum as patients with type 2 diabetes. Indeed, some of these patients will eventually develop type 2 diabetes.
2. As discussed above, this approach toward classifying patients may lead to the total disappearance of the entity of type 2 diabetes if we are successful in identifying all the causes of this syndrome. It seems arbitrary to remove a patient from the classification of type 2 diabetes simply because clinical research has succeeded in identifying the genetic locus of the patient's mutation(s).
3. In routine clinical practice, physicians lack sufficient information to classify patients with respect to etiology. For example, some patients who are heterozygous for mutations in the insulin receptor gene have a clinical syndrome that closely resembles type 2 diabetes.[237] Because it is not practical to screen all patients for mutations in the insulin receptor gene, it seems more appropriate to base a classification scheme upon information that will be routinely available to physicians caring for the patients.

In any case, what follows are some examples of syndromes presently classified as "Other specific types of diabetes."

Genetic Defects of Beta Cell Function. Several genes have been identified as loci for mutations that cause diabetes by impairing beta cell function. Mutations in the insulin gene cause disease either by inhibiting the conversion of proinsulin to insulin, or by decreasing the affinity of the insulin molecule to bind to the insulin receptor.[8] Several genes have been identified as causes of specific forms of MODY. Mutations in the glucokinase gene cause MODY2.[9] Mutations in various transcription factor genes cause other forms of MODY: hepatocyte nuclear factor (HNF) 4α in MODY1,[11] HNF1α in MODY3,[12] insulin promoter factor 1 in MODY4,[13] and HNF1β in MODY5.[14] Also, mutations in mitochondrial genes have been identified as causes of a maternally transmitted form of diabetes.[15,16] These diseases are discussed in Chaps. 104 and 105.

Genetic Defects in Insulin Action. Several distinct syndromes appear to be caused by mutations in the insulin receptor gene.[4–6] Two clinical features are commonly observed in all the syndromes: acanthosis nigricans and hyperandrogenism (in female patients). However, each distinct syndrome is defined by the presence or absence of specific clinical features. Type A extreme insulin resistance is defined by the triad of insulin resistance, acanthosis nigricans, and hyperandrogenism in the absence of obesity or lipoatrophy (Fig. 68-12).[238] Patients with leprechaunism have multiple abnormal features, including intrauterine growth retardation and fasting hypoglycemia (Fig. 68-13),[239–241] and usually die within the first year of life. The Rabson-Mendenhall syndrome is associated with short stature, abnormalities of teeth and nails, and, reportedly, pineal hyperplasia (Fig. 68-14).[242]

Patients with various forms of lipoatrophy might be included in this category because their clinical syndromes are similar in some respects—for example, the severity of the insulin resistance and the association with acanthosis nigricans and hyperandrogenism. However, the primary genetic defects appear not to be in the insulin-signaling pathway. Rather, insulin resistance is likely caused by the absence of fat.[243–246] In some respects, the situation resembles the more common association of obesity with insulin resistance. Abnormal quantities of adipose tissue (whether too much or too little) seem to cause insulin resistance although we don't fully understand either mechanism.

Disease of the Exocrine Pancreas. The clearest example of secondary diabetes is due to total surgical pancreatectomy. Similarly, other diseases such as pancreatitis or cystic fibrosis can lead to pancreatic destruction. In all of these examples, diabetes mellitus is a relatively late sign of pancreatic insufficiency, requiring the destruction or removal of most of the islet cell mass.

Endocrinopathies. Certain tumors produce counterregulatory hormones that oppose insulin action or inhibit insulin secretion. Excesses of these hormones can cause diabetes—for example,

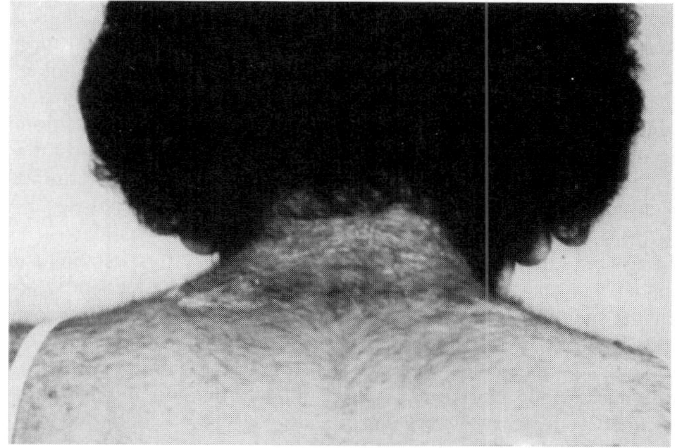

Fig. 68-12 Photograph of a patient with type A extreme insulin resistance. A photograph of patient A-5.[308,343] This photograph illustrates acanthosis nigricans on the back of her neck. The hirsutism noted on her back reflects the hyperandrogenism due to increased ovarian production of testosterone. This figure is reproduced from Taylor.[6]

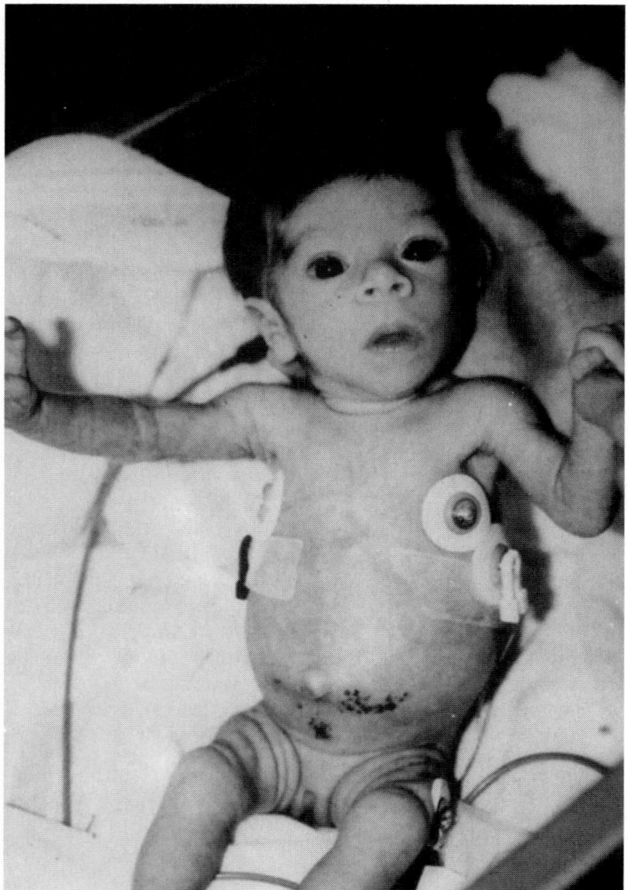

Fig. 68-13 Photograph of a patient with leprechaunism. A photograph of leprechaun/Minn-1.[298,450] This child was small for gestational age, weighing only 1.3 kg at birth. In addition, she had multiple phenotypic abnormalities including low-set ears and a depressed nasal bridge. This figure is reproduced from Taylor et al.[450]

excesses of glucagon, epinephrine, cortisol, or growth hormone in glucagonoma, pheochromocytoma, Cushing syndrome, or acromegaly, respectively.[247] Inasmuch as these endocrine diseases do not cause diabetes in every patient, the development of diabetes may reflect the presence of an underlying genetic susceptibility to develop type 2 diabetes. The excess of counterregulatory hormones presents a stress that causes the latent predisposition toward diabetes to become manifest. Similarly, islet cell tumors that produce somatostatin inhibit secretion of both insulin and glucagon.[248–251] On balance, the deficiency of insulin is more significant than the deficiency of glucagon. Thus, somatostatin excess produces diabetes. Isolated deficiency of growth hormone is also associated with impaired glucose tolerance and diabetes.[252]

Drug- or Chemical-Induced Diabetes. Many drugs can induce diabetes in susceptible individuals.[231] Therapy with glucocorticoid agents such as prednisone and cortisol can cause impaired glucose tolerance or diabetes. Induction of insulin resistance appears to be the major mechanism whereby glucocorticoids impair glucose tolerance. Many diuretics can cause diabetes by inducing a state of secondary hyperaldosteronism, leading to K^+ depletion. K^+ depletion interferes with insulin secretion, thereby leading to abnormal glucose tolerance.[253] The use of K^+-sparing diuretics or the administration of K^+ replacement will usually restore normal insulin secretion. It is beyond the scope of this chapter to discuss all the drugs that have been reported to impair glucose tolerance.

Infections. Congenital rubella triggers immune-mediated destruction of pancreatic beta cells, and leads to a disease resembling type 1 diabetes.

Uncommon Immune-Mediated Forms of Diabetes. Some patients with underlying autoimmune disease can develop spontaneous autoantibodies directed against the insulin receptor.[238,254–259] In virtually all patients there is clear clinical evidence of other autoimmune disease. Some patients have major systemic illness such as lupus erythematosus or scleroderma; other patients manifest tissue-specific autoimmunity such as Hashimoto thyroiditis or primary biliary cirrhosis; some patients have more subtle serologic abnormalities such as an elevated erythrocyte sedimentation rate or antinuclear antibodies. Antireceptor autoantibodies can cause hypoglycemia in some patients as a result of their ability to mimic the action of insulin upon the insulin receptor.[256–259] However, in most patients, the autoantibodies cause insulin-resistant diabetes as a result of their ability to inhibit insulin action.[260–262] These patients are among the most severely resistant to insulin, sometimes requiring thousands of units of intravenous insulin to elicit a detectable response. The insulin resistance is usually associated with acanthosis nigricans. In addition, premenopausal females sometimes manifest hyperandrogenism due to ovarian overproduction of testosterone.[263] At least two mechanisms appear to contribute to the ability of the antibodies to antagonize insulin action. First, the antibodies appear to down-regulate the number of insulin receptors on the cell

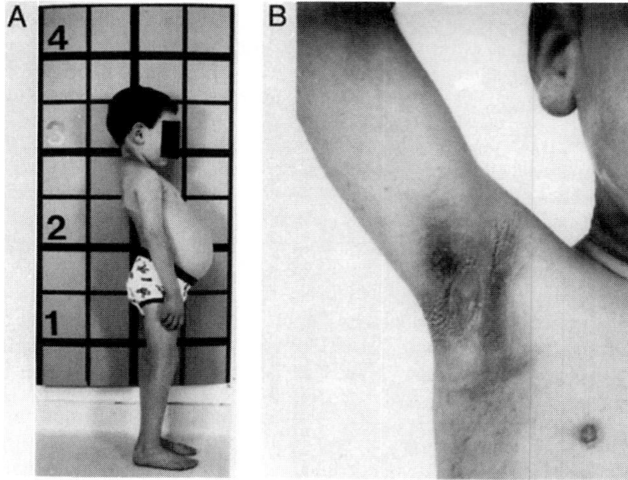

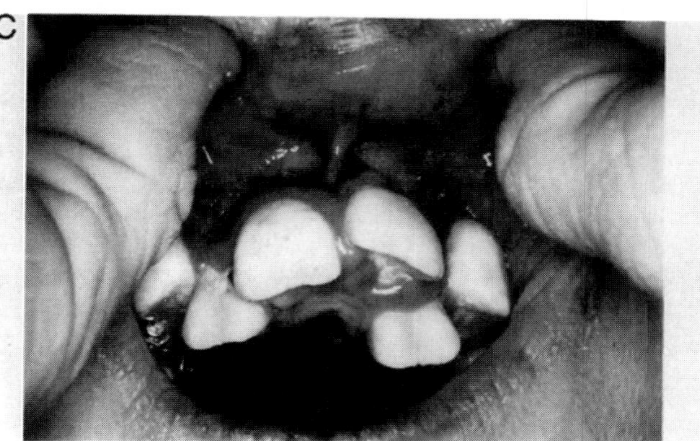

Fig. 68-14 Photographs of a patient with the Rabson-Mendenhall syndrome. Photographs of patient RM-2 with the Rabson-Mendenhall syndrome.[309] *A.* Profile of patient; note protuberant abdomen. *B.* Acanthosis nigricans in axilla. *C.* Upper jaw and mouth; note dental abnormalities. (*Reproduced from Taylor.*[6] *Used with permission.*)

surface by accelerating the rate of receptor degradation.[262] Second, the antibodies inhibit insulin from binding to the insulin receptor.[254,255] It is not completely understood why some patients develop hypoglycemia but others become insulin resistant. In some cases, patients may evolve from a picture of insulin resistance at one point in the clinical course, but develop fasting hypoglycemia at a later time.[256] The syndromes due to these antireceptor autoantibodies are usually self-limited, with the autoantibodies disappearing over a time that ranges from several month to several years. Although treatment with prednisone appears to block the hypoglycemia due to antireceptor antibodies,[257–259] there is no convincing evidence that immunosuppressive therapy has a major impact upon the titer of antireceptor autoantibodies.

Patients with "stiff man syndrome" develop antibodies to glutamic acid decarboxylase, and this can be associated with insulin deficiency due to autoimmune destruction of pancreatic beta cells (see Chap. 69).

Table 68-3 Genotypes of Patients with Genetic Forms of Insulin Resistance

Patient	Genotype
Type A extreme insulin resistance	
A-1	Amber^{133}/Ser^{462}
A-5 and A-8	Val^{382} (homozygous)
A-3	Glu^{1135}/WT (?)
A-6	Ile^{1153}/WT (?)
A-Jerusalem	$\Delta^{\text{Exon 3}}$/WT (?)
A-Saitama	$\Delta^{\text{G/Codon 1109}}$/WT (?)
A-San Diego	Gln^{993}/Opal^{1000}
A-Tokyo-1	Leu^{1178}/WT
Bl-1	Thr^{1134}/WT
Bl-2	Ser^{1200}/WT
Chiba	$\Delta^{\text{Exon 17(3')-22}}$/WT (?)
Fukuoka-1 and -2	Ser^{735} (homozygous)
Hamburg-1, -2, and -3	Ser^{462} $\Delta^{\text{10 b.p. (Exon 1)}}$
Okinawa	Val^{1008}/WT (?)
Osaka-1	Unidentified mutation/WT (?)
Osaka-2	Unidentified mutations (bis)
Sapporo-1	Val^{1008}/WT (?)
Unitad Arab Emirates	Gln^{1092}/WT (?)
Yamanashi	$\Delta^{\text{Exon 14}}$/WT (?)
Rabson-Mendenhall syndrome	
RM-1	Lys^{15}/Opal^{1000}
RM-E	AG→GG (intron 4)/$\Delta^{\text{8 b.p. (Exon 12)}}$
Leprechaunism	
Ark-1	Glu^{460}/Amber^{672}
Asahi	$\Delta^{\text{AG (Codon 955)}}$/? mutation
Atl-1	Pro^{86} (homozygous)
Geldermalsen	Pro^{233} (homozygous)
Helmond	Arg^{31}/? mutation
Minn-1	Opal^{897}/Unidentified mutation
Mt. Sinai	Opal^{1333}/Unidentified mutation
Osaka-Saitama	$\Delta^{\text{G (Codon 1109)}}$/Met^{910}
United Arab Emirates	Gln^{1092} (homozygous)
Verona-1	Ala^{28}/Arg^{366}
Winnipeg	Arg^{209} (homozygous)

Listed above are some of the mutations in the insulin receptor gene that have been identified in patients with genetic forms of insulin resistance. Missense mutations are identified by the amino acid substitution encoded by the mutation. WT refers to a wild type allele that encodes a receptor with a normal amino acid sequence. A question mark refers to an allele that is thought to be normal, but where the nucleotide sequence has been reported for only a portion of the protein-coding domain. Amber and opal refer to nonsense mutations corresponding to codons UAG and UGA, respectively. Deletion mutations are abbreviated as $\Delta^{\text{Exon 17(3')-22}}$ (a deletion beginning after codon 1012 in the 3′ part of exon 17 and extending downstream through exons 18–22), as $\Delta^{\text{Exon 14}}$ (a deletion of exon 14), and so on.

Other Genetic Syndromes Sometimes Associated with Diabetes. A large number of genetic syndromes are associated with either diabetes or impaired glucose tolerance.[264,265] Several examples will provide insight into the variety of syndromes that predispose to diabetes. In some cases (e.g., Wolfram syndrome; diabetes insipidus/diabetes mellitus/optic atrophy/deafness), diabetes mellitus is a prominent feature of the syndrome. In other cases (e.g., cystic fibrosis), impaired glucose tolerance is a relatively late complication of a major multisystem disease. While some genetic diseases (e.g., polyendocrine deficiency disease) lead to autoimmune ketosis-prone diabetes, most of the other genetic diseases predispose either to impaired glucose tolerance or to ketosis-resistant forms of diabetes. Some diseases are caused by major chromosomal abnormalities—for example, Down syndrome, Klinefelter syndrome, or Turner syndrome. Many of the diseases primarily affect the neuromuscular system—for example, myotonic dystrophy, muscular dystrophy, Huntington chorea, Friedreich ataxia. It is possible that these neuromuscular diseases impair glucose tolerance, at least in part, because they prevent normal physical activity. Just as aging predisposes to type 2 diabetes, progeroid syndromes (e.g., Werner syndrome and Cockayne syndrome) are associated with diabetes and impaired glucose tolerance. Furthermore, syndromes that predispose to endocrine tumors can lead to secondary diabetes—for example, multiple endocrine neoplasia type II leading to pheochromocytoma, and multiple endocrine neoplasia type I leading to Cushing disease, acromegaly, glucagonoma, or somatostatinoma.

Similarly, some genetic diseases are associated with risk factors that are known to predispose to the common form of type 2 diabetes. For example, Prader-Willi syndrome causes morbid obesity that predisposes to development of diabetes mellitus.[266,267] In recent years, there has been impressive progress in beginning to identify specific molecular causes of obesity. This progress in human molecular genetics has been inspired by similar investigations of genetic forms of obesity in rodents. At least six human obesity genes have been identified (Table 68-3). Leptin is a peptide secreted by adipose tissue that exerts multiple actions upon target cells, including feeding back upon the hypothalamus to suppress appetite. Thus, mutations in the leptin gene can cause obesity in both mice[268] and men.[269] Similarly, mutations in the leptin receptor gene have been demonstrated to cause obesity in both rodents[270–275] and humans.[276] Prohormone convertase-1 (PC-1), a protease involved in posttranslational processing of proteins, participates in the biosynthesis of multiple neuropeptides. Interestingly, mutations in the PC-1 gene have been reported to cause obesity in humans.[277] Similarly, mutations in the genes encoding pro-opiomelanocortin[278,279] and the melanocortin receptor 4[280] have also been identified as causes of obesity. Finally, peroxisomal activator receptor (PPAR)-γ is a ligand-regulated transcription factor that plays a key role in promoting differentiation of adipocytes.[281] Mutations that abolish a phosphorylation site required for MAP kinase-mediated inactivation of PPAR-γ have been reported to cause obesity.[282] Although somewhat less well established, polymorphisms in at least two other genes have been reported to be associated with an increased risk of developing obesity: the beta-3 adrenergic receptor[283–285] and uncoupling protein-3.[286]

Gestational Diabetes Mellitus. Gestational diabetes mellitus is a form of diabetes that has its initial onset during pregnancy, and resolves after the end of the preganancy.[287,288] In some patients, it is likely that the stress of pregnancy precipitates the decompensation of a "prediabetic" stage of type 1 diabetes. This conclusion is based upon the observation of an increased prevalence of the diabetogenic HLA antigens DR3 and DR4 as compared to racially matched pregnant women without diabetes.[289] Furthermore, in at least one study, approximately one third of women with gestational diabetes had anti-islet cell antibodies.[290] As a group, patients with gestational diabetes are at increased risk to develop type 2 diabetes later in life.[2,288,291] In summary, gestational diabetes comprises a heterogeneous group of patients, some of whom probably have a genetic predisposition to develop either type 1 or type 2 diabetes.

Modified Criteria to Diagnose Gestational Diabetes Mellitus (GDM). A different set of criteria are used to diagnose diabetes during pregnancy.[2,287,292,293] Generally, pregnant women are first screened by administering a 50 g oral glucose load, a test usually performed in the 24th to 28th weeks of gestation. Patients need not be fasting for this screening test. If the plasma glucose >140 mg/dl (7.8 mM) at 1 hr in the screening test, then it is necessary to administer another oral glucose tolerance test for definitive diagnosis. To diagnose GDM according to criteria used in the U.S., two or more values of plasma glucose must exceed the following limits during a 100 g-OGTT: fasting >105 mg/dl (5.8 mM), 1 hr >190 mg/dl (10.6 mM), 2 hr >165 mg/dl (9.2 mM), or 3 hr >145 mg/dl (8.1 mM).

Several reasons account for the use of different criteria for the diagnosis of diabetes during pregnancy. Pregnancy per se has an effect on glucose homeostasis. In addition, pregnant women are usually below 50 years of age, and the deterioration of glucose tolerance as a consequence of aging does not lead to "false positive" tests in this age group. Most importantly, in diagnosing gestational diabetes, the criteria are designed to predict adverse outcomes of the pregnancy, rather than the traditional chronic complications of diabetes. For example, inadequately controlled gestational diabetes may lead to abnormally large babies resulting in obstetric complications. In addition, infants of diabetic mothers are at increased risk to develop numerous complications during the postnatal period.

MECHANISMS OF INSULIN RESISTANCE: MUTATIONS IN THE INSULIN RECEPTOR GENE

Although insulin resistance plays a key role in the pathogenesis of type 2 diabetes (see "Insulin Resistance: Role in the Pathophysiology of Type 2 Diabetes Mellitus"), the molecular mechanisms that cause insulin resistance have not been elucidated in the majority of patients. However, there has been considerable success in identifying the cause of diabetes in several uncommon syndromes of insulin resistance due to mutations in the insulin receptor gene.

Clinical Syndromes

Leprechaunism. Leprechaunism is the most severe clinical syndrome caused by mutations in the insulin receptor gene (Fig. 68-13).[4–6,294] These patients have glucose intolerance despite having extremely high insulin levels (e.g., a hundredfold above the normal range). In addition to insulin resistance, patients have multiple abnormalities (e.g., intrauterine growth retardation and fasting hypoglycemia), and usually die within the first year of life. These patients have inactivating mutations in both alleles of the insulin receptor gene. In inbred pedigrees, the patients are truly homozygous for a single mutant allele;[295,296] in the absence of consanguinity, they are usually compound heterozygotes with two different mutant alleles.[297,298]

Type A Insulin Resistance. Type A insulin resistance is defined by the triad of insulin resistance, acanthosis nigricans, and hyperandrogenism (in female patients) in the absence of obesity or lipoatrophy (Fig. 68-12).[4–6,238,294] Acanthosis nigricans and hyperandrogenism correlate with hyperinsulinemia, and it is believed that they are caused by "toxic" effects of insulin upon the skin and the ovaries, respectively.[299] Because these patients have defects in the function of their insulin receptors, it is unlikely that the toxic effects of insulin are mediated by insulin receptors, but more likely by receptors for homologous peptides such as insulin-like growth factor-I.

Most patients with type A insulin resistance are heterozygous for a single mutant allele, most often a mutation in the tyrosine kinase domain of the receptor.[5,6,294,300–306] These patients are usually less insulin resistant than patients with two mutant alleles. Although some heterozygotes have abnormal glucose tolerance, most do not exhibit fasting hyperglycemia. However, some patients with type A insulin resistance have two mutant alleles of the insulin receptor gene.[5,6,294,295,307,308] These patients seem to develop overt diabetes with fasting hyperglycemia during childhood or adolescence, although they usually do not have fasting hyperglycemia as infants.

Rabson-Mendenhall Syndrome. The Rabson-Mendenhall syndrome is defined by the presence of several clinical features including extreme insulin resistance, acanthosis nigricans, short stature due to growth retardation, abnormalities of teeth and nails, and pineal hyperplasia (Fig. 68-14).[4–6,242] This syndrome is intermediate in clinical severity between leprechaunism and type A insulin resistance. Although the distinction between leprechaunism and the Rabson-Mendenhall syndrome may not be clear at the time of birth, it has been suggested to reserve the diagnosis of Rabson-Mendenhall syndrome for patients who survive beyond two years of life. As in leprechaunism, patients with the Rabson-Mendenhall syndrome have inactivating mutations in both alleles of the insulin receptor gene.[295,309,310]

Non-Insulin-Dependent Diabetes Mellitus. Some patients with mutations in the insulin receptor gene have syndromes that resemble the common form of type 2 diabetes. For example, in screening studies carried out in patients with the clinical syndrome of non-insulin-dependent diabetes, a low prevalence of mutations in the insulin receptor gene has been reported.[237,311] In studies of patients with mutations in the insulin receptor gene (i.e., leprechaunism and type A insulin resistance), family members (i.e., parents and siblings) have been identified who are heterozygous for mutations in the insulin receptor gene.[297,312–314] Many of these heterozygotes were insulin resistant and had significant hyperinsulinemia. Most of these family members were not diabetic. However, because most of these asymptomatic individuals were evaluated prior to the age of 40, it is possible that these heterozygotes may develop diabetes later in life as is typical for the onset of type 2 diabetes.

In summary, there are insufficient data to provide a reliable estimate of the prevalence of mutations in the insulin receptor gene. However, available data are consistent with estimates that ~1 percent of patients with non-insulin-dependent diabetes may have mutations in their insulin receptor gene.[5,6]

Mutations in the Insulin Receptor Gene

Multiple different mutations have been identified in the insulin receptor (Figs. 68-15, 68-16; Table 68-3).[5,6,294] In several instances, the same mutation has been identified in two apparently unrelated patients. However, most of the published mutations have only been identified in single kindreds. The mutations have been classified in five classes based upon the mechanisms whereby the mutations impair insulin receptor function (Fig. 68-17). This classification is a modification of the classification scheme proposed by Brown and Goldstein to describe mutations in the low density lipoprotein receptor gene.[315]

Class 1. Impaired Receptor Biosynthesis. At least one patient with leprechaunism has been reported who was homozygous for a total deletion of both insulin receptor genes,[296] and several patients were homozygous for other null alleles.[316–320]

Several types of premature chain termination mutations have been identified in the insulin receptor gene (Fig. 68-15): nonsense mutations,[295,297,298] mutations at intron-exon junctions that impair splicing of mRNA,[321] and deletion mutations that shift the reading frame.[306,322] Premature chain termination mutations interfere with receptor biosynthesis, and lead to the synthesis of truncated

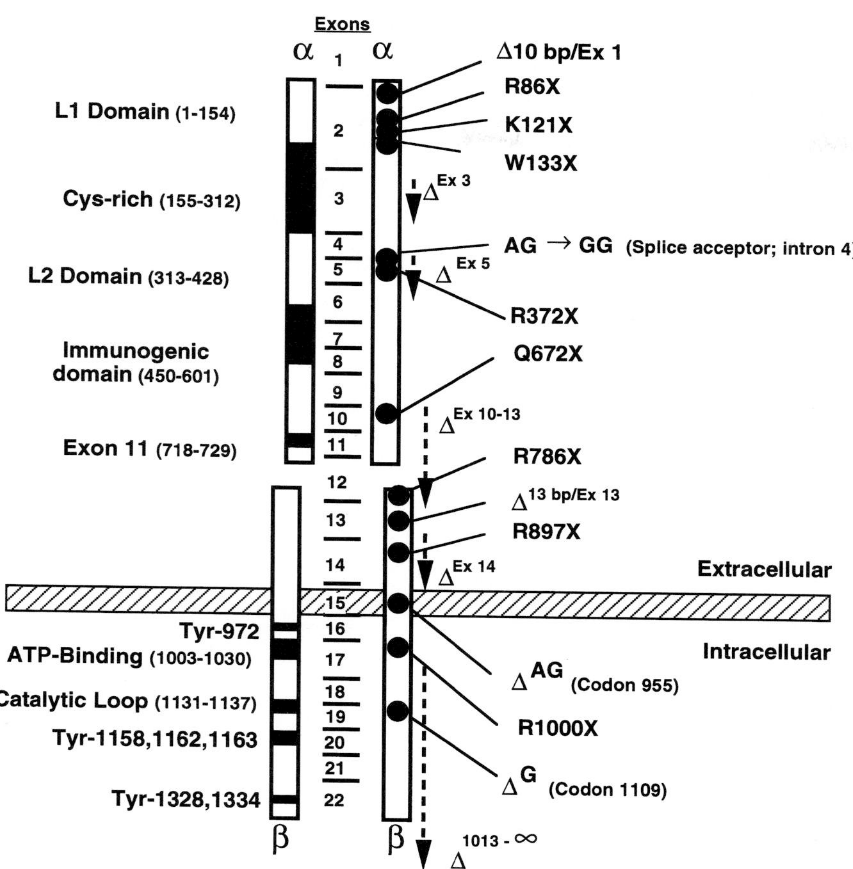

Fig. 68-15 Mutations that impair receptor biosynthesis (Class 1). In this cartoon of the receptor, the structural landmarks are indicated on the left side of the figure. Examples of Class 1 mutations are indicated on the right side of the figure. These include nonsense mutations, as well as frame shifts and splicing mutations. (In the right half of the cartoon, the tetrapeptide connecting the two subunits has not been removed in order to illustrate the sequence of the uncleaved proreceptor.) (*Modified from and based on Taylor and Arioglu.*[451])

receptor fragments. In addition, most premature chain termination mutations exert a cis-acting effect to decrease the level of mRNA transcribed from the mutant allele.[295,298] In some patients, mutant alleles have been demonstrated to decrease the level of insulin receptor mRNA, but the mutations map outside the protein coding regions, most likely in regions of the gene that regulate its level of expression.[298,323]

Class 2. Impaired Transport of Receptors to the Cell Surface. The insulin receptor precursor undergoes multiple posttranslational processing steps within the endoplasmic reticulum and Golgi.[56–58,324–326] Some mutations impair transport through the endoplasmic reticulum and Golgi to the plasma membrane, thereby reducing the number of receptors on the cell surface.[5,6,294,308,310,327–330] Because these mutations prevent the receptor from folding into its normal conformation, some Class 2 mutations also impair receptor function—for example, decreasing the affinity of insulin binding[329] or inhibiting activation of the receptor tyrosine kinase.[327] Most of the published mutations in this class are located in the N-terminal half of the α-subunit (Fig. 68-16). However, at least one mutation that inhibited posttranslational processing of the proreceptor and transport of the receptor to the plasma membrane was located in the intracellular domain and inhibited receptor tyrosine kinase activity.[305]

Class 3. Decreased Affinity of Insulin Binding. Some mutations decrease the affinity with which the receptor binds insulin (Fig. 68-16).[5,6,294] This is predicted to cause a rightward shift in the dose-response curve for insulin action—that is, to decrease the sensitivity with which the target cell responds to insulin. A mutation substituting serine for Arg[735] was the first mutation reported to decrease the affinity of insulin binding.[307,331] Arg[735] is the last amino acid in the Arg-Lys-Arg-Arg motif at the proteolytic cleavage site between the α- and β-subunits. In addition to decreasing the affinity of insulin binding, the R735S mutation inhibits cleavage of the precursor into two subunits.

Two mutations in the N-terminal half of the α-subunit have also been reported to decrease the affinity of insulin binding, consistent with the hypothesis that insulin binds to this region of the receptor.[5,6,294] For example, the N15K-mutation caused a fivefold reduction in affinity,[295,329] and the S323L mutation essentially abolished insulin binding.[309,332,333] In addition, the N15K-mutation impaired transport of the receptor to the cell surface.

Class 4. Impaired Tyrosine Kinase Activity. Many mutations have been identified in the tyrosine kinase domain that inhibit receptor tyrosine kinase activity (Fig. 68-16).[5,6,294] These observations strongly support the hypothesis that tyrosine kinase activity is required for the ability of the receptor to mediate the metabolic actions of insulin in vivo. The G1008V-mutation was among the first mutations to be identified in the tyrosine kinase domain.[301] Valine is substituted for Gly[1008], the third glycine in the highly conserved Gly-X-Gly-X-X-Gly motif in the ATP binding site. Because ATP is the phosphate donor for the tyrosine kinase reaction, it is not surprising that a mutation in the ATP binding site inactivates the tyrosine kinase. Unlike most mutations in the extracellular domain of the insulin receptor, most mutations in the tyrosine kinase domain cause insulin resistance in a dominant fashion.[5,6,294] The dominant negative effect of mutations in the tyrosine kinase domain may be related to the fact that the insulin receptor has an $\alpha_2\beta_2$ structure. Thus, in a heterozygous individual, it is possible to have a hybrid form ($\alpha_2\beta_{wt}\beta_{mut}$) in addition to the symmetrical wild type [$\alpha_2(\beta_{wt})_2$] and mutant [$\alpha_2(\beta_{mut})_2$] forms. While the symmetrical wild type receptor [$\alpha_2(\beta_{wt})_2$] is active as a tyrosine kinase, the hybrid $\alpha_2\beta_{wt}\beta_{mut}$ and the symmetrical mutant receptors [$\alpha_2(\beta_{mut})_2$] are both inactive as tyrosine kinase enzymes.[334,335] The hypothesis

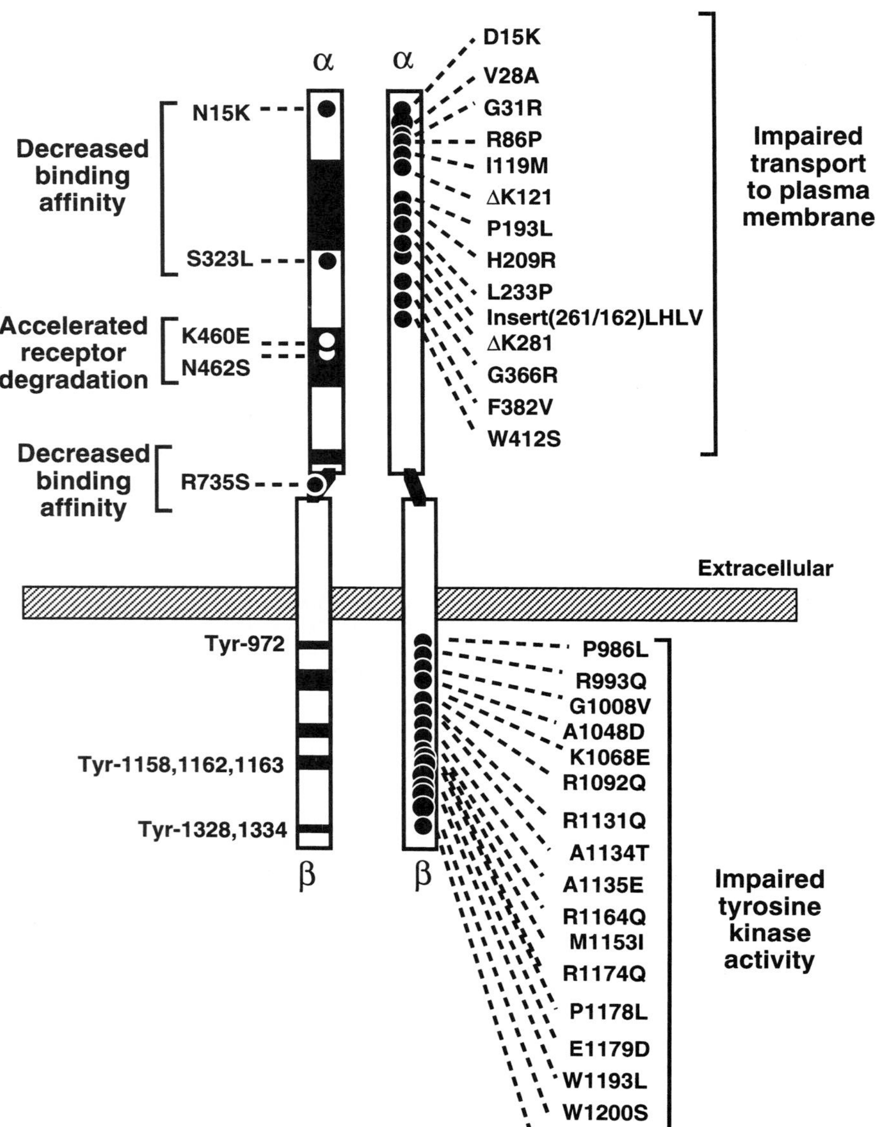

Fig. 68-16 Missense mutations in the insulin receptor gene. Examples of missense mutations in the insulin receptor gene are indicated in the figure. These mutations either impair the transport of receptors to the plasma membrane (Class 2), decrease the affinity of insulin binding (Class 3), impair tyrosine kinase activity (Class 4), or accelerate the rate at which receptors are degraded (Class 5). (*Modified from and based on Taylor and Arioglu.*[451])

that a mutation in a single allele inactivates 75 percent of the receptors provides a possible molecular explanation of the dominant pattern of inheritance observed with mutations in the tyrosine kinase domain. However, the hypothesis has remained somewhat controversial inasmuch as one study did not succeed in demonstrating the formation of heterodimers between a wild type insulin receptor and the kinase-inactive (M1153I) mutant receptor.[336]

Class 5. Accelerated Receptor Degradation. Insulin binding triggers endocytosis of the insulin-receptor complex.[179] Internalized receptors are located in endosomes with the insulin-binding site oriented on the inside of the vesicle.[337] Endosomal proton pumps acidify the interior of the endosome (pH ~5.5), and the acidic pH promotes dissociation of insulin from the receptor.[338] Subsequent to internalization, there are at least two pathways available to the receptor: recycling back to the plasma membrane for reutilization versus degradation within the lysosome. Some mutations (i.e., K460E and N462S) impair the ability of acidic pH to dissociate insulin from the receptor.[297,338,339] Both mutations are associated with an impaired recycling pathway, and preferential targeting of mutant receptors toward lysosomal degradation, thereby accelerating receptor degradation and decreasing the number of receptors on the cell surface.[297,338,340]

Correlation of Molecular Defects with Clinical Syndromes

At least three different theories have been considered to explain the fact that mutations in the insulin receptor gene can cause several distinct clinical syndromes.[4–6]

Severity of insulin resistance: According to this hypothesis, the severity of insulin resistance determines the clinical manifestations. Patients with leprechaunism have mutations in both alleles of the insulin receptor gene,[5,6] and exhibit the most extreme degree of insulin resistance. In contrast, heterozygosity for a single mutant allele causes the less severe syndrome of type A insulin resistance. Furthermore, even among patients with type A insulin resistance, the patients with two mutant alleles have a more severe form of the syndrome characterized by fasting hyperglycemia.

Existence of branched pathways: Insulin is a hormone that has multiple biologic actions. The pathways for insulin action diverge in the biochemical steps distal to the receptor. According to this hypothesis, the effect of a mutation would depend upon which biologic actions are impaired and which are preserved.[341] For

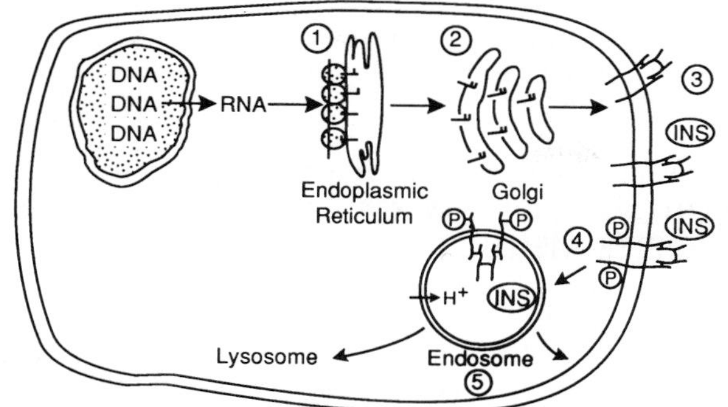

Class of Mutation	Synthesis	Transport to Plasma Membrane	Insulin Binding	Trans-membrane Signalling	Endocytosis, Recycling, Degradation
①	→ ×				
②	→	→ ×			
③	→	→	→ ×		
④	→	→	→	→ ×	
⑤	→	→	→	→	→ ×

Fig. 68-17 Classification of mutations in insulin receptor gene. This cartoon summarizes the major steps in the life of an insulin receptor. First, the gene is transcribed, and the RNA is spliced. The mature mRNA is transported from the nucleus to the cytosol where it is translated by ribosomes on the rough endoplasmic reticulum. The receptor is transported through the endoplasmic reticulum and Golgi, in which organelles it undergoes multiple posttranslational modifications. Eventually, the mature receptor is inserted in the plasma membrane. Insulin binds to the receptor on the cell surface. As a result, the receptor undergoes autophosphorylation and becomes activated as a tyrosine kinase. The interaction of insulin with its receptor initiates the various responses of the target cell to insulin. In addition, insulin binding triggers receptor endocytosis. The acid pH in the endosome dissociates insulin from its receptor. Subsequent to receptor internalization, the receptor is either transported to lysosomes for degradation or recycled back to the plasma membrane for reutilization. The five major classes of genetic defects in receptor function are summarized in the table at the bottom of the figure. This classification scheme is based upon the classification originally proposed by Brown and Goldstein[315] *for genetic defects in the function of the low-density lipoprotein receptor.* (*Reproduced from Taylor.*[6] *Used with permission.*)

example, a mutation that impairs both the metabolic actions and the growth-promoting effects of insulin might cause leprechaunism (a syndrome with growth retardation as well as abnormal glucose tolerance). If a mutation selectively impairs only the ability of the receptor to mediate the metabolic actions of insulin, this might cause type A insulin resistance (a syndrome with abnormal glucose tolerance but normal growth).

Genetic variation at different loci: According to this theory, the insulin receptor locus is the major disease gene responsible for the insulin resistance, but other genetic loci modulate the clinical syndrome. For example, defects in various growth factor receptors have been reported in patients with leprechaunism, and these defects may contribute to the growth retardation associated with the syndrome.[342] However, if the difference between type A insulin resistance and leprechaunism were due to mutations at another genetic locus, then one would predict that mutations at the two genetic loci would segregate independently. If a child inherited the insulin receptor mutations in the absence of the mutations at the other locus, the patient would manifest type A insulin resistance. If another child in the same pedigree inherited mutations in both the insulin receptor and the other locus, then he would develop leprechaunism. This pattern of inheritance has not been reported, although many kindreds have been reported with two or more siblings having the same clinical syndrome — that is, either leprechaunism or type A insulin resistance.

Nevertheless, it is likely that polygenic influences may explain some clinical variation between individuals with the same genotype at the insulin receptor locus. Two sisters with type A insulin resistance (both homozygous for the F382V mutation) illustrate this clinical variability in the syndrome.[308,343,344] Although the younger sister required treatment with several thousand units of insulin per day, the older sister responded to dietary management. The younger sister had such severe hyperandrogenism that she has never menstruated spontaneously and did not experience withdrawal bleeding when treated with estrogen + progestin, while the older sister achieved pregnancy on two occasions.

Transgenic Animal Models

Animal models of disease do not prove which genes are actually mutated in human disease. However, by inserting mutations into specific genes, one can elucidate the impact of mutations in those genes. This approach has been applied to study the effect of mutations in genes in the insulin action pathway. As expected, inactivating mutations in the genes encoding the insulin receptor,[345,346] IRS-1,[87,88] and IRS-2[89] all cause insulin resistance. However, unexpectedly, some mutations in the insulin action pathway have been reported to impair insulin secretion in some animal models.[89,347] Thus, these animal models have generated novel hypotheses that will inspire interesting approaches to study human type 2 diabetes.[348,349]

Insulin Receptor Knockout Mice. When inactivating mutations are inserted into both alleles of the insulin receptor gene, the knockout mice develop severe insulin resistance and uncontrolled diabetes.[345,346] In contrast, mice that are heterozygous for a null allele of the insulin receptor gene are hyperinsulinemic, a sign that they have some degree of insulin resistance. While not diabetic at birth, they are at increased risk to develop diabetes as they age.[350] Furthermore, the genetic background of the mouse can modulate the likelihood that diabetes will develop, as demonstrated by various breeding studies. For example, heterozygous insulin receptor knockout mice were bred with IRS-1 knockout mice to obtain double knockout mice (insr $^{-/+}$, irs1 $^{-/+}$).[350] As compared to insr $^{-/+}$ mice, the double heterozygotes (insr $^{-/+}$, irs1 $^{-/+}$) were more insulin resistant and at increased risk to develop diabetes. Because heterozygosity for a null allele of the IRS-1 gene (irs1 $^{-/+}$ mice) neither caused insulin resistance nor predisposed to diabetes, there appeared to be epistatic interactions between the two mutations that combined to increase the risk to develop diabetes. However, despite the increased risk, some of the doubly heterozygous (insr $^{-/+}$, irs1 $^{-/+}$) mice did not develop diabetes. What determined which mice escaped from developing diabetes? Interestingly, and unlike the situation in human diabetes, it was the mice with the highest insulin that developed diabetes. This suggests that it was the severity of the insulin resistance (rather than the ability of the pancreas to compensate for insulin resistance) that determined which (insr $^{-/+}$, irs1 $^{-/+}$) mice would develop diabetes. Furthermore, the insulin resistance in the (insr $^{-/+}$, irs1 $^{-/+}$) mice led to a striking degree of islet hyperplasia, presumably in an effort to compensate for the insulin resistance.

Although mice lacking insulin receptors die within the first days of life, viable mice have been obtained in which the insulin receptor knockout was limited to specific tissues.[349] Mice with skeletal muscle-specific insulin receptor knockout (MIRKO) were engineered using the technique of cre-recombinase-mediated recombination. As expected, when studied in vitro, skeletal muscle from MIRKO mice was insulin resistant.[351] Furthermore, the mice had increased body fat, presumably because glucose was shunted from insulin-resistant muscle to adipose tissue where it was converted into triglyceride for storage. Similar results were obtained in transgenic mice engineered for selective expression of a dominant negative mutant insulin receptor in skeletal muscle (Mu/A1134T-IR).[352] Interestingly, although MIRKO mice did not exhibit either hyperinsulinemia or hyperglycemia, transgenic Mu/A1134T-IR mice developed mild hyperglycemia. Thus, selective insulin resistance at the level of muscle causes little if any fasting hyperglycemia. In the fasting state when insulin levels are low, muscle oxidizes fatty acids as its principal fuel source. Muscle is responsible for a relatively small percentage of total glucose utilization during fasting, so a reduction in muscle glucose uptake does not cause a major increase in the fasting glucose level. Similarly, another transgenic mouse model, expressing a dominant negative mutant of the insulin receptor in both muscle and adipose tissue, developed mild fasting hyperglycemia and impaired glucose tolerance.[353]

The technique of cre-recombinase-mediated recombination has also been used to obtain mice in which the insulin receptor gene was selectively knocked out in pancreatic β-cells (βIRKO). These studies have yielded novel insights into the relationship between insulin action and insulin secretion. βIRKO mice exhibited impaired glucose tolerance as a result of a progressive defect in the ability of glucose to elicit insulin secretion.[347] Insulin receptors mediate at least two processes in β-cells that promote insulin secretion in vitro: insulin stimulates exocytosis of secretory vesicles,[354] and insulin feeds back to promote transcription of the insulin gene.[355] IRS-2 was shown to mediate the latter action of insulin in β-cells; this may explain the impaired insulin secretion observed in IRS-2 knockout mice (see "Knockout Mice Lacking IRS-1 and IRS-2").[89] The βIRKO mouse suggests a novel explanation for the pathogenesis of the two defects characteristic of type 2 diabetes. In this case, *insulin resistance* at the level of the beta cell directly caused *insulin deficiency.* While this hypothesis is extremely attractive, there is some evidence that the pathophysiology may not always be so simple. For example, in contrast to the insulin deficiency caused by insulin resistance at the level of the β-cell in βIRKO mice, the generalized insulin resistance in (insr $^{-/+}$, irs1 $^{-/+}$) mice led to β-cell hyperplasia and hyperinsulinemia.[350] Furthermore, patients with leprechaunism who are homozygous for inactivating mutations in the insulin receptor gene also develop hyperplastic islets.[240,349] In a heterogeneous polygenic syndrome such as type 2 diabetes, it is likely that there may not be a single unifying explanation of insulin deficiency in all patients. Nevertheless, the βIRKO mouse provides evidence of at least one simple mechanism whereby insulin resistance can lead to insulin deficiency.[347]

Knockout Mice Lacking IRS-1 and IRS-2. Knockout mice lacking IRS-1 exhibited impaired growth, but did not develop diabetes.[87,88] In fact, this was among the first clues that there was redundancy in the insulin action pathway. In fact, the absence of IRS-1 led to increased tyrosine phosphorylation of other substrates—for example, IRS-2 and IRS-3 in liver and adipose tissue, respectively. Nevertheless, the absence of IRS-1 did predispose to the ability of mutations in other genes to cause diabetes. As summarized above ("Insulin Receptor Knockout Mice"), when mice were heterozygous for mutations in two genes in the insulin action pathway (insr $^{-/+}$, irs1 $^{-/+}$), this greatly enhanced the risk of developing diabetes. Similarly, when IRS-1 knockout mice were bred with glucokinase knockout mice, the combination of a genetic defect in the insulin action pathway (IRS-1) together with a genetic defect in the insulin secretion pathway (glucokinase) produced a strong predisposition to develop diabetes.[356]

Subsequently, knockout mice lacking IRS-2 have been obtained. The absence of IRS-2 led not only to insulin resistance, but also to diabetes.[89] Why did these mice develop diabetes? The answer was both unexpected and instructive. Diabetes developed as a result of impaired insulin secretion, which interfered with the ability of the β-cell to compensate for insulin resistance.[89,357] In IRS-2 knockout mice, a single genetic defect appeared to cause both insulin resistance and insulin deficiency. This observation is consistent with the hypothesis that the β-cell requires an intact insulin action pathway in order to maintain normal insulin secretion. However, IRS-2 also functions in other signaling pathways (e.g., cytokines and insulin-like growth factors). Therefore, the role of IRS-2 in β-cells may not be limited to the insulin action pathway.

INSULIN RESISTANCE: ROLE IN THE PATHOPHYSIOLOGY OF TYPE 2 DIABETES MELLITUS

Type 2 diabetes is caused by two physiological defects: resistance to the action of insulin combined with a deficiency in insulin secretion.[344,357,358] Which is the primary cause of type 2 diabetes: insulin deficiency or insulin resistance? Some authorities conclude that insulin resistance is the primary cause of type 2 diabetes because it is easily demonstrated at an early phase of the disease when the patient has impaired glucose tolerance but has not yet developed overt diabetes.[358] However, with the exception of patients with extreme insulin resistance (e.g., patients with mutations in the insulin receptor gene), insulin resistance does not cause diabetes as long as the pancreas can secrete sufficient insulin to compensate.[359,360] Thus, some authorities conclude that insulin deficiency is the proximate cause of type 2 diabetes because insulin deficiency is the final insult that immediately precedes the development of diabetes. The most appropriate resolution of the debate is to acknowledge that both defects contribute importantly to the pathophysiology in most patients with type 2 diabetes.[344] This chapter reviews the mechanisms of insulin resistance in patients with type 2 diabetes. Issues related to insulin secretion and insulin deficiency are discussed in Chap. 67.

Progression of Physiological Defects during Development of Type 2 Diabetes

The essential defects in type 2 diabetes can be inferred from classic studies in which oral glucose tolerance tests were conducted in patients at four stages in the natural history of the disease process: normal glucose tolerance, chemical diabetes (now called impaired glucose tolerance), diabetes with minimal fasting hyperglycemia (fasting plasma glucose $<$140 mg/dl), and diabetes mellitus with overt fasting hyperglycemia (fasting plasma glucose $>$140 mg/dl) (Fig. 68-18).[361,362] The highest levels of insulin in plasma were observed in patients with impaired glucose tolerance. Despite the high levels of insulin, glucose levels were somewhat elevated, demonstrating that these patients were resistant to the action of insulin. As the patients progressed from impaired glucose tolerance to diabetes mellitus, insulin levels declined. Indeed, the lowest insulin levels were observed in the group of patients with the highest levels of plasma glucose, demonstrating a defect in insulin secretion. While this was a cross-sectional study comparing different patients at different points in the natural history of the disease,[361] longitudinal studies have obtained similar data when studying the same patient during progression from impaired glucose tolerance to overt type 2 diabetes.[363–368]

Prediabetes: Genetic Predisposition. Available evidence strongly suggests that the susceptibility to develop type 2 diabetes mellitus is determined primarily by genetic factors. For example, studies of monozygotic twins have demonstrated an extremely high concordance rate ($\sim$90 percent) for the development of type 2 diabetes, substantially higher than the concordance rate for type 1 diabetes in the same study.[369] The high concordance rate for type 2 diabetes is all the more impressive because it develops relatively late in life, at a time when the twins usually live apart and share fewer environmental factors than during childhood. However, type 2 diabetes is a complex trait that is transmitted with a pattern suggesting polygenic inheritance. It is not known which genes predispose to insulin deficiency and which to insulin resistance. Indeed, it is not certain whether it is the same or different genes that lead to the two defects.

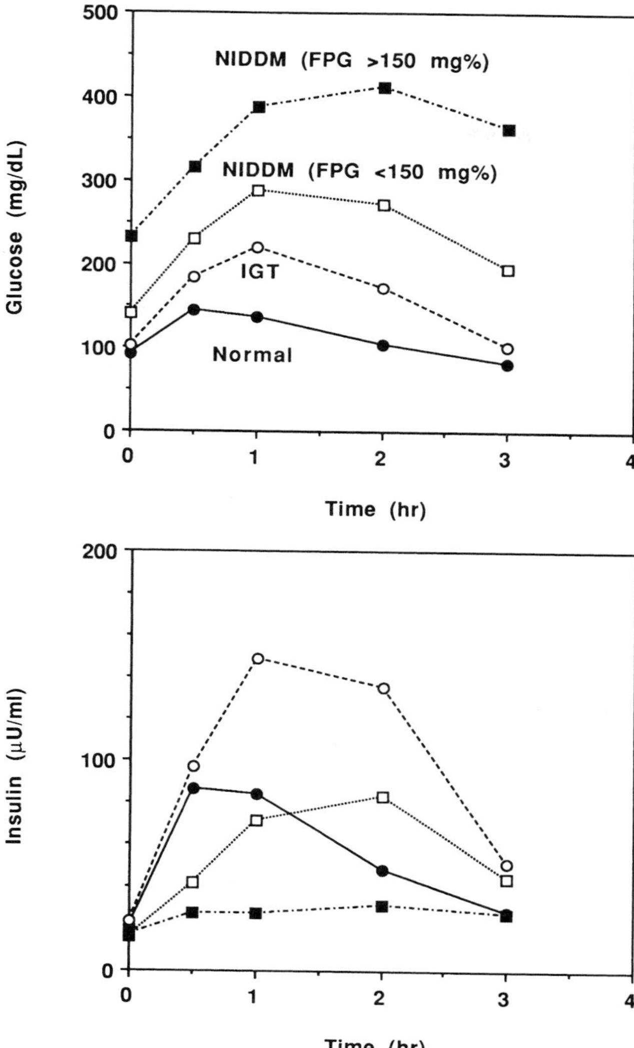

Fig. 68-18 Progressive deteriority of glucose tolerance during the evolution of type 2 diabetes. Oral glucose tolerance tests were carried out in four groups of individuals: normal individuals (solid circles), patients with impaired glucose tolerance (open circles), patients with NIDDM and fasting plasma glucose < 150 mg/dl (open squares), and patients with NIDDM and fasting plasma glucose > 150 mg/dl (closed squares). The graphs were drawn using data obtained from Reaven and Olefsky.[361]

There is considerable interest in identifying the genes that predispose to the development of type 2 diabetes. At least seven genes have been identified in which mutations cause uncommon monogenically inherited forms of diabetes: insulin, insulin receptor, glucokinase, hepatocyte nuclear factors-1α, -1β, -4α, and insulin promoter factor-1 (see above "Genetic Defects of Beta Cell Function").[4–6,8,9,11–14] However, these genes appear not to make important contributions to the genetic predisposition to develop the common form of type 2 diabetes. Efforts have been initiated to use genetic linkage methods to carry out positional cloning of type 2 diabetes genes. For example, evidence has been obtained mapping diabetes genes at the following chromosomal locations: chromosome 2q in Mexican-Americans;[370] chromosome 12q in a Finnish population;[371] chromosome 11q in Pima Indians; and chromosome 20q in another Finnish population as well as several other Caucasian populations.[372–375] These data are encouraging that the positional cloning will eventually succeed in identifying genes that predispose to type 2 diabetes. It will be a major advance when the genes causing type 2 diabetes are eventually identified.

Considerable work has also been invested in screening "candidate genes" in the insulin action pathway for mutations that might cause insulin resistance. Among the genes that have been screened are the following: IRS-1, IRS-2, and IRS-4. With one possible exception, these studies have not identified common polymorphisms or mutations associated with diabetes or insulin resistance. Although the association remains controversial, several studies have suggested that amino acid sequence polymorphisms in the IRS-1 gene may be associated with type 2 diabetes. The most common variant (i.e., substitution of Arg for Gly^{972}) has been reported to be approximately twice as prevalent in patients with type 2 diabetes as in control subjects.[376,377] Furthermore, it has been suggested that the G972R polymorphism acts synergistically with obesity. In other words, the presence of the G972R allele of IRS-1 exacerbates obesity-induced insulin resistance while not causing insulin resistance in lean subjects.[378] These studies have been extended in in vitro studies to evaluate the functional impact of the G972R substitution. The results of these studies have been equivocal. Although the G972R substitution has been reported to cause a small (~30 percent) impairment in the ability to activate PI 3-kinase,[379] this observation was not confirmed in another study.[380] In any case, studies of candidate genes published to date have not been successful in identifying common causes of type 2 diabetes.

Peripheral Insulin Resistance. Several methods have been developed to quantitate insulin action in patients.[381–383] In the insulin clamp technique, insulin is infused intravenously into a patient at a rate chosen to achieve the desired steady-state level of insulin in plasma.[358,382,384] In order to prevent hypoglycemia, glucose is infused intravenously at a rate chosen to maintain the plasma glucose level at the desired level. In the usual euglycemic clamp study, plasma glucose is maintained at a normal level (e.g., ~90 mg/dl). Under these steady-state conditions, the rate at which glucose is infused must be equal to the net total body utilization of glucose. Thus, it is possible to construct a dose-response curve for net total body utilization of glucose as a function of plasma insulin levels (Fig. 68-19). However, this analysis is oversimplified because insulin has distinct effects on different tissues. Insulin increases glucose utilization by insulin-sensitive tissues such as skeletal muscle, but it also inhibits glucose production by the liver.[358] Thus, while most of the glucose infusion during the insulin clamp study provides substrate for glucose utilization by peripheral tissues, part of the glucose is required to replace the glucose that would have been produced by the liver in the absence of insulin. Methods have been developed to quantitate the individual contributions of suppression of hepatic glucose production and stimulation of glucose utilization by peripheral tissues.[358,385,386] These methods generally involve infusing radioactively labeled glucose. By measuring the change in the specific radioactivity of the glucose molecules in plasma, it is possible to calculate the rate of endogenous hepatic glucose production and the rate of infusion of exogenous glucose. Although some controversies remain about the detailed interpretation of some of these studies, this type of approach has provided evidence that the major target tissues are resistant to biologic action of insulin in vivo.

In the postabsorptive state, insulin-independent tissues such as the brain account for ~50 percent of total body glucose utilization, and splanchnic tissue (i.e., liver plus gastrointestinal tract) account for an additional ~25 percent.[358] Under these conditions, a relatively small percentage (~25 percent) of glucose utilization occurs in insulin-dependent tissues (primarily skeletal muscle). In contrast, insulin action can dramatically increase glucose utilization by peripheral tissues. Indeed, maximally effective concentrations of insulin elicit an approximately fivefold increase in total body glucose uptake, corresponding to an ~20-fold increase in glucose utilization by insulin-sensitive tissues. Half-maximal

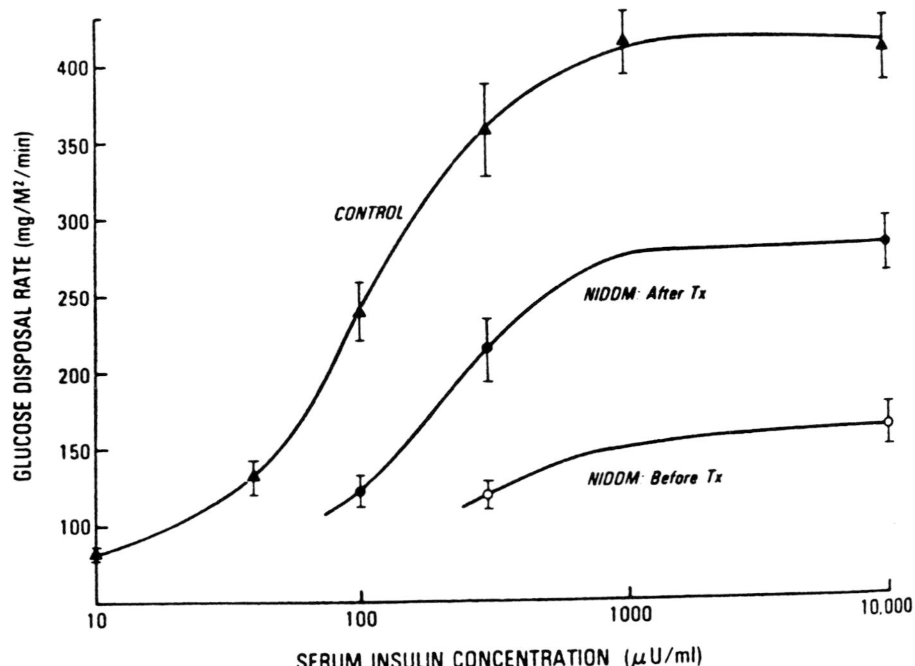

Fig. 68-19 Dose-response for insulin action in vivo. Euglycemic insulin clamps were carried out by infusing insulin intravenously at a rate chosen to achieve steady-state plasma insulin levels plotted on the horizontal axis. Glucose was infused intravenously to maintain the plasma glucose at its normal fasting level. The rate of total body glucose disposal is plotted on the vertical axis. These studies were carried out in both normal individuals (control) and in patients with poorly controlled non-insulin-dependent diabetes mellitus (NIDDM: Before Tx). In addition, the diabetic individuals were studied a second time after achieving near-normal glycemia by aggressive therapy with insulin (NIDDM: After Tx). (*Reproduced from Garvey et al.*[441] *Used with permission.*)

stimulation of glucose utilization occurs at a plasma insulin concentration of ~60 μU/ml, while maximal stimulation requires ~600–700 μU/ml.[358]

There is considerable variation in insulin-stimulated glucose utilization in the normal population. For example, if insulin action is measured in individuals with normal glucose tolerance, the average rate of glucose utilization is approximately threefold higher in the quartile with the highest rates of glucose utilization as compared to the quartile with the lowest rates of glucose utilization.[362] Furthermore, the rate of glucose utilization was almost as low in the lowest quartile of the normal population as in patients with impaired glucose tolerance or type 2 diabetes. What is the significance of peripheral insulin resistance? Epidemiologic studies have suggested that hyperinsulinemia (a biochemical marker for the presence of insulin resistance) is a risk factor that predicts future development of coronary artery disease.[387–389] In addition, in prospective studies of individuals at high risk to develop type 2 diabetes, insulin resistance has been demonstrated to predict future development of diabetes. A frequently sampled intravenous glucose tolerance test was used to quantitate insulin sensitivity in offspring of two type 2 diabetic parents.[366,367] These offspring were studied at the time when they still had normal glucose tolerance. Nevertheless, insulin resistance was the best predictor of which individuals were destined to develop type 2 diabetes. In contrast, insulin secretion was not found to be predictive in this study. A prospective study was also carried out among Pima Indians, another population at high risk to develop type 2 diabetes.[363–365] Once again, insulin resistance was found to be the best predictor of future development of diabetes. However, diminished insulin secretion was also found to be an independent risk factor.

In cross-sectional studies of patients at various stages in the development of type 2 diabetes, the rate of glucose clearance was plotted as a function of the level of fasting plasma glucose (Fig. 68-20).[358] Glucose clearance progressively decreased as fasting glucose increased from normal to a level of ~ 140 mg/dl, but there was no further decrease in glucose clearance associated with further increases in the level of plasma glucose. This suggests that insulin resistance at the level of skeletal muscle contributes to the development of impaired glucose tolerance and mild type 2 diabetes. However, the progression from mild to severe hyperglycemia is not caused by worsening of insulin resistance in muscle, but rather by an increase in hepatic glucose production (see "Increased Hepatic Glucose Production").

In patients with type 2 diabetes, there is a decrease in both insulin responsiveness (i.e., the rate of glucose utilization in the presence of maximally effective concentrations of insulin) as well as a decrease in insulin sensitivity (i.e., effective concentration of insulin required to elicit a half-maximal effect) (Fig. 68-18).[390] Both hindlimb and forearm perfusion studies have confirmed the conclusion that skeletal muscle is resistant to the action of insulin to stimulate glucose utilization.[358,391–393] Although all metabolic pathways may not be affected equally, type 2 diabetes is associated with impaired synthesis of glycogen and impaired glucose oxidation.[358,394–396] In skeletal muscle of patients with type 2 diabetes, an abnormally high proportion of glucose is metabolized to lactate, which is transported to the liver for gluconeogenesis. However, the major defect in glucose metabolism resides at the first steps in the pathway — that is, at the level of transport and/or phosphorylation of glucose.[397,398]

Insulin Deficiency. Early in the disease, pancreatic beta cells secrete enough insulin to compensate for the insulin resistance, prevent excessive hepatic glucose production, and maintain a normal level of fasting plasma glucose. What determines whether a patient will progress to develop type II diabetes? The patient's fate depends upon the fate of the pancreatic beta cell. Patients become diabetic if there is failure of the pancreatic beta cell, leading to insulin deficiency. For example, if fasting insulin levels are plotted as a function of fasting glucose levels, there is a progressive increase in fasting insulin levels until a level of fasting glucose of ~140 mg/dl.[358] Fasting insulin levels decline progressively with further increases in fasting glucose levels. Furthermore, even at lower levels of fasting glucose, there is evidence of more subtle impairment in insulin secretion. For example, it is possible to estimate insulin secretion in response to oral glucose by summing the area under the curve for insulin levels as a function of time during an oral glucose tolerance test. If the area under the curve is plotted as a function of FPG, there is a progressive increase in total insulin secretion, which achieves a maximal value at FPG = 120 mg/dl, and then begins to decline. Thus, it is around the time that a patient has become diabetic (FPG = 126 mg/dl) that there is clear evidence of impaired insulin secretion. Further increases in plasma glucose levels are

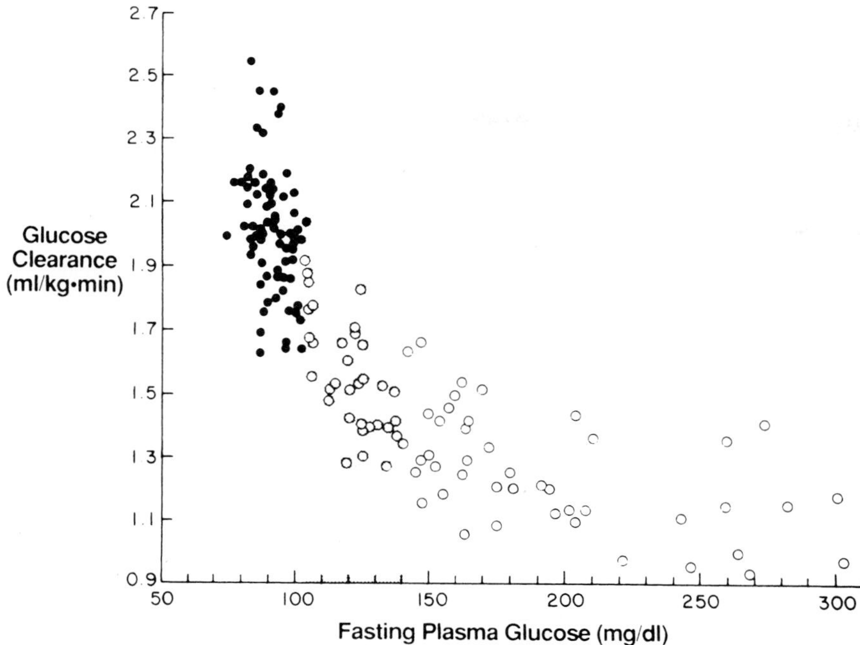

Fig. 68-20 Metabolic clearance of glucose as a function of fasting plasma glucose levels. Seventy-seven patients with non-insulin-dependent diabetes mellitus (open circles) and 72 control subjects (closed circles) were studied. The metabolic clearance rate of glucose (i.e., peripheral glucose disposal rate divided by the plasma glucose level) is plotted as a function of fasting plasma glucose (FPG). Metabolic clearance of glucose is inversely related to FPG when FPG < 180 mg/dl. For FPG > 180 mg/dl, the metabolic clearance of glucose is relatively invariant. (*Reproduced from De Fronzo.*[384] *Used with permission.*)

accompanied by progressive deterioration in insulin secretion. These issues are discussed at greater length in Chap. 67.

Increased Hepatic Glucose Production. Once patients have developed type 2 diabetes, the degree of hyperglycemia is determined by the magnitude of the increase in hepatic glucose production. In the postabsorptive state, hepatic glucose production is relatively normal in patients with impaired glucose tolerance. When plotted as a function of fasting plasma glucose, basal hepatic glucose uptake does not increase until fasting plasma glucose exceeds 140 mg/dl (Fig. 68-21).[358,384] Thus, the transition from mild diabetes (FPG < 140 mg/dl) to more severe diabetes (FPG > 140 mg/dl) is associated with a progressive increase in hepatic glucose production. However, in patients with mild hyperglycemia (FPG = 140 mg/dl), even a "normal" level of hepatic glucose production is inappropriate. There are at least two mechanisms that should have suppressed hepatic glucose output. Glucose exerts an autoregulatory effect upon the liver. In addition, the fasting hyperinsulinemia observed in patients with FPG = 140 mg/dl should suppress hepatic glucose production. These observations suggest that the liver is resistant to insulin action. In normal individuals, insulin levels of 100 μU/ml lead to a 90 percent inhibition of hepatic glucose production; half-maximal suppression is observed at an insulin concentration of ~30 to 40 μU/ml.[358,362] Although insulin can elicit the same 90 percent suppression of hepatic glucose production in patients with type 2

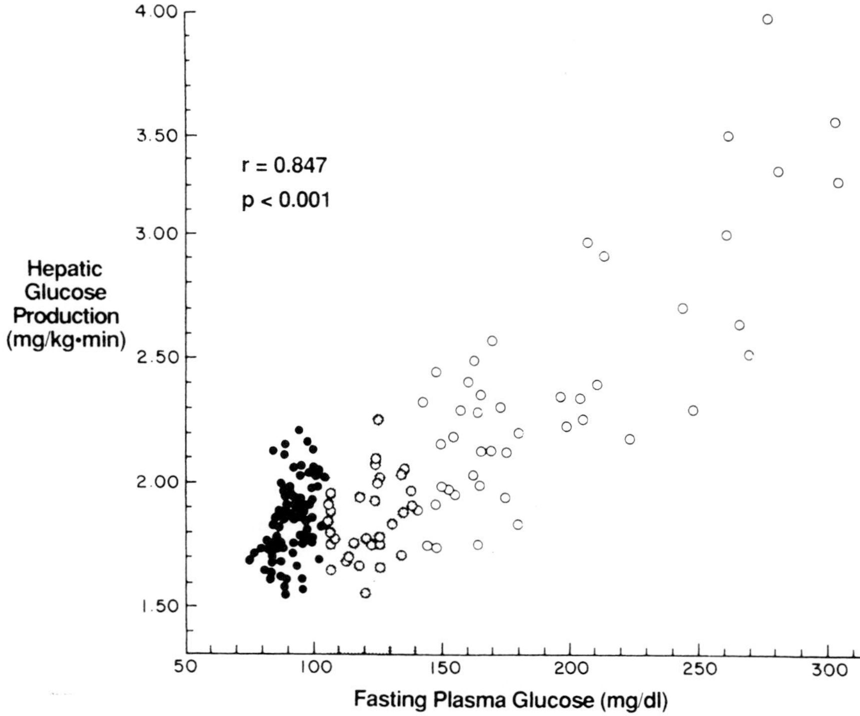

Fig. 68-21 Hepatic glucose production as a function of fasting plasma glucose levels. These studies involved the same individuals who were studied in Fig. 68-20. The rate of hepatic glucose production is plotted as a function of fasting plasma glucose (FPG). For FPG < 140 mg/dl, the rate of hepatic glucose production is relatively invariant. For FPG > 140 mg/dl, the rate of hepatic glucose production is directly related to FPG. (*Reproduced from De Fronzo.*[384] *Used with permission.*)

diabetes, higher concentrations of plasma insulin are required to achieve this degree of suppression.[358,390] Thus, the inability to restrain hepatic glucose output results from the combined defects of insulin deficiency and insulin resistance at the level of the liver.

In order to study the mechanisms of hepatic insulin resistance, it is first necessary to consider the mechanisms whereby insulin suppresses hepatic glucose production. The liver possesses insulin receptors, and also the downstream pathways that mediate insulin action. Therefore, it is tempting to assume that insulin exerts its effects directly by binding to insulin receptors in the liver. However, it has been proposed that there is an indirect mechanism whereby adipose tissue mediates the action of insulin to suppress hepatic glucose production. First, insulin acts directly upon adipose tissue to suppress lipolysis, which leads to a reduction in the level of circulating free fatty acids. Subsequently, the decrease in free fatty acid levels is hypothesized to inhibit hepatic glucose production. This indirect mechanism has been referred to as the "single gateway hypothesis."[399] If the single gateway hypothesis is correct, then insulin resistance at the level of the liver might be accounted for if adipose tissue were resistant to insulin.

One of the important functions of adipose tissue is to mobilize fatty acids from triglyceride stores through lipolysis, a biochemical process that is inhibited by insulin. In several studies, levels of free fatty acids have been used as an index of the rate of lipolysis. For example, in euglycemic insulin clamp studies, maximal (~80 percent) inhibition of lipolysis is elicited by an insulin concentration of 50 μU/ml; half-maximal inhibition is achieved at insulin concentrations of ~10–20 μU/ml. However, in patients with type 2 diabetes, the lipolytic process in adipose tissue is less sensitive to inhibition by insulin.[400,401] According to the Randle hypothesis, elevated levels of free fatty acids are thought to inhibit glucose utilization by peripheral tissue.[41] Furthermore, as summarized above, regulation of free fatty acid levels has been hypothesized to mediate insulin's ability to suppress hepatic glucose production.[399] Thus, the elevated levels of circulating free fatty acids in diabetic patients may contribute to causing fasting hyperglycemia by increasing hepatic glucose production.

MECHANISMS OF INSULIN RESISTANCE IN TYPE 2 DIABETES

Although there has been considerable progress in identifying mutations that cause maturity-onset diabetes of the young[9–13] and unusual syndromes of insulin-resistant diabetes[5,6,294] (see "Other Specific Types of Diabetes"), the disease-causing mutations have not yet been elucidated in most patients with the common form of type 2 diabetes. Nevertheless, progress is being made in using positional cloning to identify type 2 diabetes genes. Although the mechanisms causing insulin resistance in type 2 diabetes are not yet understood at the molecular level, there are several general mechanisms that have been implicated. This section outlines several important mechanisms that may contribute to the pathogenesis of insulin resistance.

Obesity

Most patients with type 2 diabetes are obese,[2] and it is generally accepted that obesity can cause insulin resistance.[387,394] Furthermore, obesity is associated with a defect in the pathway of insulin action. Specifically, insulin receptor tyrosine kinase activity was decreased in skeletal muscle from obese patients,[402] and also in multiple tissues of obese patients with type 2 diabetes.[403–406] If obese diabetic patients lose weight, this can alleviate insulin resistance. Multiple mechanisms probably contribute to this improvement in insulin action. For example, the activity of the receptor tyrosine kinase was increased by weight reduction. This demonstrated that the defect in insulin receptor function is an acquired defect,[407–410] and that it is at least partially reversible with weight loss.[406,411]

Because an increase in adipose tissue mass causes insulin resistance, it was natural to hypothesize that adipocytes secrete a substance that causes other tissues to become insulin resistant. Several candidates have been proposed to mediate the adverse effects of adipose tissue upon insulin sensitivity:

Free Fatty Acids. Each cell requires fuel in order to satisfy its need for ATP. Under aerobic conditions, oxidative metabolism provides the major source of energy for ATP synthesis. Most cells possess enzymes enabling them to oxidize a variety of fuels. Nevertheless, given a choice, most cells will oxidize fatty acids in preference to glucose. In other words, if the demand for ATP is satisfied by fatty acid oxidation, this will inhibit glucose oxidation. This phenomenon was first described by Randle and co-workers who named it the "glucose-fatty acid cycle."[41] Several molecular mechanisms have been proposed to explain the ability of fatty acid oxidation to inhibit glucose oxidation.

1. *Inhibition of pyruvate oxidation:* During glycolysis, each glucose molecule is metabolized to two pyruvate molecules. Pyruvate enters the mitochondrion, where it is oxidized to acetyl CoA plus CO_2, in a reaction catalyzed by pyruvate dehydrogenase (PDH) and yielding NADH. Fatty acid oxidation also yields NADH plus acetyl CoA, which are both competitive inhibitors of PDH.[41] Furthermore, fatty acid oxidation promotes phosphorylation of PDH.[40,42,43,412] Because it is the dephospho-form of PDH that is active, phosphorylation inhibits enzyme activity.
2. *Inhibition of glycolysis:* Fatty acid oxidation yields acetyl CoA, which condenses with oxaloacetate to form citrate. Although citrate is synthesized within the mitochondrion, some citrate is transported into the cytosol. Citrate is an important allosteric regulator of enzyme activity. For example, it is an inhibitor of phosphofructokinase (PFK), a key regulatory enzyme in glycolysis,[413] and an activator of acetyl-CoA carboxylase, an important enzyme in fatty acid biosynthesis.[414,415] Inhibition of PFK would increase the level of its substrate, glucose 6-phosphate, which is also an allosteric inhibitor (in addition to being the product) of hexokinase II. Thus, fatty acid oxidation can cause inhibition of the two kinases that catalyze important regulatory reactions in the first portion of the glycolytic pathway.
3. *Inhibition of glucose transport:* Glucose transport is the rate limiting step in glucose metabolism in several tissues, including skeletal muscle, heart, and adipose tissue. Because skeletal muscle represents the major site of peripheral glucose uptake in the presence of insulin, this has been the most extensively studied. Although the mechanism has not been elucidated, several studies suggest that elevated levels of fatty acids can lead to inhibition of glucose transport in muscle. To study the effect of fatty acids upon glucose transport, euglycemic clamp techniques to measure glucose metabolism were used in combination with magnetic resonance imaging to measure levels of intracellular metabolites.[416] This study demonstrated that fatty acids decreased the rates of glucose uptake, glucose oxidation, and glycogen synthesis. If fatty acids did not alter the rate of glucose transport, one would have predicted that the fatty acid-induced inhibition of the downstream steps of glucose metabolism would have led to an increase in intracellular glucose levels. In fact, there was no such change in the levels of intracellular glucose or glucose 6-phosphate. Thus, these data support the conclusion that glucose transport is inhibited in the face of elevated levels of fatty acids.

The previous discussion focused primarily upon the effect of free fatty acids in muscle. However, fatty acids also exert an effect upon glucose metabolism in liver—that is, to promote hepatic glucose production. In fact, according to the "single gateway hypothesis," insulin regulates hepatic glucose production indirectly: by exerting an antilipolytic action in adipose tissue, which decreases the level of fatty acids in the circulation, and in turn leads to suppression of hepatic glucose production.[399] This hypothesis—that it is necessary for insulin to decrease fatty acid levels in the circulation in order to suppress hepatic glucose production — provides a simple explanation of why elevated levels of fatty acids cause insulin resistance at the level of the liver.

Tumor Necrosis Factor (TNF)-α. Recent data have suggested a role for the cytokine tumor necrosis factor-α (TNF-α) in the pathogenesis of insulin resistance. All three animal models (i.e., *ob/ob* mice, *db/db* mice, and *fa/fa* rats) are associated with increased expression of tumor necrosis factor-α in adipose tissue.[417] Furthermore, when circulating TNF-α was neutralized by intravenous administration of a recombinant binding protein (a soluble TNF-α receptor-immunoglobulin G chimeric protein), this ameliorated the insulin resistance in *fa/fa* rats.[417] Moreover, in tissue culture models, TNF-α has been demonstrated to stimulate serine/threonine phosphorylation of IRS-1, and this in turn has led to inhibition of insulin receptor tyrosine kinase activity.[208,213] Taken together, these data suggest that elevated levels of TNF-α may have an important role in inducing the insulin resistance associated with genetic forms of obesity in rodents. However, several studies have questioned the relevance of these observations with TNF-α. For example, when knockout mice lacking TNF-α were treated with gold thioglucose, the mice became obese and developed insulin resistance despite the absence of TNF-α.[418] Thus, even in rodents, TNF-α is not required for obesity to cause insulin resistance. Furthermore, a genetically engineered anti-TNF-α antibody did not enhance insulin sensitivity in patients with type 2 diabetes.[419] Thus, at least under the conditions of this experiment, circulating TNF-α did not appear to be the principal cause of insulin resistance in these diabetic patients.

Leptin. Leptin, a peptide secreted by adipocytes, was originally discovered as the product of the *ob* gene.[268] *ob/ob* mice lack leptin, and develop the syndrome of obesity plus insulin resistance. Furthermore, *db/db* mice are homozygous for mutations in the gene encoding the leptin receptor.[270,271,275] Because they are resistant to leptin action, *db/db* mice develop essentially the same syndrome of obesity plus insulin resistance that is observed in mice lacking leptin. These observations led to the hypothesis that leptin served as a satiety factor that prevented obesity. Because insulin resistance developed in the absence of leptin and leptin receptors, there was no reason to suspect that leptin might cause insulin resistance. Thus, it was surprising when reports appeared suggesting that leptin antagonized insulin action in some cell-based in vitro models of insulin action.[420,421] Nevertheless, these observations are controversial; other reports suggest either that leptin has no effect or actually promotes insulin action in other in vitro systems.[422] Furthermore, when animals are treated either with leptin or with adenoviral expression vectors to increase leptin levels, this causes weight loss and improvement of insulin action. Thus, the dominant physiologic effects of leptin in vivo appear to promote both insulin action and insulin secretion.[423–427]

Uncontrolled Diabetes: Glucose Toxicity and Insulin Deficiency

There appear to be two components to the insulin resistance observed in patients with type 2 diabetes: a "primary" or "intrinsic" component that precedes the development of diabetes and impaired glucose tolerance (see above),[358,363–367] and an acquired component that is caused by the diabetic state, and can be reversed by a variety of anti-diabetic treatments. For example, if patients with uncontrolled diabetes are treated aggressively with insulin, this leads to significant improvement in insulin action. In fact, this improvement in insulin action occurs when insulin is administered to all diabetic patients — irrespective of whether they have type 1 or type 2 diabetes.[344] What causes the component of insulin resistance that is acquired as a consequence of the diabetic state? Also, what are the mechanisms whereby insulin alleviates insulin resistance?

Elevated circulating levels of free fatty acids. Uncontrolled diabetes is associated with accelerated lipolysis in adipose tissue, and elevated levels of free fatty acids in the circulation. This leads to insulin resistance (see "Free Fatty Acids"). By inhibiting lipolysis, insulin can alleviate this component of insulin resistance.

Insulin deficiency. Insulin regulates the expression of multiple genes. Some of the products of these genes participate in the metabolic pathways that insulin regulates. For example, insulin induces the expression of the GLUT4 glucose transporter in adipocytes.[428–430] Thus, insulin deficiency may lead to a paucity of GLUT4 in adipose tissue, thereby contributing to the insulin resistance in that tissue.

"Glucose toxicity." Hyperglycemia is associated with insulin resistance. A direct causal relationship has been suggested by studies in animal models. When pancreatectomized, diabetic rats were treated with phlorizin, an inhibitor of glucose reabsorption in renal tubules, this promoted glucosuria and normalized the level of glucose in the plasma.[431,432] Furthermore, this ameliorated the defect in glucose transport in adipocytes, and also restored in vivo insulin sensitivity to normal. Of course, unlike the situation in pancreatectomized rats, patients with type 2 diabetes have a primary defect in insulin action in addition to the acquired component. Glucose toxicity contributes only to the acquired component.

Recent evidence has suggested that it is not glucose per se that mediates this effect, but rather products of the hexosamine pathway.[433–435] Glucosamine 6-phosphate is synthesized from a reaction catalyzed by glutamine:fructose 6-phosphate amidotransferase (GFAT). Thus, elevations in the level of fructose 6-phosphate lead, by mass action, to elevated flux through the glucosamine pathway. Several studies implicate the glucosamine in the pathogenesis of insulin resistance. First, administration of glucosamine can cause insulin resistance.[436,437] Second, inhibition of GFAT alleviates insulin resistance due to hyperglycemia.[434] Third, overexpression of GFAT can cause insulin resistance in transfected cells and in transgenic mice.[435,438] Finally, in human studies, GFAT activity is elevated in muscle of patients with type 2 diabetes, and the degree of elevation correlated with the degree of insulin resistance.[439] Interestingly, increased flux through the hexosamine pathway leads to multiple defects that may contribute to insulin resistance, including decreased expression of GLUT4, inhibition of glucose transport, and inhibition of glycogen synthase activity.[358,435]

Therapeutic Implications

Just as there are multiple physiological defects in type 2 diabetes, there are multiple approaches to treating the disease.[440] For example, exogenous insulin may be administered in order to replace the insulin deficiency.[441] Alternatively, sulfonylureas work as insulin secretagogues to promote endogenous insulin secretion.[442] Other therapies function either as insulin sensitizers and/or insulinomimetic agents. For example, thiazolidinediones (e.g., troglitazone, rosiglitazone, and pioglitazone) bind to peroxisome proliferator-activated receptor-γ (PPAR-γ), a transcription factor expressed predominantly in adipose tissue. It is believed that thiazolidinediones act primarily upon adipose tissue, thereby exerting indirect actions to increase peripheral insulin sensitivity in skeletal muscle.[443–445] In contrast, metformin exerts its primary effects upon the liver to suppress hepatic glucose production, thereby ameliorating fasting hyperglycemia.[444,446] Finally, especially in obese patients, weight loss can eliminate one of the primary factors causing insulin resistance. Thus, diet and exercise have the potential to promote insulin sensitivity and improve glycemic control in patients with type 2 diabetes.[447,448]

However, as discussed ("Uncontrolled Diabetes; Glucose Toxicity and Insulin Deficiency"), uncontrolled diabetes creates a vicious cycle wherein hyperglycemia begets more hyperglycemia.[344] Therefore, successful antidiabetic therapy that improves glycemic control will lead to improved insulin sensitivity, whether or not the insulin action pathway is the direct target of the therapeutic intervention (e.g., ref. 441). Similarly, as will be discussed in Chap. 67, therapies that improve glycemic control may improve insulin secretion, whether or not the beta cell is the direct target of the therapy (e.g., ref. 441).

REFERENCES

1. National Diabetes Advisory Board: *Progress and Promise in Diabetes Research*. Washington, D.C., NIH Publication, 84–661, 1984.
2. American Diabetes Association Expert Committee: Report of the Expert Committee on the diagnosis and classification of diabetes mellitus. *Diabetes Care* **20**:1183, 1997.
3. Srikanta S, Ganda OP, Eisenbarth GS, Soeldner JS: Islet-cell antibodies and beta-cell function in monozygotic triplets and twins initially discordant for Type I diabetes mellitus. *N Engl J Med* **308**:322, 1983.
4. Taylor SI, Accili D, Cama A, Imano E, Kadowaki H, Kadowaki T: Unusual forms of insulin resistance. *Annu Rev Med* **42**:373, 1991.
5. Taylor SI, Cama A, Accili D, Barbetti F, Quon MJ, Sierra ML, Suzuki Y, Koller E, Levy Toledano R, Wertheimer E, et al.: Mutations in the insulin receptor gene. *Endocr Rev* **13**:566, 1992.
6. Taylor SI: Lilly Lecture: Molecular mechanisms of insulin resistance. Lessons from patients with mutations in the insulin-receptor gene. *Diabetes* **41**:1473, 1992.
7. Neel JV, Fajans SS, Conn JW: Diabetes Mellitus, in Neel JV, Shaw MW, Schull WJ (eds) *Genetics and the Epidemiology of Chronic Disease*. Washington, D.C., U.S. Government Printing Office, 1965, p 105.
8. Steiner DF, Tager HS, Chan SJ, Nanjo K, Sanke T, Rubenstein AH: Lessons learned from molecular biology of insulin-gene mutations. *Diabetes Care* **13**:600, 1990.
9. Bell GI, Pilkis SJ, Weber IT, Polonsky KS: Glucokinase mutations, insulin secretion, and diabetes mellitus. *Annu Rev Physiol* **58**:171, 1996.
10. Fajans SS, Bell GI, Bowden DW, Halter JB, Polonsky KS: Maturity onset diabetes of the young (MODY). *Diabet Med* **13(Suppl 6)**:S90, 1996.
11. Yamagata K, Furuta H, Oda N, Kaisaki PJ, Menzel S, Cox NJ, Fajans SS, Signorini S, Stoffel M, Bell GI: Mutations in the hepatocyte nuclear factor-4alpha gene in maturity-onset diabetes of the young (MODY1). *Nature* **384**:458, 1996.
12. Yamagata K, Oda N, Kaisaki PJ, Menzel S, Furuta H, Vaxillaire M, Southam L, Cox RD, Lathrop GM, Boriraj VV, Chen X, Cox NJ, Oda Y, Yano H, Le Beau MM, Yamada S, Nishigori H, Takeda J, Fajans SS, Hattersley AT, Iwasaki N, Hansen T, Pedersen O, Polonsky KS, Bell GI: Mutations in the hepatocyte nuclear factor-1alpha gene in maturity-onset diabetes of the young (MODY3). *Nature* **384**:455, 1996.
13. Stoffers D, Ferrer J, Clarke W, Habener J: Early-onset type-II diabetes mellitus (MODY4) linked to IPF1. *Nat Genet* **17**:138, 1997.
14. Horikawa Y, Iwasaki N, Hara M, Furuta H, Hinokio Y, Cockburn B, Lindner T, Yamagata K, Ogata M, Tomonaga O, Kuroki H, Kasahara T, Iwamoto Y, Bell G: Mutation in hepatocyte nuclear factor-1 beta gene (TCF2) associated with MODY. *Nat Genet* **17**:384, 1997.
15. Ballinger S, Shoffner JM, Hedaya EV, Trounce I, Polak MA, Koontz DA, Wallace DC: Maternally transmitted diabetes and deafness associated with a 10.4 kb mitochondrial DNA deletion. *Nature* **1**:11, 1992.
16. van den Ouweland JMW, Lemkes HHPJ, Ruitenbeek W, Sankuijl LA, de Vijlder MF, Struynenberg PAA, van de Kamp JJP Maassen JA: Mutation in mitochondrial $tRNA^{Leu(UUR)}$ gene in a large pedigree with maternally transmitted type II diabetes mellitus and deafness. *Nature Genetics* **1**:368, 1992.
17. Cahill GF Jr: Starvation in man. *N Engl J Med* **282**:668, 1970.
18. Cahill GF Jr: The Banting Memorial Lecture 1971. Physiology of insulin in man. *Diabetes* **20**:785, 1971.
19. Kimball SR, Jefferson LS: Cellular mechanisms involved in the action of insulin on protein synthesis. *Diabetes Metab Rev* **4**:773, 1988.
20. Kimball SR Jefferson LS: Regulation of initiation of protein synthesis by insulin in skeletal muscle. *Acta Diabetol* **28**:134, 1991.
21. Owen OE, Morgan AP, Kemp HG, Sullivan JM, Herrera MG, Cahill GF Jr: Brain metabolism during fasting. *J Clin Invest* **46**:1589, 1967.
22. Owen OE, Felig P, Morgan AP, Wahren J, Cahill GF Jr: Liver and kidney metabolism during prolonged starvation. *J Clin Invest* **48**:574, 1969.
23. Nilsson LH: Liver glycogen content in man in the postabsorptive state. *Scand J Clin Lab Invest* **32**:317, 1973.
24. Larner J: Insulin-signaling mechanisms. Lessons from the old testament of glycogen metabolism and the new testament of molecular biology. *Diabetes* **37**:262, 1988.
25. Cohen P, Hardie DG: The actions of cyclic AMP on biosynthetic processes are mediated indirectly by cyclic AMP-dependent protein kinase. *Biochim Biophys Acta* **1094**:292, 1991.
26. Exton JH: Mechanisms of hormonal regulation of hepatic glucose metabolism. *Diabetes Metab Rev* **3**:163, 1987.
27. El-Maghrabi MR, Claus TH, McGrane, MM Pilkis SJ: Influence of phosphorylation on the interaction of effectors with rat liver pyruvate kinase. *J Biol Chem* **257**:233, 1982.
28. Pilkis SJ, el Maghrabi MR, Claus TH: Fructose-2,6-bisphosphate in control of hepatic gluconeogenesis. From metabolites to molecular genetics. *Diabetes Care* **13**:582, 1990.
29. Pilkis SJ, Granner DK: Molecular physiology of the regulation of hepatic gluconeogenesis and glycolysis. *Annu Rev Physiol* **54**:885, 1992.
30. Newsholme EA, Crabtree B: Metabolic aspects of enzyme activity regulation. *Symp Soc Exp Biol* **27**:429, 1973.
31. Flatt JP, Ball EG: Studies on the metabolism of adipose tissue. XIX. An evaluation of the major pathways of glucose catabolism as influenced by acetate in the presence of insulin. *J Biol Chem* **241**:2862, 1966.
32. Katz J Rognstad R: The metabolism of tritiated glucose by rat adipose tissue. *J Biol Chem* **241**:3600, 1966.
33. Katz J, Landau BR, Bartsch GE: The pentose cycle, triose phosphate isomerization, and lipogenesis in rat adipose tissue. *J Biol Chem* **241**:727, 1966.
34. Katz J, Rognstad R: The labeling of pentose phosphate from glucose-^{14}C and estimation of the rates of transaldolase, transketolase, the contribution of the pentose cycle, and ribose phosphate synthesis. *Biochemistry* **6**:2227, 1967.
35. Jungas RL, Ball EG: Studies on the metabolism of adipose tissue. XII. The effects of insulin and epinephrine on free fatty acid and glycerol production in the presence and absence of glucose. *Biochemistry* **2**:383, 1963.
36. Jungas RL: Role of cyclic-3′,5′-AMP in the response of adipose tissue to insulin. *Proc Natl Acad Sci U S A* **56**:757, 1966.
37. Jungas RL: Effect of insulin on fatty acid ynthesis from pyruvate, lactage, or endogenous sources in adipose tissue: Evidence for the hormonal regulation of pyruvate dehydrogenase. *Endocrinology* **86**:1368, 1970.
38. Denton RM, Coore HG, Martin BR, Randle PJ: Insulin activates pyruvate dehydrogenase in rat epididymal adipose tissue. *Nature New Biol* **231**:115, 1971.
39. Coore HG, Denton RM, Martin BR, Randle PJ: Regulation of adipose tissue pyruvate dehydrogenase by insulin and other hormones *Biochem J* **125**:115, 1971.
40. Taylor SI, Mukherjee C, Jungas RL: Studies on the mechanism of activation of adipose tissue pyruvate dehydrogenase by insulin. *J Biol Chem* **248**:73, 1973.
41. Randle PJ, Kerbey AL, Espinal J: Mechanisms decreasing glucose oxidation in diabetes and starvation: role of lipid fuels and hormones. *Diabetes Metab Rev* **4**:623, 1988.
42. Wieland OH, Patzelt C, Löffler G: Active and inactive forms of pyruvate dehydrogenase in rat liver. Effect of starvation and refeeding and of insulin treatment on pyruvate-dehydrogenase interconversion. *Eur J Biochem* **26**:426, 1972.
43. Wieland O, Siess E, Schulze-Wethmar FH, von Funcke HG, Winton B: Active and inactive forms of pyruvate dehydrogenase in rat heart and kidney: Effect of diabetes, fasting, and refeeding on pyruvate dehydrogenase interconversion. *Arch Biochem Biophys* **143**:593, 1971.
44. Hagg SA, Taylor SI, Ruberman NB: Glucose metabolism in perfused skeletal muscle. Pyruvate dehydrogenase activity in starvation, diabetes and exercise. *Biochem J* **158**:203, 1976.
45. McGarry JD: Lilly Lecture 1978. New perspectives in the regulation of ketogenesis. *Diabetes* **28**:517, 1979.
46. Foster DW, McGarry JD: The metabolic derangements and treatment of diabetic ketoacidosis. *N Engl J Med* **309**:159, 1983.
47. Foster DW: Banting lecture 1984. From glycogen to ketones—and back. *Diabetes* **33**:1188, 1984.
48. McGarry JD: What if Minkowski had been ageusic? An alternative angle on diabetes. *Science* **258**:766, 1992.
49. O'Brien RM, Granner DK: Regulation of gene expression by insulin. *Biochem J* **278**:609, 1991.
50. Granner DK, O'Brien RM: Molecular physiology and genetics of NIDDM. Importance of metabolic staging. *Diabetes Care* **15**:369, 1992.

51. Magnuson MA, Andreone TL, Printz RL, Koch S, Granner DK: Rat glucokinase gene: structure and regulation by insulin. *Proc Natl Acad Sci U S A* **86**:4838, 1989.
52. O'Brien RM, Granner DK: PEPCK gene as model of inhibitory effects of insulin on gene transcription. *Diabetes Care* **13**:327, 1990.
53. Cheatham B, Kahn C: Insulin action and the insulin signaling network. *Endocr Rev* **16**:117, 1995.
54. White M, Yenush L: The IRS-signaling system: A network of docking proteins that mediate insulin and cytokine action. *Curr Top Microbiol Immunol* **228**:179, 1998.
55. Yang-Feng TL, Francke U, Ullrich A: Gene for human insulin receptor: localization to site on chromosome 19 involved in pre-B-cell leukemia. *Science* **228**:728, 1985.
56. Hedo JA, Kahn CR, Hayashi M, Yamada KM, Kasuga M: Biosynthesis and glycosylation of the insulin receptor. Evidence for a single polypeptide precursor of the two major subunits. *J Biol Chem* **258**:10020, 1983.
57. Ullrich A, Bell JR, Chen EY, Herrera R, Petruzzelli LM, Dull TJ, Gray A, Coussens L, Liao YC, Tsubokawa M, et al.: Human insulin receptor and its relationship to the tyrosine kinase family of oncogenes. *Nature* **313**:756, 1985.
58. Ebina Y, Ellis L, Jarnagin K, Edery M, Graf L, Clauser E, Ou JH, Masiarz F, Kan YW, Goldfine ID, Roth RA, Rutter WJ: The human insulin receptor cDNA: The structural basis for hormone-activated transmembrane signalling. *Cell* **40**:747, 1985.
59. Kasuga M, Karlsson FA, Kahn CR: Insulin stimulates the phosphorylation of the 95,000-dalton subunit of its own receptor. *Science* **215**:185, 1982.
60. Kasuga M, Zick Y, Blithe DL, Crettaz M, Kahn CR: Insulin stimulates tyrosine phosphorylation of the insulin receptor in a cell-free system. *Nature* **298**:667, 1982.
61. Morgan DO, Ho L, Korn LJ, Roth RA: Insulin action is blocked by a monoclonal antibody that inhibits the insulin receptor kinase. *Proc Natl Acad Sci U S A* **83**:328, 1986.
62. Morgan DO, Roth RA: Acute insulin action requires insulin receptor kinase activity: Introduction of an inhibitory monoclonal antibody into mammalian cells blocks the rapid effects of insulin. *Proc Natl Acad Sci U S A* **84**:41, 1987.
63. Chou CK, Dull TJ, Russell DS, Gherzi R, Lebwohl D, Ullrich A, Rosen OM: Human insulin receptors mutated at the ATP-binding site lack protein tyrosine kinase activity and fail to mediate postreceptor effects of insulin. *J Biol Chem* **262**:1842, 1987.
64. Ebina Y, Araki E, Taira M, Shimada F, Mori M, Craik CS, Siddle K, Pierce SB, Roth RA, Rutter WJ: Replacement of lysine residue 1030 in the putative ATP-binding region of the insulin receptor abolishes insulin- and antibody-stimulated glucose uptake and receptor kinase activity. *Proc Natl Acad Sci U S A* **84**:704, 1987.
65. Maegawa H, Olefsky JM, Thies S, Boyd D, Ullrich A, McClain DA: Insulin receptors with defective tyrosine kinase inhibit normal receptor function at the level of substrate phosphorylation. *J Biol Chem* **263**:12629, 1988.
66. Tornqvist HE, Pierce MW, Frackelton AR, Nemenoff RA, Avruch J: Identification of insulin receptor tyrosine residues autophosphorylated in vitro. *J Biol Chem* **262**:10212, 1987.
67. Tornqvist HE, Avruch J: Relationship of site-specific beta subunit tyrosine autophosphorylation to insulin activation of the insulin receptor (tyrosine) protein kinase activity. *J Biol Chem* **263**:4593, 1988.
68. White MF, Shoelson SE, Keutmann H, Kahn CR: A cascade of tyrosine autophosphorylation in the beta-subunit activates the phosphotransferase of the insulin receptor. *J Biol Chem* **263**:2969, 1988.
69. Hubbard S: Crystal structure of the activated insulin receptor tyrosine kinase in complex with peptide substrate and ATP analog. *EMBO J* **16**:5572, 1997.
70. Hubbard S, Wei L, Ellis L, Hendrickson W: Crystal structure of the tyrosine kinase domain of the human insulin receptor. *Nature* **372**:746, 1994.
71. Hubbard S, Mohammadi M, Schlessinger J: Autoregulatory mechanisms in protein-tyrosine kinases. *J Biol Chem* **273**:1987, 1998.
72. Blaikie P, Immanuel D, Wu J, Li N, Yajnik V, Margolis B: A region in Shc distinct from the SH2 domain can bind tyrosine-phosphorylated growth factor receptors. *J Biol Chem* **269**:32031, 1994.
73. Gustafson T, He W, Craparo A, Schaub C, O'Neill T: Phosphotyrosine-dependent interaction of SHC and insulin receptor substrate 1 with the NPEY motif of the insulin receptor via a novel non-SH2 domain. *Mol Cell Biol* **15**:2500, 1995.
74. Kavanaugh W, Williams L: An alternative to SH2 domains for binding tyrosine-phosphorylated proteins. *Science* **266**:1862, 1994.
75. Songyang Z, Shoelson S, Chaudhuri M, Gish G, Pawson T, Haser W, King F, Roberts T, Ratnofsky S, Lechleider R, et al.: SH2 domains recognize specific phosphopeptide sequences. *Cell* **72**:767, 1993.
76. Levy-Toledano R, Taouis M, Blaettler DH, Gorden P, Taylor SI: Insulin-induced activation of phosphatidyl inositol 3-kinase. Demonstration that the p85 subunit binds directly to the COOH terminus of the insulin receptor in intact cells. *J Biol Chem* **269**:31178, 1994.
77. Sun X, Rothenberg P, Kahn C, Backer J, Araki E, Wilden P, Cahill D, Goldstein B, White M: Structure of the insulin receptor substrate IRS-1 defines a unique signal transduction protein. *Nature* **352**:73, 1991.
78. Sun X, Wang L, Zhang Y, Yenush L, Myers M Jr, Glasheen E, Lane W, Pierce J, White M: Role of IRS-2 in insulin and cytokine signalling. *Nature* **377**:173, 1995.
79. Lavan B, Lane W, Lienhard G: The 60-kDa phosphotyrosine protein in insulin-treated adipocytes is a new member of the insulin receptor substrate family. *J Biol Chem* **272**:11439, 1997.
80. Sciacchitano S, Taylor S: Cloning, tissue expression, and chromosomal localization of the mouse IRS-3 gene. *Endocrinology* **138**:4931, 1997.
81. Lavan BE, Fantin VR, Chang ET, Lane WS, Keller SR, Lienhard GE: A novel 160-kDa phosphotyrosine protein in insulin-treated embryonic kidney cells is a new member of the insulin receptor substrate family. *J Biol Chem* **272**:21403, 1997.
82. Rees-Jones RW, Taylor SI: An endogenous substrate for the insulin receptor-associated tyrosine kinase. *J Biol Chem* **260**:4461, 1985.
83. Perrotti N, Accili D, Marcus SB, Rees Jones RW, Taylor SI: Insulin stimulates phosphorylation of a 120-kDa glycoprotein substrate (pp120) for the receptor-associated protein kinase in intact H-35 hepatoma cells. *Proc Natl Acad Sci U S A* **84**:3137, 1987.
84. Margolis RN, Schell MJ, Taylor SI, Hubbard AL: Hepatocyte plasma membrane ECTO-ATPase (pp120/HA4) is a substrate for tyrosine kinase activity of the insulin receptor. *Biochem Biophys Res Commun* **166**:562, 1990.
85. Fujioka Y, Matozaki T, Noguchi T, Iwamatsu A, Yamao T, Takahashi N, Tsuda M, Takada T, Kasuga M: A novel membrane glycoprotein, SHPS-1, that binds the SH2-domain-containing protein tyrosine phosphatase SHP-2 in response to mitogens and cell adhesion. *Mol Cell Biol* **16**:6887, 1996.
86. Kharitonenkov A, Chen Z, Sures I, Wang H, Schilling J, Ullrich A: A family of proteins that inhibit signalling through tyrosine kinase receptors. *Nature* **386**:181, 1997.
87. Tamemoto H, Kadowaki T, Tobe K, Yagi T, Sakura H, Hayakawa T, Terauchi Y, Ueki K, Kaburagi Y, Satoh S, et al.: Insulin resistance and growth retardation in mice lacking insulin receptor substrate-1. *Nature* **372**:182, 1994.
88. Araki E, Lipes M, Patti M, Bruning J, Haag Br, Johnson R, Kahn C: Alternative pathway of insulin signalling in mice with targeted disruption of the IRS-1 gene. *Nature* **372**:186, 1994.
89. Withers D, Gutierrez J, Towery H, Burks D, Ren J, Previs S, Zhang Y, Bernal D, Pons S, Shulman G, Bonner-Weir S, White M: Disruption of IRS-2 causes type 2 diabetes in mice. *Nature* **391**:900, 1998.
90. Quon MJ, Butte AJ, Zarnowski MJ, Sesti G, Cushman SW, Taylor SI: Insulin receptor substrate 1 mediates the stimulatory effect of insulin on GLUT4 translocation in transfected rat adipose cells. *J Biol Chem* **269**:27920, 1994.
91. Zhou L, Chen H, Lin CH, Cong LN, McGibbon MA, Sciacchitano S, Lesniak MA, Quon MJ, Taylor SI: Insulin receptor substrate-2 (IRS-2) can mediate the action of insulin to stimulate translocation of GLUT4 to the cell surface in rat adipose cells. *J Biol Chem* **272**:29829, 1997.
92. Zhou L, Chen H, Xu P, Cong LN, Sciacchitano S, Li Y, Graham D, Jacobs AR, Taylor SI, Quon MJ: Action of insulin receptor substrate-3 (IRS-3) and IRS-4 to stimulate translocation of GLUT4 in rat adipose cells. *Mol Endocrinol* **13**:505, 1999.
93. Eck MJ, Dhe-Paganon S, Trub T, Nolte RT, Shoelson SE: Structure of the IRS-1 PTB domain bound to the juxtamembrane region of the insulin receptor. *Cell* **85**:695, 1996.
94. Quon MJ, Chen H, Ing BL, Liu ML, Zarnowski MJ, Yonezawa K, Kasuga M, Cushman SW, Taylor SI: Roles of 1-phosphatidylinositol 3-kinase and ras in regulating translocation of GLUT4 in transfected rat adipose cells. *Mol Cell Biol* **15**:5403, 1995.
95. Noguchi T, Matozaki T, Horita K, Fujioka Y, Kasuga M: Role of SH-PTP2, a protein-tyrosine phosphatase with Src homology 2 domains, in insulin-stimulated Ras activation. *Mol Cell Biol* **14**:6674, 1994.
96. Chardin P, Camonis JH, Gale NW, van Aelst L, Schlessinger J, Wigler MH, Bar-Sagi D: Human Sos1: A guanine nucleotide exchange factor for Ras that binds to GRB2. *Science* **260**:1338, 1993.

97. Skolnik EY, Batzer A, Li N, Lee CH, Lowenstein E, Mohammadi M, Margolis B, Schlessinger J: The function of GRB2 in linking the insulin receptor to Ras signaling pathways. *Science* **260**:1953, 1993.
98. Sasaoka T, Draznin B, Leitner JW, Langlois WJ, Olefsky JM: Shc is the predominant signaling molecule coupling insulin receptors to activation of guanine nucleotide releasing factor and p21ras-GTP formation. *J Biol Chem* **269**:10734, 1994.
99. Vojtek AB, Hollenberg SM, Cooper JA: Mammalian Ras interacts directly with the serine/threonine kinase Raf. *Cell* **74**:205, 1993.
100. Sasaki Y, Zhang XF, Nishiyama M, Avruch J, Wands JR: Expression and phosphorylation of insulin receptor substrate 1 during rat liver regeneration. *J Biol Chem* **268**:3805, 1993.
101. Avruch J: Insulin signal transduction through protein kinase cascades. *Mol Cell Biochem* **182**:31, 1998.
102. Kyriakis JM, App H, Zhang XF, Banerjee P, Brautigan DL, Rapp UR, Avruch J: Raf-1 activates MAP kinase-kinase. *Nature* **358**:417, 1992.
103. Robinson MJ, Cobb MH: Mitogen-activated protein kinase pathways. *Curr Opin Cell Biol* **9**:180, 1997.
104. Cobb MH, Goldsmith EJ: How MAP kinases are regulated. *J Biol Chem* **270**:14843, 1995.
105. Boulton TG, Yancopoulos GD, Gregory JS, Slaughter C, Moomaw C, Hsu J, Cobb MH: An insulin-stimulated protein kinase similar to yeast kinases involved in cell cycle control. *Science* **249**:64, 1990.
106. Boulton TG, Nye SH, Robbins DJ, Ip NY, Radziejewska E, Morgenbesser SD, DePinho RA, Panayotatos N, Cobb MH, Yancopoulos GD: ERKs: A family of protein-serine/threonine kinases that are activated and tyrosine phosphorylated in response to insulin and NGF. *Cell* **65**:663, 1991.
107. Lawrence JC Jr, Roach PJ: New insights into the role and mechanism of glycogen synthase activation by insulin. *Diabetes* **46**:541, 1997.
108. Najjar SM, Philippe N, Suzuki Y, Ignacio GA, Formisano P, Accili D, Taylor SI: Insulin-stimulated phosphorylation of recombinant pp120/HA4, an endogenous substrate of the insulin receptor tyrosine kinase. *Biochemistry* **34**:9341, 1995.
109. Vanhaesebroeck B, Leevers SJ, Panayotou G, Waterfield MD: Phosphoinositide 3-kinases: A conserved family of signal transducers. *Trends Biochem Sci* **22**:267, 1997.
110. Shoelson SE, Chatterjee S, Chaudhuri M, White MF: YMXM motifs of IRS-1 define substrate specificity of the insulin receptor kinase. *Proc Natl Acad Sci U S A* **89**:2027, 1992.
111. Backer JM, Schroeder GG, Kahn CR, Myers MG Jr, Wilden PA, Cahill DA, White MF: Insulin stimulation of phosphatidylinositol 3-kinase activity maps to insulin receptor regions required for endogenous substrate phosphorylation. *J Biol Chem* **267**:1367, 1992.
112. Myers MG Jr, Backer JM, Sun XJ, Shoelson S, Hu P, Schlessinger J, Yoakim M, Schaffhausen B, White MF: IRS-1 activates phosphatidylinositol 3′-kinase by associating with src homology 2 domains of p85. *Proc Natl Acad Sci U S A* **89**:10350, 1992.
113. Rordorf-Nikolic T, Van Horn DJ, Chen D, White MF, Backer JM: Regulation of phosphatidylinositol 3′-kinase by tyrosyl phosphoproteins. Full activation requires occupancy of both SH2 domains in the 85-kDa regulatory subunit. *J Biol Chem* **270**:3662, 1995.
114. Martin SS, Haruta T, Morris AJ, Klippel A, Williams LT, Olefsky JM: Activated phosphatidylinositol 3-kinase is sufficent to mediate actin rearrangement and GLUT4 translocation in 3T3-L1 adipocytes. *J Biol Chem* **271**:17605, 1996.
115. Terauchi Y, Tsuji Y, Satoh S, Minoura H, Murakami K, Okuno A, Inukai K, Asano T, Kaburagi Y, Ueki K, Nakajima H, Hanafusa T, Matsuzawa Y, Sekihara H, Yin Y, Barrett J, Oda H, Ishikawa T, Akanuma Y, Komuro I, Suzuki M, Yamamura K, Kodama T, Suzuki H, Kadowaki T: Increased insulin sensitivity and hypoglycaemia in mice lacking the p85 alpha subunit of phosphoinositide 3-kinase. *Nat Genet* **21**:230, 1999.
116. Alessi DR, Andjelkovic M, Caudwell B, Cron P, Morrice N, Cohen P, Hemmings BA: Mechanism of activation of protein kinase B by insulin and IGF-1. *EMBO J* **15**:6541, 1996.
117. Alessi D, Deak M, Casamayor A, Caudwell F, Morrice N, Norman D, Gaffney P, Reese C, MacDougall C, Harbison D, Ashworth A, Bownes M: 3-Phosphoinositide-dependent protein kinase-1 (PDK1): Structural and functional homology with the Drosophila DSTPK61 kinase. *Curr Biol* **7**:776, 1997.
118. Alessi DR, James SR, Downes CP, Holmes AB, Gaffney PR, Reese CB, Cohen P: Characterization of a 3-phosphoinositide-dependent protein kinase which phosphorylates and activates protein kinase Balpha. *Curr Biol* **7**:261, 1997.
119. Stokoe D, Stephens LR, Copeland T, Gaffney PR, Reese CB, Painter GF, Holmes AB, McCormick F, Hawkins PT: Dual role of phosphatidylinositol-3,4,5-trisphosphate in the activation of protein kinase B. *Science* **277**:567, 1997.
120. Balendran A, Casamayor A, Deak M, Paterson A, Gaffney P, Currie R, Downes CP, Alessi DR: PDK1 acquires PDK2 activity in the presence of a synthetic peptide derived from the carboxyl terminus of PRK2. *Curr Biol* **9**:393, 1999.
121. Stephens L, Anderson K, Stokoe D, Erdjument-Bromage H, Painter GF, Holmes AB, Gaffney PR, Reese CB, McCormick F, Tempst P, Coadwell J, Hawkins PT: Protein kinase B kinases that mediate phosphatidylinositol 3,4,5- trisphosphate-dependent activation of protein kinase B [see Comments]. *Science* **279**:710, 1998.
122. Currie RA, Walker KS, Gray A, Deak M, Casamayor A, Downes CP, Cohen P, Alessi DR, Lucocq J: Role of phosphatidylinositol 3,4,5-trisphosphate in regulating the activity and localization of 3-phosphoinositide-dependent protein kinase-1. *Biochem J* **337**:575, 1999.
123. Kohn AD, Takeuchi F, Roth RA: Akt, a pleckstrin homology domain containing kinase, is activated primarily by phosphorylation. *J Biol Chem* **271**:21920, 1996.
124. Kohn AD, Kovacina KS Roth RA: Insulin stimulates the kinase activity of RAC-PK, a pleckstrin homology domain containing ser/thr kinase. *EMBO J* **14**:4288, 1995.
125. Kohn AD, Summers SA, Birnbaum MJ, Roth RA: Expression of a constitutively active Akt Ser/Thr kinase in 3T3-L1 adipocytes stimulates glucose uptake and glucose transporter 4 translocation. *J Biol Chem* **271**:31372, 1996.
126. Cong LN, Chen H, Li Y, Zhou L, McGibbon MA, Taylor SI, Quon MJ: Physiological role of Akt in insulin-stimulated translocation of GLUT4 in transfected rat adipose cells. *Mol Endocrinol* **11**:1881, 1997.
127. Tanti JF, Grillo S, Gremeaux T, Coffer PJ, Van Obberghen E, Le Marchand-Brustel Y: Potential role of protein kinase B in glucose transporter 4 translocation in adipocytes. *Endocrinology* **138**:2005, 1997.
128. Kitamura T, Ogawa W, Sakaue H, Hino Y, Kuroda S, Takata M, Matsumoto M, Maeda T, Konishi H, Kikkawa U, Kasuga M: Requirement for activation of the serine-threonine kinase Akt (protein kinase B) in insulin stimulation of protein synthesis but not of glucose transport. *Mol Cell Biol* **18**:3708, 1998.
129. Kotani K, Ogawa W, Matsumoto M, Kitamura T, Sakaue H, Hino Y, Miyake K, Sano W, Akimoto K, Ohno S, Kasuga M: Requirement of atypical protein kinase C-lambda for insulin stimulation of glucose uptake but not for akt activation in 3T3-L1 adipocytes. *Mol Cell Biol* **18**:6971, 1998.
130. Standaert ML, Galloway L, Karnam P, Bandyopadhyay G, Moscat J, Farese RV: Protein kinase C-zeta as a downstream effector of phosphatidylinositol 3-kinase during insulin stimulation in rat adipocytes. *J Biol Chem* **272**:30075, 1997.
131. Cross DA, Alessi DR, Cohen P, Andjelkovich M. Hemmings BA: Inhibition of glycogen synthase kinase-3 by insulin mediated by protein kinase B. *Nature* **378**:785, 1995.
132. Brunet A, Bonni A, Zigmond MJ, Lin MZ, Juo P, Hu LS, Anderson MJ, Arden KC, Blenis J, Greenberg ME: Akt promotes cell survival by phosphorylating and inhibiting a Forkhead transcription factor. *Cell* **96**:857, 1999.
133. Weng QP, Kozlowski M, Belham C, Zhang A, Comb MJ, Avruch J: Regulation of the p70 S6 kinase by phosphorylation in vivo. Analysis using site-specific anti-phosphopeptide antibodies. *J Biol Chem* **273**:16621, 1998.
134. Belham C, Wu S, Avruch J: Intracellular signalling: PDK1 — a kinase at the hub of things. *Curr Biol* **9**:R93, 1999.
135. Akimoto K, Nakaya M, Yamanaka T, Tanaka J, Matsuda S, Weng QP, Avruch J, Ohno S: Atypical protein kinase Clambda binds and regulates p70 S6 kinase. *Biochem J* **335**:417, 1998.
136. Hu C, Pang S, Kong X, Velleca M, Lawrence JC Jr: Molecular cloning and tissue distribution of PHAS-I, an intracellular target for insulin and growth factors. *Proc Natl Acad Sci U S A* **91**:3730, 1994.
137. Pause A, Belsham GJ, Gingras AC, Donze O, Lin TA, Lawrence JC Jr, Sonenberg N: Insulin-dependent stimulation of protein synthesis by phosphorylation of a regulator of 5′-cap function [see Comments]. *Nature* **371**:762, 1994.
138. Brunn GJ, Hudson CC, Sekulic A, Williams JM, Hosoi H, Houghton PJ, Lawrence JC Jr, Abraham RT: Phosphorylation of the translational repressor PHAS-I by the mammalian target of rapamycin. *Science* **277**:99, 1997.
139. Lawrence JC Jr, Fadden P, Haystead TA, Lin TA: PHAS proteins as mediators of the actions of insulin, growth factors and cAMP on protein synthesis and cell proliferation. *Adv Enzyme Regul* **37**:239, 1997.

140. Price DJ, Grove JR, Calvo V, Avruch J, Bierer BE: Rapamycin-induced inhibition of the 70-kilodalton S6 protein kinase. *Science* **257**:973, 1992.
141. Hara K, Yonezawa K, Kozlowski MT, Sugimoto T, Andrabi K, Weng QP, Kasuga M, Nishimoto I, Avruch J: Regulation of eIF-4E BP1 phosphorylation by mTOR. *J Biol Chem* **272**:26457, 1997.
142. Shigemitsu K, Tsujishita Y, Hara K, Nanahoshi M, Avruch J, Yonezawa K: Regulation of translational effectors by amino acid and mammalian target of rapamycin signaling pathways. Possible involvement of autophagy in cultured hepatoma cells. *J Biol Chem* **274**:1058, 1999.
143. Löpez-Aparicio P, Rascön A, Manganiello VC, Andersson KE, Belfrage P, Degerman E: Insulin-induced phosphorylation and activation of the cGMP-inhibited cAMP phosphodiesterase in human platelets. *Biochem Biophys Res Commun* **186**:517, 1992.
144. Manganiello VC, Degerman E, Smith CJ, Vasta V, Tornqvist H, Belfrage P: Mechanisms for activation of the rat adipocyte particulate cyclic-GMP-inhibited cyclic AMP phosphodiesterase and its importance in the antilipolytic action of insulin. *Adv Second Messenger Phosphoprotein Res* **25**:147, 1992.
145. Levine R, Goldstein M, Klein S, Huddlestun B: The action of insulin on the distribution of galactose in eviscerated nephrectomized dogs. *J Biol Chem* **179**:985, 1949.
146. Pessin JE, Bell GI: Mammalian facilitative glucose transporter family: structure and molecular regulation. *Annu Rev Physiol* **54**:911, 1992.
147. Mueckler M, Caruso C, Baldwin SA, Panico M, Blench I, Morris HR, Allard WJ, Lienhard GE, Lodish HF: Sequence and structure of a human glucose transporter. *Science* **229**:941, 1985.
148. Thorens B, Sarkar HK, Kaback HR, Lodish HF: Cloning and functional expression in bacteria of a novel glucose transporter present in liver, intestine, kidney, and beta-pancreatic islet cells. *Cell* **55**:281, 1988.
149. Fukumoto H, Seino S, Imura H, Seino Y, Eddy RL, Fukushima Y, Byers MG, Shows TB, Bell GI: Sequence, tissue distribution, and chromosomal localization of mRNA encoding a human glucose transporter-like protein. *Proc Natl Acad Sci U S A* **85**:5434, 1988.
150. Kayano T, Fukumoto H, Eddy RL, Fan YS, Byers MG, Shows TB, Bell GI: Evidence for a family of human glucose transporter-like proteins. Sequence and gene localization of a protein expressed in fetal skeletal muscle and other tissues. *J Biol Chem* **263**:15245, 1988.
151. James DE, Brown R, Navarro J, Pilch PF: Insulin-regulatable tissues express a unique insulin-sensitive glucose transport protein. *Nature* **333**:183, 1988.
152. James DE, Strube M, Mueckler M: Molecular cloning and characterization of an insulin-regulatable glucose transporter. *Nature* **338**:83, 1989.
153. Birnbaum MJ: Identification of a novel gene encoding an insulin-responsive glucose transporter protein. *Cell* **57**:305, 1989.
154. Charron MJ, Brosius FC 3rd, Alper SL, Lodish HF: A glucose transport protein expressed predominately in insulin-responsive tissues. *Proc Natl Acad Sci U S A* **86**:2535, 1989.
155. Fukumoto H, Kayano T, Buse JB, Edwards Y, Pilch PF, Bell GI, Seino S: Cloning and characterization of the major insulin-responsive glucose transporter expressed in human skeletal muscle and other insulin-responsive tissues. *J Biol Chem* **264**:7776, 1989.
156. Cushman SW, Wardzala LJ: Potential mechanism of insulin action on glucose transport in the isolated rat adipose cell. Apparent translocation of intracellular transport systems to the plasma membrane. *J Biol Chem* **255**:4758, 1980.
157. Suzuki K Kono T: Evidence that insulin causes translocation of glucose transport activity to the plasma membrane from an intracellular storage site. *Proc Natl Acad Sci U S A* **77**:2542, 1980.
158. Holman GD, Kozka IJ, Clark AE, Flower CJ, Saltis J, Habberfield AD, Simpson IA, Cushman SW: Cell surface labeling of glucose transporter isoform GLUT4 by bis-mannose photolabel. Correlation with stimulation of glucose transport in rat adipose cells by insulin and phorbol ester. *J Biol Chem* **265**:18172, 1990.
159. Jhun BH, Rampal AL, Liu H, Lachaal M, Jung CY: Effects of insulin on steady state kinetics of GLUT4 subcellular distribution in rat adipocytes. Evidence of constitutive GLUT4 recycling. *J Biol Chem* **267**:17710, 1992.
160. Satoh S, Nishimura H, Clark AE, Kozka IJ, Vannucci SJ, Simpson IA, Quon MJ, Cushman SW, Holman GD: Use of bismannose photolabel to elucidate insulin-regulated GLUT4 subcellular trafficking kinetics in rat adipose cells. Evidence that exocytosis is a critical site of hormone action. *J Biol Chem* **268**:17820, 1993.
161. Quon MJ: Advances in kinetic analysis of insulin-stimulated GLUT-4 translocation in adipose cells. *Am J Physiol* **266**:E144, 1994.
162. Olson A, Knight J, Pessin J: Syntaxin 4, VAMP2, and/or VAMP3/cellubrevin are functional target membrane and vesicle SNAP receptors for insulin-stimulated GLUT4 translocation in adipocytes. *Mol Cell Biol* **17**:2425, 1997.
163. Thurmond D, Ceresa B, Okada S, Elmendorf J, Coker K, Pessin J: Regulation of insulin-stimulated GLUT4 translocation by Munc18c in 3T3L1 adipocytes. *J Biol Chem* **273**:33876, 1998.
164. Krebs EG Fischer EH: The phosphorylase *b* to *a* converting enzyme of rabbit skeletal muscle. *Biochem Biophys Acta* **20**:150, 1956.
165. Friedman DL, Larner J: Studies on UDPG-α-glucan transglucosylase. III. Interconversion of two forms of muscle UDPG-α-glucan transglucosylase by a phosphorylation-dephosphorylation reaction sequence. *Biochemistry* **2**:669, 1963.
166. Rizack MA: *J Biol Chem* **239**:392, 1964.
169. O'Brien RM, Granner DK: Regulation of gene expression by insulin. *Physiol Rev* **76**:1109, 1996.
170. Alexander MC, Lomanto M, Nasrin N, Ramaika C: Insulin stimulates glyceraldehyde-3-phosphate dehydrogenase gene expression through *cis*-acting DNA sequences. *Proc Natl Acad Sci U S A* **85**:5092, 1988.
171. Nasrin N, Ercolani L, Denaro M, Kong XF, Kang I, Alexander M: An insulin response element in the glyceraldehyde-3-phosphate dehydrogenase gene binds a nuclear protein induced by insulin in cultured cells and by nutritional manipulations in vivo. *Proc Natl Acad Sci U S A* **87**:5273, 1990.
172. Croniger C, Leahy P, Reshef L, Hanson RW: C/EBP and the control of phosphoenolpyruvate carboxykinase gene transcription in the liver. *J Biol Chem* **273**:31629, 1998.
173. O'Brien RM, Noisin EL, Suwanichkul A, Yamasaki T, Lucas PC, Wang JC, Powell DR, Granner DK: Hepatic nuclear factor 3- and hormone-regulated expression of the phosphoenolpyruvate carboxykinase and insulin-like growth factor-binding protein 1 genes. *Mol Cell Biol* **15**:1747, 1995.
174. Unterman TG, Fareeduddin A, Harris MA, Goswami RG, Porcella A, Costa RH, Lacson RG: Hepatocyte nuclear factor-3 (HNF-3) binds to the insulin response sequence in the IGF binding protein-1 (IGFBP-1) promoter and enhances promoter function. *Biochem Biophys Res Commun* **203**:1835, 1994.
175. Ogg S, Paradis S, Gottlieb S, Patterson GI, Lee L, Tissenbaum HA, Ruvkun G: The Fork head transcription factor DAF-16 transduces insulin-like metabolic and longevity signals in *C. elegans*. *Nature* **389**:994, 1997.
176. Lin K, Dorman JB, Rodan A, Kenyon C: daf-16: An HNF-3/forkhead family member that can function to double the life span of *Caenorhabditis elegans*. *Science* **278**:1319, 1997.
177. Nakae J, Park BC, Accili D: Insulin stimulates phosphorylation of the Forkhead transcription factor FKHR on serine 253 through a Wortmannin-sensitive pathway. *J Biol Chem* **274**:15982, 1999.
178. Kops GJ, de Ruiter ND, De Vries-Smits AM, Powell DR, Bos JL, Burgering BM: Direct control of the Forkhead transcription factor AFX by protein kinase B. *Nature* **398**:630, 1999.
179. Carpentier JL, Paccaud JP, Gorden P, Rutter WJ, Orci L: Insulin-induced surface redistribution regulates internalization of the insulin receptor and requires its autophosphorylation. *Proc Natl Acad Sci U S A* **89**:162, 1992.
180. Rajagopalan M, Neidigh JL, McClain DA: Amino acid sequences Gly-Pro-Leu-Tyr and Asn-Pro-Glu-Tyr in the submembranous domain of the insulin receptor are required for normal endocytosis. *J Biol Chem* **266**:23068, 1991.
181. Backer JM, Kahn CR, Cahill DA, Ullrich A, White MF: Receptor-mediated internalization of insulin requires a 12-amino acid sequence in the juxtamembrane region of the insulin receptor beta-subunit [published erratum appears in *J Biol Chem* 265(34):21390, 1990]. *J Biol Chem* **265**:16450, 1990.
182. Carpentier JL, Paccaud JP, Backer J, Gilbert A, Orci L, Kahn CR, Baecker J: Two steps of insulin receptor internalization depend on different domains of the beta-subunit [published erratum appears in *J Cell Biol* 123(4):1047, 1993]. *J Cell Biol* **122**:1243, 1993.
183. Haft CR, Klausner RD, Taylor SI: Involvement of dileucine motifs in the internalization and degradation of the insulin receptor [published erratum appears in *J Biol Chem* 270(50):30235, 1995]. *J Biol Chem* **269**:26286, 1994.
184. Hamer I, Haft CR, Paccaud JP, Maeder C, Taylor S, Carpentier JL: Dual role of a dileucine motif in insulin receptor endocytosis. *J Biol Chem* **272**:21685, 1997.
185. Waelbroeck M: The pH dependence of insulin binding. A quantitative study. *J Biol Chem* **257**:8284, 1982.

186. Taylor SI, Roth J, Blizzard RM, Elders MJ: Qualitative abnormalities in insulin binding in a patient with extreme insulin resistance: Decreased sensitivity to alterations in temperature and pH. *Proc Natl Acad Sci U S A* **78**:7157, 1981.
187. Terris S, Steiner DF: Binding and degradation of 125I-insulin by rat hepatocytes. *J Biol Chem* **250**:8389, 1975.
188. Flier J, Minaker K, Landsberg L, Young J, Pallotta J, Rowe J: Impaired in vivo insulin clearance in patients with severe target-cell resistance to insulin. *Diabetes* **31**:132, 1982.
189. Hachiya HL, Treves ST, Kahn CR, Sodoyez JC, Sodoyez-Goffaux F: Altered insulin distribution and metabolism in type I diabetics assessed by [^{123}I]insulin scanning. *J Clin Endocrinol Metab* **64**:801, 1987.
190. Di Guglielmo GM, Drake PG, Baass PC, Authier F, Posner BI, Bergeron JJ: Insulin receptor internalization and signalling. *Mol Cell Biochem* **182**:59, 1998.
191. Gavin JRD, Roth J, Neville DM Jr, Meyts PD, Buell DN: Insulin-dependent regulation of insulin receptor concentrations: A direct demonstration in cell culture. *Proc Natl Acad Sci U S A* **71**:84, 1974.
192. Kasuga M, Kahn CR, Hedo JA, Van Obberghen, E Yamada KM: Insulin-induced receptor loss in cultured human lymphocytes is due to accelerated receptor degradation. *Proc Natl Acad Sci U S A* **78**:6917, 1981.
193. Shechter Y: Insulin-mimetic effects of vanadate. Possible implications for future treatment of diabetes. *Diabetes* **39**:1, 1990.
194. Goldfine AB, Simonson DC, Folli F, Patti ME, Kahn CR: In vivo and in vitro studies of vanadate in human and rodent diabetes mellitus. *Mol Cell Biochem* **153**:217, 1995.
195. Fantus IG, Tsiani E: Multifunctional actions of vanadium compounds on insulin signaling pathways: evidence for preferential enhancement of metabolic versus mitogenic effects. *Mol Cell Biochem* **182**:109, 1998.
196. Moller NP, Moller KB, Lammers R, Kharitonenkov A, Hoppe E, Wiberg FC, Sures I, Ullrich A: Selective down-regulation of the insulin receptor signal by protein- tyrosine phosphatases alpha and epsilon. *J Biol Chem* **270**:23126, 1995.
197. Chen H, Wertheimer SJ, Lin CH, Katz SL, Amrein KE, Burn P, Quon MJ: Protein-tyrosine phosphatases PTP1B and syp are modulators of insulin- stimulated translocation of GLUT4 in transfected rat adipose cells. *J Biol Chem* **272**:8026, 1997.
198. Goldstein BJ, Ahmad F, Ding W, Li PM, Zhang WR: Regulation of the insulin signalling pathway by cellular protein- tyrosine phosphatases. *Mol Cell Biochem* **182**:91, 1998.
199. Goldstein BJ, Li PM, Ding W, Ahmad F, Zhang WR: Regulation of insulin action by protein tyrosine phosphatases. *Vitam Horm* **54**:67, 1998.
200. Lammers R, Moller NP, Ullrich A: Mutant forms of the protein tyrosine phosphatase alpha show differential activities towards intracellular substrates. *Biochem Biophys Res Commun* **242**:32, 1998.
201. Elchebly M, Payette P, Michaliszyn E, Cromlish W, Collins S, Loy AL, Normandin D, Cheng A, Himms-Hagen J, Chan CC, Ramachandran C, Gresser MJ, Tremblay ML, Kennedy BP: Increased insulin sensitivity and obesity resistance in mice lacking the protein tyrosine phosphatase-1B gene [see Comments]. *Science* **283**:1544, 1999.
202. Hunter T: The Croonian Lecture 1997. The phosphorylation of proteins on tyrosine: its role in cell growth and disease. *Philos Trans R Soc Lond B Biol Sci* **353**:583, 1998.
203. Stadtmauer L, Rosen OM: Increasing the cAMP content of IM-9 cells alters the phosphorylation state and protein kinase activity of the insulin receptor. *J Biol Chem* **261**:3402, 1986.
204. Bollag GE, Roth RA, Beaudoin J, Mochly-Rosen D, Koshland DE Jr: Protein kinase C directly phosphorylates the insulin receptor in vitro and reduces its protein-tyrosine kinase activity. *Proc Natl Acad Sci U S A* **83**:5822, 1986.
205. Kellerer M, Mushack J, Seffer E, Mischak H, Ullrich A, Haring HU: Protein kinase C isoforms alpha, delta and theta require insulin receptor substrate-1 to inhibit the tyrosine kinase activity of the insulin receptor in human kidney embryonic cells (HEK 293 cells). *Diabetologia* **41**:833, 1998.
206. Dunaif A, Xia J, Book CB, Schenker E, Tang Z: Excessive insulin receptor serine phosphorylation in cultured fibroblasts and in skeletal muscle. A potential mechanism for insulin resistance in the polycystic ovary syndrome. *J Clin Invest* **96**:801, 1995.
207. Peraldi P, Hotamisligil GS, Buurman WA, White MF, Spiegelman BM: Tumor necrosis factor (TNF)-alpha inhibits insulin signaling through stimulation of the p55 TNF receptor and activation of sphingomyelinase. *J Biol Chem* **271**:13018, 1996.
208. Hotamisligil GS, Peraldi P, Budavari A, Ellis R, White MF, Spiegelman BM: IRS-1-mediated inhibition of insulin receptor tyrosine kinase activity in TNF-alpha- and obesity-induced insulin resistance. *Science* **271**:665, 1996.
209. De Fea K, Roth RA: Modulation of insulin receptor substrate-1 tyrosine phosphorylation and function by mitogen-activated protein kinase. *J Biol Chem* **272**:31400, 1997.
210. De Fea K, Roth RA: Protein kinase C modulation of insulin receptor substrate-1 tyrosine phosphorylation requires serine 612. *Biochemistry* **36**:12939, 1997.
211. Li J, DeFea K, Roth RA: Modulation of insulin receptor substrate-1 tyrosine phosphorylation by an Akt/phosphatidylinositol 3-kinase pathway. *J Biol Chem* **274**:9351, 1999.
212. Qiao LY, Goldberg JL, Russell JC, Sun XJ: Identification of enhanced serine kinase activity in insulin resistance. *J Biol Chem* **274**:10625, 1999.
213. Hotamisligil GS: Mechanisms of TNF-alpha-induced insulin resistance. *Exp Clin Endocrinol Diabetes* **107**:119, 1999.
214. Eldar-Finkelman H, Krebs EG: Phosphorylation of insulin receptor substrate 1 by glycogen synthase kinase 3 impairs insulin action. *Proc Natl Acad Sci U S A* **94**:9660, 1997.
215. Cryer PE: Glucose homeostasis and hypoglycemia, in Wilson JD, Foster DW (eds): *Williams Textbook of Endocrinology*. Philadelphia, WB Saunders, 1990, p 1223.
216. Unger RH: The Berson memorial lecture. Insulin-glucagon relationships in the defense against hypoglycemia. *Diabetes* **32**:575, 1983.
217. Schwartz NS, Clutter WE, Shah SD, Cryer PE: Glycemic thresholds for activation of glucose counterregulatory systems are higher than the threshold for symptoms. *J Clin Invest* **79**:777, 1987.
218. Clarke WL, Santiago JV, Thomas L, Ben GE, Haymond MW, Cryer PE: Adrenergic mechanisms in recovery from hypoglycemia in man: adrenergic blockade. *Am J Physiol* **236**:e147, 1979.
219. Gerich J, Davis J, Lorenzi M, Rizza R, Bohannon N, Karam J, Lewis S, Kaplan R, Schultz T, Cryer P: Hormonal mechanisms of recovery from insulin-induced hypoglycemia in man. *Am J Physiol* **236**:e380, 1979.
220. Rizza RA, Cryer PE, Gerich JE: Role of glucagon, catecholamines, and growth hormone in human glucose counterregulation. Effects of somatostatin and combined alpha- and beta-adrenergic blockade on plasma glucose recovery and glucose flux rates after insulin-induced hypoglycemia. *J Clin Invest* **64**:62, 1979.
221. Garber AJ, Cryer PE, Santiago JV, Haymond MW, Pagliara AS, Kipnis DM: The role of adrenergic mechanisms in the substrate and hormonal response to insulin-induced hypoglycemia in man. *J Clin Invest* **58**:7, 1976.
222. Spiegel AM, Shenker A, Weinstein LS: Receptor-effector coupling by G proteins: Implications for normal and abnormal signal transduction. *Endocr Rev* **13**:536, 1992.
223. Gilman AG: Nobel Lecture. G proteins and regulation of adenylyl cyclase. *Biosci Rep* **15**:65, 1995.
224. Simonds WF: G protein regulation of adenylate cyclase. *Trends Pharmacol Sci* **20**:66, 1999.
225. Iyengar R, Abramowitz J, Bordelon-Riser M, Birnbaumer L: Hormone receptor-mediated stimulation of adenylyl cyclase systems. Nucleotide effects and analysis in terms of a simple two-state model for the basic receptor-affected enzyme. *J Biol Chem* **255**:3558, 1980.
226. Exton JH: The roles of calcium and phosphoinositides in the mechanisms of alpha 1- adrenergic and other agonists. *Rev Physiol Biochem Pharmacol* **111**:117, 1988.
227. Asaoka Y, Nakamura S, Yoshida K, Nishizuka Y: Protein kinase C, calcium and phospholipid degradation. *Trends Biochem Sci* **17**:414, 1992.
228. Bennett PH, Rushforth NB, Miller M, LeCompte PM: Epidemiologic studies of diabetes in the Pima Indians. *Recent Prog Horm Res* **32**:333, 1976.
229. Jarrett RJ, Keen H: Hyperglycaemia and diabetes mellitus. *Lancet* **2**:1009, 1976.
230. Fujita Y, Chacra AR, Herron AJ, Seltzer HS: Influence of antecedent carbohydrate intake on the biphasic insulin response to intravenous glucose. *Diabetes* **24**:1072, 1975.
231. Seltzer HS: Diagnosis of diabetes, in Ellenberg M, Rifkin H: *Diabetes Mellitus: Theory and Practice*. New Hyde Park, NY: Medical Examination, 1983, p 415.
232. Harris MI, Eastman RC, Cowie CC, Flegal KM, Eberhardt MS: Comparison of diabetes diagnostic categories in the U.S. population according to the 1997 American Diabetes Association and 1980–1985 World Health Organization diagnostic criteria. *Diabetes Care* **20**:1859, 1997.

233. Harris MI, Flegal KM, Cowie CC, Eberhardt MS, Goldstein DE, Little RR, Wiedmeyer HM, Byrd-Holt DD: Prevalence of diabetes, impaired fasting glucose, and impaired glucose tolerance in U.S. adults. The Third National Health and Nutrition Examination Survey, 1988–1994 [see Comments]. *Diabetes Care* **21**:518, 1998.
235. Zimmet PZ, Tuomi T, Mackay IR, Rowley MJ, Knowles W, Cohen M, Lang DA: Latent autoimmune diabetes mellitus in adults (LADA): The role of antibodies to glutamic acid decarboxylase in diagnosis and prediction of insulin dependency. *Diabet Med* **11**:299, 1994.
236. Zimmet P, Turner R, McCarty D, Rowley M, Mackay I: Crucial points at diagnosis. Type 2 diabetes or slow type 1 diabetes. *Diabetes Care* **22(Suppl 2)**:B59, 1999.
237. Cocozza S, Porcellini A, Riccardi G, Monticelli A, Condorelli G, Ferrara A, Pianese L, Miele C, Capaldo B, Beguinot F, et al.: NIDDM associated with mutation in tyrosine kinase domain of insulin receptor gene. *Diabetes* **41**:521, 1992.
238. Kahn CR, Flier JS, Bar RS, Archer JA, Gorden P, Martin MM, Roth J: The syndromes of insulin resistance and acanthosis nigricans. Insulin-receptor disorders in man. *N Engl J Med* **294**:739, 1976.
239. Donohue WL, Uchida I: Leprechaunism: A euphuism for a rare familial disorder. *J Pediatr* **45**:505, 1954.
240. Elders MJ, Schedewie HK, Olefsky J, Givens B, Char F, Bier DM, Baldwin D, Fiser RH, Seyedabadi S, Rubenstein A: Endocrine-metabolic relationships in patients with leprechaunism. *J Natl Med Assoc* **74**:1195, 1982.
241. Rosenberg AM, Haworth JC, Degroot GW, Trevenen CL, Rechler MM: A case of leprechaunism with severe hyperinsulinemia. *Am J Dis Child* **134**:170, 1980.
242. Rabson SM, Mendenhall EN: Familial hypertrophy of pineal body, hyperplasia of adrenal cortex and diabetes mellitus. *Am J Clin Pathol* **26**:283, 1956.
243. Ross SR, Graves RA, Spiegelman BM: Targeted expression of a toxin gene to adipose tissue: Transgenic mice resistant to obesity. *Genes Dev* **7**:1318, 1993.
244. Burant CF, Sreenan S, Hirano K, Tai TA, Lohmiller J, Lukens J, Davidson NO, Ross S, Graves RA: Troglitazone action is independent of adipose tissue. *J Clin Invest* **100**:2900, 1997.
245. Moitra J, Mason MM, Olive M, Krylov D, Gavrilova O, Marcus-Samuels B, Feigenbaum L, Lee E, Aoyama T, Eckhaus M, Reitman ML, Vinson C: Life without white fat: A transgenic mouse. *Genes Dev* **12**:3168, 1998.
246. Shimomura I, Hammer RE, Richardson JA, Ikemoto S, Bashmakov Y, Goldstein JL, Brown MS: Insulin resistance and diabetes mellitus in transgenic mice expressing nuclear SREBP-1c in adipose tissue: Model for congenital generalized lipodystrophy. *Genes Dev* **12**:3182, 1998.
247. Flier JS, Roth J: Diabetes in acromegaly and other endocrine disorders, in DeGroot LJ, Cahill GF Jr, Martini L, Nelson DH, Odell WD, Potts JT Jr, Steinberger E, Winegrad AI (eds): *Endocrinology*. New York, Grune and Stratton, 1979, p 1085.
248. Axelrod L, Bush MA, Hirsch HJ, Loo SW: Malignant somatostatinoma: Clinical features and metabolic studies. *J Clin Endocrinol Metab* **52**:886, 1981.
249. Stacpoole PW, Kasselberg AG, Berelowitz M, Chey WY: Somatostatinoma syndrome: Does a clinical entity exist? *Acta Endocrinol (Copenh)* **102**:80, 1983.
250. Vinik AI, Strodel WE, Eckhauser FE, Moattari AR, Lloyd R: Somatostatinomas, PPomas, neurotensinomas. *Semin Oncol* **14**:263, 1987.
251. Gorden P, Comi RJ, Maton PN, Go VL: NIH conference. Somatostatin and somatostatin analogue (SMS 201-995) in treatment of hormone-secreting tumors of the pituitary and gastrointestinal tract and non-neoplastic diseases of the gut. *Ann Intern Med* **110**:35, 1989.
252. Merimee TJ, Fineberg SE, McKusick VA, Hall J: Diabetes mellitus and sexual ateliotic dwarfism: a comparative study. *J Clin Invest* **49**:1096, 1970.
253. Gorden P: Glucose intolerance with hypokalemia. Failure of short-term potassium depletion in normal subjects to reproduce the glucose and insulin abnormalities of clinical hypokalemia. *Diabetes* **22**:544, 1973.
254. Flier JS, Kahn CR, Jarrett DB, Roth J: Characterization of antibodies to the insulin receptor: A cause of insulin-resistant diabetes in man. *J Clin Invest* **58**:1442, 1976.
255. Flier JS, Kahn CR, Jarrett DB, Roth J: Autoantibodies to the insulin receptor. Effect on the insulin-receptor interaction in IM-9 lymphocytes. *J Clin Invest* **60**:784, 1977.
256. Flier JS, Bar RS, Muggeo M, Kahn CR, Roth J, Gorden P: The evolving clinical course of patients with insulin receptor autoantibodies: spontaneous remission or receptor proliferation with hypoglycemia. *J Clin Endocrinol Metab* **47**:985, 1978.
257. Taylor SI, Grunberger G, Marcus Samuels B, Underhill LH, Dons RF, Ryan J, Roddam RF, Rupe CE, Gorden P: Hypoglycemia associated with antibodies to the insulin receptor. *N Engl J Med* **307**:1422, 1982.
258. Moller DE, Ratner RE, Borenstein DG, Taylor SI: Autoantibodies to the insulin receptor as a cause of autoimmune hypoglycemia in systemic lupus erythematosus. *Am J Med* **84**:334, 1988.
259. Selinger S, Tsai J, Pulini M, Saperstein A, Taylor SI: Autoimmune thrombocytopenia and primary biliary cirrhosis with hypoglycemia and insulin receptor autoantibodies: A case report. *Ann Intern Med* **107**:686, 1987.
260. Grunfeld C, Van Obberghen E, Karlsson FA, Kahn CR: Antibody-induced desensitization of the insulin receptor. Studies of the mechanism of desensitization in 3T3-L1 fatty fibroblasts. *J Clin Invest* **66**:1124, 1980.
261. Dons RF, Havlik R, Taylor SI, Baird KL, Chernick SS, Gorden P: Clinical disorders associated with autoantibodies to the insulin receptor. Simulation by passive transfer of immunoglobulins to rats. *J Clin Invest* **72**:1072, 1983.
262. Taylor SI, Marcus Samuels B: Anti-receptor antibodies mimic the effect of insulin to down-regulate insulin receptors in cultured human lymphoblastoid (IM-9) cells. *J Clin Endocrinol Metab* **58**:182, 1984.
263. Taylor SI, Dons RF, Hernandez E, Roth J, Gorden P: Insulin resistance associated with androgen excess in women with autoantibodies to the insulin receptor. *Ann Intern Med* **97**:851, 1982.
264. Rotter JI, Anderson CE, Rimoin DL: Genetics of diabetes mellitus, in Ellenberg M, Rifkin h (eds): *Diabetes Mellitus: Theory and Practice*-New Hyde Park, NY, Medical Examination, 1983, p 481.
265. Rotter JI, Vadheim CM, Raffel LJ, Rimoin DL: Genetics, diabetes mellitus heterogeneity, and coronary heart disease. *Prog Clin Biol Res* **147**:445, 1984.
266. Gunay-Aygun M, Cassidy SB, Nicholls RD: Prader-Willi and other syndromes associated with obesity and mental retardation. *Behav Genet* **27**:307, 1997.
267. Khan NL, Wood NW: Prader-Willi and Angelman syndromes: update on genetic mechanisms and diagnostic complexities. *Curr Opin Neurol* **12**:149, 1999.
268. Zhang Y, Proenca R, Maffei M, Barone M, Leopold L, Friedman JM: Positional cloning of the mouse obese gene and its human homologue. *Nature* **372**:425, 1994.
269. Montague CT, Farooqi IS, Whitehead JP, Soos MA, Rau H, Wareham NJ, Sewter CP, Digby JE, Mohammed SN, Hurst JA, Cheetham CH, Earley AR, Barnett AH, Prins JB, O'Rahilly S: Congenital leptin deficiency is associated with severe early onset obesity in humans. *Nature* **387**:903, 1997.
270. Lee GH, Proenca R, Montez JM, Carroll KM, Darvishzadeh JG, Lee JI, Friedman JM: Abnormal splicing of the leptin receptor in diabetic mice. *Nature* **379**:632, 1996.
271. Chen H, Charlat O, Tartaglia LA, Woolf EA, Weng X, Ellis SJ, Lakey ND, Culpepper J, Moore KJ, Breitbart RE, Duyk GM, Tepper RI, Morgenstern JP: Evidence that the diabetes gene encodes the leptin receptor: Identification of a mutation in the leptin receptor gene in *db/db* mice. *Cell* **84**:491, 1996.
272. Phillips MS, Liu Q, Hammond HA, Dugan V, Hey PJ, Caskey CJ, Hess JF: Leptin receptor missense mutation in the fatty Zucker rat [Letter]. *Nat Genet* **13**:18, 1996.
273. Chua SC Jr, White DW, Wu-Peng XS, Liu SM, Okada N, Kershaw EE, Chung WK, Power-Kehoe L, Chua M, Tartaglia LA, Leibel RL: Phenotype of fatty due to Gln269Pro mutation in the leptin receptor (Lepr). *Diabetes* **45**:1141, 1996.
274. Takaya K, Ogawa Y, Hiraoka J, Hosoda K, Yamori Y, Nakao K, Koletsky RJ: Nonsense mutation of leptin receptor in the obese spontaneously hypertensive Koletsky rat [Letter]. *Nat Genet* **14**:130, 1996.
275. Lee G, Li C, Montez J, Halaas J, Darvishzadeh J, Friedman JM: Leptin receptor mutations in 129 db3J/db3J mice and NIH facp/facp rats. *Mamm Genome* **8**:445, 1997.
276. Clement K, Vaisse C, Lahlou N, Cabrol S, Pelloux V, Cassuto D, Gourmelen M, Dina C, Chambaz J, Lacorte JM, Basdevant A, Bougneres P, Lebouc Y, Froguel P, Guy-Grand B: A mutation in the human leptin receptor gene causes obesity and pituitary dysfunction [see Comments]. *Nature* **392**:398, 1998.
277. Jackson RS, Creemers JW, Ohagi S, Raffin-Sanson ML, Sanders L, Montague CT, Hutton JC, O'Rahilly S: Obesity and impaired prohormone processing associated with mutations in the human prohormone convertase 1 gene [see Comments]. *Nat Genet* **16**:303, 1997.

278. Hinney A, Becker I, Heibult O, Nottebom K, Schmidt A, Ziegler A, Mayer H, Siegfried W, Blum WF, Remschmidt H, Hebebrand J: Systematic mutation screening of the pro-opiomelanocortin gene: Identification of several genetic variants including three different insertions, one nonsense and two missense point mutations in probands of different weight extremes. *J Clin Endocrinol Metab* **83**:3737, 1998.
279. Krude H, Biebermann H, Luck W, Horn R, Brabant G, Gruters A: Severe early onset obesity, adrenal insufficiency and red hair pigmentation caused by POMC mutations in humans. *Nat Genet* **19**:155, 1998.
280. Yeo GS, Farooqi IS, Aminian S, Halsall DJ, Stanhope RG, O'Rahilly S: A frameshift mutation in MC4R associated with dominantly inherited human obesity [Letter]. *Nat Genet* **20**:111, 1998.
281. Ristow M, Muller-Wieland D, Pfeiffer A, Krone W, Kahn CR: Obesity associated with a mutation in a genetic regulator of adipocyte differentiation. *N Engl J Med* **339**:953, 1998.
282. Hu E, Kim JB, Sarraf P, Spiegelman BM: Inhibition of adipogenesis through MAP kinase-mediated phosphorylation of PPARgamma. *Science* **274**:2100, 1996.
283. Mitchell BD, Blangero J, Comuzzie AG, Almasy LA, Shuldiner AR, Silver K, Stern MP, MacCluer JW, Hixson JE: A paired sibling analysis of the beta-3 adrenergic receptor and obesity in Mexican Americans. *J Clin Invest* **101**:584, 1998.
284. Clement K, Vaisse C, Manning BS, Basdevant A, Guy-Grand B, Ruiz J, Silver KD, Shuldiner AR, Froguel P, Strosberg AD: Genetic variation in the beta 3-adrenergic receptor and an increased capacity to gain weight in patients with morbid obesity [see Comments]. *N Engl J Med* **333**:352, 1995.
285. Widen E, Lehto M, Kanninen T, Walston J, Shuldiner AR, Groop LC: Association of a polymorphism in the beta 3-adrenergic-receptor gene with features of the insulin resistance syndrome in Finns [see Comments]. *N Engl J Med* **333**:348, 1995.
286. Argyropoulos G, Brown AM, Willi SM, Zhu J, He Y, Reitman M, Gevao SM, Spruill I, Garvey WT: Effects of mutations in the human uncoupling protein 3 gene on the respiratory quotient and fat oxidation in severe obesity and type 2 diabetes. *J Clin Invest* **102**:1345, 1998.
287. O'Sullivan JB: Criteria for the oral glucose tolerance test in pregnancy. *Diabetes* **13**:278, 1964.
288. O'Sullivan JB: Diabetes mellitus after GDM. *Diabetes* **2**:131, 1991.
289. Freinkel N, Metzger BE, Phelps RL, Dooley SL, Ogata ES, Radvany RM, Belton A: Gestational diabetes mellitus: Heterogeneity of maternal age, weight, insulin secretion, HLA antigens, and islet cell antibodies and the impact of maternal metabolism on pancreatic B-cell and somatic development in the offspring. *Diabetes* **34(Suppl 2)**:1, 1985.
290. McEvoy RC, Franklin B, Ginsberg Fellner F: Gestational diabetes mellitus: evidence for autoimmunity against the pancreatic beta cells. *Diabetologia* **34**:507, 1991.
291. Kjos SL, Peters RK, Xiang A, Schaefer U, Buchanan TA: Hormonal choices after gestational diabetes. Subsequent pregnancy, contraception, and hormone replacement. *Diabetes Care* **21(Suppl 2)**:B50, 1998.
292. National Diabetes Data Group: Classification and diagnosis of diabetes mellitus and other categories of glucose intolerance. *Diabetes* **28**:1039, 1979.
293. Ratner R: Gestational diabetes mellitus: After three international workshops do we know how to diagnose and manage it yet? *J Clin Endocrinol Metab* **77**:1, 1993.
294. Taylor SI, Wertheimer E, Accili D, Cama A, Hone J, Roach P, Quon MJ, Suzuki Y, Levy-Toledano R, Taouis M, Sierra ML, Barbetti F, Gorden P: Mutations in the insulin receptor gene: Update 1994, in Underwood LE (ed): *Endocrine Reviews Monographs. 2. The Endocrine Pancreas, Insulin Action, and Diabetes*. Bethesda, MD, The Endocrine Society, 1994, p 58.
295. Kadowaki T, Kadowaki H, Rechler MM, Serrano Rios M, Roth J, Gorden P, Taylor SI: Five mutant alleles of the insulin receptor gene in patients with genetic forms of insulin resistance. *J Clin Invest* **86**:254, 1990.
296. Wertheimer E, Lu SP, Backeljauw PF, Davenport ML, Taylor SI: Homozygous deletion of the human insulin receptor gene. *Nat Genet* **5**:71, 1993.
297. Kadowaki T, Bevins CL, Cama A, Ojamaa K, Marcus Samuels B, Kadowaki H, Beitz L, McKeon C, Taylor SI: Two mutant alleles of the insulin receptor gene in a patient with extreme insulin resistance. *Science* **240**:787, 1988.
298. Kadowaki T, Kadowaki H, Taylor SI: A nonsense mutation causing decreased levels of insulin receptor mRNA: Detection by a simplified technique for direct sequencing of genomic DNA amplified by the polymerase chain reaction. *Proc Natl Acad Sci U S A* **87**:658, 1990.
299. Fradkin JE, Eastman RC, Lesniak MA, Roth J: Specificity spillover at the hormone receptor—exploring its role in human disease. *N Engl J Med* **320**:640, 1989.
300. Moller DE, Flier JS: Detection of an alteration in the insulin-receptor gene in a patient with insulin resistance, acanthosis nigricans, and the polycystic ovary syndrome (type A insulin resistance). *N Engl J Med* **319**:1526, 1988.
301. Odawara M, Kadowaki T, Yamamoto R, Shibasaki Y, Tobe K, Accili D, Bevins C, Mikami Y, Matsuura N, Akanuma Y, Takaku F, Taylor SI, Kasuga M: Human diabetes associated with a mutation in the tyrosine kinase domain of the insulin receptor. *Science* **245**:66, 1989.
302. Moller DE, Yokota A, White M, Pazianos, AG Flier JS: A naturally occurring mutation of insulin receptor Ala^{1134} impairs tyrosine kinase function and is associated with dominantly inherited insulin resistance. *J Biol Chem* **265**:14979, 1990.
303. Cama A, Sierra ML, Ottini L, Kadowaki T, Gorden P, Imperato McGinley J, Taylor SI: A mutation in the tyrosine kinase domain of the insulin receptor associated with insulin resistance in an obese woman. *J Clin Endocrinol Metab* **73**:894, 1991.
304. Cama A, Quon MJ, Sierra ML, Taylor SI: Substitution of isoleucine for methionine at position 1153 in the beta-subunit of the human insulin receptor. A mutation that impairs receptor tyrosine kinase activity, receptor endocytosis, and insulin action. *J Biol Chem* **267**:8383, 1992.
305. Cama A, Sierra ML, Quon MJ, Ottini L, Gorden P, Taylor SI: Substitution of glutamic acid for alanine-1135 in the putative "catalytic loop" of the tyrosine kinase domain of the human insulin receptor: A mutation that impairs proteolytic processing into subunits and inhibits receptor tyrosine kinase activity. *J Biol Chem* **268**:8060, 1993.
306. Wertheimer E, Litvin Y, Ebstein RP, Bennet ER, Barbetti F, Accili D, Taylor SI: Deletion of exon 3 of the insulin receptor gene in a kindred with a familial form of insulin resistance. *J Clin Endocrinol Metab* **78**:1153, 1994.
307. Yoshimasa Y, Seino S, Whittaker J, Kakehi T, Kosaki A, Kuzuya H, Imura H, Bell GI, Steiner DF: Insulin-resistant diabetes due to a point mutation that prevents insulin proreceptor processing. *Science* **240**:784, 1988.
308. Accili D, Frapier C, Mosthaf L, McKeon C, Elbein SC, Permutt MA, Ramos E, Lander E, Ullrich A, Taylor SI: A mutation in the insulin receptor gene that impairs transport of the receptor to the plasma membrane and causes insulin-resistant diabetes. *EMBO J* **8**:2509, 1989.
309. Roach P, Zick Y, Accili D, Taylor SI, Gorden P: A novel human insulin receptor gene mutation uniquely inhibits insulin binding without impairing post-translational processing. *Diabetes* **43**:1096, 1994.
310. Wertheimer E, Barbetti F, Muggeo M, Roth J, Taylor SI: Two mutations in a conserved structural motif in the insulin receptor inhibit normal folding and intracellular transport of the receptor. *J Biol Chem* **269**:7587, 1994.
311. O'Rahilly S, Choi WH, Patel P, Turner RC, Flier JS, Moller DE: Detection of mutations in insulin-receptor gene in NIDDM patients by analysis of single-stranded conformation polymorphisms. *Diabetes* **40**:777, 1991.
312. Taylor SI, Marcus Samuels B, Ryan Young J, Leventhal S, Elders MJ: Genetics of the insulin receptor defect in a patient with extreme insulin resistance. *J Clin Endocrinol Metab* **62**:1130, 1986.
313. Lekanne Deprez RH, Potter van Loon BJ, van der Zon GC, Möller W, Lindhout D, Klinkhamer MP, Krans HM, Maassen JA: Individuals with only one allele for a functional insulin receptor have a tendency to hyperinsulinaemia but not to hyperglycaemia. *Diabetologia* **32**:740, 1989.
314. Shimada F, Taira M, Suzuki Y, Hashimoto N, Nozaki O, Taira M, Tatibana M, Ebina Y, Tawata M, Onaya T, et al.: Insulin-resistant diabetes associated with partial deletion of insulin-receptor gene. *Lancet* **335**:1179, 1990.
315. Brown MS, Goldstein JL: A receptor-mediated pathway for cholesterol homeostasis. *Science* **232**:34, 1986.
316. Krook A, Brueton L, O'Rahilly S: Homozygous nonsense mutation in the insulin receptor gene in infant with leprechaunism [see Comments]. *Lancet* **342**:277, 1993.
317. Psiachou H, Mitton S, Alaghband-Zadeh J, Hone J, Taylor SI, Sinclair L: Leprechaunism and homozygous nonsense mutation in the insulin receptor gene [Letter; Comment]. *Lancet* **342**:924, 1993.
318. Hone J, Accili D, al-Gazali LI, Lestringant G, Orban T, Taylor SI: Homozygosity for a new mutation (Ile119 → Met) in the insulin receptor gene in five sibs with familial insulin resistance. *J Med Genet* **31**:715, 1994.

319. Hone J, Accili D, Psiachou H, Alghband-Zadeh J, Mitton S, Wertheimer E, Sinclair L, Taylor SI: Homozygosity for a null allele of the insulin receptor gene in a patient with leprechaunism. *Hum Mutat* **6**:17, 1995.
320. Jospe N, Kaplowitz PB, Furlanetto RW: Homozygous nonsense mutation in the insulin receptor gene of a patient with severe congenital insulin resistance: Leprechaunism and the role of the insulin-like growth factor receptor. *Clin Endocrinol (Oxf)* **45**:229, 1996.
321. Kadowaki H, Takahashi Y, Ando A, Momomura K, Kaburagi Y, Quin JD, MacCuish AC, Koda N, Fukushima Y, Taylor SI, Akanuma Y, Yazaki Y, Kadowaki T: Four mutant alleles of the insulin receptor gene associated with genetic syndromes of extreme insulin resistance. *Biochem Biophys Res Commun* **237**:516, 1997.
322. Taira M, Taira M, Hashimoto N, Shimada F, Suzuki Y, Kanatsuka A, Nakamura F, Ebina Y, Tatibana M, Makino H, et al.: Human diabetes associated with a deletion of the tyrosine kinase domain of the insulin receptor. *Science* **245**:63, 1989.
323. Imano E, Kadowaki H, Kadowaki T, Iwama N, Watarai T, Kawamori R, Kamada T, Taylor SI: Two patients with insulin resistance due to decreased levels of insulin-receptor mRNA. *Diabetes* **40**:548, 1991.
324. Hedo JA, Kasuga M, Van Obberghen E, Roth J, Kahn CR: Direct demonstration of glycosylation of insulin receptor subunits by biosynthetic and external labeling: Evidence for heterogeneity. *Proc Natl Acad Sci U S A* **78**:4791, 1981.
325. Hedo JA, Collier E, Watkinson A: Myristyl and palmityl acylation of the insulin receptor. *J Biol Chem* **262**:954, 1987.
326. Collier E, Gorden P: O-linked oligosaccharides on insulin receptor. *Diabetes* **40**:197, 1991.
327. Accili D, Mosthaf L, Ullrich A, Taylor SI: A mutation in the extracellular domain of the insulin receptor impairs the ability of insulin to stimulate receptor autophosphorylation. *J Biol Chem* **266**:434, 1991.
328. Accili D, Kadowaki T, Kadowaki H, Mosthaf L, Ullrich A, Taylor SI: Immunoglobulin heavy chain-binding protein binds to misfolded mutant insulin receptors with mutations in the extracellular domain. *J Biol Chem* **267**:586, 1992.
329. Kadowaki T, Kadowaki H, Accili D, Taylor SI: Substitution of lysine for asparagine at position 15 in the alpha-subunit of the human insulin receptor. A mutation that impairs transport of receptors to the cell surface and decreases the affinity of insulin binding. *J Biol Chem* **265**:19143, 1990.
330. Kadowaki T, Kadowaki H, Accili D, Yazaki Y, Taylor SI: Substitution of arginine for histidine at position 209 in the alpha-subunit of the human insulin receptor. A mutation that impairs receptor dimerization and transport of receptors to the cell surface. *J Biol Chem* **266**:21224, 1991.
331. Yoshimasa Y, Paul JI, Whittaker J, Steiner DF: Effects of amino acid replacements within the tetrabasic cleavage site on the processing of the human insulin receptor precursor expressed in Chinese hamster ovary cells. *J Biol Chem* **265**:17230, 1990.
332. Taouis M, Levy-Toledano R, Roach P, Taylor SI, Gorden P: Rescue and activation of a binding-deficient insulin receptor. Evidence for intermolecular transphosphorylation. *J Biol Chem* **269**:27762, 1994.
333. Taouis M, Levy-Toledano R, Roach P, Taylor SI, Gorden P: Structural basis by which a recessive mutation in the alpha-subunit of the insulin receptor affects insulin binding. *J Biol Chem* **269**:14912, 1994.
334. Treadway JL, Morrison BD, Soos MA, Siddle K, Olefsky J, Ullrich A, McClain DA, Pessin JE: Transdominant inhibition of tyrosine kinase activity in mutant insulin/insulin-like growth factor I hybrid receptors. *Proc Natl Acad Sci U S A* **88**:214, 1991.
335. Frattali AL, Treadway JL, Pessin JE: Transmembrane signaling by the human insulin receptor kinase. Relationship between intramolecular beta subunit *trans*- and *cis*-autophosphorylation and substrate kinase activation. *J Biol Chem* **267**:19521, 1992.
336. Levy-Toledano R, Caro LH, Accili D, Taylor SI: Investigation of the mechanism of the dominant negative effect of mutations in the tyrosine kinase domain of the insulin receptor. *EMBO J* **13**:835, 1994.
337. Hedo JA, Simpson IA: Internalization of insulin receptors in the isolated rat adipose cell. Demonstration of the vectorial disposition of receptor subunits. *J Biol Chem* **259**:11083, 1984.
338. Kadowaki H, Kadowaki T, Cama A, Marcus Samuels B, Rovira A, Bevins CL, Taylor SI: Mutagenesis of lysine 460 in the human insulin receptor. Effects upon receptor recycling and cooperative interactions among binding sites. *J Biol Chem* **265**:21285, 1990.
339. Cama A, Sierra ML, Kadowaki T, Kadowaki H, Quon MJ, Rudiger HW, Dreyer M, Taylor SI: Two mutant alleles of the insulin receptor gene in a family with a genetic form of insulin resistance: A 10 base pair deletion in exon 1 and a mutation substituting serine for asparagine-462. *Hum Genet* **95**:174, 1995.
340. McElduff A, Hedo JA, Taylor SI, Roth J, Gorden P: Insulin receptor degradation is accelerated in cultured lymphocytes from patients with genetic syndromes of extreme insulin resistance. *J Clin Invest* **74**:1366, 1984.
341. Flier JS: Lilly Lecture 1991. Syndromes of insulin resistance: From patient to gene and back again. *Diabetes* **41**:1207, 1992.
342. Reddy SS, Kahn CR: Epidermal growth factor receptor defects in leprechaunism. A multiple growth factor-resistant syndrome. *J Clin Invest* **84**:1569, 1989.
343. Barnes ND, Palumbo PJ, Hayles AB, Folgar H: Insulin resistance, skin changes, and virilization: A recessively inherited syndrome possibly due to pineal gland dysfunction. *Diabetologia* **10**:285, 1974.
344. Taylor SI, Accili D, Imai Y: Insulin resistance or insulin deficiency. Which is the primary cause of NIDDM? *Diabetes* **43**:735, 1994.
345. Accili D, Drago J, Lee E, Johnson M, Cool M, Salvatore P, Asico L, Jose P, Taylor S, Westphal H: Early neonatal death in mice homozygous for a null allele of the insulin receptor gene. *Nat Genet* **12**:106, 1996.
346. Joshi R, Lamothe B, Cordonnier N, Mesbah K, Monthioux E, Jami J, Bucchini D: Targeted disruption of the insulin receptor gene in the mouse results in neonatal lethality. *EMBO J* **15**:1542, 1996.
347. Kulkarni R, Bruning J, Winnay J, Postic C, Magnuson M, Kahn C: Tissue-specific knockout of the insulin receptor in pancreatic beta cells creates an insulin secretory defect similar to that in type 2 diabetes. *Cell* **96**:329, 1999.
348. Kahn BB: Type 2 diabetes: when insulin secretion fails to compensate for insulin resistance. *Cell* **92**:593, 1998.
349. Taylor SI: Deconstructing type 2 diabetes. *Cell* **97**:9, 1999.
350. Bruning JC, Winnay J, Bonner-Weir S, Taylor SI, Accili D, Kahn CR: Development of a novel polygenic model of NIDDM in mice heterozygous for IR and IRS-1 null alleles. *Cell* **88**:561, 1997.
351. Brüning J, Michael M, Winnay J, Hayashi T, Horsch D, Accili D, Goodyear L, Kahn C: A muscle-specific insulin receptor knockout exhibits features of the metabolic syndrome of NIDDM without altering glucose tolerance. *Mol Cell* **2**:559, 1998.
352. Moller D, Chang P, Yaspelkis Br, Flier J, Wallberg-Henriksson H, Ivy J: Transgenic mice with muscle-specific insulin resistance develop increased adiposity, impaired glucose tolerance, and dyslipidemia. *Endocrinology* **137**:2397, 1996.
353. Lauro D, Kido Y, Castle A, Zarnowski M, Hayashi H, Ebina Y, Accili D: Impaired glucose tolerance in mice with a targeted impairment of insulin action in muscle and adipose tissue. *Nat Genet* **20**:294, 1998.
354. Aspinwall C, Lakey J, Kennedy R: Insulin-stimulated insulin secretion in single pancreatic beta cells. *J Biol Chem* **274**:6360, 1999.
355. Leibiger I, Leibiger B, Moede T, Berggren P: Exocytosis of insulin promotes insulin gene transcription via the insulin receptor/PI-3 kinase/p70 s6 kinase and CaM kinase pathways. *Mol Cell* **1**:933, 1998.
356. Terauchi Y, Iwamoto K, Tamemoto H, Komeda K, Ishii C, Kanazawa Y, Asanuma N, Aizawa T, Akanuma Y, Yasuda K, Kodama T, Tobe K, Yazaki Y, Kadowaki T: Development of non-insulin-dependent diabetes mellitus in the double knockout mice with disruption of insulin receptor substrate-1 and beta cell glucokinase genes. Genetic reconstitution of diabetes as a polygenic disease. *J Clin Invest* **99**:861, 1997.
357. Kahn BB, Rossetti L: Type 2 diabetes—Who is conducting the orchestra? *Nat Genet* **20**:223, 1998.
358. De Fronzo R: Pathogenesis of type 2 diabetes: Metabolic and molecular implications for identifying diabetes genes. *Diabetes Rev* **5**:177, 1997.
359. Porte D Jr: Banting lecture 1990. Beta-cells in type II diabetes mellitus. *Diabetes* **40**:166, 1991.
360. Leahy JL, Bonner Weir S, Weir GC: Beta-cell dysfunction induced by chronic hyperglycemia. Current ideas on mechanism of impaired glucose-induced insulin secretion. *Diabetes Care* **15**:442, 1992.
361. Reaven GM, Olefsky JM: Relationship between heterogeneity of insulin responses and insulin resistance in normal subjects and patients with chemical diabetes. *Diabetologia* **13**:201, 1977.
362. Reaven GM: Banting lecture 1988. Role of insulin resistance in human disease. *Diabetes* **37**:1595, 1988.
363. Lillioja S, Mott DM, Howard BV, Bennett PH, Yki Järvinen H, Freymond D, Nyomba BL, Zurlo F, Swinburn B, Bogardus C: Impaired glucose tolerance as a disorder of insulin action. Longitudinal and cross-sectional studies in Pima Indians. *N Engl J Med* **318**:1217, 1988.

364. Saad MF, Knowler WC, Pettitt DJ, Nelson RG, Mott DM, Bennett PH: The natural history of impaired glucose tolerance in the Pima Indians. *N Engl J Med* **319**:1500, 1988.
365. Saad MF, Knowler WC, Pettitt DJ, Nelson RG, Mott DM, Bennett PH: Sequential changes in serum insulin concentration during development of non-insulin-dependent diabetes. *Lancet* **1**:1356, 1989.
366. Warram JH, Martin BC, Krolewski AS, Soeldner JS, Kahn CR: Slow glucose removal rate and hyperinsulinemia precede the development of type II diabetes in the offspring of diabetic parents. *Ann Intern Med* **113**:909, 1990.
367. Martin BC, Warram JH, Krolewski AS, Bergman RN, Soeldner JS, Kahn CR: Role of glucose and insulin resistance in development of type 2 diabetes mellitus: Results of a 25-year follow-up study. *Lancet* **340**:925, 1992.
368. Jallut D, Golay A, Munger R, Frascarolo P, Schutz Y, Jëquier E, Felber JP: Impaired glucose tolerance and diabetes in obesity: A 6-year follow-up study of glucose metabolism. *Metabolism* **39**:1068, 1990.
369. Barnett AH, Eff C, Leslie RD, Pyke DA: Diabetes in identical twins. A study of 200 pairs. *Diabetologia* **20**:87, 1981.
370. Hanis CL, Boerwinkle E, Chakraborty R, Ellsworth DL, Concannon P, Stirling B, Morrison VA, Wapelhorst B, Spielman RS, Gogolin-Ewens KJ, Shepard JM, Williams SR, Risch N, Hinds D, Iwasaki N, Ogata M, Omori Y, Petzold C, Rietzch H, Schroder HE, Schulze J, Cox NJ, Menzel S, Boriraj VV, Chen X, et al.: A genome-wide search for human non-insulin-dependent (type 2) diabetes genes reveals a major susceptibility locus on chromosome 2 [see Comments]. *Nat Genet* **13**:161, 1996.
371. Mahtani MM, Widen E, Lehto M, Thomas J, McCarthy M, Brayer J, Bryant B, Chan G, Daly M, Forsblom C, Kanninen T, Kirby A, Kruglyak L, Munnelly K, Parkkonen M, Reeve-Daly MP, Weaver A, Brettin T, Duyk G, Lander ES, Groop LC: Mapping of a gene for type 2 diabetes associated with an insulin secretion defect by a genome scan in Finnish families [see Comments]. *Nat Genet* **14**:90, 1996.
372. Bowden DW, Sale M, Howard TD, Qadri A, Spray BJ, Rothschild CB, Akots G, Rich SS, Freedman BI: Linkage of genetic markers on human chromosomes 20 and 12 to NIDDM in Caucasian sib pairs with a history of diabetic nephropathy. *Diabetes* **46**:882, 1997.
373. Ji L, Malecki M, Warram JH, Yang Y, Rich SS, Krolewski AS: New susceptibility locus for NIDDM is localized to human chromosome 20q. *Diabetes* **46**:876, 1997.
374. Zouali H, Hani EH, Philippi A, Vionnet N, Beckmann JS, Demenais F, Froguel P: A susceptibility locus for early-onset non-insulin dependent (type 2) diabetes mellitus maps to chromosome 20q, proximal to the phosphoenolpyruvate carboxykinase gene. *Hum Mol Genet* **6**:1401, 1997.
375. Ghosh S, Watanabe RM, Hauser ER, Valle T, Magnuson VL, Erdos MR, Langefeld CD, Balow J Jr, Ally DS, Kohtamaki K, Chines P, Birznieks G, Kaleta HS, Musick A, Te C, Tannenbaum J, Eldridge W, Shapiro S, Martin C, Witt A, So A, Chang J, Shurtleff B, Porter R, Boehnke M, et al.: Type 2 diabetes: Evidence for linkage on chromosome 20 in 716 Finnish affected sib pairs. *Proc Natl Acad Sci U S A* **96**:2198, 1999.
376. Almind K, Bjorbaek C, Vestergaard H, et al.: Aminoacid polymorphism of insulin receptor substrate-1 in non-insulin-dependent diabetes mellitus. *Lancet* **342**:828, 1993.
377. Imai Y, Fusco A, Suzuki Y, Lesniak MA, D'Alfonso R, Sesti G, Bertoli A, Lauro R, Accili D, Taylor SI: Variant sequences of insulin receptor substrate-1 in patients with noninsulin-dependent diabetes mellitus. *J Clin Endocrinol Metab* **79**:1655, 1994.
378. Clausen JO, Hansen T, Bjorbaek C, Echwald SM, Urhammer SA, Rasmussen S, Andersen CB, Hansen L, Almind K, Winther K, et al.: Insulin resistance: Interactions between obesity and a common variant of insulin receptor substrate-1. *Lancet* **346**:397, 1995.
379. Almind K, Inoue G, Pedersen O, Kahn CR: A common amino acid polymorphism in insulin receptor substrate-1 causes impaired insulin signaling. Evidence from transfection studies. *J Clin Invest* **97**:2569, 1996.
380. Imai Y, Philippe N, Sesti G, Accili D, Taylor SI: Expression of variant forms of insulin receptor substrate-1 identified in patients with noninsulin-dependent diabetes mellitus. *J Clin Endocrinol Metab* **82**:4201, 1997.
381. Shen SW, Reaven GM, Farquhar JW: Comparison of impedance to insulin-mediated glucose uptake in normal subjects and in subjects with latent diabetes. *J Clin Invest* **49**:2151, 1970.
382. DeFronzo RA, Tobin JD, Andres R: Glucose clamp technique: A method for quantifying insulin secretion and resistance. *Am J Physiol* **237**:e214, 1979.
383. Bergman RN: Lilly lecture 1989. Toward physiological understanding of glucose tolerance. Minimal-model approach. *Diabetes* **38**:1512, 1989.
384. DeFronzo R: Lilly lecture 1987. The triumvirate: Beta-cell, muscle, liver. A collusion responsible for NIDDM. *Diabetes* **37**:667, 1988.
385. Ferrannini E, Smith JD, Cobelli C, Toffolo G, Pilo A, DeFronzo RA: Effect of insulin on the distribution and disposition of glucose in man. *J Clin Invest* **76**:357, 1985.
386. Bell PM, Firth RG, Rizza RA: Assessment of insulin action in insulin-dependent diabetes mellitus using [6-^{14}C]glucose, [3-^{3}H]glucose, and [2-^{3}H]glucose. Differences in the apparent pattern of insulin resistance depending on the isotope used. *J Clin Invest* **78**:1479, 1986.
387. Ferrannini E, Natali A, Bell P, Cavallo-Perin P, Lalic N, Mingrone G: Insulin resistance and hypersecretion in obesity. European Group for the Study of Insulin Resistance (EGIR). *J Clin Invest* **100**:1166, 1997.
388. Liese AD, Mayer-Davis EJ, Haffner SM: Development of the multiple metabolic syndrome: An epidemiologic perspective. *Epidemiol Rev* **20**:157, 1998.
389. Haffner SM: Issues in management: The role of insulin in cardiovascular outcomes. *Diabetes Metab Rev* **14(Suppl 1)**:S51, 1998.
390. Kolterman OG, Scarlett JA, Olefsky JM: Insulin resistance in non-insulin-dependent, type II diabetes mellitus. *Clin Endocrinol Metab* **11**:363, 1982.
391. DeFronzo RA, Gunnarsson R, Björkman O, Olsson M, Wahren J: Effects of insulin on peripheral and splanchnic glucose metabolism in noninsulin-dependent (type II) diabetes mellitus. *J Clin Invest* **76**:149, 1985.
392. Capaldo B, Napoli R, Di Bonito P, Albano G, Saccä L: Glucose and gluconeogenic substrate exchange by the forearm skeletal muscle in hyperglycemic and insulin-treated type II diabetic patients. *J Clin Endocrinol Metab* **71**:1220, 1990.
393. Kelley DE, Mandarino LJ: Hyperglycemia normalizes insulin-stimulated skeletal muscle glucose oxidation and storage in non-insulin-dependent diabetes mellitus. *J Clin Invest* **86**:1999, 1990.
394. Sims EA, Danforth EJ, Horton ES, Bray GA, Glennon JA, Salans LB: Endocrine and metabolic effects of experimental obesity in man. *Recent Prog Horm Res* **29**:457, 1973.
395. Bogardus C, Lillioja S, Stone K, Mott D: Correlation between muscle glycogen synthase activity and in vivo insulin action in man. *J Clin Invest* **73**:1185, 1984.
396. Shulman GI, Rothman DL, Jue T, Stein P, DeFronzo RA, Shulman RG: Quantitation of muscle glycogen synthesis in normal subjects and subjects with non-insulin-dependent diabetes by ^{13}C nuclear magnetic resonance spectroscopy. *N Engl J Med* **322**:223, 1990.
397. Rothman D, Shulman R Shulman G: ^{31}P nuclear magnetic resonance measurements of muscle glucose 6-phosphate: Evidence for reduced insulin dependent muscle transport or phosphorylation activity in non-insulin-dependent diabetes mellitus. *J Clin Invest* **89**:1069, 1992.
398. Rothman DL, Magnusson I, Cline G, Gerard D, Kahn CR, Shulman RG, Shulman GI: Decreased muscle glucose transport/phosphorylation is an early defect in the pathogenesis of non-insulin-dependent diabetes mellitus. *Proc Natl Acad Sci U S A* **92**:983, 1995.
399. Bergman R: New concepts in extracellular signaling for insulin action: The single gateway hypothesis. *Recent Prog Horm Res* **52**:359, 1997.
400. Chen YD, Golay A, Swislocki AL, Reaven GM: Resistance to insulin suppression of plasma free fatty acid concentrations and insulin stimulation of glucose uptake in noninsulin-dependent diabetes mellitus. *J Clin Endocrinol Metab* **64**:17, 1987.
401. Swislocki AL, Chen YD, Golay A, Chang MO, Reaven GM: Insulin suppression of plasma-free fatty acid concentration in normal individuals and patients with type 2 (non-insulin-dependent) diabetes. *Diabetologia* **30**:622, 1987.
402. Caro JF, Sinha MK, Raju SM, Ittoop O, Pories WJ, Flickinger EG, Meelheim D, Dohm GL: Insulin receptor kinase in human skeletal muscle from obese subjects with and without noninsulin dependent diabetes. *J Clin Invest* **79**:1330, 1987.
403. Caro JF, Ittoop O, Pories WJ, Meelheim D, Flickinger EG, Thomas F, Jenquin M, Silverman JF, Khazanie PG, Sinha MK: Studies on the mechanism of insulin resistance in the liver from humans with noninsulin-dependent diabetes. Insulin action and binding in isolated hepatocytes, insulin receptor structure, and kinase activity. *J Clin Invest* **78**:249, 1986.
404. Comi RJ, Grunberger G, Gorden P: Relationship of insulin binding and insulin-stimulated tyrosine kinase activity is altered in type II diabetes. *J Clin Invest* **79**:453, 1987.

405. Freidenberg GR, Henry RR, Klein HH, Reichart DR, Olefsky JM: Decreased kinase activity of insulin receptors from adipocytes of non-insulin-dependent diabetic subjects. *J Clin Invest* **79**:240, 1987.
406. Freidenberg GR, Reichart D, Olefsky JM, Henry RR: Reversibility of defective adipocyte insulin receptor kinase activity in non-insulin-dependent diabetes mellitus. Effect of weight loss. *J Clin Invest* **82**:1398, 1988.
407. Moller DE, Yokota A, Flier JS: Normal insulin-receptor cDNA sequence in Pima Indians with NIDDM. *Diabetes* **38**:1496, 1989.
408. Cama A, Patterson AP, Kadowaki T, Kadowaki H, Siegel G, D'Ambrosio D, Lillioja S, Roth J, Taylor SI: The amino acid sequence of the insulin receptor is normal in an insulin-resistant Pima Indian. *J Clin Endocrinol Metab* **70**:1155, 1990.
409. Kusari J, Verma US, Buse JB, Henry RR, Olefsky JM: Analysis of the gene sequences of the insulin receptor and the insulin-sensitive glucose transporter (GLUT-4) in patients with common-type non-insulin-dependent diabetes mellitus. *J Clin Invest* **88**:1323, 1991.
410. Kusari J, Olefsky JM, Strahl C, McClain DA: Insulin-receptor cDNA sequence in NIDDM patient homozygous for insulin-receptor gene RFLP. *Diabetes* **40**:249, 1991.
411. Brillon DJ, Freidenberg GR, Henry RR, Olefsky JM: Mechanism of defective insulin-receptor kinase activity in NIDDM. Evidence for two receptor populations. *Diabetes* **38**:397, 1989.
412. Taylor SI, Mukherjee C, Jungas RL: Regulation of pyruvate dehydrogenase in isolated rat liver mitochondria. Effects of octanoate, oxidation-reduction state, and adenosine triphosphate to adenosine diphosphate ratio. *J Biol Chem* **250**:2028, 1975.
413. Mansour TE: Phosphofructokinase. *Curr Top Cell Regul* **5**:1, 1972.
414. Allred JB, Reilly KE: Short-term regulation of acetyl CoA carboxylase in tissues of higher animals. *Prog Lipid Res* **35**:371, 1996.
415. Ruderman NB, Saha AK, Vavvas D, Witters LA: Malonyl-CoA, fuel sensing, and insulin resistance. *Am J Physiol* **276**:E1, 1999.
416. Roden M, Price TB, Perseghin G, Petersen KF, Rothman DL, Cline GW, Shulman GI: Mechanism of free fatty acid-induced insulin resistance in humans. *J Clin Invest* **97**:2859, 1996.
417. Hotamisligil GS, Shargill NS, Spiegelman BM: Adipose expression of tumor necrosis factor-alpha: direct role in obesity-linked insulin resistance. *Science* **259**:87, 1993.
418. Ventre J, Doebber T, Wu M, MacNaul K, Stevens K, Pasparakis M, Kollias G, Moller DE: Targeted disruption of the tumor necrosis factor-alpha gene: Metabolic consequences in obese and nonobese mice. *Diabetes* **46**:1526, 1997.
419. Ofei F, Hurel S, Newkirk J, Sopwith M, Taylor R: Effects of an engineered human anti-TNF-alpha antibody (CDP571) on insulin sensitivity and glycemic control in patients with NIDDM. *Diabetes* **45**:881, 1996.
420. Cohen B, Novick D, Rubinstein M: Modulation of insulin activities by leptin. *Science* **274**:1185, 1996.
421. Muller G, Ertl J, Gerl M, Preibisch G: Leptin impairs metabolic actions of insulin in isolated rat adipocytes. *J Biol Chem* **272**:10585, 1997.
422. Berti L, Kellerer M, Capp E, Haring HU: Leptin stimulates glucose transport and glycogen synthesis in C2C12 myotubes: Evidence for a P13-kinase mediated effect. *Diabetologia* **40**:606, 1997.
423. Campfield LA, Smith FJ, Guisez Y, Devos R, Burn P: Recombinant mouse OB protein: evidence for a peripheral signal linking adiposity and central neural networks [see Comments]. *Science* **269**:546, 1995.
424. Halaas JL, Gajiwala KS, Maffei M, Cohen SL, Chait BT, Rabinowitz D, Lallone RL, Burley SK, Friedman JM: Weight-reducing effects of the plasma protein encoded by the obese gene [see Comments]. *Science* **269**:543, 1995.
425. Pelleymounter MA, Cullen MJ, Baker MB, Hecht R, Winters D, Boone T, Collins F: Effects of the obese gene product on body weight regulation in *ob/ob* mice [see Comments]. *Science* **269**:540, 1995.
426. Shimabukuro M, Koyama K, Chen G, Wang MY, Trieu F, Lee Y, Newgard CB, Unger RH: Direct antidiabetic effect of leptin through triglyceride depletion of tissues. *Proc Natl Acad Sci U S A* **94**:4637, 1997.
427. Zhou YT, Shimabukuro M, Koyama K, Lee Y, Wang MY, Trieu F, Newgard CB, Unger RH: Induction by leptin of uncoupling protein-2 and enzymes of fatty acid oxidation. *Proc Natl Acad Sci U S A* **94**:6386, 1997.
428. Sivitz WI, DeSautel SL, Kayano T, Bell GI, Pessin JE: Regulation of glucose transporter messenger RNA in insulin-deficient states. *Nature* **340**:72, 1989.
429. Garvey WT, Huecksteadt TP, Birnbaum MJ: Pretranslational suppression of an insulin-responsive glucose transporter in rats with diabetes mellitus. *Science* **245**:60, 1989.
430. Kahn BB, Charron MJ, Lodish HF, Cushman SW, Flier JS: Differential regulation of two glucose transporters in adipose cells from diabetic and insulin-treated diabetic rats. *J Clin Invest* **84**:404, 1989.
431. Rossetti L, Smith D, Shulman GI, Papachristou D, DeFronzo RA: Correction of hyperglycemia with phlorizin normalizes tissue sensitivity to insulin in diabetic rats. *J Clin Invest* **79**:1510, 1987.
432. Kahn BB, Shulman GI, DeFronzo RA, Cushman SW, Rossetti L: Normalization of blood glucose in diabetic rats with phlorizin treatment reverses insulin-resistant glucose transport in adipose cells without restoring glucose transporter gene expression. *J Clin Invest* **87**:561, 1991.
433. Traxinger RR, Marshall S: Coordinated regulation of glutamine:fructose-6-phosphate amidotransferase activity by insulin, glucose, and glutamine. Role of hexosamine biosynthesis in enzyme regulation. *J Biol Chem* **266**:10148, 1991.
434. Marshall S, Bacote V, Traxinger RR: Discovery of a metabolic pathway mediating glucose-induced desensitization of the glucose transport system. Role of hexosamine biosynthesis in the induction of insulin resistance. *J Biol Chem* **266**:4706, 1991.
435. McClain DA, Crook ED: Hexosamines and insulin resistance. *Diabetes* **45**:1003, 1996.
436. Rossetti L, Hawkins M, Chen W, Gindi J, Barzilai N: In vivo glucosamine infusion induces insulin resistance in normoglycemic but not in hyperglycemic conscious rats. *J Clin Invest* **96**:132, 1995.
437. Barzilai N, Hawkins M, Angelov I, Hu M, Rossetti L: Glucosamine-induced inhibition of liver glucokinase impairs the ability of hyperglycemia to suppress endogenous glucose production. *Diabetes* **45**:1329, 1996.
438. Hebert LF Jr, Daniels MC, Zhou J, Crook ED, Turner RL, Simmons ST, Neidigh JL, Zhu JS, Baron AD, McClain DA: Overexpression of glutamine:fructose-6-phosphate amidotransferase in transgenic mice leads to insulin resistance. *J Clin Invest* **98**:930, 1996.
439. Yki-Jarvinen H, Daniels MC, Virkamaki A, Makimattila S, DeFronzo RA, McClain D: Increased glutamine:fructose-6-phosphate amidotransferase activity in skeletal muscle of patients with NIDDM. *Diabetes* **45**:302, 1996.
440. Feinglos MN, Bethel MA: Treatment of type 2 diabetes mellitus. *Med Clin North Am* **82**:757, 1998.
441. Garvey WT, Olefsky JM, Griffin J, Hamman RF, Kolterman OG: The effect of insulin treatment on insulin secretion and insulin action in type II diabetes mellitus. *Diabetes* **34**:222, 1985.
442. Zimmerman BR: Sulfonylureas. *Endocrinol Metab Clin North Am* **26**:511, 1997.
443. Henry RR: Thiazolidinediones. *Endocrinol Metab Clin North Am* **26**:553, 1997.
444. Inzucchi SE, Maggs DG, Spollett GR, Page SL, Rife FS, Walton V, Shulman GI: Efficacy and metabolic effects of metformin and troglitazone in type II diabetes mellitus [see Comments]. *N Engl J Med* **338**:867, 1998.
445. Zierath JR, Ryder JW, Doebber T, Woods J, Wu M, Ventre J, Li Z, McCrary C, Berger J, Zhang B, Moller DE: Role of skeletal muscle in thiazolidinedione insulin sensitizer (PPARgamma agonist) action. *Endocrinology* **139**:5034, 1998.
446. Bell PM, Hadden DR: Metformin. *Endocrinol Metab Clin North Am* **26**:523, 1997.
447. Wing RR: Behavioral treatment of obesity. Its application to type II diabetes. *Diabetes Care* **16**:193, 1993.
448. Wing RR, Venditti E, Jakicic JM, Polley BA, Lang W: Lifestyle intervention in overweight individuals with a family history of diabetes [see Comments]. *Diabetes Care* **21**:350, 1998.
449. Bell GI, Kayano T, Buse JB, Burant CF, Takeda J, Lin D, Fukumoto H, Seino S: Molecular biology of mammalian glucose transporters. *Diabetes Care* **13**:198, 1990.
450. Taylor S, Samuels B, Roth J, Kasuga M, Hedo J, Gorden P, Brasel D, Pokora T, Engel R: Decreased insulin binding in cultured lymphocytes from two patients with extreme insulin resistance. *J Clin Endocrinol Metab* **54**:919, 1982.
451. Taylor SI, Arioglu E: Syndromes associated with insulin resistance and acanthosis nigricans. *J Basic Clin Physiol Pharmacol* **9**:1998.

CHAPTER 69

Type 1 Diabetes

Noel Keith Maclaren ▪ Anjli Kukreja

1. Diabetes is the name given to a collection of diseases that have elevations in blood glucose levels in common. Population studies have defined cutoff levels of glycemia that are eventually associated with increased microvascular disease such as retinopathy. Two replicate fasting levels that exceed 126 mg/dl (>7 mM) are diagnostic in the absence of symptoms. Persons with fasting levels between 110 and 126 mg/dl are at risk of diabetes (impaired fasting glycemia). Replicate, 2-h glycemic responses >200 mg/dl (>11.1 mM) after a standard oral glucose tolerance test indicates diabetes also. This stage is often reached, however, before the fasting glucose levels are seen to rise. Type 1 diabetes comprises those forms of diabetes that are primarily due to insulin deficiency, however a relative insulin deficiency also is part of type 2 diabetes, which is however less severe, though it is compounded by degrees of insulin resistance, often associated with obesity. Long-term type 2 diabetes is complicated by glucose (glucosamine) toxicity, which decreases the patients' abilities to secrete insulin further, leading to diagnostic confusion with type 1 diabetes. Whereas type 2 diabetes is usually strongly familial, type 1 is much less so, having only one member of the family so affected in 90 percent of cases.
2. The immune-mediated form of type 1 diabetes (IMD) is most common amongst Caucasian races and is presumed present when autoantibodies to islet cells and/or to insulin and/or to defined islet proteins are detected in the presence of diabetes. However, an insulin-deficient type of diabetes in the presence of the risk HLA phenotypes is presumptive evidence. Adult onset IMD is characterized by a gradual decline in insulin secretion compared to children, a situation readily confused with type 2 diabetes unless autoantibodies to islet cell cytoplasm (ICA) and/or to glutamic acid decarboxylase (GAD_{65}) can be detected.
3. The pathogenesis of IMD involves multiple genetic lesions affecting immunoregulation against self, coupled to strong influences from the environment affecting penetrance. Studies from rodent models of the disease suggest that there is a gene dose effect of quantitative trait loci, with accumulating numbers of susceptibility genes compounding the risk. There are protective genes also. The obligate genes, however, are those encoding DR and DQ A plus B chain heterodimers. Both loci are involved in human patients. The nonobese diabetic (NOD) mouse expresses no IE (DR homologous) molecules but only a unique recombinant b/d haplotype IA molecule (DQ homologous). This IAg^7 is a poor antigen binder, and thus may allow leakage of autoreactive T cells from the thymus into the peripheral blood. This could account for the increased propensity to develop multiple organ-specific autoimmune diseases comprising the type 2 autoimmune polyglandular syndrome of which IMD is a part. The others include Addison disease, thyroid autoimmune disease especially Hashimoto, atrophic gastritis/pernicious anemia, vitiligo, and celiac disease. Further, poor expression of islet cell antigens by the thymus may similarly lead to defective eradication of potentially autoimmune-provoking $CD4^+$ T cells. Similarly, some studies suggest that class-I major histocompatibility complex (MHC) antigens may carry some relevant genetic information in addition to the class-II MHC, perhaps by analogy resulting in defective thymic ablation of $CD8^+$ cytotoxic T cells with high-affinity receptors for islet antigens.
4. However, even in normal persons, autoreactive T cells with low-affinity receptors capable of reactivity to self escape the thymus and need multiple fail-safe mechanisms to regulate them. Such mechanisms are inherently faulty in IMD. An active down-regulation by cytokine-rich natural killer T cells (NK-T cells) is one emerging mechanism mediated by regulatory T cells that in the mouse appear to have a $CD4^+/CD25^+$ (IL-2 receptor$^+$) phenotype and be responsive to TNF-α cytokine, or be mediated by suppressor macrophages. NOD mice have near absence of NK-T cells in their early life, and humans appear to be defective in them also. Further, in NOD mice, if not in patients with IMD, there is evidence that, once activated, T cells persist abnormally. In patients there is an association with a T cell apoptosis gene (CTLA-4) that suggests that a defect in expression of this inducible molecule would lead to persistence of T cells that become activated against self. Autoimmune destruction of pancreatic insulin-secreting β-cells is promoted by T helper responses of the Th1 phenotype, which promote T cell-mediated cytolysis, promoted in part by INF-λ. Experimental procedures that create Th2 responses to islet antigens are generally protective. The Th2 pathway promotes antibody-biased responses, sometimes leading to allergies, mediated in part by IL-4. Thus autoimmune responses that are deviated to the protective Th2 type may inhibit pathogenic autoimmune responses of the Th1 type.
5. Though the inductive event in the disease remains enigmatic, immunization by an environmental antigen with molecular homology to an islet cell protein could be one such trigger. This could happen if the environmental antigen were the P2-C protein of Coxsackie B virus, because GAD has an 18-amino-acid homologous segment. Alternatively, a viral infection of pancreatic β-cells could result in a Th1 response within the islets, which could, in turn, induce a secondary bystander autoimmune reaction involving release of sequestered antigens.
6. Much progress has been made in identifying the islet cell antigens targeted by islet cell autoimmunity. Autoimmunity to insulin itself appears early in the natural history of the disease. Islet cell reactivity as islet cell autoantibodies (ICA) detectable by indirect immunofluorescence microscopy comprise multiple antigenic determinants, such as those against the two tyrosine phosphatases IA-2 and IA-2β and against GAD_{65}, and more are anticipated. These autoantibodies react to native antigens by their conformational epitopes. In the case of the transmembrane tyrosine phosphatases, only the internal domains react, which

suggests that their involvement might be secondary. One or more of these antibodies begin to appear by the first year of life and most are evident if they are going to be, before age 3. Relatives and even persons from the general population who have two or more of these autoantibodies are at high risk of impending IMD, however those with only one antibody and none of the others are at only modest risk. Thus antigenic and epitopic spreading of the autoimmune response is usually a sign that the disease is progressive.

7. **Studies on T cell reactivity in IMD are hampered by the fact that autoreactive T cells once formed will leave the blood to migrate into the pancreatic islets resulting in "insulitis" lesions. Nevertheless, peripheral blood, proliferative T cell responses to in vitro exposure to the above islet cell antigens, and their peptides have been repeatedly reported, some with a Th1 to Th2 cytokine bias. In general, T cell reactivities to nonantigen-specific stimulations in IMD appear diminished in patients with IMD.**
8. **The long natural history, and the relatively low concordance of IMD in twin pairs affected by the disease, provides a window of opportunity for disease prevention and the anticipation that protective effects from the environment appear sufficient to prevent overt diabetes and even evidence of β-cell destruction. A number of ongoing studies in academia and industry are actively exploring many approaches. Past studies with immunosuppressant agents such as azathioprine and cyclosporin A in newly diagnosed patients have documented a delay in the completion of β-cell destruction. However, the beneficial effects eventually wear off in most patients, and these drugs have the inherent risks of lymphoma induction and of infections. Several general immunosuppressants attacking accessory molecular engagements in the T cell activation sequence are under study, while antigen-based immunization procedures to block the pathogenic immune responses or deviate them to the protective Th2 type have begun.**
9. **Pancreatic transplantations in late disease, often in context of companion kidney transplants, continue to improve, and have become clinically viable in selected cases, albeit successful transplants may be associated with a worsening microvascular disease such as retinopathy. The patients must of course be chronically maintained on immunosuppressant drugs to prevent rejection. In identical twins where one is the normal donor and the other the recipient, immunosuppressants are not required to prevent rejection, although diabetes may quickly reappear due to a recurrence of islet cell autoimmunity. Recent studies have held promise for islet cell transplantation: where a companion bone marrow transplantation has resulted in a stable chimera, sometimes long-term acceptance has been reported. Furthermore, the use of therapeutic antibodies that interfere with accessory molecule interactions such as B7 and CD28/CTLA or CD40 and CD40 ligand (CD154) has been reported to extend the life of engrafted tissues in primates. However the latter have led to unwelcome thrombotic phenomena, because platelets bear the marker also. At the time of writing, the first successes in human islet cell transplants have been reported by the group in Edmonton, Canada.[259]**

INTRODUCTION

Diabetes is a collection of more than sixty diseases, which result in elevated blood glucose levels. Diabetes is defined by the American Diabetes Association (ADA) Expert Panel[1] by replicate fasting blood glucose levels exceeding 126 mg/dl (7 mM) and/or 2-h peak glucose levels after an intravenous glucose tolerance test (IVGTT) (1.75 gms/kg up to 75 gms) of 200 mg/dl (11.1 mM) in the absence of symptoms, or a random glucose level exceeding 200 mg/dl in the presence of symptoms such as polyuria, polydipsia, and weight loss suggesting underlying insulinopenia. The above cutoff values of blood glucose levels are those that in the general U.S. population,[2] in Pima Indians,[3] and in Egyptians[4] were associated with subsequent complications such as diabetic retinopathy. Under the previous criteria, the peak cutoff value of 200 mg/dl did not equate in terms of long-term risk of complications with the cutoff fasting glucose value of 140 mg/dl being used, the latter abnormality usually representing a more advanced stage of the disease. The reduction in the diagnostic fasting level to 126 mg/dl is equivalent to the peak 200 mg/dl level 2 h after a standard oral glucose tolerance test (OGTT). The classification of diabetes by the ADA moved from a clinically based one that was oriented to the treatments given to the patients, to one that is based on an understanding of the pathogenesis. This became possible after our understanding of the genetic and metabolic bases of these diseases had sufficiently advanced. The ADA also acknowledged that intra- and interphysician variations in treatment choices for patients were high, with inconsistencies in treatments for diabetic patients often arising from the belief, by some, that insulin therapies conveyed a better prognosis than did the use of oral agents in type 2 diabetes. Further, it is evident that hyperglycemia, either by itself or associated with some metabolic abnormality, can be toxic to the insulin-secreting pancreatic β-cells, and that falling levels of insulin secretion can compound a diabetes resulting primarily from decreased insulin action. Whereas the occurrence of complications of diabetes is dependent upon the duration of the disease and the severity of the blood glucose elevations, diabetic outcomes are heavily influenced by associated hypertension, hyperlipidemia, and life-style factors such as smoking, insufficient exercise, and overweight. As we enter the third millennium, diabetes has emerged as one of the most serious public health issues of our time. The prevalence rates of type 2 diabetes have risen to epidemic proportions due to increasing obesity, longevity, and physical inactivity in the population given its considerable underlying genetic predispositions, especially in persons of African and Hispanic descents. Diabetes now affects increasing numbers of children also. Children with type 2 diabetes will have to live with their disease for longer than their diabetic forebears, and will develop higher rates of diabetic complications as a consequence. However type 1 diabetes is also becoming increasingly common in Western countries of the world, and affecting more young children than ever before.

DIABETES DEFINITION AND CLASSIFICATION

The definition of diabetes adopted by the ADA expert committee and their classification schema are shown in Tables 69-1 and 69-2, respectively. This chapter focuses on type 1 diabetes, specifically those forms of the disease that result primarily from a defect in the pancreatic islet's ability to secrete adequate amounts of insulin. As shown in Table 69-3, there are a number of diseases that constitute type 1 diabetes or should be considered in the differential diagnosis of type 1 diabetes. However, because the immune-mediated type is the most common, discussion of it will occupy the majority of this chapter. Discussion of maturity-onset diabetes of the young (MODY) by Taylor can be found in Chap. 68.

Immune-Mediated (Type 1) Diabetes (IMD)

On the basis of autoantibodies to islet cells (ICA), to insulin (IAA), or to islet cell proteins ($GAD_{65}A$, IA-2A, and IA-2βA), some 90 percent of children who present with type 1 diabetes have an immune-mediated pathogenesis, as do 60 percent of such Caucasian adults.[5] Further, as many as 20 percent of Caucasian adults diagnosed to have diabetes for the first time, are found to be autoantibody positive. The natural history of IMD usually begins with autoantibody evidence of islet cell autoimmunity during

Table 69-1 Etiological Classification of Diabetes Mellitus

I. Type 1 diabetes* (β-cell destruction, usually leading to absolute insulin deficiency)
- A. Immune-mediated
- B. Idiopathic

II. Type 2 diabetes* (may range from predominantly insulin resistance with relative insulin deficiency to predominantly secretory defect with insulin resistance)

III. Other specific types
- A. Genetic defects of β-cell function
  1. Chromosome 12, HNF-1α (formerly MODY-3)
  2. Chromosome 7, glucokinase (formerly MODY-2)
  3. Chromosome 20, HNF-4α (formerly MODY-1)
  4. Mitochondrial DNA
  5. Other
- B. Genetic defects in insulin action
  1. Type A insulin resistance
  2. Leprechaunism
  3. Rabson-Mendenhall syndrome
  4. Lipoatrophic diabetes
  5. Others
- C. Diseases of the exocrine pancreas
  1. Pancreatitis
  2. Trauma/pancreatectomy
  3. Neoplasia
  4. Cystic fibrosis
  5. Hemochromatosis
  6. Fibrocalculous pancreatopathy
  7. Others
- D. Endocrinopathies
  1. Acromegaly
  2. Cushing syndrome
  3. Glucagonoma
  4. Pheochromocytoma
  5. Hyperthyroidism
  6. Somatostatinoma
  7. Aldosteronoma
  8. Others
- E. Drug- or chemical-induced
  1. Vacor
  2. Pentamidine
  3. Nicotinic acid
  4. Glucocorticoids
  5. Thyroid hormone
  6. Diazoxide
  7. β-Adrenergic agonists
  8. Thiazides
  9. Dilantin
  10. α-Interferon
  11. Others
- F. Infections
  1. Congenital rubella
  2. Cytomegalovirus
  3. Others
- G. Uncommon forms of immune-mediated diabetes
  1. "Stiff man" syndrome
  2. Anti-insulin receptor antibodies
  3. Others
- H. Other genetic syndromes sometimes associated with diabetes
  1. Down syndrome
  2. Klinefelter syndrome
  3. Turner syndrome
  4. Wolfram syndrome
  5. Friedreich ataxia
  6. Huntington chorea
  7. Lawrence Moon Beidel syndrome
  8. Myotonic dystrophy
  9. Porphyria*
  10. Prader-Willi syndrome
  11. Others

IV. Gestational diabetes mellitus (GDM)

*Patients with any form of diabetes may require insulin treatment at some stage of their disease. Such use of insulin does not, of itself, classify the patient.

Reproduced with permission from *Diabetes Care* 20(7):1053, 1998.

Table 69-2 Criteria for the Diagnosis of Diabetes Mellitus

1. Symptoms of diabetes plus casual plasma glucose concentration >200 mg/dl (11.1 mM). Casual is defined as any time of day without regard to time since last meal. The classic symptoms of diabetes include polyuria, polydipsia, and unexplained weight loss.

or

2. FPG* ≥126 mg/dl (7.0 mM). Fasting is defined as no caloric intake for at least 8 h.

or

3. 2h PG ≥200 mg/dl during an OGTT†. The test should be performed as described by WHO,[248] using a glucose load containing the equivalent of 75 g anhydrous glucose dissolved in water.

In the absence of unequivocal hyperglycemia with acute metabolic decompensation, these criteria should be confirmed by repeat testing on a different day. The third measure (OGTT) is not recommended for routine clinical use.

*Fasting Plasma Glucose
†Oral Glucose Tolerance Test

infancy, while progression of the disease to a clinically apparent outcome thereafter is quite variable. IMD results from the chronic autoimmune destruction of pancreatic β-cells in genetically prone individuals, as strongly influenced by the environment.[6] IMD is an incurable disease of children and adults that is increasing in incidence in Western countries, especially in very young children.

Epidemiological studies indicate that the natural history of IMD begins as an islet cell autoimmunity, usually during infancy and early childhood, recognizable by autoantibodies to IAA and to glutamic acid decarboxylase ($GAD_{65}A$), often appearing from 9 to 18 months of age.[7] Autoantibodies to tyrosine phosphatase, insulinoma antigen-2 (IA-2A), and IA-2βA can appear at the same time as $GAD_{65}A$ and IAA, but they often appear after IAA and $GAD_{65}A$. Destruction of the pancreatic β-cells in human and nonobese diabetic (NOD) mouse IMD is mediated through cellular immune mechanisms and a biased T helper-1 (Th1) immune pathway. Cytotoxic $CD8^+$ T cells recognize the targeted antigens of the islet cells presented in the context of class I MHC and destroy them. Cytotoxic $CD4^+$ T cells reacting to islet cell antigens in context of class II MHC may participate. It is, however, probably quite normal for $CD8^+$ T cells with low affinity receptors to islet cell antigen 9 mer peptides to escape ablation in the thymus, and enter the circulation. Whereas such autoreactive $CD8^+$ T cells are regulated in the periphery, they are capable of inducing β-cell damage and IMD only if activated by specific $CD4^+$ T helper cells in an IMD-prone individual who has multiple genetic defects in T cell immunoregulation (Fig. 69-1). The *inductive event(s)* that initiate islet cell inflammation (insulitis)

Table 69-3 Differential Diagnoses in Type 1 Diabetes

- Immune-mediated diabetes (IMD)
- Stiff man syndrome
- Transient neonatal diabetes
- Pancreatic diseases; hemochromatosis, cystic fibrosis, pancreatitis, pancreatectomy, iron overload after multiple blood transfusions for hemoglobinopathies
- Diabetes insipidus, diabetes mellitus, optic atrophy, deafness (DIDMOAD), and other mitochondrial forms of diabetes
- Pancreatic agenesis/dystrophy
- Genetic defects affecting insulin secretion: familial hyperproinsulinemia, MODY 1–6
- African diabetes (type 1.5)
- Long-standing type 2 diabetes

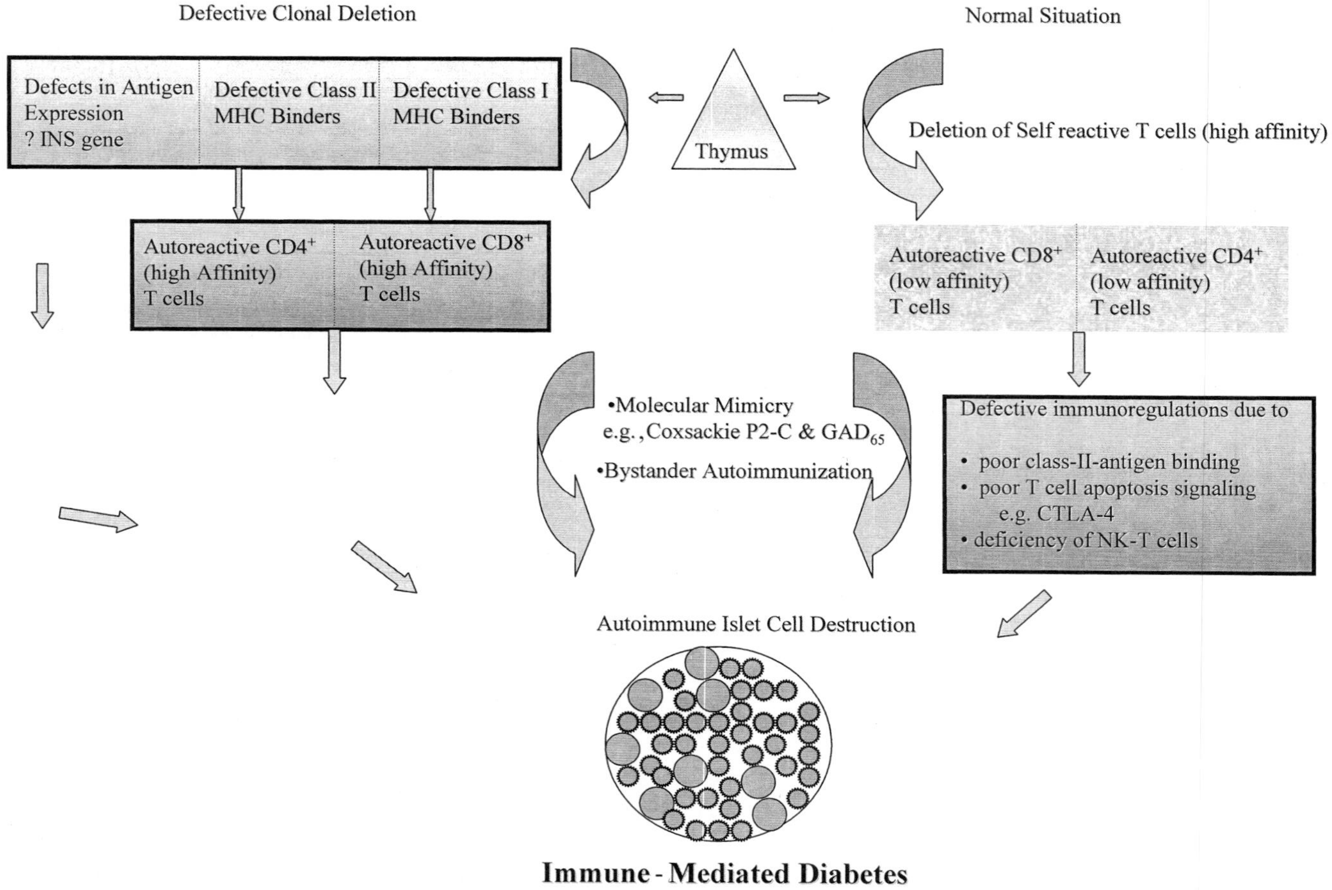

Defective Clonal Deletion

Normal Situation

Defects in Antigen Expression ? INS gene

Defective Class II MHC Binders

Defective Class I MHC Binders

Thymus

Deletion of Self reactive T cells (high affinity)

Autoreactive CD4+ (high Affinity) T cells

Autoreactive CD8+ (high Affinity) T cells

Autoreactive CD8+ (low affinity) T cells

Autoreactive CD4+ (low affinity) T cells

•Molecular Mimicry e.g., Coxsackie P2-C & GAD_{65}

•Bystander Autoimmunization

Defective immunoregulations due to

- poor class-II-antigen binding
- poor T cell apoptosis signaling e.g. CTLA-4
- deficiency of NK-T cells

Autoimmune Islet Cell Destruction

Immune - Mediated Diabetes

Fig. 69-1 The pathogenesis of immune-mediated (type 1) diabetes (IMD). The bold boxes indicate inherited/acquired defects in IMD that contribute to the pathogenesis. Escape from ablation of potentially autoreactive helper/cytotoxic T cells with high-affinity receptors for islet cell antigens can occur because of defective expression of these antigens in the thymus, which can become pathogenic due to molecular mimicry or by bystander autoactivation by viral infections. Further, escape of T cells with low-affinity receptors for islet cells can occur even in normal persons, and become activated in the periphery by these same mechanisms in persons inherently susceptible to IMD because of multiple defects in immunoregulation. For details refer to accompanying text.

and maintain autoimmune β-cell ablation leading to clinical diabetes remain poorly understood. A molecular mimicry mechanism, such as through the structural homology between the P2-C protein of Coxsackie B viruses and GAD_{65} (Fig. 69-2),[8] is one possible mechanism. Immunization against the P2-C protein of the virus thus could initiate an islet attack because of antigenic crossreactivity with GAD. Another possible mechanism is through "bystander" activation where viral infections of the islets (e.g., by Coxsackie B4) result in the incursion of activated macrophages and Th1 cells and their released cytokines, in turn triggering T cell activation for self antigens released during β-cell lysis.[9]

Metabolic Derangements of Type 1 Diabetes. As the pancreatic β-cell mass declines in an islet cell autoantibody (ICA) positive person, the first metabolic abnormality discernible is a *decline in the first phase of insulin release* (FPIR) to an IVGTT.[10] The 1 min plus 3 min level after a 3- to 4-min infusion of glucose at 0.5 gms/kg rises abruptly in normal children at about 8 years of age, perhaps coincident with the onset of adrenal puberty or adrenarche.[11] In the relatives and children from the general population with positive ICA, a decline in the FPIR is a strong predictive marker of impending diabetes.[5,11,12] Subsequently, there is a decline in the ability to keep the 2-h, post-OGTT glucose level

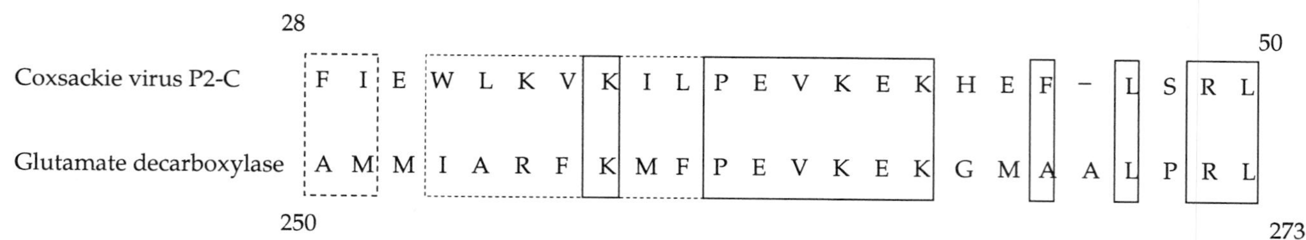

Fig. 69-2 Sequence homology between Coxsackie virus and human GAD_{65}. The solid lines denote identical amino acid residues. Dashed lines denote amino acid residues with similar charge, polarity, or hydrophobicity. The numbers refer to the number of amino acid residues from the N-terminus of each protein.

below 200 mg/dl. Often later, there is a rise in the fasting glucose levels. Transient insulin resistance is also seen which may be due to raised levels of free fatty acids (FFAs) from uncontrolled lipolysis[13] and decreased levels of hepatic glucokinase and GLUT 4 glucose transporters in adipocytes.[14–16] Later still, symptomatic diabetes manifests itself. Once insulin replacement therapy begins, there is usually some recovery in the patient's ability to secrete insulin (the "honeymoon" period), but within months and occasionally years, this partial recovery in endogenous insulin secretion ultimately fails. Initially, the glucagon-secreting cells within the pancreatic islets are relatively preserved, with excessive secretion of glucagon after protein meals.[17] These elevated glucagon levels exacerbate the effects of the insulin deficiency and promote lipolysis and ketoacidemia, effects that can be partially reversed acutely, by an infusion of somatostatin.[18] This occurs at a time when neoislet formation is seen, with regenerated islets having increased numbers of cells secreting glucagon or pancreatic polypeptide. However, over time there is continued loss of islets with eventual glucagon deficiency, making the patients susceptible to insulin-induced hypoglycemia in established, long-standing IMD.[19,20] Insulin is the hormone of "feasting," promoting deposition of ingested nutrients into body stores and having multiple anabolic effects in tissues. Insulin deficiency thus induces a starvation-like state, associated with (a) excessive hepatic and renal gluconeogenesis, (b) decreased peripheral utilization of glucose with glycosuria and loss of water and sodium salts, (c) proteolysis in muscle liberating amino acids such as alanine and glutamine for gluconeogenesis,[21–23] and (d) uncontrolled lipolysis with rapid mobilization of triglycerides with increased very low density type lipoprotein (VLDL) and fatty acids with formation of ketone bodies. Specifically, hepatic glucokinase levels fall with insulinopenia, synthesis of hepatic triglyceride and glycogen levels decline, malonyl CoA falls and thereby carnitine palmitoyltransferase-I levels rise, promoting the transport of fatty acyl CoA into mitochondria and the formation of acetyl CoA.[24–26] In the liver, acetyl CoA is converted into β-hydroxybutyrate and acetoacetate (in a proportion that depends upon the prevailing redox state), which provide additional fuel substrates for muscle and brain.[23,27,28] Lipoprotein lipases are also inactivated, leading to reduced hydrolysis of triglycerides which may turn the serum milky with increased VLDL characteristic of the type 4 lipemic phenotype.[29–31] A milky serum is characteristic of diabetes onset in NOD mice.

Autoantigens and Autoantibodies. The Doniach group in London first reported ICA in patients with autoimmune polyglandular syndromes (APSs),[32] especially in those with APS type 1 (APS-1),[33] even though such patients did not often develop diabetes. Lendrum and colleagues, having failed to find serological evidence for an autoimmune basis for chronic pancreatitis, did succeed in finding ICA detectable by indirect immunofluorescence in patients with IMD, while islet cell surface autoantibodies and reactive peripheral blood T cells were also reported.[34,35] Over the years that followed, the ICA finding in U.S. patients was confirmed but much lower frequencies of ICA were found among African American diabetic patients.[36] Insulin autoantibodies (IAA) were discovered in patients with IMD before their first dose of insulin had been received.[37] Their presence together with ICA denoted a group of nondiabetic relatives of probands with IMD that were at high risk for IMD themselves.[38] Insulin itself is not an ICA antigen. Subsequently, much of the antigenic nature of this ICA reactivity was clarified. It was recognized that many patients with "stiff man" syndrome, who were prone to develop IMD, also had ICA and autoantibodies to GAD_{65}. These GAD autoantibodies penetrated the blood brain barrier and found high concentrations of GAD in the cerebellum.[39] Lower levels of the inhibitory neurotransmitter gamma amino benzoic acid (GABA) resulted in cerebellar dysfunction, with involuntary fixation of motor movements with stiffness. That GAD was the antigen that accounted for the 64-kDa islet cell protein previously discovered by Baekkeskov to react with autoantibodies in IMD, was later confirmed by the same investigator.[40] Antibodies to recombinant GAD_{65} and GAD_{67} in IMD were soon reported.[41] The autoantibodies reacted to the antigens by three-dimensional conformational rather than linear epitopes, and therefore with native rather than denatured islet cell antigens. Thus, they were best detected by liquid-phase assays such as radioimmunoassay, rather than by ELISA. In stiff man syndrome, the predominant GAD autoantibodies reacted with linear epitopes. It became known that besides islet cell 64-kDa proteins, autoantibodies in the sera of IMD patients also precipitated islet cell proteins of 50, 40, and 37 kDa.[42] The next islet cell antigen discovered was one of the two-dozen tyrosine phosphatases expressed in islet cells, insulinoma antigen-2 (IA-2).[43] This antigen shared structural homologies with the ICA-512 antigen already reported.[44] A second tyrosine phosphatase named IA-2β was discovered next.[45] These additional tyrosine phosphatase antigens allowed for the matching of the islet cell proteins previously identifiable only by their molecular weights. Thus GAD_{65} and its tryptic fragment explained the 64- and 50-kDa proteins, while tryptic fragments of IA-2 and IA-2β were identical with the 40-kDa and the 37-kDa islet-precipitable proteins, respectively.[46] The tyrosine phosphatases are a family of transmembrane enzymes, of which only these two expressed by the pancreatic islets react with IMD autoantibodies. The reactivity is almost exclusively with the internal domains of these molecules, suggesting that they often arise as a consequence of islet cell damage from autoimmunity. Antibodies to IA-2 crossreact with those of IA-2β in about 50 percent of the patients' sera. Some unusual patient sera, however, react exclusively with IA-2β. The question of why only these two members of the tyrosine phosphatase family are targets of islet cell autoimmunity has been answered by the finding that they are relatively resistant to proteolytic enzymatic digestion, and once released from islet cells after their lysis, are insoluble and thus become better antigens for autoimmunization, than those that remain soluble and are more rapidly digested.[47] Recently, another antigen of 38-kDa size (GLIMA) was added to the islet cell group, although only a minority of patients' sera reacts to it.[48] More islet cell autoantigens yet are likely to be discovered. The detection of islet cell autoantibodies is useful for diagnosis of IMD from diabetes of other causes, and can be used to predict onset of diabetes months to years before onset of the clinical disease[5,12,49,50] in nondiabetic relatives of probands with IMD, and even in the general population.[51] Importantly, the clinical onset of the disease is often long preceded by the appearance of autoantibodies reactive to islet cells (ICA)[50] and to insulin,[38] as independent age-related variables in predicting a diabetic outcome.[52] ICA also show a strong tendency to disappear after onset of diabetes when all β-cells are destroyed.[53,54] Similar antibodies (IAA and GADA) have been reported in NOD mice but with much less consistency, unless detected as part of a recall response following exogenous immunization by those antigens, and at lower titers than seen in patients. The presence of multiple autoantibodies strikingly increases the risk of diabetes, whereas the presence of one in the absence of all the others denotes only a modestly increased risk.[5,12] The principle at work is one of antigenic epitope spreading in a sustained or accelerated autoimmune attack.[55] Besides autoimmunity to islet cell autoantigens, patients with IMD are subject to other autoimmunities. Thus IMD is a component of the autoimmune polyglandular syndromes, being unusual in APS-1, but common in APS-2 and APS-3.[33] Accordingly, patients with IMD have high rates of thyroid autoimmunity, especially if they are female,[56] and are at risk for Addison disease,[56] atrophic gastritis,[57] pernicious anemia,[58] celiac disease,[59] and vitiligo.[60] The antigens involved are shown in Table 69-4.

Antigen-Specific Cellular Immunity. Autoreactive T cells that develop in impending IMD, probably home to the pancreatic islets, where they become a component of the evolving insulitis lesions. Thus, circulating autoreactive T cells would be expected to be

Table 69-4 Autoantibody Reactive Autoantigens in Patients with Immune-Mediated (Type 1) Diabetes

IMD Specific:	Autoantibodies	References
		93
ICA Group	$GAD_{65} > GAD_{67}$	67
	IA-2	43
	IA-2β	45
	?GLIMA-38	48
Other	IAA	37, 249
	?Insulin receptors	250
	?GLUT-2	251
Associated diseases		
Hashimoto	Peroxidase, thyroglobulin	252
Graves	TSH receptors	253
Atrophic gastritis	H^+K^+ ATPase	254
Pernicious anemia	Gastrin receptors/Intrinsic factor	255
Addison	21-hydroxylase	256, 257
Vitiligo	Tyrosinase ? Others	60
Celiac	Transglutaminase	258

relatively sparse in impending IMD. Nevertheless, antigen-specific T cells, as identifiable through prolonged in vitro cultures in the presence of purified or recombinant islet cell autoantigens, such as GAD_{65}[61] and IA-2,[62] have been reported. In fact, reactivity to a large number of autoantigens has been reported in both human and murine diabetes.[63] T cell proliferative responses to insulin and GAD_{65}, and more generally to islet extracts, have been repeatedly reported both in patients with IMD[64,65] and NOD mice.[66–68] However, both in humans and NOD mice, reports of spontaneous proliferative responses have been difficult to reproduce and validate, probably because of the relative paucity of autoreactive T cells in peripheral blood samples, and the ready contamination of recombinant antigens by lymphotoxin or lipopolysaccharide (LPS) that can by itself produce proliferative responses even when present in trace amounts. Thus, a number of laboratories have reported T cell reactivities in diabetic patients against GAD and IA-2 and their peptides with variable results.[62,64,69–74] Cellular proliferative responses to GAD_{65} determinants were marked in 25 percent of 16 newly diagnosed IMD patients in one early study, but in none of the 13 healthy control subjects. A set of overlapping synthetic GAD_{65} peptides was used to study the most reactive T cell determinants in individuals at increased risk for IMD, that is, autoantibody-positive, first-degree relatives of IMD patients. Elevated in vitro T cell responses were observed to GAD_{65} peptides (amino acid 247 to 266 and amino acid 260 to 279) in newly diagnosed diabetic patients and in nondiabetic, autoantibody-positive, at-risk relatives of IMD patients. In a recent study, the epitope spanning 805 to 820 amino acid elicited maximum T cell responses in at-risk relatives, out of a total of 68 overlapping synthetic peptides encompassing the intracytoplasmic domain of IA-2[75] that were tested. T cell responses to peptide epitopes have also been shown to diversify throughout the course of the disease. These T cell responses may expand from a nested set of peptides, spreading out to include many other peptide regions. Similar phenomena have been observed in NOD mice. Tisch et al.[68] presented T cell and antibody data using various autoantigens in IMD. They concluded that immune responses were initially targeted toward the autoantigen GAD, followed by intermolecular spreading resulting in immune responses to other antigens (carboxypeptidase H, heat-shock protein). Similarly, immune responses to GAD_{65} in IMD were reported, which diversified over time to a panel of peptide epitopes derived from human GAD_{65}.[67] It was also shown that responses to multiple peptides could be blocked by inducing early tolerance to the initially autoreactive peptides. Both of these studies presented evidence that inducing tolerance early to the epitopes involved in the autoimmune process could reduce the severity of insulitis and the incidence of diabetes. This documented that progression to full-blown IMD was largely dependent on a progressive diversification of immune responses to include other protein/peptide autoantigens. This epitope-spreading phenomenon is directly related to the extent that Th1 cells are present in the inflammatory lesion, which have varied effects on antigen-presenting cells (APC), including the up-regulation of antigen processing and peptide presentation.[76] Cytokines released by T cells up-regulate cathepsins and MHC proteins in APCs, allowing for more stringent processing and presentation of the additional T cell epitopes, thus leading to epitope spreading. In doing so, a more diverse repertoire of T cells becomes activated coincident with an accelerated pace of destruction of the targeted islet cells. At this point, activated T cells reacting with multiple β-cell determinants continue to induce β-cell death, resulting in a positive feedback loop (early pathogenesis). However in established diabetes, the loss of the majority of β-cell mass resulting in associated loss of GAD_{65} and other antigens results, in turn, in the inactivation of T cells due to the loss of the peptide antigens driving the response. Thus antigenic/epitopic spreading is an undesirable phenomenon associated with progression in autoimmune diseases like IMD.

Pathology. That some patients presenting with diabetes had inflammatory lesions within their islets was probably first described by Von Meyenburg.[77] However, Gepts[78] reported that the pancreases of the majority of patients with type 1 disease but not type 2 disease had these lesions. He coined the term *insulitis*. Insulitis lesions are typically patchy in distribution. There is an increase in class I MHC expression of the islet cells, which express IFN-α and other cytokines,[79] while the infiltrate includes many $CD8^+$ T cells, suggesting that a cell-mediated cytolysis is taking place. In human and NOD insulitis, infiltrates of T cells, which express the Th1 cytokine IFN-λ, are present. One group has suggested that the T cells of such lesions have biased receptor variable gene repertoire usage in their T cell receptor (TCR) $\alpha\beta$ chain dimers, suggesting that they had been expanded by a superantigen.[80] Superantigens are those viral or bacterial antigens that bind to the exterior of many MHC molecules and outside of their binding clefts, inducing large numbers of them to expand and secrete cytokines. A local version of "toxic shock" syndrome (which results from a widespread activation of T cells bearing HLA-A2, from antigens released from staphylococci-infected tampons), was suggested by these authors. This group went on to report that a human endogenous retrovirus of the HERV-K10 family could have been responsible through expression of its envelope protein,[81] but these data could not be duplicated.[82]

Nature versus Nurture in IMD. IMD results from a chronic autoimmune destruction of pancreatic β-cells in genetically prone individuals, which is strongly influenced by the environment.[6] The rapidly increasing incidence of IMD in Western countries can only be explained by the environment and not by an accumulation of IMD predisposition genes. In identical twins affected by IMD, the frequency of discordance is relatively high at 2 of every 3 twin pairs, suggesting that there are strong environmental influences at work.[83] These influences are likely to be predominantly the removal of factors that are protective.[6] Such an environmental influence must be expressed in early life to be effective, because islet cell autoimmunity often begins then. The worldwide incidence rates vary widely, being highest in industrialized nations and lowest in countries in the tropics where infectious diseases and parasites abound.[84] BioBreeding (BB) rats and NOD mice, when reared in gnotobiotic environments, have increased, rather than decreased, frequencies of diabetes, whereas a plethora of immunization events in NOD mice can lower their diabetes rates.[85] Although the possible factors that dictate induction of islet cell autoimmunity in a genetically susceptible person are unknown, viruses remain the leading candidates through mechanisms of molecular mimicry or through bystander activation.

Genetic Defects and T Cell Immuno-Dysregulation. Individuals with IMD have inherited a number of quantitative trait loci (QTL) that encode protective and predisposing alleles which have exceeded the net genetic threshold required to predispose them to the disease. However, this genetic threshold (penetrance) is dependent in turn on chance interactions with greater net predisposing than protective environmental forces. The *multiple genetic influences* in IMD comprise a major effect from DR/DQ genotypes (<50 percent), coupled to several other QTLs with minor influences. All of the latter minor-influence QTLs are not obligatory genetic elements themselves, but they collectively conspire to create additive influences on the genetic threshold. Siblings develop IMD (5 percent) at about fifteenfold greater frequency than persons in the general population (1:250 to 300), or at a λs value of 15 (see Chap. 6). The HLA predisposition to IMD is encoded by *cis* and *trans* complementation DQA1*/DQB1* heterodimers which have an arginine at residue 52 of the A chain and a neutral amino acid (DQB1*0302, *0201) rather than a charged aspartic acid at residue 57 of the B chain (DQB1*0602/3 and DQB1*0301),[86] as modified by DRB1*04 subtypes (*0401 and 5 are susceptible and *0403 and 6 are resistant types)[87] in the HLA genotype. Further, HLA-DP alleles have also been implicated, even though they show a considerable recombination frequency from the closely linked DR/DQ loci.[88] Remarkably, NOD mice have one class II MHC (I-A) that is unique in lacking an aspartic acid at residue 57 of its B chain also. This unique I-A^{g7} is a recombinant of the IA from the d haplotype with that of the b haplotype. Like other mice of b haplotypes, the NOD encodes no IE A chain and thus can express no IE dimers. Murine MHC I-As share structural homologies with human DQs, as do their IEs with human DRs. Congenic NOD mice that have been made to express the IE of b are protected from diabetes,[89] while the substitution of a charged histidine for a proline at position 56 and a serine for aspartate at position 57 of the I-A^{g7} B chain also protects the NOD from diabetes.[89] Recent studies have suggested that the NOD MHC class II molecule, I-A^{g7}, is a poor antigenic peptide binder, forming loose complexes with peptide antigens because of its low affinities for them.[90] Thus potentially autoactive $CD4^+$ T cells cannot bind with sufficient affinity to islet autoantigens expressed in the thymus, to be destroyed before they reach the periphery. Further, they cannot be eradicated efficiently in the periphery either once they get there. Others have suggested that it is promiscuous antigenic binding to IMD-prone HLA-DQ that promotes islet cell autoimmunity,[91] which could permit the creation and defective regulation of autoreactive $CD4^+$ T cells in the periphery. This could be the reason that mice bearing the I-A^{g7} MHC have an increased complement of T cells involved in the β-cell autoimmunity leading to diabetes.[92] A combination of these pathogenic effects might be plausible, because patients with IMD are only subject to a finite number of autoimmunities (to the thyroid, gastric mucosa, adrenal cortex, intestinal epithelia, melanocytes)[36,93] and they do not react globally to all self antigens that promote autoimmune responses in other disease states. That class I MHC (HLA-A24 in Japanese IMD) also encodes susceptibility to IMD is perhaps consistent with the $CD8^+$ T cell-mediated cytolysis mechanism. However, defective thymic ablation of autoreactive $CD8^+$ T cells with high-affinity receptors for islet cell autoantigens in context of the risk alleles of class-I MHC might similarly occur.[94] Other genes involved include the variable number of tandem repeat (VNTR) alleles 5′ to the insulin (INS) gene on chromosome 11p15, where the protective class III alleles (>200 repeats) are associated with increased expression of insulin in the thymus and thus theoretically lead to a more efficient eradication of insulin autoreactive T cells.[95,96] There are also CTLA-4 gene polymorphisms on chromosome 2q that are associated with IMD. CTLA-4 is an induced accessory molecule that is expressed on activated T cells. It interacts with B 7.2 expressed by antigen-presenting macrophages, signaling apoptosis of T cells that become activated as part of an immune response, and thereby confining the response. The NOD mouse has an enlarged lymphoid mass because its T cells are resistant to apoptosis,[97] as is true in the CTLA-4 knockout mice, which readily develop lymphocytic organ infiltrates like the NOD mice. These genes collectively affect the general ability to be tolerant to "self" antigens. Another susceptibility locus, (the IDDM 4) in the genomic interval on chromosome 11q13, harbors the high-affinity IgE Fc receptor gene that has been linked to atopy and asthma, which are inherent Th2 responses that may help to protect individuals against the development of anti-islet Th1 responses and thereby protect against IMD. In our clinical experience, persons with an allergic diathesis do appear to have low frequencies of IMD. There are other genomic intervals associated with or linked to IMD that have been putatively mapped, but these mostly lack plausible candidate genes in the contained DNA region, and pathogenic mechanisms for them cannot yet be offered, even if they become unambiguously confirmed. The NOD mouse, however, has been subjected to extensive genetic mapping studies, in the hopes that genomic intervals harboring susceptibility or protective genes which are syntenic to the humans will be discovered, thus hastening the identification of equivalent defective genes.[98] However, it is equally likely that different genetic lesions will be discovered that encode functional defects that result in similar disturbances in immunoregulation in the two species. If so, then genetic synteny with NOD mice will not help to locate the human IMD genes. We find that patients, who are developing or have developed IMD, have T cells that are deficient in their abilities to secrete INF-λ and IL-4, a defect that directly correlates with low numbers of circulating natural killer-T (NK-T) cells, which are also deficient in these cytokines. These findings are in concert with those of another group studying NOD mice, who suggest that it is the secretion of INF-λ rather than IL-4 by NK-T cells that is critical to the maintenance of T cell tolerance to self.[99] In NOD mice, there is a profound deficiency of NK-T cells arising from early life and experimental transfers of these cells from F1 hybrid mice, which are not diabetes-prone, have been shown to protect the NOD mice if they become stable chimeras.[100]

The Environment. In genetically identical NOD mice, complete concordance for diabetes is never fully achieved, albeit all NOD mice have marked insulitis lesions but quite variable degrees of associated islet cell destruction. In addition, a large number of immunization events result in lowered diabetes rates.[101,102] Because of this, some investigators have actually argued against the notion that the NOD mouse is a useful model for testing preventive strategies to be tried in humans.[85] It can be argued, conversely, that successes in diabetes prevention in NOD mice provide exciting clinical opportunities, because they may prove as effective in man as in mouse. As mentioned above, in identical human twins affected by IMD, concordance for diabetes, or even islet cell autoimmunity, is the exception rather than the rule, clearly documenting the important role of the environment.[83] Further, whereas the large geographic disparities in the incidence rates of IMD probably have strong genetic bases,[103–105] it can be argued that it is the temperate zones of the world, where infectious and parasitic diseases are uncommon, that harbor populations with the highest frequencies of IMD, while those in the tropical areas have the lowest frequencies. Admittedly, African people everywhere have low incidence rates of IMD,[36] except where there has been a high rate of Caucasian genetic admixture. Several studies have reported a viral etiology associated with IMD.[8,106] The disease pathogenesis may involve multiple factors including the genetics of the host, strain of the virus, activation status of the autoreactive T cells, up-regulation of pancreatic MHC class I antigens, molecular mimicry between viral and β-cell epitopes, and direct islet cell destruction by viral cytolysis. Viruses, as one of the environmental factors affecting the induction of IMD, may act as triggering agents of autoimmunity or as primary injurious agents, which directly damage pancreatic β-cells (Fig. 69-1). Presumably, direct β-cell damage by chemicals, such as the rodenticide Vacor, might also do this.

Moreover, direct evidence for virus-induced diabetes largely comes from experiments in animals.[107] Several studies in humans also point to viruses as triggers of the disease.[106,108,109] These studies suggest that viruses play an important role in the pathogenesis of diabetes on the basis of:

- The presence of viral-specific antigens in the islets of Langerhans and destruction of β-cells in the pancreas of diabetic patients.[110]
- The presence of viral antibodies with rising titers in paired sera from newly diagnosed IMD patients.[111]
- The high frequency of Coxsackie B virus-specific IgM antibody in newly identified diabetic children.[112]
- β-Cell damage in children who died of overwhelming viral infections.[109]
- The isolation of viruses from patients with acute-onset diabetes and the demonstration that these isolated viruses can cause diabetes in mice.[113]
- The association of antibody production with certain viral infections, for example, congenital rubella and persistent cytomegalovirus infection.[114]
- Secretion of INF-γ by β-cells undergoing autoimmune destruction.

Coxsackie B virus and rubella virus have been linked with IMD and, in a few instances, Coxsackie B virus has even been isolated from pancreatic tissues of individuals with acute IMD. Inoculation of this virus into certain strains of mice but not others then produced IMD, fulfilling Koch's postulates.[113] The possibility that viruses might cause some cases of IMD by infecting and directly destroying pancreatic β-cells has received considerable attention. However, it was difficult to demonstrate in vivo that viruses replicate in human β-cells and/or produce diabetes in humans. An in vitro system was therefore developed to determine whether viruses are capable of destroying human β-cells in culture.[115,116] By this method, it was clearly shown that several common human viruses, including mumps virus, Coxsackie B_3 virus,[115] Coxsackie B_4 virus,[117] and reovirus type 3,[118] could infect human β-cells. In addition it was shown by radioimmunoassay that the infection markedly decreased the insulin content of the β-cells. A strong correlation was found between the presence of the CMV genome in the peripheral blood leukocytes and the islet cell autoantibodies in the sera from diabetic patients.[119] About 15 percent of newly diagnosed IMD patients have been reported to have persistent CMV infections, whereas an autopsy study of patients who died with CMV infections showed some with insulitis lesions. Furthermore, it has been proposed that a molecular mimicry between protein 2C (p2-C) of Coxsackie virus B_4 and the autoantigen GAD_{65} may play a role in pathogenesis of IMD. Kaufman et al.[120] and Vreugdenhil et al.[106] showed that the amino acid sequence of p2C shares a striking homology with a sequence in GAD_{65} (PEVKEK) and is highly conserved in Coxsackie virus B_4 isolates, as well as in other viruses of the subgroup of Coxsackie B-like viruses[8] as shown in Fig. 69-2. These are the most prevalent enteroviruses and therefore the exposure to the mimicry motif should be a frequent event throughout life. Furthermore, they suggested that molecular mimicry might be limited to the HLA-DR3 subpopulation of the IMD patients. In addition, this specific region of GAD_{65} contains a T cell epitope involved in the GAD cellular autoimmunity in humans with IMD[61] and this region is an early target of the cellular immunity in NOD mice.[67,68]

Increasing Incidence Rates of IMD May Be Due to Diminished Natural Stimuli of Innate Immunity. In industrialized countries, incidence rates of IMD are rising, affecting younger children than ever before.[121] Either environmental triggers of the disease are more pervasive now than in the past, with increasing numbers of susceptible persons coming in contact with them, or else protective environmental influences are becoming lost with time. The latter possibility is probably more likely.[122] Increased and earlier consumption of cow's milk[123] is another factor believed be important by some[124] but viewed more skeptically by others.[125] One report invokes the use of childhood vaccines to explain the increased incidence in IMD.[126] The author found that vaccination of NOD mice with DPT before 8 weeks of life decreased the incidence of diabetes, while it increased the incidence when given after 8 weeks of life. Our own findings are not in accord with this. We find that the vaccine promotes strong Th2 responses and protects NOD mice from diabetes. Classen proposed recently that *Haemophilus influenzae* type B vaccine is also associated with an increased incidence of diabetes.[127] An alternative and more attractive hypothesis is that, when environmental protective factors become less prevalent, then the incidence of IMD rises. NOD mice and BB rats have the highest rates of diabetes when they have been kept in sterile conditions, suggesting that "natural" immunizations from the environment can be protective. Asian Indians living in the Punjab, in India have low incidence rates of IMD, but when they move to Birmingham, England (Kochupillai, personal communication) and raise their families there, then their rates of diabetes approach those of the English. In Finns, it is speculated that control of the fish tapeworm, *Diphyllobothrium latum* in the 1960s occurred around the time that the incidence rates of type 1 diabetes began to rise dramatically (Semil, personal communication).

Cell-Mediated Immunity in IMD. IMD is a prototypic autoimmune disease of NOD mice and man, which proceeds as a chronic inflammatory process within the pancreatic islets, until sufficient numbers of β-cells are lost to result in an absolute insulin deficiency and diabetes. The destructive phase of the insulitis process may occur relatively late in the process. This cell-mediated pathological response in mice is mediated through T helper cells of Th1 phenotype. The discovery of polarized subsets of $CD4^+$ T cells that differ in their cytokine secretion patterns and effector functions has provided a basis for understanding the diversity of T-cell-dependent immune responses.[128] T helper (Th) subsets can be defined by their functions, cytokine profiles, and antigenic phenotypes into at least 2 types. Th1 cells promote delayed hypersensitivity reactions and cell-mediated cytolysis. They produce IL-2, TNF-α and -β, and IFN-λ and -α. They are driven by macrophage-secreted IL-12 and they express high-affinity IL-12 receptors, a functional ligand for P and E selectin, and selective (CXCR3 and CCR5) chemokine receptors. Th2 cells, by contrast, promote allergic or antibody-biased responses, and are strongly induced by nematode infestations. They promote antibody immune responses skewed towards IgE subtype and the IgG1 isotype. They express CCR8 and CCR4 chemokine receptors, and produce IL-4, 5, 6, 10, and 13 cytokines.[129,130] There are differences in chemokine receptors also.[131] Precursor Th0 cells express both Th1 and Th2 cytokines, and such cells are thought be a more common feature in humans than they are in mice. Uncontrolled Th1 and Th2 responses can cause chronic inflammatory autoimmune (delayed hypersensitivity) diseases and antibody-mediated autoimmunities or allergies, respectively.[132] Th3 cells, on the other hand, are part of the gut-associated lymphoid tissue (GALT) regulatory network, which secretes TGF-β. Development of antigen-specific Th1 versus Th2 responses are influenced by the cytokine milieu in which they develop.[55] Activated macrophages produce IL-12, which in turn stimulates the Th1 pathway. However, NK-T cells also greatly influence these polarizing responses by secreting Th1 or Th2 (IFN-λ or IL-4) cytokines. Thus IL-12 from macrophages and IFN-λ from NK-T cells drive the Th1 pathway, while IL-4 from NK-T and Th2 cells themselves are thought to drive the Th2 pathway.

Cytokines have been shown to play important and crucial roles in autoimmune diseases and their outcomes. Whereas anti-islet Th1 responses are generally destructive, anti-islet Th2/Th3 responses, when induced, are usually protective. These polarized Th1 versus Th2 responses are driven in turn by stimuli that provoke them. In humans, it was found that T cells from diabetic individuals preferentially produced a Th1 cytokine pattern, whereas those from their healthy siblings did not. Various studies in NOD mice have shown that the β-cell destruction was observed in conjunction with infiltrations of local IFN-λ-positive T cells, while lesions dominated by IL-4-producing T cells did not result in islet cell destruction. Furthermore, diabetes has been transferred by CD4$^+$ T cells expressing a Th1 cytokine profile, while treatments with IL-4 or IL-10 protected mice from the disease. A Th1 dominated infiltration of T cells has also been observed in type 1 diabetic patients who died at their disease onsets. This Th1/Th2 dichotomy as an explanation of predisposition to IMD is, however, too simplistic. Recent studies have shown that Th1-type cytokines (e.g., IFN-λ) can actually be protective and prevent diabetes.[133] Besides biased cytokine responses in IMD, numerous human in vitro studies have reported T cell abnormalities from patients with the disease.[134] These include elevated numbers of activated T cells, subnormal T cell production of IL-2, and defective autologous mixed lymphocyte responses (AMLRs). The latter are considered to reflect defective immunoregulatory circuits. Many of these T cell function defects could be secondary to abnormal cytokine production or responsible for them. Reduced IL-2 and IL-4 secretion, and increased or reduced IFN-λ, have all been reported. Our own recent studies have shown that T cells from IMD patients are deficient in both IFN-λ and IL-4 secretion. Such being the case, it is important to determine whether these T cells have intrinsic defects and, if so, what genes are involved. One study has reported a defect in the signal transduction pathway of the TCR/CD3 complex in response to anti-CD3 monoclonal antibody (mAb) stimulation, resulting in ineffective protein kinase C (PKC) activation, low IL-2 production, and subnormal proliferation of T cells in newly diagnosed IMD patients. The addition of exogenous IL-2 at least partially corrected the defective proliferative response in this case. Stimulation of T cells by various stimuli leads to a cascade of well-regulated intracellular transduction events, resulting in activation, proliferation, cytokine secretion and apoptosis induction. These signaling molecules ensure that the T cells can respond appropriately to the environmental stimulus that induced them. Functional defects in components of surface-receptor coupled signaling cascades may either cause immune deficiency or autoimmunity.

NK-T Cells and Autoimmunity. Natural killer-like T cells (NK-T cells) are a recently described subpopulation of T cells expressing NK 1.1,[135] many of which also highly express cytokines. They are capable of making substantial amounts of IL-4 promptly upon in vivo stimulation with anti-CD3.[136] These cells play a role in providing the cytokine environment when conventional T cells make their initial encounter with antigen and become activated. NK-T cells were first identified in mice where they can be distinguished from the conventional T cells by their expression of the NK locus-encoded C-type lectin molecule NK1. These cells have a very restricted TCR variable gene repertoire, with the great majority expressing an invariant TCR-α chain structure (Vα14-Jα281) paired preferentially with Vβ8, 7, or 2.[137,138] Recently, it has been demonstrated that the human immune system contains a population of T cells that show striking conservation of most of the key features of murine NK-T cells.[139,140] The human NK-T cells express an invariant Vα24JαQ TCR-α chain, which is highly homologous to the invariant TCR-α chain of murine NK-T cells.[140] In addition, human NK-T cells also express a restricted Vβ chain repertoire[141] and several NK locus-encoded C-type lectins including NKR-P1A (CD161), which is the homologue of murine NK1.[142] At present, the function of NK-T cells in the immune response remains incompletely resolved. Recently, some interesting findings have generated much interest in this subpopulation of T cells. Murine and human NK-T cells are able to produce large amounts of both IL-4 and IFN-λ rapidly upon activation, and it was thought that NK-T cells might represent the major source of early IL-4 in certain immune responses driving the Th2 differentiation.[143] However, Th2 responses can also develop in β_2-microglobulin- or cluster designation-1- (CD1-) deficient mice that completely lack NK-T cells.[144] They also respond to IL-12 of macrophage origin by secreting INF-λ, expressing NK1, and becoming activated. When activated, they express CD69, 94, and 161 antigens and become capable of lysing tumoral NK targets. They respond to lipid or LPS antigens in context of CD1 antigens that have binding clefts that are deep and hydrophobic, and present lipid rather than peptide antigens to respondent NK-T cells. Several mouse models of autoimmunity are characterized by decreased Vα14$^+$ T cells. Mieza et al.[145] showed that these Vα14$^+$ T cells are specifically reduced with aging in C57BL/6 *lpr/lpr* or MRL *lpr/lpr* mice, whereas no age-related changes were observed in control mice. Recent results also suggest major roles for murine NK-T cells in the rejection of malignant tumors[146] and in regulating autoimmunity.[145] As in humans, Vα24JαQ TCR expressing human NK-T cells have also been suggested to play a role in autoimmune diseases. A study by Sumida et al.[147] showed that there was a selective reduction of T cells bearing Vα24JαQ chain receptors in patients with systemic sclerosis. Similarly another study by Yanagihara et al.[148] showed that NK-T cells are depressed in the peripheral blood of patients with rheumatoid arthritis (RA), suggesting that the measurement of NK-T cells in peripheral blood may have clinical importance for a Th1-type autoimmune disease like RA.

NK-T Cell Deficiencies and IMD. Although the role of NK-T cells in the immune system is incompletely understood, it is now clear that their dysfunction correlates with the pathogenesis of T cell-mediated autoimmune diseases. NOD mice have fewer NK-T cells (CD4 Vα14$^+$ T cells) compared with immunologically normal mice, but this defect tends to improve with age.[149] This quantitative defect is associated with a reduced secretion of cytokines. NK-T cells can directly down modulate T cells in antitumor immunity,[150] graft versus host disease,[151] and rejection of allogenic bone marrow stem cells.[152] The importance of the NK-T cell defect to diabetes has been demonstrated by the complete protection of NOD mice by injection of thymic NK-T cells from nonautoimmune prone (NOD X BALB/c) F1 mice.[100,153] Lehuen et al.[154] showed that overexpression of NK-T cells protects Vα14-Jα281 transgenic NOD mice against diabetes. However, Falcone et al.[99] suggested that it is the functional defects in NK-T cells that are associated with defective immunoregulation and onset of diabetes. Diabetes-prone BB rats have also been shown to be severely deficient in NK-T cells.[155] A human study by Wilson et al.[156] showed that CD4$^-$CD8$^-$ Vα24JαQ$^+$ T cells cloned from diabetic siblings or twins/triplets secreted only IFN-λ upon stimulation, whereas clones from at-risk nonprogressers and normal controls secreted both IL-4 and IFN-λ. They postulated a model for IMD in which Th1-cell-mediated tissue damage is initially regulated by Vα24JαQ$^+$ T cells producing both cytokines and their loss of capacity to secrete IL-4 is correlated with IMD. Our data, however, indicate that both NK-T cells and their expressed cytokines INF-λ and IL-4 are low in IMD. Because NK-T cells carry strong inflammatory and cytotoxic properties, which as a component of the innate immune system are critical for the early clearance of environmental pathogens,[157] how the defect of NK-T cells relates to a propensity to autoimmunity, and the precise nature of the antigens involved when these cells become activated remain to be determined. Murine Vα14 TCR$^+$ T cells all recognize α-galactosyl ceramide in the context of CD1 antigens.[158]

Insulin Replacement Therapies. As of 1989, 40 percent of the 8 million diabetics in the United States were taking insulin (National Center for Health Statistics, 1990). Initially, insulins of bovine or porcine origin were all that were available. Porcine and bovine insulins differ from human insulin by 1 and 3 amino acids, respectively. These insulin preparations were amorphous solutions of an alcohol extraction and acid precipitation. Later, zinc was added, which promoted crystal formation and a short-acting insulin lasting 5 to 8 h. Next, the duration of action of insulin was prolonged by complexing it with protamine, a basic fish protein which made the insulin soluble and more slowly adsorbed, while the addition of zinc stabilized it. Protamine zinc insulin was improved by adding protamine in stoichiometric proportions, resulting in neutral protamine Hagedorn (NPH or isophane insulin), which had a peak action of 6 to 10 h and lasted about 24 h. An alternative development was the Lente insulins, crystalline complexes of insulin and zinc in the presence of an acetate buffer but without protamine. Of the two insulins that result, one is amorphous (Semilente) and has an action like regular insulin, and the other is crystalline (Ultralente) and has a prolonged action of up to 36 h. Lente insulin is a 30:70 mixture of Semilente and Ultralente, respectively. Beginning in the early 1980s, biosynthetic human insulin became available for the first time and currently is produced recombinantly as proinsulin, from which the C-peptide is cleaved enzymatically.[159] Insulin aggregates when given subcutaneously, delaying its absorption. Dimers of insulin form tertiary hexamer structures, which must first dissociate before they can be absorbed.[160] Thus, regular insulin, when administered for a long time, exceeds the action period of endogenous native insulin. The proline residue at position 28 of the B chain was discovered to be critical for insulin dimerization.[161] Switching the lysine at position 29 for proline and vice versa gave a molecule that did not associate, and has an action that is like that of native insulin because it does not aggregate and its biological actions are unaffected, as the COOH terminus does not bind to the insulin receptor. The Eli Lilly Co., which developed the insulin, has named it lispro. Lispro insulin acts within 15 min, its peak activity is 60 to 90 min, and its duration of action is 4 to 5 h.[162] Efforts have also been made to create longer acting or basal insulins. Proinsulin acts like NPH, but at only a quarter of the potency. One human trial suggested that proinsulin therapy might promote myocardial infarctions.[163] One insulin analogue has two additional glycines at the C-terminus of the B chain and a substitution of the A21 asparagine residue by glycine (HOE 901: Roussel), which make it relatively insoluble at normal pH levels of the body,[164] giving it a relatively peakless delivery of about 24 h. More substituted insulins are anticipated. The routes of insulin administration are also under investigation. Oral insulin is not absorbed, but attempts to get some absorption by placing it into liposomes have been partially successful. Intranasal insulin is also poorly absorbed, even when given in large doses in bile acids. However, insulin taken through the lungs is currently being evaluated, because some 25 percent of the dose given by inhaler can be absorbed. The long-term consequences of insulin inhalations on the lungs have yet to be evaluated.

Immunotherapies for IMD, Past and Future. Because the evidence for an autoimmune basis for IMD is high, a number of studies were initiated with general immunosuppressive agents, such as cyclosporin-A,[165–167] azathioprine, and prednisone[168] in patients with new clinical onset IMD. Insulin-free remission rates were increased and endogenous insulin (C-peptide) reserves were improved. However, despite continued immunotherapy with the attendant risks of renal damage and lymphomas at higher doses, relapses were the rule and such treatments were abandoned. Cyclosporin given at a prediabetic phase of the disease delayed but did not prevent diabetes.[169,170] The immunomodulator Linomide was tried in newly diagnosed children with a modest benefit lasting up to 1 year.[171] In NOD mice, BCG therapy can dramatically lower the diabetes rates.[172] This approach was tried in humans with some success reported in an earlier trial,[173] but not in subsequent trials. With the observation that nicotinamide prevents β-cell destruction from streptozotocin by raising otherwise depleted levels of islet cell NAD as a result of superoxide-induced DNA breaks and repair, the vitamin was subjected to a large European and Canadian trial (ENDIT), and the results are pending at the time of writing. One German study (DENIS) showed no effect of nicotinamide on preventing IMD.[174] Other antigen-based human trials have been built upon studies carried out in NOD mice. Daily doses of long-acting insulin in NOD mice prevent their diabetes and strongly inhibit β-cell autoimmunity.[121] The mechanism was in part due to β-cell rest with reduced islet cell expression of the autoantigens, but immunological effects are also likely. Use of close control after diagnosis by intravenous insulin in patients also gave relative remissions[175] and the combination of daily subcutaneous long-acting insulin plus intermittent intravenous insulin appeared promising in at-risk patients.[176] Thus the high risk (>50 percent) based upon ICA plus FPIR below the first percentile arm of the U.S. multicentered type 1 diabetes trial (DPT-1) was born using such a combination. Daily doses of insulin at 0.25 units/kg/day are used in the trial. Results of this trial may be available by 2002. Oral feedings of insulin to NOD mice also delay their onsets of diabetes[177] as does oral feedings of GAD, whereas feedings of the combination had the best effects. Oral feedings of 7.5 mg recombinant, regular insulin per day are being given to relatives with a moderate (20 to 50 percent) risk of IMD based upon ICA plus IAA in the face of a normal FPIR. One trial of oral insulin at 10 mg a day in newly diagnosed patients appeared to be ineffective in those who were diagnosed before 20 years of age, but may have improved endogenous insulin reserves after the initial 6 months.[178] It is clear that many interventions in NOD mice are capable of improving the diabetes rates. This provides considerable encouragement that the situation may be no different in humans. The relatively low concordance rates in identical twins affected by IMD support this. Immunizations of insulin, insulin B chain, and the 8- to 20-amino-acid peptide in IFA all dramatically reduce the diabetes rate in NOD mice,[179–181] as did the B chain peptide when given with alum or the childhood DPT vaccine. The protection was transferable to irradiated NOD recipients by $CD4^+$ T cells. A human trial using this approach is about to begin in newly diagnosed patients [Maclaren]. Interestingly, the 8- to 23-amino-acid insulin B chain peptide was the predominant epitope of T cell clones raised from the insulitis lesions of NOD mice and nasal inhalations of the peptide also reduced the NOD diabetes rate.[182] Two human trials of intranasal insulins are ongoing in Australia and Finland (Harrison and Semil, personal communication). Two peptides within this peptide were found to be targeted by $CD8^+$ T cells, which were capable of transferring diabetes to NODscid mice.[183] Immunizations by human GAD_{65} peptides or IA-2 were minimally effective or not effective in NOD mice.[102] Currently, we are aware of several other approaches in various stages of development for human trials. These include immunizations by GAD peptides and B25-Asp insulin, use of altered peptide ligands (APL) of insulin and GAD, GAD peptides in soluble class II MHC, oral insulin linked to cholera B chain carriers, immunizations by peptide 277 of the heat shock protein (hsp60), humanized anti-CD3 or anti-CD3 Fab, selective IL-4 agonists, anti-CD40L or CD80, and COX-2 inhibitors (Proceedings of The Workshop on Future Directions in Prevention of Type I Diabetes; Miami, January 9–10, 2000). This rapidly advancing field will bear watching.

Complications. The accumulation of complications in all forms of diabetes, but of type 1 diabetes in particular, makes this disease expensive to manage and psychologically burdensome to the patients. The lesions include wide-spread micro- and macrovascular disease, nephropathy, neuropathy (especially involving the peripheral sensory nerves and the sympathetic nervous system), and cataract formation. Capillary basement membranes are thickened in all tissues of the body,[184] due mostly to the accumulation of type IV collagen secreted by capillary cells.[185] Another lesion of the microvasculature is loss of pericytes.[186] Hyperglycemia may induce adverse effects through sorbitol-myoinositol flux (a long hypothesized mechanism for development of diabetic neuropathy), redox alteration resulting in increased ratios of $NADH/NAD^+$, increased levels of the cellular metabolic regulator in vascular cells,[187] or increased formation of advanced glycation endproducts (AGEs). Nonenzymatic glycation of proteins in the body appears to be a key mechanism involved in diabetic complications.[188] The amino groups of proteins, lipids, and nucleic acids react nonenzymatically with the reducing sugars, glucose, fructose, galactose, and triose phosphates forming initially reversible Schiff bases and later slowly reversible Amadori products. Fortunately, the reactions are slowest with glucose over the other monosaccharides. These Amadori products undergo auto-oxidation with generation of nonreactive end-products.[190] These products may undergo further rearrangements to form irreversible cross-linked advanced AGEs.[191] The AGEs bind to receptors on several cell types, including macrophages, endothelia, and mesangial cells, followed by AGE internalization with disturbances of cell functions.[192] Several AGEs have been recognized. These comprise p60 (a 50-kDa protein with homologies to the oligosaccharyl transferase complex OST-48 [AGE-R1]); p90 (an 80-kDa protein homologous to protein kinase 80 K-H substrate [AGE-R2]); galactin-3 (Gal-3, a 32-kDa protein known as Mac-2 [AGE-R3]); and a 35-kDa immunoglobulin receptor named RAGE. Injections of AGE-proteins in nondiabetic animals have been shown to induce up-regulation of TGF-β, type IV collagen, and laminin mRNA in the kidney, associated with the functional and structural changes characteristic of diabetes such as extracellular matrix overproduction, reduced cellular proliferation and increased expression of insulin-like growth factor-1 (IGF-1) and platelet-derived growth factor (PDGF).[193–198] AGEs have been shown to increase vascular endothelial growth factor (VEGF) in retinal cells, TNF-α, IL-1, PDGF, and IGF-1 in monocytes-macrophages, quenching of NO, activation of NF-kB, and overexpression of vascular cell adhesion molecule-1 (VCAM-1).[196] Inhibitors of nonenzymatic glycation such as aminoguanidine, which blocks AGE formation by interacting with the Amadori fragmentation products and the thiazolidine compound OPB-9195, have been shown to prevent diabetic nephropathy in experimental animals.[199–202] The most frequent late complication of type 1 diabetes is retinopathy, consisting of microaneurysms, hemorrhages, and exudates and, most seriously, proliferative retinopathy. The latter lesion, which can herald blindness, is seen first after 10 years of diabetes, and the prevalence rises to about 2 of every 3 diabetic patients after 40 years of the disease.[203,204] The recently concluded diabetes control and complication trial (DCCT) indicate that intensive glycemic control is associated with lower rates of retinopathy with a threshold of HbA1c near 8.5 percent. Diabetic nephropathy is characterized by glomerular hypertrophy and expansion of the mesangium, due to increased formation and deposition and impaired removal of types IV, V, and VI collagens, fibronectin, thrombospondin, and tenascin. TGF-β and IGF-1 are involved in the early lesions. The accumulation of periodic acid-Schiff (PAS) positive staining material becomes visible by light microscopy, with advancing lesions representing the Kimmel-Steil-Wilson disease. Clinically, microalbuminuria is followed by overt proteinuria[205] at a frequency that is related to the time of IMD after puberty.[206] After 30 years, about one-third of the patients have proteinuria and as many have microalbuminuria that has not progressed.[207] End-stage renal disease is seen in 20 percent of patients after 30 years of diabetes,[208] though it is hoped that the current patient population will improve upon this outlook.[209] Family studies suggest a clear genetic component to the nephropathy of IMD.[210] Use of angiotensin-converting enzymes (ACE) inhibitors such as captopril provides strong evidence of a protective effect from diabetic retinopathy.[211] Coronary heart disease rates have been estimated to be about 40 percent by age 55 in juvenile onset IMD.[212] Attention to hypertension and hyperlipidemia, stopping smoking, and taking of daily aspirin should lower these rates.

Animal Models of Type 1 Diabetes. In animal and human populations, the prevalence rates of circulating autoantibodies and autoreactive T cells responsive to "self" are relatively high, whereas the occurrences of overt autoimmune diseases are very much lower. Thus, most persons with detectable islet cell autoantibodies will never develop clinical IMD. Over the past 25 years, major advances have been made in understanding the pathogenesis of autoimmune diseases, by studying experimental animal models that have been induced with relative difficulty, through immunizations by "self"-tissue antigens in adjuvants. However the first animal model of spontaneous autoimmune disease, the New Zealand Black (NZB) mouse, was discovered in 1959. It was later shown that when NZB mice were crossed with the New Zealand White (NZW) strain, mice (NZB x NZW F1) with all immunopathological features of human lupus nephritis were produced.[213] Further, two major animal models of spontaneous IMD in rodents, the NOD mouse[214] and the BB rat,[215] have been discovered. Both have many features in common with human IMD. The animals spontaneously develop insulin-dependent diabetes similar to IMD, replete with insulitis lesions and autoantibodies and autoreactive T cells to islet cell antigens[85] and a propensity to develop other related autoimmune diseases such as those affecting the thyroid and gastric mucosa.[216,217] The NOD and BB rodent strains have both been inbred to homogeneity. Whereas BB rats exhibit a striking T lymphocytopenia with marked defects in T cell functioning such as allogeneic mixed lymphocyte responses (MLR) and rejection of skin grafts,[217] NOD mice have a relative lymphocytosis, suggesting that they have defective T cell apoptosis.[218] Diabetogenesis in NOD mice results from multiple immunodeficiencies that have been acquired through complex polygenic QTL defects, the most important of which is found within the MHC region on chromosome 17. In the pathogenic events leading to diabetes in NOD mice, the autoimmune process is characterized by stepwise development with two proposed critical checkpoints.[219] The first (around 4 to 6 weeks) is characterized by infiltration of islets of Langerhans with lymphoid and myeloid cells, which has been somewhat misnamed as insulitis, and the second (around 12 weeks) is marked by a phase of massive destruction of insulin-producing β cells, which rapidly leads to diabetes. The early lymphocytic infiltration of the pancreas begins as a periductal and perivascular monocytic accumulation. However, by 6 to 8 weeks of age, the lymphocytes begin to invade the islets accompanied by initial damage to the insulin-secreting β-cells. Overt diabetes is observed around 3 to 4 months of age with female mice having earlier onsets by about 1 month, and eventually significantly higher diabetes rates ($\sim$80 percent), than male mice ($\sim$20 percent). In NOD mice, autoimmunity has been reported to begin first and most critically against GAD[67,220,221] followed by epitope spreading to involve other islet cell antigens such as insulin,[222] though others have suggested that autoimmunity to insulin may represent the initial event. In humans, autoimmunity to insulin and/or GAD also develops earliest in the course of the disease, and tends to extend to IA-2/IA-2β later.[93] Autoantibodies against multiple antigens (epitope spreading) appear to be strongly associated with the risk for clinical disease.

Many groups have used transgenic mice bearing human MHC class II on the C57BL/6 (nondiabetes prone) genetic background, as well as in the NOD mouse, to investigate the pathogenic epitopes of preproinsulin[223,224] and GAD.[221] The potential value of HLA transgenic animals as "humanized" disease models was first illustrated in the HLA-B27 transgenic rat, which developed a disease resembling human spondyloarthropathy.[225] Predisposition to IMD is strongly associated with the presence of DQ8 (DQB1*0302/DQA1*0301), while DQ6 (DQB1*0602/DQA1*0102) has been found to be protective. To determine if HLA-DQ6 can protect against glycosuria and insulitis, NOD mice expressing the DQ6 transgene but no murine I-A^{g7} were created, and a lower incidence of glycosuria and insulitis was observed.[226] These studies suggest that transgenic mice can be used to define T cell epitopes to potential autoantigens that are relevant in the disease, and that a strategy to down-modulate the autoimmune response can be formulated. These humanized mice may lack the appropriate requirement for protein digestion and cleavage, however.[91] Previous studies using NOD mice have shown that insulin or insulin mid B-chain native peptide given orally,[177,180,182] subcutaneously,[102,227] or intranasally[182] can protect the animals from diabetes.

Transient Neonatal Diabetes

Insulin is a potent growth hormone in the fetus. Whereas somatic growth of infants with anencephaly and pituitary growth hormone deficiency is normal, children with neonatal diabetes are small for their gestational age. Transient neonatal diabetes is an uncommon condition in which natural insulin secretion is impaired, being responsive to caffeine or phosphodiesterase inhibitors but not to tolbutamide.[228] This implies that there is immaturity of the pancreatic β-cell in its activation by the cAMP system. Recently, it was suggested that the cell cycle control gene ZAC/PLAGLI (chromosome 6q24) is the defective gene involved, because it is a transcription regulator of the type-12 receptor for pituitary adenylate cyclase-activating polypeptide, the most potent known insulin secretagogue and an important mediator of autocrine control of insulin secretion in the pancreatic islets.[229]

Pancreatic Diabetes and DIDMOAD/Wolfram Syndrome

Wolfram syndrome (WFS) is an autosomal recessive disorder characterized by type 1 diabetes mellitus, diabetes insipidus, optic atrophy, and a number of neurological symptoms including deafness, ataxia, and peripheral neuropathy. A tendency to develop this syndrome has been related to some class II antigens of the HLA system. A study by Vendrell et al.[230] established a high frequency of the HLA-DR2 (DRB1*15) antigen in the WFS group (44.4 percent) compared to a control group (21.9 percent; relative risk 2.8) and to patients with IMD, where it is rarely found. A similar finding was previously reported for males with an onset of type 1 diabetes that was associated with pancreatic dysplasia.[231] A high frequency of HLA-DQw1 antigen (85.5 percent) was also found in this disease but without statistical significance. Recently, mitochondrial DNA deletions have been described in a few patients and a locus mapped to 4p16 (WFS1) by linkage analysis.[232,233] That group identified a gene they named wolframin that encodes a transmembrane protein expressed in pancreas and brain, among other tissues. In one of the studies on 6 WFS families, mutations in the WFS1 gene encoding a putative 890-amino acid transmembrane protein were found in all affected individuals and these mutations were associated with the disease phenotype.[234] Most of the mutations in the WFS1 gene were found in exon 8 in another study of 30 patients, but no common founder mutation was found.[232] Subsequent studies require a complete analysis of exon 8 and the upstream exons. One study found instances of optic neuropathy associated with mitochondrial tRNA (Leu9UUR), a 3243G mutation responsible for the MELAS syndrome (mitochondrial encephalopathy, lactic acidosis, and stroke-like episodes), diabetes mellitus, and progressive ophthalmoplegia.[235]

African Diabetes

A high rate of diabetes among persons of African (and Indian) descent has been long recognized in certain Caribbean islands. Indeed "J" type diabetes is so named after Jamaica, where it is very prevalent. Diabetes is increasingly common in African Americans, whereas Nigerians have well-preserved glucose tolerances.[236] Because the initial observations of lower frequencies of ICA in African American than U.S. Caucasian patients who presented with diabetes during childhood or early adulthood,[56] this strongly inherited form of diabetes, which is frequent among this racial group, became better characterized.[231] Most patients are obese and female, but some patients have acanthosis nigricans and hirsutism reminiscent of the polycystic ovary syndrome. Such patients would be likely to have primarily an increased insulin resistance. Often affecting family members in successive generations like type 2 diabetes, diabetes in African Americans may present with acute symptoms suggesting insulinopenia and type 1 diabetes. However, after the institution of insulin replacement therapy, the diabetes can improve, and the patient can go off insulin therapy until another episode is triggered by an incidental infection or stress. Immunological studies rule out this being a variant form of IMD, as ICA, $GAD_{65}A$, and IA-2A are not found, and HLA haplotypes typical of IMD are not found either unless the patients are lean with typical symptoms of insulin deficiency.[237,238] Metabolic studies suggest that the principal lesion lies in the pancreatic islet cells,[239,240] making the disease more like a form of type 1 diabetes, but compounded by the increased insulin resistance or insulinopenia and obesity. If so, then the metabolic basis of this disease has yet to be shown. However large doses of insulin may not restore normoglycemia but may worsen the associated obesity. Insulin secretogogues are the drugs of choice. There is a female bias to the disease and obesity is a distinct factor. The rising incidence of the disease is fast becoming a silent epidemic, affecting 1 in 4 black women 55 years and older in one study.[241] Children are increasingly affected also.[242]

Insulin Deficiency in Type 2 Diabetes

It is a common clinical experience that many patients who present with type 2 diabetes deteriorate over a period often measured in years, to increasing insulin deficiency and eventually to a therapeutic insulin requirement. As discussed above, an accelerated form of this is common in late onset IMD, though the deterioration is also a feature of patients with type 2 diabetes, albeit at a slower rate of progression.[243] Besides impaired insulin secretory capacity, glucose "toxicity" contributes to insulin resistance as well.[244] The two leading hypotheses for the progressive loss of endogenous insulin reserves are a glucose-mediated toxicity, and damage to the islets mediated by accumulation of lipid or FFAs.[245] In several animal models, accumulation of lipids within the islet cells can be striking. In studies in Zucker diabetic fatty rats, chronic hyperglycemia resulted in loss of insulin and the insulin transcription factor PDX-1 that was reversible through use of troglitazone to lower insulin resistance.[246] When the β-cell line (HIT-T15) was cultured in the presence of glucose at 11.1 mM in the presence of N-acetyl-L-cysteine or aminoguanidine, the decreases in insulin mRNA, insulin promoter activity, DNA binding of the insulin promoter and transcription factors PDX-1 and STF-1 were lessened. These data suggest that chronic oxidative stress could play a role in glucose toxicity.[247]

In this chapter, we have reviewed the diseases that fall under the type 1 diabetes umbrella, with particular emphasis on the most common immune-mediated (IMD) form. Whereas type 2 diabetes appears to be an increasing price to pay for societal affluence, there is evidence worldwide for a rising tide of type 1 diabetes too. With respect to the latter, an understanding of the pathogenic events has created the intellectual climate for prevention trials that are underway or will soon be initiated in the U.S. and other countries.

REFERENCES

1. Report of the Expert Committee on the Diagnosis and Classification of Diabetes Mellitus. *Diabetes Care* **20**:1183, 1997.
2. Harris MI, Hadden WC, Knowler WC, Bennett PH: Prevalence of diabetes and impaired glucose tolerance and plasma glucose levels in U.S. population aged 20–74 yr. *Diabetes* **36**:523, 1987.
3. McCance DR, Hanson RL, Charles MA, Jacobsson LT, Pettitt DJ, Bennett PH, Knowler WC: Comparison of tests for glycated haemoglobin and fasting and two hour plasma glucose concentrations as diagnostic methods for diabetes [published erratum appears in *BMJ* 309(6958):841, 1994]. *BMJ* **308**:1323, 1994.
4. Engelgau MM, Thompson TJ, Herman WH, Boyle JP, Aubert RE, Kenny SJ, Badran A, et al.: Comparison of fasting and 2-hour glucose and HbA1c levels for diagnosing diabetes. Diagnostic criteria and performance revisited. *Diabetes Care* **20**:785, 1997.

5. Maclaren N, Lan M, Coutant R, Schatz D, Silverstein J, Muir A, Clare-Salzer M, et al.: Only multiple autoantibodies to islet cells (ICA), insulin, GAD65, IA-2 and IA-2beta predict immune-mediated (Type 1) diabetes in relatives. *J Autoimmun* **12**:279, 1999.
6. Kukreja A, Maclaren NK: Commentary: Autoimmunity and diabetes. *J Clin Endocrinol Metab* **84**:4371, 1999.
7. Ziegler AG, Bachmann W, Rabl W: Prophylactic insulin treatment in relatives at high risk for type 1 diabetes. *Diabetes Metab Rev* **9**:289, 1993.
8. Maclaren NK, Atkinson MA: Insulin-dependent diabetes mellitus: The hypothesis of molecular mimicry between islet cell antigens and microorganisms. *Mol Med Today* **3**:76, 1997.
9. Horwitz MS, Sarvetick N: The pathogen connection. *Nat Med* **4**:781, 1998.
10. Ganda OP, Srikanta S, Brink SJ, Morris MA, Gleason RE, Soeldner JS, Eisenbarth GS: Differential sensitivity to beta-cell secretagogues in "early" type I diabetes mellitus. *Diabetes* **33**:516, 1984.
11. Cantor AB, Krischer JP, Cuthbertson DD, Schatz DA, Riley WJ, Malone J, Schwartz S, et al.: Age and family relationship accentuate the risk of insulin-dependent diabetes mellitus (IDDM) in relatives of patients with IDDM. *J Clin Endocrinol Metab* **80**:3739, 1995.
12. Rewers M, Norris JM, Eisenbarth GS, Erlich HA, Beaty B, Klingensmith G, Hoffman M, et al.: Beta-cell autoantibodies in infants and toddlers without IDDM relatives: Diabetes autoimmunity study in the young (DAISY). *J Autoimmun* **9**:405, 1996.
13. Randle PJ, Kerbey AL, Espinal J: Mechanisms decreasing glucose oxidation in diabetes and starvation: Role of lipid fuels and hormones. *Diabetes Metab Rev* **4**:623, 1988.
14. Exton JH: Mechanisms of hormonal regulation of hepatic glucose metabolism. *Diabetes Metab Rev* **3**:163, 1987.
15. El-Maghrabi MR, Claus TH, McGrane MM, Pilkis SJ: Influence of phosphorylation on the interaction of effectors with rat liver pyruvate kinase. *J Biol Chem* **257**:233, 1982.
16. Pilkis SJ, Granner DK: Molecular physiology of the regulation of hepatic gluconeogenesis and glycolysis. *Annu Rev Physiol* **54**:885, 1992.
17. Unger R, Foster DW: Diabetes mellitus, in Wilson JD, Foster DW (eds): *Williams Textbook of Endocrinology*. Philadelphia, WB Saunders, 1990, p 1255.
18. Gerich JE, Lorenzi M, Bier DM, Schneider V, Tsalikian E, Karam JH, Forsham PH: Prevention of human diabetic ketoacidosis by somatostatin. Evidence for an essential role of glucagon. *N Engl J Med* **292**:985, 1975.
19. Gerich JE, Langlois M, Noacco C, Karam JH, Forsham PH: Lack of glucagon response to hypoglycemia in diabetes: Evidence for an intrinsic pancreatic alpha cell defect. *Science* **182**:171, 1973.
20. Raskin P, Unger RH: Hyperglucagonemia and its suppression. Importance in the metabolic control of diabetes. *N Engl J Med* **299**:433, 1978.
21. Kimball SR, Jefferson LS: Cellular mechanisms involved in the action of insulin on protein synthesis. *Diabetes Metab Rev* **4**:773, 1988.
22. Kimball SR, Jefferson LS: Regulation of initiation of protein synthesis by insulin in skeletal muscle. *Acta Diabetol* **28**:134, 1991.
23. Cahill GF, Jr: Starvation in man. *Clin Endocrinol Metab* **5**:397, 1976.
24. Foster DW, McGarry JD: The metabolic derangements and treatment of diabetic ketoacidosis. *N Engl J Med* **309**:159, 1983.
25. McGarry JD: Lilly Lecture 1978. New perspectives in the regulation of ketogenesis. *Diabetes* **28**:517, 1979.
26. McGarry JD: What if Minkowski had been ageusic? An alternative angle on diabetes. *Science* **258**:766, 1992.
27. Owen OE, Morgan AP, Kemp HG, Sullivan JM, Herrera MG, Cahill GF Jr: Brain metabolism during fasting. *J Clin Invest* **46**:1589, 1967.
28. Owen OE, Felig P, Morgan AP, Wahren J, Cahill GF Jr: Liver and kidney metabolism during prolonged starvation. *J Clin Invest* **48**:574, 1969.
29. Ashby P, Robinson DS: Effects of insulin, glucocorticoids and adrenaline on the activity of rat adipose-tissue lipoprotein lipids. *Biochem J* **188**:185, 1980.
30. Parkin SM, Walker K, Ashby P, Robinson DS: Effects of glucose and insulin on the activation of lipoprotein lipase and on protein-synthesis in rat adipose tissue. *Biochem J* **188**:193, 1980.
31. Tavangar K, Murata Y, Pedersen ME, Goers JF, Hoffman AR, Kraemer FB: Regulation of lipoprotein lipase in the diabetic rat. *J Clin Invest* **90**:1672, 1992.
32. Bottazzo GF, Florin-Christensen A, Doniach D: Islet-cell antibodies in diabetes mellitus with autoimmune polyendocrine deficiencies. *Lancet* **2**:1279, 1974.
33. Neufeld M, Maclaren N, Blizzard R: Autoimmune polyglandular syndromes. *Pediatr Ann* **9**:154, 1980.
34. Huang W, Connor E, Rosa TD, Muir A, Schatz D, Silverstein J, Crockett S, et al.: Although DR3-DQB1*0201 may be associated with multiple component diseases of the autoimmune polyglandular syndromes, the human leukocyte antigen DR4-DQB1*0302 haplotype is implicated only in beta-cell autoimmunity. *J Clin Endocrinol Metab* **81**:2559, 1996.
35. Maclaren N, Huang S, Fogh J: Antibody to cultured human insulinoma cells in insulin-dependent diabetes. *Lancet* **1**:997, 1975.
36. Neufeld M, Maclaren NK, Riley WJ, Lezotte D, McLaughlin JV, Silverstein J, Rosenbloom AL: Islet cell and other organ-specific antibodies in U.S. Caucasians and Blacks with insulin-dependent diabetes mellitus. *Diabetes* **29**:589, 1980.
37. Palmer JP, Asplin CM, Clemons P, Lyen K, Tatpati O, Raghu PK, Paquette TL: Insulin antibodies in insulin-dependent diabetics before insulin treatment. *Science* **222**:1337, 1983.
38. Atkinson MA, Maclaren NK, Riley WJ, Winter WE, Fisk DD, Spillar RP: Are insulin autoantibodies markers for insulin-dependent diabetes mellitus? *Diabetes* **35**:894, 1986.
39. Solimena M, Folli F, Denis-Donini S, Comi GC, Pozza G, De Camilli P, Vicari AM: Autoantibodies to glutamic acid decarboxylase in a patient with stiff-man syndrome, epilepsy, and type 1 diabetes mellitus. *N Engl J Med* **318**:1012, 1988.
40. Baekkeskov S, Aanstoot HJ, Christgau S, Reetz A, Solimena M, Cascalho M, Folli F, et al.: Identification of the 64 K autoantigen in insulin-dependent diabetes as the GABA-synthesizing enzyme glutamic acid decarboxylase [published erratum appears in *Nature* 347(6295):782, 1990]. *Nature* **347**:151, 1990.
41. Atkinson MA, Kaufman DL, Newman D, Tobin AJ, Maclaren NK: Islet cell cytoplasmic autoantibody reactivity to glutamate decarboxylase in insulin-dependent diabetes. *J Clin Invest* **91**:350, 1993.
42. Christie MR, Genovese S, Cassidy D, Bosi E, Brown TJ, Lai M, Bonifacio E, et al.: Antibodies to islet 37k antigen, but not to glutamate decarboxylase, discriminate rapid progression to IDDM in endocrine autoimmunity. *Diabetes* **43**:1254, 1994.
43. Lu J, Li Q, Xie H, Chen ZJ, Borovitskaya AE, Maclaren NK, Notkins AL, et al.: Identification of a second transmembrane protein tyrosine phosphatase, IA-2β, as an autoantigen in insulin-dependent diabetes mellitus: Precursor of the 37-kDa tryptic fragment. *Proc Natl Acad Sci U S A* **93**:2307, 1996.
44. Solimena M, Dirkx R Jr, Hermel JM, Pleasic-Williams S, Shapiro JA, Caron L, Rabin DU: ICA 512, an autoantigen of type I diabetes, is an intrinsic membrane protein of neurosecretory granules. *EMBO J* **15**:2102, 1996.
45. Lan MS, Wasserfall C, Maclaren NK, Notkins AL: IA-2, a transmembrane protein of the protein tyrosine phosphatase family, is a major autoantigen in insulin-dependent diabetes mellitus. *Proc Natl Acad Sci U S A* **93**:6367, 1996.
46. Notkins AL, Lu J, Li Q, Vander Vegt FP, Wasserfall C, Maclaren NK, Lan MS: IA-2 and IA-2 beta are major autoantigens in IDDM and the precursors of the 40 kDa and 37 kDa tryptic fragments. *J Autoimmun* **9**:677, 1996.
47. Lan MS, Maclaren NK: Cryptic epitope and autoimmunity. *Diabetes Metab Rev* **14**:333, 1998.
48. Aanstoot HJ, Kang SM, Kim J, Lindsay LA, Roll U, Knip M, Atkinson M, et al.: Identification and characterization of glima 38, a glycosylated islet cell membrane antigen, which together with GAD65 and IA2 marks the early phases of autoimmune response in type 1 diabetes. *J Clin Invest* **97**:2772, 1996.
49. Bonifacio E, Bingley PJ, Shattock M, Dean BM, Dunger D, Gale EA, Bottazzo GF: Quantification of islet-cell antibodies and prediction of insulin-dependent diabetes. *Lancet* **335**:147, 1990.
50. Riley WJ, Atkinson MA, Schatz DA, Maclaren NK: Comparison of islet autoantibodies in "pre-diabetes" and recommendations for screening. *J Autoimmun* **1**:47, 1990.
51. Schatz D, Maclaren N: The natural history of pre-type 1 diabetes. *Curr Sci* **2**:31, 1995.
52. Krischer JP, Schatz D, Riley WJ, Spillar RP, Silverstein JH, Schwartz S, Malone J, et al.: Insulin and islet cell autoantibodies as time-dependent covariates in the development of insulin-dependent diabetes: A prospective study in relatives. *J Clin Endocrinol Metab* **77**:743, 1993.
53. Irvine WJ, McCallum CJ, Gray RS, Campbell CJ, Duncan LJ, Farquhar JW, Vaughan H, et al.: Pancreatic islet-cell antibodies in diabetes mellitus correlated with the duration and type of diabetes, coexistent autoimmune disease, and HLA type. *Diabetes* **26**:138, 1977.

54. Riley WJ, Maclaren NK, Krischer J, Spillar RP, Silverstein JH, Schatz DA, Schwartz S, et al.: A prospective study of the development of diabetes in relatives of patients with insulin-dependent diabetes. *N Engl J Med* **323**:1167, 1990.
55. Kumar V, Sercarz E: Induction or protection from experimental autoimmune encephalomyelitis depends on the cytokine secretion profile of TCR peptide-specific regulatory CD4 T cells. *J Immunol* **161**:6585, 1998.
56. Riley WJ, Maclaren NK, Neufeld M: Adrenal autoantibodies and Addison disease in insulin-dependent diabetes mellitus. *J Pediatr* **97**:191, 1980.
57. Riley WJ, Toskes PP, Maclaren NK, Silverstein JH: Predictive value of gastric parietal cell autoantibodies as a marker for gastric and hematologic abnormalities associated with insulin-dependent diabetes. *Diabetes* **31**:1051, 1982.
58. Irvine WJ, Clarke BF, Scarth L, Cullen DR, Duncan LJ: Thyroid and gastric autoimmunity in patients with diabetes mellitus. *Lancet* **2**:163, 1970.
59. Rapoport MJ, Bistritzer T, Vardi O, Broide E, Azizi A, Vardi P: Increased prevalence of diabetes-related autoantibodies in celiac disease. *J Pediatr Gastroenterol Nutr* **23**:524, 1996.
60. Song YH, Connor E, Li Y, Zorovich B, Balducci P, Maclaren N: The role of tyrosinase in autoimmune vitiligo. *Lancet* **344**:1049, 1994.
61. Atkinson MA, Bowman MA, Campbell L, Darrow BL, Kaufman DL, Maclaren NK: Cellular immunity to a determinant common to glutamate decarboxylase and Coxsackie virus in insulin-dependent diabetes. *J Clin Invest* **94**:2125, 1994.
62. Ellis TM, Schatz DA, Ottendorfer EW, Lan MS, Wasserfall C, Salisbury PJ, She JX, et al.: The relationship between humoral and cellular immunity to IA-2 in IDDM. *Diabetes* **47**:566, 1998.
63. Bach JF, Chatenoud L: Immunosuppression in insulin-dependent diabetes mellitus: From cellular selectivity towards autoantigen specificity. *Chem Immunol* **60**:32, 1995.
64. Atkinson MA, Kaufman DL, Campbell L, Gibbs KA, Shah SC, Bu DF, Erlander MG, et al.: Response of peripheral-blood mononuclear cells to glutamate decarboxylase in insulin-dependent diabetes. *Lancet* **339**:458, 1992.
65. Harrison LC, Honeyman MC, De Aizpurua HJ, Schmidli RS, Colman PG, Tait BD, Cram DS: Inverse relation between humoral and cellular immunity to glutamic acid decarboxylase in subjects at risk of insulin-dependent diabetes. *Lancet* **341**:1365, 1993.
66. Gelber C, Paborsky L, Singer S, McAteer D, Tisch R, Jolicoeur C, Buelow R, et al.: Isolation of nonobese diabetic mouse T-cells that recognize novel autoantigens involved in the early events of diabetes. *Diabetes* **43**:33, 1994.
67. Kaufman DL, Clare-Salzler M, Tian J, Forsthuber T, Ting GS, Robinson P, Atkinson MA, et al.: Spontaneous loss of T-cell tolerance to glutamic acid decarboxylase in murine insulin-dependent diabetes. *Nature* **366**:69, 1993.
68. Tisch R, Yang XD, Singer SM, Liblau RS, Fugger L, McDevitt HO: Immune response to glutamic acid decarboxylase correlates with insulitis in non-obese diabetic mice. *Nature* **366**:72, 1993.
69. Endl J, Otto H, Jung G, Dreisbusch B, Donie F, Stahl P, Elbracht R, et al.: Identification of naturally processed T cell epitopes from glutamic acid decarboxylase presented in the context of HLA-DR alleles by T lymphocytes of recent onset IDDM patients. *J Clin Invest* **99**:2405, 1997.
70. Honeyman MC, Stone N, de Aizpurua H, Rowley MJ, Harrison LC: High T cell responses to the glutamic acid decarboxylase (GAD) isoform 67 reflect a hyperimmune state that precedes the onset of insulin-dependent diabetes. *J Autoimmun* **10**:165, 1997.
71. Lohmann T, Leslie RD, Hawa M, Geysen M, Rodda S, Londei M: Immunodominant epitopes of glutamic acid decarboxylase 65 and 67 in insulin-dependent diabetes mellitus. *Lancet* **343**:1607, 1994.
72. Lohmann T, Leslie RD, Londei M: T cell clones to epitopes of glutamic acid decarboxylase 65 raised from normal subjects and patients with insulin-dependent diabetes. *J Autoimmun* **9**:385, 1996.
73. Panina-Bordignon P, Lang R, van Endert PM, Benazzi E, Felix AM, Pastore RM, Spinas GA, et al.: Cytotoxic T cells specific for glutamic acid decarboxylase in autoimmune diabetes. *J Exp Med* **181**:1923, 1995.
74. Weiss U, Manfras BJ, Terjung D, Eiermann T, Wolpl A, Loliger C, Kuhnl P, et al.: In vitro stimulation with glutamic acid decarboxylase (GAD65) leads to an oligoclonal response of peripheral T-cells in an IDDM patient. *Scand J Immunol* **42**:673, 1995.
75. Honeyman MC, Stone NL, Harrison LC: T-cell epitopes in type 1 diabetes autoantigen tyrosine phosphatase IA-2: Potential for mimicry with rotavirus and other environmental agents. *Mol Med* **4**:231, 1998.
76. Zechel MA, Krawetz MD, Singh B: Epitope dominance: Evidence for reciprocal determinant spreading to glutamic acid decarboxylase in non-obese diabetic mice. *Immunol Rev* **164**:111, 1998.
77. Von Meyenburg H: Uber "insulitis" bei diabetes. *Schweiz Med Wochenschr* **21**:554, 1940.
78. Gepts W, Pipeleers D: The endocrine pancreas. Functional morphology and histopathology. *Acta Med Scand (Suppl)* **205**:95, 1977.
79. Foulis AK, Farquharson MA, Meager A: Immunoreactive alpha-interferon in insulin-secreting beta cells in type 1 diabetes mellitus. *Lancet* **2**:1423, 1987.
80. Conrad B, Weidmann E, Trucco G, Rudert WA, Behboo R, Ricordi C, Rodriquez-Rilo H, et al.: Evidence for superantigen involvement in insulin-dependent diabetes mellitus aetiology. *Nature* **371**:351, 1994.
81. Conrad B, Weissmahr RN, Boni J, Arcari R, Schupbach J, Mach B: A human endogenous retroviral superantigen as candidate autoimmune gene in type I diabetes. *Cell* **90**:303, 1997.
82. Lan MS, Mason A, Coutant R, Chen QY, Vargas A, Rao J, Gomez R, et al.: HERV-K10s and immune-mediated (type 1) diabetes. *Cell* **95**:14, 1998.
83. Leslie RD, Pyke DA: Concordance between twins for beta-cell autoimmunity [Letter; Comment]. *Diabetes* **45**:1284, 1996.
84. Todd JA: From genome to aetiology in a multifactorial disease, type 1 diabetes. *Bioessays* **21**:164, 1999.
85. Atkinson MA, Leiter EH: The NOD mouse model of type 1 diabetes: As good as it gets? *Nat Med* **5**:601, 1999.
86. Todd JA: Genetics of type 1 diabetes. *Pathol Biol (Paris)* **45**:219, 1997.
87. She JX: Susceptibility to type I diabetes: HLA-DQ and DR revisited. *Immunol Today* **17**:323, 1996.
88. Noble JA, Cavalli AS, Erlich HA: DPB1*5901a: a novel HLA-DPB1 allele from a Caucasian family with insulin-dependent diabetes mellitus. *Tissue Antigens* **47**:159, 1996.
89. Lund T, O'Reilly L, Hutchings P, Kanagawa O, Simpson E, Gravely R, Chandler P, et al.: Prevention of insulin-dependent diabetes mellitus in non-obese diabetic mice by transgenes encoding modified I-A beta-chain or normal I-E alpha-chain. *Nature* **345**:727, 1990.
90. Schmidt D, Amrani A, Verdaguer J, Bou S, Santamaria P: Autoantigen-independent deletion of diabetogenic CD4+ thymocytes by protective MHC class II molecules. *J Immunol* **162**:4627, 1999.
91. Nepom GT, Kwok WW: Molecular basis for HLA-DQ associations with IDDM. *Diabetes* **47**:1177, 1998.
92. Kanagawa O, Martin SM, Vaupel BA, Carrasco-Marin E, Unanue ER: Autoreactivity of T cells from nonobese diabetic mice: An I-Ag7-dependent reaction. *Proc Natl Acad Sci U S A* **95**:1721, 1998.
93. Song YH, Li Y, Maclaren NK: The nature of autoantigens targeted in autoimmune endocrine diseases. *Immunol Today* **17**:232, 1996.
94. Nakanishi K, Kobayashi T, Inoko H, Tsuji K, Murase T, Kosaka K: Residual beta-cell function and HLA-A24 in IDDM. Markers of glycemic control and subsequent development of diabetic retinopathy. *Diabetes* **44**:1334, 1995.
95. Pugliese A, Zeller M, Fernandez A Jr, Zalcberg LJ, Bartlett RJ, Ricordi C, Pietropaolo M, et al.: The insulin gene is transcribed in the human thymus and transcription levels correlated with allelic variation at the INS VNTR-IDDM2 susceptibility locus for type 1 diabetes. *Nat Genet* **15**:293, 1997.
96. Vafiadis P, Bennett ST, Todd JA, Nadeau J, Grabs R, Goodyer CG, Wickramasinghe S, et al.: Insulin expression in human thymus is modulated by INS VNTR alleles at the IDDM2 locus. *Nat Genet* **15**:289, 1997.
97. Garchon HJ, Luan JJ, Eloy L, Bedossa P, Bach JF: Genetic analysis of immune dysfunction in non-obese diabetic (NOD) mice: Mapping of a susceptibility locus close to the Bcl-2 gene correlates with increased resistance of NOD T cells to apoptosis induction. *Eur J Immunol* **24**:380, 1994.
98. Wicker LS, Chen SL, Nepom GT, Elliott JF, Freed DC, Bansal A, Zheng S, et al.: Naturally processed T cell epitopes from human glutamic acid decarboxylase identified using mice transgenic for the type 1 diabetes-associated human MHC class II allele, DRB1*0401. *J Clin Invest* **98**:2597, 1996.
99. Falcone M, Yeung B, Tucker L, Rodriguez E, Sarvetnick N: A defect in interleukin 12-induced activation and interferon gamma secretion of peripheral natural killer T cells in nonobese diabetic mice suggests new pathogenic mechanisms for insulin-dependent diabetes mellitus. *J Exp Med* **190**:963, 1999.

100. Baxter AG, Kinder SJ, Hammond KJ, Scollay R, Godfrey DI: Association between alphabetaTCR+CD4-CD8-T-cell deficiency and IDDM in NOD/Lt mice. *Diabetes* **46**:572, 1997.
101. Qin HY, Sadelain MW, Hitchon C, Lauzon J, Singh B: Complete Freund's adjuvant-induced T cells prevent the development and adoptive transfer of diabetes in nonobese diabetic mice. *J Immunol* **150**:2072, 1993.
102. Ramiya VK, Lan MS, Wasserfall CH, Notkins AL, Maclaren NK: Immunization therapies in the prevention of diabetes. *J Autoimmun* **10**:287, 1997.
103. Dorman JS, La Porte RE, Trucco M: Genetics of diabetes. Genes and environment. *Baillieres Clin Endocrinol Metab* **5**:229, 1991.
104. Maclaren N, Atkinson M: Is insulin-dependent diabetes mellitus environmentally induced? [Editorial; Comment]. *N Engl J Med* **327**:348, 1992.
105. Karvonen M, Tuomilehto J, Libman I, La Porte R: A review of the recent epidemiological data on the worldwide incidence of type 1 (insulin-dependent) diabetes mellitus. World Health Organization DIAMOND Project Group [published erratum appears in *Diabetologia* 38(6):642, 1994]. *Diabetologia* **36**:883, 1993.
106. Vreugdenhil GR, Geluk A, Ottenhoff TH, Melchers WJ, Roep BO, Galama JM: Molecular mimicry in diabetes mellitus: The homologous domain in Coxsackie B virus protein 2C and islet autoantigen GAD65 is highly conserved in the Coxsackie B-like enteroviruses and binds to the diabetes associated HLA-DR3 molecule. *Diabetologia* **41**:40, 1998.
107. Yoon JW, Ray UR: Perspectives on the role of viruses in insulin-dependent diabetes. *Diabetes Care* **1**:39, 1985.
108. Sutkowski N, Palkama T, Ciurli C, Sekaly RP, Thorley-Lawson DA, Huber BT: An Epstein-Barr virus-associated superantigen. *J Exp Med* **184**:971, 1996.
109. Jenson AB, Rosenberg HS, Notkins AL: Pancreatic islet-cell damage in children with fatal viral infections. *Lancet* **2**:354, 1980.
110. Gladisch R, Hofmann W, Waldherr R: [Myocarditis and insulitis following Coxsackie virus infection]. *Z Kardiol* **65**:837, 1976.
111. Champsaur HF, Bottazzo GF, Bertrams J, Assan R, Bach C: Virologic, immunologic, and genetic factors in insulin-dependent diabetes mellitus. *J Pediatr* **100**:15, 1982.
112. Banatvala JE, Bryant J, Schernthaner G, Borkenstein M, Schober E, Brown D, De Silva LM, et al.: Coxsackie B, mumps, rubella, and cytomegalovirus specific IgM responses in patients with juvenile-onset insulin-dependent diabetes mellitus in Britain, Austria, and Australia. *Lancet* **1**:1409, 1985.
113. Yoon JW, Austin M, Onodera T, Notkins AL: Isolation of a virus from the pancreas of a child with diabetic ketoacidosis. *N Engl J Med* **300**:1173, 1979.
114. Ginsberg-Fellner F, Witt ME, Yagihashi S, Dobersen MJ, Taub F, Fedun B, McEvoy RC, et al.: Congenital rubella syndrome as a model for type 1 (insulin-dependent) diabetes mellitus: Increased prevalence of islet cell surface antibodies. *Diabetologia* **27**:87, 1984.
115. Yoon JW, Onodera T, Jenson AB, Notkins AL: Virus-induced diabetes mellitus. XI. Replication of Coxsackie B3 virus in human pancreatic beta cell cultures. *Diabetes* **27**:778, 1978.
116. Prince GA, Jenson AB, Billups LC, Notkins AL: Infection of human pancreatic beta cell cultures with mumps virus. *Nature* **271**:158, 1978.
117. Yoon JW, Onodera T, Notkins AL: Virus-induced diabetes mellitus. XV. Beta cell damage and insulin-dependent hyperglycemia in mice infected with Coxsackie virus B4. *J Exp Med* **148**:1068, 1978.
118. Yoon JW, Selvaggio S, Onodera T, Wheeler J, Jenson AB: Infection of cultured human pancreatic B cells with reovirus type 3. *Diabetologia* **20**:462, 1981.
119. Pak CY, Eun HM, McArthur RG, Yoon JW: Association of cytomegalovirus infection with autoimmune type 1 diabetes. *Lancet* **2**:1, 1988.
120. Kaufman DL, Erlander MG, Clare-Salzler M, Atkinson MA, Maclaren NK, Tobin AJ: Autoimmunity to two forms of glutamate decarboxylase in insulin-dependent diabetes mellitus. *J Clin Invest* **89**:283, 1992.
121. Atkinson MA, Maclaren NK: What causes diabetes? *Sci Am* **263**:62, 1990.
122. Horwitz MS, Bradley LM, Harbertson J, Krahl T, Lee J, Sarvetnick N: Diabetes induced by Coxsackie virus: Initiation by bystander damage and not molecular mimicry. *Nat Med* **4**:781, 1998.
123. Virtanen SM, Saukkonen T, Savilahti E, Ylonen K, Rasanen L, Aro A, Knip M, et al.: Diet, cow's milk protein antibodies and the risk of IDDM in Finnish children. Childhood Diabetes in Finland Study Group. *Diabetologia* **37**:381, 1994.
124. Gerstein HC: Cow's milk exposure and type I diabetes mellitus. A critical overview of the clinical literature. *Diabetes Care* **17**:13, 1994.
125. Schatz DA, Maclaren NK: Cow's milk and insulin-dependent diabetes mellitus. Innocent until proven guilty [Editorial; Comment]. *JAMA* **276**:647, 1996.
126. Classen JB: Childhood immunisation and diabetes mellitus [Letter]. *N Z Med J* **109**:195, 1996.
127. Classen JB, Classen DC: Immunisation and type 1 diabetes mellitus: Is there a link? *Drug Saf* **21**:423, 1999.
128. Abbas AK, Murphy KM, Sher A: Functional diversity of helper T lymphocytes. *Nature* **383**:787, 1996.
129. Mosmann TR, Coffman RL: TH1 and TH2 cells: Different patterns of lymphokine secretion lead to different functional properties. *Annu Rev Immunol* **7**:145, 1989.
130. Mosmann TR, Sad S: The expanding universe of T-cell subsets: Th1, Th2 and more. *Immunol Today* **17**:138, 1996.
131. Bonecchi R, Bianchi G, Bordignon PP, D'Ambrosio D, Lang R, Borsatti A, Sozzani S, et al.: Differential expression of chemokine receptors and chemotactic responsiveness of type 1 T helper cells (Th1s) and Th2s. *J Exp Med* **187**:129, 1998.
132. Segal BM, Dwyer BK, Shevach EM: An interleukin (IL)-10/IL-12 immunoregulatory circuit controls susceptibility to autoimmune disease. *J Exp Med* **187**:537, 1998.
133. Nicoletti F, Zaccone P, Di Marco R, Magro G, Grasso S, Stivala F, Calori G, et al.: Paradoxical antidiabetogenic effect of gamma-interferon in DP-BB rats. *Diabetes* **47**:32, 1998.
134. De Maria R, Todaro M, Stassi G, Di Blasi F, Giordano M, Galluzzo A, Giordano C: Defective T cell receptor/CD3 complex signaling in human type I diabetes. *Eur J Immunol* **24**:999, 1994.
135. MacDonald HR: NK1.1+ T cell receptor-alpha/beta+ cells: new clues to their origin, specificity, and function. *J Exp Med* **182**:633, 1995.
136. Yoshimoto T, Paul WE: CD4pos, NK1.1pos T cells promptly produce interleukin 4 in response to in vivo challenge with anti-CD3. *J Exp Med* **179**:1285, 1994.
137. Koseki H, Asano H, Inaba T, Miyashita N, Moriwaki K, Lindahl KF, Mizutani Y, et al.: Dominant expression of a distinctive V14+ T-cell antigen receptor alpha chain in mice. *Proc Natl Acad Sci U S A* **88**:7518, 1991.
138. Lantz O, Bendelac A: An invariant T cell receptor alpha chain is used by a unique subset of major histocompatibility complex class I-specific CD4+ and CD4-8-T cells in mice and humans. *J Exp Med* **180**:1097, 1994.
139. Exley M, Garcia J, Balk SP, Porcelli S: Requirements for CD1d recognition by human invariant Valpha24+ CD4-CD8-T cells. *J Exp Med* **186**:109, 1997.
140. Davodeau F, Peyrat MA, Necker A, Dominici R, Blanchard F, Leget C, Gaschet J, et al.: Close phenotypic and functional similarities between human and murine alphabeta T cells expressing invariant TCR alpha-chains. *J Immunol* **158**:5603, 1997.
141. Dellabona P, Padovan E, Casorati G, Brockhaus M, Lanzavecchia A: An invariant V alpha 24-J alpha Q/V beta 11 T cell receptor is expressed in all individuals by clonally expanded CD4-8- T cells. *J Exp Med* **180**:1171, 1994.
142. Exley M, Porcelli S, Furman M, Garcia J, Balk S: CD161 (NKR-P1A) costimulation of CD1d-dependent activation of human T cells expressing invariant V alpha 24 J alpha Q T cell receptor alpha chains. *J Exp Med* **188**:867, 1998.
143. Chen H, Paul WE: Cultured NK1.1+ CD4+ T cells produce large amounts of IL-4 and IFN-gamma upon activation by anti-CD3 or CD1. *J Immunol* **159**:2240, 1997.
144. Foucras G, Coureau C, Beijleveld L, Druet P, Saoudi A, Guery JC: Beta 2-microglobulin-dependent T cells are not necessary for alloantigen-induced Th2 responses after neonatal induction of lymphoid chimerism in mice. *J Immunol* **161**:1751, 1998.
145. Mieza MA, Itoh T, Cui JQ, Makino Y, Kawano T, Tsuchida K, Koike T, et al.: Selective reduction of V alpha 14+ NK T cells associated with disease development in autoimmune-prone mice. *J Immunol* **156**:4035, 1996.
146. Cui J, Shin T, Kawano T, Sato H, Kondo E, Toura I, Kaneko Y, et al.: Requirement for Valpha14 NKT cells in IL-12-mediated rejection of tumors. *Science* **278**:1623, 1997.
147. Sumida T, Sakamoto A, Murata H, Makino Y, Takahashi H, Yoshida S, Nishioka K, et al.: Selective reduction of T cells bearing invariant V alpha 24J alpha Q antigen receptor in patients with systemic sclerosis. *J Exp Med* **182**:1163, 1995.
148. Yanagihara Y, Shiozawa K, Takai M, Kyogoku M, Shiozawa S: Natural killer (NK) T cells are significantly decreased in the peripheral blood

of patients with rheumatoid arthritis (RA). *Clin Exp Immunol* **118**:131, 1999.

149. Gombert JM, Herbelin A, Tancrede-Bohin E, Dy M, Carnaud C, Bach JF: Early quantitative and functional deficiency of NK1+-like thymocytes in the NOD mouse. *Eur J Immunol* **26**:2989, 1996.
150. Tamada K, Harada M, Abe K, Li T, Tada H, Onoe Y, Nomoto K: Immunosuppressive activity of cloned natural killer (NK1.1+) T cells established from murine tumor-infiltrating lymphocytes. *J Immunol* **158**:4846, 1997.
151. Onoe Y, Harada M, Tamada K, Abe K, Li T, Tada H, Nomoto K: Involvement of both donor cytotoxic T lymphocytes and host NK1.1+ T cells in the thymic atrophy of mice suffering from acute graft-versus-host disease. *Immunology* **95**:248, 1998.
152. Tsukahara A, Kawamura H, Iiai T, Moroda T, Suzuki S, Tada T, Minagawa M, et al.: Participation of NK1.1+ T cells in the rejection of lpr alphabetaT cells when bone marrow cells of lpr mice are transplanted into B6 mice. *Microbiol Immunol* **42**:447, 1998.
153. Hammond KJL, Poulton LD, Palmisano LJ, Silveira PA, Godfrey DI, Baxter AG: alpha/beta-T cell receptor (TCR)+CD4-CD8-(NKT) thymocytes prevent insulin-dependent diabetes mellitus in nonobese diabetic (NOD)/Lt mice by the influence of interleukin (IL)-4 and/or IL-10. *J Exp Med* **187**:1047, 1998.
154. Lehuen A, Lantz O, Beaudoin L, Laloux V, Carnaud C, Bendelac A, Bach JF, et al.: Overexpression of natural killer T cells protects Valpha14-Jalpha281 transgenic nonobese diabetic mice against diabetes. *J Exp Med* **188**:1831, 1998.
155. Iwakoshi NN, Greiner DL, Rossini AA, Mordes JP: Diabetes prone BB rats are severely deficient in natural killer T cells. *Autoimmunity* **31**:1, 1999.
156. Wilson SB, Kent SC, Patton KT, Orban T, Jackson RA, Exley M, Porcelli S, et al.: Extreme Th1 bias of invariant Vα24JαQ T cells in type 1 diabetes. *Nature* **391**:177, 1998.
157. Denkers EY, Scharton-Kersten T, Barbieri S, Caspar P, Sher A: A role for CD4+ NK1.1+ T lymphocytes as major histocompatibility complex class II independent helper cells in the generation of CD8+ effector function against intracellular infection. *J Exp Med* **184**:131, 1996.
158. Kawano T, Cui J, Koezuka Y, Toura I, Kaneko Y, Motoki K, Ueno H, et al.: CD1d-restricted and TCR-mediated activation of valpha14 NKT cells by glycosylceramides. *Science* **278**:1626, 1997.
159. Burge MR, Schade DS: Insulins. *Endocrinol Metab Clin North Am* **26**:575, 1997.
160. Brange J, Owens DR, Kang S, Volund A: Monomeric insulins and their experimental and clinical implications. *Diabetes Care* **13**:923, 1990.
161. DiMarchi RD, Mayer JP, Fan L, et al.: Synthesis of a fast-acting insulin based on structural homology with insulin-like growth factor 1, in Smith JA, Rivier JE (eds): *Peptides: Chemistry and Biology. Proceedings of the Twelfth American Peptide Symposium*. Leiden, Netherlands, ESCOM, 1992, p 26.
162. Howey DC, Bowsher RR, Brunelle RL, Woodworth JR: [Lys(B28), Pro(B29)]-human insulin. A rapidly absorbed analogue of human insulin. *Diabetes* **43**:396, 1994.
163. Galloway JA, Hooper SA, Spradlin CT, Howey DC, Frank BH, Bowsher RR, Anderson JH: Biosynthetic human proinsulin. Review of chemistry, in vitro and in vivo receptor binding, animal and human pharmacology studies, and clinical trial experience. *Diabetes Care* **15**:666, 1992.
164. Seipke G, Geisen K, Neubauer HP, et al.: New insulin preparations with prolonged action profiles: A21-modified arginine insulins. *Diabetologia* **35(Suppl 1)**:A4, 1992.
165. Cyclosporin-induced remission of IDDM after early intervention. Association of 1 yr of cyclosporin treatment with enhanced insulin secretion. The Canadian-European Randomized Control Trial Group. *Diabetes* **37**:1574, 1988.
166. Stiller CR, Dupre J, Gent M, Jenner MR, Keown PA, Laupacis A, Martell R, et al.: Effects of cyclosporine immunosuppression in insulin-dependent diabetes mellitus of recent onset. *Science* **223**:1362, 1984.
167. Feutren G, Papoz L, Assan R, Vialettes B, Karsenty G, Vexiau P, Du Rostu H, et al.: Cyclosporin increases the rate and length of remissions in insulin-dependent diabetes of recent onset. Results of a multicentre double-blind trial. *Lancet* **2**:119, 1986.
168. Silverstein J, Maclaren N, Riley W, Spillar R, Radjenovic D, Johnson S: Immunosuppression with azathioprine and prednisone in recent-onset insulin-dependent diabetes mellitus. *N Engl J Med* **319**:599, 1988.
169. De Filippo G, Carel JC, Boitard C, Bougneres PF: Long-term results of early cyclosporin therapy in juvenile IDDM. *Diabetes* **45**:101, 1996.
170. Carel JC, Boitard C, Eisenbarth G, Bach JF, Bougneres PF: Cyclosporine delays but does not prevent clinical onset in glucose intolerant pre-type 1 diabetic children. *J Autoimmun* **9**:739, 1996.
171. Coutant R, Landais P, Rosilio M, Johnsen C, Lahlou N, Chatelain P, Carel JC, et al.: Low dose linomide in Type I juvenile diabetes of recent onset: A randomised placebo-controlled double blind trial. *Diabetologia* **41**:1040, 1998.
172. Singh B, Elliot JF: Can progression of IDDM be prevented in newly diagnosed patients by BCG immunotherapy? *Diabetes Metab Rev* **13**:320, 1997.
173. Shehadeh N, Calcinaro F, Bradley BJ, Bruchlim I, Vardi P, Lafferty KJ: Effect of adjuvant therapy on development of diabetes in mouse and man. *Lancet* **343**:706, 1994.
174. Lampeter EF, Klinghammer A, Scherbaum WA, Heinze E, Haastert B, Giani G, Kolb H: The Deutsche Nicotinamide Intervention Study: An attempt to prevent type 1 diabetes. DENIS Group. *Diabetes* **47**:980, 1998.
175. Shah SC, Malone JI, Simpson NE: A randomized trial of intensive insulin therapy in newly diagnosed insulin-dependent diabetes mellitus. *N Engl J Med* **320**:550, 1989.
176. Keller RJ, Eisenbarth GS, Jackson RA: Insulin prophylaxis in individuals at high risk of type I diabetes. *Lancet* **341**:927, 1993.
177. Zhang ZJ, Davidson L, Eisenbarth G, Weiner HL: Suppression of diabetes in nonobese diabetic mice by oral administration of porcine insulin. *Proc Natl Acad Sci U S A* **88**:10252, 1991.
178. Coutant R, Zeidler A, Rappaport R, Schatz D, Schwartz S, Malone J, Raskin P, et al.: Oral insulin therapy in newly diagnosed immune mediated (type 1) diabetes. Preliminary analysis of a randomized double-blind placebo-controlled study. New Orleans, LA, ADA, 1998.
179. Muir A, Peck A, Clare-Salzler M, Song YH, Cornelius J, Luchetta R, Krischer J, et al.: Insulin immunization of nonobese diabetic mice induces a protective insulitis characterized by diminished intraislet interferon-gamma transcription. *J Clin Invest* **95**:628, 1995.
180. Ramiya VK, Shang XZ, Pharis PG, Wasserfall CH, Stabler TV, Muir AB, Schatz DA, et al.: Antigen based therapies to prevent diabetes in NOD mice. *J Autoimmun* **9**:349, 1996.
181. Ramiya VK, Shang XZ, Wasserfall CH, Maclaren NK: Effect of oral and intravenous insulin and glutamic acid decarboxylase in NOD mice. *Autoimmunity* **26**:139, 1997.
182. Daniel D, Wegmann DR: Protection of nonobese diabetic mice from diabetes by intranasal or subcutaneous administration of insulin peptide B-(9-23). *Proc Natl Acad Sci U S A* **93**:956, 1996.
183. Wong FS, Karttunen J, Dumont C, Wen L, Visintin I, Pilip IM, Shastri N, et al.: Identification of an MHC class I-restricted autoantigen in type 1 diabetes by screening an organ-specific cDNA library. *Nat Med* **5**:1026, 1999.
184. Williamson JR, Kilo C: Extracellular matrix changes in diabetes mellitus, in Sarpelli DG, Migahi G (eds): *Comparative Pathobiology of Major Age-Related Diseases*. New York, Liss, 1984, p 269.
185. Federoff HJ, Lawrence D, Brownlee M: Nonenzymatic glycosylation of laminin and the laminin peptide CIKVAVS inhibits neurite outgrowth. *Diabetes* **42**:509, 1993.
186. Merimee TJ: Diabetic retinopathy. A synthesis of perspectives. *N Engl J Med* **322**:978, 1990.
187. King GL, Shiba T, Oliver J, Inoguchi T, Bursell SE: Cellular and molecular abnormalities in the vascular endothelium of diabetes mellitus. *Annu Rev Med* **45**:179, 1994.
188. King GL, Brownlee M: The cellular and molecular mechanisms of diabetic complications. *Endocrinol Metab Clin North Am* **25**:255, 1996.
189. Brownlee M, Cerami A, Vlassara H: Advanced glycosylation end products in tissue and the biochemical basis of diabetic complications. *N Engl J Med* **318**:1315, 1988.
190. Mullarkey CJ, Edelstein D, Brownlee M: Free radical generation by early glycation products: A mechanism for accelerated atherogenesis in diabetes. *Biochem Biophys Res Commun* **173**:932, 1990.
191. Vlassara H, Bucala R, Striker L: Pathogenic effects of advanced glycosylation: Biochemical, biologic, and clinical implications for diabetes and aging. *Lab Invest* **70**:138, 1994.
192. Miyata S, Monnier V: Immunohistochemical detection of advanced glycosylation end products in diabetic tissues using monoclonal antibody to pyrroline. *J Clin Invest* **89**:1102, 1992.
193. Yang CW, Vlassara H, Peten EP, He CJ, Striker GE, Striker LJ: Advanced glycation end products up-regulate gene expression found in diabetic glomerular disease. *Proc Natl Acad Sci U S A* **91**:9436, 1994.

194. Vlassara H, Striker LJ, Teichberg S, Fuh H, Li YM, Steffes M: Advanced glycation end products induce glomerular sclerosis and albuminuria in normal rats. *Proc Natl Acad Sci U S A* **91**:11704, 1994.
195. Skolnik EY, Yang Z, Makita Z, Radoff S, Kirstein M, Vlassara H: Human and rat mesangial cell receptors for glucose-modified proteins: Potential role in kidney tissue remodelling and diabetic nephropathy. *J Exp Med* **174**:931, 1991.
196. Pugliese G, Pricci F, Romeo G, Pugliese F, Mene P, Giannini S, Cresci B, et al.: Upregulation of mesangial growth factor and extracellular matrix synthesis by advanced glycation end products via a receptor-mediated mechanism. *Diabetes* **46**:1881, 1997.
197. Doi T, Vlassara H, Kirstein M, Yamada Y, Striker GE, Striker LJ: Receptor-specific increase in extracellular matrix production in mouse mesangial cells by advanced glycosylation end products is mediated via platelet-derived growth factor. *Proc Natl Acad Sci U S A* **89**:2873, 1992.
198. Crowley ST, Brownlee M, Edelstein D, Satriano JA, Mori T, Singhal PC, Schlondorff DO: Effects of nonenzymatic glycosylation of mesangial matrix on proliferation of mesangial cells. *Diabetes* **40**:540, 1991.
199. Soulis-Liparota T, Cooper M, Papazoglou D, Clarke B, Jerums G: Retardation by aminoguanidine of development of albuminuria, mesangial expansion, and tissue fluorescence in streptozocin-induced diabetic rat. *Diabetes* **40**:1328, 1991.
200. Edelstein D, Brownlee M: Mechanistic studies of advanced glycosylation end product inhibition by aminoguanidine. *Diabetes* **41**:26, 1992.
201. Nakamura S, Makita Z, Ishikawa S, Yasumura K, Fujii W, Yanagisawa K, Kawata T, et al.: Progression of nephropathy in spontaneous diabetic rats is prevented by OPB-9195, a novel inhibitor of advanced glycation. *Diabetes* **46**:895, 1997.
202. Youssef S, Nguyen DT, Soulis T, Panagiotopoulos S, Jerums G, Cooper ME: Effect of diabetes and aminoguanidine therapy on renal advanced glycation end-product binding. *Kidney Int* **55**:907, 1999.
203. Klein R, Klein BE, Moss SE, Cruickshanks KJ: Relationship of hyperglycemia to the long-term incidence and progression of diabetic retinopathy. *Arch Intern Med* **154**:2169, 1994.
204. Krolewski AS, Warram JH, Rand LI, Christlieb AR, Busick EJ, Kahn CR: Risk of proliferative diabetic retinopathy in juvenile-onset type I diabetes: A 40-yr follow-up study. *Diabetes Care* **9**:443, 1986.
205. Mogensen CE, Christensen CK, Vittinghus E: The stages in diabetic renal disease. With emphasis on the stage of incipient diabetic nephropathy. *Diabetes* **2**:64, 1983.
206. Janner M, Knill SE, Diem P, Zuppinger KA, Mullis PE: Persistent microalbuminuria in adolescents with type I (insulin-dependent) diabetes mellitus is associated to early rather than late puberty. Results of a prospective longitudinal study. *Eur J Pediatr* **153**:403, 1994.
207. Mathiesen ER, Ronn B, Storm B, Foght H, Deckert T: The natural course of microalbuminuria in insulin-dependent diabetes: A 10-year prospective study. *Diabet Med* **12**:482, 1995.
208. Krolewski M, Eggers PW, Warram JH: Magnitude of end-stage renal disease in IDDM: A 35 year follow-up study [published erratum appears in *Kidney Int* **51**(3):978, 1997]. *Kidney Int* **50**:2041, 1996.
209. Diabetes Control and Complications Trial Research Group: Progression of retinopathy with intensive versus conventional treatment in the Diabetes Control and Complications Trial. *Ophthalmology* **102**:647, 1995.
210. Quinn M, Angelico MC, Warram JH, Krolewski AS: Familial factors determine the development of diabetic nephropathy in patients with IDDM. *Diabetologia* **39**:940, 1996.
211. Laffel LM, McGill JB, Gans DJ: The beneficial effect of angiotensin-converting enzyme inhibition with captopril on diabetic nephropathy in normotensive IDDM patients with microalbuminuria. North American Microalbuminuria Study Group. *Am J Med* **99**:497, 1995.
212. Krolewski AS, Kosinski EJ, Warram JH, Leland OS, Busick EJ, Asmal AC, Rand LI, et al.: Magnitude and determinants of coronary artery disease in juvenile-onset, insulin-dependent diabetes mellitus. *Am J Cardiol* **59**:750, 1987.
213. Howie JB, Helyer BJ: The immunology and pathology of NZB mice. *Adv Immunol* **9**:215, 1968.
214. Makino S, Kunimoto K, Muraoka Y, Mizushima Y, Katagiri K, Tochino Y: Breeding of a non-obese, diabetic strain of mice. *Jikken Dobutsu* **29**:1, 1980.
215. Nakhooda AF, Like AA, Chappel CI, Wei CN, Marliss EB: The spontaneously diabetic Wistar rat (the "BB" rat). Studies prior to and during development of the overt syndrome. *Diabetologia* **14**:199, 1978.
216. Crisa L, Mordes JP, Rossini AA: Autoimmune diabetes mellitus in the BB rat. *Diabetes Metab Rev* **8**:4, 1992.
217. Elder ME, Maclaren NK: Identification of profound peripheral T lymphocyte immunodeficiencies in the spontaneously diabetic BB rat. *J Immunol* **130**:1723, 1983.
218. Serreze DV, Leiter EH: Insulin dependent diabetes mellitus (IDDM) in NOD mice and BB rats: Origins in hematopoietic stem cell defects and implications for therapy, in Shafrir E (ed): *Lessons from Animal Diabetes*, vol V. London, Smith Gordon, 1995, p 59.
219. Andre I, Gonzalez A, Wang B, Katz J, Benoist C, Mathis D: Checkpoints in the progression of autoimmune disease: Lessons from diabetes models. *Proc Natl Acad Sci U S A* **93**:2260, 1996.
220. Wong FS, Janeway CA Jr.: Insulin-dependent diabetes mellitus and its animal models. *Curr Opin Immunol* **11**:643, 1999.
221. Yoon JW, Yoon CS, Lim HW, Huang QQ, Kang Y, Pyun KH, Hirasawa K, et al.: Control of autoimmune diabetes in NOD mice by GAD expression or suppression in beta cells. *Science* **284**:1183, 1999.
222. Tisch R, McDevitt H: Insulin-dependent diabetes mellitus. *Cell* **85**:291, 1996.
223. Ignatowicz L, Kappler J, Marrack P: The repertoire of T cells shaped by a single MHC/peptide ligand. *Cell* **84**:521, 1996.
224. Miyazaki T, Wolf P, Tourne S, Waltzinger C, Dierich A, Barois N, Ploegh H, et al.: Mice lacking H2-M complexes, enigmatic elements of the MHC class II peptide-loading pathway. *Cell* **84**:531, 1996.
225. Hammer RE, Maika SD, Richardson JA, Tang JP, Taurog JD: Spontaneous inflammatory disease in transgenic rats expressing HLA-B27 and human beta 2m: An animal model of HLA-B27-associated human disorders. *Cell* **63**:1099, 1990.
226. Fukui Y, Nishimura Y, Iwanga T, Kimura A, Inamitsu T, Hanaoka Y, Kitigawa T, et al.: Glycosuria and insulitis in NOD mice expressing the HLA-DQw6 molecule. *J Immunogenet* **16**:445, 1989.
227. Hutchings P, Cooke A: Protection from insulin dependent diabetes mellitus afforded by insulin antigens in incomplete Freund's adjuvant depends on route of administration. *J Autoimmun* **11**:127, 1998.
228. Pagliara AS, Karl IE, Kipnis DB: Transient neonatal diabetes: delayed maturation of the pancreatic beta cell. *J Pediatr* **82**:97, 1973.
229. Kamiya M, Judson H, Okazaki Y, Kusakabe M, Muramatsu M, Takada S, Takagi N, et al.: The cell cycle control gene ZAC/PLAGL1 is imprinted—A strong candidate gene for transient neonatal diabetes. *Hum Mol Genet* **9**:453, 2000.
230. Vendrell J, Ercilla G, Faundez A, Soler S, Gutierrez C, Gomis R, Vilardell E, et al.: Analysis of the contribution of the HLA system to the inheritance in the Wolfram syndrome. *Diabetes Res Clin Pract* **22**:175, 1994.
231. Winter WE, Maclaren NK, Riley WJ, Clarke DW, Kappy MS, Spillar RP: Maturity-onset diabetes of youth in black Americans. *N Engl J Med* **316**:285, 1987.
232. Hardy C, Khanim F, Torres R, Scott-Brown M, Seller A, Poulton J, Collier D, et al.: Clinical and molecular genetic analysis of 19 Wolfram syndrome kindreds demonstrating a wide spectrum of mutations in WFS1. *Am J Hum Genet* **65**:1279, 1999.
233. Strom TM, Hortnagel K, Hofmann S, Gekeler F, Scharfe C, Rabl W, Gerbitz KD, et al.: Diabetes insipidus, diabetes mellitus, optic atrophy and deafness (DIDMOAD) caused by mutations in a novel gene (wolframin) coding for a predicted transmembrane protein. *Hum Mol Genet* **7**:2021, 1998.
234. Inoue H, Tanizawa Y, Wasson J, Behn P, Kalidas K, Bernal-Mizrachi E, Mueckler M, et al.: A gene encoding a transmembrane protein is mutated in patients with diabetes mellitus and optic atrophy (Wolfram syndrome). *Nat Genet* **20**:143, 1998.
235. Hwang JM, Park HW, Kim SJ: Optic neuropathy associated with mitochondrial tRNA[Leu(UUR)] A3243G mutation. *Ophthalmic Genet* **18**:101, 1997.
236. Rotimi CN, Cooper RS, Okosun IS, Olatunbosun ST, Bella AF, Wilks R, Bennett F, et al.: Prevalence of diabetes and impaired glucose tolerance in Nigerians, Jamaicans and US blacks. *Ethn Dis* **9**:190, 1999.
237. Fernandez-Vina M, Ramirez LC, Raskin P, Stastny P: Genes for insulin-dependent diabetes mellitus (IDDM) in the major histocompatibility complex (MHC) of African-Americans. *Tissue Antigens* **41**:57, 1993.
238. Umpierrez GE, Woo W, Hagopian WA, Isaacs SD, Palmer JP, Gaur LK, Nepom GT, et al.: Immunogenetic analysis suggests different pathogenesis for obese and lean African-Americans with diabetic ketoacidosis. *Diabetes Care* **22**:1517, 1999.
239. Osei K, Gaillard T, Schuster DP: Pathogenetic mechanisms of impaired glucose tolerance and type II diabetes in African-Americans. The significance of insulin secretion, insulin sensitivity, and glucose effectiveness. *Diabetes Care* **20**:396, 1997.

240. Joffe BI, Panz VR, Wing JR, Raal FJ, Seftel HC: Pathogenesis of non-insulin-dependent diabetes mellitus in the black population of southern Africa. *Lancet* **340**:460, 1992.
241. McNabb W, Quinn M, Tobian J: Diabetes in African American women: The silent epidemic. *Womens Health* **3**:275, 1997.
242. Lipton RB, Fivecoate JA: High risk of IDDM in African-American and Hispanic children in Chicago, 1985–1990. *Diabetes Care* **18**:476, 1995.
243. Rossetti L: Glucose toxicity: The implications of hyperglycemia in the pathophysiology of diabetes mellitus. *Clin Invest Med* **18**:255, 1995.
244. Rossetti L, Giaccari A, De Fronzo RA: Glucose toxicity. *Diabetes Care* **13**:610, 1990.
245. Hirose H, Lee YH, Inman LR, Nagasawa Y, Johnson JH, Unger RH: Defective fatty acid-mediated beta-cell compensation in Zucker diabetic fatty rats. Pathogenic implications for obesity-dependent diabetes. *J Biol Chem* **271**:5633, 1996.
246. Harmon JS, Gleason CE, Tanaka Y, Oseid EA, Hunter-Berger KK, Robertson RP: In vivo prevention of hyperglycemia also prevents glucotoxic effects on PDX-1 and insulin gene expression. *Diabetes* **48**:1995, 1999.
247. Tanaka Y, Gleason CE, Tran PO, Harmon JS, Robertson RP: Prevention of glucose toxicity in HIT-T15 cells and Zucker diabetic fatty rats by antioxidants. *Proc Natl Acad Sci U S A* **96**:10857, 1999.
248. World Health Organization: *Diabetes Mellitus: Report of a WHO Study Group. World Health Organ Tech Rep Ser*, 1985.
249. Maclaren NK, Riley WJ: Thyroid, gastric, and adrenal autoimmunities associated with insulin-dependent diabetes mellitus. *Diabetes Care* **1**:34, 1985.
250. Flier JS, Kahn CR, Jarrett DB, Roth J: Characterization of antibodies to the insulin receptor: A cause of insulin-resistant diabetes in man. *J Clin Invest* **58**:1442, 1976.
251. Johnson JH, Ogawa A, Chen L, Orci L, Newgard CB, Alam T, Unger RH: Underexpression of beta cell high Km glucose transporters in noninsulin-dependent diabetes [published erratum appears in *Science* 250(4985):1195, 1990]. *Science* **250**:546, 1990.
252. Roitt IM, Doniach D: A reassessment of studies on the aggregation of thyroid autoimmunity in families of thyroiditis patients. *Clin Exp Immunol* **2**:727, 1967.
253. McKenzie JM: Humoral factors in the pathogenesis of Graves' disease. *Physiol Rev* **48**:252, 1968.
254. Karlsson FA, Burman P, Loof L, Mardh S: Major parietal cell antigen in autoimmune gastritis with pernicious anemia is the acid-producing H+,K+-adenosine triphosphatase of the stomach. *J Clin Invest* **81**:475, 1988.
255. Loveridge N, Bitensky L, Chayen J, Hausamen TU, Fisher JM, Taylor KB, Gardner JD, et al.: Inhibition of parietal cell function by human gamma-globulin-containing gastric parietal cell antibodies. *Clin Exp Immunol* **41**:264, 1980.
256. Song YH, Connor EL, Muir A, She JX, Zorovich B, Derovanesian D, Maclaren N: Autoantibody epitope mapping of the 21-hydroxylase antigen in autoimmune Addison's disease. *J Clin Endocrinol Metab* **78**:1108, 1994.
257. Furmaniak J, Kominami S, Asawa T, Wedlock N, Colls J, Smith BR: Autoimmune Addison's disease — Evidence for a role of steroid 21-hydroxylase autoantibodies in adrenal insufficiency. *J Clin Endocrinol Metab* **79**:1517, 1994.
258. Dieterich W, Ehnis T, Bauer M, Donner P, Volta U, Riecken EO, Schuppan D: Identification of tissue transglutaminase as the autoantigen of celiac disease. *Nat Med* **3**:797, 1997.
259. Shapiro AMJ, Lakey JRT, Ryan EA, Korbutt GS, Toth E, Warnock GL, Kneteman NM, Rajotte RV: Islet transplantation in seven patients with type 1 diabetes mellitus using a glucocorticoid-free immunosuppressive regimen. *N Engl J Med* **343**:230, 2000.

CHAPTER 70

Disorders of Fructose Metabolism

Beat Steinmann ▪ Richard Gitzelmann
Georges Van den Berghe

1. Fructose is an important source of dietary carbohydrates. In Western societies, daily intake by adults is presently approximately 100 g. The liver, kidney, and small intestine are the main sites of fructose metabolism, but adipose tissue also participates. Fructose, given intravenously in high doses, is clearly toxic and causes hyperuricemia, hyperlactatemia, and ultrastructural alterations in liver and intestinal cells.

2. Essential fructosuria, an autosomal-recessive disorder, is a benign, asymptomatic metabolic anomaly caused by the absence of fructokinase. Alimentary hyperfructosemia and fructosuria are the principal signs. Despite the interruption of the specific fructose pathway, up to nine tenths of the administered fructose is retained by fructokinase-deficient subjects.

3. Hereditary fructose intolerance, an autosomal-recessive disorder, is characterized by severe hypoglycemia and vomiting shortly after the intake of fructose. Prolonged fructose ingestion in infants leads to poor feeding, vomiting, hepatomegaly, jaundice, hemorrhage, proximal renal tubular syndrome, and finally, hepatic failure and death. Patients develop a strong distaste for noxious food. Therefore, a chronic course is observed only in preschool-aged children. Fructaldolase B of liver, kidney cortex, and small intestine is deficient. Hypoglycemia after fructose ingestion is caused by fructose 1-phosphate–inhibiting glycogenolysis at the phosphorylase level and gluconeogenesis at the mutant aldolase level. Patients remain healthy on a fructose- and sucrose-free diet. The severity of the disease phenotype appears to be independent of the nature of the aldolase B gene mutations so far identified.

4. Hereditary fructose 1,6-bisphosphatase deficiency, an autosomal-recessive disorder, is characterized by episodic spells of hyperventilation, apnea, hypoglycemia, ketosis, and lactic acidosis, with a precipitous and often lethal course in the newborn infant. Later episodes are often triggered by fasting and febrile infections. Due to the enzyme defect, gluconeogenesis is severely impaired. Gluconeogenic precursors such as amino acids, lactate, and ketones accumulate as soon as liver glycogen stores are depleted. Patients do not vomit after fructose intake, and aversion to sweets does not develop. Their tolerance to fasting grows with age. Patients past early childhood seem to develop normally.

5. D-glyceric aciduria, erythrocyte aldolase deficiency, and incomplete fructose absorption are briefly mentioned.

Three inherited abnormalities of fructose metabolism are known. Two of these are caused by a defect of one of the enzymes of the specialized fructose pathway—essential fructosuria and hereditary fructose intolerance—the former a harmless and the latter a potentially lethal condition. Although not a defect of the specialized fructose pathway, hepatic fructose 1,6-bisphosphatase deficiency is usually classified as an error of fructose metabolism. The defect of this enzyme of the gluconeogenic pathway becomes clinically manifest through hypoglycemia and lactic acidosis on fasting and also may be life threatening. The description of the clinical symptoms and biochemical anomalies in the three inborn errors of metabolism is preceded by an outline of the metabolism of fructose. The potential toxic effects of fructose in humans also are discussed: it is essential to understand these toxic effects in order to comprehend the pathophysiology of hereditary fructose intolerance and of fructose 1,6-bisphosphatase deficiency.

METABOLISM OF FRUCTOSE

Chemical Properties and Determination of Fructose

Fructose (β-D-fructofuranose) is a 6-carbon, levorotatory ketose, hence its older name *levulose.* Although it contains no aldehyde group, its tautomeric isomerization from the keto into the enol form in basic solution results in a reducing power equivalent to that of glucose. The presence of fructose, like that of galactose, should thus be suspected in urine samples yielding a positive test result for reducing sugars and a negative reaction with glucose oxidase because both do not react with the latter enzyme. No specific method is available for measuring fructose in the presence of other sugars because even fructokinase can utilize other ketohexoses; however, a useful approach has been described.[1,2] Most colorimetric methods are derived from the Seliwanoff reaction, which is based on the conversion of fructose to hydroxymethylfurfural and condensation with resorcinol in hot acid to form a red product. As modified by Roe *et al.*,[3] or by Higashi and Peters,[4] the technique is satisfactory for the measurement of fructose in blood and urine in clinical situations. To ascertain further the presence of fructose, thin-layer,[5] gas,[6] and liquid[7] chromatography techniques are available. A D-fructose dehydrogenase has been used for measurements of seminal fructose.[8] A method has been devised that allows the measurement of picomolar concentrations of the phosphorylated metabolites of fructose, fructose 1-phosphate, and fructose 1,6-bisphosphate.[9]

A list of standard abbreviations is located immediately preceding the index in each volume. Nonstandard abbreviations used in this chapter include: GLUT5 = glucose transporter 5; ATP = adenosine triphosphate; GTP = guanosine triphosphate; ADP = adenosine diphosphate; PFK 1, 6-phosphofructo-1-kinase; PFK 2, 6-phosphofructo-2-kinase; cAMP = cyclic adenosine monophosphate; AICA = 5-amino-4-imidazole carboxamide; IMP = inosine monophosphate; MRS = magnetic resonance spectroscopy.

Sources and Uses of Fructose

Fructose is widely distributed in nature. As the free monosaccharide, it is found in honey and in numerous vegetables and fruits. As the disaccharide sucrose, it is found in many more nutrients and constitutes an important source of dietary carbohydrate. Lists of the fructose content of various foodstuffs are available.[10,11] Fructose is also a constituent of the trisaccharide raffinose, of the tetrasaccharide stachyose (e.g., in leguminosae seeds), and of inulin (a fructose polymer found in vegetables). However, these compounds play no role in human nutrition, owing to the absence of intestinal enzymes able to degrade them.[12] It should be mentioned that fructose constitutes the main sugar of seminal fluid. Its synthesis in the accessory glands by way of aldose reductase and sorbitol dehydrogenase[13] is testosterone dependent. The presence of the latter enzyme in numerous tissues explains why sorbitol is another source of fructose. Although less abundant than fructose, sorbitol is also widely distributed in fruits and vegetables. Fructose and sucrose are extensively used in human nutrition as sweetening additives for foods, medications, and even infant formulas. In Western societies, its intake has steadily increased since the beginning of this century, is currently approximately 100 g/day per adult[14] or more,[15] and is still rising.[16] The sweetening power of fructose is 1.5 to 1.7 times that of sucrose. Oral fructose has been investigated as a means to avoid hypoglycemia[17] and muscle glycogen depletion[18] during athletic exercise. The issue of fructose consumption and atherosclerosis has been discussed in several symposia[19–21] and reviews.[22,23]

Two medical uses for fructose have been advocated. The observation by Minkowski in 1893[24] that the utilization of fructose does not require insulin resulted in the still widespread belief that fructose as well as sorbitol are adequate sweetening agents for patients with diabetes mellitus. In fact, intravenous (IV) and oral fructose do produce an insulin response when blood glucose is elevated.[25] The development of IV nutrition in the early 1950s has led to the use of various compounds, among them fructose and sorbitol, as a source of energy in this therapy. Solutions of equimolar amounts of fructose and glucose, prepared by the hydrolysis of sucrose and known as *invert sugar,* as well as solutions of pure fructose (levulose) are available. The use of sorbitol is fostered by its chemical stability. As will be discussed, the infusion of fructose and sorbitol carries important risks to normal individuals and becomes life threatening in individuals with hereditary fructose intolerance and fructose 1,6-bisphosphatase deficiency. The use of these sugars as glucose substitutes in parenteral nutrition should therefore be strongly discouraged.

Utilization of Fructose by the Body as a Whole

Several studies of the utilization of fructose at the whole-body level in humans and experimental animals have shown that it is utilized mainly in the liver, kidney, and small intestine.[26] Only data obtained in humans are summarized here.

Taken by mouth, fructose is absorbed by the small intestine at a rate roughly half that of glucose and galactose.[27,28] In the small intestine, fructose is not converted to glucose, and a large proportion is absorbed unchanged.[27,29] Following the instillation of approximately 0.7 g/kg fructose into the jejunal lumen, its concentration in the portal system may reach about 2.5 mM within 5 to 15 min.[27] Once fructose reaches the bloodstream, it is utilized rapidly. Administered in a peripheral vein at the dose of 0.5 g/kg body weight over 30 min, fructose disappears from the circulation twice as fast as glucose, its half-life being about 18 min,[30] as compared with 43 min for glucose.[31] Studies of fructose utilization during prolonged perfusion in subjects with hepatic vein catheterization show that approximately half of the fructose load is taken up by the splanchnic bed, with the liver accounting for more than 75 percent and the small intestine for approximately 10 percent of this uptake.[32,33] Catheterization of the renal vein shows that about 20 percent of an IV fructose load is taken up by the kidney.[34] The prominent role played by liver, kidney, and small intestine in fructose utilization is explained by the presence of the specialized pathway of fructose metabolism described below. That this metabolism is highly efficient is evidenced by the observations that, following the oral ingestion of 1 g/kg fructose, its concentration in peripheral veins does not increase above 0.3 to 0.35 mM[35] and that, although there is virtually no renal threshold for fructose, only a small percentage of the administered dose is recovered in the urine.[30,32,36,37]

Transport of Fructose

The study of the membrane transport of fructose is complicated by its rapid intracellular utilization, particularly in tissues possessing the specialized enzymes of fructose metabolism. Investigation of the intestinal transport of fructose is further confounded by species differences. Most studies nevertheless indicate that transport of fructose through the brush-border membrane does not proceed via the Na^+-glucose cotransporter, but by facilitated diffusion via a separate carrier, the glucose transporter 5 (GLUT5), which is Na^+ independent, insensitive to phlorizin, operates more slowly, and has lower capacity.[38–41] The latter explains why, in the majority of human subjects, the oral ingestion of amounts of fructose exceeding 0.5 to 1.0 g/kg body weight induces malabsorption.[43–47] (See later section on Incomplete Fructose Absorption.) Enhancement of the intestinal absorption of fructose has been reported when the ketose is given in the form of sucrose or together with free glucose or galactose[45,48,49] or glycine.[50] This has led to the hypothesis of a joint transport of fructose with glucose or galactose by a disaccharidase-related transport system located in the intestinal brush-border membrane.[51] However, most recent studies indicate that the transporter responsible for the uptake of fructose from the lumen of the small intestine, across the apical membrane of the enterocyte, is the glucose transporter isoform GLUT5.[52] GLUT5 transports fructose with high affinity and has a much higher capacity to transport fructose than glucose. Expression of GLUT5 in the intestine is up-regulated by fructose but not by sucrose,[53,54] and displays a circadian rhythm with a several-fold increase in GLUT5 messenger RNA (mRNA) at the end of the light cycle.[55] GLUT5 is also developmentally regulated because its expression increases progressively during the postnatal period,[55,56] although it can be enhanced by precocious introduction of dietary fructose.[57] The identity of the carrier responsible for the efflux of fructose from the enterocytes into the circulation, across the basolateral membrane, is controversial: both GLUT2[56,58] and GLUT5[59] have been claimed to play this role. Expression of GLUT5 in muscle[60] and erythrocytes[61] indicates that it probably also plays a role in fructose transport in these tissues (see later section on Incomplete Intestinal Fructose Absorption).

Fructose does not enter the hepatocyte freely, as evidenced by the steep gradient between its extracellular and intracellular concentrations.[42,62] Computations from the kinetics of fructose uptake and metabolism in the perfused rat liver[62] are in accordance with a carrier-mediated transport with a K_m of 67 mM and a V_{max} of 30 µmol/min/g of tissue (Fig. 70-1). Experiments performed, to avoid interference of fructose metabolism, over less than 1 min with isolated rat hepatocytes have given an even higher K_m value of around 200 mM.[63] Competition studies indicate that fructose is transported into the liver cell, at least in part, by the same system as glucose and galactose.[63,64]

In adipose tissue, fructose is transported by at least two different carriers. A specific fructose transporter requires a concentration of about 25 mM for half-maximal saturation and is insensitive to glucose and to insulin. Fructose also can enter the adipocyte by the glucose transporter, which has a five- to tenfold lower K_m for it than the specific carrier and an approximately 50 percent lower V_{max}, which is roughly doubled by insulin. However, a participation of the latter carrier in the transport of fructose into adipocytes under physiologic conditions is unlikely, owing to the competition exerted by glucose.[65–67]

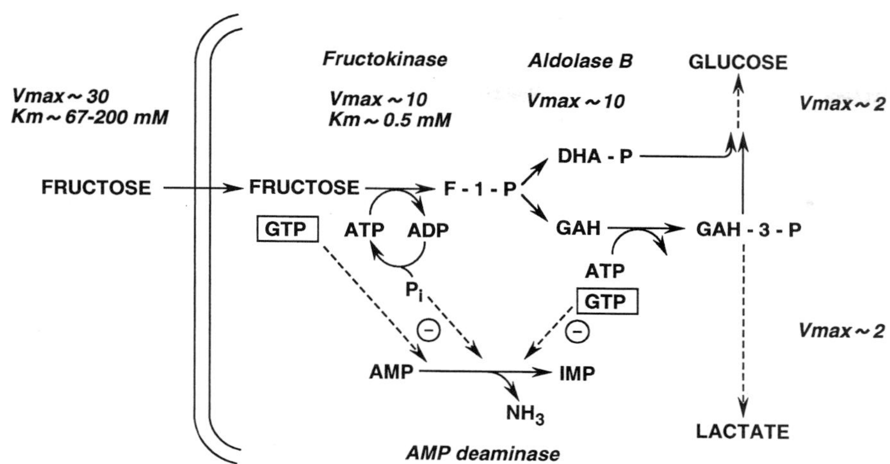

Fig. 70-1 The mechanism of fructose-induced accumulation of fructose 1-phosphate and hyperuricemia. DHA = dihydroxyacetone; GAH = glyceraldehyde; F = fructose. (−) = inhibition. Velocities are given as μmol/min per g of liver at 37°C. Further explanations are given in the text.

Enzymes of Fructose Metabolism

The predominance of liver, kidney, and small intestine is based on the presence of the three enzymes — fructokinase, aldolase type B, and triokinase — which convert fructose into intermediates of the glycolytic–gluconeogenic pathway (Fig. 70-2). A detailed account of the experiments that led to the elucidation of the fructose pathway was given by Hers.[68]

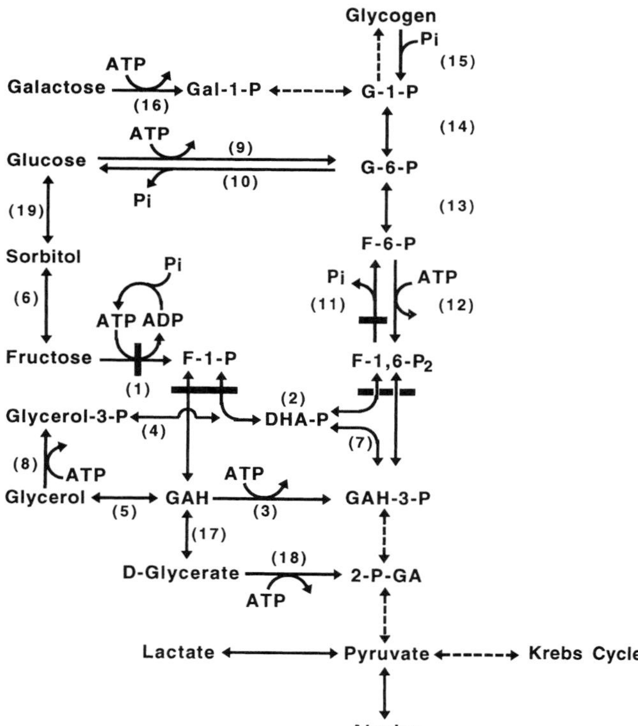

Fig. 70-2 Pathway of fructose metabolism in the liver and its defects. DHA = dihydroxyacetone; GAH = glyceraldehyde; F = fructose; G = glucose; GA = glycerate; (1) = fructokinase; (2) = fructaldolase; (3) = triokinase; (4) = glycerol 3-P-dehydrogenase; (5) = alcohol dehydrogenases and aldose reductase; (6) = sorbitol dehydrogenase; (7) = triose phosphate isomerase; (8) = glycerol kinase; (9) = hexokinase and glucokinase; (10) = glucose 6-phosphatase; (11) = fructose 1,6-bisphosphatase; (12) = 6-phosphofructose-1-kinase; (13) = phosphohexose isomerase; (14) = phosphoglucomutase; (15) = glycogen phosphorylase; (16) = galactokinase; (17) = aldehyde dehydrogenase; (18) = glycerate kinase; (19) = aldose reductase (not present in liver).

Fructokinase (Ketohexokinase, EC 2.7.1.3). Fructokinase catalyzes the phosphorylation of fructose to fructose 1-phosphate (see Fig. 70-2).[69–71] The enzyme is not specific for fructose because it also utilizes L-sorbose, D-tagatose, D-xylulose, L-galactoheptulose,[70,72–74] 5-keto-D-fructose,[75,76] and certain 2,5-anhydroalditols, such as 2,5-anhydro-D-mannitol.[77] It is therefore considered a ketohexokinase. The phosphoryl donors are adenosine triphosphate (ATP), to a minor extent 2′-dATP and 3′-dATP,[72] and guanosine triphosphate (GTP).[78] The K_m for fructose is about 0.5 mM.[70,72,74,79] Affinity constants for Mg^2-ATP, obtained by different researchers, vary between 0.2 and 2 mM.[72,74,79,80] The V_{max} in crude extracts of rat and human liver reaches 2 to 3 μmol/min/g of tissue at 22 to 25°C[42,72,81,82] or about 10 μmol/min/g at 37°C (see Fig. 70-1). Fructokinase is most abundant in the liver, where it constitutes between 0.04 and 0.6 percent of total protein; in the kidney, small intestine, and pancreas; and at much lower levels in heart, brain, and muscle.[83] Fructokinase requires high concentrations of KCl[84] and is strongly inhibited by adenosine diphosphate (ADP), one of the reaction products.[79] Rat liver fructokinase is presumably a monomer with a molecular weight of 28,000,[74] but the beef liver enzyme was reported to be a dimer with a molecular weight of 56,000.[76] Full-length complementary DNAs for the rat liver[85] and the human[86] enzyme have been obtained. Recently, the chromosomal localization of the fructokinase gene has been reassigned to 2p23.2-23.3.[87] The human genomic structure has been defined.[88] It spans 14 kb and contains nine exons (1–2, 3a, 3c, 4–8). An intragenic duplication has resulted in two similar 135-bp exons (designated 3a and 3c), separated by a short intron. Exons 3a and 3c are mutually exclusively spliced into fructokinase mRNA and produce two different mRNA types as described.[86] This exon–intron structure, as well as the pattern of alternative splicing, are conserved in both rat and mouse, suggesting distinct conserved functions for the two fructokinase isoforms. The alternative splicing is also tissue specific: in both rats and humans, tissues expressing high levels of fructokinase (i.e., liver, kidney cortex, and duodenum) utilize exclusively the 3c exon, whereas other tissues use only 3a; both isoforms are present in the pancreas. Furthermore, comparison of human fetal and adult tissues indicates a developmental shift from use of exon 3a to 3c.[88] Expression studies of both forms in *Escherichia coli* show that the A splice form has a very high K_m for fructose (approximately 10 mM) as compared with the C splice form; together with its distribution at low level in a variety of tissues, it makes it unlikely that fructose is a physiologic substrate for the fructokinase isoform A.[89]

Fructaldolase (Fructose 1,6-Bisphosphate Aldolase, Aldolase, EC 4.1.2.13). Three aldolase isozymes are known, and at least three different aldolase genes have been identified. They are related and probably derive from a single ancestral gene.[90] Aldolase of the liver, kidney, and small intestine (aldolase B; Genebank Accession No. X01098) reversibly splits fructose 1-phosphate into D-glyceraldehyde and dihydroxyacetone phosphate. Similarly to its isozymes found in muscle (aldolase A; Accession No. M11560) and in brain (aldolase C; Accession No. X07092), aldolase B also catalyzes the splitting of the glycolytic–gluconeogenic intermediate fructose 1,6-bisphosphate into D-glyceraldehyde-3-phosphate and dihydroxyacetone phosphate, and the condensation of the latter triosephosphates. The three aldolases can be distinguished by their catalytic and immunologic properties as well as by their tissue and cell distribution. Liver aldolase B has approximately the same V_{max} with fructose 1-phosphate and fructose-1,6-bisphosphate,[91,92] reaching 2 to 3 μmol/min/g of tissue at 25°C in rat[42] and human liver.[81,92] In contrast, aldolases A and C have a fifty- and tenfold lower V_{max} activity with fructose 1-phosphate than with fructose 1,6-bisphosphate.[93] The K_m of human liver aldolase B is around 1 mM for fructose 1-phosphate and 4 to 12 μM for fructose 1,6-bisphosphate.[91,94] The aldolases have a molecular weight of about 160,000 and are composed of four identical subunits that are immunologically distinct in isozymes A, B, and C.[95,96] Strikingly, the isolated aldolase A monomer retains substantial catalytic activity, indicating that the quaternary structure is not required for catalysis.[97] Evidence has been presented that liver aldolase could form a complex with fructose 1,6-bisphosphatase.[98,99] The three isoforms of human aldolase have been shown to bind in a tissue-specific fashion to the actin-containing filaments of the cytoskeleton.[100]

Interestingly, early fetal human liver, kidney, and small intestine contain mainly aldolase A[101,102] and aldolase C[103]; their subsequent replacement by aldolase B with different kinetic characteristics suggests adaptation to specific metabolic needs. Hepatoma formation, on the other hand, is associated with the repression of aldolase B and the reappearance of the A and C isoenzymes.[103,104] In the kidney, aldolase B is found mainly in the proximal tubules, whereas aldolase A is predominant in the distal tubules and glomeruli.[105–108] In small-intestinal epithelium, aldolase B predominates in the absorptive villus cells and aldolase A in the rapidly dividing crypt cells.[109] Human erythrocytes[110,111] and cultured fibroblasts[112,113] contain aldolase A.

Aldolases A and C are constitutively expressed, but the B isoform is under dietary control.[114] Under resting conditions, the expression of aldolase B mRNA is low and any functional enzyme present in the cytosol appears to associate with components of the cytoskeletal network, rendering it catalytically inactive; after feeding a carbohydrate diet, mRNA expression is induced and the enzyme is activated by dissociation of the enzyme–cytoskeletal protein complex in the presence of accumulated intermediate metabolites. During fasting, the activity of rabbit liver aldolase decreases to less than half the fed value.[115] The finding that this decrease was not accompanied by a decrease in total immunoreactive protein has led to the identification of several lysosomal proteinases that catalyze inactivation of the enzyme by limited proteolysis.[116,117] Although liver aldolase is susceptible to proteolytic degradation during its purification,[118] results obtained under conditions that avoid disruption of lysosomes during the isolation procedure[117] suggest that the modifications induced by fasting occur *in vivo*.

The molecular biology of aldolases has been extensively investigated, mainly because such study may provide insight into the regulatory mechanism of tissue-specific gene expression in eukaryotic cells.[119] The increase in liver aldolase B recorded during fetal development was linked to an increase of isozyme-specific mRNA in humans[120] and in rats.[121] Cloning and characterization of cDNA for aldolase B has been achieved in rats[122–124] and humans.[125,126] The complete structure and genomic organization of both rat and human aldolase B genes is known.[127–129] The human aldolase B gene is present in a single copy, and its chromosomal location is 9q13 → q32.[130,131] It is 14,500 bp long, contains nine exons, the first of which is not translated,[128] encoding a 364 amino acid protein.[126,128,129,132] At least four aldolase B mRNA species exist in human liver.[132] Aldolase A and C genes have been mapped to chromosomes 16 and 17, respectively.[133,134]

The most thoroughly investigated rabbit muscle aldolase (aldolase A) has been crystallized and the three-dimensional structure determined by x-ray diffraction at a resolution of 1.9 Å[135,136] (for more details, see legend to Fig. 70-12).

Triokinase (EC 2.7.1.28). This enzyme converts D-glyceraldehyde into D-glyceraldehyde-3-phosphate, allowing thereby the nonphosphorylated product of the cleavage of fructose 1-phosphate to reach the glycolytic–gluconeogenic pathway (see Fig. 70-2).[91] Triokinase preferentially utilizes ATP as phosphoryl donor, but inosine triphosphate can be utilized at 14 percent and GTP at 10 percent of the rate of utilization of the adenine nucleotide.[137] The V_{max} of the enzyme is around 2 μmol/min/g at 37°C in rat[81,138] and human[81] liver, whereas the K_m values are 0.01 mM for D-glyceraldehyde[139] and 0.8 mM for Mg^{2+}-ATP.[140]

Fructose 1,6-Bisphosphatase (EC 3.1.3.11). Fructose 1,6-bisphosphatase, also called hexose bisphosphatase, catalyzes the irreversible splitting of fructose 1,6-bisphosphate into fructose 6-phosphate and inorganic phosphate (P_i) (see Fig. 70-2). Fructose 1,6-bisphosphatase is found in many cell types and species, but its activity is highest in the gluconeogenic tissues, namely liver and kidney. In rat and human liver, its V_{max} at 25°C reaches approximately 6.5 and 4.1 μmol/min/g of tissue, respectively.[81] Liver fructose 1,6-bisphosphatase possesses complex regulatory properties.[141–143] It is Mg^{2+} dependent and, in the absence of effectors, displays hyperbolic kinetics for its substrate with a K_m in the low micromolar range. The enzyme is inhibited competitively by concentrations in the physiologic range of fructose 6-phosphate and P_i, the products of the reaction, and noncompetitively by physiologic concentrations of AMP, which binds to an allosteric site. The inhibition by AMP is markedly reinforced by low micromolar concentrations of fructose 2,6-bisphosphate, a regulatory molecule discovered in 1980.[144–146] Fructose 2,6-bisphosphate changes the substrate saturation curve from hyperbolic to sigmoidal.[147] This suggests an allosteric interaction, either at an independent site or at the AMP-binding site, although binding of fructose 2,6-bisphosphate to the active site of the enzyme also has been proposed.[148,149]

Fructose 2,6-bisphosphate is also a potent stimulator of 6-phophofructo-1-kinase (PFK 1).[150] This enzyme catalyzes the reaction which opposes that of fructose 1,6-bisphosphatase, namely the equally irreversible conversion of fructose 6-phosphate into fructose 1,6-bisphosphate, utilizing ATP as the phosphoryl donor (Fig. 70-3). Owing to its opposite effects on PFK 1 and fructose 1,6-bisphosphatase, the concentration of fructose 2,6-bisphosphate determines whether metabolic flux through the hepatic Embden-Meyerhof pathway proceeds in the direction of glycolysis or gluconeogenesis. Glucose, the main glycolytic substrate, increases fructose 2,6-bisphosphate by stimulating its synthesis from fructose 6-phosphate by 6-phosphofructo-2-kinase (PFK 2). The latter activity is exerted by a bifunctional enzyme protein, which also catalyzes the degradation of fructose 2,6-bisphosphate.[151] Elevation of fructose 2,6-bisphosphate results in stimulation of PFK 1 and in inhibition of fructose 1,6-bisphosphatase. Glucagon, the principal gluconeogenic hormone, decreases fructose 2,6-bisphosphate by activating fructose 2,6-bisphosphatase via a cyclic adenosine monophosphate (cAMP)-dependent phosphorylation. The decrease in fructose 2,6-bisphosphate suppresses both stimulation of PFK 1 and inhibition of fructose 1,6-bisphosphatase. The opposite effects of fructose 2,6-bisphosphate on PFK 1 and fructose 1,6-bisphosphatase thus theoretically avoid simultaneous operation of both enzymes, resulting in a so-called futile recycling of substrates. Nevertheless, although little or no recycling between fructose 6-phosphate and

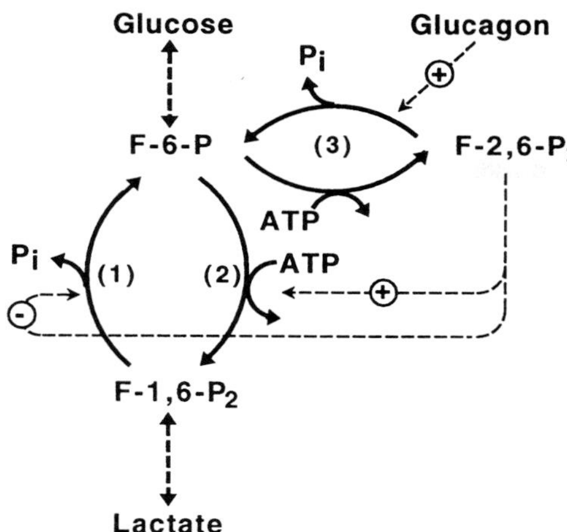

Fig. 70-3 Fructose 6-phosphate-fructose 1,6-bisphosphate substrate cycle in the liver and its regulation. (1) = fructose 1,6-bisphosphatase; (2) = 6-phosphofructose-1-kinase (PFK 1); (3) = bifunctional 6-phophofructose-2-kinase (PFK 2) and fructose 2,6-bisphosphatase. Stimulation is denoted by (+) and inhibition by (−). Further explanations are given in the text.

fructose 1,6-bisphosphate occurs in the liver of starved rats, it proceeds to a significant extent in the fed state.[152]

Liver fructose 1,6-bisphosphatase is a homotetramer with a molecular weight of around 140,000.[153] The enzyme is susceptible to proteolysis by lysosomal proteases,[154,155] rendering the enzyme more active at alkaline pH and more sensitive to stimulation by histidine, the latter effect being probably related to the chelation of inhibitory Zn^{2+} ions.[156] The long-term increase in activity of fructose-1,6-bisphosphatase in gluconeogenic conditions such as prolonged starvation, diabetes, or corticoid treatment has been attributed to this mechanism, because histidine increases in these situations. The mode of regulation of fructose 1,6-bisphosphatase by zinc seems complex.[157] Intestinal fructose 1,6-bisphosphatase of some animal species has been shown to differ from the liver enzyme in its AMP inhibition characteristics.[158] The complete amino acid sequence of fructose 1,6-bisphosphatase of pig kidney[159] and of sheep[160] and rat[161] liver has been reported. Differences in amino acid content[162] indicate that muscle fructose 1,6-bisphosphatase is a different enzyme. The enzyme from pig kidney cortex has been crystallized, and its three-dimensional molecular structure in different conformational states, induced by binding of products and effectors, has been determined by x-ray crystallography.[163–166]

The localization of fructose 1,6-bisphosphatase in rat liver and kidney was determined immunologically.[167] The study showed that the enzyme was preferentially localized in hepatocytes of the periportal region and was absent from the perivenous region. The enzyme was also preferentially localized in the proximal renal tubules and was absent in glomeruli, loops of Henle, collecting and distal tubules, and the renal medulla. The enzyme was present mainly in the perinuclear region in liver and kidney cells, as shown by confocal microscopy, and subcellular fractionation studies showed that the majority of the enzyme activity was associated with particulate structures; thus, it cannot be considered a soluble enzyme in the classic sense. As discussed by Saéz *et al.*,[167] the data support the concept of *metabolic zonation*: regulation of glycolysis and gluconeogenesis is important in organs and tissues (such as liver and kidney cortex) sharing both capabilities. It has been shown by tissue microdissection that in the liver, glucose is mainly formed periportally by gluconeogenesis and glycogenolysis, whereas in the perivenous zone liponeogenesis is linked to glycolysis. This metabolic zonation is analogous to that in the renal cortex, itself heterogeneous, with gluconeogenesis located in the proximal and glycolysis in the distal tubules.

A full-length coding cDNA[161] and the gene[168] of rat liver fructose 1,6-bisphosphatase have been cloned. The gene has a length of 23 kb, contains seven exons, encodes a 362-amino acid sequence, and has been used to express the enzyme in *E. coli*.[169] The severalfold elevation of the activity of fructose 1,6-bisphosphatase, recorded in starvation and diabetes, has been explained by a glucagon and cAMP-mediated increase in fructose 1,6-bisphosphatase mRNA. On the other hand, the insulin-induced diminution of the amount of fructose 1,6-bisphosphatase in diabetic animals has been shown to result from a decrease of the level of mRNA.[168] The cDNA of human liver fructose 1,6-bisphosphatase has been isolated and expressed in *E. coli*,[170] and the gene has been characterized and localized to chromosome bands 9q22.2-q22.3.[171] Although only a single fructose 1,6-bisphosphatase gene has been identified up to now, observations in fructose 1,6-bisphosphatase deficiency indicate the presence of at least one other gene. The molecular structure of human liver fructose 1,6-bisphosphatase and the effect of site-directed mutagenesis of active[170] and allosteric[172] site residues also have been investigated, the latter with the goal of designing inhibitors of the enzyme for therapy in non–insulin-dependent diabetes. Inhibition of fructose 1,6-bisphosphatase by ZMP, an AMP analog formed from 5-amino-4-imidazole carboxamide (AICA) riboside, has indeed been shown to inhibit gluconeogenesis in isolated rat hepatocytes[173] and to lower blood glucose in normal mice.[174]

Alternate Pathways of Fructose Metabolism

Phosphorylation of Fructose to Fructose 6-Phosphate. The marked affinity for fructose and the high activity of fructokinase explain the preferential utilization of the ketose and its phosphorylation to fructose 1-phosphate by the tissues possessing the enzyme. Nevertheless, these and other tissues theoretically also can metabolize fructose to fructose 6-phosphate using hexokinase and even glucokinase (hexokinase D).[175] However, in the presence of physiologic concentrations of glucose, this conversion will be severely restricted because the affinity of the hexokinases for fructose is several orders of magnitude lower than that for glucose.[175–177] The capacity of several tissues to metabolize fructose has been investigated in detail by Froesch and Ginsberg.[65,178] Human erythrocytes and leukocytes, incubated in the absence of glucose, metabolize fructose nearly as fast as glucose; in the presence of a physiologic concentration of glucose (approximately 5 mM), the utilization of 5 mM fructose is about 90 percent inhibited. Muscle and adipose tissue may nevertheless participate to some extent in the metabolism of fructose. In the rat diaphragm, the utilization of 5 mM fructose is only 50 percent inhibited by the addition of glucose at physiologic concentrations. This is attributed to the low concentration of free glucose inside muscle cells. Under this condition, the utilization of 5 mM fructose nevertheless reaches only 20 percent of that of a similar concentration of glucose. The utilization of fructose by adipose tissue may be more important. At a concentration of 10 mM, fructose is utilized at two thirds the rate of glucose by rat epididymal fat. When both sugars are added together, rates are nearly additive. This can be explained by the virtual absence of free glucose in the adipocyte because it is bound to its carrier.

Phosphorylation of Fructose to Fructose 3-Phosphate. This fructose ester was initially identified in the lens and sciatic nerve of diabetic rats.[179] Its presence was also demonstrated in erythrocytes of normal, diabetic, and fructosuric humans, with concentrations tending to be higher in the latter.[180,181] Incubation of erythrocytes[182] and lenses[183] with concentrations of fructose in the range of those recorded following its oral or IV administration (0.1 to 2.5 mM) has shown that these cells can phosphorylate (by a yet-to-be-defined kinase) fructose to fructose 3-phosphate. Unlike phosphorylation to fructose 6-phosphate, formation of fructose 3-phosphate is not inhibited by physiologic concentrations of glucose[182] but can be prevented by inhibitors of aldose reductase.[184] Owing to its potency as a protein-glycating and –cross-linking agent, it was hypothesized that fructose 3-phosphate may play a role in the etiology of diabetic complications, but this view has been contested.[181] How hyperglycemia results in an increased formation of fructose 3-phosphate remains to be determined.

Phosphorylation of Fructose 1-Phosphate to Fructose 1,6-Bisphosphate. It has been proposed that only 50 percent of the fructose 1-phosphate formed from fructose is split by aldolase B and that the remainder is directly converted into fructose 1,6-bisphosphate by a fructose 1-phosphate kinase.[185] This theory was based on studies performed in children who received uniformly labeled [^{13}C]fructose by gastric infusion. Whereas, owing to cleavage of [^{13}C]fructose 1-phosphate by aldolase and recombination of the resulting [^{13}C]dihydroxyacetone-phosphate and phosphorylated [^{13}C]glyceraldehyde with unlabeled triosephosphate molecules, essentially only C1-C2-C3– and C4-C5-C6–labeled glucose was expected, about 50 percent of [^{13}C]glucose found in blood was uniformly labeled. Conversion of fructose to glucose by way of phosphorylation into fructose 6-phosphate was ruled out because no uniformly labeled [^{13}C]fructose was found in patients with fructose 1,6-bisphosphatase deficiency.[186] However, no uniformly labeled [^{13}C]glucose was found following IV administration of [U-^{13}C]fructose in animals.[187] This raised the suspicion, proven by studies of the fructose-to-glucose conversion in rabbit small intestine,[188] that the results of the oral studies can be explained by incomplete dilution of the [^{13}C]triosephosphates by a smaller pool of unlabeled triosephosphates in the intestinal mucosa as compared with the liver.

Conversion of D-Glyceraldehyde to Triosephosphate. Two alternate pathways (see Fig. 70-2) to the formation of glyceraldehyde 3-phosphate by triokinase have been proposed: reduction to glycerol by NADH and alcohol dehydrogenase or by NADPH and aldose reductase, followed by phosphorylation to glycerol 3-phosphate and subsequent oxidation to dihydroxyacetone phosphate; and oxidation to D-glycerate and conversion to 2-phosphoglycerate. As was discussed by Hers,[68] studies of the randomization of the fructose carbons indicate that D-glyceraldehyde is utilized by triokinase *in vivo*. This was confirmed by a kinetic study of the glyceraldehyde-metabolizing enzymes and by experiments with [4–^{3}H,6–^{14}C]fructose.[189] The observation that in some patients with D-glyceric aciduria, a rare inborn error of metabolism (see later section on D-Glyceric Aciduria), the excretion of D-glyceric acid increases after ingestion of fructose[190] suggests that oxidation of glyceraldehyde into D-glycerate in fact occurs under certain conditions. Studies with isolated rat liver cells have indicated moreover that, at fructose concentrations exceeding 5 mM, oxidation of D-glyceraldehyde and subsequent formation of 2-phosphoglycerate might proceed inside the mitochondria.[191]

End Products of Fructose Metabolism

Controversies surround the use of fructose for parenteral nutrition and as a sweetener in healthy and diabetic subjects. It is further suspected to exert a hypertriglyceridemic effect. Therefore, its metabolic end products have been studied. In isolated rat liver perfused with fructose, about 50 to 75 percent is recovered as glucose and 20 to 25 percent as lactate plus pyruvate.[42,62,192] Similar results were obtained for human liver and kidney during IV perfusion with 0.3 g of fructose/kg/h, by sampling in the hepatic and renal veins.[34] However, with higher doses of fructose, up to 60 percent is taken up by the human liver and converted to lactic acid, whereas the release of glucose from the splanchnic area is not modified or even reduced.[193,194] Glycogen constitutes quantitatively the third most important product of fructose metabolism, accounting for 8 percent of its utilization by the perfused rat liver.[192] Studies with radioactive fructose also have shown its conversion to triglycerides,[195–198] estimated to represent 1 to 3 percent of its overall metabolism.[199] Additional data concerning the further metabolism of fructose can be found elsewhere.[22,23,26,200]

Influence of Fructose on the Hepatic Uptake of Glucose

Several long-standing observations show that fructose stimulates the hepatic uptake of glucose and the incorporation of the latter into glycogen.[68,201a,211.] Some studies[201,201b] have demonstrated that this effect is mediated by a 60-kDa protein regulator of glucokinase, and rat liver cDNAs encoding this regulator have been cloned.[202] The regulator decreases the affinity of glucokinase for glucose by forming a complex with the enzyme in the presence of physiologic (10 to 40 μM) concentrations of fructose 6-phosphate. Fructose 1-phosphate, already at 10 μM concentration, opposes the formation of the complex and thereby antagonizes the inhibition of glucokinase.[203] Intragastric administration of as little as 20 mg/kg of fructose to rats increases their hepatic concentration of fructose 1-phosphate from less than 5 nmol/g to approximately 30 nmol/g, and doubles the rate of glucose phosphorylation in their liver.[204] Fructose can thus be considered as a signal to the liver that glucose, with which it is often associated, is being absorbed from the gut.

TOXICITY OF FRUCTOSE

After the discovery of hereditary fructose intolerance, fructose toxicity was first thought to be limited to individuals with the aldolase B defect. In the late 1960s, deleterious effects of high doses of IV fructose were also recognized clinically in healthy persons. Hyperuricemia[205] and lactic acidosis[206] were the prominent findings. These observations have led to the recommendation of great caution in the use of fructose in parenteral nutrition.[207–210] Deleterious effects can be traced to the very rapid metabolism after parenteral administration by tissues possessing the specialized enzymes fructokinase, aldolase B, and triokinase, and to the resulting accumulation of fructose 1-phosphate (see Fig. 70-1). The high V_{max} of fructokinase (about 10 μmol/min/g of tissue at 37°C) is a major determinant of this rapid metabolism. For instance, in the liver the maximal rate of phosphorylation of fructose is more than 10 times higher than the glucose-phosphorylating capacity of glucokinase.[211] However, the V_{max} of fructokinase is not the only determinant of the fructose uptake rate. Because the affinity constant of the hepatic transport system for fructose (67 to 200 mM, as said before) is more than an order of magnitude higher than the K_m of fructokinase (approximately 0.5 mM), its entry rate into the cells and hence the rate of its phosphorylation is critically dependent on the blood fructose concentration. As already seen, it can reach about 2.5 mM in the portal vein after an oral load.[27] However, severalfold higher concentrations may be obtained by IV infusion. At rates of 0.5, 1.0, and 1.5 g of fructose/kg/h, fructosemia reaches 2.3, 4.8, and 7 mM in humans.[30] The mode of administration of fructose thus plays a determining role in the rate of its uptake by the liver.

The first consequence of the rapid metabolism of fructose is the accumulation of fructose 1-phosphate, initially recognized in the liver. Within minutes after a fructose load, the concentration of the fructose ester, normally undetectable, may reach 10 μmol/g.[42,80,212–218] The accumulation of fructose 1-phosphate demonstrates that its formation is much faster than its further metabolism. The limiting step has been a subject of controversy. Although inosine monophosphate (IMP) inhibits liver aldolase,[42] its accumulation cannot explain the initial buildup of fructose 1-phosphate because the latter precedes it.[217] The utilization of fructose 1-phosphate thus seems limited by triokinase and by the glycolytic and gluconeogenic pathways originating from the triosephosphates (see Fig. 70-1). Indeed, the V_{max} of triokinase reaches only 1.5 μmol/min/g of liver at 37°C,[138] and the maximal flux through each of the latter pathways does not exceed 2 mmol of C6 units per min/g of liver at 37°C,[192] so the additive rate of both is less than half the activity of fructokinase. The accumulation of fructose 1-phosphate provokes important changes in the concentration of several other metabolites, which explain the toxic effects of fructose.

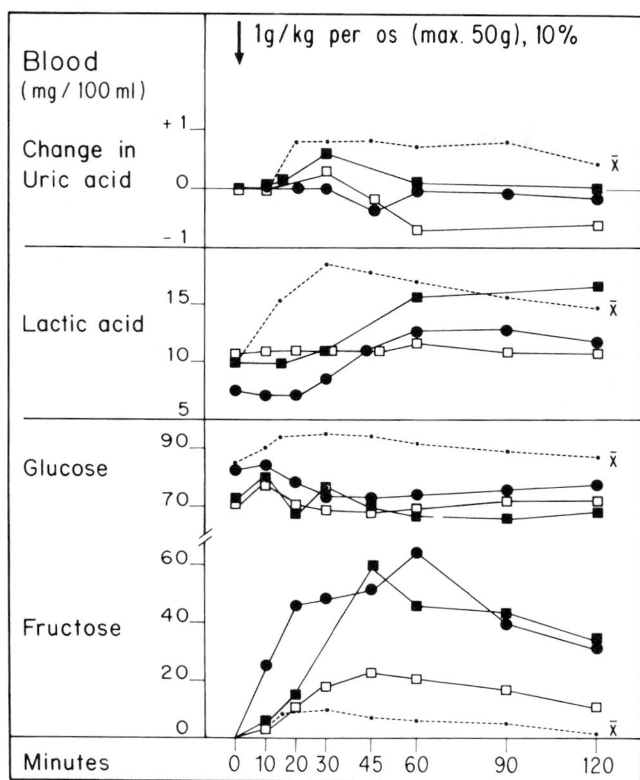

Fig. 70-4 Oral fructose and sorbitol tolerance tests in two sibs with essential fructosuria. Fructose: ■ = R.K. male, 16 years; ● = A.K. female, 19 years; ... = controls (N = 5). Sorbitol: □ = R.K. In the probands, phosphorus, magnesium, standard bicarbonate, free fatty acids, and insulin remained unchanged. [*Reprinted with permission from Steinmann B, Baerlocher K, Gitzelmann R. Nutr Metab 18 (suppl 1):115, 1975.*[224]]

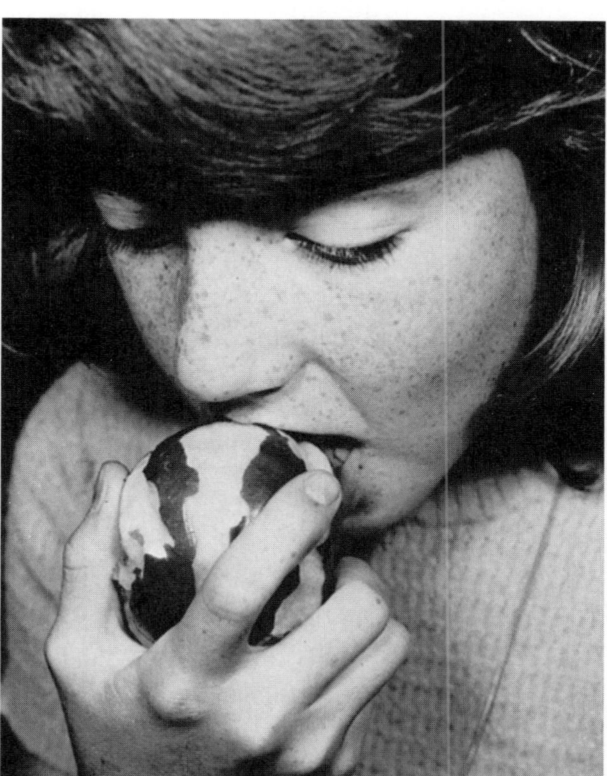

Fig. 70-5 A 12-year-old girl with hereditary fructose intolerance "eating" an apple. She had been referred by a pediatric psychiatrist for anomalous behavior at age 8 years.

Hyperuricemic Effect of Fructose

In 1967, Perheentupa and Raivio[205] reported that the IV administration of 0.5 g fructose/kg body weight provoked hyperuricemia and hyperuricosuria not only in patients with hereditary fructose intolerance but also in normal children. This observation has been repeatedly confirmed[219,220] in patients as well as in healthy adult volunteers, especially at infusion rates above 1.0 to 1.5 g/kg/h.[221] Although other researchers have not observed the effect with lower infusion rates,[222–224] an increase of serum uric acid has been found after the infusion of as little as 0.16 g/kg/h fructose in critically ill subjects.[225] A single IV test dose of 200 mg/kg fructose provokes an increase of serum uric acid in healthy children and adults (Figs. 70-10 and 70-11). The urinary excretion of uric acid, expressed as the creatinine ratio, is a more sensitive indicator of the effect of fructose than is hyperuricemia.[224,226,227] Increased urinary excretion of precursors of uric acid, namely, inosine, hypoxanthine, and xanthine, and their increase in plasma also has been reported in humans and animals.[219,228,229]

Investigations in animals by Mäenpää *et al.*[230] and later in humans[215,231] demonstrated that the hyperuricemic effect of fructose results from the degradation of adenine nucleotides. Indeed, within 2 min after a parenteral fructose load to rats, the concentration of hepatic ATP decreases to 40 percent of its normal value without an equivalent increase of ADP and AMP.[230] There is also a marked decrease in the concentration of P_i preceding that of ATP. The decrease of ATP is explained by its utilization in the fructokinase reaction. The P_i depletion results from its participation in the rephosphorylation of ADP in mitochondria (see Fig. 70-1). In recent years, the accumulation of fructose 1-phosphate and the depletion of ATP and Pi also have been documented by ^{31}P magnetic resonance spectroscopy (MRS). Studies have been performed in rat[232] and human liver[218,233–235] (Figs. 70-6 and 70-7). It is worth mentioning that in the latter studies the hepatic concentration of ATP decreased by 40 to 60 percent and that of P_i by 80 percent with the infusion of as little as 200 mg/kg fructose, a dose that did not increase plasma uric acid above the limits established for healthy controls.[92] Both the fructose-induced accumulation of fructose 1-phosphate and depletion of P_i are less marked in patients with chronic hepatitis[236] and cirrhosis.[237] This is probably due to impaired hepatic phosphorylation of fructose under these conditions.

The concentrations of several other nucleotides: uridine triphosphate, UDP-glucose,[238,239] and GTP[217] are also diminished following fructose infusion. The decrease of GTP may be due to its utilization in both the fructokinase[78] and triokinase reactions.[140] Depletion of high-energy phosphates also has been observed in other fructose-metabolizing tissues, namely, the kidney[239,240] and small intestine.[241] Studies with single rat nephrons have shown that in accordance with the localization of fructokinase and aldolase B, the effects of fructose are confined to the proximal tubule.[107] The contribution of the kidney and small intestine to the hyperuricemic effects of fructose is difficult to assess because in humans, xanthine oxidase is found only in liver and small intestinal mucosa.[242]

The catabolism of the adenine nucleotides ATP, ADP, and AMP (maintained in equilibrium by adenylate kinase) can theoretically begin either by deamination of AMP, catalyzed by AMP deaminase, followed by dephosphorylation of IMP to inosine by the cytoplasmic 5′-nucleotidase, or by dephosphorylation of AMP by the same enzyme, followed by deamination of adenosine to inosine by adenosine deaminase (Fig. 70-8). From inosine, the successive action of nucleoside phosphorylase and xanthine oxidase leads to the formation of uric acid, the end product of

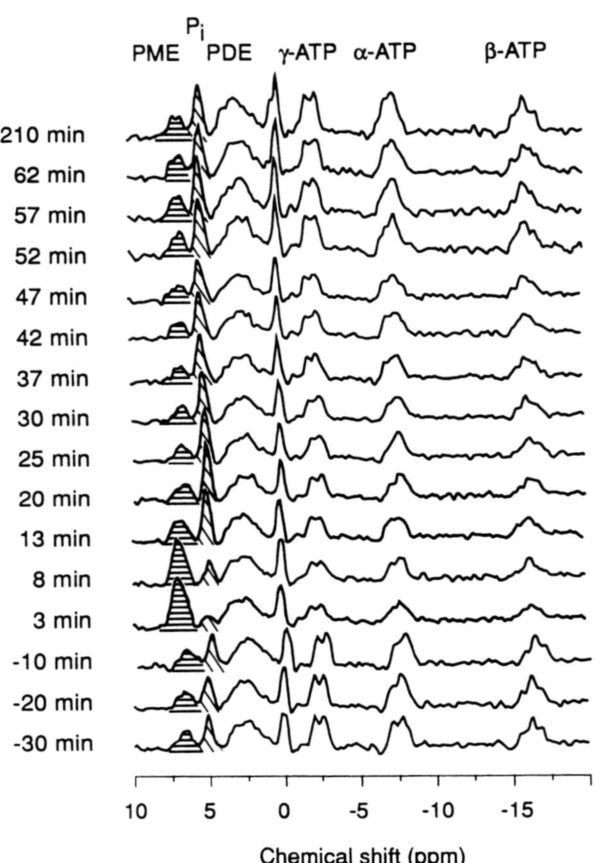

Fig. 70-6 ^{31}P-MRS of liver metabolites before (−) and after an IV bolus of fructose (200 mg/kg, in 2 min) in a healthy adult (C.G.). PME = phospomonoesters; PDE = phosphodiesters. The increase of phosphomonoesters is attributed to that of fructose 1-phosphate. (*Reprinted with permission from Boesiger P, Buchli R, Meier D, Steinmann B, Gitzelmann R. Pediatr Res 36:436, 1994.*[218])

purine nucleotide catabolism in humans and higher apes. The catabolism of the adenine nucleotides has to be kept to a minimum for two reasons: adenine nucleotides play a major role in the energy metabolism of the cell, and the low solubility of uric acid, coupled with its limited renal excretion, poses the danger of precipitation of crystals, with the damaging consequences found in gout. Studies of the catabolism of the adenine nucleotides in isolated rat hepatocytes have shown that here the initial catabolism of AMP proceeds exclusively by way of AMP deaminase under physiologic conditions.[243,244] Furthermore, dephosphorylation of AMP by the cytoplasmic 5′-nucleotidase takes place but does not contribute to the production of uric acid, because the resulting adenosine is continuously recycled by adenosine kinase.[245] AMP deaminase is the limiting step in the catabolism of the hepatic adenine nucleotides and therefore controls their breakdown. The enzyme has complex allosteric properties and is strongly influenced by various metabolites: ATP is a potent activator, whereas P_i and GTP are inhibitory. At physiologic concentrations of substrate and effectors, the enzyme is 95 percent inhibited.[217]

The mechanism of the fructose-induced degradation of the adenine nucleotide pool has been studied mainly in the liver. Studies with isolated hepatocytes have shown that, similarly to physiologic catabolism, it proceeds by way of AMP deaminase.[243] It is explained by a release of the physiologic inhibition of AMP deaminase[217] caused by the decrease of P_i and GTP concentrations during fructose metabolism (see Fig. 70-1). The accumulation of IMP following fructose administration, first recorded by Woods *et al.*,[42] is a reflection of the increased flux through AMP deaminase.

The fructose-induced hyperuricemia is thus not harmless. Rather, it indicates degradation of ATP, that is, the main "energy currency" of the cell. ATP degradation is reflected by a decrease in tissue and increase in plasma Mg^{2+} (see Figs. 70-10 and 70-11),[92,246,247] owing to the loss of this potent Mg^{2+} chelator. The degradation of another high-energy phosphate, uridine triphosphate, most likely accounts for the elevation of plasma uridine recorded following fructose infusion.[248,248a] In the fructose-metabolizing tissues, depletion of ATP results in a series of disturbances. They include inhibition of protein[215,230,247] and

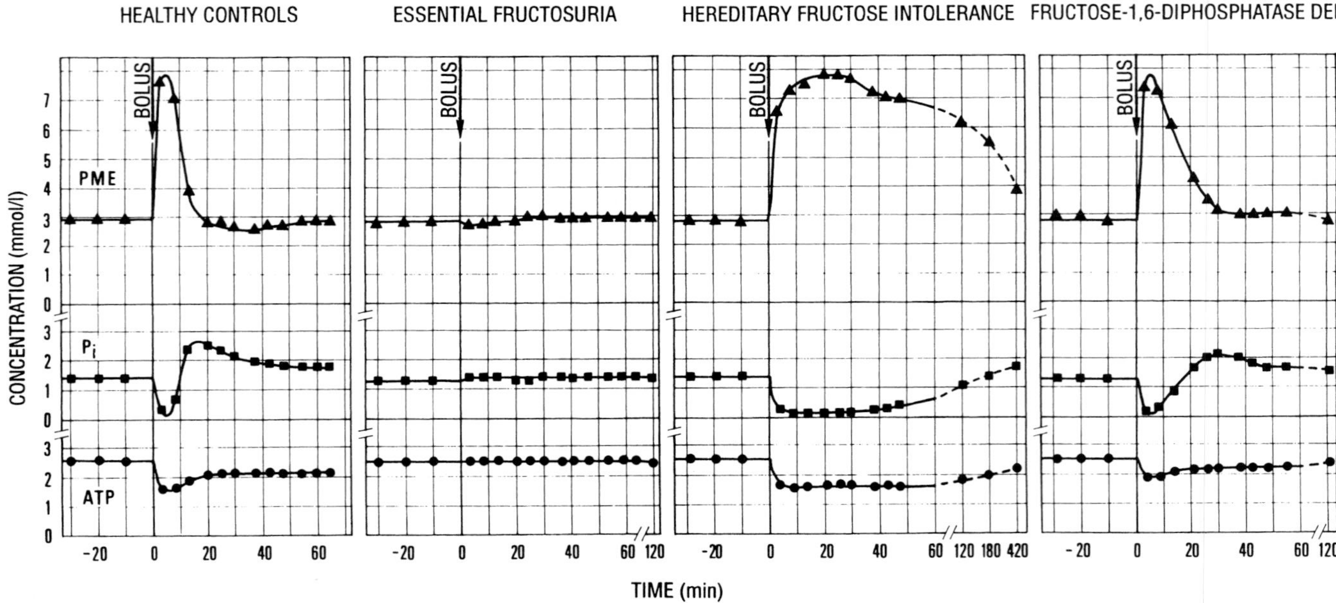

Fig. 70-7 ^{31}P-MRS of liver metabolite concentrations (mM) before (−) and after an intravenous bolus of fructose (200 mg/kg, in 2 min), in three healthy controls and in an adult proband with essential fructosuria (RK), hereditary fructose intolerance (VL), or fructose-1,6-bisphosphatase deficiency (TM). PME = phosphomonoesters; P_i = inorganic phosphate; ATP = adenosine triphosphate. Note that three fourths of the inorganic phosphorus present in liver remains invisible by MRS.[218,498] (*Reprinted with permission from Boesiger P, Buchli R, Meier D, Steinmann B, Gitzelmann R. Pediatr Res 36:436, 1994.*[218])

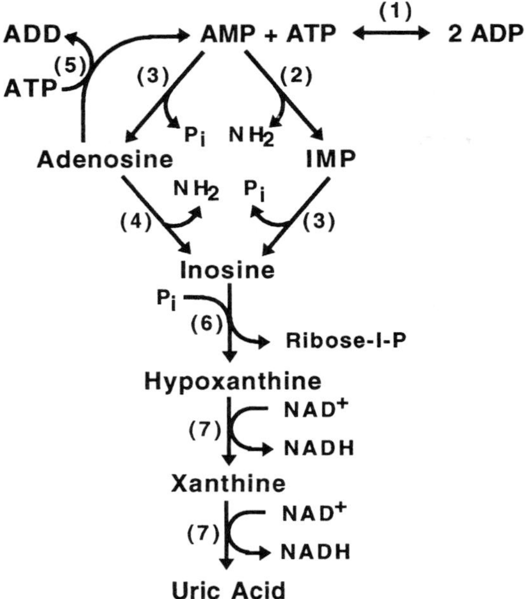

Fig. 70-8 Pathways of adenine nucleotide catabolism in the liver. (1) = adenylate kinase; (2) = AMP deaminase; (3) = cytoplasmic 5′-nucleotidase; (4) = adenosine deaminase; (5) = adenosine kinase; (6) = nucleoside phosphorylase; (7) = xanthine oxidase.

RNA[215,248] synthesis, disaggregation of ribosomes,[251] interference with the formation of cAMP,[216] and detoxification of ammonia.[249] Marked ultrastructural lesions such as loss of ribosomes in rat hepatocytes[250,251] and smooth ER proliferation in mouse jejunal absorptive cells[252] have been described.

Theoretically, the degradation of adenine nucleotides may be prevented by the administration of phosphate. Data obtained in animals indicate that, although the infusion of phosphate largely prevents the fructose-induced degradation of adenine nucleotides in the kidney cortex, it is much less effective in the liver, probably because of its limited entry into this tissue.[240] However, in transgenic mice expressing creatine kinase in the lives and fed creatine, the presence of phosphocreatine as an alternative source of phosphate markedly reduces the fructose-induced depletion of P_i and catabolism of the hepatic adenine nucleotides.[253]

The fructose-induced catabolism of the purine nucleotides is followed by a compensatory increase in their *de novo* synthesis.[254] This involves conversion of phosphoribosyl pyrophosphate amidotransferase, the limiting enzyme of the *de novo* pathway from its large, inactive, into its small, active form[255] and elevation of the concentration of phosphoribosyl pyrophosphate,[255,256] which also increases the recovery of hypoxanthine by the salvage pathway.[256]

Increase in Blood Lactate Provoked by Fructose

Whereas the IV infusion of glucose usually does not elevate the concentration of blood lactate by more than twofold, two- to fivefold increases have been reported after the infusion of fructose in healthy volunteers and in patients.[223,227,257,258] Wide individual variations and the observed bimodal distribution have led to the suggestion of genetic differences in the metabolism of fructose.[259] The faster formation of lactate from fructose than from glucose can be explained by several factors:

1. The higher activity of fructokinase compared with the capacity of hexokinase plus glucokinase to phosphorylate glucose
2. The fact that fructolysis bypasses phosphofructokinase, the first regulatory enzyme along the glycolytic pathway
3. A stimulation of pyruvate kinase, the second regulatory step of glycolysis, by fructose 1-phosphate[260] and by fructose 1,6-bisphophate[261]

Additional data concerning the effect of fructose on the glycolytic–gluconeogenic pathway can be found elsewhere.[26]

The fructose-induced increase in lactic acid may provoke metabolic acidosis in adults[206,262] and children.[263,264] Metabolic acidosis also has been reported in the fetuses of mothers receiving IV fructose during labor.[265] It may become life threatening in liver failure, as exemplified by the case reports provided by Craig and Crane[262] and by Woods and Alberti.[208] Fructose is therefore a potentially dangerous substitute for glucose in parenteral nutrition, although still stubbornly advocated by some researchers.[266] Inborn errors of fructose, lactate, and ammonia metabolism, glycogenosis type I, and acquired conditions in which the hepatic utilization of peripherally produced lactate is impaired, such as anoxia, liver disease, and diabetes mellitus, are absolute contraindications.

In recent years, a number of studies performed with perfused livers and hepatocytes from rats have shown that the addition of 5 to 20 mM fructose protects liver cells against anoxia[267–269] and a variety of mitochondrial toxins.[270–272] Protection was evidenced by a decrease of the release of lactic acid dehydrogenase and by other parameters of cell damage. This protective effect of fructose can be explained by its high rate of conversion into lactate. The resulting generation of ATP by the glycolytic pathway compensates to a certain extent the anoxia- and toxin-induced impairment of the synthesis of ATP in the mitochondria. Nevertheless, the risks of lactic acidosis outweigh the potential benefits of a therapeutic application of these experimental findings, except maybe for liver preservation prior to transplantation.

ESSENTIAL FRUCTOSURIA–HEPATIC FRUCTOKINASE DEFICIENCY (MIM 229800)

Historical Note and Definition

This rare and benign error of metabolism[273] was first described in 1876 independently by Czapek[274] and by Zimmer[275] in a man who also suffered from diabetes mellitus. In 1961 Laron[276] counted 50 published cases, and in 1969 Steinitz and Mizrahy counted fewer than 80.[277] Because the disorder is asymptomatic and harmless, many cases may remain undetected and the detected ones unpublished. The original name of the disorder, essential fructosuria, became obsolete in 1961–1962 when the fructokinase defect was discovered, but it is still in use. A nonalimentary fructosuria of obscure etiology has been observed in one child.[278]

Laboratory Findings, Biochemical Defect, and Functional Studies

Affected persons are usually discovered on routine urinalysis by the presence of a reducing substance. They are healthy and have otherwise normal liver function. Fructosuria depends on the time and amount of fructose and sucrose intake; thus, it is inconstant. After an overnight fast, fructose is measurable only in small quantities, if at all, in the blood, just as in normal persons. The misdiagnosis of diabetes mellitus[279,280] or renal diabetes[280] is avoided only when the nonglucose nature of the sugar is recognized.

The disorder is caused by the inherited deficiency of fructokinase (EC 2.7.1.3) normally present in the liver, intestine, pancreatic islets, and kidney cortex.[81,107,281–283] The deficiency was demonstrated in the liver of an adult by Schapira *et al.*[284] using the assay designed by Hers and Joassin.[285] To our knowledge, assays of intestinal or kidney cortex fructokinase have not been performed in persons with essential fructosuria. The metabolic block appears to be as follows:

$$\text{Fructose} \xrightarrow[\quad /\!/ \quad]{\text{fructokinase}} \text{Fructose 1-phosphate}$$

After an oral or IV load, for example, with 1 g/kg body weight, blood fructose increases rapidly, far beyond the level of 10 to 30 mg/100 ml seen in controls, declines slowly, and does not disappear for 6 h or longer.[224,276] Between 10 and 20 percent of the administered dose is excreted in urine,[276,286] as compared with 1 to 2 percent[276] or less[224] in normal subjects. Blood glucose, lactate, pyruvate, and urate change little, in contrast to the increase of these metabolites in normal persons; phosphorus, magnesium, standard bicarbonate, free fatty acids, and insulin remain constant[224,286–288] (see Fig. 70-4). The increase of the respiratory quotient after fructose ingestion in fasting patients with essential fructosuria is less than in normal subjects.[279,287] These findings indicate a slower than normal utilization of fructose. The nine tenths of a dose of fructose retained by fructosuric subjects after a bolus is most probably metabolized via fructose 6-phosphate in adipose tissue[65,225] and skeletal muscle. As in normal subjects, D-sorbitol is converted to fructose, which becomes measurable in blood (see Fig. 70-4)[224,289]; urinary loss as fructose is only about half that seen after a fructose load.[224,289] Almost 80 percent of a 5-g sorbose load was lost in urine by a woman with fructosuria.[279]

In an adult with essential fructosuria who lost only 10 percent of an IV test dose of fructose in 2 h in urine, ^{31}P-MRS showed no increase of fructose 1-phosphate and no decrease of ATP and P_i in liver, in accordance with his presumed fructokinase deficiency[218] (see Fig. 70-7). Thus, nine tenths of the test dose remained unaccounted for. Interestingly, he had no epigastric pain during the test, which contrasted with observations in healthy controls and patients with hereditary fructose intolerance[92,218] (see later section on Hereditary Fructose Intolerance). In the red cells of the same patient and his two affected sisters, fasting concentrations of fructose 3-phosphate were 3 to 15 times higher than in healthy controls, and sorbitol 3-phosphate was above normal albeit to a lesser degree.[181] The fact that the individual fasting levels differed considerably was taken as an effect of the varying degree of alimentary hyperfructosemia. An oral load with 50 g of fructose produced a further increase of fructose 3-phosphate in their red cells. However, it was calculated that the erythrocyte compartments retained less than 1 percent of the fructose load in this form. It is worth mentioning that these red cells had a normal capability for forming fructose 3-phosphate *in vitro*.[181]

Neither cataracts nor other diabetic complications have been reported in fructosuric subjects. Furthermore, in the three adults tested,[181] glycated hemoglobin (HbA1 and HbA1c) was normal. This finding and the benign nature of their anomaly, with high levels of fructose 3-phosphate in red cells, cast doubt on the suggested pathogenic role[179] of fructose 3-phosphate alone as the cause of the diabetic complications.[181]

A lactating affected woman (H.K.) was given 50 g of fructose in 300 ml of water by mouth. Although blood fructose reached 2.5 mM after 60 min, fructose remained undetectable thereafter in the first and last portion of breast milk during the feeding.[292] Thus, the mammary gland does not appear to secrete fructose; whether fructose reaches a primary milk stage and is reabsorbed remains undetermined.

Genetics and Molecular Biology

The most careful study of the mode of inheritance of essential fructosuria was that of Lasker.[293] After reviewing the literature and her own cases, she concluded that the anomaly was inherited as an autosomal-recessive trait and occurred perhaps once in 130,000 individuals. She gave good reasons why this was only an approximate figure and stated that the disorder may be even rarer. On the other hand, given its benign character, it may escape discovery during a lifetime, even more so in the future because clinical laboratories are abandoning tests for reducing substances in urine in favor of specific glucose tests. Marble[294] reported only four cases among 29,000 cases of mellituria seen at the Joslin Clinic. Heterozygotes appear to excrete no more fructose after an oral load than normal subjects.[295] Fructokinase has not been assayed in heterozygotes. Essential fructosuria has been reported from many parts of the world.[293] By 1961, the proportion of Jews in the known and proven cases of this disorder was 18 out of 50 cases.[276]

Full-length cDNA clones encoding human fructokinase (ketohexokinase) have been isolated.[86] In a family with three fructosuric sibs, all three were found to be compound heterozygotes for two mutations in exon 2: G40R and A43T. Both mutations result from G-A transitions, and each alters the same conserved region of the fructokinase protein. Neither mutation was seen in 52 unrelated control individuals.

HEREDITARY FRUCTOSE INTOLERANCE (MIM 229600)

Historical Note and Definition

In 1956 Chambers and Pratt[296] described an "idiosyncrasy to fructose" in a 24-year-old "spinster" who complained, apart from minor phobic symptoms, of vomiting after eating fruit or sugar. She could take glucose without ill effects, although she did not enjoy the taste. Symptoms had appeared on weaning at age 10 months. The investigators recognized that the condition differed from fructosuria, speculated that symptoms were presumably caused by a toxic intermediate, and proposed that the condition be considered as a cause of difficulty in weaning. Froesch et al.[297] reported the typical syndrome of hereditary fructose intolerance in 1957 in two sibs and two relatives and suspected a deficiency of aldolase as its cause. The defect was characterized by Hers and Joassin in 1961, on two liver biopsy specimens, as a loss of the ability of the enzyme to split fructose 1-phosphate.[285] By 1971, 100 cases from Europe and the United States had been recorded.[298] The disorder, once considered rare, is sufficiently common for certain centers to have collected the records of dozens of patients.[92,299,300]

In 1970, hereditary fructose 1,6-bisphosphatase deficiency was recognized as a separate disorder.[301] After a reinvestigation in 1972, it was determined that another disease, familial galactose and fructose intolerance, originally described in 1961, must be questioned as an entity.[302]

Clinical and Laboratory Findings

Infants and adult patients with hereditary fructose intolerance are perfectly healthy and asymptomatic as long as they do not ingest any food containing fructose or sucrose. Thus, during breast-feeding, no metabolic derangement occurs. At weaning, with the intake of fruits and vegetables, the first symptoms appear. The younger the child[303] and the higher the dietary fructose load, the more severe the reaction. The defenseless newborn infant who is not breast-fed but receives a cow's milk formula with fructose or sucrose is in danger of death.

In the infant and small child,[299,300] the leading symptoms are poor feeding, vomiting, and failure to thrive (Table 70-1). All other symptoms occur less frequently but are more specific and indicative of gastrointestinal discomfort, hypoglycemia, shock, and liver disease. Because the clinical presentation is multifaceted in the small infant, the diagnosis is easily missed. If the intake of the noxious sugar persists, hypoglycemic episodes recur, and liver and kidney failure progress, eventually leading to death. In one series,[299] clinical findings in the order of decreasing frequency were hepatomegaly; pallor; hemorrhages such as melena, hematemesis, and suffusions; trembling and jerks; shock; jaundice; edema; tachypnea; ascites; oliguria or anuria; severe shock; splenomegaly; fever; and rickets. Laboratory findings are those of liver failure, proximal renal tubular dysfunction, and certain derangements of intermediary metabolism (Table 70-2).

The child survives and symptoms regress when the formula is changed to a non-noxious one or is replaced by IV glucose infusions. If the patient escapes diagnosis at this point, the disease takes a protracted, uphill–downhill course. By experience, certain parents learn quickly how to select harmless formulas and foods for their affected child. The protracted course is also typical for the patient whose first exposure to fructose occurs at regular weaning. Here, the prominent features are abdominal distension, hepato-

Table 70-1 Symptoms and Signs in Hereditary Fructose Intolerance*

Acute Exposure	Chronic Exposure
Sweating	Poor feeding, vomiting
Trembling	Failure to thrive
Dizziness	Incessant crying, irritability
Nausea	
Vomiting	Drowsiness, apathy
Apathy, lethargy, coma	
Convulsions	Jaundice
	Abdominal distension
	Hepatomegaly
	Hemorrhages
	Diarrhea
	Tremor, jerking
	Edema, ascites
	Poor growth

* Sequelae: Protracted fibrosis, cirrhosis, steatosis of the liver; aversion to sweets and peculiar feeding habits; lack of dental caries.

megaly, and poor growth. Acute episodes become rarer as the child develops an aversion to foods and drinks that cause discomfort. Aversion to sweet food is neither general nor indiscriminate[296]; it is not innate, but acquired by learning. Children usually adopt peculiar feeding habits that protect them but are not always understood by people around them, who sometimes resort to forcing sweet foods.[304–306] Diagnosis at preschool and school age is usually made during examination for suspected storage disorder, for failure to thrive or growth delay, or sometimes for anomalous behavior[304] (see Fig. 70-5) and only after carefully taking the nutritional history. Other patients, following a self-imposed low-fructose diet, go on undiagnosed into adulthood and may be discovered by chance. Interestingly, the majority of adults with hereditary fructose intolerance report that their aversion to sweets and fruit wanes over the years.[292] Approximately half of all adults with hereditary fructose intolerance are completely free of caries,[303,305,307–309] suggesting that dietary sucrose is the chief caries-promoting agent.[310] It also leads dentists to suspect hereditary fructose intolerance.[306] Some adult patients are diagnosed during a family investigation after the discovery of an affected young relative,[306,307,311] sometimes their own child.[312,313] Several medical students have diagnosed their own hereditary fructose intolerance during pathophysiology lectures.[12,292] Yet other undiagnosed fructose-intolerant children and adults are less fortunate and receive infusions of fructose, sorbitol, or invert sugar, sometimes for unrelated health reasons,[314–317] for example, after routine surgery. Consequently, some die from acute poisoning.[318–323]

Table 70-2 Laboratory Findings in Patients with Hereditary Fructose Intolerance after Exposure to Fructose

Urine	Blood
Fructose increased	Phosphorus decreased
Glucose increased	Glucose decreased
Phosphorus increased	Urate increased
Amino acids increased	Magnesium increased
Urate increased	Potassium decreased
Bicarbonate increased	Fructose increased
Potassium increased	Lactate increased
Protein increased	pH decreased
Lactate increased	Bicarbonate decreased
	Proteins decreased
	Coagulation factors decreased
	Hepatic enzymes increased
	Bilirubin increased
	Methionine, tyrosine, etc. increased
	Anemia
	Thrombocytopenia
	Acanthocytes, fragmentocytes

It must be stressed that in the two casuistic reviews[299,300] comprising 75 children, hypoglycemia was documented only in a minority. It correlated poorly with jerking and trembling, and although it is considered a major and dangerous metabolic manifestation of hereditary fructose intolerance, it is short-lived, lasting only a limited time after each ingestion of fructose. It thus easily escapes detection.

Histology of liver examined via biopsy has shown diffuse steatosis of liver cells, necrosis of a few scattered hepatocytes, periportal and intralobular fibrosis, and, in more advanced stages of the disease, cirrhosis.[300,324,325] At autopsy, findings include hepatic dystrophy and necrosis.[325–327] In the kidney, histologic changes are remarkably discrete. They include some granulation and perhaps vacuolization of epithelial cells lining the proximal tubules, which may be slightly dilated.[326,327] In the small intestine, gross inspection and microscopic examination may reveal submucosal or serosal hemorrhages. Intracranial[300,303] and intraocular hemorrhages[299] have been reported.

Ultrastructural studies conducted by Spycher[328] on several liver biopsy specimens revealed that hepatocytes and sometimes Kupffer cells contained cytoplasmic degradation foci and polymorphous cytoplasmic inclusions of different size, partly membrane bound and probably lysosomal. Inclusions contained amorphous, electron-dense masses and numerous concentric membranous arrays varying greatly in size and often surrounded by an electron-lucent halo. Other cytoplasmic findings were smooth endoplasmic reticular proliferation and vesiculation and occasional formation of glycogen bodies (see Fig. 70-9). Similar findings had been reported earlier.[329]

Enzyme Defect

The defect (see Fig. 70-2) is that of aldolase B (fructose 1,6-bisphosphate aldolase, EC 4.1.2.13) of the liver, kidney cortex, and small intestine. Aldolases A and C,[95,96,105] prevalent in other organs such as skeletal muscle and brain, are not affected. The activity of the liver enzyme is reduced to 15 percent of normal or less with fructose 1-phosphate and to a distinctly lesser degree with fructose 1,6-bisphosphate. A representative sample of measurements on liver biopsy specimens is shown in Table 70-3. It confirms the findings of an earlier series[330] and shows that in the patients, the ratio of activities measured with fructose 1,6-bisphosphate as substrate to fructose 1-phosphate as substrate is increased, a fact of diagnostic value originally pointed out by Hers and Joassin[285] and Schapira *et al.*[284] Fructose 1-phosphate aldolase activity was undetectable in 5 of 35 biopsy specimens in one series[92] but was never absent in the 34 biopsy specimens of another series.[330] The activities of liver fructokinase[284,285,331] and fructose 1,6-bisphosphatase (see Table 70-3) are normal. A similar reduction of fructaldolase activities is found in jejunal mucosa and in kidney cortex examined via biopsy and at autopsy (Table 70-4).[322]

The significance of residual fructaldolase activities in the liver, kidney, and intestine of patients with hereditary fructose intolerance has been controversial. Mature human liver contains all three forms of fructaldolase, but type B predominates, with 98 percent of the enzyme protein.[105]Aldolase A, with less than 2 to 3 percent of the protein,[105,330] contributes 15 percent of the total activity,[330] owing to its higher specific activity. Residual liver fructose 1,6-bisphosphate aldolase has been attributed variably to a persisting fetal enzyme, shortly to be recognized as aldolase A,[285,331,332] and to aldolase C.[330] Both are unaffected by the mutation and have a higher fructose 1,6-bisphosphate aldolase/fructose 1-phosphate

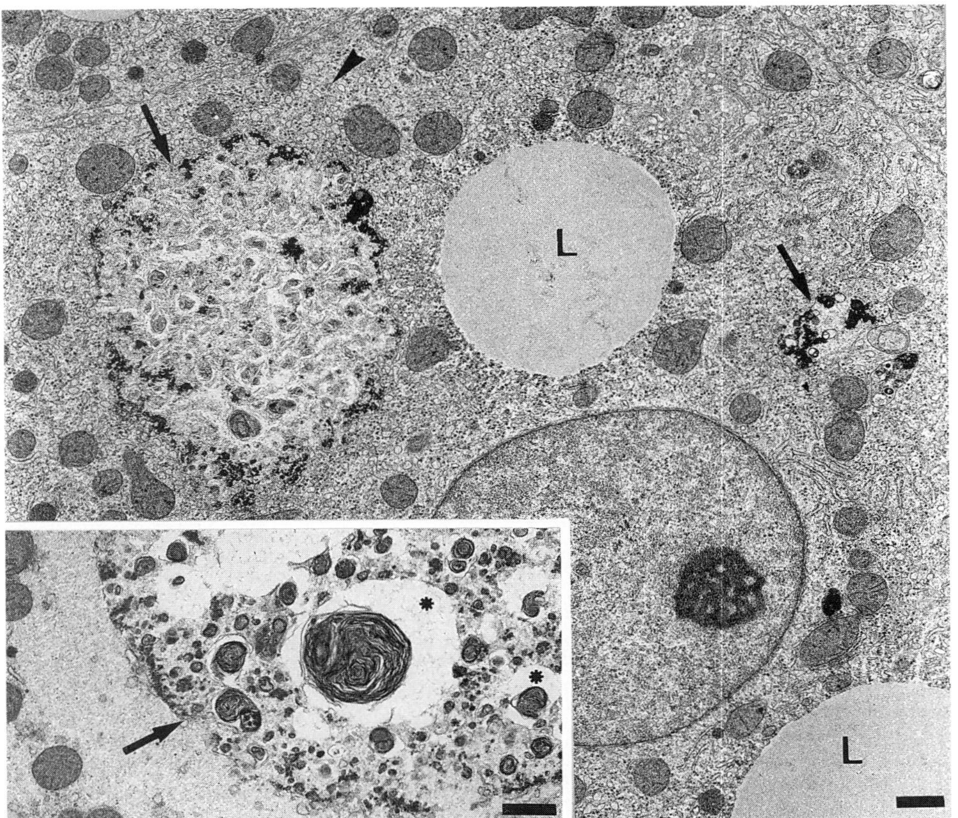

Fig. 70-9 Liver cell ultrastructure of girl M.S., 4 months of age, acutely ill from hereditary fructose intolerance; the liver biopsy was taken $3\frac{1}{2}$ weeks after fructose withdrawal. Hepatocytes show foci of cytoplasmic degradation (arrows) and lipid inclusions (L). Degradation foci are partly membrane bound and contain electron-dense granular masses, as well as numerous membranous arrays with a 4 to 4.5-nm periodicity (insert). Membranous bodies are often surrounded by an electron-lucent halo (asterisk). The smooth endoplasmic reticulum is proliferated and vesiculated (arrowhead). Bars = 1 μm. (Courtesy of Dr. Max A. Spycher, Zurich.)

aldolase activity ratio, 13 and 7, respectively, than normal aldolase B, 0.9.[333] Patients who are either homozygous or compound heterozygous carriers of functional null alleles (Table 70-5) do have residual activity in liver, a fact validating the abovementioned interpretation. Furthermore, the partially inactive mutant aldolase B itself may have an increased activity ratio, as determined by expression studies of the A149P variant.[334] In the majority of biopsy specimens studied, a cross-reacting material was present.[92,330,335–337] An abnormally high K_m for fructose 1,6-bisphosphate[94] and fructose 1-phosphate,[330] and decreased heat stability[92,337] of mutant human aldolase have been reported. Furthermore, a certain restoration of fructose 1-phosphate aldolase activity in liver biopsy specimens was achieved *in vitro* by reducing agents[330] and by antibodies to normal aldolase B.[337] The amount of residual activity has never been shown to correlate with the degree of the intolerance to fructose.

The residual aldolase activity never appears to become rate limiting in glycolysis or gluconeogenesis except after fructose loading. Normal functioning of gluconeogenesis is amply documented by the prompt increase of glucose after oral

Table 70-3 Fructaldolase Activity in Liver Biopsy Specimens of Children with Hereditary Fructose Intolerance (HFI) and Controls

	Fructaldolase*			
	FBP	F-1-P	FBP/F-1-P	FBPase
HFI				
*Mean (or median)	0.46	0.11	(3.9)	3.82
SD	0.16	0.09		1.66
Range	0.13–0.82	0.00–0.36	(1.7 up to 00)	1.71–7.20
n	35	35		24
Controls†				
*Mean	2.61	2.40	1.1	3.78
SD	0.46	0.49	0.1	0.74
Range	2.07–3.79	1.82–3.40	1.0–1.2	2.73–4.98
N	10	10	10	7

* Activity measured with the indicated substrate.
† Nine adult organ donors and one child with a histologically normal liver. Activities are in IU/g wet weight. FBPase was the control enzyme.
FDP = Fructose 1,6-bisphosphatase; F-1-P = Fructose 1-phosphate; FBPase = Fructose 1,6-bisphosphatase.
Data from Steinmann et al.[92]

Table 70-4 **Ratios of Activity of Aldolase with the Two Substrates Fructose 1,6-Bisphosphate and Fructose 1-Phosphate in Tissues of Patients with Hereditary Fructose Intolerance and Controls, at Biopsy or Autopsy, and in Purified Human Aldolases A, B, and C**

	Contols			Hereditary Fructose Intolerance			
	Mean	Range	N	Mean (or median)	Range	N	References
Liver	1.0	0.9–1.1	5	6.2;6.2		2	285
	1.1	1.0–1.2	10	(3.9)	1.8 and up	33	92
				1.7;11*		2	92
		1.0–1.2		6.6	2.9–11.0	34	330
	1.4*	1.1–1.8*	6	9.0*		1	322
	1.7		11				81
Intestine	1.9	1.0–2.5	28	(26.7)	3.1 and up	8	502
				1.8		1	303
		3.5–4.0	4				281
	1.7	1.1–2.3	7	32.6;3.5		2	503
				9.1*		1	504
Kidney cortex	2.8*		5				282
	1.3		1				505
	3.2	2.6–4	6	∞		1	506
	1.7;2.5*		2	18*		1	92
	2.7*						106
Kidney medulla	6*		4				282
	23		1				505
	5.8;9.6*		2				92
	3.4*						106
Aldolase A	13						333
Aldolase B	0.9						333
Aldolase C	7						333

*Values refer to measurements at autopsy.

Table 70-5 **Human Aldolase B Gene Mutations in Hereditary Fructose Intolerance***

Trivial Name	Systematic Designation†	Mutated Codon†	Ethnic Distribution	References
M-1T	c.2T → C	MIT	Italian (private)	384
C134R	c.403T → C	C135R	Amerindian (private)	429
W147R	c.442T → C	W148R	Angloamerican (private)	507, 520
A149P	c.448G → C	A150P	European (widespread)	420
E165V	c.497A → T	E166V	German (private)	516
A174T†	c.523G → A	A175T	Turkish (private)	516
A174D	c.524C → A	A175D	S European (widespread)	422
L256P	c.770T → C	L257P	Italian (private)	508
R303W	c.910C → T	R304W	Turkish/Italian (rare)	509, 511, 520
N334K	c.1005C → G	N335K	E European (widespread)	510
A337V	c.1013C → T	A338V	Turkish/Finnish/Swiss (rare)	511, 519, 520
R3ter	c.10C → T	R4X	Turkish (private)	517
R59ter	c.178C → T	R60X	Austria (rate)	517, 429
Y203ter	c.672T → A	Y204X	Italian (private)	384
C239ter	c.720C → A	C239X	Japanese (private)	512
IVS5nt1	IVS 5+IG → C	–	New Zealand (private)	511, 425
IVS6sas	IVS 6-IG → A	–	French (private)	517
Q20ΔA	c.62 del A	Q21 del	Italian (private)	509
L288ΔC	c.865 del C	L289 del	Sicilian (private)	422
Δ4IVS2-E3	IVS2-1G del GGTA	G38T39 del	Swiss (private)	513
Δ4E4	c.360-363 del CAAA	N120 K 121 del	W European (widespread, rare)	507, 514
Δ7+1 3′ intron 8	IVS8-1G del GGCTAAC ins G	A334 N335 del	American (private)	515
ΔE6-E7	g.9912-10836 del	N181-G267 del	Swiss (private)	513
ΔE4-E5	g.7516-9165 del	L109-5160 del	French (private)	513

*Trivial name represents the mutated sequence of the inferred translation product after cleavage of the initiator methionine residue; similarly, the codon mutation refers to the initiator methionine numbered as position (+)1.

†Mutations have been assigned according to current guidelines (Antonarakis SE[518] and website http://ariel.ucs.unimelb.edu.au:80/~cotton/antonare.htm).

† It is at present not yet clear if this represents a disease-causing mutation or a rare polymorphism[516].

Adapted and amended with permission From Ali M, Rellos P, Cox Tm. J med Genet 35: 353, 1998.

See also website "Hereditary Fructose Intolerance and Aldolase Home page" (http://www.bu.edu/aldolase)

dihydroxyacetone[224,338–340] and by the patients' normal tolerance to fasting. This indicates that aldolase B activity is not critical for gluconeogenesis in the interprandial state, that (especially convincing in cases homozygous or compound heterozygous for functional null alleles) gluconeogenesis and glycolysis principally depend upon the ubiquitous aldolase A, and that aldolase B is thus a component of an accessory pathway allowing efficient assimilation of specific dietary sugars as an adaptive response to rapid nutritional changes.

Functional Studies

In individuals with hereditary fructose intolerance, ingestion and injection of fructose cause symptoms and chemical changes, some of which are also seen in normal persons, albeit to a far lesser degree (see Fig. 70-7).[218,234] Patients and healthy persons[92,308,341,342] experience unexplained dull epigastric pain 2 to 5 min after a rapid IV load, which tapers off after 10 min. Only the patients report a nagging feeling of hunger toward and during the second hour.[92] In some healthy persons, an oral fructose load causes borborygmi and occasional diarrhea but no other ill effects (see later section on Incomplete Fructose Absorption). In contrast, patients become limp and nauseated, vomit (sometimes with blood), are covered with cold sweat, and have signs of shock and hypoglycemia. Ill effects are dose dependent[296,297] and may last for several hours. Proteinuria, generalized amino aciduria, an increase in serum transaminases, and jaundice may appear and last for several days.[324,343,344]

The chemical signs provoked by fructose in the patient consist of a rapid decrease, first of serum phosphate and then of blood glucose, and an increase of urate and magnesium (see Figs. 70-10 and 70-11). Blood alanine, lactate, glycerol, and nonesterified fatty acids increase.[306,307,345] Insulin remains constant or decreases,[303,307,308,346,347] whereas growth hormone increases,[307,347] probably in response to hypoglycemia. Effects are clearly dose dependent[340] and diminish with age,[92,297] but considerable differences in the individual patient also have been recorded.[304] Because of the ill effects of oral loads and the unreliability of results, fructose tolerance tests should not be performed orally. The small dose of 200 mg/kg is recommended. Fructose-intolerant children and adults extract fructose from the blood normally,[92] except when the administered dose is excessive.[348] One girl converted to the adult type of blood response between ages 12 and 18.5 years.[92] Adults experience a short-lived hyperkalemia[92] followed by a decline in serum potassium,[92,308] and this also was seen in one child.[92] Urinary excretion of lactate, alanine, urate, and magnesium increases after the IV load[92,224]— changes also seen after an oral load.[344]

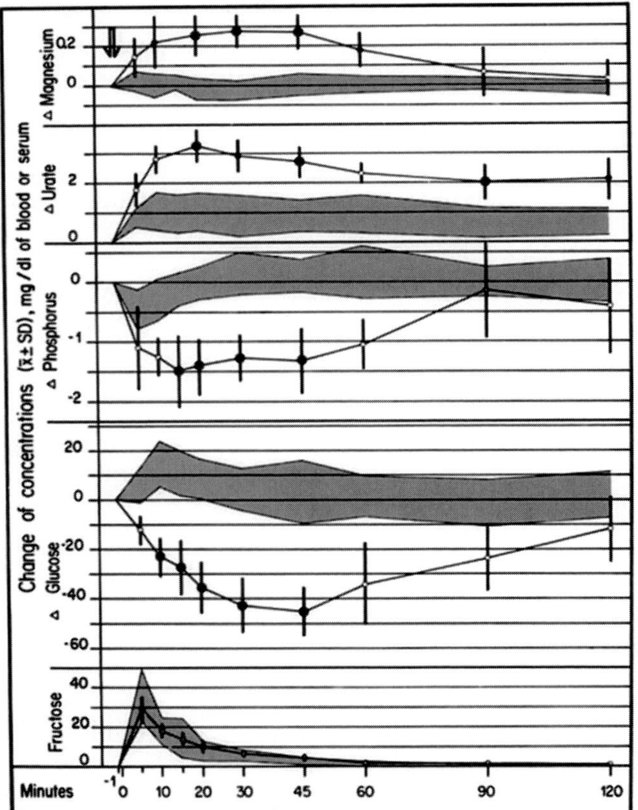

Fig. 70-10 Intravenous fructose tolerance tests (200 mg/kg; 20 percent solution) in 10 children with hereditary fructose intolerance and 16 control children. The shaded areas represent means ±1 SD of the controls; bars represent the means ±1 SD in the patients. ● = mean, no overlap between the two groups; • = mean, the extreme values of both groups coincided; ○ = mean, overlap occurred between the two groups. (*Reprinted with permission from Steinmann B, Gitzelmann R. Helv Paediatr Acta 36:297, 1981.*[92])

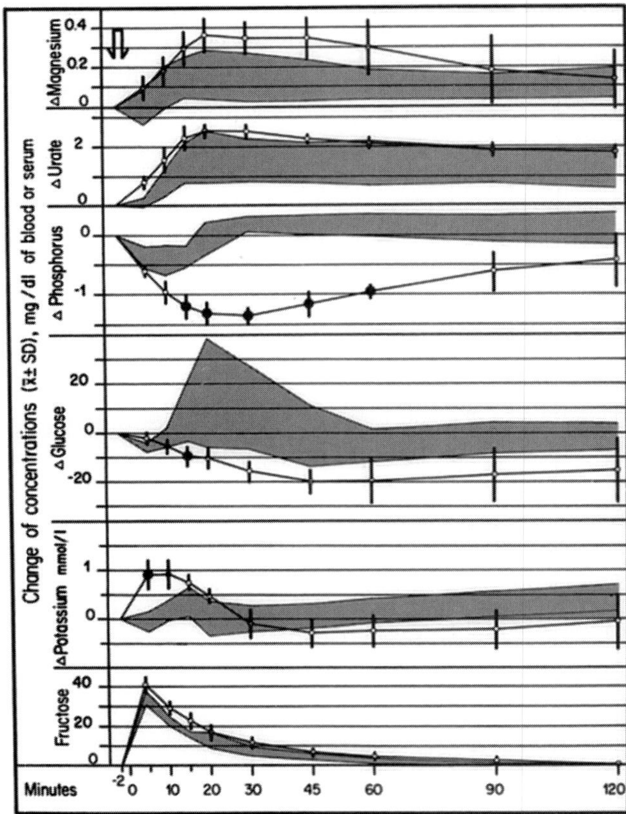

Fig. 70-11 Intravenous fructose tolerance tests (200 mg/kg; 20 percent solution) in six adults with hereditary fructose intolerance and six controls. For symbols, see Fig. 70-10. (*Reprinted with permission from Steinmann B, Gitzelmann R. Helv Paediatr Acta 36:297, 1981.*[92])

Intravenous fructose tests are not entirely harmless even when fructose is given in a small dose; a test-induced proximal renal tubular syndrome has been observed in adult patients.[92,349] Acute fructose hepatotoxicity for the fructose-intolerant subject was evident.[350] Infusions of fructose for 4 h in children caused clotting factors II, V, VII, and X to decrease after 2 to 4 h; they reverted to normal levels only after 24 to 48 h. Interesting morphologic observations in the liver and small intestine of an adult 2 h after an oral load with 50 g fructose were made by Phillips *et al.*[351] By light microscopy, there were no changes, but electron microscopy revealed striking fine structural alterations reminiscent of those seen in fructose-loaded laboratory animals[352] (see earlier section on Toxicity of Fructose). They included concentric and irregularly disposed membranous arrays in and marked rarefaction of the hyaloplasm of hepatocytes. Concentric arrays of smooth endoplasmic reticulum were visible in the supranuclear region of enterocytes.

Intravenous loading with sorbitol causes the same chemical changes in the patient, but only insignificant fructosemia[92] or none at all.[308] This supports the assertion that IV sorbitol is rapidly converted to fructose in the liver and that fructosemia is not a prerequisite for hypoglycemia and the other observed changes. It is noteworthy that the test does not appear to cause epigastric discomfort.[308]

The disappearance of L-sorbose from the blood of normal subjects is somewhat slower than that of fructose. This would be expected from the fact that liver fructokinase phosphorylates fructose faster than sorbose and in preference to it.[73] The half-life of sorbose, calculated from data of Froesch *et al.*,[308] is between 24 and 29 min. In two normal subjects, about 30 percent of the administered L-sorbose was excreted in urine, as compared with 1 to 2 percent with fructose.[308] In patients with hereditary fructose intolerance, the sorbose level rose higher and decreased more slowly, with a half-life of approximately 64 min, and accordingly these patients excreted over 80 percent in the urine within 24 h. The ability to assimilate sorbose obviously was greatly impaired, but patients had no symptoms and changes of blood glucose and inorganic phosphorus.[308,312,346] Furthermore, prior administration of sorbose did not alter or delay the response of patients with hereditary fructose intolerance to subsequent administration of fructose.[308] One might speculate that because of the small affinity of fructokinase for sorbose, only a small amount of sorbose 1-phosphate accumulates in the liver cells, too little to cause the metabolic effects attributed to fructose 1-phosphate accumulation (see later section on Pathophysiology).

Sucrose tolerance tests are not routinely performed when hereditary fructose intolerance is suspected. One 10-month-old boy suspected of having intestinal sucrose-isomaltase deficiency was given an oral sucrose load (50 g/m^2)[353]; he developed hypoglycemia, whereupon the correct diagnosis was made.[292] A fructose-intolerant woman volunteered for an oral raffinose loading test (42 g) when it was questioned whether this fructose-containing trisaccharide of vegetable origin could be hydrolyzed in the human small intestine.[354] She experienced no hypoglycemia, although with an equivalent dose of oral fructose (12 g) she did.[12] In contrast to sucrose, raffinose is not hydrolyzed in the intestine and thus is safe for consumption by fructose-intolerant persons.

Pathophysiology

Fructose intake will result in the accumulation of fructose 1-phosphate in the liver, kidney, and small intestine, owing to the inability of the defective aldolase B to split it. Fructose 1-phosphate accumulates not only after fructose loads but also after the ingestion of physiologic amounts. Nausea appears to be due to accumulation of fructose 1-phosphate in the small intestine, as was demonstrated in an affected women with a transplanted liver; she received a sorbitol infusion, had acute liver failure, but was rescued by liver transplantation.[317] After transplantation, she reported that nausea started 5 to 10 minutes after the ingestion of fructose, and its intensity and duration depended on the amount of the noxious sugar. Interestingly, relief of nausea was prompted by eating fructose-free food such as bread or milk.

The pathophysiologic effects (e.g., hyperuricemia and lactic acidosis) constitute an exaggeration of the untoward effects observed in normal individuals (see earlier section on Toxicity of Fructose). In addition, conversion of fructose to blood glucose is hampered. Direct proof that the changes in cellular metabolites observed after fructose loads in animals also occur in the patient was, until recently, scarce for ethical reasons. The accumulation of fructose 1-phosphate has been verified.[355,356] A depletion of intracellular P_i was inferred from the long-lasting decrease of serum P_i in the patients after fructose administration. For instance, it was calculated that the conversion of 6.6 mmol (1.2 g) fructose to fructose 1-phosphate by an infant weighing 8.8 kg required more P_i than the amount present in the entire extracellular fluid.[308] The increase of serum magnesium and uric acid after fructose in the patients[92,303,357] most probably reflected the loss — that is, the consumption and breakdown — of ATP from the fructose-metabolizing tissues. Indeed, ATP is a strong Mg^{2+} chelator, and a decrease in its concentration is likely to result in the release of cellular Mg^{2+}. Undoubtedly, several of the toxic effects of fructose in the patients are caused by the depletion of ATP. The loss of hepatic ATP, by its effect on protein synthesis, may explain the hyperaminoacidemia, the decrease in blood-clotting factors, and the other signs of liver failure. The complex renal tubular dysfunction resembling the Fanconi syndrome[358] may be caused by the degradation of ATP in the kidney. A modulation of the renal dysfunction by the level of parathyroid hormone has been reported.[349] The metabolic acidosis is due to both lactic acidosis and proximal renal tubular acidosis, the former being far more important.[344] The abnormally high elevation of fructose 1-phosphate in liver most likely also explains the deficient glycosylation of serum transferrin, which has been documented in a 15-month-old untreated boy with hereditary fructose intolerance.[359] Fructose 1-phosphate has indeed been shown to inhibit phosphomannomutase,[360] the deficiency of which is the cause of carbohydrate-deficient glycoprotein syndrome type I[361] .

With the advent of clinically applicable ^{31}P–MRS, the direct proof for fructose 1-phosphate accumulation, ATP breakdown, and decrease of P_i in the patients' liver has become possible,[218,233–235,342] and absolute concentrations have been measured.[218,234] After an IV fructose bolus, metabolite changes were as rapid as, but not more marked than, in the controls, but baseline concentrations were reestablished only after a tenfold delay (see Fig. 70-7).

The rapid IV infusion of fructose may exceptionally induce a slight lowering of blood glucose in normal newborn infants[362] and healthy adults.[363] Its mechanism is not immediately apparent and has been the subject of extensive investigations. It is not due to increased glucose utilization by the peripheral tissues but is caused by a block of glucose release from the liver.[348] The fructose-induced hypoglycemia seen in the patients is not due to hyperinsulinism[303,307,308,346,348] and is not corrected by exogenous glucagon[216,307,308,340,345,364] or dibutyryl-cAMP.[216] On the other hand, when administration of oral or IV fructose is accompanied[339] or followed[307,340] by oral or IV galactose, the fructose-induced hypoglycemia is prevented or corrected. Neither dihydroxyacetone[339,340] nor P_i[298,340,346,364] has a corrective effect. These facts demonstrate that during a limited time after the fructose load, hepatic glucose formation by way of glycogenolysis and gluconeogenesis is impaired.

Decreased gluconeogenesis is apparent from the fact that the fructose-induced hypoglycemia cannot be corrected by dihydroxyacetone, which enters the glycolytic-gluconeogenic pathway at the triokinase step. The hindrance of dihydroxyacetone conversion to glucose may be due to several mechanisms. Inhibition by fructose 1-phosphate of the two gluconeogenic enzymes glucose 6-phosphate isomerase[365] (phosphohexose isomerase) and liver aldolase[366] has been reported. When residual aldolase was assayed in the direction of condensation of the triose phosphates to fructose 1,6-bisphosphate, inhibition was observed in patient liver homogenate but not in control liver.[366] The inhibition of glucose 6-phosphate isomerase by fructose 1-phosphate may account for the occasional occurrence of a transient decrease in blood glucose on rapid infusion of the ketose in normal subjects.[362,363] Depletion of ATP also may explain decreased gluconeogenesis. Indeed, in perfused rat liver, its rate depends on the concentration of ATP up to the physiologic level, a half-maximal effect being observed at 0.6 mM ATP.[367] Even complete inhibition of gluconeogenesis cannot by itself explain the rapid, fructose-induced decrease in blood glucose characteristic of hereditary fructose intolerance, because several hours of fasting are required for patients with fructose 1,6-bisphosphatase deficiency to become hypoglycemic (see later section on Fructose 1,6-Bisphosphatase Deficiency).

A block of glycogenolysis during fructose-induced hypoglycemia is evidenced by the inability of glucagon to correct the blood glucose. The increase of liver glycogen measured in a biopsy sample by Cain and Ryman[368] is in keeping with this observation. Inhibition of phosphoglucomutase by fructose 1-phosphate *in vitro* was suggested by Sidbury.[369] However, fructose-induced hypoglycemia can be corrected by galactose[307]; thus, conversion of glucose 1-phosphate to glucose 6-phosphate and free glucose is not impaired *in vivo*. Therefore, breakdown of liver glycogen must be blocked at the level of phosphorylase.

The effects of fructose on the different steps of glycogenolysis have been investigated in detail.[200,216,370,371] The glucagon-induced accumulation of cAMP is markedly reduced by prior administration of fructose. This effect was observed in the urine of patients after a diagnostic dose of IV fructose and in the livers of rats receiving fructose loads, where it correlated with the decrease of ATP, the substrate of adenylate cyclase. Slowed formation of cAMP did not explain the suppression of the hormonal effect, because fructose-induced hypoglycemia was not corrected by the injection of dibutyryl-cAMP. Furthermore, the amount of cAMP formed in the livers of experimental animals was still sufficient to bring about the conversion of phosphorylase b to the active form a. Competitive inhibition of phosphorylase a from animal liver by fructose 1-phosphate has been demonstrated.[216,372–375] It is enhanced by lowering the concentration of P_i. At the concentration of fructose 1-phosphate and P_i prevailing in the livers of experimental animals after fructose administration, the inhibition seemed insufficient to account for the complete abolition of the phosphorolytic degradation of glycogen. Total inhibition of phosphorylase a could nevertheless be evidenced *in vivo*.[371,375] Van den Berghe,[371] after loading with tagatose, concluded that part of the total P_i measured may be bound and consequently unavailable for phosphorylase a, resulting in the enhancement of the inhibitory effect of fructose 1-phosphate. The absence of a corrective effect of phosphate infusions may be related to the limited entry of P_i into the liver.[240]

Despite the inability of the liver, kidney, and small intestine to metabolize fructose beyond fructose 1-phosphate, only 10 to 20 percent of the administered sugar is excreted in the patient's urine. This led to further investigations. As expected, red and white blood cells metabolized fructose normally, by way of hexokinase, in the absence of glucose; in liver tissue, oxidation of [U-^{14}C]fructose to $^{14}CO_2$ and incorporation of the label into glycogen was only 1 to 6 percent of normal.[308] Studies *in vivo* by Landau *et al.*[376] indicate that this limited metabolism occurs by phosphorylation to fructose 6-phosphate. The amount of fructose utilized by the liver of these patients is too small to explain why as much as 90 percent of the administered fructose is assimilated. It has therefore been suggested that adipose tissue is the main site of fructose utilization in patients with hereditary fructose intolerance as well as in those with essential fructosuria.[65,178] As was seen in the latter, red cell fructose 3-phosphate does not account for the missing fructose[181] (see earlier section on Essential Fructosuria).

Diagnosis, Treatment, and Course

The diagnosis of hereditary fructose intolerance can be suspected from a detailed nutritional history and the clinical picture.[299,324] A high degree of clinical awareness is often needed for prompt diagnosis, because the spectrum of symptoms and signs is wide and nonspecific.[299,300,314,350,377] Small infants are referred for vomiting of unknown etiology, pyloric stenosis or gastroesophageal reflux, or toxic disorders, whereas older infants and small children are referred for hepatomegaly, failure to thrive, or growth delay.[299,300,378] Usually, hepatitis, intrauterine infection, septicemia, hemolytic-uremic syndrome, tumor of the liver or storage disorder, galactosemia, tyrosinosis, and Wilson disease are considered. Suspicion is fostered by the presence of reducing substances in urine (glucose or fructose or both) or by hyperaminoaciduria and high blood methionine and tyrosine, discovered by selective screening. It is important to know that fructosuria may have disappeared at the time of urinalysis.

As soon as hereditary fructose intolerance is suspected, all sucrose, fructose, and sorbitol must be eliminated at once from the diet and from medications. The beneficial effect of withdrawal, usually seen within days, is the first positive element of diagnosis. It must be confirmed by DNA analysis (see Table 70-5) or, after several weeks of fructose abstinence, by an IV fructose tolerance test (200 mg/kg) (see Figs. 70-10 and 70-11) and, in case of doubt, by the assay[379] of fructaldolase in a biopsy of the liver or, perhaps, small intestine (see Tables 70-3 and 70-4). The liver is the preferred organ for biopsy.[12] Fructaldolase activities in the serum of patients are only slightly diminished and hence of no diagnostic value.[380] Enzymatic diagnosis from blood cells is not possible,[381] and the same must be said of cultured skin fibroblasts and placenta, because they appear to express predominantly aldolase A.[112,113,382,383] Diagnostic analysis of DNA from blood leukocytes has become possible and can be successfully applied (see Table 70-5). Postmortem DNA diagnosis in archival tissue preserved at autopsy allows the identification of victims of iatrogenic fructose poisoning.[384]

Treatment consists of the elimination from the diet of all sources of sucrose and fructose.[10,11,385,386] Supportive measures such as infusion of fresh-frozen plasma or exchange transfusion may alleviate the clotting disorder and restore complement deficiency.[387] Recovery of renal and hepatic function takes days. Small infants recover more slowly than older ones and may yet die of hepatic and renal failure several days after the withdrawal of fructose. Once recovery is made, the further course is uneventful, intellectual development is unimpaired, and catch-up growth proceeds.[324,388,389] A daily supplement of vitamin C is needed; the prescription should, of course, be free of any noxious sugar.

Children with hereditary fructose intolerance during their first year of life start protecting themselves by a self-imposed exclusion diet that, although sufficiently stringent to spare them intolerance symptoms, is liberal enough to cause hepatomegaly and stunted growth. Therefore, after diagnosis, the child's aversion cannot be relied on and a diet must be prescribed. Two treated preschool boys after partial relaxation of their diet to 250 mg/kg fructose per day had sustained increases in serum and urinary uric acid and magnesium, yet no symptoms of intolerance.[389]

Small children usually have hepatomegaly for months or years despite adequate treatment.[300] The reason for this is unclear, but it may be connected with a particularly high degree of intolerance during childhood[308] and with hidden sources[309] of dietary fructose and sucrose. A group of adult patients on average consumed 2.5 g sucrose daily — 5 percent of what was consumed by controls.[309] Dietary indiscretion in an adult was elegantly detected by ^{31}P-MRS.[235] A rapid disappearance of intralobular hepatic fibrosis and a decrease of periportal fibrosis were observed in serial liver biopsy specimens, but fatty vacuolization of liver cells persisted or increased, and its distribution changed from diffuse to periportal.[300,385]

The first known patient with fructose intolerance was born in 1886, and her condition was properly recognized toward the end of the nineteenth century as intolerance to sugar, although it was never reported. She had lived sugar-free and died at age 83 of an unrelated cause; the diagnosis was verified biochemically on postmortem liver examination.[390] The original patient described by Chambers and Pratt[296] is alive and in good physical health at the age of 70 and is a grandparent.[390a]

Patients, or their parents, should declare their fructose intolerance on every hospital admission. They should understand that infusion solutions containing fructose, sorbitol, or invert sugar, unfortunately still in use (e.g., after routine surgery), are an immediate threat to the health and life of the patient.[391] Instances of iatrogenic deaths, or near-miss deaths, have been published and continue to occur despite ample warnings[208,299,314–318,320–323,384,391–405]; one patient with liver failure was rescued by transplantation.[317] Indeed, the time has come for fructose, sorbitol, and invert sugar solutions to be abandoned,[405] and fructose and sucrose have no place in infant formula. A European Community Commission Directive in 1991 permitting sucrose in first infant formula is as incomprehensible as it is life-threatening to hereditary fructose-intolerant infants. Sucrose as an analgesic for newborn infants[406–408] is a new threat to the infant with hereditary fructose intolerance.

Incidence, Genetics, Molecular Biology, and Population Genetics

Cases of hereditary fructose intolerance have been reported from Europe, North America, India,[409] Australia,[396] and other parts of the world. The true incidence is not known but may be as high as 1:20,000 in Switzerland[410] and Great Britain.[411] Evidence is overwhelming that considerable numbers of children and adult patients must live undiagnosed in the general population; this is concluded from the following facts: reports of iatrogenic accidents and deaths following infusions; the surfacing of undiagnosed patients among older sibs and other relatives of young probands during extended family investigations[306,307,324,343]; the self-diagnosis of medical students during lectures on hereditary fructose intolerance[12]; and the frequent occurrence of parent–child[306,311–313,392,410,412–414] or grandparent–grandchild[415] cases.

The mode of inheritance is autosomal recessive. Sex distribution among the affected is even. Affected monozygotic twins have been observed.[309,349,403] The overwhelming majority of parents are unaffected. Consanguinity of parents is not uncommon. One pair of affected parents produced four children, all affected.[319] An apparently dominant case may be the child of an affected homozygous parent and a healthy heterozygote (pseudo-dominance).[416]

Heterozygotes for hereditary fructose intolerance can be identified by DNA analysis[384] and by ^{31}P-MRS.[235] Older conventional methods were unsuccessful. Oral or IV fructose tolerance tests yielded normal results in six sets of parents,[303,307,417] as well as in another parent and his healthy grandchild, who was the daughter of a patient.[306] In one set of parents given a continuous fructose infusion, blood clearance was diminished[418]; this could not be confirmed in 11 parents.[224,298,348] In seven, significant differences were not found, even though blood glucose, standard bicarbonate, phosphorus, lactate, urate, and urinary urate/creatinine and magnesium/creatinine ratios were determined.[224] Heterozygote detection by the estimation of immunoreactive aldolase in intestinal biopsy has been attempted.[336] All parents examined so far have had normal liver fructaldolase activity,[417] a fact yet unexplained.

Molecular heterogeneity of the aldolase B gene (for review, see Table 70-5 and Fig. 70-12) confirms what had been inferred from earlier studies of mutant proteins. Given the variations of enzyme activities[303] and the different K_m values for fructose 1-phosphate[94] between patients, it was speculated that there may be more than one genotype involved. Differences in antibody activation,[337,419] heat stability[92,337] of residual aldolase, and the finding of different structural anomalies of aldolase subunits[336,419a] in one kindred indicated the same. The demonstration of different mutations at the DNA level[420,421] and evidence for compound heterozygosity[420] was soon to follow. The aldolase B gene is located on chromosome 9 and has been cloned and sequenced (see earlier section on Enzymes of Fructose Metabolism). The direct analysis of aldolase B genes amplified by polymerase chain reaction in 50 patients, with one exception from Europe, showed three point mutations: the A149P mutation in 67 percent, the A174D mutation in 16 percent of alleles, and the L288ΔC mutation causing a frame shift, restricted to Sicilian subjects.[422] The former two point mutations and an N334K mutation are prevalent causes of hereditary fructose intolerance,[384] accounting together for 84 percent of hereditary fructose intolerance alleles in Europe.[423] Functional null alleles also have been described (see Table 70-5). Today, more than 95 percent of patients with hereditary fructose intolerance are amenable to rapid noninvasive diagnosis with the help of a limited panel of allele-specific oligonucleotides.[384,422] For interesting structure–function relationships for aldolase B and the other aldolases, and their disturbance by specific mutations, either naturally occurring or by site-specific mutagenesis, the reader is referred to Fig. 70-12 and Table 70-5.

Population genetics. The most frequent allele causing hereditary fructose intolerance is A149P, which has a wide distribution among populations in Europe, including Ashkenasi Jews and other residents of Israel, Turkey, North America,[424] The Dominican Republic, Australia, and New Zealand.[425] Haplotype linkage analysis of A149P alleles has shown absolute linkage disequilibrium with informative linked aldolase B polymorphisms in intron 8 (C → T at nucleotide 84 and A → G at nucleotide 105), which excludes a mutational hot spot but provides convincing evidence that the mutation arose on a single chromosome and spread throughout populations by a combination of mass migration and random genetic drift.[426] The occurrence of a reciprocal haplotype on all chromosomes harboring the A174D allele is further evidence for spread by genetic drift.[426] This happened early during the evolution of modern populations and possibly before the European expansion that characterized the late Bronze Age.[427] This also means that parents who appear not to be consanguineous, but give rise to offspring with the homozygous A149P genotype, are thus likely to be related by blood, albeit distantly. The original patient of Chambers and Pratt[296] was later shown to be homozygous for the A149P mutation.[390a] Neonatal screening for the A149P mutation in the British population has revealed 27 heterozygotes in a random cohort of 2050 newborns, predicting a frequency of 1 homozygote for A149P in 23,000.[411] The aldolase B allele A149P was not found in a series of 192 Norwegian victims of sudden infant death; thus, an association of sudden infant death with hereditary fructose intolerance was not evidenced.[290] Differences in the geographic distribution of mutant alleles throughout Europe are recognizable (see Table 70-5).[422,428]

Expression Studies and Model of Fructose Intolerance

So far the disease causing aldolase B variants C134R and A149P, obtained by site-directed mutagenesis, have been synthesized in *E. coli*, to understand further the effects of the natural mutations on the enzyme molecule. Brooks and Tolan[429] expressed the mutant C134R and showed that, although the mutant enzyme retained residual activity toward the fructose 1-phosphate substrate, the reduced level of expression compared with wild type in this host/vector system suggested that structural instability of the partially active mutant enzyme may be the cause of the disease phenotype. The expressed A149P mutant enzyme protein is inactive toward its specific substrate, fructose 1-phosphate, with residual activity toward fructose 1,6-bisphosphate.[520]

An interesting model of fructose intolerance has been obtained by the expression of rat liver fructokinase in yeast cells whose growth was inhibited in a dose-dependent fashion by fructose in the medium[85]; and intracellular fructose 1-phosphate accumulation was shown by ^{31}P-MRS.[430]

FRUCTOSE 1,6-BISPHOSPHATASE DEFICIENCY (MIM 229700)

Historical Note

Fructose 1,6-bisphosphatase deficiency was first described in 1970 by Baker and Winegrad.[301] Two further reports appeared within a year[338,431] and were followed by a number of observations.[432–446] By 1987, we were aware of 85 patients in published and unpublished reports, all children.[447] A variant form of fructose 1,6-bisphosphatase deficiency in a woman and her daughter[448] and combined fructose 1,6-bisphosphatase and glucose 6-phosphatase deficiency in another woman[449] have been reported.

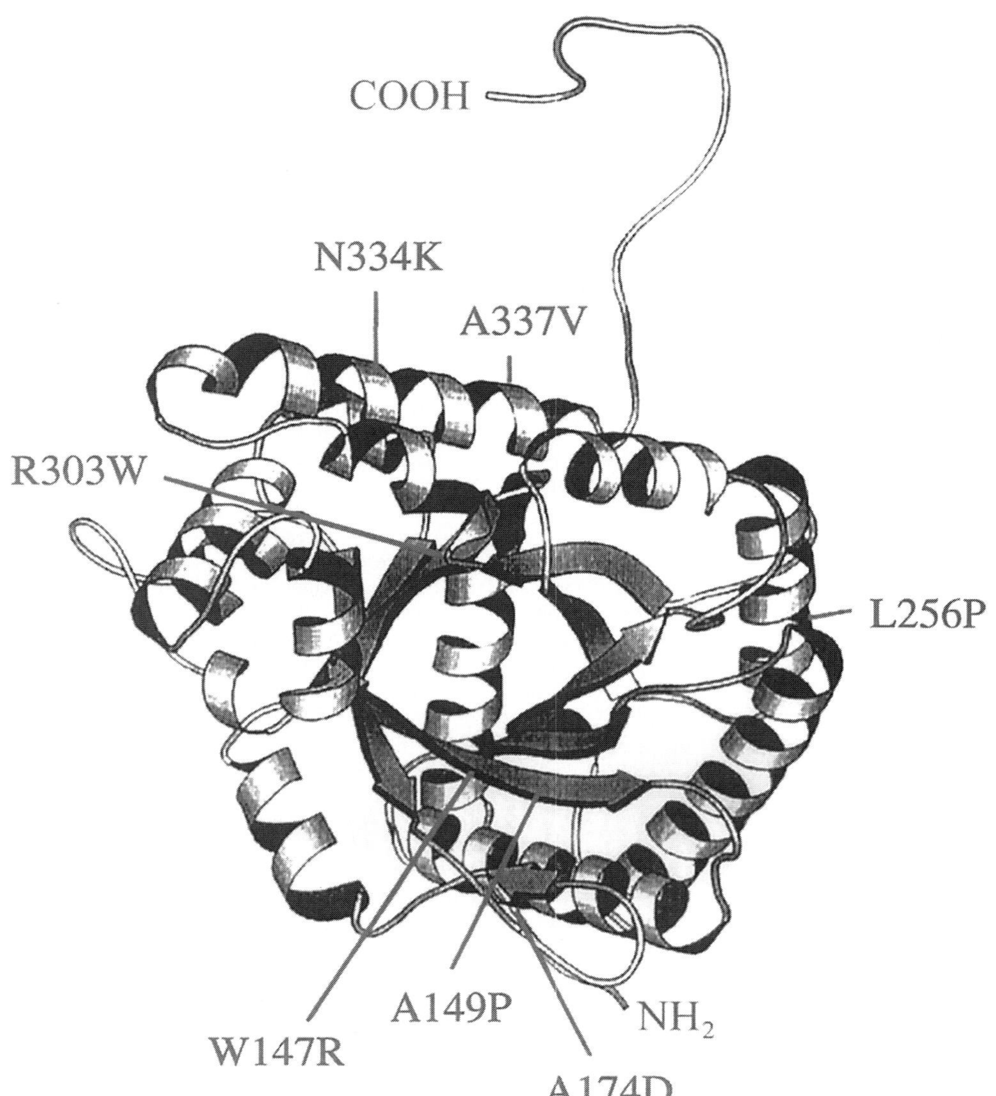

Fig. 70-12 Diagram of the three-dimensional structure of a single human aldolase A subunit with some of the amino acid substitutions of aldolase B in patients with hereditary fructose intolerance. Because the structure of human aldolase A is highly homologous to aldolase B, it can be used to model missense mutations in aldolase B associated with hereditary fructose intolerance.

The polypeptide backbone of the enzyme folds into an alternating arrangement of α helices and β sheets (arrows), which adopt a basic eight-membered β barrel type structure. The active site lies in the middle of the barrel, and the catalytically important residues are located in the β sheets that line the barrel. A recent model has indicated that the C-terminal residues (indicated here in bold) actually project into the active site[136] and that they perhaps mediate movement of the substrates in and out of the barrel structure,[135] where the substrate-binding residues Lys 146, Arg 148, and Lys 229 (which forms the Schiff base[501]) line the active site pocket encoded by exons 3, 5, 6, and 7.[423]

The mutations C134R, W147R, A149P, and A174D all appear to be located in the vicinity of the substrate-binding pocket and are likely to disrupt important residues, including C-1 phosphate-binding residues, Lys 146, and Arg 148, in the active site of the enzyme.[135,499,500] The mutations N334K and A337V occur in an α helix and may affect the mobility of the conformationally flexible C-terminal tail, which is thought to mediate access of the substrate into the active site pocket.[135] Because tetramer formation required for functional aldolase B involves close contacts between hydrophobic residues, it may be that the mutation L256P, which appears to lie on the outer surface of the molecule, disrupts this hydrophobic interaction, possibly resulting in a failure of tetrameric assembly and formation of aldolase subunits which, although catalytically active, are unstable.[97] For additional mutations, see Table 70-5. (*Reprinted with permission Rellos P, Sygusch J, Cox TM. J Biol Chem 275:1145, 2000.*[520])

Clinical and Laboratory Findings

Fructose 1,6-bisphosphatase deficiency is a severe disorder of gluconeogenesis causing life-threatening episodes in newborn infants and small children. Approximately half the afflicted children had their first symptoms between the first and fourth days of life, the remainder in equal numbers before and after their sixth month. The latest manifestation, with one exception, was at age 4 years.[444] In the newborn, hyperventilation is the most common symptom, usually caused by profound acidosis. Irritability, somnolence or coma, apneic spells, dyspnea and tachycardia, muscular hypotonia, and a moderate hepatomegaly may be observed. Hypoglycemia may be an isolated chemical sign[440] but is usually detected when sought, together with ketonuria. Attention has been drawn to the fact that in an occasional patient, ketonuria may be absent.[291,450] This can be explained by the accumulation of pyruvate, resulting in the build-up of oxaloacetate, and hence in diversion of mitochondrial acetyl-CoA away from ketone body formation into citrate synthesis. The latter results in increased synthesis of malonyl-CoA in the cytosol.

Elevated malonyl-CoA, by inhibiting carnitine palmitoyl transferase 1, prevents entry of long-chain fatty acyl-CoA into the mitochondria, thereby further reducing ketogenesis. The first hypoglycemic attacks in the newborn period are promptly overcome by the administration of glucose and sodium bicarbonate. Weeks or many months of apparent well-being can pass between the first and further attacks.

Later episodes are usually triggered by febrile infections. Refusal to feed and vomiting, which often accompany febrile infections in children, precipitate the onset. The evolution is usually dramatic: hyperventilation, trembling, lethargy, coma, and convulsions follow in short succession within a few hours and reflect profound acidosis, ketosis, and hypoglycemia. Apnea and cardiac arrest have been observed.[338] Flushing[338] and hematemesis[435,436] have occurred rarely. Lactate, ketones, alanine, and uric acid[441,443] are elevated in blood and appear in urine.[338,436] Also detected in urine are glycerol, glycerol 3-phosphate, and other phosphorylated intermediates.[451–454] Blood glucose is low, but attacks of ketoacidosis without hypoglycemia have been observed.[441–443] Hepatomegaly and muscle weakness are often present. Failure to thrive is the exception.[443] In one child, the clinical and biochemical presentation and course were suggestive of tyrosinosis,[431,432] with liver dysfunction, hyperaminoaciduria, wasting, sepsis, and death. In contrast to hereditary fructose intolerance, disturbances of liver function are the exception,[438] and renal tubular function and blood coagulation are undisturbed. Electroencephalographic tracings may be abnormal during attacks but later return to normal. A slow-wave pattern has been described.[441,442] Two sibs had a peculiar low-amplitude pattern with slowed background activity and intermittent, spindle-shaped, fast-activity bursts.[338]

Most affected children experience a number of acute attacks before the diagnosis is made. Once diagnosis is established and treatment begins, the course is favorable. The patients do not have an aversion to sweet foods; in fact, they may even enjoy eating fruits and sweets.[301] Hepatomegaly regresses slowly or more rapidly, but lapses occur[435,441,442,446] and may be related to the intake of fructose and sucrose. Somatic, psychomotor, and intellectual development seems unimpaired.

Biochemical Defect, Functional Studies, and Pathogenesis

Deficiency of fructose 1,6-bisphosphatase (hexose bisphosphatase, fructose 1,6-bisphosphatase, EC 3.1.3.11) can be demonstrated in the liver, jejunum,[434] kidney,[431,436] and probably the leukocytes (see later section on Diagnosis, Treatment, and Prognosis). In two thirds of the children, liver fructose 1,6-bisphosphatase activity was either absent or reduced to a trace, in the others reduced to one fifth or less. Anomalous kinetic behavior of the residual enzyme has been reported.[455] Inactivity of fructose 1,6-bisphosphatase in the liver and active enzyme in skeletal muscle was demonstrated in one patient[433]; in another, the enzyme activity was absent in the liver, kidney, and leukocytes but was present in skeletal muscle extract.[436] These findings, together with further biochemical evidence, demonstrate that muscle contains a distinct enzyme not involved in this disorder.

Liver glycogen was normal in four liver biopsy specimens but was increased in many others.[12,338,436] Liver glucose 6-phosphatase activity was normal, with one exception,[449] as were fructaldolase, pyruvate kinase, phosphoenolpyruvate carboxykinase, phosphorylase, phosphoglucomutase, phosphofructokinase, amylo 1,6-glucosidase, and acid maltase.

Fructose 1,6-bisphosphatase is a key enzyme of gluconeogenesis. Its inactivity prevents the endogenous formation of glucose from the precursors lactate, glycerol, and gluconeogenic amino acids such as alanine. It is not surprising that more than half the afflicted infants become symptomatic within the first week of life, when they are dependent on gluconeogenesis.[456] On subsequent days, higher milk intake and more frequent feedings seem to postpone further manifestations.

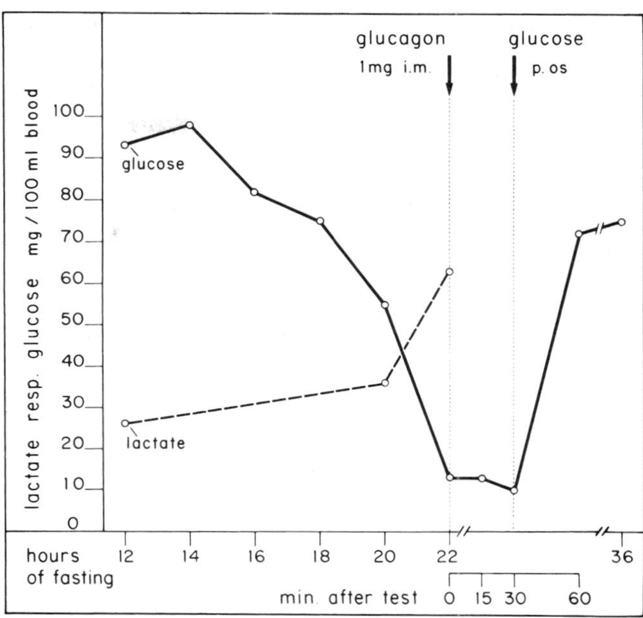

Fig. 70-13 Prolonged fasting in a 17-month-old boy (T.M.) with fructose 1,6-bisphosphatase deficiency. (*Reprinted with permission from Baerlocher K, Gitzelmann R, Nüssli R, Dumermuth G. Helv Paediatr Acta 26:489, 1971.*[338])

Dependence of fructose 1,6-bisphosphatase–deficient children on exogenous glucose can easily be demonstrated. During *fasting*, maintenance of blood glucose depends on glycogenolysis, and the duration of normoglycemia thus depends on the amount of available liver glycogen. Blood glucose may decrease within a few hours[436] or only after 14 h or more.[301,338,445] Simultaneously, lactate and pyruvate increase[301,338,436,445] and their ratio increases. Blood ketones and alanine increase also. When hypoglycemia is reached, the blood glucose level is unresponsive to injected glucagon. This indicates that liver glycogen stores have been depleted (Fig. 70-13). In the fed state, patients have a normal hyperglycemic response to glucagon. Feeding a diet excessively high in protein or fat equally provokes hypoglycemia, acidosis, and ketonemia.[433] High lactate/pyruvate and glycerol 3-phosphate/dihydroxyacetone phosphate ratios, demonstrated in liver biopsy specimens, indicate the accumulation of glyceraldehyde 3-phosphate and insufficient oxidation of NADH.[433]

Patients with fructose 1,6-bisphosphatase deficiency have reduced tolerance to *fructose and sorbitol*, but generally it is higher than in patients with hereditary fructose intolerance. In the liver of an adult with fructose 1,6-bisphosphatase deficiency, fructose 1-phosphate increased, after an IV fructose bolus, and ATP and P_i decreased, as evidenced by ^{31}P-MRS. Changes were as rapid and as important as in the control and in the patient with hereditary fructose intolerance. Restoration of baseline concentrations was, however, delayed when compared with the control, but far quicker than in the patient with hereditary fructose intolerance (see Fig. 70-7).[218,234] One infant tolerated 5 g/kg sucrose per day in his formula.[224] Fructose 1,6-bisphosphatase–deficient patients do not have gastrointestinal symptoms after an oral load.[301,338] As in hereditary fructose intolerance, blood glucose and phosphorus drop after the load, whereas lactate, urate, magnesium, and alanine increase (Fig. 70-14). Fructose-induced hypoglycemia is not related to insulin release[301,338,433,435,439,457] and cannot be corrected by injecting glucagon[301,435,440–442,] or epinephrine.[436] The response to fructose is similar when given intravenously or orally and is dose dependent.[338,440–442] Although in fructose 1,6-bisphosphatase–deficient children, fructose-induced changes of blood metabolites seem somewhat less drastic than they are in children with hereditary fructose intolerance, fructose tolerance

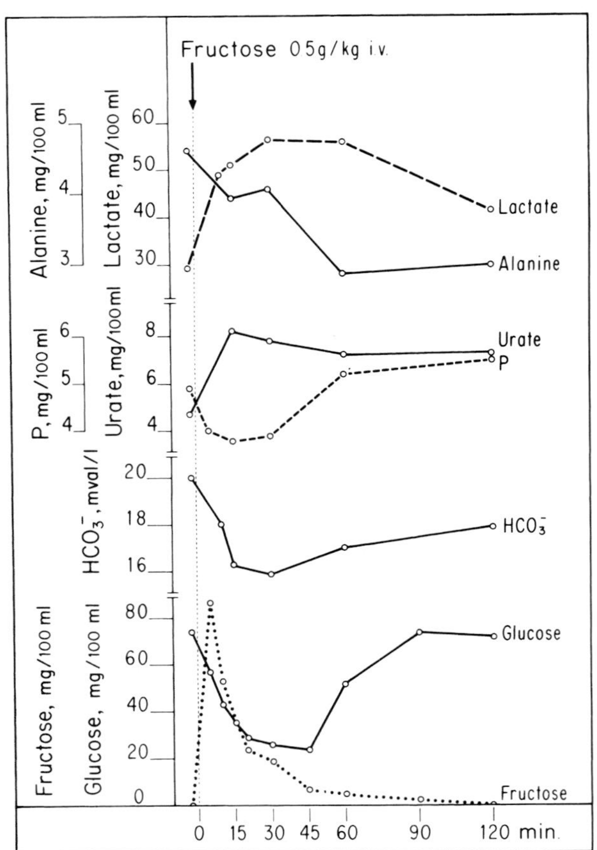

Fig. 70-14 Intravenous fructose tolerance test in a 21-month-old boy (T.M.) with fructose 1,6-bisphosphatase deficiency,[338] with the high dose of 500 mg/kg. The lower dose of 200 mg/kg is preferable.[92] *(Reprinted with permission from Steinmann B, Gitzelmann R. Int J Vitam Nutr Res Suppl 15:289, 1976.*[395]*)*

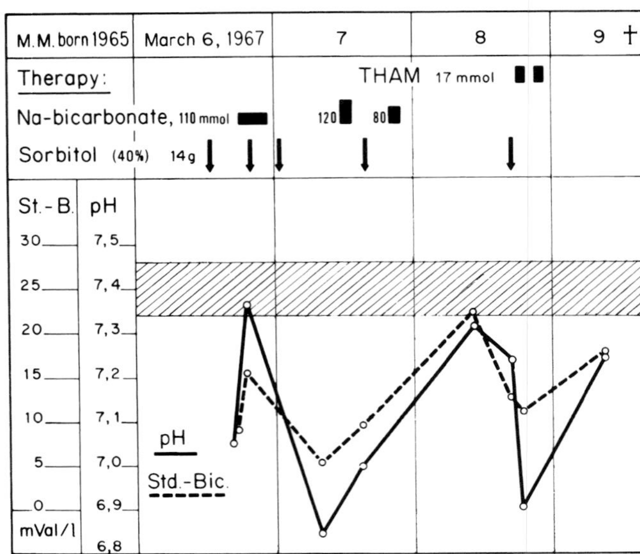

Fig. 70-15 Final course of a 2-year-old girl, M.M., older sib of T.M.,[338] with undiagnosed fructose 1,6-bisphosphatase deficiency after repeated sorbitol infusions for assumed cerebral edema. After each sorbitol dose, severe acidosis occurred and was corrected with sodium bicarbonate and buffer (THAM). *(Reprinted with permission from Gitzelmann R, Baerlocher K, Prader A. Monatsschr Kinderheilkd 121:174, 1973; and Baerlocher K, Gitzelmann R, Steinmann B. In Burman D, Holton JB, Pennock CA (eds): Inherited Disorders of Carbohydrate Metabolism. Lancaster, MTP, 1980, pp 163–190.*[459]*)*

tests are not without risk. The 20-month-old patient studied by Corbeel et al.[441,442] became comatose after the injection of 500 mg/kg fructose. Repeated therapeutic sorbitol infusions in a 2-year-old patient were deleterious[458,459] (Fig. 70-15).

Oral administration of *glycerol*[301,338,433,434,437,439,440,443,445,446] provokes a response quite similar to that seen after fructose administration. Hypoglycemia is paralleled by a drop of phosphorus and bicarbonate; lactate increases. In contrast, children with intact gluconeogenesis respond with an increase of blood glucose but not of lactic acid.[433] Hypoglycemia is again unrelated to insulin release[301,433] and is refractory to glucagon.[301] *Alanine*, given intravenously or orally, can cause a similar though milder hypoglycemic response[433,439–442] or none at all.[434,435,439,446] The responses to alanine infusion after 6 and 12 h of fasting were divergent in Pagliara's patient.[433] After a 6-h fast, alanine caused an increase of glucose, and after a 12-h fast, a late decrease. The handling of *dihydroxyacetone* (1 g/kg body weight orally) was tested in only one patient on two occasions.[224,292,338] He vomited 25 min after the ingestion; during the first half-hour, blood glucose decreased in the patient but increased in adult controls and in a child with hereditary fructose intolerance.[224] In all, blood lactate increased and phosphorus and bicarbonate decreased. The adult controls had a delayed hypoglycemic response due to hyperinsulinism[224] whereas the 5-year-old boy had prompt insulin secretion in spite of hypoglycemia (Fig. 70-16); it was concluded that hypoglycemia was complex in this patient and due to direct insulin secretion stimulated by dihydroxyacetone, to a functional block in glycogenolysis by sugar phosphates (see below), and to his basic defect in gluconeogenesis.[292]

Children with fructose 1,6-bisphosphatase deficiency have normal *galactose* tolerance. Injection or ingestion is followed by normoglycemia or mild hyperglycemia, indicating normal assimilation of this sugar.

Hypoglycemia occurs after prolonged *fasting* when glycogen stores are depleted and the liver switches from glycogen breakdown to gluconeogenesis. Tolerance to fasting, although limited (see Fig. 70-13), is not nil (Fig. 70-17). It seems to improve somewhat with age. A correlation with residual fructose 1,6-bisphosphatase activity in the liver should exist but has not been documented.

Reactive hypoglycemia after fructose, sorbitol, glycerol, dihydroxyacetone, and alanine is somewhat more complex (see Fig. 70-2). As in hereditary fructose intolerance, phosphate esters may accumulate intracellularly and inhibit glycogen phosphorylase. This presumption is supported by the glucagon refractoriness of hypoglycemia. The appearance of glycerol 3-phosphate and of other phosphorylated intermediates in urine is surprising, because organophosphates are not usually excreted; it has been confirmed[453] in the case of Dremsek *et al.*[451] during fasting but not in Baerlocher's patient[338] after recovery. The provenance of the organophosphates is obscure.

Liver phosphorylase is inhibited in various ways by fructose 1-phosphate, fructose 1,6-bisphosphate, and glycerol 3-phosphate.[216,372,373,375] Inhibition becomes stronger as inorganic phosphate decreases. Hyperuricemia and hypermagnesemia reflect adenine nucleotide breakdown (see earlier section on Pathophysiology of Hereditary Fructose Intolerance).

The cause of hepatomegaly and of fatty infiltration of the liver is uncertain. Fat deposition is likely to result from a constant flooding with amino acids and glycerol that can either be released as lactate or converted to fat and stored.

Diagnosis, Treatment, and Prognosis

The diagnosis of fructose 1,6-bisphosphatase deficiency must be suspected in full-term newborns of normal birth weight suffering from hyperventilation, convulsions, and coma accompanied by

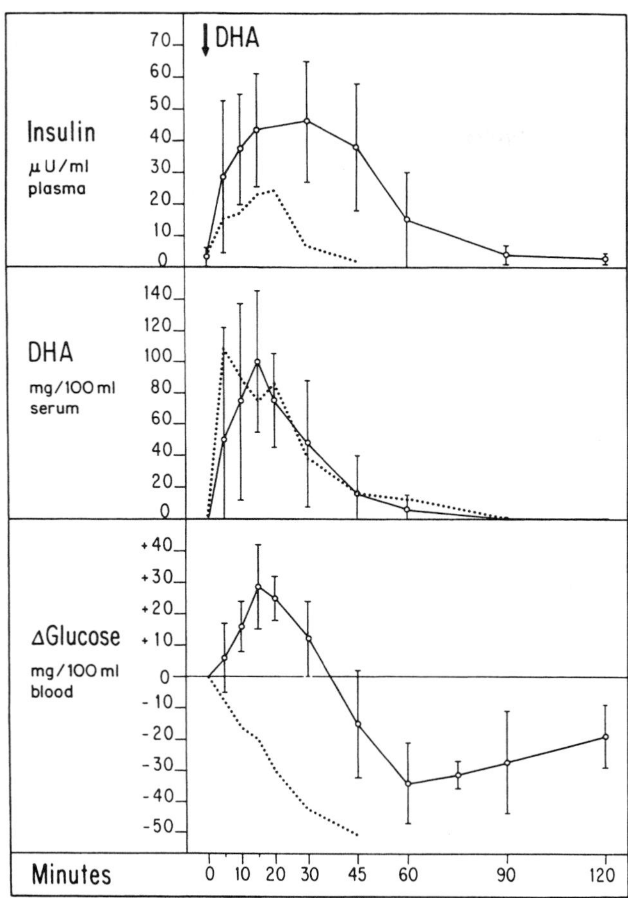

Fig. 70-16 Oral dihydroxyacetone tolerance test (1 g/kg body weight) in a 5-year-old boy (T.M.; ......) with fructose 1,6-bisphosphatase deficiency[292] and in six healthy adult volunteers (—) (mean ±1 SD).[224]

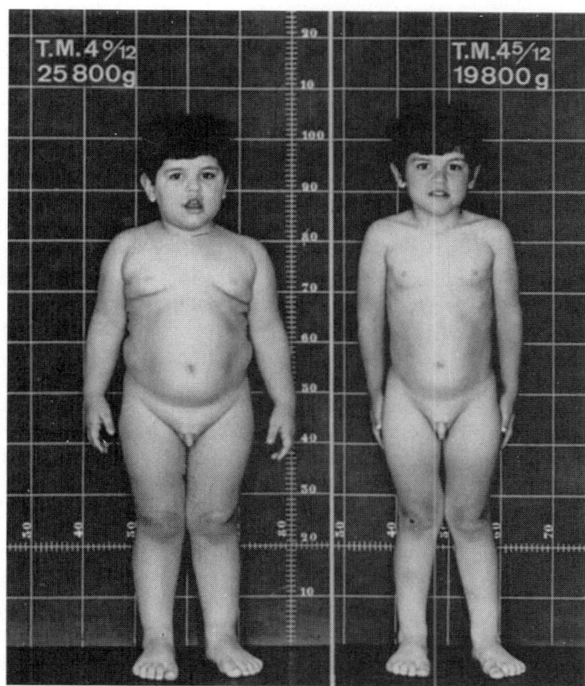

Fig. 70-17 Patient T.M.,[338] fructose 1,6-bisphosphatase-deficient, 4 years of age and obese because of overnutrition. Five months later, he had lost 6 kg by dieting (800 to 900 kcal/m^2/day; carbohydrates, 66 percent; proteins, 22 percent; fat, 12 percent). At ages 14 and 16.5 years, he dieted again and, after hard exercise, he ate insufficiently. The following mornings he suffered from life-threatening hypoglycemic attacks with lactic acidosis.[292]

hypoglycemia, ketosis, and acidosis, especially when signs of neonatal infection, cerebral hemorrhage, and left heart failure are absent. The disorder also must be suspected in small children suffering from episodic hypoglycemia triggered by febrile infection or starvation. Other causes of lactic acidosis, such as the deficiencies of glucose 6-phosphatase, pyruvate carboxylase, pyruvate dehydrogenase, and phosphoenolpyruvate carboxykinase,[460] may be difficult to exclude. Fasting tests (see Fig. 70-13) and tolerance tests with fructose (see Fig. 70-14), sorbitol, glycerol, alanine, or dihydroxyacetone[224,449] must be postponed until remission and should be performed with adequate monitoring and interpreted with caution. A fructose load should not be given by mouth unless hereditary fructose intolerance is definitely excluded. The use of a moderate dose (e.g., 200 mg/kg intravenously) is recommended[92] because higher doses may be dangerous.[441,442] Aversion to sweets and signs of proximal renal tubular syndrome after fructose (or sorbitol) exposure, as seen in hereditary fructose intolerance, are absent in fructose 1,6-bisphosphatase deficiency.

The diagnosis should be established by demonstrating an enzyme deficiency in a liver biopsy specimen[379] or by mutational analysis. Whether fructose 1,6-bisphosphatase deficiency can be diagnosed by enzyme assays in white blood cells has long been a subject of controversy. The low activity of the normal enzyme in leukocytes probably explains why some investigators have attempted this in vain,[461] or had to correct initially reported data,[436,462] whereas others[437,441,442,446,462–465] have claimed to be able to demonstrate the defect. Nowadays it can be stated that diagnosis can be attempted on leukocytes, taking into account that a deficiency is diagnostic, but that a normal activity does not rule out fructose 1,6-bisphosphatase deficiency in the liver, particularly in girls, as repeatedly observed.[466,467] Somewhat reduced leukocyte function (i.e., chemotaxis, phagocytosis, and microbial killing) has been reported in two children and attributed to lack of glucose 6-phosphate.[468] However, a tendency toward frequent microbial infections is not a recognized feature of fructose 1,6-bisphosphatase deficiency. Culturing peripheral lymphocytes[469] and monocytes[465] increased the specific fructose 1,6-bisphosphatase activity considerably; this may become of diagnostic use.[470] Fructose 1,6-bisphosphatase deficiency also has been documented in jejunal biopsy material[434] and in the kidney at autopsy.[431,436] Results of enzyme assays on tissues obtained at autopsy must be interpreted with caution, because the enzyme is rapidly inactivated owing to autolysis.[92,453] Fructose 1,6-bisphosphatase is unmeasurable in cultured skin fibroblasts and in amniotic fluid cells.[453,462] Fructose 1,6-bisphosphatase in chorionic villi biopsy samples has not been measured. Prenatal diagnosis is thus impossible. Light microscopy of liver biopsy samples and autopsy samples usually reveals fatty infiltration but neither fibrosis nor disturbed architecture, as is common in hereditary fructose intolerance. Electron microscopic findings[338,435,444] have not been revealing.

Treatment of acute attacks consists of correction of hypoglycemia and acidosis by IV infusion and is usually rapidly successful. Later, avoidance of fasting prevents further episodes. Fructose and sucrose should be limited in the diet but probably need not be eliminated. The degree of intolerance to fructose may vary considerably between patients and even in the individual.[435] Acute episodes may be precipitated by fructose or sucrose ingestion. For instance, one newborn gained weight on a sucrose-containing formula during his first and later weeks of life,[338] and another infant had her second and repeated attacks at age 7 months when weaned to baby food.[433] An 8-year-old boy, in remission for 2 years, suffered a relapse that led to diagnosis on being prescribed a fructose-containing syrup for asthenia.[444] The liver size usually diminishes, but lapses occur.[435,438,441,444,446]

Substitution of part of the dietary fat with carbohydrates and reduction of protein to the basic requirement have been recommended.[433] Treatment with folic acid was advocated[434] and repeatedly tried in typical cases[437,444] as well as in the "mild" variant,[437] but its benefit remains to be proven.[445]

Prognosis As a rule, the firstborn child with the disease dies or suffers more than the following children, who profit from the experience gained by parents and physicians with the first child. Once the diagnosis is established, the course seems benign, and growth and development are normal. Lapses during febrile infections are controlled easily by glucose, either alone or in combination with sodium bicarbonate. Baker and Winegrad[301] had the clinical impression that tolerance to fasting increases with age, and our experience supports this. It may be assumed that undiagnosed fructose 1,6-bisphosphatase–deficient adults exist in the general population. These persons, like those with undiagnosed hereditary fructose intolerance, may be endangered by the indiscriminate use of fructose, invert sugar, or sorbitol in infusion solutions.

Genetics and Molecular Biology

The mode of inheritance is autosomal recessive. Thirty years after its first description, the incidence of fructose 1,6-bisphosphatase deficiency is still unknown. Of the first known 85 patients and affected sibs, 34 were boys and 51 girls; two thirds of them were diagnosed by enzyme assay of liver biopsy samples. Most families lived in Europe, the United States, Japan,[446,470,454,457] and Lebanon.[464] One patient was a black North American[434] and one an Indian child living in England.[438] We have made the diagnosis from liver biopsies in 21 cases between 1971 and 2000; among the 20 families with affected children, 12 were of Turkish origin.[121]

Parental consanguinity was reported.[338,431,432,440,464] The parents are healthy. One couple had normal responses to IV fructose and glycerol.[433] All three parents tested had intermediate fructose 1,6-bisphosphatase activity in the liver,[435,458] but results of activity measurements in leukocytes were less than conclusive.[436,446,462] A radiochemical procedure, although apparently superior to the commonly used spectrophotometric method, still does not allow the identification of all carriers.[464] The use of cultured lymphocytes[470] or monocytes[465] may improve discrimination of heterozygotes from normal individuals.

Although there is evidence for at least two fructose 1,6-bisphosphatase genes in humans, only one, *FBP1,* has been cloned hitherto. It is localized on chromosome 9, spans about 31 kb, contains seven exons and six introns, and encodes the liver enzyme.[171] Recent studies show that liver fructose 1,6-bisphosphatase deficiency results from a variety of mutations,[471–474] among them point mutations (E30X, G164S, A177D, G261A), single nucleotide deletions of A and C at base positions 35 and 966, respectively,[474] an extensive deletion, and a G insertion at base 961 in exon 7. The latter seems to be the predominant mutation in the Japanese.[473] In two white patients, silent mutations were identified,[171] and in three other Japanese patients no mutation was found.[473] This suggests unidentified mutations in the promoter of the liver fructose 1,6-bisphosphatase gene or, more hypothetically, mutations of the bifunctional enzyme that controls the concentration of fructose 2,6-bisphosphate (see Fig. 70-3), the main physiologic inhibitor of hepatic fructose 1,6-bisphosphatase.[144–146] Interestingly, the gene controlling the bifunctional enzyme in liver is located on the X chromosome. The hypothesis that mutations of this enzyme may correlate with the apparent differences of male and female leukocyte 1,6-bisphosphatase activity has been advanced.[171]

D-(+)-GLYCERIC ACIDURIA (MIM 220120)

Abnormal urinary excretion of glyceric acid occurs in only two inherited diseases, in each of which the disorder is characterized by the presence of a specific enantiomer of glyceric acid, namely the D-(+) or L-(−) form. In D-(+)-glyceric aciduria, only glyceric acid is the dominant metabolite, whereas L-(−)-glyceric aciduria is part of oxalosis type II (see Chap. 133).

D-glyceric aciduria has been described in only a few families.[190,475–478,481,482] Symptoms appeared soon after birth. In one child, tachypnea, tachycardia, and refusal to feed led to the discovery of persistent metabolic acidosis necessitating permanent treatment with sodium bicarbonate.[478] Motor delay and a moderate degree of mental retardation was noted during the next 16 months. In other children, hypotonia, myoclonic jerks, seizures, severe developmental delay, and hyperglycinuria suggested the diagnosis of nonketotic hyperglycinemia. One infant presented with developmental delay, axial hypotonia, and spastic tetraparesis,[481] whereas in four affected sibs, clinical manifestations were mild in two and absent in the others.[482] All patients excreted D-glyceric acid, a compound not usually found in urine. One set of parents excreted only traces of D-glycerate.[190] Two children also had D-glyceric acidemia. Of three tested children, two responded to oral fructose loads with increased D-glyceric acid excretion in urine, one by an increase of both urinary and plasma D-glycerate concentrations. In the last child, oral dihydroxyacetone caused the same effect.[190] This girl responded to the restriction of dietary fructose and sucrose by the reduction of seizures and a lowering of D-glycerate excretion.

Low leukocyte D-glyceric acid dehydrogenase and only 10 percent of glycine cleavage activity in liver at autopsy was reported in one[477] and low red-cell glyceraldehyde 3-phosphate dehydrogenase and normal erythrocyte triokinase in the other patient.[190] A defect of hepatic triokinase appeared to be a reasonable theory.[190] Van Schaftingen[483] demonstrated in the liver of one child[481] a 5 percent residual activity of D-glycerate kinase, whereas activities of glycerate dehydrogenase and triokinase were normal. He concluded that D-glycerate kinase deficiency is a cause of D-glyceric aciduria. In fact, this group of patients may be heterogeneous.

The examination of urinary organic acids in an Afghan hound referred for hepatic insufficiency led to the chance observation of the first animal with D-glyceric aciduria.[484] Oral serine (200 mg/kg) and fructose (1 g/kg) loading enhanced D-glyceric acidemia and aciduria and caused an increase in plasma lactate similar to that reported in children. The animal regained full health.

At this time, it cannot be stated definitively whether the described symptoms are caused by the metabolic defect or whether the condition is harmless.

ERYTHROCYTE ALDOLASE DEFICIENCY WITH NONSPHEROCYTIC HEMOLYTIC ANEMIA (ALDOLASE A DEFICIENCY) (MIM 103850)

This defect was first observed[479,480] in a boy born to first cousins, small for gestational age, with dysmorphic facial features, short neck, and lax skin. At 6 weeks of age, nonspherocytic hemolytic anemia was noted. Urine amino acids, blood glucose, and karyotype were normal. At 4 months, a liver biopsy revealed mild elevation of glycogen content (7.2 g/100 g) and an increase of fibrous tissue judged compatible with congenital hepatic fibrosis. The boy required blood transfusions until his second year of life. When last seen at age 7 years, moderate hepatomegaly persisted. He was microcephalic, his growth was stunted, and his intellectual development was delayed. Biochemical findings included an increase of blood glucose after a fructose load (indicating normal function of hepatic aldolase B) and a marked deficiency of red cell and fibroblast aldolase. The child's parents had normal red cell aldolase activity.

Erythrocytes and fibroblasts in culture normally express aldolase A.[111,113] Because both cell types were aldolase deficient, Beutler's assumption[479] that this child suffered from a deficiency of type A aldolase, perhaps on the basis of a regulatory mutation, seemed justified. Aldolase A is the isoenzyme of fetal tissues occurring in brain, liver, and kidney. Postnatally, it is the predominant isoenzyme in muscle, presumably in red cells, and, together with aldolase C, in the brain.[90] There can be little doubt that the impairment of glycolysis due to aldolase A deficiency was the cause of hemolysis, although it remains unclear why the latter did not persist beyond the second year. As to the remainder of the phenotype, it is tempting to speculate that aldolase A deficiency caused prenatal liver damage and that it compromised brain development from fetal to postnatal life. Dysmorphism and slowing of intrauterine and postnatal growth could equally be viewed as consequences of impaired glycolysis in growing tissues. Nevertheless, because this child's parents were first cousins, the patient could have been homozygous for a number of recessive traits unrelated to aldolase activity.

Two brothers with spherocytosis and a syndrome remarkably similar to that seen in Beutler's patient were observed.[485] Because aldolase levels were reduced only by the amount predicted for the degree of hemolysis, aldolase deficiency was not judged responsible for the syndrome in the two brothers.

Two other cases of red cell aldolase deficiency were reported.[486] Two related boys — Japanese islanders 14 months and 13 years of age — had mild nonspherocytic hemolytic anemia since infancy, aggravated by infections. In contrast to Beutler's patients, they were orthomorphic and normally developed. Red cell aldolase activity was grossly reduced in the boys and intermediate in both sets of parents and in some other family members. Red cell fructose 1,6-bisphosphate was elevated in the two patients, and hexose monophosphate shunt activity was reduced, presumably due to the inhibition of glucose 6-phosphate dehydrogenase by fructose 1,6-bisphosphate. Red cell aldolase was heat labile and had reduced affinity for fructose 1,6-bisphosphate. A structural mutation of aldolase A was assumed. In one of these patients, a single nucleotide substitution was demonstrated.[487]

Recently, a fourth patient with red cell aldolase deficiency was identified.[488] In this 4-year-old boy, nonspherocytic hemolytic anemia was accompanied by pronounced myopathic symptoms, mainly muscle weakness, premature muscle fatigue, and repeat episodes of rhabdomyolysis. Routine laboratory investigations revealed markedly increased serum creatine kinase, hemoglobinuria and myoglobinuria. The activity of aldolase A was 11 percent of normal in muscle, and 4 percent of normal in erythrocytes. The aldolase A activity of erythrocytes from the patient's parents and brother was about 50 percent of normal. Molecular studies showed a single G-to-A transition, resulting in an E206K mutation in a fully conserved region of the enzyme protein. That this mutation affected the region involved in the main subunit interface of the enzyme tetramers probably explains the myopathy, which was not observed in the three other aldolase-deficient patients, in whom the mutations affected less extensive interaction sites. This report suggests that assay of aldolase A should be part of the diagnostic evaluation of myopathies characterized by exercise intolerance and rhabdomyolysis.

INCOMPLETE FRUCTOSE ABSORPTION

It has been recognized that one of three healthy adults[43,44,489] and two of three children[45] incompletely absorb fructose when administered orally at a dose of 0.7 to 2 g/kg. This finding may account for the abdominal symptoms such as bloating, rumbling, pain, flatulence, and watery diarrhea experienced by some persons after the ingestion of fructose,[25,490] fruit,[491] and other fructose-containing foods. Symptoms usually disappear after the elimination of fructose and sorbitol[492] from the diet. In only one patient was sucrose intolerance also documented. This 12-year-old girl had normal small-intestinal sucrase activity and was intolerant of as little as 1 g of oral fructose.[493] The basic defect in these persons remains to be established.

The absorption deficit is dose dependent,[46,47] apparently far more frequent than was previously believed,[46,50,490,492,] and is aggravated by physical exercise, which seems to speed intestinal transit[47] (see earlier section on Transport of Fructose). Although the functional properties and tissue distribution of GLUT5 suggest that incomplete fructose absorption might be due to mutations in the *GLUT5* gene, no mutations were found in the protein-coding region of this gene in eight patients.[494] The enhancement of fructose absorption by equimolar amounts of glucose, galactose, or glycine, observed in healthy subjects and in fructose malabsorbers,[45,48–50,490,492,497] still suggests the involvement of some common carrier in the small intestine in these persons. The fact that up to half of all fructose malabsorbers are free of symptoms and that fructose malabsorption is often seen in healthy controls led to the demonstration of somewhat higher fructose avidity of anaerobic colonic bacteria in the symptomatic persons and to the conclusion that colonic bacterial activity determines the symptoms in fructose malabsorbers.[489]

REFERENCES

1. Bernt E, Bergmeyer HU: D-Fruktose, in Bergmeyer HU (ed): *Methoden der enzymatischen Analyse*. Weinheim, Germany, Verlag Chemie, 1970, p 1266.
2. Blau N, Heizmann CW, Fischer M: Two-reagent end-point fructose assay by random-access analysis. *Clin Chem* **36**:980, 1990
3. Roe JH, Epstein JH, Goldstein NP: A photometric method for the determination of inulin in plasma and urine. *J Biol Chem* **178**:839, 1949.
4. Higashi A, Peters L: Rapid colorimetric method for determination of inulin in plasma and urine. *J Lab Clin Med* **35**:475, 1950.
5. Kraffczyk F, Helger R, Bremer HJ: Thin-layer chromatographic screening tests for carbohydrate anomalies in plasma, urine and faeces. *Clin Chim Acta* **42**:303, 1972.
6. Clamp JR, Bhatti T, Chambers RE: The determination of carbohydrate in biological materials by gas-liquid chromatography. *Methods Biochem Anal* **19**:229, 1971.
7. Palmer JK, Brandes WB: Determination of sucrose, glucose and fructose by liquid chromatography. *J Agr Food Chem* **22**:709, 1974.
8. Nakashima K, Takei H, Adachi O, Shinagawa E, Ameyama M: Determination of seminal fructose using D-fructose dehydrogenase. *Clin Chem Acta* **151**:307, 1985.
9. Niculescu L, Veiga-da-Cunha M, Van Schaftingen E: Enzymatic assays of fructose-1-phosphate and fructose-1,6-bisphosphate in the picomole range. *Anal Biochem* **235** :243, 1996.
10. Hardinge MG, Swarner JB, Crooks H: Carbohydrates in foods. *J Am Diet Assoc* **46**:197, 1965.
11. Somogyi JC, Trautner K: Der Glukose-, Fruktose- und Saccharosegehalt verschiedener Gemüsearten. *Schweiz Med Wochenschr* **104**:177, 1974.
12. Gitzelmann R, Steinmann B: Unpublished observation.
13. Hers HG: L'aldolase-réductase. Le mécanisme de la formation du fructose séminal et du fructose foetal. *Biochim Biophys Acta* **37**:127, 1960.
14. Anderson TA: Recent trends in carbohydrate consumption. *Annu Rev Nutr* **2**:113, 1982.
15. Yudkin J: Sugar and health. *Lancet* **1**:918, 1987.
16. US Department of Agriculture: Sugar and sweetener — outlook and situation. *Sugar Sweetener Rep* **6**:40, 1981.
17. Koivisto VA, Karonen SL, Nikkilä EA: Carbohydrate ingestion before exercise: Comparison of glucose, fructose and sweet placebo. *J Appl Physiol* **51**:783, 1981.
18. Levine L, Evans WJ, Cadarette BS, Fisher EC, Bullen BA: Fructose and glucose ingestion and muscle glycogen use during submaximal exercise. *J Appl Physiol* **55**:1767, 1983.
19. Nikkilä EA, Huttunen JK (eds): Clinical and metabolic aspects of fructose. *Acta Med Scand Suppl* 542, 1972.
20. Sipple HL, McNutt KW: *Sugars in Nutrition*. New York, Academic, 1974.
21. Guggenheim B: *Health and Sugar Substitutes*. Basel, Switzerland, Karger, 1979.
22. Mayes PA, Laker ME: Effects of acute and long-term fructose administration on liver lipid metabolism, in Paoletti R (ed): *Progress in Biochemical Pharmacology: Metabolic Effects of Dietary Carbohydrates*. Vol. 21. Basel, Switzerland, Karger, 1986, pp 33–58.
23. Vrána A, Kazdová L: Effects of dietary sucrose or fructose on carbohydrate and lipid metabolism. Animal studies, in Paoletti R (ed):

Progress in Biochemical Pharmacology: Metabolic Effects of Dietary Carbohydrates, Vol. 21. Basel, Switzerland, Karger, 1986, pp 59–73.

24. Minkowski O: Untersuchungen über den Diabetes mellitus nach Exstirpation des Pankreas. *Arch Exp Pathol Pharmakol* **31**:85, 1893.
25. Reiser S, Pwell AS, Yang C-Y, Canary JJ: An insulinogenic effect of oral fructose in humans during postprandial hyperglycemia. *Am J Clin Nutr* **45**:580, 1987.
26. Van Den Berghe G: Fructose: Metabolism and short-term effects on carbohydrate and purine metabolic pathways, in Paoletti R (ed): *Progress in Biochemical Pharmacology: Metabolic Effects of Dietary Carbohydrates*, Vol. 21. Basel, Switzerland, Karger, 1986, pp 1–32.
27. Holdsworth CD, Dawson AM: Absorption of fructose in man. *Proc Soc Exp Biol Med* **118**:142, 1965.
28. Mehnert H, Dietze G, Haslbeck M: Zucker und Zucker-Austauschstoffe in der Diätetik von Störungen des Kohlenhydratstoffwechsels. *Nutr Metab* **18** (suppl 1):171, 1975.
29. Cook GC: Absorption and metabolism of D(-)fructose in man. *Am J Clin Nutr* **24**:1302, 1971.
30. Smith LH, Ettinger RH, Seligson D: A comparison of the metabolism of fructose and glucose in hepatic disease and diabetes mellitus. *J Clin Invest* **32**:273, 1953.
31. Conrad V: Mesure de l'assimilation du glucose: Bases théoriques et application cliniques. *Acta Gastroenterol Belg* **18**:655, 1955.
32. Mendeloff AI, Weichselbaum TE: Role of the human liver in the assimilation of intravenously administered fructose. *Metabolism* **2**:450, 1953.
33. Wolfe BM, Ahuja SP, Marliss EB: Effects of intravenously administered fructose and glucose on splanchnic amino acid and carbohydrate metabolism in hypertriglyceridemic men. *J Clin Invest* **56**:970, 1975.
34. Björkman O, Felig P: Role of the kidney in the metabolism of fructose in 60-hour fasted humans. *Diabetes* **31**:516, 1982.
35. McDonald I, Turner LJ: Serum-fructose levels after sucrose or its constituent monosaccharides. *Lancet* **1**:841, 1968.
36. Lane HC, Dodd K: Use of glucose, invert sugar and fructose for parenteral feeding of children. *Pediatrics* **20**:668, 1957.
37. Miller M, Drucker WR, Owens JE, Craig JW, Woodward H Jr: Metabolism of intravenous fructose and glucose in normal and diabetic subjects. *J Clin Invest* **31**:115, 1952.
38. Gracey M, Burke V, Oshin A: Active intestinal transport of D-fructose. *Biochim Biophys Acta* **266**:397, 1972.
39. Honegger P, Semenza G: Multiplicity of carriers for free glucalogues in hamster small intestine. *Biochim Biophys Acta* **318**:390, 1973.
40. Macrae AR, Neudoerffer TS: Support for the existence of an active transport mechanism of fructose in the rat. *Biochim Biophys Acta* **288**:137, 1972.
41. Sigrist-Nelson K, Hopfer U: A distinct D-fructose transport system in isolated brush border membrane. *Biochim Biophys Acta* **367**:247, 1974.
42. Woods HF, Eggleston LV, Krebs HA: The cause of hepatic accumulation of fructose 1-phosphate on fructose loading. *Biochem J* **119**:501, 1970.
43. Ravich WJ, Bayless TM, Thomas M: Fructose: Incomplete intestinal absorption in humans. *Gastroenterology* **84**:26, 1983.
44. Steinmann B: Personal experience.
45. Kneepkens CMF, Vonk RJ, Fernandes J: Incomplete intestinal absorption of fructose. *Arch Dis Child* **59**:735, 1984.
46. Born P: Fructose- und Sorbit-Malabsorption. *Dtsch Med Wochenschr* **115**:598, 1990.
47. Fujisawa T, Mulligan K, Wada L, Schumacher L, et al.: The effect of exercise on fructose absorption. *Am J Clin Nutr* **58**:75, 1993.
48. Rumessen JJ, Gudmand-Hoyer E: Absorption capacity of fructose in healthy adults. Comparison with sucrose and its constituent monosaccharides. *Gut* **27**:1161, 1986.
49. Truswell AS, Seach JM, Thorburn AW: Incomplete absorption of pure fructose in healthy subjects and the facilitating effect of glucose. *Am J Clin Nutr* **48**:1424, 1988.
50. Harms HK: Personal communication.
51. Fujisawa T, Riby J, Kretchmer N: Intestinal absorption of fructose in the rat. *Gastroenterology* **101**:360, 1991.
52. Burant CF, Takeda J, Brot-Laroche E, Bell GI, Davidson NO: Fructose transporter in human spermatozoa and small intestine is GLUT5. *J Biol Chem* **267**:14523, 1992.
53. Miyamoto K, Hase K, Takagi T, et al.: Differential responses of intestinal glucose transporter mRNA transcripts to levels of dietary sugars. *Biochem J* **295**:211, 1993.
54. Burant CF, Saxena M: Rapid reversible substrate regulation of fructose transporter expression in rat small intestine and kidney. *Am J Physiol* **267**: G71, 1994.
55. Castello A, Guma A, Sevilla L, Furriols M, Testar X, Palacin M, Zorzano A: Regulation of *GLUT5* gene expression in rat intestinal mucosa: Regional distribution, circadian rhythm, perinatal development and effect of diabetes. *Biochem J* **309**:271, 1995.
56. Davidson NO, Hausmann AML, Ifkovits CA, Buse JB, Gould GW, Burant CF, Bell GI: Human intestinal glucose transporter expression and localization of GLUT5. *Am J Physiol* **262**:C795, 1992.
57. Shu R, David ES, Ferraris RP: Dietary fructose enhances intestinal fructose transport and GLUT5 expression in weaning rats. *Am J Physiol* **272**:G446, 1997.
58. Cheeseman CI: GLUT2 is the transporter for fructose across the rat intestinal basolateral membrane. *Gastroenterology* **105**:1050, 1993.
59. Blakemore SJ, Aledo JC, James J, Campbell FC, Lucocq JM, Hundal HS: The GLUT5 hexose transporter is also localized to the basolateral membrane of the human jejunum. *Biochem J* **309**:7, 1995.
60. Kristiansen S, Darakhshan F, Richter EA, Hundal HS: Fructose transport and GLUT-5 in human sarcolemmal vesicles. *Am J Physiol* **273**:E543, 1997.
61. Concha II, Velasquez FV, Martinez JM, et al.: Human erythrocytes express GLUT5 and transport fructose. *Blood* **89**:4190, 1997.
62. Sestoft L, Fleron P: Determination of the kinetic constants of fructose transport and phosphorylation in the perfused rat liver. *Biochim Biophys Acta* **345**:27, 1974.
63. Craik JD, Elliott KRF: Transport of D-fructose and D-galactose into isolated rat hepatocytes. *Biochem J* **192**:373, 1980.
64. Hooper RH, Short AH: The hepatocellular uptake of glucose, galactose and fructose in conscious sheep. *J Physiol* **264**:523, 1977.
65. Froesch ER, Ginsberg JL: Fructose metabolism of adipose tissue. I. Comparison of fructose and glucose metabolism in epididymal adipose tissue of normal rats. *J Biol Chem* **237**:3317, 1962.
66. Halperin ML, Cheema-Dhadli S: Comparison of glucose and fructose transport into adipocytes of the rat. *Biochem J* **202**:717, 1982.
67. Schoenle E, Zapf J, Froesch ER: Transport and metabolism of fructose in fat cells of normal and hypophysectomized rats. *Am J Physiol* **237**:E325, 1979.
68. Hers HG: *Le Métabolisme du Fructose*. Brussels, Editions Arscia, 1957.
69. Cori GT, Ochoa S, Slein MW, Cori CF: The metabolism of fructose in liver. Isolation of fructose-1-phosphate and inorganic pyrophosphate. *Biochim Biophys Acta* **7**:304, 1951.
70. Hers HG: La fructokinase du foie. *Biochim Biophys Acta* 8:416, 1952.
71. Leuthardt F, Testa E: Die Phosphorylierung der Fructose in der Leber. II. Mitteilung. *Helv Chiv Acta* **34**:931, 1951.
72. Adelman RC, Ballard FJ, Weinhouse S: Purification and properties of rat liver fructokinase. *J Biol Chem* **242**:3360, 1967.
73. Kuyper CMA: Studies on fructokinase. 1. Substrate specificity. *Proc K Ned Akad Wet* **62**:137, 1959.
74. Sanchez JJ, Gonzalez NS, Pontis HG: Fructokinase from rat liver. I. Purification and properties. *Biochim Biophys Acta* **227**:67, 1971.
75. England S, Berkower I, Avigad G: 5-keto-D-fructose. VII. Phosphorylation by liver fructokinase and the monophosphate ester as an inhibitor of liver aldolase. *Biochim Biophys Acta* **279**:229, 1972.
76. Raushel FM, Cleland WW: Bovine liver fructokinase: Purification and kinetic properties. *Biochemistry* **16**:2169, 1977.
77. Raushel FM, Cleland WW: The substrate and anomeric specificity of fructokinase. *J Biol Chem* **248**:8174, 1973.
78. Phillips MI, Davies DR: The mechanism of guanosine triphosphate depletion in the liver after a fructose load. The role of fructokinase. *Biochem J* **228**:667, 1985.
79. Parks RE, Ben-Gershom E, Lardy HA: Liver fructokinase. *J Biol Chem* **227**:231, 1957.
80. Sestoft L: Regulation of fructose metabolism in the perfused rat liver. Interrelation with inorganic phosphate, glucose, ketone body and ethanol metabolism. *Biochim Biophys Acta* **343**:1, 1974.
81. Heinz F, Lamprecht W, Kirsch J: Enzymes of fructose metabolism in human liver. *J Clin Invest* **47**:1826, 1968.
82. Thieden HID, Grunnet N, Damgaard SE, Sestoft L: Effect of fructose and glyceraldehyde on ethanol metabolism in human liver and rat liver. *Eur J Biochem* **30**:250, 1972.
83. Bais R, James HM, Rofe AM, Conyers RAJ: the purification and properties of human liver ketohexokinase. *Biochem J* **230**:53, 1985.

84. Sanchez JJ, Gonzalez NS, Pontis HG: Fructokinase from rat liver. II. The role of K+ on the enzyme activity. *Biochim Biophys Acta* **227**:79, 1971.
85. Donaldson A, Doyle TC, Matas N: Expression of rat liver ketohexokinase in yeast results in fructose intolerance. *Biochem J* **291**:179, 1993.
86. Bonthron DT, Brady N, Donaldson IA, Steinmann B: Molecular basis of essential fructosuria: molecular cloning and mutational analysis of human ketohexokinase (fructokinase). *Hum Mol Genet* **3**:1627, 1994.
87. Hayward BE, Fantes JA, Warner JP, et al.: Co-localization of the ketohexokinase and glucokinase regulator genes to a 500-kb region of chromosome 2p23. *Mamm Genome* **7**:454, 1996.
88. Hayward BE, Bonthron DT: Structure and alternative splicing of the ketohexokinase gene. *Eur J Biochem* **257**:85, 1998.
89. Bonthron DT: Personal communication.
90. Salvatore F, Izzo P, Paolella G: Aldolase gene and protein families: Structure, expression and pathophysiology, in Blasi F (ed): *Human Genes and Diseases: Horizons in Biochemistry and Biophysics*, Vol. 8. New York, John Wiley, 1986, pp 611–665.
91. Hers HG, Kusaka T: Le métabolisme du fructose-1-phosphate dans le foie. *Biochim Biophys Acta* **11**:427, 1953.
92. Steinmann B, Gitzelmann R: The diagnosis of hereditary fructose intolerance. *Helv Paediatr Acta* **36**:297, 1981.
93. Penhoet E, Rajkumar T, Rutter WJ: Multiple forms of fructose diphosphate aldolase in mammalian tissues. *Proc Natl Acad Sci U S A* **56**:1275, 1966.
94. Koster JF, Slee RG, Fernandes J: On the biochemical basis of hereditary fructose intolerance. *Biochem Biophys Res Commun* **64**:289, 1975.
95. Penhoet EE, Kochman M, Rutter WJ: Isolation of fructose diphosphate aldolases A, B and C. *Biochemistry* **8**:4391, 1969.
96. Penhoet EE, Kochman M, Rutter WJ: Molecular and catalytic properties of aldolase C. *Biochemistry* **8**:4396, 1969.
97. Beernink PT, Tolan DR: Disruption of the aldolase A tetramer into catalytically active monomers. *Proc Natl Acad Sci USA* **93**:5374, 1996.
98. MacGregor JS, Singh VN, Davoust S, et al.: Evidence for formation of a rabbit liver aldolase-rabbit liver fructose-1,6-bisphosphatase complex. *Proc Natl Acad Sci U S A* **77**:3889, 1980.
99. Horecker BL, MacGregor JS, Singh VN, Melloni E, Pontremoli S: Aldolase and fructose bisphosphatase: Key enzymes in the control of gluconeogenesis and glycolysis. *Curr Top Cell Regul* **18**:181, 1981.
100. Kusakabe T, Motoki K, Hori K: Mode of interactions of human aldolase isozymes with cytoskeletons. *Arch Biochem Biophys* **344**:184, 1997.
101. Lebherz HG, Rutter WJ: Distribution of fructose diphosphate aldolase variants in biological systems. *Biochemistry* **8**:109, 1969.
102. Rehbein-Thöner M, Pfleiderer G: The changes in aldolase isoenzyme pattern during development of the human kidney and small intestine — demonstrated in organ extracts and tissue sections. *Hoppe Seyler Z Physiol Chem* **358**:169, 1977.
103. Schapira F, Hatzfeld A, Weber A: Resurgence of some fetal isozymes in hepatoma, in Markert CL (ed): *Isoenzymes*, Vol. 3, New York, Academic, 1975, pp 987–1003.
104. Mukai T, Joh K, Arai Y, Yatsuki H, Hori K: Tissue-specific expression of rat aldolase A mRNAs. *J Biol Chem* **261**:3347, 1986.
105. Pfleiderer G, Dikow AL, Falkenberg F: Verteilungsmuster der Aldolase A, B und C in menschlichen Organ- und Gewebsextrakten sowie in normalen und pathologischen Seren. *Hoppe Seyler Z Physiol Chem* **355**:233, 1974.
106. Pfleiderer G, Thöner M, Wachsmuth ED: Histological examination of the aldolase monomer composition of cells from human kidney and hypernephroid carcinoma. *Beitr Pathol* **156**:266, 1975.
107. Burch HB, Choi S, Dence CN, Alvey TR, Cole BR, Lowry OH: Metabolic effects of large fructose loads in different parts of the rat nephron. *J Biol Chem* **255**:8239, 1980.
108. Hibi N, Arii S, Iizumi T, Nemoto T, Chu TM: Human monoclonal antibody recognizing liver-type aldolase B. *Biochem J* **240**:847, 1986.
109. Wachsmuth ED: Differentiation of epithelial cells in human jejunum: Localization and quantification of aminopeptidase, alkaline phosphatase and aldolase isozymes in tissue sections. *Histochemistry* **48**:101, 1976.
110. Strapazon E, Steck TL: Interaction of the aldolase and the membrane of human erythrocytes. *Biochemistry* **16**:2966, 1977.
111. Yeltman DR, Harris BG: Purification and characterization of aldolase from human erythrocytes. *Biochim Biophys Acta* **484**:188, 1977.
112. Burton BK, Chacko CM, Nadler HL: Aldolase in cultivated human fibroblasts. *Proc Soc Exp Biol Med* **146**:605, 1974.
113. Izzo P, Costanzo P, Lupo A, et al.: A new human species of aldolase A mRNA from fibroblasts. *Eur J Biochem* **164**:9, 1987.
114. Ali M, Rellos P, Cox TM: Hereditary fructose intolerance. *J Med Genet* **35**:353, 1998.
115. Pontremoli S, Melloni E, Salamino F, Sparatore B, Michetti M, Horecker BL: Changes in activity of fructose-1,6-bisphosphate aldolase in livers of fasted rabbits and accumulation of crossreacting immune material. *Proc Natl Acad Sci USA* **76**:6323, 1979.
116. Pontremoli S, Melloni E, et al.: Limited proteolysis of liver aldolase and fructose 1,6-bisphosphatase by lysosomal proteinases: Effect on complex formation. *Proc Natl Acad Sci USA* **79**:2451, 1982.
117. Pontremoli S, Melloni E, Michetti M, et al.: Characterization of the inactive form of fructose 1,6-bisphosphate aldolase isolated from livers of fasted rabbits. *Proc Natl Acad Sci U S A* **79**:5194, 1982.
118. Chappel A, Hoogenraad NJ, Holmes RB: Purification and properties of the native form of rabbit liver aldolase. Evidence for proteolytic modification after tissue extraction. *Biochem J* **175**:377, 1978.
119. Munnich A, Besmond C, Darquy S, et al.: Dietary and hormonal regulation of aldolase B gene expression. *J Clin Invest* **75**:1045, 1985.
120. Gregori C, Besmond C, Kahn A, Dreyfus JC: Characterization of messenger RNA for aldolase B in adult and fetal human liver. *Biochem Biophys Res Commun* **104**:369, 1982.
121. Numazaki M, Tsutsumi K, Tsutsumi R, Ishikawa K: Expression of aldolase isozyme mRNAs in fetal rat liver. *Eur J Biochem* **142**:165, 1984.
122. Tsutsumi K, Mukai T, Hidaka S, et al.: Rat aldolase isozyme gene. Cloning and characterization of cDNA for aldolase B messenger RNA. *J Biol Chem* **258**:6537, 1983.
123. Tsutsumi K, Mukai T, Tsutsumi R, et al.: Nucleotide sequence of rat liver aldolase B messenger RNA. *J Biol Chem* **259**:14572, 1984.
124. Simon MP, Besmond C, et al.: Molecular cloning of cDNA for rat L-type pyruvate kinase and aldolase B. *J Biol Chem* **258**:14576, 1983.
125. Besmond C, Dreyfus JC, et al.: Nucleotide sequence of a cDNA clone for human aldolase B. *Biochem Biophys Res Commun* **117**:601, 1983.
126. Rottmann WH, Tolan DR, Penhoet EE: Complete amino acid sequence for human aldolase B derived from cDNA and genomic clones. *Proc Natl Acad Sci U S A* **81**:2738, 1984.
127. Tsutsumi K, Mukai T, Tsutsumi R, et al.: Structure and genomic organization of the rat aldolase B gene. *J Mol Biol* **181**:153, 1985.
128. Tolan DR, Penhoet EE: Characterization of the human aldolase B gene. *Mol Biol Med* **3**:245, 1986.
129. Mukai T, Yatsuki H, Arai Y, et al.: Human aldolase B gene: Characterization of the genomic aldolase B gene and analysis of sequences required for multiple polyadenylations. *J Biochem* **102**:1043, 1987.
130. Henry I, Gallano P, Besmond C, et al.: The structural gene for aldolase B maps to 9q13 → 32. *Ann Hum Genet* **49**:173, 1985.
131. Lebo RV, Tolan DR, Bruce BD, Cheung MC, Kan YW: Spot-blot analysis of sorted chromosomes assigns a fructose intolerance disease locus to chromosome 9. *Cytometry* **6**:478, 1985.
132. Sakakibara M, Mukai T, Yatsuki H, Hori K: Human aldolase isozyme gene: The structure of multispecies aldolase B mRNAs. *Nucleic Acids Res* **13**:5055, 1985.
133. Serero S, Maire P, Van Cong N, et al.: Localization of the active gene of aldolase on chromosome 16, and two aldolase A pseudogenes on chromosomes 3 and 10. *Hum Genet* **78**:167, 1988.
134. Tolan DR, Niclas J, Bruce BD, Lebo RV: Evolutionary implications of the human aldolase-A, -B, -C, and -pseudogene chromosome locations. *Am J Hum Genet* **41**:907, 1987
135. Sygusch J, Beaudry D, Allaire M: Molecular architecture of rabbit skeletal muscle aldolase at 2.7-A resolution. *Proc Natl Acad Sci USA* **84**:7846, 1987
136. Blom N, Sygusch J: Product binding and role of the C-terminal region of class I D-fructose 1,6-bisphosphate aldolase. *Nature Struct Biol* **4**:36, 1997.
137. Phillips MI, Davies DR: The mechanism of guanosine triphosphate depletion in the liver after a fructose load. The role of fructokinase. *Biochem J* **228**:667, 1985.
138. Hers HG: Triokinase, in Colowick SP, Kaplan NO (eds): *Methods in Enzymology*, Vol. 5. New York, Academic, 1962, pp 362–364.
139. Sillero MAG, Sillero A, Sols A: Enzymes involved in fructose metabolism in liver and the glyceraldehyde metabolic crossroads. *Eur J Biochem* **10**:345, 1969.
140. Frandsen EK, Grunnet N: Kinetic properties of triokinase from rat liver. *Eur J Biochem* **23**:588, 1971.

141. Benkovic SJ, Demaine MM: Mechanism of action of fructose 1,6-bisphosphatase. *Adv Enzymol* **53**:45, 1982.
142. Tejwani GA: Regulation of fructose-bisphosphatase activity. *Adv Enzymol* **54**:121, 1982.
143. Dzugaj A, Kochman L: Purification of human liver fructose-1,6-bisphosphatase. *Biochim Biophys Acta* **614**:407, 1980.
144. Hers HG, Van Schaftingen E: Fructose 2,6-bisphosphate 2 years after its discovery. *Biochem J* **206**:1, 1982.
145. Van Schaftingen E: Fructose 2,6-bisphosphate. *Adv Enzymol* **59**:315, 1987.
146. Van Schaftingen E: Role of fructose-2,6-bisphosphate in the regulation of hepatic carbohydrate metabolism, in Pilkis SJ (ed): *Fructose-2,6-Bisphosphate*. Boca Raton, FL, CRC, 1990, pp 65–85.
147. Van Schaftingen E, Hers HG: Inhibition of fructose-1,6-bisphosphatase by fructose-2,6-bisphosphate. *Proc Natl Acad Sci U S A* **78**:2861, 1981.
148. Pilkis SJ, El-Maghrabi MR, Pilkis J, Claus T: Inhibition of fructose-1,6-bisphosphatase by fructose 2,6-bisphosphate. *J Biol Chem* **256**: 3619, 1981.
149. El-Maghrabi MR, Austin LR, Correia JJ, Pilkis SJ: Lysine 274 is essential for fructose-2,6-bisphosphate inhibition of fructose-1,6-bisphosphatase. *J Biol Chem* **267**:6526, 1992.
150. Van Schaftingen E, Jett MF, Hue L, Hers HG: Control of liver 6-phosphofructokinase by fructose 2,6-bisphosphate and other effectors. *Proc Natl Acad Sci U S A* **78**:3483, 1981.
151. El-Maghrabi MR, Colosia AD, Lange AJ, et al.: Liver 6-phospho-fructo-2-kinase/fructose 2,6-bisphosphatase, in Pilkis SJ (ed): *Fructose-2,6-Bisphosphate*. Boca Raton, FL, CRC, 1990, pp 87–124.
152. Hue L: The role of futile cycles in the regulation of carbohydrate metabolism in the liver. *Adv Enzymol* **52**:247, 1981.
153. Traniello S, Melloni E, Pontremoli S, et al.: Rabbit liver fructose 1,6-diphosphatase. Properties of the native enzyme and their modification by subtilisin. *Arch Biochem Biophys* **149**:222, 1972.
154. Horecker BL, Melloni E, Pontremoli S: Fructose 1,6-bisphosphatase: Properties of the neutral enzyme and its modification by proteolytic enzymes. *Adv Enzymol* **42**:193, 1975.
155. Pontremoli S, Deflora A, Salamino F, Melloni E, Horecker BL: Hormonal effects on structure and catalytic properties of fructose 1,6-bisphosphatase. *Proc Natl Acad Sci U S A* **72**:2969, 1975.
156. Tejwani GA, Pedrosa FO, Pontremoli S, Horecker BL: Dual role of Zn^2 as inhibitor and activator of fructose 1,6-bisphosphatase of rat liver. *Proc Natl Acad Sci U S A* **73**:2692, 1976.
157. Cowen LA, Bell DE, Hoadley JE, Cousins RJ: Influence of dietary zinc deficiency and parenteral zinc on rat liver fructose 1,6-bisphosphatase activity. *Biochem Biophys Res Commun* **134**:944, 1986.
158. Mizunuma H, Tashima Y: Evidence for the intestinal type of fructose 1,6-bisphosphatase in mouse, rat, and golden hamster. *Arch Biochem Biophys* **217**:512, 1982.
159. Marcus F, Edelstein I, Reardon I, Heinrikson L: Complete amino acid sequence of pig kidney fructose-1,6-bisphosphatase. *Proc Natl Acad Sci U S A* **79**:7161, 1982.
160. Fisher WK, Thompson EOP: Amino acid sequence studies on sheep liver fructose-bisphosphatase. II. The complete sequence. *Aust J Biol Sci* **36**:235, 1982.
161. El-Maghrabi MR, Pilkis J, et al.: cDNA sequence of rat liver fructose-1,6-bisphosphatase and evidence for down-regulation of its mRNA by insulin. *Proc Natl Acad Sci U S A* **85**:8430, 1988.
162. Fernando J, Enser M, Pontremoli S, Horecker BL: Purification and properties of rabbit muscle fructose1,6-diphosphatase. *Arch Biochem Biophys* **126**:599, 1968.
163. Ke H, Thorpe CM, Seaton BA, Lipscomb WN: Structure refinement of fructose-1,6-bisphosphatase and its fructose-2,6-bisphosphate complex at 2.8 A resolution. *J Mol Biol* **212**:513, 1989.
164. Ke H, Thorpe CM, Seaton BA, Marcus F, Lipscomb WN: Molecular structure of fructose-1,6-bisphosphatase at 2.8-A resolution. *Proc Natl Acad Sci U S A* **86**:1475, 1989.
165. Ke H, Zhang Y, Lipscomb WN: Crystal structure of fructose-1,6-bisphosphatase complexed with fructose 6 phosphate, AMP, and magnesium. *Proc Natl Acad Sci U S A* **87**:5243, 1990.
166. Ke H, Liang J-Y, Zhang Y, Lipscomb WN: Conformational transition of fructose-1,6-bisphosphatase: Structure comparison between the AMP complex (T form) and the fructose-6-phosphate complex (R form). *Biochemistry* **30**:4412, 1991.
167. Saéz DE, Figueroa CD, Concha II, Slebe JC: Localization of the fructose 1,6-bisphosphatase at the nuclear periphery. *J Cell Biochem* **63**:453, 1996.
168. El-Maghrabi MR, Lange AJ, Kuemmel L, Pilkis SJ: The rat fructose-1,6-bisphosphatase gene. *J Biol Chem* **266**:2115, 1991.
169. El-Maghrabi MR, Pilkis SJ: Expression of rat liver fructose1,6-bisphosphatase in *Escherichia coli. Biochem Biophys Res Commun* **176**:137, 1991.
170. El-Maghrabi MR, Gidh-Jain M, Austin LR, Pilkis SJ: Isolation of a human liver fructose-1,6-bisphosphatase cDNA and expression of the protein in *Escherichia coli. J Biol Chem* **268**:9466, 1993.
171. El-Maghrabi MR, Lange AJ, et al.: Human fructose-1,6-bisphosphatase gene Exon-intron organization, localization to chromosome bands 9q22.2-q22.3, and mutation screening in subjects with fructose-1,6-bisphosphatase deficiency. *Genomics* **27**:520, 1995.
172. Gidh-Jain M, Zhang Y, van Poelje PD, et al.: The allosteric site of human liver fructose-1,6-bisphosphatase. Analysis of six AMP site mutants based on the crystal structure. *J Biol Chem* **269**:27732, 1994.
173. Vincent MF, Marangos PJ, Gruber HE, Van den Berghe G: Inhibition by AICA riboside of gluconeogenesis in isolated rat hepatocytes. *Diabetes* **40**:1259, 1991.
174. Vincent MF, Erion MD, Gruber HE, Van den Berghe G: Hypoglycaemic effect of AICAriboside in mice. *Diabetologia* **39**:1148, 1996.
175. Cardenas ML, Rabajille E, Niemeyer H: Fructose is a good substrate for rat liver "glucokinase" (hexokinase D). *Biochem J* **222**:363, 1984.
176. Katzen HM, Schimke RT: Multiple forms of hexokinase in the rat: Tissue distribution, age dependency and properties. *Proc Natl Acad Sci U S A* **54**:1218, 1965.
177. Sols A, Crane RK: Substrate specificity of brain hexokinase. *J Biol Chem* **210**:581, 1954.
178. Froesch ER: Fructose metabolism in adipose tissue from normal and diabetic rats, in Renold AE, Cahill GF Jr (eds): *Handbook of Physiology: Adipose Tissue*, Vol. 52. Washington, DC, American Physiology Society, 1965, pp 281–293.
179. Szwergold BS, Kappler F, Brown TR: Identification of fructose 3-phosphate in the lens of diabetic rats. *Science* **247**:451, 1990.
180. Petersen A, Szwergold BS, Kappler F, Weingarten M, Brown TR: Identification of sorbitol 3-phosphate and fructose 3-phosphate in normal and diabetic human erythrocytes. *J Biol Chem* **265**:17424, 1990.
181. Petersen A, Steinmann B, Gitzelmann R: Essential fructosuria: Increased levels of fructose 3-phosphate in erythrocytes. *Enzyme* **46**:319, 1992.
182. Petersen A, Kappler F, Szwergold BS, Brown TR: Fructose metabolism in the human erythrocyte. Phosphorylation to fructose 3-phosphate. *Biochem J* **284**:363, 1992.
183. Lal S, Szwergold BS, Kappler F, Brown T: Detection of fructose-3-phosphokinase activity in intact mammalian lenses by ^{31}P NMR spectroscopy. *J Biol Chem* **268**:7763, 1993.
184. Cheng HM, Cheng FY, Xiong H, Xiong J: The further metabolism of sorbitol-3-phosphate and fructose-3-phosphate in the mature rat lens. *Ophthalmic Res* **28**: 57, 1996.
185. Gopher A, Vaisman N, Mandel H, Lapidot A: Determination of fructose metabolic pathways in normal and fructose-intolerant children: A ^{13}C NMR study using [U-^{13}C]fructose. *Proc Natl Acad Sci U S A* **87**:5449, 1990.
186. Lapidot A, Gopher A, Gutman A: Does fructose metabolize to fructose-6-P by hexokinase in human liver? *In vivo* studies of fructose metabolism in patients with fructose-1,6-diP deficiency. Society of Magnetic Resonance in Medicine, Ninth Annual Scientific Meeting and Exhibition, August 18–24, 1990, New York, Book of Abstracts, Vol. 2, p 938.
187. Gopher A, Lapidot A: The effect of mode of fructose administration on its metabolic pathways in a rhesus monkey and rabbits, studied by [U-^{13}C]fructose and ^{13}C NMR. Society of Magnetic Resonance in Medicine, Ninth Annual Scientific Meeting and Exhibition, August 18–24, 1990, New York, Book of Abstracts, Vol. 2, p 938.
188. Bismut H, Hers HG, Van Schaftingen E: Conversion of fructose to glucose in the rabbit small intestine. *Eur J Biochem* **213**:721, 1993.
189. Hue L, Hers HG: The conversion of [4-^{3}H]fructose and of [4-^{3}H]glucose to liver glycogen in the mouse. An investigation of the glyceraldehyde crossroads. *Eur J Biochem* **29**:268, 1972.
190. Duran M, Beemer FA, Bruinvis L, Ketting D, Wadman SK: D-glyceric acidemia: An inborn error associated with fructose metabolism. *Pediatr Res* **21**:502, 1987.
191. Grivell AR, Halls HJ, Berry MN: Role of mitochondria in hepatic fructose metabolism. *Biochim Biophys Acta* **1059**:45, 1991
192. Exton JH, Park CR: Control of gluconeogenesis in liver. 1. General features of gluconeogenesis in the perfused livers of rats. *J Biol Chem* **242**:2622, 1967.

193. Bergström J, Hultman E: Synthesis of muscle glycogen in man after glucose and fructose infusion. *Acta Med Scand* **182**:93, 1967.
194. Tygstrup N, Winkler K, Lundquist F: The mechanism of the fructose effect on the ethanol metabolism of the human liver. *J Clin Invest* **44**:817, 1965.
195. Bar-On H, Stein Y: Effect of glucose and fructose administration on lipid metabolism in the rat. *J Nutr* **94**:95, 1968.
196. Pereira JN, Jangaard NO: Different rates of glucose and fructose metabolism in rat liver tissue *in vitro*. *Metabolism* **20**:392, 1971.
197. Zakim D, Pardini RS, Herman RH, Sauberlich HE: Mechanism for the differential effects of high carbohydrate diets on lipogenesis in rat liver. *Biochim Biophys Acta* **114**:242, 1967.
198. Zakim D, Herman RH, Gordon WC: The conversion of glucose and fructose to fatty acids in the human liver. *Biochem Med* **2**:427, 1969.
199. Nikkilä EA: Control of plasma and liver triglyceride kinetics by carbohydrate metabolism and insulin. *Adv Lipid Res* **7**:63, 1969.
200. Van Den Berghe G: Metabolic effects of fructose in the liver. *Curr Top Cell Regul* **13**:97, 1978.
201. Van Schaftingen E. Vandercammen A, Detheux M, Davies DR: The regulatory protein of liver glucokinase. *Adv Enzyme Regul* **32**:133, 1993.
201a. Clark DG, Filseli OH, Topping DL: Effects of fructose concentration on carbohydrate metabolism, heat production and substrate cycling in isolated rat hepatocytes. *Biochem J* **184**:501, 1979.
201b. Van Schaftingen E: A protein from rat liver confers to glucokinase the property of being entagonistically regulated by fructose 6-phosphate and fructose 1-phosphate. *Eur J Biochem* **179**:179, 1989.
202. Detheux M, Vandekerckhove J, Van Schaftingen E: Cloning and sequencing of rat liver cDNAs encoding the regulatory protein of glucokinase. *FEBS Lett* **321**:111, 1993.
203. Vandercammen A, Van Schaftingen E: The mechanism by which rat liver glucokinase is inhibited by the regulatory protein. *Eur J Biochem* **191**:483, 1990.
204. Van Schaftingen E, Davies DR: Fructose administration stimulates glucose phosphorylation in the livers of anesthetized rats. *FASEB J* **5**:326, 1991.
205. Perheentupa J, Raivio K: Fructose-induced hyperuricaemia. *Lancet* **2**:528, 1967.
206. Bergström J, Hultman E, Roch-Norlund AE: Lactic acid accumulation in connection with fructose infusion. *Acta Med Scand* **184**:359, 1968.
207. Hers HG: Misuses for fructose. *Nature* **227**:241, 1979.
208. Woods HF, Alberti KGMM: Dangers of intravenous fructose. *Lancet* **2**:1354, 1972.
209. Sestoft L: Fructose-en advarsel. *Ugeskr Laeger* **134**:571, 1972.
210. Van Den Berghe G, Hers HG: Dangers of intravenous fructose and sorbitol. *Acta Paediatr Belg* **31**:115, 1978.
211. Bontemps F, Hue L, Hers HG: Phosphorylation of glucose in isolated rat hepatocytes. Sigmoidal kinetics explained by the activity of glucokinase alone. *Biochem J* **174**:603, 1978.
212. Kjerulf-Jensen K: The phosphate esters formed in the liver tissue of rats and rabbits during assimilation of hexoses and glycerol. *Acta Physiol Scand* **4**:249, 1942.
213. Günther MA, Sillero A, Sols A: Fructokinase assay with a specific spectrophotometric method using 1-phosphofructo kinase. *Enzymol Biol Clin* **8**:341, 1967.
214. Heinz F, Junghänel J: Metabolitmuster in Rattenleber nach Fructoseapplikation. *Hoppe Seyler Z Physiol Chem* **350**:859, 1969.
215. Bode JC, Zelder O, et al.: Depletion of liver adenosine phosphates and metabolic effects of intravenous infusion of fructose or sorbitol in man and in the rat. *Eur J Clin Invest* **3**:436, 1973.
216. Van Den Berghe G, Hue L, Hers HG: Effect of the administration of fructose on the glycogenolytic action of glucagon. An investigation of the pathogeny of hereditary fructose intolerance. *Biochem J* **134**:637, 1973.
217. Van Den Berghe G, Bronfman M, Vanneste R, Hers HG: The mechanism of adenosine triphosphate depletion in the liver after a load of fructose. A kinetic study of liver adenylate deaminase. *Biochem J* **162**:601, 1977.
218. Boesiger P, Buchli R, Meier D, Steinmann B, Gitzelmann R: Changes of liver metabolite concentrations in adults with disorders of fructose metabolism after intravenous fructose by ^{31}P magnetic resonance spectroscopy. *PediatrRes* **36**:436, 1994.
219. Fox IH, Kelley WN: Studies on the mechanism of fructose-induced hyperuricemia in man. *Metabolism* **21**:713, 1972.
220. Narins RG, Weisberg JS, Myers AR: Effects of carbohydrates on uric acid metabolism. *Metabolism* **23**:455, 1974.
221. Heuckenkamp PU, Zöllner N: Fructose-induced hyperuricaemia. *Lancet* **1**:808, 1971.
222. Curreri PW, Pruitt BA: Absence of fructose-induced hyperuricaemia in men. *Lancet* **1**:839, 1970.
223. Hessov I: Effects of fructose and glucose infusions on blood acid-base equilibrium in the postoperative period. *Acta Chir Scand* **140**:347, 1974.
224. Steinmann B, Baerlocher K, Gitzelmann R: Hereditäre Störungen des Fruktosestoffwechsels: Belastungsproben mit Fruktose, Sorbitol und Dihydroxyaceton. *Nutr Metab* **18** (suppl 1):115, 1975.
225. Peaston MJT: Dangers of intravenous fructose. *Lancet* **1**:266, 1973.
226. Kogut MD, Roe TF, Ng WON, Donnell GN: Fructose-induced hyperuricemia: Observations in normal children and in patients with hereditary fructose intolerance and galactosemia. *Pediatr Res* **9**:774, 1975.
227. Sahebjami DH, Scalettar R: Effects of fructose infusion on lactate and uric acid metabolism. *Lancet* **1**:366, 1971.
228. Edwards NL, Gelfand EW, Biggar D, Fox IH: Partial deficiency of purine nucleoside phosphorylase: Studies of purine and pyrimidine metabolism. *J Lab Clin Med* **91**:736, 1978.
229. Kurtz TW, Kabra PM, Booth BE, Al-Bander HA, Portale AA, Serena BG, Tsai HC, Morris RC: Liquid-chromatographic measurements of inosine, hypoxanthine and xanthine in studies of fructose-induced degradation of adenine nucleotides in humans and rats. *Clin Chem* **32**:782, 1986.
230. Mäenpää PH, Raivio KO, Kekomäki MP: Liver adenine nucleotides: Fructose-induced depletion and its effect on protein synthesis. *Science* **161**:1253, 1968.
231. Hultman E, Nilsson LH, Sahlin K: Adenine nucleotide content of human liver. Normal values and fructose-induced depletion. *Scand J Clin Lab Invest* **35**:245, 1975.
232. Iles RA, Griffiths JR, Stevens AN, Gadian DG, Porteous R: Effect of fructose on the energy metabolism and acid-base status of the perfused starved-rat liver. *Biochem J* **192**:191, 1980.
233. Oberhaensli RD, Galloway GJ, Taylor DJ, Bore PJ, Radda GK: Assessment of human liver metabolism by phosphorus-31 magnetic resonance spectroscopy. *Br J Radiol* **59**:695, 1986.
234. Boesiger P, Buchli R, Meier D, Steinmann B, Gitzelmann R: Metabolic changes in liver after intravenous fructose in adults with disorders of fructose metabolism and in healthy controls, followed by phosphorus magnetic resonance spectroscopy (Abstract). *Pediatr Res* **30**:651, 1991.
235. Oberhaensli RD, Rajagopalan B, Taylor DJ, Radda GK: Study of hereditary fructose intolerance by use of ^{31}P magnetic resonance spectroscopy. *Lancet* **2**:931, 1987.
236. Sakuma H, Itabashi K, Takeda K, et al.: Serial P-31 MR spectroscopy after fructose infusion in patients with chronic hepatitis. *J Magn Reson Imaging* **1**:701, 1991.
237. Dufour JF, Stoupis C, Lazeyras F, et al.: Alterations in hepatic fructose metabolism in cirrhotic patients demonstrated by dynamic ^{31}Phophorus spectroscopy. *Hepatology* **15**:835, 1992.
238. Burch HB, Max P, Chyu K, Lowry OH: Metabolic intermediates in liver of rats given large amounts of fructose or dihydroxyacetone. *Biochem Biophys Res Commun* **34**:619, 1969.
239. Burch HB, Lowry OH, Meinhardt L, Max P, Chyu K: Effect of fructose, dihydroxyacetone, glycerol, and glucose on metabolites and related compounds in liver and kidney. *J Biol Chem* **245**:2092, 1970.
240. Morris RC, Nigon K, Reed EB: Evidence that the severity of depletion of inorganic phosphate determines the severity of the disturbance of adenine nucleotide metabolism in the liver and renal cortex of the fructose-loaded rat. *J Clin Invest* **61**:209, 1978.
241. Lamers JMJ, Hülsmann WC: The effect of fructose on the stores of energy-rich phosphate in rat jejunum *in vivo*. *Biochim Biophys Acta* **313**:1, 1973.
242. Watts RWE, Watts JEM, Seegmiller JE: Xanthine oxidase activity in human tissues and its inhibition by allopurinol (4-hydroxypyrazolo (3,4-d) pyrimidine). *J Lab Clin Med* **66**:688, 1965.
243. Van Den Berghe G, Bontemps F, Hers HG: Purine catabolism in isolated rat hepatocytes. Influence of coformycin. *Biochem J* **188**:913, 1980.
244. Van Den Berghe G: Regulation of purine catabolism, in Hue L, Van de Werve G (eds): *Short-Term Regulation of Liver Metabolism*. Amsterdam, Elsevier/North-Holland, 1981, pp 361–376.

245. Bontemps F, Van Den Berghe G, Hers HG: Evidence for a substrate cycle between AMP and adenosine in isolated hepatocytes. *Proc Natl Acad Sci U S A* **80**:2829, 1983.
246. Mäenpää PH: Fructose-induced alterations in liver polysome profiles and Mg^{2+} levels. *FEBS Lett* **24**:37, 1972.
247. Mäenpää PH: Fructose and liver protein synthesis. *Acta Med Scand Suppl* **542**:115, 1972.
248. Lindqvist L, Nyyssönen K, Mäenpää PH: Quantitative changes in aminoacylation of transfer RNA and in free amino acids during fructose-induced depletion of adenine nucleotides in rat liver. *Biochim Biophys Acta* **763**:107, 1983.
248a. Yamamoto T, Moriwaki Y, Takahashi S, et al.: Effect of ethanol and fructose on plasma uridine and purine bases. *Metabolism* **46**:544, 1997.
249. Van Den Berghe G, Vincent MF: Effect of fructose on the metabolization of ammonia. Presented at the Annual Meeting of the European Society for Paediatric Research, Turku, Finland, June 25–29, 1978.
250. Yu DT, Burch HB, Phillips MJ: Pathogenesis of fructose hepatotoxicity. *Lab Invest* **30**:85, 1974.
251. Phillips MJ, Hetenyi G, Adachi F: Ultrastructural hepatocellular alterations induced by *in vivo* fructose infusions. *Lab Invest* **22**:370, 1970.
252. Hugon JS, Maestracci D, Menard D: Smooth endoplasmic reticulum proliferation in mouse enterocytes induced by fructose feeding. *Histochemie* **29**:189, 1972.
253. Brosnan MJ, Chen L, Wheeler CE, et al.: Phosphocreatine protects ATP from a fructose load in transgenic mouse liver expressing creatine kinase. *Am J Physiol* **260**:C1191, 1991.
254. Raivio KO, Becker MA, et al.: Stimulation of human purine synthesis *de novo* by fructose infusion. *Metabolism* **24**:861, 1975.
255. Itakura M, Sabina RL, Heald PW, Holmes EW: Basis for the control of purine biosynthesis by purine ribonucleotides. *J Clin Invest* **67**:994, 1981.
256. Vincent MF, Van Den Berghe G, Hers HG: Increase in phosphoribosyl pyrophosphate induced by ATP and Pi depletion in hepatocytes. *FASEB J* **3**:1862, 1989.
257. Ashare R, Moore R, Ellison EH: Utilization of glucose, fructose and invert sugar. Comparison in diseases of the liver and pancreas. *Arch Surg* **70**:428, 1955.
258. Kaye R, Williams ML, Barbero G: Comparative study of glucose and fructose metabolism in infants with reference to utilization and to the accumulation of glycolytic intermediates. *J Clin Invest* **37**:752, 1958.
259. Cook GC, Jacobson J: Individual variation in fructose metabolism in man. *Br J Nutr* **26**:187, 1971.
260. Eggleston LV, Woods HF: Activation of liver pyruvate kinase by fructose-1-phosphate. *FEBS Lett* **6**:43, 1970.
261. Mapungwana SW, Davies DR: The effect of fructose on pyruvate kinase activity in isolated hepatocytes. Inhibition by allantoin and alanine. *Biochem J* **208**:171, 1982.
262. Craig GM, Crane CW: Lactic acidosis complicating liver failure after intravenous fructose. *BMJ* **4**:211, 1971.
263. Andersson G, Brohult J, Sterner G: Increasing metabolic acidosis following fructose infusion in two children. *Acta Paediatr Scand* **58**:301, 1969.
264. Odièvre M, Poirier C, Levillain P, Modigliani E, Strauch G: Etude des réponses glucosémiques, lactacidémiques et insulinémiques après administration intraveineuse rapide de doses variables de fructose chez l'enfant normal. *Arch Fr Pediatr* **27**:1057, 1970.
265. Pearson JF, Shuttleworth R: The metabolic effects of a hypertonic fructose infusion on the mother and fetus during labor. *Am J Obstet Gynecol* **111**:259, 1971.
266. Adolph M, Eckart A, Eckart J: Fruktose vs. Glukose in der total parenteralen Ernährung kritisch kranker Patienten . *Anaesthesist* **44**:770, 1995.
267. Anundi I, De Groot H: Hypoxic liver cell death: Critical PO_2 and dependence of viability on glycolysis. *Am J Physiol* **257**:G58, 1989.
268. Gasbarrini A, Borle AB, Farghali H, Francavilla A, Van Thiel D: Fructose protects rat hepatocytes from anoxic injury. *J Biol Chem* **267**:7545, 1992.
269. Anundi I, Kind J, Owne DA, Schneider H, Lemaster JJ, Thurman RG: Fructose prevents hypoxic cell death in liver. *Am J Physiol* **253**:G390, 1987.
270. Di Mone D, Sandy MS, Blank L, Smith MT: Fructose prevents 1-methyl-4-phenyl-1,2,3,6-tetrahydropyridine (MPTP)-induced ATP depletion and toxicity in isolated hepatocytes. *Biochem Biophys Res Commun* **153**:734, 1988.
271. Nieminen A-L, Dawson TL, Gores GJ, et al.: Protection by acidotic pH and fructose against lethal injury to rat hepatocytes from mitochondrial inhibitors, ionophore and oxidant chemicals. *Biochem Biophys Res Commun* **167**:600, 1990.
272. Cannon JR, Harvison PJ, Rush GF: The effects of fructose on adenosine triphosphate depletion following mitochondrial dysfunction and lethal cell injury in isolated rat hepatocytes. *Toxicol Appl Pharmacol* **108**:407, 1991.
273. Krane SM: Fructosuria, in Stanbury JB, Wyngaarden JB, Fredrickson DS (eds): *The Metabolic Basis of Inherited Disease*. New York, McGraw-Hill, 1960, pp 144–155.
274. Czapek F: Eine seltene Form von Diabetes mellitus. *Prager Med Wochenschr* **1**:245, 265, 1876.
275. Zimmer K: I. Levulose im Harn eines Diabetikers. *Dtsch Med Wochenschr* **1**:329, 1876.
276. Laron Z: Essential benign fructosuria. *Arch Dis Child* **36**:273, 1961.
277. Steinitz H, Mizrahy O: Essential fructosuria and hereditary fructose intolerance. *N Engl J Med* **280**:222, 1969.
278. Khachadurian AK: Nonalimentary fructosuria. *Pediatrics* **32**:455, 1963.
279. Heeres PA, Vos H: Fructosuria. *Arch Intern Med* **44**:47, 1929.
280. Lenzner AR: Fructosuria: Report of a case. *Ann Intern Med* **45**:702, 1956.
281. Heinz F, Schlegel F, Krause PH: Enzymes of fructose metabolism in human small intestine mucosa. *Enzyme* **19**:93, 1975.
282. Heinz F, Schlegel F, Krause PH: Enzymes of fructose metabolism in human kidney. *Enzyme* **19**:85, 1975.
283. Malaisse WJ, Malaisse-Lagae F, Davies DR, Van Schaftingen E: Presence of fructokinase in pancreatic islets. *FEBS Lett* **255**:175, 1989.
284. Schapira F, Schapira G, Dreyfus J-C: La lésion enzymatique de la fructosurie bénigne. *Enzymol Biol Clin* **1**:170, 1961–1962.
285. Hers HG, Joassin G: Anomalie de l'aldolase hépatique dans l'intolérance au fructose. *Enzymol Biol Clin* **1**:4, 1961.
286. Sachs B, Sternfeld L, Kraus G: Essential fructosuria. Its pathophysiology. *Am J Dis Child* **63**:252, 1942.
287. Rynbergen HJ, Chambers WH, Blatherwick NR: Respiratory metabolism in fructosuria. *J Nutr* **21**:553, 1941.
288. Baylon H, Schapira F, Wegmann R, Dreyfus J-C, Moulias R, Poyart C, Coumel P: Note préliminaire sur l'étude clinique, biologique, histochimique et enzymatique de la fructosurie familiale essentielle. *Rev Fr Etud Clin Biol* **7**:531, 1962.
289. Silver S, Reiner M: Essential fructosuria. Report of three cases with metabolic studies. *Arch Intern Med* **54**:412, 1934.
290. Aarskog NK, Ogreid D: Aldolase B A149P mutation and hereditary fructose intolerance are not associated with sudden infant death syndrome. *Acta Paediatr* **84**:947, 1995.
291. Saudubray JM, Charpentier C: Clinical phenotypes: Diagnosis/algorithms, in Scriver CR, Beaudet AL, Sly WS, Valle D (eds): *The Metabolic and Molecular Bases of Inherited Disease*, 7th ed. New York, McGraw-Hill, 1995, pp 327–400.
292. Steinmann B: Unpublished observations, 1973–2000.
293. Lasker M: Essential fructosuria. *Hum Biol* **13**:51, 1941.
294. Marble A: The diagnosis of the less common meliturias. Including pentosuria and fructosuria. *Med Clin North Am* **31**:313, 1947.
295. Leonidas JC: Essential fructosuria. *NY State J Med* **65**:2257, 1965.
296. Chambers RA, Pratt RTC: Idiosyncrasy to fructose. *Lancet* **2**:340, 1956.
297. Froesch ER, Prader A, Labhart A, Stuber HW, Wolf HP: Die hereditäre Fructoseintoleranz, eine bisher nicht bekannte kongenitale Stoffwechselstörung. *Schweiz Med Wochenschr* **87**:1168, 1957.
298. Perheentupa J, Raivio KO, Nikkilä EA: Hereditary fructose intolerance. *Acta Med Scand Suppl* **542**:65, 1972.
299. Baerlocher K, Gitzelmann R, Steinmann B, Gitzelmann-Cumarasamy N: Hereditary fructose intolerance in early childhood: A major diagnostic challenge. Survey of 20 symptomatic cases. *Helv Paediatr Acta* **33**:465, 1978.
300. Odièvre M, Gentil C, Gautier M, Alagille D: Hereditary fructose intolerance in childhood. *Am J Dis Child* **132**:605, 1978.
301. Baker L, Winegrad AI: Fasting hypoglycaemia and metabolic acidosis associated with deficiency of hepatic fructose-1,6-diphosphatase activity. *Lancet* **2**:13, 1970.
302. Turner RC, Spathis GS, Nabarro JDN, Dormandy TL: Familial fructose and galactose intolerance. *Lancet* **2**:872, 1972.
303. Levin B, Snodgrass GJAI, Oberholzer VG, Burgess EA, Dobbs RH: Fructosaemia. Observations on seven cases. *Am J Med* **45**:826, 1968.

304. Swales JD, Smith ADM: Adult fructose intolerance. *Q J Med* **35**:455, 1966.
305. Marthaler TM, Froesch ER: Hereditary fructose intolerance. Dental status of eight patients. *Br Dent J* **123**:597, 1967.
306. Köhlin P, Melin K: Hereditary fructose intolerance in four Swedish families. *Acta Paediatr Scand* **57**:24, 1968.
307. Cornblath M, Rosenthal IM, Reisner SH, Wybregt SH, Crane RK: Hereditary fructose intolerance. *N Engl J Med* **269**:1271, 1963.
308. Froesch ER, Wolf HP, Baitsch H, Prader A, Labhart A: Hereditary fructose intolerance. An inborn defect of hepatic fructose-1-phosphate splitting aldolase. *Am J Med* **34**:151, 1963.
309. Newbrun E, Hoover C, Mettraux G, Graf H: Comparison of dietary habits and dental health of subjects with hereditary fructose intolerance and control subjects. *J Am Dent Assoc* **101**:619, 1980.
310. Howarth D: Sugar intake and dental caries. *Lancet* **1**:827, 1983.
311. Rampa M, Froesch ER: Eleven cases of hereditary fructose intolerance in one Swiss family with a pair of monozygotic and dizygotic twins. *Helv Paediatr Acta* **36**:317, 1981.
312. Wolf H, Zschocke D, Wedemeyer FW, Hübner W: Angeborene hereditäre Fructose-Intoleranz. *Klin Wochenschr* **37**:693, 1959.
313. Barry RGG, St Colum SR, Magner JW: Hereditary fructose intolerance in parent and child. *J Ir Med Assoc* **61**:308, 1968.
314. Lameire N, Mussche M, Baele G, Kint J, Ringoir S: Hereditary fructose intolerance: A difficult diagnosis in the adult. *Am J Med* **65**:416, 1978.
315. De Vroede M, Mozin M-J, Cadranel S, Loeb H, Heimann R: Découverte d'une fructosémie à l'occasion d'une insuffisance hépatique aigue chez un enfant de 16 mois. *Pediatrie* **35**:353, 1980.
316. Sachs M, Asskali F, Forster H, Encke A: Wiederholte perioperative Applikation von Fructose und Sorbit bei einer Patientin mit hereditärer Fructoseintoleranz (HFI). *Z Ernahrungswiss* **32**:56, 1993.
317. Steinmetz HT, Siedek M, Höpp HW, Baldamus CA: Akutes Leber- und Nierenversagen mit Laktatazidose nach Sorbitinfusion bei unerkannter hereditärer Fruktoseintoleranz. *Intensivmed* **27**:309, 1990.
318. Heine W, Schill H, Tessmann D, Kupatz H: Letale Leberdystrophie bei drei Geschwistern mit hereditärer Fruktoseintoleranz nach Dauertropfinfusionen mit sorbitolhaltigen Infusionslösungen. *Dtsch Gesundheitswes* **24**:2325, 1969.
319. Schulte M-J, Lenz W: Fatal sorbitol infusion in patient with fructose-sorbitol intolerance. *Lancet* **2**:188, 1977.
320. Hackl JM, Balogh D, Kunz F, Dworzak E, Puschendorf B, Decristoforo A, Maier F: Postoperative Fruktoseinfusion bei wahrscheinlich hereditärer Fruktoseintoleranz. *Wien Klin Wochenschr* **90**:237, 1978.
321. Girgensohn H: Die hereditäre Fructoseintoleranz beim Erwachsenen. *Verh Dtsch Ges Pathol* **66**:637, 1982.
322. Müller-Wiefel DE, Steinmann B, Holm-Hadulla M, Wille L, Schärer K, Gitzelmann R: Infusionsbedingtes Nieren- und Leberversagen bei undiagnostizierter hereditärer Fructose-Intoleranz. *Dtsch Med Wochenschr* **108**:985, 1983.
323. Wagner K, Wolf AS: Todesfall nach Fructose- und Sorbitinfusionen. *Anaesthetist* **33**:573, 1984.
324. Black JA, Simpson K: Fructose intolerance. *BMJ* **4**:138, 1967.
325. Roschlau G: Fruktose-Intoleranz, in *Leberbiopsie im Kindesalter.* Jena, Germany, Fischer Verlag, 1978, pp 80–83.
326. Dubois R, Loeb H, Malaisse-Lagae F, Toppet M: Etude clinique et anatomo-pathologique de deux cas d'intolérance congénitale au fructose. *Pediatrie* **20**:5, 1965.
327. Briner J, Schneider J: Personal communication.
328. Spycher MA: Unpublished observations, 1973–1998.
329. Rossner JA, Feist D: Hereditäre Fructoseintoleranz. *Verh Dtsch Ges Pathol* **55**:376, 1971.
330. Schapira F, Hatzfeld A, Gregori C: Studies on liver aldolases in hereditary fructose intolerance. *Enzyme* **18**:73, 1974.
331. Shapira F, Dreyfus J-C: L'aldolase hépatique dans l'intolérance au fructose. *Rev Fr Etud Clin Biol* **12**:486, 1967.
332. Schapira F, Nordmann Y, Grégori C: Hereditary alterations of fructose metabolizing enzymes. *Acta Med Scand Suppl* **542**:77, 1972.
333. Dikow AL, Jeckel D, Pfleiderer G: Isolierung und Charakterisierung von Aldolase A, B und C aus menschlichen Organen. *Hoppe Seyler Z Physiol Chem* **352**:1151, 1971.
334. Cox TM: Aldolase B and fructose intolerance. *FASEB J* **8**:62, 1994.
335. Grégori C, Schapira F, Kahn A, Delpech M, Dreyfus J-C: Molecular studies of liver aldolase B in hereditary fructose intolerance using blotting and immunological techniques. *Ann Hum Genet* **46**:281, 1982.
336. Cox TM, O'Donnell MW, Camilleri M, Burghes AH: Isolation and characterization of a mutant liver aldolase in adult hereditary fructose intolerance. *J Clin Invest* **72**:201, 1983.
337. Gitzelmann R, Steinmann B, Bally C, Lebherz HG: Antibody activation of mutant human fructosediphosphate aldolase B in liver extracts of patients with hereditary fructose intolerance. *Biochem Biophys Res Commun* **59**:1270, 1974.
338. Baerlocher K, Gitzelmann R, Nüssli R, Dumermuth G: Infantile lactic acidosis due to hereditary fructose-1,6 diphosphatase deficiency. *Helv Paediatr Acta* **26**:489, 1971.
339. Gentil C, Colin J, Valette AM, Alagille D, Lelong M: Etude du métabolisme glucidique au cours de l'intolérance héréditaire au fructose. Essai d'interprétation de l'hypoglucosémie. *Rev Fr Etud Clin Biol* **9**:596, 1964.
340. Rossier A, Milhaud G, Colin J, Job J-C, Brault A, Beauvais P, Lemerle J: Intolérance congénitale au fructose. Deux cas familiaux avec étude biochimique *in vitro*. *Arch Fr Pediatr* **23**:533, 1966.
341. Saxon L, Papper S: Abdominal pain occurring during the rapid administration of fructose solutions. *N Engl J Med* **256**:132, 1957.
342. Terrier F, Vock P, Cotting J, Ladebeck R, Reichen J, Hentschel D: Effect of intravenous fructose on the P-31 MR spectrum of the liver: Dose response in healthy volunteers. *Radiology* **171**:557, 1989.
343. Froesch ER, Prader A, Wolf HP, Labhart A: Die hereditäre Fructoseintoleranz. *Helv Paediatr Acta* **14**:99, 1959.
344. Richardson RMA, Little JA, Patten RL, Goldstein MB, Halperin ML: Pathogenesis of acidosis in hereditary fructose intolerance. *Metabolism* **28**:1133, 1979.
345. Perheentupa J, Pitkänen E, Nikkilä EA, Sommersalo O, Hakosalo J: Hereditary fructose intolerance. A clinical study of four cases. *Ann Paediatr Fenn* **8**:221, 1962.
346. Nivelon J-L, Mathieu M, Kissin C, Collombel C, Cotte J, Béthenod M: Intolérance au fructose. Observation et méchanisme physiopathologique de l'hypoglucosémie. *Ann Pediatr (Paris)* **43**:817, 1967.
347. Modigliani E, Strauch G, Odièvre M: Hormonal response to intravenous fructose in normal and fructosaemic children: A study of insulin and growth hormone secretion. *Rev Eur Etud Clin Biol* **15**:882, 1970.
348. Dubois R, Loeb EH, Ooms HA, Gillet P, Bartman J, Champenois A: Etude d'un cas d'hypoglycémie fonctionelle par intolérance au fructose. *Helv Paediatr Acta* **16**:90, 1961.
349. Morris RC, McSherry E, Sebastian A: Modulation of experimental renal dysfunction of hereditary fructose intolerance by circulating parathyroid hormone. *Proc Natl Acad Sci U S A* **68**:132, 1971.
350. Odièvre M: Les difficultés du diagnostic de l'intolérance héréditaire au fructose chez le nurrisson. *Arch Fr Pediatr* **26**:5, 1969.
351. Phillips MJ, Little JA, Ptak TW: Subcellular pathology of hereditary fructose intolerance. *Am J Med* **44**:910, 1968.
352. Phillips MJ, Yu DT, Burch HB: Animal model of human disease: Hereditary fructose intolerance. *Am J Pathol* **75**:591, 1974.
353. Prader A: Unpublished observation.
354. Gitzelmann R, Auricchio S: The handling of soya alpha-galactosides by a normal and a galatosemic child. *Pediatrics* **36**:231, 1965.
355. Pitkänen E, Perheentupa J: Eine biochemische Untersuchung über zwei Fälle von Fructoseintoleranz. *Ann Paediatr Fenn* **8**:236, 1962.
356. Hue L: Unpublished data.
357. Levin B, Oberholzer VG, Snodgrass GJAI, Stimmer L, Wilmers MJ: Fructosaemia. An inborn error of fructose metabolism. *Arch Dis Child* **38**:220, 1963.
358. Morris RC Jr: An experimental renal acidification defect in patients with hereditary fructose intolerance. II. Its distinction from classic renal tubular acidosis; its resemblance to the renal acidification defect associated with the Fanconi syndrome of children with cystinosis. *J Clin Invest* **47**:1648, 1968.
359. Adamowicz M, Pronicka E: Carbohydrate deficient glycoprotein syndrome–like transferrin isoelectric focusing pattern in untreated fructosaemia. *Eur J Pediatr* **155**:347, 1996.
360. Jaeken J, Pirard M, Adamowicz M, Pronicka E, Van Schaftingen E: Inhibition of phosphomannose isomerase by fructose 1-phosphate: An explanation for defective N-glycosylation in hereditary fructose intolerance. *Pediatr Res* **40**:764, 1996.
361. Van Schaftingen E, Jaeken J: Phosphomannomutase deficiency is a cause of carbohydrate-deficient glycoprotein syndrome type I. *FEBS Lett* **377**:318, 1995.
362. Schwartz R, Gamsu H, Mulligan PB, Reisner SH, Wybregt SH, Cornblath M: Transient intolerance to exogenous fructose in the newborn. *J Clin Invest* **43**:333, 1964.

363. Renold AE, Winegrad AI, Froesch ER, Thorn GW: Studies on the site of action of the arylsulfonylureas in man. *Metabolism* **5**:757, 1956.
364. Desbuquois B, Lardinois R, Gentil C, Odièvre M: Effets d'une surcharge en phosphate de sodium sur l'hypoglucosémie dans onze observations d'intolérance héréditaire au fructose. *Arch Fr Pediatr* **26**:21, 1969.
365. Zalitis J, Oliver IT: Inhibition of glucose phosphate isomerase by metabolic intermediates of fructose. *Biochem J* **102**:753, 1967.
366. Bally C, Leuthardt F: Unpublished data.
367. Wilkening J, Nowack J, Decker K: The dependence of glucose formation from lactate on the adenosine triphosphate content in the isolated perfused rat liver. *Biochim Biophys Acta* **392**:299, 1975.
368. Cain ARR, Ryman BE: High liver glycogen in hereditary fructose intolerance. *Gut* **12**:929, 1971.
369. Sidbury JB: Zur Biochemie der hereditären Fructoseintoleranz. *Helv Paediatr Acta* **14**:317, 1959.
370. Rambaud P, Joannard A, Bost M, et al.: Trouble de la glycogénolyse dans l'intolérance héréditaire au fructose. Etude de deux observations chez l'enfant. *Arch Fr Pediatr* **30**:1051, 1973.
371. Van Den Berghe G: Biochemical aspects of hereditary fructose intolerance, in Hommes FA, van den Berg CJ (eds): *Normal and Pathological Development of Energy Metabolism*. London, Academic, 1975, pp 211–228.
372. Maddaiah VT, Madsen NB: Kinetics of purified liver phosphorylase. *J Biol Chem* **241**:3873, 1966.
373. Kaufmann U, Froesch ER: Inhibition of phosphorylase-a by fructose-1-phosphate, a-glycerophosphate and fructose-1,6-diphosphate: Explanation for fructose-induced hypoglycaemia in hereditary fructose intolerance and fructose-1,6-diphosphatase deficiency. *Eur J Clin Invest* **3**:407, 1973.
374. Thurston JH, Jones EM: Decrease and inhibition of liver phosphorylase (LP) after fructose: An experimental model for the study of hereditary fructose intolerance (HFI). *Pediatr Res* **5**:392, 1971.
375. Thurston JH, Jones EM, Hauhart RE: Decrease and inhibition of liver glycogen phosphorylase after fructose. An experimental model for the study of hereditary fructose intolerance. *Diabetes* **23**:597, 1974.
376. Landau BR, Marshall JS, Craig JW, Hostetler KY, Genuth SM: Quantitation of the pathways of fructose metabolism in normal and fructose-intolerant subjects. *J Lab Clin Med* **78**:608, 1971.
377. Mercier J-C, Bourrillon A, Beaufils F, Odièvre M: Intolérance héréditaire au fructose à révélation précoce. *Arch Fr Pediatr* **33**:945, 1976.
378. Perheentupa J, Pitkänen E: Symptomless hereditary fructose intolerance. *Lancet* **1**:1358, 1962.
379. Gitzelmann R: Enzymes of fructose and galactose metabolism; galactose-1-phosphate, in Curtius H-C, Roth M (eds): *Clinical Biochemistry: Principles and Methods*. Berlin, Gruyter, 1974, pp 1236–1251.
380. Hue L, Van Hoof F, Hers H-G: Serum aldolase in Tay-Sachs disease and in fructose intolerance. *Am J Med* **51**:785, 1971.
381. Gitzelmann R, Steinmann B, Tuchschmid P: Patients with hereditary fructose intolerance have normal erythrocyte aldolase activity. *Clin Chim Acta* **181**:163, 1989.
382. Gliksman R, Ghosh NK, Cox RP: Comparison of aldolase isozymes in placenta, HeLa cells, and human fibroblast cultures. *Enzyme* **22**:416, 1977.
383. Shin YS, Rimböck H, Endres W: Fructose-1-phosphate aldolase activity in human fetal and adult tissues as well as leukocytes and cultured fibroblasts in hereditary fructose intolerance. *J Inherit Metab Dis* **5**(suppl 1):45, 1982.
384. Ali M, Rosien U, Cox TM: DNA diagnosis of fatal fructose intolerance from archival tissue. *Q J Med* **86**:25, 1993.
385. Odièvre M, Gautier M, Rieu D: Intolérance héréditaire au fructose du nourrisson. Evolution des lésions histologiques hépatiques sous traitment diététique prolongé. (Etude de huit observations.) *Arch Fr Pediatr* **26**:433, 1969.
386. Cornblath M, Schwartz R: *Disorders of Carbohydrate Metabolism in Infancy,* 2nd ed, Vol. 3. Major problems in clinical pediatrics. Philadelphia, Saunders, 1976.
387. Wyke RJ, Rajkovic IA, Eddleston ALWF, Williams R: Defective opsonization and complement deficiency in serum from patients with fulminant hepatic failure. *Gut* **21**:643, 1980.
388. Nüssli R: Das Wachstum von Patienten mit hereditärer Fruktoseintoleranz oder hereditärer Saccharose-Isomaltose-Malabsorption. *Helv Paediatr Acta* **26**:637, 1971.
389. Mock DM, Perman JA, Thaler MM, Morris RC: Chronic fructose intoxication after infancy in children with hereditary fructose intolerance: A cause of growth retardation. *N Engl J Med* **309**:764, 1983.
390. Brauman J, Kentos P, Frisque P, Gepts W, Verbanck M: Intolérance héréditaire au fructose chez une femme de 83 ans. *Acta Clin Belg* **26**:65, 1971.
390a. Cox TM: Personal communication.
391. Gitzelmann R, Steinmann B, Müller-Wiefel DE, Holm-Hadulla M, Wille L, Schärer K: Infusionslösungen. *Dtsch Med Wochenschr* **108**:1656, 1983.
392. Blom W, Fernandes J: Unpublished data.
393. Froesch ER: Unpublished data.
394. Trost C: Personal communication.
395. Steinmann B, Gitzelmann R: Fruktose und Sorbitol in Infusionsflüssigkeiten sind nicht immer harmlos. *Int J Vitam Nutr Res Suppl* **15**:289, 1976.
396. Danks DM, Connellan JM, Solomon JR: Hereditary fructose intolerance: Report of a case and comments on the hazards of fructose infusion. *Aust Paediatr J* **8**:282, 1972.
397. Ruecker AV, Endres W, Shin YS, Butenandt I, Steinmann B, Gitzelmann R: A case of fatal hereditary fructose intolerance. Misleading information on formula composition. *Helv Paediatr Acta* **36**:599, 1981.
398. Galaske RG, Burdelski M, Brodehl J: Primär polyurisches Nierenversagen und akute gelbe Leberdystrophie nach Infusion von Zuckeraustauschstoffen im Kindesalter. *Dtsch Med Wochenschr* **111**:978, 1986.
399. Locher S: Akutes Leber- und Nierenversagen nach Sorbitinfusion bei 28jährigem Patienten mit undiagnostizierter Fruktoseintoleranz. *Anasth Intensivther Notfallmed* **22**:194, 1987.
400. Otten A, Wagner F, Wolk H: Tödliche Gefahr durch Fructoseinfusionen. *Anasth Intensivmed* **29**:314, 1988.
401. Rey M, Behrens R, Zeilinger G: Fatale Folgen einer Fructose-Infusion bei undiagnostizierter Fructose-Intoleranz. *Dtsch Med Wochenschr* **113**:945, 1988.
402. Keller U: Zuckerersatzstoffe Fructose und Sorbit: Ein unnötiges Risiko in der parenteralen Ernährung. *Schweiz Med Wochenschr* **119**:101, 1989.
403. Steegmanns I, Rittmann M, Bayerl JR, Gitzelmann R: Erwachsene mit hereditärer Fructoseintoleranz: Gefährdung durch Fructoseinfusion. *Dtsch Med Wochenschr* **115**:539, 1990.
404. Wolf H, Klinge O, Otten A: Hereditäre Fructoseintoleranz. Lebensgefahr durch Fructose- und Sorbitinfusionen. *Munch Med Wochenschr* **134**:254, 1992.
405. Collins J: Time for fructose solutions to go. *Lancet* **341**:600, 1993.
406. Blass EM, Hoffmeyer LB: Sucrose as an analgesic for newborn infants. *Pediatrics* **87**:215, 1991.
407. Bucher HU, Moser T, von Siebenthal K, Keel M, Wolf M, Duc G: Sucrose reduces pain reaction to heel lancing in premature infants: A placebo-controlled, randomized and masked study. *Pediatr Res* **38**:332, 1995
408. Stevens B, Taddio A, Ohlsson A, Einarson T: The efficacy of sucrose for relieving procedural pain in neonates — a systematic review and metaanalysis. *Acta Paediatr* **86**:837, 1997.
409. Sitadevi C, Ramaiah Y, Askari Z: Fructose intolerance associated with congenital cataract. *Indian J Pediatr* **35**:496, 1968.
410. Gitzelmann R, Baerlocher K: Vorteile und Nachteile der Fructose in der Nahrung. *Paediatr Fortbildungskurse Prax* **37**:40, 1973.
411. James CL, Rellos P, Ali M, et al.: Neonatal screening for hereditary fructose intolerance: Frequency of the most common mutant aldolase B allele in the British population. *J Med Genet* **33**:837, 1996.
412. Lindén AL, Nisell I: Hereditär fruktosintolerans. *Sven Laekartidn* **61**:3185, 1964.
413. Kurz R, Hächl G, Hohenwallner W, Berger H: Hereditäre Fruktoseintoleranz mit vermutlich dominantem Erbang. *Arch Kinderheilkd* **183**:233, 1971.
414. Von Ruecker A, Endres W, Shin YS, et al.: A case of fatal hereditary fructose intolerance. Misleading information on formula composition. *Helv Paediatr Acta* **36**:599, 1981.
415. Leupold D: Unpublished data.
416. Cox TM, Camilleri M, O'Donnell MW, Chadwick VS: Pseudodominant transmission of fructose intolerance in an adult and three offspring. *N Engl J Med* **307**:537, 1982.
417. Raivio K, Perheentupa J, Nikkilä EA: Aldolase activities in the liver in parents of patients with hereditary fructose intolerance. *Clin Chim Acta* **17**:275, 1967.

418. Beyreiss K, Willgerodt H, Theile H: Untersuchungen bei heterozygoten Merkmalsträgern für Fructoseintoleranz. *Klin Wochenschr* **46**:465, 1968.
419. Schapira F: Kinetic and immunological abnormalities of aldolase B in hereditary fructose intolerance. *Biochem Soc Trans* **3**:232, 1975.
419a. Cox TM, O'Donnell MW, Camilleri M: Allelic heterogeneity in adult hereditary fructose intolerance. *Mol Biol Med* **1**:393, 1983.
420. Cross NCP, Tolan DR, Cox TM: Catalytic deficiency of human aldolase B in hereditary fructose intolerance caused by a common missense mutation. *Cell* **53**:881, 1988.
421. Grégori C, Besmond C, Odièvre M, et al.: DNA analysis in patients with hereditary fructose intolerance. *Ann Hum Genet* **48**:291, 1984.
422. Cross NCP, De Franchis R, Sebastio G, et al.: Molecular analysis of aldolase B genes in hereditary fructose intolerance. *Lancet* **335**:306, 1990.
423. Tolan DR: Molecular basis of hereditary fructose intolerance: Mutations and polymorphisms in the human aldolase B gene. *Hum Mutat* **6**:210, 1995.
424. Tolan DR, Brooks CC: Molecular analysis of common aldolase B alleles for hereditary fructose intolerance in North Americans. *Biochem Med Metab Biol* **48**:19, 1992
425. Ali M, James CL, Cox TM: A newly identified aldolase B splicing mutation (G → C, 5′ intron 5) in hereditary fructose intolerance from New Zealand. *Hum Mutat* **7**:155, 1996.
426. Brooks CC, Tolan DR: Association of the widespread A149P hereditary fructose intolerance mutation with newly identified sequence polymorphisms in the aldolase B gene. *Am J Hum Genet* **52**:835, 1993.
427. Cavalli-Sforza LL, Menozzi P, Piazza A: *The History and Geography of Human Genes*. Princeton, NJ, Princeton University Press, 1993.
428. Cross NCP, Cox TM: Hereditary fructose intolerance. *Int J Biochem* **22**:685, 1990.
429. Brooks CC, Tolan DR: A partially active mutant aldolase B from a patient with hereditary fructose intolerance. *FASEB J* **8**:107, 1994.
430. Doyle TC, Spickett CM, Donaldson IA, Ratcliffe RG: Metabolic studies of a fructose-intolerant yeast by *in vivo* ^{31}P-nuclear magnetic resonance spectroscopy. *Yeast* **9**:867, 1993.
431. Hülsmann WC, Fernandes J: A child with lactacidemia and fructose diphosphatase deficiency in the liver. *Pediatr Res* **5**:633, 1971.
432. Bakker HD, De Bree PK, Ketting D, Van Sprang FJ, Wadman SK: Fructose-1,6-diphosphatase deficiency: Another enzyme defect which can present itself with the clinical features of "tyrosinosis." *Clin Chim Acta* **55**:41, 1974.
433. Pagliara AS, Karl IE, Keating JP, Brown BI, Kipnis DM: Hepatic fructose-1,6-diphosphatase deficiency. A cause of lactic acidosis and hypoglycemia in infancy. *J Clin Invest* **51**:2115, 1972.
434. Greene HL, Stifel FB, Herman RH: "Ketotic hypoglycemia" due to hepatic fructose-1,6-diphosphatase deficiency. *Am J Dis Child* **124**:415, 1972.
435. Saudubray J-M, Dreyfus J-C, Cepanec C, et al.: Acidose lactique, hypoglycémie et hépatomegalie par déficit héréditaire en fructose-1,6-diphosphatase hépatique. *Arch Fr Pediatr* **30**:609, 1973.
436. Melançon SB, Khachadurian AK, Nadler HL, Brown BI: Metabolic and biochemical studies in fructose-1,6-diphosphatase deficiency. *J Pediatr* **82**:650, 1973.
437. De Rosas FJ, Wapnir RA, Lifshitz F, Silverberg M, Olson M: Folic acid enhanced gluconeogenesis in glycerol-induced hypoglycemia and fructose-1,6-diphosphatase deficiency. Presented at the 56th Annual Meeting of the Endocrine Society, Atlanta, 1974.
438. Eagle RB, MacNab AJ, Ryman BE, Strang LB: Liver biopsy data on a child with fructose-1,6-diphosphatase deficiency that closely resembled many aspects of glucose 6-phosphatase deficiency (von Gierke's type I glycogen-storage disease). *Biochem Soc Trans* **2**:1118, 1974.
439. Odièvre M, Brivet M, Moatti N, et al.: Déficit en fructose-1,6-diphosphatase chez deux soeurs. *Arch Fr Pediatr* **32**:113, 1975.
440. Retbi J-M, Gabilan J-C, Marsac C: Acidose lactique et hypoglycémie à début néonatal par déficit congénital en fructose-1,6-diphosphatase hépatique. *Arch Fr Pediatr* **32**:367, 1975.
441. Corbeel L, Eggermont E, Eeckels R, et al.: Recurrent attacks of ketotic acidosis associated with fructose-1,6-diphosphatase deficiency. *Acta Paediatr Belg* **29**:29, 1976.
442. Corbeel LM, Eggermont E, Bettens W, et al.: Fructose intolerance with normal liver aldolase. *Helv Paediatr Acta* **25**:626, 1970. [Note: The FBPase activity, reported to be low in the note added in proof, was later reinvestigated by more refined techniques and found deficient (De Barsy T, personal communication).]
443. Hopwood NJ, Holzman I, Drash AL: Fructose-1,6-diphosphatase deficiency. *Am J Dis Child* **131**:418, 1977.
444. De Prà M, Laudanna E: La malattia di Baker-Winegrad. *Minerva Pediatr* **30**:1973, 1978.
445. Rallison ML, Meikle AW, Zigrang WD: Hypoglycemia and lactic acidosis associated with fructose-1,6-diphosphatase deficiency. *J Pediatr* **94**:933, 1979.
446. Kinugasa A, Kusunoki T, Iwashima A: Deficiency of glucose-6-phosphate dehydrogenase found in a case of hepatic fructose-1,6-diphosphatase deficiency. *Pediatr Res* **13**:1361, 1979.
447. Borrone C, Genoa; Brown BI, St. Louis; De Barsy T, Bruseles; Endres W, München, Gitzelmann R, Zürich, Hug G, Cincinnati; Lemonnier A, Kremlin-Bicêtre; Leonard JV, London; Marsac C, Paris; Maire I, Mathieu M, Lyon; Saudubray JM, Paris; Schaub J, Kiel; Smit PA, Groningen: Personal communications.
448. Taunton OD, Greene HL, Stifel FB, Hofeldt FD, Lufkin EG, Hagler L, Herman Y, Herman RH: Fructose-1,6-diphosphatase deficiency, hypoglycemia, and response to folate therapy in a mother and her daughter. *Biochem Med* **19**:260, 1978.
449. Service FJ, Veneziale CM, Nelson RA, Ellefson RD, Go VLW: Combined deficiency of glucose-6-phosphatase and fructose-1,6-diphosphatase. Studies of glucagon secretion and fuel utilization. *Am J Med* **64**:696, 1978.
450. Morris AAM, Deshpande S, Ward-Platt MP, et al.: Impaired ketogenesis in fructose-1,6-bisphosphatase deficiency: A pitfall in the investigation of hypoglycaemia. *J Inherit Metab Dis* **18**:28, 1995.
451. Dremsek PA, Sacher M, Stögmann W, Gitzelmann R, Bachmann C: Fructose-1,6-diphosphatase deficiency: Glycerol excretion during fasting test. *Eur J Pediatr* **144**:203, 1985.
452. Krywawych S, Katz G, Lawson AM, Wyatt S, Brenton DP: Glycerol-3-phosphate excretion in fructose-1,6-diphosphatase deficiency. *J Inherit Metab Dis* **9**:388, 1986.
453. Gitzelmann R, Curtius H-C, Wirth R, Steinmann B: Unpublished observation.
454. Nakai A, Shigematsu Y, Liu YY, Kikawa Y, Sudo M: Urinary sugar phosphates and related organic acids in fructose-1,6-diphosphatase deficiency. *J Inherit Metab Dis* **16**:408, 1993.
455. Hommes FA, Campbell R, Steinhart C, Roesel RA, Bowyer F: Biochemical observations on a case of hepatic fructose-1,6-diphosphatase deficiency. *J Inherit Metab Dis* **8**:169, 1985.
456. Pagliara AS, Karl IE, Hammond M, Kipnis DM: Hypoglycemia in infancy and childhood, Parts I and II. *J Pediatr* **82**:365, 558, 1973.
457. Nagai T, Yokoyama T, Hasegawa T, Tsuchiya Y, Matsuo N: Fructose and glucagon loading in siblings with fructose-1,6-diphosphatase deficiency in fed state. *J Inherit Metab Dis* **15**:720, 1992.
458. Gitzelmann R, Baerlocher K, Prader A: Hereditäre Störungen im Fructose- und Galaktosestoffwechsel. *Monatsschr Kinderheilkd* **121**:174, 1973.
459. Baerlocher K, Gitzelmann R, Steinmann B: Clinical and genetic studies of disorders in fructose metabolism, in Burman D, Holton JB, Pennock CA (eds): *Inherited Disorders of Carbohydrate Metabolism*. Lancaster, MTP, 1980, pp 163–190.
460. Robinson BH, Taylor J, Sherwood WG: The genetic heterogeneity of lactic acidosis: Occurrence of recognizable inborn errors of metabolism in a pediatric population with lactic acidosis. *Pediatr Res* **14**:956, 1980.
461. Cahill J, Kirtley ME: FBPase activity in human leukocytes. *N Engl J Med* **292**:212, 1975.
462. Melançon SB, Nadler HL: Detection of fructose-1,6-diphosphatase deficiency with use of white blood cells. *N Engl J Med* **286**:731, 1972.
463. Schrijver J, Hommes FA: Activity of fructose-1,6diphosphatase in human leukocytes. *N Engl J Med* **292**:1298, 1975.
464. Alexander D, Assaf M, Khudr A, Haddad I, Barakat A: Fructose-1,6-diphosphatase deficiency: Diagnosis using leukocytes and detection of heterozygotes with radiochemical and spectrophotometric methods. *J Inherit Metab Dis* **8**:147, 1985.
465. Kikawa Y, Takano T, Nakai A, Shigematsu Y, Sudo M: Detection of heterozygotes for fructose-1,6-diphosphatase deficiency by measuring fructose-1,6-diphosphatase activity in monocytes cultured with calcitriol. *Clin Chim Acta* **215**:81, 1993.
466. Shin YS: Diagnosis of fructose-1,6-bisphosphatase deficiency using leukocytes: Normal leukocyte enzyme activity in three female patients. *Clin Invest* **71**:115, 1993.
467. Besley GTN, Walter JH, Lewis MA, Chard CR, Addison GM: Fructose-1,6-bisphosphatase deficiency: severe phenotype with normal leukocyte enzyme activity. *J Inherit Metab Dis* **17**:333, 1994.

468. Biasucci G, Gigliotti M, Luotti D, Bertagnolio B, Riva E: Defective neutrophil activity in fructose-1,6-diphosphatase deficiency. *J Inherit Metab Dis* **18**:162, 1995.
469. Fong W-F, Hynie I, Lee H, McKendry JBR: Increase of fructose-1,6-diphosphatase activity in cultured human peripheral lymphocytes and its suppression by phytohemagglutinin. *Biochem Biophys Res Commun* **88**:222, 1979.
470. Ito M, Kuroda Y, Kobashi H, Watanabe T, Takeda E, Toshima K, Miyao M: Detection of heterozygotes for fructose-1,6-diphosphatase deficiency by measuring fructose1,6-diphosphatase activity in their cultured peripheral lymphocytes. *Clin Chim Acta* **141**:27, 1984.
471. Kikawa Y, Inuzuka M, Takano T, et al.: cDNA sequences encoding human fructose-1,6-bisphosphatase from monocytes, liver and kidney: Application of monocytes to molecular analysis of human fructose-1,6-biphosphatase deficiency. *Biochem Biophys Res Commun* **199**:687, 1994.
472. Kikawa Y, Inuzuka M, Jin BY, et al.: Identification of a genetic mutation in a family with fructose-1,6-bisphosphatase deficiency. *Biochem Biophys Res Commun* **210**:797, 1995.
473. Kikawa Y, Inuzuka M, Jin BY, Kaji S, Koga J, Yamamoto Y, Fujisawa K, Hata I, Nakai A, Shigematsu Y, Mizunuma H, Taketo A, Mayumi M, Sudo M: Identification of genetic mutations in Japanese patients with fructose-1,6-bisphosphatase deficiency. *Am J Hum Genet* **61**:852, 1997.
474. Herzog B, Wendel U, Morris AAM, Eschrich K: Novel mutations in patients with fructose-1,6-bisphosphatase deficiency. *J Inherit Metab Dis* **22**:132, 1999.
475. Brandt NJ, Rasmussen K, Brandt S, Kolvraa S, Schonheyder F: D-glyceric-acidaemia and non-ketotic hyperglycinaemia. *Acta Paediatr Scand* **65**:17, 1976.
476. Grandgeorge D, Favier A, Bost M, Frappat P, Boujet C, Garrel S, Stoebner P: L'acidémie D-glycérique. *Arch Fr Pediatr* **37**:577, 1980.
477. Kolvraa S, Gregersen N, Christensen E: *In vivo* studies on the metabolic derangement in a patient with D-glyceric acidaemia and hyperglycinaemia. *J Inherit Metab Dis* **7**:49, 1984.
478. Wadman SK, Duran M, Ketting D, et al.: D-glyceric acidemia in a patient with chronic metabolic acidosis. *Clin Chim Acta* **71**:477, 1976.
479. Beutler E, Scott S, Bishop A, Margolis N, Matsumoto F, Kuhl W: Red cell aldolase deficiency and hemolytic anemia: A new syndrome. *Trans Assoc Am Physicians* **86**:154, 1973.
480. Lowry RB, Hanson JW: "Aldolase A" deficiency with syndrome of growth and developmental retardation, midfacial hypoplasia, hepatomegaly and consanguineous parents. *Birth Defects* **13**:223, 1977.
481. Fontaine M, Porchet N, Largilliere C, et al.: Biochemical contribution to diagnosis and study of a new case of D-glyceric acidemia/aciduria. *Clin Chem* **35**:2148, 1989.
482. Bonham JR, Stephenson TJ, Carpenter KH, et al.: D(+)-Glyceric aciduria: Etiology and clinical consequences. *Pediatr Res* **28**:38, 1990.
483. Van Schaftingen E: D-Glycerate kinase deficiency as a cause of D-glyceric aciduria. *FEBS Lett* **243**:127, 1989.
484. Sewell AC, Moritz A, Duran M: D(+)-Glyceric aciduria in an Afghan Hound. *J Inherit Metab Dis* **20**:395, 1997.
485. Hurst JA, Baraitser M, Winter RM:A syndrome of mental retardation, short stature, hemolytic anemia, delayed puberty, and abnormal facial appearance. Similarities to a report of aldolase A deficiency. *Am J Med Genet* **28**:965, 1987.
486. Miwa S, Fujii H, Tani K, et al.: Two cases of red cell aldolase deficiency associated with hereditary hemolytic anemia in a Japanese family. *Am J Hematol* **11**:425, 1981.
487. Kishi H, Mukai T, Hirono A, et al.: Human aldolase A deficiency associated with a hemolytic anemia: Thermolabile aldolase due to a single base mutation. *Proc Natl Acad Sci U S A* **84**:8623, 1987.
488. Kreuder J, Borkhardt A, Repp R, et al.: Brief report: Inherited metabolic myopathy and hemolysis due to a mutation in aldolase A. *N Engl J Med* **334**:1100, 1996.
489. Born P, Zech J, Lehn H, Classen M, Lorenz R: Colonic bacterial activity determines the symptoms in people with fructose-malabsorption. *Hepatogastroenterology* **42**:778, 1995.
490. Götze H, Mahadi A: Fruktosemalabsorption und dysfunktionelle gastrointestinale Beschwerden. *Monatsschr Kinderheilkd* **140**:814, 1992.
491. Andersson DEH, Nygren A: Four cases of long-standing diarrhoea and colic pains cured by fructose-free diet — A pathogenetic discussion. *Acta Med Scand* **203**:87, 1978.
492. Classen M, Nielinger J: Fruktosemalabsorption und dysfunktionelle abdominale Beschwerden (zur Arbeit von H Götze u. A Mahadi). *Monatsschr Kinderheilkd* **140**:276, 1993.
493. Barnes G, McKellar W, Lawrance S: Detection of fructose malabsorption by breath hydrogen test in a child with diarrhea. *J Pediatr* **103**:575, 1983.
494. Wasserman D, Hoekstra JH, Tolia V, et al.: Molecular analysis of the fructose transporter gene (GLUT5) in isolated fructose malabsorption. *J Clin Invest* **98**:2398, 1996.
495. Hyams JS, Leichtner AM: Apple juice. An unappreciated cause of chronic diarrhea. *Am J Dis Child* **139**:503, 1985.
496. Wales JKH, Primhak RA, Rattenbury J, Taylor CJ: Isolated fructose malabsorption. *Arch Dis Child* **65**:227, 1990.
497. Born P, Kamenisch W, Müller S, Paul F: Fruktosemalabsorption — Normalisierung durch Glukosezugabe. *Zeitschr Verdauungskrankheiten* **9**:239, 1991.
498. Iles RA, Stevens AN, Griffiths JR, Morris PG: Phosphorylation status of liver by ^{31}P-n.m.r. spectroscopy, and its implications for metabolic control. *Biochem J* **229**:141, 1985.
499. Gamblin SJ, Davies GJ, Grimes JM, Jackson RM, Littlechild JA, Watson HC: Activity and specificity of human aldolases. *J Mol Biol* **219**:573, 1991.
500. Morris AJ, Tolan DR: Lysine-146 of rabbit muscle aldolase is essential for cleavage and condensation of the C3-C4 bond of fructose 1,6-bis(phosphate). *Biochemistry* **33**:12291, 1994.
501. Horeker BL, Pontermoll S, Ricci C, Cheng T: On the nature of the transaldolase-dihydroxyacetone complex. *Proc Natl Acad Sci USA* **47**:1949, 1961.
502. Streb H, Posselt HG, Wolter K, Bender SW: Aldolase activities of the small intestinal mucosa in malabsorption states and hereditary fructose intolerance. *Eur J Pediatr* **37**:5, 1981.
503. Nisell J, Lindén L: Fructose-1-phosphate aldolase and fructose-1,6-diphosphate aldolase activity in the mucosa of the intestine in hereditary fructose intolerance. *Scand J Gastroenterol* **3**:80, 1968.
504. Métais P, Juif J, Sacrez R: Etude biochimique d'un cas d'intolérance héréditaire au fructose. *Ann Biol Clin* **20**:801, 1962.
505. Kranhold JF, Loh D, Morris RC: Renal fructosemetabolizing enzymes: Significance in hereditary fructose intolerance. *Science* **165**:402, 1969.
506. Morris RC, Ueki I, Loh D, et al.: Absence of renal fructose-1-phosphate aldolase activity in hereditary fructose intolerance. *Nature* **214**:920, 1967.
507. Ali M, Cox TM: Diverse mutations in the aldolase B gene that underlle the prevalence of hereditary fructose intolerance. *Am J Hum Genet* **56**:1002, 1995.
508. Ali M, Sebastio G, Cox TM: Identification of a novel mutation (Leu256 → Pro) in human aldolase B gene associated with hereditary fructose intolerance. *Hum Mol Genet* **3**:203, 1994.
509. Santamaria R, Tamasl S, Del Piano G, et al.: Molecular basis of hereditary fructose intolerance in Italy: Identification of two novel mutations in the aldolase B gene. *J Med Genet* **33**:786, 1996.
510. Cross NCP, Stojanov LM, Cox TM: A new aldolase B variant, N334K, is a common cause of hereditary fructose intolerance in Yugoslavia. *Nucleic Acids Res* **18**:1925, 1990.
511. Ali M: The molecular basis of fructose intolerance. PhD Thesis, University of Cambridge, UK, 1995.
512. Kajihara S, Mukai T, Arai Y, et al.: Hereditary fructose intolerance caused by a nonsense mutation of the aldolase B gene. *Am J Hum Genet* **47**:562, 1990.
513. Cross NCP, Cox TM: Partial aldolase B gene deletions in hereditary fructose intolerance. *Am J Hum Genet* **47**:101, 1990.
514. Dazzo C, Tolan DR: Molecular evidence for compound heterozygosity in hereditary fructose intolerance. *Am J Hum Genet* **46**:1194, 1990.
515. Brooks CC, Buist N, Tuerck J, Tolan DR: Identification of a splice-site mutation in the aldolase B gene from an individual with hereditary fructose intolerance. *Am J Hum Genet* **49**:1075, 1991.
516. Böhme H-J, personal communication.
517. Ali M, Tunman G, Cross NCP, et al.: Null alleles of the aldolase B gene in patients with heredity fructose intolerance. *J Med Genet* **31**:499, 1994.
518. Antonorakis S and the Nomenclature Working Group: Recommendations for a nomenclature system for human gene mutations. *Hum Mut* **11**:1, 1998.
519. Rellos P, Ali M, Vidallhet M, et al.: Alteration of substrate specificity by a naturally-occurring aldolase B mutation (Ala337 > Val) in fructose intolerance. *Biochem J* **340**:321, 1999.
520. Rellos P, Sygusch J, Cox TM: Expression, purification, and characterization of natural mutants of human aldolase B: Role of quaternary structure in catalysis. *J Biol Chem* **275**:1145, 2000.

CHAPTER 71

Glycogen Storage Diseases

Yuan-Tsong Chen

1. **Glycogen storage diseases are inherited disorders that affect glycogen metabolism. Virtually all proteins involved in the synthesis or degradation of glycogen and its regulation have been discovered to cause some type of glycogen storage disease. The glycogen found in these disorders is abnormal in quantity, quality, or both. The different forms of glycogen storage disease have been categorized by number in accordance with the chronological order in which these enzymatic defects were identified.**
   Liver and muscle have abundant quantities of glycogen and are the most commonly and seriously affected tissues. Because carbohydrate metabolism in the liver is responsible for plasma glucose homeostasis, glycogen storage diseases that mainly affect the liver usually have hepatomegaly and hypoglycemia as the presenting features.
   In contrast, the role of glycogen in muscle is to provide substrates for the generation of ATP for muscle contraction. The predominant clinical features of glycogen storage diseases that mainly affect the muscle are muscle cramps, exercise intolerance, susceptibility to fatigue, and progressive weakness.
2. **Type Ia glycogen storage disease, or von Gierke Disease (MIM 23220), is caused by a deficiency of glucose 6-phosphatase activity in the liver, kidney, and intestinal mucosa, with excessive accumulation of glycogen in these organs. The stored materials in the liver include both glycogen and fat. The clinical manifestations are growth retardation, hepatomegaly, hypoglycemia, lactic acidemia, hyperuricemia, and hyperlipidemia. A variant caused by a defect in the transport of glucose 6-phosphate (type Ib) (MIM 23220) has the additional findings of neutropenia and impaired neutrophil function, resulting in recurrent bacterial infections and oral and intestinal mucosa ulceration. Both type Ia and Ib genes have been cloned and mutations responsible for the diseases identified.**
   In the past, many patients with type I glycogen storage disease died, and the prognosis was guarded in those who survived. Long-term complications include gout, hepatic adenomas, osteoporosis, renal disease, and short stature. Major progress has been made in managing this disorder. The current treatment of type I glycogen storage disease is nocturnal nasogastric infusion of glucose or orally administered uncooked cornstarch. Both methods are effectively improving growth, reducing hepatomegaly and sustaining the commonly measured metabolic indexes of adequate therapy in patients with type I glycogen storage disease.
   Early diagnosis and early initiation of an effective treatment have improved the outcome of the disease, but it is not known if all long-term complications can be avoided by good metabolic control. Some early treated patients who are now adults still develop hepatic adenomas and proteinuria.
3. **Type II glycogen storage disease, also known as Pompe Disease (MIM 232300), is caused by a deficiency of lysosomal acid α-glucosidase and is the prototype of an inborn lysosomal storage disease. This disease is described in Chap. 135.**
4. **Type III glycogen storage disease (MIM 232400) is caused by a deficiency of glycogen debranching enzyme activity. A deficiency of debranching enzyme impairs the release of glucose from glycogen but does not affect glucose released from gluconeogenesis. The glycogen accumulated has a structure that resembles limit dextrin (glycogen with short outer chains).**
   Most patients with type III glycogen storage disease have both liver and muscle involvement (type IIIa). However, some patients (~15 percent of all type III cases) have only liver involvement, without apparent muscle disease (type IIIb). During infancy and childhood, both type IIIa and IIIb diseases may be almost indistinguishable from type I disease, as hepatomegaly, hypoglycemia, hyperlipidemia, and growth retardation are similar predominant features. In type III, however, blood lactate and uric acid levels are usually normal, and elevations of liver transaminases are prominent. The liver symptoms in general improve with age and disappear after puberty. Progressive liver cirrhosis and failure however may occur in adulthood. In patients with disease also involving muscle (type IIIa), muscle weakness, though minimal during childhood, can become predominant in adults; these patients show signs of neuromuscular involvement, with slowly progressive weakness and distal muscle wasting. Cardiac muscle is also involved with ventricular hypertrophy a frequent EKG finding.
   Treatment of type III disease is symptomatic; if hypoglycemia is present, frequent meals high in carbohydrates, with cornstarch supplements or nocturnal gastric drip feeding, constitute effective therapy. A high-protein diet may also be effective in preventing hypoglycemia as gluconeogenesis is intact in these patients. Currently, there is no effective treatment for the progressive myopathy or cardiomyopathy.
5. **Type IV glycogen storage disease (MIM 232500) is caused by a deficiency of branching enzyme activity, which results in the accumulation of glycogen with unbranched, long, outer chains in the tissues. This form of glycogen storage disease typically presents in the first year of life, with hepatosplenomegaly and failure to thrive. Hypoglycemia is rarely seen. Progressive liver cirrhosis with portal hypertension, ascites, esophageal varices, and death, usually occur before the age of 5 years. Liver transplantation has been performed and may be an effective treatment. However, caution should be taken in selecting patients for liver transplantation as a nonpogressive hepatic form of the**

A list of standard abbreviations is located immediately preceding the index in each volume. Additional abbreviations used in this chapter include: GLUT1-5 = glucose transporter 1–5; *PGYB, PGYL, PGYM*, gene symbols for brain, liver, and muscle isoforms of phosphorylase, respectively; *PHKA1, PHKB, PHKG2* = gene symbols for α_1, β, and α_2 subunits of phosphorylase kinase, respectively; PKA = cAMP-dependent protein kinase A; PKB = protein kinase B.

disease exists and extrahepatic manifestations of the disease may occur after transplantation. In addition to the hepatic form, there are variant forms with neuromuscular presentation.

6. **Type V glycogen storage disease, also known as McArdle Disease (MIM 232600), is caused by a deficiency of muscle phosphorylase activity. Symptoms usually appear in adulthood and are characterized by exercise intolerance with muscle cramps that can be accompanied by attacks of myoglobinuria.**
   Exercise tolerance can be augmented by aerobic training or by oral administration of glucose or fructose. Avoidance of strenuous exercise prevents the symptoms.
7. **Type VI (MIM 232700) and type IX (MIM 306000) glycogen storage diseases represent a heterogeneous group of diseases caused by a deficiency of the liver phosphorylase system. In this chapter, we refer to type VI as a defect in liver phosphorylase itself, and type IX as a defect in one of the four subunits of phosphorylase kinase. It should be noted that the latter enzyme deficiency has also been classified as VIa or VIII in the past. Patients with either phosphorylase or phosphorylase kinase deficiencies present in early childhood with hepatomegaly and growth retardation. Hypoglycemia and hyperlipidemia are variable and, if present, usually mild. There is no hyperlactic acidemia or hyperuricemia. Treatment is based on the symptoms with a high-carbohydrate diet and frequent feedings to alleviate hypoglycemia. Most patients require no specific treatment. These are, in general, benign forms of glycogen storage disease. Prognosis is good; adult patients have normal stature and minimal hepatomegaly. In contrast to the other types of glycogen storage disease, which are inherited in an autosomal recessive manner, family studies indicate an X-linked inheritance in most patients with liver phosphorylase kinase deficiency.**
   Other phosphorylase kinase deficiency variants include an autosomal recessive type that affects both liver and muscle (MIM 261750) or liver only, a myopathic form that resembles type V glycogen storage disease, and an isolated myocardial phosphorylase kinase deficiency (MIM 261740). The clinical heterogeneity can be explained by the presence of four subunits of phosphorylase kinase variably expressed in tissue-specific manners.
8. **Type VII glycogen storage disease (MIM 232800) is caused by a deficiency of muscle phosphofructokinase activity. The clinical features are very similar to those in type V glycogen storage disease with the notable exceptions of a compensated hemolytic anemia and early onset myogenic hyperuricemia. In addition to the accumulation of normal glycogen in muscle, an abnormal glycogen, resembling amylopectin, can be found in some muscle fibers.**
9. **Other glycogenoses discussed in this chapter are glycogen synthase deficiency (MIM 240600), hepatic glycogenosis with renal Fanconi Syndrome (MIM 227810), phosphoglucoisomerase deficiency, muscle phosphoglycerate kinase deficiency (MIM 311800), phosphoglycerate mutase deficiency (MIM 261670), lactate dehydrogenase deficiency (MIM 50000), fructose 1,6-bisphosphate aldolase A deficiency (MIM 103850), and muscle pyruvate kinase deficiency. All these disorders are extremely rare conditions. The latter five represent muscle glycogenoses with a defect in glycolysis and cause symptoms and signs similar to type V glycogen storage disease.**
   Hepatic glycogenosis with renal Fanconi Syndrome is now known to be caused by defects in the facilitative glucose transporter 2 (GLUT2), which transports glucose in and out of hepatocytes, pancreatic beta cells and the basolateral membranes of intestinal and renal epithelial cells.

GLYCOGEN AND ITS METABOLISM

The Proteins of Glycogen Metabolism

The genetic deficiencies of the proteins involved in both glycogen metabolism and its regulation result in a wide spectrum of clinical disorders. During the past 50 years, the study of these genetic deficiencies has been invaluable to scientists and has led to a greatly increased understanding of the proteins and their regulation. A surprisingly wide variety of types of proteins are involved in glycogen metabolism; for example, debranching enzyme is a large monomeric protein with two independent catalytic sites; phosphorylase kinase is a large, multisubunit protein complex; and glucose 6-phosphatase system is composed of at least two different membrane-bound proteins. Most of the proteins involved in glycogen metabolism are highly regulated by allosteric mechanisms and/or by covalent modification, and there is coordinated control of the pathways of carbohydrate metabolism.

Advances in understanding the molecular basis of the various genetic deficiencies, their proteins and regulation are, in turn, being used to improve both the methods of diagnosis and the prediction of the clinical outcome. In the longer term, the molecular studies will hopefully lead to the development of successful gene therapy for the more severe disorders.

Function of Glycogen

Glucose is the primary source of energy for most mammalian cells. It is, therefore, an advantage to an individual to be able to take up excess glucose from the bloodstream at times of plenty and store it in macromolecular form for future use. Glycogen is the storage form of glucose in virtually all animal cells.[1] It is most abundant in liver and muscle. In different tissues, the primary function of glycogen varies. In skeletal muscle, glycogen is a fuel source for the cells in which it is stored, and it is used for short-term, high-energy consumption. In the brain, it provides an emergency supply of energy for use during brief periods of hypoglycemia or hypoxia. In contrast, liver takes up glucose from the bloodstream at times of plenty (e.g., after a meal) and stores it as glycogen. Whenever blood glucose levels start to fall, the liver releases glucose into the blood for use by tissues that cannot themselves make significant amounts of glucose (e.g., brain, muscle, and erythrocytes).

The glycogen storage diseases are genetic deficiencies, which result in the storage of abnormal amounts and/or forms of glycogen. Some deficiencies affect only one tissue; others can affect several tissues. To understand the clinical complexity of the glycogen storage diseases, it is first necessary to understand the structure of glycogen and the properties and regulation of the proteins involved in its synthesis and degradation.

Structure of Glycogen

There are different forms of glycogen in liver and muscle. In muscle, glycogen forms β particles, which are spherical and can contain up to 60,000 glucose residues. Liver contains, in addition, rosettes of glycogen called α particles, which look like aggregated β particles. These particles represent dynamic cellular organelles called glycosomes and consist of a protein component, which provides the enzymatic machinery of the organelle, and of glycogen, which is the product of its synthetic activity. Under the electron microscope these particles interpreted as glycogen are actually the protein component stainable with uranium and lead.[2] The glucose residues in glycogen are joined in straight chains by α1–4 linkages, which are branched at intervals of 4 to 10 residues with α1–6 linkages (Fig. 71-1).

In the past 15 years, significant progress has been made toward understanding the mechanism of glycogen biosynthesis (see

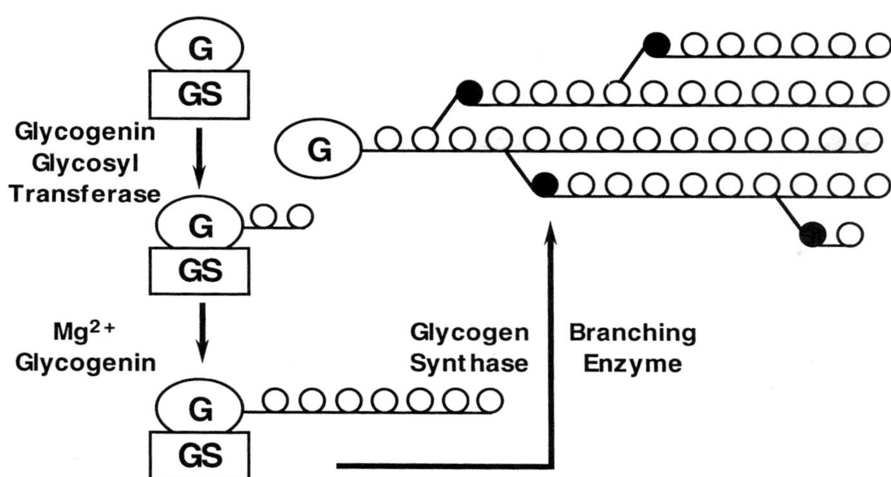

Fig. 71-1 Schematic of synthesis of a small portion of a glycogen molecule. G represents a glycogenin protein molecule and GS represents a glycogen synthase protein molecule. Each small circle represents a single glucose molecule. Open symbols represent the linear portions of glycogen with glucose molecules in a 1–4 linkage. Closed circles represent branch points with 1–6 linkages.

Fig. 71-1) (see references 3 and 4). The initiation of glycogen synthesis involves a protein "primer" which was first proposed in 1972[5] and later identified as a protein named glycogenin.[6] The first step is the attachment of one or two glucose molecules to tyrosine 194 of the glycogenin protein by autoglucosylation[6–8] (see Fig. 71-1). The second stage is the addition of six (or seven) more glucose molecules via a divalent cation-dependent autoglucosylation reaction again catalyzed by glycogenin, which is itself a uridine diphosphoglucose requiring glucosyltransferase[9] (see Fig. 71-1). Glycogenin with eight glucose residues attached is the primer for the third stage, which is the elongation of the glucose chain by glycogen synthase and branching of the chain by the branching enzyme (see Fig. 71-1). Initially glycogen synthase and glycogenin are present as a complex in a 1:1 ratio, and one molecule of each is present per β particle of glycogen. Only glycogen synthase that is complexed to glycogenin is capable of elongating the primer, although logically the glycogen synthase and glycogenin must dissociate as the glycogen molecule grows larger to allow glycogen synthase to reach the outer branches.

Glycogenin in liver and muscle is a 37-kDa protein encoded by a single gene on chromosome 3q24.[10] Recent study indicates the presence of a second glycogenin gene in the liver, which encodes 3 isoforms different in the N-terminal with molecular masses ranging from 51 to 55 kDa.[11] It has been suggested that liver glycogen α particles might be formed by the cross-linking of β particles through their glycogenin molecules, but as there appears to be only one glycogenin molecule per α particle this cannot be the explanation of the rosette structure of α particles. Glycogen is not always composed exclusively of glucose residues and glycogenin; there are reports of the presence of small and very variable quantities of bound phosphate and glucosamine.[12] The presence of glucosamine is common in liver glycogen, but it is absent in muscle glycogen. The role of these additional trace components is not clear, but the average molecular size of liver glycogen seems to increase with increasing glucosamine and phosphate content. The glucose chains of glycogen are broken down by the enzymes phosphorylase and debranching enzyme (Fig. 71-2). To date no genetic deficiencies of glycogenin have been reported.

Enzymes That Synthesize and Break Down Glycogen

Uridine Diphosphoglucose (UDP-Glc) Pyrophosphorylase. UDP-Glc pyrophosphorylase catalyzes the conversion of glucose 1-phosphate plus uridine triphosphate (UTP) to UDP-Glc and pyrophosphate (see Fig. 71-2), and it is inhibited by UDP and UDP-Glc.[13] It provides the UDP-Glc, which is needed by glycogen synthase (see Fig. 71-2) and for gluccuronide synthesis and galactose metabolism.[14] Liver UDP-Glc pyrophosphorylase is a large protein with a molecular mass of approximately 400 kDa.

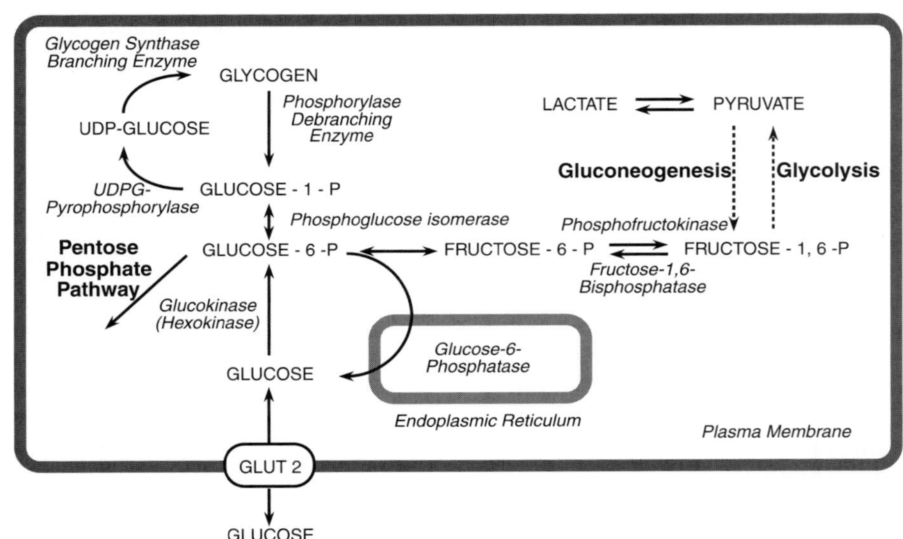

Fig. 71-2 Major pathways of synthesis and breakdown of glycogen in liver. The broken line indicates that several enzymes have been omitted between pyruvate and fructose-1,6-P_2. GLUT= glucose transport protein; UDP=uridine diphosphate; UDPG=uridine diphosphate-glucose.

It is comprised of eight identical catalytic subunits, each having a catalytic site. The enzyme has a low K_m for glucose 1-phosphate and is present in very high levels in liver, so in the vast majority of metabolic conditions, it is not the rate-limiting step in glycogen metabolism. The muscle enzyme is also comprised of eight subunits, each of which has a molecular mass of 53 kDa.[15] There have also been reports of a second smaller liver isoenzyme associated with Golgi membranes.[16] To date no human genetic deficiencies of this enzyme have been reported. A mammalian cell line with a persistent low level of UDP-glucose was found to have mutations in the UDP-glucose pyrophosphorylase gene.[17]

Glycogen Synthase. Glycogen synthase catalyzes the synthesis of glycogen by transferring glucose units from UDP-Glc to a glycogen primer (see Fig. 71-1). The initial glycogen primer is the glycogenin protein with eight glucosyl units attached (see above). Liver and muscle glycogen synthase (Gen Bank P54840, J04501) are different gene products, and they are oligomeric proteins with a subunit molecular mass of approximately 85 kDa. Both liver and muscle glycogen synthase genes have been cloned.[18,19] A distinct glycogen synthase gene from brain has also been cloned.[20]

Glycogen synthase is the rate-limiting enzyme in glycogen synthesis, and it is very highly regulated. Insulin stimulates the activity of glycogen synthase by decreasing its level of phosphorlation.[21] Epinephrine and glucagon inhibit glycogen synthase by increasing its level of phosphorylation.[22] The inhibitory action of epinephrine or glucagon is dominant, as it can override the effect of insulin.[23]

The phosphorylation of glycogen synthase is very complex, and at least nine serine residues of the protein can be phosphorylated by a wide variety of different protein kinases. In addition, the phosphorylation of different serines has distinct effects.[24] The inhibitory effects of phosphorylation on the activity of glycogen synthase are reversed by the allosteric activator glucose 6-phosphate.

The effects of glucagon and epinephrine on liver-glycogen synthase are indirect (Fig. 71-3). For example, glucagon activates

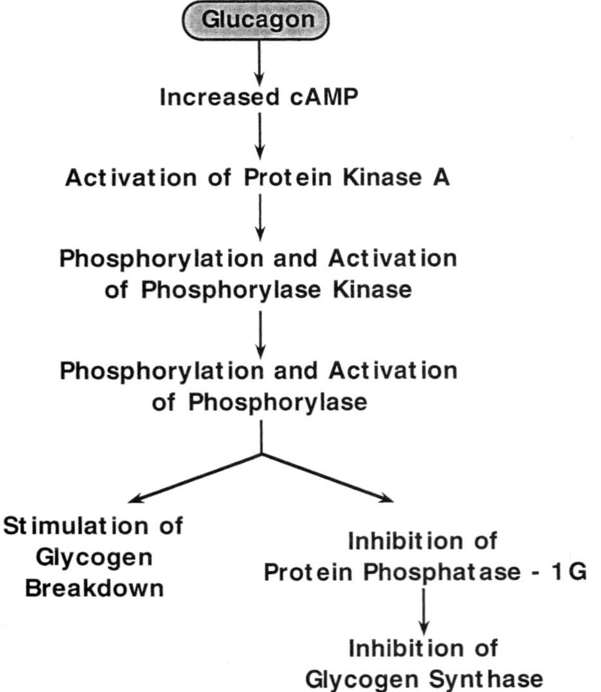

Fig. 71-3 The pathways of inhibition of glycogen synthase and activation of phosphorylase by glucagon. cAMP=cyclic adenosine monophosphate.

cAMP-dependent protein kinase in liver, which activates phosphorylase kinase, which, in turn, activates phosphorylase (see Fig. 71-3). The phosphorylated phosphorylase then inhibits the liver-glycogen-bound form of protein phosphatase 1, which is the enzyme that catalyzes the dephosphorylation of glycogen synthase. Thus, the level of phosphorylation of glycogen synthase remains high and its activity is inhibited (see Fig. 71-3).[25] The effects of insulin on liver-glycogen synthase are complicated. The direct pathway involves activation of p13 kinase through activation of the insulin receptor, which leads to a more active form of glycogen synthase. The indirect pathway involves lowering the level of cyclic AMP in liver, thereby decreasing the level of phosphorylase *a* and relieving the inhibition of the protein phosphatase 1.[25a]

In contrast, the action of insulin on muscle-glycogen synthase is directly mediated through the muscle-glycogen-bound form of protein phosphatase 1 (see reference 26). Briefly, insulin activates glycogen synthase via mitogen-activated protein (MAP) kinase-dependent phosphorylation of p90rsk which in turn phoshorylates the Ser 46 in the glycogen binding subunit (also called regulatory subunit) of potein phosphatase 1, leading to dephosphorylation and activation of the synthase.[27] An alternative pathway is that insulin activates glycogen synthase by inhibiting glycogen synthase kinase-3 (GSK-3) via the activation of protein kinase RAC/Akt, also known as protein kinase B (PKB).[28] In turn, the PKB phosphorylates and inactivates GSK-3, leading to dephosphorylation and activation of the synthase. β-Adrenergic agonists act via protein kinase A to phosphorylate Ser 65 in the glycogen-binding subunit of the protein phosphatase 1, leading to the dissociation of protein phosphatase 1 from the binding subunit, thus inhibiting protein phosphatase 1 from acting on glycogen synthase. Genetic deficiency of muscle glycogen synthase has not been reported; transgenic mice overexpressing muscle synthase gene is associated with increased glycogen accumulation.[29] Genetic deficiency of liver glycogen synthase activity causes a decrease in liver glycogen stores and fasting hypoglycemia (see "Glycogen Synthetise Deficiency," below).

Branching Enzyme. Branching enzyme transfers a minimum of six α1–4-linked glucosyl units from the outer end of a chain of glycogen into an α1–6 position on the same or a neighboring chain.[30] Branching of the chains of glucosyl units is essential to pack a very large number of glucosyl units into a relatively soluble spherical molecule; the genetic deficiency of branching enzyme activity (type IV glycogen storage disease) is a disorder that leads to the production of relatively insoluble glycogen, which may be the cause of liver cell damage. Branching enzyme has been purified from rat liver as a monomeric protein with a molecular mass of approximately 71 kDa.[31] Human branching enzyme cDNA has been cloned (GenBank L07956) and it appears to be encoded by a single copy gene located on chromosome 3p.[32] The protein deduced from the open reading frame of the cDNA consists of 702 amino acids with a predicted molecular mass of 80 kDa. Branching enzyme is much less abundant in muscle than in liver.

Debranching Enzyme. Debranching enzyme is unusual because it is one of the few known proteins with two independent catalytic activities occurring at separate sites on a single polypeptide chain.[33–35] The two active sites utilize different catalytic mechanisms (Fig. 71-4).[34] Phosphorylase degrades the glycogen chains until only four glucosyl units remain before an α1–6 branch point (see Fig. 71-4). Debranching enzyme then transfers three glucose residues from the short branch to the end of another branch using its transferase (1,4-α-D-glucan; 1,4-α-D-glucan 4-αD-glycosyltransferase) activity (see Fig. 71-4). Debranching enzyme can then hydrolyze the remaining α1–6 branch-point glucose residue using its amylo-1,6-glucosidase activity. For normal, full debranching enzyme activity, both catalytic activities are required. Phosphorylase and debranching enzyme can, therefore, completely degrade glycogen (see Fig. 71-2). Debranching enzyme has been purified from several species and shown to be a large monomeric protein with a molecular mass of 160 to 170 kDa in both muscle and liver.[35–37] Both human and rabbit debranching enzyme cDNAs have been cloned.[38,39] Asp at amino acid codon 549 has been assigned as a putative catalytic nucleophile of the transferase site via trapping of the glucosyl-enzyme intermediate.[40] The human debranching enzyme gene is a large, single copy gene (GenBank M85168) located on chromosome 1p21,[41] the same region that amylase genes are mapped. The human debranching enzyme gene spans 85 kb and contains 35 exons.[42] Six mRNA isoforms different in the 5′ untranslated region and tissue distribution result from differential transcription and alternative exon usage of a single debrancing enzyme gene.[43] The major mRNA isoform present in both muscle and liver encodes a protein of 1532 amino acid residues with a calculated molecular mass of 174 kDa.[38,43] The genetic deficiency of debranching enzyme activity is known as type III glycogen storage disease.

Phosphorylase. Phosphorylase catalyzes the sequential cleavage of glucosyl units from α-1,4-glucosyl-linked chains of glycogen, and in doing so, it liberates glucose 1-phosphate (see Fig. 71-4).[44] Three human phosphorylase isoenzymes (termed "liver," "muscle," and "brain" based on the tissues in which they are preferentially expressed) have been cloned[45–47] (GenBank AF046785, M16013 for liver and muscle, respectively), and shown to be products of separate genes which map on different chromosomes.[48,49] In addition, there is a second brain phosphorylase gene, and there have been several reports of other possible forms of mammalian phosphorylases (see reference 44). All the phosphorylase isoenzymes contain pyridoxal phosphate as a cofactor. The most active form of phosphorylase is a homodimer. Phosphorylase is highly regulated. All three characterized isoenzymes are activated by phosphorylation at Ser 14 in response to epinephrine or glucagon (see Fig. 71-3)[23] and are inhibited by dephosphorylation by protein phosphatase 1.[44] The allosteric regulation of the three phosphorylase isoenzymes is different.[50,51] For example, they are differentially activated by AMP and inhibited by glucose 6-phosphate. The muscle phosphorylase is also neurally regulated; denervation or prolonged muscle inactivity causes decreased steady-state levels of the transcript.[52] Genetic deficiency of muscle phosphorylase activity and liver phosphorylase activity each cause different forms of glycogen storage disease with different clinical manifestations.

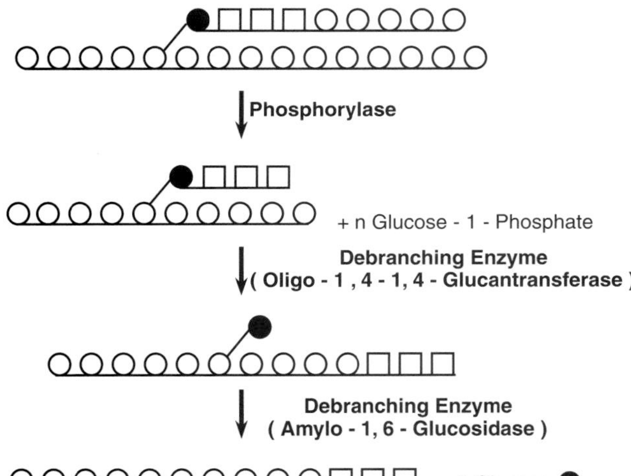

Fig. 71-4 Schematic of the degradation of a small outer portion of a glycogen molecule. Each small square or circle represents a single glucose molecule. Open symbols represent the linear portions of glycogen with the glucose molecules in a 1–4 linkage. Closed circles represent branch points with 1–6 linkages.

Acid α-Glucosidase. Glycogen can also be degraded in lysosomes by the enzyme acid α-glucosidase. This enzyme is described in Chap. 135.

Enzymes That Regulate Glycogen Phosphorylase and Synthase

Glycogen synthase and phosphorylase activities are both hormonally regulated via a variety of phosphorylation and dephosphorylation mechanisms. The hormonal signals have opposite effects on the activity of the two enzymes. Therefore, a deficiency of any of the enzymes involved in the regulation of glycogen synthase and/or phosphorylase also has the potential to cause glycogen storage disease.

Phosphorylase Kinase. Phosphorylase kinase is a protein kinase, which phosphorylates and activates phosphorylase (see Fig. 71-3), whose role is to increase glycogen breakdown in response to either neuronal or hormonal stimulation.[53] Phosphorylase kinase is itself activated by Ca^{2+} and by phosphorylation by cAMP-dependent protein kinase (see Fig. 71-3). Phosphorylase kinase is a multisubunit protein with a molecular mass of 1300 and four different subunits, α, β, γ, and δ; the subunit structure is $(\alpha\beta\gamma\delta)_4$.[54,55] The molecular masses of the four subunits are 138, 125, 43, and 17 kDa, respectively. The α- and β-subunits are regulatory subunits (regulated by phosphorylation); γ is the catalytic subunit;[56] and the δ subunit is the protein calmodulin[55] and is the subunit regulated by Ca^{2+}. Calmodulin is a Ca^{2+}-binding protein with K_d for Ca^{2+} in the micromolar range. Calmodulin is not just part of phosphorylase kinase, it also interacts and activates several other protein kinases involved in other pathways. There are different isoenzymes of phosphorylase kinase in liver and muscle, and even different isoenzymes in white and red muscle.[57] There have been descriptions of many different variants of phosphorylase kinase deficiency, some X chromosomally inherited and some autosomally inherited, with great variations in severity, and in which tissues are affected (see "Type VI and IX Glycogen Storage Disease," below). Very elegant studies involving cloning of the different subunits of phosphorylase kinase (see reference 58) have greatly increased our understanding of phosphorylase kinase and its various genetic deficiencies.

The α and β subunits of phosphorylase kinase have extensive regions of homology, but each subunit also possesses unique sequences.[59] It has been shown that the α and β subunits are encoded by a family of three genes.[60,61] What appears to have occurred in evolutionary terms is that the α and β genes diverged, and each acquired DNA sequences for subunit-specific domains that can be phosphorylated. Then later, two α-subunit genes diverged. Both α-subunit genes are on the X chromosome but in different regions.[62] One α-subunit gene encodes the predominant liver α subunit (GenBank X80497) and the other α-subunit gene encodes a predominantly muscle α subunit. Both genes are expressed in heart and brain. In addition, two differentially spliced subtypes of the muscle α subunit have been described, as well as three differentially spliced subtypes of the β subunit.[61] Only one β-subunit gene (GenBank J04120) is known to date, and it was localized to chromosome 16q12-13.[63]

The muscle γ subunit has been cloned (GenBank X80590) and it was localized to chromosome 7p12-q21.[64–66] A second isoform of the γ subunit preferentially expressed in the testis and liver has also been cloned[67] (GenBank M31606) and it was localized to chromosome 16p.[68]

The δ subunit is the protein calmodulin, and there are three human autosomal calmodulin genes located on chromosomes 2p21, 14q24-31, and 19q13.[69,70] There is no specific gene for the phosphorylase kinase δ subunit; it seems to come from the whole calmodulin mRNA pool in the cells.[71] Therefore, mutations in calmodulin genes are not likely to cause isolated phosphorylase kinase deficiency, as they would be expected to produce much more complex and severe phenotypes as calmodulin has many cellular roles.

cAMP-Dependent Protein Kinase. cAMP-dependent protein kinase (PKA) phosphorylates and activates phosphorylase kinase (see Fig. 71-3). It also phosphorylates and regulates a large number of other enzymes in other pathways, and plays an important role in the regulation of some transcriptional events.[72] cAMP-dependent protein kinase is a heterotetramer comprised of two regulatory and two catalytic subunits. The binding of cAMP to the regulatory subunits leads to dissociation of the tetramer and release of the active catalytic subunits, which are then able to phosphorylate target proteins.[73] There are multiple genes for each type of subunit of cAMP-dependent protein kinase.[74]

Protein Phosphatase. There are four major types of protein (serine/threonine) phosphatases in mammalian cells (see reference 75), but protein phosphatase 1 and protein phosphatase 2A are the only phosphatases in muscle with significant activity toward the enzymes of glycogen metabolism.[76] Protein phosphatase 1 plays the major role, as it has activity toward glycogen synthase, phosphorylase, and phosphorylase kinase. The catalytic subunit of protein phosphatase 1 has a molecular mass of 37 kDa, and it has been cloned from skeletal muscle.[77–79] In muscle, the major active forms of protein phosphatase 1 are bound to glycogen (and to sarcoplasmic reticulum) and have been termed "protein phosphatase 1G."[80] Protein phosphatase 1 binds to glycogen via a large, highly asymmetric, glycogen binding (G) subunit (also called regulatory subunit) of molecular mass 126 kDa. It is the G subunit, which is phosphorylated by insulin-sensitive protein kinase (see "Glycogen Synthase," above). Recent studies indicate other protein phosphatase 1-binding proteins with a role in glycogen metabolism are also present.[81,82] No genetic deficiencies of protein phosphatase 1 have been reported.

Protein phosphatase 2A has some activity toward glycogen synthase, phosphorylase, and phosphorylase kinase, and it is the major phosphatase acting on the α subunit of phosphorylase kinase in muscle. It has a molecular mass of 36 kDa.[76] Genes coding for catalytic and regulatory subunits of protein phosphatase 2A have been isolated from a number of different species including man (see reference 75). No genetic deficiencies of protein phosphatase 2A have been reported.

Enzymes That Catalyze Reversible Steps

Most of the irreversible steps of glycogen metabolism, gluconeogenesis, and glycolysis (see Fig. 71-2) are highly regulated. In contrast, the reversible steps are not regulated. Nevertheless, a defect in either phosphoglucomutase or phosphoglucoisomerase would, because of the enzymes' positions in the pathways (see Fig. 71-2), have the potential to cause profound disturbances in the storage of glycogen.

Phosphoglucomutase. Phosphoglucomutase is the only enzyme that catalyzes a reversible step in the pathways of glycogen synthesis and glycogen breakdown (see Fig. 71-2). It catalyzes the reversible transfer of a phosphate group between the 6 and 1 positions of glucose. The reaction involves the formation of a phosphoenzyme intermediate and uses glucose 1,6-bisphosphate as a cofactor.[83] The thermodynamic equilibrium is in favor of the formation of glucose 6-phosphate, which occurs via an exchange-type mechanism.[84] There are at least three isoenzymes of phosphoglucomutase, and their genes are located on different chromosomes.[85,86] One of the isoenzymes, phosphoglucomutase 1, which is very polymorphic, has been cloned from human muscle, and the gene localized to chromosome 1q31. This gene has achieved prominence as a key marker in linkage mapping and in forensic medicine.[86]

Phosphoglucoisomerase. Phosphoglucoisomerase (often also called "glucose 6-phosphate isomerase" or "phosphohexose isomerase") catalyzes a reversible step in the glycolytic and gluconeogenic pathways (see Fig. 71-2). It catalyzes the interconversion of glucose 6-phosphate and fructose 6-phosphate. Phosphoglucoisomerase is not thought to be a rate-limiting step in either glycolysis or gluconeogenesis. An unexpected finding of the phosphoglucoisomerase is that it is the same protein as the autocrine motility factor, a tumor-secreted cytokine which stimulates cell migration in vitro and metastasis in vivo.[87] There are several human isoforms of phosphoglucoisomerase, all of which appear to be dimers.[88–90] There are a number of reports of isolated phosphoglucoisomerase deficiency in red blood cells causing hemolytic anemia (see Chap. 182) but there have been only two reports of generalized phosphoglucoisomerase deficiency causing mental retardation, muscle fatigue, and liver glycogen accumulation (see "Phosphoglucoisomerase Deficiency," below).

Interconversion of Glucose and Glucose 6-Phosphate

The tissue-specific differences in the regulation of most of the steps in the pathways involved in the synthesis and degradation of glycogen are brought about by the existence of tissue-specific isoenzymes; for example, for phosphorylase, phosphorylase kinase (see above). The reason that most tissues cannot make significant amounts of glucose is that the conversion of glucose 6-phosphate to glucose does not take place in most cell types (and many tissues, e.g., muscle), because no glucose 6-phosphatase activity is present. There are also major differences in the conversion of glucose to glucose 6-phosphate in liver and pancreatic islet β cells; in these two organs, the major enzyme is glucokinase and all other tissues contain the hexokinase isoenzymes. A knowledge of the roles and regulation of glucose 6-phosphatase, glucokinase, hexokinase, and the plasma membrane glucose transport proteins (see Fig. 71-2) is essential to understanding the different metabolic effects that the glycogen storage diseases have in various tissues.

Hexokinase. Three hexokinase isoenzymes (types I, II, and III) have been characterized. These isoenzymes catalyze the phosphorylation of glucose, and use ATP plus glucose to form glucose 6-phosphate and adenosine diphosphate. They have a very wide tissue distribution, including muscle and brain, and have a low K_m for glucose (0.05 to 0.15 mM, which is well below normal blood glucose concentrations). These isoenzymes are allosterically inhibited by their product, glucose 6-phosphate,[91] but are not regulated by insulin or glucagon. They are relatively nonspecific as they can also phosphorylate a variety of other sugars, for example, fructose and glucosamine. The molecular mass of the hexokinase family of proteins is approximately 100 kDa. The human and rat hexokinase isoenzymes have been cloned.[92,93] A comparison of deduced amino acid sequences from various hexokinases with glucokinase (see below) suggests that the larger hexokinases I-III arise from a glucokinase-like gene through gene duplication (see reference 94). Genetic deficiency of hexokinase I causes nonspherocytic hemolytic anemia[95] (See Chap. 182).

Glucokinase. Glucokinase also known as hexokinase IV, is a member of the same gene family as the hexokinases I-III. Glucokinase is expressed in liver and in pancreatic islet β cells.[96–99] Like the hexokinases, it uses ATP to catalyze the phosphorylation of glucose to form glucose 6-phosphate plus ADP. Glucokinase is a monomer with a molecular mass of 56 kDa. There are a number of metabolically significant differences between the hexokinases (see above) and liver glucokinase. Glucokinase has a K_m of approximately 8 mM for glucose (which means that enzyme activity can be affected by blood glucose levels); it is also not inhibited by physiological levels of glucose 6-phosphate. Glucokinase activity in liver is decreased in diabetes and starvation and can be increased again by insulin or refeeding, respectively. For many years, it was assumed that there was no short-term regulation of liver glucokinase, other than via its substrate concentration. There is now considerable evidence that liver glucokinase activity is highly regulated.[100,101] In addition, it has been suggested that glucokinase is a glucose sensor, or part of the glucose sensor, in both hepatocytes and pancreatic islet β cells.[102]

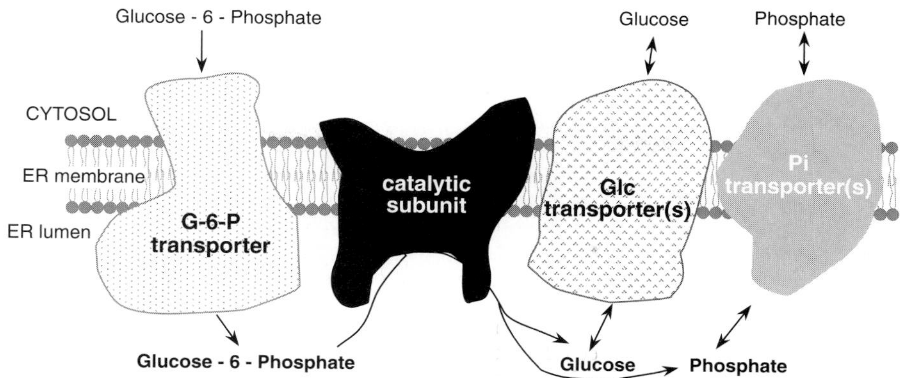

Fig. 71-5 Schematic working model of the hepatic microsomal glucose-6-phosphatase system. ER = endoplasmic reticulum. This model is not meant to represent the actual topology of the proteins in the membrane. The stoichiometry of each of the proteins is unknown, and it is unknown whether these proteins form a complex in the membrane. Phosphate transporter and glucose transporter proteins have not been unequivocally demonstrated and an alternative model that characterizes glucose 6-phosphatase as an integral channel-protein of the microsomal membrane, having both catalytic and transport functions, has been proposed.[447] In the alternative model, all transporter proteins would be missing from the diagram.

Glucokinase cDNAs have been cloned from both liver and pancreatic islets[98,99,103] and different promoters in the glucokinase gene control the tissue-specific expression in liver and islets have been shown.[97,99,104] Glucokinase is encoded by a single copy gene that has 11 exons. The transcripts present in the liver and β cell share sequences encoded by the last 9 exons but differ in the first 15 amino acids. In addition, heterogeneous expression of glucokinase in different pancreatic β cells has been reported.[105] Alternative splicing also produces different liver isoforms of glucokinase.[106] Loss of function mutations in this gene are associated with maturity onset diabetes of the young, which is characterized by decreased glucose phosphorylation and decreased insulin secretion (see reference 107). A gain of function missense mutation results in an increase of the affinity of glucokinase for glucose is a cause of an autosomal dominant form of familiar hyperinsulinism.[108]

The Glucose 6-Phosphatase System. Glucose 6-phosphatase catalyzes the final step of both gluconeogenesis and glycogen breakdown (see Fig. 71-2). It catalyzes the hydrolysis of glucose 6-phosphate to glucose and phosphate and is the only enzyme that is capable of producing significant amounts of glucose in the body; debranching enzyme (see Fig. 71-4) and acid α-glucosidase can make small amounts of glucose. Glucose 6-phosphatase is present in high levels only in liver, kidney, and pancreatic islet β cells.[109–112] Other tissues cannot produce significant levels of glucose, even though glucose 6-phosphatase is also present at low levels in human intestine,[111] gallbladder mucosa,[113] and in some cell types of the tissues, such as brain astrocytes.[114]

Glucose 6-phosphatase is unique among the enzymes described in this chapter in that its active site is situated inside the lumen of the endoplasmic reticulum,[115] whereas all other enzymes involved in glycogen metabolism are in the cytoplasm (see Fig. 71-2). This means that its substrates and products must cross the endoplasmic reticulum membrane (see Fig. 71-2) (see references 116 and 117). In vivo, four different proteins may be needed for normal glucose 6-phosphatase activity (see Fig. 71-5). The hydrolysis of glucose 6-phosphate was described in 1945,[118] and the deficiency of glucose 6-phosphatase activity in liver was first described in 1952,[119] but it is only in the past five years that the characterization of the glucose 6-phosphatase system proteins has rapidly progressed when the glucose 6-phosphatase and translocase genes were cloned.[120,121] The study of the glycogen storage diseases that result in deficiencies of liver glucose 6-phosphatase activity (i.e., glycogen storage diseases type 1a, 1b, and 1c) has been invaluable in identifying and characterizing the glucose 6-phosphatase proteins.

The Catalytic Subunit of Glucose 6-Phosphatase. The human glucose 6-phosphatase catalytic subunit gene is a single copy gene[120] (Gen Bank 401120) located on chromosome 17q21.[122] The human gene spans 12.5 kb and consists of 5 exons. The catalytic subunit consists of 357 amino acids with a calculated molecular mass of 40 kDa. This is in keeping with the apparent molecular mass of 36.5 kDa estimated by study of phosphoryl-enzyme intermediate[123] and a protein purified from rat liver.[124] The deduced protein is extremely hydrophobic and contains nine putative membrane-spanning segments[115] (Fig. 71-6), as well as the endoplasmic reticulum transmembrane protein retention signal at its C-terminus.[120] His176, located in the endoplasmic reticulum lumen, is the phosphate-acceptor site in glucose 6-phosphatase catalysis (Fig. 71-6). In addition to hydrolyzing glucose 6-phosphate, the catalytic subunit can also hydrolyze a number of other compounds (e.g., pyrophosphate and carbamyl phosphate) and can carry out a number of phosphotransferase reactions.[109] The glucose 6-phosphatase catalytic subunit mRNA and activity are both elevated in diabetes and starvation, and decreased by insulin.[125–127] The insulin effect is mediated via a cluster of insulin-responsive elements in the glucose 6-phosphatase gene promoter.[127] Thus, the gene for the catalytic unit is regulated in exactly the opposite way to glucokinase (see above). Like glucokinase, it was assumed that there is no short-term regulation of glucose 6-phosphatase activity, other than via its substrate concentration. It has become clear that both the catalytic subunit and the transport proteins of glucose 6-phosphatase can be regulated.[109,114,125–127] The genetic deficiency of the catalytic subunit is now commonly termed "type Ia glycogen storage disease" (see "Type I Glycogen Storage Disease (Glucose 6-Phosphatase Deficiency, Von Gierke Disease)" below).

Microsomal Glucose 6-Phosphate Transport. Glucose 6-phosphatase activity is latent. That is, there is more enzymatic activity in disrupted microsomal vesicles than there is in intact vesicles. To explain this phenomenon, it was proposed that there was a rate-limiting microsomal glucose 6-phosphate transport protein, termed "T1"[128,129] (see Fig. 71-5). T1 has not yet been purified to homogeneity, but its presence was demonstrated when a cDNA coding for the putative glucose 6-phosphate transporter was isolated and characterized[121] (GenBank Y15409). Mutations in this gene are responsible for genetic deficiency of microsomal glucose 6-phosphate transport termed "type Ib glycogen storage disease" (see "Glucose 6-Phosphatase Deficiency von Gierke Disease" below). The gene for glucose 6-phosphate transporter spans 5.3 kb (GenBank AF097831) and consists of 9 exons[130] located on chromosome 11q23.[130–132] The protein deduced from

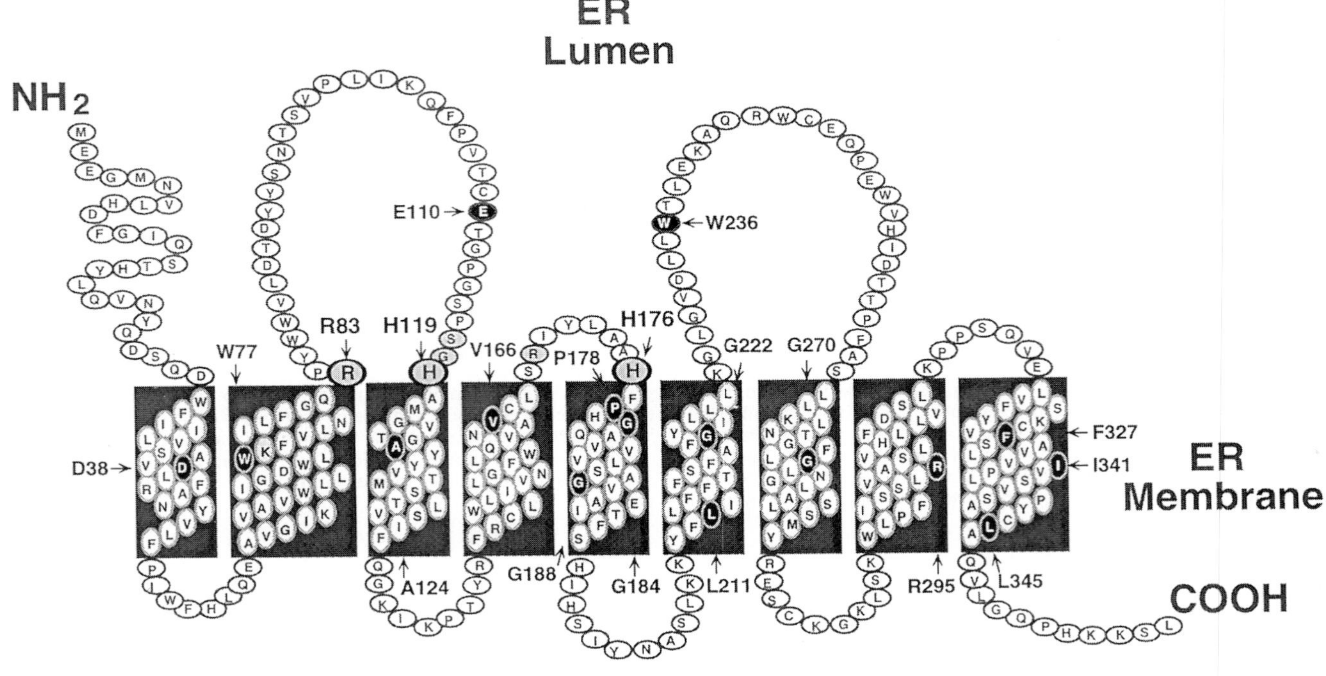

Fig. 71-6 The predicted nine-transmembrane helical structure of human glucose 6-phosphatase. The amino acids predicted to contribute to the active site of the enzyme are shaded. The locations of mutations identified in the type I glycogen storage disease patients are shown in black (*Courtesy of Janice Chou*[115] *with permission of the Journal of Biological Chemistry.*)

the open reading frame of the cDNA consists of 429 amino acids with a predicted molecular mass of 46 kDa. Like the catalytic subunit, the transporter protein also has the endoplasmic reticulum transmembrane protein retention signal, is highly hydrophobic, and contains 10 putative transmembrane domains.[121,132]

Microsomal Phosphate Transport. Phosphate is one of the products of glucose 6-phosphate hydrolysis (see Fig. 71-5). Phosphate is an inhibitor of the glucose 6-phosphatase enzyme, and if it was confined to the lumen of the endoplasmic reticulum, it would inhibit the enzyme.[133] A 37-kDa microsomal phosphate transport protein has been identified and purified.[134] It also transports pyrophosphate and carbamyl phosphate, which are both substrates of the glucose 6-phosphatase enzyme. Until recently, it was widely assumed that there was only one microsomal phosphate transport protein. If only one liver microsomal phosphate transport protein existed, phosphate should not be transported across the microsomal membrane in conditions under which the protein is completely deficient. However, in microsomes isolated from several human livers in which there is no microsomal pyrophosphate transport and no immunodetectable protein, phosphate can still be transported across the microsomal membrane.[133,134] This suggests that there may be a second microsomal phosphate transport protein. The genes for the putative phosphate transport proteins, however, have not been cloned. Thus a definitive conclusion of their presence and role in the genetic deficiency of microsomal phosphate transporter(s), also termed "type Ic glycogen storage disease" cannot be drawn at the present time.

Microsomal Glucose Transport. In the past few years, a family of plasma membrane facilitative glucose transport proteins, termed GLUTs 1–5 (and a pseudogene GLUT6), have been described.[135,136] The major liver and pancreatic islet β-cell plasma membrane glucose transport protein is GLUT2[137] (see Fig. 71-2), and the predominant muscle proteins are GLUT4 and GLUT1. The major difference between GLUT2 and GLUTs 1, 3, 4, and 5 is that GLUT2 has a much higher K_m for glucose. Deficiency of GLUT1 causes hypoglycorrhachia (low CSF glucose), infantile seizures, and developmental delay;[138] deficiency of GLUT2 (GenBank J03810) causes a syndrome termed "hepatic glycogenosis with renal Fanconi syndrome"[139] (see below). Glucose is the other product of the glucose 6-phosphatase enzyme, and it needs to cross the endoplasmic reticulum membrane (see Fig. 71-5). Genetic deficiency in microsomal glucose transporter has been termed type Id. However, the existence of the type Id defective in a glucose transporter remains to be demonstrated. An earlier suggestion that the GLUT7 cDNA encodes the microsomal glucose transporter was proven to be a cloning artifact.[140]

Glycolytic Proteins

Phosphofructokinase. Phosphofructokinase catalyzes the conversion of fructose 6-phosphate to fructose 1,6-bisphosphate. It is a key regulatory enzyme of glycolysis.[141,142]

Human phosphofructokinase is a tetramer with a subunit molecular mass of approximately 85 kDa. There are three different types of subunit, termed M (muscle), L (liver), and P (platelet).[143] Tissues may express one, two, or all three types of subunit which appear to form random tetramers to yield a wide variety of tissue-specific isoenzymes. Human muscle has homotetramers of the M-type subunit (GenBank 424183), and liver has homotetramers of the L-type subunit. In contrast, red blood cells have five different isoenzymes, and platelets have a further three different isoenzymes. This, presumably, partially explains the heterogeneous clinical manifestations of genetic deficiency of muscle phosphofructokinase activity, which is known as type VII glycogen storage disease (see "Type VII Glycogen Storage Disease (Phosphofructokinase Deficiency, Tarui Disease)" below).

The fructose 6-phosphate/fructose 1,6-bisphosphate cycle is very highly regulated.[144] Phosphofructokinase is allosterically regulated by numerous compounds; examples of negative effectors are ATP, citrate, and H^+. The most potent positive effectors are AMP and fructose 2,6-bisphosphate.[144,145] Fructose 2,6-bisphosphate levels are controlled by a bifunctional enzyme called "phosphofructokinase-2/fructose 2,6-bisphosphatase," which has two active sites, one that forms fructose 2,6-bisphosphate and the other that hydrolyzes it. This enzyme is itself regulated by cAMP-dependent protein kinase in liver (see references 143 and 144). It seems likely that genetic deficiencies of the bifunctional enzyme also exist, although none have been reported.

Regulation of Glycogen Metabolism

It is generally assumed that glycogen synthase controls the rate of glycogen synthesis. Recent in vivo NMR studies suggest, however, that at least in muscle, the control step may be at glucose transporter/hexokinase.[146] Obviously, glycogen metabolism is very tightly regulated, and there is coordinated control of the different pathways as well. Short-term hormonal control is mediated via allosteric regulation and/or covalent modification of the enzymes (via phosphorylation-dephosphorylation reactions) that catalyze most of the irreversible steps of the pathways (see Fig. 71-2). At the irreversible steps of the pathways there is constant substrate cycling,[145] for example, between glucose and glucose 6-phosphate[147,148] or between glycogen and glycogen and glucose 1-phosphate.[149] The cycling allows for very fine regulation of the direction of flux through the various pathways, and it means that even during period of rapid net glycogen synthesis, glycogen is still being degraded.[149,150] The direction of net flux through some, but not all, pathways can change rapidly in response to metabolic signals. Figure 71-7 is a diagrammatic representation of the changes that happen in liver rapidly after refeeding a starved individual. During starvation, glycogen breakdown and gluconeogenesis provide glucose 6-phosphate, which is hydrolyzed in liver to maintain blood glucose homeostasis. After refeeding, gluconeogenesis still provides glucose 6-phosphate, but now it is used for glycogen synthesis, and the liver takes up and uses glucose to make glycogen instead of making glucose.[151] There are two means by which glucose is converted into glycogen in the liver—the direct and indirect pathways. The direct pathway is glucose, glucose 6-phosphate, and glucose 1-phosphate to glycogen; the indirect pathway is glucose to gluconeogenic precursors, and then gluconeogenesis to glucose 6-phosphate and glycogen. A large amount of work has been done to quantify the relative contributions of the two pathways[151–153] and it seems that the relative importance of the two pathways varies depending on the precise metabolic conditions.

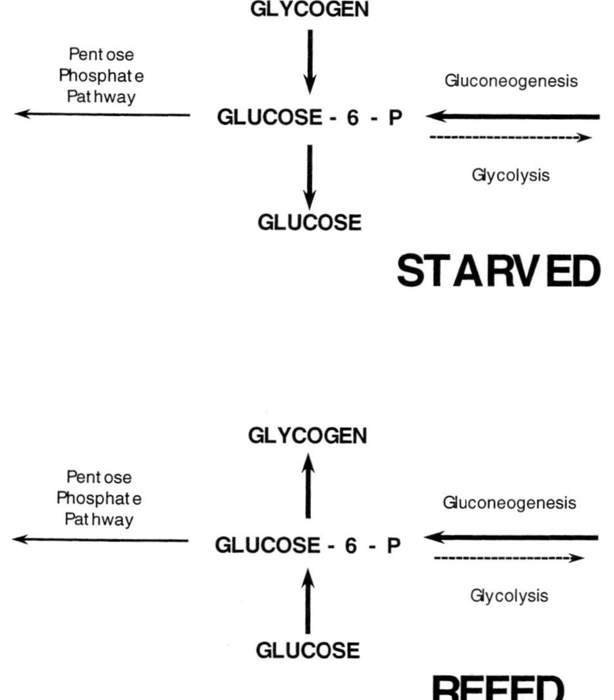

Fig. 71-7 Schematic of the way the direction of flux through the pathways of glycogen metabolism can change in response to metabolic needs.

Longer-term changes in the regulation of the expression of most of the proteins of glycogen metabolism also occur, as does tissue-specific expression. In addition, the expression of many of the enzymes varies greatly during development, and some have fetal isoforms and isoenzymes.[111,154–158]

INHERITED ABNOMALITIES IN GLYCOGEN METABOLISM

The first clinical description of a patient with a defect in glycogen mobilization was in 1928 by Snappes and Van Creveld.[159] Since then, a variety of disturbances of glycogen metabolism have been described. Biochemical classification began to be possible when the details of the pathways of glycogen metabolism were elucidated.[160] Over the past 50 years, virtually all proteins involved in the synthesis or degradation of glycogen and its regulation were discovered to cause some type of glycogen-storage disease.[1,161] There are over 12 forms of glycogen: storage disease presently known, and a wide spectrum of clinical presentations are seen. The different forms of glycogen-storage diseases have been categorized by numerical type in accord with the chronological order in which these enzymatic defects were identified. This numerical classification is still widely used, at least up to number VII. In this chapter, we follow that numerical order in the description of the various forms of glycogen-storage disease.

Liver and muscle have abundant quantities of glycogen and are the most common and seriously affected tissues. Because carbohydrate metabolism in the liver is responsible for plasma glucose homeostasis, glycogen storage diseases that mainly affect the liver have hepatomegaly and hypoglycemia as the usual presenting features. The types (and associated enzymatic deficiency) affecting the liver as the major organ are types I (glucose 6-phosphatase), III (debrancher), IV (brancher), VI (liver phosphorylase), and type IX (phosphorylase kinase), as well as glycogen synthase deficiency and glucose transporter-2 deficiency. The liver glycogen storage diseases vary in the age of onset, progression, other organ involvement, and clinical severity.

In contrast, the role of glycogen in muscle is to provide substrates, which enable the ATP generation that is necessary for muscle contraction. The glycogen storage diseases that principally affect the muscle can be divided into two groups. The first group is characterized by progressive skeletal muscle weakness and atrophy and/or cardiomyopathy, and is represented by a lysosomal enzyme deficiency (acid α-glucosidase, type II glycogen storage disease). This disease is described in Chap. 135. The second group is a muscle-energy disorder characterized by muscle pain, exercise intolerance, myoglobiuria, and susceptibility to fatigue. This group includes myophosphorylase deficiency (McArdle Disease, type V) and deficiencies of phosphofructokinase (type VII), phosphoglycerate kinase, phosphoglycerate mutase, lactate dehydrogenase, fructose 1,6-bisphosphate aldolase A, and muscle pyruvate kinase. Some of the latter enzyme deficiencies may also be associated with a compensated hemolysis, suggesting a more generalized defect in glucose metabolism (see Chap. 182.).

The overall frequency of all forms of glycogen storage diseases, based on European data, is approximately 1 in 20,000 to 25,000 live births.[161] Types I, II (lysosomal α-glucosidase

Table 71-1 Distribution of Various Types of Glycogenoses

Type	Enzyme	Number of Patients		% of Total
		Group 1*	Group 2†	
Liver glycogenoses				
Type I (Ib)	Glucose 6-phosphatase system	151 (15)	203 (33)	24.6
Type III	Glycogen debrancher enzyme	139	209	24.2
Type IV	Branching enzyme	7	40	3.3
Type VI & IX	Liver phosphorylase & phosphorylase kinase	256	176	30.0
Muscle glycogenoses				
Type II	Lysosomal α-1,4-glucosidase	104	116	15.3
Type V	Muscle phosphorylase	15	19	2.4
Type VII	Phosphofructokinase	0	3	0.2
Totals		672	766	100

*Combined European data from laboratories of Drs. Hers, Van Hoof, de Barsy, and Fernandes.[161]
†Combined U.S. data from laboratories of Drs. Barbara Brown and Y.-T. Chen.[448]

deficiency), III, VI, and IX are the most common, accounting for over 90 percent of all cases (Table 71-1). It should be recognized, however, that the muscle glycogenoses (types V and VII) are most likely underrepresented in these studies, as the data were collected from laboratories that specialized in liver glycogenosis. The majority of the glycogen storage diseases are inherited in an autosomal recessive manner. The exceptions are phosphoglycerate kinase and a common form of phosphorylase kinase deficiency, which are X-linked.

Reviews of glycogen storage diseases are available: clinical aspects and general descriptions can be found in Hers et al.,[161] Chen,[162] Fernandes and Chen,[163] Moses,[164] and Cornblath and Schwartz;[165] muscle glycogenosis in DiMauro and Bruno,[166] Moses,[167] and Tein;[168] recommendations of treatment in Moses,[164] Fernandes et al.,[169] and Chen et al;[170] description of morphologic features in McAdams et al.[171] and Jevon and Feingold;[172] useful laboratory techniques in Brown,[173] Shin,[174] and Turnbull and Sherratt;[175] description of molecular pathology in Elpeleg;[175a] and animal models of glycogen storage diseases in Walvoort.[176]

Type I Glycogen Storage Disease (Glucose 6-Phosphatase Deficiency, von Gierke Disease)

History and General Description. Type I glycogen storage disease was first described as "hepatonephromegalia glycogenica" by von Gierke in 1929, and it is still widely referred to as von Gierke Disease.[177] In 1952, Cori and Cori[119] demonstrated that the absence of glucose 6-phosphatase activity was the enzymatic defect responsible for the disease, establishing the first ever metabolic disorder in which an enzyme defect was identified. Since 1959, an increasing number of patients who had the same clinical course as type I glycogen storage disease but who were not deficient in glucose 6-phosphatase activity in frozen liver, have been described. In 1968, Senior and Loridan[178] proposed the term "glycogenosis type Ib" for these patients, and specified cases with absent activity in a frozen liver sample as type Ia. In 1977, Bialek et al.,[179] and in 1978, Narisawa et al.,[180] proposed that a defect in the microsomal membrane transport system of glucose 6-phosphate was the cause of type Ib; this was later demonstrated by Lange et al.[181] in 1980. Type Ic, a third form caused by a defect in microsomal phosphate or pyrophosphate transport, was first described by Nordlie et al. in 1983.[182] Type Ic has been reported in only a few cases. Type Id, a form with presumed defect in the microsomal glucose transporter, remains unproven.

The deficiency of glucose 6-phosphatase enzyme activity, or a deficiency in the microsomal transport proteins for glucose 6-phosphate or phosphate, results in excessive accumulation of glycogen in liver, kidney, and intestinal mucosa. The stored material in the liver also includes fat. The deficiencies lead to inadequate hepatic glucose production through normal glycogenolysis and gluconeogenesis.

Clinical and Laboratory Findings. Patients with type I glycogen storage disease may present in the neonatal period with hypoglycemia and lactic acidosis; however, they more commonly present at 3 to 4 months of age with hepatomegaly and/or hypoglycemic seizures. These children often have doll-like faces with excess adipose tissue in cheeks, relatively thin extremities, short stature, and a protuberant abdomen that is due to massive hepatomegaly (Fig. 71-8). The kidneys are also symmetrically enlarged but the spleen and heart are of normal size.

Skin xanthomas over the upper and lower extremities may be present in infancy, and retinal changes characterized by multiple, yellowish discrete paramacular lesions can be found. These changes appear to be positively correlated with the degree of hyperlipidemia.

The hallmarks of the disease are hypoglycemia, lactic acidosis, hyperuricemia, and hyperlipidemia. Hypoglycemia and lactic acidemia can occur after a short fast. In the past, many patients with unrecognized and untreated type I glycogen storage disease died in early infancy from profound hypoglycemia and acidosis. Hyperuricemia is present in young children, but gout rarely develops before puberty. Despite marked hepatomegaly, the liver transaminases are usually normal or only slightly elevated. Plasma biotinidase activity is elevated in type Ia but not Ib patients.[183,184] Intermittent diarrhea occurs in some patients; the mechanism remains unresolved. Easy bruising and epistaxis are common, and are associated with a prolonged bleeding time as a result of impaired platelet aggregation and adhesion.

The plasma may be "milky" in appearance as a result of a striking elevation of triglycerides. Cholesterol and phospholipids are also elevated, but less prominently. The lipid abnormality resembles type IV hyperlipidemia and is characterized by increased concentrations of very low density lipoprotein (VLDL), low-density lipoprotein (LDL), high density lipoprotein (HDL)-cholesterol, and a unique apolipoprotein profile consisting of increased levels of apo B, C, and E with relatively normal or reduced levels of apo A and D.[185,186] The erythrocyte aggregation index and disaggregation shear rate threshold are also elevated.[187]

The histology of the liver is characterized by a universal distension of hepatocytes by glycogen and fat. The lipid vacuoles

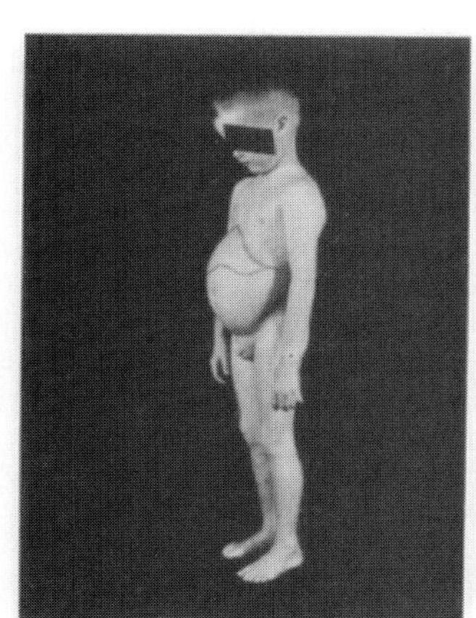
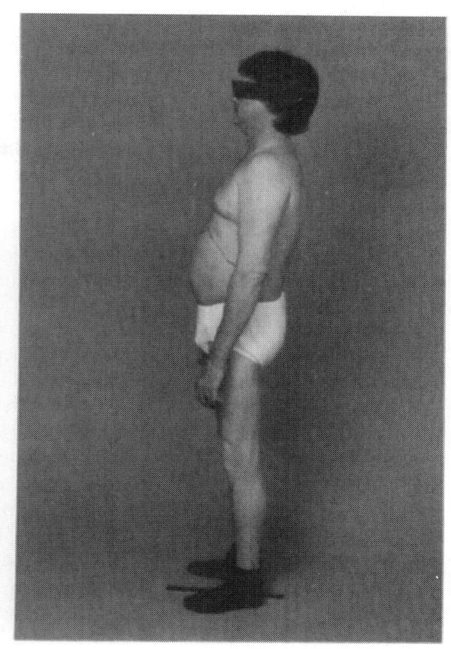

A

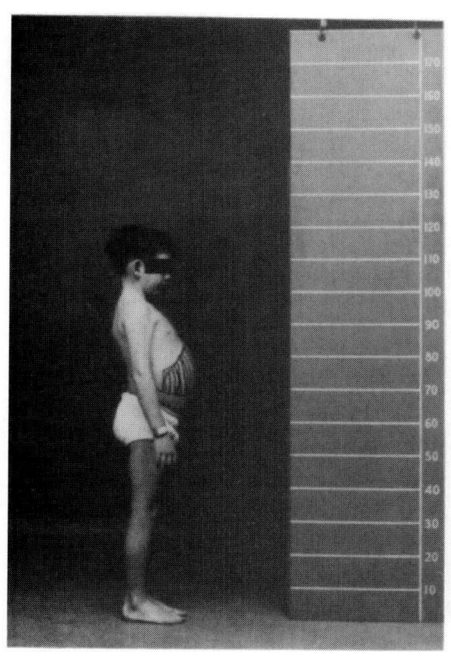
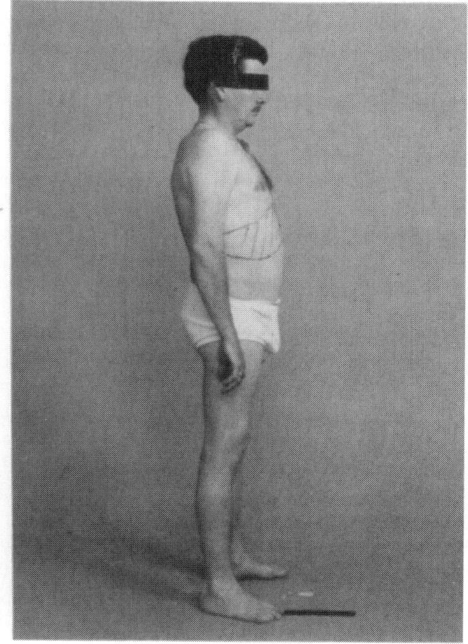

B

Fig. 71-8 Growth and development in two patients with type Ia glycogen storage disease. A, Patient (at age 7 years) originally described in a previous edition of this chapter; the patient is now 39 years old. B, Another type Ia patient at age 10 years, and follow up at age 33 years. Both patients survive despite their disease not being adequately treated. Note that the abdomen is less protuberant with age. Hypoglycemia also improves with age. In adulthood, however, both patients continue to be short, and both have gout, multiple liver adenomas, and a progressive renal disease.

are particularly large and prominent. There is little associated fibrosis.[171,172]

In rare cases, type I glycogen storage disease patients may be asymptomatic except for a noticeable hepatomegaly.[188,189]

Type Ib has a similar clinical course, with the additional findings of neutropenia and impaired neutrophil function resulting in recurrent bacterial infections.[190–192] Oral and intestinal mucosa ulceration are common, and chronic inflammatory bowel disease may occur.[192,193]

Type Ic has been reported in only a few patients.[133,182,194] There is insufficient clinical information to allow for a general description of clinical manifestations. Some Ic patients, who have been reported to have neutropenia, turned out to be Ib when molecular analysis was performed.[130,194a]

Long-Term Complications. Although type I glycogen storage disease affects mainly the liver, multiple organ systems are also involved. The long-term complications discussed here were mostly observed in adult patients whose disease had not been adequately treated (see Fig. 71-8). With early diagnosis and initiation of current effective treatment, it is hoped that these complications can be prevented (see Prognosis, below).

In adolescence, growth continues to be impaired and adult height is reduced. Puberty is often delayed. Virtually all females have ultrasound findings consistent with polycystic ovaries;[195] however, the other clinical features of polycystic ovary syndrome, such as acne and hirsutism, are not seen. It remains to be seen whether this ovarian finding actually affects ovulation and fertility. Symptoms of gout usually start around puberty owing to the

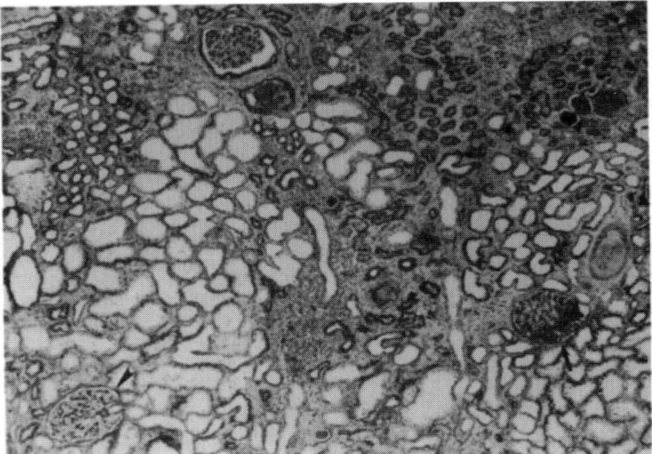

A

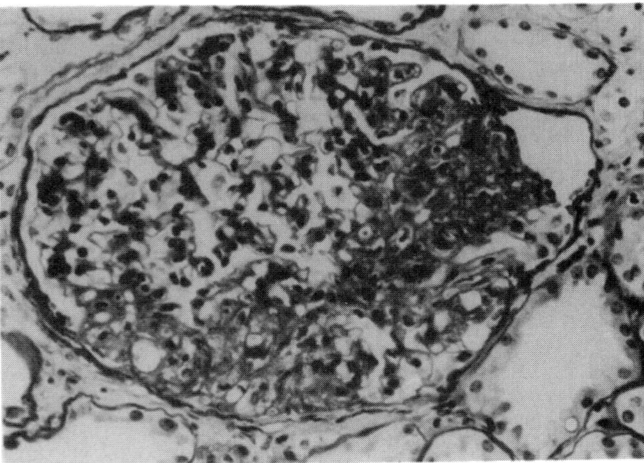

B

Fig. 71-9 Kidney-biopsy sections from patients with type I glycogen storage disease. A, Histologic section demonstrating focal segmental glomerular lesions (arrow), interstitial fibrosis, and focal tubular atrophy. Note the uninvolved glomerulus (arrowhead). The section is 3μm; periodic acid-Schiff stain, x30. B, Glomerulus with early focal segmental glomerulosclerosis, including segmental tuft collapse and partial adhesion to the capsule. The section is 3μm periodic acid-Schiff stain, x210. (From Chen et al.[202] with permission of the *New England Journal of Medicine*.)

long-term hyperuricemia. Secondary to the lipid abnormalities, there is an increased risk of pancreatitis.[196,197]

The dyslipidemia together with elevated erythrocyte aggregation, predispose these patients for atherosclerosis.[186,187] Premature atherosclerosis, however, has not yet been clearly documented except for one patient who had myocardial infarction at age 35 years and another patient died of amyloidosis-related heart failure at age 35 years who had severe atherosclerosis in his coronary arteries.[198] Impaired platelet aggregation may function as a protective mechanism to help reduce the risk of atherosclerosis.

Hepatic adenomas are known to develop in most patients with type I glycogen storage disease by the time they reach their second or third decade of life.[199] Stimulation of the liver by hepatotropic hormones responding to the hypoglycemia may play a part in the pathogenesis of the adenomas. Hemorrhage within the adenomas or malignant transformation can occur.[200,201]

Renal disease has been recognized as a late complication.[202–205] Almost all patients with type I glycogen storage disease who are more than 20 years of age have proteinuria. Many also have hypertension, renal stones, nephrocalcinosis, and altered creatinine clearance. Glomerular hyperfiltration, increased renal plasma flow, and tubular proteinuria are often found in the early stages of renal dysfunction and can occur before the onset of albuminuria.[202,206] In younger patients, hyperfiltration and hyperperfusion may be the only signs of renal abnormalities. With advancement of renal disease, focal segmental glomerulosclerosis and interstitial fibrosis are typically seen on biopsy (Fig. 71-9). In some patients, renal function has deteriorated and progressed to failure, requiring dialysis and transplantation. Other renal abnormalities seen in type I glycogen storage disease patients include amyloidosis, a Fanconi-like syndrome, and a distal renal tubular acidification defect.[207–209]

Symptoms of type I glycogen storage disease may be exacerbated by pregnancy.[210–212] The increase in renal perfusion and maternal volume which normally occurs in pregnancy can exacerbate renal problems. In addition, hypoglycemia may also become more difficult to control. Increased vaginal spotting has also been known to occur secondary to the bleeding abnormalities.

Pulmonary hypertension has been reported in six patients. Two of the six had shunt surgery involving either portacaval or intestinal vein to inferior vena cava. Four patients, however, had neither shunt surgery nor evidence of liver cirrhosis or portal hypertension. All patients died in their teens with progressive heart failure secondary to pulmonary hypertension.[213,214] A prospective study showed that 27 percent of patients have increased right ventricular pressure which may be an indication of early pulmonary hypertension.[215]

Osteoporosis has also been reported. Evidence of osteoporosis was found in a series of patients studied at postmortem.[216] Frequent fractures and radiographic evidence of osteopenia were often found in adult patients.[198] A recent study showed that radial bone mineral content was also significantly reduced in the prepubertal patients.[217]

Pathophysiology. The major biochemical findings in type I glycogen storage disease are hypoglycemia, lactic acidosis, hyperuricemia, and hyperlipidemia (Fig. 71-10).

Hypoglycemia. The deficiency of glucose 6-phosphatase activity in the liver blocks the final steps of the glycogenolytic and gluconeogenic pathways. It also interrupts the constant recycling of glucose in the liver through the glucose to glucose 6-phosphate to glucose system.[145] As expected, these patients are unable to maintain normal blood glucose levels in the fasting state, although the propensity for hypoglycemia decreases with age. As is also expected from the enzyme block, the endogenous glucose production is severely compromised. However, several studies performed on both adults and young patients clearly indicate that these patients are still capable of producing glucose.[218–220] Young patients had endogenous glucose production rates approximately half the control rates, and this rate increased in the adults and ranged from two-thirds of normal to normal values. The increased glucose production rate with age might explain why adults with glycogen storage disease are less susceptible to hypoglycemia. The impaired hepatic glucose output causes hypoglycemia, increased glucagon secretion, and chronic hypoinsulinism.

The mechanism of the endogenous glucose production remains a puzzle. Glucose isotope studies have excluded gluconeogenesis as a source of this production. Autophagy and the action of the lysosmal α-glucosidase, a process stimulated by the elevated glucagon levels, could provide a baseline glucose production. However, because it is poorly controlled, it cannot be the main mechanism. Recent studies do not support the concept of increased cycling of glucose moieties through glycogen with the action of debrancher enzyme releasing free glucose to be the sources of endogenous glucose production.[221,222] The evidence regarding residual glucose 6-phosphatase activity as a mechanism is unclear.

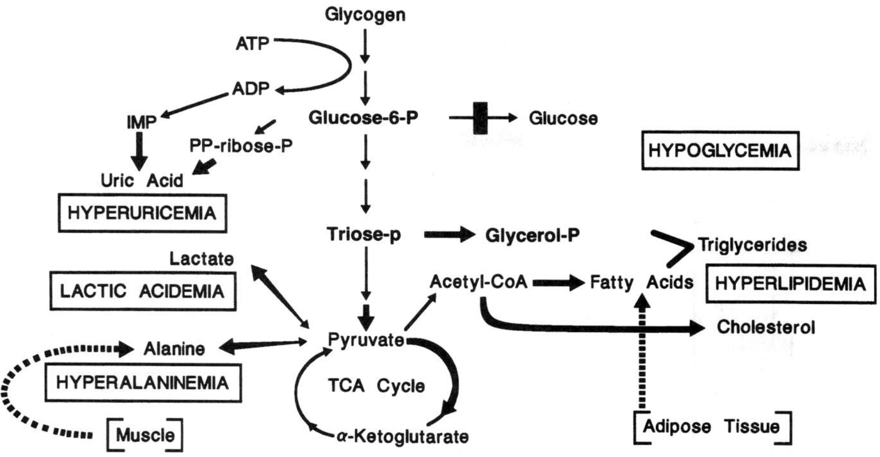

Fig. 71-10 Metabolic consequences of the type I glycogen storage disease. Acetyl-CoA = acetyl coenzyme A; IMP = inosine-5′-monophosphate; TCA = tricarboxylic acid.

Lactic Acidosis. In type I glycogen storage disease, glucose 6-phosphate formed from glycogenolysis, gluconeogenesis, or phosphorylation of glucose by glucokinase, cannot leave the liver as glucose, and it accumulates. An increase in phosphomonoesters (most likely glycolytic intermediates) during fasting, with a decrease in intracellular phosphate, has been demonstrated in type Ia patients by ^{31}P magnetic resonance spectroscopy.[223] These changes returned to normal after a glucose load. High levels of fructose 6-phosphate (in equilibrium with glucose 6-phosphate) lead to an increase in fructose 2,6-biphosphate and, hence, activation of phosphofructokinase, resulting, in increased glycolysis.[224] Glucose 6-phosphate follows the glycolytic pathway, where it can leave as the increased lactate. Chronic lactic acidosis may provide the brain with an alternative fuel in the face of a shortage of glucose.[225] Ketosis, however, is not prominent in most patients with type I glycogen storage disease, despite hypoglycemia.[226,227]

Several alternative metabolic substrates, including galactose, fructose, and glycerol, have an obligatory hepatic transformation to glucose through the glucose 6-phosphate pathway. The disaccharides sucrose and lactose result in increased blood lactate levels with little rise in blood glucose.[228] In the untreated patient, ethanol is metabolized at two to five times the normal rate, which increases the resistance to inebriation and reduces fasting blood lactate.[229]

Hyperuricemia. Hyperuricemia is caused by both decreased renal clearance and increased production. Lactate competes with uric acid for excretion in the kidney. Increased production of uric acid is evident from increased incorporation of labeled glycine.[230,231] Accumulation of phosphate esters results in decreased intrahepatic phosphate.[232] This relieves the physiological block on the hepatic AMP-deaminase; thus, degradation of adenine nucleotides increases, and uric acid is produced (see Fig. 71-10). Administration of glucagon causes depletion of ATP and phosphate and leads to marked hyperuricemia.[232,233] Synthesis of PP-ribose-P can be stimulated by the increased pentose phosphate shunt and also by the high liver phosphate levels after refeeding; however, this mechanism as a cause of hyperuricemia has not been fully investigated.

Hyperlipidemia. Hyperlipidemia is a result of both increased synthesis of triglycerides, VLDL, and LDL, and decreased peripheral lipolysis.[186] The exaggerated glycolytic pathway produces a generous supply of NADH and NADPH and abundant acetyl-CoA and glycerol; thus, both substrates and cofactors are available for hepatic triglyceride synthesis. Increased pyruvate and stimulus of pyruvate carboxylase by glucagon lead to increased oxaloacetate, which, with acetyl-CoA, forms citrate. Citrate provides a source for cytosolic acetyl-CoA, which is then carboxylated to malonyl-CoA. Malonyl-CoA inhibits carnitine palmitoyl transferase-I,[234] preventing the transfer of fatty acids into the mitochondria for β-oxidation. This could result in reduced ketone production and increased dicarboxylic acids.[235] Hypoinsulinism results in decreased activity of lipoprotein lipase and peripheral fatty acid utilization. Moreover, it induces lipolysis, leading to increased free fatty acids in plasma.

If apolipoprotein synthesis and VLDL formation cannot follow the increased synthesis of the lipids, then fat droplets form in the liver. The fatty infiltration of the liver accounts to a large extent for the marked hepatomegaly in type I glycogen storage disease.

Biochemical/Molecular Basis of the Disease. Type Ia glycogen storage disease is the deficiency of the catalytic subunit of the glucose 6-phosphatase system (see Fig. 71-5). In some patients with complete deficiency, the liver enzyme protein is completely absent, as judged by immunoblot analysis, but normal amounts of normal-molecular-weight protein are present in most of these patients.[236,237] When the glucose 6-phosphatase gene is disrupted in the type Ia mouse, the glucose 6-phosphatase activity is absent from both the liver and the kidney.[238] Thus, when the enzyme is completely deficient in the human liver, it should be also deficient in the kidney, although the activity of the glucose 6-phosphatase enzyme is rarely measured in kidney. It is not known whether patients lacking the catalytic subunit in the liver are also lacking the enzyme in pancreatic islet β cells, brain astrocytes, or the other cell types that contain the glucose 6-phosphatase enzyme. Recent evidence suggests that a glucose 6-phosphatase-related protein is present in the pancreas and is encoded by a different gene.[239,240]

A number of patients with partial deficiencies of the catalytic subunit of glucose 6-phosphatase activity in liver have been described;[188,189,237] some have low amounts of immunodetectable protein, while others have normal levels of protein. Both K_m and V_{max} defects have been described.

The cDNA encoding human liver glucose 6-phosphatase has been cloned (GenBank U01120) and mutations responsible for type Ia glycogen storage disease identified.[120] The mutations in the glucose 6-phosphatase gene appear to cluster according to the ethnic background of patients (see reference 117; see Fig. 71-6 for location of some of the common mutations). Ethnic-specific mutations have been described: R83C and Q347X are prevalent in Caucasians; 459insTA and R83C in Hispanics; R83C in Jews; R83H and G727T in Chinese; G727T in Japanese; and V166G in Muslim Arabs. Glucose 6-phosphatase is an integral membrane protein localized in endoplasmic reticulum (Fig. 71-6). It is of interest that there is no mutation in the cytoplasmic loop of the protein, and that mutations in the transmembrane helices in general cause a more severe reduction of the enzyme activity than mutations in the luminal loop. These features suggest that the structural integrity of the transmembrane helices is critical for catalysis.[115]

Type Ib glycogen storage disease is the deficiency of the hepatic microsomal glucose 6-phosphate transport protein (see Fig. 71-5). In vivo, it results in abnormally low or absent hepatic glucose 6-phosphatase activity in intact microsomes depending on whether the defect is complete or partial. A cDNA encoding the putative glucose 6-phosphate translocase was recently isolated and characterized[121] (EMBL Y15409). The putative translocase gene is localized to chromosome 11q23,[130,132,241] the same region that type Ib locus was mapped in by linkage analysis of the affected families.[131] Mutation analysis indicates that this putative glucose 6-phosphate translocase gene is the gene responsible for the type Ib disorder. Two mutations, G339C and 1211 delCT, appear to be prevalent in Caucasian patients,[130] while W118R appears to be most common in Japanese patients.[241] Interestingly, some previously diagnosed Ic and Id patients also have mutations in the glucose 6-phosphate translocase gene,[130,194a] suggesting that Ib, some Ic, and Id are the same disease and that inorganic phosphate and glucose 6-phosphate may be transported by the same translocase.

Type Ic glycogen storage disease is the deficiency of microsomal phosphate transport. It results in abnormally low glucose 6-phosphatase activity in intact microsomes. There seems to be two microsomal phosphate transport proteins, but so far all cases of type Ic in the literature have been shown to be deficiencies in only one of the proteins, which is termed T2β.[133] Some of the patients have no immunologically detectable T2β protein in their livers, while others have normal amounts of normal-molecular-weight protein.[133,242] As mentioned above, some patients previously diagnosed as type Ic had mutations in the translocase gene. The gene(s) for the phosphate transporter proteins have not been cloned. Thus a definitive conclusion regarding their status cannot be drawn at the present time.

Diagnosis. The diagnosis of type I glycogen storage disease can be suspected on the basis of clinical presentation and abnormal lactate and lipid values. In addition, administration of glucagon or epinephrine results in little or no rise in blood glucose, but the lactate level rises significantly. A functional study of the enzyme can also be performed utilizing ^{13}C nuclear magnetic resonance spectroscopy to measure hepatic glucose carbon production and recycling.[243] There is a reduction in glucose recycling, as gluconeogenesis does not produce glucose. Prior to cloning of glucose 6-phosphatase and glucose 6-phosphate translocase genes, a definitive diagnosis required a liver biopsy to demonstrate a deficiency. Gene-based mutational analyses now provide non-invasive ways of diagnosis for the majority of Ia and Ib patients.

Treatment. The treatment of type I glycogen storage disease is to maintain normal blood glucose concentrations. Normoglycemia can correct most of the metabolic abnormalities and will reduce the morbidity associated with this disease. Normoglycemia can be achieved through a number of different approaches, including total parenteral nutrition, nocturnal nasogastric infusion of glucose,[244] and orally administered uncooked cornstarch.[245] The result of long-term treatment data are now available for the latter two dietary regimens;[170,246,246a] both methods have yielded dramatic clinical improvement in these patients (see Prognosis below). Nocturnal nasogastric drip feeding can be introduced in early infancy from the time of diagnosis. It may consist of an elemental enteral formula, or it may contain only glucose or glucose polymer to provide 8 to 10 mg/kg/min of glucose in an infant, and 5 to 7 mg/kg/min in an older child.[163,247] Frequent feedings with a high complex carbohydrate content are given during the day. The distribution of calories should be approximately 65 to 70 percent carbohydrate, 10 to 15 percent protein, and 20 to 25 percent fat with one-third of the total 24-h caloric intake provided through nocturnal gastric feeding. If nocturnal nasogastric infusion is being used, the first meal of the day should be taken no longer than 15 to 30 min after stopping the infusion. Continuous feeding with infusion pump should be used with meticulous attention to detail, as hypoglycemia and death have resulted from malfunction of the pump or disconnection of the tube.[248,249]

Uncooked cornstarch acts as a slow-release form of glucose, and can be introduced at a dose of 1.6 g/kg every 4 h for infants under 2 years of age.[250] The response of young infants is variable. As the child grows older, the cornstarch regimen can be changed to every 6 h, and cornstarch can be prepared in water or diet drinks (1:2, weight in gram:volume in ml) at a dose of 1.75 to 2.5 g/kg of body weight. In young adults, a single dose of cornstarch at bedtime can maintain normoglycemia for greater than 7 h in most patients.[251] The caloric distributions with cornstarch therapy are similar to those in patients receiving gastric feeding.

Dietary intake of fructose and galactose should be restricted, as it cannot be converted to free glucose. As the diet is restricted, dietary supplements of multivitamins and calcium are required. Allopurinol is used to help reduce the levels of uric acid. The aim is to lower the serum urate concentration to below 6.4 mg/dl, the concentration at which monosodium urate saturates extracellular fluids.[252]

In type Ib glycogen storage disease, granulocyte and granulocyte-macrophage colony-stimulating factors have been used successfully to correct the neutropenia, to decrease the number and the severity of bacterial infections, and to improve the chronic inflammatory bowel disease in these patients.[253,254]

Portacaval shunts have been performed with limited benefit for patients with type I glycogen storage disease.[255,256] The shunt did not alter the metabolic status or the consequences of the abnormalities in the patients undergoing the procedures. Because good dietary management reduces or prevents most of the complications of type I glycogen storage disease, portacaval shunts should not be performed.

Liver transplantation has been performed in patients with type I disease because of multiple liver adenomas bearing the risk of malignant transformation and/or poor metabolic control. None, however, had carcinomas confirmed in the explanted livers (see references 257 and 257a). The hypoglycemia and other biochemical abnormalities were corrected after transplantation; and growth improved. Whether liver transplantation results in reversal and/or prevention of renal disease remains unclear. Neutropenia persisted in type Ib patients after liver transplantation, necessitating continuous treatment with granulocyte colony-stimulating factor. In view of the favorable response to the conventional treatment, liver transplantation should be considered only after all other methods of dietary treatment have failed, or when there is evidence of hepatocellular carcinomas.

Kidney transplantation has been performed secondary to renal failure. The renal allografts did not correct the hypoglycemia.[258,259] In one patient, the posttransplantation course was complicated by increased lactic acidemia, hyperlipidemia, and hyperglycemia.[259] Insulin resistance was also found. The increase in lactate production was thought to be the result of the gluconeogenic effect of the glucocorticoids, which were given for immunosuppression.

Surgery in type I glycogen storage disease should not be undertaken without first evaluating the patient's bleeding status and establishing good metabolic control. Prolonged bleeding time can be normalized by the use of intensive intravenous glucose infusion for 24 to 48 h prior to surgery. Use of 1-deamino-8-D-arginine vasopressin DDAVP was reported to reduce bleeding complications.[260] Lactated Ringer's solution should be avoided as it contains lactate and no glucose. Glucose levels should be maintained in the normal range throughout surgery with the use of 10 percent dextrose.

Prognosis. In the past, many patients with type I glycogen storage disease died, and the prognosis was guarded for those who survived. Maintenance of normoglycemia, through either ingestion of uncooked raw cornstarch or through continuous nocturnal nasogastric infusion of glucose, improves the metabolic abnormalities. With the prevention of hypoglycemia, growth improves, and the blood lactate, cholesterol, and triglyceride levels decrease.

In most adequately treated children, normal growth rates and ultimate adult height may be attained.[170,246] Some children may respond less favorably and may continue to be short.[246] In patients who have been adequately treated to maintain normal glucose levels since early infancy, there is less incidence of liver adenoma.[257] Many of these patients are now young adults, well into the age range in which hepatic adenomas are known to develop. The regression of adenomas after the initiation of dietary therapy has been reported.[261] Dietary therapy is effective in improving proximal renal tubular function.[207] However, it is unknown whether renal disease can be completely avoided through good metabolic control. Even with good treatment, glomerular hyperfiltration is still seen.

Genetics. Type I glycogen storage disease is inherited as an autosomal recessive genetic condition. The gene for glucose 6-phosphatase is on chromosome 17q21 and for translocase is on chromosome 11q23.[120,130] Prenatal diagnosis of type Ia has been accomplished through fetal liver biopsy.[262] DNA mutation analysis in chorionic villi or amniocytes now obviate the need of a more invasive fetal liver biopsy.[263,264]

Animal Model. A knockout type Ia mouse model generated by target disruption of the glucose 6-phosphatase gene and a naturally occurring mutant dog model have been reported.[238,265] Both models resemble human disease with failure to thrive, hepatomegaly, renomegaly, and hypoglycemia. Biochemically the mouse model does not have hyperlactic acidemia. The dog model is caused by a missense mutation (M121I) in the third transmembrane domain of the glucose 6-phosphatase gene.[266]

Type III Glycogen Storage Disease (Debrancher Deficiency; Limit Dextrinosis; Cori or Forbes Disease)

History and General Description. In contrast to patients with type I glycogen storage disease, in which no abnormality in the structure of glycogen can be demonstrated, in 1952, Illingworth and Cori[267] recognized the presence of excessive amounts of abnormally structured glycogen in liver and muscle from a patient who was studied clinically by Forbes.[268] Because the stored glycogen had very short outer chains, as in a phosphorylase-limit dextrin, a deficiency of amylo-1,6-glucosidase was predicted, which was actually demonstrated in 1956.[269] The disease is also called "limit dextrinosis," "Cori," or "Forbes" disease.

Most patients with type III glycogen storage disease survive into later life, as for example, the two patients originally reported by Snappes and Van Creveld in 1928,[159] who had hepatomegaly and an inability to mobilize liver glycogen. These patients were eventually shown by Van Creveld and Huijing, in 1964, to be deficient in debranching enzyme activity.[270] Both patients, a male and a female, had improved clinically and noted less marked hepatomegaly after puberty, a relatively common finding in affected individuals. It had long been alleged that most adult patients are asymptomatic. During the past few years, however, several reports have documented the presence of a progressive skeletal myopathy, cardiomyopathy, and/or liver cirrhosis in these patients.[271–276]

Clinical and Laboratory Findings. Genetic deficiency of glycogen debranching enzyme in humans causes hepatomegaly, hypoglycemia, short stature, variable skeletal myopathy, and cardiomyopathy. Patients with this disease vary remarkably, both clinically and enzymatically.[1,173,277] Most patients have disease involving both liver and muscle that is termed type IIIa. However, in about 15 percent of patients, the disease appears to involve only liver and is classified as type IIIb.

During infancy and childhood, the disease may be almost indistinguishable from type I glycogen storage disease, as hepatomegaly, hypoglycemia, hyperlipidemia, and growth retardation are common features of both. Splenomegaly may be present, but kidney is not enlarged in type III. Hepatomegaly and hepatic symptoms in most type III glycogen storage disease patients improve with age and are usually resolved after puberty.[278] However, progressive liver cirrhosis and failure may occur[274,276,279] and seems especially common in Japanese patients.[275] Hepatic adenomas have been reported; its prevalence may be as high as 25 percent in French patients.[280] Malignant transformation of adenomas has not been observed, although two patients developed a hepatocellular carcinoma associated with end-stage liver cirrhosis.[257,279] In patients with muscular involvement (type IIIa), muscle weakness is usually minimal during childhood, but can become severe after the third or fourth decade of life, as evidenced by slowly progressive weakness and wasting[271–273,281] (Fig. 71-11). Electromyography changes are consistent with a widespread myopathy, and nerve conduction studies may be abnormal. Ventricular hypertrophy is a frequent finding, but overt cardiac dysfunction is rare.[282–285] Hepatic symptoms in some patients may be so mild that the diagnosis is not made until adulthood, when the patients show symptoms and signs of neuromuscular disease. The initial diagnosis has been confused with Charcot-Marie-Tooth Disease.[286] Polycystic ovary appears to be a common finding in female patients with type III glycogen storage disease;[195] fertility, however, does not seem to be reduced.

Hypoglycemia and hyperlipidemia are common findings. In contrast to type I glycogen storage disease, elevation of liver transaminases and fasting ketosis are prominent, and blood lactate

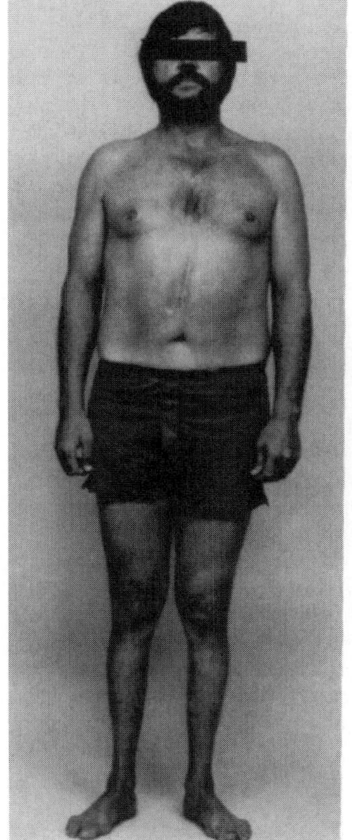

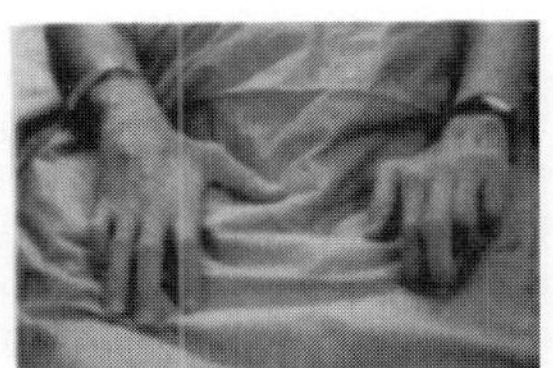

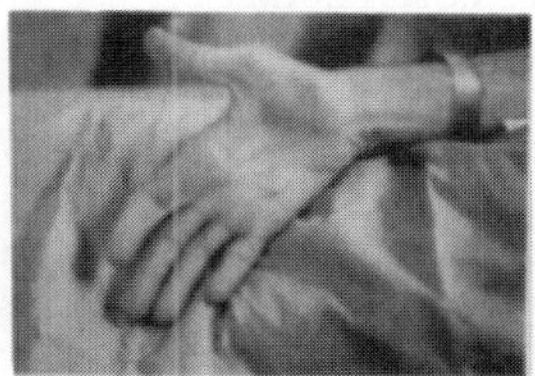

Fig. 71-11 Progressive myopathy in a patient with type IIIa glycogen storage disease. The patient has a debrancher deficiency in both liver and muscle (subtype IIIa). As a child, he had hepatomegaly, hypoglycemia, and growth retardation. After puberty, he no longer had hepatomegaly, and his final height is normal. Note the muscle wasting in the lower legs and both hands at age 44 years (left panel); this progressed to a pronounced muscle atrophy at age 53 years (two right panels).

and uric acid concentration are usually normal. The administration of glucagon 2 h after a carbohydrate meal provokes a normal rise of blood glucose, but after an overnight fast, glucagon may provoke no change in blood glucose. Serum creatine kinase levels can sometimes be useful to identify patients with muscle involvement, but normal levels do not rule out muscle enzyme deficiency.[273,287]

The histology of the liver is characterized by a universal distension of hepatocytes by glycogen and the presence of fibrous septa. The fibrosis and the paucity of fat distinguish type III glycogenosis from type I. The fibrosis, which ranges from minimal periportal fibrosis to micronodular cirrhosis, appears in most cases to be nonprogressive. However, this needs to be followed closely, as it has been reported that patients develop overt liver cirrhosis in adulthood (see above).

Biochemical/Molecular Basis of the Disease. As additional cases of type III glycogen storage disease are studied, it is apparent that not all patients lacking the debranching enzyme in liver are also missing the enzyme in the skeletal muscle.[173,277] Enzymatically, patients with both myopathy and liver symptoms have what appears to be a generalized enzyme defect (subtype IIIa). The deficient enzyme activity can be demonstrated not only in liver and muscle, but also in other tissues, such as heart, erythrocytes, and cultured fibroblasts.[173,174,288] Besides this common form, there are well-documented patients who have only hepatic symptoms without clinical or laboratory evidence of myopathy (subtype IIIb). Both liver and muscle biopsies have been performed on many of these patients and have clearly demonstrated that enzyme activity is deficient only in the liver and is retained in the muscle.[173,277] It seems logical to assume that progressive myopathy and/or cardiomyopathy develop only in patients who also show muscle debranching enzyme deficiency; indeed, this has been shown.[278] As stated above, normal creatine kinase levels do not rule out muscle enzyme deficiency. In the past, to predict accurately whether myopathy or cardiomyopathy may occur, one had to determine whether debranching enzyme was deficient in muscle. Ongoing molecular characterization of the disease can provide a noninvasive way of the subtype assignments (see below).

At the protein level, with the exception of rare cases of isolated transferase or glucosidase deficiency, all patients with type III glycogen storage disease have absent, or greatly reduced, amounts of the debrancher protein in western blot analyses.[288] There appears to be no correlation between the amount of debrancher protein and clinical severity.[289]

At the DNA level, a frameshift mutation (4529insA) in homozygous form was seen in a IIIa patient with severe phenotype;[290] an ethnic-specific mutation (4455delT) was found in all North African Jewish IIIa patients,[291] and a donor splicing-site mutation was found in a Japanese patient.[292] Two nonsense mutations, R864X and R1228X, with frequencies of 10.3 percent and 5.2 percent, respectively, were found in both IIIa and IIIb Caucasian patients, while two other mutations, 17delAG and Q6X, were exclusively found in patients with IIIb.[293] The latter two mutations reside in exon 3 at the amino acid codon 6. Both mutations result in severely truncated proteins, which are unlikely to have the debranching enzyme activity. The mechanism for how the exon 3 mutations retain the debranching enzyme activity in muscle is not clear.

Diagnosis. Definitive diagnosis rests on the demonstration of abnormal glycogen (short outer branch) and a deficiency of the debranching enzyme activity in liver and/or muscle. Skin fibroblasts or lymphocytes have been used for diagnosis, either by measuring enzyme activities with a qualitative assay or by a western blot analysis showing low levels or absence of the debrancher protein.[288,294] In some patients, excess glycogen and deficient debranching enzyme can be demonstrated in erythrocytes.[295,296] In the past, definitive assignment of subtype of type III glycogen storage disease required both liver and muscle biopsies. The striking and specific association of exon 3 mutations with IIIb now allows subtyping of the type III in a blood sample using a DNA-based diagnosis.[293]

Treatment. Dietary management is less demanding than in type I glycogen storage disease. If hypoglycemia is present, frequent meals, that are high in carbohydrates and with cornstarch supplements or nocturnal gastric drip feedings, constitute effective therapy.[297,298] Overtreatment may result in symptomatic hypoglycemia caused by hyperinsulinism.[299] A high-protein diet during the daytime plus overnight protein enteral infusion may also be effective in preventing hypoglycemia, as protein can be used as substrate for gluconeogenesis, a pathway which is intact in type III glycogen storage disease. Currently, there is no satisfactory treatment for the progressive myopathy. Patients do not need to restrict dietary intake of fructose and galactose, as do patients with type I glycogen storage disease. Liver transplantation has been performed in patients with end-stage cirrhosis and/or carcinoma.[257,279]

Genetics. Type III glycogenosis is inherited in an autosomal recessive manner. The disease has been reported in those of Caucasian, African, Hispanic, and Asian ethnicity. The frequency of the disease is relatively high in non-Ashkenazi Jews of North African extraction (prevalence 1 in 5400). Prenatal diagnosis and carrier detection is technically difficult with enzyme assays,[300–302] but is possible using a DNA-based method by mutation analysis or linkage study.[303]

Animal Model. Type III glycogenosis has been observed in dogs. The disease is much more severe in dogs than in humans.[304]

Type IV (Branching Enzyme Deficiency, Amylopectinosis, or Andersen Disease)

History and General Description. Type IV glycogen storage disease is also known as Andersen Disease, or amylopectinosis, in recognition of Andersen's 1956 clinical description of a patient with a progressive hepatosplenomegaly who stored an abnormal polysaccharide with poor solubility in the liver.[305] The abnormal glycogen had fewer branch points, more α1–4-linked glucose units, and longer outer chains than normal glycogen, resulting in a structure resembling amylopectin.[267] Because of the structure of this abnormal glycogen, the deficiency of a branching enzyme activity was suspected and was later demonstrated by Brown and Brown in 1966.[306]

Clinical and Laboratory Findings. Type IV glycogen storage disease most frequently presents in the first few months of life, with hepatosplenomegaly and failure to thrive. This is followed by a progressive liver cirrhosis with portal hypertension, ascites, esophageal varices, and death by 5 years of age. Hypoglycemia is rarely seen but can occur when liver cirrhosis progresses, as few hepatocytes are available for glucose mobilization. There are, though less frequently, patients with liver dysfunction who survive without evidence of progression of the liver disease.[307,308] In addition to the hepatic presentation, a neuromuscular form of the disease has been reported. These patients may present at birth with severe hypotonia, muscle atrophy, and neuronal involvement with death in the neonatal period;[309–311] present in late childhood with myopathy or cardiomyopathy;[312,313] or present as adults with diffuse central and peripheral nervous system dysfunction accompanied by accumulation of polyglucosan body disease in the nervous system (so-called adult polyglucosan body disease).[314,315]

In most cases, tissue deposition of amylopectin-like materials are generalized and have been demonstrated in liver, heart, muscle, skin, intestine, brain, spinal cord, and peripheral nerve.[316–318] The histologic findings of the liver in this disease are characteristic. Light microscopy shows a distorted architecture with diffuse

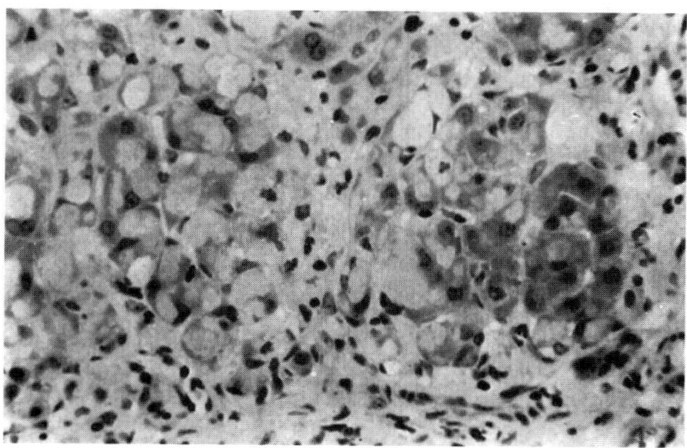

Fig. 71-12 Liver biopsy from a patient with type IV glycogen storage disease. The hepatocytes are enlarged and contain faintly stained basophilic inclusions in their cytoplasm. Note also, extensive intralobular fibrosis (hematoxylin-eosin stain, x400). (Courtesy of Milton J. Finegold, M.D., Baylor College of Medicine, Houston, Texas.)

interstitial fibrosis and wide fibrous septa surrounding micronodular areas of parenchyma. The hepatocytes are enlarged to two or three times normal and contain faintly stained basophilic inclusions within their cytoplasm (Fig. 71-12). These inclusions consist of coarsely clumped, stored material that is periodic acid-Schiff-positive and partially resistant to diastase digestion. Electromicroscopy shows, in addition to the conventional α and β glycogen particles, accumulation of the fibrillar aggregations that are typical of amylopectin. The distinct staining properties of the cytoplasmic inclusions, as well as electromicroscopic findings, could be diagnostic. However, polysaccharidoses with histologic features reminiscent of type IV disease, but without enzymatic correlation, have been observed.[319] The definitive diagnosis rests on the demonstration of the deficient branching enzyme activity.

The pathogenesis of the liver injury is not clear. The stored material with abnormal glycogen structure and/or insolubility may be the origin of the cellular injury.

Biochemical/Molecular Basis of the Disease. Branching enzyme is a monomeric protein with a molecular mass of 80 kDa encoded by a gene located on chromosome 3p14[32] (GenBank L07956). Mutational analysis reveals that both hepatic and neuromuscular forms of the type IV disease are caused by mutations in the same glycogen-branching enzyme gene.[320] A 210-bp deletion in the cDNA caused by a 3′ acceptor splice-site mutation was found in a patient with the fatal neonatal neuromuscular presentation. A point mutation, Y329S, was found in patients with the nonprogressive hepatic form. This mutant allele results in significant retention of the branching enzyme activity and may be the reason for the mild disease. Interestingly, the Y329S mutation was also found in Ashkenazi Jewish patients with adult polyglucosan body disease.[320a] Three other point mutations (R515C, F257L, and R524X) were found in patients with the classical progressive liver cirrhosis presentation.[320]

Diagnosis. The clinical and biochemical picture of the disease cannot be distinguished from other causes of cirrhosis in infancy. The diagnosis of type IV requires biopsy for demonstration of abnormal glycogen (long outer chains, an amylopectin-like polysaccharide) and a deficiency of branching enzyme in liver, muscle, leukocytes, erythrocytes, or fibroblasts.[306,321,322] Two enzyme assays have been developed and could be used for diagnosis of branching enzyme deficiency. The original assay measures the stimulating effect of the branching enzyme on the synthetic activity of glycogen phosphorylase in polymerizing glucose from glucose 1-phosphate;[306] a newer assay uses glycogen synthase as the indicating enzyme and UDP-Glc as substrate.[323] By these methods, affected patients have 1 to 10 percent of the activities in the tissues. Both assays are indirect and are not suitable for quantitation of a residual branching activity, as might be expected in the variant forms of type IV disease without apparent progressive liver disease. For adult polyglucosan body disease, leukocytes or nerve biopsy is needed to establish the diagnosis as the branching enzyme deficiency is limited to those tissues.[314,315]

Treatment. There is no specific treatment for type IV glycogen storage disease. Maintenance of normoglycemia and adequate nutrient intake improve liver function and muscle strength, and extend the time for growth in some patients. For progressive hepatic failure, liver transplantation has been performed and may be an effective treatment[324,325] (see Matern[257] for a review). Of 14 patients who underwent liver transplantation, 2 died immediately after transplantation (3 days and 36 days) and 2 died posttransplantation (9 months and 2.5 years) from heart failure with heavy infiltration of amylopectin in the myocardium;[325,326] 1 died 5.5 years posttransplant from meningococcal sepsis; 9 surviving patients have not had neuromuscular or cardiac complications during followup periods for as long as 13.5 years,[257] with reduction in the amount of amylopectin on myocardial biopsy in some of these patients.[324] Caution should be taken in selecting type IV patients for liver transplantation because of the variable phenotype, which include a nonprogressive form of the liver disease and extrahepatic manifestations of the disease.

Genetics. Type IV glycogen storage disease is inherited as an autosomal recessive trait. Carrier detection is possible by enzyme assay or DNA analysis. Partial enzyme deficiency has been observed in obligate carriers by measurement of enzyme activity in leukocytes, erythrocytes, or skin fibroblasts. Prenatal diagnosis by enzyme assay is available for the fatal form of glycogenosis, by using cultured amniocytes or chorionic villi.[327] Ongoing characterization of mutations will allow a DNA-based diagnosis.

Animal Model. Type IV glycogen storage disease has been reported in a family of purebred domestic cats. The disease resembles the neuromuscular form of human disease with a progressive skeletal and cardiac myopathy that starts around 5 months of age; hepatic cirrhosis and failure are not seen.[328] The disease in cats is due to a 6-kb deletion in the feline branching enzyme gene.[329]

Type V (Muscle Phosphorylase Deficiency, McArdle Disease, Myophosphorylase Deficiency)

History and General Description. Type V glycogen storage disease is also known as McArdle Disease, in recognition of McArdle's clinical description, in 1951, of a 30-year-old patient who suffered from muscle pain, weakness, and stiffness following slight exercise.[330] Blood lactate in this patient fell during exercise instead of rising normally, suggesting that the patient was unable to convert muscle glycogen into lactate. The biochemical lesion due to the deficiency of muscle phosphorylase was not identified until 1959.[331–333]

Clinical and Laboratory Findings. Clinical symptoms usually appear in young adulthood and are characterized by exercise intolerance with muscle cramps. About half of the patients have had burgundy color of urine after exercise. The burgundy color is due to rhabdomyolysis, which results in myoglobinuria. There are also a few reports of acute renal failure secondary to intense myoglobinuria.[334,335] These episodes occur after vigorous exercise. Although the majority of patients present with symptoms in the second or third decade, many report weakness and lack of endurance since childhood. In rare cases, electromyographic findings may be indistinguishable from those of an inflammatory myopathy, and the diagnosis may be confused with polymyositis.[336] Later in adult life, persistent weakness and muscle wasting may develop with fatty replacement.[337]

There are two types of activity that tend to cause symptoms: brief exercise of great intensity, such as sprinting or carrying heavy loads, and less intense but sustained activity, such as climbing stairs or walking uphill. Moderate exercise, such as walking on level ground, can be performed by most patients at their own pace, even for long periods. Many patients experience a characteristic "second wind" phenomenon. If they slow down or pause briefly at the first appearance of muscle pain, they can resume exercise with more ease.

Serum creatine kinase is usually elevated at resting, with further increase seen after exercise. The blood ammonia, inosine, hypoxanthine, and uric acid also increase with exercise.[338,339] These elevations are attributed to accelerated recycling of muscle purine nucleotides when there is insufficient ATP production.

Rare Variants. Clinical heterogeneity is not common in type V glycogen storage disease, as the majority of patients present with symptoms in the second or third decade of life. However, there are reports of late-onset type V glycogen storage disease with no symptoms until the age of 74 years.[340] There have also been reports of an early-onset, fatal presentation of type V glycogen storage disease.[341–343] The presenting features were hypotonia, generalized muscle weakness, and progressive respiratory insufficiency. One preterm infant also had congenital joint contracture;[343] death occurred before 4 months of age. In addition, phosphorylase deficiency was reported in a 4-year-old boy presenting with delayed psychomotor development, proximal weakness, elevated creatine kinase levels, and myopathic electromyographic changes.[344] Biochemical studies have failed to show any differences in the severity of the enzyme defect or in the concentration of muscle glycogen in the different variants.[344,345] Genetic analysis has also failed to provide an explanation; a child with fatal infantile myopathy was homozygous for the common mutation (R49X, see below) seen in adults with typical McArdle Disease.[346]

Pathophysiology. Resting or minimally active muscle derives most of its energy from the oxidation of fatty acids.[347] During the early phase of moderate exercise, energy comes mostly from glycogen breakdown and anaerobic glycolysis. As exercise continues for more than 10 to 15 min, bloodborne substrates (glucose and fatty acids) become increasingly important sources of energy; finally, for sustaining exercise for long duration, the fatty acids represent the most important fuel. Thus, mobilization of fatty acids and increased blood flow to exercising muscle underlie the mechanisms of the "second-wind" phenomenon. On the other hand, for intense exercise, muscle seems to depend almost exclusively on endogenous glycogen, and fatigue coincides with glycogen depletion. This explains why patients with McArdle Disease can usually tolerate moderate exercise but intense exercise produces symptoms. Another factor that contributes to exercise intolerance is an impairment of the exercise-induced increase in muscle perfusion.[348] A reduced level of skeletal muscle sodium-potassium ATPase pump has been reported.[348a] This finding explains several previous observations in McArdle disease patients including the excessive rise of plasma potassium with exercise and the decline in the compound muscle action potential with repetitive stimulation.

Biochemical/Molecular Basis of the Disease. Phosphorylase exists in multiple tissue-specific isoforms, the muscle, liver, and brain forms, and each is encoded by a separate gene. The muscle form is the only isozyme present in mature muscle; it represents about half the total enzyme in the heart, about 20 to 30 percent in the brain, and none in the liver. This probably explains why, clinically, muscle phosphorylase deficiency does not affect organs other than muscle.[349]

Biochemically, phosphorylase activity is extremely low or undetectable in muscle. Glycogen concentration is increased; the accumulated glycogen is of normal structure. The excess glycogen can be found in subsarcolemmal and intermyofibrillar spaces with disruption of myofibrillar structure at the level of the I band.[350] At the protein level, the majority of patients have absent or greatly reduced amounts of phosphorylase protein, a circumstance similar to debranching enzyme deficiency. The gene for muscle phosphorylase has been cloned and mapped to chromosome 11q13-qter[49] (GenBank M16013). At the gene level, there is extensive genetic heterogeneity with at least 14 different mutations causing McArdle Disease identified to date.[346,351–353] A nonsense mutation changing arginine to a stop at codon 49 (R49X) and a deletion of a single codon in exon 17 are prevalent in Caucasian and Japanese patients, respectively.

Diagnosis. An ischemic exercise test offers rapid diagnostic screening for metabolic myopathies. Lack of an increase in blood lactate concentration and exaggerated blood ammonia elevations are indicative of muscle glycogenoses in which a defect in the conversion of glycogen, or glucose, to lactate may be found. The abnormal ischemic exercise response, however, is not limited to type V glycogen storage disease. Other muscle defects along the pathways of glycogenolysis or glycolysis can produce similar results; for example, deficiencies of muscle phosphofructokinase or debranching enzyme (when the test is done after fasting).

Phosphorus magnetic resonance imaging (^{31}P MRI) allows for the noninvasive evaluation of muscle metabolism. Patients with type V glycogen storage disease have no decrease in intracellular pH and have excessive reduction in phosphocreatine in response to exercise.[354] The diagnosis should be confirmed by enzymatic evaluation of muscle or molecular analysis of mutations using DNA isolated from any readily available tissue such as leukocytes.[355]

Treatment. The ability to tolerate exercise can be augmented by aerobic training[355a] or by oral administration of glucose or fructose, or by injection of glucagon. A high-protein diet appears to increase muscle endurance in some patients.[356] Vitamin B6 supplementation has been shown to reduce exercise intolerance and muscle cramps.[356a] In general, avoidance of strenuous exercise prevents the symptoms. Longevity does not appear to be affected.

Genetics. Type V glycogen storage disease is inherited as an autosomal recessive trait. In most cases, heterozygous carriers are clinically unaffected; however, there are reports of heterozygotes manifesting with this disease.[357,358] An unusual family in which clinical manifestations could be traced in four generations has also been reported.[359] Carrier studies have been performed in type V disease by measurement of enzyme activity in biopsied muscle, use of ^{31}P MRI to study muscle metabolism,[360] or a DNA-based diagnosis.[355] There appears to be no indication for prenatal diagnosis of this relatively benign metabolic disorder. Prenatal diagnosis for the rare and fatal infantile form is of greater interest and may be possible by fetal muscle biopsy, by ultrasound assessment of fetal movement, or by a DNA-based test. However, there are no reports that these have been done.

Animal Model. A breed of cattle and a flock of sheep that exhibited exercise intolerance and/or myoglobinuria were found to have muscle phosphorylase deficiency. The cattle model is caused by a missense mutation and the sheep model by a splice-site mutation.[361,362]

Type VI Glycogen Storage Disease (Liver Phosphorylase Deficiency, Hers Disease)

History and General Description. In the 1950s and 1960s, a large proportion of patients with glycogen storage disease could not be classified as belonging to any of the types which had been previously described. These patients had hepatomegaly, mild hypoglycemia, and markedly increased glycogen content in the liver. In 1959, Hers described three such patients with normal activities of the glucose 6-phosphatase catalytic subunit and debranching enzyme, but greatly diminished activity of phosphorylase in their livers.[363] This was classified as type VI glycogen storage disease by Stetten and Stetten.[364]

Clinical and Laboratory Findings. The number of patients with enzymatically documented liver phosphorylase deficiency is small. Whereas analyses of liver phosphorylase activity were performed in the presence and absence of an activating system, most patients proved to be deficient in phosphorylase kinase activity rather than to have a primary defect in phosphorylase. It appears that patients with liver phosphorylase deficiency have a benign course.[365,366] These patients present with hepatomegaly and growth retardation early in childhood. Hypoglycemia, hyperlipidemia, and hyperketosis are usually mild if present. Lactic acid and uric acid are normal. The heart and skeletal muscles are not involved. The hepatomegaly improves with age and usually disappears around puberty. The liver phosphorylase gene has been cloned and mapped to chromosome 14.[48]

Treatment. Treatment is symptomatic. A high-carbohydrate diet and frequent feeding are effective in preventing hypoglycemia, but most patients require no specific treatment.

Genetics. Three phosphorylase isoforms are known: the muscle (M), liver (L), and brain (B) isoforms. They are encoded by separate genes—*PGYM*, *PGYL*, and *PGYB*—which have been mapped to chromosomes 11, 14, and 20, respectively. Mutations in *PGYL* (GenBank AF046785) cause type VI glycogen storage disease; a splicing-site mutation in intron 13 has been identified in a large Mennonite kindred and four other mutations were found in patients with different ethnic background.[367,368]

Type VII Glycogen Storage Disease (Muscle Phosphofructokinase Deficiency, Tarui Disease)

History and General Description. Type VII glycogen storage disease is also known as Tarui disease, in recognition of Tarui's clinical and enzymatic description in 1965 of a family with three affected sibs, one female and two males in their twenties, who presented with easy fatigability and exercise intolerance similar to that seen in type V glycogen storage disease.[369] Muscle glycogen was increased, but the level of phosphorylase activity was normal. Levels of glucose 6-phosphate and fructose 6-phosphate were elevated, and assays for phosphofructokinase revealed almost undetectable activity. Erythrocyte phosphofructokinase was also decreased by about 50 percent.

Clinical and Laboratory Findings. The clinical features are very similar to those in type V glycogen storage disease (see reference 370). The patients experienced early onset of fatigue and pain with exercise. Vigorous exercise causes severe muscle cramps and myoglobinuria. There are, however, five features that may differentiate type VII from type V. In type VII, (a) for most patients, the exercise intolerance is evident in childhood and symptoms are more severe than those seen in type V glycogen storage disease, and the attack may be associated with nausea and vomiting; (b) a compensated hemolytic anemia occurs as evidenced by an increased level of serum bilirubin and reticulocyte count, and erythrocyte 2,3-biphosphoglycerate is also decreased secondary to blockage of glycolysis at the phosphofructokinase step[371] (see Chap. 182); (c) hyperuricemia is often seen and exaggerated by muscle exercise to a more severe degree than that observed in type V or III glycogen storage disease;[339] (d) an abnormal polysaccharide is present in muscle fibers and is periodic acid-Schiff-positive but resistant to diastase digestion;[372,373] and (e) exercise intolerance is particularly acute following meals that are rich in carbohydrates.[374]

The abnormal polysaccharide in muscle has a fine fibrillar appearance resembling amylopectin, as seen in type IV glycogen storage disease. It has been hypothesized that this may be due to activation of glycogen synthase by the elevated concentration of glucose 6-phosphate in the muscle. Glycogen synthase elongates the polysaccharide chain of glycogen. The exercise intolerance after carbohydrate meals can be attributed to the fact that the glucose not only cannot be utilized in muscle of type VII glycogenosis patients because of the enzymatic block, but because the administered glucose actually lowers blood levels of fatty acids—the primary source of muscle fuel. In contrast, patients with type V glycogen storage disease can metabolize bloodborne glucose derived from either liver glycogenolysis or exogenous glucose. Glucose infusion improves the exercise tolerance in type V glycogen storage disease.

Rare Variants. In addition to the typical form of muscle phosphofructokinase deficiency, two other variants have been reported. One presents with onset in infancy with hypotonia, limb weakness, and/or joint contractures, and proceeds to a rapidly progressive myopathy and death.[375–378] The other variant presents in middle or late adult life and is characterized by a slowly progressive, fixed muscle weakness rather than cramps and myoglobinuria.[373,379,380]

Biochemical/Molecular Basis of the Disease. Phosphofructokinase is a tetrameric enzyme derived from three genetic loci that code for muscle (M), liver (L), and platelet (P) subunits.[142] The platelet enzyme is the same as the fibroblast type. The genes for the muscle, liver, and platelet types are assigned to chromosomes 12, 21, and 10, respectively.[142,143,381,382] These subunits are variably expressed in different tissue. Mature muscle expresses only the M subunit and contains only the homotetramer M4. Erythrocytes express both the M and L subunits, and random tetramer formation produces five isozymes, the M_4 and L_4 and three hybrid forms (M_3L, M_2L_2, and ML_3). In classical muscle phosphofructokinase deficiency, a genetic defect of the M subunit (GenBank U24183) causes a total lack of the enzyme activity in muscle, whereas erythrocytes lack the M_4 and hybrid isozymes but still express the L_4, which accounts for about 50 percent of normal erythrocyte phosphofructokinase activity. In contrast, patients with late-onset myopathic form of phosphofructokinase deficiency have both M-containing hybrid isozymes and L_4 in their erythrocytes.[383] The residual M subunit may explain the mild symptoms and late onset of this variant form of phosphofructokinase deficiency.

Multiple mutations, including splicing defects, frameshifts, and missense mutations, have been identified.[384–386] There is no obvious genotype-phenotype correlation. Muscle phosphofructokinase deficiency appears to be prevalent among people of Ashkenazi Jewish descent. Molecular diagnosis is now feasible for Ashkenazi Jewish patients who share two common mutations in the gene; the more frequent is an exon 5 splicing defect, which accounts for ~68 percent of mutant alleles in this population.

Diagnosis. The molecular diagnosis is practical only in limited patient populations or in families with known mutations. For most patients, diagnosis requires biochemical or histochemical demonstration of the enzymatic defect in the muscle. The absence of the M isoenzyme of phosphofructokinase can also be demonstrated in blood cells and fibroblasts.[386]

Treatment. There is no specific treatment for this condition. Avoidance of strenuous exercise is advisable to prevent acute attacks of muscle cramps and myoglobinuria. Clinical benefit of a ketogenic diet has been reported in an infant with infantile phosphofructokinase deficiency with arthrogryposis.[387]

Genetics. Type VII glycogen storage disease is inherited as an autosomal recessive trait. The disease appears to be prevalent among people of Ashkenazi Jewish descent. Prenatal diagnosis is not of great interest for this relatively benign disorder, except for the rare fatal form of the disease. There are no reports that prenatal diagnosis has been accomplished.

Animal Model. The deficiency of the M isoenzyme of phosphofructokinase has been observed in dogs.[388] The lack of the enzyme activity in the dog is caused by a nonsense mutation leading to rapid degradation of a truncated protein.[389] Dogs manifest primarily a chronic hemolytic anemia without much of muscle symptoms; this could be accounted for by both the high oxidative potential of the canine muscle and the presence of L isoenzyme in the muscle.[388] The dog model is caused by a nonsense mutation in the phosphorylase kinase M gene.[388a]

Type IX Glycogen Storage Disease (Phosphorylase Kinase Deficiency)

History and General Description. Hug et al., in 1966,[390] and Huijing, in 1967,[391] reported that the activation system for phosphorylase was defective in the liver and leukocytes from some of their patients with liver glycogenoses. Later Huijing and Fernandes[392] described a series of patients with X-linked liver glycogenosis in whom a deficiency of phosphorylase b kinase could be demonstrated in leukocytes and erythrocytes; this group of patients was designated as type VIa. Hug, however, studied a group of patients with phosphorylase kinase deficiency and concluded that their disease was not X-linked; he classified this presumably autosomal recessive form of phosphorylase kinase deficiency as type IX glycogenosis and a form of phosphorylase deficiency with brain involvement as type VIII.[393] McKusick, in the *Online Mendelian Inheritance in Man*, classified X-linked liver phosphoralase kinase as type VIII. The confusing numerical classification was in part due to a lack of understanding of the complicated phosphorylase activating system.

The genetic complexity now is clearer—knowing that phosphorylase kinase consists of four subunits encoded by different genes on different chromosomes (X chromosome as well as autosomes) and differentially expressed in different tissues. In this chapter, we refer to all phosphorylase kinase deficiencies as type IX glycogen storage disease. Based on the gene/subunit involved, tissues that are primarily affected and the mode of inheritance, phosphorylase kinase deficiency in man is further divided into six subtypes (see references 58 and 394) Table 71-2. Two rodent models, which differ in affected tissues and modes of inheritance, are included for comparison.

X-Linked Liver Phosphorylase Kinase Deficiency (Type IXa). This is the most common form of type IX glycogen storage disease (about 75 percent of all cases). Besides liver, enzyme activity may be also deficient in erythrocytes, leukocytes, and fibroblasts, but normal in muscle. A longitudinal study of 41 patients characterized the typical case history as "that of a youngster aged 1–5 years, presenting with protuberant abdomen due to hepatomegaly; growth retardation; slight delay in motor development; mild elevation of cholesterol, triglycerides, AST, and ALT; and fasting hyperketosis."[395] These abnormalities gradually disappear with age, and most adult patients are practically asymptomatic, despite a persistent phosphorylase kinase deficiency. Growth retardation, most pronounced during early childhood, is a major concern to patients and their parents, but most growth-retarded patients achieve a normal final height. Hypoglycemia is variable and is usually mild, if present. Patients respond normally to the hyperglycemic action of glucagon. X-linked liver phosphorylase kinase deficiency is generally considered a benign condition, although clinical severity may vary substantially.[396,397] Asymptomatic males carrying the deficiency, as well as heterozygotic females with mild symptoms, have been observed.[395]

Liver histology shows glycogen-distended hepatocytes. The accumulated glycogen (α particles, rosette form) has a frayed or burst appearance and is less compact than the glycogen seen in type I or type III glycogen storage disease. Remarkably, fibrous septal formation and low-grade inflammatory changes may also be seen.[171,397] Cirrhosis of the liver has been reported in several female patients who had a presumably autosomal recessive form of phosphorylase kinase deficiency.[398,399] (See below type IXc.)

X-linked liver phosphorylase kinase deficiency has been mapped by linkage analysis to Xp22.[400] The structural gene for the liver isoform of the phosphorylase kinase α subunit is localized in the same region[62] (GenBank X80497). Several missense, nonsense, and splice-site mutations in this gene have been identified in familiar and sporadic cases of liver phosphorylase kinase deficiency.[401–403] A few patients with X-linked liver phosphorylase kinase deficiency and normal, or even elevated, red blood cell phosphorylase kinase levels have been reported. These patients also have mutations in the same α gene. The mutations however tend to be subtle, causing the substitution, deletion, or insertion of one or two amino acids, and seem to be clustered at a few sites.[404,405] This is in contrast to the many nonsense mutations seen in the typical X-linked glycogenosis having phosphorylase kinase deficiency in both liver and blood cells. The patients with X-linked phosphorylase kinase deficient in both liver and blood cells are designated as subtype IXa-1, or termed X-linked liver glycogenosis-I (XLG1) with phosphorylase kinase deficiency in liver but normal in blood cells as subtype IXa-2, or XLG2.

Autosomal Liver and Muscle Phosphorylase Kinase Deficiency (Type IXb). Several patients with phosphorylase kinase deficiency in liver and blood cells and an autosomal mode of inheritance have been reported.[390,406–408] As with the X-linked form, hepatomegaly and growth retardation apparent in early childhood are the predominant symptoms. Some of these patients also exhibited muscle hypotonia. In a few of these cases, reduced

Table 71-2 Glycogen Storage Disease Caused by Phosphorylase Kinase Deficiency (Type IX Glycogen Storage Disease)

Subtype	Species	Affected Tissues	Inheritance	Mutant Gene/Subunit
IXa-1	Human	Liver, blood cells	X chromosomal	PHKA2/α_L
IXa-2	Human	Liver (in blood cells, normal or high)	X chromosomal	PHKA2/α_L
IXb	Human	Liver, blood cells, muscle	autosomal	PHKB/β
IXc	Human	Liver, blood cells	autosomal	PHKG2/γ_{TL}
IXd	Human	Muscle	X chromosomal	PHKA1/α_M
IXe	Human	Muscle	autosomal	?
IXf	Human	Heart	autosomal?	?
	I-Mouse*	Muscle	X chromosomal	PHKA1/α_M
	gsd-Rat†	Liver	autosomal	PHKG2/γ_{TL}

SOURCE: Courtesy of Dr. Manfred W. Kiliman, Ruhr-Universitat, Bochum, Germany
*Resembles human IXd.
†Resembles human IXc.

activity of the enzyme was also demonstrated in muscle. In other cases, the enzyme activity was not measured in muscle; therefore, muscle involvement has not been excluded. This autosomal recessive phosphorylase kinase deficiency in both liver and muscle is caused by mutations in the β subunit of phosphorylase kinase gene (*PHKB*) (GenBank J04120). Several nonsense mutations, a single-base insertion, a splice-site mutation, and a large intragenic mutation have been identified.[409] A missense mutation A117P was observed in an atypical patient who had normal blood cell phosphorylase kinase activity.[410]

Autosomal Liver Phosphorylase Kinase Deficiency (IXc). The occurrence of autosomal phosphorylase kinase deficiency restricted to liver is certainly possible, as reported by Hug[393] and as illustrated by the rat gsd strain (Table 71-2). In both human and rat, this form of phosphorylase kinase deficiency is due to mutations in the testis/liver isoform of the γ subunit of the gene (*PHKG2*)[411] (GenBank M31606). In contrast to the benign course of X-linked phosphorylase kinase deficiency, patients with mutations in the *PHKG2* gene have more severe phenotypes and often develop a liver cirrhosis.[412,413]

Muscle-Specific Phosphorylase Kinase Deficiency (IXd). A few cases of phosphorylase kinase deficiency restricted to muscle have been reported. Four male patients presented either with cramps and pigmenturia on exercise, or with progressive muscle weakness and atrophy.[414,415] Phosphorylase kinase activity was decreased in muscle but (when determined) normal in liver and blood cells. Characteristically, onset of symptoms was late (adolescence or adulthood). In addition, two female patients exhibited muscle weakness during infancy and childhood, respectively.[416,417] Glycogen deposition and phosphorylase kinase deficiency was observed in muscle biopsies from both. Phosphorylase kinase activity in other tissues was not determined, but there was no hepatomegaly or cardiomyopathy. The muscle isoform of the α subunit (*PHKA1*) gene and the muscle-specific exon of the *PHKB* gene would be plausible candidates for these presumably autosomal recessive muscle-specific phosphorylase kinase deficiency. A single male patient presented at 46 years of age with progressive fatigability, weakness, and atrophy, but no exertional pain or cramps was found to have a nonsense mutation in the *PHKA1* gene.[418] The mutation in this same gene is responsible for the phosphorylase kinase deficiency in the I strain of mouse.[419]

Phosphorylase Kinase Deficiency Limited to Heart. Several sporadic cases with cardiac-specific phosphorylase kinase deficiency have been reported. All died during infancy from cardiac failure due to massive glycogen deposition in the myocardium.[420–422a] The molecular basis has not been defined.

Diagnosis. Definitive diagnosis of phosphorylase b kinase deficiency requires demonstration of the enzymatic defect in affected tissues. Phosphorylase b kinase can be measured in leukocytes and erythrocytes but, as the enzyme has many isozymes, the diagnosis can be missed without studies of liver, muscle, or heart. Molecular genetic analysis provides further subtyping of the disease.

Treatment. The treatment for liver phosphorylase kinase deficiency is symptomatic. A high-carbohydrate diet and frequent feedings are effective in preventing hypoglycemia, but most patients require no specific treatment. Prognosis is usually good; adult patients have normal stature and minimal hepatomegaly. There is currently no treatment for the fatal form of isolated cardiac phosphorylase kinase deficiency.

Animal Model. A mouse strain with X-linked phosphorylase kinase deficiency in muscle, intermediate level in heart but normal in liver, has been intensively studied. Affected mice do not have clinical symptoms other than being less agile than normal laboratory mice. The trait maps on the X chromosome to the same region as the muscle α-subunit structural gene (*PHKA1*) and a frameshift mutation of this gene is responsible for the muscle phosphorylase kinase deficiency.[419] A rat strain, gsd, displays hepatomegaly, increased glycogen in the liver, and an autosomal recessive phosphorylase kinase deficiency in liver but not muscle[423] that is caused by mutations in the testis/liver isoform of the phosphorylase kinase γ subunit (*PHKG2*).[411]

Other Glycogenoses

Glycogen Synthase Deficiency. Genetic deficiency of glycogen synthase activity in humans appears to be very rare.[424–426] Strictly speaking, this is not a type of glycogen storage disease, as the deficiency of the enzyme leads to decreased glycogen stores. The patients present in early infancy with early morning drowsiness and fatigue and sometimes with convulsions associated with hypoglycemia and hyperketonemia. There is no hepatomegaly or hyperlipidemia. Hyperglycemia and a rise of blood lactate concentration may occur after meals. This can be attributed to the glucose being preferentially converted to lactate in the absence of glycogen synthesis. During fasting, administration of glucagon has no effect on blood glucose, lactate, or alanine concentrations, whereas after a meal, glucagon causes a rise in glucose and a fall in lactate and alanine. Treatment is symptomatic and involves frequent feedings rich in protein and nighttime supplementation with uncooked cornstarch to alleviate hypoglycemia. Prognosis seems good as patients survive to adulthood with resolution of hypoglycemia except during pregnancy.[427]

Because glycogen synthase deficiency is not expressed in muscle, erythrocytes, or cultured fibroblasts, a definitive diagnosis requires liver biopsy. Under normal conditions of nutrition, the hepatic glycogen content of normal individuals is 3.3 ± 1.7 percent of wet liver weight (range: 1 to 6 percent). The affected patients have decreased glycogen stores (< 1.5 percent) and deficient glycogen synthase activity. The disease is inherited in an autosomal recessive manner. Carrier detection has not been done. The liver glycogen synthase gene is located on chromosome 12p12.2 (GenBank P54840). Mutations in this gene that cause glycogen synthase deficiency have been identified.[428]

Hepatic Glycogenosis with Renal Fanconi Syndrome (Fanconi-Bickel Syndrome). This rare autosomal recessive disease is caused by defects in the facilitative glucose transporter 2 (GLUT2) (GenBank J03810), which transports glucose in and out of hepatocytes, pancreatic β cells and the basolateral membranes of intestinal and renal epithelial cells.[139,429] The disease is characterized by proximal renal tubular dysfunction, impaired glucose and galactose utilization, and accumulation of glycogen in liver and kidney.[430–432] The disease is also known as Fanconi-Bickel syndrome, in recognition of their clinical description of the first patient in 1949.[430] The disease may be confused with type I glycogen storage disease, as a Fanconi-like syndrome can develop in type I patients.[207]

The affected child presents in the first year of life with failure to thrive, rickets, and a protuberant abdomen due to hepato- and renomegaly. Laboratory findings include glucosuria, phosphaturia, generalized aminoaciduria, bicarbonate wasting, hypophosphatemia, increased serum alkaline phosphatase levels, and radiologic findings of rickets. Mild fasting hypoglycemia and hyperlipidemia may be present. Liver transaminases, plasma lactate, and uric acid are usually normal. Oral galactose or glucose tolerance tests show intolerance to these sugars which could be explained by the functional loss of GLUT2 preventing liver uptake of these sugars.

Tissue biopsies show marked accumulation of glycogen in hepatocytes and proximal renal tubular cells, presumably due to the altered glucose transport out of these organs. Diffuse glomerular mesangial expansion accompanied by glomerular hyperfiltration and microalbuminuria similar to nephropathy in glycogen storage disease type Ia and diabetes have been reported.[433]

There is no specific therapy. Growth retardation persists through adulthood. Symptomatic replacement of water, electrolytes, and vitamin D, restriction of galactose intake, and a diabetes mellitus-like diet, presented in frequent and small meals with cornstarch supplement and an adequate caloric intake, may improve growth.[434]

The low prevalence of Fanconi-Bickel syndrome (less than 100 cases reported worldwide) is underlined by the finding of consanguinity of the parents in 72% of reported families and in 70% of the cases with a detectable GLUT2 mutation. Most mutations detected so far predicted a premature termination of translation; the resulting loss of the C-terminal end of the GLUT2 protein predicts a nonfunctioning glucose transporter (with an inward-facing substrate binding site).[139–429] A mouse model of GLUT2 inactivation generated by homologous recombination shows symptoms characteristic of noninsulin-dependent diabetes mellitus.[435]

Phosphoglucoisomerase Deficiency. The hereditary disorder of phosphoglucoisomerase deficiency in humans usually is limited to erythrocytes and is manifested by a congenital nonspherocytic hemolytic anemia[436] (see Chap. 182). Two patients with mental retardation, muscle weakness, and/or hepatomegaly were found to have a generalized phosphoglucoisomerase deficiency with excessive amounts of glycogen in the muscle, liver, and erythrocytes.[437,438] There was no hypoglycemia. Frequent meals with a diet low in carbohydrate normalized the liver size in one patient.

Other Muscle Glycogenoses with Muscle-Energy Impairment. Five additional enzyme defects, phosphoglycerate kinase (GenBank V00572), phosphoglycerate mutase (GenBank M18172), lactate dehydrogenase (GenBank S66853), fructose 1,6-bisphosphate aldolase A deficiency (GenBank NM 000034),[438a] and muscle pyruvate kinase deficiency,[438b] in the pathway of the terminal glycolysis also cause symptoms and signs of muscle energy impairment similar to type V or VII glycogen storage disease. Phosphoglycerate kinase deficiency, an X-linked disease can cause hemolytic anemia, central nervous system dysfunction, and/or myopathy.[439,440] So far, six missense mutations and one splice-junction mutation have been identified in seven patients, two of whom had myopathy.[441] Human phosphoglycerate mutase comprises M, B, and MB-types isozymes. Deficiency of muscle phosphoglycerate mutase M subunit is associated with exercise intolerance, muscle cramps, and myoglobinuria.[440,442] A point mutation resulting in a stop codon at codon position 78 of the muscle phosphoglycerate mutase protein is responsible for phosphoglycerate mutase deficiency in patients with an African-American background.[443] Lactate dehydrogenase M-subunit deficiency was first reported in 1980 as an exertional myoglobinuria, some patients also have skin lesions.[444–446] Fructose 1,6-bisphosphate aldolase A deficiency causes exercise intolerance, muscle weakness, and hemolytic anemia. The disease is due to mutation in the aldolase A gene located on chromosome 16q22-q24.[338a] Deficiency of the muscle isoform of pyruvate kinase is associated with muscle cramps and fixed weakness. The molecular defect has not been defined.[348b]

The failure of blood lactate to increase in response to exercise is a useful diagnostic test for these disorders and can be used to differentiate muscle glycogenoses from disorders of lipid metabolism, such as carnitine palmitoyl transferase II deficiency and very long chain acyl-CoA dehydrogenase deficiency, which also cause muscle cramps and myoglobinuria[168] (see Chap. 101). Muscle glycogen levels may be normal in these disorders affecting terminal glycolysis, and definite diagnosis is made by assaying the enzyme activity in muscle tissues. There is no specific treatment. As in other muscle glycogenoses, avoidance of strenuous exercise prevents acute attacks of muscle cramps and myoglobinuria.

ACKNOWLEDGMENTS

I thank Janice Chou for discussion and critical review of the section on glucose 6-phosphatase systems, and Ann Burchell for providing the updated figures. Studies contributing to the information in this chapter were supported in part by the National Institutes of Health DK 39078 and M01-RR30, National Centers for Research Sources, General Clinical Research Centers Program.

REFERENCES

1. Howell R, Williams J, The glycogen storage diseasess, in Stanbury JB, Fredrickson DS, Goldstein JL, Brown MS (Eds): *The Metabolic Basis of Inherited Disease*. 5th Edition. New York, McGraw-Hill, 1983, p. 141.
2. Rybicka KK: Glycosomes — The organelles of glycogen metabolism. *Tissue Cell* **28**:254, 1996.
3. Roach P, Skurat A: Self-glucosylating initiator proteins and their role in glycogen biosynthesis. *Prog Nucleic Acid Res Mol Biol* **57**:289, 1997.
4. Alonso M, Lomako J, Lomako W, Whelan W: A new look at the biogenesis of glycogen. *FASEB J* **9**:1126, 1995.
5. Krisman C: A possible intermediate in the initiation of glycogen biosynthesis. *Biochem Biophys Res Commun* **46**:1206, 1972.
6. Rodriguez I, Whelan W: A novel glycogsyl-amino acid linkage: Rabbit muscle glycogen is covalently linked to a protein via tyrosine. *Biochem Biophys Res Commun* **132**:829, 1985.
7. Smythe C, Cohen P: The discovery of glycogenin and the priming mechanism for glycogen biogenesis. *Eur J Biochem* **200**:625, 1991.
8. Lomako J, Lomako W, Whelan W: The biogenesis of glycogen: Nature of the carbohydrate in the protein primer. *Biochem Int* **21**:251, 1990.
9. Pitcher J, Smythe C, Cohen P: Glycogenin is the priming glucosyltransferase required for the initiation of glycogen biogenesis in rabbit skeletal muscle. *Eur J Biochem* **176**:391, 1988.
10. Lomako J, Mazuruk K, Lomako W, Alonso M, Whelan W, Rodriguez I: The human intron-containing gene for glycogenin maps to chromosome 3, band q24. *Genomics* **33**:519, 1996.
11. Mu J, Skurat A, Roach P: Glycogenin-2, a novel self-glucosylating protein involved in liver glycogen biosynthesis. *J Biol Chem* **272**:27589, 1997.
12. Kirkman B, Whelan W, Bailey J: The distribution of glucosamine in mammalian glycogen from different species, organs, and tissues. *Biofactors* **2**:123, 1989.
13. Roach P, Warren K, Atkinson D: Uridine diphosphate glucose synthase from calf liver: Determinants of enzyme activity in vitro. *Biochemistry* **14**:5445, 1975.
14. Albrecht G, Bass S, Seifert L, Hansen R: Crystallization and properties of uridine diphosphate glucose pyrophosphorylase from liver. *J Biol Chem* **241**:2968, 1966.
15. Bergamini C, Signorini M, Ferrari C, Dallocchio F: Purification of muscle uridine diphosphoglucose pyrophosphorylase by hydrophobic chromatography. *Anal Biochem* **143**:35, 1984.
16. Azzar G, Persat F, Degiuli A, Got R: Purification of a UTP: D-Glucose-1-phosphate uridylyl-transferase from Golgi apparatus of cat liver by affinity chromatography on UTP-agarose. *Anal Biochem* **142**:518, 1984.
17. Flores-Diaz M, Alape-Giron A, Persson B, Pollesello P, Moos M, von Eichel-Streiber C, Thelestam M, et al. Cellular UDP-glucose deficiency caused by a single point mutation in the UDP-glucose pyrophosphorylase gene. *J Biol Chem* **272**:23784, 1997.
18. Bai G, Zhang Z, Werner R, Nuttall F, Tan A, Lee E: The primary structure of rat liver glycogen synthase deduced by cDNA cloning. *J Biol Chem* **265**:7845, 1990.
19. Browner M, Nakano K, Bang A, Fletterick R: Human muscle glycogen synthetase cDNA sequence: A negatively charged protein with an asymmetric charge distribution. *Pro Natl Acad Sci U S A* **86**:1443, 1989.
20. Pellegri G, Rossier C, Magistretti P, Martin J: Cloning, localization, and induction of mouse brain glycogen synthase. *Br Res Mol Br Res* **38**:191, 1996.
21. Dent P, Lavoinne A, Nakielny S, Caudwell F, Watt P, Cohen P: The molecular mechanism by which insulin stimulates glycogen synthesis in mammalian skeletal muscle. *Nature* **348**:302, 1990.
22. Stalmans W: Glucagon and liver glycogen metabolism, in Liefebvre PJ (ed): *Handbook of Experimental Pharmacology*. Springer Verlag, 1983, p. 291.

23. Nakielny S, Campbell D, Cohen P: The molecular mechanism by which adrenaline inhibits glycogen synthesis. *Eur J Biochem* **199**:713, 1991.
24. Cohen P, Hardie D: The actions of cyclic AMP on biosynthetic processes are mediated indirectly by cyclic AMP-dependent protein kinase. *Biochem Biophys Acta* **1094**:292, 1991.
25. Stalmans W, De Wulf H, Hers H: The control of liver glycogen synthetase phosphatase by phosphorylase. *Eur J Biochem* **18**:582, 1971.
25a. Bollen M, Keppens S, Stalmans W: Specific features of glycogen metabolism in the liver. *Biochem J* **336**:19, 1998.
26. Lawrence J, Roach P: New insights into the role and mechanism of glycogen synthase activation by insulin. *Diabetes* **46**:541, 1997.
27. Hubbard M, Cohen P: On target with a new mechanism for the regulation of protein phosphorylation. *Trends Biochem Sci* **18**:172, 1993.
28. Cross D, Alessi D, Cohen P, Andjelkovich M, Hemmings B: Inhibition of glycogen synthase kinase-3 by insulin mediated by protein kinase B. *Nature* **378**:785, 1995.
29. Manchester J, Skurat A, Roach P, Hauschka S, Lawrence J: Increased glycogen accumulation in transgenic mice overexpressing glycogen synthase in skeletal muscle. *Proc Natl Acad Sci U S A* **93**:10707, 1996.
30. Verhue W, Hers H: A study of the reaction catalyzed by the liver branching enzyme. *Biochem J* **93**:222, 1966.
31. Zimmerman C, Gold A: Isolation and characterization of glycogen branching enzyme from rabbit liver. *Biochemistry* **22**:3387, 1983.
32. Thon V, Khalil M, Cannon J: Isolation of human glycogen branching enzyme cDNAs by screening complementation in yeast. *J Biol Chem* **268**:7509, 1993.
33. Bates E, Heaton G, Taylor C, Kernohan J, Cohen P: Debranching enzyme from rabbit skeletal muscle: Evidence for the location of the two active centres on a single polypeptide chain. *FEBS Lett* **58**:181, 1975.
34. Liu W, Madsen N, Braun C, Withers S: Reassessment of the catalytic mechanism of glycogen debranching enzyme. *Biochemistry* **30**:1419, 1991.
35. Brown D, Gordon R, Brown B: Studies on the structure and mechanism of action of the glycogen debranching enzymes of muscle and liver. *Ann N Y Acad Sci* **210**:238, 1973.
36. Taylor C, Cox A, Kernohan J, Cohen P: Debranching enzyme from rabbit skeletal muscle: Purification, properties, and physiological role. *Eur J Biochem* **51**:105, 1975.
37. Chen Y-T, He J-K, Ding J-H, Brown B: Glycogen debranching enzyme: Purification, antibody characterization, and immunoblot analyses of type III glycogen storage disease. *Am J Hum Genet* **41**:1002, 1987.
38. Yang B-Z, Ding J-H, Enghild J, Bao Y, Chen Y-T: Molecular cloning and nucleotide sequence of cDNA encoding human muscle glycogen debranching enzyme. *J Biol Chem* **267**:9294, 1992.
39. Liu W, de Castro M, Takrama J, Bilous P, Vinayagamoorthy T, Madsen N, Bleackley R: Molecular cloning, sequencing and analysis of the cDNA for rabbit muscle glycogen debranching enzyme. *Arch Biochem Biophy* **306**:232, 1993.
40. Braun C, Lindhorst T, Madsen N, Withers S: Identification of Asp 549 as the catalytic nucleophile of glycogen-debranching enzyme via trapping of the glycosyl-enzyme intermediate. *Biochemistry* **35**:5458, 1996.
41. Yang-Feng T, Zheng K, Yu J, Yang B-Z, Chen Y-T: Assignment of the human glycogen debrancher gene to chromosome Ip21. *Genomics* **13**:931, 1992.
42. Bao Y, Dawson T, Chen Y-T: Human glycogen debranching enzyme gene: Complete structural organization and characterization of the 5′ flanking region. *Genomics* **38**:155, 1996.
43. Bao Y, Yang B-Z, Dawson T, Chen Y: Isolation and nucleotide sequence of human liver glycogen debranching enzyme mRNA: Identification of multiple tissue-specific isoforms. *Gene* **197**:389, 1997.
44. Newgard C, Hwang P, Fletterick R: The family of glycogen phosphorylases: Structure and function. *Crit Rev Biochem Mol Biol* **24**:69, 1989.
45. Newgard C, Nakano K, Hwang P, Fletterick R: Sequence analysis of the cDNA encoding human liver glycogen phosphorylase reveals tissue-specific codon usage. *Pro Natl Acad Sci U S A* **83**:8132, 1986.
46. Newgard C, Littman D, van Genderen C, Smith M, Fletterick R: Human brain glycogen phosphorylase. Cloning, sequence analysis, chromosomal mapping, tissue expression, and comparison with the human liver and muscle isozymes. *J Biol Chem* **263**:3850, 1988.
47. Hwang P, See Y, Vincentini A, Powers M, Fletterick R, Crerar M: Comparative sequence analysis of rat, rabbit, and human muscle glycogen phosphorylase cDNAs. *Eur J Biochem* **152**:267, 1985.
48. Newgard C, Fletterick R, Anderson L, Lebo R: The polymorphic locus for glycogen storage disease VI (liver glycogen phophorylase) maps to chromosome 14. *Am J Hum Genet* **40**:351, 1987.
49. Lebo R, Gorin F, Fletterick R, Kao F-T, Cheung M, Bruce B, Kan Y: High resolution chromosome sorting and DNA spot-blot analysis localize McArdle's Syndrome to Chromosome 11. *Science* **225**:57, 1984.
50. Rath V, Newgard C, Sprang S, Goldsmith E, Fletterick R: Modelling the biochemical differences between rabbit muscle and human liver phosphorylase. *Proteins* **2**:225, 1987.
51. Coats W, Browner M, Fletterick R, Newgard C: An engineered liver glycogen phosphorylase with AMP allosteric activation. *J Biol Chem* **266**:16113, 1991.
52. Matthews C, Carlsen R, Froman B, Tait R, Gorin F: Nerve-dependent factors regulating transcript levels of glycogen phosphorylase in skeletal muscle. *Cell Mol Neurobiol* **18**:319, 1998.
53. Pickett-Gies C, Walsh D: Phosphorylase kinase, in Boyer KE (Ed): *The Enzymes*. Orlando, FL; Academic, 1986, p. 395.
54. Cohen P: The subunit structure of rabbit-skeletal-muscle phosphorylase kinase, and the molecular basis of its activation reactions. *Eur J Biochem* **34**:1, 1973.
55. Cohen P, Burchell A, Foulkes J, Cohen P: Identification of the Ca^{2+} dependent modulator protein as the fourth subunit of rabbit skeletal muscle phosphorylase kinase. *FEBS Lett* **92**:287, 1978.
56. Shuster J, Chan K, Graves D: Isolation and properties of the catalytically active subunit of phosphorylase β kinase. *J Biol Chem* **255**:2203, 1980.
57. Burchell A, Cohen P, Cohen P: Distribution of isoenzymes of the glycogenolytic cascade in different types of muscle fibre. *FEBS Lett* **67**:17, 1976.
58. Kilimann M: Glycogen storage disease due to phosphorylase kinase deficiency, in Swallow EY (Ed.): *Protein Dysfunction and Human Genetic Disease*. Oxford, BIOS Scientific Publishers, 1997.
59. Kilimann M, Zander N, Kuhn C, Crabb J, Meyer H, Heilmeyer LJ: The α and β subunits of phosphorylase kinase are homologous: cDNA cloning and primary structure of the β subunit. *Proc Natl Acad Sci U S A* **85**:9381, 1988.
60. Zander N, Meyer H, Hoffmann-Posorske E, Crabb J, Heilmeyer LJ, Kilimann M: cDNA cloning and complete primary structure of skeletal muscle phosphorylase kinase (α-subunit). *Proc Natl Acad Sci U S A* **85**:2929, 1988.
61. Harmann B, Zander N, Kilimann M: Isoform diversity of phosphorylase kinase α and β subunits generated by alternative RNA splicing. *J Biol Chem* **266**:15631, 1991.
62. Davidson J, Ozcelik T, Hamachar C, Willems P, Francke U, Kilimann M: cDNA cloning of a liver isoform of the phosphorylase kinase α subunit and mapping of the gene to Xp22.2-p22.1, the region of human X-linked liver glycogenosis. *Proc Natl Acad U S A* **89**:2096, 1992.
63. Francke U, Darras B, Zander N, Kilimann M: Assignment of human genes for phosphorylase kinase subunits α (PHKA) to Xq12-q13 and β (PHKB) to 16q12-q13. *Am J Hum Genet* **45**:276, 1989.
64. da Cruz e Silva E, Cohen P: Isolation and sequence analysis of a cDNA clone encoding the entire catalytic subunit of phosphorylase kinase. *FEBS Lett* **220**:36, 1987.
65. Chamberlain J, Van Tuinen P, Reeves A, Philip B, Caskey C: Isolation of cDNA clones for the catalytic subunit of mouse phosphorylase kinase: Expression of mRNA in normal and mutant PHK mice. *Proc Natl Acad Sci U S A* **84**:2886, 1987.
66. Jones T, da Cruz E, Spurr N, Sheer D, Cohen P: Location of the gene encoding the catalytic γ subunit of phosphorylase kinase to human chromosome bands 7p12-q21. *Biochim Biophys Acta* **1048**:24, 1990.
67. Calalb M, Fox D, Hanks S: Molecular cloning and enzymatic analysis of the rat homolog of "PhK-γT," an isoform of phosphorylase kinase catalytic subunit. *J Biol Chem* **267**:1455, 1992.
68. Whitmore S, Apostolou S, Lane S, Nancarrow J, Phillips H, Richards R, Sutherland G, et al: Isolation and characterization of transcribed sequences from a chromosome 16 hn-cDNA library and the physical mapping of genes and transcribed sequences using a high-resolution somatic cell panel of human chromosome 16. *Genomics* **20**:169, 1994.

69. Fischer R, Koller M, Flura M, Mathews S, Strehler-Page M, Krebs J, Pennisten J, et al: Multiple divergent mRNA's code for a single human calmodulin. *J Biol Chem* **263**:17055, 1988.
70. Berchtold M, Egli R, Rhyner J, Hameister H, Strehler E: Localization of the human bona fide calmodulin genes CALM1, CALM2, and CALM3 to chromosomes 14q24-q31, 2p21.1-21.3, and 19q13.2-q13.3. *Genomics* **16**:461, 1993.
71. Bender P, Dedman J, Emerson C: The abundance of calmodulin mRNAs is regulated in phosphorylase kinase-deficient skeletal muscle. *J Biol Chem* **263**:9733, 1988.
72. Cohen P, Foulkes J: The hormonal control of gene transcription, in Cohen H, Foulkes JG (Ed) *The Molecular Aspects of Cellular Regulation*. Amsterdam, Elsevier, 1991.
73. McKnight G, Clegg C, Uhler M, Chrivia J, Cadd G, Correll L, Otten A: Analysis of the cAMP-dependent protein kinase system using molecular genetic approaches. *Recent Prog Horm Res* **44**:307, 1988.
74. Cohen P, Foulkes J, Goris J, Hemmings B, Ingebritsen T, Stewart A, Strada S: Classification of protein phosphatases involved in cellular regulation, in Holzer H (Ed): *Metabolic Interconversion of Enzymes*. Heidelberg, Springer-Verlag, 1980, p. 28.
75. Cohen P: Novel protein serine/threonine phosphatases: Variety is the spice of life. *Trends Biochemi Sci* **22**:245, 1997.
76. Cohen P: The structure and regulation of protein phosphatases. *Ann Rev Biochem* **58**:453, 1989.
77. Bai G, Zhang Z, Amin J, Deans-Zirattu S, Lee E: Molecular cloning of a cDNA for the catalytic subunit of rabbit muscle phosphorylase phosphatase. *FASEB J* **2**:3010, 1988.
78. Zhang Z, Bai G, Deans-Zirattu S, Browner M, Lee E: Expression of the catalytic subunit of phosphorylase phosphatase (protein phosphatase-1) in *Escherichia coli*. *J Biol Chem* **267**:1484, 1992.
79. Berndt N, Campbell D, Caudwell F, Cohen P, da Cruz e Silva E, da Cruz e Silva O, Cohen P: Isolation and sequence analysis of a cDNA clone encoding a type-1 protein phosphatase catalytic subunit: Homology with protein phosphatase 2. *FEBS Lett* **223**:340, 1987.
80. Mvumbi L, Stalmans W: High-affinity binding of glycogen-synthase phosphatase to glycogen particles in the liver. Role of glycogen in the inhibition of synthase phosphatase by phosphorylase. *Biochem J* **246**:367, 1987.
81. Printen J, Brady M, Saltie A: PTG, a protein phosphatase 1-binding protein with a role in glycogen metabolism. *Science* **275**:1475, 1997.
82. Doherty M, Young P, Cohen P: Amino acid sequence of a novel protein phosphatase 1 binding protein (R5) which is related to the liver- and muscle-specific glycogen binding subunits of protein phosphatase 1. *Fed Eur Biochem Soc* **399**:339, 1996.
83. Leloir L, Trucco R, Cardini C, Paladini A, Caputto R: The coenzyme of phosphoglucomutase. *Arch Biochem* **19**:339, 1948.
84. Percival M, Withers S: ^{19}F NMR investigations of the catalytic mechanism of phosphoglucomutase using fluorinated substrates and inhibitors. *Biochemistry* **31**:505, 1992.
85. Whitehouse D, Putt W, Lovegrove J, Morrison K, Hollyoake M, Fox M, Hopkinson D, et al: Phosphoglucomutase 1: Complete human and rabbit mRNA sequences and direct mapping of this highly polymorphic marker on human chromosome 1. *Proc Natl Acad Sci U S A* **89**:411, 1992.
86. Edwards Y, Putt W, Fox M, Ives J: A novel human phosphoglucomutase (PGM5) maps to the centromeric region of chromosome 9. *Genomics* **30**:350, 1995.
87. Watanabe H, Takehana K, Date M, Shinozaki T, Raz A: Tumor cell autocrine motility factor is the neuroleukin/phosphohexose isomerase polypeptide. *Cancer Res* **56**:2960, 1996.
88. Sun A-Q, Yuksel K, Jacobson T, Gracy R: Isolation and characterization of human glucose-6-phosphate isomerase isoforms containing two different size subunits. *Arch Biochem* **283**:120, 1990.
89. Baumann M, Brand K: Purification and characterization of phosphohexose isomerase from human gastrointestinal carcinoma and its potential relationship to neuroleukin. *Cancer Res* **48**:7018, 1988.
90. Carter N, Yoshida A: Purification and characterization of human phosphoglucose isomerase. *Biochim Biophys Acta* **181**:12, 1969.
91. Fujii S, Beutler E: High glucose concentrations partially release hexokinase from inhibition by glucose 6-phosphate. *Proc Natl Acad Sci U S A* **82**:1552, 1985.
92. Schwab D, Wilson J: Complete amino acid sequence of rat brain hexokinase, deduced from the cloned cDNA, and proposed structure of a mammalian hexokinase. *Proc Natl Acad Sci U S A* **86**:2563, 1989.
93. Nishi S, Seino S, Bell G: Human hexokinase: Sequences of amino- and carboxyl-terminal halves are homologous. *Biochem Biophys Res Commun* **157**:937, 1988.
94. Cardenas M, Cornish-Bowden A, Ureta T: Evolution and regulatory role of the hexokinases. *Biochim Biophys Acta* **1401**:242, 1998.
95. Bianchi M, Crinelli R, Serafini G, Giammarini C, Magnani M: Molecular bases of hexokinase deficiency. *Biochim Biophys Acta* **1360**:211, 1997.
96. Iynedjian P, Mobius G, Seitz H, Wollheim C, Renold A: Tissue-specific expression of glucokinase: Indentification of the gene product in liver and pancreatic islets. *Proc Natl Acad Sci U S A* **83**:1998, 1986.
97. Magnuson M, Shelton K: An alternative promoter in the glucokinase gene is active in the pancreatic β cell. *J Biol Chem* **264**:15936, 1989.
98. Newgard C, Quaade C, Hughes S, Milburn J: Glucokinase and glucose transporter expression in liver and islets: Implications for control of glucose homeostasis. *Biochem Soc Tran* **18**:851, 1990.
99. Iynedjian P, Pilot P-R, Nouspikel T, Milburn J, Quaade C, Hughes S, Ucla C, et al: Differential expression and regulation of the glucokinase gene in liver and islets of Langerhans. *Proc Natl Acad Sci U S A* **86**:7838, 1989.
100. Detheux M, Vandercammen A, Van Schaftingen E: Effectors of the regulatory protein acting on liver glucokinase: A kinetic investigation. *Eur J Biochem* **200**:553, 1991.
101. Van Schaftingen E, Vandercammen A: Mechanism of the stimulatory effect of a potassium-rich medium on the phosphorylation of glucose in isolated rat hepatocytes. *Eur J Biochem* **204**:363, 1992.
102. Matschinsky F: Glucokinase as glucose sensor and metabolic signal generator in pancreatic β-cells and hepatocytes. *Diabetes* **39**:647, 1990.
103. Iynedjian P, Ucla C, Mach B: Molecular cloning of glucokinase cDNA: Developmental and dietary regulation of glucokinase mRNA in rat liver. *J Biol Chem* **262**:6032, 1987.
104. Magnuson M, Andreone T, Printz R, Koch S, Granner D: Rat glucokinase gene: Structure and regulation by insulin. *Proc Natl Acad Sci U S A* **86**:4838, 1989.
105. Jetton T, Magnuson M: Heterogeneous expression of glucogkinase among pancreatic β cells. *Proc Natl Acad Sci U S A* **89**:2619, 1992.
106. Hayzer D, Iynedjian P: Alternative splicing of glucokinase mRNA in rat liver. *Biochem J* **270**:261, 1990.
107. Froguel P: Glucokinase and MODY: From the gene to the disease. *Diabe Med* **13**:S96, 1996.
108. Glaser B, Kesavan P, Heyman M, Davis E, Cuesta A, Buchs A, Stanley C, et al: Familial hyperinsulinism caused by an activating glucokinase mutation. *N Engl J Med* **338**:226, 1998.
109. Nordlie R, Sukalski K: Multifunctional glucose-6-phosphatase: A critical review, in An M (Ed): *The Enzymes of Biological Membranes*. New York, Plenum Press, 1985, p. 349.
110. Burchell A, Waddell I: The molecular basis of the hepatic microsomal glucose-6-phosphatase system. *Biochim Biophys Acta* **1092**:129, 1991.
111. Pan C-J, Lei K-J, Chen H, Ward J, Chou J: Ontogeny of the murine glucose-6-phosphatase system. *Arch Biochem Biophy* **358**:17, 1998.
112. Khan A, Hong-Lie C, Landau B: Glucose-6-phosphatase activity in islets from ob/ob and lean mice and the effect of dexamethasane. *Endocrinology* **136**:1934, 1995.
113. Hill A, Waddell I, Hopwood D, Burchell A: The microsomal glucose-6-phosphatase enzyme of human gallbladder. *J Pathol* **158**:53, 1989.
114. Burchell A: The molecular basis of the type I glycogen storage diseases. *Bioessays* **14**:395, 1992.
115. Pan C, Kei K, Annabi B, Hemrika W, Chou J: Transmembrane topology of glucose-6-phosphatase. *J Biol Chem* **273**:6144, 1998.
116. Foster J, Pederson B, Nordlie R: Glucose-6-phosphatase structure, regulation, and function: An update. *Proc Soc Exp Biol Med* **214**:314, 1997.
117. Chou J, Mansfield B: Molecular Genetics of type I glycogen storage disease. *Trends Endocrinol Metab* **10**:104, 1999.
118. Fantl P, Rome M: Dephosphorylation in liver extracts. *Aust J Exper Biol Med Sci* **23**:21, 1945.
119. Cori G, Cori C: Glucose-6-phosphatase of the liver in glycogen storage disease. *J Biol Chem* **199**:661, 1952.
120. Lei K, Shelly L, Pan C, Sidbury J, Chou J: Mutations in the glucose 6-phosphatase gene that cause glycogen storage disease type Ia. *Science* **262**:580, 1993.
121. Gerin I, Veiga-da-Cunha M, Achouri Y, Collet J-F, Van Schaftingen E: Sequence of a putative glucose 6-phosphate translocase, mutated in glycogen storage disease type Ib. *Fed Eur Biochem Soc* **419**:235, 1997.

122. Lei K-J, Pan C-J, Shelly L, Liu J-L, Chou J: Identification of mutations in the gene for glucose-6-phosphatase, the enzyme deficient in glycogen storage disease type Ia. *J Clin Invest* **93**:1994, 1994.
123. Countaway J, Waddell I, Burchell A, Arion W: The Phosphohydrolase component of the hepatic microsomal glucose-6-phosphatase system is a 36.5 kilodalton polypeptide. *J Biol Chem* **263**:2673, 1988.
124. Speth M, Schulze H-U: The purification of a detergent-soluble glucose-6-phosphatase from rat liver. *Eur J Biochem* **208**:643, 1992.
125. Liu Z, Barrett E, Dalkin A, Zwart A, Chou J: Effect of acute diabetes on rat hepatic glucose-6-phosphatase activity and its messenger RNA level. *Biochem Biophys Res Commun* **205**:680, 1994.
126. Minssian C, Zitoun C, Mithieux G: Differetial time cource of liver and kidney glucose-6-phosphatase activity during long-term fasting in rat correlates with differential time course of messenger RNA level. *Mol Cell Biochem* **155**:37, 1996.
127. Streeper R, Svitek C, Chapman S, Greenbaum L, Taub R, O'Brien R: A multicomponent insulin response sequence mediates a strong repression of mouse glucose-6-phosphatase gene transcription by insulin. *J Biol Chem* **272**:11698, 1997.
128. Arion W, Ballas L, Lange A, Wallin B: Microsomal membrane permeability and the hepatic glucose-6-phosphatase system. *J Biol Chem* **251**:4901, 1976.
129. Arion W, Canfield W, Callaway E, Burger H-J, Hemmerle H, Schubert G, Herling A, et al: Direct evidence for the involvement of two glucose 6-phosphate-binding sites in the glucose-6-phosphatase activity of intact liver microsomes. *J Biol Chem* **273**:6223, 1998.
130. Veiga-da-Cunha M, Gerin I, Chen Y-T, de Barsy T, de Lonlay P, Dionisi-Vici C, Fenske C, et al: A gene on Chromosome 11q23 coding for a putative glucose 6-phosphate translocase is mutated in glycogen storage disease type Ib and type Ic. *Am J Hum Genet* **63**:976, 1998.
131. Annabi B, Hiraiwa H, Mansfield B, Lei K-J, Ubagai T, Polymeropoulos M, Moses S, et al: The gene for glycogen storage disease type Ib maps to chromosome 11q23. *Am J Hum Genet* 1998.
132. Pan CJ, Lin B, Chou JY: Transmembrane topology of human glucose 6-phosphate transporter. *J Biol Chem* **274**:13865, 1999.
133. Nordlie R, Scott H, Waddell I, Hume R, Burchell A: Analysis of human hepatic microsomal glucose-6-phosphatase in clinical conditions where the T2 pyrophosphate/phosphate transport protein is absent. *Biochem J* **281**:859, 1992.
134. Waddell I, Lindsay J, Burchell A: The identification of T2; the phosphate/pyrophosphate transport protein of the hepatic microsomal glucose-6-phosphatase system. *FEBS Lett* **229**:179, 1988.
135. Kayamo T, Burant C, Fukumoto H, Gould G, Fan Y, Eddy R, Byers M, et al: Human facilitative glucose transporters. *J Biol Chem* **265**:13276, 1990.
136. Devaskar S, Meuckler M: The mammalian glucose transporters. *Pediatr Res* **31**:1, 1992.
137. Thorens B: Cloning and functional expression in bacteria of a novel glucose transporter present in liver, intestine, kidney, and β pancreatic islet cells. *Cell* **55**:281, 1988.
138. Seidner G, Alvarez M, Yeh J, O'Driscoll K, Klepper J, Stump T, Wang D, et al: GLUT-1 deficiency syndrome caused by haploinsufficiency of the blood-brain barrier hexose carrier. *Nat Genet* **18**:188, 1998.
139. Santer R, Schneppenheim R, Dombrowski A, Gotze H, Steinmann B, Schaub J: Mutations in *GLUT2*, the gene for the liver-type glucose transporter, in patients with Fanconi-Bickel syndrome. *Nat Genet* **17**:324, 1997.
140. Burchell A: A re-evaluation of GLUT 7. *Biochem J* **331**:973, 1998.
141. Uyeda K: Phosphofructokinase. *Adv Enzymol* **48**:193, 1979.
142. Vora S: Isozymes of phosphofructokinase. *Isozymes Curr Top Biol Med Res* **6**:119, 1982.
143. Vora S, Durham S, De Martinville B, George D, Francke U: Assignment of the human gene for muscle-type phosphofructokinase (PFKM) to chromosome 1 (region cen-q32) using somatic cell hybrids and monoclonal anti-M antibody. *Somat Cell Genet* **8**:95, 1982.
144. Pilkis S, El-Maghrabi M, McGrane M, Pilkis J, Fox E, Claus T: Fructose 2,6-biphosphate: A mediator of hormone action at the fructose 6-phosphate/fructose 1,6-biphosphate substrate cycle. *Mol Cell Endocrinol* **25**:245, 1982.
145. Hue L: The role of futile cycles in the regulation of carbohydrate metabolism in the liver. *Adv Enzymol* **52**:247, 1981.
146. Shulman R, Bloch G, Rothman D: In vivo regulation of muscle glycogen synthase and the control of glycogen synthesis. *Proc Natl Acad Sci U S A* **92**:8535, 1995.
147. Khan A, Chandramouli V, Ostenson C-G, Berggren P, Low H, Landau B, Efendic S: Glucose cycling is markedly enhanced in pancreatic islets of obese hyperglycaemic mice. *Endocrinology* **126**:2413, 1990.
148. Shulman G, Ladenson P, Wolfe M, Ridgway E, Wolfe R: Substrate cycling between gluconeogenesis and glycolysis in euthyroid, hypothyroid, and hyperthyroid man. *J Clin Invest* **76**:757, 1985.
149. Wajngot A, Chandramouli V, Schumann W, Efendic S, Landau B: Quantitation of glycogen/glucose-1-P cycling in liver. *Metabolism* **40**:877, 1991.
150. David M, Petit W, Laughlin M, Shulman R, King J, Barrett E: Simultaneous synthesis and degradation of rat liver glycogen: An in vivo nuclear magnetic resonance spectroscopic study. *J Clin Invest* **86**:612, 1990.
151. Katz J, Kuwajima M, Foster D, MGarry J: The glucose paradox. New perspectives on hepatic carbohydrate metabolism. *Trends Biochem Sci* **11**:136, 1986.
152. Shulman G, Cline G, Schumann W, Chandramouli V, Kumaran K, Landau B: Quantitative comparison of pathways of hepatic glycogen repletion in fed and fasted humans. *Am J Physiol* **259:E335, 1990.**
153. Landau B, Wahren J: Quantification of the pathways followed in glycogen formation from glucose. *FASEB J* **2**:2368, 1988.
154. Burchell A, Arion W, Smith I, Hume R: Perinatal expression of elevated hepatic protein phosphatase type I activity levels. *J Inherit Metab Dis* **13**:255, 1990.
155. Newgard C, Norkiewicz B, Hughes S, Frenkel R, Coats W, Martiniuk F, Johnston J: Developmental expression of glycogenolytic enzymes in rabbit tissues: Possible relationship to fetal lung maturation. *Biochim Biophy Acta* **1090**:333, 1991.
156. Warburton D, Cohen P: Ontogeny of protein phosphatases 1 and 2A in developing rat lung. *Pediat Res* **24**:25, 1988.
157. Gold A: Structural studies on neonatal rat liver glycogen synthase: A comparison between adult and newborn synthase phosphopeptides. *Arch Biochem Biophys* **256**:202, 1987.
158. Dunaway G, Kasten T, Crabtree S, Mhaskar Y: Age-related changes in subunit composition and regulation of hepatic 6-phosphofructo-1-kinase. *Biochem J* **266**:823, 1990.
159. Snappes I, Van Creveld S: Un cas d'hypoglycemie avec acetonemie chez un enfant. *Bull Mem Soc Med Hop* **52**:1315, 1928.
160. Cori G: Glycogen structure and enzyme deficiencies in glycogen storage disease. *Harvey Lec* **48**:145, 1954.
161. Hers H, Van Hoof F, De Barsy T: Glycogen storage diseases, in Scriver CR, Sly WS, Valle D (Eds): *The Metabolic Basis of Inherited Disease*, 6th edition. New York, McGraw-Hill, 1989, p. 425.
162. Chen Y-T: Glycogen storage diseases, in *Harrison's Principles of Internal Medicine*, 14th Edition. New York, McGraw Hill, 1998, p. 2176.
163. Fernandes J, Chen Y-T: The glycogen storage diseases, in *Inborn Metabolic Diseases: Diagnosis and Treatment*. 1995, p. 71.
164. Moses S: Pathophysiology and dietary treatment of the glycogen storage diseases. *J Pediat Gastroenterol Nutr* **11**:155, 1990.
165. Cornblath M, Schwartz R: Disorders of glycogen metabolism, in *Disorders of Carbohydrate Metabolism in Infancy*, 3rd ed. Boston, Blackwell Scientific, 1991, p. 247.
166. DiMauro S, Bruno C: Glycogen storage diseases of muscle. *Curr Opin Neurol* **11**:477, 1998.
167. Moses S: Muscle glycogenosis. *J Inherit Metab Dis* **13**:452, 1990.
168. Tein I: Metabolic myopathies. *Sem Pediatr Neurol* **3**:59, 1996.
169. Fernandes J, Leonard J, Moses S, Odievre M, di Rocco M, Schaub J, Smith G, et al:[RHA26] Glycogen storage disease: Recommendations for treatment. *Eur J Pediatr* **147**:226, 1988.
170. Chen Y-T, Bazarre C, Lee M, Sidbury J, Coleman R: Type I glycogen storage disease: Nine years of management with cornstarch. *Eur J Pediatr* **152**:S56, 1993.
171. McAdams A, Hug G, Bove K: Glycogen storage disease, types I to X: Criteria for morphologic diagnosis. *Hum Pathol* **5**:463, 1974.
172. Jevon G, Finegold M: Reliability of histological criteria in glycogen storage disease of the liver. *Pediat Pathol* **14**:709, 1994.
173. Brown B: Diagnosis of glycogen storage disease, in Raw (Ed): *Congential Metabolic Disease, Diagnosis and Treatment*. Basel, Switzerland, Dekker, 1985, p. 227.
174. Shin Y: Diagnosis of glycogen storage disease. *J Inherit Metab Dis* **13**:419, 1990.
175. Turnbull D, Sherratt S, Metabolic studies using isolated skeletal-muscle. Investigation of metabolic myopathies, in Alberti HP, Taylor

R (Eds): *Technical Metabolic Investigations of Man.* Sussex, UK, Baillieres, Tindall and WB Saunders, 1987, p. 967.

175a. Elpeleg ON: The molecular background of glycogen metabolism disorders. *J. Pediatr Endocrinol Metab* **12**:363, 1999.

176. Walvoort HC: Glycogen storage diseases in animals and their potential value as models of human disease. *J Inherit Metab Dis* **6**:3, 1983.

177. von Gierke E: Hepato-nephro-megalia glycogenica (Glykogenspeicher-krankheit der Leber und Nieren). *Beitr Pathol Anat* **82**:497, 1929.

178. Senior B, Loridan L: Studies of liver glycogeneses, with particular reference to the metabolism of intravenously administered glycerol. *N Engl J Med* **279**:958, 1968.

179. Bialek D, Sharp H, Kane W, Elders J, Nordlie R: Latency of glucose 6-phosphatase in type Ib glycogen storage disease. *J Pediatr* **91**:838, 1977.

180. Narisawa K, Igarashi Y, Otomo H, Tada K: A new variant of glycogen storage disease type I probably due to a defect in the glucose 6-phosphate transport system. *Biochem Biophys Res Commun* **83**:1360, 1978.

181. Lange A, Arion W, Beaudet A: Type Ib glycogen storage disease is caused by a defect in the glucose 6-phosphate translocase of the microsomal glucose 6-phosphatase system. *J Biol Chem* **255**:8381, 1980.

182. Nordlie R, Sukalski K, Munoz J, Baldwin J: Type Ic, a novel glycogenosis. Underlying mechanisms. *J Biol Chem* **258**:9739, 1983.

183. Hug G, Chuck G, Tsoras M: Increased serum biotinidase activity in glycogen storage disease type Ia. *Pediatr Res* **35**:203A, 1994.

184. Burlina A, Dermikol M, Mantau A, Piovan S, Grazian L, Zacchello F Y S: Increased plasma biotinidase activity in patients with glycogen storage disease type Ia: Effect of biotin supplementation. *J Inherit Metab Dis* **19**:209, 1996.

185. Alaupovic P, Fernandes J: The serum apolipoprotein profile of patients with glucose 6-phosphatase deficiency. *Pediatr Res* **19**:380, 1985.

186. Levy E, Thibault L, Roy C, Bendayan M, Lepage G, Letarte J: Circulating lipids and lipoproteins in glycogen storage disease type I with nocturnal intragastric feeding. *J Lipid Res* **29**:215, 1988.

187. Keddad K, Razavian S, Baussan C, Chalas J, Abella A, Levenson J, Simon A, et al: Blood lipids and rheological modifications in glycogen storage disease. *Clin Biochem* **29**:73, 1996.

188. Keller K, Schutz M, Podskarbi T, Bindl L, Lentze M, Shin Y: A new mutation of the glucose-6-phosphatase gene in a 4-year-old girl with oligosymptomatic glycogen storage disease type Ia. *J Pediatr* **132**:360, 1998.

189. Stamm W, Webb D: Partial deficiency of hepatic glucose-6-phosphatase in an adult patient. *Arch Intern Med* **135**:1107, 1975.

190. Beaudet A, Anderson D, Michels V, Arion W, Lange A: Neutropenia and impaired neutrophil migration in type Ib glycogen storage disease. *J Pediatr* **97**:906, 1980.

191. Bartram C, Przyrembel H, Wendel U, Bremer H, Schaub J, Haas J: Glycogenosis type Ib complicated by severe granulocytopenia resembling inherited neutropenia. *Eur J Pediatr* **137**:81, 1981.

192. Ambruso D, McCabe E, Anderson D, Beaudet A, Ballas L, Brandt I, Brown B, et al: Infectious and bleeding complications in patients with glycogenosis Ib. *Am J Dis Child* **139**:691, 1985.

193. Roe T, Thomas D, Gilsanz V, Isaacs HJ, Atkinson J: Inflammatory bowel disease in glycogen storage disease type Ib. *J Pediatr* **109**:55, 1986.

194. Burchell A, Jung R, lang C, Bennett W, Sheperd A: Diagnosis of type Ia and type Ic glycogen storage diseases in adults. *Lancet* **1**:1059, 1987.

194a. Veiga-da-Cunha M, Gerin I, Chen Y-T, Lee PJ, Leonard JV, Maire I, Wendel U, et al: The putative glucose 6-phosphate translocase gene is mutated in essentially all cases of glycogen storage disease type I non-a. *Eur J Hum Genet* **7**:717, 1999.

195. Lee P, Patel A, Hindmarsh P, Mowat A, Leonard J: The prevalence of polycystic ovaries in the hepatic glycogen storage diseases: Its association with hyperinsulinism. *Clin Endocrinol* **42**:601, 1995.

196. Michels V, Beaudet A: Hemorrhagic pancreatitis in a patient with glycogen storage disease type I. *Clin Genet* **17**:220, 1980.

197. Kikuchi M, Hasegawa K, Handa I, Watabe M, Narisawa K, Tada K: Chronic pancreatitis in a child with glycogen storage disease type I. *Eur J Pediatr* **150**:852, 1991.

198. Talente G, Coleman R, Alter C, Baker L, Brown B, Cannon R, Chen Y-T, et al: Glycogen storage disease in adults: A retrospective study of clinical and laboratory findings in types Ia, Ib, and III. *An Intern Med* **120**:218, 1994.

199. Howell R, Stevenson R, Ben-Menachem Y, Phyliky R, Berry D: Hepatic adenomata with type I glycogen storage disease. *JAMA* **236**:1481, 1976.

200. Fink A, Appelman H, Thompson N: Hemorrhage into a hepatic adenoma and type Ia glycogen storage disease: A case report and review of the literature. *Surgery* **97**:117, 1985.

201. Limmer J, Fleig W, Leupold D, Bittner R, Ditschuneit H, Beger H: Hepatocellular carcinoma in type I glycogen storage disease. *Hepatology* **8**:531, 1988.

202. Chen Y-T, Coleman R, Scheinman J, Kolbeck P, Sidbury J: Renal disease in type I glycogen storage disease. *N Engl J Med* **318**:7, 1988.

203. Baker L, Dahlem S, Goldfarb S, Kern E, Stanley C, Egler J, Olshan J, et al: Hyperfiltration and renal disease in glycogen storage disease, type I. *Kidney Int* **35**:1345, 1989.

204. Reitsma-Bierens W, Smith G, Troelstra J: Renal function and kidney size in glycogen storage disease type I. *Pediatr Nephrol* **6**:236, 1992.

205. Chen Y-T: Type I glycogen storage disease, kidney involvement, pathogenesis and its treatment. *Pediat Nephrol* **5**:71, 1991.

206. Lee P, Dalton R, Shah V, Hindmarsh P, Leonard J: Glomerular and tubular function in glycogen storage disease. *Pediatr Nephrol* **9**:705, 1995.

207. Chen Y-T, Scheinman J, Park H, Coleman R, Roe C: Amelioration of proximal renal tubular dysfunction in type I glycogen storage disease with dietary therapy. *N Engl J Med* **323**:590, 1990.

208. Kikuchi M, Haginoya K, Miyabayashi S, Igarashi Y, Narisawa K, Tada K: Secondary amyloidosis in glycogen storage disease type Ib. *Eur J Pediatr* **149**:344, 1990.

209. Restaino I, Kaplan B, Stanley C, Baker L: Nephrolithiasis, hypocitraturia, and a distal renal tubular acidification defect in type I glycogen storage disease. *J Pediatr* **122**:392, 1993.

210. Farber M, Knuppel R, Binkiewicz A, Kennison R: Pregnancy and Von Gierke's disease. *Obstet Gynecol* **47**:226, 1976.

211. Johnson M, Compton A, Drugan A, Evans M: Metabolic control of Von Gierke disease (glycogen storage disease type Ia) in pregnancy: Maintenance of euglycemia with cornstarch. *Obstet Gynecol* **75**:507, 1990.

212. Decker-Phillips M, Chen Y-T, Disorders of carbohydrate metabolism, in Gleicher N (Ed): *Principles of Practice of Medical Therapy in Pregnancy.* 3rd edition Stamford, CT, Appleton & Lange, 1998, pp. 377–382.

213. Pizzo C: Type I glycogen storage disease with focal nodular hyperplasia of the liver and vasoconstrictive pulmonary hypertension. *Pediatrics* **65**:341, 1980.

214. Hamaoka K, Nakagawa M, Furukawa N, Sawada T: Pulmonary hypertension in type I glycogen storage disease. *Pediatr Cardiol* **11**:54, 1990.

215. Kishnani P, Bengur A, Chen Y-T: Pulmonary hypertension in glycogen storage disease type I. *J Inher Metab Dis* **19**:213, 1996.

216. Soejima K, Landing B, Roe T, Swanson V: Pathologic studies of the osteoporosis of von Gierke disease (glycogenosis Ia). *Pediatr Pathol* **3**:307, 1985.

217. Lee P, Patel J, Fewtrell M, Leonard J, Bishop N: Bone mineralisation in type I glycogen storage disease. *Eur J Pediatr* **154**:483, 1995.

218. Kalhan S, Gilfillan C, Tserng K, Savin S: Glucose production in type I glycogen storage disease. *J Pediatr* **101**:159, 1982.

219. Tsalikian E, Simmons P, Gerich J, Howard C, Haymond M: Glucose production and utilization in children with glycogen storage disease type I. *Am J Physiol* **247**:E513, 1984.

220. Collins J, Bartlett K, Leonard J, Aynsley-Green A: Glucose production rates in type I glycogen storage disease. *J Inher Metab Dis* **13**:195, 1990.

221. Lapidot A: Inherited disorders of carbohydrate metabolism in children studied by ^{13}C-labelled precursors, NMR and GC-MS. *J Inher Metab Dis* **13**:466, 1990.

222. Rother K, Schwenk W: Glucose production in glycogen storage disease I is not associated with increased cycling through hepatic glycogen. *Am J Physiol* **269**:E774, 1995.

223. Oberhaensli R, Rajagopalan B, Taylor D, Radda G, Collins J, Leonard J: Study of liver metabolism in glucose 6-phosphatase deficiency (glycogen storage disease type Ia) by P-31 magnetic resonance spectroscopy. *Pediatr Res* **23**:375, 1988.

224. Hers H-G: Mechanisms of blood glucose homeostasis. *J Inher Metab Dis* **13**:395, 1990.

225. Fernandes J, Berger R, Smit G: Lactate as a cerebral metabolic fuel for glucose 6-phosphatase deficient children. *Pediatr Res* **18**:335, 1984.
226. Fernandes J, Pikaar N: Ketosis in hepatic glycogenosis. *Arch Dis Child* **47**:41, 1972.
227. Binkiewicz A, Senior B: Decreased ketogenesis in von Gierke's disease (type I glycogenosis). *J Pediatr* **83**:973, 1973.
228. Fernandes J: The effect of disaccharides on the hyperlactic acidemia of glucose 6-phosphatase-deficient children. *Acta Paediatr Scand* **63**:695, 1974.
229. Greene H, Parker P, Hoyumpa A, Hall S: Rapid ethanol elimination in patients with type I glycogen storage disease is an adaptive change resulting from recurrent hypoglycemia. *J Lab Clin Invest* **107**:118, 1986.
230. Jakovcic S, Sorensen L: Studies of uric acid metabolism in glycogen storage disease associated with gouty arthritis. *Arthritis Rheum* **10**:129, 1967.
231. Kelley W, Rosenbloom F, Seegmiller J, Howell R: Excessive production of uric acid in type I glycogen storage disease. *J Pediatr* **72**:488, 1968.
232. Greene H, Wilson F, Hefferan P, Terry A, Moran J, Slonim A, Claus T, et al: ATP depletion, a possible role in the pathogenesis of hyperuricemia in glycogen storage disease type I. *J Clin Invest* **62**:321, 1978.
233. Cohen J, Vinik A, Faller J, Fox I: Hyperuricemia in glycogen storage disease type I. Contributions by hypoglycemia and hyperglucagonemia to increased urate production. *J Clin Invest* **75**:251, 1985.
234. McGarry J, Foster D: Regulation of hepatic fatty acid oxidation and ketone body production. *Annu Rev Biochem* **49**:395, 1980.
235. Dosman J, Crawhall J, Klassen G, Mamer O, Neumann P: Urinary excretion of C6-C10 dicarboxylic acids in glycogen storage diseases types I and III. *Clin Chim Acta* **51**:93, 1974.
236. Burchell A: Molecular pathology of glucose-6-phosphatase. *FASEB J* **4**:2978, 1990.
237. Pears J, Jung R, Jankowski J, Waddell I, Burchell A: Glucose-6-phosphatase in normal adult human intestinal mucosa. *Clin Sci* **83**:683, 1992.
238. Lei K, Chen H, Pan C, Ward J, Mosinger B, Lee E, Westphal H, et al: Glucose-6-phosphatase dependent substrate transport in the glycogen storage disease type Ia mouse. *Nat Genet* **13**:203, 1996.
239. Arden SD, Zahn T, Steegers S, Webb S, Bergman B, O'Brien RM, Hutton JC: Molecular cloning of a pancreatic islet-specific glucose-6-phosphatase catalytic subunit-related protein. *Diabetes* **48**:531, 1999.
240. Ebert DH, Bischof LJ, Streeper RS, Chapman SC, Svitek CA, Goldman JK, Mathews CE, et al: Structure and promoter activity of an islet-specific glucose-6-phosphatase catalytic subunit-related gene. *Diabetes* **48**:543, 1999.
241. Kure S, Suzuki Y, Matsubara Y, Sakamoto O, Shintaku H, Isshiki G, Hoshida C, et al: Molecular analysis of glycogen storage disease type Ib: Identification of a prevalent muatation among Japanese patients and assignment of a putative glucose-6-phosphate translocase gene to chromosome 11. *Biochem Biophy Res Commun* **248**:426, 1998.
242. Burchell A, Waddell I: The molecular basis of the genetic deficiencies of 5 of the components of the glucose-6-phosphatase system: Improved diagnosis. *Eur J Pediatr* **152**:518, 1993.
243. Kalderon B, Korman S, Gutman A, Lapidot A: Estimation of glucose carbon recycling in children with glycogen storage disease: A ^{13}C NMR study using [^{13}C] glucose. *Proc Natl Acad Sci U S A* **86**:4690, 1989.
244. Greene H, Slonim A, O'Neil J, Burr I: Continuous nocturnal intragastric feeding for management of type I glycogen storage disease. *N Engl J Med* **294**:423, 1976.
245. Chen Y-T, Cornblath M, Sidbury J: Cornstarch therapy in type I glycogen storage disease. *N Engl J Med* **310**:171, 1984.
246. Fernandes J, Alaupovic P, Wit J: Gastric drip feeding in patients with glycogen storage disease type I: Its effects on growth and plasma lipids and apolipoproteins. *Pediatr Res* **25**:327, 1989.
246a. Wolfsdorf JI, Crigler JF Jr: Effect of continuous glucose therapy begun in infancy on the long-term clinical course of patients with type I glycogen storage disease. *J Pediatr Gastrol Nutr* **29**:136, 1999.
247. Schwenk W, Haymond M: Optimal rate of enteral glucose administration in children with glycogen storage disease type I. *N Engl J Med* **314**:682, 1986.
248. Leonard J, Dunger D: Hypoglycaemia complicating feeding regimens for glycogen storage disease. *Lancet* **12**:1203, 1978.
249. Dunger D, Sutton P, Leonard J: Hypoglycaemia complicating treatment regimens for glycogen storage disease. *Arch Dis Child* **72**:274, 1995.
250. Wolfsdorf J, Keller R, Landy H, Crigler J: Glucose therapy for glycogenosis type I in infants: Comparison of intermittent uncooked cornstarch and continuous overnight glucose feedings. *J Pediat* **117**:384, 1990.
251. Wolfsdorf J, Crigler J: Cornstarch regimens for nocturnal treatment of young adults with type I glycogen storage disease. *Am J Clin Nutr* **65**:1507, 1997.
252. Fox I, Kelley W: Management of gout. *JAMA* **242**:361, 1979.
253. Wang W, Crist W, Ihle L, Arnold B, Keating J: Granulocyte colony-stimulating factor corrects the neutropenia associated with glycogen storage disease type Ib. *Leukemia* **5**:347, 1991.
254. Schroten H, Roesler J, Breidenbach T, Wendel U, Elsner J, Schweitzer S, Zeidler C, et al: Granulocyte and granulocyte-macrophage colony-stimulating factors for treatment of neutropenia in glycogen storage disease type Ib. *J Pediatr* **119**:748, 1991.
255. Starzl T, Putnam C, Porter K, Benichou J: Portacaval shunt for glycogen storage disease and hyperlipidaemia. *Ciba Found Symp* **55**:311, 1977.
256. Borowitz S, Greene H, Gay J, Neblett W: Comparison of dietary therapy and portacaval shunt in the management of a patient with type ib glycogen storage disease. *J Pediatr Gastroenterol Nutr* **6**:635, 1987.
257. Matern D, Starzl T, Arnaout W, Barnard J, Bynon J, Dhawan A, Emond J, et al: Liver transplantation for glycogen storage disease types I, III, and IV. *Eur J Pediatr* **158(Suppl 2)**:543, 1999.
257a. Faivre I, Houssin D, Valayer J, Brouard J, Hadchouel M, Bernard O: Long-term outcome of liver transplantation in patients with glycogen storage disease type Ia. *J Inheit Metab Dis* **22**:723, 1999.
258. Emmett M, Narins R: Renal transplantation in type I glycogenesis: Failure to improve glucose metabolism. *JAMA* **239**:1642, 1978.
259. Chen Y-T, Scheinman J: Hyperglycaemia associated with lactic acidaemia in a renal allograft recipient with type I glycogen storage disease. *J Inher Metab Dis* **14**:80, 1991.
260. Marti G, Rick M, Sidbury J, Gralnick H: DDAVP infusion in five patients with type Ia glycogen storage disease and associated correction of prolonged bleeding times. *Blood* **68**:180, 1986.
261. Parker P, Burr I, Slonim A, Ghishan F, Greene H: Regression of hepatic adenomas in GSD-Ia with dietary therapy. *Gastroenterology* **81**:534, 1981.
262. Golbus M, Simpson T, Koresawa M, Appelman Z, Alpers C: The prenatal determination of glucose-6-phosphatase activity by fetal liver biopsy. *Prenat Diagn* **8**:401, 1988.
263. Wong LJ: Prenatal diagnosis of glycogen storage disease type Ia by direct mutation detection. *Prenat Diagn* **16**:105, 1996.
264. Parvari R, Hershkovitz E, Carmi R, Moses S: Prenatal diagnosis of glycogen storage disease type Ia by single stranded conformation polymorphism (SSCP). *Prenat Diagn* **16**:862, 1996.
265. Brix A, Howerth E, McConkie-Rosell A, Peterson D, Egnor D, Wells M, Chen Y-T: Glycogen storage disease type Ia in two littermate maltese puppies. *Vet Pathol* **32**:460, 1995.
266. Kishnani P, Bao Y, Wu J-Y, Brix A, Lin J: Isolation and nucleotide sequence of canine glucose-6-phosphatate mRNA. *Biochem Mol Med* **61**:168, 1997.
267. Illingworth B, Cori G: Structure of glycogens and amylopectins, III. *Biol Chem* **199**:653, 1952.
268. Forbes G: Glycogen storage disease. Report of a case with abnormal glycogen structure in liver and skeletal muscle. *J Pediatr* **42**:645, 1953.
269. Illingworth B, Cori G, Cori C: Amylo-1, 6-glucosidase in muscle-tissue in generalized glycogen storage disease. *J Biol Chem* **218**:123, 1956.
270. Van Creveld S, Huijing F: Differential diagnosis of the type of glycogen disease in two adult patients with long history of glycogenosis. *Metabolism* **13**:191, 1964.
271. Brunberg J, McCormick W, Schochet S: Type III glycogenosis: An adult with diffuse weakness and muscle wasting. *Arch Neurol* **25**:171, 1971.
272. DiMauro S, Hartwig G, Hays A, Eastwood A, Franco R, Olarte M: Debrancher deficiency: Neuromuscular disorder in 5 adults. *Ann Neurol* **5**:422, 1979.
273. Coleman R, Winter H, Wolf B, Gilchrist J, Chen Y-T: Glycogen storage disease type III (glycogen debranching enzyme deficiency): Correlation of biochemical defects with myopathy and cardiomyopathy. *Ann Intern Med* **116**:896, 1992.

274. Fellows I, Lowe J, Ogilvie A, Stevens A, Toghill P, Atkinson M: Type III glycogenosis presenting as liver disease in adults with atypical histological features. *J Clin Pathol* **36**:431, 1983.
275. Momoi T, Sano H, Yamanaka C, Sasaki H, Mikawa H: Glycogen storage disease type III with muscle involvement: Reappraisal of phenotypic variability and prognosis. *Am J Med Genet* **42**:696, 1992.
276. Markowitz A, Chen Y-T, Muenzer J, DelBuono E, Lucey M: A man with type III glycogenosis associated with cirrhosis and portal hypertension. *Gastroenterology* **105**:1882, 1993.
277. Van Hoof F, Hers H: The subgroups of type III glycogenosis. *Eur J Biochem* **2**:265, 1967.
278. Coleman R, Winter H, Wolf B, Chen Y-T: Glycogen debranching enzyme deficiency: Relationship of serum enzyme activities to biochemical diagnosis and clinical features. *J Inherit Metab Dis* **15**:869, 1992.
279. Haagsma E, Smit G, Niezen-Koning K, Gouw A, Meerman L, Slooff M: Type IIIb glycogen storage disease associated with end-stage cirrhosis and hepatocellular carcinoma. The Liver Transplant Group. *Hepatology* **25**:537, 1997.
280. Labrune P, Trioche P, Duvaltier I, Chevalier P, Odievre M: Hepatocellular adenomas in glycogen storage disease type I and III: A series of 43 patients and review of the literature. *J Pediatr Gastroenterol Nut* **24**:276, 1997.
281. Moses S, Gadoth N, Bashan N, Ben-David E, Slonim E, Wanderman K: Neuromuscular involvement in glycogen storage disease type III. *Acta Paediatr Scand* **75**:289, 1986.
282. Labrune P, Huguet P, Odievre M: Cardiomyopathy in glycogen storage disease type III: Clinical and echographic study of 18 patients. *Pediatr Cardiol* **12**:161, 1991.
283. Miller C, Alleyne G, Brooks S: Gross cardiac involvement in glycogen storage disease type III. *Br Heart J* **34**:862, 1972.
284. Moses S, Wanderman K, Myroz A, Frydman M: Cardiac involvement in glycogen storage disease type III. *Eur J Pediatr* **148**:764, 1989.
285. Lee P, Deanfield J, Burch M, Baig K, McKenna W, Leonard J: Comparison of the functional significance of left ventricular hypertrophy in hypertrophic cardiomyopathy and glycogenosis type III. *Am J Cardiol* **79**:834, 1997.
286. Cornelio F, Bresolin N, Singer P, DiMauri S, Rowland L: Clinical varieties of neuromuscular disease in debrancher deficiency. *Arch Neurol* **41**:1027, 1984.
287. Lee P, Burch M, Leonard J: Plasma creatine kinase and cardiomyopathy in glycogen storage disease type III. *J Inherit Metab Dis* **18**:751, 1995.
288. Ding J-H, de Barsy T, Brown B, Coleman R, Chen Y-T: Immunoblot analyses of glycogen debranching enzyme in different subtypes of glycogen storage disease type III. *J Pediatr* **116**:95, 1990.
289. Yang B-Z, Stewart C, Din J-H, Chen Y-T: Type III glycogen storage disease: An adult case with mild disease but complete absence of debrancher protein. *Neuromuscul Disord* **1**:173, 1991.
290. Shen J, Bao Y, Chen Y-T: A nonsense mutation due to a single base insertion in the 3′ coding region of glycogen debranching enzyme gene is associated with a severe phenotype in a patient with glycogen storage disease type IIIa. *Hum Mutat* **9**:352, 1997.
291. Parvari R, Moses S, Shen J, Hershkovitz E, Chen Y-T: A single base deletion in the 3′ coding region of glycogen debranching enzyme gene is prevalent in glycogen storage disease type IIIa in a population of North African Jewish patients. *Eur J Hum Genet* **5**:266, 1998.
292. Okubo M, Aoyama Y, Murase T: A novel donor splice-site mutation in the glycogen debranching enzyme gene is associated with glycogen storage disease type III. *Biochem Biophysi Res Commun* **225**:695, 1996.
293. Shen J, Bao Y, Liu H-M, Lee P, Leonard J, Chen Y-T: Mutations in exon 3 of the glycogen debranching enzyme gene are associated with glycogen storage disease type III that is differentially expressed in liver and muscle. *J Clin Invest* **98**:352, 1996.
294. Brown B, Brown D: Definitive assays for glycogen debranching enzyme in human fibroblasts, in *Diseases of the Motor Unit*. New York, John Wiley, 1982, p. 667.
295. Sidbury JJ, Gitzelmann R, Fisher J: The glycogenoses: Further observations on glycogen in erythrocytes of patients with glycogenosis. *Helv Paediatr Acta* **16**:506, 1961.
296. Shin Y, Ungar R, Rieth M, Endres W: A simple assay for amylo-1-6-glucosidase to detect heterozygotes for glycogenosis type III in erythrocytes. *Clin Chem* **30**:1717, 1984.
297. Borowitz S, Greene H: Cornstarch therapy in a patient with type III glycogen storage disease. *Pediatr Gastroenterol Nutr* **6**:631, 1987.
298. Gremse D, Bucuvalas J, Balistreri W: Efficacy of cornstarch therapy in type III glycogen storage disease. *Am J Clin Nutr* **52**:671, 1990.
299. Lee P, Ferguson C, Alexander F: Symptomatic hyperinsulinism reversed by dietary manipulation in glycogenosis type III. *J Inherit Metab Dis* **20**:612, 1997.
300. Yang B-Z, Ding J-H, Brown B, Chen Y-T: Definitive prenatal diagnosis for type III glycogen storage disease. *Am J Hum Genet* **47**:735, 1990.
301. Maire I, Mandon G, Mathieu M: First trimester prenatal diagnosis of glycogen storage disease type III. *J Inherit Metab Dis* **12**:292, 1989.
302. Van Diggelen O, Janse H, Smit G: Debranching enzyme in fibroblasts, amniotic fluid cells and chorionic villi: Pre and postnatal diagnosis of glycogenosis type III. *Clin Chim Acta* **149**:129, 1985.
303. Shen J, Liu H, McConkie-Rosell A, Chen Y-T: Prenatal diagnosis and carrier detection for glycogen storage disease type III using polymorphic DNA markers. *Prenat Diagn* **18**:61, 1998.
304. Ceh L, Hauge J, Svenkerud R, Strande A: Glycogenosis type III in the dog. *Acta Vet Scand* **17**:210, 1976.
305. Andersen D: Familial cirrhosis of the liver with storage of abnormal glycogen. *Lab Invest* **5**:11, 1956.
306. Brown B, Brown D: Lack of an α-1, 4-glucan:α-1, 4-glucan 6-glycosyl transferase in a case of type IV glycogenosis. *Pro Natl Acad Sci U S A* **56**:725, 1966.
307. Greene HL BB, McClenathan DT, Agostini RM Jr, Taylor SR: A new variant of type IV glycogenosis: Deficiency of branching enzyme activity without apparent progressive liver disease. *Hepatology* **8**:302, 1988.
308. McConkie-Rosell A, Wilson C, Piccoli D, Boyle J, DeClue T, Kishnani P, Shen J-J, et al: Clinical and laboratory findings in four patients with the non-progressive hepatic form of type IV glycogen storage disease. *J Inherit Metab Dis* **19**:51, 1996.
309. Zellweger H, Mueller S, Ionasescu V, Schochet S, McCormick W: Glycogenosis IV: A new cause of infantile hypotonia. *J Pediatr* **80**:842, 1972.
310. McMaster K, Powers J, Hennigar G, Wohltmann H, Farr G: Nervous system involvement in type IV glycogenosis. *Arch Pathol Lab Med* **103**:105, 1979.
311. Tang T, Segura A, Chen Y-T, Ricci L, Franciosi R, Splaingard M, Lubinsky M: Neonatal hypotonia and cardiomyopathy secondary to type IV glycogenosis. *Acta Neuropathol* **87**:531–536, 1994.
312. Servidei S, Riepe R, Langston C, Tani L, Bricker J, Crisp-Lindgren N, Travers H, et al.: Severe cardiopathy in branching enzyme deficiency. *J Pediatr* **111**:51, 1987.
313. Nase S, Kunze K, Sigmund M, Schroeder J, Shin Y, Hanrath P: A new variant of type IV glycogenosis with primary cardiac manifestation and complete branching enzyme deficiency. In vivo detection by heart muscle biopsy. *Eur Heart J* **16**:1698–1704, 1995.
314. Lossos A, Barash V, Soffer D, Argov Z, Gomori M, Ben-Nariah Z, Abramsky O, et al.: Hereditary branching enzyme dysfuntion in adult polyglucosan body disease: A possible metabolic cause in two patients. *Ann Neurol* **30**:655, 1991.
315. Bruno C, Servidei S, Shanske S, McKee D, Karpati G, DiMauro S: Glycogen branching enzyme in adult polyglucosan body disease. *Neurology* **42**:230, 1992.
316. Schochet S, McCormick W, Zellwerger H: Type IV glycogenosis (amylopectinosis) light and electron microscopic observations. *Arch Pathol* **90**:354, 1970.
317. Bannayan G, Dean W, Howell R: Type IV glycogen storage disease: Light-microscopic, electron-microscopic and enzymatic study. *Am J Clin Pathol* **66**:702, 1976.
318. Ishihara T, Yokota T, Yamashita Y, Takahashi M, Kawano H, Uchino F, Kamei T, et al.: Comparative study of the intracytoplasmic inclusions in Lafora disease and type IV glycogenosis by electron microscopy. *Acta Pathol Jpn* **37**:1591, 1987.
319. Greene G, Weldon D, Ferrans V, Cheatham J, McComb R, Brown B, Gumbiner C, et al.: Juvenile polysaccharidosis with cardioskeletal myopathy. *Arch Pathol Lab Med* **111**:977, 1987.
320. Bao Y, Kishnani P, Wu J, Chen Y: Hepatic and neuromuscluar forms of glycogen storage disease type IV caused by mutation in the same glycogen branching enzyme gene. *J Clin Invest* **97**:941–948, 1996.
320a. Lossos A, Meiner Z, Barash V, Soffer D, Schlesinger I, Abramsky O, Argov Z: Adult polyglucosan body disease in Ashkenazi Jewish patients carrying the Tyr329Ser mutation in the glycogen-branching enzyme gene. *Ann Neurol* **44**:867, 1998.
321. Howell R, Kaback M, Brown B: Type IV glycogen storage disease: Branching enzyme deficiency in skin fibroblasts and possible heterozygote detection. *J Pediatr* **78**:638, 1971.

322. Shin Y, Steiguber H, Klemm P, Endres W, Schwab O, Wolff G: Branching enzyme in erythrocytes: Detection of type IV glycogenosis homozygotes. *J Inherit Metab Dis* **11**:252, 1988.
323. Brown D, Brown B: Studies of the residual glycogen branching enzyme activity present in human skin fibroblasts from patients with type IV glycogen storage disease. *Biochem Biophys Res Commun* **111**:636, 1983.
324. Selby R, Starzl T, Yunis E, Brown B, Kendall R, Tzakis A: Liver transplantation for type IV glycogen storage disease. *N Engl J Med* **324**:39, 1991.
325. Sokal E, Van Hoof F, Alberti D, de Ville de Goyet J, de Barsy T, Otte J: Progressive cardiac failure following orthotopic liver transplantation for type IV glycogenosis. *Eur J Pediatr* **151**:200, 1992.
326. Rosenthal P, Podesta L, Grier R, Said J, Sher L, Cocjin J, Watanabe F, et al: Failure of liver transplantation to diminish cardiac deposits of amylopectin and leukocyte inclusions in type IV glycogen storage disease. *Liver Transplant Surg* **1**:373, 1995.
327. Brown B, Brown D: Branching enzyme activity of cultured amnicytes and chroionic villi: Prenatal testing for type IV glycogen storage disease. *Am J Hum Genet* **44**:378, 1989.
328. Fyfe J, Giger U, Van Winkle T, Haskins M, Steinberg S, Wang P, Patterson D: Glycogen storage disease type IV: Inherited deficiency of branching enzyme activity in cats. *Pediatr Res* **32**:719, 1992.
329. Fyfe J, Kurzhals R, Henthorn P, Patterson D: Feline glycogenosis type IV is caused by a complex rearrangement deleting 6 kb of the branching enzyme gene and eliminating an exon. *Am J Hum Genet* **61**:A251, 1997.
330. McArdle B: Myopathy due to a defect in muscle glycogen breakdown. *Clin Sc* **10**:13, 1951.
331. Mommaerts W, Illingworth B, Pearson C, Guillory R, Seraydarian K: A functional disorder of muscle associated with the absence of phosphorylase. *Proc Natl Acad Sci* U S A 45:791, 1959.
332. Larner J, Villar-Palasi C: Enzymes in a glycogen storage myopathy. *Proc Natl Acad Sci* U S A 45:1234, 1959.
333. Schmid R, Mahler R: Chronic progressive myopathy with myoglobinuria: Demonstration of a glycogenolytic defect in the muscle. *J Clin Invest* **38**:2044, 1959.
334. Grunfeld J, Ganeval D, Chanard J, Fardeau M, Dreyfus J: Acute renal failure in McArdle's disease: Reports of two cases. *N Engl J Med* **286**:1237, 1972.
335. Bank W, DiMauro S, Rowland L: Renal failure in McArdles's disease. *N Engl J Med* **287**:1102, 1972.
336. Higgs J, Blaivas M, Albers J: McArdle's disease presenting as treatment resistant polymyositis. *J Rheumatol* **16**:1588, 1989.
337. De Kerviler E, Leroy-Willig A, Duboc D, Eymard B, Syrota A: MR quantification of muscle fatty replacement in McArdle's disease. *Magn Reson Imaging* **14**:1137, 1996.
338. Brooke M, Patterson V, Kaiser K: Hypoxanthine and McArdle disease: A clue to metabolic stress in the working forearm. *Muscle Nerve* **6**:204, 1983.
339. Mineo I, Kono N, Hara N, Shimizu T, Yamada Y, Kawachi M, Kiyokawa H, et al: Myogenic hyperuricemia: A common pathophysiologic feature of glycogenosis types III, V, and VII. *N Engl J Med* **317**:75, 1987.
340. Hewlett R, Gardner-Thorpe C: What limit to the age of onset? *S Afr Med J* **53**:60, 1978.
341. DiMauro S, Hartlage P: Fatal infantile form of muscle phosphorylase deficiency. *Neurology* **28**:1124, 1978.
342. De La Marza M, Patten B, Williams J, Chambers J: Myophosphorylase deficiency: A new cause of infantile hypotonia simulating muscular atrophy. *Neurology* **30**:402, 1980.
343. Milstein J, Herron T, Haas J: Fatal infantile muscle phosphorylase deficiency. *Child Neurol* **4**:186, 1989.
344. Cornelio F, Bresolin N, DiMauro S, Mora M, Balestrini M: Congenital myopathy due to phosphorylase deficiency. *Neurology* **33**:1383, 1983.
345. Servidei S SS, Zeviani M, Lebo R, Fletterick R, DiMauro S: McArdle's disease: Biochemical and molecular genetic studies. *Ann Neurol* **24**:774, 1988.
346. Tsujino S, Shanske S, DiMauro S: Molecular genetic heterogeneity of myophospharylase deficiency (McArdle's disease). *N Engl J Med* **329**:241, 1993.
347. McArdle WD, Katch FI, Katch VL (Eds): *Exercise Physiology: Energy, Nutrition and Human Perfomance*, 4th ed. Baltinore, Williams & Wilkins, 1996.
348. Jehenson P, Leroy-Willig A, de Kerviler E, Merlet P, Duboc D, Syrota A: Impairment of the exercise-induced increase in muscle perfusion in McArdle's disease. *Eur J Nucl Med* **22**:1256, 1995.
348a. Haller RG, Clausen T, Vissing J: Reduced levels of skeletal muscle Na+K+-ATPase in McArdle disease. *Neurology* **50**:37, 1998.
349. DiMauro S, Bresolin N: Phosphorylase deficiency, in Engel BB (Ed): *Myology*. New York, McGraw-Hill, 1986, p. 1585.
350. Schotland D, Spiro D, Rowland L, Carmel P: Ultrastructural studies of muscle in McArdle's disease. *J Neuropathol Exp Neurol* **24**:629, 1965.
351. Vorgerd M, Kubisch C, Burwinkel B, Reichmann H, Mortier W, Tettenborn B, Pongratz D, et al: Mutation analysis in myophosphorylase deficiency (McArdle's disease). *Am Neurol Assoc* **43**:326, 1998.
352. Bartram C, Edwards R, Beynon R: McArdle's disease: Muscle glycogen phosphorylase deficiency. *Biochim Biophys Acta* **1272**:1, 1995.
353. Sugie H, Sugie Y, Ito M, Fukuda T, Nonaka I, Igarashi Y: Genetic analysis of Japanese patients with myophosphorylase deficiency (McArdle's disease): Single-codon deletion in exon 17 is the predominant mutation. *Clin Chim Acta* **236**:81, 1995.
354. Ross B, Radda G, Gadian D, Rocker G, Esiri M, Falconer-Smith J: Examination of a case of suspected McArdle's syndrome by ^{31}P nuclear magnetic resonance. *N Engl J Med* **304**:1338, 1981.
355. el-Schahawi M, Tsujino S, Shanske S, DiMauro S: Diagnosis of McArdle's disease by molecular genetic analysis of blood. *Neurology* **47**:579, 1996.
356. Slonim A, Goans P: Myopathy in McArdle's syndrome: Improvement with a high-protein diet. *N Engl J Med* **312**:355, 1985.
356a. Phoenix J, Hopkins P, Bartram C, Beynon RJ, Quinlivan RC, Edwards RH: Effect of vitamin B6 supplementation in McArdle's disease: A strategic case study. *Neuromuscul Disord* **8**:210, 1998.
357. Manfredi G, Silvestri G, Servidei S, Ricci E, Mirabella M, Bertini E, Papacci M, et al: Manifesting heterozygotes in McArdle's disease: Clinical, morphological, and biochemical studies in a family. *J Neurol Sci* **115**:91, 1993.
358. Schmidt B, Servidei S, Gabbai A, Silva A, de Sousa Bulle de Oliveira A, DiMauro S: McArdle's disease in two generations: Autosomal recessive transmission with manifesting heterozygote. *Neurology* **37**:1558, 1987.
359. Chui L, Munsat T: Dominant inheritance of McArdle's syndrome. *Arch Neurol* **33**:636, 1976.
360. Bogusky R, Taylor R, Anderson L, Angelos K, Lieberman J, Walsh D: McArdle's disease heterozygotes: Metabolic adaption assessed using 31P-nuclear magnetic resonance. *J Clin Invest* **77**:1881, 1986.
361. Tsujino S, Shanske S, Valberg S, Cardinet G, Smith B, DiMauro S: Cloning of bovine muscle glycogen phosphorylase cDNA and identification of a mutation in cattle with myophosphorylase deficiency, an animal model for McArdle's disease. *Neuromuscul Disord* **6**:19, 1996.
362. Tan P, Allen J, Wilton S, Akkari P, Huxtable C, Laing N: A splice-site mutation causing ovine McArdle's disease. *Neuromuscul Disord* **7**:336, 1997.
363. Hers H: Etudes enzymatiques sur fragments hepatiques. Application a la classification des glycogenoses. *Rev Int Hepatol* **9**:35, 1959.
364. Stetten DJ, Stetten M: Glycogen metabolism. *Physiol Rev* **40**:505, 1960.
365. Ockerman P, Jelke H, Kaijser K: Glycogenosis type 6 (liver phosphorylase deficiency): A case followed for ten years with normal phosphorylase activity in white blood cells and jejunal mucosa. *Acta Paediatr Scand* **55**:10, 1966.
366. Fernandes J, Koster J, Grose W, Sorgedrager N: Hepatic phosphorylase deficiency: Its differentiation from other hepatic glycogenoses. *Arch Dis Child* **49**:186, 1974.
367. Chang S, Rosenberg M, Morton H, Francomano C, Biesecker L: Identification of a mutation in liver glycogen phosphorylase in glycogen storage disease type VI. *Hum Mol Genet* **7**:865, 1998.
368. Burwinkel B, Bakker H, Herschkovitz E, Moses S, Shin Y, Kilimann M: Mutations in the liver glycogen phosphorylase gene *(PYGL)* underlying glycogenosis type VI (Hers disease). *Am J Hum Genet* **62**:785, 1998.
369. Tarui S, Okuno G, Ikura Y, Tanaka T, Suda M, Nishikawa M: Phosphofructokinase deficiency in skeletal muscle: A new type of glycogenosis. *Biochem Biophys Res Common* **19**:517, 1965.
370. Rowland L, DiMauro S, Layzer R: Phosphofructokinase deficiency, in Engel BB (ed): *Myology: Basic and Clinical*. New York, McGraw-Hill; 1986, p. 1986.

371. Shimizu T, Kono N, Kiyokawa H, Yamada Y, Hara N, Mineo I, Kawachi M, et al: Erythrocyte glycolysis and its marked alternations by muscular exercise in type VII glycogenosis. *Blood* **71**:1130, 1988.
372. Agamanolis D, Askari A, DiMauro S, Hays A, Kumar K, Lipton M, Raynor: Muscle phosphofructokinase deficiency: Two cases with unusual polysaccharide accumulation and immunologically active enzyme protein. *Muscle Nerve* **3**:456, 1980.
373. Hays A, Hallet M, Delfs J, Morris J, Sotrel A, Shevchuk M, DiMauro S: Muscle phosphofructokinase deficiency: Abnormal polysaccharide in a case of late-onset myopathy. *Neurology* **31**:1077, 1981.
374. Haller R, Lewis S: Glucose-induced exertional fatigue in muscle phosphofructokinase deficiency. *N Engl Med* **324**:364, 1991.
375. Guibaud P, Carrier H, Mathieu M, Dorche C, Parchoux B, Bethenod M, Larbre F: Observation familiale de dystrophie musculaire congenitale par deficit en phosphofructokinase. *Arch Fr Pediatr* **35**:1105, 1978.
376. Servidei S, Bonilla E, Diedrich R, Kornfield M, Oates J, Davidson M, Vora S, et al: Fatal infantile form of muscle phosphofructokinase deficiency. *Neurology* **36**:1465, 1986.
377. Danon M, Carpenter S, Manaligod J, Schliselfeld L: Fatal infantile glycogen storage disease: Deficiency of phosphofructokinase and phosphorylase b kinase. *Neurology* **31**:1303, 1981.
378. Moerman P, Lammens M, Fryns J, Lemmens F, Lauweryns J: Fetal akinesia sequence caused by glycogenosis type VII. *Genet Couns* **6**:15, 1995.
379. Serratrice G, Monges A, Roux H, Aquaron R, Gambarel-li D: Forme myopathique du deficit en phosphofructokinase. *Rev Neurol* **120**:271, 1969.
380. Danon M, Servidei S, DiMauro S, Vora S: Late-onset muscle phosphofructokinase deficiency. *Neurology* **38**:956, 1988.
381. Van Keuren M, Drabkin H, Hart I, Harker D, Patterson D, Vora S: Regional assignment of human liver-type 6-phosphofructokinase to chromosome 21q.22.3 by using somatic cell hybrids and a monoclonal anti-L-antibody. *Hum Genet* **74**:34, 1986.
382. Howard T, Akots G, Bowden D: Physical and genetic mapping of the muscle phosphofructokinase gene (PFKM): Reassignment to human chromosome 12q. *Genomics* **34**:122, 1996.
383. Vora S, DiMauro S, Spear D, Harker D, Danon M: Characterization of the enzymatic defect in late-onset muscle phosphofructokinase deficiency. *J Clin Invest* **80**:1479, 1987.
384. Nakajima H, Kono N, Yamasaki T, Hotta K, Kawachi M, Kuwajima M, Noguchi T, et al: Genetic defect in muscle phosphofructokinase deficiency: Abnormal splicing of the muscle phosphofructokinase gene due to a point mutation at the 5′ splice site. *J Biol Chem* **365**:9392, 1990.
385. Raben N, Sherman J, Miller F, Mena H, Poltz H: A 5′ splice junction mutation leading to exon deletion in an Ashkenazic Jewish family with phosphofructokinase deficiency (Tauri disease). *J Biol Chem* **268**:4963, 1993.
386. Kahn A, Weil D, Cottreau D, Dreyfus J: Muscle phosphofructokinase deficiency in man: Expression of the defect in blood cells and cultured fibroblasts. *Ann Hum Genet* **45**:5, 1981.
387. Swoboda K, Specht L, Jones H, Shapiro F, DiMauro S, Korson M: Infantile phosphofructokinase deficiency with arthrogryposis: Clinical benefit of a ketogenic diet. *J Pediatr* **131**:932, 1997.
388. Vora S, Giger U, Turchen S, Harvey J: Characterization of the enzymatic lesion in inherited phosphofructokinase deficiency in the dog: An animal analogue of human glycogen storage disease type VII. *Proc Natl Acad Sci U S A* **82**:8109, 1985.
388a. Smith BF, Stedman H, Rajpurohit Y, Henthorn PS, Wolfe JH, Patterson DF, Giger U: Molecular basis of canine muscle type phosphofructokinase deficiency. *J Biol Chem* **271**:20070, 1998.
389. Smith B, Stedman H, Rajpurohit Y, Henthorn P, Wolfe J, Patterson D, Giger U: Molecular basis of canine muscle type phosphofructokinase deficiency. *J Biol Chem* **271**:20070, 1996.
390. Hug G, Schubert W, Chuck G: Phosphorylase kinase of the liver: Deficiency in a girl with increased hepatic glycogen. *Science* **153**:1534, 1966.
391. Huijing F: Phosphorylase kinase in leucocytes of normal subjects and of patients with storage disease. *Biochim Biophys Acta* **148**:601, 1967.
392. Huijing F, Fernandes J: X-chromosomal inheritance of liver glycogenoses with phosphorylase kinase deficiency. *Am J Hum Genet* **21**:275, 1969.
393. Hug G: Nonbilirubin genetic disorders of the liver, in *International Academy of Pathology*. Baltimore, MD, Williams and Wilkins, 1973.
394. Van den Berg I, Berger R: Phosphorylase b kinase deficiency in man: A review. *J Inherit Metab Dis* **13**:442, 1990.
395. Willems P, Gerver W, Berger R, Fernandes J: The natural history of liver glycogenosis due to phosphorylase kinase deficiency: A longitudinal study of 41 patients. *Eur Pediat* **149**:268, 1990.
396. Lederer B, Van Hoof F, Van Den Berghe G, Hers H: Glycogen phosphorylase and its converter enzymes in haemolysates of normal human subjects and of patients with type VI glycogen storage disease. *Biochem J* **147**:23, 1975.
397. Tuchman M, Brown B, Burke B, Ulstrom R: Clinical and laboratory obserations in a child with hepatic phosphorylase kinase deficiency. *Metabolism* **35**:627, 1986.
398. Shiomi S, Saeki Y, Kim K, Nishiguchi S, Seki S, Kuroki T, Kobayashi K, et al: A female case of type VIII glycogenosis who developed cirrhosis of the liver and hepatocellular tumor. *Gastroenterol Jpn* **24**:711, 1989.
399. Kagalwalla A, Kagalwalla Y, Al Ajaji S, Gorka W, Ali M: Phosphorylase b kinase deficiency glycogenosis with cirrhosis of the liver. *J Pediatr* **127**:602, 1995.
400. Willems P, Hendrickx J, Van der Auwera B, Vits L, Raeymaekers P, Coucke P, Van den Bergh I, et al: Mapping of the gene for X-linked liver glycogenosis due to phosphorylase kinase deficiency to human chromosome region Xp22. *Genomics* **9**:565, 1991.
401. Hendrickx J, Coucke P, Dams E, Lee P, Odievre M, Corbeel L, Fernandez J, et al: Mutations in the phosphorylase kinase gene PHKA2 are responsible for X-linked liver glycogen storage disease. *Hum Mol Genet* **4**:77, 1995.
402. Hirono H, Hayasaka K, Sato W, Takahashi T, Takada G: Isolation of cDNA encoding the human liver phosphorylase kinase alpha subunit (PHKA2) and identification of a missense mutation of the *PHKA2* gene in a family with liver phosphorylase kinase deficiency. *Biochem Mol Biol Intern* **36**:505, 1995.
403. van den Berg I, van Beurden E, Malingre H, Ploos van Amstel H, Poll-The B, Smeitink J, Lamers W, et al.: X-linked liver phosphorylase kinase deficiency is associated with mutations in the human liver phosphorylase kinase α subunit. *Am J Hum Genet* **56**:381, 1995.
404. Burwinkel B, Shin Y, Bakker H, Deutsch J, Lozano M, Maire I, Kilimann M: Mutation hotspots in the PHKA2 gene in X-linked liver glycogenosis due to phosphorylase kinase deficiency with atypical activity in blood cells (XLG2). *Hum Mol Genet* **5**:653, 1996.
405. Hendrickx J, Dams E, Coucke P, Lee P, Fernandes J, Willems P: X-linked liver glycogenosis type II (XLG II) is caused by mutations in PHKA2, the gene encoding the liver alpha subunit of phosphorylase kinase. *Hum Mol Genet* **5**:649, 1996.
406. Lederer B, Van de Werve G, de Barsy T, Hers H: The autosomal form of phosphorylase kinase deficiency in man: Reduced activity of the muscle enzyme. *Biochem Res Commun* **92**:169, 1980.
407. Bashan N, Iancu T, Lerner A, Fraser D, Potashnik R, Moses S: Glycogenosis due to liver and muscle phosphorylase kinase deficiency. *Pediatric Res* **15**:299, 1981.
408. Sovik O, deBarsy T, Maehle B: Phosphorylase kinase deficiency: Severe glycogen storage disease with evidence of autosomal recessive mode of inheritance. *Eur J Pediatr* **139**:210, 1982.
409. Burwinkel B, Maichele A, Aagenaes O, Bakker H, Lerner A, Shin Y, Kilimann M: Autosomal glycogenosis of liver and muscle due to phosphorylase kinase deficiency is caused by mutations in the phosphorylase kinase β subunit (PHKB). *Hum Mol Genet* **6**:1109, 1997.
410. Burwinkel B, Moses S, Kilimann M: Phosphorylase-kinase-deficient liver glycogenosis with an unusual biochemical phenotype in blood cells associated with a missense mutation in the β subunit gene (PHKB). *Hum Genet* **101**:170, 1997.
411. Maichele A, Burwinkel B, Maire I, Sovik O, Kilimann M: Mutations in the testis/liver isoform of the phophorylase kinase γ subunit (PHKG2) cause autosomal liver glycogenosis in the *gsd* rat and in humans. *Nat Genet* **14**:337, 1996.
412. van Beurden E, de Graaf M, Wendel U, Gitzelmann R, Berger R, van den Berg I: Autosomal recessive liver phosphorylase kinase deficiency caused by a novel splice-site mutation in the gene encoding the liver gamma subunit (PHKG2). *Biochem Biophy Res Commun* **236**:544, 1997.
413. Burwinkel B, Shiomi S, Al Zaben A, Kilimann M: Liver glycogenosis due to phosphorylase kinase deficiency: PHKG2 gene structure and mutations associated with cirrhosis. *Hum Mol Genet* **7**:149, 1998.

414. Abarbanel J, Bashan N, Potashnik R, Osimani A, Moses S, Herishanu Y: Adult muscle phosphorylase kinase deficiency. Abstract 7, session on genetics I. *Neurology* **37**:139, 1986.
415. Clemens P, Yamamoto M, Engel A: Adult phosphorylase b kinase deficiency. *Ann Neurol* **28**:529, 1990.
416. Ohtani Y, Matsuda I, Iwamasa T, Tamari H, Origuchi Y, Miike T: Infantile glycogen storage myopathy in a girl with phosphorylase kinase deficiency. *Neurology* **32**:833, 1982.
417. Iwamasa T, Fukuda S, Tokumitsu S, Ninomiya N, Matsuda I, Osame M: Myopathy due to glycogen storage disease: Pathological and biological studies in relationship to glycogenosome formation. *Expe Mol Pathol* **38**:405, 1983.
418. Wehner M, Clemens P, Engel A, Kilimann M: Human muscle glycogenosis due to phosphorylase kinase deficiency associated with a nonsense mutation in the muscle isoform of the α subunit. *Hum Mol Genet* **3**:1983, 1994.
419. Schneider A, Davidson J, Wullrich A, Kilimann M: Phosphorylase kinase deficiency in I-strain mice is associated with a frameshift mutation in the α subunit muscle isoform. *Nat Genet* **5**:381, 1993.
420. Eishi Y, Takemura T, Sone R, Yamamura H, Narisawa K, Ichinohasama R, Tanaka M, et al: Glycogen storage disease confined to the heart with deficient activity of cardiac phosphorylase kinase: A new type of glycogen storage disease. *Hum Pathol* **16**:193, 1985.
421. Servidei S, Metlay L, Chodosh J, DiMauro S: Fatal infantile cardiopathy caused by phosphorylase b kinase deficiency. *J Pediatr* **113**:82, 1988.
422. Elleder M, Shin Y, Zuntova A, Vojtovic P, Chalupecky V: Fatal infantile cardiomyopathy secondary to deficiency of heart specific phosphorylase β kinase. *Virch Arch A Pathol Anat* **423**:303, 1993.
422a. Regalado JJ, Rodriguez MM, Ferrer PL: Infantile hypertrophic cardiomyopathy of glycogenosis type IX: Isolated cardiac phosphorylase kinase deficiency. *Pediatr Cardiol* **20**:304, 1999.
423. Malthus R, Clark D, Watts C, Sneyd J: Glycogen storage disease in rats, a genetically determined deficiency of liver phosphorylase kinase. *Biochem J* **188**:99, 1980.
424. Lewis G, Spencer-Peet J, Stewart K: Infantile hypoglycaemia due to inherited deficiency of glycogen synthetase in liver. *Arch Dis Child* **38**:40, 1963.
425. Aynsley-Green A, Williamson D, Gitzelmann R: Hepatic glycogen synthetase deficiency. *Arch Dis Child* **52**:573, 1977.
426. Gitzelmann R, Spycher M, Feil G, Muller J, Seilnacht B, Stahl M, Bosshard N: Liver glycogen synthase deficiency: A rarely diagnosed entity. *Eur J Pediat* **155**:561, 1996.
427. Byrne B, Gillmer M, Turner R, Aynsley-Green A: Glucose homeostasis in adulthood and in pregnancy in a patient with hepatic glycogen synthetase deficiency. *Br J Obs Gynaecol* **102**:931, 1995.
428. Orho M, Bosshard N, Buisl N, Gilzelmann R, Aynsley-Croon A, Blumel P, Cannon M, et al: Mutations in the liver glycogen synthase gene in children with hypoglycemia due to glycogen storage disease type 0. *J Clin Invest* **102**:507, 1998.
429. Santer R, Schneppenheim R, Suter D, Schaub J, Steinmann B: Fanconi-Bickel syndrome—the original patient and his natural history, historical steps leading to the primary defect, and a review of the literature. *Eur J Pediatr* **157**:783, 1998.
430. Fanconi G, Bickel H: Die chronische aminoacidurie (Aminosaurediabetes oder nephrotisch-glukosurischer Zwergwuchs) bei der glykogenose und der cystinkrankheit. *Helv Paediatr Acta* **4**:359, 1949.
431. Garty R, Cooper M, Tabachnik E: The Fanconi syndrome associated with hepatic glycogenosis and abnormal metabolism of galactose. *J Pediatr* **85**:821, 1974.
432. Manz F, Bicket H, Brodehl J, Feist D, Gellissen K, Gescholl-Bauer B, Gilli G, et al: Fanconi-Bickel syndrome. *Pediatr Nephrol* **1**:509, 1987.
433. Berry G, Baker L, Kaplan F, Witzleben C: Diabetes-like renal glomerular disease in Fanconi-Bickel syndrome. *Pediatr Nephrol* **9**:287, 1995.
434. Lee P, Van't Hoff W, Leonard J: Catch-up growth in Fanconi-Bickel syndrome with uncooked cornstarch. *J Inherit Metab Dis* **18**:153, 1995.
435. Guillam M-T, Hummler E, Schaerer E, Wu J-Y, Birnbaum M, Beermann F, Schmidt A, et al: Early diabetes and abnormal postnatal pancreatic islet development in mice lacking Glut-2. *Nat Genet* **17**:327, 1997.
436. Paglia D, Valentine W: Hereditary glucosephosphate isomerase deficiency. *Am J Clin Pathol* **62**:740, 1974.
437. Van Biervliet J, Staal G: Excessive hepatic glycogen storage in glucosephosphate isomerase deficiency, a review. *Acta Paediatr Scand* **66**:311, 1977.
438. Schroter W, Eber S, Bardosi A, Gahr M, Gabriel M, Sitzmann F: Generalized glucosephosphate isomerase (GPI) deficiency causing haemolytic anaemia, neuromuscular symptoms and impairment of granulocytic function: A new syndrome due to a new stable GPI variant with diminished specific activity (GPI Homburg). *Eur J Pediatr* **144**:301, 1985.
438a. Kreuder J, Borkhardt A, Repp R, Pekrun A, Gottsche B, Gottschalk U, Reichmann H: et al: Brief report: inherited metabolic myopathy and hemolysis due to a mutation in aldolase A. *N Engl J Med* **334**:1100, 1996.
438b. Poulton KR, Curtis EM, Rossi ML: Muscle pyruvate kinase deficiency: Glycogen storage disease or mitochondrial myopathy? *Funct Neurol* **12**:25, 1997.
439. Rosa R, George C, Fardeau M, Calvin M, Rapin M, Rosa J: A new case of phosphoglycerate kinase deficiency: PGK Creteil associated with rhabdomyolysis and lacking hemolytic anemia. *Blood* **60**:84, 1982.
440. DiMauro S, Miranda A, Khan S, Gitlin K, Friedman R: Human muscle phosphoglycerate mutase deficiency: Newly discovered metabolic metabolic myopathy. *Science* **212**:1277, 1981.
441. Tsujino S, Shanske S, DiMauro S: Molecular genetic heterogeneity of phosphoglycerate kinase (PGK) deficiency. *Muscle Nerve* **3:S45, 1995.**
442. Bresolin N, Ro Y, Reyes M, Miranda A, DiMauro S: Muscle phosphophosphoglycerate mutase (PGAM) deficiency: A second case. *Neurology* **33**:1049, 1983.
443. Tsujino S, Shanske S, Sakoda S, Feniche G, DiMauro S: The molecular genetic basis of muscle phosphoglycerate mutase (PGAM) deficiency. *Am J Hum Genet* **52**:472, 1993.
444. Kanno T, Sudo K, Takeuchi I, Kanda S, Honda N, Nishimura Y, Oyama K: Hereditary deficiency of lactate dehydrogenase-M subunit. *Neuropediatrics* **13**:103, 1980.
445. Nagata N, Miike T, Matsuda I, Shikama H, Tokumitsu Y, Ui M: Glycogen storage myopathy with abnormal lactate dehydrogenase. *Neuropediatrics* **13**:103, 1982.
446. Kanno T, Maekawa M: Lactate dehydrogenase M-subunit deficiencies: Clinical features, metabolic background, and genetic heterogeneities. *Muscle Nerve* **3:S54, 1995.**
447. Berteloot A, St-Denis J, van de Werve G: Evidence for a membrane exchangeable glucose pool in the functioning of rat liver glucose 6-phosphatase. *J Biol Chem* **270**:21098, 1995.
448. Chen Y-T: The glycogenoses, in Rudolph A (ed): *Rudolph's Pediatrics*. Norwalk, CT, Appleton and Lange, 1991, p. 331.

CHAPTER 72

Galactosemia

J. B. Holton ▪ J. H. Walter ▪ L. A. Tyfield

1. The main sources of galactose are milk and milk products. Galactose is present as the disaccharide lactose, but lactose is hydrolyzed to its constituent monosaccharides prior to absorption from the intestine. Galactose is an essential energy source in infants, but it is necessary that it is first metabolized to glucose. The principal pathway for the metabolism of galactose involves three enzymes: galactokinase, galactose-1-phosphate uridyltransferase, and uridine diphosphate galactose 4′-epimerase. There are genetic diseases due to disorders of all these enzymes.

2. The biochemical consequences of the genetic disorders of galactose metabolism are abnormally high concentrations of galactose and its metabolites in body tissues and fluids. The clinical consequences range from life-threatening crises in the neonatal period and severe long-term complications to complete normality.

3. The first enzyme in the galactose pathway is galactokinase. The gene encoding galactokinase has been mapped to chromosome 17p24. It consists of 8 exons spanning about 7.3 kb of genomic DNA and shows many of the features of a housekeeping gene. The enzyme is a monomer containing 392 amino acids with a molecular weight of 42.

4. The main clinical feature of galactokinase deficiency is cataracts that are usually bilateral and detectable in the early weeks of life, although they have been observed at birth and in a fetus at 20 weeks' gestation. Pseudotumor cerebri has been described in several cases of galactokinase deficiency and is considered to be a true consequence of the disorder. These features resolve when a galactose-restricted diet is introduced.

5. The gene encoding galactose-1-phosphate uridyltransferase is located on the short arm of chromosome 9 in the p13 region and consists of 11 exons. The cDNA is 1295 bases in length and codes a polypeptide of 379 amino acids and an estimated molecular weight of 44. The active enzyme is a dimer of the polypeptide. More than 150 base changes have been characterized at the gene. A few are common, but most are rare; the distribution of several mutations has been studied in a number of major human groups. Q188R is the most common one in Europe and in individuals of European descent. S135L is found almost exclusively in individuals of African descent.

6. Severe galactose-1-phosphate uridyltransferase deficiency (classical galactosemia) presents in the first weeks of life as poor feeding and weight loss, vomiting, diarrhea, lethargy, and hypotonia. Liver dysfunction, bleeding tendencies, cataracts, and septicemia may be found on examination. These features usually resolve dramatically provided treatment is started early; however, it is now recognized that the majority of cases will have serious long-term complications.

7. The human uridine diphosphate galactose 4′-epimerase gene has been mapped to the short arm of chromosome 1 at 1p36. The gene spans 4 kb of genomic DNA, consists of 11 exons encoding a polypeptide of 348 amino acids and has a molecular weight of 38. The active enzyme is a dimer. Several mutations have been described at the *GALE* locus in affected individuals.

8. The majority of patients described with uridine diphosphate galactose 4′-epimerase deficiency have an enzyme defect principally in their erythrocytes and have normal growth and development. A generalized, severe form of enzyme deficiency has been described in only five cases from two families. Patients with this form present similarly to those with classical galactosemia and respond to the removal of galactose from their diets. There may be long-term complications in these patients, but because of the high degree of consanguinity in their families it is possible that other loci are also involved in their clinical abnormalities.

9. Neonatal screening for classical galactosemia has been introduced in some areas in order to promote early treatment, although the efficacy of this practice has been questioned. Prenatal diagnosis has been possible for all three enzyme disorders for a number of years.

10. There has been a large volume of research into the pathogenesis of the galactose disorders, and many hypotheses have been put forward. It is probable that cataract formation is caused by galactitol accumulation in the lens of the eye, but the mechanisms of all other features of these disorders remain to be elucidated.

BACKGROUND

Individuals intolerant of ingested galactose were described in the medical literature as early as 1908.[1] Since that time, numerous publications have elaborated the symptoms and signs of the disorder commonly referred to as "classical" galactosemia.[2] In most normal diets the principal sources of galactose are mammalian milks and milk-containing food products. Milks contain lactose, a disaccharide in which galactose is combined with glucose, its carbon 4 epimer (Fig. 72-1). Ingested lactose is hydrolyzed rapidly to galactose and glucose by a lactase contained within the brush border.[3] Although galactose has been found free in many fruits and vegetables and in glycosidic linkage in other plant and animal products,[4] there is no evidence that these sources, or potential sources, of galactose make a significant contribution to the dietary galactose load.[5]

Galactose and glucose are absorbed in the intestine by a sodium-coupled, energy-dependent system.[6] In normal individuals galactose loads are absorbed and cleared from the blood very rapidly[7]. Studies using ^{14}C-labeled galactose have shown that the label soon appears in the glucose pool and subsequently in the CO_2 of expired air.[8] The close correlation between the rate of galactose

A list of standard abbreviations is located immediately preceding the index in each volume. Nonstandard abbreviations used in this chapter include: GALE = Uridine diphosphate galactose-4′-epimerase; GALK = Galactokinase; GALT = Gal-1-P uridyltransferase; Gal-1-P = Galactose-1-phosphate; Glc-1-P = Glucose-1-phosphate.

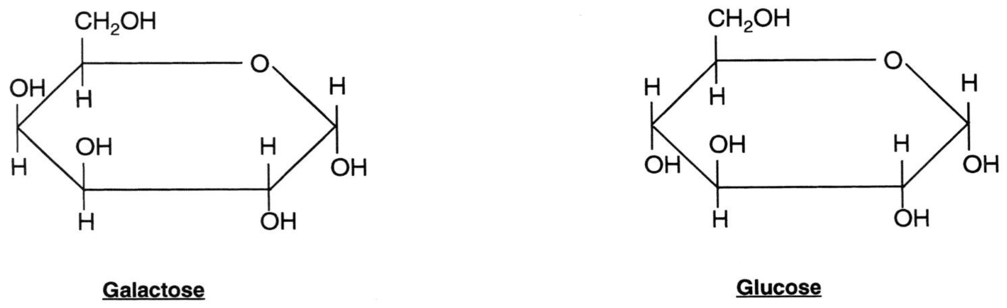

Galactose Glucose

Fig. 72-1 The structure of galactose and glucose.

clearance and that of hepatic blood flow,[9] and the early successful use of galactose tolerance tests to assess liver function,[7] indicated that the liver is the major organ involved in galactose metabolism. This conclusion is relevant in considering the clinical significance of the results of diagnostic enzyme tests for galactosemia, which are usually done on erythrocytes or amniotic fluid cells. The degree of enzyme deficiency in these cells does not necessarily reflect accurately the situation in the liver.

It was suggested many years ago that a further source of galactose was endogenous synthesis from glucose.[10] Recently it was established beyond any doubt that this is the case.[11] Although endogenous galactose production is small compared to the galactose intake of those ingesting high levels of milk and milk products, it may be very significant in the pathogenesis of the long-term complications of the galactose disorders.

It has been suggested that glucose has emerged as the primary metabolic fuel because of its stability and its limited potential for formation of glycosylated protein conjugates. Galactose, on the other hand, is much less favorable in this respect, and it is very advantageous that a pathway for the rapid conversion of galactose to glucose has evolved.[12]

The important metabolic pathway for the conversion of galactose to glucose was elucidated initially in yeasts and bacteria between 1949 and 1953[13,14] and was named after Leloir, who had made a major contribution to this work (Fig. 72-2). The pathway involves three enzymes: a galactose-specific kinase (GALK, EC 2.7.1.6); galactose-1-phosphate (Gal-1-P) uridyltransferase (GALT, EC 2.7.7.10), which, with UDP-glucose (UDP-Glc) as cofactor, incorporates the galactose into UDP-galactose (UDP-Gal) while releasing glucose-1-phosphate (Glc-1-P); and an epimerase, uridine diphosphate galactose 4′-epimerase (GALE, EC 5.1.3.2), which maintains an equilibrium between UDP-Gal and UDP-Glc, enabling galactose to make a major contribution to the energy requirements of the organism. Subsequently, it was shown that red cells from patients with classical galactosemia accumulated galactose-1-phosphate (Gal-1-P), one of the intermediary metabolites in the Leloir pathway.[15] It was soon demonstrated that the Leloir pathway was functional in the red cell[16] and that the second enzyme in the pathway (GALT) was deficient in classical galactosemia. More recently, deficiencies of both GALK[17] and GALE[18] have been described in association with characteristic clinical disorders.

PATHWAYS OF GALACTOSE METABOLISM

The Leloir Pathway

The Leloir, or main, pathway of galactose metabolism to Glc-1-P, as described in "Background" above, is essential for the utilization of galactose as an energy source. However, in addition, one of the intermediate products of the pathway, UDP-Gal, is an essential cofactor for the galactose transferases that are involved in the incorporation of galactose into glycoproteins and glycolipids,[19] (Fig. 72-2). Although the liver is the major organ of galactose metabolism, the enzymes of the Leloir pathway have been found in many cell types and tissues in which they have been

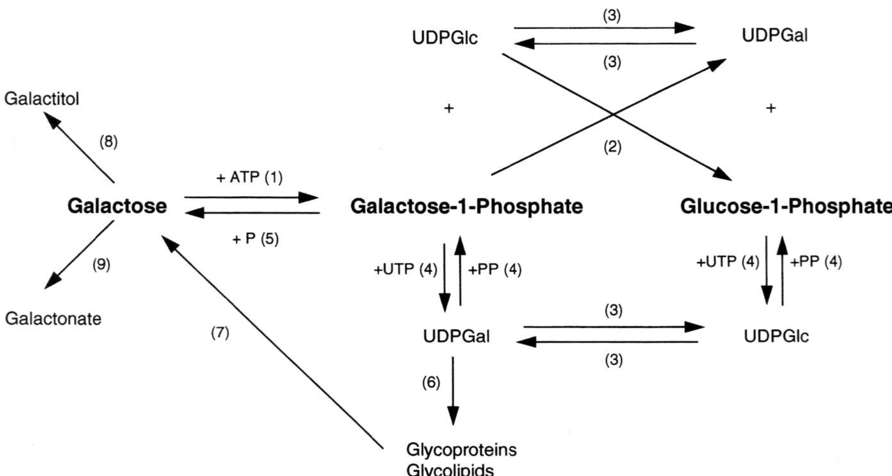

Fig. 72-2 The metabolic pathways of galactose. The main pathway of galactose metabolism, from galactose to glucose-1-phosphate, involves three enzymes, galactokinase (GALK) (1), galactose-1-phosphate uridyltransferase (GALT) (2), and uridine diphosphate galactose-4′-epimerase (GALE) (3). The pyrophosphorylase pathway, which is believed to operate mainly in the endogenous synthesis of galactose from glucose-1-phosphate, requires a UDP-Glc pyrophosphorylase (4); GALE (3); UDP-Gal pyrophosphorylase, considered to be the same enzyme as 4; and a phosphatase (5). UDP-Gal is incorporated into glycoproteins and glycolipids requiring a galactosyltransferase (6); the turnover of these compounds contributes to the free galactose pool (7). Particularly when its levels are increased, galactose may be metabolized to galactitol by aldose reductase (8) and to galactonic acid by galactose dehydrogenase (9).

Table 72-1 Enzymes of the Leloir pathway in human peripheral cells, skin fibroblasts, and tissues

	References		
Source	GALK	GALT	GALE
Red cells	45, 46, 320	320–322	78, 320
Leukocytes	323	323	
Fibroblasts	323, 324	323	324
Liver	325	321, 322, 325, 326	287
Kidney and skeletal muscle	325	325	
Intestinal mucosa	327	327	
Ovaries and testes	320	320	320

sought (Table 72-1). Galactose-1-phosphate uridyltransferase and galactokinase are present in fetal red cells, liver, lung, spleen, and cardiac muscle from at least 10 weeks' gestation, and their activities are higher in the second and third trimesters than at any time postnatally.[20] This suggests the possibility that damage may occur in utero in GALT deficiency.

Accessory Pathways

1) The pyrophosphorylase pathway. In 1957, Isselbacher postulated the existence of an alternative to the Leloir pathway of galactose metabolism in humans.[21] The alternative pathway was proposed as an explanation for the perceived ability to tolerate an increasing intake of galactose with age in some cases of GALT deficiency.[22] This pathway had already been described in yeast by Kalckar and co-workers.[23] The pyrophosphorylase pathway (Fig. 72-2) involves the phosphorylation of galactose to Gal-1-P, catalyzed by GALK, followed by a UTP-dependent pyrophosphorylase reaction in which the galactose moiety is incorporated into UDP-Gal. UDP-Gal is then converted into its epimer, UDP-Glc, from which a second pyrophosphorylase reaction generates Glc-1-P and UTP.

The two reactions that are unique to this alternative pathway are the UDP-Gal and UDP-Glc pyrophosphorylations. Although there is good evidence that a specific UDP-Gal pyrophosphorylase exists,[24,25] it has very low activity, and it is most probable that both of the pyrophosphorylation reactions are catalyzed by the enzyme designated UDP-Glc pyrophosphorylase.[26,27] Pyrophosphorylase activity has been detected in human adult and fetal liver, kidney, and skeletal muscle.[25]

A study of the rate of galactose pyrophosphorylation in human liver from newborn infants and adults of all ages from 20 to 70 years suggests that the pyrophosphorylase pathway can metabolize galactose at a rate only 1 percent of that of the Leloir pathway and could not account for an increase in galactose tolerance with age in GALT-deficient patients.[28] On the contrary, Gitzelmann considered that the main importance of the pyrophosphorylase pathway is in the reverse direction to that described by Isselbacher.[10] This ensures that the cell can synthesize the important UDP-Gal from Glc-1-P in the event that it is not produced by the metabolism of galactose through the main pathway, either because of a deficiency of free galactose or, more probably, due to a GALK or GALT disorder. In addition, however, Gal-1-P and, through the action of phosphatases, free galactose may be generated by the pyrophosphorylase pathway (Fig. 72-2), and this explains why in GALT deficiency high levels of Gal-1-P accumulate in spite of careful dietary galactose restriction. The magnitude of this endogenous galactose synthesis has now been measured in normal and GALT-deficient adults as 0.53–1.05 mg/kg/h.[11]

2) Reduction of galactose to galactitol. Galactose is a substrate for the enzymes that catalyze the first stage of the so-called polyol pathway of carbohydrate metabolism, which was described initially to explain the production of fructose from glucose in the seminal vesicles.[29] This first reaction in the pathway, from the hexose to the corresponding hexitol, may be catalyzed by either of two enzymes, aldose reductase (polyol:NADP$^+$ oxidoreductase, EC 1.1.1.21) and L-hexonate dehydrogenase (L-gulonate:NADP$^+$ oxidoreductase, EC 1.1.1.19).[30] On the basis of the tissue distribution of each enzyme and their affinities for different substrates, it was concluded that the former is the more important in metabolizing galactose.

Galactitol, the product of the reduction of galactose by aldose reductase (Fig. 72-3), is not a substrate for the subsequent enzyme in the polyol pathway and, consequently, may accumulate in tissues and is excreted in the urine. Abnormally high urinary concentrations of galactitol have been found in both untreated and galactose-restricted cases of GALT[31] and GALK[32] deficiencies.

The significance of the metabolism of galactose to galactitol is thought to be not as an alternative means of excreting the hexose in disorders of the Leloir pathway but in the possible involvement of the hexitol in the pathogenesis of both the acute and the long-term effects of galactosemia. These aspects are discussed in a later section of the chapter.

3) Oxidation of galactose to galactonate. Patients with GALT deficiency given a 35-g/m^2 load of galactose have been shown to excrete six times as much galactonate in their urine as normal subjects exposed to the same experimental conditions (Fig. 72-3).[33] More recently, using nuclear magnetic resonance spectroscopy to quantitate galactonate, it was demonstrated that galactosemic infants and adults on a galactose-restricted diet excreted the metabolite without being given an additional galactose load.[33a] A postmortem liver sample from a patient with classic galactosemia contained an increased amount of the metabolite compared to control liver samples.[34] Rats[34] and guinea pigs[35] fed experimental diets containing large amounts of galactose accumulated galactonate in a number of tissues and excreted increased levels of the metabolite in urine.

It has been proposed that the production of galactonate occurs through the activity of a soluble NAD$^+$-dependent galactose dehydrogenase, catalyzing the conversion of galactose to D-galactonolactone (D-galactose:NAD$^+$ oxidoreductase, EC 1.1.1.48). The enzyme in rat liver has been purified a hundredfold.[36,37] In the experimental system it is supposed that D-galactonolactone is changed to galactonate spontaneously, but it is possible that *in vivo* this reaction is controlled enzymatically. The existence of the highly active, soluble, NAD$^+$-dependent galactose dehydrogenase has been questioned and considered to be an artifact of the analytic system used.[38,39] A microsomal enzyme has been described that catalyzes the production of galactonic acid from galactose. This enzyme was not NAD$^+$- or NADP$^+$-dependent but was associated with H_2O_2 formation.

Although the mechanism of the metabolism of galactose to galactonate may be controversial, that this conversion occurs in GALT-deficient patients is unquestionable. However, there is no evidence to associate the accumulation of galactonate with the pathology of galactosemia; on the contrary, it is probable that its synthesis is the first step in an alternative pathway of galactose metabolism.[40] In this putative metabolic sequence, D-galactonic acid is converted to β-keto-D-galactonic acid and thence to D-xylose and D-xylose phosphate, which then enters the pentose phosphate oxidative pathway (Fig. 72-4). It was proposed that this could account for the significant amounts of galactose that appear to be metabolized in patients without an active Leloir pathway.[41]

Enzymes of the Leloir pathway

The enzymes of the Leloir pathway have been studied in humans (Table 72-1), in some animal species, and in microorganisms, in particular yeasts and *Escherichia coli*. It should be appreciated that, in general, enzymes which catalyze the same reaction have

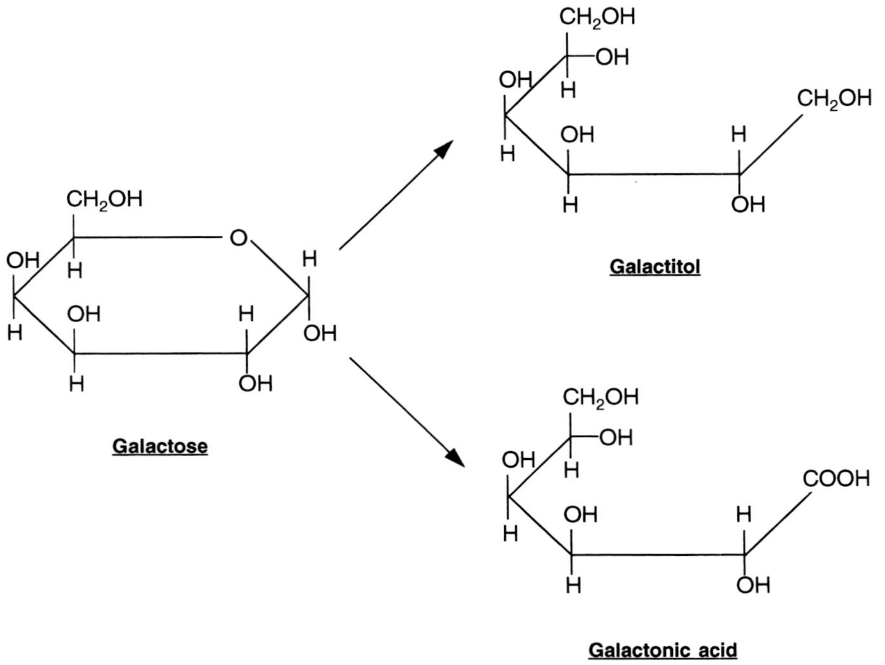

Galactose

Galactitol

Galactonic acid

Fig. 72-3 The conversion of galactose to galactitol by a nonspecific aldose reductase and to galactonic acid by aldehyde dehydrogenase.

similar characteristics in tissues and cells from the same species but differ from one species to another.[42]

Galactokinase Galactokinase has been studied in humans, in rat and pig, and in yeast and *E.coli*. One area that has attracted considerable attention, is the developmental aspects of the enzyme. Cuatrecasas and Segal[43] considered that differences in the activity and properties of the enzymes in the newborn and adult rat could be explained by a change in its molecular structure with age. On the other hand, Walker and Khan, also using rat liver, could find no evidence of enzyme heterogeneity with age.[44] In human beings it has been suggested that differences in the kinetic and inhibition characteristics of GALK between erythrocytes in umbilical cord blood and in adult blood are a result of molecular changes in the enzyme.[45] Other authors' work does not support this concept.[20,46]

Recent work on the molecular genetics of GALK, reviewed later ("Location and Structure of *GALK*, *GALT* and *GALE* Genes"), has not resolved completely the question of whether more than one type of galactokinase exists in humans. It is clear that the *GALK* gene mapping to chromosome 17q 21–22 codes for the enzyme GK1, which is the most significant in terms of activity. Patients with clinical GALK deficiency have mutations in this gene.[47] However, a second *GALK* (*GK2*) cDNA has been described, which is located on chromosome 15.[48] Although only *GK1* cDNA produced significant amounts of GALK when both cDNAs were expressed in COS cells,[49] some role of *GK2*, possibly at a developmental stage, cannot be excluded.

Determination of the structure and molecular weight of GALK by classic biochemical methods has had varying results; some appear to show it is a monomer with a molecular weight of 38,[51] others a dimer with a molecular weight of 55.[52] Calculations from the relevant DNAs suggest that GK1 is a polypeptide of 392 amino acids, molecular weight 42.271[48] and that GK2 has 458 amino acids and a molecular weight of 50.386.[49]

Some biochemical studies carried out on GALK in *in vitro* systems, sometimes with nonhuman material, may be relevant in understanding the deficiency disease. First, studies of the equilibrium constant for GALK in yeast indicate that the reaction it catalyzes is reversible but confirm that the equilibrium point is far over toward the product, Gal-1-P.[52] Second, studies in rat liver[43] and in human red cells[45] have indicated that GALK is inhibited by both its substrate and its product. This may limit the accumulation of Gal-1-P in GALT or GALE deficiency. Finally, fractionation of red cells from a patient with a new variant of GALK deficiency revealed higher levels of enzyme activity in reticulocytes than in older red cell.[53] This indicates that a mutation in the *GK1* gene exists that causes synthesis of an unstable product. The most notable factor in this situation is that tissues with high cell turnover could have significant levels of GALK activity.

Gal-1-P uridyltransferase. Gal-1-P uridyltransferase, the second enzyme in the Leloir pathway, has been found in microorganisms[54] and in mammalian cells and tissues[55] particularly in humans (Table 72-1). In contrast to the case with GALK, there has

The Metabolism of Galactose via Galactonate

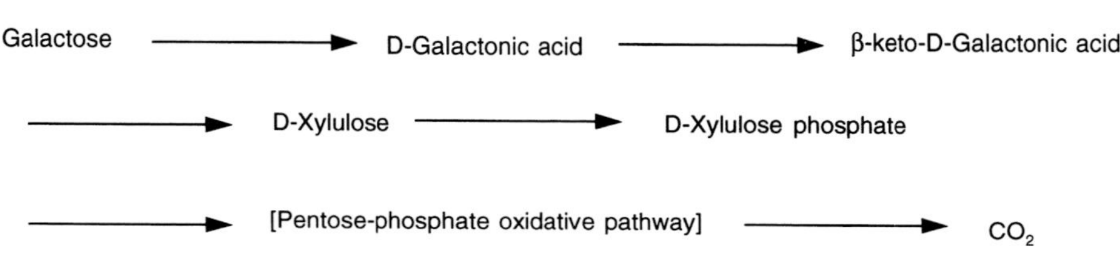

Fig. 72-4 An alternative oxidative pathway of galactose metabolism via galactonate.

been no suggestion that there is any heterogeneity in human GALT, even during development.[20] The gene for GALT, located on chromosome 9p13 in humans, codes for a protein with a molecular weight of 43. The active enzyme is a dimer,[55] and hence has a calculated molecular weight of 86. By classic biochemical methods, values of 69[56] and 88[57] have been found, the latter agreeing more closely with the calculated result.

It is of some significance that subjects who were heteroallelic at the *GALT* gene, possessing a wild-type and a mutant null gene (Q188R or R333W), made wild-type and mutant homodimer GALT products but also heterodimers.[58]. It appeared that wild-type and mutant monomers combined in a completely random fashion and, moreover, that heterodimers had enzyme activity levels somewhere between those of the homodimers. When the activity levels of the wild-type and mutant enzyme monomers vary in their homodimer and heterodimer combinations, the total GALT activity in heterozygotes for these genes will differ from the mean value in homozygote subjects for the two genes.

The mechanism of GALT activity has been investigated in great detail. Early work suggested the probability that the kinetics of the reaction are of the "ping-pong" type,[59] and this has been confirmed by the combined research of many workers, summarized recently by Frey.[60] The essential aspect of the reaction kinetics is the binding of the uridyl (UMP) group to a histidine molecule within the active site of the enzyme. In *E. coli* the binding occurs on a histidine at position 166 of the *GALT* gene, which is part of a His-Pro-His sequence. This sequence is highly conserved in evolution and is found in the human enzyme.[61] The presence of a cystine residue within the active site was also suggested by early experiments.[62] This has been confirmed and is consistent with GALT's being a Zn/Fe metalloprotein in which the metal ions stabilize the structure.[60] The sequence of the reactions of GALT are shown in the following two equations, in which E is the enzyme molecule:

$$\text{E-His} + \text{UDP-Glc} \leftrightarrow \text{E-His.UDP-Glc} \leftrightarrow \text{E-His-UMP} + \text{Glc-1-P} \quad \text{(Eq. 72-1)}$$

$$\text{E-His-UMP} + \text{Gal-1-P} \leftrightarrow \text{E-His-UMP} \cdot \text{Gal-1-P} \leftrightarrow \text{E-His} + \text{UDP-Gal} \quad \text{(Eq. 72-2)}$$

Other experimental work on galactosemic subjects and in rats has indicated a possibility of enhancing galactose oxidation, partly through an increase in GALT activity. In one paper[63] it was shown that three prepubertal boys with classic galactosemia given progesterone 10–20 mg/day for 6 days had up to tenfold enhancement of galactose oxidation, as measured by their ability to convert [1-^{14}C]galactose to $^{14}CO_2$. The same study showed that the formation of cataracts in young male rats fed a high-galactose diet could be delayed by the administration of progesterone. More recently it has been shown that GALT activity can be increased by administration of folic acid.[64] Seven-day-old suckling rats were given 1 mg/day folic acid for the next 7 days. Liver perfusion experiments carried out after folic acid administration showed a very rapid rate of galactose uptake for 35 minutes compared to the rate in control rats. GALT activity was shown to be elevated in the livers of test rats. These experiments have suggested some therapeutic possibilities, particularly in patients who have some residual GALT activity, but they have not been pursued.

Uridine diphosphate galactose-4′-epimerase. The main function of uridine diphosphate galactose 4-epimerase (GALE) is usually seen as being the final enzyme in the Leloir pathway, inverting the hydroxyl and hydrogen groups at the 4 carbon in the galactose molecule. The enzyme occurs widely in microorganisms and mammalian cells, human cells in particular (Table 72-1). However, epimerase is essentially a reversible enzyme. This is important in situations in which galactose is not available and UDP-Gal cannot be synthesized via the Leloir pathway, because both UDP-Gal and UDP-Glc are necessary cofactors for the incorporation of galactose and glucose into essential complex polysaccharides.

The properties and mechanism of action of GALE have been studied most intensively in microorganisms, and work in *E. coli* has been reviewed recently.[60] However, there are very important differences between the enzyme in microorganisms and that in the mammal. The most significant of these is that UDP-N-acetylgalactosamine and UDP-N-acetylglucosamine are substrates for mammalian GALE,[65] whereas these compounds are not metabolized by the enzyme from microorganisms–yeasts, for example.[66]

The importance of GALE in ensuring the availability of both UDP-Gal and UDP-Glc for complex polysaccharide synthesis was stressed earlier, and an analogous situation occurs for the UDP-N-acetylglucosamine and UDP-N-acetylgalactosamine derivatives that are required for the incorporation of the hexosamines into some polysaccharides. This has been demonstrated in studies of LDL receptor synthesis in cultured cells of normal and GALE-deficient mutants of Chinese hamster ovarian cell lines with only glucose as substrate.[67] It has also been shown that GALE in normal human skin fibroblast cultures accepts the UDP-N-acetylhexosamines as substrates and that LDL receptor can be synthesized in the absence of galactose, but the fibroblasts from a GALE-deficient patient were deficient in activity toward both UDP hexoses and UDP-N-acetylhexosamines and synthesized a minimal amount of LDL receptor.[68]

A further difference in the epimerases from microorganisms and mammalian sources has been suggested with respect to the binding of NAD^+, which is a cofactor in all of the enzymes. The epimerases of *E. coli*[69] and yeast[70] appear to bind NAD^+ extremely strongly, as the purified enzymes demonstrate catalytic activity without an added cofactor. In addition, NADH does not inhibit these enzymes. On the other hand, purified calf liver enzyme was found to be inhibited by NADH,[71] although it has been predicted that NAD^+ dissociates from the apoenzyme only once in every 9000 catalytic events.[72]

Regardless of the differences in substrate specificity and the possible variation in NAD^+ binding between the mammalian and microorganism enzymes, the mechanism of the reaction that inverts the OH and the H groups at C-4 in the hexose molecule appears to be the same. Maxwell[71] was the first to propose that this is an oxidation/reduction process. Confirmation that this is the case and that the intermediate in the reaction is uridine diphosphate-4-ketoglucose has come from several sources.[73–75] The importance of the loose attachment of the hexose to the enzyme through the nucleotide group for the epimerization reaction has become apparent.[60] Attempts to determine the structure of mammalian tissue epimerase have produced some conflicting results. Bovine liver and mammary gland enzymes were both found to contain molecules of with a molecular weight of 40,000 or 37,000, depending on the purification methods used, and the enzyme was not considered to be polymeric.[76] On the other hand, calf liver enzyme was considered to be a dimer with a molecular weight of 70,000.[72] The latter figure agrees well with the molecular genetic data suggesting that *GALE* cDNA codes for a subunit of 348 amino acids with a molecular weight of 38.266 and with the evidence that the enzyme is a dimer.[77]

There are interesting developmental changes in human red blood cells, which have implications with regard to the assay of GALE.[78] GALE activity in hemolysates from adults is negligible unless NAD^+ is added. This is in contrast to the case in the newborn, in whom hemolysate activity levels are optimal without exogenous cofactor. The reason for the difference is that in adults there is a stromal nucleosidase that destroys NAD^+ when the red cells are lysed. The nucleosidase is not present in red cells from newborn children. The destruction of NAD^+ in the adult leading to loss of red cell GALE activity may be another manifestation of weak enzyme-cofactor binding in mammals. Using optimal conditions for the enzyme assay, it would appear that red cell GALE concentrations are higher in newborn infants than in adults.[78] Cohn and Segal[79] found that GALE activities were highest in postnatal rats before 2 days of age, with levels declining to adult values at 20 days.

Substances that affect the cellular NAD^+:NADH ratio tend to alter the activity of GALE. The effect of alcohol has been studied *in vitro* using the soluble fraction of rat liver homogenate and measuring the oxidation of [1-^{14}C]galactose to $^{14}CO_2$. The oxidation of alcohol is accompanied by a reduction of the NAD^+:NADH ratio and an effect on epimerase activity that decreases galactose oxidation. NADH concentration in liver was increased up to twofold after administration of alcohol to rats. The effect of alcohol on NADH concentration is not found in red cells, because they lack aldehyde dehydrogenase. Stimulation of galactose oxidation in rat liver and intestine on administration of progesterone is considered to be due to a decrease in NADH concentration as a result of aldehyde dehydrogenase inhibition by the steroid.[80]

Location and structure of the *GALK, GALT,* and *GALE* genes

GALK. The human galactokinase gene, termed *GALK1*, was originally mapped to chromosome 17 by Elsevier et al. in 1974[81] and has since been localized to 17p24 by Stambolian et al. through isolation of a human cDNA.[47] The gene predicts an mRNA transcript of 1.35 kb and a protein of 392 amino acids. Alignment of the predicted protein with galactokinases from other organisms[82–84] shows only low to moderate degrees of overall sequence homology, the greatest level of conservation being with *E. coli* at almost 45 percent.[84] Analysis of the predicted protein sequence shows a conserved galactokinase signature sequence in exon 1 that may be required for functional activity and separate ATP-binding motifs in exons 3 and 7 that are also conserved among all the galactokinases.[84,85]

The full-length gene consists of 8 exons and spans about 7.3 kb of genomic DNA[86] (GenBank L76927). The promoter has many features in common with other housekeeping genes, including the absence of TATA- and CCAAT-box motifs and a high GC content, which reflects in part potential binding sites for the Sp1 transcription factor. The *GALK1* mRNA is heterogeneous at the 5′ terminus, with transcription sites occurring at many locations between 21 and 61 bases upstream of the ATG start site of the coding region. Multiple transcription initiation sites in the promoter are another characteristic of a housekeeping gene. The organization of the human galactokinase gene is given in Table 72-2.

Another human galactokinase cDNA, which maps to chromosome 15 and is denoted *GK2*, had already been isolated.[48] This gene, showing 29 percent sequence homology to galactokinase of *Saccharomyces*, was cloned by complementation in yeast and had been a promising candidate galactokinase gene. However, its role in galactose metabolism could not be established, because its galactokinase activity had not been functionally demonstrated[48,49] and mutations at this locus could not be identified in patients with galactokinase deficiency. Nevertheless, the *GK2* gene shows approximately 35 percent amino acid identity with the *GALK1* gene and 25–39 percent amino acid sequence homology with the other galactokinases. It is interesting to speculate that this gene might function only at specific stages of development.

GALT. After some early conflicting reports regarding its chromosome location, the *GALT* locus was correctly assigned to chromosome 9[87–92] and localized to the short arm in the region 9p13.[93]

The *GALT* cDNA was cloned and characterized in 1988 by Reichardt and Berg[94] and a corrected sequence subsequently published.[95] The cDNA is 1295 bases in length and encodes a polypeptide of 379 amino acids with an estimated molecular weight of 44 kDa. The open reading frame starts with ATG at base 29 and ends with a TGA stop codon at base 1166.

The availability of the human *GALT* cDNA enabled cloning of the full-length human *GALT* gene.[96] The sequence originally published[96] and submitted to GenBank under Accession No.

Table 72-2 Exon/intron organization of the human galactokinase (*GALK*) gene

Region		Number of nucleotides	Nucleotide number from first Met (ATG) in cDNA	Exon border type[a]	Amino acid numbers[b]
	exon 1	179-227[c]	1–165	3/	1–55
intron 1		886			
	exon 2	190	166–355	1/	56–119
intron 2		459			
	exon 3	120	356–475	1/	119–159
intron 3		170			
	exon 4	136	476–611	2/	159–204
intron 4		127			
	exon 5	182	612–793	1/	204–265
intron 5		4107			
	exon 6	151	794–944	2/	265–315
intron 6		76			
	exon 7	163	945–1107	3/	315–369
intron 7		82			
	exon 8	189	1108–1179	3/	370–392
Total			1179		392

[a] The border type describes whether the exon ends after the first (1/), second (2/), or third (3/) nucleotide of the codon.
[b] The amino acid number is included in two exons when the border type is 1 or 2.
[c] This suggests multiple starting sites.
Submitted under GenBank accession number L76927[86]

M96264 has also been updated.[97] The gene spans 4.3 kb of DNA arranged into 11 exons. Comparison of the amino acid sequences of GALT from *E. coli*,[98] yeast,[99] and mouse (N, Leslie, GenBank Accession No. M96265) reveals overall amino acid identities of 46, 39, and 87 percent, respectively, with respect to human GALT.[96] Some exons, notably 6, 9, and 10, have been highly conserved through evolution, whereas others, such as exons 1, 2, 5, and 7, are poorly conserved. The promoter region of the human *GALT* gene contains two GC-rich Sp1 sites, three AP-1 sequences, and a CCAAT sequence. There is no consensus TATA box. Thus, the gene may be expressed as a "housekeeping" gene, but the regulatory domains could play a role in tissue-specific and development-specific gene expression.

The structure of the gene is graphically depicted in Fig. 72-5. The full-length nucleotide sequence has been transcribed from Leslie et al.,[96] incorporating appropriate corrections in intron sequences[97] to a database available on a website at http://www.ich.bris.ac.uk/galtdb/.[100] The total number of nucleotides is 4321, including the promoter region. The cDNA sequence is numbered from the first nucleotide of the initiator methionine codon according to the recommendations of Antonarakis.[101] Thus, the full-length cDNA is 28 bases shorter than initially reported.[94]

GALE. The human *GALE* gene was mapped to a single locus on chromosome 1 using somatic cell hybrids,[102,103] and fluorescent *in situ* hybridization has subsequently localized the gene more precisely to the short arm at 1p36.[102] The cDNA, originally cloned by Daude et al.,[78] is 1488 bp in length and predicts a protein of 348 amino acids with a molecular weight of 38 kDa. The predicted protein has an extraordinary degree of sequence identity with that from rat (87 percent) and to the GAL10 protein from the yeast *Kluyveromyces lactis* (53 percent) as well as to the galE polypeptide of the prokaryote *E. coli* (51 percent).[98]

The full-length genomic *GALE* gene has been cloned and characterized by Maceratesi et al.[104] and the sequence submitted to GenBank under Accession No. A1022382. The gene consists of 11 exons extending over about 4 kb of genomic DNA (Table 72-3). The first exon contains the 5′-untranslated region, and the last exon harbors the last 54 bases of the protein-coding sequence, the termination codon, and the 3′-untranslated sequence. Interestingly, at the boundary between the first exon and the first intron, the splice site donor sequence is GC and not the usual consensus GT sequence.

GALK DEFICIENCY

Clinical presentation

The only consistent clinical finding in GALK deficiency (OMIM 230200) is cataracts.[17,105–112] These are morphologically identical to those in GALT deficiency and characteristically are bilateral. They have been reported in GALK-deficient children as young as 4 weeks of age.[109] Although other abnormalities have been described in individual patients, including macular deposits,[113] mental retardation,[114] complement deficiency,[115] and seizures with neurologic deterioration,[107] these are most likely to be coincidental. Pseudotumor cerebri has been reported in more than one infant.[116,117] Since it has been postulated that pseudotumor cerebri occurs by the same mechanism responsible for cataract formation.[118] it is possible that this is a true, albeit rare, complication of GALK deficiency.

Although the relationship between homozygosity for GALK deficiency and cataracts is well established, there remains controversy as to whether heterozygotes are at risk of developing this complication. A number of studies have supported such an association,[119–125] but others have not.[126–128] Stambolian,[129] in a review of galactose and cataracts, concluded that the relationship between a partial reduction of GALK activity and cataracts was also dependent upon the dietary intake of galactose. In heterozygous GALK deficiency, presenile cataracts may become manifest only if galactose intake is sufficiently high to cause excess production of galactitol. It is also suggested that adults who are neither homozygotes nor heterozygotes for GALK deficiency may be at greater risk for developing senile cataracts if they consume large quantities of milk.[130]

Mutations at the *GALK* locus

The first two mutations reported at the *GALK* gene were a nonsense mutation of Glu to stop in exon 2 (designated E80X) and a missense mutation of Val to Met in exon 1 (designated V32M), which were characterized in two families with cataracts and GALK deficiency.[47] Transfection of the mutant V32M sequence into a mammalian expression system confirmed its effect on reducing enzyme activity.

As of July 1999, at least 13 different mutations, including deletions, insertions, and missense and nonsense mutations, have been characterized at the *GALK* gene in individuals who had GALK deficiency.[47,131,132] Only one, a Gly to Ser substitution, designated G349S, involves a hypermutable site and the base substitution that would be expected from deamination of a methylated cytosine.[133] Several individuals are known to be homozygous for a specific mutation but it is not clear whether this has occurred because of consanguinity or through an identity by descent. The nonsense mutation of Gln to stop, designated Q382X, has been reported in at least six Costa Rican individuals.[131] Further analysis of the genetic background of this mutation would provide some insights into its relatively high frequency in this population. Details of some of these are given in Appendix 72-1.

The enzyme defect

Gitzelmann[134] was the first to confirm the position of the enzyme defect in a patient with juvenile cataracts associated with galactosuria. The red cells of the patient were shown to have normal GALT and GALE activity and respired normally with Gal-1-P as substrate. The level of GALK was shown to be indistinguishable from zero. A further study in the same patient in which [1-^{14}C]galactose was injected intravenously[135] showed that only 5 percent of the label appeared in his expired air over a 5-hour period. It was concluded that the GALK deficiency was most probably common to all cells and tissues of the body.

The incidence of the enzyme deficiency appears to be very low and cannot be assessed with any accuracy. Heterozygotes for the condition have approximately 50 percent of normal enzyme activity in their red cells,[134] the inheritance of the disease being autosomal recessive. A study of a North American population[136] found that 1 percent were heterozygotes, suggesting a disease frequency of 1 in 40,000. However, a screening study for the complete deficiency carried out in Massachusetts detected no positives in 177,000 newborns.[137]

The possibility of racial polymorphism in GALK levels was concluded from a study of red cell GALK and GALT levels in 1082 black and 618 white pregnant women in Philadelphia.[138] The results showed that the black females had significantly lower mean levels of GALK than the whites and that the distribution of the enzyme levels was not normal. The existence of a low-activity GALK variant in the black population was postulated. Three subjects in the study had enzyme levels above the normal range, suggesting the possibility of a high-activity variant in this population.

Metabolic abnormality

Gitzelmann's initial study of a GALK-deficient patient[134] showed that when he was drinking milk large amounts of galactitol were excreted in his urine. On a galactose intake of 360 g/day, corresponding to a milk intake of 3 liters/day, two thirds of the load could be accounted for as galactose and galactitol in urine. The fate of the remainder was unclear. The molar ratio of galactose

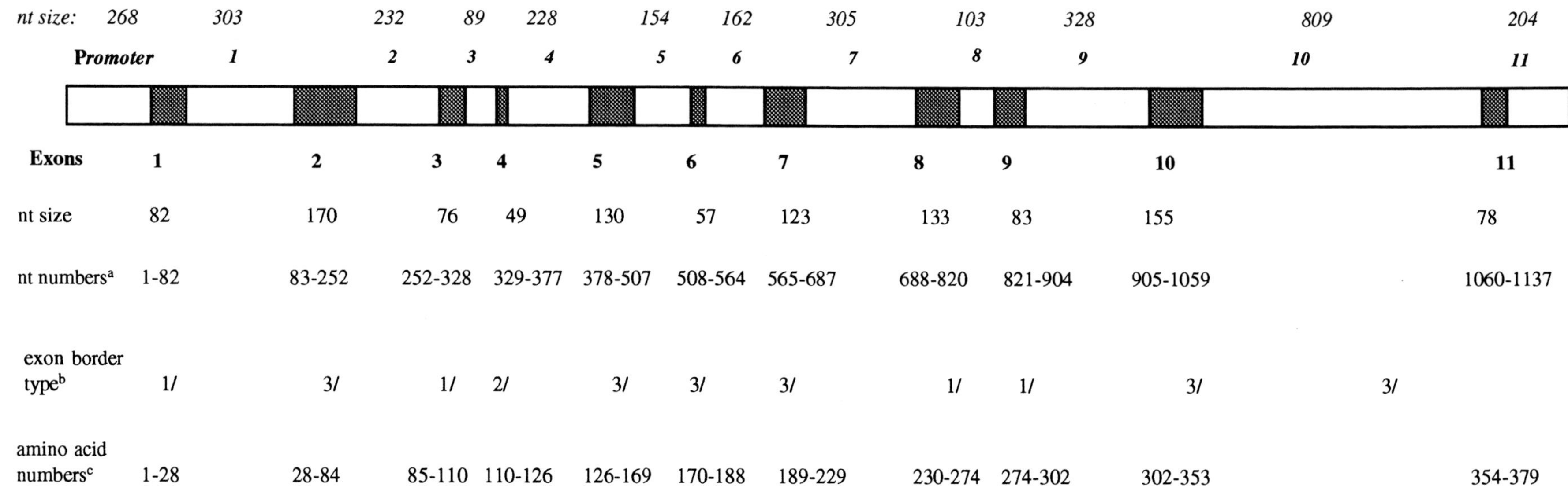

Exons	1	2	3	4	5	6	7	8	9	10	11
nt size	82	170	76	49	130	57	123	133	83	155	78
nt numbers[a]	1-82	83-252	252-328	329-377	378-507	508-564	565-687	688-820	821-904	905-1059	1060-1137
exon border type[b]	1/	3/	1/	2/	3/	3/	3/	1/	1/	3/	3/
amino acid numbers[c]	1-28	28-84	85-110	110-126	126-169	170-188	189-229	230-274	274-302	302-353	354-379

[a] The nucleotide number is determined from the first nucleotide of the first Methionine (ATG) codon of the cDNA.
[b] The border type describes whether the exon ends after the first (1/), second (2/) or third nucleotide (3/) of the codon.
[c] The amino acid number is included in two exons when the border type is 1/ or 2/.

Fig. 72-5 Structure and organization of the human *GALT* gene. Relative sizes of introns and exons are drawn to scale.

Table 72-3 Exon/intron organization of the human UDP-Galactose 4′-epimerase (*GALE*) gene

Region		Number of nucleotides	Nucleotide number from first Met (ATG) in cDNA	Exon border type[a]	Amino acid numbers[b]
	exon 1	70	(−93)		
intron 1		350–355			
	exon 2	121	1–121	1/	1–41
intron 2		156			
	exon 3	116	122–237	3/	41–79
intron 3		385			
	exon 4	114	238–351	3/	80–117
intron 4		245			
	exon 5	177	352–528	3/	118–176
intron 5		544			
	exon 6	114	529–642	3/	177–214
intron 6		90			
	exon 7	67	643–709	1/	215–237
intron 7		93			
	exon 8	86	710–795	3/	237–265
intron 8		137			
	exon 9	78	796–873	3/	266–291
intron 9		235			
	exon 10	120	874–993	3/	292–331
intron 10		144			
	exon 11	401	994–1097		332–348
intron 11			1098–1395		
Total			1488[c]		348

[a] The border type describes whether the exon ends after the first (1/), second (2/), or third (3/) nucleotide of the codon.
[b] The amino acid number is included in two exons when the border type is 1 or 2.
[c] Including the 5-untranslated region of exon 1.
Submitted under GenBank accession number A1022382[104]

to galactitol in the urine was 1:4. It was proposed that the galactose that could not be accounted for was metabolized to galactonate and subsequently, by oxidation of this compound, to CO_2. There is some doubt about this, however, since the studies in the same patient using carbon-14-labeled galactose[135] found only 5 percent of the injected label appearing in CO_2. Moreover, it was shown that injected ^{14}C-labeled galactonate was not metabolized to CO_2. Experimental data in the GALK-deficient patient supported the proposal that galactose was metabolized to CO_2, but not via galactonate.

Diagnosis

The diagnosis of GALK deficiency has usually followed the investigation of infants and children with unexplained cataracts. Even though GALK deficiency is a rare cause of congenital cataracts, since prevention is possible, all infants presenting with this phenomenon should be investigated for it. GALK deficiency may also be found by newborn screening programs that identify galactose in blood or urine. Screening tests for galactosemia include microbiologic and fluorometric assays for galactose and a fluorescent spot screening test for GALT activity (Beutler test). Most screening laboratories include a combination of the Beutler test and the fluorometric assay for galactose.[139] These should therefore identify and differentiate between infants with GALK deficiency and those with GALT deficiency. GALK deficiency will not be detected if only the Beutler test is undertaken.

Treatment

As in GALT deficiency, cataracts may be reversible provided a galactose-free diet is started in early infancy. After a few months of age, permanent changes occur that are not corrected by diet.[105,111] Galactose restriction has also been recommended for heterozygotes,[129] but there are insufficient data to determine how strict this restriction needs to be or whether it is really necessary. It has been suggested that in addition to homozygotes, heterozygotes should also be offered regular slit-lamp examination of the lens.[129]

GALT DEFICIENCY

Clinical presentation

GALT deficiency (OMIM 230400) most often presents within the first weeks after birth as a life-threatening illness. Initial symptoms include poor feeding with poor weight gain, vomiting and diarrhea, lethargy, and hypotonia. On physical examination, infants are jaundiced, have hepatomegaly, may have a full fontanelle, and show prolonged bleeding after venous or arterial sampling, or excessive bruising. The results of initial investigations indicate liver disease (unconjugated or combined hyperbilirubinemia; raised liver transaminases; raised plasma amino acids, particularly phenylalanine, tyrosine, and methionine); and renal tubular disease (metabolic acidosis, galactosuria, glycosuria, albuminuria, aminoaciduria). In addition, hematologic abnormalities are common; disordered clotting results from liver disease, and hemolytic anemia may occur. Septicemia is not uncommonly associated with the early presentation of galactosemia (particularly *E. coli*) and may cause diagnostic confusion. Cataracts are usually seen at presentation but in the first weeks of life are mostly mild and may be detected only on slit lamp examination.

Less frequently, patients present with a more chronic illness with persistent poor feeding and vomiting, failure to thrive, and developmental delay. This phenotypic variability may be due either to environmental factors, for example, those related to galactose intake, or to genetic heterogeneity with residual GALT activity.[140]

Long-term complications. Late effects are common in patients with GALT deficiency and occur despite early diagnosis and treatment. These include effects on cognitive development, ovarian failure in females, and an ataxic neurologic disease.

Neuropsychological outcome. Although it was initially hoped that with dietary treatment the outcome for patients with galactosemia would be good, concerns that this was not the case were first raised over a quarter of a century ago by Komrower, based on the findings of follow-up studies in Manchester.[141] It is now generally accepted that, even with early diagnosis and good dietary treatment, neuropsychological development is significantly impaired. Age at start of diet, except after 2 months; milk restriction during pregnancy; and Gal-1-P levels do not correlate with DQ or IQ.[142–144] In most studies of cognitive development in older children and adults, mean IQ for patients has been in the range of 70–90, although normal and above-average intelligence in individual patients is possible.[141–143,145,146]

Formal developmental and intelligence testing at different ages suggests that intelligence may fall during childhood.[142,143,146]. In a number of studies the mean IQ for patients was lower in older age groups.[141–143,146,147] In the international survey by Waggoner et al.[142] decreases of 6.2 points in 42 children who had an assessment at 3–5 years of age, repeated at 6–9 years, and of 4.4 points in 46 children tested at 6–9 years, repeated at 10–16 years, were reported. There was not, however, a consistent fall in children tested with the same IQ test, and in other studies no decrease in cognitive ability over time has been demonstrated.[148] Endogenous galactose production with continuing toxicity to the central nervous system might account for a fall in intelligence with age. However, whether there is a true reduction in cognitive ability can be questioned on the basis of inadequate longitudinal testing in individuals, the wide variety of IQ measures used, and the lack of control data. Speech and language defects are particularly frequent in patients with galactosemia, with delayed vocabulary and articulation problems reported in over 90 percent of children.[142,149] Verbal dyspraxia, an unusual speech disorder due to a sensory motor disturbance of articulation, has been reported as occurring relatively frequently.[150,151] Additionally, a number of children have visual-perceptual dysfunction.[141,153] Patients with the most severe speech disorders or visual-perceptual difficulties generally have lower IQs.[142,150] It is not clear whether these particular impairments are specific deficits or part of the global cognitive disorder; some studies have found speech defects in line with general cognitive abilities.[146] There is some evidence to suggest that adults with GALT deficiency have a particular personality trait; individuals are described as having shy and timid personalities, being anxious and fearful in interpersonal relationships, and developing into overdependent adults.[141,147,153]

Growth. Although height in late childhood and in adolescents may be lower than that of the normal population, the final height in patients is usually within normal limits. Growth is often delayed in childhood and early adolescence but often continues beyond the age of 18 and into the early twenties.[142,154] This pattern of growth may be related to early ovarian failure but has also occurred in male patients.[154] Whether it is a consequence of inadequate nutrient intake in childhood or a feature of the galactosemia itself is unclear.

Ataxia and other late neurologic complications. Progressive neurologic disease developing after early childhood in galactosemia patients who have been treated from infancy was first described in 1973.[155] Since then there have been a number of case reports confirming this association.[143,155–159] Hypotonia, resting tremor, intention tremor, dysdiadochokinesis, and ataxic gait; dystonic, choreic, and ballistic movements; uncoordinated facial movements; and scanning dysarthric speech have all been described. The similar clinical presentation in these reports suggests a specific neurologic syndrome due primarily to cerebellar dysfunction, although extrapyramidal disturbance may also play a part.[159] The age of onset has varied from early to mid-childhood to middle age. Early signs have included truncal ataxia and hypotonia, which have then proceeded to more florid cerebellar disease. Only a proportion of individuals with classic galactosemia have developed this complication. In the international survey by Waggoner et al., 18 percent of patients over 3.5 years old were reported to have problems with coordination or gait.[142] In a retrospective study in Germany, 22 percent of patients had evidence of cerebellar dysfunction; intention tremor was found in 11 out of 78 patients, mild ataxia in three, and severe ataxia in three.[143] Kaufman et al.[146] reported that 12 of 45 (27 percent) patients had tremor, ataxia, or dysmetria. Early dietary treatment has not protected individuals from late neurologic disease.[157]

Brain imaging. Abnormalities on brain imaging are common in classical galactosemia. Computerized tomography and magnetic resonance imaging in patients with late neurologic disease have demonstrated abnormal white matter, ventricular enlargement, diffuse cortical atrophy with basal ganglia and brainstem involvement, and cerebellar atrophy.[156–161] Nelson et al. have reported the results of magnetic resonance brain imaging in 67 transferase-deficient patients, of whom 63 had classic galactosemia.[162] T1-weighted images showed normal myelination for age in all patients. However, the reduction in peripheral white matter attenuation on T2- and intermediate-weighted images that occurs normally in infancy was not present in 52 of 55 patients with classical galactosemia over the age of 1 year. This abnormality was postulated to represent a failure of normal myelination.Twenty-two patients had mild lateral ventricular enlargement compatible with cerebral atrophy and eight had enlargement of the 4th ventricle and cerebellar sulci, suggesting cerebellar atrophy. In six of these eight patients the cerebellar atrophy was moderately severe. Ten of the 63 patients were ataxic on examination, but only two of these had moderate cerebellar atrophy. In addition to these findings, 11 patients had two or more discrete focal white matter lesions on T2-weighted images scattered through the cerebral white matter, most commonly near the corners of the lateral ventricles. The basal ganglia nuclei and brainstem were normal in all patients.

Ovarian failure. Hypergonadotropic hypogonadism is common in galactosemia occurring in over 90 percent of GALT-deficient females in some series.[163] It may be manifested as delayed puberty, primary amenorrhea, secondary amenorrhea, or oligomenorrhea. The first biochemical evidence for ovarian failure may be an abnormal (increased) release of follicle-stimulating hormone (FSH) and LH following an LRH stimulation test, although most patients will have raised basal FSH and LH when investigated. Estradiol concentration may initially be normal with high gonadotropin levels, indicating continued follicular development, but fall as ovarian failure progresses.[163] As with other late complications, ovarian failure appears to be independent of the age at which treatment is started and of dietary compliance. The etiology is unknown. Prenatal damage is suggested by reduced oocyte numbers in rats subjected to prenatal exposure to high levels of galactose,[164] and streak ovaries have been reported on laparoscopy.[165,166] However, postnatal damage is supported by the report of normal ovarian tissue in a girl who died from *E. coli* sepsis at 5 days of age[167] and by the finding that in some patients gonadal function may be initially normal but can become abnormal with time.[163] Ovarian histology in galactosemic women with ovarian failure has been variable.[168] Oocyte numbers have generally been absent or low, with the stroma reported as fibrous or streaky in appearance. Possible mechanisms for the ovarian dysfunction include the production of abnormal FSH,[169] abnormal receptor activity, and a direct toxic effect of galactose, Gal-1-P, or other metabolites on ovarian tissue. Gonadal dysfunction in galactosemia and its various possible etiologies have been reviewed by Gibson.[168]

In the study by Waggoner et al., 8 out of 34 women over 17 years of age had primary amenorrhea.[142] The mean age of menarche in the remaining patients was 14 years (range 10–18 years), and the majority of these developed secondary amenorrhea or oligomenorrhea after a relatively short period. Although most female patients are infertile by the time they reach childbearing age, a small number of women have given birth (14 pregnancies in nine women in the Waggoner study); the majority had normal infants.[142,170] Gal-1-P levels were not significantly raised in the cord blood in two infants from two sisters with galactosemia[154] despite high maternal levels, confirming that Gal-1-P does not cross the placenta. However, maternal Gal-1-P levels have been reported to rise toward the end of pregnancy and after delivery, possibly due to endogenous lactose production and subsequent catabolism to glucose and galactose.[154,171] In addition to unassisted conception, a single pregnancy has been reported after oocyte donation.[172] In this case an ovarian biopsy had demonstrated a fibrotic stoma with no intermediate or graafian follicles present. The endometrium responded to exogenous hormone replacement, allowing embryo implantation. A normal infant was born by cesarean section at 37 weeks with a birth weight of 3090 g. In contrast to gonadal dysfunction in females with galactosemia, testicular function appears to be normal in males.

Mutations of *GALT* have been linked with an increased incidence of Müllerian fusion defects. Müllerian aplasia and streaklike ovaries have been reported in one girl, whose mother had a Müllerian fusion anomaly.[173] The girl, her mother, and her maternal grandmother were all heterozygous for classic galactosemia. Heterozygosity for an allele with an Asn to Asp substitution at codon 314, designated N314, was more common in a series of 33 women with endometriosis than in controls (30 percent compared with 14 percent) and in 13 females with vaginal agenesis (46 percent compared with 14 percent).[174,175] It was postulated that decreased fetal or maternal GALT activity with increased exposure to galactose *in utero* had led to defects in canalization of the cervix, predisposing to endometriosis or to vaginal agenesis. There have, however, been no reports of Müllerian fusion defects in infants born to mothers homozygous for the N314D galactosemia allele. (See "N314D, vaginal agenesis and endometriosis" below for further discussion of this subject.)

Ovarian function in heterozygotes. There is limited evidence that ovarian function may be abnormal in women who are heterozygous for classical galactosemia. Women heterozygous for the Q188R or the N314D mutation and those with *GALT* polymorphisms associated with low GALT activity have been found to have significantly higher basal FSH levels.[176] Possession of a *GALT* polymorphism was found to be an independent predictive factor for high FSH. However, time to pregnancy, a measure of fecundity; menstrual cycle patterns; and natural menopause were no different in a retrospective study comparing 103 mothers of galactosemic children with 116 mothers of children with phenylketonuria.[177] In this study, however, it was not possible to determine whether menopause was earlier in the carriers of galactosemia, since the number of women over the age of 45 was small.

Mutations at the *GALT* locus

The first collection of disease-causing mutations and polymorphisms at the *GALT* gene was characterized by Reichardt and colleagues in 1991.[61,178] As of July 1999, over 150 different base changes had been documented.[178a] Details about individual base changes and up-to-date information are available on two websites at the following addresses: http://www.ich.bris.ac.uk/galtdb/[100] and http://www.cc.emory.edu/PEDIATRICS/medgen/research/db.htm. More than 260 entries from 26 different populations and ethnic groups in 18 different countries were documented by July 1999.[100]

A few of the base changes are nonsense mutations (9 percent), small deletions or insertions (10 percent), and splice site mutations (5 percent), but, as predicted,[178] most (almost 61 percent) are missense mutations that are scattered along the length of the gene (see Table 72-4 and Fig. 72-6). Twenty-nine mutations are at CpG hypermutable sites[133] (see Table 72-4), and two thirds of these have resulted in base changes that would be predicted from a C $\rightarrow$ T transition of a methylated cytosine on either the sense or the antisense strand. Of the hypermutable sites, multiple mutations have been reported at four of them, arginine 123 (resulting in R123G and R123Q); arginine 148 (resulting in R148W, R148Q, and R148G); arginine 333 (resulting in R333W, R333Q, and R333G); and nucleotides c.957–958, where the CpG site spans two codons (resulting in H319Q and A320T). Several individual mutations at hypermutable sites have multiple entries through citings in different populations or ethnic groups.[100]

The effects of nonsense mutations, frameshift insertions/deletions, and splice site mutations on protein structure and function can be anticipated. The biochemical consequences of apparent missense mutations, on the other hand, are not easy to predict, but some information about their effects can usually be established through *in vitro* expression analysis. Two *in vitro* systems have been used to examine effects of mutations at the *GALT* locus: a mammalian cell transfection system[61] and a yeast expression system.[180] Occasionally, the two systems have produced inconsistent results for individual mutations, with the yeast system generally yielding lower *in vitro* enzyme activities than the COS cell system. Nevertheless, both have their merits, and they should be used in parallel, particularly when either system alone fails to model the human biochemical phenotypes faithfully.

There are 11 exonic single nucleotide polymorphisms (SNPs), or 'silent' mutations, and 13 intronic base changes at sequences other than the donor or acceptor splice sites (Table 72-4 and Fig. 72-6).[100] One of the former and three of the latter are known to be in linkage disequilibrium with N314D in the Duarte 1 (Los Angeles) or the Duarte 2 allele, respectively (see "N314D and the Duarte Alleles," below), and their influence on the Duarte phenotypes is discussed in a later section ("The Duarte Alleles"). The others, which are mostly rare, have all been reported on chromosomes from affected individuals. Whether these base changes are truly the disease-causing mutations or simply polymorphisms without effect can only be established only by using *in vivo* or *in vitro* functional assays. For example, the C $\rightarrow$ T transition 56 bases from the 5′ donor splice site of intron 10 (IVS10nt + 56C $\rightarrow$ T) has been shown through mRNA extraction to be a disease-causing mutation and not a polymorphism. The base change activates a cryptic splice site, which results in the insertion of 18 amino acids in a highly conserved part of the protein.[181]

Most Common Mutations. As with other common genetic disorders, notably cystic fibrosis (see chapter 201) and phenylketonuria (see chapter 77), a few mutations at the *GALT* gene are frequent, but most are rare. About 67 percent of the base changes have been documented in only one study, and except for the base changes in linkage disequilibrium with N314D, fewer than 10 percent of mutations have been reported in multiple ethnic groups

Table 72-4 Classification of mutations at the *GALT* gene according to type

Missense						Nonsense	Deletions	Insertions	Splice site	?Silent	?Polymorphism
D28Y[b]	F117S	R148Q[a]	I198T	R262P[b]	P325L[a]	Q54X	5′UTR-119delGTCA[c]	L74fsinsG	V85–N97fsdel38bp	R11R	IVS3nt + 29G → C
I32N	Q118H	R148G[b]	A199T	R272G[b]	R328H[a]	R80X[a]	Exons 1–10	S112fsinsA	IVS3nt − 2 A → C	D39D	IVS4nt − 27G → C[c]
Q38P	R123G[b]	V150L	R201H[a]	L282V	S329F	W154X	L74fsdelCT		IVS4nt + 1G → T	G110G	IVS5nt + 62G → A[c]
V44L	R123Q[a]	V151A[d]	E203K[d]	K285N	A330V	Q164X			IVS5nt + 2T → C	Y165Y	IVS5nt − 38T → C
V44M	V125A	W154G	R204P[b]	L289R	R333W[a]	R204X[a,d]	W134fsdelT		IVS6nt − 2A → G	L195L	IVS5nt − 24G → A[c]
R51L[b]	K127E	W167R	Y209C	E291K	R333Q[a]	Q212X	L256–P257delGCC		IVS6nt + 1G → A	L218L	IVS5nt − 11C → G
G55C	M129T	Q169K	Y209S	F294Y	R333G[b]	W249X	L275fsdelT		IVS7nt + 2T → C	V233V	IVS5nt − 11C → A
L62M	C130Y	F171S	Q212H	E308K	K334R	W316X[d]	F294fsdelT		IVS10nt + 56C → T[a]	G302G	IVS5nt − 5G → C
P66L	H132Y	G179D	L217P	N314D	M336L	L264X	Q317fsdelC			H315H	IVS6nt + 32T → A
R67C[a]	S135L[a]	P183T	L226P	Q317H	E340K[a]	E340X[b,e]	L318fsdelC			L318L	IVS8nt + 13A → G
L74P	T138M[a]	H184Q	R231H[a]	Q317R	Q344K	Q353X	H260 R263del12bp			P324P	IVS8nt + 23T → G
A81T	L139P	Q188R	W249R	H319Q[b]	T350A	Y366X	L326fsdelC			G338G	IVS8nt + 58G → T
F95L	M142V	S192N	Y251C	A320T[a]	X380R	Q370X	L327fsdelC				IVS10nt + 36T → A
D98N[a]	M142K	F194L	Y251S	Y323D			L349fsdelC				
D113N	S143L[a]	L195P	R258C[a]	Y323H			P351fsdelC				
H114L	R148W[a]	I198M	R259W[a]	P324S							

[a]CpG hypermutable site.
[b]CpG site but not a mutation commonly associated with hypermutable site.
[c]Intron polymorphisms associated with N314D on Duarte 2 alleles in European populations.
[d]Associated with Duarte 2 allele.
[e]Associated with Duarte 1 allele, including N314D and L218L.

or geographic areas throughout the world.[100] The mutations most frequently reported are Q188R, K285N, S135L, and N314D, of which only S135L is at a CpG hypermutable site.

Q188R, a Glu to Arg substitution at amino acid position 188 of the GALT protein, results from an A → G transition at nucleotide c.563* in exon 6. First reported in 1991 by Reichardt et al.[61] by July 1999 it had 22 citations in the *GALT* database[100] and is certainly the most common *GALT* mutation in Europe and North America (see below). This mutation is located in a domain highly conserved across species and is in close proximity to the putative enzyme catalytic site, which is a histidine-proline-histidine triad.[182] *In vitro* expression analysis using either a mammalian[61] or a yeast expression system[180] has confirmed that the mutation results in a substantial, if not complete, loss of GALT activity. The effect of the Glu to Arg substitution on the normal biochemical mechanism of GALT, described earlier by Frey and his associates[60] has been studied using an *E. coli* GALT model. It has been concluded that the usual hydrogen bonding of the glutamine to a histidine in the active site of the enzyme is compromised by the substitution of arginine for glutamine, destabilizing the UMP-GALT complex. This impairs the latter stage of the GALT reaction, in which Gal-1-P displaces UDP-Gal from the uridylyl complex.[182a,182b]

*The nucleotide position is recorded here as c.563 and not nt591 as originally reported in the paper by Reichardt et al. in 1991.[61] The numbering system used is based on that recommended by Antonarakis,[101] in which the first nucleotide is numbered from the first base of the first methionine codon in the cDNA. This is nt position +29 in the original sequence. See sequence and annotation at http://www.ich.bris.ac.uk/galtdb/.[100]

K285N, a Lys to Asp substitution in exon 9, results from a G → T transversion at nucleotide c.855 and was first reported by Leslie et al.[96] The amino acid substitution is not in a region of the protein that is highly conserved across species, and the effects of the substitution have not been determined through expression analysis. Nevertheless, its high relative frequency on mutant chromosomes in some populations makes it almost certain that it is a disease-causing mutation.

The third mutation is N314D, a base change first reported by Reichardt and Woo.[178] Originally thought to be a polymorphism, it is now known to be associated with the so-called Duarte alleles and in linkage disequilibrium with other base changes (see "The Duarte Alleles" below). The mutation is in exon 10 and has been reported to occur in many populations and major human groups.[100]

Mutation Frequencies and Population Variation

Europe and North America. Q188R is the most frequently occurring *GALT* mutation in European populations and in those of predominantly European descent. Although it was originally thought to account for as few as 25 percent of mutant alleles in North American galactosemic individuals (of multiple racial and ethnic backgrounds),[62] subsequent studies have established that its relative frequency in North American Caucasians is between 60 and 70 percent of mutant chromosomes.[96,183–185]

Ng et al.[140] and Wong et al.[186] recorded the mutation's relative frequency in North American Caucasians more precisely by differentiating between Q188R alleles in individuals principally of European descent (63.5 percent) and those in Hispanics of Mexican origin (50–58 percent). In fact, taking Europe as a whole, the overall frequency of Q188R on more than 700 mutant

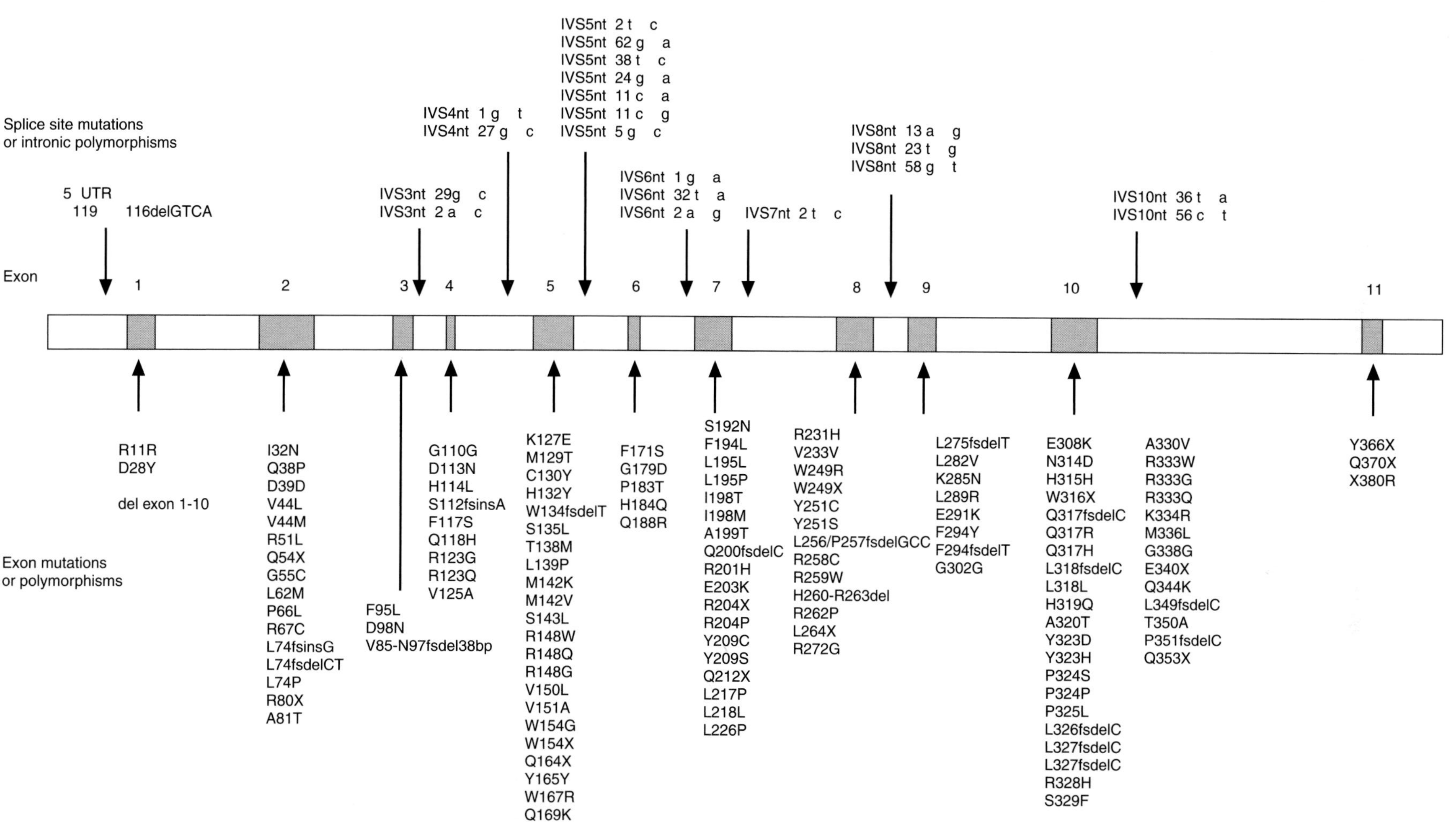

Fig. 72-6 Mutations characterized at the *GALT* gene as of July 1999. Appropriate references for each citation are given in a database at http://www.ich.bris.ac.uk/galtdb.[100] Except for Ito et al.[331] and Reichardt et al.,[332] all publications are referred to elsewhere in this chapter.

chromosomes is indeed 64 percent, but there is considerable variation in the relative frequency in individual European populations (Table 72-5). The highest frequencies are in the Republic of Ireland[187,188] (in both the Traveller and non-Traveller population groups[188]) and Great Britain,[189] and it decreases in continental Europe moving through populations in an eastern direction (Fig. 72-7). In view of the predominant Spanish and Portuguese ancestries of inhabitants of Central and South America, the slightly lower relative frequency of Q188R in North American Hispanics (50–58 percent)[140,186] is in keeping with that seen currently for Q188R (48 percent) in the Iberian peninsula[189] (Boleda, personal communication).

Globally, K285N is much rarer than Q188R. Its overall frequency in Europe is about 8 percent but, as for Q188R, there are large differences in its relative frequency in different populations. In many, it is the second most common disease-causing *GALT* mutation, and in some countries of east and central Europe, it accounts for 25–35 percent of mutant chromosomes[190],[191],[191a] (Table 72-5 and Figure 72-8). This suggests that the center of diffusion for K285N lies farther to the east than that for Q188R. The relative frequency of the mutation in studies from North America has not yet been documented.

Black Africans and Americans of African descent. One mutation, a Ser to Leu substitution at codon 135, designated S135L, is almost exclusive to black Africans and African-Americans. The mutation was originally reported by Reichardt et al.,[192] and additional studies[186,193] have established that S135L accounts for almost 50 percent of mutant GALT-related chromosomes in this major population group in America (Table 72-5). A second mutation, a Phe to Ser substitution at codon 171, designated F171S, also first reported by Reichardt et al.,[192] is much rarer, accounting for only about 4 percent of mutant alleles in African-Americans.[186]

In the only study of negroid people in Africa, Manga et al.[193a] reported that S135L accounted for 91 percent of mutant *GALT* chromosomes in galactosemic patients in South Africa. The frequency of this allele in 600 healthy black South Africans was 1 in 150 (the carrier frequency being 1 in 75). Although the sample number was low in other ethnic groups, the mutation was not found in the Khoisin population of other southern African countries, including Angola, Botswana, and Namibia. Two out of 292 individuals screened from countries in central Africa (including Cameroon and the Central African Republic) and one of 199 individuals from western Africa (including Guinea, Sierra Leone, Ivory Coast, Ghana, and Senegal) carried the S135L mutation.

Q188R, found in three white galactosemics in South Africa, was not detected in the black population.[193a] In African-Americans, on the other hand, this mutation is found at relative frequencies varying from 12 to 21 percent.[140,185,186,193] This is the result of Caucasian admixture and occurs at a frequency approaching that expected.[194]

Approximately 30–35 percent of mutant chromosomes have not been characterized in African-Americans. It is probable that, as with other major human groups and other disorders, these mutations are multiple and varied.

Japan. The common European mutations, Q188R and K285N, are rare in galactosemic individuals whose ancestries are non-European.[140,195] In Japan, for example, where galactosemia affects only one person per million, 14 different mutations have been characterized on 23 mutant chromosomes. Nine of the mutations have been found only once, and 10 appear to be uniquely

Table 72-5 Relative frequency of Q188R, S135L and K285N alleles in different geographic areas and major population groups

	North America Ethnic Group						
	Hispanic		Caucasoid		African American		
	n = 14	n = 48	n = 191	n = 402	n = 26	n = 104	n = 33
Q188R (%)	58	50	64	64	12	21	–
S135L (%)	–	0	–	1.5	–	47	48
Ref	140	186	140	186	140	186	193

	Europe Region										
	Western			Northern and Central					Southern		
Country	Ireland Non-Travellers	Travellers	British Isles	Denmark	Germany	Austria	Czech & Slovak Republics	Poland	Spain	Italy	Turkey
	n = 46	n = 32	n = 276	n = 78	n = 132	n = 60	n = 66	n = 58	n = 44	n = 22	n = 32
Q188R (%)	89	100	77	83	65	60	45	51	47	18	57
K285N (%)	0		3	0	9	28	28	34	9	14	6
Ref	188	188	199	Salaman personal communication	214	190	191	191a	Boleda, personal communication	198	196a, 197

Region Major Population Group	South Africa	
	Negroid	Caucasoid
	n = 53	n = 6
Q188R	0	100
S135L (%)	91	0
Ref	193a	193a

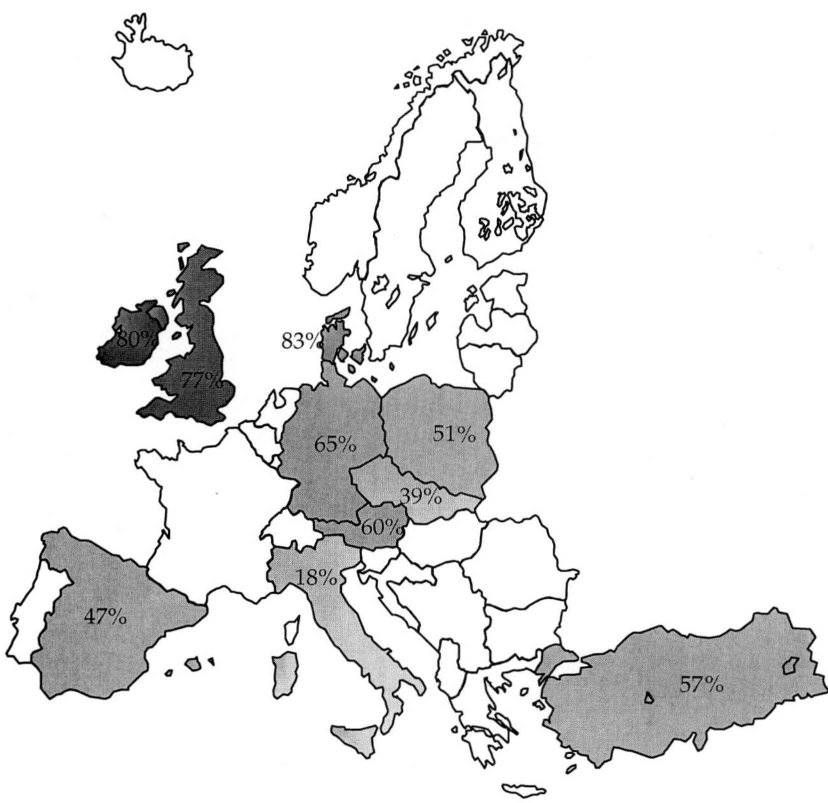

Fig. 72-7 Relative frequencies of the Q188R mutation at the *GALT* gene in different European populations. See Table 72-5 for appropriate references.

Japanese[195,196] (Okano, personal communication). Q188R and K285N have not been reported, but N314D has been reported on two mutant chromosomes.

Turkey. In Turkey, eight different base changes have been characterized on 32 mutant alleles.[196a]. Q188R is by far the most common *GALT* mutation, accounting for 57 percent of mutant chromosomes,[197] a relative frequency considerably higher than that seen in Italy[198] and even higher than that seen in the Czech and Slovak Republics[191] (Table 72-5). Four of the remaining seven mutations have been reported in German patients, and one mutation, a Phe to Tyr substitution at codon 294, designated F294Y, is novel.[100,196a] Whether this mutation is unique to a Turkish population is not known. Nevertheless, it is certain that admixture between Turkish and Germanic populations is responsible for the appearance of rare mutations in both populations.

Other Populations and Major Groups. In the Traveller population of the Republic of Ireland, in which the incidence of transferase-deficient galactosemia is estimated to be 1 in 550, Q188R is the sole mutation present.[188] The relative frequency of the Q188R allele in this group is an order of magnitude higher than that in the non-Traveller population (0.046 compared to 0.005). Evidence does not support population inbreeding as a cause of this high frequency in the Travellers. Rather, founder effect combined with demographic factors similar to those that have acted in the Saguenay population[198a] has been proposed as a possible explanation.

In individuals of Indian and Pakistani ancestry, Q188R is very rare,[140] and in the British Isles, only "private" mutations have been found in affected individuals of Arab or Indian ancestry.[199] The only large deletions of genomic DNA have been reported in individuals of Ashkenazi Jewish origin.[200] (Tyfield, personal communication).

History of the Mutations. Significant differences in the distribution and frequency of mutations in various major population groups enable some speculation about the possible origins of the mutations and the history of the disorder in different populations. The almost exclusive occurrence of S135L in individuals of African origin suggests that this mutation is relatively new and that it arose after the first wave of migration of *Homo sapiens sapiens* out of Africa more than 100,000 years ago. The C $\rightarrow$ T transition resulting in S135L is at a hypermutable site, but the paucity of polymorphic markers at this locus precludes the determination of single or multiple origins of the mutation. In African negroids it is found at varying frequencies, and it appears to be rare or absent in southwestern Africa.[193a] The ancestors of most present-day African-Americans originated from a variety of geographic locales in western Africa.[194] The high relative frequency of S135L in southern African negroid peoples suggests that they could have been a source of slaves in North America or that they have close affinities with the populations from which most of those slaves were taken.[193a] Genetic drift and subsequent range expansion could also have contributed to the high relative frequency of S135L in African-Americans.

The high relative frequencies of Q188R in populations of European descent and its absence in Asians indicates that this mutation arose after the migration out of Africa and after the subsequent divergence between Caucasian and Asian populations. Although a single ancestral origin cannot be proved because of the lack of genetic diversity at the *GALT* gene, its high relative frequency in Ireland and the British Isles suggests that at least one point of origin of Q188R is in northwestern Europe, possibly in Ireland, and that the observed gradient seen in Europe has occurred through migration and admixture.

On the other hand, the occurrence of N314D in Asians and Caucasians but not in individuals of African descent suggests that this mutation arose after the migration out of Africa but before the divergence and radiation east and west.[195]

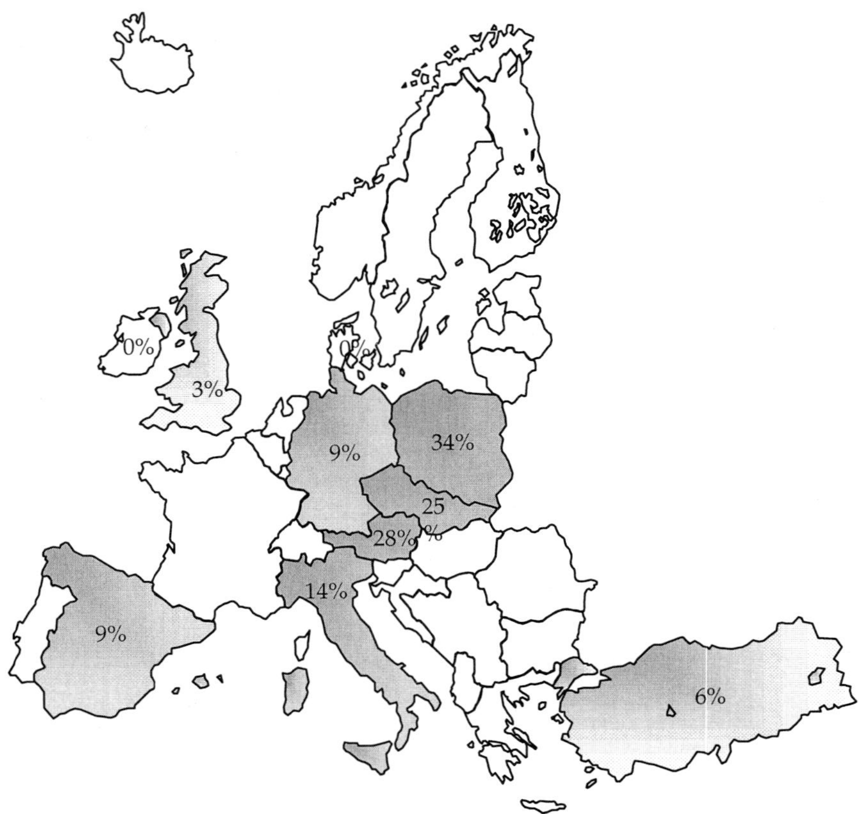

Fig. 72-8 Relative frequencies of the K285N mutation at the *GALT* gene in different European populations. See Table 72-5 for appropriate references.

N314D and the Duarte Alleles. The Duarte variant (D2) has been defined biochemically by reduced enzyme activity and by an isoform distinguishable by gel electrophoresis and isoelectric focusing.[25,201,202] Another GALT enzyme, the Los Angeles variant (D1), exists, with isoforms and immunochemical reactions identical to those of Duarte 2 except that it is associated with increased activity compared with controls.[203] It is now known that both variants carry the A → G transition at c.940 of the *GALT* gene, which results in a substitution of aspartic acid for asparagine at amino acid 314 of the GALT protein (N314D).[96,204,205]

N314D is in linkage disequilibrium with other base changes, some of which are different on the (D1) and (D2) alleles. Gathof et al.[206] first reported the coexistence of N314D with the "silent" mutation, L218L, in exon 7, but Greber et al.[207] and Podskarbi et al.[208] independently reported that N314D/L218L coexisted on Duarte 1 alleles and that two base changes in introns 4 and 5 (IVS4nt − 27G → C and IVS5nt − 24G → A)† were in linkage disequilibrium with N314D on Duarte 2 alleles. It is clear that the intron 5 *SacI* polymorphism reported to be in linkage disequilibrium with N314D[209] is the G → A transition at IVS5nt − 24. An additional intron change, IVS5nt + 62G → A,[191,210] and a 4-bp deletion in the 5′ untranslated region 116–119 bases upstream from the first methionine codon have also been reported on Duarte 2 alleles.[191] Finally, both D1 and D2 alleles are reported to have an extended sequence of 28 adenine nucleotides in intron 10 instead of 17 adenine nucleotides in the corresponding sequence of the normal allele.[210a]

The intron polymorphisms have been found in linkage disequilibrium with Duarte 2 alleles in European populations in countries including Germany,[208] Austria,[190] the Czech and Slovak Republics,[191] England,[199] and Scotland.[199] In view of the European ancestries of many North Americans, it is curious that in some studies no other sequence variation has been reported when the entire D2 *GALT* gene is sequenced.[211] Whether the N314D mutation has arisen on several genetic backgrounds and whether the ancestral origin of the Duarte 2 allele in specific geographic areas of North America is different from that seen in northern European populations remain to be determined. A hypermutable site is not involved.

On rare occasions, N314D has been found to occur in *cis* on galactosemia chromosomes that carry another mutation.[204] In studies from Germany, all galactosemia chromosomes carrying a Glu to stop mutation at codon 340, designated E340X, are found in *cis* with N314D/L218L,[206,208,210a] and a Trp to stop mutation at codon 316, designated W316X, is reported exclusively on chromosomes carrying N314D/IVS4nt − 27G → C/IVS5nt − 24G → A.[208,210a] An Arg to stop mutation at codon 204, designated R204X, in England[212] and a Val to Ala substitution at codon 151, designated V151A, in the Czech and Slovak Republics[191] have also been reported only in association with N314D and the polymorphisms in introns 4 and 5. Each mutation has been found on a relatively small number of chromosomes, very often in a single population. It is possible that each one arose only once on the more common genetic backgrounds that define Duarte 1 or Duarte 2 alleles and that their appearance on these limited numbers of chromosomes represents an identity by descent. Interestingly, R204X has been found on a single chromosome in the Czech Republic, and unlike those in the English population, this mutation is not on a Duarte 2 haplotype background (Kozak, personal communication). The fact that it occurs at a CpG hypermutable site would suggest that the mutation has arisen independently on two haplotype backgrounds.

A Glu to Lys substitution at codon 203, designated E203K, is another rare mutation that has been found to occur in *cis* with N314D, once in a galactosemic male in America[213] and once in a young woman in England (Tyfield, unpublished results). The latter was originally investigated because of Müllerian aplasia and was

†The base changes are originally reported as g1105c and g1391a, where the nt numbers are taken from the genomic sequence published by Leslie et al.[96] The nomenclature used here is taken from the cDNA sequence as recommended by Antonarakis.[101]

found to have erythrocyte GALT enzyme activity in the heterozygous range. In her, N314D is associated with the intron polymorphisms. The appearance of these rare alleles in two apparently unrelated families may represent an identity by descent.

E203K has also been reported on an allele that does not carry N314D[213] in an affected individual who carried N314D on the opposite allele. As with R204X, the appearance of this rare mutation on two different genetic backgrounds is unusual, but unlike that for R204X, the G → A transition yielding E203K does not involve a hypermutable site. Further investigation of additional base changes associated with both alleles could help to determine whether the mutation is likely to have arisen as two separate events on different genetic backgrounds or whether gene conversion or recombination transferred the mutation from an allele carrying N314D to another that did not, or vice versa.

It has been known for some time, particularly through neonatal screening programs that include galactosemia, that the Duarte allele is not uncommon in Caucasians. The prevalence of N314D in the nongalactosemic population is about 5–6 percent in North America.[204,205] In Germany, Podskarbi et al.[214] differentiated between D1 and D2 alleles and reported a relative frequency of 5.4 percent for N314D/L218L and 9.5 percent for N314D/IVS4/IVS5 alleles. In the Czech and Slovak Republics, the relative frequencies are slightly lower, with the D1 mutations occurring on 2.8 percent of 1008 control chromosomes and D2 mutations occurring on 5.4 percent.[191] In Japan, the prevalence of the Duarte allele is 2 percent.[215]

Phenotypic effects of various mutations. Dietary restriction of galactose results in rapid clinical improvement in the neonate. However, the neurologic and intellectual prognosis of galactosemic patients is often poor, and ovarian failure is frequently observed. Although only two or three mutations may account for 70–80 percent of mutant chromosomes in some populations, the identification of more than 120 mutations at the *GALT* gene suggests that some phenotypic variability is related, at least in part, to allelic heterogeneity.

The most common mutation, Q188R, is generally associated with a more severe biochemical phenotype. Erythrocyte GALT activity in individuals homoallelic for Q188R are undetectable,[140,210,216] a finding that is compatible with the results of *in vitro* expression analysis. Some attempts have been made to determine the effects of these mutations on long-term clinical complications. One study had suggested that homozygosity for Q188R alone was a significant determinant of poor clinical outcome,[183] whereas another showed that there was no statistically significant difference in long-term outcome among galactosemic individuals who were Q188R-homoallelic, Q188R-heteroallelic or Q188R-negative.[217]

Although homozygosity for Q188R is the most common mutant genotype in most European populations or those predominantly of European descent, it is now clear that many other mutations are also associated with long-term clinical complications. Twenty-two percent of base changes at the *GALT* gene are nonsense mutations, splice site mutations, and frameshift deletions or insertions (Table 72-4).[100] Although they are individually rare, when one of these occurs in a homoallelic or heteroallelic state with Q188R, a more severe clinical phenotype would be anticipated and indeed has been reported.[206,218] Another missense mutation, K285N, which is relatively common in some European populations, is invariably associated with a total loss of erythrocyte GALT activity[216,218] and a more severe phenotype.[199,218] The phenotype associated with a Lys to Pro mutation at codon 195, designated L195P, may be variable. Although the results of expression analysis have demonstrated an almost complete loss of enzyme activity,[219] patients homozygotic for L195P have been reported to show a milder clinical course,[210a] whereas those heteroallelic for Q188R and L195P have shown a more severe phenotype.[199] In some populations these mutations account for 5–30 percent of mutant alleles.[190,191,198,199,214] Thus, assuming Hardy-Weinberg equilibrium, homozygosity for these mutations and heterozygosity with Q188R would be expected to account for 30–40 percent of affected individuals.

Other mutations have been reported to be associated with a milder biochemical phenotype.[216,218,220,210a,220a] For example, some erythrocyte GALT activity, varying between 1.5 and 2 percent of normal, is detectable in individuals homoallelic for S329F or IVS8nt + 13 A → G and in those heteroallelic for T138M, T350A, R259W, or A330V, and a "null" mutation.[220a] Their plasma Gal-1-P concentrations are reported to decrease much faster than those of other galactosemic patients with two "null" alleles, and late-onset complications have not been observed even among adult patients carrying these mutations.[220a] Other mutations are associated with erythrocyte GALT activity between 15 and 25 percent of normal when they occur in combination with a "null" allele; these include IVS3nt + 29G → C (Schonstadt), IVS8nt + 58G → T (Munich 2), R333G (Marburg),[220a] and R333Q.[210a] After the neonatal period, individuals carrying the first three mutations required no treatment for normal development.[220a] *In vitro* expression analysis of R333Q has revealed residual activity similar to that of the Duarte 2 allele.[196]

S135L in black Africans and African-Americans. For some mutations, correlations between *in vitro* expression results and biochemical and clinical phenotypes are more enigmatic. For example, it has been known for some time that galactosemia in African-Americans (the originally "Negro" variant[221]) is often a milder disorder than in Caucasians. It is now known that S135L accounts for almost 50 percent of mutant alleles in this 'major population' group. *In vitro* expression analysis in mammalian COS cells showed S135L to have near-normal enzyme activity,[178] whereas when it was expressed in a yeast-model system, enzyme activity was reduced to ~5% of the wild-type levels.[222] The reduction in enzyme activity in the yeast expression system appears to be brought about by a reduction by a factor of two in abundance of the mutant compared to the wild-type protein as well as a reduction by a factor of 10 in specific activity.[223a] Taken together, these account for the reduction to one twentieth of normal activity that has been observed in the yeast expression system. It is still unclear, however, why individuals carrying S135L appear to exhibit some tissue specificity in GALT activity[223a] and why some patients homozygous for this mutation are able to oxidize a substantial amount of galactose to CO_2 *in vivo*.[193]

The Duarte Alleles. One amino acid change, N314D, is found on both Duarte alleles, D1 (or LA), associated with an increase in enzyme activity, and D2, associated with reduced activity. *In vitro* studies[178,224] have shown that N314D alone does not impair GALT activity. Thus, the widely differing levels of enzyme activity may be influenced, at least in some measure, by additional base changes that differ on D1 and D2 alleles.

Podskarbi et al., who first reported the additional base changes in association with N314D on D1 and D2 alleles, proposed that the intron base changes on D2 may be involved in regulation of *GALT* gene expression.[208] However, results of subsequent studies by Lai et al.[211] suggest that the intron base changes are polymorphisms that do not significantly affect rates of transcription. Consistent with the earlier work of Anderson et al.,[224a] Lai et al. reported reduced abundance of the GALT dimer in lymphoblastoid cell lines from individuals homozygous for D2.[211] A concomitant reduction in *GALT* mRNA was not observed, but the GALT enzyme demonstrated thermal instability and a reduced biologic half-life. It would appear, then, that the reduced enzyme activity associated with the N314D mutation in the Duarte 2 allele is brought about through biologic instability of the active enzyme. Although the significance of the 4-base pair (GTCA) deletion in the 5′ promoter region of the Duarte 2 allele has yet to be established, Kozak et al[191] have reported that a computer search[224b] showed that two binding factors (activator proteins AP1 Q2 and AP1 Q4) would lose their binding motifs in the Duarte 2 alleles.

In the D1 (LA) allele, on the other hand, there are two nucleotide substitutions in coding regions, both of which are transcribed into mRNA. Since the exon 7 base change is a "silent" mutation (L218L), the enzyme protein will carry only one amino acid change, N314D, the same as that found in D2. Despite this, lymphoblastoid cell lines from individuals who are heteroallelic for the D1 variant appear to have an *increased* abundance in GALT protein. Once again, this is consistent with the earlier work of Anderson et al.[224a] No increase in transcription or in thermal stability of the enzyme in D1 compared to that in D2 was observed.[97] A molecular mechanism involving an increased rate of translation through "codon bias"[225] in the altered mRNA has been postulated.[97] The altered codon is CTA → TTA, the latter being rarer than CTA leucine codon in human *GALT* mRNA. The hypothesis that increased availability of TTA tRNA in the human cell produces more efficient translation of the altered mRNA remains to be tested. In this regard, it is interesting that another base change in exon 7, a C → T transition at nt c.583 that results in the "silent" mutation L195L (Munich 1), is also associated with an increase in GALT activity compared to that in controls.[210a]

Compound effects of mutations on D1 and D2 alleles. The compound effects of additional mutations occurring in *cis* with N314D are variable and are probably influenced by the type and position of the second mutation. Individually, these alleles are rare; nevertheless, biochemical and clinical phenotypes that have been reported in affected individuals carrying multiple mutations are worthy of mention. For most of the mutations, biochemical effects in association with D1 or D2 alleles have not been investigated *in vitro*.

Three nonsense mutations have been reported on either D1 or D2 alleles. R204X, found in association with D2, is upstream from the N314D mutation and is a nonsense mutation that would result in synthesis of a truncated protein. The phenotype of individuals carrying this mutation would be expected to be consistent with one of hemizygosity for the mutation on the other allele. In fact, all four children with these mutations in the British Isles are heteroallelic for R204X and either Q188R or L195P. They have negligible erythrocyte enzyme activity and one infant (R204X/L195P) died in the neonatal period with severe sepsis[199] (J. Holton, personal communication). E340X, on the other hand, is downstream of N314D and occurs on D1 alleles that also carry the L218L mutation. One Turkish patient is homoallelic for E340X on D1 alleles, and although erythrocyte GALT activity is negligible, there was no evidence of developmental or neurologic impairment at the age of 8 years.[206] The third nonsense mutation is W316X, which is two amino acids downstream from N314D on D2 alleles. Some residual enzyme activity (1.5 percent of normal) was detected in the erythrocytes of the affected individual in whom this mutation was first reported.[216] The patient has a rare missense mutation, Arg to Cys at codon 67, designated R67C, on the other allele, so the impact of the individual mutations on the phenotype are difficult to ascertain.

When N314D occurs in *cis* with a missense mutation, some anomalies in the compound effect in different individuals may be observed. E203K, for example, has been reported on chromosomes both with and without N314D in *cis*.[213] It is clear that the mutation on its own effects a reduction in enzyme activity, but when it occurs in *cis* with N314D, the overall effects on biochemical phenotype are more abstruse and may be influenced by the genotype of the other allele. It has been proposed that E203K acts as a "revertant" to N314D in *cis*, restoring thermal stability and enzyme activity to normal.[211] Nevertheless, an affected individual heterozygous for the E203K/N314D allele and a splice site mutation (IVS3nt − 2A → C) is reported to have virtually undetectable erythrocyte GALT activity.[213]

N314D, vaginal agenesis and endometriosis. In view of the fact that gonadal dysfunction is an almost universal finding in females with galactosemia, it is interesting that defects in galactose metabolism specifically involving N314D and the D2 allele have also been implicated in causes of infertility brought about by canalization defects.[174,175]

In two parallel studies, Cramer et al. reported, first, a significantly higher frequency of heterozygosity for N314D in daughters with vaginal agenesis and in their mothers than in controls[174] and, second, that women with endometriosis were more likely to carry at least one N314D allele than controls.[175] In these studies, although the *GALT* gene was screened for only two mutations, N314D and Q188R, erythrocyte activity and electrophoretic patterns indicated that individuals carried no other mutation at the *GALT* gene locus either in *cis* or in *trans* with N314D.

By reference to rodent experiments in which high-galactose feeding of pregnant animals caused delayed vaginal opening and oocyte depletion in female offspring,[164] it had been proposed that equivalent canalization defects in humans could also be related to high intra-uterine exposure to galactose. Although it is an interesting hypothesis, it is clear that this alone would not account for the specific association with N314D and not with other, more severe *GALT* mutations that effect a greater loss in enzyme activity. Further, a recent study in the UK on the frequency of N314D in women with sporadic familial endometriosis found no statistically significant difference compared with controls.[225a]

The enzyme defect

It was mentioned earlier that Isselbacher et al.[16] confirmed that the deficient enzyme in classic galactosemia was GALT. It would now appear to be established that, within the limits of the accuracy and precision of the methods for assaying GALT, the levels of enzyme in the red cells of classical galactosemia patients are zero, and these patients have the most severe and comprehensive manifestation of the defect. The complete enzyme deficiency has also been demonstrated in white blood cells,[226] skin fibroblasts,[227] intestinal mucosa,[68] and liver.[185]

Most of the variants of GALT deficiency have subnormal, though more than zero, enzyme activity in some or all of their cells or tissues, and in rare cases above-normal enzyme levels are found. The low-activity variants are most often detected as the result of newborn screening programs that are dependent on GALT measurement or when patients who present with neonatal signs of galactosemia are shown subsequently to have GALT levels above zero or to have unexpectedly high tolerance of galactose.

The defect in the variants may predominantly affect the active site of the enzyme and may affect equally all cells and tissues in which the enzyme is found. This is the case for the Duarte variant, for example.[201] Otherwise the main effect may be on the stability of the enzyme molecule, and cells with a long life span, erythrocytes, for example, will have lower enzyme levels than those with a higher rate of turnover, such as liver cells. In the variant originally called "Negro,"[228] the GALT activity is zero in erythrocytes but liver and intestine have 10 percent of normal enzyme activity. The Indiana variant[229] also shows evidence of an unstable GALT molecule, showing 35 percent of normal activity in red blood cells when assayed immediately after the blood is obtained but zero enzyme levels if the blood is kept in the phosphate incubation buffer for a short time. Table 72-6 summarizes the characteristics of some of the known GALT variants. Since the variant genes are allelic with the normal GALT gene, subjects may be found who are homozygous for the variant and others who have inherited it in combination with a normal or classical galactosemia gene.

It is probable that the incidence of variant genes is much greater than the published data on the named types would suggest. Hammersen et al.[230] have described white patients with characteristics similar to those of patients with the Rennes variant, and other white patients with approximately 10 percent of normal

Table 72-6 Galactose-1-phosphate uridyltransferase variants

Variant forms (Ref)	RBC, Activity (% of Normal)	Mobility on Starch Gel	Neonatal signs
Homozygous forms			
Classical[16]	0	No bands	Yes
Duarte[201]	50	Faster than normal	No
Negro[228]	0[a]	No bands	Yes
Munster[328]	30[b]	No bands	Yes
Los Angeles[203]	140	Faster than normal	No
Heterozygous forms			
Duarte/Classical[201]	25	Faster than normal	Yes[232] No[233]
Rennes/Classical[329]	7	Slower than normal	Yes
Chicago/Classical[330]	27	Faster than normal	?
Indiana[229]	0–35	Slower than normal	Yes

[a]10 percent activity in liver and intestine.
[b]Enzyme inactivated by product of GALT reaction (Glc-1-P).

Table 72-7 Galactose and galactitol excretion in untreated classic galactosemia (muscle/mol creatinine)

	Galactitol	Galactose	Galactitol: Glucose ratioα
Controls (Age >1 year)	31	140	
Range	3–81	10–380	
N	20	20	
Case 1	8000	3000	2.7
2	30,000	16,000	1.9
3	30,000	7000	4.3
4	47,000	227,000	0.21
5	52,000	43,000	1.2
6	69,000	96,000	0.72

SOURCE: From Jacobs et al.[31]

GALT activity in erythrocytes are known (J.T. Allen, personal communication). Xu et al.,[231] using a method which it is claimed can measure minute amounts of GALT activity (on the order of 0.1 percent of control levels) with the necessary accuracy and precision, have studied 423 patients with galactosemia. Of these, 363 had zero erythrocyte GALT levels and 10 of these also had zero activity in leukocytes. The remaining 60 had erythrocyte GALT levels between 0.02 and 5 percent of normal and were designated galactosemia-variant (G/V) patients. Two of the G/V patients had comparable GALT levels in leukocytes, and it has been suggested that even this low enzyme activity may confer an advantage in escaping some of the complications associated with the deficiency.[232] In earlier studies, it was found that patients with some GALT activity showed no signs of ovarian failure[233] and that no G/V patient had a homozygous Q188R genotype.[140]

Metabolic abnormality

Complete deficiency of GALT has a profound effect on many metabolic pathways, particularly when normal galactose intake continues. Galactose itself accumulates in the tissues and blood and is excreted in excess. Gal-1-P also accumulates in blood cells and tissues but is not excreted in the urine. Increased amounts of the products of the alternative galactose metabolic pathways, galactitol and galactonic acid, are excreted in the urine, and galactitol accumulates in many parts of the body. In addition, there is significant lowering of red blood cell UDP-Gal levels and a disturbance of the UDP-Gal/UDP-Gal equilibrium catalyzed by epimerase. There is also some effect on glucose metabolism.

Galactose. Normal newborn infants given a standard milk feed show very much greater increases in venous blood glucose than in blood galactose, in absolute terms.[234] This demonstrates the rapid conversion of galactose to glucose in normal circumstances. In comparison, galactosemic infants have very large increases in blood galactose following a lactose or galactose load,[41,235] and a fall in blood glucose to hypoglycemic levels may occur.[41]

Recent results using gas-liquid chromatographic analytical techniques[236] have shown urinary concentrations of galactose rising to 227 mol/mol creatinine in untreated galactosemic patients,[31] (Table 72-7). The galactose excretion rate has been compared to that of galactitol excretion in six patients, and the results have demonstrated their limited capacity to remove galactose from the body as galactitol. The effectiveness of the galactitol pathway in this respect is seen to be much more significant in patients with a lesser overall load of galactose to remove.

Gal-1-P. Gal-1-P, excessive levels of which in red blood cells were the key to the identifying the position of the metabolic block in classic galactosemia,[15] is also increased in the disease in liver, kidney, brain, tongue, adrenal gland, heart,[237] ocular lens,[238] and cultured skin fibroblasts.[239] Two galactosemic fetuses at 20 weeks' gestation had levels of Gal-1-P in the liver comparable to those of infants who died of the disorder in the neonatal period.[239,240] Galactose and galactitol levels were similarly raised.

Blood Gal-1-P is the most commonly measured metabolite in galactosemic patients. Numerous technical methods are used, and many different units are employed to express the results. Gitzelmann[241] found concentrations of 2.5–6.5 mM in packed red cells in untreated patients from birth to 9 days of age. Although the levels of Gal-1-P fell dramatically on the galactose-restricted diet, values remained significantly raised (0.1–0.2 mM) compared to those in normal infants on a normal diet, which are immeasurable by most assay methods. If the levels of the metabolite do fall to zero on starting the diet, it is probably an indication that the patient has a GALT variant with some enzyme activity.

Galactitol. Similarly to the case for Gal-1-P, numerous tissues from a galactosemic infant have been shown to accumulate galactitol.[242] A further study has confirmed that brain concentrations are particularly high.[243] Wells et al.[244] were the first to demonstrate the significant urinary excretion of galactitol in galactosemia, and raised levels in amniotic fluid at 10 (J. T. Allen, personal communication) and 20[245] weeks' gestation indicate that the affected fetus accumulates galactitol early in pregnancy. The study of Jakobs et al. referred to earlier ("Reduction of galactose to galactitol"),[31] indicated that while galactitol excretion decreased in galactosemic patients on a galactose-restricted diet, the level was still 20–30 times higher than in control subjects, although excretion of the metabolite tends to decrease with age. This pattern is similar to that of red blood cell Gal-1-P, although no correlation between blood Gal-1-P and galactitol excretion has been found. Berry et al. set out to determine whether galactose in fruit and vegetables could be the cause of continuing increased galactitol excretion in galactosemic patients on a standard galactose restricted diet.[5] They concluded that the galactose content of these foods was not sufficient to explain the problem. Endogenous production of galactose was postulated, and the production rate required to explain the known galactitol excretion rate was calculated. The resulting figure agreed very closely with that determined by more direct means.[11]

Sugar nucleotides. Shin et al.[246] were the first to claim that there is a decreased level of UDP-Gal in the red blood cells of galactosemic patients, and it was postulated that this could have an adverse effect on the synthesis of galactosides. This concept was developed by Ng et al.,[247] who concluded that UDP-Gal levels were reduced specifically in patients with zero GALT activity as determined by the method mentioned earlier ("The enzyme defect")[231] and that were correlated with some long-term complications of the disorder. A deficit of UDP-Gal was also found in liver and skin fibroblasts.[247] This early work was carried out using enzyme assay methods for UDP-Gal and UDP-Glc. Subsequent investigations by two groups using high-performance liquid chromatography (HPLC) methods[248,249] and by a researcher using an enzyme technique,[250] confirmed that there was a reduction in red blood cell UDP-Gal relative to UDP-Glc, but their absolute levels of both metabolites were approximately 300 percent lower than those reported in the initial studies. The accuracy of one of the HPLC methods[248] and the more recent enzyme technique[250] was validated by comparison to a ^{31}P-NMR assay. There was good correlation among all three methods[251] The validity of this work, particularly of the enzyme methods, needs to be confirmed.

The pathologic significance of reduced UDP-Gal levels has been questioned, partly because of the inaccuracy of the early work but also because subsequent research, although confirming a statistically significant reduction in UDP-Gal levels, found a large overlap between normal and galactosemic results. In addition, no abnormality in UDP-Gal levels has been found in fibroblast cultures[252,253] and leukocytes[252] from galactosemic patients. However, more recent work from Ng et al. using an HPLC method has apparently shown that classic galactosemic patients, defined as having zero GALT activity detected by the sensitive enzyme technique cited earlier ("Sugar nucleotides"),[231] have a clear-cut reduction in red blood cell UDP-Gal concentrations and that and galactosemia variant (G/V) patients have completely normal levels.[254]

Attempts have been made to define factors that determine the levels of sugar nucleotides in the red cells of normals, galactosemics, and other patients with metabolic disorders who have a low galactose intake.[255] A high proportion of the patients had a high UDP-Glc:UDP-Gal ratio, which was attributed to a perturbation of GALE. The proportion of galactosemic patients with UDP-Gal levels within the normal range appeared to be higher than would be expected if this occurred only in GV patients. Further work on nongalactosemic metabolic disorder patients[256] has shown that a high red cell UDP-Glc:UDP-Gal ratio on a limited-galactose diet is readily corrected by galactose supplements. It appears that in the absence of dietary galactose, GALE cannot maintain the accepted equilibrium of nucleotide sugars, which is achieved only when galactose is being metabolized through the Leloir pathway.

Diagnosis

The diagnosis of GALT deficiency may be made following the results of newborn screening or from the investigation of clinical illness.

Classic galactosemia should be suspected in all infants with liver disease, jaundice, recurrent vomiting, and failure to thrive. The early clinical presentation of galactosemia is by no means specific, and a high index of suspicion is necessary, particularly in countries where galactosemia is not included in the newborn screening program. The presence of reducing substances or galactose in urine is neither sensitive nor specific and should not be used to either confirm or refute a diagnosis. Small quantities of galactose are commonly found in the urine of any patient with liver disease, and galactose may disappear rapidly from the urine of patients with galactosemia who are on intravenous fluids.

A fluorescent spot test (Beutler test) for GALT activity is now widely used for the diagnosis of galactosemia.[257] In this assay, whole blood is added to a reaction mixture containing UDP-Glc, Gal-1-P, and nicotinamide adenine dinucleotide phosphate (NADP). After a period of incubation, the reaction mixture is spotted onto filter paper. If GALT activity is normal, NADPH is produced, as demonstrated by fluorescence under ultraviolet light (wavelength approximately 360 nm). Fluorescence after incubation for 1 h is normal. No fluorescence after 2 h of incubation indicates GALT (or glucose-6-phosphate dehydrogenase) deficiency. False positive results may occur if blood is collected into EDTA tubes or stored at warm temperatures. Due to GALT activity in transfused red cells, this test is not reliable if a blood transfusion has been given up to 120 days previously.

An abnormal Beutler test must be followed by further biochemical or molecular confirmation of the diagnosis. The most commonly used quantitative measurement of GALT activity is based on the consumption of UDP-Glc by transferase with measurement of residual UDP-Glc by a UDP-Glc dehydrogenase/ NAD^+ assay by absorbance at 340 nm. Other assays are also available.[258] Although these quantitative enzyme assays are more reliable, they can, like the Beutler assay, give false negative results following blood transfusion. In such situations the diagnosis can usually be confirmed by DNA analysis for the common Q188R mutation. However, since the diagnosis cannot be excluded by mutation analysis, for patients who are not found to be homozygous for the Q188R mutation, it is necessary to measure plasma Gal-1-P. In this assay, the level of galactose, released from Gal-1-P by alkaline phosphatase, is determined by the fluorimetric measurement of NADH following incubation with galactose dehydrogenase and NAD^+. Gal-1-P levels are invariably high at diagnosis and fall only slowly, over a period of weeks to months.

Newborn screening

Screening is provided as part of newborn care in many parts of the world. Most laboratories use a microbiologic or fluorometric assay that detects an increase in blood galactose and/or fluorescent spot testing using the Beutler enzyme method. The advantage of the Beutler test is that it is independent of ingestion of galactose-containing milk. False negative results are very infrequent for homozygotes, but Duarte or Duarte/galactosemia compound heterozygotes may not be detected. As stated above, false negatives may occur up to 3 months following blood transfusions if the Beutler method is used. False positive results are also common with the Beutler test if samples are stored at high temperatures.[259]

Newborn screening is available in the great majority of states within the USA and in a number of countries within Europe. In the UK only about 9 percent of newborn infants are screened for galactosemia, and the case for its inclusion is not generally accepted.[260] In assessing the value of screening a number of questions must be addressed: Does screening result in earlier diagnosis, reduce early morbidity and mortality, or prevent or reduce late complications? Unfortunately, there are no prospective studies that have answered all these questions satisfactorily.

In the retrospective survey by Waggoner et al.,[142] 80 percent of patients who had newborn screening were diagnosed by 14 days of age, compared with only 35 percent in those who were not screened. Of the screened group, 20 percent were said to be without symptoms at the time of diagnosis. The British Paediatric Surveillance Unit ascertained new cases of classical galactosemia in the UK and the Republic of Ireland prospectively over a 3-year period.[261] Sixty affected children were identified, giving an incidence of 1 in 44,000 in the UK as a whole and 1 in 23,500 in the Republic of Ireland. Because there is screening for galactosemia in Scotland and the Republic of Ireland but not in England and Wales, it was possible to compare infants with galactosemia born where such screening was available to those born where the diagnosis could be made only after the onset of clinical illness. Of 14 affected children who underwent neonatal screening, one was diagnosed after 3 weeks, compared with four out of 45 of those not screened. Of these four children, one was diagnosed at 90 days and another at 120 days. In this study, one infant died in the non-screened group, compared with none in those screened. However, this death occurred at 4 days and would not have been prevented by screening. Furthermore, morbidity was no more frequent in the latter group. The authors concluded that, provided clinical vigilance were maintained, galactosemia could be diagnosed in an acceptable time without screening.

Not surprisingly, in view of the rarity of the disorder, there is evidence that clinical vigilance does fail on occasions. For example, two infants diagnosed on newborn screening in Canada were in the hospital with an undiagnosed acute illness at the time.[262] It seems very probable that there are infants with GALT deficiency in unscreened populations who have died from gram-negative sepsis or other complications without their underlying diagnosis having been recognized. The result of newborn screening in Ireland from 1972 to 1992 has been reviewed.[263] Over this 20-year period, 1.2 million infants were screened, with 55 cases of classical galactosemia (incidence of 1:23,000) found and seven Duarte variants diagnosed. Of the patients, 39 were detected by routine newborn screening, with a mean age of diagnosis of 8 days, and 15 on high-risk screening (previous sibling affected). Seven patients (11 percent) had false negative results, and five of them had classical galactosemia. Three of these five infants were feeding poorly at the time of screening, whereas the other two were on lactose-free milk. Seven older siblings of the index patients had died unexpectedly in infancy. Six of these had been born before newborn screening was introduced. The authors thought their deaths to be probably due to galactosemia and consequently concluded that newborn screening had prevented deaths. The importance of newborn screening in preventing early morbidity and mortality is a view that is also supported by Schweitzer.[264]

As stated above, there is evidence that the long-term complications associated with galactosemia are not prevented or reduced by early diagnosis or by a galactose-restricted diet. The confirmation by Berry et al[11] that there is significant endogenous production of galactose regardless of diet provides an attractive hypothesis as a cause of this continuing morbidity. Waggoner et al.[142] found no relationship between IQ at 6–9 years and age when treatment was begun. Those infants who were diagnosed before the onset of clinical illness had an incidence of developmental delay, speech delay, and ovarian dysfunction similar to that in probands diagnosed and started on treatment within the first 2 days of life when compared to their older siblings. Although this study is retrospective, it provides no evidence to support newborn screening as a means of preventing long-term complications.

In conclusion, reliable methods for newborn screening are available for galactosemia. Available evidence suggests that although screening may result in earlier diagnosis and limit early morbidity and mortality, it probably has no effect on long-term complications.

Treatment

Initial management. Infants who are suspected on a clinical basis to have galactosemia and those detected on newborn screening who are symptomatic should have galactose excluded from their diets immediately; it is inappropriate to wait for the results of diagnostic investigations. Breast feeding and cow's milk formulas must therefore be stopped. Many children will be seriously ill at the time of diagnosis and require considerable supportive care. Vitamin K and fresh-frozen plasma may be necessary to correct clotting abnormalities. In order to prevent false negative results on enzyme analysis, samples should be taken before any blood transfusion is given. Gram-negative sepsis should be assumed and an appropriate intravenous antibiotic given. Unconjugated hyperbilirubinemia is usually not severe enough to warrant phototherapy or exchange transfusion, but infants may be at increased risk of kernicterus if albumin levels are particularly low secondary to liver disease. If the infant is too sick to tolerate enteral feeding for more than 1 or 2 days, then parenteral feeding should be considered but prescribed cautiously if there is significant liver disease or thrombocytopenia. Most children at diagnosis will, however, be able to tolerate enteral feedings, although these may initially have to be given by nasogastric tube due to poor sucking. Infant soy formulas are most appropriate unless there is significant liver disease, in which case a medium-chain triglyceride containing casein hydrolysate, such as Pregestimil, should be used until this has resolved. However, casein hydrolysates contain small amounts of galactose (in the range of 60–90 mg/100 ml) and, in the absence of significant liver disease, are not the first choice as an infant formula. After dietary galactose has been excluded, most infants show rapid clinical improvement. Features such as hepatomegaly, abnormal liver function, and renal tubular disease usually resolve fully within 1–2 weeks. Cataracts, if present, may take longer to disappear but in the majority of infants do so completely.

Newborn infants known to be at risk for galactosemia, such as siblings of known patients, should not be given breast milk or cow's milk formulas until galactosemia has been excluded. This can be done most easily by collecting cord blood for either analysis of GALT activity or, if the genotype within the family has been characterized, mutation analysis. The results of these assays should be available within as short a time as possible in order to allow those mothers who wish to breast-feed to do so without undue delay.

Partial GALT deficiency. Infants at no known risk who appear well but who have a positive result on newborn screening should be carefully assessed for any symptoms and signs of galactosemia. In such cases, provided that the screening procedure has been carried out correctly, it is most likely that such infants are Duarte/galactosemia compound heterozygotes with partial GALT deficiency, although Duarte homozygotes and galactosemia heterozygotes may also have positive results on screening.[265] The treatment of infants with partial enzyme deficiencies has been reviewed by Gitzelmann and Bosshard.[265] They recommend dietary treatment for all infants with GALT levels of 9 μmol/h per g Hb or lower and Gal-1-P levels greater than 10 mg/dl. If at 4 months of age, after a 1-week trial of 2–3 dl of cows' milk, there is no aminoaciduria and Gal-1-P has fallen to less than 2 mg/dl, the infant is put on a normal diet. As Gitzelmann and Bosshard point out, because partial GALT deficiencies may be up to 10 times more common than classic galactosemia, this approach to treatment generates considerable work and expense, and the necessity of such intervention remains unknown. Partial GALT deficiencies with significant remaining enzyme activity are only rarely detected in the investigation of sick infants and children in centers where there is no newborn screening program, suggesting that they do not contribute to significant morbidity, at least in childhood. (See "Phenotypic effects of various mutations," above, for discussion on the phenotypic effects of particular mutations).

Subsequent treatment. Dietary restriction of galactose remains the only effective long-term treatment for galactosemia, despite its limited efficacy in preventing long-term complications. Patients should continue to exclude milk or milk products from their diets indefinitely, since significant ingestion of galactose at any age is likely to lead to toxic effects. However, many adults with galactosemia probably comply poorly, if at all, with such a diet and do not show evidence of liver or renal disease. Milk is often a minor component of the diet after childhood, and this probably explains the lack of manifestations of the disorder in some of these older patients, although it remains a possibility that, in galactosemia, galactose is more toxic in infants and children than in adults.

It is clear from the analysis of many different foods that a diet free of dairy products will still contain some galactose. These findings led to the statement by Acosta and Gross, "It is certain that no patients with GALT deficiency have ever ingested a galactose-free diet."[4] Small amounts of free soluble galactose are present in most fresh fruit and vegetables and in larger quantities in some legumes, such as peas and dried beans.[4] Bound galactose, with glycosidic linkages, is an important component of a number of plant compounds, such as the raffinose oligosaccharides, arabinogalactan type I and type II, and galactan. In addition, galactocerebrosides and gangliosides are found in offal. The extent to which bound galactose can be broken down in the gut is not known, but most studies suggest the effect of reducing intake is likely to be minimal.[266–268]

A number of medications also contain lactose, and this should be checked before prescribing them to patients with galactosemia. However, in most cases, the amount of galactose (compared with endogenous production) is unlikely to be significant, particularly if the medication is not given for a prolonged period.

Soy-based infant formulas normally provide adequate calcium in infancy. However, by 1 year of age, the volume of soy formula taken begins to fall. It is then necessary to change to commercially available calcium-enriched soy milk or to give adequate calcium supplementation. Poor calcium intake, in addition to other factors, particularly ovarian failure, may lead to a decrease in bone density.[269] The nutritional adequacy of the diet should be reviewed at least annually.

Monitoring Patients with Classical Galactosemia

The mistaken belief that, following diagnosis, galactosemia could be treated easily and successfully by dietary restriction of milk and milk products has resulted in many patients' being followed in nonspecialist centres, if they are seen at all. Careful review is important, however, in order to monitor development, provide specialist dietary assessment and advice, and recognize late complications, particularly ovarian failure. Regular assessment of development and cognitive function using standardized tests is useful to provide an objective measure of outcome. Early assessment of speech is particularly important. Recognition of disabilities allows appropriate help to be offered to a child and his or her family.

A plan for outpatient review and standardized assessments has been recommended by the UK galactosemia steering group.[2] Under this protocol, patients are seen by a specialist team every three months to 1 year, every four months to 2 years, every six months to 14 years, and annually thereafter. More frequent monitoring is necessary for girls in late childhood and adolescence to monitor pubertal development. Specialist speech assessments are made at 1 and 2 years, a standardized developmental assessment at 4 years, and intelligence assessments at 8, 14, and 18 years.

Biochemical monitoring. Measurement of Gal-1-P in red cells is the most common method used to monitor dietary compliance. Concentrations of Gal-1-P are often very high at diagnosis and fall progressively after the introduction of galactose restriction. Acceptable values following the introduction of the diet are usually achieved within a few weeks, but even with good dietary compliance, in rare cases it takes up to a year. Even on such a diet, levels never decline to those found in normal individuals. The units used to express Gal-1-P concentrations and target levels vary among different laboratories. The difference in the Gal-1-P concentrations recommended by different centers is related in part to methodology. However, as a general rule, the upper limit usually considered acceptable, given in different units, is as follows: 150 μmol/liter of red cells; 50 μg/ml packed red cells; 5 mg/100 ml red blood cells, 0.5 μmol/g Hb.

There is no evidence of a relationship between red cell Gal-1-P concentration and long-term outcome. Frequent measurement as a means of monitoring patients with classical galactosemia is consequently difficult to justify. Poor dietary control may lead to significantly raised levels, but some patients have high values even with very good compliance. A suggested schedule for testing Gal-1-P levels is every three months to 1 year, every six months from 1 to 14 years, and yearly thereafter.[2]

Urinary galactitol has also been investigated as a means of monitoring diet but is available in only a few centers. Its value has not been validated, although it may have some practical and theoretical advantages compared to Gal-1-P. Hutchesson et al. found intra- and interindividual coefficients of variation of 37 percent and 42 percent, respectively, for urinary galactitol, with an analytical coefficient of only 5.5 percent, indicating that the major source of variability was biologic.[269a] They concluded that the high intraindividual variability for galactitol (and similar variability for Gal-1-P) limited the usefulness of both urinary galactitol and Gal-1-P as means of biochemical monitoring.

Treatment with uridine. Uridine has not been shown to prevent or reverse long-term complications. One study of oral treatment has now been published.[148] Uridine powder at a dose of 150 mg/kg/day was given to 29 patients and their cognitive function compared that of with six other patients who did not receive uridine. The period of the study for each patient was 2 to 5 years, with a mean of 3.9 years. No significant difference was found between the two groups, both of which showed a small increase in cognitive abilities.

Pubertal development in females with galactosemia. Since hypergonadotropic hypogonadism occurs in the majority of galactosemic females, recognition and treatment of this complication should be a routine part of managing females with galactosemia. Raised gonadotropin levels in infancy may be an indication of early ovarian failure, but their measurement thereafter in early childhood is not helpful. Recommendations for the ages at which endocrine assessment should be undertaken have been published. Walter et al.[2] suggest measurement of FSH, LH, and estradiol at 6 months, then at 10 and 12 years, and, if necessary, yearly thereafter, with referral to a pediatric endocrinologist by 10 years. The age when hormone therapy should be started is debated. Some groups have recommended treatment from the age of 16,[270] whereas others suggest starting earlier. The recommendation from the UK galactosemia steering group and the British Society for Paediatric Endocrinology and Diabetes is that hormone therapy be given to patients with elevated basal gonadotropin levels and low estradiol beginning at 12 years of age, or at 13 years if the girl is short.[2] Their suggested regimen is given in Table 72-8. All oral hormone preparations contain small quantities of lactose, but the total dose is very small in comparison to endogenous production.

Management during pregnancy

Pregnancy in women with classical galactosemia. No specific additional treatment during pregnancy has been necessary for the small number of women with galactosemia who have conceived normally. Gal-1-P is not transported across the placenta and is found at normal levels in cord blood from heterozygous infants.[170,271]. Infants born to mothers with galactosemia have been healthy at birth and have shown normal development.[142,170,271] The synthesis of lactose for breast milk is increased in the latter stages of pregnancy and during lactation. Maternal Gal-1-P levels have been reported to be raised toward the end of pregnancy and after delivery.[170,171] It has been suggested that this is due to endogenous breakdown of lactose, since suppression of lactation has resulted in a fall in Gal-1-P, which reaches basal levels only after 2 months.[171] There are no reports of continued breast-feeding in mothers with galactosemia, and it is therefore difficult to know whether Gal-1-P continues to rise and whether this would eventually cause clinical manifestations in the mother.

Pregnancy in heterozygous women. Galactose ingestion in heterozygous pregnant women at risk for having an affected fetus has not been shown to have any harmful effects. Some clinics recommend limiting milk intake to no more than 1 pint a day, but there is no evidence to suggest that this is necessary. Dietary

Table 72-8 Recommendations for the treatment of hypergonadotropic hypogonadism in females with galactosemia. From Walter et al. [2] See text for details

Year of treatment	Treatment
1	Ethinyl estradiol at a dose of 2 mg/day. If pubertal advance is particularly slow, then the time at this dose should be reduced to 6 months.
2	Ethinyl estradiol at a dose of 5 mg/d.
3	Ethinyl estradiol 10 mg/d. The patient and parents should be informed that vaginal spotting or withdrawal bleeds may occur during this year. If vaginal spotting or withdrawal bleeds occur, a progestogen should be added at the start of each month.
4 and thereafter	Loestrin (an oral contraceptive preparation containing 20 mg ethinyl estradiol and a progestogen) given in the usual way, ie, daily for 21 days followed by 7 days off). This preparation should be adequate for most young women. If there is breakthrough bleeding or any other symptoms of estrogen deficiency, then a preparation containing 30 mg of ethinyl estradiol can be used. (Natural estrogens would be an acceptable alternative to synthetic estrogen.)
Notes	Outpatient review should be every 4 months during the first 2 years of hormone treatment and every 6 months thereafter. Monitor • Physical development and growth throughout these years of pubertal induction. • Bone age yearly from the start of treatment. • Pelvic ultrasound (for uterine dimensions) at the start of treatment; and repeat after 2 and 4 years. • Blood pressure. Special care and advice should be given to those with a family history or past history of venous thrombosis and to those who are overweight or who smoke.

restriction of maternal lactose intake does not prevent accumulation of galactitol in the amniotic fluid of affected fetuses.[272] In the international survey by Waggoner et al., the outcome for those infants whose mothers followed milk-restricted diets during the pregnancies was no better than than that of babies for whom no such restriction was reported.[142]

GALE DEFICIENCY

Clinical presentation

The great majority of patients with galactase diphosphate galactose-4′-epimerase deficiency (OMIM 230350) confined to erythrocytes have been asymptomatic. This includes the original patient described by Gitzelmann et al. and children subsequently detected on newborn screening.[273–278] These individuals, despite raised red cell Gal-1-P levels, have shown normal growth and development and have not developed renal disease or cataracts. One girl, with a unilateral zonular cataract diagnosed at the age of $5\frac{1}{2}$ years, was found to have a partial deficiency of epimerase in red cells.[279] However, the absence of cataracts in other children with erythrocyte epimerase deficiency suggests that this was probably a coincidental finding. A further patient has been reported with severe but transient disease that was stated to be related to galactose ingestion.[280] This infant presented at the age of 48 hours with seizures, vomiting, and hypoglycemia. He improved following withdrawal of lactose from the diet but became ill again on two occasions following its reintroduction. While on a galactose-free diet he had a high Gal-1-P in blood level of 0.81 mg/dl (control < 0.6 mg/dl) and his UDP-Gal was slightly increased. Erythrocyte GALT and GK activity were normal but GALE activity just below the normal range at 9 months of age. He remained well following the reintroduction of a normal diet at the age of 1 year. The authors postulated that his transient severe galactose-dependent disease was due to low-normal epimerase activity. In contrast to this, Alano et al.[280a] reported a male patient of mixed Pakistani/Caucasian ancestry with what may be an intermediate phenotype. This child was diagnosed in the neonatal period and remained clinically well on a lactose-containing diet throughout the first year of life. Developmental delay first became apparent during the second year of life, and by the age of 5 the patient exhibited global delays in language and cognitive abilities.

Generalized GALE deficiency appears to be an exceptionally rare disorder, with only five patients from two families described.[18,281–283] Both families are of Asian origin, and in each case the parents of the affected individuals are consanguineous. The first child described was born in 1980 and presented soon after birth with jaundice, weight loss, hypotonia, and vomiting. She was found to have generalized aminoaciduria and galactosuria. Her symptoms improved on a low-lactose formula, and she started to gain weight, but she had persistent hypotonia, developmental delay, and severe sensorineural deafness. She has some facial dysmorphism, with an inner canthus distance below the 3rd centile, palpebral fissure length above the 97th centile, posteriorly rotated ears, and a short philtrum. She has had normal pubertal development, with no evidence of ovarian failure. The mother had another affected child in 1990. This infant had been diagnosed prenatally and started on a low-galactose diet from birth. A galactose challenge at 12 months of age led to evidence of liver damage with increased liver transaminases and a raised bilirubin level. Unlike her sister, this child is not significantly dysmorphic and does not have sensorineural deafness, but she does have poor growth and moderate learning difficulties.

The first affected child from the second family was born in 1984. She fed poorly, became irritable and developed corneal opacities and liver disease within the first week of life. She improved on dietary treatment but subsequently showed moderate learning difficulties and severe sensorineural deafness. She has some mild facial dysmorphism, with micrognathia, ligamentous laxity, and posteriorly rotated ears; persistent femoral anteversion;

internal tibial torsion; and short stature and poor growth. Her pubertal development and ovarian function have also been normal. A brother, born in 1995, was found to have epimerase deficiency. He has more severe dysmorphic features, with marked micrognathia and fixed flexion deformities of his fingers. Although he has had recurrent middle ear disease, he does not have sensorineural deafness. He is hypotonic and has moderate developmental delay. His weight gain and growth have been poor. Epimerase deficiency was also found in a first cousin of these children, born in 1994. She has similar dysmorphic features, sensorineural deafness, poor growth, and global developmental delay. Another cousin from this family had severe congenital deformities but did not have epimerase deficiency. In view of the high degree of consanguinity over many generations, it is thought probable that there are other recessive disorders within this second family. As a consequence, it is difficult to determine which features are due to epimerase deficiency. All five affected children from both families have learning difficulties, developmental delay, hypotonia, and poor growth, and three have sensorineural deafness. In contrast to the picture in GALT deficiency, ovarian failure has not occurred in the two girls who are old enough to have entered puberty.

Mutations at the *GALE* locus

As of July 1999, fewer than 10 mutations have been characterized at the *GALE* gene (Appendix 72-2). Most mutations are individually rare, having been reported only on single alleles[104,278,284] or in a homoallelic state in one individual.[104,284] Only a Val to Met substitution at codon 94, designated V94M, characterized by Wohlers et al.[284a] in the Asian patient first reported by Holton et al.,[18] was found in another extended consanguineous family[283] which was not known to be related to the first. A large number of mutations have yet to be characterized. For example, the five mutations characterized by Maceratesi et al. in 35 patients with a biochemical diagnosis of epimerase enzyme deficiency accounted for fewer than 13 percent of mutant chromosomes.[104,284] Structural abnormalities in the *GALE* gene have not been detected as a significant cause of GALE deficiency,[77] so it has been postulated that other mutations may be in promoter sequences, such as transcription factor binding sites that are involved in regulation of gene expression.

A null-background yeast expression system for the human GALE enzyme has been developed to enable structural and functional studies of wild-type and mutant alleles.[278] In an elegant series of experiments, Quimby et al.[278] and Wohlers et al.[284a] investigated six mutations using this system, and although the numbers are small, their results suggest that some naturally occurring *GALE* substitution mutations result in severe catalytic impairment, while others have little effect on enzyme function.

With respect to UDP-Gal as substrate, the mutations associated with an almost complete loss of enzyme activity were V94M, G90E, and L183P, the first being the mutation found in a homoallelic state in the Pakistani children with generalized epimerase deficiency. D103G, L313M, and N34S, on the other hand, demonstrated near-normal activity. Coexpression studies suggest that allelic interaction, as either partial dominant negative or partial dominant positive, may be allele specific.[278,284a]

UDP-N-acetylgalactosamine (UDP-GalNAc) was also used as a substrate, and it was evident that some patient mutations (Gly to Glu at codon 90, designated G90E, and Asp to Gly at codon 103, designated D103G) disrupt GALE activity equally with respect to both substrates, whereas others do not. V94M in particular exhibited considerably higher activity with respect to UDP-GalNAc (24 percent) than with respect to UDP-Gal (5 percent). UDP-GalNAc and UDP-GlcNAc play key roles in the assembly of complex polysaccharides and other glycosylated macromolecules, especially in the brain, and Wohlers et al. have considered that the impact of patient mutations on this reaction may be as relevant as the interruption of the Leloir pathway in the pathogenesis of epimerase-deficiency galactosemia.[284a]

The enzyme defect

It can be seen from Table 72-9 that both of the GALE deficiency disorders, benign[285] and severe,[18,282] are identified by a complete absence of the enzyme in red blood cells. On the other hand, epimerase activity was present in both forms of the disorder in liver[286,287] and skin fibroblasts.[68,286] However, the finding of epimerase in the fibroblasts of the severely affected patient was not confirmed by Gillett.[287] Phytohemagglutinin treatment of leukocytes from a patient with the benign form of the condition resulted in the production of epimerase, and a long-term lymphoblast cell line had control levels of the enzyme.[288]

The findings in both forms of GALE deficiency are consistent with gene mutations' resulting in the production of unstable enzyme forms. Cells with a long lifespan, like red blood cells, are devoid of enzyme activity, but tissues and cells with a fast turnover may show significant levels of enzyme activity. The mutant enzyme in the benign form of the disorder is clearly more stable than that in the severe form, as shown by almost normal epimerase levels in liver and fibroblasts from patients with the former compared with 10 percent activity in the liver of the patient with the latter.

GALE purified from fibroblast and lymphocyte cell lines in the benign form was shown to have reduced heat stability and an increased requirement for the NAD^+ coenzyme, although the pH optimum and K_m for UDP-Gal were the same as those found in cells with the normal enzyme.[289] The liver enzyme from a patient with the severe form of the disorder also had a normal pH optimum and K_m, but its activity was not enhanced by increased NAD^+ concentrations.[287]

The metabolic abnormality

It has been demonstrated that Gal-1-P accumulates in the erythrocytes of subjects with both forms of epimerase deficiency receiving some dietary galactose.[18,282,290] Erythrocyte UDP-Gal levels have been investigated only in a severely affected patient, in

Table 72-9 Levels of enzyme activity in cells and tissues of patients with benign and severe forms of UDP-galactose 4′-epimerase deficiency

	Benign			Severe		
Origin	N	% of Normal	Ref	N	% of Normal	Ref
RBC	9	0	252	2	0	18, 253
Leukocytes	7	0	252			
Lymphocytes	1/3	6	254			
Liver	2	60	254	1	10	287
Fibroblasts	4	70	254	1	0	287
				1	2 (UDP-Gal) 11 (UDP-N-acetyl galactosamine)	68

whom they were increased.[281] UDP-Gal levels rose rapidly to a plateau of around 180 μmol/L on galactose intakes of as little as 1 g/day (Fig. 72-9). Whereas Gal-1-P levels were raised minimally on this galactose supplement, they appeared to increase linearly with galactose intake up to the maximum given (4 g/day). It has been suggested that the level of UDP-Gal in red blood cells is limited in this patient by the availability of UDP-Glc from the pyrophosphorylase pathway for the operation of the transferase reaction. Once this supply of UDP-Glc is exhausted, Gal-1-P will accumulate and become the major galactose metabolite.[281]

Treatment

No treatment appears to be required for peripheral epimerase deficiency. Treatment for children with generalized epimerase deficiency, as for those with GALT deficiency, consists of restriction of dietary galactose. If epimerase deficiency is absolute, then there should, in theory, be no production of galactoproteins and galactolipids. It has therefore been suggested that a small amount of exogenous galactose should be prescribed in the diet to allow these essential compounds to be manufactured. However, production of low-density lipoproteins, which are themselves galactoproteins, was normal in fibroblasts from one of the patients with generalized epimerase deficiency.[68] This finding is presumably related to residual enzyme activity in liver, and possibly other tissues, and suggests that such supplementation may not be necessary.

PRENATAL DIAGNOSIS

The disorders of galactose metabolism are particularly amenable technically to prenatal diagnosis. However, as discussed later in this section, prenatal diagnosis is requested quite rarely for this group of metabolic disorders.

GALK has been assayed in skin fibroblasts and cultured amniotic fluid cells (amniocytes) using a method that is a modification of the red cell enzyme assay of Beutler et al.[201] The results[291] suggest that prenatal diagnosis of galactokinase deficiency would be possible, but the one "at risk" pregnancy investigated turned out to have a normal outcome.

Prenatal diagnosis of GALT deficiency was first achieved by the assay of amniocytes produced from fluid obtained at 16–18 weeks' gestation and subsequently at 8–10 weeks' gestation. The analytic methods used[239,292,293] have been modifications of the sensitive erythrocyte assay of Ng et al.[294] The method of Monk and Holton[293] proved particularly reliable in that amniocytes from the same subject gave constant GALT results whether harvested from 1 to 7 days after subculture; the results for a classical galactosemia/Duarte variant heterozygote was clearly distinguished from those for a classical galactosemia homozygote. More recently, direct assay of GALT from chorionic villus biopsy samples obtained in the first trimester has been achieved.[295] This provides a very rapid result, as cell culture is not needed, although chorionic villus cells can be cultured as a back-up or as confirmation of the direct assay.

A different approach to the prenatal diagnosis of GALT deficiency was suggested by the work of Allen et al., which showed increased galactitol levels in amniotic fluid obtained in two affected pregnancies.[240] This technique was developed by the same group using fluid samples obtained between 15 and 20 weeks of gestation[245] and by Jakobs et al.[296] Differentiation of pregnancies with a galactosemic fetus from those not at risk of the clinical disorder has been successfully achieved in 50 cases using gas chromatography/mass spectrometry to assay galactitol in amniotic fluid.[297] The method has now been validated in an affected pregnancy using amniotic fluid obtained at 10 weeks' gestation (J. T. Allen, personal communication).

Prenatal diagnosis of GALT deficiency is now possible by DNA analysis, provided the mutations on the genes on both chromosomes have been established.[298] Chorionic villus biopsy is an excellent and rapid source of fetal DNA. Failing this, DNA can be extracted from amniocytes, although this does impose a delay of 2–3 weeks in the result's becoming available.

One paper has been concerned with the prenatal diagnosis of GALE deficiency by means of assaying the enzyme in amniocytes.[299] A prenatal diagnosis was performed in the second pregnancy of a woman whose first child suffers from the severe form of GALE deficiency. The result suggested that the fetus was heterozygous for the deficiency, and erythrocyte epimerase levels at 14 days of age supported this conclusion. The baby suffered none of the neonatal problems associated with epimerase deficiency and has developed normally.

The only disorder in which there has been a significant number of prenatal diagnoses is GALT deficiency, and even for this condition it appears, certainly in the experience of European

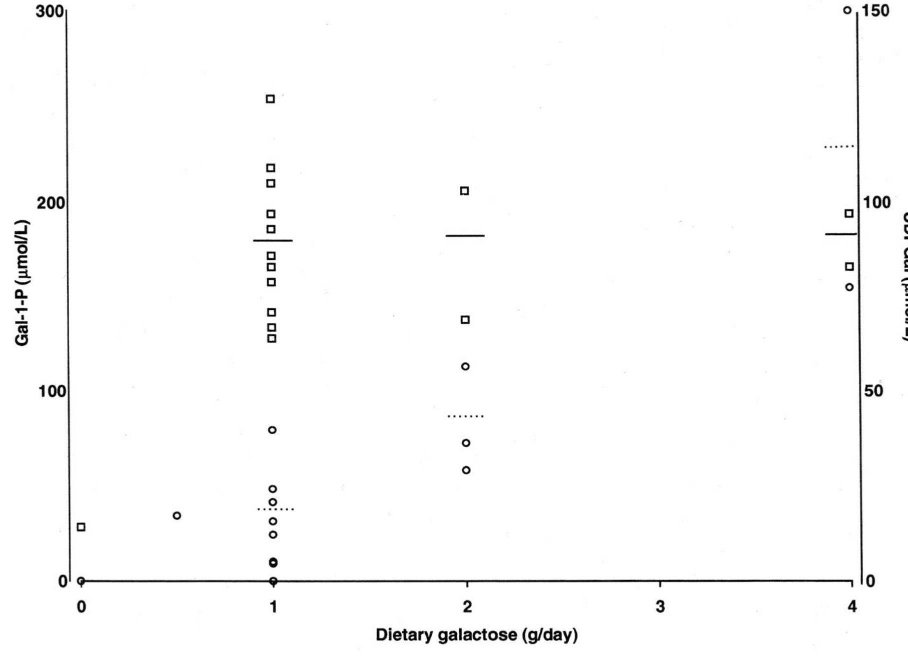

Fig. 72-9 Accumulation of galactose metabolites in a child with the severe form of epimerase deficiency given various galactose supplements: O = levels of Gal-1-P in packed red cells, — = mean levels of Gal-1-P in blood samples collected when the galactose intake is the same, open squares = levels of UDP-Gal in packed red cells, ··· = levels of UDP-Gal in blood samples collected when the galactose intake is the same.

workers,[291,297] that it is rarely requested. Also, it is considered that many of the diagnoses that are carried out do not have a valid reason, or that the reason does not justify the risk of carrying out an amniocentesis or chorionic villus biopsy. In the absence of any studies into these aspects of prenatal diagnosis, it is unclear why it is so rarely carried out with the aim of preventing the birth of another galactosemic child into the family. It has been postulated[291,297] that counseling is not offered or does not include advising the prospective parents on the serious, long-term complications of classical galactosemia. It is possible that there is some reluctance to emphasize these complications when the index case is being treated with apparent success. This conclusion is supported by the observation of Holton and Raymont[300] that in four out of five unrelated cases in which termination of the pregnancy was being considered, the index patient in the family had died in the neonatal period.

PATHOGENESIS

General considerations

Some tentative conclusions can be drawn regarding the pathogenetic mechanisms involved in the features of the disorders of galactose metabolism. Cataracts are a complication of all these enzyme deficiency disorders in the neonatal period but are probably the sole abnormality in GALK deficiency. The main biochemical feature of GALK deficiency is galactitol accumulation,[134] so this is considered to be the primary cause of cataracts in the galactosemias.

The acute neonatal complications of GALT and severe epimerase-deficiency galactosemias are similar, and very high levels of Gal-1-P are present in both disorders at this stage. Consequently, this metabolite has been considered to be the cause of the acute neonatal toxicity.[241] It is difficult to extend this comparison of biochemical and clinical features further, as the long-term outcome of epimerase deficiency is not known with any certainty. However, attempts to correlate long-term outcome in GALT deficiency as measured by IQ with average Gal-1-P levels on treatment have been unsuccessful.[142,144]

An alternative hypothesis to explain the long-term complications in GALT deficiency involves the reduced level of UDP-Gal, which may lead to abnormal glycoprotein and glycolipid synthesis.[247] The nucleotide deficiency is not a feature of severe GALE deficiency, in which UDP-Gal levels tend to be raised. In fact, high UDP-Gal concentrations have been postulated to be the cause of the sensorineural deafness that was considered to be a unique feature of severe GALE deficiency, although this has now been questioned.[283]

The time when the damage leading to the long-term complications of GALT deficiency occurs has also been considered. IQ did not correlate with age when treatment was begun.[142] This negative result was emphasized in a study of affected siblings in which the older siblings, treated beginning 1 to 11 months after birth, performed as well in psychometric tests as the younger siblings treated starting at birth.[301]

The failure to correlate outcome with length of exposure to abnormal metabolites before treatment and with residual level of Gal-1-P after treatment suggests the possibility that damage might occur in utero. The clear evidence that the pathways of galactose metabolism normally develop around the tenth week of gestation[20] and that the galactosemic fetus has abnormal levels of metabolites from about that time[239,240] suggests that damage could be sustained *in utero* and become progressively apparent with age. The only real evidence that clinical features of galactosemia may have their origins '*in utero*' however, is the finding of cataracts at birth[302] and in a fetus at 20 weeks' gestation.[303] Otherwise, histologic studies of the livers of infants who died of galactosemia have concluded that cirrhosis has originated *in utero*,[304] and there is good reason to surmise that ovarian failure is also determined prenatally.[168]

Possible pathogenetic mechanisms

There has been much experimental work with possible relevance to the pathogenesis of galactosemia, both in *in vitro* systems and in animals, but little of this is known to be of any real consequence.

Gal-1-P. Gitzelmann[241] has summarized data on the inhibition of glucose-metabolizing enzymes by Gal-1-P. The enzymes considered were glucose-6-phosphatase, glucose-6-phosphate dehydrogenase, phosphoglucomutase, glycogen phosphorylase, and UDP-Glc-pyrophosphorylase. There is evidence that high concentrations of Gal-1-P inhibit galactosyl transferase[19] and this may be relevant to the defects in the galactosylation of glycoproteins and glycolipids that are discussed in "Galactitol accumulation" below.

One other proposed mechanism that may be very significant is involvement of Gal-1-P in a futile phosphorylation cycle in which ATP is trapped in Gal-1-P, which may be dephosphorylated to metabolites that have no energy-generating capability.[305] Support for this hypothesis, which has a parallel in the metabolism of fructose in hereditary fructose intolerance, comes from animal model systems in which liver necrosis is induced by galactose analogues.[306] In 1975, confirmation of the existence of this futile phosphorylation cycle in galactosemia was forthcoming from two groups of workers.[307,308] It was shown that a galactose load given to adult galactosemic patients induced hyperuricemia. This provided indirect evidence for increased catabolism and depletion of hepatic nucleotides due to Gal-1-P accumulation and trapping of ATP.

Galactitol accumulation. As mentioned previously, patients with any of the defects in the Leloir pathway have neonatal cataracts, the cause of which has been related to the accumulation of galactitol in the ocular lens, resulting in osmotic swelling. A similar mechanism may be the cause of cerebral edema, a rare complication of GALK and GALT deficiency.[309]

There is a large volume of literature on experimental galactosemia in animals, which is pertinent to the effect of galactitol accumulation. The work has been performed in rats and mice in particular, the galactosemia being induced by diets containing as much as 50 percent galactose.[310] This produces damage to a wide range of organs, including the ocular lens, retina, cornea, kidney, ovary and peripheral nerves. The pathologic abnormalities that these organs demonstrate are associated with significant galactitol accumulation, together with myoinositol depletion. Confirmation that galactitol accumulation is the primary cause of the pathology is provided by the prevention of the abnormalities with the concurrent administration of an aldose reductase inhibitor.

Since the pathologic features found in the animal feeding studies could be equated to some of the long-term complications of GALT deficiency, and since galactitol levels remain elevated in galactosemic patients on galactose-restricted diets, it seems reasonable to consider the possibility that galactitol accumulation could be the cause of the problems in the human disorder. Unfortunately, this hypothesis appears to be completely incompatible with the fact that no features other than cataract have been established in GALK deficiency. It seems probable that experimental galactosemia in rats and mice may not be a good model for the study of the disorder in humans. On the other hand, experiments in which dogs were fed a high-galactose diet have suggested that they may have a sensitivity to galactitol accumulation that is more akin to that in humans, the retina being particularly affected.[310a,310b]

Galactosylation defects. Haberland et al.,[311] while examining the brain of a galactosemic child at autopsy, found an abnormality in its glycoproteins, and it was suggested that the cause could be a defect in galactose incorporation. The same biochemical defect was considered a possibility as a consequence of the reduction in

UDP-Gal concentrations found in GALT-deficient patients.[246,247] More recently, Petry et al.[312] reported a deficiency of normal galactose and N-acetyl galactosamine-containing glycolipids and an accumulation of their precursors in the brains and lymphocytes of galactosemic patients. Dobbie et al.[313] and Ornstein et al.[314] have shown, by quite different approaches, that there is a low uptake of galactose into the glycoproteins of cultured skin fibroblasts from GALT-deficient patients compared to those from controls.

Two groups of workers have described abnormalities in hexose metabolism and cell growth in skin fibroblasts from galactosemic patients that they postulate could be related to long-term neurologic problems. Kadhom et al.[315] have demonstrated low efficiency of [^{14}C]-galactose incorporation into GALT-deficient cells. Wolfrom et al.[316] studied the growth and morphology of cells from both GALT- and GALK-deficient patients in medium containing glucose as the energy source and homologous serum. Although the medium was adequate to support normal growth in control fibroblasts, the uptake of glucose in the galactosemic cells was 65–70 percent of control levels and cell growth was subnormal. However, the suggestion that this phenomenon could be related to long-term neurologic problems has to be questioned in view of the lack of any significant evidence that this clinical feature occurs in galactokinase deficiency.

Jaeken et al[317] have suggested that the pathogenetic mechanisms in classical galactosemia may be similar to those in carbohydrate-deficient glycoprotein (CDG) syndrome, a major group of abnormalities with nervous system involvement and ovarian failure in some of its forms. The similarities they observed included decreased thyroid-binding globulin and abnormalities in the isoelectric focusing pattern of the sialo transferrins. Since abnormal lysosomal enzymes have been found in CDG syndrome, the authors went on to study two newborn galactosemic babies and found them to have abnormal isoelectric focusing patterns of serum β-N-acetylhexosaminidase and α-fucosidase before treatment. It may be very significant that the patterns normalized after a week of treatment. It was postulated that in classic galactosemia increased Gal-1-P levels interfere with carbohydrate processing at the Golgi galactosyltransferase step, leading to partial deficiency of the terminal disaccharide (sialic acid + galactose). In this context, the work of Bonham et al.,[318] showing a correlation between urinary transferrin/creatinine ratio and blood Gal-1-P levels in galactosemic patients on treatment, is of some interest. Recently, Prestoz et al.[169] have demonstrated abnormal isoforms of FSH in classic galactosemic patients. It appeared that N-acetyl galactosamine sites on the abnormal FSH were waiting to be galactosylated, which would suggest that a galactosylation defect in the pituitary is a likely cause of ovarian dysfunction in female galactosemic patients.

A genetically engineered GALT-deficient animal model

The most recent tool in attempts to understand the pathogenesis of classic galactosemia is the genetically engineered mouse model.[319] The mice, created by gene targeting, have liver GALT levels that are indistinguishable from zero and comparable to tissue levels in humans who are homozygous for the common Q188R mutation. Furthermore, tissue and erythrocyte levels of Gal-1-P and galactose are extremely high. It is surprising, therefore, that the GALT-deficient mice show none of the toxic signs associated with the enzyme deficiency in humans. It is hoped that a deeper understanding of galactose metabolism in the mouse model may provide some clues to why GALT-deficient humans, in particular, are affected by the metabolic abnormality. One hypothesis that has been suggested already is that the early toxic signs of classic galactosemia are due to a combined effect of Gal-1-P and galactitol accumulation. Mice, possessing only weak aldose reductase activity, accumulate less galactitol and hence would escape the early toxic presentation.[319a]

Further studies may be aided by modeling human mutations onto the three-dimensional structure of the crystallized *E. coli* galT protein[182a] or of the human GALT protein itself. Although no reports on extensive GALT modeling have been published to date, the feasibility of this approach has been demonstrated by modeling the human GALE protein on the *E. coli* galE three-dimensional structure.[77]

ACKNOWLEDGMENTS

We gratefully acknowledge our many colleagues who have assisted us in preparing this work. We are particularly indebted to Dr. Juergen Reichardt for his generosity in sharing ideas and information. We also thank Mrs. Christine Caveney for secretarial help with the manuscript.

APPENDIX 72-1 Details of mutations characterized at the *GALK* gene

Region	Nucleotide	Systematic name	Nucleotide Nomenclature	Trivial Name	Ethnic Origin	Reference
Exon 1	3	c. 3 G → T	ATG/ATT	MII	African American	131
Exon 1	82	c. 82 C → A	CCC/ACC	P28T	Turkish, Bulgarian Romani	131,131a
Exon 1	94	c. 94 G → A	GTG/ATG	V32M		47
Exon 1	106	c. 106 G → A	GGC/AGC	G36R	Swiss	131
Exon 1	130	c. 130 C → T	CAC/TAC	H44Y	German	131
Exon 2	228	c. 228ins67bp	CTC^ACCins67bpfs	L76ins67bpfs	Hispanic	131
Exon 2	238	c. 238 G → T	GAG/TAG	E80X		47
Exon 2	280	c. 280insACTGCCC	A^CAinsACTGCCCfs	T94ins7bpfs		131
Exon 4	610	c. 610insG	A^GGinsGfs	R204insGfs	Swiss	131
Exon 5	761	c. 761delG	AGCdelGfs	S254delGfs		131
Exon 7	1012	c. 1012insG	G^TTinsGfs	V338insGfs	Swiss Gypsy	131
Exon 7	1036	c. 1036 G → A	GGT/AGT	G346S		131
Exon 7	1045	c. 1045 G → A	GGT/AGT	G349S	Japanese, German	132
Exon 8	1144	c. 1144 C → T	CAA/TAA	Q382X	Costa Rican	131

APPENDIX 72-2 Details of mutations characterized at the *GALE* gene

Region	Nucleotide	Systematic name	Nucleotide Nomenclature	Trivial Name	Ethnic Origin	Reference
Exon 2	194	c. 194 A → G	AAC/AGC	N34S	Caucasian	278
Exon 4	362	c. 362 G → A	GGG/GAG	G90E	Asian	284
Exon 4	369	c. 369 G → A	GTT/ATT	V94M	Pakistani	284a
Exon 4	401	c. 401 A → G	GAT/GGT	D103G	Asian	284
Exon 6	641	c. 641 T → C	CTG/CCG	L183P	Pakistani	278
Exon 8	863	c. 863 A → G	AAG/AGG	K257R	African-American	284
Exon 10	1030	c. 1030 C → A	CTG/ATG	L313M	Asian	284
Exon 10	1049	c. 1049 G → A	GGG/GAG	G319E	African-American	284

REFERENCES

1. von Reuss A: Zuckerausscheidung im Sauglingsalter. *WIEN Med Wochenschr* **58**:799, 1908.
2. Walter JH, Collins J, Leonard JV: Recommendations for the management of galactosaemia. *Arch Dis Childhood* **80**:93, 1999.
3. Gray GM, Santiago NA: Intestinal beta-galactosidases: I. Separation and characterization of three enzymes in normal human intestine. *J Clin Invest* **48**:716, 1969.
4. Acosta PB, Gross KC: Hidden sources of galactose in the environment. *Eur J Pediatr* **154**:S87, 1995.
5. Berry GT, Palmieri M, Gross KC, et al.: The effect of dietary fruits and vegetables on urinary galactitol excretion in galactose-1-phosphate uridyltransferase deficiency. *J Inherit Metab Dis* **16**:91, 1993.
6. Gray GM: Carbohydrate digestion and absorption: Role of the small intestine. *N Engl J Med* **292**:1225, 1975.
7. Stenstam T: Peroral and intravenous galactose tests: Comparative study of their significance in different conditions. *Acta Med Scand* **177**:1, 1946.
8. Segal S, Blair A: Some observations on the metabolism of D-galactose in normal man. *J Clin Invest* **40**:2016, 1961.
9. Tygstrup N, Winkler K: Galactose blood clearance as a measure of hepatic blood flow. *Clin Sci* **17**:1, 1961.
10. Gitzelmann R: Formation of galactose-1-phosphate from uridine diphosphate galactose in erythrocytes from patients with galactosemia. *Pediatr Res* **3**:279, 1969.
11. Berry GT, Nissim I, Lin Z, Mazur AT, Gibson JB, Segal S: Endogenous synthesis of galactose in normal man and patients with hereditary galactosaemia. *Lancet* **346**:1073, 1995.
12. Bunn BH, Higgins PJ: Reaction of monosaccharides with protein: Possible evolutionary significance. *Science* **213**:222, 1981.
13. Caputto R, Leloir LF, Gardini CE, Paladini AC: Isolation of the coenzyme of galactose phosphate-glucose phosphate transformation. *J Biol Chem* **184**:333, 1950.
14. Leloir LF: The enzymatic transformation of uridine diphosphate glucose into a galactose derivative. *Arch Biochem* **33**:186, 1951.
15. Schwarz V, Goldberg L, Komrower GM, Holzel A: Some disturbance of erythrocyte metabolism in galactosaemia. *Biochem J* **62**:34, 1956.
16. Isselbacher KJ, Anderson EP, Kurahashi K., Kalckar HM: Congenital galactosaemia, a single enzymatic block in galactose metabolism. *Science* **123**:635, 1956.
17. Gitzelmann R: Deficiency of erythrocyte galactokinase in a patient with galactose diabetes. *Lancet* **2**:670, 1965.
18. Holton JB, Gillett MG, MacFaul R, Young R: Galactosaemia: A new severe variant due to uridine diphosphate galactose-4-epimerase deficiency. *Arch Dis Child* **56**:885, 1981.
19. Roth S, McGuire EJ, Roseman S: Evidence for cell-surface glycosyltransferases: Their potential role in cellular recognition. *J Cell Biol* **51**:536, 1971.
20. Shin-Buehring YS, Beier T, Tan A, Osang M, Schaub J: The activity of galactose-1-phosphate uridyltransferase and galactokinase in human fetal organs. *Paediat Res* **11**:1045, 1977.
21. Isselbacher KJ: Evidence for an accessory pathway of galactose metabolism in mammalian liver. *Science* **126**:652, 1957.
22. Townsend EH, Mason HH, Strong PS: Galactosemia and its relation to Laennec's cirrhosis. *Pediatrics* **7**:760, 1951.
23. Kalckar HM, Braganca B, Munch-Petersen A: Uridyl transferase and the formation of uridine diphosphate galactose. *Nature* **172**:1038, 1953.
24. Isselbacher KJ: A mammalian uridine diphosphate galactose pyrophosphorylase. *J Biol Chem* **232**:429, 1958.
25. Shin YS, Niedermeier HP, Endres W, Schaub J, Weidinger S: Agarose gel isoelectrofocusing of UDP-galactose pyrophosphorylase and galactose-1-phosphate uridyltransferase. Developmental aspect of UDP-galactose pyrophosphorylase. *Clin Chim Acta* **166**:27, 1987.
26. Knop J, Hansen R: Uridine diphosphate glucose pyrophosphorylase: IV. Crystallization and properties of the enzyme from human liver. *J Biol Chem* **245**:2499, 1970.
27. Turnquist RL, Turnquist MM, Bachmann RC, Hansen RG: Uridine diphosphate glucose pyrophosphorylase: Differential heat inactivation and further characterization of human liver enzyme. *Biochim Biophys Acta* **364**:59, 1974.
28. Abraham H, Howell R: Human hepatic uridine diphosphate galactose pyrophosphorylase. *J Biol Chem* **244**:545, 1969.
29. Hers HG: L'aldose reductase. *Biochim Biophys Acta* **37**:120, 1969.
30. Hayman S, Lou MF, Merola LO, Kinoshita JH: Aldose reductase in the lens and other tissues. *Biochim Biophys Acta* **128**:474, 1996.
31. Jakobs C, Schweitzer S, Dorland B: Galactitol in galactosemia. *Eur J Pediatr* **154**:(7 Suppl 2)S50, 1995.
32. Gitzelmann R, Curtius HC, Muller M: Galactitol excretion in the urine of a galactokinase deficient man. *Biochem Biophys Res Commun* **22**:437, 1966.
33. Bergren W, Ng W, Donnell G: Galactonic acid in galactosaemia: Identification in urine. *Science* **176**:683, 1972.

33a. Wehrli SL, Berry GT, Palmieri M, Mazur A, Elsas L, Segal S: Urinary galactonate in patients with galactosaemia: Quantitation by nuclear magnetic resonance spectroscopy. *Pediatr Res* **42**:855,1997.

34. Rancour NJ, Hawkins ED, Wells WW: Galactose oxidation in liver. *Arch Biochem Biophys* **193**:232, 1979.
35. Wada E: r-Galactonolactone in experimental galactosemic animals. *Arch Biochem Biophys* **251**:215, 1986.
36. Cuatrecasas P, Segal S: Mammalian galactose dehydrogenase: I. Identification and purification in rat liver. *J Biol Chem* **241**:5904, 1966.
37. Cuatrecasas P, Segal S: Mammalian galactose dehydrogenase: II. Properties, substrate specificity, and developmental changes. *J Biol Chem* **241**:5910, 1966.
38. Srivastava SK, Beutler E: Identification of reaction products of hexose-6-phosphate dehydrogenase and of galactose dehydrogenase. *J Biol Chem* **244**:6377, 1969.
39. Shaw CR, Koen AL: "Galactose dehydrogenase", "nothing dehydrogenase", and alcohol dehydrogenase: Interrelation. *Science* **156**:1517, 1967.
40. Cuatrecasas P, Segal S: Galactose conversion to D-xylulose: An alternate route of galactose metabolism. *Science* **153**:549, 1966.
41. Komrower GM, Schwarz V, Holzel A, Goldberg L: A clinical and biochemical study of galactosaemia. A possible explanation of the nature of the biochemical lesion. *Arch Dis Child* **31**:254, 1956.
42. Stambolian D, Scarpino-Meyers , Harris H: Isoelectric-focussing of galactokinase in lens and other tissues. *Exp Eye Res* 38:231, 1984.
43. Cuatrecasas P, Segal S: Mammalian galactokinase: Developmental and adaptive characteristics in the rat liver. *J Biol Chem* **240**:2382, 1962.

44. Walker DG, Khan HH: Some properties of galactokinase in developing rat liver. *Biochem J* **108**:169, 1968.
45. Mathai C, Beutler E: Biochemical characteristics of galactokinase from adult and fetal human red cells. *Enzymologia* **33**:224, 1965.
46. Ng WG, Donnell GN, Bergren WR: Galactokinase activity in human erythrocytes of individuals at different ages. *J Lab Clin Med* **66**:115, 1965.
47. Stambolian D, Ai Y, Sidjanin D, et al.: Cloning of the galactokinase cDNA and identification of mutations in two families with cataracts. *Nat Genet* **10**:307, 1995.
48. Lee RT, Peterson CL, Calman AF, Herskowitz I, O'Donnell JJ: Cloning of a human galactokinase gene (GK2) on chromosome 15 by complementation in yeast. *Proc Natl Acad Sci U S A* **89**:10887, 1992.
49. Ai Y, Basu M, Bergsma DJ, Stambolian D: Comparison of the enzymatic activities of human galactokinase GALK1 and a related human galactokinase protein GK2. *Biochem Biophys Res Commun* **212**:687, 1995.
50. Stambolian D, Scarpino-Meyers V, Harris H: Purification of human galactokinase and evidence for its existence as a monomer form. *Biochim Biophys Acta* **831**:306, 1985.
51. Blume KG, Beutler E: Purification and properties of galactokinase from human red blood cells. *J Biol Chem* **246**:6507, 1971.
52. Atkinson M, Barton R, Morton R: Equilibrium constant of phosphoryl transfer from adenosine triphosphate to galactose in the presence of galactokinase. *Biochem J* **78**:813, 1961.
53. Magnani M, Cucchiarini L, Dacha M, Fornaini G: A new variant of galactokinase. *Hum Hered* **32**:329, 1982.
54. Kurahashi K, Sugimura A: Purification and properties of galactose-1-phosphate uridyltransferase from *E. coli*. *J Biol Chem* **235**:940, 1960.
55. Bertoli D, Segal S: Developmental aspects and some characteristics of mammalian galactose 1-phosphate uridyltransferase. *J Biol Chem* **241**:4023, 1966.
56. Dale GL, Popjak G: Purification of normal and inactive galactosemic galactose-1-phosphate uridylyltransferase from human red cells. *J Biol Chem* **251**:1057, 1976.
57. Williams VP: Purification and some properties of galactose 1-phosphate uridylyltransferase from human red cells. *Arch Biochem Biophys* **191**:182, 1978.
58. Elsevier JP, Wells L, Quimby BB, Fridovich Keil JL: Heterodimer formation and activity in the human enzyme galactose-1-phosphate uridylyltransferase. *Proc Natl Acad Sci U S A* **93**:7166, 1996.
59. Marcus HB, Wu LJW, Boches FS, Tedesco TA, Mellman WJ, Kallen RG: Human erythrocyte galactose-1-phosphate uridyl transferase: Evidence for a uridylyl-enzyme intermediate by kinetic and exchange reaction studies. *J Biol Chem* **252**:5363, 1977.
60. Frey PA: The Leloir pathway: A mechanistic imperative for three enzymes to change the stereochemical configuration of a single carbon in galactose. *FASEB J* **10**:461, 1996.
61. Reichardt JK, Packman S, Woo SL: Molecular characterization of two galactosemia mutations: Correlation of mutations with highly conserved domains in galactose-1-phosphate uridyl transferase. *Am J Hum Genet* **49**:860, 1991.
62. Williams VP, Fried C, Popjak G: Human red cell galactose 1-phosphate uridylyltransferase: Effects of site-specific reagents on catalytic activity. *Arch Biochem Biophys* **206**:353, 1981.
63. Pesch LA, Segal S., Topper YJ: Progesterone effects on galactose metabolism in prepubertal patients with congenital galactosaemia and in rats maintained on high galactose diets. *J Clin Invest* **39**:178, 1960.
64. Rogers S, Segal S: Enhanced galactose metabolism in isolated perfused livers of folate-treated suckling rats. *Metabolism* **33**:634, 1984.
65. Piller F, Hanlon MH, Hill RL: Co-purification and characterization of UDP-glucose 4-epimerase and UDP-N-acetylglucosamine 4-epimerase from porcine submaxillary glands. *J Biol Chem* **258**:10774, 1983.
66. Salo W, Nordin J, Peterson D, Bevill R, Kirkwood S: The specificity of UDP-glucose 4-epimerase from the yeast *Saccharomyces fragilis*. *Biochim Biophys Acta* **151**:484, 1968.
67. Kingsley DM, Kozarsky KF, Hobbie L, Krieger M: Reversible defects in O-linked glycosylation and LDL receptor expression in a UDP-Gal/UDP-GalNAc 4-epimerase deficient mutant. *Cell* **44**:749, 1986.
68. Kingsley DM, Krieger M, Holton JB: Structure and function of low-density-lipoprotein receptors in epimerase-deficient galactosemia [letter]. *N Engl J Med* **314**:1257, 1986.
69. Wilson DB, Hogness DS: The enzymes of the galactose operon in *Escherichia coli*: I. Purification and characterization of uridine diphosphate galactose-4-epimerase. *J Biol Chem* **239**:2469, 1964.
70. Darrow RA, Rodstrom R: Purification and properties of uridine diphosphate galactose 4-epimerase from yeast. *Biochemistry* **7**:1645, 1968.
71. Maxwell E: The enzymatic interconversion of uridine diphosphogalactose and uridine diphosphoglucose. *J Biol Chem* **229**:139, 1957.
72. Langer R, Glaser L: Interaction of nucleotides with liver uridine diphosphate-glucose-4′-epimerase. *J Biol Chem* **249**:1126, 1974.
73. Maitra US, Ankel H: Uridine diphosphate-4-keto-glucose, an intermediate in the uridine diphosphate galactose-4-epimerase reaction. *Proc Natl Acad Sci U S A* **68**:2660, 1971.
74. Adair WL Jr, Gabriel O, Ullrey D, Kalckar HM: 4-Uloses as intermediates in enzyme-nicotinamide adenine dinucleotide-mediated oxidoreductase mechanisms: I. Uridine diphosphate-galactose-4-epimerase. *J Biol Chem* **248**:4635, 1973.
75. Nelsestuen GL, Kirkwood S: Mechanisms of action of uridine diphosphoglucose 4-epimerase. *Fed Proc* **29**:337, 1970.
76. Geren CR, Ebner KE: Purification and characterization of UDP-galactose-4-epimerase from bovine tissues. *J Biol Chem* **252**:2082, 1977.
77. Daude N, Gallaher TK, Zeschnigk M, et al.: Molecular cloning, characterization, and mapping of a full-length cDNA encoding human UDP-galactose 4′-epimerase. *Biochem Mol Med* **56**:1, 1995.
78. Bergren WG, Ng WG, Donnell GN: Uridine diphosphate galactose-4′-epimerase in human and other mammalian haemolysates. *Biochim Biophys Acta* **315**:464, 1973.
79. Cohn R, Segal S: Some characteristics and developmental aspects of rat uridine diphosphogalactose 4-epimerase. *Biochim Biophys Acta* **171**:333, 1969.
80. Isselbacher KJ, Krane SM: Studies on the mechanism of the inhibition of galactose oxidation by ethanol. *J Biol Chem* **236**:2394, 1961.
81. Elsevier SM, Kucherlapati RS, Nichols EA, et al.: Assignment of the gene for galactokinase to human chromosome 17 and its regional localisation to band q21–22. *Nature* **251**:633, 1974.
82. Citron BA, Donelson JE: Sequence of the *Saccharomyces GAL* region and its transcription *in vivo*. *J Bacteriol* **158**:269, 1984.
83. Adams CW, Fornwald JA, Schmidt FJ, Rosenberg M, Brawner ME: Gene organization and structure of the *Streptomyces lividans*gal operon. *J Bacteriol* **170**:203, 1988.
84. Debouck C, Riccio A, Schumperli D, et al.: Structure of the galactokinase gene of *Escherichia coli*, the last (?) gene of the *gal* operon. *Nucleic Acids Res* **13**:1841, 1985.
85. Ai Y, Jenkins NA, Copeland NG, Gilbert DH, Bergsma DJ, Stambolian D: Mouse galactokinase: Isolation, characterization, and location on chromosome 11. *Genome Res* **5**:53, 1995.
86. Bergsma DJ, Ai Y, Skach WR, et al.: Fine structure of the human galactokinase *GALK1* gene [letter]. *Genome Res* **6**:980, 1996.
87. Mohandas T, Sparkes RS, Sparkes MC, Shulkin JD: Assignment of the human gene for galactose-1-phosphate uridyltransferase to chromosome 9: Studies with Chinese hamster-human somatic cell hybrids. *Proc Natl Acad Sci U S A* **74**:5628, 1977.
88. Mohandas T, Sparkes RS, Sparkes MC, Shulkin JD, Toomey KE, Funderburk SJ: Regional localization of human gene loci on chromosome 9: Studies of somatic cell hybrids containing human translocations. *Am J Hum Genet* **31**:586, 1979.
89. Mohandas T, Sparkes RS, Sparkes MC, Shulkin JD, Toomey KE, Funderburk SJ: Assignment of GALT to chromosome 9 and regional localization of GALT, AK1, AK3, and ACONS on chromosome 9. *Cytogenet Cell Genet* **22**:456, 1978.
90. Aitken DA, Ferguson-Smith MA: Intrachromosomal assignment of the structural gene for GALT to the short arm of chromosome 9 by gene dosage studies. *Cytogenet Cell Genet* **25**:131, 1979.
91. Sparkes RS, Sparkes MC, Funderburk SJ, Moedjono S: Expression of GALT in 9p chromosome alterations: Assignment of GALT locus to 9cen leads to 9p22. *Ann Hum Genet* **43**:343, 1980.
92. Dagna-Bricarelli F, Magnani M, Arslanian A, et al.: Expression of GALT in two unrelated 9p-patients: Evidence for assignment of the GALT locus to the 9p21 band. *Hum Genet* **59**:112, 1981.

93. Shih LY, Suslak L, Rosin I, Searle BM, Desposito F: Gene dosage studies supporting localization of the structural gene for galactose-1-phosphate uridyl transferase (GALT) to band p13 of chromosome 9. *Am J Med Genet* **19**:539, 1984.
94. Reichardt JK, Berg P: Cloning and characterization of a cDNA encoding human galactose-1-phosphate uridyl transferase. *Mol Biol Med* **5**:107, 1988.
95. Flach JE, Reichardt JK, Elsas LJ: Sequence of a cDNA encoding human galactose-1-phosphate uridyl transferase. *Mol Biol Med* **7**:365, 1990.
96. Leslie ND, Immerman EB, Flach JE, Florez M, Fridovich-Keil JL, Elsas LJ: The human galactose-1-phosphate uridyltransferase gene. *Genomics* **14**:474, 1992.
97. Langley SD, Lai K, Dembure PP, Hjelm LN, Elsas LJ: Molecular basis for Duarte and Los Angeles variant galactosemia. *Am J Hum Genet* **60**:366, 1997.
98. Lemaire HG, Muller HB: Nucleotide sequences of the *gal E* gene and the *gal T* gene of *E. coli*. *Nucleic Acids Res* **14**:7705, 1986.
99. Tajima M, Nogi Y, Fukasawa T: Primary structure of the *Saccharomyces cerevisiae GAL7* gene. *Yeast* **1**:67, 1985.
100. Tyfield, L.: *GALT* database. http://www.ich.bris.ac.uk/galtdb/.
101. Antonarakis SE: Recommendations for a nomenclature system for human gene mutations: Nomenclature Working Group. *Hum Mutat* **11**:1, 1998.
102. Lin MS, Oizumi J, Ng WG, Alfi OS, Donnell GN: Regional mapping of the gene for human UDPGal 4-epimerase on chromosome 1 in mouse-human hybrids. *Cytogenet Cell Genet* **24**:217, 1979.
103. Benn PA, Shows TB, D'Ancona GG, Croce CM, Orkwiszewski KG, Mellman WJ: Assignment of a gene for uridine diphosphate galactose-4-epimerase to human chromosome 1 by somatic cell hybridization, with evidence for a regional assignment to 1pter yields 1p21. *Cytogenet Cell Genet* **24**:138, 1979.
104. Maceratesi P, Daude N, Dallapiccola B, et al.: Human UDP-galactose 4′ epimerase (*GALE*) gene and identification of five missense mutations in patients with epimerase-deficiency galactosemia. *Mol Genet Metab* **63**:26, 1998.
105. Oberman AE, Wilson WA, Frasier SD, Donnell GN, Bergren WR: Galactokinase-deficiency cataracts in identical twins. *Am J Ophthalmol* **74**:887, 1972.
106. Levy NS, Krill AE, Beutler E: Galactokinase deficiency and cataracts. *Am J Ophthalmol* **74**:41, 1972.
107. Pickering WR, Howell RR: Galactokinase deficiency: Clinical and biochemical findings in a new kindred. *J Pediatr* **81**:50, 1972.
108. Cook JG, Don NA, Mann TP: Hereditary galactokinase deficiency. *Arch Dis Child* **46**:465, 1971.
109. Kerr MM, Logan RW, Cant JS, Hutchison JH: Galactokinase deficiency in a newborn infant. *Arch Dis Child* **46**:864, 1971.
110. Dahlqvist A, Gamstorp I, Madsen H: A patient with hereditary galactokinase deficiency. *Acta Paediatr Scand* **59**:669, 1970.
111. Anand VR, Sindhi JC: Kinase defect in galactosaemia: A case report. *Indian Pediatr* **16**:379, 1979.
112. Verma KC, Jamwal DS, Gupta S: A variant of galactosemia presenting as larger bilateral lenticular opacities in an older child. *Indian Pediatr* **16**:375, 1979.
113. Hodes BL, Schietroma JM, Lane SS, Sadeghi J, Cunningham D, Stambolian D: Macular deposits in galactokinase deficiency. *Metab Pediatr Syst Ophthalmol* **8**:39, 1985.
114. Segal S, Rutman JY, Frimpter GW: Galactokinase deficiency and mental retardation. *J Pediatr* **95**:750, 1979.
115. Borzy MS, Wolff L, Gewurz A, Buist NR, Lovrien E: Recurrent sepsis with deficiencies of C2 and galactokinase. *Am J Dis Child* **138**:186, 1984.
116. Litman N, Kanter AI, Finberg L: Galactokinase deficiency presenting as pseudotumor cerebri. *J Pediatr* **86**:410, 1975.
117. Colin J, Voyer M, Thomas D, Schapira F, Satge P: [Cataract due to galactokinase deficiency in a premature infant] Cataracte par déficit en galactokinase chez un premature. *Arch Fr Pediatr* **33**:77, 1976.
118. Huttenlocher PR, Hillman RE, Hsia YE: Pseudotumor cerebri in galactosemia. *J Pediatr* **76**:902, 1970.
119. Skalka HW, Prchal JT: Presenile cataract formation and decreased activity of galactosemic enzymes. *Arch Ophthalmol* 98:269, 1980.
120. Monteleone JA, Beutler E, Monteleone PL, Utz CL, Casey EC: Cataracts, galactosuria and hypergalactosemia due to galactokinase deficiency in a child: Studies of a kindred. *Am J Med* **50**:403, 1971.
121. Prchal JT, Conrad ME, Skalka HW: Association of presenile cataracts with heterozygosity for galactosaemic states and with riboflavin deficiency. *Lancet* **1**:12, 1978.
122. Winder AF, Claringbold LJ, Jones RB, et al.: Partial galactose disorders in families with premature cataracts. *Arch Dis Child* **58**:362, 1983.
123. Stambolian D, Scarpino-Myers V, Eagle RC Jr, Hodes B, Harris H: Cataracts in patients heterozygous for galactokinase deficiency. *Invest Ophthalmol Vis Sci* **27**:429, 1986.
124. Elman MJ, Miller MT, Matalon R: Galactokinase activity in patients with idiopathic cataracts. *Ophthalmology* **93**:210, 1986.
125. Simonelli F, Giovane A, Frunzio S, et al.: Galactokinase activity in patients with idiopathic presenile and senile cataract. *Metab Pediatr Syst Ophthalmol* **15**:53, 1992.
126. Stevens RE, Datiles MB, Srivastava SK, Ansari NH, Maumenee AE, Stark WJ: Idiopathic presenile cataract formation and galactosaemia. *Br J Ophthalmol* **73**:48, 1989.
127. Beutler E, Matsumoto F, Kuhl W, et al.: Galactokinase deficiency as a cause of cataracts. *N Engl J Med* **288**:1203, 1973.
128. Magnani M, Cucchiarini L, Stocchi V, Dacha M: Red blood cell galactokinase activity and presenile cataracts. *Enzyme* **29**:58, 1983.
129. Stambolian D: Galactose and cataract. *Surv Ophthalmol* **32**:333, 1988.
130. Simoons FJ: A geographic approach to senile cataracts: Possible links with milk consumption, lactase activity, and galactose metabolism. *Dig Dis Sci* **27**:257, 1982.
131. Kolosha V, Anoia E, deCespedes C, Gitzelmann R, Shih L, Casco T, Sabori M, Trejos R, Buist N, Tedesco T, Skach W, Mitelmann O, Ledee D, Huang K, Stambolian D: Novel mutations in 13 probands with galactokinase deficiency. *Hum Mutat* **15**:447, 2000.
131a. Kalaydjieva L, Perez-Lezaun A, Angelicheva D, Onengut S, Dye D, Bosshard NU, Jordanova A, Savov A, Yanakiev P, Kremensky I, Radeva B, Halimayer J, Markov A, Nedkova V, Tournev I, Aneva L, Gitzelmann R: A founder mutation in the GK1 gene is responsible for galactokinase deficiency in Rome (Gypsies). *Am J Hum Genet* **65**:1299, 1999.
132. Hazeyama A, Ohtake A, Harashima H, et al.: cDNA analysis of a male case with galactokinase deficiency. *International Congress of Inborn Errors of Metabolism* W130,1997. (abstr.)
133. Cooper DN, Youssoufian H: The CpG dinucleotide and human genetic disease. *Hum Genet* **78**:151, 1988.
134. Gitzelmann R: Hereditary galactokinase deficiency: A newly recognized cause of juvenile cataracts. *Pediatr Res* **1**:14, 1967.
135. Gitzelmann R, Wells HJ, Segal S: Galactose metabolism in a patient with hereditary galactokinase deficiency. *Eur J Clin Invest* **4**:79, 1974.
136. Mayes JS, Guthrie R: Detection of heterozygotes for galactokinase deficiency in a human population. *Biochem Genet* **2**:219, 1968.
137. Shih VE, Levy HI, Karolkewicz V, et al.: Galactosemia screening of newborns in Massachusetts. *N Engl J Med* **284**:753, 1971.
138. Tedesco TA, Miller KL, Rawnsley BE, Mennuti MT, Spielman RS, Mellman WJ: Human erythrocyte galactokinase and galactose-1-phosphate uridylyltransferase: A population survey. *Am J Hum Genet* **27**:737, 1975.
139. Newborn screening fact sheets. American Academy of Pediatrics. Committee on Genetics. *Pediatrics* **98**:473, 1996.
140. Ng WG, Xu YK, Kaufman FR, et al.: Biochemical and molecular studies of 132 patients with galactosemia. *Hum Genet* **94**:359, 1994.
141. Komrower GM, Lee DH: Long-term follow-up of galactosaemia. *Arch Dis Child* **45**:367, 1970.
142. Waggoner DD, Buist NR, Donnell GN: Long-term prognosis in galactosaemia: Results of a survey of 350 cases. *J Inherit Metab Dis* **13**:802, 1990.
143. Schweitzer S, Shin Y, Jakobs C, Brodehl J: Long-term outcome in 134 patients with galactosemia. *Eur J Pediatr* **152**:36, 1993.
144. Cleary MA, Heptinstall LE, Wraith JE, Walter JH: Galactosaemia: Relationship of IQ to biochemical control and genotype. *J Inherit Metab Dis* **18**:151, 1995.
145. Donnell GN, Collado M, Koch R: Growth and development of children with galactosemia. *J Pediatr* **58**:836, 1961.
146. Kaufman FR, McBride-Chang C, Manis FR, Wolff JA, Nelson MD: Cognitive functioning, neurologic status and brain imaging in classical galactosemia. *Eur J Pediatr* **154**:S2, 1995.
147. Fishler K, Donnell GN, Bergren WR, Koch R: Intellectual and personality development in children with galactosemia. *Pediatrics* **50**:412, 1972.

148. Manis FR, Cohn LB, McBride-Chang C, Wolff JA, Kaufman FR: A longitudinal study of cognitive functioning in patients with classical galactosaemia, including a cohort treated with oral uridine. *J Inherit Metab Dis* **20**:549, 1997.
149. Waisbren SE, Norman TR, Schnell RR, Levy HL: Speech and language deficits in early-treated children with galactosemia. *J Pediatr* **102**:75, 1983.
150. Nelson CD, Waggoner DD, Donnell GN, Tuerck JM, Buist NR: Verbal dyspraxia in treated galactosemia. *Pediatrics* **88**:346, 1991.
151. Hansen TW, Henrichsen B, Rasmussen RK, Carling A, Andressen AB, Skjeldal O: Neuropsychological and linguistic follow-up studies of children with galactosaemia from an unscreened population. *Acta Paediatr* **85**:1197, 1996.
152. Fishler K, Koch R, Donnell GN, Wenz E: Developmental aspects of galactosemia from infancy to childhood. *Clin Pediatr (Philadelphia)* **19**:38, 1980.
153. Fishler K, Koch R, Donnell G, Graliker BV: Psychological correlates in galactosemia. *Am J Ment Defic* **71**:116, 1966.
154. Sardharwalla IB, Wraith JE: Galactosaemia. *Nutr Health* **5**:175, 1987.
155. Jan JE, Wilson RA: Unusual late neurological sequelae in galactosaemia. *Dev Med Child Neurol* **15**:72, 1973.
156. Bohu PA, Hannequin D, Hemet C, Brivet M, Samson Y, Augustin P: [Late neurologic complications of galactosemia: Study of 3 cases] Complications neurologiques tardives de la galactosemie: Etude de trois cas. *Rev Neurol (Paris)* **151**:136, 1995.
157. Koch TK, Schmidt KA, Wagstaff JE, Ng WG, Packman S: Neurologic complications in galactosemia. *Pediatr Neurol* **8**:217, 1992.
158. Friedman JH, Levy HL, Boustany RM: Late onset of distinct neurologic syndromes in galactosemic siblings. *Neurology* **39**:741, 1989.
159. Bohles H, Wenzel D, Shin YS: Progressive cerebellar and extrapyramidal motor disturbances in galactosaemic twins. *Eur J Pediatr* **145**:413, 1986.
160. Lo W, Packman S, Nash S, et al.: Curious neurologic sequelae in galactosemia. *Pediatrics* **73**:309, 1984.
161. Choulot JJ, Brivet M, Virlon P, et al.: [Severe neurologic course of galactosemia. Default of myelinization caused by deficient synthesis of UDP-galactose?] Evolution neurologique severe d'une galactosemie: Defaut de myelinisation par synthese insuffisante en UDP galactose? *Arch Fr Pediatr* **48**:267, 1991.
162. Nelson MD Jr, Wolff JA, Cross CA, Donnell GN, Kaufman FR: Galactosemia: Evaluation with MR imaging. *Radiology* **184**:255, 1992.
163. Kaufman FR, Donnell GN, Roe TF, Kogut MD: Gonadal function in patients with galactosaemia. *J Inherit Metab Dis* **9**:140, 1986.
164. Chen YT, Mattison DR, Feigenbaum L, Fukui H, Schulman JD: Reduction in oocyte number following prenatal exposure to a diet high in galactose. *Science* **214**:1145, 1981.
165. Hoefnagel D, Wurster-Hill D, Child EL: Ovarian failure in galactosaemia [letter]. *Lancet* **2**:1197, 1979.
166. Morrow RJ, Atkinson AB, Carson DJ, Carson NA, Sloan JM, Traub AI: Ovarian failure in a young woman with galactosaemia. *Ulster Med J* **54**:218, 1985.
167. Levy HL, Driscoll SG, Porensky RS, Wender DF: Ovarian failure in galactosemia [letter]. *N Engl J Med* **310**:50, 1984.
168. Gibson JB: Gonadal function in galactosemics and in galactose-intoxicated animals. *Eur J Pediatr* **154**:S14, 1995.
169. Prestoz LL, Couto AS, Shin YS, Petry KG: Altered follicle stimulating hormone isoforms in female galactosaemia patients. *Eur J Pediatr* **156**:116, 1997.
170. Sardharwalla IB, Komrower GM, Schwarz V: Pregnancy in classical galactosaemia, in Burman D, Holton JB, Pennock CA (eds): *Inherited disorders of carbohydrate metabolism*. Lancaster, UK, MTP Press, 1980, p 125.
171. Brivet M, Raymond JP, Konopka P, Odievre M, Lemonnier A: Effect of lactation in a mother with galactosemia. *J Pediatr* **115**:280, 1989.
172. Sauer MV, Kaufman FR, Paulson RJ, Lobo RA: Pregnancy after oocyte donation to a woman with ovarian failure and classical galactosemia. *Fertil Steril* **55**:1197, 1991.
173. Aughton DJ: Mullerian duct abnormalities and galactosaemia heterozygosity: Report of a family. *Clin Dysmorphol* **2**:55, 1993.
174. Cramer DW, Goldstein DP, Fraer C, Reichardt JK: Vaginal agenesis (Mayer-Rokitansky-Kuster-Hauser syndrome) associated with the N314D mutation of galactose-1-phosphate uridyl transferase (GALT). *Mol Hum Reprod* **2**:145, 1996.
175. Cramer DW, Hornstein MD, Ng WG, Barbieri RL: Endometriosis associated with the N314D mutation of galactose-1-phosphate uridyl transferase (GALT). *Mol Hum Reprod* **2**:149, 1996.
176. Cramer DW, Barbieri RL, Xu H, Reichardt JK: Determinants of basal follicle-stimulating hormone levels in premenopausal women. *J Clin Endocrinol Metab* **79**:1105, 1994.
177. Sayle AE, Cooper GS, Savitz DA: Menstrual and reproductive history of mothers of galactosemic children. *Fertil Steril* **65**:534, 1996.
178. Reichardt JK, Woo SL: Molecular basis of galactosemia: Mutations and polymorphisms in the gene encoding human galactose-1-phosphate uridylyltransferase [published erratum appears in *Proc Natl Acad Sci U S A* 88:7457, 1991]. *Proc Natl Acad Sci U S A* **88**:2633, 1991.
178a. Tyfield L, Reichardt J, Fridovich-Keil J, et al: Classical galactosaemia and mutations at the galactose-1-phosphate uridyl transferase (GALT) gene. *Hum Mutat* **13**:417, 1999,
179. Reichardt JK: Molecular analysis of 11 galactosemia patients. *Nucleic Acids Res* **19**:7049, 1991.
180. Fridovich-Keil JL, Jinks-Robertson S: A yeast expression system for human galactose-1-phosphate uridylyltransferase. *Proc Natl Acad Sci U S A* **90**:398, 1993.
181. Wadelius C, Lagerkvist A, Molin AK, Larsson A, von Dobeln U, Pettersson U: Galactosemia caused by a point mutation that activates cryptic donor splice site in the galactose-1-phosphate uridyltransferase gene. *Genomics* **17**:525, 1993.
182. Field TL, Reznikoff WS, Frey PA: Galactose-1-phosphate uridylyltransferase: Identification of histidine-164 and histidine-166 as critical residues by site-directed mutagenesis. *Biochemistry* **28**:2094, 1989.
182a. Geeganage S, Frey PA: Transient kinetics of formation and reaction of the uridylyl-enzyme form of galactose-1-phosphate uridyltransferase and its Q168R variant: Insight into the molecular basis of galactosaemia. *Biochemistry* **37**:14500,1998.
182b. Lai K, Willis AC, Elsas U: The biochemical role of glutamine 188 in human galactose-1-phosphate uridyl transferase. *J Biol Chem* **274**: 6559, 1999.
183. Elsas LJ, Fridovich-Keil JL, Leslie ND: Galactosemia: A molecular approach to the enigma. *Int Pediatr* **8**:101, 1993.
184. Reichardt J: The molecular genetic basis of galactosemia. *Int Pediatr* **8**:110, 1993.
185. Elsas LJ, Langley S, Paulk EM, Hjelm LN, Dembure PP: A molecular approach to galactosemia. *Eur J Pediatr* **154**:S21–S27, 1995.
186. Wong LJ, Xu YK, Want BT, Williams J, Kaufman F, Ng WG: Genotyping of 277 galactosemia patients. *Am J Hum Genet* **59(suppl)**:A295, 1996. (abstr.)
187. Murphy M, Sexton D, O'Neill C, Croke DT, Mayne PD, Naughten ER: Frequency distribution of the Q188R mutation in the Irish galactosaemic population. *J Inherit Metab Dis* **19**:217, 1996.
188. Murphy M, McHugh B, Tighe O, Mayne P, O'Neill C, Naughten E, Croke D: The genetic basis of transferase-deficient galactosaemia in Ireland and the population history of the Irish Travellers. *Eur J Hum Genet* **7**:549, 1999.
189. Tyfield L, Stephenson A, Carmichael D, et al.: A database of genetic variation at the GALT gene: Preliminary evidence on 500 chromosomes for stratification by population and region in Europe, in *Proceedings of the European Science Foundation Conference on Inherited Disorders and Their Genes in Different European Populations 1998.* (abstr.)
190. Greber-Platzer S, Guldberg P, Scheibenreiter S, et al.: Molecular heterogeneity of classical and Duarte galactosemia: Mutation analysis by denaturing gradient gel electrophoresis. *Hum Mutat* **10**:49, 1997.
191. Kozak L, Francova H, Pijackova A, et al: Presence of a deletion in the 5′ upstream region of the GALT gene in Duarte (D2) alleles. *J Med Genet***36**:576, 1999.
191a. Zekanowski C, Radomyska B, Bal J: Molecular characterization of Polish patients with classical galactosemia. *J Inher Metab Dis* **22**:679, 1999.
192. Reichardt JK, Levy HL, Woo SL: Molecular characterization of two galactosemia mutations and one polymorphism: Implications for structure-function analysis of human galactose-1-phosphate uridylyltransferase. *Biochemistry* **31**:5430, 1992.

193. Lai K, Langley SD, Singh RH, Dembure PP, Hjelm LN, Elsas LJ: A prevalent mutation for galactosemia among black Americans. *J Pediatr* **128**:89, 1996.

193a. Manga N, Jenkins T, Jackson DA, Whittaker DA, Lane AB: The molecular basis of transferase galactosaemia in South African negroids. *J Inherit Metab Dis* **22**:37, 1999.

194. Chakraborty R, Kamboh MI, Nwankwo M, Ferrell RE: Caucasian genes in American blacks: New data [see comments]. *Am J Hum Genet* **50**:145, 1992.

195. Ashino J, Okano Y, Suyama I, et al.: Molecular characterization of galactosemia (type 1) mutations in Japanese. *Hum Mutat* **6**:36, 1995.

196. Hirokawa H, Okano Y, Asada M, Fujimoto A, Suyama I, Isshiti G.: Molecular basis for phenotypic heterogeneity in galactosaemia: predication of clinical phenotype from genotype in Japanese patients. *Eur J Hum Genet* **7**:757, 1999.

196a. Seyrantepe V, Ozguc M, Coskun T, Ozalp I, Reichardt JK: Identification of mutations in the galatose-1-phosphate uridyltransferase (GALT) gene in 16 Turkish patients with galactosemia, including a novel mutation of F294Y. *Hum Mutat* **13**:339, 1999.

197. Coskun T, Erkul E, Seyrantepe V, Ozguc M, Tokatli A, Ozalp I: Mutational analysis of Turkish galactosaemia patients. *J Inherit Metab Dis* **18**:368, 1995.

198. Maceratesi P, Sangiuolo F, Novelli G, et al.: Three new mutations (P183T, V150L, 528insG) and eleven sequence polymorphisms in Italian patients with galactose-1-phosphate uridyltransferase (GALT) deficiency. *Hum Mutat* **8**:369, 1996.

198a. Heyer E: Genetic consequences of differential demographic behaviour in the Saguenay region, Quebec. *Am J Phys Anthropol* **98**:1, 1995.

199. Tyfield L, Stephenson A, Holton JB: Mutation analysis and psychometric assessments in the galactosaemic population of the British Isles. *J Med Genet* **34**:S18, 1997. (abstr.)

200. Muralidharan K, Zhang W, Dembure PP, et al.: A naturally occurring, 'knock-out' mutation of human galactose-1-phosphate uridyl transferase gene reveals an alternate pathway for galactose metabolism. *Am J Hum Genet* **59(suppl)**:A204, 1996. (abstr.)

201. Beutler E, Baluda MC, Sturgeon P, Day RW: A new genetic abnormality resulting in galactose-1-phosphate uridyltransferase deficiency. *Lancet* **1**:353, 1965.

202. Kelley RI, Harris H, Mellman WJ: Characterization of normal and abnormal variants of galactose-1-phosphate uridylyltransferase (EC 2.7.7.12) by isoelectric focusing. *Hum Genet* **63**:274, 1983.

203. Ng WG, Bergren WR, Donnell GN: A new variant of galactose-1-phosphate uridyltransferase in man. *Ann Hum Genet* **37**:1, 1972.

204. Lin HC, Kirby LT, Ng WG, Reichardt JK: On the molecular nature of the Duarte variant of galactose-1-phosphate uridyl transferase (GALT). *Hum Genet* **93**:167, 1994.

205. Elsas LJ, Dembure PP, Langley S, Paulk EM, Hjelm LN, Fridovich-Keil J: A common mutation associated with the Duarte galactosemia allele. *Am J Hum Genet* **54**:1030, 1994.

206. Gathof BS, Sommer M, Podskarbi T, et al.: Characterization of two stop codon mutations in the galactose-1-phosphate uridyltransferase gene of three male galactosemic patients with severe clinical manifestation. *Hum Genet* **96**:721, 1995.

207. Greber S, Guldberg P, Scheibenreiter S, Strobl W: Mutations in classical and Duarte 2 galactosemia. *Ped Res* **38**:434,1995. (abstr.)

208. Podskarbi T, Kohlmetz T, Gathof BS, et al.: Molecular characterization of Duarte-1 and Duarte-2 variants of galactose-1-phosphate uridyltransferase. *J Inherit Metab Dis* **19**:638, 1996.

209. Lin HC, Reichardt JK: Linkage disequilibrium between a *Sac*I restriction fragment length polymorphism and two galactosemia mutations. *Hum Genet* **95**:353, 1995.

210. Podskarbi T, Shin YS: Neonatal screening and differential diagnosis of galactosemia, in *Proceedings of the 3rd Meeting of the International Society for Neonatal Screening*, Boston, p 317, 1998.

210a. Shin YS, Koch HG, Kohler M, Hoffman G, Patsoura A, Podskarbi T: Duarte-1 (Los Angeles) and Duarte-1 (Duarte) variants in Germany: Two new mutations in the GALT gene which cause GALT activity decrease by 40–50% of normal in red cells. *J Inherit Metab Dis* **21**:232, 1998.

211. Lai K, Langley SD, Dembure PP, Hjelm LN, Elsas LJ: Duarte allele impairs biostability of galactose-1-phosphate uridyltransferase in human lymphoblasts. *Hum Mutat* **11**:28, 1998.

212. Tyfield LA, Holton JB, Stephenson A, Marlow N: Mutation analysis and psychometric assessments in the galactosaemia population of the British Isles. *International Congress of Inborn Errors of Metabolism* W121,1997. (abstr.)

213. Elsas LJ, Langley S, Steele E, et al.: Galactosemia: A strategy to identify new biochemical phenotypes and molecular genotypes. *Am J Hum Genet* **56**:630, 1995.

214. Podskarbi T, Bieger WP, Shin YS: Allelic heterogeneity of the galactose-1-phosphate uridyltransferase gene: Biochemical and clinical phenotypes. *Eur J Clin Chem Clin Biochem* **35**:A27,1997. (abstr.)

215. Ichiba Y: The variant of galactosemia. *Jpn J Pediatr* **42**:579, 1989.

216. Sommer M, Gathof BS, Podskarbi T, Giugliani R, Kleinlein B, Shin YS: Mutations in the galactose-1-phosphate uridyltransferase gene of two families with mild galactosaemia variants. *J Inherit Metab Dis* **18**:567, 1995.

217. Kaufman FR, Reichardt JK, Ng WG, et al.: Correlation of cognitive, neurologic, and ovarian outcome with the Q188R mutation of the galactose-1-phosphate uridyltransferase gene. *J Pediatr* **125**:225, 1994.

218. Podskarbi T, Franzmann H, Kleinlein B, Gathof BS, Shin YS: A genotype-phenotype correlation in classical galactosemia, in *Diagnosis and Treatment of Inborn Errors of Metabolism*. Turkish Society for PKU, 1996, p 56.

219. Reichardt JK, Belmont JW, Levy HL, Woo SL: Characterization of two missense mutations in human galactose-1-phosphate uridyltransferase: Different molecular mechanisms for galactosemia. *Genomics* **12**:596, 1992.

220. Shin YS, Gathof BS, Podskarbi T, Sommer M, Giugliani R, Gresser U: Three missense mutations in the galactose-1-phosphate uridyltransferase gene of three families with mild galactosaemia. *Eur J Pediatr* **155**:393, 1996.

220a. Shin YS, Zschocke J, Das AM, Podskarbi T: Molecular and biochemical basis for variants and deficiency forms of galactose-1-phosphate uridyltransferase. *J Inher Metab Dis* **22**:327, 1999.

221. Baker L, Mellman WJ, Tedesco TA, Segal S: Galactosemia: Symptomatic and asymptomatic homozygotes in one Negro sibship. *J Pediatr* **68**:551, 1966.

222. Fridovich-Keil JL, Langley SD, Mazur LA, Lennon JC, Dembure PP, Elsas JL: Identification and functional analysis of three distinct mutations in the human galactose-1-phosphate uridyltransferase gene associated with galactosemia in a single family. *Am J Hum Genet* **56**:640, 1995.

223. Wells L, Fridovich-Keil JL: Biochemical characterization of the S135L allele of galactose-1-phosphate uridylyltransferase associated with galactosaemia. *J Inherit Metab Dis* **20**:633, 1997.

223a. Topper V, Laster L, Segal S: Galactose metabolism: Phenotype differences among tissues of a patient with congenital galactosemia. *Nature* **196**:1006, 1962.

224. Fridovich-Keil JL, Quimby BB, Wells L, Mazur LA, Elsevier JP: Characterization of the N314D allele of human galactose-1-phosphate uridylyltransferase using a yeast expression system. *Biochem Mol Med* **56**:121, 1995.

224a. Anderson M, Williams V, Sparkes M, Sparkes R: Transferase deficiency galactosemia: Immunochemical studies of the Duarte and Los Angeles variants. *Hum Genet* **65**:287, 1984.

224b. Heinemeyer T, Wingender E, Reuter I, et al: Databases on transcriptional regulation: TRANSFAC, TRRD, and COMPEL. *Nucleic Acids Res* **26**:362, 1998.

225. Kurland CG: Codon bias and gene expression. *FEBS Lett.* **285**:165, 1991.

225a. Hadfield RM, Manek S, Nakago S, Mukherjee S, Weeks DE, Mardon HJ, Barlow DH, Kennedy SH. Absence of a relationship between endometriosis and the N324D polymorphism of galactose-1-phosphate uridyl transferase in a UK population. *Mol Hum Reprod* **5**:990, 1999.

226. Inouye T, Nadler HL, Hsia YY: Galactose-I-phosphate uridyltransferase in red and white blood cells. *Clin Chim Acta* **19**:169, 1968.

227. Krooth R, Winberg AN: Studies on cell lines developed from the tissues of patients with galactosaemia. *J Exp Med* **113**:1155, 1964.

228. Segal S, Blair A, Roth H: The metabolism of galactose by patients with congenital galactosemia. *Am J Med* **38**:62, 1965.

229. Chacko CM, Christian JC, Nadler HL: Unstable galactose-1-phosphate uridyl transferase: A new variant of galactosemia. *J Pediatr* **78**:454, 1971.

230. Hammersen G, Houghton S, Levy HL: Rennes-like variant of galactosemia: Clinical and biochemical studies. *J Pediatr* **87**:50, 1975.

231. Xu YK, Kaufman FR, Donnell GN, Ng WG: Radiochemical assay of minute quantities of galactose-1-phosphate uridyltransferase activity in erythrocytes and leukocytes of galactosemia patients. *Clin Chim Acta* **235**:125, 1995.

232. Ng WG, Xu YH, Kaufman FR, Lefauconnier JM, Donnell GN: Biochemical and clinical heterogeneity among 358 galactosaemic patients. *Neonatal Screening in the Nineties* 181, 1991.

233. Kaufman FR, Xu YK, Ng WG, Donnell GN: Correlation of ovarian function with galactose-1-phosphate uridyl transferase levels in galactosemia [published erratum appears in *J Pediatr* 1989 115:329]. *J Pediatr* **112**:754, 1988.

234. Siegel CD, Sparks JW, Battaglia FC: Patterns of serum glucose and galactose concentrations in term newborn infants after milk feeding. *Biol Neonate* **54**:301, 1988.

235. Greenman L, Rathbun JC: Galactose studies in an infant with idiopathic galactose intolerance. *Paediatrics* **2**:666, 1948.

236. Jansen G, Muskiet FA, Schierbeek H, Berger R, van der Slik W: Capillary gas chromatographic profiling of urinary, plasma and erythrocyte sugars and polyols as their trimethylsilyl derivatives, preceded by a simple and rapid prepurification method. *Clin Chim Acta* **157**:277, 1986.

237. Schwarz V: The value of galactose-1-phosphate determinations in the treatment of galactosaemia. *Arch Dis Child.* **35**:428, 1960.

238. Gitzelmann R, Curtius HC, Schneller I: Galactitol and galactose-1-phosphate in the lens of a galactosemic infant. *Exp Eye Res* **6**:1, 1967.

239. Ng WG, Donnell GN, Bergren WR, Alfi O, Golbus MS: Prenatal diagnosis of galactosemia. *Clin Chim Acta* **74**:227, 1977.

240. Allen JT, Gillett M, Holton JB, King GS, Pettit BR: Evidence for galactosaemia in utero [letter]. *Lancet* **1**:603, 1980.

241. Gitzelmann R: Galactose-1-phosphate in the pathophysiology of galactosemia. *Eur J Pediatr* **154**:S45, 1995.

242. Quan-Ma R, Wells HJ, Wells WW, Sherman FE, Egan TJ: Galactitol in the tissues of a galactosemic child. *Am J Dis Child* **112**:477, 1966.

243. Wells WW, Pitzalis MV, Egan TJ: The isolation and identification of galactitol from the brains of galactosemic patients. *J Biol Chem* **240**:1002, 1965.

244. Wells WW, Pittman TA: The isolation and identification of galactitol from the urine of patients with galactosemia. *J Biol Chem* **239**:3192, 1964.

245. Allen JT, Holton JB, Gillett MG: Gas-liquid chromatographic determination of galactitol in amniotic fluid for possible use in prenatal diagnosis of galactosaemia. *Clin Chim Acta* **110**:59, 1981.

246. Shin YS, Reith S, Hover S, Endres W: Uridine diphosphogalactose, galactitol and galactose-1-phosphate concentration in patients with classical galactosemia. *Proceedings of the Annual Symposium of the SSIEM* **23**:34, 1985.

247. Ng WG, Xu YK, Kaufman FR, Donnell GN: Deficit of uridine diphosphate galactose in galactosaemia. *J Inherit Metab Dis* **12**:257, 1989.

248. Berry GT, Palmieri MJ, Heales S, Leonard JV, Segal S: Red blood cell uridine sugar nucleotide levels in patients with classic galactosemia and other metabolic disorders. *Metabolism* **41**:783, 1992.

249. Keevill NJ, Holton JB, Allen JT: The investigation of UDPGlucose and UDPGalactose concentration in red blood cells of patients with classical galactosaemia. *Clin Chim Acta* **221**:135, 1993.

250. Kirkman HN: Uridine diphosphate glucose and uridine diphosphate galactose in galactosemia. *J Pediatr* **117**:838, 1990.

251. Wehrli SL, Palmieri MJ, Reynolds RA, Segal S: 31P NMR spectra of intact red blood cells: Quantitation of UDPGlucose and UDPGalactose. *Magn Reson Med* **30**:494, 1993.

252. Gibson JB, Reynolds RA, Palmieri MJ, States B, Berry GT, Segal S: Uridine diphosphate hexoses in leukocytes and fibroblasts of classic galactosemics and patients with other metabolic diseases. *Pediatr Res* **36**:613, 1994.

253. Keevill NJ, Holton JB, Allen JT: UDP-glucose and UDP-galactose concentrations in cultured skin fibroblasts of patients with classical galactosaemia. *J Inherit Metab Dis* **17**:23, 1994.

254. Xu YK, Kaufman FR, Donnell GN, Giudici T, Alfi O, Ng WG: HPLC analysis of uridine diphosphate sugars: Decreased concentrations of uridine diphosphate galactose in erythrocytes and cultured skin fibroblasts from classical galactosemia patients. *Clin Chim Acta* **240**:21, 1995.

255. Gibson JB, Reynolds RA, Palmieri MJ, et al.: Comparison of erythrocyte uridine sugar nucleotide levels in normals, classic galactosemics, and patients with other metabolic disorders. *Metabolism* **44**:597, 1995.

256. Gibson JB, Berry GT, Palmieri MJ, Reynolds RA, Mazur AT, Segal S: Sugar nucleotide concentrations in red blood cells of patients on protein- and lactose-limited diets: Effect of galactose supplementation. *Am J Clin Nutr* **63**:704, 1996.

257. Beutler E, Baluda MC: A simple spot screening test for galactosemia. *J Lab Clin Med* **68**:137, 1966.

258. Beutler E: Galactosemia: Screening and diagnosis. *Clin Biochem* **24**:293, 1991.

259. Mathias D, Bickel H: Follow-up study of 16 years neonatal screening for inborn errors of metabolism in West Germany. *Eur J Pediatr* **145**:310, 1986.

260. Frey C: [Klinefelter syndrome: is early diagnosis by screening study necessary?] Klinefelter-Syndrom: Ist eine Fruhdiagnose durch Screeninguntersuchung anzustreben? *Monatsschr Kinderheilkd* **134**:78, 1986.

261. Honeyman MM, Green A, Holton JB, Leonard JV: Galactosaemia: Results of the British Paediatric Surveillance Unit Study, 1988–90. *Arch Dis Child* **69**:339, 1993.

262. Kirby LT, Norman MG, Applegarth DA, Hardwick DF: Screening of newborn infants for galactosemia in British Columbia. *Can Med Assoc J* **132**:1033, 1985.

263. Badawi N, Cahalane SF, McDonald M, et al.: Galactosaemia–a controversial disorder: Screening & outcome: Ireland 1972-1992. *Ir Med J* **89**:16, 1996.

264. Schweitzer S: Newborn mass screening for galactosemia. *Eur J Pediatr* **154**:S37, 1995.

265. Gitzelmann R, Bosshard NU: Partial deficiency of galactose-1-phosphate uridyltransferase. *Eur J Pediatr* **154**:S40, 1995.

266. Wiesmann UN, Rose-Beutler B, Schluchter R: Leguminosae in the diet: The raffinose-stachyose question. *Eur J Pediatr* **154**:S93, 1995.

267. Koch R, Acosta P, Ragsdale N: Nutrition in the treatment of galactosemia. *J Am Diet Assoc* **43**:216, 1963.

268. Gitzelmann R, Auricchio S: The handling of soy alpha-galactosides by a normal and a galactosemic child. *Pediatrics* **36**:231, 1965.

269. Kaufman FR, Loro ML, Azen C, Wenz E, Gilsanz V: Effect of hypogonadism and deficient calcium intake on bone density in patients with galactosemia. *J Pediatr* **123**:365, 1993.

269a. Hutchesson ACJ, Murdoch-Davis C, Green A, Preece MA, Allen J, Holton JB, Rylance G: Biochemical monitoring of treatment for galactosaemia: Biological variability in metabolite concentrations. *J Inher Metab Dis* **22**:139, 1999.

270. Gitzelmann R: Disorders of galactose metabolism, in Fernandes J, Saudubray JM, Tada K (eds): *Inborn Metabolic Diseases* 1st ed. Berlin, Springer-Verlag, 1990, p 95.

271. Roe TF, Hallatt JG, Donnell GN, Ng WG: Childbearing by a galactosemic woman. *J Pediatr* **78**:1026, 1971.

272. Jakobs C, Kleijer WJ, Bakker HD, Van Gennip AH, Przyrembel H, Niermeijer MF: Dietary restriction of maternal lactose intake does not prevent accumulation of galactitol in the amniotic fluid of fetuses affected with galactosaemia. *Prenat Diagn* **8**:641, 1988.

273. Misumi H, Wada H, Kawakami M, et al.: Detection of UDP-galactose-4-epimerase deficiency in a galactosemia screening program. *Clin Chim Acta* **116**:101, 1981.

274. Oyanagi K, Nakata F, Hirano S, et al.: Uridine diphosphate galactose 4-epimerase deficiency. *Eur J Pediatr* **135**:303, 1981.

275. Ichiba Y, Namba N, Misumi H: Uridine diphosphate galactose 4-epimerase deficiency. *Am J Dis Child* **134**:995, 1980.

276. Gitzelmann R, Steinmann B, Mitchell B, Haigis E: Uridine diphosphate galactose 4′-epimerase deficiency: IV. Report of eight cases in three families. *Helv Paediatr Acta* **31**:441, 1976.

277. Bowling FG, Fraser DK, Clague AE, Hayes A, Morris DJ: A case of uridine diphosphate galactose-4-epimerase deficiency detected by neonatal screening for galactosaemia. *Med J Aust* **144**:150, 1986.

278. Quimby BB, Alano A, Almashanu S, DeSandro AM, Cowan TM, Fridovich-Keil JL: Characterization of two mutations associated with epimerase-deficiency galactosemia, by use of a yeast expression system for human UDP- galactose-4-epimerase. *Am J Hum Genet* **61**:590, 1997.

279. Schulpis KH, Papaconstantinou ED, Koidou A, et al.: UDP galactose-4-epimerase deficiency in a 5.5-year-old girl with unilateral cataract. *J Inherit Metab Dis* **16**:903, 1993.

280. Boleda MD, Giros ML, Briones P, et al.: Severe neonatal galactose-dependent disease with low-normal epimerase activity. *J Inherit Metab Dis* **18**:88, 1995.

280a. Alano A, Almashanu S, Chinsky JM, Costeas P, Blitzer MG, Wulfsberg EA, Cowan TM: Molecular characterization of a unique patient with epimerase-deficiency galactosaemia. *J Inher Metab Dis* **21**:341, 1998.

281. Henderson MJ, Holton JB, MacFaul R: Further observations in a case of uridine diphosphate galactose-4-epimerase deficiency with a severe clinical presentation. *J Inherit Metab Dis* **6**:17, 1983.

282. Sardharwalla IB, Wraith JE, Bridge C, Fowler B, Roberts SA: A patient with severe type of epimerase deficiency galactosaemia. *J Inherit Metab Dis* **11**(suppl 2):249, 1988.

283. Walter JH, Roberts REP, Besley GTN, Wraith JE, Holton JB, MacFaul R: Generalised uridine diphosphate-4-epimerase deficiency. *Arch Dis Child* **80**:374, 1999.

284. Maceratesi P, Dallapiccola B, Novelli G, Okano Y, Isshiki G, Reichardt J: Missense mutations in Japanese patients with epimerase-deficiency galactosemia. *Am J Hum Genet* **59(suppl)**:A204, 1996. (abstr.)

284a. Wohlers TM, Christacos NC, Harrman MT, Fridovich-Keil JL: Identification and characterization of a mutation, in the human UDP-galactose-4-epimerase gene, associated with generalized epimerase-deficiency galactosemia. *Am J Hum Genet* **64**:462, 1999.

285. Gitzelmann R, Steinmann B: Uridine diphosphate galactose 4-epimerase deficiency: II. Clinical follow-up, biochemical studies and family investigation. *Helv Paediatr Acta* **28**:497, 1973.

286. Gitzelmann R, Steinmann B, Mitchell B, Haigis E: Uridine diphosphate galactose-4′-epimerase deficiency: IV. Report of 8 cases in 3 families. *Helv Paediatr Acta* **31**:441, 1976.

287. Gillett MG: Investigation of human uridine 5′ diphosphate galactose 4′ epimerase. *MSc Thesis*, University of Bath, UK, p 193, 1985.

288. Mitchell B, Haigis E, Steinmann B, Gitzelmann R: Reversal of UDP-galactose 4-epimerase deficiency of human leukocytes in culture. *Proc Natl Acad Sci U S A* **72**:5026, 1975.

289. Gitzelmann R, Haigis E: Appearance of active UDP-galactose 4′-epimerase in cells cultured from epimerase-deficient persons. *J Inherit Metab Dis* **1**:41, 1978.

290. Gitzelmann R, Hansen RG: Galactose metabolism, hereditary defects and their clinical significance, in Burman D, Holton JB, Pennock CA, (eds): *Inherited Disorders of Carbohydrate Metabolism*. Lancaster, MTP Press, 1980, p 92.

291. Holton JB, Allen JT, Gillett MG: Prenatal diagnosis of disorders of galactose metabolism. *J Inherit Metab Dis* 12(suppl **1**):202, 1989.

292. Fensom AH, Benson PF, Blunt S: Prenatal diagnosis of galactosaemia. *Br Med J* **4**:386, 1974.

293. Monk AM, Holton JB: Galactose-1-phosphate uridyltransferase in cultured cells. *Clin Chim Acta* **73**:537, 1976.

294. Ng WG, Bergren WR, Donnell GN: An improved procedure for the assay of hemolysate galactose-1-phosphate uridyl transferase activity by the use of ^{14}C-labeled galactose-1-phosphate. *Clin Chim Acta* **15**:489, 1967.

295. Kleijer WJ, Janse HC, Van Diggelen OP, et al.: First-trimester diagnosis of galactosaemia [letter]. *Lancet* **1**:748, 1986.

296. Jakobs C, Warner TG, Sweetman L, Nyhan WL: Stable isotope dilution analysis of galactitol in amniotic fluid: An accurate approach to the prenatal diagnosis of galactosemia. *Pediatr Res* **18**:714, 1984.

297. Jakobs C, Kleijer WJ, Allen J, Holton JB: Prenatal diagnosis of galactosemia. *Eur J Pediatr* **154**:S33, 1995.

298. Holton JB, Tyfield L: Prenatal diagnosis of inherited metabolic diseases, in Williams D, Marks V (eds): *Scientific Foundations of Biochemistry in Clinical Practice*. Oxford, Butterworth Heinemann Ltd, 1994, p 237.

299. Gillett MG, Holton JB, MacFaul R: Prenatal determination of uridine diphosphate galactose-4-epimerase activity. *Prenat Diagn* **3**:57, 1983.

300. Holton JB, Raymont CM: Prenatal diagnosis of classical galactosaemia, in Burman D, Holton JB, Pennock CA (eds): *Inherited Disorders of Carbohydrate Metabolism*. Lancaster, MTP Press, 1980, p 141.

301. Donnell GN, Koch R, Fishler K, Ng WG: Clinical aspects of galactosaemia, in Burman D, Holton JB, Pennock CA (eds): *Inherited Disorders of Carbohydrate Metabolism*. Lancaster, MTP Press, 1980, p 114.

302. Donnell GN, Koch R, Bergren WR: Observations on results of management of galactosemic patients, in Hsia DY (ed): *Galactosemia*. Springfield, Illinois, CC Thomas, 1969, p 247.

303. Vannas A, Hogan MJ, Golbus MS, Wood I: Lens changes in a galactosemic fetus. *Am J Ophthalmol* **80**:726, 1975.

304. Komrower GM: Galactosaemia thirty years on: The experience of a generation. *J Inherit Metab Dis* **5**:96, 1982.

305. Mayes JS, Miller LR: The metabolism of galactose by galactosemic fibroblasts *in vitro*. *Biochim Biophys Acta* **313**:9, 1973.

306. Starling JJ, Keppler DO: Metabolism of 2-deoxy-D-galactose in liver induces phosphate and uridylate trapping. *Eur J Biochem* **80**:373, 1977.

307. Kogut MD, Roe TF, Ng W, Nonnel GN: Fructose-induced hyperuricemia: Observations in normal children and in patients with hereditary fructose intolerance and galactosemia. *Pediatr Res* **9**:774, 1975.

308. Forster J, Schuchmann L, Hans C, Niederhoff H, Kunzer W, Keppler D: Increased serum urate in galactosemia patients after a galactose load: A possible role of nucleotide deficiency in galactosemic liver injury. *Klin Wochenschr* **53**:1169, 1975.

309. Welch RJ, Milligan DW: Cerebral edema and galactosemia [letter]. *Pediatrics* **80**:597, 1987.

310. Berry GT: The role of polyols in the pathophysiology of hypergalactosemia. *Eur J Pediatr* **154**:S53, 1995.

310a. Kobayashi I, Kubo E, Takahashi Y, Yonezawa H, Akagi Y: Retinal vessel changes in galactose fed dogs. *Arch Ophthalmol* **116**: 785,1998.

310b. Sugimoto K, Kasahara I, Yonezawa H, Yagihashi S: Peripheral nerve structure and function in long-term galactosemic dogs: Morphometric and electron microscopic analyses. *Acta Neuropathol* (Berlin) **97**:369,1999.

311. Haberland C, Perou M, Brunngraber EG, Hof H: The neuropathology of galactosemia: A histopathological and biochemical study. *J Neuropathol Exp Neurol* **30**:431, 1971.

312. Petry K, Greinix HT, Nudelman E, et al.: Characterization of a novel biochemical abnormality in galactosemia: Deficiency of glycolipids containing galactose or N-acetylgalactosamine and accumulation of precursors in brain and lymphocytes. *Biochem Med Metab Biol* **46**:93, 1991.

313. Dobbie JA, Holton JB, Clamp JR: Defective galactosylation of proteins in cultured skin fibroblasts from galactosaemic patients. *Ann Clin Biochem* **27**:274, 1990.

314. Ornstein KS, McGuire EJ, Berry GT, Roth S, Segal S: Abnormal galactosylation of complex carbohydrates in cultured fibroblasts from patients with galactose-1-phosphate uridyltransferase deficiency. *Pediatr Res* **31**:508, 1992.

315. Kadhom N, Baptista J, Brivet M, Wolfrom C, Gautier M: Low efficiency of [14C]-galactose incorporation by galactosemic skin fibroblasts: Relationship with neurological sequelae. *Biochem Med Metab Biol* **52**:140, 1994.

316. Wolfrom C, Raynaud N, Kadhom N, Poggi J, Soni T, Gautier M: Impaired hexose uptake by diploid skin fibroblasts from galactosaemic patients: Connection with cell growth and amino acid metabolism, and possible bearing on late-onset clinical symptoms. *J Inherit Metab Dis* **16**:78, 1993.

317. Jaeken J, Kint J, Spaapen L: Serum lysosomal enzyme abnormalities in galactosaemia [letter]. *Lancet* **340**:1472, 1992.

318. Bonham JR, Allen JT, Chapman C: Increased urinary transferrin excretion in galactosemia: A possible indicator of control, in *Abstracts of Society for the Study of Inborn Errors of Metabolism Annual Symposium*, 1994, 136.

319. Leslie ND, Yager KL, McNamara PD, Segal S: A mouse model of galactose-1-phosphate uridyl transferase deficiency. *Biochem Mol Med* **59**:7, 1996.

319a. Segal S: Komrower Lecture: Galactosaemia today: The enigma and the challenge. *J Inher Metab Dis* **21**:455,1998.

320. Xu YK, Ng WG, Kaufman FR, Lobo RA, Donnell GN: Galactose metabolism in human ovarian tissue [published erratum appears in *Pediatr Res* 1990 27:117]. *Pediatr Res* **25**:151, 1989.

321. Tedesco TA: Human galactose 1-phosphate uridyltransferase: Purification, antibody production, and comparison of the wild type, Duarte variant, and galactosemic gene products. *J Biol Chem* **247**:6631, 1972.

322. Banroques J, Gregori C, Dreyfus JC: Purification of human liver uridylyl transferase and comparison with the erythrocyte enzyme. *Biochimie* **65**:7, 1983.

323. Tedesco TA, Mellman WJ: Galactose-1-phosphate uridyltransferase and galactokinase activity in cultured human diploid fibroblasts and

peripheral blood leukocytes: I. Analysis of transferase genotypes by the ratio of the activities of the two enzymes. *J Clin Invest* **48**:2390, 1969.

324. Chacko CM, McCrone L, Nadler HL: A study of galactokinase and glucose 4-epimerase from normal and galactosemic skin fibroblasts. *Biochim Biophys Acta* **284**:552, 1972.
325. Shin-Buehring YS, Stuempfig L, Pouget E, Rahm P, Schaub J: Characterization of galactose-1-phosphate uridyl-transferase and galactokinase in human organs from the fetus and adult. *Clin Chim Acta* **112**:257, 1981.
326. Segal S, Rogers S, Holtzapple PG: Liver galactose-1-phosphate uridyl transferase: Activity in normal and galactosemic subjects. *J Clin Invest* **50**:500, 1971.
327. Rogers S, Holtzapple PG, Mellman WJ, Segal S: Characteristics of galactose-1-phosphate uridyl transferase in intestinal mucosa of normal and galactosemic humans. *Metabolism* **19**:701, 1970.
328. Lang A, Groebe H, Hellkuhl B, von FK: A new variant of galactosemia: Galactose-1-phosphate uridylyltransferase sensitive to product inhibition by glucose 1-phosphate. *Pediatr Res* **14**:729, 1980.
329. Schapira F, Kaplan JC: Electrophoretic abnormality of galactose-1-phosphate uridyl transferase in galactosemia. *Biochem Biophys Res Commun* **35**:451, 1969.
330. Chacko CM, Wappner RS, Brandt IK, Nadler HL: The Chicago variant of clinical galactosemia. *Hum Genet* **37**:261, 1977.
331. Reichardt JK, Novelli G, Dallapiccola B: Molecular characterization of the H319Q galactosemia mutation. *Hum Mol Genet* **2**:325, 1993.

CHAPTER 73

Pentosuria

Howard H. Hiatt

1. **Essential pentosuria is an inborn error of metabolism in which 1.0 to 4 g of the pentose L-xylulose is excreted in the urine each day. It is a benign disturbance that occurs principally in Jews and behaves genetically as an autosomal-recessive characteristic.**
2. **This disorder bears no relationship to diabetes mellitus and is easily distinguished from several other varieties of pentosuria in which milligram quantities of a number of pentoses other than L-xylulose appear in the urine.**
3. **Essential pentosuria is the result of a defect in the glucuronic acid oxidation pathway. In this route of carbohydrate metabolism the carboxyl carbon atom of D-glucuronic acid is removed in a series of reactions, giving rise to the pentose L-xylulose. The latter may then be converted to its stereoisomer, D-xylulose, which, in turn, may be phosphorylated. D-xylulose-5-phosphate may participate in reactions of the pentose phosphate pathway which lead to its conversion to hexose phosphate. (Glucuromic acid → gulonic acid → L-xylulose→ xylitol → D-xylulose → pentose phosphate pathway → hexose phosphate.) The glucuronic acid oxidation pathway serves no essential function in humans.**
4. **The block results from reduced activity of the nicotinamide adenine dinucleotide phosphate (NADP)-linked xylitol dehydrogenase, the enzyme that catalyzes the conversion of L-xylulose to xylitol.**
5. **The heterozygote can be recognized by demonstrating either an intermediate level of erythrocyte activity of xylitol dehydrogenase or increased urinary or serum L-xylulose, or both, in a glucuronolactone loading test.**

The first six decades that followed the original description by Salkowski and Jastrowitz in 1892 of an individual with essential pentosuria[1] yielded much information concerning the clinical aspects of this condition but virtually none that cast light on the nature of the biochemical lesion. Clinical and laboratory studies in the ensuing 18 years, however, led to identification of the metabolic defect. As a result, and perhaps even more significantly, important information was uncovered concerning the operation in normal individuals of a previously unknown pathway of carbohydrate metabolism. Such an elucidation of a normal mechanism by studies of an accident of nature led Garrod[2] in 1928 to stress "the lesions of rare maladies," and prompted Harvey[3] 300 years earlier to note that "nature is nowhere accustomed more openly to display her secret mysteries than in cases where she shows traces of her workings apart from the beaten path."

A consideration of essential pentosuria requires its separation from other conditions in which a five-carbon sugar is excreted in the urine. Essential pentosuria, or chronic essential pentosuria, is the only member of the group in which a genetic defect accounts for the melituria. It may be further defined as an innocuous condition, presumably present from birth, in which a relatively constant amount of the pentose L-xylulose appears in the urine. It has no apparent relation to diabetes mellitus and has been described almost exclusively in Jews. It is the result of an impairment in the metabolism of glucuronic acid (Fig. 73-1) and may easily be distinguished from several other situations in which much smaller quantities of certain pentoses other than L-xylulose are found in the urine (Table 73-1). The structure of some of the urinary pentoses follows:

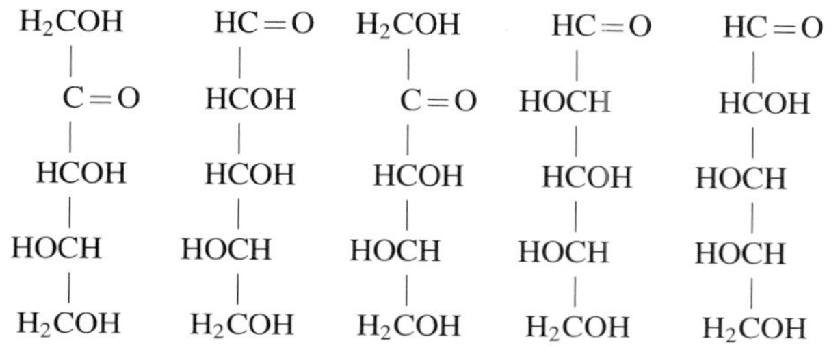

L-Xylulose	D-Ribose	D-Ribulose	L-Xylose	L-Arabinose
H_2COH	HC=O	H_2COH	HC=O	HC=O
C=O	HCOH	C=O	HOCH	HCOH
HCOH	HCOH	HCOH	HCOH	HOCH
HOCH	HOCH	HOCH	HOCH	HOCH
H_2COH	H_2COH	H_2COH	H_2COH	H_2COH

Alimentary pentosuria is the term applied to the excretion of small amounts of arabinose or xylose* following the ingestion of unusually large quantities of such fruits as plums, cherries, and grapes and fruit juices.[4–6] Small amounts of D-ribose are often present in urine from healthy persons, and slightly larger quantities may be found in the urine of some patients with muscular dystrophy,[7] presumably as a result of the excessive breakdown of ribose-containing nucleotide in degenerating muscle. Finally, traces of L-xylulose[8,9] and of D-ribulose[9] may be found in the urine of normal individuals. It is essential pentosuria with which this chapter is primarily concerned.

HISTORICAL SURVEY

In 1887 Kiliani[10] demonstrated that arabinose, the sugar of gum arabic, was a member of a hitherto undescribed class of sugars containing, in contrast to the hexoses, only five carbon atoms. Shortly thereafter, the wood sugar xylose was identified as another member of this group. The biologic significance of this class of sugars was strengthened by the report of Salkowski and Jastrowitz of a human being in whose urine a pentose was consistently excreted.[1] This sugar was not fermented by yeast, was optically inactive, and yielded an osazone with a melting point of 159°C. The latter observation led these researchers to suggest that the sugar was a pentose. Several similar case reports appeared in the German literature during the next decade, and in 1906 Janeway,[11] in a paper entitled "Essential Pentosuria in Two Brothers," recorded the first instances in an American publication. Although Janeway acknowledged that in many of the previous reports in the literature neurasthenic symptoms were prominent, he stressed that no harmful effects of the disorder were known. He emphasized that the most important responsibility of the physician was to

This chapter is reprinted from the fourth edition with an addendum by the editors as there have not been substantial developments in the area.

A list of standard abbreviations is located immediately preceding the index in each volume. Nonstandard abbreviations used in this chapter include: NADP = nicotinamide adenine dinucleotide phosphate.

* Although L-xyloses are said to be the alimentary pentoses,[4,5] the evidence for this chemical identification is not convincing.

Table 73-1 Types of Pentosuria

Type	Urine pentose	Amount excreted, g/24 *h*	Cause	Origin of pentose
Essential	L-Xylulose	1.0–4.0	Metabolic error	D-Glucuronic acid
Alimentary	L-Arabinose, L-Xylose	Less than 0.100	Excessive fruit intake	Dietary fruit
"Ribosuria"	D-Ribose	Up to 0.030	Muscular dystrophy	Muscle coenzymes (?)
Normal	L-Xylulose	Up to 0.060		
	D-Ribose	Up to 0.015		
	D-Ribulose	Traces		

explain carefully to the patient the difference between the patient's ailment and diabetes mellitus and to effect "the removal of any dietetic restrictions he may have been subjected to." Although more than a half century has elapsed since Janeway's report, his advice still points out an essential function of any physician confronted by a person with pentosuria. Two years after Janeway's paper, in his classic Croonian lectures of 1908, Garrod[12] reviewed 30 recorded cases of essential pentosuria, and he assigned this abnormality along with cystinuria, alcaptonuria, and albinism to a category that he labeled as "inborn errors of metabolism." He stressed the differences between essential pentosuria and the alimentary variety. Garrod noted the incidence of essential pentosuria in Jews, and the tendency for the condition to occur in several members of the same family. A prevalent early impression that pentosuria frequently accompanies diabetes mellitus[13] has not been borne out.

Much of the present knowledge concerning the clinical aspects of pentosuria, its genetic transmission, and the nature of the urinary sugar is derived from the careful observations of Enklewitz and Lasker.[14–20] More than half of their 70 subjects with pentosuria were followed for more than 16 years. Fifty years following the first description of pentosuria, Derivaux[21] was able to collect 163 case reports from the literature, and in a 1958 review of the subject this figure exceeded 200.[22]

For many years controversy existed concerning the nature of the sugar in pentosuric urine. The first chemical identification was that of Neuberg,[23] who in 1900 reported that the sugar present in the urine of one person with pentosuria was racemic arabinose. Five additional individuals with arabinosuria were subsequently described by Cammidge and Howard,[24] and single cases of similar patients were presented by a number of other researchers, including Aron,[25] Luzzatto,[26] and Schuler.[27] Zerner and Waltuch[28] in 1913 presented convincing evidence that the urinary pentose was optically active and that it was not arabinose. The following

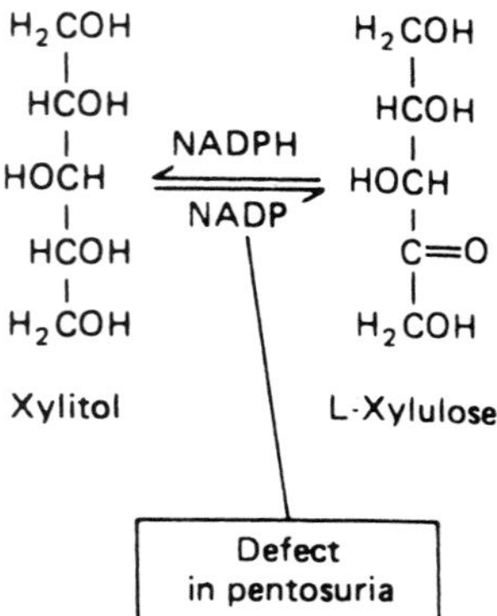

Fig. 73-1 The metabolic defect in pentosuria caused by deficiency in NADP-linked xylitol dehydrogenase.

year Levene and LaForge showed that the urinary sugar of a person with pentosuria was L-xylulose.[†29] Their identification was based on the following observations:

1. An osazone of the urinary sugar had a melting point of 160 to 163°C; when it was mixed with an osazone of D-xylose, the melting point was increased by 40°C.
2. The initial optical rotation of the osazone was lower than the equilibrium rotation; this is characteristic of xylosazone but not of arabinosazone.
3. The foregoing observations indicated that the urinary pentosazone was a xylosazone. On the basis of the optical rotation of the urinary sugar ($\alpha_D^{20} = +33.1°$), the character of its *p*-bromphenylhydrazone, and its behavior in oxidation experiments, Levene and LaForge concluded that the urinary pentose could only have been L-xylulose.

In the same year Zerner and Waltuch[30] isolated the sugar from the urine of two patients with pentosuria and also concluded that it was L-xylulose. A similar conclusion concerning the pentose in their patients' disease was reached by Hiller,[31] Greenwald,[32] and Lasker and Enklewitz.[15] Some of the early reports of arabinosuria were subsequently corrected. For example, a patient of Solis Cohen was first described in 1909 as having arabinosuria.[33] At that time Solis Cohen assumed from previously reported cases that arabinose was the urinary sugar excreted in pentosuria. However, his patient was followed for almost three decades, and in a follow-up report that appeared in 1936,[34] the same researcher indicated that he had identified the patient's urinary sugar as L-xylulose and that his earlier impression had been in error. Similarly, a patient reported as having arabinosuria in 1913[25] was reexamined 40 years later; paper chromatography of his urine revealed the major sugar component to be L-xylulose; no evidence of arabinose was found.[35]

The question of arabinosuria was considered at length in 1950 by Lasker,[19] who indicated that she had identified L-xylulose in the urine of 72 individuals with pentosuria but had never seen a patient with arabinosuria. She further stated that no case of arabinosuria had been reported since 1928 and that since in early reports the arabinose was always identified by the same method, this impression may have been in error. Studies with paper chromatographic techniques have provided further corroboration that L-xylulose is the only sugar excreted in substantial amounts in pentosuria. In addition to L-xylulose, a small quantity of L-arabitol has been isolated from the urine of one pentosuric patient[36]; other reports that pentosuric patients excrete more than one pentose[35,37] are considered below.

The constancy of the amount of urine pentose excreted by individuals with pentosuria has long been recognized. Enklewitz and Lasker[16] found that the excretion in five adults varied from 1.1

†The early reports of "D-xyloketose" excretion were published prior to the adoption of the current practice of classifying sugars according to their structural relation to D- and L-glyceraldehyde. Throughout this chapter the present convention is followed, regardless of the terminology applied in the original reports.

to 3.7 g per 24 h, but that the daily variation in any given subject never exceeded 0.9 g. The excretion is independent of dietary variations: Early reports by Janeway[11] and Klercker[13] that the amount of urinary pentose can be altered by changes in dietary nucleic acid or protein have not been substantiated. Margolis noted a marked increase in pentose excretion in pentosuric subjects following aminopyrine ingestion.[38] When Enklewitz and Lasker observed a similar stimulation not only following the intake of certain other drugs, including borneol, antipyrine, and menthol, but also after the administration of glucuronic acid,[16] they ascribed the effect of the drugs to their glucuronogenic action. The metabolic interrelations of glucuronic acid and L-xylulose, however, remained obscure, and there was no experimental evidence for Everett's postulate that an abnormal enzyme system existed in pentosuric patients that decarboxylated glucuronic acid to L-xylulose.[39] The identification of L-xylulose as an intermediate in the metabolism of glucuronic acid,[40,41] the elucidation of the reactions involved in the further metabolism of L-xylulose,[42,43] and the demonstration of xylitol metabolism by erythrocytes[44,45] were followed by the localization of the biochemical defect.[46] Much of the present concept stems from the careful studies of Touster and his associates.[40–43] Further contributions have come from the laboratories of Ashwell,[47–51] Burns,[52] Ul Hassan and Lehninger,[53] the author,[54–57] Wang and van Eys,[46] and others. Not only have these studies permitted insight into the biochemical aberration in pentosuria, but they also have provided important information concerning the operation of the glucuronic acid oxidation pathway in normal individuals.

PENTOSE METABOLISM IN HUMAN BEINGS

Several five-carbon sugars are known to be present in human beings. Some, such as ribose and deoxyribose, are present as part of more complex substances, including the nucleic acids and certain coenzymes. Others, including D-xylulose, D-ribulose, and L-xylulose, are intermediates in metabolic pathways and normally are not detectable in body fluids or are present only in trace quantity. Finally, there are those that are not known to be synthesized by humans but that occasionally may be ingested and thereafter are excreted in the urine. These include arabinose and xylose.

Many pathways of carbohydrate metabolism involve pentoses as key intermediates.[58] A consideration of these pathways is essential to understanding the several varieties of pentosuria that have been described, including essential pentosuria.

The Pentose Phosphate Pathway

Ribose, the sugar moiety found in all ribonucleic acids and several coenzymes, may be synthesized from glucose by either the oxidative or the nonoxidative reactions of the pentose phosphate pathway (Fig. 73-2).[59] In the oxidative reactions, glucose-6-phosphate is converted successively to 6-phosphogluconolactone, 6-phosphogluconic acid, and, following oxidative removal of its first carbon atom, ribulose-5-phosphate. The latter may be isomerized to ribose-5-phosphate. In this series of reactions, for every molecule of pentose phosphate synthesized from hexose phosphate, two molecules of nicotinamide adenine dinucleotide phosphate (NADP) are reduced to NADPH. Much information has accumulated indicating that the conversion of the coenzyme from its oxidized to its reduced form is as important a function of these reactions as pentose production.[58] This conclusion is based on the evidence for the NADPH requirement of a variety of reductive synthetic reactions and on observations that suggest that the oxidative reactions of the pentose phosphate pathway are the principal means available to the cell for NADP reduction.

Ribose also may be produced nonoxidatively from hexose phosphate via the transketolase and transaldolase reactions. In these reactions the first two carbon atoms of one molecule of fructose-6-phosphate may be cleaved and condensed with a molecule of triose phosphate, under the influence of the enzyme transketolase. This results in the formation of one molecule of xylulose-5-phosphate and one of erythrose-4-phosphate. The latter, together with another molecule of fructose-6-phosphate, may then participate in the transaldolase reaction, resulting in the production of a molecule of sedoheptulose-7-phosphate and one of triose phosphate. In another reaction catalyzed by transketolase, these products may undergo conversion to xylulose-5-phosphate and ribose-5-phosphate. The xylulose-5-phosphate may be epimerized to ribulose-5-phosphate, which, as already noted, can be isomerized to ribose-5-phosphate. Thus, in this series of reactions there is no net loss of carbon, and two molecules of hexose phosphate and one of triose phosphate may be converted to three molecules of pentose phosphate. Available data indicate that in animals[60,61] and in human beings[62] ribose is normally synthesized from hexose by way of both the oxidative and the nonoxidative reactions of the pentose phosphate pathway. The fact that thiamine pyrophosphate is a cofactor for the enzyme transketolase[63] accounts for the block in ribose synthesis by way of the nonoxidative sequence of reactions in the thiamine-deficient animal.[64]

In contrast to the oxidative reactions, which afford only a mechanism for pentose production from hexose, the transketolase–transaldolase sequence is reversible and provides a means for the interconversion of hexose and pentose.[65] Evidence has been presented demonstrating that the nonoxidative reactions mediate the conversion of ribose to hexose in human beings.[66] It also has been shown that ribose may participate directly in riboside[64] and nucleic acid[67] synthesis. Thus, mechanisms exist for the disposition of any ribose released in nucleic acid or coenzyme breakdown.

Small quantities [up to 2.8 μmol/(24 h · kg body weight)] of ribose have been reported in normal human urine.[7] This presumably represents either newly synthesized ribose or pentose released from nucleic acids or coenzymes that escapes further metabolism. It has been asserted that ribose excretion is slightly but significantly increased in patients with myopathies, presumably because of the increased breakdown of ribose-containing compounds in diseased muscle,[7] but this observation has not met universal acceptance.[68] A metabolite of histamine, imidazoleacetic acid, is excreted by the rat[69,70] and by human beings[62] in part as the riboside. Ribulose, a trace constituent of normal urine,[9] is presumably excreted following hydrolysis of the phosphate ester, which is an intermediate in the pentose phosphate pathway.

Deoxyribose, the sugar component of deoxyribonucleic acid, is apparently synthesized by way of direct reduction of the ribose molecule at the nucleoside diphosphate level.[71]

The Glucuronic Acid Oxidation Pathway

The pentoses L-xylulose and D-xylulose and the pentitol xylitol are intermediates in the glucuronic acid oxidation pathway (Fig. 73-3). The carbon skeleton of D-glucuronic acid is known to originate in glucose,[72,73] and uridine nucleotides are involved as intermediates.[74,75] As has been noted, the studies of Touster,[40–43] Ashwell,[47–51] Burns,[52] and Lehninger,[53] and their associates have provided much information concerning the further metabolism of D-glucuronic acid. A reductive reaction involving NADPH as a cofactor results in the conversion of D-glucuronic acid to L-gulonic acid. L-Gulonolactone has been shown to be an intermediate in the synthesis of ascorbic acid in most animal species, but in primates and in the guinea pig this transformation cannot take place. However, L-gulonic acid, in all animal species examined, may be oxidized to β-keto-L-gulonic acid,[50] which, in turn, is enzymatically decarboxylated to L-xylulose.[59,51] In the latter reaction the atom corresponding to the sixth carbon atom of the parent glucose molecule is oxidized to CO_2. Carbon atom 1 of L-xylulose is derived from the fifth carbon atom of glucose. Touster has prepared two enzymes from guinea pig liver, one of which catalyzes the reduction of L-xylulose to the sugar alcohol xylitol and the other of which promotes the oxidation of xylitol to D-xylulose.[42,43] These reactions require NADPH and NAD, respectively. It is noteworthy that in contrast to other schemes of intermediary carbohydrate metabolism in which only phosphate

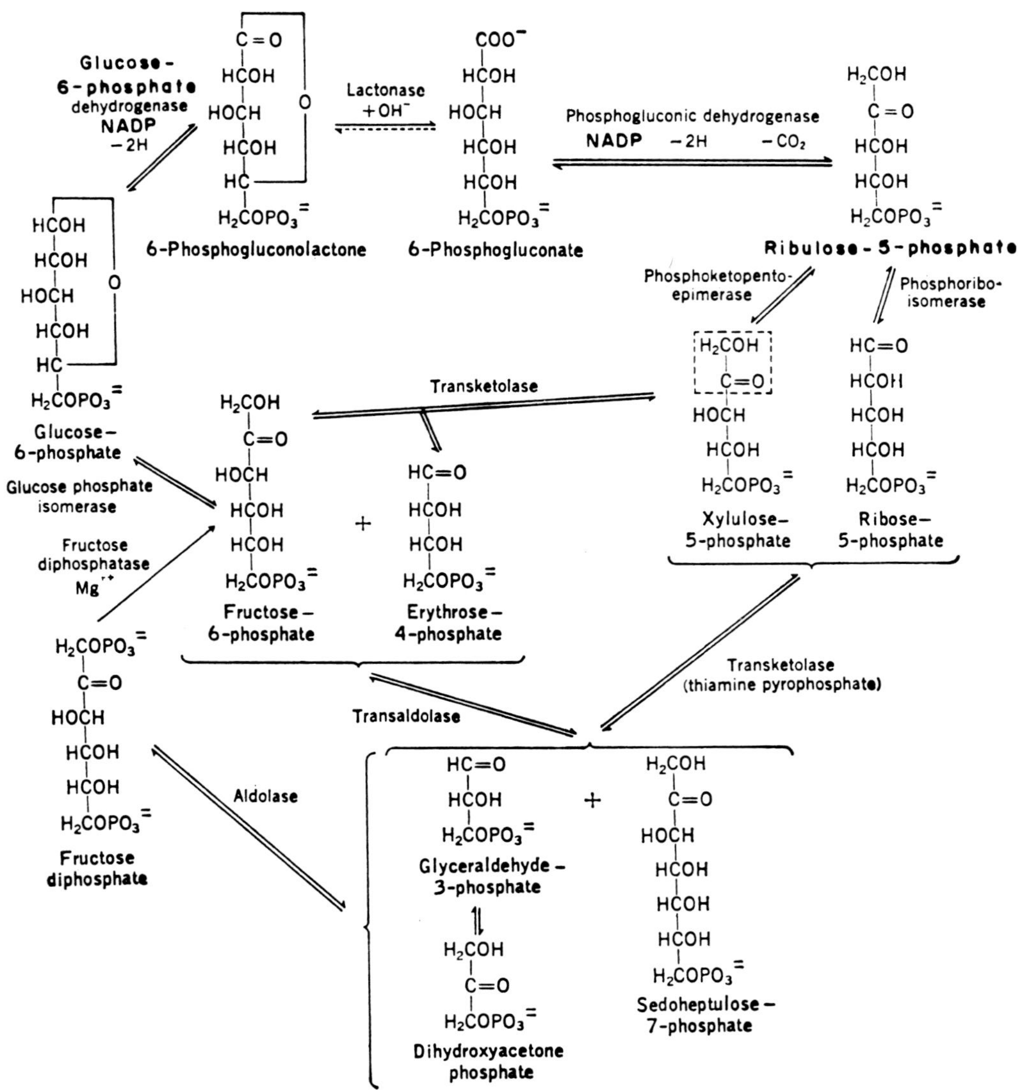

Fig. 73-2 The phosphogluconate-oxidative pathway. (*Reprinted with permission from Horecker BL, Hiatt H: New Engl J Med 258:177, 255, 1958.*)

esters participate, these reactions involve the free sugars. Hickman and Ashwell[48] have described a kinase for D-xylulose in mammalian liver. D-xylulose-5-phosphate will be recognized as an intermediate in the pentose phosphate pathway and may be converted to ribose-5-phosphate and to hexose phosphate. A kinase for L-xylulose has been purified from bacteria,[76] but there is no evidence for this enzyme in mammalian tissues. Evidence has been presented[77] suggesting that the pathway is operative in rat adipose tissue and that activity is increased in tissue from starved or diabetic animals and in human diabetic patients.[78]

The elucidation of the reactions involved in glucuronic acid metabolism provides insight not only into the origin of the L-xylulose found in trace amounts in normal urine, but also into the site of the defect in individuals with chronic essential pentosuria. Furthermore, it explains the hitherto poorly understood increase in L-xylulose excretion by pentosuric subjects given glucuronic acid.

The glucuronic acid oxidation pathway does not play an indispensable role in human metabolism—individuals with pentosuria, in whom the pathway is blocked, suffer no ill effects from the abnormality. It does appear to be responsible for myoinositol catabolism.[79] Although the reactions of the glucuronic acid oxidation pathway together with those of the pentose phosphate pathway provide a potential mechanism for ribose biosynthesis from hexose (i.e., hexose phosphate → glucuronic acid → xylulose → xylulose phosphate → ribose phosphate), animal studies indicate that little ribose is normally produced by way of this sequence of reactions.[54] In most mammalian species the early reactions of the pathway are required for the production of L-gulonic acid, a precursor of ascorbic acid.[80] In primates and the guinea pig, however, ascorbic acid cannot be synthesized.‡ Thus, in humans the pathway serves to return a portion of glucuronic acid carbon to the mainstream of carbohydrate metabolism.

Effects of Drugs. The basis for the effect of drugs and hormones on the glucuronic acid oxidation pathway remains a fascinating but poorly understood area. Margolis' early observation that aminopyrine stimulates the excretion of L-xylulose by individuals with pentosuria[38] was followed by reports indicating that this drug and others, such as chloretone and barbital, stimulate free glucuronic acid[82] and ascorbic acid[83] excretion in animals. The drug effect is apparently not related to any known detoxification mechanism because barbital is excreted unchanged. Studies of Burns and his

‡A report of the urinary excretion of radioactive ascorbic acid following administration of radioactive glucuronolactone[81] requires confirmation and amplification.

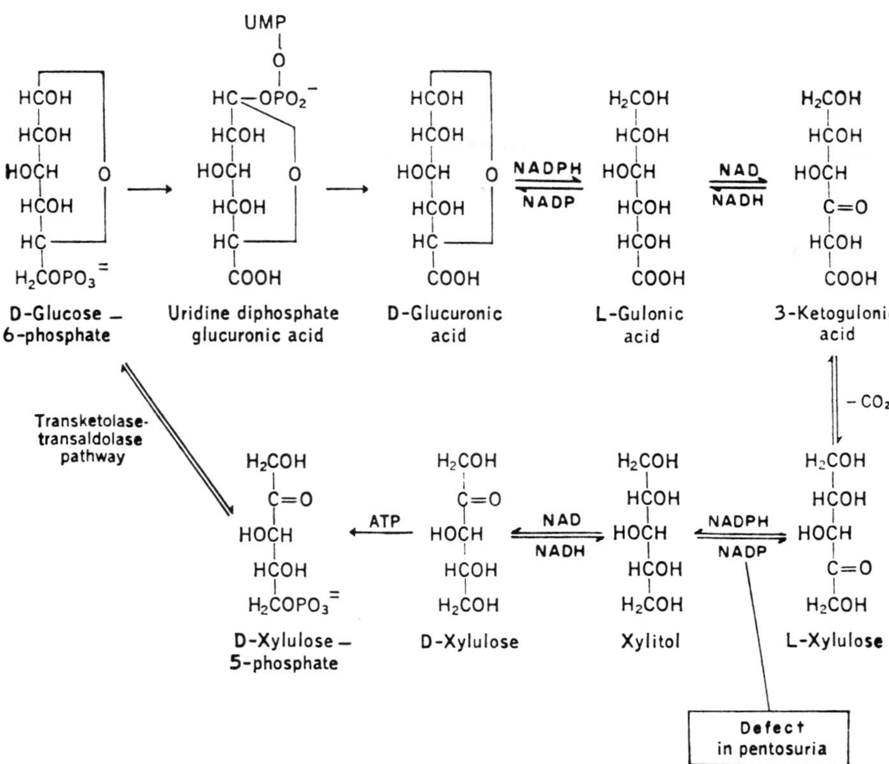

Fig. 73-3 The glucuronic acid oxidation pathway.

associates indicate that the drugs enhance the production of glucuronic acid, as well as ascorbic acid (and presumably L-xylulose in pentosuria), from glucose[84] and from galactose.[85] Increased levels of uridine diphosphate glucose dehydrogenase have been found in livers of animals treated with some[86,87] but not all[87] of the drugs known to stimulate ascorbic acid production. Hormonal involvement in this process is indicated by the observation of Burns and his associates that the administration of chloretone or barbital to hypophysectomized rats is not followed by an increase in ascorbic acid excretion.[82] It also has been observed that thyroid hormone stimulates pentose excretion in the rat,[88] and that the increase in pentose excretion that results from exposure to low temperatures is prevented by the administration of thyroid-blocking agents.[89] An increase in L-xylulose excretion by normal human beings given triiodothyronine has been reported.[90]

THE BIOCHEMICAL ABNORMALITY IN ESSENTIAL PENTOSURIA

Nature of the Urinary Sugar

As has been pointed out, there is now conclusive evidence that the urinary sugar excreted by pentosuric persons is L-xylulose (L-xyloketose, L-threopentulose). In the light of present knowledge, one must conclude that the early purported demonstrations of urinary arabinose either were in error because of deficiencies in the experimental methods used or else were concerned with patients who do not fit into this category. L-xylulose is excreted in fairly constant amounts, ranging from 1.0 to 4.0 g per 24 h. The excretion is increased following the intake of glucuronic acid and of certain drugs, but it is unaffected by diet and is not altered by insulin administration.

Much smaller quantities of other sugars in addition to L-xylulose have been reported in pentosuric urine. Touster and Harwell[36] found arabitol and suggested that this sugar alcohol may be derived from L-xylulose reduction. Wolfson, Cohn, and Devaney[37] observed a second unidentified component following chromatography of pentosuric urine, and Barnes and Bloomberg[35] found small amounts of several substances in addition to large quantities of L-xylulose following chromatography of deionized urine from several pentosuric subjects.

Because one substance that appeared in all the urines examined by Barnes and Bloomberg had a chromatographic mobility similar to that of xylose, some of my unpublished observations seem pertinent. Following the procedure of Barnes and Bloomberg, I, too, found a xylose-like component in the urine of two pentosuric subjects. This material was eluted from paper chromatograms and was found by Ashwell[91] to behave like L-xylose in several enzymatic reactions. However, this substance was not present in pentosuric urine subjected to paper chromatography *without* prior exposure to ion-exchange resins. In addition, normal urine to which only L-xylulose was added and which was then deionized and chromatographed on paper also exhibited the xylose spot. Accordingly, I have concluded that the appearance of L-xylose in chromatograms of pentosuric urine is an artifact attributable to the preparative procedure.

Site of the Defect

Although Enklewitz and Lasker[16] demonstrated more than 20 years earlier that glucuronic acid administration greatly enhanced the excretion of L-xylulose, it was not until the elucidation of the glucuronic acid oxidation pathway that a plausible hypothesis could be advanced concerning the biochemical abnormality in pentosuria. Even before the recent work that established the site of the metabolic lesion,[46] evidence was available to support the following propositions:

1. Glucuronic acid is a direct precursor of the urinary pentose.
2. Glucuronic acid is incompletely metabolized in pentosuric individuals.
3. Although the pentosuric person can convert glucuronic acid to L-xylulose, a block exists in the further metabolism of the pentose.

Touster and his associates[40] confirmed the observation of Enklewitz and Lasker that the ingestion of glucuronolactone is followed by an increased excretion of L-xylulose by pentosuric

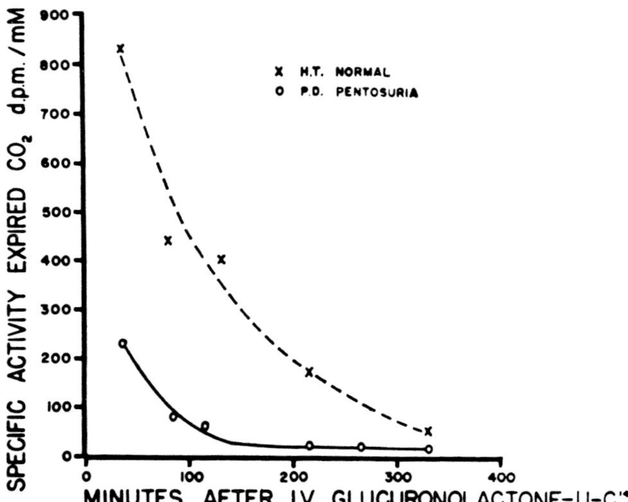

Fig. 73-4 $^{14}CO_2$ excretion in the expired air following the intravenous administration of glucuronolactone uniformly labeled with ^{14}C to a normal subject and to a pentosuric individual.

persons, and they postulated that the conversion of glucuronolactone to xylulose is direct. They substantiated this hypothesis by two studies of a pentosuric subject.[41] First, they demonstrated that the administration of glucuronolactone labeled with ^{13}C in its sixth carbon atom (the carboxyl carbon) was followed by the excretion of nonisotopic L-xylulose. Second, they showed that the ingestion of [1-^{13}C]glucuronolactone was followed by the urinary excretion of heavily labeled pentose, the isotope of which was predominantly in the fifth carbon atom. These data indicate that the carboxyl carbon of glucuronic acid is lost in the conversion to L-xylulose but that the rest of the molecule is preserved intact. Touster also demonstrated that some normal human beings and guinea pigs excrete traces of L-xylulose and that this excretion is slightly augmented following glucuronolactone ingestion. These observations strengthened the concept that L-xylulose is a metabolic intermediate in normal subjects.

The following study from Hiatt's laboratory supported the hypothesis that a defect in glucuronic acid metabolism exists in pentosuria. Let us postulate that a pentosuric person can remove carbon atom 6 of glucuronolactone with unimpaired efficiency but is incapable of metabolizing the remainder of the carbon chain. Then, following the administration of glucuronolactone uniformly labeled with ^{14}C, there should be six times as much $^{14}CO_2$ in the expired air of a normal person as in that of the pentosuric person. These expectations were fulfilled in an experiment (Fig. 73-4) in which 5 μCi of glucuronolactone uniformly labeled with ^{14}C was given intravenously to a 16-year-old boy with essential pentosuria and to a 22-year-old woman with no abnormality of carbohydrate metabolism. Samples of expired air were collected at intervals for 6 h thereafter and were analyzed for CO_2 and for radioactivity. In this period, 16 percent of the administered ^{14}C appeared in the expired air of the normal subject and 2.6 percent in that of the pentosuric subject, almost exactly the sixfold difference that was predicted. In the first 12 h, 57 percent of the administered radioactivity appeared in the urine of the normal individual and 76 percent in that of the pentosuric person. Thus, the total ^{14}C excretion in urine and expired air of the normal and pentosuric subjects during the intervals measured was in excess of 73 and 79 percent, respectively.

Further Isotope Experiments

The foregoing study strongly supports the view that glucuronic acid metabolism is impaired in pentosuria. Some information concerning the site of the defect was deduced from the results of a published experiment,[55] which will be briefly summarized. Using a "ribose-trapping" technique suggested by the observations of Tabor and Hayaishi[69] and Karjala[70] that imidazoleacetic acid is excreted in the urine in part as a riboside, Hiatt demonstrated ribose synthesis from hexose in humans by way of the oxidative and nonoxidative reactions of the pentose phosphate pathway.[62] If the glucuronic acid oxidation pathway were operative in normal individuals, it would afford a mechanism for the conversion of glucuronolactone carbon to ribose in this way: glucuronolactone → L-xylulose → D-xylulose → D-xylulose-5-phosphate → D-ribose-5-phosphate. (For an outline of the reactions involved, see Fig. 73-3.) Thus, the administration of imidazoleacetic acid and of glucuronolactone uniformly labeled with ^{14}C should be followed by the excretion of imidazoleacetic acid riboside containing [^{14}C]ribose. On the other hand, if this pathway were blocked in pentosuria at a site beyond L-xylulose, then a pentosuric subject might be expected to excrete radioactive L-xylulose but nonisotopic riboside ribose. (Because there is no reason to postulate an impairment in the pentose phosphate pathway in pentosuria, the synthesis and excretion of the riboside ribose should proceed normally.) The results of such an experiment are described in Table 73-2. The significant ^{14}C incorporation in the urinary riboside ribose of the normal subject is consistent with the conversion of glucuronolactone to ribose by way of the reactions of the glucuronic acid oxidation and the pentose phosphate pathways (Fig. 73-3). The pentosuric subject excreted ribose in an amount comparable with that excreted by the normal individual, but the virtual absence of radioactivity indicated that it was derived from sources other than glucuronolactone. The large quantity of isotope in the urinary L-xylulose is in agreement with Toustor's demonstration that glucuronic acid is a direct precursor of the pentose. This experiment not only provides information concerning the impairment in pentosuria, but also helps to establish the concept that the glucuronic acid oxidation pathway is operative in normal individuals.

Knox pointed out that impaired L-xylulose reabsorption by the renal tubule could be the defect present in pentosuria.[22] An experiment cited in support of this possibility is that of Enklewitz and Lasker,[14] who gave 5 g L-xylulose by mouth to a pentosuric subject and found only 0.5 g "additional" L-xylulose in the urine. This suggested metabolism of the pentose. However, in the absence of information concerning the efficiency of L-xylulose absorption from the human gastrointestinal tract, the Enklewitz and Lasker experiment cannot be thus interpreted. Indeed, other

Table 73-2 Urinary L-Xylulose and Ribose in Normal and Pentosuric Subjects Given Imidazoleacetic Acid (ImAA) and D-Glucuronolactone Uniformly Labeled with ^{14}C

Test	Normal person	Pentosuric subject
D-Glucuronolactone administered, counts/min	1.57×10^7	7.85×10^6
μmol	370	185
ImAA hydrochloride administered, μmol	2000	1000
Urinary L-xylulose (0–10 h), μmol	0.5	3950
Relative molar activity, counts/(min · μmol)		85
Total ^{14}C content, counts/min	300*	3.36×10^5
Percent administered ^{14}C	0.002*	4.3
Ribose from urinary ImAA riboside (0–10 h), μmol	275	208
Percent administered ImAA	14	21
Relative molar activity, counts/(min · μmol)	33	
Total ^{14}C content, counts/(min · μmol)	9100	190*
Percent administered ^{14}C	0.058	0.002*

*Significance doubtful because of small quantity of radioactivity.

Table 73-3 Serum and Urine L-Xylulose Levels Before and After Oral Administration of D-glucuronolactone

		Serum L-xylulose			Urine L-xylulose		
Subject	Amount of glucurono-lactone, g	Fasting, mg/dl	Maximal, mg/dl	Time after glucurono-lactone, min	Fasting, mg/h	Maximal, mg/h	Time after glucurono-lactone, h
Pentosuric subjects:							
A	5	1.2	7.2	60		320	1–2
B	10	1.3	9.9	60	106	549	1–2
C	10	1.7	14.7	30	88	450	1–2
Relative of pentosuric subjects:							
D	25	*	1.26	60	*		
E	25	*	3.9	30	*		
F	25	0.18	0.71	30	*	81	0–1
G	25	*	1.41	30	0.1	63	0–1
H	25	*	0.77	30			
Control subjects:							
I	25	*	*		*	9	0–1
J	25	*	*		*	22	0–1
K	25	*	0.22	90	*	16	0–1
L	25	*	0.29	90	0.6	13	0–1
M	25	*	0.15	60	0.3	18	1–2

*Less than 0.1 mg/dl.

published studies indicate that although parenteral administration of L-xylulose to animals is followed by extensive metabolism,[40,92,93] the pentose orally administered is not glycogenic in rats.[94] Moreover, even if considerable absorption takes place, the possibility exists that the absorbed pentose might inhibit endogenous L-xylulose production by way of a feedback mechanism.

Following the publication of Knox's review, three studies appeared that convincingly excluded the renal abnormality hypothesis. Bozian and Touster[95] found in the plasma of a pentosuric subject, but not of two normal individuals, a sugar that was identified as xylulose by paper chromatographic techniques. (Flynn[96] had previously demonstrated xylulose in pentosuric plasma by chromatography.) After glucuronolactone administration, the serum xylulose level in a pentosuric subject of Bozian and Touster reached 11 mg/dl. Simultaneous with the Bozian and Touster study, Freedberg, Feingold, and Hiatt[57] used the specific enzymatic assay of Hickman and Ashwell[97] to measure L-xylulose levels in the serum and urine of several non-Jewish controls, three pentosuric persons, and four close relatives of pentosuric persons (Table 73-3). This work was later extended,[56] and one additional relative is included in Table 73-3. From the latter work, several points merit emphasis. Fasting serum L-xylulose levels in all three pentosuric persons were in excess of 1 mg/dl, whereas in the serums of all but one of the other individuals no L-xylulose was detectable in the fasting state. In all but two subjects, D-glucuronolactone led to an increase in serum L-xylulose levels, with a peak generally reached within 1 h of feeding. The increase in serum pentose level was accompanied by a marked increase in urinary pentose in the pentosuric persons and by the appearance of urinary pentose in all other subjects tested. The serum levels of four heterozygotes (D and H in Table 73-3 are the parents of A; E is the mother of B; G's mother has pentosuria) and of a fifth individual, F, with three pentosuric sibs, were considerably greater than those of the control individuals reported here and of the large number described elsewhere.[56] On the basis of his serum level and his family history, F is considered to be heterozygous. The urine levels of the two heterozygous subjects tested were considerably greater than those of the control subjects. Assuming normal glomerular filtration rates for these subjects, one can calculate that virtually all L-xylulose entering the renal glomeruli appears in the urine of normal, as well as of heterozygous and pentosuric, subjects. Thus, a "defect" in renal tubular reabsorption of L-xylulose appears to exist in all subjects, but it is clearly not the metabolic error that distinguishes the pentosuric from the normal person.

Unequivocal proof that a block in the glucuronic acid oxidation pathway is the metabolic lesion in pentosuria was provided by Wang and van Eys in 1970.[46] These workers found in the erythrocytes of three subjects homozygous for pentosuria a marked decrease in activity of the NADP-linked xylitol dehydrogenase, the enzyme involved in the conversion of L-xylulose to xylitol. Two activities, one "normal" and one "abnormal," were found in the erythrocytes of a heterozygous subject. In contrast, activity of the NAD-linked xylitol dehydrogenase, which catalyzes the interconversion of xylitol and D-xylulose, was normal in both homozygous and heterozygous subjects.

CLINICAL CONSIDERATIONS

Manifestations

Pentosuria can be classified with those inborn errors of metabolism in which no disturbance of function has been demonstrated to result from the genetic abnormality. Indeed, the most frequent difficulty encountered by pentosuric subjects is consequent to a mistaken diagnosis of diabetes mellitus and the institution thereafter of dietary and insulin "therapy." A number of reports in the literature indicate that only after an episode of insulin-induced hypoglycemia has the correct diagnosis been made. No abnormality of glucose metabolism is demonstrable, except in those rare instances in which pentosuria and diabetes mellitus coincide. Several researchers have commented on the frequency and severity of psychological disturbances encountered in subjects with pentosuria, but a causal relationship between such disturbances and the error in carbohydrate metabolism has not been established, and the suggestion is often made that at least some neurotic complaints may be related to the conflicting medical opinions to which many patients have been subjected. Lasker has followed 40 pentosuric individuals for periods in excess of 16 years and has found no decrease in life expectancy as compared with normal individuals.[20] Some typical clinical considerations may best be presented by citing a report of a case of pentosuria first diagnosed in 1958.

Patient A. P.D., a 16-year-old high school sophomore, was first seen in the Outpatient Department of the Beth Israel Hospital in February 1958. One year previously, a physician had found a reducing substance in the patient's urine and had placed him on a low carbohydrate diet. Despite his faithful adherence to this regimen, the urine continued consistently to yield a 1+ reaction in the Benedict test. For this reason, his physician suggested instituting insulin therapy, and the patient's father brought him to the Beth Israel Hospital to seek an additional opinion. The patient had never noted polydipsia, polyuria, or polyphagia, and during the 6 months prior to admission he had gained 8 pounds. The father could not recall a single negative urine sugar test result during this period, but at no time did the patient produce more than a 1+ reduction. There was a family history of diabetes mellitus in a paternal great uncle but not of other known disturbances of carbohydrate metabolism. The patient was an only child of Austrian-born Jewish parents, who were not consanguine and whose forebears had come from Poland. His past medical history was not contributory except in two important respects. Ten years and six years previously the patient had been seen in the Pediatric Clinic of the Beth Israel Hospital for upper respiratory infections. Urinalyses carried out on both occasions were recorded as having yielded a 1+ Benedict test result. In addition, he had frequently been seen by psychiatrists during the previous decade because of problems of behavior. During the year prior to admission his emotional disturbances were apparently magnified by his concern over his condition and also by his resentment at the dietary restrictions to which he had been subjected.

Physical examination revealed a well-developed, well-nourished boy who appeared in good health. Vital signs were normal, and no significant abnormalities were found on examination. Laboratory studies revealed a normal hemogram, a 2-h postprandial blood sugar of 95 mg/dl, and a urinalysis result that was normal except for a 1+ test result for a reducing substance. The urine, however, did not give a positive reaction with Testape (an enzyme-impregnated paper that reacts specifically with glucose). The urine sugar was shown to be L-xylulose by preparation of the osazone and by paper chromatography in n-butanol-ethanol-water (50:10:40) with authentic L-xylulose as a standard, followed by staining with the orcinol–trichloroacetic acid reagent.[98] A glucose tolerance test (50 g glucose by mouth) showed a fasting blood sugar level of 80 mg/dl and blood glucose levels at 30, 60, 120, 180, and 240 min of 120, 110, 95, 80, and 60 mg/dl, respectively. The patient's 24-h urinary excretion of L-xylulose was found to be 2 g, and this increased to 4 g during the 24 h following the ingestion of 5 g of D-glucuronolactone. Studies of L-xylulose levels in the patient (A in Table 73-3), his mother (D), and his father (H) before and after glucuronolactone administration strengthen the assumption that the parents are heterozygous for the aberration apparent in the son. The patient and his parents were reassured concerning the benign nature of this disturbance in carbohydrate metabolism and specifically concerning the absence of any relationship of his condition to diabetes mellitus. He was returned to an unrestricted diet and, according to his parents, within a month many of the behavioral disturbances which had been present during the previous year were greatly diminished.

Diagnostic Measures

A diagnosis of pentosuria should be suspected in any person, particularly in a Jewish person, who has none of the symptoms of diabetes mellitus but in whose urine a small quantity of a reducing substance is consistently found. This possibility is strengthened in those instances in which the urine does not give a positive test with any of the enzymatic methods specific for glucose. The measures that have proved most useful in establishing the diagnosis of pentosuria may be summarized as follows:

1. *Reduction of Benedict's reagent at low temperature.*[15] L-xylulose is a strong reducing substance and in contrast to glucose and most other urinary sugars will reduce Benedict's reagent at 55°C in 10 min or at room temperature in 3 h. (Fructose also will reduce Benedict's reagent at low temperature.)
2. *Paper chromatography.* On paper chromatography L-xylulose can be readily distinguished from other sugars. For example, with a mixture of *n*-butanol, ethanol, and water (50:10:40) as the solvent, L-xylulose has a characteristic mobility ($R_F = 0.26$) exceeding those of other commonly observed urinary sugars[98] and gives a red color on staining with the orcinol–trichloroacetic acid reagent.[99] Chromatography is the most convenient means of establishing an unequivocal diagnosis.
3. *Cysteine-carbazole test.*[100]
4. *Behavior of osazone.*[29] The phenylosazone of L-xylulose has a melting point of about 160°C. When it is mixed with the osazone of D-xylose, the crystalline appearance is radically altered, and the melting point increases by approximately 40°.
5. *Demonstration of the enzymatic defect in erythrocytes.*[46] This can be carried out only in a laboratory in which special facilities are available.

GENETICS

Estimates of the incidence of pentosuria vary. The most widely accepted figure, 1 in 40,000 to 50,000, is derived from examinations of applicants for life insurance in the United States.[94,101] All these cases were found in Jews; thus, the occurrence in American Jews is considered to be about 1:2000 to 2500. Mizrahi and Ser reported an incidence of pentosuria of 1:5000 in Israeli Jews; their 18 cases, 8 males and 10 females, were all born in Eastern European countries.[102] The vast majority of pentosuric persons are Jews resident in widely dispersed areas, but the antecedents of a substantial number have been traced to Eastern Europe.[103] Two sisters of Lebanese descent with xylulosuria have been found in South Africa,[35] and further study of four generations of the same family revealed an additional 8 cases in 127 members.[104] In this study individuals were reported to show pentosuria weeks to years after negative urine examinations. Twelve cases of pentosuria were found in 60 members of three other well-studied Lebanese families, these in Lebanon.[105] Among them was an infant with xylulosuria from at least the second week of life. The earlier reports that pentosuria occurs predominantly in males[12] are not substantiated by studies of the families of pentosuric persons, in which the incidence seems evenly divided between the sexes.

Garrod first proposed that a homozygous state was required for the expression of pentosuria,[12] and this thesis has been amply supported by the very careful family studies of Lasker.[18,103] The latter[103] has found 31 of 122 sibs (excluding propositi) to have pentosuria when both parents tested negative. When one parent had the disturbance, however, 17 of 31 sibs were afflicted. The incidence of consanguinity in 79 marriages that produced pentosuric offspring was 12.6 percent.

The sensitivity of the enzymatic assay for L-xylulose, which permits measurement of serum levels far below those found in individuals with pentosuria, has made possible the demonstration of a partial lesion in parents and children of pentosuric individuals.[57] This provides unequivocal confirmation of the theories of Garrod and Lasker concerning a homozygous genotype in pentosuria. Relatives of pentosuric individuals with one normal and one abnormal gene apparently have sufficient competent enzyme to deal with the products of normal metabolism. However, when the glucuronic acid oxidation pathway is stressed, as occurs during the "loading test" with glucuronolactone, the pentosuria heterozygote is not able to metabolize the extra L-xylulose produced as efficiently as in the normal individual. The data in Table 73-3 demonstrate that following glucuronolactone administration, both parents of one person with pentosuria, the mother of a second, and the child of a third all had serum levels of L-xylulose significantly higher than those of control subjects, but far below those of pentosuric patients. Thus, it is apparent that although the presence of two abnormal genes is required to produce the clinical picture of essential pentosuria, the consequences of one abnormal gene are recognizable not only by enzyme studies[46] but also under the special conditions which prevail following glucuronolactone administration.

ACKNOWLEDGMENTS

This work was supported in part by funds from the American Cancer Society, Inc., and the Public Health Service. I am most grateful to Dr. Margaret W. Lasker and Dr. F. H. Renwick for their very helpful suggestions.

EDITORS' ADDENDUM

The proper nomenclature for the deficient enzyme in pentosuria is L-xylulose reductase (EC 1.1.1.10).[106] The enzyme deficiency described by Wang and van Eys[46] (termed NADP-linked xylitol dehydrogenase by them) has been confirmed by numerous investigators. Although pentosuria had been described primarily in Ashkenazi Jews and among the Lebanese, a Japanese case of pentosuria with L-xylulose reductase deficiency was identified.[107] In agreement with the original report of Wang and van Eys,[46] these investigators reported an increased $K_m$for NADP in the pentosuric subject.[107] Pentosuria was reported in three cousins in a highly inbred family from Andhra Pradesh, India.[108]

In 1985, Lane reported the separation of a major and a minor isozyme for L-xylulose reductase in human erythrocytes.[109] The major isozyme had a cathodal position and was absent from patients with pentosuria. The minor or anodal band was present in pentosuric and normal subjects. The separation of the two isozymes was confirmed using carboxymethyl CM-cellulose chromatography. Lane[109] did not confirm the increased K_m for NADP reported by Wang and van Eys.[46] The difference in results may be related to the fact that Wang and van Eys measured the production of NADPH when xylitol is converted to L-xylulose, while Lane measured the production of $NADP^+$ when L-xylulose is converted to xylitol, the latter being the predominant direction *in vivo*. The more recent studies found a similar K_m for NADP from normal and pentosuric subjects. Significant increases in K_m were found for xylitol and L-xylulose in pentosuric subjects, but the data indicated that the differences were due to the selective preservation of the minor isozyme in these individuals. Cellular fractionation studies indicated that the major isoenzyme is present in mitochondria and cytosol, whereas the minor isoenzyme occurs only in the cytosol.[110]

Using the newer assay method, Lane and Jenkins[110] restudied a Lebanese family previously reported to show dominant inheritance of pentosuria.[104] The reanalysis convincingly documented the presence of a single pentosuric individual. Other family members previously reported to be affected were heterozygotes. These investigators also surveyed a population of Ashkenazi Jewish students and found L-xylulose reductase activity in erythrocytes to be more than two standard deviations below the mean in 7 of 237 individuals. Six of these seven individuals underwent a loading test with D-glucuronolactone, and five showed a major increase in serum L-xylulose, although one did not. These results suggested a heterozygote frequency of 0.0127 in this Ashkenazim population.

A search of the literature did not identify any significant publications regarding pentosuria from 1986 to Aug. 2000.

REFERENCES

1. Salkowskie, Jastrowitz M: Ueber eine bisher nicht beobachtete Zuckerart im Harn. *Zentralbl Med Wiss* **30**:337, 1892.
2. Garrod AE: The lessons of rare maladies. *Lancet* **1**:1055, 1928.
3. *The Works of William Harvey, M.D.* [translated by Robert Willis]. Sydenham, London, 1847, p 616 (cited in ref. 1).
4. Peters JP, Van Slyke DD: *Quantitative Clinical Chemistry. Interpretations*. Vol. I. Baltimore, Williams & Wilkins, 1946.
5. Hawk PB, Oser BL, Summerson WH: Practical Physiological Chemistry, McGraw-Hill, New York, 1954, pp 844–845.
6. Johnstone RW: Pentosuria: Chronic and alimentary. *Edinb Med F* **20**:138, 1906.
7. Tower DB, Peters EL, Pogorelskin MA: Nature and significance of pentosuria in neuromuscular disease. *Neurology* **6**:125, 1956.
8. Touster O, Hutcheson RM, Reynolds VH: The formation of L-xylulose in mammals and its utilization by liver preparations. *Fam Chem Soc* **76**:5005, 1954.
9. Futterman S, Roe JH: The identification of ribulose and L-xylulose in human and rat urine. *F Biol Chem* **215**:257, 1955.
10. Kiliani H: Ueber die Zusammensetzung and Constitution der Arabinose carbonsure bezw. der Arabinose. *Berl Dtsch Chem Ges* **20**:339, 1887.
11. Janeway TC: Essential pentosuria in two brothers. *Am J Med Sci* **132**:423, 1906.
12. Garrod AE: Inborn errors of metabolism. *Lancet* **2**:217, 1908.
13. Klercker KO: Studien uber die Pentosurie. *Nord Med Ark* **38**:1, 1905.
14. Englewitz M, Lasker M: Studies in pentosuria: A report of 12 cases. *Am J Med Sci* **186**:539, 1933.
15. Lasker M, Enklewitz M: A simple method for the detection and estimation of L-xyloketose in urine. *F Biol Chem* **101**:289, 1933.
16. Enklewitz M, Lasker M: The origin of L-xyloketose (urine pentose). *F Biol Chem* **110**:443, 1935.
17. Enklewitz M, Lasker M: Pentosuria in twins. *JAMA* **105**:958, 1935.
18. Lasker M, Enklewitz M, Lasker GW: The inheritance of L-xyloketosuria (essential pentosuria). *Hum Biol* **8**:243, 1936.
19. Lasker M: The question of arabinosuria. *Am J Clin Pathol* **20**:485, 1950.
20. Lasker M: Mortality of persons with xyloketosuria. *Hum Biol* **27**:294, 1955.
21. Derivaux RC: Essential pentosuria (xyloketosuria). *South Med J* **36**:587, 1943.
22. Knox WE: Sir Archibald Garrod's inborn errors of metabolism. IV. Pentosuria *Am J Hum Genet* **10**:385, 1958.
23. Neuberg C: Ueber die Harnpentose ein optisch inactives naturlich vorkommendes Kohlehydrat. *Berl Dtsch Chem Ges* **33**:2243, 1900.
24. Cammidge PJ, Hah H: Seven cases of essential pentosuria. *Br Med J* **2**:777, 1920.
25. Aron H: Einfall von Pentosuria im fruhen Kindesalter. *Monatsschr Kinderheilk* **1**:177, 1913.
26. Luzzatto R: Recherches dans un can de pentosurie chronique. *Arch Ital Biol* **51**:469, 1909.
27. Schuler L: Ueber inaktive and rechtsdrehende Arabinose ausscheidung im Harn. *Berl Klin Wochenschr* **47**:1322, 1910.
28. Zerner E, Waltuch R: Ein Beitrag zur Kenntnis der Pentosurie vom chemischen Standpunkt. *Monatsschr Chem* **34**:1639, 1913.
29. Levene PA, Laforge FB: Note on a case of pentosuria. *J Biol Chem* **18**:319, 1914.
30. Zerner E, Waltuch R: Zur Frage des Pentosuriezuckers. *Biochem Z* **58**:410, 1913.
31. Hiller A: The identification of the pentose in a case of pentosuria. *J Biol Chem* **30**:129, 1917.
32. Greenwald I: The nature of the sugar in four cases of pentosuria. *J Biol Chem* **88**:1, 1930.
33. Solis Cohen S: Essential pentosuria. *Am J Med Sci* **139**:349, 1910.
34. Solis Cohen S, Gershenfeld L: Supplemental report of a case of essential pentosuria of twenty-eight years' standing. *Am J Med Sci* **192**:610, 1936.
35. Barnes HD, Bloomberg BM: Paper chromatography of the urinary sugar in essential pentosuria. *S Afr J Med Sci* **18**:93, 1953.
36. Touster O, Harwell S: The isolation of L-arabitol from pentosuric urine. *J Biol Chem* **230**:1031, 1958.
37. Wolfson WG, Cohn C, Devaney WA: An improved apparatus and procedure for ascending chromatography on large size filter paper sheets. *Science* **109**:541, 1949.
38. Margolis JI: Chronic pentosuria and migraine. *Am J Med Sci* **177**:348, 1929.
39. Everett MR: *Medical Biochemistry*. New York, Hoeber-Harper, 1942, p 312.
40. Touster O, Hutcheson RM, Rice L: The influence of D-glucuronolactone on the excretion of L-xylulose by humans and guinea pigs. *J Biol Chem* **215**:677, 1955.

41. Touster O, Mayberry RH, McCormick DB: The conversion of 1-13C-D-glucuronolactone to 5-13C-L-xylulose in a pentosuric human. *Biochim Biophys Acta* **24**:196, 1957.
42. Touster O, Reynolds VH, Hutcheson RM: The reduction of L-xylulose to xylitol by guinea pig liver mitochondria. *J Biol Chem* **221**:697, 1956.
43. Hollman S, Touster O: The L-xylulose-xylitol enzyme and other polyol dehydrogenases of guinea pig liver mitochondria. *J Biol Chem* **225**:87, 1957.
44. Bassler KH, Reimold WV: Lactatbildung aus Zuckern and Zuckeralkoholen in Erythrocyten. *Klin Wochenschr* **43**:169, 1965.
45. Asakura T, Adachi K, Minakami S, Yoshikawa H: Nonglycolytic sugar metabolism in human erythrocytes. I. Xylitol metabolism. *J Biochem* **62**:184, 1967.
46. Wang YM, Van Eys J: The enzymatic defect in essential pentosuria. *New Engl J Med* **282**:892, 1970.
47. Ashwell G: Enzymatic degradation of D-galacturonic and D-glucuronic acid. *Fed Proc* **16**:146, 1957.
48. Hickman J, Ashwell G: Purification and properties of D-xylulokinase in liver. *J Biol Chem* **232**:737, 1958.
49. Ashwell G, Kanfer J, Burns JJ: Studies of the mechanism of L-xylulose formation by kidney enzymes. *J Biol Chem* **234**:472, 1959.
50. Smiley JD, Ashwell G: Purification and properties of β-L-hydroxy acid hydrogenase. II. Isolation of β-keto-L-gulonic acid, an intermediate in L-xylulose biosynthesis. *J Biol Chem* **236**:357, 1961.
51. Winkelman J, Ashwell G: Enzymic formation of L-xylulose from β-keto-L-gulonic acid. *Biochim Biophys Acta* **52**:170, 1961.
52. Burns JJ, Kanfer J: Formation of L-xylulose from L-gulonolactone in rat kidney. *J Am Chem Soc* **79**:3604, 1957.
53. Ul Hassan M, Lehninger AL: Enzymatic formation of ascorbic acid in rat liver extracts. *J Biol Chem* **223**:123, 1956.
54. Hiatt HH, Lareau J: Studies of ribose metabolism. VII. An assessment of ribose biosynthesis from hexose by way of the C-6 oxidation pathway. *J Biol Chem* **233**:1023, 1958.
55. Hiatt HH: Studies of ribose metabolism. IV. The metabolism of D-glucuronolactone in normal and pentosuric subjects. *Biochim Biophys Acta* **28**:645, 1958.
56. Kumahara Y, Feingold DS, Freedberg IM, Hyatt HH: Studies of pentose metabolism in normal subjects and in patients with pentosuria and pentosuria trait. *J Clin Endocrinol Metab* **21**:887, 1961.
57. Freedberg IM, Fringold DS, Hiatt HH: Serum and urine L-xylulose in pentosuric and normal subjects and in individuals with pentosuria trait. *Biochem Biophys Res Commun* **1**:328, 1959.
58. Horecker BL, Hiatt HH: Pathways of carbohydrate metabolism in normal and neoplastic cells. *New Engl J Med* **258**:177, 255, 1958.
59. Horecker BL, Mehler AH: Carbohydrate metabolism. *Annu Rev Biochem* **24**:207, 1955.
60. Marks PA, Feigelson P: Biosynthesis of nucleic acid ribose and of glycogen glucose in the rat. *J Biol Chem* **226**:1001, 1957.
61. Hiatt HH: Studies of ribose metabolism. II. A method for the study of ribose synthesis *in vivo*. *J Biol Chem* **229**:725, 1957.
62. Hiatt HH: Studies of ribose metabolism. VI. Pathways of ribose synthesis in man. *J Clin Invest* **37**:1461, 1958.
63. Horecker BL, Smyrniotis PZ: The coenzyme function of thiamine pyrophosphate in pentose phosphate metabolism. *J Am Chem Soc* **75**:1009, 1953.
64. Hiatt HH: Studies of ribose metabolism. V. Factors influencing *in vivo* ribose synthesis in the rat. *J Clin Invest* **37**:1453, 1958.
65. Horecker BL, Gibbs M, Klenow H, Smyrniotis PZ: The mechanism of pentose phosphate conversion to hexose monophosphate. I. With a liver enzyme preparation. *J Biol Chem* **207**:393, 1954.
66. Hiatt HH: Studies of ribose metabolism. III. The pathway of ribose carbon conversion to glucose in man. *J Clin Invest* **37**:651, 1958.
67. Hiatt HH: Studies of ribose metabolism. I. The pathway of nucleic acid ribose synthesis in a human carcinoma cell in tissue culture. *J Clin Invest* **36**:1408, 1957.
68. Perkoff GT, Tyler FH: Studies in disorders of muscle. XI. The problem of pentosuria in progressive muscular dystrophy. *Metabolism* **5**:563, 1956.
69. Tabor H, Hayaishi O: The excretion of imidazoleacetic acid riboside following the administration of imidazoleacetic acid or histamine to rats. *J Am Chem Soc* **77**:505, 1955.
70. Karjala SA: The partial characterization of a histamine metabolite from rat and mouse urine. *J Am Chem Soc* **77**:504, 1955.
71. Reichard P: Enzymatic synthesis of deoxyribonucleotides. I. Formation of deoxycytidine diphosphate from cytidine diphosphate with enzymes from *Escherichia coli*. *J Biol Chem* **237**:3513, 1962.
72. Mosbach EH, King CG: Tracer studies of glucuronic acid biosynthesis. *J Biol Chem* **185**:491, 1950.
73. Eisenberg F Jr, Gurin S: The biosynthesis of glucuronic acid from 1-C-14-glucose. *J Biol Chem* **195**:317, 1952.
74. Ginsburg V, Weissbach A, Maxwell ES: Formation of glucuronic acid from uridinediphosphate glucuronic acid. *Biochim Biophys Acta* **28**:649, 1958.
75. Pogell BM, Leloir LF: Nucleotide activation of liver microsomal glucuronidation. *J Biol Chem* **236**:293, 1961.
76. Anderson RL, Wood WA: Purification and properties of L-xylulokinase. *J Biol Chem* **237**:1029, 1962.
77. Winegrad AI, Shaw WN: Glucuronic acid pathway activity in adipose tissue. *Am J Physiol* **206**:165, 1964.
78. Winegrad AI, Burden CL: Hyperactivity of the glucuronic acid pathway in diabetes mellitus. *Trans Assoc Am Physicians* **78**:158, 1965.
79. Hankes LV, Politzer WM, Touster O, Anderson L: Myoinositol catabolism in human pentosurics: The predominant role of the glucuronate-xylulose-pentose phosphate pathway. *Ann NY Acad Sci* **165**:564, 1969.
80. Isherwood FA, Chen YT, Mapson LW: Synthesis of L-ascorbic acid in plants and animals. *Biochem J* **56**:1, 1954.
81. Baker EM, Sauberlich HE, Wolfskill SJ, Wallace WT, Dean EE: Tracer studies of vitamin C utilization in men: Metabolism of D-glucuronolactone-6-C14, D-glucuronic-6-C14 acid, and L-ascorbic-1-C14 acid. *Proc Soc Exp Biol Med* **109**:737, 1962.
82. Burns JJ, Evans C, Trousof N, Kaplan J: Stimulatory effect of drugs on excretion of L-ascorbid acid and non-conjugated D-glucuronic acid. *Fed Proc* **16**:286, 1957.
83. Longenecker HF, Fricke HH, King CG: The effect of organic compounds upon vitamin C synthesis in the rat. *J Biol Chem* **135**:497, 1940.
84. Burns JJ, Evans C, Trousof N: Stimulatory effect of barbital on urinary excretion of L-asorbic acid and non-conjugated D-glucuronic acid. *J Biol Chem* **227**:785, 1957.
85. Evans C, Conney AH, Trousof N, Burns JJ: Metabolism of D-galactose to D-glucuronic acid, L-gulonic acid, and L-ascorbic acid in normal and barbital-treated rats. *Biochim Biophys Acta* **41**:9, 1960.
86. Conney AH, Bray GA, Evans C, Burns JJ: Metabolic interactions between L-ascorbic acid and drugs. *Ann NY Acad Sci* **92**:115, 1961.
87. Hollmann S, Touster O: Alterations in tissue levels of uridine diphosphate glucose dehydrogenase, uridine diphosphate glucuronic acid pyrophosphatase, and glucuronyl transferase induced by substances influencing the production of ascorbic acid. *Biochim Biophys Acta* **62**:338, 1962.
88. Roe JH, Coover MO: Role of the thyroid gland in urinary pentose excretion in the rat. *Proc Soc Exp Biol Med* **75**:818, 1950.
89. Coover MO, Feinberg LJ, Roe JH: Effect of cold, adrenocorticotropic, and thyroid hormones on urinary excretion of pentose in the rat. *Proc Soc Exp Biol Med* **74**:146, 1950.
90. Baker EM, Plough IC, Bierman EL: Alternate pathways of glucose metabolism in man: Factors influencing the excretion of ketopentose. *Clin Res Proc* **6**:406, 1958.
91. Ashwell G: Personal communication.
92. Greenwals I: The possible significance of L-xyloketose (urine pentose) in normal metabolism. *J Biol Chem* **91**:731, 1931.
93. Larson HW, Chambers WH, Blatherwick NR, Ewing ME, Sawyer SD: The metabolism of D- and L-xylulose in the depancreatized dog. *J Biol Chem* **129**:701, 1939.
94. Larson HW, Blatherwick NR, Bradshaw PJ, Ewing ME, Sawyer SD: The metabolism of L-xylulose. *J Biol Chem* **138**:353, 1941.
95. Bozian RC, Touster O: Essential pentosuria: Renal or enzymic disorder. *Nature* **184**:463, 1959.
96. Flynn FV: Essential pentosuria. *BMJ* **1**:391, 1955.
97. Hickman J, Ashwell G: A sensitive and stereospecific enzymatic assay for xylulose. *J Biol Chem* **234**:758, 1957.
98. Lederer E, Lederer M: *Chromatography*. Amsterdam, Elsevier, 1955.
99. Hough L, Jones JKN, Wadman WH: Quantitative analysis of mixtures of sugars by the method of partition chromatography. Part V. Improved methods for the separation and detection of the sugars and their methylated derivatives on the paper chromatogram. *J Chem Soc* 1702, 1950.
100. Dische Z, Borenfreund E: A new spectrophotometric method for the detection and determination of keto sugars and trioses. *J Biol Chem* **192**:583, 1951.
101. Wright WT: Incidence of pentosuria. *New Engl J Med* **265**:1154, 1961.

102. Mizrahi O, Ser I: Essential pentosuria, in Goldschmidt E (ed): *Genetics of Migrant and Isolate Populations*. Baltimore, Williams & Wilkins, 1963, p 300.
103. Lasker M: Personal communication.
104. Politzer WM, Fleischmann H: L-xylulosuria in a Lebanese family. *Am J Hum Genet* **14:**256, 1962.
105. Khachadurian AK: Essential pentosuria. *Am J Hum Genet* **14:**249, 1962.
106. Webb EC: *Enzyme Nomenclature*. New York, Academic, 1984.
107. Soyama K, Furukawan: A Japanese case of pentosuria. *J Inherit Metab Dis* **8:**37, 1985.
108. Reddi OS, Reddy SV, Reddy KR: Familial incidence of L-xylulosuria. *Hum Genet* **39:**143, 1977.
109. Lane AB: On the nature of L-xylulose reductase deficiency in essential pentosuria. *Biochem Genet* **23:**61, 1985.
110. Lane AB, Jenkins T: Human L-xylulose reductase variation: Family and population studies. *Ann Hum Genet* **49:**227, 1985.

CHAPTER 74

Defects of *N*-Glycan Synthesis

Jaak Jaeken ▪ Gert Matthijs
Hubert Carchon ▪ Emile Van Schaftingen

1. **Many proteins undergo posttranslational modifications. Most membrane proteins and most extracellular proteins as well as several intracellular proteins, like lysosomal enzymes, are glycosylated. The structures of these oligosaccharides or glycans present on proteins are basically of two types defined by their linkage to the protein: O linked and N linked. N-linked glycans are bound to the amide group of asparagine via an *N*-acetylglucosamine residue. The biosynthetic pathway for the assembly of these *N*-glycans involves numerous glycosyltransferases that sequentially attach monosaccharides to the growing glycan unit using nucleotide-linked sugars or dolichol phosphate-linked sugars as donors. Subsequently a series of glycosidases and Golgi glycosyltransferases intervene in the further processing of the glycan moiety. The glycan units of glycoproteins serve a great number of diverse functions particularly in relation to the function and metabolism of the underlying proteins.**
2. **Type-I CDG syndromes have a type-I serum sialotransferrin pattern on isoelectrofocusing (IEF) characterized by increased di- and asialotransferrin bands. They are mostly due to defects in the *N*-glycan synthesis in the cytosol or in the endoplasmic reticulum (ER); some may be due to an *N*-glycan processing defect in the Golgi apparatus. Two pre-ER defects have been well characterized: phosphomannomutase (PMM) deficiency (CDGS type IA) and phosphomannose isomerase (PMI) deficiency (CDGS type IB) Evidence has been presented in one family for deficient glucosylation of the dolichol-oligosaccharide ER intermediate.**

   Type-II CDG syndromes have a type-II serum sialotransferrin pattern on IEF, i.e., besides increased di- and asialotransferrin bands there is also an increase of the tri- and/or monosialotransferrin bands. They are probably all due to defects of the N-linked glycan processing in the Golgi apparatus. Only one defect has been identified: *N*-acetylglucosaminyltransferase (GnT) II deficiency (CDGS type IIA).
3. **PMM (EC 5.4.2.28) deficiency (CDGS type IA) results in an autosomal recessive disease reported in at least 124 patients. It is a multisystem disease including specific dysmorphy in most patients and moderate to severe nervous system involvement. It is caused by mutations in the *PMM2* gene (MIM 601785) on chromosome 16p13.**

   PMI (EC 5.3.1.8) deficiency (CDGS type IB) results in an autosomal recessive disease and has been reported in six patients belonging to four families. Two of them suffered from severe protein-losing enteropathy and three others (siblings) from recurrent vomiting. These five patients also had liver fibrosis. One patient had only transient liver disease. Oral mannose, given to one patient with protein-losing enteropathy, had a strikingly beneficial effect. The patient who showed only liver disease recovered completely after the introduction of solid food without extra mannose. In two patients, mutations were found in the *PMI* gene (MIM 602579) located on chromosome 15q22.

   Deficient glucosylation of the dolichol-oligosaccharide intermediate in the ER was found in five members of an inbred family with mild to moderate psychomotor retardation and epilepsy. The basic defect is most probably in an ER-localized glucosyltransferase or in the synthesis of dolichyl-phosphoglucose.

   GnT II (EC 2.4.1.143) deficiency (CDGS type IIA) is an autosomal recessive disease. The two reported patients had craniofacial dysmorphy and severe encephalopathy. They were homozygous for different point mutations of the GnT II gene that is located on chromosome 14q21.

   Leukocyte adhesion deficiency syndrome type II is probably an autosomal recessive disease and has been described in two unrelated patients who suffered from recurrent bacterial infections without pus formation and showed typical facial features, short stature, and an encephalopathy. This phenotype appears to result from a general deficiency of fucose (*N*-glycans as well as *O*-glycans contain fucose) possibly due to a defect in the transformation of guanosine diphosphomannose (GDP-mannose) into GDP-fucose.
4. **A number of patients with an unexplained *N*-glycosylation defect have been reported or are known to the authors. The majority of them have a type-I serum sialotransferrin pattern; it is proposed to name these CDGS type I-X for the time being. Some of these patients have only a mild nervous system involvement. Studies are under way to unravel the basic defects in these patients.**
5. **Deficient *N*-glycosylation has been demonstrated in two well-known genetic diseases of carbohydrate metabolism: galactosemia and hereditary fructose intolerance. The hypoglycosylation in galactosemia is possibly due, at least in part, to a disturbed transport of uridine**

This review is on genetic defects of *N*-glycan synthesis (carbohydrate-deficient glycoconjugate syndromes or CDGS; MIM 212065).

A list of standard abbreviations is located immediately preceding the index in each volume. Additional abbreviations used in this chapter include: CDGS = carbohydrate-deficient; glycoconjugate syndrome; GDP = guanosine diphosphate; GC = guanosine-cytosine; CpG = cytidine-phosphate-guanine; GnT = *N*-acetylglucosaminyltransferase; GPI = glycosyl phosphatidylinositol; IEF = isoelectrofocusing; LAD = leukocyte adhesion deficiency; M-1-P = mannose 1-phosphate; M-6-P = mannose 6-phosphate; PMM = phosphomannomutase; PMI = phosphomannose isomerase; TBG = thyroxine-binding globulin.

diphosphogalactose into the Golgi; in hereditary fructose intolerance, it is secondary to inhibition of PMI by the accumulated fructose 1-phosphate.

INTRODUCTION AND HISTORY

The carbohydrate-deficient glycoprotein (CDG) or, more accurately, glycoconjugate syndromes are a family of genetic diseases characterized by a deficiency of the carbohydrate moiety (glycan) of glycoproteins and other glycoconjugates. In humans, only defects in the synthesis of asparagine-linked glycans (*N*-glycans) have been well characterized. The synthesis of the *N*-glycans is one of the longest metabolic pathways known, consisting of some 40 (enzymatic and transport) steps and encompassing three cellular compartments: a pre-endoplasmic reticulum (ER) (cytosolic) compartment, the ER, and the Golgi apparatus (Fig. 74-1). In the first part of this pathway, nucleotide diphosphate sugars, including guanosine diphosphomannose (GDP-mannose), are synthesized from intermediates of the glycolytic pathway. On the cytoplasmic side and subsequently on the lumenal side of the ER, a dolichyl-pyrophosphate oligosaccharide (Dol-pyrophosphate-$GlcNAc_2$-Man_9-Glc_3) precursor is assembled stepwise. Subsequently, the oligosaccharide moiety is transferred en bloc to selected asparagines of nascent proteins by the oligosaccharyltransferase complex. In the third part of the *N*-glycan synthesis, the three glucoses and next six mannoses are trimmed off and are replaced by two residues each of *N*-acetylglucosamine, galactose, and finally sialic acid in the Golgi apparatus. These *complex* N-linked glycoproteins are secreted into body fluids (secretory glycoproteins) or incorporated in cell membranes (membranous glycoproteins such as receptors and transporters). Some glycoproteins (lysosomal enzymes) undergo only trimming of the three glucose residues and retain a high number of mannoses on some of their glycans. This is followed by phosphorylation of end-standing mannoses, binding of the glycoproteins to mannose 6-phosphate (M-6-P) insulin-like growth factor II receptors and uptake in the lysosomes (*high-mannose* glycoproteins). *Hybrid* glycans have high-mannose as well as "complex" sugar branches.[1–5]

The glycans play very important and diverse roles in the metabolism, structure, and function of glycoproteins and other glycoconjugates.[3,6,7] This is dramatically illustrated by the severe diseases that result from defects in the synthesis of *N*-glycans. The basis for the discovery of these diseases has been the observation, by one of the authors (J.J.), of unusual serum protein abnormalities in the two princeps patients, viz. a decrease of thyroxine-binding globulin (TBG) and an increase of arylsulfatase A.[8] This led to a search for a defect in the common feature of these and other proteins, i.e., the glycan moiety. Substantial evidence for this "carbohydrate deficiency" was generated by the demonstration of a sialic acid deficiency in serum transferrin by isoelectrofocusing (IEF).[9] The important steps in the elucidation and delineation of these diseases are summarized in Table 74-1. Together with the mitochondrial diseases, they are among the most complex metabolic diseases. One can wonder why these diseases were not discovered earlier. Probably, because the serum glycoprotein abnormalities are generally not pronounced, they were disregarded or considered as unimportant. Also, because very different proteins are involved, a common cause is not apparent. Finally, there is no simple diagnostic test available. As of June 1998, about 270 patients worldwide (published and unpublished) were known to the authors.[10–28] The diagnosis of these multisystem diseases is usually made by IEF of serum transferrin.[29] Each of these defects causes somehow a deficiency of the end-standing sialic acid. Since this sugar is negatively charged, the IEF pattern shows a cathodal shift (Fig. 74-2). Three diseases have been well characterized at the enzymatic level: phosphomannomutase (PMM) deficiency, phosphomannose isomerase (PMI) deficiency (pre-ER disorders), and *N*-acetylglucosaminyltransferase (GnT) II deficiency (Golgi

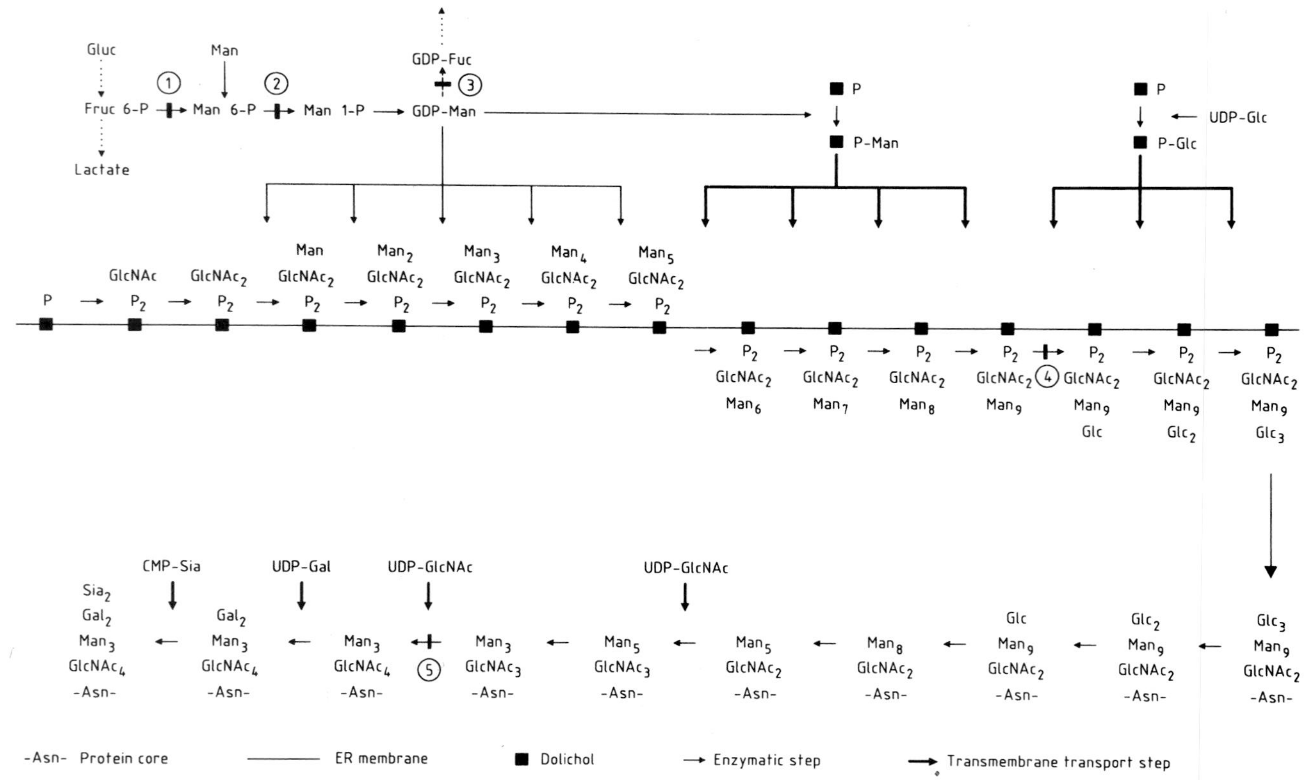

Fig. 74-1 Simplified scheme of the N-linked glycosylation pathway. Synthesis of glycosyl phosphatidylinositol (GPI) anchor formation has been omitted. Known defects are indicated by *bars* and *circled figures*: (1) phosphomannose isomerase (PMI) deficiency, (2) phosphomannomutase (PMM) deficiency, (3) defect in leukocyte adhesion deficiency (LAD II), (4) probable defect in hypoglycosylation syndrome, and (5) *N*-acetylglucosaminyltransferase (GnT) II deficiency.

Table 74-1 Chronology of Important Steps in the Delineation and Elucidation of Genetic Defects of N-Glycan Synthesis

Chronology		References
1980	Princeps description of patients (Belgian monozygotic twin sisters).	8
1984	Evidence for sialic acid deficiency in serum transferrin of patients (type-I isoelectrofocusing pattern).	9
1987	Description of abnormal subcutaneous fat distribution in patients.	47
1989	First report on non-Belgian patients (from Sweden).	36
1990	Demonstration that not only sialic acid but also galactose and *N*-acetylglucosamine are deficient in serum transferrin of patients.	73
1991	Introduction of the name *carbohydrate-deficient glycoprotein (CDG) syndrome.*	24
	Report of a new CDGS (type II).	198
1992	Evidence for an early glycosylation defect in CDGS type I.	117
	Report of LAD II.	206, 207
1993	Report of CDGS type III.	213
	Evidence for normal glycosylation of serum glycoproteins in the fetus with CDGS type I.	33
	CDG syndromes show a unique pattern of coagulation abnormalities.	65
1994	*N*-Acetylglucosaminyltransferase II deficiency is a cause of CDGS type II (type IIA).	197
	Linkage of CDGS type I to chromosome 16p13.3-13.12.	138
1995	Report of CDGS type IV.	214
	PMM deficiency is a cause of CDGS type I (type IA).	48
	CDGS type IA shows a unique pattern of endocrinologic abnormalities.	35
	Mannose corrects altered N-glycosylation in fibroblasts of PMM-deficient patients.	123
1996	PMM2 deficiency is a major cause of CDGS type I.	75
	Mutations in the *MGAT2* gene in CDGS type IIA.	204
1997	Mutations in the *PMM2* gene in CDGS type IA.	57
	Oral or intravenous mannose has no beneficial effect in patients with PMM deficiency.	22, 167
1998	Phosphomannose isomerase deficiency is a cause of CDGS type I and represents a new CDGS phenotype (hepatic-intestinal presentation) (type IB).	174,175, 177
	Description of a new type-I CDGS with unusually mild neurological involvement and hypoglucosylation.	195

ABBREVIATIONS: CDGS = carbohydrate-deficient glycoconjugate syndrome; GDP = guanosine diphosphate; LAD = leukocyte adhesion deficiency; PMM = phosphomannomutase.

disorder). The first two diseases show a type-I IEF pattern of serum sialotransferrins (called types IA and IB, respectively) whereas the third shows a type-II pattern (type IIA). In a considerable number of patients, the basic defect remains to be determined.

Mucolipidosis II (I-cell disease) and mucolipidosis III—lysosomal diseases due to UDP-GlcNAc:*N*-acetylglucosamine-1-phosphotransferase deficiency—can also be considered as disorders of N-linked glycan processing[30] (see the section "I-Cell Disease" in Chap. 138).

PHOSPHOMANNOMUTASE DEFICIENCY (CDGS TYPE IA) (MIM 601785)

Clinical Spectrum and Variability

The disease has a worldwide occurrence: patients have been identified from Austria, Australia, Belgium, Denmark, Ecuador, France, Germany, Italy, Japan, Norway, Peru, Poland, Portugal, Spain, Sweden, the Netherlands, the United Kingdom, and the United States.[8,9,24,31–77] However, its prevalence is unknown. Both sexes are equally affected.[78] In a number of cases, it can be reasonably accepted that they had (or have) CDG syndrome (CDGS) type IA on the basis of the clinical picture and the serum transferrin IEF pattern, in some combined with the result of linkage studies.[79,80] The patients described by Agamanolis et al in 1986[81] and by Chang et al in 1993[82] most probably also had CDGS type IA.[83] At least 124 patients are known with proven PMM deficiency (Table 74-3).

The clinical presentation comprises three main features: moderate to severe neurologic disease, more or less typical dysmorphy, and variable involvement of different organs. A somewhat artificial and partly overlapping but useful classification according to age has been proposed: the infantile multisystem stage, the childhood ataxia-mental retardation stage, the teenage leg atrophy stage, and the adult hypogonadal stage.[84] The diagnosis can be made in the first days of life. The neurologic picture comprises abnormal slow-rolling vertical or horizontal eye movements combined with slow head movements in the neonatal period, alternating internal strabismus, axial hypotonia, and hyporeflexia. A few patients have been reported with neonatal cerebral hemorrhage.[42,67,85] Later, a marked psychomotor retardation generally becomes obvious (IQ usually 40 to 60), as well as ataxia. Deafness has exceptionally been reported.[86] After infancy, retinitis pigmentosa,[38,46,87–89] joint contractures, strokelike episodes (in about 50 percent), and sometimes epilepsy develop. The strokelike episodes may be stupor or coma, and convulsions, as well as hemiplegia usually recovering in hours, days, or weeks. Two patients were blind for months after an episode (J. Jaeken et al, unpublished).[90]

Several patients developed deep venous thromboses, and one patient had an arterial thrombosis in a hand.[85,91–93] Only rarely do these patients achieve walking without support, but as a rule there is no regression. They mostly have an extrovert and cheerful personality. Growth tends to slow after infancy, and microcephaly develops in about half of the patients[84] (Fig. 74-3). During the first year(s) of life, there are variable feeding problems (anorexia, vomiting, diarrhea) that can result in severe failure to thrive and that can necessitate nasogastric tube feeding or feeding via gastrostomy.[94]

Other symptoms are mild facial dysmorphism (in particular, large, more or less dysplastic ears), abnormal subcutaneous adipose tissue distribution (fat pads, "orange peel" skin, "tallow," nipple retraction), skeletal abnormalities, dystrophic extremities, mild to moderate hepatomegaly, and mild to moderate tubular proteinuria (Fig. 74-4). It is important to note that dysmorphism can be minimal or absent. Some infants develop pericardial effusion (even before birth)[20,41,66,68,86,95–97] and/or cardiomyopathy.[66,69] There exists a great variability in clinical expression even among affected siblings.[98] One patient has been recently identified with a very mild clinical picture (slight to moderate psychomotor retardation and no dysmorphy) and normal levels of serum glycoproteins associated with an unusually high residual PMM activity (J. Jaeken et al, unpublished). A minority of infants develop a severe organ failure such as liver failure, cardiac insufficiency, nephrotic syndrome, or multiorgan failure.[20,64,69,86] Together with severe infections, these are the main causes of death. The overall mortality rate is about 20 percent, occurring

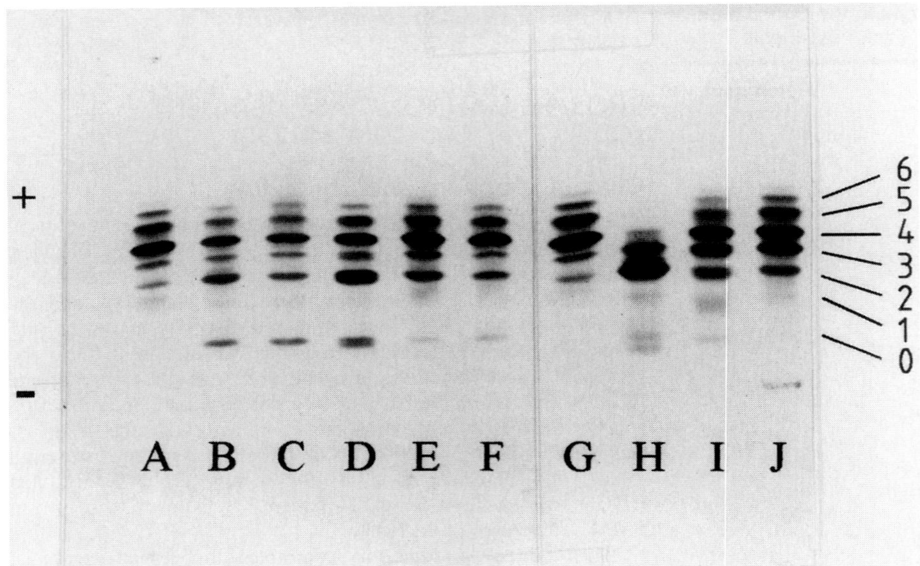

Fig. 74-2 Isoelectrofocusing of serum sialotransferrins. Figures on the *right* indicate the sialotransferrin fractions. *Lanes A and G* are from controls, *lanes B to F* show the type-I pattern [*B*, phosphomannomutase (PMM) deficiency; *C*, phosphomannose isomerase (PMI) deficiency; *D*, hypoglucosylation defect; *E*, unidentified defect with mild neurologic phenotype; and *F*, unidentified defect with severe neurologic phenotype], and *lanes H to J* show the type-II pattern [*H*, *N*-acetylglucosaminyltransferase (GnT II) deficiency; *I*, unidentified defect with mild liver disease; and *J*, unidentified defect with severe neurologic phenotype].

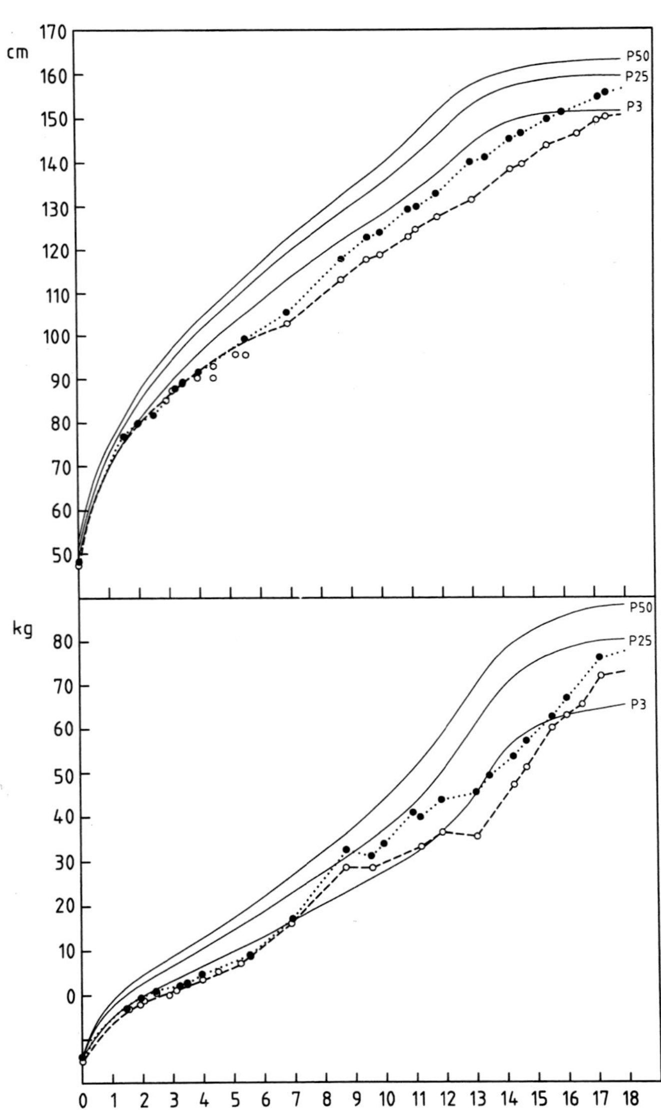

Fig. 74-3 Growth curves of the princeps patients with phosphomannomutase (PMM) deficiency (monozygotic twin sisters).[8]

mostly in the first years of life. In adulthood, the disease is compatible with a socially functioning but dependent, wheelchair-bound lifestyle.[25] Hypogonadism is common in females, but testicular atrophy has also been seen.[72,84] There is nonprogressive ataxia, strabismus, stable mental retardation, and variable peripheral neuropathy. Some adults show striking premature aging.[84]

Postmortem findings comprise olivopontocerebellar hypoplasia, loss of neurons, and gliosis in the cerebral cortex, the basal ganglia, the thalamus, and the spinal cord.[72] The peripheral nerves show decreased myelin and multivacuolar inclusions in the Schwann cells.[70] Renal cysts, fibrosis of the testes, and lymph node abnormalities have been observed.[72,74] Liver pathology is characterized by fibrosis, steatosis, and glycogen storage; electron microscopy shows myelin-like inclusions in the lysosomes of the hepatocytes but not in the Kupffer cells[71] (Fig. 74-5). Histologic examination of the skin shows abnormalities of the dermis consisting of increased and thickened bundles of collagen and elastic fibers in different directions. Cultured fibroblasts show features of premature aging (inclusions and ballooning) and dilated ER.[99,100]

Electrophysiologic investigations reveal decreased sensory and motor nerve conduction velocities (polyneuropathy) and abnormal somatosensory (and sometimes auditory and visual) evoked potentials.[41,101] Radiologic examination of the skeleton shows osteopenia, dysostosis multiplex,[102] and metaphalangeal dysplasia,[68] and computed tomographic scan of the brain shows mostly cerebellar atrophy of early onset. In some patients, the cerebellum initially looks rather normal but subsequently develops progressive hypoplasia (SI. Pascual-personal, communication). Other abnormalities include Dandy-Walker malformation; atrophy of the pons, brainstem, and olives; frontotemporal cortical atrophy; dilated ventricles; corpus callosum hypoplasia; and small cysts in the white matter.[24,40,103–105] Some children seem to develop supratentorial atrophy following episodes of neurologic deterioration.[105]

Biochemical Features

A large number of serum glycoproteins are abnormal, including transport proteins, glycoprotein hormones, lysosomal and other enzymes, and other glycoproteins (Table 74-2). These patients have a unique coagulopathy, with mainly a marked factor XI deficiency, as well as deficiencies of the anticlotting factors antithrombin, protein C, protein S, and heparin cofactor II.[54,65,85,91,106] Transient coagulation factor deficiencies have also been observed.[42] Analysis of platelet function reveals an

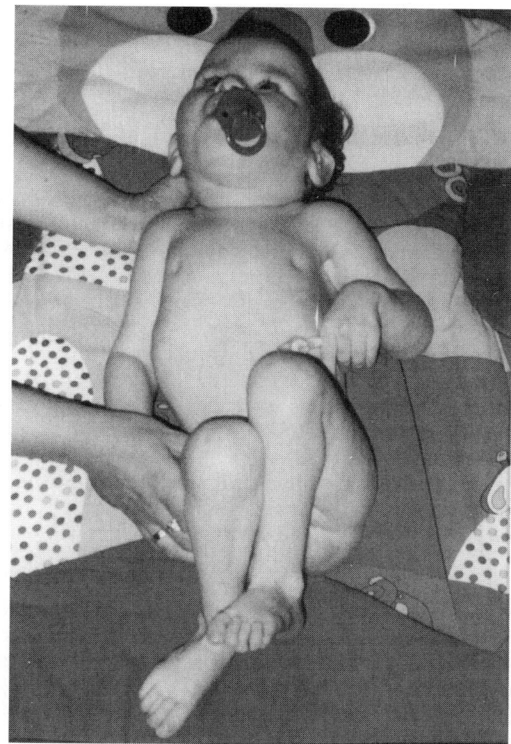

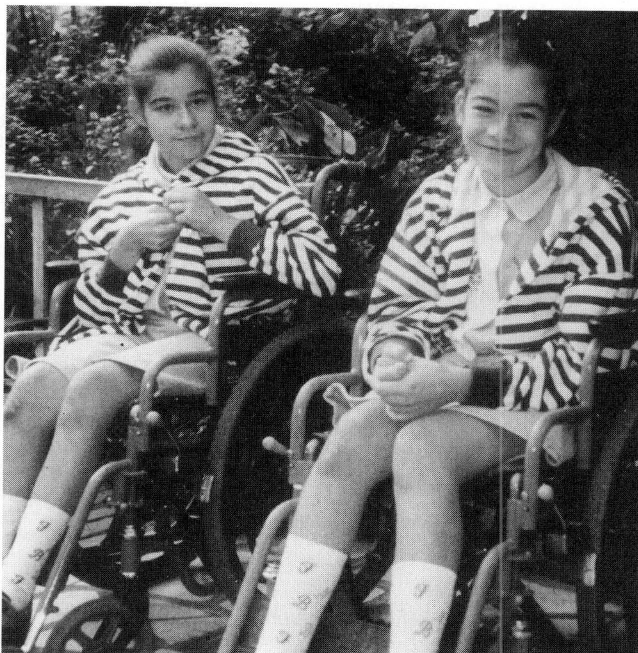

Fig. 74-4 A: Girl aged 2 years with phosphomannomutase (PMM) deficiency. Note the abnormal subcutaneous fat distribution, large ears, and button-gastrostomy necessitated by severe anorexia. B: Monozygotic twin sisters aged 22 years with PMM deficiency. As a rule, these patients are wheelchair bound.

increased reactivity resulting in spontaneous aggregation and in strong ristocetin-induced agglutination. This is compatible with the lower level of platelet membrane glycoprotein sialalation, demonstrated by flow cytometric analysis using several lectins.[107]

Besides, these patients have a peculiar age-dependent constellation of endocrinologic abnormalities, including hypergonadotropic hypogonadism with deficient follicle-stimulating hormone rather than luteinizing hormone action, transient hyperthyrotropinemia,

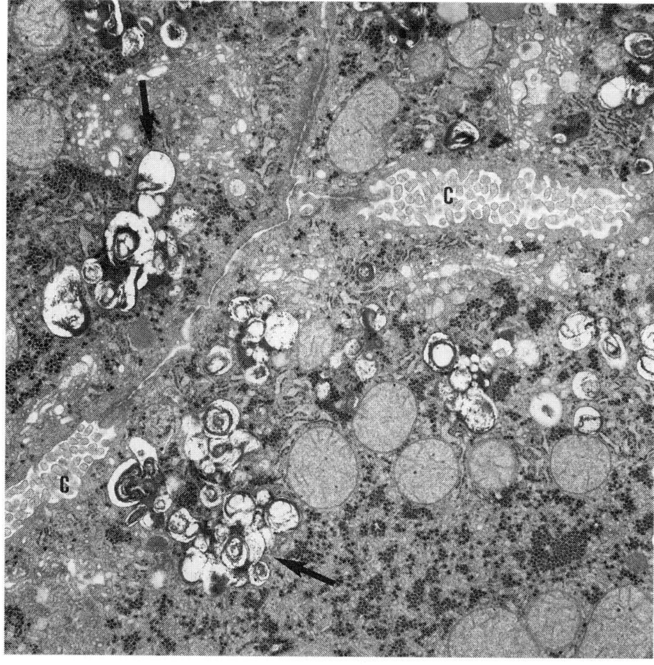

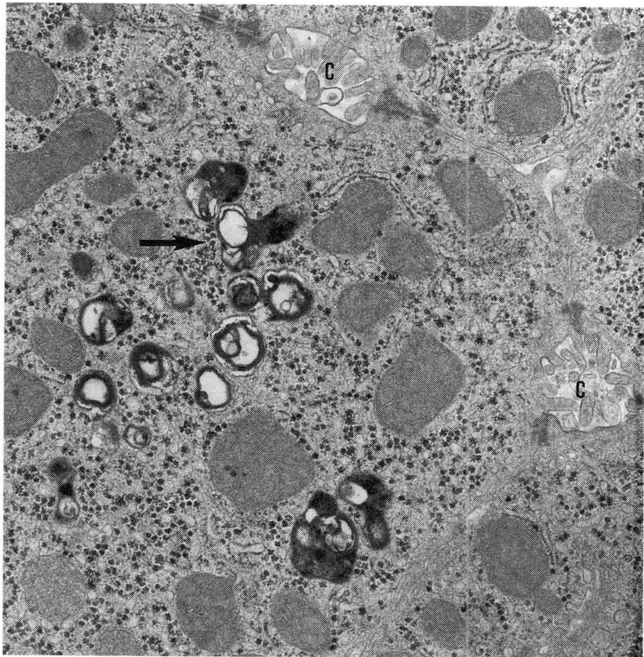

Fig. 74-5 Electron micrographs showing part of adjacent hepatocytes. A: A patient with phosphomannomutase (PMM) deficiency. The cytoplasm contains numerous lysosomal inclusions composed of concentrically arranged electron-dense membranes alternating with lucent content (*arrows*) (magnification, × 15,000). B: A patient with hereditary fructose intolerance before the start of the diet. The cytoplasm contains a moderate number of lysosomal inclusions composed of concentrically arranged electron-dense membranes alternating with lucent content (*arrow*) (magnification, × 23,000). (Courtesy of Prof. R. De Vos, Leuven, Belgium.)

Table 74-2 Glycoproteins Reported to Be Abnormal in Phosphomannomutase Deficiency and Showing an Abnormal Pattern on Isoelectrofocusing, Two-dimensional Electrophoresis, Western Blotting, and/or Decreased or Increased Concentration or Enzymatic Activity

Serum

Transport Proteins[8,9,54,65,111]

Apoprotein B, apoprotein CII, apoprotein E, ceruloplasmin, haptoglobin, α_2-macroglobulin, retinol-binding protein, sex hormone-binding globulin, thyroxine-binding globulin, transcobalamin II, transcortin, transferrin, vitamin D-binding globulin

Coagulation and Anticoagulation Factors[39,54,65,85,92,94,106,111]

Antithrombin, α_2-antiplasmin, coagulation factors II, V, VI, VIII, IX, X, XI, and XII, heparin cofactor II, plasminogen, protein C, protein S

Hormones[8,35,108,147]

Follicle-stimulating hormone, luteinizing hormone, prolactin, thyroid-stimulating hormone

Lysosomal Enzymes[8,109,240,241]

Arylsulphatase A, α-fucosidase, β-galactosidase, β-glucuronidase, β-hexosaminidase

Other Enzymes[160,242,243]

N-Acetylglucosaminidase, carboxypeptidase, cholinesterase

Other Glycoproteins[111–113,151,244–246]

Amyloid P, α_1-acid glycoprotein, α_1-antichymotrypsin, α_1-antitrypsin, α_1-B glycoprotein, clusterin, complement C3a, complement C4a, complement C1 esterase inhibitor, α_2-HS-glycoprotein, immunoglobulin G, orosomucoid, peptide PLS:29, peptide PLS:34, Zn-α_2-glycoprotein

Cerebrospinal Fluid[9,23,247]

β-Trace protein, transferrin

Leukocytes

Lysosomal Enzymes[109]

α-Fucosidase, β-glucuronidase, α-iduronidase, α-mannosidase, β-mannosidase

Sialoglycoproteins on B lymphocytes[248]

Fibroblasts[249]

Biglycan, decorin

Liver[113]

α_1-Acid glycoprotein, α_1-antitrypsin, haptoglobin, transferrin

inconsistent hyperprolactinemia, hyperglycemia-induced growth hormone release, deficiencies of hormone-binding glycoproteins, and possibly decreased insulin sensitivity.[8,35,108] Some of these endocrinologic abnormalities suggest defects in receptors (membrane glycoproteins) or postreceptor glycoproteins. Most glycoprotein concentrations or enzyme activities in serum are decreased; the others are increased (e.g., several lysosomal enzyme activities[109]) or normal (e.g., transferrin and immunoglobulins[110]). IEF of serum glycoproteins shows a cathodal shift with, in the case of transferrin, prominent a- and disialotransferrins, and decreased tetra-, penta- and hexasialotransferrins[9,73,111–113] (Fig. 74-2). These patients have to various extents decreased serum levels of copper, iron, zinc, cholesterol, total thyroxine, and triiodothyronine[114] as a consequence of decreased levels of the corresponding transport proteins. A rather constant and unexplained finding is the frequent hypoalbuminemia, which may contribute to the tendency of extravascular fluid effusion.[47] In cerebrospinal fluid, protein is often increased in infancy (and may subsequently normalize, or the opposite may occur), as well as some amino acids, particularly threonine, glycine, methionine, and histidine.[42,115] Proton magnetic resonance spectroscopy shows a reduction of *N*-acetylaspartate and an increase of glutamine and γ-aminobutyrate in white matter.[116]

Wada et al[117] and Yamashita et al[118,119] made a decisive contribution to the elucidation of this disease by showing that serum disialotransferrin from these patients completely lacks one or the other or both glycans and that serum asialotransferrin completely misses both glycans. Subsequently it was found that fibroblasts from these patients incorporate less [^{3}H]mannose into glycoprotein glycans and contain truncated dolichol-linked oligosaccharide precursors.[60,120–122] These data strongly suggested a defect in an early glycosylation step, namely, in the synthesis or the transfer of dolichol-linked oligosaccharide precursors. Defects in the synthesis of M-6-P from glucose[123] and in the synthesis of dolichyl-phosphate and *N*-acetylglucosaminyl pyrophosphoryl-dolichol,[124] as well as a deficiency of *N*-oligosaccharyltransferase activity,[125] were excluded. Finally, Van Schaftingen and Jaeken were able to identify the basic defect as PMM deficiency[48] (Fig. 74-1). This defect is associated with a reduction in mannose 1-phosphate (M-1-P), GDP-mannose, GDP-fucose, and dolichyl-phosphomannose in fibroblasts of these patients but not with an increase of the substrate M-6-P.[122,126] Moreover, mannose levels are reduced in serum of these patients.[127]

Remarkably, in serum of preterm infants with PMM deficiency (postmenstrual age less than 37 weeks), a normal IEF pattern of α_1-antitrypsin, β-hexosaminidase, and transferrin was observed.[33]

Properties of the Normal Enzyme

The involvement of an enzyme distinct from phosphoglucomutase in the conversion of M-6-P to M-1-P was first demonstrated by Guha and Rose.[128] It is now known that two different PMM isozymes exist in human tissues: PMM1, encoded by a gene at 22q13[129–131] and PMM2, encoded by a gene at 16p13,[57] respectively. They share about 66 percent sequence identity and are homologous to PMMs from *Saccharomyces cerevisiae* (also known as SEC53) and *Candida albicans*. There is also biochemical evidence for the existence of two different isozymes in rat tissues (M. Pirard et al, unpublished).[132]

Human PMM1 and PMM2 have been overexpressed in *Escherichia coli*, and their kinetic properties have been investigated (M. Pirard et al, unpublished).[129,132] Like most phosphomutases, eukaryotic PMMs require a bisphosphate cofactor (mannose 1,6-bisphosphate or glucose 1,6-bisphosphate in the case of PMM), which serves to phosphorylate the catalytic site. Conversion of M-6-P to M-1-P involves two successive phosphoryl transfer reactions with the intermediary formation of mannose 1,6-bisphosphate. The phosphorylated residue in eukaryotic PMM is the first aspartate in an extremely conserved DXDXT/V motif that is close to the N-terminus of the enzyme.[133] This motif is also found in a series of other phosphatases and phosphomutases, including L-3-phosphoserine phosphatase, which together make up a new protein family distantly related to ATPases of the Na^+/K^+ ATPase family.[133,134] In marked contrast, prokaryotic PMMs belong to the same protein family as eukaryotic phosphoglucomutases,[135] which are phosphorylated on a serine residue.

Human PMM1 and PMM2, as well as yeast PMM, are homodimers with subunits of 30 kDa.[132,137] PMM1 and the yeast enzyme are approximately as active in converting glucose 1-phosphate to glucose 6-phosphate as in converting M-1-P to M-6-P, whereas PMM2 acts 20 times more rapidly as a PMM than as a phosphoglucomutase (M. Pirard et al, unpublished). In addition, PMM1, though not PMM2, acts as a hexose 1,6-bisphosphatase, which hydrolyses both mannose 1,6-bisphosphate and glucose 1,6-bisphosphate at a rate corresponding to about 3 percent of its mutase activity. Thus, both in terms of substrate recognition and in the kind of reaction that is catalyzed, PMM2 is more specific than PMM1. PMM2 also displays a significantly higher affinity for its hexose bisphosphate cofactor than PMM1.

The tissue distributions of PMM1 and PMM2 have been studied in rats, based both on differences in their kinetic properties as well as in their reactivity to antibodies raised against the two human isozymes. PMM2 is more widely distributed than PMM1, which is restricted to the brain and the lungs, where it makes up about 65 percent and 10 percent, respectively, of the total PMM activity (M. Pirard et al, unpublished). PMM2 appears to be responsible for more than 97 percent of the activity in other tissues, including cerebellum. The finding that the PMM activity of one patient with CDGS type IA was below the detection level both in liver and in skeletal muscle argues also for PMM2 being the only isozyme expressed in these two tissues in humans (E. van Schaftingen, unpublished).

Properties of the Mutant Enzyme

The finding of very low activities (less than 5 percent of the normal activity) in liver, leukocytes, fibroblasts, or lymphoblasts of most patients with CDGS type IA indicates that most of the mutations identified in patients are particularly severe, a finding that appears to be confirmed by observations on mutant proteins expressed in bacterial systems (M. Pirard et al, unpublished). Significantly higher activity (up to 25 percent of the normal activity) has been recorded in fibroblasts or in lymphoblasts from some patients, whereas, in striking contrast, low activity (less than 5 percent) was observed in leukocytes of the same patient or of other patients with the same mutations.[52,75] It is not known presently whether this high activity in fibroblasts or lymphoblasts results from abnormal expression of PMM1 or from overexpression of a partially active enzyme.

Northern analysis of human tissues showed highest expression of the PMM2 gene in pancreas and liver, two organs with an important production of secreted proteins. The gene is also expressed in kidney and placenta, to a lesser extent in skeletal muscle and heart, and weakly in brain. On Northern blots, no expression is detected in lung.[57] The expression pattern of PMM1 is different from the pattern obtained for PMM2: expression of the latter is remarkably low in the brain.[129] It is not clear at present how these levels of expression would correlate with the clinical picture, in which the brain is one of the most severely affected organs. Immunohistologic data are not available yet. It could be worthwhile to look also at expression in fetal or infant brain.

The *PMM2* Gene

CDGS type IA is inherited in an autosomal recessive manner. Previous suggestions of X-linkage[47] have not been further substantiated. By using DNA samples from 25 small nuclear families for linkage analysis, the CDGS type-IA gene had been localized to chromosome 16p13, with a Lod score above 8.[138] The linkage to the region between D16S406 and D16S500 was later confirmed in 10 of 11 informative families.[56] In one family with two affected siblings, the disease was, however, not linked to chromosome 16p, indicating genetic heterogeneity for CDGS type IA.[56] Fine mapping of the disease locus by haplotype and linkage disequilibrium analysis in Scandinavian families[139] defined a region of less than 1 cM between markers D16S513 and D16S502. By observing critical crossovers in carriers, identified by measuring PMM activities in siblings of patients, the minimal region was contained in the region between markers D16S404 and D16S406.[140] The difference was caused by inconsistencies in the available physical maps, which have now been rectified.[141] There is a clear founder effect in Scandinavian families with CDGS type IA.[139] Of 25 CDGS type-IA chromosomes, originating from the southwestern Sweden, southern Norway, and eastern Denmark, 15 had a common haplotype (A haplotype). In two families, the CDGS type-IA children were homozygous for this haplotype.

The identification of the *PMM2* gene on chromosome 16p13 and the identification of mutations in this gene that segregate with the disease[57] gave conclusive support to the biochemical evidence that PMM deficiency is the basis for CDGS type IA.[48,49] The human *PMM2* gene[57] and the *PMM1* gene (OMIM 601786)[129] were identified on the basis of the sequence similarity of a number of expressed sequence tags in the public database with the sequence of yeast PMM or SEC53. The cDNA of PMM2 has an open reading frame of 738 base pairs (bp) and encodes a protein of 246 amino acids. The protein has been expressed in vitro and shown to have PMM activity. The degree of identity with yeast SEC53 is higher for PMM2 than for PMM1.[57,129] Evidence that the *PMM2* gene mapped to the CDGS type-IA minimal candidate region on the short arm of chromosome 16 was obtained by fluorescence in situ hybridization (FISH) analysis and by hybridizing a *PMM2* probe to DNA from yeast artificial chromosomes (YACs) in a contig that spanned this region.[140,141] The gene is located between D16S3020 and D16S502/D16S406.[140,141] Marker D16S3020 is close to (within 20 kb) and upstream (5′) of the *PMM2* gene. The chromosomal orientation of the gene has not been determined.

The *PMM2* gene consists of eight exons spanning approximately 20 kb of genomic DNA.[57,137] The sizes of the coding exons range from 66 to 116 bp. An analysis of the sequence of the 5′ region of the gene suggests that *PMM2* has a housekeeping promoter: the region upstream of the first ATG is characterized by a high guanosine-cytosine (GC) content and contains many cytosine-phosphate-guanosine (CpG) dinucleotides and several potential binding sites for transcription factor Sp1. This is expected for an enzyme with a very fundamental role in posttranslational processing. However, the variable expression suggests that the basal expression can be modulated in a tissue-specific manner. Thus, specific elements must be present in the promoter or in enhancers, to more precisely regulate the expression in tissues with an important production of glycosylated (secreted) proteins and a corresponding high expression of the gene.

Phosphomannomutase Deficiency and Mutations in the *PMM2* Gene

In a first survey of *PMM2* mutations in patients with CDGS type IA, 56 patients from 13 countries were included, all except two of Caucasian origin.[52] The PMM deficiency was documented biochemically in 47 patients from whom fibroblasts, lymphoblasts, or fresh leukocytes were available. In two of these patients, a partial deficiency of PMM was found in fibroblasts, and, in one family, intermediate values were measured in the patients' lymphoblasts. In total, mutations were found on 111 (99 percent) of 112 disease chromosomes. In one Japanese patient, heterozygous for one mutation at the genomic level, a second mutation was not found even though all exons were scrutinized by sequencing. This mutation is probably in a regulatory region of the gene.

Molecular analysis of the *PMM2* gene has led to the identification of a large number of mutations that are generally of the missense type. A total of 36 different mutations detected in 124 patients by investigators from Belgium, Denmark, Germany, France, the United Kingdom, and Japan have been compiled in Table 74-3. The mutations are numbered according to their position in the cDNA (GenBank accession number HSU 85773).[57]

The most intriguing observation is the total lack of patients homozygous for the most frequent mutation: R141H (T. Martinsson, personal communication).[142] On the other hand, patients homozygous for the relatively frequent F119L mutation were found[52,141,143] as well as one patient homozygous for the D65Y mutation.[52] The latter is a rare mutation, and the disease allele was probably inherited from a common ancestor of the parents. Thus, it is suggested that the R141H mutation is a severe mutation, and homozygosity may not be compatible with life.

CDGS type IA is pan-ethnic, but different populations have their own set of mutations (Table 74-3). R141H is by far the most frequent in Caucasians. F119L is very frequent in Western Europe and particularly in Scandinavia due to a founder effect (Sweden and Denmark).[141,142] D188G seems to be restricted to Belgian (Flemish) and Dutch patients. V44A is probably of Spanish origin, whereas D65Y, homozygous in a Portuguese patient, is also found in a French patient (with Portuguese ancestors). V129M may well be of Italian origin. In Japanese patients, three specific mutations have been found: F144L, R238P, and Y229S.[52,144] It seems that some mutations are old mutations that have been present in the different populations for centuries. For instance, R141H is caused by a CGC-to-CAC transition, but the equally likely CGC-to-TGC transition (R141C, which is found in a processed pseudogene,

Table 74-3 Mutations in the *PMM2* Gene

Exon	Mutation	Codon Change	Amino Acid Change	*N**	Status†	Origin‡	References
1	26 G>A	TGC>TAC	C9Y	2	SC	F	V. Cormier-Daire et al., in preparation
2	131 T>C	GTA>GCA	V44A	3	C	E, Sp	52
3	193 G>T	GAT>TAT	D65Y	3	C	F, Po	52
4	303 C>G	AAC>AAG	N101K	1	NC	G	52
4	317 A>G	TAC>TGC	Y106C	1	C	B	52, 57
4	324 delG	Frameshift	. . .	1	. . .	G	52
4	323 C>T	GCG>GTG	A108V	1	C	F	52,57
4	338 C>T	CCG>CTG	P113L	15	C	B, F, G, N, Po, Sp	52, 57, 259
5	349 G>C	GGT>CGT	G117R	1	C	D	142
5	357 C>A	TTC>TTA	F119L	47	C	D, F, G, N, Sw, UK	52, 57, 141, 142, T. Marquardt et al., personal communication
5	368 G>A	CGA>CAA	R123Q§	8	C	F, J, N, Sp	52, V. Cormier-Daire et al., in preparation
5	385 G>A	GTG>ATG	V129M	3	SC	F, I, USA	52, 57, V. Comier-Daire et al., in preparation
5	389 delC	Frameshift	. . .	1	. . .	USA	260
5	391 C>G	CCT>GCT	P131A	1	C	F	52
5	395 T>C	ATT>ACT	I132T	4	C	F, I	52, V. Cormier-Daire et al., in preparation
5	396T>A	ATT>AAT	I132N	1	C	UK	F. Imtiaz, et al., personal communication
5	422 G>A	CGC>CAC	R141H	96	C	B, D, E, F, G, N, Po, Sp, Sw, UK, USA	52, 57, 142, 250, V. Cormier-Daire et al., in preparation; T. Marquardt et al., unpublished
5	430 C>T	TTC>CTC	F144L	2	C	J	144
6	452 A>G	GAA>GGA	E151G	1	SC	N	G. Matthijs et al., unpublished
6	458T>C	ATA>ACA	I153T	1	C	US	250
6	470 T>C	TTT>TCT	F157S	1	SC	Sp	G. Matthijs et al., unpublished
6	484 C>T	CGG>TGG	R162W	2	C	N, UK	52, 57
6	523 G>C	GGA>CGA	G175R	1	C	B	52
7	563 A>G	GAC>GGC	D188G	5	C	B, N	52
7	623 G>C	GGA>GCA	G208A	2	C	UK, USA	52
8	647 A>T	AAT>ATT	N216I	1	C	I	52
8	653 A>T	CAT>CTT	H218L	1	SC	G	G. Matthijs et al., unpublished
8	669 C>G	GAC>GAG1	D223E	1	C	D	142
8	677 C>G	ACC>AGC	T226S	2	C	F	V. Cormier-Daire et al., in preparation
8	686 A>C	TAC>TCC	Y229S	2	C	J	52, 144
8	691 G>A	GTG>ATG	V231M	15	C	B, F, I, Pe, UK, USA	52, 57, V. Cormier-Daire et al., in preparation
8	697 G>A	GCG>ACG	A233T¶	2	C	F, G	52
8	710 C>T	ACG>ATG	T237M	4	C	F, UK, USA	52
8	710 C>T	ACG>AGG	T237R	2	C	F, G	52
8	713 G>C	CGC>CCC	R238P	2	SC	J	52
8	722 G>C	TGT>TCT	C241S	1	NC	B	G. Matthijs et al., unpublished

* Number of times observed in the series of 248 disease alleles (compiled up to June 1998).

† Conservation status compared with the human PMM1, yeast PMM (SEC53), and *C. albicans* PMM. C = conserved; NC=not conserved; SC=semiconserved.

‡ Geographic origin: B = Belgium; D = Denmark; E = Ecuador; F = France; G = Germany; I = Italy; J = Japan; N = The Netherlands; Pe = Peru; Po = Portugal; Sw = Sweden; Sp = Spain; UK = United Kingdom; USA = United States.

§ The R123Q mutation was mistakenly labeled R123G in reference.[109]

¶ A233T is observed in combination with either the T237R or the T237M mutation (patients 46 and 53).

At the time of submittal of these data, mutations were not yet detected on the following numbers of disease chromosomes: 1/16 (T. Marquardt et al., personal communication), 2/36,[142] 3/146 (G. Matthijs et al., unpublished),[52] 3/26 (V. Cormier-Daire et al., in preparation), 2/18 (F. Imtiaz et al., personal communication).

NOTE: The Internet addresses of the parent organizations on CDGS are http://www.cdgs.com/ for the CDGS Family Network, Inc. in the United States and http://www.emu.lu.se/cdg/indexeng.shtml for the CDG Societies in Scandinavia.

derived from *PMM2* and located on chromosome 18q) has not been observed in patients. Thus, R141H may be a very old mutation, like the frequent ΔF508 in cystic fibrosis,[145] unless R141C is a dominant, lethal mutation. On the other hand, some mutations must have occurred independently in the different populations. For instance, R123Q, shared by one Spanish and two Dutch patients, is syntenic with a polymorphism at nucleotide 324 in the coding region and was also identified in a Japanese patient and a French patient but without the polymorphism.[52,140] It is remarkable that only two frameshift mutations have been observed, while the remaining are missense mutations. Perhaps, only mutations that retain residual protein and enzyme activity are tolerated in patients because more severe mutations might not be compatible with life. G175R might also affect splicing. The 25 mutations found to date affect residues that are strictly conserved among PMMs (Table 74-3).

The mutation analysis has revealed extensive allelic heterogeneity. Hence, very limited inferences can be made from the genotype-phenotype comparison. There is no clear correlation between the PMM activities and the genotype in 6 and 14 patients with the R141H/P113L and R141H/F119L combinations, respectively. It has previously been remarked that a great variability exists in the clinical expression, even among affected siblings.[98] One significant observation is the high mortality rate among patients with the D188G/R141H genotype: four of five patients died before the age of 2, whereas the fifth patient, now 10 years of age, is severely affected. The twin patients, described originally, are now 22 years old and relatively well, and have an R141H/

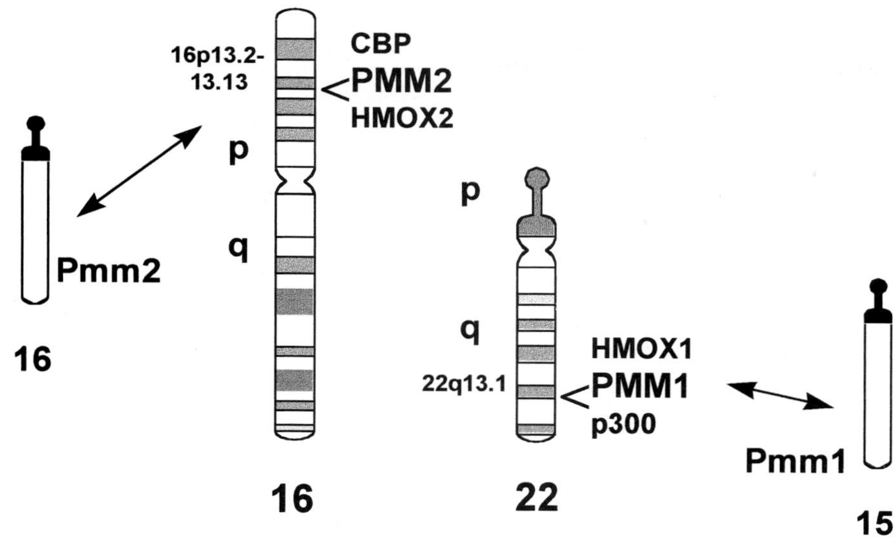

Fig. 74-6 The orthologues of the human *PMM1* and *PMM2* genes have been cloned and mapped in the mouse. *Pmm1* is located on mouse chromosome 15, and *Pmm2* is located on mouse chromosome 16.

P113L genotype. R123G is present in two Spanish patients with pubertal development, which is not normally seen in CDGS type IA. There is a relatively high residual PMM activity in fibroblasts of the D65Y/D65Y patient.[52] However, the same D65Y mutation, in combination with R141H, was found in a patient with a severe phenotype, who died at a very young age.[52] There is emerging data on adult cases of CDGS type IA. A 35-year-old patient with a typical history of CDGS type IA was homozygous for F119L.[52,143] French investigators identified two patients (30 and 33 years old) with the C9Y/R141H genotype (V. Cormier-Daire, in preparation).

The search for the CDGS type-I gene has revealed the existence of a family of *PMM* genes in humans. At least two genes in the human genome—*PMM1* and *PMM2* located on chromosome 22q13 and 16p13, respectively—encode active PMMs. An alignment was published in Matthijs et al.[57] *PMM2* is shorter than *PMM1* and yeast and *C. albicans PMM*, and the difference is mainly due to a deletion of seven amino acids in the N-terminal part of the protein. An insertion of two amino acids, after position 63 and between conserved domains, is unique to PMM1.

Comparison of the genomic structure of *PMM1* and *PMM2* indicates that these genes must have arisen by gene duplication.[137] There are 78 differences at the amino acid level between *PMM1* and *PMM2*, not including the four mutational events that have led to difference in length of the proteins. At the DNA level, the silent sites vary in over 50 percent of the positions, suggesting that the ancestral gene was duplicated before the mammalian radiation that occurred 75 to 110 million years ago. We have cloned *Pmm1* and *Pmm2*, the orthologues of *PMM1* and *PMM2* in the mouse, and these genes are indeed located on syntenic chromosomal regions in the human genome and in the mouse genome (L. Heykants et al, unpublished) (Fig. 74-6).

During the mapping experiments, a processed pseudogene was identified on chromosome 18.[140] It is more closely related to *PMM2*. When compared with *PMM2*, several base substitutions and single-base insertions or deletions are present, suggesting that this processed pseudogene (*PMM2ψ*) has been inactivated by mutations. Remarkably, several base substitutions in *PMM2* that are associated with disease are also present at the corresponding positions in the *PMM2ψ*. Thus, mutations that occur at a slow rate in the active gene in the population have also accumulated in the processed pseudogene. It is an important observation, because these mutations might interfere with certain mutation detection strategies, e.g., dot-blot analysis. Therefore, probes need to be designed carefully.

Pathogenesis

Theoretically, an accumulation of substrate, a deficiency of reaction product(s), or a combination of both might be responsible for the symptoms and signs of PMM deficiency. No accumulation of substrate has been demonstrated: normal levels of M-6-P were found in fibroblasts of PMM-deficient patients.[126] On the other hand, evidence has been presented for decreased levels, in PMM-deficient fibroblasts, of M-1-P and its metabolites GDP-mannose, GDP-fucose, and dolichyl-phosphomannose,[122,126] and hence underglycosylation of (mainly N-linked) glycoproteins. Deficiency and/or dysfunction of an innumerable number of glycoproteins (extracellular, membranous, and intracellular) due to under-glycosylation undoubtedly plays a major role in the phenotypical expression of this disorder. For example, the lysosomal storage of heterogeneous material[71] and the elevated levels of lysosomal enzymes in the plasma can be easily explained by the early and generalized hypoglycosylation of these proteins causing a deficiency of the M-6-P signal necessary for their uptake in the lysosomes. Moreover, GDP-mannose and dolichyl-phosphomannose are essential for the biosynthesis of glycosyl phosphatidyl-inositol (GPI) anchors, and, thus, membrane-bound enzymatic and receptor functions, cell-to-cell signaling, and cell adhesion might also be affected.

Glycosylation plays a role in determining the circulatory lifetime of proteins, and the low serum levels of a number of glycoproteins in this disease can be easily explained by enhanced clearance from the circulation.[7,146] The hypogonadism could be tentatively attributed to hypoglycosylation of pituitary gonadotropins possibly associated with hypoglycosylation of gonadal receptor and/or postreceptor glycoproteins.[35,108] However, Kristiansson et al[147] were unable to demonstrate a deficiency of the terminal charged carbohydrate portion of gonadotropins. It is suggested that hypoglycosylation of peripheral myelin glycoproteins such as P_o is, at least in part, responsible for the peripheral neuropathy.[148] Cerebellar hypoplasia is a well-known feature of many metabolic diseases but is particularly pronounced and usually present at a very early age in PMM deficiency. Since inhibition of N-linked glycosylation induces early apoptosis at least in some cells,[149] we hypothesize that this mechanism might also be involved in this cerebellar hypoplasia.

The dilatation of the ER in liver[71] and fibroblasts[122] of these patients probably results from deficient glycosylation of glycoproteins causing their accumulation in this cell organelle.[150] We hypothesize that this ER dilatation also causes ER dysfunction and hence possibly the hypoalbuminemia of this disease, due to disturbed protein synthesis.

Diagnosis

PMM deficiency should be considered in any child or adult with unexplained psychomotor retardation, whether isolated or associated with various combinations of the aforementioned clinical and biochemical abnormalities. Especially suggestive features are unusual subcutaneous fat distribution, retracted nipples, feeding problems with failure to thrive, liver fibrosis, and decreased coagulation factor XI and antithrombin. Owing to the partial TBG deficiency, some patients are detected through neonatal screening for congenital hypothyroidism by T4 measurement.

The clinical suspicion of PMM deficiency can be substantiated by IEF and immunofixation of a serum glycoprotein, usually transferrin,[9,73] or any other method measuring charge or mass changes of glycoproteins.[112,113,151–153] Normal serum transferrin is mainly composed of tetrasialotransferrin besides small amounts of mono-, di-, tri-, penta-, and hexasialotransferrin.[154] The partial deficiency of sialic acid in PMM deficiency causes a cathodal shift resulting in a marked increase of both asialo- and disialotransferrin, and a decrease of tetra-, penta-, and hexasialotransferrin (type-I pattern) (Fig. 74-2). These changes can be measured by densitometry. It has to be noted that cord sera from controls show increased a-, mono-, and disialotransferrin fractions.[155] Percentile values of the different serum sialotransferrin fraction in controls and in patients have been published.[21] It is important to use serum for the IEF since EDTA plasma can produce pseudopathologic patterns.[22] Dried blood spots can also be used.[156] When an abnormal pattern is obtained, IEF of another glycoprotein (e.g., hexosaminidase, TBG) should be performed to rule out a protein variant of transferrin. The determination of carbohydrate-deficient transferrin in serum uses microanion-exchange chromatography followed by a transferrin radioimmunoassay of the eluate.[157,158] This method, initially developed for diagnosing alcohol abuse, measures the concentration of cathodal isotransferrins in serum, while the normal components are retained by the anion exchanger. Except when rare genetic D variants of transferrin are present, increased concentrations of carbohydrate-deficient transferrin indicate a reduction in its sialic acid content.[159,160] The diagnosis is confirmed by finding decreased PMM activity in leukocytes or fibroblasts.[48,60,75]

This diagnosis should be completed by mutational analysis. The methods and primers for the mutation analysis of the eight exons of the PMM2 gene by single strand conformation polymorphism (SSCP) have been described.[52] Given the frequency of the R141H, F119L, and P113L mutations, the obvious approach is to search for these mutations first. SSCP analysis represents a fairly simple, reliable, and cost-effective approach for further molecular analysis of CDGS type-IA patients. Recent work shows that PMM deficiency is found in a majority, but not in all, of patients with CDGS type I. In these patients, there is no reason to search for mutations in the *PMM2* gene. Accordingly, in the family in which the linkage to chromosome 16 could be excluded,[56] no PMM deficiency was found in the propositus. Due to this heterogeneity, PMM assays are still useful for diagnosis. The only drawback of these measurements is that in some cases the residual activity in fibroblasts or in lymphoblasts may be as high as 30 percent of the control value, whereas, in other samples derived from the same patients or from other patients with the same genotype, the activity was less than 5 percent of the control activity.[52] This problem has not been encountered in assays performed with fresh material such as leukocytes or liver. In the latter cases, a profound deficiency has nearly always been observed. We have at present no explanation for these discordant findings. One possibility is that *PMM1* or the mutant forms of *PMM2* become overexpressed after several passages in culture. PMM measurements are also useful for the identification of carriers. If cells from an affected child are not available, indirect evidence can be obtained from the PMM activities in leukocytes from the parents. This has proven worthwhile in two cases with an urgent request for prenatal diagnosis, in which we derived information on the PMM deficiency from the parents, before initiating the molecular analysis.[161] In view of the genetic heterogeneity, prenatal testing should be offered only to families with a documented PMM deficiency and mutations in *PMM2*. Thus far, we have combined enzymatic measurements and mutation analysis for prenatal diagnosis.[161] The molecular analysis is the most dependable test for prenatal diagnosis. Remarkably, for an unknown reason, abnormal glycosylation of serum proteins cannot be detected during pregnancy in fetuses affected by PMM deficiency.[33,162,163]

Treatment and Prognosis

No efficient treatment is available, although the finding that mannose is able to correct glycosylation in fibroblasts with PMM deficiency raised some hope.[122,164,165] Trials with oral and intravenous mannose did not cause clinical or biochemical improvement.[22,166,167] The reason why mannose is active in vitro is not fully understood; maybe it stimulates the residual PMM activity by increasing the concentration of the substrate M-6-P (Fig. 74-2).

Since mannose is effective in vitro, why has it no effect in vivo? There are only few studies regarding the bioavailability, absorption, fate, and incorporation of mannose into glycoproteins in higher animals.[168] One study in humans concluded that oral mannose was inefficiently absorbed by the gut.[169] Recent work indicated that mannose is efficiently taken up by control fibroblasts,[170,171] possibly via a specific mannose transporter, but not by PMM-deficient fibroblasts.[172] On the other hand, it has been shown, at least in cultured hepatoma cells, that radiolabeled mannose is a better precursor for glycan synthesis than radiolabeled glucose.[173] This is, however, no proof that the cells depend on exogenous mannose for correct glycosylation, as the preferential labeling from mannose may simply reflect the lack of isotopic equilibration of the M-6-P and glucose 6-phosphate pools.

Prognosis is discussed in the section "Clinical Spectrum and Variability."

PHOSPHOMANNOSE ISOMERASE DEFICIENCY (CDGS TYPE IB) (MIM 602579)

Clinical Spectrum and Variability

The clinical presentation is very different from that of PMM deficiency, since it is mainly hepatic-intestinal without dysmorphic features and with no or only minor neurologic involvement.[45,174–178] Six patients (four boys and two girls) have been reported, belonging to four families and four nationalities (Lebanese, German, Italian, and Turkish) The histories of these patients are summarized below. Symptoms started at ages between 1 and 11 months. The Lebanese patient was admitted at 5.5 months for diarrhea since the age of 3 months, as well as for symptomatic hyperinsulinemic hypoglycemia. The liver was enlarged (6 cm) and firm. Liver biopsy revealed fibrosis of the portal spaces and microvesicular steatosis. Reevaluation at 10 months showed dwarfism and generalized edema due to hypoalbuminemia. Gross motor development was moderately retarded. Serum bilirubin and glutamate-oxaloacetate transaminase were slightly increased. Prothrombin time was 63 percent. There was intermittent slight proteinuria and moderate hyperaminoaciduria (particularly of glycine) Radiologic examination of the intestine showed fragmentation and flocculation of the contrast substance and suggested malabsorption. On endoscopy, there was easy bleeding of the intestinal mucosa. Histology of duodenal biopsy samples showed partial villus atrophy with hypercellularity and only rare and discrete lymphangiectasias. Repeat liver biopsy at 1 year revealed a more pronounced picture of congenital hepatic fibrosis with proliferation of biliary canaliculi without any inflammation and without parenchymal alteration. Renal hyperechogenicity was found on ultrasound examination. The patient was fed a hydrolyzed, medium-chain triglyceride-supplemented milk via nasogastric tube. He suffered from frequent bacterial as well as viral gastroenteritis. Evaluation at 26 months showed a large abdomen with pronounced collateral circulation, numerous disseminated angiomas, and persistent hepatomegaly. A gastrostomy was performed. Psychomotor development and neurologic examination were normal. He died at the age of 4 years from an unknown cause.[45,59,175]

The German patient, a boy, started vomiting with diarrhea at the age of 11 months. Protein-losing enteropathy was diagnosed. Ultrastructural analysis of a small bowel biopsy sample showed lysosomal inclusions and a dilated ER filled with tubular bundles. In addition, he had recurrent thromboses of the extremities and the forehead, and episodes of severe abdominal pain and vomiting due to microthromboses of the jejunum. During prophylaxis with vitamin-K antagonists, several life-threatening, diffuse gastrointestinal bleedings occurred.[174,176] The Italian patient, a boy, was admitted at the age of 1.5 months for recurrent vomiting since the age of 1 month, lipodystrophy, and hypotonia. He was breast-fed. He showed megaloblastic anemia and disturbed liver function test results. No liver infection was demonstrated. Computed tomographic scan of the brain showed diffuse white-matter hypodensity and a normal cerebellum. At the age of 3 months, solid food was introduced and, from then on, he progressively improved and eventually completely normalized.[175,178]

In the consanguineous Turkish family, three siblings were affected. The oldest patient, a 19-year-old girl, was admitted 24 times from the age of 10 months with episodic vomiting sometimes associated with pronounced diarrhea. During the attacks, her liver was mildly enlarged and the serum transaminases were slightly to moderately elevated. There was no renal or gastrointestinal protein loss. At 11 years, she presented with severe liver failure. Liver biopsy at 14 years showed minimal histologic abnormalities consistent with "ductal plate malformation." Her sister, now 18 years old, presented at 2 months with an acute multiorgan failure. Otherwise, she had a very similar clinical history. In the 14-year-old brother, symptoms started at the age of 10 months. Liver biopsies performed in both at the ages of 18 months and 3 years, respectively, were consistent with congenital hepatic fibrosis.[177]

In 1985, four infants were reported with a very similar syndrome called "secretory diarrhea with protein-losing enteropathy, enterocolitis cystica superficialis, intestinal lymphangiectasia, and congenital hepatic fibrosis."[179] They originated from the same northeastern part of Quebec and consanguinity was found in two kindreds. Hypoglycemia, present in all, was symptomatic only in two. One also had seizures and hemiplegia secondary to cerebral thromboses and infarcts, and another had a nonfunctional multicystic kidney. All died between 4 and 21 months of age, most probably also of the same disease, the more since antithrombin measured in one patient was deficient.

Biochemical Features

The blood biochemical abnormalities were indistinguishable from those found in PMM deficiency, including decrease of albumin,[45,174–178] low-density lipoprotein (LDL)-cholesterol, TBG, cholinesterase,[178] antithrombin,[45,174,175,178] protein C, protein S,[175] and factor XI;[175,178] hypoglycosylation of transferrin with type-I IEF pattern[174,175,177] and of α_1-antitrypsin;[174,178] normal structure of transferrin glycans, which were partially absent;[174,177] and decreased mannose levels[174] (Fig. 74-2). Contrary to PMM deficiency, there was an increased incorporation of [2-^{3}H]mannose into newly synthesized glycoproteins in fibroblasts.[174] PMI deficiency was demonstrated in leukocytes,[174,177] fibroblasts[174,175,177] and liver.[177]

Properties of the Normal Enzyme

PMI catalyzes the first committed step in the synthesis of the nucleotide sugar GDP-mannose. The enzyme was initially isolated from yeast[180] and shown to contain 1 mol Zn^{2+}/mol enzyme. Implication of this divalent cation in catalysis is supported by the observation that various metal-ion chelators cause the inactivation of the enzyme, which is reversed upon Zn^{2+} addition, as well as from the observation that Zn^{2+} promotes the nonenzymatic conversion of M-6-P to fructose 6-phosphate.[182] The x-ray three-dimensional structure of the *C. albicans* enzyme shows that this ion is bound to the side chains of two histidines, a glutamate and a glutamine, as well as to water, which presumably occupies the place of the substrate.[183] PMI is a candidate target for fungicidal therapy, e.g., in *C. albicans* infections; hence the significant interest in this gene.

The cDNA encoding the human PMI has previously been cloned and shown to encode a 423-amino-acid protein homologous to the enzymes from yeast, *C. albicans*, and *E. coli*, although not to those of several bacteria.[184] Northern blots indicated that the enzyme is widely distributed in human tissues. Refolding of the heterologously expressed human enzyme was shown to be dependent on Zn^{2+}, further proving the importance of this ion.[185]

PMI can be easily measured spectrophotometrically through the conversion of M-6-P to fructose 6-phosphate.[182] The presence of metal chelators in the extraction buffer should be minimized, as they cause progressive inactivation of the enzyme.[186]

Properties of the Mutant Enzyme

The mutated PMIs have not yet been isolated in pure form, and therefore the precise effect of the mutations on the enzymatic activity is not known. Residual PMI activities ranging between about 3 percent and 20 percent of the control values have been observed in extracts of leukocytes, fibroblasts, and liver from the patients that have been analyzed.[174,175,177] It is not known if this residual activity is contributed by the mutated enzyme. No increase in PMI activity was observed when the Arg219Gln mutant was expressed in COS cells, whereas a 10-fold increase was observed in cells transfected with the wild-type enzyme. This suggests that the mutated enzyme is either poorly active or extremely unstable.

The *PMI* Gene

The human *PMI* cDNA sequence is published (GenBank accession number 602579).[184] The genomic structure of the *PMI* gene is not available. The gene has been localized to human chromosome 15q22.[184]

Properties of the Mutant Gene

The Lebanese patient[13,59] was a compound heterozygote for a C-to-T mutation at position 304 (codon 102), causing a Ser-to-Leu substitution, and a T-to-C mutation at position 413 (codon 138), replacing a Met by Thr.[175] Both mutations involve residues that are conserved from *S. cerevisiae* and *C. albicans* to human PMI.[184] The corresponding amino acids are situated near the active site of the *C. albicans* enzyme.[183] The Glu residue adjacent to Met135 (Glu135 in *C. albicans* corresponding to Glu134 in human PMI) is one of the four residues involved in binding the catalytic Zn^{2+} ion. The Lys residue at position 100 in *C. albicans* (corresponding to Lys98 in human PMI) points inward into the active site, and the mutation at Ser101 may well affect this orientation. Thus, the mutations in the *PMI* gene are likely to explain the lack of activity of this enzyme in this patient.

In another patient with PMI deficiency,[174,175] one mutation affects Arg219 (R219Q), but a second mutation was not found. Niehues et al[174] found evidence for a reduced expression of the second allele, whereas we found that, on the second allele, one exon is spliced out at the cDNA level. However, we have not been able to pinpoint the defect at the genomic level: the splice sites of the corresponding exon are normal. There is only a polymorphism at position +9 in the intron, which may well affect splicing and for which the patient is homozygous (E. Schollen et al, unpublished). Another patient with deficiency of PMI is known: the mutations are Y255C/I399T.[187]

Except for a polymorphism at codon 377 (GTA/GTG, both coding for Val), no other sequence variations were detected in cDNA amplification from the patient with the very mild phenotype.[175] Since there is no mutation in the structural gene, the low activity in fibroblasts could be due to a decrease in the transcription of the gene because of mutations either in the promoter or in a transcription factor required for the expression of the enzyme. The finding of a normal activity in leukocytes of the parents argues for this second possibility, if at least the same isozyme is expressed in fibroblasts and leukocytes.

There may exist different isozymes of PMI, as is the case for PMM.[57,129,132] The cDNA that has been identified and sequenced by Proudfoot et al[184] appears to be derived from a gene that is only poorly expressed in liver, as shown by Northern blot analysis. However, all human expressed sequence tags found in databanks seem to be derived from this gene, except maybe one that could possibly encode an isozyme. However, we have not been able to amplify human liver and leukocyte cDNA by polymerase chain reaction using primers designed on the basis of the latter sequence. So, at present, there is no evidence for a second PMI gene.

Pathogenesis

Several explanations can be provided for the differences in tissue involvement between PMI and PMM deficiency and for the fact that the clinical manifestations of PMI deficiency are mainly hepatic and intestinal:[175]

- The possible existence of different isozymes of PMI, as is the case for PMM.[57,129,132]
- Possible differences in expression of the specific, low-K_m mannose transporter,[171] which appears to be involved in the preferential utilization of mannose over glucose in cultured fibroblasts.[188]
- PMI, but not PMM, can be bypassed by the low-K_m hexokinases. These enzymes can convert mannose to M-6-P, displaying for this substrate a rather high affinity in the case of the brain hexokinase[189] (Fig. 74-1). In contrast, glucokinase, the major, if not the only, hexokinase present in hepatocytes,[190] has a very low affinity for mannose[191] and is therefore rather inefficient in phosphorylating this substrate at the concentrations prevailing in plasma (± 50 μM in controls[192]). Blood mannose, which is derived from glycoprotein degradation and alimentary mannose in unknown proportion, is therefore most likely sufficient to support *N*-glycosylation in brain (and other tissues) but probably not in liver.
- GDP-mannose requirements of rat intestinal mucosa seem to be remarkably high, as evidenced by the specific activity of PMM, which is four times higher than that of other tissues.[133]
- Intestinal mucosa has a high glucose concentration due to active absorption from the intestinal lumen through the GluT 2 transporter.[193] Glucose can therefore competitively inhibit the phosphorylation of mannose.

Diagnosis

Based on the clinical spectrum present in the small number of patients known, PMI deficiency should be considered in unexplained liver disease, in protein-losing enteropathy particularly when associated with thromboses and/or liver disease, in recurrent vomiting with increased transaminases during the attacks, and in hyperinsulinemic hypoglycemia in otherwise healthy children or adults. Measurement of blood or serum levels of glycoproteins such as antithrombin is helpful. The diagnosis is made by IEF of serum sialotransferrins showing the type-I pattern. It is confirmed by PMI activity measurement in leukocytes, fibroblasts, or liver, and by mutation analysis. Evidence obtained in one patient[175,178] indicates that some individuals with PMI deficiency can be clinically normal and have normal serum glycoproteins, including a normal sialotransferrin pattern. It is hypothesized that the mannose content of normal food is sufficient to sustain their *N*-glycosylation needs.

Treatment and Prognosis

Unlike PMM deficiency (and, theoretically, all defects in further steps of the *N*-glycosylation pathway), PMI deficiency, a potentially lethal disease, should be treatable by administration of mannose. This is a logical consequence of the fact that hexokinase phosphorylates mannose to M-6-P, thus bypassing the defect. It is corroborated by the successful experience in one of the patients.[174] In this patient, mannose therapy was initiated at the age of 6 years, before the diagnosis of PMI deficiency was known, starting from the observation that mannose could correct abnormal glycosylation in some type-I fibroblasts.[122] Mannose was given orally in a dose of 100 mg/kg body weight, three times a day, and 8 months later the dose was increased to 150 mg/kg five times a day. Serum mannose levels reached a maximum of 490 μM 90 min after ingestion of the latter dose. Gastrointestinal bleeding and the chronic diarrhea disappeared within a few weeks, and blood antithrombin levels normalized. IEF of serum transferrin, performed 6 months after the start of therapy, showed a partial correction and, after 11 months of therapy, a near normalization. The Lebanese patient unfortunately died before trials with mannose could be attempted.[175] Mannose treatment has been similarly successful in another patient who was diagnosed with a PMI deficiency at 1 month of age.[187]

CDGS TYPE I DUE TO ENDOPLASMIC RETICULUM-LOCALIZED HYPOGLUCOSYLATION

Four children from an inbred Dutch family showed a mild to moderate psychomotor retardation associated with a type-I serum sialotransferrin pattern, and very low blood levels of factor XI, antithrombin, and protein C, but normal activities of PMI, PMM, and GDP-mannose synthetase in fibroblasts (Fig. 74-7). Analysis of the dolichol-linked oligosaccharides in fibroblasts revealed a major fraction consisting of nine mannose- and two *N*-acetylglucosamine residues ($Man_9GlcNAc_2$) instead of the fully assembled dolichol-linked oligosaccharide ($Glc_3Man_9GlcNAc_2$) predominantly found in controls. These data indicated that fibroblasts from these patients had a strongly reduced capacity to glucosylate dolichol-linked oligosaccharides. This defect explained the hypoglycosylation of their serum glycoproteins, because non-glucosylated oligosaccharides are a suboptimal substrate for the oligosaccharyltransferase and are therefore transferred to proteins with a reduced efficiency. The primary defect in these patients is not yet known. In yeast cells, both a deficiency in the dolichyl-phosphoglucose-synthesizing enzyme or in the first dolichyl-phosphoglucose-dependent glucosyltransferase lead to accumulation of dolichol-linked $Man_9GlcNAc_2$. Interestingly, the activities of different Golgi-localized glycosyltransferases were differently affected in the patients: there was a 50 percent reduction of fibroblast α-2,6-sialyltransferase and a 30 percent increase of β-1,4-galactosyltransferase. The reason why the clinical picture of these patients is much milder and more restricted than that of PMM deficient patients might be that a deficiency in glucosylation of the dolichol-linked oligosaccharides does not affect the biosynthesis of GDP-mannose and hence not the biosynthesis of GDP-fucose nor the biosynthesis of GPI anchors.[194,195]

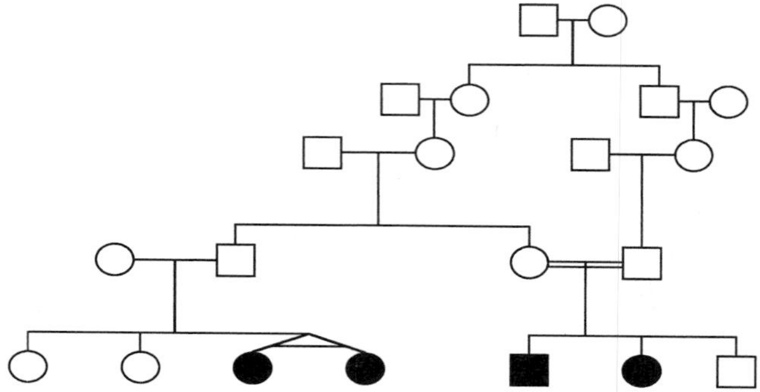

Fig. 74-7 The family tree of an inbred family with a type-I sialotransferrin pattern and evidence of a hypoglucosylation defect. (Courtesy of Dr. J. de Rijk-van Andel, Breda, The Netherlands.)

N-ACETYLGLUCOSAMINYLTRANSFERASE II DEFICIENCY (CDGS TYPE IIA) (MIM 212066)

Clinical Spectrum and Variability

Among the known defects of the *N*-glycan synthesis, this seems to be the most severe. Only two patients have been reported: an Iranian girl and a Belgian boy.[196–199] The sister of the girl died at the age of 43 days from a clinically similar disorder, and recently another sibling was born with CDGS type IIA. As to the boy, a brother of his grandfather died at the age of 3 months from what might have been the same disease. Both patients had facial dysmorphy: high forehead, long eyelashes, beaked nose with prominent base, upturned alae nasi, receding chin, protruding upper incisivae, and dysplastic, large, and low-set ears in oblique position (Fig. 74-8). They also had a short neck, hollowed chest, increased internipple distance, proximal implantation of the thumbs, and irregular implantation of the toes. Both had a ventricular septal defect. There was a prominent stereotypic behavior, including hand-washing movements and, by the boy, head turning and knocking on his cheeks. They showed a growth retardation after the first years (at 10 years of age, the boy was 11 cm below the 3rd centile) and a relative macrocephaly. They showed generalized hypotonia, but deep tendon reflexes were normal. Psychomotor development was severely retarded: the boy could take a few steps only at the age of 7 years, and at 10 years he uttered only some monotonous sounds. Visual contact always remained poor. In addition, the boy suffered from regurgitation due to volvulus of the stomach, and, after the age of 1 year, gum hypertrophy, thoracolumbar kyphoscoliosis, hypotrophic distal limbs, and flat feet were also noted. At the age of 6 years, he developed poorly manageable epilepsy. The diagnosis of CDGS type II was made in the boy at 9.5 years when, during an investigation for gum bleeding, the typical coagulopathy of CDGS was observed. Clinical examination at that age also revealed hypogonadism. Laboratory investigation showed in both an increase in the serum aspartate aminotransferase level [88 U/L and 80 to 160 U/liter, respectively (normal, less than 40)] but a normal alanine aminotransferase level. The thrombin time in the girl was normal and slightly decreased in the boy. Concentration of cerebrospinal fluid proteins was slightly increased in the girl. The results of chromosomal analysis in lymphocytes were normal. Lymphocyte culture in the boy was successful only at the seventh attempt! Radiologic examination of the skeleton showed osteopenia and gracile long bones and, in the boy, also luxation of the left radius, bilateral coxa valga, and hemivertebra of C6. Nerve conduction velocity, evoked potentials, and findings on electromyography were normal. Electroencephalography in the boy showed a slow basal rhythm and paroxysmal activity, and ophthalmologic examination at 9 years revealed somewhat pale and hazy papillae and decreased amplitude of the electroretinogram. Magnetic resonance imaging of the girl's brain showed symmetric hypointense signals for myelin particularly in the corpus callosum, internal capsule, and fronto-occipital white matter. There was also global cortical atrophy, and small focal lesions were scattered over the white matter of both hemispheres. In the boy, brain imaging was normal. Electron-microscopic examination of a liver biopsy sample was performed only in the girl and the findings were normal. Recently, a third patient with CDGS type IIA was identified (V. Cormier-Daire et al, in preparation).

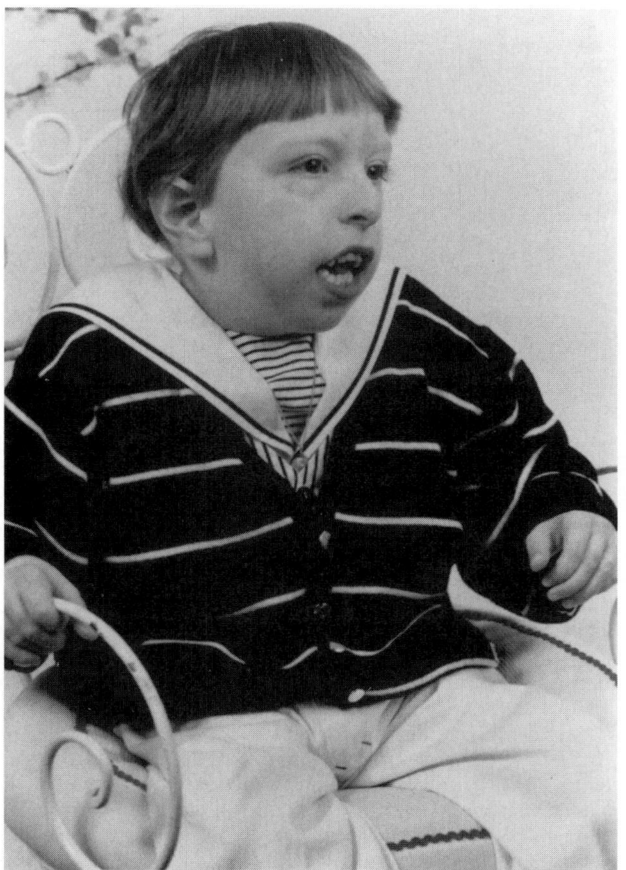

Fig. 74-8 A boy aged 10 years with *N*-acetylglucosaminyltransferase (GnT) II deficiency. Note the dysmorphic facial features (beaked nose, protruding upper incisivae, receding chin, and large dysplastic ears in oblique position) and short neck.

Biochemical Features

Decreased blood or serum values were found for a large number of glycoproteins. Unlike in PMM deficiency, there was no decrease of serum albumin and cholesterol and no increase of arylsulfatase A, and analysis of platelet function revealed reduced platelet adhesion under shear stress controlled flow conditions. No sialic acid residues were detected on platelet membrane glycoproteins during flow cytometric analysis using several lectins.[107] IEF of serum transferrin showed a markedly abnormal pattern different from the type I in that tetrasialotransferrin was nearly absent, disialotransferrin was more increased, and the trisialo- and monosialotransferrins were also increased (type-II pattern)[197,198] (Fig. 74-2). Carbohydrate analysis of serum transferrin of the boy showed a deficiency of 2 mol of sialic acid, galactose, and *N*-acetylglucosamine per mole of transferrin. The primary structure of his transferrin glycans, analyzed by 400 MHz [^{1}H] NMR spectroscopy, corresponded to a truncated di-antennary glycan, missing the terminal trisaccharide on one antenna[196,200] (Fig. 74-9). The accumulation of this structure suggested a deficiency of the Golgi-localized GnT II (*N*-acetylglucosaminyltransferase II). This was confirmed in fibroblasts of both patients and in mononuclear cells of the boy.[197,201]

Properties of the Normal Enzyme

GnT II is a medial Golgi type-II transmembrane glycoprotein. It has a typical glycosyltransferase domain structure, namely, a short N-terminal cytoplasmic domain, a lumenal stem region, and a large lumenal C-terminal catalytic domain besides the transmembrane domain. The enzyme catalyzes incorporation of a GlcNAc residue in β-1,2 linkage to the Man-α-1,6-arm of the *N*-glycan core and is therefore essential for the biosynthesis of complex from hybrid *N*-glycans. It shows no sequence homology to any previously cloned glycosyltransferase.[5]

Properties of the Mutant Enzyme

GnT II activities in fibroblast extracts from the two patients were 0.9 percent and 1.4 percent, respectively, of the mean activity in controls (2.2 $\pm$ 1.0 nmol/mg prot.hour).[197] GnT II activity in mononuclear cell extracts, assayed only in the boy, was undetectable, whereas his parents had levels consistent with

A

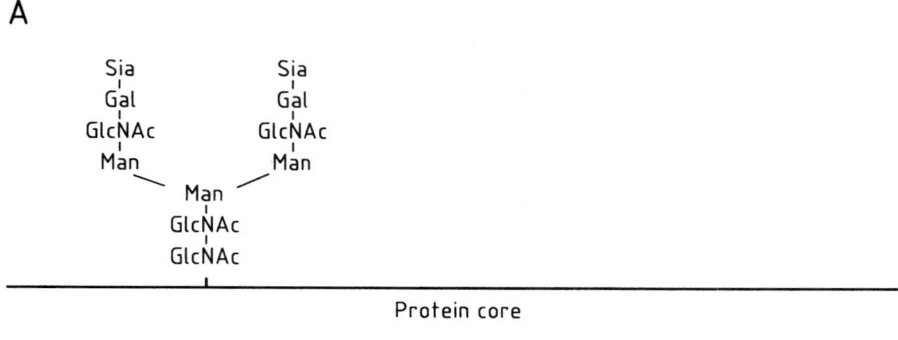

B

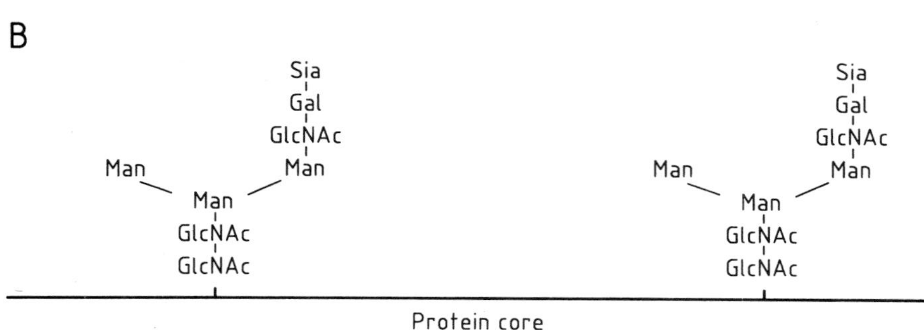

Fig. 74-9 Schematic glycan structures of serum disialotransferrins from (A) a phosphomannomutase (PMM)-deficient patient and (B) an *N*-acetylglucosaminyltransferase (GnT) II-deficient patient.

heterozygosity.[201] The presence of an enzyme inhibitor was ruled out.

The *N*-Acetylglucosaminyltransferase II Gene

The gene for human GnT II (*MGAT2*) has been cloned and localized to chromosome 14q21.[202] Southern analysis indicated that there is only a single copy of *MGAT2*. The entire coding region was shown to be on a single exon. It is a typical housekeeping gene (e.g., multiple transcription start sites, GC-rich nature of the promotor region).[203] However, some characteristics of the 5′ and 3′ flanking regions suggest that regulation of GnT II gene expression may play a role in development and differentiation.

Genetics and Molecular Bases

CDGS type IIA is an autosomal recessive disease. In the first reported patients, the lack of GnT II activity was due to point mutations: C1551T (Ser290Phe) in the girl, and A1467G (His262Arg) in the boy.[204] Both patients were homozygous for their respective mutations, and both mutations occurred in the C-terminal catalytic domain. One patient had two different mutations: N318D/C399X (V. Cormier-Daire et al, in preparation).

Pathogenesis

Patients with inactivating mutations of the GnT II gene develop severe multisystem developmental abnormalities especially in the brain. Mice embryos homozygous for the *Mgat2* deletion (targeted inactivation) show a very similar clinical picture: most die perinatally, are small, and exhibit delayed and abnormal skeletal maturation as well as congenital heart malformations.[205] These data provide the first direct evidence that complex glycans are essential for normal development. A great deal of evidence suggests that mediation of cell-cell interactions is the basis for the role of cell-surface glycoconjugates in embryogenesis and development.[204] However, the detailed mechanisms of these processes remain to be determined.

Diagnosis

Since only three patients with this disease are known, the extent of its clinical spectrum is at present unknown. Therefore, it seems worthwhile to perform IEF of serum sialotransferrins in any child or adult with an unexplained association of neurologic disease and craniofacial dysmorphy. The serum sialotransferrin pattern is very typical (type-II pattern) but conceivably might be less so in patients with milder defects. (Fig. 74-2) The diagnosis is confirmed by GnT II activity measurement in fibroblasts or mononuclear blood cells, and by mutation analysis. Prenatal diagnosis has not yet been performed but should be possible.

Treatment and Prognosis

No efficient treatment is available. Prognostic expectations have to be inferred from only three patients who had a severely handicapping disease and from the knowledge that in two families a child with most probably the same disease died at an early infantile age.

LEUKOCYTE ADHESION DEFICIENCY SYNDROME TYPE II (MIM 266265)

Leukocyte adhesion deficiency syndrome type II was first reported in 1992 in two unrelated boys with a syndrome comprising recurrent bacterial infections besides other features.[206,207] Infections were typically accompanied by high leukocyte counts (up to 150,000 cells/μl) but surprisingly never by pus. In addition, the patients had an unusual facial appearance, short stature, and encephalopathy. Their neutrophils showed a lack of sialyl-Lewis X, a fucose-containing carbohydrate ligand of the selectin family of cell adhesion molecules required for normal recruitment of neutrophils to sites of inflammation.[208] Other fucose-containing carbohydrate sequences were also absent, such as A, B, O, and Lewis A blood groups. It was subsequently reported that the biochemical basis of this disease possibly is a failure to convert GDP-mannose to GDP-fucose, resulting in a general deficiency of fucose.[28] Which of the two steps of this pathway is involved remains to be determined. Fucose is found in *N*- and *O*-glycans and glycolipids, attached to Gal or GlcNAc residues in α-linkage to carbons 2, 3, 4, or 6.[5] The study of these patients undoubtedly will yield further insights into the biologic roles of fucose-containing glycans of glycoproteins and glycolipids.

UNEXPLAINED DEFECTS OF *N*-GLYCAN SYNTHESIS

At least 10 patients (belonging to seven families) have been reported with a type-I CDGS but normal activities of PMM and PMI in fibroblasts.[50,56,77,209–212] One of them had a relatively mild clinical phenotype consisting of moderate psychomotor retardation and (decreasing) ataxia and episodes of apathy,[211] whereas the others had a severe phenotype including dysmorphy, failure to thrive,[50,77] epilepsy,[77,209,210,212] and cardiomyopathy.[50,212] Four died at an early age (from 2 days to 5 months).[50,209,212] Features previously not reported in CDG syndromes were cataract,[209,210] involvement of the spinal cord,[209] and nonimmunologic *hydrops fetalis*.[212] Furthermore, Stibler et al reported a type-III[213] and a type-IV[214] CDGS. The two (unrelated) patients with type III had severe neurologic disease with pronounced psychomotor retardation, hypsarrhythmia, cerebral and optic atrophy, and dysmyelination, as well as depigmented skin areas. The serum transferrin IEF showed increased tetrasialotransferrin and approximately equal increases of tri-, di-, mono-, and asialotransferrin. Since this pattern is also seen in nongenetic diseases, such as infectious diseases,[196] and since the serum levels of other glycoproteins were normal, it is doubtful whether these patients had a primary glycosylation disease. The increase of tri- and monosialotransferrin permits the classification of this pattern as type II.[198,199] The two (unrelated) patients with CDGS type IV were also severely neurologically handicapped and showed minimal psychomotor development, spastic tetraparesis, intractable epilepsy, and microcephaly. They had multiple serum glycoprotein abnormalities, and their serum transferrin IEF pattern showed mainly an increase of disialotransferrin. Since there was no increase of tri- and monosialotransferrin, we propose reclassifying these patients as having type-I CDGS and the consideration of a pre-ER or ER-localized glycosylation defect.

Another glycosylation disorder waiting for elucidation is congenital dyserythropoietic anemia type II or hereditary erythroblastic multinuclearity with a positive acidified serum lysis test (HEMPAS). This is an autosomal recessive anemia due to ineffective erythropoiesis and associated with decreased glycosylation of erythrocyte membrane protein bands 3 and 4.5. In some patients, α-mannosidase deficiency was found in mononuclear blood cells.[215] In other patients, GnT II was found to be deficient,[216] although the clinical picture is totally different from CDGS type IIA and erythrocytes of the latter patients have neither the serology nor the band-3 glycan structure typical for HEMPAS.[201] Mice lacking a functional α-mannosidase gene exhibited a loss of complex glycans limited to the erythroid lineage and showed a phenotype similar to human HEMPAS disease.[217] These data revealed a widely used alternative pathway in complex N-linked glycan biosynthesis that involves a distinct Golgi α-mannosidase termed *α-mannosidase III* or IIx.[217,218] Conclusive evidence has been presented for linkage of HEMPAS to the long arm of chromosome 20q11.2,[219] excluding GnT II, α-mannosidase II, and α-mannosidase III as candidates for the disease.[220] One hypothesis is that the disease is due to a defect of a transcription factor regulating both α-mannosidase II and GnT II.[220]

The number of patients with an unidentified glycosylation defect is steadily growing. They have various clinical phenotypes. The majority of them show a type-I serum sialotransferrin pattern (J. Jaeken et al, unpublished). The following abbreviated case report is an example. This girl had, since infancy, feeding problems, psychomotor retardation, ichthyosis, growth retardation with partial growth hormone deficiency, and hypo-β-lipoproteine-

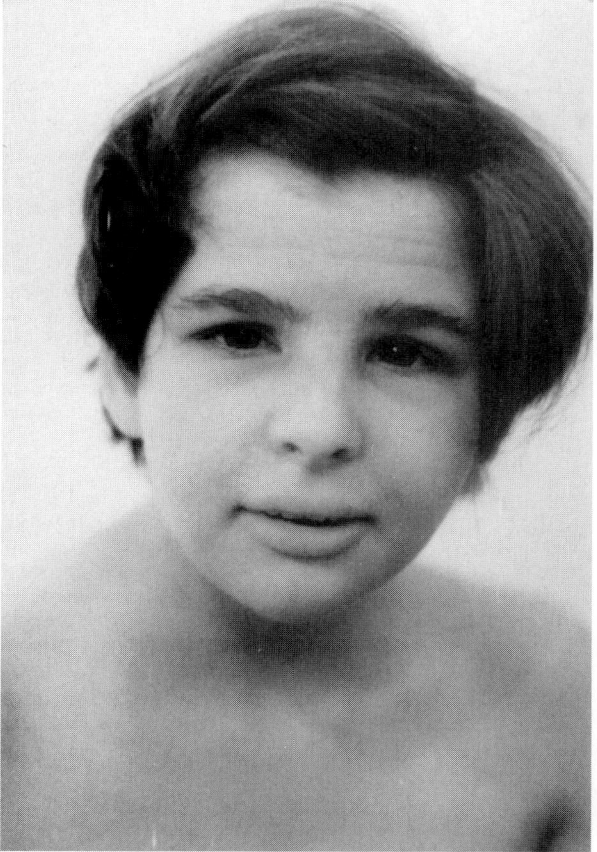

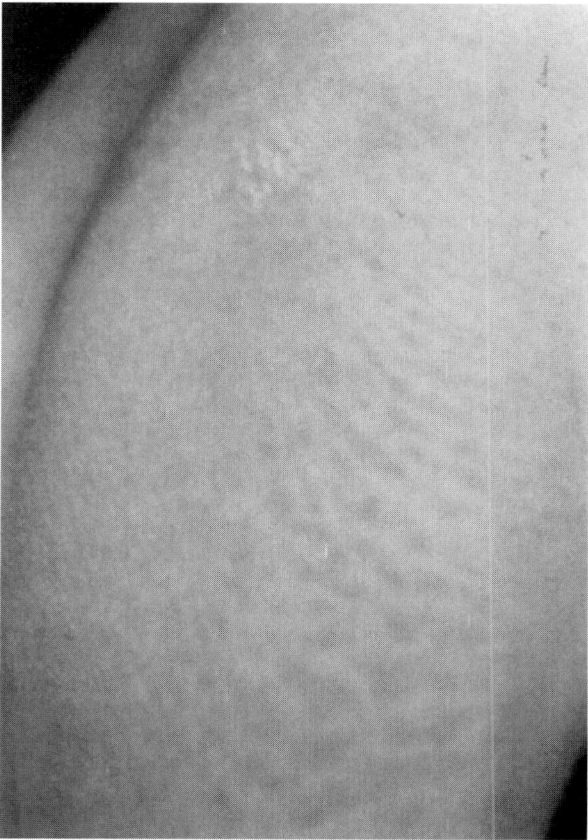

Fig. 74-10 A girl aged 16 years with unidentified glycosylation defect. Note the generalized skin lesions with ichthyosis on the legs.

mia. A sibling had died at 3 months with a similar syndrome. The patient was lost from follow-up and seen again at the age of 16 years with the following problems: an impressive scaly and itching skin disease particularly of the face with ichthyosis of the lower legs, night blindness and, during the day, sight problems changing in parallel with the severity of the skin lesions (Fig. 74-10). Pubertal development was normal. She showed dwarfism [height 134 cm ($< P3 = 150$ cm), weight 40.9 kg ($P3 = 40$ kg), and head circumference 52 cm (P3)]. She could slowly walk without support and speak a few words. She grasped for objects with gross movements. She had very dry, erythematous and scaly skin, dry hair, and very convex nails. The results of neurologic examination were normal. Laboratory investigation showed a type-I serum sialotransferrin pattern and decreased values of serum LDL-cholesterol (52 mg/dl), cholinesterase (2.6 kU/liter), progesterone (0.07 mg/dl), estradiol (29 pg/ml), and of blood factor XI (34 percent), antithrombin (49 percent), protein C (34 percent), and protein S (69 percent). Serum levels of haptoglobin, transaminases, TBG, growth hormone, and insulin-like growth factor I were normal. The findings on vaginoscopy and hysteroscopy were normal, as were the findings on echocardiography and magnetic resonance imaging of the brain, and nerve conduction velocity was normal. Activities of PMI, PMM, and GDP-mannose synthase in fibroblasts were normal.

DEFICIENT *N*-GLYCOSYLATION IN GENETIC DISEASES OF CARBOHYDRATE METABOLISM

The galactosemias due to galactose 1-phosphate uridyltransferase deficiency and UDP-galactose 4′ epimerase deficiency, as well as hereditary fructose intolerance (aldolase B deficiency), are associated with secondary glycosylation disturbances. In untreated galactose 1-phosphate uridyltransferase deficiency, evidence has been presented for deficient glycosylation of serum transferrin,[221–223] TBG,[224] lysosomal enzymes,[225] and follicle-stimulating hormone,[226] and more specifically for deficient galactosylation of lymphocytes and brain glycolipids,[227] serum,[226] and fibroblast[228,229] glycoproteins, and serum transferrin glycans.[230] Also, UDP-galactose 4′ epimerase deficiency shows a CDGS type-I pattern.[231] These data point to a defect at the level of the Golgi-localized galactosylation, but its mechanism is still unclear. There is published evidence in favor of a galactosyltransferase inhibition (discussion in Charlwood et al[230]), as well as against it.[222,229] It is generally agreed that there is no decreased synthesis of the donor UDP-galactose.[232] A disturbed transport of UDP-galactose into the Golgi, possibly due to competition with galactose 1-phosphate, has been proposed.[230]

In hereditary fructose intolerance, the situation is more clear-cut. As in galactosemia, serum transferrin of these patients shows the CDGS type-I pattern.[233] There are a number of other features in common with early glycosylation defects, including myelin-like and other lysosomal inclusions in liver[234] (Fig. 74-5). This has been attributed to a secondary deficiency of PMI, since fructose 1-phosphate, a structural analogue of M-6-P, is a potent competitive inhibitor of this enzyme.[235]

Although there is some doubt whether this disturbed glycosylation completely normalizes under adequate dietary treatment of these diseases, IEF of serum transferrin or analysis of the glycans of serum transferrin has been proposed as a measure of dietary compliance[230,236] analogous to measurement of glycated hemoglobin rather than blood glucose in the follow-up of diabetes. It remains to be determined whether this hypoglycosylation contributes to the clinical picture of these diseases, particularly the long-term complications in galactosemia.

CONCLUSION AND OUTLOOK

Genetic defects of *N*-glycan synthesis are a large and rapidly growing family of diseases with different phenotypes. Most probably, only the tip of the iceberg is known. The identification of new members of this group will be greatly facilitated by the availability of yeast glycosylation mutants[237] but particularly of knockout mice.[217,238,239]

A broad screening is recommended by performing serum sialotransferrin analysis in any unexplained clinical disorder. As to nomenclature, we propose to continue to make a first classification into either type I (on the basis of increased serum di- and/or asialotransferrin; mainly pre-Golgi defects) or type II [when there is also increased tri- and /or monosialotransferrin; mainly (or only?) Golgi defects, followed by -X, or when the basic defect is known, followed by the name of the enzyme or transporter involved]. Once the gene defect is identified, the name of the enzyme or transporter can be replaced by the name of the gene involved.

ADDENDUM

Since submission of this manuscript (June 1998) the nomenclature of this group of diseases has been updated [carbohydrate-deficient glycoprotein syndromes became congenital defects of glycosylation (CDG)][251] and four new defects have been identified: alpha 1,3 mannosyltransferase deficiency (CDG-ld, MIM 601110),[252] dolichyl-P-mannose synthase 1 deciency (CDG-le, MIM 603503),[253,254] glucosidase I deficiency (CDG-llb, MIM 601336),[255] and deficient import of GDP-fucose in the Golgi apparatus[256] as a cause of leukocyte adhesion deficiency II syndrome.[206,207] The basis of CDG with hypoglucosylation has been identified as the ER localized alpha 1,3 glucosyltransferase deficiency (CDG-lc).[257]

REFERENCES

1. Kornfeld R, Kornfeld S: Assembly of asparagine-linked oligosaccharides. *Annu Rev Biochem* **54**:631, 1985.
2. Schachter H: The "yellow brick road" to branched complex *N*-glycans. *Glycobiology* **1**:453, 1991.
3. Kobata A: Structures and functions of the sugar chains of glycoproteins. *Eur J Biochem* **209**:483, 1992.
4. Rudd PM, Dwek RA: Glycosylation: Heterogeneity and the 3D structure of proteins. *Crit Rev Biochem Mol Biol* **32**:1, 1997.
5. Brockhausen I, Schachter H: Glycosyltransferases involved in *N*- and *O*-glycan biosynthesis, in Gabius H-J, Gabius S (eds): *Glycosciences*. Weinheim, Germany, Chapman and Hall, 1997, p 79.
6. Rademacher TW, Parekh RB, Dwek RA: Glycobiology. *Annu Rev Biochem* **57**:785, 1988.
7. Varki A: Biological roles of oligosaccharides: All of the theories are correct. *Glycobiology* **3**:97, 1993.
8. Jaeken J, Vanderschueren-Lodeweyckx M, Casaer P, Snoeck L, Corbeel L, Eggermont E, Eeckels R: Familial psychomotor retardation with markedly fluctuating serum proteins, FSH and GH levels, partial TBG-deficiency, increased serum arylsulphatase A and increased CSF protein: A new syndrome? *Pediatr Res* **14**:179, 1980.
9. Jaeken J, van Eijk HG, van der Heul C, Corbeel L, Eeckels R, Eggermont E: Sialic acid-deficient serum and cerebrospinal fluid transferrin in a newly recognized genetic syndrome. *Clin Chim Acta* **144**:245, 1984.
10. Holzbach U, Hanefeld F: Das klinische Spectrum des CDG-Syndroms, in Rating D (ed): *Aktuelle Neuropädiatrie*. Basel, Ciba-Geigy, Verlag, 1994, p 113.
11. Winchester B, Clayton P, Mian N, Di Tomaso E, Dell A, Reason A, Keir G: The carbohydrate-deficient glycoprotein syndrome: An experiment of nature in glycosylation. *Biochem Soc Trans* **23**:185, 1995.
12. Yamashita K, Ohno K: Carbohydrate-deficient glycoprotein syndrome type I, in Montreuil J, Vliegenthart JFG, Schachter H (eds): *Glycoproteins and disease*, Amsterdam, Elsevier Science, 1996, p 445.
13. Amiel J, Poggi F, Lacombe D, Billette T, Jaeken J, Saudubray JM: CDG syndromes: Un nouveau chapitre des maladies métaboliques. *Prog Néonatol* **15**:136, 1995.
14. Hagberg BA, Blennow G, Kristiansson B, Stibler H: Carbohydrate-deficient glycoprotein syndromes: Peculiar group of new disorders. *Pediatr Neurol* **9**:255, 1993.
15. Hagberg B, Blennow G, Kristiansson B, Stibler H: Carbohydrate-deficient glycoprotein syndromes, in Moser HW (ed): *Handbook for Clinical Neurology, Neurodystrophics and Neurolipidoses*, vol 22. Amsterdam, Elsevier Science, 1996, p 623.

16. Hagberg B, Blennow G, Stibler H: The birth and infancy of a new disease: The carbohydrate-deficient glycoprotein syndrome. *Fetal Perinat Neurol* **314**:15, 1992.
17. Gahl WA: Carbohydrate-deficient glycoprotein syndrome: Hidden treasures. *J Lab Clin Med* **129**:394, 1997.
18. Heyne K, Weidinger S: Diagnostik und Nosologie der Glykanose CDG [Carbohydrate-deficient glycoprotein syndrome]. *Monatsschr Kinderheilkd* **140**:822, 1992.
19. Jaeken J, Carchon H: The carbohydrate-deficient glycoprotein syndromes: An overview. *J Inherited Metab Dis* **16**:813, 1993.
20. Jaeken J, Carchon H: The carbohydrate-deficient glycoprotein syndromes: Recent developments. *Int Pediatr* **8**:60, 1993.
21. Jaeken J, Carchon H, Stibler H: The carbohydrate-deficient glycoprotein syndromes: Pre-Golgi and Golgi disorders? *Glycobiology* **3**:423, 1993.
22. Jaeken J, Casaer P: Carbohydrate-deficient glycoconjugate (CDG) syndromes: A new chapter of neuropaediatrics. *Eur J Paediatr Neurol* **2/3**:61, 1997.
23. Jaeken J, Pohl S, Hoffmann A, Carchon H, Conradt HS: Looking at brain glycosylation in carbohydrate-deficient glycoconjugate (CDG) syndromes by isoelectrofocusing of cerebrospinal fluid (CSF) β-trace protein. *Amino Acids* **12**:388, 1997.
24. Jaeken J, Stibler H, Hagberg B: The carbohydrate-deficient glycoprotein syndrome: A new inherited multisystemic disease with severe nervous system involvement. *Acta Paediatr Scand Suppl* **375**:1991.
25. Stibler H, Blennow G, Kristiansson B, Lindehammer H, Hagberg B: Carbohydrate-deficient glycoprotein syndrome: Clinical expression in adults with a new metabolic disease. *J Neurol Neurosurg Psychiatry* **57**:552, 1994.
26. Vidailhet M: Des maladies du réticulum endoplasmique et de l'appareil de Golgi: Les déficits de glycosylation des glycoprotéines. *Arch Pédiatr* **2**:509, 1995.
27. McDowell G, Gahl WA: Inherited disorders of glycoprotein synthesis: Cell biological insights. *Proc Soc Exp Biol Med* **215**:145, 1997.
28. Kornfeld S: Diseases of abnormal protein glycosylation: An emerging area. *J Clin Invest* **11**:1293, 1998.
29. de Jong G, van Dijk JP, van Eijk HG: The biology of transferrin. *Clin Chim Acta* **190**:1, 1990.
30. Kornfeld S, Sly WS: I-cell disease and pseudo-Hurler polydystrophy: Disorders of lysosomal enzyme phosphorylation and localization, in Scriver CR, Beaudet AL, Sly WS, Valle D (eds): *The Metabolic and Molecular Bases of Inherited Disease*, vol 2, 7th ed. New-York, McGraw-Hill, 1995, p 2495.
31. Vilharinho L, Mota C, Barbosa C, et al: Carbohydrate deficient glycoprotein (CDG) syndrome type I: A Portuguese case. *Amino Acids* **12**:391, 1997.
32. Ohkura T, Fukushima K, Kurisaki A, et al: A partial deficiency of dehydrodolichol reduction is a cause of carbohydrate-deficient glycoprotein syndrome type I. *J Biol Chem* **272**:6868, 1997.
33. Clayton P, Winchester B, Di Tomaso E, Young E, Keir G, Rodeck C: Carbohydrate-deficient glycoprotein syndrome: Normal glycosylation in the fetus. *Lancet* **341**:956, 1993.
34. De Bont ESJM, Van Spronsen FJ, Kimpen JLL, Stolte-Dijkstra I, Smit GPA: Pasgeborenen met fatty pads die onvoldoende groeien en braken: Het syndroom van Jaeken? *Tijdschr Kindergeneeskd* **62**:33, 1994.
35. De Zegher F, Jaeken J: Endocrinology of the carbohydrate-deficient glycoprotein syndrome type 1 from birth through adolescence. *Pediatr Res* **37**:395, 1995.
36. Kristiansson B, Andersson M, Tonnby B, Hagberg B: Disialotransferrin developmental deficiency syndrome. *Arch Dis Child* **64**:71, 1989.
37. Di Rocco M, Gatti R, Veneselli E, Tortori-Donati P, Barabino A, Jaeken J, Borrone C: Carbohydrate deficient glycoprotein (CDG) syndrome: The first two Italian patients. *Riv Ital Pediatr* **19**:179, 1993.
38. Fiumara A, Barone R, Buttitta P, Di Pietro M, Scuderi A, Nigro F, Jaeken J: Carbohydrate deficient glycoprotein syndrome type I: Ophthalmic aspects in four Sicilian patients. *Br J Ophthalmol* **78**:845, 1994.
39. Fiumara A, Barone R, Buttitta P, Musso R, Pavone L, Nigro F, Jaeken J: Haemostatic studies in carbohydrate-deficient glycoprotein syndrome type I. *Thromb Haemost* **76**:502, 1996.
40. Fiumara A, Barone R, Nigro F, Sorge G, Pavone L: Familial Dandy-Walker variant in CDG syndrome. *Am J Med Genet* **63**:412, 1996.
41. Horslen SP, Clayton PT, Harding BN, Hall NA, Keir G, Winchester B: Olivopontocerebellar atrophy of neonatal onset and disialotransferrin developmental deficiency syndrome. *Arch Dis Child* **66**:1027, 1991.
42. Jaeken J, Stibler H: A newly recognized inherited neurological disease with carbohydrate-deficient secretory glycoproteins, in Wetterberg L (ed): *Genetics of Neuropsychiatric Diseases*. Wenner-Gren Center International Symposium Series, vol 51. New York, Macmillan, 1989, p 69.
43. Macchia PE, Harrison HH, Scherberg NH, Sunthornthepvarakul T, Jaeken J, Refetoff S: Thyroid function tests and characterization of thyroxine-binding globulin in the carbohydrate-deficient glycoprotein syndrome type I. *J Clin Endocrinol Metab* **80**:3744, 1995.
44. Artigas J, Cardo E, Pineda M, Nosas R, Jaeken J: Phosphomannomutase deficiency and normal pubertal development. *J Inherited Metab Dis* **21**:78, 1998.
45. Billette de Villemeur T, Poggi-Travert F, Laurent J, Jaeken J, Saudubray JM: Le syndrome d'hypoglycosylation des protéines: Un nouveau groupe de maladies héréditaires à expression multisystémique, in Arthuis M, Beaufils F, Caille B, et al (eds): *Journées Parisiennes de Pédiatrie 1995*. Paris, Médecine-Sciences Flammarion, 1995, p 119.
46. Casteels I, Spileers W, Leys A, Lagae L, Jaeken J: Evolution of ophthalmic and electrophysiological findings in identical twin sisters with the carbohydrate deficient glycoprotein syndrome type 1 over a period of 14 years. *Br J Ophthalmol* **80**:900, 1996.
47. Jaeken J, Eggermont E, Stibler H: An apparent homozygous X-linked disorder with carbohydrate-deficient serum glycoproteins. *Lancet* **2**:1398, 1987.
48. Van Schaftingen E, Jaeken J: Phosphomannomutase deficiency is a cause of carbohydrate-deficient glycoprotein syndrome type I. *FEBS Lett* **377**:318, 1995.
49. Jaeken J, Artigas J, Barone R, et al: Phosphomannomutase deficiency is the main cause of carbohydrate-deficient glycoprotein syndrome with type I isoelectrofocusing pattern of serum sialotransferrins. *J Inherited Metab Dis* **20**:447, 1997.
50. Charlwood J, Clayton P, Johnson A, Keir G, Mian N, Winchester B: A case of the carbohydrate-deficient glycoprotein syndrome type 1 (CDGS type 1) with normal phosphomannomutase activity. *J Inherited Metab Dis* **20**:817, 1997.
51. Krasnewich D, Bernardini I, Rouhani F, et al: Three biochemical subtypes in type I carbohydrate-deficient glycoprotein syndrome. *Pediatr Res* **41**:105A, 1997.
52. Matthijs G, Schollen E, Van Schaftingen E, Cassiman J-J, Jaeken J: Lack of homozygotes for the most frequent disease allele in carbohydrate-deficient glycoprotein syndrome type 1A. *Am J Hum Genet* **62**:542, 1998.
53. Jaeken J: The carbohydrate-deficient glycoprotein syndromes. *Mol Chem Neuropathol* **27**:84, 1996.
54. Stibler H, Holzbach U, Kristiansson B: Isoforms and levels of transferrin, anti-thrombin, α_1-antitrypsin and thyroxine-binding globulin in 48 patients with carbohydrate-deficient glycoprotein syndrome type I. *Scand J Clin Lab Invest* **58**:55, 1998.
55. Matthijs G, Legius E, Jaeken J, Cassiman J-J: Refinement of the candidate region for carbohydrate-deficient glycoprotein syndrome type I (CDG1) on chromosome 16p. *Am J Hum Genet* **27**:A22, 1995.
56. Matthijs G, Legius E, Schollen E, et al: Evidence for genetic heterogeneity in the carbohydrate-deficient glycoprotein syndrome type I (CDG1). *Genomics* **35**:597, 1996.
57. Matthijs G, Schollen E, Pardon E, Veiga-Da-Cunha M, Jaeken J, Cassiman J-J, Van Schaftingen E: Mutations in *PMM2*, a phosphomannomutase gene on chromosome 16p13, in carbohydrate-deficient glycoprotein type I syndrome (Jaeken syndrome). *Nature Genet* **16**:88, 1997.
58. Mayatepek E, Schröder M, Kohlmüller D, Bieger WP, Nützenadel W: Continuous mannose infusion in carbohydrate-deficient glycoprotein syndrome type I. *Acta Paediatr* **86**:1138, 1997.
59. Ogier de Baulny H, Poggi-Travert F, Besnard M, Saudubray JM: Déficit de glycosylation des protéines: Présentation clinique. *Arch Pédiatr* **3**(suppl 1):158S, 1996.
60. Orvisky E, St John E, Parker M, et al: Carbohydrate-deficient glycoprotein syndrome. Correlation of in vitro 2[^{3}H]mannose metabolic labelling studies with phosphomannomutase activity (PMM) determined by direct analysis of mannose-1-phosphate to mannose-6-phosphate interconversion. *Glycobiology* **7**:1037, 1997.
61. Pavone L, Fiumara A, Barone R, Rizzo R, Buttitta P, Dobyns WB, Jaeken J: Olivopontocerebellar atrophy leading to recognition of carbohydrate-deficient glycoprotein syndrome type I. *J Neurol* **243**:700, 1996.
62. Pineda M, Pavia C, Vilaseca MA, et al: Normal pubertal development in a female with carbohydrate deficient glycoprotein syndrome. *Arch Dis Child* **74**:242, 1996.

63. Schlüter B, Bürk G, Jaeken J, Aksu F, Andler W: Manifestation des CDG-Syndroms Typ I im jungen Säuglingsalter. *Monatsschr Kinderheilkd* **142**:755, 1994.
64. Van der Knaap MS, Wevers RA, Monnens L, Jakobs C, Jaeken J, van Wijk JAE: Congenital nephrotic syndrome: A novel phenotype of type I carbohydrate-deficient glycoprotein syndrome. *J Inherited Metab Dis* **19**:787, 1996.
65. Van Geet C, Jaeken J: A unique pattern of coagulation abnormalities in carbohydrate-deficient glycoprotein syndrome. *Pediatr Res* **33**:540, 1993.
66. Kristiansson B, Stibler H, Conradi N, Ericksson BO, Ryd W: The heart and pericardial effusions in CDGS-I (carbohydrate-deficient glycoprotein syndrome type I). *J Inherited Metab Dis* **21**:112, 1998.
67. Póo P, Escofet C, Pineda M, Vilaseca MA, Ferrer I: Sindrome de glycoproteinas deficientes en carbohydratos tipo I con hemorragia cerebral neonatal, in *Abstracts of the II Congreso Nacional Errores Congenitones del Metabolismo*. Barcelona, 1998, p 42.
68. Roche MC, Salas S, Maties M, Vilaseca MA, Jaeken J, Chabas A, Morales YC: Forma neonatal de sindrome CDG tipo I, in *Abstracts of the II Congreso Nacional Errores Congenitos del Metabolismo*. Barcelona, 1998, p 41.
69. Clayton PT, Winchester BG, Keir G: Hypertrophic obstructive cardiomyopathy in a neonate with the carbohydrate-deficient glycoprotein syndrome. *J Inherited Metab Dis* **15**:857, 1992.
70. Nordborg C, Hagberg B, Kristiansson B: Sural nerve pathology in the carbohydrate-deficient glycoprotein syndrome. *Acta Paediatr Scand Suppl* **375**:39, 1991.
71. Conradi N, De Vos R, Jaeken J, Lundin P, Kristiansson B, Van Hoof F: Liver pathology in the carbohydrate-deficient glycoprotein syndrome. *Acta Paediatr Scand Suppl* **375**:50, 1991.
72. Strømme P, Maehlen J, Strøm EH, Torvik A: Postmortem findings in two patients with the carbohydrate-deficient glycoprotein syndrome. *Acta Paediatr Scand Suppl* **375**:55, 1991.
73. Stibler H, Jaeken J: Carbohydrate deficient serum transferrin in a new systemic hereditary syndrome. *Arch Dis Child* **65**:107, 1990.
74. Strøm EH, Strømme P, Westvik J, Pedersen SJ: Renal cysts in the carbohydrate-deficient glycoprotein syndrome. *Pediatr Nephrol* **7**:253, 1993.
75. Jaeken J, Besley G, Buist N, et al: Phosphomannomutase deficiency is the major cause of carbohydrate-deficient glycoprotein syndrome type I. *J Inherited Metab Dis* **19**(suppl 1):6, 1996.
76. Spada M, Dionisi-Vici C, Fiumara A, et al: Carbohydrate-deficient glycoprotein syndrome type I: The Italian experience. *Amino Acids* **12**:390, 1997.
77. Midro AT, Hanefeld F, Zadrozna Tolwińska B, Stibler H, Olchowik B, Stasiewicz-Jarocka B: Jaeken's (CDG) syndrome in siblings. *Pediatr Pol* **71**:621, 1996.
78. Eedebol Eeg-Olofsson K, Wahlström J: Genetic and epidemiological aspects of the carbohydrate-deficient glycoprotein syndrome. *Acta Paediatr Scand Suppl* **375**:63, 1991.
79. Hassing JM, Wiltse H, Huseman CA: Hypoketotic hypoglycemia in the carbohydrate deficient glycoprotein syndrome (CDGS). *Pediatr Res* **35**:100A, 1994.
80. Heyne K, Marg W, Walther F, Harms D, Janssen FW, Weidinger S: Glykanose CDG Typ I — Puzzle — Teile des Multisystemstadiums. *Monatsschr Kinderheilkd* **142**:748, 1994.
81. Agamanolis DP, Potter JL, Naito HK, Robinson HB Jr, Kulasekaran T: Lipoprotein disorder, cirrhosis, and olivopontocerebellar degeneration in two siblings. *Neurology* **36**:674, 1986.
82. Chang Y, Twiss JL, Horoupian DS, Caldwell SA, Johnston KM: Inherited syndrome of infantile olivopontocerebellar atrophy, micronodular cirrhosis, and renal tubular microcysts: Review of the literature and a report of an additional case. *Acta Neuropathol* **86**:399, 1993.
83. Clayton P, Mian N: Concerning "Agamanolis disease." *Am J Med Genet* **56**:289, 1995.
84. Jaeken J, Hagberg B, Strømme P: Clinical presentation and natural course of the carbohydrate-deficient glycoprotein syndrome. *Acta Paediatr Scand Suppl* **375**:6, 1991.
85. Stephani U, Hahn A, von Zimmermann W, Mehdorn M: CDG-Syndrom und Gerinnungsstörungen. *Monatsschr Kinderheilkd* **142**:759, 1994.
86. Hutchesson ACJ, Gray RGF, Spencer DA, Keir G: Carbohydrate deficient glycoprotein syndrome: Multiple abnormalities and diagnostic delay. *Arch Dis Child* **72**:445, 1995.
87. Di Rocco M: On Saraiva and Baraitser and Joubert syndrome: A review. *Am J Med Genet* **46**:732, 1993.
88. Andréasson S, Blennow G, Ehinger B, Strömland K: Full-field electroretinograms in patients with the carbohydrate-deficient glycoprotein syndrome. *Am J Ophthalmol* **112**:83, 1991.
89. Strömland K, Hagberg B, Kristiansson B: Ocular pathology in disialotransferrin developmental deficiency syndrome. *Ophthalmic Paediatr Genet* **11**:309, 1990.
90. Blennow G, Jaeken J, Wiklund LM: Neurological findings in the carbohydrate-deficient glycoprotein syndrome. *Acta Paediatr Scand Suppl* **375**:14, 1991.
91. Stibler H, Holzbach U, Tengborn L, Kristiansson B: Complex functional and structural coagulation abnormalities in the carbohydrate-deficient glycoprotein syndrome type I. *Blood Coagul Fibrinolysis* **7**:118, 1996.
92. Funk M, Becker S, Pötzsch B, Kreuz W, Böhles H: Thrombophilia in a child with CDG-syndrome type I. *Thromb Haemost* **74**:1199, 1995.
93. Iijima K, Murakami F, Nakamura K, et al: Hemostatic studies in patients with carbohydrate-deficient glycoprotein syndrome. *Thromb Res* **76**:193, 1994.
94. Petersen MB, Brostrøm K, Stibler H, Skovby F: Early manifestations of the carbohydrate-deficient glycoprotein syndrome. *J Pediatr* **122**:66, 1993.
95. García Silva MTG, De Castro J, Stibler H, et al: Prenatal hypertrophic cardiomyopathy and pericardial effusion in carbohydrate-deficient glycoprotein syndrome. *J Inherited Metab Dis* **19**:257, 1996.
96. Harding B, Dunger DB, Grant DB, Erdohazi M: Familial olivopontocerebellar atrophy with neonatal onset: A recessively inherited syndrome with systemic and biochemical abnormalities. *J Neurol Neurosurg Psychiatry* **51**:385, 1988.
97. Heyne K, Mayatepek E, Walther F, Weidinger S, Pahl HL: Pericardial effusion in glycanosis CDG type I (MIM 212 065): An inflammatory endoplasmic reticulum overload response? *Eur J Pediatr* **157**:168, 1998.
98. Ramaekers VT, Reul J, Thron A, Heimann G: Phenotypische Heterogenität beim CDG-Syndrom Typ I. *Monatsschr Kinderheilkd* **142**:759, 1994.
99. Jaeken J, Matthijs G, Barone R, Carchon H: Carbohydrate deficient glycoprotein (CDG) syndrome type I. *J Med Genet* **34**:73, 1997.
100. Marquardt T, Ullrich K, Zimmer P, Hasilik A, Deufel T, Harms E: Carbohydrate-deficient glycoprotein syndrome (CDGS): Glycosylation, folding and intracellular transport of newly synthesized glycoproteins. *Eur J Cell Biol* **66**:268, 1995.
101. Itoh M, Ohno K, Tomita Y, Takeshita K: Abnormal short-latency somatosensory evoked potentials in two patients with carbohydrate-deficient glycoprotein syndrome. *Acta Paediatr* **82**:607, 1993.
102. Garel C, Baumann C, Besnard M, Ogier H, Jaeken J, Hassan M: Carbohydrate-deficient glycoprotein syndrome type I: A new cause of dysostosis multiplex. *Skeletal Radiol* **27**:43, 1998.
103. Chitayat D: Dandy-Walker malformation syndromes: Reply to Fiumara, et al. *Am J Med Genet* **63**:413, 1996.
104. Akaboshi S, Ohno K, Takeshita K: Neuroradiological findings in the carbohydrate-deficient glycoprotein syndrome. *Neuroradiology* **37**:491, 1995.
105. Jensen PR, Hansen FJ, Skovby F: Cerebellar hypoplasia in children with the carbohydrate-deficient glycoprotein syndrome. *Neuroradiology* **37**:328, 1995.
106. Okamoto N, Wada Y, Kobayashi M, et al: Decreased blood coagulation activities in carbohydrate-deficient glycoprotein syndrome. *J Inherited Metab Dis* **16**:435, 1993.
107. Van Geet C, Jaeken J, Lenaerts T, Arnout J, Vermylen J, Hoylaerts MF: Underglycosylation of platelet membrane proteins in patients with carbohydrate deficient glycoprotein syndrome type IA and type IIA leads to different haemostatic patterns. (Submitted.)
108. Ohzeki T, Motozumi H, Hanaki K, et al: Carbohydrate-deficient glycoprotein syndrome in a girl with hypogonadism due to inactive follicle stimulating hormone. *Horm Metab Res* **25**:646, 1993.
109. Barone R, Carchon H, Jansen E, et al: Lysosomal enzyme activities in serum and leukocytes from patients with carbohydrate-deficient glycoprotein syndrome type IA (phosphomannomutase deficiency). *J Inherited Metab Dis* **21**:167, 1998.
110. Björklund JEM, Stibler H, Kristiansson B, Johansson SGO, Magnusson CGM: Immunoglobulin levels in patients with carbohydrate-deficient glycoprotein syndrome type I. *Int Arch Allergy Immunol* **114**:116, 1997.
111. Yuasa I, Ohno K, Hashimoto K, Iijima K, Yamashita K, Takeshita K: Carbohydrate-deficient glycoprotein syndrome: Electrophoretic study of multiple serum glycoproteins. *Brain Dev* **17**:13, 1995.
112. Harrison HH, Miller KL, Harbison MD, Slonim AE: Multiple serum protein abnormalities in carbohydrate-deficient glycoprotein syndrome: Pathognomonic finding of two-dimensional electrophoresis? *Clin Chem* **38**:1390, 1992.

113. Henry H, Tissot J-D, Messerli B, et al: Microheterogeneity of serum glycoproteins and their liver precursors in patients with carbohydrate-deficient glycoprotein syndrome type I: Apparent deficiencies in clusterin and serum amyloid P. *J Lab Clin Med* **129**:412, 1997.
114. Heyne K, Marg W, Walther F, Stephani U, Hermanussen M, Weidinger S: Hypothyroidism phenocopy in glycanosis CDG (carbohydrate-deficient glycoprotein syndrome). *Eur J Pediatr* **153**:866, 1994.
115. Subhedar NV, Isherwood DM, Davidson DC: Hyperglycinaemia in a child with carbohydrate-deficient glycoprotein syndrome type I. *J Inherited Metab Dis* **19**:796, 1996.
116. Holzbach U, Hanefeld F, Helms G, Hänicke W, Frahm J: Localized proton magnetic resonance spectroscopy of cerebral abnormalities in children with carbohydrate-deficient glycoprotein syndrome. *Acta Paediatr* **84**:781, 1995.
117. Wada Y, Nishikawa A, Okamoto N, Inui K, Tsukamoto H, Okada S, Taniguchi N: Structure of serum transferrin in carbohydrate-deficient glycoprotein syndrome. *Biochem Biophys Res Commun* **189**:832, 1992.
118. Yamashita K, Ohkura T, Ideo H, Ohno K, Kanai M: Electrospray ionization-mass spectrometric analysis of serum transferrin isoforms in patients with carbohydrate-deficient glycoprotein syndrome. *J Biochem* **114**:766, 1993.
119. Yamashita K, Ideo H, Ohkura T, Fukushima K, Yuasa I, Ohno K, Takeshita K: Sugar chains of serum transferrin from patients with carbohydrate deficient glycoprotein syndrome: Evidence of asparagine-N-linked oligosaccharide transfer deficiency. *J Biol Chem* **268**:5783, 1993.
120. Krasnewich DM, Holt GD, Brantly M, Skovby F, Redwine J, Gahl WA: Abnormal synthesis of dolichol-linked oligosaccharides in carbohydrate-deficient glycoprotein syndrome. *Glycobiology* **5**:503, 1995.
121. Powell LD, Paneerselvam K, Vij R, et al: Carbohydrate-deficient glycoprotein syndrome: Not an N-linked oligosaccharide processing defect, but an abnormality in lipid-linked oligosaccharide biosynthesis? *J Clin Invest* **94**:1901, 1994.
122. Panneerselvam K, Freeze HH: Mannose corrects altered *N*-glycosylation in carbohydrate-deficient glycoprotein syndrome fibroblasts. *J Clin Invest* **97**:1478, 1996.
123. Panneerselvam K, Freeze HH: Enzymes involved in the synthesis of mannose-6-phosphate from glucose are normal in carbohydrate deficient glycoprotein syndrome fibroblasts. *Biochem Biophys Res Commun* **208**:517, 1995.
124. Yasugi E, Nakasuji M, Dohi T, Oshima M: Major defect of carbohydrate-deficient-glycoprotein syndrome is not found in the synthesis of dolichyl phosphate or *N*-acetylglucosaminyl-pyrophosphoryl-dolichol. *Biochem Biophys Res Commun* **200**:816, 1994.
125. Knauer R, Lehle L, Hanefeld F, von Figura K: Normal *N*-oligosaccharyltransferase activity in fibroblasts from patients with carbohydrate-deficient glycoprotein syndrome. *J Inherited Metab Dis* **17**:541, 1994.
126. Körner C, Lehle L, von Figura K: Abnormal synthesis of mannose 1-phosphate derived carbohydrates in carbohydrate-deficient glycoprotein syndrome type I fibroblasts with phosphomannomutase deficiency. *Glycobiology* **8**:165, 1998.
127. Panneerselvam K, Etchison JR, Skovby F, Freeze HH: Abnormal metabolism of mannose in families with carbohydrate-deficient glycoprotein syndrome type 1. *Biochem Mol Med* **61**:161, 1997.
128. Guha SK, Rose ZB: The synthesis of mannose 1-phosphate in brain. *Arch Biochem Biophys* **243**:168, 1985.
129. Matthijs G, Schollen E, Pirard M, Budarf ML, Van Schaftingen E, Cassiman J-J: PMM (PMM1), the human homologue of SEC53 or yeast phosphomannomutase, is localized on chromosome 22q13. *Genomics* **40**:41, 1997.
130. Wada Y, Sakamoto M: Isolation of the human phosphomannomutase gene (*PMM1*) and assignment to chromosome 22q13. *Genomics* **39**:416, 1997.
131. Hansen SH, Freank SR, Casanova JE: Cloning and characterization of human phosphomannomutase, a mammalian homologue of yeast SEC53. *Glycobiology* **7**:829, 1997.
132. Pirard M, Collet JF, Matthijs G, Van Schaftingen E: Comparison of PMM1 with the phosphomannomutases expressed in rat liver and in human cells. *FEBS Lett* **411**:251, 1997.
133. Collet JF, Stroobant V, Pirard M, Delpierre G, Van Schaftingen E: A new class of phosphotransferases phosphorylated on an aspartate residue in a DXDXT/V motif. *J Biol Chem* **273**:14,107, 1998.
134. Aravind L, Galperin MY, Koonin EV: The catalytic domain of the P-type ATPase has the haloacid dehalogenase fold. *Trends Biochem Sci* **23**:127, 1998.
135. Zielinski NA, Chakrabarty AM, Berry A: Characterization and regulation of the *Pseudomonas aeruginosa algC* gene encoding phosphomannomutase. *J Biol Chem* **266**:9754, 1991.
136. Ray WJ Jr, Peck EJ Jr: Phosphomutases, in Boyer P (ed): *The Enzymes*, vol 6, 3d ed. New York, Academic, 1972, p 407.
137. Kepes F, Schekman R: The yeast *SEC53* gene encodes phosphomannomutase. *J Biol Chem* **263**:9155, 1988.
138. Martinsson T, Bjursell C, Stibler H, et al: Linkage of a locus for carbohydrate-deficient glycoprotein syndrome type I (CDG1) to chromosome 16p, and linkage disequilibrium to microsatellite marker D16S406. *Hum Mol Genet* **3**:2037, 1994.
139. Bjursell C, Stibler H, Wahlström J, et al: Fine mapping of the gene for carbohydrate-deficient glycoprotein syndrome, type I (CDG1): Linkage disequilibrium and founder effect in Scandinavian families. *Genomics* **39**:247, 1997.
140. Schollen E, Pardon E, Heykants L, et al: Comparative analysis of the phosphomannomutase genes *PMM1, PMM2* and *PMM2*(PSI): The sequence variation in the processed pseudogene is a reflection of the mutations found in the functional gene. *Hum Mol Genet* **7**:157, 1998.
141. Bjursell C, Wahlström J, Berg K, Stibler H, Kristiansson B, Matthijs G, Martinsson T: Detailed mapping of the phosphomannomutase 2 (PMM2) gene and mutation detection enable improved analysis for Scandinavian CDG type I patients. *Eur J Hum Genet* **6**:603, 1998.
142. Kjaergaard S, Skovby F, Schwartz M: Absence of homozygosity for predominant mutations in PMM2 in Danish patients with carbohydrate-deficiency glycoprotein syndrome type 1. *Eur J Hum Genet* **6**:331, 1998.
143. Van Tintelen P, Matthijs G, Braam W, Cassiman J-J, Duran M, Poll-The BT: Homozygosity for the F119L mutation in the PMM2 gene in an adult with CDG syndrome type Ia. *Eur J Hum Genet* **6**(suppl 1):62, 1998.
144. Kondo I, Mizugishi K, Yamanaka K, Shigemoto K, Yuasa I, Kuwajima K: Phosphomannomutase 2 (PMM2) mutations in Japanese siblings with carbohydrate deficient glycoprotein syndrome 1(CDG1). *Am J Hum Genet* **61**(suppl):A255, 1997.
145. Morral N, Nunes V, Casals V, Chillón X, Giménez J, Bertranpetit J, Estrivill X: Microsatellite haplotypes for cystic fibrosis: Mutation frameworks and evolutionary tracers. *Hum Mol Genet* **2**:1015, 1993.
146. Kronman C, Velan B, Marcus D, Ordentlich A, Reuveny S, Shafferman A: Involvement of oligomerization, *N*-glycosylation and sialylation in the clearance of cholinesterases from the circulation. *Biochem J* **311**:959, 1995.
147. Kristiansson B, Stibler H, Wide L: Gonadal function and glycoprotein hormones in the carbohydrate-deficient glycoprotein (CDG) syndrome. *Acta Paediatr* **84**:655, 1995.
148. Burger D, Perruisseau G, Simon M, Steck AJ: Comparison of the N-linked oligosaccharide structures of the two major human myelin glycoproteins MAG and P_o: Assessment and relative occurrence of oligosaccharide structures by serial lectin affinity chromatography of ^{14}C-glycopeptides. *J Neurochem* **58**:845, 1992.
149. Pérez-Sala D, Mollinedo F: Inhibition of N-linked glycosylation induces early apoptosis in human promyelocytic HL-60 cells. *J Cell Physiol* **163**:523, 1995.
150. Buscà R, Pujana MA, Pognonec P, Auwerx J, Deeb SS, Reina M, Vilaro S: Absence of *N*-glycosylation at asparagine 43 in human lipoprotein lipase induces its accumulation in the rough endoplasmic reticulum and alters this cellular compartment. *J Lipid Res* **36**:939, 1995.
151. Seta N, Barnier A, Hochedez F, Besnard MA, Durand G: Diagnostic value of Western blotting in carbohydrate-deficient glycoprotein syndrome. *Clin Chim Acta* **254**:131, 1996.
152. Iourin O, Mattu TS, Mian N, Keir G, Winchester B, Dwek RA, Rudd PM: The identification of abnormal glycoforms of serum transferrin in carbohydrate deficient glycoprotein syndrome type I by capillary zone electrophoresis. *Glycoconjugate J* **13**:1031, 1996.
153. Wada Y, Gu J, Okamoto N, Inui K: Diagnosis of carbohydrate-deficient glycoprotein syndrome by matrix-assisted laser desorption time-of-flight mass spectrometry. *Biol Mass Spectrom* **23**:108, 1994.
154. Spik G, Bayard B, Fournet B, Strecker G, Bouquelet S, Montreuil J: Studies on glycoconjugates: LXIV. Complete structure of two carbohydrate units of human serotransferrin. *FEBS Lett* **50**:296, 1975.
155. Spaapen LJM, Bakker JA, Van der Meer SB, Velmans MH, van Pelt J: Sialotransferrin patterns and carbohydrate-deficient transferrin values in neonatal and umbilical cord blood, in *Abstracts of the 33rd SSIEM Annual Symposium*. Lancaster: Kluwer Academic, 1995, p 171.

156. Stibler H, Cederberg B: Diagnosis of the carbohydrate-deficient glycoprotein syndrome by analysis of transferrin in filter paper blood spots. *Acta Paediatr* **82**:55, 1993.
157. Stibler H, Borg S, Allgulander C: Clinical significance of abnormal heterogeneity of transferrin in relation to alcohol consumption. *Acta Med Scand* **206**:275, 1979.
158. Foo Y, Rosalki SB: Carbohydrate deficient transferrin measurement. *Ann Clin Biochem* **35**:345, 1998.
159. Wevers RA, Rusch H, Huyben K, Vreken P: Underestimation of the a-, mono- and disialotransferrin isoforms using the Pharmacia CDTect kit does not lead to misdiagnosing carbohydrate deficient glycoprotein syndrome type I. *J Inherited Metab Dis* **20**(suppl 1):90, 1997.
160. Stibler H, Jaeken J, Kristiansson B: Biochemical characteristics and diagnosis of the carbohydrate-deficient glycoprotein syndrome. *Acta Paediatr Scand Suppl* **375**:21, 1991.
161. Matthijs G, Schollen E, Cassiman J-J, Cormier-Daire V, Jaeken J, Van Schaftingen E: Prenatal diagnosis in CDG1 families: Beware of heterogeneity. *Eur J Hum Genet* **6**:99, 1998.
162. Stibler H, Skovby F: Failure to diagnose carbohydrate-deficient glycoprotein syndrome prenatally. *Pediatr Neurol* **11**:71, 1994.
163. Stibler H, Kristiansson B: Analysis of transferrin and α_1-fetoprotein in amniotic fluid and neonatal serum: A possible means for indirect prenatal diagnosis of the carbohydrate-deficient glycoprotein syndrome. *Acta Paediatr Scand Suppl* **375**:32, 1991.
164. Freeze HH, Panneerselvam K: Mannose corrects underglycosylation in carbohydrate deficient glycoprotein syndrome cells. *Glycoconjugate J* **12**:575, 1995.
165. Körner C, Lehle L, von Figura K: Carbohydrate-deficient glycoprotein syndrome type 1: Correction of the glycosylation defect by deprivation of glucose or supplementation of mannose. *Glycoconjugate J* **15**:499, 1998.
166. Freeze H, Niehues R, Hasilik M, Marquardt T, Etchison J, Panneerselvam K, Harms K: Initial results of mannose therapy in *N*-glycosylation disorders. *Glycobiology* **7**:1020, 1997.
167. Marquardt T, Hasilik M, Niehues R, et al: Mannose therapy in carbohydrate-deficient glycoprotein syndrome type 1: First results of the German multicenter study. *Amino Acids* **12**:389, 1997.
168. Herman RH: Mannose metabolism. *Am J Clin Nutr* **24**:488, 1971.
169. Wood FC Jr, Cahill GF Jr: Mannose utilization in man. *J Clin Invest* **42**:1300, 1963.
170. Alton G, Kjaergaard S, Etchison JR, Skovby F, Freeze HH: Oral ingestion of mannose elevates blood mannose levels: A first step toward a potential therapy for carbohydrate-deficient glycoprotein syndrome type I. *Biochem Mol Med* **60**:127, 1997.
171. Panneerselvam K, Freeze HH: Mannose enters mammalian cells using a specific transporter that is insensitive to glucose. *J Biol Chem* **271**:9417, 1996.
172. Dupré T, Ogier-Denis E, Cormier-Daire V, et al: Mannose facilitative transport in type I carbohydrate-deficient glycoprotein syndrome fibroblasts. *Glycoconjugate J* **14**(suppl 1):S44, 1997.
173. Alton G, Hasilik M, Niehues R, Panneerselvam K, Etchison JR, Fana F, Freeze HH: Direct utilization of mannose for mammalian glycoprotein biosynthesis. *Glycobiology* **8**:285, 1998.
174. Niehues R, Hasilik M, Alton G, et al: Carbohydrate-deficient glycoprotein syndrome type Ib: Phosphomannose isomerase deficiency and mannose therapy. *J Clin Invest* **101**:1414, 1998.
175. Jaeken J, Matthijs G, Saudubray J-M, et al: Phosphomannose isomerase deficiency: A carbohydrate-deficient glycoprotein syndrome with hepatic-intestinal presentation. *Am J Hum Genet* **62**:1535, 1998.
176. Marquardt T, Hasilik M, Niehues R, Körner C, Freeze H, Harms K, Harms E: Carbohydrate-deficient glycoprotein syndrome type Ib: Phosphomannose isomerase deficiency. *Eur J Pediatr* **157**:174, 1998.
177. de Koning TJ, Dorland L, van Diggelen OP, et al: A novel disorder of *N*-glycosylation due to phosphomannose isomerase deficiency. *Biochem Biophys Res Commun* **245**:38, 1998.
178. Dionisi-Vici C, Bermli A, Bertini E, et al: Phosphomannomutase isomerase deficiency: A novel, potentially treatable CDG syndrome variant. *Pediatr Res* **43**:123A, 1998.
179. Pelletier VA, Galeano N, Brochu P, Morin CL, Weber AM, Roy CC: Secretory diarrhea with protein-losing enteropathy, enterocolitis cystica superficialis, intestinal lymphangiectasia, and congenital hepatic fibrosis: A new syndrome. *J Pediatr* **108**:61, 1986.
180. Gracy RW, Noltmann EA: Studies on phosphomannose isomerase: I. Isolation, homogeneity measurements, and determination of some physical properties. *J Biol Chem* **243**:3161, 1968.
181. Gracy RW, Noltmann EA: Studies on phosphomannose isomerase: II. Characterization as a zinc metalloenzyme. *J Biol Chem* **243**:4109, 1968.
182. Gracy RW, Noltmann EA: Studies on phosphomannose isomerase: 3. A mechanism for catalysis and for the role of zinc in the enzymatic and the nonenzymatic isomerization. *J Biol Chem* **243**:5410, 1968.
183. Cleasby A, Wonacott A, Skarzynski T, et al: The x-ray crystal structure of phosphomannose isomerase from *Candida albicans* at 1.7 Å resolution. *Nature Struct Biol* **3**:470, 1996.
184. Proudfoot AE, Turcatti G, Wells TN, Payton MA, Smith DJ: Purification, cDNA cloning and heterologous expression of human phosphomannose isomerase. *Eur J Biochem* **219**:415, 1994.
185. Proudfoot AEI, Goffin L, Payton MA, Wells TNC, Bernard AR: In vivo and in vitro folding of a recombinant metalloenzyme, phosphomannose isomerase. *Biochem J* **318**:437, 1996.
186. Saunders SA, Gracy RW, Schnackerz KD, Noltmann EA: Are honey-bees deficient in phosphomannose isomerase? *Science* **164**:858, 1969.
187. De Lonlay P, Cuer M, Vuillaumiet-Barrot S, et al: Hyperinsulinemic hypoglycemia as a presenting sign in phosphomannose isomerase deficiency: A new manifestation of carbohydrate deficient glycoprotein syndrome treatable with mannose. *J Pediatr* **135**:379, 1999.
188. Panneerselvam K, Etchison JR, Freeze HH: Human fibroblasts prefer mannose over glucose as a source of mannose for *N*-glycosylation: Evidence for the functional importance of transported mannose. *J Biol Chem* **272**:23,123, 1997.
189. Sols A, Crane RK: Substrate specificity of brain hexokinase. *J Biol Chem* **210**:581, 1954.
190. Reyes A, Cardenas ML: All hexokinase isoenzymes coexist in hepatocytes. *Biochem J* **221**:303, 1984.
191. Weinhouse S: Regulation of glucokinase in liver. *Curr Top Cell Regul* **11**:1, 1976.
192. Etchison JR, Freeze HH: Enzymatic assay of D-mannose in serum. *Clin Chem* **43**:533, 1997.
193. Thorens B, Sarkar HK, Kaback HR, Lodish HF: Cloning and functional expression in bacteria of a novel glucose transporter present in liver, intestine, kidney and β-pancreatic islet cells. *Cell* **55**:281, 1988.
194. Borsig L, Jaeken J, De Rijk-van Andel JF, Van Schaftingen E, Wevers R, Berger EG: CDG-syndrome type I with normal PMM activity: Is α 2,6 *N*-sialyltransferase affected? *Amino Acids* **12**:387, 1997.
195. Burda P, Borsig L, de Rijk-van Andel J, et al: A novel carbohydrate-deficient glycoprotein syndrome characterized by a deficiency in glucosylation of the dolichol-linked oligosaccharide. *J Clin Invest* **102**:647, 1998.
196. Jaeken J, Spik G, Schachter H: Carbohydrate-deficient glycoprotein syndrome. Type II: An autosomal recessive disease due to mutations in the N-acetylglucosaminyltransferase II gene, in Montreuil J, Vliegenthart JFG, Schachter H (eds): *Glycoproteins & Disease*. Amsterdam, Elsevier Science, 1996, p 457.
197. Jaeken J, Schachter H, Carchon H, De Cock P, Coddeville B, Spik G: Carbohydrate deficient glycoprotein syndrome type II: A deficiency in Golgi localised *N*-acetyl-glucosaminyltransferase II. *Arch Dis Child* **71**:123, 1994.
198. Ramaekers VT, Stibler H, Kint J, Jaeken J: A new variant of the carbohydrate deficient glycoproteins syndrome. *J Inherited Metab Dis* **14**:385, 1991.
199. Jaeken J, De Cock P, Stibler H, Van Geet C, Kint J, Ramaekers V, Carchon H: Carbohydrate-deficient glycoprotein syndrome type II. *J Inhe. Metab Dis* **16**:1041, 1993.
200. Coddeville B, Carchon H, Jaeken J, Briand G, Spik G: Determination of glycan structures and molecular masses of the glycovariants of serum transferrin from a patient with carbohydrate deficient syndrome type II. *Glycoconjugate J* **15**:265, 1998.
201. Charuk JHM, Tan J, Bernardini M, Haddad S, Reithmeier RAF, Jaeken J, Schachter H: Carbohydrate-deficient glycoprotein syndrome type II: An autosomal recessive *N*-acetylglucosaminyltransferase II deficiency different from typical hereditary erythroblastic multinuclearity, with a positive acidified-serum lysis test (HEMPAS). *Eur J Biochem* **230**:797, 1995.
202. Tan J, d'Agostaro GAF, Bendiak B, et al: The human UDP-*N*-acetylglucosamine:α-6-D-mannoside-β-1,2-*N*-acetylglucosaminyltransferase II gene (MGAT2): Cloning of genomic DNA, localization to chromosome 14q21, expression in insect cells and purification of recombinant protein. *Eur J Biochem* **231**:317, 1995.
203. Chen S-H, Zhou S, Tan J, Schachter H: Transcriptional regulation of human UDP-GlcNAc:α-6-D-mannoside β-1-2-*N*-acteylglucosaminyltransferase II gene (*MGAT2*) which controls complete *N*-glycan synthesis. *Glycoconjugate J* **14**:758, 1997.

204. Tan J, Dunn J, Jaeken J, Schachter H: Mutations in the MGAT2 gene controlling complex N-glycan synthesis cause carbohydrate-deficient glycoprotein syndrome type II, an autosomal recessive disease with defective brain development. *Am J Hum Genet* **59**:810, 1996.
205. Campbell R, Tan J, Schachter H, Bendiak B, Marth J: Targeted inactivation of the murine UDP-GlcNAc:α-6-D-mannoside β-1-2-*N*-acetylglucosaminyltransferase II gene. *Glycobiology* **7**:1050, 1997.
206. Etzioni A, Frydman M, Pollack S, Avidor I, Phillips ML, Paulson JC, Gershoni-Baruch R: Recurrent severe infections caused by a novel leukocyte adhesion deficiency. *N Engl J Med* **327**:1789, 1992.
207. Frydman M, Etzioni A, Eidlitz-Markus, et al: Rambam-Hasaron syndrome of psychomotor retardation, short stature, defective neutrophil motility, and Bombay phenotype. *Am J Med Genet* **44**:297, 1992.
208. Phillips ML, Schwartz BR, Etzioni A, Bayer R, Ochs HD, Paulson JC, Harlan JM: Neutrophil adhesion in leukocyte adhesion deficiency syndrome type 2. *J Clin Invest* **96**:2898, 1995.
209. Eyskens F, Ceuterick C, Martin J-J, Janssens G, Jaeken J: Carbohydrate-deficient glycoprotein syndrome with previously unreported features. *Acta Paediatr* **83**:892, 1994.
210. Skladal D, Sperl W, Henry H, Bachmann C: Congenital cataract and familial brachydactyly in carbohydrate-deficient glycoprotein syndrome. *J Inher Metab Dis* **19**:251, 1996.
211. Assmann B, Hoffmann GF, Köhler M, Hackler R, Kleine TO, Jaeken J: CDG-syndrome type I with normal phosphomannomutase activity and unusually mild clinical manifestations. *Amino Acids* **12**:387, 1997.
212. Dorland L, de Koning TJ, Toet M, de Vries LS, van den Berg IET, Poll-The BT: Recurrent non-immune hydrops fetalis associated with carbohydrate-deficient glycoprotein syndrome. *J Inher Metab Dis* **20**(suppl 1):88, 1997.
213. Stibler H, Westerberg B, Hanefeld F, Hagberg B: Carbohydrate-deficient glycoprotein (CDG) syndrome: A new variant, type III. *Neuropediatrics* **24**:51, 1993.
214. Stibler H, Stephani U, Kutsch U: Carbohydrate-deficient glycoprotein syndrome: A fourth subtype. *Neuropediatrics* **26**:235, 1995.
215. Fukuda MN, Masri KA, Dell A, Luzzatto L, Moremen KW: Incomplete synthesis of *N*-glycans in congenital dyserythropoietic anemia type II caused by a defect in the gene encoding α-mannosidase II. *Proc Natl Acad Sci USA* **87**:7443, 1990.
216. Fukuda MN, Dell A, Scartezzini P: Primary defect of congenital dyserythropoietic anemia type II: Failure in glycosylation of erythrocyte lactosaminoglycan proteins caused by lowered *N*-acetylglucosaminyltransferase II. *J Biol Chem* **262**:7195, 1987.
217. Chui D, Oh-Eda M, Liao YF, et al: Alpha-mannosidase-II deficiency results in dyserythropoiesis and unveils an alternate pathway in oligosaccharide biosynthesis. *Cell* **90**:157, 1997.
218. Oh-Eda M, Misago M, Moremen KW, Fukuda M, Fukuda MN: Characterization of human α-mannosidase IIx and its potential involvement in an alternative pathway for complex *N*-glycan biosynthesis. *Glycoconjugate J* **14**(suppl 1):S29, 1997.
219. Gasparini P, Miraglia del Giudice E, Delaunay J, et al: Localization of the congenital dyserythropoietic anemia II locus to chromosome 20q11.2 by genomewide search. *Am J Hum Genet* **61**:1112, 1997.
220. Iolascon A, Miraglia del Giudice E, Perrotta S, Granatiero M, Zelante L, Gasparini P: Exclusion of three candidate genes as determinants of congenital dyserythropoietic anemia type II (CDA-II). *Blood* **90**:4197, 1997.
221. Spaapen LJM, Vulsma T, Theunissen PMVM, Van der Meer SB, Jaeken J: Galactosaemia, a carbohydrate-deficient glycoprotein syndrome, in *Abstracts of the 30th SSIEM Annual Meeting*. Lancaster: Kluwer Academic, 1992, p 10.
222. Stibler H, Von Döbeln U, Kristiansson B, Guthenberg C: Carbohydrate-deficient transferrin in galactosaemia. *Acta Paediatr* **86**:1377, 1997.
223. Van Pelt J, van der Meer SB, Bakker JA, Spaapen LJM: Carbohydrate deficient transferrin (CDT) and galactosemia. *J Inher Metab Dis* **19**(suppl 1):65, 1996.
224. Rubio-Gozalbo E, Worm P, Otten B, Smeitink J, Noordam K, De Jong J: Abnormal TBG glycosylation and decreased total T4 concentrations in classical galactosaemia patients with normalisation after diet. *J Inher Metab Dis* **20**(suppl 1):89, 1997.
225. Jaeken J, Kint J, Spaapen L: Serum lysosomal enzyme abnormalities in galactosaemia. *Lancet* **340**:1472, 1992.
226. Prestoz LLC, Couto AS, Shin YS, Petry KG: Altered follicle stimulating hormone isoforms in female galactosaemia patients. *Eur J Pediatr* **156**:116, 1997.
227. Petry K, Greinix HT, Nudelman E, Eisen H, Hakomori S, Levy HL, Reichardt JKV: Characterization of a novel biochemical abnormality in galactosemia: Deficiency of glycolipids containing galactose or *N*-acetylgalactosamine and accumulation of precursors in brain and lymphocytes. *Biochem Med Metab Biol* **46**:93, 1991.
228. Dobbie JA, Holton JB, Clamp JR: Defective galactosylation of proteins in cultured skin fibroblasts from galactosaemic patients. *Ann Clin Biochem* **27**:274, 1990.
229. Ornstein KS, McGuire EJ, Berry GT, Roth S, Segal S: Abnormal galactosylation of complex carbohydrates in cultured fibroblasts from patients with galactose-1-phosphate uridyltransferase deficiency. *Pediatr Res* **31**:508, 1992.
230. Charlwood J, Clayton P, Keir G, Mian N, Winchester B: Defective galactosylation of serum transferrin in galactosemia. *Glycobiology* **8**:351, 1998.
231. Besley GTN, Bridge C, Marsh LM, Wraith JE, Walter JH: Two new cases of generalised UDP-galactose-4-epimerase deficiency: Abnormal transferrin patterns at presentation, in *Abstracts of the 33rd SSIEM Annual Symposium*. Lancaster: Kluwer Academic, 1995, p 160.
232. Petry KG, Reichardt JKV: The fundamental importance of human galactose metabolism: Lessons from genetics and biochemistry. *Trends Genet* **14**:98, 1998.
233. Adamowicz M, Pronicka E: Carbohydrate deficient glycoprotein syndrome-like transferrin isoelectric focusing pattern in untreated fructosaemia. *Eur J Pediatr* **155**:347, 1996.
234. Rossner JA, Feist D: Hereditäre Fructoseintolerantz. *Verh Dtsch Ges Pathol* **55**:376, 1971.
235. Jaeken J, Pirard M, Adamowicz M, Pronicka E, Van Schaftingen E: Inhibition of phosphomannose isomerase by fructose 1-phosphate: An explanation for defective *N*-glycosylation in hereditary fructose intolerance. *Pediatr Res* **40**:764, 1996.
236. Pronicka E, Adamowicz M, Rogaszewska M, Socha P, Kowalik A, Jaeken J: Decreased transferrin glycosylation as a possible marker of insufficient compliance of fructose restricted diet in young patients with inherited fructose intolerance. *J Inher Metab Dis* **20**(suppl 1):87, 1997.
237. Stanley P, Ioffe E: Glycosyltransferase mutants: Key to new insights in glycobiology. *FASEB J* **9**:1436, 1995.
238. Hennet T, Chui D, Paulson JC, Marth JD: Immune regulation by the ST6Gal sialyltransferase. *Proc Nat Acad Sci USA* **95**:4504, 1998.
239. Asano M, Furukawa K, Kido M, Matsumoto S, Umesaki Y, Kochibe N, Iwakura Y: Growth retardation and early death of beta-1,4-galactosyltransferase knockout mice with augmented proliferation and abnormal differentiation of epithelial cells. *EMBO J* **16**:1850, 1997.
240. Jaeken J, Kint J: Abnormal serum lysosomal isoenzymes in a neurological disease with carbohydrate deficient glycoproteins, in *Abstracts 25th SSIEM Annual Symposium*. Sheffield, SSIEM, 1987, p 83.
241. Heyne K, Schlüter B, Weidinger S: Arylsulfatase A bei Glykanose CDG Typ I. *Monatsschr Kinderheilkd* **144**:1024, 1996.
242. Ohno K, Yuasa I, Akaboshi S, et al: The carbohydrate deficient glycoprotein syndrome in three Japanese children. *Brain Dev* **14**:30, 1992.
243. Jaeken J: The carbohydrate deficient glycoproteins syndrome: A genetic multisystemic disease with major nervous system involvement. *Int Pediatr* **6**:56, 1991.
244. Gu J, Kondo A, Okamoto N, Wada Y: Oligosaccharide structures of immunoglobulin G from two patients with carbohydrate-deficient glycoprotein syndrome. *Glycosylation Dis* **1**:247, 1994.
245. Heyne K, Henry H, Messerli B, Bachmann C, Stephani U, Tissot J-D, Weidinger S: Apolipoprotein J deficiency in types I and IV carbohydrate-deficient glycoprotein syndrome (glycanosis CDG). *Eur J Pediatr* **156**:247, 1997.
246. Heyne K, Weidinger S: Drei neue biochemische Marker bei Glykanose CDG [carbohydrate deficient glycoprotein syndrome]. *Monatsschr Kinderheilkd* **142**:199, 1994.
247. Pohl S, Hoffmann A, Rüdiger A, Nimtz M, Jaeken J, Conradt HS: Hypoglycosylation of a brain glycoprotein (β-trace protein) in CDG syndromes due to phosphomannomutase deficiency and *N*-acetylglucosaminyl-transferase II deficiency. *Glycobiology* **7**:1077, 1997.
248. Bergmann M, Gross H-J, Abdelatty F, Jaeken J, Schwartz-Albiez R: Abnormal surface expression of sialoglycans on B lymphocyte cell lines from patients with carbohydrate deficient glycoprotein syndrome type IA (CDGS IA) (phosphomannomutase deficiency). *Glycobiology* **8**:963, 1998.
249. Gu J, Wada Y: Aberrant expressions of decorin and biglycan genes in the carbohydrate-deficient glycoprotein syndrome. *J Biochem* **117**:1276, 1995.

250. Tayebi N, Reissner K, Orvisky E, et al: Analysis of a phosphomannomutase 2 gene in American patients with type 1 carbohydrate-deficient glycoprotein syndrome (CDGS). *Am J Hum Genet* **61**(suppl):A348, 1997.
251. Aebi M, Helenius A, Schenk B, et al: Carbohydrate-Deficient Glycoprotein Syndromes become Congenital Disorders of Glycosylation: an updated nomenclature for CDG. *Glycobiology* **10**:iii, 2000.
252. Körner C, Knauer R, Stephani U, Marquardt T, Lehle L, von Figura K: Carbohydrate deficient glycoprotein syndrome type IV: deficiency of dolichyl-P-Man: $Man_5GlcNAc_2$-PP-dolichyl mannosyltransferase. *EMBO J* **18**:6816, 1999.
253. Imbach T, Schenk B, Schollen E, et al: Deficiency in dolichol-phosphate-mannose synthase-1 causes congenital disorder of glycosylation type Ie. *J Clin Invest* **105**:233, 2000.
254. Kim S, Westphal V, Strikishna G, et al: Dolichol phosphate mannose synthase (DPM1) mutations define congenital disorder of glycosylation Ie. *J Clin Invest* **105**:191, 2000.
255. De Praeter CM, Gerwig GJ, Bause E, et al: A novel disorder caused by defective biosynthesis of N-linked oligosaccharides due to glucosidase Ie deficiency. *Am J Hum Genet* **66**:1744, 2000.
256. Lübke T, Marquardt T, von Figura K, Körner C: A new type of carbohydrate-deficient glycoprotein syndrome due to a decreased import of GDP-fucose into the Golgi. *J Biol Chem* **274**:25986, 1999.
257. Grünewald S, Imbach T, Huyben K, et al: Clinical and biochemical characteristics of congenital disorder of glycosylation type Ie, the first recognized endoplasmic reticulum defect in N-glycan synthesis. *Ann Neurol* **47**:771, 2000.

CHAPTER 75

Small-Intestinal Disaccharidases

Giorgio Semenza ▪ Salvatore Auricchio ▪ Ned Mantei

1. **The brush-border membrane of the human small intestine is endowed with a total of seven glycosidases,* which give rise to free monosaccharides by splitting dietary disaccharides and oligosaccharides that arise in the intestinal lumen from the α-amylolysis of starch. The four "maltases" occur as two heterodimers (i.e., the glucoamylase complex and the sucrase-isomaltase complex); the β-glycosidase complex, which is composed of a single type of polypeptide, has two catalytic sites (lactase and glycosylceramidase). Trehalase is composed of a single type of subunit(s) (Table 75-1). These glycosidases are stalked intrinsic proteins of the membrane; the body of the protein mass, including the catalytic sites, protrudes toward the small-intestinal lumen.**
2. **The glycosidases, with the exception of trehalase, are synthesized as very large polypeptide chains, each of which has an apparent molecular weight in the range of 200,000 to 250,000. These pro forms are each split into the final forms either extracellularly (as are the α-glucosidase complexes) or mostly intracellularly (the β-glycosidase complex; see Table 75-2). Since the two catalytic domains in each of these complexes belong to a single translational unit, they are subject to the same biologic control mechanism(s).**
3. **Mammals other than humans are equipped at birth with the β-glycosidase and the glucoamylase complexes. Sucrase-isomaltase and trehalase develop at the time of weaning, when the β-glycosidase complex begins to decline, eventually reaching a level as low as 5 to 10 percent of that at birth. In contrast, in humans, the brush-border disaccharidases develop before birth, beginning prior to week 10 of gestation, with a developmental burst (particularly in the β-glycosidase complex) a few weeks before birth. The level of the β-glycosidase complex—in effect, the level of lactase activity—remains high throughout adulthood in most white people and a few other races.**
4. **The primary site of control in the spontaneous physiological development of sucrase-isomaltase is in all likelihood at the level of transcription. Dietary and hormonal factors also control the levels of disaccharidase activities.**
5. **Both secondary and primary (genetic) disaccharidase deficiencies are known, which may lead to malabsorption and intolerance of the corresponding disaccharide(s) but not of the constituent monosaccharides. Diagnosis depends on determination of enzyme activities through small-intestinal biopsies and/or on an oral tolerance test with the corresponding disaccharides. Among the latter, the breath hydrogen test is particularly reliable.**
6. **All genetic variants of intestinal disaccharidases are monofactorial and autosomal. The most common polymorphic variant is adult-type hypolactasia, in which intestinal lactase declines in childhood or shortly thereafter to 10 percent or less of the level at birth. It should be considered the normal situation, since it occurs in the majority of human populations (and in essentially all mammals other than humans). The genetic basis of human adult-type hypolactasia is discussed in Chap. 76.**
7. **Sucrase-isomaltase deficiency is much rarer and is also genetically heterogeneous.**
8. **Congenital lactase deficiency and trehalase deficiency are very rare, and little is known about their molecular basis.**

LUMINAL HYDROLYSIS OF STARCH

In the average Western diet, starch provides approximately 50 percent of absorbable carbohydrates, but disaccharides (mainly sucrose and lactose) are also important nutrients. In addition, small amounts of free fructose, of the disaccharide trehalose (which is hydrolyzed into two molecules of glucose), and of nonabsorbable carbohydrates, including dietary fiber, stachyose, and raffinose, are ingested.[1–3] Starch is a mixture of two types of polysaccharides: amylose and amylopectin. *Amylose* has a linear structure and is made up of 1-4-α-linked glucose units. *Amylopectin* has a branched structure: the majority of the glucose residues are connected by 1,4-α-glucosidic bonds (the linear chains); the branch points are made by 1,6-α-glucosidic linkages. In the digestive tract, starch is eventually hydrolyzed to yield free glucose by the cumulative action of both the salivary and pancreatic α-amylases, the latter being present in solution in the intestinal lumen (but also adsorbed at the surface of the brush-border membrane), and of the α-glucosidases of the intestinal mucosa.

The hydrolysis in vitro of amylose by salivary or pancreatic α-amylase starts as a random hydrolysis of the internal 1,4 bonds. As it proceeds, it becomes more and more selective, as a result of the greater resistance to enzymatic attack of the last and next-to-last 1,4-α-glucopyranosyl bonds at the nonreducing end of the small linear 1,4-α-glucans and of the 1,4-α bond adjacent to the reducing end.[4–10] The final (limit) products resulting from amylose hydrolysis in vitro are maltose and maltotriose.[11] Those from amylopectin are glucose (in small amounts), maltose, maltotriose, and branched dextrins (Fig. 75-1).[12–16]

In humans older than 1 year, the α-amylase activity of duodenal juice after a test meal is very high, so the intestinal hydrolysis of starch in vivo is very rapid. The amylopectin of a test meal consisting of more than 5000 glucose units is digested at the end of the duodenum into oligosaccharides composed of an average of 3 glucose units.[17] The major components of this carbohydrate

A list of standard abbreviations is located immediately preceding the index in each volume. Additional abbreviations used in this chapter include: HNF-1 = hepatocyte nuclear factor 1; SIF = sucrase-isomaltase footprint.

*In this chapter, we use the term ***disaccharidases*** to refer to the enzymes listed in Tables 75-1 and 75-2. The term is used even in cases in which the substrates of interest are oligosaccharides or glycosides other than disaccharides.

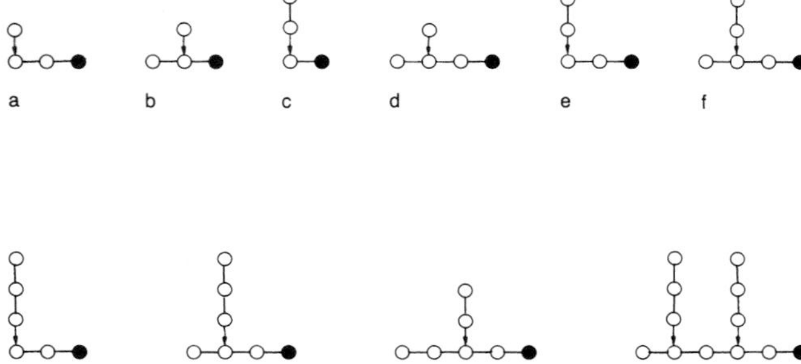

Fig. 75-1 Branched limit dextrins from the α-amylolysis of amylopectin in vitro: ○ = nonreducing glucose unit; • = reducing glucose unit; — = 1,4-α-glucopyranosidic bond; → = 1,6-α-glucopyranosidic bond. (*From Auricchio et al.*[500] *Used by permission.*)

mixture are maltose, maltotriose, and branched dextrins with both 1,4-α and one or more 1,6-α branching links. (Isomaltose is not produced in the digestion of starch by α-amylase.[17]) Maltose, maltotriose, and at least some of these branched dextrins must be considered limit products of the α-amylolysis in vivo, which are further hydrolyzed into free glucose by brush-border α-glucosidases [see the section "Intestinal (Membrane Surface) Hydrolysis of Oligosaccharides"].

Although the intraluminal hydrolysis of free starch does proceed rapidly in vivo, the starch in most staple foods (wheat, corn, oats, and potatoes) may escape *complete* digestion and absorption in the small intestine, and thus some may reach the colon.[18,19] From the amount of hydrogen excreted in the breath[20] (see the section "Diagnosis of Disaccharidase Deficiency, Carbohydrate Malabsorption, and Carbohydrate Intolerance") after an oral load of 100 g flour from different sources, the proportion of starch not absorbed by the healthy small bowel was estimated to be 5 to 20 percent.[18,19] These values were then confirmed by measuring directly the ileal recovery of carbohydrates after ingestion of starch.[21,22] The type of starch and the protein content of the flour appear to be important, because starch from all-purpose wheat flour and from potato is absorbed by the small intestine less completely than that from rice flour or low-gluten wheat flour.[18,19] With other foods, such as legumes or rices rich in amyloses,[23] the percentage of carbohydrates reaching the colon may be even higher. It has been calculated that a substantial amount of dietary starch, perhaps as much as 40 g/day, may reach the colon.[21]

The diarrhea that would otherwise ensue from the delivery of such large quantities of carbohydrates to the large intestine is prevented by the action of the colonic flora. Inadequately absorbed carbohydrates are in fact salvaged through fermentation to gases (hydrogen, methane, and carbon dioxide) and to acetic, propionic, and butyric acids; these acids are readily absorbed from and/or metabolized in the colon. This organ, therefore, makes an important contribution to the absorption of carbohydrates escaping small-intestinal digestion,[24] so that, as a rule, sugars are absent from the stool. As a matter of fact, after the first year of life, children are able to absorb, almost completely, 170 g/m^2 body surface of cooked wheat or potato starch, administered in biscuits and macaroni.[25] The human colon can metabolize anaerobically up to 50 g of unprocessed wheat starch without changing the stool content of volatile fatty acids and lactic acid or its bacterial mass.[26,27]

DIGESTION OF STARCH AND GLUCOSE POLYMERS IN HUMAN INFANTS

α-Amylase activity in the duodenal lumen does not reach normal adult levels until well after birth.[17] There is practically no α-amylase activity in the duodenal fluid of premature and term infants at birth.[28] After the first month of life, amylase activity can be increased on stimulation by pancreozymin and secretin and in response to ingested starch.[29] As a consequence of the low levels of α-amylase activity in duodenal juice, in most infants younger than 6 months of age the duodenal hydrolysis of amylopectin is incomplete, with large amounts of dextrin composed of more than 30 glucose units and, in comparison with older infants, less maltose and more maltotetrose in the luminal fluid; maltotetrose accounts for only 1 to 3 percent of total carbohydrates in the duodenal juice by the end of the first year of life.[17]

This does not mean that young infants may not absorb even sizable quantities of starch and glucose polymers almost completely.[25,30–32] One-month-old infants may tolerate up to 100 g/m^2 rice starch per day, whereas larger quantities cause fermentative diarrhea.[25] Healthy young infants, however, do not absorb glucose polymers longer than 43 glucose units as completely as short-chain glucose polymers (e.g., 3 to 8 glucose units).[33] The capability of young infants to digest limited amounts of starches and glucose polymers in spite of low levels of pancreatic α-amylase may depend on various factors. First of all, the low levels of salivary[34] and of pancreatic α-amylase activity in duodenal juice may still be sufficient if the quantities of starch or glucose polymers are small. Furthermore, the glucoamylase of the small-intestinal mucosa probably plays an important role in digestion of dextrins and glucose polymers during the first few months of life, even if this enzyme is best suited for the hydrolysis of oligomers smaller than 10 glucose residues.[35,36] Finally, at this age also the colonic flora undoubtedly plays a significant role in salvaging unabsorbed starch and glucose polymers.[31]

INTESTINAL (MEMBRANE SURFACE) HYDROLYSIS OF OLIGOSACCHARIDES

The elaborate structure of the brush border greatly expands the surface area of the intestinal apical plasma membrane (to some 200 m^2 in a normal man!), making it better suited to carry out the final steps in digestion and to absorb the resulting products. The tight packing of microvilli, however, also results in thick, unstirred layers, to which mucus also contributes. The limiting factor in membrane digestion in vivo is often the diffusion of the substrate from the lumen to the membrane surface. It seems very appropriate, therefore, that large molecules such as starch and glycogen are first split by enzymes present in solution in the lumen (through *cavital digestion*) and that their smaller, partial degradation products diffuse onto the brush-border membrane to be split further (*membrane digestion*[37]).

Table 75-1 lists the essentials of the substrate specificities of brush-border glycosidases (more can be found in the original literature cited). Considering only the digestion of the oligosaccharides and disaccharides commonly occurring as such in the diet, or arising during the digestion of starch and glycogen, the β-glycosidase complex accounts for all the lactase activity; trehalase for all the trehalase activity; the sucrase-isomaltase complex for all the sucrase activity, for almost all or all of the isomaltase (1,6-α-oligosaccharidase) activity, and for about 80 percent of the maltase activity; and the maltase-glucoamylase complex for a few percent (if any) of the isomaltase activity, for about 20 percent of the maltase activity, and for all the glucoamylase activity.†

†Pancreatic α-amylase and brush-border glucoamylase hydrolyze only 1,4-α-glucopyranosidic bonds, as they occur, for example, in starch and other 1,4-α-glucans. They differ, however, in several respects. α-Amylase prefers long chains and does not split maltose, whereas glucoamylase prefers short chains and does split maltose. The end products of the action of α-amylase on linear chains are maltose and maltotriose, whereas the end product of glucoamylase is glucose only. (It is set free progressively from the nonreducing ends.) Finally, different compounds are known that activate or inhibit either α-amylase or glucoamylase without affecting the other; they enable the quantitative determination of either enzyme in the presence of the other (see, e.g., Schlegel-Haueter et al[195] and Messer and Kerry[327]).

Table 75-1 Major Intestinal Disaccharidases

Enzyme or Complex	Representative Data on Substrate Specificities
Glucoamylase complex (EC 3.2.1.20; the "heat-stable" maltases): glucoamylase (maltase) 1 + glucoamylase (maltase) 2	See Fig. 75-2. In detail, the two catalytic sites have similar but probably not quite identical substrate specificities.[36,501] They split 1,4-α-glucopyranosidic bonds from the nonreducing ends of amylose, amylopectin, glycogen, and straight-chain 1,4-α-glucopyranosyl oligomers, including maltose.[40,502] Minor 1,6-α-glucopyranosidase activity.[39,324,502,503]
Sucrase-isomaltase complex (the "heat-labile" maltases): sucrase (maltase) (EC 3.2.1.48) + isomaltase (maltase) (EC 3.2.1.10)	See Fig. 75-2. In addition, both subunits split maltose (see, for example, refs. 324, 493, and 503), maltotriose,[327] maltitol (G. Semenza, and A.K. Balthazar, unpublished), α-F-glucopyranoside,[504] and (less well) aryl-α-glucopyranosides.[143] In addition, the sucrase subunit splits sucrose and turanose;[505] the isomaltase subunit splits the 1,6-α-glucopyranosyl bonds in isomaltose, isomaltulose (palatinose), and panose, and in a number of branched limit α-dextrins.[38,324,503,506–508]
Trehalase (EC 3.2.1.28)	α,α′-Trehalose and 6,6′-dideoxy-α-α′-trehalose;[509] α- and β-F-glucopyranoside (tested on renal trehalase).[156]
β-Glycosidase complex: lactase (EC 3.2.1.23) + glycosylceramidase (EC 3.2.1.45–46; also called phlorizin hydrolase, EC 3.2.1.62)	A number of β-glycosides: α- and β-lactose, 3-(β-D-galactosido)-D-glucose, 6-(β-D-galactosido)-D-glucose, aryl-β-galactopyranosides, aryl-β-glucopyranosides, methyl-β-galactopyranoside.[510,511] The "lactase" site preferentially splits β-glycosides with hydrophilic aglycons, typically lactose, but also cellobiose,[195,480,492–494] cellotriose, and cellotetrose, and also, but much less, cellulose;[494] some aryl-β-glycopyranosides, e.g., o-nitrophenyl-β-glucopyranoside and -galactopyranoside, are mainly split by the "lactase" site.[495] So are (dietary) flavonoid and isoflavone glycosides.[495a] The "glycosylceramidase" site preferentially splits β-glycosides with a large, hydrophobic aglycon (typically galactosyl- and glucosyl-β-ceramides,[492] phlorizin,[491] and some other aryl-β-glycosides.[495,511]

Hence, the limit dextrins arising from the α-amylolysis of starch in the lumen are completely split to free glucose by the combined action of the glucoamylase and the sucrase-isomaltase complexes (Fig. 75-2).[38–40] The linear 1,4-α-glucans are split, with different V_{max} and K_m values, by the four maltases listed in Table 75-2. The 1,6-α-branched dextrins are split almost exclusively by the isomaltase subunit of the sucrase-isomaltase complex. It should be noted that these branched dextrins can be as much as 25 percent of the original starch.

In adult human small intestine, lactase-glycosylceramidase and sucrase-isomaltase activities are highest in the jejunum and lower at the proximal and distal ends. In contrast, glucoamylase activity increases along the small intestine and reaches maximal values in the ileum, or distal end.[41,42] Similar distribution patterns have been demonstrated in the intestine of human newborns.[43,44]

The capacity for digestion of most oligosaccharides of α-glucose exceeds the capacity for absorption of the component monosaccharides. The anatomic structure of the brush-border

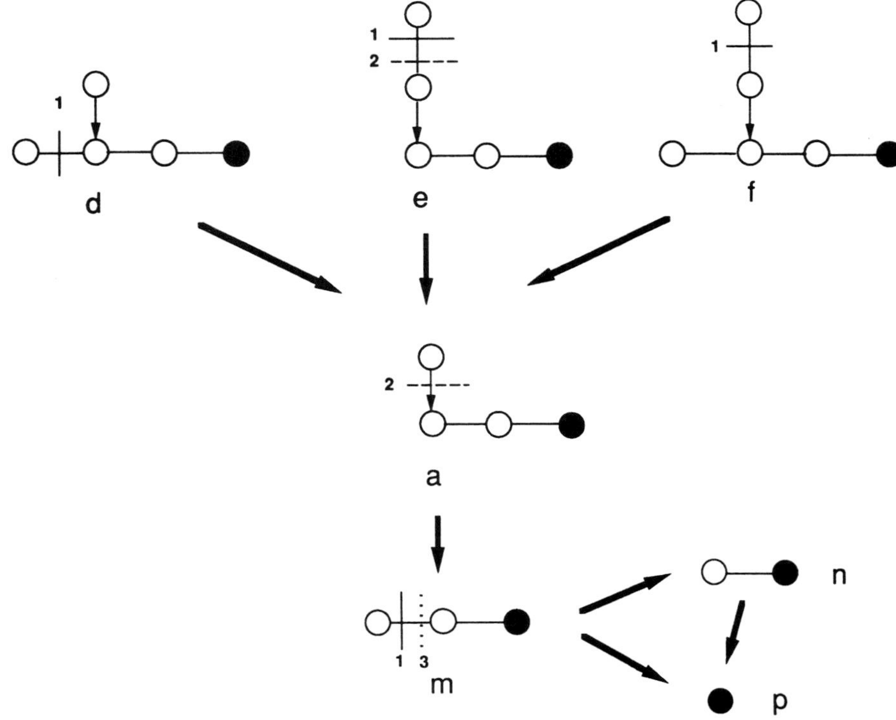

Fig. 75-2 Hydrolysis by glucoamylases and by sucrase-isomaltase of the shortest limit dextrins resulting from exhaustive digestion of starch by α-amylase: ○ = nonreducing glucose unit; • = reducing glucose unit; — = 1,4-α-glucopyranosidic bond; → = 1,6-α-glucopyranosidic bond; *d* = 6-α-D-glucopyranosylmaltotetrse; *e* = 6-α-D-maltopyranosylmaltotriose; *f* = 6-α-D-maltopyranosyl-maltotetraose; *a* = 6-α-D-glucopyranosyl-maltotriose; *m* = maltotriose; *n* = maltose; *p* = D-glucose; 1– = bond hydrolyzed by a glucoamylase; 2— = bond hydrolyzed by isomaltase; 3 = bond hydrolyzed by sucrase. Hence, glucoamylases hydrolyze the pentasaccharides *d* and *e* and hexasaccharide *f* to the tetrasaccharide *a*. The further degradation of α (6-α-D-glucopyranosyl-maltotriose) to maltotriose (*m*), maltose (*n*), and eventually to glucose (*p*) is accomplished mainly by the sucrase-isomaltase complex. (*Data from Auricchio.*[500] *Used by permission.*)

Table 75-2 Molecular Weights of the Small-Intestinal Disaccharidases and of Their Precursors*

Enzyme	Species	M_r (Thousands) of the Primary Translation Product, Nonglycosylated Form†	Brush-Border Form [in Parentheses, the M_r (thousands) of Proteolytically Cleaved Mature Forms]	References
Glucoamylase complex (maltases-glucoamylases)	Pig	200	~245 (125, 135)	68, 120
	Human	209,702	~335	67
Sucrase-isomaltase complex	Rabbit	210,139	~275 (120, 140)‡	55, 60, 65, 71, 128
	Human	209, 974	~235 (145, 150)	79, 121
	Rat		~240 (140, 160)	512
	Pig	225	~265 (140, 150)	119, 120
Trehalase	Rabbit	65, 516	~66	153
β-Glycosidase complex (lactase-phlorizin hydrolyse; lactase-glycosylceramidase)	Rabbit	215, 629	121, 221§	84
	Human	216,393	120,0.68§	84, 97, 98, 106, 121
	Rat	217,266	225(130)	85, 96, 99, 227
	Pig	210	245 (160)	96

*During their migration from the endoplasmic reticulum through the Golgi stacks to the brush-border membrane, these membrane proteins are first *N*-glycosylated (to high-mannose, endo-H-sensitive forms), trimmed, and eventually complex-glycosylated (see the text). The glycosylated forms naturally have larger molecular weights than the nonglycosylated forms. Trehalase exchanges its transient C-terminal hydrophobic peptide sequence for the final phosphatidylinositol anchor in the endoplasmic reticulum. Pre-pro-lactase-phlorizin hydrolase is subjected to extensive proteolytic processing (see the text).

†The M_r values are either estimates from SDS-PAGE or have been deduced from the cDNA sequences. In the latter case, the M_r values of the primary translation products have been calculated for the amino acid sequence alone, from the initiation methionine to the stop codon; they therefore include the cleavable or noncleavable signal sequence, and, in the case of trehalase, the transient hydrophobic anchor sequence that is exchanged in the endoplasmic reticulum for a phosphatidylinositol anchor.

‡The smaller subunit is sucrase; the larger one is isomaltase and carries the hydrophobic anchor not far from the N-terminus.[59,66] Sucrase stems from the C-terminal and isomaltase from the N-terminal portion of pro-sucrase-isomaltase.[64]

§Calculated from the cDNA sequence and from the position of the secondary amino terminus.

¶The differences in apparent molecular sizes (by SDS-PAGE) between human and rat lactase-phlorizin hydrolases are real,[512] and are probably due to different extents of glycosylation.

region provides a diffusion barrier to the movement of monosaccharides (liberated by the disaccharidases) back from the outer surface of the brush-border membrane into the intestinal lumen. It thus favors the absorption of monosaccharides originating from the disaccharides.[45–49] In spite of this, some of the monosaccharides liberated do appear in the intestinal lumen;[50,51] that is, for most oligosaccharides, hydrolysis is not rate limiting. However, the glucose itself inhibits intestinal maltases somewhat.[52]

In contrast to the hydrolysis of other oligosaccharides, that of lactose is the rate-limiting step for the absorption of this sugar.[53] Even in individuals with persistent high lactase activity, mucosal activity of lactase is the lowest of all the disaccharidase activities. (Indeed, the capacity of this enzyme can be exceeded easily, which results in the presence of unsplit lactose in the lumen.) The monosaccharides arising from the hydrolysis of lactose never appear in significant amounts at the luminal side of the brush border, indicating that the transport system or systems for its component monosaccharides, glucose, and galactose are capable of completely absorbing the hydrolysis products presented to them.[54]

MEMBRANE ANCHORING AND BIOSYNTHESIS OF DISACCHARIDASES

The mode of anchoring and the biosynthesis of brush-border glycosidases have been the object of some reviews,[55–58] to which readers are referred for details. See also Table 75-2.

The Sucrase-Isomaltase, Maltase-Glucoamylase, and β-Glycosidase (Lactase-Phlorizin Hydrolase) Complexes§

The α-glucosidase complexes are heterodimers, each composed of two similar but not identical subunits (but see more below on maltase-glucoamylase): each subunit consists of a single glycosylated polypeptide chain with an apparent molecular weight in the 120,000 to 160,000 range (see Table 75-2). The sucrase-isomaltase[59,60] and the glucoamylase[61,62] complexes are anchored to the membrane via one subunit only. The anchoring segment in

§The β-glycosidase activity associated with lactase was initially described as phlorizin hydrolase (β-glucosidase).[491] It was later recognized[492] that the "natural" substrates of β-glycosidase are β-glucosyl and β-galactosyl ceramides. These substrates, however, are costly and are so little soluble in water that they are impractical in routine determinations. In this chapter, we refer interchangeably to this β-glycosidase activity as *phlorizin hydrolase* activity or *glycosylceramidase activity*. That two catalytic sites, and not a single one, exist in the mature lactase-phlorizin hydrolase of the brush-border membrane and after its isolation therefrom is demonstrated by differential heat inactivation,[195,480,492–494] differential inactivation by active-site directed inhibitor,[91,495] incorporation of 2 mol of active-site directed inhibitor per mole of protein,[91,495] lack of mutual inhibition by the two substrates,[480,492,495] etc., and by site-directed mutagenesis.[90] In the single report[496] attributing to one active site alone both lactase and phlorizin hydrolase activity, the authors determined their "phlorizin hydrolase" activity by using *o*-nitro-phenyl-β-galactopyranoside, a substrate that has long been known to be split by 80 percent by *lactase* rather than by phlorizin hydrolase.[495] It is the *meta*-isomer that is split almost exclusively by phlorizin hydrolase.[66,495]

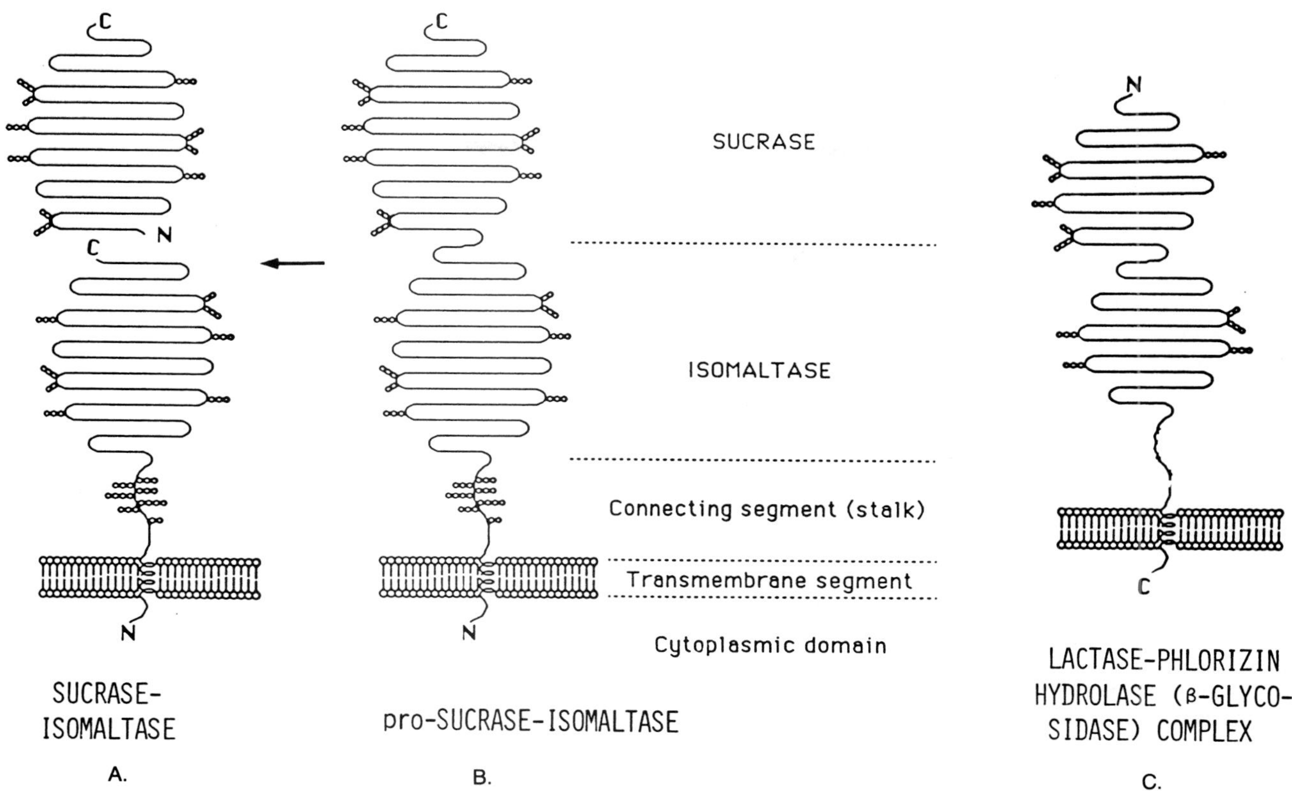

Fig. 75-3 Position of sucrase-isomaltase (A) and of pro-sucrase-isomaltase (B) in the small-intestinal brush-border membrane. The (unspecified) interactions within and between the sucrase and isomaltase domains (or subunits) are not indicated. OOO = sugar chains. (*From Semenza.*[56] *Used by permission.*) Maltase-glucoamylase is positioned in the brush-border membrane in a manner similar to that of pro-sucrase-isomaltase (if not split) or of sucrase-isomaltase (if split).[67,68] (*C*) Position of the lactase-phlorizin hydrolase (β-glycosidase) complex. Note the opposite direction of the polypeptide chain spanning the brush-border membrane, and also that this "complex" consists of a *single* polypeptide chain, with the two catalytic activities associated with different domains. (*Adapted from Mantei et al.*[84] *Used by permission.*) The domain more remote from the membrane is phlorizin hydrolase, and the other, closer to the membrane, is lactase.[90,91]

the transmembrane subunit is located not far from the N-terminus of the subunit.

The positioning of the sucrase-isomaltase complex is now known in a fair amount of detail (reviewed in Wacker et al,[55] Semenza,[56] and Spiess et al;[57] see Fig. 75-3*A*). The N-terminus of the isomaltase subunit is located at the *cytosolic* side of the membrane[60] (and can be phosphorylated by protein kinase A[63]); a number of positive charges occur in the first four amino acid residues; an extremely hydrophobic stretch of approximately 20 residues[60,64] crosses the membrane once[60] in a helical configuration;[65] and most of the protein mass of isomaltase, including the C-terminus, protrudes to the outer, luminal side of the membrane. The sucrase subunit has a peripheral positioning,[66] interacting with the membrane fabric solely via isomaltase;[59] the only hydrophobic segment present in the whole complex is the one that occurs at the N-terminal region of the isomaltase subunit[60] and accounts for approximately 1 percent of the total protein mass.

Human maltase-glucoamylase is composed of a single polypeptide chain[67] which is apparently not split in two "subunits" by (luminal?) protease(s). In those species in which it is split, but often not completely, the "anchor" is confined to one subunit only;[61,62] it is located not far from the N-terminal region of that subunit[68] (see Fig. 75-3*A* and *B*).

Both the sucrase-isomaltase[69] and the glucoamylase[68] complexes dimerize further, thus forming homo-heterotetramers of the type $(\alpha\beta)_2$ in the brush-border membrane.

The major lines in the biosynthesis of these heterodimers have been originally established in some detail for sucrase-isomaltase and more recently for maltase-glucoamylase.[67]

As discussed in later sections, sucrase and isomaltase activities develop simultaneously, respond identically to hormonal and dietary stimuli, and in most cases are equally affected by genetic defects. Their identical or closely related biologic control mechanism(s), *plus* a very close similarity in the functional (and, where known, structural) properties of the two subunits,[70–72] *plus* the mode of membrane insertion of sucrase-isomaltase (in Fig. 75-3*A*, notice the peripheral positioning of sucrase and the anchoring of isomaltase via the N-terminal region) prompted one of us to formulate the *one polypeptide chain, two active sites* precursor hypothesis,[73–75] as follows: (1) An ancestral gene existed, coding for a one-polypeptide chain, one-active site enzyme that split both maltose and isomaltose (a simple isomaltase). (2) The gene was partially duplicated, resulting in a gene coding for a long single polypeptide chain with two identical active sites (a double isomaltase). (3) Point mutation(s) and/or deletion(s) changed one of these active sites from an isomaltase-maltase into a sucrase-maltase. Thereby, a long polypeptide chain was formed, carrying two similar, but not identical, active sites (the pro-sucrase-isomaltase). (4) Posttranslational modification of this single long polypeptide chain by pancreatic proteases leads to the two subunits that make up the final sucrase-isomaltase complex. The subunits remain associated with one another via interactions formed during the folding of the original single-chain pro-sucrase-isomaltase.

When sucrase-isomaltase is synthesized unexposed to pancreatic juice — whether in vivo or in vitro and whether produced in cultivated tissue or cells or translated in a cell-free system — it is always in the form of a 260,000-Da single-chain polypeptide, that is, of pro-sucrase-isomaltase.[55,56] Furthermore, the total sequence of the 1827 amino acid residues of this pro-sucrase-isomaltase (inferred from a cDNA sequence[60]) has revealed a 41 percent identity between the isomaltase and sucrase portions, with another 40 percent of nonidentical but conservative changes, 28 percent of which result from single-base mutations of the codons. This has brought final evidence, therefore, for the partial gene duplication postulated by the "one polypeptide chain, two active sites" mechanism. Finally, the characteristics and mode of membrane insertion of fowl (pro-)sucrase-isomaltase, which are very similar to those of the mammalian enzyme, strongly suggest that the mutation of double isomaltase into pro-sucrase-isomaltase took place prior to the separation of mammals from reptiles and birds, that is, more than 350 million years ago.[62]

This phylogenetic pedigree of sucrase-isomaltase has been enriched by two more observations. The membrane-spanning domains of (1) pro-sucrase-isomaltase, maltase-glucoamylase, and endopeptidase 24.11[76] (all three are brush-border enzymes) and (2) the asialoglycoprotein receptors (proteins of the basolateral membrane)[77] show significant homology to one another and may have evolved from an exon unrelated to those of the glucosidase portions.

The sequence identity between human maltase-glucoamylase and sucrase-isomaltase is 59 percent.[67] (It is 100 percent in the catalytic sites.) Furthermore, lysosomal α-glucosidase (the enzyme whose absence leads to glycogenosis type II, Pompe disease) also has a highly significant homology with brush-border sucrase and isomaltase.[78] The lysosomal enzyme lacks both the stalk and the N-terminal hydrophobic anchor of pro-sucrase-isomaltase and is synthesized with an N-terminal *cleavable* signal. Lysosomal α-glucosidase is thus likely to have evolved from the same ancestral gene as brush-border isomaltase before it acquired the hydrophobic anchor and the stalk portion. These mammalian α-glucosidases are homologous to a yeast glucoamylase.[79]

The maltase-glucoamylase complex also is synthesized as a single polypeptide chain of 220 kDa or more,[67,80,81] which can be split into the "final" unequal subunits (see above).

The individual steps in biosynthesis and membrane insertion of these polypeptides are less well understood. It is clear, however, that pro-sucrase-isomaltase, is synthesized *without* a cleavable signal; that is, that the hydrophobic stretch at the N-terminal region of isomaltase has a dual function: that of the signal ("leading sequence") during biosynthesis and insertion into the membrane of the endoplasmic reticulum, and that of the anchor in the final protein (Fig. 75-3A,B). This was demonstrated by the pro-sucrase-isomaltase cDNA sequence, which showed no signal prior to the N-terminus of the final polypeptide,[60] and directly by N-terminal sequencing of the primary translation product (synthesized in a cell-free system, without microsomal membranes), which yielded a sequence corresponding exactly to that of mature pro-sucrase-isomaltase.[82] Judging from its amino acid sequence, in maltase-glucoamylase also the leading sequence is not split and serves as final membrane anchor.[67] Thus, pro-sucrase-isomaltase and maltase-glucoamylase are type II integral membrane proteins.

A novel kind of α-glucosidase complex has been purified and partially characterized from frog intestine (*R. japonica*).[83] It is composed of two subunits, one with maltase-glucoamylase activity, and the other with isomaltase, but no sucrase or maltase activity.

The complete primary structure of the β-glycosidase complex (lactase-phlorizin hydrolase) and of its pre-pro form has been established in three species.[84,85] It shows no homology with the α-glycosidases, but it does with a soluble cytosolic protein of mammalian liver,[86] with a membrane protein of the intestinal tract of chicken and mussel[87] (perhaps a phylogenetic precursor?), with the *klotho* enzyme (surprisingly),[88] and with bacterial β-glycosidases.[89] The long pre-pro-lactase-phlorizin hydrolase (1927 amino acid residues for the human enzyme, and 1926 for the rabbit and 1928 for the rat homologue; the fraction of identical amino acids among the three pre-pro-lactase-phlorizin hydrolases is 75 to 80 percent) comprises five domains: (1) a putative cleaved signal of 19 amino acids (21 in rats); (2) a large pro portion of 847 amino acids (in the rabbit), or 849 amino acids (in humans), none of which appears in the mature brush-border lactase-phlorizin hydrolase; (3) the mature enzyme, which contains both catalytic sites in a single polypeptide chain,[66] lactase being closer and phlorizin hydrolase being more distant from the brush-border membrane;[90,91] (4) a membrane-spanning hydrophobic segment near the C-terminus, which serves as the membrane anchor; and (5) a short hydrophilic segment at the C-terminus, which is cytosolic and can be phosphorylated in vivo by protein kinase A.[92] The positioning of "final" lactase-phlorizin hydrolase in the brush-border membrane is shown in Fig. 75-3*C*.

Whereas pro-sucrase-isomaltase shows a twofold internal homology, pro-lactase-phlorizin hydrolase shows a fourfold internal homology (which indicates that partial gene duplications have occurred twice)—two of the homologous regions occur in the "pro" portion and two in mature lactase-phlorizin hydrolase. Pre-pro-lactase-phlorizin hydrolase, therefore, in addition to not showing any homology with α-glucosidases, differs from them in several respects: the degree of internal homology is different; its mode of anchoring in the brush-border membrane is different; and its mode of biosynthesis is also different in part, since it is endowed with a cleavable, rather than an uncleavable, signal.[93]

Of the more than 1920 amino acid residues in pre-pro-lactase, only the 60 to 65 percent C-terminal ones eventually constitute mature lactase. The sites of conversion of pre-pro-lactases to pro-lactase (i.e., sites of the cleavage of the signal sequences taking place in the endoplasmic reticulum) were predicted[84,85] (on the basis of von Heijne's algorithm) and actually found to take place after G19 in human[94,95] pre-pro-lactase and after G21 in the rat enzyme. (The rabbit pre-pro-lactase is also presumed to be cleaved after G19, ref. 84). The N-terminal sequences of pro-lactase are thus SDWESD... in all three species.

Most, if not all, of the degradation of the pro sequence takes place intracellularly,[96–101] in the *trans*-Golgi network or in a later compartment,[102] as shown in small-intestinal cultures, where the progress of pro-lactase to the Golgi is blocked by either brefeldin A or low temperature.

The pro sequence is cleaved in various steps, which differ in the three species (and which are probably not all known yet). Responsible for the differences are minor differences in the primary sequences, which produce—or fail to produce—consensus sequences for furin-like pro-hormone convertases and/or still unspecified differences in the tertiary structure. A conspicuous 180-kDa intermediate appears in the biosynthesis of the rabbit, but not of the human, enzyme. It is due to a furin consensus sequence R-A-A-R[349] that occurs within the homologous region I in rabbits, but not in humans.[103,104] (Curiously, two other furin-like consensus sequences in the same region, at R^{114} and R^{192}, also occurring in rabbits but not in humans, are not used.) The mRNAs of furin, PC1/3 and PC6A, have both been detected in the enterocytes by in situ hybridization.[103]

In humans, pro-lactase is processed by furin (or by another furin-like convertase) to a smaller intermediate ("mature-like" lactase) of a size very similar to that of "mature," brush-border lactase by a cleavage after the consensus motif R-T-P-R[832] (see Mesonero et al[94]). The intermediate reported by Jacob et al is some 3 to 4 kDa larger.[105] (Incidentally, these "mature-like lactases" have been mistaken for "mature lactases" in the past by all groups, including our own.)

What happens next? That is, which protease or proteases cleave after the motif R/K-X-R that precedes the N-terminus of final, "mature" brush-border lactase? In vitro trypsin can easily produce lactase from pro-lactase,[106] and some[107] have even suggested that this is the major mechanism whereby lactase is formed from pro-lactase. This is certainly not so, because, for example, in vitro cultures do produce a lactase of a size similar to or identical with that of "mature" lactase; even if in many cases this in vitro lactase

Table 75-3 Sequences of Pro-Lactase Hydrolases near the N-Terminus of Mature Lactase, and N-Terminal Amino Sequences of Mature Rat Lactases Either Exposed (Mature Brush-Border Lactase) or Not (Lactase from Thiry-Vella Loop) to Pancreatic Proteases

Human pro-lactase	...TVNLPSKVR^{868}AFTFPS...
Rabbit pro-lactase	...SAHLPSKTR^{866}ASALPS...
Rat pro-lactase	...RADFTSRAR^{869}VTDSLP...
Mature brush-border lactase*	VTDSLP...
Lactase from Thiry-Vella Loop	XR^{869}VXDX...

*The same N-terminal sequence was found for lactase isolated from normal rats, from sham-operated rats, or from the jejunumileum anastomosis (which is exposed to pancreatic juice) of rats carrying a Thiry-Vella loop.

SOURCE: From Zecca et al.[90] Used by permission.

may be the "mature-like" one, the fact is that most of the trimming does take place in the absence of pancreatic juice. One arrives at the same conclusion when investigating the lactase prepared from the intestinal mucosa of Thiry-Vella loops (in rats) that have not been exposed to pancreatic juice for weeks.[108] Trypsin, however, does have some role: first of all, is it quite possible that the processing of pro-lactase may (under some physiological or pathologic conditions) not keep up with its migration to the brush-border membrane. These "leftover" large lactases may well be cleaved to "mature" lactase after they have reached the intestinal lumen. Secondly, careful comparisons between "mature" lactase and the "mature-like" lactase synthesized in vitro [e.g., by N-terminal sequencing or very accurate determination of the molecular size by sodium dodecyl sulfate-polyacrylamide gel electrophoresis (SDS-PAGE)][105] do show that the work of intracellular proteases requires "finishing" by trypsin. Finally, the "mature-like" lactase in the brush-border membrane of the small intestinal mucosa of Thiry-Vella loops is two amino acid residues longer than regular "mature" lactase[90] (Table 75-3).

It is still not completely clear which enterocytic proteases trim "mature-like" lactases prior to the final cleavage by luminal trypsin. Additional furin-like proteases, perhaps cathepsins and/or aminopeptidases (on their way to or in the very brush-border membrane) are reasonable candidates, as is especially granzyme A, which splits after a K or an R residue.[109] The N-terminal sequences of "mature," brush-border lactase-phlorizin hydrolases are: AFTFP... (humans[95,110]), ASALP... (rabbits[84]) and VTDSL... (rats[93]), respectively. Summing up, it seems most likely that the details in the processing of pro-lactase to lactase differ in the different species, mainly due to the presence or absence of the R-X-X-R furin (and furin-like) consensus sequences in the pro-lactases. These species differences are probably related to the lack of selective pressure in this process.[104]

What is the role of the pro sequence? It certainly does not have glycosidase activity (at least not of the configuration-retaining type), because it lacks the catalytically critical glutamate (which occurs in both the lactase and phlorizin hydrolase active sites in mature lactase);[66] because pro-lactase has the same specific activity as mature lactase using either lactose of phlorizin as substrates;[106] and because no such activity has been found in preparations of the pro sequence.[111] The only known function of this pro sequence is that it is necessary for (pro)lactase to exit the endoplasmic reticulum and reach the brush-border membrane: in fact, lactase if expressed in COS cells alone (i.e., as pre-lactase, rather than pre-pro-lactase) is retained in the endoplasmic reticulum.[111,112] A number of reasons and a combination thereof can be conceived why the pro sequences (which are homologous but not identical in the three species for which the primary structures are known) are needed for pro-lactase to exit the endoplasmic reticulum: they might form a necessary intramolecular heterodimer with other, homologous region(s) of pro-lactase,[112] and/or they may be needed for pro-lactase to dimerize[113] (but see Naim and Naim[114])—in general, to pass the quality control in the secretory pathway (see Danielson,[115] Helenius et al,[116] and Zhang et al[117]).

In the endoplasmic reticulum and in the subsequent compartments, brush-border proteins undergo the usual sequence of mannosylation, glycosylation, trimming, and complex glycosylation. It should perhaps be mentioned that some of them, including pro-sucrase-isomaltase and pro-glucoamylase are tyrosine-sulfated in the *trans*-Golgi network,[118] a process previously reported for secreted proteins alone. Its biologic significance, if any, is still obscure.

The in vivo turnover of both sucrase-isomaltase and lactase-phlorizin hydrolase has been determined in adult rats.[93] Interestingly, the mean residence time in the brush-border membrane is as short as 5.8 h for sucrase and 7.8 h for lactase. The fractional synthesis rates were more than 400 percent per day for sucrase and more than 300 percent per day for lactase.

In tissue cultures and in Caco-2 cells, movement of the glycosidases from the endoplasmic reticulum through the Golgi membranes takes 60 to 90 min (see Danielson,[119] Danielson et al,[120] and Hauri et al,[121] and others), which is much longer than for peptidases. This asynchronous transport to the cell surface is likely to be due to differential transit through the Golgi apparatus.[117,122,123] Pro-sucrase-isomaltase seems to be transferred to the brush-border membrane directly from the *trans*-Golgi complex, apparently without passing transiently through the basolateral membrane[124–127] (see, however, Hauri et al[128]). But pro-lactase-phlorizin hydrolase and processed lactase-phlorizin hydrolase (at least in transfected MDCK cells) appear in the basolateral membrane.[129] This may indicate that (some?) pro-lactase-phlorizin hydrolase passes transiently through the basolateral membrane before reaching the brush border. For a discussion on the trafficking of brush-border enzymes, and in particular on the question of whether any of them reaches the final destination via basolateral membrane, or directly from the *trans*-Golgi network, see the review by Danielsen et al.[130]

In cultures in vitro, microvillar proteins are arrested in their high-mannose form by lowering the temperature to 20°C (e.g., see Danielson et al[131]). Some sucrase-isomaltase[132] and some pro-lactase[133] reach the lysosomes, either via the brush-border membrane or directly.[134] The sugar moieties of these glycoproteins may have some effect on their enzymatic activities [and, when they have some effect, it is still unclear whether the effect is direct or indirect (e.g., via effects on stability)]. "Mature" human lactase-phlorizin hydrolase, both *N*- and *O*-glycosylated, is reported to have a fourfold higher lactase activity than the solely *N*-glycosylated form.[135] On the other hand, the high-mannose form of human pro-lactase-phlorizin hydrolase has the same specific activities as mature lactase that has undergone, in addition to proteolytic processing, complex glycosylation.[106] Pig pro-sucrase-isomaltase also is about twice as active in the fully glycosylated as in the high-mannose form.[136]

The sugar chains are often responsible for the blood group specificity of these enzymes.[137] They are likely to be responsible, also, for the high-affinity binding of *Clostridium difficile* toxin A to sucrase-isomaltase.[138] Electrophoretic microheterogeneity may be related to the extent of sialylation (e.g., see Cousineau and Green[139] and Kraml et al[140,141]).

Sucrase-isomaltase, glucoamylases, and lactase-phlorizin hydrolase are all configuration-retaining glycosidases. Readers interested in their catalytic mechanism are referred to the reviews in Semenza[72,142] (see also Cogoli and Semenza[143]).

The genes for sucrase-isomaltase and for lactase-phlorizin hydrolase have been assigned to different human chromosomes, the former to chromosome 3q25-26[144,145] and the latter to chromosome 2q21.[146–148]

The human chromosomal lactase-phlorizin hydrolase gene is approximately 50 kb long and has 17 exons. All exons and their intron borders, as well as 1 kb of 5′ flanking region, have been sequenced.[149] The polymorphism of the lactase gene in humans is discussed in Chap. 76. In rabbits (but not in rats or in humans), three chromosomal lactase-phlorizin hydrolase genes exist; they are expressed differently along the small intestine.[150]

Trehalase

Trehalase is unique among intestinal brush-border glycosidases in several respects. It is a very minor component, accounting for about 0.1 percent of the intrinsic protein,[151] but has a far larger turnover number. As a result, trehalase and sucrase activities are at comparable levels in the brush-border membrane. Trehalase occurs either as a monomer or as a homo-oligomer.[151,152] Its apparent monomer size is approximately 75 kDa[151,152] or 65 kDa (from its 578 amino acid residues, including the cleavable leading sequence and the transient hydrophobic C-terminal anchor, as deduced from the cDNA of rabbit intestinal pretrehalase[153]). Trehalase is thus considerably smaller than the other brush-border glycosidases (see Table 75-2). Among the glycosidases, it alone is anchored to the membrane via phosphatidylinositol.[153,154]

The amino acid sequence of rabbit intestinal trehalase is known.[153] It has no homology with any other known glycosidase, except for other trehalase, including that of *Escherichia coli* trehalase[155] (38 percent identical residues). Like other phosphatidylinositol-anchored proteins, its primary translation product begins with a cleavable signal sequence (19 to 22 amino acids long) and ends with a hydrophobic stretch located not far from the (cytosolic) C-terminal segment. This hydrophobic stretch is exchanged for the final phosphatidylinositol anchor while still in the endoplasmic reticulum. Other than this, very little is known about trehalase biosynthesis; also, the exact location of the junction between the polypeptide chain and the phosphatidylinositol anchor, or the exact structure of the latter, is not known. Trehalase can be expressed in *Xenopus laevis* oocytes, where it appears at the membrane surface, again anchored via phosphatidylinositol.[153]

Little is known of the catalytic mechanism of trehalase; it leads to inversion of the configuration at C1, liberating the "α-glucosyl" moiety as β-glucopyranose[156] (H. Wacker and G. Semenza, unpublished observations, 1991). Therefore, in this respect also trehalase differs from all other brush-border glycosidases. The trehalase gene is located on human chromosome 11 (T. Kruse et al, unpublished observations, 1992).

DEVELOPMENT AND REGULATION OF THE DISACCHARIDASES

In Mammals Other Than Humans

At birth, the small-intestinal brush-border membrane of most mammals is endowed with lactase-phlorizin hydrolase and the glucoamylase complex only. The other α-glucosidases develop during extrauterine life—in rats (see, e.g., Rubino et al[157]) and rabbits (see Dubs et al[158]) from days 15 to 18 and approximately days 25 to 30, respectively, that is, during weaning. At the same time, lactase (see, e.g., Doell and Kretchmer[159] and a great many others) and phlorizin hydrolase[160] activities begin to decline. Their levels in adulthood are eventually approximately 10 percent of those at birth. Initiation of the postnatal ontogenic events in the rat gastrointestinal tract is probably determined by the genetic program,[161,162] whereas the terminal phase of intestinal development seems to be influenced by environmental factors such as nutrients and hormones.[163–165]

Enterocytes arising in the crypts acquire the ability to digest and absorb during subsequent migration along the intestinal villi. Interestingly, columnar cells may display a nonhomogeneous pattern of differentiation along the villus, as indicated by the variable expression of the lactase protein in adult animals.[166] The basic program describing this differentiation is carried within the enterocyte, but the signal(s) to differentiate depends on the interactions taking place between crypts, enterocytes, and underlying fibroblasts.[167,168]

On weaning in suckling rats, an enzymatically active sucrase-isomaltase first appears in crypt cells and then progresses gradually to uniform distribution along the villus.¶[169–171]

The primary site of control in spontaneous development of brush-border disaccharidases is most probably at the level of transcription, because in rats and rabbits the enzyme activities appear concordantly with the cognate mRNAs (sucrase-isomaltase, at weaning;[172,173] lactase, in fetal life[174]). Also, studies along the crypt-villus axis (in rats) agree with the site of control of sucrase-isomaltase biosynthesis being at the level of transcription,[175,176] as the bulk of sucrase-isomaltase mRNA is located at the crypt-villus junction and proximal villus.

The expression of α-glucosidase activities responds to hormonal administration—cortisone-like steroids,[177–180] thyroxine,[178] insulin,[181] and epidermal growth factor[182]—which can induce their appearance (in rats, rabbits, and mice) if administered approximately 1 week before the time of their spontaneous development. Glucocorticosteroid-induced precocious development of rat intestinal epithelium and increased turnover rate (see below) may be mediated, at least in part, through alterations in the synthesis of extracellular matrix proteins by differential regulation of their gene expression.[183] The response of sucrase-isomaltase mRNA to hydrocortisone administration parallels that of enzyme activity,[184,185] as does that of trehalase mRNA and activity (J. Riby and N. Kretchmer, and G. Galand, personal communications). The glucocorticoid receptor occurs at high concentrations in the small intestine during the suckling period and decreases thereafter;[186] after weaning, hydrocortisone fails to elicit an increase in sucrase activity.[187] This does not necessarily mean, though, that the physiological trigger of development of sucrase during weaning is a glucocorticosteroid, because an antagonist of these hormones for their receptor does not prevent the normal development of sucrase.[188] Readers will find a discussion of this complicated topic and of the equally complicated dietary regulation of disaccharidases in other reviews and papers.[164,189–194]

At weaning, intestinal lactase-phlorizin hydrolase declines to very low levels in most mammals, including most human populations (see Chap. 76).

What factor triggers this decline? Since weaning is accompanied by the progressive removal of lactose from the diet, it was suggested more than 30 years ago that dietary lactose may be necessary to "sustain" the presence of high levels of lactase in enterocytes. However, the large amount of work (carried out in a number of species, under a number of experimental conditions, and testing a variety of β-glycosides) has produced comparatively disappointing results—administering even large amounts of lactose could achieve only a moderate delay in the onset and a less steep decline in lactase activity.[191–200] Dietary lactose, therefore, does not seem to have more than a marginal effect.

A similar statement can probably be made about the effects of hormones on the decline of lactase at weaning; glucocorticosteroids increase lactase activity only little (see Yeh et al[201] and literature quoted therein), which is in keeping with the observation that the consensus sequence for the glucocorticosteroid-receptor binding was not found in 1000 bp upstream in the human lactase gene.[149] Thyroxine, at pharmacologic dose levels,[201–210] does produce a decline in lactase, particularly if it follows cortisone

¶This pro-sucrase-isomaltase should not be confused with the enzymatically inactive protein cross-reacting with sucrase-isomaltase that has been obtained in homogeneous or highly purified form from the intestine of baby rats[497] or rabbits.[158] The kind and amount of information on these cross-reacting proteins is somewhat different for the two species, but perhaps what is known for one species complements what is known for the other. The protein from rabbit intestine appears at about day 6 of life, reaches a maximum at about day 80, and decreases thereafter, still remaining detectable in adult life, particularly at the apical pole of crypt cells. It has a somewhat larger molecular weight ($S_{20,w}$ = 9.8 S) than sucrase-isomaltase ($S_{20,w}$ = 9.2 S). The cross-reacting proteins from rats are, unlike sucrase-isomaltase, periodic acid-Schiff negative. These proteins may derive from endocytosed, partially degraded sucrase-isomaltase or from incompletely or nonglycosylated (pro-)sucrase-isomaltase, or they may have another origin.

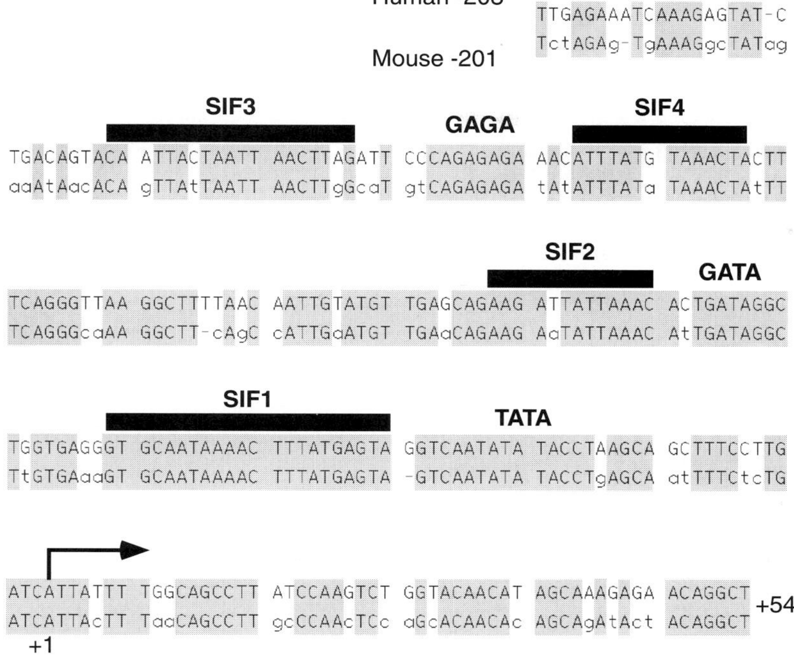

Fig. 75-4 Comparison of the sequences of the mouse and human promoters of the sucrase-isomaltase gene. Nucleotides identical in the two sequences are *shaded*. The *arrow* indicates the start of transcription. The *black bars* labeled SIF1 to SIF4 indicate regions shown to produce DNase footprints (SIF is an abbreviation for sucrase-isomaltase footprint); TATA indicates the putative TATA box; GATA and GAGA indicate further potential binding sites for transcription factors. (*Adapted from Traber and Silberg*[234] *Used by permission.*)

administration.[201] Much, if not all, of the effect of thyroxine on the steady-state levels of intestinal lactase is due to posttranslational mechanism(s).[202,203]

Parallel to the decline of lactase activity at the time of weaning, the life span of the enterocyte also decreases.[165,211–215] Indeed, the correlation between the decline of lactase and shortened life span of enterocytes is reported to be so close[213,214] that the former has been suggested to derive from the latter. Accurate cytokinetic measurements by another group[216] have also led to the conclusion that accelerated cell migration can contribute to the decline of lactase, at least during a part of the weaning time. But pathologic conditions have also been identified in experimental animals, under which crypt-cell hyperplasia correlates with an increase of intestinal lactase.[217,218]

In suckling rats and rabbits, lactase protein and activity can be visualized along the whole length of the small intestine and in all enterocytes along the villus: contrary to this, in adult animals, some populations of enterocytes in the proximal and distal segments of the small intestine do not express lactase, whereas other, neighboring ones do. This patchy expression of lactase (which, incidentally, is not observed for sucrase, for example) undoubtedly contributes to the low average lactase in these intestinal segments.[219]

The levels of lactase-phlorizin hydrolase mRNA are typically some two- to fourfold lower in adult compared with suckling mammals, as shown for rats,[174,205,220–223] rabbits,[174] pigs,[205] and other species. A substantial fraction of the decline in lactase activity can therefore be explained by reduced accumulation of mRNA. In sheep, the drop in both mRNA and enzymatic activity is particularly drastic.[221]

Shortly before birth, lactase appears also in the colon and declines thereafter. In the colon, the levels of the enzyme and those of the mRNA parallel each other.[224,225]

In vivo studies on the rate of biosynthesis and processing of lactase using pulse and chase of methionine in preweaning and postweaning rats[214,226,227] have indicated that its velocity of synthesis does not significantly change at weaning. (Although previous authors[215] reported that lactase biosynthesis decreases at weaning.) In vitro cultures of small intestine from adult rabbits synthesize less lactase precursor than cultures from suckling rabbits.[228]

Genetic elements involved in regulation of sucrase-isomaltase and lactase genes have been studied in transgenic mice carrying sequences of the respective promoter regions coupled to a reporter gene (Fig. 75-4). Relatively short stretches of 5′ flanking sequence, ca. 200 and 1000 bp for sucrase-isomaltase and lactase, respectively, were able to direct developmentally regulated, intestine-specific transcription.[229,230] However, even sequences up to 8000 bp in length could not completely reproduce the complex patterns of expression of the endogenous genes. Aberrant expression in cell types other than enterocytes was observed,[229,231,232] as well as differences along the length of the intestine[231–233] or during the course of development.[233] Since the deviations were in the direction of too much rather than too little expression, negative elements or repressors are likely to play a role in the fine regulation (see the discussion by Traber and Silberg[234]).

Further study of the proximal promoter regions has begun to reveal some of the transcription factors and binding sites involved in regulating transcription of the sucrase-isomaltase and lactase genes. DNase footprinting of the sucrase-isomaltase promoter region enabled identification of three binding sites: sucrase-isomaltase footprint (SIF) 1, SIF2, and SIF3.[235] The SIF2 and SIF3 sites were later shown[236] to bind the transcription factors hepatocyte nuclear factor 1 (HNF-1) α and β, and HNF-1α could activate the sucrase-isomaltase promoter in cotransfection experiments. SIF1 was found to bind and to be activated by the product of the homeobox gene *cdx2*, which is related to the *caudal* gene family of *Drosophila melanogaster*.[237] In the adult, Cdx proteins are expressed at high levels only in the intestinal epithelium:[237–239] they may be involved in specifying the intestinal epithelium per se,[240] and Cdx2 may determine at least in part the tissue specificity of expression of sucrase-isomaltase and other genes.[240–242] Other aspects of the sucrase-isomaltase promoter are discussed in Traber and Silberg.[234]

Troelsen et al[243] identified a nuclear factor in pig enterocytes that binds within a 14-bp sequence (called CE-LPH1) in the lactase promoter near the TATA box. Binding to this site is competed out by the aforementioned SIF1 site,[244] and indeed Cdx2 can bind to and activate the lactase promoter at this site.[245] However, other factors can also bind,[246] including the homeodomain protein HOXC11.[247] Cdx2 and HNF-1 synergistically activate the lactase promoter.[247a] It has been suggested that

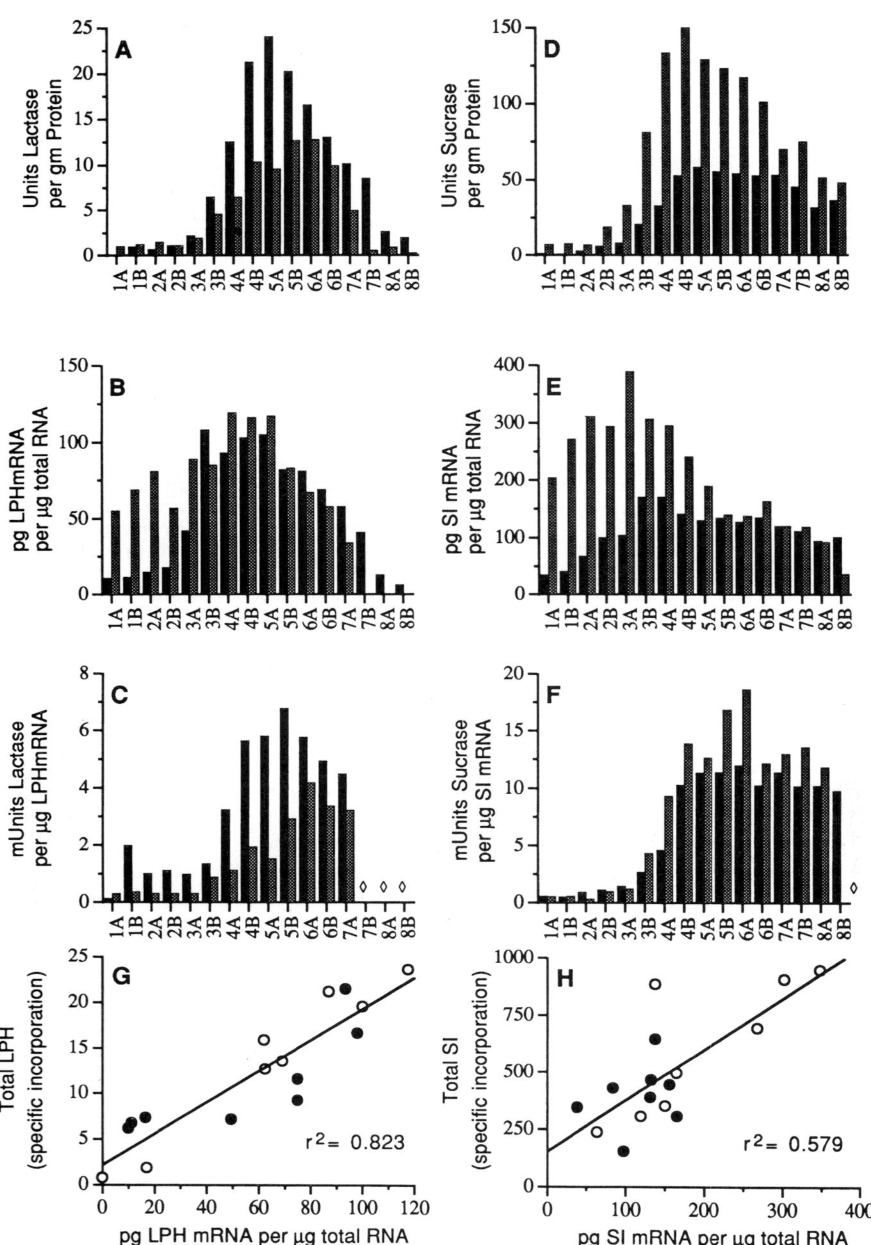

Fig. 75-5 Lactase-phlorizin hydrolase (LPH; A, B, C, and G) and sucrase-isomaltase (SI; D, E, F, and H) along the small intestine of rabbits. A and D: Lactase and sucrase enzymatic activities, respectively. B and E: Their cognate mRNAs. C and F: ratios between the enzymatic activities and the cognate mRNAs. Note that these ratios, being independent of total protein or total RNA, are not confounded by irrelevant variables and thus enable estimation of the importance of mechanisms affecting the steady-state levels of mRNA. G and H: Correlation between the in vitro biosynthesis of LPH (G) and SI (H) and the respective mRNA levels. The enzymatic and mRNA levels were determined in 16 segments from the pylorus to the ileal-cecal valve; the rates of biosynthesis were in eight samples in between. *Black bars* and *black dots* = 36-day-old rabbit; *shaded bars* and *open circles* = 3.5-year-old rabbit. *Diamonds* = ratios (not reported) that were too inaccurate, due to the small magnitudes involved. (*Reproduced from Keller et al.*[252] *Used by permission.*)

factors binding to CE-LPH1 may regulate the level of lactase mRNA during development, because binding is higher in extracts of pig enterocytes with high lactase activity than in those with low activity.[243] Conflicting results have been reported for rats.[248,249] A GATA motif ca. 60 bp upstream of the TATA box is required for activity of the lactase promoter when transfected in to Caco-2 cells, and transcription mediated by this element can be stimulated by coexpression of the zinc-finger transcription factor GATA-6.[250] GATA-family transcription factors may also influence the activity of the sucrase-isomaltase promoter.[234]

Additional reasons may blur the reported observations on mRNA levels. Relatively little attention has been paid, for example, to individual variability, which we find remarkable, even among animals with similar pedigrees. Also, prior to the report by Freund et al,[220] little attention was paid to the fact that the lactase/lactase-mRNA ratios change along the intestine, and that the pattern of these ratios is modulated by the diet during weaning.[251] The former observation was expanded in the experiment referred to in Fig. 75-5 on rabbit small intestine:[252] the rates of in vitro biosynthesis correlated well with the lactase-mRNA levels (Fig. 75-5*G*), but the lactase/lactase-mRNA ratios (a very important criterion! see the figure legend) were much smaller in the proximal third of the intestine than in more distal segments (Fig. 75-5*C*). (Similar observations were made for sucrase; see the right-hand panels in Fig. 75-5.) It is quite possible, therefore, that pancreatic proteases may act locally as a "posttranslational" factor degrading in part intestinal brush-border enzymes; they are probably the reason why lactase, for example, is often absent from the tip of the villi.[219] But the role of pancreatic proteases is certainly not essential in the decline of lactase at weaning (see Keller et al[108] and references therein). Studies with rats[223,253] have shown that in sucklings the lactase gene is transcribed actively in distal duodenum, jejunum, and proximal ileum, but much less so in proximal duodenum and nearly not at all in distal ileum. After weaning, neither mRNA nor lactase were detected in distal ileum, while mosaicism appeared in duodenum.

The decisive factors deciding the decline of lactase must reside primarily in the small intestine itself (and/or in the animal's hormonal setup), because isografts of fetal or newborn mouse[254] or rat[255] small intestine do show this decline, albeit with some delay, as compared with the controls (and develop sucrase at the same time as the controls).

It may well be that the origin of the decline of intestinal lactase at weaning has multiple causes and may differ in different species. As has been pointed out,[256] past the weaning age, mammals as a rule do not come across lactose in their diets. No special advantage arises from persistent intestinal lactase, and no major disadvantage from its disappearance. The postweaning decline may thus have evolved after the mammalian radiation, and the relative importance of various mechanisms—transcriptional, translational, posttranslational—could therefore differ from one species to another.

As will be mentioned below, brush-border glycoproteins are richer in terminal sialic acid residues before than after weaning. It would be conceivable, therefore, that, for example, postweaning lactase-phlorizin hydrolase, which is poorer in or even devoid of sialic acid residues, would be more prone to be degraded by intracellular (processing?) proteases. It seems, however, that the switch in glycosylation does not exactly correlate with the decline of lactase.[257]

In Humans

The developmental pattern of disaccharidases is different in humans from that in other mammals. In humans, both α- and β-glycosidase activities develop during fetal life. Newborns are therefore able to digest not only lactose but also α-glucosides; thus, with due precautions, newborns can be precociously weaned. This contrasts with other mammalian species, which survive infancy on mother's milk only.

Intestinal lactase activity is detectable in human fetal intestine by week 8 of gestation. Mucosal enzyme activity rises gradually between weeks 8 and 34 of gestation and more rapidly shortly before birth, so that lactase activity in term neonates is two to four times higher than that in infants 2 to 11 months of age (Fig. 75-6).[44,258–262]

Within the first week of life, enterally fed preterm infants show a rapid postnatal rise in lactase activity.[44,263] Most premature infants do not experience lactose intolerance. Although the absorption of this disaccharide in the small bowel is incomplete in both preterm and term infants,[264] adequate colonic salvage of malabsorbed carbohydrates is achieved by colonic flora.[265–271] In human fetuses, the biosynthesis of lactase is most probably controlled by the level of their mRNA.[272]

α-Glucosidase activities appear between weeks 8 and 10 of gestation. Thereafter, they increase sharply just before birth.[258,259] The primary site of control is likely to be again at the level of transcription, since the appearance of sucrase-isomaltase mRNA parallels that of the enzymatic activities.[184] The immediate promoter region of the sucrase-isomaltase gene is highly conserved between mice and humans,[229] and the previous discussion of promoter elements applies to both.

Established cell lines derived from human colonic cancer show an "enterocyte-like" differentiation similar to that which occurs in fetal colon. Glucose is a powerful negative modulator of the biosynthesis of sucrase-isomaltase in these cells.[273–276]

GLYCOSYLATION OF DISACCHARIDASES AND CHANGES DURING DEVELOPMENT

Before weaning, the sugar moieties of brush-border disaccharidases are rich in sialic acid residues; after weaning, they are nearly or totally devoid of them and rich in fucosyl residues.[140,257,277–280] This change in composition of the sugar moieties corresponds to changes in the levels of two sugar transferases: sialyltransferase is high before and low after weaning; fucosyltransferase is the opposite.[281,282]

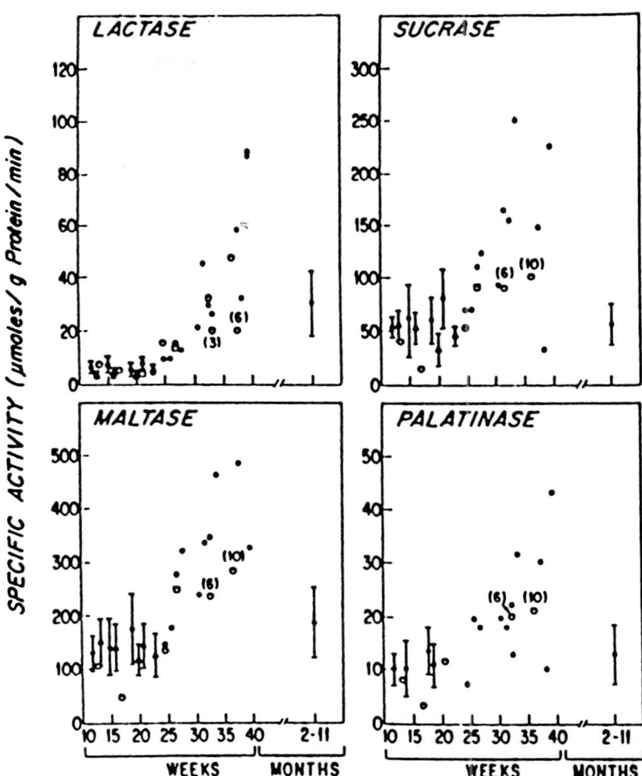

Fig. 75-6 Development of disaccharidase activities in human fetal jejunum. Values in *parentheses* are numbers of observations. For infants 2 to 11 months of age *n* = 25. Where possible, data are means ± SD (*bars*). (*From Mobassaleh et al.*[262] *Original data from Antonovicz et al.,*[258] *Dahlqvist and Lindberg,*[260] *and Jiřsová et al.*[261] *Used by permission.*)

The increase of fucosyltransferase at the time of weaning, as in other organs, is probably under transcriptional control,[283] but the process in the small intestine seems to be more complex, involving an inhibitor of this enzyme,[284] which declines in rat small intestine between days 18 and 23 of extrauterine life.[285,286]

Treatment of rats with hydrocortisone during the suckling period (but not after weaning) leads to a precocious increase in fucosyltransferase activity. However, administration of an antagonist of glucocorticosteroids to suckling rats does not prevent the normal increase in fucosyltransferase activity at weaning.[287,288] This response of fucosyltransferase activity to hormone is thus reminiscent of the aforementioned response of sucrase. Dexamethasone treatment of cultured rat jejunum induces a parallel increase of α-2,6-sialyltransferase and its cognate mRNA,[289] which suggests that this hormonal regulation occurs at the level of transcription; an anti-glucocorticosteroid, onapristone, inhibits the effect of dexamethasone.

Dietary manipulations at weaning can modulate the levels of small-intestinal transglycosidase activities and hence the composition of the glycosyl moieties of these glycoproteins.[282] For an important review, see Biol et al.[288]

CHANGES OF DISACCHARIDASES IN ACQUIRED DISEASES

Several factors such as dietary components, hormones, and endoluminal enzymes may alter the activity of brush-border oligosaccharidases by varying the rates of their synthesis, their degradation, or both, and may also lead to a change in their covalent structure. The turnover of disaccharidases is much faster than cell turnover. In fact, rather than being simply synthesized once and for all by an intestinal cell, a particular membrane protein is turned over repeatedly during the cell's life cycle: whereas the life of rat intestinal villous enterocytes is about 36 h, that of sucrase can vary from 2.5 to 14 h, depending on the experimental conditions.[290,291] Turnover of brush-border proteins is also heterogeneous. Large-molecular-weight proteins, including disaccharidases, have a more rapid turnover than lower-molecular-weight proteins.[292,293] The sucrase and the isomaltase parts of the sucrase-isomaltase complex appear to be degraded at different rates (see below), and the carbohydrate moiety may be selectively removed at least in part, whereas the protein core remains attached to the membrane.[294] Altered degradation rate is an important mechanism controlling levels of brush-border enzymes in various pathologic and physiological conditions.

In the following, we briefly discuss some representative conditions in which changes of disaccharidase activities are brought about by a variety of mechanisms.

Diabetes

Diabetes, either in humans or in experimental animals, is accompanied by an increase in activity of membrane transport systems (for a review, see Karasov and Diamond[295]) and in hydrolytic enzyme activities, including those of disaccharidases; the enhanced sucrase in diabetic animals reflects a selective increase in sucrase-isomaltase *protein,* which is due (mainly) to a decreased rate of degradation,[291] perhaps related to altered glycosylation of intestinal microvillus[296] and of the sucrase-isomaltase itself.[297] The turnover of brush-border proteins as a whole and of the enterocyte is either normal or increased. In congenital diabetic BioBreed rats, but not in streptozotocin-induced diabetic rats, changes in the glycosylation of sucrase-isomaltase have been observed.

The increased disaccharidase activity in diabetic rats appears to be the result of insulin deficiency: it is independent of intraluminal factors, such as food intake or pancreatobiliary secretions[298] (for a review, see Koldovský[191]).

Exocrine Pancreatic Insufficiency

In addition to processing some "pro" forms to the final heterodimers (see the earlier section on biosynthesis of disaccharidases), luminal proteases, particularly pancreatic, seem to play an important role in the degradation and inactivation of intestinal microvillous membrane proteins. In distal rat small intestine, the sucrase part of the sucrase-isomaltase complex is (preferentially) broken down by pancreatic enzymes.[299] Reduction of pancreatic enzymes in intestinal lumen in rats[300,301] and genetic exoc pancreatic insufficiency in mice[302] cause decreased degradation rates and thereby lead to increases in several disaccharidases (maltase, sucrase, and lactase). Administration of elastase restores to normal the enzyme activity levels and the turnover rates.[300] In humans, pancreatic insufficiency caused by chronic pancreatitis or by cystic fibrosis also leads to increased levels of sucrase and maltase, which are also ascribed to a decrease in degradation of these enzymes. Oral administration of pancreatic proteases in patients causes a decrease in sucrase, maltase, and lactase activities.[303]

Secondary Generalized Glycosidase Deficiency

In a number of intestinal diseases with various degrees of mucosal atrophy of the small intestine, there is a generalized decrease in glycosidase activity of varying severity. In atrophic intestinal mucosa from proximal small intestine of children with active celiac disease or cow's milk protein intolerance[304] or of patients with infectious diarrheas (particularly those accompanied by malnutrition and/or small-intestinal lesion[305]), glycosidase activities are significantly reduced as compared with those of normal controls. In all these conditions, lactase is usually the first glycosidase affected, is the one to reach the lowest level, and is the last to recover. Malnutrition suppresses the lactase gene transcription or mRNA stability in infants[306] and also affects posttranslational processing in young pigs.[307] Glucoamylase activity is usually only slightly reduced.[308–312]

In aging rats, the ileum has higher lactase, sucrase, and maltase activities than that in young animals, which is due a higher proliferation index and a larger number of enterocytes.[313] Also, it responds to malnutrition with a further increase in lactase activity.

Various mechanisms may underlie the decrease in disaccharidase activities mentioned in a previous paragraph: atrophy of small-intestinal mucosa, with reduced surface; reduced microvillus surface area;[314] presence on the villi of immature enterocytes with low levels of digestive enzymes;[315] altered cell kinetics; or increased degradation of proteins of the brush-border membrane by luminal enzymes of bacterial origin, either proteases or deglycosylating enzymes, with partially deglycosylated disaccharidases then becoming more susceptible to luminal proteolysis.[316] The last mechanism could be the cause of decreased disaccharidase activity in contaminated small-bowel syndrome[317] or in giardiasis.[318]

DIAGNOSIS OF DISACCHARIDASE DEFICIENCY, CARBOHYDRATE MALABSORPTION, AND CARBOHYDRATE INTOLERANCE

Disaccharidase Deficiency

Disaccharidase activity is usually measured in homogenates of small-intestinal biopsy samples obtained only from the proximal small intestine and therefore gives little information on the ability of the total bowel mucosa to hydrolyze disaccharide.*

Assay of disaccharidases in biopsy specimens involves use of D-glucose-oxidase[319,320] or D-glucose-dehydrogenase[321] to measure glucose released from the substrate. Lactase activity should be assayed in the presence of *p*-chloromercuribenzoate, so that only the relevant brush-border enzyme is measured.[322] Alternatively, brush-border lactase can be selectively determined by using cellobiose as the substrate,[323] since cellobiose is not hydrolyzed by the other β-glycosidases present in the cell homogenate. For the assay of glucoamylase with glycogen or high-molecular-weight soluble starch as the substrate, it is necessary to inactivate the pancreatic α-amylase adsorbed on the small-intestinal mucosa; with maltose as the substrate, the sucrase-isomaltase complex must first be heat inactivated.[324–326] Appropriate inhibitors can also be used.[195,327]

Disaccharidases may also be measured by quantitative immunoelectrophoresis of proteins from individual small-intestinal biopsy specimens by using specific antisera.[328]

Enzymatic activity is usually expressed either in units per gram of wet mucosa or in units per gram of protein (1 g wet weight of mucosa contains approximately 100 mg protein). There are no advantages in one way of expressing the results over another. (For a discussion on this point, see also Karasov and Diamond.[295])

Most investigators agree satisfactorily on the mean values and the standard deviations of normal α-glucosidase activities (e.g., see Dahlqvist[319] and Auricchio et al,[320] as well as Lebenthal et al,[329] Newcomer et al,[330] and Eggermont et al[331]). Normal enzymatic values are usually defined as those of histologically normal small-intestinal mucosa.[332–334] Disaccharidase *deficiency* is defined as the reduction of an enzyme activity to levels lower than the normal mean by at least 2 standard deviations.[331,334]

Most studies carried out in the past investigated disaccharidase activities present in the *jejunal* mucosa at some distance from the ligament of Treitz, that is, within the jejunal plateau of maximum disaccharidase activities. This segment of the small intestine is most appropriate (biochemically speaking), because it has the highest activities and is less dependent on the exact location from

*One source of error, often not recognized, is the circadian rhythm in disaccharidase activities. Activity may vary by a factor of 2 between minimum and maximum (for a review, see Koldovský[191]). The reader's attention is drawn also to an important review on the biology of the circadian rhythm in the digestive system.[318a]

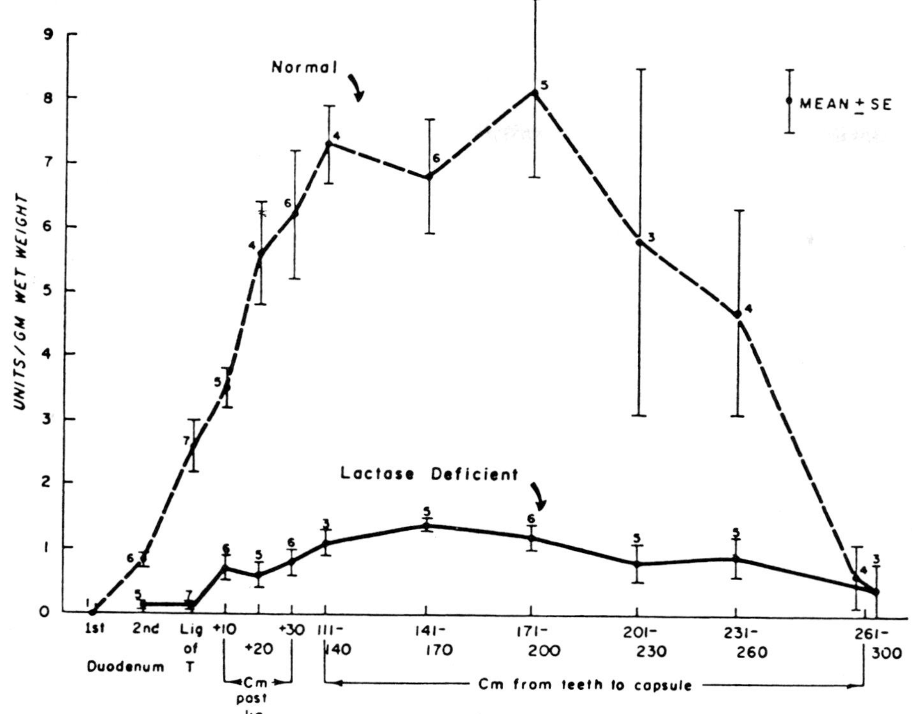

Fig. 75-7 Distribution of lactase activity in the small bowel of seven normal and seven hypolactasic adults. ***(From Newcomer and McGill.[355] Used by permission. See also Triadou et al.[42])***

which the samples are taken. However, biopsy samples from this part of the jejunum can be obtained only during operations (e.g., of the Billroth II type) or perorally using the Crosby capsule. Using the latter, Newcomer and McGill[335] investigated the longitudinal distribution of maltase, sucrase, and lactase activities (for the latter, see Fig. 75-7) in multiple samples from the same individuals. This classic study demonstrated a very steep oral-aboral gradient for the disaccharidase activities (particularly for lactase) from the beginning of the duodenum until 20 to 40 cm *after* the ligament of Treitz. Newcomer and McGill's main results were confirmed in 1983 in kidney donors by Triadou et al.[42]

For ethical reasons, the Crosby capsule and the fluoroscopic control its use entails were some years ago replaced by endoscopy. However, this procedure only gives access to the duodenum and, at the most, to the very beginning of the jejunum. Unfortunately, it is these segments of the small intestine that show the steepest oral-aboral gradient of disaccharidase expression (see Fig. 75-7 for lactase). Hence, samples from proximal duodenum may mimic a transcriptionally regulated lactase deficiency; moreover, the steep gradient artificially increases the individual variability in enzyme activities.

On the other hand, the end of the duodenum and the beginning of the jejunum are exposed to high concentrations of pancreatic juice, which undoubtedly degrades in part the ectoenzymes of the intestinal brush border. In the experiment shown in Fig. 75-5, for example, the low enzyme activities are accompanied by high levels of the cognate mRNAs in proximal small intestine of rabbit and may be mistaken for a "posttranscriptional" lactase deficiency.

In sum, the very part of the small intestine that is accessible to peroral endoscopy is a very treacherous one, and data obtained therefrom must be interpreted with great caution. In particular, conclusions should not be extrapolated to the rest of the small intestine. A minimum, albeit gross, complement to the enzymatic activities in a peroral biopsy may be provided by one of the various lactose tolerance tests. This need for caution cannot be overstressed, also because it has become apparent from the work of Freund's group,[253] as mentioned previously, that the lactase gene is transcribed more or less actively along the (rat) small intestine (see Fig. 75-5 for rabbits).

In congenital sucrase-isomaltase deficiency, sucrase activity is absent or nearly so, isomaltase activity is either absent or heavily reduced, and maltase activity is severely reduced (see the section "Molecular Defects").[336]

In heterozygotes for congenital sucrase-isomaltase deficiency, sucrase and isomaltase levels are intermediate between those of affected patients and normal controls,[336,337] and the sucrase/lactase ratio is abnormal (the normal value for the ratio having been determined for subjects with persistent high lactase activity in adult life).[338] Heterozygotes are best identified by comparing the activity of the relevant enzyme with a weighted average of other enzymatic activities in their own brush-border membrane.[339] The polymorphism of the human lactase gene is discussed in Chap. 76.

In humans, lactase activity varies widely according to age and ethnic group (see Chap. 76). It is conventional to regard levels of lactase activity less than 8 U/g of protein or 0.7 U/g wet weight as diagnostic of primary adult hypolactasia (i.e., of decline of lactase in adulthood).[340–342]

Carbohydrate Malabsorption

Sugar malabsorption is the failure to digest and absorb carbohydrates adequately, with or without signs of clinical intolerance. *Intolerance* and *malabsorption* should thus not be used as synonyms.

The oral absorption tests used routinely in humans are based either on the extent of the blood glucose increase following oral administration of the sugar,‡ on the appearance of gases (mainly hydrogen) in the expired air, or on the presence in feces of

‡Mention should also be made of the oral tolerance test with 3-*O*-methyllactose. This substituted disaccharide is split by small-intestinal lactase to yield galactose and 3-*O*-methylglucose. The latter is absorbed in the small intestine (but not in the colon) and is not metabolized to any significant extent. Hence, the appearance of 3-*O*-methylglucose in urine following oral administration of 3-*O*-methyllactose is an indirect measure of total small-intestinal lactase activity.[498]

the malabsorbed carbohydrates and/or of their fermentation products created by the colonic flora. The first two tests measure the capacity of the small bowel to digest and absorb a carbohydrate load; the third one includes information on the efficiency of colonic mechanisms to compensate for small-bowel failure.

The amount of sugar administered in oral tolerance tests is usually much larger than that present in a physiologically balanced diet.

Blood samples are obtained at chosen times after ingestion of the load (2 g sugar per kilogram of body weight; maximum, 50 g). After sucrose and lactose are administered, a peak rise in serum glucose of less than 20 to 25 mg/dl (during the first 90 min) is diagnostic of sugar malabsorption.[320,340,343] The rise in blood glucose following administration of the disaccharide is best compared with that observed after administration of the component monosaccharides.[320,340]

Whereas this oral load test is reliable in adults, it is not so reliable in children, for whom both false-positive and false-negative results are reported with either lactose or sucrose in 20 to 30 percent of cases.[344] It is imperative that the child have no diarrhea at the time of the test.

The extent of rise in blood glucose following oral administration of a sugar provides no information, however, as to whether the sugar has been absorbed *completely*. Incomplete absorption can be deduced only by measuring parameters directly related to the carbohydrates reaching the colon, such as the increase in breath hydrogen after ingesting a sugar load.

The breath hydrogen test is the least invasive procedure for measuring carbohydrate malabsorption, even in children.[345–348] A peak rise in breath hydrogen greater than 20 parts per million (10 parts, according to Kneepkens et al[349]) over the fasting baseline value after ingestion of a carbohydrate load or a carbohydrate-containing meal indicates sugar malabsorption. When the test meal consists of solids, breath hydrogen collection should be continued for 8 h in recognition of the delayed orocecal transit of solids as compared with liquids.[350] No antibiotic should be given before or during the test. False-negative hydrogen breath tests due to the inability of colonic bacterial flora to produce hydrogen from unabsorbed carbohydrates amount to 2 to 9 percent.[351–354] Excretion of hydrogen in breath after a test meal may be quantitated by comparing it with hydrogen excretion after a dose of lactulose, which is not split by lactase[18,19] and can thus be used as a reference for totally nonabsorbable sugar. This method has been validated in vivo in humans.[26] The lactose breath hydrogen test gives the best discrimination between lactose absorbers and malabsorbers.[330,342] The specificity and sensitivity of this test, however, have not been studied accurately. For a critical review of the value of this test to measure lactose malabsorption, see Suarez and Levitt.[355]

Acetate is another product of the bacterial colonic fermentation of unabsorbed carbohydrate. Venous blood acetate in the nonfasting state can be quantitatively related to carbohydrate breakdown in the colon, although the concentration of acetate in blood may vary with different types of malabsorbed carbohydrates. Breath hydrogen and blood acetate correlate with each other.[24]

When the colon fails to compensate fully for the carbohydrate malabsorption in the small intestine, the sugars themselves and the products of their bacterial breakdown (such as lactic acid or volatile fatty acids) appear in a liquid stool. Detection of reducing substances in feces by using copper sulfate tablets (Clinitest)[356] is useful as a screening test for lactose malabsorption in infants after a milk-containing meal or after administration of an oral lactose load but is relatively unreliable in newborns[357] and adults.[358]

Malabsorbed carbohydrates can be also detected in feces by chromatographic methods[359] or by measuring fecal excretion of ^{13}C-enriched sugars.[32,33]

A new test for assessment of lactose absorption is based on the measurement of urinary galactose after ingestion of 50 g lactose in adults. The ratio between urinary galactose and urinary creatinine completely separates lactose absorbers from lactose malabsorbers.[360]

Carbohydrate Intolerance

Sugar intolerance refers to abdominal symptoms (such as flatulence, borborygmi, abdominal distension, pain, and diarrhea) that result from sugar malabsorption. Final confirmation of the role of disaccharide intolerance in producing these symptoms in an individual patient requires resolution of symptoms after the foods containing the offending disaccharide are eliminated from the diet.

Clinical intolerance of lactose may correlate poorly with the levels of intestinal lactase activity[361] or with the results of oral tolerance tests[362] or of the breath hydrogen test[363,364] (see the next section).

PATHOGENESIS OF CARBOHYDRATE INTOLERANCE

General

Whether sugar malabsorption produces symptoms[18,26,365–367] depends not only on the intestinal digestive and absorptive capacity, but also on factors such as the quantity of the ingested sugar, the rate of gastric emptying, the response of the small intestine to the osmotic load, the metabolic activity of colonic bacteria, and the absorptive capacities of the colon, mainly for water and short-chain fatty acids.[368] We will discuss some of these factors, one at a time.

Gastric emptying is delayed and duodenal-ileal transit is accelerated by the insufficient digestion of the sugar itself: The unabsorbed carbohydrate, when present in the distal small intestine, inhibits gastric emptying by an ill-defined mechanism; at the same time, it stimulates duodenal-ileal transit, because of the decreased water and sodium absorption.[27,369–373] (The delayed gastric emptying thus partially compensates for the effects of the high sugar levels in the intestine.[344])

As a consequence, the reduced digestion per se, the delayed gastric emptying, and the accelerated duodenal-ileal transit all concur in reducing monosaccharide absorption.[27,374] The ensuing flattened blood glucose profile elicits, in turn, little or no increase in the plasma levels of insulin, C peptide, and gastric inhibitory polypeptide.

Accelerated duodenal-ileal transit may entail the malabsorption of unrelated nutrients, such as starch or fat.[375–377] Furthermore, ileal flow rates may exceed the critical values above which the right colon propels fluid onward.[378–380]

The colonic bacterial flora salvages some of the dietary carbohydrate not digested and absorbed by the small bowel[20] and, in so doing, limits both colonic wastage and diarrhea. In normal adults, it has been calculated that the colon may salvage up to 20 to 25 g lactose (or lactulose) and up to 50 g starch.[26,381,382] Adaptation of the colonic flora to a particular dietary carbohydrate may further increase this salvaging capacity.[383–385] Diarrhea ensues either when this capacity is exceeded because the amount of unsplit carbohydrates is excessive or when it is reduced for one reason or another. The latter mechanism has been suggested as the cause of lactose intolerance in milk-fed infants treated with antibiotics.[386]

Individual differences in intestinal microflora are a reason for variation in severity of abdominal symptoms in lactose malabsorption. The fecal concentrations and the relative contributions of isobutyric and isovaleric acids in fecal short-chain fatty acids of lactose-tolerant lactose malabsorbers are significantly higher than those of the intolerant ones. This is probably due to larger colonization of the small bowel of lactose-tolerant malabsorbers with anaerobes such as the *Bacteroides* species. The fermentation of unabsorbed lactose by bacteria colonizing the small intestine may act as a complementary protective mechanism reducing the osmotic load of the sugar and avoiding the development of diarrhea.[387]

In Sucrase-Isomaltase Deficiency

The intolerance of sugars in congenital sucrase-isomaltase deficiency deserves a special comment. The clinical symptoms are mainly those of intolerance of ingested sucrose — abdominal distension and osmotic-fermentative diarrhea with liquid feces containing sucrose and glucose (see, e.g., Auricchio et al[359]). This correlates well with the lack of sucrase activity in this disease.

The situation with respect to 1,6-α-glucopyranosides is more complex. The oral tolerance of substrates of isomaltase [e.g., palatinose (i.e., 1,6-α-glucopyranosylfructose) and 1,6-α-glucose oligomers] may be as poor as that of sucrose;[388] that of dextrins, amylopectin, or starch may also be reduced.[388] When present in the diet, the latter glucans may nevertheless elicit diarrhea to a much milder degree than sucrose, particularly during the first year of life.[343,359,388] The milder symptoms are due to the low content of 1,6-α-glucosyl bonds in these glucans (as compared with the oligosaccharides used in the oral tolerance tests just mentioned); to the reduced, but not necessarily absent, 1,6-α-glucosidase (isomaltase) activity (see the section "Molecular Defects"); to the salvaging role of colonic flora; and to a sufficient residual capacity to hydrolyze 1,4-α-glucopyranosidic bonds.

The last point must be discussed further. The hydrolysis of amylopectin and of starch by α-amylase(s) is, as a rule, normal in these patients (but see below).[389] The capacity to hydrolyze completely the 1,4-α-glucans arising from α-amylolysis is severely reduced in patients with sucrase-isomaltase deficiency, yet the level is still sufficient to ensure adequate digestion. This level is mainly due to the glucoamylase complex (see Table 75-1), which is generally unaffected (but see Eggermont and Hers,[390] Hadorn et al,[391] and Skovbjerg and Krasilnikoff:[392] in some cases of sucrase-isomaltase deficiency, glucoamylase also is affected, which can lead to reduced starch tolerance); also, the maltase activity of the "residual, altered isomaltase" present in some patients with sucrase-isomaltase deficiency (see the section "Molecular Defects") may contribute an adequate digestion of 1,4-α-glucopyranosidic bonds.

Finally, as mentioned in the foregoing section "Digestion of Starch and Glucose Polymers in Human Infants," in *normal* infants younger than 6 months of age the α-amylolytic digestion of starch in the lumen is either nil (during the first month of life) or incomplete. Infants of this age, if affected by sucrase-isomaltase deficiency, therefore show a very poor tolerance to starch.[361,389]

TYPES OF HEREDITARY CARBOHYDRATE INTOLERANCE

Primary Adult-Type Hypolactasia

Primary adult-type hypolactasia is the most common form of genetically determined disaccharidase deficiency. Isolated low lactase activity in adults was first described in Caucasians,[393,394] a population in which the majority typically have persistent high lactase activity in adult life. The latter phenotype was considered "normal" until it was realized that, in the majority of the world's human populations, intestinal lactase declines during childhood and adolescence to about 5 to 10 percent of the level at birth,[395] as it does in most mammals after weaning (see Chap. 76). Subjects with primary adult hypolactasia have no feeding problems during infancy, since the enzyme deficiency is not present at birth.

Clinical and Nutritional Consequences of Hypolactasia. Shortly after drinking milk, most persons with low lactose digestive capacity experience borborygmi and abdominal symptoms such as meteorism, abdominal fullness, loose stools or diarrhea, and abdominal pain.[365,396–399] The clinical effects of lactose ingestion are related to dose, with a wide variation in response among individuals.[397,400,401] The relationship of symptoms to milk ingestion may even go unrecognized by some patients. The conventional lactose load used in the tolerance test, 50 g, will produce symptoms in 70 to 90 percent of malabsorbers, whereas 10 to 15 g lactose or half a pint of milk will produce abdominal symptoms in only 30 to 60 percent.[366,401,402]

Lactose intolerance due to lactase deficiency should be considered as the possible cause of gastrointestinal complaints in a number of patients with "idiopathic" diarrhea, irritable bowel syndrome, or recurrent abdominal pain, particularly in children[349,403] and in gastrectomized adults. A coincident lactose intolerance may modify the pattern of clinical presentation of gastrointestinal or other disease, and a period on a lactose-free diet may often be of diagnostic value in patients with abdominal complaints.[404] However, well-controlled trials have recently shown that moderate doses of milk (one or two cups per day) or lactose do not produce symptoms in most lactose malabsorbers, and that subjects who believe themselves to be intolerant to small doses of lactose may in reality have an underlying gastrointestinal disturbance (such as irritable bowel) that they misattribute to lactose intolerance.[405–408] Further medical implications of adult-age lactase decline or persistence are discussed in Chap. 76.

Diagnosis. The diagnosis of lactose intolerance relies first of all on objective measurements of the clinical effects of the withdrawal and reintroduction of lactose. If the symptoms are due solely to lactose intolerance, response to a lactose-poor diet is excellent. Partial resolution of symptoms may suggest a coincidental problem of lactose malabsorption with another disorder, most often irritable bowel syndrome.[404] When gastrointestinal symptoms occur after ingestion of cow's milk, they need not be due to late-onset lactase deficiency. They may relate to a secondary lactase deficiency resulting from some gastrointestinal disease, to malabsorption of the monosaccharides deriving from the intestinal hydrolysis of lactose (glucose and galactose), to an allergic reaction to cow's milk protein,[409,410] or to some other cause.

Thus, the diagnosis of lactose intolerance and lactase deficiency should be secured by appropriate tests (i.e., an oral tolerance test, a breath hydrogen test, and/or an assay of lactase in a jejunal biopsy specimen); see the foregoing section on diagnosis of malabsorption and intolerance.

Genetics and the Geographic Hypothesis. Lactase activity in human jejunum after infancy is genetically determined. This subject is discussed in detail by Swallow in Chap. 76, to which the readers are referred.

Therapy. In most cases, it is sufficient to avoid foods rich in lactose (fresh milk, powdered milk, and milk puddings), whereas foods containing small amounts of lactose are usually well tolerated. Some individuals with hypolactasia can drink small amounts of milk without symptoms.

Lactose malabsorbers do not have symptoms when they ingest appreciable quantities of lactose in yogurt, since the lactase of the yogurt microorganism itself markedly contributes to the digestion of the disaccharide in vivo.[411–414] In children, mechanisms other than enhanced lactose absorption may lead to improved tolerance of the lactose present in yogurt.[415] The calcium in the yogurt is absorbed normally by lactose malabsorbers; thus, yogurt is an excellent source of dietary calcium for them.[416]

Pretreatment of milk with β-galactosidase makes it well tolerated. In some countries, milk previously percolated through immobilized β-galactosidase, and thus made poor in lactose, is available to the general public. The addition of microbial β-galactosidase directly to milk at mealtime also represents an effective enzyme replacement therapy.[417]

Congenital Lactase Deficiency

Congenital lactase deficiency is a very rare disease.[418–421] It is relatively more frequent in Finland, where 16 cases have been described.[422] Not more than 40 cases have been reported altogether.

A severe diarrhea starts during the first hours or days of life, with dehydration, malnutrition, and large amounts of lactose in the feces. Hypercalcemia and nephrocalcinosis may be present.[423] On a lactose-free diet, children show good growth and psychomotor development. The disease appears in sibs and seems to have an autosomal recessive inheritance mode.[422] On a lactose-free diet, jejunal biopsy samples are morphologically normal. Lactase was originally thought to be totally absent in this disease,[424,425] even when a very sensitive assay method was used,[426] but most probably lactase is present, albeit at trace levels[422,427] much lower than in adult hypolactasia.

Congenital lactase deficiency should not be confused with severe infantile lactose intolerance, first described by Durand.[428] In the latter disease, infants are critically ill, suffering from vomiting and failure to thrive on a lactose-containing diet, with lactosuria, aminoaciduria, and acidosis.[429–432] Cataract may also be present.[429,430,432] This disorder is not a mucosal enzyme deficiency, because substantial evidence exists that jejunal lactase activity is normal. It is probably due to an abnormal permeability of the intestinal mucosa.[431]

Congenital Sucrase-Isomaltase Deficiency

Hereditary sucrose malabsorption was first described by Weijers et al[433] in 1960. Shortly thereafter, it was realized that, in this condition, isomaltose malabsorption is also present,[359,388,434] because of an absence of or severe reduction in not only sucrase but also isomaltase activity.[336,435–437] The disease occurs in families and is inherited as an autosomal recessive trait.[337,437]

Symptoms appear when sucrose or starch dextrins[438] are added to the diet. Breast-fed infants or infants fed formulas containing only lactose remain well. The clinical manifestations are watery, osmotic-fermentative diarrhea, which may lead to dehydration and malnutrition, and even to occasional vomiting and milk steatorrhea. Failure to thrive and other symptoms are severe in the young child, but there is a tendency toward spontaneous improvement of symptoms with age; starch tolerance improves after the first years of life.[439] Delay of introduction of sucrose and its decrease in infants' diets have modified the symptomatology in the last two decades.[440] Symptoms, if they persist into adult life, may be limited to some increase in frequency of bowel movement and to minor abdominal distension, although episodes of diarrhea associated with high sucrose intake may still occur. In spite of this spontaneous favorable evolution, it is important that this condition be recognized as early as possible, so that the normal development of the child can be secured by removal of sucrose from the diet.[441]

The diagnosis can be missed in children with chronic diarrhea,[441,442] particularly in older children with a mild clinical presentation and normal growth and development.[443] In adults, the disease is a possible cause of refractory diarrhea or gastrointestinal complaints.[444] Many adults with this disorder have symptoms dating back to childhood, but occasionally the symptoms may appear as late as puberty.[367,445–448]

Hereditary sucrase-isomaltase deficiency is probably rare in most human populations: only some 200 cases were reported up to 1984.[449] Welsh et al found a 2 percent frequency of heterozygotes in a large series of small-intestinal biopsy specimens from white American subjects.[338] The disease is more common among Greenland and Canadian Inuit, and among Canadian Amerindians the reported incidence of homozygotes varies between 4 and 10 percent.[450–452] It is not known whether the high frequency of the disease in these populations is the result of the high degree of inbreeding or whether this mutation produced an unidentified biologic advantage in populations that do not traditionally eat foods containing sucrose. Such an advantage might be related to some role of sucrase-isomaltase other than its digestive function. In rabbits, the sucrase-isomaltase complex may serve as an intestinal receptor for an enteropathogenic *E. coli*[453] and (along with other membrane glycoproteins) as a high-affinity receptor of *C. difficile* toxin A.[351]

The diagnosis is based on the demonstration that osmotic-fermentative diarrhea, with increased fecal excretion of lactic acid, is elicited by sucrose and starch dextrins in the diet. A sucrose-tolerance test will produce a flat blood glucose curve and result in acid watery diarrhea and the presence of sucrose in the feces, whereas the absorption of a mixture of glucose and fructose will be normal. The sucrose hydrogen breath test demonstrates excessive H_2 excretion in the breath.[347,454,455] The final diagnosis is based on the demonstration of deficiencies of α-glucosidase enzymes typical of the disease.

Treatment in the first years of life consists of the elimination of sucrose, glucose polymers, and starch from the diet. Symptoms subside within a few days. Restriction of starch intake is usually unnecessary after 2 to 3 years of age, although excessive amounts should be avoided. Enzyme replacement therapy with lyophilized bakers' yeast (*Saccharomyces cerevisiae*), or with a liquid preparation derived from bakers' yeast and which is very rich in invertase, has been used for successful treatment of children affected by this disease.[456]

Trehalase Deficiency

Trehalose is a disaccharide that occurs mainly in insects and in mushrooms.[457] Isolated trehalase malabsorption has been reported in an elderly woman[458] and in a family.[459] In the latter case, a 24-year-old man developed diarrhea and vomiting after ingestion of a large amount of *edible* mushrooms. Peroral biopsy specimens from the patient and of his father showed a lack of trehalase activity: both subjects had trehalose malabsorption on oral tolerance test with the disaccharide. Trehalase deficiency appears to be an autosomal recessive phenotype.[459]

Trehalase deficiency is likely to go undetected, since ingestion of large quantities of foods containing trehalose is not common; therefore, its real frequency is unknown. Studies on disaccharidase activities in intestinal biopsy samples suggest that this defect is rare in adult white Americans,[338] whereas it is very frequent (10 to 15 percent) in Greenland Inuit,[449,460] and not infrequent among Finns.[460a]

MOLECULAR DEFECTS

Congenital Sucrase-Isomaltase Deficiency

In the complex chain of events coding for the expression and hormonal regulation of a polypeptide chain of nearly 2000 amino acid residues, its membrane insertion, and its glycosylation, its homing to the brush-border membrane (see the foregoing section on disaccharidase biosynthesis and anchoring), many steps can conceivably be affected by mutations. The result may be a lack of sucrase-isomaltase, or the appearance of an abnormal sucrase-isomaltase. Indeed, it was realized fairly early that sucrose-isomaltose malabsorption is a heterogeneous condition: whereas all patients lack sucrase, some have only traces of isomaltase activity and others have reduced but still conspicuous isomaltase activity.[336,391,392,427,461–463] The reports on the molecular defects in cases of sucrose-isomaltose malabsorption differ widely; they certainly agree with the concept that this condition has molecular genetic heterogeneity. But it is unfortunate that most of the papers dealing with this infrequent condition have investigated only a few patients (mostly belonging to a single pedigree) and considered only a few properties. What follows is a list of reported and/or potential molecular defects.

1. Absence of sucrase-isomaltase activity and of immunologically cross-reacting material in total homogenates of jejunal biopsy samples was reported by Gray's group.[462] These conditions could be the consequence of mutations in the sucrase-isomaltase gene, in its promoter, or in a regulatory gene.

2. Absence of sucrase-isomaltase activity and of the corresponding protein band in SDS-PAGE of brush-border *membranes* was reported by Crane's group[464] and by others.[392,461,463] This finding would be compatible with that mentioned in the preceding

paragraph and also with a defective homing mechanism of pro-sucrase-isomaltase into the brush border.

3. Defective homing of pro-sucrase-isomaltase en route to the brush-border membrane[117,465–470] has been reported (for a review, see Sterchi et al[471]): various phenotypes were identified by the combined use of electrophoresis, monoclonal antibodies, and electron microscopy. In one, the sucrase-isomaltase protein accumulated probably in the endoplasmic reticulum as a high-mannose precursor; in another, the intracellular transport was apparently blocked in the Golgi apparatus, and sucrase-isomaltase displayed an "immature" conformation;[117] in a third, a catalytically altered enzyme was transported to the cell surface; in a fourth, pro-sucrase-isomaltase did not undergo normal glycosylation in the Golgi apparatus and was mistargeted to the basolateral membrane;[472] and, in a fifth, high-mannose pro-sucrase-isomaltase was slowly and incompletely complex-glycosylated and cleaved intracellularly, with an isomaltase-like subunit being transferred to the brush-border membrane.[472] In some patients with defective homing, the high-mannose form is reported to be more easily degraded.[467] In most of these phenotypes, the block along the route was shown in pulse-chase in vitro experiments using peroral biopsy specimens.

4. A glutamine-to-proline mutation at position 1098 has been found to cause retention of pre-sucrase-isomaltase in the endoplasmic reticulum/*cis*-Golgi compartments and to lead to sucrase-isomaltase deficiency.[469] (Interestingly, an analogous mutation in lysosomal α-glucosidase, which is homologous to sucrase-isomaltase, leads to a similar block in transport.[470]) Other mutations in the same position do not impede transfer and give normal homing of pre-sucrase-isomaltase.[468]

5. Absence of the sucrase and isomaltase bands in SDS-PAGE of the brush-border membranes and presence of abnormal band(s) have been reported. In one case, a high-molecular-weight single-chain isomaltase was found that cross-reacted with anti–sucrase-isomaltase antisera.[473] Is it a "back-mutated" protease-resistant double isomaltase? (See the preceding section on disaccharide biosynthesis for the "one polypeptide chain, two active sites" hypothesis.) Is it a mutated pro-sucrase-isomaltase with enzymatically inactive sucrase portion and with resistance to proteolytic processing?

6. Absence of the sucrase subunit and presence of a low-activity isomaltase subunit have been reported.[392,463] This may indicate a mutated isomaltase subunit with (evidently) lower enzymatic activity and impaired capacity to interact normally with sucrase. It may be due, also, to a stop in the expression of the pro-sucrase-isomaltase polypeptide chain somewhere near the end of the isomaltase portion, which prevents synthesis of the sucrase portion (and hence of the sucrase subunit). Ito et al. have cloned the sucrase-isomaltase cDNA of the house musk shrew *S. murinus* and of a mutant devoid of sucrase and with very much reduced maltase activity. Most interestingly, the "pro-sucrase-isomaltase" in this sucrase-deficient shrew stops at amino acid position 922: it thus lacks the sucrase portion completely; its isomaltase is 69 amino acids shorter[473a]. Both "normal" sucrase-isomaltase and the sucrase-free isomaltase have been isolated and characterized; the activity splitting maltose and its higher homologues is essentially confined to the "sucrase" site, for which they are actually far better substrates that sucrase itself.[473b]

7. Presence of an immunologically cross-reacting, enzymatically inactive protein was reported by Dubs et al[474] in patients with nonzero isomaltase activity.

8. Reduction in the amount[391,392,461,463] and/or change in the sedimentation properties[390] of the maltase-glucoamylase complex, present in some cases of sucrose-isomaltose malabsorption, may indicate that the biologic regulation of mechanisms of the two α-glucosidase heterodimeric complexes are related.

9. A possible regulatory gene controlling the expression of sucrase-isomaltase and its response to diet has been demonstrated in mice,[475] which may indicate that mutations in the regulatory gene are potentially responsible for (human) sucrose-isomaltose malabsorption: the sucrase and isomaltase activities in the brush-border membranes can indeed be equally and severely reduced.[476] The regulatory gene demonstrated in mice does not influence either maltase-glucoamylase or trehalase.

Congenital Lactase Deficiency

In a Finnish subject with this condition, the coding region of the lactase-phlorizin hydrolase gene has been sequenced[477,477a] and found to be identical with that reported in lactase persistence,[84] save for minor allelic differences. The locus for this lactase deficiency has been assigned to 2q21, close to, but separate from the lactase-phlorizin hydrolase gene.[447b]

Primary Adult-Type Hypolactasia

The β-glycosidase complex present in the small intestine of subjects affected with primary adult-type hypolactasia seems to be indistinguishable from that present in lactose digesters: it has the same electrophoretic mobility,[339,478] the same immunologic properties,[478,479] and the same specific lactase[478,479] and phlorizin hydrolase activities[480] (although individual enterocytes may have inactive, or inactivated, lactase; see below). Sequence analysis (at the mRNA level) has shown that subjects with hypolactasia and persistence of lactase can code for identical pre-pro-lactase enzymes.[149] The genetic defect(s) leading to the adult-type human hypolactasia are described in Chap. 76. As in the case of the decline of lactase at weaning in experimental animals, various, sometimes contradictory, observations have been reported; thus, different molecular mechanisms have been suggested. Some contradictions may well eventually turn out to be apparent only. For example, different sites of control may be operative in different regions of the small intestine. If this is so, it may well be misleading to derive conclusions from samples obtained from the duodenum alone (the only segment of small intestine accessible to peroral duodenal endoscopy), even more so because in the duodenum the oral-aboral gradient of lactase is the steepest (see Fig. 75-7) and its variability the largest, as it has been shown in the classic study by Newcomer and McGill[335] (see also Triadou et al[42]). Furthermore, in distal duodenum, lactase and other brush-border enzymes are exposed to massive amounts of pancreatic proteases. Care should also be taken not to base one's work only on samples derived from upper duodenum where, even in lactase-persistent subjects, this enzyme is not expressed. Finally, the proximal-distal gradient of lactase activity in lactose absorbers need not be identical with that of Fig. 75-7 in all ethnic or age groups (as discussed in the section "Diagnosis"). Hence, studies carried out on endoscopic duodenal biopsy specimens alone,[481] for example, without independent information on the capacity of the individual to digest lactose (say, via breath hydrogen tests), may be subject to question. Naturally, reliable studies have been carried out using duodenal samples.

But genetic variability may well be real; that is, the molecular mechanism operating in different pedigrees may well be different, depending on the ethnic group and perhaps other factors. Keeping these limitations in mind, we will try to summarize below the present state of knowledge (see also Auricchio and Semenza[482]).

At the cellular level, the proximal small intestine of hypolactasic subjects is characterized by the existence of two types of populations of enterocytes — one expressing and the other not expressing lactase.[483] This is undoubtedly (one of) the mechanism(s) that can lead to the hypolactasia in the proximal small intestine of some adult humans. In fact, it agrees with the biochemical findings that the proximal small intestines of hypolactasic adults often synthesize lactase at reduced rates: reduced synthesis is observed in surviving in vitro cultures of peroral biopsy specimens.[484–486] Also, markedly reduced mRNA levels are found in endoscopic duodenal biopsy samples[481,487,488] and in several (but not all; see below) surgical biopsy specimens from proximal jejunum.[174,489]

On the other hand, in the jejunal specimen of many Neapolitan adults we have studied[174,489] and also of North American subjects,[490] some decrease in the level of lactase mRNA was found but less conspicuous than that of the lactase activity. Indeed, in a few subjects, the levels of mRNA were comparable to those of adults with persistent high lactase activity, suggesting a posttranscriptional control of lactase in the intestinal tissue of these subjects with adult-type hypolactasia.

Delayed maturation of lactase[484,486] associated with the accumulation of immunoreactive material in the Golgi region on immunoelectron microscopy[484] has been observed in some hypolactasic adults.[484] Furthermore, in the intestinal tissue of one subject, lactase biosynthesis was characterized by normal synthesis of high-molecular-weight precursors, followed by reduced conversion of these precursors to mature enzyme.[485]

There is therefore no doubt that multiple mechanisms are responsible for the loss of lactase in adult mammals. The 10-fold reduction in the steady-state levels of lactase activity may result from the combined, indeed multiplicative, effects of such factors — increased cell kinetics, decreased transcription (see also Chap. 76), and posttranslational degradation of the synthesized protein. Different factors act in the same individual, indeed in the very same villus, and some may be more prominent in some individuals than in others. The multiplicity of factors causing the decline of lactase also explains why lactase, even in adult persistent subjects, shows the highest variability of all disaccharidases.

In the intestine of sucklings, on the contrary, high levels of lactase mRNA, the commitment of all enterocytes emerging from the crypts to produce lactase, the low enterocyte turnover, and the low intraluminal pancreatic (and bacterial) proteolysis favor high expression of lactase activity. *Persistence* of high lactase activity in the weaned human subject is most probably primarily due to increased biosynthesis of lactase; whereas a variety of factors lead to the *decline* of lactase activity, a single overriding factor in *lactase persistence* is the high rate of its synthesis.[489] Indeed, when it became advantageous to some human populations to retain intestinal lactase activity in adulthood, it was probably biologically "simpler" to act on a single biologic event (i.e., to increase the rate of lactase biosynthesis via increased transcription) rather than to act on the host of factors causing lactase decline (see also the section "Development and Regulation of the Disaccharidases, in Mammals Other Than Humans"). The concept that lactase decline may be due to various factors, even acting in the very same individual, whereas lactase persistence is due to a single overriding factor (i.e., increased transcription) simplifies, therefore, our present understanding of these phenomena by focusing on persistence rather on the decline of the enzyme.

REFERENCES

1. McMichael HB: Disorders of carbohydrate digestion and absorption. *Clin Endocrinol Metab* **5**:627, 1976.
2. Gray GM: Carbohydrate absorption and malabsorption, in Johnson LR (ed): *Gastrointestinal Disease*. New York, Raven, 1981, p 1063.
3. Gitzelmann R, Auricchio S: The handling of soya alpha-galactosides by a normal and a galactosemic child. *Pediatrics* **36**:231, 1965.
4. Pazur JH, French D, Knapp DW: Mechanism of salivary amylase action. *Proc Iowa Acad Sci* **57**:203, 1950.
5. Pazur JH: The hydrolysis of amylotriose and amylotetraose by salivary amylase. *J Biol Chem* **205**:75, 1953.
6. Pazur JH, Budovich T: Hydrolysis of amylotriose by crystalline salivary amylase. *Science* **121**:702, 1955.
7. Pazur JH: Radioisotopes and enzymatic transformation of oligosaccharides, in *Abstracts of the 134th American Chemical Society Meeting*. New York, 1958.
8. Nordin PH: Action pattern of salivary amylase. Ph-D. Thesis, Iowa State College, 1953.
9. Bird R, Hopkins RH: The action of some alpha-amylases on amylose. *Biochem J* **56**:86, 1954.
10. Walker GJ, Whelan WJ: The action patterns of alfa-amylases. *Starke* **12**:358, 1960.
11. Whelan WJ, Roberts PJP: The mechanism of carbohydrase action: Part II. Alfa-amylolysis of linear substrate. *J Chem Soc* 1298, 1953.
12. Whelan WJ: The action patterns of alfa-amylases. *Starke* **12**:358, 1960.
13. Roberts PJP, Whelan WJ: The mechanism of carbohydrase action: 5. Action of human salivary alpha-amylase on amylopectin and glycogen. *Biochem J* **76**:246, 1960.
14. Bines J, Whelan WJ: The mechanism of carbohydrase action: 6. Structure of a salivary alpha-amylase limit dextrin from amylopectin. *Biochem J* **76**:253, 1960.
15. Heller J, Schramm M: Alpha-amylase limit dextrins of high molecular weight obtained from glycogen. *Biochim Biophys Acta* **81**:96, 1964.
16. Nordin PH, French D: I-phenyl-flavazole derivates of starch dextrins. *J Am Chem Soc* **80**:1445, 1958.
17. Auricchio S, Della Pietra D, Vegnente A: Studies on intestinal digestion of starch in man: II. Intestinal hydrolysis of amylopectin in infants and children. *Pediatrics* **39**:853, 1967.
18. Anderson IH, Levine AS, Levitt MD: Incomplete absorption of the carbohydrate in all-purpose wheat flour. *N Engl J Med* **304**:891, 1981.
19. Levine AS, Levitt MD: Malabsorption of starch moiety of oats, corn, and potatoes. *Gastroenterology* **80**:1209, 1981.
20. Bond JH, Levitt MD: Use of pulmonary hydrogen (H_2) measurements to quantitate carbohydrate absorption: Study of partially gastrectomized patients. *J Clin Invest* **51**:1219, 1972.
21. Stephen AM, Haddad AC, Phillips SF: Passage of carbohydrate into the colon. *Gastroenterology* **85**:589, 1983.
22. Chapman RW, Sillery JK, Graham MM, Saunders DR: Absorption of starch by healthy ileostomates: Effect of transit time and carbohydrate load. *Am J Clin Nutr* **41**:1244, 1985.
23. Goddard MS, Young G, Marcus R: The effect of amylose content on insulin and glucose responses to ingested rice. *Am J Clin Nutr* **39**:388, 1984.
24. Pomare EW, Branch WJ, Cunnings JH: Carbohydrate fermentation in the human colon and its relation to acetate concentration in venous blood. *J Clin Invest* **75**:1448, 1985.
25. De Vizia B, Ciccimarra F, De Cicco N, Auricchio S: Digestibility of starches in infants and children. *J Pediatr* **86**:50, 1975.
26. Flourie B, Florent C, Jouany JP, Thivend P, Etanchaud F, Rambaud JC: Colonic metabolism of wheat starch in healthy humans. *Gastroenterology* **90**:111, 1986.
27. Layer P, Zinsmeister AR, Di Magno E: Effects of decreasing intraluminal amylase activity on starch digestion and postprandial gastrointestinal function in humans. *Gastroenterology* **91**:41, 1986.
28. Lebenthal E, Lee PC: Development of functional response in human exocrine pancreas. *Pediatrics* **66**:556, 1980.
29. Zoppi G, Andreotti G, Pajno-Ferrara F, Njai DM, Gaburro D: Exocrine pancreas function in premature and full-term neonates. *Pediatr Res* **6**:880, 1972.
30. Senterre J: Net absorption of starch in low birth weight infants. *Acta Paediatr Scand* **69**:653, 1980.
31. Shulman RJ, Wong WW, Irving CS, Nichols BL, Klein PD: Utilization of dietary cereal by young infants. *J Pediatr* **103**:23, 1983.
32. Klein PD, Klein ER: Application of stable isotopes to pediatric nutrition and gastroenterology: Measurement of nutrient absorption and digestion using ^{13}C. *J Pediatr Gastroenterol Nutr* **4**:19, 1985.
33. Shulman RJ, Kerzner B, Sloan HR, Boutton TW, Wong WW, Nichols BL, Klein PD: Absorption and oxidation of glucose polymers of different lengths in young infants. *Pediatr Res* **20**:740, 1986.
34. Murray RD, Kerzner B, Sloan HR, McClung J, Gilbert M, Ailabouni A: The contribution of salivary amylase to glucose polymers hydrolysis in premature infants. *Pediatr Res* **20**:186, 1986.
35. Kerzner B, Sloan HR, McClung HJ, Ailabouni A: The jejunal absorption of glucose oligomers in the absence of pancreatic enzymes. *Pediatr Res* **15**:250, 1981.
36. Kelly JJ, Alpers DH: Properties of human intestinal glucoamylase. *Biochem Biophys Acta* **315**:113, 1981.
37. Ugolev AM: Membrane (contact) digestion. *Physiol Rev* **45**:555, 1965.
38. Gray GM, Lally BC, Conklin KA: Action of intestinal sucrase-isomaltase and its free monomers on an alpha-limit dextrin. *J Biol Chem* **254**:6038, 1979.
39. Taravel FR, Datema R, Woloszczuk W, Marshall JJ, Whelan WJ: Purification and characterization of a pig intestinal alpha-limit dextrinase. *Eur J Biochem* **130**:147, 1983.
40. Rodriguez IR, Taravel FR, Whelan WJ: Characterization and function of pig intestinal sucrase isomaltase and its separate subunits. *Eur J Biochem* **143**:575, 1984.

41. Skovbjerg H: Immunoelectrophoretic studies on human small intestinal brush border proteins: The longitudinal distribution of peptidases and disaccharidases. *Clin Chim Acta* **112**:205, 1981.
42. Triadou N, Bataille J, Schmitz J: Longitudinal study of the human intestinal brush border membrane proteins: Distribution of the main disaccharidases and peptidases. *Gastroenterology* **85**:1326, 1983.
43. Raul F, Lacroix B, Aprahamian M: Longitudinal distribution of brush border hydrolases and morphological maturation in the intestine of the preterm infant. *Early Hum Dev* **13**:225, 1986.
44. Auricchio S, Rubino A, Mürset G: Intestinal glycosidase activities in the human embryo, fetus and newborn. *Pediatrics* **35**:944, 1965.
45. Miller D, Crane RK: The digestive function of the epithelium of the small intestine: 1. An intracellular locus of disaccharide and sugar phosphate ester hydrolysis. *Biochim Biophys Acta* **52**:281, 1961.
46. Parson DS, Pritchard JS: Hydrolysis of disaccharides during absorption by the perfused small intestine of amphibia. *Nature* **208**:1097, 1965.
47. Hamilton JD, McMichael HB: Role of microvillous in the absorption of disaccharides. *Lancet* **2**:154, 1968.
48. Malathi P, Ramaswamy K, Caspary WF, Crane RK: Studies on the transport of glucose from disaccharides by hamster small intestine in vitro: 1. Evidence for a disaccharidase-related transport system. *Biochim Biophys Acta* **307**:613, 1973.
49. Ramaswamy K, Malathi P, Caspary WF, Crane RK: Studies on the transport of glucose from disaccharides by hamster small intestine in vitro: II. Characteristics of the disaccharidase-related transport system. *Biochim Biophys Acta* **345**:39, 1974.
50. Gray GM, Ingelfinger FJ: Intestinal absorption of sucrose in man: The site of hydrolysis and absorption. *J Clin Invest* **44**:390, 1965.
51. McMichael HB, Webb J, Dowson AM: The absorption of maltose and lactose in man. *Clin Sci* **33**:135, 1967.
52. Alpers DH, Cote MN: Inhibition of lactose hydrolysis by dietary sugars. *Am J Physiol* **221**:865, 1971.
53. Dawson DJ, Lobley RW, Burrows PC, Miller W, Holmes R: Lactose digestion by human jejunal biopsies: The relationship between hydrolysis and absorption. *Gut* **27**:521, 1986.
54. Gray GM, Santiago N: Disaccharide absorption in normal and diseased human intestine. *Gastroenterology* **51**:489, 1966.
55. Wacker H, Jaussi R, Sonderegger O, Dokow M, Ghersa P, Hauri HP, Christen PH, et al: Cell-free synthesis of the one-chain precursor of a major intrinsic protein complex of the small-intestinal brush border membrane (pro-sucrase-isomaltase). *FEBS Lett* **136**:329, 1981.
56. Semenza G: Anchoring and biosynthesis of stalked brush border membrane proteins: Glycosidases and peptidases of enterocytes and renal tubuli. *Annu Rev Cell Biol* **2**:255, 1986.
57. Spiess M, Hunziker W, Lodish HF, Semenza G: Molecular cell biology of brush border hydrolases: Sucrase isomaltase and gamma-glutamyl transpeptidase, in Kenny AJ, Turner AJ (eds): *Ectoenzymes*. Amsterdam, Elsevier, 1987, p 87.
58. Semenza G: The insertion of stalked proteins of the brush border membranes: The state of the art in 1988. *Biochem Int* **18**:15, 1989.
59. Brunner J, Hauser H, Braun H, Wilson KJ, Wacker H, O'Neill B, Semenza G: The mode of association of the enzyme complex sucrase-isomaltase with the intestinal brush border membrane. *J Biol Chem* **254**:1821, 1979.
60. Hunziker W, Spiess M, Semenza G, Lodish H: The sucrase-isomaltase complex: Primary structure, membrane orientation and evolution of a stalked intrinsic brush border protein. *Cell* **46**:227, 1986.
61. Lee L, Forstner G: Hydrophobic binding domains of rat intestinal maltase-glucoamylase. *Biochem Cell Biol* **64**:782, 1986.
62. Hu C, Spiess M, Semenza G: The mode of anchoring and precursor forms of sucrase-isomaltase and maltase-glucoamylase in chicken intestinal brush border membrane: Phylogenetic implications. *Biochim Biophys Acta* **896**:275, 1987.
63. Keller P, Semenza G, Shaltiel S: Phosphorylation of the N-terminus tail of sucrase-isomaltase by cAMP-dependent protein kinase. *Eur J Biochem* **233**:963, 1995.
64. Sjöström H, Norén O, Christiansen LA, Wacker H, Spiess M, Bigler-Meier B, Rickli EE, et al: N-terminal sequences of pig intestinal sucrase-isomaltase and pro-sucrase-isomaltase: Implications for the biosynthesis and membrane insertion of pro-sucrase-isomaltase. *FEBS Lett* **148**:321, 1982.
65. Spiess M, Brunner J, Semenza G: Hydrophobic labeling, isolation and partial characterization of the NH_2-terminal membranous segment of sucrase-isomaltase complex. *J Biol Chem* **257**:2370, 1982.
66. Wacker H, Keller P, Falchetto R, Legler G, Semenza G: Location of the two catalytic sites in intestinal lactase-phlorizin hydrolase: Comparison with sucrase-isomaltase and with other glycosidases—The membrane anchor of lactase-phlorizin hydrolase. *J Biol Chem* **267**:18,744, 1992.
67. Nichols BL, Eldering J, Avery S, Hahn D, Quaroni A, Sterchi EE: Human small intestinal maltase-glucoamylase cDNA cloning: Homology to sucrase-isomaltase. *J Biol Chem* **273**:3076, 1998.
68. Norén O, Sjöström H, Cowell G, Tranum-Jensen J, Hansen OC, Welinder KG: Pig intestinal microvillar maltase-glucoamylase: Structure and membrane insertion. *J Biol Chem* **261**:12,306, 1986.
69. Cowell GM, Sjöström H, Norén O, Tranum-Jensen J: Topology and quaternary structure of pro-sucrase-isomaltase and final forms of sucrase isomaltase. *Biochem J* **237**:455, 1986.
70. Semenza G: Intestinal oligo- and disaccharides, in Randle PJ, Steiner DF (eds): *Carbohydrate Metabolism and Its Disorders*. London, Academic, 1981, p 425.
71. Hauser H, Semenza G: Sucrase-isomaltase: A stalked intrinsic protein of the brush border membrane. *Crit Rev Biochem* **14**:319, 1983.
72. Semenza G: Glycosidases, in Kenny AJ, Turner AJ (eds): *Ectoenzymes*. Amsterdam, Elsevier, 1987, p 265.
73. Semenza G: The sucrase-isomaltase complex, a large dimeric amphipathic protein from the small intestinal brush border membrane: Emerging structure-function relationships, in Ahlberg P, Sundelöf LO (eds): *Structure and Dynamics of Chemistry*. Symposium, 500th Jubilee, University of Uppsala, Sweden. Stockholm, Almquist and Wiksell, 1977, p 226.
74. Semenza G: Mode of insertion of the sucrase-isomaltase complex in the intestinal brush border membrane: Implications for the biosynthesis of this stalked intrinsic membrane protein. *Ciba Found Symp* **70**:133, 1979.
75. Semenza G: The mode of anchoring of sucrase-isomaltase to the small-intestinal brush border membrane and its biosynthetic implications, in Rapoport S, Schewe T (eds): *Proceedings of the 12th FEBS Meeting, Dresden*, vol 53. Oxford, Pergamon, 1978, p 21.
76. Fulcher IS, Pappin JC, Kenny AJ: The N-terminal amino acid sequence of pig kidney endopeptidase 24.11 shows homology with pro-sucrase-isomaltase. *Biochem J* **240**:305, 1986.
77. Spiess M, Mantei N, Semenza G: Unpublished observations, 1989.
78. Hoefsloot LH, Hoogeveen-Westerveld M, Kroos MA, Van Beeumen J, Reuser AJJ, Oostra BA: Primary structure and processing of lysosomal alpha-glucosidase: Homology with the intestinal sucrase-isomaltase complex. *EMBO J* **7**:1697, 1988.
79. Chantret I, Lacasa M, Chevalier G, Ruf J, Islam I, Mantei N, Edwards Y, et al: Sequence of the complete cDNA and the 5′ structure of the human sucrase isomaltase gene: Homology with a yeast glucoamylase. *Biochem J* **285**:915, 1992.
80. Naim HY, Sterchi EE, Lentze MJ: Structure, biosynthesis, and glycosylation of human small intestinal maltase-glucoamylase. *J Biol Chem* **263**:19,709, 1988.
81. Danielsen EM, Sjöström H, Norén O: Biosynthesis of microvillar proteins: Pulse-chase labeling studies on maltase-glucoamylase, aminopeptidase A and dipeptidyl peptidase IV. *Biochem J* **210**:389, 1983.
82. Ghersa P, Huber P, Semenza G, Wacker H: Cell-free synthesis, membrane integration and glycosylation of pro-sucrase-isomaltase. *J Biol Chem* **261**:7969, 1986.
83. Takesue Y, Takesue S: Purification and characterization of alpha-glucosidase complex from the intestine of the frog, *Rana japonica*. *Biochim Biophys Acta* **1296**:152, 1996.
84. Mantei N, Villa M, Enzler T, Wacker H, Boll W, James P, Hunziker H, et al: Complete primary structure of human and rabbit lactase-phlorizin hydrolase: Implications for biosynthesis, membrane anchoring and evolution of the enzyme. *EMBO J* **7**:2705, 1988.
85. Duluc I, Boukamel R, Mantei N, Semenza G, Raul F, Freund JN: Sequence of the precursor of intestinal lactase-phlorizin hydrolase from fetal rat. *Gene* **103**:275, 1991.
86. Hays WS, Jenison SA, Yamada T, Pastuszyn A, Glew RH: Primary structure of the cytosolic beta-glucosidase of guinea pig. **319**:829, 1996.
87. Freund JN, Jost B, Lorentz O, Duluc I: Identification of homologues of the mammalian intestinal lactase gene in non-mammals (birds and molluscs). *Biochem J* **322**:491, 1997.
88. Kuro-o M, Matsumara Y, Aizawa H, Kawaguchi H, Suga T, Utsugi T, Ohyama Y, et al: Mutation of the mouse *klotho* gene leads to a syndrome resembling ageing. *Nature* **390**:45, 1997.

89. Gräbnitz F, Seiss M, Rücknagel KP, Staudenbauer WL: Structure of the β-glucosidase gene *bglA* of *Clostridium thermocellum*. *Eur J Biochem* **200**:301, 1991.
90. Zecca L, Mesonero JE, Stutz A, Poirée JC, Giudicelli J, Cursio R, Gloor SM, et al: Intestinal lactase-phlorizin hydrolase (LPH): The two catalytic sites — The role of the pancreas in pro-LPH maturation. *FEBS Lett* **435**:225, 1998.
91. Díaz Arriba JC, García Herrero A, Martín-Lomas M, Cañada FJ, He S, Withers SG: Differential mechanism-based labeling and unequivocal assignment of the two active sites of intestinal lactase-phlorizin hydrolase. *Eur J Biochem* (in press, 2000).
92. Keller P, Semenza G, Shaltiel S: Disposition of carboxy-terminus tail of rabbit lactase-phlorizin hydrolase elucidated by phosphorylation with protein kinase A in vitro and in tissue culture. *FEBS Lett* **368**:563, 1995.
93. Dudley MA, Hachey DL, Quaroni A, Hutchens TW, Nichols BL, Rosenberger J, Perkinson JS, et al: In vivo sucrase-isomaltase and lactase-phlorizin hydrolase turnover in fed adult rat. *J Biol Chem* **268**:13,609, 1998.
94. Mesonero JE, Gloor SM, Semenza G: Human intestinal pro-lactase is processed to an intermediate form by furin-like PC(s). *J Biol Chem* **273**:29,430, 1995.
95. Wüthrich M, Grünberg J, Hahn D, Jacob R, Radebach I, Naim HY, Sterchi EE: Proteolytic processing of human lactase-phlorizin hydrolase is a two-step event: Identification of the cleavage sites. *Arch Biocham Biophys* **336**:27, 1996.
96. Danielsen EM, Skovbjerg H, Norén O, Sjöström H: Biosynthesis of intestinal microvillar proteins: Intracellular processing of lactase-phlorizin hydrolase. *Biochem Biophys Res Commun* **122**:82, 1984.
97. Skovbjerg H, Danielsen EM, Norén O, Sjöström H: Evidence for biosynthesis of lactase-phlorizin hydrolase as a single-chain high-molecular weight precursor. *Biochim Biophys Acta* **789**:247, 1984.
98. Naim HY, Sterchi EE, Lentze MJ: Biosynthesis and maturation of lactase-phlorizin hydrolase in the human small intestinal epithelial cells. *Biochem J* **241**:427, 1987.
99. Büller HA, Montgomery RK, Sasak WV, Grand RJ: Biosynthesis, glycosylation and intracellular transport of intestinal lactase-phlorizin hydrolase in rat. *J Biol Chem* **262**:17,206, 1987.
100. Witte J, Lloyd M, Lorenzsonn V, Korsmo H, Olsen WA: The biosynthetic basis of adult lactase deficiency. *J Clin Invest* **86**:1338, 1990.
101. Rossi M, Maiuri L, Russomanno C, Auricchio S: In vitro biosynthesis of lactase in preweaning and adult rabbit. *FEBS Lett* **313**:260, 1992.
102. Lottaz D, Oberholzer T, Bähler P, Semenza G, Sterchi EE: Maturation of human lactase-phlorizin hydrolase: Proteolytic cleavage of precursor occurs after passage through the Golgi complex. *FEBS Lett* **313**:270, 1992.
103. Keller P, Zecca L, Boukamel R, Zwicker E, Gloor S, Semenza G: Furin, PC1/3, and PC6A process rabbit, but not human, pro-lactase-phlorizin hydrolase to the 180 kDa intermediate. *J Biol Chem* **270**:25,722, 1995.
104. Zecca L, Mesonero JE, Gloor SM, Semenza G: Species differences in the sites of cleavage of pro-lactase to lactase supports lack of selective pressure. *Biochim Biophys Acta* **1435**:51, 2000.
105. Jacob R, Radebach I, Wüthrich M, Grünberg J, Sterchi EE, Naim HY: Maturation of human intestinal lactase-phlorizin hydrolase: Generation of the brush border form of the enzyme involves at least two proteolytic cleavage steps. *Eur J Biochem* **236**:789, 1996.
106. Naim HY, Lacely SW, Sambrook JF, Gething MJH: Expression of a full-length cDNA coding for human intestinal lactase-phlorizin hydrolase reveals an uncleaved, enzymatically active and transport-competent protein. *J Biol Chem* **266**:12,313, 1991.
107. Yeh KY, Yeh M, Pan PC, Holt PR: Posttranslational cleavage of rat intestinal lactase occurs at the luminal side of the brush border membrane. *Gastroenterology* **101**:312, 1991.
108. Keller P, Poirée JC, Giudicelli G, Semenza G: Do pancreatic proteases play a role in the processing of pro-lactase and/or in the post-weaning decline of lactase? *Am J Physiol* **268**:G41, 1995.
109. Haddad P, Jenne DE, Krähenbühl O, Tschopp J: Structure and possible functions of lymphocyte granzymes, in Sitkovsky MV, Henkart PA (eds): *Cytotoxic Cells: Recognition, Effector Function, Generation, and Methods*. Boston, Birkhäuser, 1993.
110. Montgomery RK, Büller HA, Rings EHHM, Grand RJ: Lactose intolerance and the genetic regulation of intestinal lactase-phlorizin hydrolase. *FASEB J* **5**:2824, 1991.
111. Naim HY, Jacob R, Naim H, Sambrook JF, Gething MJH: The pro region of human intestinal lactase-phlorizin hydrolase. *J Biol Chem* **269**:26,933, 1994.
112. Oberholzer T, Mantei N, Semenza G: The pro sequence of lactase-phlorizin hydrolase is required for the enzyme to reach the plasma membrane: An intramolecular chaperone? *FEBS Lett* **333**:127, 1993.
113. Grünberg J, Sterchi EE: Human lactase-phlorizin hydrolase: Evidence of dimerization in the endoplasmic reticulum. *Arch Biochem Biophys* **323**:367, 1995.
114. Naim HY, Naim H: Dimerization of lactase-phlorizin hydrolase occurs in the endoplasmic reticulum, involves the putative membrane spanning domain and is required for an efficient transport of the enzyme to the cell surface. *Eur J Cell Biol* **70**:198, 1996.
115. Danielsen EM: Biosynthesis of intestinal microvillar proteins: Dimerization of aminopeptidase N and lactase-phlorizin hydrolase. *Biochemistry* **29**:305, 1990.
116. Helenius A, Trombetta ES, Hebert DN, Simons JF: Calnexin, calreticulin and the folding of glycoproteins. *Trends Cell Biol* **7**:193, 1997.
117. Zhang JX, Braakman I, Matlack KES, Helenius A: Quality control in the secretory pathway: The role of celreticulin, calnexin and BiP in the retention of glycoproteins with C-terminal truncations. *Mol Biol Cell* **8**:1943, 1997.
118. Danielsen EM: Tyrosine sulfation, a post-translational modification of microvillar enzymes in the small intestinal enterocyte. *EMBO J* **6**:2891, 1987.
119. Danielsen EM: Biosynthesis of intestinal microvillar proteins: Pulse-chase labeling studies on aminopeptidase N and sucrase-isomaltase. *Biochem J* **204**:639, 1982.
120. Danielsen EM, Cowell GM, Norén O, Sjöström H: Biosynthesis of microvillar proteins. *Biochem J* **221**:1, 1984.
121. Hauri HP, Sterchi EE, Bienz D, Fransen JAM, Marxer A: Expression and intracellular transport of microvillus membrane hydrolases in human intestinal epithelial cells. *J Cell Biol* **101**:838, 1985.
122. Danielsen EM, Cowell GM: Biosynthesis of intestinal microvillar proteins: The intracellular transport of aminopeptidase N and sucrase-isomaltase occurs at different rates pre-Golgi but at the same rate post-Golgi. *FEBS Lett* **190**:69, 1985.
123. Stieger B, Matter K, Baur B, Höchli M, Hauri HP: Dissection of the asynchronous transport of intestinal microvillar hydrolases to the cell surface. *J Cell Biol* **106**:1853, 1988.
124. Danielsen EM, Cowell GM: Biosynthesis of intestinal microvillar proteins: Evidence for an intracellular sorting taking place in, or shortly after, exit from the Golgi complex. *Eur J Biochem* **152**:493, 1985.
125. Hansen G, Dabelsteen E, Sjöström H, Norén O: Immunomicroscopic localization of aminopeptidase N in the pig enterocyte: Implication for the route of intracellular transport. *Eur J Cell Biol* **43**:53, 1987.
126. Matter K, Brauchbar M, Bucher K, Hauri HP: Sorting of endogenous plasma membrane proteins occurs from two sites in cultured human intestinal epithelial cells (Caco-2). *Cell* **60**:429, 1990.
127. LeBivic A, Quaroni A, Nichols B, Rodriguez-Boulan E: Biogenetic pathways of plasma membrane proteins in Caco-2, a human intestinal epithelial cell line. *J Cell Biol* **111**:1351, 1990.
128. Hauri HP, Quaroni A, Isselbacher K: Biogenesis of intestinal plasma membrane: Posttranslational route and cleavage of sucrase-isomaltase. *Proc Natl Acad Sci USA* **76**:5183, 1979.
129. Grünberg J, Luginbühl U, Sterchi EE: Proteolytic processing of human intestinal lactase-phlorizin hydrolase precursor is not a prerequisite for correct sorting in Madin Darby canine kidney (MDCK) cells. *FEBS Lett* **314**:224, 1992.
130. Danielsen EM, Vogel LK, Sjöström H: Trafficking and sorting of cell-surface peptidases in epithelial cells, in Kenny AJ, Turner AJ (eds): *Cell-Surface Peptidases in Health and Disease*. Oxford, UK, BIOS Sci Publ. Oxford, UK, 1997, p 47.
131. Danielsen EM, Hansen GH, Cowell GM: Biosynthesis of intestinal microvillar proteins: Low temperature arrests both processing and intracellular transport. *Eur J Cell Biol* **49**:123, 1989.
132. Fransen JAM, Ginsel LA, Hauri HP, Sterchi EE, Blok J: Immunoelectromicroscopical localization of a microvillus membrane disaccharidase in the human small-intestinal epithelium with monoclonal antibodies. *Eur J Cell Biol* **38**:6, 1985.
133. Wüthrich M, Sterchi EE: Human lactase-phlorizin hydrolase expressed in COS-1 cells is proteolytically processed by the lysosomal pathway. *FEBS Lett* **405**:321, 1997
134. Matter K, Stieger B, Klumperman J, Ginsel L, Hauri HP: Endocytosis, recycling, and lysosomal delivery of brush border

hydrolases in cultured human intestinal epithelial cells (Caco-2). *J Biol Chem* **265**:3503, 1990.

135. Naim HY, Lentze MJ: Impact of *O*-glycosylation on the function of human intestinal lactase-phlorizin hydrolase. *J Biol Chem* **267**:25,494, 1992.
136. Sjöström H, Norén O, Danielsen EM: The enzymatic activity of "high mannose" glycosylated forms of intestinal microvillar hydrolases. *J Pediatr Gastroenterol Nutr* **4**:980, 1985.
137. Kelly JJ, Alpers DH: Blood group antigenicity of purified human intestinal disaccharidases. *J Biol Chem* **248**:8216, 1973.
138. Pothoulakis C, Gilbert RJ, Cladaras C, Castagliuolo I, Semenza G, Hitti Y, Montcrief JS, et al: Rabbit sucrase-isomaltase contains a functional intestinal receptor for *Clostridium difficile* toxin A. *J Clin Invest* **98**:641, 1996.
139. Cousineau J, Green JR: Isolation and characterization of the proximal and distal forms of lactase-phlorizin-hydrolase from the small intestine of the suckling rat. *Biochim Biophys Acta* **615**:147, 1980.
140. Kraml J, Kolínská J, Kodlecová L, Zákostelecká M, Lojda Z: Analytical isoelectric focusing of rat intestinal brush border enzymes: Postnatal changes and effect of neuraminidase in vitro. *FEBS Lett* **151**:193, 1983.
141. Kraml J, Kolínská J, Kodlecová L, Zákostelecká M, Lojda Z: Effect of hydrocortisone on the desialylation of intestinal brush border enzymes of the rat during postnatal development. *FEBS Lett* **172**:25, 1984.
142. Semenza G: The minimum catalytic mechanism of intestinal sucrase and isomaltase. *Indian J Biochem Biophys* **28**:331, 1991.
143. Cogoli A, Semenza G: A probable oxocarbonium ion in the reaction mechanism of small intestinal sucrase and isomaltase. *J Biol Chem* **250**:7802, 1975.
144. Green F, Edwards Y, Hauri HP, Povey S, Ho WM, Pinto M, Swallow D: Isolation of a cDNA probe for a human jejunum brush-border hydrolase, sucrase-isomaltase, and assignment of the gene locus to chromosome 3. *Gene* **57**:101, 1987.
145. West LF, Davis MB, Green FR, Lindenbaum RH, Swallow D: Regional assignment of the gene coding for human sucrase-isomaltase (SI) to chromosome 3q25-26. *Ann Hum Genet* **52**:57, 1988.
146. Kruse TA, Bolund L, Grzeschik KH, Ropers HH, Sjöström H, Norén O, Mantei N, et al: The human lactase-phlorizin hydrolase gene is located on chromosome 2. *FEBS Lett* **240**:123, 1988.
147. Kruse TA, Bolund L, Byskov A, Sjöström H, Norén O, Mantei N, Semenza G: Mapping of the human lactase-phlorizin hydrolase gene to chromosome 2. *Cytogenet Cell Genet* **51**:1026, 1989.
148. Harvey CB, Fox MF, Jeggo PA, Mantei N, Povey S, Swallow DM: Regional localization of the lactase-phlorizin hydrolase gene, *LCT*, to chromosome 2q21. *Ann Hum Genet* **57**:179, 1993.
149. Boll W, Wagner P, Mantei N: Structure of the chromosomal gene and cDNAs coding for lactase-phlorizin hydrolase in humans with adult-type hypolactasia or persistence of lactase. *Am J Hum Genet* **48**:889, 1991.
150. Villa M, Brunschwiler D, Gächter T, Boll W, Semenza G, Mantein N: Region-specific expression of multiple lactase-phlorizin hydrolase genes in intestine of rabbit. *FEBS Lett* **336**:70, 1993.
151. Galand G: Purification and characterization of kidney and intestinal brush-border membrane trehalases from the rabbit. *Biochim Biophys Acta* **789**:10, 1984.
152. Yokota K, Nishi Y, Takesue Y: Purification and characterization of amphiphilic trehalase from rabbit small intestine. *Biochim Biophys Acta* **881**:405, 1986.
153. Ruf J, Wacker H, James P, Maffia M, Seiler P, Galand G, Von Kieckebush A, et al: Rabbit small intestinal trehalase: Purification, cDNA cloning, expression, and verification of glycosylphosphatidylinositol anchoring. *J Biol Chem* **265**:15,034, 1990.
154. Takesue Y, Yokota K, Nishi Y, Taguchi R, Ikesawa H: Solubilization of trehalase from rabbit renal and intestinal brush-border membranes by a phosphoinositol-specific phospholipase C. *FEBS Lett* **201**:5, 1986.
155. Gutierrez C, Ardourel M, Bremer E, Middendorf A, Boos W, Ehmann U: Analysis and DNA sequence of the osmoregulated *treA* gene encoding the periplasmic trehalase of *Escherichia coli* K12. *Mol Gen Genet* **217**:347, 1989.
156. Hehre EJ, Sawai T, Brewer CF, Nakano M, Kanda T: Trehalase: Stereocomplementarity hydrolytic and glucosyl transfer reactions with alpha- and β-D-glucosyl fluoride. *Biochemistry* **21**:3090, 1982.
157. Rubino A, Zimbalatti F, Auricchio S: Intestinal disaccharidase activities in adult and suckling rats. *Biochim Biophys Acta* **92**:305, 1964.
158. Dubs R, Gitzelman R, Steinmann B, Lindenmann J: Catalytically inactive sucrase antigen of rabbit small intestine: The enzyme precursor. *Helv Paediatr Acta* **30**:89, 1975.
159. Doell RG, Kretchmer N: Studies of small intestine during development: I. Distribution and activity of β-galactosidase. *Biochim Biophys Acta* **62**:353, 1962.
160. Colombo V, Lorenz-Meyer H, Semenza G: Small-intestinal phlorizin hydrolase: The "β-glycosidase complex." *Biochim Biophys Acta* **327**:412, 1973.
161. Lee PC, Lebenthal E: Early weaning and precocious development of small intestine in rats: Genetic, dietary or hormonal control. *Pediatr Res* **17**:645, 1983.
162. Yeh KJ, Holt PR: Ontogenic timing mechanism initiates the expression of rat intestinal sucrase activity. *Gastroenterology* **90**:520, 1986.
163. Henning SJ: Postnatal development: Coordination of feeding, digestion and metabolism. *Am J Physiol* **241**:G199, 1981.
164. Henning SJ: Ontogeny of enzymes in the small intestine. *Annu Rev Physiol* **47**:231, 1985.
165. Klein RM, McKenzie JC: The role of cell renewal in the ontogeny of the intestine: I. Cell proliferation patterns in adult, fetal and neonatal intestine. *J Pediatr Gastroenterol Nutr* **2**:204, 1983.
166. Maiuri L, Garipoli V, Norén O, Dabelsteen E, Swallow D, Auricchio S: Mosaic pattern of expression of lactase protein and mRNA by villus enterocytes in adult rabbit. *Gastroenterology* **100**:A227, 1991.
167. Kedinger M, Simon PM, Grenier JF, Haffen K: Role of epithelial mesenchymal interactions in the ontogenesis of intestinal brush border enzymes. *Dev Biol* **86**:339, 1981.
168. Haffen K, Lacroix B, Kedinger M, Simon-Assmann PM: Inductive properties of fibroblastic cell cultures derived from rat intestinal mucosa on epithelial differentiation. *Differentiation* **23**:226, 1983.
169. Simon PM, Kedinger M, Raul F, Grenier JF, Haffen K: Developmental pattern of rat intestinal brush border enzymic proteins along the villous-crypt axis. *Biochem J* **178**:407, 1979.
170. Boyle JT, Kokonos M, Koldovský O: Developmental profile of jejunal lactase and sucrase activity along the villous-crypt in the rat. *Pediatr Res* **16**:157A, 1982.
171. Lund EK, Smith MW: Rat jejunal disaccharidase activity increases biphasically during early development. *J Physiol (Lond)* **391**:487, 1987.
172. Sebastio G, Hunziker W, Ballabio A, Auricchio S, Semenza G: On the primary site of control in the spontaneous development of small intestinal sucrase isomaltase after birth. *FEBS Lett* **208**:460, 1986.
173. Leeper LL, Henning SJ: Development and tissue distribution of sucrase-isomaltase mRNA in rats. *Am J Physiol* **258**:652, 1990.
174. Sebastio G, Villa M, Sartorio R, Guazzetta V, Poggi V, Auricchio S, Boll W, et al: Control of lactase in human adult-type hypolactasia and in weaning rabbits and rats. *Am J Hum Genet* **45**:489, 1989.
175. Traber PG: Regulation of sucrase-isomaltase gene expression along the crypt-villus axis of rat small intestine. *Biochem Biophys Res Commun* **173**:765, 1990.
176. Lorenzsonn V, Lloyd M, Olsen WA: Transcription of mRNA for sucrase-isomaltase peaks before the protein on the crypt-villus axis of rat small intestine. *J Cell Biol* **109**:124A, 1989.
177. Doell RG, Kretchmer N: Intestinal invertase: Precocious development of activity after injection of hydrocortisone. *Science* **143**:42, 1964.
178. Malo CH, Ménard D: Hormonal control of intestinal glucoamylase activity in suckling and adult mice. *Comp Biochem Physiol [B]* **65**:169, 1980.
179. Kedinger M, Simon PM, Raul F, Grenier JF, Haffen K: The effect of dexamethasone on the development of rat intestinal brush border enzymes in organ culture. *Dev Biol* **74**:9, 1980.
180. Beaulieu JF, Calvert R: Influences of dexamethasone on the maturation of fetal mouse intestinal mucosa in organ culture. *Comp Biochem Physiol [A]* **82**:91, 1985.
181. Ménard D, Malo CH, Calvert R: Insulin accelerates the development of intestinal brush border hydrolytic activities of suckling mice. *Dev Biol* **85**:150, 1981.
182. Malo CH, Ménard D: Influence of epidermal growth factor on the development of suckling mouse intestinal mucosa. *Gastroenterology* **83**:28, 1982.
183. Walsh MJ, Leleiko NS, Sterling KM: Glucocorticoid-induced development of the rat small intestine is associated with differential regulation of intestinal and basement membrane collagen in RNA synthesis. *Gastroenterology* **90**:1683A, 1986.
184. Sebastio G, Hunziker W, O'Neill B, Malo C, Ménard D, Auricchio S, Semenza G: The biosynthesis of intestinal sucrase-isomaltase in

human embryo is most likely controlled at the level of transcription. *Biochem Biophys Res Commun* **149**:830, 1987.
185. Sebastio G, Hunziker W, Ballabio A, Maiuri S, Auricchio S, Semenza G: On the primary site of control in spontaneous and glucocorticoid-triggered precocious development of small-intestinal sucrase-isomaltase complex [abstr]. *Pediatr Res* **22**:99, 1987.
186. Henning SJ, Ballard PL, Kretchmer N: A study on the cytoplasmic receptors for glucocorticoid in intestine of pre- and postweaning rats. *J Biol Chem* **250**:2073, 1975.
187. Henning SJ, Leeper LL: Coordinate loss of glucocorticoid responsiveness by intestinal enzymes during postnatal development. *Am J Physiol* **242**:G89, 1982.
188. Galand G: Effect of an antiglucocorticoid (RU-38486) on hydrocortisone induction of maltase-glucoamylase, sucrase-isomaltase and trehalase in brush border membranes of suckling rats. *Experientia* **44**:516, 1988.
189. Kedinger M, Haffen K, Simon-Assman P: Control mechanisms in the ontogenesis of villus cells, in Desnuelle P, Sjöström H, Norén O (eds): *Molecular and Cellular Biology of Digestion*. Amsterdam, Elsevier, 1986, p 323.
190. Moog F: Perinatal development of the enzymes of the brush border membrane, in Lebenthal E (ed): *Textbook of Gastroenterology and Nutrition*. New York, Raven, 1981, p 139.
191. Koldovský O: Developmental, dietary and hormonal control of intestinal disaccharidases in mammals (including man), in Randle PJ, Steiner DF, Whelan WJ (eds): *Carbohydrate Metabolism and Its Disorders*, vol 3. London, Academic, 1981, p 418.
192. Enck P, Whitehead WE: Lactase deficiency and lactose malabsorption: A review. *Z Gastroenterol* **24**:125, 1986.
193. Galand G: Brush border membrane sucrase-isomaltase, maltase-glucoamylase and trehalase in mammals: Comparative development, effects of glucocorticoids, molecular mechanisms, and phylogenetic implications. *Comp Biochem Physiol [B]* **94**:1, 1989.
194. Hamr A, Delannoy P, Verbert A, Kolínská J: The hydrocortisone-induced transcriptional down-regulation of beta-galactoside alpha-2,6-sialyltransferase in the small intestine of suckling rats is suppressed by mefipristone (RU-38.486). *J Steroid Biochem Mol Biol* **60**:59, 1997.
195. Schlegel-Haueter S, Hore P, Kerry KR, Semenza G: The preparation of lactase and glucoamylase of rat small intestine. *Biochim Biophys Acta* **258**:506, 1971.
196. Leichter J: Effect of dietary lactose on intestinal lactase activity in young rats. *J Nutr* **103**:392, 1973.
197. Ferguson A, Gerskowitch VP, Russell RI: Pre- and postweaning disaccharidase patterns in isografts of fetal mouse intestine. *Gastroenterology* **64**:292, 1973.
198. Bolin TD, McKern A, Davis AE: The effect of diet on lactase activity in the rat. *Gastroenterology* **60**:432, 1971.
199. Bolin TD, Pirola RC, Davis AE: Adaptation of intestinal lactase in the rat. *Gastroenterology* **57**:406, 1969.
200. Montgomery RK, Sybicki MA, Grand RJ: Autonomous biochemical and morphological differentiation in the fetal rat intestine transplanted at 17 and 20 days of gestation. *Dev Biol* **87**:76, 1981.
201. Yeh KY, Yeh M, Holt PR: Intestinal lactase expression and epithelial cell transit in hormone-treated suckling rats. *Am J Physiol* **260**:G379, 1991.
202. Liu T, Reisenauer AM, Castillo RO: Ontogeny of intestinal lactase: Posttranslational regulation by thyroxine. *Am J Physiol* **263**:G538, 1992.
203. Galluser M, Belkhou R, Freund JN, Duluc I, Torp N, Danielsen M, Raul F: Adaptation of intestinal hydrolases to starvation in rats: Effect of thyroid function. *J Comp Physiol [B]* **161**:357, 1991.
204. Nsi-Emvo E, Launay JF, Raul F: Is adult-type hypolactasia in the intestine of mammals related to changes in the intracellular processing of lactase? *Cell Mol Biol* **33**:335, 1987.
205. Freund JN, Duluc I, Raul F: Discrepancy between the intestinal lactase enzymatic activity and the mRNA accumulation in suckling and adults: Effect of starvation and thyroxine treatment. *FEBS Lett* **248**:39, 1989.
206. Freund JN, Duluc I, Foltzer-Jourdainne C, Gosse F, Raul F: Specific expression of lactase in the jejunum and colon during postnatal development and hormone treatments in the rat. *Biochem J* **268**:99, 1990.
207. Moog F: The functional differentiation of the small intestine: II. The differentiation of alkaline phosphomonoesterases in the duodenum of the mouse. *J Exp Zool* **118**:187, 1951.
208. Moog F: The functional differentiation of the small intestine: III. The influence of the pituitary-adrenal system on the differentiation of phosphatase in the duodenum of the suckling mouse. *J Exp Zool* **124**:329, 1953.
209. Yeh K, Moog F: Intestinal lactase activity in the suckling rat: Influence of hypophysectomy and thyroidectomy. *Science* **183**:77, 1974.
210. Malo CH, Ménard D: Opposite effects of one and three injections of cortisone or thyroxine on intestinal lactase activity in suckling mice. *Experientia* **35**:493, 1979.
211. Buts JP, De Meyer R: Postnatal proximodistal development of the small bowel mucosal mass in growing rats. *Biol Neonate* **40**:62, 1981.
212. Buts JP, De Meyer R: Intestinal development in the suckling rat: Effects of weaning, diet composition and glucocorticoids on thymidine kinase activity and DNA synthesis. *Pediatr Res* **18**:145, 1984.
213. Tsuboi KK, Kwong LK, Neu J, Sunshine P: A proposed mechanism of normal intestinal lactase decline in the postweaned mammal. *Biochim Biophys Res Commun* **101**:645, 1981.
214. Tsuboi KK, Kwong LK, d'Harlingue AE, Stevenson DK, Kerner JA, Sunshine P: The nature of maturational decline of intestinal lactase activity. *Biochim Biophys Acta* **840**:69, 1985.
215. Jonas MM, Montgomery RK, Grand RJ: Intestinal lactase synthesis during postnatal development in the rat. *Pediatr Res* **19**:956, 1985.
216. Smith MW, James PS: Cellular origin of lactase decline in postweaning rats. *Biochim Biophys Acta* **905**:503, 1987.
217. Smith MW, Lloyd S: Intestinal infection with *Nematospiroides dubius* selectively increases lactase expression in mouse jejunal enterocytes. *Clin Sci* **77**:139, 1989.
218. Smith MW, Lloyd S, James PS: Testing the hypothesis that crypt cell hyperplasia inhibits lactase expression by mouse jejunal enterocytes. *Q J Exp Physiol* **73**:777, 1988.
219. Maiuri L, Rossi M, Raia V, Swallow D, Quaroni A, Auricchio S: Patchy expression of lactase protein in adult rabbit and rat intestine. *Gastroenterology* **103**:1739, 1992.
220. Freund JN, Duluc I, Raul F: Lactase expression is controlled differently in the jejunum and ileum during development in rats. *Gastroenterology* **100**:388, 1991.
221. Lacey SW, Naim HY, Magness RR, Gething MJ, Sambrook JF: Expression of lactase-phlorizin hydrolase in sheep is regulated at the RNA level. *Biochem J* **302**:929, 1994.
222. Büller HA, Kothe MJC, Goldman DA, Grubman SA, Sasak WV, Madsudaira PT, Montgomery RK, et al: Coordinate expression of lactase-phlorizin hydrolase mRNA and enzyme levels in rat intestine during development. *J Biol Chem* **265**:6978, 1990.
223. Krasinski SD, Estrada G, Yeh KY, Yeh M, Traber PG, Rings EH, Buller HA, et al: Transcriptional regulation of intestinal hydrolase biosynthesis during postnatal development in rats. *Am J Physiol* **267**:G584, 1994.
224. Freund JN, Duluc I, Foltzer-Jourdainne C, Gosse F, Raul F: Specific expression of lactase in the jejunum and colon during postnatal development and hormone treatments in the rat. *Biochem J* **268**:99, 1990.
225. Foltzer-Jourdainne C, Kedinger M, Raul F: Perinatal expression of brush-border hydrolases in rat colon: Hormonal and tissue regulations. *Am J Physiol* **257**:G496, 1989.
226. Quan R, Santiago NA, Tsuboi KT, Gray GM: Intestinal lactase: Shift in intracellular processing to altered, inactive species in the adult rat. *J Biol Chem* **265**:15,882, 1990.
227. Castillo RO, Reisenauer AM, Kwong LK, Tsuboi KT, Quan R, Gray GM: Intestinal lactase in the neonatal rat: Maturational changes in intracellular processing and brush-border degradation. *J Biol Chem* **256**:15,889, 1990.
228. Rossi M, Maiuri L, Salvati VM, Russomanno C, Capparelli R, Auricchio S: In vitro biosynthesis of lactase in suckling and adult rabbits: Regulatory mechanisms involved in the decline of the lactase activity. *FEBS Lett* **329**:106, 1993.
229. Tung J, Markowitz AJ, Silberg DG, Traber PG: Developmental expression of SI is regulated in transgenic mice by an evolutionarily conserved promoter. *Am J Physiol* **273**:G83, 1997.
230. Troelsen JT, Mehlum A, Olsen J, Spodsberg N, Hansen GH, Prydz H, Noren O, et al: 1 kb of the lactase-phlorizin hydrolase promoter directs post-weaning decline and small intestinal-specific expression in transgenic mice. *FEBS Lett* **342**:291, 1994.
231. Markowitz AJ, Wu GD, Birkenmeier EH, Traber PG: The human sucrase-isomaltase gene directs complex patterns of gene expression in transgenic mice. *Am J Physiol* **265**:G526, 1993.
232. Markowitz AJ, Wu GD, Bader A, Cui Z, Chen L, Traber PG: Regulation of lineage-specific transcription of the sucrase-isomaltase gene in transgenic mice and cell lines. *Am J Physiol* **269**:G925, 1995.

233. Krasinski SD, Upchurch BH, Irons SJ, June RM, Mishra K, Grand RJ, Verhave M: Rat lactase-phlorizin hydrolase/human growth hormone transgene is expressed on small intestinal villi in transgenic mice. *Gastroenterology* **113**:844, 1997.
234. Traber PG, Silberg DG: Intestine-specific gene transcription. *Annu Rev Physiol* **58**:275, 1996.
235. Traber PG, Wu GD, Wang W: Novel DNA-binding proteins regulate intestine-specific transcription of the sucrase-isomaltase gene. *Mol Cell Biol* **12**:3614, 1992.
236. Wu GD, Chen L, Forslund K, Traber PG: Hepatocyte nuclear factor-1 alpha (HNF-1 alpha) and HNF-1 beta regulate transcription via two elements in an intestine-specific promoter. *J Biol Chem* **269**:17,080, 1994.
237. Suh E, Chen L, Taylor J, Traber PG: A homeodomain protein related to caudal regulates intestine-specific gene transcription. *Mol Cell Biol* **14**:7340, 1994.
238. James R, Kazenwadel J: Homeobox gene expression in the intestinal epithelium of adult mice. *J Biol Chem* **266**:3246, 1991.
239. James R, Erler T, Kazenwadel J: Structure of the murine homeobox gene *cdx-2*: Expression in embryonic and adult intestinal epithelium. *J Biol Chem* **269**:15,229, 1994.
240. Suh E, Traber PG: An intestine-specific homeobox gene regulates proliferation and differentiation. *Mol Cell Biol* **16**:619, 1996.
241. Taylor JK, Boll W, Levy T, Suh E, Siang S, Mantei N, Traber PG: Comparison of intestinal phospholipase A/lysophospholipase and sucrase-isomaltase genes suggests a common structure for enterocyte-specific promoters. *DNA Cell Biol* **16**:1419, 1997.
242. Lambert M, Colnot S, Suh E, l'Horset F, Blin C, Calliot ME, Raymondjean M, et al: *cis*-Acting elements and transcription factors involved in the intestinal specific expression of the rat calbindin-D9K gene: Binding of the intestine-specific transcription factor Cdx-2 to the TATA box. *Eur J Biochem* **236**:778, 1996.
243. Troelsen JK, Olsen J, Norén O, Sjöström H: A novel intestinal *trans*-factor (NF-LPH1) interacts with the lactase-phlorizin hydrolase promoter and co-varies with the enzymatic activity. *J Biol Chem* **267**:20,407, 1992.
244. Troelsen JT, Olsen J, Mitchelmore C, Hansen GH, Sjöström H, Norén O: Two intestinal specific nuclear factors binding to the lactase-phlorizin hydrolase and sucrase-isomaltase promoters are functionally related oligomeric molecules. *FEBS Lett* **342**:297, 1994.
245. Troelsen JT, Mitchelmore C, Spodsberg N, Jensen AM, Norén O, Sjöström H: Regulation of lactase-phlorizin hydrolase gene expression by the caudal-related homeodomain protein Cdx-2. *Biochem J* **322**:833, 1997.
246. Boukamel R, Freund JN: The *cis*-element CE-LPH1 of the rat intestinal lactase gene promoter interacts in vitro with several nuclear factors present in endodermal tissues. *FEBS Lett* **353**:108, 1994.
247. Mitchelmore C, Troelsen JT, Sjöström H, Norén O: The HOXC11 homeodomain protein interacts with the lactase-phlorizin hydrolase promoter and stimulates HNF1 alpha-dependent transcription. *J Biol Chem* **273**:13,297, 1998.
247a. Mitchelmore C, Troelsen JT, Spodsberg N, Sjöström H, Norén O: Interaction between the homeodomain proteins Cdx2 and HNF1α mediates expression of the lactase-phlorizin hydrolase gene. *Biochem J* **346**:529, 2000.
248. Tanaka T, Takase S, Goda T: A possible role of a nuclear factor NF-LPH1 in the regional expression of lactase-phlorizin hydrolase along the small intestine. *J Nutr Sci Vitaminol (Tokyo)* **43**:565, 1997.
249. Hecht A, Torbey CF, Korsmo HA, Olsen WA: Regulation of sucrase and lactase in developing rats: Role of nuclear factors that bind to two gene regulatory elements. *Gastroenterology* **112**:803, 1997.
250. Fitzgerald K, Bazar L, Avigan MI: GATA-6 stimulates a cell line-specific activation element in the human lactase promoter. *Am J Physiol* **274**:G314, 1998.
251. Duluc I, Galluser M, Raul F, Freund JF: Dietary control of the lactase mRNA distribution along the rat small intestine. *Am J Physiol* **262**:G954, 1992.
252. Keller P, Zwicker E, Mantei N, Semenza G: The levels of lactase and of sucrase-isomaltase along the rabbit small intestine are regulated both at the mRNA level and post-translationally. *FEBS Lett* **313**:265, 1992.
253. Duluc I, Jost B, Freund JF: Multiple levels of control of the stage- and region-specific expression of rat intestinal lactase. *J Cell Biol* **123**:1577, 1993.
254. Ferguson A, Gerskowich VP, Russel RI: Pre- and postweaning disaccharidase patterns in isografts of fetal mouse intestine. *Gastroenterology* **64**:292, 1973.
255. Yeh KY, Holt PR: Ontogenic timing mechanism initiates the expression of rat intestinal sucrase activity. *Gastroenterology* **90**:520, 1986.
256. Mantei N: Afterthought: How did the decline of lactase in adults evolve? *Dyn Nutr Res* **3**:208, 1993.
257. Büller HA, Rings EHHM, Pajkrt D, Montgomery RK, Grand RJ: Glycosylation of lactase-phlorizin hydrolase in rat small intestine during development. *Gastroenterology* **98**:667, 1990.
258. Antonovicz I, Chang SK, Grand RJ: Development and distribution of lysosomal enzymes and disaccharidases in human fetal intestine. *Gastroenterology* **67**:51, 1974.
259. Antonovicz I, Lebenthal E: Development pattern of small intestinal enterokinase and disaccharidase activity in the human fetus. *Gastroenterology* **72**:1299, 1977.
260. Dahlqvist A, Lindberg T: Fetal development of the small intestinal disaccharidase and alkaline phosphatase activities in the human. *Biol Neonate* **9**:24, 1965.
261. Jiřsová V, Heringov, Uher J, Jodl J: Development of invertase activity in the intestines of human fetuses: Appearance of jejunoileal differences. *Biol Neonate* **13**:143, 1968.
262. Mobassaleh M, Montgomery RK, Büller HA, Grand RJ: Development of carbohydrate absorption in the fetus and neonate. *Pediatrics* **75**(suppl):160, 1985.
263. Mayne A, Hughes CA, Sule D, Brown GA, McNeish AS: Development of intestinal disaccharidases in preterm infants. *Lancet* **2**:622, 1983.
264. Kien CL, McClead RE, Cordero L Jr: In vivo lactose digestion in preterm infants. *Am J Clin Nutr* **64**:700, 1996.
265. MacLean WC Jr, Fink BB: Lactose malabsorption by premature infants: Magnitude and clinical significance. *J Pediatr* **97**:383 1980.
266. MacLean WC, Fink BB, Schoeller DA, Wong W, Klein PD: Lactose assimilation by full-term infants: Relations of (^{13}C) and H_2 breath test with fecal (^{13}C) excretion. *Pediatr Res* **17**:629, 1983.
267. Schoeller DA, Kelin PD, MacLean WC, Watkins JB, Van Santen E: Fecal ^{13}C analysis for the detection and quantitation of intestinal malabsorption: Limits of detection to disorders of intestinal cholylglycine metabolism. *J Lab Clin Med* **97**:439, 1981.
268. Lifshitz CH, O'Brian SE, Garza C: Delayed complete functional lactase sufficiency in breast-fed infants. *J Pediatr Gastroenterol Nutr* **2**:478, 1983.
269. Chiles C, Watkins JB, Barr RG, Tsaj PY, Goldman DA: Lactose utilization in the newborn: Role of colonic flora. *Pediatr Res* **13**:365, 1979.
270. Bond JH, Currier BE, Buchwald H, Levitt MD: Colonic conservation of malabsorbed carbohydrate. *Gastroenterology* **78**:444, 1980.
271. Murray RD, Boutton TW, Klein PD, Gilbert M, Paule CL, MacLean WC: Comparative absorption of [^{13}C]glucose and [^{13}C]lactose by premature infants. *Am J Clin Nutr* **51**:59, 1990.
272. Villa M, Ménard D, Semenza G, Mantei N: The expression of lactase enzymatic activity and mRNA in human fetal jejunum: Effect of organ culture and of treatment with hydrocortisone. *FEBS Lett* **301**:202, 1992.
273. Trugnan G, Rousset M, Chantret I, Barbat A, Zweibaum A: The posttranslational processing of sucrase-isomaltase in HT-29 cells is a function of their state of enterocytic differentiation. *J Cell Biol* **104**:1199, 1987.
274. Zweibaum A, Pinto M, Chevalier G, Dussaulx E, Triadou N, Lacroix B, Haffen K, et al: Enterocytic differentiation of a subpopulation of the human colon tumor cell line HT-29 selected for growth in sugar-free medium and its inhibition by glucose. *J Cell Biol* **100**:118, 1985.
275. Chantret I, Trugnan G, Dussaulx E, Zweibaum A, Rousset M: Monensin inhibits the expression of sucrase-isomaltase in Caco-2 cells at the mRNA level. *FEBS Lett* **235**:125, 1988.
276. Rousset M, Chantret I, Darmoul D, Trugnan G, Sapin C, Green F, Swallow D, et al: Reversible forskolin-induced impairment of sucrase-isomaltase mRNA levels, biosynthesis, and transport to the brush border membrane in Caco-2 cells. *J Cell Physiol* **141**:627, 1989.
277. Auricchio S: "Fetal" forms of brush border enzymes in the intestine and meconium. *J Pediatr Gastroenterol Nutr* **2**(suppl):164, 1983.
278. Auricchio S, Caporale C, Santamaria F, Skovbjerg H: Fetal forms of oligoaminopeptidase, dipeptidylaminopeptidase IV and sucrase in human intestine and meconium. *J Pediatr Gastroenterol Nutr* **3**:28, 1984.
279. Triadou N, Zweibaum A: Maturation of sucrase-isomaltase complex in human fetal small and large intestine during gestation. *Pediatr Res* **19**:136, 1985.

280. Kraml J, Kolínská J: Sialylated forms of intestinal brush-border enzymes: Lecture presented at the 14th International Congress of Biochemistry, Prague, 1988 [abstr TU:C18-3].
281. Chu SW, Walker WA: Developmental changes in the activities of sialyl- and fucosyltransferases in rat small intestine. *Biochim Biophys Acta* **883**:496, 1986.
282. Biol MC, Pintori S, Mathian B, Louisot P: Dietary regulation of intestinal glycosyl-transferase activities: Relation between developmental changes and weaning in rats. *J Nutr* **121**:114, 1991.
283. Paulson JC, Colley KJ: Glycosyltransferases. *J Biol Chem* **264**:17,615, 1989.
284. Martin A, Ruggiero-Lopez D, Biol MC, Louisot P: Evidence for the presence of an endogenous cytosolic protein inhibitor of intestinal fucosyltransferase activities. *Biochem Biophys Res Commun* **166**:1024, 1990.
285. Ruggiero-Lopez D, Biol MC, Louisot P, Martin A: Participation of an endogenous inhibitor of fucosyltransferase activities in the developmental regulation of intestinal fucosylation process. *Biochem J* **279**:801, 1991.
286. Ruggiero-Lopez D, Martin A, Louisot P: Caractérisation et évolution post-natale d'un inhibiteur protéique endogène des fucosyl-transférases intestinales. *Gastroenterol Clin Biol* **15**:939, 1991.
287. Biol MC, Lenoir D, Hugueny I, Louisot P: Hormonal regulation of glycosylation process in rat small intestine: Responsiveness of fucosyl-transferase activity to hydrocortisone during the suckling period, unresponsiveness after weaning. *Biochim Biophys Acta* **1133**:206, 1992.
288. Biol MC, Martin A, Louisot P: Nutritional and developmental regulation of glycosylation processes in digestive organs. *Biochimie* **74**:13, 1992.
289. Kolínská J, Zákostelecká M, Hamr A, Baudyšová M: Coordinate expression of beta-galactoside alpha-2,6-sialyltransferase mRNA and enzyme activity in suckling rat jejunum cultured in different media: Transcriptional induction by dexamethasone. *J Steroid Biochem Mol Biol* **58**:289, 1996.
290. James WPT, Alpers DH, Gerber JE, Isselbacher KJ: The turnover of disaccharidases and brush border proteins in rat intestine. *Biochim Biophys Acta* **230**:194, 1971.
291. Olsen WA, Korsmo H: The intestinal brush border membrane in diabetes: Studies of sucrase-isomaltase metabolism in rats with streptozotocin diabetes. *J Clin Invest* **60**:181, 1977.
292. Alpers DH: The relation of size to the relative rates of degradation of intestinal brush border proteins. *J Clin Invest* **51**:2621, 1972.
293. Forstner G, Galand G: The influence of hydrocortisone on the synthesis and turnover of microvillus membrane glycoproteins in suckling rat intestine. *Can J Biochem* **54**:224, 1976.
294. Ahnen DJ, Santiago NA, Yoshioka C, Gray GM: Intestinal sucrase-alpha-dextrinase: Differential degradation of its protein and carbohydrate components in vivo. *Gastroenterology* **82**:1006, 1982.
295. Karasov WH, Diamond JM: Adaptive regulation of sugar and amino acid transport by vertebrate intestine. *Am J Physiol* **245**:G443, 1983.
296. Jacobs LR: Alterations in labeling of cell-surface glycoproteins from normal and diabetic rat intestinal microvillus membranes. *Biochim Biophys Acta* **649**:155, 1981.
297. Najjar S, Hampp LT, Rabkin R, Gray GM: Sucrase-alpha-dextrinase in diabetic BioBreed rats: Reversible alteration of subunit structure. *Am J Physiol* **260**:G275, 1991.
298. Schedl HP, Al-Jurf AS, Wilson DH: Elevated intestinal disaccharidase activity in the streptozotocin diabetic rat is independent of enteral feeding. *Gastroenterology* **82**:1171, 1982.
299. Goda T, Koldovský O: Evidence of degradation process of sucrase-isomaltase in jejunum of adult rats. *Biochem J* **229**:751, 1985.
300. Alpers DH, Tedesco FJ: The possible role of pancreatic proteases in the turnover of the intestinal brush border proteins. *Biochim Biophys Acta* **401**:28, 1975.
301. Riby JE, Kretchmer N: Participation of pancreatic enzymes in the degradation of intestinal sucrase-isomaltase. *J Pediatr Gastroenterol Nutr* **4**:971, 1985.
302. Kwong WKL, Seetharam B, Alpers DH: Effect of exocrine pancreatic insufficiency on small intestine in the mouse. *Gastroenterology* **74**:1277, 1978.
303. Seetharam B, Perrillo R, Alpers DH: Effect of pancreatic proteases on intestinal lactase activity. *Gastroenterology* **79**:827, 1980.
304. Smith MW, Phillips AD, Walker-Smith JA: Selective inhibition of brush border hydrolase development in coeliac disease and cow's milk protein intolerance [abstr]. *Pediatr Res* **20**:693, 1986.
305. Lifshitz F: Perspectives of carbohydrate intolerance in infants with diarrhea, in Lifshitz F (ed): *Carbohydrate Intolerance in Infancy.* New York, Marcel Dekker, 1982, p 3.
306. Nichols BL, Dudley MA, Nichols VN, Putman M, Avery SE, Fraley JK, Quaroni A, et al: Effect of malnutrition on expression and activity of lactase in children. *Gastroenterology* **112**:742, 1997.
307. Dudley MA, Wykes L, Dudley AW, Fiorotto M, Burrin DG, Rosenberger J, Jahoor F, et al: Lactase-phlorizin hydrolase synthesis is decreased in protein-malnourished pigs. *J Nutr* **127**:687, 1997.
308. Shmerling DH, Auricchio S, Rubino A, Hadorn B, Prader A: Der sekundäre Mangel an intestinalen Disaccharidaseakvität bei der Coeliakie: Quantitative Bestimmung der Enzymaktivität und klinische Beurteilung. *Helv Paediatr Acta* **19**:507, 1964.
309. Lebenthal E, Lee P: Possible alternative pathway for starch digestion in infants and mucosal glucamylase activity in small intestinal atrophy. *Pediatr Res* **29**:504, 1980.
310. Gray GM, William MW Jr, Eugene H: Persistent deficiency of intestinal lactase in apparently cured tropical sprue. *Gastroenterology* **54**:552, 1968.
311. Romer H, Urbach R, Gomez MA, Lopez A, Perozo-Ruggeri G, Vegas ME: Moderate and severe protein energy malnutrition in childhood: Effects of jejunal mucosae morphology and disaccharidase activities. *J Pediatr Gastroenterol Nutr* **2**:459, 1983.
312. Greene HL, McCabe DR, Merenstein GB: Protracted diarrhea and malnutrition in infancy: Changes in intestinal morphology and disaccharidase activities during treatment with total intravenous nutrition or oral elemental diets. *J Pediatr* **87**:695, 1975.
313. Thoreux K, Balas D, Senegas-Balas F: Vieillissement des epitheliums digestifs chez le rat (pancréas, intestin): Influence des conditions nutritionelles. *Gastroenterol Clin Biol* **21**:A182, 1997.
314. Phillips AD, Avigad S, Sacks J, Rice SJ, France NE, Walker-Smith SA: Microvillous surface area in secondary disaccharidase deficiency. *Gut* **21**:44, 1980.
315. Boyle JT, Celano R, Koldovský O: Demonstration of a difference in expression of maximal lactase and sucrase activity along the villus in the adult rat jejunum. *Gastroenterology* **79**:503, 1980.
316. Alpers DH, Seetharam B: Pathophysiology of diseases involving intestinal brush border proteins. *N Engl J Med* **296**:1047, 1977.
317. Sherman P, Wesley A, Forstner G: Sequential disaccharidase loss in rat intestinal blind loops: Impact of malnutrition. *Am J Physiol* **248**:626, 1985.
318. Welsh JD, Poley JR, Hensley J, Bathia M: Intestinal disaccharidase and alkaline phosphatase activity in giardiasis. *J Pediatr Gastroenterol Nutr* **3**:37, 1984.
318a. Scheving LA: Biological clocks and the digestive system. *Gastroenterology* **119**:536, 2000.
319. Dahlqvist A: Method for assay of intestinal disaccharidases. *Anal Biochem* **7**:18, 1964.
320. Auricchio S, Rubino A, Tosi R, Semenza G, Landolt M, Kistler HJ, Prader A: Disaccharidase activities in human intestinal mucosa. *Enzymol Biol Clin* **3**:193, 1963.
321. Banauch D, Brummer W, Ebeling W, Metz H, Rindfrey M, Land H: Eine Glucose-Dehydrogenase für die Glucose-Bestimmung in Körperflüssigkeiten. *Z Klin Chem Klin Biochem* **13**:101, 1975.
322. Asp NG, Dahlqvist A: Human small-intestinal β-galactosidases: Specific assay of three different enzymes. *Anal Biochem* **47**:527, 1972.
323. Tsuboi KK, Schwarz SM, Burrill PH, Kwong LK, Sunshine P: Sugar hydrolases of the infant rat intestine and their arrangement on the brush border membrane. *Biochim Biophys Acta* **554**:234, 1979.
324. Dahlqvist A: Specificity of the human intestinal disaccharidases and implications for hereditary disaccharide intolerance. *J Clin Invest* **41**:463, 1962.
325. Eggermont E: The hydrolysis of the naturally occurring alpha-glucosides by the human intestinal mucosa. *Eur J Biochem* **9**:483, 1969.
326. Auricchio S, Ciccimarra F, Starace E, Vegnente A, Giliberti P, Provenzale L: Glucamylase activity of human intestinal mucosa. *Rend Gastroenterol* **3**:1, 1971.
327. Messer M, Kerry KR: Intestinal digestion of maltotriose in man. *Biochim Biophys Acta* **132**:432, 1967.
328. Skovbjerg H, Sjöström A, Norén O, Gudmand-Høyer E: Immunoelectrophoretic studies on human small intestinal brush border proteins: A quantitative study from single, small intestinal biopsies. *Clin Chim Acta* **92**:315, 1979.
329. Lebenthal E, Antonowicz I, Shwachman H: Correlation of lactase activity, lactose tolerance and milk consumption in different age groups. *Am Clin Nutr* **28**:595, 1975.

330. Newcomer AD, McGill DB, Thomas PM, Hofmann AF: Prospective comparison of indirect methods for detecting lactase deficiency. *N Engl J Med* **293**:1232, 1975.
331. Eggermont E, Carchon H, Eeckels R: Centile values of small intestinal mucosal enzymatic activities in Caucasian children. *Pediatr Res* **15**:1205A, 1981.
332. Niessen KH, Schmidt K, Bruggmann G: Disaccharidasen der Dünndarmschleimhaut bei Säuglingen und Kindern. *Z Gastroenterol* **13**:565, 1975.
333. McMichael WB, Webb J, Dawson AM: Jejunal disaccharidases and some observations on the cause of lactase deficiency. *BMJ* **2**:1037, 1966.
334. Calvin RT, Klish WJ, Nichols BL: Disaccharidase activities, jejunal morphology, and carbohydrate tolerance in children with chronic diarrhea. *J Pediatr Gastroenterol Nutr* **4**:949, 1985.
335. Newcomer AD, McGill DB: Distribution of disaccharidase activity in the small bowel of normal and lactase-deficient subjects. *Gastroenterology* **51**:481, 1966.
336. Auricchio S, Rubino A, Prader A, Rey J, Jos J, Frézal J, Davidson M: Intestinal glycosidase activities in congenital malabsorption of disaccharides. *J Pediatr* **66**:555, 1965.
337. Kerry KR, Townley RRW: Genetic aspects of intestinal sucrase-isomaltase deficiency. *Aust Pediatr J* **1**:223, 1965.
338. Welsh JD, Poley JR, Bhatia M, Stevenson DE: Intestinal disaccharidase activities in relation to age, race, and mucosal damage. *Gastroenterology* **75**:855, 1978.
339. Crane RK, Ménard D, Preiser H, Cerda J: The molecular basis of brush border membrane disease, in Bolis L, Hoffman JF, Leaf A (eds): *Membranes and Disease*. New York, Raven, 1976, p 229.
340. Haemmerli UP, Kistler HJ, Ammann R, Marthaler T, Semenza G, Auricchio S, Prader A: Acquired milk intolerance in the adult caused by lactose malabsorption due to a selective deficiency of intestinal lactase activity. *Am J Med* **38**:7, 1965.
341. Newcomer AD, McGill DB: Disaccharidase activity in the small intestine: Prevalence of lactase deficiency in 100 healthy subjects. *Gastroenterology* **53**:881, 1967.
342. Forget P, Lambet J, Grandfils C, Dandrifosse G, Genbelle F: Lactase insufficiency revisited. *J Pediatr Gastroenterol Nutr* **4**:868, 1985.
343. Weijers HA, Van de Kamer JH, Dicke WK, Ijsseling J: Diarrhoea caused by deficiency of sugar-splitting enzymes: I. *Acta Paediatr Scand* **50**:55, 1961.
344. Krasilnikoff PA, Gudmand-Høyer E, Moltke HH: Diagnostic value of disaccharide tolerance tests to children. *Acta Paediatr Scand* **64**:693, 1975.
345. Fernandes J, Vos CE, Douwes AC, Slotema E, Degenhart HJ: Respiratory hydrogen excretion as a parameter for lactose malabsorption in children. *Am J Clin Nutr* **31**:597, 1978.
346. Maffei HVL, Metz G, Bampoe V, Shiner M, Herman S, Brook CGD: Lactose intolerance, detected by breath hydrogen test in infants and children with chronic diarrhoea. *Arch Dis Child* **52**:766, 1977.
347. Perman JA, Barr RG, Watkins JB: Sucrose malabsorption in children: Non-invasive diagnosis by interval breath hydrogen determination. *J Pediatr* **93**:17, 1978.
348. Robb TA, Davidson GP: Advances in breath hydrogen quantitation in paediatrics: Sample collection and normalization to constant oxygen and nitrogen levels. *Clin Chim Acta* **111**:281, 1981.
349. Kneepkens CMF, Bijleveld CMA, Vonk RJ, Fernandes J: The daytime breath hydrogen profile in children with abdominal symptoms and diarrhoea. *Acta Paediatr Scand* **75**:632, 1986.
350. Kerlin P, Phillips SF: Differential transit of liquids and solid residue through the ileum of man. *Am J Physiol* **245**:G38, 1983.
351. Douwes AC, Schaap C, van der Klei-van Moorsel JM: Hydrogen breath test in schoolchildren. *Arch Dis Child* **60**:333, 1985.
352. Levitt MD, Donaldson RM: Use of respiratory hydrogen to detect carbohydrate malabsorption. *J Lab Clin Med* **75**:937, 1970.
353. Bjorneklett A, Jenssen E: Relationship between hydrogen (H_2) and methane (CH_4) in man. *Scand J Gastroenterol* **17**:985, 1982.
354. Gardiner AJ, Tarlow MJ, Symonds J, Hutchinson GJP, Shuterland JT: Failure of the hydrogen breath test to detect primary sugar malabsorption. *Arch Dis Child* **56**:368, 1981.
355. Suarez F, Levitt MD: Should we test for lactose malabsorption? *J Gastroenterol Hepatol* **29**:113, 1997.
356. Kerry KR, Anderson CM: A ward test for sugar in faeces. *Lancet* **1**:981, 1964.
357. Davidson AGF, Mullinger M: Reducing substances in neonatal stool detected by Clinitest. *Pediatrics* **46**:632, 1970.
358. McMichael HB, Webb J, Dawson AM: Lactase deficiency in adult: A cause of functional diarrhoea. *Lancet* **1**:717, 1965.
359. Auricchio S, Prader A, Mürset G, Witt G: Saccharoseintoleranz: Durchfall infolge hereditären Mangels an intestinaler Saccharaseaktivität. *Helv Paediatr Acta* **16**:483, 1961.
360. Grant JD, Bezerra JA, Thompson SH, Lemen RJ, Koldovský O, Udall JN: Assessment of lactose absorption by measurement of urinary galactose. *Gastroenterology* **97**:895, 1989.
361. Harrison M, Walker-Smith JA: Reinvestigation of lactose intolerant children: Lack of correlation between continuing lactose intolerance and small intestinal morphology, disaccharidase activity and lactose tolerance tests. *Gut* **18**:48, 1977.
362. Dawson DJ, Newcomer AD, McGill DB: Lactose tolerance tests in adults with normal lactase activity. *Gastroenterology* **50**:340, 1966.
363. Davidson GP, Robb TA: Value of breath hydrogen analysis in management of diarrheal illness in childhood: Comparison with duodenal biopsy. *J Pediatr Gastroenterol Nutr* **4**:381, 1985.
364. Lifshitz CH, Bautista A, Gapalachrishna GS, Stuff J, Garza C: Absorption and tolerance of lactose in infants recovering from diarrhea. *J Pediatr Gastroenterol Nutr* **4**:942, 1985.
365. Welsh JD: Isolated lactase deficiency in humans: Reports on 100 patients. *Medicine (Baltimore) 4* **9**:257, 1970.
366. Bayless TM, Rothfeld B, Massa C, Wise L, Paige D, Bedine MS: Lactose and milk intolerance: Clinical implications. *N Engl J Med* **292**:1156, 1975.
367. Ringrose RE, Preiser H, Welsh JD: Sucrase-isomaltase (Palatinase) deficiency diagnosed during adulthood. *Dig Dis Sci* **25**:384, 1980.
368. Ravich WJ, Bayless TM: Carbohydrate absorption and malabsorption. *Clin Gastroenterol* **12**:335, 1983.
369. Launiala K: The effect of unabsorbed sucrose and mannitol on small intestinal flow rate and mean transit time. *Scand J Gastroenterol* **3**:665, 1968.
370. Launiala K: The effect of unabsorbed sucrose- or mannitol-induced accelerated transit on absorption in the human small intestine. *Scand J Gastroenterol* **4**:25, 1969.
371. Goda T, Bustamante S, Edmond J, Grimes J, Koldovský O: Precocious increase of sucrase activity by carbohydrates in the small intestine of suckling rats: II. Role of digestibility of sugars, osmolality, and stomach evacuation in producing diarrhea. *J Pediatr Gastroenterol Nutr* **4**:634, 1985.
372. Caspary WF, Kalish H: Effect of alpha-glucosidehydrolase inhibition on intestinal absorption of sucrose, water, and sodium in man. *Gut* **20**:750, 1979.
373. Azpiroz F, Malagelada JR: Luminal nutrients in the proximal and distal small intestine elicit gastric relaxation. *Dig Dis Sci* **29**:564, 1984.
374. Jenkins DFA, Taylor RH, Goff WD: Scope and specificity of acarbose in slowing carbohydrate absorption in man. *Diabetes* **31**:951, 1981.
375. Holgate AM, Read NW: Relationship between small bowel transit time and absorption of a solid meal. *Dig Dis Sci* **28**:812, 1983.
376. Chapman RW, Graham MM: Absorption of starch by healthy ileostomatoses: Effect of transit time and of carbohydrate load. *Am J Clin Nutr* **41**:1244, 1985.
377. Auricchio S, Ciccimarra F, De Vizia B: Starch malabsorption, in *13th International Congress of Pediatrics*, Vienna, Aug. 29–Sept. 4, 1971 p 139.
378. Chauve A, Devroede G, Bastin E: Intraluminal pressures during perfusion of the human colon in situ. *Gastroenterology* **70**:336, 1976.
379. Debongnie JC, Philips FS: Capacity of the human colon to absorb fluid. *Gastroenterology* **74**:698, 1978.
380. Palma R, Vidon N, Bernier JJ: Maximal capacity for fluid absorption in human bowel. *Dig Dis Sci* **26**:929, 1981.
381. Newcomer AD, McGill DB, Thomas PM, Hoffman AF: Tolerance to lactose among lactase deficient American Indians. *Gastroenterology* **74**:44, 1978.
382. Saunders DR, Wiggins HS: Conservation of mannitol, lactulose and raffinose by the human colon. *Am J Physiol* **241**:G387, 1981.
383. Argenzio RA, Southworth M: Sites of organic acid production and absorption in gastrointestinal tract of the pig. *Am J Physiol* **228**:454, 1975.
384. Orskov ER, Frase C, Mason WC, Mann SO: Influence of starch digestion in the large intestine of sheep on caecal fermentation, caecal microflora and faecal nitrogen excretion. *Br J Nutr* **24**:671, 1970.
385. Florent CH, Flourie B, Leblond A, Rautureau M, Bernier JJ, Rambaud JC: Influence of chronic lactulose ingestion on the colonic metabolism of lactulose in man (an in vivo study). *J Clin Invest* **75**:608, 1985.

386. Bhatia J, Prihoda AR, Richardson CJ: Parenteral antibiotics and carbohydrate intolerance in term neonates. *Am J Dis Child* **149**:111, 1986.
387. Siigur U, Tamm A, Tammur R: The fecal SCFAs and lactose tolerance in lactose malabsorbers. *Eur J Gastroenterol* **3**:321, 1991.
388. Auricchio S, Dahlqvist A, Mürset G, Prader A: Isomaltose intolerance causing decreased ability to utilize dietary starch. *J Pediatr* **62**:165, 1963.
389. Auricchio S, Ciccimarra F, Moauro L, Rey F, Jos J, Rey J: Intraluminal and mucosal starch digestion in congenital deficiency of intestinal sucrase and isomaltase activities. *Pediatr Res* **6**:832, 1972.
390. Eggermont E, Hers HG: The sedimentation properties of the intestinal alpha-glucosidases of normal human subjects and of patients with sucrose intolerance. *Eur J Biochem* **9**:488, 1969.
391. Hadorn B, Green JR, Sterchi EE, Hauri HP: Biochemical mechanism in congenital enzyme deficiencies of the small intestine. *Clin Gastroenterol* **10**:671, 1981.
392. Skovbjerg H, Krasilnikoff PA: Maltase-glucoamylase and residual isomaltase in sucrose intolerant patients. *J Pediatr Gastroenterol Nutr* **5**:365, 1986.
393. Auricchio S, Rubino A, Landolt M, Semenza G, Prader A: Isolated intestinal lactase deficiency in the adult. *Lancet* **2**:324, 1963.
394. Dahlqvist A, Hammond JD, Crane RK, Dunphy JV, Littman A: Intestinal lactase deficiency and lactose intolerance in adults: Preliminary report. *Gastroenterology* **45**:488, 1963.
395. Simoons FJ: The geographic hypothesis and lactose malabsorption: A weighing of the evidence. *Dig Dis* **23**:963,
396. Jussila J, Launiala K, Gorbatow O: Lactase deficiency and a lactose-free diet in patients with "unspecific abdominal complaints." *Acta Med Scand* **186**:217, 1969.
397. Gudmand-Høyer E, Dahlqvist A, Jarnum S: The clinical significance of lactose malabsorption. *Am J Gastroenterol* **53**:460, 1970.
398. Mitchell KJ, Bayless TM, Huang SS, Paige DM, Goodgame RW, Rothfeld B: Intolerance of a glass of milk in healthy teenagers. *Gastroenterology* **64**:773, 1973.
399. Sahi T: Dietary lactose and aetiology of human small intestinal hypolactasia. *Gut* **19**:1074, 1978.
400. Keusch GT, Troncale FJ, Miller LH, Promadhat V, Anderson PR: Acquired lactose malabsorption in Thai children. *Pediatrics* **43**:540, 1969.
401. Bedine MS, Bayless TM: Intolerance of small amount of lactose by individuals with low lactase levels. *Gastroenterology* **65**:735, 1973.
402. Jones DW, Latham MC, Kosikowski FW, Woodward G: Symptom response to lactose-reduced milk in lactose-intolerant adults. *Am J Clin Nutr* **29**:633, 1976.
403. Webster RB, Di Palma AJ, Gremse DA: Lactose maldigestion and recurrent abdominal pain in children. *Dig Dis Sci* **40**:1506, 1995.
404. Ferguson A: Diagnosis and treatment of lactose intolerance. *BMJ* **283**:1423, 1981.
405. Malagelada JR: Lactose intolerance. *N Engl J Med* **333**:53, 1995.
406. Suarez FL, Savaiano DA, Levitt MD: A comparison of symptoms after the consumption of milk or lactose-hydrolyzed milk by people with self-reported severe lactose intolerance. *N Engl J Med* **333**:1, 1995.
407. Vesa TH, Korpela RA, Sahi T: Tolerance to small amounts of lactose in lactose maldigesters. *Am J Clin Nutr* **64**:197, 1996.
408. Suarez FL, Savaiano D, Arbisi P, Levitt MD: Tolerance to the daily ingestion of two cups of milk by individuals claiming lactose intolerance. *Am J Clin Nutr* **65**:1502, 1997.
409. Jackson W: Clinical manifestations, in Jackson W (ed): *Proceedings of the First Food Allergy Workshop*. Oxford, Medical Education Service, 1980, p 41.
410. Lessoff MH, Wraith DG, Merrett TG, Merrett J, Buisseret PD: Food allergy and intolerance in 100 patients—Local and systemic effects. *Q J Med* **49**:259, 1980.
411. Kolars JC, Levitt MD, Aouji M, Savaiano DA: Yoghurt: An autodigesting source of lactose. *N Engl J Med* **310**:1, 1984.
412. Lerebours E, Djitoyap NCN, Lavoine A, Hellot MF, Antoine JM, Colin R: Yogurt and fermented-then-pasteurized milk: Effects of short-term and long-term ingestion on lactose absorption and mucosal lactase activity in lactase-deficient subjects. *Am J Clin Nutr* **49**:823, 1989.
413. Onwulata CI, Rao DR, Vankineni P: Relative efficiency of yogurt, sweet acidophilus milk, hydrolyzed-lactose milk, and a commercial lactase tablet in alleviating lactose maldigestion. *Am J Clin Nutr* **49**:1233, 1989.
414. Marteau P, Flourie B, Pochart P, Chastang C, Desjeux JF, Rambaud JC: Effect of the microbial lactase (EC 3.2.1.23) activity in yoghurt on the intestinal absorption of lactose: An in vivo study in lactase-deficient humans. *Br J Nutr* **64**:71, 1990.
415. Shermak MA, Saavegra JM, Jackson TL, Huang SS, Bayless TM, Perman JA: Effect of yogurt on symptoms and kinetics of hydrogen production in lactose-malabsorbing children. *Am J Clin Nutr* **62**:1003, 1995.
416. Smith TM, Kolars JC, Savaiano DA: Absorption of calcium from milk and yoghurt. *Am J Clin Nutr* **42**:1197, 1985.
417. Rosado JL, Solomons NW, Lisker R, Bourges H, Anrubio G, Garcia A, Perez-Briceno R, et al: Enzyme replacement therapy for primary adult lactase deficiency: Effective reduction of lactose malabsorption and milk intolerance by direct addition of beta-galactosidase to milk at mealtime. *Gastroenterology* **87**:1072, 1984.
418. Holzel A, Schwarz V, Sutcliffe KW: Defective lactose absorption causing malnutrition in infancy. *Lancet* **1**:1126, 1959.
419. Lifshitz F: Congenital lactase deficiency. *J Pediatr* **69**:229, 1966.
420. Launiala K, Kuitunen P, Visakorpi J: Disaccharidases and histology of duodenal mucosa in congenital lactose malabsorption. *Acta Paediatr Scand* **55**:257, 1966.
421. Levin B, Abraham JM, Burgess EA, Wallis PG: Congenital lactose malabsorption. *Arch Dis Child* **45**:173, 1975.
422. Savilathi E, Launiala K, Kuitunen P: Congenital lactase deficiency: A clinical study on 16 patients. *Arch Dis Child* **58**:246, 1983.
423. Saarela T, Simila S, Koivisto M: Hypercalcemia and nephrocalcinosis in patients with congenital lactase deficiency. *J Pediatr* **127**:920, 1995.
424. Asp NG, Dahlqvist A: Intestinal β-galactosidases in adult low lactase activity and in congenital lactase deficiency. *Enzyme* **18**:84, 1974.
425. Asp NG, Dahlqvist A, Kuitunen P, Launiala K, Visakorpi JK: Complete deficiency of brush border lactase in congenital lactose malabsorption. *Lancet* **2**:329, 1973.
426. Dahlqvist A, Asp NG: Accurate assay of low intestinal lactase activity with a fluorimetric method. *Anal Biochem* **44**:654, 1971.
427. Freiburghaus AU, Schmitz J, Schindler M, Rotthauwe HW, Kuitunen P, Launiala K, Hadorn B: Protein patterns of brush border fragments in congenital lactose malabsorption and in specific hypolactasia of the adult. *N Engl J Med* **294**:1030, 1976.
428. Durand P: Lattosuria idiopatica in una paziente con diarrea cronica ed acidosi. *Minerva Pediatr* **1**:706, 1958.
429. Russo G, Molica F, Mazzone D, Santonocito B: Congenital lactose intolerance of gastrogen origin associated with cataracts. *Acta Paediatr Scand* **63**:457, 1974.
430. Hirashima Y, Shinozuka S, Ieiri T, Matsuda I, Ono Y, Murata T: Lactose intolerance associated with cataracts. *Eur J Pediatr* **130**:41, 1979.
431. Berg NO, Dahlqvist A, Lindberg T: A boy with severe infantile gastrogen lactose intolerance and acquired lactase deficiency. *Acta Paediatr Scand* **68**:751, 1979.
432. Hoskova A, Sabacky J, Mrskos A, Pospisil R: Severe lactose intolerance with lactosuria and vomiting. *Arch Dis Child* **55**:304, 1980.
433. Weijers HA, Van de Kamer JH, Mosel DAA, Dick WK: Diarrhoea caused by deficiency of sugar splitting enzymes. *Lancet* **2**:296, 1960.
434. Prader A, Auricchio S, Mürset G: Durchfall infolge hereditären Mangels an intestinaler Saccharaseaktivität (Saccharoseintoleranz). *Schweiz Med Wochenschr* **91**:465, 1961.
435. Anderson CM, Messer M, Townley RRW, Freeman M, Robinson RJ: Intestinal isomaltase deficiency in patients with hereditary sucrose and starch intolerance. *Lancet* **2**:556, 1962.
436. Anderson CM, Messer M, Townley RRW, Freeman M: Intestinal sucrase and isomaltase deficiency in two siblings. *Pediatrics* **31**:1003, 1963.
437. Burgess EA, Levin B, Mahalanabis D, Tonge RE: Hereditary sucrose intolerance: Levels of sucrase activity in jejunal mucosa. *Arch Dis Child* **39**:431, 1964.
438. Newton T, Murphy SM, Booth IW: Glucose polymer as a cause of protracted diarrhea in infants with unsuspected congenital sucrase-isomaltase deficiency. *J Pediatr* **128**:753, 1996.
439. Prader A, Auricchio S: Defects of intestinal disaccharide absorption. *Annu Rev Med* **13**:345, 1965.
440. Baudon JJ, Veinberg F, Thioulouse E, Morgant G, Aymard P, Charritat JL: Sucrase-isomaltase deficiency: Changing pattern over two decades. *J Pediatr Gastroenterol Nutr* **22**:284, 1996.

441. Gudmand-Høyer E, Krasilnikoff PA: The effect of sucrose malabsorption on the growth pattern in children. *Scand J Gastroenterol* **12**:103, 1977.
442. Ament ME, Perera DR, Esther LJ: Sucrase-isomaltase deficiency, a frequently misdiagnosed disease. *J Pediatr* **83**:721, 1973.
443. Antonovicz I, Lloyd JD, Khaw KT, Shwachman H: Congenital sucrase isomaltase deficiency: Observation over a period of 6 years. *Pediatrics* **49**:847, 1972.
444. Sonntag WM, Brill ML, Troyer WE, Welsh JD, Semenza G, Prader A: Sucrose-isomaltose malabsorption in an adult female. *Gastroenterology* **47**:18, 1964.
445. Neale G, Clark M, Levin B: Intestinal sucrase deficiency presenting as sucrose intolerance in adult life. *BMJ* **2**:1223, 1965.
446. Starnes CW, Welsh JD: Intestinal sucrase-isomaltase deficiency and renal calculi. *N Engl J Med* **202**:1023, 1970.
447. Jansen W, Que CS, Veeger W: Primary combined saccharase and isomaltase deficiency. *Arch Intern Med* **116**:1125, 1972.
448. Cooper BT, Scott J, Hopkins J, Peters TJ: Adult onset sucrase-isomaltase deficiency with secondary disaccharidase deficiency resulting from severe dietary carbohydrate restriction. *Dig Dis Sci* **28**:473, 1983.
449. Gudmand-Høyer E, Krasilnikoff PA, Skovbjerg H: Sucrose-isomaltose malabsorption. *Adv Nutr Res* **6**:233, 1984.
450. Ellestead-Sayed JJ, Haworth JC, Hildes JA: Disaccharide consumption and malabsorption in Canadian Indians. *Am J Clin Nutr* **30**:698, 1977.
451. Ellestead-Sayed JJ, Haworth JC, Hildes JA: Disaccharide malabsorption and dietary patterns in two Canadian Eskimo communities. *Am J Clin Nutr* **31**:1473, 1978.
452. Gudmand-Høyer E: Sucrose malabsorption in children: A report of thirty-one Greenlanders. *J Pediatr Gastroenterol Nutr* **4**:873, 1985.
453. Cheney CP, Boedeker EC: Evidence that the sucrase/isomaltase complex may serve as an intestinal receptor for an enteropathogenic *Escherichia coli. Gastroenterology* **82**:1032, 1982.
454. Metz G, Jenkins DJA, Newman A, Blendis LM: Breath hydrogen in hyposucrasia. *Lancet* **1**:119, 1976.
455. Douwes AC, Fernandes J, Jongbloed AA: Diagnostic value of sucrose tolerance test in children evaluated by breath hydrogen measurement. *Acta Paediatr Scand* **69**:79, 1980.
456. Treen WR: Clinical heterogeneity in congenital sucrase-isomaltase deficiency. *J Pediatr* **128**:727, 1996.
457. Birch JB: Trehalose. *Adv Carbohydr Chem* **18**:201, 1963.
458. Bergoz R: Trehalose malabsorption causing intolerance to mushrooms. *Gastroenterology* **5**:909, 1971.
459. Madzarovová-Nohejilov J: Trehalase deficiency in a family. *Gastroenterology* **65**:130, 1973.
460. McNair A, Gudmand-Høyer E, Jarnum S, Orrild L: Sucrose malabsorption in Greenland. *BMJ* **2**:19, 1972.
460a. Arola H, Koivula T, Karvonen AL, Jokela H, Ahola T, Isokoski M: Low trehalase activity is associated with abdominal symptoms caused by edible mushrooms. *Scand J Gastroenterol* **39**:898, 2000.
461. Schmitz J, Bresson JL, Triadou N, Bataille J, Rey J: Analyse en electrophorèse sur gel de polyacrylamide des protéines de la membrane microvillositaire et d'une fraction cytoplasmique dans 8 cas d'intolérance congénitale au saccharose. *Gastroenterol Clin Biol* **4**:251, 1980.
462. Gray GM, Conklin KA, Townley RRW: Sucrase-isomaltase deficiency: Absence of an inactive enzyme variant. *N Engl J Med* **294**:750, 1976.
463. Skovbjerg H, Krasilnikoff PA: Immunoelectrophoretic studies on human small intestinal brush border protein: The residual isomaltase in sucrose intolerant patients. *Pediatr Res* **15**:214, 1981.
464. Preiser H, Ménard D, Crane RK, Cerda JJ: Deletion of enzyme protein from brush border membrane in sucrase-isomaltase deficiency. *Biochim Biophys Acta* **363**:279, 1974.
465. Naim HY, Roth J, Sterchi EE, Lentze M, Milla P, Schmitz J, Hauri HP: Sucrase-isomaltase deficiency in humans: Different mutations disrupt intracellular transport, processing and function of an intestinal brush border enzyme. *J Clin Invest* **82**:667, 1988.
466. Naim HY, Sterchi EE, Hauri HP, Schmitz J, Lentze MJ: Defective posttranslational processing of sucrase-isomaltase (SI) in congenital sucrase-isomaltase deficiency. Presented at the 19th Annual Meeting of the European Society for Paediatric Gastroenterology and Nutrition (ESPAGN), Edinburgh, June 25–27, 1986 [abstr 26].
467. Lloyd ML, Olsen WA: A study of the molecular pathology of sucrase-isomaltase deficiency: A defect in the intracellular processing of the enzyme. *N Engl J Med* **316**:438, 1987.
468. Ouwendijk J, Peters WJM, Te Morsche RHM, Van de Vorstenbosch RA, Ginsel LA, Naim HY, Fransen JAM: Analysis of a naturally occurring mutation in sucrase-isomaltase: Glutamine 1098 is not essential for transport to the surface of COS-1 cells. *Biochim Biophys Acta* **1406**:299, 1998
469. Ouwendijk J, Moolenaar CE, Peters WJ, Hollenberg CP, Ginsel LA, Fransen JA, Naim HY: Congenital sucrase-isomaltase deficiency: Identification of a glutamine to proline substitution that leads to a transport block of sucrase-isomaltase in a pre-Golgi compartment. *J Clin Invest* **97**:633, 1996.
470. Moolenaar CE, Ouwendijk J, Wittpoth M, Wisselaar HA, Hauri HP, Ginsel LA, Naim HY, et al: A mutation in a highly conserved region in brush-border sucrase-isomaltase and lysosomal alpha-glucosidase results in Golgi retention. *J Cell Sci* **110**:557 1997.
471. Sterchi EE, Lentze MJ, Naim HY: Molecular aspects of disaccharidase deficiencies. *Baillieres Clin Gastroenterol* **4**:79, 1990.
472. Fransen JAM, Hauri HP, Ginsel LA, Naim HY: Naturally occurring mutations in intestinal sucrase-isomaltase provide evidence for the existence of an intracellular sorting signal in the isomaltose subunit. *J Cell Biol* **115**:45, 1991.
473. Freiburghaus AU, Dubs R, Hadorn B, Gaze H, Hauri HO, Gitzelmann R: The brush border membrane in hereditary sucrase-isomaltase deficiency: Abnormal protein pattern and presence of immunoreactive enzyme. *Eur J Clin Invest* **7**:455, 1977.
473a. Ito T, Hayashi Y, Ohmori S, Oda S, Seo H: Molecular cloning of surcase-isomaltase cDNA in the house musk shrew *Suncus murinus* and identification of a mutant responsible for isolated surcase deficiency. *J Biol Chem* **273**:16464, 1998.
473b. Takesue Y, Yokota K, Oda S, Takesue S: Comparison of surcase-free isomaltase with surcase-isomaltase purified from the house musk shrew *Suncus murinus. Biochim Biophys Acta* in press, 1998.
474. Dubs R, Steinmann B, Gitzelmann R: Demonstration of an inactive enzyme antigen in sucrase-isomaltase deficiency. *Helv Paediatr Acta* **28**:187, 1973.
475. James PS, Smith MW, Butcher GW, Brown D, Lund EK: Evidence for a possible regulatory gene (*Suc-1*) controlling sucrase expression in mouse intestine. *Biochem Genet* **24**:169, 1986.
476. Cooper BT, Candy DCA, Harries JT, Peters TJ: Subcellular fractionation studies of the intestinal mucosa in congenital sucrase-isomaltase deficiency. *Clin Sci Mol Med* **57**:181, 1979.
477. Poggi V, Savilhati E, Sebastio G, Mantei N, Boll W, Congia H, Santantonio AA, et al: Primary sequence of coding region of lactase-phlorizin hydrolase gene in congenital human lactase deficiency. *J Pediatr Gastroenterol Nutr* **13**:A17, 1991.
477a. Poggi V, Sebastio G: Molecular analysis of the lactase gene in the congenital lactase deficiency. *Am J Hum Genet* **49**:105, 1991.
477b. Järvelä I, Sabri Enattah N, Kokkenen J, Varilo T, Savilahti E, Peltonen L: Assignment of the locus for congenital lactase deficiency to 2q21, in the vicinity of but separate from the lactase-phlorizin hydrolase gene. *Am J Hum Genet* **63**:1078, Oct. 1998.
478. Skovbjerg H, Gudmand-Høyer E, Fenger HJ: Immunoelectrophoretic studies on human small intestinal brush border proteins: The amount of lactase protein in adult-free hypolactasia. *Gut* **21**:360, 1980.
479. Potter J, Ho MW, Bolton H, Eurth AJ, Swallow DM, Griffith B: Human lactase and the molecular basis of lactase persistence. *Biochem Genet* **23**:432, 1985.
480. Lorenz-Meyer H, Blum AL, Haemmerli HP, Semenza G: A second enzyme defect in acquired lactase deficiency: Lack of small-intestinal phlorizin-hydrolase. *Eur J Clin Invest* **2**:326, 1972.
481. Escher JC, De Koning ND, Van Engen CGJ, Arora S, Büller H, Montgomery RK, Grand RJ: Molecular basis of lactase levels in adult humans. *J Clin Invest* **89**:480, 1992.
482. Auricchio S, Semenza G (eds): Common food intolererances 2: Milk in human nutrition and adult-type hypolactasia. *Dyn Nutr Res* 3, 1993
483. Maiuri L, Raia V, Potter J, Swallow D, Ho MW, Fiocca R, Finzi G, et al: Mosaic pattern of lactase expression by villous enterocytes in human small adult-type hypolactasia. *Gastroenterology* **100**:359, 1991.
484. Sterchi EE, Mills RP, Fransen JAM, Hauri HP, Lentze MJ, Naim HI, Ginsel L, et al: Biogenesis of intestinal lactase-phlorizin hydrolase in adults with lactase intolerance. *J Clin Invest* **86**:1329, 1990.

485. Witte J, Lloyd M, Lorenzsonn V, Korsmo H, Olsen W: The biosynthetic basis of adult lactase deficiency. *J Clin Invest* **86**:1338, 1990.
486. Rossi M, Maiuri L, Fusco MI, Danielsen EM, Auricchio S: The human adult-type hypolactasia is a heterogeneous condition in vitro biosynthetic studies. *Dyn Nutr Res* **3**:174, 1993.
487. Lloyd M, Mevissen, Fischer M, Olsen W, Goodspeed D, Genini M, Boll W, et al: Regulation of intestinal lactase in adult hypolactasia. *J Clin Invest* **89**:524, 1992.
488. Fajardo O, Naim HY, Lacey SW: The polymorphic expression of lactase in adults is regulated at the messenger RNA level. *Gastroenterology* **106**:1233, 1994.
489. Rossi M, Maiuri L, Fusco MI, Salvati VM, Fuccio A, Auricchio S, Mantei N, et al: Lactase persistence versus decline in human adults: Multifactorial events are involved in down-regulation after weaning. *Gastroenterology* **112**:1506, 1997.
490. Musy P, Kastern W, Cerda J, Neu J: Maturational decline of lactase-phlorizin hydrolase is not due to decreased mRNA synthesis. *Pediatr Res* **29**:109A, 1991.
491. Malathi P, Crane RK: Phlorizin hydrolase: A β-glucosidase of hamster intestinal brush border membrane. *Biochim Biophys Acta* **173**:245, 1969.
492. Leese HJ, Semenza G: On the identity between the small-intestinal enzymes phlorizin-hydrolase and glycosylceramidase. *J Biol Chem* **248**:8170, 1973.
493. Semenza G, Auricchio S, Rubino A: Multiplicity of human intestinal disaccharidases: 1. Chromatographic separation of maltases and of two lactases. *Biochim Biophys Acta* **96**:487, 1965.
494. Skovbjerg H, Norén O, Sjöström H, Danielsen EM, Enevoldsen BS: Further characterization of intestinal lactase-phlorizin hydrolase. *Biochim Biophys Acta* **707**:89, 1982.
495. Colombo V, Lorenz-Meyer H, Semenza G: Small-intestinal phlorizin hydrolase: The β-glycosidase complex. *Biochim Biophys Acta* **327**:412, 1973.
495a. Day AJ, Cañada FJ, Díaz JC, Kroon PA, Mclauchlan R, Faulds CB, Plumb GW, Morgan MRA, Williamson G: Dietary flavonoid and isoflavon glycosides are hydrolysed by the lactase site of lactase-phlorizin hydrolase. *FEBS Lett* **468**:166, 2000.
496. Neele AM, Einerhand AWC, Dekker J, Büller HA, Freund JN, Verhave M, Grand RJ, et al: Verification of the lactase site of rat lactase-phlorizin hydrolase by site-directed mutagenesis. *Gastroenterology* **109**:1234, 1995.
497. Kolínská J, Kraml J, Zákostelecká M, Lojda Z: Low molecular weight antigens of sucrase-isomaltase in the intestinal mucosa of suckling rats. *Mol Physiol* **5**:133, 1984.
498. Martinez-Pardo M, Montes PG, Marin-Lomas M, Sols A: Intestinal lactase evaluation in vivo with 3-methyllactose. *FEBS Lett* **98**:99, 1979.
499. Auricchio S, Ciccimarra F, Della PD, Vegnente A: Intestinal hydrolysis of starch. *Mod Probl Pediatr* **11**:23, 1968.
500. Auricchio S: Brush border enzymes, in Anderson GM, Burke V, Gracey M (eds): *Paediatric Gastroenterology*, 2d ed. Australia, Melbourne, Blackwell, 1987, ch 5, pt 3, p 185.
501. Sjöström H, Norén O, Danielsen EM, Skovbjerg H: Structure of microvillar enzymes in different phases of their life cycles. *Ciba Found Symp* **95**:50, 1983.
502. Sørensen SH, Norén O, Sjöström H, Danielsen EM: Amphiphilic pig intestinal microvillus maltase/glucoamylase: Structure and specificity. *Eur J Biochem* **126**:559, 1982.
503. Auricchio S, Semenza G, Rubino A: Multiplicity of human intestinal disaccharidases: II. Characterization of the individual maltases. *Biochim Biophys Acta* **96**:498, 1965.
504. Barnett JEG, Jarvis WTS, Munday KA: Enzymic hydrolysis of the carbon-fluorine bond of a alpha-d-glucosyl fluoride by rat intestinal mucosa. *Biochem J* **103**:699, 1967.
505. Dahlqvist A: Characterization of hog intestinal invertase as a glucosidoinvertase: III. Specificity of purified invertase. *Acta Chem Scand* **14**:63, 1960.
506. Kolínská J, Semenza G: Studies on intestinal sucrase and on intestinal sugar transport: V. Isolation and properties of sucrase-isomaltase from rabbit small intestine. *Biochim Biophys Acta* **146**:181, 1967.
507. Larner J, McNickle CM: Gastrointestinal digestion of starch: I. The action of oligo-1,6-glucosidase on branched saccharides. *J Biol Chem* **215**:723, 1955.
508. Seiji M: Studies on digestion of starch by alpha-limit-dextrinase. *J Biochem* **40**:519, 1953.
509. Labat-Robert J, Baumann FC, Bar-Guilloux E, Robic D: Comparative specificities of trehalases from various species. *Comp Biochem Physiol* [B] **61**:111, 1978.
510. Wallenfels K, Fischer J: Untersuchungen über milchzuckerspaltende Enzyme: X. Die Laktase des Kälberdarms. *Z Physiol Chem* **321**:223, 1960.
511. Kraml J, Kolínská J, Elledérová H, Hiršová D: β-Glucosidase (phlorizin hydrolase) activity of the lactase fraction isolated from the small intestinal mucosa of infant rat and the relationship between β-glucosidases and β-galactosidases. *Biochim Biophys Acta* **258**:520, 1972.
512. Castillo RO, Kwong LK, Reisenauer AM, Tsuboi KK: Human intestinal lactase-phlorizin hydrolase: Isolation and preparation of a specific antiserum. *Biochem Biophys Res Commun* **164**:94, 1989.

CHAPTER 76

Genetic Polymorphism of Intestinal Lactase Activity in Adult Humans*

Dallas M. Swallow ▪ Edward J. Hollox

1. **Dietary lactose is hydrolyzed by the enzyme lactase which is located in the brush border of small intestinal enterocytes. Lactase activity is high during infancy, when milk is the main nutrient. As in other mammals, lactase activity declines after the weaning phase in the majority of humans and remains low throughout life (phenotype: *lactase nonpersistence*, also known as restriction or adult-type hypolactasia; OMIM 223100). In other healthy humans, lactase activity persists at a high level (phenotype: *lactase persistence*). Subjects with lactase nonpersistence have a low lactose digestion capacity (low LDC); those with lactase persistence can hydrolyze large amounts of lactose (high LDC). The adult lactase phenotypes can be diagnosed through small-intestinal biopsy or lactose-tolerance tests.**
2. **Family studies, measurement of relative lactase activity, and a study of lactose digestion in twins show that the lactase phenotypes are genetically determined and can be explained by a Mendelian system of two autosomal alleles. The lactase persistence allele is dominant to the lactase nonpersistence (or *restriction*) allele: the individuals with low LDC are homozygous for the nonpersistence allele.**
3. **The distribution of the lactase phenotypes in human populations is highly variable. In most tropical and subtropical countries and in all East Asian populations, lactase nonpersistence is predominant. In the Old World, lactase persistence predominates in only two human population groups: northwestern Europeans and milk-dependent nomads of the Afro-Arabian desert zone. Natural selection in favor of the lactase persistence gene due to improved utilization of animal milk in the nutrition of older children and adults with high LDC is a likely cause of the unusual lactase phenotype distribution in Europeans and Afro-Arabian nomads, but the age of the polymorphism and the relative roles of selection and genetic drift are not yet clear.**
4. **The role of lactase nonpersistence in irritable bowel syndrome in adults and osteoporosis in postmenopausal women and the role of lactase persistence in promoting coronary heart disease and premature cataract are controversial. However, the genetically determined down-regulation of lactase expression may contribute to malabsorption and abdominal complaints, particularly in young children.**
5. **So far, studies have not revealed a difference in the DNA sequence of the structural gene for lactase (*LCT* at the LAC locus), between subjects with lactase persistence and nonpersistence, but a number of nucleotide polymorphisms have been detected both in the coding and noncoding regions. These polymorphisms are associated with each other to form very few haplotypes in Europeans. Studies on the expression of lactase mRNA transcripts that made use of these polymorphisms as markers have demonstrated that a *cis*-acting element is likely to be responsible for this activity polymorphism. Lactase persistence is associated with a particular haplotype (A) in Europeans.**

A list of standard abbreviations is located immediately preceding the index in each volume. Additional abbreviations used in this chapter include: LAC = locus controlling lactase expression in adults (*cis*-acting to *LCT*); *LCT* = structural gene (symbol) for lactase; *P = *LCT* persistence allele; *R = *LCT* nonpersistence allele; LDC = lactose digestion capacity.

*This chapter is derived & updated from Gebhard Flatz in the 7th edition of this work.

INTRODUCTION

The utilization of lactose for human nutrition requires the hydrolysis of this disaccharide in the intestinal tract. This hydrolysis is catalyzed by the enzyme lactase-phlorizin hydrolase, herein called *lactase*, a β-galactosidase (E.C. 3.2.1.108) located in the brush border of small-intestinal enterocytes (see Chap. 75). A difference in lactase activity between suckling and adult animals has been known since 1895, when Röhmann and Nagano[1] showed that cows and adult dogs have a much lower small-intestinal lactose digestion capacity (LDC) than calves and puppies. The developmental rule derived from this observation was not applied to humans for a long time, probably because medical research was most active in countries where the majority of the population retain high small-intestinal lactase activity throughout life. Constitutionally low lactase activity ("lactase deficiency") in healthy adult humans was discovered independently by two groups of researchers in 1963.[2,3] Since it is now known that the majority of adult humans have this phenotype, the term lactase deficiency is inappropriate, because it suggests a pathologic or abnormal condition. The idea that the variability of lactase activity represented a normal genetic polymorphism (OMIM 223100) was first clearly expressed by Bayless and Rosensweig.[4]

This chapter describes the progress of our understanding of the genetically determined causes of lactase variability in adults and discusses the evolutionary origin of this polymorphism and its significance in relation to disease.

LOW AND HIGH ADULT LACTASE ACTIVITY AS PHYSIOLOGICAL TRAITS

When lactase activity is determined in biopsies of morphologically normal small intestine, a wide variation of activities is observed in different adult humans. In Central and Northern Europeans and their overseas descendants, the mean lactase activity is not much lower than that of normal infants of the same population. Some individuals, however, exhibit a distinctly low lactase activity. Depending on the method of analysis, the two ranges of lactase activity may be separate or overlapping. The overlapping of low and high lactase activities is probably caused in part by variations of the reference parameters (net weight of tissue, protein or DNA content, or another disaccharidase activity). Experience has shown that the ratios of disaccharidase activities are fairly constant in a given individual, and maltase-lactase or sucrase-lactase ratios are more effective than simple lactase activities in resolving a distinct group of adults with low lactase activity.[5–7] In several studies, a clear trimodality of activity distribution has been observed (discussed in the next section, "Genetic Determination of the Lactase Phenotypes").[8–10] The difference in lactase activity is evident throughout the length of the intestine (see Fig. 5 of Chap. 75[7]).

The physiological difference between individuals who are lactase persistent and those who are lactase nonpersistent can be demonstrated by a lactose-tolerance test. Subjects with high lactase activity can completely digest the usual test dose of 50 g lactose. They have a significant rise in blood glucose concentration within 15 to 45 min following lactose administration, and since no undigested lactose reaches the colon, they lack colonic hydrogen formation and hydrogen excretion in their breath. In contrast, the LDC of subjects in the group with low lactase activity is usually exceeded by a single dose of 50 g lactose. There is no increase or only a small increase in blood glucose concentration; lactose reaching the colon is fermented by colonic bacteria; the hydrogen produced in this process is partially excreted in the expired air; and the osmotic effects of undigested lactose, the acidification of the colonic contents by short-chain fatty acids, and the formation of copious amounts of gas cause symptoms of lactose intolerance, such as nausea, meteorism, flatulence, borborygmi, and diarrhea. Comparative studies have shown that the lactose-tolerance test with breath hydrogen determination and the lactose-ethanol test[11] with urinary galactose determination most reliably separate the two phenotypic groups of adults with high and low lactase activity.[12,13] Most enzyme activity studies have to be done using biopsy material collected as part of clinical investigations. The biopsies are first assessed for histologic normality, but measurement of a second brush-border disaccharide is particularly useful to assist in excluding secondary disaccharidase deficiency.[10,14,15]

Having low lactase as an adult appears to be the normal phenotype in other mammals. In all mammals tested that produce milk containing lactose, a characteristic developmental pattern of lactase activity has been observed[16–20] (Chap. 75). Lactase activity is high in the newborn and suckling period, declines after the species-specific weaning phase, and remains low in adolescent and adult animals, though it should be stressed that, in the main, very few individuals of each species have been tested. As in other mammals, all healthy human newborns and infants have high lactase activity. In adult life, however, some people have high lactase and some have very little. In humans with low adult lactase activity, the decrease occurs during childhood. It appears that, in general, the onset of lactose intolerance begins between the age of 2 and 3 years and is usually complete by the age of 5 to 10 years.[15,21–23] However, exceptions to this timing have been reported; for example, a conversion from high to low lactase

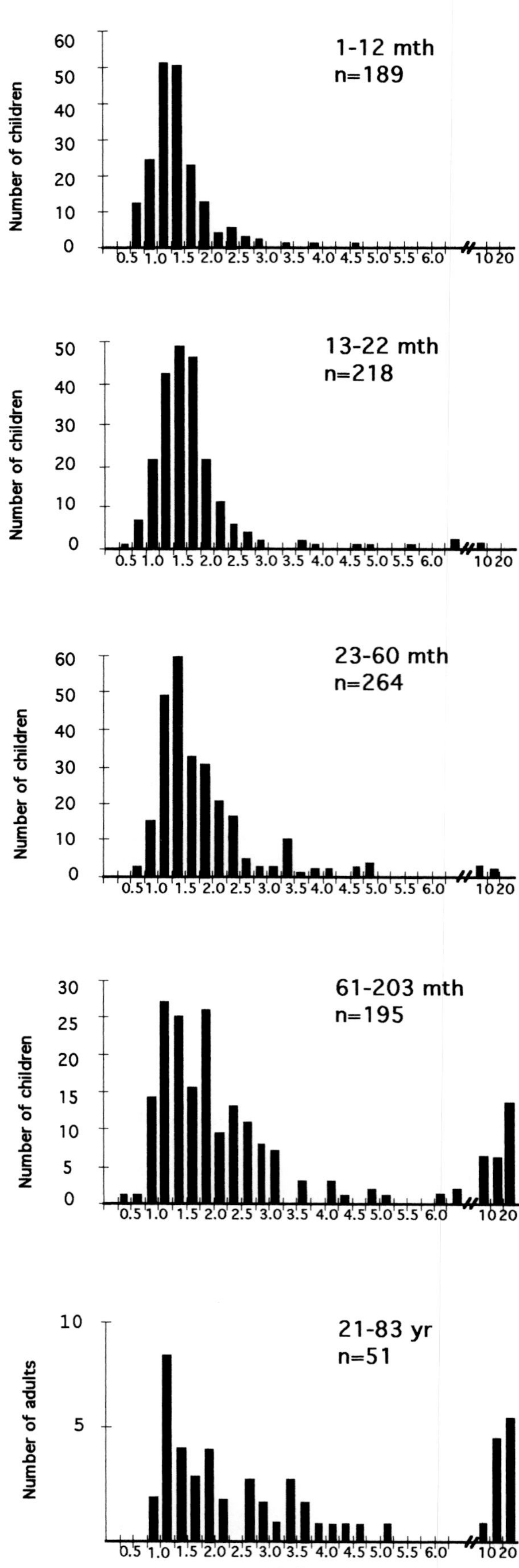

Fig. 76-1. Distribution of sucrase/lactase (S/L) ratios in five different age groups shown in histogram form. The ratios are shown along the *x*-axis and the numbers of individuals in each class on the *y*-axis. All four histograms are to the same scale along the *x*-axis although the *y*-axes are on different scales: The scale of the end of the *x*-axis is condensed from the position marked (6.5 and above—lactase nonpersistent) with the highest ratio group containing all with ratios above 20. (Adapted from Wang et al.[15] Used by permission.) All samples were collected in London[10,15] and are of mixed ethnic origin.

activity during adolescence is observed in Finland.[24] In other healthy humans, this decline in lactase activity does not occur, and LDC remains high throughout life. Examination of the distribution of lactase activities in children of different ages shows evidence of the adult trimodal distribution in children of 5 years of age and over[15] (Fig. 76-1), as is discussed in more detail in the next section, "Genetic Determination of the Lactase Phenotypes." There is ample evidence of the independence of these developmental patterns and the resulting phenotypes, from nutritional factors such as the amount of milk in the diet.[25–27]

GENETIC DETERMINATION OF THE LACTASE PHENOTYPES

A genetic basis for the two physiological adult lactase phenotypes was suspected soon after the discovery of low lactase activity ("lactase deficiency") as a common trait among healthy adult humans.[28] Family studies were conducted in different parts of the world, including families in which the parents differed in ethnic or racial origin. The quality of these data was patchy, but by 1973 convincing evidence of Mendelian inheritance of the two adult lactase phenotypes was obtained using large families.[29] This work was facilitated by the relatively high frequency of low lactase activity among Finns, but also by the fact that this author was first to apply a reliable diagnostic procedure — the lactose-ethanol tolerance test with blood galactose determination[30] — to a sufficiently large number of large informative families. This showed convincingly that healthy adult subjects with low lactase activity are homozygous for an autosomal recessive allele that causes the physiological postweaning decline of lactase activity (low LDC, lactase nonpersistence or restriction, which is also referred to as adult type hypolactasia; see Chap. 75), whereas subjects with high adult lactase activity are either heterozygous or homozygous for a dominant allele *LAC*P* (the persistence allele) that prevents the normal decline of lactase activity. Table 76-1 shows a summary of these and other published families from different parts of the world. Only eight cases have been reported in which individuals with high LDC were found in the progeny of parents who both had low LDC.[31,32] In neither study was nonpaternity excluded.

Further evidence of the genetic etiology of low and high adult lactase activity and their Mendelian segregation came from two other sources. The first evidence concerned the relationship between lactase phenotype and genotype: using disaccharidase activity ratios, a trimodal distribution of sucrase-lactase or maltase-lactase activity ratios was observed. The frequencies were compatible with predictions from the Hardy-Weinberg equation for the existence of three activity genotypes at the *LAC* locus: **P/*P*, **P/*R* and **R/*R*[8,9] where **P* is the persistence allele and **R* is the nonpersistence or lactase "restriction" allele

Table 76-1 Inheritance of Lactose Intolerance*

Type of Mating	Number of Matings	Progeny: High LDC	Progeny: Low LDC	Country (Ethnic Origin)	Test method†	Ref.
High LDC × high LDC	1	2	3	Great Britain	B, L, G	115
Low LDC × low LDC	2	0	7	U.S.A. (2 black and 1 white)	L, G	116
High LDC × low LDC	1	2	1			
High LDC × high LDC	1	2	1	Great Britain	R	117
High LDC × low LDC	1	2	0			
High LDC × low LDC	2	4	4	Thailand	L	118
High LDC × low LDC	4	10	2	U.S.A. (2 black and 4 white)	L,	119
Low LDC × low LDC	2	—	3		Probands B	
High LDC × high LDC	3	5	2	Israel	L 6B	31
High LDC × low LDC	16	20	30			
Low LDC × low LDC	11	4	26			
High LDC × high LDC	27	53	15	Finland	L, G, E	29, 120
High LDC × low LDC	18	29	20			
Low LDC × low LDC	2	—	6			
High LDC × high LDC	3	7	2	Mexico	L	32
High LDC × low LDC	22	30	42			
Low LDC × low LDC	36	4	92			
High LDC × low LDC	10	18	11	Nigeria (Yoruba and European)	L	121
Low LDC × low LDC	10	0	21			
Summary						
Low LDC × low LDC *(LAC*R/LAC*R × LAC*R/LAC*R)*	63	8	148			
High LDC × low LDC *(LAC*P/LAC*R × LAC*R/LAC*R)* *(LAC*P/LAC*P × LA*R/LAC*R)*	73	113	110			
High LDC × high LDC *(LAC*P/LAC*R × LAC*P/LAC*P)*	34	67	22			

*LDC, lactose digestion capacity; *LAC*R* and *LAC*P* are allele at the *LAC* locus.

†B, intestinal biopsy; E, tolerance tests were performed with ethanol; G, glucose-tolerance test; L, lactose-tolerance test; R, radiographic determination.

SOURCE: Adapted from Swallow and Harvey.[114] Used by permission.

Table 76-2 Relationship of the Adult Lactase Phenotypes, the Lactose Digestion Capacity (LDC) Phenotypes, and Putative Genotypes

Enzymatic Phenotype	Digestive Phenotype	Genotype
Lactase nonpersistence (restriction)	Low LDC	*LAC*R/LAC*R*
Lactase persistence	High LDC	*LAC*P/LAC*R* *LAC*P/LAC*P*

The designations *LAC*P* and *LAC*R* may represent groups of alleles with similar physiological action.

(Table 76-2). The observation of a trimodal distribution also implied that *cis*-acting differences (i.e., within or neighboring the lactase gene) are responsible for the polymorphism. The distribution of lactase activities shown as a sucrase/lactase ratio in children and adults is shown in Fig. 76-1. The second piece of evidence of monogenic inheritance of the lactase phenotypes was from a study of lactose digestion in twins. Concordance of the lactase phenotypes was complete in monozygous twins, and the distribution of dizygous twin pairs corresponded with Hardy-Weinberg predictions.[13]

In view of occasional doubts concerning the simple genetic etiology of the lactase phenotypes, it is important to note that diagnosis requires the administration of nonphysiological doses of lactose. Therefore, low LDC and lactase nonpersistence are not synonymous with lactose intolerance: many healthy subjects with low lactase activity experience no symptoms or only minimal symptoms with ordinary amounts of milk or other lactose-containing foods. Many genetic and nutritional factors influence lactose tolerance in a single individual,[25] so that family studies in which lactose tolerance is assessed by personal nutritional history will not necessarily show Mendelian segregation.[33]

It should be noted that lactase persistence behaves as a dominant trait because half levels of lactase activity are sufficient to digest 50 g lactose. However, the levels of lactase are the rate-limiting step for absorption of this sugar, as discussed in Chap. 75, so under conditions of physiological stress or in certain mildly pathologic situations, heterozygotes may become intolerant.

DISTRIBUTION OF THE LACTASE PHENOTYPES IN HUMAN POPULATIONS: THE LACTASE PERSISTENCE POLYMORPHISM

The data on the distribution of the lactase phenotype in the world population are not as reliable as those on other monogenic traits. This is due mainly to the difficulties in performing lactose-tolerance tests (in comparison with serologic or electrophoretic tests) and to the inadequacy of the methods of lactose tolerance testing in earlier studies. Even if specific enzymatic methods for the glucose assay are used, the lactose-tolerance test based solely on blood glucose determination is unreliable. Despite these limitations, the available data of lactose-tolerance tests on more than 20,000 subjects give quite a good description of the distribution of the lactase phenotypes in the world population. Table 76-3 shows the worldwide lactase-phenotype distribution.

As is evident from the data summarized in Table 76-3, low LDC (lactase nonpersistence) is the predominant phenotype in the native populations of Australia and the Pacific, East and Southeast Asia, tropical Africa, and the Americas. The opposite distribution—predominance of the lactase persistence allele—is found in two separate groups of populations: (1) Central and Northern Europeans (the Scandinavian countries, Germany, Austria, Switzerland, northern France, the Netherlands, Britain, and Ireland), and (2) nomadic, milk-dependent populations in the arid zones of North and Central Africa and Arabia (e.g., the Tuareg, Fulbe, Beja, and Bedouin peoples). In these populations, it is clear that the lactase persistence allele is more frequent than the nonpersistence allele. The two regions of high frequency of lactase persistence are separated by a wide peri-Mediterranean belt inhabited by peoples in whom lactase nonpersistence is the most common phenotype. This includes the littoral of North Africa, the Near East, Turkey, the Balkans, Italy, and southern France—areas where the frequency of low LDC is between 45 and 95 percent. In the eastern part of Central Europe (Hungary and Poland), 30 to 40 percent of the people have low LDC, and there may be a continuous west-east gradient extending from this region to the Far East, where 76 percent of the Kasakhs of northwestern China, 88 percent of Mongols in China, and 95 to 100 percent of southern Chinese have low lactase activity. A similar gradient has been noted by Kozlov and colleagues[34] across the Ural region. A north-south gradient is evident in Europe, with a very high frequency of nonpersistence in southern Italy. Lactase nonpersistence is also the predominant phenotype in Southeast Asia and in South Asia (Iran, Afghanistan, Pakistan, India, and Sri Lanka), but there is evidence of regional gene-frequency differences within the Indian subcontinent (Table 76-3), lactase persistence being quite prevalent in the north. As expected, the frequencies of the lactase phenotypes found in groups who have migrated to other continents reflect those of their native populations, and intermediate frequencies are found in populations originating from recent mixing of peoples with high and low frequencies of low LDC. In some of these, for example, American Indians[35] and Eskimos,[36] the frequency of lactase persistence is correlated with the number of European ancestors.

Overall, it is clear that postweaning decline of lactase occurs in the majority of humans and conforms to the developmental pattern in most other mammalian species. Lactase persistence is the "unusual" or even "abnormal" condition, and its high prevalence in some populations requires explanation.[37]

EXPLANATIONS FOR THE VARIABLE DISTRIBUTION OF THE LACTASE PHENOTYPES IN HUMAN POPULATIONS

High frequencies of adult lactase persistence are found only in populations with a tradition of substantial production and consumption of animal milk. It is generally assumed that the lactase persistence gene has reached high frequency by natural selection in pastoralist populations that developed dairying during the Neolithic period.[38] Milk provides an important source of adult nutrition in those who can digest it, but milk consumption has been adopted by populations with a predominantly low LDC, for example, the Mongols, the Herero, the Nuer, and the Dinka. Even in populations with generally high milk intake, subjects with low LDC rarely experience severe symptoms of lactose intolerance. It appears that people adjust their dietary intake of milk and milk products consciously or unconsciously to their individual lactose-tolerance threshold. Milk is also often fermented to products such as yogurt and cheese, which have a reduced lactose content.

Another possible selective advantage of the ability to digest fresh milk may be that it provides an important source of water in desert climates.[39,40] Furthermore, additional selective forces may have applied in Northern Europe where a tradition of mixed farming meant that there was less dependence on milk. The frequency of the lactase persistence allele does not correspond to the known genetic gradient caused by the migratory settlement of Europe from the Near East in the postglacial period.[41] Indeed, the highest frequency of *LAC*P* is found in Scandinavia, where agriculture and dairying were introduced late, probably not more than 4000 years ago.[42] To explain the relatively rapid establishment of high frequencies of a lactase persistence allele in Northern Europe in the absence of milk dependence, Flatz and Rotthauwe[25] suggested the hypothesis that the selective benefit was improved calcium absorption. This was based on the observation that lactose increases the absorption of calcium in subjects with high LDC in the absence of monosaccharides[43] and on the assumption that

Table 76-3 Distribution of Adult Lactase Phenotypes in Human Populations

Continent and Nation	Population	Groups	*N*	% Low LDC	*LAC*P*	Ref.
Americas						
Greenland	Eskimo		119	85	0.08	√
	Eskimo/European		108	**38**	**0.38**	
American	Amerindians	Apache	22	100	0	√
		Chippewa	33	97	0.02	√
		Hopi	21	100	0	√
		Papago	14	93	0.04	√
		Pima	62	95	0.03	√
Canada	Whites		16	**6**	**0.76**	
	Polish		21	**29**	**0.46**	
	Czech		17	**18**	**0.58**	
	Chinese		48	98	0.01	123
	Amerindians		30	63	0.21	
U.S.A.	Whites		913	**22**	**0.53**	
	North Europeans		188	**7**	**0.74**	
	Blacks		390	65	0.19	
	Mexicans		305	52	0.28	
	Vietnamese		31	100	0	
Mexico	Mexicans		401	83	0.09	
Puerto Rico			50	54	0.27	
Guatemala			20	83	0.09	124
Colombia	Amerindians	Chami	24	100	0	
Bolivia	Amerindians	Aymara	31	77	0.12	
Brazil	Whites		53	**49**	**0.30**	
	Japanese		20	100	0	125
Africa						
North Africa	Tunisia		43	83	0.09	√
	Morocco, Tunisia	Maghrebi	55	78	0.17	
	Egypt	Sinai Desert	72	**11**	**0.67** }	
		Other	670	70	0.16* }	√
West Africa	Niger	Tuareg (Aullimenden)	118	**13**	**0.64**	P√
	Nigeria	Hausa	17	76	0.13	√
		Fulani (pastoralist)	9	**22**	**0.53**	P√
		Fulani (sedentary)	24	71	0.16	√
		Yoruba	100	91	0.05	√
		Igbo	16	81	0.10	√
	Senegal	Peuhl (Fulbe)	29	**0**	**1.00**	
		Famers	131	35	0.41	
	Gabon		20	60	0.23	126
Gentral Africa	Sudan	Shilluk	8	63	0.21	√
Sudan	Baggara	Habbania	19	53	0.27	√
	Baggara	Messiria	20	60	0.23	P√
	Beja	Amarar	82	**13**	**0.64**	P√
	Beja	Beni Amir	40	**13**	**0.64**	P√
	Beja	Haddendoa	137	**20**	**0.55**	P√
	Beja	Bisharin	22	**14**	**0.62**	P√
		Dinka	213	76	0.13	√
	Nubians	Midobi	21	67	0.18	P√
	Nubians	Nuer	23	78	0.17	√
Somalia	Somali		244	76	0.13	
Uganda/Rwanda		Tutsi	59	**7**	**0.74**	√
		Hutu	51	51	0.29	√
	Bantu	Ganda	27	96	0.20	√
South Africa	San	!Kung and # hua	65	95	0.03	√
	Nama		18	**50**	**0.29**	√
	Herero		37	97	0.02	P√
	Bantu	Zulu	32	81	0.10	√
	Bantu	Xhosa	17	82	0.09	√
	Bantu	Tswana	24	83	0.09	√
	Bantu	Swazi	12	75	0.13	√
	Bantu	Sotho	23	65	0.19	√
Near/Middle East						
Jordan	Bedouin		162	**24**	**0.51**	P√
	Other Arabs		204	75	0.13	√

(Continued on next page)

Table 76-3 (Continued)

Continent and Nation	Population	Groups	*N*	% Low LDC	*LAC*P*	Ref.
Saudi Arabia	Bedouin		35	**17**	**0.59**	P√
Iran	Iranians		40	83	0.09	√
Syria			75	91	0.05	
Israel	General		151	61	0.22	
	Jews		276	68	0.17	
Lebanon	Lebanese		225	79	0.11	√
Europe						
Russian Federation	Russians		103	57	0.25	√
	Kola Peninsula	Kildin Saami	50	**48**	**0.31**	127
	Permian Finn	Komi Permiak	112	**50**	**0.29**	127
Estonia	Estonians		902	**27**	**0.48**	12, 67 8
Finland	Lapps		519	**41**	**0.36**	P√
	Swedish speakers		91	**8**	**0.72**	
	Finnish speakers		449	**17**	**0.59**	
Sweden	Swedish		400	**1**	**0.90**	
U.K.	White		163	**5**	**0.78**	129
	Afro-Caribbean		50	82	0.09	129
	Indian		55	55	0.25	129
Ireland	Irish		50	**4**	**0.80**	√
Denmark	Danes		761	**3**	**0.83**	
Netherlands	Dutch		14	**0**	**1.00**	
Germany			646	**15**	**0.61**	
	Germans–NW		441	**8**	**0.72**	
	Germans–NE		246	**22**	**0.53**	
	Germans–W		182	**14**	**0.62**	
	Bavarians		221	**14**	**0.62**	
	Germans–SW		136	**23**	**0.52**	
	French		22	**32**	**0.43**	
France	French–north		62	**23**	**0.52**	
	French–south		71	**44**	**0.34**	
Austria			528	**20**	**0.55**	
Switzerland			64	**16**	**0.60**	
Czech Republic	Czechs		200	**13**	**0.64**	√
Hungary	Hungarians		262	**41**	**0.36**	√
	Hungarians–NE		103	**42**	**0.35**	130
	Hungarians–E		70	**29**	**0.46**	130
	Hungarians–W		100	**28**	**0.47**	130
	Matyo		172	**37**	**0.39**	130
	Roma/Sinti		113	56	0.25	130
Poland			275	**37**	**0.39**	
Slovenia	Slovenians		153	**35**	**0.41**	
Spain	Spaniards–NW		338	**34**	**0.42**	131
			265	**15**	0.61	√
Greece	Greeks		800	52	0.28	√
Italy	Italians–north		383	**50**	**0.29**	
	Italians–south		197	67	0.18	√
	Sicilians		100	71	0.16	
Turkey	Turks		470	71	0.16	√
Indian Subcontinent						
Pakistan	Kashmir		27	70	0.16	
	Punjabis		384	56	0.25	√
	Sindhi		45	**42**	**0.35**	√
	Other		66	**35**	**0.41**	
India	North		264	**27**	**0.48**	
	Central		125	63	0.21	
	South		60	67	0.18	
Sri-Lanka	Sinhalese		158	73	0.15	√
	Tamils		31	71	0.16	√
Asia						
Russian Federation	Ob River basin	Komi Izhem	56	63	0.21	127
	Sub-Arctic	Mansi	58	71	0.16	127
	Sub-Arctic	Khanty	115	72	0.15	127
	West Siberia	Nenets	9	78	0.12	127
Afghanistan	Pashtun		71	79	0.11	
	Tajik		79	82	0.09	

Table 76-3 (Continued)

Continent and Nation	Population	Groups	*N*	% Low LDC	*LAC*P*	Ref.
	Uzbek		16	100	0	
	Hazara		10	80	0.11	
	Pasha-i		60	87	0.07	
China	North (Han)		314	88	0.06	√
	Mongols		198	88	0.06	**P**√
	Kasakhs		195	76	0.12	132
Taiwan			71	100	0	
Japan			66	81	0.10	√
Myanmar	Burmese		31	93	0.04	133
Thailand	Thais		339	98	0.01	
Pacific Rim						
Fiji	Fijians		12	100	0	√
Papua	Tribal groups		123	90	0.05	
Singapore	Chinese		77	95	0.03	123
Indonesia	Javanese		53	91	0.05	√
Australasia						
Australia		Aborigines	45	84	0.08	√
		Aborigines, other	100	59	0.23	
		Whites	133	**5**	**0.78**	
New Zealand		Maoris	30	64	0.20	134
		Samoans	26	54	0.26	134
		Europeans	44	**9**	**0.70**	134

Most of the data were collected using lactose-tolerance tests; thus frequencies are shown as % low LDC (low lactose digestion capacity—or lactase nonpersistence). The calculated lactase persistence allele frequency (**P*) is also shown. Results are shown in **bold** for those populations that are less than 50 percent low LDC. For references see Holden and Mace[44] and Flatz[122] and additional references where indicated. A checkmark (√) indicates populations analyzed in the Holden and Mace study, and **P** indicates populations, used in the Holden and Mace study, with milk-based pastoralism as greater than 55 percent of total subsistence activity.[45]

rickets and osteomalacia were strong selective forces in the conditions of low solar irradiation that are characteristic of Northwestern Europe.

Holden and Mace[44] recently attempted to reevaluate the possible selective forces. A major problem with the interpretation of the population data is that the relationships between variable environmental factors and LDC are confounded by the very different degree of relatedness of the populations under consideration. In their study, Holden and Mace attempted to address this issue by making direct comparisons between the genetic relatedness and the cultural relatedness. Their study was restricted to populations that fulfilled certain stringent criteria, such as presence in the *Ethnographic Atlas*[45] and lack of migration since 1492, and thus only 7000 individuals could be included. Their analysis supports the hypothesis that lactase persistence is an adaptation to pastoralism (i.e., pastoralism developing before lactase persistence), but no evidence was obtained for the added selective effect of highly arid environments or high latitudes (global solar irradiation). Rather few Northern European populations could be included (see Table 76-3), however, and the measure of global solar irradiation may not be an accurate assessment of sunshine, because of the complexity of variable cloud cover.

Several authors have attempted to make mathematical models, often assuming coevolution of the cultural trait of milk drinking,[44] to explain how modern gene frequencies of lactase persistence were reached within 6000 to 9000 years, the period since humans first domesticated livestock and practiced milk-based pastoralism. Most of the models require high selection coefficients, typically 5 percent, and a reasonable starting gene frequency to reach a frequency of 0.70 in 6000 to 9000 years. However, other investigators[46] claim that genetic drift can explain present-day frequencies if the relevant mutation originated before the geographical expansion of modern humans. These authors suggested that populations in which the lactase persistence gene attained high frequencies by chance (genetic drift) were able to utilize the benefit of animal milk in adult nutrition. Subsequent selection in favor of the lactase persistence gene was possible but not essential to explain the present distribution of the lactase phenotypes.

Most models involving selection make the tacit assumption that lactase nonpersistence is the phenotype of all nonhuman adult primates. One study shows clear evidence of down-regulation of lactase in baboons (*Papio papio*)[47] but, in another study, 9 of 10 adult Cebus monkeys (*Macaca fascicularis*) were shown to be lactose tolerant.[48] We have been unable to find references to studies on the lactase persistence in chimpanzees, gorillas, or orangutans. Adult chimpanzees (*Pan troglodytes*) and gorillas (*Gorilla gorilla*) at London Zoo are given occasional milk shakes without adverse effects (A.W. Sainsbury, personal communication), but the lactose load may not be enough to cause symptoms. Weaning is very late in the great apes, being 1460 days in the common chimpanzee and 1583 days in gorillas as compared with 720 days in hunter-gatherer humans.[49] It is therefore possible that lactase persistence may have evolved as part of the changes that enabled higher primates to delay weaning and protect their young for longer, and space their births. Indeed, one group have put forward the hypothesis that selection against lactase persistence and late weaning, by malaria, might account for the near absence of this allele in much of Africa.[50]

Ultimately, analysis of the causal mutation(s) and haplotype background may tell us whether Afro-Arabian and European lactase persistence have a common or a separate origin and together with the analysis of primates will indicate which of these explanations is likely.

NUTRITIONAL AND MEDICAL IMPLICATIONS

The majority of humans with genetically determined low adult LDC live in countries where animal milk is not used in the normal diet. Consequently, lactose intolerance is not likely to occur. Even in milk-consuming societies, lactose intolerance is not a frequent medical problem, because individuals with low lactase seem to adjust milk intake to their individual tolerance level. Lactose intolerance is most likely to develop when people with low LDC change their dietary habits—for example, following the move from a country with low milk consumption to an area where milk use is high, or when nutrients with high lactose concentration, such as powdered milk, are distributed for famine relief in communities where the majority of people have low LDC. In these cases, the pharmacologic action of lactose in subjects with lactase nonpersistence should be kept in mind. Friends in Southern Europe indicate that a glass of cold milk can be a convenient and inexpensive laxative for people with low lactase activity, and that milk is not consumed in the evenings!

Lactose intolerance in children is, however, a common problem in pediatric gastroenterology clinics.[51] Though this is often secondary to disease, the normal genetically determined down-regulation should not be forgotten. Our own studies have shown evidence of very variable down-regulation in clinic patients with normal histology.[15] It will be of great interest to elucidate the factors that account for this variability.

Several associations between the adult lactase phenotypes and diseases have been reported,[52] but the evidence is controversial. Only a few of these studies are satisfactory with respect to matching in ethnicity between the patient and control groups, which seems mandatory in view of the great variation in the distribution of the lactase phenotypes. Even in those cases, hidden population stratification cannot be excluded.

Low LDC may play a role in recurrent abdominal pain in children and in irritable bowel syndrome in adults but this is not shown in all studies, and psychological factors, such as the possible placebo, have been claimed and there are other reports that do not support this association.[53–56] Lactose intolerance may also be secondary to changes in bowel transit time or inflammation as occurs in inflammatory bowel disease.[57,58]

Several reports describe a significantly higher frequency of lactase nonpersistence in osteoporotic women in comparison with control groups,[59–62] and increased fractures of weight-bearing bones and altered bone density,[63,64] and a reduction of calcium availability by milk avoidance[52] and by reduced absorption, is claimed to be a causative factor. Indeed, recommended intakes of calcium have been increased in some countries[65] and advice given to substitute lactase-treated milk or yogurt for fresh milk as a source of calcium. However, the etiology of osteoporosis is complex and not primarily due to calcium deficiency.

Lactase persistence is not devoid of possible disease associations. There is some conflicting evidence for a role of milk consumption by lactase-persistent subjects in the causation of hyperlipidemia,[66] coronary heart disease,[67,68] and cataract.[69] Since the cataracts observed in genetic disorders of galactose metabolism are attributed to galactitol, physiological differences in galactose metabolism and milk consumption may play a role in the development of cataracts. A study in Naples demonstrated, in a population with a high prevalence of lactose malabsorption, a high frequency of lactose absorbers in adults with idiopathic[70] and diabetic[70] senile and presenile cataract. These results have been confirmed in northern Italy,[70] in Sardinia,[70] and in France.[70] In another study, high milk intake correlated with cortical cataracts.[70] Similar surveys in populations with a high prevalence of lactose absorption in Sweden and Mexico showed no correlation;[71,72] however, one study revealed a high risk of cataract formation in subjects with high lactose intake and low activities of galactokinase.[73] Association with ovarian cancer has also been claimed[74] but not supported.[75,76]

MOLECULAR STUDIES OF THE LACTASE PHENOTYPES

At present, the molecular mechanisms of this ontogenetic switch (nonpersistence of lactase activity) and its failure (persistence of lactase activity throughout life) are unknown. Early studies showed that the lactase enzyme present in the small intestine of lactase-nonpersistent subjects was indistinguishable from that present in lactase-persistent individuals, having the same electrophoretic mobility,[77,78] the same immunologic properties, and the same specific lactase[78,79] and the same phlorizin hydrolase activities.[79,80] Cloning and sequencing of the lactase structural gene *LCT* [accession numbers M81834 and M6185 (GenBank/EMBL)] and cDNA (accession number X07994) has revealed polymorphisms within the coding sequence, some of which alter amino acids[15,81,82] (Fig. 76-2), but none of these sequence differences is unique to lactase-persistent or lactase-nonpersistent individuals.[83] The structural locus for intestinal lactase (*LCT*) is located on chromosome 2,[84,85] and all the available evidence (cloning,[81,86] family studies,[82] and expression studies[15,87]) supports the notion that just a single gene encodes human lactase.

Particularly in the early studies, findings concerning lactase mRNA levels were conflicting,[88–90] but it is now generally agreed that lactase-nonpersistent individuals have lower levels of lactase messenger RNA[10,91,92] (Fig. 76-3). The difference in mRNA level is more marked in some studies than others, relatively higher levels of lactase mRNA being found in lactase-nonpersistent

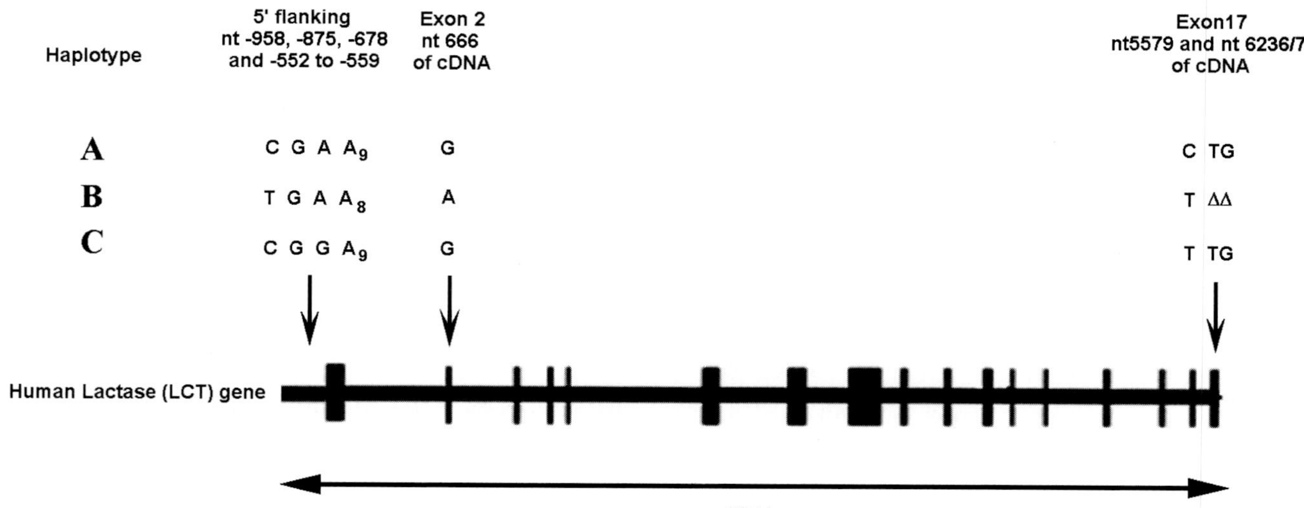

Fig. 76-2. Diagram of the human lactase gene (*LCT*) showing the positions of the 17 exons and the polymorphic sites used in the association and haplotype studies.[82,83] Several other polymorphisms have been identified in the exons[15,81] but do not appear to break up these haplotypes in Europeans (Poulter, Hollox and Swallow, unpublished data).

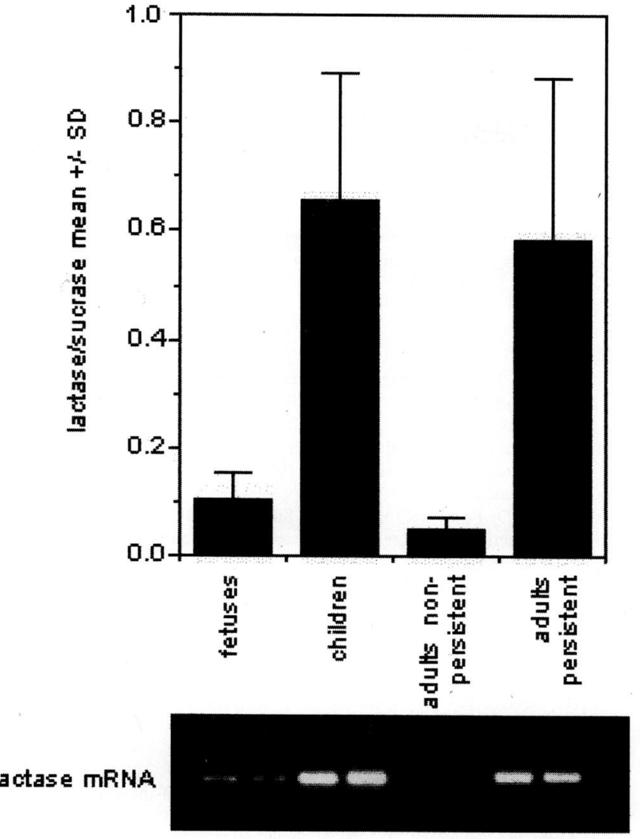

Fig. 76-3. Correspondance of lactase activities (lactase/sucrase ratio) and lactase mRNA levels determined by semiquantitative reverse transcriptase-polymerase chain reaction (RT-PCR).[94] Data from fetuses, $n = 10$; children, $n = 29$; lactase-persistent adults, $n = 36$; and lactase-nonpersistent adults, $n = 11$. RT-PCR products from two representative individuals are shown in each case. Data are taken from our own studies on the London population. Further RNA data are shown in Harvey et al.[10] and Wang et al.[15,94]

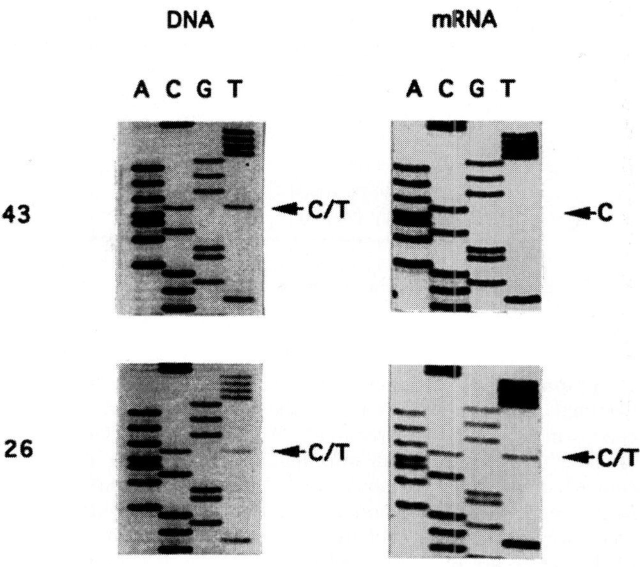

Fig. 76-4. Sequencing of genomic DNA and cDNA from two lactase-persistent individuals across the polymorphic site in exon 2 (on the antisense strand). One individual (no. 26) is homozygous for high expression of the lactase gene and is thus homozygous persistent (*P/*P), whereas the other (no. 43) shows high expression of one allele and low expression of the other (T on the antisense strand or A on the sense strand) and is heterozygous (*P/*R). (From Wang et al.[87] Used by permission.)

individuals from Naples.[87,92] Genetic, or just conceivably environmental/dietary, differences may be responsible for this, but it seems most likely that the discrimination between the two phenotypes is clearer in duodenal samples, as used in most studies, than it is in jejunal samples used in Naples, even though this would not have been predicted by the early studies by Newcomer and McGill[7] (see Fig. 5 of Chap. 75).

Studies on mRNA levels that made use of polymorphisms within the exons of the gene have demonstrated clearly that in some lactase-persistent individuals only one of the two *LCT* homologues is expressed at high levels, with the other accounting for 10 percent or less of the total lactase message[87] (Fig. 76-4). Such individuals are interpreted as lactase-persistent heterozygotes who carry one lactase-persistent and one lactase-nonpersistent allele. This observation demonstrates unequivocally a *cis*-acting effect and suggests that the relevant sequence differences reside within or near the *LCT* gene. Informative fetuses showed low expression[93,94] (Fig. 76-3) of both transcripts,[15,87] whereas young babies showed high equal expression of two transcripts.[15] Evidence of progressive but variable downregulation of expression of certain lactase transcripts was observed in children aged 20 months to 11 years.[15]

The polymorphism can thus be best described as due to a failure in a regular genetic switch that controls a developmental program that is characteristic of almost all species of mammals. However, despite overwhelming evidence that the lactase persistence/nonpersistence polymorphism operates through variation in the steady-state level of lactase mRNA, there is no direct evidence as to whether this effect is transcriptional or due to RNA stability. Furthermore, a number of observations require clarification. In the Neapolitan studies, lactase nonpersistent individuals have different populations of enterocytes, some expressing, and some not expressing lactase.[95] *In situ* hybridization shows that lactase mRNA is present in rather more cells than the protein.[96] The mosaic patches of cells give the appearance that groups of related cells have escaped the transcriptional control or silencing, and that the gene is reexpressed. However, the spatial relationship of these cells is not consistent with the known clonal origin of intestinal villus cells, which would be expected to appear as ribbons emerging from a single crypt stem cell.[97] Patches of lactase-expressing cells have been less evident in other studies,[10] and this might also reflect a difference between duodenum and jejunum, but clear evidence of patchiness has also been found in one study that used duodenal biopsy specimens,[98] although two types of immunohistologic patterns were observed in that study. This and other evidence suggests some variability in posttranslational processing in different samples. Measuring lactase in relation to lactase mRNA (but not in relation to sucrase), Rossi and colleagues[92] found several lactase-nonpersistent individuals with high lactase enzymatic activity in relation to their mRNA level. In some cases, evidence has been presented for abnormal or slower processing[99,100] and abnormal electrophoretic mobility[10] (C.B. Harvey and D.M. Swallow, unpublished data). At this stage, it is not really clear whether these differences reflect additional genetic variability or epigenetic effects such as cellular turnover and mosaicism. It is clear, however, that some of the glycosylation of lactase is genetically polymorphic, since lactase carries the ABH and Lewis blood group determinants in secretors but not nonsecretors[101] and this normal variation may affect the properties of the residual protein in lactase-nonpersistent individuals. Indeed, some studies have suggested that *O*-glycosylation affects lactase activity.[102] In addition, two of the polymorphisms detected within the coding region alter amino acids, which may likewise affect the properties of the protein.[15,81,82] Whatever the explanation for the heterogeneity, it is clear that the major effect operates through the level of mRNA transcripts. Together the data suggest sequence differences in a *cis*-acting regulatory element.

Table 76-4 Comparision of the Frequencies of the Lactase Persistence Allele *LAC*P* (from Table 76-3) and the Frequency of C at nt 5579*

Population	*LAC*P*	*N* (Individuals Tested; from Table 76-3)	nt 5579 C	*N* (Individuals Tested; Own Data)
U.K. whites	0.78	163	0.86	52
France (north)	0.52	62	0.62	24
Italy (south)	0.18	67	0.47	29

*This discriminates the A haplotype from B and C haplotypes in Europeans (the Italians tested for nt 5579 were all from the Naples area).

Information is accumulating, both in humans and other mammals, as to the mechanism of the down-regulation of lactase gene which occurs on weaning[92,103–109] (and see Chap. 75). Perhaps the most critical information comes from the work conducted on the pig promoter, work that has shown that just 1 kb of upstream sequence enables the normal developmental down-regulation in pigs.[110] Regulatory elements identified include CE-LPH1 (at −40 to −54), which binds the intestine specific transcription factor Cdx-2 and also HOXC11, and HNF1α elements.[111,112]

Although it would be surprising if the genetic switch were not common to almost all mammals, the parallels should be treated with caution. To date, the *cis* element that is responsible for the polymorphism in humans has not been identified, despite sequencing of a panel of at least five individuals in extensive regions of the lactase gene, which includes all of the regions upstream from the start of transcription[81,113] (M. Poulter, E.J. Hollox, and D.M. Swallow, unpublished data) which is homologous to the pig region needed for normal developmental down-regulation. A very large number of polymorphic sites have now been characterized[15] (Poulter, Hollox, and Swallow, unpublished data), and a high level of linkage disequilibrium is observed over more than 60 kb — at least in Europeans.[82,83] Very few haplotypes are detected in Europeans, and the frequencies of these differ in a north-south gradient in Europe in a similar way to lactase persistence and nonpersistence (Table 76-4). Furthermore, population studies, a few limited families, and analysis of mRNA transcript expression show significant association with a single haplotype — the A haplotype, which is most frequent in Europeans (Fig. 76-2), accounting for 87 percent of Northern European chromosomes. Recent work on Finnish families has suggested that a region approximately 2 Mb upstream of lactase is responsible for congenital alactasia (see Chap. 76).[135] The same *cis* element might be involved in congenital alactasia and in the lactase persistence polymorphism. Such an element may be essential for lactase expression as well as being involved in lactase down-regulation. The observations so far might suggest that lactase persistence is the result of a single mutation, at least in Europeans, which occurred on an A-haplotype background, but this mutation may not necessarily be a point mutation and may be located at some distance from the *LCT* gene.

Studies in Africans show much more haplotype diversity, and the common European A haplotype is probably rare (Hollox, Poulter, and Swallow, unpublished data). It will be interesting to see whether lactase persistence in African pastoralists resides on the same haplotype background as found in Europeans.

REFERENCES

1. Röhmann F, Nagano J: Über die Resorption und die fermentative Spaltung der Disaccharide im Dünndarm des ausgewachsenen Hundes. *Arch Ges Physiol* **95**:533, 1903.
2. Auricchio S, Rubino A, Semenza G, Landolt M, Prader A: Isolated intestinal lactase deficiency in the adult. *Lancet* **2**:324, 1963.
3. Dahlqvist A, Hammond B, Crane R, Dunphy J, Littman A: Intestinal lactase deficiency and lactose intolerance in adults: Preliminary report. *Gastroenterology* **45**:488, 1963.
4. Bayless T, Rosensweig N: A racial difference in the incidence of lactase deficiency: A survey of milk intolerance and lactase deficiency in healthy adult males. *JAMA* **197**:968, 1966.
5. Maiuri L, Rossi M, Raia V, Paparo F, Coletta S, Mazzeo F, Breglia A, et al: Morphological method for the diagnosis of human adult type hypolactasia. *Gut* **35**:1042, 1994.
6. Welsh JD, Poley JR, Bhatia M, Stevenson DE: Intestinal disaccharidase activities in relation to age, race, and mucosal damage. *Gastroenterology* **75**:847, 1978.
7. Newcomer A, McGill D: Distribution of disaccharidase activity in the small bowel of normal and lactase-deficient subjects. *Gastroenterology* **51**:481, 1966.
8. Flatz G: Gene dosage effect on intestinal lactase activity demonstrated in vivo. *Am J Hum Genet* **36**:306, 1984.
9. Ho MW, Povey S, Swallow DM: Lactase polymorphism in adult British natives: Estimating allele frequencies by enzyme assays in autopsy samples. *Am J Hum Genet* **34**:650, 1982.
10. Harvey CB, Wang Y, Hughes LA, Swallow DM, Thurrell WP, Sams VR, Barton R, et al: Studies on the expression of intestinal lactase in different individuals. *Gut* **36**:28, 1995.
11. Arola H, Koivula T, Jokela H, Isokoski M: Simple urinary test for lactose malabsorption. *Lancet* **2**:524, 1982.
12. Newcomer A, McGill D, Thomas P, Hofmann A: Prospective comparison of indirect methods for detecting lactase deficiency. *N Engl J Med* **293**:1232, 1975.
13. Metneki J, Czeizel A, Flatz S, Flatz G: A study of lactose absorption capacity in twins. *Hum Genet* **67**:296, 1984.
14. Phillips AD, Avigad S, Sacks J, Rice SJ, France NE, Walker-Smith JA: Microvillous surface area in secondary disaccharidase deficiency. *Gut* **21**:44, 1980.
15. Wang Y, Harvey CB, Hollox EJ, Phillips AD, Poulter M, Clay P, Walker-Smith JA, et al: The genetically programmed down-regulation of lactase in children. *Gastroenterology* **114**:1230, 1998.
16. Blaxter K: Lactation and the growth of the young, in Kow S, Cowie A (eds): *Milk: The Mammary Gland and Its Secretion*. New York, Academic, 1961, p 329.
17. Hore P, Messer M: Studies on disaccharidase activities of the small intestine of the domestic cat and other carnivorous mammals. *Comp Biochem Physiol* **24**:717, 1968.
18. Koldovsky O, Heringova A, Jisrova V, Chytil F, Hoskova J: Postnatal changes in β-galactosidase activity in the jejunum and ileum of mice, rabbits, and guinea pigs. *Can J Biochem* **44**:523, 1966.
19. Plimmer RA: On the presence of lactase in the intestine of animals and on the adaptation of the intestine to lactose. *J Physiol* **35**:20, 1906.
20. Welsh JD, Walker A: Intestinal disaccharidase and alkaline phosphatase activity in the dog. *Proc Soc Exp Biol Med* **120**:525, 1965.
21. Wittenberg D, Moosa A: Lactose maldigestion: Age specific prevalence in black and Indian children. *S Afr Med J* **78**:470, 1990.
22. Thomas S, Walker-Smith JA, Senewiratne B, Hjelm M: Age dependency of the lactase persistence and lactase restriction phenotypes among children in Sri Lanka and Britain. *J Trop Pediatr* **36**:80, 1990.
23. Simoons F: Age of onset of lactose malabsorption. *Pediatrics* **66**:646, 1980.
24. Sahi T, Launiala K, Laitinen H: Hypolactasia in a fixed cohort of young Finnish adults: A follow-up study. *Scand J Gastroenterol* **18**:865, 1983.
25. Flatz G, Rotthauwe HW: Evidence against nutritional adaption to tolerance to lactase. *Humangenetik* **13**:118, 1971.
26. Lebenthal E, Sunshine P, Kretchmer N: Effect of prolonged nursing on the activity of intestinal lactase. *Gastroenterology* **64**:1136, 1973.

27. Knudsen K, Welsh M, Kronenberg R, Vanderveen J, Heidelbauch N: Effect of a nonlactose diet on human intestinal disaccharidase activity. *Am J Dig Dis* **13**:593, 1968.
28. Cuatrecasas P, Lockwood H, Caldwell J: Lactase deficiency in the adult: A common occurrence. *Lancet* **1**:14, 1965.
29. Sahi T: The inheritance of selective adult-type lactose malabsorption. *Scand J Gastroenterol* **9**:1, 1974.
30. Isokoski M, Jussila J, Sarna S: A simple screening method for lactose malabsorption. *Gastroenterology* **62**:28, 1972.
31. Gilat T, Benaroya Y, Gelman-Malachi E, Adam A: Genetics of primary adult lactase deficiency. *Gastroenterology* **64**:562, 1973.
32. Lisker R, Gonzalez B, Daltabuit M: Recessive inheritance of the adult type of intestinal lactase deficiency. *Am J Hum Genet* **27**:662, 1975.
33. Johnson R, Schwitters S, Cole R, Ahern F, Au K: A family study of lactose intolerance. *Behav Genet* **11**:369, 1981.
34. Kozlov AI, Balanovskaya EV, Nurbaev SD, Balanovsky OI: Gene geography of primary hypolactasia in populations of the Old World. *Russian J Genet* **34**:445, 1998.
35. Newcomer A, Gordon H, Thomas P, McGill D: Family studies of lactase deficiency in the American Indian. *Gastroenterology* **73**:985, 1977.
36. Gudmand-Hoyer E, McNair A, Jarnum S, Broersma L, McNair J: Laktosemalabsorption in Vestgronland. *Ugeskr Laeger* **135**:169, 1973.
37. Dahlqvist A: The basic aspects of the chemical background of lactase deficiency. *Postgrad Med J* **53**:57, 1977.
38. Simoons F: The geographic hypothesis and lactose malabsorption: A weighing of the evidence. *Am J Dig Dis* **23**:963, 1978.
39. Cook GC: Did persistence of intestinal lactase into adult life originate in the Arabian peninsula? *Man* **13**:418, 1978.
40. Cook GC, Al-Torki MT: High intestinal lactase concentrations in adult Arabs in Saudi Arabia. *BMJ* **3**:135, 1975.
41. Piazza A, Menozzi P, Cavalli-Sforza LL: The HLA-A,B gene frequencies in the world: Migration or selection? *Hum Immunol* **4**:297, 1971.
42. Ammermann A, Cavalli-Sforza L: Measuring the rate of spread of early farming in Europe. *Man* **6**:674, 1971.
43. Birlouez-Aragon I: Effect of lactose hydrolysis on calcium absorption during duodenal milk perfusion. *Reprod Nutr Dev* **28**:1465, 1988.
44. Holden C, Mace R: Phylogenetic analysis of the evolution of lactose digestion in adults. *Hum Biol* **69**:605, 1997.

44a. Feldman MW, Cavalli-Sforza LL: On the theory of evolution under genetic and cultural transmission with application to the lactose absorption problem, in Feldman MW (ed): *Mathematical Evolutionary Theory*. Princeton, Princeton University Press, 1989, p 145.

45. Murdock GP: *Ethnographic Atlas*. Pittsburgh, PA, University of Pittsburgh Press, 1967.
46. Nei M, Saitou N: Genetic relationship of human populations and ethnic differences in relation to drugs and food, in Kalow W, Goedde HW, Agarwal DP (eds): *Ethnic Differences in Reactions to Drugs and Other Xenobiotics*. New York, Alan R Liss, 1986, p 21.
47. Welsh JD, Russell LC, Walker AW: Changes in intestinal lactase and alkaline phosphatase activity levels with age in the Baboon (*Papio papio*). *Gastroenterology* **66**:993, 1974.
48. Wen C-P, Antonowicz PHI, Tovar E, McGandy RB, Gershoff SN: Lactose feeding in lactose-intolerant monkeys. *Am J Clin Nutr* **26**:1224, 1973.
49. Harvey PH, Martin RD, Clutton-Brock TH: Life histories in comparative perspective, in Smuts BB, Cheney DL, Seyfarth RM, Wrangham RW, Struhsaker TT (eds): *Primate Societies*. Chicago, University of Chicago Press, 1987, p 181.
50. Anderson B, Vullo C: Did malaria select for primary adult lactase deficiency? *Gut* **35**:1487, 1994.
51. Büller HA, Rings EHHM, Montgomery RK, Grand RJ: Clinical aspects of lactose intolerance in children and adults. *Scand J Gastroenterol Suppl* **188**:73, 1991.
52. Gudmand-Hoyer E: The clinical significance of disaccharide maldigestion. *Am J Clin Nutr* **59**:735S, 1994.
53. Lebenthal E, Rossi TM, Nord KS, Branski D: Recurrent abdominal pain and lactose absorption in children. *Pediatrics* **67**:828, 1981.
54. Tolliver BA, Jackson MS, Jackson KL, Barnett ED, Chastang JF, DiPalma JA: Does lactose maldigestion really play a role in the irritable bowel? *J Clin Gastroenterol* **23**:15, 1996.
55. Bohmer CJ, Tuynman HA: The clinical relevance of lactose malabsorption in irritable bowel syndrome. *Eur J Gastroenterol Hepatol* **8**:1013, 1996.
56. Lisker R, Solomons NW, Perez Briceno R, Ramirez Mata M: Lactase and placebo in the management of the irritable bowel syndrome: A double-blind, cross-over study. *Am J Gastroenterol* **84**:756, 1989.
57. Mishkin S: Dairy sensitivity, lactose malabsorption and elimination diets in inflammatory bowel disease. *Am J Clin Nutr* **65**:564, 1997.
58. Mishkin B, Yalovsky M, Mishkin S: Increased prevalence of lactose malabsorption in Crohn's disease patients at low risk for lactose malabsorption based on ethnic origin. *Am J Gastroenterol* **92**:1148, 1997.
59. Birge SJ, Keutmann HT, Cuatrecasas P, Whedon GD: Osteoporosis, intestinal lactase deficiency and low dietary calcium intake. *N Engl J Med* **276**:445, 1967.
60. Velebit L, Cochet B, Courvoisier B: Incidence de l'intolerance au lactose dans l'osteoporose post-menopausique. *Schweiz Med Wochenschr* **108**:2061, 1978.
61. Kocian J, Vulterianova M, Beijblova O, Skala I: Influence of lactose intolerance on the bones of patients after partial gastrectomy. *Digestion* **8**:324, 1973.
62. Newcomer AD, Hodgson SF, McGill DB, Thomas PJ: Lactase deficiency: Prevalence in osteoporosis. *Ann Intern Med* **89**:218, 1978.
63. Honkanen R, Kroger H, Alhava E, Turpeinen P, Tuppurainen M, Saarikoski S: Lactose intolerance associated with fractures of weight-bearing bones in Finnish women aged 38–57 years. *Bone* **21**:473, 1997.
64. Honkanen R, Pulkkinen P, Jarvinen R, Kroger H, Lindstedt K, Tupurainen M, Uusitupa M: Does lactose intolerance predispose to low bone density? A population based study of perimenopausal Finnish women. *Bone* **19**:23, 1996.
65. Murray TM: Prevention and management of osteoporosis: Consensus statements from the Scientific Advisory Board of the Osteoporosis Society of Canada. 4. Calcium nutrition and osteoporosis. *Can Med Assoc J* **155**:935, 1996.
66. Sahi T, Jussila J, Penttilü I, Sarna S, Isokoski M: Serum lipids and proteins in lactose malabsorption. *Am J Clin Nutr* **30**:476, 1977.
67. Lember M, Tamm A: Lactose absorption and milk drinking habits in Estonians with myocardial infarction. *BMJ* **296**:95, 1988.
68. Segall JJ: Dietary lactose as a possible risk factor for ischaemic heart disease: Review of epidemiology. *Int J Cardiol* **46**:197, 1994.
69. Simoons F: A geographic approach to senile cataracts: Possible links with milk consumption, lactase activity and galactose metabolism. *Dig Dis Sci* **27**:257, 1982.
70. Rinaldi E, Albini L, Costagliola C, Derosa G, Auricchio G, Devizia B, Auricchio S: High frequency of lactose absorbers among adults with idiopathic senile and presenile cataract in a population with a high prevalence of primary adult lactose malabsorption. *Lancet* **1**:355, 1984.

70a. Auricchio S, Costagliola C, De Rosa G, De Vizia B, Rinaldi E, Simonelli F: High frequency of lactose absorbers among adults with idiopathic and diabetic cataract in a population with high prevalence of primary adult type hypolactasia (Abstract). *Gastroenterology* **96**:A18, 1989.

70b. Spinelli D, Vota MG, Formenti F, Accetta S, Careddu P, Ruggero T, Lubriano A, Volpe C: Idiopathic presenile and senile cataract formation and changes in lactose activity. *Fortschr Ophthalmol* **84**:666, 1987.

70c. Meloni G, Ogana A, Mannazzu MC, Meloni T, Carta F, Carta A: High prevalence of lactose absorbers in patients with presenile cataract from Northern Sardinia. *Br J Ophthalmol* **79**:709, 1995.

70d. Birlouez-Aragon I, Stevenin L, Rouzier C, Brivet M: Consommation de lactose et activité lactasique: Deux facteurs de risque de la cataracte senile et diabetique. *Age Nutr* **1**:74, 1990.

70e. Bhatnagar R, Sharma YR, Vajpayee RB, Madan M, Chbabra VK, Ram N, et al: Does milk have a cataractogenic effect? Weighing of clinical evidence. *Dig Dis Sci* **34**:1745, 1989.

71. Bengtsson B, Steen B, Dahlqvist A, Jagerstad M: Does lactose intake induce cataract in man? *Lancet* **1**:1293, 1984.
72. Lisker RL, Cervantes G, Perez-Briceno R, Alva G: Lack of relationship between lactose absorption and senile cataracts. *Ann Ophthalmol* **20**:436, 1988.
73. Jacques PF, Phillips J, Hartz SC, Chylack LT: Lactose intake, galactose metabolism and senile cataracts. *Nutr Res* **10**:255, 1990.
74. Cramer DW: Lactase persistence and milk consumption as determinants of ovarian cancer risk. *Am J Epidemiol* **130**:904, 1989.
75. Risch HA, Jain M, Marrett LD, Howe GR: Dietary lactose intake, lactose intolerance, and the risk of epithelial ovarian cancer in southern Ontario (Canada). *Cancer Causes Control* **5**:540, 1994.
76. Herrinton LJ, Weiss NS, Beresford SA, Stanford JL, Wolfla DM, Feng Z, Scott CR: Lactose and galactose intake and metabolism in relation to the risk of epithelial ovarian cancer. *Am J Epidemiol* **141**:407, 1995.

77. Crane RK, Ménard D, Preiser H, Cerda J: *The Molecular Basis of Brush Border Membrane Disease*. New York, Raven, 1965.
78. Skovbjerg H, Gudmand-Hfyer E, Fenger H: Immunoelectrophoretic studies on human small intestinal brush border proteins: Amount of lactase protein in adult-type hypolactasia. *Gut* **21**:360, 1980.
79. Potter J, Ho M-W, Bolton H, Furth AJ, Swallow DM, Griffiths B: Human lactase and the molecular basis of lactase persistence. *Biochem Genet* **23**:432, 1985.
80. Lorenz-Meyer H, Blum AL, Haemmerli HP, Semenza G: A second enzyme defect in acquired lactase deficiency: Lack of small intestine phlorizin-hydrolase. *Eur J Clin Invest* **2**:326, 1972.
81. Boll W, Wagner P, Mantei N: Structure of the chromosomal gene and cDNAs coding for lactase-phlorizin hydrolase in humans with adult-type hypolactasia or persistence of lactase. *Am J Hum Genet* **48**:889, 1991.
82. Harvey CB, Pratt W, Islam I, Whitehouse DB, Swallow DM: DNA polymorphisms in the lactase gene: Linkage disequilibrium across the 70kb region. *Eur J Hum Genet* **3**:27, 1995.
83. Harvey CB, Hollox EJ, Poulter M, Wang Y, Rossi M, Auricchio S, Iqbal TH, et al: Lactase haplotype frequencies in Caucasians: Association with the lactase persistence/non-persistence polymorphism. *Ann Hum Genet* **62**(Pt 3):215, 1998.
84. Kruse T, Bolund L, Grzeschik K, Ropers H, Sjöström H, Norén O, Mantei N, et al: The human lactase-phlorizin hydrolase gene is located on chromosome 2. *FEBS Lett* **240**:123, 1988.
85. Harvey CB, Fox MF, Jeggo PA, Mantei N, Povey S, Swallow DM: Regional localization of the lactase-phlorizin hydrolase gene, *LCT*, to chromosome 2q21. *Ann Hum Genet* **57**:179, 1993.
86. Mantei N, Villa M, Enzler T, Wacker H, Boll W, James P, Hunziker W, et al: Complete primary structure of human and rabbit lactase-phlorizin hydrolase: Implications for biosynthesis, membrane anchoring and evolution of the enzyme. *EMBO J* **7**:2705, 1988.
87. Wang Y, Harvey CB, Pratt WS, Sams VR, Sarner M, Rossi M, Auricchio S, et al: The lactase persistence/non-persistence polymorphism is controlled by a *cis*-acting element. *Hum Mol Genet* **4**:657, 1995.
88. Escher JC, De Koning N, Van Engen C, Arora S, Büller HA, Montgomery RK, Grand RJ: Molecular basis of lactase levels in adult humans. *J Clin Invest* **89**:480, 1992.
89. Montgomery RK, Büller HA, Rings EHHM, Grand RJ: Lactose intolerance and the genetic regulation of intestinal lactase-phlorizin hydrolase. *FASEB J* **5**:2824, 1991.
90. Sebastio G, Villa M, Sartorio R, Guzzetta V, Poggi V, Auricchio S, Boll W, et al: Control of lactase in human adult-type hypolactasia and in weaning rabbits and rats. *Am J Hum Genet* **45**:489, 1989.
91. Fajardo O, Naim HY, Lacey SW: The polymorphic expression of lactase in adults is regulated at the mRNA level. *Gastroenterology* **106**:1233, 1994.
92. Rossi M, Mauiri L, Fusco MI, Salvati VM, Fuccio A, Auricchio S, Mantei N, et al: Lactase persistence versus decline in human adults: Multifactorial events are involved in downregulation after weaning. *Gastroenterology* **112**:1506, 1997.
93. Villa M, Ménard D, Semenza G, Mantei N: The expression of lactase enzymatic activity and mRNA in human fetal jejunum: Effect of organ culture and of treatment with hydrocortisone. *FEBS Lett* **301**:202, 1992.
94. Wang Y, Harvey C, Rousset M, Swallow D: Expression of intestinal mRNA transcripts during development: Analysis by a semi-quantitative RNA PCR method. *Pediatr Res* **36**:514, 1994.
95. Maiuri L, Raia V, Potter J, Swallow DM, Ho MW, Fiocca R, Finzi G, et al: Mosaic pattern of lactase expression in villous enterocytes in human adult-type hypolactasia. *Gastroenterology* **100**:359, 1991.
96. Maiuri L, Rossi M, Raia V, Garipoli V, Hughes L, Swallow D, Norén O, et al: Mosaic regulation of lactase in human adult-type hypolactasia. *Gastroenterology* **107**:54, 1994.
97. Hamano Y, Kodama H, Fujikawa Y, Tanaka Y, Nishimura K, Yanagisawa M: Use of immunocytochemical analysis of a duodenal biopsy specimen to identify a carrier of ornithine transcarbamylase deficiency. *N Engl J Med* **318**:1521, 1988.
98. Lorenzsonn V, Lloyd M, Olsen WA: Immunocytochemical heterogeneity of lactase-phlorizin hydrolase in adult lactase deficiency. *Gastroenterology* **105**:51, 1993.
99. Witte J, Lloyd M, Lorenzsonn V, Korsmo H, Olsen W: The biosynthetic basis of adult lactase deficiency. *J Clin Invest* **86**:1338, 1990.
100. Sterchi E, Mills P, Fransen J, Hauri H, Lentze M, Naim H, Ginsel L, et al: Biogenesis of intestinal lactase-phlorizin hydrolase in adults with lactose intolerance: Evidence for reduced biosynthesis and slowed-down maturation in enterocytes. *J Clin Invest* **86**:1329, 1990.
101. Green FR, Greenwell P, Dickson L, Griffiths B, Noades J, Swallow DM: Expression of the ABH, Lewis and related antigens on the glycoproteins of the human jejunal brush border, in Harris RJ (ed): *Subcellular Biochemistry: Immunological Aspects*. New York, Plenum, 1988, p. 119.
102. Naim HY, Lentze MJ: Impact of *O*-glycosylation on the function of human intestinal lactase-phlorizin hydrolase: Characterization of glycoforms varying in enzyme activity and localization of *O*-glycoside addition. *J Biol Chem* **267**:25,494, 1992.
103. Duluc I, Jost B, Freund J-N: Multiple levels of control of the stage- and region-specific expression of rat intestinal lactase. *J Cell Biol* **123**:1577, 1993.
104. Boukamel R, Freund J-N: The *cis*-element CE-LPH1 of the rat intestinal lactase gene promoter interacts in vitro with several nuclear facts present in endodermal tissues. *FEBS Lett* **353**:108, 1994.
105. Krasinski SD, Upchurch BH, Irons SJ, June RM, Mishra K, Grand RJ, Verhave M: Rat lactase-phlorizin hydrolase/human growth hormone transgene is expressed on small intestinal villi in transgenic mice. *Gastroenterology* **113**:844, 1997.
106. Lacey SW, Naim HY, Magness RR, Gething M-J, Sambrook JF: Expression of lactase-phlorizin hydrolase in sheep is regulated at the RNA level. *Biochem J* **302**:929, 1994.
107. Hecht A, Torbey CF, Korsmo HA, Olsen WA: Regulation of sucrase and lactase in developing rats: Role of nuclear factors that bind to two gene regulatory elements. *Gastroenterology* **112**:803, 1997.
108. Verhave M, Krasinski SD, Maas SM, Smiers FJW, Mishra K, Breeuwsma NG, Naim HY, et al: Further characterisation of the 5′-flanking region of the rat lactase-phlorizin hydrolase gene. *Biochem Biophys Res Commun* **209**:989, 1995.
109. Van Beers EH, Al RH, Rings EHHM, Einerhand AWC, Dekker J, Büller HA: Lactase and sucrase-isomaltase gene expression during Caco-2 cell differentiation. *Biochem J* **306**:769, 1995.
110. Troelsen JT, Mehlum A, Olsen J, Spodsberg N, Hansen GH, Prydz H, Norén O, et al: 1 kb of the lactase-phlorizin hydrolase promoter directs post-weaning decline and small intestinal-specific expression in transgenic mice. *FEBS Lett* **342**:291, 1994.
111. Troelsen JT, Olsen J, Mitchelmore C, Hansen GH, Sjöström H, Norén O: Two intestinal specific nuclear factors binding to the lactase-phlorizin hydrolase and sucrase-isomaltase promoters are functionally related oligomeric molecules. *FEBS Lett* **342**:297, 1994.
112. Mitchelmore C, Troelsen JT, Sjöström H, Norén O: The HOXC11 homeodomain protein interacts with the lactase-phlorizin hydrolase promoter and stimulates HNF1α-dependent transcription. *J Biol Chem* **273**:13297, 1998.
113. Lloyd M, Mevissen G, Fischer M, Olsen W, Goodspeed D, Genini M, Boll W, et al: Regulation of intestinal lactase in adult hypolactasia. *J Clin Invest* **89**:524, 1992.
114. Swallow DM, Harvey CB: Genetics of adult-type hypolactasia, in Auricchio S, Semenza G (eds): *Common Food Intolerances: 2. Milk in Human Nutrition and Adult-Type Hypolactasia*. Basel, Karger, 1993, p 85.
115. Ferguson A, Maxwell J: Genetic aetiology of lactose intolerance. *Lancet* **2**:188, 1967.
116. Welsh JD, Zschiesche OM, Willits VL, Russell L: Studies of lactose intolerance in families. *Arch Intern Med* **122**:315, 1968.
117. Neale G: The diagnosis, incidence and significance of disaccharidase deficiency in adults. *Proc R Soc Med* **61**:1099, 1968.
118. Flatz G, Saengudom C: Lactose tolerance in Asians: A family study. *Nature* **224**:915, 1969.
119. Welsh JD: Isolated lactase deficiency in humans: Report on 100 patients. *Medicine (Baltimore)* **49**:257, 1970.
120. Sahi T, Isokoski M, Jussila J, Launiala K, Pyörülü K: Recessive inheritance of adult-type lactose malabsorption. *Lancet* **2**:823, 1973.
121. Ransome-Kuti O, Kretchmer N, Johnson JD, Gribble JT: A genetic study of lactose digestion in Nigerian families. *Gastroenterology* **68**:431, 1975.
122. Flatz G: Genetics of lactose digestion in humans, in Harris H, Hirschhorn K (eds): *Advances in Human Genetics*. New York, Plenum, 1987, p 1.
123. Yap I, Berris B, Kang JY, Math M, Chu M, Miller D, Pollard A: Lactase deficiency in Singapore-born and Canadian-born Chinese. *Dig Dis Sci* **34**:1085, 1989.
124. Goldman B, Corcino JJ: Adult lactose malabsorption in Puerto Rico. *Ann Clin Lab Sci* **6**:352, 1976.

125. Seva-Pereira A, Magalhaes FN, Pereura-Filho RA, Beiguelman B: Primary adult lactose malabsorption, a common genetic trait among southeastern Brazilians. *Rev Brazil Genet* **4**:747, 1983.
126. Gendrel D, Dupont C, Richard-Lenoble D, Gendrel C, Nardou M, Chaussain M: Milk lactose malabsorption in Gabon measured by the breath hydrogen test. *J Pediatr Gastroenterol Nutr* **8**:545, 1989.
127. Kozlov AI: Hypolactasia in the indigenous populations of Northern Russia. *Int J Circumpolar Health* **57**:18, 1998.
128. Lember M, Tamm A, Villako K: Lactose malabsorption in Estonians and Russians. *Eur J Gastroenterol Hepatol* **3**:479, 1991.
129. Iqbal TH, Wood GM, Lewis KO, Leek JP, Cooper BT: Prevalence of primary lactase deficiency in adult residents of west Birmingham. *BMJ* **306**:1303, 1993.
130. Czeizel A, Flatz G, Flatz SD: Prevalence of primary adult lactose malabsorption in Hungary. *Hum Genet* **64**:398, 1983.
131. Leis R, Tojo R, Pavón P, Douwes A: Prevalence of lactose malabsorption in Galicia. *J Pediatr Gastroenterol Nutr* **25**:296, 1997.
132. Wang Y, Yan Y, Xu JJ, Du RF, Flatz SD, Kuhnau W, Flatz G: Prevalence of primary adult lactose malabsorption in three populations of northern China. *Hum Genet* **67**:103, 1984.
133. Batu A-T, Hla-Pe U, Aye Aye C: Lactose intolerance in the Burmese. *Union of Burma J Life Sci* **5**: 133–135, 1971.
134. Abbott WGH, Tasman-Jones C: Incidence of acquired primary hypolactasia in three New Zealand racial groups. *NZ Med J* **98**:228, 1985.
135. Jarvela I, Enattah NS, Kokkonen J, Varilo T, Savilahti E, Peltonen L: Assignment of the locus for congenital lactase deficiency to 2q21, in the vicinity of but separate from the lactase-phlorizin hydrolase gene. *Am J Hum Genet* **63**:1078, 1998.

STANDARD ABBREVIATIONS

Abbreviation	Name
ACTH	corticotropin (adrenocorticotropin, adrenocorticotropic hormone)
ADA	adenosine deaminase
AdoMet	s-adenosylmethionine
Ag	antigen
AIDS	acquired immunodeficiency syndrome
ALT	alanine aminotransferase
AMP, ADP, and ATP*	adenosine 5′-mono-, di-, and triphosphates
AP1, AP2	activator protein 1, 2; transcription factors
apo A-I	apolipoprotein A-I
apo A-II	apolipoprotein A-II
apo A-III	apolipoprotein A-III
apo B	apolipoprotein B
apo C-I	apolipoprotein C-I
apo C-II	apolipoprotein C-II
apo C-III	apolipoprotein C-III
apo D	apolipoprotein D
apo E	apolipoprotein E
APRT	adenine phosphoribosyltransferase
ASO	allele-specific oligonucleotide
AST	aspartate aminotransferase
ATPase	adenosine triphosphate
α_1AT	α_1-antitrypsin
B cell	B lymphocyte
BAC	bacterial artificial chromosome
cAMP, cGMP, etc.	cyclic AMP (adenosine 3′: 5′-monophosphate), etc.
CAT	chloramphenicol acetyltransferase
CD	cluster of differentiation or cluster determinant (e.g., CD34)
cDNA	complementary DNA
CHO cells	Chinese hamster ovary cells
CoA (or CoASH)	coenzyme A
CoASAc	acetyl coenzyme A
cM	centimorgan
Cm-cellulose	O-(carboxymethyl)cellulose
CMP, CDP, and CTP*	cytidine 5′-mono-, di-, and triphosphates
CNS	central nervous system
COS cells	CV-I origin, SV40; cells widely used for transfection studies
CPK	creatine phosphokinase
CRM, CRM$^+$, CRM$^-$	cross-reacting material, CRM positive, CRM negative
CT	computerized tomography
CVS	chorionic villus sampling
DEAE-cellulose	O-(diethylaminoethyl)cellulose
DNA	deoxyribonucleic acid
DNase	deoxyribonuclease
DOPA	3,4-dihydroxyphenylalanine
DPN, DPN$^+$, DPNH$^+$	diphosphopyridine nucleotide and its oxidized and reduced forms
DPT	diphtheria, pertussis, tetanus vaccine
dTMP, dTDP, and dTTP*	thymidine 5′-mono-, di-, and triphosphates
DTT	dithiothreitol
EBV	Epstein-Barr virus
EDTA	ethylenediaminetetraacetate
EEG	electroencephalogram
EGF	epidermal growth factor
EGTA	[ethylenebis(oxyethylenenitrilo)] tetraacetic acid
EKG	electrocardiogram
ELISA	enzyme-linked immunosorbent assay
EM	electron microscopy or microscopic
ER	endoplasmic reticulum
ES cells	embryonic stem cells
FAD and $FADH_2$	flavin-adenine dinucleotide and its fully reduced form
FISH	fluorescence *in situ* hybridization
FITC	fluorescein isothiocyanate
FMN	riboflavin 5′-phosphate
G, G_i, G_s	guanine nucleotide binding protein, inhibitory form, stimulatory form
G-6-PD	glucose 6-phosphate dehydrogenase
GABA	γ-aminobutyric acid
GC	gas chromatography
GC/MS	gas chromatography/mass spectroscopy
GERL	Golgi endoplasmic reticulum-like
GFR	glomerular filtration rate
GMP, GDP, and GTP*	guanosine 5′-mono-, di-, and triphosphates
GSH and GSSG	glutathione and its oxidized form
Hb, HbCO, HbO_2	hemoglobin, carbon monoxide hemoglobin, oxyhemoglobin
HDL	high density lipoprotein
HEPES	4-(2-hydroxyethyl)-1-piperazine ethanesulfonic acid
Hep G2	hepatocellular carcinoma human cell line
HIV	human immunodeficiency virus
HLA	human leukocyte antigens
HMG-CoA	3-hydroxy-3-methylglutaryl-coenzyme A
HPLC	high performance (or pressure) liquid chromotography
HPRT	hypoxanthine-guanine phosphoribosyltransferase
IDDM	insulin-dependent diabetes mellitus
IFN	interferon
Ig	immunoglobulin
IgA	gamma A immunoglobulin
IgG	gamma G immunoglobulin
IgM	gamma M immunoglobulin
IL	interleukin, including IL-1, IL-2, etc.
IM or i.m.	intramuscular
IMP, IDP, and ITP*	inosine 5′-mono-, di, and triphosphates
LDH	lactate dehydrogenase
LDL	low density lipoproteins
LINE	long interspersed repeat element
lod	logarithm of the odds
MCH	erythrocyte mean corpuscular hemoglobin
MCHC	erythrocyte mean corpuscular hemoglobin concentration
MCV	erythrocyte mean corpuscular volume
MHC	histocompatibility complex
MPS	mucopolysaccharide or mucopolysaccharidosis
MRI	magnetic resonance imaging
mRNA	messenger RNA
MS	mass spectrometry
mtDNA, mtRNA	mitochondrial DNA, RNA
Myc	oncogene homologous to avian myelocytomatosis virus including c-*myc*, N-*myc*, and L-*myc*
NAD, NAD$^+$, and NADH†	nicotinamide adenine dinucleotide and its oxidized and reduced forms
NADP, NADP$^+$, and NADPH†	nicotinamide adenine dinucleotide phosphate and its oxidized and reduced forms
NIDDM	non-insulin-dependent diabetes mellitus

(Continues)

STANDARD ABBREVIATIONS (*Cont.*)

Abbreviation	Name	Abbreviation	Name
NK cells	natural killer cells	SE	standard error
NMN	nicotinamide mononucleotide	SEM	standard error of mean
NMR	nuclear magnetic resonance	SER	smooth endoplasmic reticulum
p	probability	SH1, SH2, SH3	Src homology domains 1, 2, 3
p_i	inorganic phosphate	SNP	single nucleotide polymorphism
PAC	P1-derived artificial chromosome	*src*	oncogene homologous to Rous sarcoma virus
PAS	periodic acid Schiff	SSCP	single strand conformational polymorphism
PCR	polymerase chain reaction	STR	short tandem repeat
PEG	polyethylene glycol	SV40	Simian virus 40
PFGE	pulsed-field gel electrophoresis	T_3	triiodothyronine
PKA	protein kinase A	T_4	thyroxine
PKC	protein kinase C	T cell	T lymphocyte
PKU	phenylketonuria	TMP, TDP, and TTP*	ribosylthymine 5′-mono-, di-, and triphosphates
PP_i	inorganic pyrophosphate	TNF	tumor necrosis factor (e.g. TNF-1)
PP-ribose-P	phosphoribosylpyrophosphate	TPN, TPN^+, $TPNH^†$	triphosphopyridine nucleotide and its oxidized and reduced forms
ras	oncogenes homologous to sarcoma retroviruses including HRAS, KRAS, and NRAS, H-*ras*, K-*ras*, and N-*ras*	Tris	tris(hydroxymethyl)aminomethane
RER	rough endoplasmic reticulum	tRNA	transfer RNA
RFLP	restriction fragment length polymorphism	UDP-Gal	uridine diphosphogalactose
RIA	radioimmunoassay	UDP-Glc	uridine diphosphoglucose
rRNA	ribosomal RNA	UMP, UDP, and UTP*	uridine 5′-mono-, di-, and triphosphates
RNase	ribonuclease	UV	ultraviolet light
RT-PCR	reverse transcription-polymerase chain reaction	VLDL	very low density lipoprotein
SD	standard deviation	VNTR	variable number tandem repeat
SDS	sodium dodecyl sulfate	YAC	yeast artificial chromosome
SDS-PAGE	sodium dodecyl sulfate polyacrylamide gel electrophoresis		

*The d prefix may be used to represent the corresponding deoxyribonucleoside phosphates, e.g., dADP.
†Note that DPN = NAD and TPN = NADP.

AMINO ACID SYMBOLS

Name	Symbols		Name	Symbols	
alanine	Ala	A	leucine	Leu	L
arginine	Arg	R	lysine	Lys	K
asparagine	Asn	N	methionine	Met	M
aspartic acid	Asp	D	phenylalanine	Phe	F
cysteine	Cys	C	proline	Pro	P
glutamic acid	Glu	E	serine	Ser	S
glutamine	Gln	Q	threonine	Thr	T
glycine	Gly	G	tryptophan	Trp	W
histidine	His	H	tyrosine	Tyr	Y
isoleucine	Ile	I	valine	Val	V

CARBOHYDRATE SYMBOLS

Name	Symbols	Name	Symbols
fructose	Fru	N-acetylgalactosamine	GalNAc
fucose	Fuc	N-acetylglucosamine	GlcNAc
galactose	Gal	N-acetylneuraminic acid	NeuAc
glucosamine	GlcN	ribose	Rib
glucose	Glc	sialic acid	Sia
glucuronic acid	GlcA	xylose	Xyl
mannose	Man		

INDEX

Page numbers followed by an "f" indicate figures; numbers followed by a "t" indicate tables.

ISBN 0-07-913035-6

90000

9 780079 130358

SCRIVER/MMBID, 8E SET

ISBN 0-07-136319-X

90000

9 780071 363198

SCRIVER/MMBID, 8E VOLI

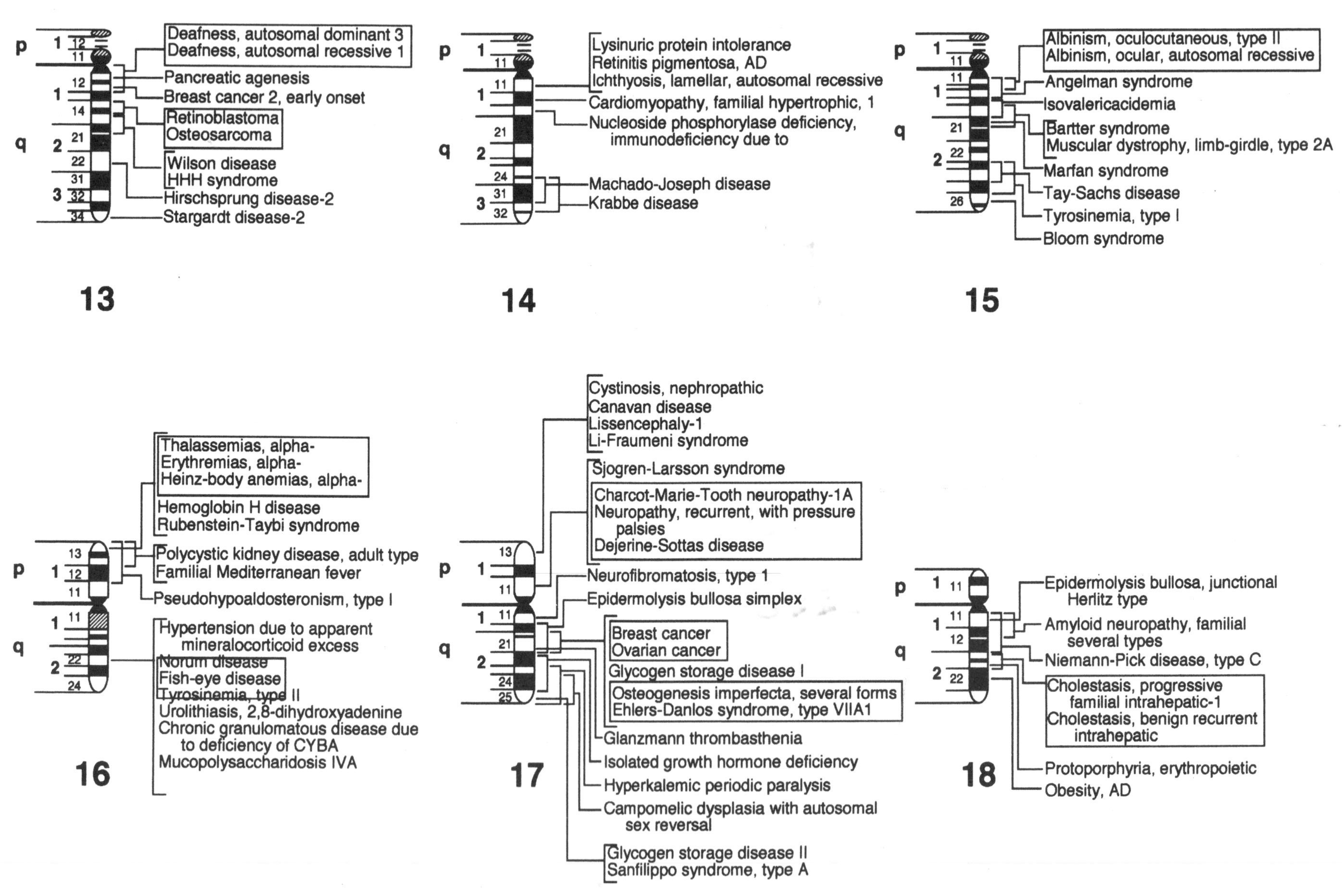

13
Deafness, autosomal dominant 3
Deafness, autosomal recessive 1
Pancreatic agenesis
Breast cancer 2, early onset
Retinoblastoma
Osteosarcoma
Wilson disease
HHH syndrome
Hirschsprung disease-2
Stargardt disease-2
14
Lysinuric protein intolerance
Retinitis pigmentosa, AD
Ichthyosis, lamellar, autosomal recessive
Cardiomyopathy, familial hypertrophic, 1
Nucleoside phosphorylase deficiency, immunodeficiency due to
Machado-Joseph disease
Krabbe disease
15
Albinism, oculocutaneous, type II
Albinism, ocular, autosomal recessive
Angelman syndrome
Isovalericacidemia
Bartter syndrome
Muscular dystrophy, limb-girdle, type 2A
Marfan syndrome
Tay-Sachs disease
Tyrosinemia, type I
Bloom syndrome
16
Thalassemias, alpha-
Erythremias, alpha-
Heinz-body anemias, alpha-
Hemoglobin H disease
Rubenstein-Taybi syndrome
Polycystic kidney disease, adult type
Familial Mediterranean fever
Pseudohypoaldosteronism, type I
Hypertension due to apparent mineralocorticoid excess
Norum disease
Fish-eye disease
Tyrosinemia, type II
Urolithiasis, 2,8-dihydroxyadenine
Chronic granulomatous disease due to deficiency of CYBA
Mucopolysaccharidosis IVA
17
Cystinosis, nephropathic
Canavan disease
Lissencephaly-1
Li-Fraumeni syndrome
Sjogren-Larsson syndrome
Charcot-Marie-Tooth neuropathy-1A
Neuropathy, recurrent, with pressure palsies
Dejerine-Sottas disease
Neurofibromatosis, type 1
Epidermolysis bullosa simplex
Breast cancer
Ovarian cancer
Glycogen storage disease I
Osteogenesis imperfecta, several forms
Ehlers-Danlos syndrome, type VIIA1
Glanzmann thrombasthenia
Isolated growth hormone deficiency
Hyperkalemic periodic paralysis
Campomelic dysplasia with autosomal sex reversal
Glycogen storage disease II
Sanfilippo syndrome, type A
18
Epidermolysis bullosa, junctional Herlitz type
Amyloid neuropathy, familial several types
Niemann-Pick disease, type C
Cholestasis, progressive familial intrahepatic-1
Cholestasis, benign recurrent intrahepatic
Protoporphyria, erythropoietic
Obesity, AD